Holland – Frei

Cancer 7 Medicine ONLINE

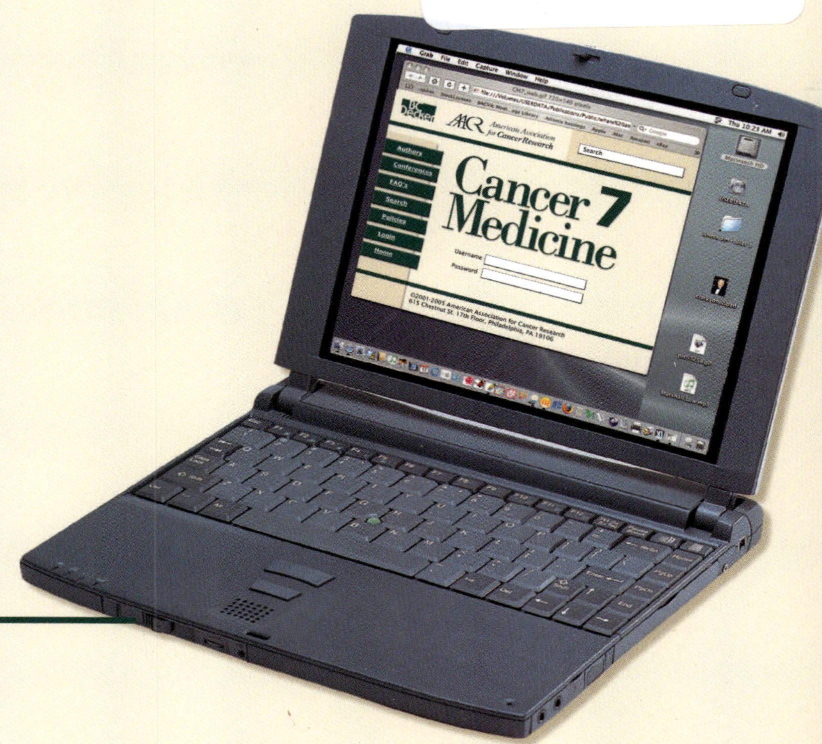

Cancer Medicine 7 Online Edition * is a database resource that includes the full text as well as monthly updates and fully downloadable illustrations. Purchasers of the printed text can access the online edition by simply entering a user name and password.

Additional features:

- Emerging Therapies in Oncology
- Patient Management Problems in Oncology
- Board Review in Oncology
- Need to Know Oncology
- Links to AACR journals

To access *Cancer Medicine 7* Online click:

www.bcdecker.com/cm7

***Available March 31, 2006**

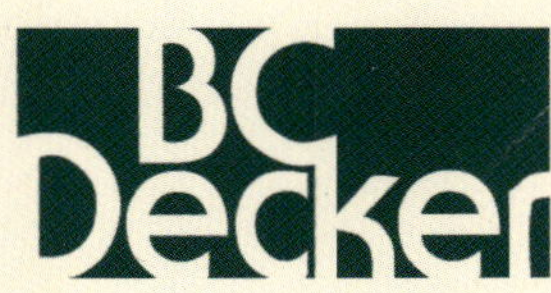

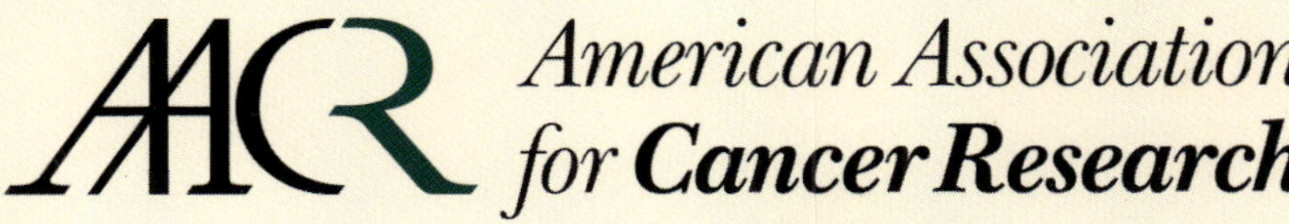

Holland – Frei Cancer Medicine 7

Editors

Donald W. Kufe, MD
Professor of Medicine
Dana-Farber Cancer Institute
Harvard Medical School
Boston, Massachusetts

Robert C. Bast Jr, MD
Internist and Professor of Medicine
Vice President for Translational Research
Harry Carothers Wiess Chair for Cancer Research
University of Texas
MD Anderson Cancer Center
Houston, Texas

William N. Hait, MD, PhD
Professor and Director
UMDNJ/Robert Wood Johnson Medical School
Department of Pharmacology
The Cancer Institute of New Jersey
New Brunswick, New Jersey

Waun Ki Hong, MD
American Cancer Society Professor
Samsung Distinguished University Chair in Cancer Medicine
Professor and Head, Division of Cancer Medicine
University of Texas
MD Anderson Cancer Center
Houston, Texas

Raphael E. Pollock, MD, PhD
Head, Division of Surgery
Professor and Chair, Department of Surgical Oncology
Senator A.M. Aiken Jr, Distinguished Chair
University of Texas
MD Anderson Cancer Center
Houston, Texas

Ralph R. Weichselbaum, MD
Daniel K. Ludwig Professor
Chair, Department of Radiation and Cellular Oncology
University of Chicago Hospital
Director, Chicago Tumor Institute
University of Chicago
Chicago, Illinois

James F. Holland, MD, ScD (hc)
Distinguished Professor of Neoplastic Diseases
Director Emeritus, Derald H. Ruttenberg Cancer Center
Mount Sinai School of Medicine
New York, New York

Emil Frei III, MD
Physician-in-Chief, Emeritus
Dana-Farber Cancer Institute
Richard and Susan Smith Distinguished Professor of Medicine
Harvard Medical School
Boston, Massachusetts

Holland – Frei

Cancer Medicine 7

An approved publication of the

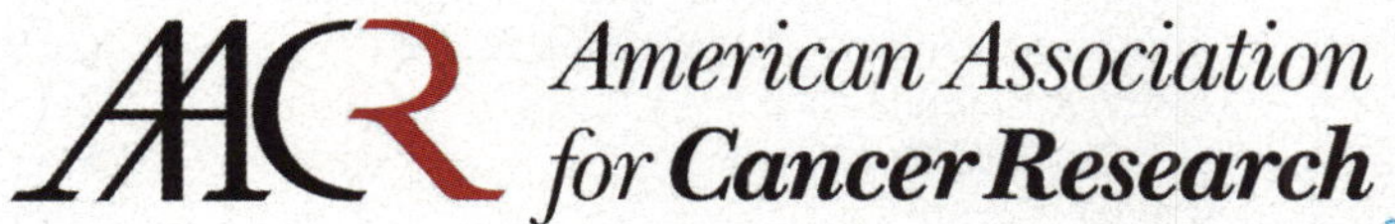

2006
BC Decker Inc
Hamilton • London

BC Decker Inc
P.O. Box 620, L.C.D. 1
Hamilton, Ontario L8N 3K7
Tel: 905-522-7017; 800-568-7281
Fax: 905-522-7839; 888-311-4987
E-mail: info@bcdecker.com
www.bcdecker.com

Fifth edition, 2000. Sixth edition, 2003.

05 06 07 08/QWB/9 8 7 6 5 4 3 2 1

ISBN 1-55009-307-X
Printed in Colombia by Quebecor World Bogotá S. A.
Production Editors: Larissa Byj & Petrice Custance; Typesetter: Silverchair Science + Communications, Inc.; Cover Designer: Doug Hesseltine

Sales and Distribution

United States
BC Decker Inc
P.O. Box 785
Lewiston, NY 14092-0785
Tel: 905-522-7017; 800-568-7281
Fax: 905-522-7839; 888-311-4987
E-mail: info@bcdecker.com
www.bcdecker.com

Canada
BC Decker Inc
50 King Street East
P.O. Box 620, LCD 1
Hamilton, Ontario L8N 1A6
Tel: 905-522-7017; 800-568-7281
Fax: 905-522-7839; 888-311-4987
E-mail: info@bcdecker.com
www.bcdecker.com

Foreign Rights
John Scott & Company
International Publishers' Agency
P.O. Box 878
Kimberton, PA 19442
Tel: 610-827-1640
Fax: 610-827-1671
E-mail: jsco@voicenet.com

Japan
Igaku-Shoin Ltd.
Foreign Publications Department
3-24-17 Hongo
Bunkyo-ku, Tokyo, Japan 113-8719
Tel: 3 3817 5680
Fax: 3 3815 6776
E-mail: fd@igaku-shoin.co.jp

UK, Europe, Scandinavia, Middle East
Elsevier Science
Customer Service Department
Foots Cray High Street
Sidcup, Kent
DA14 5HP, UK
Tel: 44 (0) 208 308 5760
Fax: 44 (0) 181 308 5702
E-mail: cservice@harcourt.com

Singapore, Malaysia, Thailand, Philippines, Indonesia, Vietnam, Pacific Rim, Korea
Elsevier Science Asia
583 Orchard Road
#09/01, Forum
Singapore 238884
Tel: 65-737-3593
Fax: 65-753-2145

Australia, New Zealand
Elsevier Science Australia
Customer Service Department
STM Division
Locked Bag 16
St. Peters, New South Wales, 2044
Australia
Tel: 61 02 9517-8999
Fax: 61 02 9517-2249
E-mail: stmp@harcourt.com.au
www.harcourt.com.au

Mexico and Central America
ETM SA de CV
Calle de Tula 59
Colonia Condesa
06140 Mexico DF, Mexico
Tel: 52-5-5553-6657
Fax: 52-5-5211-8468
E-mail: editoresdetextosmex@prodigy.net.mx

Brazil
Tecmedd Importadora E Distribuidora De Livros Ltda.
Avenida Maurílio Biagi, 2850
City Ribeirão, Ribeirão Preto – SP – Brasil
CEP: 14021-000
Tel: 0800 992236
Fax: (16) 3993-9000
E-mail: tecmedd@tecmedd.com.br

India, Bangladesh, Pakistan, Sri Lanka
Elsevier Health Sciences Division
Customer Service Department
17A/1, Main Ring Road
Lajpat Nagar IV
New Delhi – 110024, India
Tel: 91 11 2644 7160-64
Fax: 91 11 2644 7156
E-mail: esindia@vsnl.net

Front cover: The colon cancer cell line HCT116 was transfected with GFP-Bax, a pro-apoptosis molecule and then treated with a protease inhibitor, MG132. Cells were then stained with the DNA dye Hoeschst 33342. Normal cells have large round nuclei (*blue*) and the GFP-Bax signals (*green*) are diffusive indicating a cytoplasmic distribution. Apoptotic cells have small, condensed or fragmented nuclei (*blue*) and the GFP-Bax signals are punctate indicating the translocation of Bax from the cytoplasm to the mitochondria, where it initiated the apoptotic program. (Images provided by Drs. Xiao-Ming Yin and Wen-Xing Ding, Department of Pathology, University of Pittsburgh School of Medicine, Pittsburgh, PA 15261, USA.)

CONTRIBUTORS

Stuart A. Aaronson, MD
Department of Oncological Sciences
Mount Sinai School of Medicine
New York, New York

James L. Abbruzzese, MD, FACP
Department of Gastrointestinal Medical Oncology
MD Anderson Cancer Center
Houston, Texas

Scott I. Abrams, PhD
Laboratory of Immunology and Biology
National Cancer Institute
Bethesda, Maryland

David H. Abramson, MD, FACS
Department of Surgery
Memorial Sloan-Kettering Cancer Center
New York, New York

Roberto Adachi, MD
Department of Pulmonary Medicine
MD Anderson Cancer Center
Houston, Texas

Ranjana Advani, MD
Department of Medicine
Stanford University
Stanford, California

Sunil J. Advani, MD
Department of Radiation and Cellular Oncology
University of Chicago
Chicago, Illinois

Joseph Aisner, MD
Department of Medicine
The Cancer Institute of New Jersey
New Brunswick, New Jersey

Jaffer A. Ajani, MD
Department of Gastrointestinal Medical Oncology
MD Anderson Cancer Center
Houston, Texas

Karen Albritton, MD
Departments of Internal Medicine and Pediatrics
University of Utah
Salt Lake City, Utah

Edward P. Ambinder, MD
Department of Medicine
Mount Sinai School of Medicine
New York, New York

Kenneth C. Anderson, MD
Division of Hematologic Malignancy
Dana-Farber Cancer Institute
Boston, Massachusetts

Michael Andreeff, MD, PhD
Department of Blood and Marrow Transplantation
MD Anderson Cancer Center
Houston, Texas

Anne L. Angiolillo, MD
Department of Hematology/Oncology
Children's National Medical Center
Washington, District of Columbia

Narin Apisarnthanarax, MD
Department of Dermatology
Case Western Reserve University School of Medicine
Cleveland, Ohio

Richard Aplenc, MD, MSCE
Division of Oncology
Children's Hospital of Philadelphia
Philadelphia, Pennsylvania

James O. Armitage, MD
Department of Oncology/Hematology
University of Nebraska Medical Center
Omaha, Nebraska

Anna Bafico, PhD
Department of Oncological Sciences
Mount Sinai School of Medicine
New York, New York

Anna D. Barker, PhD
Department of Strategic Initiatives
National Cancer Institute
Bethesda, Maryland

Lara Bashoura, MD
Department of Pulmonary Medicine
MD Anderson Cancer Center
Houston, Texas

Lawrence W. Bassett, MD, FACR
Department of Radiological Sciences
University of California Los Angeles
Los Angeles, California

Robert C. Bast Jr, MD
Department of Medicine
MD Anderson Cancer Center
Houston, Texas

Norman Beauchamp Jr, MD, MHS
Department of Radiology
University of Washington School of Medicine
Seattle, Washington

Robert S. Benjamin, MD
Department of Sarcoma Medical Oncology
MD Anderson Cancer Center
Houston, Texas

Jonathan S. Berek, MD, MMSc
Division of Gynecologic Oncology
UCLA Center for Health Sciences
Los Angeles, California

Ross S. Berkowitz, MD
Division of Gynecologic Oncology
Harvard Medical School
Boston, Massachusetts

Leslie Bernstein, PhD
Department of Preventative Medicine
University of Southern California
Los Angeles, California

Mark L. Bernstein, MD, FRCP(C)
Department of Pediatrics
University of Montreal
Montreal, Québéc

Donald A. Berry, PhD
Department of Biostatics and Applied Mathematics
MD Anderson Cancer Center
Houston, Texas

Joseph R. Bertino, MD
Department of Medicine
Robert Wood Johnson Medical School
New Brunswick, New Jersey

Smita Bhatia, MD, MPH
Division of Pediatric Oncology
City of Hope Cancer Center
Duarte, California

Charles D. Blanke, MD
Division of Hematology and Medical Oncology
Oregon Health Science University
Portland, Oregon

W. Archie Bleyer, MD
Department of Community Oncology
MD Anderson Cancer Center
Houston, Texas

Gerald P. Bodey, MD
Department of Infection Control and Employee Health
MD Anderson Cancer Center
Houston, Texas

Ernest C. Borden, MD
Center for Cancer Drug Discovery and Development
Taussig Cancer Center
Cleveland, Ohio

Robert S. Bresalier, MD
Department of Gastrointestinal Medicine and Nutrition
MD Anderson Cancer Center
Houston, Texas

Marcia S. Brose, MD, PhD
Division of Hematology/Oncology
University of Pennsylvania Cancer Center
Philadelphia, Pennsylvania

Thomas A. Buchholz, MD
Department of Radiation Oncology
MD Anderson Cancer Center
Houston, Texas

Aman U. Buzdar, MD
Department of Breast Medical Oncology
MD Anderson Cancer Center
Houston, Texas

Mitchell S. Cairo, MD
Division of Pediatric Oncology
Columbia University
New York, New York

Michele Carbone, MD, PhD
Department of Pathology
Loyola University
Chicago, Illinois

Alan C. Carver, MD
Department of Neurology
Mount Sinai School of Medicine
New York, New York

Barrie R. Cassileth, PhD, MS
Department of Medicine
Memorial Sloan-Kettering Cancer Center
New York, New York

A. Philippe Chahinian, MD
Division of Medical Oncology
Mount Sinai School of Medicine
New York, New York

Richard Champlin, MD
Department of Blood and Marrow Transplantation
MD Anderson Cancer Center
Houston, Texas

Joe Y. Chang, MD, PhD
Department of Radiation Oncology
MD Anderson Cancer Center
Houston, Texas

Yung-Chi Cheng, MD
Department of Pharmacology
Yale University School of Medicine
New Haven, Connecticut

Haesun Choi, MD
Department of Radiology
MD Anderson Cancer Center
Houston, Texas

Stephen Chui, MD
Department of Medicine
Duke University
Durham, North Carolina

Theodore D. Chung, MD, PhD
Department of Radiation Oncology
Massey Cancer Center
Richmond, Virginia

John A. Cidlowski, PhD
Laboratory of Signal Transduction
National Institute of Environmental Health Sciences
Research Triangle Park, North Carolina

Margie L. Clapper, PhD
Department of Population Science
Fox Chase Cancer Center
Philadelphia, Pennsylvania

Timothy M. Clay, PhD
Duke University
Durham, North Carolina

Gary L. Clayman, DDS, MD, FACS
Department of Head and Neck Surgery
MD Anderson Cancer Center
Houston, Texas

Lewis Clayman, DMD, MD
Department of Oral and Maxillofacial Surgery
University of Detroit
Detroit, Michigan

James E. Cleaver, PhD
Professor of Dermatology
University of California San Francisco Cancer Center
San Francisco, California

Steven K. Clinton, MD, PhD
Department of Internal Medicine
Ohio State University
Columbus, Ohio

Carmel J. Cohen, MD
Department of Obstetrics and Gynecology
Columbia University
New York, New York

Harvey J. Cohen, MD
Department of Medicine
Duke University
Durham, North Carolina

Jeffrey I. Cohen, MD
Laboratory of Clinical Investigation
National Institute of Allergy and Infectious Diseases
Bethesda, Maryland

Peter D. Cole, MD
Department of Pediatric Hematology/Oncology
Cancer Institute of New Jersey
New Brunswick, New Jersey

R. Edward Coleman, MD
Division of Nuclear Medicine
Duke University Medical Center
Durham, North Carolina

Michael Colvin, MD
Comprehensive Cancer Center
Duke University
Durham, North Carolina

Ana Maria Comaru-Schally, MD, MS*
Department of Medicine
Veterans Affairs Medical Center
New Orleans, Louisiana

James L. Connolly, MD
Department of Pathology
Beth Israel Deaconess Medical Center
Boston, Massachusetts

Christopher L. Corless, MD, PhD
Department of Pathology
Oregon Health Sciences University
Portland, Oregon

Jorge Cortes, MD
Department of Leukemia
MD Anderson Cancer Center
Houston, Texas

R. Lee Cothran, MD
Department of Radiology
Duke University Medical Center
Durham, North Carolina

Kenneth H. Cowan, MD, PhD
Eppley Institute for Cancer Research
University of Nebraska Medical Center
Omaha, Nebraska

Christopher H. Crane, MD
Department of Radiation Oncology
MD Anderson Cancer Center
Houston, Texas

*deceased

Carlo M. Croce, MD
Department of Medicine
Ohio State University
Columbus, Ohio

Chistopher P. Crum, MD
Department of Pathology
Harvard Medical School
Boston, Massachusetts

John Cunningham, MD
Department of Surgery
Columbia University
New York, New York

Steven A. Curley, MD, FACS
Department of Pathology
MD Anderson Cancer Center
Houston, Texas

Anthony V. D'Amico, MD
Department of Radiation Oncology
Harvard Medical School
Boston, Massachusetts

Marta L. Davila, MD
Department of GI Medicine & Nutrition
MD Anderson Cancer Center
Houston, Texas

Lisa M. DeAngelis, MD
Department of Neurology
Memorial Sloan-Kettering Cancer Center
New York, New York

Gary Deng, MD, PhD
Department of Medicine
Memorial Sloan-Kettering Cancer Center
New York, New York

Samuel R. Denmeade, MD
Department of Oncology
Johns Hopkins University
Baltimore, Maryland

Maria T. DeSancho, MD
Division of Hematology/Oncology
Mount Sinai Medical Center
New York, New York

Mark W. Dewhirst, DVM, PhD
Department of Radiation Oncology
Duke University Medical Center
Durham, North Carolina

Robert B. Diasio, MD
Department of Medicine
University of Alabama
Birmingham, Alabama

Eduardo M. Diaz Jr, MD, FACS
Department of Head and Neck Surgery
MD Anderson Cancer Center
Houston, Texas

Burton F. Dickey, MD
Department of Pulmonary Medicine
MD Anderson Cancer Center
Houston, Texas

Jeffrey S. Dome, MD
Department of Hematology and Oncology
St. Jude Children's Research Hospital
Memphis, Tennessee

Brian J. Druker, MD
Department of Medicine
Oregon Health Sciences Center
Portland, Oregon

Stephen W. Duffy, MSc
Department of Cancer Screening
Cancer Research UK Centre for Epidemiology, Mathematics and Statistics
London, United Kingdom

Ira J. Dunkel, MD
Department of Pediatrics
Weill Medical College of Cornell University
New York, New York

Madeleine M. Duvic, MD
Department of Dermatology
MD Anderson Cancer Center
Houston, Texas

Ann M. Dvorak, MD
Department of Pathology
Beth Israel Deaconess Medical Center
Boston, Massachusetts

Harold F. Dvorak, MD
Department of Pathology
Harvard Medical School
Boston, Massachusetts

George A. Eapen, MD
Department of Pulmonary Medicine
MD Anderson Cancer Center
Houston, Texas

Joseph Paul Eder, MD
Department of Adult Oncology
Dana-Farber Cancer Institute
Boston, Massachusetts

Patricia J. Eifel, MD
Professor of Radiation Oncology
MD Anderson Cancer Center
Houston, Texas

Lawrence H. Einhorn, MD
Department of Hematology/Oncology
Indiana University
Indianapolis, Indiana

Andrew J. Einstein, MD, PhD
Department of Cardiology
Mount Sinai School of Medicine
New York, New York

Suhendan Ekmekcioglu, PhD
Department of Experimental Therapeutics
MD Anderson Cancer Center
Houston, Texas

Ezekiel J. Emanuel, MD, PhD
Department of Clinical Bioethics
Warren G. Magnuson Clinical Center
Bethesda, Maryland

Paul F. Engstrom, MD
Department of Population Science
Fox Chase Cancer Center
Philadelphia, Pennsylvania

Jeremy J. Erasmus, MD
Department of Diagnostic Radiology
MD Anderson Cancer Center
Houston, Texas

Carmen P. Escalante, MD
Division of Internal Medicine
MD Anderson Cancer Center
Houston, Texas

Laura Esserman, MD
Departments of Surgery and Radiology
University of California
San Francisco, California

Richard Essner, MD, FACS
John Wayne Cancer Institute
Santa Monica, California

David S. Ettinger, MD
Department of Oncology
Johns Hopkins University School of Medicine
Baltimore, Maryland

Alison A. Evans, ScD
Division of Population Science
Fox Chase Cancer Center
Philadelphia, Pennsylvania

Douglas B. Evans, MD
Department of Surgical Oncology
MD Anderson Cancer Center
Houston, Texas

Michael S. Ewer, MD, MPH
Department of Medicine
MD Anderson Cancer Center
Houston, Texas

Harmon J. Eyre, MD
Cancer Control Sciences Department
American Cancer Society
Atlanta, Georgia

Stefan Faderl, MD
Department of Leukemia
MD Anderson Cancer Center
Houston, Texas

Mark K. Ferguson, MD
Department of Thoracic Surgery
University of Chicago Hospitals
Chicago, Illinois

Marshall S. Flam, MD, FACP
Department of Medicine
University of California
San Francisco, California

Kathleen M. Foley, MD
Department of Neurology
Memorial Sloan-Kettering Cancer Center
New York, New York

Judah Folkman, MD
Department of Surgery and Cell Biology
Harvard University
Boston, Massachusetts

Yuman Fong, MD
Department of Surgery
Memorial Sloan-Kettering Cancer Center
New York, New York

Richard S. Foster, MD
Department of Urology
Indiana University
Indianapolis, Indiana

Arthur E. Frankel, MD
Professor of Cancer Biology and Medicine
Wake Forest University School of Medicine
Winston-Salem, North Carolina

Janet L. Franklin, MD
Division of Hematology/Oncology
Children's Hospital Los Angeles
Los Angeles, California

Milo Frattini, PhD
Department of Experimental Oncology
National Institute for Tumor Study and Treatment
Milan, Italy

Arnold S. Freedman, MD
Department of Medicine
Dana-Farber Cancer Institute
Boston, Massachusetts

Emil Frei III, MD
Department of Medicine
Harvard Medical School
Boston, Massachusetts

Valentin Fuster, MD, PhD
Department of Cardiology
Mount Sinai School of Medicine
New York, New York

Robert F. Gagel, MD
Professor of Medicine
MD Anderson Cancer Center
Houston, Texas

Michael A. Gallo, PhD
Toxicology Division
Environmental and Occupational Health Sciences Institute
Piscataway, New Jersey

Robert C. Gallo, MD
Institute of Human Virology
University of Maryland
Baltimore, Maryland

Chirag D. Gandhi, MD
Department of Neurosurgery
Mount Sinai School of Medicine
New York, New York

Paul S. Gaynon, MD
Department of Clinical Oncology Research
Children's Hospital Los Angeles
Los Angeles, California

Mark C. Gebhardt, MD
Department of Orthopedic Surgery
Harvard University
Boston, Massachusetts

Teresa Ann Gilewski, MD
Department of Clinical Medicine
Weill Medical College-Cornell University
New York, New York

Ann Marie Gillenwater, MD
Department of Head and Neck Surgery
MD Anderson Cancer Center
Houston, Texas

Timothy D. Gilligan, MD
Lank Center for Genitourinary Oncology
Dana-Farber Cancer Institute
Boston, Massachusetts

Edward L. Giovannucci, MD, ScD, DPH
Department of Nutrition
Harvard School of Public Health
Boston, Massachusetts

Jeffrey D. Goldsmith, MD
Department of Pathology and Laboratory Medicine
Harvard Medical School
Boston, Massachusetts

Donald P. Goldstein, MD
Department of Obstetrics, Gynecology and Reproductive Biology
Harvard Medical School
Boston, Massachusetts

David W. Goodrich, PhD
Department of Pharmacology Therapeutics
Roswell Park Cancer Institute
Buffalo, New York

Richard G. Gorlick, MD, FAAP
Department of Molecular Pharmacology and Pediatrics
Albert Einstein College of Medicine
Bronx, New York

David J. Grdina, PhD
Department of Radiation and Cellular Oncology
University of Chicago
Chicago, Illinois

F. Anthony Greco, MD
Medical Director
Sarah Cannon Cancer Center
Nashville, Tennessee

Elizabeth A. Grimm, PhD
Department of Experimental Therapeutics
MD Anderson Cancer Center
Houston, Texas

Sean Grimm, MD
Department of Neurology
Memorial Sloan-Kettering Cancer Center
New York, New York

Elizabeth G. Grubbs, MD
Department of Surgery
Duke University
Durham, North Carolina

Paul E. Grundy, MD
Department of Pediatrics
University of Alberta
Edmonton, Alberta

Sanjay Gupta, MD
Department of Diagnostic Radiology
MD Anderson Cancer Center
Houston, Texas

John D. Hainsworth, MD
Director of Clinical Research
Sarah Cannon Cancer Center
Centennial Medical Center
Nashville, Tennessee

William N. Hait, MD, PhD
Director
Cancer Institute of New Jersey
New Brunswick, New Jersey

Axel-R Hanauske, MD, PhD
Abteilung Haematologie und Onkologie
Klinik Rechts der Isar
Munich, Germany

Curtis C. Harris, MD
Laboratory of Human Carcinogenesis
National Cancer Institute
Bethesda, Maryland

Harold A. Harvey, MD
Department of Hematology/Oncology
Penn State College of Medicine
Hershey, Pennsylvania

Tayyaba Hasan, PhD
Department of Dermatology
Harvard Medical School
Boston, Massachusetts

Michael C. Heinrich, MD
Department of Medical Oncology
Oregon Health Sciences University
Portland, Oregon

Clyde A. Helms, MD
Department of Radiology and Orthopedics
Duke University School of Medicine
Durham, North Carolina

Brian E. Henderson, MD
Department of Preventative Medicine
University of Southern California
Los Angeles, California

Roy S. Herbst, MD, PhD
Department of Thoracic/Head and Neck Medical Oncology
MD Anderson Cancer Center
Houston, Texas

Pamela A. Hershberger, PhD
Department of Pharmacology
University of Pittsburgh
Pittsburgh, Pennsylvania

Diana M. Hey, PharmD
Pharmacy-PC Operations Department
MD Anderson Cancer Center
Houston, Texas

John Heymach, MD, PhD
Department of Thoracic/Head and Neck Medical Oncology
MD Anderson Cancer Center
Houston, Texas

Marshall E. Hicks, MD
Department of Diagnostic Radiology
MD Anderson Cancer Center
Houston, Texas

Teru Hideshima, MD, PhD
Department of Medicine
Dana-Farber Cancer Institute
Boston, Massachusetts

Amy C. Hobeika, PhD
Department of Surgery
Duke University
Durham, North Carolina

James W. Hodge, PhD
Laboratory of Tumor Immunology and Biology
National Cancer Institute
Bethesda, Maryland

Paulo Hoff, MD
Department of Medicine
MD Anderson Cancer Center
Houston, Texas

James F. Holland, MD, ScD (hc)
Department of Medicine
Mount Sinai School of Medicine
New York, New York

Jimmie C. Holland, MD
Department of Psychiatry and Behavioral Sciences
Memorial Sloan-Kettering Cancer Center
New York, New York

Waun Ki Hong, MD
Division of Thoracic/Head & Neck Medical Oncology
MD Anderson Cancer Center
Houston, Texas

Richard T. Hoppe, MD
Department of Radiation Oncology
Stanford University School of Medicine
Stanford, California

Gabriel N. Hortobagyi, MD, FACP
Department of Breast Medical Oncology
MD Anderson Cancer Center
Houston, Texas

Robert A. Hromas, MD
Department of Internal Medicine
University of New Mexico
Albuquerque, New Mexico

Arthur Hung, MD
Department of Radiation Oncology
Oregon Health & Science University
Portland, Oregon

Arti Hurria, MD
Department of Medicine
Memorial Sloan-Kettering Cancer Center
New York, New York

Christopher J. Hurt, MD
Johns Hopkins University School of Medicine
Baltimore, Maryland

Mark Hurwitz, MD
Department of Radiation Oncology
Brigham and Women's Hospital
Boston, Massachusetts

Ahmedin Jemal, DVM, PhD
Department of Epidemiology and Surveillance Research
American Cancer Society
Atlanta, Georgia

Anuja Jhingran, MD
Department of Radiation Oncology
MD Anderson Cancer Center
Houston, Texas

Carlos A. Jimenez, MD
Department of Pulmonary Medicine
MD Anderson Cancer Center
Houston, Texas

Steven Joffe, MD, MPH
Department of Pediatric Oncology
Harvard Medical School
Boston, Massachusetts

Eric Jonasch, MD
Department of Genitourinary Medical Oncology
MD Anderson Cancer Center
Houston, Texas

Ellen Jones, MD, PhD
Department of Radiation Oncology
Duke University Medical Center
Durham, North Carolina

Roy Jones, PhD, MD
Department of Blood and Marrow Transplantation
MD Anderson Cancer Center
Houston, Texas

V. Craig Jordan, OBE, PhD, DSc
Medical Science Division
Fox Chase Cancer Center
Philadelphia, Pennsylvania

Hamilton Jordan
Atlanta, Georgia

John A. Kalapurakal, MD
Department of Radiation Oncology
Northwestern University
Chicago, Illinois

Raghu Kalluri, PhD
Department of Medicine
Beth Israel Deaconess Medical Center
Boston, Massachusetts

Barton A. Kamen, MD, PhD
Department of Pediatric Hematology/Oncology
Cancer Institute of New Jersey
New Brunswick, New Jersey

Hagop M. Kantarjian, MD
Department of Leukemia
MD Anderson Cancer Center
Houston, Texas

Philip W. Kantoff, MD
Department of Medical Oncology
Dana-Farber Cancer Institute
Boston, Massachusetts

Anne G. Kasmar, MD, MSc
Department of Medicine
Harvard Medical School
Boston, Massachusetts

Richard M. Kaufman, MD
Department of Pathology
Harvard Medical School
Boston, Massachusetts

Harmeet Kaur, MD
Department of Radiology
MD Anderson Cancer Center
Houston, Texas

Michael J. Keating, MD
Department of Medicine
MD Anderson Cancer Center
Houston, Texas

Nancy E. Kemeny, MD
Department of Medicine
Memorial Sloan-Kettering Cancer Center
New York, New York

Samuel Kenan, MD
Department of Orthopedics
New York University School of Medicine
New York, New York

Merrill S. Kies, MD
Department of Thoracic/Head and Neck Medical Oncology
MD Anderson Cancer Center
Houston, Texas

Youn H. Kim, MD
Department of Dermatology
Stanford University School of Medicine
Stanford, California

John M. Kirkwood, MD
Department of Medicine
University of Pittsburgh School of Medicine
Pittsburgh, Pennsylvania

Catherine E. Klein, MD
Department of Medicine
University of Colorado Health Sciences Center
Denver, Colorado

H. Phillip Koeffler, MD
Division of Hematology/Oncology
Cedars-Sinai Medical Center
Los Angeles, California

Elise C. Kohn, MD
Molecular Signaling Section
National Cancer Institute
Bethesda, Maryland

Ritsuko K. Komaki, MD
Department of Radiation Oncology
MD Anderson Cancer Center
Houston, Texas

Robert J. Kreitman, MD
Laboratory of Molecular Biology
National Cancer Institute
Bethesda, Maryland

Donald W. Kufe, MD
Department of Medicine
Dana-Farber Cancer Institute
Boston, Massachusetts

Joy H. Kunishige, MD
Department of Dermatology
University of Texas Health Science Center
Houston, Texas

Joanne Kurtzberg, MD
Department of Pediatrics
Duke University Medical Center
Durham, North Carolina

Razelle Kurzrock, MD
Department of Experimental Therapeutics
MD Anderson Cancer Center
Houston, Texas

Beverly Lange, MD
Division of Oncology
University of Philadelphia
Philadelphia, Pennsylvania

Olegario Jay Lara, DO
Department of Radiological Sciences
University of California, Los Angeles
Los Angeles, California

George E. Laramore, PhD, MD
Department of Radiation Oncology
University of Washington Medical Center
Seattle, Washington

Nancy Lewis, MD
Department of Medical Oncology
Fox Chase Cancer Center
Philadelphia, Pennsylvania

Chuan Y. Li, PhD
Department of Radiation Oncology
Duke University Medical Center
Durham, North Carolina

Donghui Li, PhD
Department of Medical Oncology
MD Anderson Cancer Center
Houston, Texas

Tara L. Lin, MD
Department of Oncology
Johns Hopkins University School of Medicine
Baltimore, Maryland

Scott M. Lippman, MD
Department of Clinical Cancer Prevention
MD Anderson Cancer Center
Houston, Texas

John B. Little, MD
Laboratory of Radiobiology
Harvard School of Public Health
Boston, Massachusetts

Christopher J. Logothetis, MD
Department of Genitourinary Medical Oncology
MD Anderson Cancer Center
Houston, Texas

Janina A. Longtine, MD
Department of Pathology
Brigham and Women's Hospital
Boston, Massachusetts

Evelyne M. Loyer, MD
Department of Radiology
MD Anderson Cancer Center
Houston, Texas

H. Kim Lyerly, MD
Department of Oncology
Duke University
Durham, North Carolina

Donald F. Lynch Jr, MD
Department of Urology
Eastern Virginia School of Medicine
Norfolk, Virginia

Henry T. Lynch, MD
Department of Preventative Medicine
Creighton University School of Medicine
Omaha, Nebraska

Tobey J. MacDonald, MD
Department of Hematology-Oncology
Children's National Medical Center
Washington, District of Columbia

Robert G. Maki, MD, PhD
Memorial Sloan-Kettering Cancer Center
New York, New York

Paul F. Mansfield, MD
Department of Surgical Oncology
MD Anderson Cancer Center
Houston, Texas

Neyssa Marina, MD
Division of Hematology-Oncology
Stanford University School of Medicine
Palo Alto, California

John M. Maris, MD
Department of Pediatrics
Children's Hospital of Philadelphia
Philadelphia, Pennsylvania

Peter M. Mauch, MD
Department of Radiation Oncology
Harvard Medical School
Boston, Massachusetts

H. Page McAdams, MD
Department of Radiology
Duke University Medical Center
Durham, North Carolina

Justin C. McCarty
Department of Medicine
University of Pittsburgh
Pittsburgh, Pennsylvania

Kenneth S. McCarty Jr, MD, PhD
Department of Pathology and Medicine
University of Pittsburgh Cancer Institute
Pittsburgh, Pennsylvania

Kenneth S. McCarty Sr, PhD *
Department of Biochemistry
Duke University
Durham, North Carolina

Beryl McCormick, MD
Department of Radiation Oncology
Memorial Sloan-Kettering Cancer Center
New York, New York

Lorraine I. McKay, PhD
Department of Immunology
Bristol Myers Squibb Pharmaceutical Research Institute
Princeton, New Jersey

Catherine M. McLachlin, MD
Department of Medicine
University of Western Ontario
London, Ontario

Anna T. Meadows, MD
Department of Medicine
Children's Hospital of Philadelphia
Philadelphia, Pennsylvania

Jeffrey I. Mechanick, MD
Department of Medicine
Mount Sinai Hospital
New York, New York

William H. Meyer, MD
Department of Pediatrics
University of Oklahoma
Oklahoma City, Oklahoma

Matthew Meyerson, MD
Department of Pathology
Dana-Farber Cancer Institute
Boston, Massachusetts

Elizabeth C. Miller, MS, RD
Department of Internal Medicine
Ohio State University
Columbus, Ohio

David L. Mitchell, PhD
Department of Carcinogenesis
MD Anderson Cancer Center
Science Park Research Division
Smithville, Texas

Rodolfo C. Morice, MD
Department of Pulmonary Medicine
MD Anderson Cancer Center
Houston, Texas

Charles S. Morrow, MD, PhD
Department of Biochemistry
Wake Forest University School of Medicine
Winston-Salem, North Carolina

Phuong Khanh H. Morrow, MD
Department of Medical Oncology
MD Anderson Cancer Center
Houston, Texas

Michael A. Morse, MD
Department of Medicine
Duke University
Durham, North Carolina

Donald L. Morton, MD, FACS
Department of Surgery
John Wayne Cancer Institute
Santa Monica, California

Natalie Moryl, MD
Department of Neurology
Memorial Sloan-Kettering Cancer Center
New York, New York

Jeffrey A. Moscow, MD
Department of Pediatrics
University of Kentucky
Lexington, Kentucky

Arno J. Mundt, MD
Department of Radiation and Cellular Oncology
University of Chicago
Chicago, Illinois

Hyman B. Muss, MD
Department of Hematology/Oncology
University of Vermont School of Medicine
Burlington, Vermont

Piero Mustacchi, MD, ScD
Department of Medicine and Epidemiology
University of California
San Francisco, California

James Nachman, MD
Division of Hematology and Oncology
University of Chicago
Chicago, Illinois

Lee M. Nadler, MD
Department of Medicine
Harvard Medical School
Boston, Massachusetts

Victor A. Neel, MD, PhD
Division of Dermatological Surgery
Massachusetts General Hospital
Boston, Massachusetts

Alfred I. Neugut, MD, PhD
Department of Medical Oncology
Columbia University
New York, New York

Craig R. Nichols, MD
Division of Hematology and Medical Oncology
Oregon Health Sciences University
Portland, Oregon

Mark D. Nichols, PhD
Department of Pharmacology
University of Pittsburgh
Pittsburgh, Pennsylvania

Larry Norton, MD
Department of Medicine
Memorial Sloan-Kettering Cancer Center
New York, New York

Lauretta Odogwu-Oti, MD
Department of Medicine
Duke University
Durham, North Carolina

William K. Oh, MD
Department of Medicine
Harvard Medical School
Boston, Massachusetts

Takao Ohnuma, MD, PhD
Department of Medical Oncology
Mount Sinai School of Medicine
New York, New York

Amir Onn, MD
Department of Pulmonary Medicine
MD Anderson Cancer Center
Houston, Texas

Bernhard Ortel, MD
Department of Dermatology
Harvard Medical School
Boston, Massachusetts

Brian O'Sullivan, MD, FRCPI
Department of Medicine
University of Toronto
Toronto, Ontario

Alberto S. Pappo, MD
Division of Hematology/Oncology
The Hospital for Sick Children
Toronto, Ontario

David M. Parham, MD
Department of Pathology
University of Arkansas
Little Rock, Arkansas

*deceased

Ben Ho Park, MD, PhD
Department of Oncology
Johns Hopkins University
Baltimore, Maryland

Harvey I. Pass, MD
Department of Surgery and Oncology
Harper Hospital
Detroit, Michigan

Edward F. Patz Jr, MD
Department of Radiology
Duke University Medical Center
Durham, North Carolina

C. Leigh Pearce, PhD
Department of Preventative Medicine
University of Southern California
Los Angeles, California

Sherrie Perkins, MD, PhD
Department of Pathology
University of Utah
Salt Lake City, Utah

Elizabeth J. Perlman, MD
Department of Pathology
Northwestern University
Chicago, Illinois

Marco A. Pierotti, PhD
Department of Experimental Oncology
National Institute for Tumor Study and Treatment
Milan, Italy

Peter W.T. Pisters, MD, FACS
Department of Surgical Oncology
MD Anderson Cancer Center
Houston, Texas

Giuseppe Pizzorno, PhD, PharmD
Department of Internal Medicine
Yale University School of Medicine
New Haven, Connecticut

William K. Plunkett Jr, PhD
Department of Therapeutics
MD Anderson Cancer Center
Houston, Texas

Brian W. Pogue, PhD
Thayer School of Engineering
Dartmouth College
Hanover, New Hampshire

Raphael E. Pollock, MD, PhD, FACS
Department of Surgical Oncology
MD Anderson Cancer Center
Houston, Texas

Kornelia Polyak, MD, PhD
Department of Medical Oncology
Dana-Farber Cancer Institute
Boston, Massachusetts

Kalmon D. Post, MD
Department of Neurosurgery
Mount Sinai School of Medicine
New York, New York

Michael D. Prados, MD
Department of Neurosurgery
University of California
San Francisco, California

S. Egbert Pravinkumar, MD, FRCP
Department of Critical Care
MD Anderson Cancer Center
Houston, Texas

Leonard Prosnitz, MD
Department of Radiation Oncology
Duke University Medical Center
Durham, North Carolina

Martin N. Raber, MD
Department of Medicine
MD Anderson Cancer Center
Houston, Texas

Elizabeth A. Raetz, MD
Department of Pediatrics
Mount Sinai School of Medicine
New York, New York

Kristjan T. Ragnarsson, MD
Department of Rehabilitation Medicine
Mount Sinai School of Medicine
New York, New York

Jamal Rahaman, MD
Department of Reproductive Science
Mount Sinai School of Medicine
New York, New York

Kanti R. Rai, MD
Division of Hematology/Oncology
Long Island Jewish Center
New Hyde Park, New York

Noopur Raje, MD, MB, BS
Department of Medicine
Brigham and Women's Hospital
Boston, Massachusetts

Jacob H. Rand, MD, FACP
Departments of Pathology and Medicine
Albert Einstein College of Medicine
Bronx, New York

R. Lor Randall, MD, FACS
Department of Orthopedics
University of Utah
Salt Lake City, Utah

Mark J. Ratain, MD
Department of Medicine
University of Chicago
Chicago, Illinois

Gregory H. Reaman, MD
Department of Pediatrics
George Washington University
Washington, District of Columbia

John C. Reed, MD, PhD
President and CEO
The Burnham Institute
La Jolla, California

Marvin S. Reitz Jr, PhD
Institute of Human Virology
University of Maryland
Baltimore, Maryland

Susan R. Rheingold, MD
Department of Oncology
University of Pennsylvania
Philadelphia, Pennsylvania

David C. Rice, MD
Department of Thoracic and Cardiovascular Surgery
MD Anderson Cancer Center
Houston, Texas

Jerome P. Richie, MD
Department of Surgery
Harvard Medical School
Boston, Massachusetts

Paula Trahan Rieger, RN, MSN, AOCN, FAAN
American Society of Clinical Oncology
Alexandria, Virginia

Michael L. Ritchey, MD
Department of Surgery
University of Texas Medical School
Houston, Texas

Leslie L. Robison, PhD
Division of Epidemiology and Clinical Research
University of Minnesota
Minneapolis, Minnesota

Miguel A. Rodriguez-Bigas, MD
Department of Surgical Oncology
MD Anderson Cancer Center
Houston, Texas

Carlos Rodriguez-Galindo, MD
Department of Hematology-Oncology
St. Jude Children's Research Hospital
Memphis, Tennessee

John C. Roeske, PhD
Department of Radiation Oncology
University of Chicago Hospitals
Chicago, Illinois

Kenneth V.I. Rolston, MD, FACP
Section of Infectious Diseases
MD Anderson Cancer Center
Houston, Texas

Brian R. Rood, MD
Department of Hematology and Oncology
George Washington University
Washington, District of Columbia

Gerald Rosen, MD
Medical Director
Cedar-Sinai Comprehensive Cancer Center
Los Angeles, California

Robert W. Ross, MD
Department of Medicine
Harvard Medical School
Boston, Massachusetts

Ronald K. Ross, MD
Department of Preventative Medicine
University of South California
Los Angeles, California

Bruce J. Roth, MD
Department of Medicine
Vanderbilt University Medical Center
Nashville, Tennessee

Jack A. Roth, MD
Department of Thoracic and Cardiovascular Surgery
MD Anderson Cancer Center
Houston, Texas

Jacob H. Rotmensch, MD
Department of Gynecologic Oncology
University of Chicago
Chicago, Illinois

Eric K. Rowinsky, MD
Chief Medical Officer
Senior Vice President
ImClone Systems
New York, New York

Eric H. Rubin, MD
Department of Medicine
Cancer Institute of New Jersey
New Brunswick, New Jersey

Raymond W. Ruddon, MD, PhD
Departments of Research and Graduate Studies
University of Michigan
Ann Arbor, Michigan

Alexandra Sacks, BA
Medical Student
Mount Sinai School of Medicine
New York, New York

Amar Safdar, MD, FACP
Department of Infectious Diseases
MD Anderson Cancer Center
Houston, Texas

Thaddeus Samulski, PhD
Department of Radiation Oncology
Duke University Medical Center
Durham, North Carolina

Kadria Sayed, MD
Department of Pathology
University of Arkansas
Little Rock, Arkansas

David T. Scadden, MD
Division of Hematology & Medical Oncology
Massachusetts General Hospital Cancer Center
Boston, Massachusetts

Andrew V. Schally, PhD, DSc, MD (hc)
Department of Research
Veterans Affairs Medical Center
New Orleans, Louisiana

Amy C. Schefler, MD
Resident in Ophthalmology
University of Miami
Miami, Florida

Charles A. Schiffer, MD
Departments of Medicine and Oncology
Wayne State University
Detroit, Michigan

Jeffrey Schlom, PhD
Laboratory of Tumor Immunology and Biology
National Cancer Institute
Bethesda, Maryland

Erasmus Schneider, PhD
Department of Biomedical Sciences
University at Albany
Albany, New York

Robert A. Schnoll, PhD
Department of Health Education and Administration
Arcadia University
Glenside, Pennsylvania

David E. Schteingart, MD
Department of Internal Medicine
University of Michigan
Ann Arbor, Michigan

Kitt Shaffer, MD, PhD
Department of Radiology
Dana-Farber Cancer Center
Boston, Massachusetts

Brenda Shank, MD, PhD, FACR
Department of Radiation Oncology
University of California
San Francisco, California

Vickie R. Shannon, MD
Department of Pulmonary Medicine
MD Anderson Cancer Center
Houston, Texas

Steven I. Sherman, MD
Department of Endocrine Neoplasia and Hormonal Disorders
MD Anderson Cancer Center
Houston, Texas

Elizabeth Shpall, MD
Department of Blood and Marrow Transplantation
MD Anderson Cancer Center
Houston, Texas

Suzanne Shusterman, MD
Department of Pediatrics
Harvard Medical School
Boston, Massachusetts

Branimir I. Sikic, MD
Department of Medicine – Oncology
Stanford University
Stanford, California

Elin R. Sigurdson, MD
Medical Science Division
Fox Chase Cancer Center
Philadelphia, Pennsylvania

Richard T. Silver, MD
Division of Hematology-Oncology
Weill Medical College of Cornell University
New York, New York

Lewis R. Silverman, MD
Department of Medicine
Mount Sinai School of Medicine
New York, New York

Paul M. Silverman, MD
Department of Diagnostic Radiology
MD Anderson Cancer Center
Houston, Texas

Robert A. Smith, PhD
Cancer Control Sciences Department
American Cancer Society
Atlanta, Georgia

Thomas C. Smyrk, MD
Department of Pathology
Mayo Clinic
Rochester, Minnesota

Arthur J. Sober, MD
Department of Dermatology
Harvard Medical School
Boston, Massachusetts

Nicolas Solban, PhD
Department of Dermatology
Harvard Medical School
Boston, Massachusetts

Stephen T. Sonis, DMD, DMSc
Department of Surgery Research
Brigham and Women's Hospital
Boston, Massachusetts

Gabriella Sozzi, PhD
Department of Experimental Oncology
National Institute for Tumor Study and Treatment
Milan, Italy

Michael B. Sporn, MD
Department of Pharmacology
Dartmouth Medical School
Hanover, New Hampshire

Dempsey Springfield, MD
Department of Orthopedics
Mount Sinai School of Medicine
New York, New York

Graeme S. Steele, MD
Division of Urologic Surgery
Brigham and Women's Hospital
Boston, Massachusetts

David P. Steensma, MD
Department of Internal Medicine
Mayo Medical School
Rochester, Minnesota

Richard M. Stone, MD
Department of Medicine
Dana-Farber Cancer Institute
Boston, Massachusetts

Erich M. Sturgis, MD, FACS
Department of Head and Neck Surgery/Epidemiology
MD Anderson Cancer Center
Houston, Texas

Max W. Sung, MD
Department of Medicine
Mount Sinai School of Medicine
New York, New York

Stephen G. Swisher, MD
Department of Thoracic and Cardiovascular Surgery
MD Anderson Cancer Center
Houston, Texas

James A. Talcott, MD, SM
Department of Medicine
Harvard Medical School
Boston, Massachusetts

Joseph M. Taraska, JD
Jacobs & Goodman PA
Altamont Springs, Florida

Ayalew Tefferi, MD
Department of Medicine
Mayo Medical School
Rochester, Minnesota

Lisa A. Teot, MD
Department of Pathology
University of Pittsburgh
Pittsburgh, Pennsylvania

Richard L. Theriault, DO, MBA, FACP
Department of Breast Medical Oncology
MD Anderson Cancer Center
Houston, Texas

David C. Thomas, MD, MS
Department of Medicine
Mount Sinai School of Medicine
New York, New York

Michael J. Thun, MD, MS
Epidemiology and Surveillance Research
American Cancer Society
Atlanta, Georgia

Swan N. Thung, MD
Department of Pathology
Mount Sinai School of Medicine
New York, New York

Jeffrey A. Toretsky, MD
Department of Oncology and Pediatrics
Georgetown University
Washington, District of Columbia

Guillermo Tortolero-Luna, MD, PhD
Department of Gynecologic Oncology
MD Anderson Cancer Center
Houston, Texas

Elizabeth L. Travis, PhD
Department of Experimental Radiation Oncology
MD Anderson Cancer Center
Houston, Texas

Mylene T. Truong, MD
Department of Thoracic Radiology
MD Anderson Cancer Center
Houston, Texas

Douglas Tyler, MD
Department of Surgery
Duke University
Durham, North Carolina

Samir D. Undevia, MD
Department of Internal Medicine
University of Chicago
Chicago, Illinois

Ara A. Vaporciyan, MD
Department of Thoracic and Cardiovascular Surgery
MD Anderson Cancer Center
Houston, Texas

Bert Vogelstein, MD
Department of Oncology
Johns Hopkins University
Baltimore, Maryland

Daniel D. Von Hoff, MD, FACP
Department of Medicine
University of Arizona
Tucson, Arizona

Evan Vosburgh, MD
Department of Medicine
Yale University
New Haven, Connecticut

Zeljko Vujaskovic, MD, PhD
Department of Radiation Oncology
Duke University Medical Center
Durham, North Carolina

Michael J. Wallace, MD
Department of Diagnostic Radiology
MD Anderson Cancer Center
Houston, Texas

Ronald S. Walters, MD
Division of Medical Oncology
MD Anderson Cancer Center
Houston, Texas

Helen H. Wang, MD, DrPH
Department of Pathology
Harvard Medical School
Boston, Massachusetts

Ralph R. Weichselbaum, MD
Department of Radiation and Cellular Oncology
University of Chicago
Chicago, Illinois

Lawrence Weiss, MD
Division of Pathology
City of Hope Medical Center
Duarte, California

Ainsley Weston, MD
Toxicology and Molecular Biology Branch
National Institute for Occupational Safety and Health
Morgantown, West Virginia

J. Taylor Wharton, MD
Department of Gynecologic Oncology
MD Anderson Cancer Center
Houston, Texas

Cheryl L. Willman, MD
Department of Medicine
University of New Mexico
Albuquerque, New Mexico

Suzanne Wolden, MD
Department of Radiation Oncology
Memorial Sloan-Kettering Cancer Center
New York, New York

Robert A. Wolff, MD
Department of Gastrointestinal Medical Oncology
MD Anderson Cancer Center
Houston, Texas

Robert C. Wollman, MD
Department of Radiation Oncology
Saint John's Health Center
Santa Monica, California

James C. Yao, MD
Department of Gastrointestinal Medical Oncology
MD Anderson Cancer Center
Houston, Texas

Edward T.H. Yeh, MD
Department of Cardiology
MD Anderson Cancer Center
Houston, Texas

K. Simon Yeung, RPh, MBA, LAc
Memorial Sloan-Kettering Cancer Center
New York, New York

Sai-Ching Jim Yeung, MD, PhD
Division of Internal Medicine
MD Anderson Cancer Center
Houston, Texas

Michael R. Zalutsky, PhD
Department of Radiology
Duke University
Durham, North Carolina

Anthony L. Zietman, MD
Department of Radiation Oncology
Massachusetts General Hospital
Boston, Massachusetts

PREFACE

Cancer medicine has begun to harvest the fruits of the molecular biological revolution. An understanding of the complex interaction of molecules outside and inside a living cell has elucidated many of the qualitative and quantitative differences between cancer cells and normal cells. The progression of increasing abnormality that punctuates the itinerary from normal to precancerous, to noninvasive cancer, to invasive cancer, and to metastasis are now more readily understandable in molecular terms. Somatic genetic differences derived from over- and underexpression of genes and their derivative pathways have clarified the fundamentals of pathogenesis for many tumors. Specific therapies crafted for identified molecular targets of particular tumors have emerged. Particular enzyme inhibitors and antibodies have allowed for the exploitation of recognizable qualitative differences between cancer cells and normals. Minimally invasive surgery has improved the contributions of this discipline, much as intensity-modulated radiation therapy has contributed to patient welfare. Multidisciplinary care is the norm, and science-based decisions often inform evidence-based clinical decisions for cancer management. Society has come to grips with cancer prevention: Smoke-free zones, increased taxation, and publicity have begun to crack the impervium of the tobacco industry, and thus impact the most preventable cancers. Cancer prevention is within our intellectual reach, if not our immediate grasp.

The editors have selected authors whose expertise is recognized by their accomplishments and their special interests in and understanding of the topics on which they write. In every chapter we have sought to present a scientific basis for clinical implementation. The implementation of knowledge about cancer requires an understanding of the clinical character of neoplasia and of cancer patients. The compleat oncologist is one who can incorporate fundamental understanding into clinical use. We are proud that *Cancer Medicine 7* accomplishes this synthesis of principles and practice. The third of a century since the first edition of *Cancer Medicine* has seen more progress in understanding, treating, and preventing cancer than in the eons that preceded. We believe the momentum is unstoppable. The aging of the United States population and the decline of cardiovascular mortality will soon make cancer the leading cause of death. Cancer research and cancer prevention will even more persuasively become everybody's business. The trajectory of the current advances will make even more evident the already declining annual mortality from cancer. Old age appears inevitable.

The editors are grateful to the authors whose chapters establish the quality of this work. They are also grateful to their families, colleagues, and staff for the often unrecognized contributions that they have made in producing this edition. We are proud that the American Association for Cancer Research has adopted *Cancer Medicine 7* as an authorized publication. The editors are firmly committed to the proposition that most of the diseases we classify as cancer are preventable or curable. That we have not yet reached this achievement does not invalidate the concept. Preventing cancer, and curing it when it is not prevented, is a challenge that will be surmounted by greater understanding through research, and by conscientious application of what is already known.

This work is dedicated to physicians, scientists, nurses, and health workers who will use it to help prevent and cure cancer. We offer our hopes to those patients and their families whose care may be improved by the knowledge contained herein.

The Editors
March 2006

CONTENTS

Part I CARDINAL MANIFESTATIONS OF CANCER

1 Cardinal Manifestations of Cancer 3
James F. Holland, MD, ScD (hc), Emil Frei III, MD, Donald W. Kufe, MD, Robert C. Bast Jr, MD, Raphael E. Pollock, MD, PhD, Ralph R. Weichselbaum, MD, Waun Ki Hong, MD, William N. Hait, MD, PhD

Part II SCIENTIFIC FOUNDATIONS OF CANCER

Section 1: CANCER BIOLOGY

2 Molecular Biology, Genomics, and Proteomics, and Mouse Models of Human Cancer 9
Kornelia Polyak, MD, PhD, Matthew Meyerson, MD, PhD

3 Cell Proliferation and Differentiation 27
Michael Andreeff, MD, PhD, David W. Goodrich, PhD, H. Phillip Koeffler, MD

4 Apoptosis and Cancer 41
John C. Reed, MD, PhD

5 Growth Factors and Signal Transduction in Cancer 53
Anna Bafico, PhD, Stuart A. Aaronson, MD

6 Oncogenes 68
Marco A. Pierotti, PhD, Milo Frattini, PhD, Gabriella Sozzi, PhD, Carlo M. Croce, MD

7 Tumor Supressor Genes 85
Ben Ho Park, MD, PhD, Bert Vogelstein, MD

8 Genomic Alterations and Chromosomal Aberrations in Human Cancer 104
Cheryl L. Willman, MD, Robert Hromas, MD

9 Biochemistry of Cancer 135
Raymond W. Ruddon, MD, PhD, Donald W. Kufe, MD, William N. Hait, MD, PhD

10 Invasion and Metastases 148
Elsie C. Kohn, MD

11 Tumor Angiogenesis 157
Judah Folkman, MD, John Heymach, MD, PhD, Raghu Kalluri, PhD

Section 2: CANCER IMMUNOLOGY

12a Tumor Antigens 193
Michael A. Morse, MD

12b Cancer Biomarkers 199
Stephen Chui, MD

12c Effectors of Immunity 205
Timothy M. Clay, PhD, H. Kim Lyerly, MD, Lauretta Odogwu-Oti, MD, Michael A. Morse, MD

12d Defects in Antitumor Immunity 209
Michael A. Morse, MD

12e Monitoring the Immune Response to Cancer Vaccines 213
Amy C. Hobeika, PhD, Timothy M. Clay, PhD, H. Kim Lyerly, MD, Michael A. Morse, MD

Section 3: CANCER ETIOLOGY

13 Genetic Predisposition to Cancer 216
Marcia S. Brose, MD, PhD, Thomas C. Smyrk, MD, Henry T. Lynch, MD

14 Chemical Carcinogenesis 246
Ainsley Weston, PhD, Curtis C. Harris, MD

15 Hormones and the Etiology of Cancer 259
Leslie Bernstein, PhD, C. Leigh Pearce, PhD, Ronald K. Ross, MD, Brian E. Henderson, MD

16 Ionizing Radiation 270
John B. Little, MD, David J. Grdina, PhD

17 Ultraviolet Radiation Carcinogenesis 283
James E. Cleaver, PhD, David L. Mitchell, PhD

18 Inflammation, Trauma, and Physical Agents in Cancer 292
Michael A. Gallo, PhD, Joseph Aisner, MD

19 Tumor Viruses 297
Robert C. Gallo, MD, Marvin S. Reitz Jr, PhD

20 Herpesviruses 310
Jeffrey I. Cohen, MD

21 Papillomaviruses and Cervical Neoplasia 318
Christopher P. Crum, MD, Catherine M. McLachlin, MD

22 Hepatitis Viruses 323
Max W. Sung, MD, Swan N. Thung, MD

23 Parasites 332
Piero Mustacchi, MD, ScD, Anne G. Kasmar, MD, MSc

Section 4: CANCER EPIDEMIOLOGY, PREVENTION, and SCREENING

24 Cancer Epidemiology 339
Michael J. Thun, MD, MS, Ahmedin Jemal, DVM, PhD

25 Prevention of Tobacco-Related Cancers 354
Paul F. Engstrom, MD, Margie L. Clapper, PhD, Robert A. Schnoll, PhD

26 Nutrition in the Etiology and Prevention of Cancer 363
Steven K. Clinton, MD, PhD, Edward L. Giovannucci, MD, ScD, DPH, Elizabeth C. Miller, MS, RD, LD

27 Chemoprevention of Cancer 377
Michael B. Sporn, MD, Scott M. Lippman, MD

28 Cancer Screening and Early Detection 389
Robert A. Smith, PhD, Steven W. Duffy, MSc, Harmon J. Eyre, MD

Section 5: CLINICAL TRIALS AND OUTCOMES ASSESSMENT

29 Statistical Innovations in Cancer Research 411
Donald A. Berry, PhD

30 Cancer Outcomes 426
James A. Talcott, MD, SM

Part III PRINCIPLES OF CANCER DIAGNOSIS

Section 6: CANCER PATHOLOGY

31 Principles of Cancer Pathology 437
James L. Connolly, MD, Jeffrey D. Goldsmith, MD, Helen H. Wang, MD, DrPH, Janina A. Longtine, MD, Ann M. Dvorak, MD, Harold F. Dvorak, MD

Section 7: IMAGING

32 Principles of Imaging 455
Edward F. Patz Jr, MD

32a Imaging Cancer of Unknown Primary Site 456
Kitt Shaffer, MD, PhD

32b Imaging Neoplasms of the Central Nervous System, Head, and Neck 460
Christopher J. Hurt, MD, Norman J. Beauchamp Jr, MD, MHS

32c Imaging Neoplasms of the Thorax 468
Jeremy J. Erasmus, MD, Mylene T. Truong, MD, H. Page McAdams, MD

32d Imaging Neoplasms of the Abdomen and Pelvis 474
Haesun Choi, MD, Harmeet Kaur, MD, Evelyne M. Loyer, MD, Paul M. Silverman, MD

32e Imaging of Musculoskeletal Neoplasms 479
R. Lee Cothran, MD, Clyde A. Helms, MD

32f Imaging the Breast 482
Lawrence W. Bassett, MD, FACR, Olegario Jay Lara, DO

32g Radionuclide Imaging in Cancer Medicine 488
R. Edward Coleman, MD

33 Interventional Radiology for the Cancer Patient 492
Marshall E. Hicks, MD, Michael J. Wallace, MD, Sanjay Gupta, MD

Part IV PRINCIPLES OF THERAPEUTIC MODALITIES

Section 8: SURGICAL ONCOLOGY

34 Principles of Surgical Oncology. 503
Raphael E. Pollock, MD, PhD, FACS, Donald L. Morton, MD, FACS

Section 9: RADIATION ONCOLOGY

35 Principles of Radiation Oncology 517
Arno J. Mundt, MD, John C. Roeske, PhD, Theodore D. Chung, MD, PhD, Ralph R. Weichselbaum, MD

35a Photodynamic Therapy of Cancer 537
Tayyaba Hasan, PhD, Bernhard Ortel, MD, Nicolas Solban, PhD, Brian W. Pogue, PhD

35b Hyperthermia 549
Mark W. Dewhirst, DVM, PhD, Ellen Jones, MD, PhD, Thaddeus Samulski, PhD, Zeljko Vujaskovic, MD, PhD, Chuan Y. Le, PhD, Leonard Prosnitz, MD

Section 10: MEDICAL ONCOLOGY

36 Principles of Medical Oncology. 562
William N. Hait, MD, PhD, James F. Holland, MD, ScD (hc), Emil Frei III, MD, Donald W. Kufe, MD, Robert C. Bast Jr, MD, Waun Ki Hong, MD

Section 11: CHEMOTHERAPY

37 Cytokinetics. 570
Teresa Ann Gilewski, MD, Larry Norton, MD

38 Principles of Dose, Schedule, and Combination Therapy 590
Emil Frei III, MD, Joseph Paul Eder, MD

39 Preclinical and Early Clinical Development of New Anticancer Agents 600
Daniel D. Von Hoff, MD, FACP, Axel-R. Hanauske, MD, PhD

40 Pharmacology 617
Samir D. Undevia, MD, Mark J. Ratain, MD, William Plunkett, PhD

41 Drug Resistance and its Clinical Circumvention. 630
Jeffrey Moscow, MD, Erasmus Schneider, PhD, Branimir I. Sikic, MD, Charles S. Morrow, MD, PhD, Kenneth H. Cowan, MD, PhD

Section 12: CHEMOTHERAPEUTIC AGENTS

42 Folate Antagonists 648
Peter D. Cole, MD, Barton A. Kamen, MD, PhD, Joseph R. Bertino, MD

43 Pyrimidine and Purine Antimetabolites. 661
Giuseppe Pizzorno, PhD, PharmD, Robert B. Diasio, MD, Yung-Chi Cheng, PhD

44 Alkylating Agents and Platinum Antitumor Compounds 675
Michael Colvin, MD

45 Drugs That Target DNA Topoisomerases 688
Eric H. Rubin, MD, William N. Hait, MD, PhD

46 Microtubule-Targeting Natural Products. 699
Eric K. Rowinsky, MD

47 Small-Molecule Inhibitors of Protein Kinases in the Treatment of Human Cancer 722
Michael C. Heinrich, MD, Charles D. Blanke, MD, Christopher L. Corless, MD, PhD, Brian J. Druker, MD

Section 13: BIOTHERAPEUTICS

48 Interferons 733
Ernest C. Borden, MD

49 Cytokines and Hematopoietic Growth Factors 744
Suhendan Ekmekcioglu, PhD, Elizabeth Ann Grimm, PhD, Razelle Kurzrock, MD

50 Monoclonal Serotherapy 770
Robert C. Bast Jr, MD, Michael R. Zalutsky, PhD, Robert J. Kreitman, MD, Arthur E. Frankel, MD

51 Vaccines and Immunostimulants 786
James W. Hodge, PhD, Jeffrey Schlom, PhD, Scott I. Abrams, PhD

Section 14: ENDOCRINE THERAPY

52 Hypothalamic and Other Peptide Hormones. 802
Andrew V. Schally, PhD, DSc, MD (hc), Ana Maria Comaru-Schally, MD, MS

53 Corticosteroids. 817
Lorraine I. McKay, PhD, John A. Cidlowski, PhD

54 Estrogens, Antiestrogens and Aromatase Inhibitors 828
Aman U. Buzdar, MD, Harold A. Harvey, MD, V. Craig Jordan, OBE, PhD, DSc

55 Progestins 843
Kenneth S. McCarty Jr, MD, PhD, Mark D. Nichols, PhD, Pamela A. Hershberger, PhD, Justin C. McCarty, Kenneth S. McCarty, PhD

56 Androgens 850
Samuel R. Denmeade, MD

Section 15: GENE THERAPY

57 Cancer Gene Therapy 860
Sunil J. Advani, MD, Ralph R. Weichselbaum, MD, Donald W. Kufe, MD

Section 16: BONE MARROW TRANSPLANTATION

58 Hematopoietic Cell Transplantation 879
Roy Jones, PhD, MD, Elizabeth Shpall, MD, Richard Champlin, MD

Part V PRINCIPLES OF MULTIDISCIPLINARY MANAGEMENT

Section 17: PSYCHO-ONCOLOGY

59 Principles of Psycho-Oncology 901
Jimmie C. Holland, MD, Alexandra Sacks, BA

Section 18: ONCOLOGY NURSING

60 Principles of Oncology Nursing 915
Paula Trahan Rieger, RN, MSN, AOCN, FAAN

Section 19: CANCER REHABILITATION MEDICINE

61 Principles of Cancer Rehabilitation Medicine 922
David C. Thomas, MD, Kristjan T. Ragnarsson, MD

Section 20: MULTIDISCIPLINARY MANAGEMENT

62 Principles of Multidisciplinary Management 935
James F. Holland, MD, ScD (hc), Emil Frei III, MD, Donald W. Kufe, MD, Robert C. Bast Jr, MD, Raphael E. Pollock, MD, PhD, Ralph R. Weichselbaum, MD, Waun Ki Hong, MD, William N. Hait, MD, PhD

63 Cancer and Pregnancy 941
Phuong Khanh H. Morrow, MD, Richard L. Theriault, DO, MBA, FACP, Gabriel N. Hortobagyi, MD, FACP

64 Cancer and Aging 949
Arti Hurria, MD, Hyman B. Muss, MD, Harvey J. Cohen, MD

65 Integrative Oncology: Complementary Therapies in Cancer Care 957
Barrie R. Cassileth, PhD, MS, Gary Deng, MD, PhD, K. Simon Yeung, RPh, MBA, LAc

Section 21: PAIN AND PALLIATION

66 Palliative Care 966
Natalie Moryl, MD, Alan C. Carver, MD, Kathleen M. Foley, MD

67 Management of Cancer Pain 979
Natalie Moryl, MD, Alan C. Carver, MD, Kathleen M. Foley, MD

Section 22: SOCIETAL ONCOLOGY

68 Ethics in Oncology 998
Ezekiel J. Emanuel, MD, PhD, Steven Joffe, MD, MPH

69 Legal Aspects of Cancer 1015
Joseph Taraska, JD

70 The Government and Cancer Medicine 1021
Anna D. Barker, PhD, Hamilton Jordan

71 Delivering High-Quality Cancer Care in a Changing Health Care Environment 1031
Martin N. Raber, MD, Ronald S. Walters, MD

Part VI CANCER MANAGEMENT

Section 23: CENTRAL NERVOUS SYSTEM

72 Primary Neoplasms of the Central Nervous System in Adults 1037
Michael D. Prados, MD

73 Brain Metastases 1065
Sean Grimm, MD, Lisa M. DeAngelis, MD

Section 24: THE EYE

74 Neoplasms of the Eye 1071
David H. Abramson, MD, FACS, Amy C. Schefler, MD, Ira J. Dunkel, MD, Beryl McCormick, MD

Section 25: ENDOCRINE GLANDS

75 Neoplasms of the Endocrine Glands: Pituitary Neoplasms 1084
Chirag D. Gandhi, MD, Kalmon D. Post, MD

76 Neoplasms of the Thyroid 1093
Steven I. Sherman, MD, Ann Marie Gillenwater, MD

77 Neoplasms of the Adrenal Cortex 1103
David E. Schteingart, MD

78 Neoplasms of the Diffuse Endocrine System 1109
Evan Vosburgh, MD

Section 26: HEAD AND NECK

79 Neoplasms of the Head and Neck 1131
Eduardo M. Diaz Jr, MD, FACS, Merrill S. Kies, MD, Erich M. Sturgis, MD, FACS, Lewis Clayman, DMD, MD, George E. Laramore, PhD, MD, Scott M. Lippman, MD, Gary L. Clayman, DMD, MD, FACS

Section 27: THE THORAX

80 Cancer of the Lung 1179
Amir Onn, MD, Ara A. Vaporciyan, MD, Joe Y. Chang, MD, PhD, Ritsuko Komaki, MD, Jack A. Roth, MD, Roy S. Herbst, MD, PhD

81 Malignant Mesothelioma 1225
Harvey I. Pass, MD, Michele Carbone, MD, PhD, A. Philippe Chahinian, MD

82 Thymomas and Thymic Tumors 1237
A. Philippe Chahinian, MD

83 Tumors of the Heart and Great Vessels 1245
A. Philippe Chahinian, MD, Andrew J. Einstein, MD, PhD, Valentin Fuster, MD, PhD

84 Primary Germ Cell Tumors of the Thorax 1249
John D. Hainsworth, MD, F. Anthony Greco, MD

Section 28: GASTROINTESTINAL TRACT

85 Neoplasms of the Esophagus 1255
Stephen G. Swisher, MD, David C. Rice, MD, Jaffer A. Ajani, MD, Ritsuko K. Komaki, MD, Mark K. Ferguson, MD

86 Carcinoma of the Stomach 1268
James C. Yao, MD, Christopher H. Crane, MD, Paul F. Mansfield, MD

87 Primary Neoplasms of the Liver 1292
Paul F. Engstrom, MD, Elin R. Sigurdson, MD, PhD, Alison A. Evans, ScD, Nancy Lewis, MD

88 Treatment of Liver Metastases 1302
Nancy E. Kemeny, MD, Yuman Fong, MD

89 Gallbladder and Bile Duct Cancer 1318
Steven A. Curley, MD

90 Neoplasms of the Exocrine Pancreas 1331
Robert A. Wolff, MD, Christopher H. Crane, MD, Donghui Li, PhD, James L. Abbruzzese, MD, FACP, Douglas B. Evans, MD

91 Neoplasms of the Small Intestine, Vermiform Appendix, and Peritoneum 1359
Elizabeth G. Grubbs, MD, Douglas S. Tyler, MD

92 Carcinoma of the Colon and Rectum 1369
Miguel A. Rodriguez-Bigas, MD, Paulo Hoff, MD, Christopher H. Crane, MD

93 Neoplasms of the Anus 1392
Brenda Shank, MD, PhD, FACR, Marshall S. Flam, MD, FACP, John Cunningham, MD

Section 29: GENITOURINARY TRACT

94 Renal Cell Carcinoma 1401
Jerome P. Richie, MD, Eric Jonasch, MD, Philip W. Kantoff, MD

95 Neoplasms of the Renal Pelvis and Ureter 1410
Jerome P. Richie, MD, Philip W. Kantoff, MD

96 Bladder Cancer 1415
Timothy D. Gilligan, MD, Graeme Steele, MD, Anthony L. Zietman, MD, Philip W. Kantoff, MD

97 Neoplasms of the Prostate 1431
Robert W. Ross, MD, William K. Oh, MD, Mark Hurwitz, MD, Anthony V. D'Amico, MD, Jerome P. Richie, MD, Philip W. Kantoff, MD

98 Tumors of the Penis and Urethra 1462
Donald F. Lynch Jr, MD

99 Testis Cancer 1468
Craig R. Nichols, MD, Arthur Hung, MD, Christopher Corless, MD, Richard S. Foster, MD, Bruce J. Roth, MD, Lawrence H. Einhorn, MD

Section 30: FEMALE REPRODUCTIVE ORGANS

100 Neoplasms of the Vulva and Vagina 1488
Jacob H. Rotmensch, MD

101 Neoplasms of the Cervix 1497
Anuja Jhingran, MD, Patricia J. Eifel, MD, J. Taylor Wharton, MD, Guillermo Totolero-Luna, MD, PhD

102 Endometrial Cancer 1522
Jamal Rahaman, MD, Carmel J. Cohen, MD

103 Neoplasms of the Fallopian Tube 1537
Carmel J. Cohen, MD, Jamal Rahaman, MD

104 Ovarian Cancer 1543
Jonathan S. Berek, MD, MMSc, Robert C. Bast Jr, MD

105 Gestational Trophoblastic Disease 1569
Ross S. Berkowitz, MD, Donald P. Goldstein, MD

106 Gynecologic Sarcomas 1576
Jamal Rahaman, MD, Carmel J. Cohen, MD

Section 31: THE BREAST

107 Neoplasms of the Breast 1584
Gabriel N. Hortobagyi, MD, FACP, Laura Esserman, MD, Thomas A. Buchholz, MD

Section 32: THE SKIN

108 Malignant Melanoma 1644
Donald L. Morton, MD, Richard Essner, MD, John M. Kirkwood, MD, Robert C. Wollman, MD

109 Other Skin Cancers 1663
Victor A. Neel, MD, PhD, Arthur J. Sober, MD

Section 33: BONE AND SOFT TISSUE

110 Bone Tumors 1675
Dempsey Springfield, MD, Gerald Rosen, MD

111 Soft Tissue Sarcomas 1694
Peter W.T. Pisters, MD, Brian OiSullivan, MD, Robert G. Maki, MD, PhD

Section 34: HEMATOPOIETIC SYSTEM

112 The Myelodyplastic Syndrome 1721
Lewis R. Silverman, MD

113 Acute Myeloid Leukemia in Adults Mast Cell Leukemia and Other Mast Cell Neoplasms 1739
Charles A. Schiffer, MD, Richard M. Stone, MD

114 Chronic Myeloid Leukemia 1761
Jorge Cortes, MD, Richard T. Silver, MD, Hagop Kantarjian, MD

115 Acute Lymphocytic Leukemia in Adults 1772
Stefan Faderl, MD, Hagop M. Kantarjian, MD

116 Chronic Lymphocytic Leukemia 1786
Kanti R. Rai, MD, Michael J. Keating, MD

117 Hodgkin Disease 1802
Peter M. Mauch, MD, Lawrence Weiss, MD, James O. Armitage, MD

118 Non-Hodgkin Lymphoma 1825
Arnold S. Freedman, MD

119 Mycosis Fungoides and the Sézary Syndrome 1839
Richard T. Hoppe, MD, Youn H. Kim, MD, Ranjana Advani, MD

120 Plasma Cell Tumors 1848
Noopur Raje, MD, MB, BS, Teru Hideshima, MD, PhD, Kenneth C. Anderson, MD

121 Chronic Myeloproliferative Disorders: Essential Thrombocythemia, Myelofibrosis with Myeloid Metaplasia, and Polycythemia Vera 1874
David P. Steensma, MD, Ayalew Tefferi, MD

Section 35: NEOPLASMS IN AIDS

122 Neoplasms in Acquired Immunodeficiency Syndrome....... 1887
David T. Scadden, MD

Section 36: UNKNOWN PRIMARY SITE

123 Neoplasms of Unknown Primary Site.................... 1904
John D. Hainsworth, MD, F. Anthony Greco, MD

Section 37: PEDIATRIC ONCOLOGY

124 Pediatric Oncology: Principles and Practice............... 1914
Gregory H. Reaman, MD

124a Incidence, Origins, and Epidemiology 1917
Leslie L. Robison, PhD

124b Late Effects of Cancer in Children and Adolescents 1921
Smita Bhatia, MD, MPH

124c Childhood Acute Lymphoblastic Leukemia 1934
Paul S. Gaynon, MD, Anne L. Angiolillo, MD, Janet L. Franklin, MD, Gregory H. Reaman, MD

124d Acute Myeloid Leukemia in Children 1944
Richard Aplenc, MD, MSCE, Beverly Lange, MD

124e Central Nervous System Tumors of the Infant and Child.. 1951
Tobey J. MacDonald, MD, Brian R. Rood, MD

124f Hodgkin Disease.................................. 1959
James Nachman, MD

124g Non-Hodgkin Lymphoma in Children 1962
Mitchell S. Cairo, MD, Elizabeth Raetz, MD, Sherrie Perkins, MD, PhD

124h Less-Frequently Enountered Tumors of Childhood 1976
Carlos Rodriguez-Galindo, MD, Alberto S. Pappo, MD

124i Renal Tumors of Childhood 1983
Paul E. Grundy, MD, Jeffrey S. Dome, MD, John A. Kalapuakal, MD, Elizabeth J. Perlman, MD, Michael L. Ritchey, MD

124j Neuroblastoma 1990
John M. Maris, MD, Suzanne Shusterman, MD

124k Soft Tissue Sarcomas of Childhood 2007
William H. Meyer, MD

124l Unique Pathologic Features of Childhood Cancer 2013
Kadria Sayed, MD, David M. Parham, MD

124m Pediatric Bone Tumors 2019
Richard G. Gorlick, MD, FAAP, Mark L. Bernstein, MD, FRCP(C), Jeffrey A. Toretsky, MD, R. Lor Randall, MD, FACS, Mark C. Gebhardt, MD, Lisa A. Teot, MD, Suzzane Wolden, MD, Neyssa Marina, MD

Section 38: COMPLICATIONS OF CANCER AND THEIR TREATMENT

125 Cancer in Young Adults and Older Adolescents 2028
W. Archie Bleyer, MD, Karen Albritton, MD

126 Cancer Anorexia and Cachexia......................... 2037
Takao Ohnuma, MD, PhD

127 Antiemetic Therapy 2055
David S. Ettinger, MD, Tara L. Lin, MD

128 Neurologic Complications 2061
Lisa M. DeAngelis, MD

129 Dermatologic Complications of Cancer Chemotherapy...... 2077
Joy H. Kunishige, MD, Narin Apisarnthanarax, MD, Madeline M. Duvic, MD

130 Skeletal Complications.............................. 2085
Samuel Kenan, MD, Jeffrey I. Mechanick, MD

131 Hematologic Complications and Blood Bank Support 2095
Richard M. Kaufman, MD, Kenneth C. Anderson, MD

132 Coagulopathic Complications of Cancer Patients 2113
Maria T. DeSancho, MD, Jacob H. Rand, MD

133 Urologic Complications.............................. 2123
Christopher J. Logothetis, MD, Diana M. Hey, PharmD

134 Cardiac Complications.............................. 2131
Michael S. Ewer, MD, MPH, JD, Robert S. Benjamin, MD, Edward T.H. Yeh, MD

135 Respiratory Complications........................... 2150
Vickie R. Shannon, MD, George A. Eapen, MD, Carlos A. Jimenez, MD, Rodolfo C. Morice, MD, Elizabeth L. Travis, PhD, Lara Bashoura, MD, Amar Safdar, MD, FACP, Roberto Adachi, MD, S. Egbert Pravinkumar, MD, FRCP, Burton F. Dickey, MD

136 Gastrointestinal and Hepatic Complications in Cancer Patients..................................... 2174
Marta L. Davila, MD, Robert S. Bresalier, MD

137 Oral Complications of Cancer and Their Treatment......... 2184
Stephen T. Sonis, DMD, DMSc

138 Gonadal Complications 2194
Catherine E. Klein, MD

139 Endocrine Complications and Paraneoplastic Syndromes.... 2204
Sai-Ching Jim Yeung, MD, PhD, Robert F. Gagel, MD

140 Treatment-Related Secondary Cancers 2216
Susan R. Rheingold, MD, Alfred I. Neugut, MD, PhD, Anna T. Meadows, MD

Section 39: INFECTION IN THE CANCER PATIENT

141 Infections in Patients with Cancer 2222
Kenneth V.I. Rolston, MD, FACP, Gerald P. Bodey, MD

Section 40: ONCOLOGIC EMERGENCIES

142 Oncologic Emergencies 2246
Sai-Ching Jim Yeung, MD, PhD, Carmen P. Escalante, MD

Section 41: ONCOLOGY AND INFORMATICS

143 Oncology Informatics................................ 2266
Edward P. Ambinder, MD

Index.. 2283

Part I

Cardinal Manifestations of Cancer

1

Cardinal Manifestations of Cancer

James F. Holland, MD, ScD (hc)
Emil Frei III, MD
Donald W. Kufe, MD
Robert C. Bast Jr, MD
Raphael E. Pollock, MD, PhD
Ralph R. Weichselbaum, MD
Waun Ki Hong, MD
William Hait, MD, PhD

Cancer is a singular word that embraces a vast diversity of diseases that can occur in any organ system throughout the animal kingdom. The unique characteristic of cancer is the proliferation of cells of a type different from, if ever so slightly, the normal complement of the organism. The proliferation may be rapid or slow, the accumulation of cells may be massive or miniscule. The essence of the matter, however, is that aberrant cells, distinct from the ordinary evolution of cell types, appear and accumulate. Thus, a cancer differs from hypertrophy and hyperplasia, which involve normal cells.

A cancer cell does not obey the complex rules of architecture and function that govern the usual placement and behavior of cells within a tissue. The wondrous coexistence of cells and tissues of multiple types that make up the eye, the finger, or the kidney, for example, each with appropriate anatomic location, all connections intact to fulfill their appointed tasks, is part of the miracle we call life. The explanation for this marvelous organization is the field of continuing exploration seeking the messages and exquisite controls that exist in multicellular organisms. Some believe the ultimate explanations will be discovered not in science, but in the field of religion.

Cancer is distinguished from other abnormal cellular growths that lead to benign tumors in its characteristic independence from the restrictions present in normal tissues. Benign tumors expand and compress, but do not attack or invade adjacent tissues. Accumulated cancer cells make a tissue that ignores the anatomic barriers of adjacent cell membranes and basement membranes. Through chemical and mechanical means, the cancer cell insinuates itself between and into the space of the normal cells, killing them by chemical and physical means, the grand usurper. Even though the placenta in mammals shows this behavior, there is self-limitation in location and in survival of the placental invasion. Although leukocytes normally extravasate and permeate tissues, they do not share the other characteristics of cancer. The cancer cell is partially or absolutely insensitive to such normal constraints, and may continue its invasiveness indefinitely.

Upon reaching a circulatory conduit, either a lymphatic or capillary vessel, a process that may not be entirely haphazard, cancer cells often penetrate the wall as part of their invasive behavior. They then may be carried by the lymphatic or venous circulation to remote sites where the possibility of adherence, extravasation, and colonization can occur, establishing metastases. In the absence of an intervening event, and given enough time, with few exceptions, the cancer process, as described, can lead to such anatomic or functional distortions that death ensues.

The cancer process does not start with a fully invasive cancer cell. A disorder in molecular instructions for protein synthesis is the common precursor lesion, nearly always because of qualitatively or quantitatively aberrant ribonucleic acid (RNA) messages transcribed from nuclear deoxyribonucleic acid (DNA). This occurs because of a mutation of the DNA, or because of overexpression of particular genes that encode for proteins important as catalysts in pathways for stimulating growth, or because of underexpression of genes whose coded proteins control and inhibit growth. Portions of genes may be lost, translocated, or amplified. Indeed, entire chromosomes may be deleted, replicated, or fused in abnormal ways. All such distortions of DNA can give rise to abnormal or unbalanced RNA messages, leading to qualitative or quantitative differences in proteins that result in disordered cellular function. Sometimes the functional abnormality is so extreme as to be lethal, initiating the suicidal mechanism of apoptosis. In other instances, the functional abnormality results in disease. Some of these diseases display the characteristics of cancer. Mutation, overexpression, and underexpression of genes can result from a wide spectrum of intrinsic and extrinsic causes, with various pathways that lead not to one final common pathway, but by several converging routes to cells with the phenotypic characteristics of cancer. When these cells are limited to an epithelial layer above the basement membrane, they are called *carcinoma-in-situ* or *intraepithelial neoplasia.* Similar changes probably occur, but are more difficult to recognize, in the mesenchymal tissues. Even cancer cells that do not penetrate the basement membrane, and thus lack one of the cardinal features of true cancer, represent a long series of antecedent molecular abnormalities that eventually lead to this optically recognizable cellular change. Furthermore, these evolving cancer cells are the common, if not the exclusive, precursor of invasive cancer.

In their earliest stages, as proliferating cells accumulate, cancers are almost always asymptomatic. Cancers cause symptoms as they advance as a consequence of their mass, because they ulcerate on an epithelial surface, or because of change in function of the affected structure or organ. Nearly all the symptoms that can be caused by cancer can also be caused more commonly by noncancerous diseases. The astute clinician must include cancer in the differential diagnosis of virtually every symptom, albeit a benign disease may usually explain it. Doctors never diagnose diseases they do not think of. Cancers occur at any age. A longer life span provides greater opportunity for intrinsic organic events or an encounter with environmental carcinogens, however, and greater opportunity for initial DNA mutations to be fully realized as invasive cancers. Thus, age is the principal risk factor for most, but not all, cancers.

Such common symptoms as sore throat, runny nose, or a chest cold can sometimes be a result of cancers of pharynx, sinuses, or bronchi, respectively. Indeed, patients with these cancer diagnoses usually have been treated, often repeatedly and for extended periods, for the benign disease because cancer was not considered in the differential diagnosis, and appropriate observations were not made. Cancer symptoms such as diarrhea, constipation, or mild pain often seem commonplace. Cancer symptoms may be intermittent, with spontaneous temporary improvement, a phenomenon that is usually misinterpreted by patients and often by physicians as evidence against the diagnosis of cancer. In fact, recurrent appearance or chronicity of a symptom, which in short duration is characteristic of a common benign disease, markedly heightens the possibility of an underlying dysfunction caused by cancer.

Cancers cause their symptoms by a few readily understandable mechanisms.

Occlusion of an essential conduit, partial or complete, can be caused by tumor. A tumor mass grows to such size that it partially or completely occludes an essential conduit. Classic presentations are cancer of the bronchus where partial bronchial occlusion causes cough, diminishes ciliary clearance of secretion, and sometimes leads to bronchopneumonia. Complete bronchial occlusion leads to atelectasis and chronic pneumonia. Compromise of the esophageal lumen by tumor mass or muscular dysfunction resulting from infiltration causes dysphagia, which, in its early presentation, is far too often attributed to benign cause. Gastric tumors rarely cause complete obstruction, but often impair normal gastric motility. This defect may lead to easy satiety, anorexia, indigestion, and nausea. Decrease in caliber of the transverse and descending colon, sigmoid or rectum by tumor mass can lead to change in bowel habit, including diminished caliber of stools, constipation, and bouts of cramps and/or diarrhea from peristaltic efforts of the proximal gut. Compromise of the lumen of the common bile duct by carcinoma of the head of the pancreas or of the bile duct itself produces obstructive jaundice, not infrequently after minor antecedent digestive complaints or unexplained pruritus ascribed to accumulated bile salts.

Ureteral obstruction by compression from retroperitoneal masses or bladder tumor leads to hydroureter and hydronephrosis, often asymptomatic or revealed by vague discomfort in flank or loin, or by urinary tract infection. Bilateral obstruction leads to uremia with its protean symptomatology. Compromise of the urethra as it courses through the prostate causes diminished urinary stream, inadequate bladder emptying, frequency, urgency, nocturia, and when severe, obstructive uropathy and uremia.

Tumors in the cecum and ascending colon and in the urinary bladder, because their content is not solid and because of greater luminal diameter, uncommonly cause obstruction, but may distort normal function enough to alter bowel or urinary habits.

A mass discovered by palpation or x-ray may be a presenting finding, as in breast carcinoma. Dysfunction from replacement of the substance of a parenchymatous organ by tumor is a subset of mass presentation. The classic example is primary or, more commonly, metastatic brain tumor, which becomes identified by abnormal brain function. Seizure or paralysis, sensory or coordination abnormality, memory defect, and personality change may all be consequences of space occupation. These changes may occur not only because a specific area of the brain is affected, but since the calvarium is not distensible, because of increased intracranial pressure. Headache may be the only symptom of increased intracranial pressure. Similar dysfunction of the spinal cord with distal motor and sensory phenomena can reflect space occupation by a mass within or impinging on the cord or cauda equina. Hepatic dysfunction by space occupation from primary or metastatic tumor, often with related intrahepatic bile duct compression, can present as jaundice. Sometimes the liver enlarges to enormous size, causing digestive disorders, pain, and a visible and palpable mass in the upper abdomen. Thyroid cancer usually presents as a mass, and uncommonly this results in hypothyroid laboratory values, but rarely in clinical hypothyroidism.

A sarcoma of the soft tissues usually presents as a palpable mass. Testicular cancer ordinarily presents as a mass: the testicle may only be slightly larger than its fellow, but harder and heavier in the examiner's hand. Ovarian cancer may be detected as an adnexal mass.

A new lump or mass, or a changing one, requires exclusion of cancer based on clinical examination, imaging studies, or a biopsy. Most lipomas, and self-discovery of the xiphoid, are two types of lumps that can usually be dismissed on clinical grounds. A dominant breast mass or even a questionable one, requires assessment by appropriate imaging, and often by cytologic means. A thyroid nodule, an enlarged lymph node that is hard, a node that remains enlarged without infectious explanation for 2 weeks, a skin mass with the characteristics of melanoma or carcinoma, especially if ulcerated, a new subcutaneous or abdominal or scrotal mass all require consideration of cancer and appropriate diagnostic study.

Ulceration on the skin or on an epithelial surface, can lead to blood loss and occasionally can serve as a portal of infection. Skin ulcerations are commonly ignored for weeks or months and are often interpreted as a common injury of unremembered origin that did not heal. Bronchial ulceration results in hemoptysis, usually blood-tinged sputum, and only rarely massive bleeding. Any of the upper alimentary canal cancers can ulcerate and bleed. Usually the bleeding is slow, intermittent, and silent, leading to iron-deficiency anemia. Hematemesis or massive melena is uncommon. Carcinomas of the cecum and ascending colon often present with the symptoms of anemia because of ulceration and bleeding.

Carcinoma of the bladder and carcinoma of the kidney commonly manifest hematuria. Sometimes this is fortuitously discovered as a microscopic or chemical abnormality on routine urinalysis. Clots from renal bleeding can lead to ureteral colic. Hematuria less often heralds prostate cancer, but hematospermia implies prostate disease, benign or malignant, because carcinoma of the seminal vesicle is exceedingly rare.

Endometrial carcinoma most often presents as postmenopausal vaginal bleeding, although any vaginal bleeding outside the normal menstrual cycle is worthy of suspicion. Contact bleeding during intercourse is suggestive of cervical ulceration, most commonly a result of cancer.

Pain is commonly thought of as a surrogate for early cancer, although this is mistaken. Most cancers are initially painless. Pain occurs when a tumor invades, presses on, or stretches a nerve, or when proximal smooth muscle contracts in an attempt to bypass an obstructed or dysfunctional distal segment of a conduit. Most pains of short duration that disappear are not caused by cancer. Cancer must enter the differential diagnosis, however, when pain is recurrent or persistent without ready explanation, or atypical, or present when there is no other recognizable cause. New pain, not necessarily severe, must be carefully interpreted. Abdominal pain and skeletal pain distinct from joint symptomatology deserve particular attention, and early rather than late studies to establish a cause. Pain in a breast mass does not exclude its being cancer.

Weight loss may first indicate an unsuspected cancer, and when combined with grumbling low-grade discomforts, malaise, and fatigue, is a cause for particular scrutiny. A wide variety of other diseases can also cause these common symptoms, but cancer should not be at the bottom of the list. If a diagnosis is not established after initial studies a second complete history and physical examination after a short interval is imperative.

Effusion caused by cancer in the pleural or pericardial, or peritoneal cavities can lead to dyspnea and discomfort. Increasing abdominal girth, often with malaise, oliguria, constipation, and weight gain, is a cardinal symptom of ascites. In the thorax, bronchogenic carcinoma, mesothelioma, metastatic breast, or ovarian cancer, and primary carcinoma of serous membranes are the frequent causes of malignant effusion. Ascites as a presenting symptom is characteristic of ovarian cancer and cancer of the serous membranes. Pancreatic cancer, mesothelioma, metastatic carcinoma of the liver, and several non-neoplastic diseases also enter the differential diagnosis.

Perforation caused by invasion of the wall of a hollow viscus causes pain, usually sudden. Cancer is not suspected in most cases when this rare event occurs. Pneumothorax from perforation of the pleura by a primary or metastatic pulmonary tumor is an uncommon emergency. Fistulization of gastric cancer into the transverse colon leads to vague abdominal discomfort, which is misinterpreted or neglected, and then sudden onset of diarrhea with prominent gastrocolic reflex. Appendiceal cancer, albeit a rare tumor, frequently presents as acute appendicitis with peritonitis because of rupture. Perforation of the colon is more frequently caused by diverticulitis than by colon cancer. Ruptured ectopic pregnancy due to choriocarcinoma has been reported. Tracheoesophageal fistulization in the course of esophageal or bronchogenic carcinomas occurs late.

Fever of unknown origin that persists for more than one week must include cancer among its possible causes. Hodgkin disease, other lymphomas, acute leukemia, cancer of the kidney, and cancers of the liver are high on the list of neoplasms that can cause fever. Certain cancers predispose to infections because of ulceration, obstruction, or disordered leukopoiesis.

Endocrine hyperactivity syndromes may occasionally turn out to be caused by cancer. Hyperadrenalism, sometimes first manifest as hirsutism, can indicate adrenal cancer. Cushing's syndrome can also result from small-cell carcinoma of the lung. Hyperparathyroidism rarely comes from parathyroid cancer but can be mimicked by ovarian cancer and squamous carcinomas. Tumors that secrete thyroid hormone, estrogens, insulin, glucagon, aldosterone, epinephrine, or norepinephrine are usually benign tumors of the parent endocrine organ, but cancer must always be considered. Functional neuroendocrine tumors may secrete serotonin and other vasoactive principles that cause the carcinoid syndrome.

Paraneoplastic syndromes may be early symptoms of cancer. Myasthenia gravis, Raynaud's syndrome, hypertrophic osteoarthropathy and clubbing, and refractory anemia may herald thymoma, myeloma, lung cancer, and hematologic dyscrasia (and thymoma) respectively. A diligent search must be made for these and other causes.

Absence of cardinal manifestations is usual for cancers detected by screening by Pap smears, mammography, prostate-specific antigen (PSA) determinations, colonoscopy, computed tomography (CT) lung scanning, and total skin examination. Asymptomatic cancers discovered by these methods are generally far less advanced than those that cause symptoms. Occasionally, routine chemical or hematologic laboratory data in asymptomatic patients suggest cancer or leukemia. Such incidental discovery reinforces the proposition that early in their pathogenesis, cancers are almost always asymptomatic.

Predisposition to cancer characterizes a broad spectrum of diseases, exposures, and lifestyle behaviors. Patients who have had inflammatory bowel disease, human papilloma virus infection of the cervix, hepatitis B or C infection, those with prior radiation exposure, alkylating agent treatment, or specific environmental exposures such as asbestos; those who have smoked, heavily imbibed alcohol, or sun worshipped, and those with a strong family history of cancer all are in groups that deserve special consideration for the particular cancers that occur in them at a higher frequency than normal.

Cancerophobia does not predispose to cancer. Depression occurs more frequently with carcinoma of the pancreas than with gastric carcinoma, however, and may be an early symptom of pancreatic neoplasia.

By the time cancer is diagnosed, it is often past the stage of easy curability. Frequently the earliest symptoms were ignored or rationalized. Mammography has decreased mortality from breast cancer, cytology and early treatment have diminished cervical cancer mortality, and colonoscopy and polypectomy have decreased colon cancer mortality. Other screening programs portend similar promise by diagnosing cancers before they become symptomatic. Cancer has replaced syphilis as the great imitator. Many symptomatic patients with cancer are still curable with today's therapies. However, delay cannot possibly help once an early symptom occurs that eventually proves to be caused by cancer. Inclusion of cancer as a possibility in every differential diagnosis can save lives.

The expansion of diagnostic techniques based on genomics and proteomics augurs well for earlier identification of cancers. Not only is it reasonable to believe that clinical diagnosis will be accelerated, but these two disciplines are likely to alter our understanding of the cancer process as it occurs in humans. It is hoped that the consequent impact of this knowledge on cancer prevention and on cancer therapy will be revolutionary. The cardinal manifestations of cancer may then become laboratory abnormalities that are instrumentally detectable well before clinical presentation. Indeed departure from a population norm may be less significant than departure from one's prior proteomic profile taken as a baseline during health. If such a blue sky future ever unfolds, public understanding and compliance will still be critical determinants of cancer prevention and early diagnosis.

Part II

Scientific Foundations of Cancer

Section 1

CANCER BIOLOGY

2

Molecular Biology, Genomics, Proteomics, and Mouse Models of Human Cancer

Kornelia Polyak, MD, PhD
Matthew Meyerson, MD, PhD

Cancer is a genetic disease. Abnormalities in genes that control cellular proliferation lead to the unrestrained growth that characterizes the malignant cell. Thus, to gain the initiative in cancer detection and treatment, oncologists must begin to understand the molecular roots of the disease: genes, their messenger ribonucleic acids (mRNAs), and the proteins they produce. In short, oncologists should be conversant with the tools of molecular biology.

This chapter is a basic survey of molecular biology and is directed toward the clinician or trainee who wants a fundamental understanding of this discipline. It is "methods oriented" and will serve as a frame of reference for other chapters in this section. It describes the principles that underlie the procedures used most commonly by molecular biologists and provides examples of clinically relevant situations that draw on particular techniques. It will become apparent that molecular biology already plays an important role in clinical cancer medicine, from the analysis of tumors for prognostic or pathogenetic information to the production of pharmacologic agents, such as colony-stimulating factors, interleukins, and erythropoietin.

We begin with an overview of genes, gene expression, and gene cloning. Our discussion of techniques will follow the flow of genetic information as we explain the procedures used to analyze gene expression at the levels of deoxyribonucleic acid (DNA), ribonucleic acid (RNA), and protein. Good general overviews can be found in several books.[1–3]

OVERVIEW: GENE STRUCTURE

Genes and Gene Expression The gene is the fundamental unit of inheritance and the ultimate determinant of all phenotypes. The DNA of a normal human cell contains an estimated 30,000 to 120,000 genes, but only a fraction of these are used (or expressed) in any particular cell at any given time. For example, genes specific for erythroid cells, such as the hemoglobin genes, are not expressed in brain cells. The identity of each gene expressed in a particular cell at a given time and its level of expression are defined as the transcriptome.

According to the central dogma of molecular biology, a gene exerts its effects by having its DNA transcribed into an mRNA, which, in turn, is translated into a protein, the final effector of the gene's action. Thus, molecular biologists often investigate gene expression or activation, by which is meant the process of transcribing DNA into RNA or translating RNA into protein. The process of transcription involves creating a perfect RNA copy of the gene using the DNA of the gene as a template. Translation of mRNA into protein is a somewhat more complex process because the structure of the gene's protein is encoded in the mRNA and that structural message must be decoded during translation.

Functional Components of the Gene Every gene consists of several functional components, each involved in a different facet of the process of gene expression (Figure 2-1). Broadly speaking, however, there are two main functional units: the promoter region and the coding region.

The promoter region controls when and in what tissue a gene is expressed. For example, the promoter of the hemoglobin gene is responsible for its expression in erythroid cells and not in brain cells. How is this tissue-specific expression achieved? In the DNA of the gene's promoter region, there are specific structural elements, nucleotide sequences (see Structural Considerations below) that permit the gene to be expressed only in an appropriate cell. These are the elements in the hemoglobin gene that instruct an erythroid cell to transcribe hemoglobin mRNA from that gene. These structures are referred to as "*cis*"-acting elements because they reside on the same molecule of DNA as the gene. In some cases, other tissue type–specific *cis*-acting elements, called *enhancers*, reside on the same DNA molecule but at great distances from the coding region of the gene.[4,5] In the appropriate cell, the *cis*-acting elements bind protein factors that are physically responsible for transcribing the gene. These proteins are called *trans*-acting factors because they reside in the cell's nucleus separate from the DNA molecule bearing the gene. For example, brain cells would not have the right *trans*-acting factors that bind to the hemoglobin promoter; therefore, brain cells would not express hemoglobin. They would, however, have *trans*-acting factors that bind to neuron-specific gene promoters.

The structure of a gene's protein is specified by the gene's coding region. The coding region contains the information that directs an erythroid cell to assemble amino acids in the proper order to make the hemoglobin protein. How is this order of amino acids specified? As described in detail below, DNA is a linear polymer consisting of four distinguishable subunits called *nucleotides*. In the coding region of a gene, the linear sequence of nucleotides encodes the amino acid sequence of the protein. This genetic code is in triplet form so that every group of three nucleotides encodes a single amino acid. The 64 triplets that can be formed by four nucleotides exceed the 20 distinct amino acids used to make proteins.

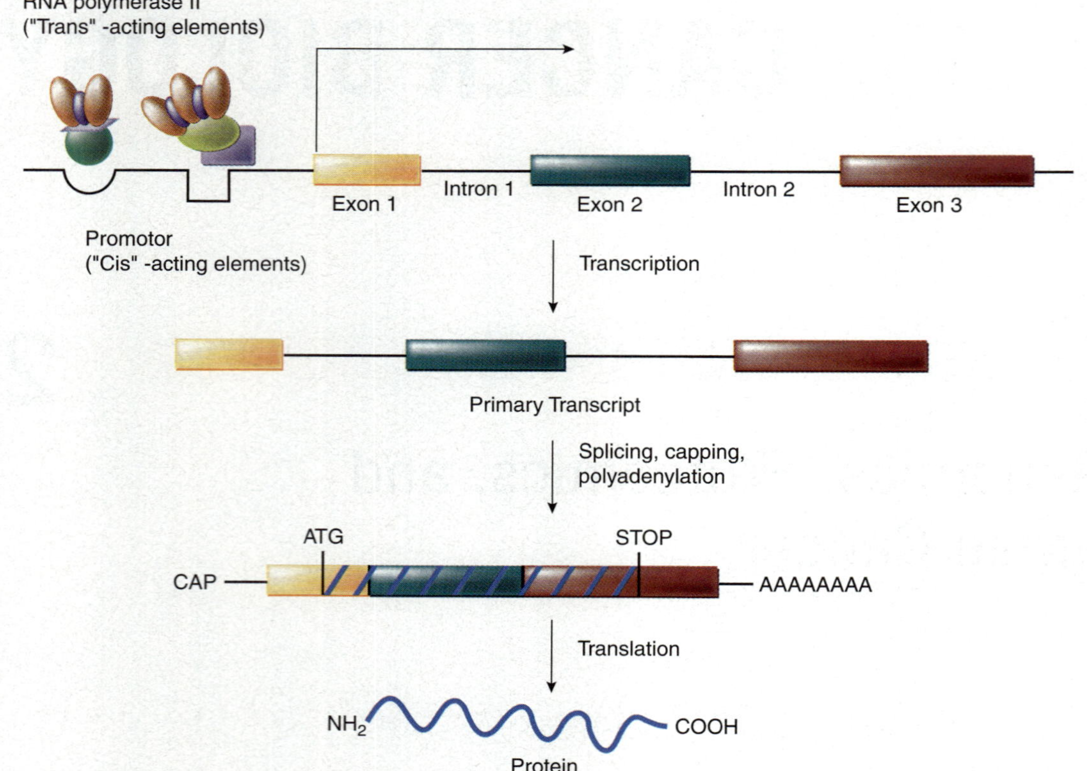

Figure 2-1 Gene expression. A gene's deoxyribonucleic acid (DNA) is transcribed into messenger ribonucleic acid (mRNA), which, in turn, is translated into protein. The functional components of a gene are schematically diagrammed here. Areas of the gene destined to be represented in mature mRNA are called *exons*, and intervening areas of DNA between exons are called *introns*. The portion of the gene that controls transcription, and therefore expression, is the promoter. This control is exerted by specific nucleotide sequences in the promoter region (so-called "*cis*"-acting factors) and by proteins (so-called "*trans*"-acting factors) that must interact with promoter DNA and/or ribonucleic acid (RNA) polymerase II for transcription to occur. The primary transcript is the RNA molecule made by RNA polymerase II that is complementary to the entire stretch of DNA containing the gene. Before leaving the nucleus, the primary transcript is modified by splicing together exons (thus removing intron sequences), adding a cap to the 5' end and adding a poly(A) tail to the 3' end. Once in the cytoplasm, mature mRNA undergoes translation to yield a protein.

This makes the code degenerate and allows some amino acids to be encoded by several different triplets.[6] The nucleotide sequence of any gene can now be determined (see below). By translating the code, one can derive a predicted amino acid sequence for the protein encoded by a gene.

Structural Considerations **Fine Structure** The basic repeating units of the DNA polymer are nucleotides (Figure 2-2). Nucleotides consist of an invariant portion, a five-carbon deoxyribose sugar with a phosphate group, and a variable portion, the base. Of the four bases that appear in the nucleotides of DNA, two are purines, adenine (A) and guanine (G), and two are pyrimidines, cytosine (C) and thymine (T). Nucleotides are connected to each other in the polymer through their phosphate groups, leaving the bases free to interact with each other through hydrogen bonding. This base-pairing is specific, so that A interacts with T and C interacts with G. DNA is ordinarily double-stranded, that is, two linear polymers of DNA are aligned so that the bases of the two strands face each other. Base-pairing makes this alignment specific so that one DNA strand is a perfectly complementary copy of the other. This complementarity means that each DNA strand carries the information needed to make an exact replica of itself.

In every strand of a DNA polymer, the phosphate substitutions alternate between the 5' and 3' carbons of the deoxyribose molecules. Thus, there is directionality to DNA: the genetic code reads in the 5' to 3' direction. In double-stranded DNA, the strand that carries the translatable code in the 5' to 3' direction is called the *sense strand*, whereas its complementary partner is the *antisense strand*.

Gross Structure In eukaryotes, the coding regions of most genes are not continuous. Rather, they consist of areas that are transcribed into mRNA, the exons, which are interrupted by stretches of DNA that do not appear in mature mRNA, the introns (see Figure 2-1). The functions of introns are not known with certainty. A purpose of some sort is implied by their conservation in evolution. However, their overall physical structure might be more important than their specific nucleotide sequences because the nucleotide sequences of introns diverge more rapidly in evolution than do the sequences of exons. Overall, DNA that contains genes comprises a minority of total DNA. Between genes, vast stretches of untranscribed DNA are assumed to play an important structural role.

In the nucleus, DNA is not present as naked nucleic acid. Rather, DNA is found in close association with a number of accessory proteins, such as the histones, and in this form is called *chromatin*.[7] Although many of DNA's accessory proteins have no known specific function, they generally appear to be involved in the correct packaging of DNA. For example, DNA's double helix is ordinarily twisted on itself to form a supercoiled structure.[8] This structure must unwind partially during DNA replication and transcription.[9] Some of the accessory proteins, for example, topoisomerases and histone acetylases, are involved in regulating this process.

Summary Genes specify the structure of proteins that are responsible for the phenotype associated with a particular gene. Although the nucleus of every human cell contains 30,000 to 120,000 genes, only a fraction of them are expressed in any given cell at any given time. The promoter (with or without an enhancer) is the part of the gene that determines when and where it will be expressed. The coding region is the part of the gene that dictates the amino acid sequence of the protein encoded by the gene. DNA is a linear polymer of nucleotides. Ordinarily, the nucleotide bases of one strand of DNA interact with those of another strand (A with T, C with G) to make double-stranded DNA. In the cell's nucleus, DNA is associated with accessory proteins to make the structure called *chromatin*.

GENERAL TECHNIQUES

Restriction Endonucleases and Recombinant DNA In eukaryotic chromosomes, individual molecules of DNA are several million base pairs long. Because these molecules are far too large to analyze directly, scientists are usually interested in cutting DNA into fragments of manageable size. Fortunately, for molecular biologists, bacteria have evolved a highly diverse set of enzymes, the restriction endonucleases, which cleave DNA internally within the polymer.[10]

In nature, these enzymes have evolved to protect the bacteria from invasion by foreign DNA molecules, such as phage. To discriminate between "domestic" and "foreign" DNA, these enzymes recognize specific nucleotide sequences. DNA without such specific sequences is left undisturbed by the enzymes. However, when a restriction endonuclease spots a recognition site, it binds to the site and cleaves both strands of the DNA to which it has bound. Individual restriction endonucleases recognize specific sequences, usually in the order of four to six bases in length, and these sequences are often palindromes, that is, the 5' to 3' sequence in the upper strand is identical to the 5' to 3' sequence in the lower strand (Figure 2-3).[11]

Although restriction endonucleases cut DNA into smaller fragments, there is a lower limit to

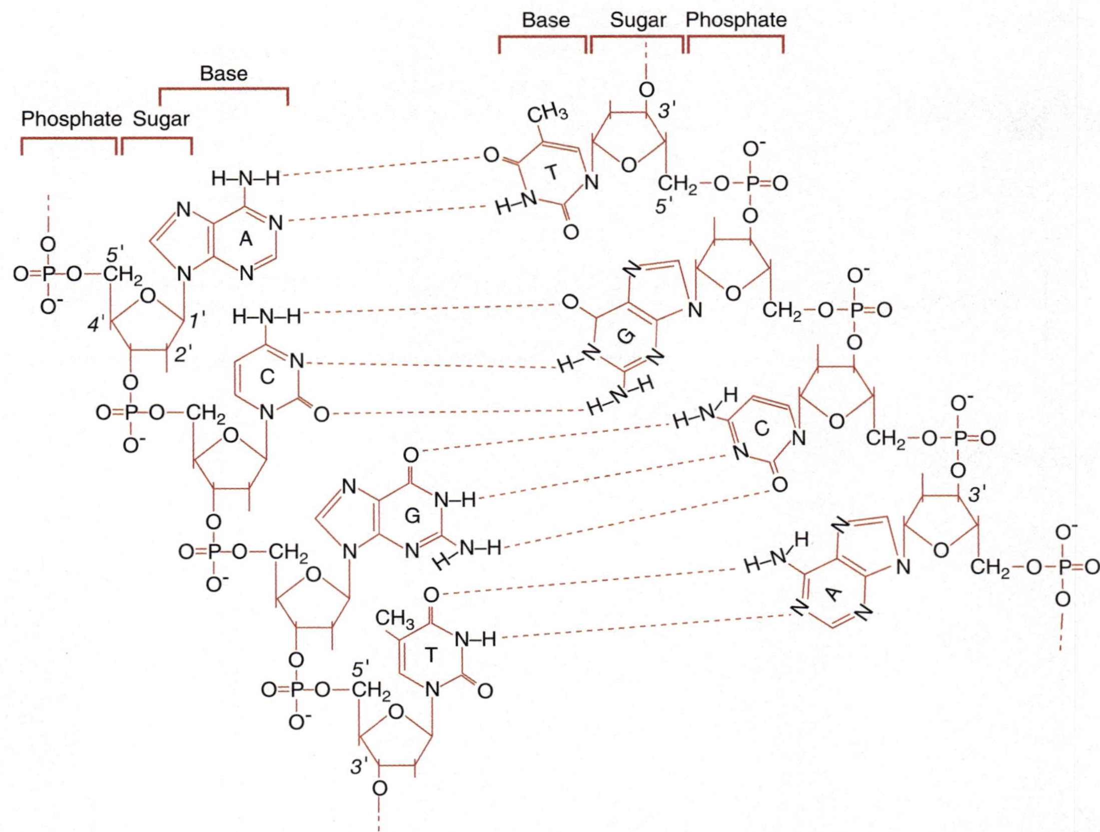

Figure 2-2 Structure of base-paired, double-stranded deoxyribonucleic acid (DNA). Each strand of DNA consists of a backbone of five-carbon deoxyribose sugars connected to each other through phosphate bonds. Note that as one follows the sequence down the left-hand strand (A to C to G to T), one is also following the carbons of the deoxyribose ring, going from the 5' carbon to the 3' carbon. This is the basis for the 5' to 3' directionality of DNA. The 1' carbon of each deoxyribose is substituted with a purine or pyrimidine base. In double-stranded DNA, bases face each other in the center of the molecule and base pair via hydrogen bonds (*dotted lines*). Base-pairing is specific so that adenine pairs with thymine and guanine pairs with cytosine.

the size of useful fragments. One would not want to cut DNA into such small pieces that the informational content of each piece is negligible. Statistically, the longer a restriction endonuclease's recognition sequence, the less frequently this sequence will occur in a stretch of DNA. Therefore, the enzymes most commonly used to cut DNA into usefully large fragments are those that recognize a six-nucleotide recognition site (so-called "six-base cutters"). For example, an endonuclease isolated from *Escherichia coli*, called EcoRI, recognizes the sequence GAATTC, and wherever this occurs in double-stranded DNA, it will cleave between the G and A (see Figure 2-3). (Note that the antisense strand, which reads CTTAAG in the 3' to 5' direction, will also read GAATTC in the 5' to 3' direction. This is what is meant by a palindromic sequence.)

Gene Cloning Mechanics The most powerful technique available for gene analysis, the one technique that is the cornerstone for all others, is gene cloning (see Figure 2-3). In the gene cloning process, a discrete piece of DNA is faithfully replicated in the laboratory. Cloning provides quantities of specific DNA sufficient for biochemical analysis or for any other manipulation, including joining to a foreign piece of DNA. In the early 1970s, Cohen and Boyer drew on two fundamental properties of bacteria and their viruses (phages) that made this innovation possible: plasmids and DNA ligases.[12]

Plasmids are circular molecules of DNA that replicate in the cytoplasm of bacterial cells, separate from the bacteria's own DNA. In nature, plasmids often carry genetic information useful to the host bacterium, such as genes that confer resistance to antibiotics. For the purposes of gene cloning, plasmids are important because they contain all of the information necessary for directing bacterial enzymes to replicate the plasmid DNA, in some cases, to many thousands of copies per bacterium.

DNA ligases are enzymes produced by bacteria (and some phages when they infect bacteria) that can link or ligate together separate pieces of DNA. The nucleotide sequence in a piece of DNA does not influence the activity of a DNA ligase so that a DNA ligase can join two pieces of DNA that are not ordinarily connected to each other in nature.

In gene cloning, one uses a restriction endonuclease to cut open the circular plasmid DNA in a region of the plasmid not necessary for replication (see Figure 2-3). Suppose, for example, that the enzyme EcoRI cuts open the plasmid in such a nonessential area. EcoRI recognizes the sequence GAATTC and cuts both DNA strands between the G and the A nucleotides. Protruding from the cut ends will be single-stranded DNA "tails" with the sequence AATT. (Note that the tail's sequence in the sense strand is the same as the sequence in the antisense strand when the nucleotides are read in the 5' to 3' direction.) Any other piece of DNA that has been cut with EcoRI will also have single-stranded AATT tails, and the AATT tails on this foreign piece of DNA can base-pair with the complementary TTAA tails (reading 3' to 5') on the cut plasmid. When this happens, the foreign DNA piece physically closes the gap in the plasmid, forming a closed circular plasmid again (which is necessary for plasmid propagation).

Although the nucleotides at the ends of the plasmid and foreign DNA now abut each other, they are not covalently connected. This is an unstable situation that the DNA ligase rectifies. The DNA ligase covalently joins the plasmid and foreign DNA to create a recombinant plasmid, which still has all of the information needed to be replicated in a bacterium but which also contains a foreign DNA insert. Obviously, the EcoRI-cut ends of the plasmid can also base-pair with themselves again to reform the native plasmid, but molecular biologists have developed a number of tricks to suppress this phenomenon. It should be pointed out that single-stranded tails are not always necessary for making recombinant DNA. Under certain conditions, the DNA ligase can join together two fragments of blunt-ended DNA without these tails.

When a recombinant plasmid is reintroduced into a host bacterium (by a process called *transformation*), the plasmid will replicate normally. Now, however, its foreign DNA insert is replicated along with the plasmid into which it was inserted. The transformed bacteria can then be grown to large numbers in liquid culture. With each bacterial cell division, the progeny bacteria contain plasmid molecules that continue to replicate. When the bacterial culture contains the desired quantity of this plasmid (this may be milligrams of plasmid DNA in a 1 L culture), it can be reisolated as pure DNA. The cloned foreign piece of DNA can then be cut out (with EcoRI, in our example) for further analysis or manipulation. One can also use bacterial viruses (or phages) in the same manner by infecting host bacteria with recombinant phage-bearing foreign DNA sequences. In all of these experiments, the plasmid or phage that houses the foreign DNA is called a *vector* because it is the vehicle that directs the foreign DNA into the host bacterium.

These extraordinarily powerful tools, which are now part of the standard armamentarium of all molecular biology laboratories, have been responsible for the development of nearly all of the analytic techniques described below. Several excellent manuals have been published that describe these techniques in detail.[13,14]

Gene Probes and Hybridization We shall see in the following sections that what lies at the heart of gene analysis is the ability to identify a

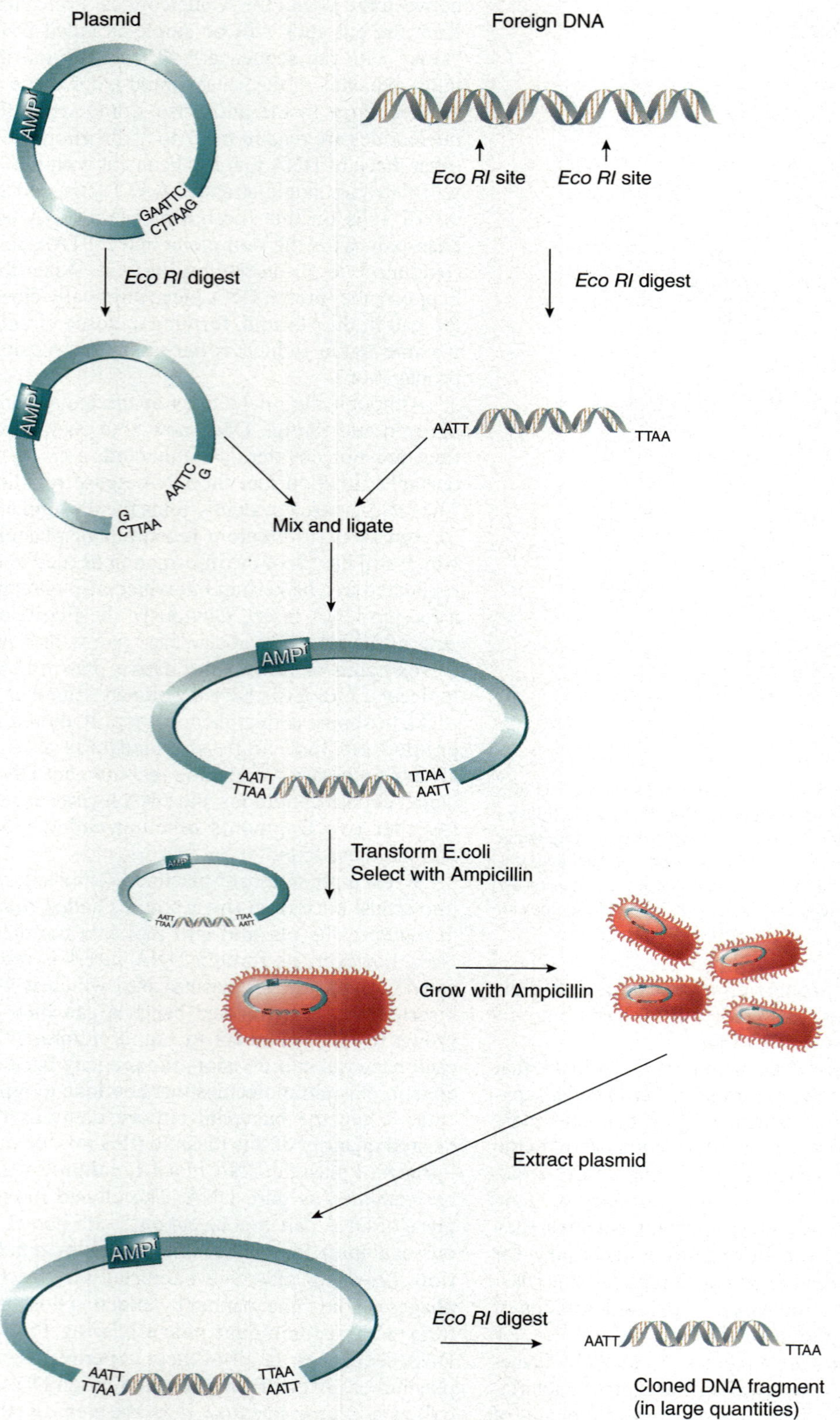

Figure 2-3 Digestion of deoxyribonucleic acid (DNA) with the restriction endonuclease EcoRI and gene cloning. In this example, a small amount of foreign DNA (a few nanograms) is digested with EcoRI. The nucleotide sequence of this stretch of DNA contains the recognition sequence for EcoRI, GAATTC (*boxed*). EcoRI cuts the DNA in both strands between the indicated nucleotides, resulting in fragments with 5' single-stranded tails. This foreign DNA can come from any source, the only requirement being that it contains the same restriction endonuclease recognition sites as the vector. Plasmid vector is also digested with EcoRI to create a linear DNA molecule. The "sticky" single-stranded ends of the foreign DNA can align and base-pair with the complementary "sticky ends" of the plasmid, after which DNA ligase covalently bonds foreign DNA to plasmid DNA. This recombinant DNA is introduced into *Escherichia coli* by a process called transformation. Because the bacteria themselves are not resistant to ampicillin, growth in ampicillin will select only those bacteria that have taken up the plasmid DNA (which carries an ampicillin resistance gene). The plasmid contains a bacterial origin of replication so that as the bacterial culture grows, plasmids replicate, resulting in several copies in each bacterium. When the culture has grown to sufficient size, plasmid DNA can be isolated biochemically, foreign DNA can be cut from the plasmid using EcoRI, and the resulting yield will often be milligrams of DNA, that is, greater than a 10^6-fold amplification.

specific gene (or mRNA) in a complex mixture of all of the DNA (or RNA) in a cell or tissue. This can be done only when one already has a cloned fragment of DNA from the gene of interest. Such fragments are usually obtained from gene libraries constructed from genomic DNA or cDNA or generated using polymerase chain reaction (PCR, to be described below). These DNA fragments can be almost any size, from a fraction of the size of the gene (a few hundred or even fewer nucleotides) to the size of an entire gene (several thousand nucleotides). These cloned gene fragments are called *probes* because they are used to probe native DNA or RNA for the gene of interest.

To be useful, a gene probe must contain a sufficient number of nucleotides so that it will recognize the sequences of its corresponding gene. Recognition occurs by a process called *nucleic acid hybridization*, in which two pieces of DNA can align themselves (or anneal) by base-pairing. Hybridization occurs by the specific pairing of A to T bases and of G to C bases (see Figure 2-2). Perfectly matched sequences pair more tightly than sequences containing mismatches, and long matched sequences pair more tightly than shorter matched sequences. Hybridization is the concept that underlies molecular biology methods, such as Southern blotting, microarray analysis, and PCR (see below).

Summary Genes can be cut from total genomic DNA using restriction endonucleases that recognize specific nucleotide sequences. Individual genes can be captured and replicated in bulk for detailed analysis. This process is called *cloning* and employs bacterial plasmids and viruses (phage) as carriers for the cloned genes. Enzymes called DNA ligases join foreign DNA to plasmid or phage vectors, which can then replicate within bacterial cells to create gene libraries. Using nucleic acid hybridization, cloned genes act as probes to detect the presence of their native counterparts in complex mixtures of DNA or RNA.

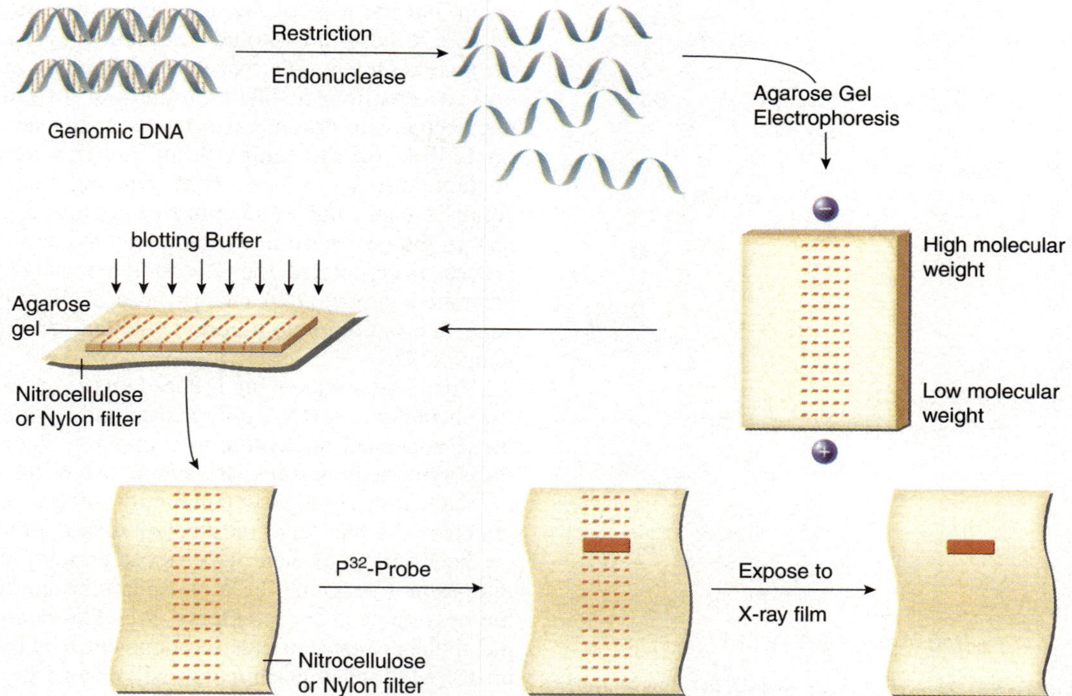

Figure 2-4 Genomic Southern blotting. Genomic deoxyribonucleic acid (DNA) is digested with a single restriction endonuclease, resulting in a complex mixture of DNA fragments of different sizes, that is, molecular weights. Digested DNA is arrayed by size using electrophoresis through a semisolid agarose gel. Because DNA is negatively charged, fragments will migrate toward the anode, but their progress is variably impeded by interactions with the agarose gel. Small fragments interact less and migrate farther; large fragments interact more and migrate less. The arrayed fragments are then transferred to a sheet of nitrocellulose or nylon-based filter paper by forcing buffer through the gel as shown. The DNA fragments are carried by capillary action and can be made to bind irreversibly to the filter. Now the DNA fragments, still arrayed by size on the filter, can be probed for specific nucleotide sequences using a ^{32}P-radiolabeled nucleic acid probe. The probe will hybridize to complementary sequences in the DNA, and the position of the fragment that contains these sequences can be revealed by exposing the filter to x-ray film.

GENE ANALYSIS: DNA

Southern Blotting One of the most useful techniques for analyzing a gene at the level of genomic DNA is Southern blotting, named for its originator, E. M. Southern.[15] In general, it allows one to determine whether specific nucleotide sequences in a cloned probe are present in a sample of genomic DNA. The presence of these sequences usually means that the gene itself is present in the genomic DNA. Figure 2-4 diagrams the technique. Purified genomic DNA is digested with a specific restriction endonuclease, which, as described above, will produce an array of differently sized DNA fragments. Electrophoresis through an agarose gel then separates these fragments according to size. (Because the phosphate groups in DNA make the molecules negatively charged, they will migrate toward the anode in an electric field. The semiporous agarose will allow molecules of DNA to pass with varying degrees of ease, at a rate inversely proportional to their size. At any time after electrophoresis begins, small molecules will be closer to the anode than large molecules.) The agarose gel is usually cast in the form of a flat rectangle a few millimeters thick.

The final goal of Southern blotting is to identify specific fragments of cut DNA using nucleic acid hybridization. Because the agarose gel used in electrophoresis is thick and the DNA fragments can move within it, DNA in the gel is not in a suitable form for further analysis. The DNA fragments must be transferred to a solid support to which they are irreversibly bound to carry out nucleic acid hybridization studies. Thus, after electrophoresis, a paper-thin membrane microfilter (made of nitrocellulose or nylon) is placed over the flat portion of the gel. Liquid is then forced through the agarose gel in a direction perpendicular to the direction in which the DNA moved during electrophoresis. As the liquid perfuses the gel, it carries DNA fragments with it, depositing them on the membrane filter, to which the DNA sticks. After transfer, the DNA fragments are arrayed by size on the solid support.

At this point, a fragment of cloned DNA (the probe) is radiolabeled by using any of a variety of techniques. The membrane containing the transferred DNA is then soaked in a solution containing the radiolabeled probe. If there are any sequences in the genomic DNA that are complementary to those in the probe, the probe will hybridize to those sequences on the filter. The unbound probe can be washed away, and the remaining specifically hybridized probe can be visualized by exposing the filter to x-ray film.

What results from these studies is a pattern of one or more bands on x-ray film. Each band corresponds to a restriction endonuclease–generated DNA fragment containing nucleotide sequences complementary to those in the radioactive probe. For any particular gene probe, the size (ie, length) of the band it identifies will be the same from individual to individual (although see below for a discussion of restriction fragment length polymorphisms [RFLPs], an important exception). Therefore, if a gene has undergone a structural rearrangement, as, for example, when the c-*abl* oncogene is translocated from chromosome 9 to 22, the pattern may change. Suppose, for example, that the c-*abl* probe ordinarily recognizes a 2,000-base EcoRI fragment in normal genomic DNA. If the translocation break point in a Chronic Myelogenous Leukemia (CML) patient occurs within that fragment, part of the c-*abl* gene and one of its EcoRI sites will move to chromosome 22. Southern blot analysis of the patient's DNA may now detect either (1) a larger fragment

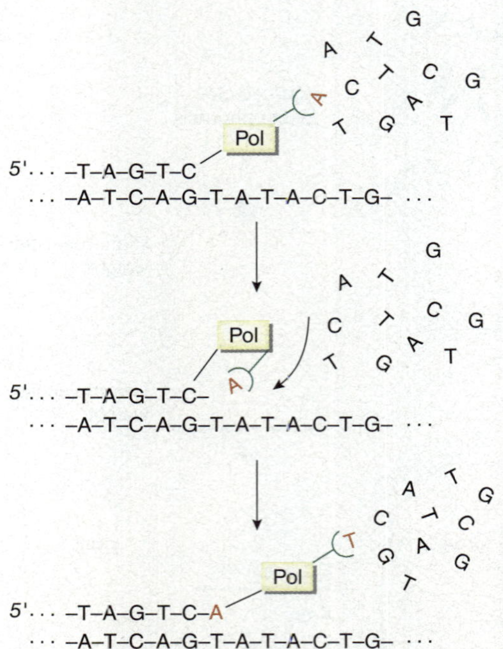

Figure 2-5 Deoxyribonucleic acid (DNA) polymerase. In this schematic, the enzyme DNA polymerase is creating a new DNA chain (*upper strand*) using a template (*lower strand*). Specific nucleotides are added from the 5' to the 3' direction as determined by the next nucleotide in the template.

than normal if the recipient chromosome has an EcoRI site farther away than the old EcoRI site or (2) a smaller fragment if it has an EcoRI site closer than the old one. Southern blotting is thus a sensitive technique for detecting large structural rearrangements in the genome, such as those that are occasionally associated with malignancy.

Because the amount of the radiolabeled probe that hybridizes to a Southern blot is proportional to the number of copies of the specific gene present in the target DNA, this technique can be used quantitatively. For example, in an analysis of primary breast cancer tissue, Southern blotting was used to determine that 30% of these samples contained multiple copies of c-*neu* oncogene DNA, that is, the gene was amplified.[16]

Nucleotide Sequencing The nucleotide sequence of a gene's coding region encodes the amino acid sequence of its protein. This means that even in the absence of any knowledge about a gene's protein, we can predict the structure of that protein given the nucleotide sequence of the gene. How can the nucleotide sequence of a gene be determined? The major method used for sequencing DNA is the "enzymatic chain termination" method devised by Sanger and colleagues.[17]

The chain termination method relies on properties of enzymes called *DNA polymerases* (Figure 2-5). These are enzymes that create new DNA polymers starting from individual nucleotides. However, for a DNA polymerase to work, it needs a template of single-stranded DNA on which to create the new polymer. DNA polymerase adds a new nucleotide to the 3' end of a growing DNA chain, but the base of the new nucleotide must be able to base-pair (ie, be complementary) to the base on the template over which the polymerase is positioned. After the addition of that nucleotide, the polymerase moves to the next nucleotide on the template and adds a new nucleotide to the 3' end of the growing chain. Again, the new nucleotide must be complementary to the next base in the template. When the process is completed, the DNA polymerase will have made a new DNA chain whose nucleotide sequence is completely complementary to the template DNA.

Nucleotide sequencing is based on the observation that when DNA polymerase adds a synthetic abnormal nucleotide to a growing chain, the polymerization stops. The synthetic terminating nucleotides used most commonly are dideoxynucleotides that have no alcohol substitutions on the 3' carbon of their deoxyribose groups and thus cannot be joined by a phosphate bridge to the next nucleotide (see Figure 2-2). For example, in the presence of dideoxyadenosine triphosphate (ATP), chain termination will occur wherever an A appears in the new DNA sequence (a T in the template) (Figure 2-6). These reactions are performed in vitro in a test tube, where millions of new DNA molecules are being made at once. If normal deoxy-ATP is mixed with dideoxy-ATP in the proper proportion, only a few of these molecules will terminate at each T in the template. This will generate a series of new DNA polymers, each one stretching from the beginning of the chain to the position of an A (ie, a T in the template). If the newly formed DNA is fluorescently labeled, the products can be separated electrophoretically in a polyacrylamide gel or capillary gel (see below). Each step of the ladder is a fragment of DNA that stretches from the start of the new polymer to the position of an A. Four separate reactions are performed using each of the four dideoxynucleotides, each coded with a distinct fluorescent color. The four reactions are run together in a capillary gel, and the order of nucleotides is read by the order of the different colors.

Following the completion of the human genome sequence, genome researchers shifted their efforts from de novo to comparative sequencing. Large-scale sequencing projects have been initiated aimed at comparing groups of healthy and diseased individuals with the aim of understanding genetic variation associated with a particular disorder. The successful completion of these projects

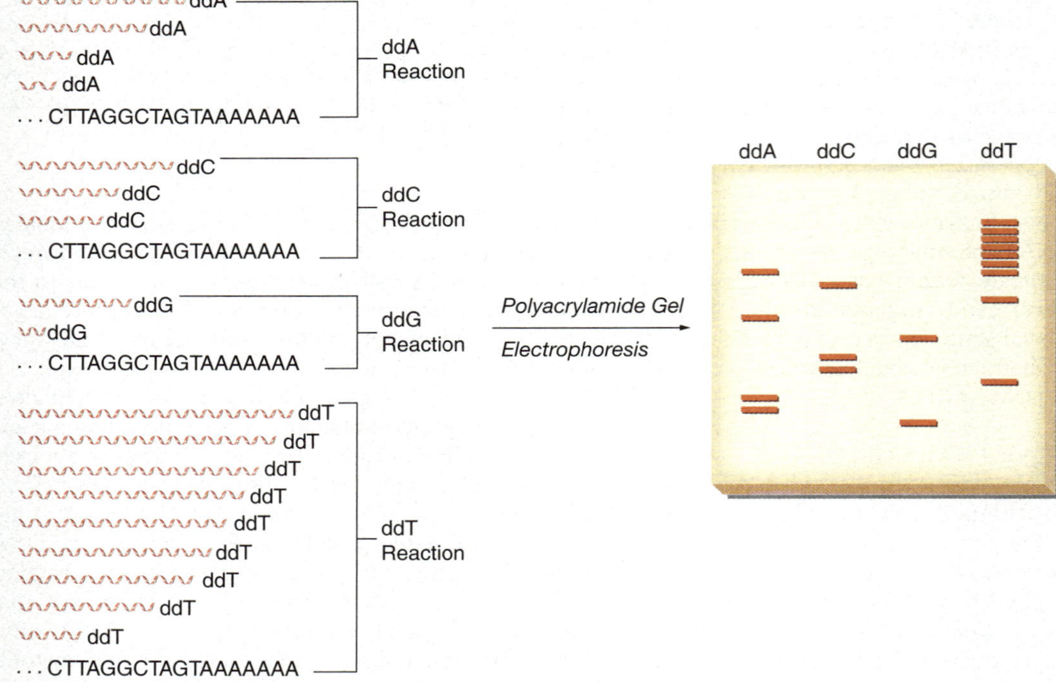

Figure 2-6 Deoxyribonucleic acid (DNA) sequencing using the chain termination method. In this example, DNA ending with the sequence . . .CTTAGGCTAGTAAAAAAA is being analyzed. Four reactions are performed, each using this DNA as a template for a DNA polymerase reaction and each containing one of the four dideoxynucleotides (dideoxyadenosine triphosphate [ddA], dideoxycytidine triphosphate [ddC], dideoxyguanosine triphosphate [ddG], and dideoxythymidine triphosphate [ddT]). In each reaction, chain elongation will terminate when the dideoxynucleotide is incorporated at the position of its complementary nucleotide in the template. This will result in a family of chains of differing lengths that correspond to the position at which polymerization terminated. In this example, these chains can be resolved by electrophoresis through a urea-containing polyacrylamide gel, in which longer chains run near the top of the gel and shorter chains near the bottom. Each new chain is radioactively labeled, and after autoradiography, the pattern of bands can be read from x-ray film. By noting the order in which bands appear, starting at the bottom of the gel, one can read the sequence of the template by substituting the complement of each dideoxynucleotide at every position. Reading from the bottom yields GAATCCGATCATTTTTTT, and substituting the complementary base at each position yields CTTAGGCTAGTAAAAAAA, the sequence of the template. The use of fluorescent labels in capillary gel electrophoresis is conceptually similar.

requires new sequencing technologies that allow fast, affordable, and accurate sequencing. A variety of array-oriented methods, including oligonucleotide array hybridization, fluorescent detection of the sequencing extension of arrayed PCR products, and chemiluminescent detection of the sequence extension of arrayed PCR products, now offer the potential of increased sequencing throughput and decreased cost.

The applications of DNA sequencing for cancer diagnosis and treatment selection are increasing as our knowledge of cancer-causing mutations continues to grow. In general, tumor suppressor genes are inactivated by loss-of-function mutations in cancer, whereas oncogenes are activated by amplification, translocation, or gain-of-function mutations. A specific example with clinical relevance is the discovery of mutations in the c-kit protein tyrosine kinase gene by DNA sequencing of gastrointestinal stromal tumors (GISTs).[18] This led to the successful treatment of GIST with the c-kit inhibitor STI-571 or Gleevec.[19]

With the completion of the human genome sequence, targeted sequencing studies of particular gene families have now led to the identification of common cancer-associated mutations. To date, these systematic studies have focused on enzyme families such as protein kinases, protein phosphatases, and lipid kinases. Of note, activating mutations in the *BRAF* serine-threonine kinase gene were found in over half of all melanomas [20] and subsequently in other cancer types, including colorectal, lung, and thyroid carcinomas. Mutations in the phosphatidylinositol 3-kinase catalytic subunit gene *PIK3CA* mutations have been discovered in colorectal carcinoma and glioblastoma,[21] as well as breast carcinomas. In lung adenocarcinoma, activating mutations in the epidermal growth factor receptor (*EGFR*) tyrosine kinase gene are common, especially in East Asian populations.[22–24] The discovery of *EGFR* mutations in lung adenocarcinoma sheds light on the mechanism of response to the kinase inhibitors gefitinib and erlotinib,[22–24] whereas the *BRAF* and *PIK3CA* mutation discoveries highlight candidate targets for anticancer chemotherapy. The analysis of *EGFR* mutation is now a useful diagnostic tool for lung carcinoma patients. One can anticipate that many different DNA sequencing tests will become part of cancer diagnostics in the setting of treatment with targeted therapies.

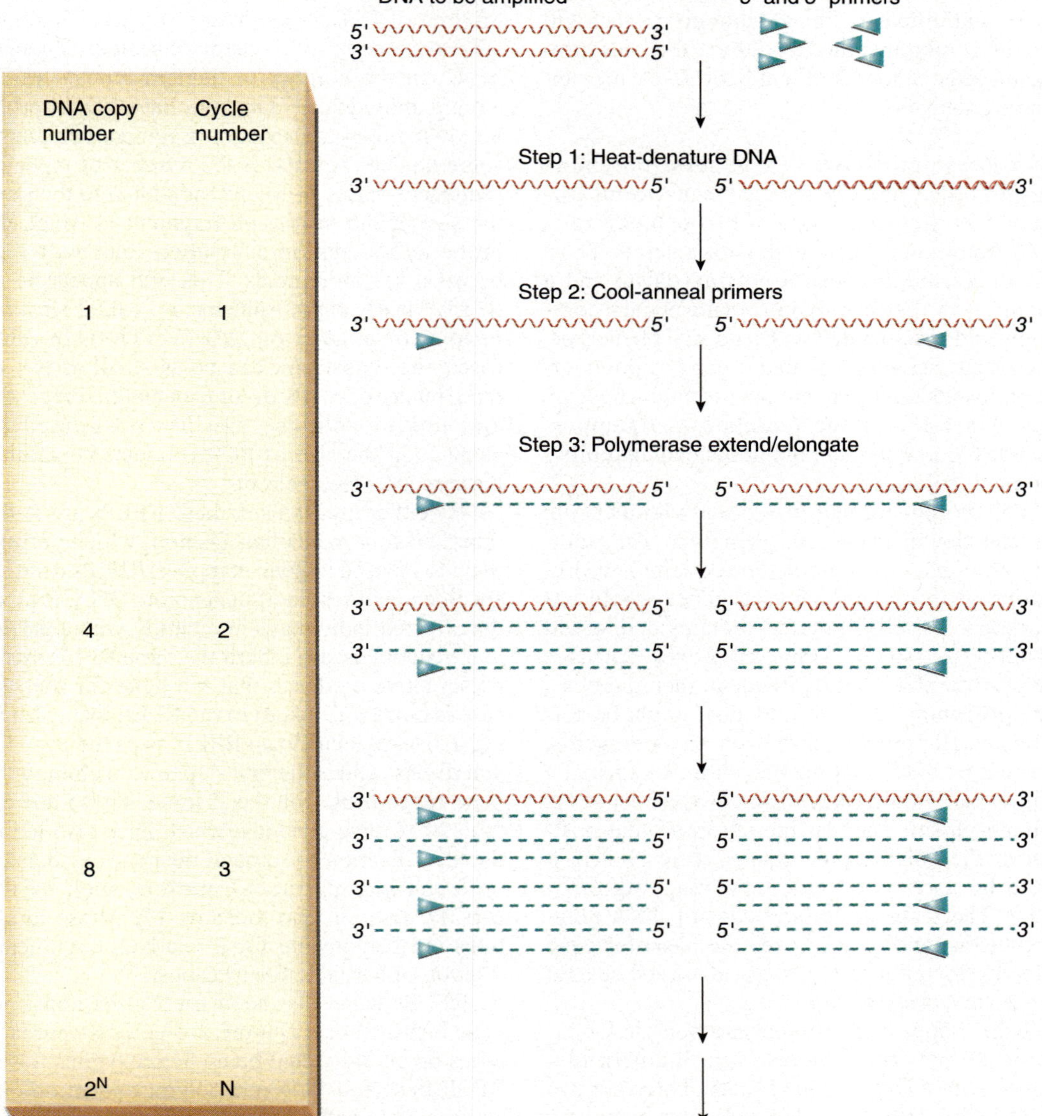

Figure 2-7 Polymerase chain reaction. Deoxyribonucleic acid (DNA) is mixed with short (10–20 base) single-stranded oligonucleotide primers that are complementary to the 5' and 3' ends of the sequence to be amplified. The mixture is heated to denature or "melt" all double-stranded DNA and then cooled to permit the primers to anneal to their complementary sequences on the DNA to be amplified. Note that the 5' primer will anneal to the lower strand and the 3' primer will anneal to the upper strand. A heat-resistant (thermostable) DNA polymerase (*Taq* polymerase; see text) was present in the original mixture, and it now synthesizes DNA by starting at the primers and using the strands to which the primers are annealed as a template. This results in the formation of two double-stranded DNA copies for every molecule of double-stranded DNA in the original mixture. The reaction is then heated to melt double-stranded DNA and cooled to allow reannealing, and the polymerase makes new double-stranded DNA again. There are now four double-stranded DNA copies for each original DNA molecule. This process can be repeated n times (usually 20–50) to result in 2^n copies of double-stranded DNA.

Polymerase Chain Reaction To detect gene sequences by Southern blotting, at least 1 to 2 µg of genomic DNA is required. This translates into milligram quantities of tissue that must be used fresh or freshly frozen. By amplifying specific fragments of DNA, the PCR lowers the theoretic limit of detectable DNA sequences in a sample to a single molecule of DNA. With some advance knowledge of the nucleotide sequences in the DNA to be detected, microscopically small amounts of tissue, even a single cell, contain enough DNA to be amplified, and the amplified DNA can be easily analyzed. Even fixed tissue in paraffin blocks or on slides can yield sufficient DNA for analysis using PCR.[25] The concepts underlying PCR are diagrammed in Figure 2-7. Two short single-stranded DNA fragments, called primers, have sequences complementary to those that flank the stretch of DNA to be amplified. They are added to the target DNA, the mixture is heated to dissociate the paired double strands of target DNA, and then the temperature is lowered to permit hybridization, or annealing, of the primers to their complementary sequences on the target DNA. A DNA polymerase enzyme is added to the mixture, which will add nucleotides to the 3' end of the primers using the target DNA as a sequence template. This step generates one copy of each of the strands of one target DNA molecule. The mixture is heated again to dissociate the strands and then cooled to allow more primers to anneal to the target sequences on both the original and new pieces of DNA. DNA polymerase is added again and now generates four copies of the target sequences. These steps are repeated, resulting in a geometrically increasing amount of target DNA, that is, a chain reaction.[26,27] With the discovery and cloning of the DNA polymerase from the thermophilic bacterium *Thermus aquaticus* (the Taq polymerase), which retains activity after being heated to 95°C, heating and cooling steps could be carried out on the same mixture without adding a new enzyme.[28] This allowed the procedure to be automated. There are now automated thermal cyclers in every molecular biology laboratory and in many clinical laboratories that will take PCR mixtures through 20 to 50 cycles, producing large amounts of synthetic DNA for subsequent analysis.

DNA Polymorphisms A genetic polymorphism (which literally means "many forms") is defined as the occurrence of two or more relatively common normal alleles for a single locus. The difference between a polymorphism and a mutation is that a polymorphism occurs commonly and is associated with a normal phenotype. The usual distinction is that a gene is polymorphic when its least frequent manifestation appears in at least 1% of the population. Examples include blood types and major histocompatibility complex molecules.

Polymorphisms may also occur without being associated with an obvious phenotype. For example, changes in nucleotide sequence within introns or in regions between genes would not necessarily result in altered proteins and would therefore be "silent." However, if these changes are polymorphic, that is, frequent, then there is a high probability that an individual might be heterozygous for the polymorphism. In other words, it would be likely that the two chromosomes of a diploid pair would carry different versions of the polymorphism. Then, if the chromosomal position of the polymorphic change were known, it could be used as a marker for mapping other genes. There are several varieties of DNA polymorphisms, and they provide the basis for gene mapping techniques that have identified several important cancer genes.

RFLPs appear as differences among individuals in the pattern of bands on a Southern blot probed with a single-cloned DNA. There are two mechanisms whereby DNA polymorphisms are detectable by Southern blotting. First, a single nucleotide change might either create or destroy the recognition site for a restriction endonuclease. This would cause an alteration in the Southern blot pattern of that gene when the DNA is digested with a particular restriction endonuclease. For example, if a stretch of DNA with the sequence …AGGA**T**TTCGA… in one individual contained a single nucleotide change in a second individual so that the sequence was …AGGAA**T**TCGA…, the recognition site for EcoRI (GAATTC) would be created (see Figure 2-3). Digesting the second individual's DNA with EcoRI would generate two new restriction fragments and remove one old one when compared with the first individual's DNA.

The second mechanism involves one of the more mysterious features of genomic DNA in eukaryotes, namely, that it is replete with repeated sequences of unknown function. The sequences often stretch themselves along the DNA polymer, one set of sequences after the other, in so-called tandem repeats. In humans, the best known repetitive sequence is called *alu* (because it contains recognition sites for the restriction endonuclease AluI), and its nucleotide sequence is so specific that it can be used to identify human DNA in a mixture of DNAs from many species. There are several examples of tandemly repeated sequences in which the number of tandem repeats varies among individuals.[29] One may have a DNA probe that recognizes a restriction fragment containing some tandem repeats. If the number of repeated sequences varies from one individual to the next, the size of the restriction fragment to which the probe hybridizes on a Southern blot will vary between the individuals. This will appear as an RFLP. These polymorphisms are called *variable number of tandem repeats* (VNTRs). In other cases, the repeat unit can be as small as two or three nucleotides (ie, di- or trinucleotide repeats), and polymorphisms can be recognized by changes in the size of PCR products containing these repeats (see below).

By either mechanism, these RFLPs are stably inherited in a mendelian fashion, which permits them to be used in gene mapping. RFLPs occur at specific positions (loci) in genomic DNA. If all of the affected individuals in a family with a particular genetic disease inherit the same RFLP, this is presumptive evidence that the gene for the disease is close (or linked) to the RFLP locus. Linking a disease locus to an RFLP maps the gene for that disease and is the first step toward cloning the gene responsible for the disease. These are the tools of reverse genetics, which have also led to the identification of some of the genes associated with malignant transformation, such as the *BRCA1* gene on chromosome 17, whose mutations are responsible for a relatively significant fraction of heritable breast cancer.[30]

RFLPs have also been used to demonstrate gene loss in cancer (Figure 2-8A). This approach relies on an individual being heterozygous for an RFLP, that is, having one polymorphism on one chromosome and another polymorphism on the other. If an individual with cancer is heterozygous for a particular RFLP (termed an *informative individual*), his or her tumor can be analyzed by Southern blotting, using the probe that recognizes the polymorphism, and compared with normal tissue analyzed the same way. If one of the RFLPs present in the heterozygous individual's normal DNA is missing from the tumor cell DNA, the tumor is said to have undergone a reduction to homozygosity or a loss of heterozygosity (LOH). This implies a loss of genetic material from the tumor, specifically the DNA that includes the missing RFLP. This is the hallmark of a tumor suppressor gene.[31] It was in this way that the involvement of the suppressor gene *TP53* was found in human colon cancers.[32,33]

A particularly interesting polymorphism is known as a microsatellite. For unknown reasons, about 50,000 copies of the repetitive sequence dC-dA (tandemly repeated 10 to 60 times) are dispersed throughout the human genome.[34] Because the longer tandem repeats (VNTRs, as mentioned above) have been called minisatellite DNA, the shorter dC-dA repeats are called microsatellite DNA. (The term *satellite* refers to the fact that the buoyant density of repetitive DNA is different from the majority of genomic DNA. This leads to the appearance of small satellite bands distinct from the main DNA band when genomic DNA is purified by density gradient centrifugation.) The number of repeats at a particular locus varies in a polymorphic way among individuals, and because these sequences are stably inherited, they can serve as polymorphic markers. The difference in the number of repeat units between two polymorphic microsatellites can be as small as a few nucleotides. These differences cannot be detected by Southern blotting, which has a resolution of 100 nucleotides. However, these differences can easily be resolved using PCR. Primers that flank the repeat region are used in a PCR reaction in the presence of radiolabeled deoxynucleotides, and the products are separated on a DNA sequencing-style polyacrylamide gel. Mini- and microsatellite polymorphic markers are much more useful in gene mapping than RFLPs because, unlike RFLPs, which usually have only two alleles, the variable number of repeats creates multiple alleles for each locus, significantly raising the likelihood that an individual will be heterozygous for the marker.

Although the number of repeats in a microsatellite marker is usually stable, in some cancers, most notably colorectal cancer, the number of microsatellite repeats in the tumors differs from that in normal colorectal tissue from the same patient. Because the variability in repeat number occurs at all positions throughout the genome of the tumor, this suggests that the tumors experience overall genetic instability.[35,36] The basis of this instability is believed to be a mutation in the human homologues of DNA "proofreading" genes that, when mutated in yeast, lead to the appearance of unstable numbers of dC-dA repeats. One of these human genes, *MSH2*, which maps to chromosome 2, is responsible for hereditary nonpolyposis colorectal cancer.[37,38]

Single nucleotide polymorphisms (SNPs) are the most common polymorphism within the human genome.[39] SNPs are single base variations within a coding or noncoding DNA sequence; they occur approximately once every 1,350 base pairs in the average individual.[40–42] Analysis of SNPs has several uses in human cancer genetics. SNP analysis can be used to localize genes causing familiar cancers by linkage analysis.

SNP analysis is a powerful method to determine LOH in human cancers. The major approach for LOH is the use of microarrays (see below) that contain large numbers of human SNPs. PCR amplification of genomic DNA and hybridization to arrays permits the detection of chromosomal regions of LOH (Figure 2-8B). This provides a high-throughput and automatable method for large-scale LOH analysis.[43,44] Furthermore, SNP analysis of LOH can be performed on laser-capture microdissected cells from paraffin-embedded tissue specimens,[45] thereby allowing genomic studies on standard pathologic specimens.

In addition to predicting LOH, SNP arrays can also be used for assaying overall genome-

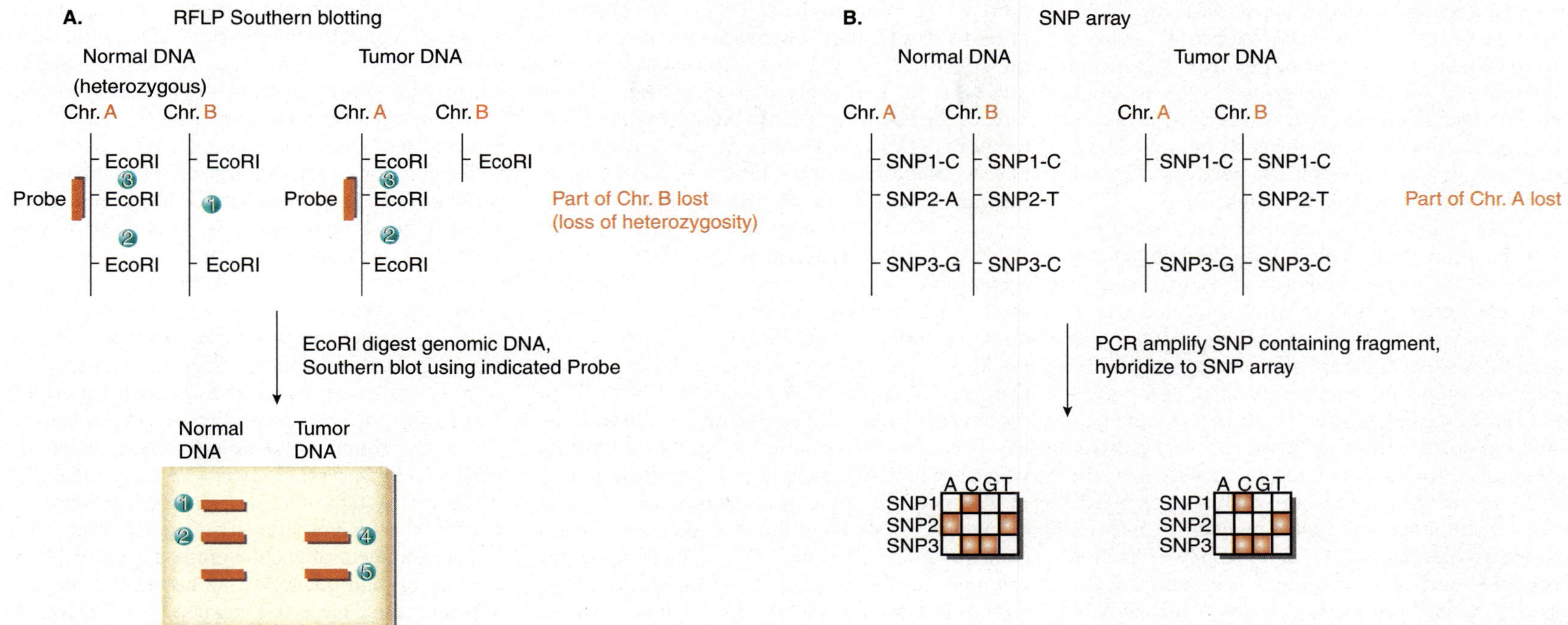

Figure 2-8 Methods to detect loss of heterozygosity in tumor tissue. **A,** Restriction fragment length polymorphism (RFLP) and Southern blotting. In this example, an individual is heterozygous for an EcoRI recognition site: the second EcoRI site on chromosome A is absent on its diploid partner, chromosome B. The individual's tumor is assumed to be clonal and to have arisen from a cell that lost the region of chromosome B displayed in the figure. Southern blotting can then be performed using genomic deoxyribonucleic acid (DNA) from the individual's normal DNA and tumor DNA in separate lanes of the agarose gel. Probing the DNA with the probe (indicated on the figure) reveals a heterozygous banding pattern in normal DNA (reflecting the presence of both polymorphisms, one on each chromosome pair) and a loss of that pattern in the tumor DNA. This is one of the hallmarks of a tumor suppressor gene. **B,** Single nucleotide polymorphism (SNP) array. In this example, an individual is heterozygous for SNPs 2 and 3 and homozygous for SNP 1. Following the polymerase chain reaction (PCR) amplification of genomic fragments containing each SNP individually, these fragments are hybridized to an array composed of oligonucleotides complementary to the ones amplified. The loss of a heterozygous SNP signal on the array indicates loss of the chromosomal region containing this SNP.

wide copy number changes and identify amplified chromosomal areas that frequently harbor oncogenes.[46] For example, *HER2/neu*, *EGFR1*, *MYC*, and *CCDN1* are oncogenes that are commonly overactivated owing to a significant increase in their copy number.

Comparative genomic hybridization, employed using whole-chromosome spreads or array-based platforms, is another method used for the detection of chromosomal copy number changes based on the comparison of the hybridization intensity of tumor and normal control DNA samples.[47,48] The resolution of the best available array comparative genomic hybridization is comparable to that of currently used SNP arrays (30 kb average across the genome). However, SNP arrays can more accurately predict LOH, thus allowing the quantitative determination of both chromosomal losses and gains and allelic changes in a single experiment.

Summary Genomic DNA is too large to be analyzed easily in the laboratory, but it can be cut into manageable fragments using restriction endonucleases isolated from bacteria. Electrophoresis through an agarose gel can separate these fragments by size. Pulsed-field gel electrophoresis is a variation of this technique that allows the separation of extremely large DNA molecules. Fragments that carry nucleotide sequences corresponding to a gene of interest can then be detected by Southern blotting. Specific nucleotide changes (mutations) that give rise to stable genetic differences can be determined by DNA sequencing. PCR technology permits the detection of specific genes in extremely small amounts of tissue or in tissue that has been fixed for histologic analysis. There are polymorphic sites throughout genomic DNA; some create or destroy restriction endonuclease sites leading to RFLPs; others contain a variable number of tandemly repeated sequences and are called mini- or microsatellites; a third group, SNPs, represents single base variations. Polymorphisms can be used for gene mapping or cancer diagnostics.

GENE EXPRESSION: mRNA TRANSCRIPT ANALYSIS

Structural Considerations The first step in gene expression is transcription of the genetic information in DNA into RNA. The individual building blocks of RNA, ribonucleotides, have the same structure as the deoxyribonucleotides in DNA, except that (1) the 2' carbon of the ribose sugar is substituted with an OH group instead of H and (2) there are no thymine bases in RNA, only uracil (demethylated thymine), which also pairs with adenine by hydrogen bonding. Just like the DNA polymerases described above, the enzyme RNA polymerase II uses the nucleotide sequence of the gene's DNA as a template to form a polymer of ribonucleotides with a sequence complementary to the DNA template.

For transcription to be "correct," RNA polymerase II must (1) use the antisense strand of DNA as a template, (2) begin transcription at the start of the gene, and (3) end transcription at the end of the gene. The signals that ensure correct transcription are provided to the RNA polymerase II by DNA in the form of specific nucleotide sequences in the promoter of the gene. After reading and interpreting these signals, the RNA polymerase generates a primary RNA transcript that extends from the initiation site to the termination site in a perfect complementary match to the DNA sequence used as a template. However, not all transcribed RNA is destined to arrive in the cytoplasm as mRNA. Rather, by an incompletely understood process, sequences complementary to introns (see above) are excised from the primary transcript, and the ends of exon sequences are joined together in a process termed *splicing*.[49]

In addition to splicing, the primary transcript is further modified by the addition of a methylated guanosine triphosphate "cap" at the 5' end[50] and the addition of a stretch of anywhere from 20 to 40 A bases at the 3' end.[51] These modifications appear to promote the translatability[52,53] and relative stability of mRNAs and help direct the subcellular localization of mRNAs destined for translation.

Northern Blotting The fundamental question in the analysis of gene expression at the RNA level is whether RNA sequences derived from a gene of interest are present in cells or tissues. Detecting specific RNA sequences can be accomplished by Northern blotting, the whimsically named analogue of Southern blotting, when applied to RNA analysis. RNA can be isolated from cells in its intact form, free from significant amounts of DNA.[54] Messenger RNA is much smaller than genomic DNA, so it can be analyzed by agarose gel electrophoresis without the enzymatic digestion steps that are necessary for the analysis of high-molecular-weight DNA.

RNA is single stranded and has a tendency to fold back on itself. This allows complementary bases on the same stretch of RNA to base-pair with each other and form what is termed *secondary structure*. Because secondary structure can lead to aberrant electrophoretic behavior, RNA is electrophoretically separated by size in the presence of a denaturing agent, such as formaldehyde or glyoxal/dimethyl sulfoxide. After electrophoresis through a denaturing agarose gel, the RNA is transferred to a nitrocellulose or nylon-based membrane in the same manner as DNA for Southern blotting (see Figure 2-4). Hybridization schemes and blot washing are essentially the same for Northern blotting as for Southern blotting. In this manner, specific RNA sequences corresponding to those in cloned DNA probes can easily be identified.

There is a lower limit to the sensitivity of Northern blotting so that only moderately abundant mRNAs can be detected using this technique. One way to increase the sensitivity of Northern blotting is to enrich the RNA preparation for mRNA. Ordinarily, mRNA makes up less than 10% of the total RNA content of a cell or tissue. When RNA is isolated from these sources, all RNA species are being isolated, that is, ribosomal and transfer RNA as well as mRNA. As noted above, most mRNAs destined for the cytoplasm and translation are modified by the addition of a 3' poly(A) tract. An RNA preparation can, therefore, be greatly enriched for mRNA species by removing all RNA molecules that lack the 3' poly(A) tail.[55] This can be done by exposing the RNA preparation to a tract of poly(U) or poly(T) bound to an immobilized support, such as a plastic bead. The poly(A) portion of mRNA will bind to the poly(U) or poly(T) material, and non–poly(A)-containing RNA can be washed away. After washing, the poly(A)-containing mRNA can be recovered from the solid support and used in Northern blot analysis. This procedure improves the sensitivity of Northern blotting by nearly two orders of magnitude.

A dramatic use of Northern blotting in cancer research has been the demonstration of oncogene expression in some human tumors. RNA was isolated from human tumor samples and analyzed by Northern blotting using cloned DNA probes derived from various oncogenes. The earliest observations included expression of c-*abl* and c-*myc* in human tumor cell lines and leukemic blasts.[56,57] Since then, however, a large number of proto-oncogenes have been shown to be transcribed in primary human tumor tissue.

Complementary DNA The flow of genetic information usually runs from DNA to RNA to protein, according to the so-called central dogma of molecular biology. There are, however, exceptions to this rule, the most prominent of which involves the life cycle of retroviruses. These viruses encode their genetic information in RNA rather than DNA. When they invade a susceptible host cell, they direct the synthesis of a DNA intermediate that is a complementary copy of their genomic RNA. The enzyme that accomplishes this task, reverse transcriptase, is a DNA polymerase (see above) that uses RNA, rather than DNA, as a template to form a complementary deoxyribonucleic acid (cDNA) copy of the RNA.[58,59] This enzyme can be used in vitro to make cDNA copies of any available RNA.

One important application of cDNA synthesis has been the construction of cDNA libraries, which are basically gene libraries consisting only of the genes that are expressed in a cell or tissue of interest.[60,61] Most of the time, one is not really concerned with all of the DNA in the genome, for example, intron sequences, promoters, and vast regions of "uninformative" DNA that lie between genes. Furthermore, if one were interested in analyzing the genes expressed in a brain cell, why bother making a library that contained sequences for the hemoglobin gene? One way to construct a library comprising only tissue-specific expressed genes would be to clone all of the mRNA in a specific cell or tissue of interest. Unfortunately, there is no way to ligate single-stranded RNA to a double-stranded DNA cloning vector. However, one can use all of the mRNA in a cell as a template for making double-stranded cDNA, which can then be inserted into a cloning vector.

To make a cDNA library, one isolates all of the mRNA from a cell or tissue. Then, using this mRNA as a template, reverse transcriptase makes cDNA copies of each mRNA molecule in the mixture. The cDNA is ligated into a plasmid or phage vector as described above (see Figure 2-3), and the recombinant vectors are introduced into bacteria. After growth on agar plates, each bacterial colony or phage plaque of a cDNA library houses a unique recombinant vector containing the cDNA copy of a single mRNA. Desired clones can be detected by nucleic acid hybridization to the plaques or colonies using a radiolabeled gene probe.[62,63] Alternatively, if the vector containing the cDNA molecules can direct transcription of mRNA by host bacterial cells, mRNA will be synthesized, and that mRNA will be translated. In this case, each bacterial colony or plaque will produce a different protein, and each protein will have been encoded by an mRNA from the original cell or tissue being investigated. If an antibody directed against a protein of interest is available, the cDNA clone corresponding to the mRNA that encodes that protein can be identified by binding the antibody to the colonies or plaques of the cDNA library.[64] This technique, called *expression cloning*, often employs the bacteriophage λgt11 as the cloning vector.

cDNA libraries can be used to clone cDNA for a known gene to discover the sequence of the mRNA it encodes. One application of this is the generation of expressed sequence tag databases by sequencing clones of various cDNA libraries. Alternatively, cDNA libraries can also be used to identify previously unknown genes. In a process called *differential screening*, cDNAs can be discovered that owe their existence to a particular differentiation or activation state in the cell of origin. For example, this technique has been used to identify genes whose expression is turned on by hormones or by growth factors.[65]

Serial Analysis of Gene Expression The most comprehensive way to display a unique pattern of gene expression that determines the identity of a cell or tissue would be to construct a cDNA library from it and sequence every clone. This is obviously an impossible task. Rather, a technique called *serial analysis of gene expression* (SAGE) achieves the same end in a practical manner. In SAGE, the investigator sequences a small and unique fragment of each expressed gene (called a SAGE tag) and quantifies the number of times it appears (called the SAGE tag number). The SAGE tag numbers, therefore, directly reflect the abundance of the corresponding transcript.

The sensitivity and the quantitative accuracy of SAGE are theoretically unlimited. The generation of a SAGE library does not require any prior knowledge of what genes are expressed in the cell of interest. Therefore, SAGE is able to detect and quantify the expression of previously uncharacterized genes. SAGE is based on two fundamental principles:

1. A short (10–17 base pair) oligonucleotide fragment (SAGE tag) is sufficient to uniquely identify a specific mRNA transcript or its cognate cDNA. A 10 bp oligonucleotide sequence has a complexity of 4^{10} different combinations. Because there are only about 30,000 to 120,000 genes encoded by the human genome, a 10 bp sequence tag corresponding to a defined position of a cDNA is sufficient to uniquely identify any transcribed human gene.
2. Multiple 10 bp SAGE tags can be concatenated in a single plasmid, thereby greatly compressing the number of actual plasmid preparations and DNA sequencing reactions that are required to analyze a large number of genes. In practice, a single sequencing reaction can provide information on 30 to 35 different SAGE tags and therefore 30 to 35 different cDNAs.

The generation of a SAGE library is a technically challenging multistep procedure that has been described in detail.[66] Figure 2-9 outlines the essence of the method.

SAGE has been used to characterize the yeast transcriptome and monitor alterations in gene expression patterns following ionizing radiation during apoptosis induced by the tp53 and the APC tumor suppressor proteins.[67–70] In all of these cases, the ability to measure the expression levels of thousands of different transcripts simultaneously was extremely useful for the understand-

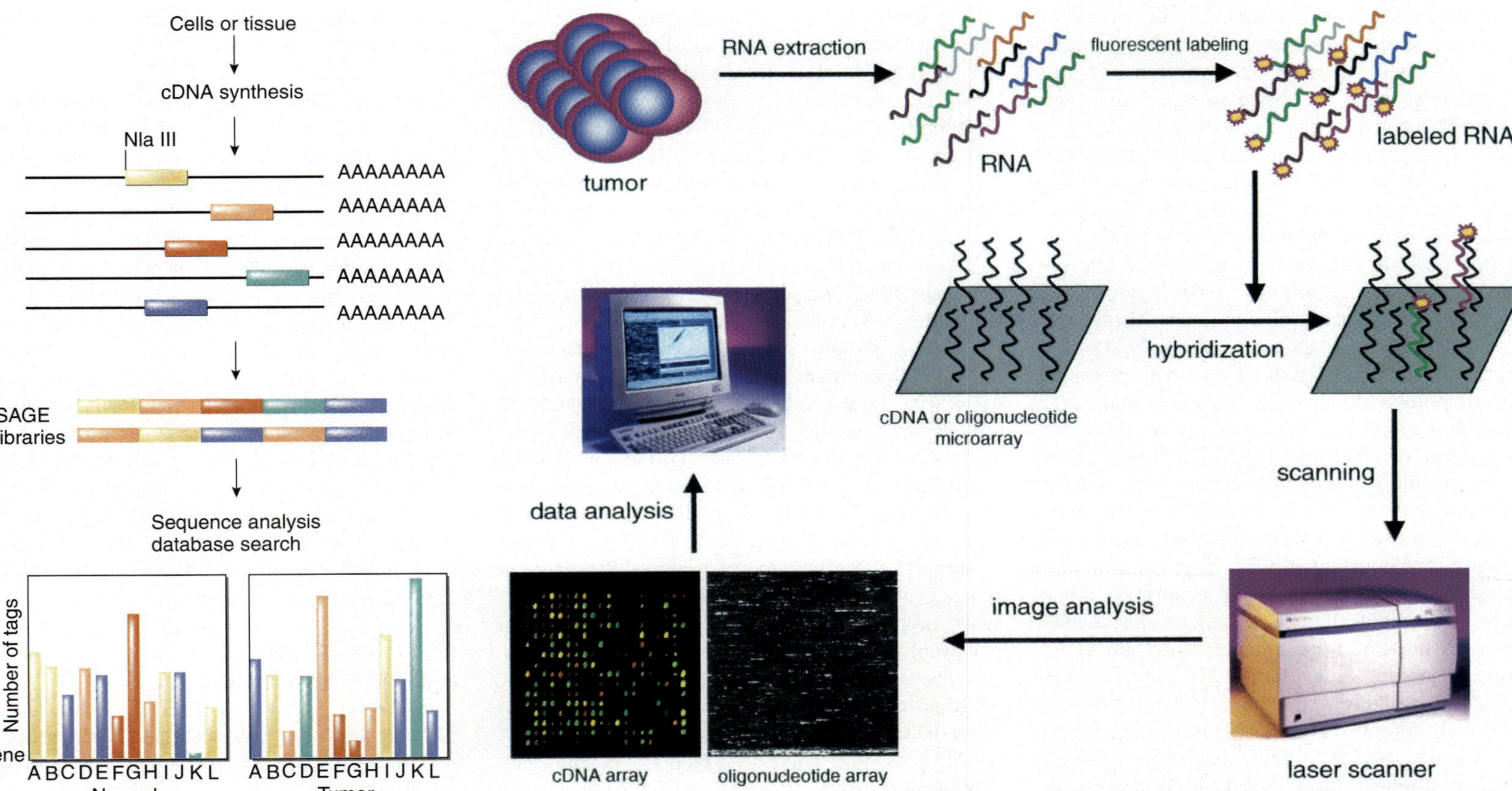

Figure 2-9 Construction and analysis of serial analysis of gene expression (SAGE) libraries. In step 1, a complementary deoxyribonucleic acid (cDNA) library is constructed from the cells or tissue of interest, and the cDNAs are immobilized on magnetic beads at their 3' ends. In step 2, the cDNAs are subjected to restriction enzyme digestion with a so-called anchoring enzyme. This anchoring enzyme is a frequent cutter restriction endonuclease (usually NlaIII) that ensures that all of the cDNAs are cut at least once. In step 3, cleaved cDNAs are divided into two pools. Short oligonucleotide linkers are ligated to the newly cut 5' ends of the tags. A different linker is used for each pool (linkers A and B as shown). These oligonucleotide linkers contain a recognition site for a tagging enzyme. This tagging enzyme is a type two restriction endonuclease (usually BsmfI) that cuts at some distance to the 3' side of the actual recognition site. In step 4, SAGE tags are released by cleavage with the tagging enzyme and further processed to yield blunt ends. In step 5, the free, blunt-ended SAGE tags are dimerized to yield ditags. These ditags are amplified by polymerase chain reaction using linker A and B primers. Note that each ditag is flanked by the recognition site for the frequent cutter anchoring enzyme used in step 2. These flanking recognition sites serve as punctuation marks for sequence analysis of the concatenated SAGE tags. Once sufficient amounts of ditags are generated, they are ligated together in linear arrays containing several ditags (ie, they are concatemerized) and subcloned into a plasmid that can be used as a template for automated sequencing. Each sequenced plasmid can yield data on 30 to 35 SAGE tags. Data are analyzed by using the SAGE software that reads the sequence obtained, derives the SAGE tags, matches them to their cognate cDNA, and gives the gene expression profile in a numeric format.

Figure 2-10 Deoxyribonucleic acid (DNA) microarray analysis. In this example, ribonucleic acid (RNA) extracted from a tumor is end-labeled with a fluorescent marker and then allowed to hybridize to a chip derivatized with complementary deoxyribonucleic acids (cDNAs) or oligonucleotides, as described in the text. The precise location of RNA hybridization to the chip can be determined using a laser scanner. Because the position of each unique cDNA or oligonucleotide is known, the presence of a cognate RNA for any given unique sequence can be determined.

ing of the underlying physiologic processes. The application of SAGE to the comparison of the expression profiles of normal and tumor tissues is probably the most attractive one because by comparing the expression profiles of normal and cancer cells in a comprehensive way, it is possible to identify genes or subsets of genes that could be used as potential diagnostic or prognostic markers or therapeutic targets.[71–74] SAGE is one of the techniques used by the National Cancer Institute–funded Cancer Gene Anatomy Project (CGAP).[75] A goal of this project is to create a catalogue of genes expressed in various normal and cancerous tissue types. To date, more than 120 different SAGE libraries have been deposited on the National Center for Biotechnology Education/CGAP SAGEmap Web site (<http://cgap.nci.nih.gov/SAGE>), which is now the largest source of public SAGE data.[75,76]

DNA Microarray Analysis Another approach to comparative gene expression profiling employs the use of DNA microarrays, often referred to as DNA chips. Two basic types of DNA microarrays are currently available: oligonucleotide arrays[77,78] and cDNA arrays.[79,80] Both approaches involve the immobilization of DNA sequences in a gridded array on the surface of a solid support, such as a glass microscope slide or silicon wafer. In the case of oligonucleotide arrays, 25 nucleotide–long fragments of known DNA sequence are synthesized in situ on the surface of the chip using a series of light-directed coupling reactions similar to photolithography. Using this method, as many as 400,000 distinct sequences representing over 18,000 genes can be synthesized on a single 1.3 × 1.3 cm microarray. In the case of cDNA microarrays, cDNA fragments are deposited onto the surface of a glass slide using a robotic spotting device. For both microarray approaches, the next step involves the purification of RNA from the source of interest (eg, from a tumor), enzymatic fluorescent labeling of the RNA, and hybridization of the fluorescently labeled material to the microarray. Hybridization events are then captured by scanning the surface of the microarray with a laser scanning device and measuring the fluorescence intensity at each position in the microarray. The fluorescence intensity of each spot on the array is proportional to the level of expression of the gene represented by that spot. This process is illustrated in Figure 2-10.

DNA microarray technology is evolving rapidly, with improvements in miniaturization, reproducibility, production capabilities, and the development of alternative approaches to microarray synthesis. The application of gene expression profiling methods to important questions in biology and medicine is also emerging. The ability to monitor the expression levels of thousands of genes simultaneously offers the potential opportunity to expand the analysis of cancer genetics beyond single–candidate gene approaches toward considering genetic networks. It is becoming increasingly clear that whereas some tumors appear to be caused by mutations in a single gene (eg, oncogene or tumor suppressor gene), most cancers likely arise through the collaboration of multiple genes, none of which, when considered alone, are sufficient for transformation. Until recently, the analysis of such genetic networks has been impractical in that methods for measuring the expression levels of multiple genes in parallel have not been available. The development of DNA microarrays may, in large part, have solved this problem. Microarrays capable of monitoring the expression levels of the entire human genome (estimated to contain approximately 30,000 to 120,000 genes) are likely to become available in the near future.

Microarray analysis has proven to be a powerful method for the analysis of gene expression patterns in human cancer and for cancer classification. Gene expression profiles have been used for class prediction, or determining which samples belong to which tumor class, and for class discovery of new tumor types. The first proof of principle for gene expression analysis in cancer was the demonstration that acute myeloid leukemias and acute lymphoid leukemias could be accurately distinguished.[81] Since then, new cancer classes have been discovered in leukemias,[82] lymphomas,[83,84] brain cancers,[85] breast cancer,[86,87] prostate cancers,[88–90] and lung cancers,[91,92] among others. Although gene expression analysis of cancer has not yet been used for clinical diagnosis, it is likely that such applications will be developed during the next several years.

The challenge now is not so much how to generate complex gene expression data but rather how to interpret it. The key is to develop methods for recognizing meaningful gene expression patterns and distinguishing those patterns from noise. Such noise (random gene expression levels) can be generated by (1) variability among microarrays, (2) variability in RNA labeling and hybridization methods, and, perhaps most importantly, (3) biologic variability among samples. It is likely that all of the above sources of variability are significant. It has become clear that the successful elucidation of genetic networks through expression profiling will require the expertise of a new generation of scientists, namely, computational biologists. Improvements in DNA microarray fabrication will become valuable only if pattern recognition algorithms are similarly developed. Nonetheless, it is likely that the future of cancer diagnostics will include the analysis of gene expression profiles that might help guide treatment planning of individual patients.

Polymerase Chain Reaction Another important use of cDNA technology has allowed PCR to be applied to RNA. Because the *Taq* polymerase is a DNA polymerase (see above), it cannot use RNA as a template. Simply adding primers and *Taq* polymerase to an RNA preparation will not result in amplification. However, if an RNA of interest could be made into DNA, then PCR would proceed as usual.

The first step in this analysis is generating a cDNA copy of the mRNA of interest using reverse transcriptase. This can be done using a primer consisting of Ts [complementary to the poly(A) tail] or of a sequence complementary to some portion of the 3' region of the mRNA. The 5' primer can then be added along with *Taq* polymerase, and the single-stranded cDNA made in the first step will be amplified as described above (see Figure 2-7). In one of the first applications of this technique, Philadelphia chromosome–positive leukemias were diagnosed by identifying chimeric *bcr-abl* mRNA species in clinical material using PCR. Since then, so-called reverse transcriptase PCR has come into widespread use.[93]

One inherent problem in using PCR to monitor mRNA expression is quantitation of the amplified PCR products. In Northern blotting or nuclease protection analysis, the intensity of the hybridization signal is directly proportional to the amount of target RNA in the sample. Thus, one can compare the number of RNA molecules in one sample with another. With PCR, a slight change in the efficiency of polymerization in an early cycle in one sample will lead to a geometrically increasing discrepancy between the amount of amplified product in that sample compared with another sample, and the amounts of PCR product when the reaction reaches saturation can also differ significantly. Fortunately, a number of techniques have been described for normalizing the products of PCRs to allow quantitative comparisons. Most notably, quantitative real-time PCR[94] is a method for continuous monitoring of amplification. This method makes quantitative comparisons of amplifications during the unbiased linear range in which each cycle gives a constant increase in amplification. In brief, quantitative real-time PCR takes advantage of a fluorogenic probe within the amplified region containing a fluorescent tag on one end and a quencher on the other end. Amplification also leads to digestion of the probe, now liberating a free fluorescent molecule; the increase in fluorescence is proportional to the amplification.

Ribozymes and RNA Interference Some RNA molecules, in addition to proteins, have enzymatic activity. These RNAs, called ribozymes, can cleave RNA at sequence-specific sites.[95] They were originally discovered in *Tetrahymena* when it appeared that some of the primary RNA molecules in that species were capable of splicing out their introns without the aid of any protein enzymes. Ribozymes have also recently been described in higher organisms, and it is likely that they will be found to play a universal and important role in RNA processing. Sequence-specific ribozymes that will destroy specific mRNAs can be synthesized. One application of this technology is the introduction into malignant cells of ribozymes directed against activated oncogenes.

A different method to disrupt cellular RNA molecules is RNA interference. In RNA interference, double-stranded RNA molecules can lead to the degradation of specific cellular messenger RNA species.[96] This method has now been applied to mammalian cells using 21 bp RNA duplexes[97] or plasmids, permitting stable expression of RNA interference.[98]

Summary The genetic information in DNA is copied, or transcribed, into mRNA by the enzyme RNA polymerase II. Before being transported to the cytoplasm, primary transcripts in the nucleus are modified by splicing out introns, adding a 5' cap, and adding a 3' poly(A) tract. Cytoplasmic mRNA can be detected by Northern blotting, nuclease protection assays, or modified PCR. Although nuclease protection assays are technically somewhat more demanding than Northern blotting, they are more sensitive and can provide structural information about mRNA transcripts. A retroviral enzyme called reverse transcriptase can make cDNA copies of mRNA transcripts. These cDNAs can be cloned into cDNA libraries, which are useful for isolating and analyzing expressed genes. In the future, ribozymes and/or RNA interference may be useful for the selective elimination of specific mRNA species.

GENE EXPRESSION: PROTEIN ANALYSIS

Structural Considerations Proteins are polymeric molecules consisting of amino acids linked by peptide bonds. The sequence of amino acids in a protein is dictated by the sequence of nucleic acids in the mRNA that encodes the protein. Because amino acids are joined to each other in a linear polymer, there is directionality to proteins, just as there is to DNA and RNA. The 5' end of the mRNA corresponds to the amino end of its cognate protein and the 3' end corresponds to the carboxy end (see Figure 2-1).

For many proteins, the linear polymer of amino acids must undergo a number of alterations to be functional. These alterations are referred to as *post-translational modifications*. For example, proteins destined to be secreted from a cell initially exist as propeptides with a 20– to 30–amino acid sequence at their amino ends. This highly hydrophobic tail, called a *leader sequence*, remains embedded in the membranes of the endoplasmic reticulum and secretory granule until the protein is to be secreted, at which point, the leader sequence is cleaved. There are many examples of propeptides that undergo cleavage of specific amino acids before they become mature, functional proteins.

Other post-translational modifications include the addition of various nonpeptide substituents to the side chains of amino acids. These include simple and complex carbohydrate chains, sulfate groups, and phosphate groups. Phosphorylation of intracellular proteins, usually on serine, threonine, or tyrosine residues, plays an important regulatory role in protein function. For example, many of the cell surface receptors for growth factors, such as the platelet-derived growth factor (PDGF) receptor[99] and the receptor for macrophage colony-stimulating factor (M-CSF),[100,101] are themselves protein tyrosine kinases. When this type of receptor binds its ligand, the receptor undergoes a conformational change that activates its kinase activity. The activated receptor then adds phosphate groups to some of its own tyrosine residues and to tyrosines in other proteins. These phosphorylations are part of the signal transduction process, whereby a message is sent from the cell surface receptor to the nucleus. The importance of tyrosine phosphorylation in cell growth may be reflected in the fact that tyrosine kinases form the largest functional subset of oncogenes. Recently, tyrosine kinase inhibitors, such as imatinib mesylate or Gleevec, which blocks the action of the c-abl and c-kit tyrosine kinases, have been proven as effective anticancer chemotherapeutic treatments.[19,102]

Sodium Dodecyl Sulfate–Polyacrylamide Gel Electrophoresis As with nucleic acids, the most common analytic technique applied to proteins is separation by size using electrophoresis. However, unlike nucleic acids, not all proteins are anionic, and they do not have a uniform charge-to-mass ratio. In the presence of an electric field, a mixture of unmodified and uncharacterized proteins would migrate in an unpredictable way, providing little or no information about their structures. This problem has been overcome by performing protein electrophoresis in the presence of the anionic detergent sodium dodecyl sulfate (SDS). SDS binds to proteins in a uniform way, approximately one molecule of SDS for every two amino acids. Thus, all proteins become polyanions in the presence of SDS, and the number of negative charges (supplied by the sulfate group in SDS) is directly proportional to the size, or molecular weight, of the protein.

Because proteins are generally smaller than the most commonly analyzed nucleic acids, electrophoresis is performed through a solid support made of polyacrylamide, which resolves low-molecular-weight molecules better than agarose. In the presence of an electric field, proteins in SDS will migrate toward the anode at a rate inversely proportional to the log of their molecular weights.[103] Proteins can be analyzed by sodium dodecyl sulfate–polyacrylamide gel electrophoresis (SDS-PAGE) in the presence or absence of β-mercaptoethanol (β-ME), which reduces sulfhydryl groups on the side chains of cysteines that can bind two separate protein chains together. Electrophoresis in the presence of β-ME permits the analysis of protein subunits, whereas electrophoresis in the absence of β-ME can reveal multimeric protein associations. SDS-PAGE is routinely employed to test the purity of a protein preparation. It is also an integral component of the techniques of immune precipitation and Western blotting.

Immunoblotting One of the most valuable immunologic identification techniques is immunoblotting (Figure 2-11A).[104] A mixture of proteins can be electrophoretically separated by SDS-PAGE, and the separated proteins can be transferred to a nitrocellulose or nylon-based filter by electrophoresis in a direction perpendicular to that of the first electrophoresis. The proteins will remain bound to the membrane support. By analogy to Southern blotting for DNA and Northern blotting for RNA, this technique for protein transfer has been called Western blotting. The protein blot can be soaked in a solution that contains a specific antibody that binds to the protein of interest. The presence of the bound antibody on the blot can then be detected if the antibody is labeled. The label can be an enzyme that reveals its presence by catalyzing a color or light-emitting reaction, or it can be a radionuclide, such as ^{125}I, that can be detected by autoradiography. Alternatively, an unlabeled antibody can be detected by washing the blot in a solution that contains a labeled anti-immunoglobulin antibody. This technique has been used to demonstrate overexpression of the HER2/*neu* protein in some breast cancers in which Southern blotting revealed no gene amplification.[105] Because the protein is the effector of gene function and the determinant of phenotype, overexpression of the protein can be highly significant and is often considered to be the "gold standard" of overexpression.

Immune Precipitation A primary goal of molecular biology is to use gene probes to detect the presence of a particular gene in a complex mixture of DNAs or RNAs. In a similar way, a specific antibody can be used as a probe to detect the presence of a particular protein in a complex mixture of proteins. An antibody directed against a protein of interest can be added to a mixture of proteins under conditions that allow the antibody to bind to its target protein (Figure 2-11B). One can then collect all of the immunoglobulins in that mixture by adding a protein that binds to immunoglobulins, such as anti-immunoglobulin antibodies or staphylococcal protein A. These proteins are often bound to a solid support, such as polystyrene beads, which can be removed from the solution by gentle centrifugation. As the beads collect at the bottom of the centrifuge tube, their attached immunoglobulin and target proteins collect there as well. When boiled in SDS and β-ME, the protein complexes dissociate, and they can be electrophoretically separated by SDS-PAGE. This process is called immune precipitation. To document the specificity of the antibody, a second immune precipitation is usually performed with a control antibody that does not bind the protein of interest. The two precipitations can be run side by side on SDS-PAGE, and the protein of interest can be identified by its presence in the experimental lane and its absence from the control lane. The proteins can be identified by staining reactions or, if the protein preparation is radiolabeled, by autoradiography.

An important application of this technique was the demonstration that the protein product of the retinoblastoma susceptibility gene (*Rb*) binds to proteins encoded by DNA tumor viruses. Antibodies directed against adenovirus proteins were used in an immune precipitation of proteins from cells transformed or infected by adenovirus. In addition to the adenovirus proteins, the precipitated proteins contained another protein that was proven to be the protein encoded by the retinoblastoma susceptibility gene.[106] Similar experiments using antibodies directed against the large T antigen of SV40 revealed an interaction between the T antigen protein and the Rb protein.[107] In both cases, these interactions appear to be central to the mechanisms whereby these viruses oncogenically transform susceptible host cells.

Enzyme-Linked Immunosorbent Assay Measurement of serum protein levels can be a valuable tool in cancer screening, cancer diagnosis, and monitoring the results of therapy. One of the most important applications of this approach is the measurement of prostate-specific antigen (PSA) levels for the detection and follow-up of prostate cancer.[108,109] The method used to measure PSA and other serum protein levels is ELISA.[110] This method is diagrammed in Figure 2-11C. The principle is essentially the same as immune precipitation, except that instead of binding the antibody to protein A beads, the specific antibody is immobilized onto the surface of a transparent plastic plate. The specific test protein then binds to the antibody (this is the immunosorbent part of the assay), and other proteins are washed away. A second antibody, which recognizes a distinct epitope or antigenic region of the same antigenic protein, is then added. This antibody is covalently coupled to an enzyme (hence the enzyme-linked part). Specific binding of the second antibody leads to an enzyme concentration proportional to the amount of protein. The addition of a substrate for a fluorescent, chemiluminescent, or colorimetric reaction then gives a signal proportional to the amount of enzyme and hence the amount of antigenic protein. Small molecule concentrations (eg, drug levels) can be measured in the same way if there are two independent antibodies, which can both bind to the molecule at the same time.

Sequencing The ultimate in protein identification is direct determination of amino acid sequence. Automated sequenators are now available that have considerably simplified this technically demanding analysis. In addition, recent advances in protein chemistry have permitted sequencing to be performed on mere picomoles of protein. In fact, Western blotting can be used to purify small amounts of protein, and the fragment of the blot containing the stained protein of interest can be used directly in an automated sequenator.[111]

Direct protein sequencing was responsible for ushering in the modern era of molecular oncology. The protein encoded by the oncogene v-*sis*, the transforming gene of the simian sarcoma virus, was found to be nearly identical to the empirically determined amino acid sequence of the B chain of human PDGF.[112,113] This was the first demonstration of a connection between oncogenes and the components involved in normal cellular proliferation.

Mass Spectrometry Dramatic advances in mass spectrometric methods in recent years have made mass spectrometry a preferred method for protein analysis and offer promise for use in diag-

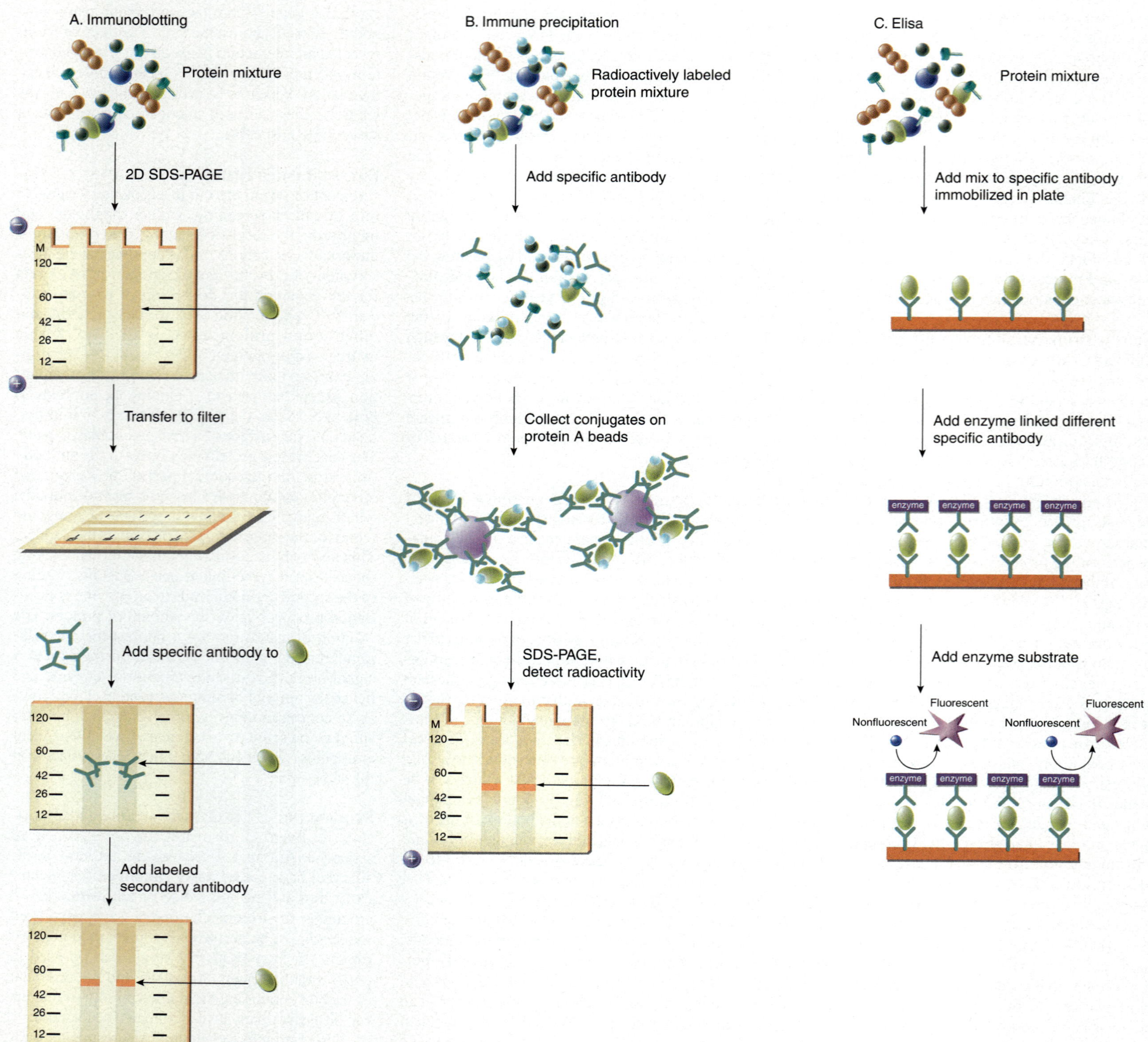

Figure 2-11 Methods of protein identification and detection. **A,** Immune (Western) blotting. A complex mixture of proteins can be separated by size using electrophoresis (sodium dodecyl sulfate–polyacrylamide gel electrophoresis [SDS-PAGE]). The separated proteins are then transferred to a nitrocellulose or nylon filter in an electric field, maintaining their size-specific spatial orientation on the filter. Antibodies directed against one specific protein (in this case, the *gray ellipsoid*) in the original mixture are added to the filter and bind to the specific protein. Bound antibodies can be radiolabeled or enzymatically labeled themselves, or they can be visualized by incubating the filter with labeled anti-immunoglobulin antibodies. **B,** Immunoprecipitation. A complex mixture of radiolabeled proteins (indicated by *different geometric shapes*) is incubated with antibodies specific for one of those proteins (in this case, the *gray ellipsoid*). After the antibodies have bound to their protein, small polystyrene or agarose beads containing staphylococcal protein A are added to the mixture. Protein A binds to the antibodies, and when centrifuged, the beads to which the protein A is bound will sediment to the bottom of the centrifuge tube, taking along the antibodies and the specific protein to which they have bound. The unbound proteins remain in the supernatant and can be removed. After boiling to dissociate the protein A/antibody/protein complex, specifically precipitated radiolabeled protein can be visualized by electrophoresis (SDS-PAGE) and autoradiography. **C,** Enzyme-linked immunosorbent assay (ELISA). To perform ELISA, one needs to develop two independent antibodies that bind to the protein to be detected (*gray ellipsoid* in this example) with high specificity and affinity. One of these antibodies is then coupled to a plate, which is then incubated with the protein mix to be analyzed (this can be tissue, blood, or another body fluid). The specifically bound protein is retained on the plate and is detected with the second antibody generated against it that is coupled to an enzyme or isotope, allowing quantitation of the bound protein. ELISAs are usually very sensitive and can detect picomolar amounts of proteins.

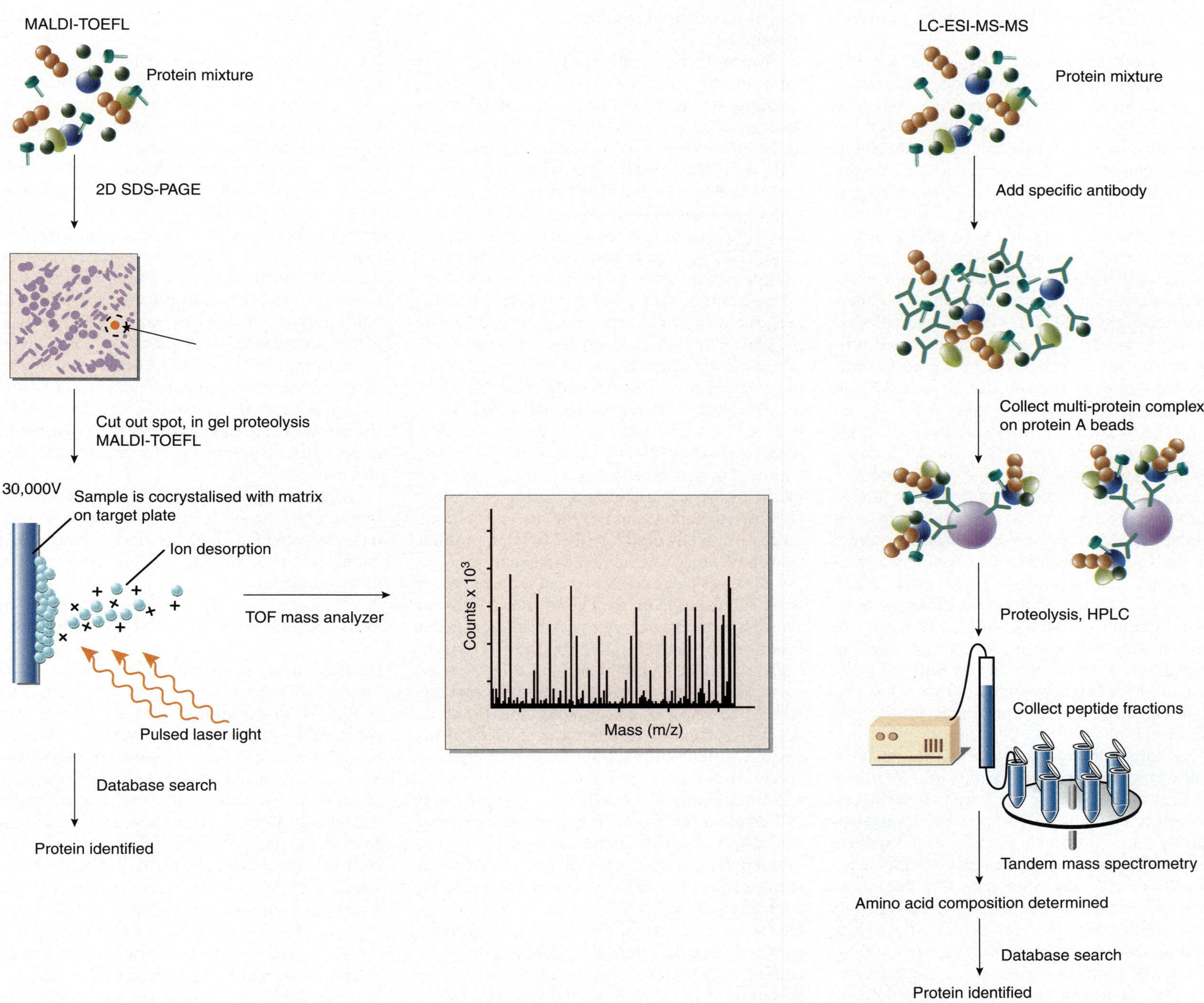

Figure 2-12 Mass spectrometry. **A,** Matrix-assisted laser desorption ionization time-of-flight mass spectrometry (MALDI-TOF). For organisms whose genome sequence is known, the identification of "interesting" protein spots from a two-dimensional gel is routinely performed using MALDI-TOF. A complex mixture of proteins is separated by size and charge using two-dimensional electrophoresis. Protein spots are excited from the gel, digested with a protease, mixed with a matrix solution, and allowed to cocrystallize on a target plate. When a laser is fired at the target plate, the matrix absorbs the laser light's energy and vaporizes, carrying some of the sample with it into a vacuum space. At the time the laser is fired, a high voltage is applied to the target plate to accelerate the ionized sample's movement toward the time-of-flight (TOF) mass analyzer. The resulting peptide fingerprint can then be used to search databases to determine the identity of the protein. **B,** The liquid chromatography electrospray ionization tandem mass spectrometry (LC-ESI-MS-MS) can be used to obtain amino acid sequence information, allowing highly refined database searches. The approach employs capillary high-performance liquid chromatography (HPLC), which allows very slow (submicroliter/min) flow rates that are essential for obtaining high-sensitivity ESI-MS-MS of peptides. Following the liquid chromatography and electrospray ionization, the ions are analyzed by linearly linked tandem mass spectrometers that yield amino acid composition information.

nostic analysis as well. Mass spectrometry is a technique to convert molecules into ions and then to measure their mass. The distinct mass of a given protein is a method to identify that protein in a mixture. Furthermore, proteins can be identified unambiguously by tandem mass spectrometry, in which the proteins are first fragmented into peptides and separated, and then the peptides are fragmented further for sequencing.[114,115] Mass spectrometry is summarized briefly in Figure 2-12. An excellent review article is available.[116]

Engineered Protein Expression The final goal of many experiments in molecular biology is the use of biologic systems to synthesize the protein encoded by the gene being studied. This process, called engineered protein expression, can be an experimental end in itself. When the expressed protein synthesized by recombinant DNA methods can be shown to have all of the properties of the natural protein, this is considered to be proof that the proper gene has been cloned. Alternatively, expression can be an end in itself when one wants to produce large amounts of a particular protein that might be difficult to obtain from natural sources.

In Vitro Translation One very simple expression method is in vitro translation, in which translation occurs entirely in a test tube. All of the components necessary for translating mRNA can be obtained from cells that are highly efficient in protein synthesis, such as reticulocytes (usually from rabbits) or wheat germ. Under the appropriate conditions, and in the presence of all 20 amino acids, a synthetic or purified RNA added to such a system will be efficiently translated into protein. If a radioactive amino acid, such as [^{35}S]methionine, is included in the mix, the reaction products can be analyzed by SDS-PAGE and autoradiography. Demonstrating an appropriately sized protein or one that is recognized by a specific antibody constitutes good evidence that the mRNA in hand is the one the investigator desires.

Large-Scale Production of Recombinant Proteins In vitro translation can be applied only at a small-scale analytic level. To produce large amounts of protein, one must turn to in vivo expression systems. One of the simplest involves cloning the cDNA for the desired protein into a bacterial plasmid or phage that contains a transcriptional promoter active in bacteria. When introduced into the appropriate bacterial host, large amounts of mRNA will be transcribed, which, in turn, will be translated into protein. The recombinant protein can then be purified away from all of the bacterial proteins. This is the way in which some clinically available interferons have been produced.[117–119]

As noted above, many eukaryotic proteins require post-translational modifications for maximal activity. Bacteria do not have the machinery required to accomplish complex modifications, such as the addition of specific carbohydrate groups. Moreover, the interior milieu of a bacterial cell is a reducing environment so that disulfide bonds essential to the structure and function of many eukaryotic proteins cannot form. When these modifications are required, mammalian cells can be used for expression. The basic concept is the same as in bacterial systems: a cDNA is cloned into a vector with a eukaryotic transcriptional promoter, and the resulting recombinant DNA is introduced into mammalian cells.[120] However, there are still significant disadvantages in the use of mammalian cells for large-scale recombinant protein production. Mammalian cells are expensive to grow in vitro because they require a medium rich in nutrients and growth factors. Yeast cells, insect cells, and even plant cells are being exploited as an attractive compromise between mammalian cell culture and bacterial culture for protein expression. These eukaryotic cells can execute most of the post-translational modifications required by mammalian proteins, including disulfide bonding. At the same time, these cells are easier and more economical to grow in vitro. A number of expression vectors analogous to those described here for bacteria and animal cells have been developed for these alternative eukaryotic hosts. Interested readers are referred to other sources for in-depth descriptions.[121,122]

Methods for Analyzing Protein-Protein Interactions An important and challenging task in postgenomic biology is to understand the function of proteins encoded by the genome and to determine their involvement in signaling pathways and cellular networks. One approach to understanding protein function is to investigate its interaction with other proteins of known function. By performing such analysis at a genome-wide level, one can create protein-protein physical interaction networks.[123] These networks can be combined with gene expression or other genomic data to generate regulatory and signaling networks at the cellular level. Several methods allow the characterization of protein-protein interactions at a genome-wide scale.[123] These include comprehensive protein pull-down assays, protein chips, and two-hybrid screens. Comprehensive protein pull-down assays use the combination of immunoprecipitation and mass spectrometric methods discussed above, whereas protein chips are the application of the microarray technology originally used for DNA or RNA profiling (see above) for protein interaction analysis.

The classic two-hybrid screen is performed in yeast and is based on the Gal4 system. Gal4 is a yeast transcriptional factor with well-defined and functionally distinct DNA-binding (DB) and *trans*-activator (TA) domains and a DNA target sequence. In the two-hybrid screen, the two proteins to be analyzed are fused to the DB and TA domains of Gal4, respectively. The resulting fusion proteins are referred to as "bait" and "prey." If the two proteins interact, then the DB and TA domains are brought into close proximity and create a functional transcriptional activator, the activity of which can be monitored using various reporter genes. The two-hybrid screen can be performed at three different levels: (1) testing the interaction of two known proteins, (2) testing the interaction of a known protein with all proteins, and (3) testing the interaction among all proteins. Unlike other approaches used for analyzing protein-protein interactions, the yeast two-hybrid screen does not require the expression and purification of any recombinant proteins. Thus, it is fairly straightforward to perform at a genome-wide scale and is applicable for nearly all protein interaction studies. A few such genome-wide studies were recently performed, and the resulting "interactome" maps greatly facilitate the functional annotation of the genome.[124–126]

Summary The genetic information in DNA is transcribed into RNA, and the information in RNA is ultimately translated into protein. Like DNA and RNA, proteins are also directional. The amino and carboxy termini of proteins are specified by the 5' and 3' ends, respectively, of their cognate mRNAs. After translation, proteins may require further modification to be fully functional.

Proteins can be fractionated by size using electrophoresis through polyacrylamide gels in the presence of the anionic detergent SDS (SDS-PAGE). SDS-PAGE is an integral component of the analytic techniques of immune precipitation and Western blotting. Automated analyzers are now available that can directly determine the amino acid sequence of a protein using vanishingly small amounts of material.

The mRNA that encodes a protein can be translated in vitro using cellular extracts of rabbit reticulocytes or wheat germ. The DNA that encodes a protein can be transcribed and the RNA translated in vivo by using appropriate vector and host cell combinations in culture. Bacterial cells are simple and economical vehicles for expressing foreign genes, but they cannot perform many of the post-translational modifications required by mammalian proteins. Vectors have been designed that permit mammalian cells to express foreign proteins with great efficiency and fidelity. Eukaryotic expression systems using yeast cells, insect cells, or plant cells also provide excellent alternatives.

Global analysis of protein interactions is used for the generation of interactome maps that reveal regulatory and functional networks, greatly facilitating our understanding of cellular function at the systemic level.

MOUSE MODELS OF HUMAN CANCER

Despite advances in our understanding of the biology of cancer at the molecular level, the application of this knowledge to the clinical management of cancer patients has been lagging behind. One of the factors limiting the translation of discoveries made in the laboratory to the clinic has been the availability of in vivo animal models of cancer that faithfully reproduce the human disease. Animals, particularly rodents, have been used in cancer research for decades for understanding physiologically relevant pathways necessary for tumorigenesis and the preclinical testing of anticancer or chemopreventive drugs.[127] Initially, these studies were limited to the transplantation of murine or human tumor cells into mice or analyzing spontaneously developing tumors. In the early 1980s, a new era of animal models built on genetically engineered mice opened up, enabling in vivo testing of the role of individual genes in tumorigenesis. The first-generation mouse models included transgenic mice carrying activated oncogenes in the form of transgenes driven by general or tissue-specific promoters; these transgenes are randomly inserted in the genome and are present in every cell of the animal (although expression can be restricted by the promoter). Similarly, "knockout" mice have been generated in which endogenous tumor suppressor genes in each cell of the animal have been replaced with exogenous sequences (such as neomycin resistance gene) on one (heterozygous) or both (homozygous) strands of the DNA. A detailed description of the basic methodologies required for the generation of transgenic and knockout mice can be found in an excellent manual on the manipulation of the mouse embryo.[128]

These early mouse models were very powerful in validating the cancer-relevant role of particular genes or their combination in tumorigenesis and allowed the identification of cooperating genetic alterations by insertional mutagenesis. However, a major drawback of these early mouse models is that genetically engineered mutations are present in every cell of the mouse. This is problematic for multiple reasons. First, it can lead to embryonic lethality or abnormalities if the affected oncogene or tumor suppressor gene is required for normal development. Second, with the exception of hereditary cancer predisposition syndromes, the modus operandi of these mutational events does not reproduce the human disease because the majority of human tumors evolve owing to acquired somatic genetic changes. Third, it did not allow the interrogation of the role of cancer-relevant genes in a particular organ type or stage of tumorigenesis. Recognizing these deficiencies, investigators have been developing ever more sophisticated mouse models that more and more faithfully reflect the human disease.

Currently used state-of-the-art mouse models are very different from those first-generation ones.[129] Constitutive and generalized expression systems have been replaced with inducible and cell type–specific platforms, and conditional gene targeting strategies are usually favored over germline loss-of-function mutations. At present, tetracycline (TET), tamoxifen (TAM), and Cre/loxP and their various combinations are the most popular choices for conditional gene expression and targeting. The TET system allows both temporally and cell type–specific gene expression. It has two different variations, TET-OFF and TET-ON, depending on whether the expression of the targeted gene (regulated by a TET-responsive transactivator) is expressed in the presence (TET-ON) or absence (TET-OFF) of TET.[130] The Cre/loxP system is used for the conditional inactivation (tumor suppressor genes) or activation (oncogenes) of gene function.[131,132] This approach is based on the use of a bacterial enzyme (Cre recombinase) that specifically catalyzes the recombination of loci flanked by its recognition sites (LoxP). For example, when a tumor suppressor gene of interest is flanked by two loxP sites, expression of the Cre recombinase will lead to the deletion of that gene.[131,132] Because the Cre expression can be regulated, for example, by the TET system, spatially and temporally, inactivation of such a tumor suppressor can now be achieved at will, in a specific cell compartment and at specific times during development or tumorigenesis.

Although significant progress has been made, several critical hurdles remain for preclinical uses of genetically engineered mice. Among these, one important one relates to intrinsic species difference between the mouse and the human. Unlike humans, genetically engineered mice harboring genetic mutations found in human cancers do not appear to manifest a similar spectrum of cancer phenotypes, particularly with respect to progression; mouse tumors rarely metastasize. Another important unanswered question relates to the predictive value of genetically engineered mice for preclinical drug testing. Finally, genetically engineered mice should be viewed not only as models trying to recapitulate human disease but also as genetic platforms themselves, enabling the discovery and validation of novel cancer susceptibility and modifier genes.

Summary Animal models are fundamental for the preclinical testing of novel cancer therapeutic and preventive compounds. Therefore, the development of models that faithfully recapitulate the human disease is one of the major important areas of current cancer research. Despite problems in part owing to interspecies differences, their use has been useful for deciphering tumorigenic pathways and identifying ways to interfere with them.

REFERENCES

1. Alberts B, Johnson A, Lewis J, et al. Molecular biology of the cell. Garland Press; Oxford, 2002.
2. Lewin B. Genes VII Oxford (UK): Oxford University Press; 1999.
3. Watson JD, Gilman M, Witkowski J. Recombinant DNA. W. H. Freeman; 1992.
4. Atchison ML. Enhancers: mechanisms of action and cell specificity. Annu Rev Cell Biol 1988;4:127–53.
5. McKnight S, Tjian R. Transcriptional selectivity of viral genes in mammalian cells. Cell 1986;46:795–805.
6. Nirenberg MW, Leder P. RNA code words and protein synthesis. Science 1964;145:1399.
7. Laskey RA, Earnshaw WC. Nucleosome assembly. Nature 1980;286:763–7.
8. Bauer WR, Crick FHC, White JH. Supercoiled DNA. Sci Am 1980;243:100–13.
9. Wang JC. DNA topoisomerases. Annu Rev Biochem 1985;54:665–97.
10. Smith HO. Nucleotide sequence specificity of restriction endonucleases. Science 1979;205:455–62.
11. Roberts RJ. Restriction and modification enzymes and their recognition sequences. Nucleic Acids Res 198210:r117–44.
12. Cohen SN, Chang AC, Boyer HW, Helling RB. Construction of biologically functional bacterial plasmids in vitro. Proc Natl Acad Sci U S A 1973;70:3240–4.
13. Ausubel FM, Brent R, Kingston RE, et al. Current protocols in molecular biology. John Wiley and Sons; 1998.
14. Sambrook J, Russell D. Molecular cloning: a laboratory manual. Cold Spring Harbor (NY): Cold Spring Harbor Laboratory Press; 2001.
15. Southern EM. Detection of specific sequences among DNA fragments separated by gel electrophoresis. J Mol Biol 1975;98:503–17.
16. Slamon DJ, Clark GM, Wong SG, et al. Human breast cancer: correlation of relapse and survival with amplification of the HER-2/neu oncogene. Science 1987;235:177–82.
17. Sanger F, Nicklen S, Coulson AR. DNA sequencing with chain-terminating inhibitors. Proc Natl Acad Sci U S A 1977;74:5463–7.
18. Nakahara M, Isozaki K, Hirota S, et al. A novel gain-of-function mutation of c-kit gene in gastrointestinal stromal tumors. Gastroenterology 1998;115:1090–5.
19. Joensuu H, et al. Effect of the tyrosine kinase inhibitor STI571 in a patient with a metastatic gastrointestinal stromal tumor. N Engl J Med 2001;344:1052–6.
20. Davies H, Bignell GR, Cox C, et al. Mutations of the BRAF gene in human cancer. Nature 2002;417:949–54.
21. Samuels Y, Wang Z, Bardelli A, et al. High frequency of mutations of the PIK3CA gene in human cancers. Science 2004;304:554.
22. Lynch TJ, Bell DW, Sordella R, et al. Activating mutations in the epidermal growth factor receptor underlying responsiveness of non-small-cell lung cancer to gefitinib. N Engl J Med 2004;350:2129–39.
23. Pao W, Miller V, Zakowski M, et al. EGF receptor gene mutations are common in lung cancers from “never smokers” and are associated with sensitivity of tumors to gefitinib and erlotinib. Proc Natl Acad Sci U S A 2004;101:13306–11.
24. Paez JG, Janne PA, Lee JC, et al. EGFR mutations in lung cancer: correlation with clinical response to gefitinib therapy. Science 2004;304:1497–500.
25. Impraim CC, Saiki RK, Erlich HA, Teplitz RL. Analysis of DNA extracted from formalin-fixed, paraffin-embedded tissues by enzymatic amplification and hybridization with sequence-specific oligonucleotides. Biochem Biophys Res Commun 1987;142:710–6.
26. Mullis KB, Faloona FA. Specific synthesis of DNA in vitro via a polymerase-catalyzed chain reaction. Methods Enzymol 11987;155:335–50.
27. Saiki RK, et al. Primer-directed enzymatic amplification of DNA with a thermostable DNA polymerase. Science 1988;239:487–91.
28. Saiki RK, et al. Enzymatic amplification of beta-globin genomic sequences and restriction site analysis for diagnosis of sickle cell anemia. Science 1985;230:1350–4.
29. Nakamura Y, Leppert M, O'Connell P, et al. Variable number of tandem repeat (VNTR) markers for human gene mapping. Science 1987;235:1616–22.
30. Miki Y, Swensen J, Shattuck-Eidens D, et al. A strong candidate for the breast and ovarian cancer susceptibility gene BRCA1. Science 1994;266:66–71.
31. Cavenee WK, Dryja TP, Phillips RA, et al. Expression of recessive alleles by chromosomal mechanisms in retinoblastoma. Nature 1983;305:779–84.
32. Baker SJ, Fearon ER, Nigro JM, et al. Chromosome 17 deletions and p53 gene mutations in colorectal carcinomas. Science 1989;244:217–21.
33. Vogelstein B, Fearon ER, Kern SE, et al. Allelotype of colorectal carcinomas. Science 1989;244:207–11.
34. Litt M, Luty JA. A hypervariable microsatellite revealed by in vitro amplification of a dinucleotide repeat within the cardiac muscle actin gene. Am J Hum Genet 1989;44:397–401.
35. Aaltonen LA, Peltomaki P, Leach FS, et al. Clues to the pathogenesis of familial colorectal cancer. Science 1993;260:812–6.
36. Thibodeau SN, Bren G, Schaid D. Microsatellite instability in cancer of the proximal colon. Science 1993;260:816–9.
37. Fishel R, Lescoe MK, Rao MR, et al. The human mutator gene homolog MSH2 and its association with hereditary nonpolyposis colon cancer. Cell 1993;75:1027–38.
38. Leach FS, Nicolaides NC, Papadopoulos N, et al. Mutations of a mutS homolog in hereditary nonpolyposis colorectal cancer. Cell 1993;75:1215–25.
39. Wang DG, Fan JB, Siao CJ, et al. Large-scale identification, mapping, and genotyping of single-nucleotide polymorphisms in the human genome. Science 1993;280:1077–82.
40. Mullikin JC, et al. An SNP map of human chromosome 22. Nature 2000;407:516–20.
41. Altshuler D, et al. An SNP map of the human genome generated by reduced representation shotgun sequencing. Nature 2000;407:513–6.
42. Sachidanandam R, Weissman D, Schmidt SC, et al. A map of human genome sequence variation containing 1.42 million single nucleotide polymorphisms. Nature 2001;409:928–33.
43. Mei R, Galipeau PC, Prass C, et al. Genome-wide detection of allelic imbalance using human SNPs and high-density DNA arrays. Genome Res 2000;10:1126–37.
44. Lindblad-Toh K, Winchester E, Daly MJ, et al. Large-scale discovery and genotyping of single-nucleotide polymorphisms in the mouse. Nat Genet 2000;24:381–6.
45. Primdahl H, Wikman FP, von der Maase H, et al. Allelic imbalances in human bladder cancer: genome-wide detection with high-density single-nucleotide polymorphism arrays. J Natl Cancer Inst 2002;94:216–23.
46. Zhao X, Li C, Paez JG, et al. An integrated view of copy number and allelic alterations in the cancer genome using single nucleotide polymorphism arrays. Cancer Res 2004;64:3060–71.
47. Mantripragada KK, Buckley PG, de Stahl TD, Dumanski JP. Genomic microarrays in the spotlight. Trends Genet 2004;20:87–94.
48. Albertson DG, Pinkel D. Genomic microarrays in human genetic disease and cancer. Hum Mol Genet 2003;12:R145–52.
49. Sharp PA. Split genes and RNA splicing. Cell 1994;77:805–15.
50. Shatkin AJ. Capping of eukaryotic mRNAs. Cell 1976;9:645–53.
51. Birnstiel ML, Busslinger M, Strub, K. Transcription termination and 3' processing: the end is in site! Cell 1985;41:349–59.

52. Filipowicz W. Functions of the 5'-terminal m7G cap in eukaryotic mRNA. FEBS Lett 1978;96:1–11.
53. Shatkin AJ. mRNA cap binding proteins: essential factors for initiating translation. Cell 1985;40:223–4.
54. Chirgwin JM, Przybyla AE, MacDonald RJ, Rutter WJ. Isolation of biologically active ribonucleic acid from sources enriched in ribonuclease. Biochemistry 1979;18:5294–9.
55. Aviv H, Leder P. Purification of biologically active globin messenger RNA by chromatography on oligothymidylic acid-cellulose. Proc Natl Acad Sci U S A 1972;69:1408–12.
56. Westin EH, Wong-Staal F, Gelmann EP, et al. Expression of cellular homologues of retroviral onc genes in human hematopoietic cells. Proc Natl Acad Sci U S A 1982;79:2490–4.
57. Eva A, Robbins KC, Andersen PR, et al. Cellular genes analogous to retroviral onc genes are transcribed in human tumour cells. Nature 1982;295:116–9.
58. Baltimore D. RNA-dependent DNA polymerase in virions of RNA tumour viruses. Nature 1970;226:1209–11.
59. Temin HM, Mizutani S. RNA-dependent DNA polymerase in virions of Rous sarcoma virus. Nature 1970;226:1211–3.
60. Efstratiadis A, Kafatos FC, Maniatis T. The primary structure of rabbit beta-globin mRNA as determined from cloned DNA. Cell 1977;10:571–85.
61. Rougeon F, Mach B. Stepwise biosynthesis in vitro of globin genes from globin mRNA by DNA polymerase of avian myeloblastosis virus. Proc Natl Acad Sci U S A 1976;73:3418–22.
62. Grunstein M, Hogness DS. Colony hybridization: a method for the isolation of cloned DNAs that contain a specific gene. Proc Natl Acad Sci U S A 1975;72:3961–5.
63. Benton WD, Davis RW. Screening lambda gt recombinant clones by hybridization to single plaques in situ. Science 1977;196:180–2.
64. Young RA, Davis RW. Efficient isolation of genes by using antibody probes. Proc Natl Acad Sci U S A 1983;80:1194–8.
65. Cochran BH, Reffel AC, Stiles CD. Molecular cloning of gene sequences regulated by platelet-derived growth factor. Cell 1983;33:939–47.
66. Velculescu VE, Zhang L, Vogelstein B, Kinzler KW. Serial analysis of gene expression. Science 1995;270:484–7.
67. He TC, Sparks AB, Rago C, et al. Identification of c-myc as a target of the APC pathway. Science 1998;281:1509–12.
68. Hermeking H, Lengauer C, Polyak K, et al. 14-3-3 sigma is a p53-regulated inhibitor of G2/M progression. Mol Cell 1997;1:3–11.
69. Polyak K, Xia Y, Zweier JL, et al. A model for p53-induced apoptosis. Nature 1997;389:300–5.
70. Velculescu VE, Zhang L, Zhou W, et al. Characterization of the yeast transcriptome. Cell 1997;88:243–51.
71. Zhang L, Zhou W, Velculescu VE, et al. Gene expression profiles in normal and cancer cells. Science 1997;276:1268–72.
72. Zhou W, Sokoll LJ, Bruzek DJ, et al. Identifying markers for pancreatic cancer by gene expression analysis. Cancer Epidemiol Biomarkers Prev 1998;7:109–12.
73. Porter D, Lahti-Domenici J, Keshaviah A, et al. Molecular markers in ductal carcinoma in situ of the breast. Mol Cancer Res 2003;1:362–75.
74. Polyak K, Riggins GJ. Gene discovery using the serial analysis of gene expression technique: implications for cancer research. J Clin Oncol 2001;19:2948–58.
75. Lal A, Lash AE, Altschul SF, et al. A public database for gene expression in human cancers. Cancer Res 1999;59:5403–7.
76. Lash AE, Tolstoshev CM, Wagner L, et al. SAGEmap: a public gene expression resource. Genome Res 2000;10:1051–60.
77. Chee M, Yang R, Hubbell E, et al. Accessing genetic information with high-density DNA arrays. Science 1996;274:610–4.
78. Lockhart DJ, Dong H, Byrne MC, et al. Expression monitoring by hybridization to high-density oligonucleotide arrays. Nat Biotechnol 1996;14:1675–80.
79. Schena M, Shalon D, Davis RW, Brown PO. Quantitative monitoring of gene expression patterns with a complementary DNA microarray. Science 1995;270:467–70.
80. Schena M, Shalon D, Heller R , et al. Parallel human genome analysis: microarray-based expression monitoring of 1000 genes. Proc Natl Acad Sci U S A 1996;93:10614–9.
81. Golub TR, Slonim DK, Tamayo P, et al. Molecular classification of cancer: class discovery and class prediction by gene expression monitoring. Science 1999;286:531–7.
82. Armstrong SA, Staunton JE, Silverman LB, et al. MLL translocations specify a distinct gene expression profile that distinguishes a unique leukemia. Nat Genet 2002;30:41–7.
83. Alizadeh AA, Eisen MB, Davis RE, et al. Distinct types of diffuse large B-cell lymphoma identified by gene expression profiling. Nature 2000;403:503–11.
84. Shipp MA, Ross KN, Tamayo P, et al. Diffuse large B-cell lymphoma outcome prediction by gene-expression profiling and supervised machine learning. Nat Med 2002;8:68–74.
85. Pomeroy SL, Tamayo P, Gaasenbeek M, et al. Prediction of central nervous system embryonal tumour outcome based on gene expression. Nature 2002;415:436–42.
86. Perou CM, Sorlie T, Eisen MB, et al. Molecular portraits of human breast tumours. Nature 2000;406:747–52.
87. van de Vijver MJ, He YD, van't Veer LJ, et al. A gene-expression signature as a predictor of survival in breast cancer. N Engl J Med 2002;347:1999–2009.
88. Dhanasekaran SM, et al. Delineation of prognostic biomarkers in prostate cancer. Nature 2001;412:822–6.
89. Singh D, Febbo PG, Ross K, et al. Gene expression correlates of clinical prostate cancer behavior. Cancer Cell 2002;1:203–9.
90. Welsh JB, Zarrinkar PP, Sapinoso LM, et al. Analysis of gene expression profiles in normal and neoplastic ovarian tissue samples identifies candidate molecular markers of epithelial ovarian cancer. Proc Natl Acad Sci U S A 2001;98:1176–81.
91. Bhattacharjee A, Richards WG, Staunton J, et al. Classification of human lung carcinomas by mRNA expression profiling reveals distinct adenocarcinoma subclasses. Proc Natl Acad Sci U S A 2001;98:13790–5.
92. Garber ME, Troyanskaya OG, Schluens K, et al. Diversity of gene expression in adenocarcinoma of the lung. Proc Natl Acad Sci U S A 2001;98:13784–9.
93. Kawasaki ES, Clark SS, Coyne MY, et al. Diagnosis of chronic myeloid and acute lymphocytic leukemias by detection of leukemia-specific mRNA sequences amplified in vitro. Proc Natl Acad Sci U S A 1988;85:5698–702.
94. Livak KJ, Flood SJ, Marmaro J, et al. Oligonucleotides with fluorescent dyes at opposite ends provide a quenched probe system useful for detecting PCR product and nucleic acid hybridization. PCR Methods Appl 1995;4:357–62.
95. Zaug AJ, Been MD, Cech TR. The *Tetrahymena* ribozyme acts like an RNA restriction endonuclease. Nature 1986;324:429–33.
96. Fire A, Xu S, Montgomery MK, et al. Potent and specific genetic interference by double-stranded RNA in *Caenorhabditis elegans*. Nature 1998;391:806–11.
97. Elbashir SM, Harborth J, Lendeckel W, et al. Duplexes of 21-nucleotide RNAs mediate RNA interference in cultured mammalian cells. Nature 2001;411:494–8.
98. Brummelkamp TR, Bernards R, Agami R. A system for stable expression of short interfering RNAs in mammalian cells. Science 2002;296:550–3.
99. Ek B, Westermark B, Wasteson A, Heldin CH. Stimulation of tyrosine-specific phosphorylation by platelet-derived growth factor. Nature 1982;295:419–20.
100. Sherr CJ, Rettenmier CW, Sacca R, et al. The c-fms proto-oncogene product is related to the receptor for the mononuclear phagocyte growth factor, CSF-1. Cell 1985;41:665–76.
101. Rettenmier CW, Chen JH, Roussel MF, Sherr CJ. The product of the c-fms proto-oncogene: a glycoprotein with associated tyrosine kinase activity. Science 1985;228:320–2.
102. Druker BJ, Sawyers CL, Kantarjian H, et al. Activity of a specific inhibitor of the BCR-ABL tyrosine kinase in the blast crisis of chronic myeloid leukemia and acute lymphoblastic leukemia with the Philadelphia chromosome. N Engl J Med 2001;344:1038–42.
103. Laemmli UK. Cleavage of structural proteins during the assembly of the head of bacteriophage T4. Nature 1970;227:680–5.
104. Towbin H, Staehelin T, Gordon J. Electrophoretic transfer of proteins from polyacrylamide gels to nitrocellulose sheets: procedure and some applications. Proc Natl Acad Sci U S A 1979;76:4350–4.
105. Slamon DJ, Godolphin W, Jones LA, et al. Studies of the HER-2/neu proto-oncogene in human breast and ovarian cancer. Science 1989;244:707–12.
106. Whyte P, Buchkovich KJ, Horowitz JM, et al. Association between an oncogene and an anti-oncogene: the adenovirus E1A proteins bind to the retinoblastoma gene product. Nature 1988;334:124–9.
107. DeCaprio JA, Ludlow JW, Figge J, et al. SV40 large tumor antigen forms a specific complex with the product of the retinoblastoma susceptibility gene. Cell 1988;54:275–83.
108. Kuriyama M, Wang MC, Papsidero LD , et al. Quantitation of prostate-specific antigen in serum by a sensitive enzyme immunoassay. Cancer Res 1980;40:4658–62.
109. Kuriyama M, Wang MC, Lee CI, et al. Use of human prostate-specific antigen in monitoring prostate cancer. Cancer Res 1981;41:3874–6.
110. Engvall E, Perlman P. Enzyme-linked immunosorbent assay (ELISA). Quantitative assay of immunoglobulin G. Immunochemistry 1971;8:871–4.
111. Matsudaira P. Sequence from picomole quantities of proteins electroblotted onto polyvinylidene difluoride membranes. J Biol Chem 1987;262:10035–8.
112. Doolittle RF, Hunkapiller MW, Hood LE, et al. Simian sarcoma virus onc gene, v-sis, is derived from the gene (or genes) encoding a platelet-derived growth factor. Science 1983;221:275–7.
113. Waterfield MD, Scrace GT, Whittle N, et al. Platelet-derived growth factor is structurally related to the putative transforming protein p28sis of simian sarcoma virus. Nature 1983;304:35–9.
114. Wilm M, Shevchenko A, Houthaeve T, et al. Femtomole sequencing of proteins from polyacrylamide gels by nano-electrospray mass spectrometry. Nature 1996;379:466–9.
115. Shevchenko A, Chernushevich I, Wilm M, Mann M. De novo peptide sequencing by nanoelectrospray tandem mass spectrometry using triple quadrupole and quadrupole/time-of-flight instruments. Methods Mol Biol 2000;146:1–16.
116. Mann M, Hendrickson RC, Pandey A. Analysis of proteins and proteomes by mass spectrometry. Annu Rev Biochem 2001;70:437–73.
117. Goeddel DV, Yelverton E, Ullrich A, et al. Human leukocyte interferon produced by *E. coli* is biologically active. Nature 1980;287:411–6.
118. Derynck R, Remaut E, Saman E, et al. Expression of human fibroblast interferon gene in *Escherichia coli*. Nature 1980;287:193–7.
119. Nagata S, Taira H, Hall A, et al. Synthesis in *E. coli* of a polypeptide with human leukocyte interferon activity. Nature 1980;284:316–20.
120. Kaufman RJ, Murtha P, Davies MV. Translational efficiency of polycistronic mRNAs and their utilization to express heterologous genes in mammalian cells. EMBO J 1987;6:187–93.
121. Ailor E, Betenbaugh, MJ. Modifying secretion and post-translational processing in insect cells. Curr Opin Biotechnol 1999;10:142–5.
122. Sudbery PE. The expression of recombinant proteins in yeasts. Curr Opin Biotechnol 1996;7:517–24.
123. Xia Y, Yu H, Jansen R, et al. Analyzing cellular biochemistry in terms of molecular networks. Annu Rev Biochem 2004;73:1051–87.
124. Fromont-Racine M, Rain JC, Legrain P. Toward a functional analysis of the yeast genome through exhaustive two-hybrid screens. Nat Genet 1997;16:277–82.
125. Uetz P, Giot L, Cagney G, et al. A comprehensive analysis of protein-protein interactions in *Saccharomyces cerevisiae*. Nature 2000;403:623–7.
126. Ito T, Chiba T, Yoshida M. Exploring the protein interactome using comprehensive two-hybrid projects. Trends Biotechnol 2001;19:S23–7.
127. Hansen K, Khanna C. Spontaneous and genetically engineered animal models; use in preclinical cancer drug development. Eur J Cancer 2004;40:858–80.
128. Nagy A, Gertsensenstein M, Vintersten K, Behringer R. Manipulating the mouse embryo: a laboratory manual. Cold Spring Harbor (NY): Cold Spring Harbor Laboratory Press; 2002.
129. Giuriato S, Rabin K, Fan AC, et al. Conditional animal models: a strategy to define when oncogenes will be effective targets to treat cancer. Semin Cancer Biol 2004;14:3–11.
130. Albanese C, Hulit J, Sakamaki T, Pestell RG. Recent advances in inducible expression in transgenic mice. Semin Cell Dev Biol 2002;13:129–41.
131. Tuveson DA, Jacks T. Technologically advanced cancer modeling in mice. Curr Opin Genet Dev 2002;12:105–10.
132. Van Dyke T, Jacks T. Cancer modeling in the modern era: progress and challenges. Cell 2002;108:135–44.

3

Cell Proliferation and Differentiation

Michael Andreeff, MD, PhD
David W. Goodrich, PhD
H. Phillip Koeffler, MD

The biology of cell division, differentiation, and apoptosis is exceedingly similar in both normal and cancer cells. The cancer cell differs from its normal counterpart in that it is aberrantly regulated. Cancer cells generally contain the full complement of biomolecules that are necessary for survival, proliferation, differentiation, cell death, and expression of many cell-type-specific functions. Failure to regulate these functions properly, however, results in an altered phenotype and cancer.

Four cellular functions tend to be inappropriately regulated in a neoplasm. First, the normal constraints on cellular proliferation are ineffective. Second, the differentiation program can be distorted. The tumor cells may be blocked at a particular stage of differentiation, or they may differentiate into an inappropriate or abnormal cell type. Third, chromosomal and genetic organization may be destabilized such that variant cells arise with high frequency. Some variants may have increased motility or enzyme production that permits invasion and metastases. Finally, the tightly regulated cell death program (apoptosis) may be dysregulated.[1]

To comprehend the biology of cancer, it is necessary to understand how these functions are controlled in normal cells and how they become uncontrolled in cancer cells. This chapter focuses on the biology of cell proliferation and differentiation and how these functions are linked in the development of neoplasia. Pathways describing the regulation of apoptosis are discussed in Chapter 4.

PROLIFERATION

Tumor Growth and Cell Proliferation In Vivo Fundamentally, cancer is a disease of abnormally excessive cell proliferation. It is the increase in tumor cell number, and thus tumor burden that ultimately accounts for the adverse effects on the host. Indeed, the goal of most current cancer therapy is to reduce the number of tumor cells and to prevent their further accumulation. To better accomplish this goal, a more complete description of the unique characteristics of tumor cell proliferation is required. This task is made difficult by the fact that the mechanisms that underlie tumor and normal cell proliferation are very similar. In this section, we will review current understanding of the complex molecular mechanisms involved in the regulation of cell proliferation with particular emphasis on the aberrations in this system that occur in malignant cells.

One hallmark feature of cancer is that most are genetically clonal, suggesting they arise from the progeny of a single cell. In cancers where preneoplastic lesions can be identified, however, the preneoplastic cells are likely to be genetically distinct from the overtly neoplastic cells. These observations suggest a model for the genesis of cancer through continual genetic evolution of mutant cells by a process of natural selection. Genetically abnormal cells are generated as a result of environmental insult or normal errors in replication. Some small fraction of these cells escapes normal controls on cell proliferation and increases their number. As this pool of mutant cells proliferates, additional mutant variants are continuously generated. If the result of these additional mutations provides a selective growth advantage, then the mutant variant will increase its relative number. Through multiple rounds of proliferation, mutation, and selection, a neoplastic variant evolves to cause cancer (Figure 3-1). The model predicts that two parameters will critically affect the rate of this clonal evolution, the mutation rate, and the rate of proliferation. It follows that mutations that increase the rates of proliferation or mutation rate will increase the rate of neoplastic transformation. Such mutations are, therefore, more likely to be detected in cancer cells than other types of mutations. Further, if such a mutation is inherited, the incidence of cancer within such a family is expected to be significantly higher than normal. As we shall discuss below, both of these predictions are generally confirmed by available observations.

A key assumption of this model is that the genetic potential to form cancer cells exists within the deoxyribonucleic acid (DNA) of normal cells. This assumption has been validated upon the discovery that the cancer genes of acutely transforming retroviruses are captured from the genomes of their hosts. Previously, it had been assumed that cancer genes evolved de novo in viruses. In retrospect, that normal cells have the genetic potential to evolve into cancer cells is logical based on bio-

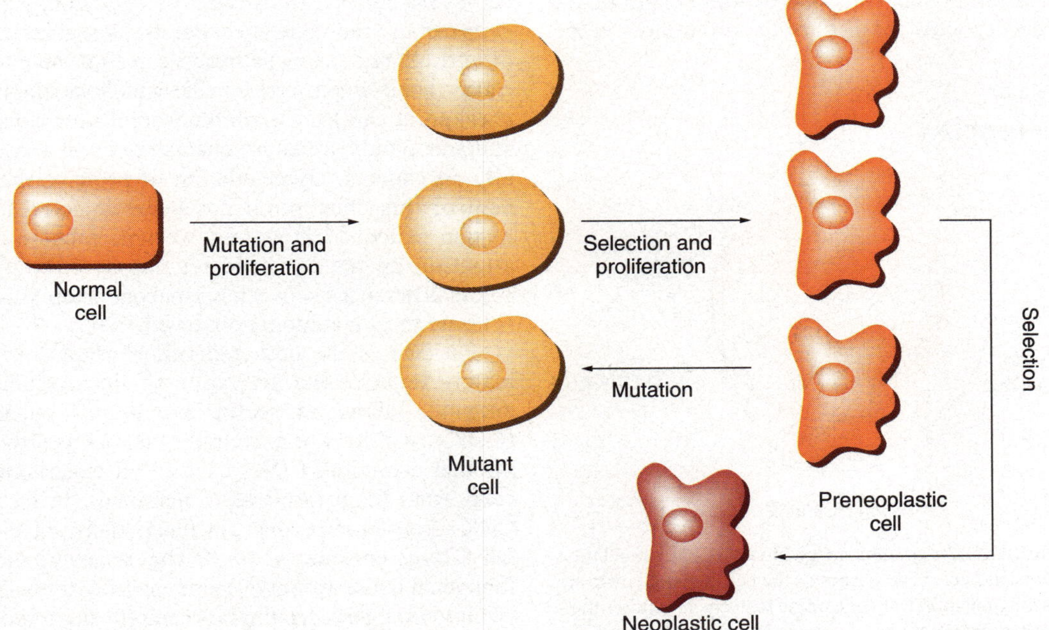

Figure 3-1 Evolution of neoplastic cells. Genetic analysis of cancer suggests that neoplastic cells arise through an accumulation of mutations. The genetic clonality observed in most cancers suggests they arise from a single neoplastic cell that has undergone multiple rounds of mutation, proliferation, and selection. This hypothesis is summarized in the diagram above. Normal cells undergo random mutagenesis generating several distinct variants. Variants that survive undergo additional rounds of mutation and selection. Subvariants escaping normal growth controls can expand to form preneoplastic lesions. Additional mutations within the population of preneoplastic cells gives rise to clonal variants that proliferate into cancer.

logical arguments. For example, it is clear that human cells possess an intrinsic proliferative capacity that is in vast excess of that required to meet the needs of normal growth and development. Normal human cells can divide as often as once or twice a day in vivo. A cell dividing at this rate would generate a cell number equal to the total number of cells in an adult human in less than 2 months. We have evolved highly regulated mechanisms to restrain this proliferative capacity to appropriate times and places. It is this excess proliferative capacity that provides the genetic foundation on which a cancer cell is built. The key in understanding tumor cell proliferation, then, is to characterize the mechanisms that are normally used to restrain the proliferation of normal cells and to understand how they fail during cancer.

Cell-Cycle Control The cell division cycle can be divided into two functional phases, S and M phases, and two preparatory phases, G1 and G2 (Figure 3-2). S phase is defined as the phase in which the DNA is replicated. The time it takes a typical human cell to complete S phase is about 8 hours and is invariant under normal circumstances. Fully replicated chromosomes are segregated to each of the two daughter nuclei by the process of mitosis during M phase. The length of M phase is about 1 hour and is also normally invariant. G1 phase precedes S phase, whereas G2 phase precedes M phase. G1 and G2 phases are required for the synthesis of cellular constituents needed to support the following phase and ultimately to complete cell division. In mammalian cells, the length of G2 phase is about 2 hours. The length of G1 phase is highly variable and can range from about 6 hours to several days or longer. In human cells, the varying length of G1 phase accounts for most of the differences in the

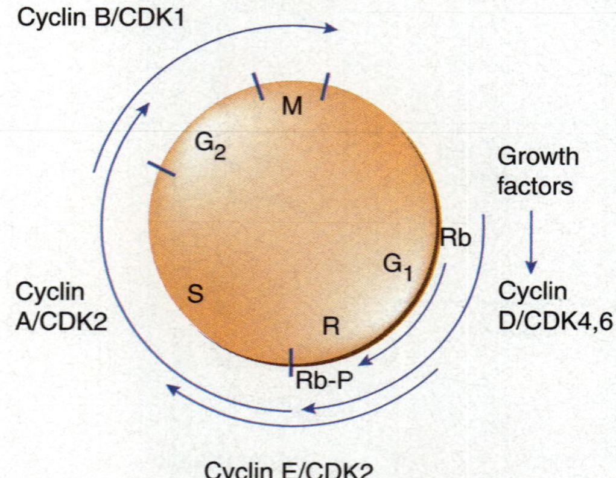

Figure 3-2 Cyclin-dependent kinase (CDK) regulation of the cell cycle. The phases of the cell division cycle are shown. Transition from one phase to the next requires transit of a checkpoint like the restriction point (R) during the G0/G1 to S-phase transition. Transit of the checkpoint is mediated by activation of cyclin-dependent kinases. The timing of activation of individual CDKs during the cell cycle is shown by the respective arrows. Activation of cyclin D/CDK4,6 is coincident with phosphorylation of the retinoblastoma tumor suppressor protein (Rb) and transit of the R checkpoint.

time it takes to execute a cell division cycle between different cell types or between cells growing under different conditions. Cells that persist in G1 phase for extended periods of time enter a distinct state called G0. Although such cells are metabolically active, they are not actively proliferating. Cells in G0 can reenter the cell cycle or they can remain in G0 indefinitely.[2]

A successful cell division cycle requires the orderly and unidirectional transition from one cell-cycle phase to the next. Certain events must be completed before others are begun. For example, beginning mitosis before the completion of DNA replication would obviously be deleterious to the cell. In theory, the ordering of cell-cycle events may be accomplished in a manner analogous to the substrate-product relationship of a metabolic pathway. The product of one reaction serves as the substrate for the next. The rate of the first reaction, therefore, limits that of the next. Hence, regulation of the system is inherent in the biochemical events of the process itself. The prevailing view, however, is that the timing and ordering of cell-cycle transitions is dependent on separate positive and negative regulatory circuits.[3] The regulatory circuits enforce a series of checkpoints, allowing passage only after completion of critical cell-cycle events. Two classes of regulatory circuits exist, intrinsic and extrinsic. Intrinsic regulatory pathways are responsible for the precise ordering of cell-cycle events. Since the length of S, G2, and M phases in mammalian cells is relatively invariant, the transitions between these phases are controlled predominantly by intrinsic regulatory pathways. Extrinsic regulatory pathways function in response to environmental conditions or in response to detected cell-cycle defects. Both types of regulatory circuits can use the same checkpoints. Deregulation of intrinsic regulatory pathways can contribute to cancer. For example, errors in the spindle-assembly checkpoint can lead to chromosomal imbalance and aneuploidy, a feature characteristic of virtually all cancers. Dysregulation of proteins that control this checkpoint has been detected in human cancer.[4,5] However, we will focus our attention on the extrinsic regulatory circuits, where differences between normal and neoplastic cells are most commonly observed.

Passage of the cell-cycle checkpoints ultimately requires the activation of intracellular enzymes known as cyclin-dependent kinases (CDKs). CDKs are extremely well conserved through evolution. CDKs exist in all eukaryotic cells, from fungi to plants to mammals. In fact, CDKs from human cells can functionally substitute for the enzymes in yeast. The structural and functional conservation of these enzymes through evolution suggests that they are centrally important for the cell cycle in all eukaryotic cells. The requirement for these enzymes for cell-cycle transitions has been amply documented, particularly in organisms like yeast that are amenable to genetic manipulation.[3] Since activation of CDKs is the central event in cell-cycle transitions, it is not surprising that their activity is exquisitely regulated at

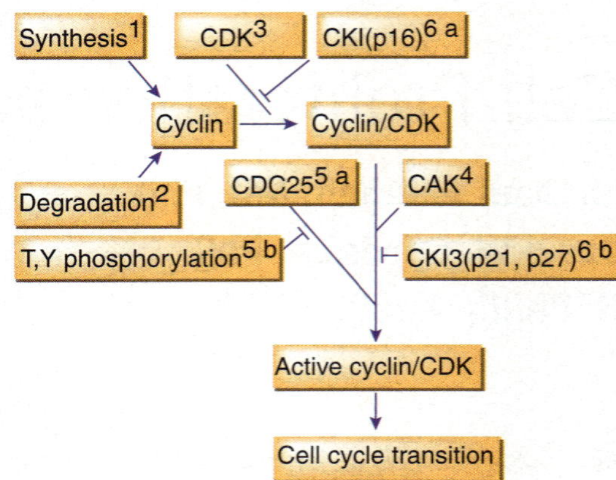

Figure 3-3 Regulation of cyclin-dependent kinases (CDKs). The activity of CDKs is controlled at several levels. (1) Synthesis of cyclins occurs at specific times during the cell cycle or in response to certain growth factors (see Figure 3-2). (2) Degradation of cyclins occurs at specific times during the cell cycle and is mediated by ubiquitin-dependent proteolysis. (3) The cyclin subunit must complex with the catalytic CDK subunit. (4) The assembled complex requires phosphorylation by CDK-activating kinase (CAK) to reach maximum specific activity. (5) The assembled complex is inactivated by phosphorylation on specific residues in the ATP binding sight of the enzyme (5b) and can be reactivated by dephosphorylation of these residues by cdc25 (5a). (6) CKIs can inhibit assembly of the cyclin/CDK complex (6a) or the activation of the assembled complex (6b).

several levels (Figure 3-3).[6–8] The active CDK holoenzyme is composed of a catalytic subunit and the cyclin regulatory subunit. Each cyclin is synthesized at a particular stage of the cell cycle. For example, cyclin E is synthesized in late G1 and early S phase, cyclin A is synthesized during S and G2 phases, and cyclin B is synthesized in G2 and M phases. Therefore, a given catalytic subunit cannot become active until an appropriate cyclin is synthesized. Upon synthesis, a cyclin can assemble with an appropriate catalytic subunit. However, this complex requires phosphorylation on threonine by another regulated kinase, the CDK-activating kinase or CAK. CAK is itself a CDK composed of cyclin H and CDK7 proteins. Hence the levels of CAK influence the activity of assembled CDKs. Another level of regulation is deactivation of the CDK by phosphorylation of its ATP binding site by yet another regulated kinase activity. This kinase activity is unusual in that it has dual specificity for both tyrosine and threonine. A CDK deactivated by phosphorylation of its ATP binding site can be reactivated by a dual specificity phosphatase of the Cdc25 family. In fact, dephosphorylation by these phosphatases may be the rate-limiting step in triggering cell-cycle transitions. Another level of regulation is the presence of a diverse family of proteins known as cyclin-dependent kinase inhibitors, or CKIs, that can block activation of CDKs. Two distinct classes of CKIs have been described. One class inhibits multiple CDKs and includes p21CIP1, p27KIP1, and p57KIP2. The other class specifically inhibits cyclin D/CDK4 or 6 CDKs and includes p16INK4, p15INK4B, p18INK4C, and p19INK4D. The synthesis, degradation, and activity of these CKIs are regulated in response to both mitogenic and antimitogenic signals. For example, cell-cycle regulation by cell-cell contact or transforming growth factor-β (TGF-β) is mediated by p27KIP1.[9,10] Once activated, the CDKs that drive the transition into a particular cell-cycle phase often need to be deactivated before completion of that phase and transition to the ensuing phase. For example, the CDKs required for initiation of mitosis also prevent exit from mitosis and into G1 phase. The final level of CDK regulation involves their specific degradation in precise order. It is now generally understood that ubiquitin-mediated proteolysis is responsible for this regulation as well as the regulation of a host of other cell-cycle regulators.[11,12] Hence, synthesis, post-translational modification, and programmed degradation all contribute to the regulation of CDKs.

The G0 to S Checkpoints As discussed above, the time it takes to progress through the S, G2, and M phases of the cell cycle is relatively invariant. The length of G1 phase on the other hand is variable. In addition, cells can exit the cell cycle for extended periods of time and mammalian cells do so during the G1 phase of the cell cycle. Cells that have exited the cell cycle are said to be in a G0 state, or "quiescent." Most cells in adults are in G0. This absence from the cell division cycle can be temporary or permanent as in terminally differentiated cells, for example. Cells in G0 can be very active functionally and metabolically, and proliferation of G0 cells can be initiated by changes in cell density, the presence of mitogens or growth factors, or the supply of nutrients. These cells then reenter the cell cycle, beginning a sequence of events that culminates in cell division. Hence, the G0/G1 to S-phase transition is highly regulated, and the result of this regulation, by and large, determines the growth fraction of a population of cells.

The transition from G0/G1 to S phase is regulated by two major checkpoints called competence and the restriction point (R). These checkpoints are located approximately 12 and 2 hours before the start of the S phase, respectively. At least three growth factors, provided in serum, are required sequentially to transit these checkpoints following resumption of proliferation of fibroblasts in vitro: platelet-derived growth factor (PDGF), epidermal growth factor (EGF), and insulin-like growth factor (IGF-1). As mentioned above, extracellular TGF-β has the opposite effect. It inhibits the growth of various epithelial cells by modulating expression of CKIs. Paracrine production of TGF-β could limit growth of both normal and cancer cells, and experimental models suggest that it may play a role in the regression of breast cancers in response to hormonal or drug therapies.[13,14] Once the R point has been passed, the cell is committed to a round of cell division. The cell now completes S, G2, and M phases without the need for additional growth factors or even additional protein synthesis. Once initiated, the cell cycle is not free running; the competence and restriction checkpoints must be passed in each subsequent G1 phase, thus requiring the continued presence of growth factors. The switching of cells back and forth between quiescence and cycling depends on extracellular conditions and is regulated differently in normal and tumor cells.

Growth factor receptors are complex, large proteins that span the plasma membrane. They have a specific domain that recognizes the growth factor on the outside of the cell, and their cytoplasmic portion may have an enzymatic function, such as a protein tyrosine kinase. Binding of a growth factor or ligand to its receptor can induce transmission of a signal to the cytoplasm through activation of the kinase.[15,16] The next step is a transduction of the cytoplasmic signal to the cell nucleus. This is accomplished by a heterogeneous group of molecules known as second messengers and includes various proteins that are phosphorylated by kinases, small molecules such as inositol phosphates and cyclic AMP, and ions, including Ca++, H+, and Zn++. Within the nucleus, genes are then activated in response to these second messengers. As an illustration of this general scheme, upon binding of EGF to the extracellular domains of its receptor, autophosphorylation occurs in the intracellular domain of the protein. This phosphorylated domain facilitates the formation of a protein complex containing Grb2 and Sos. This complex activates the Ras protein by catalyzing exchange of Ras-bound GDP for GTP. The GTP-bound form of Ras activates the c-Raf kinase. This kinase then triggers a phosphorylation cascade, ultimately activating mitogen-activated protein kinase. This kinase may phosphorylate and regulate transcription factors such as Jun, Fos, and Myc.

A variety of proteins are produced during G1 after cells leave quiescence. Some are enzymes that expand metabolic functions lost by G0 cells, such as those providing energy, and more ribosomes are made for rapid protein synthesis. Others have so-called housekeeping functions that keep both quiescent and growing cells in metabolic balance. Only a few proteins appear to be key regulatory molecules. For example, enzymes are required for the synthesis of isoprenoids, which are necessary for activity of the Ras oncogene, and for the synthesis of polyamines, which have many functions, including ionic binding to nucleic acids. The Ras oncogene product is synthesized as a precursor protein that requires post-translational processing to become biologically active and capable of transforming mammalian cells. Farnesylation appears to be a critical modification of the Ras protein, and drugs that inhibit farnesyl-protein transferase can block Ras-dependent transformation. These agents have been proposed as a potential new class of therapy for cancer.[17,18] Enzymes involved in the synthesis of DNA, such as thymidine kinase and DNA polymerase, as well as histones, are synthesized just prior to the S phase. These enzyme molecules relocate at the beginning of DNA synthesis, moving from the cytoplasm into the nucleus. A variety of experiments show that DNA is made by a high-molecular-weight, multienzyme complex.[19–21] This complex contains many enzymes known to be involved in the process of DNA replication, but its size and other features are still a matter of debate. After DNA synthesis has commenced, cell growth becomes relatively independent of external controls. The daughter cells, now in the G1 phase, will then either pass through another cycle or arrest in a quiescent G0 state, depending, once more, on external conditions. If these conditions are not adequate, the cell will become arrested before it reinitiates DNA synthesis.

How is reentry into the cell cycle from G0 ultimately controlled? Like other cell-cycle transitions, activation of CDKs are required. G0 cells are devoid of significant CDK activity. In the presence of mitogenic growth factors, expression of D-type cyclins (cyclins D1, D2, and D3) is stimulated and continues throughout G1 phase as long as the growth factors are present.[22] D-type cyclins complex with either CDK4 or CDK6 catalytic subunits to form a holoenzyme modified by CAK. All of the relevant substrates for cyclin D/CDK4 or 6 have probably not been enumerated. However, one important substrate is likely the retinoblastoma tumor-suppressor protein (Rb) and the other members of its gene family p107 and p130. Rb is constitutively expressed and constrains cells from progressing through the G1 phase of the cell cycle (Figure 3-4).[23] Rb complexes with many cellular proteins including the E2F transcription factors. When in complex with E2F, Rb represses transcription from E2F-dependent promoters. Upon phosphorylation by cyclin D/CDK4 or 6,[24] Rb loses its ability to restrain the cell cycle.[25] This response is presumably because it can no longer complex with E2F and/or repress E2F-dependent transcription.[26] The E2F family contains at least six members (E2F-1 through E2F-6).[27] The E2F proteins function as transcriptional activators when in heterodimeric complex with one of the E2F-related proteins DP-1, 2, or 3. The heterodimeric complex binds a specific DNA sequence and activates transcription from the promoters of many genes important for S phase, including dihydrofolate reductase, DNA polymerase α, and thymidine kinase.[28] Perhaps most importantly, E2F influences the expression of cyclin E.[29] In fact, of many E2F-dependent genes, cyclin E is the only one deregulated upon loss of Rb in normal cells.[30] Cyclin E expression begins in late G1 phase and complexes with CDK2. Cyclin E/CDK2 activity is necessary and sufficient for the start of S phase.[31] Forced expression of cyclin E/CDK2 activity can trigger the start of S phase in the absence of Rb phosphorylation and derepression of other E2F-dependent genes, suggesting that cyclin E is a primary target for regulation by cyclin D/CDK4 or 6, Rb, and E2F.[32,33]

DNA Damage-Induced Checkpoints Upon nuclear DNA damage, normal cells initiate a response that includes cell-cycle checkpoint activation, apoptotic cell death, and transcriptional

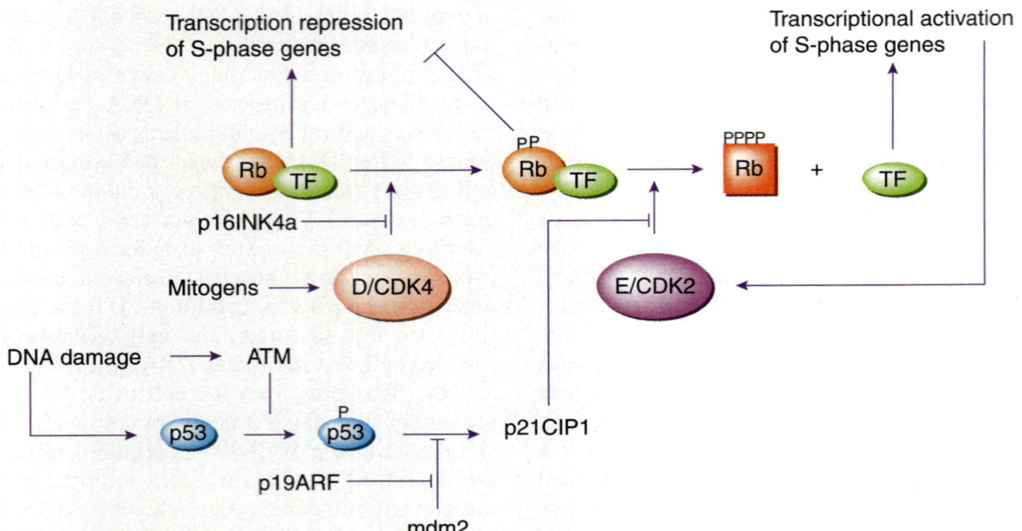

Figure 3-4 G1 phase checkpoints mediated by TP53 and Rb. The figure depicts how Rb can enforce a G1 checkpoint by association with transcription factors (TF) and repression of genes containing the relevant TF DNA binding site. The genes regulated by Rb/TF complexes include cyclin-dependent kinases (CDKs) thereby comprising a positive feedback loop. This feedback is damped by the presence of CKIs like p16INK4a and p21CIP1. CKI expression can be modulated by the TP53 DNA damage response pathway as indicated. Phosphorylation status of proteins is indicated by "P" where relevant.

induction of genes involved in DNA repair. Induction of apoptosis is an important response to DNA damage and is discussed in detail in a separate chapter. Normal cells in G1 phase prior to the R point will arrest in G1 phase upon sensing DNA damage. This arrest is presumably induced to prevent the replication of damaged DNA. Replication of damaged DNA can result in the incorporation of heritable genetic mutations. If cells are past the R point or within S phase, DNA replication is slowed, again to allow time for DNA repair. If cells sense DNA damage while in G2 phase, a G2 cell-cycle arrest will occur. Different types of DNA damage can interfere with normal mitosis, resulting in heritable genetic mutations or cell death.

The tumor-suppressor genes *ATM* and *TP53* play an important part in responses to damaged DNA.[34,35] For example, cells containing mutations in *TP53* fail to arrest in G1 or undergo apoptosis efficiently upon irradiation. Cells containing mutations in *ATM* are also deficient for cell-cycle arrest as well as some forms of DNA repair. The TP53 protein functions as a transcription factor by binding specific DNA sequences and regulating transcription from promoters containing those sequences. In normal cells, DNA damage induces an increase in TP53 levels by inhibiting the normal rapid turnover of the protein. The TP53 protein is normally targeted for ubiquitin-dependent proteolysis by association with the MDM2 protein. This association is inhibited by phosphorylation of TP53 on specific amino-terminal residues that is triggered by DNA damage.[36] Phosphorylation on these amino-terminal residues also facilitates dephosphorylation or acetylation of TP53 carboxy-terminal residues. These modifications increase the affinity of TP53 for its DNA binding site by distinct mechanisms[37,38] and, hence, increase its ability to activate transcription. The transcription of a number of genes can be affected by activation of TP53. However, the ability of TP53 to directly increase expression of p21CIP1 is probably important for TP53-dependent G1 cell-cycle arrest observed upon DNA damage. As discussed above, p21CIP1 is a CKI that can inhibit the activity of multiple CDKs, including cyclin D/CDK4 or 6 as well as cyclin E/CDK2. In summary, DNA damage generates a signal that can activate TP53 by post-translational modification. Increased TP53 activity up-regulates p21CIP1, which prevents activation of CDKs, required for the G1 to S transition (see Figure 3-4).

ATM is the gene whose mutation is responsible for ataxia telangiectasia. Immunodeficiency, progressive cerebellar ataxia, radiosensitivity, cell-cycle checkpoint defects, and cancer predisposition characterize this disease. *ATM* encodes a protein containing a phosphatidyl-inositol 3-kinase-like domain, implicating it in signal transduction. Like TP53 mutant cells, mutant ATM cells are defective in the G1/S checkpoint activated after radiation-induced DNA damage. This defect is attributable to the lack of TP53 activation that normally occurs, suggesting that ATM may participate in the same pathway as TP53. ATM protein, and the related ATR protein, can, in fact, associate with and phosphorylate TP53 at its amino-terminal sites.[39,40] The TP53-directed kinase activity of the ATM protein is itself activated by DNA damage. ATM protein, therefore, contributes to the activation and stabilization of TP53 by phosphorylating amino-terminal sites during the radiation-induced DNA damage response. ATM protein may play a role in sensing DNA damage and generating the DNA damage signal.

Environmental agents like radiation or DNA-damaging chemicals most commonly induce DNA damage. Rarely, DNA damage can be generated by mistakes in the normal execution of the cell cycle or as a consequence of normal metabolic activity through the generation of reactive oxygen species. However, a form of DNA damage eventually occurs in all normal cells as they suffer replicative senescence. Normal cells have a limited replicative lifespan both in vivo and in vitro; a cell can undergo only a finite number of cell divisions. This limit is thought to be imposed, at least in part, by levels of telomerase activity.[41] Telomerase is an enzymatic activity within cells that is required to maintain the integrity of DNA ends.[42] DNA polymerases involved in DNA replication synthesize DNA in the 5' to 3' direction and require a primer and template. The requirement for a primer ensures that some genetic information will be lost from the 5' end of DNA during each round of DNA replication. Telomerase adds DNA of a particular sequence to the ends of DNA without the need for a separate primer or template, thus protecting cells from loss of genetic information. Telomeric DNA also protects chromosomes from degradation or recombination. Without telomeric DNA, chromosomes become unstable. As normal cells become senescent, they lose telomerase activity and their cell division cycle is arrested. This cell-cycle arrest may be mediated by the DNA damage checkpoint since shortened telomeric DNA is associated with DNA strand breaks that may be sensed as damaged DNA. Consistent with this hypothesis, shortening of telomeric DNA triggers a TP53-dependent cell-cycle arrest by accumulation of single stranded DNA.[43] However, there is some controversy as to whether telomere shortening itself is a trigger for replicative senescence.[44]

Checkpoint Defects in Tumor Cells To maintain tissue homeostasis and to support normal development, each organ maintains tight controls over Tc, growth fraction, and cell loss. Physiologic stimuli can alter these parameters in normal tissues, leading to increased tissue growth, but this growth will cease when the stimulus is withdrawn or a new steady state is achieved. In contrast to normal cells, however, tumor cells continue to proliferate even in the absence of proliferative signals. Although tumor cells proliferate under inappropriate conditions, they do not necessarily proliferate faster than normal cells. In fact, some normal tissues grow faster than cancers under physiologic conditions (Table 3-1). Biopsy samples from normal, inflammatory, and neoplastic lesions of the lung, cervix, vocal cord, or pharynx have been analyzed for the rate of cell proliferation; these studies showed that benign inflammatory lesions can grow over 20 times faster than cancer in a discrete time and place.[45–47] Similarly, rapid proliferation of human lymphoid cells is induced by immunostimulants, and growth kinetics of these cells are similar to those observed in high-grade lymphomas.[48] So, it is not simply rapid growth at a single time and place that distinguishes neoplasia but rather growth that is not restrained to appropriate times and places.

Table 3-1 Growth Parameters of Human Neoplasms and Normal Tissues

Cell Type	Labeling Index (%)	Estimated Cell Doubling Time (d)
Normal bone marrow myeloblasts	32–75	0.7–1.1
Acute myeloid leukemia	8–25	0.5–8.0
Normal B-cell lymphocytes	0–1	14–21+
High-grade lymphoma	19–29	2–3
Normal intestinal crypts	12–18	1–2
Colon adenocarcinoma	3–35	1.6–5.0
Normal epithelium/pharynx	2–3	—
Squamous cell carcinoma of the nasopharynx	5–16	2–4
Normal epithelium/bronchus	—	9–10
Epidermoid carcinoma of the lung	5–8	8–10
Normal epithelium/cervix	4–8	—
Ovarian carcinoma	3–20	5–6
Benign mole of skin	0.3	—
Malignant melanoma of skin	12.8	—

It generally is believed that neoplastic cells multiply exponentially during the early phases of tumor cell growth. As the tumor mass increases, however, the rate of growth declines. Measuring tumor growth over time describes a curve with an exponential increase in the early period, then a flattening out of the growth rate over time (ie, Gompertzian curve).[49] Several mechanisms have been invoked to explain this change in growth rate with larger tumors: (1) decrease in the growth fraction; (2) increase in cell loss (ie, exfoliation, necrosis); (3) nutritional depletion of tumor cells resulting from outgrowth of available blood supply; or (4) lengthening of Tc. Experimental tumor models suggest that cell-cycle time changes only slightly when tumor growth decreases.[50] Under adverse conditions, tumor cells often leave the growth fraction and enter a nongrowing state (G0 or prolonged G1) (see Figure 3-1), although these same cells can reenter the division cycle when conditions improve or when stimulated by growth factors. Therefore, the mass doubling time of tumors is correlated with the growth fraction (Table 3-2).

The biochemistry of growth appears to be very similar qualitatively in tumor and normal cells.[51] Despite numerous efforts, universal differences in biochemical machinery have not yet been discovered between normal and tumor cells. The fundamental difference probably lies in a relaxation of the regulation of cell growth.[50,52] For example, normal cells generally are quiescent at physiologic levels of growth factors, whereas related tumor cells are able to proliferate under these conditions. In some experimental models, tumor cells proliferate in the absence of or at very low levels of growth factors. Further, fibroblast-derived tumor cells are less sensitive than normal cells to the presence of other cells in their immediate vicinity. Normal cells typically cease proliferation when the in vitro culture becomes confluent, but tumor cells can reach severalfold higher densities in culture. Also, cells of normal solid tissue lie on a secreted extracellular matrix (ECM) that is composed of various proteins that stimulate cell growth.[53] Tumor cells often are partly or completely independent of ECM for optimal growth, and they may secrete little matrix material.[54]

Table 3-2 Correlation between Mass Doubling Time and Growth Fraction

Cell Type	Growth Fraction (%)	Doubling Time (d)
Experimental tumors		
L1210 (mouse)	86	0.5
B 16 (mouse)	55	1.9
LL (mouse)	38	2.9
DMBA (rat)	10	7.4
Human tumors		
Embryonal carcinoma	90	27
Lymphoma (high grade)	90	29
Squamous cell carcinoma	25	58
Adenocarcinoma	6	83

What molecular defects bring about the relaxed growth requirements in neoplastic cells? Defects can occur at several levels. For example, limiting growth factors may not be needed because tumor cells inappropriately produce their own (ie, an autocrine mechanism). Alternatively, receptors may be produced in excess, as is the case for EGF receptors in numerous clinical tumors, leading to adequate stimulation at the low growth factor concentrations found in vivo. Moreover, mutations that alter intracellular signaling mechanisms may bypass growth factor dependence. Mutated forms of proto-oncogenes and inactivated tumor-suppressor genes can activate growth in these ways. We will focus here on defects that occur in cell-cycle regulatory proteins that enforce the checkpoints discussed above.

Like normal cells, the transit of cell-cycle checkpoints in cancer cells ultimately requires the activation of CDKs. Due to the complexity of CDK regulation, defects leading to inappropriate activation of CDKs can occur at several levels. The overexpression of cyclin D1 has been detected in many human cancers due to gene amplification or translocation of the cyclin D1 gene.[55] The cyclin D1 gene is located on chromosome 11q13. This chromosomal region is amplified in a wide variety of human cancers including small-cell lung tumors (10%), primary breast cancers (13%), bladder cancer (15%), esophageal carcinoma (34%), and squamous cell carcinoma of the head and neck (43%) among others.[56] Of course, other potential oncogenes could be contained within the amplified region. However, cyclin D1 is likely important since its expression is consistently elevated in these tumors. Cyclin D1 overexpression can also be observed in tumors, such as sarcomas, colorectal tumors, and melanomas, without amplification of the gene. In some cases, cyclin D1 expression is activated by chromosomal translocation. In parathyroid adenoma, Motokura and colleagues[57] have identified cyclin D1 as being translocated to the parathyroid hormone gene, thereby deregulating cyclin D1 expression. Translocation of the cyclin D1 gene with immunoglobulin heavy chain gene transcriptional control elements has also been observed in B-cell lineage mantle cell lymphomas. Cyclin D1 is a growth factor responsive cyclin that plays an important role in regulating the G0/S checkpoint. Deregulated expression of cyclin D1 could inappropriately increase cyclin D1/CDK4 activity and drive transit of the checkpoint even in the absence of appropriate growth factors. Direct evidence that forced expression of cyclin D1 can facilitate tumorigenesis has been obtained from transgenic mice in which overexpression of cyclin D1 has been targeted to the mammary epithelium. These mice develop ductal hyperproliferation and eventual mammary tumor formation.[58]

CDK activation can also be accomplished by inactivation of CKIs. Genetic mutation of CKI genes has also been observed frequently in human cancer. In this scenario, loss of a CKI relieves one constraint on the activation of CDKs and provides a proliferation stimulus. In particular, the INK4 locus within chromosomal region 9p21 is one of the most frequently mutated areas in human cancers.[59] This locus is also frequently methylated in some tumor types including bladder cancer and leukemia. Extensive methylation of DNA prevents efficient transcription of genes within the methylated region, thus silencing gene expression. Three proteins are encoded by the INK4 locus, including the CKIs, p16INK4a, and p15INK4b, as well as p19ARF (see below). It is likely that p16INK4a is a bona fide tumor-suppressor gene since many of the mutations detected in tumors specifically target expression of this protein, and because germline mutations that specifically map to p16INK4a have been detected in kindreds with familial melanoma and pancreatic adenocarcinoma. In addition, mutations in CDK4 that prevent binding with p16INK4a, thus relieving it of p16-mediated inhibition, have also been found in melanoma-prone families. Loss of p16INK4a may facilitate activation of cyclin D1/CDK4 or 6, which is likely to affect regulation of the G0/S checkpoint. Mutation of other CKIs in human cancer is rare, suggesting that they may be required for execution of the cell cycle. However, expression of p27KIP1 is inversely correlated with clinical outcome in a limited number of cancers, including melanoma and carcinoma of the oral cavity.

CDK activation also requires dephosphorylation of inhibitory threonine/tyrosine phosphory-

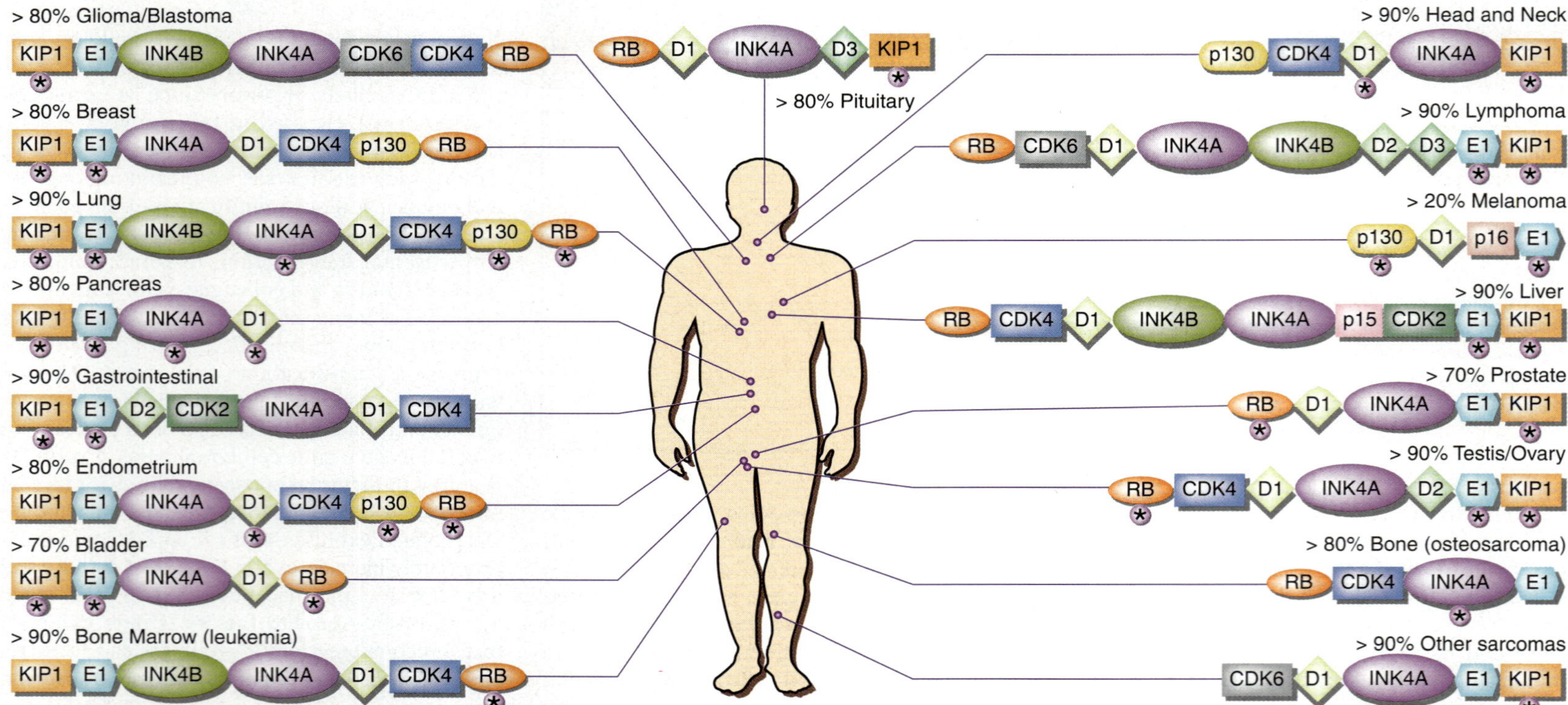

Figure 3-5 Deregulation of the Rb growth control pathway in human cancer. The figure depicts several clinically important human cancers and the genetic or epigenetic alterations of the Rb growth control pathway that have been identified in such cancers. Members of this pathway include CKIs, cyclins, cyclin-dependent kinases (CDKs), and the Rb family of proteins. The percentages given indicate fraction of cases where alteration in any of the indicated pathway components has been detected. Alterations with a demonstrated correlation with prognosis are indicated with an asterisk. Adapted from Malumbres and Barbacid, 2001.

lation sites by the Cdc25 family of dual specificity phosphatases. In vitro evidence exists that the Cdc25 family members are potential oncogenes.[60] Forced expression of Cdc25 can cooperate with Ha-Ras or loss of Rb to induce oncogenic transformation of primary cells. Overexpression of Cdc25 has also been detected in some primary human tumors. Cdc25A may be a direct transcriptional target for the *myc* oncogenes.[61] Inappropriately high Cdc25 levels may provide an oncogenic stimulus by inappropriately activating CDK activity.

One of the most important genes involved in human cancer is the Rb tumor-suppressor gene. An interesting feature of retinoblastoma is that close to 40% of cases are hereditary, and susceptibility to retinoblastoma is inherited as a simple autosomal dominant trait with high (90%) penetrance. The simple genetics of retinoblastoma has provided the means to molecularly clone the gene responsible; mutational inactivation of both alleles of Rb is necessary and sufficient for retinoblastoma.[62] Mutation of Rb is observed at high frequency in osteosarcoma and soft-tissue sarcoma as well. Rb mutations can also be detected in a wide variety of clinically important cancers including carcinoma of the breast, prostate, bladder, kidney, liver, pancreas, cervix, and lung, as well as leukemia. Further, expression of wild-type Rb cDNA in cancer cells can inhibit their tumorigenicity.[63] As mentioned above, cyclin D/CDK4 or 6 phosphorylation, which, in turn, is regulated by p16INK4a, inhibits Rb function. This finding suggests that these three proteins function in the same biochemical pathway (see Figure 3-4). Support for this functional interrelation comes from the observation that deregulation of any one of these proteins greatly decreases the likelihood of detecting defects in the other proteins. For example, tumor cells that lose p16INK4a or overexpress cyclin D1 generally retain wild-type Rb. Cells lacking wild-type Rb typically express normal levels of cyclin D1 and p16INK4a. In addition, induction of cell-cycle arrest by forced expression of p16INK4a only occurs in cells that contain functional Rb. If mutations in any of the members of this pathway are considered, disruption of this p16INK4a/cyclin D1/CDK4 or 6/Rb pathway may occur in most human cancers (Figure 3-5).[62] Since this pathway is important for regulation of the G0 to S-phase transition, it has a major influence on the growth fraction of normal tissues.

The *TP53* gene is the most frequently mutated gene in human cancer.[64] Germ line *TP53* mutation is involved in the cancer-prone Li-Fraumeni syndrome.[65] Mice lacking *TP53* because of genetically engineered disruption are also cancer prone. Wild-type TP53 is critically important for operation of the DNA damage-induced checkpoint (see above). Upon sensing DNA damage, TP53 is activated, resulting in either G1 cell-cycle arrest or apoptosis. These responses either allow time for the cell to repair the damage or to rid the body of cells with damaged DNA. Loss of TP53 function, therefore, decreases genomic stability. Loss of genomic stability can increase the accumulation of additional genetic mutations required for neoplastic transformation. The MDM2 gene encodes a protein that binds TP53 and targets it destruction by the ubiquitin-proteosome pathway. Too much MDM2 protein may be analogous to TP53 inactivation since any TP53 synthesized would be rapidly degraded. MDM2 was originally identified as an oncogene amplified in a spontaneously transformed mouse cell line. Overexpression of MDM2 mediated by gene amplification can also be detected in human cancer, particularly sarcoma.[66] Interestingly, the p19ARF protein encoded by the INK4a locus also regulates TP53 function.[67] The p19ARF protein can bind MDM2 and prevent MDM2 from targeting TP53 for degradation. Consistent with the ability of p19ARF to activate TP53, forced expression of p19ARF can cause a TP53-dependent cell-cycle arrest. As discussed previously, mutations of the INK4 locus that inactivate p19ARF, as well as p16INK4a, are commonly observed in human cancer. Inactivation of p19ARF may contribute to tumorigenesis since MDM2-mediated degradation of TP53 would be unimpeded. The functional interrelation between p19ARF, MDM2, and TP53 defines another cell-cycle checkpoint control pathway (see Figure 3-5). Deficiencies in this pathway also play a vital role in neoplastic transformation.

Although cancer cells use the same cell-cycle machinery as normal cells, the cell-cycle checkpoints in tumor cells are relaxed. Of the scores of proto-oncogenes and tumor-suppressor genes that have been identified to date, most function in signal transduction pathways that mediate mitogenic stimulation. These signal transduction pathways eventually converge on the cell-cycle checkpoint that controls the G0/G1 to S-phase transition and activate appropriate CDKs. Influencing the transit of this checkpoint has a major influence on the proliferation of normal and tumor cells by affecting both Tc and growth fraction. Increased proliferation, in turn, increases the rate of evolution toward neoplasia (see above). Despite the number and variety of genes involved in signal transduction, relaxation of the G1/G0 to S checkpoint controls in tumor cells is mediated, for the most part, by disruption of two pathways, the Rb and TP53 growth control pathways. These two genes, individually, are the most frequently mutated in human cancer cells. Disruption of the Rb or TP53 pathways probably occurs in virtually every human cancer.

Insights into the mechanisms of cell-cycle control have provided entirely new approaches to cancer therapy. Kinase inhibitors such as flavopiridol, UCN-01, proteosome inhibitors (eg, bortezomib), and others are being tested in clinical trials and are quickly becoming part of the therapeutic armamentarium.[68–70] TP53, which can be inactivated in cancer by complex formation of overexpressed MDM2, can be reactivated by Nutlins,[71,72] which disrupt MDM2/TP53, resulting in apoptosis.[73]

APOPTOSIS AND PROLIFERATION

There are at least two interesting connections between regulators of cell proliferation and apoptosis. One is based on the observation that many slowly proliferating tumors, such as chronic lymphocytic leukemias,[74] low-grade non-Hodgkin's lymphomas,[75] multiple myelomas,[76] and colon[77] and breast cancers,[78] overexpress the antiapoptotic proteins Bcl-2 and Bcl-X_L. The interaction between Bcl-2 and calcineurin may be relevant to the inhibition by Bcl-2 of cell proliferation because NF-AT-inducible genes are important for proliferation in some types of cells. There is emerging evidence that Bcl-2 and its close relatives exert at least two distinct functions: They not only inhibit apoptosis, but also restrain cell-cycle entry.[79–81] These two functions can be genetically separated because mutation of a conserved tyrosine residue (Y28) at the C-terminal end of the BH4 region of Bcl-2 does not affect its antiapoptotic activity, but markedly reduces its ability to restrain reentry of quiescent cells into the cell cycle.[81] The inhibitory effect of Bcl-2 on entry into the cell cycle may contribute to the better prognosis of patients whose breast cancer tissue shows abnormally high levels of Bcl-2.[82] Delayed cell-cycle entry could result in longer times to relapse. Quiescent leukemic progenitor cells also overexpressed Bcl-X_L and Bcl-2 compared to their proliferating counterparts.[83] When Bcl-2 antisense oligonucleotides were used in vitro in primary acute myelogenous leukemia (AML) samples, recruitment of leukemic cells into the cell cycle was observed.[84] The precise mechanism by which Bcl-2 affects cell-cycle progression remains to be determined. Another Bcl-2 family member Mcl-1 was recently found to be essential for the survival of hematopoietic stem cells.[85]

Downstream of Bcl-2, a member of caspase-inhibitors termed "Inhibitors-of-Apoptosis" (IAP) proteins, may also affect cell-cycle regulation; survivin itself is expressed in a cell-cycle-dependent manner and is regulated by the MAPK and PI3K signaling pathways.[86] Maximal expression is in G_2/M and recent studies suggest that survivin plays a role in cell cytokinesis. Its down-regulation can cause G_2 block and polyploidization. For details of survivin's antiapoptotic function, see Chapter 4. Down-regulation of survivin expression with antisense oligonucleotides or MAPK and PI3K inhibitors[86] has resulted in cell-cycle arrest, and to a lesser degree, in apoptosis, confirmed its dual function.

DIFFERENTIATION

All tumors show abnormalities in differentiation (ie, anaplasia). The presence of immature and the lack of mature, terminally differentiated cells is a hallmark of cancer, with rare exceptions. In chronic myelogenous leukemias (CML), the number of mature granulocytes is actually increased, at least at early stages of the disease, and it takes several years and additional genetic alterations of immature blast cells until they predominate. Similarly, in myelodysplastic syndromes, mature-appearing granulocytes can be clonal.[87] Hence, the differentiation block characteristic for most cancers is not absolute. The anaplasia of tumors can provide insights into their etiology, degree of malignancy, prognosis, and sensitivity to therapeutic intervention by differentiation- or maturation-inducing agents. These differences in phenotype arise from differences in gene expression, not in gene content. The genes expressed by a particular cell comprise only approximately 10 to 20% of the coding capacity of the genome. In humans, there are over 100,000 genes that code for proteins; however, an individual cell generally expresses only 10,000 to 20,000 genes. Genes expressed by a particular cell depend on its embryonic lineage, developmental stage of the organism, tissue and cellular environment, and functions that the cell must fulfill. The mechanisms that regulate gene expression are incompletely understood; however, they most certainly entail the sequential action of cell-type-specific or cell-lineage-specific transcription factors that repress or activate the differentiation-specific genes. The transcription of genes itself is regulated by a complex enzymatic machinery. Histone acetylation/deacetylation and methylation/demethylation of target genes have recently been the focus of detailed studies and provide the basis for "transcription therapy."[88] Programs of gene expression generally are instituted early in embryogenesis and sequentially altered as development proceeds.[89,90] Post-transcriptional modifications, such as phosphorylation and ubiquination of many genes, add further complexity to the regulation of gene expression. Messenger RNA transcripts can be silenced by short "interference" RNAs (siRNAs),[91] short hairpin RNAs (shRNAs), or cDNA/RNAi hybrid molecules.[92–95]

Some genes are expressed by many, if not all, cell types. These "housekeeping" genes generally encode proteins that participate in basic or universal cellular functions. Other genes that are expressed only in specific cell types and/or stages of development are said to be cell-type- or differentiation-specific genes. Thus, the expression of specific gene products marks both the cell lineage and the stage of differentiation.

Differentiation and Cell Proliferation Differentiation begins shortly after the first few cell divisions that follow fertilization. Throughout development, and in adult organisms, the ability of a cell to proliferate is intimately connected to its state of differentiation. Adult tissues generally express a variety of factors that act to maintain both the proliferation and the differentiation status of the cells. These include secreted molecules, transmembrane receptors, intracellular signaling molecules, and transcription factors. For example, myoD[96] and c/EBP-α[97] are nuclear factors that activate the transcription of muscle- and adipocyte-specific genes, respectively; in addition, both proteins are potent inhibitors of cell proliferation.

Transcription factors are the engines that drive proliferation and differentiation of cells. Their disruption is associated with cancer.[98,99] One of the earliest revelations of this fact was the identification of retroviral oncogenes that were associated with the development of cancer. For example, the avian myeloblastosis virus causes myeloblastic leukemia in chickens. The virus overexpresses the transcription factor *myb*. Likewise, avian myelocytomatosis virus produces a variety of cancers in chickens. This virus has a dysregulated *myc* oncogene. Both *myc* and *myb* have subsequently been identified as dysregulated in a variety of human cancers. A second manner in which cancer-related dysregulated transcription factors were discovered, was by analysis of chromosomal translocations. One of the genes at the chromosomal rearrangement is often a transcription factor that becomes dysregulated, such as the fusion of the *PML* and *RAR* (retinoic acid receptor) genes in acute promyelocytic leukemia. *RAR* is a transcription factor often involved in differentiation; however, when fused to *PML*, the fusion product behaves as a repressor of differentiation-related target genes.

Some transcription factors are necessary for differentiation of stem cells to their mature progeny. Dysfunction of these transcription factors can be associated with a block in differentiation, resulting in the cell remaining in the proliferative pool. This provides them with a growth advantage compared to their normal counterpart, thus setting the stage for the development or progression of cancer. For example, the CCAAT/enhancer binding protein-alpha (C/EBPα) is a transcription factor mutated in approximately 7 to 15% of AMLs.[100–102] Also, members of a family with an increased proclivity to develop AML were found to have a germline mutation of one allele of C/EBPα.[103] Another leukemia-prone syndrome has a germline mutation of one allele of the transcription factor RUNX1. These individuals with the germline C/EBPα and RUNX1 mutation have a long latency period (10–30 years) before developing leukemia, suggesting additional mutations are necessary for progression to leukemia.[104] In addition, these families suggest that haploinsufficiency of either of these transcription factors increases the risk of development of AML. Besides mutations, expression and/or activity of C/EBPα can be disrupted in a variety of cancers. For example, the AML-1/ETO and the PML/RARα leukemia-associated fusion proteins can inappropriately sequester C/EBPα in the cytoplasm, as well as blunt its transcription.[105] The BCR-ABL fusion product found in chronic myelogenous leukemia, inhibits the efficient translation of C/EBPα. Also, tumors derived from the lung, liver, and breast have a low expression of C/EBPα compared to surrounding normal tissue. The mechanism of gene silencing in these cancers is not clear.

Besides acting as a transcription factor, C/EBPα can bind and block the activity of E2F and the cyclin-dependent kinase-2 (CDK-2) and CDK-4, and it can increase levels of $p21^{WAF1}$, a cyclin-dependent kinase inhibitor. Thus, C/EBPα can directly slow proliferation, independent of its transcriptional activity. These antigrowth effects are lost with dysregulation of C/EBPα. Taken together, an altered C/EBPα can foster aberrant cell growth at the same time as it loses its capacity to induce differentiation. Experimental forced expression of C/EBPα in leukemia cells induces their terminal differentiation, suggesting that induction of expression of C/EBPα may be a worthwhile therapeutic target in selected cancers and leukemias.

In early embryos, cell proliferation is the primary means by which the cell mass increases. As the organism develops, however, proliferation becomes restricted. Some differentiated cells continue to proliferate, but others irreversibly lose this ability. Embryonic cells often display traits that confer on them a selective growth advantage over that of an adult cell. They proliferate vigorously,[106] are capable of extensive migration, secrete factors that increase the local supply of blood, and produce enzymes capable of degrading basement membranes.[107] These traits also are characteristic of tumor cells, including the ability to increase local blood supply (ie, angiogenesis).[108] Recent data suggest that tumor angiogenesis is an important, negative prognostic indicator for carcinomas and leukemias.[109,110] Angiogenesis is now being extensively investigated as a potential target for cancer therapy.[111] Thus, in adult organisms, mutations or conditions that activate portions of embryonic programs for gene expression or inactivate portions of the adult program can produce cells with many properties of malignant tumor cells.[112]

Stem Cells Stem cells have the capacity for both self-renewal (ie, proliferation without a change in phenotype) and differentiation (ie, changing into a new phenotype). Some stem cells have already undergone considerable differentiation, so further differentiation is restricted to a single cell type or lineage. Other stem cells are multipotent and differentiate into a variety of cell types (ie, hematopoietic stem cells). It has been difficult to demonstrate cells in adults that are totipotent (ie, capable of differentiating into most or all of the cell types that comprise the organism), but the recent cloning of animals from mature cells demonstrates the persistence of stem cell characteristics even in fully differential cells.[113] Also, recently, neuronal stem cells were shown to produce a variety of blood cell types,[114] and adult human mesenchymal stem cells that are present in adult marrow were shown to have the potential to differentiate to lineages of mesenchymal tissues, including bone, cartilage, fat, tendon, muscle, marrow stroma, neuronal cells, and myocytes.[115–118] Conversely, primitive hematopoietic stem cells were reported to give rise to muscle,[119] liver,[120,121] intestinal,[121,122] pulmonary epithelial,[123,124] and neuronal cells.[125,126] Engraftment and differentiation by a single, bone marrow-derived stem cell in liver, lungs, GI tract, and skin were reported.[123] Some of these data were obtained from experiments where hematopoietic cells or whole bone marrow cell populations, including stromal cells being transplanted into sex mismatched hosts, and sex-chromosome differences were used to determine the origin of immune histochemically identified organ cells.[127–129] However, co-localization of markers is technically challenging, and recent reports have explained some of the published data as results of cell fusions rather than of "transdifferentiation"[130,131] or have failed to confirm previous reports. Wagers and colleagues, transplanting single green fluorescent protein-marked hematopoietic stem cells into lethally irradiated nontransgenic mice, did not find convincing evidence of bone marrow-derived neuronal cells, liver, kidney, gut, skeletal muscle, cardiac muscle, or lung cells.[132] Another recent report was unable to confirm the ability of bone marrow cells to differentiate into neuronal cells.[133]

While dedifferentiation or "transdifferentiation" of adult stem cells remain uncertain or very rare, embryonic stem (ES) cells have great value for the study of differentiation, for the elucidation of organ-specific coordinated gene expression programs, and for the development of regenerative medicine applications.[134] These studies have now been extended to cells of human origin.[135,136] ES cells are pluripotent cell lines derived from the inner cell mass (ICM) of blastocyst stage embryos[106] and have been successfully gene marked.[137] They have the ability to differentiate into myocytes with structural and functional properties of cardiomyocytes[138] and into many other cell types.[138–143] Their therapeutic utility for cancer and degenerative disease is presently under investigation in preclinical model systems.

Mesenchymal stem cells (MSC) can be isolated from bone marrow samples and subsequently expanded over a millionfold in culture. MSC differentiate into adipocytes, osteocytes, chondrocytes, tenocytes, marrow stromal cells, muscle cells, and perhaps neuronal cells[118,144] and are being used in early clinical trials to enhance bone marrow grafting and to suppress graft-versus-host disease in allogeneic bone marrow transplants.[145] An intriguing finding is the observation that MSC can contribute to the formation of stroma in solid tumors and tumor metastases and that they can deliver therapeutic genes such as interferon-beta and induce tumor regressions.[71,146,147]

In general, stem cell differentiation results in two types of changes: the expression of specialized, differentiation-specific gene products and a partial or complete restriction of the cell's capacity for further proliferation. It then follows that another mechanism by which tumor cells might arise is through mutations that render a stem cell partly or wholly unable to differentiate.

Some cells, particularly in adults, are terminally differentiated. These cells are irreversibly blocked in their ability to proliferate, although they may perform specialized functions for a long period of time, perhaps with the exception of CML. Tumors of terminally differentiated cells are not found. Thus, tumors of mature muscle or nerve cells do not occur, although tumors of less differentiated myoblastic or neuronal stem cells do. Cell proliferation appears to be incompatible with the expression of a terminally differentiated program of gene expression. Thus, irreversible arrest of cell division and expression of the terminally differentiated phenotype are interdependent.

In many tissues, continuous proliferation is restricted to a subpopulation of cells, the stem cells, which undergo self-renewal, as well as differentiation into cell types with a more restrictive proliferative potential. It then follows that mutations or conditions that interfere with the differentiation of stem cells will result in unbalanced proliferation and, thus, uncontrolled growth of the tissue. Mutations that drive proliferation are associated with an accumulation and overgrowth of less-differentiated cells in the tissue. A common feature of tumor cells is their failure to differentiate terminally under appropriate conditions either in vivo or in culture.[148–150]

Extracellular Factors That Control Differentiation During embryogenesis and in a number of adult tissues, differentiation depends on external factors. These include insoluble factors, such as ECM, and both the proximity and type of neighboring cells as well as a growing list of soluble factors. In model systems, differentiation can be induced by a variety of biologic agents and drugs (Table 3-3). Both the ECM and differentiation-promoting soluble factors may be produced in an autocrine or paracrine fashion.

Cell-cell and cell-ECM interactions are important for both the induction and maintenance of differentiation in several cell lineages. Although our understanding at a molecular level of insoluble factors is still incomplete, progress has been made in identifying key molecules and pathways through which these factors act. In the case of the ECM, specific cell surface receptors

Table 3-3 Induction of Differentiation in Culture

Stem Cell	Differentiation Markers	Inducers
Preadipocyte	Adipocyte	Insulin, cort, cell density
Basal keratinocyte	Cornified envelope	RA deficiency, cell density
Myoblast	Myotube	GF deficiency, cell density
Squamous cell carcinoma	Cornified envelope	GF deficiency, cort
Embryonal carcinoma	Endoderm, mesoderm, ectoderm	RA, ara-C, mito, HMBA, co-culture with blastocyst
Neuroblastoma	Neuron, neurotransmitter, action potential	PI, 6TG, ara-C, MTX, dox, bleo, RA, GF deficiency
Melanoma	Dendrite, melanin, tyrosinase	PI, dox, DMSO, TPA, RA, MSH
Colon adenocarcinoma	Mucus, dome formation, CEA, columnar cell	NMF, DMSO, butyrate, low glucose, IFN, HMBA, cell density
Breast adenocarcinoma	Casein, dome formation	RA, PGE, DMSO
Bladder transitional cell carcinoma	Keratin filament, loss of surface antigen	HMBA
Erythroleukemia	Mature erythroid cell, hemoglobin	Dox, ara-C, 6TG, mito, dact, aza, hemin, DMSO, HMBA, CSF, RA, IFN
Promyelocytic	Granulocyte, macrophage	IFN, CSF, vitD, TPA, DMSO, NMF, dact, HMBA, aza, ara-C, RA
Myelocytic leukemia	Granulocyte, macrophage	CSF, RA, vitD, ara-C, dact, DMSO, TPA, cort, dox

ara-C = Cytarabine; aza = 5-azacytidine; bleo = bleomycin; CEA = carcinoembryonic antigen; cort = glucocorticoids; CSF-colony stimulating factor; dact = dactnomycin; DMSO = dimethylsulfoxide; dox = doxorubicin; GF = growth factor; hemin; HMBA = hexamethylbisacetamide; IFN = alpha- or gamma-interferon; mito = mitomycin C; MSH = melanocyte-stimulating hormone; MTX = methotrexate; NMF = *N,N*-dimethylformamide; PGE = prostaglandin E; PI = phosphodiesterase inhibitor; RA = retinoic acid; TPA = 12-0-tetradecanoylphorbol-13-acetate; vitD = 1,25-dihydroxy vitamin D; 6TG = 6-thioguanine. Data from Cheson BD et al.,[207] Reiss M et al.,[199] and Waxman S et al.[200]

bind to particular components of the ECM.[151] It now appears that the binding of an ECM component to its cellular receptor activates an intracellular signal transduction pathway that is analogous to the signaling pathways that have been identified for polypeptide GFs and growth inhibitors. Tumor cells often lose their ability to sense the ECM or neighboring cells.[152]

The soluble factors that regulate differentiation can be broadly classified into those that bind to cell surface receptors and those that freely cross the plasma membrane and bind to cytoplasmic or nuclear receptors. The first class includes molecules such as the fibroblast growth factors (FGFs) (TGF-β, IGF-1 and b-FGF) and hematopoietic factors such as colony-stimulating factor-1 (CSF-1), granulocyte colony-stimulating factor (G-CSF), granulocyte-macrophage colony-stimulating factor (GM-CSF), stem cell factor (SCF), Flt-3 Ligand, and the interleukins. These are all polypeptides, and many were first identified as GFs or growth inhibitors. It now is clear, however, that these factors have a multitude of effects depending on the target cells and the cellular microenvironment.[153]

For example, basic FGF was identified as a fibroblast mitogen in brain and pituitary extracts, but recent data suggest that FGF induces mesodermal differentiation in early embryos, is angiogenic, and is a survival factor for endothelial cells.[154,155] FGF also inhibits the differentiation of some cells. Terminal differentiation into mature myotubes cannot occur unless it is withdrawn from proliferating myoblasts. Similarly, TGF-β was first identified as a stimulator of anchorage-independent growth in mesenchymal cells and later as an inhibitor of epithelial cell proliferation.[156,157] Like FGF, TGF-β stimulates the differentiation of some cells (ie, keratinocytes or intestinal epithelial cells) but inhibits differentiation in others (ie, myoblasts or preadipocytes). In some human tumor cells cultured in vitro or in athymic mice, TGF-β both inhibits tumor growth and promotes a more differentiated phenotype in the remaining cells. Other studies suggest that TGF-β induces the expression of one or more inhibitors of cyclin-dependent protein kinases (eg, p21, p27, p16); inhibition of these kinases, in turn, prevents the phosphorylation and, thus, inactivation of the RB protein, thereby inhibiting cell proliferation.[158–161]

Another family of extracellular proteins is the CCN protein family, which is composed of six members: Cyr61, CTGF, NOV, WISP-1, WISP-2, and WISP-3 (officially known as CCN1-6, respectively).[162] The CCN genes contain four conserved modular domains that share sequence similarity with other protein families: IGF-binding protein (IGFBP), Von Willebrand type C (VWC), thrombospondin type 1 (TSP1), and a C-terminal domain (CT). Cyr61 (CCN1) is a secreted, cysteine-rich, heparin-binding protein that associates with the extracellular matrix and the cell surface. Integrins, including $\alpha_v\beta_3$, $\alpha_v\beta_5$, $\alpha_6\beta_1$, and $\alpha_{IIb}\beta 3$, have been identified as receptors of Cyr61. Through these receptors, Cyr61 probably exerts its effects on cellular activity in a variety of tissue types. It is highly expressed in many breast and brain cancers and melanomas, and high expression has been associated with a worse prognosis.[163–165] Furthermore, forced expression of Cyr61 in "normal" cell lines from these same tissues allows them to form tumors in immunodeficient mice. Dysregulation of various cellular signaling pathways, such as the receptor tyrosine kinases (eg, epidermal growth factor receptor), can cause a cascade of signaling that induces expression and secretion of CCN1 (Cyr61), which, in a paracrine and autocrine fashion, stimulates integrins to provide growth signals for the cancer and precancer cells.

The membrane-permeable regulators of differentiation include retinoic acid (ie, vitamin A) and its derivatives (RA).[166] There is strong evidence that concentration gradients of RA are critical for the morphogenesis of some tissues in the early embryo.[113] RA can stimulate or inhibit growth and differentiation depending on the cell type. In general, RA is required for the differentiation of many epithelial cells. It diffuses freely into cells, whereupon it binds to specific nuclear protein receptors (ie, the retinoic acid receptors [RARs]). In addition, other nuclear proteins, called RAR coregulators, have been found that interact with RARs and modulate their actions in various cell types.[167] These differences may explain why specific cells and tissues differ in their responses to RA. Some differentiation-specific genes that are regulated by RA contain sequences specific to the initiation of transcription,[168] to which RA-RAR complexes bind and thereby activate transcription.[113,169] In acute promyelocytic leukemia (APL), RAR fuses with the *PML* gene in the reciprocal translocation t(15;17) and with PLZF in t(11;17).[170] The ensuing fusion proteins PML/RARα and PLZF/RARα inhibit transcription by inducing the N-Cor/sin3A/HDAC1 corepressor complex (Figure 3-6). This transcriptional silencing in APL is mediated through deacetylation of the core proteins of nucleosomes, histones H2A, H2B, H3, and H4 (Figure 3-7). Lysines (k) in the amino-terminal tails of H2A, H2B, H3, and H4 are acetylation/deacetylation sites for histone acetyltransferases (HATs) and histone deacetylases (HDACs).[171–173] With inhibition of HDACs by HDAC inhibitors such as suberoylanilide hydroxamic acid (SAHA),[174] histones are acetylated, and the DNA that is tightly wrapped around a deacetylated histone core relaxes (Figure 3-8). Other HDAC inhibitors include trichostatin A and depsipeptide; SAHA and depsipeptide are in clinical trials. In RA-resistant PLZF-RARα leukemias, the combined exposure to ATRA and SAHA resulted in therapeutic effects. This therapeutic concept has been termed "transcription therapy."[88,174–177]

The sex steroids estrogen and testosterone may regulate differentiation by similar mechanisms. Another nuclear receptor, the peroxisome proliferator-activated receptor-γ (PPARγ) has recently been identified as a potential target for cancer therapy. It is highly expressed in normal adipose tissues, monocytes, leukemias, and epithelial malignancies. PPARγ ligands signal differentiation, growth arrest, and apoptosis. PPARγ

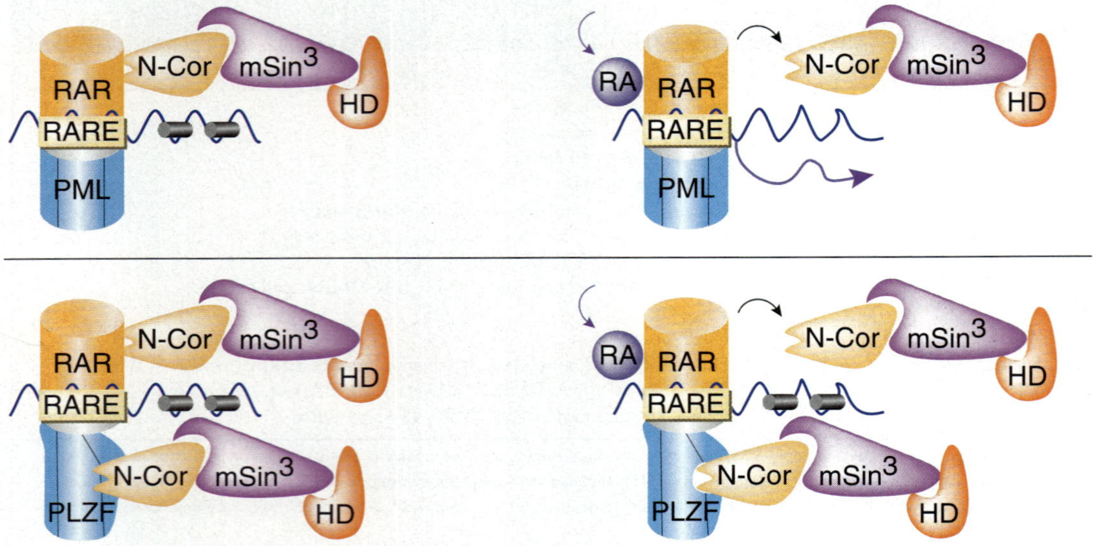

Figure 3-6 RARα fusion proteins induce N-CoR/Sin3A/HDAC1, corepressor complex and inhibit transcription. A model for the interactions of APL fusion proteins with the N-CoR–mSin3–histone deacetylase complex. PML–RARα interacts with N-CoR (or SMRT) and recruits the mSin3–HD complex, decreasing histone acetylation and producing repressive chromatin organization and transcriptional repression. Retinoic acid (RA) induces dissociation of the N-CoR–mSin3-HD complex, recruitment of coactivators with histone acetyltransferase activity (not shown), increased levels of histone acetylation, chromatin remodeling and transcriptional activation. PLZF–RARα has two N-CoR binding sites that, even in the presence of RA, recruit the N-CoR–mSin3–HD complex and maintain transcription repression. Redrawn from Grignani F, et al.[170]

must form a heterodimer with RXR to bind DNA and activate transcription. In the absence of ligand, the heterodimer associates with a complex of corepressor proteins that silence target promoters by deacetylating histones in the adjacent chromatin. Ligand binding induces a conformational change in the receptor, which dissociates the corepressor complex, and permits the heterodimer to interact with coactivator complexes (p160/CBP and DRIP). The complexes acetylate histones and allow transcription (reviewed by Konopleva and Andreeff[178]). Somatic loss-of-function PPARγ mutations were found in colon cancers and a PAX8-PPARγ fusion was recently identified in human thyroid follicular carcinomas carrying the translocation t(2;3)(q13;p25). PPARγ ligation may affect tumor growth indirectly through regulation of the tumor suppressor gene PTEN.[178,179] In a clinical trial, PPARγ ligation resulted in the induction of differentiation in liposarcomas.[180]

Tumor cells often produce factors that affect both growth and differentiation. Basic FGF can confer neoplastic properties when expressed in an inappropriate cell type (eg, a fibroblast). In addition, inappropriate expression of FGF by one cell may stimulate the growth and affect the differentiation of neighboring cell types.[155]

Intracellular Regulators External factors and intrinsic programs of gene expression control cellular differentiation. In either case, the expression of differentiation-specific genes generally is under the control of a small number of master regulatory genes. Genes recently have been identified that are potential "master regulators" of developmental stages and differentiation-specific gene expression. The most globally acting master regulatory genes are known as homeotic genes, which were first identified as genetic loci that determined the developmental and spatial fates of cells in embryos of the fruit fly *Drosophila*. Similar genes have been identified in the genomes of higher organisms, including humans. Individual homeotic genes are expressed at different times during development and also are expressed in different adult tissues. Some homeotic genes code for extracellular factors, whereas others code for nuclear proteins that are probably transcriptional regulatory factors. Homeotic genes regulate programs of differentiation as opposed to individual differentiation-specific genes. They appear to act by initiating cascades of gene expression that involve regulatory genes having a more restricted range of actions.[181,182] Some homeotic genes may function as tumor suppressors in normal tissues; others may promote tumorigenesis when mutated or deregulated. Mutations in homeotic genes may reactivate portions of an embryonic program of gene expression or suppress portions of an adult program of gene expression.[183–185]

DNA Methylation In many cases, cells must go through one or more rounds of DNA replication before they can differentiate. This requirement may be because there often is a need to modify the pattern of DNA methylation before differentiation begins. DNA methylation in eukaryotes involves addition of a methyl group to the carbon/5 position of the cytosine ring.[186] Changes in DNA methylation commonly are introduced during DNA replication. DNA methylation is essential for development in the mouse and plays an important role in inactivation of the X-chromosome and genomic imprinting.[187] It may also contribute to the control of tissue-specific gene expression. The most direct mechanism by which DNA methylation can interfere with transcription is to prevent the binding of basal transcriptional machinery or ubiquitous transcription factors that require contact with cytosine in the major groove of the double helix. Most mammalian transcription factors have GC-rich binding sites and many have CpGs in their

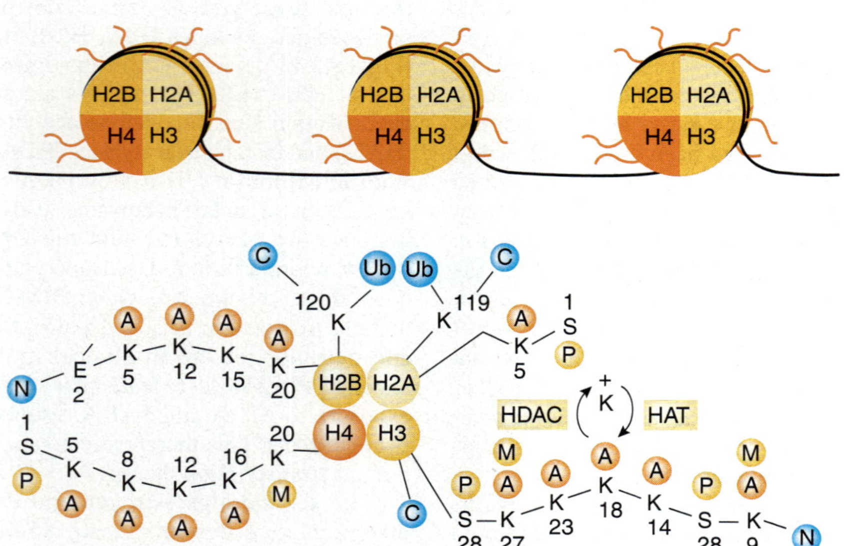

Figure 3-7 Schematic of the structure of histones in nucleosomes. **A,** The core proteins of nucleosomes are designated H2A (histone 2A), H2B (histone 2B), H3 (histone 3) and H4 (histone 4). Each histone is present in two copies, so the DNA (black) wraps around an octomer of histones-the core nucleosome. **B,** The amino-terminal tails of core histones. Lysines (K) in the amino-terminal tails of histones H2A, H2B, H3 and H4 are potential acetylation/deacetylation sites for histone acetyltransferases (HATs) and histone deacetylases (HDACs). Acetylation neutralizes the charge on lysines. A, acetyl; C, carboxyl terminus; E, glutamic acid; M, methyl; N, amino terminus; P, phosphate; S, serine, Ub, ubiquitin. Reproduced with permission from Marks PA, et al.[171]

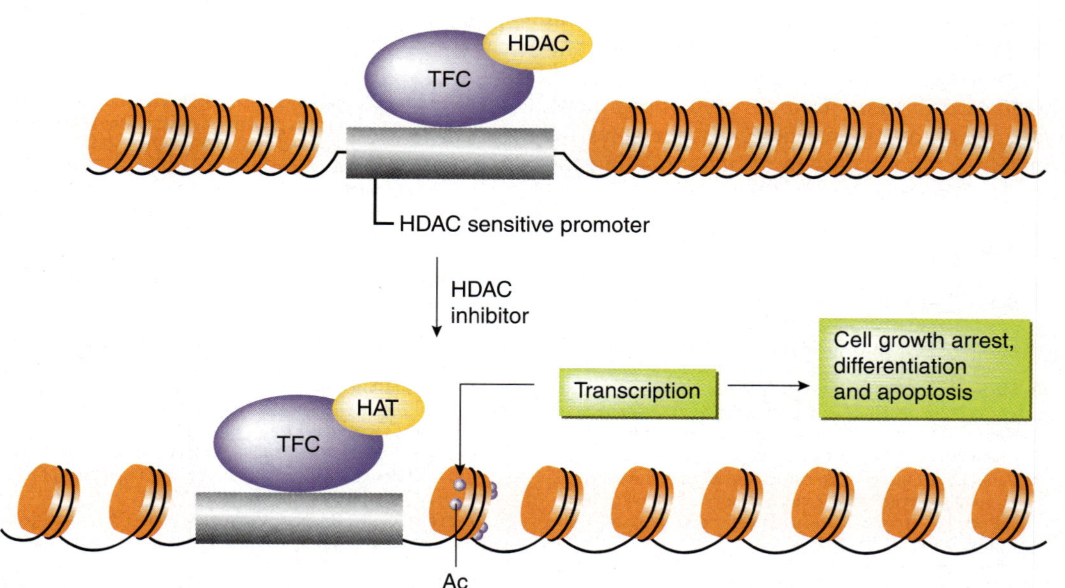

Figure 3-8 Proposed mechanism of action of histone deacetylase inhibitors. With inhibition of histone deacetylases (HDACs) by HDAC inhibitors such as suberoylanilide hydroxamic acid, histones are acetylated, and the DNA that is tightly wrapped around a deacetylated histone core relaxes. It has been proposed that there are specific sites in the promoter region of a subset of genes (eg, SP1 sites) that recruit the transcription factor complex (TFC) with HDAC and that the accumulation of acetylated histones in nucleosomes leads to increased transcription of this subset of genes (for example, *CDKN1A*, which encodes WAF1), which, in turn, leads to downstream effects that result in cell-growth arrest, differentiation and/or apoptotic cell death acetyltransferase. Reproduced with permission from Marks PA, et al.[171]

DNA recognition elements. Binding by several of these factors is indeed impeded or abolished by methylation of CpG, though some factors, notably Sp1, are indifferent to methylation status. The highest density of nonmethylated CpGs in the vertebrate genome are found in CpG islands, which usually contain promoter or other regulatory DNA that is required for active transcription of a gene. CpG island chromatin is enriched in hyperacetylated histones and deficient in linker histones. These are essential features of transcriptionally competent chromatin templates. In contrast, chromatin assembled on artificially methylated DNA becomes associated with hypoacetylated histones, refractory to nuclease or restriction endonuclease digestion, and transcriptionally silent. Many tumor-suppressor and other cancer-related genes have been found to be hypermethylated in human cancer cells and primary tumors (Table 3-4).[188] The different classes of genes that are silenced by DNA methylation include tumor suppressor genes, genes that suppress tumor invasion and metastasis, DNA repair genes, genes for hormone receptors, and genes that inhibit angiogenesis. The methylation of DNA on specific cytosine residues is believed to contribute to the changes in gene expression that occur during development. Presumably, DNA methylation affects gene expression because the transcriptional regulatory proteins that bind to methylated DNA differ from those that bind to unmethylated DNA. Many neoplastic tissues have hypermethylated genes relative to their normal counterparts[189–193] and, indeed, pharmacologic agents that alter the pattern of DNA methylation induce differentiation in a number of cultured cell lines: 5-azacytidine and recently deoxyazacytidine (DAC) have shown promise in vitro and in clinical trials in leukemias.[187,188] Gene silencing by hypermethylation of promoter genes has been recognized as an important mechanism of carcinogenesis that has great promise for cancer prevention and therapy ("epigenetic therapy"). In breast cancer, demethylating agents have been proposed to reactivate silenced genes, including the estrogen receptor and RARβ genes. As discussed above, the first described alteration in the retinoid pathway was the leukemogenic role of the PML-RAR fusion protein. Later, evidence supported the role of RARβ2 as a tumor suppressor gene: the induction of RARβ2 related to the chemopreventive effects of retinoids, the loss of RARβ2 expression in human neoplasms, frequent chromosomal losses at 3p21–3p24, where RARβ2 is located, and the methylation-mediated silencing of RARβ2.[194] Subsequently, the epigenetic silencing of the cellular retinol-binding protein-1 gene (*CRBP1*) was reported as a common alteration in human cancer.[195] The loss of CRBP1 may compromise retinoic acid metabolism by diminishing retinol transport and blocking the formation of retinyl esters and may increase the activity of the β-catenin-LEF/T-cell factor signaling pathway, a central element in malignant cell transformation. Until now, the use of retinoids to prevent or treat human cancer has achieved only modest success. The disruption of CRBP1 and RARβ2 by promoter hypermethylation in many human neoplasms may in part explain this resistance. However, in colorectal tumors, 30% of malignancies did not present any apparent lesion in the retinoid pathway and it was therefore postulated that these tumors may be extremely sensitive to treatment with retinoids. In order to maximize the induction of differentiation in cancer, combinations of HDAC inhibitors and demethylating agents have been proposed.[187] DNA methylation is probably not a universal mechanism for differentiation, however, and some cells can be induced to differentiate with either minimal or no change in cell-cycle progression.[196] DNA methylation and gene silencing are also not always strictly correlated.

Table 3-4 Genes Silenced by Aberrant DNA Methylation

Gene
Tumor suppressor
p15 INK4B (cyclin kinase inhibitor)
p16 INK4A (cyclin kinase inhibitor)
p73 (TP53 homology)
ARF/INK4A (regulate level TP53)
Wilms tumor
Von Hippel Lindau (VHL)
Retinoic acid receptor-β (RARβ)
Estrogen receptor
Androgen receptor
Mammary-derived growth inhibitor
Hypermethylated in cancer (HIC1)
Retinoblastoma (Rb)
Invasion/metastasis inhibitor
E-cadherin
Tissue inhibitor metalloproteinases-3 (TIMP-3)
mts-1
CD-44
DNA repair/detoxify carcinogens
Methylguanine methyltransferase
HMLH1 (mismatch DNA repair)
Glutathione S-transferase
BRCA-1
Angiogenesis inhibitor
Thrombospondin-1 (TSP-1)
TIMP-3
Tumor antigen
MAGE-1

Data from Momparler RL, et al.[188]

Differentiation and Cancer Therapy Analysis of differentiation by tumor cells often provides valuable information for both the diagnosis and therapy of human cancers. As tumor cells grow and die, they can release glycoproteins and other products similar to those of fetal tissues, and these oncofetal products can be detected in serum or other body fluids to assist in diagnosis, follow-up, and selection of therapies. Examples include estrogen receptors and α-lactalbumin in breast cancer, prostate-specific antigen and prostatic acid phosphatase in prostate cancers, and myoglobin and desmin in sarcomas.[197]

Elevations of these markers in the serum often predict relapse of the neoplasm before any sign by routine examination or radiographic tests. In general, the specificity of such markers for a given neoplasm is poor because minor elevations also occur with inflammatory and other benign conditions or with several types of neoplasms. In carcinoma of unknown primary site, tissue markers for neuroendocrine differentiation select for a subgroup of patients with improved response to chemotherapy.[198]

Some tumor cells can be induced to differentiate terminally. This has been shown most extensively in cultured cell lines (see Table 3-3) but also in experimental animals.[161,199,200] After tumor cells have been induced to undergo terminal differentiation, their ability to grow as a tumor often is stably suppressed. In contrast to most anticancer drugs, which have nonspecific toxicity to both normal and cancer cells, drug-induced differentiation can be demonstrated with agents (or drug levels) that exert minimal effects on normal cells.[199] These observations have stimulated increased interest in clinical applications of differentiating agents to provide therapeutic gain with minimal toxicity.[201]

A number of agents known to induce differentiation in various model systems have been used clinically (see Table 3-3). Some are useful only in a particular type of tumor; for example, estrogens and androgens have been useful in treating some breast, prostate, and gynecologic tumors, providing that tumor cells express the appropriate nuclear receptor. Other differentiation-inducing drugs have been more widely studied. For example, high doses of RA, hexamethylene bisacetamide (HMBA), or 5-azacytidine, an inhibitor of DNA methylation, can induce differentiation and inhibit the growth of several types of tumors in laboratory models.[200] HMBA was found to induce differentiation in patients with myelodysplastic syndromes,[202] and complete remission was achieved with direct evidence of terminal differentiation of leukemic cells to clonal granulocytes.

Combinations of HDAC inhibitors (eg, valproic acid) and demethylating agents (5-Azacytidine, deoxyazacytidine) are being investigated in leukemias. In fresh cultures of human promyelocytic leukemia, retinoid-induced differentiation, similar to the effects seen in passaged leukemia cell lines, has been observed.[203] All-*trans*-retinoic acid has been used in clinical therapy of promyelocytic leukemia with promising results,[204,205] and retinoids have been used in combination with interferon-α to produce responses in patients with squamous cell cancer of the skin or cervix.[206] Because differentiating agents may inhibit tumor cell growth by multiple mechanisms, it is difficult to prove specific differentiating actions of these agents when used in patients.[205,207] For example, retinoids not only induce differentiation in leukemia, but they also down-regulate antiapoptotic genes.[208] An exception are studies in leukemias where sequential samples are readily available, differentiation markers are well established, and the clonality of differentiated cells can be ascertained by methods such as molecular cytogenetics (FISH).[203]

Retinoids and other differentiating agents also are used in clinical trials to prevent cancer in patients with premalignant lesions or a high risk of developing cancer of the breast, cervix, colon, skin, lung, or oral cavity. Early results are encouraging, including the reversal of oral leukoplakia and prevention of second neoplasms in patients with treated squamous cell carcinoma of the head and neck.[207,209] Greater knowledge about the molecular basis for the control of differentiation should lead to more accurate predictions, however, as well as rational design of therapies for controlling tumor growth by manipulating the state of differentiation.[200,210,211]

REFERENCES

1. Evan GI, Vousden KH. Proliferation, cell cycle and apoptosis in cancer. Nature 2001;411:342–8.
2. Malumbres M, Barbacid M. To cycle or not to cycle: a critical decision in cancer. Nat Rev Cancer 2001;1:222–31.
3. Hartwell LH, Weinert TA. Checkpoints: controls that ensure the order of cell cycle events. Science 1989;246:629–34.
4. Nigg EA. Mitotic kinases as regulators of cell division and its checkpoints. Nat Rev Mol Cell Biol 2001;2:21–32.
5. Cahill DP, Lengauer C, Yu J, et al. Mutations of mitotic checkpoint genes in human cancers. Nature 1998;392:300–3.
6. Harper JW, Adams PD. Cyclin-dependent kinases. Chem Rev 2001;101:2511–26.
7. Obaya AJ, Sedivy JM. Regulation of cyclin-Cdk activity in mammalian cells. Cell Mol Life Sci 2002;59:126–42.
8. Ortega S, Malumbres M, Barbacid M. Cyclin D-dependent kinases, INK4 inhibitors and cancer. Biochim Biophys Acta 2002;1602:73–87.
9. Polyak K, Lee M-H, Erdjument-Bromage H, et al. Cloning of p27Kip1, a cyclin-dependent kinase inhibitor and a potential mediator of extracellular antimitogenic signals. Cell 1994;78:59–66.
10. Polyak K, Kato JY, Solomon MJ, et al. p27Kip1, a cyclin-Cdk inhibitor, links transforming growth factor-beta and contact inhibition to cell cycle arrest. Genes Dev 1994;8:9–22.
11. Harper JW. Protein destruction: adapting roles for Cks proteins. Curr Biol 2001;11:R431–5.
12. Koepp DM, Harper JW, Elledge SJ. How the cyclin became a cyclin: regulated proteolysis in the cell cycle. Cell 1999;97:431–4.
13. Zugmaier G, Lippman ME. Effects of TGF beta on normal and malignant mammary epithelium. Ann N Y Acad Sci 1990;593:272–5.
14. Wakefield LM, Roberts AB. TGF-beta signaling: positive and negative effects on tumorigenesis. Curr Opin Genet Dev 2002;12:22–9.
15. Favoni RE, de Cupis A. The role of polypeptide growth factors in human carcinomas: new targets for a novel pharmacological approach. Pharmacol Rev 2000;52:179–206.
16. Druker BJ, Mamon HJ, Roberts TM. Oncogenes, growth factors, and signal transduction. N Engl J Med 1989;321:1383–91.
17. Purcell WT, Donehower RC. Evolving therapies: farnesyltransferase inhibitors. Curr Oncol Rep 2002;4:29–36.
18. Adjei AA. Blocking oncogenic Ras signaling for cancer therapy. J Natl Cancer Inst 2001;93:1062–74.
19. Jaunin F, Fakan S. DNA replication and nuclear architecture. J Cell Biochem 2002;85:1–9.
20. Gerbi SA, Bielinsky AK. DNA replication and chromatin. Curr Opin Genet Dev 2002;12:243–8.
21. Blow JJ, Hodgson B. Replication licensing—defining the proliferative state? Trends Cell Biol 2002;12:72–8.
22. Matsushime H, Roussel MF, Ashmun RA, Sherr CJ. Colony-stimulating factor 1 regulates novel cyclins during the G1 phase of the cell cycle. Cell 1991;65:701–13.
23. Goodrich DW, Wang NP, Qian YW, et al. The retinoblastoma gene product regulates progression through the G1 phase of the cell cycle. Cell 1991;67:293–302.
24. Matsushime H, Ewen ME, Strom DK, et al. Identification and properties of an atypical catalytic subunit (p34PSK-J3/cdk4) for mammalian D type G1 cyclins. Cell 1992;71:323–34.
25. Connell-Crowley L, Harper JW, Goodrich DW. Cyclin D1/Cdk4 regulates retinoblastoma protein-mediated cell cycle arrest by site-specific phosphorylation. Mol Biol Cell 1997;8:287–301.
26. Nevins JR, Leone G, DeGregori J, Jakoi L. Role of the Rb/E2F pathway in cell growth control. J Cell Physiol 1997;173:233–6.
27. Trimarchi JM, Lees JA. Sibling rivalry in the E2F family. Nat Rev Mol Cell Biol 2002;3:11–20.
28. Wu CL, Zukerberg LR, Ngwu C, et al. In vivo association of E2F and DP family proteins. Mol Cell Biol 1995;15:2536–46.
29. Geng Y, Eaton EN, Picon M, et al. Regulation of cyclin E transcription by E2Fs and retinoblastoma protein. Oncogene 1996;12:1173–80.
30. Hurford RKJ, Cobrinik D, Lee MH, Dyson N. pRB and p107/p130 are required for the regulated expression of different sets of E2F responsive genes. Genes Dev 1997;11:1447–63.
31. Ohtsubo M, Theodoras AM, Schumacher J, et al. Human cyclin E, a nuclear protein essential for the G1-to-S phase transition. Mol Cell Biol 1995;15:2612–24.
32. Leng X, Connell-Crowley L, Goodrich D, Harper JW. S-phase entry upon ectopic expression of G1 cyclin-dependent kinases in the absence of retinoblastoma protein phosphorylation. Curr Biol 1997;7:709–12.
33. Lukas J, Herzinger T, Hansen K, et al. Cyclin E-induced S-phase without activation of the pRb/E2F pathway. Genes Dev 1997;11:1479–92.
34. Amundson SA, Myers TG, Fornace AJ Jr. Roles for p53 in growth arrest and apoptosis: putting on the brakes after genotoxic stress. Oncogene 1998;17:3287–99.
35. Hoekstra MF. Responses to DNA damage and regulation of cell cycle checkpoints by the ATM protein kinase family. Curr Opin Genet Dev 1997;7:170–5.
36. Unger T, Juven-Gershon T, Moallem E, et al. Critical role for Ser20 of human p53 in the negative regulation of p53 by Mdm2. EMBO J 1999;18:1805–14.
37. Sakaguchi K, Herrera JE, Saito S, et al. DNA damage activates p53 through a phosphorylation-acetylation cascade. Genes Dev 1998;12:2831–41.
38. Waterman MJ, Stavridi ES, Waterman JL, Halazonetis TD. ATM-dependent activation of p53 involves dephosphorylation and association with 14-3-3 proteins. Nat Genet 1998;19:175–8.
39. Banin S, Moyal L, Shieh S, et al. Enhanced phosphorylation of p53 by ATM in response to DNA damage. Science 1998;281:1674–7.
40. Khanna KK, Keating KE, Kozlov S, et al. ATM associates with and phosphorylates p53: mapping the region of interaction. Nat Genet 1998;20:398–400.
41. de Lange T. Activation of telomerase in a human tumor. Proc Natl Acad Sci U S A 1994;91:2882–5.
42. Buchkovich KJ. Telomeres, telomerase, and the cell cycle. Prog Cell Cycle Res 1996;2:187–95.
43. Saretzki G, Sitte N, Merkel U, et al. Telomere shortening triggers a p53-dependent cell cycle arrest via accumulation of G-rich single stranded DNA fragments. Oncogene 1999;18:5148–58.
44. Stewart SA, Weinberg RA. Senescence: does it all happen at the ends? Oncogene 2002;21:627–30.
45. Fabrikant JI, Cherry J. The kinetics of cellular proliferation in normal and malignant tissues. V. Analysis of labeling indices and potential tissue doubling times in human tumor cell populations. J Surg Oncol 1969;1:23–47.
46. Fukuda K, Iwasaka T, Hachisuga T, et al. Immunocytochemical detection of S-phase cells in normal and neoplastic cervical epithelium by anti-BrdU monoclonal antibody. Anal Quant Cytol Histol 1990;12:135–8.
47. Teodori L, Trinca ML, Goehde W, et al. Cytokinetic investigation of lung tumors using the anti-bromodeoxyuridine (BUdR) monoclonal antibody method: comparison with DNA flow cytometric data. Int J Cancer 1990;45:995–1001.
48. Carlsson M, Totterman TH, Matsson P, Nilsson K. Cell cycle progression of B-chronic lymphocytic leukemia cells induced to differentiate by TPA. Blood 1988;71:415–21.
49. Tannock I. Cell kinetics and chemotherapy: a critical review. Cancer Treat Rep 1978;62:1117–33.
50. Fingert HJ, Campisi J, Pardee AB. Molecular Biology and Biochemistry of Cancer. In: Knapp R, Berkowitz R, editors. Gynecologic oncology. New York: Macmillan; 1991. p. 30.
51. Weber G. Biochemical strategy of cancer cells and the design of chemotherapy: G. H. A. Clowes Memorial Lecture. Cancer Res 1983;43:3466–92.
52. Pardee AB. G1 events and regulation of cell proliferation. Science 1989;246:603–8.
53. Juliano R. Cooperation between soluble factors and integrin-mediated cell anchorage in the control of cell growth and differentiation. Bioessays 1996;18:911–7.
54. Liotta LA. Tumor invasion and metastases—role of the extracellular matrix: Rhoads Memorial Award lecture. Cancer Res 1986;46:1–7.
55. Hall M, Peters G. Genetic alterations of cyclins, cyclin-dependent kinases, and Cdk inhibitors in human cancer. Adv Cancer Res 1996;68:67–108.
56. Sherr CJ. Cancer cell cycles. Science 1996;274:1672–7.
57. Motokura T, Bloom T, Kim HG, et al. A novel cyclin encoded by a bcl1-linked candidate oncogene. Nature 1991;350:512–5.
58. Wang TC, Cardiff RD, Zukerberg L, et al. Mammary hyperplasia and carcinoma in MMTV-cyclin D1 transgenic mice. Nature 1994;369:669–71.

59. Kamb A. Cyclin-dependent kinase inhibitors and human cancer. Curr Top Microbiol Immunol 1998;227:139–48.
60. Galaktionov K, Lee AK, Eckstein J, et al. CDC25 phosphatases as potential human oncogenes. Science 1995;269:1575–7.
61. Galaktionov K, Chen X, Beach D. Cdc25 cell-cycle phosphatase as a target of c-myc. Nature 1996;382:511–7.
62. Goodrich DW, Lee WH. The molecular genetics of retinoblastoma. Cancer Surv 1990;9:529–54.
63. Lee W-H. The molecular basis of cancer suppression by the retinoblastoma gene. Princess Takamatsu Symp 1989;20:159–70.
64. Prives C, Hall PA. The p53 pathway. J Pathol 1999;187:112–26.
65. Akashi M, Koeffler HP. Li-Fraumeni syndrome and the role of the p53 tumor suppressor gene in cancer susceptibility. Clin Obstet Gynecol 1998;41:172–99.
66. Oliner JD, Kinzler KW, Meltzer PS, et al. Amplification of a gene encoding a p53-associated protein in human sarcomas. Nature 1992;358:80–3.
67. Sharpless NE, DePinho RA. The INK4A/ARF locus and its two gene products. Curr Opin Genet Dev 1999;9:22–30.
68. Swanton C. Cell-cycle targeted therapies. Lancet Oncol 2004;5:27–36.
69. Dai Y, Grant S. Cyclin-dependent kinase inhibitors. Curr Opin Pharmacol 2003;3:362–70.
70. Senderowicz AM. Targeting cell cycle and apoptosis for the treatment of human malignancies. Curr Opin Cell Biol 2004;16:670–8.
71. Vermeulen K, Van Bockstaele DR, Berneman ZN. The cell cycle: a review of regulation, deregulation and therapeutic targets in cancer. Cell Prolif 2003;36:131–49.
72. Yu H, Jove R. The STATs of cancer—new molecular targets come of age. Nat Rev Cancer 2004;4:97–105.
73. Vassilev LT, Vu BT, Graves B, et al. In vivo activation of the p53 pathway by small-molecule antagonists of MDM2. Science 2004;303:844–8.
74. Robertson LE, Plunkett W, McConnell K, et at. Bcl-2 expression in chronic lymphocytic leukemia and its correlation with the induction of apoptosis and clinical outcome. Leukemia 1996;10:456–9.
75. Winter JN, Andersen J, Reed JC, et al. BCL-2 expression correlates with lower proliferative activity in the intermediate- and high-grade non-Hodgkin's lymphomas: an Eastern Cooperative Oncology Group and Southwest Oncology Group cooperative laboratory study. Blood 1998;91:1391–8.
76. Puthier D, Pellat-Deceunynck C, Barille S, et al. Differential expression of Bcl-2 in human plasma cell disorders according to proliferation status and malignancy. Leukemia 1999;13:289–94.
77. Sinicrope FA, Hart J, Michelassi F, Lee JJ. Prognostic value of bcl-2 oncoprotein expression in stage II colon carcinoma. Clin Cancer Res 1995;1:1103–10.
78 Berardo MD, Elledge RM, de Moor C, et al. bcl-2 and apoptosis in lymph node positive breast carcinoma. Cancer 1998;82:1296–302.
79. Mazel S, Burtrum D, Petrie HT. Regulation of cell division cycle progression by bcl-2 expression: a potential mechanism for inhibition of programmed cell death. J Exp Med 1996;183:2219–26.
80. O'Reilly LA, Huang DC, Strasser A. The cell death inhibitor Bcl-2 and its homologues influence control of cell cycle entry. EMBO J 1996;15:6979–90.
81. Vairo G, Innes KM, Adams JM. Bcl-2 has a cell cycle inhibitory function separable from its enhancement of cell survival. Oncogene 1996;13:1511–19.
82. Lipponen P, Pietilainen T, Kosma VM, et al. Apoptosis suppressing protein bcl-2 is expressed in well-differentiated breast carcinomas with favourable prognosis. J Pathol 1995;177:49–55.
83. Konopleva M, Zhao S, Hu W, et al. The anti-apoptotic genes Bcl-X(L) and Bcl-2 are over-expressed and contribute to chemoresistance of non-proliferating leukaemic CD34+ cells. Br J Haematol 2002;118:521–34.
84. Konopleva M, Tari AM, Estrov Z, et al. Liposomal Bcl-2 antisense oligonucleotides enhance proliferation, sensitize acute myeloid leukemia to cytosine-arabinoside, and induce apoptosis independent of other antiapoptotic proteins. Blood 2000;95:3929–38.
85. Opferman JT, Iwasaki H, Ong CC, et al. Obligate role of anti-apoptotic MCL-1 in the survival of hematopoietic stem cells. Science 2005;307:1101–4.
86. Carter BZ, Milella M, Altieri DC, Andreeff M. Cytokine-regulated expression of *survivin* in myeloid leukemia. Blood 2001;97:2784–90.
87. Andreeff M, Stone R, Michaeli J, et al. Hexamethylene bisacetamide in myelodysplastic syndrome and acute myelogenous leukemia: a phase II clinical trial with a differentiation-inducing agent. Blood 1992;80:2604–9.
88. Pandolfi PP. Histone deacetylases and transcriptional therapy with their inhibitors. Cancer Chemother Pharmacol 2001;48 Suppl 1:S17–9.
89. Jan YN, Jan LY. HLH proteins, fly neurogenesis, and vertebrate myogenesis. Cell 1993;75:827–30.
90. Gurdon JB. Embryonic induction—molecular prospects. Development 1987;99:285–306.
91. Yu JY, DeRuiter SL, Turner DL. RNA interference by expression of short-interfering RNAs and hairpin RNAs in mammalian cells. Proc Natl Acad Sci U S A 2002;99:6047–52.
92. Paddison PJ, Caudy AA, Bernstein E, et al. Short hairpin RNAs (shRNAs) induce sequence-specific silencing in mammalian cells. Genes Dev 2002;16:948–58.
93. McCaffrey AP, Meuse L, Pham TT, et al. RNA interference in adult mice. Nature 2002;418:38–9.
94. Miyagishi M, Taira K. U6 promoter-driven siRNAs with four uridine 3' overhangs efficiently suppress targeted gene expression in mammalian cells. Nat Biotechnol 2002;20:497–500.
95. Lin SL, Chuong CM, Ying SY. A Novel mRNA-cDNA interference phenomenon for silencing bcl-2 expression in human LNCaP cells. Biochem Biophys Res Commun 2001;281:639–44.
96. Sorrentino V, Pepperkok R, Davis RL, et al. Cell proliferation inhibited by MyoD1 independently of myogenic differentiation. Nature 1990;345:813–5.
97. Umek RM, Friedman AD, McKnight SL. CCAAT-enhancer binding protein: a component of a differentiation switch. Science 1991;251:288–92.
98. Tenen DG. Disruption of differentiation in human cancer: AML shows the way. Nat Rev Cancer 2003;3:89–101.
99. Kelly LM, Gilliland DG. Genetics of myeloid leukemias. Annu Rev Genomics Hum Genet 2002;3:179–98. Epub 2002 Apr 15:179–98.
100. Nerlov C. C/EBPalpha mutations in acute myeloid leukaemias. Nat Rev Cancer 2004;4:394–400.
101. Pabst T, Mueller BU, Zhang P, et al. Dominant-negative mutations of CEBPA, encoding CCAAT/enhancer binding protein-alpha (C/EBPalpha), in acute myeloid leukemia. Nat Genet 2001;27:263–70.
102. Gombart AF, Hofmann WK, Kawano S, et al. Mutations in the gene encoding the transcription factor CCAAT/enhancer binding protein alpha in myelodysplastic syndromes and acute myeloid leukemias. Blood 2002;99:1332–40.
103. Smith ML, Cavenagh JD, Lister TA, Fitzgibbon J. Mutation of CEBPA in familial acute myeloid leukemia. N Engl J Med 2004;351:2403–7.
104. Song WJ, Sullivan MG, Legare RD, et al. Haploinsufficiency of CBFA2 causes familial thrombocytopenia with propensity to develop acute myelogenous leukaemia. Nat Genet 1999;23:166–75.
105. Park DJ, Chumakov AM, Vuong PT, et al. CCAAT/enhancer binding protein epsilon is a potential retinoid target gene in acute promyelocytic leukemia treatment. J Clin Invest 1999;103:1399–408.
106. Amit M, Carpenter MK, Inokuma MS, et al. Clonally derived human embryonic stem cell lines maintain pluripotency and proliferative potential for prolonged periods of culture. Dev Biol 2000;227:271–8.
107. Smith AG. Embryo-derived stem cells: of mice and men. Annu Rev Cell Dev Biol 2001;17:435–62.
108. Risau W, Sariola H, Zerwes HG, et al. Vasculogenesis and angiogenesis in embryonic-stem-cell-derived embryoid bodies. Development 1988;102:471–8.
109. Weidner N, Carroll PR, Flax J, et al. Tumor angiogenesis correlates with metastasis in invasive prostate carcinoma. Am J Pathol 1993;143:401–9.
110. Weidner N, Semple JP, Welch WR, Folkman J. Tumor angiogenesis and metastasis—correlation in invasive breast carcinoma. N Engl J Med 1991;324:1–8.
111. Bernstein LR, Liotta LA. Molecular mediators of interactions with extracellular matrix components in metastasis and angiogenesis. Curr Opin Oncol 1994;6:106–13.
112. Mintz B, Fleischman RA. Teratocarcinomas and other neoplasms as developmental defects in gene expression. Adv Cancer Res 1981;34:211–78.
113. Dolle P, Ruberte E, Kastner P, et al. Differential expression of genes encoding alpha, beta and gamma retinoic acid receptors and CRABP in the developing limbs of the mouse. Nature 1989;342:702–5.
114. Bjornson CR, Rietze RL, Reynolds BA, et al. Turning brain into blood: a hematopoietic fate adopted by adult neural stem cells in vivo [comments]. Science 1999;283:534–7.
115. Kocher AA, Schuster MD, Szabolcs MJ, et al. Neovascularization of ischemic myocardium by human bone-marrow-derived angioblasts prevents cardiomyocyte apoptosis, reduces remodeling and improves cardiac function. Nat Med 2001;7:430–6.
116. Orlic D, Kajstura J, Chimenti S, et al. Bone marrow cells regenerate infarcted myocardium. Nature 2001;410:701–5.
117. Orlic D, Kajstura J, Chimenti S, et al. Mobilized bone marrow cells repair the infarcted heart, improving function and survival. Proc Natl Acad Sci U S A 2001;98:10344–9.
118. Pittenger MF, Mackay AM, Beck SC, et al. Multilineage potential of adult human mesenchymal stem cells. Science 1999;284:143–7.
119. Ferrari G, Cusella-De Angelis G, Coletta M, et al. Muscle regeneration by bone marrow-derived myogenic progenitors. Science 1998;279:1528–30.
120. Tamura H, Okamoto S, Iwatsuki K, et al. In vivo differentiation of stem cells in the aorta-gonad-mesonephros region of mouse embryo and adult bone marrow. Exp Hematol 2002;30:957–66.
121. Danet GH, Luongo JL, Butler G, et al. C1qRp defines a new human stem cell population with hematopoietic and hepatic potential. Proc Natl Acad Sci U S A 2002;99:10441–5.
122. Brittan M, Hunt T, Jeffery R, et al. Bone marrow derivation of pericryptal myofibroblasts in the mouse and human small intestine and colon. Gut 2002;50:752–7.
123. Krause DS, Theise ND, Collector MI, et al. Multi-organ, multi-lineage engraftment by a single bone marrow-derived stem cell. Cell 2001;105:369–77.
124. Kotton DN, Ma BY, Cardoso WV, et al. Bone marrow-derived cells as progenitors of lung alveolar epithelium. Development 2001;128:5181–8.
125. Mezey E, Chandross KJ, Harta G, et al. Turning blood into brain: cells bearing neuronal antigens generated in vivo from bone marrow. Science 2000;290:1779–82.
126. Eglitis MA, Mezey E. Hematopoietic cells differentiate into both microglia and macroglia in the brains of adult mice. Proc Natl Acad Sci U S A 1997;94:4080–5.
127. Korbling M, Katz RL, Khanna A, et al. Hepatocytes and epithelial cells of donor origin in recipients of peripheral-blood stem cells. N Engl J Med 2002;346:738–46.
128. Quaini F, Urbanek K, Beltrami AP, et al. Chimerism of the transplanted heart. N Engl J Med 2002;346:5–15.
129. Theise ND, Badve S, Saxena R, et al. Derivation of hepatocytes from bone marrow cells in mice after radiation-induced myeloablation. Hepatology 2000;31:235–40.
130. Ying QL, Nichols J, Evans EP, Smith AG. Changing potency by spontaneous fusion. Nature 2002;416:545–8.
131. Terada N, Hamazaki T, Oka M, et al. Bone marrow cells adopt the phenotype of other cells by spontaneous cell fusion. Nature 2002;416:542–5.
132. Wagers AJ, Sherwood RI, Christensen JL, Weissman IL. Little evidence for developmental plasticity of adult hematopoietic stem cells. Science 2002;297:2256–9.
133. Castro RF, Jackson KA, Goodell MA, et al. Failure of bone marrow cells to transdifferentiate into neural cells in vivo. Science 2002;297:1299.
134. Lebkowski JS, Gold J, Xu C, et al. Human embryonic stem cells: culture, differentiation, and genetic modification for regenerative medicine applications. Cancer J 2001;7 Suppl 2:S83–93.
135. Reubinoff BE, Pera MF, Fong CY, et al. Embryonic stem cell lines from human blastocysts: somatic differentiation in vitro. Nat Biotechnol 2000;18:399–404.
136. Lagasse E, Shizuru JA, Uchida N, et al. Toward regenerative medicine. Immunity 2001;14:425–36.
137. Eiges R, Schuldiner M, Drukker M, et al. Establishment of human embryonic stem cell-transfected clones carrying a marker for undifferentiated cells. Curr Biol 2001;11:514–8.
138. Kehat I, Kenyagin-Karsenti D, Snir M, et al. Human embryonic stem cells can differentiate into myocytes with structural and functional properties of cardiomyocytes. J Clin Invest 2001;108:407–14.
139. Odorico JS, Kaufman DS, Thomson JA. Multilineage differentiation from human embryonic stem cell lines. Stem Cells 2001;19:193–204.
140. Assady S, Maor G, Amit M, et al. Insulin production by human embryonic stem cells. Diabetes 2001;50:1691–7.
141. Kaufman DS, Hanson ET, Lewis RL, et al. Hematopoietic colony-forming cells derived from human embryonic stem cells. Proc Natl Acad Sci U S A 2001;98:10716–21.
142. Reubinoff BE, Itsykson P, Turetsky T, et al. Neural progenitors from human embryonic stem cells. Nat Biotechnol 2001;19:1134–40.
143. Zhang SC, Wernig M, Duncan ID, et al. In vitro differentiation of transplantable neural precursors from human embryonic stem cells. Nat Biotechnol 2001;19:1129–33.

144. Haynesworth SE, Goshima J, Goldberg VM, Caplan AI. Characterization of cells with osteogenic potential from human marrow. Bone 1992;13:81–8.
145. Lazarus HM, Haynesworth SE, Gerson SL, et al. Ex vivo expansion and subsequent infusion of human bone marrow-derived stromal progenitor cells (mesenchymal progenitor cells): implications for therapeutic use. Bone Marrow Transplant 1995;16:557–64.
146. Studeny M, Marini FC, Champlin RE, et al. Bone marrow-derived mesenchymal stem cells as vehicles for interferon-beta delivery into tumors. Cancer Res 2002;62:3603–8.
147. Studeny M, Marini FC, Dembinski J, et al. Mesenchymal stem cells: potential precursors for tumor stroma and targeted-delivery vehicles for anti-cancer agents. J Natl Cancer Inst 2004;96:1593–603.
148. Wille JJ Jr., Maercklein PB, Scott RE. Neoplastic transformation and defective control of cell proliferation and differentiation. Cancer Res 1982;42:5139–46.
149. Yuspa SH, Lichti U, Strickland J, et al. Aberrant regulation of differentiation in epidermal carcinogenesis. In: Colburn NH, Moses HL, Stanbridge EJ, editors. Growth factors, tumor promoters and cancer genes. New York: Liss; 1988. p. 183–9.
150. Rheinwald JG, Beckett MA. Defective terminal differentiation in culture as a consistent and selectable character of malignant human keratinocytes. Cell 1980;22:629–32.
151. Ekblom P, Vestweber D, Kemler R. Cell-matrix interactions and cell adhesion during development. Annu Rev Cell Biol 1986;2:27–47.
152. Petersen OW, Ronnov-Jessen L, Howlett AR, Bissell MJ. Interaction with basement membrane serves to rapidly distinguish growth and differentiation pattern of normal and malignant human breast epithelial cells [published erratum appears in Proc Natl Acad Sci U S A 1993;90(6):2556]. Proc Natl Acad Sci U S A 1992;89:9064–8.
153. Varticovski L, Druker B, Morrison D, et al. The colony stimulating factor-1 receptor associates with and activates phosphatidylinositol-3 kinase. Nature 1989;342:699–702.
154. Lemmon SK, Riley MC, Thomas KA, et al. Bovine fibroblast growth factor: comparison of brain and pituitary preparations. J Cell Biol 1982;95:162–9.
155. Rifkin DB, Moscatelli D. Recent developments in the cell biology of basic fibroblast growth factor. J Cell Biol 1989;109:1–6.
156. Rozengurt E. Early signals in the mitogenic response. Science 1986;234:161–6.
157. Todaro GJ, De Larco JE, Fryling C, et al. Transforming growth factors (TGFs): properties and possible mechanisms of action. J Supramol Struct Cell Biochem 1981;15:287–301.
158. Moses HL, Yang EY, Pietenpol JA. TGF-beta stimulation and inhibition of cell proliferation: new mechanistic insights. Cell 1990;63:245–7.
159. Peter M, Herskowitz I. Joining the complex: cyclin-dependent kinase inhibitory proteins and the cell cycle [comment]. Cell 1994;79:181–4.
160. Sherr CJ. G1 phase progression: cycling on cue [comments]. Cell 1994;79:551–5.
161. Twardzik DR, Ranchalis JE, McPherson JM, et al. Inhibition and promotion of differentiated-like phenotype of a human lung carcinoma in athymic mice by natural and recombinant forms of transforming growth factor-beta. J Natl Cancer Inst 1989;81:1182–5.
162. Perbal B. CCN proteins: multifunctional signalling regulators. Lancet 2004;363:62–4.
163. Xie D, Miller CW, O'Kelly J, et al. Breast cancer. Cyr61 is overexpressed, estrogen-inducible, and associated with more advanced disease. J Biol Chem 2001;276:14187–94.
164. Xie D, Yin D, Tong X, et al. Cyr61 is overexpressed in gliomas and involved in integrin-linked kinase-mediated Akt and beta-catenin-TCF/Lef signaling pathways. Cancer Res 2004;64:1987–96.
165. Xie D, Yin D, Wang HJ, et al. Levels of expression of CYR61 and CTGF are prognostic for tumor progression and survival of individuals with gliomas. Clin Cancer Res 2004;10:2072–81.
166. Sporn MB, Roberts AB, Goodman DS. The retinoids. New York: Academic; 1984. p. 56.
167. Glass CK, Devary OV, Rosenfeld MG. Multiple cell type-specific proteins differentially regulate target sequence recognition by the alpha retinoic acid receptor. Cell 1990;63:729–38.
168. Bennington JL. Cellular kinetics of invasive squamous carcinoma of the human cervix. Cancer Res 1969;29:1082–8.
169. Vasios GW, Gold JD, Petkovich M, et al. A retinoic acid-responsive element is present in the 5' flanking region of the laminin B1 gene. Proc Natl Acad Sci U S A 1989;86:9099–103.
170. Grignani F, De Matteis S, Nervi C, et al. Fusion proteins of the retinoic acid receptor-alpha recruit histone deacetylase in promyelocytic leukaemia. Nature 1998;391:815–8.
171. Marks P, Rifkind RA, Richon VM, et al. Histone deacetylases and cancer: causes and therapies. Nat Rev Cancer 2001;1:194–202.
172. Wang C, Fu M, Mani S, et al. Histone acetylation and the cell-cycle in cancer. Front Biosci 2001;6:D610–29.
173. Timmermann S, Lehrmann H, Polesskaya A, Harel-Bellan A. Histone acetylation and disease. Cell Mol Life Sci 2001;58:728–36.
174. He LZ, Guidez F, Tribioli C, et al. Distinct interactions of PML-RARalpha and PLZF-RARalpha with co-repressors determine differential responses to RA in APL. Nat Genet 1998;18:126–35.
175. Salomoni P, Pandolfi PP. Transcriptional regulation of cellular transformation. Nat Med 2000;6:742–4.
176. Warrell RP Jr., He LZ, Richon V, et al. Therapeutic targeting of transcription in acute promyelocytic leukemia by use of an inhibitor of histone deacetylase. J Natl Cancer Inst 1998;90:1621–5.
177. McLaughlin F, Finn P, La Thangue NB. The cell cycle, chromatin and cancer: mechanism-based therapeutics come of age. Drug Discov Today 2003;8:793–802.
178. Konopleva M, Andreeff M. Role of peroxisome proliferator-activated receptor-gamma in hematologic malignancies. Curr Opin Hematol 2002;9:294–302.
179. Patel L, Pass I, Coxon P, et al. Tumor suppressor and anti-inflammatory actions of PPARgamma agonists are mediated via upregulation of PTEN. Curr Biol 2001;11:764–8.
180. Demetri GD, Fletcher CD, Mueller E, et al. Induction of solid tumor differentiation by the peroxisome proliferator-activated receptor-gamma ligand troglitazone in patients with liposarcoma. Proc Natl Acad Sci U S A 1999;96:3951–6.
181. Holland PW, Hogan BL. Expression of homeo box genes during mouse development: a review. Genes Dev 1988;2:773–82.
182. Gehring WJ. Homeo boxes in the study of development. Science 1987;236:1245–52.
183. Castronovo V, Kusaka M, Chariot A, et al. Homeobox genes: potential candidates for the transcriptional control of the transformed and invasive phenotype. Biochem Pharmacol 1994;47:137–43.
184. Deschamps J, Meijlink F. Mammalian homeobox genes in normal development and neoplasia. Crit Rev Oncog 1992;3:117–73.
185. McCormick A, Campisi J. Cellular aging and senescence. Curr Opin Cell Biol 1991;3:230–4.
186. Singal R, Ginder GD. DNA methylation. Blood 1999;93:4059–70.
187. Bird AP, Wolffe AP. Methylation-induced repression—belts, braces, and chromatin. Cell 1999;99:451–4.
188. Momparler RL, Bovenzi V. DNA methylation and cancer. J Cell Physiol 2000;183:145–54.
189. Jones PA, Baylin SB. The fundamental role of epigenetic events in cancer. Nat Rev Genet 2002;3:415–28.
190. Esteller M, Corn PG, Baylin SB, Herman JG. A gene hypermethylation profile of human cancer. Cancer Res 2001;61:3225–9.
191. Baylin SB, Belinsky SA, Herman JG. Aberrant methylation of gene promoters in cancer—concepts, misconcepts, and promise. J Natl Cancer Inst 2000;92:1460–1.
192. Garcia-Manero G, Daniel J, Smith TL, et al. DNA methylation of multiple promoter-associated CpG islands in adult acute lymphocytic leukemia. Clin Cancer Res 2002;8:2217–24.
193. Issa JP. The epigenetics of colorectal cancer [discussion 153–5]. Ann N Y Acad Sci 2000;910:140–53.
194. Widschwendter M, Berger J, Hermann M, et al. Methylation and silencing of the retinoic acid receptor-beta2 gene in breast cancer. J Natl Cancer Inst 2000;92:826–32.
195. Esteller M, Guo M, Moreno V, et al. Hypermethylation-associated inactivation of the cellular retinol-binding-protein 1 gene in human cancer. Cancer Res 2002;62:5902–5.
196. Carlsson M, Totterman TH, Matsson P, Nilsson K. Cell cycle progression of B-chronic lymphocytic leukemia cells induced to differentiate by TPA. Blood 1988;71:415–21.
197. Gorstein F, Thor A. Tumor markers in diagnostic pathology. In: Gorstein F, Thor A, editors. Clinics in laboratory medicine. Philadelphia: Saunders; 1990.
198. Hainsworth JD, Johnson DH, Greco FA. Poorly differentiated neuroendocrine carcinoma of unknown primary site. A newly recognized clinicopathologic entity. Ann Intern Med 1988;109:364–71.
199. Reiss M, Gamba-Vitalo C, Sartorelli AC. Induction of tumor cell differentiation as a therapeutic approach: preclinical models for hematopoietic and solid neoplasms. Cancer Treat Rep 1986;70:201–18.
200. Waxman S, Rossi GB, Takaku F. The status of differentiation therapy of cancer. New York: Raven Press; 1988.
201. Grandgirard D, Studer E, Monney L, et al. Alphaviruses induce apoptosis in Bcl-2-overexpressing cells: evidence for a caspase-mediated, proteolytic inactivation of Bcl-2. EMBO J 1998;17:1268–78.
202. Andreeff M, Stone R, Michaeli J, et al. Hexamethylene bisacetamide in myelodysplastic syndrome and acute myelogenous leukemia: a phase II clinical trial with a differentiation-inducing agent. Blood 1992;80(10):2604–9.
203. Breitman TR, Collins SJ, Keene BR. Terminal differentiation of human promyelocytic leukemic cells in primary culture in response to retinoic acid. Blood 1981;57:1000–4.
204. Castaigne S, Chomienne C, Daniel MT, et al. All-trans retinoic acid as a differentiation therapy for acute promyelocytic leukemia. I. Clinical results. Blood 1990;76:1704–9.
205. Warrell RP Jr, Frankel SR, Miller WH Jr, et al. Differentiation therapy of acute promyelocytic leukemia with tretinoin (all-trans-retinoic acid). N Engl J Med 1991;324:1385–93.
206. Chabner BA. Biological basis for cancer treatment [comment]. Ann Intern Med 1993;118:633–7.
207. Cheson BD, Jasperse DM, Chun HG, Friedman MA. Differentiating agents in the treatment of human malignancies. Cancer Treat Rev 1986;13:129–45.
208. Andreeff M, Jiang S, Zhang X, et al. Expression of Bcl-2-related genes in normal and AML progenitors: changes induced by chemotherapy and retinoic acid. Leukemia 1999;13:1881–92.
209. Hong WK, Lippman SM, Itri LM, et al. Prevention of second primary tumors with isotretinoin in squamous-cell carcinoma of the head and neck [comments]. N Engl J Med 1990;323:795–801.
210. Meyskens FL Jr. Coming of age—the chemoprevention of cancer [editorial and comments]. N Engl J Med 1990;323:825–7.
211. Rowley JD, Aster JC, Sklar J. The clinical applications of new DNA diagnostic technology on the management of cancer patients. JAMA 1993;270:2331–7.

4

Apoptosis and Cancer

John C. Reed, MD, PhD

Programmed cell death plays critical roles in a wide variety of physiologic processes during fetal development and in adult tissues. In most cases, physiologic cell death occurs by a process known as "apoptosis." Defects in apoptotic cell death contribute to neoplastic diseases, by preventing or delaying normal cell turnover, thus promoting cell accumulation. Defects in apoptosis also facilitate tumor progression, by rendering cancer cells resistant to death mechanisms relevant to metastasis, hypoxia, growth factor-deprivation, chemotherapy, and irradiation. Knowledge of the molecular mechanisms responsible for the regulation and execution of apoptosis has provided insights into the pathobiology of cancer and has suggested a variety of novel therapeutic strategies that may eventually improve the efficacy of cancer treatment.

It is now well established that defects in the normal mechanisms that control programmed cell death (PCD) occur commonly in cancers. Cell numbers in the body are governed not only by cell division, which determines the rate of cell production, but also by cell death, which sets the rate of cell loss. In the course of a typical day, an average adult produces, and in parallel eradicates ~50 to 70 billion cells, representing approximately 1 million cells per second. Normally, these two processes of cell division and cell death are tightly coupled so that no net increase in cell numbers occurs, or so that such increases represent only temporary responses to environmental stimuli. However, alternations in the expression or function of the genes that control PCD can upset this delicate balance, contributing to the expansion of neoplastic cells.[1,2]

Defects in normal programmed cell death mechanisms play a major role in the pathogenesis of tumors (Table 4-1), allowing neoplastic cells to survive beyond their normally intended lifespans, subverting the need for exogenous survival factors, providing protection from hypoxia and oxidative stress as tumor mass expands, and allowing time for accumulative genetic alterations that deregulate cell proliferation, interfere with differentiation, promote angiogenesis, and increase cell motility and invasiveness during tumor progression. In fact, apoptosis defects are recognized as an important complement to proto-oncogene activation, as many deregulated oncoproteins that drive cell division also trigger apoptosis (eg, Myc; E1a; cyclinD1).[3] Defects in apoptosis facilitate metastasis by allowing epithelial cells to survive in a suspended state, without attachment to extracellular matrix.[4] They also promote resistance to the immune system, in as much as many of the weapons cytolytic T cells (CTL) and natural killer (NK) cells use for attacking tumors depend on integrity of the apoptosis machinery.[5] Finally, cancer-associated defects in apoptosis play a role in chemoresistance and radioresistance, increasing the threshold for cell death, and thereby requiring higher doses for tumor killing.[6,7] Thus, defective apoptosis regulation is a fundamental aspect of the biology of cancer.

Table 4-1 Cancer and Apoptosis: Pathogenesis, Progression, Therapy Resistance

Cell accumulation (cell death < cell division)
Longevity (accumulation of genetic lesions)
Proto-oncogene tolerance (nullify pro-apoptotic effects)
Genomic instability (tolerate DNA mistakes)
Immune surveillance (resistance to immune attack)
Growth factor/hormone-independence (survival without paracrine/endocrine growth factors)
Angiogenesis (resistance to hypoxia; hypoglycemia)
Metastasis (survival without attachment)
Chemoresistance/radioresistance (increased threshold for cell death)

Apoptosis is defined by its morphologic features. As viewed with the assistance of the light- (or preferably electron-) microscope, the characteristics of the apoptotic cell include chromatin condensation and nuclear fragmentation (pyknosis), plasma membrane blebbing, and cell shrinkage. Eventually, the cell breaks into small membrane-surrounded fragments (apoptotic bodies), which are cleared by phagocytosis, without inciting an inflammatory response. The release of apoptotic bodies is what inspired the term "apoptosis" from the Greek, meaning "to fall away from" and conjuring notions of the falling of leaves in the autumn from deciduous trees.[8]

In recent years, the molecular machinery responsible for apoptosis has been elucidated, revealing a family of intracellular proteases, caspases, which are responsible directly or indirectly for the morphologic and biochemical changes that characterize the phenomenon of apoptosis.[9,10] Diverse regulators of the caspases have also been discovered, including activators and inhibitors of these cell death proteases. Inputs from signal transduction pathways into the core of the cell death machinery have also been identified, demonstrating ways of linking environmental stimuli to cell death responses or cell survival maintenance. Knowledge of the molecular mechanisms of apoptosis is providing insights into the pathogenesis and progression of cancer, and is beginning to suggest new approaches to the treatment of neoplastic diseases.

In this chapter, some of the genes involved in apoptosis regulation are described, and examples of cancer-associated defects in the expression or regulation of those genes or their encoded proteins are provided. In addition, some of the emerging strategies for restoring apoptosis sensitivity to tumors based on pharmacologic manipulation of cell death proteins are explained.

APOPTOSIS CAUSED BY CASPASES

What causes the morphologic changes that we recognize as "apoptosis" and the biochemical changes often associated with this phenomenon? The answer is proteases. Specifically, activation of a family of intracellular cysteine proteases which cleave their substrates at aspartic acid residues, known as "caspases" for cysteine aspartyl-specific proteases.[11] These proteases are present as inactive zymogens in essentially all animal cells, but can be triggered to assume active states, generally involving their proteolytic processing at conserved aspartic acid (Asp) residues. During activation, the zymogen pro-proteins are cleaved to generate the large (~ 20 kDa) and small (~10 kDa) subunits of the active enzymes, typically liberating an N-terminal prodomain from the processed polypeptide chain. The active enzymes consist of heterotetramers composed of two large and two small subunits, with two active sites per molecule.[9,10]

The observation that Caspases cleave their substrates at Asp residues, and that they are also activated by proteolytic processing at Asp residues, makes evident that these proteases collaborate in proteolytic cascades, where Caspases activate themselves and each other. Humans contain 11 Caspases. They can be subgrouped according to either their amino-acid sequence similarities or their protease specificities. From a functional perceptive, it is useful to view the Caspases as either upstream "initiator" Caspases or downstream "effector" Caspases.[12] The zymogen forms of upstream initiator Caspases possess large N-terminal pro-domains, which function as protein interaction modules, allowing them to interact with various proteins that trigger Caspase activation. In contrast, the proforms of downstream effector Caspases contain only short N-terminal pro-domains, serving no apparent function. Downstream Caspases are largely dependent on upstream Caspases for their proteolytic processing and activation. The substrates of effector Caspases include protein kinases (often separating the auto-repressing regulatory domains from catalytic domains) and other signal transduction proteins, cytoskeletal and nuclear matrix proteins, chromatin-modifying (eg, poly-ADP-ribose polymerase) and DNA repair proteins, and inhibitory subunits of endonucleases (CIDE-family proteins).[9,10,12]

Inactivating mutations in genes encoding Caspases in human malignancies have been reported. For example, homozygous deletions of the *CASPASE-3* gene were identified in MCF7 cells, a breast cancer cell line commonly employed as an experimental model.[13] Similarly, missense mutations in the *CASPASE-8* gene have been documented, as well as gene silencing in association with hyper-methylation of CpG islands, in neuroblastomas and some other types of solid tumors.[14,15] Frame-shift mutations that disrupt the reading-frame of the *Caspase-5* gene have been cited in colon cancers that have microsatellite instability (MSI), a DNA mismatch repair enzyme defect associated with mutations in homopolymeric stretches of nucleotides throughout the genome.[16] Thus, precedence exists for cancer-associated mutations in Caspase-encoding genes, presumably contributing to apoptosis-resistance states. However, because of redundancy in the 11 member Caspase-family of humans, these defects do not prevent apoptosis altogether, leaving alternative routes to apoptosis intact.

Caspase Activation Pathways: an Overview Several pathways for activating Caspases exist, although details remain sketchy for some of them (Figure 4-1). The simplest is exploited by CTL cells and NK cells, which introduce apoptosis-inducing proteases, particularly granzyme B, into effective intracellular compartments of target cells via perforin-dependent mechanisms.[17] Unlike the Caspases, granzyme B is a serine protease. However, similar to the Caspases, granzyme B specifically cleaves its substrates at Asp residues. Granzyme B is capable of cleaving and activating multiple Caspases and some Caspase substrates.[18] Endogenous and viral inhibitors of granzyme B have been identified, accounting for resistance to this apoptosis inducer.[19–21]

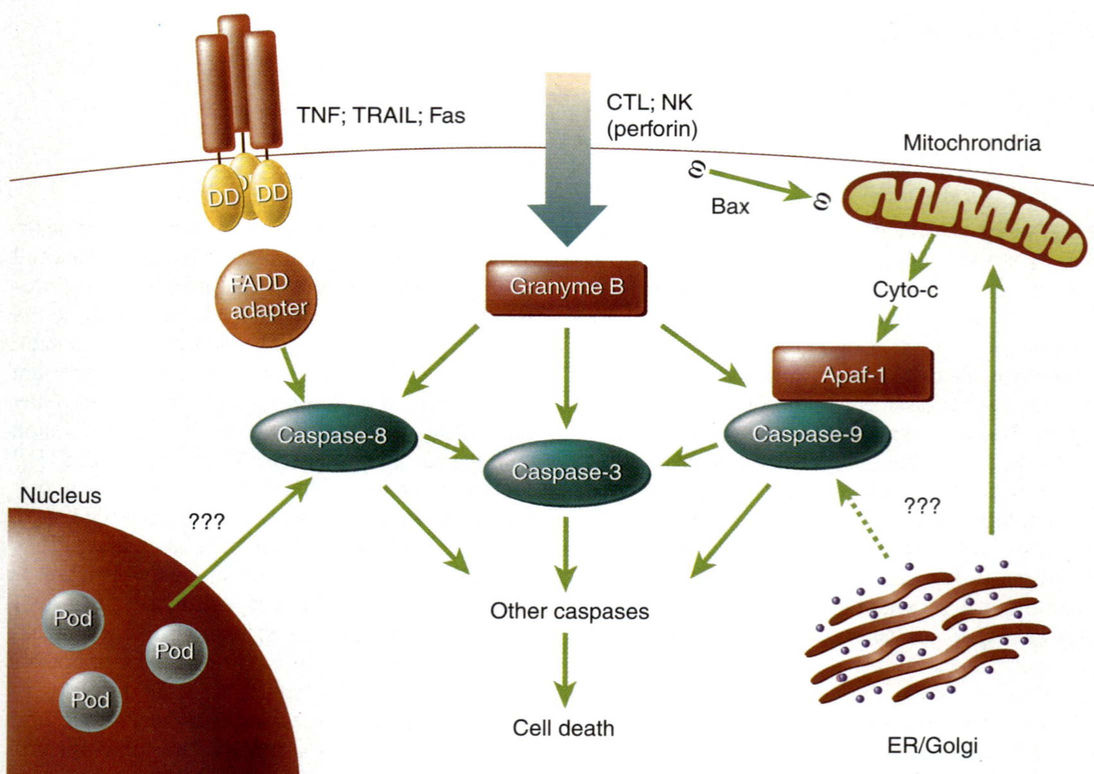

Figure 4-1 Pathways for Caspase activation. The major pathways for Caspase activation in mammalian cells are presented. The extrinsic (*left*) is induced by members of the TNF-family of cytokine receptors such as TNFR1, Fas, and the TRAIL receptors. These proteins recruit adapter proteins to their cytosolic death domains, including FADD, which then bind death effector domain-containing pro-Caspases, particularly pro–Caspase-8, inducing their activation. Cytolytic T cells and natural killer cells introduce the protease granzyme B into target cells (*middle*). This protease cleaves and activates multiple members of the Caspase family. The intrinsic pathway (*right*) is initiated by release of cytochrome *c* from mitochondria, induced by various stimuli, including elevations in the levels of pore-forming pro-apoptotic Bcl-2 family proteins such as Bax. In the cytosol, cytochrome *c* binds and activates APAF-1, allowing it to be associated with and activate pro–Caspase-9. Active Caspase-9 (intrinsic) and Caspase-8 (extrinsic) have been shown to directly cleave and activate the effector protease, Caspase-3. Other Caspases also become involved in these pathways (not shown), thus the schematic represents an over simplification of the events that occur in vivo. Poorly defined pathways linking nuclear structures called PML oncogenic domains (PODs) (*lower left*) and stress in the Golgi and endoplasmic reticulum (ER) (*lower right*) to Caspase activation have also been described.

Another Caspase-activation pathway is represented by tumor necrosis factor (TNF)-family receptors. Eight of the ~30 known members of the TNF family in humans contain a so-called death domain (DD) in their cytosolic tails.[22] Several of these DD-containing TNF-family receptors use Caspase-activation as a signaling mechanism, including TNFR1/CD120a; Fas/APO1/CD95; DR3/Apo2/Weasle; DR4/TrailR1; DR5/TrailR2; and DR6. Ligation of these receptors at the cell surface results in receptor clustering and recruitment of several intracellular proteins, including certain pro-Caspases, to the cytosolic domains of these receptors, forming a "death-inducing signaling complex" (DISC) that triggers Caspase activation and leads to apoptosis.[23,24] The specific Caspases summoned to the DISC are Caspase-8 and, in some cases, Caspase-10. These Caspases contain so-called death effector domains (DEDs) in their N-terminal prodomains that bind to a corresponding DED in FADD, a bipartite adapter protein containing a DD and a DED. FADD functions as a molecular bridge between the DD and DED domain families, and is in fact the only protein in the human genome with this dual domain structure.[25] Consequently, cells from mice in which the *FADD* gene has been knocked out are resistant to apoptosis induction by TNF-family cytokines and their receptors.[26] Cells derived from *Caspase-8* knock-out mice also fail to undergo apoptosis in response to ligands or antibodies that activate TNF-family death receptors, demonstrating an essential role for this Caspase in this pathway.[27] However, mice lack the highly homologous protease, Caspase-10, which is found in humans, having arisen from an apparent gene duplication on chromosome.[2,25] Thus, it is presently unclear to what extent Caspase-8 and -10 display redundancy in human cells.

Mitochondria also play important roles in apoptosis, releasing cytochrome *c* (cyt *c*) into the cytosol, which then causes assembly of a multiprotein Caspase-activating complex, referred to as the "apoptosome."[28,29] The central component of the apoptosome is APAF1, a Caspase-activating protein that oligomerizes upon binding cyt *c* and which specifically binds pro–Caspase-9. APAF1 and pro–Caspase-9 interact with each other via their caspase recruitment domains (CARDs). Such CARD-CARD interactions play important roles in many steps in apoptosis pathways. In addition to cyt *c,* mitochondria also release several other proteins of relevance to apoptosis, including endonuclease G, AIF (an activator of nuclear endonucleases), and Smac (Diablo) and Omi (HtrA2), antagonists of a family of Caspase-inhibitory proteins known as the IAPs (see below). However, the central importance of the cyt *c*–dependent pathway for apoptosis is underscored by the observation that cells derived from mice in which either the *apaf1* or *pro–Caspase-9* genes have been ablated are incapable of undergoing apoptosis in response to agents that trigger cyt *c* release from mitochondria.[30] Nevertheless, such cells can die by nonapoptotic routes, demonstrating that mitochondria control both Caspase-dependent and Caspase-independent cell death pathways.[31] The mitochondrial pathway for apoptosis is activated by myriad stimuli, including growth factor deprivation, oxidants, $Ca2^{+}$ over-load, DNA-damaging agents, and microtubule-modifying drugs.[29,32]

Mitochondria can also participate in cell death pathways induced via TNF-family death receptors, through cross-talk mechanisms involving proteins such as Bid, BAR, and Bap31.[33–36] However, mitochondrial ("intrinsic") and death receptor ("extrinsic") pathways for Caspase activation are fully capable of independent operation in most types of cells.[37]

A Caspase activation pathway linked to endoplasmic reticulum (ER)/Golgi stress has been proposed. In the mouse, evidence has been presented, based on gene ablation studies, that suggests the possibility that Caspase-12 represents the apical Caspase linked to this pathway.[38] However, humans lack a functional Caspase-12 ortholog, due to the presence of a stop codon early in the open reading frame.[39] A connection between Caspase-2 and the Golgi has also been suggested but details are unclear.[40] Both Caspase-2 and -12 are CARD-carrying proteins, but little is known presently about the adapter proteins that bind their CARDs and that control activation of these proteases.

Finally, a nuclear pathway for apoptosis regulation may exist which centers on discrete nuclear organelles, called PML oncogenic domains (PODs) or nuclear bodies (NBs). Targeted ablation of the *pml* gene in mice results in general resistance to apoptosis through an unknown mechanism.[41] Several proteins that can promote apoptosis have been localized to PODs, including Daax, Zip Kinase, and Par4.[42–46] How these nuclear structures are linked to Caspase activation pathways is unknown. PML was first identified because of its fusion to the retinoic acid receptor (*RAR*) gene in t(15;17) chromosomal translocations found in acute promyelomonocytic leukemias, where it disrupts PODs and creates an apoptosis-resistant state.[47]

Although diverse mechanisms exist for activating initiator Caspases, as outlined above, in most instances the biochemical mechanisms appear to be remarkably similar. Much of Caspase activation and can be explained by the "induced proximity model".[48] The induced-proximity model is predicated on the empiric observation that the zymogen forms of unprocessed Caspases are not entirely inactive but rather possess weak protease activity (measured in some cases at ~1% of the fully active enzymes). When brought into close apposition through protein interactions, the zymogens can trans-process each other, producing the fully active proteases. This mechanism is clearly operative in the Caspase-activation pathways induced by TNF-family receptors (extrinsic pathway) and cyt *c*/mitochondria ("intrinsic pathway").

PROTEIN DOMAINS INVOLVED IN APOPTOSIS REGULATION

The proteins that directly control the intrinsic, extrinsic, and other less understood Caspase activation pathways often exist as families that can be recognized based on their amino acid sequences and/or structural similarity. Moreover, interactions among these proteins are commonly mediated by domains that are intimately associated with apoptosis regulation, including CARDs, DDs, DEDs, Bcl-2 Homology (BH) domains of Bcl-2 family proteins, and Baculovirus IAP Repeat (BIR) domains of IAP-family proteins. A summary of some of the proteins that constitute these families of apoptosis regulators follows, along with information about their mechanisms; examples of alterations in cancer, and strategies for exploiting the information for devising new cancer therapies.

Death Domain Proteins The DD is a protein interaction module consisting of a compact bundle of six helices.[49] DDs bind each other, probably forming oligomers of unknown stoichiometry. Specificity for partner selection among DDs is dictated by differences in surface residues. Several of the members of the TNF-family of cytokine receptors contain DDs in their cytosolic regions, including TNFR1, Fas [Apo1], DR3 [Apo2], DR4 [Trail-R1], DR5 [Trail-R2], DR6 in humans, mice, and probably other mammals. The p75 nerve growth factor receptor (p75-NGFr) also contains a modified ("type II") DD,[50] and has been reported to induce apoptosis under some circumstances.[51]

The TNF-family receptors, TNFR1, DR3, and DR6 are known to bind an adapter protein TRADD, via its homologous DD.[52–55] The DD of TRADD is capable of binding certain other DD-containing proteins, including the adapter protein FADD. The FADD (Mort1) protein contains two protein interaction modules, a DD and a DED. FADD links TNF-family death receptors to Caspases, using its DD to bind TRADD or to interact directly with the cytosolic DD of the TNFR-family member Fas, and employing its DED to bind DED-containing Caspases. Experimental evidence has demonstrated the presence of FADD within the receptor complexes of all known DD-containing members of the TNF-family except p75-NGFr. Thus, this protein plays a central role in linking Caspases to TNF-family death receptors, a notion borne out by gene ablation studies in mice, which have demonstrated an inability of TNFR1, Fas, and other death receptors tested thus far to induce apoptosis in the absence of FADD.[26,56–58]

The TNF family receptors member, Fas (Apo1; CD95) is a potent inducer of apoptosis. Fas plays a critical role in immune system homeostasis, eradicating potentially autoreactive lymphocytes and down-regulating immune responses after elimination of foreign antigen by reducing the numbers of expanded clones of antigen-specific T-cells and B cells in peripheral lymphoid organs.[22,59,60] Germ line mutations in Fas and Fas-Ligand (FasL) have been discovered as the underlying basis for the lymphoproliferative autoimmune phenotype of *lpr/lpr* and *gdl/gdl* strain mice, respectively.[61,62] Similarly, causative mutations have been identified in the *FAS* gene of humans in patients with autoimmune lymphoproliferative syndrome (ALPS). Thus, the Fas/FasL system plays a critical role in lymphocyte homeostasis in vivo. FasL is also a principal weapon used by cytolytic T cells for inducing apoptosis of virus-infected, tumorigenic, and allogenic cells.[60] Unfortunately, pre-clinical liver toxicity has precluded attempts to apply FasL or agonistic anti-Fas antibodies for the treatment of cancer.[63]

At least some of the mutant Fas proteins found in humans with ALPS have been shown to operate as trans-dominant inhibitors of wild-type Fas, probably explaining the dominant inheritance pattern of this disorder. In contrast, mutations in the *fas* gene of *lpr*-strain mice produce a similar autoimmune lymphoproliferative disorder with a recessive inheritance pattern.[61] FasL, like most TNF family members, is a trimer, and the receptor probably also forms trimers and perhaps higher-order oligomers, thus explaining why some Fas mutants display dominant-negative effects on wild-type Fas whereas others do not. Indeed, mutant versions of Fas from some patients with hereditary ALPS have been demonstrated to antagonize wild-type Fas, probably forming mixed oligomers of wild-type and mutant molecules.[64]

Somatic mutations in the *FAS* gene have been found in multiple myelomas and non-Hodgkin lymphomas. In a study of 150 cases of non-Hodgkin lymphomas (NHLs) where the coding regions of the gene were systematically sequenced, *FAS* gene mutations were found in 16 (11%) of the tumors.[65] Missense mutations within the death domain of the receptor were associated with retention of the wild-type allele, suggesting a dominant-negative mechanism, whereas missense mutations outside the death domain were associated with allelic loss.[65]

Fas expression confers important prognostic information for some patients with leukemia. The *FAS* gene encodes two protein isoforms through alternative mRNA splicing: full-length Fas which has a transmembrane domain and a soluble form of Fas that lacks this transmembrane domain.[66] Soluble Fas is secreted into the extracellular environment where it acts as a decoy and binds FasL. As such, soluble Fas is an inhibitor of apoptosis. In a study of 59 patients with adult T-cell leukemia, increased serum levels of soluble Fas were associated with reduced survival and remained an important predictor in multivariate analysis even after accounting for other clinical risk factors.[67] Higher levels of soluble Fas in serum have also been correlated with disease progression and advanced clinical stage in B-CLL.[68,69] In addition to squelching Fas-induced apoptosis through secretion of soluble Fas, another suppressor of Fas, called DcR3, has been identified that is overexpressed in some tumors. DcR3 represents a member of the TNF-family that competes with Fas for binding to Fas L but which lacks a DD and does not transduce apoptotic signals, functioning as a "decoy" receptor.[70]

TRAIL is a TNF-family ligand that has shown promise for the treatment of cancer. Unlike many other TNF-family cytokines, TRAIL does not induce inflammatory reactions and appears to be well tolerated in preclinical animal models, provided the recombinant protein is prepared in a careful manner.[71] The version of TRAIL that seems likely to be used in humans is a soluble trimer, representing the extracellular domain of TRAIL. TRAIL induces apoptosis via two DD-containing receptors, TRAIL-R1 (DR4) and TRAIL-R2 (DR5). In addition to these death receptors, however, at least three TNF-family proteins have been identified that compete for binding to TRAIL, but which do not deliver death signals into cells. These "decoy" receptors, include DcR1, DcR2, and osteoprotegerin (OPG) (Figure 4-2).[70] It has been speculated that differences in the ratios of death and decoy receptors explain the selective toxicity of TRAIL to tumor cells versus normal cells, although this is probably not always true, representing an over-simplification of the mechanisms that account for the observed differential sensitivity to TRAIL. Agonistic antibodies to the TRAIL-receptor, DR4, have recently completed phase I clinical trials for cancer (<http:/hgs.com>), and similar antibodies that bind DR5 and that trigger tumor cell apoptosis have demonstrated promising results in preclinical animal models.[72] The observation that tumor suppressor p53 can induce transcription of the death receptors Fas and DR5 in some types of tumor cells,[73,74] may explain in part the synergistic antitumor activity in mouse models reported when combining cytotoxic anticancer drugs with TNF-family death ligands or agonistic antibodies that bind TNF-family death receptors.[75]

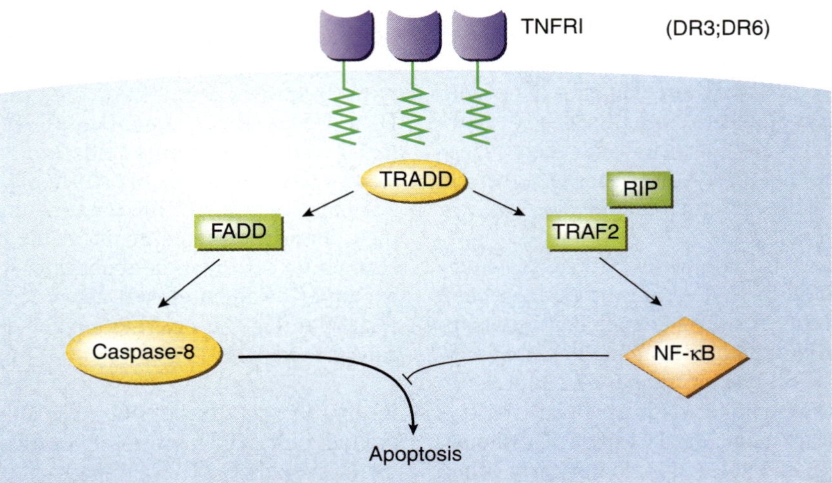

Figure 4-3 Opposing pathways for cell death and cell survival are induced by tumor necrosis factor (TNF)-family receptors. Several TNF-family receptors simultaneously engage parallel pathways for apoptosis and apoptosis-suppression, including TNFR1, DR3, and DR6. The death domain (DD)-containing adapter protein TRADD binds DDs in the cytosolic domains of TNF-family receptors. TRADD can associate with FADD, which in turn binds Caspase-8 and -10, triggering their activation. However, TRADD can also bind RIP and TRAFs, inducing activation of protein kinases that leads to NFκB activation. NFκBii family transcription factors induce expression of several anti-apoptotic genes. Some TNF-family receptors activate only one of these two pathways. For example, Fas and TRAIL-receptors induce Caspase activation but fail to interact with the proteins required for NFκB responses. Conversely, multiple TNF-family receptors, including TNFR2, CD30, and CD40 activate the NFκB pathway, but do not recruit TRADD or FADD to their cytosolic domains (not shown).

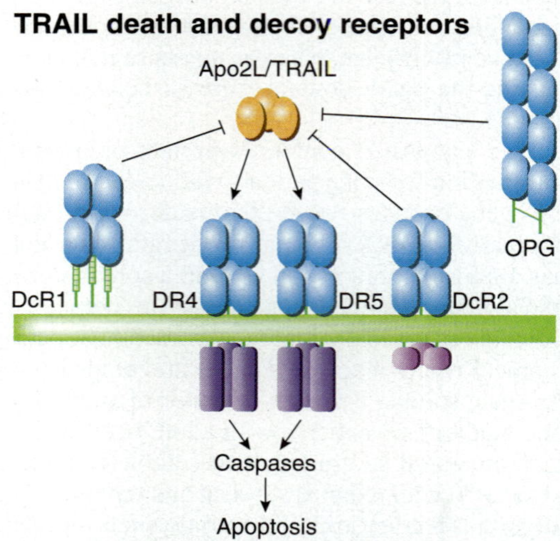

Figure 4-2 TRAIL receptors. In humans, five receptors have been identified for TRAIL. Two of these, DR4 (TRAIL-R1) and DR5 (TRAIL-R2), are transmembrane proteins containing cytosolic death domains (DDs) that engage the Caspase activation machinery. The others function as "decoys," competing for binding to TRAIL but lacking the capacity to signal into the cell death pathway. DcR1 is a GPI-linked protein, attached to the membrane via lipid modification. DcR2 is a transmembrane protein containing a non-function, truncated DD. Osteoprotegerin is a secreted protein. Differences in the ratios of TRAIL-binding death and decoy receptors may account in some cases for differential sensitivity of normal and tumor cells to this death-ligand.

Besides the DD-containing TNF-family receptors, additional DD-containing proteins have been implicated in apoptosis, such as the DAP kinase, which modulates apoptosis induction by TNF-family death receptors through unclear mechanisms.[76] This kinase has been implicated in suppression of metastasis. Several cytoskeleton-associated ankyrin-family proteins contain DDs, but their relevance to apoptosis remains uncertain. Given evidence however that Caspase-8 activation is triggered by suspension of adherent epithelial cells,[77,78] an event that disturbs the cytoskeleton, it is intriguing to speculate a possible role in the phenomenon of "anoikis" (ie, apoptosis induced by depriving cells of integrin-mediated attachments to extracellular matrix). Avoidance of anoikis represents an important aspect of tumor invasion, metastasis, and angiogenesis.[79] It is also fundamental to correct positioning of cells during development, possibly accounting for the embryonic lethality of *fadd* and *Caspase-8* gene ablation in mice.

Death domains, however, are not always involved in Caspase activation. In fact, some of the signal transduction pathways in which non-Caspase-activating DD-proteins are involved indirectly regulate apoptosis through effects on NFκB, suppressing rather than inducing apoptosis. For example, the RIP protein, binds TRADD and activates kinases that induce degradation of IκB, thus releasing NFκB so that it can translocate to the nucleus and fulfill its function as a transcription factor.[80–82] Among NFκB-inducible genes are several that block apoptosis, including anti-apoptotic Bcl-2 family members Bfl-1 (A1) and Bcl-X, and IAP (inhibitor of apoptosis proteins)-family member cIAP2 and possibly cIAP1 and XIAP, and FLIP, an endogenous antagonist of Caspase-8 and -10.[51,83–87] The dual function of TRADD, as a partner for both Caspase-activator FADD and NFκB activator RIP, causes many of the TNF-family receptors to self-nullify their apoptosis-inducing activity (Figure 4-3). Thus, TNFR1, DR3, and DR6 are uncertain apoptosis inducers, unless NFκB induction is inhibited, in which case they typically elicit robust apoptotic responses.[88,89] In contrast, Fas and the Trail-receptors DR4 and DR5 only rarely activate NFκB, probably because these receptors complexes contain FADD but not TRADD.[57,58,90,91] In fact, it is because TRAIL receptors (DR4; DR5) do not induce NFκB-mediated pro-inflammatory

TNF induces apoptotic and anti-apoptotic pathways responses in vivo that TRAIL is under consideration for clinical use in the treatment of cancer, whereas NFκB-inducing TNF proved to be unacceptable.

Death Effector Domain (DED) Proteins

The structure of the DED is similar to the DD, comprised of 6 helices.[92] DEDs are found in Caspase-8 and -10 in humans. The pro-domain regions of pro–Caspase-8 and -10 contain two tandem DEDs, which are responsible for their interactions with the DED of FADD, thus mediating their recruitment to death receptor complexes. Multiple DED-containing modulators of apoptosis have been identified, some of which enhance and others that inhibit Caspase-activation by TNF-family death receptors.[93] Among these, the DED-containing protein FLIP (also known as Flame, CASH, Clarp, MRIT, Casper, I-Flice, Usurpin) has emerged as an important suppressor

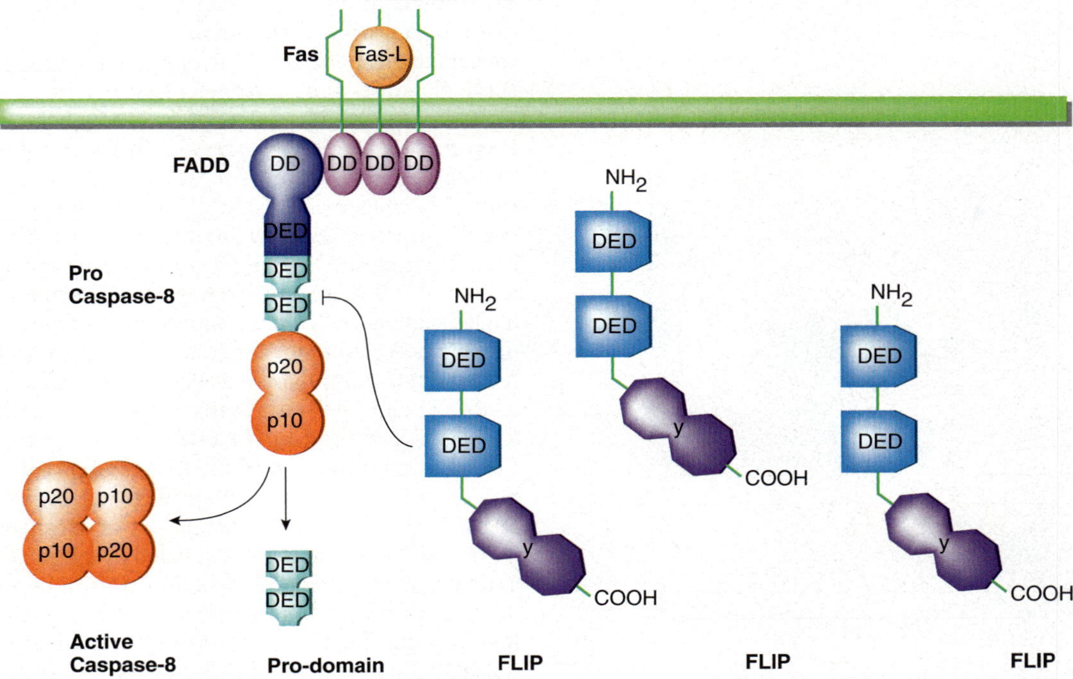

Figure 4-4 Suppression of Fas-signaling by FLIP. The tumor necrosis factor (TNF)-family receptor Fas contains a cytosolic death domain (DD) that binds the bipartite adapter protein, FADD. The DD of FADD interacts with Fas, and its death effector domain (DED) binds the DEDs in pro–Caspase-8. Recruitment of pro–Caspase-8 to clustered receptors on the plasma membrane induces proteolytic processing and activation of pro–Caspase-8, releasing the active protease into the cytosol. FLIP contains DED domains that compete for binding to pro–Caspase-8 and FADD, squelching signaling by Fas. Over-expression of FLIP occurs in many cancers.

of apoptosis in cancer (Figure 4-4). FLIP shares extensive amino-acid sequence similarity with pro–Caspase-8 and -10, containing two N-terminal DEDs followed by a pseudo-Caspase domain that lacks critical residues required for protease activity, including the catalytic cysteine.[94,95] FLIP associates with pro–Caspase-8 and also competes with pro–Caspase-8 and -10 for binding to FADD, thus squelching death receptor signaling. Interestingly, some tumors have been reported to contain inappropriately elevated levels of FLIP, rendering them resistant to apoptosis induction by Fas-expressing cytolytic T cells.[96] FLIP-mediated resistance to Fas may even allow tumor cells to tolerate expressing FasL, using this death ligand as a weapon against neighboring normal cells and triggering apoptosis of immune cells.[97–99] Down-regulation of FLIP using antisense oligonucleotides or drugs that reduce FLIP protein levels can restore sensitivity of tumor cell lines to apoptosis induced by TRAIL or FasL,[100,101] suggesting opportunities for improved cancer therapy. The mechanisms responsible for increased expression of FLIP in tumors are unknown. Because FLIP is an NFκB-inducible gene,[102] tumor-associated increases in NFκB activity may play a role.

CARD-Family Proteins Several pro-Caspases contain N-terminal CARDs in their prodomains, including Caspase-1, -2, -4, -5, -9 in humans. The overall structure of the CARD is similar to DDs and DEDs, comprised of 6 helices.[103–106] Homotypic interactions among CARD-carrying proteins play important roles in Caspase activation throughout animal evolution. One of the paradigms used for Caspase activation is embodied in CED-4/Apaf-1 family proteins. These proteins contain a CARD domain in combination with a nucleotide-binding oligomerization domain, known as an NBARC[107] domain (Nucleotide-Binding domain homologous to Apaf-1, CED-4 and plant R gene products).[108] The N-terminal CARDs of Apaf-1 in humans and CED-4 in the nematode *Caenorhabditis elegans (C. elegans)* mediate interactions with the CARDs of specific initiator caspases, pro–Caspase-9 and pro–CED-3, respectively.[109–111] Oligomerized APAF-1 and CED-4 activate Caspases by the induced proximity mechanism.[112–114]

With the CED-4 protein of *C. elegans,* binding and activation of the Caspase pro–CED-3 is spontaneous. In contrast, the human APAF-1 protein contains, in addition, regulatory domain comprised of several WD repeat domains, which renders it dependent on cyt *c*.28, [115] Biochemical analysis of human Apaf-1 using in vitro reconstituted systems with purified components indicates that cyt *c,* in combination with dATP, induces oligomerization of APAF-1 molecules, followed by binding to and activation of pro–Caspase-9.[113,114] Several mechanisms for suppressing Caspase-activation by APAF-1 have been identified in tumors, including: (1) expression of a splice variant that produces a shorter, non-catalytic isoform of pro–Caspase-9 that can compete with full-length pro–Caspase-9 for binding APAF-1; (2) phosphorylation of human Caspase-9 by the kinases Akt or Erk1/2; (3) over-expression of heat shock proteins, that bind either APAF-1 or pro–Caspase-9; (4) over-expression of TUCAN, a CARD-containing antagonist of Caspase-9 that prevents its association with APAF1; (5) Caspase-9-binding IAP-family proteins; (6) over-expression of heat shock proteins; (7) silencing of the *APAF1* gene by methylation; and (8) alkalinization of the cytosol, induced probably by the Na^+-H^+ exchanger in response to protein kinases activated by growth factors.[116–122]

Besides regulating Caspase activation, several CARD-family proteins have been reported to induce or inhibit NFκB activation. For example, *BCL-10* (also known as huE10 and CIPER) is a gene initially identified because of its involvement in chromosomal translocations found in lymphomas that arise in mucosal areas (MALTomas).[123] Bcl-10 induces NFκB activation, and ablation of the *bcl-10* gene in mice precludes NFκB activation via antigen receptors in T- and B-lymphocytes.[124] Mutant versions of Bcl-10 have been reported in cancers, although the frequency of such gene mutations is debated.[123,125,126] These truncated forms of Bcl-10 display NFκB-inducing activity and manifest transforming activity in classic rodent cell-based assays in vitro.[123]

IAP Family Proteins The IAPs (inhibitor of apoptosis proteins) represent a family of evolutionarily conserved apoptosis suppressors.[127–129] Although these proteins can interact with a variety of biochemical pathways in cells, the fundamental mechanisms of action of IAP-family proteins is direct suppression of Caspases—acting as endogenous inhibitors of the cell death proteases.[127]

IAPs are found in the genomes of mammals, insects, and certain animal viruses. All members of this family, by definition, contain at least one copy of a so-called BIR *(baculovirus iap repeat)* domain, a zinc-binding fold,[130–132] which is important for their anti-apoptotic activity. In addition to 1 to 3 copies of a BIR domain, many IAP family proteins also contain other domains, including RING zinc-fingers, CARDs, ubiquitin-conjugating enzyme (E2s) domains, or putative nucleotide-binding domains. Interestingly, the RINGs of IAPs have recently been implicated in interactions with the cellular components of the ubiquitination machinery,[133] thus controlling turnover of these proteins and other proteins with which they associate. Also, the BIR-containing protein, Apollon (Bruce), contains a domain with ubiquitin-conjugating enzyme (E2) activity, further suggesting links of BIR-family proteins to the cellular ubiquitination machinery.[134] Although IAP-family proteins all contain BIR domains, the mere presence of a BIR domain does not necessarily indicate anti-apoptotic activity. For example, BIR-containing proteins which regulate mitosis and meiosis, but which have no apparent effect on cell death regulation, have been described in yeast and *C. elegans*.[135,136]

Several IAPs have been shown to bind and potently inhibit activated Caspases. Among the Caspases inhibited by human IAP family members XIAP, cIAP1, and cIAP2 are the effector Caspase-3 and -7, as well as the initiator Caspase-9.[137–139] (Figure 4-5) In the case of XIAP, it was shown that the second BIR domain and the linker

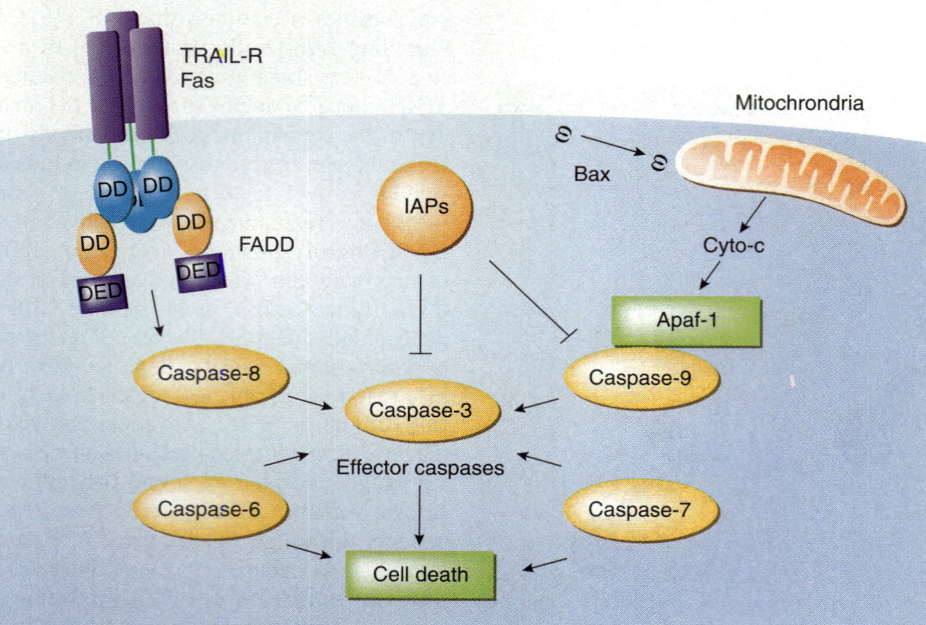

Figure 4-5 Caspase-suppression by inhibitor of apoptosis proteins (IAP) family proteins. Several IAP-family proteins in humans have been shown to directly bind and inhibit Caspases. XIAP, cIAP1, and cIAP2, for example, can inhibit active Caspase-3 and Caspase-7, representing downstream effector Caspases that function at the convergence of apoptosis pathways. XIAPs, cIAP1, cIAP2, and Livin also inhibit active Caspase-9, the apical protease in the mitochondrial pathway for apoptosis.

region between BIR1 and BIR2 are required for binding and suppressing Caspase-3 and -7, whereas the third BIR domain binds Caspase-9.[130,140–142] Thus, different domains in the multi-BIR containing IAPs are responsible for suppression of different Caspases. IAP family member, Livin (ML-IAP), contains a single BIR and inhibits Caspase-9 but not Caspase-3 and -7.[143] Survivin also contains a single BIR and reportedly associates with Caspase-9, although its mechanism of Caspase suppression is poorly defined.[144] IAPs are selective Caspase inhibitors, and lack activity against many members of the Caspase-family of cell death proteases. Thus, over-expression of IAPs may block some apoptosis pathways but not others. This stands in marked contrast to the baculovirus p35 protein, an apoptosis suppressor that displays broad activity against Caspases, but for which no cellular homolog has been identified.[19] Nevertheless, human IAPs such as XIAP can arrest apoptosis induced via either the intrinsic (mitochondrial) or extrinsic (death receptor) pathways, probably because they target effector caspases which are common to both pathways (see Figure 4-5).[142]

Over-expression of IAP-family gene has been documented in cancers. For example, over-expression of the IAP-member *Survivin* has been observed in many common types of cancer.[145] Survivin is highly expressed in the developing fetus but largely absent from normal adult tissues.[146] Through unclear mechanisms, Survivin becomes over-expressed in cancers. Indeed, genome-wide transcription profiling suggests that *Survivin* is among the most tumor-specific genes thus far identified.[147] The promoter of the *Survivin* gene is normally cell cycle-regulated, becoming activated specifically in late G2/M-phase.[148] Moreover, the Survivin protein is associated with the chromosomes during mitosis and the mitotic spindle apparatus, where it appears to play a critical role in ensuring proper control chromosome segregation during anaphase and in the final execution of cytokinesis. Suppression of *Survivin* expression using antisense methods or dominant-inhibitory mutants results in polyploidy, aneuploidy, and apoptosis.[149] Apparent Survivin orthologs in yeast and *C. elegans* also participate in cell cycle regulation but lack effects on cell life/death,[136,150] suggesting that *Survivin* evolved this function later as a possible way of creating a cell cycle checkpoint that ensures apoptotic elimination of cells, which fail to properly sort their genetic material during cell division.

Elevated expression of other IAP-family members in cancer also occurs.[151] For example, Livin (ML-IAP; KIAP; Ts-IAP; ILP2) is scarcely expressed in normal tissues but reportedly found at high levels in melanomas or renal cancers.[143,152,153] Examples of over-expression of XIAP, cIAP1, and cIAP2 in cancers have also been reported, sometimes in association with adverse clinical outcome.[127,128] Antisense-mediated reductions on XIAP or cIAP1 can induce apoptosis of tumor cell lines in culture, or sensitize cells to cytotoxic anticancer drugs. Although its overall relevance to apoptosis remains uncertain, antisense-mediated down-regulation of IAP-family member Apollon can sensitize tumor cell lines to apoptosis induced by anticancer drugs.[154] These types of antisense experiments provide proof of concept evidence that the pathological elevations of IAPs found in cancers are important for maintaining tumor cell survival and resistance to chemotherapy.

Endogenous antagonists of the IAPs help to keep these apoptosis-suppressors in check, promoting apoptosis. Two of these naturally-occurring IAP-antagonists, SMAC (Diablo) and HtrA2 (Omi), are sequestered inside mitochondria, becoming released into the cytosol during apoptosis.[155,156] SMAC and HtrA2 have N-terminal leader sequences that are removed by proteolysis upon import into mitochondria, exposing a novel tetra-peptide motif that binds the BIR domains of IAPs. These IAP-antagonists compete with Caspases for binding to IAPs, thus freeing Caspases from the grip of the IAPs and promoting apoptosis. Synthetic peptides that mimic SMAC and HtrA2 induce apoptosis or sensitize tumor cell lines to apoptosis induced by cytotoxic anticancer drugs.[157–159] Structural information derived from high-field NMR and x-ray crystallography indicate that a tetra-peptide motif is sufficient to bind the BIRs of IAPs, suggesting a path to drug discovery where small-molecule chemical compounds that occupy the same tetra-peptide–binding motif on BIRs can be envisioned as new apoptosis-sensitizing agents for cancer. It remains to be determined whether tumors down-regulate expression of their endogenous IAP-antagonists such as SMAC and HtrA2 as a strategy for achieving apoptosis resistance.

BCL-2 Family Proteins The mitochondria-dependent pathway for apoptosis is governed by Bcl-2-family proteins. Bcl-2, Bcl-X^L, Bak, and many other members of the Bcl-2-family have a hydrophobic stretch of amino-acids near their carboxyl-terminus that anchors them in the outer mitochondrial membrane.[29] In contrast, other Bcl-2-family members such as Bid, Bim, and Bad lack these membrane-anchoring domains, but target to mitochondria in response to specific stimuli. Still others have the membrane-anchoring domain but keep it latched against the body of the protein, until stimulated to expose it (eg, Bax).[160]

Bcl-2 family proteins are conserved throughout metazoan evolution, with homologs found in vertebrate and invertebrate animal species. Several types of animal viruses also harbor Bcl-2 family genes within their genomes, including herpes simplex viruses implicated in cancer such as the Epstein-Barr Virus (EBV) and Kaposi sarcoma herpes virus (KSHV). Both pro-apoptotic and anti-apoptotic Bcl-2 family proteins have been delineated.[161–165] The relative ratios of anti- and pro-apoptotic Bcl-2 family proteins dictate the ultimate sensitivity or resistance of cells to various apoptotic stimuli, including growth factor deprivation, hypoxia, radiation, anticancer drugs, oxidants, and $Ca2^+$ overload.

Alterations in the amounts of these proteins have been associated with cancer, including excess expression of anti-apoptotic and reduced expression of pro-apoptotic *BCL-2*-family genes.[166] For example, the *BCL-2* gene (anti-apoptotic) is activated by chromosomal translocations in the majority of non-Hodgkin lymphomas[167,168] and is also inappropriately over-expressed in many solid tumors, contributing to resistance to chemotherapy- and radiation-induced apoptosis.[169] Conversely, loss-of-function mutations have been identified in the *BAX* genes (pro-apoptotic) of human tumors[170] and analysis of *bax* -/- knock-out mice indicates that *bax* is a tumor suppressor in vivo.[171] Transcription of the human *BAX* gene is also directly regulated by p53, thus providing another connection of this important tumor suppressor to apoptosis pathways.[172]

In humans, 26 members of the Bcl-2 family gene family have been identified (<http://apoptosis-db.org>). These genes encode the anti-apoptotic proteins, Bcl-2, Bcl-X^L, Mcl-1, Bfl-1 (A1), Bcl-W, and Bcl-B (Boo;Diva), as well as the pro-apoptotic proteins Bax, Bak, Bok (Mtd), Bad, Bid, Bim, Bik, Hrk, Bcl-X^S, APR (Noxa), PUMA, p193, Bcl-Gs, Bcl-rambo (Mil), Nip3, and Nix (BNIP). Some of the Bcl-2 family genes produce two or more proteins through alternative mRNA splicing, sometimes exerting opposing effects on cell death regulation (eg Bcl-X^L versus Bcl-X^S). Gene ablation studies in mice suggest that each of the Bcl-2 family members plays unique roles in controlling cell survival in vivo, reflecting their tissue-specific patterns of expression or cell-context-dependent requirements for these proteins.

Based on their predicted (or experimentally determined) 3-dimensional structures, Bcl-2 family proteins can be broadly divided into two groups. One subset of these proteins is probably similar in structure to the pore-forming domains of bacterial toxins, such as the colicins and diphtheria toxin.[173–176] These helical pore-like proteins include both anti-apoptotic proteins (Bcl-2, Bcl-X^L, Mcl-1, Bfl-1, Bcl-W, and possibly Boo), as well as pro-apoptotic proteins (Bax, Bak, Bok, and Bid). Most of the proteins in this subcategory can be recognized by conserved stretches of amino-acid sequence homology, including the presence of Bcl-2 Homology (BH) domains, BH1, BH2, BH3, and sometimes BH4. However, this is not uniformly the case, as the Bid protein contains only a BH3 domain but has been determined to share the same overall protein-fold with Bcl-X^L, Bcl-2, and Bax.[174,175] Where tested to date, these proteins have all been shown to form ion-conducting channels in synthetic membranes in vitro, including Bcl-2, Bcl-X^L, Bax, and Bid.[177–181]

The other subset of Bcl-2 family proteins appears to have in common only the presence of the BH3 domain, including Bad, Bik, Bim, Hrk, Bcl-GS, p193, APR (Noxa), and PUMA. These "BH3-only" proteins are uniformly pro-apoptotic. Their cell death-inducing activity depends, in most cases, on their ability to dimerize with anti-apoptotic Bcl-2 family members, functioning as trans-dominant inhibitors of proteins such as Bcl-2 and Bcl-X^L.[165,182] However, one of these proteins (eg, Bid) can also dimerize with pro-apoptotic proteins (eg, Bax; Bak), functioning as an agonist of the killers, in addition to dimerizing with anti-apoptotics (eg, Bcl-2; Bcl-X^L), functioning as an antagonist (Figure 4-

Functional and physical interactions of Bcl-2 family proteins

BH3 only — Bcl-2 Bcl-X_L — Bax Bak → Cell death

Bid Bim

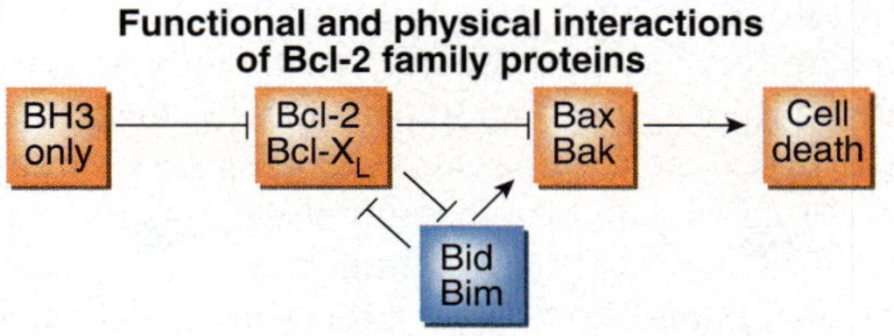

Figure 4-6 Network of interactions among Bcl-2-family proteins. The functional and physical interactions among Bcl-2-family proteins are depicted.

6).[183,184] Binding of Bid to Bax or Bak promotes their insertion into and oligomerization in membranes, apparently forming large pores through which molecules such as cyt *c*, SMAC, and Omi can escape from mitochondria.[185,186]

The BH3 domain has been shown to mediate dimerization among Bcl-2 family proteins. This domain consists of an amphipathic a-helix of ~16 amino-acids length that inserts into a hydrophobic crevice on the surface of anti-apoptotic proteins such as Bcl-X^L.[187] Thus, mutations in the BH3 domain of proteins such as Bad, Bik, Bim, Bcl-GS, and Hrk that abolish their ability to bind other Bcl-2 family members also abrogate their capacity to induce apoptosis. Proof-of-concept experiments performed with synthetic peptides representing the BH3 domain have suggested a path forward in terms of drug discovery. For example, BH3 peptides directed against anti-apoptotic proteins over-expressed in cancers (eg, Bcl-2; Bcl-X^L) can restore sensitivity to apoptosis, at least in vitro.[188] Accordingly, small-molecule chemical compounds have been delineated that interact with the same BH3-binding pocket on Bcl-2 and Bcl-X^L, nullifying their cytoprotective actions, and promoting tumor cell apoptosis.[189–191] It remains to be determined whether these BH3 mimicking compounds can be sufficiently optimized to take them forward into clinical trials.

The BH3-only proteins link a wide-variety of environmental stimuli to the mitochondrial pathway for apoptosis (Figure 4-7). For example, the transcription factor p53 directly induces expression of BH3-only proteins Noxa (APR) and PUMA,[192–194] thus linking p53 to the death machinery. The BH3-only protein BFM is associated with the actin cytoskeleton.[195] Circumstances that perturb the cytoskeleton, such as cell detachment from extracellular matrix, release BFM, allowing it to dimerize with anti-apoptotic proteins on the surface of mitochondria and induce apoptosis. Thus, BFM may represent an important defense mechanism against metastasis. Bid is cleared by Caspase-8 in the context of signaling by apoptosis-inducing TNF-family receptors, removing the N-terminal 52 amino-acids and exposing both the BH3 dimerization domain, as well as generating a novel N-terminus that becomes myristoylated, facilitating targeting of the Bid protein into membranes.[34,181,196,197]

This Caspase-8-mediated activation of Bid represents an important mechanism accounting for cross-talk between the death receptor (extrinsic) and mitochondrial (intrinsic) pathways. Isoforms

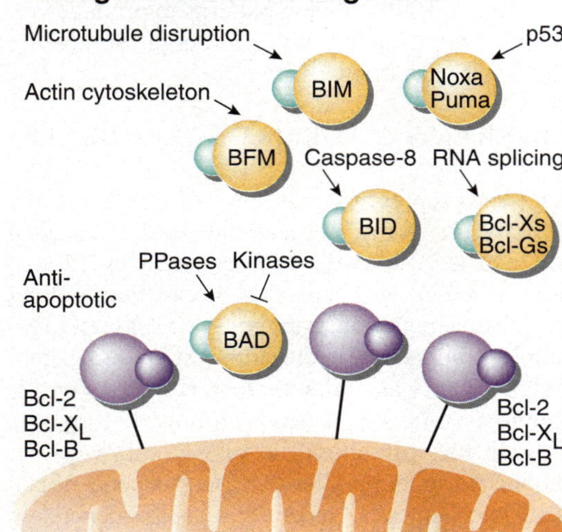

Figure 4-7 BH3-only proteins link cell-death stimuli to the mitochondrial pathway for apoptosis. Multiple proapoptotic BH3-only proteins have been identified that dimerize with and antagonize anti-apoptotic Bcl-2 family proteins such as Bcl-2 and Bcl-X^L on the surface of mitochondria. BFM associates with the actin cytoskeleton but is released when the cytoskeleton is disrupted, translocating to mitochondria. BFM may be important therefore for apoptosis that results when cells detach from extracellular matrix. This cause of apoptosis has been termed "anoikis." Longer isoforms of BIM associate with proteins that bind microtubules. Disruption of microtubules therefore may release BIM. The BAD protein is regulated by phosphorylation. Several kinases, including Akt, have been reported to phosphorylate and thereby inhibit dimerization of BAD with Bcl-X^L. Phosphatases counteract this effect, and activate BAD, allowing it to induce apoptosis. BID is cleaved by Caspase-8 in the context of apoptosis induction by tumor necrosis factor (TNF)-family death receptors. The uncleaved BID protein is inactive in the cytosol, whereas cleavage produces a truncated protein that targets mitochondrial membranes and dimerizes with other Bcl-2 family proteins. NOXA and PUMA are proteins whose expression is induced by p53. The activation of p53 is induced by DNA damage, thus linking DNA-damage (caused for example by anticancer drugs or x-irradiation) to apoptotic responses. Bcl-Gs and Bcl-X^S are apoptosis-inducing apoptosis proteins produced as a results of alternative mRNA splicing. Longer forms of these proteins lack pro-apoptotic activity. Switching to production of the short forms promotes apoptosis.

of the BH3-only protein, Bim, associate with microtubules via direct binding to microtubule-associated dynein light-chain (DLC).[198] Disruption of these protein interactions frees microtubule-associated isoforms of Bim, allowing them to dimerize via the BH3 domain with anti-apoptotic Bcl-2 family proteins on the surface of mitochondria. The BH3-only protein Bad translocates between the cytosol and mitochondria, depending on whether it is phosphorylated. Several protein kinases, including Akt (PKB), PKA, Raf1, Rsk1, and Pak1 have been reported to phosphorylate BAD, thus inactivating the protein so that it cannot dimerize with and antagonize Bcl-2 or Bcl-X^L.[199,200] Evidence has been presented that BAD is inactivated by this phosphorylation mechanism in many cancers. Finally, expression of some pro-apoptotic Bcl-2 family proteins is controlled at the level of mRNA splicing, with specific signals switching mRNA splicing patterns to produce versions of the proteins with pro-apoptotic activity (eg, Bcl-X^S; Bcl-Gs).[201,202]

ALTERNATIVE FORMS OF CELL DEATH

Apoptosis represents only one cell death mechanism. Necrosis is a Caspase-independent route of cell demise, typically characterized by loss of osmotic stability of cells, with organellar swelling and plasma membrane rupture. The release of intracellular components to the extracellular milieu generally triggers an inflammatory response, unlike apoptosis. Many cell death stimuli that operate through the mitochondrial or ER pathways for apoptosis trigger parallel caspase-independent cell death mechanisms. Generally, Caspase-dependent kills faster than the Caspase-independent mechanisms, but Caspase-suppressors (either pharmacological or endogenous) can unmask the latter, and thus result in non-apoptotic cell death. Caspase-independent mediators of non-apoptotic cell death that are released by mitochondria include the endonuclease endo-G, the flavoprotein apoptosis inducing factor (AIF), a modulator of transcription factors called Bit, and other proteins.[203] How the ER induced Caspase-independent cell death is uncertain, but liberation of $Ca2^+$ from the lumen of this organelle is likely to be involved, which can have several downstream consequences, including activation of calpain-family cysteine proteases and induction of $Ca2^+$—dependent swelling and rupture of mitochondria.[204]

Besides apoptosis and necrosis, autophagic cell death has recently been recognized as a route of cellular demise with relevance to cancer. Autophagy is an evolutionarily conserved process whereby intracellular macromolecules and organelles are encased in a membranous vesicle (the autophagosome) for delivery to lysosomes, where the sequestered cargo undergoes degradation and recycling into anabolic pathways. At least in yeast for which the genetics of this pathway have been worked out in some detail, autophagy is induced under times of nutrient deprivation, allowing cells to generate ATP through catabolism of organelles and other cellular structures. Although autophagy evolved in eukaryotes as a survival mechanism, autophagy has been associated with nonapoptotic cell death.[205] Malignant cells often display abnormally low levels of autophagy.[206,207]The connection between cancer and decreased autophagy was solidified with the discovery that the *BECLIN1* gene locus, which is mutated in 40 to 75% of prostate, breast, and ovarian cancers,[206,207] encodes an evolutionarily conserved component of the autophagic machinery.[208,209]Unlike many tumor suppressors, biallelic inactivation of the *BECLIN1* locus has not been observed, suggesting that partial loss (ie, haploinsufficiency) of the Beclin-1 protein is positively selected during tumorigenesis but that complete loss of Beclin-1 function is not compatible with tumor progression. Interestingly, Beclin binds Bcl-2,[210] and several other proteins of the apoptotic and autophagic cell death machinery. In this regard, recent data suggest that autophagy and apoptosis may be antagonistic processes, because caspases have been reported to suppress the autophagic program in tumor cells.[211] If true, then it may be important to understand how cancer therapies predicated on induction of apoptosis interact with the autophagy machinery of cells.

SIGNAL TRANSDUCTION AND APOPTOSIS DYSREGULATION IN CANCER

In addition to genes that encode "core" components of the apoptosis machinery, tumor-associated alterations have been identified in genes that provide important regulatory inputs into the expression of apoptosis genes or the regulation of their encoded proteins. This includes many transcription factors and growth factor receptors. However, ultimately, many of these signaling molecules funnel into common pathways linked to the apoptosis machinery. Two prominent examples are described here, namely, NFκB and Akt. For more comprehensive summaries of signal transduction inputs into the core apoptosis machinery, the reader is referred to recent reviews.[182,212–215]

NFκB NFκB represents a family of transcription factors, comprising the REL gene family. NFκB directly binds the promoters and induces expression of several anti-apoptotic genes, including the *BCL-2* family members *BCL-X* and *BFL-1,* the IAP-family member *C-IAP2,* and the DED-family gene *C-FLIP.*[216] Thus, elevations in NFκB activity can increase cellular resistance to apoptosis, affecting (1) the Intrinsic (mitochondrial) pathway through elevations in anti-apoptotic Bcl-2 family proteins, (2) the Extrinsic (TNF-family death receptor) pathway through upregulation of FLIP, and (3) downstream common pathways involving effector Caspases, as a result of over-expression of cIAP2. Recent data demonstrate hyperactivity of NFκB in many solid and hematopoietic malignancies.[217]

The first example of NFκB involvement in malignancy was provided by studies of the avian Rev-T retrovirus, a transforming retrovirus that causes rapidly fatal lymphomas in young chickens and that carries the v-Rel oncogene. The cellular homolog of this viral oncogene is *C-REL,* which encodes the p65 subunit of NFκB. Amplification of the *C-REL* gene has been reported in NHLs, occurring in ~23% of diffuse large B-cell lymphoma and commonly associated with extranodal presentation.[218] Other genetic alterations associated with dysregulation of NFκB include chromosomal translocations involving the IκB family member *BCL-3* in B-CLL.[219] IκB family proteins bind and sequester NFκB complexes, preventing the transcription factor from entering the nucleus. Typically, IκB is regulated by ubiquitin-mediated turnover by the 26s proteasome. Mutations in IκB thus may enhance NFκB activity, either by producing unstable proteins or reducing the affinity of IκB for NFκB. The anticancer

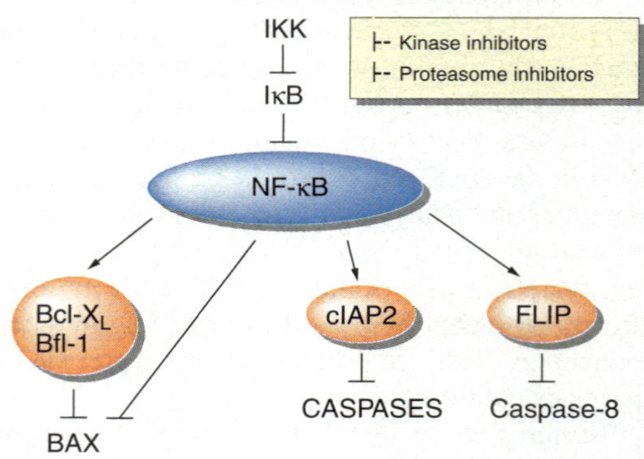

Figure 4-8 Apoptosis-suppressing mechanisms of NFκB. NFκB-family transcription factors induce the expression of multiple anti-apoptotic genes, including *BCL-2* family members *BCL-X and BFL1 (A1)*, inhibitor of apoptosis proteins (IAP) family member *C-IAP2,* and Caspase-8 antagonist, *FLIP.* NFKB can also suppress expression of pro-apoptotic gene *BAX,* in some tumor cells. NFκB activation can be induced by at least two pathways. The "classical" pathway is presented, showing NFκB under suppression by IκB-family proteins. IκBs are targeted for ubiquitination and proteasome-dependent degradation when phosphorylated by IκB kinases (IκKs). Several types of upstream kinases can activate the IκKs. Drugs that inhibit IκKs, as well as proteasome inhibitory drugs, represent novel approaches for interfering with NFκB activation in tumor cells.

activity of drugs that inhibit the proteasome, currently in human clinical trials, may be attributable in part to suppression of IκB degradation, thereby inhibiting NFκB induction.[220] Kinases that induce phosphorylation of IκB, a prerequisite for ubiquitination and subsequent degradation, also have emerged as attractive drug-discovery targets (Figure 4-8).

AKT The protein kinase Akt (PKB) plays important roles in linking growth factor receptors and oncoproteins to apoptosis pathways (Figure 4-9). The murine gene encoding Akt was first discovered by virtue of its similarity to the *v-akt* oncogene found in some murine leukemia viruses and through its activation in thymomas caused by retrovirus insertions near the *c-akt* gene.[221] Humans contain three *AKT* genes. Akt can phosphorylate multiple proteins within the core apoptosis machinery, some of which have been mentioned above. For example, the pro-apoptotic Bcl-2 family member BAD is a target of Akt, where phosphorylation of BAD inhibits its ability to heterodimerize with Bcl-X^L.[200] Akt also can phosphorylate human Caspase-9, blocking apoptosis down-stream of mitochondria.[117] Another substrate of Akt that is relevant to apoptosis is forkhead transcription factors (FKHD). Some FKHD family members appear to control apoptosis, perhaps by affecting transcription of the gene encoding FasL.[222] Phosphorylation of FKHD by Akt prevents its entry into the nucleus. Akt may also play a role in NFκB activation.[223] Moreover, Akt has been implicated in suppression of Nur77 (TR3), an orphan member of the retinoid/steroid family of transcription factors implicated in apop-

Akt (PKB) suppresses apoptosis by multiple mechanisms

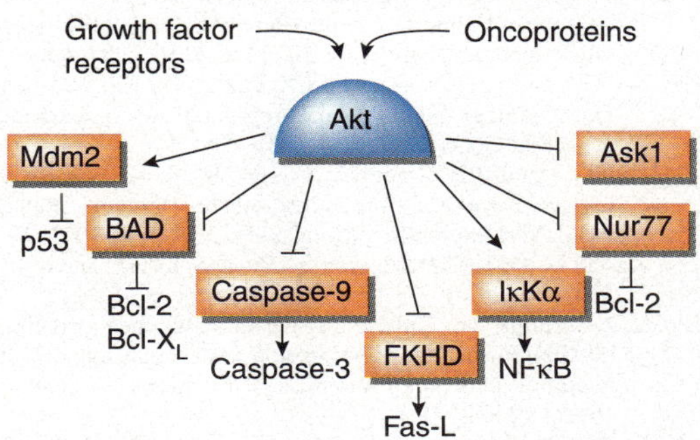

Figure 4-9 Apoptosis substrates of Akt. The protein kinase Akt (PKB) is activated in response to second-messagers produced by PI3K, a lipid kinase that is activated by many growth factor receptors and oncoproteins. PTEN is a lipid phosphatase that prevents accumulation of these second messagers, the expression of which is lost in many tumors through gene deletions, gene mutations, and other mechanisms.[227] Akt can phosphorylate and either activate (*arrows*) or inactivate (⊥) multiple proteins directly or indirectly relevant to apoptosis[226]. Phosphorylation of BAD prevents dimerization with Bcl-X^L. Phosphorylation of human pro–Caspase-9 suppresses its activation, as well as reducing cellular activity of processed (active) Caspase-9. Phosphorylation of forkhead family transcription factors by Akt results in their sequestration in the cytosol, preventing their transcriptional induction of pro-apoptotic gene such as *FasL*. Akt may also phosphorylate and suppress Nur77 (TR3), an orphan member of the retinoid/steroid family of transcription factors implicated in apoptosis induction. Akt may also enhance NFκB activity, through poorly understood mechanisms, in some types of cells. Akt opposes activation of Ask1, a protein kinase implicated in apoptosis. Finally, phosphorylation of Mdm2 by Akt promotes its entry into the nucleus, where it binds and induces ubiquitination and proteasome-dependent degradation of p53.

tosis induction.[224] Akt also opposes apoptosis induced by the kinase Ask1[225] and promotes p53 degradation through effects on Mdm2.[226]

In recent years, evidence of hyper-activity of kinase Akt has been found for many types of human cancers.[200,227] The Akt protein contains a PH domain which binds phospholipid second-messengers produced by phosphatidyl-inositol 3' kinase (PI3K). Elevations in the levels of these lipid second-messengers result in recruitment of Akt to the plasma membrane, where it becomes activated by phosphorylation.[227] These phospholipid second-messengers are destroyed by PTEN, a lipid phosphatase and important tumor suppressor. Deletions and somatic point mutations that inactivate PTEN occur commonly in cancers.[228] Other mechanisms for deregulating Akt activity have also been described in cancers, including amplification of the *AKT2* gene in breast and ovarian cancers, and over-production of an Akt-binding protein called Tcl1, as a result of chromosomal translocations in T-cell pro-lymphocytic leukemia (T-PLL). Consequently, Akt has emerged as an attractive candidate for drug discovery, using small-molecule compounds to target the ATP-binding site of the kinase, thereby inhibiting its catalytic activity.

THERAPEUTIC OPPORTUNITIES FROM APOPTOSIS RESEARCH

Emerging knowledge about the proteins that constitute the apoptosis core machinery and their upstream inputs has revealed multiple new opportunities for therapeutic intervention, some of which are already under investigation in clinical trials. These opportunities include both discovery and development of new agents (many of which were mentioned above), as well as the potential for more effective exploitation of existing anticancer agents through a deeper understanding of their effects on apoptosis pathways. With respect to new agents in clinical trials, a prominent example of a new strategy for attacking apoptosis resistance mechanisms in cancer is found in nuclease-resistant (phosphorothioate) antisense oligonucleotides directed against *BCL-2* mRNA, currently in phase III trials for patients with multiple myeloma, melanoma, CLL, and AML, and in phase II for several solid tumors (<http://genta.com>). Agonistic antibodies directed against the TRAIL receptors, TRAIL-R1 (DR4), have also recently completed phase I clinical trials (<http://hgs.com>), and may one day provide new arrows for the quivers of medical oncologists.

A wide variety of existing and emerging anticancer agents that alter transcriptional mechanisms also indirectly regulate the expression of apoptosis genes, and provide opportunities for modulating apoptosis-resistance. Prominent among these are members of the retinoid/steroid family of transcription factors that require small ligands for their transcriptional activation. For example, it has been shown that expression of *BCL-2* in mammary epithelium is estrogen-dependent. By negating the transcriptional activity of the ER, antiestrogens such as Tamoxifen reduce *BCL-2* expression and promote apoptosis of breast cancer cells,[228] probably explaining in part the beneficial effects of anti-hormonal agents in the treatment of ER-positive breast cancers. Similarly, vitamin D (1,25 (OH)2-cholcalcitriol), and more potent synthetic analogues lacking hypercalcemic effects, activate the vitamin D receptor (VDR) and suppress expression of several anti-apoptotic *BCL-2* family genes, including *BCL-2, BCL-X^L*, and *MCL-1,* restoring apoptosis-sensitivity.[229,230] High-dose vitamin D is currently in clinical trials for prostate cancer. The retinoid, *all-trans* retinoic-acid (ATRA), and newer retinoic acid receptor-X (RXR)-selective compounds (eg, Bexaretinone) also suppress expression of anti-apoptotic *BCL-2* family genes *(BCL-2; BCL-X^L)* in leukemias and some types of solid tumors. Thiazolidinedione drugs (currently in use for treatment of type 2 diabetes) that bind PPARγ, another member of the steroid/retinoid family of transcription factors, also reduce expression of *BCL-2* or other anti-apoptotic *BCL-2* family proteins in some breast, prostate, or colon cancer cell lines.[231] Some PPARγ modulatory drugs also seem to reduce levels of FLIP, the Caspase-8 antagonist, thereby sensitizing tumor cells to the TNF-family death ligands.[100]

Many additional agents can indirectly modulate apoptosis pathways. Histone deacetylase (HDAC) inhibitors, for example, can reduce transcription of anti-apoptotic *BCL2* family genes in cancers, and are currently under investigation in clinical trials.[206] Upstream of Akt, a compound that inhibits the kinase activity of BCR/ABL (STI-571 [Gleevec]) has recently been approved for chronic myelogenous leukemia, providing a powerful weapon in the armamentarium of agents for combating this leukemia. Similarly, small-molecule drugs and monoclonal antibodies directed against various cell-surface growth factors receptors that possess protein tyrosine kinase activity (eg, HER-2; EGFR; IGFR) are expected to shut-down the Akt pathway, and thus should render tumor cells more sensitive to apoptosis.

Altogether therefore, prospects are bright for translation of concepts emerging from apoptosis research into more efficacious therapies for the treatment of malignancy. This effort will benefit from a more detailed understanding of the cellular pathways that control expression of apoptosis-regulatory genes, and from knowledge of the tumor-specific lesions that dictate sensitivity or resistance to chemical modulators of these pathways. In this way, treatment strategies can be optimized for individual patients based on the genetic characteristics of their tumors, with the goal of restoring apoptosis sensitivity and encouraging cancer cells to commit suicide by activating their endogenous pathways for programmed cell death.

ACKNOWLEDGMENTS

The author thanks J. Valois and R. Cornell for manuscript preparation, and gratefully acknowledge the generous support of the National Cancer Institute (NCI).

REFERENCES

1. Reed J. Dysregulation of apoptosis in cancer. J Clin Oncol 1999;17:2941.
2. Reed JC. Dysregulation of apoptosis in cancer. Cancer J Sci Am 1998;4:S8–13.
3. Evan G, Littlewood T. A matter of life and cell death. Science 1998;281:1317–22.
4. Frisch SM, Screaton RA. Anoikis mechanisms. Curr Opin Cell Biol 2001;13:555–62.
5. Tschopp J, Martinon F, Hofmann K. Apoptosis: silencing the death receptors. Curr Biol 1999;9:R381–4.
6. Reed JC. Apoptosis and cancer: strategies for integrating programmed cell death. Semin Hematol 2000;37:9–16.
7. Makin G, Hickmann JA. Apoptosis and cancer chemotherapy. Cell Tissue Res 2000;301:143.
8. Kerr JF, Wyllie AH, Currie AR. Apoptosis: a basic biological phenomenon with wide-ranging implications in tissue kinetics. Br. J. Cancer 26:239–57.
9. Thornberry NA, Lazebnik Y. Caspases: enemies within. Science 1998;281:1312–6.
10. Cryns V, Yuan Y. Proteases to die for. Genes Dev 1999;12:1551–70.
11. Alnemri ES, Livingston DJ, Nicholson DW, et al. Human ICE/CED-3 Protease Nomenclature. Cell 1996;87:171.
12. Salvesen GS, Dixit VM. Caspases: Intracellular signaling by proteolysis. Cell 1997;91:443–6.
13. Blane C, Deveraux QL, Krajewski S, et al. Caspase-3 is essential for procaspase-9 processing and cisplatin-induced apoptosis of MCF-7 breast cancer cells. Cancer Res 2000;60:4386–90.
14. Teitz T, Wei T, Valentine MB, et al. Caspase-8 is deleted or silenced preferentially in childhood neuroblastomas with *MYCN* amplification. Nat Med 2000;6:529–35.

15. Takita J, Yang HW, Chen YY, et al. Allelic imbalance on chromosome 2q and alterations of the caspase 8 gene in neuroblastoma. Oncogene 2001;20:4424–32.
16. Schwartz S Jr, Yamamoto H, Navarro M, et al. Frameshift mutations at mononucleotide repeats in caspase-5 and other target genes in endometrial and gastrointestinal cancer of the microsatellite mutator phenotype. Cancer Res 1999;59:2995–3002.
17. Motyka B, Korbutt G, Pinkoski MJ, et al. Mannose 6-phosphate/insulin-like growth factor II receptor is a death receptor for granzyme B during cytotoxic T cell-induced apoptosis. Cell 2000;103:491–500.
18. Martin SJ, Amarante-Mendes GP, Shi L, et al. The cytotoxic cell protease granzyme B initiates apoptosis in a cell-free system by proteolytic processing and activation of the ICE/CED-3 family protease, CPP32, via a novel two-step mechanism. EMBO J 1996;15:2407–16.
19. Zhou Q, Krebs J, Snipas S, et al. Interaction of the baculovirus antiapoptotic protein p35 with caspases. Specificity, kinetics, and characterization of the caspase/p35 complex. Biochemistry 1998;37:10757–65.
20. Quan LT, Caputo A, Bleackley RC, et al. Granzyme B is inhibited by the cowpox virus serpin cytokine response modifier A. J Biol Chem 1995;270:10377–9.
21. Sun J, Ooms L, Bird CH, et al. A new family of 10 murine ovalbumin serpins includes two homologs of proteinase inhibitor 8 and two homologs of the granzyme B inhibitor (proteinase inhibitor 9). J Biol Chem 1997; 272:15434–41.
22. Locksley RM, Killeen N, Lenardo MJ. The TNF and TNF receptor superfamilies: integrating mammalian biology. Cell 2001;104:487–501.
23. Wallach D, Varfolomeev EE, Malinin NL, et al. Tumor necrosis factor receptor and Fas signaling mechanisms. Ann Rev Immunol 1999;17:331–67.
24. Yuan J. Transducing signals of life and death. Curr Opin Cell Biol 1997;9:247–51.
25. Reed JC, Doctor K, Rojas A, et al. Comparative analysis of apoptosis and inflammation genes of mice and humans. 2002. [In press]
26. Zhang J, Cado C, Chen A, et al. Fas-mediated apoptosis and activation-induced T-cell proliferation are defective in mice lacking FADD/Mort 1. Nature 1998;392:296–9.
27. Varfolomeev E, Schuchmann M, Luria V, et al. Targeted disruption of the mouse caspase 8 gene ablates cell death inductation by the TNF receptors, Fas/Apo1, and DR3 and is lethal prenatally. Immunity 1998;9:267–76.
28. Reed JC. Cytochrome C: Can't live with it; Can't live without it. Cell 1997;91:559–62.
29. Green DR, Reed JC. Mitochondria and apoptosis. Science 1998;281:1309–12.
30. Hakem R, Hakem A, Duncan GS, et al. Differential requirement for caspase 9 in apoptotic pathways in vivo. Cell 1998;94:339–52.
31. Haraguchi M, Torii S, Matsuzawa S, et al. Apoptotic protease activating factor (Apaf-1)-independent cell death suppression by Bcl-2. J Exp Med 2000;191:1709–20.
32. Kroemer G, Reed JC. Mitochondrial control of cell death. Nature Med 2000;6:513–9.
33. Gross A, Yin X-M, Wang K, et al. Caspase cleaved BID targets mitochondria and is required for cytochrome c release, while BCL-X^L prevents this release but not TNF-R1/Fas death. 1998. [In press]
34. Li H, Zhu H, Xu C, Yuan J. Cleavage of BID by caspase 8 mediates the mitochondrial damage in the Fas pathway of apoptosis. Cell 1998;94:491–501.
35. Zhang H, Xu Q, Krajewski S, et al. BAR: An apoptosis regulator at the intersection of caspase and bcl-2 family proteins. Proc Natl Acad Sci U S A 2000;97:2597–602.
36. Ng FWH, Nguyen M, Kwan T, et al. p28 Bap31, a Bcl-2/Bcl-X^L-and procaspase-8-associated protein in the endoplasmic reticulum. J Cell Biol 1997;39:327–38.
37. Vaux DL, Strasser A. The molecular biology of apoptosis. Proc Natl Acad Sci U S A 1996;93:2239–44.
38. Nakagawa T, Zhu H, Morishima N, et al. Caspase-12 mediates endoplasmic-reticulum-specific apoptosis and cytotoxicity by amyloid-(3. Nature 2000;403:98–103.
39. Fischer H, Koenig U, Eckhart L, Tschachler E. Human caspase-12 has acquired deleterious mutations. Biochem Biophys Res Commun 2002;293:722–6.
40. Mancini M, Machamer CE, Roy S, et al. Caspase-2 is localized at the Golgi complex and cleaves golgin-160 during apoptosis. J Cell Biol 2000;149:603–12.
41. Wang Z-G, Ruggero D, Ronchetti S, et al. Pml is essential for multiple apoptotic pathways. Nat Genet 1998;20:266–72.
42. Torii S, Egan DA, Evans RA, Reed JC. Human daxx regulates fas-induced apoptosis from nuclear pml oncogenic domains (pods). EMBO J 1999;18:6037–49.
43. Zhong S, Salomoni P, Ronchetti S, et al. Promyelocytic leukemia protein (PML) and daxx participate in a novel nuclear pathway for apoptosis. J Exp Med 2000;191:631–9.
44. Mattson MP, Duan W, Chan SL, Camandola S. Par-4: an emerging pivotal player in neuronal apoptosis and neurodegenerative disorders. J Mol Neurosci 2000;13:17–30.
45. Page G, Kogel D, Rangnekar V, Scheidtmann KH. Interaction partners of Dlk/ZIP kinase: co-expression of Dlk/ZIP kinase and Par-4 results in cytoplasmic retention and apoptosis. Oncogene 1999;18:7265–73.
46. Sells SF, Han SS, Muthukkumar S, et al. Expression and function of the leucine zipper protein Par-4 in apoptosis. Mol Cell Biol 1997;17:3823–32.
47. Salomoni P, Pandolfi PP. The role of PML in tumor suppression. Cell 2002;108:165–70.
48. Salvesen GS, Dixit VM. Caspase activation: the induced-proximity model. Proc Natl Acad Sci U S A 1999;96: 10964–7.
49. Huang B, Eberstadt M, Olejniczak ET, et al. NMR structure and mutagenesis of the Fas (APO-1/CD95) death domain. Nature 1996;384:638–41.
50. Liepinsh E, Ilag LL, Otting G, Ibanez CF. NMR structure of the death domain of the p75 neurotrophin receptor. EMBO J 1997;16:4999–5005.
51. Lee HH, Dadgostar H, Cheng Q, et al. NFκB-mediated upregulation of bcl-x and bfl-1/a1 is required for CD40 survival signaling in B lymphocytes. Proc Natl Acad Sci U S A 1999;96:9136–41.
52. Hsu H, Xiong J, Goeddel DV. The TNF receptor 1-associated protein TRADD signals cell death and NFkappaB activation. Cell 1995;81:495–504.
53. Chinnaiyan AM, O'Rourke K, Yu G-L, et al. Signal transduction by DR3, a death domain-containing receptor related to TNFR-1 and CD95. Science 1996;274.
54. Pan G, Bauer JH, Haridas V, et al. Identification and functional characterization of DR6, a novel death domain-containing TNF receptor. FEBS Lett 1998;431:351–6.
55. Pan G, Humke EW, Dixit VM. Activation of caspases triggered by cytochrome c in vitro. FEBS Lett 1998;426:151–4.
56. Yeh W, De La Pompa J, El-Deiry W, et al. FADD: essential for embryo development and signaling from some, but not all, inducers of apoptosis. Science 1998;279:1954–8.
57. Sprick MR, Weigand MA, Rieser E, et al. FADD/MORT1 and caspase-8 are recruited to TRAIL receptors 1 and 2 and are essential for apoptosis mediated by TRAIL receptor 2. Immunity 2000;12:599–609.
58. Kischkel FC, Lawrence DA, Chuntharapai A, et al. Apo2L/TRAIL-dependent recruitment of endogenous FADD and caspase-8 to death receptors 4 and 5. Immunity 2000;12:611–20.
59. Nagata S. Apoptosis by death factor. Cell 1997;88:355–65.
60. Krammer PH. CD95's deadly mission in the immune system. Nature 2000;407:789–95.
61. Watanabe-Fukunaga R, Brannan CI, Copeland NG, et al. Lymphoproliferation disorder in mice explained by defects in Fas antigen that mediates apoptosis. Nature 1992;356:314–7.
62. Takahashi T, Tanaka M, Brannan CI., et al. Generalized lymphoproliferative disease in mice, caused by a point mutation in the Fas ligand. Cell 1994;76:969–76.
63. Ogasawara J, Watanabe-Fukunaga R, Adachi M, et al. Lethal effect of the anti-Fas antibody in mice. Nature 1993;364:8069.
64. Fisher GH, Rosenberg FJ, Straus SE, et al. Dominant interfering fas gene mutations impair apoptosis in a human autoimmune lymphoproliferative syndrome. Cell 1995;81:935–46.
65. Gronbaek K, Straten PT, Ralfkiaer E, et al. Somatic Fas mutations in non-Hodgkin's lymphoma: association with extranodal disease and autoimmunity. Blood 1998;92:3018–24.
66. Cheng J, Zhou T, Liu C, et al. Protection from fas-mediated apoptosis by a soluble form of the fas molecule. Science 1994;263:1759–62.
67. Kamihira S, Yamada Y, Tomonaga M, et al. Discrepant expression of membrane and soluble isoforms of Fas (CD95/APO-1) in adult T-cell leukaemia: soluble Fas isoform is an independent risk factor for prognosis. Br J Haematol 1999;107:851–60.
68. Osorio LM, Aguilar-Santelises M, De Santiago A, et al. Increased serum levels of soluble Fax in progressive B-CLL. Eur J Haematol 2001;66:342–6.
69. Niitsu N, Sasaki K, Umeda M. A high serum soluble Fas/APO-1 level is associated with a poor outcome of aggressive non-Hodgkin's lymphoma. Leukemia 1999;13:1434–40.
70. Ashkenazi A, Dixit VM. Apoptosis control by death and decoy receptors. Curr Opin Cell Biol 1999;11:255–60.
71. Kelley SK, Harris LA, Xie D, et al. Preclinical studies to predict the disposition of Apo2L/tumor necrosis factor-related apoptosis-inducing ligand in humans: characterization of in vivo efficacy, pharmacokinetics, and safety. J Pharmacol Exp Ther 2001;299:31–8.
72. Ichikawa K, Liu W, Wang Z, et al. Tumoricidal activity in the absence of hepatocyte cytotoxicity of a novel anti-human DR5 monoclonal antibody. Nat Med 2001;7:954–60.
73. Wu GS, Burns TF, McDonald ER, et al. KILLER/DR5 is a DNA damage-inducible p53-regulated death receptor gene. Nat Genet 1997;17:141–3.
74. Owen-Schaub LB, Zhang W, Cusack JC, et al. Wild-type human p53 and a temperature-sensitive mutant induce Fas/APO-1 expression. Mol Cell Biol 1995;15:3032–40.
75. Kastan M. On the TRAIL from p53 to apoptosis? Nat Genet 1997;17:130–1.
76. Levy-Strumpf N, Kimchi A. Death associated proteins (DAPs): From gene identification to the analysis of their apoptotic and tumor suppressive functions. Oncogene 1998;17:3331–40.
77. Frisch S. Evidence for a function of death-receptor-related, death-domain-containing proteins in anoikis. Curr Biol 1999;9:1047–9.
78. Rytomaa M, Martins L, Downward J. Involvement of FADD and caspase-8 signaling in detachment-induced apoptosis. Curr Biol 1999;9:1043–6.
79. Frisch SM, Ruoslahti E. Integrins and anoikis. Curr Opin Cell Biol 1997;9:701–6.
80. Stanger BZ, Leder P, Lee T-H, et al. RIP: A novel protein containing a death domain that interacts with Fas/APO-1 (CD95) in yeast and causes cell death. Cell 1995;81:513–23.
81. Hsu H, Huang J, Shu H, et al. TNF-dependent recruitment of the protein kinase RIP to the TNF receptor-1 signaling complex. Immunity 1996;4:387–96.
82. Ting AT, Pimentel-Muinos FX, Seed B. RIP mediates tumor necrosis factor receptor 1 activation of NFκB but not Fas/APO-1-initiated apoptosis. EMBO J 1996;15:6189–96.
83. Stroka D, Badrichani A, Bach F, Ferran C. A1: An NFκB-inducible, anti-apoptotic Bcl gene that inhibits endothelial cell activation. Blood [In press]
84. Grumont R, Rourke I, Gerondakis S. Rel-dependent induction of A1 transcription is required to protect B cells from antigen receptor ligation-induced apoptosis. Genes Dev 1998;13:400–11.
85. Stehlik C, de Martin R, Kumabashiri I, et al. Nuclear Factor (NF)-κB-regulated X-chromosome-linked iap gene expression protects endothelial cells from tumor necrosis factor a-induced apoptosis. J Exp Med 1998;188:211–6.
86. Stehlik C, de Martin R, Binder B, Lipp J. Cytokine induced expression of porcine inhibitor of apoptosis protein (iap) family member is regulated by NFκB. Biochem Biophys Res Commun 1998;243:827–32.
87. Wang C, Mayo M, Korneluk R, et al. NFκB antiapoptosis: induction of TRAF1 and TRAF2 and c-IAP1 and c-IAP2 to suppress capase-8 activation. Science 1998;281:1680–3.
88. Antwerp DJ, Martin SJ, Kafri T, et al. Suppression of TNF-a-induced apoptosis by NFκB. Science 1996;274:787–9.
89. Liu Z-G, Hsu H, Goeddel DV, Karin M. Dissection of TNF receptor 1 effector functions: JNK activation is not linked to apoptosis while NFκB activation prevents cell death. Cell 1996;87:565–76.
90. Sabbatini P, Han J, Chiou S-K, et al. Interleukin 1b converting enzyme-like proteases are essential for p53-mediated transcriptionally dependent apoptosis. Cell Growth Differ 1997;8:643–53.
91. Muzio M, Chinnaiyan AM, Kischkel FC, et al. FLICE, a novel FADD-homologous ICE/CED-3-like protease, is recruited to the CD95 (Fas/APO-1) death—inducing signaling complex. Cell 1996;85:817–27.
92. Eberstadt M, Huang B, Chen Z, et al. NMR structure and mutagenesis of the FADD (Mort1) death-effector domain. Nature 1998;392:941–5.
93. Reed JC. Mechanisms of apoptosis (Warner/Lambert Award). Am J Pathol 2000;157:1415–30.
94. Wallach D. Placing death under control. Nature 1997;388:123–6.
95. Tschopp J, Irmler M, Thome M. Inhibition of Fas death signals by FLIPs. Curr Opin Immunol 1998;10:552–8.
96. French L, Tschopp J. Inhibition of death receptor signaling by FLICE-inhibitory protein as a mechanism for immune escape of tumors. J Exp Med 1999;190:891–3.
97. O'Connell J, O'Sullivan GC, Collins JK, Shanahan F. The Fas counterattack: Fas-mediated T cell killing by colon cancer cells expressing Fas ligand. J Exp Med 1996;184:1075–82.
98. Bennett M, O'Connell J, O'Sullivan et al. The Fas counterattack in vivo: apoptotic depletion of tumor-infiltrating lym-

phocytes associated with Fas ligand expression by human esophageal carcinoma. J Immunol 1998;160:5669–75.
99. OConnell J, Bennett M, O'Sullivan G, et al. Fas ligand expression in primary colon adenocarcinomas: evidence that the Fas counterattack is a prevalent mechanism of immune evasion in human colon cancer. J Pathol 1998;186:240–6.
100. Kim Y, Suh N, Sporn M, Reed JC. An inducible pathway for degradation of FLIP protein sensitizes tumor cells to TRAIL-induced apoptosis. J Biol Chem 2002;277:22320–9.
101. Hyer ML, Sudarshan S, Kim Y, et al. Down-regulation of c-FLIP sensitizes DU145 prostate cancer cells to Fas-mediated apoptosis. Cancer Biol Ther 2002;4:405–10.
102. Micheau O, Lens S, Gaide O, et al. NFκB signals induce the expression of c-FLIP. Mol Cell Biol 2001; 21:5299–305.
103. Chou J, Matsuo H, Duan H, Wagner G. Solution structure of the RAIDD CARD and model for CARD/CARD interaction in caspase-2 and caspase-9 recruitment. Cell 1998;94:171–80.
104. Zhou P, Chou J, Olea RS, et al. Solution structure of Apaf-1 CARD and its interaction with caspase-9 CARD: a structural basis for specific adaptor/caspase interaction. Proc Natl Acad Sci U S A 1999;96:11265–70.
105. Vaughn DE, Rodriguez J, Lazebnik Y, Joshua-Tor L. Crystal structure of Apaf-1 caspase recruitment domain: an alpha-helical Greek key fold for apoptotic signaling. J Mol Biol 1999;293:439–47.
106. Day CL, Dupont C, Lackmann M, et al. Solution structure and mutagenesis of the caspase recruitment domain (CARD) from Apaf-1. Cell Death Differ 1999;6:1125–32.
107. Hsieh J-K, Chan F, O'Connor D, et al. RB regulates the stability and the apoptotic function of p53 via MDM2. Mol Cell 1999;3:181–93.
108. Koonin EV, Aravind L. The NACHT family-a new group of predicted NTPases implicated in apoptosis and MHC Transcription activation. Trends Biol Sci 2000;25:223–4.
109. Li P, Nijhawan D, Budihardjo I, et al. Cytochrome c and dATP-dependent formation of Apaf-1/Caspase-9 complex initiates an apoptotic protease cascade. Cell 1997;91:479–89.
110. Chinnaiyan A, Chaudhary D, O'Rourke K, et al. Role of CED-4 in the activation of CED-3. Nature 1997;388:728–9.
111. Seshagiri S, Miller LK. *Caenorhabditis elegans* CED-4 stimulates CED-3 processing and CED-3-induced apoptosis. Curr Biol 1997;7:455–60.
112. Yang X, Chang H, Baltimore D. Essential role of CED-4 oligomerization in CED-3 activation and apoptosis. Science 1998;281:1355–7.
113. Zou H, Li Y, Liu X, Wang X. An APAF-1 cytochrome c multimeric complex is a functional apoptosome that activates procaspase-9. J Biol Chem 1999;274:11549–56.
114. Saleh A, Srinivasula S, Acharya S, et al. Cytochrome c and dATP-mediated oligomerization of Apaf-1 is a prerequisite for procaspase-9 activation. J Biol Chem 1999;274:17941–5.
115. Abrams JM. An emerging blueprint for apoptosis in Drosophila. Trends Cell Biol 1999;9:435–40.
116. Srinivasula SM, Ahmad M, Guo Y, et al. Identification of an endogenous dominant-negative short isoform of caspase-9 that can regulate apoptosis. Cancer Res 1999;59:999–1002.
117. Cardone MH, Roy N, Stennicke HR, et al, Regulation of cell death protease caspase-9 by phosphorylation. Science 1998;282:1318–20.
118. Pandey P, Saleh A, Nakazawa A, et al. Negative Regulation of Cytochrome c-mediated Oligomerization of Apaf-1 and Activation of Procaspase-9 by Heat Shock Protein 90b. 2000. [In Press]
119. Beere HM, Wolf BB, Cain K, et al. Heat-shock protein 70 inhibits apoptosis by preventing recruitment of procaspase-9 to the Apaf-1 apoptosome. Nat Cell Biol 2000;2:469–75.
120. Matsuyama S, Llopi J, Deveraux QL, et al. Changes in intramitochondrial and cytosolic pH: Early events that modulate caspase activation during apoptosis. Nat Cell Biol 2000;2:318–25.
121. Pathan N, Marusawa H, Krajewska M, et al. TUCAN: An anti-apoptotic CARD family protein over-expressed in cancer. J Biol Chem 2001;276:32220–9.
122. Soengas MS, Capodieci P, Polsky D, et al. Inactivation of the apoptosis effector Apaf-1 in malignant melanoma. Nature 2001;409:207–11.
123. Willis TG, Jadayel DM, Peng H, et al. Bcl10 is involved in t(1;14) (p22;q32) of MALT B cell lymphoma and mutated in multiple tumor types. Cell 1999;96:35–45.
124. Ruland J, Duncan GS, Elia A, et al. Bcl10 is a positive regulator of antigen receptor-induced activation of NFκB and neural tube closure. Cell 2001;104:33–42.
125. Zhang Q, Siebert R, Yan M, et al. Inactivating mutations and overexpression of BCL-10, a caspase recruitment domain-containing gene, in MALT lymphoma with t(1;14)(p22;q32). Nat Genet 1999;22:63–8.
126. Lee SH, Shin MS, Kim HS, et al. Point mutations and deletions of the *Bcl-10* gene in solid tumors and malignant lymphomas. Cancer Res 1999;59:5674–7.
127. Deveraux QL, Reed JC. IAP family proteins: suppressors of apoptosis. Genes Dev 1999;13:239–52.
128. La Casse EC, Baird S, Korneluk RG, MacKenzie AE. The inhibitors of apoptosis (IAPs) and their emerging role in cancer. Oncogene 1998;17:3247–59.
129. Miller L. An exegesis of IAPs: salvation and surprises from BIR motifs. Trends Cell Biol 1999;9:323–8.
130. Sun C, Cal M, Gunasekera A, et al. NMR structure and mutagenesis of the inhibitor-of-apoptosis protein XIAP. Nature 1999;401:818–21.
131. Hinds MG, Norton RS, Vaux DL, Day CL. Solution structure of a baculoviral inhibitor of apoptosis (IAP) repeat. Nat Struct Biol 1999;6:648–51.
132. Verdecia MA, Huang H-k, Dutil E, et al. Structure of the human anti-apoptotic protein survivin reveals a dimeric arrangement. Nat Struct Biol 2000;7:602–8.
133. Yang Y, Fang S, Jensen JP, et al. Ubiquitin protein ligase activity of IAPs and their degradation in proteasomes in response to apoptotic stimuli. Science 2000;288:874–7.
134. Hauser H, Bardroff M, Pyrowolakis G, Jentsch S. A giant ubiquitin-conjugating enzyme related to IAP apoptosis inhibitors. J Cell Biol 1998;141:1415–22.
135. Fraser A, James C, Evan G, Hengartner M. Caenorhabditis elegans inhibitor of apoptosis protein (IAP) homologue BIR-1 plays a conserved role in cytokinesis. Curr Biol 1999;9:292–301.
136. Vaux DL, Uren AG, Beilharz T, et al. Role for yeast inhibitor of apoptosis (IAP)-like proteins in cell division. Proc Natl Acad Sci U S A 1999;96:10170–5.
137. Deveraux QL, Takahashi R, Salvesen GS, Reed JC. X-linked IAP is a direct inhibitor of cell death proteases. Nature 1997;388:300–4.
138. Roy N, Deveraux QL, Takashashi R, et al. The c-IAP-1 and c-IAP-2 proteins are direct inhibitors of specific caspases. EMBO J 1997;16:6914–25.
139. Deveraux QL, Leo E, Stennicke HR, et al. Cleavage of human inhibitor of apoptosis protein XIAP results in fragments with distinct specificities for caspases. EMBO J 1999;18:5242–51.
140. Takahashi R, Deveraux QL, Tamm I, et al. A single BIR domain of XIAP sufficient for inhibiting caspases. J Biol Chem 1998;273:7787–90.
141. Liu Z, Sun C, Olejniczak ET, et al. Structural basis for binding of Smac/DIABLO to the XIAP BIR3 domain. Nature 2000;408:1004–8.
142. Deveraux QL, Roy N, Stennicke HR, et al. IAPs block apoptotic events induced by caspase-8 and cytochrome c by direct inhibition of distinct caspases. EMBO J 1998;17:2215–23.
143. Vucic D, Stennicke HR, Pisabarro MT, et al. ML-IAP, a novel inhibitor of apoptosis that is preferentially expressed in human melanomas. Curr Biol 2000; 10:1359–66.
144. Reed JC. The survivin saga goes in vivo. J Clin Invest 2001;108:965–9.
145. Ambrosini G, Adida C, Altieri DC. A novel anti-apoptosis gene, Survivin, expressed in cancer and lymphoma. Nat Med 1997;3:917–21.
146. Adida C, Crotty PL, McGrath J, et al. Developmentally regulated expression of the novel cancer anti-apoptosis gene survivin in human and mouse differentiation. Am J Pathol 1998;152:43–9.
147. Madden SL, Zhang L, Lash AE, et al, Analysis of human transcriptomes. Nat Genet 1999;23:387–8.
148. Li F, Ambrosini G, Chu EY, et al. Cell cycle control of apoptosis and mitotic spindle checkpoint by survivin. 1998. [In Press]
149. Li F, Ackermann E, Bennett C, et al. Pleiotropic cell-division defects and apoptosis induced by interference with survivin function. Nat Cell Biol 1999;1:461–6.
150. Li F, Flanary PL, Altieri DC, Dohlman HG. Cell division regulation by BIR1, a member of the inhibitor of apoptosis family in yeast. J Bio Chem 2000;275:6707–11.
151. Tamm I, Kornblau SM, Segall H, et al. Expression and prognostic significance of iap-family genes in human cancers and myeloid leukemias. Clin Cancer Res 2000;6:1796–803.
152. Kasof GM, Gomes BC. Livin, a novel inhibitor-of-apoptosis (IAP) family member. J Biol Chem 2001; 276:3238–46.
153. Lin JH, Deng G, Huang Q, Morser J. KIAP, a novel member of the inhibitor of apoptosis protein family. Biochem Biophys Res Commun 2000;279:820–31.
154. Chen Z, Naito M, Hori S, et al. A human IAP-family gene, apollon, expressed in human brain cancer cells. Biochem Biophys Res Commun 1999;264:84754.
155. Du C, Fang M, Li Y, et al. SMAC, a mitochondrial protein that promotes cytochrome c-dependent caspase activation by eliminating IAP inhibition. Cell 2000;102:33–42.
156. Verhagen AM, Ekert PG, Pakusch M, et al. Identification of DIABLO, a mammalian protein that promotes apoptosis by binding to and antagonizing IAP proteins. Cell 2000;102:43–53.
157. Chai J, Du C, Wu JW, et al. Structural and biochemical basis of apoptotic activation by Smac/DIABLO. Nature 2000;406:855–62.
158. Srinivasula SM, Hegde R, Saleh A, et al. A conserved XIAP-interaction motif in caspase-9 and Smac/DIA BLO regulates caspase activity and apoptosis. Nature 2001;410:112–6.
159. Herr I, Debatin K-M. Cellular stress response and apoptosis in cancer therapy. Blood 2001;98:2603–14.
160. Nechushtan A, Smith C, Hsu Y-T, Youle R. Conformation of the Bax C-terminus regulates subcellular location and cell death. EMBO J 1999;18:2330–41.
161. Reed JC. Double identity for proteins of the Bcl-2 family. Nature 1997;387:773–6.
162. Adams J, Cory S. The Bcl-2 protein family: arbiters of cell survival. Science 1998;281:1322–6.
163. Reed JC. Bcl-2 family proteins. Oncogene 1998;17:3225–36.
164. Gross A, McDonnell JM, Korsmeyer SJ. BCL-2 family members and the mitochondria in apoptosis. Genes Dev 1999;13:1899–911.
165. Kelekar A, Thompson CB. Bcl-2-family proteins—the role of the BH3 domain in apoptosis. Trends Cell Biol 1998;8:324–30.
166. Reed JC. Mechanisms of Bcl-2 family protein function and dysfunction in health and disease. Behring Inst Mitt 1996;97:72–100.
167. Tsujimoto Y, Cossman J, Jaffe E, Croce C. Involvement of the Bcl-2 gene in human follicular lymphoma. Science 1985;228:1440–3.
168. Weiss LM, Warnke RA, Sklar J, Cleary ML. Molecular analysis of the t(14;18) chromosomal translocation in malignant lymphomas. N Engl J Med 1987;317:1185–9.
169. Reed JC, Miyashita T, Takayama S, et al. Bcl-2 family proteins: regulators of cell death involved in the pathogenesis of cancer and resistance to therapy. J Cell Biochem 1996;60:23–32.
170. Rampino N, Yamamoto H, Ionov Y, et al. Somatic frameshift mutations in the BAX gene in colon cancers of the microsatellite mutator phenotype. Science 1997;275:967–9.
171. Yin C, Knudson CM, Korsmeyer SJ, Van Dyke T. Bax suppresses tumorigenesis and stimulates apoptosis in vivo. Nature 1997;385:637–40.
172. Miyashita T, Reed JC. Tumor suppressor p53 is a direct transcriptional activator of human Bax gene. Cell 1995;80:293–9.
173. Muchmore SW, Sattler M, Liang H, et al. X-ray and NMR structure of human Bcl-X^L, an inhibitor of programmed cell death. Nature 1996;381:335–41.
174. Chou J, Li H, Salvesen G, et al. Solution structure of BID, an intracellular amplifier of apoptotic signaling. Cell 1999;96:615–24.
175. McDonnell JM, Fushman D, Milliman CL, et al. Solution structure of the pro-apoptotic molecule BID: a structural basis for apoptotic agonists and antagonists. Cell 1999;96:625–34.
176. Schendel S, Montal M, Reed JC. Bcl-2 family proteins as ion-channels. Cell Death Differ 1998;5:372–80.
177. Minn AJ, Velez P, Schendel SL, et al. Bcl-x^L forms an ion channel in synthetic lipid membranes. Nature 1997;385:353–7.
178. Schendel SL, Xie Z, Montal MO, et al. Channel formation by antiapoptotic protein Bcl-2. Proc Natl Acad Sci U SA 1997;94:5113–8.
179. Antonsson B, Conti F, Ciavatta A, et al. Inhibition of Bax channel-forming activity by Bcl-2. Science 1997;277:370–2.
180. Schlesinger P, Gross A, Yin X-M, et al. Comparison of the ion channel characteristics of pro-apoptotic BAX and antiapoptotic BCL-2. Proc Natl Acad Sci U S A 1997;94:11357–62.
181. Schendel S, Azimov R, Pawlowski K, et al. Ion channel activity of the BH3 only Bcl-2 family member, BID. J Biol Chem 1999;274:21932–6.

182. Huang DC, Strasser A. BH3-only proteins-essential initiators of apoptotic cell death. Cell 2000;103:839–42.
183. Wang K, Yin W-M, Chao DT, et al. BID: a novel BH3 domain-only death agonist. Genes Dev 1996;10:2859–69.
184. Desagher S, Osen-Sand A, Nichols A, et al. Bid-induced conformational change of Bax is responsible for mitochondrial cytochrome c depletion during apoptosis. J Cell Biol 1999;144:891–901.
185. Kuwana T, Mackey MR, Perkins G, et al. Bid, bax, and lipids cooperate to form supramolecular openings in the outer mitochondrial membrane. Cell 2002;111:331–42.
186. Korsmeyer SJ, Wei MC, Saito M, et al. Pro-apoptotic cascade activates BID, which oligomerizes BAK or BAX into pores that result in the release of cytochrome *c*. Cell Death Differ 2000;7:1166–73.
187. Sattler M, Liang H, Nettesheim D, et al. Structure of Bcl-x^{L}-Bak peptide complex: recognition between regulators of apoptosis. Science 1997;275:983–6.
188. Holinger E, Chittenden T, Lutz R. Bak BH3 peptides antagonize Bcl-xL function and induce apoptosis through cytochrome c-independent activation of Caspases. J Biol Chem 1999;274:13298–304.
189. Wang J-L, Liu D, Zhang Z-J, et al. Structure-based discovery of an organic compound that binds Bcl-2 protein and induces apoptosis of tumor cells. Proc Natl Acad Sci U S A 2000;97:7124–9.
190. Tzung S, Kim KM, Basanez G, et al. Antimycin A mimics a cell-death-inducing Bcl-2 homology domain 3. Nat Cell Biol 2001;3:183–92.
191. Degterev A, Lugovskoy A, Cardone M, et al. Identification of small-molecule inhibitors of interaction between the BH3 domain and Bcl-x^{L}. Nat Cell Biol 2001;3:173–82.
192. Oda E, Ohki R, Murasawa H, et al. Noxa, a BH3-only member of the Bcl-2 family and candidate mediator of p53-induced apoptosis. Science 2000;288:1053–8.
193. Nakano K, Vousden KH. *PUMA,* a novel pro-apoptotic gene, is induced by p53. Mol Cell 2001;7:683–94.
194. Yu J, Zhang L, Hwang PM, et al. PUMA induces the rapid apoptosis of colorectal cancer cells. Mol Cell 2001;7:673–82.
195. Puthalakath H, Villunger A, L.A., et al. Bmf: a pro-apoptotic BH3-only protein regulated by interaction with the myosin V actin motor complex, activated by anoikis. Science 2001;293:1829–32.
196. Luo X, Budihardjo I, Zou H, et al. Bid, a Bcl2 interacting protein, mediates cytochrome c release from mitochondria in response to activation of cell surface death receptors. Cell 1998;94:481–90.
197. Zha J, Weiler S, Oh KJ, et al. Posttranslational N-myristoylation of BID as a molecular switch for targeting mitochondria and apoptosis. Science 2000;290:1761–5.
198. Puthalakath H, Huang D, O'Reilly L, et al. The pro-apoptotic activity of the Bcl-2 family member bim is regulated by interaction with the dynein motor complex. Mol Cell 1999;3:287–96.
199. Franke TF, Cantley LC. A bad kinase makes good. Nature 1997;390:116–7.
200. Datta S, Brunet A, Greenberg M. Cellular survival: a play in three Akts. Genes Dev 1999;13:2905–27.
201. Boise L, Gonzalez-Garcia M, Postema C, et al. Bcl-x, a Bcl-2-related gene that functions as a dominant regulator of apoptotic cell death. Cell 1993;74:597–608.
202. Guo B, Godzik A, Reed JC. Bcl-G, a novel pro-apoptotic member of the Bcl-2 family. J Biol Chem 2001;276:2780–5.
203. Reed JC. Apoptosis-based therapies. Nature Reviews Drug Disc 2002;1:111–21.
204. Demaurex N, Distelhorst C. Apoptosis—the calcium connection. Science 2003;300:65–7.
205. Edinger AL, Thompson CB. Death by design: apoptosis, necrosis and autophagy. Curr Opin Cell Biol 2004;16:663–9.
206. Otsuka H, Moskowitz M. Differences in the rates of protein degradation in untrasformed and transformed cell lines. Exp Cell Res 1978;112:127–35.
207. Futreal PA, Soderkvist P, Marks JR, et al. Detection of frequent allelic loss on proximal chromosome 17q in sporadic breast carcinoma using microsatellite length polymorphisms. Cancer Res 1992;52:2624–7.
208. Yue Z, Jin S, Yang C, et al. Beclin 1, an autophagy gene essential for early embryonic development, is a haploinsufficient tumor suppressor. Proc Natl Acad Sci U S A 2003;100:15077–82.
209. Kamada Y, Funakoshi T, Shintani T, et al. Tor-mediated induction of autophagy via an Apg1 protein kinase complex. J Cell Biol 2000;150:1507–13.
210. Liang XH, Kleemen LK, Jiang HH, et al. Protection against fatal Sindbis virus encephalitis by beclin, a novel Bcl-2-interacting protein. J Virol 1998;72:8586–96.
211. Yu L, Alva A, Su H, et al. Regulation of an ATG7-beclin 1 program of autophagic cell death by caspase-8. Science 2004;304:1500–2.
212. Kitada S, Pedersen IM, Schimmer A, Reed JC. Dysregulation of apoptosis genes in hematopoietic malignancies. Oncogene 2002;21:3459–74.
213. Reed JC. Apoptosis-regulating proteins as targets for drug discovery. Trends Mol Med 2001;7:314–9.
214. Reed JC, Tomaselli K. Drug discovery opportunities from apoptosis research. Curr Opin Biotechnol 2000;11:586–92.
215. Reed JC. Apoptosis-based therapies. Nat Rev Drug Discov 2002;1:111–21.
216. Karin M, Lin A. NFkappaB at the crossroads of life and death. Nat Immunol 2002;3:221–7.
217. Karin M, Cao Y, Greten FR, Li Z-W. NFκB in cancer: from innocent bystander to major culprit. Nat Rev Genet 2002;2:301–10.
218. Houldsworth J, Mathew S, Rao PH, et al. REL proto-oncogene is frequently amplified in extranodal diffuse large cell lymphoma. Blood 1996;87:25–9.
219. Karnolsky IN. Cytogenetic abnormalities in chronic lymphocytic leukemia. Folia Med (Plovdiv) 2000;42:5–10.
220. Hayashi T, Faustman D. Essential role of human leukocyte antigen-encoded proteasome subunits in NFκB activation and prevention of tumor necrosis factor-a-induced apoptosis. J Biol Chem 2000;275:5238–47.
221. Ahmed NN, Franke TF, Bellacosa A, et al. The proteins encoded by c-akt and v-akt differ in post-translational modification, subcellular localization and oncogenic potential. Oncogene 1993;8:1957–63.
222. Brunet A, Bonn, A, Zigmond MJ, et al. Akt promotes cell survival by phosphorylating and inhibiting a forkhead transcription factor. Cell 1999;96:857–68.
223. Ozes ON, Mayo LD, Gustin JA, et al. NFkappaB activation by tumour necrosis factor requires the Akt serine-threonine kinase [see comments]. Nature 1999;401:82–5.
224. Pekarsky Y, Hallas C, Palamarchuk A, et al. Akt phosphorylates and regulates the orphan nuclear receptor Nur77. Proc Natl Acad Sci U S A 2001;98:3690–4.
225. Kim AH, Khursigara G, Sun X, et al. Akt1 phosphorylates and negatively regulates ASK1. Mol Cell Biol 2001;21:893–901.
226. Testa JR, Bellacosa A. AKT plays a central role in tumorigenesis. Proc Nat Acad Sci U S A 2001;98:10983–5.
227. Cantley L, Neel BG. New insights into tumor suppression: PTEN suppresses tumor formation by restraining the phosphoinositide 3-kinase/AKT pathway. Proc Natl Acad Sci U S A 1999;96:4240–5.
228. Teixeira C, Reed JC, Pratt MAC. Estrogen promotes chemotherapeutic drug resistance by a mechanism involving Bcl-2 proto-oncogene expression in human breast cancer cells. Can Res 1995;55:3902–7.
229. Blutt SE, McDonnell TJ, Polek TC, Weigel NL. Calcitriol-induced apoptosis in LNCaP cells is blocked by overexpression of Bcl-2. Endocrinol 2000;141:10–7.
230. Guzey M, Kitada S, Reed JC. Apoptosis induction by 1a225(OH)2 in vitamin-D3 prostate cancer cell lines. Mol Cell Ther 2002;1:667–77.
231. Elstner E, Linker-Israeli M, Umiel T, et al. Combination of a potent 20-epi-vitamin D3 analogue (KH 1060) with 9-cis-retinoic acid irreversibly inhibits clonal growth, decreases bcl-2 expression, and induces apoptosis in HL-60 leukemic cells. Can Res 1996;56:3570–6.

5

Growth Factors and Signal Transduction in Cancer

Anna Bafico, PhD
Stuart A. Aaronson, MD

The evolution of multicellular organisms has involved the development of intercellular communication required for such processes as embryonic development, tissue differentiation, and as systemic responses to wounds and infections. These complex signaling networks are in large part mediated by growth factors, cytokines, and hormones. Such factors can influence cell proliferation in positive or negative ways, as well as induce a series of differentiated responses in appropriate target cells. The interaction of a growth factor with its receptor by specific binding, in turn, activates a cascade of intracellular biochemical events that are ultimately responsible for the biologic responses observed. Cytoplasmic molecules that mediate these responses have been termed second messengers. The eventual transmission of biochemical signals to the nucleus leads to effects on the expression of cassettes of genes involved in mitogenic and differentiation responses.

The pathogenic expression of critical genes in growth factor signaling pathways can also contribute to altered cell growth associated with malignancy. The v-*sis* oncogene of simian sarcoma virus, which encodes a growth factor homologous to the B chain of human platelet-derived growth factor (PDGF-B), is the paradigm for such genes.[1] The normal counterparts of other oncogenes have been shown to encode membrane-spanning growth factor receptors.[2,3] Other genes that act early in intracellular pathways of growth factor signal transduction have been implicated as oncogenes as well. Present knowledge indicates that the constitutive activation of growth factor signaling pathways through genetic alterations affecting these genes contributes to the development and progression of most, if not all, human cancers.

This chapter focuses on normal aspects of growth factor signaling, particularly those mediated by growth factor receptors possessing intrinsic protein tyrosine kinase activity. In addition, examples are provided where abnormalities in early steps in these pathways involving alterations in growth factor expression and/or receptor signaling have been implicated in the etiology of human malignancies. Finally, we will discuss how this knowledge may be useful in efforts to design new approaches toward therapeutic intervention with the malignant process. The limitation of space precludes a discussion of several important families of ligands and their receptors. These include the cytokines and their receptors, which lack intrinsic tyrosine kinase activity but associate with cytoplasmic tyrosine kinases. Other ligand/receptor families will not be discussed.

BACKGROUND

Hormones that act at great distances from the cells producing them have been known for many years. Hormones as signaling molecules were isolated from tissue fluids and readily characterized by their in vivo effects. In contrast, knowledge of growth factors is relatively recent. Growth factor activity capable of stimulating the growth of chicken embryonic nerve cells was found to be released by mouse sarcoma cells.[4] During purification of this nerve growth factor (NGF), a second activity that promoted eyelid opening and incisor eruption in newborn mice and rats was discovered. Because of recognition of its effects on epithelial cells, this factor was designated epidermal growth factor (EGF).[5]

An important discovery concerning growth factors came from the demonstration of a unique enzymologic activity associated with binding of EGF to its receptor.[5] Studies of the product of the viral oncogene v-*src* had led to the demonstration of its ability to act as a protein kinase.[6,7] Many protein kinases had been previously identified, but these had the capacity to phosphorylate serine and/or threonine residues. Moreover, it was well established that phosphorylations and dephosphorylations affected the activities of a variety of proteins. However, the Src product was subsequently shown to have a unique specificity as a protein kinase in that it was capable of phosphorylating tyrosine residues.[8] Cohen then showed that addition of EGF led to phosphorylation of its purified receptor on tyrosine residues.[5] Subsequent studies have demonstrated that tyrosine kinase activity is central to the functions of a large number of mitogenic signaling molecules.

Several major modes of action for growth factors have been described. Sporn and Todaro[9] defined autocrine and paracrine as major modes of action for growth factors in addition to the classic means by which hormones travel great distances from their sites of production (Figure 5-1). The autocrine mode refers to the ability of growth factor to act on the same cell releasing it. In the paracrine mode, the released growth factor from one cell acts on a nearby or adjacent cell. Certain growth factors also exist as membrane-anchored forms, which can bind and activate membrane receptors only on adjacent cells. This process, considered a variant of the paracrine mode, has been termed juxtacrine[10] and is capable of delivering spatially localized intercellular stimuli. A number of researchers have observed that factors that are produced in cells but are not detectably secreted nevertheless can induce observable phenotypic changes in those cells. The suggestion has been made that this represents an "intracrine" mode of action, whereby the factor interacts with its receptor, for example, within the Golgi apparatus.[11] A sixth mode of action, in which the growth factor is bound to and stored within the extracellular matrix before presentation to the receptor on the cell surface, has also been demonstrated.[12]

GROWTH FACTOR RECEPTORS WITH TYROSINE KINASE ACTIVITY

Growth factors mediate their diverse biologic responses by binding to and activating cell-surface receptors with intrinsic protein kinase activity.[13] To date, more than 50 receptor tyrosine kinases (RTKs), which belong to at least eighteen different receptor families, have been identified. All RTKs contain a large, glycosylated, extracellular ligand-binding domain, a single transmembrane region, and a cytoplasmic portion with a conserved protein tyrosine kinase domain. In addition to the catalytic domain, a juxtamembrane region and a carboxyl-terminal tail can be identified in the cytoplasmic portion. Because of their structure, RTKs can be visualized as membrane-

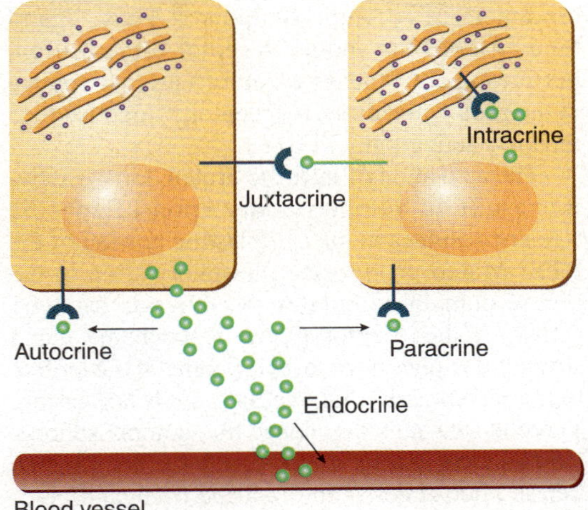

Figure 5-1 Modes of action for growth factors.

associated allosteric enzymes with the ligand binding and protein tyrosine kinase domains separated by the plasma membrane. Their role is to catalyze the transfer of the γ-phosphate of adenosine triphosphate (ATP) to tyrosine residues within their own polypeptide chain and to that of exogenous substrates. Tyrosine phosphorylation represents the language that these receptors use to transduce the information carried by the growth factor.

On the basis of sequence similarity, it is possible to classify these receptors into related groups.[14] Characteristic structural features of their extracellular domains include cysteine-rich motifs, immunoglobulin-like repeats (Ig-like), fibronectin type III repeats (FNIII), and EGF motifs that can be present singly or in different combinations. These different domains help to determine specificity for ligand binding.

There is substantial evidence that ligand-induced activation of the kinase domain and its signaling potential are mediated by receptor oligomerization.[15] This event stabilizes interactions between adjacent cytoplasmic domains and controls the activation of kinase activity. Dimerization can take place between two identical receptors (homodimerization), between different members of the same receptor family, or, in some cases, between a receptor and an accessory protein (heterodimerization).[15] Heterodimerization of RTKs has been shown, on the one hand, to increase the repertoire of ligands that can be recognized by each receptor alone and, on the other hand, to expand the diversity of signaling pathways that can be recruited by a given receptor.

How ligands bind to the receptors and induce oligomerization seems specific for each class of RTKs.[16] PDGF, for example, induces receptor dimerization by virtue of its dimeric nature.[17] EGF, instead, possesses two binding sites for its receptor. In the proposed model, the ligand uses one site to bind monovalently to the receptor and the other to bridge two ligand/receptor complexes.[18] Fibroblast growth factor (FGF), which is a monomeric ligand like EGF, needs instead an accessory molecule to induce receptor dimerization.[19] Interestingly, the insulin receptor (IR) family exists as disulfide-bonded homo- or heterodimers of receptor subunits.[20] Thus, ligand binding does not induce receptor dimerization, but presumably causes a conformational change in the preformed dimeric receptor, which leads to receptor activation.

The activation of intrinsic protein kinase activity results in autophosphorylation of specific tyrosine residues in the cytoplasmic portion of the RTK. Moreover, tyrosine phosphorylation in the kinase domain stimulates the intrinsic catalytic activity of the receptor. Recently, biochemical and structural studies have revealed some of the molecular mechanisms that mediate such activation. There is substantial evidence that autophosphorylation occurs in *trans* by a second receptor tyrosine kinase after dimerization induced by ligand binding. In the unphosphorylated state, the receptor possesses a low catalytic activity because of the particular conformation of a specific domain in the kinase region, which interferes with the phosphotransfer event. Phosphorylation of the kinase domain removes this inhibition, and the catalytic activity is enhanced and persists for some time independently of the presence of the ligand. Although kinase activity is at a low basal level in the monomeric state, this activity is sufficient to induce transautophosphorylation once the dimer forms. Autophosphorylation also occurs outside the kinase domain and serves the important function of creating docking sites for downstream signal transduction molecules (see below).

The main function of the transmembrane domain is to anchor the receptor in the plane of the plasma membrane, thereby connecting the extracellular environment with internal compartments of the cell. It was initially thought that this domain represented a passive anchor of the receptor to the membrane;[15] however, point mutations in the transmembrane domain of one receptor, the neu/erbB-2, enhance its transforming properties. The transmembrane mutation in neu may have a stabilizing effect on the conformation, which results in dimerization and constitutive activation of receptor signaling.[21] Genetic alterations in this domain have, in fact, demonstrated an active role of this region in RTK dimerization and demonstrated that dimerization is not sufficient, but proper alignment must also occur for activation and signaling.[22]

The juxtamembrane sequence that separates the transmembrane and cytoplasmic domains is not well conserved between different families of receptors. However, juxtamembrane sequences are highly similar among members of the same receptor family. Studies indicate that this domain plays a role in modulation of receptor functions by heterologous stimuli, a process termed "receptor transmodulation."[15] For example, addition of PDGF to many types of cells causes a rapid decrease in high-affinity binding of EGF to its receptor. This has been shown to be a downstream effect of PDGF receptor activation in which protein kinase C, itself a serine protein kinase, is activated and, in turn, phosphorylates a site in the juxtamembrane domain of the EGF receptor.[15] This region may also play a role in signaling, as has been suggested by the capacity to bind specific substrates in a ligand-dependent manner. For example, it has been shown that *eps8* directly binds to the juxtamembrane domain of EGFR in a phosphotyrosine- and SH2-independent manner.[23]

The tyrosine kinase domain is the most conserved among tyrosine kinase receptors, and an intact protein tyrosine kinase domain is absolutely required for receptor signaling. For example, mutation of a single lysine in the ATP binding site, which blocks the ability of the receptor to phosphorylate tyrosine residues, completely inactivates receptor biologic function. The kinase domain of some receptor tyrosine kinases (eg, PDGF and FGF receptors) is split by insertions of up to 100 mostly hydrophilic amino acid residues. Kinase insertion sequences are highly conserved between species, suggesting an important role of this domain in receptor function. In fact, this region contains important autophosphorylation sites that have the function of coupling with signal-transducing molecules. Thus, it appears that the role of the kinase insert region is to mediate receptor interactions with second messengers.[15]

The carboxyl-terminal tail sequences are among the most divergent between known RTKs.[13] The carboxy terminal domain of the receptor is thought to play an important role in regulating kinase activity. This region typically contains several tyrosine residues, which are phosphorylated by the activated kinase. In fact, the receptor itself is often the major tyrosine phosphorylated species observed following ligand stimulation. Specific amino acid sequences in this domain play an important role in determining activation of specific signal-transducing molecules by RTKs as described in the section "Growth Factor Receptor Signaling" later in this chapter. The ability to molecularly clone related genes based on the conserved nature of their kinase domains has led to the identification of a number of structurally related members of several receptor families as listed below.

CLASSIFICATION OF GROWTH FACTORS AND THEIR RECEPTORS

Platelet-Derived Growth Factor Family PDGF is the major protein growth factor in human serum and is a markedly heat-stable, cationic protein that consists of two related but nonidentical (36.7% amino acid sequence identity) polypeptide chains designated A and B (also called PDGF-1 and PDGF-2).[1] PDGF molecules exist as AA and BB homodimers, as well as an AB heterodimer.[17] All of the ligands of the PDGF family exhibit similar dimeric structure and spacing of cysteines. PDGF-AB is the major PDGF form found in platelets and is released into serum upon blood clotting. However, there is evidence for the natural occurrence of each of the other forms. Connective tissue and glial cells in culture are highly sensitive to the mitogenic effects of PDGF,[17] and these cells express PDGF receptors. As shown in Figure 5-2, receptors of the PDGF family exhibit several distinctive features. Their extracellular regions show primary sequence characteristics and the same spacing of cysteine residues, consistent with the organization of five immunoglobulin-like domains.[24] Another feature of the PDGF receptor family is the presence of a large kinase insert within the tyrosine kinase domain. These 80 to 100 amino acid stretches are highly divergent among different family members. There are reports that the kinase insert is required for interaction with certain substrates,[25] and deletions in this domain impair receptor mitogenic signaling.[26] The α and β PDGF receptors are encoded by distinct genes,[24] and there is evidence that they exist as receptor subunits that differentially interact with the three dimeric PDGF ligands.[17] Thus, PDGF-AA can bind only the α receptor dimer, whereas PDGF-BB can interact with α, αβ, and β receptor dimers. The

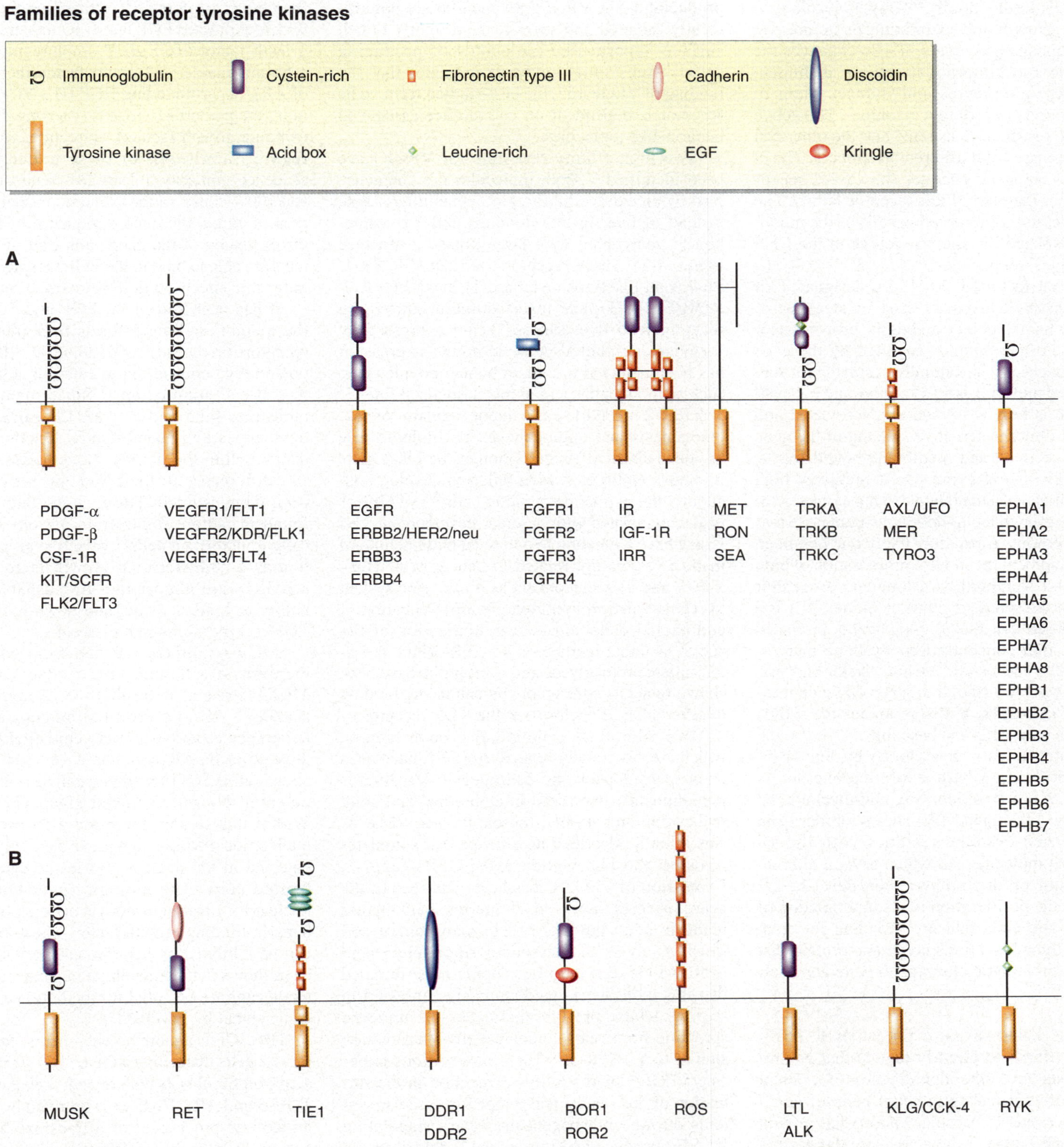

Families of receptor tyrosine kinases

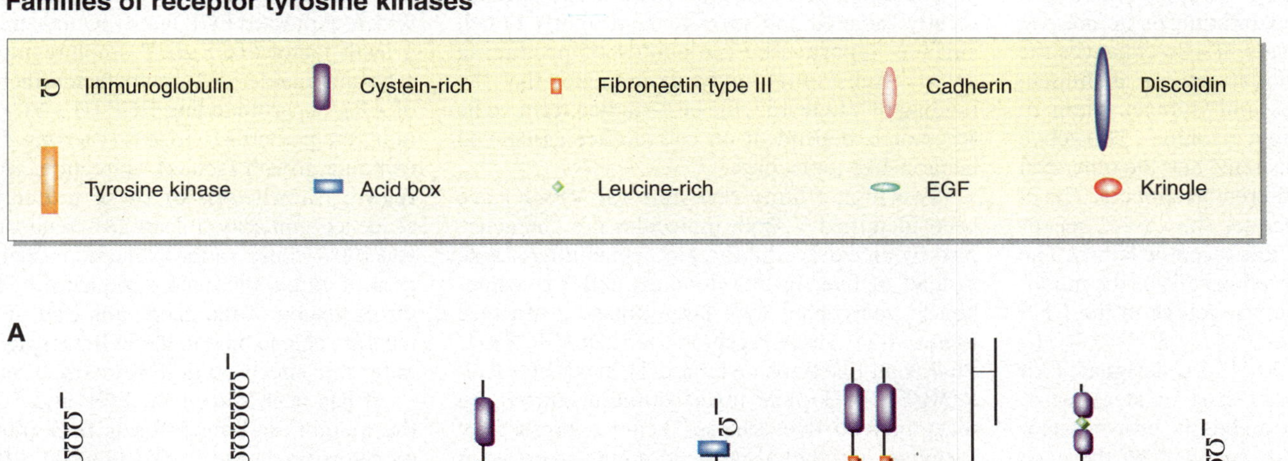

Figure 5-2 Families of receptor tyrosine kinases.

PDGF-AB heterodimer preferentially interacts with and triggers α and αβ receptors and would bind the β receptor without, however, inducing its dimerization. This is an example of the fine degree of regulation that can evolve in the interactions of ligands with their receptors. Presumably, in the case of PDGF, this relates to quantitative regulation of responses based on differential availability in tissues of ligands and receptors, since there is evidence that the two PDGF receptors themselves are each capable of mediating the major known PDGF responses including mitogenic signaling and chemotaxis.[24]

The transforming protein expressed by SSV shares close structural similarities with PDGF-B chain homodimers.[27] PDGF-B has been detected in human tumor cells[28] that also possess PDGF receptors. These findings, taken together with the demonstration that the normal PDGF-B gene can act as an oncogene when expressed at high levels[29] suggest that PDGF-B plays a role in the development of certain human cancers. The PDGF-A chain is frequently expressed by human tumor cells, and AA homodimers are produced by osteosarcoma, melanoma, and glioblastoma cells.[30] Recently, PDGF-C and -D, related ligands, which interact with PDGF receptors have been identified and isolated using bioinformatics approaches and mining of genome databases. The recently discovered PDGF-C and -D ligands have been reported to play an autocrine transforming role in some glioblastomas.[31]

Colony stimulating factor 1 (CSF-1) or macrophage-colony stimulating factor (M-CSF) also belongs to this family.[32] This molecule promotes the growth and maturation of monocytes and macrophage precursors. It also enhances the phagocytic and tumoricidal activity of human macrophage/monocytes and induces them to secrete a variety of different cytokines. Two active forms, one of which is secreted and the other cell associated, arise from differential splicing. The c-fms proto-oncogene encodes the CSF-1 receptor,[3] another member of this receptor family. The CSF-1 receptor is expressed in cells of the monocyte/macrophage lineage, as well as in the CNS and placental trophoblasts.[33]

Stem cell factor (SCF),[34] also designated kit ligand, mast cell growth factor, or steel factor (SLF), is a hematopoietic and tissue growth factor that binds to the receptor encoded by the c-kit proto-oncogene.[33] The naturally occurring form of this secreted molecule is a 165 amino acid polypeptide, which is heavily N- and O-glycosylated and exists as a dimer. Alternative splicing of the gene results in secreted and membrane-bound forms. The SCF/kit ligand is present at relatively high levels in human plasma relative to most other cytokines. This growth factor does not stimulate hematopoietic colony formation itself but has been shown to augment the in vitro proliferation of both myeloid and lymphoid hematopoietic progenitor cells in the presence of other cytokines.[34] It has been proposed that the SCF/kit ligand, produced locally at high concentrations by bone marrow stromal cells, acts as an "anchor" factor and permits stem cells to respond to physiologic concentrations of cytokines. It also promotes the activation of skin mast cells and basophils.

The Flt3 receptor was cloned by low stringency hybridization with a c-fms probe and is expressed in pre-B, monocytic, and myeloid cell lines.[33] The Flt3 ligand (Fl) shows similarity in the conserved cysteine residues with the kit ligand. This molecule, for which several alternative splicing products have been described,[35] stimulates the proliferation of a subpopulation of hematopoietic cells that are enriched for stem cells. The ligand is a transmembrane protein that undergoes proteolytic cleavage to generate a soluble factor.

Vascular Endothelial Growth Factor Family Efforts to identify factors that control angiogenesis led to the identification of a potent mitogen for vascular endothelial cells of small and large vessels.[36] Vascular endothelial growth factor (VEGF), also designated "vascular permeability factor" (VPF), is a glycosylated, dimeric heparin-binding protein (mol. wt. 45,000 Da) able to stimulate angiogenesis and to increase the permeability of capillary vessels to different macromolecules. The potent mitogenic effects of VEGF are restricted to cells of vascular endothelial origin.

VEGF 121, 165, 189, and 206 correspond in amino acid length to the four known isoforms. These arise from the alternative splicing of the primary transcriptional product. Whereas VEGF 121 and 165 are secreted into the medium from producing cells, VEGF 189 and 206 are not efficiently secreted and seem to bind tightly to cell surface heparin-like molecules of producing cells.[37] Substantial evidence indicates that the binding of VEGF 165, the best-studied form, to its receptor is dependent on cell surface-associated heparin-like molecules.

Two high-affinity receptors for VEGF have been identified.[37] Both molecules are characterized by an extracellular region containing seven, instead of five, Ig-like domains and a tyrosine-kinase interrupted by a large kinase insert (see Figure 5-2). These receptors, termed VEGFR-1/Flt-1 (fms-like tyrosine kinase-1), and VEGFR-2/KDR/Flk-1 (kinase insert domain containing receptor/fetal liver kinase-1), are expressed by vascular endothelial cells, although expression has been detected in certain hematopoietic cells, such as monocytes, and in melanoma cell lines.[37] VEGFR-2 is reported as a major regulator of vasculogenesis and angiogenesis. Its biologic role has been clarified by disruption of the Flk-1 gene in mouse embryos, which failed to develop both endothelial and hematopoietic cells.[38] VEGFR-1 is also associated with vascular development, and it may have a function in quiescent endothelium of mature vessels not related to cell growth. Thus, VEGF and its receptors act as a paracrine system to regulate the proliferation and differentiation of endothelial cells and neovascularization of tissues.[37] Another member is VEGFR-3/Flt4. Heparan sulfate proteoglycan and neurophilin have been shown to act as coreceptors by enhancing binding of several VEGF isoforms to the KDR receptor.[37]

Two additional endothelial growth factors, which are structurally related to VEGF, have been reported by Joukov and colleagues.[39] VEGF-B is predominantly expressed in embryonal and adult myocardial and skeletal muscle tissues. VEGF-C was initially identified as a factor that stimulates tyrosine phosphorylation of VEGFR-2 and -3. Expression of VEGF-C has been described in the heart, placenta, ovary, small intestine, and thyroid gland in adult humans and in many tumor cell lines. Analysis of messenger ribonucleic acid (mRNA) expression in developing mice revealed that this molecule is predominantly expressed in regions where the lymphatic vessels undergo sprouting from veins, with a pattern of expression similar to VEGFR-3.[40] These observations implicate VEGF-C and VEGFR-3 function in the formation of the venous and lymphatic vascular systems during embryogenesis.[39] Paracrine-acting VEGFs produced by tumor cells contribute to neoangiogenesis and lymphangiogenesis.[41]

Placenta-derived growth factor (PlGF)[42] is another member of this family, whose expression appears limited to placenta. Two isoforms, of which one, PlGF-2, shows high-affinity binding to heparin, arise from the same gene.

Epidermal Growth Factor Family EGF consists of 53 amino acids constrained by three internal disulfide bonds and is generated from a 1,200 residue precursor which contains eight units similar to EGF and is detected as a glycosylated membrane protein.[43,44] Other members of this widely expressed EGF family include transforming growth factor (TGF)-α,[45] amphiregulin (AR) or schwannoma-derived growth factor (rat homologue of AR), heparin-binding EGF (HB-EGF), betacellulin, the poxvirus mitogens (vaccinia, Shope, and myxoma growth factors), epiregulin, and the neuregulin family. All of these molecules share sequence similarity, at least 28% sequence identity, and 100% conservation of the six cysteine residues present within the mature sequence of EGF. With the exception of the neuregulins, all of these proteins are able to bind to the EGF receptor and show mitogenic effects on EGF-responsive cells.[46]

It has been shown for EGF and TGF-α, that the membrane-bound forms may interact with receptors on the surface of adjacent cells, thereby potentially contributing to cell-cell adhesion and to cell-cell stimulation.[45] Since many of these molecules bind and activate the same receptor, there appears to be substantial functional redundancy within this family. Nonetheless, quantitative differences in their biologic activities have been demonstrated. The findings that TGF-α is found in culture fluids from various oncogenically transformed cells[47] gave rise to its designation as a "transforming growth factor." TGF-α and EGF are almost indistinguishable in their ability to bind, activate, and down-modulate the EGF receptor in mammalian cells.[47]

AR was initially purified from conditioned medium of a human breast adenocarcinoma, MCF-7, treated with phorbol 12-myristate 13-acetate.[48] AR is a potent stimulator of normal keratinocytes and mammary epithelial cells. Relative to EGF, AR contains a very basic 40 αα stretch at its NH2 terminus, which is also rich in potential N- and O-linked glycosylation sites. Within this region, there are also two putative nuclear localization signals. In fact, AR has been detected in the nucleus and in the cytoplasm of treated cells. The biologic importance of its nuclear localization is not yet understood. AR is a heparin-binding growth factor, whose bioactivity can be inhibited by heparin sulfate.[48] It has also been shown that extracellular heparan sulfate proteoglycans are essential for mediation of its mitogenic signal by EGFR.[49]

HB-EGF is a more potent mitogen for smooth-muscle cells than either EGF or TGF-α.[50] It is also active on fibroblasts but not endothelial cells. Like TGF-α and AR, HB-EGF is secreted by means of proteolytic processing of a transmembrane precursor. At least five different forms with amino-terminal heterogeneity have been identified.[51] It has also been demonstrated recently that the membrane-anchored form of HB-EGF acts as the diphtheria toxin receptor.[52] Betacellulin is a potent mitogen for retinal pigment epithelial cells and vascular smooth-muscle cells.[53] Epiregulin was identified as a novel EGFR ligand, which stimulates the proliferation of fibroblasts, hepatocytes, and smooth-muscle cells.[54]

Purification of rat and human stimulatory proteins for the second member of the EGF receptor family (see below) led to the isolation of cDNAs encoding novel EGF-related proteins. The 44-kDa rat factor, termed neu differentiation factor (NDF), stimulates p185neu tyrosine phosphorylation and induces the production of milk components in certain breast carcinoma cell lines. The homologous human factors, termed heregulins (HRGs) or neuregulins (NRGs), were found to be mitogenic for certain mammary tumor cells.[55] At least 14 different NRG-1 isoforms have been described, including the acetylcholine receptor inducing activity (ARIA), and glial growth factors (GGF). NRG isoforms are encoded by the same gene through alternative splicing and are classified into two groups, α and β, that differ in their EGF-like domains.[55] Like TGF-α, NRGs display a wide distribution in many tissues and organs. Moreover, the expression patterns of some isoforms are tissue specific. For example, the α2 isoform is the predominant form in mesenchymal tissues, whereas the β1 isoform is enriched in brain tissue and spinal cord. Neuronal and non-neuronal tissues differ also in splicing of additional putative exons. Several other genes with a high degree of homology to NRG-1 have been identified. NRG-2 and NRG-3 are expressed predominantly in neural tissues both in embryos and adults, while NRG-4 was detected in adult pancreas and weakly in muscle.[55]

EGF family ligands have been classified based on their affinity for one of four members of the EGF/ErbB receptor family, which includes the EGFR (see review by Yarden[46]), ErbB-2, (also known as HER-2, for homologue of the human EGF receptor, or c-neu for homologue of the rat proto-oncogene neu), ErbB-3, and ErbB-4. The first group of ligands binds to the EGFR and includes EGF, TGF-α, AR, HB-EGF, betacellulin and epiregulin. The second group, represented by betacellulin, HB-EGF, and epiregulin, binds the EGFR and ErbB4. All NRGs bind to ErbB3 and ErbB4. Although no direct ligand for ErbB2 has been identified, it has been shown that this receptor is the preferred heterodimerization partner of the other ErbB receptors. In the case of ErbB3, heterodimerization is essential for NRG signaling since this unique receptor possesses an impaired kinase activity.[56] ErbB receptor heterodimerization allows the receptors to work synergistically by expanding the array of signaling events that can be activated by a single molecule.[46]

The EGFR was identified and isolated by biochemical techniques and shown to be the cellular homologue of the v-*erbB*, a retroviral oncogene.[2] The other members were isolated from genomic DNAs and cDNA libraries by low-stringency hybridization techniques using conserved tyrosine kinase domain probes. The extracellular domains of each of these molecules contain cysteine-rich motifs in two distinct regions and an uninterrupted tyrosine kinase domain. Whereas the EGFR and ErbB-2 are expressed in a wide variety of cell types, the expression of ErbB-3 is restricted to cells of epithelial or neuroectodermal origin.[46]

Fibroblast Growth Factor Family FGFs comprise a 22-member family that exhibits mitogenic activity toward a wide variety of cells of mesenchymal, neuronal, and epithelial origin.[19,57] These proteins can bind to and have their biologic activities modulated by heparin. The family includes acidic FGF (aFGF, FGF-1), basic FGF (bFGF, FGF-2), int-2 (FGF-3), hst/KS3 (FGF-4), FGF-5, FGF-6, keratinocyte growth factor (FGF-7), androgen-induced growth factor (AIGF or FGF-8), and glia activating factor (GAF or FGF-9).

The first to be isolated, bFGF, was recognized in certain hormone preparations by its mitogenicity for fibroblasts and chondrocytes and was later purified from bovine pituitary. aFGF was purified independently from acidic extracts of bovine brain.[57] Both acidic and basic FGF are angiogenic in vivo and are thought to function during embryogenesis. Both are single-chain polypeptides of about 17,000 daltons with 55% amino acid sequence identity. A striking feature of their structures, in contrast to those of many other family members, is the lack of a consensus secretory signal peptide. This has generated a great deal of speculation regarding their mode of release from cells. It has been argued that they are liberated by lysis or escorted out of intact cells by other proteins. The presence of a nuclear translocation signal and detection of aFGF and bFGF in the nuclei of endothelial and mesenchymal cells, respectively,[58,59] have suggested that these growth factors may also act internally without requiring a secretory signal sequence.

Analysis of DNA of mammary tumors induced by mouse mammary tumor virus (MMTV) revealed that the viral genome frequently integrates within a genetic locus termed int-2, and thereby activates expression of this gene by insertional mutagenesis. The protein encoded by int-2, renamed FGF3, is predicted to be 245 amino acids long and highly similar to aFGF and bFGF. The normal expression of int-2 is apparently limited to embryonic tissues.[57]

FGF-4 and FGF-5 were uncovered during searches for oncogenes in human tumor cells.[19,57] FGF-4 was isolated independently from a human stomach tumor (hst) and a Kaposi's sarcoma (KS3). It is mitogenic for vascular endothelial cells, human melanocytes, and mouse NIH/3T3 fibroblasts. The FGF-5 gene was isolated by DNA transfection using a selection system in which cell proliferation was dependent on abrogation of growth factor requirements.

FGF-6 was isolated by low stringency hybridization and was shown to act as a transforming gene for NIH/3T3 cells by transfection analysis.[19] KGF (FGF-7) was isolated from media conditioned by a human embryonic lung fibroblast cell line and was found to be a potent mitogen for epithelial cells, but to lack activity on fibroblasts or endothelial cells.[60] Thus, KGF was distinct in its target cell specificity, not only from other members of the FGF family, but from other known polypeptide growth factors as well. KGF is expressed by stromal, but not epithelial, cells of most major epithelial tissues. There is evidence that KGF plays a role in epithelial renewal during wound repair and as a stromal mediator of epithelial cell proliferation/differentiation in sex hormone-responsive tissues.[61] All of these findings support the concept that this factor is important in the normal mesenchymal stimulation of epithelial cell growth.

AIGF (FGF-8) was isolated from media conditioned by a cell line derived from a testosterone-dependent mouse mammary tumor cell line.[57] Target cells include epithelial and fibroblast cells and its expression appears to be restricted to the testes in the adult, and during the period of embryonic reproductive tract development.

GAF (FGF-9)[57] was purified from supernatants of a human glioma cell line. Little information is as yet available concerning most of the more recently identified FGF family members.

FGF-10 was identified by homologous-based PCR and has target cell specificity most similar to FGF-7. Other FGF family members have been recently identified by degenerate PCR or by homology searches of genome databases. Several lack secretory signal peptides and/or possess nuclear localization signals, and their functions remain to be defined.[57]

The prototype FGF receptor closely resembles the PDGF receptor family, but instead contains extracellular domain variants with two or three immunoglobulin-like motifs instead of five. Moreover, the kinase insert within the tyrosine-kinase domain of this receptor family is shorter (14 amino acids) than in members of the PDGF receptor (see Figure 5-2). Four distinct but related genes, FGFR1, FGFR2, FGFR3, and FGFR4, have been identified.[19] Adding to this complexity are findings of alternatively spliced forms of FGF receptors expressed in different cell types. In the case of the FGFR1 and FGFR2 genes, multiple forms of the FGF receptor are generated via alternative splicing. The second half of Ig domain III represents one site of alternative splicing in both FGFR1 and -2. Binding studies have shown that alternative splicing in this domain is important in determining ligand-binding specificities.

Tissue-specific alternative splicing in the third Ig domain and tissue-specific differential gene expression occur in vivo and regulate responsiveness to different FGF ligands. The complexity of heterodimeric interactions among different FGFRs remains to be elucidated.[19,57]

The Insulin Family The diversity of metabolic effects of insulin has been studied intensively for decades.[62] Its primary in vivo functions involve the regulation of rapid anabolic responses such as glucose uptake, lipogenesis, and amino acid and ion transport. In addition to its effects on metabolism, insulin stimulates DNA synthesis and cell growth. The insulin-like growth factors, IGF-I and IGF-II, were first recognized as serum factors, antigenically distinct from insulin. These molecules are induced by growth hormone and serve as its effectors in stimulating growth of skeletal tissues.[63]

IGFs are bound to carrier proteins and are maintained at steady concentrations in the bloodstream. The carrier proteins belong to a recently recognized class of proteins that have high affinity and specificity for the IGFs and are designated as insulin-like growth factor binding proteins (IGFBP). Five different IGFBPs have been identified in humans, and it seems that they are well conserved among mammals. The IGFBPs are involved in modulation of the proliferative and mitogenic effects of the IGFs at endocrine, paracrine, and autocrine levels.[64]

IGF-I, insulin, and IGF-II share around 50% amino acid sequence similarity.[63] Insulin is synthesized as a 109 amino acid precursor (preproinsulin), which is processed to a 6 kilodalton protein consisting of two chains (A and B) linked by two disulfide bonds. The structures of IGF-I and IGF-II are analogous to proinsulin in that they consist of a single polypeptide chain. In vivo studies indicate that IGF-I acts in an autocrine or paracrine mode, since infusion of IGF-I does not give rise to its growth-promoting actions.[63] Although it is not known whether overexpression of insulin family members can lead to transformation, addition of exogenous IGF-I or supraphysiologic levels of insulin to mouse NIH/3T3 cells overexpressing IGF-I receptors induced morphologic transformation and enabled the cells to grow in soft agar and form tumors in nude mice.[65]

The insulin receptor, IR, is the prototype for a family of RTKs, whose distinctive structural feature is to function as a heterotetrameric aggregation of two α and two β subunits (see Figure 5-2). The extracellular ligand-binding subunit, which contains a single cysteine-rich cluster, is disulfide linked to the transmembrane β subunit, which contains the cytoplasmic tyrosine kinase domain.[66] The IR binds insulin with approximately 100-fold greater affinity than it does IGF-I or IGF-II (100 pM v 10 nM). The IGF-I receptor is closely related to the IR in sequence and structure but binds IGF-I with highest affinity (100 pM), followed by IGF-II and insulin.[66] IGF-II is also bound by another receptor, which has been shown to be identical to the cation-independent mannose-6-phosphate receptor. The IGF-II receptor binds IGF-II and IGF-I with high affinity but does not bind insulin, and it appears to have a role in limiting IGF-II bioavailability. IGF-II growth effects during embryonic development occur earlier than those of IGF-I. A third member of the insulin receptor family, the insulin receptor-related receptor (IRR), shares their structural features. However, the ligand for IRR has not been identified.[67]

Hepatocyte Growth Factor Hepatocyte growth factor (HGF) was isolated from plasma[68] or platelets.[69] HGF levels were found to increase dramatically following acute liver injury, thus, HGF was reasoned to play an important role in liver regeneration. The biochemical and biologic properties of HGF were found to differ from those of other known growth factors. The molecular weight of native HGF is around 90,000 daltons and consists of two polypeptide chains of about 70,000 and 34,000 daltons linked by disulfide bonds. HGF cDNA is encoded as a single 728 amino acid protein, which is processed by proteolytic cleavage into heavy and light chains.[70] HGF is structurally related to plasminogen, containing serine-protease domains and disulfide bond-linked intrachain structures known as "kringles." Neither plasminogen nor plasmin have HGF-like activity, and HGF is not likely to be a protease since the histidine and serine residues in the region corresponding to the catalytic site are replaced by other amino acids.[70] HGF is mitogenic for a variety of epithelial cells, as well as endothelial cells and melanocytes and is also capable of inducing certain cell types to undergo morphogenesis when suspended in a semisolid matrix. Thus, HGF/scatter factor is a mitogen, motogen, and a morphogen.[71] The HGF gene knockout is an embryonic lethal, leading to obvious abnormalities in liver and placenta development.[72]

A ligand related to HGF, termed "HGF-like" or macrophage-stimulating protein (MSP),[73] is a heterodimer of a heavy chain of 53 kDa (α) and a light chain of 25 kDa (β). MSP shares with HGF the overall four kringle/protease domain-like structure. Liver appears to be the main source of MSP, and its major activity to date is stimulating macrophage migration.

C-met was initially identified as a rearranged oncogene in a human osteogenic sarcoma cell line transformed in vitro with a chemical carcinogen.[74] This proto-oncogene encodes a 190-kDa glycoprotein that is processed to form a heterodimer composed of a 50-kDa β-chain and 145-kDa α-chain. The extracellular, membrane spanning, and tyrosine kinase domains are located on the β-chain (see Figure 5-2). MET is expressed in a variety of tissues, but the highest levels are found in epithelial cells. The expression of HGF is detected in mesenchymal cells of various organs and in particular in stromal and non parenchymal cells neighboring epithelia.[74]

Ron/Stk was isolated as a c-met–related gene by means of degenerate oligonucleotides.[75] Ron cDNA encodes a glycosylated protein, which shares overall similar topology with the HGF receptor, displays 63% sequence identity in its catalytic domain and has a similar tissue distribution. The ligand for RON is MSP.[76]

Neurotrophin Family In addition to NGF,[4] which was discovered several decades ago, the neurotrophin family includes brain-derived neurotrophic factor (BDNF), neurotrophin-3 (NT-3), neurotrophin-4 (NT-4), neurotrophin-5 (NT-5), and neurotrophin-6 (NT-6). These factors mediate cell interactions regulating neuron survival during development and function in the adult nervous system as well.[77]

NGF is a basic 118 amino acid protein that acts in sensory and sympathetic neurons in the peripheral nervous system.[4] NGF is also present in the brain, where it serves a trophic function in the development and maintenance of cholinergic neurons of the basal forebrain. BDNF supports the survival of neural crest-derived embryonic sensory neurons in vitro, and is expressed mainly in the central nervous system (CNS). NT-3 shows a strong sequence similarity to both NGF and BDNF and displays a high degree of regional specificity. It is expressed in a subset of pyramidal and granular neurons in the hippocampus. NT-4 was isolated from Xenopus as a molecule showing the capacity to stimulate sensory neurons in culture. Thus, although members of the NGF family share considerable sequence similarity, they have unique biologic activities and cooperate to support the development and maintenance of the vertebrate nervous system.

The neurotrophins interact with two distinct classes of receptors.[77,78] One is represented by the p75/p80 low-affinity NGF receptor (p75NTR) protein. This receptor is a glycoprotein that is highly conserved across species and is broadly expressed in neuronal and non-neuronal tissues. Its extracellular region contains a cysteine-rich domain, whereas the intracellular domain is not related to any known protein and has no known enzymatic function. Low-affinity binding (Kd of 10-9 M) of all tested neurotrophins is mediated via this p75NTR, although its physiologic functions are not yet well understood.[78] The second class of neurotrophin receptors is encoded by the trk genes (see Figure 5-2). Trk or trkA was discovered in efforts to isolate oncogenes from human tumor cells.[79] The other two members of the family, trkB and trkC, were isolated by screening mammalian cDNA libraries with the trkA proto-oncogene as probe.[78] In contrast to the p75NTR, the cytoplasmic regions of p140 trkA, p140 trkB, and p145 trkC contain tyrosine kinase catalytic domains.

Whereas p140 trkA binds and becomes activated by NGF and NT-3, p140 trkB is activated by BDNF, NT-3 and NT-4. The trkC product is activated by NT-3.[78]

Ligands for the Axl/SKY/MER Family Protein S acts by indirectly inhibiting proteases involved in the coagulation cascade, although the precise mechanism remains unclear. Other functions, not directly involving coagulation, had been proposed for protein S.[80] This 70-kDa protein contains several modules, including an N-terminal region containing vitamin K-dependent α-carboxylation sites, a thrombin-sensitive module, a series of EGF-like repeats that undergo hydroxylation modification, and a module with homology to steroid-binding globulin. Gas6 was cloned as a growth arrest-specific gene[81] and shares all but the thrombin-sensitive module with protein S. Coagulation factors such as thrombin are able to activate intracellular signaling via G protein-coupled cell surface receptors. Thus some proteases and protease regulators may serve to integrate coagulation with associated cellular responses required for tissue repair and growth. Protein S and Gas6 serve as ligands for a subfamily of RTKs comprising Sky/Tyro3, Axl/Ufo and Mer (see Figure 5-2). Axl was identified as a transforming gene from patients with chronic myelogenous leukemia and myeloproliferative disorders, respectively, by DNA transfection-tumorigenicity analysis.[82] Axl expression has been detected in the majority of cell types examined. Sky is expressed predominantly in brain and it has been proposed that it may be involved in cell adhesion and/or survival, particularly in the CNS.[82,83]

A third family member, c-mer, was isolated from a human B-lymphoblastoid cDNA expression library.[82] The designation c-mer was based on its expression pattern in monocytes and tissues of epithelial and reproductive origin. Gas6 activates all three receptors, while Protein S is specific for Sky.[83] There is evidence that this family of receptors plays a role in regulation of macrophage activation and that compromised signaling results in a hyperactive immune system and may contribute to autoimmune diseases.[82] Their expression in neural tissues argues for neurotrophic roles as well.[83]

The Ephrin Family Ligands named ephrins do not function as typical soluble ligands but as membrane-bound molecules. The ephrins are divided into two groups: ephrin-A subclass, which is anchored to the membrane by a GPI linkage, and ephrin-B, which possesses a transmembrane domain.[84] The EPH receptors are the largest subfamily of RTKs (see Figure 5-2). These genes encode proteins of approximately 130 to 135 kDa, classified into two groups (A and B) based on relatedness of their extracellular domain sequences. With few exceptions, ephrin-A binds to EPHA receptors, whereas ephrin-B binds to EPHB receptors.[84] Although the mechanism by which membrane attachment participates in receptor activation has not been established, the activity of clustered soluble forms of these ligands suggests that membrane anchorage somehow facilitates their dimerization or aggregation. Moreover, recently it has been shown that the transmembrane ephrin-B molecules can signal bidirectionally following binding and activation of receptors in a neighboring cell.[84]

Although the EPH receptors and their ligands are differentially expressed, all members are expressed with a specific distribution in both the developing and adult nervous system, implicating a possible role in a variety of developmental processes. It is now clear that these receptors and their ligands mediate contact-dependent cell interactions. In particular, it has been shown that they play a role in the repulsion mechanisms that guide migrating cells and neuronal growth cones to their specific targets. This ligand-receptor system plays an important role in patterning of embryonic structure of the brain and somites. Repulsive interactions and complementary expression patterns have also been shown in the vasculature systems where EPH receptors are implicated in a demarcation between arterial and venous systems and vasculature remodeling.[84]

Agrin Family Agrin, named from the Greek word *agrein* (to aggregate), is a heparin Sepharose proteoglycan that is capable of inducing aggregation of acetylcholine receptors (AchRs) in myotubes at the postsynaptic membrane.[85] Agrin is a component of the extracellular matrix that is also capable of inducing aggregation of several other synaptic proteins. MuSK (muscle-specific kinase) is a novel RTK characterized by an extracellular portion containing four immunoglobulin-like domains (see Figure 5-2). MuSK knockout mice have established its central role in the AchR clustering. MuSK is crucial for agrin signaling at the neuromuscular junction, but evidence indicates that agrin does not directly bind MuSK. Thus, other components of the receptor complex must exist.[85]

GDNF Family Glial cell line-derived neurotrophic factor (GDNF), neurturin (NRTN), artemin (ART), and persephin (PSP) are members of the GDNF family of neurotrophic factors that, based on their cysteine knot structure, represent a subgroup of the TGF-β protein superfamily.[86] GDNF was initially identified as a trophic factor for midbrain dopaminergic neurons. GDNF is the most potent survival factor for motor neurons yet identified and has received attention as a potential therapeutic agent for the treatment of neurogenerative diseases.[87] GDNF also acts as a morphogen in kidney development. NRTN and ART have similar biologic properties to GDNF, whereas PSP is expressed at low levels in most tissues and is not a trophic factor for peripheral neurons.[86] GDNF acts through a receptor complex that consists of the c-ret proto-oncogene[88] encoded RTK (see Figure 5-2) and a ligand-binding component, the GDNF-family receptor α (GFRα). GFRα was identified by expression cloning as a novel glycosyl phosphatidylinositol (GPI)-linked protein.[89] Current evidence suggests that dimeric GDNF first binds to GFRα and this complex then interacts with RET to induce its dimerization and activation. Each GDNF family member ligand appears to bind preferentially to a different GFRα, but all signal through RET.[86]

The RET extracellular domain shows a unique feature: the presence of sequences similar to cadherin repeats. This motif is known to play an important role in Ca2+-dependent homophilic binding in other proteins.[90] So far, only RET, among all RTKs, is known to contain this sequence (see Figure 5-2). RET is essential for the development of the sympathetic, parasympathetic, and enteric nervous systems and the kidney.[90]

Angiopoietins The TIE (tyrosine kinase with immunoglobulin and epidermal growth factor homology domains) family of RTKs includes two receptors that are exclusively expressed in endothelial cells[91] (see Figure 5-2). Ang1 through -4 bind to the TIE2 receptor. Recent studies suggest that Ang ligands can also trigger TIE1 and that activation is amplified via TIE2.[92] Whereas Ang1 and -4 are activators of the TIE2 kinase, Ang2 and -3 are receptor antagonists.[91] Analysis of mice lacking Ang1 has shown that this molecule is critical for normal remodeling, maturation, and stabilization of the developing vasculature. Ang1 seems to mediate interactions between endothelial cells and supporting smooth muscle in a paracrine fashion.[91]

DDR Ligands Discoidin domain receptors (DDRs) are now referred to as DDR1 and DDR2.[93] As shown in Figure 5-2, these receptors possess several features that are shared with the TRK family in their kinase domains. However, the extracellular domains contain a motif with homology to discoidin-1, a lectin found in *Dictyostelium discoideum*, where it is involved in cell aggregation.[94] These receptors are widely and differentially expressed during development and in adulthood.[93] A unique feature of DDR1 and DDR2 is the fact that both receptors have collagens as ligands. Whereas DDR1 activation is achieved by type I to typeVI and type VIII collagens, DDR2 is only activated by fibrillar collagens.[93] Stimulation of DDR kinase activity requires the native triple-helical structure of collagen and occurs over an extended period of time. DDR1 null mice are viable but small and have mammary gland defects,[95] and the knockout of DDR2 leads to dwarfism and shortening of long bones.[96]

Other RTKs The identification of new RTKs implies the existence of new growth factors as well. Several RTKs await the assignment of ligands. ROR1 and ROR2[97] were originally identified based on similarity of their TK domains to the Trk family of neurotrophin receptors (see Figure 5-2). Both are widely expressed at high levels during early embryonic development. Dror, the corresponding gene in *Drosophila*,[98] is expressed specifically in the developing nervous system.[97] The ROR extracellular domains also show sequence similarity with the cysteine-rich domain of frizzled proteins, which acts as Wnt receptors, and there is evidence that ROR2 is involved in noncanonical Wnt signaling.[99]

Ros is the cellular counterpart of v-ros, originally identified in the avian sarcoma virus UR2.[100] This RTK has an unusually large extracellular domain of nearly 2,000 amino acids, and is closely related to the product of the sevenless gene from *Drosophila*. Ros is expressed during mammalian embryonic development and persists in the male reproductive tract. Male mice homozygous for deletion of this gene are sterile.[101]

Leukocyte tyrosine kinase (LTK) is expressed in B lymphocyte precursors, forebrain neurons in the mouse, as well as in placenta and hematopoietic cells in human.[102] A related gene identified as rearranged with the NPM nucleolar phosphoprotein gene in most anaplastic large-cell non-Hodgkin's lymphomas[103] is termed anaplastic lymphoma kinase (ALK). Alk is normally expressed in the small intestine, testis, and brain, but not in normal lymphoid cells. The *Drosophila* homologue of Alk is the receptor for the secreted molecule jelly belly.[104]

KLG (for kinase-like gene) was isolated from a cDNA library prepared from embryonic chicken tissues using as a probe the v-*sea* oncogene.[105] KLG is a member of the immunoglobulin gene superfamily, with seven Ig-like loops in its extracellular domain (see Figure 5-2). Its human homologue, CCK-4/PTK7, was isolated from a colon carcinoma.[106] Recent studies indicate that this receptor is a regulator of planar cell polarity in vertebrates.[107]

Table 5-1 Genetic Alterations of Growth Factor Signaling in Cancer

Growth Factor Receptor	Oncogenic Activation Mechanism	Cancer
PDGFR (and)	Autocrine activation	Osteosarcoma, melanoma, glioblastoma
	Tel-PDGFR– t(5;12) translocation	Chronic myelomonocytic leukemia (CMML)
CSF-1R/fms	Extracellular domain mutations	AML, myelodysplastic syndrome (MDS)
CSFR/kit	Point mutations and deletions	AML, mastocytomas, gastrointestinal stromal tumors
Flk2/Flt3	Internal tandem duplication (juxtamembrane domain)	AML, MDS, PML
VEGFR1, -2, -3	Paracrine activation	Tumor angiogenesis and lymphangiogenesis
EGFR	Autocrine activation, amplification/overexpression (amplification)	Squamous cell carcinoma, glioblastoma, other cancers
	Extracellular domain deletions	Glioblastoma
ErbB-2	Amplification/overexpression, amplification	Breast and ovarian carcinoma
FGFR1	Chromosomal translocations (ZNF198-FGFR1, FOP-FGFR1, CEP110-FGFR1, BCR-FGFR1)	Myeloid malignancies
FGFR3	IGH/MMSET t(4;14)-FGFR3 translocation	Multiple myelomas
c-met	Gene rearrangement: Tpr-met t(1;7)	Gastric carcinomas
	Amplification/overexpression	Thyroid, ovarian and colorectal cancers
	Point mutations	Hereditary and sporadic papillary renal carcinoma
TrkA	Gene rearrangement: Tpm-TrkA t(1;1)	Papillary thyroid carcinoma
TrkC	Gene rearrangement: Tel-TRKC t(12;15)	Congenital fibrosarcoma, acute myeloid leukemia, human breast carcinoma
Ret	Gene rearrangements: Ret/PTC (at least 10 PTC loci)	Papillary thyroid carcinomas
	Germline point mutations	Men2A, Men2B, FMTC
Tie1, Tie2	Paracrine activation	Tumor angiogenesis and lymphangiogenesis
Alk	Gene rearrangement: NPM-Alk t(2;5)	Anaplastic large-cell lymphomas

AML = acute myeloid leukemia; PML = promyelocytic leukemia; tpr = translocated promoter region.

RYK (for related to tyrosine kinase)[108] is ubiquitously expressed and encodes a protein consisting of a WIF (Wnt Inhibitory Factor) containing extracellular domain, and an atypical tyrosine kinase lacking kinase function.[109] Recent evidence indicates that Ryk binds canonical Wnts and is involved in Wnt signaling.[110]

ABNORMALITIES ASSOCIATED WITH GROWTH FACTORS IN CANCER CELLS

The role of growth factors in transformation was demonstrated by findings that the v-*sis* oncogene encoded a protein closely related to human PDGF-B.[1] MMTV induction of mammary carcinoma in mice correlated with integration of the provirus in the region of the int-2 (FGF-3) gene. Moreover, the FGF-4 and FGF-5 genes were isolated by their ability to cause transformation of mouse fibroblasts in vitro.[19,57] The expression of any growth factor and its specific receptor by the same cell might establish an autocrine loop that contributes to tumor progression. Autocrine transforming interactions have been identified in a number of human malignancies. At least one PDGF chain and one of its receptors have been detected in a high fraction of sarcomas and in glial-derived neoplasms.[30,111,112] In tissue culture, such tumor cells exhibit evidence of a functional autocrine loop, in which chronic PDGF receptor activation can be demonstrated by the detection of tyrosine phosphorylated receptors and/or down-regulation of the receptor protein. TGF-α is often detected in carcinomas that express high levels of EGF receptors.[113] Since many more ligands for tyrosine kinase receptors have recently been identified, the contribution of autocrine loops to human malignancies is probably much more extensive than is presently documented.

Growth factors also contribute to tumor progression by a paracrine mode. For example, continuous stimulation by growth factors in paracrine as well as autocrine modes during chronic tissue damage and repair associated with cirrhosis and inflammatory bowel disease may predispose to tumors.[114] Paracrine-acting angiogenic growth factors such as the VEGFs are produced by some tumor cells. Such growth factors cause the paracrine stimulation of endothelial cells inducing neoangiogenesis and lymphangiogenesis, which contribute to tumor progression.[41]

ABERRATIONS AFFECTING GROWTH FACTOR RECEPTORS IN TUMOR CELLS

Although growth factor receptors can be constitutively activated by autocrine loops, a number of other mechanisms have been identified by which growth factor receptors can become transforming. The paradigm for such alterations is v-*erbB*, the oncogenic counterpart of the EGFR receptor, transduced as the viral oncogene of avian erythroblastosis virus.[2] The mechanism of v-*erbB* activation involved deletion of its ligand binding domain, resulting in a truncated EGFR. More subtle mutational changes are responsible for oncogenic activation of v-fms, whose normal homologue is the CSF-1 receptor.[3] Here, a small genetic alteration affecting the external domain of the molecule was responsible for constitutive activation of this receptor as an oncogene.[115] V-ros and v-kit (see sections above) represent other examples.[33] Neu was initially identified as an oncogene by NIH/3T3 transfection analysis[116] of cDNA from ethylnitroso urea-induced rat neuroblastomas. The transforming gene was identified as having a specific mutation in its transmembrane domain responsible for oncogenic activation.[117]

Alterations affecting a large number of RTKs have been implicated in human malignancies as summarized in Table 5-1. One mechanism involves the amplification or overexpression of a normal receptor. As shown in Table 5-1 examples include the EGFR, ERBB-2, and c-met (see Birchmeier and colleagues[74] and Roskoski[118] for reviews). *ErbB-2* was initially identified as an amplified gene in a primary human breast carcinoma and a salivary gland tumor. Moreover, *erbB-2* overexpression beyond some critical threshold level in NIH/3T3 fibroblasts was shown to be sufficient to induce the malignant phenotype. Clinical studies have indicated that the normal *erbB-2* gene is frequently amplified and/or overexpressed in human breast carcinomas and in ovarian carcinomas, and detection in breast carcinomas of high *erbB-2* levels is a prognostic indicator of poor survival.[46,118]

Whereas *erbB-2* overexpression has been observed primarily in adenocarcinomas, overexpression of an apparently normal EGFR has been reported frequently in squamous cell carcinomas and glioblastomas. In many cases, the EGFR appears to be activated by autocrine stimulation by one of its ligands, most commonly TGF-α. Genomic alterations such as mutation or rearrangement have also been shown to activate the transforming capacity of receptor tyrosine kinases in human malignancies (see Table 5-1). In some human tumors, deletions within the external domain of the EGFR receptor or mutations in its tyrosine kinase domain[119,120] are associated with its constitutive activation.[46] The *ret* gene is activated by rearrangement, as a somatic event, in about one-third of papillary thyroid carcinomas. Germline mutations affecting the cysteine residues in the extracellular region are responsible for multiple endocrine neoplasia (MEN) 2A and for the familial medullary thyroid (FMTC) carcinoma syndrome. In contrast, a substitution of methionine by threonine at codon 918 in the catalytic region of the tyrosine kinase has been reported in MEN 2B.[121] These mutations have been shown to up-regulate RET catalytic function, resulting in its genetic transmission as an oncogene.

Met is overexpressed and/or mutationally activated in a variety of human tumors. A direct role of Met in hereditary papillary renal carcinoma (HPRC) has also been established.[74] This hereditary disease is characterized by multiple, bilateral renal papillary tumors, in which mutations activate constitutive kinase activity and transforming properties. Somatic mutations in MET have also been detected in some sporadic renal papillary tumors.[74] Several other receptors, including the PDGF-β, TrkA, TrkC, and Alk, have been shown to be oncogenically activated in human malignancies by gene rearrangements that lead to fusion products containing the activated TK domain.[33,122–124]

SIGNALING PATHWAYS OF TYROSINE KINASE RECEPTORS

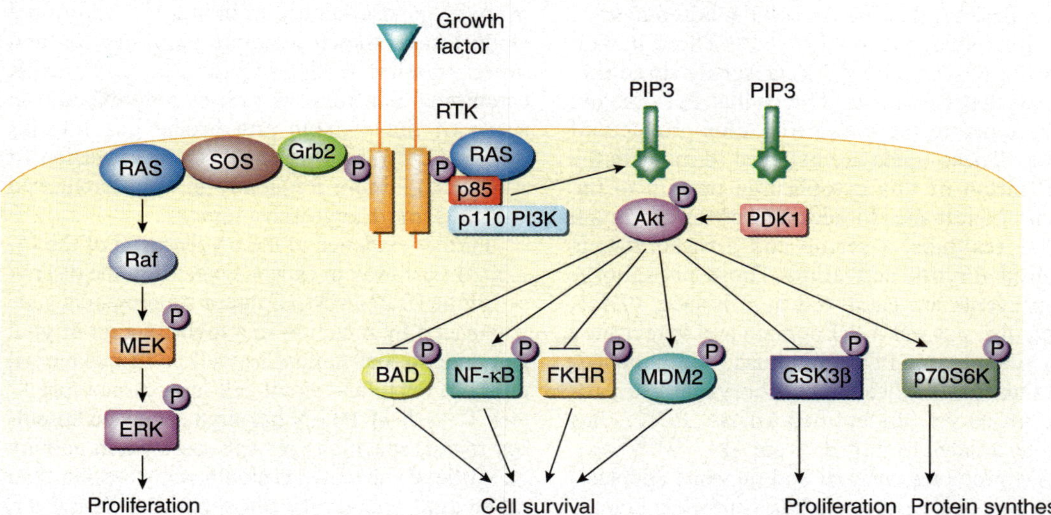

Figure 5-3 Intracellular effectors of receptor tyrosine kinases.

Molecules known as adaptor and scaffolding proteins[125] play an integral role in intracellular signaling by both recruiting various proteins to specific locations, and by assembling networks of proteins particular to RTK cascades. One such adaptor, Grb2, is important in the activation of the small G-protein Ras (Figure 5-3). These adaptor proteins often contain a variety of motifs that mediate protein-protein interactions. Src homology 2 (SH2) domains are protein motifs that bind to specific phosphorylated tyrosine containing sequences, dictating particular binding partners. SH3 domains recognize and bind to proline-rich sequences in target proteins.[126] Thus, in the case of an adaptor protein such as Grb2, which contains both SH2 and SH3 sequences, an adaptor protein can bring a cytoplasmic protein via its SH3 domain to an activated RTK via an SH2 domain binding to phosphorylated tyrosine residues of the receptor.

Another form of adapter, a docking protein, provides multiple binding sites on which effector molecules can attach, thereby expanding the magnitude of responses from an activated RTK. One such docking protein, IRS-1, is a substrate of the IR.[127] It contains tyrosine phosphorylation sites and two other important domains: a pleckstrin homology domain (PH) that binds to specific phosphoinositides and a phosphotyrosine-binding (PTB) domain that, like the SH2 domains, binds to phosphorylated tyrosine-containing sequences. These two domains are believed to properly position IRS-1 adjacent to the receptor. Proteins that attach to the phosphorylated tyrosine residues phosphorylated in response to IR activation include PI3-K, Shp-2, Nck, and Grb-2.

Another concept that has surfaced in mammalian signaling is the importance of so-called scaffolding proteins in signaling cascades. Scaffolding proteins allow the formation of multienzyme complexes. The activation of a signaling cascade by a growth factor is an extremely rapid process and is not likely to occur as a result of two proteins randomly floating in the intracellular milieu. Scaffolding proteins ensure the close proximity of the necessary components. Moreover several enzymatic components of a particular signaling cascade may be shared, although the substrates of each may differ. Thus, scaffolding proteins ensure the proper routing of signals by preventing unwanted cross talk between pathways.[125]

The PDGF system has served as the prototype for identification of the components of signaling cascades. Certain molecules become physically associated and/or phosphorylated by the activated PDGF receptor kinase. Those identified to date include phospholipase C (PLC)-γ,[128] phosphatidylinositol-3'-kinase (PI-3-K) regulatory subunit (p85),[129] NCK,[130] the phosphatase SHP-2,[131] Grb2,[132] CRK,[133] *RAS* p21 GTPase-activating protein (GAP),[134] *SRC,* and *SRC*-like tyrosine kinases.[135] Many of these molecules contain SH2 or SH-3 domains.

PLC-γ is one of several PLC isoforms and is involved in the generation of two important second messengers, inositol triphosphate and diacylglycerol.[136] The former causes release of stored intracellular calcium and the latter activates protein kinase C (PKC). These second messengers appear rapidly in cells following stimulation by growth factors such as PDGF. The relative increase in their synthesis in vivo correlates reasonably well with the ability of a particular receptor kinase to induce tyrosine phosphorylation of PLC-γ.[128] The actions of a number of tumor promoters are thought to be mediated by PKC,[136] and PKC overexpression or gene alteration has been reported to increase cell proliferation in culture.[137]

PI-3-Kinase and Survival Signaling The regulation of cell survival and cell death is of extreme importance. During development, certain cells are eliminated by apoptosis (programmed cell death) and others permitted to survive. This is essential for organs and systems to form correctly. The deregulation of these processes can lead to a variety of malformations resulting in deformities or, in extreme cases, incompatibility with life. In adulthood, regulation of cell survival is equally important for proper homeostasis. Damaged cells must be removed and terminally differentiated cells must be sustained. A failure for this to occur may result in either the accumulation of mutations leading to cancer or, alternatively, to degenerative diseases.

PI-3-K is a lipid kinase that catalyzes the transfer of the γ-phosphate from ATP to the D3 position of the phosphoinositide (PtdIns) generating PtdIns3P, 4P2, and PtdIns3, 4, 5P3. These lipids can act in a variety of cascades, promoting the activation of several proteins[138] (see Figure 5-3). PI-3-K activation has been demonstrated to play an important role in cell survival signaling in a number of cell types.[139] There are three classes of PI-3-Ks, which exhibit variability with respect to their method of activation or their preferred lipid substrate.

The prototypical class 1 PI-3-K consists of two subunits encoded by two distinct loci: a regulatory and a catalytic subunit. The regulatory subunit is a 50–85 kDa protein that is tightly associated with the p110 catalytic subunit. The most well studied regulatory subunit is p85. This subunit has several characteristic protein domains, including two SH2 domains, which can bind to the phosphorylated tyrosines of several RTKs, thereby facilitating its activation,[139] an SH3 domain that binds to proline-rich regions of several proteins, and an inter SH2 region that is essential for its association with the p110 catalytic subunit. As is evident, p85 is a complex molecule and the exact functions of each domain have not been completely elucidated.

The classic mode of PI-3-K activation involves its binding to the phosphorylated tyrosine residues of RTKs, including PDGFR, EGFR, bFGFR, and TRK A via the two SH2 domains of p85. This results in a conformational change that is believed to facilitate activation of p110 catalytic activity. PI-3-K activates PtdIns by a phosphorylation event. There are several known downstream effectors of PI-3-K. These include RaC, $p70^{s6k}$, certain isoforms of PKC, and, most relevant to cell survival, Akt/PKB.[139] Akt has been shown to be responsible for PI-3-K–dependent cell survival and is the cellular homologue of the viral oncogene v-Akt.[139,140] Three human homologues encode 57-kDa serine/threonine kinases that contain an N-terminal PH domain, which binds to the activated PtdIns products of PI-3-K. These lipids are believed to mediate the localization of this cytoplasmic protein to the plasma membrane. In addition, phosphorylation of two residues, a serine and a threonine, is required for full activation. These phosphorylation events are catalyzed by a kinase, PDK1, which also possess a PH domain and is recruited to the membrane. PDK1 (PtdIns3, 4, 5P3 dependent kinase) specifically phosphorylates Thr307 of Akt. An as yet unidentified kinase, PDK2, has been postulated to fully activate Akt.[139,140]

Akt promotes survival and prevents apoptosis in various cell types including cerebellar granule neurons, superior cervical neurons, myeloid cells, and myc-overexpressing fibroblasts. The mechanism of Akt-induced survival has begun to be understood. Akt phosphorylates the proapoptotic Bcl-2 family member, BAD. When BAD is phosphorylated, it gains affinity for the cytosolic protein 14-3-3 and forms a complex with this protein. Nonphosphorylated BAD can heterodimerize with the antiapoptotic Bcl-2 family member Bcl-X_L. Upon phosphorylation of BAD, its binding to 14-3-3 decreases formation of the BAD-Bcl-X_L heterodimer, thus permitting free Bcl-X_L to protect the cell from apoptosis[139,140] (see Figure 5-3). However, the expression of BAD is not ubiquitous, and in certain cell types in which PI-3-K/Akt prevents apoptosis, BAD is not expressed. Akt also phosphorylates the Forkhead-related transcription factor (FKHR), creating a binding site for 14-3-3, which retains FKHR in the cytoplasm and inhibits its transcriptional gene targets including proapoptotic proteins such as BIM and FAS ligand. There is also evidence that Akt can indirectly increase the function of the NFκB transcription-factor complex, which has prosurvival functions. Akt has been reported to activate IκB kinase (IKK), which induces degradation of the NFκB inhibitor, IκB. Recent studies indicate that Akt may increase TP53 degradation through phosphorylation of MDM2.[139,140] Thus, Akt has multiple prosurvival functions. There is also evidence that activated Akt and/or PDK1 exert positive effects on cell growth through phosphorylation of proteins such as p70S6K, involved in protein synthesis, and inhibitory phosphorylation of GSK3, which normally targets cyclin D1 for degradation. Thus, the functions of PI3 kinase are complex and extend beyond prosurvival functions in the coordinated responses of a cell to growth factor signaling (see Figure 5-3).[139,140]

PI-3-Kinase Signaling in Cancer PIK3CA, which encodes the p110α catalytic subunit, was found to be amplified in a high percentage of ovarian tumors and ovarian tumor cell lines.[141] Recent studies have shown that PIK3CA is mutationally activated in more than 25% of colon, brain, and gastric tumors.[142] There is also evidence of Akt involvement in human malignancies. Akt1 was found to be amplified 20-fold in a primary gastric adenocarcinoma.[143] Additional studies have shown genomic amplification and overexpression of Akt2 in pancreatic and ovarian carcinoma cell lines, as well as amplification in some of the ovarian and breast carcinomas examined[140] (see Table 5-1). Overexpression of Akt2 occurs more frequently in undifferentiated and, thus, more aggressive tumors.

Further evidence of the involvement of the PI-3-K/Akt pathway in cancer stems from the discovery of the PTEN/MMAC tumor suppressor, a gene inactivated by mutation in a high fraction of glial and endometrial tumors as well as in melanoma, prostate, renal, and small-cell lung carcinomas[144] (see Table 5-1). PTEN has high sequence homology to dual specificity phosphatases but its activity on artificial substrates is significantly weaker than other dual specificity phosphatases. However, PTEN was shown to dephosphorylate the 3 position of phosphatidylinositol both in vitro and in vivo. Thus, PTEN directly opposes PI-3-K activity by dephosphorylating its activated lipid products. Therefore, the tumor suppressor activity of PTEN is mediated via its ability to oppose both PI-3-K and Akt, both of which have been shown to be themselves oncogenic.[144]

Ras Ras proteins are a major point of convergence in RTK signaling and are an important component of the cellular machinery necessary to transduce extracellular signals[145] (see Figure 5-3). Ras small GTP-binding proteins are membrane-bound intracellular signaling molecules that mediate a wide variety of cellular functions including proliferation, differentiation, and survival. This family consists of 10 highly conserved proteins, including H-, N-, and K-Ras, R-Ras, Rap1(A and B), TC21 (R-Ras2), and R-RAS3.[145,146] Ras proteins are synthesized in the cytosol and become associated with the inner leaflet of the plasma membrane via post-translational modifications, including a form of fatty acid lipidation, isoprenylation, on Cys-186. The C-terminal CAAX box (Cys, two aliphatic amino acids, followed by any residue) is the motif required for this essential post-translational modification.[147] Ras acts as a molecular switch alternating from an inactive GDP-bound state to an active GTP-bound state. The paradigm for Ras activation involves the recruitment of a guanine nucleotide exchange factor (GNEF) to the membrane in response to growth factor binding and subsequent activation of an RTK.[145] GNEFs promote the release of GDP from the catalytic pocket of Ras, and the relative abundance of intracellular GTP as compared to GDP ensures preferential binding of GTP. The best example of a Ras GNEF is SOS (son of sevenless), which is brought to the membrane by its stable association with the adaptor protein Grb2.[148] Additional Ras GNEFs have been cloned and include GRF1 and 2 and Ras GRP. The exact specificity of their interactions with different Ras family members and the nature of the stimuli that activate these various exchange factors is presently under investigation.[149]

Although Ras is a GTPase, its intrinsic GTPase activity is actually quite low and requires additional proteins known as GTPase-activating proteins (GAPs) to promote GTP hydrolysis. GAPs can accelerate GTP hydrolysis by several orders of magnitude and are, thus, negative regulators of Ras functions.[150] The mechanism by which GAP accelerates the GTPase reaction is complex and not completely understood. Currently, several GAPs for Ras have been identified, including p120 GAP, NF1-GAP/neurofibromin, and GAP1^m, as well as GAPs with preferential activity on related proteins such as R-Ras.[150] Of particular interest is NF1 as it is found to be frequently inactivated by mutation in patients with the familial tumor syndrome, neurofibromatosis type I.

Ras Function Ras mediates important cellular processes such as proliferation, survival, and differentiation. The exact contribution of H-, N-, and K-Ras isoforms is not clear, as targeted knockouts to H- and N-Ras genes resulted in mice that did not exhibit an abnormal phenotype, whereas a K-Ras knockout is an embryonic lethal and exhibits liver and hematopoietic defects.[147] Therefore, there may be a certain degree of redundancy between these three Ras proteins.

Ras and Cancer Ras is involved in a high fraction of human cancers (see Table 5-1). Ras has been shown to be oncogenically activated by mutations in over 15% of all human tumors, and in some cancers, such as pancreatic carcinoma, the frequency is as high as 90%.[151] The initial evidence for Ras involvement in cancer came from the discovery of transforming retroviruses, Harvey and Kirsten sarcoma viruses, which contained H- and K-ras cellular-derived oncogenes. The first human oncogenes were identified by transfecting genomic DNA from human tumor cell lines into NIH3T3 mouse fibroblasts and isolating the DNA fragments from the transformed foci. These were shown to be the human homologues of the viral *ras* genes.[152]

The major hotspots for activating *ras* mutations are all located near the bound nucleotide, particularly in proximity to the nucleotide phosphate groups. Naturally occurring mutations in human tumors have been found at residues 12, 13, 59, and 61, with positions 12 and 61 being the most common.[147,151] The majority of these mutations decrease the intrinsic rate of GTP hydrolysis by Ras and make the molecule significantly less sensitive to GAP-stimulated GTP hydrolysis. Thus, the outcome is a predominantly GTP-bound form that is constitutively active and essentially independent of growth factor stimulation. Ras-transformed cells appear refractile and spindle shaped, have disorganized actin filaments, and have a decreased affinity for the substratum. They can proliferate in the absence of adhesion (anchorage independence) or in the presence of low serum concentration. Of note, Ras alone is unable to transform primary mouse or human fibroblasts.[152] When oncogenic Ras is introduced into such cells by retroviral mediated gene transfer, the cells undergo permanent growth arrest, also termed senescence, characteristic of primary cells passed for multiple generations in culture.[153] This senescence response appears to be dependent on the function of certain genes such as *p16*^{INK4a} and *TP53,* which act as tumor suppressor genes. The inactivation of these tumor suppressor genes plays a critical role in cancer development. In fact, inactivation of *TP53* or *p16*^{INK4a} allows Ras to transform cells, which may help to explain the selective pressure for loss of these tumor suppressor genes in tumors containing *ras* oncogenic mutations.[153]

Additional members of the Ras family of GTP-binding proteins can cause cellular transformation when overexpressed in rodent fibroblasts. These include R-Ras,[154] TC21/R-Ras2,[155] and R-Ras3.[156] In fact, TC21 has been found to be mutated infrequently in cancers. The other transforming members have not been shown to be oncogenically activated in human tumors.

Signaling Downstream of Ras Ras mediates its multitude of biologic effects via several downstream effectors. Several proteins have been shown to directly bind to Ras either in vivo or in vitro in a GTP-dependent manner by such methods as yeast 2-hybrid or co-immunoprecipitation. These include A, B, and C-Raf, Ral GDS, RGL II, the PI-3-K, MEKK1, AF6, and PKC.[145] Whether they are all true physiologic effectors of Ras remains uncertain. It has been demonstrated that PI-3-K can be activated independently of RTKs by Ras, providing a direct connection between Ras and PI-3-K prosurvival signaling.[157]

Ras>Raf>MAPKinase Cascade The most well studied effector of Ras is the serine/threonine kinase Raf. Raf has been shown to bind to Ras and in many cases has been demonstrated to be indispensable for Ras functions such as cellular transformation.[158] In fact, activated Raf or v-Raf, a truncated form of Raf, was initially isolated as a retroviral oncogene. There are three known mammalian Raf isoforms, designated A-, B-, and C-Raf (also known as Raf-1). C-Raf is ubiquitous in its tissue expression, whereas A-Raf and B-Raf expression are more restricted. A-Raf is expressed mainly in steroid-responsive tissues, particularly in urogenital tissues, whereas B-Raf is restricted to neural-derived tissues.[159] The N-terminus of the protein has a negative regulatory role in Raf activation, while the C-terminus contains the kinase domain. Ras-mediated activation of Raf requires its binding to the amino terminus.

It is believed that interaction of Ras with Raf allows translocation of Raf to the membrane (see Figure 5-3), where additional steps leading to its full activation can occur.[145] Several phosphorylation events on both serine/threonine and tyrosine residues are believed to have a role in the full activation of Raf, and major differences in certain phosphorylation sites between B-Raf and C-Raf, indicate that regulation of these two isoforms may differ significantly.[159]

Once activated, Raf can phosphorylate MEK (mitogen/extracellular-signal regulated kinase kinase), also known as Map Kinase Kinase (MKK), a dual specificity kinase, on Ser_{218} and Ser_{222} leading to its activation[160] (see Figure 5-3). There are two isoforms of MEK, designated MEK1 and 2, both of which are expressed ubiquitously with an approximate sequence identity of 80%. MEK, once activated, can, in turn, activate MAP Kinase or extracellular signal regulated kinase (ERK).[160] Activation occurs via tandem phosphorylations on both threonine and tyrosine (Thr_{183}-Glu-Tyr_{185}) with the phosphorylation on tyrosine occurring first. There are two ERK isoforms (1 and 2), ubiquitously expressed and with very similar sequence (90%). These proteins, 44 kDa and 42 kDa, respectively, translocate to the nucleus where they can activate a variety of proteins through phosphorylation on serine or threonine. ERK can phosphorylate several of the members of the ETS family of transcription factors, explaining its ability to activate transcription of certain genes.[160] The ETS transcription factors are helix-turn-helix proteins. A member of this family, p62^{TCF}/Elk-1, in complex with the serum response factor (SRF), transactivates the serum response element (SRE), which can be found in several promoters, including that of c-fos. Phosphorylation of ElK-1 by ERK dramatically increases c-fos transcription. ERK can also activate a variety of protein kinases via phosphorylation. For example, p90 RSK is a serine/threonine kinase that has a role in protein translation and is a substrate for the ERKs.[160]

In addition to positive regulation of the MAP kinase pathway by phosphorylation, there are negative regulatory mechanisms that serve to attenuate activation of this cascade. A principal mode of this negative regulation is through a variety of phosphatases, a majority of which have a dual specificity, meaning that they can dephosphorylate both serine/threonine and tyrosine residues.[160] This is consistent with the knowledge that ERK must be phosphorylated on both threonine and tyrosine to achieve maximal activation. There are several known MAP Kinase phosphatases that differ in terms of substrate specificity.

ERK activation can lead to increased DNA synthesis and cell proliferation. In fact, cyclin D1 expression is induced by activated forms of Ras, Raf, and MEK.[161] Dominant negative mutants of members of this cascade can also block this induction in response to growth factor stimulation. Of particular interest is the fact that cyclin D1 can be rearranged or amplified in human tumors and tumor cell lines (see Table 5-1), thus implicating a role for this G1 cyclin in human cancer.[162]

Raf and Cancer Knowledge of the importance of RTK signal transduction in cancer has recently led to screening of tumor cell lines for mutations in these pathways. Davies and colleagues[163] identified B-raf mutations in around 66% of human melanoma cell lines and primary tumors (see Table 5-1). Of note, the nucleotide changes observed were not consistent with mutations typically induced by UV. Lower frequencies of analogous mutations were observed in colon carcinoma and small-cell lung cancer (SCLC)[163] (see Table 5-1). These mutations were further shown to oncogenically activate B-raf as determined by NIH3T3 transfection analysis, although the transforming efficiency was significantly lower than observed with Ras. These findings increase the number of human tumors that exhibit mutational activation of growth factor signal transduction pathways.[163]

Other MAP Kinases In addition to the ERKs, there are other MAP kinases belonging to distinct MAPK cascades with both different upstream activators and downstream effectors. The c-Jun N-terminal kinase (JNK)/stress-activated protein kinase (SAPK) and p38 MAP kinase have been demonstrated to modulate cellular responses to a wide variety of extracellular stimuli including mitogens, inflammatory cytokines, and UV irradiation.[164] In contrast to its ability to activate the MAPK/ERK cascade, H-Ras only minimally perturbs JNK/SAPK. However, overexpression of the constitutively activated mutants of the small G-proteins, Rac, and Cdc42, leads to the robust stimulation of JNK/SAPK activity.[164] The pathways leading to JNK activation mirror those seen for ERK. Thus, a variety of MKKs have been discovered that can phosphorylate the various JNK isoforms.[164]

As with the ERKs, the end result of JNK activation is the phosphorylation of certain transcription factors within their activation domains, increasing the transcriptional activity of promoters containing response elements for these factors. JNK can phosphorylate ATF2, ATFa, c-Jun, and Jun-d, as well as ElK-1 and SAP1.[164] Phosphorylation of c-Jun by JNK increases its half-life, preventing ubiquitin mediated degradation of this shortly-lived protein.[165] Evidence from experiments performed using knockout cells of an upstream activator of JNK (MKK4) have demonstrated that JNK plays a role in AP-1 transcriptional-dependent events in response to stress.[166]

MAP kinase cascades also activate transcription factors such as c-*fos* and c-*jun*. Of note, these genes were initially discovered as retroviral oncogenes in mice and chickens, respectively. The FBJ and FBR murine viruses contain the *fos* sequence under the viral LTR promotor and exhibit changes in regulatory phosphorylation sites that make them more active than the proto-oncogene.[167] ASV17 is a chicken retrovirus containing a Jun oncogene fused to the viral Gag sequence and has lost regulatory phosphorylation sites.[168] Overexpression of c-*fos* can cause cell transformation[169] as well. Fos and Jun together comprise the AP-1 transcription factor. This dimer, in response to UV irradiation, environmental stresses, and PKC activation, binds to AP-1 target sequences such as 12-O-tetradecanoylphorbol-13-acetate (TPA) responsive elements.[170]

IMPLICATIONS FOR CANCER THERAPY

Since many of the signaling pathways involved in cellular transformation by oncogenes have been elucidated, efforts are underway to develop treatment strategies that target these specific signaling molecules or their downstream effectors. This type of therapy has great potential because it relies on blocking specific molecules rather than traditional chemo- or radiation therapy. One possible point at which to intervene is the initial interaction between the growth factor and its cognate receptor at the surface of tumor cells whose growth is dependent on autocrine or paracrine mechanisms. Specific antagonists can be developed based on knowledge of ligand-receptor binding interactions. In some cases, such molecules are produced naturally and presumably have a physiologic role in modulating growth factor signaling.[171,172]

One approach is based on the application of monoclonal antibodies that specifically neutralize the activities of growth factors or interfere with ligand receptor interactions. Monoclonal antibodies directed against receptors have been applied against tumors with receptor overexpression.[173] For example, administration of certain monoclonal ERBB2/HER2/neu or EGFR receptor antibodies was shown to inhibit tumor cell growth.[174,175] Such studies led to the development of Herceptin (trastuzumab), a humanized monoclonal antibody against the extracellular domain of ERBB2. Experimental evidence further indicated that Herceptin enhances the responsiveness of ERBB2 overexpressing breast cancer cells to taxanes, anthracyclines, and platinum compounds.[176] Moreover, a phase III trial indicating that Herceptin added to first-line therapy for metastatic breast cancer provided a significant benefit with respect to survival[177] led to regulatory approval for its use with paclitaxel in first-line therapy. A further recent trial showed its great advantage in breast cancers with ERBB2 overexpression in combination with chemotherapy for treatment in the adjuvant setting. A chimeric monoclonal directed against the extracellular domain of the EGFR,[178] cetuximab (IMC-C225; Erbitux), has been approved for use in patients with metastatic colorectal tumors exhibiting EGFR overexpression.

A related strategy uses receptor monoclonals or growth factors to deliver cytotoxic agents, such as toxins or radioisotopes, to tumor cells that overexpress a particular RTK.[179] In addition to targeting an overexpressed receptor on which tumor proliferation is dependent, this approach could provide a means of targeting chemotherapeutic agents internalized by the receptor to sites within the tumor cell. As with other receptor targeting strategies, the efficacy of this approach would be expected to depend on the differential magnitude of receptor expression by the tumor as opposed to normal cells, as well as accessibility of tumor cells to the systematic administration of such agents.

Increased understanding of the important role of growth factor signal transduction in cancer has also led to intensive efforts focused on the development of small molecule inhibitors of specific target molecules including receptor tyrosine kinases and their downstream effectors. The most exciting progress to date has come from investigations of Gleevec (imatinib; STI571; Glivec), a low molecular weight inhibitor of the tyrosine kinase activity of the PDGFR, c-kit, and the nonreceptor tyrosine kinase Abl, developed by Novartis. Abl is translocated in chronic myelogenous leukemia (CML) as part of the Philadelphia chromosome to create the Bcr-Abl oncogene.[180] Gleevec blocks ATP binding to the Abl tryosine kinase, preventing phosphorylation reactions involved in signaling.[173,181] Clinical trials rapidly confirmed the efficacy of Gleevec in CML and, therefore, Bcr-Abl as a target in this disease. Remarkable responses were observed in the chronic phase of the disease with complete clearing of Ph+ cells from the circulation in 95% of patients who had failed standard therapy. Only 9% of patients relapsed over a median follow-up of 18 months,[181] leading to regulatory approval. Gleevec is most effective in the chronic phase; fewer responses and more relapses occur with patients in myeloid blast crisis. As might be expected, de novo resistance correlated with accumulation of resistance conferring mutations during disease progression.[181] The success of Gleevec has been extended to gastrointestinal stromal tumors (GIST) in which activating mutations in c-kit or the PDGFR have been identified. Remarkable clinical activity was observed in this chemotherapy-refractory tumor, leading to approval for use of Gleevec in such patients.[182] Other tumors with c-kit or PDGFR activating mutations are currently being evaluated for treatment efficacy by Gleevec.[173,181]

Small molecule inhibitors, which target the ATP binding site of the EGFR, are being developed by a number of pharmaceutical companies. Iressa (gefitinib) developed by AstraZeneca, exhibited activity as a single agent in preclinical studies and enhanced the antitumor effects of taxanes and platinum compounds.[183] Although phase III clinical trials with NSCLC in both settings did not show striking benefits, regulatory approval was provided for metastatic NSCLC patients, who have failed standard therapy. Recent studies indicate that a minority of NSCLC possess EGFR tyrosine kinase activating mutations and that this subset of tumors is sensitive to the EGFR kinase inhibitors.[119,120] More recently Tarceva (erlotinib), developed by OSI/Genentech, was shown to increase survival in advanced NSCLC in phase III clinical trials leading to its approval for this indication. Preclinical development and/or clinical trials for other small molecule inhibitors of the EGFR or the EGFR and ERBB2 are ongoing. Other RTKs against which small molecule inhibitors are currently under development include the PDGF receptor, which is commonly activated in glioblastomas by an autocrine mechanism, and c-met, which is involved in a number of cancers.[173,184]

Downstream components of growth factor signaling pathways activated in cancer cells are also potential therapeutic targets. There has been extensive preclinical and clinical evaluation of inhibitors of activated Ras. Most approaches have focused on efforts to inhibit ras membrane localization required for its function through inhibition of farnesylation or geranylation steps. To date, clinical trials have involved farynesyl transferase inhibitors. Unfortunately, most of these agents have shown toxicities, limiting enthusiasm for this class of agent. However, most of these agents are not specific for ras farnesylation, and the prenylation pathway through generanylgeranyl transferase is a known alternative pathway for K- and N-ras membrane targeting. Thus, whether agents, which target ras through this alternative pathway, will lead to new anticancer agents remains to be resolved.[185]

Raf and MEK have also emerged as key targets for anticancer drug design based on the fact that a broad array of solid tumors use this important pathway. The development of agents has largely focused on the design of small molecule inhibitors of enzyme function. There are as yet few studies on the use of selective Raf inhibitors, although the patent literature has identified several classes of substituted ureas with specific activity against Raf. BAY-43-9006, which inhibits Raf, was shown to have antitumor activity in xenograft models of colon, pancreatic, and ovarian cancer.[186] BAY-43-9006 is undergoing clinical evaluation with several ongoing trials. This is an area of increased emphasis with the recent discovery that B-raf oncogenic mutations commonly occur in melanoma, colon, and NSLCs.[186] An orally active MEK inhibitor, PD184352, has been reported to be active in preclinical in vivo tumor growth models.[187] This agent is a non-ATP–competitive, highly selective MEK inhibitor. Since the RAS/RAF/MAPK pathway has pleiotropic effects on proliferation, motility, and cell survival, inhibitors of this pathway might be expected to exert multiple adverse effects on tumor cells. It is likely that therapeutic efficacy will be tested both in the single agent setting and in increasing therapeutic efficacy of standard therapeutic agents. Another obvious therapeutic strategy is to inhibit Akt antiapoptotic functions. The ultimate therapeutic potential of signaling antagonists directed against the MAPK[187] and Akt[188] pathways can only be determined by human testing. One of the important advantages of rationally based targets is that reagents are generally available with which to monitor in vivo inhibition of the target molecule. This makes correlation of clinical response with pharmacodynamic analyses of target suppression feasible and should speed the process of clinical testing. Another advantage is that some of these agents appear to have less inherent toxicities than standard chemotherapeutic regimens.

Neoangiogenesis can also be a limiting factor in tumor growth and, thus, play an important role in tumor progression. Targeting neoangiogenesis has several theoretical advantages in that drug resistance is less likely to develop in normal endothelial cells than in the genetically unstable tumor cell. Moreover, such therapy might be applicable to a wide range of tumors as well as complementing existing therapies. In fact, Avastin (bevacizumab), developed by Genentech, is a humanized monoclonal antibody directed against VEGF that was initially approved for treatment of advanced colon carcinoma. Clinical trials for its use in first- as well as second-line therapy look very promising in several tumors. Other agents are under investigation with several directed against VEGF or its major receptor, VEGFR2. For example, VEGFR2 expression is specific for endothelial cells. Other targets include angiogenesis-related RTKs, VEGFR3, FGF receptors, and Tie2, as well as integrins used by endothelial cells.[173] Although paracrine acting growth factors involved in angiogenesis are the most obvious targets, other paracrine acting growth factors may be targets as well.

Although attacking growth factor signal transduction is becoming an increasing focus of cancer drug development, growth factors themselves have also been applied clinically in efforts to ameliorate the toxicities of conventional therapies to rapidly proliferating normal tissues. For example, Amgen has successfully developed erythropoietin and granulocyte stimulating factor (G-CSF), which specifically stimulate erythrocyte and granulocyte production, as the drugs, Epogen (epoetin alfa) and Neupogen (filgrastim), respectively. Moreover, second generation versions of each that require less frequent administration have been developed and approved for clinical use. Toxicity to the normal gastrointestinal tract is a complication of a number of cancer therapies. Oral mucositis associated with increased need for pain medication and parenteral nutrition can be debilitating to patients as can bowel irritation associated with bleeding or diarrhea. As discussed above, FGF7 (KGF) is a growth factor that acts specifically on epithelial cells. Amgen has developed KGF as a drug, Kepivance (palifermin), recently approved for use clinically in ameliorating oral mucositis associated with bone marrow transplantation for hematopoietic tumors.[189] Conceivably, the ability to protect normal rapidly proliferating cells of the bone marrow and gastrointestinal tract from the toxicities of certain cancer therapies may allow the use of more intensive treatment with greater likelihood of cure.

It is anticipated that future therapies will likely involve a combination of target-specific agents tailored to particular tumors. The recent advances in targeting specific growth factor signaling aberrations in human cancer cells argue strongly that the knowledge that has been gained concerning the important role of growth factor signal transduction in cancer is leading to a promising new era in cancer therapeutics.

REFERENCES

1. Doolittle RF, Hunkapiller MW, Hood LE, et al. Simian sarcoma virus onc gene, v-sis, is derived from the gene (or genes) encoding a platelet-derived growth factor. Science 1983;221:275–7.
2. Downward J, Yarden Y, Mayes E, et al. Close similarity of epidermal growth factor receptor and v-erb-B oncogene protein sequences. Nature 1984;307:521–7.
3. Sherr CJ, Rettenmier CW, Sacca R, et al. The c-fms proto-oncogene product is related to the receptor for the mononuclear phagocyte growth factor, CSF-1. Cell 1985;41:665–76.
4. Levi-Montalcini R. The nerve growth factor 35 years later. Science 1987;237:1154–62.
5. Cohen S. Nobel lecture. Epidermal growth factor. Biosci Rep 1986;6:1017–28.
6. Brugge JS, Erikson RL. Identification of a transformation-specific antigen induced by an avian sarcoma virus. Nature 1977;269:346–8.
7. Levinson AD, Oppermann H, Levintow L, et al. Evidence that the transforming gene of avian sarcoma virus encodes a protein kinase associated with a phosphoprotein. Cell 1978;15:561–72.
8. Collett MS, Erikson RL. Protein kinase activity associated with the avian sarcoma virus src gene product. Proc Natl Acad Sci U S A 1978;75:2021–4.
9. Sporn MB, Todaro GJ. Autocrine secretion and malignant transformation of cells. N Engl J Med 1980;303:878–80.
10. Bosenberg MW, Massague J. Juxtacrine cell signaling molecules. Curr Opin Cell Biol 1993;5:832–8.
11. Logan A. Intracrine regulation at the nucleus—a further mechanism of growth factor activity? J Endocrinol 1990:125:339–43.
12. Yayon A, Klagsbrun M, Esko JD, et al. Cell surface, heparin-like molecules are required for binding of basic fibroblast growth factor to its high affinity receptor. Cell 1991;64:841–8.
13. Aaronson SA. Growth factors and cancer. Science 1991;254:1146–53.
14. Blume-Jensen P, Hunter T. Oncogenic kinase signalling. Nature 2001;411;355–65.
15. Schlessinger J. Cell signaling by receptor tyrosine kinases. Cell 2000;103:211–25.
16. Heldin C-H, Ostman A. Ligand-induced dimerization of growth factor receptors: variation on the theme. Cytokine Growth Factor Rev 1996;**7**:3–10.
17. Fredriksson L, Li H, Eriksson U. The PDGF family: four gene products form five dimeric isoforms. Cytokine Growth Factor Rev 2004;15:197–204.
18. Lemmon MA, Bu Z, Ladbury JE, et al. Two EGF molecules contribute additively to stabilization of the EGFR dimer. EMBO J 1997;16:281–94.
19. Wilkie AO, Patey SJ, Kan SH, et al. FGFs, their receptors, and human limb malformations: clinical and molecular correlations. Am J Med Genet 2002;112:266–78.
20. LeRoith D, Roberts CT Jr. The insulin-like growth factor system and cancer. Cancer Lett 2003;195:127–37.
21. Weiner DB, Liu J, Cohen JA, et al. A point mutation in the neu oncogene mimics ligand induction of receptor aggregation. Nature 1989;339:230–1.
22. Burke CL, Lemmon MA, Coren BA, et al. Dimerization of the p185*neu* transmembrane domain is necessary but not sufficient for transformation. Oncogene 1997;14:687–96.
23. Castagnino P, Biesova Z, Wong WT, et al. Direct binding of *eps8* to the juxtamembrane domain of EGFR is phosphotyrosine- and SH2-independent. Oncogene 1995;10:723–9.
24. Tallquist M, Kazlauskas A. PDGF signaling in cells and mice. Cytokine Growth Factor Rev 2004;15:205–13.
25. Kazlauskas A, Cooper JA. Autophosphorylation of the PDGF receptor in the kinase insert region regulates interactions with cell proteins. Cell 1989;58:1121–33.
26. Escobedo JA, Williams LT. A PDGF receptor domain essential for mitogenesis but not for many other responses to PDGF. Nature 1988;335:85–7.
27. Robbins KC, Antoniades HN, Devare SG, et al. Structural and immunological similarities between simian sarcoma virus gene product(s) and human platelet-derived growth factor. Nature 1983;305:605–8.
28. Igarashi H, Rao CD, Siroff M, et al. Detection of PDGF-2 homodimers in human tumor cells. Oncogene 1987;1:79–85.
29. Gazit A, Igarashi H, Chiu IM, et al. Expression of the normal human sis/PDGF-2 coding sequence induces cellular transformation. Cell 1984;39:89–97.
30. Pietras K, Sjoblom T, Rubin K, et al. PDGF receptors as cancer drug targets. Cancer Cell 2003;3:439–43.
31. Lokker NA, Sullivan CM, Hollenbach SJ, et al. Platelet-derived growth factor (PDGF) autocrine signaling regulates survival and mitogenic pathways in glioblastoma cells: evidence that the novel PDGF-C and PDGF-D ligands may play a role in the development of brain tumors. Cancer Res 2002;62:3729–35.
32. Rettenmier CW, Sherr CJ. The mononuclear phagocyte colony-stimulating factor (CSF-1, M-CSF). Hematol Oncol Clin North Am 1989;3:479–93.
33. Scheijen B, Griffin JD. Tyrosine kinase oncogenes in normal hematopoiesis and hematological disease. Oncogene 2002;21:3314–33.
34. Martin FH, Suggs SV, Langley KE, et al. Primary structure and functional expression of rat and human stem cell factor DNAs. Cell 1990;63:203–11.
35. Lyman SD, James L, Vanden Bos T, et al. Molecular cloning of a ligand for the flt3/flk-2 tyrosine kinase receptor: a proliferative factor for primitive hematopoietic cells. Cell 1993;75:1157–67.
36. Leung DW, Cachianes G, Kuang WJ, et al. Vascular endothelial growth factor is a secreted angiogenic mitogen. Science 1989;246:1306–9.
37. Neufeld G, Cohen T, Gengrinovitch S, Poltorak Z. Vascular endothelial growth factor (VEGF) and its receptors. FASEB J 1999;13:9–22.
38. Shalaby F, Rossant J, Yamaguchi TP, et al. Failure of blood-island formation and vasculogenesis in Flk-1-deficient mice. Nature 1995;376:62–6.
39. Joukov V, Kaipainen A, Jeltsch M, et al. Vascular endothelial growth factors VEGF-B and VEGF-C. J Cell Physiol 1997;173:211–5.
40. Joukov V, Pajusola K, Kaipainen A, et al. A novel vascular endothelial growth factor, VEGF-C, is a ligand for the Flt4 (VEGFR-3) and KDR (VEGFR-2) receptor tyrosine kinases [published erratum appears in EMBO J 1996;15:1751]. EMBO J 1996;15:290–8.
41. Korpelainen EI, Alitalo K. Signaling angiogenesis and lymphangiogenesis. Curr Opin Cell Biol 1998;10:159–64.
42. Maglione D, Guerriero V, Viglietto G, et al. Isolation of a human placenta cDNA coding for a protein related to the vascular permeability factor. Proc Natl Acad Sci U S A 1991;88:9267–71.
43. Gray A, Dull TJ, Ullrich A. Nucleotide sequence of epidermal growth factor cDNA predicts a 128,000-molecular weight protein precursor. Nature 1983;303:722–5.
44. Mroczkowski B, Reich M, Chen K, et al. Recombinant human epidermal growth factor precursor is a glycosylated membrane protein with biological activity. Mol Cell Biol 1989;9:2771–8.
45. Massague J. Transforming growth factor-alpha. A model for membrane-anchored growth factors. J Biol Chem 1990;265:21393–6.
46. Yarden Y. The EGFR family and its ligands in human cancer: signalling mechanisms and therapeutic opportunities. Eur J Cancer 2001;37 Suppl 4:S3–8.
47. Todaro GJ, Fryling C, De Larco JE. Transforming growth factors produced by certain human tumor cells: polypeptides that interact with epidermal growth factor receptors. Proc Natl Acad Sci U S A 1980;77:5258–62.
48. Shoyab M, Plowman GD, McDonald VL, et al. Structure and function of human amphiregulin: a member of the epidermal growth factor family. Science 1989;243:1074–6.
49. Johnson GR, Wong L. Heparan sulfate is essential to amphiregulin-induced mitogenic signaling by the epidermal growth factor receptor. J Biol Chem 1994;269:27149–54.
50. Higashiyama S, Abraham JA, Miller J, et al. A heparin-binding growth factor secreted by macrophage-like cells that is related to EGF. Science 1991;251:936–9.
51. Higashiyama S, Lau K, Besner GE, et al. Structure of heparin-binding EGF-like growth factor. Multiple forms, primary structure, and glycosylation of the mature protein. J Biol Chem 1992;267:6205–12.
52. Mitamura T, Higashiyama S, Taniguchi N, et al. Diphtheria toxin binds to the epidermal growth factor (EGF)-like domain of human heparin-binding EGF-like growth factor/diphtheria toxin receptor and inhibits specifically its mitogenic activity. J Biol Chem 1995;270:1015–9.
53. Shing Y, Christofori G, Hanahan D, et al. Betacellulin: a mitogen from pancreatic beta cell tumors. Science 1993;259:1604–7.
54. Taylor DS, Cheng X, Pawlowski JE, et al. Epiregulin is a potent vascular smooth muscle cell-derived mitogen induced by angiotensin II, endothelin-1, and thrombin. Proc Natl Acad Sci U S A 1999;96:1633–8.
55. Falls DL. Neuregulins: functions, forms, and signaling strategies. Exp Cell Res 2003;284:14–30.
56. Pinkas-Kramarski R, Shelly M, Guarino BC, et al. ErbB tyrosine kinases and the two neuregulin families constitute a ligand-receptor network [published erratum appears in Mol Cell Biol 1998;18:7602]. Mol Cell Biol 1998;18:6090–101.
57. Powers CJ, McLeskey SW, Wellstein A. Fibroblast growth factors, their receptors and signaling. Endocr Relat Cancer 2000;**7**:165–97.
58. Bouche G, Gas N, Prats H, et al. Basic fibroblast growth factor enters the nucleolus and stimulates the transcription of ribosomal genes in ABAE cells undergoing G0–G1 transition. Proc Natl Acad Sci U S A 1987;84:6770–4.
59. Sano H, Forough R, Maier JA, et al. Detection of high levels of heparin binding growth factor-1 (acidic fibroblast growth factor) in inflammatory arthritic joints. J Cell Biol 1990;110:1417–26.
60. Rubin JS, Osada H, Finch PW, et al. Purification and characterization of a newly identified growth factor specific for epithelial cells. Proc Natl Acad Sci U S A 1989;86:802–6.

61. Finch PW, Rubin JS. Keratinocyte growth factor/fibroblast growth factor 7, a homeostatic factor with therapeutic potential for epithelial protection and repair. Adv Cancer Res 2004;91:69–136.
62. Espinal J. Mechanism of insulin action [news]. Nature 1987;328:574–5.
63. Clemmons DR. Structural and functional analysis of insulin-like growth factors. Br Med Bull 1989;45:465–80.
64. Clemmons DR. Insulin-like growth factor binding proteins and their role in controlling IGF actions. Cytokine Growth Factor Rev 1997;8:45–62.
65. Kaleko M, Rutter WJ, Miller AD. Overexpression of the human insulinlike growth factor I receptor promotes ligand-dependent neoplastic transformation. Mol Cell Biol 1990;10:464–73.
66. Foulstone E, Prince S, Zaccheo O, et al. Insulin-like growth factor ligands, receptors, and binding proteins in cancer. J Pathol 2005;205:145–53.
67. Klammt J, Garten A, Barnikol-Oettler A, et al. Comparative analysis of the signaling capabilities of the insulin receptor-related receptor. Biochem Biophys Res Commun 2005;327:557–64.
68. Gohda E, Tsubouchi H, Nakayama H, et al. Purification and partial characterization of hepatocyte growth factor from plasma of a patient with fulminant hepatic failure. J Clin Invest 1988;81:414–9.
69. Nakamura T, Nawa K, Ichihara A, et al. Purification and subunit structure of hepatocyte growth factor from rat platelets. FEBS Lett 1987;224:311–6.
70. Nakamura T, Nishizawa T, Hagiya M, et al. Molecular cloning and expression of human hepatocyte growth factor. Nature 1989;342:440–3.
71. Tamagnone L, Comoglio PM. Control of invasive growth by hepatocyte growth factor (HGF) and related scatter factors. Cytokine Growth Factor Rev 1997;8:129–42.
72. Schmidt C, Bladt F, Goedecke S, et al. Scatter factor/hepatocyte growth factor is essential for liver development. Nature 1995;373:699–702.
73. Yoshimura T, Yuhki N, Wang MH, et al. Cloning, sequencing, and expression of human macrophage stimulating protein (MSP, MST1) confirms MSP as a member of the family of kringle proteins and locates the MSP gene on chromosome 3. J Biol Chem 1993;268:15461–8.
74. Birchmeier C, Birchmeier W, Gherardi E, Vande Woude GF. Met, metastasis, motility and more. Nat Rev Mol Cell Biol 2003;4:915–25.
75. Ronsin C, Muscatelli F, Mattei MG, Breathnach R. A novel putative receptor protein tyrosine kinase of the met family. Oncogene 1993;8:1195–202.
76. Gaudino G, Follenzi A, Naldini L, et al. RON is a heterodimeric tyrosine kinase receptor activated by the HGF homologue MSP. EMBO J 1994;13:3524–32.
77. Maness LM, Kastin AJ, Weber JT, et al. The neurotrophins and their receptors: structure, function, and neuropathology. Neurosci Biobehav Rev 1994;18:143–59.
78. Segal RA. Selectivity in neurotrophin signaling: theme and variations. Annu Rev Neurosci 2003;26:299–330.
79. Klein R, Jing SQ, Nanduri V, et al. The trk proto-oncogene encodes a receptor for nerve growth factor. Cell 1991;65:189–97.
80. Phillips DJ, Greengard JS, Fernandez JA, et al. Protein S, an antithrombotic factor, is synthesized and released by neural tumor cells. J Neurochem 1993;61:344–7.
81. Schneider C, King RM, Philipson L. Genes specifically expressed at growth arrest of mammalian cells. Cell 1988;54:787–93.
82. Lemke G, Lu Q. Macrophage regulation by Tyro 3 family receptors. Curr Opin Immunol 2003;15:31–6.
83. Funakoshi H, Yonemasu T, Nakano T, et al. Identification of Gas6, a putative ligand for Sky and Axl receptor tyrosine kinases, as a novel neurotrophic factor for hippocampal neurons. J Neurosci Res 2002;68:150–60.
84. Surawska H, Ma PC, Salgia R. The role of ephrins and Eph receptors in cancer. Cytokine Growth Factor Rev 2004;15:419–33.
85. Bezakova G, Ruegg MA. New insights into the roles of agrin. Nat Rev Mol Cell Biol 2003;4:295–308.
86. Airaksinen MS, Saarma M. The GDNF family: signalling, biological functions and therapeutic value. Nat Rev Neurosci 2002;3:383–94.
87. Grondin R, Gash DM. Glial cell line-derived neurotrophic factor (GDNF): a drug candidate for the treatment of Parkinson's disease. J Neurol 1998;245:35–42.
88. Takahashi M, Buma Y, Iwamoto T, et al. Cloning and expression of the ret proto-oncogene encoding a tyrosine kinase with two potential transmembrane domains. Oncogene 1988;3:571–8.
89. Robertson K, Mason I. The GDNF-RET signalling partnership. Trends Genet 1997;13:1–3.
90. Santoro M, Melillo RM, Carlomagno F, et al. Minireview: RET: normal and abnormal functions. Endocrinology 2004;145:5448–51.
91. Loughna S, Sato TN. Angiopoietin and Tie signaling pathways in vascular development. Matrix Biol 2001;20:319–25.
92. Saharinen P, Kerkela K, Ekman N, et al. Multiple angiopoietin recombinant proteins activate the Tie1 receptor tyrosine kinase and promote its interaction with Tie2. J Cell Biol 2005;169:239–43.
93. Vogel W. Discoidin domain receptors: structural relations and functional implications. FASEB J 1999;13 Suppl:S77–82.
94. Springer WR, Cooper DN, Barondes SH. Discoidin I is implicated in cell-substratum attachment and ordered cell migration of Dictyostelium discoideum and resembles fibronectin. Cell 1984;39:557–64.
95. Vogel WF, Aszodi A, Alves F, Pawson T. Discoidin domain receptor 1 tyrosine kinase has an essential role in mammary gland development. Mol Cell Biol 2001;21:2906–17.
96. Labrador JP, Azcoitia V, Tuckermann T, et al. The collagen receptor DDR2 regulates proliferation and its elimination leads to dwarfism. EMBO Rep 2001;2:446–52.
97. Forrester WC. The Ror receptor tyrosine kinase family. Cell Mol Life Sci 2002;59:83–96.
98. Wilson C, Goberdhan DC, Steller H. Dror, a potential neurotrophic receptor gene, encodes a Drosophila homolog of the vertebrate Ror family of Trk-related receptor tyrosine kinases. Proc Natl Acad Sci U S A 1993;90:7109–13.
99. Oishi I, Suzuki H, Onishi N, et al. The receptor tyrosine kinase Ror2 is involved in non-canonical Wnt5a/JNK signalling pathway. Genes Cells 2003;8:645–54.
100. Matsushime H, Wang LH, Shibuya M. Human c-ros-1 gene homologous to the v-ros sequence of UR2 sarcoma virus encodes for a transmembrane receptorlike molecule. Mol Cell Biol 1986;6:3000–4.
101. Cooper TG, Wagenfeld A, Cornwall GA, et al. Gene and protein expression in the epididymis of infertile c-ros receptor tyrosine kinase-deficient mice. Biol Reprod 2003;69:1750–62.
102. Maru Y, Hirai H, Takaku F. Human ltk: gene structure and preferential expression in human leukemic cells. Oncogene Res 1990;5:199–204.
103. Morris SW, Kirstein MN, Valentine MB, et al. Fusion of a kinase gene, ALK, to a nucleolar protein gene, NPM, in non-Hodgkin's lymphoma [published erratum appears in Science 1995;267:316–7]. Science 1994;263:1281–4.
104. Englund C, Loren CE, Grabbe C, et al. Jeb signals through the Alk receptor tyrosine kinase to drive visceral muscle fusion. Nature 2003;425:512–6.
105. Chou YH, Hayman MJ. Characterization of a member of the immunoglobulin gene superfamily that possibly represents an additional class of growth factor receptor. Proc Natl Acad Sci U S A 1991;88:4897–901.
106. Mossie K, Jallal B, Alves F, et al. Colon carcinoma kinase-4 defines a new subclass of the receptor tyrosine kinase family. Oncogene 1995;11:2179–84.
107. Lu X, Borchers AG, Jolicoeur C, et al. PTK7/CCK-4 is a novel regulator of planar cell polarity in vertebrates. Nature 2004;430:93–8.
108. Hovens CM, Stacker SA, Andres AC, et al. RYK, a receptor tyrosine kinase-related molecule with unusual kinase domain motifs. Proc Natl Acad Sci U S A 1992;89:11818–22.
109. Halford MM, Stacker SA. Revelations of the RYK receptor. Bioessays 2001;23:34–45.
110. Lu W, Yamamoto V, Ortega B, Baltimore D. Mammalian Ryk is a Wnt coreceptor required for stimulation of neurite outgrowth. Cell 2004;119:97–108.
111. Maxwell M, Naber SP, Wolfe HJ, et al. Coexpression of platelet-derived growth factor (PDGF) and PDGF-receptor genes by primary human astrocytomas may contribute to their development and maintenance. J Clin Invest 1990;86:131–40.
112. Nister M, Liberman TA, Betsholtz C, et al. Expression of messenger RNAs for platelet-derived growth factor and transforming growth factor-alpha and their receptors in human malignant glioma cell lines. Cancer Res 1988;48:3910–8.
113. Di Marco E, Pierce JH, Fleming TP, et al. Autocrine interaction between TGF alpha and the EGF-receptor: quantitative requirements for induction of the malignant phenotype. Oncogene 1989;4:831–8.
114. Marra F. Chemokines in liver inflammation and fibrosis. Front Biosci 2002;**7**:d1899–914.
115. Roussel MF, Downing JR, Rettenmier CW, Sherr CJ. A point mutation in the extracellular domain of the human CSF-1 receptor (c-fms proto-oncogene product) activates its transforming potential. Cell 1988;55:979–88.
116. Schechter AL, Stern DF, Vaidyanathan L, et al. The neu oncogene: an erb-B-related gene encoding a 185,000-Mr tumour antigen. Nature 1984;312:513–6.
117. Bargmann CI, Hung MC, Weinberg RA. Multiple independent activations of the neu oncogene by a point mutation altering the transmembrane domain of p185. Cell 1986;45:649–57.
118. Roskoski R Jr. The ErbB/HER receptor protein-tyrosine kinases and cancer. Biochem Biophys Res Commun 2004;319:1–11.
119. Lynch TJ, Bell DW, Sordella R, et al. Activating mutations in the epidermal growth factor receptor underlying responsiveness of non-small-cell lung cancer to gefitinib. N Engl J Med 2004;350:2129–39.
120. Paez JG, Janne PA, Lee JC, et al. EGFR mutations in lung cancer: correlation with clinical response to gefitinib therapy. Science 2004;304:1497–500.
121. Santoro M, Melillo RM, Carlomagno F, et al. Molecular mechanisms of RET activation in human cancer. Ann N Y Acad Sci 2002;963:116–21.
122. Carroll M, Tomasson MH, Barker GF, et al. The TEL/platelet-derived growth factor beta receptor (PDGF beta R) fusion in chronic myelomonocytic leukemia is a transforming protein that self-associates and activates PDGF beta R kinase-dependent signaling pathways. Proc Natl Acad Sci U S A 1996;93:14845–50.
123. Greco A, Pierotti MA, Bongarzone I, et al. TRK-T1 is a novel oncogene formed by the fusion of TPR and TRK genes in human papillary thyroid carcinomas. Oncogene 1992;7:237–42.
124. Greco A, Mariani C, Miranda C, et al. The DNA rearrangement that generates the TRK-T3 oncogene involves a novel gene on chromosome 3 whose product has a potential coiled-coil domain. Mol Cell Biol 1995;15:6118–27.
125. Pawson T, Scott JD. Signaling through scaffold, anchoring, and adaptor proteins. Science 1997;278:2075–80.
126. Sudol M. From Src Homology domains to other signaling modules: proposal of the 'protein recognition code.' Oncogene 1998;17:1469–74.
127. Ogawa W, Matozaki T, Kasuga M. Role of binding proteins to IRS-1 in insulin signalling. Mol Cell Biochem 1998;182:13–22.
128. Meisenhelder J, Suh PG, Rhee SG, Hunter T. Phospholipase C-gamma is a substrate for the PDGF and EGF receptor protein-tyrosine kinases in vivo and in vitro. Cell 1989;57:1109–22.
129. Escobedo JA, Navankasattusas S, Kavanaugh WM, et al. cDNA cloning of a novel 85 kd protein that has SH2 domains and regulates binding of PI3-kinase to the PDGF beta-receptor. Cell 1991;65:75–82.
130. Nishimura R, Li W, Kashishian A, et al. Two signaling molecules share a phosphotyrosine-containing binding site in the platelet-derived growth factor receptor. Mol Cell Biol 1993;13:6889–96.
131. Kazlauskas A, Feng GS, Pawson T, Valius M. The 64-kDa protein that associates with the platelet-derived growth factor receptor beta subunit via Tyr-1009 is the SH2-containing phosphotyrosine phosphatase Syp. Proc Natl Acad Sci U S A 1993;90:6939–43.
132. Arvidsson AK, Rupp E, Nanberg E, et al. Tyr-716 in the platelet-derived growth factor beta-receptor kinase insert is involved in GRB2 binding and Ras activation. Mol Cell Biol 1994;14:6715–26.
133. Anderson D, Koch CA, Grey L, et al. Binding of SH2 domains of phospholipase C gamma 1, GAP, and Src to activated growth factor receptors. Science 1990;250:979–82.
134. Kaplan DR, Morrison DK, Wong G, et al. PDGF beta-receptor stimulates tyrosine phosphorylation of GAP and association of GAP with a signaling complex. Cell 1990;61:125–33.
135. Ralston R, Bishop JM. The product of the protooncogene c-src is modified during the cellular response to platelet-derived growth factor. Proc Natl Acad Sci U S A 1985;82:7845–9.
136. Berridge MJ, Irvine RF. Inositol phosphates and cell signalling. Nature 1989;341:197–205.
137. Housey GM, Johnson MD, Hsiao WL, et al. Overproduction of protein kinase C causes disordered growth control in rat fibroblasts. Cell 1988;52:343–54.
138. Rameh LE, Cantley LC. The role of phosphoinositide 3-kinase lipid products in cell function. J Biol Chem 1999;274:8347–50.

139. Cantley LC. The phosphoinositide 3-kinase pathway. Science 2002;296:1655–7.
140. Vivanco I, Sawyers CL. The phosphatidylinositol 3-Kinase AKT pathway in human cancer. Nat Rev Cancer 2002;2:489–501.
141. Shayesteh L, Lu Y, Kuo WL, et al. PIK3CA is implicated as an oncogene in ovarian cancer [comments]. Nat Genet 1999;21:99–102.
142. Samuels Y, Wang Z, Bardelli A, et al. High frequency of mutations of the PIK3CA gene in human cancers. Science 2004;304:554.
143. Staal SP. Molecular cloning of the akt oncogene and its human homologues AKT1 and AKT2: amplification of AKT1 in a primary human gastric adenocarcinoma. Proc Natl Acad Sci U S A 1987;84:5034–7.
144. Cantley LC, Neel BG. New insights into tumor suppression: PTEN suppresses tumor formation by restraining the phosphoinositide 3-kinase/AKT pathway. Proc Natl Acad Sci U S A 1999;96:4240–5.
145. Campbell SL, Khosravi-Far R, Rossman KL, et al. Increasing complexity of Ras signaling. Oncogene 1998;17:1395–413.
146. Bos JL. All in the family? New insights and questions regarding interconnectivity of Ras, Rap1 and Ral. EMBO J 1998;17:6776–82.
147. Santos E, Nebreda AR. Structural and functional properties of ras proteins. FASEB J 1989;3:2151–63.
148. Buday L, Downward J. Epidermal growth factor regulates p21ras through the formation of a complex of receptor, Grb2 adapter protein, and Sos nucleotide exchange factor. Cell 1993;73:611–20.
149. Marshall CJ. Ras effectors. Curr Biol 1996;8:197–204.
150. Wittinghofer A, Scheffzek K, Ahmadian MR. The interaction of Ras with GTPase-activating proteins. FEBS Lett 1997;410:63–7.
151. Bos JL. ras Oncogenes in human cancer: a review [published erratum appears in Cancer Res 1990;50:1352]. Cancer Res 1989;49:4682–9.
152. Barbacid M. ras Genes. Annu Rev Biochem 1987;56:779–827.
153. Serrano M, Lin AW, McCurrach ME, et al. Oncogenic ras provokes premature cell senescence associated with accumulation of p53 and p16INK4a. Cell 1997;88:593–602.
154. Saez R, Chan AM, Miki T, Aaronson SA. Oncogenic activation of human R-ras by point mutations analogous to those of prototype H-ras oncogenes. Oncogene 1994;9:2977–82.
155. Chan AM, Miki T, Meyers KA, Aaronson SA. A human oncogene of the RAS superfamily unmasked by expression cDNA cloning. Proc Natl Acad Sci U S A 1994;91:7558–62.
156. Kimmelman A, Tolkacheva T, Lorenzi MV, et al. Identification and characterization of R-ras3: a novel member of the RAS gene family with a non-ubiquitous pattern of tissue distribution. Oncogene 1997;15:2675–85.
157. Rodriguez-Viciana P, Warne PH, Vanhaesebroeck B, et al. Activation of phosphoinositide 3-kinase by interaction with Ras and by point mutation. EMBO J 1996;15:2442–51.
158. Van Aelst L, Barr M, Marcus S, et al. Complex formation between RAS and RAF and other protein kinases. Proc Natl Acad Sci U S A 1993;90:6213–7.
159. Wellbrock C, Karasarides M, Marais R. The RAF proteins take centre stage. Nat Rev Mol Cell Biol 2004;5:875–85.
160. Lewis TS, Shapiro PS, Ahn NG. Signal transduction through MAP kinase cascades. Adv Cancer Res 1998;74:49–139.
161. Kerkhoff E, Rapp UR. Cell cycle targets of Ras/Raf signalling. Oncogene 1998;17:1457–62.
162. Donnellan R, Chetty R. Cyclin D1 and human neoplasia. Mol Pathol 1998;51:1–7.
163. Davies H, Bignell GR, Cox C, et al. Mutations of the BRAF gene in human cancer. Nature 2002;417:949–54.
164. Davis RJ. Signal transduction by the JNK group of MAP kinases. Cell 2000;103:239–52.
165. Musti AM, Treier M, Bohmann D. Reduced ubiquitin-dependent degradation of c-Jun after phosphorylation by MAP kinases. Science 1997;275:400–2.
166. Yang D, Tournier C, Wysk M, et al. Targeted disruption of the MKK4 gene causes embryonic death, inhibition of c-Jun NH2-terminal kinase activation, and defects in AP-1 transcriptional activity. Proc Natl Acad Sci U S A 1997;94:3004–9.
167. Van Beveren C, van Straaten F, Curran T, et al. Analysis of FBJ-MuSV provirus and c-fos (mouse) gene reveals that viral and cellular fos gene products have different carboxy termini. Cell 1983;32:1241–55.
168. Maki Y, Bos TJ, Davis C, et al. Avian sarcoma virus 17 carries the jun oncogene. Proc Natl Acad Sci U S A 1987;84:2848–52.
169. Miller AD, Curran T, Verma IM. c-fos protein can induce cellular transformation: a novel mechanism of activation of a cellular oncogene. Cell 1984;36:51–60.
170. Hill CS, Treisman R. Transcriptional regulation by extracellular signals: mechanisms and specificity. Cell 1995;80:199–211.
171. Chan AM, Rubin JS, Bottaro DP, et al. Identification of a competitive HGF antagonist encoded by an alternative transcript. Science 1991;254:1382–5.
172. Duan DS, Werner S, Williams LT. A naturally occurring secreted form of fibroblast growth factor (FGF) receptor 1 binds basic FGF in preference over acidic FGF. J Biol Chem 1992;267:16076–80.
173. Madhusudan S, Ganesan TS. Tyrosine kinase inhibitors in cancer therapy. Clin Biochem 2004;37:618–35.
174. Hudziak RM, Lewis GD, Winget M, et al. p185HER2 monoclonal antibody has antiproliferative effects in vitro and sensitizes human breast tumor cells to tumor necrosis factor. Mol Cell Biol 1989;9:1165–72.
175. Kasprzyk PG, Song SU, Di Fiore PP, King CR. Therapy of an animal model of human gastric cancer using a combination of anti-erbB-2 monoclonal antibodies. Cancer Res 1992;52:2771–6.
176. Yu D. Mechanisms of ErbB2-mediated paclitaxel resistance and trastuzumab- mediated paclitaxel sensitization in ErbB2-overexpressing breast cancers. Semin Oncol 2001;28:12–7.
177. Slamon DJ, Leyland-Jones B, Shak S, et al. Use of chemotherapy plus a monoclonal antibody against HER2 for metastatic breast cancer that overexpresses HER2. N Engl J Med 2001;344:783–92.
178. Kawamoto T, Sato JD, Le A, et al. Growth stimulation of A431 cells by epidermal growth factor: identification of high-affinity receptors for epidermal growth factor by an anti-receptor monoclonal antibody. Proc Natl Acad Sci U S A 1983;80:1337–41.
179. Pastan I, FitzGerald D. Recombinant toxins for cancer treatment. Science 1991;254:1173–7.
180. de Klein A, van Kessel AG, Grosveld G, et al. A cellular oncogene is translocated to the Philadelphia chromosome in chronic myelocytic leukaemia. Nature 1982;300:765–7.
181. Druker BJ. Perspectives on the development of a molecularly targeted agent. Cancer Cell 2002;1:31–6.
182. van Oosterom AT, Judson I, Verweij J, et al. Safety and efficacy of imatinib (STI571) in metastatic gastrointestinal stromal tumours: a phase I study. Lancet 2001;358:1421–3.
183. Ciardiello F, Caputo R, Bianco R, et al. Antitumor effect and potentiation of cytotoxic drugs activity in human cancer cells by ZD-1839 (Iressa), an epidermal growth factor receptor- selective tyrosine kinase inhibitor. Clin Cancer Res 2000;6:2053–63.
184. Shawver LK, Slamon D, Ullrich A. Smart drugs: tyrosine kinase inhibitors in cancer therapy. Cancer Cell 2002;1:117–23.
185. Downward J. Targeting RAS signalling pathways in cancer therapy. Nat Rev Cancer 2003;3:11–22.
186. Garnett MJ, Marais R. Guilty as charged: B-RAF is a human oncogene. Cancer Cell 2004;6:313–9.
187. Sebolt-Leopold JS, Herrera R. Targeting the mitogen-activated protein kinase cascade to treat cancer. Nat Rev Cancer 2004;4:937–47.
188. Luo J, Manning BD, Cantley LC. Targeting the PI3K-Akt pathway in human cancer: rationale and promise. Cancer Cell 2003;4:257–62.
189. Spielberger R, Stiff P, Bensinger W, et al. Palifermin for oral mucositis after intensive therapy for hematologic cancers. N Engl J Med 2004;351:2590–8.

6

Oncogenes

Marco A. Pierotti, PhD
Milo Frattini, PhD
Gabriella Sozzi, PhD
Carlo M. Croce, MD

Since the early proposals of Boveri more than a century ago, multiple experimental evidences have confirmed that at the molecular level, cancer is due to lesions in the cellular DNA. First, it has been observed that a cancer cell transmits to its daughter cells the phenotypic features characterizing the "cancerous" state. Second, most of the recognized mutagenic compounds are also carcinogenic, having as a target cellular DNA. Finally, the karyotyping of several types of human tumors, particularly those belonging to the hematopoietic system, led to the identification of recurrent qualitative and numerical chromosomal aberrations, reflecting pathologic rearrangements of the cellular genome. Taken together, these observations suggest that the molecular pathogenesis of human cancer is due to structural and/or functional alterations of specific genes whose normal function is to control cellular growth and differentiation or, in different terms, cell birth and cell death.[1,2]

The identification and characterization of the genetic elements playing a role in the scenario of human cancer pathogenesis have been made possible by the development of DNA recombinant techniques during the last two decades. One milestone was the use of the DNA transfection technique that helped clarify the cellular origin of the "viral oncogenes." The latter were previously characterized as the specific genetic elements capable of conferring the tumorigenic properties to the RNA tumor viruses also known as retroviruses.[3,4] Further, the transfection technique led to the identification of cellular transforming genes that do not have a viral counterpart. Besides the source of their original identification, viral or cellular genome, these transforming genetic elements have been designated as proto-oncogene in their normal physiologic version and oncogene when altered in cancer.[5,6] A second relevant experimental approach has regarded the identification and characterization of clonal and recurrent cytogenetic abnormalities in cancer cells, especially those derived from the hematopoietic system. Several oncogenes have been thus defined by molecular cloning of the chromosomal breakpoints including translocations, inversions, etc. Additional oncogenes have been identified through the analysis of chromosomal regions anomalously stained (homogeneously staining regions [HSR]), representing gene amplification. Finally, the detection of chromosome deletions has been instrumental in the process of identification and cloning of a second class of cancer-associated genes, the tumor suppressors. Contrary to the oncogenes that are activated by dominant mutations and whose activity is to promote cell growth, tumor suppressors act in the normal cell as negative controllers of cell growth and are inactive in tumor cells. In general, therefore, the mutations inactivating tumor suppressor genes are of the recessive type. More recently, using the high-throughput technologies, several genes have been demonstrated to be altered (mainly due to hyperactivating mutations) in human cancers. One of these, *BRAF*, represents the most relevant gene in melanoma development.[7] In the last subgroup, we can also number those obtained by the analysis of the protein kinases (kinome)[8] or phosphatases (phosphatome)[9] of the human genome or of several isoforms of a relevant protein involved in cancer development such as PI3K.[10]

Furthermore, a third class of cancer-associated genes has been defined thanks to the analysis of tumors of a particular type, that is, tumors in which an inherited mutated predisposing gene plays a significant role. These tumors include cancers in patients suffering from hereditary nonpolyposis colorectal cancer (HNPCC) syndromes.[11]

The genes implicated in these tumors have been defined as mutator genes or genes involved in the DNA-mismatch repair process. Although not directly involved in the carcinogenesis process, these genes, when inactivated, expose the cells to a very high mutagenic load that eventually may involve the activation of oncogenes and the inactivation of tumor suppressors.[12]

In this chapter, the methods by which oncogenes were discovered will be first described. The various functions of cellular proto-oncogenes will then be presented, and the genetic mechanisms of proto-oncogene activation will be summarized. Finally, the role of specific oncogenes in the initiation and progression of human tumors will be discussed.

DISCOVERY AND IDENTIFICATION OF ONCOGENES

The first oncogenes were discovered through the study of *retroviruses*, RNA tumor viruses whose genomes are reverse-transcribed into DNA in infected animal cells.[13] During the course of infection, retroviral DNA is inserted into the chromosomes of host cells. The integrated retroviral DNA, called the provirus, replicates along with the cellular DNA of the host.[14] Transcription of the DNA provirus leads to the production of viral progeny that bud through the host cell membrane to infect other cells. Two categories of retroviruses are classified by their time course of tumor formation in experimental animals. Acutely transforming retroviruses can rapidly cause tumors within days after injection. These retroviruses can also transform cell cultures to the neoplastic phenotype. Chronic or weakly oncogenic retroviruses can cause tissue-specific tumors in susceptible strains of experimental animals after a latency period of many months. Although weakly oncogenic retroviruses can replicate in vitro, these viruses do not transform cells in culture.

Retroviral oncogenes are altered versions of host cellular proto-oncogenes that have been incorporated into the retroviral genome by recombination with host DNA, a process known as retroviral *transduction*.[15] This surprising discovery was made through study of the Rous sarcoma virus (RSV) (Figure 6-1). RSV is an acutely transforming retrovirus first isolated from a chicken sarcoma over 80 years ago by Payton Rous.[16] Studies of RSV mutants in the early 1970s revealed that the transforming gene of RSV was not required for viral replication.[17–19] Molecular hybridization studies then showed that the RSV transforming gene (designated v-*src*) was homologous to a host cellular gene (c-*src*) that was widely conserved in eukaryotic species.[20] Studies of many other acutely transforming retroviruses from fowl, rodent, feline, and nonhuman primate species have led to the discovery of dozens of different retroviral oncogenes (see below and Table 6-1). In every case, these retroviral oncogenes are derived from normal cellular genes captured from the genome of the host. Viral oncogenes are responsible for the rapid tumor formation and efficient in vitro transformation activity characteristic of acutely transforming retroviruses.

In contrast to acutely transforming retroviruses, weakly oncogenic retroviruses do not carry viral oncogenes. These retroviruses, which

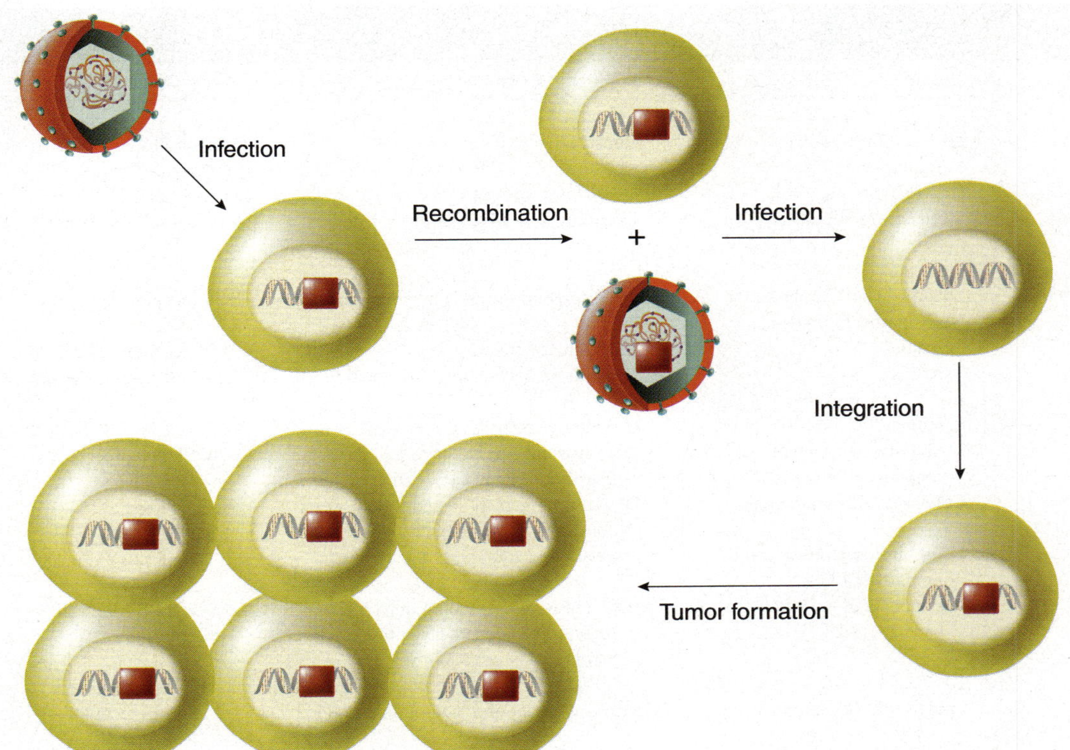

Figure 6-1 Retroviral transduction. An RNA tumor virus infects a human cell carrying an activated *src* gene (*red box*). After the process of recombination between retroviral genome and host DNA, the oncogene *c-src** is incorporated into the retroviral genome and is re-named *v-src*. When the retrovirus carrying *v-src* infects a human cell, the viral oncogene is rapidly transcribed and is responsible for the rapid tumor formation.

include mouse mammary tumor virus (MMTV) and various animal leukemia viruses, induce tumors by a process called *insertional mutagenesis* (Figure 6-2).[12] This process results from integration of the DNA provirus into the host genome in infected cells. In rare cells, the provirus inserts near a proto-oncogene. Expression of the proto-oncogene is then abnormally driven by the transcriptional regulatory elements contained within the long terminal repeats of the provirus.[21,22] In these cases, proviral integration represents a mutagenic event that activates a proto-oncogene. Activation of the proto-oncogene then results in transformation of the cell, which can grow clonally into a tumor. The long latent period of tumor formation of weakly oncogenic retroviruses is therefore due to the rarity of the provirus insertional event that leads to tumor development from a single transformed cell. Insertional mutagenesis by weakly oncogenic retroviruses, first demonstrated in bursal lymphomas of chickens, frequently involves the same oncogenes (such as *myc*, *myb*, and *erb B*) that are carried by acutely transforming retroviruses.[23–25] In many cases, however, insertional mutagenesis has been used as a tool to identify new oncogenes, including *int-1*, *int-2*, *pim-1*, and *lck*.[26]

The demonstration of activated proto-oncogenes in human tumors was first shown by the DNA-mediated transformation technique.[27,28] This technique, also called *gene transfer* or *transfection assay*, verifies the ability of donor DNA from a tumor to transform a recipient strain of rodent cells called NIH 3T3, an immortalized mouse cell line[29] (Figure 6-3).[30] This sensitive assay, which can detect the presence of single-copy oncogenes in a tumor sample, also enables the isolation of the transforming oncogene by molecular cloning techniques. After serial growth of the transformed NIH 3T3 cells, the human tumor oncogene can be cloned by its association with human repetitive DNA sequences. The first human oncogene isolated by the gene transfer technique was derived from a bladder carcinoma.[31,32] Overall, approximately 20% of individual human tumors have been shown to induce transformation of NIH 3T3 cells in gene-transfer assays. The value of transfection assay was recently reinforced by the laboratory of Robert Weinberg, which showed that the ectopic expression of the telomerase catalytic subunit (hTERT), in combination with the simian virus 40 large T product and a mutated oncogenic H-*ras* protein, resulted in the direct tumorigenic conversion of normal human epithelial and fibroblast cells.[33] Many of the oncogenes identified by gene-transfer studies are identical or closely related to those oncogenes transduced by retroviruses. Most prominent among these are members of the *ras* family that have been repeatedly isolated from various human tumors by gene transfer.[34,35] A number of new oncogenes (such as *neu*, *met*, and *trk*) have also been identified by the gene-transfer technique.[36,37] In many cases, however, oncogenes identified by gene transfer were shown to be activated by rearrangement during the experimental procedure and are not activated in the human tumors that served as the source of the donor DNA,[38] as in the case of *ret* that was subsequently found genuinely rearranged and activated in papillary thyroid carcinomas.[39,40]

Chromosomal translocations have served as guideposts for the discovery of many new oncogenes.[41,42] Consistently recurring karyotypic abnormalities are found in many hematologic and solid tumors. These abnormalities include chromosomal rearrangements as well as the gain or loss of whole chromosomes or chromosome segments. The first consistent karyotypic abnormality identified in a human neoplasm was a characteristic small chromosome in the cells of patients with chronic myelogenous leukemia (CML).[43] Later identified as a derivative of chromosome 22, this abnormality was designated the Philadelphia chromosome, after its city of discovery. The application of chromosome banding techniques in the early 1970s enabled the precise cytogenetic characterization of many chromosomal translocations in human leukemia, lymphoma, and solid tumors.[44] The subsequent development of molecular cloning techniques then enabled the identification of proto-oncogenes at or near chromosomal breakpoints in various neoplasms. Some of these proto-oncogenes, such as *myc* and *abl*, had been previously identified as retroviral oncogenes. In general, however, the cloning of chromosomal breakpoints has served as a rich source of discovery of new oncogenes involved in human cancer.

More recently, the use of high-throughput sequencing technologies and bioinformatics from the Human Genome Project led to the discovery of new genes involved in cancer development, such as *BRAF* and *PI3K*.[7,10]

Oncogenes, Proto-oncogenes, and Their Functions Proto-oncogenes encode proteins that are involved in the control of cell growth. Alteration of the structure and/or expression of proto-oncogenes can activate them to become oncogenes capable of inducing in susceptible cells the neoplastic phenotype. Oncogenes can be classified into five groups based on the functional and biochemical properties of protein products of their normal counterparts (proto-oncogenes). These groups are (1) growth factors, (2) growth factor receptors, (3) signal transducers, (4) transcription factors, and (5) others, including programed cell death regulators. Table 6-1 lists examples of oncogenes according to their functional categories.

Growth Factors Growth factors are secreted polypeptides that function as extracellular signals to stimulate the proliferation of target cells.[45,46] Appropriate target cells must possess a specific receptor in order to respond to a specific type of growth factor. A well-characterized example is platelet-derived growth factor (PDGF), an approximately 30-kd protein consisting of two polypeptide chains.[47] PDGF is released from platelets during the process of blood coagulation. PDGF stimulates the proliferation of fibroblasts, a cell growth process that plays an important role in wound healing. Other well-characterized examples of growth factors include nerve growth factor, epidermal growth factor, and fibroblast growth factor.

Table 6-1 Oncogenes

Oncogene	Chromosome	Method of Identification	Neoplasm	Mechanism of Activation	Protein Function
Growth factors					
v-sis	22q12.3–13.1	Sequence homology	Glioma/fibrosarcoma	Constitutive production	B chain PDGF
int2	11q13	Proviral insertion	Mammary carcinoma	Constitutive production	Member of FGF family
KS3	11q13.3	DNA transfection	Kaposi's sarcoma	Constitutive production	Member of FGF family
HST	11q13.3	DNA transfection	Stomach carcinoma	Constitutive production	Member of FGF family
Growth factor receptors					
Tyrosine kinases: integral membrane proteins					
EGFR	7p1.1–1.3	DNA amplification/DNA sequencing	Squamous cell carcinoma Non-small cell lung cancer	Gene amplification/protein/point mutation	EGF receptor
v-fms	5q33-34 (FMS)	Viral homologue	Sarcoma	Constitutive activation	CSF1 receptor
v-kit	4q11-21 (KIT)	Viral homologue/DNA sequencing	Sarcoma/GIST	Constitutive activation/point mutation	Stem cell factor receptor
v-ros	6q22 (ROS)	Viral homologue	Sarcoma	Constitutive activation	?
MET	7p31	DNA transfection	MNNG-treated human osteocarcinoma cell line	DNA rearrangement/ligand-independent constitutive activation (fusion proteins)	HGF/SF receptor
TRK	1q32–41	DNA transfection	Colon/thyroid carcinomas	DNA rearrangement/ligand-independent constitutive activation (fusion proteins)	NGF receptor
NEU	17q11.2–12	Point mutation/DNA amplification	Neuroblastoma/breast carcinoma/NSCLC	Gene amplification/point mutation	?
RET	10q11.2	DNA transfection	Carcinomas of thyroid Men 2A. Men 2B	DNA rearrangement/point mutation (ligand-independent constitutive activation/fusion proteins)	GDNF/NTT/ART/PSP receptor
Receptors lacking protein kinase activity					
mas	6q24–27	DNA transfection	Epidermoid carcinoma	Rearrangement of 5' non-coding region	Angiotensin receptor
Signal transducers					
Cytoplasmic tyrosine kinases					
SRC	20p12–13	Viral homologue	Colon carcinoma	Constitutive activation	Protein tyrosine kinase
v-yes	18q21–3 (YES)	Viral homologue	Sarcoma	Constitutive activation	Protein tyrosine kinase
v-fgr	1p36.1–36.2 (FGR)	Viral homologue	Sarcoma	Constitutive activation	Protein tyrosine kinase
v-fes	15q25–26 (FES)	Viral homologue	Sarcoma	Constitutive activation	Protein tyrosine kinase
ABL	9q34.1	Chromosome translocation	CML	DNA rearrangement (constitutive activation/fusion proteins)	Protein tyrosine kinase
Membrane-associated G proteins					
H-RAS	11p15.5	Viral homologue/DNA transfection	Colon, lung, pancreas carcinomas	Point mutation	GTPase
K-RAS	12p11.1–12.1	Viral homologue/DNA transfection	AML, thyroid carcinoma, melanoma/colon/lung	Point mutation	GTPase
N-RAS	1p11–13	DNA transfection	Carcinoma, melanoma	Point mutation	GTPase
BRAF	6	DNA sequencing	Melanoma, thyroid, colon, ovary	Point mutation	Ser/Thr kinase
gsp	20	DNA sequencing	Adenomas of thyroid	Point mutation	Gs alpha
gip	3	DNA sequencing	Ovary, adrenal carcinoma	Point mutation	Gi alpha
GTPase exchange factor (GEF)					
Dbl	Xq27	DNA transfection	Diffuse B-cell lymphoma	DNA rearrangement	GEF for Rho and Cdc42Hs
Vav	19p13.2	DNA transfection	Hematopoietic cells	DNA rearrangement	GEF for Ras?
Serine/threonine kinases: cytoplasmic					
v-mos	8q11 (MOS)	Viral homologue	Sarcoma	Constitutive activation	Protein kinase (ser/thr)
v-raf	3p25 (RAF-1)	Viral homologue	Sarcoma	Constitutive activation	Protein kinase (ser/thr)
pim-1	6p21 (PIM-)	Insertional mutagenesis	T-cell lymphoma	Constitutive activation	Protein kinase (ser/thr)
Cytoplasmic regulators					
v-crk	17p13 (CRK)	Viral homologue		Constitutive tyrosine phosphorylation of cellular substrates (eg, paxillin)	SH-2/SH-3 adaptor
Transcription factors					
v-myc	8q24.1 (MYC)	Viral homologue	Carcinoma myelocytomatosis	Deregulated activity	Transcription factor
N-MYC	2p24	DNA amplification	Neuroblastoma: lung carcinoma	Deregulated activity	Transcription factor
L-MYC	1p32	DNA amplification	Carcinoma of lung	Deregulated activity	Transcription factor
v-myb	6q22–24	Viral homologue	Myeloblastosis	Deregulated activity	Transcription factor
v-fos	14q21–22	Viral homologue	Osteosarcoma	Deregulated activity	Transcription factor API
v-jun	p31–32	Viral homologue	Sarcoma	Deregulated activity	Transcription factor API
v-ski	1q22–24	Viral homologue	Carcinoma	Deregulated activity	Transcription factor
v-rel	2p12–14	Viral homologue	Lymphatic leukemia	Deregulated activity	Mutant NF-kappa B
v-ets-1	11p23–q24	Viral homologue	Erythroblastosis	Deregulated activity	Transcription factor
v-ets-2	21q24.3	Viral homologue	Erythroblastosis	Deregulated activity	Transcription factor
v-erbA1	17p11–21	Viral homologue	Erythroblastosis	Deregulated activity	T3 Transcription factor
v-erbA2	3p22–24.1	Viral homologue	Erythroblastosis	Deregulated activity	T3 Transcription factor
Others					
BCL2	18q21.3	Chromosomal translocation	B-cell lymphomas	Constitutive activity	Antiapoptotic protein
MDM2	12q14	DNA amplification	Sarcomas	Gene amplification/increased protein	Complexes with p53

AML = acute myeloid leukemia; CML = chronic myelogenous leukemia; GTPase = guanosine triphosphatase; PDGF = platelet-derived growth factor.

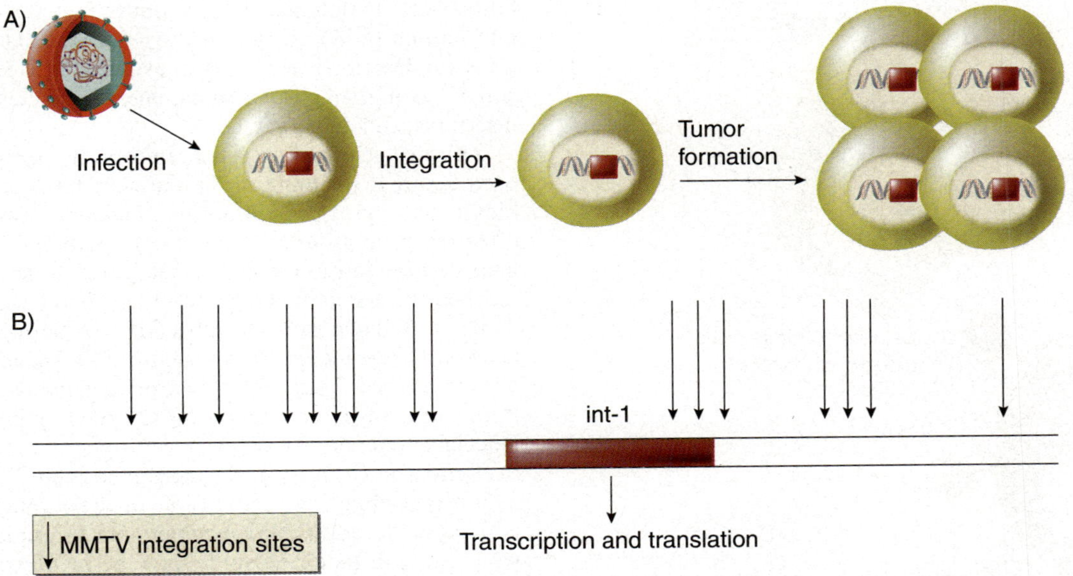

Figure 6-2 Insertional mutagenesis. **A,** The process is independent from genes carried by the retrovirus. Retrovirus, for example MMTV, infects a human cell. The proviral DNA is integrated into the host genome in infected cells. Rarely, the provirus inserts near a proto-oncogene (for example *int-1*) and activates the proto-oncogene. Activated proto-oncogene results in cell transformation and in tumor formation. **B,** Sites of integration of MMTV retrovirus near the proto-oncogene *int-1*. All sites determine *int-1* activation.

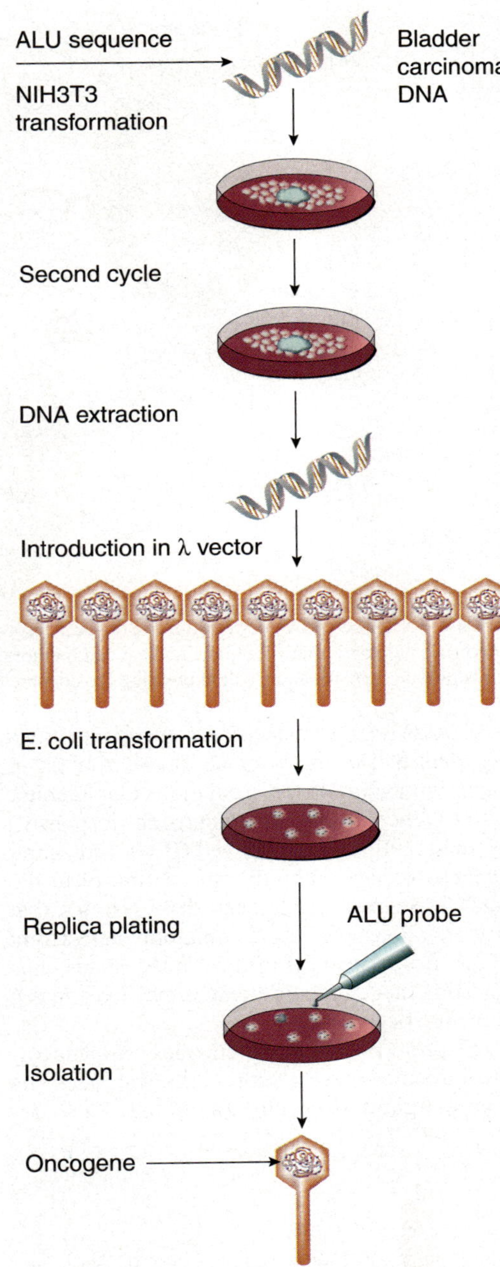

Figure 6-3 Transfection assay. DNA from a tumor (for example bladder carcinoma) is used to transform a rodent immortalized cell line (NIH3T3). After serial cycles, DNA from transformed cells was extracted and then inserted into λ vector, that was subsequently used to transform an appropriate *Escherichia coli* strain. Using a specific probe (*Alu* in the figure) it was possible to isolate and then characterize the involved human oncogene.

The link between growth factors and retroviral oncogenes was revealed by study of the *sis* oncogene of simian sarcoma virus, a retrovirus first isolated from a monkey fibrosarcoma. Sequence analysis showed that *sis* encodes the beta chain of PDGF.[48] This discovery established the principle that inappropriately expressed growth factors could function as oncogenes. Experiments demonstrated that the constitutive expression of the *sis* gene product (PDGF-*b*) was sufficient to cause neoplastic transformation of fibroblasts but not of cells that lacked the receptor for PDGF.[49] Thus, transformation by *sis* requires interaction of the *sis* gene product with the PDGF receptor. The mechanism by which a growth factor affects the same cell that produces it is called *autocrine stimulation*[50] (Figure 6-4). The constitutive expression of the *sis* gene product appears to cause neoplastic transformation by the mechanism of autocrine stimulation, resulting in self-sustained aberrant cell proliferation. This model, derived from experimental animal systems, has been recently demonstrated in a human tumor. Dermatofibrosarcoma protuberans (DP) is an infiltrative skin tumor that was demonstrated to present specific cytogenetic features: reciprocal translocation and supernumerary ring chromosomes, involving chromosomes 17 and 22.[51,52] Molecular cloning of the breakpoints revealed a fusion between the collagen type Ia1 (COL1A1) gene and PDGF-β gene. The fusion gene resulted in a deletion of PDGF-β exon 1 and a constitutive release of this growth factor. Subsequent experiments of gene transfer of DP's genomic DNA into NIH 3T3 cells directly demonstrated the occurrence of an autocrine mechanism by the human rearranged PDGF-beta gene involving the activation of the endogenous PDGF receptor.[53,54] Another example of a growth factor that can function as an oncogene is *int-2*, a member of the fibroblast growth factor family. *Int-2* is sometimes activated in mouse mammary carcinomas by MMTV insertional mutagenesis.[55]

Growth Factor Receptors Some viral oncogenes are altered versions of normal growth factor receptors that possess intrinsic tyrosine kinase activity.[56] Receptor tyrosine kinases, as these growth factor receptors are collectively known, have a characteristic protein structure consisting of three principal domains: (1) the extracellular ligand-binding domain, (2) the transmembrane domain, and (3) the intracellular tyrosine kinase catalytic domain (Figure 6-5). Growth factor receptors are molecular machines that transmit information in a unidirectional fashion across the cell membrane. The binding of a growth factor to the extracellular ligand-binding domain of the receptor results in the activation of the intracellular tyrosine kinase catalytic domain. The recruitment and phosphorylation of specific cytoplasmic proteins by the activated receptor then trigger a series of biochemical events generally leading to cell division.

Because of the role of growth factor receptors in the regulation of normal cell growth, it is not surprising that these receptors constitute an important class of proto-oncogenes. Examples include *erb B*, *erb B-2*, *fms*, *kit*, *met*, *ret*, *ros*, and *trk*. Mutation or abnormal expression of growth factor receptors can convert them into oncogenes.[57] For example, deletion of the ligand-binding domain of *erb B* (the epidermal growth factor receptor) is thought to result in constitutive activation of the receptor in the absence of ligand binding.[58] Point mutation in the tyrosine kinase domain or of the extracellular domain and deletion of intracellular regulatory domains can also result in the constitutive activation of receptor tyrosine kinases. Relevant examples are represented by *erb B-2*, *erb B* and *kit*. By the sequencing of *erb B-2* gene, it has been found that mutations occur in 4% of primary lung cancers and, more in detail, in 10% of the adenocarcinoma subtype. These mutations are within the kinase domain. More rarely somatic hyperactivating mutations were also detected in gastric and ovarian tumors, and in glioblastoma. Interestingly, immunohistochemical staining for *erb B-2* revealed no differences between tumors with or without *erb B-2* mutations, indicating that overexpression probably does not accompany the mutation.[59]

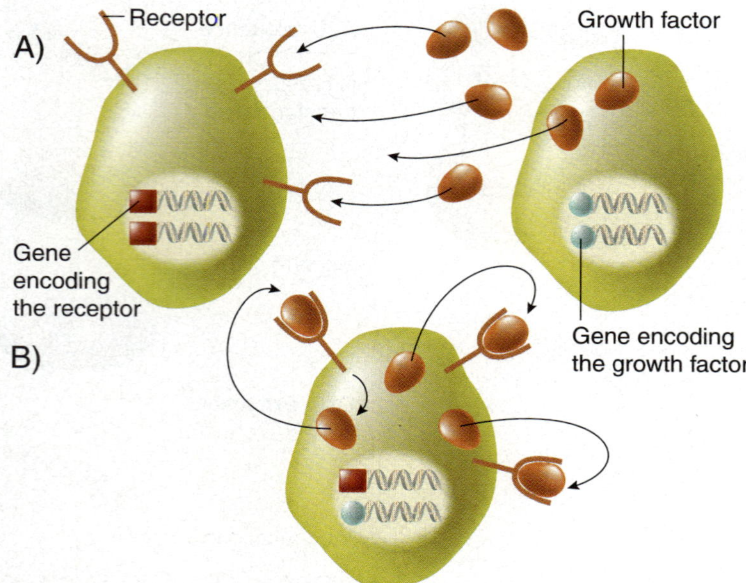

Figure 6-4 Paracrine and autocrine stimulation. **A,** A growth factor produced by the cell on the right stimulates another cell carrying the appropriate receptor (*left*) on cell membrane. This process is named paracrine stimulation. **B,** A growth factor is produced by the same cell expressing the cognate receptor. This process is designated autocrine stimulation.

As far as *erb B* is concerned, somatic mutations were identified in the tyrosine kinase domain in patients with gefitinib (an *erb B* molecular inhibitor used in a chemotherapeutic approach)-responsive non–small-cell lung cancer (NSCLC), indicating that these mutations confer susceptibility to the drug.[60] Moreover, it has been demonstrated that *erb B* mutations were more commonly detected in NSCLC from Japan than from United States, thus suggesting that ethnic differences may exist in *erb B* mutation occurrence.[61]

The proto-oncogene *kit* encodes a transmembrane tyrosine kinase glycoprotein. Binding of its cognate ligand stem-cell factor (SCF) to *kit* results in receptor homodimerization, activation of *kit* tyrosine kinase activity and resultant phosphorylation of a variety of substrates, including Akt and STAT3. Three general mechanisms of *kit* activation in tumor cells have been described: (1) autocrine and/or paracrine stimulation of the receptor by its ligand, SCF; (2) cross-activation by other kinases and/or loss of regulatory phosphatase activity; and (3) acquisition of activating mutations of several different exons of the *kit* gene. *Kit* mutations (typically in exon 17) are most commonly found in mastocytosis/mast cell leukemia, acute myelogenous leukemia (AML), seminoma/dysgerminoma, and sinosal natural killer/T-cell lymphoma. In gastrointestinal stromal tumors (GIST), more heterogeneous mutations are described, occurring in exons 9, 11, 13, and 17, comprising point mutations, "in-frame" insertions, and deletions.

Of great relevance, it has been recently demonstrated that imatinib, an inhibitor of tyrosine kinase activity in *bcr-abl*-positive leukemia was effective in treating GIST.[62] In this pathology, gain of function mutations result in the ligand independent receptor activation. It has then been demonstrated that patients with a GIST harboring an exon 11 *kit* mutation had a significantly higher partial response rate (72%) than patients whose tumor had an exon 9 mutation (31.6%) or no detectable mutation (11.8%).[63]

Increased expression through gene amplification and abnormal expression in the wrong cell type are additional mechanisms through which growth factor receptors may be involved in neoplasia. The identification and study of altered growth factor receptors in experimental models of neoplasia have contributed much to our understanding of the normal regulation of cell proliferation.

Signal Transducers Mitogenic signals are transmitted from growth factor receptors on the cell surface to the cell nucleus through a series of complex interlocking pathways collectively referred to as the signal transduction cascade.[64] This relay of information is accomplished in part by the stepwise phosphorylation of interacting proteins in the cytosol. Signal transduction also involves guanine nucleotide-binding proteins and second messengers such as the adenylate cyclase system.[65] The first retroviral oncogene discovered, *src*, was subsequently shown to be involved in signal transduction.

Many proto-oncogenes are members of signal transduction pathways.[66,67] These consist of two main groups: nonreceptor protein kinases and guanosine triphosphate (GTP)-binding proteins. The nonreceptor protein kinases are subclassified into tyrosine kinases (eg, *abl*, *lck*, and *src*) and serine/threonine kinases (eg, *raf-1*, *mos*, and *pim-1*). GTP-binding proteins with intrinsic GTPase activity are subdivided into monomeric and heterotrimeric groups.[68] Monomeric GTP-binding proteins are members of the important *ras* family of proto-oncogenes that includes H-*ras*, K-*ras*, and N-*ras*.[69] Heterotrimeric GTP-binding proteins (G proteins) implicated as proto-oncogenes currently include *gsp* and *gip*. Signal transducers are often converted to oncogenes by mutations that lead to their unregulated activity, which in turn leads to uncontrolled cellular proliferation.[70] (For a review on signal transduction, see *Oncogene*, issue 1, Vol. 17, N. 11, September 1998.)

Transcription Factors Transcription factors are nuclear proteins that regulate the expression of target genes or gene families.[71] Transcriptional regulation is mediated by protein binding to specific DNA sequences or DNA structural motifs, usually located upstream of the target

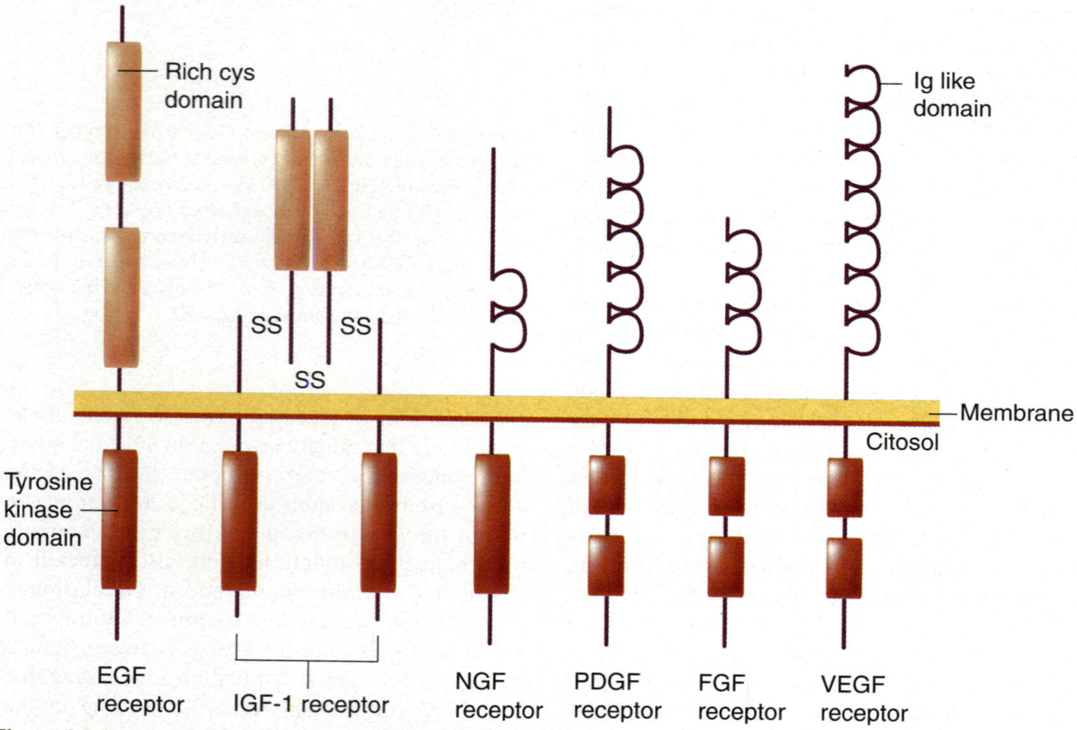

Rich cys domain
Ig like domain
SS
SS
SS
Membrane
Citosol
Tyrosine kinase domain
EGF receptor
IGF-1 receptor
NGF receptor
PDGF receptor
FGF receptor
VEGF receptor

Figure 6-5 Representative examples of tyrosine kinase receptor families.

gene. Transcription factors often belong to multigene families that share common DNA-binding domains such as zinc fingers. The mechanism of action of transcription factors also involves binding to other proteins, sometimes in heterodimeric complexes with specific partners. Transcription factors are the final link in the signal transduction pathway that converts extracellular signals into modulated changes in gene expression.

Many proto-oncogenes are transcription factors that were discovered through their retroviral homologues.[72] Examples include *erb A*, *ets*, *fos*, *jun*, *myb*, and c-*myc*. Together, *fos* and *jun* form the AP-1 transcription factor, which positively regulates a number of target genes whose expression leads to cell division.[73,74] *Erb A* is the receptor for the T3 thyroid hormone, triiodothyronine.[75] Proto-oncogenes that function as transcription factors are often activated by chromosomal translocations in hematologic and solid neoplasms.[76] In certain types of sarcomas, chromosomal translocations cause the formation of fusion proteins involving the association of *EWS* gene with various partners and resulting in an aberrant tumor-associated transcriptional activity. Interestingly, a role of the adenovirus *E1A* gene in promoting the formation of fusion transcript fli1/ews in normal human fibroblasts was recently reported.[77] An important example of a proto-oncogene with a transcriptional activity in human hematologic tumors is the c-*myc* gene, which helps to control the expression of genes leading to cell proliferation.[78] As will be discussed later in this chapter, the c-*myc* gene (which is encoded for a nuclear DNA-binding protein belonging to the helix-loop-helix/leucine zipper superfamily, involved in transcriptional regulation) is frequently activated by chromosomal translocations in human leukemia and lymphoma.

Programed Cell Death Regulation Normal tissues exhibit a regulated balance between cell proliferation and cell death. Programed cell death is an important component in the processes of normal embryogenesis and organ development. A distinctive type of programed cell death, called apoptosis, has been described for mature tissues.[79] This process is characterized morphologically by blebbing of the plasma membrane, volume contraction, condensation of the cell nucleus, and cleavage of genomic DNA by endogenous nucleases into nucleosome-sized fragments. Apoptosis can be triggered in mature cells by external stimuli such as steroids and radiation exposure. Studies of cancer cells have shown that both uncontrolled cell proliferation and failure to undergo programed cell death can contribute to neoplasia and insensitivity to anticancer treatments.

The first proto-oncogene shown to regulate programmed cell death is *bcl-2*. It was the study of chromosomal translocations in human lymphoma that lead to the discovery of *bcl-2*.[80,81] Experimental studies show that *bcl-2* activation inhibits programed cell death in lymphoid cell populations.[82] The dominant mode of action of activated *bcl-2* led to classify it as an oncogene.

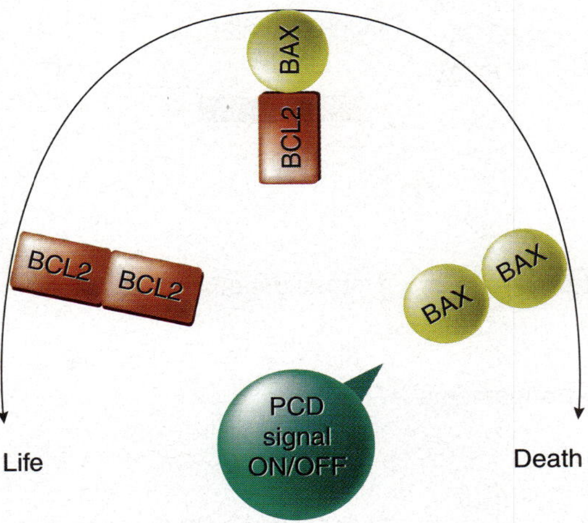

Figure 6-6 Effect of bcl-2 activity on the control of the cell life. In the presence of BAX only, the cell goes to apoptosis. bcl-2 Regulates the cycle of the cell by the interaction with BAX. When bcl-2 is overexpressed, the cell cycle is deregulated and the apoptosis is prevented, eventually leading to tumor formation. This is an important cause for tumor formation. PCD = program cell death or apoptosis.

The *bcl-2* gene encodes a protein localized to the inner mitochondrial membrane, endoplasmic reticulum, and nuclear membrane. The mechanism of action of the bcl-2 protein has not been fully elucidated, but studies indicate that it functions in part as an antioxidant that inhibits lipid peroxidation of cell membranes.[83,84] Moreover, bcl-2 homologues, some of which bind to bcl-2, have been identified, suggesting that bcl-2 functions at least in part through protein-protein interaction. Site-directed mutagenesis of bcl-2 protein BH1 and BH2 domains showed that these two regions are important for binding of bcl-2 to bax, a member of the bcl-2-family that promotes cell death and whose interaction with bcl-2 is necessary to regulate the apoptotic pathway.[11] (Figure 6-6) Although translocation is the main mechanism of *bcl-2* gene activation, *bcl-2* point mutations and amplification also have been reported. Mutations clustering in the *bcl-2* open-reading frame occur in high-grade B-cell lymphomas transformed from low grade follicular lymphomas carrying *bcl-2* gene rearrangement.[85] The amplification of the *bcl-2* gene, which leads to increased protein production, has been detected in about 30% of high-grade diffuse large cell lymphomas (DLCL) lacking bcl-2 translocation.[86] Clinical relevance of bcl-2 expression has been shown in solid tumors, such as breast, prostate, thyroid, and lung.[87–90] The down-regulation of bcl-2 protein expression by antisense oligonucleotides (ASO) which induce bcl-2 mRNA degradation may offer a new therapeutic approach for treatment improvements in patients with neoplasms resistant to traditional therapies. The results on in vitro[91,92] and in vivo[93] models are promising, especially when a combination of bcl-2 ASO (G3139) with a cytotoxic agent is used. In humans, G3139 has entered phase I trials.[94]

The second oncogene more recently shown to be involved in apoptosis is caspase-9, which is activated by the following intrinsic pathway. Release of cytochrome c into the cytosol results in activation of the caspase adaptor Apaf-1 and pro-caspase-9, which form a holoenzyme complex named apoptosome. Caspase-9, in turn, activates downstream caspases, most importantly caspase-3 and also caspase-6, 7, and 8, which results in DNA fragmentation and apoptosis.[11,95] It has been demonstrated that Akt may regulate apoptosome function by phosphorylation of caspase-9 at the Ser-196 level.[96] This phosphorylation event has relevant functional consequences, leading to the suppression of apoptosis caspase-9-mediated. The Akt suppression is specific for caspase-9 and probably is due to the inactivation of the intrinsic catalytic activity.[97] More recently it has been demonstrated that bax is also involved, leading to caspase-9 stimulation (through Apaf-1) in response to mitochondrial membrane damage.[98]

MECHANISMS OF ONCOGENE ACTIVATION

The activation of oncogenes involves genetic changes to cellular proto-oncogenes. The consequence of these genetic alterations is to confer a growth advantage to the cell. Four genetic mechanisms activate oncogenes in human neoplasms: (1) mutation, (2) gene amplification, (3) chromosome rearrangements, and (4) overexpression. The first three mechanisms result in either an alteration of proto-oncogene structure or an increase in proto-oncogene expression (Figure 6-7). Because neoplasia is a multistep process, more than one of these mechanisms often contribute to the genesis of human tumors by altering a number of cancer-associated genes. Full expression of the neoplastic phenotype, including the capacity for metastasis, usually involves a combination of proto-oncogene activation and tumor suppressor gene loss or inactivation.

Mutation Mutations activate proto-oncogenes through structural alterations in their encoded proteins. These alterations, which usually involve critical protein regulatory regions, often lead to the uncontrolled, continuous activity of the mutated protein. Various types of mutations, such as base substitutions, deletions, and insertions, are capable of activating proto-oncogenes.[99] Retroviral oncogenes, for example, often have deletions that contribute to their activation. Examples include deletions in the amino-terminal ligand-binding domains of the *erb B*, *kit*, *ros*, *met*, and *trk* oncogenes.[6] In human tumors, however, most characterized oncogene mutations are base substitutions (point mutations) that change a single amino acid within the protein.

Point mutations are frequently detected in the *ras* family of proto-oncogenes (K-*ras*, H-*ras*, and N-*ras*).[100] The human *ras* genes encode for similar membrane-bound 21 kd proteins (189 amino acids) involved in signal transduction, with a guanine

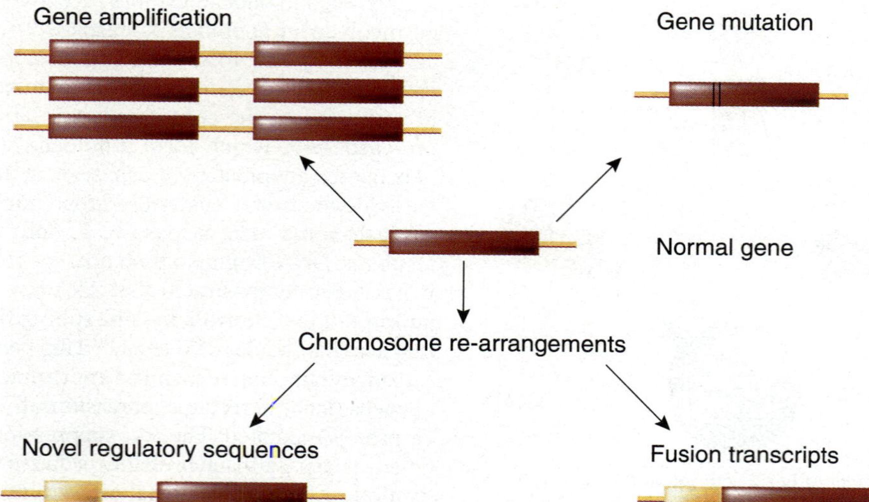

Figure 6-7 Schematic representation of the main mechanisms of oncogene activation (from proto-oncogenes to oncogenes). The normal gene (proto-oncogene) is depicted with its transcribed portion (*rectangle*). In the case of gene amplification, the latter can be duplicated 100-fold, resulting in an excess of normal protein. A similar situation can occur when following chromosome rearrangements such as translocation, the transcription of the gene is now regulated by novel regulatory sequences belonging to another gene. In the case of point mutation, single amino acid substitutions can alter the biochemical properties of the gene product, causing, in the example, its constitutive enzymatic activation. Chromosome rearrangements, such as translocation and inversion, can then generate fusion transcripts resulting in chimeric oncogenic proteins.

nucleotide-binding activity as well as an intrinsic guanosine triphosphatase (GTP) activity. When activated, ras proteins transduce the signal by linking tyrosine kinases to downstream serine/threonine kinases, such as raf, and mitogen-activated protein kinases (MAPK)[69] (Figure 6-8). Stabilization of ras proteins in their active state causes a continuous flow of signal transduction, which results in malignant transformation. This status can be achieved after point mutation, mainly at codon 12 level, with a smaller number involving other regions such as codons 13 or 61.[101] Mutations of *ras* in human tumors have been linked to carcinogen exposure. It has been estimated that as many as 15 to 20% of unselected human tumors may contain a *ras* mutation. Mutations in K-*ras* predominate in carcinomas. Studies have found K-*ras* mutations in about 30% of lung adenocarcinomas, 50% of colorectal carcinomas, and 90% of carcinomas of the pancreas.[102] N-*ras* mutations are preferentially found in hematologic malignancies, with up to a 25% incidence in acute myeloid leukemias and myelodysplastic syndromes.[103,104] The majority of thyroid carcinomas have been found to have *ras* mutations distributed among K-*ras*, H-*ras*, and N-*ras*, without preference for a single *ras* family member, but showing an association with the follicular type of differentiated thyroid carcinomas.[105,106] Moreover, K-*ras* mutations could be identified in stool specimens, thus representing a noninvasive presymptomatic indicator of colonic adenomas (mostly adenomas larger than 1 cm)[107] or early colorectal tumors.[108,109] This finding acquires more relevance since some evidence suggests a link between poor outcome and specific types of K-*ras* mutations (codon 12 G-T transversions) in colorectal cancer.[110] Demonstration of such a prognostic effect, not yet firmly established, otherwise may allow appropriate targeting of intensive follow-up and adjuvant therapy.[111,112]

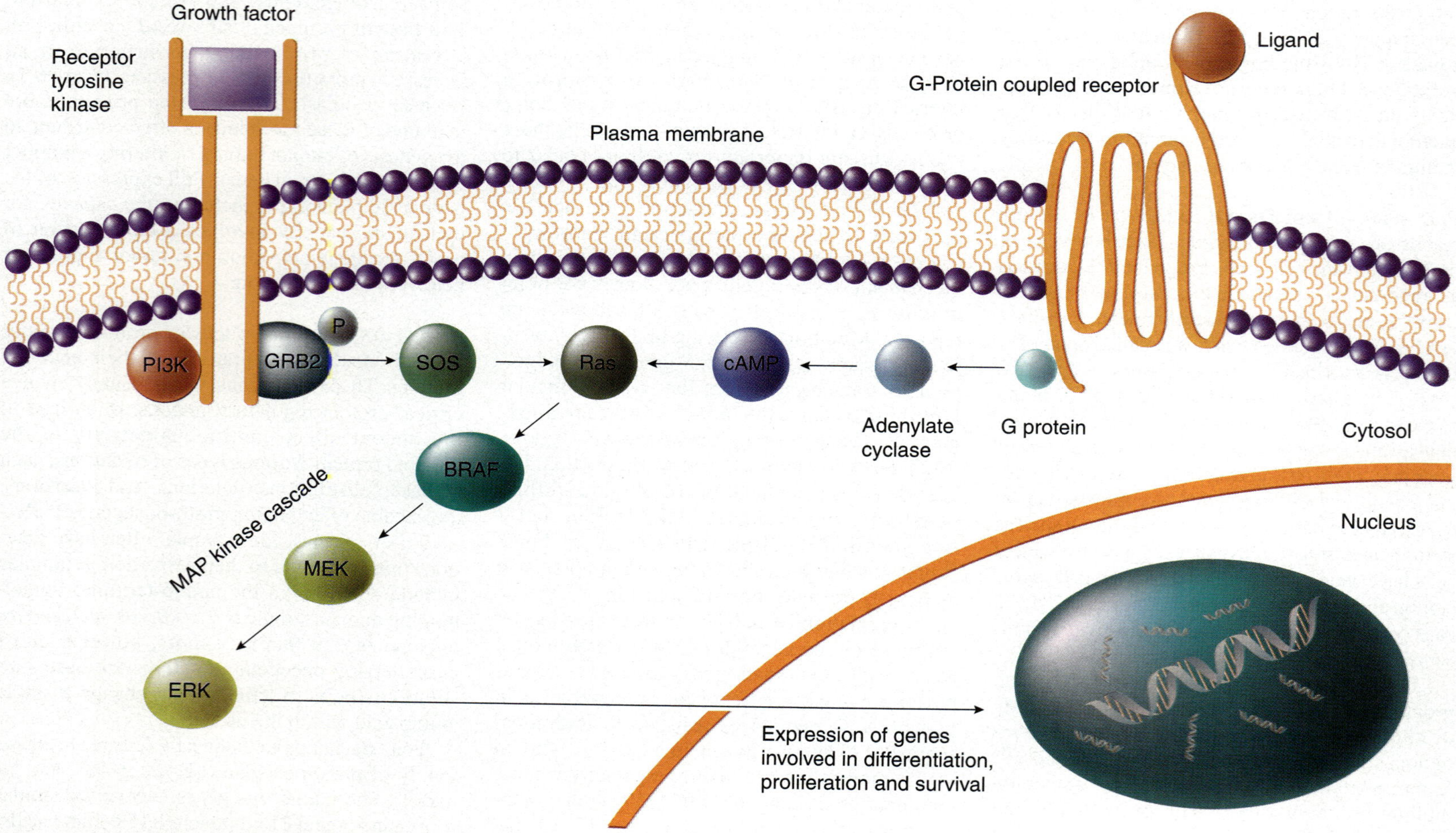

Figure 6-8 The ras-raf-MAPK signaling pathway.

Another example of activating point mutations is represented by those occurring in *BRAF* gene, the first result of the human genome project in the screening of cancer genes using high-throughput genomic technologies.[7] The *BRAF* sequence contains the three conserved regions CR1, which encodes for the putative zinc finger domain, CR2, where several serine/threonine-rich regions are located, and CR3, which corresponds to the kinase domain. BRAF is recruited to the plasma membrane upon binding to ras-GTP and represents a key point in the signal transduction through the mitogen-activated protein (MAP) kinase pathway (see Figure 6-8). The most common oncogenic mutation of *BRAF*, occurring in more than 90% of cases, changes the valine residue at position 599 within the BRAF kinase domain to glutamic acid (V599E), thus mimicking the phosphorylation of threonine 598 and serine 601, two major points of BRAF regulation which lead to a protein with high activity, able to constitutively activate ERK protein.[11] In cell lines, *BRAF* alterations were mostly detected in melanoma (59%) and then in colorectal cancer (18%), liver cancer (14%), and gliomas (11%).[7] In tissue specimens, *BRAF* mutations were found in melanomas (75%), thyroid (45%), colorectal (12%), and ovarian cancer (14%).[7,113] Furthermore, it has been shown that *BRAF* mutations occur in colorectal cancer only when tumors do not carry mutations in the K-*ras* gene and such a mutual exclusion has led to the assumption that *BRAF* and K-*ras* alterations could have the same functional effect in colorectal carcinogenesis.[11,114] Moreover, again in colorectal cancer, it seems that *BRAF* mutations could be related to the mismatch-repair status.[114] In melanoma, *BRAF* mutations may even precede the neoplastic transformation, since all types of nevi besides Spitz and Blue nevi show *BRAF* alterations at a high frequency, with dysplastic nevi showing a notably lower frequency.[115] BRAF now provides a critical new target for drugs treating malignant melanoma are developing, including antisense oligonucleotides and small molecules. These inhibitors block the expression of BRAF protein, block the BRAF/ras interaction, block its kinase activity or the kinase activity of the BRAF target protein MAP kinase. One of these, BAY-43-9006, recently entered phase III clinical trials.[94]

Another significant example of activating point mutations is represented by those affecting the *ret* proto-oncogene in multiple endocrine neoplasia type 2A syndrome (MEN2A).

Germline point mutations affecting one of the cysteines located in the juxtamembrane domain of the *ret* receptor have been found to confer an oncogenic potential to the latter as a consequence of the ligand-independent activation of the tyrosine kinase activity of the receptor. Experimental evidences have pointed out that these cysteine residue-involving mutations promote *ret* homodimerization via the formation of intermolecular disulfide bonding, most likely as a result of an unpaired number of cysteine residues.[116,117]

Gene Amplification Gene amplification refers to the expansion in copy number of a gene within the genome of a cell. Gene amplification was first discovered as a mechanism by which some tumor cell lines can acquire resistance to growth-inhibiting drugs.[118] The process of gene amplification occurs through redundant replication of genomic DNA, often giving rise to karyotypic abnormalities called double-minute chromosomes (DMs) and homogeneous staining regions (HSRs).[119] DMs are characteristic minichromosome structures without centromeres. HSRs are segments of chromosomes that lack the normal alternating pattern of light and dark staining bands. Both DMs and HSRs represent large regions of amplified genomic DNA, containing up to several hundred copies of a gene. Amplification leads to the increased expression of genes, which in turn can confer a selective advantage for cell growth.

The frequent observation of DMs and HSRs in human tumors suggested that the amplification of specific proto-oncogenes may be a common occurrence in neoplasia.[120] Studies then demonstrated that three proto-oncogene families—*myc*, *erb B*, and *ras*—are amplified in a significant number of human tumors (Table 6-2). About 20 to 30% of breast and ovarian cancers show c-*myc* amplification, and an approximately equal frequency of c-*myc* amplification is found in some types of squamous cell carcinomas.[121] N-*myc* was discovered as a new member of the *myc* proto-oncogene family through its amplification in neuroblastomas.[122] Amplification of N-*myc* correlates strongly with advanced tumor stage in neuroblastoma[123] (Table 6-3), suggesting a role for this gene in tumor progression.[124] L-*myc* was discovered through its amplification in small-cell carcinoma of the lung, a neuroendocrine-derived tumor, and in bladder neoplasia.[125] Furthermore, c-*myc* activation may be mediated by APC and/or β-catenin alterations in several tumors, leading to an increase of c-*myc* transcription through an accumulation of β-catenin into the cytoplasm and the nucleus.[126] A nuclear accumulation of c-*myc* may identify high-risk subsets of patients with synovial sarcoma of the extremities.[127] Amplification and overexpression of c-*myc*, in combination with *erb B-2* alterations, have been reported to be associated with tumor progression from noninvasive to invasive[128] and with poor prognosis[129] in patients with breast carcinoma. In melanoma[130] and in medulloblastoma,[131,132] c-*myc* expression seems to be a useful prognostic marker able to identify high-risk patients. Amplification of *erb B*, the epidermal growth factor receptor, is found in up to 50% of glioblastomas, in 10 to 20% of squamous carcinomas of the head and neck, and in about 50% of colorectal cancer.[100,133] Gene amplification and overexpression of *erb B-2* have been reported in approximately 25% of breast, ovarian, endometrial, gastric, and salivary gland carcinomas.[134] It was detected also in 16% of non–small-cell lung carcinoma (NSCLC)[135] and in a subset of malignant pancreatic endocrine tumor (gastrinoma).[11,136] Overexpression of the *erb B-2*, performed at immunohistochemical level, was detected in thick melanoma,[137] in pancreatic carcinoma,[138] and in prostatic tumors.[139]

Table 6-2 Oncogene Amplification in Human Cancers

Tumor Type	Gene Amplified	Percent
Neuroblastoma	MYCN	20–25
Small cell lung cancer	MYC	15–20
Glioblastoma	ERB B-1 (EGFR)	33–50
Breast cancer	MYC	20
	ERB B-2 (EGFR2)	~20
	FGFR1	12
	FGFR2	12
	CCND1 (cyclin d1)	15–20
Esophageal cancer	MYC	38
	CCND1 (cyclin d1)	25
Gastric cancer	K-RAS	10
	CCNE (cyclin e)	15
Hepatocellular cancer	CCND1 (cyclin d1)	13
Sarcoma	MDM2	10–30
	CDK4	11
Cervical cancer	MYC	25–50
Ovarian cancer	MYC	20–30
	ERB B-2 (EGFR2)	15–30
	AKT2	12
Head and neck cancer	MYC	7–10
	ERB B-1(EGFR)	10
	CCND1(cyclin d1)	~50
Colorectal cancer	MYB	15–20
	H-RAS	29
	K-RAS	22

Table 6-3 Correlation of N-myc Copy Number with Stage and Survival in Neuroblastoma

Tumor Type	Number of Cases	Percent
Benign ganglioneuromas	0/64	(0%)
Low stages	31/772	(4%)
Stage 4-S	15/190	(8%)
Advanced stages	612/1.974	(31%)
Total	658/3000	(22%)

In breast cancer, *erbB-2* amplification correlates with advanced stage and poor prognosis.[140] Members of the *ras* gene family, including K-*ras* and N-*ras*, are sporadically amplified in various carcinomas.

Chromosomal Rearrangements Recurring chromosomal rearrangements are often detected in hematologic malignancies as well as in some solid tumors.[41,141,142] These rearrangements consist mainly of chromosomal translocations and, less frequently, chromosomal inversions. Chromosomal rearrangements can lead to hematologic malignancy by two different mechanisms: (1) the transcriptional activation of proto-oncogenes or (2) the creation of fusion genes. Transcriptional activation, sometimes referred to as gene activation, results from chromosomal rearrangements that move a proto-oncogene close to an immunoglobulin or T-cell receptor gene (see Figure 6-7). Transcription of the proto-oncogene then falls under the control of regulatory elements from the immunoglobulin or T-cell receptor locus. This circumstance causes deregulation of proto-oncogene expression, which can then lead to neoplastic transformation of the cell.

Fusion genes can be created by chromosomal rearrangements when the chromosomal breakpoints fall within the loci of two different genes.

Table 6-4 Molecularly Characterized Chromosome Rearrangements in Tumors

Affected Gene	Rearrangements	Disease	Protein Type
Hematopoietic tumor			
Gene fusion			
c-ABL (9q34)	t(9:22) (q34:q11)	Chronic myelogenous leukemia and acute leukemia	Tyrosine kinase activated by BCR
BCR (22q11)			
PBX-1(1q23)	t(1:19)(q23:p13.3)	Acute pre-B-cell leukemia	Homeodomain
E2A(19p13.3)			HLH
PML(15q21)	t(15:17) (q21:q11–22)	Acute myeloid leukemia	Zn finger
RAR(17q21)			
CAN(6p23)	t(6:9) (p23:q34)	Acute myeloid leukemia	No homology
DEK(9q34)			
REL	ins(2:12) (p13:p11.2–14)	Non-Hodgkin's lymphoma	NF-κB family
NRG			No homology
Oncogenes juxtaposed with IG loci			
c-MYC	t(8:14) (q24:q32) t(2:8) (p12:q24) t(8:22) (q24:q11)	Burkitt's lymphoma. BL-ALL	HLH domain
BCL1 (PRADI?)	t(11:14) (q13:q32)	B-cell chronic lymphocyte leukemia	PRADI-GI cyclin
BCL-2	t(14:18) (q32:21)	Follicular lymphoma	Inner mitochondrial membrane
BCL-3	t(14:19) (q32:q13.1)	Chronic B-cell leukemia	CDC10 motif
IL-3	t(5:14) (q31:q32)	Acute pre-B-cell leukemia	Growth factor
Oncogenes juxtaposed with TCR loci			
c-MYC	t(8:14) (q24:q11)	Acute T-cell leukemia	HLH domain
LYLA	t(7:19) (q35:p13)	Acute T-cell leukemia	HLH domain
TALA/SCL/TCL-5	t(1:14) (q32:q11)	Acute T-cell leukemia	HLH domain
TAL-2	t(7:9) (q35:q34)	Acute T-cell leukemia	HLH domain
Rhombotin 1/Ttg-1	t(11:14) (p15:q11)	Acute T-cell leukemia	LIM domain
Rhombotin 2/Ttg-2	t(11:14) (p13:q11) t(7:11) (q35:p13)	Acute T-cell leukemia	LIM domain
HOX 11	t(10:14) (q24:q11) t(7:10) (q35:q24)	Acute T-cell leukemia	Homeodomain
TAN-1	t(7:9) (q34:q34.3)	Acute T-cell leukemia	Notch homologue
TCL-1	t(7q35-14q32.1) or inv t(14q11-14q32.1) or inv	B-cell chronic lymphocyte leukemia	
Solid tumors			
Gene fusions in sarcomas			
FLI1,EWS	t(11:22) (q24:q12)	Ewing's sarcoma	Ets transcription factor family
ERG,EWS	t(21:22) (q22:q12)	Ewing's sarcoma	Ets transcription factor family
ATV1,EWS	t(7:21) (q22:q12)	Ewing's sarcoma	Ets transcription factor family
ATF1,EWS	t(12:22) (q13:q12)	Soft-tissue clear cell sarcoma	Transcription factor
CHN,EWS	t(9:22) (q22 31:q12)	Myxoid chondrosarcoma	Steroid receptor family
WT1,EWS	t(11:22) (p13:q12)	Desmoplastic small round cell tumor	Wilms' tumor gene
SSX1,SSX2,SYT	t(X:18) (p11.2:q11.2)	Synovial sarcoma	HLH domain
PAX3,FKHR	t(2:13) (q37:q14)	Alveolar	Homeobox homologue
PAX7,FKHR	t(1:13) (q36:q14)	Rhabdomyosarcoma	Homeobox homologue
CHOP,TLS	t(12:16) (q13:p11)	Myxoid liposarcoma	Transcription factor
var,HMG1-C	t(var:12) (var:q13-15)	Lipomas	HMG DNA-binding protein
HMG1-C?	t(12:14) (q13-15)	Leiomyomas	HMG DNA-binding protein
Gene fusions in thyroid carcinomas			
RET/ptc1	inv(10) (q11.2:q2.1)	Papillary thyroid carcinomas	Tyrosine kinase activated by H4
RET/ptc2	t(10:17) (q11.2:q23)	Papillary thyroid carcinomas	Tyrosine kinase activated by RIa(PKA)
RET/ptc3	inv(10) (q11.2)	Papillary thyroid carcinomas	Tyrosine kinase activated by ELE1
TRK	inv(1) (q31:q22-23)	Papillary thyroid carcinomas	Tyrosine kinase activated by TPM3
TRK –T1(T2)	inv(1) (q31:q25)	Papillary thyroid carcinomas	Tyrosine kinase activated by TPR
TRK –T3	t(1q31:3)	Papillary thyroid carcinomas	Tyrosine kinase activated by TFG
Haematopoietic and solid tumors			
Oncogenes juxtaposed with other loci			
PTH deregulates PRAD1	inv(11)(p15:q13)	Parathyroid adenoma	PRADI-GI cyclin
BTG1 deregulates MYC	t(8:12)(q24:q22)	B-cell chronic lymphocytic	MYC-HLH domain

IG = immunoglobulin; TCR = T-cell receptor; HLH = helix loop helix structural domain; zn = zinc; HMG = high mobility group; H4; ELE1; TPR and 1TFG = partially uncharacterized genes with a dimerizing coiled-coil domain; RIa = regulatory subunit of PKA enzyme; TPM3 = isoform of non-muscle tropomyosin.

The resultant juxtaposition of segments from two different genes gives rise to a composite structure consisting of the head of one gene and the tail of another gene. Fusion genes encode chimeric proteins with transforming activity. In general, both genes involved in the fusion contribute to the transforming potential of the chimeric oncoprotein. Mistakes in the physiologic rearrangement of immunoglobulin or T-cell receptor genes are thought to give rise to many of the recurring chromosomal rearrangements found in hematologic malignancy.[143] Examples of molecularly characterized chromosomal rearrangements in hematologic and solid malignancies are given in Table 6-4. In some cases, the same proto-oncogene is involved in several different translocations (ie, c-*myc*, *ews*, and *ret*).

Gene Activation The t(8;14)(q24;q32) translocation, found in about 85% of cases of Burkitt's lymphoma, is a well-characterized example of the transcriptional activation of a proto-oncogene. This chromosomal rearrangement places the c-*myc* gene, located at chromosome band 8q24, under control of regulatory elements from the immunoglobulin heavy-chain locus located at 14q32.[144] The resulting transcriptional activation of c-*myc*, which encodes a nuclear protein involved in the regulation of cell proliferation, plays a critical role in the development of Burkitt's lymphoma.[145] The c-*myc* gene is also activated in some cases of Burkitt's lymphoma by translocations involving immunoglobulin light-chain genes.[146,147] These are t(2;8)(p12;q24), involving the κ locus located at 2p12, and t(8;22)(q24;q11), involving the λ locus at 22q11 (Figure 6-9). Although the position of the chromosomal breakpoints relative to the c-*myc* gene may vary considerably in individual cases of Burkitt's lymphoma, the consequence of the translocations is the same—deregulation of c-*myc* expression, leading to uncontrolled cellular proliferation. Moreover, again in lymphoma, c-*myc* gene mutations can occur in the gene transactivation domain and in the coding region after translocation into the *Ig* gene.[148] Mutations can occur in the noncoding gene exon 1 and at the exon 1/intron 1 boundary with or without c-*myc* gene translocation.[148] This region is considered the c-*myc* regulatory region and is responsible for its mRNA stability. In Burkitt's lymphoma, mutations frequently occur at sites of phosphorylation, a finding that suggests that they may have a pathogenetic role.

In some cases of T-cell acute lymphoblastic leukemia (T-ALL), the c-*myc* gene is activated by the t(8;14)(q24;q11) translocation. In these cases, transcription of c-*myc* is placed under the control of regulatory elements within the T-cell receptor α locus located at 14q11.[149] In addition to c-*myc*, several proto-oncogenes that encode nuclear proteins are activated by various chromosomal translocations in T-ALL involving the T-cell receptor α or β locus. These include *HOX11*, *TAL1*, *TAL2*, and *RBTN1/Tgt1*.[150–152] The proteins encoded by these genes are thought to function as transcription factors through DNA-binding and protein-protein interactions. Overexpression or inappropriate expression of these proteins in T cells is thought to inhibit T-cell differentiation and lead to uncontrolled cellular proliferation.

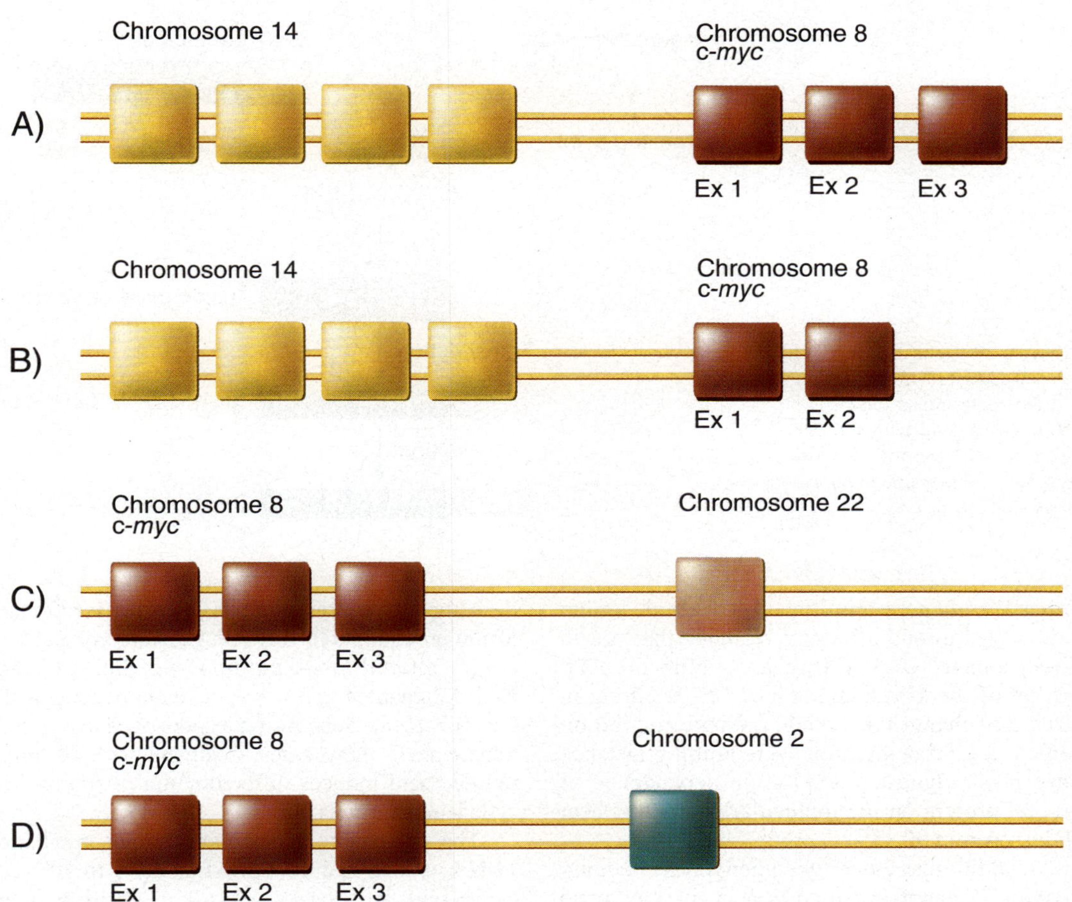

Figure 6-9 c-*myc* Translocations found in Burkitt's lymphoma. **A,** t(8;14)(q24;q32) Translocation involving the locus of immunoglobulin heavy chain gene located at 14q32. **B,** t(8;14)(q24;q32) Translocation where only 2 exons of c-myc are translocated under regulatory elements from the immunoglobulin heavy chain locus located at 14q32. **C,** t(8;22)(q24;q11) Translocation involving the *l* locus of immunoglobulin light chain gene at 22q11. **D,** t(2;8)(p12;q24) Translocation involving the *k* locus of immunoglobulin light chain gene located at 2p12.

A number of other proto-oncogenes are also activated by chromosomal translocations in leukemia and lymphoma. In most follicular lymphomas and some large cell lymphomas, the bcl-2 gene (located at 18q21) is activated as a consequence of t(14;18)(q32;q21) translocations.[80,81] Overexpression of the bcl-2 protein inhibits apoptosis, leading to an imbalance between lymphocyte proliferation and programed cell death.[82] Mantle cell lymphomas are characterized by the t(11;14)(q13;q32) translocation, which activates the cyclin D1 (bcl-1) gene located at 11q13.[153,154] cyclin D1 is a G1 cyclin involved in the normal regulation of the cell cycle. In some cases of T-cell chronic lymphocytic leukemia and prolymphocytic leukemia, the *tcl-1* gene at 14q32.1 is activated by inversion or translocation involving chromosome 14.[155] The tcl-1 gene product is a small cytoplasmic protein whose function is not yet known.

Gene Fusion The first example of gene fusion was discovered through the cloning of the breakpoint of the Philadelphia chromosome in chronic myelogenous leukemia (CML).[156] The t(9;22)(q34;q11) translocation in CML fuses the c-*abl* gene, normally located at 9q34, with the *bcr* gene at 22q11 (Figure 6-10).[157] The *bcr/abl* fusion, created on the der(22) chromosome, encodes a chimeric protein of 210 kD with increased tyrosine kinase activity and abnormal cellular localization.[158] The precise mechanism by which the *bcr/abl* fusion protein contributes to the expansion of the neoplastic myeloid clone is not yet known. The t(9;22) translocation is also found in up to 20% of cases of acute lymphoblastic leukemia (ALL). In these cases, the breakpoint in the *bcr* gene differs somewhat from that found in CML, resulting in a 185-kD bcr/abl fusion protein.[159] It is unclear at this time why the slightly smaller bcr/abl fusion protein leads to such a large difference in neoplastic phenotype. Inhibition of bcr/abl tyrosine kinase activity has been introduced as a chemotherapeutic approach in patients with CML. Administration of imatinib resulted in an antileukemic effect in CML patients in whom treatment with standard chemotherapy had failed.[160] However, cases of imatinib-resistance have also been recently documented.[161] Cause of such a failure is due to

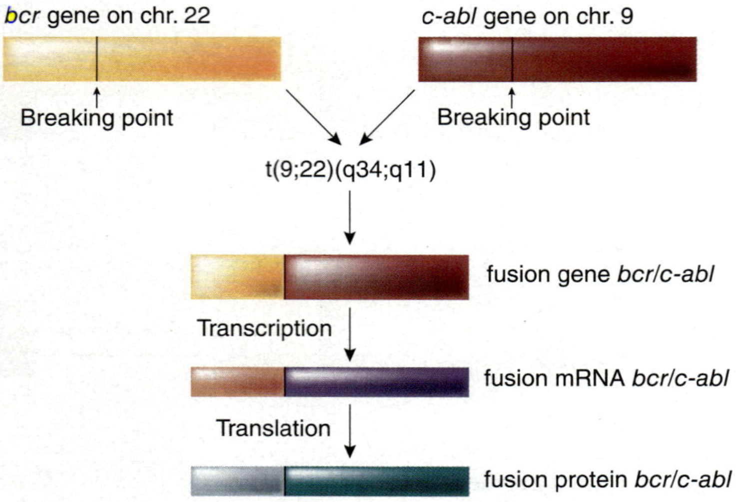

Figure 6-10 Gene fusion. The t(9;22)(q34;q11) translocation in CML determines the fusion of the c-*abl* gene with the *bcr* gene. Such a gene fusion encodes an oncogenic chimeric protein of 210 KD.

either *bcr/abl* gene amplification or single amino acid substitutions affecting residues that are in direct contact with ATP or are within the ATP pocket of the kinase domain of abl, resulting in structural changes that could influence inhibition sensitivity. Strategies for overcoming resistance have been suggested, exploiting dependence of bcr/abl protein on the molecular chaperone heat shock protein 90.[162]

In addition to c-*abl*, two other genes encoding tyrosine kinases are involved in distinct gene fusion events in hematologic malignancy. The t(2;5)(p23;q35) translocation in anaplastic large-cell lymphomas fuses the *NPM* gene (5q35) with the *ALK* gene (2p23).[163] *ALK* encodes a membrane-spanning tyrosine kinase similar to members of the insulin growth factor receptor family. The NPM protein is a nucleolar phosphoprotein involved in ribosome assembly. The *NPM/ALK* fusion creates a chimeric oncoprotein in which the ALK tyrosine kinase activity may be constitutively activated. The t(5;12)(q33;p13) translocation, characterized in a case of chronic myelomonocytic leukemia (CMML), fuses the *tel* gene (12p13) with the tyrosine kinase domain of the platelet-derived growth factor receptor *b* gene (PDGFR-*b* at 5q33).[164] The *tel* gene is thought to encode a nuclear DNA-binding protein similar to those of the *ets* family of proto-oncogenes.

Gene fusions sometimes lead to the formation of chimeric transcription factors.[76,141] The t(1;19)(q23;p13) translocation, found in childhood pre-B-cell ALL, fuses the *E2A* transcription factor gene (19p13) with the *PBX1* homeodomain gene (1q23).[165] The E2A/PBX1 fusion protein consists of the amino-terminal transactivation domain of the E2A protein and the DNA-binding homeodomain of the PBX1 protein. The t(15;17)(q22;q21) translocation in acute promyelocytic leukemia fuses the *PML* gene (15q22) with the *RARA* gene at 17q21.[166] The PML protein contains a zinc-binding domain called a RING finger that may be involved in protein-protein interactions. *RARA* encodes the retinoic acid alpha-receptor protein, a member of the nuclear steroid/thyroid hormone receptor superfamily. Although retinoic acid binding is retained in the fusion protein, the PML/RARA fusion protein may confer altered DNA-binding specificity to the RARA ligand complex.[167] Leukemia patients with the *PML/RARA* gene fusion respond well to retinoid treatment. In these cases, treatment with all-*trans* retinoic acid induces differentiation of promyelocytic leukemia cells.

The *ALL1* gene, located at chromosome band 11q23, is involved in approximately 5 to 10% of acute leukemia cases overall in children and adults.[168,169] These include cases of ALL, acute myeloid leukemia (AML), and leukemias of mixed cell lineage. Among leukemia genes, *ALL1* (also called *MLL* and *HRX*) is unique because it participates in fusions with a large number of different partner genes on the various chromosomes. Over 20 different reciprocal translocations involving the *ALL1* gene at 11q23 have been reported, the most common of which are those involving chromosomes 4, 6, 9, and 19.[170] In approximately 5% of cases of acute leukemia in adults, the *ALL1* gene is fused with a portion of itself.[171] This special type of gene fusion is called self-fusion.[172] Self-fusion of the *ALL1* gene, which is thought to occur through a somatic recombination mechanism, is found in high incidence in acute leukemias with trisomy 11 as a sole cytogenetic abnormality. The *ALL1* gene encodes a large protein with DNA-binding motifs, a transactivation domain, and a region with homology to the *Drosophila trithorax* protein (a regulator of homeotic gene expression).[173,174] The various partners in *ALL1* fusions encode a diverse group of proteins, some of which appear to be nuclear proteins with DNA-binding motifs.[175,176] The ALL1 fusion protein consists of the aminoterminus of ALL1 and the carboxylterminus of one of a variety of fusion partners. It appears that the critical feature in all ALL1 fusions, including self-fusion, is the uncoupling of the ALL1 amino-terminal domains from the remainder of the ALL1 protein.

Solid tumors, especially sarcomas, sometimes have consistent chromosomal translocations that correlate with specific histologic types of tumors.[177] In general, translocations in solid tumors result in gene fusions that encode chimeric oncoproteins. Studies thus far indicate that in sarcomas, the majority of genes fused by translocations encode transcription factors.[178] In myxoid liposarcomas, the t(12;16)(q13;p11) fuses the *FUS* (*TLS*) gene at 16p11 with the *CHOP* gene at 12q13.[179] The FUS protein contains a transactivation domain that is contributed to the FUS/CHOP fusion protein. The CHOP protein, which is a dominant inhibitor of transcription, contributes a protein-binding domain and a presumptive DNA-binding domain to the fusion. Despite knowledge of these structural features, the mechanism of action of the FUS/CHOP oncoprotein is not yet known. A variant transcript, consisting of exons 1–10 of *EWS* and exons 2–4 of *CHOP*, was recently described.[180] In Ewing's sarcoma, the t(11;22)(q24;q12), fuses the *EWS* gene at 22q12 with the *FLI1* gene at 11q24.[181] Like FUS, the EWS protein contains three glycine-rich segments and an RNA-binding domain. The FLI1 protein contains an *ets*-like DNA-binding domain. The EWS/FLI1 fusion protein combines a transactivation domain from EWS with the DNA-binding domain of FLI1. In alveolar rhabdomyosarcoma, the t(2;13)(q35;q14) fuses the *PAX3* gene at 2q35 with the *FKHR* gene at 13q14.[182] The PAX3 protein, a transcription factor that activates genes involved in development, is a paired-box homeodomain protein with two distinct DNA-binding domains. The FKHR protein encodes a conserved DNA-binding motif (the fork head domain) similar to that first identified in the *Drosophila* fork head homeotic gene. The PAX3/FKHR fusion protein is a chimeric transcription factor containing the PAX3 DNA-binding domains, a truncated fork head domain, and the carboxy-terminal FKHR regions.

In dermatofibrosarcoma protuberans (DP), an infiltrating skin tumor, both a reciprocal translocation t(17;22)(q22;q13) and supernumerary ring chromosomes derived from the t(17;22), have been described.

Although early successful studies in this field have been performed with lymphomas and leukemia, as we have discussed before, the first chromosomal abnormality in solid tumors to be characterized at the molecular level as a fusion protein was an inversion of chromosome 10 found in papillary thyroid carcinomas.[183] In this tumor, two main recurrent structural changes have been described, including inv(10) (q112.2; q21.2), as the more frequent alteration, and a t(10;17)(q11.2; q23). These two abnormalities represent the cytogenetic mechanisms which activate the proto-oncogene *ret* on chromosome 10, forming the oncogenes *ret/ptc1* and RET/*ptc2*, respectively. Moreover, other chromosomal rearrangements leading to *ret* activation were recently described. The *ret/ptc3* and *ret/ptc4* oncogenes are generated by the fusion of the tyrosine kinase domain of *ret* and a gene named *ELE1a-ARA70* (or *RFG*), located in the same region 10q11.2.[184,185] In this case a paracentric inversion of the long arm of chromosome 10 occurs. Translocations of *ret/ptc4* are very frequent events in thyroid cancerogenesis of children of the Chernobyl-contaminated areas. That accident led to the occurrence of new forms of *ret* rearrangements in papillary thyroid cancers, named *ret/ptc5-9*, *ret/PCM1*, and *ELKS/ret*. For instance, ret/ptc5 fusion partner protein is a coiled-coil protein expressed on the Golgi surface. The fusion partner proteins ret/ptc6 and 7 display rearrangements with the transcriptional intermediary factor 1-alpha and gamma, respectively. RET/ptc8 fusion partner protein is kinectin, whereas in *ret/ptc9 ret* rearranges with a putative cytoplasmic protein possibly involved in intracellular-transport processes. *ret/PCM1* lead to a centrosomal protein production, displaying distinct cell-cycle distribution. The *ELKS/ret* oncogene is retrotranscribed into an ubiquitously expressed mRNA with unknown function.[186-191] Alterations of chromosome 1 in the same tumor type have then been associated to the activation of NTRK1 (chromosome 1), an NGF receptor, which, like RET, forms chimeric fusion oncogenic proteins in papillary thyroid carcinomas.[192] A comparative analysis of the oncogenes originated from the activation of these two tyrosine kinase receptors has allowed the identification and characterization of common cytogenetic and molecular mechanisms of their activation. In all cases, chromosomal rearrangements fuse the tK portion of the two receptors to the 5' end of different genes that, because of their general effect, have been designated as "activating genes." In the majority of cases, the latter belong to the same chromosome where the related receptor is located, 10 for *RET* and 1 for NTRK1.

Furthermore, although functionally different, the various activating genes share the following three properties:

1. They are ubiquitously expressed.
2. They display domains demonstrated or predicted to be able to form dimers or multimers.
3. They translocate the tK-receptor-associated enzymatic activity from the membrane to the cytoplasm.

These characteristics can explain the mechanism(s) of oncogenic activation of *ret* and *NTRK1* proto-oncogenes. In fact, following the fusion of their tK domain to the activating gene (1) *ret* and *NTRK1*, whose tissue-specific expression is restricted to subsets of neural cells, become expressed in the epithelial thyroid cells; (2) their dimerization triggers a constitutive, ligand-independent transautophosphorylation of the cytoplasmic domains and, as a consequence, the latter can recruit SH2- and SH3-containing cytoplasmic effector proteins, such as Shc and Grb2 or phospholipase C gamma (PLCγ), thus inducing a constitutive mitogenic pathway; and (3) the relocalization in the cytoplasm of *ret* and *NTRK1* enzymatic activity could allow their interaction with unusual substrates, perhaps modifying their functional properties.

In conclusion, in PTCs, the oncogenic activation of *ret* and *NTRK1* proto-oncogenes following chromosomal rearrangements occurring in breakpoint cluster regions of both proto-oncogenes could be defined as an ectopic, constitutive, and topologically abnormal expression of their associated enzymatic (tK) activity.[193]

Protein overexpression and constitutive phosphorylation Protein overexpression refers to a general deregulation driven by a mechanism not understood or not investigated. An example is Akt, a serine-threonine kinase that represents a major effector-mediating survival signal. Akt possesses 6 sites of phosphorylation: Ser124 and Thr450 are basally phosphorylated, Tyr315 and Tyr316 depend on Src, Thr308 represents the major site of regulation and is phosphorylated by 3-phosphoinositides-dependent protein kinase 1 (PDK1), Ser473 is only required for maximal Akt activity but the mechanism by which it is phosphorylated remains controversial.[194] Akt is phosphorylated and therefore activated after cell stimulation from different growth factors and from a series of interleukins (reviewed by Shi and colleagues[97]), while its action is inhibited by PTEN, which dephosphorylates PIP_3 and PIP_2. Once activated, Akt dissociates from the plasma membrane and translocates to both the cytoplasm and the nucleus.[97,195] Akt inhibits directly, through phosphorylation of Bad and caspase-9, indirectly, by inducing de novo gene expression of IKK protein kinase and transcription factors.[97,194] Akt determines cell survival also by virtue of its involvement in cell-cycle progression.[97,194–196] Akt is overexpressed and/or constitutively phosphorylated in several human tumors such as ovarian, pancreatic, thyroid, colorectal, prostate, and breast,[197–200] and these alterations are related to worse prognosis. Finally, deregulation of Akt expression seems to be involved in Akt drug response and radioresistance in several tumors.[201]

NEW MARKERS FROM LARGE-SCALE GENOMIC ANALYSIS

Kinases A recent analysis organized the protein kinase complement of the human genome (the so-called "kinome") into a dendrogram containing nine broad groups of genes.[202] Using high-throughput sequencing technologies and bioinformatics from the human genome project, one major branch of the histogram, containing three of the nine major groups, was selected for mutational analysis. The selected groups included the 90 tyrosine kinase genes (TK group), the 43 tyrosine kinase-like genes (TKL group), and the 5 receptor guanylate cyclase genes (RGC group). The analysis took into consideration all exons encoding their predicted kinase domains in 35 colorectal cancer cell lines and in 147 colorectal specimens.[203] Thirty-five different types of somatic mutations were identified in 7 genes (*NTRK3*, *FES*, *KDR*, *EPHA3*, *NTRK2* belonging to the TK group, *MLK4* to TKL and *GUCY2F* to RGC) and the data suggest that a minimum of 30% of colorectal cancers contain at least one mutation in the tyrosine kinome, whose members represent an attractive target for chemotherapeutic intervention.[203]

Phosphatases The protein tyrosine phosphatases (PTPs), gene superfamily (the so-called "phosphatome") is composed of three main families: (1) the classic PTPs, including the receptor PTPs (RPTPs) and the nonreceptor PTPs (NRPTPs); (2) the dual specificity phosphatases (DSPs), which can dephosphorylate serine and threonine in addition to tyrosine residues; and (3) the low molecular weight phosphatases (LMPs).[204] Using high-throughput technologies, a mutational analysis of all the coding exons of 53 classic PTPs (21 RPTPs and 32 NRPTPs), 32 DSPs and 1 LMP was performed in 175 colorectal cancers.[9] Six genes containing somatic mutations were identified, including three members of the RPTP subfamily (*PTPRF*, *PTPRG*, and *PTPRT*), and three members of the NRPTP subfamily (*PTPN3*, *PTPN13*, and *PTPN14*). Overall, 77 mutations were identified, in aggregate, affecting 26% of colorectal tumors analyzed. The great majority of the mutations would result in proteins devoid of phosphatase catalytic activity.[9] The identification of protein phosphatases mutated could lead to reactivation of their activity through new targeted pharmacologic treatments or, better, inactivate the corresponding kinases that phosphorylate substrates normally regulated by the mutant phosphatases.

PI3K isoforms Phosphatidylinositol 3-kinases (PI3K) belong to the lipid kinase family that regulate signal transduction.[205] Hidden Markov models identified eight *PI3K* and *PI3K*-like genes, including two uncharacterized genes, in the human genome. By the analysis of the predicted kinase domains of these genes in 234 colorectal cancers, it has been found that *PIK3CA* was the only gene with somatic mutations,[10] which affect 32% of colorectal cancers. A *PIK3CA* mutation was also observed in a very advanced tubulovillous adenoma greater than 5 cm in diameter, suggesting that *PIK3CA* mutations arise late in colorectal tumorigenesis. Hyperactivating *PIK3CA* mutations were also identified in 27% of glioblastoma, 25% of gastric cancers, up to 40% of breast tumors, and 4% of lung cancers. No mutations were observed in pancreatic cancers and medulloblastoma.[10,206]

Finally, the clustering of mutations in the *PIK3CA* gene makes the gene an excellent marker for early detection of cancer or for monitoring tumor progression.

ONCOGENES IN THE INITIATION AND PROGRESSION OF NEOPLASIA

Human neoplasia is a complex multistep process involving sequential alterations in proto-oncogenes (activation) and in tumor suppressor genes (inactivation). Statistical analysis of the age incidence of human solid tumors indicates that five or six independent mutational events may contribute to tumor formation.[207] In human leukemias, only

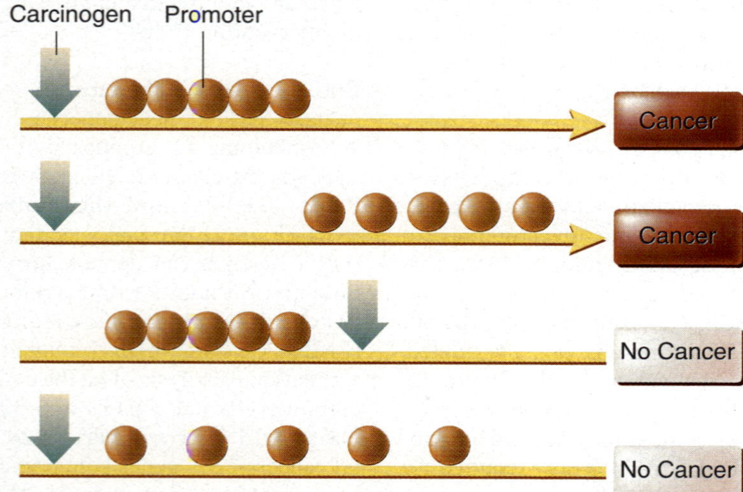

Figure 6-11 Some possible ways of exposure to a mutagen and to a tumor promoter and their effects. Cancer develops exclusively when the exposure to promoter follows the exposure to carcinogen (mutagen, for example 7,12-dimethyl-benzanthracene) and only when the intensity of the exposure to promoter is higher than a threshold.

three or four mutational events may be necessary, presumably involving different genes.

The study of chemical carcinogenesis in animals provides a foundation for our understanding of the multistep nature of cancer.[208] In the mouse model of skin carcinogenesis, tumor formation involves three phases, termed *initiation*, *promotion*, and *progression*. Initiation of skin tumors can be induced by chemical mutagens such as 7,12-dimethyl-benzanthracene (DMBA). (Figure 6-11) After application of DMBA, the mouse skin appears normal. If the skin is then continuously treated with a promoter, such as the phorbol ester TPA, precancerous papillomas will form. Chemical promoters such as TPA stimulate growth but are not mutagenic substances. Over a period of months of continuous application of the promoting agent, some of the papillomas will progress to skin carcinomas. Treatment with DMBA or TPA alone does not cause skin cancer. Mouse papillomas initiated with DMBA usually have H-*ras* oncogenes with a specific mutation in codon 61 of the H-*ras* gene. The mouse skin tumor model indicates that initiation of papillomas is the result of mutation of the H-*ras* gene in individual skin cells by the chemical mutagen DMBA. For papillomas to appear on the skin, however, growth of mutated cells must be continuously stimulated by a promoting agent. Additional unidentified genetic changes must then occur for papillomas to progress to carcinoma.

Although a single oncogene is sufficient to cause tumor formation by some rapidly transforming retroviruses such as RSV, transformation by a single oncogene is not usually seen in experimental models of cancer. Other rapidly transforming retroviruses carry two different oncogenes that cooperate in producing the neoplastic phenotype. One well-characterized example of this type of cooperation is the avian erythroblastosis virus, which carries the *erb A* and *erb B* oncogenes.[209] Cooperation between oncogenes can also be demonstrated by in vitro transformation studies using nonimmortalized cell lines. For example, studies have shown cooperation between the nuclear myc protein and the cytoplasmic-membrane-associated ras protein in the transformation of rat embryo fibroblasts.[210] As previously reported, a cooperation between SV40 large T product and mutated H-*ras* gene also has been found necessary to transform normal human epithelial and fibroblast cells, provided that they constitutively expressed the catalytic subunit of telomerase enzyme, indicating a more complex pattern in the neoplastic conversion of human cells.

Collaboration between two different general categories of oncogenes (eg, nuclear and cytoplasmic) can often be demonstrated but is not strictly required for transformation.[211] These transgenic mice strains, in fact, generally show an increased incidence of neoplasia and the tumors that result frequently are clonal, implying that other events are necessary. The production of transgenic mice expressing a single oncogene such as *myc* has also demonstrated that multiple genetic changes are necessary for tumor formation.[212] (For a review on the mouse model of cancer, see *Oncogene*, Vol. 18, issue 2, N. 38, September 1999.)

Cytogenetic studies of the clonal evolution of human hematologic malignancies have provided much insight into the multiple steps involved in the initiation and progression of human tumors.[213] The evolution of CML from chronic phase to acute leukemia is characterized by an accumulation of genetic changes seen in the karyotypes of the evolving malignant clones. The early chronic phase of CML is defined by the presence of a single Philadelphia chromosome. The formation of the *bcr/abl* gene fusion as a consequence of the t(9;22) translocation is thought to be the initiating event in CML.[157] The biologic progression of CML to a more malignant phenotype corresponds with the appearance of additional cytogenetic abnormalities such as a second Philadelphia chromosome, isochromosome 17, or trisomy 8.[214] These karyotypic changes are thought to reflect additional genetic changes involving an increase in oncogene dosage and loss or inactivation of tumor suppressor genes. Although the karyotypic changes in evolving CML are somewhat variable from patient to patient, the accumulation of genetic changes always correlates with progression from differentiated cells of low malignancy to undifferentiated cells of high malignancy.

The initiation and progression of human neoplasia involve the activation of oncogenes and the inactivation or loss of tumor suppressor genes. The mechanisms of oncogene activation and the time course of events, however, vary among different types of tumors. In hematologic malignancies, soft-tissue sarcomas, and the papillary type of thyroid carcinomas, initiation of the malignant process predominantly involves chromosomal rearrangements that activate various oncogenes.[141] Many of the chromosomal rearrangements in leukemia and lymphoma are thought to result from errors in the physiologic process of immunoglobulin or T-cell receptor gene rearrangement during normal B-cell and T-cell development. Late events in the progression of hematologic malignancies involve oncogene mutation, mainly of the *ras* family, inactivation of tumor suppressor genes such as *TP53*, and sometimes additional chromosomal translocations.[215]

In lung cancers, the initiation of neoplasia has been shown to involve oncogene and tumor suppressor gene mutations. These mutations are generally thought to result from chemical carcinogenesis, especially in the case of tobacco-related lung cancer, where a novel tumor suppressor gene (designated *FHIT*) has been found to be inactivated in the majority of cancers, particularly in those from smokers.[216,217] Later, K-*ras* (especially in the adenocarcinoma subtype) and *TP53* alterations drive the malignant transformation of lung cancer.[218]

As far as colorectal cancer is concerned, intensive screening for genetic alteration led to the identification of two major types of colorectal cancer that are distinct by their carcinogenic process. One is characterized by normal karyotype, normal DNA index,[219] and genetic instability at microsatellite loci (MSI) and was called RER-positive tumor for replicative error-positive phenotype and now is called MSI-positive cancer.[220] The second one is represented by alterations of *APC*, K-*ras* and *TP53* genes and genetic losses at microsatellite loci.[221] The second type led to the association between the stepwise progression from normal to dysplastic epithelium to carcinoma and the accumulation of multiple clonally selected genetic alterations. This model, first proposed by Vogelstein in 1990,[222] suggests that APC (or, better, the APC-β-catenin pathway) represents the initial mutational event that determines hyperplastic proliferation and then early adenoma formation. The stage of late adenoma is achieved with K-ras protein stabilization. Loss of tumor suppressor genes at chromosome 18q (such as *DCC*) and mutations in the *TP53* gene lead to carcinoma in situ formation (Figure 6-12).

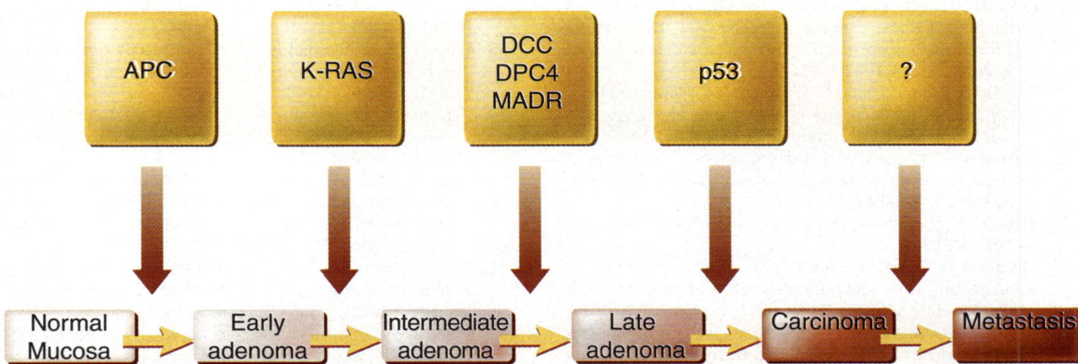

Figure 6-12 Colorectal cancer development. Colorectal cancer results from a series of pathological changes that transform normal colonic epithelium into invasive carcinoma. Specific genetic events, shown by vertical arrows, accompany this multistep process.

However, this stepwise model of colorectal tumorigenesis has been mainly validated conceptually, and there is mounting evidence that alternative genetic events may occur during colorectal carcinogenesis, sometimes preferentially, sometimes randomly, sometimes with an overlap.[220] An extensive analysis of the four molecular markers showed a wide spectrum of combination of mutations with a prevalence of two pathways, which cumulatively encompass about 40% of analyzed cases: the *APC-K-Ras-TP53-DCC* and the *APC-TP53-DCC* pathway. These results strongly support the existence of two preferential pathways followed by sporadic colorectal cancer with microsatellite stability: a K-ras dependent, in agreement with the Vogelstein model, and a K-ras independent one, respectively. Moreover, significant differences between colon and rectal tumors could be outlined: the K-ras dependent pathway is preferentially followed by colon cancer, while the K-Ras independent is predominant in rectal tumors.[223]

In melanoma, *BRAF* mutations occur in the vast majority of cases and represent a very early event, since they were also detected in prenoeplastic lesions such as nevi besides Spitz and Blue nevi.[7,115]

Gene amplification is often seen in the progression of some carcinomas and other types of tumors. Amplification of the *erb B-2* oncogene may be a late event in the progression of breast cancer.[140] Members of the *myc* oncogene family are frequently amplified in small-cell carcinoma of the lung.[125] As mentioned previously, amplification of N-*myc* strongly correlates with the progression and clinical stage of neuroblastoma.[124] Although there is variability in the pathways of human tumor initiation and progression, studies of various types of malignancy have clearly confirmed the multistep nature of human cancer.

SUMMARY AND CONCLUSIONS

The initiation and progression of human neoplasia is a multistep process involving the accumulation of genetic changes in somatic cells. These genetic changes then consist of the activation of cooperating oncogenes and the inactivation of tumor suppressor genes, which both appear necessary for a complete neoplastic phenotype. Oncogenes are altered versions of normal cellular genes called proto-oncogenes. Proto-oncogenes are a diverse group of genes involved in the regulation of cell growth. The functions of proto-oncogenes include growth factors, growth factor receptors, signal transducers, transcription factors, and regulators of programed cell death. Proto-oncogenes may be activated by mutation, chromosomal rearrangement, or gene amplification. Chromosomal rearrangements that include translocations and inversions can activate proto-oncogenes by deregulation of their transcription (eg, transcriptional activation) or by gene fusion. Tumor suppressor genes, which also participate in the regulation of normal cell growth, are usually inactivated by point mutations or truncation of their protein sequence coupled with the loss of the normal allele.

The discovery of oncogenes represented a breakthrough for our understanding of the molecular and genetic basis of cancer. Oncogenes have also provided important knowledge concerning the regulation of normal cell proliferation, differentiation, and programed cell death. The identification of oncogene abnormalities has provided tools for the molecular diagnosis and monitoring of cancer. Most important, oncogenes represent potential targets for new types of cancer therapies. It is more than a hope that a new generation of chemotherapeutic agents directed at specific oncogene targets will be developed. The goal of these new drugs will be to kill cancer cells selectively while sparing normal cells. One promising approach entails using specific oncogene targets to trigger programed cell death. One example of the accomplishment of such a goal is represented by the inhibition of the tumor-specific tyrosine kinase bcr/abl in CML, by imatinib[224] (Figure 6-13). The same compound has been proven active also in a different tumor type, GIST (gastrointestinal stromal tumor) where it inhibits the tyrosine kinase receptor c-kit[225] and in chordomas, where it switches off the PDGFR.[226] Another example is represented by gefitinib and C-225, which inhibit the intracellular tyrosine kinase and the extracellular domain, respectively, of *erb B*. The use of high-throughput technologies for the identification of new oncogenes and the rapidly expanding knowledge of the molecular mechanisms of cancer hold great promise for the development of better combined methods of cancer therapy in the near future.

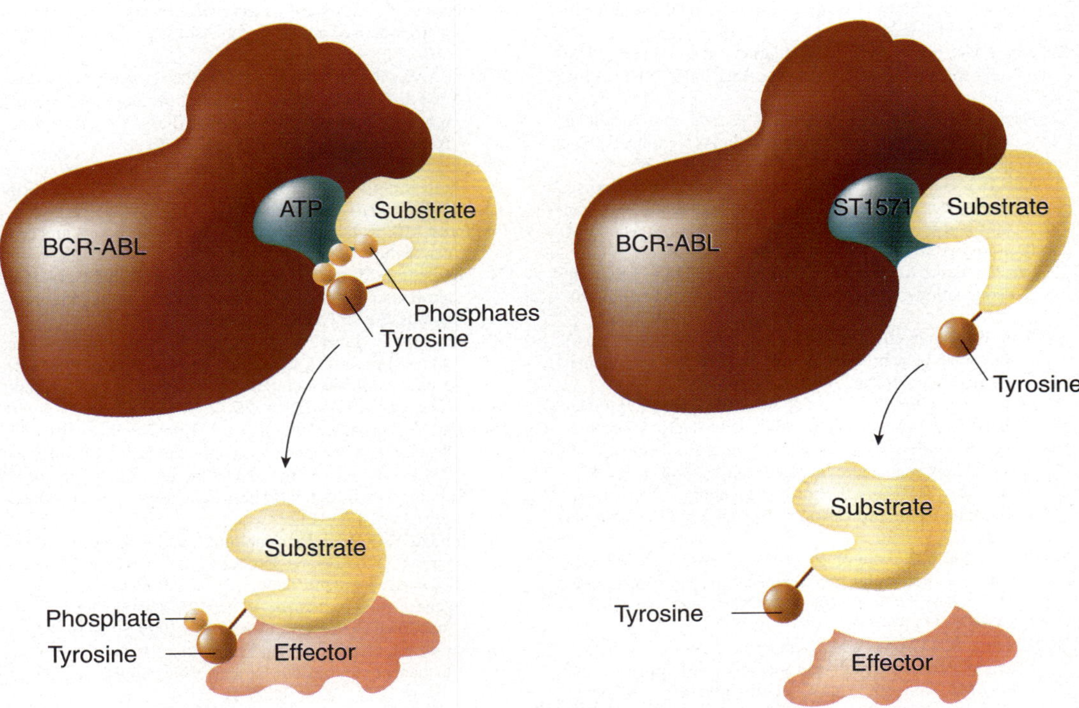

Figure 6-13 Mode of action of imatinib. In the left panel the effect of ATP binding on the oncoprotein BCR-ABL is depicted. The fusion protein binds the molecule of ATP in the kinase pocket. Afterward, it can phosphorylate a substrate, that can interact with the downstream effector molecules. When imatinib is present (*right panel*), the oncoprotein binds imatinib in the kinase pocket (competing with ATP) and then the substrate cannot be phosphorylated.

REFERENCES

1. Yokota J. Tumor progression and metastasis. Carcinogenesis 2000;21(3):497–503.
2. Bernards R, Weinberg RA. A progression puzzle. Nature 2002;418(6900):823.
3. Bishop JM. Retroviruses and oncogenes II. In: Almqvist and Wiksell, editor. Les Prix Nobel. Stockholm; 1989. p. 220–38.
4. Varmus HE. Retroviruses and oncogenes I. In: Almqvist and Wiksell, editor. Les Prix Nobel. Stockholm; 1989. p. 194–212.
5. Butel JS. Viral carcinogenesis: revelation of molecular mechanisms and etiology of human disease. Carcinogenesis 2000;21(3):405–26.
6. Todd R, Wong DT. Oncogenes. Anticancer Res 1999;19(6A):4729–46.
7. Davies H, Bignell GR, Cox C, et al. Mutations of the BRAF gene in human cancer. Nature 2002;417(6892):949–54.
8. Bardelli A, Parsons DW, Silliman N, et al. Mutational analysis of the tyrosine kinome in colorectal cancers. Science 2003;300(5621):949.
9. Wang Z, Shen D, Parsons DW, et al. Mutational analysis of the tyrosine phosphatome in colorectal cancers. Science 2004;304(5674):1164–6.
10. Samuels Y, Wang Z, Bardelli A, et al. High frequency of mutations of the PIK3CA gene in human cancers. Science 2004;304(5670):554.
11. Vogelstein B, Kinzler KW. Cancer genes and the pathways they control. Nat Med 2004;10(8):789–99.
12. Boland CR. Hereditary nonpolyposis colorectal cancer. In: Vogelstein B, Kinzler KW, editors. The genetic basis of human cancer. Mc-Graw-Hill;, 1998.
13. Varmus H. Retroviruses. Science 1988;240(4858):1427–35.
14. Mahalingam S, Meanger J, Foster PS, Lidbury BA. The viral manipulation of the host cellular and immune environments to enhance propagation and survival: a focus on RNA viruses. J Leukoc Biol 2002;72(3):429–39.
15. Varmus HE. Form and function of retroviral proviruses. Science 1982;216(4548):812–20.
16. Rous P. A transmissible avian neoplasm. (Sarcoma of the common fowl) by Peyton Rous, M.D. Experimental Medicine for Sept. 1, 1910, vol. 12, p. 696–705. J Exp Med 1979;150(4):738–53.
17. Duesberg PH, Vogt PK. Differences between the ribonucleic acids of transforming and nontransforming avian tumor viruses. Proc Natl Acad Sci U S A 1970;67(4):1673–80.
18. Martin GS. Rous sarcoma virus: a function required for the maintenance of the transformed state. Nature 1970;227(262):1021–3.
19. Baker SJ, Fearon ER, Nigro JM, et al. Chromosome 17 deletions and p53 gene mutations in colorectal carcinomas. Science 1989;244:217–21.
20. Frame MC. Src in cancer: deregulation and consequences for cell behaviour. Biochim Biophys Acta 2002;1602(2):114–30.
21. Hayward WS, Neel BG, Astrin SM. Activation of a cellular onc gene by promoter insertion in ALV-induced lymphoid leukosis. Nature 1981;290(5806):475–80.
22. Neel BG, Hayward WS, Robinson HL, et al. Avian leukosis virus-induced tumors have common proviral integration sites and synthesize discrete new RNAs: oncogenesis by promoter insertion. Cell 1981;23(2):323–34.
23. Sanchez-Beato M, Sanchez-Aguilera A, Piris MA. Cell cycle deregulation in B-cell lymphomas. Blood 2002;101:1220-35.
24. Jiang W, Kanter MR, Dunkel I, et al. Minimal truncation of the c-myb gene product in rapid-onset B-cell lymphoma. J Virol 1997;71(9):6526–33.
25. Zhou H, Chen WD, Qin X, et al. MMTV promoter hypomethylation is linked to spontaneous and MNU associated c-neu expression and mammary carcinogenesis in MMTV c-neu transgenic mice. Oncogene 2001;20(42):6009–17.
26. Buckley AR, Buckley DJ. Prolactin regulation of apoptosis-associated gene expression in T cells. Ann N Y Acad Sci 2000;917:522–33.
27. Shih C, Shilo BZ, Goldfarb MP, et al. Passage of phenotypes of chemically transformed cells via transfection of DNA and chromatin. Proc Natl Acad Sci U S A 1979;76(11):5714–8.
28. Krontiris TG, Cooper GM. Transforming activity of human tumor DNAs. Proc Natl Acad Sci U S A 1981;78(2):1181–4.
29. Murray MJ, Shilo BZ, Shih C, et al. Three different human tumor cell lines contain different oncogenes. Cell 1981;25(2):355–61.
30. Perucho M, Goldfarb M, Shimizu K, et al. Human-tumor-derived cell lines contain common and different transforming genes. Cell 1981;27(3 Pt 2):467–76.
31. Pulciani S, Santos E, Lauver AV, et al. Oncogenes in human tumor cell lines: molecular cloning of a transforming gene from human bladder carcinoma cells. Proc Natl Acad Sci U S A 1982;79(9):2845–9.
32. Parada LF, Tabin CJ, Shih C, Weinberg RA. Human EJ bladder carcinoma oncogene is homologue of Harvey sarcoma virus ras gene. Nature 1982;297(5866):474–8.
33. Hahn WC, Counter CM, Lundberg AS, et al. Creation of human tumour cells with defined genetic elements. Nature 1999;400(6743):464–8.
34. Manser E. Small GTPases take the stage. Dev Cell 2002;3(3):323–8.
35. Macaluso M, Russo G, Cinti C, et al. Ras family genes: an interesting link between cell cycle and cancer. J Cell Physiol 2002;192(2):125–30.
36. Indo Y. Molecular basis of congenital insensitivity to pain with anhidrosis (CIPA): mutations and polymorphisms in *TRKA* (*NTRK*) gene encoding the receptor tyrosine kinase for nerve growth factor. Hum Mutat 2001;18:462–71.
37. Lohrisch C, Piccart M. An overview of HER2. Semin Oncol 2001;28(6 Suppl 18):3–11.
38. Takahashi M, Ritz J, Cooper GM. Activation of a novel human transforming gene, ret, by DNA rearrangement. Cell 1985;42:581–8.
39. Fusco A, Grieco M, Santoro M, et al. A new oncogene in human papillary thyroid carcinomas and their lymph-nodal metastases. Nature 1987;328:170–2.
40. Grieco M, Santoro M, Berlingieri MT, et al. PTC is a novel rearranged form of the ret proto-oncogene and is frequently detected in vivo in human thyroid papillary carcinomas. Cell 1990;60:557–63.
41. Falini B, Mason DY. Proteins encoded by genes involved in chromosomal alterations in lymphoma and leukemia: clinical value of their detection by immunocytochemistry. Blood 2002;99(2):409–26.
42. Tomescu O, Barr FG. Chromosomal translocations in sarcomas: prospects for therapy. Trends Mol Med 2001;7(12):554–9.
43. Nowell PC, Croce CM. Chromosomal approaches to the molecular basis of neoplasia. Symp Fundam Cancer Res 1986;39:17–29.
44. Nowell PC. Progress with chronic myelogenous leukemia: a personal perspective over four decades. Annu Rev Med 2002;53:1–13.
45. Hanahan D, Weinberg RA. The hallmarks of cancer. Cell 2000;100:57–70.
46. Pupa SM, Menard S, Forti S, Tagliabue E. New insights into the role of extracellular matrix during tumor onset and progression. J Cell Physiol 2002;192(3):259–67.
47. Betsholtz C, Karlsson L, Lindahl P. Developmental roles of platelet-derived growth factors. Bioessays 2001;23(6):494–507.
48. Liu J, Xu R, Jin Y, Wang D. Triplex targeting of human PDGF-B (c-sis, proto-oncogene) promoter specifically inhibits factors binding and PDGF-B transcription. Nucleic Acids Res 2001;29(3):783–91.
49. Heldin CH, Westermark B. Mechanism of action and in vivo role of platelet-derived growth factor. Physiol Rev 1999;79(4):1283–316.
50. Sporn MB, Roberts AB. Autocrine growth factors and cancer. Nature 1985;313(6005):745–7.
51. Minoletti F, Miozzo M, Pedeutour F, et al. Involvement of chromosomes 17 and 22 in dermatofibrosarcoma protuberans. Genes Chrom Cancer 1995;13:62–5.
52. Pedeutour F, Simon MP, Minoletti F, et al. Translocation, t(17;22)(q22;q13), in dermatofibrosarcoma protuberans: a new tumor-associated chromosome rearrangement. Cytogenet Cell Genet 1996;72:171–4.
53. Greco A, Fusetti L, Villa R, et al. Transforming activity of the chimeric sequence formed by the fusion of collagene gene COL1A1 and the platelet derived growth factor B-chain gene in dermatofibrosarcoma protuberans. Oncogene 1998;17:1313–9.
54. Shimizu A, O'Brien KP, Sjoblom T, et al. The dermatofibrosarcoma protuberans-associated collagen type Iα1/platelet-derived growth factor (PDGF) B-chain fusion gene generates a transforming protein that is processed to functional PDGF-BB. Cancer Res 1999;59:3719–23.
55. Grimm SL, Nordeen SK. Mouse mammary tumor virus sequences responsible for activating cellular oncogenes. J Virol 1998;72(12):9428–35.
56. Zwick E, Bange J, Ullrich A. Receptor tyrosine kinase signalling as a target for cancer intervention strategies. Endocr Relat Cancer 2001;8(3):161–73.
57. Miranda C, Zanotti G, Pagliardini S, et al. Gain of function mutations of RTK conserved residues display differential effects on NTRK1 kinase activity. Oncogene 2002;21(54):8334–9.
58. Arteaga CL. Epidermal growth factor receptor dependence in human tumors: more than just expression? Oncologist 2002;7 Suppl 4:31–9.
59. Stephens P, Hunter C, Bignell G, et al. Lung cancer: intragenic ERBB2 kinase mutations in tumours. Nature 2004;431(7008):525–6.
60. Lynch TJ, Bell DW, Sordella R, et al. Activating mutations in the epidermal growth factor receptor underlying responsiveness of non-small-cell lung cancer to gefitinib. N Engl J Med 2004;350(21):2129–39.
61. Paez JG, Janne PA, Lee JC, et al. EGFR mutations in lung cancer: correlation with clinical response to gefitinib therapy. Science 2004;304(5676):1497–500.
62. Joensuu H, Dimitrijevic S. Tyrosine kinase inhibitor imatinib (STI571) as an anticancer agent for solid tumours. Ann Med 2001;33(7):451–5.
63. Tamborini E, Bonadinam L, Greco A, et al. A new mutation in the KIT ATP pocket causes acquired resistance to imatinib gastrointestinal stromal tumor patient. Gastroenterology 2004;127:294–9.
64. Pollock PM, Meltzer PS. Lucky draw in the gene raffle. Nature 2002;417(6892):906–7.
65. Vallar L. Oncogenic role of heterotrimeric G proteins. Cancer Surv 1996;27:325–38.
66. Cantley LC, Auger KR, Carpenter C, et al. Oncogenes and signal transduction. Cell 1991;64:281–302.
67. Bourne HR, De Franco AL. Signal transduction and intracellular messengers. In: Weinberg RA, editor. Oncogenes and the molecular origins of cancer. Cold Spring Harbor (NY): Cold Spring Harbor Laboratory Press; 1989. p. 97–124.
68. Kaziro Y, Itoh H, Kozasa T, et al. Structure and function of signal-transducing GTP-binding proteins. Annu Rev Biochem 1991;60:349–400.
69. Salgia R, Skarin AT. Molecular abnormalities in lung cancer. J Clin Oncol 1998;16(3):1207–17.
70. Rodrigues GA, Park M. Oncogenic activation of tyrosine kinases. Current Opinion Genet Develop 1994;4:15–24.
71. Mitchell PJ, Tjian R. Transcriptional regulation in mammalian cells by sequence-specific DNA binding proteins. Science 1989;245(4916):371–8.
72. Darnell JE Jr. Transcription factors as targets for cancer therapy. Nat Rev Cancer 2002;2(10):740–9.
73. Shaulian E, Karin M. AP-1 in cell proliferation and survival. Oncogene 2001;20(19):2390–400.
74. Shaulian E, Karin M. AP-1 as a regulator of cell life and death. Nat Cell Biol 2002;4(5):E131–6.
75. Thormeyer D, Baniahmad A. The v-erbA oncogene (review). Int J Mol Med 1999;4(4):351–8.
76. Cleary ML. Oncogenic conversion of transcription factors by chromosomal translocations. Cell 1991;66(4):619–22.
77. Sanchez-Prieto R, de Alava E, Palomino T, et al. An association between viral genes and human oncogenic alterations: the adenovirus E1A induces the Ewing tumor fusion transcript EWS-FLI1. Nat Med 1999;5(9):1076–9.
78. Boxer LM, Dang CV. Translocations involving c-myc and c-myc function. Oncogene 2001;20(40):5595–610.
79. Konopleva M, Zhao S, Xie Z, et al. Apoptosis. Molecules and mechanisms. Adv Exp Med Biol 1999;457:217–36.
80. Tsujimoto Y, Finger LR, Yunis J, et al. Cloning of the chromosomal breakpoint of neoplastic B-cells with the t(14;18) chromosome translocation. Science 1984;226:1097–9.
81. Cleary ML, Smith SD, Sklar J. Cloning and structural analysis of cDNAs for bcl-2 and a hybrid bcl-2/immunoglobulin transcript resulting from the t(14;18) translocation. Cell 1986;47:19–28.
82. Baliga BC, Kumar S. Role of Bcl-2 family of proteins in malignancy. Hematol Oncol 2002;20(2):63–74.
83. Huang Z. The chemical biology of apoptosis. Exploring protein-protein interactions and the life and death of cells with small molecules. Chem Biol 2002;9(10):1059–72.
84. Willis S, Day CL, Hinds MG, Huang DC. The Bcl-2-regulated apoptotic pathway. J Cell Sci 2003;116(Pt;):4053–6.
85. Matolcsy A, Casali P, Warnke RA, Knowles DM. Morphologic transformation of follicular lymphoma is associated with somatic mutation of the translocated Bcl-2 gene. Blood 1996;88(10):3937–44.
86. Monni O, Joensuu H, Franssila K, et al. BCL2 overexpression associated with chromosomal amplification in diffuse large B-cell lymphoma. Blood 1997;90(3):1168–74.
87. Pilotti S, Collini P, Rilke F, et al. bcl-2 Protein expression in carcinomas originating from the follicular epithelium of the thyroid gland. J Pathol 1994;172:337–42.

88. Pollina L, Pacini F, Fontanini G, et al. bcl-2, p53 and proliferating cell nuclear antigen expression is related to the degree of differentiation in thyroid carcinomas. Br J Cancer 1996;73(2):139–43.
89. Viale G, Roncalli M, Grimelius L, et al. Prognostic value of bcl-2 immunoreactivity in medullary thyroid carcinoma. Hum Pathol 1995;26(9):945–50.
90. Hwang JH, Lim SC, Kim YC, et al. Apoptosis and bcl-2 expression as predictors of survival in radiation-treated non-small-cell lung cancer. Int J Radiat Oncol Biol Phys 2001;50(1):13–8.
91. Hong JH, Lee E, Hong J, et al. Antisense Bcl2 oligonucleotide in cisplatin-resistant bladder cancer cell lines. BJU Int 2002;90(1):113–7.
92. Shi XB, Gumerlock PH, Muenzer JT, deVere White RW. BCL2 antisense transcripts decrease intracellular Bcl2 expression and sensitize LNCaP prostate cancer cells to apoptosis-inducing agents. Cancer Biother Radiopharm 2001;16(5):421–9.
93. Klasa RJ, Bally MB, Ng R, et al. Eradication of human non-Hodgkin's lymphoma in SCID mice by BCL-2 antisense oligonucleotides combined with low-dose cyclophosphamide. Clin Cancer Res 2000;6(6):2492–500.
94. Bollag G, Freeman S, Lyons JF, Post LE. Raf pathway inhibitors in oncology. Curr Opin Investig Drugs 2003;4(12):1436–41.
95. Dlamini Z, Mbita Z, Zungu M. Genealogy, expression, and molecular mechanisms in apoptosis. Pharmacol Ther 2004;101(1):1–15.
96. Cardone MH, Roy N, Stennicke HR, et al. Regulation of cell death protease caspase-9 by phosphorylation. Science 1998;282(5392):1318–21.
97. Datta SR, Brunet A, Greenberg ME. Cellular survival: a play in three Akts. Genes Dev 1999;13:2905–27.
98. Cory S, Huang DC, Adams JM. The Bcl-2 family: roles in cell survival and oncogenesis. Oncogene 2003;22(53):8590–607.
99. Bishop JM. Molecular themes in oncogenesis. Cell 1991;64:235–48.
100. Rodenhuis S. ras and human tumors. Semin Cancer Biol 1992;3(4):241–7.
101. Oudejans JJ, Slebos RJ, Zoetmulder FA, et al. Differential activation of ras genes by point mutation in human colon cancer with metastases to either lung or liver. Int J Cancer 1991;49(6):875–9.
102. Minamoto T, Mai M, Ronai Z. K-ras mutation: early detection in molecular diagnosis and risk assessment of colorectal, pancreas, and lung cancers—a review. Cancer Detect Prev 2000;24(1):1–12.
103. Beaupre DM, Kurzrock R. RAS and leukemia: from basic mechanisms to gene-directed therapy. J Clin Oncol 1999;17(3):1071–9.
104. Padua RA, West RR. Oncogene mutation and prognosis in the myelodysplastic syndromes. Br J Haematol 2000;111(3):873–4.
105. Wynford-Thomas D. Origin and progression of thyroid epithelial tumours: cellular and molecular mechanisms. Horm Res 1997;47(4–6):145–57.
106. Motoi N, Sakamoto A, Yamochi T, et al. Role of ras mutation in the progression of thyroid carcinoma of follicular epithelial origin. Pathol Res Pract 2000;196(1):1–7.
107. Tomlinson I, Ilyas M, Johnson V, et al. A comparison of the genetic pathways involved in the pathogenesis of three types of colorectal cancer. J Pathol 1998;184(2):148–52.
108. Lev Z, Kislitsin D, Rennert G, Lerner A. Utilization of K-ras mutations identified in stool DNA for the early detection of colorectal cancer. J Cell Biochem Suppl 2000;34:35–9.
109. Imperiale TF, Ransohoff DF, Itzkowitz SH, et al. Fecal DNA versus fecal occult blood for colorectal-cancer screening in an average-risk population. N Engl J Med 2004;351(26):2704–14.
110. Cerottini JP, Caplin S, Saraga E, et al. The type of K-ras mutation determines prognosis in colorectal cancer. Am J Surg 1998;175(3):198–202.
111. Esteller M, Gonzalez S, Risques RA, et al. K-ras and p16 aberrations confer poor prognosis in human colorectal cancer. J Clin Oncol 2001;19(2):299–304.
112. Font A, Abad A, Monzo M, et al. Prognostic value of K-ras mutations and allelic imbalance on chromosome 18q in patients with resected colorectal cancer. Dis Colon Rectum 2001;44(4):549–57.
113. Frattini M, Ferrario C, Bressan P, et al. Alternative mutations of *BRAF*, *RET* and *NTRK1* are associated with similar but distinct gene expression patterns in papillary thyroid cancer. Oncogene 2004;23:7436–40.
114. Rajagopalan H, Bardelli A, Lengauer C, et al. Tumorigenesis: RAF/RAS oncogenes and mismatch-repair status. Nature 2002;418(6901):934.
115. Rodolfo M, Daniotti M, Vallacchi V. Genetic progression of metastatic melanoma. Cancer Lett 2004;214(2):133–47.
116. Pasini B, Ceccherini I, Romeo G. *RET* mutations in human disease. TIG 1996;12:138–44.
117. Ponder BAJ, Pierotti MA. Mutations in RET in MEN2. In: Nelkin BD, editor. Genetic mechanisms in multiple endocrine neoplasia type 2. Landes Company; 1996.
118. Alt FW, Kellems RE, Bertino JR, Schimke RT. Selective multiplication of dihydrofolate reductase genes in methotrexate-resistant variants of cultured murine cells. J Biol Chem 1978;253(5):1357–70.
119. Cowell JK. Double minutes and homogeneously staining regions: gene amplification in mammalian cells. Annu Rev Genet 1982;16:21–59.
120. Keung YK, Cobos E, Morgan D, et al. Double minute chromosomes and myelodysplastic syndrome: a case report and literature review. Cancer Genet Cytogenet 1997;97(2):94–6.
121. Brison O. Gene amplification and tumor progression. Biochim Biophys Acta 1993;1155(1):25–41.
122. Schwab M, Alitalo K, Klempnauer KH, et al. Amplified DNA with limited homology to myc cellular oncogene is shared by human neuroblastoma cell lines and a neuroblastoma tumour. Nature 1983;305(5931):245–8.
123. Brodeur GM, Hogarty MD. Gene amplification in human cancer: biological and clinical significance. In: Vogelstein B, Kinzler K, editors. The genetic basis of human cancer. McGraw-Hill; 1998: p. 161–72.
124. Kruidering M. N-MYC overexpression and neuroblastomas. Trends Pharmacol Sci 2002;23(10):452.
125. Zajac-Kaye M. Myc oncogene: a key component in cell cycle regulation and its implication for lung cancer. Lung Cancer 2001;34 Suppl 2:S43–6.
126. You Z, Saims D, Chen S, et al. Wnt signaling promotes oncogenic transformation by inhibiting c-Myc-induced apoptosis. J Cell Biol 2002;157(3):429–40.
127. Shen J, Scotlandi K, Baldini N, et al. Prognostic significance of nuclear accumulation of c-myc and mdm2 proteins in synovial sarcoma of the extremities. Oncology 2000;58(3):253–60.
128. Naidu R, Wahab NA, Yadav M, Kutty MK. Protein expression and molecular analysis of c-myc gene in primary breast carcinomas using immunohistochemistry and differential polymerase chain reaction. Int J Mol Med 2002;9(2):189–96.
129. Persons DL, Borelli KA, Hsu PH. Quantitation of HER-2/neu and c-myc gene amplification in breast carcinoma using fluorescence in situ hybridization. Mod Pathol 1997;10(7):720–7.
130. Chana JS, Grover R, Wilson GD, et al. The prognostic importance of c-myc oncogene expression in head and neck melanoma. Ann Plast Surg 2001;47(2):172–7.
131. Aldosari N, Bigner SH, Burger PC, et al. MYCC and MYCN oncogene amplification in medulloblastoma. A fluorescence in situ hybridization study on paraffin sections from the Children's Oncology Group. Arch Pathol Lab Med 2002;126(5):540–4.
132. Herms J, Neidt I, Luscher B, et al. C-MYC expression in medulloblastoma and its prognostic value. Int J Cancer 2000;89(5):395–402.
133. McKay JA, Murray LJ, Curran S, et al. Evaluation of the epidermal growth factor receptor (EGFR) in colorectal tumours and lymph node metastases. Eur J Cancer 2002;38(17):2258–64.
134. Press MF, Bernstein L, Thomas PA, et al. HER-2/neu gene amplification characterized by fluorescence in situ hybridization: poor prognosis in node-negative breast carcinomas. J Clin Oncol 1997;15(8):2894–904.
135. Hirsch FR, Varella-Garcia M, Franklin WA, et al. Evaluation of HER-2/neu gene amplification and protein expression in non-small cell lung carcinomas. Br J Cancer 2002;86(9):1449–56.
136. Goebel SU, Iwamoto M, Raffeld M, et al. Her-2/neu expression and gene amplification in gastrinomas: correlations with tumor biology, growth, and aggressiveness. Cancer Res 2002;62(13):3702–10.
137. Eliopoulos P, Mohammed MQ, Henry K, Retsas S. Overexpression of HER-2 in thick melanoma. Melanoma Res 2002;12(2):139–45.
138. Koka V, Potti A, Koch M, et al. Role of immunohistochemical identification of Her-2/neu and detection of variability in overexpression in pancreatic carcinoma. Anticancer Res 2002;22(3):1593–7.
139. Jorda M, Morales A, Ghorab Z, et al. Her2 expression in prostatic cancer: a comparison with mammary carcinoma. J Urol 2002;168(4 Pt 1):1412–4.
140. Eccles SA. The role of c-erbB-2/HER2/neu in breast cancer progression and metastasis. J Mammary Gland Biol Neoplasia 2001;6(4):393–406.
141. Mitelman F. Recurrent chromosome aberrations in cancer. Mutat Res 2000;462(2–3):247–53.
142. Heerema NA. Chromosomes in lymphomas and solid tumors. Cancer Invest 1998;16(3):183–7.
143. Flajnik MF. Comparative analyses of immunoglobulin genes: surprises and portents. Nat Rev Immunol 2002;2(9):688–98.
144. Siebert R, Matthiesen P, Harder S, et al. Application of interphase fluorescence in situ hybridization for the detection of the Burkitt translocation t(8;14)(q24;q32) in B-cell lymphomas. Blood 1998;91(3):984–90.
145. Mann G, Trebo MM, Haas OA, et al. Philadelphia chromosome-positive mature B-cell (Burkitt cell) leukaemia. Br J Haematol 2002;118(2):559–62.
146. Martin-Subero JI, Harder L, Gesk S, et al. Interphase FISH assays for the detection of translocations with breakpoints in immunoglobulin light chain loci. Int J Cancer 2002;98(3):470–4.
147. Yamamoto K, Hamaguchi H, Nagata K, Taniwaki M. A variant Burkitt-type translocation (8;22)(q24;q11) in multiple myeloma. Report of a new case and review of the literature. Cancer Genet Cytogenet 1998;104(2):98–103.
148. Johnston JM, Carroll WL. c-myc hypermutation in Burkitt's lymphoma. Leuk Lymphoma 1992;8(6):431–9.
149. Glassman AB, Hopwood V, Hayes KJ. Cytogenetics as an aid in the diagnosis of lymphomas. Ann Clin Lab Sci 2000;30(1):72–4.
150. Hatano M, Roberts CW, Minden M, et al. Deregulation of a homeobox gene, HOX11, by the t(10;14) in T cell leukemia. Science 1991;253(5015):79–82.
151. Baer R. TAL1, TAL2 and LYL1: a family of basic helix-loop-helix proteins implicated in T cell acute leukaemia. Semin Cancer Biol 1993;4(6):341–7.
152. Sanchez-Garcia I, Rabbitts TH. LIM domain proteins in leukaemia and development. Semin Cancer Biol 1993;4(6):349–58.
153. Elnenaei MO, Jadayel DM, Matutes E, et al. Cyclin D1 by flow cytometry as a useful tool in the diagnosis of B-cell malignancies. Leuk Res 2001;25(2):115–23.
154. Drexler HG, MacLeod RA. Malignant hematopoietic cell lines: in vitro models for the study of mantle cell lymphoma. Leuk Res 2002;26(9):781–7.
155. Pekarsky Y, Hallas C, Croce CM. Molecular basis of mature T-cell leukemia. JAMA 2001;286(18):2308–14.
156. Groffen J, Stephenson JR, Heisterkamp N, et al. Philadelphia chromosomal breakpoints are clustered within a limited region, bcr, on chromosome 22. Cell 1984;36:93–4.
157. Shtivelman E, Lifshitz B, Gale RP, Canaani E. Fused transcript of abl and bcr genes in chronic myelogenous leukaemia. Nature 1985;315(6020):550–4.
158. Druker BJ. Current treatment approaches for chronic myelogenous leukemia. Cancer J 2001;7 Suppl 1:S14–8.
159. Ottmann OG, Druker BJ, Sawyers CL, et al. A phase 2 study of imatinib in patients with relapsed or refractory Philadelphia chromosome-positive acute lymphoid leukemias. Blood 2002;100(6):1965–71.
160. Druker BJ, Talpaz M, Resta DJ, et al. Efficacy and safety of a specific inhibitor of the BCR-ABL tyrosine kinase in chronic myeloid leukemia. N Engl J Med 2001;344(14):1031–7.
161. Druker BJ, Sawyers CL, Kantarjian H, et al. Activity of a specific inhibitor of the BCR-ABL tyrosine kinase in the blast crisis of chronic myeloid leukemia and acute lymphoblastic leukemia with the Philadelphia chromosome. N Engl J Med 2001;344(14):1038–42.
162. Roche-Lestienne C, Soenen-Cornu V, Grardel-Duflos N, et al. Several types of mutations of the Abl gene can be found in chronic myeloid leukemia patients resistant to STI571, and they can pre-exist to the onset of treatment. Blood 2002;100(3):1014–8.
163. Duyster J, Bai RY, Morris SW. Translocations involving anaplastic lymphoma kinase (ALK). Oncogene 2001;20(40):5623–37.
164. Dierov J, Xu Q, Dierova R, Carroll M. TEL/platelet-derived growth factor receptor beta activates phosphatidylinositol 3 (PI3) kinase and requires PI3 kinase to regulate the cell cycle. Blood 2002;99(5):1758–65.
165. Uckun FM, Sensel MG, Sather HN, et al. Clinical significance of translocation t(1;19) in childhood acute lymphoblastic leukemia in the context of contemporary therapies: a report from the Children's Cancer Group. J Clin Oncol 1998;16(2):527–35.
166. Salomoni P, Pandolfi PP. The role of PML in tumor suppression. Cell 2002;108(2):165–70.

167. Wang ZG, Delva L, Gaboli M, et al. Role of PML in cell growth and the retinoic acid pathway. Science 1998;279(5356):1547–51.
168. Whitman SP, Strout MP, Marcucci G, et al. The partial nontandem duplication of the MLL (ALL1) gene is a novel rearrangement that generates three distinct fusion transcripts in B-cell acute lymphoblastic leukemia. Cancer Res 2001;61(1):59–63.
169. Armstrong SA, Staunton JE, Silverman LB, et al. MLL translocations specify a distinct gene expression profile that distinguishes a unique leukemia. Nat Genet 2002;30(1):41–7.
170. Thirman MJ, Gill HJ, Burnett RC, et al. Rearrangement of the MLL gene in acute lymphoblastic and acute myeloid leukemias with 11q23 chromosomal translocations. N Engl J Med 1993;329(13):909–14.
171. Schichman SA, Caligiuri MA, Gu Y, et al. ALL-1 partial duplication in acute leukemia. Proc Natl Acad Sci U S A 1994;91:6236–9.
172. Schichman SA, Canaani E, Croce CM. Self-fusion of the ALL1 gene. A new genetic mechanism for acute leukemia. JAMA 1995;273(7):571–6.
173. Breen TR. Mutant alleles of the Drosophila trithorax gene produce common and unusual homeotic and other developmental phenotypes. Genetics 1999;152(1):319–344.
174. Cimino G, Rapanotti MC, Sprovieri T, Elia L. ALL1 gene alterations in acute leukemia: biological and clinical aspects. Haematologica 1998;83(4):350–7.
175. Cimino G, Elia L, Rapanotti MC, et al. A prospective study of residual-disease monitoring of the ALL1/AF4 transcript in patients with t(4;11) acute lymphoblastic leukemia. Blood 2000;95(1):96–101.
176. Prasad R, Leshkowitz D, Gu Y, et al. Leucine-zipper dimerization motif encoded by the AF17 gene fused to ALL-1 (MLL) in acute leukemia. Proc Natl Acad Sci U S A 1994;91(17):8107–11.
177. Skapek SX, Chui CH. Cytogenetics and the biologic basis of sarcomas. Curr Opin Oncol 2000;12(4):315–22.
178. Barr FG. Gene fusions involving PAX and FOX family members in alveolar rhabdomyosarcoma. Oncogene 2001;20(40):5736–46.
179. Panagopoulos I, Mertens F, Isaksson M, Mandahl N. A novel FUS/CHOP chimera in myxoid liposarcoma. Biochem Biophys Res Commun 2000;279(3):838–45.
180. Hosaka T, Nakashima Y, Kusuzaki K, et al. A novel type of EWS-CHOP fusion gene in two cases of myxoid liposarcoma. J Mol Diagn 2002;4(3):164–71.
181. Arvand A, Welford SM, Teitell MA, Denny CT. The COOH-terminal domain of FLI-1 is necessary for full tumorigenesis and transcriptional modulation by EWS/FLI-1. Cancer Res 2001;61(13):5311–17.
182. Anderson J, Ramsay A, Gould S, Pritchard-Jones K. PAX3-FKHR induces morphological change and enhances cellular proliferation and invasion in rhabdomyosarcoma. Am J Pathol 2001;159(3):1089–96.
183. Pierotti MA, Santoro M, Jenkins RB, et al. Characterization of an inversion on the long arm of chromosome 10 juxtaposing D10S170 and ret and creating the oncogenic sequence ret/ptc. Proc Natl Acad Sci U S A 1992;89:1616–20.
184. Bongarzone I, Butti MG, Coronelli S, et al. Frequent activation of *ret* protooncogene by fusion with a new activating gene in papillary thyroid carcinomas. Cancer Res 1994;54:2979–85.
185. Santoro M, Dathan NA, Berlingieri MT, et al. Molecular characterization of *RET*/PTC3; a novel rearranged version of the *RET* proto-oncogene in a human thyroid papillary carcinoma. Oncogene 1994;9 (2):509–16.
186. Klugbauer S, Demidchik EP, Lengfelder E, Rabes HM. Detection of a novel type of RET rearrangement (PTC5) in thyroid carcinomas after Chernobyl and analysis of the involved RET-fused gene RFG5. Cancer Research 1998;58(2):198–203.
187. Klugbauer S, Rabes HM. The transcription coactivator HTIF1 and a related protein are fused to the RET receptor tyrosine kinase in childhood papillary thyroid carcinomas. Oncogene 1999;18(30):4388–93.
188. Salassidis K, Bruch J, Zitzelsberger H, et al. Translocation t(10;14)(q11.2:q22.1) fusing the kinetin to the RET gene creates a novel rearranged form (PTC8) of the RET proto-oncogene in radiation-induced childhood papillary thyroid carcinoma. Cancer Res 2000;60:2786–9.
189. Klugbauer S, Jauch A, Lengfelder E, et al. A novel type of RET rearrangement (PTC8) in childhood papillary thyroid carcinomas and characterization of the involved gene (RFG8). Cancer Res 2000;60(24):7028–32.
190. Corvi R, Berger N, Balczon R, Romeo G. RET/PCM-1: a novel fusion gene in papillary thyroid carcinoma. Oncogene 2000;19:4236–42.
191. Nakata T, Kitamura Y, Shimizu K, et al. Fusion of a novel gene, ELKS, to RET due to translocation t(10;12)(q11;p13) in a papillary thyroid carcinoma. Genes, Chromosomes & Cancer 1999;25(2):97–103.
192. Russell JP, Powell DJ, Cunnane M, et al. The *TRK-T1* fusion protein induces neoplastic transformation of thyroid epithelium. Oncogene 2000;19(50):5729–35.
193. Pierotti MA, Bongarzone I, Borrello MG, et al. Cytogenetics and molecular genetics of the carcinomas arising from the thyroid epithelial follicular cells. Genes Chrom Cancer 1996;16:1–14.
194. Nicholson KM, Anderson NG. The protein kinase B/Akt signalling pathway in human malignancy. Cell Signal 2002;14(5):381–95.
195. Lawlor MA, Alessi DR. PKB/Akt: a key mediator of cell proliferation, survival and insulin responses? J Cell Sci 2001;114(Pt 16):2903–10.
196. Testa JR, Bellacosa A. AKT plays a central role in tumorigenesis. Proc Natl Acad Sci U S A 2001;98(20):10983–5.
197. Yuan ZQ, Sun M, Feldman RI, et al. Frequent activation of AKT2 and induction of apoptosis by inhibition of phosphoinositide-3-OH kinase/Akt pathway in human ovarian cancer. Oncogene 2000;19(19):2324–30.
198. Ringel MD, Hayre N, Saito J, et al. Overexpression and overactivation of Akt in thyroid carcinoma. Cancer Res 2001;61(16):6105–11.
199. Roy HK, Olusola BF, Clemens DL, et al. AKT proto-oncogene overexpression is an early event during sporadic colon carcinogenesis. Carcinogenesis 2002;23(1):201–5.
200. Sun M, Wang G, Paciga JE, et al. AKT1/PKBalpha kinase is frequently elevated in human cancers and its constitutive activation is required for oncogenic transformation in NIH3T3 cells. Am J Pathol 2001;159(2):431–7.
201. Perez-Tenorio G, Stal O. Activation of AKT/PKB in breast cancer predicts a worse outcome among endocrine treated patients. Br J Cancer 2002;86(4):540–5.
202. Manning G, Whyte DB, Martinez R, et al. The protein kinase complement of the human genome. Science 2002;298(5600):1912–34.
203. Bardelli A, Parsons DW, Silliman N, et al. Mutational analysis of the tyrosine kinome in colorectal cancers. Science 2003;300(5621):949.
204. Neel BG, Tonks NK. Protein tyrosine phosphatases in signal transduction. Curr Opin Cell Biol 1997;9(2):193–204.
205. Vivanco I, Sawyers CL. The phosphatidylinositol 3-Kinase AKT pathway in human cancer. Nat Rev Cancer 2002;2(7):489–501.
206. Campbell IG, Russell SE, Choong DY, et al. Mutation of the PIK3CA gene in ovarian and breast cancer. Cancer Res 2004;64(21):7678–81.
207. Peto R. Epidemiology, multistage models and short-term mutagenicity models. Cold Spring Harbor Conf Cell Prolif 1977;4:1404–28.
208. Weinberg RA. Oncogenes and multistep carcinogenesis. In: Weinberg RA, editor. Oncogenes and the molecular origins of cancer. New York: Cold Spring Harbor; 1989. p. 307–26.
209. Lobmayr L, Sauer T, Killisch I, et al. Transferrin receptor hyperexpression in primary erythroblasts is lost on transformation by avian erythroblastosis virus. Blood 2002;100(1):289–98.
210. Land H, Parada LF, Weinberg RA. Tumorigenic conversion of primary embryo fibroblasts requires at least two cooperating oncogenes. Nature 1983;304(5927):596–602.
211. Ruley HE. Transforming collaborations between ras and nuclear oncogenes. Cancer Cells 1990;2(8–9):258–68.
212. Pelengaris S, Khan M, Evan G. c-MYC: more than just a matter of life and death. Nat Rev Cancer 2002;2(10):764–76.
213. Nowell PC. The clonal evolution of tumor cell populations. Science 1976;194(4260):23–8.
214. Rowley JD. Chromosome abnormalities in human cancer. In: De Vita VT, Hellman S, Rosenberg SA, editors. Principles and practice of oncology. Philadelphia: Lippincott; 1989. p. 81–7.
215. Stirewalt DL, Kopecky KJ, Meshinchi S, et al. FLT3, RAS, and TP53 mutations in elderly patients with acute myeloid leukemia. Blood 2001;97(11):3589–95.
216. Sozzi G, Veronese ML, Negrini M, et al. The FHIT gene at 3p14.2 is abnormal in lung cancer. Cell 1996;85:17–26.
217. Sozzi G, Sard L, De Gregorio L, et al. Association between cigarette smoking and *FHIT* gene alterations in lung cancer. Cancer Res 1997;57(11):2121–3.
218. Bearzatto A, Conte D, Frattini M, et al. p16(INK4A) Hypermethylation detected by fluorescent methylation-specific PCR in plasmas from non-small cell lung cancer. Clin Cancer Res 2002;8(12):3782–7.
219. Remvikos Y, Vogt N, Muleris M, et al. DNA-repeat instability is associated with colorectal cancers presenting minimal chromosome rearrangements. Genes Chromosomes Cancer 1995;12(4):272–6.
220. Ilyas M, Straub J, Tomlinson IP, Bodmer WF. Genetic pathways in colorectal and other cancers. Eur J Cancer 1999;35(3):335–51.
221. Laurent-Puig P, Blons H, Cugnenc PH. Sequence of molecular genetic events in colorectal tumorigenesis. Eur J Cancer Prev 1999;8 Suppl 1:S39–47.
222. Fearon ER, Vogelstein B. A genetic model for colorectal tumorigenesis. Cell 1990;61:759–67.
223. Frattini M, Balestra D, Suardi S, et al. Different genetic features associated with colon and rectal carcinogenesis. Clin Cancer Res 2004;15(10):4015–21.
224. Goldman JM, Melo JV. Targeting the BCR-ABL tyrosine kinase in chronic myeloid leukemia. N Engl J Med 2001;344(14):1084–6.
225. Heinrich MC, Blanke CD, Druker BJ, Corless CL. Inhibition of KIT tyrosine kinase activity: a novel molecular approach to the treatment of KIT-positive malignancies. J Clin Oncol 2002;20(6):1692–703.
226. Casali PG, Messina A, Stacchiotti S, et al. Imatinib mesylate in chordoma. Cancer 2004;101(9):2086–97.

7

Tumor Suppressor Genes

Ben Ho Park, MD, PhD
Bert Vogelstein, MD

A genetic basis for the development of cancer has been hypothesized for a century, with support provided by familial, epidemiologic, and cytogenetic studies. Nevertheless, only in the past 30 years has definitive evidence emerged that cancer is a genetic disease. It is now known that cancers arise through a multistage process in which inherited and somatic mutations of cellular genes lead to repeated waves of clonal selection in which cells with the most robust and aggressive growth properties prevail. Two classes of genes, proto-oncogenes and tumor suppressor genes, are primary targets for the mutations, because these genes control the ratio of cell birth and cell death. In all normal tissues of the adult, the ratio between cell birth and cell death is exactly 1.0; mutations increase that ratio. A third class of genes, called genomic stability genes, do not alter the ratio when mutated, but can indirectly contribute to tumorigenesis through an acceleration of mutations in proto-oncogenes and tumor suppressor genes.

The vast majority of the mutations that contribute to the development and behavior of cancer cells are somatic (ie, arising during tumor development) and are present only in the neoplastic cells of the patient. A small fraction of mutations in cancer cells are constitutional and thus present in all somatic cells of affected individuals. Such mutations not only predispose to cancer, but can also be passed on to future generations.

The identification and function of proto-oncogenes and their oncogenic variants are reviewed in other chapters in this book. However, we briefly mention their general properties in an effort to compare them with tumor suppressor genes. More than 100 different proto-oncogenes have been identified through various experimental strategies. In general, proto-oncogenes have critical roles in a variety of growth regulatory pathways, and their protein products are distributed throughout many subcellular compartments. The mutant alleles present in cancers have sustained gain-of-function alterations resulting from point mutations, chromosomal rearrangements, or gene amplifications of the proto-oncogene sequences. In the overwhelming majority of cancers, mutations in proto-oncogenes arise somatically in the tumor cells, although germline mutations activating the function of the rearranged during transfection (*RET*) gene have been identified in those with multiple endocrine neoplasia type 2 and in familial medullary thyroid cancer. In analogous fashion, germline mutations in the metastasis (*MET*) gene have been found in affected members of families with hereditary papillary renal cell carcinoma.

Whereas oncogenic alleles harbor activating mutations, tumor suppressor genes are defined by their inactivation in human cancer. As reviewed below, many tumor suppressor genes have been hypothesized to exist. Thus far, approximately 30 tumor suppressor genes have been identified and definitively implicated in cancer development. As in the case of the proto-oncogenes, the cellular functions of the tumor suppressor genes appear to be diverse.

Defects in genomic stability genes have also been implicated in a broad spectrum of human cancers. Like other tumor suppressor genes, the genomic stability genes are inactivated in human cancers. However, unlike the mutations in tumor suppressor genes, mutations in genomic stability genes are much more often inherited in mutant form. For example, inherited mutations in the breast cancer 1 early onset (*BRCA1*) or breast cancer 2 early onset (*BRCA2*) genes play a role in hereditary breast and ovarian cancers, but these genes are never mutated somatically in nonfamilial forms of breast cancers. Similarly, inherited mutations of nucleotide excision repair (NER) genes give rise to xeroderma pigmentosa, but somatic mutations of the genes have only rarely been reported in non-familial forms of cancer.

Enormous progress has been made in the identification of inherited and somatic mutations in proto-oncogenes, tumor suppressor genes, and genomic stability genes in human cancers. Concomitantly, the function of these genes has been elucidated, in part, through the analysis of a variety of model systems employing mice, flies, worms, and other organisms, and through the investigation of human cancer cell lines. The principal aims of this chapter are to review the somatic cell genetic and epidemiologic studies that established the existence of tumor suppressor genes; to describe the identification and cloning of representative tumor suppressor genes, such as the retinoblastoma and *TP53* genes; to call attention to selected studies of the function of tumor suppressor genes in the regulation of cell birth and cell death; and to describe an example of a genomic stability gene that plays a role in common human cancers.

GENETIC BASIS FOR TUMOR DEVELOPMENT

The inherited basis of human cancer has been appreciated for more than a century. In 1866, Broca described a family in which many members developed breast or liver cancer, and he proposed that an inherited abnormality within the affected tissue allowed tumor development.[1] Following the rediscovery of Mendel's work, studies of the rates of spontaneous mammary tumor formation in various inbred strains of mice led Haaland to argue that tumorigenesis could behave in a formal sense as a Mendelian genetic trait.[2] Similarly, Warthin's analysis of the pedigrees of cancer patients at the University of Michigan Hospital between 1895 and 1913 identified four multi-generational families with susceptibilities to specific cancer types that appeared to be transmitted as autosomal dominant Mendelian traits (Figure 7-1).[3] Although these and other studies suggested the existence of an inherited genetic basis for some cancers, other explanations for familial clustering were possible (eg, shared exposure to a carcinogenic agent in the environment or diet). Furthermore, it was argued that most cancers in humans appeared to arise as sporadic, isolated cases.

A role for somatic mutations in the development of cancer was first proposed by Boveri, who noted that, in sea urchin eggs fertilized by two sperm, abnormal mitotic divisions leading to the

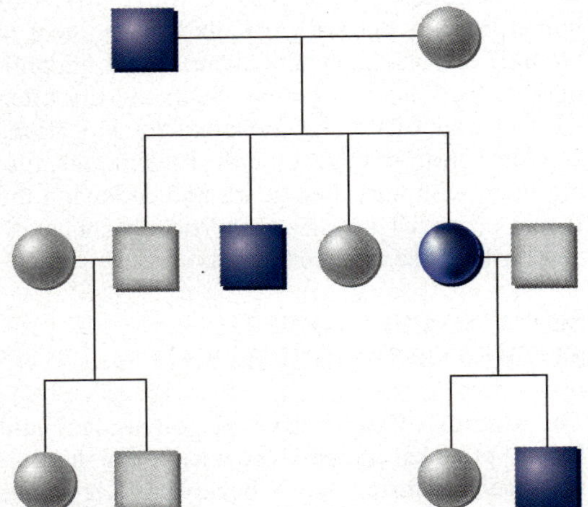

Figure 7-1 The inheritance of cancer in a family. The affected members with cancer are indicated by shaded squares (males) or circles (females). This family demonstrates a dominant pattern of inheritance, meaning that each offspring has a 50% chance of inheriting a germline mutation that predisposes to a high probability of developing cancer.

loss of chromosomes occurred in daughter cells, and atypical tissue masses could be seen in the resulting gastrula.[4] He believed that these abnormal tissues appeared physically similar to the poorly differentiated tissue masses seen in tumors and hypothesized that cancer arose from a cellular aberration producing abnormal mitotic figures. Boveri's hypothesis apparently did not gain favor at the time, initially because of the lack of direct experimental support from studies of the karyotypes of animal and human tumors. Such karyotypes were impossible to obtain with the technology available at that time. Once such karyotypic studies were performed decades later, Boveri's hypothesis was still doubted because of uncertainty about whether the changes in chromosome number in tumors were a cause or an effect of the neoplastic process.

A landmark observation in the search to identify a genetic basis for cancer was reported by Rous in 1911, when he showed that sarcomas could be reproducibly induced in chickens by cell-free filtrates of a sarcoma that had previously arisen in another chicken.[5] Although this observation provided strong evidence that neoplasms could be virally induced, the observation also provided support for the view that cancer could be attributed to discrete genetic elements. Sixty years after Rous's initial report, the oncogenic region of the Rous sarcoma virus was identified. Further characterization and cloning of the transforming sequences demonstrated that the oncogenicity of the virus depended on v-*src*, a transduced and mutated copy of the c-*src* cellular proto-oncogene. Subsequently, all oncogenes of acutely transforming ribonucleic acid (RNA) tumor viruses have been found to be transduced cellular genes. (In fact, they were defined as proto-oncogenes.) The viral oncogenes cause transformation because they are mutated versions of cellular proto-oncogenes or are expressed at abnormally high levels. In human cancers, somatic mutations generate oncogenic alleles from proto-oncogenes.

Oncogenes play a role in most forms of human cancer, but are particularly prominent in "liquid" tumors, such as leukemias and lymphomas, as well as in sarcomas. Such cancers often have characteristic chromosomal translocations that alter proto-oncogenes at the breakpoints, fusing them with unrelated genes and endowing the fusion product with new properties that increase cell birth or decrease cell death.

SOMATIC CELL GENETIC STUDIES OF TUMORIGENESIS

The studies of Ephrussi and colleagues[6] and Harris[7] provided compelling evidence that the ability of cells to form a tumor behaves as a recessive trait at the cellular level. They observed that the growth of murine tumor cells in syngeneic animals could be suppressed when the malignant cells were fused to nonmalignant cells, although reversion to tumorigenicity often occurred when the hybrids were propagated for extended periods in culture. The reappearance of malignancy was found to be associated with specific chromosome losses. The interpretation of those authors, that malignancy can be suppressed in somatic cell hybrids, was subsequently supported by additional studies of mouse, rat, and hamster intraspecies somatic cell hybrids, as well as by interspecies hybrids between rodent tumor cells and normal human cells.[8,9] The karyotypic instability of the rodent–human hybrids, however, complicated the analysis of the human chromosomes involved in the suppression process. Stanbridge and his colleagues overcame this problem by studying hybrids made by fusing human tumor cell lines to normal, diploid human fibroblasts.[10,11] Their analysis confirmed that hybrids retaining both sets of parental chromosomes were suppressed, with tumorigenic variants arising only rarely after chromosome losses in the hybrids. Moreover, it was demonstrated that the loss of specific chromosomes, and not simply chromosome loss in general, correlated with the reversion to tumorigenicity. Tumorigenicity could be suppressed even if activated oncogenes, such as mutant *ras* genes, were expressed in the hybrids.[11,12]

The observation that the loss of specific chromosomes was associated with the reversion to malignancy suggested that a single chromosome (and perhaps even a single gene) might be sufficient to suppress tumorigenicity. To directly test that hypothesis, the technique of microcell-mediated chromosome transfer was used to transfer single chromosomes from normal cells to tumor cells. It was found that the transfer of a single chromosome 11 into the HeLa cervical carcinoma cell line suppressed the tumorigenic phenotype of the cells.[13] Similarly, transfer of chromosome 11 into a Wilms tumor cell line was found to suppress tumorigenicity, whereas the transfer of several other chromosomes had no effect.[14] Many studies have demonstrated that transfer of even very small chromosome fragments will specifically suppress the tumorigenic properties of certain cancer cell lines.

Although tumorigenic growth in immunocompromised animals can often be suppressed in hybrids resulting from fusion between malignant and normal cells or by transfer of unique chromosome fragments, other traits characteristic of the parental tumor cells, such as immortality and anchorage-independent growth in vitro, may be retained. This observation is consistent with the notion that most malignant tumors arise as a result of multiple genetic alterations. Suppression of tumorigenicity following cell fusion or microcell chromosome transfer might thus represent correction of only one of many alterations.

In summary, somatic cell genetic approaches provided early and persuasive evidence for the existence of critical growth-regulating genes in normal cells that can suppress phenotypic traits of immortal or even fully cancerous cells.

RETINOBLASTOMA: A PARADIGM FOR TUMOR SUPPRESSOR GENE FUNCTION

Essentially concurrent with the initial cell fusion experiments of Harris and colleagues, Knudson's analysis of the age-specific incidence of retinoblastoma led him to propose that two "hits" or mutagenic events were necessary for retinoblastoma development.[15] Retinoblastoma occurs sporadically in most cases, but, in some families, it displays an autosomal dominant inheritance. In an individual with the inherited form of the disease, Knudson proposed that the first hit is present in the germline, and thus in all cells of the body. However, the presence of a mutation at the susceptibility locus was argued to be insufficient for tumor formation, and a second somatic mutation was hypothesized to be necessary for promoting tumor formation. Given the high likelihood of a somatic mutation occurring in at least one retinal cell during development, the dominant inheritance pattern of retinoblastoma in some families could be explained. In the nonhereditary form of retinoblastoma, both mutations were proposed to arise somatically within the same cell. Although each of the two hits could theoretically have been in different genes, subsequent studies (see below) led to the conclusion that both hits were at the same genetic locus, ultimately inactivating both alleles of the retinoblastoma 1 (*RB1*) susceptibility gene. Knudson's hypothesis served not only to illustrate mechanisms through which inherited and somatic genetic changes might collaborate in tumorigenesis, but also to link the notion of recessive genetic determinants for human cancer to somatic cell genetic findings on the recessive nature of tumorigenesis.

The first clue to the location of a putative gene responsible for inherited retinoblastoma was obtained from karyotypic analyses of patients with retinoblastoma. Constitutional deletions of chromosome 13 were observed in some cases.[16] Subsequent cytogenetic studies of patients with retinoblastoma identified detectable germline deletions of chromosome 13 in only about 5% of all patients. However, in cases where deletions were observed, the common region of deletion was centered around chromosome band 13q14.[17] When compared with karyotypically normal family members, patients with deletions of 13q14 were found to have reduced levels of esterase D, an enzyme of unknown physiologic function.[18] This finding implied that the esterase D gene might be contained within chromosome band 13q14. Indeed, analysis of the segregation patterns of esterase D isozymes and retinoblastoma development in families with inherited retinoblastoma established that the esterase D and *RB1* loci were genetically linked.[19]

Subsequently, a child with inherited retinoblastoma was found to have esterase D levels approximately one-half of normal, although no deletion of chromosome 13 was seen in karyotype studies of his blood cells and skin fibroblasts.[20] Interestingly, tumor cells from this patient had a complete absence of esterase D activity, despite harboring one apparently intact copy of chromosome 13. Based on these findings, it was proposed that the copy of chromosome 13 retained in the tumor cells had a submicroscopic deletion of both the esterase D and *RB1* loci.

Moreover, it was concluded that the initial *RB1* mutation in the child was recessive at the cellular level (ie, cells with inactivation of one *RB1* allele had a normal phenotype). However, the effect of the predisposing mutation could be unmasked in the tumor cells by a second event, such as the loss of the chromosome 13 carrying the wild-type *RB1* allele. This proposal was entirely consistent with Knudson's two-hit hypothesis.[15,21]

To establish the generality of these observations, Cavenee and colleagues undertook studies of retinoblastomas, both inherited and sporadic, by using deoxyribonucleic acid (DNA) probes from chromosome 13. Probes detecting DNA polymorphisms were used, so that the two parental copies of chromosome 13 in the cells of the patient's normal and tumor tissues could be distinguished from one another. By using such markers to compare paired normal and tumor samples from each patient, the Cavenee group were able to demonstrate that loss of heterozygosity (LOH—ie, the loss of one parental set of markers) for chromosome 13 alleles had occurred during tumorigenesis in more than 60% of the cases studied.[22] LOH for chromosome 13, and specifically for the region of chromosome 13 containing the *RB1* gene, occurred via a number of different mechanisms (Figure 7-2). In addition, through study of inherited cases, it was shown that the copy of chromosome 13 retained in the tumor cells was derived from the affected parent and that the chromosome carrying the wild-type *RB1* allele had been lost.[22,23] These data established that the unmasking of a predisposing mutation at the *RB1* gene, whether the initial mutation had been inherited or had arisen somatically in a single developing retinoblast, occurred by the same chromosomal mechanisms.

Patients with the inherited form of retinoblastoma were known to be at an increased risk for the development of a few other cancer types, particularly osteosarcomas. LOH for the chromosome 13q region containing the *RB1* locus was seen in osteosarcomas arising in patients with the inherited form of retinoblastoma, suggesting that inactivation of both *RB1* alleles was critical to the development of osteosarcomas in those with inherited retinoblastoma.[24,25] Chromosome 13q LOH was also frequently observed in sporadic osteosarcomas. These molecular studies of retinoblastomas and osteosarcomas provided strong support for Knudson's two-hit hypothesis and suggested that a variety of tumors might arise through the inactivation of various tumor suppressor loci.[11,21,23] In addition, the studies demonstrated that the inherited and sporadic forms of a specific tumor type both appeared to arise as a result of genetic alterations in the same gene.

Cloning and Analysis of the *RB1* Gene

The molecular cloning of the *RB1* gene was facilitated by the identification in the chromosome 13q14 region of an anonymous DNA marker that detected DNA rearrangements in retinoblastomas.[26] Analysis of the DNA sequences flanking this DNA marker revealed a gene with the properties expected of *RB1*.[27–29] The *RB1* gene has a complex organization, with 27 exons spanning more than 200 kb of DNA, and an RNA transcript of about 4.7 kb. The *RB1* gene appears to be expressed ubiquitously rather than to be restricted to retinoblasts and osteoblasts.

Cloning of *RB1* allowed study of mutations that inactivate the gene. Although gross deletions of *RB1* sequences have been observed in a small subset of retinoblastoma and osteosarcoma cases, most tumors appear to express full-length *RB1* transcripts and lack detectable gene rearrangements when analyzed by Southern blotting.[30–33] Hence, the detection of inherited and somatic mutations in the *RB1* gene in most cases has required detailed characterization of its sequence. Mutant *RB1* alleles from both constitutional cells of individuals with the inherited

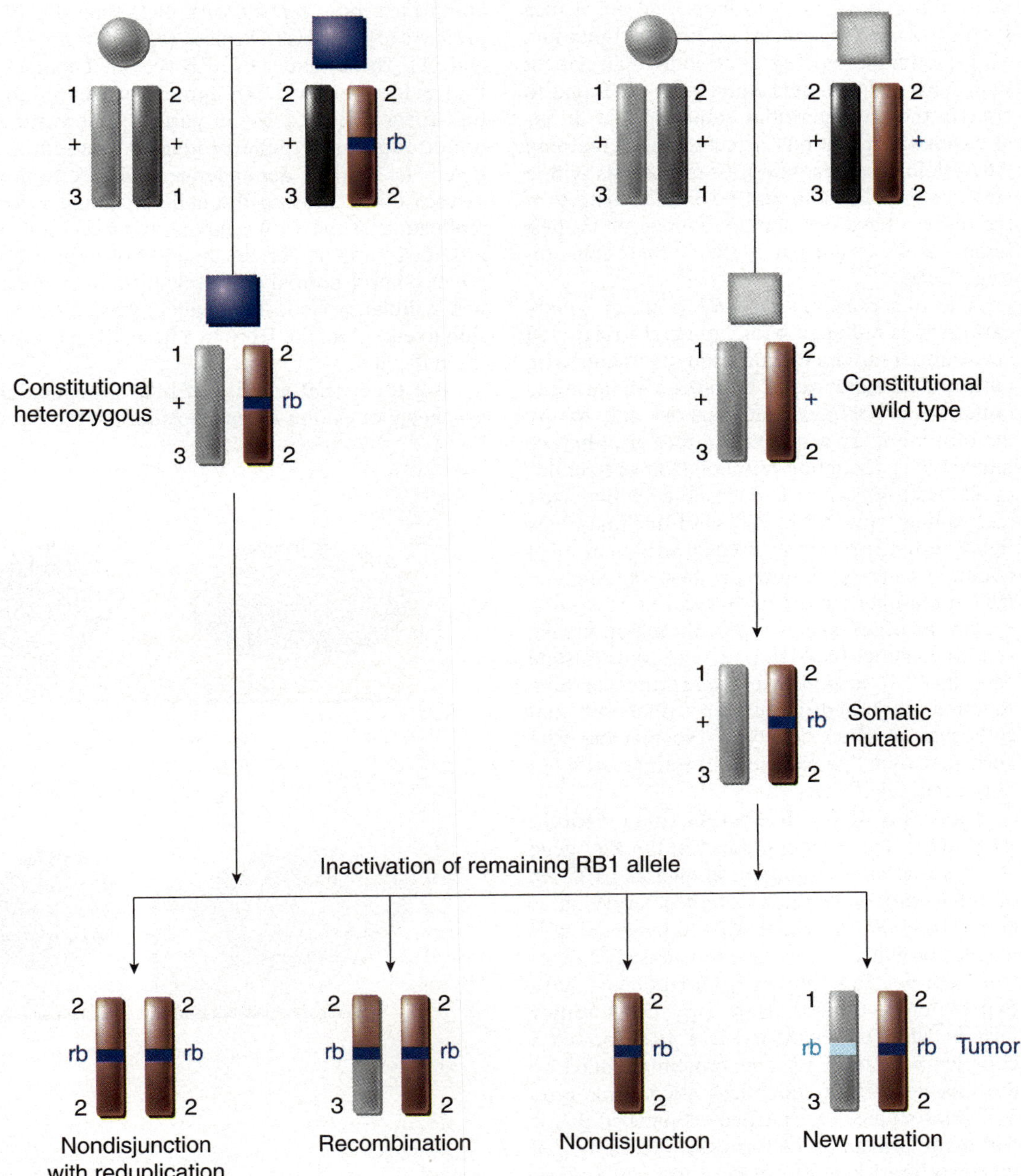

Figure 7-2 Chromosomal mechanisms that result in loss of heterozygosity for alleles at the retinoblastoma predisposition (*RB1*) locus at chromosomal band 13q14. In the inherited form of the disease (*top left*), the affected son inherits a mutant *RB1* allele (*rb*) from his affected father and a normal *RB1* allele (+) from his mother. Thus, he has one wild-type and one mutant *RB1* allele in all his cells (ie, constitutional genotype for *RB1* is *rb* /+). The two copies of chromosome 13 in his normal cells (one from each parent) can be distinguished using polymorphic DNA markers flanking the *RB1* locus (the polymorphic alleles are designated by number). A retinoblastoma can arise after inactivation of the remaining wild-type *RB1* allele. Among the genetic mechanisms found to inactivate the remaining wild-type *RB1* allele during tumor development are chromosome nondisjunction and reduplication of the remaining copy of chromosome 13, mitotic recombination, nondisjunction, and new RB mutations that inactivate the remaining *RB1* allele. Shown at the *top right* is the situation in the non-inherited (sporadic) form of the disease. A somatic mutation arises in a developing retinal cell and inactivates one of the *RB1* alleles. A retinoblastoma will develop if the remaining *RB1* allele is inactivated by one of the mechanisms shown.

form of the disease and from retinoblastomas of both the inherited and sporadic types have now been quite extensively analyzed. The analysis has provided definitive molecular evidence supporting Knudson's two-hit model. As predicted, patients with inherited retinoblastoma have been found to have one mutated and one normal allele in their constitutional (blood) cells. In retinoblastomas of such individuals, the remaining *RB1* allele has been found to be inactivated by somatic mutation, usually by loss of the normal allele through a gross chromosomal event (see Figure 7-2), but in some cases by point mutation. Multiple tumors arising in an individual patient with inherited retinoblastoma were all found to contain the same germline mutation, but different somatic mutations affected the remaining *RB1* allele. The vast majority of patients with a single retinoblastoma and no family history of the disease have two somatic mutations in their tumors and two normal alleles in their constitutional cells.

The observation that *RB1* is ubiquitously expressed is rather puzzling, given the restricted spectrum of tumors that develop in patients with germline *RB1* mutations. Patients with germline mutations of *RB1* are at elevated risk only for the development of a rather limited number of tumor types, including retinoblastomas in childhood, osteosarcomas, soft-tissue sarcomas, and melanomas later in life. *RB1* germline mutations fail to provide a strong predisposition to most common cancers, despite the fact that somatic *RB1* mutations have been observed in a wide variety of other cancer types, including breast, small cell lung, bladder, pancreas, and prostate cancers.[34] It is possible that retinoblastoma functions slightly differently in retinal epithelial cells than in other cell types, so that the *RB1* gene acts as a "gatekeeper" in retinal cells but not in other cell types.

Function of the Retinoblastoma Protein P105-RB The protein product of the *RB1* gene is a nuclear phosphoprotein known as p105-Rb or, more commonly, pRB. Its molecular weight is about 105,000 Da. Studies by Whyte and colleagues provided critical insights into pRB function, connecting human tumorigenesis with experimental tumors caused by DNA tumor viruses. They demonstrated that pRB formed a complex with the E1A oncoprotein encoded by the murine DNA tumor virus adenovirus type 5.[35] Prior studies of E1A had established that it had many effects on cell growth, including cell immortalization and cooperation with other oncogenes (eg, mutated *ras* oncogene alleles) in neoplastic transformation. It was thus hypothesized that functional inactivation of pRB through its interaction with E1A might contribute to some of E1A's transforming functions. Additional support for that proposal was provided by data establishing that mutations inactivating the ability of E1A to bind to pRB also inactivated E1A's transforming function.[36,37]

The significance of physical interaction between pRB and a DNA tumor virus oncoprotein was further supported by the subsequent demonstration that other DNA tumor virus oncoproteins also formed complexes with pRB, including SV40 T antigen and the E7 proteins of human papillomavirus (HPV) types 16 and 18 (Figure 7-3).[38,39] Many of the mutations that inactivated the transforming activities of these oncoproteins also inactivated their ability to interact with pRB. Furthermore, E7 proteins from "high-risk" HPVs (ie, those linked to cancer development), such as HPV 16 and 18, formed complexes more tightly with pRB than did E7 proteins of "low-risk" viruses (eg, HPV types 6 and 11). These studies of pRB provided compelling evidence that DNA tumor viruses might transform cells at least in part by inactivating tumor suppressor gene products. In addition, given the critical dependence of DNA tumor viruses on harnessing the cell's machinery for replication of the viral genome, the studies also provided support for the hypothesis that pRB might control normal cell growth by interacting with cellular proteins that regulate the cell's decision to enter into the DNA synthesis (S) phase of the cell cycle.

The functional activity of pRB is regulated by phosphorylation during normal progression through the cell cycle. Accordingly, pRB appears to be predominantly unphosphorylated or hypophosphorylated in the G1 phase of the cell cycle and maximally phosphorylated in G2 (Figure 7-4). The critical phosphorylation events regulating the function of pRB are likely to be mediated at the boundary between the G1 and S phases of the cell cycle by cyclin and cyclin-dependent kinase (Cdk) protein complexes.[34,40] Presumably, phosphorylation of pRB, particularly at the G1–S boundary, inactivates its ability to interact with cellular proteins that regulate entry into S phase. For example, when it is not phosphorylated, pRB forms complexes with proteins in the E2F family and inhibits transcription by recruiting proteins involved in transcriptional repression.[40] When phosphorylated, pRB can no longer efficiently form complexes with E2Fs (see Figure 7-4). The E2F proteins, when dimerized with their differentiation-regulated transcription factor (DP) partner proteins, are then capable of activating the expression of a number of genes that are likely to regulate or promote entry into S phase, including DNA polymerase α, thymidylate synthase, ribonucleotide reductase, cyclin E, and dihydrofolate reductase.[40] That E2F family members directly

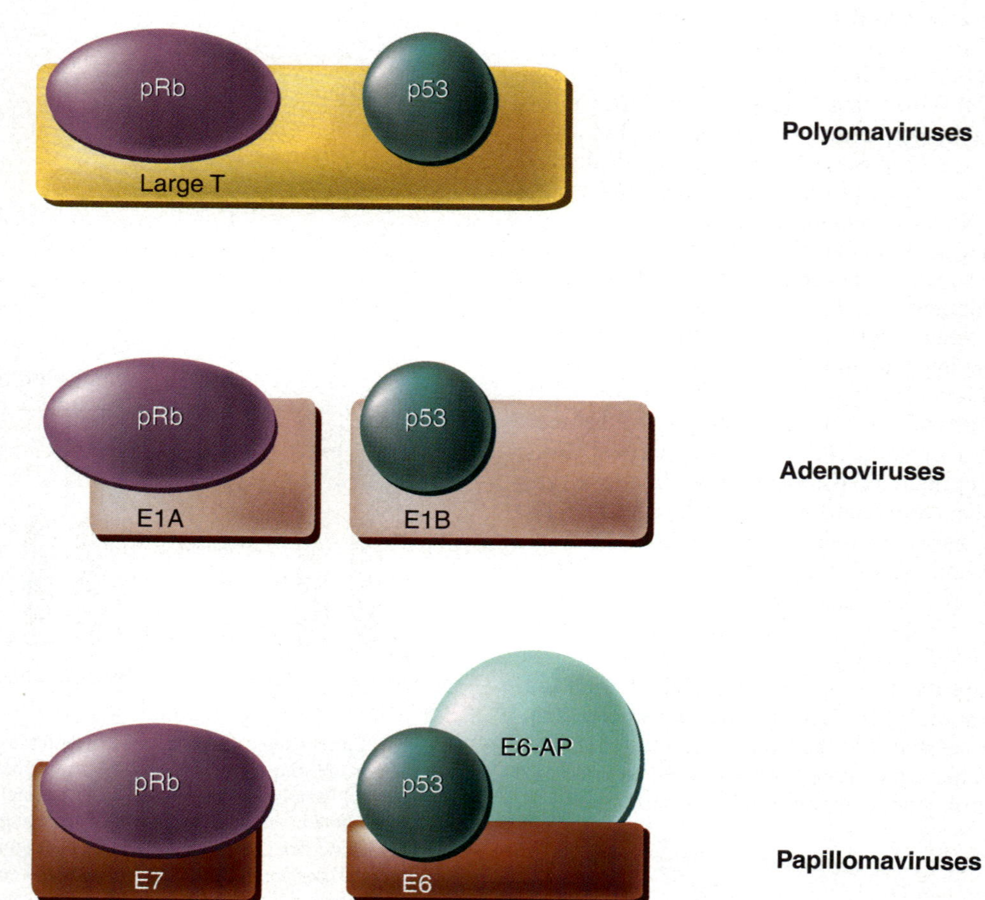

Figure 7-3 Schematic representation of interactions between tumor suppressor gene products and proteins encoded by DNA tumor viruses. Large T antigen from polyomaviruses (such as simian virus 40 [SV40]) bind both the retinoblastoma (pRB) and TP53 proteins. For the adenoviruses and the high-risk human papillomaviruses (HPV types 16 and 18), various viral protein products complex with pRB and TP53. A cellular protein known as E6-associated protein (E6-AP) cooperates with the HPV E6 protein to complex and degrade TP53.

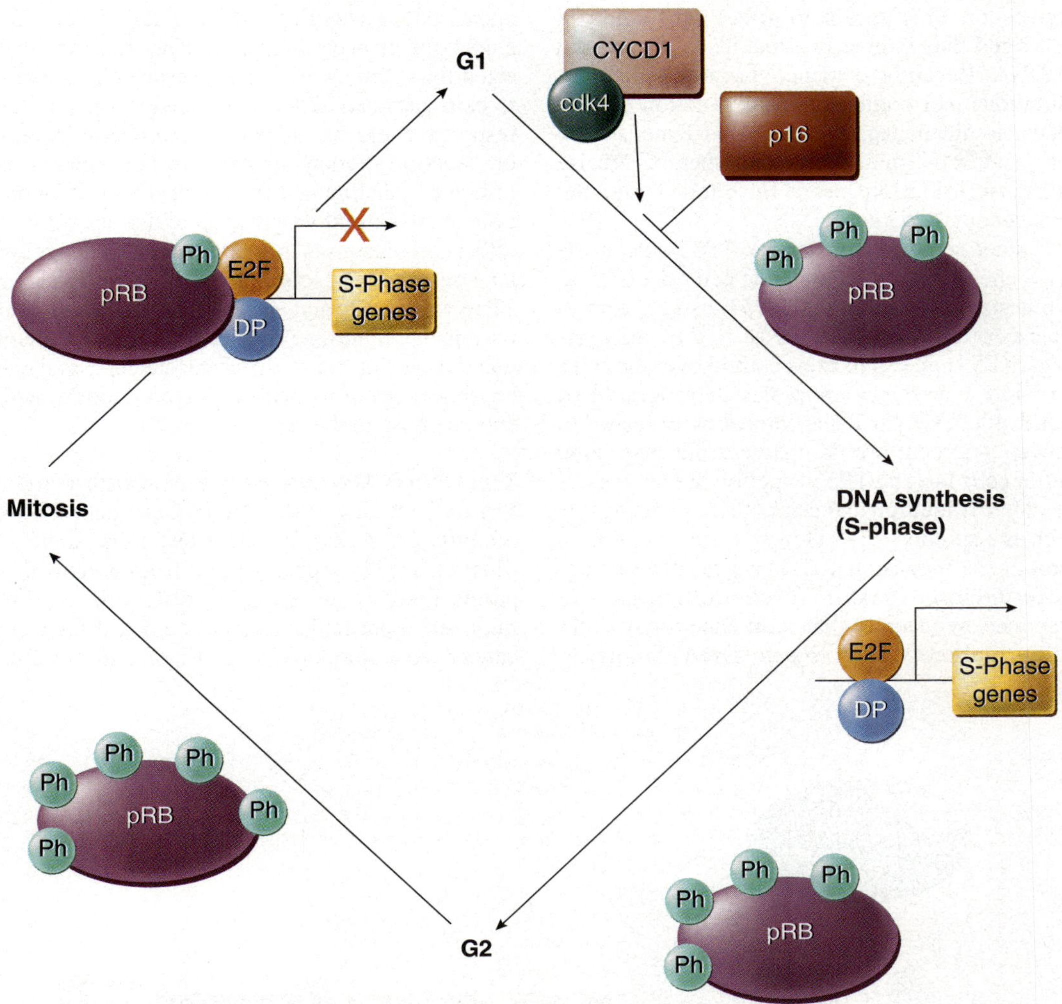

Figure 7-4 The function of the retinoblastoma protein (pRB) is regulated during the cell cycle by phosphorylation. The pRB protein is hypophosphorylated in the G1 phase of the cell cycle, and phosphorylation (Ph) of specific sites appears to increase during progression through the cell cycle. A protein complex that appears to phosphorylate pRB prior to DNA synthesis (S-phase) includes a cyclin (Cyc) and a cyclin-dependent kinase (Cdk)—for example, cyclin D1 and Cdk4. The CycD1/Cdk4 complex is regulated by the p16 inhibitor protein, which is itself the product of a tumor suppressor gene on chromosome 9p, known as *CDKN2* (see text). In its hypophosphorylated state, pRB binds to E2F transcriptional regulatory proteins. When pRB is brought to the promoter regions of genes via its interaction with E2F proteins, pRB represses the expression of the E2F/DP target genes. Phosphorylation of pRB releases it from the E2F/DP protein complex and results in gene activation, including those genes involved in DNA synthesis. The figure also indicates that pRB phosphorylation increases in G2 with pRB dephosphorylated at or near anaphase.

affect cellular proliferation was recently shown in conditional mouse knockout models.[41] Several other cellular proteins that bind to pRB have been identified, but their functions and the significance of their interactions with pRB remain less-well characterized than the interactions of pRB with E2Fs. Future studies will undoubtedly shed further light on the means by which loss of pRB function contributes to cancer development.

***TP53* Gene** Studies in the late 1970s revealed that a cellular phosphoprotein with a relative molecular mass of about 53,000 Da formed a tight complex with SV40 T antigen—hence, the name of the TP53 protein.[42–44] Further work established that TP53 also formed a complex with other viral oncogene products, including the adenovirus E1B protein, and that TP53 was present at low levels in normal cells and high levels in many tumors and tumor cell lines.[44–47] These initial findings suggested that increased levels of TP53 might contribute to cancer. Consistent with that notion, gene transfer studies provided data demonstrating that *TP53* functioned as an oncogene in in vitro experiments.[47–50] However, subsequent studies showed that *TP53* was in reality a tumor suppressor gene. The first definitive evidence for that conjecture came from studies of human tumors.[51]

The rationale for the human cancer studies was the observation that chromosome 17p LOH was common in a number of tumor types, including colorectal, bladder, breast, and lung cancer.[52,53] Detailed mapping showed that region 17p that was lost in colorectal cancers included the *TP53* gene.[51] Analysis of the sequence of the *TP53* alleles retained in those cancers with 17p LOH demonstrated that the remaining *TP53* allele was mutated,[51] in perfect accord with Knudson's hypothesis for the alterations expected in tumor suppressor genes. These observations were soon extended to other cancer types, and they explained many previous observations concerning TP53 that had been confusing when TP53 was believed to be an oncogene.[54–58] Additional evidence that *TP53* functions as a tumor suppressor gene in human cancer is provided by gene transfer studies, but such overexpression studies cannot be easily interpreted, because many genes with no role in neoplasia can inhibit the growth of transfected cells.[59–62] Based on the types of tumors in which *TP53* mutations have been found, and the prevalence of *TP53* mutations in those tumor types, *TP53* is believed to be the most frequently mutated gene in human cancer.[63]

Detailed characterization of the particular base substitutions in the *TP53* gene revealed distinctly different spectra of *TP53* mutations in various types of cancer. For example, most *TP53* mutations in colorectal cancers appear to have arisen spontaneously as a result of deamination of methylated cytosine bases, leading to C → T transition mutations. By contrast, many of the *TP53* mutations seen in lung cancers are transversion mutations (eg, G → T) that may have arisen as result of direct interactions of *TP53* gene sequences with carcinogens present in tobacco smoke. Furthermore, some of the most compelling data to link mutagenic and carcinogenic agents with cancer induction come from study of the *TP53* mutations seen in squamous cell cancers of the skin or in hepatocellular cancers. In squamous cell cancers arising in ultraviolet light–exposed skin, a sizable fraction of the *TP53* mutations appear to have arisen from the generation of pyrimidine dimer premutagenic lesions. Similar studies of the *TP53* gene in hepatocellular cancers arising in individuals from geographic areas with very high exposures to aflatoxin identified mutations that are similar to those generated by aflatoxin in in vitro studies.[63]

Germline mutations in the *TP53* gene have been seen in those affected by Li–Fraumeni syndrome (LFS) and in a small subset of pediatric patients with sarcomas or osteosarcomas that do not meet the more strict criteria for diagnosis of LFS.[64–66] Those with LFS are at risk of developing a number of tumors, including soft-tissue sarcomas, osteosarcomas, brain tumors, breast cancers, and leukemias. Between one-half and two-thirds of patients with LFS have germline mutations in the central core domain of the *TP53* coding sequences that resemble the somatic mutations frequently seen in the *TP53* gene in various sporadic cancers.[67] Some LFS patients and families with phenotypic features of LFS have germline mutations in a gene termed *hCHK2* that phosphorylates *TP53* and controls the cell's response to DNA-damaging events.[68]

In addition to somatic and inherited mutations in the gene, *TP53* function can be inactivated by other mechanisms. As noted above, most cervical cancers contain high-risk or cancer-associated HPV genomes (ie, HPV type 16 or 18). The E6 gene product of high-risk, but not low-risk, HPV types binds to a cellular protein known as E6AP (for E6-associated protein) and stimulates TP53 degradation.[69–73] A cellular TP53-binding protein known as mouse double minute 2 (MDM2) is overexpressed in a subset of soft-tissue sarcomas as a result of gene amplification involving chromosome 12q sequences.[74] DNA transfection studies have shown that the *MDM2* gene can function as an oncogene when overexpressed. The oncogenic function of MDM2 is presumably mediated through its binding to and inactivation of TP53. MDM2 masks TP53's transcriptional activation domain and promotes TP53's ubiquitination and subsequent degradation by the proteasome.[75–77] Consistent with the notion that MDM2 is a critical inhibitor of TP53 function, sarcomas with *MDM2* amplification and overexpression rarely harbor somatic mutations in *TP53*.[78] Disruption of the *MDM2* gene in the germline of mice is lethal, probably because such disruption allows unregulated activity of TP53. Accordingly, disruption of the murine *TP53* gene rescues MDM2-deficient mice from embryonic lethality.[79] Other mechanisms of regulating TP53 function have also been described, including mutation of a nuclear-cytoplasmic shuttle protein called nucleophosmin in almost 100% of adult acute myelogenous leukemias (except the FAB M3 subtype) that demonstrate cytoplasmic localization of this protein.[80]

TP53 Function The TP53 protein has been shown to function as a transcriptional regulatory protein.[81,82] In its wild-type state, the TP53 protein is capable of binding to specific DNA sequences with its central core domain (Figure 7-5). The amino terminal sequences of TP53 function as a transcriptional activation domain, and the carboxyl terminal sequences appear to be required for TP53 to form dimers and tetramers with itself. TP53 activates transcription of a number of genes with roles in the control of the cell cycle, including *WAF1/CIP1/p21* (which encodes a regulator of Cdk activity),[83] *MDM2* (as noted above, encoding a protein that is a known negative regulator of TP53), and 14–3–3σ (a regulator of G2/M progression),[84] and various genes that likely function in apoptosis, including *PUMA* and *NOXA*. Experimental disruption of these genes by targeted homologous recombination can recreate some of the phenotypes associated with TP53 inactivation.[85,86]

The vast majority of the somatic mutations in *TP53* are missense mutations leading to amino acid substitutions in the central portion of the protein (exons 5 to 9).[63] Consistent with the structure of the TP53 protein, these missense mutations have marked effects on the TP53 protein's ability to bind to its cognate DNA recognition sequence through either of two mechanisms.[87] Some mutations (eg, mutations at codons 248 or 273) alter TP53 sequences that are directly responsible for sequence-specific DNA binding. Other mutations (eg, codon 175) appear to affect the folding of TP53 and thus indirectly affect its ability to bind to DNA. Recently, evidence that these missense mutations can confer "gain of function" rather than a dominant negative effect was demonstrated via "knock in" mouse models, whereby precise missense mutations were introduced into the endogenous *TP53* gene.[88–92]

Under some circumstances, TP53 acts at the G1/S checkpoint to regulate the cell's decision to synthesize DNA, although TP53 also appears to have a critical function at G2/M.[93,94] In other settings, TP53 appears to exert control over the cell's decision to undergo apoptosis or programmed cell death.[81] Of particular interest with regard to cancer treatment are data suggesting that some tumor cells lacking TP53 function are less sensitive to γ-irradiation and chemotherapeutic agents such as cisplatin.[91,95,96] However, studies of other tumor cells suggest that TP53 status shows a very different relationship to chemotherapeutic response, with cells that lack functional TP53 being markedly sensitive to DNA-damaging agents but resistant to 5-fluorouracil.[97] Thus far, studies of primary human cancers have emphasized that a rather complex relationship is likely to exist between *TP53* mutational status and the responsiveness of cancer cells to chemotherapy or radiation therapy, or both. In particular, it is difficult to distinguish the effects of *TP53* mutation on the natural progression of disease from its effects on responses to treatment and other cellular stresses.[98,99] Hopefully, further research on TP53 will clarify and enrich our understanding of its normal functions, the basis for its frequent inactivation in many different cancers, and the consequences of its inactivation on tumor growth and response to therapy.

The Cyclin-Dependent Kinase Inhibitor 2A Locus Studies of the cyclin-dependent kinase inhibitor 2A (*CDKN2A*) locus on chromosome 9p illustrate well how observations from initially disparate lines of investigation often converge to implicate a particular locus as a critical factor in cancer development. The LOH of chromosome

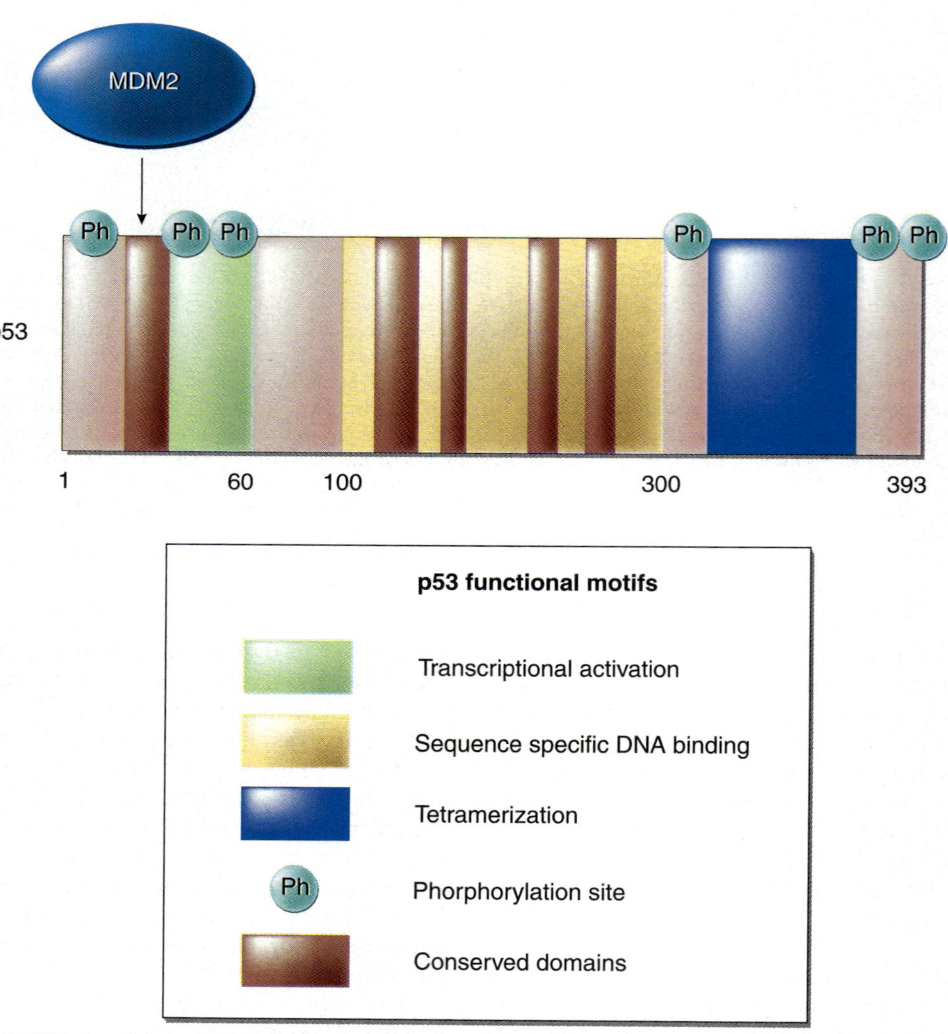

Figure 7-5 TP53 functional motifs. Sequences of TP53 involved in transcriptional activation, sequence-specific DNA binding, tetramerization, and binding by the MDM2 protein are indicated. The five distinct regions of TP53 sequence that are highly conserved between TP53 proteins of diverse species are indicated. In addition, the locations of several sites in the protein that are phosphorylated (Ph) and that regulate TP53 function are indicated.

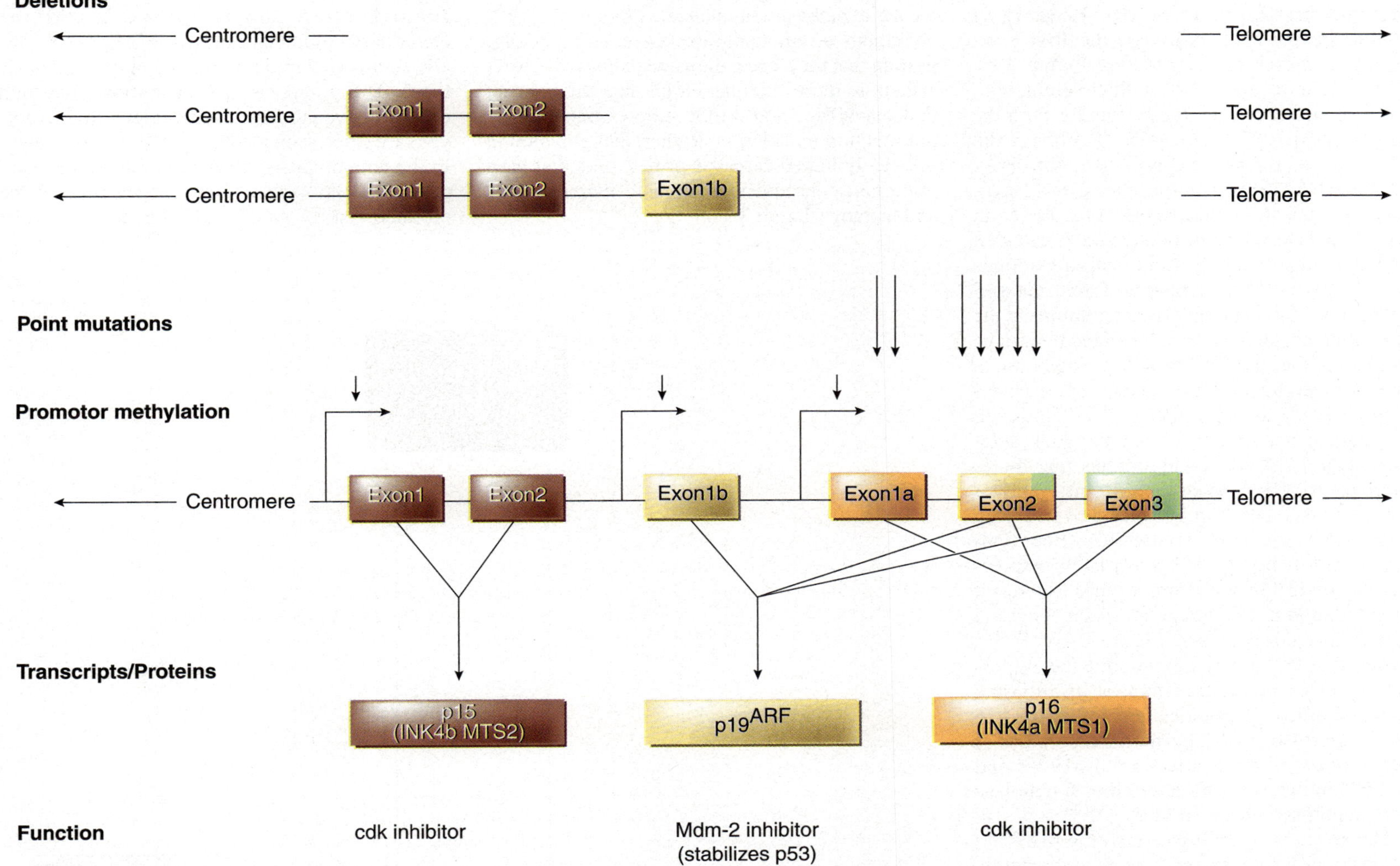

Figure 7-6 Genomic structure, mutations, and transcripts of the *CDKN2B* (p15) and *CDKN2A* (p16/p19^{ARF}) locus. The origins of the p15, p16, and p19^{ARF} transcripts are shown schematically, along with a representative depiction of genomic deletions, point mutations (*arrows*), and promoter methylation (*arrowheads*) noted in human cancers. The exons of the *CDKN2B* and *CDKN2A* loci are shown as *rectangles*. The transcripts/proteins and presumed functions of the transcripts/proteins are indicated. The *red rectangles* indicate the open reading frame in transcripts encoding p15; the *yellow rectangles* indicate the open reading frame present in transcripts encoding p19^{ARF}; and the *lavender rectangles* indicate the open reading frame present in transcripts encoding p16. The size of the locus, exons, and transcripts are not shown to scale.

9p was frequently found in many different tumor types, including melanomas, gliomas, and non-small cell lung, bladder, and head and neck cancers, as well as leukemias.[100–103] Of considerable interest were observations establishing that a subset of such tumors had homozygous (complete) deletions affecting the 9p21 region,[104–106] strongly supporting the existence of a tumor suppressor gene in the region. In addition to the frequent somatic alterations of chromosome 9p sequences in cancers, linkage studies of some families with inherited melanoma indicated a melanoma predisposition gene mapped to essentially the same region of 9p.[107] These observations stimulated great interest in the chromosome 9p region presumed to contain the tumor suppressor gene or genes. One of the genes identified in the region as a result of positional cloning efforts was initially termed multiple tumor suppressor 1(*MTS1*).[108] Sequence analysis of *MTS1* showed that it was identical to a previously described gene that encoded the Cdk inhibitor protein known as p16.[109] Because the p16 protein functioned by inhibiting Cdk4 and Cdk6, it was termed an inhibitor of cyclin dependent kinase 4 (INK4) protein. Another highly related gene, mapping immediately next to the *p16*/*MTS1* gene on chromosome 9p, was found to encode a second INK4 protein, known as p15 (Figure 7-6). The gene encoding the p16 protein is most often termed *INK4A*, and the gene for p15 is *INK4B*.[110,111] The approved symbols are *CDKN2A* and *CDKN2B* respectively.

Subsequent studies show that heterozygous mutations in *CDKN2A* are present in some patients with inherited melanoma and in some families with inherited melanoma and pancreatic cancer.[112–115] Somatic mutations in *CDKN2A* are present in a significant fraction of many different cancer types, including but not limited to melanomas, gliomas, pancreatic and bladder cancers, and leukemias. In some tumors, deletions affecting the *CDKN2A* gene also involve the *CDKN2B* gene. In rare tumors, deletions inactivate *CDKN2B* but not *CDKN2A*.[116] The prevalence and specific nature of *CDKN2A* mutations vary markedly from one tumor type to another. In contrast to other tumor suppressor genes, such as *RB1* and *TP53*, homozygous deletion is a fairly common mechanism of *CDKN2A* inactivation in cancer.[117]

Detailed studies of the *CDKN2A* locus led to the identification of a novel alternative transcript containing nucleotide sequences identical to those in transcripts for the p16^{INK4A} protein, but with unique 5' sequences (see Figure 7-6).[110,111,118] The alternative *CDKN2A* locus transcript encodes a protein known as p19 alternative reading frame (p19^{ARF}), with p19 denoting its apparent weight. The human version of the mouse p19^{ARF} protein is sometimes called p14^{ARF} because of its smaller apparent molecular weight in gel electrophoresis studies. However, both proteins appear to have identical functions, and the discussion below uses the p19^{ARF} terminology because that is the term found more frequently in the literature.

The p19^{ARF} protein contains sequences from a distinct first exon (exon 1β). Exon 1β is located upstream of exon 1α, the first exon present in transcripts for p16 (see Figure 7-6). Exon 1β is spliced to exon 2, which, along with exon 3, is present in the transcripts for both the p19^{ARF} and p16^{INK4A} proteins. However, the p19^{ARF} protein shares no sequence similarity with the p16^{INK4A} protein because p19^{ARF} synthesis initiates at a unique methionine codon in exon 1β and continues through exon 2, using an alternative open reading frame with no similarity to the p16^{INK4A} open reading frame. Careful studies of somatic and inherited mutations at the *CDKN2A* locus indicate that localized mutations inactivating the p16^{INK4A} protein are common in human cancer, but that localized mutations inactivating p19^{ARF} are uncommon.[110,111] However, the frequent occurrence of homozygous deletions at the *CDKN2A* locus implies that mutational inactivation of both proteins—and of p15^{INK4B}—may be strongly selected for during tumor development (see Figure 7-6). Other findings suggest that p16^{INK4A} and p19^{ARF} expression may be lost in some tumor types as a result of methylation of DNA regulatory sequences at the *CDKN2A* locus (see Figure 7-6).[119–121] Recent studies have demonstrated the importance of DNA methyltransferases in initiating and maintaining epigenetic silencing of the p16 tumor suppressor.[122,123] Furthermore, studies of mice with germline inactivation of p19^{ARF} and p16^{INK4A} indicate that these proteins function as tumor suppressor genes in vivo.[124–126]

The mechanism through which the p16^{INK4A} protein controls tumorigenic growth is apparently through its inhibition of Cdk4 activity. As indicated above, phosphorylation of pRB impedes its ability to transcriptionally regulate E2F-target genes (see Figure 7-4). The cyclin D1/Cdk4 complex has a critical role in regulating pRB phosphorylation and function.[121] Hence, the p16^{INK4A} protein, by virtue of its regulation of Cdk4 activity, is, in turn, a critical factor in regulating pRB phosphorylation. Presumably, inactivation of p16^{INK4A} results in inappropriate phosphorylation of pRB and a subsequent inability of hyperphosphorylated pRB to bind E2Fs and appropriately regulate gene expression at the G1–S transition.

Initially, insights into the means by which p19^{ARF} functioned as a growth regulator and tumor suppressor in vitro and in vivo were lacking, in part because the p19^{ARF} protein lacks significant similarity to proteins with well-established function. It is now clear that p19^{ARF} binds directly to the MDM2 protein, and its binding blocks both MDM2-induced degradation of TP53 and the effects of MDM2 on TP53-mediated transcriptional activation of genes.[111] Hence, p19^{ARF} function may be important for maintaining the appropriate function of TP53 in cells, much as p16^{INK4A} function is critical for appropriate pRB function.

Arguing against this idea, however, is the fact that alterations of p19^{ARF} and TP53 often coexist in cancer cells, suggesting that they do not alter the same pathway. In contrast, Rb and p16^{INK4A} alterations are mutually exclusive, strongly suggesting that they affect the same pathway.[127] Nevertheless, these findings emphasize the concept that oncogenes and tumor suppressor genes do not function in isolation. Rather, they function in intricately linked cascades or networks that have important consequences for both tumorigenesis and therapy (Figure 7-7).[81,128]

The Adenomatosis Polyposis Coli Gene

Identification and Germline Mutations

Hereditary colorectal cancer syndromes are usually subdivided into polyposis and nonpolyposis types. The polyposis types are those in which dozens or even thousands of benign tumors (polyps) are often seen prior to cancer development. In the nonpolyposis types, few if any polyps are noted prior to cancer formation, in spite of the elevated risk of cancer and the fact that most

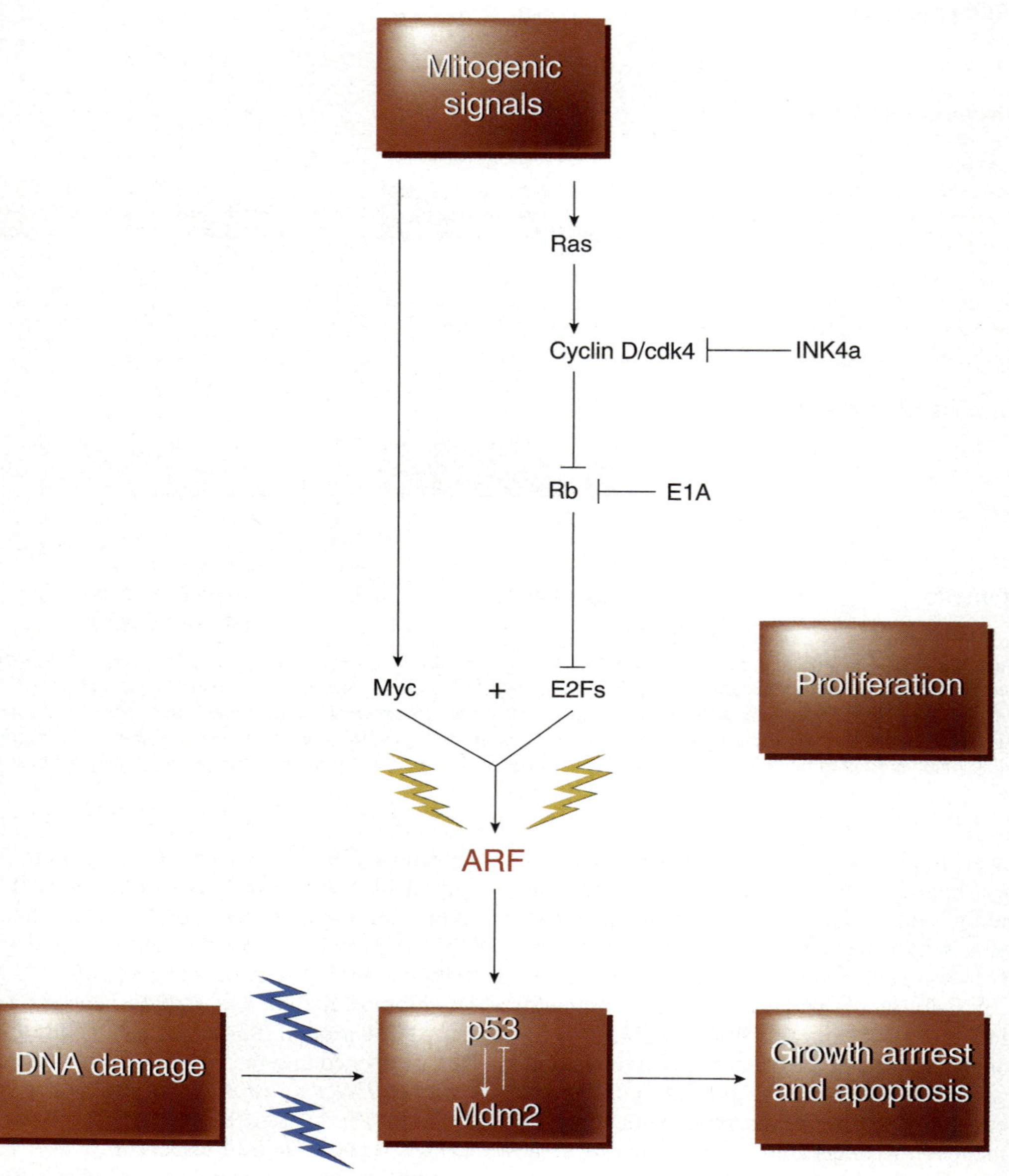

Figure 7-7 Role of the p19^{ARF} protein in checkpoint control. The p19^{ARF} protein (ARF) responds to proliferative signals normally required for cell proliferation. When these signals exceed a critical threshold, the ARF-dependent checkpoint (*yellow lightning bolts*) is activated, and ARF triggers a TP53-dependent response that induces growth arrest or apoptosis, or both. Signals now known to induce signaling via the ARF– TP53 pathway include Myc, E1A, and E2F-1. In principle, "upstream" oncoproteins, such as products of mutated *ras* alleles, constitutively activated receptors, or cytoplasmic signal transducing oncoproteins, might also trigger ARF activity via the cyclin D-Cdk4-RB-E2F or Myc-dependent pathways, both of which are normally necessary for S-phase entry. In inhibiting cyclin D-dependent kinases, p16^{INK4A} can dampen the activity of mitogenic signals. In the figure, E1A is shown to work, at least in part, by opposing RB function. For simplicity, Myc and E2F-1 are shown to activate only TP53 via the effects on ARF, though highly over-expressed levels of these proteins can activate TP53 in ARF-negative cells, albeit with an attenuated efficiency. ARF activation of TP53 likely depends on inactivation of Mdm2-specific function(s). DNA damage signals (eg, ionizing and ultraviolet radiation, hypoxic stress) activate (*blue lightning bolts*) TP53 through multiple signaling pathways.

colorectal cancers are believed to arise from adenomatous precursor lesions. The nonpolyposis colorectal cancer syndromes are addressed below in the context of defects in DNA repair pathway genes.

One of the polyposis syndromes is known as familial adenomatous polyposis (FAP) or adenomatosis polyposis coli (APC). FAP is an autosomal dominant disorder affecting about 1 in 7,000 individuals in the United States. The syndrome is characterized by the development of hundreds of adenomatous polyps in the colon and rectum of affected individuals by early adulthood. The lifetime risk of colorectal cancer in those with the classic form of FAP is extremely high, approaching nearly 100% by age 60 years.

An observation that greatly aided localization of the *APC* gene was the demonstration by Herrera and Sandberg, in 1986, of an interstitial deletion of chromosome 5q in a patient with features of FAP, but without any family history of the syndrome.[129] Subsequent DNA linkage studies confirmed that, in multiple kindreds with FAP or the related condition known as Gardner syndrome, the polyposis phenotype segregated with DNA markers near 5q21.[130,131] In 1991, positional cloning efforts identified the *APC* gene as the specific gene responsible for FAP.[132–135] The *APC* gene is large, with more than 15 exons, and alternative splicing affects the 5' untranslated portion of transcripts. The predominant *APC* transcript encodes a 2,843–amino acid protein expressed in many adult tissues.

In the great majority of individuals with FAP, heterozygous germline mutations can be identified in the *APC* gene.[136–138] All of the germline *APC* mutations in those with FAP appear to inactivate APC protein function. The overwhelming majority of these germline mutations are localized nonsense or frameshift mutations in the 5' half of the coding region of *APC* (Figure 7-8). Consistent with Knudson's two-hit hypothesis, inactivation of the remaining wild-type *APC* allele by somatic mutation in those carrying a germline *APC* mutation is observed in the cancers that arise.[139,140] Correlations between the location of a particular germline *APC* mutation and clinical features have been found, although clear insights into the molecular basis for the predisposition to extracolonic tumors (eg, jaw osteomas and desmoid tumors) in FAP patients with variant phenotypes are lacking. However, some light has been shed on the variability in polyp number seen in families with polyposis.[140,141] Mutations in the 5' region of the *APC* gene appear to be correlated with an attenuated phenotype attributable to reentry of the ribosome on the APC transcript downstream of the premature stop codon, resulting in an APC protein that retains some of its normal activity.[141] Mutations in 3' third of the *APC* gene are also associated with a milder polyposis phenotype than are mutations in the central third of the gene, perhaps because the mutated APC proteins similarly retain some tumor suppressor activity. Unexpectedly, extracolonic features such as desmoid tumors appear to be more common in patients with 3' mutations.[140] Finally, a missense mutation in the middle of the *APC* gene has been found to predispose to colorectal cancers in Ashkenazi Jewish families.[142] This mutation does not alter the function of the gene product, but creates a "hot-spot" that appears to be highly mutable, resulting in somatic deletions or insertions of surrounding nucleotides that produce truncations.

Somatic Mutations in Sporadic Colon Tumors Whereas germline *APC* mutations are an uncommon cause of colorectal cancer in the general population and are present in only about 0.5% of all colon cancers, somatic *APC* mutations are present in the vast majority of sporadic colorectal adenomas and carcinomas.[143] The initial observation suggesting that *APC* inactivation might be common in colon tumors was the observation that the chromosome 5q region containing the *APC* gene was affected by LOH in many sporadic colorectal adenomas and carcinomas.[53,144] Since the identification of the *APC* gene, detailed analyses of the somatic mutations inactivating the *APC* gene in colorectal tumors have been carried out. The somatic *APC* mutations in sporadic tumors are similar in nature and location to the germline *APC* mutations found in those with FAP (see Figure 7-8). Present findings suggest that more than 90% of colorectal tumors, regardless of their size or particular histopathologic features, harbor somatic mutations that inactivate *APC*.[140]

Function The *APC* gene encodes a large protein of roughly 300 kDa that is hypothesized to regulate cell adhesion, cell migration, or apoptosis in the colonic crypt. The localization of the APC protein in the basolateral membrane of colonic epithelial cells, with an apparent increase in APC expression in cells near the top of the crypt implies that APC may regulate shedding or apoptosis of cells as they reach the crypt apex.[145] Perhaps consistent with this view, restoration of APC protein expression in colorectal cancer cells lacking endogenous APC expression has been reported to promote apoptosis.[146]

The APC protein binds to a number of proteins, including β-catenin, γ-catenin (also known as plakoglobin), glycogen synthase kinase 3β (GSK3β), end-binding protein 1 (EB1), human Drosophila large discs (hDLG), microtubules, and the related proteins axin and conductin.[147] With the exception of β-catenin, GSK3β, and the conductin and axin

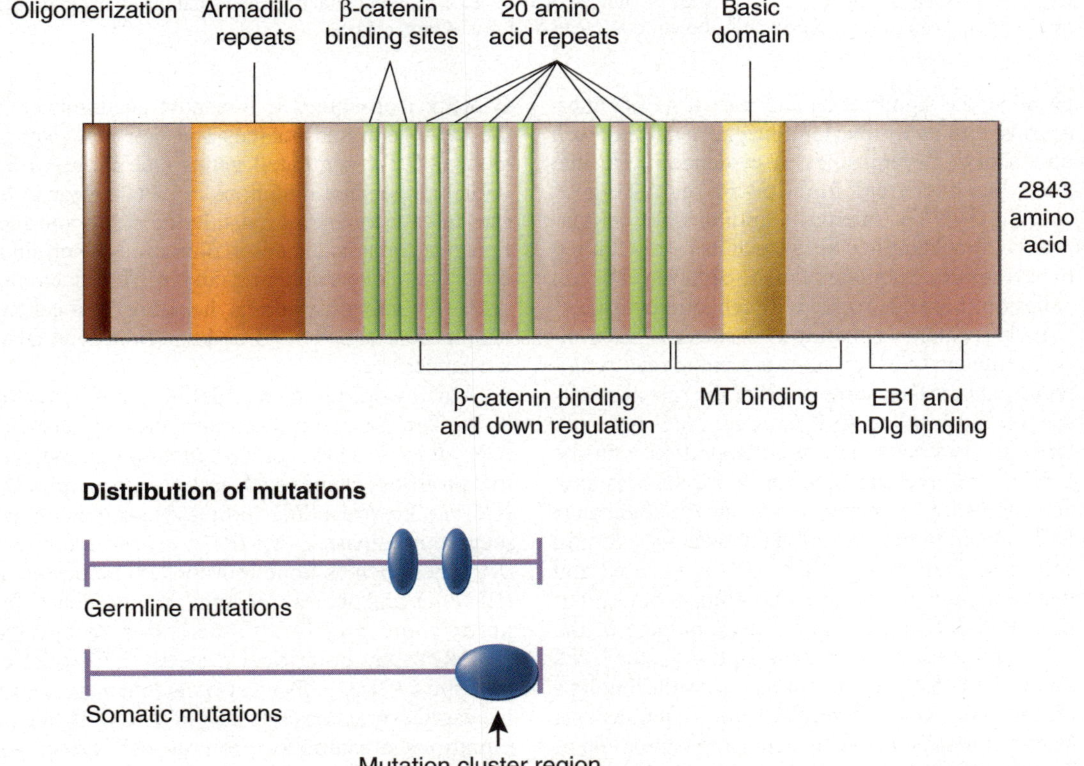

Figure 7-8 Schematic representation of Apc protein domains with respect to mutational analysis results. The relative positions of various Apc domains. A putative domain involved in homo-oligomerization of Apc is located at the amino-terminus. Also noted are a series of repeats of unknown function with similarity to the *Drosophila* armadillo protein, sequences known to mediate binding to β-catenin and its down-regulation, a basic domain in the carboxy-terminal third of the protein that appears to facilitate complexing with microtubules (MT), and sequences near the carboxy-terminus of Apc that are known to interact with the EB1 and human homolog of the *Drosophila* disc large (hDlg) protein. Germline mutations in the *APC* gene (predominantly chain terminating) are dispersed throughout the 5' half of the sequence, with two apparent "hot spots" at codons 1061 and 1309. Somatic mutations in the *APC* gene in colorectal cancer appear to cluster in a region termed the "mutation cluster region," and mutations at codons 1309 and 1450 are most common.

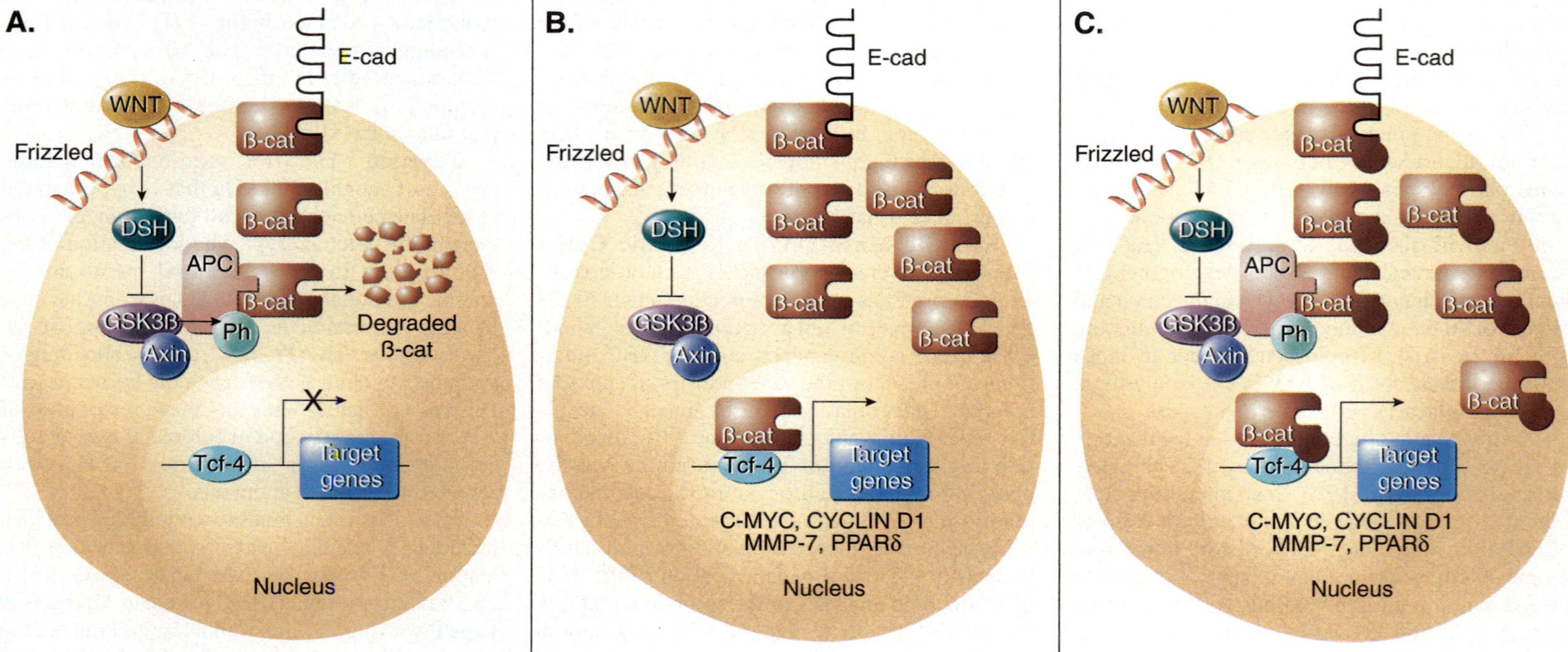

Figure 7-9 A model indicating the function of the Apc, axin, and Gsk3β proteins in the regulation of β-catenin (β-cat) in normal cells, and the consequence of Apc or β-cat defects in cancer cells. β-Cat is an abundant cellular protein, and much of it is often bound to the cytoplasmic domain of the E-cadherin (E-cad) cell–cell adhesion protein. **A,** In normal cells, the proteins glycogen synthase kinase 3β (Gsk3β), Apc, and axin function to promote degradation of free cytosolic β-cat, probably as a result of phosphorylation of the N-terminal sequences of β-cat by Gsk3β. Gsk3β activity and β-cat degradation are inhibited by activation of the wingless (Wnt) pathway, as a result of the action of the Frizzled receptor and disheveled (Dsh) signaling protein. **B,** Mutation of Apc in colorectal and other cancer cells results in accumulation of β-cat, binding to Tcf-4, and transcriptional activation of Tcf-4 target genes, such as c-*myc*, cyclin D1, *MMP-7*, and *PPARδ* (see text). **C,** Point mutations and small deletions in β-cat in cancer cells inhibit phosphorylation and degradation of β-cat by Gsk3β and Apc, with resultant activation of c-*myc* and other Tcf-4 target genes.

proteins, the significance and role of APC's interactions with its various binding partners is not well understood. Several lines of evidence imply that APC has a critical function in regulating β-catenin.[147,148] β-Catenin is an abundant cellular protein, first identified because of its role in linking the cytoplasmic domain of the E-cadherin cell–cell adhesion molecule to the cortical actin cytoskeleton, via β-catenin's binding to α-catenin. The truncated (mutant) APC proteins present in many colorectal cancers lack some or all of the repeat motifs crucial for binding to β-catenin. APC not only binds to β-catenin, but, in collaboration with the GSK3β enzyme and other proteins, such as axin and conductin, it appears to regulate the abundance of β-catenin in the cytosol via phosphorylation. In colorectal cancers in which *APC* is mutated and unable to bind or effectively coordinate the regulation of β-catenin, β-catenin accumulates in the cell, complexes with the transcription factor T cell factor-4 (Tcf-4) and translocates to the nucleus (Figure 7-9). Once there, β-catenin functions as a transcriptional coactivator, activating expression of Tcf-4–regulated genes. Consistent with the notion that β-catenin is a critical target of *APC* regulation, somatic mutations in β-catenin have been found in many of the small fraction of colorectal cancers lacking *APC* mutations.[149–151] These mutations consistently alter GSK3β phosphorylation consensus sites near the amino terminus of the β-catenin protein, and the mutations presumably render the defective β-catenin proteins oncogenic as a result of their resistance to degradation by APC and GSK3β. Consequently, β-catenin accumulates in the cytoplasm and nucleus and activates expression of Tcf-4–regulated genes (see Figure 7-9). Although somatic mutations in *APC* appear to be rare in cancers arising outside the colon and rectum, oncogenic mutations in β-catenin's N-terminus have been observed in many different cancer types, including melanoma, hepatocellular cancer, endometrial cancer, and endometrioid-type ovarian cancer.[152]

Much work remains to define genes activated by the Tcf/ β-catenin complex in cancer cells with *APC* defects. However, recent findings indicate that proto-oncogenes such as c-*myc* and cyclin D1 (*CCND1*), extracellular proteases such as matrix metalloproteinase 7 (MMP-7), growth inhibitory cytokines such as bone morphogenetic protein 4 (BMP-4), and nuclear receptor factors such as the peroxisome proliferator–activator receptor δ (PPARδ) may be critical targets.[153–159] Like c-*myc* and *CCND1*, other Tcf/β-catenin targets with increased expression as a result of *APC* or β-catenin mutations presumably promote cell growth or inhibit cell death, or both. Further work on APC function should offer crucial insights into the development of colon and other cancers and novel strategies and targets for chemotherapy and perhaps even chemoprevention.

Wilms Tumor Gene Wilms tumors are the most common renal neoplasm in children, accounting for approximately 6% of all pediatric cancers.[160] Wilms tumors are similar to retinoblastomas in a number of ways: both can occur bilaterally or unilaterally, with single or multiple foci, and in a sporadic or inherited fashion. The two-mutation model originally proposed for retinoblastoma was also proposed to explain Wilms tumor.[161] However, hereditary cases are not as common among Wilms tumor patients as they are in retinoblastoma patients. Almost all patients inheriting a mutation at the *RB1* locus develop a retinoblastoma, but only approximately 50% of individuals carrying a germline mutation predisposing to Wilms tumor develop the disease (ie, lower penetrance).[160]

Perhaps the first finding to offer insight into an inherited genetic basis for Wilms tumor was a report in 1964 describing six patients with Wilms tumor and sporadic aniridia (ie, congenital absence of the iris).[162] It was proposed that the simultaneous occurrence of these two very rare conditions might result from chromosomal aberrations affecting two or more loci, a situation now often called a contiguous gene syndrome—mutation of one locus presumably leading to aniridia and mutation of another leading to Wilms tumor. This hypothesis was subsequently supported by the discovery of interstitial deletions of chromosome 11p13 in peripheral blood samples from children with the WAGR syndrome (Wilms tumor with aniridia, genitourinary abnormalities, and mental retardation) of Wilms tumor.[163] Cytogenetic studies of tumor tissues in a few cases of sporadic-type Wilms tumors revealed deletions or translocations of chromosome band 11p13.[164,165]

Subsequent studies of paired samples of Wilms tumor and normal cells from patients, using probes that detect restriction fragment length polymorphisms (RFLPs) on chromosome 11p, revealed that LOH of 11p occurred frequently in Wilms tumors of both the inherited and sporadic types.[166–169]

The Wilms tumor 1 (*WT1*) gene was identified in 1990 by virtue of mutations inactivating the gene in patients with the WAGR syndrome and by analysis of somatic mutations in the gene in tumors from a minority of patients with unilateral Wilms tumor and no associated congenital malformation.[170] *WT1* is encoded by 10 exons and its transcripts are subject to alternative splicing.[171,172] In contrast to the rather ubiquitous expression of the *RB1*, *TP53*, and *APC* genes, expression of the *WT1* gene appears to be restricted to embryonic kidney and a small subset of other tissues.[173,174] *WT1* messenger ribonucleic acids (mRNAs) encode proteins with molecular masses of 45,000 to 49,000 Da and 4 zinc-finger motifs. Based on its predicted amino acid sequence, the WT1 proteins were suspected from the outset to function in transcriptional regulation.[174] Several studies provide evidence to support that notion, although some WT1 isoforms may have a role in RNA processing, rather than in transcription regulation.[172,174] WT1 proteins suppress the transcriptional activity of promoter elements from a number of growth-inducing genes, including the genes for early growth response (EGR1), insulin-like growth factor-2 (IGF-2), and platelet-derived growth factor A chain (PDGFA), suggesting that WT1 may function in gene repression.[175] Other studies suggest that WT1 can activate or repress gene expression, depending on the cell type and promoter context.[176] Consistent with the notion that WT1 may have a physiologic function in transcriptional activation, recent work indicates that WT1 activates expression of amphiregulin, a member of the epidermal growth factor family.[177] Loss of amphiregulin expression may contribute to loss of appropriate differentiation during Wilms tumor development. Adding to the complex nature of WT1's role as a transcriptional regulator, recent studies suggest that certain *WT1* splice variants have dramatically different effects in their ability to regulate gene expression.[178]

WT1 inactivation clearly contributes to Wilms tumor development in those with the WAGR syndrome. Moreover, approximately 10% of apparently sporadic Wilms tumors harbor detectable somatic mutations in the *WT1* gene.[179] Nevertheless, much evidence indicates that Wilms tumors arise through mutations in genes other than *WT1*. First, the chromosome 11p allelic losses seen in Wilms tumor frequently involve band 11p15, but not band 11p13, where the *WT1* gene resides.[179–181] Second, the 11p15 region harbors a gene responsible for Beckwith-Wiedemann syndrome (BWS), a congenital disorder in which affected individuals manifest hyperplasia of the kidneys, endocrine pancreas, and other internal organs; macroglossia; and hemihypertrophy.[182,183] Those affected by BWS are also at increased risk of developing embryonic tumors, such as hepatoblastoma and Wilms tumor. Finally, linkage studies of three families with dominant inheritance of Wilms tumor exclude linkage of the susceptibility locus in those families to any part of chromosome 11p.[184,185] On the whole, the data suggest that germline mutations in any one of at least three different genes (ie, *WT1*, the BWS gene, and at least one gene not on chromosome 11p) predispose to Wilms tumor. Whether a combination of inherited and somatic mutations in more than one of those genes is ultimately required for the transformation of a developing kidney cell into a Wilms tumor, or whether alternative genetic pathways for the development of Wilms tumors exist, remains to be established. The genetic heterogeneity observed among Wilms tumors provides an important contrast to the apparently less complex genetic pathway of retinoblastoma.

NEUROFIBROMATOSIS 1 AND 2 GENES **Neurofibromatosis 1 Gene** Von Recklinghausen's disease, also called neurofibromatosis 1 (NF1), is a dominantly inherited syndrome with variable disease manifestations. The consistent feature is that tissues derived from the neural crest are commonly affected. In addition to the nearly uniform development of neurofibromas, NF1 patients are at elevated risk of developing pheochromocytomas, schwannomas, neurofibrosarcomas, and primary brain tumors.[186–188] The *NF1* gene was initially localized to the pericentromeric region of chromosome 17q by linkage analyses.[189,190] Subsequently, karyotype studies of two NF1 patients identified germline chromosomal rearrangements involving band 17q11.[191,192] In further work, both patients were found to have genetic alterations of a localized region of band 17q11. Intensive positional cloning efforts in this chromosome region led to the identification of the *NF1* gene in 1991.[193–195] The *NF1* gene is large, spanning roughly 350 kb of DNA, and it encodes a protein product with a molecular mass of about 300 kDa.[187,188,196] Although germline mutations in the *NF1* gene are believed to underlie the development of the associated disease features in all or very nearly all NF1 patients, specific germline *NF1* mutations have been identified in approximately one-half to two-thirds of NF1 patients.[187,188,196,197] Difficulties in identifying germline mutations in the *NF1* gene in the remaining NF1 patients may be a result of the inherent inefficiencies and insensitivity associated with mutation detection strategies in such a large gene.

In addition to germline *NF1* mutations in those patients with NF1, the *NF1* gene is affected by somatic mutations in a fraction of colon cancers, melanomas, neuroblastomas, and bone marrow cells from patients with the myelodysplastic syndrome.[188,196,198–200] Consistent with its presumed tumor suppressor role, the mutations inactivate *NF1*. Studies of leukemias arising in pediatric neurofibromatosis patients provide the clearest evidence that both copies of the *NF1* gene are inactivated during tumorigenesis,[201] as predicted by the Knudson model. Like the *RB1*, *TP53*, and *APC* genes, the *NF1* gene is expressed ubiquitously. Thus, as for other inherited cancer syndromes, the basis for the tissue specificity of the malignant tumors observed in neurofibromatosis patients is puzzling. The NF1 protein product, termed neurofibromin, is a member of the guanosine triphosphate (GTPase)–activating protein family (GAPs).[188,202–204] Perhaps the best-studied GAP is Ras-GAP, which markedly enhances the GTPase activity of the wild-type K-Ras, H-Ras, and N-Ras proteins. Although the means through which *NF1* defects alter cell growth is not well understood, it is likely that inactivation of neurofibromin function leads to alterations in signaling pathways regulated by small Ras-like GTPase proteins.

Neurofibromatosis 2 Gene Neurofibromatosis 2 (NF2—also known as central neurofibromatosis) is an autosomal dominant disorder that is distinct from NF1 on both genetic and clinical grounds.[188,205,206] A hallmark of NF2 is the occurrence of bilateral schwannomas that affect the vestibular branch of the eighth cranial nerve (acoustic neuromas). NF2 patients are also at elevated risk for meningiomas, spinal schwannomas, and ependymomas. The neurofibromatosis 2 (*NF2*) gene was mapped to chromosome 22q by a combination of linkage analyses and LOH studies[207–209] and was cloned in 1993 using positional cloning approaches.[210,211] Germline mutations inactivating the *NF2* gene were observed in those patients with NF2, and somatic *NF2* mutations were also observed in a subset of sporadic schwannomas and meningiomas. Somatic *NF2* mutations in most other tumor types appear to be infrequent. However, preliminary studies indicate that the *NF2* gene may be frequently affected by somatic mutations in malignant mesotheliomas[212] despite this tumor type not being seen at increased frequency in patients with NF2.[205] The *NF2* gene encodes a protein with strong similarity to a cytoskeletal protein family thought to act as linker proteins between integral membrane proteins and scaffolding proteins of the filamentous submembrane lattice.[211] Consequently, *NF2* gene alterations might contribute to tumor development, at least in part, by effects on cell shape, cell–cell interactions, or cell movement (or a combination). Mouse studies confirm the importance of *NF2* in tumor development. Although *NF2* null mice typically develop osteosarcomas and not schwannomas, recent studies that used a conditional NF2 inactivation system in mouse Schwann cells appear to recapitulate the disease phenotype observed in humans.[213]

VON HIPPEL-LINDAU GENE Von Hippel-Lindau (VHL) syndrome is a rare dominant disorder predisposing affected individuals to the development of hemangioblastomas of the central nervous system and retina, to renal carcinomas of clear cell type, and to pheochromocytomas.[214–216] The *VHL* gene was mapped to chromosome 3p by linkage analysis. As with many other inherited cancer genes, LOH studies established that the

VHL gene behaves as a typical tumor suppressor gene, with both alleles inactivated during tumorigenesis.[216,217] Positional cloning efforts identified the *VHL* gene in 1993.[218] Germline mutations inactivating one *VHL* allele are seen in the majority of individuals in families displaying features of the VHL syndrome.[214–216] As with some other inherited cancer syndromes, preliminary genotype–phenotype relationships have been observed. Specifically, a certain class of *VHL* germline mutations is associated with the development of renal cancer only, a second class is linked to predisposition to both renal cancer and pheochromocytoma, and yet a third mutation class is associated only with pheochromocytoma.[216] Somatic mutations in the *VHL* gene are also seen in more than 80% of sporadic renal cell carcinomas of the clear cell type, but not in renal cell carcinomas of other histopathologic types (eg, papillary type).[214,216] Approximately 20% of sporadic clear cell renal cancers do not carry a detectable mutation in the *VHL* gene. However, in many of these cases, the *VHL* gene may be inactivated by epigenetic silencing,[219] a mechanism noted earlier in this chapter in connection with inactivation of the *CDKN2A* locus. In tumor types other than clear cell renal cancer, inactivation of the *VHL* gene appears to be uncommon.[216]

The *VHL* gene encodes a 213–amino acid protein whose major function appears to be in the regulation of angiogenesis through protein degradation. The protein encoded by *VHL* is part of a ubiquitin ligase complex that degrades hypoxia-induced factor 1α (HIF-1α) in the presence of oxygen. In the absence of oxygen in normal cells, or when *VHL* is mutated in tumor cells, the HIF-1α transcription factor is stabilized, leading to the expression of cytokines such vascular endothelial growth factor and the stimulation of angiogenesis. Further biochemical and cell biology studies on *VHL* and renal cell carcinomas are likely to offer definitive insights into angiogenesis, one of the most important stromal processes associated with neoplasia.[220]

Genomic Stability Genes Several recessive cancer predisposition syndromes resulting from inactivation of genes that function in DNA damage recognition and repair have been described, including ataxia-telangiectasia (AT), Bloom syndrome, xeroderma pigmentosum, and Fanconi anemia. In each case, the specific cancer type and the DNA-damaging agents that increase cancer risk are distinct. Although AT heterozygotes may subtly increase the risk of breast cancer,[221] in other recessive cancer syndromes, only homozygotes appear to clearly increase cancer risk. That observation contrasts sharply with the picture in the dominant cancer predisposition syndromes discussed earlier (eg, inherited retinoblastoma, familial adenomatous polyposis, NF1, and NF2), where heterozygotes have a clearly elevated cancer risk. Homozygotes for tumor suppressor gene mutations rarely if ever exist, probably because the condition is lethal during embryogenesis. It is important to remember that the tumor suppressor genes do not only function as guardians against cancer; their main function is the control of normal cell balance, and their inactivation is expected to be incompatible with normal embryonic development.

Because recessive cancer syndromes are quite rare, this discussion of the role of genomic stability genes in cancer will focus on syndromes that are inherited in autosomal dominant fashion. These syndromes include the most common types of familial cancers, predisposing to tumors of the colon, breast, and other organs.

DNA Mismatch Repair Gene Defects and Hereditary Nonpolyposis Colorectal Cancer Familial clustering of colon cancer has long been recognized, with approximately 5% of all colon cancers attributable to inheritance of a gene defect with a strong effect on cancer risk and another 10 to 15% with a moderate effect on risk. Germline *APC* mutations are responsible for 0.5 to 1% of colorectal cancer cases in the Western world, and hereditary nonpolyposis colorectal cancer (HNPCC) is responsible for 2 to 4%.[222–224]

Diagnosis of HNPCC is problematic when only clinical criteria are used. First, overt clinical findings prior to cancer diagnosis, such as the florid intestinal polyposis seen in individuals with FAP, are lacking in individuals with HNPCC. Second, for a common malignancy such as colorectal cancer, a likelihood of chance clustering always exists within a family. Nevertheless, diagnostic criteria for identifying those individuals and families most likely to be affected by HNPCC have been determined.[222–225] Representative diagnostic criteria include (1) exclusion of familial polyposis; (2) colorectal cancer in at least three relatives, one of them being a first-degree relative of the others; (3) two or more successive generations affected; and (4) at least one of the affected individuals being younger than 50 years of age at the time of diagnosis. Even though not all individuals affected by HNPCC meet those criteria, the criteria are useful for excluding familial aggregations of colorectal cancer that are likely to have a genetic basis distinct from that underlying the majority of HNPCC cases.[223,224]

Several genes responsible for HNPCC have been identified, including two on chromosome 2p (mutS homologs 2 and 6 [*MSH2*, *MSH6*]) and another on chromosome 3p (mutS homolog 1 [*MLH1*]). Together, germline mutations in these three genes account for virtually all classic HNPCC cases.[223–227] The protein products of the *MSH2* and *MLH1* genes appear to have critical roles in the recognition and repair of DNA mismatches (Figure 7-10). A number of other gene-encoding proteins that function in mismatch repair have been identified, and mutations inactivating the postmeiotic segregation increased 2 (*PMS2*) genes have been seen in a small fraction of those with HNPCC-like disease.[223–228]

In cells with one normal and one mutant allele of a DNA mismatch repair gene, DNA repair is minimally impaired, if at all. However, inactivation of the remaining allele can occur as a result of somatic mutation in a normal epithelial cell. This "second hit" abrogates mismatch repair function, and from hundreds to thousands of mutations may thereby occur during each subsequent cell-division cycle. Because these mutations preferentially arise in mononucleotide, dinucleotide, and trinucleotide repeat tracts (ie, microsatellite sequence tracts), the phenotype is often called the microsatellite instability (MSI) phenotype.

Germline mutations in the known multimerin (MMR) genes have been detected in only 2 to 4% of colorectal cancer patients, although approximately 10 to 15% of all colon cancers display the MSI phenotype.[224–227,229–231] Clearly, only a small fraction of the sporadic colorectal cancers with the MSI phenotype develop as the result of a germline mutation in a known mismatch repair gene. Somatic mutations in mismatch repair genes have been found in some sporadic colorectal cancers with the MSI phenotype.[232] In most sporadic cases, however, inactivation of the *MLH1* gene occurs as a result of epigenetic inactivation.[233,234] The basis for this inactivation and the molecular mechanism or mechanisms underlying the accompanying methylation of the *MLH1* gene promoter are unknown.

Many of the mutations arising in cells with MMR deficiency are likely to be detrimental to cell growth. A small fraction of the total mutations that arise presumably activate oncogenes or inactivate tumor suppressor genes. Some genes are preferentially mutated in MMR-deficiency cancers, presumably because the mutations confer a selective growth advantage. For instance, genes that contain repetitive DNA sequences, such as microsatellite tracts, might be expected to be targets of mutation in these cancers, and data support this prediction. An example of a gene that contains a mononucleotide repeat tract in its coding sequence, and that is frequently inactivated in colorectal cancers with MMR-deficiency, is the type II receptor for transforming growth factor-β (TGF-β).

The TGF-β type II receptor is a compelling candidate tumor suppressor gene, because both copies of the gene are inactivated by mutations in more than 90% of MSI colorectal cancers.[235,236] The TGF-β cytokine is known to inhibit the growth of many epithelial cells. Intriguingly, a recent study has suggested that germline mutations in the cytoplasmic domain of the TGF-β type II receptor is associated with HNPCC,[237] although it will be important to confirm this observation in additional HNPCC kindreds. Finally, a downstream effector of the TGF-β pathway, SMAD mothers against DPP homolog 4 (*SMAD4*, also called *DPC4*), has been identified as a tumor suppressor gene. *SMAD4* is somatically mutated in 45 to 50% of pancreatic cancers, in 10 to 20% of colorectal cancers, and in a very small fraction of other cancers.[238–240] Germline inactivating mutations in *SMAD4* are found in a major fraction of patients with juvenile polyposis syndrome (JPS).[241] Patients with JPS develop benign (hamartomatous, not adenomatous) pol-

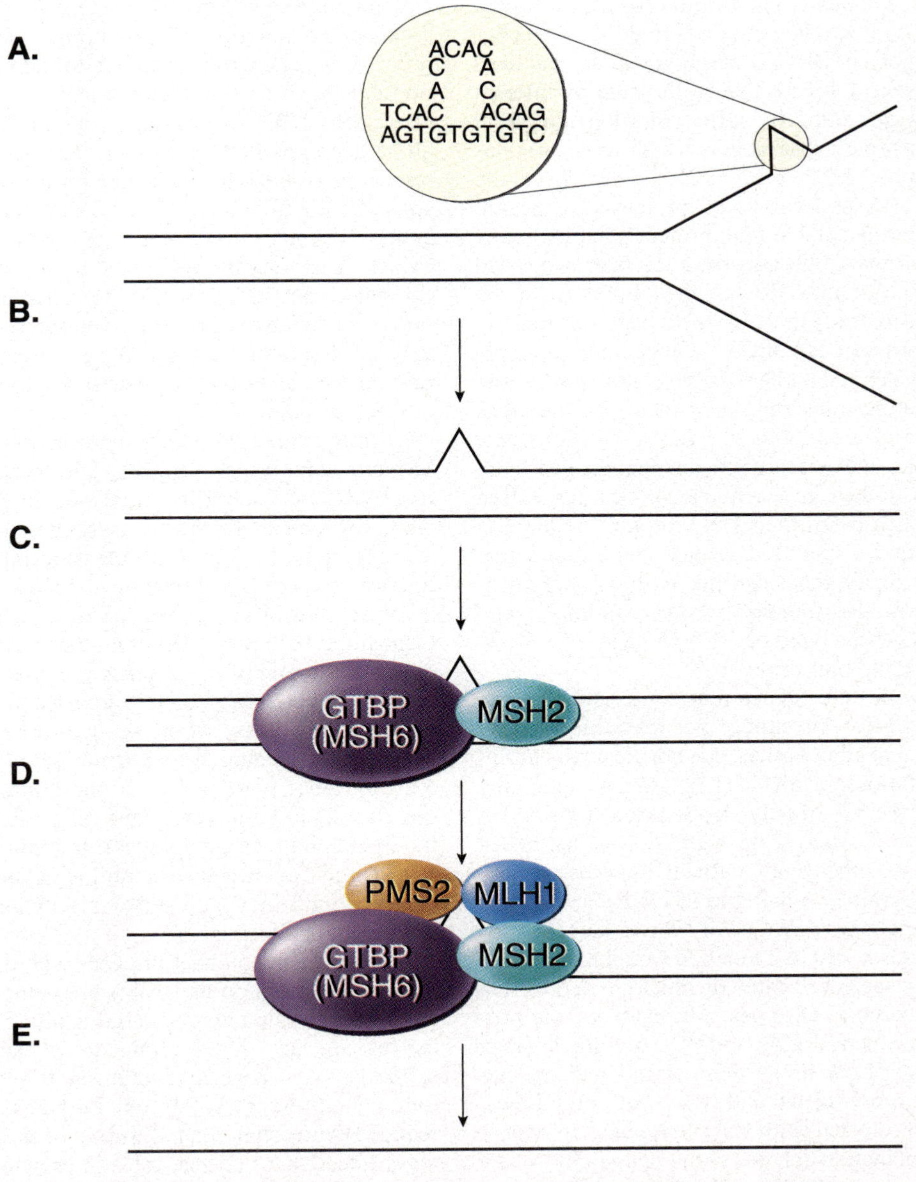

Figure 7-10 Mismatch repair pathway in human cells. **A, B,** During DNA replication, DNA mismatches may arise, such as from strand slippage (shown) or misincorporation of bases (not shown). **C,** The mismatch is recognized by MutS homologs, perhaps most often Msh2 and GTBP/Msh6, although another MutS homolog, Msh3, may substitute for GTBP/Msh6 in some cases. **D, E,** MutL homologs, such as Mlh1 and Pms2, are recruited to the complex and the mismatch is repaired through the action of a number of proteins, including an exonuclease, helicase, DNA polymerase, and ligase.

yps of the intestinal tract and are at increased risk of colorectal and gastric cancer. And germline mutations of a receptor for BMP, a TGF-β family member, have also been described to lead to JPS.[242]

Another recently suggested candidate for somatic inactivation in MMR-deficient colorectal cancers is the B cell lymphoma 2 (BCL-2)—associated X protein (*BAX*) gene,[243] which is a potential TP53-regulated gene encoding a BCL-2–related proapoptotic protein. Finally, there are data suggesting that gain-of-function mutations in β-catenin arise preferentially in MSI colon cancers,[149,150,244] although the β-catenin mutations are not present in a microsatellite tract. These mutation comparisons emphasize that it is the *pathways* rather than the specific genes that are best considered targets of mutations. In MMR-proficient cancers, *APC* is much more frequently mutated than is β-catenin, while the reverse is true for MMR-deficient cancers. These mutations have similar effects on the pathways through which APC and β-catenin control growth. Similarly, in MMR-proficient cancers, *TP53* is more often mutated than *BAX*, c-Ki-*ras*-2 is more often mutated than v-*raf* murine sarcoma viral oncogene homolog B1 (*BRAF*), and *SMAD4* is more often mutated than TGF-β RII, while the reverse is true for MMR-deficient cancers.[245] These provide excellent examples of the ways in which the spectrum of somatic mutations in specific cancers can provide important clues to pathogenesis.

***BRCA1* AND *BRCA2* GENES** As in the case of colorectal cancers, family history has long been hypothesized to be a major risk factor in breast cancer. The greatest risk is seen in those who have a history of breast cancer in multiple first-degree relatives. However, only in the late 1980s was evidence obtained that pre-disposition to breast cancer in some families could be attributed to a highly penetrant autosomal dominant allele. Subsequently, in 1990, Hall and colleagues reported the localization of one such breast cancer predisposition gene, *BRCA1*, on chromosome 17q21.[246] Others found that germline *BRCA1* mutations substantially increase the risk not only of breast cancer but also of ovarian cancer.[247,248] Intensive research efforts were focused on the region of chromosome 17q harboring *BRCA1*, and the gene was ultimately identified by positional cloning approaches in 1994.[249,250]

Studies of germline *BRCA1* mutations in breast cancer patients have yielded important results. In studies of families with four or more cases of breast or ovarian cancer (or both) diagnosed before age 60 years, germline *BRCA1* mutations were identified in nearly 50% of families studied.[251–253] In fact, germline *BRCA1* mutations may account for cancer predisposition in roughly 75% of families who manifest both breast and ovarian cancer.[251,253] Many distinct germline *BRCA1* mutations have been identified, although most of the mutations result in the synthesis of a truncated *BRCA1* protein.[251,253] Whereas most germline *BRCA1* mutations have been identified in only one or a few families, some mutations have been found recurrently. The 11 most common mutations account for about 45% of the total *BRCA1* mutations observed.[252,253] In fact, the two most common mutations in *BRCA1* (185delAG and 5382insC) account for approximately 10% of the total. Of note, the 185delAG frameshift mutation at codon 185 of *BRCA1*, involving a deletion of two bases (adenine and guanine), has been identified in more than 20 Jewish families with familial breast or ovarian cancer. Moreover, population surveys of Ashkenazi Jews, chosen without regard to a family history of cancer, indicate that approximately 1% carry the 185delAG mutation.[252–254] Based on studies of families with germline *BRCA1* mutations, the lifetime risks of breast cancer and ovarian cancer in those carrying an inactivating mutation are estimated to be 85% and 50%, respectively.[251,253,255] Whether specific germline *BRCA1* mutations confer a greater risk of breast and ovarian cancer than do other mutations remains uncertain.

As with most tumor suppressor genes and their associated familial cancer syndromes, germline mutations of *BRCA1* lead to the presence of a mutant allele in every cell of the body. Cancers then arise through inactivation of the second wild-type allele by the mechanisms outlined in Figure 7-2. In the case of *BRCA1* (and *BRCA2*), LOH of the remaining wild-type allele is usually responsible for the second "hit" leading to inactivation of the *BRCA1* gene. Additionally, LOH of the *BRCA1* locus was found in approximately 50% of unselected breast cancers and 65 to 80% of unselected ovarian cancers.[253,256] Because most breast and ovarian cancers are not associated with a hereditary predisposition (ie, they are sporadic), these studies of unselected cancers led investigators to hypothesize that *BRCA1* would play an important role in the development of sporadic breast and ovarian cancers. However, despite these LOH data, sporadic breast and ovarian cancers rarely, if ever, harbor mutations in the *BRCA1* gene, demonstrating that at least one-wild type allele is still present in most of these sporadic cancers.[253,256] Somewhat surprisingly, that finding would suggest that *BRCA1* does not have a role in the genesis of the more common, nonfamilial forms of breast and ovarian cancers. However, it is still possible that downstream effectors of the BRCA1 protein are altered in sporadic breast and ovarian cancers, suggesting that the pathway, rather than the gene, is an important contributor to the carcinogenic process of these cancers.

Although germline mutations in the *BRCA1* gene underlie cancer predisposition in roughly 40 to 50% of families with multiple breast cancer cases, another highly penetrant autosomal dominant susceptibility gene termed *BRCA2* plays a critical role in a significant fraction of the families with multiple breast cancer cases lacking *BRCA1* mutations. The *BRCA2* gene was mapped to chromosome 13q12–13 in 1994,[257] and identified by positional cloning strategies in 1995.[258] At the time of writing, many uncertainties about the nature, spectrum, prevalence, and significance of germline and somatic mutations in the *BRCA21* gene remain. However, several points have been fairly well established. First, although germline mutations in *BRCA1* and *BRCA2* appear to confer essentially similar lifetime risks of female breast cancer (ie, approximately 80%), the risk of ovarian cancer is reduced to approximately 10% in those with *BRCA2* mutations as compared with approximately 40 to 50% in those with *BRCA1* mutations. The risk of male breast cancer is markedly elevated in *BRCA2* mutation carriers, with a lifetime risk of approximately 6%. In contrast, no obvious risk of male breast cancer is found in *BRCA1* mutation carriers. There also appears to be an elevated risk of pancreatic and perhaps several other cancers in both male and female *BRCA2* mutation carriers.[253] As is the case for *BRCA1*, LOH of the *BRCA2* locus at 13q12, but not at the *RB1* locus at 13q14, has been observed in some sporadic breast, pancreatic, head and neck, and other cancers, suggesting that *BRCA2* may be a target for somatic mutations in cancer. However, as with *BRCA1*, detections of somatic *BRCA2* mutations in sporadic cancers have been few,[253] once again suggesting that perhaps the pathway, rather than the gene, is the target of genetic alteration in sporadic forms of these cancers.

The *BRCA1* and *BRCA2* genes each encode a large nuclear protein. The amino acid sequences of the two proteins have only short regions of similarity with one another or other well-characterized proteins. Although their lack of obvious functional motifs stymied initial attempts to define the cellular functions of BRCA1 and BRCA2, several lines of evidence indicate that both proteins interact directly or indirectly with homologs of yeast Rad51, a protein that functions in the repair of double-stranded DNA breaks.[259–266] Moreover, the BRCA1, BRCA2, and Rad51 proteins all appear to be present in a stable multiprotein complex in the cell's nucleus. Consequently, it has been suggested that BRCA1 and BRCA2 may function in the response to or repair of DNA damage, particularly double-strand DNA breaks. Other findings imply that BRCA1 and perhaps BRCA2 may have a role in regulating transcription.[267] Although the DNA repair and transcription regulation functions may be distinct, it is entirely possible that the two functions are linked in a process sometimes called transcription-coupled DNA repair.[263] There is precedent for this idea, in that some nucleotide excision repair genes causing xeroderma pigmentosum can also function in transcription,[268] and repair of certain types of DNA damage is known to be coupled to transcription.[269]

As with other genes that confer site-specific predisposition to cancer yet are ubiquitously expressed in adult tissues, it is not clear why germline mutations in *BRCA1* and *BRCA2* markedly increase the risk of only selected cancer types (eg, breast and ovarian). One suggestion is that breast and certain other epithelial cells may be particularly susceptible to the type of DNA damage that arises in cells with *BRCA1* or *BRCA2* defects. Loss of BRCA1 or BRCA2 function would then lead to markedly increased rates of mutation acquisition only in certain cell types. Alternatively, the processes in which BRCA1 and BRCA2 function may have many back-up systems or fail-safe mechanisms in most normal cell types, but not in breast and other selected epithelial cell types. A third possible explanation for the tissue specificity of the cancers seen in *BRCA1* and *BRCA2* mutation carriers is that inactivation of either BRCA1 or BRCA2 is most often associated with a detrimental or even a lethal effect in stem cells other than those of the breast or ovary. Finally, although the observations thus far have implicated BRCA1 and BRCA2 predominantly in maintenance of genome integrity, other functions for the proteins are possible. For example, a recent report suggests a link between the estrogen receptor and BRCA1 function, and another study demonstrates BRCA1 interaction with inactivated X chromosomes found only in female cells, thus providing another potential explanation for this tumor suppressor's tissue and gender specificity.[270,271]

Candidate Tumor Suppressor Genes The tumor suppressor genes discussed above and others summarized in Table 7-1 are distinguished by the fact that germline-inactivating mutations in the genes are associated with inherited cancer predisposition. The link between germline mutation and elevated cancer risk provides incontrovertible evidence of the gene's role in tumorigenesis. By analogy, this is akin to knockout mice, in which germline deletion of a single gene leads to a cancer phenotype thus providing unequivocal proof of a gene's role in tumor initiation. Other findings, such as the demonstration in sporadic cancers of LOH of one tumor suppressor gene allele accompanied by somatic mutation of the remaining allele, offer evidence for a more widespread role for many of the inherited cancer genes. Although the tumor suppressor genes in Table 7-1 are definitively linked to inherited cancer syndromes, it is possible that germline mutations in other bona fide tumor suppressor genes may be associated with a more modest cancer risk, as has already been demonstrated for the I1307K mutation in *APC*.

Tumor suppressor genes that are not found to be mutated in the germline may still frequently be inactivated by somatic mutations in sporadic forms of cancer. In these cases, their principal role may relate to tumor progression rather than tumor initiation. Because the evidence in favor of involvement of these genes does not include predisposition by inheritance in mutant form, confidence in the role of these genes in human tumorigenesis is not as high as for those listed in Table 7-1. Nevertheless, when such a gene can be shown to be mutated in a large number of cases of a given tumor type, and when the mutations are clearly inactivating (eg, truncating mutations), the likelihood that they play a role in tumorigenesis is high. A complete accounting of such genes can be found in Vogelstein and Kinzler[127] and Futreal and colleagues.[272]

An increasing number of genes with decreased or absent expression in cancers are being discovered through microarrays, serial analysis of gene expression, and other global gene expression techniques.[127] These genes are sometimes termed tumor suppressors solely on the basis of their reduced expression. A small subset of these genes may, indeed, have critical roles in growth regulation, but expression data provide insufficient evidence to invoke causality. The altered expression of genes in cancers more often reflects the effect than the cause of the neoplastic process (ie, the altered growth and differentiation properties of cancer cells and their abnormal microenvironment as compared with normal cells in the tissue or organ from which the cancer arose). Moreover, many genes that play no role in cancer can dramatically alter cell growth when expressed exogenously at a high, unphysiologic level, rendering functional analyses of such candidates problematic. In the end, the mutational and functional evidence should be carefully weighed before a conclusion can be drawn that a gene has a causal role in tumorigenesis and that it should appropriately be designated a tumor suppressor gene.

SUMMARY

There is now overwhelming evidence that mutations in tumor suppressor genes are major molecular determinants for most common human cancers. In the last 15 years, more than 30 tumor suppressor genes have been identified by molec-

Table 7-1 Tumor Suppressor and Stability Genes Associated with Inherited Cancer Predisposition Syndromes

Gene*	Syndrome	Hereditary Pattern	Second Hit	Pathway**	Major Hereditary Tumor Types***
Tumor Suppressor Genes					
APC	FAP	Dominant	Inactivation of wt allele	APC	Colon, thyroid, stomach, intestine
AXIN2	Attenuated polyposis	Dominant	Inactivation of wt allele	APC	Colon
CDH1 (E-cadherin)	Familial gastric carcinoma	Dominant	Inactivation of wt allele	APC	Stomach
GPC3	Simpson-Golabi-Behmel syndrome	X-linked	?	APC	Embryonal
CYLD	Familial cylindromatosis	Dominant	Inactivation of wt allele	APOP	Pilotrichomas
EXT1, EXT2	Hereditary multiple exostoses	Dominant	Inactivation of wt allele	GLI	Bone
PTCH	Gorlin	Dominant	Inactivation of wt allele	GLI	Skin, medulloblastoma
SUFU	Medulloblastoma predisposition	Dominant	Inactivation of wt allele	GLI	Skin, medulloblastoma
FH	Hereditary leiomyomatosis	Dominant	Inactivation of wt allele	HIF1	Leiomyomas
SDHB, SDHC, SDHD	Familial paraganglioma	Dominant	Inactivation of wt allele	HIF1	Paragangliomas, pheochromocytomas
VHL	Von Hippel-Lindau	Dominant	Inactivation of wt allele	HIF1	Kidney
TP53 (p53)	Li-Fraumeni	Dominant	Inactivation of wt allele	TP53	Breast, sarcoma, adrenal, brain, …
WT1	Familial Wilms tumor	Dominant	Inactivation of wt allele	TP53	Wilms
STK11 (LKB1)	Peutz-Jeghers	Dominant	Inactivation of wt allele	PI3K	Intestinal, ovarian, pancreatic
PTEN	Cowden	Dominant	Inactivation of wt allele	PI3K	Hamartoma, glioma, uterus
TSC1, TSC2	Tuberous sclerosis	Dominant	Inactivation of wt allele	PI3K	Hamartoma, kidney
CDKN2A ($p16^{INK4A}$, $p14^{ARF}$)	Familial malignant melanoma	Dominant	Inactivation of wt allele	RB	Melanoma, pancreas
CDK4	Familial malignant melanoma	Dominant	?	RB	Melanoma
RB1	Hereditary retinoblastoma	Dominant	Inactivation of wt allele	RB	Eye
NF1	Neurofibromatosis	Dominant	Inactivation of wt allele	RTK	Neurofibroma
BMPR1A	Juvenile polyposis	Dominant	Inactivation of wt allele	SMAD	Gastrointestinal
MEN1	Multiple endocrine neoplasia type I	Dominant	Inactivation of wt allele	SMAD	Parathyroid, pituitary, islet cell, carcinoid
SMAD4 (DPC4)	Juvenile polyposis	Dominant	Inactivation of wt allele	SMAD	Gastrointestinal
BHD	Birt-Hogg-Dube	Dominant	Inactivation of wt allele	?	Renal, hair follicle
HRPT2	Hyperparathyroidism jaw-tumor	Dominant	Inactivation of wt allele	?	Parathyroid, jaw fibroma
NF2	Neurofibromatosis	Dominant	Inactivation of wt allele	?	Meningioma, acoustic neuromas
Stability Genes					
MUTYH	Attenuated polyposis	Recessive	None required	BER	Colon
ATM	Ataxia-telangiectasia	Recessive	None required	CIN	Leukemias, lymphomas, brain
BLM	Bloom	Recessive	None required	CIN	Leukemias, lymphomas, skin
BRCA1, BRCA2	Hereditary breast cancer	Dominant	Inactivation of wt allele	CIN	Breast, ovary
FANCA, FANCC, FANCD2, FANCE, FANCF, FANCG	Fanconi anemia A, C, D2, E, F, and G	Recessive	None required	CIN	Leukemias
NBS1	Nijmegen breakage	Recessive	None required	CIN	Lymphomas, brain
RECQL4	Rothmund-Thomson	Recessive	None required	CIN	Bone and skin
WRN	Werner	Recessive	None required	CIN	Bone and brain
MSH2, MLH1, MSH6, PMS2	HNPCC	Dominant	Inactivation of wt allele	MMR	Colon, uterus
XPA, XPC; ERCC2, ERCC3, ERCC4, ERCC5; DDB2	Xeroderma pigmentosum	Recessive	None required	NER	Skin

Adapted from Vogelstein and Kinzler.[127]

* Representative genes of all the major pathways and hereditary cancer predisposition types are listed. Approved gene symbols are provided for each entry. Alternative names appear in parentheses.

** In many cases, the gene has been implicated in several pathways. The single pathway that is listed for each gene represents a "best guess" (when one can be made) and should not be regarded as conclusive.

*** In most cases, the non-familial tumor spectrum caused by somatic mutations of the gene includes those occurring in familial cases but also additional tumor types. For example, mutations of *TP53* and *CDKN2A* are found in many more tumor types than those to which Li-Fraumeni and familial malignant melanoma patients, respectively, are predisposed.

APC = adenomatous polyposis coli; APOP = apoptotic pathway; BER = base excision repair; CIN = chromosomal instability; FAP = familial adenomatous polyposis; GLI = glioma associated oncogene; HIF1 = hypoxia inducing factor 1; MMR = mismatch repair; NER = nucleotide excision repair; PI3K = phosphatidylinositol 3-kinase; RB = retinoblastoma; RTK = receptor tyrosine kinase pathway; SMAD = SMA and MAD related protein 4; wt = wild type.

ular cloning techniques. In some cases, these genes are inactivated in the germline, and their inactivation predisposes to cancer. Far more frequently, these same tumor suppressor genes are inactivated by somatic mutations during tumor development. Although much has been learned about tumor suppressor genes, a great deal of work remains. A more complete description of tumorigenesis will undoubtedly emerge with the identification of additional tumor suppressor genes, the detailed characterization of their normal cellular functions, and the elucidation of the frequency and spectrum of mutations and other mechanisms that inactivate these genes and their protein products in human tumors. The findings will not only provide new insights into cancer pathogenesis, but should also prove critical in improving the diagnosis and management of patients with cancer.

REFERENCES

1. Broca P. Etiologie des productions accidentelles. Traite des Tumerus 1866;147–57.
2. Haaland M. Spontaneous tumors in mice. Sci Rep Invest Imp Cancer Res Fund 1911;4:1.
3. Warthin A. Heredity with reference to carcinoma as shown by the study of the cases examined in the pathological library of the University of Michigan, 1895-1913. Arch Intern Med 1913;12:546.
4. Boveri T. The origin of malignant tumors. Baltimore (MD): Williams and Wilkins; 1929.
5. Rous P. A transmissible Avian neoplasm, (sarcoma of the common fowl). J Exp Med 1910;12:696–705.
6. Ephrussi B, Davidson RL, Weiss MC, et al. Malignancy of somatic cell hybrids. Nature 1969;224:1314–6.
7. Harris H. The analysis of malignancy by cell fusion: the position in 1988. Cancer Res 1988;48:3302–6.
8. Amundson SA, Myers TG, Fornace AJ Jr. Roles for *P53* in growth arrest and apoptosis: putting on the brakes after genotoxic stress. Oncogene 1998;17:3287–99.
9. Versteege I, Sevenet N, Lange J, et al. Truncating mutations of *hSNF5/INI1* in aggressive paediatric cancer. Nature 1998;394:203–6.

10. Stanbridge EJ, Der CJ, Doersen CJ, et al. Human cell hybrids: analysis of transformation and tumorigenicity. Science 1982;215:252–9.
11. Stanbridge EJ, Cavenee WK. Heritable cancer and tumor-suppressor genes: a tentative connection. In: Weinberg R, editor. Oncogenes and the molecular origins of cancer. Cold Spring Harbor (NY): Cold Spring Harbor Laboratory; 1989. p. 281–306.
12. Geiser AG, Der CJ, Marshall CJ, Stanbridge EJ. Suppression of tumorigenicity with continued expression of the c-Ha-*ras* oncogene in EJ bladder carcinoma–human fibroblast hybrid cells. Proc Natl Acad Sci U S A 1986;83:5209–13.
13. Saxon PJ, Srivatsan ES, Stanbridge EJ. Introduction of human chromosome 11 via microcell transfer controls tumorigenic expression of HeLa cells. EMBO J 1986;5:3461–6.
14. Weissman BE, Saxon PJ, Pasquale SR, et al. Introduction of a normal human chromosome 11 into a Wilms' tumor cell line controls its tumorigenic expression. Science 1987;236:175–80.
15. Knudson AG Jr. Mutation and cancer: statistical study of retinoblastoma. Proc Natl Acad Sci U S A 1971;68:820–3.
16. Orye E, Delbeke MJ, Vandenabeele B. Retinoblastoma and long arm deletion of chromosome 13. Attempts to define the deleted segment. Clin Genet 1974;5:457–64.
17. Francke U. Retinoblastoma and chromosome 13. Birth Defects Orig Artic Ser 1976;12:131–4.
18. Sparkes RS, Sparkes MC, Wilson MG, et al. Regional assignment of genes for human esterase D and retinoblastoma to chromosome band 13q14. Science 1980;208:1042–4.
19. Sparkes RS, Murphree AL, Lingua RW, et al. Gene for hereditary retinoblastoma assigned to human chromosome 13 by linkage to esterase D. Science 1983;219:971–3.
20. Benedict WF, Murphree AL, Banerjee A, et al. Patient with 13 chromosome deletion: evidence that the retinoblastoma gene is a recessive cancer gene. Science 1983;219:973–5.
21. Knudson AG Jr. Hereditary cancer, oncogenes, and antioncogenes. Cancer Res 1985;45:1437–43.
22. Cavenee WK, Dryja TP, Phillips RA, et al. Expression of recessive alleles by chromosomal mechanisms in retinoblastoma. Nature 1983;305:779–84.
23. Cavenee WK, Hansen MF, Nordenskjold M, et al. Genetic origin of mutations predisposing to retinoblastoma. Science 1985;228:501–3.
24. Hansen MF, Koufos A, Gallie BL, et al. Osteosarcoma and retinoblastoma: a shared chromosomal mechanism revealing recessive predisposition. Proc Natl Acad Sci U S A 1985;82:6216–20.
25. Hansen MF, Cavenee WK. Genetics of cancer predisposition. Cancer Res 1987;47:5518–27.
26. Dryja TP, Rapaport JM, Joyce JM, Petersen RA. Molecular detection of deletions involving band q14 of chromosome 13 in retinoblastomas. Proc Natl Acad Sci U S A 1986;83:7391–4.
27. Friend SH, Bernards R, Rogelj S, et al. A human DNA segment with properties of the gene that predisposes to retinoblastoma and osteosarcoma. Nature 1986;323:643–6.
28. Lee WH, Bookstein R, Hong F, et al. Human retinoblastoma susceptibility gene: cloning, identification, and sequence. Science 1987;235:1394–9.
29. Fung YK, Murphree AL, T'Ang A, et al. Structural evidence for the authenticity of the human retinoblastoma gene. Science 1987;236:1657–61.
30. Dunn JM, Phillips RA, Zhu X, et al. Mutations in the *RB1* gene and their effects on transcription. Mol Cell Biol 1989;9:4596–604.
31. Goddard AD, Balakier H, Canton M, et al. Infrequent genomic rearrangement and normal expression of the putative *RB1* gene in retinoblastoma tumors. Mol Cell Biol 1988;8:2082–8.
32. Weichselbaum RR, Beckett M, Diamond A. Some retinoblastomas, osteosarcomas, and soft tissue sarcomas may share a common etiology. Proc Natl Acad Sci U S A 1988;85:2106–9.
33. Yandell DW, Campbell TA, Dayton SH, et al. Oncogenic point mutations in the human retinoblastoma gene: their application to genetic counseling. N Engl J Med 1989;321:1689–95.
34. Sellers WR, Kaelin WG Jr. Role of the retinoblastoma protein in the pathogenesis of human cancer. J Clin Oncol 1997;15:3301–12.
35. Whyte P, Buchkovich KJ, Horowitz JM, et al. Association between an oncogene and an anti-oncogene: the adenovirus E1A proteins bind to the retinoblastoma gene product. Nature 1988;334:124–9.
36. Moran E, Mathews MB. Multiple functional domains in the adenovirus *E1A* gene. Cell 1987;48:177–8.
37. Whyte P, Williamson NM, Harlow E. Cellular targets for transformation by the adenovirus E1A proteins. Cell 1989;56:67–75.
38. DeCaprio JA, Ludlow JW, Figge J, et al. SV40 large tumor antigen forms a specific complex with the product of the retinoblastoma susceptibility gene. Cell 1988;54:275–83.
39. Dyson N, Howley PM, Munger K, Harlow E. The human papilloma virus-16 E7 oncoprotein is able to bind to the retinoblastoma gene product. Science 1989;243:934–7.
40. Kaelin WG Jr. Functions of the retinoblastoma protein. Bioessays 1999;21:950–8.
41. Wu L, Timmers C, Maiti B, et al. The E2F1-3 transcription factors are essential for cellular proliferation. Nature 2001;414:457–62.
42. Lane DP, Crawford LV. T antigen is bound to a host protein in SV40-transformed cells. Nature 1979;278:261–3.
43. Linzer DI, Levine AJ. Characterization of a 54K dalton cellular SV40 tumor antigen present in SV40-transformed cells and uninfected embryonal carcinoma cells. Cell 1979;17:43–52.
44. DeLeo AB, Jay G, Appella E, et al. Detection of a transformation-related antigen in chemically induced sarcomas and other transformed cells of the mouse. Proc Natl Acad Sci U S A 1979;76:2420–4.
45. Sarnow P, Ho YS, Williams J, Levine AJ. Adenovirus E1b-58kd tumor antigen and SV40 large tumor antigen are physically associated with the same 54 kd cellular protein in transformed cells. Cell 1982;28:387–94.
46. Crawford LV, Pim DC, Lamb P. The cellular protein P53 in human tumours. Mol Biol Med 1984;2:261–72.
47. Lane DP, Benchimol S. P53: oncogene or anti-oncogene? Genes Dev 1990;4:1–8.
48. Eliyahu D, Raz A, Gruss P, et al. Participation of P53 cellular tumour antigen in transformation of normal embryonic cells. Nature 1984;312:646–9.
49. Jenkins JR, Rudge K, Currie GA. Cellular immortalization by a cDNA clone encoding the transformation-associated phosphoprotein P53. Nature 1984;312:651–4.
50. Parada LF, Land H, Weinberg RA, et al. Cooperation between gene encoding P53 tumour antigen and *ras* in cellular transformation. Nature 1984;312:649–51.
51. Baker SJ, Fearon ER, Nigro JM, et al. Chromosome 17 deletions and *P53* gene mutations in colorectal carcinomas. Science 1989;244:217–21.
52. Fearon ER, Hamilton SR, Vogelstein B. Clonal analysis of human colorectal tumors. Science 1987;238:193–7.
53. Vogelstein B, Fearon ER, Hamilton SR, et al. Genetic alterations during colorectal-tumor development. N Engl J Med 1988;319:525–32.
54. Wolf D, Rotter V. Major deletions in the gene encoding the P53 tumor antigen cause lack of P53 expression in HL-60 cells. Proc Natl Acad Sci U S A 1985;82:790–4.
55. Mowat M, Cheng A, Kimura N, et al. Rearrangements of the cellular *P53* gene in erythroleukaemic cells transformed by Friend virus. Nature 1985;314:633–6.
56. Masuda H, Miller C, Koeffler HP, et al. Rearrangement of the *P53* gene in human osteogenic sarcomas. Proc Natl Acad Sci U S A 1987;84:7716–9.
57. Ahuja H, Bar-Eli M, Advani SH, et al. Alterations in the *P53* gene and the clonal evolution of the blast crisis of chronic myelocytic leukemia. Proc Natl Acad Sci U S A 1989;86:6783–7.
58. Eliyahu D, Goldfinger N, Pinhasi-Kimhi O, et al. Meth A fibrosarcoma cells express two transforming mutant *P53* species. Oncogene 1988;3:313–21.
59. Eliyahu D, Michalovitz D, Eliyahu S, et al. Wild-type *P53* can inhibit oncogene-mediated focus formation. Proc Natl Acad Sci U S A 1989;86:8763–7.
60. Finlay CA, Hinds PW, Levine AJ. The *P53* proto-oncogene can act as a suppressor of transformation. Cell 1989;57:1083–93.
61. Hinds P, Finlay C, Levine AJ. Mutation is required to activate the *P53* gene for cooperation with the *ras* oncogene and transformation. J Virol 1989;63:739–46.
62. Baker SJ, Markowitz S, Fearon ER, et al. Suppression of human colorectal carcinoma cell growth by wild-type *P53*. Science 1990;249:912–5.
63. Hollstein M, Hergenhahn M, Yang Q, et al. New approaches to understanding *P53* gene tumor mutation spectra. Mutat Res 1999;431:199–209.
64. Malkin D, Li FP, Strong LC, et al. Germ line *P53* mutations in a familial syndrome of breast cancer, sarcomas, and other neoplasms. Science 1990;250:1233–8.
65. Srivastava S, Zou ZQ, Pirollo K, et al. Germ-line transmission of a mutated *P53* gene in a cancer-prone family with Li-Fraumeni syndrome. Nature 1990;348:747–9.
66. Birch JM, Hartley AL, Tricker KJ, et al. Prevalence and diversity of constitutional mutations in the *P53* gene among 21 Li-Fraumeni families. Cancer Res 1994;54:1298–304.
67. Malkin D. *P53* and the Li-Fraumeni syndrome. Biochim Biophys Acta 1994;1198:197–213.
68. Bartek J, Falck J, Lukas J. CHK2 kinase—a busy messenger. Nat Rev Mol Cell Biol 2001;2:877–86.
69. Werness BA, Levine AJ, Howley PM. Association of human papillomavirus types 16 and 18 E6 proteins with *P53*. Science 1990;248:76–9.
70. Scheffner M, Huibregtse JM, Vierstra RD, Howley PM. The HPV-16 E6 and E6-AP complex functions as a ubiquitin–protein ligase in the ubiquitination of *P53*. Cell 1993;75:495–505.
71. Scheffner M, Munger K, Byrne JC, Howley PM. The state of the *P53* and retinoblastoma genes in human cervical carcinoma cell lines. Proc Natl Acad Sci U S A 1991;88:5523–7.
72. Kessis TD, Slebos RJ, Han SM, et al. *P53* gene mutations and *MDM2* amplification are uncommon in primary carcinomas of the uterine cervix. Am J Pathol 1993;143:1398–405.
73. Crook T, Vousden KH. Properties of *P53* mutations detected in primary and secondary cervical cancers suggest mechanisms of metastasis and involvement of environmental carcinogens. EMBO J 1992;11:3935–40.
74. Oliner JD, Kinzler KW, Meltzer PS, et al. Amplification of a gene encoding a *P53*-associated protein in human sarcomas. Nature 1992;358:80–3.
75. Momand J, Zambetti GP, Olson DC, et al. The MDM-2 oncogene product forms a complex with the P53 protein and inhibits P53-mediated transactivation. Cell 1992;69:1237–45.
76. Haupt Y, Maya R, Kazaz A, Oren M. Mdm2 promotes the rapid degradation of P53. Nature 1997;387:296–9.
77. Juven-Gershon T, Oren M. Mdm2: the ups and downs. Mol Med 1999;5:71–83.
78. Leach FS, Tokino T, Meltzer P, et al. *P53* mutation and *MDM2* amplification in human soft tissue sarcomas. Cancer Res 1993;53:2231–4.
79. Montes de Oca Luna R, Wagner DS, Lozano G. Rescue of early embryonic lethality in MDM2-deficient mice by deletion of *P53*. Nature 1995;378:203–6.
80. Falini B, Mecucci C, Tiacci E, et al. Cytoplasmic nucleophosmin in acute myelogenous leukemia with a normal karyotype. N Engl J Med 2005;352:254–66.
81. Vogelstein B, Lane D, Levine AJ. Surfing the P53 network. Nature 2000;408:307–10.
82. el-Deiry WS. Regulation of *P53* downstream genes. Semin Cancer Biol 1998;8:345–57.
83. el-Deiry WS, Tokino T, Velculescu VE, et al. *WAF1*, a potential mediator of *P53* tumor suppression. Cell 1993;75:817–25.
84. Hermeking H, Lengauer C, Polyak K, et al. 14-3-3 sigma is a P53-regulated inhibitor of G2/M progression. Mol Cell 1997;1:3–11.
85. Yu J, Wang Z, Kinzler KW, et al. *PUMA* mediates the apoptotic response to P53 in colorectal cancer cells. Proc Natl Acad Sci U S A 2003;100:1931–6.
86. Waldman T, Kinzler KW, Vogelstein B. P21 is necessary for the P53-mediated G1 arrest in human cancer cells. Cancer Res 1995;55:5187–90.
87. Cho Y, Gorina S, Jeffrey PD, Pavletich NP. Crystal structure of a P53 tumor suppressor–DNA complex: understanding tumorigenic mutations. Science 1994;265:346–55.
88. Lang GA, Iwakuma T, Suh YA, et al. Gain of function of a *P53* hot spot mutation in a mouse model of Li-Fraumeni syndrome. Cell 2004;119:861–72.
89. Olive KP, Tuveson DA, Ruhe ZC, et al. Mutant P53 gain of function in two mouse models of Li-Fraumeni syndrome. Cell 2004;119:847–60.
90. Topley GI, Okuyama R, Gonzales JG, et al. P21(WAF1/Cip1) functions as a suppressor of malignant skin tumor formation and a determinant of keratinocyte stem-cell potential. Proc Natl Acad Sci U S A 1999;96:9089–94.
91. Jeffers JR, Parganas E, Lee Y, et al. *PUMA* is an essential mediator of P53-dependent and -independent apoptotic pathways. Cancer Cell 2003;4:321–8.
92. Villunger A, Michalak EM, Coultas L, et al. P53- and drug-induced apoptotic responses mediated by BH3-only proteins *PUMA* and *NOXA*. Science 2003; 302:1036–8.
93. Bunz F, Dutriaux A, Lengauer C, et al. Requirement for *P53* and *p21* to sustain G2 arrest after DNA damage. Science 1998;282:1497–501.

94. Chan TA, Hermeking H, Lengauer C, et al. 14-3-3Sigma is required to prevent mitotic catastrophe after DNA damage. Nature 1999;401:616–20.
95. Lowe SW, Ruley HE, Jacks T, Housman DE. P53-dependent apoptosis modulates the cytotoxicity of anticancer agents. Cell 1993;74:957–67.
96. Lowe SW, Bodis S, McClatchey A, et al. *P53* status and the efficacy of cancer therapy in vivo. Science 1994;266:807–10.
97. Bunz F, Hwang PM, Torrance C, et al. Disruption of P53 in human cancer cells alters the responses to therapeutic agents. J Clin Invest 1999;104:263–9.
98. Graeber TG, Osmanian C, Jacks T, et al. Hypoxia-mediated selection of cells with diminished apoptotic potential in solid tumours. Nature 1996;379:88–91.
99. Wahl GM, Linke SP, Paulson TG, Huang LC. Maintaining genetic stability through TP53 mediated checkpoint control. Cancer Surv 1997;29:183–219.
100. Merlo A, Gabrielson E, Askin F, Sidransky D. Frequent loss of chromosome 9 in human primary non-small cell lung cancer. Cancer Res 1994;54:640–2.
101. Olumi AF, Skinner EC, Tsai YC, Jones PA. Molecular analysis of human bladder cancer. Semin Urol 1990;8:270–7.
102. Sidransky D, Messing E. Molecular genetics and biochemical mechanisms in bladder cancer. Oncogenes, tumor suppressor genes, and growth factors. Urol Clin North Am 1992;19:629–39.
103. van der Riet P, Nawroz H, Hruban RH, et al. Frequent loss of chromosome 9p21-22 early in head and neck cancer progression. Cancer Res 1994;54:1156–8.
104. Diaz MO, Rubin CM, Harden A, et al. Deletions of interferon genes in acute lymphoblastic leukemia. N Engl J Med 1990;322:77–82.
105. Fountain JW, Karayiorgou M, Taruscio D, et al. Genetic and physical map of the interferon region on chromosome 9p. Genomics 1992;14:105–12.
106. Olopade OI, Jenkins RB, Ransom DT, et al. Molecular analysis of deletions of the short arm of chromosome 9 in human gliomas. Cancer Res 1992;52:2523–9.
107. Goldstein AM, Tucker MA. Genetic epidemiology of familial melanoma. Dermatol Clin 1995; 13:605–12.
108. Kamb A, Gruis NA, Weaver-Feldhaus J, et al. A cell cycle regulator potentially involved in genesis of many tumor types. Science 1994;264:436–40.
109. Serrano M, Hannon GJ, Beach D. A new regulatory motif in cell-cycle control causing specific inhibition of cyclin D/CDK4. Nature 1993;366:704–7.
110. Haber DA. Splicing into senescence: the curious case of *p16* and *p19*^{ARF}. Cell 1997;91:555–8.
111. Sherr CJ. Tumor surveillance via the ARF–P53 pathway. Genes Dev 1998;12:2984–91.
112. Hussussian CJ, Struewing JP, Goldstein AM, et al. Germline p16 mutations in familial melanoma. Nat Genet 1994;8:15–21.
113. Kamb A, Shattuck-Eidens D, Eeles R, et al. Analysis of the *p16* gene (*CDKN2*) as a candidate for the chromosome 9p melanoma susceptibility locus. Nat Genet 1994;8:23–6.
114. Wainwright B. Familial melanoma and p16—a hung jury. Nat Genet 1994;8:3–5.
115. Whelan AJ, Bartsch D, Goodfellow PJ. Brief report: a familial syndrome of pancreatic cancer and melanoma with a mutation in the *CDKN2* tumor-suppressor gene. N Engl J Med 1995; 333:975–7.
116. Walker GJ, Flores JF, Glendening JM, et al. Virtually 100% of melanoma cell lines harbor alterations at the DNA level within *CDKN2A*, *CDKN2B*, or one of their downstream targets. Genes Chromosomes Cancer 1998;22:157–63.
117. Cairns P, Polascik TJ, Eby Y, et al. Frequency of homozygous deletion at *p16/CDKN2* in primary human tumours. Nat Genet 1995;11:210–2.
118. Quelle DE, Zindy F, Ashmun RA, Sherr CJ. Alternative reading frames of the *INK4A* tumor suppressor gene encode two unrelated proteins capable of inducing cell cycle arrest. Cell 1995;83:993–1000.
119. Herman JG, Merlo A, Mao L, et al. Inactivation of the *CDKN2/p16/MTS1* gene is frequently associated with aberrant DNA methylation in all common human cancers. Cancer Res 1995; 55:4525–30.
120. Merlo A, Herman JG, Mao L, et al. 5' CpG island methylation is associated with transcriptional silencing of the tumour suppressor *p16/CDKN2/MTS1* in human cancers. Nat Med 1995;1:686–92.
121. Jacobs JJ, Kieboom K, Marino S, et al. The oncogene and Polycomb-group gene *BMI-1* regulates cell proliferation and senescence through the *INK4A* locus. Nature 1999;397:164–8.
122. Rhee I, Bachman KE, Park BH, et al. DNMT1 and DNMT3B cooperate to silence genes in human cancer cells. Nature 2002;416:552–6.
123. Bachman KE, Park BH, Rhee I, et al. Histone modifications and silencing prior to DNA methylation of a tumor suppressor gene. Cancer Cell 2003;3:89–95.
124. Kamijo T, Zindy F, Roussel MF, et al. Tumor suppression at the mouse *Ink4a* locus mediated by the alternative reading frame product p19ARF. Cell 1997;91:649–59.
125. Sharpless NE, Bardeesy N, Lee KH, et al. Loss of *p16*^{Ink4a} with retention of *p19*^{Arf} predisposes mice to tumorigenesis. Nature 2001;413:86–91.
126. Krimpenfort P, Quon KC, Mooi WJ, et al. Loss of *p16*^{Ink4a} confers susceptibility to metastatic melanoma in mice. Nature 2001;413:83–6.
127. Vogelstein B, Kinzler KW. Cancer genes and the pathways they control. Nat Med 2004;10:789–99.
128. Schmitt CA, Fridman JS, Yang M, et al. A senescence program controlled by *P53* and *p16*^{INK4A} contributes to the outcome of cancer therapy. Cell 2002;109:335–46.
129. Herrera L, Kakati S, Gibas L, et al. Gardner syndrome in a man with an interstitial deletion of 5q. Am J Med Genet 1986;25:473–6.
130. Bodmer WF, Bailey CJ, Bodmer J, et al. Localization of the gene for familial adenomatous polyposis on chromosome 5. Nature 1987;328:614–6.
131. Leppert M, Dobbs M, Scambler P, et al. The gene for familial polyposis coli maps to the long arm of chromosome 5. Science 1987;238:1411–3.
132. Groden J, Thliveris A, Samowitz W, et al. Identification and characterization of the familial adenomatous polyposis coli gene. Cell 1991;66:589–600.
133. Joslyn G, Carlson M, Thliveris A, et al. Identification of deletion mutations and three new genes at the familial polyposis locus. Cell 1991;66:601–13.
134. Kinzler KW, Nilbert MC, Su LK, et al. Identification of *FAP* locus genes from chromosome 5q21. Science 1991;253:661–5.
135. Nishisho I, Nakamura Y, Miyoshi Y, et al. Mutations of chromosome 5q21 genes in FAP and colorectal cancer patients. Science 1991;253:665–9.
136. Miyoshi Y, Ando H, Nagase H, et al. Germ-line mutations of the *APC* gene in 53 familial adenomatous polyposis patients. Proc Natl Acad Sci U S A 1992;89:4452–6.
137. Nagase H, Miyoshi Y, Horii A, et al. Correlation between the location of germ-line mutations in the *APC* gene and the number of colorectal polyps in familial adenomatous polyposis patients. Cancer Res 1992;52:4055–7.
138. Powell SM, Petersen GM, Krush AJ, et al. Molecular diagnosis of familial adenomatous polyposis. N Engl J Med 1993;329:1982–7.
139. Levy DB, Smith KJ, Beazer-Barclay Y, et al. Inactivation of both *APC* alleles in human and mouse tumors. Cancer Res 1994;54:5953–8.
140. Kinzler KW, Vogelstein B. Lessons from hereditary colorectal cancer. Cell 1996;87:159–70.
141. Spirio L, Olschwang S, Groden J, et al. Alleles of the *APC* gene: an attenuated form of familial polyposis. Cell 1993;75:951–7.
142. Gruber SB, Petersen GM, Kinzler KW, Vogelstein B. Cancer, crash sites, and the new genetics of neoplasia. Gastroenterology 1999;116:210–2.
143. Powell SM, Zilz N, Beazer-Barclay Y, et al. *APC* mutations occur early during colorectal tumorigenesis. Nature 1992;359:235–7.
144. Solomon E, Voss R, Hall V, et al. Chromosome 5 allele loss in human colorectal carcinomas. Nature 1987;328:616-9.
145. Smith KJ, Johnson KA, Bryan TM, et al. The APC gene product in normal and tumor cells. Proc Natl Acad Sci U S A 1993;90:2846–50.
146. Morin PJ, Vogelstein B, Kinzler KW. Apoptosis and APC in colorectal tumorigenesis. Proc Natl Acad Sci U S A 1996;93:7950–4.
147. Bienz M. APC: the plot thickens. Curr Opin Genet Dev 1999;9:595–603.
148. Willert K, Nusse R. Beta-catenin: a key mediator of Wnt signaling. Curr Opin Genet Dev 1998;8:95–102.
149. Morin PJ, Sparks AB, Korinek V, et al. Activation of beta-catenin-Tcf signaling in colon cancer by mutations in beta-catenin or *APC*. Science 1997;275:1787–90.
150. Sparks AB, Morin PJ, Vogelstein B, Kinzler KW. Mutational analysis of the APC/beta-catenin/Tcf pathway in colorectal cancer. Cancer Res 1998;58:1130–4.
151. Iwao K, Nakamori S, Kameyama M, et al. Activation of the beta-catenin gene by interstitial deletions involving exon 3 in primary colorectal carcinomas without adenomatous polyposis coli mutations. Cancer Res 1998;58:1021–6.
152. Polakis P. The oncogenic activation of beta-catenin. Curr Opin Genet Dev 1999;9:15–21.
153. Crawford HC, Fingleton BM, Rudolph-Owen LA, et al. The metalloproteinase matrilysin is a target of beta-catenin transactivation in intestinal tumors. Oncogene 1999;18:2883–91.
154. He TC, Sparks AB, Rago C, et al. Identification of c-*myc* as a target of the Apc pathway. Science 1998;281:1509–12.
155. Tetsu O, McCormick F. Beta-catenin regulates expression of cyclin D1 in colon carcinoma cells. Nature 1999;398:422–6.
156. Shtutman M, Zhurinsky J, Simcha I, et al. The cyclin D1 gene is a target of the beta-catenin/LEF-1 pathway. Proc Natl Acad Sci U S A 1999;96:5522–7.
157. Park BH, Vogelstein B, Kinzler KW. Genetic disruption of *PPAR*delta decreases the tumorigenicity of human colon cancer cells. Proc Natl Acad Sci U S A 2001;98:2598–603.
158. Kim JS, Crooks H, Dracheva T, et al. Oncogenic beta-catenin is required for bone morphogenetic protein 4 expression in human cancer cells. Cancer Res 2002;62:2744–8.
159. Sancho E, Batlle E, Clevers H. Signaling pathways in intestinal development and cancer. Annu Rev Cell Dev Biol 2004;20:695–723.
160. Coppes MJ, Haber DA, Grundy PE. Genetic events in the development of Wilms' tumor. N Engl J Med 1994;331:586–90.
161. Knudson AG Jr, Strong LC. Mutation and cancer: a model for Wilms' tumor of the kidney. J Natl Cancer Inst 1972;48:313–24.
162. Miller RW, Fraumeni JF Jr, Manning MD. Association of Wilms's tumor with aniridia, hemihypertrophy and other congenital malformations. N Engl J Med 1964;270:922–7.
163. Francke U, Holmes LB, Atkins L, Riccardi VM. Aniridia-Wilms' tumor association: evidence for specific deletion of 11p13. Cytogenet Cell Genet 1979;24:185–92.
164. Kaneko Y, Egues MC, Rowley JD. Interstitial deletion of short arm of chromosome 11 limited to Wilms' tumor cells in a patient without aniridia. Cancer Res 1981;41:4577–8.
165. Slater RM, de Kraker J. Chromosome number 11 and Wilms' tumor. Cancer Genet Cytogenet 1982;5:237–45.
166. Fearon ER, Vogelstein B, Feinberg AP. Somatic deletion and duplication of genes on chromosome 11 in Wilms' tumours. Nature 1984;309:176–8.
167. Koufos A, Hansen MF, Lampkin BC, et al. Loss of alleles at loci on human chromosome 11 during genesis of Wilms' tumour. Nature 1984;309:170–2.
168. Orkin SH, Goldman DS, Sallan SE. Development of homozygosity for chromosome 11p markers in Wilms' tumour. Nature 1984;309:172–4.
169. Reeve AE, Housiaux PJ, Gardner RJ, et al. Loss of a Harvey *ras* allele in sporadic Wilms' tumour. Nature 1984;309:174–6.
170. Call KM, Glaser T, Ito CY, et al. Isolation and characterization of a zinc finger polypeptide gene at the human chromosome 11 Wilms' tumor locus. Cell 1990;60:509–20.
171. Haber DA, Sohn RL, Buckler AJ, et al. Alternative splicing and genomic structure of the Wilms tumor gene *WT1*. Proc Natl Acad Sci U S A 1991;88:9618–22.
172. Larsson SH, Charlieu JP, Miyagawa K, et al. Subnuclear localization of *WT1* in splicing or transcription factor domains is regulated by alternative splicing. Cell 1995;81:391–401.
173. Reddy JC, Licht JD. The *WT1* Wilms' tumor suppressor gene: how much do we really know? Biochim Biophys Acta 1996;1287:1–28.
174. Rauscher FJ 3rd. The WT1 Wilms tumor gene product: a developmentally regulated transcription factor in the kidney that functions as a tumor suppressor. FASEB J 1993;7:896–903.
175. Englert C, Hou X, Maheswaran S, et al. WT1 suppresses synthesis of the epidermal growth factor receptor and induces apoptosis. EMBO J 1995; 14:4662–75.
176. Hosono S, Gross I, English MA, et al. E-cadherin is a WT1 target gene. J Biol Chem 2000;275:10943–53.
177. Lee SB, Huang K, Palmer R, et al. The Wilms tumor suppressor *WT1* encodes a transcriptional activator of amphiregulin. Cell 1999;98:663–73.
178. Hammes A, Guo JK, Lutsch G, et al. Two splice variants of the Wilms' tumor 1 gene have distinct functions during sex determination and nephron formation. Cell 2001;106:319–29.

179. Haber DA, Housman DE. The genetics of Wilms' tumor. Adv Cancer Res 1992;59:41–68.
180. Mannens M, Slater RM, Heyting C, et al. Molecular nature of genetic changes resulting in loss of heterozygosity of chromosome 11 in Wilms' tumours. Hum Genet 1988;81:41–8.
181. Reeve AE, Sih SA, Raizis AM, Feinberg AP. Loss of allelic heterozygosity at a second locus on chromosome 11 in sporadic Wilms' tumor cells. Mol Cell Biol 1989;9:1799–803.
182. Koufos A, Grundy P, Morgan K, et al. Familial Wiedemann-Beckwith syndrome and a second Wilms tumor locus both map to 11p15.5. Am J Hum Genet 1989;44:711–9.
183. Ping AJ, Reeve AE, Law DJ, et al. Genetic linkage of Beck-with-Wiedemann syndrome to 11p15. Am J Hum Genet 1989;44:720–3.
184. Grundy P, Koufos A, Morgan K, et al. Familial predisposition to Wilms' tumour does not map to the short arm of chromosome 11. Nature 1988;336:374–6.
185. Huff V, Compton DA, Chao LY, et al. Lack of linkage of familial Wilms' tumour to chromosomal band 11p13. Nature 1988;336:377–8.
186. Ponder B. Human genetics. Neurofibromatosis gene cloned. Nature 1990;346:703–4.
187. Shen MH, Harper PS, Upadhyaya M. Molecular genetics of neurofibromatosis type 1 (NF1). J Med Genet 1996;33:2–17.
188. Gutman DH, Collins FS. Neurofibromatosis type 1. In: Kinzler KW, Vogelstein B, editors. The genetic basis of human cancer. New York: McGraw-Hill; 1998. p. 423–42.
189. Barker D, Wright E, Nguyen K, et al. Gene for von Recklinghausen neurofibromatosis is in the pericentromeric region of chromosome 17. Science 1987;236:1100–2.
190. Seizinger BR, Rouleau GA, Ozelius LJ, et al. Genetic linkage of von Recklinghausen neurofibromatosis to the nerve growth factor receptor gene. Cell 1987;49:589–94.
191. Fountain JW, Wallace MR, Bruce MA, et al. Physical mapping of a translocation breakpoint in neurofibromatosis. Science 1989;244:1085–7.
192. O'Connell P, Leach R, Cawthon RM, et al. Two *NF1* translocations map within a 600-kilobase segment of 17q11.2. Science 1989;244:1087–8.
193. Cawthon RM, Weiss R, Xu GF, et al. A major segment of the neurofibromatosis type 1 gene: cDNA sequence, genomic structure, and point mutations. Cell 1990;62:193–201.
194. Viskochil D, Buchberg AM, Xu G, et al. Deletions and a translocation interrupt a cloned gene at the neurofibromatosis type 1 locus. Cell 1990;62:187–92.
195. Wallace MR, Marchuk DA, Andersen LB, et al. Type 1 neurofibromatosis gene: identification of a large transcript disrupted in three NF1 patients. Science 1990;249:181–6.
196. Viskochil D, White R, Cawthon R. The neurofibromatosis type 1 gene. Annu Rev Neurosci 1993;16:183–205.
197. Park VM, Pivnick EK. Neurofibromatosis type 1 (NF1): a protein truncation assay yielding identification of mutations in 73% of patients. J Med Genet 1998;35:813–20.
198. Johnson MR, Look AT, DeClue JE, et al. Inactivation of the *NF1* gene in human melanoma and neuroblastoma cell lines without impaired regulation of GTP.Ras. Proc Natl Acad Sci U S A 1993;90:5539–43.
199. Seizinger BR. *NF1*: a prevalent cause of tumorigenesis in human cancers? Nat Genet 1993;3:97–9.
200. The I, Murthy AE, Hannigan GE, et al. Neurofibromatosis type 1 gene mutations in neuroblastoma. Nat Genet 1993;3:62–6.
201. Shannon KM, O'Connell P, Martin GA, et al. Loss of the normal *NF1* allele from the bone marrow of children with type 1 neurofibromatosis and malignant myeloid disorders. N Engl J Med 1994;330:597–601.
202. DeClue JE, Papageorge AG, Fletcher JA, et al. Abnormal regulation of mammalian p21*ras* contributes to malignant tumor growth in von Recklinghausen (type 1) neurofibromatosis. Cell 1992;69:265–73.
203. Wigler MH. Oncoproteins. GAPs in understanding *ras*. Nature 1990;346:696–7.
204. Xu GF, O'Connell P, Viskochil D, et al. The neurofibromatosis type 1 gene encodes a protein related to GAP. Cell 1990;62:599–608.
205. MacCollin M, Gusella J. Neurofibromatosis type 2. In: Kinzler KW, Vogelstein B, editors. The genetic basis of human cancer. New York: McGraw-Hill; 1998. p. 443–54.
206. Evans DG, Huson SM, Donnai D, et al. A genetic study of type 2 neurofibromatosis in the United Kingdom. I. Prevalence, mutation rate, fitness, and confirmation of maternal transmission effect on severity. J Med Genet 1992;29:841–6.
207. Seizinger BR, Martuza RL, Gusella JF. Loss of genes on chromosome 22 in tumorigenesis of human acoustic neuroma. Nature 1986;322:644–7.
208. Seizinger BR, de la Monte S, Atkins L, et al. Molecular genetic approach to human meningioma: loss of genes on chromosome 22. Proc Natl Acad Sci U S A 1987;84:5419–23.
209. Seizinger BR, Rouleau G, Ozelius LJ, et al. Common pathogenetic mechanism for three tumor types in bilateral acoustic neurofibromatosis. Science 1987;236:317–9.
210. Rouleau GA, Merel P, Lutchman M, et al. Alteration in a new gene encoding a putative membrane-organizing protein causes neuro-fibromatosis type 2. Nature 1993;363:515–21.
211. Trofatter JA, MacCollin MM, Rutter JL, et al. A novel moesin-, ezrin-, radixin-like gene is a candidate for the neurofibromatosis 2 tumor suppressor. Cell 1993;72:791–800.
212. Bianchi AB, Mitsunaga SI, Cheng JQ, et al. High frequency of inactivating mutations in the neurofibromatosis type 2 gene (*NF2*) in primary malignant mesotheliomas. Proc Natl Acad Sci U S A 1995;92:10854–8.
213. Giovannini M, Robanus-Maandag E, van der Valk M, et al. Conditional biallelic *Nf2* mutation in the mouse promotes manifestations of human neurofibromatosis type 2. Genes Dev 2000;14:1617–30.
214. Maher ER, Webster AR, Moore AT. Clinical features and molecular genetics of von Hippel-Lindau disease. Ophthalmic Genet 1995;16:79–84.
215. Gnarra JR, Duan DR, Weng Y, et al. Molecular cloning of the von Hippel-Lindau tumor suppressor gene and its role in renal carcinoma. Biochim Biophys Acta 1996;1242:201–10.
216. Linehan WM, Klausner R. Renal carcinoma. In: Kinzler KW, Vogelstein B, editors. The genetic basis of human cancer. 2nd ed. New York: McGraw-Hill; 1998. p. 455–74.
217. Seizinger BR, Rouleau GA, Ozelius LJ, et al. Von Hippel-Lindau disease maps to the region of chromosome 3 associated with renal cell carcinoma. Nature 1988;332:268–9.
218. Latif F, Tory K, Gnarra J, et al. Identification of the von Hippel-Lindau disease tumor suppressor gene. Science 1993;260:1317–20.
219. Herman JG, Latif F, Weng Y, et al. Silencing of the *VHL* tumor-suppressor gene by DNA methylation in renal carcinoma. Proc Natl Acad Sci U S A 1994;91:9700–4.
220. Kerbel R, Folkman J. Clinical translation of angiogenesis inhibitors. Nat Rev Cancer 2002;2:727–39.
221. Gatti RA. Ataxia-telangiectasia. In: Kinzler KW, Vogelstein B, editors. The genetic basis of human cancer. New York: McGraw-Hill; 1998. p. 275–300.
222. Lynch HT, Smyrk TC, Watson P, et al. Genetics, natural history, tumor spectrum, and pathology of hereditary nonpolyposis colorectal cancer: an updated review. Gastroenterology 1993;104:1535–49.
223. Park JG, Vasen HF, Park KJ, et al. Suspected hereditary nonpolyposis colorectal cancer: International Collaborative Group on Hereditary Non-Polyposis Colorectal Cancer (ICG-HNPCC) criteria and results of genetic diagnosis. Dis Colon Rectum 1999;42:710–5; discussion 715–6.
224. Boland CR. Hereditary nonpolyposis colorectal cancer. In: Kinzler KW, Vogelstein B, editors. The genetic basis of human cancer. New York: McGraw-Hill; 1998. p. 333–46.
225. Lynch HT, de la Chapelle A. Genetic susceptibility to nonpolyposis colorectal cancer. J Med Genet 1999;36:801–18.
226. Aaltonen LA. Hereditary intestinal cancer. Semin Cancer Biol 2000;10:289–98.
227. Yan H, Papadopoulos N, Marra G, et al. Conversion of diploidy to haploidy. Nature 2000;403:723–4.
228. Muller A, Fishel R. Mismatch repair and the hereditary nonpolyposis colorectal cancer syndrome (HNPCC). Cancer Invest 2002;20:102–9.
229. Ionov Y, Peinado MA, Malkhosyan S, et al. Ubiquitous somatic mutations in simple repeated sequences reveal a new mechanism for colonic carcinogenesis. Nature 1993;363:558–61.
230. Thibodeau SN, Bren G, Schaid D. Microsatellite instability in cancer of the proximal colon. Science 1993;260:816–9.
231. Aaltonen LA, Peltomaki P, Leach FS, et al. Clues to the pathogenesis of familial colorectal cancer. Science 1993;260:812–6.
232. Liu B, Nicolaides NC, Markowitz S, et al. Mismatch repair gene defects in sporadic colorectal cancers with microsatellite instability. Nat Genet 1995;9:48–55.
233. Kane MF, Loda M, Gaida GM, et al. Methylation of the hMLH1 promoter correlates with lack of expression of hMLH1 in sporadic colon tumors and mismatch repair-defective human tumor cell lines. Cancer Res 1997;57:808–11.
234. Herman JG, Umar A, Polyak K, et al. Incidence and functional consequences of hMLH1 promoter hypermethylation in colorectal carcinoma. Proc Natl Acad Sci U S A 1998;95:6870–5.
235. Markowitz S, Wang J, Myeroff L, et al. Inactivation of the type II TGF-beta receptor in colon cancer cells with microsatellite instability. Science 1995;268:1336–8.
236. Parsons R, Myeroff LL, Liu B, et al. Microsatellite instability and mutations of the transforming growth factor beta type II receptor gene in colorectal cancer. Cancer Res 1995;55:5548–50.
237. Lu SL, Kawabata M, Imamura T, et al. HNPCC associated with germline mutation in the TGF-beta type II receptor gene. Nat Genet 1998;19:17–8.
238. Hahn SA, Schutte M, Hoque AT, et al. *DPC4*, a candidate tumor suppressor gene at human chromosome 18q21.1. Science 1996;271:350–3.
239. Moskaluk CA, Kern SE. Cancer gets Mad: *DPC4* and other TGFbeta pathway genes in human cancer. Biochim Biophys Acta 1996;1288:M31–3.
240. Thiagalingam S, Lengauer C, Leach FS, et al. Evaluation of candidate tumour suppressor genes on chromosome 18 in colorectal cancers. Nat Genet 1996;13:343–6.
241. Howe JR, Roth S, Ringold JC, et al. Mutations in the *SMAD4/DPC4* gene in juvenile polyposis. Science 1998;280:1086–8.
242. Howe JR, Bair JL, Sayed MG, et al. Germline mutations of the gene encoding bone morphogenetic protein receptor 1A in juvenile polyposis. Nat Genet 2001;28:184–7.
243. Rampino N, Yamamoto H, Ionov Y, et al. Somatic frameshift mutations in the *BAX* gene in colon cancers of the microsatellite mutator phenotype. Science 1997;275:967–9.
244. Mirabelli-Primdahl L, Gryfe R, Kim H, et al. Beta-catenin mutations are specific for colorectal carcinomas with microsatellite instability but occur in endometrial carcinomas irrespective of mutator pathway. Cancer Res 1999;59:3346–51.
245. Lengauer C, Kinzler KW, Vogelstein B. Genetic instabilities in human cancers. Nature 1998;396:643–9.
246. Hall JM, Lee MK, Newman B, et al. Linkage of early-onset familial breast cancer to chromosome 17q21. Science 1990;250:1684–9.
247. Easton DF, Bishop DT, Ford D, Crockford GP. Genetic linkage analysis in familial breast and ovarian cancer: results from 214 families. The Breast Cancer Linkage Consortium. Am J Hum Genet 1993;52:678–701.
248. Narod SA, Feunteun J, Lynch HT, et al. Familial breast-ovarian cancer locus on chromosome 17q12-q23. Lancet 1991;338:82–3.
249. Futreal PA, Liu Q, Shattuck-Eidens D, et al. *BRCA1* mutations in primary breast and ovarian carcinomas. Science 1994;266:120–2.
250. Miki Y, Swensen J, Shattuck-Eidens D, et al. A strong candidate for the breast and ovarian cancer susceptibility gene *BRCA1*. Science 1994;266:66–71.
251. Collins FS. *BRCA1*–lots of mutations, lots of dilemmas. N Engl J Med 1996;334:186–8.
252. Couch FJ, Weber BL. Mutations and polymorphisms in the familial early-onset breast cancer (*BRCA1*) gene. Breast Cancer Information Core. Hum Mutat 1996;8:8–18.
253. Couch FJ, Weber BL. In: Vogelstein B, Kinzler KW, editors. The genetic basis of human cancer. New York: McGraw-Hill; 1998. p. 537–64.
254. Szabo CI, King MC. Inherited breast and ovarian cancer. Hum Mol Genet 1995;4 Spec No:1811–7.
255. King MC, Marks JH, Mandell JB. Breast and ovarian cancer risks due to inherited mutations in *BRCA1* and *BRCA2*. Science 2003;302:643–6.
256. Merajver SD, Pham TM, Caduff RF, et al. Somatic mutations in the *BRCA1* gene in sporadic ovarian tumours. Nat Genet 1995;9:439–43.
257. Wooster R, Neuhausen SL, Mangion J, et al. Localization of a breast cancer susceptibility gene, *BRCA2*, to chromosome 13q12-13. Science 1994;265:2088–90.
258. Wooster R, Bignell G, Lancaster J, et al. Identification of the breast cancer susceptibility gene *BRCA2*. Nature 1995;378:789–92.
259. Sharan SK, Morimatsu M, Albrecht U, et al. Embryonic lethality and radiation hypersensitivity mediated by Rad51 in mice lacking *Brca2*. Nature 1997;386:804–10.

260. Welcsh PL, Schubert EL, King MC. Inherited breast cancer: an emerging picture. Clin Genet 1998;54:447–58.
261. Feunteun J. Breast cancer and genetic instability: the molecules behind the scenes. Mol Med Today 1998; 4:263–7.
262. Chen J, Silver DP, Walpita D, et al. Stable interaction between the products of the *BRCA1* and *BRCA2* tumor suppressor genes in mitotic and meiotic cells. Mol Cell 1998;2:317–28.
263. Gowen LC, Avrutskaya AV, Latour AM, et al. *BRCA1* required for transcription-coupled repair of oxidative DNA damage. Science 1998;281:1009–12.
264. Scully R, Chen J, Plug A, et al. Association of *BRCA1* with Rad51 in mitotic and meiotic cells. Cell 1997; 88:265–75.
265. Scully R, Chen J, Ochs RL, et al. Dynamic changes of *BRCA1* subnuclear location and phosphorylation state are initiated by DNA damage. Cell 1997;90:425–35.
266. Marmorstein LY, Ouchi T, Aaronson SA. The Brca2 gene product functionally interacts with P53 and Rad51. Proc Natl Acad Sci U S A 1998;95:13869–74.
267. Scully R, Anderson SF, Chao DM, et al. Brca1 is a component of the RNA polymerase II holoenzyme. Proc Natl Acad Sci U S A 1997;94:5605–10.
268. Bootsma D, Kraemer KH, Cleaver JE, Hoeijmakers JHJ. Nucleotide excision repair syndromes: xeroderma pigmentosum, Cockayne syndrome, and trichothiodystrophy. In: Kinzler KW, Vogelstein B, editors. The genetic basis of human cancer. 2nd ed. New York: McGraw-Hill; 2002. p. 211–38.
269. Hanawalt PC, Ford JM, Lloyd DR. Functional characterization of global genomic DNA repair and its implications for cancer. Mutat Res 2003;544:107–14.
270. Fan S, Wang J, Yuan R, et al. Brca1 inhibition of estrogen receptor signaling in transfected cells. Science 1999;284:1354–6.
271. Ganesan S, Silver DP, Greenberg RA, et al. Brca1 supports Xist RNA concentration on the inactive X chromosome. Cell 2002;111:393–405.
272. Futreal PA, Coin L, Marshall M, et al. A census of human cancer genes. Nat Rev Cancer 2004;4:177–83.

8

Genomic Alterations and Chromosomal Aberrations in Human Cancer

Cheryl L. Willman, MD
Robert A. Hromas, MD

INTRODUCTION

Since the dawn of the new millennium in 2000, we have entered a technological revolution in biomedical research. Rapid advances in genomics, proteomics, cell biology, bioengineering, imaging, and computational sciences are providing extraordinary new tools for probing the genetics and biology of cancer cells and tissues, both *in vitro* and *in vivo*. Increasingly, cancer is recognized as a heterogeneous collection of diseases whose initiation and progression are promoted by the aberrant function of genes that regulate DNA repair, genome stability, cell proliferation, cell death, adhesion, angiogenesis, invasion, and metastasis in complex cell and tissue microenvironments.[1,2] Of the 25,000 genes in the human genome, over 1%, or approximately 350 genes have been causally linked to the development of cancer to date (please see online edition for Table 8-1).[3–5] Variant or aberrant function of these so-called cancer genes may result from naturally occurring DNA polymorphisms, changes in genome copy number (through amplification, deletion, chromosome loss, or duplication), changes in gene and chromosome structure (through chromosomal translocation, inversion, or other rearrangement that leads to chimeric transcripts or deregulated gene expression), and point mutations (including base substitutions, deletions, or insertions in coding regions and splice sites) (Table 8-2). Beyond perturbations of the DNA sequence itself, heritable epigenetic modifications of the genome, including DNA methylation, genomic imprinting, and histone modification by acetylation, methylation, or phosphorylation, have also been shown to play a critical role in tumorigenesis.[6–7] Inactivation of genes that normally suppress the cancer phenotype (tumor suppressor genes) have been shown to occur through mutation, deletion, and epigenetic modifications, while activation of genes that promote the cancer phenotype (oncogenes) may occur through mutation, amplification, epigenetic modifications, and structural chromosomal rearrangements.[1,2] Strikingly, the function of the same cancer-promoting gene may be disrupted through different molecular mechanisms in tumors of different lineages (see Table 8-1). Although the vast majority (90%) of cancer genes identified to date are mutated or altered through chromosomal aberrations in somatic tissues, 10%

Table 8-2 Glossary

Alu Element:	Alu sequences are a family of short interspersed repeats and are the most abundant repeat sequences in the human genome, comprising 5–10% of the total human genome sequence. Alu sequences can be found at sites of chromosome aberrations in human cancer and may foster chromosomal rearrangements.
BAC:	Bacterial artificial chromosome; a cloning vector that contains very large (45–70 kb) human genomic DNA fragments; BAC clones covering > 98% of the human genome are now available for FISH chromosomal studies.
Centromere:	The constriction along the length of the chromosome that is the site of the spindle fiber attachment. The position of the centromere determines whether chromosomes are metacentric (X-shaped, such as chromosomes 1, 3, 16, 19 20) or acrocentric (inverted V-shaped, such as chromosomes 13–15, 21, 22, Y).
CGH:	Comparative genomic hybridization. CGH is a fluorescent molecular cytogenetic technique for determining copy number gains and losses and amplifications between two samples of DNA, by competitively hybridizing differentially labeled DNA from these samples to normal metaphase chromosomes (Figure 7A and 7B).
Clone:	In traditional chromosomal banding studies and analysis of metaphase chromosome spreads, a "clone" is defined as two cells with the same additional or structurally rearranged chromosome or three cells with loss of the same chromosome.
Deletion:	A segment of a chromosome is missing as the result of two breaks and loss of the intervening piece (Figure 8-3).
Diploid:	Normal chromosome number and composition of chromosomes.
Epigenetic:	Epigenetics is the study of the heritable changes in gene function that result from modifications to the genome (such as methylation or chromatin remodeling), rather than changes in the primary DNA sequence itself.
FISH:	FISH is a technique in which DNA probes are labeled with various fluorochromes (e.g., rhodamine), followed by hybridization to either metaphase spreads or interphase cells and detected using fluorescence microscopy (Figures 8-1B and 8-4).
Hyperdiploid:	Additional chromosomes therefore the modal number is 47 or greater.
Hypodiploid:	Loss of chromosomes with modal number 45 or less.
Haploid:	Only one-half the normal complement, ie, 23 chromosomes.
Inversion:	Two breaks occur in the same chromosome with rotation of the intervening segment. If both the breaks are on the same side of the centromere, it is called a paracentric inversion. If they are on opposite sides, it is called a pericentric inversion (Figure 8-3).
Isochromosome:	A chromosome that consists of identical copies of one chromosome arm with loss of the other arm. Thus, an isochromosome for the long arm of No. 17 [i(17q)] contains two copies of the long arm (separated by the centromere) with loss of the short arm of the chromosome.
Karyotype:	Arrangement of chromosomes from a particular cell according to a well-established system such that the largest chromosomes are first and the smallest ones are last. Normal female karyotype is 46,XX; normal male karyotype is 46,XX.
DNA Polymorphism:	One of two or more alternate forms (alleles) of a chromosomal locus that differ in nucleotide sequence or have variable numbers of repeated nucleotide units.
Single Nucleotide Polymorphism (SNP):	SNPs (pronounced "snips") are heritable DNA sequence variations that occur when a single nucleotide (A,T,C,or G) in the genome sequence is changed. Most SNPs involve the replacement of cytosine (C) with thymine (T). Occurring every 100 to 300 bases along the human genome, SNPs are the most frequent type of human DNA polymorphism. They are heritable and stable from generation to generation.
SKY:	SKY (Figure 8-5) and M-FISH (Figure 8-6) are molecular cytogenetic techniques that permit the simultaneous visualization of all human chromosomes in different colors, facilitating karyotype analysis. For these techniques, chromosome-specific probe pools (referred to as "chromosome painting" probes) generated from flow cytometric-sorted chromosomes, are amplified and then fluorescently labeled and hybridized to metaphase chromosomes.
Translocation:	A break in at least two chromosomes with exchange of material; in a reciprocal translocation, such that there is no obvious loss of chromosomal material. (Figure 8-3).
YAC:	Yeast artificial chromosome; a yeast cloning vector that contains large human genomic DNA fragments.

are altered in the germline, thereby transmitting heritable cancer susceptibility through successive generations (see Table 8-1).[3]

From the discovery of the first chromosomal abnormality in human cancer in 1960 by Nowell—the "Philadelphia chromosome" fragment associated with chronic myelogenous leukemia (CML)[8]—and the determination by Rowley in 1973, using newly developed chromosomal banding techniques, that the Philadelphia chromosome was actually a balanced reciprocal translocation between chromosomes 9 and 22 (Figure 8-1),[9–10] the study and cataloguing of genomic and chromosomal aberrations in cancer has accelerated at a rapid pace. Today, in addition to high resolution chromosome banding and advanced chromosomal imaging technologies, chromosome aberrations in cancer cells can be analyzed with an increasing number of large-scale, comprehensive genomic and molecular genetic technologies discussed and illustrated throughout this chapter. These techniques include fluorescence in situ hybridization (FISH),[11–14] spectral karyotyping (SKY),[11] comparative genomic hybridization (CGH),[15–19] and other high-throughput methods that detect loss of heterozygosity (LOH),[2,18,20] in cancer cells such as the new single nucleotide polymorphism arrays (SNP Chips)[21] that detect comprehensive genome-wide copy number changes. Extensive catalogues of the cytogenetic aberrations observed in over 48,000 human tumors have been compiled and are now maintained and regularly updated online (see The Mitelman Database of Chromosome Aberrations in Cancer at the US National Cancer Institute [NCI] Cancer Genome Anatomy Project [CGAP] Web site: <http://cgap.nci.nih.gov>).[22] The NCI Cancer Genome Anatomy Project is focused on integrating cytogenetic and physical maps of the human cancer genome, through the generation of a repository of human BAC clones (see Table 8-2) from the entire genome that can be fluorescently labeled and used as probes to localize genes and identify chromosomal regions involved in cancer chromosome aberrations, and through the maintenance of online databases of SKY, CGH, and FISH studies of chromosome aberrations in human cancer (see <http://cgap.nci.nih.gov>). Large-scale DNA sequencing projects focused on high throughput sequencing of selected gene families in human tumors, such as those underway by the Wellcome Trust Sanger Institute Cancer Genome Project (<http://www.sanger.ac.uk>), have identified novel point mutations in cancer genes.[3,4,23] Other clinically significant cancer gene mutations have recently been identified, such as those in *EGFR*, because they are associated with striking responses in subsets of patients treated with targeted therapeutic agents.[24,25] The Wellcome Trust Sanger Institute Cancer Genome Project maintains a highly useful detailed online "Cancer Gene Census" of all human genes that have been causally linked to tumorigenesis (see Table 8-1; <http://www.sanger.ac.uk/genetics/CGP/Census/>)[3,4] as well as the COSMIC (Catalogue Of Somatic Mutations in Cancer) database of somatic mutations in human cancer (<http://www.sanger.ac.uk/genetics/

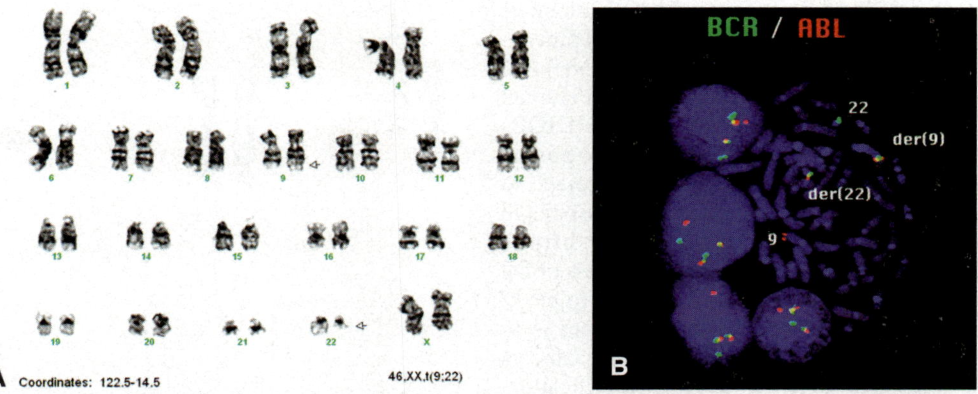

Figure 8-1 **A,** Chromosome G banded karyotype of metaphase chromosomes from a case of chronic myelogenous leukemia (CML): 46,XX, t(9;22). **B,** Interphase and metaphase FISH detection of the t(9;22) BCR-ABL gene fusion using fluorescently-labeled genomic probes for the BCR (green) and ABL (red). Note that the fusion of BCR and ABL probes results in a yellow signal indicating co-localization of the red and green probes as a result of the t(9;22). Figures courtesy of Dr. Susana Raimondi of St. Jude Children's Research Hospital.

CGP/cosmic/>). Interestingly, the most common functional domain in the 347 cancer genes identified to date (see Table 8-1) is the protein kinase domain, followed by functional domains involved in DNA binding or transcriptional regulation.[3,4] Given the rapid proliferation, enormous complexity, and sheer quantity of data on chromosomal aberrations and mutations in human cancer, frequently updated Web-based catalogues have become one of the most important vehicles for data dissemination.

Paralleling the rapid pace of discovery in human cancer genetics and genomics, although proceeding at a much slower pace, is the development and testing of novel therapies targeted to specific cancer gene mutations and chromosomal aberrations. It is particularly fitting that one of the first successful targeted cancer therapies was developed to the first reported chromosomal abnormality in human cancer (see Figure 8-1). The seminal discovery of the t(9;22) Philadelphia chromosome translocation[8–10] laid the foundation for the subsequent cloning and characterization of the *BCR-ABL* chimeric fusion gene arising from the t(9;22), the determination that *BCR-ABL* encoded a constitutively active tyrosine kinase, and the ultimate development of one of the first successfully targeted cancer therapies by Drucker and colleagues—the selective tyrosine kinase inhibitor imatinib, or Gleevec, for the treatment of cell-mediated lympholysis (CML).[26–28] This paradigm has been repeated with dramatic success. Several newly introduced cancer drugs targeted to specific genomic lesions have shown clinical efficacy: imatinib/Gleevec, not only for the selective inhibition of the ABL kinase in CML, but also the PDGFR and KIT tyrosine kinases altered by genomic changes in gastrointestinal stromal tumors and hypereosinophilic syndromes[29–31]; trastuzumab/Herceptin, the neutralizing antibody targeted to Her2/ErbB2 tyrosine kinase receptor whose encoding gene *ERBB2* is amplified and overexpressed in 25 to 30% of breast carcinomas[32,33]; and gefitinib/Iressa or erlotinib/Tarceva, recently shown to have striking effectiveness in the 5 to 10% of lung adenocarcinomas in patients with European ancestry and 25 to 30% of Japanese patients who harbor activating mutations in the *EGFR* gene.[24,25] Clinical trials are underway with many novel therapeutic agents directed against genomic targets in cancer, including *FLT3* mutations in leukemia,[34,35] *VHL* mutations in renal cell carcinoma,[36] and *B-RAF* mutations in melanoma.[37,38]

Despite the initial success of therapies targeted to single gene mutations in human cancers, the therapeutic effectiveness of these agents is frequently not sustained, and tumors evolve molecular mechanisms and acquire additional mutations that ultimately lead to therapeutic resistance. Overwhelming evidence supports the hypothesis that cancer is caused by the stepwise accumulation of numerous genetic and epigenetic aberrations.[1] Even in CML, where the *BCR-ABL* fusion is essential for initiation, maintenance, and disease progression, the transformation of CML from chronic to blast phase is associated with the acquisition of additional genetic and epigenetic abnormalities.[26] Studies of the recurrent cytogenetic abnormalities associated with the acute leukemias, such as the t(15;17) in acute promyelocytic leukemia, the t(8;21) and inv(16) in acute myeloid leukemia (AML), and the recurrent translocations that are the hallmarks of pediatric acute lymphoblastic leukemia (ALL), have shown that these signature fusion genes are not sufficient for tumorigenesis and that additional genomic changes are required.[39] Thus, comprehensive discovery and the functional analysis of the full spectrum of genomic changes in each human cancer is not only essential for continued advances in cancer research, but also is paramount for improved cancer diagnosis and treatment and the development of new and more effective therapies with curative intent. A detailed understanding of the genomic lesions underlying cancer will facilitate the identification of the cellular pathways and networks perturbed by genomic mutations, improve cancer diagnosis through molecular classification, enhance the selection of therapeutic targets for drug development, promote the development of faster and more efficient clinical trials using agents targeted to specific genomic abnormalities, and create markers for early detection and prevention. To meet these challenges, the US National Cancer Institute and National Institute for Human Genome Research Genome Institute (NIHGR) are planning to launch a new collaborative project in 2006, the Human Cancer Genome Project, to identify all of the genomic alterations associated with all major cancer types (see <http://cgap.nci.nih.gov>). Building on the success of the highly collaborative Human Genome Project,[40] the intent of this comprehensive program is to completely characterize the major human cancers for all regions of genomic loss and amplification, all mutations in coding genes, all chromosome rearrangements, all regions of aberrant methylation, and to derive complete gene expression profiles from each tumor. The ultimate success of such comprehensive, large-scale projects will continue to rapidly advance our understanding of cancer genetics and genomics and will potentially revolutionize our approach to the diagnosis and treatment of cancer.

CHROMOSOME NOMENCLATURE AND CANCER CYTOGENETIC ABERRATIONS

Normal human diploid cells have 22 pairs of autosomes (nonsex chromosomes), numbered from chromosome 1 (the longest human chromosome) to 22 (the smallest double-stranded DNA fragment), and two sex chromosomes (X or Y) (Figure 8-2). Traditional cytogenetic analyses are performed on metaphase chromosomes spreads (karyotypes) and, hence, can be obtained only from actively dividing normal or cancer cells. This essential characteristic has complicated the cytogenetic analysis of many tumors, particularly solid tumors, which may be difficult to adapt to short-term *in vitro* cultures to derive metaphases. Cells under analysis must be suspended and exposed to a hypotonic solution, fixed, and stained according to a variety of protocols. Brief exposure of metaphase chromosomes to mitotic inhibitors, DNA-binding agents to elongate chromosomes, or amethopterin or fluorodeoxyuridine to synchronize cells has resulted in longer, more distinct chromosomes. To enhance the likelihood of obtaining acceptable metaphases from hematopoietic as well as solid tumors, PHA-stimulated conditioned medium, recombinant colony-stimulating factors, and other lineage-specific growth factors are frequently added to the culture medium.

Banding of human chromosomes is essential for traditional cytogenetic investigations because it allows the identification of individual chromosomes and creates regional markers for physical mapping and topography. A band is defined as a chromosome area that is distinguished from adjacent segments by appearing darker or lighter through one or more banding techniques, including quinacrine-mustard (Q bands) and trypsin-Giemsa (G bands) staining (see Figure 8-2). Typically, approximately 600 bands can be discerned under high-power microscopy in a metaphase spread using chromosome banding techniques. Each chromosome band and subband is numbered from the centromere to the telomere of each arm, allowing investigators to be able to consistently refer to specific chromosomal bands and regions. International standards have been developed and are applied to the descriptive nomenclature that defines chromosome topography and karyotypic aberrations (insertions, deletions, translocations, amplifications) in cancer cells (Table 8-3).[41] This cytogenetic nomenclature is under constant refinement with the use of newer state of the art means of chromosome analysis, including SKY, CGH, and FISH (see <http://cgap.nci.nih.gov>). The longest arm from the centromere of each chromosome is termed the q arm, and the short arm is termed the p arm (see Table 8-3). Visual karyotypes, derived from chromosome metaphases of actively dividing cells, are usually displayed with the long arm of each chromosome on the bottom (see Figure 8-2). When a karyotype is displayed in written form, the total number of chromosomes (the modal number) is followed by the sex chromosomes.

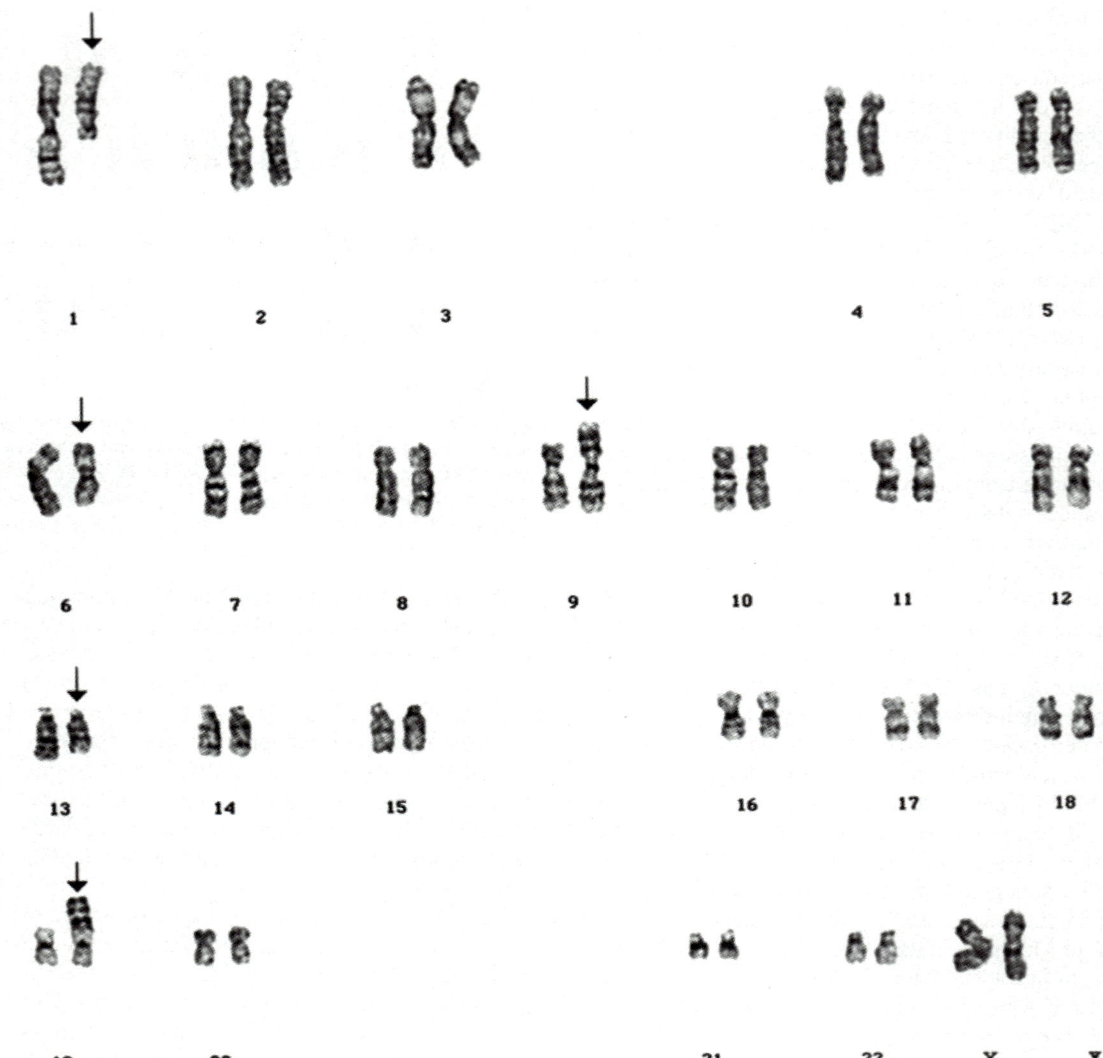

Figure 8-2 Chromosome G banded karyotype of metaphase chromosomes from a case of pediatric B precursor acute lymphocytic leukemia (ALL) with the recurrent t(1;19)46,XX,t(1;19)(q23;p13.3),del(6)(q21q25),i(9)(q10),del(13)(q22q32). Figure courtesy of Dr. Andrew Carroll, University of Alabama at Birmingham.

There is considerable variability in the degree to which cancer genomes are aberrant at the chromosomal level in different human tumors. Some cancers are characterized by a single signature chromosomal abnormality, such as a recurrent translocation, while others have numerous aberrations and very complex karyotypes. In solid epithelial-derived tumors, cytogenetic analyses have identified many structural chromosomal aberrations, but in contrast to hematopoietic and mesenchymal tumors, very few are recurrent.[1,22] The sheer number and variety of chromosome aberrations in many tumors has led some to assert that many aberrations are "noise," but the majority of the evidence supports the view that the seemingly random aberrations generated by failures in the maintenance of genomic integrity are the result of selection in the evolution of a tumor.[1,2] In contrast, recurrent structural aberrations are frequent transforming events in sarcomas, leukemias, and lymphomas. Indeed, the majority of cancer genes identified to date (see Table 8-1) reside at the break point of recurrent cytogenetic abnormalities in hematopoietic neo-

Table 8-3 ISCN Abbreviated Terms and Symbols

Term (Symbol)	Description
add	Additional material of unknown origin
approximate sign (-)	Denotes intervals and boundaries of a chromosome segment
C	Constitutional anomaly
comma (,)	Separates chromosome numbers, sex chromosomes, chromosome abnormalities
Cp	Composite karyotype
Del	Deletion
Der	Derivative chromosome
Dic	Dicentric
Dmin	Double minute
Dup	Duplication
Fis	Fission, at the centromere
Hsr	Homogeneously staining region
I	Isochromosome
Idem	Denotes the stemline karyotype in subclones
Ider	ISO derivative chromosome
Idic	ISO dicentric chromosome
Inc	Incomplete karyotype
Ins	Insertion
Inv	Inversion
Mar	Marker chromosome
minus sign (–)	Loss
multiplication sign (×)	Multiple copies of rearranged chromosomes
Or	Alternative interpretation
P	Short arm of chromosome
parentheses ()	Surround structurally altered chromosome and breakpoints
plus sign (+)	Gain
Q	Long arm of chromosome
Qpd	Quadruplication
question mark (?)	Questionable identification of a chromosome or chromosome structure
R	Ring chromosome
semicolon (;)	Separates altered chromosomes and breakpoints in structural rearrangements involving more than one chromosome
Slant line (/)	Separates clones
T	Translocation
Tas	Telomeric association
Trc	Tricentric chromosome
Trp	Triplication

plasms, despite the fact that hematopoietic tumors constitute only 10% of human cancers.[3–5] Although there is wide agreement that recurrent aberrations are particularly important for cancer development,[1,2] identifying the important cancer-related genes in many recurrent cytogenetic abnormalities is not always straightforward because aberrations may contain multiple genes and more than one may be involved in different structural aberrations and contribute to the cancer phenotype.

One of the simplest and most common abnormalities in cancer cells is a gain or a loss of a whole chromosome resulting from defective chromosome segregation during telophase in mitosis or defective cytokinesis. Gains or losses of whole chromosomes or individual chromosome arms are displayed in written karyotypes as a plus sign (+) or a minus sign (–) before the designated number of the chromosome gained or lost (see Table 8-3). The functional consequence of these chromosome aberrations, which occur particularly frequently in solid tumors, may be hard to establish because the aberrations may extend over tens of thousands of megabases and may affect hundreds to thousands of genes. It has been easier to establish the cancer relevance of more limited regions of chromosomal gain and loss, created by amplification or deletion, as these smaller aberrations have been shown to alter the dosage of known oncogenes or tumor suppressor genes. Deletions are indicated by the abbreviation "del" and insertions by "ins" (see Table 8-3), with each abbreviation coming before the number of the chromosome involved. Restricted regions of the genome may also be amplified and the amplified fragments may be present in small extrachromosomal acentric fragments (so-called double minutes or dmin), integrated into chromosomes in homogeneous staining regions (HSRs), or dispersed throughout the genome (see Table 8-3). Adding to the complexity, amplified DNA fragments may contain DNA from different chromosomal regions.[2] Classic examples of oncogene activation in solid tumors include *ERBB2* in breast cancers and *MYC* in many tumors (see Table 8-1). The amplification of several cancer genes has been associated with therapeutic resistance, such as amplification of the *BCR-ABL* gene in CML patients resistant to imatinib/Gleevec,[26,42] amplification of *DHFR* in patients resistant to methotrexate,[43] and amplification of the androgen receptor AR in prostate cancers resistant to endocrine therapy.[44] Loss of specific regions of the genome are often associated with loss of tumor suppressor genes, such as *TP53*, *RB1*, *PTEN*, and *CDKN4* (see Table 8-1). Elimination of the remaining normal alleles of carriers of inherited mutations of *RB1*, *BRCA1*, *BRCA2*, *TP53*, and *PTPRJ*, or, in somatic cancer cells that have acquired mutations in one allele of these genes, is critical for the promotion of tumorigenesis (see Table 8-1). Based on these data, it is reasonable to expect that many more critical "cancer genes" will soon be identified in other less well studied regions of chromosome gain and loss in human cancers.

As previously described, recurrent structural chromosomal rearrangements occur frequently in hematopoietic neoplasms, sarcomas, and in some epithelial solid tumors. These structural changes may involve equal exchange of material between two chromosomes (referred to as "balanced") or may be nonreciprocal, in which portions of the genome are gained or lost as a consequence of the genomic alteration. One of the most common cytogenetic alterations in cancer is "translocation," where material between two or more chromosomes is exchanged (see Tables 8-2 and 8-3; Figure 8-3). Translocations are identified by the abbreviation t, with the chromosomes involved noted in the first set of parentheses and the break points in the second set of parentheses (see Table 8-3). Translocations may occur as a consequence of abnormal double-strand break (DSB) repair or through other means of intra- or interchromosomal recombination.[2] Translocations may result if DSBs occur in two distinct chromosomes simultaneously and the DSBs are aberrantly repaired; if the free end of one chromosome is ligated to another chromosome rather than its cognate free chromosome fragment, a translocation may result. In balanced reciprocal translocations (see Figure 8-3), both chromosomes ligate each other's free ends, resulting in two abnormal chromosomes that are reciprocal products of each other. In an unbalanced translocation, only one set of DSBs is ligated, resulting in one abnormal chromosome; the unligated free chromosome fragments are often unstable and lost in the next mitosis. Another structural cytogenetic defect seen in cancer is an inversion (inv) (see Tables 8-2 and 8-3 and Figure 8-3). Chromosome inversions may occur if two DSBs occur simultaneously in the same chromosome; instead of repairing the proper free ends to each other, the middle fragment of the chromosome inverts and is ligated to the opposite free ends.

In traditional cytogenetic analysis using chromosome banding techniques, structural abnormalities such as a translocation are required to be seen in at least two of 20 metaphase chromosome spreads using light microscopy to be recognized as "clonal" for that tumor.[22,41] Gain or loss of a chromosome must occur in at least three cells to be recognized as a clonal abnormality. Clearly, examination of such few cells, even with high resolution technologies, does not adequately allow for studies of the clonal heterogeneity and genetic complexity of most human tumors. Thus, the challenge for the future is to develop automated, high throughput methods for the analysis of structural chromosome defects in large numbers of dividing and nondividing cancer cells.

NEWER METHODS OF CHROMOSOME AND GENOME ANALYSIS

In the late 1980s and continuing to the present day, advances in the development of fluorescence in situ hybridization (FISH) technologies and advances in microscopic imaging of human chromosomes have revolutionized and increased the sensitivity and specificity of cancer chromosome analysis. Three technologies have particularly revolutionized state-of-the-art cytogenetic analyses: fluorescence in situ hybridization (FISH) in interphase cells; spectral karyotyping (SKY) or multiplex FISH (M-FISH) in tumor metaphases; and comparative genomic hybridization (CGH) in metaphase cells. Each of these technologies is briefly described below and in Table 8-2. In the research laboratory, new high throughput methods have been developed for detection of loss of heterozygosity (LOH) and for the mapping of fine regions of chromosome gain and loss, including array CGH and single nucleotide polymorphism arrays (so-called SNP Chips). Other highly sensitive but complex methods, including restriction landmark genome scanning (RLGS),[21] represen-

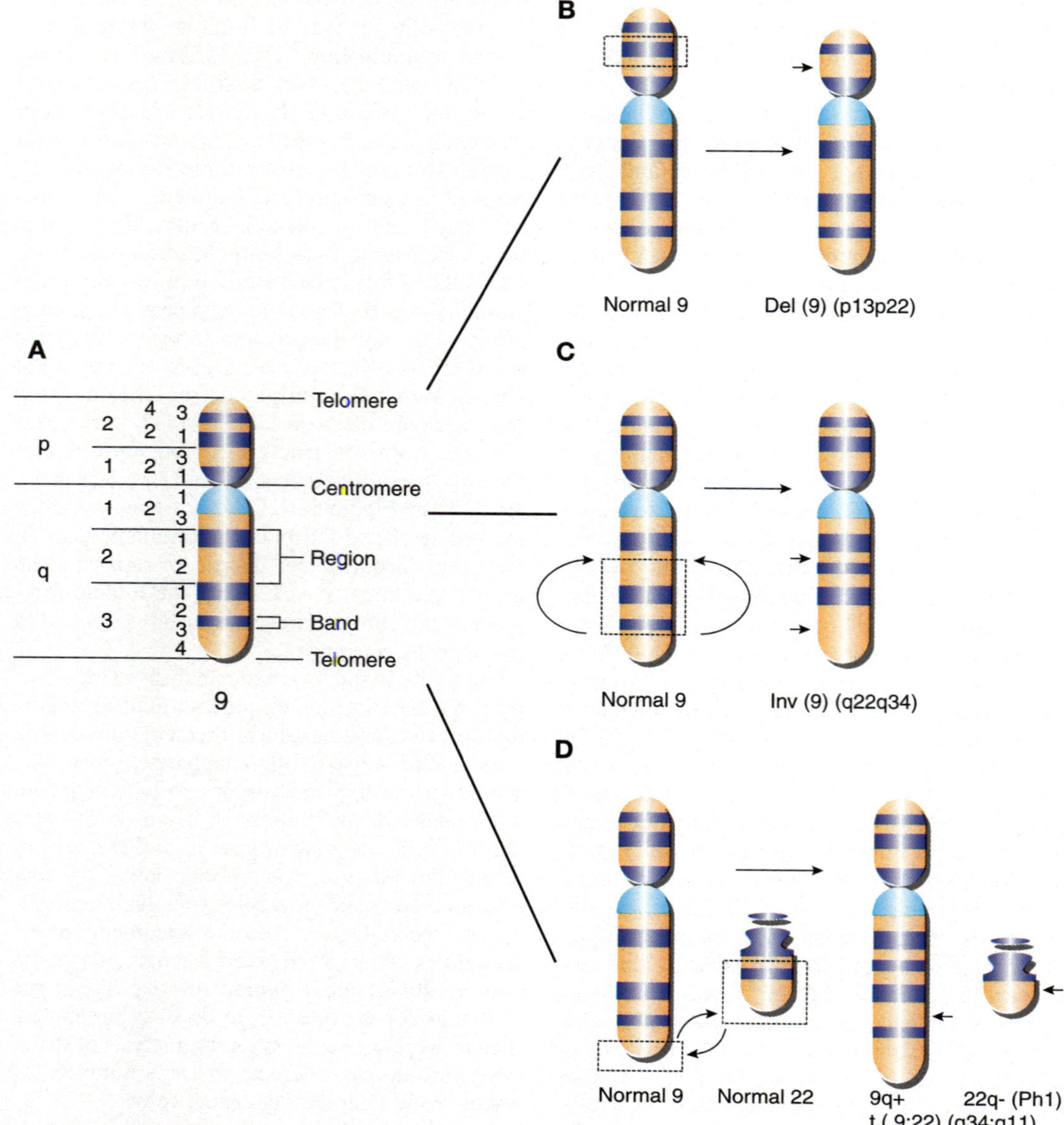

Figure 8-3 Schematic diagram illustrating a normal chromosome and three chromosomal abnormalities observed in human neoplasms. **A,** Diagram of the banding pattern of a normal chromosome 9. The chromosome arms (p, short arm; q, long arm), regions, and band numbers are indicated on the left of the chromosome; specific chromosome structures are indicated on the right of the chromosome. **B,** Diagram of the mechanism of an interstitial deletion of the short arm of chromosome 9, a common abnormality in acute lymphoblastic leukemia. Chromosome breaks occur in bands 9p13 and 9p22, and the intervening chromosomal segment (band 9p21 and parts of bands 9p13 and 9p22) is lost [del(9)(p13p22)]. **C,** Diagram of the mechanism of a paracentric inversion. Chromosome breaks occur in two bands within a single chromosome arm, in this case, within 9p22 and 9q34; the intervening segment is inverted and the chromosome breaks are repaired [inv(9)(q22q34)]. **D,** Diagram of the mechanism of the reciprocal translocation involving chromosomes 9 and 22, t(9;22)(q34;q11), which gives rise to the Philadelphia (Ph1) chromosome in the malignant cells of patients with chronic myelogenous leukemia. Breaks occur in bands q34 and q11 of chromosomes 9 and 22, respectively, followed by a reciprocal exchange of chromosomal material. This rearrangement results in the translocation of the ABL oncogene, normally located at 9q34, adjacent to the BCR gene on chromosome 22, giving rise to a chimeric BCRABL gene, whose protein product plays a role in the transformation of myeloid cells.

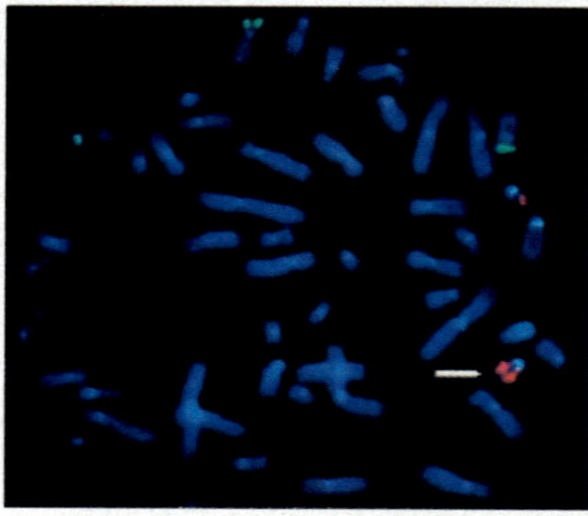

Figure 8-4 FISH analysis of gene amplification in acute myeloid leukemia using BAC probes to TEL and RUNX1. The green fluorescence shows the TEL gene located on chromosome 12 and the red fluorescence shows the RUNX1 gene on chromosome 21. Note the amplification of RUNX1 on one chromosome 21 indicated by the arrow. Figure courtesy of Dr. Kathy Richkind, Genzyme Genetics.

tational difference analysis (RDA),[21] and end sequence profiling (ESP), are in investigative use and are refining both the sensitivity and specificity of chromosome analysis.[2]

FISH FISH[11–14,45] is a technique in which DNA probes are labeled with various fluorochromes (eg, rhodamine), followed by hybridization to either metaphase spreads or interphase cells and detected using fluorescence microscopy (see Figures 8-1B and 8-4). FISH has had a dramatic impact on the sensitivity, detection, and analysis of chromosome aberrations in cancer cells and has been rapidly adapted to the clinical diagnostic setting. The ability to detect chromosomal aberrations in interphase cells has been a particularly dramatic advance and has facilitated the analysis of genomic aberrations in all cancers, but particularly in solid tumors that have been less adaptable to *in vitro* culture and metaphase analysis. A large number of commercially available probes are now available for FISH analysis of chromosome aberrations in metaphase spreads and interphase nuclei. These probes include chromosome-specific centromere probes that unequivocally detect the number of copies of a specific chromosome presents in interphase and metaphase; whole chromosome paints that color an entire chromosome; large DNA probes (derived from YAC or BAC clones, see Table 8-2) from specific regions of the genome that can be used to screen for regional aberrations, such as amplifications or structural chromosomal aberrations, such as recurring translocations; and genomic DNA probes for specific human genes. Particularly useful for the detection of structural rearrangements are new "split-apart" probes for the specific chromosomal aberrations seen in hematopoietic malignancies and sarcomas.[46–48] Split-apart FISH probes are derived from two adjacent regions of the genome and are differentially labeled; these two probes move apart only in the event of a structural chromosomal rearrangement in the interval normally flanked by the probes. Such probes are independent of the partner gene and are particularly useful in detecting structural rearrangements in "promiscuous" cancer genes that may be translocated to many different partner genes on different chromosomes (see Table 8-1: *ALK*, *BCL6*, *ETV6* [*TEL*], *EVI1*, *EWSR1*, *IGH*, *MLL*, *MYC*, *NUP98*, *PDGFR*, *RARA*, *RET*, and *RUNX1* [*AML1*]). FISH technologies have also been shown to be highly useful for the detection of specific gene amplifications, such as *ERBB2* in breast cancer, in both interphase cells and metaphase chromosomes. Another highly interesting application of FISH techniques is the integration of FISH and immunophenotyping (called FICTION).[48] FICTION is useful for mapping the actual cells that carry specific chromosomal abnormalities. A particularly striking recent discovery with this technique was that lymphoma-associated endothelial cells contain the same specific translocation as the surrounding tumor cells,[49] suggesting that lymphoma may arise in a multipotent progenitor cell capable of both lymphoid and endothelial differentiation. Although other explanations include cell fusion or the uptake of apoptotic material, this observation is very intriguing.

Given suitable probes, interphase FISH enhances cytogenetic analysis in specimens with a low mitotic index, such as in myeloma or chronic lymphocytic leukemia (CLL), and in specimens that tend to have poor chromosome morphology in metaphase spreads, such as in ALL. Interphase FISH can be scaled up to analyze hundreds of cells and thereby increase the sensitivity of analysis and the detection of clonal chromosomal abnormalities in far greater numbers of cells than traditional chromosome banding techniques and metaphase analysis. FISH also increases the sensitivity of detection of cytogenetic abnormalities—particularly cryptic translocations or smaller structural rearrangements—and is useful for monitoring the response to treatment and low sensitivity minimal residual disease detection. The current sensitivity of interphase FISH is approximately 5% abnormal cells. FISH analysis of metaphase chromosomes is particularly useful for detection of cryptic translocations (such as the *BCR-ABL* translocation in CML or the recently discovered inv(7)(p15q34) cryptic translocation in T-ALL resulting in aberrant *HOX* gene expression[50]), resolving complex chromosomal rearrangements, and identifying the origin of "marker" chromosomes, which are unknown chromosome fragments in metaphase spreads.

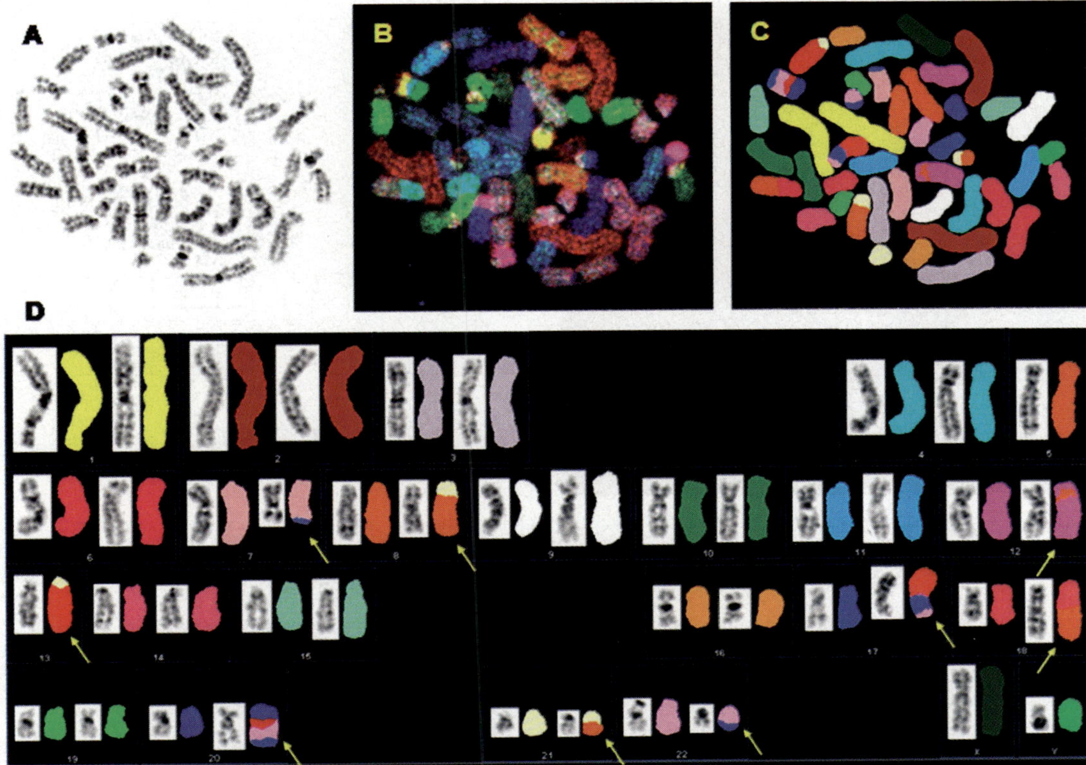

Figure 8-5 Complex karyotype detected in a patient with acute myeloid leukemia, analyzed using spectral karyotyping (SKY). **A,** Inverted and contrast-enhanced DAPI image of the metaphase cell. **B** and **C,** The same metaphase cell with chromosomes shown in SKY display colors (**B**) and SKY classification colors (**C**). **D,** Karyotype of the same cell with each chromosome represented twice, by its inverted DAPI-stained image on the left and SKY image shown in classification colors on the right. Arrows denote structurally rearranged chromosomes. The karyotype interpretation is as follows: 44,XY,-5, der(7)t(7;17)(q22;?),der(8)(8qter→8q21?.2::8p21→cen→8q21?.2::21q21→21q21::21q21→21qter),der(12)ins(12;5)(p12;?q31?q22),-13,der(13)ins(13;21)(q11;q?q?),der(17)(13qter→13q14::17p11→cen→17q21::17?→17?::22q?→22q?), der(18)(18pter→cen→18q21.3~22::5?q22→5?q11.2),der(20)(20pter→cen→20q11::13q12→13q14 or 13q14→13q12::22q11 →22q13 or 22q13→22q11::17q2?3→17qter), der(21)t(8;21)(?p21;q11),der(22)t(20;22)(q1?;q11). Figures courtesy of Dr. Krzysztof Mrózek, The Ohio State University.

Spectral Karyotyping and Multiplex Fluorescence In Situ Hybridization SKY (Figure 8-5) and M-FISH (Figure 8-6) are molecular cytogenetic techniques that permit the simultaneous visualization of all human chromosomes in different colors, facilitating karyotype analysis. For these techniques, chromosome-specific probe pools (referred to as "chromosome painting" probes) generated from flow cytometric-sorted chromosomes are amplified and then fluorescently labeled using degenerate oligonucleotide-primed polymerase chain reaction. Both SKY and M-FISH use a combinatorial labeling scheme with different fluorochromes that can be spectrally distinguished, but use different fluorescence detection methods. In SKY, image acquisition is performed using epifluorescence microscopy, CCD imaging, and Fourier transform spectroscopy.[11] With this approach, the entire fluorescence emission spectrum can be analyzed with a single exposure. In M-FISH, separate images are captured for each of the five fluorochromes using filters, and then computer software is used to combine the images. In both M-FISH and SKY, unique pseudocolors are ultimately assigned to each individual chromosome based on their overall specific fluorescence signature (see Figures 8-5 and 8-6).

SKY and M-FISH are useful in detecting and mapping structural chromosomal rearrangements, detecting unknown "marker" chromosomes, detecting cryptic translocations, and in characterizing complex chromosomal rearrangements. With the advent of M-FISH and SKY, it is clear that many malignancies have a far greater fraction of cytogenetic abnormalities than was previously thought. For example, previously, 50% of AML could be found to have cytogenetic abnormalities by careful conventional cytogenetics. Using M-FISH and SKY, the percentage of AML that have cytogenetic abnormalities is 80% (see Figure 8-5).[51] However, SKY and M-FISH may not have high enough resolution to identify the exact chromosomal region involved in abnormalities.

Comparative Genomic Hybridization CGH is a fluorescent molecular cytogenetic technique for determining copy number gains and losses and amplifications between two samples of DNA by competitively hybridizing differentially labeled DNA from these samples to normal metaphase chromosomes (Figure 8-7). It is a powerful tool for screening chromosomal copy number changes in tumor genomes and has the advantage of analyzing entire genomes in a single experiment. As it is dependent on DNA for analysis, it is particularly applicable to the study of tumors that do not yield sufficient metaphases for chromosome analysis, and it can be applied to small numbers of microdissected cells, fixed or frozen samples, as well as paraffin-embedded tissues. CGH is based on quantitative two-color fluorescence in situ hybridization; equal amounts of tumor DNA and normal reference DNA that are labeled with distinct fluorochromes are mixed together and competitively hybridized to normal metaphase spreads (see Figure 8-7A). The fluorescence intensity ratio between labeled tumor DNA and normal chromosome DNA is measured by scanning along each chromosomal region in the metaphase spread. This provides information about the relative copy number of tumor versus normal DNA by chromosomal region. Thus, gains and losses can be digitally visualized. CGH is limited by the fact that it will only detect gains or losses present in a large fraction of the tumor cells and cannot detect balanced chromosomal transloca-

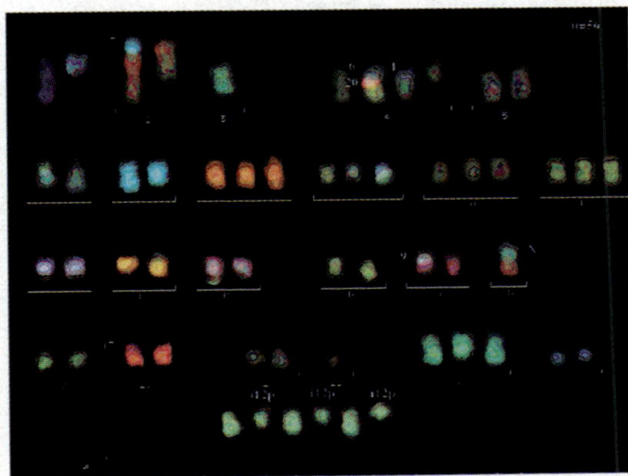

Figure 8-6 M-FISH studies performed on a germ cell tumor, demonstrating both the isochromosome 12p and also the general amplification of 12p material that is very common in all germ cell tumors. The amplified oncogene on 12p has not yet been identified. Figure courtesy of Dr. Octavian Henegariu.

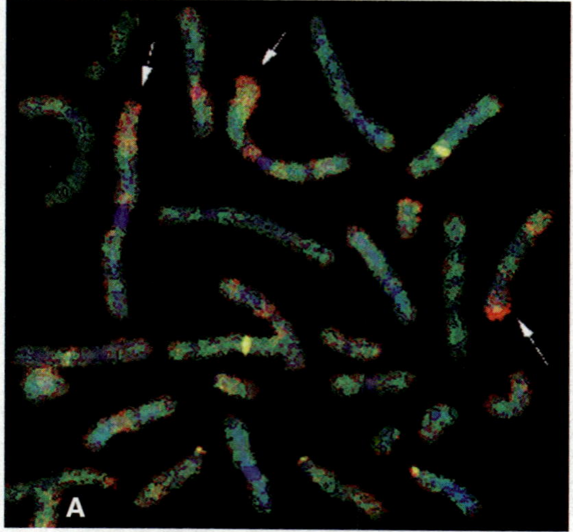

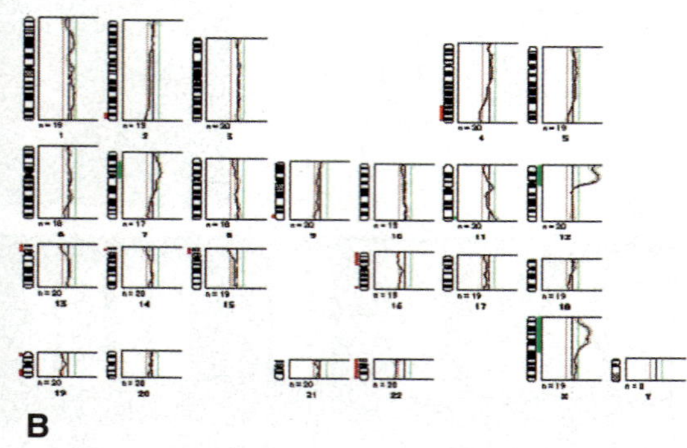

Figure 8-7 CGH on a germ cell tumor sample. The arrows indicate the amplification of 12p material common in these tumors. **A,** The photomicrograph on the left demonstrates the annealing of fluorescently labeled normal chromosomes to a tumor specimen. **B,** The diagram on the right demonstrates the computer analysis of gains or losses of tumor DNA compared to normal DNA. Right of the line indicates gain and left of the line indicates loss of chromosomal material relative to normal. Note the marked gain of material on chromosome 12. Figures courtesy of Dr. Octavian Henegariu.

tions or other aberrations. This limits its effectiveness, especially in hematologic malignancies, where most translocations are balanced. The use of CGH is mostly investigational, and it is rarely used in the clinical diagnostic setting. However, this technique is powerful because it does not require advance knowledge of cytogenetic abnormalities. It also precludes the selection of a subpopulation of the tumor under analysis during the short-term in vitro culture necessary to obtain metaphases. CGH has been applied to many tumor types and revealed novel regions of chromosome gain and loss in cancers of the colon, breast (gains on chromosomes 1, 8, 17, 20, 13q, and 17p), prostate, cervix, glioblastomas (identifying chromosome 7 gain and chromosome 10 loss), and lymphomas.[52]

Array CGH[16,17,19] Traditional CGH methodology has been recently enhanced and largely replaced by microarray-based platforms using large insert genomic DNA clones, cDNAs, or oligonucleotides in place of metaphase chromosomes. Compared with traditional CGH, array CGH provides many advantages, including easier standardization, higher resolution, and the ability to directly and precisely map copy number changes to the genome sequence. The first arrays contained clones spaced at approximately 1 Mb across the genome. However, high resolution tiling path arrays, consisting of overlapping BAC clones, are now available and increase the resolution of this approach even further.[53,54] Recent array CGH studies of mantle cell lymphoma have detected a 50% higher number of chromosome aberrations than traditional CGH, in addition to the identification of several novel consensus critical regions of DNA deletion—one on 8p contains a number of candidate genes, including the TRAIL receptor regulating apoptosis.[54,55]

Single Nucleotide Polymorphism Arrays (SNP Chips)[21,56–58] Oligonucleotide arrays allowing the genotyping of thousands of single nucleotide polymorphisms (SNPs), the most abundant form of variation in the genome, are now being used to very sensitively assess loss of heterozygosity (LOH) in human tumors (Figure 8-8).[56–58] These recently introduced "SNP Chips" are also being used in the rapidly evolving field of cancer pharmacogenomics to determine individual polymorphisms in genes involved in specific metabolism pathways in order to predict therapeutic responsiveness, resistance, and undue toxicity to specific pharmacologic agents. New Affymetrix Gene Chip Human Mapping 100K Sets (<www.affymetrix.com>) facilitate the rapid genotyping of over 100,000 human SNPs in a single experiment.[59] Many novel discoveries are likely with this platform in the coming years. One of the most interesting recent discoveries was the finding by Raghavan and colleagues,[60] in which a 10K SNP Chip was used to study AML cases with a presumably "normal" karyotype. Surprisingly, 20% of the AML cases studied had large, nonrandom regions of homozygosity that could not be accounted for by chromosome gain or loss using FISH. The most likely explanation of this finding is somatic recombination resulting in large chromosomal regions of uniparental disomy (UPD): the circumstance where the chromosomal material is uniparental (or derived from one parent) in origin. One possible effect of UPD would be to unmask the effect of mutated genes or reduce the gene dosages to homozygosity. Thus, SNP Chips have already facilitated the discovery of a novel mechanism of tumorigenesis as well as defined new regions of chromosome gain and loss in hematopoietic neoplasms and solid tumors.

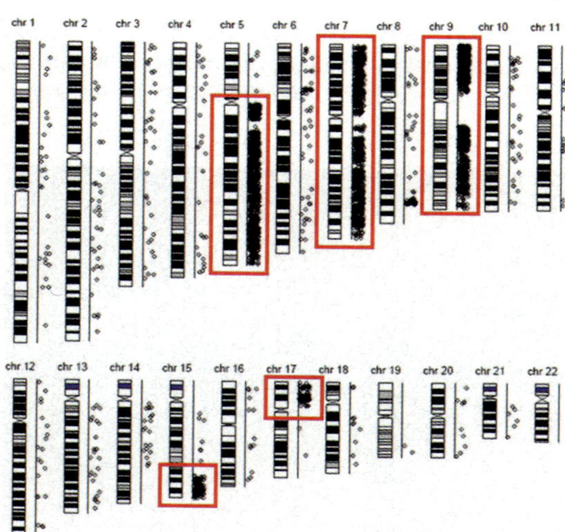

Figure 8-8 SNP Chip arrays were used to determine loss of heterozygosity (LOH) in a genome wide scan using Affymetrix GeneChip Human Mapping 100K Array, comparing germline DNA with paired DNA from diagnostic bone marrow samples in 13 cases of therapy related AML. Highlighted areas were also areas of chromosomal loss detected cytogenetically. Figure courtesy of Dr. Mary V. Relling, Chair of Pharmacology, St. Jude Children's Research Hospital.

Gene Expression Profiling Cancer research was revolutionized in the late 1990s by another advance in biotechnology—the development of the cDNA or oligonucleotide microarrays that allowed the simultaneous profiling and quantitative assessment of the expression of thousands of genes (RNAs) in the human genome.[61–73] Similar to the competitive hybridization process in CGH, labeled RNA (either total RNA or mRNA) isolated from tumor cells may be competitively hybridized with a labeled reference standard to an array containing thousands of cDNA elements, or alternatively, tumor RNA may be directly hybridized to oligonucleotide arrays. Current oligonucleotide arrays available from Affymetrix (see <www.affymetrix.com>) have complete coverage of the human genome, capable of the simultaneous analysis of over 47,000 human transcripts. The computational and statistical analysis of comprehensive array datasets must be carefully considered and may be very complex. Nonetheless, since the late 1990s, over 5,000 manuscripts have been published reporting the various gene expression profiles in human cancer. Gene expression profiles of most human cancers are now available online (see the National Library of Medicine Gene Expression Omnibus <http://www.ncbi.nlm.nih.gov/geo>, the National Cancer Institute Gene Expression Data Portal <http://gedp.nci.nih.gov/dc/index.jsp>, and the Stanford Microarray Database <http://genome-www5.stanford.edu>). Gene expression profiling has led to the development of novel molecular classification schemes for human cancers—particularly solid tumors such as lymphomas, breast cancer, prostate cancer, and brain tumors—where distinct subgroups have been identified with expression profiling that were not detected using traditional histopathologic or cytogenetic techniques; the derivation of gene expression "classifiers" or list of genes that are predictive of patient outcome to particular therapies; the identification of novel genes and pathways that are being further developed as therapeutic targets; the identification of sets of genes associated with disease progression or predictive of metastasis; and the derivation of gene expression profiles associated with or predictive of many recurrent cytogenetic abnormalities in human cancer. As large gene expression profile datasets are integrated with data from high resolution cytogenetic studies from SKY/M-FISH, CGH, and SNP Chips, and proteomic studies on well-defined cancer patients who are uniformly treated with specific therapies, we will undoubtedly dramatically alter cancer diagnosis, classification, outcome prediction, and the development of novel targeted therapies.

ETIOLOGY AND MECHANISMS OF CANCER CHROMOSOMAL ABERRATIONS

Although the majority of human cancers progress through the stepwise accumulation of genomic and epigenetic alterations, the etiology and genetic mechanisms that initiate the earliest stages of carcinogenesis and the acquisition of the very first genomic aberrations are not well understood. Furthermore, it is not clear whether there are distinct mechanisms for the initiation of cancer in different human tissues, particularly in hematopoietic and mesenchymal tissues versus solid epithelial cancers. The majority (74%) of the recurrent chromosomal aberrations reported to date have been found in hematopoietic and mesenchymal neoplasms, in contrast to solid tumors, where only 26% of those cases reported to date have recurring cytogenetic aberrations.[3,5,22] In contrast, deletion and amplification are more characteristic of solid tumors, along with progressive genetic instability and the acquisition of a complex panoply of genomic aberrations. Although many human tumors appear to be genetically unstable and acquire an increasing burden of genomic aberrations with tumor progression, the role of genomic instability in the initiation of tumorigenesis remains controversial.[2,5,74,75] Using colorectal cancer as a model, Sieber and colleagues[75] suggest that although genomic instability might promote tumorigenesis, it does not initiate it. The prevailing view is that hematopoietic neoplasms are initiated by signature recurrent chromosomal rearrangements, while deregulation of tumor suppressor genes and progressive genetic instability is the mechanism of initiation in solid tumors. A recent perspective by Mitelman and colleagues[5] challenges this view. Mitelman and colleagues demonstrate that the difference in the reported frequency of recurrent cytogenetic abnormalities in hematopoietic and mesenchymal tumors versus solid epithelial cancers may simply be a consequence of the smaller number of epithelial tumors studied to date. In every tumor type, the number of recurrent balanced chromosomal aberrations is simply a function of the number of reported cases with abnormal karyotypes.[5] Thus, Mitelman suggests that there may not be an intrinsically different mechanism for the initiation of epithelial versus mesenchymal/hematopoietic cancers, but rather, that solid tumors are simply understudied. The lower frequency of reported chromosomal rearrangements in solid tumors may be reflective of their advanced age and stage of development at disease presentation, or the failure of many solid tumors to adapt to *in vitro* culture and yield sufficient metaphases for study. Modeling of the recurrent translocations and inversions characteristic of hematopoietic neoplasms has repeatedly demonstrated that these genomic aberrations are not sufficient for tumorigenesis and that secondary genomic mutations are required for full tumor progression, similar to epithelial cancers.[26,39] Thus, whether there are different mechanisms of tumorigenesis in different tissues, or whether different types of initiating mutations initiate intrinsically different genetic mechanisms of tumorigenesis remains unresolved. Comprehensive detection and functional analysis of the full spectrum of genomic changes in each human cancer, as proposed by the new NCI/NIHGR Cancer Genome Project, may ultimately resolve this controversy.

Human cells are subject to constant DNA damage from both extrinsic (radiation, chemicals) and intrinsic (reactive oxygen species, stalling at DNA replication forks) sources. As many as 10 double-strand DNA breaks occur per cell cycle, providing ample opportunity for the acquisition of mutations and formation of chromosomal aberrations, raising the intriguing question of whether defective DNA repair is an essential first step in oncogenesis.[76–78] As a consequence of this high mutation frequency, human cells have evolved elaborate systems to monitor genome integrity and coordinate DNA repair with cell-cycle progression. More than 70 genes have been identified to date that play critical roles in DNA damage surveillance and repair (see Table 8-1), including genes involved in mismatch repair (*MSH2*, *MLH1*), nonhomologous end joining (*XRCC5*, *XRCC4*, *PRKDC*), homologous recombination (*RAD51*, *BRCA1*, *BRCA2*), and signaling cascades that respond to DNA damage (*ATM*, *ATR*, *CHEK1*, *TP53*, *BRCA1*, *BRCA2*, *BLM*). Different patterns of genomic change have been associated with perturbations in different DNA repair pathways. Disruption of *MLH1* or *MSH2* results in tumors with few chromosomal aberrations, but significant microsatellite alterations and somatic mutations. Of the two alternative DNA repair pathways for DSB repair in mammalian cells, nonhomologous end-joining (NHEJ) appears to more frequently lead to chromosomal aberrations—particularly translocations—than homologous recombination (HR) (see Table 8-2).[2,39,76–78] DNA DSBs occur normally during the development of certain cell lineages, such as rearrangement of the V(D)J exons of the B and T cell receptor genes (*BCR*, *TCR*) during development of B and T lymphoid cells, or during resolution of stalled replication forks (Holliday junctions). DSBs may also be induced by exposure to external agents, such as radiation or oxidizing agents; some DNA sites are more fragile than others and sustain DSBs at a greater frequency when exposed to DSB-inducing agents. Although controversial, genes located at these "fragile sites" may have more frequent deletions in malignancy, such as the *FHIT* tumor suppressor gene located at a fragile site at 3p14.[79] Alu elements (see Table 8-2) occur at a greater frequency in chromosomal regions that are altered in solid tumors compared with other regions of the genome, and aberrant recombination of Alu elements has been linked to the formation of both *BCR-ABL* and *MLL* duplication.[80] However, NHEJ is the dominant repair mechanism in mammalian cells and sequencing of the genomics break points of several recurrent translocations such as t(4;11) *MLL-AF4*, t(12;21) *ETV* (*TEL*)-*RUNX1* (*AML1*), t(15;17) *PML-RARα*, and t(8;21) *RUNX1* (*AML1*)-*ETO* implicate aberrant NHEJ.[39] Thus, it appears that error-prone NEHJ is the main repair mechanism involved in chromosomal translocation. Promoting proper DNA repair and preventing aberrant joining of free chromosomal ends would be beneficial in preventing malignancy, yet this is an area of remarkably little research.

In hematopoietic neoplasms, defective function of topoisomerase II combined with aberrant NHEJ has also been shown to promote the formation of translocations. Topoisomerase II relaxes DNA and unknots tangled chromosome strands, playing a crucial role in normal DNA replication. During this process, topoisomerase II creates DSBs that are resealed following the unwinding of DNA. Drugs (such as the cancer therapeutic drugs in the epidophyllotoxin and anthracycline classes) that target topoisomerase II stabilize the complexes of topoisomerase II with the DSBs, thereby slowing ligation and leaving free DNA ends that may participate in interchromosomal translocations through imprecise NHEJ.[39] Interestingly, consensus topoisomerase II-binding sites have been shown to correlate with the location of DNA break points in experimental systems and in patients with therapy-related secondary leukemias who were previously exposed to epidophyllotoxins or anthracyclines for the treatment of their primary cancer.[81–83] Rowley and Olney have recently published a review of the specific chromosomal translocations that have been linked to antecedent chemotherapy exposure.[82] Interestingly, the *MLL* gene on chromosome 11q23 (see Table 8-1), which contains consensus topoisomerase II binding sites, is very frequently involved in chromosomal rearrangements in therapy-related leukemias.[82–84] Furthermore, it is striking that some of the chromosomal translocations that are common in therapy-related leukemias (such as *MLL* fusions, see Table 8-1) are particularly common in *de novo* acute leukemias arising in infants, indicating a possible role for exposure to naturally occurring topoisomerase II inhibitors (such as dietary bioflavonoids, pesticides, and the drug dipyrone) in the etiology of these leukemias.[39,84,85]

At the earliest stages of development of B and T lymphoid cells, V(D)J recombination occurs to establish the immunologic repertoire. Directed by the recombination-activating gene (RAG) proteins, V(D)J recombination sequentially assembles exonic cassettes of the immunoglobulin or T cell receptor (*TCR*) genes to produce functional antigen receptors and immunoglobulins. Several investigators, notably Croce and Babbitts, first proposed that translocations that arise in tumors of B and T lymphoid origin accidentally result from errors in the complex genomic rearrangements that are essential to produce the immunoglobulin and TCR repertoire.[86,87] The error rate of V(D)J recombination may be particularly high in the development of the TCR, as the T-cell–associated translocations t(11;14) *LMO2-TCR*, and t(7;9) *TCR-TAL2* are found in the peripheral blood of a high proportion of normal individuals.[39,88–90] Interestingly, although aberrant V(D)J recombination appears to play a significant role in the development of the translocations and chromosome aberrations associated with pediatric and adult T-cell leukemias and with mature B-cell lymphomas, the translocations associated with the most common form of pediatric leukemia—B precursor ALL—appear to result from aberrant NHEJ, similar to myeloid leukemias and other cancers.[39]

Finally, two additional mechanisms play a role in genome instability and the development of genomic aberrations in cancer. Chromosome gains or losses may occur when genes involved in chromosome segregation of cytokinesis are deregulated.[2] Aberrant centrosome behavior, such as centrosome amplification, has been associated with mutation or loss of function of *TP53*, *STK15*, *RB1*, and *BRCA1* and has been proposed as a primary source of genetic instability in human tumors. Centrosome amplification is characterized by the presence of abnormally large centrosomes, which may have more than four centrioles, which are abnormal in both orientation and function. Another form of genomic instability occurs because of inactive telomerase; continued proliferation of somatic cells with inactive telomerase results in progressive shortening of telomeres.[91–93] If surveillance mechanisms are intact, cells with shortened telomeres should cease to proliferate; such function provides a barrier to the further development of cancer and may explain why clinically benign tumors fail to progress. However, if cell-cycle regulatory checkpoints are compromised, then the chromosomes of cells with shortened, dysfunctional telomeres become susceptible to end-to-end fusions and breakage during cell division. Cells containing such chromosomes may undergo aberrant cell division and genome reorganization.[2]

GENOMIC ALTERATIONS AND CHROMOSOMAL ABERRATIONS IN HUMAN CANCER

A comprehensive and detailed review of all of the recurrent genomic and chromosomal aberrations in human cancer, the structure and function of the genes that are altered or disrupted by each of these aberrations, the functional consequences of these aberrations on cellular networks and pathways and their mechanisms of transformation, their various means of detection, and their use in cancer diagnosis and therapy would necessitate an entire textbook. Progress in this field is so rapid and evolves in such constantly surprising directions that remaining up to date is a true challenge. Thus, the reader is directed to the many online repositories, catalogues, and resources mentioned throughout this chapter (see the full listing of URLs at the end of the chapter) and to each of the disease-oriented chapters in this book for a more thorough discussion and review of the various cancer-associated genomic and chromosomal abnormalities and their clinical significance. In the subsequent sections of this chapter, we provide brief overviews of the more frequently recurring genomic and chromosomal aberrations in both hematopoietic and solid cancers, particularly focusing on those abnormalities that illustrate specific paradigms.

HEMATOPOIETIC CANCERS: MALIGNANCIES OF THE MYELOID LINEAGE

The acute myeloid leukemias (AML), the myelodysplastic syndromes (MDS), and the chronic myeloproliferative diseases (CMPD), including chronic myelogenous leukemia (CML), have traditionally been diagnosed and classified by histopathologic, cytochemical, and immunophenotypic features, first using the French-American-British (FAB) classification system,[94] and now the World Health Organization (WHO) classification scheme.[95] However, the recurrent chromosomal aberrations and genomic changes associated with these diseases (Table 8-4) provide critical information for diagnosis, prognostication, and disease management, including risk stratification and therapeutic targeting. Over the past 25 years, the majority of the frequently recurring balanced chromosomal rearrangements in myeloid diseases have been cloned and characterized, providing both valuable insights into mechanisms of leukemogenesis and carcinogenesis in many cell lineages, as well as powerful new molecular genetic tools for more diagnosis, detection of residual disease, and monitoring of therapeutic response.

Primary Myelodysplastic Syndrome The myelodysplastic syndromes (MDS) are a highly heterogeneous group of disorders, including primary idiopathic MDS and secondary or therapy-related MDS that develop after antecedent exposure to chemotherapy or radiation. Primary MDS arises primarily in older individuals, and the incidence appears to increase significantly with age. Unfortunately, in contrast to other hematologic neoplasms, accurate population-based incidence and mortality data are lacking in MDS in the United States, as this disease has not been previously monitored and reported by the United States NCI Surveillance, Epidemiology, and End Results (SEER) Program (<http://seer.cancer.gov>). Nonetheless, the overall annual population-based incidence is currently estimated to be 5 cases per 100,000, rising to 20 to 50 cases per 100,000 in individuals greater than 60 years of age.[96] Approximately 15,000 to 20,000 new cases of MDS are expected each year in the United States, revealing that MDS is at least as common as chronic lymphocytic leukemia (CLL), the most prevalent form of leukemia in the United States.

Although still controversial, the prevailing view is that MDS is a heterogeneous group of clonal neoplastic disorders arising from hematopoietic stem cells. However, only 10 to 15% of MDS cases progress to acute leukemia. Families with an inherited genetic predisposition to MDS and AML have been reported, including families with germline mutations in *AML1/RUNX1* (see Table 8-1), but such inherited predisposition appears to be very rare.[97] Further providing evidence of a disease continuum between MDS and AML, many mouse models of leukemia demonstrate an initial MDS-like phase of disease prior to the development of frank acute leukemia.[39] Yet, whether all forms of MDS are truly clonal proliferations of multipotent stem cells remains unclear. The actual biologic hallmark of MDS is a defective capacity for stem cell self-renewal and differentiation, leading many investigators to implicate the marrow microenvironment and the aging of marrow stem cells, particularly in individuals with occupational or environmental exposures, as disease initiators. Thus, like the controversy surrounding the etiology and mechanisms of initiation of carcinogenesis in solid tumors discussed in previous sections of this chapter, it remains to be determined whether MDS arises because of initiating genomic mutations and the emergence of a clonal population of stem cells, or whether the marrow microenvironment and perturbed interactions between hematopoietic stem cells and marrow stromal cells leads to ineffective hematopoiesis and the secondary emergence of MDS clones.

Although the WHO classification system[95] has been a useful tool for defining MDS subtypes, the eight histopathologic variants recognized by WHO (refractory anemia [RA], RA with ringed sideroblasts, RA with multilineage dysplasia, RA with multilineage dysplasia and ringed sideroblasts, RA with excess blasts: Type 1 [< 5% blasts], RA with excess blasts: Type 2 [5–19% blasts], MDS with isolated del(5q), and MDS unclassified) still demonstrate striking clinical and genetic heterogeneity, spanning from diseases with more limited mortality to diseases that are barely distinguishable from AML. Clonal chromosomal abnormalities have now been reported in more than 2,000 patients with MDS, the significant majority of whom have clonal karyotypic abnormalities at diagnosis.[22,98,99] In contrast to the balanced chromosomal rearrangements characteristic of the acute leukemias, most cases of MDS are characterized by recurring patterns of chromosomal gain or loss (see Table 8-4). The recurring chromosomal aberrations most frequently associated with MDS include the following associated with a good prognosis: normal karyotype, loss of Y, del(11q), del(12p), del(20q); those associated with an intermediate prognosis: rearrangements of 3q21q26, +8, +9, del(17p), and translocations involving 11q; and those associated with a poor prognosis: complex karyotypes, –7/7q–, and i(17q).[99,100] Loss of chromosome 5 or 5q– has a variable prognosis depending upon the MDS subtype and the constellation of other cytogenetic abnormalities with which it is frequently associated. Interstitial deletions of chromosome 5 have been shown to occur in two distinct "minimally deleted regions": a 1.5 Mb region of 5q31 and a 3 Mb region of 5q33 between *ADRB2* and *IL12B*.[101] Similarly, two critical minimal regions of deletion have been defined

Table 8-4 Most Frequent Recurrent Chromosomal Abnormalities in Myeloid Disorders

Acute Myeloid Leukemias			
Cytogenetic Abnormality	**Frequency in Children**	**Frequency in Adults**	**Critical Fusion Genes**
t(8;21)(q22;q22)	12%	5–12% (<45 years) Rare (> 45 years)	AML1/ETO
Inv(16)(p13q22) t(16;16)(p13;q22)	12%	10% (<45 years) Rare (> 45 years)	CBFβ/MYH11
t(15;17)(q21;q11)	7%	15% (<45 years) Rare (> 45 years)	PML-RARα
Variants:			
t(11;17)(q23;q11)			PLZF-RARα
t(5;17)(q35;q12–21)			NPM-RARα
t(11;17)(q13;q21)			RARα-NUMA
t(17;17)(q11;q21)			RARα-STAT5b
11q23 Translocations, del(11)(q23)	>80% of infant AML cases have 11q abnormalities; most frequently t(4;11) 7% t(9;11)	5–7%	MLL
Common Variants:			
t(4;11)(q21;q23)			MLL/AF4
t(9;11)(p22;q23)			MLL/AF9
t(11;19)(q23;p13.1)			MLL/AFX
t(11;19)(q23;p13.3)			MLL/ELL MLL/ENL
t(8;16)(p11;q13)	Rare	<1%	MOZ/CBP
t(11;16)			MLL/CBP
t(11;22)			MLL/p300
t(6;9)(p23;q34)	Rare	Rare	DEK/CAN
Inv(3)(q21q26), t(3;3)(q21;q26)	3%	3–5%	Ribophorin/EVI1
t(1;22)(p13;q13)	Rare; Frequent in M7	Rare	
Poor prognosis and complex abnormalities: 5/5q-, -7/7q-, 17p abn or i(17q),del(20q), dmins hsrs,+13, complex	Rare	10–15% (< 45 years) 30–40% (> 45 years)	Unknown

Myelodysplastic Syndromes	
Cytogenetic Abnormalities	**Prognosis**
Normal karyotype loss of Y, del(11q), del(12p), del(20q)	More favorable prognosis
Rearrangements of 3q21q26, +8, +9, del(17p), and translocations involving 11q	Intermediate prognosis
Complex karyotypes, -7/7q–, and i(17q)	Poor prognosis
Loss of chromosome 5 or 5q–	Variable; depending on whether it is a sole abnormality or is within a more complex karyotype

Chronic Myeloproliferative Diseases	
Chronic myelogenous leukemia	t(9;22) BCR-ABL
Chronic myelomonocytic leukemia (CMML)	TEL-PDGFRB, TEL-JAK2, TEL-ABL, HIP1-PDGFRB, H4-PDGFRB, RBTN5-PDGFRB, PDE4DIP-PDGFRB, NIN-PDGFRB, TP53BP1-PDGFRB, HCMOGT1-PDGFRB, BCR-PDGFRB, KIAA1509-PDGFRB
Stem cell–like myeloproliferative diseases	ZNF198-FGFR1, FOP-FGFR1, CEP110-FGFR1, TIAF1-FGFR1, HERVK-FGFR1, BCR-FGFR1
Juvenile myelomonocytic leukemia (JMML)	NF1 Loss, SHP2 (PTPN11) mutations, RAS mutations

on 7q: 7q22 or 7q32–33.[102] Yet, despite intensive efforts over the past 15 years, particularly focused on chromosomes 5, 7, and 20, the molecular mechanisms of transformation and the critical genes involved in the majority of the recurring genetic aberrations in MDS remain unidentified.

Interestingly, with the exception of the isolated del(5q)/5q– and 17p– syndromes, the recurrent chromosomal abnormalities associated with MDS do not show a particularly close association with the distinct disease categories as defined by the WHO MDS classification scheme; several of the recurrent cytogenetic aberrations may be found in each morphologically defined disease category. MDS with isolated del(5q) or the "5q– syndrome" is a distinct entity that occurs in a subset of older patients, frequently women, with refractory macrocytic anemia, low blast counts, and normal or elevated platelet counts. The dominant finding in the bone marrow is the presence of abnormalities in the megakaryocytic lineage, particularly micromegakaryocytes. The "17p– syndrome" also has a distinct morphology involving a dysgranulopoiesis, which combines pseudo-Pelger–Huët hypolobulation with frequent cytoplasmic vacuoles and a reduced number of granules in granulocytes. The break point on chromosome 17 appears variable, but is always proximal to *TP53* (see Table 8-1). In addition to WHO, other classification schemes have been developed to direct clinical intervention in MDS. The International Prognostic Scoring System (IPSS),[100] uses the recurring cytogenetic aberrations in MDS, the percent of marrow blasts, and the number and degree of cytopenias to predict disease survival, the risk of transformation to acute leukemia, and to direct therapeutic intervention. Recent therapeutic advances in MDS make this classification scheme and the identification of recurring genomic abnormalities in MDS particularly important. List and colleagues have recently shown that lenalidomide, a thalidomide analogue, has a significant therapeutic benefit in MDS, particularly in the one-third of MDS patients who have pure RA with isolated erythroid abnormalities, MDS with isolated del(5q), and MDS patients with a low (more favorable) IPSS score.[103]

Acute Myeloid Leukemias Following a small peak in children aged less than 5 years, AML incidence rates in the United States increase continuously from adolescence through early adulthood and begin to rise exponentially after 45 years of age. The age-specific incidence rate for AML in adolescents and young adults less than 45 years of age at diagnosis is 3.5 per 100,000, increasing to 15 at age 70 and 35 at age 90 (see <http://seer.cancer.gov>). Importantly, the mean age of AML in the United States has risen to 68 years, indicating that AML in the United States is primarily a disease of the elderly. Importantly, the chromosomal aberrations associated with AML in younger individuals (including balanced reciprocal translocations with a more favorable prognosis, such as the t(8;21), inv(16), t(15;17), see Table 8-4), and those in elderly AML patients (sharing the recurring regions of chromosome gain and loss seen in MDS that portend a poorer outcome) are quite distinct, suggesting that the etiology and mechanisms of leukemogenesis in younger versus older AML patients are different.

Over 150 recurrent cytogenetic abnormalities have been described in AML to date and the genes involved in many of these aberrations have been cloned and characterized.[22] The most common structural aberrations seen in AML in individuals less than 45 years of age are balanced reciprocal chromosome translocations or inversions, the vast majority of which target genes encoding transcription factors. These translocations or inversions result in chimeric fusion proteins that disrupt the normal function of transcriptional regulators, thereby perturbing the gene expression programs that regulate normal hematopoiesis (see Table 8-4; Figure 8-9). One set of transcription factors frequently targeted by AML-associated translocations includes core binding factor (CBFα/β), the retinoic acid receptor alpha (RARA), and members of the HOX family of transcriptional regulators (see Tables 8-1 and 8-4). The chimeric leukemogenic fusions involving these transcription factors interfere with the normal recruitment of the nuclear corepressor/histone deacetylase (HDAC) complex, leading to constitutive repression of genes whose expression is essential for normal hematopoiesis (see Figure 8-9). In contrast, another set of genes frequently targeted by AML-associated translocations serve as coactivators of transcription; these genes include the CREB binding protein (CBP), p300, MOZ, TIF2, and MLL (see Figure 8-8 and Tables 8-1 and 8-4). Perturbation of the function of these genes by chimeric fusions leads to persistent transcriptional activation and altered gene expression programs that promote leukemogenesis. Thus, a common molecular mechanism for leukemogenesis is disruption of the transcriptional regulatory programs that underpin normal hematopoiesis, either through transcriptional repression or persistent transcriptional activation (see Figure 8-9). These insights into the molecular mechanisms of leukemogenesis have already led to the development of new biologically targeted therapies, including HDAC inhibitors.

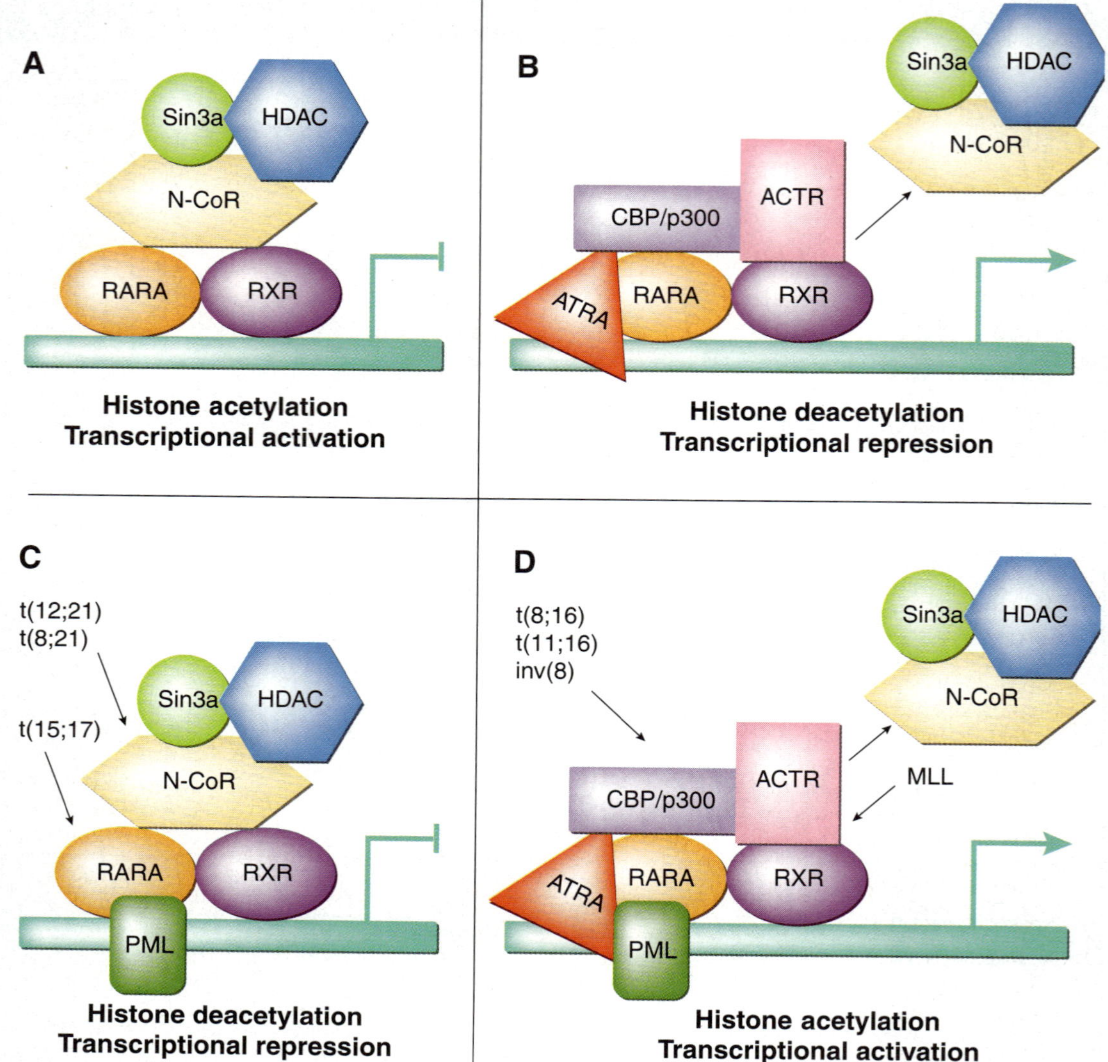

Figure 8-9 Perturbation of transcriptional regulation and chromatin modification in acute promyelocytic leukemias (APL) and other acute leukemias: a paradigm for leukemogenesis. **A,** In normal cells, the RARA protein forms a heterodimer with other retinoic acid binding proteins (RXR) and this heterodimer binds the promoters of critical retinoic acid (vitamin A)-responsive target genes to activate transcriptional programs that promote normal hematopoietic differentiation. In the absence of retinoic acid, RARA-RXR recruits a transcriptional repressor complex including N-CoR, Sin3a, and the histone deacetylase (HDAC) enzyme. Once recruited, HDAC acetylates regional histones leading to an altered chromatin state and the repression of transcription. **B,** In the presence of retinoic acid (or ATRA: all *trans* retinoic acid), there is a conformational change in RARA-RXR that leads to the removal of the transcriptional repressor complex and the recruitment of a transcriptional activation complex including CBP, its p300 homologue, and the histone acetyl transferase (ACTR) enzymatic activity. ACTR acetylates regional histones, allowing for chromatin modification and transcriptional activation from retinoic acid-responsive genes. **C,** Numerous leukemogenic fusion proteins, as well as fusion proteins in mesenchymal and other solid tumors, have been shown to recruit and maintain the transcriptional repressor complex on the promoters of target genes, leading to a persistent repression of the normal transcription program. In APL, fusion of the PML domain to RARA as a result of the t(15;17) alters the affinity of RARA for ATRA, requiring higher doses of retinoic acid (ATRA) to overcome the transcriptional repression. The ETO and TEL components of the t(8;21) AML-ETO and t(12;21) TEL-AML1 fusions also recruit the transcriptional repressor complex, promoting persistent transcriptional repression for leukemogenesis. **D,** With high doses of ATRA, the transcriptional repression of the PML-RARA fusion can be overcome and subsequent recruitment of a transcriptional activation complex can re-activate the normal transcriptional program. Interestingly, other leukemogenic fusions act by interfering with the normal function of the transcriptional activation complex (such as the t(8;16), t(11;16) and inv(8) which alter the normal function of CBP) or promote an inappropriately sustained pattern of transcriptional activation (such as the many leukemic translocations involving MLL).

Translocations Involving Core Binding Factors More than a dozen chromosomal translocations target CBF in the acute leukemias (see Tables 8-1 and 8-4). Two of the most frequent are the t(8;21)(q22;q22) AML1-ETO and the inv(16)(p13;q22) CBFβ-SMMHC that occur primarily in de novo AML; together these two translocations account for 20 to 25% of the AML cases in individuals less than 45 years of age. These two cytogenetic abnormalities target two different genes: *AML1* (see *RUNX1* also known as CBFα; see Table 8-1) and CBFβ, each of which encodes a component of the heterodimeric core-binding factor transcription factor complex termed CBFα/β or simply CBF.[104] In normal hematopoietic cells, CBF regulates the transcription of a number of genes important for hematopoiesis including *IL-1*, *IL-3*, *GM-CSF*, the CSF-1 receptor, myeloperoxidase, *BCL2*, the immunoglobulin heavy chain and T-cell receptor genes, and the multidrug resistance gene *MDR1* encoding P-glycoprotein. Further evidence for the critical role of CBF in hematopoiesis comes from studies of mice engineered to lack either CBFα or CBFβ alleles. In CBFα -/- knockout mice, fetal liver hematopoiesis is completely blocked and embryos die by day 12 of gestation owing to central nervous system hemorrhage; a similar phenotype is seen in CBFβ -/- mice, confirming that the CBFβ subunit is essential for normal CBFα function.[104–107] The transcriptional activation function of CBF and induction of the expression of critical target genes is disrupted by several leukemia-associated translocations, including the t(8;21), inv(16) and related t(16;16), the complex t(3;21)(q21;q22), and the t(12;12)(p13;q22) in pediatric ALL.

In the t(8;21), the amino terminal DNA binding domain of AML1/RUNX1/CBFα becomes fused to the carboxy terminus of ETO (eight twenty one), a zinc-binding protein that appears to function as a nuclear repressor. By binding to the same DNA binding site as normal CBF, but failing to activate the transcription of critical target genes, the AML1-ETO fusion protein acts as a "dominant negative" inhibitor or a constitutive transcriptional repressor of normal CBF function.[128,132–140] AML-ETO functions as a transcriptional repressor through recruitment of multiple corepressors (N-CoR, Sin3a) and histone deacetylases (see Figure 8-9).[104] A single AML1-ETO transcription factor fusion mRNA can be consistently detected in all AML patients with t(8;21).[108] Expression of a knocked-in *AML1-ETO* gene inhibits the establishment of definitive hematopoiesis and generates dysplastic progenitors.[109,110] The inv(16) and molecularly identical t(16;16) result in an unusual chimeric fusion of the amino terminus of the CBFβ transcription factor to the carboxy terminus of the cytoplasmic smooth muscle myosin heavy chain (*SMMHC*) gene.[111,112] The result of this fusion is to sequester a large amount of CBFβ protein in the cytoplasm, effectively excluding it from the nucleus, and thereby functionally inactivating CBF. AML cases with inv(16) and t(16;16) have a distinct morphologic appearance with acute myelomonocytic leukemia and frequent abnormal bone marrow eosinophilic precursors (FAB AML-M4Eo). In contrast to the t(8;21), the CBFβ-MYH11 fusion yields a number of different fusion transcripts arising both because of different genomic break points and alternative splicing. Although the type "A" CBFβ-MYH11 fusion (fusing CBFβ nucleotide 495 with MYH11 nucleotide 1921) is the most common and occurs in greater than 90% of AML cases with inv(16) or t(16;16), at least seven other fusion transcripts have been reported (types B-H).[112,113]

Translocations Involving the Retinoic Acid Receptor Alpha: Acute Promyelocytic Leukemia Translocations involving the retinoic acid receptor alpha (RARA; see Tables 8-1 and 8-4) include the classic hallmark translocation associated with acute promyelocytic leukemia (APL)—the t(15;17)(q22;q11–12) PML-RARA—as well as several rarer variants: t(11;17)(q23;q12) PLZF-RARA, t(5;17)(q35;q12–21) NPM-RARA, t(11;17)(q13;q21) RARA-NUMA, and the t(17;17)(q11;q21) RARA-STAT5b (see Table 8-4).[114–117] The vast majority of AML cases with morphologic and clinical features of APL, including both the hypergranular (FAB AML-M3) or microgranular (FAB AML-M3v) morphologic variants, usually have an associated t(15;17). The t(15;17) results in the fusion of PML (promyelocytic leukemia gene) on chromosome 15q with RARA on chromosome 17q. Although chromosome 17q break points invariably occur in the second intron of RARA, three different genomic break points may occur in the *PML* gene: (1) PML intron 3 to RARA intron 2, yielding a PML exon 3—RARA exon 3 fusion transcript (variably referred to as the "bcr3" or "S" [short] form of the fusion transcript); (2) PML intron 6 to RARA intron 2, yielding a PML exon 6—RARA exon 3 fusion transcript (variably referred to as the "bcr1" or "L" [long] form); and (3) PML exon 6 to RARA intron 2, yielding a PML partial exon 6—RARA exon 3 fusion transcript (variably referred to as the "bcr2" or "V" [variable form]). The reciprocal RARA-PML transcript is also expressed in the majority of APL cases. The PML-RARA fusion protein acts as a dominant negative inhibitor of both the wild-type PML, RARA, and other retinoic acid binding proteins (RXR).[118,119]

Transcriptional Repression and Chromatin Acetylation: An Evolving Paradigm in the Acute Leukemias APL was the first human leukemia to be successfully treated with a differentiation agent, all-*trans*-retinoic acid (ATRA), although ultimate cure in this disease requires the concomitant administration of chemotherapy.[120] More recent clinical trials have also employed arsenic in combination with ATRA.[121] ATRA therapy overcomes the dominant negative effect of PML-RARA by disrupting the interaction of the PML-RARα protein with the nuclear corepressor/histone deacetylase complex that promotes transcriptional repression (see Figure 8-9).[118,119] High levels of acetylation of DNA-associated histones are associated with transcriptionally active chromatin and activation of gene expression, while histone deacetylation is associated with transcriptional repression. In 1998, several laboratories first reported that PML-RARA suppressed transcription of target genes by recruitment of a histone deacetylase complex (see Figure 8-9)[118,119,122] The retinoic acid receptors consist of two distinct families, the RARs and RXRs, which likely mediate their effects by binding to the promoter elements of critical target genes as RAR-RXR heterodimers.[155,161] In the absence of the ATRA ligand, the RAR-RXR heterodimer recruits a large ubiquitous nuclear corepressor protein (N-CoR), which mediates transcriptional repression through its interaction with other proteins, particularly mSin3a and histone deacetylase (HDAC) (see Figure 8-9). With the addition of ATRA, there is a distinct conformational change in the RAR-RXR complex, resulting in the release of the repressor complex and the recruitment of transcriptional coactivators, including the CBP protein discussed above and a histone acetyltransferase, leading to chromatin acetylation and activation of gene expression.[118] Thus, the addition of ATRA converts the normal RAR-RXR and leukemic PML-RARA/RXR heterodimers from transcriptional "repressors" to transcriptional activators. Although the APL-associated PML-RARA appears to act as a dominant negative mutant and interferes with wild-type RAR for binding to RXR, exposure to high levels of ATRA can overcome the transcriptional repression of PML-RARA, which contains a single N-CoR binding site. In contrast, the relative ATRA resistance of the related PLZF-RARA fusion arising from the t(11;17) can now be explained, as PLZF contains two NCoR binding sites. Interestingly, recent studies have shown that mutation of the N-CoR binding site in PML-RARA abolishes the ability of PML-RARA to block differentiation in *in vitro* models, providing further proof that the ability of the PML-RARA fusion protein to recruit the NCoR complex is critical for transcriptional repression and leukemogenesis.[119]

Translocations Involving Chromatin Remodeling Proteins: MLL The MLL (mixed lineage leukemia) gene on human chromosome 11q23 is involved in an astonishing number of recurrent chromosomal abnormalities in the acute leukemias and MDS (see Tables 8-1, 8-4, and 8-5).[22] To date, MLL has been reported to be involved in

Table 8-5 Most Frequent Recurrent Genetic Subtypes of B and T Cell ALL

Subtype	Associated Genetic Abnormalities	Frequency in Children	Frequency in Adults
B-Precursor ALL	Hyperdiploid DNA content	35% of B precursor cases	0%
	t(12;21)(p13;q22): TEL-AML1	20% of B precursor cases	<1%
	t(9;22)(q34;q11): BCR-ABL	4% of B precursor cases	30%
	11q23/MLL rearrangements; particularly t(4;11)(q21;q23)	5% of B precursor cases; >80% of infant ALL	Rare
	t(1;19)9q23;p13)–E2A/PBX1	5% of all B lineage ALL cases	<1%
B-ALL	t(8;14)(q24;q32)–IgH/MYC	5% of all B lineage ALL cases	Rare
T-ALL	Numerous translocations involving the TCR ab (7q35) or TCR gd (14q11) loci	7% of all ALL cases	Rare
	1q deletions; t(1;14)(p32;q11) SIL-SCL	25% of T ALL	Unknown
	NOTCH mutations	50% of pediatric T-ALL cases	Unknown

nearly 60 different translocations involving distinct partner genes on different chromosomes, the majority of which have been cloned. In spite of the large size of the gene, spanning over 100 kb, the translocation break points in *MLL* cluster around an 8.3 kb region just 5' of the PHD domain. The clustering of the breaks makes it possible to detect virtually all *MLL* rearrangements with a 0.74 kb complementary DNA (cDNA) probe on Southern blot analysis or with genomic DNA probes in FISH. The fusion genes that result consist of 5' *MLL* and 3' partner genes, but the reciprocal fusion transcript (3' partner gene and 5' *MLL*) is also frequently expressed. The role of the partner genes in MLL-mediated leukemogenesis has been the subject of much debate. The fact that they lack a common motif and are so varied suggests that they may be interchangeable and play only a minor role in leukemogenesis. However, the biologic and clinical phenotypes associated with each different MLL-associated translocation are quite distinct, implying that the partner gene plays a significant role. For example, the most common MLL translocation, t(4;11)(q21;q23), which generates the MLL-AF4 (MLLT2; see Table 8-1) fusion is found in 2 to 7% of ALL cases and more than 80% of the ALL cases arising in infants less than 1 year of age. The t(11;19)(q23;p13.3) MLL-ENL fusion is also seen predominantly in ALL, while the t(9;11)(q22;q23) MLL-AF9 (MLLT3; see Table 8-1), the t(6;11)(q27;q23) MLL-AF6 (MLLT4; see Table 8-1), and the t(11;19)(q23;p13.1) MLL-ELL fusion are seen in AML. In addition to reciprocal translocations, MLL may undergo other types of aberration in the leukemias, including partial tandem duplications and amplification.[123,124]

MLL, a homologue of the *Drosophila melanogaster* trithorax, displays histone methyltransferase activity (mediated by the SET domain) and functions genetically to maintain HOX gene expression, critical for normal hematopoiesis.[123,125] *HOX* genes are important determinants of the mammalian body plan and are also differentially expressed in subsets of hematopoietic progenitor cells. *MLL* amplification is associated with up-regulation of *HOX* gene expression and a block in hematopoietic differentiation, while *MLL* loss of function is associated with a loss of *HOX* gene expression and is embryonically lethal. *MLL* regulates *HOX* gene expression by direct promoter binding and by histone H3 Lys 4 methylation mediated by the intrinsic methyltransferase activity of the SET domain. A closely related homologue, MLL2, has been reported to be amplified in solid tumors. Recent studies by Cleary and colleagues[125] have demonstrated that MLL associates with a number of proteins shared with the yeast and human SET1 histone methyltransferase complexes, including the transcriptional coregulator (HCF-1) and the related HCF-2, both of which specifically interact with a conserved binding motif in the MLL(N) (p300) subunit of MLL. MENIN, the MEN1 tumor suppressor gene, is also a component of the 1-MDa MLL complex. Interestingly, abrogation of MENIN phenocopies loss of MLL and reveals a critical role for MENIN in HOX gene expression. Oncogenic forms of MLL retain their ability to bind to MENIN, but not other components of the histone methyltransferase complex. These recent studies indicate that disruption of MLL function interferes with chromatin modeling and histone modification through methylation. Thus, in contrast to the RARA, AML1/RUNX1, and CBF leukemic fusion proteins discussed above that promote leukemogenesis through transcriptional repression and recruitment of the nuclear corepressor/histone deacetylase complex, MLL appears to transform hematopoietic cells by two distinct mechanisms. A subset of the MLL fusion partners display transcriptional activation and appear to inappropriately *maintain* (rather than repress) transcription, likely by recruiting or tethering transcriptional coactivators or chromatic modeling factors at MLL target genes through the fusion portion of the MLL chimera. A second set of MLL fusion partners consist of cytoplasmic proteins that do not have inherent transcriptional activities, but which have dimerization or oligomerization domains; these fusions appear to lead to MLL dimerization and strong transcriptional activation. Both of these pathways appear to lead to the inappropriate maintenance, rather than the repression, of transcription.

Translocations Involving Transcriptional Coactivators and Chromatin Modification: The CREB Binding Protein (CBP) Transcriptional coactivators interact with the basal transcription machinery and with transcription factors such as the cyclic AMP response element binding protein (CREB) and nuclear hormone receptors to activate transcription from target genes (see Figure 8-9). Many of these coactivators also have histone acetyl transferase (HAT) activity, which is important in chromatin remodeling and transcriptional activation (see Figure 8-9). CBP, located on chromosome band 16p13.3, is one of the best studied of these transcriptional coactivators to date. Through its binding to the phosphorylated form of CREB and its direct interactions with TFIIB and RNA polymerase II, it functions as a global transcriptional coactivator. CBP also contains a bromodomain, which is a motif that is conserved in humans, *Drosophila*, and the yeast SWI2/SNF2 complex. Several bromodomain-containing proteins, including CBP, SWI2/SNF2, TAF250, and GCN5, are involved in transcriptional regulation as mediators or coactivators. Several of these proteins also have HAT activity, are present in large multiprotein complexes, and are important in chromatin modification. CBP and its homologue p300 serve as a bridge between the transcriptional machinery and transcription factors; although they do not bind directly to DNA, they recruit multiple transcription factors (see Figure 8-9). Both CBP and p300 also contain intrinsic HAT activity, which promotes an open chromatin state and the activation of gene expression (see Figure 8-9).[126] Disruption of the critical function of CBP or p300 would presumably lead to a failure of transcriptional activation of the large number of target genes regulated by CBP and p300. Strikingly, both CBP and p300 are involved in a number of AML-associated chromosomal abnormalities that disrupt their function, including the t(11;16)(q23;p13.3) MLL-CBP, the t(8;16)(p11;p13) MOZ-CBP, and the t(11;22)(q23;q13) MLL-P300 fusion.[127–129] Another coactivator that is potentially important in leukemogenesis is TIF2, which was cloned from the inv(8)(p11q13) that generates the MOZ-TIF2 fusion protein.[130] Interestingly, in addition to its role in transcriptional coactivation and leukemogenesis, CBP is also the gene responsible for the Rubinstein-Taybi syndrome,[169] in which loss of one functional CBP allele results in a well-defined syndrome characterized by facial abnormalities, broad thumbs, and mental retardation, as well as the propensity for malignancy (see Table 8-1).

Point Mutations of the Pathogenesis of AML Although chromosomal translocations and inversions are the hallmark of AML arising in younger individuals, an increasing number of point mutations in cancer genes have also been identified (see Table 8-1; see the COSMIC database: <http://www.sanger.ac.uk/genetics/CGP/cosmic/>). Interestingly, mutations in a few of these genes may serve to initiate leukemogenesis. Positional cloning of the disease allele for the familial platelet disorder with propensity to develop AML (FPD/AML) demonstrated germline loss of function mutations in AML1/RUNX1 (see Table 8-1).[97] Loss of function point mutations in AML1 have also been identified in about 3 to 5% of sporadic AML and MDS.[170] In addition, function mutations in another hematopoietic transcription factor C/EBPα results in expression of a dominant negative C/EBPα allele that would be predicted to impair hematopoietic development.[131] However, other point mutations frequently seen in AML are not sufficient for leukemogenesis; point mutations in these genes may promote disease progression and further complement initiating genetic lesions. The most frequently mutated gene in AML is the *FLT3* tyrosine kinase, which may be mutated through internal tandem duplication (ITD) or activating mutations in the ATP binding loop.[34,35] The overall frequency of FLT3-ITD is 24% of AML cases, occurring at the highest frequencies in older AML patients; in patients with APL; and in secondary AML, where it may be associated with disease progression. The overall frequency of activating loop mutations appears to be 6 to 7%. Several studies have demonstrated biallelic mutations in *FLT3*, as well as patients in whom the residual wild-type allele is lost.[132–133] Selective inhibitors of the activated *FLT3* kinase are now being tested in clinical trials.[42] Like *FLT3*, activation loop mutations have been reported at position D816 of c-KIT in about 5% of AML patients and at the corresponding position in other receptor tyrosine kinases (RTK's), including MET and RET.

Activating mutations at codons 12, 13, or 61 of N-*ras* and K-*ras* are associated with AML and MDS, The reported incidence varies widely between studies, but is generally found in 25 to 44% of patients.[134] There has been considerable effort devoted to develop small molecule inhibitors of RAS activation, with a focus on farnesyl transferase and geranylgeranyl transferase (prenyl transferase) inhibitors that preclude appropriate targeting of activated RAS to the plasma membrane. Mutations in the nucleophosmin gene *NPM* have recently been reported to occur in AML at high frequency (see Tables 8-1 and 8-4).[136,137] *NPM* was initially discovered fused to RARA in the t(5;17) (see Table 8-4). Nucleophosmin mutations are seen in 85% of AML patients with a normal karyotype, often in concert with a FLT3-ITD; mutation in *NPM* appears to be associated with aberrant *NPM* localization in the cytoplasm rather than the nucleus.

AML in the Elderly and Secondary AML and MDS As discussed earlier in this chapter, the median age at diagnosis of AML in the United States is currently 68 years, making AML arising in the elderly the largest group of AML cases. In contrast to the molecular mechanisms of leukemogenesis in children and younger adults (see Table 8-4), recent studies indicate that the majority of cases of AML in the elderly have quite distinct biologic and molecular genetic features. The biologic, morphologic, and genetic features of AML in the elderly are strikingly similar to (1) cases of AML that arise from antecedent MDS; (2) cases of AML that arise secondary to prior therapy, particularly alkylating agent exposure; (3) cases of AML that arise from documented environmental or occupational exposures to agents such as benzene, petroleum, organic solvents, and arsenical pesticides; and (4) cases of MDS, particularly those with chromosome 7 abnormalities and defective DNA repair. These common features include trilineage dysplasia in residual myeloid elements, complex "unfavorable" cytogenetic abnormalities that are primarily large gains and losses rather than translocation (involving particularly chromosomes 5 and/or 7, del(5q), del(7q), abnormalities of 11q, inv(3), and complex or multiple abnormalities), the potential for clonal remissions and reversion to a myelodysplastic marrow picture at remission, and a high incidence of a "drug resistant" phenotype mediated by MDR-1/p-glycoprotein or other members of the ABC transporter family.[138] The similar biologic features of AML arising in older patients and MDS and secondary AML have led to the hypothesis that AML in the elderly may arise from cumulative environmental exposures in susceptible or predisposed individuals. Furthermore, the etiology and pathogenesis of AML in the elderly may be quite distinct from AML in younger patients.

The development of therapy-related MDS (t-MDS) or AML (t-AML) is one of the most serious late consequences of successful treatment of a prior malignant disease. In 1977, it was first reported that patients with prior lymphoma treated with alkylating agent chemotherapy, with or without radiation therapy, developed t-AML with a high frequency of del(5q), –7/7q–, or both.[139] Such patients may have a very complex karyotype with frequent deletion of 12p, 17p, 20q, and –18 as well.[140] t-AML arising because of alkylating agent exposure, frequently seen in breast cancer, Hodgkin's lymphoma, and myeloma following alkylating agent therapy, typically have a long latency period of greater than 5 years and are often prec\eded by a t-MDS. The response of these patients to antileukemic therapy is generally very poor. As described in earlier sections of this chapter, exposure to drugs that target topoisomerase II, such as the epipodophyllotoxins or anthracyclines promote t-MDS and t-AML associated with balanced translocations involving the *MLL* gene at 11q23 or, less often, the *AML1* gene at 21q22. These leukemias have a shorter latency period, frequently less than 2 years from initiation of therapy, lack a preceding MDS phase, and generally have a better response to chemotherapy.

Chronic Myeloproliferative Disorders In striking contrast to the recurrent chromosomal translocations and inversions seen in AML in younger patients that target the chromatin and transcriptional regulatory machinery (see Figure 8-9), chromosomal translocations in chronic myeloproliferative diseases (CMPD) almost invariably result in expression of constitutively activated fusion tyrosine kinases (see Table 8-4). The hallmark of these diseases is CML, where the *BCR-ABL*-activated tyrosine kinase results from the balanced reciprocal Philadelphia chromosome translocation t(9;22).

CML The cytogenetic, molecular genetic, and clinical features of CML were briefly discussed in earlier sections of this chapter, and excellent recent reviews are available.[26,28] Three predominant forms of the *BCR-ABL* fusion have been associated with different manifestations of disease. Depending upon the precise break point in the *BCR* gene and differential BCR exon splicing, the t(9;22) may give rise to multiple *BCR-ABL* chimeric RNAs and at least three different fusion proteins: the p210 Bcr-Abl fusion protein, most frequently associated with CML; the p185 Bcr-Abl fusion protein, more frequently associated with ALL; and the p230 Bcr-Abl fusion, which is associated with a CML-like CMPD.[26] However, the simultaneous occurrence of the p185 and p210 Bcr-Abl proteins in CML is not infrequent. The majority of patients with chronic phase CML have t(9;22), or a related variant, as their sole chromosomal abnormality. However, even though the *BCR-ABL* fusion is essential for initiation, maintenance, and disease progression, the transformation of CML from chronic to blast phase is associated with the acquisition of additional genetic and epigenetic abnormalities. During the transformation phase to CML-blast crisis, different chromosomal abnormalities occur either singly or in combination, in a distinctly nonrandom pattern. In patients with secondary chromosomal changes, the most common abnormalities are +8 (34% of cases with additional changes), +Ph (30%), i(17q) (20%), +19 (13%), –Y (8% of males), +21 (7%), +17 (5%), and monosomy 7 (5%).[141] The frequency of secondary cytogenetic abnormalities has been shown to vary in relation to the therapy given during chronic phase. Frequencies of secondary chromosomal abnormalities also vary in relation to the morphology of the blast crisis cells. A higher incidence of i(17q) is seen with myeloid blast crisis, and higher frequencies of monosomy 7, and hypodiploidy are seen in lymphoid blast crisis.[141] With widespread use of imatinib/Gleevec, resistance to this drug is more widely seen. Interestingly, several genomic aberrations are now being described in imatinib-resistant CML patients, including point mutations in the *BCR-ABL* kinase that overcome the imatinib inhibition and *BCR-ABL* amplification.[26]

Other Myeloproliferative Diseases Although rare, a number of translocations involving the PDGFRB transmembrane tyrosine kinase receptor on chromosome 5q35, the FGFR1 tyrosine kinase, and ABL have recently been cloned and characterized in Chronic Myelomonocytic Leukemia (CMML), stem cell-like myeloproliferative diseases, and hypereosinophilic syndromes (see Table 8-4). Like the ABL kinase in CML, translocation and frequent dimerization of these kinase domains by the chimeric fusions leads to inappropriate tyrosine kinase activation and signaling.

HEMATOPOIETIC CANCERS: MALIGNANCIES OF THE LYMPHOID LINEAGES

Acute Lymphoblastic Leukemia Mathematical modeling of the very sharp peak in ALL incidence seen in children 2 to 3 years old (> 80 cases per million; see <http://seer.cancer.gov>) has suggested that ALL may arise from two primary events, the first of which occurs in utero and the second after birth.[39,142] Interestingly, the detection of certain ALL-associated genetic abnormalities in cord blood samples taken at birth from children who are ultimately affected by disease supports this hypothesis.[39] Among children < 15 years of age, the incidence of ALL is consistently higher among males (20%) relative to females and among whites (threefold) as compared with blacks. Although the incidence of ALL is increasing overall, the most significant increases are in children of Hispanic origin (see <http://seer.cancer.gov>). In contrast to children and adolescents, ALL is relatively rare in adults, and AML is by far the most prevalent form of disease.

Although the use of modern combination chemotherapy has produced long-term remissions in 75% of children with ALL, nearly 25% ultimately relapse with disease that is highly refractory to conventional therapy. To prospectively categorize patients with such high relapse potential, several "risk classification" schemata have been established. The Children's Oncology Group (COG) has developed a new risk classification scheme from a detailed analysis of over 8,600 patients enrolled on legacy CCG (Children's Cancer Study Group) and POG (Pediatric Oncology Group) clinical trials. The most robust variables predictive of outcome were identified. As these variables were independent of the specific therapeutic regimens employed, they are likely to be fundamental for the biology of the disease. Children with newly diagnosed ALL are now assigned to one of four initial treatment groups at the time of diagnosis based on age, WBC, and lineage: T-cell, infant, higher risk B-precursor, and standard risk B-precursor ALL (see Table 8-5). Using clinical and laboratory parameters (age, WBC, and the presence or absence of specific cytogenetic abnormalities), patients with B-precursor ALL are further stratified into "low," "standard," "high," and "very high" risk categories. The major recurring cytogenetic abnormalities that currently define these risk groups, including t(12;21) *TEL-AML1*, t(1;19) *E2A-PBX*, t(4;11) *AF4-MLL*, t(9;22) *BCR-ABL*, hyperdiploidy (or trisomy of chromosomes 4, 10, and 17), and hypodiploidy are known to confer some of the most powerful prognostic information for the disease (see Table 8-5).[142] In a small minority of children with B-cell lineage ALL (5–7%), a poor outcome has been associated with certain "poor prognosis" cytogenetic abnormalities [t(4;11) *MLL-AF4*, t(9;22) *BCR-ABL*, and hypodiploid DNA content < 45 chromosomes]. Conversely, in nearly 25% of pediatric B-precursor ALL cases, the t(12;21) TEL-AML1 has been associated with a very favorable outcome. In addition, a hyperdiploid DNA content (defined as a modal chromosome number > 52, particularly with trisomies of chromosomes 4 and 10) occurs very frequently.

The t(12;21)(p13;q22) that results in the *TEL-AML1* fusion transcript is the most common gene rearrangement in childhood ALL, being found in about 25% of cases. It is a cryptic translocation detected only rarely by standard cytogenetics because of the similarity of the banding pattern, but easily detectable by molecular techniques such as FISH or RT-PCR. Interestingly, it is found in only 3% of adult ALL patients. *TEL*, which is also known as *ETV6* (see Table 8-1), is an ETS-related transcription factor and is associated with over 40 other genes at different translocation break points in both ALL and AML. *TEL-AML1* appears to act as a dominant negative transcriptional repressor, similar to the *AML1-ETO* fusion described extensively in previous sections of this chapter. Recent studies have suggested that *TEL* may function as a tumor suppressor; leukemic cells with one disruption of one *TEL* allele by the *TEL-AML1* translocation were found to also have the other *TEL* allele deleted, abolishing all normal *TEL* function within the cells.[143] It is intriguing, however, that dysregulation of the same transcriptional regulatory pathway involving many AML-associated translocations (see Figure 8-9) also plays a central role in *TEL-AML1*–mediated leukemogenesis in ALL. The t(1;19) ALL-associated translocation fuses the E2A basic helix-loop-helix transcription factor to PBX1 (see Figure 8-2). PBX1 is the human homolog of the *Drosophila* extradenticle protein and is thought to assist in regulation of cell differentiation through its interaction with *HOX*. Cytogenetic abnormalities involving the *MLL* gene on chromosome 11q23 are common in patients with ALL, involving 60 to 70% of infants with ALL, and approximately 10% of older children and adults. The mechanism of *MLL*-mediated transformation has been discussed extensively in prior sections of this chapter. Gene expression profiling studies by Yeoh and colleagues and Ross and colleagues have demonstrated that although heterogeneity may exist, each of the recurrent ALL translocations is associated with a distinctive gene expression profile.[70,71]

In addition to the balanced reciprocal translocations that characterize 35 to 40% of newly diagnosed pediatric ALL patients, hyperdiploidy (defined as a modal chromosome number > 52, particularly with trisomies of chromosomes 4, 10, and 17) is one of the most frequent genomic aberrations in pediatric ALL. Although not well understood, hyperdiploidy appears to confer marked therapeutic sensitivity, as children with this genetic aberration have the best outcomes in this disease. Unlike hyperdiploidy, chromosome losses or deletions are less frequent in ALL and involve chromosomes 6q, 9p, 11q, and 12p; deletions of 9p occur as a secondary change in approximately 20% of ALL cases. Homozygous deletions of 9p lead to deletion of genes encoding the IFN gene cluster, methylthioadenosine phosphorylase (MTAP), CDKN2 ($p16^{INK4A}$), and CDKN2B.[144] Homozygous deletions of p16 occur in as many as 30% of B lineage ALL cases, particularly ALL cases in adults, and 95% of T lineage cases.[145]

In contrast to pediatric ALL where the incidence of t(9;22) is quite rare, up to 20% of adult ALL cases contain the t(9;22) *BCR-ABL* fusion and continue to have a very poor clinical outcome with a high risk of relapse. ALL patients with t(9;22) have not obtained a significant sustained therapeutic benefit with Gleevec, perhaps because the p185 Bcr-Abl fusion is less sensitive, because the p185 Bcr-Abl fusion transforms a more committed B-cell progenitor that is inherently less sensitive, or because of the presence of additional genomic aberrations that accompany the development of acute leukemia.

T-Cell Acute Leukemias Recurring chromosomal translocations and inversions typically seen in T-cell ALL (see Table 8-5) in adults and children usually involve the fusion of a proto-oncogene (MYC, LYL1, TAL1, TAL2, OLIG2 [BHLHB1], LMO1, LMO2, HOX genes HOX11 [TLX1] and HOX11L2 [TLX3] [see Table 8-1] to one of the TCR loci [either TCRα {TCRA} on chromosome 14q11.2, TCRβ {TCRB} on chromosome 7q35, or TCRδ on chromosome 14q11]).[146,147] Chromosomal rearrangements only rarely involve the TCRγ locus on chromosome 7p15. The molecular mechanisms and clinical significance of these translocations in T-ALL have been recently reviewed.[146–148] One translocation of special interest in T-ALL is the t(1;14)(p32;q11). This translocation, occurring in 3% of ALL patients, juxtaposes the *TAL1* gene with TCRD.[146–148] Using probes for *TAL1*, several groups discovered a 90 kb deletion involving the 5' region of the *TAL1* gene in up to 25% of patients. Translocation or deletion of *TAL1*, not normally expressed in lymphoid cells, leads to its inappropriate expression and perturbation of the normal gene expression program associated with T-cell differentiation. Analysis of *TAL1* gene expression in T-ALL revealed expression of *TAL1* in 35% of patients whose cells have neither a translocation nor a deletion. Another very rare, although interesting t(9;14) fuses the *NOTCH1* gene that regulates T-cell development to the TCRB locus. Interestingly, recent studies by Weng and colleagues[149] have found that over 50% of T-ALL cases have *NOTCH1* mutations. Therapies targeted to *NOTCH1* are now in development for the treatment of T-ALL.

Ferrando and Look[150] recently used gene expression profiling to develop outcome predictors and improved classification schemes for T-ALL. They identified five different multistep molecular pathways that lead to T-ALL, involving activation of different T-ALL oncogenes: (1) *HOX11*, (2) *HOX11L2*, (3) *TAL1* plus *LMO1/2*, (4) *LYL1* plus *LMO2*, and (5) *MLL-ENL*. Gene expression studies indicate activation of a subset of these genes—*HOX11*, *TAL1*, *LYL1*, *LMO1*, and *LMO2*—in a much larger fraction of T-ALL cases than those harboring activating chromosomal translocations. In many such cases, the abnormal expression of one or more of these oncogenes is biallelic, implicating upstream regulatory mechanisms. Among these molecular subtypes, overexpression of the *HOX11* orphan homeobox gene occurs in approximately 5 to 10% of childhood and 30% of adult T-ALL cases. Patients with HOX11-positive lymphoblasts have an excellent prognosis when treated with modern combination chemotherapy, while cases at high risk of early failure are included largely in the TAL1- and LYL1-positive groups. Supervised learning approaches applied to microarray data further identified a group of genes whose expression is able to distinguish high-risk cases. Based on the rapid pace of research in T-ALL, made possible in large part through microarray technology, deep analysis of molecular pathways should lead to new and much more specific targeted therapies.

CHRONIC LYMPHOPROLIFERATIVE LEUKEMIA CLL is the most common form leukemia in the United States and Europe, accounting for 30% of all cases. Using newer FISH, CGH, and array CGH techniques, distinct clonal chromosomal abnormalities may be identified in up to 90% of CLL cases of the B-cell lineage.[55,151,152] Recurrent translocations seen in CLL include t(11;14)(q13;q32) fusing CCND1 (CYCLIN D1) to the IGH locus (this translocation is also characteristic of mantle cell lymphoma), t(14;19)(q32;q13) involving BCL3. Using FISH and CGH, the most common clonal chromosomal changes in CLL and their frequencies are del(13q): 55%, del(11q): 18%, trisomy 12q: 16%, del(17p): 7%, del(6q): 6%, trisomy 8: 5%, and t(14q32): 4%. Array CGH studies have also revealed two additional recurrent aberrations: trisomy 19 and N-MYC gain of copy number.[152] CLL patients with

Table 8-6 Genetic Alterations and Pathogenesis of B-Cell Lymphoma

Lymphoma	Chromosomal Translocations	Tumor-Suppressor Gene Mutations	Viruses	Other Alterations
B-Cell CLL	—	ATM (30), TP53 (15)	—	Deletion on 13q14 (60)
Mantle-cell lymphoma	CCND1-IgH (95)	ATM (40)	—	Deletion on 13q14 (50–70)
Follicular lymphoma	BCL2-IgH (90)	—	—	—
Diffuse large B cell lymphoma	BCL6-various (35) BCL2-IgH (15–30) MYC-IgH or MYC-IgL (15)	CD95 (10–20), ATM (15), TP53 (25)	—	Aberrant hypermutation of multiple proto-oncogenes (50)
Primary mediastinal B-cell lymphoma	—	SOCS1 (40)	—	Aberrant hypermutation of multiple proto-oncogenes (70)
Burkitt's lymphoma	MYC-IgH or MYC-IgL (100)	TP53 (40), RB2 (20–80)	EBV (endemic, 95; sporadic, 30)	—
MALT lymphoma	API2-MALT1 (30) BCL10-IgH (5) MALT1-IgH (15–20) FOXP1-IgH (10)	CD95 (5–80)	Indirect role of *Helicobacter pylori* in gastric MALT lymphomas	—
Hodgkin's lymphoma	—	IKBA (10–20), IKBE (10), CD95 (<10)	EBV (40)	REL amplifications (50)
Primary effusion lymphoma	—	—	HHV8 (95), EBV (70)	—
Multiple myeloma	CCND1-IgH (15–20), FGFR3-IgH (10), MAF-IgH (5–10)	CD95 (10)		Various MYC alterations (40), RAS mutations (40), deletion on 13q14 (50)

The numbers in parenthesis indicate the percentage of cases known to harbor the genetic change.
Adapted from Reference 155.

sole del(13q) have the longest median survival (133 months), while patients with +12 have longer median survival (114 months) than patients with normal karyotypes (11 months).[151] CLL patients with the poorest median survivals also included those with del(17p).

Mature B-Cell Lymphomas In the Western world, approximately 20 new cases of lymphoma per 100,000 are diagnosed each year (see <http://seer.cancer.gov>), and the incidence of particular subsets of this disease appears to be increasing. Over 95% of the lymphomas in the United States are mature B-cell lymphomas, the remainder are derived from the T-cell lineage. Like the acute leukemias, mature B-cell lymphomas have been classified in the WHO classification scheme, and 15 subtypes have been formally recognized (Table 8-6).[153] Cytogenetic, molecular genetic, and gene expression profiling studies have revealed that each of these morphologically defined subsets still has tremendous cytogenetic and clinical heterogeneity. In the past 20 years, tremendous progress has been made in elucidating the cellular origin, mechanisms of transformation, and the recurrent chromosomal translocations and genomic changes in lymphoma. Superb reviews of the recurrent cytogenetic abnormalities associated with the lymphomas and the various mechanisms of B-cell lymphomagenesis are available.[154,155] Like the lymphoid leukemias, many of the recurrent chromosomal rearrangements in lymphoma involve fusion of an oncogene to the immunoglobulin or TCR locus, leading to inappropriate and sustained transcriptional activation of the oncogene (see Table 8-6). Recent studies using gene expression profiling have also provided new insights for the molecular classification of the lymphomas, as well as for novel insights into lymphomagenesis and the development of new targeted therapies.[63–67] Many studies have revealed that B-cell lymphomas are not as autonomous as tumors in other lineages. Many B-cell lymphomas are dependent on BCR engagement and signaling for survival, as are their normal counterpart cells.[155] Both antigen activation through the BCR (stimulated by viruses, autoantigens or other triggers) and the cellular microenvironment contribute to the etiology and pathogenesis of the B-cell lymphomas.

The hallmark reciprocal translocations that activate the expression of an oncogene by fusing it into the immunoglobulin (Ig) locus can occur through three different mechanisms, all involving aberrant recombination events that are associated with various stages in the normal development of B cells (see Table 8-6). Translocations such as the t(14;18) BCL2-IGH translocation characteristic of follicular lymphoma have genomic break points that are directly adjacent to the IgH J_H or D_H regions. As these break points often show a loss of nucleotides at the end of the J_H and D_H segments and the addition on nongermline encoded nucleotides, features that are typical of V(D)J recombination, it is likely that these translocations occur as a result of mistakes in V(D)J joining.[155] In other translocations, genomic break points are found within or adjacent to V(D)J regions that have already gone through somatic hypermutation, which occurs in the normal germinal center (GC) of lymph nodes. These features suggest that these translocations are a consequence of the aberrations in the somatic hypermutation process. Finally a third type of chromosomal translocation has genomic break points within or near the sequences that regulate immunoglobulin class switching, suggesting that these translocations are formed during class-switch recombination events. Although chromosome translocations are clearly associated with many forms of B-cell lymphoma; mutations in tumor suppressor genes, such as *TP53*, *SOCS1*, *IκBα*, and *ATM*; genomic amplifications, such as REL; and translocations not involving Ig loci also occur (Table 8-6).[155] One of the most intriguing aspects of lymphomagenesis is the role of viruses, including EBV that is found in nearly all endemic Burkitt's lymphomas, many transplant lymphomas, and in about 40% of cases of Hodgkin's lymphoma.[155–157] HHV8 has also been linked to primary effusion lymphomas and the viral encoded protein FLIP activates NK-κB, which is critical for survival.[155] Hepatitis C virus (HCV)-associated B-cell lymphomagenesis has been linked to persistent exposure to viral antigens.[158,159] Finally, persistent antigenic stimulation by *Helicobacter pylori* is associated with the development of gastric mucosa-associated lymphoid tissue (MALT) lymphomas.[155]

Mantle Cell Lymphoma The malignant cells in mantle cell lymphoma (MCL) arise from cells that populate the mantle zone of lymphoid follicles, express CD5, and characteristically overexpress *CCND1* (cyclin D1; *BCL1*) as a consequence of the t(11;14)(q13;q32) translocation seen in virtually all MCL cases. FISH and CGH have also demonstrated that additional chromosomal abnormalities are found in the majority of MCL cases; the most frequent regions of chromosome gain and loss include loss of 13q, 6q, 1p, and 11q, and gain of 3q, 8q, 7p, and 18p. Recent gene expression profiling studies in this disease have shown that the proliferation gene signature is a quantitative integrator of oncogenic events and is highly predictive of survival in MCL.[160] Higher expression of cyclin D1 was correlated with an increased proliferation signature and shorter survivals. High expression of the proliferation signature was also associated with deletion of the INK4a/ARF locus, which contains two structurally unrelated tumor suppressors: $p16^{INK4a}$ and $p14^{ARF}$.[160] Interestingly, these investigators also identified a subtype of MCL that lacked expression of *CCND1*; they were morphologically indistinguishable from MCL, shared the MCL gene signature, and had similar survivals to CCND1+ MCL patients. Interestingly, these MCL cases expressed other D type cyclins, suggesting that they may substitute for CCND1 function.[160]

Follicular Lymphoma Follicular lymphoma (FL) is a low-grade lymphoma of B-cell origin that comprises 35 to 40% of the adult non-Hodgkin's lymphomas in the Western world. These nodal lymphomas have a follicular growth pattern and FL cells resemble germinal center (GC) B cells. Follicular lymphoma is characterized by the hallmark t(14;18)(q32;q21), seen in 80 to 90% of cases (see Table 8-6). This translocation fuses the *BCL2* oncogene to the IGH locus, leading to constitutive expression of *BCL2*, aberrant regulation of apoptosis, and prolonged survival. Using FISH and CGH, Hoglund and colleagues[161] analyzed the most frequent secondary genomic aberrations in a group of 336 cases of FL. These investigators determined that FL may be classified into distinct cytogenetic subgroups determined by the presence or absence of del(6q), +7, and der(18)t(14;18). The presence of a del(17p) or +12 were associated with a poorer outcome. In one of the most fascinating gene expression profiling studies to date, Dave and colleagues[65] used gene expression profiling to develop a molecular classifier that was predictive of survival in FL. A survival predictor identified four patient subgroups ranging in survival from 13.6 to 3.9 years. Strikingly, however, the gene expression profiles predictive of outcome in FL were not derived from tumor FL cells, but rather nonmalignant immune T cells and other infiltrating cells in the tumor. These studies again demonstrate the exquisite dependence of lymphomas on their microenvironment.

Diffuse Large B-Cell Lymphoma Diffuse large B-cell lymphoma (DLBCL) is a very heterogeneous subgroup of lymphoma cases that account for 40% of all adult non-Hodgkin's lymphomas. Over 50% of these cases have translocations involving 14q32, the IgH locus. The most frequently recurring translocations involve BCL2 locus on 18q21 in (20% of cases), the MYC locus at 8q24 (10% of cases), and the BCL6 locus on 3q27 (6.5% of cases) (Table 8-6). Staudt and colleagues,[63,66,67] Shipp and colleagues,[64] and Rosenwald and colleagues[162] have used gene expression profiling to develop an improved molecular classification scheme for DLBCL. These investigators have defined three groups of DLBCL with distinct gene expression profiles: (1) germinal center B-cell–like (CGB) lymphoma, (2) activated B-cell–like (ABC) lymphoma, and (3) primary mediastinal DLBLC (PMBCL). These three gene expression groups of DLBCL arise from different stages of B cell development, have distinctive mechanisms of transformation, and have different rates of overall survival. The GCB form of DLBCL has a 5-year survival rate of 60%, compared with a rate of 39% in PMBCL, and 35% in the ABC DLBCL. Key regulatory factors and their target genes are differentially expressed in these groups. APC-DLBCL and PMBCL depend on constitutive activation of the NF-κB pathway for their survival, while GCB-DLBCL does not.[67] Using CGH, Bea and colleagues[66] have recently determined the frequency of specific chromosomal aberrations in these three groups and found that each group also had distinctive patterns of chromosome gain and loss. ABC-DLBCL was characterized by +3, gains of 3q and 18q21–q22, and losses of 6q21–q22. In contrast, GCB-DLBCL had frequent gains of 12q12 and PMBCL had gains of 9p21-pter and 2p14–p16.

Burkitt Lymphoma Burkitt lymphoma is an aggressive lymphoma of B-cell origin that occurs endemically in East Africa and sporadically in the West. The t(8;14)(q24;q32) noted in Burkitt lymphoma was the first recurrent chromosomal aberration reported in lymphoma and is also seen in mature B-cell ALL (see Table 8-4). In all cases of Burkitt lymphoma, the *MYC* gene, located on chromosome 8q24, is fused to the Ig loci. In 70 to 80% of cases, the translocation involved the IgH heavy chain on chromosome 14q32, while the remainder of the translocations involve either the Ig kappa light chain on 2p12 or the Ig lambda locus on 22q11.

Mucosa-Associated Lymphoid Tissue Lymphoma The low-grade gastric MALT lymphomas depend on the interaction with tumor-infiltrating T cells and are closely associated with *H. pylori* infection.[155] Interestingly, *in vitro*, *H. pylori* stimulates the proliferation of the tumor-infiltrating T cells but not the clonal B cells. The fact that elimination of *H. pylori* by antibiotic treatment often leads to the regression of MALT lymphomas highlights the importance of these interactions in lymphoma progression.[163] Some recent studies have also demonstrated that a significant fraction of MALT lymphomas recognize autoantigens and a significant fraction express autoantibodies with specificity for IgG (rheumatoid factor).[155] Thus, foreign and autoantigens play a critical role in the pathogenesis of this most interesting cancer. Cytogenetic studies reveal chromosomal abnormalities in 60% of MALT cases (see Table 8-6). The most common recurring translocation is the t(11;18)(q21;q21), seen in approximately 30% of cases. This translocation, which results in the juxtaposition of API2 at 11q21 with the *MALT1* gene on 18q21, has been associated with a decreased response to *H. pylori* eradication therapy, suggesting it is a critical marker for disease progression.[164] Several other translocations and chromosomal aberrations may be seen in MALT lymphoma (see Table 8-6).

Multiple Myeloma Multiple myeloma (MM) is a neoplastic proliferation of cells with a differentiated plasma cell phenotype in the bone marrow. The disease has a highly variable clinical course; it can be preceded by a premalignant condition called monoclonal gammopathy of undetermined significance (MGUS) and may progress from a truly overt intramedullary form to an extramedullary plasma cell leukemia (PCL). Chromosomal translocations in this disease usually involve the IgH heavy chain locus on chromosome 14q32; this locus may be fused to *CCND1* at 11q13, *FGFR3* at 4p16.3, *WHSC1* (MMSET) on 16q23, *CCND3* on 6p21, and *MAFB* on 20q12 (see Table 8-6).[165] Interestingly, like AML, Ross and colleagues[166] used high throughput FISH assays to study recurring regions of chromosome gain and loss in 228 MM patients and determined that the incidence of various chromosomal abnormalities in MM was dependent on patient age. Deletion of chromosome 13 was determined to be associated with shorter survival and the t(14;16) involving WHSC1 was found to have a particularly poor prognosis. Interestingly however, both –13 and t(14;16) only conferred a poor prognosis in patients over 70 years of age. In contrast, in younger patients, a poorer prognosis was associated with the t(4;14) involving *FGFR3* and deletion of *TP53*.[166] Several investigators have used gene expression arrays to attempt to improve MM molecular classification and outcome prediction.[167,168]

GENOMIC ALTERATIONS AND CHROMOSOMAL ABERRATIONS IN HUMAN CANCER

Solid Tumors Perhaps the single most important advance in solid tumor cytogenetics has been the availability of computer software to aid in the laborious analysis of the complex karyotypes. Also, newer culturing and banding techniques have resulted in more consistent patterns of chromosomal rearrangements. Finally, applications of the techniques described previously in this chapter, such as CGH, M-FISH, and SKY, using computer analysis, have allowed rapid advances in the systematic analysis of solid tumor cytogenetics. During the last decade, the number of cytogenetic abnormalities in solid tumors has risen exponentially. This is best demonstrated in the Catalog of Chromosome Aberrations in Cancer (<www.ncbi.nlm.nih.gov/CCAP>). The largest advances have occurred in mesenchymal tumors, where the genes that are involved in many of the chromosomal abnormalities have been cloned and their biological role in oncogenesis has been studied.

Benign Solid Tumors Clonal cytogenetic abnormalities are not necessarily equivalent to a malignant phenotype. Clonal chromosomal aberrations can occur in benign masses that have no potential for metastasis. However, they can also signify the transformation of a benign mass to one of more malignant potential. Indeed, in the best studied example of this, detailed below, the study of the progression of colonic adenomas to adenocarcinoma has been greatly aided by serially following cytogenetic abnormalities, which lead to the identification of the genes involved. In addition, normal fibroblasts sampled from within malignant tumor masses have been shown to occasionally contain an extra chromosome 7. This chromosome carries the epidermal growth factor receptor (EGFR) and the *MET* oncogene. These fibroblasts could influence malignant tumor growth, perhaps by increasing angiogenesis or by elucidating cytokine growth factors. Table 8-7 provides a list of the recurrent chromosomal rearrangements and genes involved for benign solid tumors. This section on chromo-

Table 8-7 Recurrent Chromosomal Abnormalities in Malignant Solid Tumors

Tumor Type	Chromosome Abnormality	Involved Gene
Epithelial tumors		
Bladder cancer, squamous cell	monosomy 9	CDKN2/P16
	trisomy 7	
Bladder cancer, transitional cell	monosomy 9, del9p	CDKN2A
	trisomy 7	EGFR
	del(13q)	RB
	del(1p)	
	monosomy 11, del(11p)	HRAS1
	del(17p13)	P53
	11p mut	WT1
Breast	i(1q)	
	t(1;16)	
	+7	
	add(8q)	MYC
	add(11q)	CCND1
	del(16q)	E-cadherin
	add(17q)	ERBB2
	13q12 mut	BRCA2
	17q21 mut	BRCA1
	add(20q)	ZNF217/NABC1
	add(17q)	TBX2/RPS6KB1
Cervical	add(3q)	?FHIT
	add(4p16)	FGF4
	del(18q21)	SMAD4
Colon	del(17p)	TP53
	del(18q)	DCC/DPC4
	del(5q)	APC
	del/mut(2q)	MSH2
	del/mut(3q)	MLH1
	del/mut(7p)	PMS1/2
Endometrial–endometrioid type	add(1q)	
	+10	
	t(7;17)	JAZF1/JAZ1
Endometrial–serous type	add(3q26.1)	
add(8q)	?MYC	
Esophagus	del(8q22)	FEZ1
	del(13q)	ING1/WWOX
	del(13q)	RB
	del(17p)	P53
	del(3p21)	DLC1
Head/neck	amp(11q13)	CCND1/PRAD1
	del(18q)	
	del(13q)	ING1
	del/mut10q23	PTEN
Lung carcinoma, small cell	del(3p14–23)	FHIT
Lung cancer, non-small cell	del (3p)	VHL/FHIT/PTPRG
	del (9p21)	CDKN2A
	del(13q14)	RB
	del(17p13)	P53
	amp(11q22)	CIAP1/2
	amp(7p)	EGRFR
Prostate	del(10q24–25)	MXI1
	del(10q22-qter)	
	del(17q21)	BRCA1
	+7, del(7q)	
	loss of Y	
	del(8p), add8q	
	del(11p)	KAI1
	del(1q)	HPC1/PCAP/PRCA1
Renal cell carcinoma, papillary	t(X;1)(p11.2;q21.2)	PRCC-TFE3
	+7	MET
	Del(7q)	HPRC
Renal carcinoma	del(3p25)	VHL
	t(3;8)(p21;q24)	HRCA1
	t(6;11)	Alpha/TFE3
	t(3;8)	FHIT/TCR8
	t(2;3)	DIRC2
Renal ASPCR1-TFE3 tumor	t(X;17)(p11.2;q25)	ASPSCR1-TFE3
Thyroid cancer	inv10(q11.2;q21.2)	RET-H4(PTC1)
	t(10;12)	RET-ELK4
	t(10;17)	RET-ELK5
	inv(1q22)	NTRK1-TPM3
	t(1;3)	NTRK1-TPR/TFG
Mesenchymal tumors		
Lipoma	add(12q)	MDM2
	t(12;16)	CHOP-FUS
	t(12;22)	CHOP-EWS
Alveolar soft part sarcoma	t(X;17)	TFE3-ASPSCR1
Chondrosarcoma	trisomy 7	
	add(20p)	
	add(20q)	
Synovial sarcoma	t(X;18)(p11.2;q11.2)	SYT-SSX1/SSX2
Rhabdomyosarcoma (alveolar type)	t(2;13)(q35;q14)	PAX3-FKHR
	t(1;13)(p36;q14)	PAX7-FKHR
Infantile fibrosarcoma	+8,+11,+17,+20	
Extraskeletal myxoid chondrosarcoma	t(9;22)(q22;q12)	EWS-CHN/TEC
Fibrosarcoma	add(12q)	MDM2
	add(14q21–24)	
	add(7q31)	
	add(8q)	?MYC
Fibromyxoid sarcoma	t(7;16)	FUS-CREB3L2
Central nervous system tumors		
Anaplastic astrocytoma	trisomy 7	EGFR
	−10,−22	
	partial del 9p	CDKN2A
	del13q	RB
Glioblastoma	+7	
	−10, del(10q)	PTEN/MXI1
	del(9p)	CDKN2A
	del(22q)	NF2
Schwannoma	loss of 22, partial del(22q)	NF2
Malignant peripheral nerve sheath tumors	gain of 17q	NF1
Embryonic tumors		
Desmoplastic small round cell tumor	t(11;22)(p13;q12)	EWS-WT1
Ewing tumors	t(11;22)(q24;q12)	EWSR1-FLI1
Medulloblastoma	i(17q)	
	del17p	REN
Neuroblastoma	del(1)(p32 to p36)	
	amp(2p)	MYCN
Wilms' tumor	del(11p13)	WT1
	1q+	
Retinoblastoma	del(13q14)	RB
	gain of 1q	
	i(6p)	
Clear cell sarcoma of soft parts	t(12;22)(q13;q12)	EWSR1-ATF1
Malignant melanoma of soft parts	del(1p11–22)	
	del(6q11–q27)	
	del(9p)	CDKN2A
Germ cell tumors		
Testicular tumors	i(12p), add12p	?CyclinD2
Other tumors		
Rhabdoid tumor	t(var;22)(–;11.2)	hSNF5/INI1
Dermatofibrosarcoma protuberans	+ring chromosome	
	t(17;22)(q2;q13)	COL1A1-PDGFB

somal abnormalities in benign solid tumors is divided into subsections on benign epithelial tumors, benign mesenchymal tumors, benign nervous system tumors, and other types of benign cytogenetic abnormalities.

BENIGN EPITHELIAL TUMORS Colonic Adenomas Trisomy of chromosome 7 is the most common recurring abnormality in colon adenomas, seen in 37% of cases.[169] However, +7 does not correlate with size or degree of dysplasia of the adenoma. Using molecular techniques, loss of a portion of 5q has been seen in 30% of colonic adenomas. In familial adenomatous polyposis (FAP), which has a very high incidence of transformation to malignancy, there are also abnormalities of 5q.

This led to the cloning of the gene that was mutated in this inherited syndrome, termed adenomatous polyposis coli, or *APC*, at 5q21.[170] Mutations in this gene can also be screened for by assessing protein truncation in an adenoma biopsy. *APC* binds to the transcription factor beta-catenin and mediates its degradation. However, mutated forms of *APC* allow beta-catenin to bind to its partner *TCF4* and activate transcription of proliferation genes such as cyclin D1 and *MYC*.[171] Beta-catenin has also been shown to be important in specifying cell fates during embryogenesis. *APC* is also frequently mutated in nonfamilial adenomas. *MYH* has been found to be homozygously mutated in another autosomal recessive familial colon adenoma syndrome that maps to 1p32–34. *MYH* encodes a protein involved in base excision repair, an important DNA repair pathway, and this syndrome has a high rate of progression to colon adenocarcinoma.[172]

Benign Ovarian Tumors Trisomy 12 is the most common abnormality in benign ovarian tumors.[173] Indeed, this was the sole abnormality in five benign epithelial ovarian tumors, either thecomas or fibromas. Seven of nine cytogenetically abnormal benign ovarian tumors also contained this abnormality. Given that it was the sole abnormality in a high fraction of these tumors, the gene(s) involved in this amplification might play a role in the initiation of this benign growth.

Salivary Gland Adenomas Over 200 abnormal karyotypes have been reported in benign salivary adenomas. Of 100 cases of parotid adenoma, 47 had abnormal chromosomal changes.[174] Of these 47 adenomas with abnormal karyotypes, 34 had involvement of one of three specific chromosomal regions: 8q12, 12q13–15, and 3p21. A specific translocation, t(3;8)(p21;q12), is the most frequent abnormality seen, occurring in 27% of cases. Another translocation, t(11;19)(q21;p13), has also been described in adenolymphoma of the salivary gland (also termed Warthin's tumor). These abnormalities are not present in malignant salivary gland tumors, but the number of malignant salivary gland tumors reported remains smaller than benign tumors. Recently, the t(3;8)(p21;q12) seen in the salivary gland adenomas was shown to result in promoter swapping between *PLAG1*, a developmentally regulated zinc finger gene at 8q12 and the constitutively expressed gene for beta-catenin *CTNNB1*.[175] Thus, deregulation of the beta-catenin pathway may be an important common denominator in adenoma formation in multiple tissues. However, there are important differences between salivary gland and colon adenomas. The salivary gland adenoma translocation results in the increased expression of *PLAG1* from the beta-catenin promoter, and decreased expression of beta-catenin. Interestingly, *PLAG1* is also activated in another translocation in salivary gland adenomas, the t(8;15)(q12;q14). These reports demonstrate that activation of *PLAG1* is a critical event in the origin of salivary gland adenomas. The gene involved in the translocations involving 12q13–15 has also been isolated.[175] It is the nuclear structural protein HMGIC (also termed High Mobility Group AT-Hook Protein 2, and HMGA2). These translocations appear to either truncate HMIC protein or increase its expression. Translocations involving this gene are also seen in other benign tumors such as lipomas and uterine leiomyomas, as well as in AML. In addition, fusion transcripts between PLAG1 and HMIC have been detected in rare salivary gland adenomas, indicating that these proteins may function together to form salivary gland adenomas.

Benign Mesenchymal Tumors **Chondroid Tumors** Chondroid tumors represent a family of histologically related benign growths whose tissue of origin is cartilage or bone. There are a number of types of chondroid tumors, including osteochondroma, chondroblastoma, chondromyxoid fibroma, chondroma, chondrosarcoma, and chordoma. A large multicenter group effort, termed the Chromosomes and Morphology Collaborative Study Group (CHAMP) analyzed 117 karyotypes from 100 different individuals with chondroid tumors. Karyotypic abnormalities were seen in 46 of the 100 patients.[176,177] There were, however, striking differences related to the site of origin. All primary chondromas of bone (enchondroma or periosteal chondroma) had normal karyotypes. Chromosomal changes were only seen in chondromas arising from the soft tissue, cartilage, or juxtacortical area. Recent studies have reported a fusion of the *HMGA2* gene on chromosome 12q13–15 in soft tissue chondromas.[178] Among solitary primary well-differentiated cartilaginous lesions of the bone, an abnormal karyotype was statistically associated with grade 1 chondrosarcoma, as opposed to chondroma. Among the abnormal karyotypes seen, loss of distal 8q was associated with osteochondroma. Trisomy 5 was associated with synovial chondroma and soft tissue chondroma. Changes in 6q were associated with chondromyxoid fibroma. Trisomy 7 was associated with bone chondrosarcoma. Alterations in 17p1 were seen in grade 3 chondrosarcoma, a tumor with more malignant potential. Finally, changes in 12q13–15 were seen in synovial chondromas and myxoid chondrosarcomas.

Lipomas Lipomas are a family of benign tumors arising from adipose tissue, including lipomas, angiolipomas, spindle-cell lipomas, and atypical lipomas. There has been extensive investigation of the cytogenetics of benign (and also malignant) adipose tumors. There are abnormal karyotypes on over 200 lipomas that have been reported.[22] Interestingly, when all karyotypes from lipomas are compared, only one-fourth of these tumors have normal cytogenetics. The majority of lipomas show simple structural chromosomal changes. Balanced abnormalities are far more frequent than unbalanced changes. In one series of 26 lipomas, 70% had consistent chromosome rearrangements, and 50% had a reciprocal translocation involving 12q13–15. This break point has also been observed in liposarcomas. Analysis of 91 cases allowed a classification of lipomas into four cytogenetic subgroups: (1) those with normal karyotypes, (2) those with hyperdiploidy with ring chromosomes, (3) those with pseudodiploidy and rearrangement of 12(q13–15), and (4) those with hypodiploid or pseudodiploid karyotypes and other aberrations.[179] As described above, the gene involved in the 12q13–15 abnormalities has been isolated, as shown to be *HMGIC* (*HMGA2*). This gene can be fused to *RDC1*, *LPP*, or *LHFP1* in lipoma translocations.[180,181] These fusion partners bear little resemblance to each other in structure or function, suggesting that disruption of *HMGIC* is the important consequence of these translocations.

Pulmonary Chondroid Hamartoma Pulmonary chondroid hamartomas are benign growths of lung tissue that are made up of mixtures of undifferentiated mesenchymal cells, and differentiated cartilage, fat, and epithelium. A study of 191 pulmonary chondroid hamartomas revealed that over 70% have either a 12q14–15 or 6p21 abnormality. The genes that are rearranged in these cytogenetic lesions have been isolated. As seen so frequently in benign solid tumors, the gene for HMGIC is involved in the 12q abnormalities. The most frequent translocations involving the 12q and 6p regions were t(12;14)(q15;q24) and t(6;14)(p21.3;q24). These translocations disrupted *HMGIC* and *HMGIY*, respectively.[182] Compared with many other benign tumors that have 12q abnormalities involving *HMGIC* (including cartilage chondromas, leiomyomas, lipomas, and salivary gland adenomas), pulmonary chondroid hamartomas seem to have the highest frequency of these abnormalities, with 50% of the tumors analyzed containing this recurrent aberration.

Uterine Leiomyomas Leiomyomas of the uterus are very common benign smooth muscle tumors. There has been extensive cytogenetic analysis of these tumors.[22] The most common chromosomal changes include t(12;14)(q14–15;q22–24), del(7)(q22–32), trisomy 12, and rearrangements of 6p21.[183,184] As seen above, disruption of the *HMGIC* gene at 12q13–15 and the *HMGIY* gene at 6p21 have been observed in leiomyomas. Analyzing these translocations provided more insight into the mechanism of HMGIC's role in the origins of these benign growths. HMGIC is a nuclear protein that helps provide the architecture for the appropriate spatial scaffolding for chromosomes. Translocations involving HMGIC all result in separation of the DNA-binding domains of HMGIC from the acidic C-terminal regulatory domain. Thus, the fragmented HMGIC protein can bind chromosomes without proper regulation, and produce not only aberrant gene expression, but also affect DNA synthesis and mitosis. In addition, it has also been hypothesized that the expression of *HMGIC* and *HMGIY* is governed by negatively acting regulatory sequence elements. Rearrangements that delete these negative regulatory elements will abnormally increase expression of *HMGIC* and *HMGIY*, also affecting chromatin architecture.

Benign Central Nervous System Tumors **Meningiomas, Schwannomas, and Neurofibromas** There is a long history of cytogenetic investigation in meningioma.[185] Monosomy 22 or del(22q12.3) has now been reported in 70% of all meningioma cases and 95% of tumors with abnormal karyotypes. This region also is deleted in schwannomas and neurofibromas. Cloning of the gene deleted in these neuroepithelial tumors was facilitated by genetic mapping studies of families affected by neurofibromatosis type 2. When the gene deleted in this region was cloned, it was termed NF2 for this disease (also termed Merlin or Schwannomin). Inactivation of NF2 occurs through the classic Knudson two hit mechanism, where one gene is lost in the chromosomal deletion, and the other allele acquires a mutation.[186] NF2 functions as a tumor suppressor by inhibiting downstream *ras* proliferative signals, through blocking ralGDS activity.[187]

In neurofibromatosis type 1, frequent benign and malignant tumors of the neural sheath occur, similar to the schwannomas and neurofibromas above. There are frequent deletions of 17q in these patients, and again using genetic mapping and cloning studies from these patient families, the gene involved in the del(17q) was isolated.[188] Termed NF1, this gene and its encoded protein also functions as an inhibitor of the *ras* signaling pathway, similar to but upstream of NF2. Using FISH, 96% of patients with type I neurofibromatosis have deletions in NF1. Significantly, some patients with neurofibromatosis type 2 develop hematologic malignancies; additionally patients with juvenile myelomonocytic leukemia (JMML) have NF1 mutations.[189] NF1-/- mice also have myeloid proliferations similar to JMML, indicating that normal blood cell development requires NF1. Thus, molecular cytogenetics linked a common molecular mechanism in completely different tumor types.

Other Benign Tumors **Inflammatory Myofibroblastic Tumor** Inflammatory myofibroblastic tumors, which are also known as fibromyxoid tumors, are rare benign soft tissue tumors of controversial origin. These tumors usually occur in parenchyma of the lung, mesentery, retroperitoneum, or pelvis. The molecular cytogenetics of these tumors has been well characterized. Half the cases involve a 2p23 rearrangement involving the *ALK* gene. A number of translocations involving this gene have been cloned and characterized, such as the t(1;2)(q25;p23), t(2;17)(p23;q23), and t(2;19)(p23;p13.1). These translocations involve fusions of the *ALK* gene on 2p23 to *TPM3* in 1q25, *CLTC* in 17q23, or*TPM4* in 19p13.[190] These translocations all result in the fusion of the N-terminus of the partner gene to the C-terminus of the ALK protein. This deletes negative regulatory portions of the ALK tyrosine kinase protein. Thus, these gene fusions produce a constitutively activated chimeric ALK tyrosine kinase.

Interestingly, the *TPM3-ALK* gene fusion seen in these tumors is identical to that seen in a much more aggressive tumor, anaplastic large cell lymphoma (ALCL). This was the first example of the same translocation fusion product resulting in two completely different tumor phenotypes, which probably resulted from the fact that their translocation arose in different cellular lineages of origin.[190]

MALIGNANT SOLID TUMORS

This section provides a brief discussion of the most frequently recurring clonal cytogenetic abnormalities in solid tumors. The genes involved in many of these cytogenetic abnormalities have now been cloned and characterized, providing new insights into the molecular mechanisms of tumorigenesis, new diagnostic and prognostic tools, and new insights for the development of improved therapies. In many instances, animal models of these human tumors have been generated by introducing these genetic abnormalities into mouse models. Thus, cytogenetics has played a major role, if not the most important role, in determining the molecular origins of many solid tumors. This section on chromosomal abnormalities in malignant solid tumors is divided into subsections on malignant epithelial tumors, malignant mesenchymal tumors, malignant nervous system tumors, and other types of benign cytogenetic abnormalities. For many of these recurring chromosomal abnormalities the genes involved have also been identified (see Tables 8-1 and 8-7).

Malignant Epithelial Tumors By far, the vast majority of cases of malignancies in the Western world occur in tumors of epithelial origin. Unfortunately, studies of epithelial tumors in the past using traditional cytogenetic tools were hampered by many factors, including difficulties on obtaining adequate biopsies; difficulties in adapting disaggregated cells to short-term in vitro cultures to obtain metaphases for standard karyotypic analysis, the late stage of disease presentation; and the sheer complexity of the karyotypes obtained. Another important reason that cytogenetic studies of the common epithelial tumors may not have yielded as much insight into their etiology and mechanism of transformation is that the genetic mechanisms of tumorigenesis in solid tumors, compared with mesenchymal tumors and hematologic malignancies, may be distinct. These issues were discussed extensively in the introduction to this chapter. Epithelial solid tumors are characterized by genetic instability and multiple tumor suppressor gene deletions or mutations in contrast to the more frequent balanced reciprocal chromosomal translocations and inversions seen more frequently in hematologic and mesenchymal tumors, though this remains highly controversial.[5] As detailed in the introduction to this chapter, newer technologies for genomic analysis (CGH, M-FISH or SKY, and array technologies) hold great promise for detailed analysis of solid tumor genetic and biology.

Bladder Cancer The vast majority of bladder cancers in North America are transitional cell carcinomas. The most common chromosomal abnormalities detected in transitional cell carcinomas are +7, –9, 11, del(11p), del(13q), del(17p), and translocations of chromosomes 1, 5, and 10.[191] Monosomy 9 also appears to be a very early event in the origins of transitional cell carcinoma as it is often detected at the dysplastic stage or as the sole abnormality in early-stage tumors. Monosomy 9 is present in approximately 44% of bladder cancer cases.[192,193] Interest has focused on loss of 9p21, which contains the gene *CDKN2A*, which codes for two distinct tumor suppressors, $p14^{ARF}$ and $p16^{INK4a}$. These tumor suppressor genes are often mutated or lost in bladder cancer. Loss of 17p likely represents loss of the tumor suppressor *TP53*, as the remaining *TP53* is often mutated in this and many other malignancies.[194,195] In addition, there is frequent loss of the tumor suppressor gene *RB1* in bladder cancer.[194]

Breast Cancer Breast cancers have frequent and complex cytogenetic abnormalities. Despite the complexity of the majority of karyotypes in breast cancer, analysis of the recurrent chromosomal alterations has lead to great advances in our understanding of not only breast cancer etiology, but also new insights for the development of novel therapeutic approaches. Mitelman has reported aberrant karyotypes on more than 400 breast cancer specimens.[22] These include both complex and simple chromosomal changes; alterations of chromosome arms 1q, 3p, 6q, and 8p are often seen. Trisomies of chromosomes 7, 8, and 20 are also reported in Mitelman's survey.[22] In addition, i(1q) and der(1;16) are seen commonly and can be the sole abnormality detected. Amplification of chromosomal segments is observed frequently in breast carcinoma, most commonly associated with 8p. Der(1;16)(q10;p10), and del(3p) can be seen in benign fibroadenomas, fibrocystic disease, and carcinomas.

In a study where the karyotype of primary breast cancers was compared with the karyotype of metastatic breast cancer, random whole chromosome gains or losses were seen in the primary cancers, while structural alterations and amplifications were more commonly observed in the metastatic breast cancers.[196] In advanced breast cancer, gains of 8q were the most common cytogenetic event. The vast majority of breast cancers (80%) have gains of 1q, 8q, or both, and three changes (+1q, +8q, or –13q) occur in over 90% of tumors with an abnormal karyotype.[197]

Genomic studies of the recurrent gains and losses in breast cancer using CGH and FISH have revealed multiple regions of chromosomal gain and loss. One of the most intensely studied amplified regions is 17q11–12, containing the epidermal growth factor receptor ERBB2. ERBB2 is amplified in 20 to 30% of breast cancers and these cancers have a worst overall prognosis.[198] This finding led to the development of a monoclonal antibody, Herceptin, directed against ERBB2 that has been effective in treating high-risk breast cancer cases.[32,33] This is another example of how genomic studies in cancer have led to the development of a novel targeted therapy. Other amplicons map to 11q13 (where *CCND1* is a possible candidate), 20q13, 8q24 (where c-*MYC* is located) and 20q (ZNF217 and NABC1).[199] Analyzing 55 unselected primary breast cancer specimens with CGH, gains of 1q (67%) and 8q (49%) were the most frequent aberrations.[197] Recurrent losses of heterozygosity involved 8p, 16q, 13q, 17p, 9p, Xq, 6q, 11q, and 18q. The total number of aberrations per tumor was highest in the more undifferentiated tumors. The high frequency of 1q gains and presence of +1q as a sole abnormality in some cases suggest that gain of 1q material may be an early genetic event in breast cancers.

Genetic mapping studies, cytogenetic studies, and molecular genetic tools have been used in hereditary breast cancer to identify the genes mutated in this disease. The majority of hereditary breast cancer is due to germ line mutations in either *BRCA1* (81% of inherited cases) or *BRCA2* (14% of inherited cases). The breast cancers arising from *BRCA1* mutations are more aggressive than sporadic or *BRCA2*-associated breast cancers, have a higher pathologic grade, and are more likely to be estrogen or progesterone receptor negative.[2,200,201] Both BRCA1 and BRCA2 proteins have been shown to function as components of DNA repair pathways. Therefore, one would hypothesize that tumors arising from mutations in these proteins night have more genomic instability and more cytogenetic abnormalities. This hypothesis has indeed been confirmed using CGH; *BRCA1*- or *BRCA2*-associated tumors have twice the number of chromosomal gains or losses compared with sporadic tumors.[2,202] Some specific genes have been found to be amplified in *BRCA*-associated tumors as compared with sporadic tumors. For example, the *HER2/neu* gene is amplified in 20% of sporadic and *BRCA2*-associated tumors, but not in *BRCA1*-associated tumors. In contrast, the *myb* oncogene is amplified in 30% of *BRCA1*-associated tumors, but not in sporadic or *BRCA2*-associated tumors.[203] In addition, *CCND1* is amplified in one-third of sporadic cases, but not at all in *BRCA*-associated tumors.[204] The 17q22–24 chromosomal region is amplified more frequently in both *BRCA1*- and *2*-associated tumors compared with sporadic cases of breast cancer; this region is amplified in 50% of *BRCA1*-associated breast cancer and 87% of *BRCA2*-associated breast cancer, but only 15% of sporadic tumors. The *RPS6KB1* and *TBX2* genes are located in this region and are frequently amplified in human breast cancer cases. They have also been shown to be oncogenic in some model systems.[205–208] Using FISH, the frequency of *RPS6KB1* and *TBX2* amplification in *BRCA*-associated and sporadic tumors was recently compared and it was found that *TBX2* was preferentially amplified in *BRCA*-associated tumors as compared with sporadic tumors. This suggests that *TBX2* amplification might play a role in the development of *BRCA*-associated breast neoplasia.[205,206] Thus, hereditary *BRCA1* and *BRCA2* breast tumors appears to develop by specific and distinct evolutionary paths, because their gene expression profiles and genomic aberrations differ from each other and from sporadic breast cancers.[2,202]

Inflammatory breast cancer is an aggressive form of disease and is pathologically and clinically distinct from other types of breast cancer. The genetics of inflammatory breast cancer are poorly understood. Using gene expression profiling, comparing an inflammatory breast cancer cell line to normal mammary epithelial cells, 17 transcripts were either under- or overexpressed in the inflammatory breast cancer cell line compared with normal cells.[209] Further study of archival inflammatory breast cancer specimens led to the observation that overexpression of RhoC GTPase and loss of expression of a novel gene on 6q22 were consistent findings in inflammatory breast cancer. *WISP3*, a gene located on chromosome 6q21–22, is amplified in 80% of inflammatory breast cancers compared with only 20% of stage-matched, noninflammatory breast cancers, suggesting that *WISP3* may play a role in the etiology of inflammatory breast cancer.[209]

Colorectal Carcinomas Colorectal adenocarcinomas have been well studied for chromosomal and genomic aberrations. Common recurrent structural abnormalities include iso(8q), iso(13q), del(1p22), iso(17q), and iso(1q). The most common numeric gains of chromosomes have been in 7, 13, and X, and the most common losses in Y, 18, 14, 21, 4, 8, and 15; trisomy 7 is especially common. The most common rearrangements involve gains of material from chromosome arms 8q, 13q, 17q, and 1q and loss of material from 1p, 8p, 13p, and 17p. Translocations between 1 and 17 are especially common. Loss of segments from 5q, 17p, and 18q. CGH confirmed many of these karyotypic findings.[210]

The recurrent loss of 5q, 17p, and 18q prompted study of these regions using specific FISH probes. Starting from these initial cytogenetic studies, in a tour de force of molecular genetics, Vogelstein, Kinzler, and colleagues worked out the genetic progression of colon cancer.[201] Using DNA probes, loss of heterozygosity for chromosome regions 5q21, 17p, and 18q21 was found in a high percentage of colorectal carcinomas.[211,212] Vogelstein and colleagues proposed that colorectal tumorigenesis progresses through a series of genetic alterations that lead a colonic mucosal cell through adenoma formation to adenocarcinoma. The initiating event for adenoma formation may be the combination of the loss of *APC* on 5q and the gain of a K-*RAS* mutation.[210] *APC* is mutated in the germline of many patients with the familial adenomatous polyposis syndrome and with Gardner syndrome. For transformation from adenoma to adenocarcinoma, loss of the tumor suppressor *TP53* on 17q occurs followed by loss of the tumor suppressor DCC (deleted in colorectal cancer) on 18q.[210–212] Colon cancers with 18q loss appear to have a worse prognosis than those lacking this genomic aberration. These cytogenetic studies led directly to the isolation of both the *APC* and *DCC* tumor suppressor genes. As previously described, *APC* plays a critical role in sporadic and inherited adenoma formation, while *DCC* deletion and/or mutation is seen in a high fraction of adenocarcinoma and is thought to be important for progression to aggressive adenocarcinoma.

However, the genetic model for colon cancer has become increasingly complex, as with more sophisticated genomic studies and detailed analysis, more than one tumor suppressor gene may be deleted in the recurrent genomic aberrations in colon cancer. For example, the loss of segments from 18q21 can also delete another tumor suppressor gene *DPC4/SMAD4* as well as *DCC*. In about one-third of cases, *DPC4/SMAD4* is the deletion target, and in the remaining majority of cases *DCC* is deleted.[212] Similarly, loss of the 5q21 chromosomal region not only leads to deletion of *APC*, but also a novel gene *MCC* (mutated in colon cancer); *MCC* has also been found to be deleted in some inherited adenomatous polyposis families as well.[213] Other chromosomal regions have also been identified as being deleted in families with hereditary nonpolyposis colon cancer (HNPCC), and the tumor suppressor genes deleted in these regions have been identified. These regions and their deleted genes include: 2q (*MSH2*), 3q (*MLH1*), and chromosome 7p (*PMS1* and *PMS2*).[214,215] In HNPCC, 76% of cases have deletions and/or mutations in one of these genes. These proteins are also important in DNA repair, like the BRCA1 and BRCA2 proteins in hereditary breast cancer. However, whereas the BRCA1 and BRCA2 proteins function more in sensing DNA double-strand breaks and initiating homologous recombination of those breaks, the HNPCC mutated proteins function in nucleotide mismatch repair. Cancers in patients with HNPCC can also have mutations of the same genes that are involved in noninherited colorectal oncogenesis (such as K-*RAS*, *APC*, *TP53*, *DCC*). Consistent with the function of the mutated genes in HNPCC, tumors in these families have remarkable instability of genomic repeat sequences during cell division (termed microsatellites). This microsatellite variation can be easily evaluated using PCR, and this can serve as a rapid screening test for mutations in these genes in colon cancer. This instability results from the reduced nucleotide mismatch repair caused by germline mutations in the *MSH2*, *MLH1*, *PMS1*, or *PMS2* genes.[215] It also appears that different mutations can be used to predict poor response to therapy. In one study of six different colorectal cancer cell lines, mutations in *TP53* and loss of expression of GML, a target of TP53, were associated with decreased sensitivity to 5-fluorouracil and mitomycin C.[216] Other studies have shown that mutant K-*RAS* confers resistance to radiation and *cis*-platinum.

Esophageal Carcinoma The most common histologic type of esophageal carcinoma is squamous cell carcinoma. Esophageal cancer, like colon cancer, proceeds to carcinoma through a stepwise acquisition of specific genomic and chromosomal alterations. These step-wise alterations result in a specific sequence of changes in the histology of the esophageal mucosa, from inflammation to mucosal atypia to carcinoma in situ to invasive carcinoma, recently reviewed by Kuwano and colleagues.[217] These alterations are likely responsible for the sequence of histopathological changes seen in the progression from esophagitis to atrophy to dysplasia and then on to carcinoma in situ and subsequently invasive carcinoma. Several groups have assessed LOH in esophageal cancers using microsatellite markers. These studies found frequent losses of material on chromosomes 1p, 3p, 5q, 9, 11q, 13q, 17q, and 18q.[218] The 13q and 17q abnormalities often represent loss of *RB1* and *TP53*, respectively (see Table 8-1). These genes are commonly deleted and/or mutated as an early event in esophageal cancer.[217] Another novel tumor suppressor gene at 17q that is deleted in esophageal carcinoma is termed envoplakin.[219]

Progression of esophageal dysplasia to carcinoma likely also requires other more tissue-specific mutations in tumor suppressor genes. Using CGH to assess LOH, a number of putative tumor suppressor genes for esophageal cancer have been cloned. Two of these are *FEZ-1* at 8q22 and *DLC1* at 3p21.[220,221] In addition, loss of 13q is a recurrent abnormality. This deletion was hypothesized to involve loss of the known tumor suppressor gene *ING1*.[222] Indeed, molecular analysis found mutations in the PHD finger domain and nuclear localization motif in *ING1* and immunohistochemical studies found that all esophageal cancers had loss of expression of *ING1*. Given that there are deletions of one allele and mutations in the remaining allele of *ING1*, and that its expression is lost in all esophageal cancer, the loss of its function may be critical for the development of esophageal cancer. Another putative tumor suppressor gene, termed *WWOX*, was also isolated from 13q12.[223] Thus, *FEZ-1*, *DLC1*, *WWOX*, and *ING1* are candidates for tumor suppressor genes for progression of esophageal cancer.

The frequent loss of heterozygosity in sporadic esophageal tumors in 17q25 has been noted in several studies. The gene responsible for tylosis, an autosomal dominant syndrome with skin abnormalities, which has a high risk of progression to esophageal cancer, has also been mapped to this region. This putative gene, termed TOC (tyolysis with oesophageal cancer) has been mapped to a 500 kb region on chromosome 17q, which contains one gene, called cytoglobin. However, no cytoglobin mutations have been found to date in this syndrome, so the role of this gene is presently unclear.[224]

Head and Neck Cancer Cancers of the head and neck are characterized by recurrent regions of gain and loss. Loss of 3p13–24, 5q12–23, 8p22–23, 9p21–24, and 18q22–23 are present in nearly 50% of tumors, while gain of 3q21-qter, 5p, 7p, 8q, and 11q13–23 are present in about 33% of tumors.[225] These abnormalities may occur in isolation and combination. The gain at 11q13 may involve amplification of the *CCNDI/PRADI* gene. CGH has been used to analyze chromosomal alterations in primary head and neck squamous cell carcinomas in order to genetically classify progression of these tumors. Changes observed in over 50% of the tumors analyzed included deletions of 1p, 4, 5q, 6q, 8p, 9p, 11, 13q, 18q, and 21q, and additions of 11q13 as well as 3q, 8q, 16p, 17q, 19, 20q, and 22q. Many of these changes are seen in the karyotypic analysis mentioned above. By using ratios of gains and losses compared with tumor grade, this analysis revealed that well-differentiated carcinomas (Grade 1) were defined by the deletions of 3p, 5q, and 9p, and gains of 3q. This suggests that these regions are associated with early tumor development and less aggressive clinical behavior. Undifferentiated tumors (Grade 3) were characterized by deletions of chromosomes 4q, 8p, 11q, 13q, 18q, and 21q, and gains of 1p, 11q13, 19, and 22q.[225]

Loss of 18q has been associated with a poor outcome in squamous cell carcinomas of the head and neck. In one study of 67 patients, 40% had loss of heterozygosity of 18q. Those who lacked one 18q allele had a statistically significant worse 2-year survival as compared with those who did not (30% vs 63%, p = .008). This correlation between clinical outcome and loss of 18q implies that a tumor suppressor gene resides in that location that may play an important role in the progression of this disease.[226] Like esophageal cancer, mutations have been found in *ING1* in a small but significant number of head and neck squamous cell carcinomas.[227] In addition, somatic mutations in *PTEN* have been found in head and neck squamous cell carcinoma; 13% of carcinomas analyzed had missense mutations accompanied by loss of chromosome 10.[228]

Lung Cancer Both small-cell lung cancer (SCLC) and non–small cell lung cancer (NSCLC) have recurrent cytogenetic aberrations associated with frequently complex karyotypes.[229] Nearly all SCLC have a deletion of 3q arising in a background of complex aberrations.[230] In addition, del(3p) is frequently seen in NSCLC in a complex karyotypic background. The minimally deleted region common to all of these deletions was 3p14–23. Assessment of LOH of 3p in lung cancer has shown that LOH for markers on 3p occurs consistently in SCLC and occasionally in NSCLC. This 3p region has been the focus of intense investigation and several candidate tumor suppressor genes have been proposed, including the von Hippel–Lindau (VHL) gene at 3p25, the ubiquitin-activating enzyme homolog (UBE1L) at 3p21, dinucleoside polyphosphate hydrolase (FHIT) and the receptor protein-tyrosine phosphatase gamma (PTPRG) at 3p14.2.

Deletions of chromosome regions 3p, 5q, 13q, and 17p are also commonly seen in SCLC, in addition to double minute chromosomes (see Table 8-2) that usually represent amplification of various members of the *MYC* oncogene family.[229] In NSCLC, deletions of 3p, 9p, and 17p, +7, iso(5p10), and iso(8q10) are commonly seen. These recurrent deletions often occur at sites of known tumor suppressor genes, including *CDKN2A* (9p21), *RB1* (13q14), and *TP53* (17p13). As seen in other solid tumors, there is a report of consistent 9p abnormalities in 9 of 10 NSCLC lung cancers examined.[231] This report described nonreciprocal translocations or deletions resulting in loss of material from 9p, with a minimally deleted region at 9p11–14, suggesting the presence of a tumor suppressor gene in this region. A strong candidate for such a tumor suppressor is *CDKN2* (*p16*^{INK4a}), which is in inhibitory regulation of the cell cycle. This gene was shown to be homozygously deleted in a significant percentage of all types of lung cancer cell lines.[232] Loss of *CDKN2* (*p16*) is more common is NSCLC, with up to 70% of NSCLC tumors lacking any *p16* expression. Interestingly, in those few (11%) SCLC that had loss of *p16*, none showed *RB1* loss. In addition, of the 48 SCLC samples with no expression or mutant *RB1*, all showed detectable levels of p16 protein. Thus, there appears to be an inverse correlation in SCLC between *RB1* inactivation and *p16* inactivation, implying that in this tumor, inactivation of just one of these cell-cycle regulatory pathways may be required.

Alternative cytogenetic approaches, such as CGH, have provided new insights in lung cancer. Initial CGH studies confirm the existence of many of the karyotypic imbalances described above, and have also found several previously unrecognized recurrent abnormalities, such as 10q– in SCLC.[233] Using M-FISH and CGH, several common gains and deletions of chromosomal material were seen in NSCLC. CGH revealed gains at 5p, 3q, 8q, 11q, 2q, 12p, and 12q, and losses at 9p, 3p, 6q, 17p, 22q, 8p, 10p, 10q, and 19p. M-FISH revealed numerous complex chromosomal rearrangements. Translocations were seen commonly between 5 and 14, 5 and 11, and 1 and 6. Loss of the Y chromosome and gains of chromosomes 20 and 5p were also frequent. Using the new SNP-Chip methodology, Janne and colleagues have found that variations in single nucleotide polymorphisms can be useful in diagnosis and prognosis of lung cancer.[234]

Recently, using a combination of genetic and molecular techniques, Bailey-Wilson and colleagues mapped a major lung cancer susceptibility locus to 6q23–q25.[235] Using DNA markers, Dai and colleagues identified an amplified region on chromosome 11q22, 6q21, and 3q26.[236] Immunohistochemistry and Western blot analysis identified the apoptosis proteins CIAP1 and CIAP2 as potential oncogenes in the 11q22 region, since both are overexpressed in multiple lung cancers with or without higher copy numbers.

Adenocarcinomas that respond to the EGFR tyrosine kinase inhibitors gefitinib or erlotinib were recently found to harbor mutations in *EGFR* (located at 7p) that produced gain of function. Mutations were found in 7 of 10 tumors that responded and none of 18 tumors that were refractory to these drugs.[24,25,237] Such mutations also appear generally more common in adenocarcinomas as compared with other NSCLC and in Japanese patients compared with those of European descent.

Prostate Cancer By conventional karyotyping, recurrent chromosomal changes included trisomy 7, loss of Y, and deletions of 7q and 10q, and the appearance of double minutes. Using FISH, gains of chromosomes 1, 7, 8, 8q, 17, X, and Y, and loss of chromosomes 1, 7, 8, 8p, 10, 10q, 16q, 17q, 17, and Y have been seen.[238] Using CGH, gains of chromosome material in regions from 1q, 2p, 3q, 7q, 9q, 11p, 16p, 20, 22, and X, and loss of segments from 2q, 5q, 6q, 9p, 13q, 15q, 17p, and 18q were observed.[239] Consistency within these complex findings can be found. Although many chromosomal abnormalities are seen, alterations in four chromosomes (7, 8, 10, and 17) appear to be the most recurrent changes. Trisomy 7 has been seen in both conventional karyotyping and using FISH, and thus appears to be a common recurrent chromosomal alteration and is associated with tumor progression.[240] Chromosome 8 abnormalities are not usually seen in conventional cytogenetics; however, FISH and CGH analysis revealed an increased copy number of chromosome 8q in both primary and metastatic prostate cancer.[241] Conversely, LOH studies suggested that 8p is often deleted in prostate cancer.[242]

Deletions at 10q24–25 are also seen recurrently in prostate cancer. A candidate for the tumor suppressor gene in this region is *MXII*, which is a negative regulator of C-*MYC*.[243] Finally, deletions of chromosome 17 are seen in over 50% of primary prostate cancer specimens.[244] Male members of families with *BRCA1* germline mutations have prostate cancer at an increased frequency. Therefore, since *BRCA1* is located in the region most commonly lost, it is a strong candidate for a tumor suppressor gene in prostate cancer on chromosome 17. Indeed, loss of heterozygosity of the *BRCA1* locus has been seen in up to 70% of prostate cancers.[245] Genetic mapping of several high-risk families with an apparent predisposition to prostate cancer have been identified, one that maps to 20q13, one to 1q24, and one to Xq27–28. However, no gene candidates have been definitively identified for any of these syndromes (<www.ncbi.nlm.nih.gov\omim>).

Renal Cell Carcinoma The two primary histologic types of renal cell carcinoma are clear-cell carcinoma (nonpapillary renal cell carcinoma) and papillary renal carcinoma. Clear-cell carcinomas are the most common, comprising 80% of renal cancers. Each of these histologic types of cancer has distinct chromosomal aberrations and pathways for tumorigenesis. Inherited syndromes of renal carcinoma have provided insight into the origins of clear-cell carcinoma. A somatic translocation, t(3;8)(p21;q24), was seen in the lymphocytes of 10 members of a family who had bilateral clear-cell renal carcinoma. This translocation segregated in an autosomal dominant fashion.[246] Other families that had clear-cell carcinoma with break points in 3p were also found.[247] Using samples from these families, a gene termed *HRCA1* (also *TCR8*) from this break point was cloned. Rearrangements and deletions of 3p distinct from 3p21 have also been seen in sporadic clear-cell carcinoma. Chromosome 3p deletions may also be found as the sole abnormality in some cases. These observations suggest that del(3p) may be an initiating event in the development of clear cell carcinoma. Further investigation found several distinct regions of 3p that appear relevant to renal cell cancer development. First, patients with Von Hippel–Lindau syndrome develop clear-cell carcinoma at a high frequency. The *VHL* gene was mapped to 3p25–26 on the basis of DNA studies of 28 pedigrees that had a total of 164 affected persons. The gene was cloned and mutations were demonstrated in sporadic kidney cancer cases as well as familial cases.[248,249] The *VHL* gene was found to be mutated in a high percentage of clear-cell renal carcinomas, whereas it was not mutated in papillary renal cancer, thus suggesting a fundamental genetic difference between clear-cell and papillary renal carcinoma.[249] Mutation of *VHL* in sporadic clear-cell carcinoma is thought to be a late event in renal oncogenesis. Second, another gene on chromosome 3, *FHIT*, located at 3p21, is also disrupted in hereditary clear-cell renal cancer.[250] In rare clear-cell carcinomas, *FHIT* is fused to a patched-related gene on chromosome 8 called *TCR8*. A third region on 3p is implicated in a recurring translocation in clear-cell renal carcinoma, the t(3;5)(p13;q22). Another gene on 3p has also been identified that is implicated in clear-cell oncogenesis. This gene is termed *DIRC2*, located at 3q21 in the familial t(2;3)(q35;q21).[251] The translocation break points on chromosome 3 affect different regions of the chromosome. However, the different genes involved appear to be involved in the same genetic pathway of renal oncogenesis.

In contrast to clear cell-carcinomas, papillary carcinomas have trisomy 7 in over 50% of cases and t(X;1)(p11.2;q21) in 20% of cases.[252] The t(X;1)(p11.2;q21) rearrangement has been cloned and results in the fusion of the *PRCC* gene on the X chromosome to the *TFE3* gene on chromosome 1. The PRCC/TFE3 fusion protein includes the helix-loop-helix DNA binding domain and the leucine zipper transcriptional regulatory domains of TFE3. However, fusion of these domains to PRCC would produce a different set of genes that would be transcriptionally activated by the fusion protein than either transcription factor alone, possibly producing the oncogenic phenotype. In addition, there is a tyrosine kinase consensus site present, indicating that this protein may be regulated by phosphorylation during signaling cascades.

A highly distinctive subset of clear-cell carcinoma in pediatric patients contains a t(6;11)(p21;q12). This translocation has recently been shown to produce a fusion of alpha, a gene on 11q12, and the transcription factor gene *TFEB* on 6p21.[253] Alpha is a ubiquitously expressed RNA that does not code for a protein. As such, it may represent a micro-RNA that regulates the expression of other genes by binding to their mRNA and blocking translation.[254] This translocation may not only alter the activity of the transcription factor TFEB, but also alter the activity of an unknown miRNA. In addition, the genetic defect implicated in hereditary papillary renal carcinoma (HPRC) has been mapped to chromosome 7q, and germline mutations of *MET* at 7q31 have been detected in patients with HPRC.[255] In a study of 16 tumors from two patients with germline mutations in exon 16 of *MET*, FISH analysis revealed trisomy 7 in all tumors. Furthermore, PCR analysis of microsatellite markers revealed that the chromosome bearing the mutant *MET* allele was the one that was duplicated. This suggests that the nonrandom duplication of the mutated *MET* allele is an initiating event in renal cell cancer.[256]

Gene expression microarrays have been used to define two prognostic subgroups in papillary renal carcinoma. A 7 gene signature defines the two subgroups, with high expression of cytokeratin 7 in class 1 good prognosis tumors and high expression of topoisomerase II alpha in class 2 poor prognosis tumors.[257]

Thyroid Carcinoma Roque and colleagues reported recurrent clonal chromosomal alterations in a series of 94 tumors.[258] Of these tumors, 63 were papillary thyroid cancers, 19 were follicular cell carcinomas, and 7 were tall cell carcinomas. Clonal chromosomal abnormalities were seen in 37 (40%) of these tumors and structural cytogenetic abnormalities were detected in 18 of 37 tumors. Chromosomes 1, 3, 7, and 10 were the most often involved in these rearrangements. The most common break points involved in these rearrangements were 1p32–36, 1p11–13, 1q, 3p25–26, 7q34–36, and, especially, 10q11.2. Rearrangements of chromosome 10q were the most frequent alterations detected in these tumors. Further study found that the different translocations that involved the 10q11.2 break point all resulted in the activation of the *RET* proto-oncogene on chromosome 10. This occurred by fusion of the tyrosine kinase domain of *RET* with the 5' domain of different genes that produced constitutive activation of the tyrosine kinase activity of *RET*. For example, *RET* fuses with *H4* in the inv10(q11;q21.2), with *PKAR1A* in the t(10;17)(q11.2;q23), with *ELE1* in the inv(10q11), and *ELKS* in the t(10;12)(q11;p13).[259] There are other less frequent rearrangements of *RET* in papillary carcinoma that result in the fusion of *RET* with *PCAM1*, *GOLGA5*, *TIF1A*, and *TIF1G*.[259,260] These *RET* fusions have been numbered PTC1-7, respectively. These oncogenic fusions of *RET* can occur in familial thyroid cancer syndromes including the multiple endocrine neoplasia (MEN) syndromes, or in sporadic papillary thyroid cancer.

Approximately 15% of follicular carcinomas have rearrangements involving 1q22. These chromosomal translocations and inversions involving 1q22 also resulted in the activation of another receptor tyrosine kinase gene important in thyroid cancer, termed *NTRK1* (also *TRK*). This gene can be fused to 1q neighboring genes *TPM3* and *TPR*, and *TFG* located on chromosome 3.[260,261] Like *RET* in thyroid cancer and the classic example of *ABL* in CML, these fusions result in the constitutive activation of the tyrosine kinase activity of *NTRK1*. Another aberration frequently observed in thyroid cancer is trisomy 7, similar to prostate cancer. In follicular thyroid carcinomas, it has been shown that a gain of this chromosome is associated with dysplasia of the follicular epithelium. In papillary carcinoma, it has been correlated with a poor prognosis.[262] Significantly, there is a report of an association between increased expression of the *MET/HGF* receptor gene mapped at 7q31 with a poor outcome, indicating that this may be a candidate for amplification in trisomy 7.[263]

Uterine Carcinoma Uterine carcinomas originate from either the cervix or the endometrium.

Cervical carcinoma usually originates in the transitional zone between the squamous and columnar cell epithelium. Infection with certain serotypes of human papillomavirus (HPV) is a major factor for initiation of cervical oncogenesis. Recurrent chromosomal aberrations have been described in cervical carcinoma using conventional karyotyping. These include structural changes in chromosomes 1, 3, 5, 11, and 17.[264,265] Using CGH, a gain on 3q has been found in 90% of cervical carcinomas. This gain probably occurs at the transition from cervical dysplasia to invasive carcinoma. Recent studies suggest involvement of the *hTR* gene at 3q, which encodes the RNA component of telomerase.[266] Other studies have shown that 4p16 may be important in cervical cancer progression. This region contains the *FGFR3* gene, and mutations in this gene were found in 3 of 3 cervical cancers.[267]

Loss of heterozygosity studies in cervical cancer indicate that there are two regions on 3p where tumor suppressor genes may be situated: at 3p14 and at 3p21.[268] The gene located at 3p14 may be the *FHIT* tumor suppressor gene. Another chromosomal abnormality in cervical cancer, ani(5p), is associated with advanced disease and poor prognosis.[269] Loss of material from chromosome 18q is a frequent cytogenetic alteration in cervical cancer and is associated with a poor prognosis. Since the tumor suppressor gene *SMAD4* is located at 18q21, alterations in the *SMAD4* gene in cervical cancer was examined.[270] *SMAD4* deficiency was present in 4 of 13 cervical cancer cell lines as a result of an intronic rearrangement and deletion of 3' exons. Deletion of *SMAD4* activity would decrease responsiveness to the growth inhibitory effects of TGF-β, increasing proliferation.

Endometrial carcinoma of the uterus is heterogeneous, including many different histologic subtypes, such as endometrioid, serous, clear-cell, mucinous, mixed, and undifferentiated carcinomas. The two most common types are endometrioid (70% of cases) and serous (20% of cases). These two types are distinguished by different cytogenetic features, based on conventional karyotypes and CGH. Endometrioid carcinomas have simple chromosomal alterations, whereas those aberrations found in serous carcinomas are more complex. Endometrioid carcinomas are generally hyperdiploid, with the most common alterations being gain of the long arm of chromosome 1 (70% of cases) and trisomy 10 (40% of cases). Gain of chromosome 1q and iso(1q) can also be observed as sole abnormalities.[271] Owing to their low incidence and to the complexity of their karyotypes, the chromosomal abnormalities of serous endometrial carcinomas are not as well documented. One study of 24 tumors by CGH found a very high rate of chromosomal abnormalities. The most frequent regions of gain were 3q26 (50% of cases) and 8q (33%). High-level amplifications were detected in over 30% of the cases and involved 2q, 3q, 5p, 6p, 8q, 15q, 18p, 18q, and chromosome 20.[272]

Endometrial stromal sarcoma is a rare and aggressive uterine cancer. Cytogenetic aberrations have been reported in 22 cases of this sarcoma, and they mostly involve rearrangements of chromosomes 6, 7, and 17. The most characteristic translocation of this tumor type, t(7;17)(p15;q21), was recently shown to generate a *JAZF1/JJAZ1* fusion gene.[273,274] This fusion protein plays a role in altering transcriptional control of proliferation. This fusion has been confirmed in several other cases of this uterine sarcoma, indicating that it plays a significant role in the origins of that tumor.

Familial endometrial cancer can be seen in the Lynch syndromes, which have mutations in the mismatched repair genes *MLH1* and *MSH2*, discussed in the sections "Colorectal Carcinomas" and "Colonic Adenomas" above.[275]

Malignant Mesenchymal Tumors Solid malignancies that arise from mesenchymal tissues are rare, making up less than 1% of all human cancers. Malignant mesenchymal tumors are often histopathologically diverse, even within the same group, and can be difficult to diagnose pathologically.[276] Cytogenetic studies have greatly assisted in defining diagnostic tumor types and, therefore, future therapy in some cases. In other cases cytogenetic aberrations have helped distinguish between benign and malignant tumors. Occasionally the benign and malignant tumors from a given tissue share related cytogenetic changes and shed light on the progression of disease from atypia to metastases. The molecular genetics of these soft tissue mesenchymal tumors have provided a model for how cytogenetics can contribute to a more clear understanding of the origins of these specific diseases and assist in diagnosis and therapy.

Alveolar Soft Part Sarcoma Alveolar soft part sarcoma is an uncommon mesenchymal malignancy with a characteristic histopathology. Recent cytogenetic studies have found a recurrent nonreciprocal t(X;17)(p11.2;q25) in most cases of this sarcoma. This translocation results in an *ASPL/TFE3* gene fusion.[277] YAC and BAC probes from the break point region helped define the *TFE3* gene on Xp11. Probes of *TFE3* found that part of its sequence was present on 17q25. This transcription factor was known to be involved in translocations in papillary renal cell carcinoma. PCR then was used to define the gene that *TFE3* was fused to, and this novel gene was termed *ASPL*, which was located normally on 17q25. *ASPL* is widely expressed in all adult tissues. It encodes a predicted protein of unknown function, containing a conserved domain that may function in ubiquitylation pathway. *ASPL* was fused in-frame to *TFE3* exon 4 (type 1 fusion) or exon 3 (type 2 fusion). The reciprocal fusion transcript, TFE/ASPL was detected in only 1 of the 12 cases studied, consistent with the nonreciprocal nature of the translocation. The lack of a reciprocal product indicates that the ASPL/TFE3 and not the reciprocal protein is the key oncogenic fusion product.

Chondrosarcoma There is a large amount of cytogenetic data for skeletal chondrosarcoma, a malignancy arising from bone. Mandahl and colleagues investigated the genomic abnormalities in 59 chondrosarcomas of various size and grade.[278] Frequent hypodiploid karyotypes were seen. Although no recurrent structural aberrations were observed, nonrandom patterns of additions and deletions were found. Losses of chromosomal material most often came from 1p36, 1p13–22, 1, 5q13–31, 6q22-qter, 9p22-pter, 10p, 10q24-pter, 11p13-pter, 11q25, 13q21-qter, 14q24-qter, 18p, 18q22-qter, and 22q13. Gains commonly observed were from 7p13-pter, 12q15-qter, 19, 20pter-q11, and 21q. In addition, univariate analysis revealed that loss of material from 6q, 10p, 11p, 11q, 13q, and 22q was associated with metastatic potential. In a Cox regression model, however, only loss of material from 13q was a statistically significant independent prognostic factor for metastasis. With loss of 13q, there was a relative risk of 5.2 for metastases to be present.

Extraskeletal myxoid chondrosarcoma, a variant of chondrosarcoma that can arise from extraskeletal tissue, closely resembles embryonic cartilage. Specific chromosomal translocations define these malignancies, particularly the t(9;22)(q22;q12), which occurs in 75% of these tumors.[279] This translocation results in the formation of the fusion of EWS on 22q12 to CHN (also termed TEC) on 9q22. The chimeric protein consists of the amino-terminal domain of EWS linked to the entire CHN protein. EWS, which was originally identified as the gene rearranged in Ewing's sarcoma, encodes a putative RNA-binding protein that has transcriptional activation properties when fused to a DNA binding domain. The *CHN* gene encodes a novel orphan nuclear receptor belonging to the steroid receptor superfamily[280] and supplies the DNA binding domain to this fusion protein. Thus, this EWS/CHN fusion protein would produce aberrant activation of genes not normally activated in this tissue, and this abnormal gene expression pattern is likely the key event in myxoid chondrosarcoma oncogenesis.

Although most myxoid chondrosarcomas are characterized by the t(9;22), a minority have other translocations, such as a t(9;17)(q22;11) or a t(9;15)(q22;q21). These translocations result in chimeric proteins involving fusion of *CHN* to *TAF2N* (also *RBP56*) or *TCF12*, respectively. The common involvement of the *CHN* gene in each case indicates that it is the critical transcriptional regulatory pathway for this malignancy to develop. In these cases, also *TAF2N* and *TCF12* supply a transactivation domain to *CHN*. Thus, in comparison with skeletal chondrosarcomas, which have complex and variable cytogenetic abnormalities that have not lent themselves well to dissection of molecular oncogenesis, the cytogenetics extraskeletal chondrosarcomas have provided great insight into the disease origins.[281]

Fibrosarcoma Like skeletal chondrosarcoma, fibrosarcomas have complex and variable cytogenetic patterns. Nonetheless, cytogenetics in fibrosarcomas have provided more insight into the etiology and progression of these tumors. Using CGH, the majority of patients with fibrosarcoma had chromosome copy number changes. The most frequent gain of material was at 12q21, which was detected in 18 of 34 patients. Other recurring gains were at 12q14–15, 14q22, 4q22, 7q31, 14q23–24, 4q21, 4q23–24, 8q22, and 12q22.[282] Losses of material were much less common than gains. Changes seen in early-stage tumors included gains of 2, 4q, and 14q. Gains of chromosomes 7 and 8q were associated with more advanced disease presentation. In addition, fibrosarcomas from patients who failed therapy and died of their disease, independent of presenting stage, showed more frequent gains of 8q, 12q, 13q, and 15q compared with those who were cured of their disease.[282] A gain of material from 12q14–22 was the most common genomic imbalance in patients who did poorly. This probably reflects *MDM2* gene amplification. Thus, this gene may play a role in promoting aggressive disease in these tumors.

Low-grade fibromyxoid sarcoma is a distinct variant of fibrosarcoma. Like the extraskeletal myxoid chondrosarcomas, this tumor has a distinct translocation, the t(7;16)(q33;p11). This resulted in a fusion of the *FUS* and *CREB3L2* (also known as *BBF2H7*).[283] To define the spectrum of fibrosarcomas that had the *FUS/CREB3L2* fusion gene, 45 low-grade spindle-cell sarcomas were analyzed using RT-PCR and FISH.[283] None of these tumors were originally diagnosed as low-grade fibromyxoid sarcoma. In addition, there were also two benign soft tissue tumors and nine high-grade sarcomas with supernumerary ring chromosomes or 7q3 rearrangement and three tumors diagnosed as low-grade fibromyxoid sarcomas that were analyzed. Twelve of the 59 tumors analyzed were positive for FUS/CREB3L2, and all of these were diagnosed as low-grade myxoid fibrosacroma after histopathologic re-examination. Thus, these findings indicate that this fusion is diagnostic of this tumor type, and plays a key role in the origin of this tumor. FUS (also cloned as TLS in liposarcoma) is involved in other translocations in hematologic malignances, such as acute myeloid leukemia, indicating that diverse tumors share similar molecular mechanisms. Interestingly, another rare fibrosarcoma variant has a translocation that has a gene involved that is also involved in translocations in hematologic malignancies. In the rare form of fibrosarcoma, dermatofibrosarcoma protuberans, there is a clonal recurrent t(17;22)(q2;q13). This break point has been isolated and results in a chimeric protein COL1A1/PDGFB.[284] PDGFB, the receptor of platelet-derived growth factor, is also involved in other oncogenic translocations in MDS and AML (see Table 8-4).

Liposarcoma Myxoid liposarcoma, the most common histopathologic subtype of the malignant adipose tumors, is characterized by recurrent translocations, such as the t(12;16) or, more rarely, a t(12;22). Both of these translocations result in chimeric genes involving a fusion of the *CHOP* gene at 12q13 with the 5' end of either *TLS/FUS* on chromosome 16 or *EWS* on chromosome 22.[285] *FUS* is also involved in recurrent translocations in fibrosarcoma, while *EWS* is also disrupted by chromosomal translocations in chondrosarcoma and Ewing's sarcoma. The chimeric TLS/CHOP or EWS/CHOP proteins function as abnormal transcription factors, which activate a pattern of gene expression that produces the specific malignant phenotype of liposarcoma. CHOP has been shown to play an essential role in normal adipocyte differentiation. Thus, the translocation of CHOP and the resultant abnormal gene expression pattern alters the normal genetic regulation of differentiation, contributing to the development of malignances involving adipose tissues. Translocations of CHOP have not been demonstrated in benign adipose tumors such as lipomas, even if they have cytogenetic abnormalities in the 12q13 region where CHOP is located, further suggesting that CHOP is critical for malignant transformation.[286–288]

Other abnormalities, including ring chromosomes, are frequently observed in well-differentiated liposarcomas.[289] Further investigation of these ring chromosomes found that they were complex, containing amplicons of nonadjacent chromosomal segments. The mechanism by which these complex structures form is not understood, but it appears that they consist of amplification structures related to double minutes and homogenously staining regions within chromosomes.[290] Other genomic aberrations seen in well-differentiated liposarcomas include loss of 13q and abnormalities of the 11p telomere.

Rhabdomyosarcoma The t(2;13)(q35;q14) is seen as the sole abnormality in more 50% of alveolar rhabdomyosarcomas. This translocations results in a fusion between *PAX3* on chromosome 2 and *FKHR* on chromosome 13, in which the amino terminus of *PAX3*, including an intact DNA-binding domain, is fused to the carboxy terminus of the *FKHR* gene and its transcriptional regulatory domain.[291] Another translocation seen less commonly in alveolar rhabdomyosarcoma, a t(1;13)(p36;q14), has a similar clinical outcome as the t(2;13). This translocation results in the fusion of another member of the *PAX* gene family, PAX7, to the *FKHR* gene on chromosome 13.[292] Detection of these chimeric transcripts is a useful diagnostic and monitoring tool for these tumors. Interestingly, *PAX3* and *PAX7* are normally specifically expressed in the dorsal neural tube and the developing somites during embryonic development. Mutations of *PAX3* in Splotch mice and in Waardenburg's syndrome in man show that *PAX3* is necessary for the proper formation of the caudal neural crest and for the migration of myoblasts into limbs. Mice with a mutated *PAX7* gene suffer from defects in the formation of cephalic neural crest derivatives. These data imply that after translocation, the abnormal PAX3 and PAX7 fusion products may trigger neoplastic development by maintaining cells closer to the embryonic state, as undifferentiated and proliferative cells.[293]

Synovial Sarcoma Synovial sarcomas are associated with a hallmark translocation, the t(X;18)(p11.2;q11.2).[294] The t(X;18) results in the fusion of the *SYT* gene on chromosome 18 to either of two distinct genes, *SSX1* or *SSX2*, on the X chromosome. *SSX1* and *SSX2* encode closely related proteins, with 81% amino acid identity among 188 amino acids. The amino-terminal portion of each SSX protein exhibits homology to the Kruppel-associated box (KRAB), a transcriptional repressor domain previously found only in Kruppel-type zinc finger transcriptional regulators. PCR analysis has detected the presence of SYT/SSX1or SYT/SSX2 fusion transcripts in 29 of 32 of synovial sarcomas tested. This not only demonstrated the importance of these fusion products in this disease, but also showed that detection of these products could be a useful diagnostic tool. Furthermore, it has been observed that there is a correlation between the presence of either STY/SSX1 and STY/SSX2 fusion transcripts and survival. Patients with an STY/SSX1 fusion had a 5-year survival of 42% versus that of 89% for patients with an STY/SSX2 fusion. This same study found that patients with the STY/SSX1 fusion had higher proliferation rates. Thus, the presence of the STY/SSX1 fusion transcript is an important prognostic factor.[295]

Malignant Germ Cell Tumors Although several histopathologic types of testicular germ cell tumors are recognized, all share a common cytogenetic abnormality: an isochromosome derived from 12p. Iso(12p) has been detected in all germ cell tumor lineages, including seminomas, teratomas, and embryonal carcinomas.[296] Thus, i(12p) appears to be a consistent and specific chromosomal abnormality in testicular germ cell tumors, as it is present in 80% of these cases. Interestingly, the other 20% of testicular tumors that are negative for iso(12p) have 12p amplification, suggesting that the short arm of chromosome 12 contains gene(s) whose increased expression is required for the development of testicular cancers.[297] However, finding the exact gene or genes involved has proved very difficult. A potential candidate gene is *CCND1* (cyclin D), although its definitive role in testicular tumorigenesis remains unproven. Although initial reports suggested that the degree of 12p amplification correlated with disease outcome,[298] this finding was not confirmed in subsequent studies.[299] Nonetheless, the presence of an iso(12p) has been useful in the differential diagnosis of metastatic germ cell tumors in neoplasms of unknown origin.

MALIGNANT NERVOUS SYSTEM TUMORS **Gliomas** The most frequently recurring genomic and chromosomal abnormalities in gliomas include double minute chromosomes; structural abnormalities of chromosome 9, such as del(9p) or translocations fusing 9p to many different partner chromosomes; trisomy 7; and loss of chromosomes 10, 18, and 22.[300] The most prevalent finding involved chromosome 9 with break points either at the centromere or in 9p. With the increasing use of CGH to study chromosome gain and loss in solid tumors, the genetic changes associated with one type of glioma, primary astrocytoma, have been defined better. Chromosomal gains and losses are frequent in astrocytoma, and the average number of chromosomal losses was significantly higher in high-grade astrocytoma as compared with low-grade tumors ($p < .01$). Frequent changes included gains of 7p12–13, 7q31, 8q24.1–24.2, and 20q13.1–13.2, and losses of 9p21, 10p11–12, 10q22-qter, and 13q21–22. Similar losses of 9p, 10p, and 10q, and gain of 7p were observed in over 50% of the glioblastomas.[301] The tumor-suppressor gene *CDKN2* ($p16^{INK4a}$) is located within the 9p21 chromosomal aberration and has been reported to be deleted in 70% of glioma cell lines and primary glioma tumor samples.[302] Mutations of *TP53*, deletions of 9p and of *CKDN2*, loss of chromosome 10, and *EGFR* amplification are critical genetic events in the development of gliomas.[302,303]

The consistent loss of chromosome 10q suggested that a tumor suppressor gene was located in this region and a candidate gene, *PTEN/MMAC1*, was cloned and characterized. *PTEN* encodes a protein with homology to the catalytic domain of protein phosphatases, and also to the cytoskeletal proteins, tensin and auxilin. Further studies have determined that *PTEN* is mutated in a large number of human cancers, including glioblastoma, the most aggressive form of glioma, prostate cancer, and breast cancer.[304] Another tumor suppressor gene on 10q, *MXI1*, could also play a role in the growth of human glioblastoma because it is also lost in most 10q deletions.[305] *MXI1* codes for a protein that regulates *MYC* family members. *MYC* activates transcription and stimulates cell proliferation, while *MXI1* inhibits those activities. Using polymorphic CA microsatellite repeats, it has been demonstrated that 7 of 11 glioblastomas had loss of *MXI1*. A final candidate tumor suppressor gene on 10q is *LGI1*.[306]

Medulloblastoma Medulloblastomas are malignant tumors of the cerebellum, most commonly seen in children. Nonrandom chromosome gains and losses were frequent; nonrandom losses were seen on 10q, 11, 16q, 17p, and 8p, while regions of chromosomal gain most often included 17q and 7.[307] An isochromosome for the long arm of 17, iso(17q), is found in 30% of medulloblastomas. This isochromosome is not easily detected by conventional cytogenetics, and in cases where conventional methods fail to detect this aberration, FISH on interphase nuclei can be used to detect this abnormality. Detecting this aberration is of clinical importance as the presence of iso(17q) has been associated with a poor response to therapy and shorter survival.[308] Recently, the signaling protein REN (KCTD11) mapping to 17p13, has been hypothesized to be the tumor suppressor gene deleted in medulloblastoma.[309] REN is often deleted in medulloblastoma and ectopically expressing REN inhibits medulloblastoma cell proliferation and colony formation in vitro. It also suppresses xenograft tumor growth in vivo. REN may inhibit medulloblastoma proliferation by negatively regulating the Hedgehog pathway by antagonizing the Gli-mediated transactivation of Hedgehog target genes.[309]

Neuroepitheliomas In 1984, Whang-Peng and colleagues described a t(11;22)(q24;q12) in two cases of peripheral neuroepithelioma.[310] This seminal report was the first to demonstrate this translocation, which is also reported in more than 90% of Ewing's sarcoma tumors.[311] Neuroepithelioma and Ewing's sarcoma are closely related histologically; both appear to be derived from the same embryonic neural crest tissue. The difference appears to be the age and location at presentation of these tumors, with Ewing's sarcoma occurring at a younger age in peripheral tissue. The t(11;22) translocation results in the fusion of the amino portion of the RNA binding protein *EWS* gene at 22q12 with the carboxy fragment ETS family transcription factor Fli-1 on 11q24.[312] This translocation is also seen in pediatric small round blue tumors as described below. EWS-Fli results in the activation of genes not normally expressed in these tissues, as Fli is not normally expressed in these tissues; this aberrant pattern of gene expression is the mechanism of transformation in these tumors. The discovery that neuroepithelioma and Ewing's sarcoma both have the same translocation and fusion gene has changed the treatment modality in neuroepithelioma. Use of Ewing's sarcoma-like therapy has resulted in a marked improvement in the response of neuroepithelioma. This further solidified the concept that both neuroepithelioma and Ewing's sarcoma arise from cells of the neural crest.

Peripheral Nerve Sheath Tumor Peripheral nerve sheath tumors (PNST) include schwannomas, neurofibromas, perineuromas, and malignant peripheral nerve sheath tumors.[313] Several hereditary disorders predispose to benign and malignant peripheral nerve sheath tumors, most notably neurofibromatosis type I and type II (NF1 and NF2). As previously mentioned, NF1, also known as von Recklinghausen's disease, is an autosomal dominant disorder caused by mutations in the *NF1* gene, which functions to inhibit the *ras* signaling pathway, located on 17q. This syndrome is characterized by a propensity to develop neurofibromas and malignant nerve sheath tumors. Germline mutations in the *NF2* gene, located on chromosome 22, predispose to schwannomas, predominantly those affecting the spine and intracranial nerves. CGH analysis of both sporadic and *NF2*-associated schwannomas has revealed that loss of 22q is a frequent and recurrent abnormality. This suggests that *NF2* inactivation is important not only in the formation of hereditary schwannomas, but in sporadic cases as well.

Desmoplastic Small Round-Cell Tumor Desmoplastic small round-cell tumor is a rare and aggressive malignant tumor that usually occurs in adolescents or young adults. The cell of origin remains unknown, but it is speculated that these tumors arise from serosal lining cells in the abdomen. A specific translocation, t(11;22)(p13;q12), has been documented in this tumor. Since this tumor is histologically indistinct, this translocation may be used to confirm the diagnosis.[314–316] Gerald and colleagues found that this translocation results in the fusion of the *EWS* and *WT1* genes. *EWS* is the gene involved in Ewing's sarcoma and neuroepithelioma translocations, while *WT1* is involved in translocations in Wilms' tumor, described below. Analysis of *EWS/WT1* chimeric transcripts from these tumors revealed that the transcripts represent in-frame fusion of the amino-terminal domain of EWS to the last three zinc fingers of the DNA-binding domain of WT1. This chimeric protein produces an aberrant transcription factor, using the DNA-binding domain of WT1 and the EWS amino terminal as a transcriptional activation domain. WT1 is normally a transcriptional repressor but this novel fusion protein abnormally activates WT1 target sites, thereby contributing to the development of this tumor.[316]

Ewing's Sarcoma The t(11;22)(q24;q12) is the hallmark of Ewing's sarcoma detected in more than 90% of these tumors. As mentioned above, this translocation results in the fusion of the amino terminal transcriptional activation domain of EWS from chromosome 22 to the DNA-binding domain of the ETS family transcription factor *FLI1* on chromosome 11.[311,312] *FLI1* is usually expressed only in early hematopoietic cells and is a weak transcriptional activator. Because of this translocation, it is abnormally expressed and is a very strong transcriptional activator, leading to abnormal activation of a pattern of gene expression that leads to the development of Ewing's sarcoma. This translocation has been described in peripheral neuroepitheliomas as well in as in Ewing's sarcoma. In 5% of cases of Ewing's sarcoma, however, the *EWS* gene is involved in the variant translocations t(21;22)(q12;q12) and t(7;22)(p22;q12) that result in the fusion of EWS with the ETS family transcriptional factors ERG and ETV1, respectively.[313–317] These fusions therefore produce very similar aberrant transcriptional activators to EWS/FLI1.

Neuroblastoma A deletion of the short arm of chromosome 1 is the most frequent chromosomal aberration in neuroblastomas. In addition, gene amplifications are seen—detected either as double minutes or homogenously staining regions. In some cell lines, these have been shown to represent amplification of *MYCN*. *MYCN* amplification can be seen using DNA probes in tumor samples, and is highly correlated with advanced stage (III and IV) and a worse survival.[318]

Retinoblastoma Although retinoblastoma can be sporadic, it is the familial cases that have produced the greatest insight into the molecular mechanisms of tumorigenesis. Retinoblastomas have characteristic deletions of chromosome 13 that always includes 13q14. Using familial cases, the gene consistently deleted in retinoblastoma was cloned, and termed *RB1*.[319] The inherited deletion in chromosome 13q14 deleted one copy of *RB1*, and the remaining allele was found to be mutated. Retinoblastoma developed when the function of both copies of *RB1* were abrogated. This seminal advance not only demonstrated the existence of tumor suppressor genes, but also validated Knudson's classic two-hit hypothesis for the development of neoplasia. *RB1* has been found to be mutated in a large number of other tumors (see Table 8-1). *RB1* functions by binding to *E2F* and inhibiting the expression of genes that activate cell-cycle progression. When *RB1*'s function is deleted, cells can progress through the cell cycle without repression.[320]

Wilms' Tumor (Nephroblastoma) The most common cytogenetic abnormality in Wilms' tumors is trisomy of the long arm of chromosome 11 (11q). Deletions of 11p13 or unbalanced translocations occur in 25% of cases. Recent studies suggest that three distinct genetic loci are implicated in the development of Wilms' tumor. One locus, which is associated with the WAGR (Wilms' tumor, aniridia, genitourinary dysplasia, and mental retardation) syndrome, maps to 11p13.[321,322] A second locus, which is associated with the Beckwith-Wiedemann syndrome, maps to 11p15. The third locus, which may be involved in familial predisposition to Wilms' tumor, was not genetically linked to any of the markers on 11p and may be on another chromosome. Two groups independently isolated a candidate gene (*WT1*) for Wilms' tumor at 11p13.[323,324] Study of the mutations of *WT1* in Wilms' tumor suggests that it plays an important role in the pathogenesis of this disease. Translocations involving *WT1* are also seen in desmoplastic small round-cell tumor, described above.

Melanoma The most common recurring cytogenetic abnormalities in melanoma are deletions or rearrangements in chromosomes 1p, multiple abnormalities in 6, and extra copies of 7.[325] A translocation involving the terminal region 10q24–26 has also been seen in some premalignant lesions, and abnormalities of chromosome 10 have been seen in both early and late melanoma, suggesting that this may be a primary event in the malignant process.[326] Iso(1q) or del(1p) occurs in approximately 60% of all melanomas, while chromosome 6 is rearranged in more than 80% of cases. Trent and colleagues showed that the insertion of a normal chromosome 6 into melanoma cells could revert some features of the malignant phenotype.[327] In addition, the tumor suppressor gene *CDKN2* (*p16*), which inhibits cell cycle progression, is often deleted in melanoma cell lines.[328,329] In addition, germline mutations of this gene have been demonstrated in cases of familial melanoma that were mapped to 9p.[328] In one study, seven different *CDKN2A* germline mutations were sequenced in 17 patients (16% of the total number of patients examined). The age of onset of the melanoma was lower and the number of primary melanomas higher in patients with mutations. *CDKN2A* mutations were more frequent in patients with familial history of melanoma (35%) compared with patients without (8%). There has been a consensus statement on the counseling and cytogenetic testing of individuals that have a high incidence of melanoma in their families.[330]

Using SNP array-based genetic maps and microarray gene expression profiling, the melanocyte master regulator MITF (microphthalmia-associated transcription factor) was identified as being amplified in melanoma.[331] *MITF* amplification was more often seen in metastatic disease compared with local disease and was also correlated with poor patient survival. Also, mutations in the tumor suppressors *BRAF* and *p16* were associated with MITF amplification in melanoma cell lines. Forcing *MITF* and mutant *BRAF* (V600E) expression transformed primary human melanocytes. Thus, *MITF* is a novel melanoma oncogene. Reducing *MIT*F activity increases the sensitivity of melanoma cells to chemotherapeutic agents.[331] Therefore, reducing *MITF* function could increase the response of melanoma to chemotherapy.

SUMMARY

In conclusion, with the use of comprehensive molecular technologies, the discovery of the recurrent chromosomal aberrations in cancer is proceeding at a very rapid pace. The comprehensive discovery and functional analysis of the full spectrum of genomic changes in each human cancer will be essential for improved cancer diagnosis and treatment and will facilitate our fundamental understanding of the cellular pathways and networks perturbed by genomic mutations. With full knowledge of the chromosomal aberrations in hand, we can improve cancer diagnosis through more and more sophisticated molecular classification, enhance the selection of therapeutic targets for drug development, promote the development of faster and more efficient clinical trials using agents targeted to specific genomic abnormalities, and create markers for early detection and prevention. Yet, significant challenges remain. The task of integrating enormous data sets of the chromosomal aberrations, gene mutations, genetic predispositions, gene expression and proteomic profiles, and epigenetic changes in each human tumor will indeed be challenging. Yet the willingness of the National Cancer Institute and National Institute for Human Genome Research Genome Institute to launch comprehensive projects towards this goal is inspiring. An area ripe for more intensive investigation is a determination of how humans acquire the earliest lesions that initiate cancer and whether tumors of different lineages have different mechanisms of carcinogenesis. Furthermore, while the tools for characterizing and analyzing the genomic aberrations that initiate and promote cancer are increasingly in hand, we are less well equipped to measure and investigate the environmental exposures and social behaviors that in addition to genetic abnormalities, undoubtedly play a role in the development of most human cancers. Nonetheless, the ultimate success of comprehensive, large scale human cancer genome projects will continue to rapidly advance our understanding of cancer genetics and genomics and will potentially revolutionize our approach to the diagnosis and treatment of cancer.

URLS REFERENCED IN THIS CHAPTER

Cancer Cytogenetic Databases. The Mitelman Database of Chromosome Aberrations in Cancer at the U.S. National Cancer Institute (NCI) Cancer Genome Anatomy Project (CGAP). Website: http://cgap.nci.nih.gov.

The NCI Cancer Genome Anatomy Project: CGH, FISH, SKY Databases; the NCI NIHFR Cancer Genome Project. Website: http://cgap.nci.nih.gov.

The Wellcome Trust Sanger Institute Cancer Genome Project. Website: http://www.sanger.ac.uk.

Cancer Gene Census Lists. The Wellcome Trust Sanger Institute Cancer Genome Project Cancer Gene Census. Website: http://www.sanger.ac.uk/genetics/CGP/census.

Catalogue of Human Cancer Gene Mutations: The "COSMIC" (Catalogue Of Somatic Mutations in Cancer) Database. Website: http://www.sanger.ac.uk/genetics/CGP/cosmic).

ACKNOWLEDGMENTS

CLW is supported by D.H.H.S. NIH grants CA114762, CA118100, CA86780, CA30969, and CA32102 and a Specialized Center of Research (SCOR) grant from the Leukemia and Lymphoma Society. RH is supported by D.H.H.S. NIH grants CA102283, HL66308, CA118100, HL075783 and a Specialized Center of Research (SCOR) grant from the Leukemia and Lymphoma Society. The authors would like to thank Dr. Janet Rowley and her colleagues for developing the foundation for this chapter in prior editions of *Cancer Medicine* and for her mentorship as the premier cytogeneticist in the United States. The authors would like to thank the following colleagues for providing data and figures for the chapter: Dr. Andrew Carroll from University of Alabama, Drs. Mary Relling and Susana Raimondi of St. Jude Children's Hospital, Dr. Kathleen Richkind of Genzyme Genetics, and Dr. Octavian Henegariu.

REFERENCES

1. Hanahan D, Weinberg RA. The hallmarks of cancer. Cell 2000;100:57–70.
2. Albertson DG, Collins C, McCormick F, Gray JW. Chromosome aberrations in solid tumors. Nat Gen 2003;34(4):369–76.
3. Futreal PA, Coin L, Marshall M, et al. A census of human cancer genes. Nature Reviews Cancer 2004;4:177–83.
4. The Wellcome Trust Sanger Institute Cancer Genome Project. 2005. http://www.sanger.ac.uk/genetics/CGP.
5. Mitelman F, Johansson B, Mertens F. Fusion genes and rearranged genes as a linear function of chromosome aberrations in cancer. Nat Genet 2004;36:331–4.
6. Feinberg AP, Tycko B. The history of cancer epigenetics. Nature Reviews Cancer 2004;4:143–153.
7. Ushijima T. Detection and interpretation of altered methylation patterns in cancer cells. Nature Reviews Cancer 2005;5:223–31.
8. Nowell PC. A minute chromosome in human granulocytic leukemia. Science 1960;132:1497.
9. Caspersson T, Farber S, Foley GE, et al. Chemical differentiation along metaphase chromosomes. Exp Cell Research 1968;49:219–22.
10. Rowley JD. A new consistent chromosomal abnormality in chronic myelogenous leukaemia identified by quinacrine fluorescence and Giemsa staining. Nature 1973;243:290–3.
11. Schrock E, et al. Multicolor spectral karyotyping of human chromosomes. Science 1996;273:494–497.
12. Speicher MR, Ballard SG, Ward DC. Karyotyping human chromosomes by combinatorial multi-fluor FISH. Nat Gen 1996;12:368–75.
13. Fauth C, Speicher MR. Classifying by colors: FISH-based genome analysis. Cytogenet Cell Genet 2001;93:1–10.

14. Lichter P. Multicolor FISHing: what's the catch? Trends Genet 1997;13:475–9.
15. Kallioniemi A, et al. Comparative genomic hybridization for molecular cytogenetic analysis of solid tumors. Science 1992;258:818–21.
16. Pinkel D, et al. High resolution analysis of DNA copy number variation using competitive genomic hybridization to microarrays. Nat Gen 1998;20:207–11.
17. Solinas-Toldo S, et al. Matrix-based comparative genomic hybridization: biochips to screen for genomic imbalances. Genes Chromosomes Cancer 1997;20:399–407.
18. Knuutila S, Autio K, Aalto Y. Online access to CGH data of DNA sequence copy number changes. Am J Pathol 2000;157:689.
19. Menten B, Pattyn F, De Preter K, et al. arrayCGHbase: an analysis platform for comparative genomic hybridization microarrays. BMC Bioinformatics 2005;6:124–42.
20. Hampton GM, et al. Simultaneous assessment of loss of heterozygosity at multiple Microsatellite loci using semi-automated fluorescence-based detection: subregional mapping of chromosome 4 in cervical carcinoma. PNAS 1996;93: 6704–9.
21. Zhao X, Cheng L, Paez G, et al. An integrated view of copy number and allelic alterations in the cancer genome using single nucleotide polymorphism arrays. Cancer Res 2004;64:3060–71.
22. Mitelman database of chromosome aberrations in cancer. 2005. Mitelman F, Johansson B, Mertens F, (Eds.). http://cgap.nci.nih.gov/chromosomes/mitelman.
23. Davis H, Hunter C, Smith R, et al. Somatic mutations of the protein kinase gene family in human lung cancer. Cancer Res 2005;65:7591–5.
24. Paez JG, Janne PA, Lee JC, et al. EGFR mutations in lung cancer: correlation with clinical response to gefitinib therapy. Science 2004;304:1497–1500.
25. Lynch TJ, Bell DW, Sordella R, et al. Activating mutations in the epidermal growth factor receptor underlying responsiveness of non-small cell lung cancer to gefitinib. N Engl J Med 2004;350:2129–39.
26. Ren R. Mechanisms of BCR-ABL in the pathogenesis of chronic myelogenous leukemia. Nature Reviews Cancer 2005;5:172–83.
27. Druker BJ. et al. Efficacy and safety of a specific inhibitor of the BCR-ABL tyrosine kinase in chronic myeloid leukemia. N Engl J Med 2001;344:1031–7.
28. Deininger M, Buchdunger E, Drucker BJ. The development of imatinib as a therapeutic agent for chronic myeloid leukemia. Blood 2004;Dec 23.
29. Clark MA, Fisher C, Judson I, Thomas JM. Soft-tissue sarcomas in adults. N Engl J Med 2005;7:701–11.
30. van der Zwan SM, Dematteo RP. Gastrointestinal stromal tumors: 5 years later. Cancer 2005; August 31 (epub).
31. Muller AM, Martens UM, Hofmann SC, et al. Imatinib mesylate as a novel treatment option for hypereosinophilic syndrome: two cases and a comprehensive review of the literature. Ann Hematol 2005; Sept 1 (epub).
32. Marty M, Cognetti F, Maraninchi D, et al. Randomized phase II trial of the efficacy and safety of trastuzumab combined with docetaxel in patients with human epidermal growth factor receptor 2-positive metastatic breast cancer administered as first-line treatment: the M770001 study group. J Clin Oncol 2005;23:4265–74.
33. Buzdar AU, Ibrahim NK, Francis D, et al. Significantly higher pathologic complete remission rate after neoadjuvant therapy with trastuzumab, paclitaxel, and epirubicin chemotherapy : results of a randomized trial in human epidermal growth factor receptor 2-positive operable breast cancer. J Clin Oncol 2005;23:3676–85.
34. Stirewalt DL, Radich JR. The role of FLT3 in hematopoietic malignancy. Nature Reviews Cancer 2003;3:650–65.
35. Levis M, Small D. FLT3 tyrosine kinase inhibitors. Int J Hematol 2005;82:100–7.
36. Kim WY, Kaelin WG. Role of VHL gene mutation in human cancer. J Clin Oncol 2004;22:4991–5004.
37. Brose MS, Volpe P, Feldman M, et al. BRAF and RAS mutations in human lung cancer and melanoma. Cancer Res 2002;62:6997–7000.
38. Chang DZ, Panageas KS, Osman I, et al. Clinical significance of BRAF mutations in metastatic melanoma. J Translational Medicine 2004;2:46.
39. Greaves M,F Wiemels J. Origins of chromosome translocations in childhood acute leukaemia. Nature Reviews Cancer 2003;3:639–49.
40. Collins FS, Morgan M, Patrinos A. The Human Genome Project: lessons from large-scale biology. Science 2003;300(5617):286–90.
41. Mitelman F (ed). ISCN 1995: an international system for human cytogenetic nomenclature. Basel, Switzerland: S. Karger; 1995.
42. Gorre ME, et al. Clinical resistance to STI-571 cancer therapy caused by BCR-ABL gene mutation or amplification. Science 2001;876–80.
43. Banerjee D, et al. Novel aspects of resistance to drugs targeted to dihydrofolate reductase and thymidylate synthetase. Biochim Biophys Acta 2002;1587:164–73.
44. Koivisto P, et al. Androgen receptor amplification: a possible molecular mechanism for androgen deprivation therapy failure in prostate cancer. Cancer Res 1997; 57:314–319.
45. Jain KK. Current status of fluorescent in-situ hybridisation. Med Device Technol 2004;15:14–7.
46. van de Burg M, Poulsen TS, Hunger SP, et al. Split-signal FISH for the detection of chromosome aberrations in acute lymphoblastic leukemia. Leukemia 2004;18:895–908.
47. van Zuten LG, Velthuizen SC, Wolvers-Tettero IL, et al. Two dual-color split signal fluorescence in situ hybridization assays to detect t(5;14) involving HOX11L2 and CSX in T-cell acute lymphoblastic leukemia. Haematologica 2004;89:671–8.
48. Kearney L, Horsley SW. Molecular cytogenetics in haematologic malignancy: current technologies and future prospects. Chromosoma 2005;
49. Streubel B, Chott A, Huber D, et al. Lymphoma-specific genetic aberrations in microvascular endothelial cells in B-cell lymphomas. N Engl J Med 2004;351:250–9.
50. Speleman F, Cauweiler B, Dastugue N, et al. A new recurrent inversion, inv(7)(p15q34), leads to transcriptional activation of HOX A10 and HOX A11 in a subset of T cell acute lymphoblastic leukemias. Leukemia 2005;19:358–66.
51. Rowley JD. The role of chromosomal translocations in leukemogenesis. Semin Hematol 1999;36:494–7.
52. Lichter P, Joos S, Bentz M, et al. Comparative genomic hybridization: uses and limitations. Semin Hematol 2000;37:348–57.
53. Ishkanian AS, Malloff CA, Watson SK, et al. A tiling resolution DNA microarray with complete coverage of the human genome. Nat Genet 2004;36:299–303.
54. de Leeuw RJ, Davies JJ, Rosenwald A, et al. Comprehensive whole genome CGH array profiling of mantle cell lymphoma model genomes. Hum Mol Genet 2004;13:1827–37.
55. Kohlhammer H, Schwaenen C, Wessendorf S, et al. Genomic DNA chip hybridization of t(11;14) mantle cell lymphomas shows a high frequency of aberrations and allows a refined characterization of consensus regions. Blood 2004; 104:795–801.
56. Bignell GR, Huang J, Greshock J, et al. High resolution analysis of DNA copy number using oligonucleotide microarrays. Genome Research 2004;14:287–95.
57. Matsuzaki H, Loi H, Dong S, et al. Parallel genotyping of over 10,000 SNPs using a one primer assay on a high density oligonucleotide array. Genome Research 14:414–25.
58. Janne PA, Li C, Zhao X, et al. High-resolution single-nucleotide polymorphism array and clustering analysis of loss of heterozygosity in human lung cancer cell lines. Oncogene 2004;23(15):2716–26.
59. Matsuzaki H, Dong S, Loi H, et al. Genotyping over 100,000 SNPs on a pair of oligonucleotide arrays. Nature Methods 2004;1:109–11.
60. Raghavan M, Lillington DM, Skoulakis S, et al. Genome-wide single nucleotide polymorphism analysis reveals frequent partial uniparental isodisomy due to somatic recombination in acute myeloid leukemia. Cancer Res 2005;65:375–8.
61. Shena M, Shalon D, Davis RW, Brown PO. Quantitative monitoring of gene expression patterns with a complementary DNA microarray. Science 1995;270:467–70.
62. DeRisi J, Penland L, Brown PO, et al. Use of a cDNA microarray to analyze gene expression patterns in human cancer. Nat Genet 1996;14:457–60.
63. Alizadeh A, Eisen MB, Davis RE, et al. Distinct types of large B cell lymphoma identified by gene expression profiling. Nature 2000;403:503–11.
64. Shipp MA, Ross KN, Tamayo P, et al. Diffuse large B cell lymphoma outcome prediction by gene expression profiling and supervised machine learning. Nat Med 2002;8:68–74.
65. Dave SS, Wright G, Tan B, et al. Prediction of survival in follicular lymphoma based on molecular features of tumor-infiltrating cells. N Engl J Med 2004; 351:2159–69.
66. Bea S, Zettl A, Wright G, et al. Diffuse large cell B cell lymphoma subgroups have distinct genetic profiles that influence tumor biology and improve gene expression-based survival prediction. Blood 2005; July 26 (epub).
67. Staudt LM, Dave SS. The biology of human lymphoid malignancies revealed by gene expression profiling. Adv Immunol 2005;87:163–208.
68. van't Veer LJ, Dai H, van de Vijver MJ, et al. Gene expression profiling predicts outcome of breast cancer. Nature 2002:415:530–6.
69. van de Vijver MJ, He YD, van't Veer LJ et al. A gene expression signature as a predictor of survival in breast cancer. N Engl J Med 2002;19:1999–2009.
70. Yeoh EJ, Ross ME, Shurtleff SA, et al. Classification, subtype, discovery, and prediction of outcome in pediatric acute lymphoblastic leukemia by gene expression profiling. Cancer Cell 2002;1:1133–43.
71. Ross ME, Zhou X, Song G, et al. Classification of pediatric acute lymphoblastic leukemia by gene expression profiling. Blood 2003; 102:2951–9.
72. Valk PJ, Verhaak RF, Beijen MA, et al. Prognostically useful gene expression profiles in acute myeloid leukemia. N Engl J Med 2004;350:1617–28.
73. Bullinger L, Dohner K, Bair R, et al. Use of gene expression profiling to identify prognostic subclasses in adult acute myeloid leukemia. N Engl J Med 2004:350:1605–16.
74. Nowak MA. The role of chromosomal instability in tumor initiation. PNAS 2002; 99:16226–16231.
75. Sieber OM, Heinimann K, Tomlinson IPM. Genomic instability – the engine of tumorigenesis? Nature Reviews Cancer 2003;3:701–8.
76. Wood RD, et al. Human DNA repair genes. Science 2001;291:1284–9.
77. Sancar A, et al. Molecular mechanisms of mammalian DNA repair and the DNA damage checkpoints. Annu Rev Biochem 2004;73:39–85.
78. Khanna KK, Jackson SP. DNA double strand breaks: signaling, repair, and the cancer connection. Nat Gen 2001;27:247–54.
79. Le Beau MM, et al. An FHIT tumor suppressor gene? Genes Chromosomes Cancer 1998;21:281–9.
80. Kolomietz E, et al. The role of Alu repeat clusters as mediators of recurrent chromosomal rearrangements in tumors. Genes Chromosomes Cancer 2002;35:97–112.
81. Felix CA. Secondary leukemias induced by topoisomerase-targeted drugs. Biochim Biophys Acta 1998;1400:233–55.
82. Rowley JD, Olney HJ. International workshop on the relationship of prior therapy to balanced chromosomal aberrations in therapy-related myelodysplastic syndromes and acute leukemias. Genes Chromosomes Cancer 2002;33:331–45.
83. Felix CA, et al. Chromosome band 11q23 translocation breakpoints are DNA topoisomerase II cleavage sites. Cancer Res 1995; 55:4287–92.
84. Ross JA, Potter JD, Robinson LL. Infant leukemia, topoisomerase II inhibitors, and the MLL gene. J Natl Cancer Inst 1994; 86:1678–80.
85. Alexander FE, et al. Transplacental chemical exposure and risk of infant leukemia with MLL gene fusion. Cancer Res 2001;61:2542–6.
86. Croce CM, et al. Gene for alpha-chain of human T-cell receptor. Location on chromosome 14 region involved in T-cell neoplasms. Science 1985;227:1044–7.
87. Brown L, et al. Site-specific recombination of the tal-1 gene is a common occurrence in human T cell leukemia. EMBO J 1990;9:3343–51.
88. Marculescu R, et al. V(D)J-mediated recombination in lymphoid neoplasms: a functional assessment of genomic instability by cryptic sites. J Exp Med 2002; 195:85–98.
89. Liu Y, et al. BCL2 translocation frequency rises with age in humans. Proc Natl Acad Sci U S A 1994;91:8910–4.
90. Marculescu R, et al. Distinct t(7;9)(q34;q32) breakpoints in healthy individuals and individuals with T-ALL. Nat Genet 2003; 33:342–4.
91. Hastie ND, et al. Telomere reduction in human colorectal carcinoma with aging. Nature 1990;346:866–8.
92. Maser RS, DePinho RA. Connecting chromosomes, crisis, and cancer. Science 2002;297:565–9.
93. Artandi SE, DePinho RA. A critical role for telomeres in suppressing and facilitating carcinogenesis. Curr Opin Genet Dev 2000;10:39–46.
94. Bennett JM, et al. Proposed revised criteria for the classification of acute myeloid leukemia. A report of the French-American-British group. Ann Intern Med 1985;103:620–5.
95. Vardiman JW, Harris NL, Brunning RD. The WHO classification of myeloid neoplasms. Blood 2002;100:2292–302.
96. Cazzola M, Malcovati L. Myelodysplastic syndromes – coping with ineffective hematopoiesis. N Engl J Med 2005;352:536–538.
97. Song WJ, Sullivan MG, Legare RD, et al. Haploinsufficiency of CBFA2 causes familial thrombocytopenia with propensity to develop acute myeloid leukemia. Nature Genetics 1999;23:166–75.

98. Olney HJ, Le Beau MM. The cytogenetics of myelodysplastic syndromes. Best Pract Res Clin Haematol 2001;14:479–95.
99. Sole F, Luno E, Sanzo C, et al. Identification of novel cytogenetic markers with prognostic significance in a series of 968 patients with primary myelodysplastic syndromes. Haematologica 2005;90:1168–78.
100. Greenberg P, Cox C, LeBeau MM, et al. International scoring system for evaluating prognosis in the myelodysplastic syndromes. Blood 1997;89:2079–88.
101. Zhao N, et al. Molecular delineation of the smallest commonly deleted region of chromosome 5 in malignant myeloid diseases to 1–1.5 Mb and preparation of a PAC-based physical map. Proc Natl Acad Sci U S A 1997;94:6948–53.
102. Le Beau MM, et al. Cytogenetic and molecular delineation of a region of chromosome 7 commonly deleted in malignant myeloid diseases. Blood 1996;88:1930–5.
103. List AF, Kurtin S, Roe DJ, et al. Efficacy of lenalidomide in myelodysplastic syndromes. N Engl J Med 2005;352:549–57.
104. Speck, NA, Gilliland DG. Core binding factors in hematopoiesis and leukemia. Nature Reviews Cancer 2002;7:502–13.
105. Okuda T, van Deursen J, Hiebert SW, et al. AML1, the target of multiple chromosomal translocations in human leukemia, is essential for normal fetal liver hematopoiesis. Cell 1996;84:321–30.
106. Wang Q, Stacy T, Binder M, et al. Disruption of the Cbfa2 gene causes necrosis and hemorrhaging in the central nervous system and blocks definitive hematopoiesis. Proc Natl Acad Sci U S A 1996;93:3444–49.
107. Castilla LH, Wijmenga C, Wang Q, et al. Failure of embryonic hematopoiesis and lethal hemorrhages in mouse embryos heterozygous for a knocked-in leukemia gene CBFB-MYH11. Cell 1996;87:687–96.
108. Downing JR, Head DR, Curcio-Brent MG, et al. An AML1/ETO fusion transcript is consistently detected by RNA-based polymerase chain reaction in acute myelogenous leukemia containing the (8;21)(q22;q22) translocation. Blood 1993;81:2860–5.
109. Yergeau DA, Hetherington CJ, Wang Q, et al. Embryonic lethality and impairment of hematopoiesis in mice heterozygous for an AML1-ETO fusion gene. Nature Genetics 1997;15:303–6.
110. Okuda T, Cai Z, Yang S, et al. Expression of a knocked-in AML1-ETO leukemia gene inhibits the establishment of normal definitive hematopoiesis and directly generates dysplastic hematopoietic progenitors. Blood 1998;91:3134–43.
111. Liu P, Tarle SA, Hajra A, et al. Fusion between transcription factor CBFB/PEBP2B and a myosin heavy chain in acute myeloid leukemia. Science 1993;261:1041–4.
112. Liu PP, Hajra A, Wijmenga C, et al. Molecular pathogenesis of the chromosome 16 inversion in the M4eo subtype of acute myeloid leukemia. Blood 1995; 85:2289–302.
113. Downing J, Shurtleff S, Meyers S, et al. Molecular heterogeneity and identification of a new breakpoint in CBFβ/MYH11 fusions transcripts encoded by inv(16) and t(16;16) in acute myelogenous leukemia. Blood 1995;85:3697–703.
114. de The H, et al. The t(15;17) translocation of acute promyelocytic leukemia fuses the retinoic acid receptor alpha gene to a novel transcribed locus. Nature 1990;347:558–61.
115. Licht JD, Chen A, Goy A, et al. Clinical and molecular characterization of acute promyelocytic leukemia with translocation t(11;17). Blood 1995;85:1083–94.
116. Redner RL, Rush EA, Faas S, et al. The t(5;17) variant of acute promyelocytic leukemia expresses a nucleophosmin-retinoic acid receptor fusion. Blood 1996;87:882–6.
117. Arnould C, et al. The signal transducer and activator of transcription stat 5b gene is a new partner of retinoic acid receptor alpha in acute promyelocytic leukemia-like leukemia. Hum Mol Genet 1999;8:1741–9.
118. Collins SJ. Acute promyelocytic leukemia: relieving repression induces remission. Blood 1998;91:2631–3.
119. Grignani F, De Matteis S, Nervi C, et al. Fusion proteins of the retinoic acid receptora recruit histone deacetylase in promyelocytic leukemia. Nature 1998;391:815–8.
120. Tallman M, Andersen J, Schiffer, CA, et al. All-trans retinoic acid in acute promyelocytic leukemia. Blood 1997;85:2643.
121. Shen Z, Shen Z, Fang J, et al. Induction/maintenance with ATRA/As_2O_3 combination yields a high quality clinical/molecular remission and disease free survival in newly diagnosed patients with APL [abstract]. Blood 2003;102:141a.
122. Lin RJ, Nagy L, Inoue S, et al. Role of the histone deacetylase complex in acute promyelocytic leukemia. Nature 1998;391:811–4.
123. So CW, Cleary M. Dimerization: a versatile switch for oncogenesis. Blood 2004;15:919–22.
124. Hess JL. Mechanisms of transformation by MLL. Crit Rev Eukaryot Gene Expr 2004;14:235–54.
125. Yokoyama A, Wang Z, Wysocka J, et al. Leukemia proto-oncogene MLL forms a SET1-like histone Methyltransferase complex with menin to regulate HOX gene expression. Mol Cell Biol 2004;24:5639–49.
126. Ait-Si-Ali S, Ramirez S, Barre, FX, et al. Histone acetyltransferase activity of CBP is controlled by cell cycle dependent kinases and oncoprotein E1a. Nature 1998;396:184–6.
127. Borrow J, et al. The translocation t(8;16)(p11;q13) of acute myeloid leukemia fuses a putative acetyltransferase to the CREB-binding protein. Nat Genet 1996;14;33–41.
128. Rowley JD, et al. All patients with t(11;16)(q23;p13.3) that involves MLL and CBP have treatment related hematology disorders. Blood 1997;90:535–41.
129. Ida K, et al. Adenoviral E1a associated protein p300 is involved in acute myeloid leukemia with t(11;22)(q23;q13). Blood 1997;90:4699–704.
130. Carapeti M, et al. A novel fusion between MOZ and the nuclear receptor coactivator TIF2 in acute myeloid leukemia. Blood 1998;91:3127–33.
131. Pabst T, Mueller BU, Harakawa N, et al. AML1-ETO downregulates the granulocytic differentiation factor C/EBPalpha in t(8;21) myeloid leukemia. Nat Med 2001;7:444–51.
132. Kottaridis PD, Gale RE, Frew ME, et al. The presence of a FLT3 internal tandem duplications in patients with acute myeloid leukemia (AML) adds important prognostic information to cytogenetic risk group and response to the first cycle of chemotherapy: analysis of 854 patients from the United Kingdom Medical Research Council AML 10 and 12 trials. Blood 2001;98:1752–9.
133. Whitman SP, Archer KJ, Feng L, et al. Absence of the wild-type allele predicts poor prognosis in adult de novo acute myeloid leukemia with normal cytogenetics and the internal tandem duplication of FLT3: a cancer and leukemia group B study. Cancer Res 2001; 61: 7233–9.
134. Beaupre DM, Kurzrock R. RAS and leukemia: from basic mechanisms to gene-directed therapy. J Clin Oncol 1999;17:1071–9.
135. Karp JE. Farnesyl protein transferase inhibitors as targeted therapies for hematologic malignancies. Semin Hematol 2001;38:16–23.
136. Falini B, Mecucci C, Tiacci E, et al. Cytoplasmic nucleophosmin in acute myelogenous leukemia with a normal karyotype. N Engl J Med 2005;352:254–66.
137. Alcalay M, Tiacci E, Bergomas R, et al. Acute myeloid leukemia bearing cytoplasmic nucleophosmin (NPMc+ AML) shows a distinct gene expression profile characterized by up-regulation of genes involved in stem-cell maintenance. Blood 2005;106:899–905.
138. Willman CL. The prognostic significance of the expression and function of multidrug resistance transporter proteins in acute myeloid leukemia: Studies of the Southwest Oncology Group Leukemia Research Program. Semin Hematol 1997;34:25–33.
139. Rowley JD, Golomb HM, Vardiman J. Acute leukemia after treatment of lymphoma. N Engl J Med 1997;297:1013.
140. Smith SM, et al. Clinical-cytogenetic associations in 306 patients with therapy-related myelodysplasia and myeloid leukemia: The University of Chicago series. Blood 2003;102:43–52.
141. Johansson B, Fioretos T, Mitelman F. Cytogenetic and molecular genetic evolution of chronic myeloid leukemia. Acta Hematol 2002;107:76–94.
142. Pui CH, Relling MV, Downing JR. Acute lymphoblastic leukemia. N Engl J Med 2004;350:1535–48.
143. Raynaud S, et al. The t(12;21) translocation involving TEL and deletion of the other allele. Two frequently associated alterations found in childhood acute lymphoblastic leukemia. Blood 1996;2891–9.
144. Sixth International Workshop on Chromosomes in Leukemia. London, England, May 11–18, 1987.
145. Cayuela JM, et al. Multiple tumor suppressor gene 1 inactivation in is the most frequent genetic alteration in T cell acute lymphoblastic leukemia. Blood 1996;87:2180–6.
146. Look AT. Molecular pathways in T cell acute lymphoblastic leukemia: ramifications for therapy. Clin Adv Hematol Oncol 2004;2:779–80.
147. Armstrong SA, Look AT. Molecular genetics of acute lymphoblastic leukemia. J Clin Oncol. 2005;23:6306–15.
148. Ferrando AA, Neuberg DS, Dodge RK, et al. Prognostic importance of TLX1 (HOX11) oncogene expression in adults with T cell acute lymphoblastic leukemia. Lancet 2004;363:535–6.
149. Weng AP, Ferrando AA, Lee W, et al. Activating mutations of NOTCH1 in human T cell acute lymphoblastic leukemia. Science 2004;306:269–71.
150. Ferrando AA, Look AT. Gene expression profiling in T cell acute lymphoblastic leukemia. Semin Hematol 2003;40:274–80.
151. Dohner H, et al. Genomic aberrations and survival in chronic lymphocytic leukemia. N Engl J Med. 2000;343:1910–16.
152. Schwaenen C, et al. Automated array-based genomic profiling in chronic lymphocytic leukemia: development of a clinical tool and discovery of recurrent genomic alterations. Proc Natl Acad Sci U S A 2004;101:1039–44.
153. Jaffe ES, Harris NL, Stein H, Vardiman JW. World Health Organization classification of tumors. In: Kleihuis P, Sobin L, eds. Pathology and genetics of tumors of hematopoietic and lymphoid tissues. Lyon: IARC; 2001.
154. Chaganti RS, et al. Recurring chromosomal abnormalities in non-Hodgkin's lymphoma. Biologic and clinical significance. Semin Hematol 2000;37:396–411.
155. Kuppers R. Mechanisms of B cell lymphoma pathogenesis. Nature Reviews Cancer 2005;5:251–62.
156. Thorley-Lawson DA, Gross A. Persistence of the Epstein-Barr virus and the origins of associated lymphomas. N Engl J Med 2004;350:1328–37.
157. Young LS, Rickinson AB. Epstein-Barr virus: 40 years. Nature Reviews Cancer 2004;4:757–68.
158. Quinn ER, et al. The B cell receptor of a hepatitis C virus (HCV)-associated non-Hodgkin's lymphoma binds the viral E2 envelope protein, implicating HCV in lymphomagenesis. Blood 2001;98:3745–9.
159. Hermine O, et al. Regression of splenic lymphoma with villous lymphocytes after treatment of hepatitis C virus infection. N Engl J Med 2002;347:89–94.
160. Rosenwald A, Wright G, Wiestner A, et al. The proliferation gene expression signature is a quantitative integrator of oncogenic events that predicts survival in mantle cell lymphoma. Cancer Cell 2003;3:185–97.
161. Hoglund M, Sehn L, Connors JM, et al. Identification of cytogenetic subgroups and karyotypic pathways of clonal evolution in follicular lymphomas. Genes Chromosomes Cancer 2004:39:194–204.
162. Rosenwald A, et al. The use of molecular profiling to predict survival after chemotherapy for diffuse large cell B cell lymphoma. N Engl J Med 2002;346:1937–47.
163. Wotherspoon AC, et al. Regression of primary low-grade B cell gastric lymphoma of mucosa- associated lymphoid tissue after eradication of *Helicobacter pylori*. Lancet 1993;342:575–7.
164. Alpen B, et al. Translocation t(11;18) absent in early gastric marginal zone B cell lymphoma of MALT type responding to eradication of *Helicobacter pylori* infection. Blood 2000;95:4014–15.
165. Mattioli M, Agnelli L, Fabris S, et al. Gene expression profiling of plasma cell dyscrasias reveals molecular patterns associated with distinct IGH translocations in multiple myeloma. Oncogene 2005;24:2461–73.
166. Ross FM, et al. Age has a profound effect on the incidence and significance of chromosome abnormalities in myeloma. Leukemia 2005; June 30 (epub).
167. Zhan F, et al. Blood 2003;101:1128–40.
168. Davies FE, et al. Blood 2003;102:4504–11.
169. Meijer GA, et al. Progression from colorectal adenoma to carcinoma is associated with non- random chromosomal gains as detected by comparative genomic hybridisation. J Clin Pathol 1998;51:901–9.
170. Kinzler KW, et al. Identification of FAP locus genes from chromosome 5q21. Science 1991;253:661–5.
171. Clevers H. Wnt breakers in colon cancer. Cancer Cell 2004;5:5–6.
172. Helt CE, Wang W, Keng PC, Bambara RA. Evidence that DNA damage detection machinery participates in DNA repair. Cell Cycle 2005;4:529–32.
173. Pejovic T, et al. Trisomy 12 is a consistent chromosomal aberration in benign ovarian tumors. Genes Chromosomes Cancer 1990;2:48–52.
174. Mark J, Dahlenfors R, Ekedahl C. Cytogenetics of the human benign mixed salivary gland tumour. Hereditas 1983;99:115–29.
175. Kas K, et al. Promoter swapping between the genes for a novel zinc finger protein and beta-catenin in pleiomorphicadenomas with t(3;8)(p21;q12) translocations. Nat Genet 1997;15:170–4.
176. Enlund F, Nordkvist A, Sahlin P, Mark J, Stenman G. Expression of PLAG1 and HMGIC proteins and fusion transcripts in radiation-associated pleomorphic adenomas. Int J Oncol 2002;20:713–6.
177. Tallini G, et al. Correlation between clinicopathological features and karyotype in 100 cartilaginous and chordoid

tumours. A report from the Chromosomes and Morphology (CHAMP) Collaborative Study Group. J Pathol 2002;196:194–203.
178. Dahlen A, Mertens F, Rydholm A, et al. Fusion, disruption, and expression of HMGA2 in bone and soft tissue chondromas. Mod Pathol 2003;16:1132–40.
179. Mandahl N, et al. Three major cytogenetic subgroups can be identified among chromosomally abnormal solitary lipomas. Hum Genet 1988;79:203–8.
180. Petit, et al. LHFP, a novel translocation partner gene of HMGIC in a lipoma, is a member of a new family of LHFP-like genes. Genomics 1999 May 1;57(3):438–41.
181. Broberg, et al. Fusion of RDC1 with HMGA2 in lipomas as the result of chromosome aberrations involving 2q35–37 and 12q13–15. Int J Oncol 2002;21:321–6.
182. Kazmierczak B, et al. A high frequency of tumors with rearrangements of genes of the HMGI family in a series of191 pulmonary chondroid hamartomas. Genes Chromosomes Cancer 1999;26:125–33.
183. Mine N, et al. Gene fusion involving HNGIC is a frequent aberration in uterine leiomyomas. J Hum Genet 2001;46:408–12.
184. Klotzbucher M, Wasserfall A, Fuhrmann U. Mis-expressionof wild-type and truncated isoforms of the high-mobility group I proteins HMGI-C and HMGI(Y) in uterine leiomyomas. Am J Pathol 1999;155:1535–42.
185. Ruttledge MH, et al. Evidence for the complete inactivation of the NF2 gene in the majority of sporadic meningiomas. Nat Genet 1994;6:180–4.
186. Knudson AG. Chasing the cancer demon. Annu Rev Genet 2000;34:1–19.
187. Ryu CH, Kim SW, Lee KH, et al. The Merlin tumor suppressor interacts with Ral guanine nucleotide dissociation stimulator and inhibits its activity. Oncogene 2005;Jun 27.
188. Ward BA, Gutmann DH. Neurofibromatosis 1: from lab bench to clinic. Pediatr Neurol 2005;32:221–8.
189. Emanuel PD. Juvenile myelomonocytic leukemia. Curr Hematol Rep 2004;3:203–9.
190. Ladanyi M. Aberrant ALK tyrosine kinase signaling. Different cellular lineages, common oncogenic mechanisms. Am J Pathol 2000;157:341–5.
191. Hopman AH, et al. Numerical chromosome 1, 7, 9, and 11aberrations in bladder cancer detected by in situ hybridization. Cancer Res 1991;51:644–51.
192. Matsuyama H, et al. Nonrandom numerical aberrations of chromosomes 7, 9, and 10 in DNA-diploid bladder cancer. Cancer Genet Cytogenet 1994;77:118–24.
193. Sauter G, et al. Chromosome-9 loss detected by fluorescence in situ hybridization in bladder cancer. Int J Cancer1995;64:99–103.
194. Knowles MA. Molecular genetics of bladder cancer: pathways of development and progression. Cancer Surv 1998;31:49–76.
195. Greenblatt MS, et al. Mutations in the p53 tumor suppressor gene. Clues to cancer etiology and molecular pathogenesis. Cancer Res 1994;54:4855–78.
196. Thompson F et al. Clonal chromosome abnormalities inhuman breast carcinomas. I. Twenty- eight cases with primary disease. Genes Chromosomes Cancer1993;7:185–93.
197. Tirkkonen M, Tanner M, Karhu R, et al. Molecular cytogenetics of primary breast cancer by CGH. Genes Chromosomes Cancer 1998;21:177–84.
198. Pegram MD, Pauletti G, Slamon DJ. HER-2/neu as a predictive marker of response to breast cancer therapy. Breast Cancer Res Treat 1998;52:65–77.
199. Collins C, Rommens JM, Kowbel D, et al. Positional cloning of ZNF217 and NABC1: genes amplified at20q13.2 and overexpressed in breast carcinoma. Proc Natl Acad Sci U S A 1998;95:8703–8.
200. Armes JE, et al. Distinct molecular pathogeneses of early onset breast cancers in BRCA1 and BRCA2 mutation carriers. A population-based study. Cancer Res1999;59:2011–7.
201. Lakhani SR, et al. Multifactorial analysis of differences between sporadic breast cancers and cancers involving BRCA1 and BRCA2 mutations. J Natl Cancer Inst 1998;90:1138–45.
202. Tirkkonen M, et al. Distinct somatic genetic changes associated with tumor progression in carriers of BRCA1 and BRCA2 germ-line mutations. Cancer Res 1997;57:1222–7.
203. Kauraniemi P, et al. MYB oncogene amplification in hereditary BRCA1 breast cancer. Cancer Res 2000;60:5323–8.
204. Vaziri SA, et al. Absence of CCND1 gene amplification in breast tumours of BRCA1 mutation carriers. Mol Pathol 2001;54:259–63.
205. Sinclair CS, et al. TBX2 is preferentially amplified inBRCA1- and BRCA2-related breast tumors. Cancer Res 2002;62:3587–91.
206. Wu GJ, et al. 17q23 amplifications in breast cancer involve the PAT1, RAD51C, PS6K, and SIGma1B genes. Cancer Res 2000;60:5371–5.
207. Jacobs JJ, et al. Senescence bypass screen identifies TBX2,which represses Cdkn2a (p19(ARF)) and is amplified in a subset of human breast cancers. Nat Genet 2000;26:291–9.
208. Monni O, et al. Comprehensive copy number and gene expression profiling of the 17q23 amplicon in human breast cancer. Proc Natl Acad Sci U S A 2001;98:5711–6.
209. Kleer CG, et al. WISP3 is a novel tumor suppressor gene of inflammatory breast cancer. Oncogene 2002;21:3172–80.
210. Vogelstein B, et al. Genetic alterations during colorectal tumor development. N Engl J Med 1988;319:525–32.
211. Jen J, et al. Allelic loss of chromosome 18q and prognosis in colorectal cancer. N Engl J Med 1994;331:213–21.
212. Thiagalingam S, Lengauer C, Leach FS, et al. Evaluation of candidate tumour suppressor genes on chromosome 18 in colorectal cancers. Nat Genet 1996;13:343–6.
213. Lindgren V, Bryke CR, Ozcelik T, et al. Phenotypic, cytogenetic, and molecular studies of three patients with constitutional deletions of chromosome 5 in the region of the gene for familial adenomatous polyposis. Am J Hum Genet 1992 May;50:988–97.
214. Nicolaides NC, Papedopulos N, Liu B, et al. Mutations of two PMS homologues in hereditary nonpolyposis colon cancer. Nature 1994;328:614.
215. Bronner CE, et al. Mutation in the DNA mismatch repair gene homologue hMLH1 is associated with hereditary nonpolyposis colon cancer. Nature 1994;368:258–61.
216. Hashimoto Y, et al. The potential clinical value of GML and the p53 gene as a predictor of chemosensitivity for colorectal cancer. Int J Clin Oncol 2001;6:90–6.
217. Kuwano H, Kato H, Miyazaki T, et al. Genetic alterations in esophageal cancer. Surg Today 2005;35:7–18.
218. Iwaya T, et al. Tylosis esophageal cancer locus on chromosome 17q25.1 is commonly deleted in sporadic human esophageal cancer. Gastroenterology 1998;114:1206–10.
219. Risk JM, et al. Envoplakin, a possible candidate gene for focal NEPPK/esophageal cancer (TOC). The integration of genetic and physical maps of the TOC region on17q25. Genomics 1999;59:234–42
220. Ishii H, et al. The FEZ1 gene at chromosome 8p22 encodes a leucine-zipper protein, and its expression is altered in multiple human tumors. Proc Natl Acad Sci U S A 1999;96:3928–33.
221. Daigo Y, et al. Molecular cloning of a candidate tumor suppressor gene, DLC1, from chromosome 3p21.3. Cancer Res 1999;59:1966–72.
222. Chen L, et al. Genetic alterations of candidate tumor suppressor ING1 in human esophageal squamous cell cancer. Cancer Res 2001;61:4345–9.
223. Kuroki T, Trapasso F, Shiraishi T, et al. Genetic alterations of the tumor suppressor gene WWOX in esophageal squamous cell carcinoma. Cancer Res 2002;62:2258–60.
224. Risk JM, Evans KE, Jones J, et al. Characterization of a 500 kb region on 17q25 and the exclusion of candidate genes as the familial tylosis oesophageal cancer (TOC) locus. Oncogene 2002;21:6395–402.
225. Bockmuhl U, et al. Genomic alterations associated with malignancy in head and neck cancer. Head Neck 1998;20:145–51.
226. Pearlstein RP, et al. Loss of 18q predicts poor survival of patients with squamous cell carcinoma of the head and neck. Genes Chromosomes Cancer 1998;21:333–9.
227. Gunduz M, Ouchida M, Fukushima K, et al. Genomic structure of the human ING1 gene and tumor-specific mutations detected in head and neck squamous cell carcinomas. Cancer Res 2000;60:3143–6.
228. Poetsch M, Lorenz G, Kleist B. Detection of new PTEN/MMAC1 mutations in head and neck squamous cell carcinomas with loss of chromosome 10. Cancer Genet. Cytogenet 2002;132:20–4.
229. Testa JR, et al. Advances in the analysis of chromosome alterations in human lung carcinomas. Cancer Genet Cytogenet 1997;95:20–32.
230. Naylor SL, et al. Loss of heterozygosity of chromosome 3p markers in small-cell lung cancer. Nature1987;329:451–4.
231. Lukeis R, et al. Cytogenetics of non-small cell lung cancer. Analysis of consistent non-random abnormalities. Genes Chromosomes Cancer 1990;2:116–24.
232. Okamoto A, et al. Mutations and altered expression of p16INK4 in human cancer. Proc Natl Acad Sci U S A 1994;91:11045–9.
233. Berrieman HK, Ashman JN, Cowen ME, Greenman J, Lind MJ, Cawkwell L. Chromosomal analysis of non-small-cell lung cancer by multicolour fluorescent in situ hybridisation. Br J Cancer 2004 Feb 23;90:900–5.
234. Janne PA, Li C, Zhao X, et al. High-resolution single-nucleotide polymorphism array and clustering analysis of loss of heterozygosity in human lung cancer cell lines. Oncogene 2004;23:2716–26.
235. Bailey-Wilson JE, Amos CI, Pinney SM, et al. A major lung cancer susceptibility locus maps to chromosome 6q23–25. Am J Hum Genet 2001;75:460–74.
236. Dai Z, Zhu W-G, Morrison CD, et al. A comprehensive search for DNA amplification in lung cancer identifies inhibitors of apoptosis cIAP1 and cIAP2 as candidate oncogenes. Hum Mol Genet 2003;l12:791–801.
237. Pao W, Miller V, Zakowski M, et al. EGF receptor gene mutations are common in lung cancers from 'never smokers' and are associated with sensitivity of tumors to gefitinib and erlotinib. Proc Natl Acad Sci 2004;101:13306–11.
238. Sandberg AA. Chromosomal abnormalities and related events in prostate cancer. Hum Pathol 1992;23:368–80.
239. Brothman AR, et al. Frequency and pattern of karyotypic abnormalities in human prostate cancer. Cancer Res 1990;50:3795–803.
240. Bandyk MG, et al. Trisomy 7. A potential cytogenetic marker of human prostate cancer progression. Genes Chromosomes Cancer 1994;9:19–27.
241. Cher ML, et al. Comparative genomic hybridization, allelic imbalance, and fluorescence in situ hybridization on chromosome 8 in prostate cancer. Genes Chromosomes Cancer 1994;11:153–62.
242. Visakorpi T, et al. Genetic changes in primary and recurrent prostate cancer by comparative genomic hybridization. Cancer Res 1995;55:342–7.
243. Eagle LR, et al. Mutation of the MXI1 gene in prostate cancer. Nat Genet 1995;9:249–55.
244. Brothman AR et al. Loss of chromosome 17 loci in prostate cancer detected by polymerase chain reaction quantitation of allelic markers. Genes Chromosomes Cancer 1995;13:278–84.
245. Gao X, et al. Loss of heterozygosity of the BRCA1 and other loci on chromosome 17q in human prostate cancer. Cancer Res 1995;55:1002–5.
246. Cohen AJ, et al. Hereditary renal-cell carcinoma associated with a chromosomal translocation. N Engl J Med 1979;301:592–5.
247. Pathak S, et al. Familial renal cell carcinoma with a 3;11chromosome translocation limited to tumor cells. Science1982;217:939–41.
248. Latif F, et al. Identification of the von Hippel-Lindau disease tumor suppressor gene. Science 1993;260:1317–20.
249. Gnarra JR, et al. Mutations of the VHL tumour suppressor gene in renal carcinoma. Nat Genet 1994;7:85–90.
250. Gemmill RM, West JD, Boldog F, et al. The hereditary renal cell carcinoma 3;8 translocation fuses FHIT to a patched-related gene, TRC8. Proc Natl Acad Sci U S A 1998;95:9572–7
251. Bodmer D, Eleveld M, Kater-Baats E, et al. Disruption of a novel MFS transporter gene, DIRC2, by a familial renal cell carcinoma-associated t(2;3)(q35;q21). Hum Mol Genet 2002;11:641–9.
252. Weterman MA, Wilbrink M, Geurts van Kessel A. Fusion of the transcription factor TFE3 gene to a novel gene, PRCC, in t(X;1)(p11;q21)-positive papillary renal cell carcinomas. Proc Natl Acad Sci U S A 1996;93:15294–8.
253. Davis IJ, Hsi BL, Arroyo JD, et al. Cloning of an *Alpha-TFEB* fusion in renal tumors harboring the t(6;11)(p21;q13) chromosome translocation. Proc Natl Acad Sci U S A 2003;100:6051–6056.
254. Bartel D. MicroRNAs: genomics, biogenesis, mechanism, and function. Cell 2004;116:281–97.
255. Schmidt L, et al. Germline and somatic mutations in the tyrosine kinase domain of the MET proto-oncogene in papillary renal carcinomas. Nat Genet 1997;16:68–73.
256. Zhuang Z, et al. Trisomy 7-harbouring non-random duplication of the mutant MET allele in hereditary papillary renal carcinomas. Nat Genet 1998;20:66–9.
257. Yang XJ, et al. A molecular classification of papillary renal cell carcinoma. Cancer Res 2005 Jul 1;65:5628–37.
258. Roque L, et al. Karyotypic characterization of papillary thyroid carcinomas. Cancer 2001;92:2529–38.
259. Santoro M, Melillo RM, Carlomagno F, et al. Minireview: RET: normal and abnormal functions. Endocrinology 2004 Dec;145:5448–51.

260. Bongarzone I, et al. Age-related activation of the tyrosine kinase receptor protooncogenes RET and NTRK1 in papillary thyroid carcinoma. Oncogene 2004;23:7436–40.
261. Said S, Schlumberger M, Suarez HG. Oncogenes and anti-oncogenes in human epithelial thyroid tumors. J Endocrinol Invest 1994;17:371–9.
262. Teyssier JR, et al. Chromosomal changes in thyroid tumors. Relation with DNA content, karyotypic features, and clinical data. Cancer Genet Cytogenet 1990;50:249–63.
263. Di Renzo MF, et al. Overexpression of the c-MET/HGF receptor gene in human thyroid carcinomas. Oncogene 1992;7:2549–53.
264. Kersemaekers AM, et al. Loss of heterozygosity for defined regions on chromosomes 3, 11 and 17 in carcinomas of the uterine cervix. Br J Cancer 1998;77:192–200.
265. Atkin NB. Cytogenetics of carcinoma of the cervix uteri. A review. Cancer Genet Cytogenet 1997;95:33–9.
266. Jarboe EA, Liaw KL, Thompson LC, et al. Analysis of telomerase as a diagnostic biomarker of cervical dysplasia and carcinoma. Oncogene 2002 Jan 21;21:664–73.
267. Cappellen D, De Oliveira C, Ricol D, et al. Frequent activating mutations of FGFR3 in human bladder and cervix carcinomas. (Letter) Nat Genet 1999;23:18–20.
268. Mitra AB. Genetic deletion and human papilloma virus infection in cervical cancer. Loss of heterozygosity sites at 3p and 5p are important genetic events. Int J Cancer 1999;82:322–4.
269. Klaes R, et al. Detection of high-risk cervical intra-epithelial neoplasia and cervical cancer by amplification of transcripts derived from integrated papillomavirus oncogenes. Cancer Res 1999;59:6132–6.
270. Baldus SE, Schwarz E, Lohrey C, et al.Smad4 deficiency in cervical carcinoma cells. Oncogene. 2005 Jan 27;24:810–9.
271. Pere H, et al. Distinct chromosomal imbalances in uterine serous and endometrioid carcinomas. Cancer Res 1998;58:892–5.
272. Fletcher JA, et al. Diagnostic relevance of clonal cytogenetic aberrations in malignant soft-tissue tumors. N Engl J Med 1991;324:436–42.
273. Micci F, Walter CU, Teixeira MR, et al. Cytogenetic and molecular genetic analyses of endometrial stromal sarcoma: nonrandom involvement of chromosome arms 6p and 7p and confirmation of JAZF1/JJAZ1 gene fusion in t(7;17). Cancer Genet Cytogenet 2003;144:119–24.
274. Nakajima T, Fujino S, Nakanishi G, et al. Molecular detection of JAZF1-JJAZ1 gene fusion in endometrial stromal neoplasms with classic and variant histology: evidence for genetic heterogeneity. Am J Surg Pathol 2004;28:224–32.
275. Banno K, et al. Association of HNPCC and endometrial cancers. Int J Clin Oncol 2004;9(4):262–9.
276. Hedinger C, Ed W, Lh S. WHO international histological classification of tumors. Berlin: Springer Verlag; 1988. p. 9–11.
277. Ladanyi M, et al. The dert(X;17)(p11;q25) of human alveolar soft part sarcoma fuses the TFE3 transcription factor gene to ASPL, a novel gene at 17q25. Oncogene 2001;20:48–57.
278. Mandahl N, et al. Cytogenetic aberrations and their prognostic impact in chondrosarcoma. Genes Chromosomes Cancer 2002;33:188–200.
279. Stenman G, et al. Translocation t(9;22)(q22;q12) is a primary cytogenetic abnormality in extraskeletal myxoid chondrosarcoma. Int J Cancer 1995;62:398–402.
280. Labelle Y, et al. Oncogenic conversion of a novel receptor by chromosome translocation. Hum Mol Genet 1995;4:2219–26.
281. Sandberg AA. Genetics of chondrosarcoma and related tumors. Curr Opin Oncol 2004;16(4):342–54.
282. Schmidt H, et al. Gains of 12q are the most frequent genomic imbalances in adult fibrosarcoma and are correlated with a poor outcome. Genes Chromosomes Cancer 2002;34:69–77.
283. Panagopoulos I, Storlazzi CT, Fletcher CD, et al. The chimeric FUS/CREB3l2 gene is specific for low-grade fibromyxoid sarcoma. Genes Chromosomes Cancer 2004;40:218–28.
284. Simon MP, Navarro M, Roux D, Pouyssegur J. Structural and functional analysis of a chimeric protein COL1A1-PDGFB generated by the translocation t(17;22)(q22;q13.1) in Dermatofibrosarcoma protuberans (DP). Oncogene 2001;20:2965–75.
285. Thelin–Jarnum S, et al. Identification of genes differentially expressed in TLS-CHOP carrying myxoid liposarcomas. Int J Cancer 1999;83:30–3.
286. Orndal C, et al. Supernumerary ring chromosomes in soft tissue tumors. Cancer Genet Cytogenet 1992; 60:170–5.
287. Fletcher CD, et al. Correlation between clinicopathological features and karyotype in lipomatous tumors. A report of 178 cases from the Chromosomes and Morphology (CHAMP) Collaborative Study Group. Am J Pathol 1996;148:623–30.
288. Pedeutour F, et al. Structure of the supernumerary ring and giant rod chromosomes in adipose tissue tumors. Genes Chromosomes Cancer 1999;24:30–41.
289. Mandahl N, et al. Nonrandom pattern of telomeric associations in atypical lipomatous tumors with ring and giant marker chromosomes. Cancer Genet Cytogenet 1998;103:25–34.
290. Barr FG, et al. Localization of the t(2;13) breakpoint of alveolar rhabdomyosarcoma on a physical map of chromosome2. Genomics 1992;13:1150–6.
291. Barr FG, et al. Rearrangement of the PAX3 paired box gene in the paediatric solid tumour alveolar rhabdomyosarcoma. Nat Genet 1993;3:113–7.
292. Anderson J, et al. Genes, chromosomes, and rhabdomyosarcoma. Genes Chromosomes Cancer 1999;26:275–85.
293. Chi N, Epstein JA. Getting your Pax straight: Pax proteins in development and disease. Trends Genet 2002;18:41–7.
294. Crew AJ, et al. Fusion of SYT to two genes, SSX1 andSSX2, encoding proteins with homology to the Kruppel-associated box in human synovial sarcoma. EMBOJ 1995;14:2333–40.
295. Nilsson G, et al. The SYT-SSX1 variant of synovial sarcoma is associated with a high rate of tumor cell proliferation and poor clinical outcome. Cancer Res 1999;59:3180–4.
296. Mostert MM, et al. Comparative genomic hybridization of germ cell tumors of the adult testis. Confirmation of karyotypic findings and identification of a 12p- amplicon. Cancer Genet Cytogenet 1996;89:146–52.
297. Suijkerbuijk RF, et al. Over-representation of chromosome 12p sequences and karyotypic evolution in i(12p)-negative testicular germ-cell tumors revealed by fluorescence in situ hybridization. Cancer Genet Cytogenet 1993;70:85–93.
298. Rosenberg C, et al. Over-representation of the short arm of chromosome 12 is related to invasive growth of human testicular seminomas and non-seminomas. Oncogene 2000;19:5858–62.
299. Bosl GJ, Ilson DH, Rodriguez E, et al. Clinical relevance of the i(12p) marker chromosome in germ cell tumors. J Natl Cancer Inst 1994;86:349–55.
300. Bigner SH, et al. Specific chromosomal abnormalities in malignant human gliomas. Cancer Res 1988;48:405–11.
301. Nishizaki T, et al. Investigation of genetic alterations associated with the grade of astrocytic tumor by comparative genomic hybridization. Genes Chromosomes Cancer 1998;21:340–6.
302. Venter DJ, Thomas DG. Multiple sequential molecular abnormalities in the evolution of human gliomas. Br J Cancer 1991;63:753–7.
303. Steck PA, et al. Identification of a candidate tumour suppressor gene, MMAC1, at chromosome 10q23.3 that is mutated in multiple advanced cancers. Nat Genet 1997;15:356–62.
304. Li J, et al. PTEN, a putative protein tyrosine phosphatase gene mutated in human brain, breast, and prostate cancer. Science 1997;275:1943–7.
305. Wechsler DS, et al. MXI1, a putative tumor suppressor gene, suppresses growth of human glioblastoma cells. Cancer Res 1997;57:4905–12.
306. Chernova OB, Somerville RP, Cowell JK. A novel gene, LGI1, from 10q24 is rearranged and down-regulated in malignant brain tumors. Oncogene 1998;17:2873–81.
307. Reardon DA, et al. Extensive genomic abnormalities in childhood medulloblastoma by comparative genomic hybridization. Cancer Res 1997;57:4042–7.
308. McLendon RE, et al. Diagnostic markers in paediatric medulloblastoma. A Paediatric Oncology Group Study. Histopathology 1999;34:154–62.
309. Di Marcotullio L, et al. REN(KCTD11) is a suppressor of Hedgehog signaling and is deleted in human medulloblastoma. Proc Natl Acad Sci U S A. 2004;101(29):10833–8.
310. Whang-Peng J, Triche TJ, Knutsen T, et al. Chromosome translocation in peripheral neuroepithelioma. N Engl J Med 1984;311:584–5.
311. Delattre O, Zucman J, Merlot T, et al. The Ewing family of tumors–a subgroup of small-round-cell tumors defined by specific chimeric transcripts. N Engl J Med 1994;331:294–9.
312. Delattre O, et al. Gene fusion with an ETS DNA-binding domain caused by chromosome translocation in human tumours. Nature 1992;359:162–5.
313. Mertens F, et al. Cytogenetic characterization of peripheral nerve sheath tumours. A report of the CHAMP study group. J Pathol 2000;190:31–8.
314. Sawyer JR, Tryka AF, Lewis JM. A novel reciprocal chromosome translocation t(11;22)(p13;q12) in an intra abdominal desmoplastic small round-cell tumor. Am J Surg Pathol 1992;16:411–6.
315. Biegel JA, Conard K, Brooks JJ. Translocation (11;22)(p13;q12). Primary change in intra-abdominal desmoplastic small round cell tumor. Genes Chromosomes Cancer 1993;7:119–21.
316. Gerald WL, Rosai J, Ladanyi M. Characterization of the genomic breakpoint and chimeric transcripts in the EWS/WT1gene fusion of desmoplastic small round cell tumor. Proc Natl Acad Sci U S A 1995;92:1028–32.
317. Jeon IS, et al. A variant Ewing's sarcoma translocation(7;22) fuses the EWS gene to the ETS gene ETV1. Oncogene 1995;10:1229–34.
318. Bown N. Neuroblastoma tumour genetics: clinical and biological aspects. J Clin Pathol 2001 Dec;54:897–910.
319. Lee WH, Bookstein R, Hong F, et al. Human retinoblastoma susceptibility gene. Cloning, identification, and sequence. Science 1987;235:1394–9.
320. DeCaprio JA, Ludlow JW, Lynch D, et al. The product of the retinoblastoma susceptibility gene has properties of a cell cycle regulatory element. Cell 1989;58:1085–95.
321. Bonetta L, Kuehn SE, Huang A. Wilms tumor locus on 11p13 defined by multiple CpG island-associated transcripts. Science 1990;250:994.
322. Koufos A, Aleck KA, Cavenee WK, et al. Familial Wiedemann-Beckwith syndrome and a second Wilms tumor locus both map to 11p15.5. Am J Hum Genet 1989;44:711–9.
323. Call KM, Glaser T, Ito CY, et al. Isolation and characterization of a zinc finger polypeptide gene at the human chromosome 11 Wilms' tumor locus. Cell 1990;60:509–20.
324. Gessler M, Poustka A, Cavene W, et al. Homozygous deletion in Wilms tumours of a zinc-finger gene identified by chromosome jumping. Nature 1990;343:774–8.
325. Cowan JM, Halaban R, Francke U. Cytogenetic analysis of melanocytes from premalignant nevi and melanomas. J Natl Cancer Inst 1988;80:1159–64.
326. Parmiter AH, Balaban G, Clark WH Jr, Nowell PC. Possible involvement of the chromosome region 10q24–q26in early stages of melanocytic neoplasia. Cancer Genet Cytogenet 1988;30:313–7.
327. Trent JM, Stanbridge EJ, McBride HL. Tumorigenicity in human melanoma cell lines controlled by introduction of human chromosome 6. Science 1990;247:568–71.
328. Hussussian CJ, Struewing JP, Goldstein AM, et al. Germline p16 mutations in familial melanoma. Nat Genet 1994;8:15–21.
329. Puig S, Malvehy J, Badenas C, et al. Role of the CDKN2A locus in patients with multiple primary melanomas. J Clin Oncol 2005;23:3043–51.
330. Kefford RF, Newton Bishop JA, Bergman W, Tucker MA. Counseling and DNA testing for individuals perceived to be genetically predisposed to melanoma. A consensus statement of the Melanoma Genetics Consortium. J Clin Oncol 1999;17:3245–51.
331. Garraway LA, Widlund HR, Rubin MA, et al. Integrative genomic analyses identify MITF as a lineage survival oncogene amplified in malignant melanoma. Nature 2005;436:117–22.

9

Biochemistry of Cancer

Raymond W. Ruddon, MD, PhD
Donald W. Kufe, MD
William N. Hait, MD, PhD

BIOCHEMISTRY OF CANCER IN CONTEXT

The field of cancer biochemistry evolved from a number of disciplines, through information developed down parallel timelines, in some cases based on work initiated a century or more ago. In others, knowledge evolved over a much shorter and more recent time span. Eventually, this information converged into a matrix supporting our current understanding of cancer.

There has been a flow of genetic information into this database, starting with Gregor Mendel and the discovery of the principle of inherited traits, and leading through Theodor Boveri's work on the chromosomal mode of heredity and chromosomal damage in malignant cells,[1] to Avery's discovery of deoxyribonucleic acid (DNA) as the hereditary principle,[2] Watson and Crick's determination of the structure of DNA,[3] the human genome project, and DNA microarrays (with, of course, several other important steps along the way).

Once cell culture techniques were developed,[4] it became possible to test which genes are involved in malignant transformation and progression. This field of research led to the discovery of oncogenes[5] and tumor-suppressor genes.[6] Hereditary studies led to the two-hit theory[7] and the concept of the hereditary nature of some cancers.[8] Chromosomal staining techniques enabled Nowell and Hungerford[9] and Rowley[10] to identify chromosomal translocation as a tumor-initiating event.

Studies in yeast produced the concept of cell-cycle checkpoints,[11] and investigations with *Caenorhabditis elegans* found genes involved in apoptosis.[12] The cell cycle began to be studied in great detail in lower organisms, and organisms such as clams, yeast, and fruit flies have contributed greatly to our understanding of the cell-cycle events.[13]

The findings that simple molecules such as cyclic adenosine 3',5'-monophosphate could direct many cellular functions[14] led to the discovery of altered enzymes of cyclic nucleotide metabolism in cancer cells.[15] Today, signal-transduction pathways are favored molecular targets for anticancer drug discovery.

The biochemical differences between normal and malignant cells were originally discovered through studying patterns of enzymatic activity. In the 1920s, Warburg studied glycolysis in a wide variety of human and animal tumors and found a general trend toward increased glycolysis over oxidative phosphorylation in tumor cells.[16] He noted that when normal tissue slices were incubated in a nutrient medium containing glucose, but without oxygen, there was a high rate of lactic acid production (anaerobic glycolysis); however, if the normal tissue slices were incubated with oxygen, lactic acid production stopped. In tumor tissue slices, the rate of lactic acid production was higher in the absence of oxygen than in normal tissues, and the presence of oxygen slowed, but did not eliminate lactic acid formation in the tumor slices. Warburg concluded that cancer cells have an irreversible injury to their respiratory mechanism, which increases the rate of lactic acid production even in the presence of oxygen. He regarded the persistence of glycolysis as the crucial biochemical lesion in neoplastic transformation. This idea is supported by the presence of hypoxic areas in the core of tumors, where anaerobic metabolism predominates.

It remains unexplained why cancer cells prefer glycolysis, which generates only 2 mols of ATP per molecule of glucose, over oxidative phosphorylation, which when coupled to glycolysis produces 30 mols of ATP per molecule of glucose. Thompson's group has demonstrated that cancer cells increase the ability to transport glucose through upregulation of glucose transporters.[17] This allows cancer cells to spare pyruvate, which during oxidative phosphorylation is converted to lactate. This excess pyruvate is then available for fatty acid synthesis for new membrane production. Recent advances in clinical oncology take advantage of the Warburg principle. That tumor cells have a greater avidity for glucose than normal cells forms the basis for positron emission scanning (PET), whereby radiolabeled glucose accumulates to a greater extent in cancer than in normal tissues, thereby allowing sensitive nuclear imaging.

Because mitochondria contain the enzymatic cascades for oxidative phosphorylation, it has been suggested that damage to mitochondria may be involved in the disruptions of oxidative metabolism seen in malignant tumors. Mutations of mitochondrial DNA (mtDNA) have recently been observed in a variety of human cancers, including bladder, head and neck, lung,[18] and ovarian[19] cancers. Interestingly, in the bladder cancers, the mutation hot spots were primarily in a nicotinamide adenine dinucleotide dehydrogenase (NADH) subunit,[18] a key component of the electron transfer machinery, supporting a mechanism for the alterations in oxidative metabolism seen in malignant cells. Because mitochondrial DNA is exposed to high levels of reactive oxygen species generated during oxidative phosphorylation, it is not surprising that mtDNA is highly susceptible to mutational events. The mutational rate of mtDNA is estimated to be 10 times higher than that of nuclear DNA.[19] Mitochondria also play a key role in apoptosis, and alterations in those mitochondria-mediated events are seen in cancer cells.

On the basis of work done approximately 50 years ago on the production of hepatic cancer by feeding aminoazo dyes, the Millers advanced the "deletion hypothesis" of cancer.[20] This hypothesis was based on the observation that a carcinogenic aminoazo dye covalently bound liver proteins in animals undergoing carcinogenesis, whereas little or no dye binding occurred with the protein of tumors induced by the dye. They suggested that carcinogenesis resulted from "a permanent alteration or loss of protein essential for the control of growth."

Approximately 10 years later, Potter suggested that the proteins lost during carcinogenesis may be involved in the feedback control of enzyme systems required for cell division,[21] and he proposed the "feedback deletion hypothesis."[22] Potter postulated that "repressors" crucial to the regulation of genes involved in cell proliferation are lost or inactivated by the action of oncogenic agents, either by interacting with DNA to block repressor-gene transcription or by reacting directly with repressor proteins and inactivating them. This prediction anticipated the discovery of tumor-suppressor proteins, such as p53 and RB, by about 25 years.

Biochemical studies of cancer were also aided by the "minimal-deviation" hepatomas developed by Morris.[23] These tumors were induced in rats by feeding them the carcinogens fluorenylphthalamic acid, fluorenylacetamide, or trimethylaniline. These hepatocellular carcinomas are transplantable in an inbred host strain of rats and have a variety of growth rates and degrees of differentiation. The term, *minimal deviation* was coined by Potter[22] to convey the idea that some of these neoplasms differ only slightly from normal hepatic parenchymal cells. He reasoned that if the biochemical lesions present in the most minimally deviated neoplasm could be identified, the crucial changes defining the malignant phenotype could be determined. As Weinhouse[24] has indicated, studies of these tumors greatly advanced our knowledge of the biochemical characteristics of the malignant phenotype, and they have ruled out many secondary or nonspecific changes that relate more to tissue growth rate than to malignancy.

The extensive biochemical analyses of the Morris minimal-deviation hepatomas led Weber to formulate the "molecular correlation concept" of cancer that states that "the biochemical strategy of the genome in neoplasia could be identified by elucidation of the pattern of gene expression as revealed in the activity, concentration, and isozymic pattern of key enzymes and their linking with neoplastic transformation and progression."[25] Weber proposed three general types of biochemical alterations associated with malignancy: (1) transformation-linked alterations that correlate with the events of malignant transformation and that are probably altered in the same direction in all malignant cells; (2) progression-linked alterations that correlate with tumor growth rate, invasiveness, and metastatic potential; and (3) coincidental alterations that are secondary events and do not correlate strictly with transformation or progression. He maintained that enzymes involved in the regulation of rate and direction of flux of competing synthetic and catabolic pathways would be the enzymes most likely to be altered in the malignant process (see "Metabolomics'). In contrast, enzymes that are not rate limiting and that do not regulate reversible equilibrium reactions, would be of lesser importance. As one would expect, a number of enzyme activities that Weber and others have found to be altered in malignant cells are those involved in nucleic acid synthesis and catabolism. In general, the key enzymes in the de novo and salvage pathways of purine and pyrimidine biosynthesis are increased and the opposing catabolic enzymes are decreased during malignant transformation and tumor progression. Weber noted that the degree of neoplasia was related to the concentrations of certain regulators of key metabolic pathways. The question of why anaplastic, rapidly growing tumors tend to be biochemically alike, whereas more well-differentiated tumors display a vast array of phenotypic characteristics was approached by Knox.[26] He thought that the majority of biochemical components in tumor tissues are "normal," in the sense that they are produced by certain specialized adult normal cells or by normal cells at some stage of their differentiation. In cancer cells, it is the combination and proportions of these normal components that are abnormal. The biochemical diversity of cancer cells, then, would depend on the cell of origin of the neoplasm and its degree of neoplasticity.[26] All too frequently, in the histopathologic or biochemical characterization of cancer, a biochemical component that is present or absent, or increased or decreased, is not considered in relation to the particular cell of origin of a tumor, its differentiation state, or its degree of neoplasticity.

The data on enzyme patterns of cancer cells indicate that undifferentiated, highly malignant cells tend to resemble one another and fetal tissues more than their adult normal counterparts, whereas well-differentiated tumors tend to resemble their cell of origin more than other tumors. Between these two extremes lie several levels of neoplastic gradation leading to the vast biochemical heterogeneity of tumors. This heterogeneity also exists for tumors of the same tissue type arising in different patients or even in the same patient at different stages of the disease. The advent of global transcriptional profiling using microarray technologies confirms these observations and has had major impact on our thinking about diagnosis, prognosis and treatment.

Undifferentiated tumors tend to converge to a more fetal-like state as demonstrated by the frequent production of oncodevelopmental gene products. A number of cancer-cell characteristics, such as invasiveness and metastasis, are also seen in embryonic tissues. For example, the developing trophoblast invades the uterine wall during the implantation step of embryonic development. During organogenesis, embryonic cells dissociate themselves from the surrounding cells and migrate to new locations, a process not unlike metastasis. Thus, it is not surprising that fetal-like stem cells may exist in cancer, and that these "cancer stem cells" may be the ultimate progenitor of the entire malignancy.

BIOCHEMICAL BASIS OF MALIGNANT TRANSFORMATION

Treatment of animals or cells in culture with carcinogenic agents is a means of studying discrete biochemical events that lead to malignant transformation. Studies of cell transformation in vitro, however, have many pitfalls. For example, "tissue-culture artifacts" include overgrowth of cells not characteristic of the original population of cultured cells (eg, overgrowth of fibroblasts in cultures that were originally primarily epithelial cells), selection for a small population of variant cells with continued passage in vitro, or appearance of cells with an abnormal chromosomal number or structure (karyotype). Changes in the characteristics of cultured cell populations can lead to "spontaneous" transformation that mimics some of the changes seen in populations of cultured cells treated with oncogenic agents. Thus, it is often difficult to distinguish the critical malignant events from the noncritical ones.

Malignant transformation can also be induced by treatment of susceptible experimental animals with carcinogenic chemicals, oncogenic viruses, or irradiation. Identification of critical biochemical changes in vivo is even more complex because it is difficult to discriminate toxic from malignant events and to determine what role a myriad of factors, such as the nutritional state of the animal, hormone levels, or endogenous infections with microorganisms or parasites, might play. Moreover, tissues are a mixture of cell types, and it is difficult to determine in which cells the critical transformation events are occurring and what role the microenvironment of the tissue plays.

Most studies that are designed to identify discrete biochemical events occurring in cells during malignant transformation have therefore been done with cultured cells, because clones of relatively homogeneous cell populations can be studied and the cellular environment defined and manipulated. Recent evidence suggests the existence of cancer stem cells, that is, cancer cells of embryonic stem cell origin that generate progeny that can differentiate and populate the entire population. This has been most clearly demonstrated in certain forms of leukemia by Weissman's group,[27] and it has been suggested that similar cells exist in solid tumors such as breast and gliomas.[28,29]

The ultimate criterion that establishes whether or not cells have been transformed is their ability to form a tumor in an appropriate host animal. The ability to generate immortalized "normal" cell lines of a given differentiated phenotype from human embryonic stem cells has enhanced the ability to study cells of a normal genotype from a single source.[30]

Over the past 60 years, scientists aimed at identifying the phenotypic characteristics of in vitro–transformed cells that correlate with the growth of a cancer in vivo. This approach has tremendously increased our knowledge of the biochemistry of cancer cells. However, many of the biochemical characteristics initially thought to be closely associated with the malignant phenotype of cells in culture were subsequently found to be dissociable from the ability of those cells to produce tumors in animals. Furthermore, individual cells of malignant tumors growing in animals or in humans exhibit marked biochemical heterogeneity, as reflected in their cell surface composition, enzyme levels, immunogenicity, response to anticancer drugs, and so on. This has made it extremely difficult to identify the essential changes that produce the malignant phenotype. Recently, however, Hahn and colleagues[31] showed that ectopic expression of the human telomerase catalytic subunit (human telomerase reverse transcriptase [hTERT]) in combination with the oncogenes *H-ras* and SV40 virus large-T antigen can induce tumorigenic conversion in normal human epithelial and fibroblast cells, suggesting that disruption of the intracellular pathways regulated by these gene products is sufficient to produce a malignant cell. Additional work indicates the importance of the stroma to this process, because cancer cells of epithelial origin require specific interactions with blood vessels (angiogenesis) and matrix proteins.[32]

Table 9-1 lists the properties of transformed malignant cells growing in cell culture or in vivo.[33] Some of these characteristics may be seen both in transformed cells in culture and in tumors growing in experimental animals or patients. In addition, hyperproliferative conditions in patients, such as inflammatory bowel disease or psoriasis, may display some of these characteristics. Thus, for diagnostic purposes, it is important to use a number of characteristics that define the malignant state.

Immortality of Transformed Cells in Culture Normal diploid mammalian cells have a limited life expectancy in culture. For example,

Table 9-1 Properties of Transformed Malignant Cells Growing in Cell Culture and/or In Vivo

A. In vitro alterations

1. Cytologic changes resembling those of cancer cells in vivo, including increased cytoplasmic basophilia, increased number and size of nuclei, increased nucleus:cytoplasmic ratio, and formation of clusters and cords of cells.
2. Alteration in growth characteristics:
   - "Immortality" of transformed cells in culture. Transformed malignant cells become "immortal" in that they can be passaged indefinitely.
   - Decreased density-dependent inhibition of growth or loss of "contact inhibition." Transformed cells frequently grow to a higher density than their normal counterparts, and they may "pile up" in culture rather than stop growing when they make contact.
   - Decreased serum requirement. Transformed cells usually require lower concentrations of serum or growth factors to replicate in culture than nontransformed cells require.
   - Loss of anchorage dependence and acquisition of ability to grow in soft agar. Transformed cells may lose their requirement to grow attached to surfaces and can grow as free colonies in a semisolid medium.
   - Loss of cell-cycle control. Transformed cells fail to stop at cell-cycle checkpoints in the cell cycle when they are subject to metabolic restriction of growth.
   - Resistance to cell death.
3. Changes in cell membrane structure and function, including increased agglutinability by plant lectins; alteration in composition of cell surface glycoproteins, proteoglycans, glycolipids, and mucins; appearance of tumor-associated antigens; and increased uptake of amino acids, hexoses, and nucleosides.
4. Loss of cell–cell and cell–extracellular matrix interactions that foster cell differentiation.
5. Loss of response to differentiation-inducing agents and altered cellular receptors for these agents.
6. Altered signal-transduction mechanisms, including constitutive rather than regulated function of growth factor receptors, phosphorylation cascades, and dephosphorylation mechanisms.
7. Ability to produce tumors in experimental animals. This is the sine qua non that defines malignant transformation in vitro. If the cells believed to be transformed do not produce tumors in appropriate animal hosts, they cannot be defined as "malignant." However, failure to grow in an animal model does mean that they may not be tumorigenic in a different type of animal (eg, syngeneic vs allogeneic).

B. In vivo alterations

- Increased expression of oncogene proteins as a consequence of chromosomal translocation, amplification, or mutation.
- Loss of tumor-suppressor gene protein products because of deletion, mutation, or silencing.
- Activation of telomerase
- Alterations in DNA methylation patterns.
- Genetic imprinting errors that lead to overproduction of growth-processing substances (eg, IGF-2).
- Increased or unregulated production of growth factors (eg, TGF-α), tumor angiogenesis factors, PDGF, hematopoietic growth factors (eg, CSFs, interleukins).
- Genetic instability leading to progressive loss of regulated cell proliferation, increased invasiveness, and increased metastatic potential. "Mutator" genes may be involved in this effect.
- Alteration in enzyme patterns. Malignant cells have increased levels of enzymes involved in nucleic acid synthesis and produce higher levels of lytic enzymes (eg, proteases, collagenases, glycosidases).
- Production of oncodevelopmental gene products. Many cancers produce increased amounts of oncofetal antigens (eg, carcinoembryonic antigen), placental hormones (eg, human chorionic gonadotropin), or placental-fetal type isoenzymes (eg, placental alkaline phosphatase).
- Ability to avoid the host's antitumor immune response.

normal human fibroblast lines may live for 50 to 60 population doublings[34] (the "Hayflick index"), but then viability begins to decrease rapidly unless they transform spontaneously or are transformed by oncogenic agents. However, malignant cells, once they become established in culture, will generally live for an indefinite number of population doublings, provided the right nutrients and growth factors are present. This fundamental difference may be related to the continual shortening of chromosomal telomeres each time cells divide. In human cells, telomeres are made up of an average of 5,000 to 15,000 base-pair repeats containing the sequence $(TTAGGG)_n$ together with telomere-binding proteins.[35] Younger cells have longer telomeres. Every time a cell divides, 50 to 100 base pairs are lost, and a cellular signal is eventually triggered to stop cell division. Cells of higher eukaryotic organisms maintain telomere length by the activity of telomerase. This is a ribonucleoprotein complex that contains several proteins and ribonucleic acid (RNA). The catalytic component of this complex is a reverse transcriptase, hTERT, that uses the RNA contained in the complex as a template for reverse transcription to replicate the DNA sequences in the telomere. Germ cells and pluripotent tissue stem cells have telomerase activity; however, telomerase is turned off in cells from most tissues as they differentiate. Most human cancers appear to be able to reactivate telomerase activity, thus rejuvenating their proliferative capacity[36]; however, 10 to 15% of human cancers do not express telomerase and apparently maintain telomere length by a different mechanism.[37] Telomerase has been a target of interest for both diagnostic and therapeutic approaches to cancer. A potential problem with the use of telomerase inhibitors for cancer therapy is their slow onset of action because tumor cells can continue to proliferate until telomere length reduces to a critical length. Moreover, normal stem cells, such as those involved in hematopoiesis and wound healing, are negatively affected by telomerase inhibition.[37] There are also data indicating that restoring telomerase in human cells extends their lifespan,[38] suggesting that senescence can be overcome and perhaps providing a way to maintain human stem cells for replacement of aging or damaged tissues.

Transformed cells that become established in culture also frequently undergo karyotypic changes, usually marked by an increase in chromosomes (polyploidy). This suggests that cells with increased amounts of certain growth-promoting genes are generated and/or selected during passage in culture. The more undifferentiated cells from cancers of animals or patients also often have an atypical karyotype, suggesting that the same selection process may occur in vivo with progression over time of malignancy from a lower to a higher grade. In fact, it is highly unusual for a metastatic deposit from a recurrent cancer to be more differentiated than the primary tumor.

Decreased Requirement for Growth Factors Other properties that distinguish transformed cells from their non-transformed counterparts are decreased density-dependent ("contact") inhibition of proliferation[39] and the requirement for growth factors for replication in culture. Cells transformed by oncogenic viruses require lower serum concentrations for growth than do normal cells.[40] For example, 3T3 fibroblasts transformed by SV40,[41] polyoma,[42] murine sarcoma virus,[42] or Rous sarcoma virus[43] are all able to grow in a culture medium that lacks certain serum growth factors, whereas uninfected cells are not.

Cancer cells can produce their own growth factors that may be secreted and activate proliferation in neighboring cells (paracrine effect), or, if the same malignant cell type has both the receptor for a growth factor and the means to produce the factor, self-stimulation of cell proliferation (autocrine effect) may occur. One example of such an autocrine loop is the production of tumor necrosis factor (TNF) and its receptor TNFR1 by diffuse large cell lymphoma.[44] Coexpression of TNF-α and its receptor are negative-prognostic indicators of survival, suggesting that autocrine loops can be powerful stimuli for tumor aggressiveness and thus potentially important diagnostic and therapeutic targets.

Loss of Anchorage Dependence Most freshly isolated normal animal cells and cells from cultures of normal diploid cells do not grow well when they are suspended in fluid or a semisolid agar gel. If these cells make contact with a suitable surface, however, they attach, spread, and proliferate, a process termed *anchorage-dependent growth.* When removed from this attachment the cells rapidly undergo a form of programmed cell death termed "anoikis" (*gr.* homeless). In contrast, many cell lines derived from tumors and cells transformed by oncogenic agents exhibit *anchorage-independent growth* and proliferate without attachment to a surface. This property of transformed cells has been used to develop clones of malignant cells.[45] The ability to grow cancer cells derived from human tumors in soft agar allowed investigators to test their sensitivity to chemotherapeutic agents and to screen for potential new anticancer drugs.[46] However, because a very low percentage of cells in a human cancer are clonogenic, the usefulness of these assays has been limited.

Loss of Cell-Cycle Control and Resistance to Cell Death Normal cells respond to a variety of suboptimal growth conditions by entering a quiescent (G0) phase of the cell cycle. There appears to be a decision point in the G1 phase of the cell cycle, at which time the cell must make a commitment to continue into the S-phase, the DNA synthesis step, or to stop in G1 and wait until conditions are more optimal for cell replication to occur. If this waiting period is prolonged, the cells are said to be in a G0 phase. Once cells make a commitment to divide, they must continue through S, G2, and M to return to G1. If normal cells are blocked in S, G2, or M for any length of time, they die. The events that regulate the cell cycle are referred to as *cell-cycle checkpoints*. This loss of cell-cycle checkpoint control by cancer cells may contribute to their increased susceptibility to anticancer drugs. Normal cells use these checkpoints to protect themselves from exposure to growth-limiting conditions or toxic agents. In contrast, cancer cells can continue through these checkpoints into cell-cycle phases that make them more susceptible to the cytotoxic effects of certain drugs that require movement through the cell cycle. For example, if the DNA of normal cells is damaged, they arrest in G1 so that the DNA can be repaired prior to replication. If irreparable damage occurs, normal cells will activate cell death pathways mediated by p53 or Rb. Another checkpoint in the G2 phase allows repair of chromosome breaks before chromosomes are segregated at mitosis. A post-mitotic checkpoint prevents endoreduplication, that is, cytokinesis without adequate segregation of duplicated chromosomes to daughter cells. Cancer cells exhibiting poor or absent checkpoint controls replicate the damaged DNA, thus accounting for persisting and accumulating mutations.

Protein Synthesis, Bioenergetics, and Cell Survival Abnormal regulation of protein synthesis can transform cells through changes in the expression and activity of translation factors such as elongation initiation factor-2 alpha (eIF2 alpha) and its specific protein kinase, PKR.[47,48] There is also abundant evidence suggesting that the effect of growth factors requires transient inhibition of protein synthesis.[49] In fact, a variety of processes important to cell proliferation are stimulated by inhibitors of protein synthesis including RNA synthesis,[50] polyamine transport,[51] ATP turnover,[52] expression of early growth response genes such as *c-fos* and *c-jun*,[52,53] activation of ribosomal protein S6 kinase,[54] MAP kinases,[55] and JNK/SAPK kinases.[56] In addition, exposure of 3T3 cells to cycloheximide or puromycin results in induction of DNA synthesis and cell division.[57] These effects are linked to signal transduction pathways through the activation of phospholipase C, an enzyme that mediates the release of intracellular calcium from the endoplasmic reticulum by generating inositol tris phosphates. Intracellular calcium activates a series of calmodulin-dependent enzymes, including elongation factor-2 kinase, a ubiquitous enzyme frequently activated in transformed cells[58] that regulates protein elongation.[59]

Protein synthesis accounts for a major percentage of energy consumption. In the presence of adequate nutrients, protein synthesis is stimulated and cell death pathways such as autophagy (see below) are inhibited (Figure 9-1). The mammalian target of rapamycin (mTOR) pathway integrates the cellular response to growth factors and nutrients through regulation of protein synthesis.[60] In yeast, TOR provides a link between cellular growth and the availability of extracellular nutrients. In mammals, mTOR is also regulated by growth factors through the PI3K/Akt pathway.[61] Substantial cross talk exists between the PI3K/AKT pathway and the Ras/Raf/ERK1/2 pathways. For example, EGF activation of both ERK1/2 and Akt blocked the induction of autophagy, whereas PTEN, a negative regulator of Akt, stimulated autophagy in HT-29 colon cancer.[62] Activating Ras mutations also induced autophagy in colon cancer cells, and this was blocked by feeding amino acids.[63,64] The importance of this pathway to sustaining cancer viability makes the individual components attractive for drug development.

In the absence of nutrients, protein synthesis is inhibited and autophagy is activated. Nutrient/growth factor deprivation and ATP depletion activates autophagy by inhibiting mTOR (via activation of TSC2 by 5'AMP kinase) and decreasing phosphorylation of S6 kinase and 4EBP1.[65,66] Under these conditions, initiation of translation is repressed by the reformation of the 4EBP4/eIF4E inhibitory complex, and elongation is inhibited through activation of eEF-2 kinase. Thus, eukaryotic cells have evolved a mechanism to withstand starvation by decreasing energy use through inhibiting protein synthesis and increasing energy production through autophagic recycling of amino acids produced from digestion of cellular organelles and proteins.

Alterations in biochemical balance ("bioenergetics") can ultimately lead to cell death. Cells die through several mechanisms including apoptosis, necrosis, or autophagy. Necrosis and autophagy are tightly linked to the state of nutrient-dependent cellular bioenergetics. For example, autophagy is a mechanism by which cells respond to nutrient deprivation and is known to occur in yeast, plants, worms, flies, mice, and man.[67] In yeast, nutrient deprivation activates a programmed genetic response that results in two outcomes: (1) self-digestion of cytoplasm and organelles and the recycling of amino acids for energy use and; (2) the budding of an immortal spore. This form of self-digestion in unicellular organisms leads to self-preservation in times of famine. Not surprisingly, autophagy finds its counterpart in multicellular organisms, as high up the animal kingdom as *Homo sapiens*. At the cellular level, nutrient deprivation prompts cells to exit the cell cycle, shrink, autodigest long-lived proteins and damaged organelles, and recycle the components for synthesis of macromolecules or oxidation in mitochondria to maintain cellular ATP. Autophagy may thus result in cellular destruction or alternatively cellular "hibernation" until the supply of nutrients is restored.

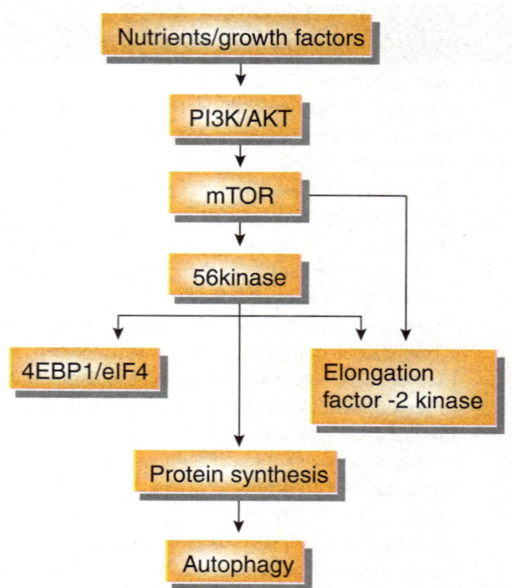

Figure 9-1 In the presence of nutrients (glucose, amino acids, growth factors) protein synthesis is stimulated and autophagy is inhibited This is mediated through activation of mTOR (via activation of PI3 kinase and AKT and inactivation of the tuberous sclerosis complex [TSC1 and 2]). mTOR phosphorylates S6 kinase and increases the translation of mRNAs that encode ribosomal and other proteins involved in translation. This initiates translation by phosphorylating 4EBP1, an inhibitor of initiation, causing its disassociation from eIF4E. Active eIF4 promotes cell proliferation by increasing translation of cyclin D1, c-Myc, and VEGF. mTOR and S6 kinase also release the cellular check on peptide elongation by phosphorylating and inactivating eEF-2 kinase. eEF2-kinase phosphorylates eEF-2, a 100kDa protein that mediates the translocation step in peptide-chain elongation by inducing the transfer of peptidyl-tRNA from the ribosomal A to P site. Phosphorylation of eEF-2 at Thr56 by eEF-2 kinase decreases the affinity of the elongation factor for ribosomes and terminates elongation. Activation of TOR in yeast inhibits induction of autophagy via phosphorylation of the APG1-APG-13 complex a process inhibited by rapamycin in both yeast and mammalian cells.

Three recent papers highlight aspects of autophagy relevant to cancer biology. For example, Kuma and colleagues[68] asked, "How do newborns survive after being cut off from the maternal blood supply and before adequate nutrients are available through suckling?" In this remarkable set of experiments, it was shown that at birth there is upregulation of autophagy in several organs most notably heart, diaphragm, alveolar cells, and skin. Mice lacking *Atg5*, a gene whose product is critical for the formation of autophagosomes, appear normal at birth but die within 24 hours of delivery. The animals have reduced circulating amino acids and die secondary to energy depletion. Electrocardiograms performed on the newborns pups revealed cardiac ischemia. Thompson's laboratory[69] looked at the role of autophagy in the survival of immortalized hematopoietic precursors and primary bone marrow cultures deprived of an obligate growth factor (IL-3). They found that cells in which apoptosis was inactivated by deleting *bax* and *bak* survived for > six weeks in the absence of IL-3 by using autophagy to supply precursors for ATP. Upon re-addition of IL-3, cells increased glucose transport and recovered size and ability to proliferate. Finally, Boya and colleagues[70] found that nutrient deprived HeLa cells underwent autophagy and prevented apoptosis (believed to occur through sequestration of damaged mitochondria). However, blocking the autophagic pathway with either small interfering RNAs against key autophagy genes (*beclin1*, *Atg10*, or *Atg12*) or with drugs (3-methyladenine, hydroxychloroquine, bafilomycin A1, or monensin) triggered apoptosis.

Eventually, cells deprived of nutrients will deplete ATP below a critical concentration compatible with life. When this occurs, cellular transporters will no longer function, electrochemical gradients will collapse, and cells ultimately undergo necrosis.[71] Thompson's group has suggested that necrotic cell death can be programmatically activated in response to overwhelming DNA damage. In this model, DNA damage activates poly-ADP ribose polymerase (PARP), which in turn ADP-ribosylates nucleosomal proteins to allow more efficient DNA repair. This reaction depletes NAD and inhibits glycolysis. Because cancer cells are reliant on glycolysis for ATP generation, PARP activation will ultimately initiate necrotic cell death.

CHANGES IN CELL MEMBRANE STRUCTURE AND FUNCTION The plasma membrane plays an important role in the "social" behavior of cells, including communication with other cells, cell movement and migration, adherence to other cells or structures, access to nutrients in the microenvironment, and recognition by the body's immune system. Alterations of the plasma membrane in malignant cells may be inferred from a variety of properties that characterize their growth and behavior, for example, the loss of density-dependent inhibition of growth, decreased adhesiveness, loss of anchorage dependence, and invasiveness through normal tissue barriers. In addition, a number of changes in the biochemical characteristics of the surfaces of malignant cells have been observed. These include appearance of new surface antigens, proteoglycans, glycolipids, and mucins, and altered cell–cell and cell–extracellular matrix communication.

Alterations in Cell Surface Glycolipids, Glycoproteins, Proteoglycans, and Mucins Aberrant glycosylation was first suggested as the basis for the tumor-associated determinants of glycolipids by the finding of a remarkable accumulation of fucose-containing glycolipids in human adenocarcinomas[72] These identifications were confirmed once monoclonal antibodies were used to identify antigens definitively. A number of monoclonal antibodies with preferential reactivity for tumor cells over normal cells react with Lewis blood group antigens, such as Le^x, Le^a, Le^b, or their analogues.[72]

The presence of high-molecular-weight glycopeptides with altered glycosylation patterns on transformed cells was detected before they were chemically identified.[73,74] Later, the chemical basis for some of the changes in tumor cell glycoproteins was attributed to the fact that the N-linked oligosaccharides of tumor cells contain more multiantennary structures than the oligosaccharides derived from normal cells.[75]

Tumor-associated carbohydrate antigens can be classified into three groups[72]: (1) epitopes expressed on both glycolipids and glycoproteins; (2) epitopes expressed only on glycolipids; and (3) epitopes expressed only on glycoproteins. To the first group belongs the lacto series structure that is found in the most common human cancers, such as lung, breast, colorectal, liver, and pancreatic cancers. The common backbone structure for these epitopes is GalP13GlcNAcP13Gal (type 1 blood group) or Gal014GlcNacP13Gal (type 2 blood group). The second group of epitopes, expressed exclusively on glycolipids, is mostly on the ganglio or globo series structures. This series of epitopes are expressed abundantly only on certain types of human cancers, such as melanoma, neuroblastoma, small-cell lung carcinoma, and Burkitt lymphoma. The third group of epitopes, seen only on glycoproteins, is the multiantennary branches of N-linked carbohydrates and the alterations of O-linked carbohydrate chains seen in some mucins.

Tumor-associated carbohydrate antigens can also be classified by the cell types expressing them as those (1) expressed on only certain types of normal cells (often only in certain developmental stages) and greatly accumulated in tumor cells; (2) expressed only on tumor cells, for example, altered blood group antigens or mucins; and (3) expressed commonly on normal cells but present in much higher concentrations on tumor cells, for example, the GM3 ganglioside in melanoma and Le^x in gastrointestinal cancer.[72]

A variety of chemical changes in tumor cells have been identified that can explain altered glycosylation patterns. These result from three kinds of altered processes: (1) incomplete synthesis and/or processing of normally existing carbohydrate chains and accumulation of the resulting precursor form; (2) activation of glycosyltransferases that are absent or have low activity in normal cells; and (3) organizational rearrangement of tumor cell membrane glycolipids.[76]

Moreover, the glycosyl epitopes found in glycolipids and glycoproteins make up microdomains that are involved in cell adhesion and signal-transduction events. They function as a "glycosynapse" in mediating these events.[43] The cell motility, altered adhesive properties, and invasiveness observed in cancer cells are regulated by these glycosynapse complexes.[77]

Interest in the carbohydrate components of the cell surface has been heightened by the fact that many monoclonal antibodies developed to tumor-associated antigens recognize these carbohydrate moieties or peptide epitopes exposed by altered glycosylation. Moreover, many of these blood group–specific antigens are seen at certain stages of embryonic development and thus fit the definition of oncodevelopmental antigens. Thus, the field of "chemical glycobiology" is making significant contributions to our understanding of the cell surface biochemistry of normal and malignant cells.[78]

Role of Glycosyl Transferases and Oligosaccharide-Processing Enzymes The substitution of additional carbohydrate moieties on blood group-related structures is not the only aberrant modification of glycoproteins or glycolipids observed in cancer cells. Increased branching of asparagine-linked oligosaccharides and incomplete processing of these oligosaccharides have also been noted in certain cell surface as well as secretory glycoproteins.[79,80] The increased activity of specific *N*-acetylglucosaminyl transferases in tumor cells appears to be responsible for the appearance of tri- and tetra-antennary structures, whereas the analogous glycoprotein in normal cells is often a biantennary structure. Unusually high expression of *N*-acetylglucosaminyltransferase IVa has been observed in human choriocarcinoma cell lines and may be the enzymatic basis for the formation of abnormal biantennary sugar chains on hCG (human chorionic gonadotropin).[81] Similarly, the extra fucosylations that appear on membrane glycoproteins and glycolipids are associated with the induction of an unusual α-fucosyltransferase in chemical carcinogen-induced precancerous rat liver and in the resulting hepatomas.[82] These investigations strongly suggest that the regulation of glycosyltransferase genes is important in malignant transformation.[83]

The use of inhibitors of glycosylation inhibitors and oligosaccharide-processing supports the importance of glycosylation patterns of cell surface glycoproteins and glycolipids in the malignant phenotype. For example, tunicamycin, an inhibitor of addition of N-linked glycans to nascent polypeptide chains, castanospermine, an inhibitor of glucosidase, and KI-8110, an inhibitor of sialyltransferase activity, all reduce the number of lung metastases in murine experimental tumor models.[84–86] In addition, swainsonine was shown to reduce the rate of growth of human melanoma xenografts in athymic nude mice,[87] and castanospermine was observed to inhibit the growth of v-*fms* oncogene-transformed rat cells in vivo.[88] These results support the hypothesis that the synthesis of highly branched complex-type oligosaccharides is associated with the malignant phenotype and may provide tumor cells with a growth advantage.

Mucins Mucins are a type of highly glycosylated proteins that contain over 50% of their molecular mass as O-linked oligosaccharides. A feature common to the mucins is a domain with tandem repeats that are rich in serines, threonines and prolines. The serine and threonine residues function as sites for the extensive *O*-glycosylation. Twenty mucins have been identified to date. There are two classes of mucins; the secreted mucins and the membrane bound (transmembrane) mucins. The secreted mucins contribute to the formation of a physical barrier that affords protection to epithelia in the respiratory system, gastrointestinal tract, and other specialized organs with secretory functions. The membrane bound mucins also contribute to this protective mucous gel through glycosylated ectodomains that are tethered to transmembrane subunits at the apical cell surface. The mucous gel protects the epithelia from diverse forms of stress that include low pH (gastric mucosa), toxins, proteases, microorganisms, and reactive oxygen species. The membrane bound mucins also signal the presence of external stress to the interior of epithelial cells to activate a repair and survival response.

The membrane bound mucins MUC1 (CA15-3), MUC4, and MUC16 (CA125) are aberrantly overexpressed in diverse human tumors. For example, with transformation and loss of polarity, carcinoma cells express MUC1 at high levels over the entire cell surface and in the cytoplasm.[89] At the cell membrane, MUC1 associates with members of the ErbB family of receptor tyrosine kinases and integrates ErbB receptor signaling with the Wnt pathway.[90,91] MUC1 is over-expressed in most carcinomas of the breast, prostate, lung, pancreas, ovary, and other transformed epithelia. Multiple myeloma cells, lymphomas, and certain leukemias also express MUC1 at high levels. Estimates indicate that of the 1.3 million tumors diagnosed annually in the United States, greater than 800,000 exhibit MUC1 over-expression. Notably, over-expression of MUC1 is sufficient to induce anchorage-independent growth and tumorigenicity.[92] Over-expression of MUC1 is also sufficient to confer resistance to induction of cell death by genotoxic anticancer agents.[93,94] How MUC1 contributes to these characteristics of the transformed phenotype is not precisely known. However, the MUC1 transmembrane subunit is targeted to the nucleus where it contributes to the regulation of gene expression.[92,95–97] MUC1 is also targeted to mitochondria where it attenuates activation of the intrinsic apoptotic pathway.[93] Moreover, MUC1 directly interacts with β-catenin and c-Src, effectors that have been linked to transformation.[98–100]

MUC4 is a transmembrane mucin that is over-expressed by pancreatic cancers. Like MUC1, MUC4 consists of a heavily *O*-glycosylated ectodomain with tandem repeats that is non-covalently tethered to a transmembrane subunit.[101] However, unlike MUC1, the extracellular region of the MUC4 transmembrane subunit contains EGF-like domains that can function as intramembrane ligands for ErbB2.[102] Over-expression of MUC4 has been correlated with pancreatic tumor progression.[103] Moreover, silencing of MUC4 has been associated with decreased pancreatic tumor cell growth and metastasis.[104] MUC4 expression is upregulated in pancreatic cancer cells by diverse signals induced by TGF-α, TGF-β, interferon-γ, TNF-α and retinoic acid.[105–107] In contrast to MUC4, MUC16 is over-expressed in ovarian cancer. Also known as CA125, MUC16 was first identified as a serum marker that is used to monitor the clinical course of women with ovarian cancer.[108] Cloning of the gene encoding CA125 demonstrated that this glycoprotein is a mucin family member and was designated MUC16.[109] The functional role of MUC16 in ovarian cancer remains unclear, although like MUC1 and MUC4, MUC16 has a transmembrane domain that may contribute to the malignant phenotype.

The over-expression of MUC1, MUC4, and MUC16 in human cancers has generated interest in these mucins as attractive targets for antibody serotherapy and for anticancer vaccines. These topics are covered in Chapter 50, "Monoclonal Serotherapy," and Chapter 51, "Vaccines and Immunostimulants," in this text.

Proteoglycans The proteoglycans are high molecular weight glycoproteins that have a protein core to which are covalently attached large numbers of side chains of sulfated glycosaminoglycans as well as N-linked and/or O-linked oligosaccharides. They are categorized on the basis of their glycosaminoglycans into several types, including heparan sulfate, chondroitin sulfate, dermatan sulfate, and keratan sulfate.[110] The glycosaminoglycans have different repetitive disaccharide units bound to the core protein through a common glycosaminoglycan linkage region: GlcNAcP 13Ga10 13Ga10 14Xy10 1-OSer. The structure of the sulfated glycopeptides from the carbohydrate-protein linkage region of some of the proteoglycans has been determined.[111]

Proteoglycans interact via their multiple binding domains with many other structural macromolecules, giving them the capacity "to function as a multipurpose 'glue' in cellular interactions."[112] They bind together extracellular matrix (ECM) components, such as hyaluronic acid, collagen, laminin, and fibronectin; mediate binding of cells to the ECM; act as a reservoir for growth factors; and "present" growth factors to growth factor receptors on cells. The proteoglycans also act as cell adhesion factors by promoting organization of actin filaments in the cell's cytoskeleton. Proteoglycans have been shown to undergo both quantitative and qualitative changes during malignant transformation, and alterations have been reported in breast, colon, and liver carcinomas, in glioma cells, and in transformed murine mammary cells and 3T3 fibroblasts.

Two putative tumor-suppressor genes are glycosyl transferases required for the biosynthesis of the proteoglycan heparan sulfate.[113] Mutations of these genes, called *ext1* and *ext2,* have been associated with the development of skeletal dysplasias, and these findings suggest that alterations in the synthesis of heparan sulfate precursor polysaccharide are involved in dysregulation of heparan sulfate production and function in tumor formation.

Modification of Extracellular Matrix

The ECM plays a key role in regulating cellular proliferation and differentiation. In the case of tumors, it is now clear that development of a blood supply and interaction with the mesenchymal stroma on which tumor cells grow are involved in their growth, invasive properties, and metastatic potential. This topic is covered n detail in Chapter 10, "Invasion and Metastases." Here, we focus only on some of the key biochemical features.

The ECM components include collagen, proteoglycans, and glycoproteins, such as fibronectin, laminin, and entactin. Basement membranes are a specialized type of ECM. These membranes serve as a support structure for cells, act as a "sieving" mechanism for transport of nutrients, cellular metabolic products, and migratory cells (eg, lymphocytes), and play a regulatory role in cell proliferation and differentiation.[114] Basement membranes also prevent the free passage of cells across them, but there are mechanisms that permit the passage of inflammatory cells. It is also clear that basement membranes act as regulators of cell attachment, through cellular receptors called integrins (see below). There is also "cross talk" between epithelial cells and their ECM to create a microenvironment for accurate signal transduction for growth factors and other regulatory molecules. It has been shown, for example, that exogenous reconstituted basement membranes stimulate specific differentiation of a variety of cell types, including mammary cells, hepatocytes, endothelial cells, lung alveolar cells, uterine epithelial cells, Sertoli cells, and Schwann cells.[115]

Cell–ECM and Cell–Cell Adhesion

Cells in tissues are attached to one another and to the ECM. Disruption of these adhesion events leads to increased cell motility and potential invasiveness of cells through the ECM. In addition, most cell types require attachment to the ECM for normal growth, differentiation, and function. This attachment is responsible for what was termed "anchorage dependence." Normal cells that are detached from their binding to the ECM undergo apoptosis, whereas tumor cells that are less dependent on this attachment are free to proliferate and invade tissues.

Cell adhesion to the ECM is mediated by cell surface receptors called *integrins.* Integrins are a family of proteins consisting of heterodimers that are integral membrane proteins with a specific arginine, glycine, aspartic acid (RGD) amino acid sequence involved in binding to the ECM.[116] Integrins also link the external ECM cytoskeleton to the intracellular actin cytoskeleton, and via this connection a linkage to control of gene expression in the cell nucleus is established. In this way, cell–ECM interactions can control gene read-out involved in cell differentiation and function. Cell–ECM interactions occur via focal adhesions that consist of clusters of ECM-bound integrins, and these, in turn, connect to actin fibrils and the signal-transduction machinery inside the cell. These signaling pathways include the focal adhesion kinase (FAK) pathway that participates in the control of anchorage dependence, and growth factor signaling pathways, such as the *ras-raf*–mitogen-activated kinase, protein kinase C, and phosphatidylinositol

3-kinase pathways.[117] Thus, integrins cooperate with growth factors to enhance mitogenic signaling. Alterations in integrin receptor expression have been observed in cell–cell interactions are also important for the normal regulation of cell proliferation and differentiation. These interactions are mediated by a family of cell adhesion molecules (CAMs), which act as both receptors (on one cell) and ligands (for another cell). The expression of CAMs is programmed during development to provide positional and migratory information for cells. A large family of CAMs has been identified. One group of these, called cadherins, comprise a superfamily of Ca^{2+}-dependent transmembrane glycoproteins that play an essential role in the initiation and stabilization of cell–cell contacts. Regulation of cadherin-mediated cell–cell adhesion is important in embryonic development and maintenance of normal tissue differentiation.[118,119]

The extracellular domain of various cadherins is responsible for cell–cell homotypic binding (a given cadherin domain for a given cell type), and the conserved cytoplasmic domains interact with cytoplasmic proteins called *catenins*. Each cadherin molecule can bind to either α-catenin or β-catenin, which, in turn, bind α-catenin. α-Catenin links the cadherin complex to the actin cytoskeleton. Cell lines that lack α-catenin lose normal cell–cell adhesiveness and have increased invasiveness.[120]

E-cadherin is the predominant type of cadherin expressed in epithelial tissue. Alterations of E-cadherin expression and function have been observed in human cancers.[121] In addition, downregulation of E-cadherin correlates with increased invasiveness, metastasis, and poor prognosis in cancer patients. Suppression of this invasive phenotype can be achieved by transfection of E-cadherin cDNA (complementary deoxyribonucleic acid) into carcinoma cells, and contrarily, invasiveness of E-cadherin gene-transfected cells can be restored by exposure of the cells to E-cadherin antibodies or an E-cadherin antisense RNA.[121] Germ line mutations of the E-cadherin gene (*cdh1*) have been found in New Zealand Maori families with a dominantly inherited susceptibility to gastric cancer.[122]

The cellular binding protein for E-cadherin is β-catenin, the intracellular location of which can be cell membrane associated, cytoplasmic, or nuclear. Early mutations in the human colon cancer progression pathway affect the cellular distribution of β-catenin. In patients with colon cancer, the normal colonic epithelial cells adjacent to neoplastic lesions had mostly cell surface membrane-associated expression of β-catenin, whereas cytoplasmic expression of β-catenin was observed in aberrant crypt foci.[123] Nuclear expression was observed in more advanced dysplasias and increased as adenomas progressed to carcinomas. These latter changes are also observed in less-well-differentiated areas of tumors and are accompanied by loss of E-cadherin expression at the invasive front of breast carcinomas, possibly as a consequence of hypermethylation of the E-cadherin promoter.[124]

Production of Lytic Enzymes Transformed malignant cells in culture and human cancer cells in vivo produce a variety of lytic enzymes that degrade the ECM and allow cancer cells to invade tissues, lymphatic channels, and the vasculature. These proteases include plasminogen activator, cathepsins, adamalysin-related membrane proteases, and a number of matrix metalloproteases (MMPs).[125] The MMPs are a large family of proteases that includes collagenases (MMPs 1, 2, and 9) and stromelysins (MMPs 3 and 11). Collagenases have been found at elevated levels in melanoma and in cancers of the colon, breast, lung, prostate, and bladder. Usually, these elevated levels correlate with higher tumor grade and invasiveness. MMP-2 and MMP-9 levels are significantly elevated in the serum of patients with metastatic lung cancer, and in those patients with high levels, response to chemotherapy is diminished.[126] The production of MMPs by tumor cells appears to be mediated, at least in part by "extracellular matrix metalloproteinase inducer," (EMMPRIN; CD147), a member of the immunoglobulin superfamily that is enriched on the surface of cancer cells.[127] Overexpression of EMMPRIN can promote anchorage-independent cell growth and render cells less sensitive to chemotherapy.[128]

BIOCHEMICAL BASIS OF CANCER EPIGENTICS

Cancer cells have altered gene expression that includes chromosomal translocations and inversions, gene deletions, gene amplifications, point mutations, and duplications or losses of whole chromosomes. Alternatively, much of the malignant phenotype is produce by epigenetic changes, whose biochemical basis we discuss herein.

Alterations in Chromatin Structure and Function Chromatin in higher organisms is organized into nucleosomes that are tuna fish can-shaped structures made up of two molecules each of the core histones H2A, H2B, H3, and H4, forming an octamer core around which approximately two turns of DNA are wrapped. In a tightly wrapped conformation, DNA transcription into messenger ribonucleic acid (mRNA) is inhibited. The initiation of gene transcription requires a partial unwrapping of this octamer core, which is regulated by biochemical alteration of the core histones. This involves chemical modifications that regulate the acetylation, methylation, phosphorylation, and ubiquitination of histones. Combinations of these covalent histone modifications have been called the "histone code," by which is meant that specific alterations of histones at specific times in the cell cycle "mark" histone tails by these chemical modifications in a way that enables them to recruit or "de-recruit" other chromatin modifying proteins such as transcriptional coactivators or repressors to promoter regions.[129] Some of the histone modifications appear to involve reciprocal alterations that affect DNA transcription. For example, Nakayama and colleagues[130] have shown in fission yeast that histone H3 methylation on lysine-9 is linked to H3 deacetylation on lysine-14, both of which events are necessary for formation of heterochromatin, the form that is inactive in transcription. In contrast, the "on" state of chromatin active in gene transcription is related to acetylation of lysine-14 and phosphorylation of serine-10.[128]

Other similar reciprocal chromatin activating and deactivating events have been observed in mammalian (HeLa) cells, in which methylation of arginine-3 of histone H4 facilitates subsequent acetylation of H4 amino acid "tails," leading to transcriptional activation of nuclear hormone receptor.[131]

Some gene-silencing events require both histone deacetylation and DNA methylation. Methylation of DNA by DNA methyltransferase recruits methyl-binding proteins and histone deacetylases. This coupling of DNA methylation and histone deacetylation correlates with silent transcriptional regions in chromatin.[132] These processes of controlling chromatin structure and function are key to understanding cell differentiation and the altered gene expression that occurs in malignant transformation.

Some of the genes involved in the acetylation and deacetylation of histones have been identified.[133] There are two categories of acetylation genes: *hat1* and *hat2*. Acetylation of histone H4, for example, reduces the affinity of the histone amino-terminal tail for DNA and allows a reduction of DNA wrapping around the histone octamer and a subsequent decrease in the tightness of nucleosome packaging. This makes more DNA sequences available for transcription. Deacetylation of histone H4 by deacetylases (HDAC1 and HDAC2), on the other hand, increases affinity of H4 for DNA and results in tighter packing of nucleosomes and less transcription. Mutations in yeast deacetylases have been identified that allow H3 and H4 acetylation to be maintained. This would be expected to result in constitutively unfolded regions of chromatin and increased gene transcription. Disruption of deacetylase activity that alters expression of many genes in yeast, as well as in mammalian cells, has been observed. Mutations in histone acetylases, deacetylases, and components of these complexes have significant effects in yeast, and similar mutations may have implications for human disease, including cancer. Recent data have shown that members of the HDAC1 and HDAC2 family of genes belong to a network of genes coordinately regulated and involved in chromatin remodeling during cell differentiation.[134]

In addition to acetylation, phosphorylation of histones is also important for chromatin structure and function.[135] A fifth histone, H1, interacts with DNA, links adjacent nucleosome cores, and further condenses chromatin structure. Phosphorylation of H1 is thought to play a role in increased gene transcription. Phosphorylation of histone H3, on the other hand, is required for proper chromosome condensation and segregation during mitosis.[135] In addition, during the immediate-early response of mammalian cells to mitogens, histone H3 is rapidly and transiently phosphorylated by a kinase called Rsk-2.[136] This suggests that chromatin remodeling is part of the cascade involved in mitogen-activated protein kinase-regulated gene expression.

A "cancer-chromatin connection" is implicated by the observations relating to the role of the tumor-suppressor gene *rb* in the regulation of the histone deacetylase HDAC1.[137] RB acts as a strong transcriptional repressor by forming a complex with the transcriptional activating factor E2F and HDAC1, tethering these activities to E2F-responsive promoters, including the cyclin E promoter region. Repression of E2F-bound promoters by RB is released by mitogenic signals that activate cyclin-dependent kinase phosphorylation of RB, thereby releasing RB from the complex and allowing histone acetylation to occur. This increases accessibility of gene promoter sequences to transcriptional activators. Point mutations of the *rb* gene observed in some tumors abolish RB-induced repression and RB-associated deacetylase activity, allowing increased E2F-mediated gene expression. Viral oncoproteins can disrupt the interaction between RB and HDAC1. In addition, unoccupied retinoic acid receptors (RARs) have been shown to repress transcription of target genes by recruiting the histone deacetylase complex to these genes.[138] Mutant forms of RAR-α result from chromosomal translocations seen in human acute promyelocytic leukemia (APL). These mutant forms prevent appropriate deacetylase activity and result in gene activation. This deregulation can be diminished by all-*trans*-retinoic acid, at doses that induce APL cell differentiation suggesting that oncogenic alterations in RARs mediate leukemogenesis via aberrant regulation of histone acetylation.

DNA Methylation Methylation of DNA on cytosine in CpG islands is another mechanism for regulating gene expression. Hypermethylated DNA sequences are usually less expressed, and hypomethylated sequences are more expressed. CpG islands are short sequences rich in CpG dinucleotides found in the 5'-regulatory regions of about half of all human genes. Alterations in DNA methylation patterns have been observed in tumor cell lines, animal tumor models, and primary human cancers. Feinberg and colleagues[139] observed an average of 8 to 10% reduction in genomic 5-methylcytosine content in colon adenomas and adenocarcinomas. Interestingly, three patients with the highest 5-methylcytosine content in their normal colon appeared to have a germ line predisposition to cancer (Lynch syndrome). Hypermethylation of DNA is postulated to be involved in the loss of tumor-suppressor gene function. Hypermethylation of the regulatory sequences of some of those genes, including *TP53, p15, p16,* E-cadherin, *vhl,* and *hmlh1,* has been observed, but whether this is a cause of tumor-suppressor gene silencing is still unclear. Aberrantly methylated CpG sequences have been detected in serum and tissue of patients with colorectal,[140] non–small-cell lung,[141] liver,[142] and prostate[143] cancers.

DNA methyltransferase activity has been reported to be over-expressed in a number of human cancer cell lines and tissues, although the incidence and extent of this is still being debated.[144] So far, three DNA methyltransferases have been detected in mammalian cells,[95] and the activity of one of these, DNMT1, is threefold higher in *fos* oncogene-transformed fibroblasts than in normal fibroblasts, and the transformed cells contain more 5-methylcytosine than normal fibroblasts.[145] Transfection of the *dnmt1* gene into fibroblasts induces transformation, whereas inhibition of *dnmt1* expression by an antisense oligonucleotide reverses *fos*-induced transformation. These results suggest that oncogene-induced malignant transformation is mediated through alterations in DNA methylation.

Genomic imprinting is an epigenetic modification of the genome that allows only the maternal or paternal allele of a gene to be expressed. Approximately 30 mammalian genes are known to be imprinted.[146] In a number of human cancers, loss of imprinting (LOI) occurs, allowing both the maternal and paternal alleles to be expressed. If this affects a growth factor, such as insulin-like growth factor-2 (IGF-2), cells obtain a double dose of a growth stimulatory signal. LOI of IGF-2 has been observed in approximately 45% of patients with colorectal cancer.[147] Interestingly, this LOI could also be detected in the circulating leukocytes of affected patients, suggesting that this is an alteration that precedes the onset of neoplasia and could be used as a screening test for cancer susceptibility. Somewhat paradoxically, LOI can be reversed by drugs that are DNA methyltransferase inhibitors, such as 5-aza-2-deoxycytidine, suggesting that an aberrant DNA methylation event induces LOI.[148] LOI of the *igf2* gene appears to be involved in tumor progression, leading to a more invasive phenotype.[149]

DNA Repair DNA repair mechanisms are covered extensively in Chapter 2, "Molecular Biology, Genomics, and Proteomics" and Chapter 5, "Signal Transduction." It is sufficient to note here that a number of biochemical mechanisms are invoked by human cells when their DNA is damaged by internal metabolic events (eg, oxidative stress, cytosine deamination) or exogenous factors (eg, chemical carcinogens, irradiation). These repair mechanisms include (1) photoactivation repair for removal of UV-induced pyrimidine dimers; (2) strand-break repair for excision and repair of a length of DNA sequence; (3) base-excision repair producing apurinic or apyrimidinic sites in DNA; (4) nucleotide excision repair; and (5) O6-alkylguanine-DNA alkyltransferase that recognizes and removes small alkyl adducts from DNA.

DNA repair is usually very accurate, but if repair cannot occur prior to or during DNA replication, it may be error prone, potentially leading to a mutagenic and carcinogenic event. A number of inherited defects in DNA repair systems predispose individuals to getting cancer. These syndromes include xeroderma pigmentosum, ataxia telangiectasia, Fanconi anemia, Bloom syndrome, and Cockayne syndrome.

BIOCHEMISTRY OF CELLULAR DIFFERENTIATION

All tissues in the body contain cells that can divide and renew themselves. A subset of the cell population in any tissue can differentiate into the functional cells of that tissue. The normal process of cellular differentiation ultimately leads to an adult, "terminally" differentiated cell that cannot, under ordinary circumstances, divide again. These fully differentiated cells carry out the recognizable functions of most tissues in the body. Carcinogenesis alters cells to produce a state of increased proliferation and decreased differentiation; the genes controlling cell proliferation are inappropriately expressed and the genes controlling differentiation are repressed.

As tissues develop, some cells retain the capacity to divide, whereas others divide and then differentiate into cells with a more restricted phenotype.[150] These latter cells are then said to be pluripotent rather than totipotent, that is, they are now committed to develop into one of the cell types peculiar to their tissue of origin. Embryologists have traditionally defined the commitment of a cell to one general pathway of differentiation rather than another as *determination.* They reserve the term *differentiation* for the final events in which a terminally differentiated cell arises from a pluripotent one. However, biochemically, this is probably an artificial distinction because the total process most likely represents a continuum of biochemical and molecular events leading from a totipotential cell to a terminally differentiated one. The final characterization of differentiation requires the identification of the particular biochemical events that led to the uniquely specialized adult cell.

By definition, the process of differentiation requires a heritable alteration in the pattern of gene readout in one of the two progeny cells arising from the same parent cell. Because all the cells in the body are derived from a single cell, the fertilized ovum, this process must entail the expression of characteristics in one progeny cell that are not expressed in the other progeny cell from the same parent cell. This process must continue to occur throughout embryonic development to generate the wonderful diversity of cell types present in the adult organism.

The discovery of human embryonic stem cells[27] and embryonic germ cells,[151] and recent data showing that even adult tissues such as brain, liver, and muscle contain stem cells that can be induced to differentiate into a variety of cell types,[152] has drastically altered the question: What is a stem cell? These findings indicate that the plasticity of certain cells in adult tissues is far beyond what was imagined a few years ago. It also raises the question of what is the target cell for the malignant transformation process. If these pluripotent stem cells are present in all tissues in the body, why are not all tissues equally susceptible to carcinogenesis? Yet we know that brain tumors and sarcomas, although not rare, occur much less often than epithelial cell tumors (carcinomas) and that cancers of heart muscle are very rare. One explanation is that muscle cells and brain cells are less exposed to environmental agents and hormonal influences that can activate the carcinogenic process. There are data, however, that damage to these tissues can activate endogenous stem cells to proliferate and move to areas of the lesion.[153] These data imply that these same cells would also be susceptible to carcinogenic damage because they are the cells that have the proliferative capacity to undergo mutagenic damage as they replicate their DNA. This also raises the question of the ability of cells in adult tissues to de-differentiate in response to tissue damage and the question of whether stem cells in adult tissues are really de-differentiated adult cells. The answer to these questions will affect how one approaches the field of cancer prevention, initiation, progression, and treatment because it depends on the cell type being targeted. If we learn that the origin of cancer is a stem cell, then this cell must be isolated, studied, and characterized for treatments to be effective.

Induction of Differentiation in Cancer Cells There are a number of examples of animal malignant tumors or human cancer cells in culture that can be induced to lose their malignant phenotype by treatment with certain differentiation-inducing agents. These include induction of differentiation of the Friend virus-induced murine erythroleukemia by dimethyl sulfoxide (DMSO); differentiation of murine embryonal carcinoma cells by exposure to retinoic acid, cAMP analogues, hexamethylene bisacetamide, or sodium butyrate; and differentiation of human acute promyelocytic (HL-60) cells in culture by a number of anticancer drugs, sodium butyrate, DMSO, vitamin D3, phorbol esters, or retinoic acid analogues.[154]

Being able to treat cancer through induction of cellular differentiation is an attractive idea, because the therapy could be target-cell specific and most likely be much less toxic than standard chemotherapeutic agents. The best example of this is the treatment of APL in patients with all-*trans*-retinoic acid. A more recent example is induction of solid tumor differentiation by the peroxisome proliferator–activated receptor γ (PPARγ) ligand troglitazone in patients with liposarcoma.[155] PPARγ is a nuclear receptor that forms a heterodimeric complex with the retinoid X receptor (RXR). This complex binds to specific recognition sequences on DNA and, after binding ligands for either receptor, enhances transcription differentiation-inducing genes, including those for the adipocyte-specific pathway. PPARγ appears to act as a tumor suppressor in the prostate and thyroid gland, but not in the colon, where its actions are more complex.[156] Nevertheless, agents that can exploit the proliferation-inhibiting effects of PPARγ in cancer tissue and have minimal metabolic side effects may be good targets for drug discovery.

BIOCHEMISTRY OF SIGNAL-TRANSDUCTION

This topic is covered in further detail in Chapter 5. A large number of growth factors, cytokines, hormones, and exogenous chemicals can trigger cellular responses via receptor-mediated events that foster cellular proliferation and/or differentiation. Sometimes these factors do both. The intracellular signaling pathways that accomplish this are varied and complex. Frequently, these pathways are inappropriately activated in cancer cells by either inappropriate expression of an oncogene coding for a growth factor, a growth factor receptor, or components of intracellular signaling pathways. There is significant cross talk between these signaling pathways such that up- or downregulation of one of them may trigger responses in another one. Thus, inhibition of one component of a signal-transduction pathway may be compensated by upregulation of another. This has important therapeutic implications because a drug that blocks an early or upstream component of a given pathway may be circumvented by activation of another parallel pathway. A goal, then, is to try to target the downstream events where transduction pathways converge in their ability to stimulate gene activation events. Alternatively, if a cancer is driven by a single or limited alteration in signal transduction (eg, bcr-abl kinase in chronic phase CML), targeting an upstream signaling mechanism can be effective.

An example of the cross talk among ligand-receptor triggered events is the binding of platelet-derived growth factor (PDGF) to its receptor R-PDGFR.[157] This induces dimerization of the receptor, which, in turn, triggers signal-transduction pathways. The PDGF receptor becomes autophosphorylated on multiple tyrosines by activation of its receptor tyrosine kinase. This fosters binding to specific Src homology 2 domain (SH2)-containing proteins that are part of the Grb2-Sos-Ras-Raf-Mek-Erk pathway. In addition, there is cross talk with the phosphatidyl inositol kinase (PI3K) pathway. PI3K can also stimulate Rac guanosine triphosphatase (GTPase), which can activate JAK/STAT signaling events. Activation of the SH2 domain protein PLC-γ1 can also potentially stimulate protein kinase C (PKC) signaling pathways. Thus, cytoplasmic signaling proteins form networks of interactions rather than simple linear pathways.[157] These diverse signaling pathways, in turn, induce broadly overlapping sets of genes.[158]

Guanosine triphosphate (GTP)-binding protein (G-protein) signaling events are another ubiquitous pathway for gene activation, some of which are mediated by cAMP and have protean effects on cellular processes.[159] Mutations in components of G-protein coupled pathways have been observed, some of which appear to be involved in a number of human diseases, including tumor formation.[159,160]

Alterations of other signal-transduction pathways also correlate with malignant transformation. For example, cellular transforming events induced by the viral oncogene v-*fps* correlate with activation of the endogenous STAT3 signal-transduction pathway.[161] TGF-β signaling is mediated via the SMAD family of transducer proteins, and somatic mutations of one of these, SMAD4, are frequently observed in pancreatic cancers and, less frequently, in colon, breast, and lung cancers.[162] Functionally disruptive mutations of SMAD2 have been observed in colorectal and lung cancers.

These observations increase the long list of signal-transduction components that are known to be altered in cancer, such as Ras, Myc, Src, and Erb B.[159] Thus, it is clear that disruption of signal-transduction pathways is a commonly observed event in human cancer and provides a target for therapeutic intervention.

Many signal transduction events involve phosphorylation steps including (1) receptors coupled to tyrosine kinase activity; (2) receptors coupled to guanine nucleotide-binding proteins, which, in turn, may activate or inhibit adenylate cyclase, activate phosphoinositide hydrolysis leading to protein kinase C activation and intracellular Ca^{2+} release, or modulate cell membrane ion channels; and (3) intracellular receptors, such as those for steroid hormones, thyroid hormone, and retinoic acid, all of which have DNA-binding domains, as well as ligand-binding domains, and can interact directly with DNA to modulate gene transcription. All of these receptor-mediated signal transduction mechanisms are potential sites for upregulation or deregulation in cancer cells, for example, by oncogene activation or overexpression or by tumor-suppressor gene inactivation.

Protein Kinases Both tyrosine- and serine/threonine-protein kinases play critical roles in cancer. Prototypes include the mitogen activated protein kinases (serine/threonine) and receptor coupled/oncogene kinases (tyrosine). Many growth factor receptors mediate their cellular effects by intrinsic tyrosine kinase activity, which, in turn, may phosphorylate other substrates involved in mitogenesis. A number of transforming oncogene products have growth factor or growth factor receptor–like activities that work via a tyrosine kinase–activating mechanism. For example, the *v-src* gene product is itself a cell membrane associated tyrosine kinase. The *v-sis* oncogene product is virtually homologous to the β chain of PDGF. The *v-erb* product is a truncated form of the epidermal growth factor (EGF) receptor. The *fms* gene product is analogous to the receptor for CSF-1. The *met* and *trk* proto-oncogene products are receptors for hepatocyte growth factor (HGF) and nerve growth factor (NGF), respectively. In chronic myelogenous leukemia (CML), the BCR-ABL translocation that causes activation of this RTK in CML can be inhibited by imatinib (Gleevec).[163] Because this agent has relatively specific activity versus BCR-ABL and *c-kit,* this has led to the development of other specific, targeted agents that promise to improve the therapeutic index of anticancer chemotherapy.

Some of the key substrates for receptor–tyrosine kinase-coupled activity are (1) phospholipase Cγ (PLCγ), which activates phosphatidyl inositol hydrolysis, releasing the second messengers diacylglycerol (DAG) and inositol triphosphate (INSP3) that activate PKC and mobilize intracellular calcium release, respectively (a number of tumor promoters also activate PKC); (2) the GTPase-activating protein (GAP) that modulates *ras* proto-oncogene protein function; (3) *src*-like tyrosine kinases; (4) PI3K that associates with and may modulate the transforming activity of polyoma middle T antigen and the *v-src and v-abl* gene products; and, (5) the *raf* proto-oncogene product that is itself a serine/threonine protein kinase.

Thus, activation of protein kinases is a key mechanism in regulating signals for cell proliferation. The substrates of these kinases include transcription regulatory factors, such as those linked to mitogenic signaling pathways, for example, proteins encoded by the *jun, fos, myc, myb, rel,* and *ets* proto-oncogenes.

The ErbB (HER) family of receptor tyrosine kinases (RTKs) are important therapeutic targets.[164–166] Four members of this family of RTKs have been identified: epidermal growth factor receptor (EGFR, or ErbB1, HER1), ErbB2 (HER2, Neu), ErbB3 (HER3), and ErbB4 (HER4). These receptors share an amino acid homology of 40 to 50% and have common functional characteristics, yet differences in expression in various tissues and different phenotypes observed in knockout mice indicate that they have non-redundant functions. At least 25 ligands, with different binding affinities, are known for various members of this family. However, no high-affinity ligand specific for ErbB2 is known. When these RTKs are activated, they, in turn, activate a number of downstream signaling partners (eg, the MAP kinases ERK1/2) that induce a variety of cellular events that regulate cell proliferation and differentiation.

Dysregulated function and/or overexpression of the ErbB family are observed in a wide variety of human cancers, including breast, prostate, lung, ovarian, and renal cancers, as well as glioblastomas. Therapeutic modalities aimed at blocking the dysregulated activities of these receptors include small molecules such as erlotinib (Tarceva) and gefitinib (Iressa)[164,165] and antibodies such as trastuzumab (Herceptin) and cetuximab (Eribtiux), targeted at ErbB2 in breast cancer and EGFR in colon cancer.[167]

A recent observation links various levels of activation of EGFR to different cellular functions. It was observed that the EGFR-mediated effects on DNA synthesis, cell adhesion, and cell motility differ depending on levels of saturation of the receptor.[166] For example, even though exogenously added EGF has no additional effects on DNA synthesis that is already maximally stimulated by subsaturating levels of EGFR occupation by endogenous ligand, added EGF can still induce integrin expression, integrin-mediated adhesion, and motility in cultured human colon cancer cells. These data suggest that these activities may be additional targets for EGFR-modulating agents.

Lipid Kinases PI3-kinase catalyzes the conversion of phosphatidylinositol 4-phosphate and phosphatidylinositol (4,5)-bisphosphate to phosphatidylinositol (3,4)-bisphosphate and phosphatidylinositol (3,4,5)-trisphosphate, respectively, thereby generating phosphoinosides that can signal and/or attract enzymes such as Akt to the plasma membrane. The activation of PI3-kinase in normal cells is dependent on the control of growth factor: receptor interactions, but can be autonomous in cancers. The phosphorylation of Akt by PI3-kinase can activate pathways that promote cell growth and inhibit cell death. The activity of PI3-kinase and Akt are normally balanced by the opposing effects of protein phosphatases.

Protein Phosphatases Protein phosphatases (PTPases) play a regulatory role in certain cellular metabolic functions such as the activation–inactivation steps for glycogen synthase and phosphorylase. PTPases also play a role in the activity of various receptors and in the function of certain cell-cycle regulating genes. For example, expression of a truncated, abnormal protein tyrosine phosphatase in BHK cells produces multinucleated cells, possibly by dephosphorylating the cyclin-dependent kinase $p34^{cdc2}$. Activation of $p34^{cdc2}$ requires dephosphorylation of a tyrosine residue, and this activation drives the cell from the G2 into the M phase. The truncated phosphatase apparently interferes with the normal synchrony between nuclear formation and cell division.

PTPases are a diverse family of enzymes that exist in cell membranes and in intracellular locations. Some are associated with receptors that have tyrosine kinase activity. The aberrant phosphorylation state of tyrosine in certain key proteins, such as c-Src or c-Raf, that can lead to cellular transformation could theoretically come about as a result of deregulation of a protein kinase or underexpression of a protein phosphatase. For example, cells treated with vanadate, a PTPase inhibitor, have increased protein phosphotyrosine levels and a transformed phenotype.[168] Further evidence that PTPases are involved in cancer is the observation that a receptor-linked PTPase located on chromosome 3, which has a deletion in renal cell and lung carcinomas, suggesting that this PTPase gene may act as a tumor-suppressor gene. Thus, one could predict that a high level of expression of specific PTPases may be able to reverse the malignant phenotype, and one can think of strategies, then, to transfect these genes into tumor cells or deliver inducers of the enzymes to tumor cells.

The PTPase PTEN is mutated in human brain, breast, and prostate cancers.[169] This was discovered by mapping homozygous deletions on human chromosome 10q23 that occur at high frequency in human cancers. Mutations of the *pten* gene were detected in 17% of primary glioblastomas, as well as in human-derived cancer cell lines and xenografts of glioblastoma (31%), prostate cancer (100%), and breast cancer (6%). PTEN is a protein tyrosine phosphatase that dephosphorylates PIP3 in the phosphatidyl inositol pathway (AKT/PI3 kinase). Loss of PTEN activity increases PIP3 phosphorylation and leads to cellular transformation. Thus, PTEN is considered to have tumor suppressor function, and this protein and its substrates are potential targets for new therapeutic agents.

An effect of PTPases opposite to that of PTEN has been observed in metastatic human colon cancer. Saha and colleagues[170] have observed that the PRL-3 protein tyrosine phosphatase gene was overexpressed in each of 18 colon cancer metastases, as compared to non-metastatic tumors and normal colorectal epithelium. This somewhat counterintuitive observation reminds us that the dysregulated state of phosphorylation events can have inhibitory or stimulatory effects on the cancer process depending on the cell type and the microenvironment. Nevertheless, it does suggest that enzymes such as that encoded by PRL-3 can be targets for another approach to anticancer drug discovery.

BIOCHEMISTRY OF THE CELL CYCLE

Cell-cycle checkpoints provide “go/no-go” decision points that determine whether a cell progresses to the next cell-cycle phase. Many of the biochemical mechanisms involved in these checkpoint controls have been identified. Most of what we know about cell-cycle regulation originally came from lower organisms, including yeast.[171] One of the first genes identified as an important cell-cycle regulator in yeast was *cdc2/cdc28.* Activation of this kinase requires association with a regulatory subunit called cyclin A. It is now known that sequential activation and inactivation of cyclin-dependent kinases (cdks) is the primary means of cell-cycle regulation.

The role of various cdks, cyclins, and other gene products in regulating checkpoints at G1 to S, G2 to M, and mitotic spindle segregation have been described in detail elsewhere[171–173] and in Chapter 3, “Cell Proliferation and Differentiation”. Alterations of one or more of these checkpoint controls occur in most, if not all, human cancers at some stage in their progression to invasive cancer.

Alteration of the G1/S checkpoint occurs in many human cancers. Cyclin D1 gene amplification occurs in a subset of breast, esophageal, bladder, lung, squamous cell carcinomas, and certain lymphomas. Cyclins D2 and D3 are overexpressed in some colorectal carcinomas. In addition, the cyclin D–associated kinases cdk4 and cdk6 are over-expressed or mutated in some cancers. Mutations or deletions in the cdk4 and cdk6 inhibitor INK4 have been observed in familial melanomas, and in biliary tract, esophageal, pancreatic, head and neck, non–small-cell lung, and ovarian carcinomas. Inactivating mutations of cdk4 inhibitory modulators p15, p16, and p18 have been observed in a wide variety of human cancers. Cyclin E is also amplified and overexpressed in some breast and colon carcinomas and leukemias.

The retinoblastoma gene is an important regulator of the G1/S checkpoint. Phosphorylation of RB by cyclin D–dependent kinase releases RB from the transcriptional regulator E2F and activates E2F function. Inactivation of *rb* by genetic alterations occurs in retinoblastoma and is also observed in other human cancers, for example, small-cell lung carcinomas and osteogenic sarcomas. Mutations in *Rb* increase the expression of enzymes involved in DNA synthesis (dihydrofolate reductase, thymidylate synthase, ribonucleotide reductase) and in experimental systems affect sensitivity to antimetabolite chemotherapeutic drugs.[174]

The *TP53* gene product is an important cell-cycle checkpoint regulator at both the G1/S and G2/M checkpoints but does not appear to be important at the mitotic spindle checkpoint because gene knockout of *TP53* does not alter mitosis. The *TP53* tumor-suppressor gene is the most frequently mutated gene in human cancer, indicating its important role in conservation of normal cell-cycle progression.[175] One of the essential roles of p53 is to arrest cells in G1 or G2 after genotoxic damage, to allow for DNA repair prior to DNA replication and cell division. In response to massive DNA damage, p53 triggers apoptosis. Preclinical evidence also suggests that p53 status can affect the sensitivity to drugs and radiation. In most cases, cell lines with wild-type p53 are more sensitive to DNA-damaging drugs.[176] Using homologous recombination to delete p53, it was shown that p53 affected sensitivity to fluoropyrimidines.[177] Because p53 transcriptionally regulates numerous genes through activation or repression, the status of p53 can also have effects on antimicrotubule drugs and irradiation.[178]

The spindle assembly checkpoint machinery involves genes called *bub* (budding uninhibited by benomyl) and *mad* (mitotic arrest-deficient).[173] There are three *bub* genes and three *mad* genes involved in the formation of this checkpoint complex. A protein kinase called Mps1 also functions in this checkpoint function. The chromosomal instability, leading to aneuploidy in many human cancers, appears to be caused by defective control of the spindle assembly checkpoint. Mutant alleles of the human *bub1* gene have been observed in colorectal tumors displaying aneuploidy. Mutations in these spindle checkpoint genes may also result in increased sensitivity to drugs that affect microtubule function because drug-treated cancer cells do not undergo mitotic arrest and go on to die.

FUTURE DIRECTIONS OF CANCER BIOCHEMISTRY

The ability to generate robust data from cells, tissues, and whole organisms will inevitably lead to further integration of biochemistry with other areas of science. Efforts are underway to understand the entire spectrum of enzyme reactions through identifying and characterizing all protein kinases at the genetic, biochemical, and structural levels. Understanding how the cell integrates these reactions to convert substrate to product and how the steady-state is disrupted in disease will be the challenge of the future. The direction that biochemistry is moving is exemplified by the new area of metabolomics.

METABOLOMICS Genomics is the global study of gene expression, transcriptomics the genome wide study of mRNA, and proteomics the study of protein expression. Metabolomics is the study of the metabolome, the repertoire of biochemicals, or small molecules that are produced by cells and tissues. The metabolome represents the final products of interactions among gene expression, protein expression, and the environment. Estimates indicate that there may be as few as 2,500 small molecules in the human metabolome. Metabolite profiles are often generated by high-throughput NMR and mass spectroscopy. Stable isotope-based dynamic metabolic profiling is also used to study metabolic fluxes (fluxomics). Metabolomics is being applied to tumor cells and to biofluids (blood and urine) from patients with cancer with a goal of attempting to link genetic alterations associated with transformation to downstream metabolic changes. For example, recent studies have demonstrated that K-Ras mutations at codon 12 are associated with increased glycolysis, whereas codon 13 mutants increase oxidative pentose phosphate pathway activity and pyruvate dehydrogenase flux.[179] In other studies, functional genomics has been combined with metabolomics to identify features of neuroendocrine cancers that have a poor outcome.[180] Metabolomics is also being used to study the effects of anticancer agents. In this context, treatment of myeloid leukemia cells with imatinib is associated with increased glucose carbon flow toward nucleic acid and fatty acid synthesis.[181] Although still at the earliest of stages, metabolomics has the potential to provide new biomarkers for the diagnosis and monitoring of cancer, and to identify new therapeutic targets for anticancer drug discovery.

REFERENCES

1. Balmain A. Cancer genetics: from Boveri and Mendel to microarrays. Nat Rev 2001;1:77–82.
2. Avery OT, MacLeod CM, McCarty M. Studies on the chemical nature of the substance inducing transformation of pneumococcal types. Induction of transformation by a deoxyribonucleic acid fraction isolated from *Pneumococcus* type III. J Exp Med 1944;79:137–58.
3. Watson JD, Crick FHC. Molecular structure of nucleic acids. A structure for deoxyribose nucleic acid. Nature 1953;171:964–9.
4. Earle WR. Production of malignancy in vitro. IV. The mouse fibroblast cultures and changes in the living cells. J Natl Cancer Inst 1943;4:165–212.
5. Stehelin D, Guntaka RV, Varmus HE, Bishop JM. Purification of DNA complementary to nucleotide sequences required for neoplastic transformation of fibroblasts by avian sarcoma viruses. J Mol Biol 1976;101:349–65.
6. Cavenee WK, Dryja TP, Phillips RA, et al. Expression of recessive alleles by chromosomal mechanisms in retinoblastoma. Nature 1983;305:779–84.
7. Knudson AG. Two genetic hits (more or less) to cancer. Nat Rev 2001;1:157–62.
8. Lynch HT, Harris RE, Guirgis HA, et al. Familial association of breast/ovarian carcinomas. Cancer 1978;41:1543–9.
9. Nowell PC, Hungerford DA. A minute chromosome in human chronic granulocytic leukemia. Science 1960; 132:1497–503.
10. Rowley JD. A new consistent chromosomal abnormality in chronic myelogenous leukemia identified by quinacrine fluorescence and Giemsa staining. Nature 1973;243:290–3.
11. Hartwell L, Weinert T. Checkpoints: controls that ensure the order of cell cycle events. Science 1989;246:629–34.
12. Hengartner MO, Horvitz HR. Programmed cell death in *C. elegans*. Curr Opin Genet Dev 1994;4:581–6.
13. Norburg C, Nurse P. Animal cell cycles and their control. Ann Rev Biochem 1992;61:441–70.
14. Sutherland EW. Studies on the mechanism of hormone action. Science 1972;177:401–8.
15. Hait WN, Weiss B. Increased cyclic nucleotide phosphodiesterase activity in leukaemic lymphocytes. Nature 1979;259:321–3.
16. Warburg O. The metabolism of tumors. London: Arnold Constable; 1930.
17. Edinger AL, Thompson CB. Akt maintains cell size and survival by increasing mTOR-dependent nutrient uptake. Mol Biol Cell 2002;13:2276–88.
18. Fliss MS, Henning U, Caballero OL, et al. Facile detection of mitochondrial DNA mutations in tumors and bodily fluids. Science 2000;287:2017–9.
19. Liu VWS, Shi HH, Cheung ANY, et al. High incidence of somatic mitochondrial DNA mutations in human ovarian carcinomas. Cancer Res 2001;61:5998–6001.
20. Miller EC, Miller JA. The presence and significance of bound aminoazo dyes in the livers of rats fed *p*-dimethylaminoazobenzene. Cancer Res 1947;7:468–80.
21. Potter VR. The biochemical approach to the cancer problem. Fed Proc 1958;17:691–8.
22. Potter VR. Biochemical perspectives in cancer research. Cancer Res 1964;24:1085–98.
23. Morris HP. Studies in the development, biochemistry, and biology of experimental hepatomas. Adv Cancer Res 1965;9:227–42.
24. Weinhouse S. Glycolysis, respiration, and anomalous gene expression in experimental hepatomas: G.H.A. Clowes memorial lecture. Cancer Res 1972;32:2007–17.
25. Weber G. Enzymology of cancer cells (part one). N Engl J Med 1977;296:486–93.
26. Knox WE. Enzyme patterns in fetal, adult, and neoplastic rat tissues. 2nd ed. Basel: S. Karger; 1976.
27. Reya T Morrison, SJ, Clarke, MF, Weissman IL. Stem cells, cancer, and cancer stem cells. Nature 2001;414:105–11.
28. Kondo T, Setoguchi T, Taga T. Persistence of a small subpopulation of cancer stem-like cells in the C6 glioma cell line. Proc Natl Acad Sci U S A 2004;101:781–6.
29. Dontu G, Abdallah WM, Foley JM, et al. In vitro propagation and transcriptional profiling of human mammary stem/progenitor cells. Genes Dev 2003;17:1253–70
30. Thomson JA, Itskovitz-Eldor J, Shapiro SS, et al. Embryonic stem cell lines derived from human blastocysts. Science 1998;282:1145–7.
31. Hahn WC, Counter CM, Lundberg AS, et al. Creation of human tumor cells with defined genetic elements. Nature 1999;400:464–8.
32. Bissell MJ, Radisky D. Putting tumours in context. Nat Rev Cancer 2001;1:46–54.
33. Ruddon RW. Cancer biology. 3rd ed. New York: Oxford University Press; 1995. p. 96–140.
34. Hayflick L. The limited in vitro lifetime of human diploid cell strains. Exp Cell Res 1965;37:614–36.
35. Blackburn EH. Switching and signaling at the telomere. Cell 2001;106:661–73.
36. Shay JW, Bacchetti S. A survey of telomerase in human cancer. Eur J Cancer 1997;33:787–91.
37. Hodes R. Molecular targeting of cancer: telomeres as targets. Proc Natl Acad Sci U S A 2001;98:7649–51.
38. Bodnar AG, Ouellette M, Frolkis M, et al. Extension of life span by introduction of telomerase into normal human cells. Science 1998;279:349–52.
39. Abercrombie M, Heaysman JEM. Social behavior of cells in tissue culture II. Monolayering of fibroblasts. Exp Cell Res 1954;6:293–306.
40. Dulbecco R. Topo inhibition and serum requirement of transformed and untransformed cells. Nature 1970;227:802–6.
41. Holley RW, Kiernan JA. Contact inhibition of cell division in 3T3 cells. Proc Natl Acad Sci U S A 1968;60:300–4.
42. Jainchill J, Todaro GJ. Stimulation of cell growth in vivo by serum with and without growth factor; relation to contact

inhibition and viral transformation. Exp Cell Res 1970;59:137–46.
43. Smith HS, Scher CD, Todaro GJ. Induction of cell division in medium lacking serum growth factor by SV40. Virology 1971;44:359–70.
44. Graeber TG, Eisenberg D. Bioinformatic identification of potential autocrine signaling loops in cancers from gene expression profiles. Nat Genet 2001;29:295–300.
45. Sanders FK, Burford BO. Ascites tumours from BHK 21 cells transformed in vitro by polyoma virus. Nature 1964;201:786–9.
46. Alley MC, Pacula-Cox CM, Hursey ML, et al. Morphometric and colorimetric analyses of human tumor cell line growth and drug sensitivity in soft agar culture. Cancer Res 1991;51:1247–56.
47. Donze O, Jagus R, Koromilas AE, et al. Abrogation of translation initiation factor eIF-2 phosphorylation causes malignant transformation of NIH 3T3 cells. EMBO J 1995;14: 3828–34.
48. Edwards DR, Mahadevan LC. Protein synthesis inhibitors differentially superinduce c-fos and c-jun by three distinct mechanisms: lack of evidence for labile repressors. EMBO J 1992;11:2415–24.
49. Herschman HR. Primary response genes induced by growth factors and tumor promoters. Annu Rev Biochem 1991;60:281–319.
50. Savinova O, Joshi B, Jagus R. Abnormal levels and minimal activity of the dsRNA-activated protein kinase, PKR, in breast carcinoma cells. Int J Biochem Cell Biol 1999;31:175–89.
51. Pohjanpelto P. Cycloheximide elicits in human fibroblasts a response characteristic for initiation of cell proliferation. Exp Cell Res 1976;102:138–42.
52. Talha Harel L. Anisomycin and cycloheximide, like growth factors, stimulate rapidly ATP turnover in 3T3 cells. Cell Biol Int Rep 1986;10:249–55.
53. Cano E, Hazzalin CA, Mahadevan LC. Anisomycin-activated protein kinases p45 and p55 but not mitogen-activated protein kinases ERK-1 and -2 are implicated in the induction of c-fos and c-jun. Mol Cell Biol 1994;14: 7352–62.
54. Gressner AM, Wool IG. The stimulation of the phosphorylation of ribosomal protein S6 by cycloheximide and puromycin. Biochem Biophys Res Commun 1974;60:1482–90.
55. Zinck R, Cahill MA, Kracht M, et al. Protein synthesis inhibitors reveal differential regulation of mitogen-activated protein kinase and stress-activated protein kinase pathways that converge on Elk-1. Mol Cell Biol 1995;15:4930–8.
56. Sidhu JS, Omiecinski CJ. Protein synthesis inhibitors exhibit a nonspecific effect on phenobarbital-inducible cytochrome P450 gene expression in primary rat hepatocytes. J Biol Chem 1998;273:4769–75.
57. Kaczmarek L, Surmacz E, Baserga R. Cycloheximide or puromycin can substitute for PDGF in inducing cellular DNA synthesis in quiescent 3T3 cells. Cell Biol Int Rep 1986;10:455–63.
58. Bagaglio DM, Cheng EH, Gorelick FS, et al. Phosphorylation of elongation factor 2 in normal and malignant rat glial cells. Cancer Res 1993;53:2260–4.
59. Ryazanov AG, Shestakova EA, Natapov PG. Phosphorylation of elongation factor 2 by EF-2 kinase affects rate of translation. Nature 1988;334:170–3.
60. Kamada Y, Sekito T, Ohsumi Y. Autophagy in yeast: a TOR-mediated response to nutrient starvation. Curr Top Microbiol Immunol 2004;279:73–84.
61. Inoki K, Corradetti MN, Guan KL. Dysregulation of the TSC-mTOR pathway in human disease. Nat Genet 2005;37:19–24.
62. Arico S, Petiot A, Bauvy C, et al. The tumor suppressor PTEN positively regulates macroautophagy by inhibiting the phosphatidylinositol 3-kinase/protein kinase B pathway. J Biol Chem 2001;276:35243–6.
63. Furuta S, Hidaka E, Ogata A, et al. Ras is involved in the negative control of autophagy through the class I PI3-kinase. Oncogene 2004;23:3898–3904.
64. Pattingre S, Bauvy C, Codogno P. Amino acids interfere with the ERK1/2-dependent control of macroautophagy by controlling the activation of Raf-1 in human colon cancer HT-29 cells. J Biol Chem 2003;278:16667–74.
65. Hardie DG, Carling D, Carlson M. The AMP-activated/SNF1 protein kinase subfamily: metabolic sensors of the eukaryotic cell? Annu Rev Biochem 1998;67:821–55.
66. Inoki K, Zhu T, Guan KL. TSC2 mediates cellular energy response to control cell growth and survival. Cell 2003;115:577–90.
67. Shintani T, Klionsky DJ. Autophagy in health and disease: a double-edged sword. Science 2004;306:990–5.
68. Kuma A, Hatano M, Matsui M, et al. The role of autophagy during the early neonatal starvation period. Nature 2004;432:1032–6.
69. Lum JJ, Bauer DE, Kong M, et al. Growth factor regulation of autophagy and cell survival in the absence of apoptosis. Cell 2005;120:237–48.
70. Boya P, Gonzalez-Polo RA, Casares N, et al. Inhibition of macroautophagy triggers apoptosis. Mol Cell Biol 2005; 25:1025–40.
71. Edinger AL, Thompson CB. Death by design: apoptosis, necrosis, and autophagy. Curr Opin Cell Biol 2004;16: 663–9.
72. Hakomori S-I. Biochemical basis of tumor-associated carbohydrate antigens. Current trends, future perspectives, and clinical applications. Immunol Allergy Clin North Am 1990;10:781–802.
73. Wu HC, Meezan E, Black PH, et al. Comparative studies on the carbohydrate-containing membrane components of normal and virus-transformed mouse fibroblasts. I. Glucosamine-labeling patterns in 3T3, spontaneously transformed 3T3, and SV-40–transformed 3T3 cells. Biochemistry 1969;8:2509–16.
74. Warren L, Fuhrer JP, Buck CA. Surface glycoproteins of normal and transformed cells: a difference determined by sialic acid and a growth-dependent sialyl transferase. Proc Natl Acad Sci U S A 1972;69:1838–42.
75. Ogata S, Muramatsu T, Kobata A. New structural characteristic of the large glycopeptides from transformed cells. Nature 1976;259:580–2.
76. Hakomori S-I. Aberrant glycosylation in cancer cell membranes as focused on glycolipids: overview and perspectives. Cancer Res 1985;45:2405–17.
77. Hakomori S-I. The glycosynapse. Proc Natl Acad Sci U S A 2002;99:225–32.
78. Bertozzi CR, Kressling LL. Chemical glycobiology. Science 2001;291:2357–64.
79. Yamashita K, Tachibana Y, Ohkura T, Kobata A. Enzymatic basis for the structural changes of asparagine-linked sugar chains of membrane glycoproteins of baby hamster kidney cells induced by polyoma transformation. J Biol Chem 1985;260:3963–9.
80. Mizuochi T, Nishimura R, Derappe C, et al. Structures of the asparagine-linked sugar chains of human chorionic gonadotropin produced in choriocarcinoma: appearance of triantennary sugar chains and unique biantennary sugar chains. J Biol Chem 1983;258:14126–9.
81. Takamatsu S, Oguri S, Minowa MT, et al. Unusually high expression of *N*-acetylglucosaminyltransferase-IVa in human choriocarcinoma cell lines: a possible enzymatic basis of the formation of abnormal biantennary sugar chain. Cancer Res 1999;59:3949–53.
82. Holmes EH, Hakomori S-I. Enzymatic basis for changes in fucoganglioside during chemical carcinogenesis: induction of specific alpha-fucosyltransferase and status of an alpha-galactosyltransferase in precancerous rat liver and hepatoma. J Biol Chem 1983;258:3706–13.
83. Salvini R, Bardoni A, Valli M, Trinchera M. beta 1,3-Galactosyltransferase beta3Gal-T5 acts on the GlcNAcbeta 1→3Galbeta 1→4GlcNAcbeta 1→R sugar chains of carcinoembryonic antigen and other N-linked glycoproteins and is down-regulated in colon adenocarcinomas. J Biol Chem 2001;276:3564–73.
84. Bolscher JGM, Schaller DCC, von Rooy H, et al. Modification of cell surface carbohydrates and invasive behavior by an alkyl lysophospholipid. Cancer Res 1988;48:977–82.
85. Kijima-Suda I, Miyamoto Y, Toyoshima S, et al. Inhibition of experimental pulmonary metastasis of mouse colon adenocarcinoma 26 sublines by a sialic-nucleoside conjugate having sialyltransferase inhibiting activity. Cancer Res 1986;46:858–62.
86. Wagner HE, Thomas P, Wolf BC, et al. Inhibition of sialic acid incorporation prevents hepatic metastases. Arch Surg 1990;125:351–4.
87. Dennis JW, Koch K, Yousefi S, VanderElst I. Growth inhibition of human melanoma tumor xenografts in athymic nude mice by swainsonine. Cancer Res 1990;50:1867–72.
88. Ostrander GK, Scribner NK, Rohrschneider LR. Inhibition of v-*fms*-induced tumor growth in nude mice by castanospermine. Cancer Res 1988;48:1091–4.
89. Kufe D, Inghirami G, Abe M, et al. Differential reactivity of a novel monoclonal antibody (DF3) with human malignant versus benign breast tumors. Hybridoma 1984;3:223–32.
90. Li Y, Kuwahara H, Ren J, et al. The c-Src tyrosine kinase regulates signaling of the human DF3/MUC1 carcinoma-associated antigen with GSK3β and β-catenin. J Biol Chem 2001;276:6061–4.
91. Li Y, Ren J, Yu W-H., et al. The EGF receptor regulates interaction of the human DF3/MUC1 carcinoma antigen with c-Src and β-catenin. J Biol Chem 2001;276:35239–242.
92. Schroeder J, Thompson M, Gardner M, Gendler S. Transgenic MUC1 interacts with epidermal growth factor receptor and correlates with mitogen-activated protein kinase activation in the mouse mammary gland. J Biol Chem 2001;276:13057–64.
93. Li Y, Liu D, Chen D, et al. Human DF3/MUC1 carcinoma-associated protein functions as an oncogene. Oncogene 2003;22:6107–10.
94. Ren J, Agata N, Chen D, et al. Human MUC1 carcinoma-associated protein confers resistance to genotoxic anticancer agents. Cancer Cell 2004;5:163–75.
95. Raina D, Kharbanda S, Kufe D. The MUC1 oncoprotein activates the anti-apoptotic PI3K/Akt and Bcl-xL pathways in rat 3Y1 fibroblasts. J Biol Chem 2004;279:20607–12.
96. Li Y, Yu, W-H, Ren J, et al. Heregulin targets γ-catenin to the nucleolus by a mechanism dependent on the DF3/MUC1 protein. Mol Cancer Res 2003;1:765–75.
97. Yin L, Huang L, Kufe D, et al. MUC1 oncoprotein activates the FOXO3a transcription factor in a survival response to oxidative stress. J Biol Chem 2004;279:45721–7.
98. Wei X, Xu H, Kufe D. Human MUC1 oncoprotein regulates p53-responsive gene transcription in the genotoxic stress response. Cancer Cell 2005;7:167–78.
99. Yamamoto M, Bharti A, Li Y, Kufe D. Interaction of the DF3/MUC1 breast carcinoma-associated antigen and β-catenin in cell adhesion. J Biol Chem 1997;272:12492–4.
100. Li Y, Bharti A, Chen D, et al. Interaction of glycogen synthase kinase 3β with the DF3/MUC1 carcinoma-associated antigen and β-catenin. Mol Cell Biol 1998;18: 7216–24.
101. Carraway KL, Price-Schiavi SA, Komatsu, M, et al Muc4/sialomucin complex in the mammary gland and breast cancer. J Mammary Gland Biol Neoplasia 2001;6: 323–37.
102. Carraway K, Pamsuer V, Haq B, Carraway C. Cell signaling through membrane mucins. Bioassays 2002;25:66–71.
103. Swartz MJ, Batra SK, Varshney GC, et al. MUC4 expression increases progressively in pancreatic intraepithelial neoplasia. Am J Clin Pathol 2002;117:791–6.
104. Singh AP, Moniaux N, Chauhan SC, et al. Inhibition of MUC4 expression suppresses pancreatic tumor cell growth and metastasis. Cancer Res 2004;64:622–30.
105. Perrais M, Pigny P, Ducourouble MP, et al. Characterization of human mucin gene MUC4 promoter: importance of growth factors and proinflammatory cytokines for its regulation in pancreatic cancer cells. J Biol Chem 2001;276:30923–33.
106. Jonckheere N, Perrais M, Mariette C, et al. A role for human MUC4 mucin gene, the ErbB2 ligand, as a target of TGF-beta in pancreatic carcinogenesis. Oncogene 2004;23:5729–38.
107. Andrianifahanana M, Agrawal A, Singh AP, et al. Synergistic induction of the MUC4 mucin gene by interferon-gamma and retinoic acid in human pancreatic tumour cells involves a reprogramming of signalling pathways. Oncogene 2005; in press.
108. Bast RC Jr, Feeney M, Lazarus H, et al. Reactivity of a monoclonal antibody with human ovarian carcinoma. J Clin Invest 1981;68:1331–7.
109. Yin BW, Lloyd KO. Molecular cloning of the CA125 ovarian cancer antigen: identification as a new mucin, MUC16. J Biol Chem 2001;276:27371–5.
110. Hardingham TE, Sosang AJ. Proteoglycans: many forms and many functions. FASEB J 1992;6:861–70.
111. Sugahara K, Yamashina I, De Waard P, et al. Structural studies on sulfated glycopeptides from the carbohydrate-protein linkage region of chondroitin 4-sulfate proteoglycans of swamp rat chondrosarcoma. J Biol Chem 1988;263:10168–74.
112. Ruoslahti E. Proteoglycans in cell regulation. J Biol Chem 1989;264:13369–72.
113. Lind T, Tufaro F, McCormick C, et al. The putative tumor suppressors EXT1 and EXT2 are glycosyltransferases required for the biosynthesis of heparan sulfate. J Biol Chem 1998;273:26265–8.
114. Yurchenco PD, Schittny JC. Molecular architecture of basement membranes. FASEB J 1990;4:1577–90.
115. Streuli CH, Bissell MJ. Expression of extracellular matrix components is regulated by substratum. J Cell Biol 1990;110:1405–15.
116. Ruoslahti E, Pierschbacher MD. New perspectives in cell adhesion: RGD and integrins. Science 1987;238:491–7.

117. Giancotti FG, Ruoslahti E. Integrin signaling. Science 1999;285:1028–32.
118. Stewart DB, Nelson WJ. Identification of four distinct pools of catenins in mammalian cells and transformation-dependent changes in catenin distributions among these pools. J Biol Chem 1997;272:29652–62.
119. Uemura T. The cadherin superfamily at the synapse: more members, more missions. Cell 1998;93:1095–8.
120. Vermeulen SJ, Bruyneel J, Bracke EA, et al. Cell-cell interactions. Cancer Res 1995;55:4722–8.
121. Guilford P. E-cadherin downregulation in cancer: fuel on the fire? Mol Med Today 1999;5:172–7.
122. Guilford P. E-cadherin germline mutations in familial gastric cancer. Nature 1998;392:402–5.
123. Hao XP, Pretlow TG, Rao JS, Pretlow TP. Beta-Catenin expression is altered in human colonic aberrant crypt foci. Cancer Res 2001;61:8085–8.
124. Brabletz T, Jung A, Reu S, et al. Variable beta-catenin expression in colorectal cancers indicates tumor progression driven by the tumor environment. Proc Natl Acad Sci U S A 2001;98:10356–61.
125. Liotta LA, Kohn EC. The microenvironment of the tumour-host interface. Nature 2001;411:375–9.
126. Ruddon RW. Cancer biology. 3rd ed. New York: Oxford University Press; 1995. p. 410–2.
127. Yan L, Zucker S, Toole BP. Roles of the multifunctional glycoprotein, emmprin (basigin; CD147), in tumour progression. Thromb Haemost 2005;93:199–204.
128. Yang JM, Xu Z, Wu H, et al. Overexpression of extracellular matrix metalloproteinase inducer in multidrug resistant cancer cells. Mol Cancer Res 2003;1:420–7.
129. Berger SL. The histone modification circus. Science 2001;292:64–5.
130. Nakayama J-I, Rice JC, Strahl BD, et al. Role of histone H3 lysine 9 methylation in epigenetic control of heterochromatin assembly. Science 2001;292:110–3.
131. Wang H, Huang Z-Q, Xia L, et al. Methylation of histone H4 at arginine 3 facilitating transcriptional activation by nuclear hormone receptor. Science 2001;293:853–7.
132. Rice JC, Allis CD. Gene regulation: code of silence. Nature 2001;414:258–9.
133. Grunstein M. Histone acetylation in chromatin structure and transcription. Nature 1997;389:349–52.
134. Verdel A, Khochbin S. Identification of a new family of higher eukaryotic histone deacetylases. J Biol Chem 1999;274:2440–5.
135. Wei Y, Yu L, Bowen J, et al. Phosphorylation of histone H3 is required for proper chromosome condensation and segregation. Cell 1999;97:99–109.
136. Sassone-Corsi P, Mizzen CA, Cheung P, et al. Requirement of Rsk-2 for epidermal growth factor-activated phosphorylation of histone H3. Science 1999;285:886–91.
137. DePinho RA. The cancer-chromatin connection. Nature 1998;391:533–6.
138. Lin RJ, Nagy L, Inoue S, et al. Role of the histone deacetylase complex in acute promyelocytic leukaemia. Nature 1998;391:811–4.
139. Feinberg AP, Gehrke CW, Kuo KC, Ehrlich M. Reduced genomic 5-methylcytosine content in human colonic neoplasia. Cancer Res 1988;48:1159–61.
140. Toyota M, Ho C, Ahuja N, et al. Identification of differentially methylated sequences in colorectal cancer by methylated CpG island amplification. Cancer Res 1999;59:2307–12.
141. Esteller M, Sanchez-Cespedes M, Rosell R, et al. Detection of aberrant promoter hypermethylation of tumor suppressor genes in serum DNA from non-small cell lung cancer patients. Cancer Res 1999;59:67–70.
142. Wong IHN, Lo YMD, Zhang J, et al. Detection of aberrant *p16* methylation in the plasma and serum of liver cancer patients. Cancer Res 1999;59:71–3.
143. Goessl C, Krause H, Muller M, et al. Fluorescent methylation-specific polymerase chain reaction for DNA-based detection of prostate cancer in bodily fluids. Cancer Res 2000;60:5941–5.
144. Eads CA, Danenberg KD, Kawakami K, et al. CpG island hypermethylation in human colorectal tumors is not associated with DNA methyltransferase overexpression. Cancer Res 1999;59:2302–6.
145. Bakin AV, Curran T. Role of DNA 5-methylcytosine transferase in cell transformation by *fos*. Science 1999; 283:387–90.
146. Tilghman SM. The sins of the fathers and mothers: genomic imprinting in mammalian development. Cell 1999;96:185–93.
147. Cui H, Horon IL, Ohlsson R, et al. Loss of imprinting in normal tissue of colorectal cancer patients with microsatellite instability. Nat Med 1998;4:1276–80.
148. Barletta J, Rainier S, Feinberg A. Reversal of loss of imprinting in tumor cells by 5-aza-2-deoxycytidine. Cancer Res 1997;57:48–50.
149. Christofori G, Naik P, Hanahan D. Deregulation of both imprinted and expressed alleles of the insulin-like growth factor 2 gene during beta-cell tumorigenesis. Nat Genet 1995;10:196–201.
150. Rutter WJ, Pictet RL, Morris PW. Toward molecular mechanisms of developmental processes. Ann Rev Biochem 1973;42:601–12.
151. Shamblott MJ, Axelman J, Wang S, et al. Derivation of pluripotent stem cells from cultured human primordial germ cells. Proc Natl Acad Sci U S A 1998;95:13726–31.
152. Blau HM, Brazelton TR, Weimann JM. The evolving concept of a stem cell: entity or function? Cell 2001;105:829–41.
153. Temple S. The development of neural stem cells. Nature 2001;414:112–7.
154. Ruddon RW. Cancer biology. 3rd ed. New York: Oxford University Press; 1995. p. 211–20.
155. Demetri GD, Fletcher CDM, Mueller E, et al. Induction of solid tumor differentiation by the peroxisome proliferator-activated receptor-γ ligand troglitazone in patients with liposarcoma. Proc Natl Acad Sci U S A 1999;96:3951–6.
156. Rosen ED, Spiegelman BM. PPARγ: a nuclear regulator of metabolism, differentiation, and cell growth. J Biol Chem 2001;276:37731–4.
157. Pawson T, Saxton TM. Signaling networks—do all roads lead to the same genes? Cell 1999;97:675–8.
158. Fambrough D, McClure K, Kazlauskas A, Lander ES. Diverse signaling pathways activated by growth factor receptors induce broadly overlapping, rather than independent, sets of genes. Cell 1999;97:727–41.
159. Ruddon RW. Cancer biology. 3rd ed. New York: Oxford University Press; 1995. p. 369–73.
160. Farfel Z, Bourne HR, Iiri T. The expanding spectrum of G protein diseases. N Engl J Med 1999;340:1012–20.
161. Nelson KL, Rogers JA, Bowman TL, et al. Activation of STAT3 by the c-Fes protein-tyrosine kinase. J Biol Chem 1998;273:7072–7.
162. Heldin CH, Miyazono K, ten Dijke P. TGF-β signaling from cell membrane to nucleus through SMAD proteins. Nature 1997;390:465–71.
163. Druker BJ, Sawyers CL, Kantarjian H, et al. Activity of a specific inhibitor of the BCR-ABL tyrosine kinase in the blast crisis of chronic myeloid leukemia and acute lymphoblastic leukemia with the Philadelphia chromosome. N Engl J Med 2001;344:1038–163.
164. Moasser MM, Basso A, Averbuch SD, Rosen N. The tyrosine kinase inhibitor ZD1839 ("Iressa") inhibits HER2-driven signaling and suppresses the growth of HER2-overexpressing tumor cells. Cancer Res 2001;61:7184–8.
165. Moulder SL, Yakes FM, Muthuswamy SK, et al. Epidermal growth factor receptor (HER1) tyrosine kinase inhibitor ZD1839 (Iressa) inhibits *HER2/neu* (*erb*B2)-overexpressing breast cancer cells in vivo and in vitro. Cancer Res 2001;61:8887–95.
166. Sawhney RS, Zhou G-HK, Humphrey LE, et al. Differences in sensitivity of biological functions mediated by epidermal growth factor receptor activation with respect to endogenous and exogenous ligands. J Biol Chem 2002;277:75–86.
167. Cobleigh MA, Vogel CL, Tripathy D, et al. Multinational study of the efficacy and safety of humanized anti-HER2 monoclonal antibody in women who have HER2-overexpressing metastatic breast cancer that has progressed after chemotherapy for metastatic disease. J Clin Oncol 1999;17:2639–48.
168. Klarlund JK. Transformation of cells by an inhibitor of phosphatases acting on phosphotyrosine in proteins. Cell 1985;41:707–17.
169. Li J, Yen C, Liaw D, et al. *PTEN,* a putative protein tyrosine phosphatase gene mutated in human brain, breast, and prostate cancer. Science 1997;275:1943–7.
170. Saha S, Bardelli A, Buckhaults P, et al. A phosphatase associated with metastasis of colorectal cancer. Science 2001;294:1343–6.
171. Johnson DG, Walker CL. Cyclins and cell cycle checkpoints. Ann Rev Pharmacol Toxicol 1999;39:295–312.
172. Sherr CJ. Cancer cell cycles. Science 1996;274:1672–7.
173. Orr-Weaver TL, Weinberg RA. A checkpoint on the road to cancer. Nature 1998;392:223–4.
174. Li W, Fan J, Hochhauser D, et al. Lack of functional retinoblastoma protein mediates increased resistance to antimetabolites in human sarcoma cell lines. Proc Natl Acad Sci U S A 1995;92:10436–40.
175. Levine AJ. p53, the cellular gatekeeper for growth and division. Cell 1997;88:323–31.
176. Lowe SW, Ruley HE, Jacks T, Housman DE. p53-dependent apoptosis modulates the cytotoxicity of anticancer agents. Cell 1993;74:957–67.
177. Bunz F, Hwang PM, Torrance C, et al. Disruption of p53 in human cancer cells alters the responses to therapeutic agents. J Clin Invest 1999;104:263–9.
178. Zhang CC, Yang JM, White E, et al. The role of MAP4 expression in the sensitivity to paclitaxel and resistance to vinca alkaloids in p53 mutant cells. Oncogene 1998;16:1617–24.
179. Vizan P, Boros LG, Figueras A, et al. K-ras codon-specific mutations produce distinctive metabolic phenotypes in human fibroblasts. Cancer Res 2005,65:5512–5.
180. Ippolito JE, Xu J, Jain S, et al. An integrated functional genomics and metabolomics approach for defining poor prognosis in human neuroendocrine cancers. Proc Natl Acad Sci U S A 2005;102:9901–6.
181. Boren J, Cascante M, Marin S, et al. Gleevec (STI571) influences metabolic enzyme activities and glucose carbon flow toward nucleic acid and fatty acid synthesis in myeloid tumor cells. J Biol Chem 2001;276:37747–53.

10

Invasion and Metastases

Elise C. Kohn, MD

Invasion and metastasis are the most insidious and life-threatening aspects of cancer.[1–3] The capacity for invasion may not be expressed initially or in all tumors. Those tumors with minimal or no invasion may be extirpated successfully leading to cure in some patients, but this only occurs in tumors with minimal or no invasion. Most cancers, however, gradually unmask their invasive potential: progressing over time to frank malignancy from preexisting carcinoma in situ, adenomas, or disorders of epithelial proliferation. Once the neoplasm becomes invasive, it can disseminate via the lymphatics and/or vascular channels that it induces through tumor-stimulated lymphangiogenesis and angiogenesis and other perturbations of the local micro-environment.[4] Invasion and metastases kill hosts through two processes: local invasion and distant organ colonization and injury. Local invasion can compromise the function of involved tissues by local compression, local destruction, or prevention of normal organ function. The most significant turning point in cancer, however, is the establishment of distant organ colonization. The patient can no longer be cured by local therapy alone at this point.

Our understanding of invasion and metastases continues to improve, but our ability to detect occult metastatic disease or metastatic potential prior to development of occult disease still lags. Commensurate with this is the poor improvement in survival of advanced solid tumor patients. Some patients with cancer have benefited from improved screening techniques that detect early stage cancer. Examples are Papanicolaou (Pap) screening for cervical cancer and mammography for breast cancer. Despite advances in screening, approximately 30% of patients will have clinically detectable metastases at the time of initial diagnosis, and a further 30% of patients will harbor occult metastases. In breast cancer, the relapse rate in stage I disease in patients with less than 1 cm tumors remains 20%, indicating that the development of metastatic potential is an early event. Improved classification of early stage tumors will encourage aggressive treatment for those patients who need it, while withholding treatment from those women for whom it is not necessary (Figure 10-1). Variation in the size and duration of metastases, their dispersed anatomic locations, and their heterogeneous composition over time reflect the dynamic nature of metastasis, hinder complete surgical extirpation of disease, and can limit the effectiveness of many systemic anticancer drugs.

Tumors of comparable size and histology can have widely divergent metastatic potential, depending on their genotype and local environmental influences. Cancer is a disease of signaling. Aberrant signaling is induced by the genetic changes of mutation and transformation and by the local tumor microenvironment. Metastatic potential is influenced by the local microenvironment, angiogenesis, stroma–tumor interactions, elaboration of cytokines by the local tissue, and by the molecular phenotype of the tumor and host cells. This complexity underscores the importance of understanding the molecular events of the metastatic process and using that understanding to develop biomarker panels, through which to predict presence and location of active metastatic disease and occult metastases, and to identify and develop therapeutic targets. The malignant phenotype is thus the culmination of a series of genetic changes in the primary tumor and its metastases through which investigation of the activation, regulation, and manipulation of regulatory elements can be exploited as a new frontier for metastases research. Golub and colleagues postulated that the metastatic phenotype was pre-existent in a tumor. Evidence was obtained using gene expression arrays.[5–7]

Tumor-induced neovascularization and invasion are obligate early events.[1] The angiogenic switch has been shown to precede actual malignant transformation in some cancers.[8] Local micro-invasion can occur early, even though distant dissemination may not be evident or may not yet have begun. Invasion is a more efficient process than metastasis where microinvasion may be ongoing without subsequent entry into the vascular portals of dissemination. Millions of cells are shed into the circulation daily from locally invasive cancer, but only a small fraction (0.01%) are successful at initiating colonies.[1,9,10] Thus, further understanding and molecular dissection of the processes of invasion and metastasis are needed (Table 10-1).

TUMOR–HOST AND TUMOR–STROMAL INTERACTIONS

Cancer is a derangement in the proper sorting of cell populations causing a violation of normal tissue boundaries. Tissue architecture, normally maintained by basement membrane delineation of tissue boundaries and cell–cell communication, suppresses inappropriate intermixing of cells from different tissue types. Normal cells remain confined to their home territory because they are held in check by intercommunication with neighboring cells and the surrounding extracellular matrix. Appropriate sorting of parenchymal tissue cells during morphogenesis and wound healing is tightly regulated by soluble and solid phase stimuli. In contrast, successful malignant tumor cells are resistant to the regulatory signals because they appropriate, misinterpret, or disregard these signals.[4] The process of metastasis is a cascade of linked sequential steps involving multiple host–tumor interactions (Table 10-2). Metastasis is a highly selective competition, favoring the survival of minor subpopulation(s) of tumor cells that pre-exist within the primary tumor.

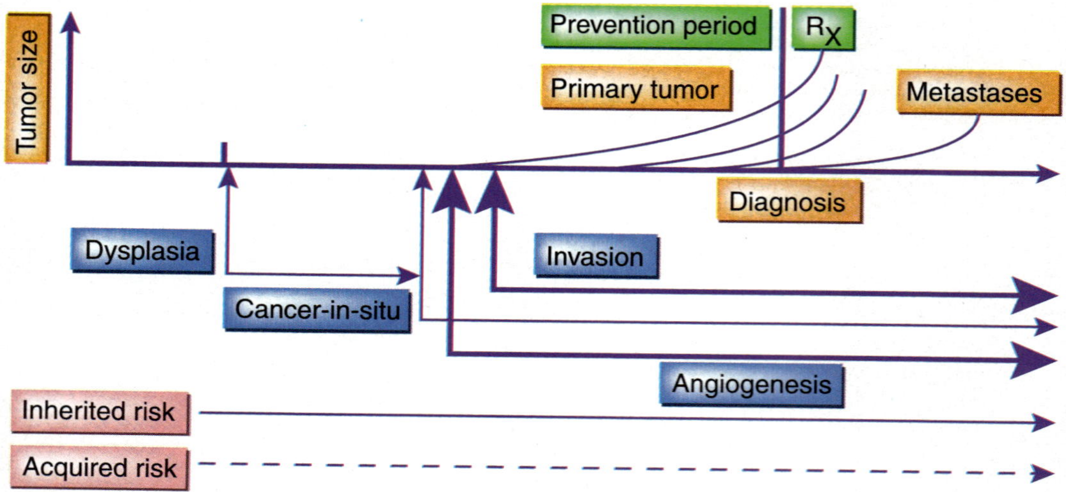

Figure 10-1 Temporal progression of cancer. Diagnosis and treatment of cancer occurs generally late in the course of disease. At this time, a high proportion of patients have obvious or occult metastases. Acquisition of the invasive and angiogenic phenotypes occur very early, in some cancers, perhaps more than 5 to 10 years prior to presentation. This demonstrates a window of opportunity to intervene with anti-invasive and antimetastasis therapies.

Table 10-1 Metastasis Facts

Up to 60% of patients with invasive cancer have overt or occult metastases at diagnosis.
Acquisition of the invasive phenotype is an early event in cancer progression.
Millions of tumor cells are shed daily into the circulation.
Less than 0.01% of circulating tumor cells successfully initiate a metastatic focus.
Angiogenesis is a ubiquitous and early event that is necessary for and promotes metastatic dissemination.
Invasion and angiogenesis use the same signal transduction programs and gene expression cassettes.
Circulating tumor cells can be detected in patients who do not develop overt metastatic disease.
Metastases may be as susceptible to anticancer therapy as their primary tumors.

The distribution of metastases varies widely depending on the histologic type and anatomic location of the primary tumor and the characteristics of the local microenvironment.[1,10] On the one hand, the most frequent organ location of distant metastases in many types of cancers still appears to be the first capillary bed or lymphatic tree encountered by the circulating cells. This explains why lung and liver metastases are the first parenchymal metastases seen from most systemic cancers. On the other hand, there are many metastatic sites that cannot be predicted on the basis of anatomic considerations alone and might be considered examples of organ tropism. The mechanisms for this homing are becoming understood as we learn more about the local microenvironment of the tumor and secondary sites. The predilection of breast and prostate cancers for bone may also reflect a degree of organ tropism and may, in part, be a result of the production and sequestration of osteopontin by the tumor cells.[11,12] This behavior was correlated with tumor aggressiveness and poor prognosis. There are several hypotheses to explain differences in organ tropism. First, tumor cells disseminate equally in all organs but grow selectively only in specific organs where the microenvironment is favorable in the cytokines and growth factors present from the tumor and the stroma.[1,4] Data to support this can be found in the different patterns of growth and dissemination that are observed when subcutaneously implanted xenografts are compared to orthotopic implants.[10] Preferential growth and homing may be induced by the local microenvironment. Second, circulating tumor cells may adhere specifically to the endothelial luminal surface only in the targeted organ and the recent recognition of tissue and tumor-specific endothelium and tumor endothelium specific proteins supports this hypothesis.[13–15] Lastly, immune regulation can regulate local behavior. Increasing evidence shows that bone marrow hemangiogenic precursor cells, CD34 positive marrow cells, can be the source of new vascular cells identified within tumor vasculature.[16] A new role for the immune system is in regulating the microenvironment of the tumor and vasculature. A new mechanism of tumor vasculogenesis is mediated by dendritic cell (DC) precursors through the cooperation of β-defensins and vascular endothelial growth factor-α (VEGF-α).[17] This finding identified a subset of dendritic cell precursors having both leukocyte and endothelial cell markers. Further, this cell subset had a plasticity, the ability to form vascular precursors, for which outcome was microenvironment-specific. This transition into vascular cells and structures was dependent on CCR6 stimulation followed by VEGF action through VEGFR-2, a receptor for which therapeutic interventions have been developed successfully. Accumulating evidence also indicates a more complex role of the immune system in regulating the development of local tumor vasculature.[18] The role of the microenvironment for both stromal cells and the tumor cells is increasingly complex and important and will have an important role in how we rethink therapeutic intervention for invasive and metastatic disease.

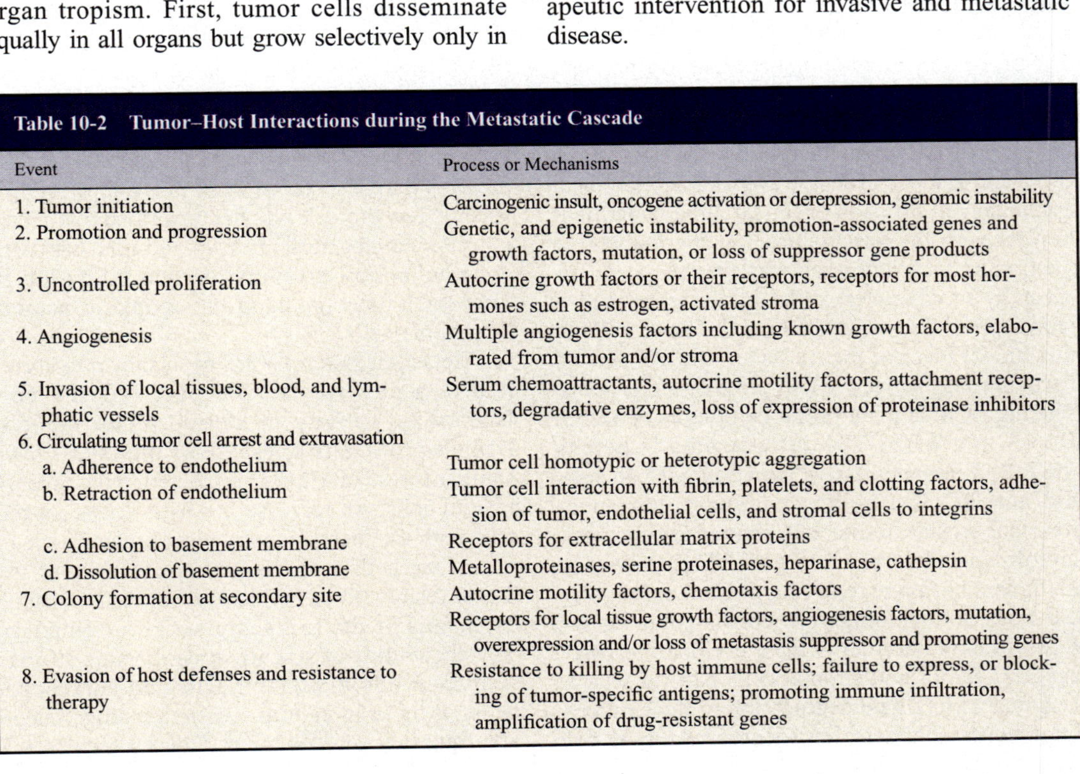

Table 10-2 Tumor–Host Interactions during the Metastatic Cascade

Event	Process or Mechanisms
1. Tumor initiation	Carcinogenic insult, oncogene activation or derepression, genomic instability
2. Promotion and progression	Genetic, and epigenetic instability, promotion-associated genes and growth factors, mutation, or loss of suppressor gene products
3. Uncontrolled proliferation	Autocrine growth factors or their receptors, receptors for most hormones such as estrogen, activated stroma
4. Angiogenesis	Multiple angiogenesis factors including known growth factors, elaborated from tumor and/or stroma
5. Invasion of local tissues, blood, and lymphatic vessels	Serum chemoattractants, autocrine motility factors, attachment receptors, degradative enzymes, loss of expression of proteinase inhibitors
6. Circulating tumor cell arrest and extravasation	
a. Adherence to endothelium	Tumor cell homotypic or heterotypic aggregation
b. Retraction of endothelium	Tumor cell interaction with fibrin, platelets, and clotting factors, adhesion of tumor, endothelial cells, and stromal cells to integrins
c. Adhesion to basement membrane	Receptors for extracellular matrix proteins
d. Dissolution of basement membrane	Metalloproteinases, serine proteinases, heparinase, cathepsin
7. Colony formation at secondary site	Autocrine motility factors, chemotaxis factors
	Receptors for local tissue growth factors, angiogenesis factors, mutation, overexpression and/or loss of metastasis suppressor and promoting genes
8. Evasion of host defenses and resistance to therapy	Resistance to killing by host immune cells; failure to express, or blocking of tumor-specific antigens; promoting immune infiltration, amplification of drug-resistant genes

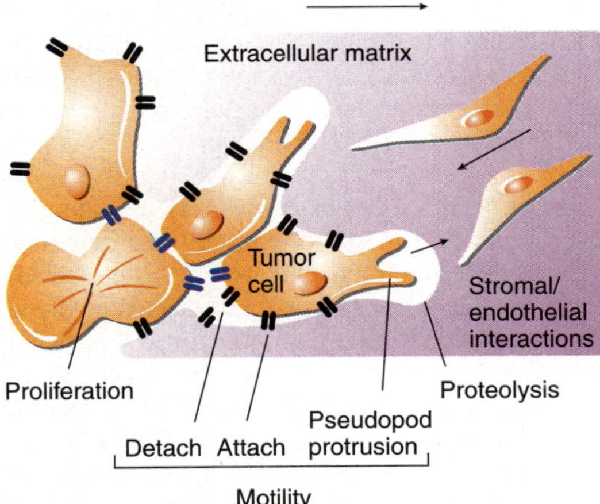

Figure 10-2 Cell invasion of the extracellular matrix. Physiologic or malignant invasion is motility coupled to adhesion and proteolysis. The advancing pseudopod, extended through calcium-regulated actin polymerization, may focus the action of cell surface proteinases, receptors, and activators. Matrix degradation is balanced by endogenous inhibitors of proteolysis to provide adhesive traction and to contain the event to the local microenvironment. Signal-transduction pathways cycle the individual invading cell through pseudopod protrusion, proteolysis, antiproteolysis, adhesion, and detachment.

What constitutes the microenvironment? It is a network of scaffolding made out of collagens, glycoproteins, growth factors, and glycans coupled with the cellular component consisting of the normal stromal elements, fibroblasts, endothelial cells, and immune cells into which the tumor cells invade and grow.[1] The scaffolding materials form structures, such as the basement membrane surrounding epithelial and endothelial structures, that separate tissue compartments. Tumor cells penetrate the basement membrane to enter the underlying interstitial stroma during a transition from in situ to invasive carcinoma.[2,19] This process of invasive behavior and the phenotypic and genotypic changes associated with it is often called epithelial-mesenchymal transition, one with involvement of the transforming growth factor-β/SMAD family of cytokines.[20,21] The basement membrane is a dense meshwork of type IV collagen, glycoproteins, such as laminin, fibronectin, proteoglycans, and embedded growth factors. Loss of continuity of the basement membrane is the distinguishing feature for malignancy. Benign proliferative disorders may have disorganized epithelial-stromal architecture without clear disruption. Extreme forms can mimic the appearance of invasive carcinoma. Thus, the sine qua non of cancer is its capacity for invasion, not unchecked proliferation (Figure 10-2).

ADHESION

Both cell–cell interactions and cell–stroma interactions play an important role during invasion. Connections through cell-adhesion molecules stabilize tissue integrity, whereas loss or alteration of these cell surface proteins is associated with increased metastatic potential. Cell polarity and organization during spreading and migration is regulated by cell interaction with extracellular matrix proteins through the integrin family, and with other cells through the transmembrane glycoprotein cadherins. Activation of these cell surface receptors transmits external signals into the cell and thus directs cell behavior.

Cadherins Cadherins are transmembrane glycoproteins that mediate extracellular calcium-dependent cell–cell interactions.[22–24] E-(epithelial) cadherin, the most extensively studied, is involved in epithelial cell–cell communication. It is found at the cell membrane in adherens junctions in complex with a family of distinct but related cytoplasmic proteins, α and β catenins, and plakoglobin and armadillo.[24,25] Cadherin–catenin complexes are linked to the cytoskeleton through direct interactions between α-catenin and α-actinin.[26,27] E-cadherin functions as a metastasis suppressor molecule in several cell lines and cancer types.[28,29] In these studies, loss of gene expression was correlated with increased invasiveness and metastatic potential, and replacement or augmentation of gene expression resulted in suppression of the invasive phenotype. Loss of E-cadherin in ovarian surface epithelial cells is associated with loss of cell–cell contact and increase in motile and metastatic potential during progression of the transformation of ovarian surface epithelium to ovarian carcinoma.[30] Human breast adenocarcinoma cells (MCF-7), but not normal mammary epithelial cells, induced endothelial cell dissociation, which correlated with the loss of E-cadherin expression at the site of tumor cell–endothelial cell contact.[31]

There are situations in which E-cadherin is normal, but other members of the complex are not. For example, when E-cadherin was expressed in invasive breast cancer MCF-7-10A cells, they exhibited the ability to aggregate, but their morphology was unaltered and the cells remain invasive. These cells had reduced expression of plakoglobin and reduced phosphorylation of β-catenin as compared with the less invasive MCF-7 human breast cancer cells.[32] β-Catenin, under normal conditions, binds to the tumor-suppressor gene product, adenomatous polyposis coli (APC).[33] APC–β-catenin interactions promote APC hyperphosphorylation, resulting in targeted degradation of β-catenin. Alternatively, β-catenin, if not degraded and when not involved in the APC cell adhesion complex, can move into the nucleus where it interacts with T Cell Factor (TCF) family members, stimulating gene transcription and promoting cell proliferation. This complex process also involves the WNT/frizzled pathway.[34,35] Thus, intercellular adhesion mediated by cadherin–catenin complexes or the release of the catenins plays a role in both structural morphology and functional differentiation. Any loss of this control mechanism may facilitate the invasive process.

Integrins The integrins are a family of transmembrane glycoproteins that are expressed by the cell as alpha-beta heterodimers.[36,37] Although originally identified as cell adhesion molecules, integrins are major signaling molecules for inhibition of apoptosis,[38–41] induction of gene expression,[42] and stimulation of cell proliferation,[43] invasion and metastasis,[37,39] and angiogenesis.[44,45] Integrin ligands include a variety of extracellular molecules, such as collagens, laminin, tenascin, fibronectin, vitronectin, von Willebrand factor, and thrombospondin.[26] Integrin signaling depends on the dynamic formation of cellular focal adhesions, specialized sites at which cells form outside-in signaling complexes. These signaling complexes regulate cell shape, migration, and proliferation, and create a framework for the association of important signaling molecules.[46] Protein phosphorylation, mobilization of calcium, and guanosine triphosphate (GTP) exchange are common signals involved in propagation of integrin-mediated information.[47] Integrins also have extensive cross-talk with different classes of transmembrane receptors, such as the receptor tyrosine kinases, allowing propagation of proliferation and invasion messages through multiple mechanisms.[48–51] Further, these proteins have been targeted successfully for therapeutic manipulation.[52]

The integrin αvβ3 plays a fundamental role in angiogenesis and invasion.[53] It mediates cellular adhesion to extracellular matrix proteins and cross-talks with receptor tyrosine kinases, such as the vascular endothelial growth factor (VEGF) receptor-2 and Ephrin A2.[54,55] Activation of this integrin can initiate a calcium-dependent signaling pathway leading to increased endothelial cell motility and proteolysis.[56] Integrin αvβ3 is expressed minimally in normal or resting blood vessels, but is up-regulated significantly on the endothelium of neovessels.[57] It has been targeted for the development of molecular therapeutics.

PROTEOLYSIS

The process of invasion is not a passive process, but rather an active, dynamic process that requires protein synthesis and degradation. Degradation of basement membrane collagen is an early and critical invasion event either for local epithelial cell invasion or for sarcoma dissemination through the vasculature.[2] A chorioallantoic membrane invasion assay was first used experimentally to characterize the importance of proteolysis in the invasive process.[58] Tumor cells in this model invaded the mesenchymal connective tissue through an active and progressive process. The highly malignant breast carcinoma cell lines Hep-3 and MDA-231 intravasated, whereas MCF-7, a less-aggressive breast tumor cell line, did not. PC-3, a highly malignant, hormone-resistant prostate tumor cell, entered the chorioallantoic vasculature, whereas LNCaP, a weakly malignant hormone requiring prostate tumor cell, did not. Both findings are consistent with the more invasive behavior of these hormone-resistant cancers. Tumor and stromal cells have to secrete enzymes to facilitate degradation of the extracellular matrix barriers for successful tumor cell intravasation.[59] Degradation of the basement membrane is not dependent solely on the amount of proteolytic enzymes present but on the balance of activated proteases and their naturally occurring inhibitors. A positive correlation with tumor aggressiveness has been shown for a variety of degradative enzymes, including heparinases, seryl-, thiol- (cathepsins), and metal-dependent enzymes.

Matrix metalloproteases (MMPs) are a family of more than 20 neutral metalloenzymes secreted as latent proenzymes. They require activation through proteolytic cleavage of the amino terminal domain, and their activity depends on the presence of Zn^{2+} or Ca^{2+}.[60,61] Five MMP subclasses have been defined and grouped according to substrate specificity: interstitial collagenases, gelatinases, stromelysins, membrane-type MMPs (MT-MMPs), and elastases.[62] Increased MMP activity has been detected and shown to correlate with invasion and metastatic potential in a wide range of cancers, including ovary, lung, prostate, breast, and pancreatic cancers.[60,63] Type IV collagen is a critical component of the basement membrane architectural scaffolding, on which laminin, heparan sulfate, proteoglycan, and minor components of the basement membrane are assembled. It is classically degraded by MMP-2 (gelatinases) and this was the logic behind using these MMPs as the first therapeutic protease targets.

These enzymes are inhibited by members of the endogenous tissue inhibitor of metalloproteinase (TIMP) family.[64–68] The relationship between the levels of activated MT-MMPs, MMPs, and free TIMPs is a major determinant of the balance between matrix degradation and matrix formation or stabilization in the tumor microenvironment. A positive correlation among MMP-2 activity, TIMP, and tumor cell invasion has been known for a long time.[70] Selectivity can be shown by the example of the action of TIMP-2 but not TIMP-1 on basic fibroblastic growth factor (βFGF)-induced stimulation of endothelial cell proliferation that is independent of its ability to inhibit MMP.[69] TIMPs have now been shown to have multiple MMP-independent activities. These proteins may also act as cytokines and recognize specific receptors. It was demonstrated that TIMP inhibited angiogenesis in vivo and both capillary endothelial cell proliferation and migration in vitro and it functions as an anti-apoptotic factor in lymphoma cells.[69,71,72]

Metastatic potential has been shown to correlate in a positive fashion with type IV collagenolytic activity in murine tumor models. Benign proliferative lesions of the breast have some increase in MMP-2 restricted to the myoepithelial cells. An increase in MMP-2 was associated with the increasing amounts of dysplastic or neoplastic cells with progressive severity of the breast lesions from atypical hyperplasia through carcinoma in situ to frankly invasive carcinoma. This dichotomy of activity is also seen in stroma. Activated fibroblasts and activated endothelial cells, or those in culture secrete a readily detectable quantity of MMP-2.[73] Thus, proteolysis is more a function of local microenvironment remodeling, whether that be due to cancer invasion, immune response, wound healing, or other benign invasive activities.[1] Other metalloproteases, such as stromelysin, matrilysin, and interstitial collagenases, are also important in physiologic and malignant invasion; they proteolyze other matrix proteins and may degrade type IV collagen in the pepsin-sensitive nonhelical domains in a less-specific fashion.

Plasminogen activators (PAs) are serine-specific proteases that convert inactive plasminogen to active plasmin, a trypsin-like enzyme that degrades a variety of proteins, including fibrin, fibronectin, type IV collagen, vitronectin, and laminin. PA exists as tissue-type plasminogen activator (tPA) and urokinase plasminogen activator (uPA). uPA is involved primarily in cell-mediated proteolysis during macrophage invasion, wound healing, embryogenesis, invasiveness, and metastasis, where it has the ability to activate latent collagenases and proplasminogen activators, and to degrade TIMPs.[74,75] uPA directly activates latent growth factors, such as the precursor form of hepatocyte growth factor/scatter factor (pro-HGF/SF) and indirectly latent transforming growth factor (TGF)-β through activation of plasminogen.[76,77] The ability of uPA to activate growth factors suggests its role in modulating extracellular matrix degradation and in tumor cell migration and proliferation. The interaction of uPA and its receptor plays an important role in direct and indirect extracellular matrix degradation, thus potentiating invasive events. uPA binds to specific cell surface receptors (uPAR).[78] Both uPA and its inactive zymogen (pro-uPA) bind with high affinity to uPAR. Expression of uPAR has been shown to be upregulated by a variety of growth factors and tumor promoters.[79–81] High levels of uPA have been observed in human tumors and a multitude of carcinoma cell lines. Elevated expression of uPA and plasminogen activator inhibitor-1 (PAI-1) in tumor extracts has been show to correlate with increased invasion, increased incidence of relapse, and shorter overall survival.[82] Breast cancer expressing high uPA levels has an increased risk for early recurrence and had a poor prognosis, whereas in primary breast cancer, metastasis-free survival can be predicted by uPA levels.[83,84]

The action of uPA can be counteracted by naturally occurring inhibitors including members of the SERPIN (serine protease inhibitor) family, PAI-1, PAI-2, and protease nexin-1 (PN-1).[85] Receptor-bound active uPA is inhibited by PAI-1, PAI-2, and PN-1.[86] Unlike the uPAR–uPA complex which remains stable at the cell surface, the uPAR–uPA-inhibitor complex is internalized quickly by the cell and degraded. PAI-1 is produced primarily by endothelial cells but also by a number of other cell types.[87] Inhibition of endothelial cell migration indicates a role for PAI-1 in blocking neoangiogenesis.[88,89] Cancer cells that overexpress PAI-1 have a decreased ability to degrade ECM (extracellular matrix) and reduced invasive potential. Although a provocative therapeutic target, no agents interrupting the uPA system have been brought to clinical testing.

TUMOR CELL MIGRATION

Migration is necessary early in invasion, whether physiologic or malignant.[1] Immune cells must exit the vasculature and migrate to the site of infection or inflammation, similarly, endothelial cells must migrate from their quiescent home for vascular budding and neoangiogenesis, and tumor cells must migrate from their primary site. The invading cell couples local proteolysis with coordinated and temporally-limited attachment and detachment to achieve forward locomotion. Tumor cells have a motile response to many agents, including host-derived motility and growth factors and cytokines, extracellular matrix components, and tumor-secreted factors.[90–92] Pseudopodia protruding in response to chemoattractants may serve multiple functions, including acting as sense organs for the migrating cell to locate directional clues, to secrete motility-stimulating factors, to provide propulsive traction for locomotion, and to induce matrix proteolysis to assist in the penetration of the matrix.[93,94] Tumor cell migration is dynamic and complex allowing the responding cell(s) to respond to multiple stimuli in additive or synergistic fashions to dictate the direction, location, and magnitude of the migratory response.

Tumor cells secrete factors that function as autocrine motility factors. The first described autocrine motility factor is autotaxin, also known as lysophospholipase D.[95] Autotaxin stimulates tumor cell motility and also was found to induce angiogenesis in xenograft systems. LPA is a potent growth, motility, and angiogenic factor and its pathway the target of many molecular therapeutics.[96–98] LPA is produced, in part, by autotaxin cleavage of lysophosphatidic acid. LPA is therefore a mechanism through which the pro-invasive and pro-angiogenic activity of autotaxin is propagated.

A wide variety of cytokines and growth factors stimulate tumor cell and endothelial cell motility, including the insulin-like growth factors (IGF), HGF, FGF, TGF-β, and cytokines of the CCR and CXC family.[99,100] HGF/SF is a paracrine motility factor that stimulates motility of epithelial and endothelial cells.[101] HGF/SF, the preferred ligand for the *c-met* proto-oncogene product, induces the scatter or chemokinetic locomotion of epithelial colonies, resulting in an invasive phenotype in vivo.[91,102,103] HGF/SF and its receptor *c-met* can play an important role during tumor progression.[104] These factors primarily stimulate chemotactic, or directed, or chemokinetic, random motility and may thus play a role in the tumor cell homing to secondary sites. Therefore, the response of the tumor cell to motility stimulation by autocrine factors, matrix components and host-derived growth factors is important in the initiation of tumor cell locomotion, its directedness, and the determination of the metastatic focus and are thus a potentially important target for molecular therapeutic intervention.

ANGIOGENESIS

Neovascularization, or angiogenesis, covered in more detail elsewhere in this compendium, is a prerequisite for the local expansion of tumor colonies beyond the size restricted by oxygen and nutrient diffusion. Tumor vascularization is, thus, one of the rate-limiting steps for tumor metastasis and growth.[104,105] New capillaries provide cancer cells with conduits for entry into the circulation, nutrition, and exposure to stimulants and modifiers. Angiogenesis is necessary at the beginning and end of the metastatic cascade. The process of blood vessel formation is functionally similar to tumor cell invasion and can be considered as a form of regulated invasion,[1,3] using the same software and hardware as invading tumor cells. Many autocrine and paracrine cytokines and growth factors discussed above for tumors are also important in the local microenvironment as angiogenic factors causing a pleiotropic response of enzyme production, migration, and/or proliferation in endothelial cells. It has been argued that nonvascularized primary tumors may be maintained as dormant, small tumor nodules, kept constant by a balance of cell proliferation and apoptosis,[106] a concept not yet proven clinically. A tumor mass larger than 0.125 mm^3 has outgrown its capacity to acquire nutrients by simple diffusion and must initiate angiogenesis through host vessel initiation of capillary sprouts in the direction of the tumor.[107] Neovascularization is thus a permissive event that allows metastatic dissemination of invasion-competent cells. The parallel between the cellular and molecular biology of angiogenic physiologic invasion and malignant invasion stresses how therapeutics targeted at invasion may have benefits as anti-angiogenic agents.

GENETIC REGULATION OF INVASION AND METASTASIS

Invasion and subsequent metastasis are very complicated multistep processes and not monogenic in molecular origin. Both loss of function/loss of suppressor and gain of function/oncogenic overexpression or overactivation of physiologically important signals combine to regulate invasion and metastasis. The metastatic phenotype requires gain of function pro-invasive and pro-angiogenic events for success. Two classes of invasion and metastasis-associated gene products can be identified: (1) those that regulate outside-in events, and (2) those that provide intracellular regulation.

METASTASIS-SUPPRESSOR GENES The existence of tumor-suppressor genes led to the hypothesis of metastasis-suppressor genes.[70,108–110] The first metastasis suppressor gene was described by Pozzatti and colleagues.[110] Rat embryo fibroblasts transfected with *c-Ha-ras* were highly metastatic on intravenous injection, but cotransfection of rat embryo fibroblasts with *c-Ha-ras* and adenovirus *2 EIA* resulted in transformed, but virtually non-metastatic, cells. *EIA* has been shown to be inhibitory to tumor growth and progression in other preclinical models and was advanced for clinical study. It antagonizes the Akt pathway in its induction of apoptosis.[111,112] Furthermore, studies of TIMP-1 and TIMP-2 show that they have metastasis suppressor and some tumor-suppressor activity.[70]

A major method of identification of candidate suppressor genes has been global unbiased search studies such as differential genomic and genetic expression techniques using invasion and metastasis as the driver.[8,113,114] Two metastasis-suppressor genes identified using these technologies are *nm23* and *KiSS-1*.[108,109,115] Expression of the *nm23* gene encoding a nucleotide diphosphate kinase, has been shown to have a consistent relationship with reduction in metastatic potential. A second example is the *KiSS* gene, encoding the metastatin gene, was identified through somatic chromosome fusion followed by differential gene expression.[116,117] Other genes have been found to have additional function as metastasis suppressor genes, for example mitogen-activated kinase kinase-4.[118,119]

NOVEL TECHNOLOGIES ADVANCE IDENTIFICATION OF METASTASIS AND INVASION-PROMOTING GENES AND GENE PRODUCTS

A major scientific challenge in the study of invasion and metastasis is to mine the physiologic events in situ, thus avoiding the bias caused by culturing cells and animal models. This was difficult prior to the development of new microdissection technologies, such as laser capture microdissection (LCM) (Figure 10-3).[120,121] The scientific community has developed and vetted standardized protocols for fixation, sectioning, LCM procurement, and molecular analysis of DNA, RNA, and protein have been developed and are broadly available. Standardized cell procurement is an advance that has allowed a more clean discrimination and collection of cells of normal, premalignant progression, malignant, invasive, and metastatic disease from which to isolate RNA, DNA, and protein. This has permitted a unique opportunity to compare gene and protein expression, and now, with protein microarrays, the activation state of proteins, at different stages of malignant transformation and invasive progression.[122] The advent of protein microarray technology with both antibody arrays and protein lysate arrays[123,124] has furthered this process, now allowing dissection of the biochemical signaling pathways underlying the progression to the invasive, angiogenic, and malignant phenotype. These may provide crucial clues for etiology, diagnostic markers, and novel therapies tailored individual patients.

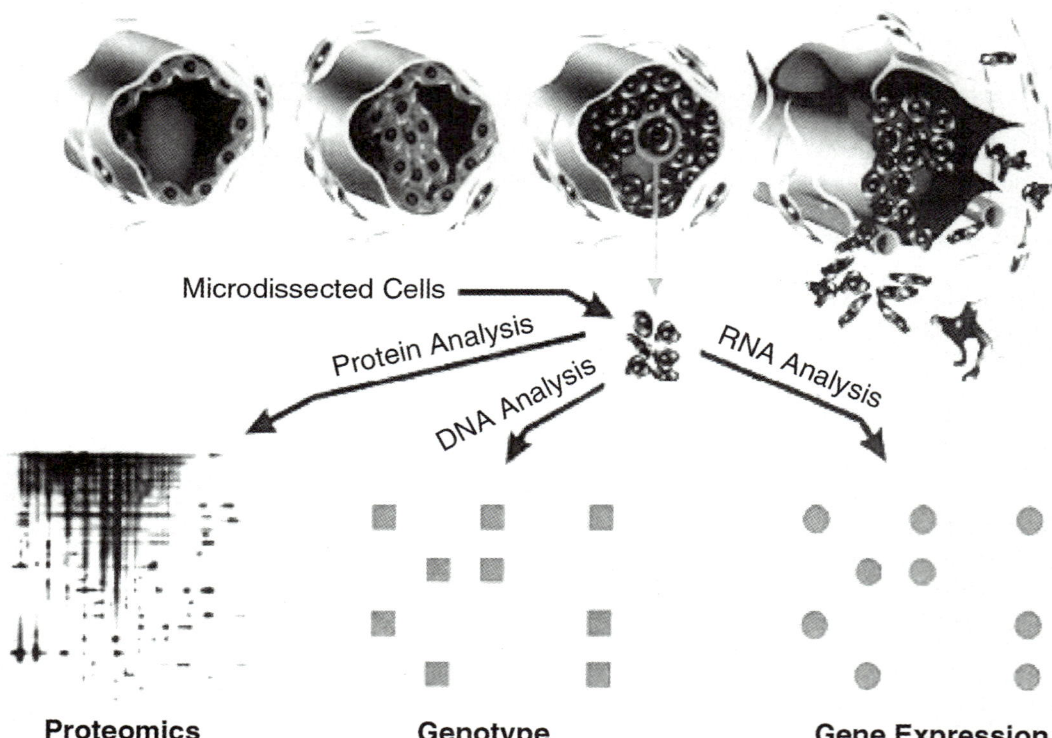

Figure 10-3 Application of microdissection to the study of invasion and metastases. Isolation of involved and stromal cells independently can allow for dissection of the genotypic, gene expression, and proteomic events underlying acquisition of invasive behavior and its use for metastatic dissemination. DNA, RNA, and protein can be retrieved from selectively microdissected cells and applied to two-dimensional electrophoresis, oligonucleotide arrays for genomic analysis, and for cDNA microarrays and establishment of cDNA libraries. Differential analysis of these tools using invasive and metastatic versus noninvasive or nonmetastatic cell materials has already yielded new information in the regulation of cancer dissemination.

INVASION AS A THERAPEUTIC MOLECULAR TARGET

Acquisition of invasive potential is an early event in the malignant process, occurring in both the host and malignant components of the tumor, and is often preceded by local angiogenesis at the in situ cancer. The biochemical events underlying invasion are shared in the different proinvasive cells and thus are logical molecular targets for therapeutic application (Table 10-3 and Figure 10-4).[1,4] Some putative targets of interest previ-

Table 10-3 Metastasis Therapeutic Targets and Agents

A. Target Metastasis Therapeutic Targets and Agents		
Target	Example Agents	Effects
Growth factors	cetuximab (anti-EGFR) erlotinib and gefitinib	Block EGFR signaling, proliferation invasive behavior
	bevacizumab	Block VEGFR signaling by complexing the ligand, reduced vascular proliferation, and remodeling
	Multi target kinase inhibitors such as imatinib, sorafenib	Block PDGFR, kit, abl, raf, VEGFR RTK signaling, vascular and stromal proliferation and invasive behavior
Cell adhesion	Anti-αvβ3 (Vitaxin) αvβ3 peptidomimetics	Blocks endothelial cell interaction with matrix, may regulate MMP activation
Motility	Taxanes	Blockade of microtubule cycling
Signaling	[See below]	Blockade of signals necessary for angiogenesis, invasion, and metastasis
B. Non-Kinase Inhibitor Signal Inhibitors		
Agent	Target	Activity
CAI	Calcium influx	Inhibits tumor and stromal cell adhesion, motility, angiogenesis
Squalamine	Inhibits NHE-3 Na exchange	Anti-angiogenic
LY294002 and analogs	PI3kinase signaling node inhibitor	Inhibits motility, proliferation, survival, angiogenesis
MAPK inhibitors	MAPK signaling node	Inhibit invasion, proliferation

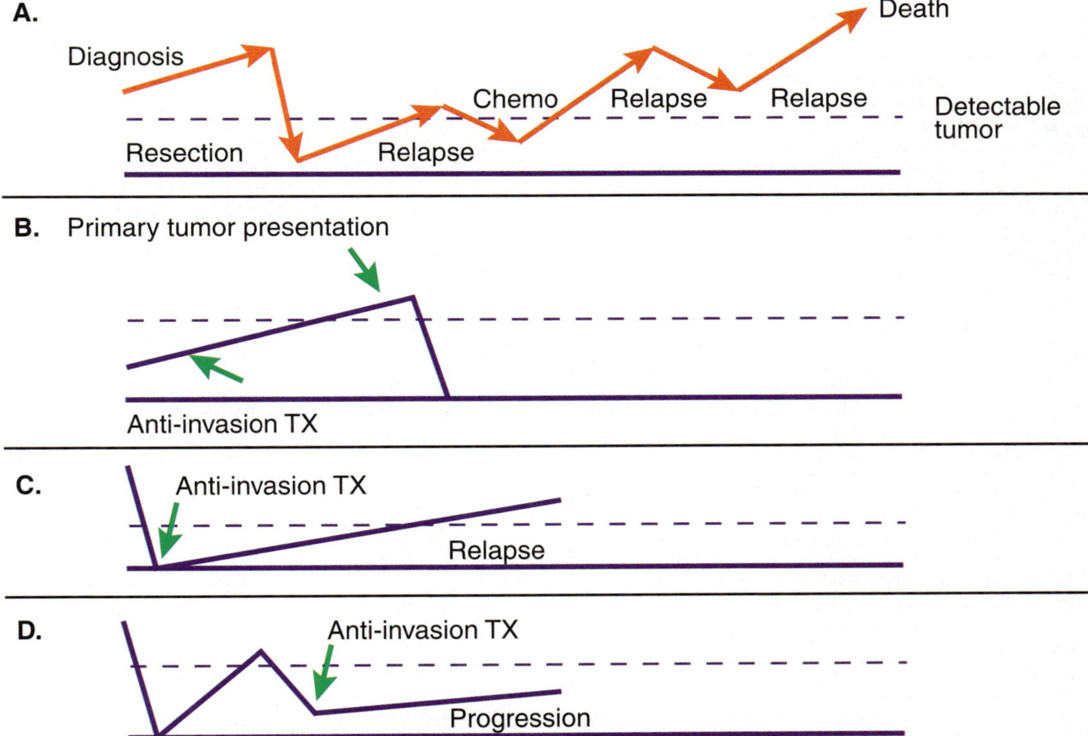

Figure 10-4 Therapeutic uses of anti-invasion therapies. **A,** Time course of solid tumor presentation, response, and progression. **B,** Prevention. Invasion and angiogenesis, which use the same molecular and biochemical processes as malignant invasion, occur early. As such, a preventative intervention can be approached in high-risk individuals. **C,** Adjuvant therapy. At the completion of diagnosis, optimal cytoreduction by surgery and therapies, and anti-invasive therapy may be applied as adjuvant treatment to slow the time to relapse or prevent relapse entirely. **D,** Maintenance. Invasion and angiogenesis are dynamic processes, ongoing throughout the cancer process. Thus, intervention with anti-invasive therapy after optimal treatment or after treatment for relapse may prolong the time to the next relapse and maintain the tumor in a more dormant or slowly progressing state.

ously have been shown not to be effective and are not discussed below.

RECEPTOR TYROSINE KINASE METASTASIS TARGETS AND OTHER KINASE TARGETS

Kinases that lie at nodal intersection points in signaling pathways regulating invasion and angiogenesis are recognized as targetable entities. One of the largest classes of biochemical molecular targets is the family of receptor tyrosine kinases (RTKs). These kinases have been successfully inhibited therapeutically with small molecules that mimic ATP and thus bind at the ATP binding pocket and abrogates kinase function. Another approach to block this class of agents has used monoclonal antibodies to block the receptor or ligand. Receptor tyrosine kinases targeted to date include the EGF receptor, vascular endothelial growth factor (VEGF) ligand and receptor[125,126]; the type III receptor tyrosine kinases (c-kit, abl) and platelet-derived growth factor receptors.[127] Several small molecule EGF receptor (HER1) and EGF receptor family (HER2, 3, 4) kinase inhibitors have been developed and some have been approved for use by the US Food and Drug Administration. These include gefitinib, erlotinib, cetuximab, and trastuzumab.[125,126,128,129] Imatinib mesylate has been shown to be remarkably successful in its inhibition of the bcr-abl fusion kinase in chronic myelogenous leukemia, as well as inhibition of c-kit in gastrointestinal stromal tumors, and dermatofibrosarcoma protuberans.[130–132] A key finding in the studies of imatinib was the rapid reduction in vascular circulation in the tumor bed as imaged using positron emission tomography and dynamic contrast enhanced magnetic resonance imaging. VEGF ligand binding with bevacizumab, and receptor kinase inhibition with sorafenib and other investigational agents has yielded success in several difficult cancers, such as the very vascular clear cell carcinoma of the kidney.[133]

Antiadhesive Agents A limited number of agents that affect tumor or endothelial cell adhesion have entered clinical trials, but several are under development. These include peptidomimetics and monoclonal antibodies that target integrins. Both types of agents have been used against $\alpha v\beta 3$, the vitronectin receptor integrin. $\alpha v\beta 3$ is particularly important because it is selectively present in immature blood vessels.[45,134] Antagonists of $\alpha v\beta 3$ include humanized monoclonal neutralizing antibodies and cyclic peptide derivatives. Blockade of $\alpha v\beta 3$ function causes vascular apoptosis, reducing neovascularization and regulating vascular maturation in preclinical models. This is related to the ability of these antagonists to selectively promote programmed cell death of newly sprouting blood vessels.[135]

Antiagiogenesis Therapies Activated endothelial cells use similar mechanisms for neovascularization of cancers and for vascular remodeling during wound healing but each process has selective components as well. These have been targeted with success and some anti-angiogenic agents are now FDA approved for use in selected cancers. Thalidomide, a cause of profound birth defects when used as a sedative, has shown promise for the treatment of both prostate cancer and multiple myeloma.[136,137] Although described as an anti-angiogenic agent, its actual mechanism of action in patients in these settings is still unclear. Imatinib mesylate, described above as an inhibitor of receptor tyrosine kinases, has clinically evident anti-angiogenic activity. Fluoro-deoxyglucose positron emission tomography (FDG-PET) and dynamic contrast-enhanced magnetic resonance imaging (DCE-MRI) are two techniques that are used to monitor and quantitate vascular flow.[138] Endothelial cell-specific reagents include those targeted at VEGF, including monoclonal anti-VEGF antibody (bevacizumab) and the small molecules directed against the VEGF receptor(s). Bevacizumab has been approved for use in second line therapy in colon cancer.[139] It and other agents, alone and in combination with chemotherapies, are in advanced phase clinical trials against cancers at several sites including lung, renal cell, and ovarian carcinomas. Highly selective inhibitors of VEGF receptors have been studied clinically for some time, but the response has been disappointing. However, a newer series of inhibitors that are more promiscuous in their activity, inhibiting several targets, are more promising. Sorafenib (BAY 43-9006) touted initially as a raf kinase inhibitor has similar activity against VEGFR2.[141] Clinical responses and disease stabilization have been observed in multiple cancer types, especially renal cell carcinoma. Enthusiasm has been renewed with the advent of these newer agents for targeting the vasculature along with improved clinical assessment tools such as FDG-PET and DCE-MRI. These new results have proven that components of the activated local microenvironment within cancers provide druggable targets.

Antimetastasis Signal-Transduction Therapy Therapeutic efforts in cancer prevention and treatment are being focused at the level of signaling pathways or selective modulatory proteins. Protein kinase activities, calcium homeostasis, and oncoprotein activation are driving signals and therefore may be key regulatory sites for therapeutic intervention. Protein kinases C (PKCs) form a family of serine/threonine kinases that mediate phosphorylation events involved in the pathway of many growth factors, matrix components, and neurotransmitters.[142,143] PKC activity has been linked to metastasis in many ways.[144–146] Staurosporine, with general protein kinase inhibitory activity, was shown to inhibit PKC and secondarily inhibit metastasis but was too toxic for clinical application.[147] An analogue of staurosporine, UCN-01,[148] that inhibits a broad range of kinases including cyclin dependent kinases[149] is now in clinical trials and has shown promise as an anticancer agent. Intracellular calcium homeostasis is a common regulator of transmembrane signal transduction and the process of invasion, metastasis, and angiogenesis.[1,150] An inhibitor of non–voltage-gated calcium mobilization and its downstream pathways, CAI (carboxyamido-triazole), was identified through a screen for anti-motility agents and shown also to inhibit angiogenesis.[151–154] Orally administered CAI was well tolerated and cytostatic, with disease stabilization seen in almost half the patients treated, with minor or partial remissions observed in single agent trials and in combination with paclitaxel.[155–157] Consistent with the anti-invasive and anti-angiogenic targets of CAI, more than 80% of patients progressed at sites of existing disease at the time of progression.

Chronic Low-Dose Chemotherapy Treatment A new application of chemotherapy has been proposed to be a more selective anti-vascular therapy with little or no effect on the tumor.[158,159] Benefits have been seen in preclinical models. Some data exist in the literature in small clinical trials to suggest that low-dose chronic applications of anticancer agents may be biologically active in patients, for example, low dose weekly administration of docetaxel or paclitaxel. Whether the clinical trial activity is a result of antiangiogenic activity has not yet been determined.

SUMMARY

The study of molecular mechanisms underlying invasion and its subsequent association with angiogenesis and metastasis has led to dramatic advances in our understanding of cancer and has identified multiple therapeutic targets. Neovascularization, for example, uses the same cassettes of genes and proteins in vascular sprout formation that cancer cells use for invasions, consistent with the observation that anti-invasive drugs can also be antiangiogenic. The dissection of the invasive and metastatic processes has created new directions for cancer marker development and application. Importantly, molecular advances have allowed confirmation that invasion and acquisition of the metastatic phenotype are early events in cancer progression. Further application of this critical knowledge will advance our ability to identify those patients at highest risk for disseminated disease, to better develop therapeutics for those key patients, and, perhaps, to prevent many patients from receiving treatment that they might not have needed.

REFERENCES

1. Kohn EC, Liotta LA. Molecular insights into cancer invasion: strategies for prevention and intervention. Cancer Res 1995;51:1865–2.
2. Liotta LA, Stetler-Stevenson WG. Tumor invasion and metastasis: an imbalance of positive and negative regulation. Cancer Res 1991;51:5054–9.
3. Duffy MJ. Inhibiting tissue invasion and metastasis as targets for cancer therapy. Biotherapy 1992;4:45–52.
4. Liotta LA, Kohn EC. The microenvironment of the tumor-host invasion field. Nature 2001:411:375–9.
5. Ramaswamy S, Ross KN, Lander ES, Golub TR. A molecular signature of metastasis in primary solid tumors. Nat Genet. 2003;33:49–54.
6. Wang Y, Klijn JG, Zhang Y, et al. Gene-expression profiles to predict distant metastasis of lymph-node-negative primary breast cancer. Lancet 2005;365:671–9.
7. Roepman P, Wessels LF, Kettelarij N, et al. An expression profile for diagnosis of lymph node metastases from primary head and neck squamous cell carcinomas. Nat Genet. 2005;37:182–6.
8. Hanahan D, Folkman J. Patterns and emerging mechanisms of the angiogenic switch during tumorigenesis. Cell 1996;86:353–64.
9. Woodhouse EC, Chuaqui RF, Liotta LA. General mechanisms of metastasis. Cancer 1997;80:1529–37.
10. Fidler IJ, Hart IR. Biologic diversity in metastatic neoplasms: origins and implications. Science 1982;217:998.
11. Tuck AB, O'Malley FP, Singhal H, et al. Osteopontin expression in a group of lymph node negative breast cancer patients. Int J Cancer 1998;79:502–8.
12. Tuck AB, Arsenault DM, O'Malley FP, et al. Osteopontin induces increased invasiveness and plasminogen activator expression of human mammary epithelial cells. Oncogene 1999;18:4237–46.
13. Hardwick JS, Yang Y, Zhang C, et al. Identification of biomarkers for tumor endothelial cell proliferation through gene expression profiling. Mol Cancer Ther 2005;4:413–25.
14. Arap W, Pasqualini R. The human vascular mapping project. Selection and utilization of molecules for tumor endothelial targeting. Haemostasis 2001;31:30–1.
15. St Croix B, Rago C, Velculescu V, et al. Genes expressed in human tumor endothelium. Science 2000;289:1197–202.
16. Peters BA, Diaz LA, Polyak K, et al. Contribution of bone marrow-derived endothelial cells to human tumor vasculature. Nat Med 2005;11:261–2.
17. Conejo-Garcia JR, Benencia F, Courreges MC, et al. Tumor-infiltrating dendritic cell precursors recruited by a β-defensin contribute to vasculogenesis under the influence of VEGF-A. Nat Med 2004;10:950–8.
18. Naldini A, Carraro F. Role of inflammatory mediators in angiogenesis. Curr Drug Targets Inflamm Allergy 2005;4:3–8.
19. Liotta LA. Tumor invasion: role of the extracellular matrix. Cancer Res 1986;46:1–7.
20. Valcourt U, Kowanetz M, Niimi H, Heldin CH, Moustakas A. TGF-β and the Smad signaling pathway support transcriptomic reprogramming during epithelial-mesenchymal cell transition. Mol Biol Cell 2005;16:1987–2002.
21. Gershengorn MC, Hardikar AA, Wei C, et al. Epithelial-to-mesenchymal transition generates proliferative human islet precursor cells. Science 2004;306:2261–4.
22. Knudsen KA, Frankowski C, Johnson KR, Wheelock MJ. A role for cadherins in cellular signaling and differentiation. J Cell Biochem 1998;30:168–76.
23. Vleminckx K, Kemler R. Cadherins and tissue formation: integrating adhesion and signaling. Bioessays 1999; 21:211–20.
24. Jou TS, Stewart DB, Stappert J, et al. Genetic and biochemical dissection of protein linkages in the cadherin-catenin complex. Proc Natl Acad Sci U S A 1995;92:5067–71.
25. Chen YT, Stewart DB, Nelson WJ. Coupling assembly of the E-cadherin/β-catenin complex to efficient endoplasmic reticulum exit and basal-lateral membrane targeting of E-cadherin in polarized MDCK cells. J Cell Biol 1999;144:687–99.
26. Pignatelli M. Integrins, cadherins, and catenins: molecular cross-talk in cancer cells. J Pathol 1998;186:1–2.
27. Sandig M, Negrou E, Rogers KA. Changes in the distribution of LFA-1, catenins, and F-actin during transendothelial migration of monocytes in culture. J Cell Sci 1997;110:2807–18.
28. Semb H, Christofori G. The tumor-suppressor function of E-cadherin. Am J Hum Genet 1998;63:1588–93.
29. Vleminckx K, Vakaet L, Mareel M, et al. Genetic manipulation of E-cadherin expression by epithelial tumor cells reveals an invasion suppressor role. Cell 1991;66:107–19.
30. Hoffman AG, Burghardt RC, Tilley R, Auersperg N. An in vitro model of ovarian epithelial carcinogenesis: changes in cell–cell communication and adhesion occurring during neoplastic progression. Int J Cancer 1993;54:828–38.
31. Lewalle JM, Bajou K, Desreux J, et al. Alterations of inter-endothelial adherens junctions following tumor cell–endothelial cell interaction in vitro. Exp Cell Res 1997;237:347–56.
32. Sommors CL, Gelmann EP, Kemler R, et al. Alterations in β-catenin phosphorylation and plakoglobin expression in human breast cancer cells. Cancer Res 1994:54:3544–52.
33. Rubinfeld B, Souza B, Albert I, et al. Association of the APC gene product with β-catenin. Science 1993;262:1731–4.
34. Hu MC, Rosenblum ND. Smad1, β-catenin and Tcf4 associate in a molecular complex with the Myc promoter in dysplastic renal tissue and cooperate to control Myc transcription. Development 2005;132:215–25.
35. Hamada F, Bienz M. The APC tumor suppressor binds to C-terminal binding protein to divert nuclear beta-catenin from TCF. Dev Cell 2004;7:677–85.
36. Hynes RO. Integrins: versatility, modulation, and signaling in cell adhesion. Cell 1992;69:11–25.
37. Gille J, Swerlick RA. Integrins: role in cell adhesion and communication. Ann N Y Acad Sci 1996;797:93–107.
38. Schwartz MA, Schaller MD, Ginsberg MH. Integrins: emerging paradigms of signal transduction. Ann Rev Cell Dev Biol 1995;11:549–99.
39. Varner AJ, Cheresh DA. Integrins and cancer. Curr Opin Cell Biol 1996;8:724–30.
40. Frisch SM, Ruoslahti E. Integrins and anoikis. Curr Opin Cell Biol 1997;9:701–6.
41. Meredith JE, Schwartz M. Integrins, adhesion, and apoptosis. Trend Cell Biol 1997;7:146–50.
42. Chicurel ME, Singer RH, Meyer CJ, Ingber DE. Integrin binding and mechanical tension induce movement of mRNA and ribosomes to focal adhesions. Nature 1998;392:730–3.
43. Giancotti FG. Integrin signaling: specificity and control of cell survival and cell cycle progression. Curr Opin Cell Biol 1997;9:691–700.
44. Friedlander M, Brooks PC, Shaffer RW, et al. Definition of two angiogenic pathways by distinct av integrins. Science 1995;27:1500–2.
45. Brooks PC, Clark RAF, Cheresh DA. Requirement of vascular integrin avP3 for angiogenesis. Science 1994; 264:569–71.
46. Schwartz MA. Transmembrane signalling by integrins. Trend Cell Biol 1992;2:304–8.
47. Keely P, Parise L, Juliano R. Integrins and GTPases in tumor cell growth, motility and invasion. Trend Cell Biol 1998;8:101–6.
48. Majumdar M, Tarui T, Shi B, et al. Plasmin-induced migration requires signaling through protease-activated receptor 1 and integrin α(9)β(1). J Biol Chem 2004;279:37528–34.
49. Hintermann E, Yang N, O'Sullivan D, et al. Integrin α6β4-erbB2 complex inhibits haptotaxis by up-regulating E-cadherin cell-cell junctions in keratinocytes. J Biol Chem 2005;280:8004–15.
50. Reynolds AR, Reynolds LE, Nagel TE, et al. Elevated Flk1 (vascular endothelial growth factor receptor 2) signaling mediates enhanced angiogenesis in beta3-integrin-deficient mice. Cancer Res 2004;64:8643–50.
51. Guo W, Giancotti FG. Integrin signalling during tumour progression. Nat Rev Mol Cell Biol 2004;5:816–26.
52. Danen EH. Integrins: regulators of tissue function and cancer progression. Curr Pharm Des 2005;11:881–91.
53. Seftor REB. Role of the (33 integrin subunit in human primary melanoma progression. Am J Pathol 1998;153:1347–51.
54. Gu C, Park S. The EphA8 receptor regulates integrin activity through p110gamma phosphatidylinositol-3 kinase in a tyrosine kinase activity-independent manner. Mol Cell Biol. 2001;21:4579–97.
55. Borges E, Jan Y, Ruoslahti E. Platelet-derived growth factor receptor beta and vascular endothelial growth factor receptor 2 bind to the beta 3 integrin through its extracellular domain. J Biol Chem 2000;275:39867–73.
56. Brooks PC, Stromblad S, Sanders LC, et al. Localization of matrix metalloproteinase MMP-2 to the surface of invasive cells by interactions with integrin avP3. Cell 1996;85:683–93.
57. Eliceiri BP, Cheresh DA. The role of alpha integrins during angiogenesis. Mol Med 1998;4:741–50.
58. Kim J, Yu W, Kovalski K, Ossowski L. Requirement for specific proteases in cancer cell intravasation as revealed by a novel semiquantitative PCR-based assay. Cell 1998;94:353–62.
59. Nagase H, Woessner JF. Matrix metalloproteinases. J Biol Chem 1999;274:21491–4.
60. Coussens LM, Werb Z. Matrix metalloproteinases and the development of cancer. Chem Biol 1996;3:895–904.
61. Kelly T, Yan Y, Osborne RL, et al. Proteolysis of extracellular matrix by invadopodia facilitates human breast cancer cell invasion and is mediated by matrix metalloproteinases. Clin Exp Metastasis 1998;16:501–12.
62. Chambers AF, Matrisian LM. Changing views of the role of matrix metalloproteinases in metastasis. J Natl Cancer Inst 1997;89:1260–70.
63. Liotta LA, Tryggvason K, Garbisa S, et al. Metastatic potential correlates with enzymatic degradation of basement membrane collagen. Nature 1980;248:67–8.

64. Stetler-Stevenson WG, Krutzsch HC, Liotta LA. Tissue inhibitor of metalloproteinase (TIMP-2): a new member of the metalloproteinase inhibitor family. J Biol Chem 1989;264:17374–8.
65. Goldberg GI, Marmer BL, Grant GA, et al. Human 72-kilodalton type IV collagenase forms a complex with a tissue inhibitor of metalloproteinases designated TIMP-2. Proc Natl Acad Sci U S A 1989;86:8207.
66. Apte SS, Olsen BR, Murphy G. The gene structure of tissue inhibitor of metalloproteinases (TIMP)-3 and its inhibitory activities define the distinct TIMP gene family. J Biol Chem 1995;270:14313–8.
67. Leco KJ, Apte SS, Taniguchi GT, et al. Murine tissue inhibitor of metalloproteinases-4 (TIMP-4): cDNA isolation and expression in adult mouse tissues. FEBS Lett 1997;401:213–7.
68. Gomez DE, Alonso DF, Yoshiji H, Thorgeirsson UP. Tissue inhibitor of metalloproteinases: structure, regulation and biological functions. Eur J Cell Biol 1997;74:111–22.
69. Murphy AN, Unsworth EJ, Stetler-Stevenson WG. Tissue inhibitor of metalloproteinases-2 inhibits bFGF-induced human microvascular endothelial cell proliferation. J Cell Physiol 1993;157:351–8.
70. Ray JM, Stetler-Stevenson WG. TIMP-2 expression modulates human melanoma cell adhesion and motility. Ann N Y Acad Sci 1994;732:233–47.
71. Schnaper HW, Grant DS, Stetler-Stevenson WG, et al. Type IV collagenase(s) and TIMPs modulate endothelial cell morphogenesis in vitro. J Cell Physiol 1993;156:235–46.
72. Guedez L, McMarlin AJ, Kingma DW, et al. Tissue inhibitor of metalloproteinase-1 alters the tumorigenicity of Burkitt's lymphoma via divergent effects on tumor growth and angiogenesis. Am J Pathol 2001;158:1207–15.
73. Kohn EC, Alessandro R, Spoonster J, et al. Angiogenesis: role of calcium-mediated signal transduction. Proc Natl Acad Sci U S A 1995;92:1307–11.
74. Gottesman, M. The role of proteases in cancer. Semin Cancer Biol 1990;1:97–100.
75. Conese M, Blasi F. The urokinase/urokinase-receptor system and cancer invasion. Baillieres Clin Haematol 1995;8:365–89.
76. Odekon LE, Blasi F, Rifkin DB. Requirement for receptor-bound urokinase in plasmin-dependent cellular conversion of latent TGF-β to TGF-β. J Cell Physiol 1994;158:398–407.
77. Naldini L, Tamagnone L, Vigna E, et al. Extracellular proteolytic cleavage by urokinase is required for activation of hepatocyte growth factor/scatter factor. EMBO J 1992;11:4825–33.
78. Nielsen LS, Kellerman GM, Behrendt N, et al. A 55,000–60,000 Mr receptor protein for urokinase-type plasminogen activator. Identification in human tumor cell lines and partial purification. J Biol Chem 1988; 263:2358–63.
79. Lund LR, Ellis V, Ronne E, et al. Transcriptional and post-transcriptional regulation of the receptor for urokinase-type plasminogen activator by cytokines and tumour promoters in the human lung carcinoma cell line A549. Biochem J 1995;310:345–52.
80. Picone R, Kajtaniak EL, Nielsen LS, et al. Regulation of urokinase receptors in monocyte-like U937 cells by phorbol ester phorbol myristate acetate. J Cell Biol 1989;108:693–702.
81. Pepper MS, Matsumoto K, Nakamura T, et al. Hepatocyte growth factor increases urokinase-type plasminogen activator (u-PA) and u-PA receptor expression in Madin-Darby canine kidney epithelial cells. J Biol Chem 1992;267:20493–6.
82. Schmitt M, Wilhelm O, Janicke F, et al. Urokinase-type plasminogen activator (uPA) and its receptor (CD87): a new target in tumor invasion and metastasis. J Obstet Gynaecol 1995;21:151–65.
83. Duffy MJ, Reilly D, O'Sullivan C, et al. Urokinase-plasminogen activator, a new and independent prognostic marker in breast cancer. Cancer Res 1990;50:6827–9.
84. Spyratos F, Martin PM, Hacene K, et al. Multiparametric prognostic evaluation of biological factors in primary breast cancer. J Natl Cancer Inst 1992;84:1266–72.
85. Potempa J, Korzus E, Travis J. The serpin superfamily of proteinase inhibitors: structure, function, and regulation. J Biol Chem 1994;269:15957–60.
86. Ellis V, Dano K, Ellis V, et al. Plasminogen activation by receptor-bound urokinase: inhibition of receptor-bound urokinase by plasminogen-activator inhibitors. Semin Thromb Hemost 1991;17:194–200.
87. Dano K, Behrendt N, Brunner N, et al. The urokinase receptor: protein structure and role in plasminogen activation and cancer invasion. Fibrinolysis 1994;8:189–203.
88. Fazioli F, Blasi F. Urokinase-type plasminogen activator and its receptor: new targets for anti-metastatic therapy? Trend Pharmacol Sci 1994;15:25–9.
89. Montesano R, Pepper MS, Mohle-Steinlein U, et al. Increased proteolytic activity is responsible for the aberrant morphogenetic behavior of endothelial cells expressing the middle T oncogene. Cell 1990;62:435–45.
90. Aznavoorian S, Stracke ML, Krutzsch HC, et al. Signal transduction for chemotaxis and haptotaxis by matrix macromolecules in tumor cells. J Cell Biol 1990;110:1427–38.
91. Rong S, Segal S, Anver M, et al. Invasiveness and metastasis of NIH 3T3 cells induced by Met-hepatocyte growth factor/scatter factor autocrine stimulation. Proc Natl Acad Sci U S A 1994;91:4731–5.
92. Eccles SA. Targeting key steps in metastatic tumour progression. Curr Opin Genet Dev 2005;15:77–86.
93. Borm B, Requardt RP, Herzog V, Kirfel G. Membrane ruffles in cell migration: indicators of inefficient lamellipodia adhesion and compartments of actin filament reorganization. Exp Cell Res 2005;302:83–95.
94. Chodniewicz D, Klemke RL. Guiding cell migration through directed extension and stabilization of pseudopodia. Exp Cell Res 2004;301:31–7.
95. Stracke ML, Krutzsch HC, Unsworth EJ, et al. Identification, purification, and partial sequence analysis of autotaxin, a novel motility-stimulating protein. J Biol Chem 1991;267:2524–9.
96. Umezu-Goto M, Kishi Y, Taira A, et al. Autotaxin has lysophospholipase D activity leading to tumor cell growth and motility by lysophosphatidic acid production. J Cell Biol 2002;158:227–33.
97. Mills GB, Moolenaar WH. The emerging role of lysophosphatidic acid in cancer. Nat Rev Cancer 2003;3:582–91.
98. Clair T, Lee HY, Liotta LA, Stracke ML. Autotaxin is an exoenzyme possessing 5'-nucleotide phosphodiesterase/ATP pyrophosphatase and ATPase activities. J Biol Chem 1997;272:996–1001.
99. Cardones AR, Murakami T, Hwang ST. CXCR4 enhances adhesion of B16 tumor cells to endothelial cells in vitro and in vivo via β(1) integrin. Cancer Res 2003;63:6751–7.
100. Murakami T, Cardones AR, Hwang ST. Chemokine receptors and melanoma metastasis. J Dermatol Sci 2004;36:71–8.
101. Stoker M, Gherardi E. Regulation of cell movement: the motogenic cytokines. Biochim Biophys Acta 1991;1072:81–102.
102. Naldini L, Weidner KM, Vigna E, et al. Scatter factor and hepatocyte growth factor are indistinguishable ligands for the MET receptor. EMBO J 1991;10:2867–78.
103. Hartmann G, Naldini L, Weidner KM, et al. A functional domain in the heavy chain of scatter factor/hepatocyte growth factor binds the c-Met receptor and induces cell dissociation but not mitogenesis. Proc Natl Acad Sci U S A 1992;89:11574–8.
104. Ma PC, Jagadeeswaran R, Jagadeesh S, et al. Functional expression and mutations of c-Met and its therapeutic inhibition with SU11274 and small interfering RNA in non-small cell lung cancer. Cancer Res 2005;65:1479–88.
105. Folkman J, Hochberg M, Knighton D. Self-regulation of growth in three dimensions: the role of surface area limitations. In: Clarkson B, Baserga R, editors. Control of proliferation in animal cells. Cold Spring Harbor (CA): 1974. p. 833–42.
106. Liotta LA, Kleinerman J, Saidel G. Quantitative relationships of intravascular tumor cells: tumor vessels and pulmonary metastases following tumor implantation. Cancer Res 1974;34:997–1003.
107. Holmgren L, O'Reilly MS, Folkman J. Dormancy of micrometastases: balanced proliferation and apoptosis in the presence of angiogenesis suppression [see comments]. Nat Med 1995;1:149–53.
108. Folkman J. Tumor angiogenesis: therapeutic implications. N Engl J Med 1971;285:1182.
109. Steeg PS, Bevilacqua G, Kopper L. Evidence for a novel gene associated with low tumor metastatic potential. J Natl Cancer Inst 1988;80:200–4.
110. Lee JH, Welch DR. Suppression of metastasis in human breast carcinoma MDA-MB-435 cells after transfection with the metastasis. Cancer Res 1997;57:2384–7.
111. Pozzatti R, Muschel R, Williams J, et al. Primary rat embryo cells transformed by one or two oncogenes show different metastatic potentials. Science 1986;232:223–7.
112. Lee WP, Wen Y, Varnum B, Hung MC. Akt is required for Axl-Gas6 signaling to protect cells from E1A-mediated apoptosis. Oncogene 2002;21:329–36.
113. Ueno NT, Yu D, Hung MC. E1A: tumor suppressor or oncogene? Preclinical and clinical investigations of E1A gene therapy. Breast Cancer 2001;8:285–93. :10–1.
114. Khanna C, Khan J, Nguyen P, et al. Metastasis-associated differences in gene expression in a murine model of osteosarcoma. Cancer Res 2001;61:3750–9.
115. Lee JH, Miele ME, Hicks DJ, et al. KiSS-1, a novel human malignant melanoma metastasis-suppressor gene. J Natl Cancer Inst 1996;88:1731–7.
116. Stafford LJ, Xia C, Ma W, et al. Identification and characterization of mouse metastasis-suppressor KiSS1 and its G-protein-coupled receptor. Cancer Res 2002;62:5399–404.
117. Takino T, Koshikawa N, Miyamori H, et al. Cleavage of metastasis suppressor gene product KiSS-1 protein/metastin by matrix metalloproteinases. Oncogene 2003;22:4617–26.
118. Ohtaki T, Shintani Y, Honda S, et al. Metastasis suppressor gene KiSS-1 encodes peptide ligand of a G-protein-coupled receptor. Nature 2001;411:613–7.
119. Robinson VL, Hickson JA, Vander Griend DJ, et al. MKK4 and metastasis suppression: a marriage of signal transduction and metastasis research. Clin Exp Metastasis 2003;20:25–30.
120. Yamada SD, Hickson JA, Hrobowski Y, et al. Mitogen-activated protein kinase kinase 4 (MKK4) acts as a metastasis suppressor gene in human ovarian carcinoma. Cancer Res 2002;62:6717–23.
121. Emmert-Buck MR, Bonner RF, Smith PD, et al. Laser capture microdissection. Science 1996;274:998–1001.
122. Bonner RF, Emmert-Buck M, Cole K, et al. Laser capture microdissection: molecular analysis of tissue. Science 1997;278:1481–3.
123. Petricoin EF, Zoon KC, Kohn EC, et al. Clinical proteomics: translating benchside promise into bedside reality. Nat Rev Drug Discov 2002;1:683–95.
124. Petricoin EF 3rd, Bichsel VE, Calvert VS, et al. Mapping molecular networks using proteomics: a vision for patient-tailored combination therapy. J Clin Oncol 2005;23:3614–21.
125. Dufva M, Christensen CB. Diagnostic and analytical applications of protein microarrays. Expert Rev Proteomics 2005;2:41–8.
126. Perrotte P, Matsumoto T, Inoue K, et al. Anti-epidermal growth factor receptor antibody C225 inhibits angiogenesis in human transitional cell carcinoma growing orthotopically in nude mice. Clin Cancer Res 1999;5:257–65.
127. Huang SM, Bock JM, Harari PM. Epidermal growth factor receptor blockade with C225 modulates proliferation, apoptosis, and radiosensitivity in squamous cell carcinomas of the head and neck. Cancer Res 1999;59:1935–40.
128. Buchdunger E, Cioffi CL, Law N, et al. Abl protein-tyrosine kinase inhibitor STI571 inhibits in vivo signal transduction mediated by c-kit and platelet-derived growth factor receptors. J Pharm Exp Ther 2000;295:139–45.
129. Sirotnak F, Zakowski M, Miller V, et al. Efficacy of cytotoxic agents against human tumor xenografts is markedly enhanced by coadministration of ZD1839 (Iressa), an inhibitor of EGFR tyrosine kinase. Clin Cancer Res 2000;6:4885–92.
130. Ciardello F, Caputo R, Bianco R, et al. Antitumor effect and potentiation of cytotoxic drugs activity in human cancer cells by ZD1839 (Iressa), an epidermal growth factor receptor-selective tyrosine kinase inhibitor. Clin Cancer Res 2000;6:2053–63.
131. Druker BJ, Talpaz M, Resta DJ et al. Efficacy and safety of a specific inhibitor of the Bcr-Abl tyrosine kinase in chronic myeloid leukemia. N Engl J Med 2001; 344:1031–7.
132. Demetri GD, von Mehren M, Blanke CD, et al. Efficacy and safety of imatinib mesylate in advanced gastrointestinal stromal tumors. N Engl J Med 2002;347:472–80.
133. McArthur GA, Demetri GD, van Oosterom A, et al. Molecular and clinical analysis of locally advanced dermatofibrosarcoma protuberans treated with imatinib: Imatinib Target Exploration Consortium Study B2225.J Clin Oncol 2005:;23:866–73.
134. Rini BI, Small EJ. Biology and clinical development of vascular endothelial growth factor-targeted therapy in renal cell carcinoma. J Clin Oncol 2005;23:1028–43
135. Gasparini G, Brooks PC, Biganzoli E, et al. Vascular integrin α(V)β3: a new prognostic indicator in breast cancer. Clin Cancer Res 1998;4:2625–34.
136. Pluda JM. Tumor-associated angiogenesis: mechanisms, clinical implications, and therapeutic strategies. Semin Oncol 1997;24:203–18.
137. Dahut WL, Gulley JL, Arlen PM, et al. Randomized phase II trial of docetaxel plus thalidomide in androgen-independent prostate cancer. J Clin Oncol 2004;22:2532–9
138. Bartlett JB, Dredge K, Dalgleish AG. The evolution of thalidomide and its IMiD derivatives as anticancer agents. Nat Rev Cancer 2004;4:314–22.

139. Rajendran JG, Krohn KA. Imaging hypoxia and angiogenesis in tumors. Radiol Clin North Am. 2005 Jan;43(1):169-87.
140. Wiedmann MW, Caca K. Molecularly targeted therapy for gastrointestinal cancer. Curr Cancer Drug Targets 2005;5:171–93.
141. Ellis LM. Bevacizumab. Nat Rev Drug Discov 2005;(Suppl):8–9.
142. Ahmad T, Eisen T. Kinase inhibition with BAY 43-9006 in renal cell carcinoma. Clin Cancer Res 2004;10(Suppl):6388–92.
143. Hofmann J. Protein kinase C isozymes as potential targets for anticancer therapy. Curr Cancer Drug Targets 2004;4:125–46.
144. Hata A, Akita Y, Suzuki K, Ohno S. Functional divergence of protein kinase C (PKC) family members. J Biol Chem 1993;268:9122–9.
145. Dumont J, Jones W, Bitonti A. Inhibition of experimental metastasis and cell adhesion of V16F1 melanoma cells by inhibitors of protein kinase C. Cancer Res 1992;52:1195–200.
146. Liu B, Renaud C, Nelson K, et al. Protein kinase C inhibitor calphostin C reduces B16 amelanotic melanoma cell adhesion to endothelium and lung colonization. Int J Cancer 1992;52:147–52.
147. Stanwell C, Gescher A, Bradshaw T, Pettit G. The role of protein kinase C isoenzymes in the growth inhibition caused by bryostatin 1 in human 549 hung and MCF-7 breast carcinoma. Int J Cancer 1994;56:585–92.
148. Schwartz GK, Redwood SM, Ohnuma T, et al. Inhibition of invasion of invasive human bladder carcinoma cells by protein kinase C inhibitor staurosporine. J Natl Cancer Inst 1990;82:1753–6.
149. Schwartz GK, Ward D, Saltz L, et al. A Phase 1 study of the protein kinase c (pkc) specific inhibitor safingol (Saf) alone and in combination with doxorubicin (Dox) [abstract]. Proc Ann Meet Am Soc Clin Oncol 1995;14:.
150. Kortmansky J, Shah MA, Kaubisch A, et al. Phase I trial of the cyclin-dependent kinase inhibitor and protein kinase C inhibitor 7-hydroxystaurosporine in combination with fluorouracil in patients with advanced solid tumors. J Clin Oncol 2005;23:1875–84.
151. Kohn EC, Alessandro R, Spoonster J, et al. Angiogenesis: role of calcium-mediated signal transduction. Proc Natl Acad Sci U S A 1995;92:1307–11.
152. Kohn EC, Felder CC, Jacobs W, et al. Structure-function analysis of signal and growth inhibition by carboxyamido-triazole, CAI. Cancer Res 1994;54:935–42.
153. Kohn EC, Jacobs W, Kim Y, et al. Calcium influx modulates expression of matrix metalloproteinases-2 (72-kDa type IV collagenase, gelatinase A). J Biol Chem 1994;269:21505–11.
154. Alessandro R, Spoonster J, Wersto RP, Kohn EC. Signal transduction as a therapeutic target. Curr Topic Microbiol Immunol 1996;213:167–88.
155. Luzzi KJ, Varghese HJ, MacDonald IC, et al. Inhibition of angiogenesis in liver metastases by carboxyamidotriazole (CAI): computer assisted analysis [citation]. Angiogenesis 1999.
156. Kohn EC, Figg WD, Sarosy GA, et al. Phase I trial of micronized formulation carboxyamidotriazole in patients with refractory solid tumors: pharmacokinetics, clinical outcome, and comparison of formulations. J Clin Oncol 1997;15:1985–93.
157. Berlin J, Tutsch K, Hutson P, et al. Phase I clinical and pharmacokinetic study of oral carboxyamidotriazole, a signal transduction inhibitor. J Clin Oncol 1997; 15:781–9.
158. Kohn EC, Reed E, Sarosy GA, et al. A Phase I trial of CAI (carboxyamido-triazole) and paclitaxel for relapsed solid tumors: potential efficacy of the combination, and demonstration of pharmacokinetic interaction. Clin Cancer Res 2001;7:1600–9.
159. Kerbel R, Folkman J. Clinical translation of angiogenesis inhibitors. Nat Rev Cancer 2002;2:727–39.
160. Kerbel RS, Klement G, Pritchard KI, Kamen B. Continuous low-dose anti-angiogenic/metronomic chemotherapy: from the research laboratory into the oncology clinic. Ann Oncol 2002;13:12–5.

11

Tumor Angiogenesis

Judah Folkman, MD
John Heymach, MD, PhD
Raghu Kalluri, PhD

Angiogenesis, the growth of new capillary blood vessels, is central to the growth of cancer. An understanding of the cellular and molecular basis of tumor angiogenesis is therefore important for clinicians who diagnose and treat cancer by whatever modalities. This chapter is focused on certain general principles of tumor angiogenesis that are intrinsic to the behavior of human cancer. Rapid progress in understanding molecular and genetic events that underlie the transformation of a normal cell to a cancer cell is reflected in many chapters in this book. These studies provide strong evidence for the hope that, eventually, there will be molecular solutions to the cancer problem. However, in virtually all scenarios of current or future therapy, the target is the cancer cell.

Experimental evidence indicates that it is prudent to develop cancer therapies against another target, the microvascular endothelial cell, with the understanding that the two targets are not mutually exclusive. This concept has now been validated in cancer patients. Angiogenesis inhibitors have been approved by the US Food and Drug Administration (FDA) and have received approval in 27 other countries (Table 11-1). The FDA commissioner, Mark McClellan, announced in February 2004 that "angiogenesis inhibitors can now be considered as the fourth modality of cancer therapy." In May 2004, Andrew C. von Eschenbach, director of the National Cancer Institute, and Allen M. Spiegel, director of the National Institute of Diabetes and Digestive and Kidney Disease, said, "We can unequivocally say that angiogenesis is not only a critical factor for cancer, but for a host of other diseases."

Consider a cancer cell that has progressed through a series of mutations so that by activation of certain oncogenes and by loss of specific suppressor genes, it has become self-sufficient in growth signals, insensitive to antigrowth signals, unresponsive to apoptotic signals, capable of limitless replicative potential, and tumorigenic.[1] Current evidence argues that these neoplastic properties may be necessary but not sufficient for a cancer cell to expand into a population that is symptomatic, clinically detectable, metastatic, and lethal. For a tumor to develop a metastatic and/or a lethal phenotype, it must first recruit and sustain its own private blood supply, a process called tumor angiogenesis.[1]

NONANGIOGENIC TUMORS ARE HARMLESS

There is an early stage of neoplastic development when tumors are not yet able to recruit new microvascular endothelial cells and cannot induce angiogenesis. As a result, most human tumors remain in situ and dormant at a microscopic size and are harmless to the host.[2] Nonangiogenic human tumors in mice are not only harmless throughout the normal life span of a mouse but usually cannot expand beyond a volume of ~1 to 2 mm^3.

CANCER WITHOUT DISEASE

Nonangiogenic tumors in humans also stop expanding at a microscopic size of ~1 mm or less. For over 100 years, pathologists performing autopsies on individuals who died of automobile accidents or other trauma have documented the presence of in situ carcinomas. These findings, summarized by Black and Welch in 1993, reveal that for a given age group, a large number of individuals harbor in situ carcinomas but a very small percentage in that age group are diagnosed with cancer during life. For example, carcinoma in situ is found in the breasts of 39% of women age 40 to 50 years who died of trauma, but only 1% are ever diagnosed with cancer in this age range. Carcinoma in situ of the prostate is diagnosed in 46% of men age 60 to 70 years who died of trauma, but only 1% are diagnosed during life. Carcinoma in situ is found in more than 98% of individuals age 50 to 70 years who died of trauma but is diagnosed in only 0.1% during life. What keeps these in situ carcinomas in check? One explanation is the potential contribution of host-derived factors that prevent in situ carcinomas from switching to the angiogenic phenotype. Among factors that could offer such protection, the role of physiologic levels of endogenous angiogenesis inhibitors is intriguing (see the sections on endogenous angiogenesis inhibitors).[2a]

DISEASE OF CANCER REQUIRES EXPANSION OF TUMOR MASS

The *disease* brought about by cancer is not manifest until after continuous expansion of a tumor mass takes place, beyond the microscopic size of the restricted nonangiogenic tumor in situ cancer. However, expansion of the tumor mass beyond the initial microscopic size of a nonangiogenic tumor is absolutely dependent on recruitment of endothelial cells. Such endothelial cell recruitment begins when tumor cells undergo a switch to the angiogenic phenotype.[45,46] The angiogenic phenotype is driven by (1) increased expression by tumor cells of angiogenic proteins such as vascular endothelial growth factor (VEGF) and basic fibroblast growth factor (bFGF); (2) increased expression of angiogenic proteins from stromal cells (ie, stromal fibroblasts), a process induced by the tumor itself; (3) decreased expression of endogenous angiogenesis inhibitors (ie, thrombospondin [TSP]-1) by the tumor and by stromal fibroblasts; and (4) recruitment of bone marrow–derived endothelial cell precursors (see below for a detailed discussion of the switch to the angiogenic phenotype). Expansion of the tumor mass can produce symptomatic, detectable, and potentially lethal cancer either from a local mass that mechanically interferes with function (ie, a brain tumor or an intestinal obstruction from ovarian cancer), from a dispersed mass (ie, multiple metastases), from release of cytokines that interfere with hemostasis and result in abnormal clotting or bleeding (the two most common causes of death in cancer patients), or from cytokines that produce cachexia (ie, tumor necrosis factor [TNF]-α) or interfere with other functions (ie, inappropriate hormone release). In summary, in its simplest terms, absence of tumor angiogenesis = no expansion of the tumor mass beyond a microscopic size = no symptoms, no metastases, and no mortality = "cancer without disease."[2a] Recruitment of microvascular endothelial cells is also necessary for expansion of a normal tissue mass and for expansion of an organ mass, for example, after partial hepatectomy. In fact, angiogenesis is fundamental to reproduction, development, and repair, but such physiologic angiogenesis occurs mainly as short-lived capillary blood vessel growth that usually lasts only days (ovulation angiogenesis), weeks (wound healing angiogenesis), or months (fetal and placental angiogenesis) but then is always down-regulated spontaneously and on a predictable timetable.[3–5]

PERSISTENCE OF PATHOLOGIC ANGIOGENESIS

In contrast to physiologic angiogenesis, a hallmark of pathologic angiogenesis is persistent

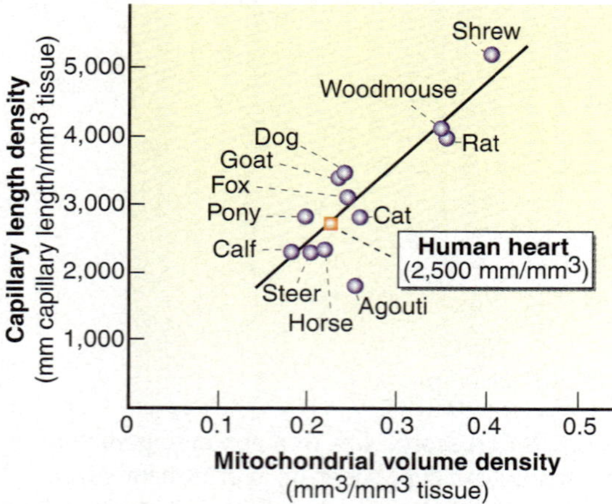

Figure 11-1 A cubic millimeter of human cardiac muscle contains approximately 2,500 millimeters of capillary blood vessels.[4]

growth of blood vessels (ie, sustained neovascularization). Tumor angiogenesis is rarely, if ever, down-regulated spontaneously. Angiogenesis that continues for months or years supports the progression of many neoplastic and non-neoplastic diseases.[9,10] However, both physiologic angiogenesis and pathologic angiogenesis are usually focal. An angiogenic focus appears as only a tiny fraction or a small "hot spot" of proliferating and migrating endothelial cells that arise from a monolayer of resting endothelium of approximately 1,000 m^2, an area the size of a tennis court. A cubic millimeter of human cardiac muscle contains approximately 2,500 mm of capillary blood vessels (as determined by stereologic methods).[4] The fundamental objectives of all antiangiogenic therapy are to inhibit the progression of pathologic angiogenesis, to return a pathologic neovascular focus to its normal resting state, to prevent its initiation (Figure 11-1). In contrast, the goal of antivascular therapy is to rapidly occlude new blood vessels so that blood flow stops. (see below, antiangiogenic versus antivascular therapy).

HISTORIC BACKGROUND

For more than 100 years, tumors had been observed to be more vascular than normal tissues.[11] This tumor hyperemia observed during surgery was generally explained by simple dilation of existing host blood vessels.[12] Vasodilation was thought to be a side effect of metabolites or of necrotic tumor products escaping from the tumor. Three reports, although largely overlooked, suggested that tumor hyperemia could be related to new blood vessel growth, that is, to neovascularization and not solely to vasodilation. A 1939 article showed that whereas neovascularization of a wound in a transparent chamber in a rabbit ear regressed completely after the wound healed,[13] a tumor implant in the chamber was associated with accelerated growth of new capillary blood vessels. The other two reports, in 1945 and 1947, demonstrated that new vessels in the neighborhood of a tumor implant arose from host vessels and not from the tumor itself.[14,15] These articles notwithstanding, debate continued in the literature for two more decades about whether a tumor could expand to a large size (centimeters) by simply living on preexisting vessels.[16] Even among the few investigators who accepted the concept of tumor-induced neovascularization, it was generally assumed that this vascular response was an inflammatory reaction, a side effect of tumor growth, not a requirement for tumor growth.[17]

BEGINNING OF ANGIOGENESIS RESEARCH

Hypothesis: Tumor Growth Depends on Angiogenesis In 1971, Folkman proposed a new view of the role of blood vessels in tumor growth. He hypothesized that tumor growth is angiogenesis dependent.[18] This hypothesis suggested that tumor cells and vascular endothelial cells within a neoplasm may constitute a highly integrated ecosystem and that endothelial cells may be switched from a resting state to a rapid growth phase by a "diffusible" chemical signal from tumor cells. An additional speculation was that angiogenesis could be a relevant target for tumor therapy (ie, antiangiogenic therapy). Folkman proposed these ideas from experiments he performed with Frederick Becker in the early 1960s, which revealed that tumor growth in isolated perfused organs was severely restricted in the absence of vascularization of the tumors.[19–24]

These concepts were not accepted at the time. Although a few investigators in the early 1970s perceived that tumors could actually induce neovascularization, the belief persisted that such neovascularization was an inflammatory host response to necrotic tumor cells or possibly a host defense detrimental to the tumor. Another obstacle to research on tumor angiogenesis was the conventional wisdom at that time that any new vessels induced by a tumor, like new vessels in a wound, would become established and thus could not be made to involute. From this assumption, scientists concluded that antiangiogenic therapy could never regress a tumor; therefore, it would be fruitless to try to discover angiogenesis inhibitors. In this pessimistic atmosphere, it took many years for compelling evidence to be generated that would convince scientists that tumor growth depended on neovascularization. Eventual acceptance of Folkman's 1971 hypothesis was slow because it would be 2 more years before the first vascular endothelial cells were successfully cultured in vitro, 8 years before it was possible to grow capillary endothelial cells in vitro, 11 years before the discovery of the first angiogenesis inhibitor, and 13 years before the purification of the first angiogenic protein.[25–29]

Throughout the 1970s, laboratory studies were devoted to demonstrating that tumor vessels were new proliferating capillaries; the sequential steps of the angiogenic process could be identified; qualitative and quantitative bioassays for angiogenesis could be developed; viable tumor cells released diffusible angiogenic factors that stimulated new capillary growth and endothelial mitosis in vivo, despite the arrest of tumor cell proliferation by irradiation; necrotic tumor products were not angiogenic per se; and angiogenesis itself could be inhibited.[30–35] Because of these efforts to provide supporting evidence that tumor growth was angiogenesis dependent, the field of angiogenesis research began. Today the field has broadened to include a wide spectrum of basic science disciplines, from developmental biology to molecular genetics, as well as a variety of clinical specialties, which include, in addition to oncology, cardiology, dermatology, gynecology, ophthalmology, and rheumatology. Approximately 70 publications on the subject of angiogenesis appear every week.

Experimental Evidence By the mid-1980s, considerable experimental evidence had been assembled to support the hypothesis that tumor growth is angiogenesis dependent. The idea could now be stated in its simplest terms: "Once tumor take has occurred, every further increase in tumor cell population must be preceded by an increase in new capillaries that converge upon the tumor."[32] The hypothesis predicted that if angiogenesis could be completely inhibited, tumors would become dormant at a small, possibly microscopic, size.[22] It forecast that whereas the presence of neovascularization would be necessary but not sufficient for expansion of a tumor, the absence of neovascularization would prevent expansion of a primary tumor mass beyond 1 to 2 mm^3 and restrict a metastasis to a microscopic dormant lesion.

The hypothesis that tumors are angiogenesis dependent is supported by biologic and pharmacologic evidence and proved by genetic evidence. The three types of evidence are summarized below because they provide a scientific basis for current clinical trials of angiogenesis inhibitors[36,37] and because they offer valid mechanisms of action for certain angiogenesis inhibitors that have recently received FDA approval since the sixth edition of *Cancer Medicine*. Also, new data since the sixth edition are included.

Biologic Evidence

1. In two-dimensional flat cultures, a population of tumor cells expands indefinitely as long as fresh medium is added and unlimited cell-free surface is provided (ie, passage of cells to a new flask). In contrast, three-dimensional spheroids of the same cells, suspended in soft agar or methylcellulose, stop enlarging at a diameter of a few millimeters, despite repeated passage of the spheroids to fresh media.[38] In these "steady-state" spheroids, cell proliferation is balanced by cell death.[39–41] This in vitro model is analogous to a dormant micrometastasis in which angiogenesis is blocked.[42]

2. Tumors implanted into subcutaneous transparent chambers grow slowly before vascularization, and tumor volume increases linearly. After vascularization, tumor growth is rapid and tumor volume may increase exponentially.[15,43]
3. Tumor growth in the avascular rabbit cornea proceeds slowly at a linear rate but converts to exponential growth after neovascularization.[44]
4. Tumors suspended in the aqueous fluid of the anterior chamber of the rabbit eye remain in a dormant state: viable, avascular, and limited in size (< 1 mm^3). These tumors induce neovascularization of iris vessels, but the new vessels are out of reach of the tumors floating in the aqueous fluid. Once a tumor spheroid is apposed to the proliferating iris vessels, the tumor becomes neovascularized and can enlarge up to 16,000 times its original volume within 2 weeks.[45] A current interpretation of this experiment is that the tumor spheroid had already switched[46] to the angiogenic phenotype but that angiogenesis was blocked by separation of the floating tumor from the nearest vascular bed.
5. Tumors grown in the vitreous of the rabbit eye remain viable but are restricted to diameters of less than 0.50 mm for as long as 100 days. Once such a tumor reaches the retinal surface, it becomes neovascularized and within 2 weeks can undergo a 19,000-fold increase in volume over the avascular tumor.[47] Cross-sectional histology of the avascular tumors reveals proliferating cells at the periphery of the tumor and necrotic tumor cells in its center.
6. Human retinoblastomas that have metastasized to the vitreous are viable and avascular, and tumor expansion is restricted.[48]
7. Within a solid tumor, the [H^3]thymidine labeling index of tumor cells decreases with increasing distance from the nearest open capillary vessel.[49] The tissue oxygen tension also decreases with increasing distance of a tumor cell from the center of a capillary vessel.[50] Because the limit of oxygen diffusion is 100 to 200 μm, tumor cells that exceed these distances from a capillary vessel become anoxic (as determined by infrared spectroscopy of tumors in transparent skin chambers in mice).[51]
8. Tumors implanted into the chorioallantoic membrane of the chick embryo remain restricted in growth during the avascular phase but enlarge rapidly once they are vascularized.[52]
9. Vascular casts of metastases in the rabbit liver reveal that tumors of up to 1 mm in diameter are usually avascular but beyond that size are vascularized.[53]
10. Human ovarian carcinomas metastasize to the peritoneal membrane as tiny avascular seeds. These implants rarely grow beyond a limited diameter of a few millimeters until after vascularization. This "avascular" state of peritoneal implants has also been demonstrated in mice with four different tumor types and is independent of whether the mice are immunocompetent or immunodeficient. The avascular peritoneal implants are less than 0.5 mm diameter and are of uniform size (C. Chen, personal communication).
11. In transgenic mice that develop carcinomas of the beta cells in the pancreatic islets, large tumors arise from a subset of preneoplastic hyperplastic islets but only after they have become vascularized.[54]
12. Neoplastic cells injected subcutaneously develop into tumors that become vascularized at about 0.4 mm^3.[55] As tumor size increases, blood vessels continue to proliferate and are enveloped by tumor cells that appear to grow toward and around the new vessels. The vessels eventually occupy up to 1.5% of the tumor volume. This is a 400% increase in vascular density over normal subcutaneous tissue.[55] In this model, new microvascular sprouts that converge on a tumor are enveloped by tumor cells, giving the appearance that the tumor has been penetrated by vessels.
13. In colon carcinomas arising in rats after carcinogen exposure, there is an early phase (tumor diameter < 3.5 mm) during which the tumor is temporarily supplied by preexisting host microvessels that are dilated and widened.[56] This stage is similar to "cooption" of blood vessels recently reported.[57] Subsequently, new capillary vessels sprout and proliferate (angiogenesis), which leads to increasing microvessel density and rapid tumor growth.

Pharmacologic Evidence By the late 1980s, it became possible to inhibit tumor angiogenesis by biochemical and molecular methods. These experiments were based on (1) administration of molecules that inhibited angiogenesis specifically or selectively, (2) blockade of tumor-derived angiogenic factors,[58] and (3) the development of spontaneous tumors in transgenic mice. Some examples are listed below:

1. An angiogenesis inhibitor, TNP-470 (AGM-1470), a synthetic analogue of fumagillin, selectively inhibited proliferating endothelial cells in vitro and in vivo.[59] It potently inhibited tumor growth in vivo but did not inhibit tumor cells in vitro. In preclinical studies, it has a broader spectrum of antitumor activity than any known anticancer drug. There are more than 60 reports from different laboratories of inhibition of 33 different types of human, mouse, rat, hamster, and rabbit primary tumors in animals and of 23 different types of metastatic tumors, including human tumor metastases in mice and rat and hamster tumor metastases. Tumor growth was inhibited at an average of 65%, with a range of 43 to 100% (ie, complete regression). All of these reports employed the same dose, 30 mg/kg every other day. Complete regression was observed in seven tumor types in mice, including neurofibrosarcoma, neurofibroma, breast cancer, gastric cancer, and choriocarcinoma, as well as mouse reticulum sarcoma and gastric carcinoma.[60,552b] Because TNP-470 inhibits microvascular endothelial cells at a concentration 3 logs lower than tumor cells, this angiogenesis inhibitor is virtually a specific inhibitor of endothelial proliferation and migration. These studies provided the first clue that angiogenesis inhibitors could be broad-spectrum anticancer agents that are relatively independent of tumor type. The appearance of different therapeutic responses by different tumor types (eg, 43–100%) was more adequately explained by the total angiogenic output of each tumor type matched against a fixed dose of angiogenesis inhibitor (see below for improvements in TNP-470.)
2. In another experiment, antibody against bFGF secreted by a tumor administered to mice bearing the tumor resulted in a dramatic reduction in neovascularization and in tumor volume.[61] To engineer bFGF that was secreted from the tumor, the complementary deoxyribonucleic acid (cDNA) for human bFGF hybridized to a signal sequence was transfected into normal mouse fibroblasts.[61] Furthermore, the structure of the bFGF was modified by site-specific mutagenesis in which two serines were substituted for cysteines. Thus, the bFGF released by the tumor could be neutralized by a specific antibody that had no effect on natural bFGF. The transfected fibroblasts became tumorigenic, exported bFGF, and were highly angiogenic. They formed large lethal tumors when implanted into mice. Tumor angiogenesis was mediated solely by bFGF released from these tumors.
3. In an analogous experiment, a neutralizing antibody to another angiogenic protein, VEGF, was administered to mice bearing tumors that induced angiogenesis solely by VEGF.[62] Tumor growth was inhibited by more than 90%. The antibody had no effect on the tumor cells in vitro. VEGF can also upregulate its receptors on endothelial cells.[63]
4. Specific immunologic inhibition of overexpression of the integrin $\alpha v \beta_3$ on capillary endothelial cells resulted in apoptosis of proliferating endothelial cells, blocked neovascularization, and induced tumor regression.[64]
5. Endogenous specific inhibitors of endothelial proliferation and of angiogenesis include angiostatin, a 38 kDa internal fragment of plasminogen (generated by Lewis lung carcinoma); endostatin, a 20 kDa internal fragment of collagen XVIII (generated from a murine hemangioendothelioma); a 53 kDa conformationally changed fragment of antithrombin III (generated

Table 11-1 Angiogenesis Inhibitors Approved for Clinical Use

Date Approved	Drug	Place	Disease
December 2003	Thalidomide	Australia	Multiple myeloma
February 2004	Avastin	US (FDA)	Colorectal cancer
November 2004	Tarceva	US (FDA)	Lung cancer
December 2004	Avastin	Switzerland	Colorectal cancer
December 2004	Macugen	US (FDA)	Macular degeneration
January 2005	Avastin	European Union (25 countries)	Colorectal cancer
September 2005	Endostatin (Endostar)	China (SFDA)	Lung cancer

from human small cell lung cancer); and tumstatin, a 28 kDa internal fragment of collagen IV (α_3 noncollagenous 1 [NC1] domain) (Table 11-2).[65–71a] They do not inhibit proliferation of resting confluent endothelial cells, epithelial cells, smooth muscle cells, fibroblasts, or tumor cells in vitro. These proteins inhibit angiogenesis in the chick chorioallantoic membrane or in the mouse cornea. Both primary and metastatic tumors are markedly inhibited, and tumor regression is achieved without toxicity or drug resistance.[69]

6. In severe combined immunodeficient (SCID) mice bearing human pancreatic cancer, human recombinant endostatin was injected into the peritoneal cavity once daily or delivered continuously by an implanted micro-osmotic pump that released 1 μL/h.[72] Continuous dosing inhibited tumor growth 10-fold more effectively than once-a-day bolus dosing and induced tumor regression, whereas bolus dosing did not (Figure 11-2).
7. An antibody to two receptors of VEGF, called VEGF-Trap, inhibits the growth of VEGF-producing tumors in mice.[73]

Genetic Evidence Genetic evidence that tumors are angiogenesis dependent began to be reported by the mid-1990s and provides the most compelling proof that tumors and their metastases cannot grow beyond a microscopic in situ size without recruiting new microvessels. These experiments are based on (1) transfection of dominant-negative receptors for a proangiogenic protein into endothelial cells in the tumor bed, (2) transfection of genes for antiangiogenic proteins into tumor cells, (3) regulation of the expression of angiogenic oncogenes, and (4) manipulation of developmental genes. Some examples are listed below:

1. The growth of brain tumors in nude mice was significantly inhibited or prevented when tumor angiogenesis was suppressed by a strategy in which a dominant-negative mutant of the receptor Flk-1 for the angiogenic protein VEGF was introduced into host endothelial cells (carried by a retrovirus). This signaling-defective receptor mutant formed an inactive dimer with the native Flk-1 receptor on endothelial cells and prevented the formation of new capillary blood vessels in response to VEGF released by the tumor.[74]
2. Transformed cells were not tumorigenic until after they had become angiogenic by down-regulating expression of TSP-1, a process that was p53 dependent.[75]
3. Transfection of normal human endothelial cells with the SV40 large T oncogene generated immortalized cells in vitro. However, when these cells were inoculated into mice, they formed microscopic nonangiogenic tumors that did not grow beyond approximately 1 mm in diameter.[76] A subsequent transfection with the *ras* oncogene switched the cells to the angiogenic phenotype, up-regulated VEGF production, down-regulated production of tissue inhibitors of metalloproteinases, and generated highly neovascularized, rapidly growing tumors.
4. Down-regulation of the *ras* oncogene in a melanoma driven by doxycycline-inducible ras led to massive apoptosis of microvascular endothelium in the tumor bed starting within 6 hours. Tumor cells began to die days later, and large tumors had completely disappeared by 12 days.[77] At the time of this 1999 publication, the authors entertained the possibility that inactivation of the *ras* oncogene directly caused tumor regression, mainly by restoring the high apoptotic rate of tumor cells within the tumor. They felt that the vascular collapse was secondary to a reduced output of angiogenic factors from the regressing tumor. However, in a subsequent article,[77a] they reported that loss of vascular integrity upon inactivation of Ras is an active process, rather than a loss of tumor cell viability. This is consistent with Watnick's recent finding that ras induces an increase in endothelial cell proliferation in a dose-dependent manner in vitro.[77b]
5. When tumor cells were transfected with the cDNA for angiostatin and implanted into mice, the higher the secretion of angiostatin, the slower the growth of the tumors. However, tumor cell proliferation in vitro was not affected by angiostatin transfection.[78]
6. When tumors were transfected with the secretable antiangiogenic protein TSP-1 and/or TSP-2, tumor growth was directly proportional to suppression of angiogenesis. Tumor growth was inhibited up to 100% (ie, microscopic dormant tumor or no tumor) when angiogenesis was suppressed completely. Tumor cell proliferation was independent of the level of TSP-1 or TSP-2 production.[79]
7. Id1 and Id3 are helix-loop-helix proteins that may control differentiation by interfering with deoxyribonucleic acid (DNA) binding of transcription factors. After targeted disruption of one allele of Id1 and two alleles of Id3, three different types of implanted tumors failed to induce angiogenesis, their growth was severely restricted, and they did not metastasize.[80] However, when these mice were injected with bone marrow from wild-type mice containing normal Id1 and Id3 markers, progenitor endothelial cells expressing Id1 and Id3 circulated from the bone marrow to the tumor vascular bed. The increase in progenitor endothelial cells correlated with and permitted the tumors to undergo increased tumor neovascularization and tumor growth.[81]
8. In collagen XVIII null mice depleted of endostatin, tumors grew 200 to 300% more rapidly than in wild-type mice. In contrast, when endostatin was overexpressed by endothelium in mice, tumors grew 300% more slowly than in wild-type mice.[81a]

A similar result was obtained when a different endogenous inhibitor, tumstatin, was eliminated from mice in which the α_3 chain of collagen was knocked out.[512a] Tumors grew up to 200 to 300% more quickly than in wild-type mice. However, when tumstatin was replaced to physiologic levels by injection of the protein, tumor growth was decreased to the wild-type rate (see the section below on endogenous angiogenesis inhibitors).

Table 11-2 Endogenous Inhibitors of Angiogenesis

Matrix Derived	Non-Matrix Derived
Arrestin	Growth factors and cytokines
Canstatin	Interferons
Collagen fragments	Interleukins
EFC-XV	PEDF
Endorepellin	Platelet factor-4
Endostatin	Other
Fibronectin fragments	Angiostatin
	Antithrombin III (cleaved)
Fibulin	Chondromodulin
Thrombospondin-1 and -2	2-Methoxyestradiol
	PEX
Tumstatin	Plasminogen Kringle 5
	Prolactin fragments
	Prothrombin Kringle 2
	sFlt-1
	TIMPs
	Troponin I
	Vasostatin

Metastasis Is Also Angiogenesis Dependent Experimental and clinical evidence suggests that the process of metastasis is also

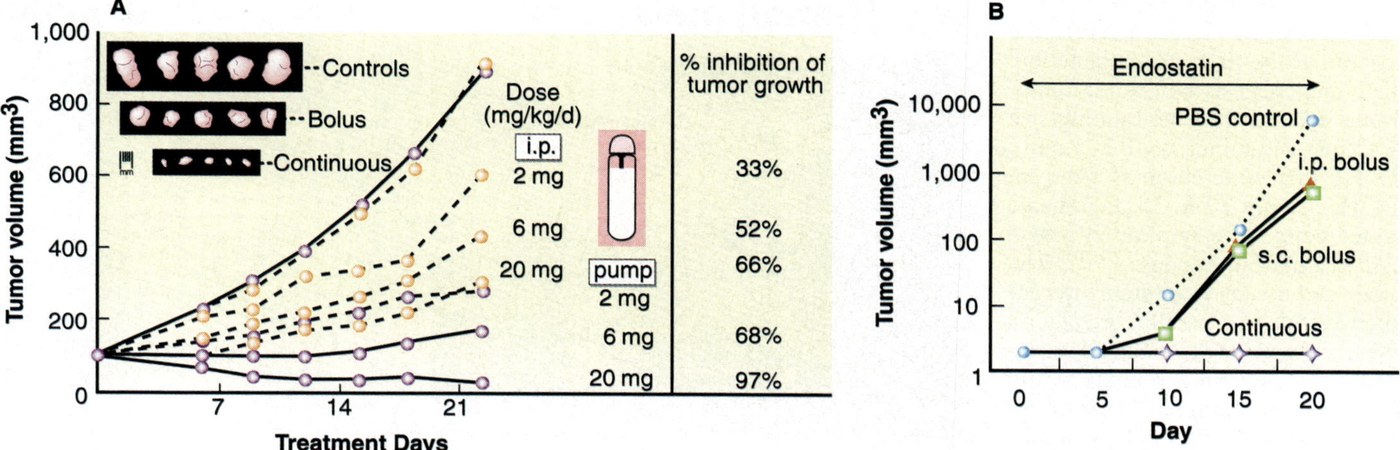

Figure 11-2 Continuous administration of endostatin is ten times more effective than the same dose given once a day as a bolus. Continuous dosing can regress tumors whereas bolus dosing does not. In this paper the pharmacokinetics show that bolus dosing gives a high peak of endostatin with a rapid fall below effective therapeutic levels. In contrast, continuous dosing provides constant therapeutic levels of 200 ng/mL up to 250 ng/mL. The implication of this study is that in order to stop tumor growth or to induce tumor regression, endothelial cells in the tumor bed must be continuously exposed to therapeutic levels of inhibitor to counteract stimulators of endothelial growth which constantly bathe the endothelium.[72]

angiogenesis dependent. For a tumor cell to metastasize successfully, it must breach several barriers and respond to specific growth factors.[82–86] Recent studies by Watnick[86a] suggest that one of the earliest events in the metastatic process is that stromal fibroblasts in a prospective metastatic site, such as the lung, may be induced to become proangiogenic by a primary tumor prior to the arrival of metastatic cells at that site. Watnick and colleagues showed that a primary tumor with a predilection to metastasize to the lung can induce the suppression of TSP-1 specifically in lung fibroblasts but not in fibroblasts of other organs that will not become future sites of metastases. Lyden showed that vascular endothelial growth factor receptor (VEGFR)-1–positive cells from bone marrow arrive at a specific future site of metastasis before the metastatic cells themselves arrive (D. Lyden, personal communication). Subsequently, tumor cells must gain access to the vasculature in the primary tumor, survive the circulation, arrest in the microvasculature of the target organ exit from this vasculature, grow in the target organ, and induce angiogenesis.[84–90] In fact, primary tumors that are not yet angiogenic are not metastatic. The most compelling experimental evidence for this statement is that nonangiogenic tumor cells isolated and cloned from human tumors and implanted into SCID mice will grow to a tumor of ~1 mm^3 and will proliferate similar to angiogenic tumor cells but will not spontaneously metastasize during the life of the host animal (T. Udagawa et al, personal communication, 2005). Transfection of these nonangiogenic tumor cells with the gene for green fluorescent protein permits the constant visualization of these microscopic tumors. If angiogenic tumor cells expressing red fluorescent protein are mixed with the nonangiogenic tumor cells, the microscopic tumor becomes neovascularized and both green and red microscopic tumor colonies appear in the lung as spontaneous metastases. However, the green nonangiogenic metastases remain at the same size limit (< 0.8 mm^3), whereas the red angiogenic metastases grow beyond this size limit and kill the mice. If the green nonangiogenic tumor cells are injected into the tail vein (unaccompanied by angiogenic tumor cells), they will form microscopic lung metastases but remain harmless at the same size limit of < 0.8 mm^3. These experimental results indicate that nonangiogenic human tumor cells are capable of completing the metastatic process once they have entered the circulation. They are, however, unable to enter the circulation from a nonangiogenic tumor.[91,92] Therefore, angiogenesis appears to be necessary at the beginning and at the completion of the metastatic cascade.

Tumor cells can enter the circulation by penetrating through proliferating capillaries that have fragmented basement membranes and are leaky.[92,93] Further, angiogenic factors from tumors such as bFGF and vascular permeability factor (VPF)/VEGF induce increased production of plasminogen activator and collagenases in proliferating endothelial cells, thus further contributing to degradation of basement membranes.[94–96] These degradative enzymes may facilitate the entry of tumor cells into the circulation. Tumor cells may not immediately become neovascularized after reaching the target organ. Such a metastasis lacking angiogenic activity for a variety of reasons may remain as a microscopic tumor of 100 to 200 μm diameter indefinitely.[42,97,98] It has been the conventional wisdom that in human dormant micrometastases (eg, metastases appearing 5 to 10 years after removal of a breast cancer), tumor cells are not cycling or are in G_0 phase. However, increasing experimental evidence indicates that micrometastases can be held dormant by blocked angiogenesis that results in a balance of tumor cell proliferation and apoptosis.[42,97] Finally, experimental metastases are as susceptible as primary tumors to control by specific angiogenesis inhibitors.[65,66] However, the relative efficacy of a given angiogenesis inhibitor can be affected by differences in metastatic sites and by the presence or absence of the primary tumor.[65]

Prevascular Phase Limits Tumor Expansion During the prevascular phase, when angiogenic activity is absent or insufficient, nonangiogenic tumors remain small, with volumes measured in a few cubic millimeters. Growth of the whole tumor is slow, and doubling times for the whole tumor may be years. However, this does not mean that the tumor cells are proliferating slowly. Experimental studies show that tumor cells in a nonangiogenic tumor may have a [^{3}H]thymidine labeling index as high as that of a large vascularized tumor. However, the nonangiogenic tumor reaches a steady state in which generation of new tumor cells is balanced by tumor cell apoptosis.[99]

When a nonangiogenic bladder cancer, cervical cancer, or cutaneous melanoma is first detected, these lesions are usually thin, slowly growing, stable for months to years, asymptomatic, and rarely metastatic.[100–103] For the majority of tumors, however, the nonangiogenic stage is clinically undetectable and can be observed only microscopically. For example, in breast and prostate cancer, carcinomas in situ can be observed before and after neovascularization in the same specimen.[89,104,105]

The size limits of experimental tumors when angiogenesis is blocked or absent are between approximately 0.2 mm (eg, for lung metastases in mice) and 2 mm (eg, for vascular chondrosarcomas in rats,[106] with a tumor population of 10^5 to 10^6 cells) in diameter.[42,106] The differences in size of prevascular (nonangiogenic) tumors may be due in part to the capacity of tumor cells to survive under differing degrees of hypoxia (Figure 11-3).[51,107] However, if cancer cells are already angiogenic at the time of implantation, they can initiate angiogenesis before the tumor population would have reached the limiting size of a non-neovascularized tumor (ie, 0.2–2 mm). The evidence for this conclusion is from an experiment in which only 20 to 30 angiogenic mammary tumor cells were implanted into a transparent skin chamber in a mouse.[108,109] The tumor cells elongated by day 2, migrated toward the nearest microvessels in a parallel orientation by day 4, divided undirectionally, induced vascular dilation and tortuosity in the neighboring microvessels by day 6, and stimulated new vascular sprouts and loops with intermittent blood flow by day 8. By this time, a microscopic colony of up to 300 to 400 cells was visible. Tumor cells preferentially grew contiguous to the microvessel sprouts, and by day 20, the tumor was filled with a newly formed vasculature. When angiogenesis was prevented by injection into the chamber of a truncated soluble receptor (Flk-1) for VEGF, some tumor cells underwent apoptosis and microscopic tumors regressed or became dormant within 5 days (ie, before the appearance of neovascular sprouts). The soluble receptor potently inhibited endothelial cell proliferation in vitro but had no effect on tumor cells. This result provides evidence for the operation of a two-way paracrine exchange of growth factors and survival factors between tumor cells and neighboring vascular endothelial cells (see below). In this model, tumor cells secrete angiogenic proteins that activate endothelial cells to elaborate chemoattractants for tumor cells. Simultaneously, the activated endothelium forms new vascular sprouts directed toward the tumor. Vascular endothelial cells can produce at least 20 mitogens and antiapoptotic factors.[110] Many of these proteins, such as bFGF and heparin-binding epithelial growth factor, are stored in the extracellular matrix and could be mobilized by proteases secreted by VEGF-stimulated endothelial cells.[106]

It is also possible that VEGF elaborated from tumor cells increases the permeability of local microvessels so that the tumor microcolony is bathed in nutrients even before neovascularization begins. The diffusion of nutrients (and oxygen) into the tumor bed would also be facilitated by loss of pericytes from microvessels owing to endothelial elaboration of angiopoietin 2.[111] Endothelial cells up-regulate expression of angiopoietin 2 in the presence of tumor cells. Further, plasma and fibrin leakage from the microvessels could facilitate chemotaxis and alignment of tumor cells, as well as subsequent migration of endothelial cells.[112,113] VEGF also up-regulates synthesis of nitric oxide in vascular endothelium.[114–116] Vasodilation and vessel tortuosity permit endothelial elongation and thus may be a prerequisite for endothelial cells to undergo mitosis and migration in response to angiogenic factors such as VEGF.[117] Even highly transformed neoplastic cells respond more efficiently to mitogens when the cells are elongated or spread than when they are rounded.[118,119] Furthermore, when well-vascularized tumors in mice were treated with anti-VEGF monoclonal antibodies, there was a dramatic reduction in diameter, tortuosity, and vascular permeability in the tumor vessels.[58]

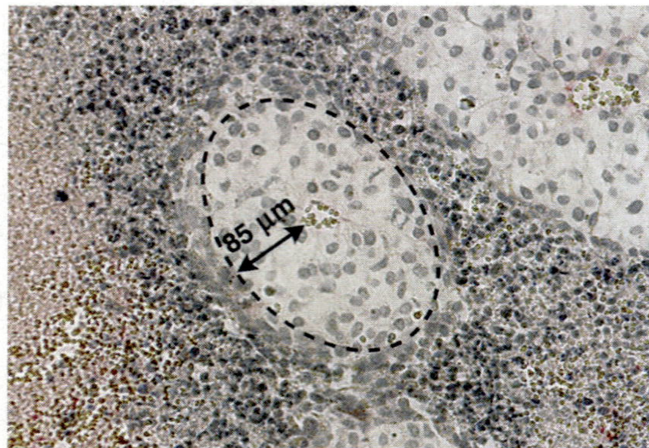

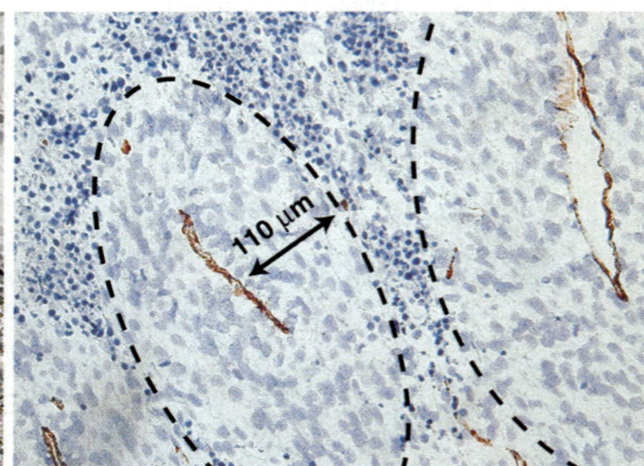

Figure 11-3 Left Panel: A cuff of live tumor cells around a microvessel in a human melanoma growing in a SCID mouse has an average radius of 85 microns. The appearance of an ellipsoid is due to the way the section is cut. Right Panel: A cuff of rat prostate cancer cells around a microvessel has an average radius of 110 microns.[558]

In summary, when a microscopic population of tumor cells emerges in avascular epidermis or mucosa—before becoming angiogenic—it may remain dormant as an in situ carcinoma separated from its vascular bed by a basement membrane.[46] If a nonangiogenic tumor emerges in vascularized tissue (ie, an islet cell carcinoma) or as a micrometastasis, it may form a microcylinder of tumor cells around preexisting capillary vessels (also called cooption).[42,46,57,58,98] In all of these situations, the preangiogenic tumor is restricted in size to a range of approximately 0.2 to 2 mm in diameter.[42,106] In contrast, a microscopic population of angiogenic tumor cells may begin to modify microvessels in the neighborhood by inducing an increase in vascular permeability, dilation, and tortuosity even before the induction of new vascular sprouts.[5]

Human Tumors and Spontaneous Animal Tumors Switch to an Angiogenic Phenotype **Mechanisms of the Angiogenic Switch** Normal cells that have been transformed to neoplastic cells are not usually angiogenic at the outset. Experimental studies of spontaneous tumors in transgenic mice reveal that the angiogenic switch is a discrete event that develops during progressive stages of tumorigenesis, beginning with the premalignant stage in these mouse models.[46,120,121] By the time most human tumors are detected, for example, by a positive mammogram, neovascularization has usually occurred. However, these tumors arise without angiogenic activity, exist in situ without neovascularization for months to years, and then switch to an angiogenic phenotype.[121] Although the angiogenic phenotype usually appears after the expression of the malignant phenotype, some human tumors (ie, carcinoma of the cervix) become neovascularized in the preneoplastic or dysplastic stage, before the malignant tumor appears.[102] At least four mechanisms of the angiogenic switch have been identified in both human tumors and spontaneous tumors in mice.

Prevascular Tumors Recruit Their Own Blood Supply This is the most common mechanism of the angiogenic switch. Approximately 95% of human cancers are carcinomas that originate as microscopic in situ lesions in an avascular epithelial layer separated by a basement membrane from underlying vasculature in the dermis or submucosa, respectively. In microscopic ductules of the breast or prostate containing in situ carcinoma that has switched to the angiogenic phenotype, one can observe a ring of new microvessels encircling the ductule. However, these vessels remain temporarily separated from the tumor cells by an intact basement membrane. The basement membrane is a physical and molecular barrier to migrating endothelial cells. For example, tumstatin, a potent inhibitor of endothelial cell migration and proliferation, is found in collagen IV.[71] After the basement membrane has been breached by new vessel sprouts, tumor cells form multiple cell layers around each new capillary blood vessel.[122] The radius of these microcylinders is restricted to the oxygen diffusion limit for a given tumor type, as originally defined by Thomlinson and Gray.[37,50] For example, for a human melanoma, the oxygen diffusion limit is approximately 85 μm. Beyond that distance from a capillary blood vessel, virtually all tumor cells are apoptotic (or necrotic). Within that radius, most tumor cells are viable (see Figure 11-3). For a prostate carcinoma, the oxygen diffusion limit is approximately 110 μm, and it may be greater for certain tumors, such as for a chondrosarcoma or a tumor in which p53 is mutated or absent, but rarely would 200 μm be exceeded.

Circulating Endothelial Stem Cells in Tumor Angiogenesis Recent experimental and clinical evidence reveals that circulating endothelial progenitor cells derived from stem cell reservoirs in the postnatal bone marrow can be recruited to the vascular bed of tumors and contribute to tumor growth.[81,123–135] Functional VEGFR-1 is expressed on hematopoietic stem cells (CD34$^+$ in humans and Lin$^-$Sca-1$^+$c-Kit$^+$ in mice).[133] Functional VEGFR-2 is expressed on CD34$^+$ AC133$^+$ progenitor human endothelial cells. VEGF elaborated by a variety of tumor signals through both VEGFR-1 (Flt-1) and VEGFR-2 (Flk-1) can mobilize progenitor endothelial cells into the circulation, where they are recruited into the vascular bed of certain tumor types but not others.[81]

Before endothelial progenitor cells can leave the bone marrow, they must transfer (along with hematopoietic stem cells) from the quiescent to the proliferative niche within the marrow. Mobilization of hematopoietic stem cells and progenitor endothelial cells necessary for their transfer to the proliferative niche is dependent on release of soluble Kit ligand, which itself depends on up-regulation of metalloproteinase 9.[134] Thus, the microvascular endothelial cells in the vascular bed of a tumor may be recruited from both the local neighborhood and the bone marrow. Rafii showed that the ratio of these endothelial cells from different sources may differ by tumor type (S. Rafii, personal communication). At this writing, the ratios of bone marrow–derived endothelium and local endothelium have not been elucidated for a wide variety of tumors. The contribution of bone marrow–derived endothelial cells to human tumors may be significantly lower than for mouse tumors.[134a]

First, the efficacy of conventional chemotherapy may turn out to correlate with the percentage of bone marrow–derived endothelial cells in a tumor. Second, during conventional chemotherapy, the off-therapy intervals necessary to rescue bone marrow may result in a surge of progenitor endothelial cells that could traffic to the tumor (S. Rafii, personal communication). Third, certain angiogenesis inhibitors may suppress the release of bone marrow–derived progenitor endothelial cells. Angiostatin targets progenitor endothelial cells, endostatin induces apoptosis in circulating endothelial cells in tumor-bearing mice, and thalidomide decreases circulating endothelial cells by 10-fold in multiple myeloma.[136–138] Endothelial cells (P1H1-12) in the circulation may be shed from the vascular bed of a tumor, especially after therapy, when apoptotic endothelial cells may appear in the circulation. Some of these cells may be apoptotic. Quantification of these two populations of circulating endothelial cells, bone marrow–derived progenitor endothelial cells and endothelial cells shed from the vascular bed of a tumor, is currently being evaluated as a potential surrogate marker for efficacy of antiangiogenic therapy or perhaps for chemotherapy.

Circulating VEGF may be one of the angiogenic signals by which tumors recruit endothelial cells from bone marrow. Subcutaneously implanted collagen gels embedded with VEGF are invaded by endothelial cells from bone marrow and from the local neighborhood.[81] VEGF serum concentrations closely correlate with platelet counts in cancer patients. VEGF is stored in platelets, transported, and released from them.[355,356,445a] Furthermore, Verheul and Pinedo and their colleagues reported that platelet counts have prognostic significance for cancer patients: higher platelet counts correlate with a worse prognosis.[357–359] Therefore, it is possible that for those types of tumors that recruit bone marrow–derived endothelial cells, communication from tumor to bone marrow may be mediated in part by the VEGF in circulating platelets. At this writing, these results have as yet no direct impact on clinical cancer therapy. However, oncologists should be aware of a potential role for platelets in cancer growth and in tumor angiogenesis. For example, bone marrow–supportive agents, currently used in high-dose chemotherapy, contribute to platelet production and thereby may influence the response to therapy.[357]

Nonendothelial Host Cells May Amplify Tumor Angiogenesis In addition to recruiting vascular endothelium from the host, certain tumors may also attract mast cells, macrophages, and inflammatory cells.[139–142] These cells can amplify tumor angiogenesis by releasing proangiogenic molecules such as bFGF or by releasing metalloproteinases that can mobilize VEGF and other angiogenic proteins.[106,113,139,143] Tumor angiogenesis and tumor growth are significantly diminished in mice deficient in metalloproteinase 9.[141] Certain tumor cells may also trigger host stromal cells (especially fibroblasts) in the tumor bed to overexpress the angiogenic protein VEGF.[144] This is another mechanism of amplification of the angiogenic phenotype once it has been initiated. Watnick has shown that c-myc elaborated from tumor cells down-regulates TSP-1 expression by stromal fibroblasts.

Vessel Cooption In certain metastases (eg, the mouse brain), it has been shown that tumor cells exit from microvessels in the target organ, begin to grow around these vessels, cause the endothelial cells to undergo apoptosis, and, finally, induce neovascular sprouts from neighboring vessels. This process, called cooption, may represent an intermediate or alternative step in the switch to the angiogenic phenotype.[57,58]

The general hypothesis that tumors are angiogenesis dependent and that antiangiogenic therapy is a method of controlling tumor growth operates for any or all of these mechanisms of angiogenic switching.

Molecular Components of the Angiogenic Switch The first proteins that regulate angiogenesis were discovered in the early 1980s.

Promoters of Angiogenesis The observation in the 1970s that tumors implanted into the avascular cornea or onto the vascularized chick chorioallantoic membrane induced an ingrowth of new capillaries indicated that tumors released diffusible angiogenic factors.[46] This result motivated the development of in vitro and in vivo bioassays to guide the search for tumor-derived angiogenic factors.[147–149]

Fibroblast Growth Factors bFGF or fibroblast growth factor (FGF) 2 was the first angiogenic protein to be isolated and purified from a tumor (1982), followed shortly by acidic fibroblast growth factor (aFGF or FGF-1).[29,150–152] There is extensive literature on the FGFs and their receptors (reviewed in Amalric and colleagues).[153] aFGFs and bFGFs stimulate endothelial cell mitosis and migration in vitro and are among the most potent angiogenic proteins in vivo. They have high affinity for heparin and heparan sulfate and are stored in extracellular matrix but lack a signal sequence for secretion.[154] The expression of bFGF receptors is very low. Although many different cells synthesize bFGF, including tumor cells of the central nervous system, sarcomas, genitourinary tumors, and even endothelial cells in the tumor vasculature, it is not clear how bFGFs, in the absence of a signal sequence, are exported from tumors, unless proteinases or heparanases mediate release of FGF from the extracellular matrix.[143,154–158] Recent work on identification of an FGF-binding protein secreted by tumors into the extracellular matrix may illuminate a mechanism of tumor mobilization of stored FGFs.[159–161] Furthermore, some tumors recruit macrophages[140] and activate them to secrete bFGF,[143] whereas others attract mast cells,[162] which, because of their high content of heparin, could sequester bFGF. In spontaneous tumors that arise in transgenic mice, aFGF and bFGF are exported into conditioned medium by angiogenic tumor cells but not by preangiogenic cells in earlier stages of tumor progression.[54,120] bFGF is not a specific endothelial mitogen but has several cell targets, including fibroblasts, smooth muscle cells, and neurons. Therefore, it is puzzling why experimental tumors transfected with bFGF containing an engineered signal sequence stimulate mainly endothelial proliferation almost to the exclusion of smooth muscle and fibroblast proliferation.[61,163] However, the ability of endothelium-derived angiopoietin 2 to repel smooth muscle or to prevent smooth muscle or pericytes from intimate contact with endothelial cells may explain this phenomenon in part (see Angiopoietins below).[164–166]

bFGF interferes with adhesion of leukocytes to endothelium, and it has been suggested that tumors that elaborate bFGF may produce a form of local immunologic tolerance.[167–169]

Abnormally elevated levels of bFGF are found in the serum and urine of some cancer patients and in the cerebrospinal fluid of patients with different types of brain tumors.[170,171] High bFGF levels in renal carcinoma correlated with a poor outcome.[172] Also, bFGF levels in the urine of children with Wilms' tumor correlate with the stage of disease and tumor grade.[173]

VEGF/VPF Dvorak first proposed that tumor angiogenesis is associated with increased microvascular permeability.[174] This led to the identification of VPF.[175–177] VPF was subsequently sequenced by Ferrara and in 1989 was reported to be a specific inducer of angiogenesis called VEGF.[176–179] At the same time, a novel angiogenic protein was first isolated and purified from a tumor (sarcoma 180) in the Folkman laboratory and in a collaboration with Ferrara was shown to be VEGF.[179] Since then, more than 15 angiogenic inducers have been identified, most of them as tumor products.[180] VEGF is an endothelial cell mitogen and motogen that is angiogenic in vivo.[181–183] Its expression correlates with blood vessel growth during embryogenesis and is essential for development of the embryonic vascular system.[184–186] VEGF expression also correlates with angiogenesis in the female reproductive tract and in tumors.[187–190] VEGF is a 40 to 45 kDa homodimeric protein with a signal sequence secreted by a wide variety of cells and the majority of tumor cells. VEGF exists as five different isoforms of 121, 145, 165, 189, and 206 amino acids, of which $VEGF_{165}$ is the predominant molecular species, produced by a variety of normal and neoplastic cells. Two receptors for VEGF are found mainly on vascular endothelial cells: the 180 kDa fms-like tyrosine kinase (Flt-1)[191] and the 200 kDa human kinase insert domain-containing receptor (KDR) and its mouse homologue, Flk-1.[192] VEGF binds to both receptors, but KDR/Flk-1 transduces the signals for endothelial proliferation and chemotaxis.[7,193–196] Other structural homologues of the VEGF family include VEGF-B, VEGF-C, VEGF-D, and VEGF-E.[197,198] VEGF-C binds to Flt-4, which is preferentially expressed on lymphatic endothelium.[199,200]

Klagsbrun and colleagues discovered that neuropilin 1, a neuronal guidance molecule, is a receptor for $VEGF_{165}$ but not for VEGF.[121,201] This finding provides a molecular mediator that coordinates growth in the vascular system with the nervous system. Other neuronal guidance proteins and/or their receptors are also angiogenesis regulators. For example, neuropilin is a receptor for VEGF and for semaphorin. Semaphorin repels neurite outgrowth and is also an angiogenesis inhibitor. Ephrins are neural guidance molecules but also genetically determined arteries and veins during embryogenesis. Ephrin B2 is expressed by tumor vascular endothelium. The receptor for slit is roundabout (Robo). The receptors for netrin are Unc 5 and DCC.

Neuropilin is not a tyrosine kinase receptor and is expressed on nonendothelial cells, including tumor cells. This allows VEGF, which is synthesized by tumor cells to bind to their surface. Surface-bound VEGF could make endothelial cells chemotactic to tumor cells, or it could act in a juxtacrine manner to mediate cooption of microvessels by tumor cells. Neuropilin also binds placental growth factor 2 (PlGF-2), and heparin is essential for the binding of $VEGF_{165}$ and PlGF-2 to neuropilin 1.[57,202] The natural cell surface polysaccharide in vivo is heparan sulfate, not heparin. Heparan sulfate may act as a template to accelerate the interaction of VEGF or PlGF-2 with VEGF. VEGF expression by tumors is up-regulated by hypoxia and is often elevated near areas of tumor necrosis.[203–207] Hypoxia activates a hypoxia-inducible factor 1 (HIF-1) binding sequence in the VEGF promoter, which leads to VEGF messenger ribonucleic acid (mRNA) transcription and stability.[7,205]

VEGF expression is also up-regulated by the *ras* oncogene. The farnesyl transferase inhibitors inhibit ras expression. It has been suggested that at least one mechanism of their antitumor effect may be to inhibit angiogenesis by inhibiting VEGF expression.[208]

VEGF expression is inhibited by the von Hippel-Lindau (VHL) protein.[209] The VHL tumor suppressor gene is inactivated in patients with VHL disease and in most sporadic clear cell renal carcinomas.[210,211] The VHL gene negatively regulates a series of hypoxia-inducible genes, including the VEGF, platelet-derived growth factor (PDGF) B, and glucose transporter 1 genes.[209,212] When VHL is mutated or deleted, these genes are overexpressed even under normoxic conditions. A recent important therapeutic advance employed an inhibitor (SU5416) of VEGFR-2 to restore sight in a patient with VHL disease who had a hemangioblastoma in the retina of her only eye.[213]

VEGF also induces fenestrations in endothelium of small venules and capillaries and even in tissues in which microvessels are not normally fenestrated.[212,214] The increased permeability of tumor vessels as revealed, for example, by the edema of brain tumors, may be partly mediated by VEGF.[215]

It is possible that certain other positive regulators of angiogenesis may operate through VEGF or be VEGF dependent. It remains to be seen whether the high angiogenic activity of bFGF is somehow acting indirectly through another endothelial mitogen, such as VEGF (see below), because of the following observations. First, bFGF induces the expression of VEGF.[216] Second, the two endothelial mitogens act synergistically[216–218] to stimulate capillary tube formation in vitro. Third, systemic administration of a soluble receptor for VEGF (Flk-1) completely blocks cornea angiogenesis induced by implanted bFGF (R. D'Amato and C. Kuo, unpublished data). Another positive regulator of angiogenesis, transforming growth factor (TGF)-α, may also be dependent on VEGF. VEGF mRNA and protein are induced in fibroblasts and epithelial cells by TGF-α[220] In contrast, mRNA for placental growth factor, an angiogenic protein related to VEGF, is not induced by TGF-α.

These recent findings suggest that the angiogenic effect of TGF-α is mediated partly by its induction of VEGF in tissues. A clinical implication of these studies is that angiogenesis inhibitors that block VEGF may inhibit other angiogenic promoters as well.

Angiopoietins Angiopoietin 1 is a 70 kDa ligand that binds to a specific tyrosine kinase expressed only on endothelial cells, called Tie2 (also called Tek). A ligand for Tie1 has not been elucidated.[221–225] Like VEGF, angiopoietin 1 is an endothelial cell–specific growth factor. Angiopoietin 1, however, is not a direct endothelial mitogen in vitro. Rather, it induces endothelial cells to recruit pericytes and smooth muscle cells to become incorporated in the vessel wall. Pericyte and smooth muscle recruitment is mediated by endothelial production of PDGF-BB (and probably other factors) when Tie2 is activated by angiopoietin 1.[226] There is increased vascularization in mice that overexpress angiopoietin 1 in the skin.[224] The vessels are significantly larger than normal, and the skin is reddened. The vessels are not leaky, and there is no skin edema, in contrast to the dermal vessels of mice overexpressing VEGF. In double transgenic mice expressing both angiopoietin 1 and VEGF in the skin, dermal angiogenesis is increased in an additive manner, but the vessels do not leak.[227] This model closely approximates angiogenesis in healing wounds (ie, relatively nonleaky vessels with pericytes and some perivascular smooth muscle cells contained in the vascular wall). In contrast, tumor vessels are leaky and thin walled, with a paucity of pericytes. Angiopoietin 2, produced by vascular endothelium in a tumor bed, blocks the Tie2 receptor and acts to repel pericytes and smooth muscle.[225] Nevertheless, tumor vessels remain thin "endothelium-lined tubes" even though some of these microvessels reach the diameter of venules. A key point is that angiopoietin 2 and VEGF together increase angiogenesis. However, if VEGF is antagonized or withdrawn at this point, endothelial cells may undergo apoptosis and new microvessels can regress.[227]

It is useful for clinicians to think of two classes of angiogenesis inhibitors: direct and indirect.[37]

Indirect Angiogenesis Inhibitors Indirect angiogenesis inhibitors generally decrease or block expression of a tumor cell product, neutralize the tumor product itself, or block its receptor on endothelial cells (Figure 11-4). Many of these tumor cell proteins are the products of oncogenes that drive the angiogenic switch. Rak and Kerbel and their colleagues reviewed the impact of 15 different oncogenes on tumor angiogenesis.[37,228–230] In vitro assays were originally employed to elucidate the activities of oncogene and tumor suppressor gene products, including proliferation of cancer cells, resistance to apoptosis, immortalization, and anchorage independence.[228,229] In these in vitro assays, increased cancer cell proliferation and decreased apoptosis associated with oncogene mutations correlated so well with tumor growth in vivo that there was at first no indication that oncogenes could also up-regulate angiogenic activity in tumor cells,[231] nor was there any basis to predict that novel anticancer drugs, which inhibit oncogene activity by inhibition of its signal transduction (eg, signal transduction inhibitors such as trastuzumab [Herceptin]), could also block proangiogenic products of tumor cells.[231] Only recently has it been recognized that many oncogenes are proangiogenic

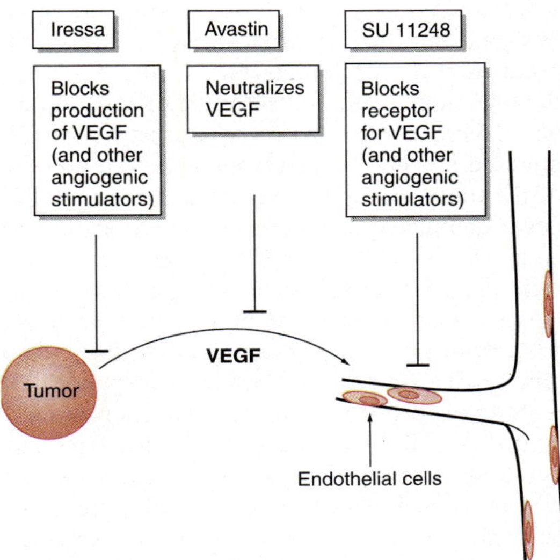

Figure 11-4 Examples of indirect angiogenesis inhibitors that can block production of a tumor cell angiogenic protein (Iressa), or neutralize a pro-angiogenic factor in the blood (Avastin), or block a receptor for a tumor cell produced angiogenic factor (SU11248).

and that this may be a major component of their tumorigenic activity.

Other experimental studies in which transfection with oncogenes increases tumor cell output of proangiogenic proteins and/or decreases expression of negative regulators of angiogenesis support this concept.[76,77,99,230] For example, when the *bcl-2* oncogene was transfected into prostate cancer cells that were already capable of developing large neovascularized tumors, VEGF expression and microvessel density both increased significantly.[232] Therefore, drugs that target oncogenes, their products, or the receptors of those products not only inhibit proliferation of tumor cells and increase their susceptibility to apoptosis, they also, most importantly, disrupt production of tumor angiogenesis. Even reactivation of the tumor suppressor *p53* can inhibit angiogenesis by at least four different mechanisms, which are discussed below.[75,161,233,234] It is not surprising, then, that certain anticancer drugs developed for their capacity to block an oncogene product (eg, inhibitors of the epidermal growth factor receptor tyrosine kinase) may have significant antiangiogenic activity and that it will be "indirect."[228,231,235] For example, ras farnesyl transferase inhibitors block oncogene signaling pathways, which up-regulate tumor cell production of VEGF and down-regulate production of the angiogenesis inhibitor TSP-1.[208]

Why emphasize in this chapter that anticancer drugs originally developed to target an oncogene product may also inhibit tumor angiogenesis? A clinician armed with this knowledge should be better able to optimize the dose and schedule of an "antioncogene drug" or a "signal transduction inhibitor" by following antiangiogenic guidelines.[37] For example, mutant tumor cells may begin to express "redundant" angiogenic proteins that differ from those angiogenic proteins blocked by an "indirect" angiogenesis inhibitor. As a result, the indirect angiogenesis inhibitor may be discontinued prematurely because of the assumption that the tumor had become drug resistant and because conventional chemotherapy is traditionally discontinued in the presence of acquired drug resistance (see Figure 11-4). However, a clinician may find it prudent to continue a drug with significant antiangiogenic activity, especially if it is not toxic, and add a second angiogenesis inhibitor. For example, trastuzumab, an antibody that blocks *HER2/neu* receptor tyrosine kinase signaling, suppresses cancer cell production of angiogenic factors such as TGF-α, angiopoietin 1, and plasminogen activator inhibitor 1 (PAI-1) and possibly VEGF.[231,235] Trastuzumab also up-regulates expression of an endogenous angiogenesis inhibitor, TSP, which may be the important basis of its antiangiogenic activity.[235] If tumor cells begin to express a different angiogenic protein, such as bFGF, or interleukin-8, the tumor under treatment may appear to have become "resistant" to trastuzumab.[236,237] A similar speculation may apply to certain EGF receptor inhibitors, such as gefitinib (Iressa).[237,238]

Of interest is that certain tumors, such as giant cell bone tumors and angioblastomas, generate only or mainly bFGF and rarely express additional angiogenic proteins. When patients with these tumors were treated with interferon-α at low daily doses, drug resistance was not observed with therapy that was continued for up to 3.5 years' duration.[239–242] Interferon-α at low doses inhibits bFGF production by tumor cells and would therefore be considered an indirect angiogenesis inhibitor.[243] However, interferon also inhibits endothelial cell motility directly and therefore can be considered to have both direct and indirect antiangiogenic activity.[244]

Direct Angiogenesis Inhibitors Direct angiogenesis inhibitors block vascular endothelial cells from proliferating, migrating, or increasing their survival in response to a spectrum of proangiogenic proteins, including VEGF, bFGF, interleukin-8, PDGF, PD-ECGF, and others. Direct angiogenesis inhibitors are less likely to induce acquired drug resistance because they target genetically stable endothelial cells rather than unstable mutating tumor cells.[245] Tumors in mice treated with antiangiogenic therapy did not develop drug resistance.[69] This does not mean that angiogenesis inhibitors are less susceptible to metabolic degradation, increased clearance from the bloodstream, or development of neutralizing antibodies than other systemically administered drugs.

Direct angiogenesis inhibitors include (1) certain synthetic inhibitors or peptides designed to interfere with various steps in the angiogenic process (eg, antagonists of the integrin $\alpha_v\beta_3$ or $\alpha_5\beta_1$ or inhibitors of metalloproteinases); (2) low-molecular-weight compounds (eg, TNP-470 and Caplostatin, thalidomide, angiostatic steroids such as tetrahydrocortisol, 2-methoxyestradiol, and squalamine; and (3) endogenous (natural) proteins, which generally prevent vascular endothelial cells from responding to a wide spectrum of angiogenic promoters (eg, interferon-α, interleukin-12, platelet factor 4, TSP-1, angiostatin, endostatin, arrestin, canstatin, tumstatin, PEX (matrix metalloproteinase 2), pigment epithelium–derived factor, and antiangiogenic antithrombin III (an internal fragment of antithrombin III, named aaAT).[28,59,64,65,67,70,246–266]

Angiostatin, endostatin, tumstatin, arrestin, canstatin, and aaAT are specific angiogenesis inhibitors. The rationale that led to their discovery is discussed here in detail because (1) these proteins have profoundly changed our thinking about how primary tumors and metastases regulate their own growth; (2) the method of their discovery provides a unique strategy that is leading to the elucidation of an enlarging family of endogenous angiogenesis inhibitors, which, under physiologic conditions, may act to limit or prevent angiogenesis; and (3) endostatin, Abbott 510 (a fragment of TSP-1), and tetrahydrocortisol are currently in phase II clinical trials.[267] Tumstatin is a candidate for future clinical trials (see the sections on clinical trials below).

The first clue to the existence of endogenous angiogenesis inhibitors came from the discovery that interferon-α inhibited endothelial cell migration and that platelet factor 4 inhibited endothelial proliferation.[244,260,268] Both were subsequently shown to inhibit angiogenesis.[244,260,268–270]

However, Bouck was the first to show that a tumor could generate an angiogenesis inhibitor. Bouck and her colleagues subsequently proposed that the angiogenic phenotype was the result of a net balance of endogenous inhibitors and stimulators of angiogenesis.[271] A nontumorigenic hamster cell line became tumorigenic in association with the loss of a suppressor gene and concomitant with the onset of angiogenic activity. The nontumorigenic line secreted high levels of an angiogenesis inhibitor, a truncated form of TSP-1, that decreased by about 96% in the tumorigenic cells.[261] TSP-1 was shown to be regulated by the wild-type tumor suppressor *p53* in fibroblasts and in mammary epithelial cells.[75,272] Loss of p53 function in the transformed derivatives of these cells dramatically decreased the level of the angiogenesis inhibitor. Restoration of p53 up-regulated TSP-1 and raised the antiangiogenic activity of the tumor cells. Deletion of TSP-1 led to accelerated growth of breast cancers that arise spontaneously in neu-transgenic mice.[273] The demonstration by Rastinejad and colleagues that the switch to an angiogenic phenotype involved a negative regulator of angiogenesis generated by the tumor per se suggested to Folkman a unifying angiogenic mechanism to explain a well-recognized but previously unsolved clinical and experimental phenomenon: the inhibition of tumor growth by the tumor mass. A description of this phenomenon is quoted from the introduction of Folkman's article[65]: "The removal of certain tumors, eg, breast carcinomas, colon carcinomas, and osteogenic sarcomas can be followed by rapid growth of distant metastases."[274–277] Postoperative chemotherapy was introduced mainly to prevent or delay the growth of secondary metastases. Several studies in terminally ill patients demonstrated the suppression of a secondary tumor by a primary tumor.[278,279] A primary tumor can suppress metastases originating from a different type of tumor (eg, a breast cancer can inhibit melanoma metastases). In melanoma, partial spontaneous regression of the primary tumor may be followed by rapid growth of metastases. When ionizing radiation is employed to regress a small cell lung cancer, distant metastases may undergo rapid growth.[70,280] If one portion of a primary tumor is removed (eg, cytoreductive surgery for testicular cancer), the residual tumor increases its rate of expansion.[281] The same phenomenon is observed in several different animal tumors, that is, that some primary tumors may inhibit the growth but not the number of their metastases.[282–286] Partial removal of a primary tumor increases the growth rate of the residual tumors similar to that in humans.[287,288] Furthermore, metastatic growth can suppress the growth of a primary tumor (analogous to the occult primary tumor in a cancer patient).[289] Many primary tumors can suppress the growth of a second tumor inoculation.[290–297] A threshold size of the primary tumor appears to be necessary for the inhibitory effect to occur, and some primary tumors can inhibit a secondary tumor of a different type.[295,297]

At least three hypotheses have been advanced to explain these diverse observations and experiments: (1) concomitant immunity, in which a primary tumor induces an immunologic response against a secondary tumor or a metastasis in the same host; (2) depletion of nutrients by the primary tumor; or (3) production of antimitotic factors from the primary tumor that directly inhibit the proliferation of the secondary tumor.[291,295,298–300] None of these concepts, however, offered a molecular mechanism to explain all of the experiments cited above, in which tumor growth is suppressed by the tumor mass.

Once it was demonstrated that a tumor could generate a negative regulator of angiogenesis, then it became clear that a primary tumor, while stimulating angiogenesis in its own vascular bed, could possibly inhibit angiogenesis in the vascular bed of a distant metastasis.[261] However, at least two conditions would be necessary: first, the primary tumor (ie, the first tumor to grow) would need to generate an angiogenic promoter in excess of an inhibitor in its own vascular bed, and, second, the putative inhibitor would need to have a longer half-life in the circulation than the angiogenic promoter. After arriving in the Folkman laboratory in 1991, O'Reilly and his colleagues validated this hypothesis by discovering angiostatin, endostatin, and antiangiogenic antithrombin over the next 8 years.[65–67,69,70,301]

Angiostatin Angiostatin is a 38 kDa internal fragment of plasminogen that was purified from the serum and urine of mice bearing a subcutaneous Lewis lung carcinoma that suppressed growth of its lung metastases by inhibiting their angiogenesis (Figure 11-5).[65] Lung metastases remained microscopic and did not grow beyond approximately 200 μm in diameter. They were not neovascularized and usually formed a microcylinder around a single microvessel. In these dormant metastases, 38% of the tumor cells were proliferating (DNA synthesis was determined by bromodeoxyuridine [BrdU]) and 7 to 8% were undergoing apoptosis.[45] The presence of a circulating angiogenesis inhibitor was evidenced by the almost complete inhibition of bFGF-stimulated corneal neovascularization in these mice. Further, serum from these tumor-bearing mice specifically inhibited capillary endothelial cell proliferation in vitro by more than 70% (but not fibroblast, smooth muscle cell, epithelial cell, or tumor cell proliferation). The tumor-bearing serum also inhibited angiogenesis on the chick chorioallantoic membrane compared with serum from mice without tumors (which stimulated endothelial cells). After removal of the primary tumor, serum endothelial inhibitory activity disappeared by 6 days (half-maximal 2.5 days), lung metastases were neovascularized by 5 days, and by 15 days, the mice were dying of large vascularized metastases. There was no change in tumor cell proliferation (approximately 38% BrdU-labeled cells), but tumor cell apoptosis fell to 2%. Systemic administration of angiostatin purified from mouse urine significantly inhibited angiogenesis in lung metastases and restricted their growth to a microscopic dormant size,[65] and recombinant angiostatin potently inhibited growth of other tumor types.[66] Again, tumor cell proliferation remained as high as in the tumor-bearing mice, and apoptosis was significantly reduced.[45,48] Angiogenesis inhibitor in the urine of tumor-bearing mice was completely removed by angiostatin neutralizing antibodies. A subline of Lewis lung carcinoma incapable of inhibiting metastatic growth did not generate angiostatin or inhibit corneal angiogenesis, nor did its serum inhibit endothelial cell growth. VEGF, the major angiogenic promoter in Lewis lung carcinoma, has a half-life of approximately 3 minutes in the circulation.

Angiostatin is not secreted by tumor cells but is generated through proteolytic cleavage of circulating plasminogen by a series of enzymes released from the tumor cells. At least one of these tumor-derived enzymes, urokinase plasminogen activator (uPA), converts plasminogen to plasmin, whereas a phosphoglycerate kinase from hypoxic tumor cells then reduces the plasmin so that it can be converted to angiostatin by one of several different metalloproteinases.[302] Other types of tumors have since been reported to generate angiostatin (eg, human prostate cancer).[303–305] Human prostate carcinoma cells express enzymatic activity that converts human plasminogen to the angiogenesis inhibitor angiostatin.[302] Prostate-specific antigen generates angiostatin-like fragments from plasminogen.[307]

Furthermore, when murine fibrosarcoma cells were transfected with angiostatin, primary subcutaneous tumors formed whose growth was slowed in proportion to increased levels of angiostatin production by the tumor cells. In these tumors, the total angiogenic output of the primary tumor was decreased by transfected angiostatin, which opposed in a dose-dependent manner the activity of the tumor's secreted angiogenic promoter but never completely counteracted it.[78] It should be emphasized that the rate of tumor growth (expansion of tumor mass) was directly proportional to the total angiogenic output of the tumor, inversely proportional to angiostatin production and to tumor cell apoptosis, and virtually independent of tumor cell proliferation. This result was confirmed in a different tumor model, Kaposi's sarcoma subjected to angiostatin gene transfer, which resulted in sustained angiostatin expression, delayed tumor growth, and reduced tumor vascularization.[360] Gene transfer with a different angiogenesis inhibitor, TSP-1, gave similar results. Streit and colleagues reported (in an experiment discussed above) that when tumor cells were transfected with the angiogenesis inhibitors TSP-1 and/or TSP-2, the proliferation rate (as determined by staining for the proliferating cell nuclear antigen), also remained relatively constant, despite the decreased angiogenesis and suppressed tumor growth.[79]Angiostatin and its isoforms induce cell arrest and apoptosis of endothelial cells and inhibit endothelial migration, angiogenesis in vitro, and angiogenesis in the quail chorioallantoic membrane.[308–317] Angiostatin can also be generated by different enzymes and by other cell types; can inhibit other tumor types by its antiangiogenic action; can decrease activity of the mitogen-activated protein kinases (MAPKs) ERK-1 and ERK-2 in endothelial cells; can up-regulate E-selectin in proliferating endothelial cells; and can be delivered in vivo by gene therapy.[302–304,313–333] Angiostatin also binds specifically to adenosine triphosphate (ATP) synthase, a transmembrane protein expressed by vascular endothelial cells, and to a fragment of vitronectin.

Angiostatin can potentiate radiation therapy of experimental tumors.[334–337] Angiostatin also appears to inhibit proliferation of circulating precursor endothelial cells derived from bone marrow.[136] Angiostatin effectively blocks endothelial cell migration induced by plasmin binding to $\alpha_v\beta_3$-integrin.[346,362] Angiostatin may act at least in part by transiently increasing ceramide, a sphingolipid second messenger implicated in a proapoptotic pathway, and by increasing RhoA, an effector of cytoskeletal structure.[361]

Other mechanisms of angiostatin have been reported. Angiostatin, but not plasminogen, specifically binds to tyrosine kinase substrate annexin II through the lysine-binding domain in endothelial cells.[338] This affinity appears to be specific for endothelial cells and does not occur with fibroblasts. Annexin II on endothelial cells organizes assembly of plasminogen on its surface and produces plasmin at maximum efficiency in the vascular bed.[338–341] Plasmin is a serine pro-

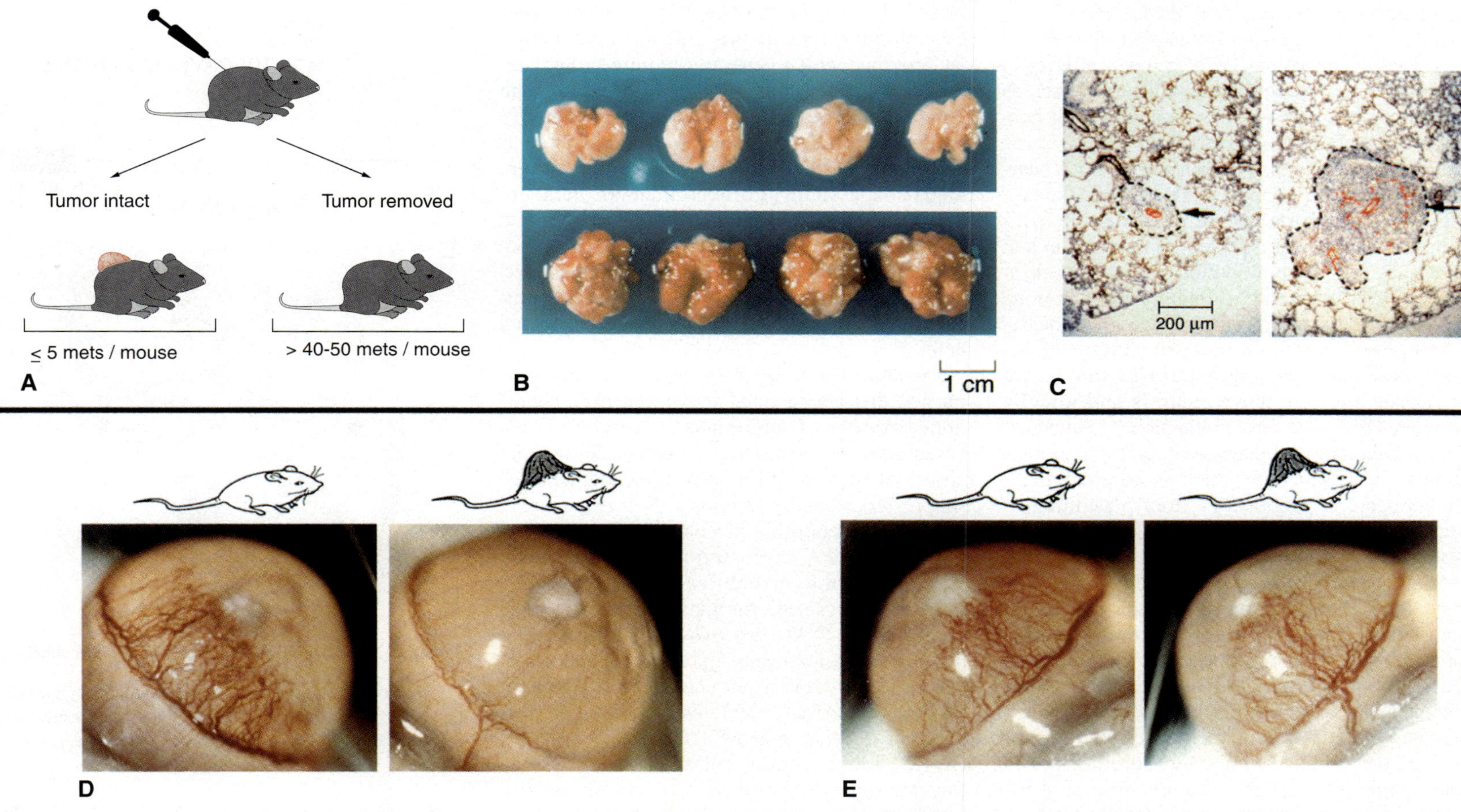

Figure 11-5 **A,** Animals bearing Lewis Lung carcinoma. Tumors were surgically removed when tumor size reached 1.5 - 2 cm^2 and the animals were killed 5 days or 15 days later. **B,** Upper panel: lungs removed from animals still bearing the primary tumor. Lower panel: lungs removed at the same time from animals in which the tumor had been removed and the animals killed 15 days later. **C,** Left panel: microscopic metastasis in the lung of an animal in which a primary tumor is in place at the same time as the right panel. This shows no angiogenesis and only a single central microvessel stained with antibody to von Willebrand factor. This dormant metastasis is approximately 200 microns in its longest diameter. Right panel: lung metastasis from an animal killed 5 days after removal of the primary tumor, showing 8 or 9 new vessels in an enlarging metastasis.[42] **D,** A human prostate carcinoma (LNCaP) growing on the dorsum of a SCID immunodeficient mouse almost completely inhibits cornea neovascularization induced by an implanted sustained release pellet of bFGF (80 ng) (right panel). Left panel shows bFGF-induced corneal neovascularization at 5 days in the absence of a primary tumor. LNCaP prostate cancer generates angiostatin. **E,** A human colon cancer that does not generate an angiogenesis inhibitor, growing on the dorsum of a SCID mouse as a control for **D**.

tease that degrades fibrin and several endothelial cell matrix proteins, such as laminin, TSP, and collagens, and facilitates capillary sprouting during angiogenesis and endothelial migration.[338,346,362] In fact, angiostatin inhibits endothelial and melanoma cellular invasion by blocking matrix-enhanced plasminogen activation.[326] However, because hypoxic tumor cells produce a phosphoglycerate kinase that enzymatically reduces plasmin, this mechanism contributes to the generation of angiostatin, which can then block plasmin organization on the endothelial surface and interfere with angiogenesis.[302,363] The gene for annexin II is also up-regulated in endothelial cells during angiogenesis. Annexin II is a central molecule in signal transduction mechanisms, and disruption of its function affects calcium signaling, tyrosine phosphorylation, cell proliferation, and apoptosis.[342–344] Angiostatin mediation of endothelial cell death appears to operate through a calcium signaling mechanism.[345] Therefore, annexin II may act as an endogenous angiogenic switch, and its blockade may be at least one potential mechanism for angiostatin.

Three other binding proteins have been suggested as putative receptors for angiostatin: (1) ATP synthase on the endothelial surface, (2) $\alpha v \beta_3$-integrin, and (3) angiomotin, which belong to a novel protein family with conserved coiled-coil and PDZ binding domains.[334,346–348] Together, annexin II and angiostatin may bind to multiple receptors and could mediate a cascade of events leading to inhibition of angiogenesis.[338] Angiostatin also inhibits signaling of hepatocyte growth factor (HGF) in endothelial cells (and in smooth muscle cells) by blocking HGF-induced signaling of c-met, Akt, and ERK-1/2.[349] However, angiostatin does not block VEGF or bFGF signaling events in endothelial cells. Angiostatin also induces intracellular acidosis and anoikis (loss of cell attachment) in endothelial cells that are incubated under conditions resembling the low pH in a tumor.[350] Angiostatin down-regulates expression of VEGF expression in tumor cells.[351] This implies that angiostatin may act as a direct and an indirect inhibitor of angiogenesis. Analysis of the x-ray crystallographic structure of angiostatin reveals that kringles 1, 2, and 3 produce a central cavity, suggesting a unique domain where they may function in concert.[352,364] The enzymatic mobilization of angiostatin is facilitated by tumor-derived matrix metalloproteinases (MMPs).[353] Other laboratories confirmed Folkman's report that circulating angiostatin generated by a primary tumor decreases significantly after certain primary tumors are removed and that this is followed by growth of remote metastases.[35,65]

Angiostatin gene therapy shows efficacy in tumor-bearing mice against a variety of tumors and their metastases, including breast cancer, renal cell cancer, gliomas, melanoma, Kaposi's sarcoma, squamous cell carcinoma, and leukemia.[310,360,365–375] Of interest is that viral vector–mediated antiangiogenic therapy using an angiostatin-endostatin fusion protein demonstrated significant down-regulation of ascites, tumor growth, vascularity, and prolongation of animal survival in three different ascites tumor models.[376] Angiostatin has been transfected into canine eyes as a preclinical model for the treatment of human uveal melanoma.[377] Long-term expression of angiostatin and endostatin from lentivirus-transduced human bladder carcinoma cells inhibited proliferation of endothelial cells cocultured with the tumor cells, the first use of a lentiviral vector for antiangiogenic gene delivery.[378] Angiostatin gene therapy has also shown efficacy in non-neoplastic mouse models of disease, such as arthritis, retinal neovascularization, choroidal neovascularization, and endometriosis.[379–382]

When angiostatin was delivered to mice bearing a variety of tumors, it showed significant efficacy either alone or in combination with endostatin, as a fusion protein of angiostatin and endostatin, or in combination with interleukin-12.[351,383–387] When three different types of murine tumors were engineered to produce granulocyte-macrophage colony-stimulating factor (GM-CSF), the level of angiostatin in the serum increased fourfold above controls and directly correlated with GM-CSF production.[388] Angiostatin levels directly correlated with macrophage metalloelastase production, which appeared to mediate cleavage of angiostatin from plasminogen. Metastases were suppressed in all three tumor systems.

Replacement of Angiostatin after Radiotherapy Radiotherapy of primary Lewis lung carcinomas in mice induced regression of the primary tumor but led to the disappearance of angiostatin from the blood and rapid growth of lung metastases.[280] Angiostatin replacement therapy prevented growth of lung metastases after regression of the primary tumor by radiotherapy. In some patients, successful radiotherapy of a primary tumor, for example, non–small cell lung cancer, is followed by growth of distant metastases. It may eventually be possible to determine if a tumor is generating an endogenous angiogenesis inhibitor prior to radiotherapy and then administer that inhibitor in combination with the radiotherapy.

Angiostatin protein also inhibits angiogenesis in non-neoplastic states. For example, angiostatin inhibits corneal neovascularization, corpus luteum development in the preovulatory follicle, and pathologic retinal angiogenesis but not physiologic retinal neovascularization.[389–392] Although the original report of 38 kDa angiostatin included kringles 1 to 4 of plasminogen, a recent report revealed the generation of a novel plasminogen fragment of 22 kDa generated by enzymatic activity from tumor cells.[65,393] The p22 plasminogen fragment includes kringle 1 plus additional N- and C-terminal residues, but circular dichroism and intrinsic fluorescence analysis define structural differences between it and recombinant kringle 1. Angiogenesis and tumor growth are potently inhibited by p22.

When a strategy similar to the one that uncovered angiostatin (eg, suppression of tumor growth by tumor mass) was employed by O'Reilly and colleagues with murine hemangioendothelioma and human small cell lung cancer, endostatin and aaAT were discovered.[67,69,70] Both endostatin and aaAT are generated from larger parent proteins by enzymes released by the tumor cells.

Endostatin Endostatin is a 20 to 22 kDa internal fragment of collagen XVIII.[67,69,394,395] It is the first of a group of endogenous angiogenesis inhibitors that are predominantly extracellular proteins, which generally require proteolytic processing to become active.[396,397] More than 760 reports on endostatin have been published in the 7 years since its isolation and identification as an angiogenesis inhibitor.[67] These range from mechanistic studies to experimental therapeutics. A variety of new findings have been reported on mechanism of action, physiologic function, structure-activity relationships, experimental therapeutics, including gene therapy, and early clinical studies. A few of these studies are reviewed here.

Structure-Activity Relationships Endostatin was first isolated and sequenced from conditioned medium of murine hemangioendothelioma based on the same strategy employed for the discovery of angiostatin (ie, hemangioendothelioma-suppressed secondary tumors).[398] It is a specific inhibitor of endothelial cell proliferation and migration, like angiostatin. High-resolution crystallographic structures have been determined for mouse and for human endostatin (Figure 11-6).[399,400] At least two enzymes produced by tumor cells are necessary to cleave endostatin from collagen XVIII: an elastase and a cathepsin.[401,402] Endostatin is derived from the nontriple helical C-terminal NC1 domain of collagen XVIII. Subsequently, collagen XV was also found to share a C-terminal NC1 domain containing the endostatin molecule, which has not been found to date in any other proteins.[403] Endostatin is released proteolytically in trimeric form and further converted to monomeric forms of about 20 kDa. Both endostatin isoforms share a compact globular fold but differ in binding properties for proteins and cells.[403] Tissue distributions are also different. Differences in activity have been found between NC1 domains, and endostatin activity may be related to its oligomerization state.

Endostatin is present in basement membranes and vessel walls and is especially rich in elastic fibers of the aorta and sparse elastic fibers of veins.[404] Some, but not all, capillaries or arterioles show weak labeling for endostatin. Within the elastic fibers, endostatin is colocalized and has been reported to bind to fibulins 1 and 2, nidogens 1 and 2, laminin 1, and perlecan.[405] Recombinant mouse endostatin binds to heparin with a K_d of 0.3 μM.[406] A major site of four clustered arginines, 155, 158, 184, and 270, and a second site (R193, R 194) are essential for binding to heparin and to heparan sulfate and sulfatides but not to fibulins 1 and 2. A minimum heparin size of 12-mer (dodecasaccharide) is necessary for efficient binding, and there is a crucial role for 2-O and 6-O sulfation. A synthetic arginine-rich dendrimer that mimicked the surface of endostatin and had high affinity for heparin had similar antiangiogenic activity in the chick embryo. This experiment demonstrates the important role of heparin affinity for the inhibitory activity of endostatin.[407] A decreased inhibitory activity after mutation of the zinc-binding site was reported for insoluble

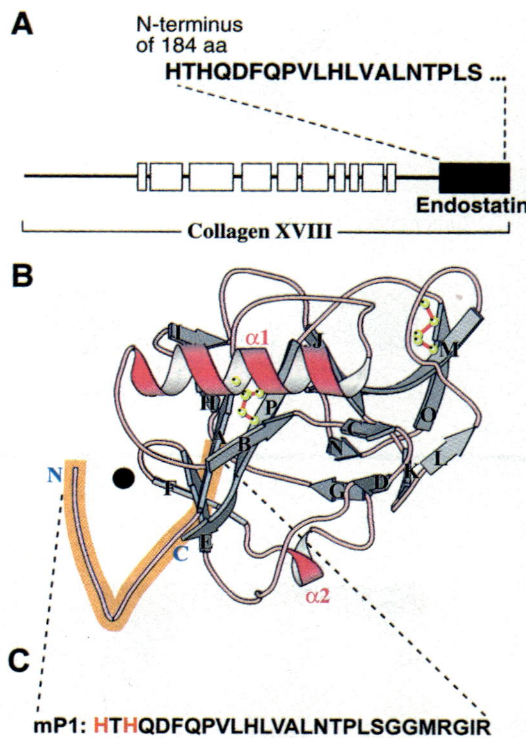

Figure 11-6 **A,** Amino acid sequence of human endostatin. **B,** Crystal structure of human endostatin resolved to 3.5 angstroms. **C,** Peptide sequence.[404a]

recombinant endostatin from *Escherichia coli*.[408] Despite two early reports that suggest that recombinant endostatin maintains its antiangiogenic and antitumor activity when zinc binding at the N-terminus is disrupted,[406,409] subsequent studies revealed that zinc binding (to a complex of three histidines in the N-terminus of endostatin) is critical for the antiangiogenic and antitumor activity of this protein.

It should not be overlooked that the original insoluble recombinant zinc-containing endostatin from *E. coli* induced more rapid tumor regression in different tumor types than has been obtained to date with soluble forms with or without zinc.[67,69] About 50% of human recombinant endostatin from yeast (produced by Entremed) binds zinc, as revealed by a doublet of protein bands on a Western gel, in contrast to recombinant *E. coli* endostatin, ~100% of which bound zinc. One possibility is that zinc is required to maintain folding of the insoluble protein.[403] Javaherian, in the Folkman laboratory, also reported that a 27–amino acid peptide in the N-terminus of endostatin retains all of the antitumor activity of the full-length protein and binds zinc.[404a] Site-specific mutations that delete one or more of the N-terminal histidines and thus prevent zinc binding inactivate the peptide. The original insoluble recombinant endostatin from *E. coli* (which was endotoxin free) is now understood to slowly release the active peptide in a nondenatured form following a subcutaneous injection. This "sustained release" of an endostatin peptide most likely accounts for the ease with which tumor regression could be achieved by once/day or twice/day subcutaneous injections of recombinant *E. coli* endostatin, in contrast to soluble yeast recombinant endostatin, which could inhibit tumor growth but could not regress it unless the endostatin was administered continuously by an implantable osmotic pump.

Furthermore, under physiologic conditions, endostatin exists mainly as a fragment of an insoluble matrix protein, collagen XVIII. It appears that only a small fraction of endostatin circulates in the soluble form (ie, in the range of 30 ng/mL).

Of the 26 collagen isoforms that have been identified so far in mammalian species, collagens IV, XV, and XVIII (which possess C-terminal globular domains) have been implicated in the regulation of angiogenesis.[410] Homologues of these three collagens have also been identified in the worm *Caenorhabditis elegans*, where the endostatin domain of type XVIII collagen and type IV collagen–like molecules control migration of neuronal cells and axon guidance instead of vascular endothelial cells.[411] The evolutionary age of endostatin and type IV collagen fragments of approximately 600 million years may be responsible, in part, for its lack of toxicity in animals and patients.[67,69,267] It is also of interest from an evolutionary perspective that certain regulators of endothelial cell migration have (or had) control of axon migration, for example, endostatin, ephrins, neuropilin, and semaphorins, among others.[412–415] This relationship provides insight into how the development of nerves and blood vessels may be coordinated.

MECHANISMS Novel mechanisms have recently been reported for the antiangiogenic action of endostatin, although we are a long way from a complete picture.

INHIBITION OF VEGFR Endostatin blocks the binding of $VEGF_{121}$ and $VEGF_{165}$ to the KDR/Flk-1 receptor, blocks tyrosine phosphorylation of this receptor, and blocks activation of its intracellular signaling events, ERK, p38 MAPK, and p125FAK.[416] This receptor mediates endothelial cell motility and proliferation. Endostatin also blocks VEGF.

DOWN-REGULATION OF VEGF EXPRESSION Although endostatin does not bind to VEGF,[416] it does down-regulate VEGF expression in tumor cells (similar to the effect of angiostatin).[351] Endostatin can therefore be considered to act as both a direct and an indirect angiogenesis inhibitor. In bFGF-treated endothelial cells, endostatin induces endothelial cell apoptosis, in part by activating tyrosine kinase signaling of the Shb adaptor protein.[417] However, endostatin does not compete with binding of bFGF to tissues and does not affect bFGF receptor signaling.[418] This result is consistent with the observation that bFGF (FGF-2) stimulation of endothelial cell proliferation in vitro and angiogenesis in vivo is mediated by VEGF.[419]

PREVENTION OF BFGF-INDUCED OR VEGF-INDUCED LOSS OF ENDOTHELIAL CELL–CELL ADHESION OR ENDOTHELIAL CELL ADHESION TO BASEMENT MEMBRANE Endothelial cell migration, which is critical for new sprout formation during angiogenesis, requires continuous turnover of cell–cell interactions and of cell–matrix interactions.[420] Cell–cell interactions between endothelial cells are maintained in part by β-catenin localized at cell–cell junctions in cadherin complexes of capillary endothelial cells in vitro. Treatment of these cells with bFGF shifts β-catenin to the cytoplasm, which loosens cell–cell adhesion and facilitates endothelial migration.[421] However, cotreatment with endostatin transiently blocks this shift.[421] Cell–matrix interactions are maintained in part by formation of focal adhesions and actin stress fibers. Either bFGF or endostatin alone induced tyrosine phosphorylation of focal adhesion kinase and paxillin, which promoted formation of focal adhesions and actin stress fibers. However, when microvascular endothelial cells were cotreated with bFGF and endostatin, focal adhesion and actin stress fibers were decreased, which decreased migration of endothelial cells. In an in vivo situation, the entire vascular bed would be exposed to circulating endostatin. But its antiangiogenic effect would become evident only in areas of high growth factor stimulation, such as those present in the tumor endothelium.[421] Taken together, these results provide a plausible mechanism to explain clinical trial data (see below) in which antiangiogenic effects of endostatin are observed in the absence of systemic toxicity.

VESSEL STABILIZATION: REVERSAL OF BFGF-INDUCED OR VEGF-INDUCED LOSS OF ENDOTHELIAL CELL–CELL ADHESION OR ENDOTHELIAL CELL ADHESION TO BASEMENT MEMBRANE Another antiangiogenic mechanism of endostatin in addition to its antiproliferative and antimotility effect on angiogenic endothelial cells is the stabilization of newly formed endothelial tubes. Endostatin decreases formation of VEGF-induced microvessels sprouting from aortic rings in vitro. By immunohistochemistry, administered endostatin localizes to endothelial cell–cell junctions and to adhesion sites between endothelial cells and their basement membrane, thus anchoring endothelial cells to each other and to their basement membrane.[422] Endostatin does not localize to quiescent vasculature. High concentrations of endostatin were detected by immunohistology in rat and human brain tumors in and around endothelial cells, in tumor cells, and in macrophages and leukocytes in the tumor's vascular bed, but normal brain showed no endostatin reactivity.[447] This unique localization of endostatin only in newly formed angiogenic microvessels appears to reverse the loosening of endothelial cells to each other and to their basement membrane, which was necessary for them to form angiogenic sprouts in the first place. Similar "stabilizing" effects of endostatin were observed in tumors in vivo, where administered endostatin was more abundant in association with angiogenic vessels undergoing maturation, mainly at the tumor marginal zone, where angiogenesis was highly active. Endostatin immunostaining is present during vascular formation up to the stage exhibiting one layer of periendothelial cells but disappears in further stabilized vessels that have more than one layer of these cells in their wall.[422] This suggests that the vascular stabilizing effect of endostatin occurs earlier than the integration of periendothelial cells into the vascular wall. A subsequent step of vascular stabilization by recruitment and integration of periendothelial cells (pericytes and smooth muscle cells) is mediated by angiopoietin 1, TGF-β, and PDGF.[226] Of interest is that during endothelial tube formation induced by VEGF, endostatin plus VEGF-treated tubes became so stable that after cessation of endostatin, the survival time of these tubes was approximately doubled in comparison with VEGF alone. Furthermore, incubation of endothelial cells with an antibody to endostatin prevented formation of stable VEGF-induced tubes and disrupted existing tubes. The role of endostatin in modulating endothelial cell interaction with the extracellular matrix is also revealed by experiments in which oligomeric endostatin (from the NC1 domain of collagen XVIII) induces motility and morphogenesis of tube-forming endothelial cells in Matrigel, whereas monomeric endostatin inhibits these effects.[423] Endostatin down-regulates the uPA system on the endothelial cell surface.[424] Proangiogenic proteins such as bFGF increase the secretion of uPA and PAI-1, leading to an overall increase in the proteolytic activity prerequisite for endothelial cell sprouting and tube formation. Endostatin treatment of endothelial cells markedly decreases their production of uPA and PAI-1. In the chick embryo, angiogenesis induced by bFGF is inhibited by endostatin but not by an endostatin mutant that does not bind to heparin.

INHIBITION OF METALLOPROTEINASE Endostatin also binds and inhibits the catalytic activity of MMP-2.[425,426] As a result, endothelial cell invasion is inhibited and tumor cell invasion may also be decreased. Tumor progression and angiogenesis are reduced in MMP-2-deficient mice, and MMP-2 is required for the switch to the angiogenic phenotype.[106,427]

BINDING OF ENDOSTATIN TO ENDOTHELIAL CELL SURFACE INTEGRINS AND OTHER PROTEINS THAT MODULATE MOTILITY AND MORPHOGENESIS Endostatin also inhibits integrin-dependent endothelial cell migration because it binds to α_5- and α_v-integrins on the endothelial cell surface, in particular $\alpha_5\beta_1$.[428] It has been proposed that $\alpha_5\beta_1$-integrin may be a functional receptor for endostatin.[37] High concentrations of endostatin also interact with tropomyosin to interrupt microfilament integrity, which inhibits endothelial motility and may participate in part in endothelial apoptosis.[429] Endostatin binds to glypicans on the endothelial cell surface at concentrations that suggest that glypicans may be low-affinity endostatin receptors.[430] Endostatin also binds to E-selectin on endothelial cells, and endostatin's antiangiogenic activity is abrogated in E-selectin–null mice.

INHIBITION OF CYCLIN D1 CAUSING G_1 ARREST OF ENDOTHELIAL CELLS Endostatin causes G_1 arrest in endothelial cells by decreasing the hyperphosphorylated retinoblastoma gene product and down-regulating cyclin D1 mRNA and protein.[431] Transcription through the LEF1 site in the cyclin D1 promoter is essential for endostatin's inhibitory activity. Others report that endostatin arrests proliferation and causes apoptosis of endothelial cells.[432,433]

Dephosphorylation of Endothelial Nitric Oxide Human recombinant endostatin dose-dependently blocks VEGF-induced endothelial cell migration, with complete inhibition at 100 ng/mL.[434] VEGF stimulates endothelial nitric oxide synthesis (eNOS). In endothelial cells, sphingosine-1 phosphate activates the serine/threonine kinase Akt and stimulates phosphorylation of eNOS to release nitric oxide.[435] VEGF-stimulated eNOS is abolished by endostatin (although VEGF-induced formation of prostacyclin is not significantly affected by endostatin). Endostatin interfered with activation of eNOS downstream of Akt by specifically inhibiting phosphorylation of eNOS at Ser 1177 by stimulating activation of the phosphatase PP2A.[434] Nitric oxide synthesis also appears to be critical for the mitogenic effect of VEGF on endothelial cells.[114–116] Inhibition of nitric oxide synthesis also blocks tumor angiogenesis.[436] Another role for nitric oxide synthesis in angiogenesis is early vasodilation of preexisting quiescent vessels, a prerequisite for sprout formation.[116]

Hypoxic Down-Regulation of Endostatin Production by Endothelial Cells and Pericytes Collagen XVIII is converted to endostatin, which is secreted from endothelial cells and pericytes in vitro at a constant rate.[437] The rate of conversion is higher in pericytes. During hypoxia, production of endostatin is significantly decreased (30–40% of this hypoxia-induced 43% degradation of endostatin occurs in pericytes and approximately 10% in endothelial cells). Exogenous endostatin is more rapidly degraded when incubated with conditioned media from hypoxic endothelial cells or pericytes. The mechanism of endostatin degradation by the conditioned medium is unknown. These results imply that (1) decreased endostatin production by hypoxic pericytes and/or endothelial cells may be another mechanism to facilitate the angiogenic switch in a tumor; (2) pericytes may employ endostatin as one of the strategies to inhibit endothelial proliferation under normal conditions; and (3) the treatment of a patient with a large tumor burden or with a tumor with a large hypoxic center (eg, glioblastoma) may require high doses of endostatin at the beginning of therapy because of endostatin degradation.

Physiologic Functions Physiologic functions for endostatin are gradually being elucidated.

Regulation of Development of Retinal Vasculature Endogenous endostatin in the eye may contribute in part to the normal development of vasculature in the retina. During development of the eye, hyaloid vessels supply the vitreous and the lens. Subsequently, these vessels regress, leaving a transparent vitreous and lens. Endostatin is thought to play a key role in regression of the hyaloid vessels because they fail to regress in endostatin's absence. In a rare disease called Knobloch syndrome, the hyaloid vessels fail to regress, retinal vasculature fails to develop, and patients suffer retinal degeneration and blindness, among other abnormalities.[438,439] In this syndrome, a splice mutation in human collagen XVIII leads to a truncated protein lacking the endostatin fragment. A proposed mechanism of retinal degeneration is that persistent hyaloid vessels increase oxygen in the retina, which suppresses HIF-1α and VEGF, both of which drive normal vascular growth in the normal developing retina. Retinal vasculature also fails to develop in a collagen XVIII–deficient mouse model.[440] Thus, a pathologic deficiency of endostatin in humans and mice reveals that endostatin is an endogenous inhibitor of angiogenesis under normal physiologic conditions. Kalluri reported that endostatin is also an endogenous inhibitor of tumor angiogenesis that acts as a natural tumor suppressor, analogous to p53. In collagen XVIII–deficient mice, tumors grew two- to threefold faster than in wild-type mice (see sections below on endogenous angiogenesis inhibitors).

When endostatin was overexpressed on endothelial cells in vivo by approximately 1.6-fold, tumors grew 300% more slowly.

Endostatin in Platelets We initially reported that platelets contain at least 14 positive regulators and approximately 12 negative regulators of angiogenesis.[441] At this writing, there are at least 30 angiogenesis regulators in platelets, of which approximately half are positive regulators of angiogenesis and the others negative angiogenesis regulators. The positive regulators include VEGF-A, VEGF-C, bFGF, HGF, angiopoietin 1, PDGF, heparanase, and sphingosine-1 phosphate, among others. The negative regulators include endostatin, platelet factor 4, TSP, plasminogen (angiostatin), high-molecular-weight kininogen (domain 5), and α_2-antiplasmin, among others. These stimulators and inhibitors of endothelial cell migration and proliferation may be released into a blood clot in a wound in an orchestrated sequence to regulate neovascularization.[442] For example, thrombin induces the release of the proangiogenic protein VEGF from platelets.[356] Thrombin also induces the release of endostatin from platelets.[443]

Thrombin induction of endostatin release is mediated by proteinase-activated receptor (PAR)-4, a mechanism that is independent of platelet aggregation and of the action of adenosine diphosphate (ADP). Positive regulators of angiogenesis, such as VEGF, are released by PAR-1. Recently, Italiano, of the Brigham and Women's Hospital, demonstrated two types of alpha granules in platelets: those that contain only angiogenesis stimulators (eg, VEGF) and those that contain only angiogenesis inhibitors (eg, endostatin).

When a clot forms in a wound, invasion by microvascular endothelial cells is initially inhibited, which avoids premature clot lysis.[442] Subsequently, endothelial cells are recruited into the clot during its neovascularization (granulation tissue). It is not known how the release of negative and positive regulators of endothelial migration from platelets is orchestrated in a wound. Recent evidence, however, reveals that if a thrombus in a large vessel is recanalized, the neovasculature harbors varying proportions of bone marrow–derived endothelial cells.[444] This is analogous to certain tumors (eg, lymphomas) that recruit the majority of their endothelial cells from bone marrow. Recent evidence reported by Raffi indicates that bone-derived endothelial precursor cells recruited to a tumor may transmigrate across the endothelial lining of tumor vessels and come to rest in the layer occupied by percicytes.

Endostatin is also released from platelets by certain drugs, such as ticlopidine, which inhibits platelet aggregation by blocking the action of ADP with its receptor.[445] The nonsteroidal anti-inflammatory drugs celecoxib and flurbiprofen, or HCT-1026 (a nitric oxide–releasing derivative of flurbiprofen), all of which are cyclooxygenase inhibitors, also release endostatin from platelets and elevate the plasma level of endostatin.[446] From these findings, one can ask whether the anti-angiogenic activity of celecoxib (Celebrex) operates in part by releasing endostatin from its stores and making it available to endothelial cells in an angiogenic site. Also, future research will be necessary to answer other questions. What is the turnover rate of endostatin in platelets? Do cancer patients on long-term celecoxib therapy deplete their platelet stores of endostatin? Can platelets be loaded with endostatin that is administered systemically or in vitro? Would cancer patients treated with celecoxib benefit from periodic endostatin therapy? Would patients on long-term endostatin benefit from celecoxib therapy? Taken together, these findings indicate that endostatin is normally distributed among three compartments: (1) stored as a cryptic fragment in collagen XVIII in basement membranes, (2) stored in platelets, and (3) circulating as low levels of free endostatin. A fourth compartment can be considered as the concentration of endostatin in and around angiogenic vessels in tumors and possibly at other angiogenic sites. Klement and Folkman[445a] recently reported that in mice, radioactive VEGF released from a subcutaneously implanted Matrigel pellet is mainly sequestered by circulating platelets and no VEGF appears in the plasma. In mice bearing microscopic human tumors of ~1 mm^3, circulating platelets endocytose VEGF and endostatin, as well as other angiogenesis regulators produced by the tumor cells.

Control of Vascular Permeability Endostatin decreases vascular permeability. bFGF treatment increases permeability of [^{3}H]inulin through confluent monolayers of capillary endothelial cells in a transwell assay, an effect that is counteracted by cotreatment with endostatin.[421] In mice that have received an intravenous injection of Evans blue dye, a large blue stain appears at the site of a subcutaneous injection of VEGF or platelet-activating factor (Miles test). Pretreatment with endostatin blocks the permeability induced by these proteins. These results imply that systemic administration of endostatin to patients may decrease edema in brain tumors.

Experimental Therapeutics Including Gene Therapy ***Insoluble Protein Administered Systemically*** Systemic administration of endostatin can inhibit or regress different tumors. The first recombinant endostatin was from *E. coli* in an insoluble form because this had previously been successful with angiostatin and because refolding of the inclusion body to a soluble form by urea, guanidine HCl, and glutathione gave a low yield (1%).[65,67,69] When this endostatin preparation was administered subcutaneously every day for prolonged periods of time in mice (185 days for Lewis lung carcinoma, 160 days for T241 fibrosarcoma, and 80 days for B-16 melanoma), there was no drug resistance. After discontinuation of endostatin at these time periods, tumors did not recur. They remained dormant at a microscopic size.[65] This was not due to an immunologic mechanism. Wounding the tumor site or moving the tumor to another site in the same mouse initiated tumor neovascularization and growth. Another possibility is preferential storage of endostatin in the matrix at the site of the regressed tumor.[448] We have observed this same dormancy after 40 days of endostatin therapy of rat mammary cancer induced by oral carcinogen.[449] Other investigators have reported successful tumor inhibition with insoluble endostatin from *E. coli*.[450] Also, soluble endostatin from *E. coli* has inhibited tumor growth.[451]

Soluble Recombinant Endostatin A wide variety of other tumors in many different laboratories have been inhibited by endostatin in mice and rats without evidence of toxicity or drug resistance.[466] These include lung adenocarcinoma, thyroid carcinoma, colon carcinoma, leukemia, human non–small cell lung cancer, human pancreatic cancer, human neuroblastoma, mammary cancer (soluble endostatin from *E. coli*), colon cancer metastases to the liver, spontaneous mouse mammary carcinoma (delayed onset, decreased tumor burden, and prolonged survival), and spontaneous pancreatic islet carcinomas.[72,452–460] Mammary carcinomas were more potently inhibited by a mutated form of endostatin in which an alanine residue was substituted for a proline at position 125 (P125A) than by the wild-type endostatin.[458] Gliosarcoma, both orthotopic and ectopic, in rats was markedly inhibited (~50%) after only 10 days of treatment by a relatively low dose of murine endostatin (0.3 mg/kg).[461] Inhibition of tumor growth persisted after cessation of therapy. Yamaguchi and colleagues reported that endostatin administered into a tumor will inhibit tumor growth at significantly lower doses than systemic administration.[461a]

Bolus versus Continuous Administration A general characteristic of optimal antiangiogenic therapy is that angiogenesis inhibitors should be at effective levels in the blood continuously. Endothelial cells in the vascular bed of a tumor are constantly exposed to a proangiogenic stimulus from the tumor cells and local stroma. This stimulus needs to be continuously opposed by inhibitors in the blood. An analogy would be titration of blood glucose by insulin, where endothelium is glucose. In a compelling experiment, 24-hour continuous parenteral administration of human endostatin was 10-fold more effective than the same dose administered as a bolus once every day against human pancreatic cancer in SCID mice (see Figure 11-3).[72] Tumor growth was inhibited in a dose-dependent manner, but only continuous administration caused tumor regression. It should be noted that continuous administration of endostatin in vitro (by a floating micro-osmotic pump in 24-well plates) inhibited endothelial proliferation more significantly than once-daily addition of endostatin.

Combinations of Endostatin with Angiostatin Reports of endostatin administered in combination with angiostatin, whether as separate proteins, separate genes, or as fusion protein of angiostatin and endostatin in tumor-bearing animals, all show a synergistic increase in efficacy.[69,375,386,462] Although the mechanism of synergy is unclear at this writing, one possibility is that endostatin and angiostatin each up-regulate TSP expression or protect it from enzymatic destruction.

Combination of Endostatin with Chemotherapy, Radiotherapy, or Immunotherapy Endostatin (and angiostatin) potentiate radiotherapy in tumor-bearing mice when the inhibitor is administered at the same time as the ionizing radiation.[463] Tumors regress when treated with a combination of ionizing radiation and endostatin but not with either modality alone, even when the endostatin dose is lowered below the effective dose and the tumor cells are radioresistant. It can be speculated that radiation damage to active endothelium in a tumor bed may not be repaired in the presence of an angiogenesis inhibitor. This experiment also suggests that radiotherapy may be, in part, endothelium dependent. The optimal schedule of radiotherapy and antiangiogenic therapy for cancer patients is unclear.

Endostatin may also potentiate immunotherapy. In an elegant experiment by Davidoff and colleagues, the gene for the potent immunogen green fluorescent protein and the gene for endostatin were transferred together to murine neuroblastoma cells prior to inoculation into syngeneic immunocompetent mice.[464] Prevention of formation of appreciable tumors was effected in 63% of mice, whereas tumor cells expressing endostatin alone or green fluorescent protein alone revealed only a modest delay in tumor growth. Mice treated with the combination were protected against subsequent tumor challenge with unmodified cells. Endostatin also potentiates conventional chemotherapy in tumor-bearing animals.[465]

Endostatin Gene Therapy Endostatin gene therapy in tumor-bearing mice has generally been successful when administered locally but problematic when administered systemically (Table 11-3).[466]

Local Gene Therapy In an example of local gene therapy, mouse liver tumor cells transfected with a retroviral vector containing the murine endostatin gene were injected subcutaneously or into the peritoneal cavity.[467] After 63 days, control tumors (vector without endostatin) reached 2,400 mm^3 compared with 30 mm^3 for endostatin-transduced tumor cells ($p < .001$). After 123 days, all 16 mice given an intraperitoneal injection of control tumor cells had died compared with only 3 of 32 mice given an injection of the endostatin-expressing tumor cells (91% survival).[467] Increased levels of endostatin were detected in tumor lysates but not in the serum of mice with subcutaneous tumors. Other reports of local gene therapy with endostatin show effective tumor inhibition in animals. Examples are inhibition of human liver carcinoma, renal cell carcinoma (RCC), and mouse melanoma.[468–471] A human breast carci-

Table 11-3 Tumors Significantly Inhibited by Recombinant Endostatin Protein Therapy[466]

Murine tumors
Ovarian
Acute myelogenous leukemia (chloroma)
Colorectal carcinoma
Spontaneous mammary carcinoma
B-16 melanoma
Transplantable mammary carcinoma
Hepatoma
Lung Adenocarcinoma
Lewis lung carcinoma
Rat glioma in brain (continuous endostatin + PKC)
Murine colorectal liver metastases
B-16 melanoma + endostatin fusion with angiostatin
Human myeloid leukemia in SCID rats
Lewis lung carcinoma
Rat carcinogen induced mammary cancer
Pancreatic insulinoma
Murine metastatic tumors
Lung adenocarcinoma (completely inhibited)
Human tumors in mice
Human ovarian carcinoma
Laryngeal squamous cell carcinoma
Glioblastoma
Prostate carcinoma
Neuroblastoma
Testicular carcinoma
Breast carcinoma
Head and neck squamous cell carcinoma
Kaposi's sarcoma
Pancreatic carcinoma
Human non-small cell lung cancer
Human pancreatic carcinoma
Brain tumors (U87)
Non-Hodgkin lymphoma (high grade)
Renal cell carcinoma
Bladder cancer
Tumors significantly inhibited by endostatin gene therapy
Murine primary tumors
Renal cell carcinoma
Brain tumors
Breast cancer and brain tumors (FM3A P-15) metastasis
Breast cancer
Lewis lung carcinoma
Leukemia (L1210)
Myeloproliferative disease (resembling human chronic myelogenous leukemia)

For 23 others, see Experimental Cell Research.[466]

noma, MDA-MB435, was markedly inhibited when the cells were transduced with endostatin, but another breast cancer MCF7 was not inhibited.[365] (However, angiostatin gene transfer inhibited MCF7 but not MDA MB435.[365]) Gliomas were inhibited by gene transfers to tumor cells, which were then implanted into rat brains.[472] Gliomas were also inhibited by intratumoral implantation of alginate-encapsulated beads containing packaging cells transfected with endostatin.[473–475]

Of interest is that intratumoral gene transfer of endostatin inhibited mouse mammary tumors (MidT2-1) but had a minimal effect in human breast MDA-MD-231 in SCID mice.[476] Despite many successes of endostatin gene transfer into tumor cells, unsolved problems remain. The fact that one author can report marked and sustained tumor inhibition with endostatin transduction of a mouse breast cancer but minimal effect in a human breast cancer MDA-MD-231 highlights the problem.[476] A third author reported marked inhibition by endostatin gene transfer into a human breast cancer MDA-MBA335 but minimal effect in MCF7, yet angiostatin gene transfer into MCF7 was very inhibitory but had only minimal effect on MDA-MB435 breast cancer cells.[365] For unknown reasons, the inhibitor may lose activity when produced by one type of tumor cell but not by another. Whether this is a protein-folding problem or results from excess local levels of endostatin at the endothelial receptor site is not clear. A fourth author reported that breast cancer (MCA-4) transduced with endostatin is significantly inhibited.[477]

Systemically Administered Gene Therapy Systemically administered gene therapy (by an intravenous or intramuscular vector in mice or rats) significantly inhibited tumor growth in RCC, Lewis lung carcinoma adenocarcinoma MC38, hemangioendothelioma, spontaneous breast cancer and its metastases, and colon cancer (when the gene was injected intramuscularly and endostatin serum levels were only moderately elevated [35–40 ng/mL]).[367,469,478–481] Adenoviral gene transfer of endostatin delayed the growth of breast cancer implants and retarded their growth by 67% after the tumors appeared.[478a]

However, other reports of systemically administered endostatin gene therapy failed to inhibit tumor growth. For example, either local or systemic endostatin gene therapy failed to inhibit rat tumors despite the achievement of serum levels more than 10 to 200 times above normal levels of endostatin (eg, 500 ng/mL up to 10 m/mL).[482] However, these tumors were significantly suppressed when an inhibitor of plasmin was administered together with endostatin by gene therapy but not when the plasmin inhibitor was administered alone.[482] This result suggests that very high levels of plasmin in a tumor bed may interfere with endostatin activity. It is interesting that angiostatin, by binding to annexin II when it is overexpressed by endothelial cells in an angiogenic site, decreases plasmin production on the endothelial surface.[326,338–341] It remans to be demonstrated if this mechanism plays a role in the synergy of angiostatin and endostatin combinations.[69,375,386,462] We also were unable to demonstrate significant inhibition of tumor growth and only 23 to 33% ($p < .002$ and .0001, respectively) inhibition of corneal angiogenesis when viruses encoding angiostatin or endostatin were administered as a single intravenous injection, despite the fact that peak serum levels of endostatin reached 400 to 599 times above the normal level.[485] In contrast, viruses encoding soluble forms of Flk-1 or Flt-1, the receptors for VEGF, resulted in approximately 80% growth inhibition of the same tumor and strong inhibition of corneal neovascularization (74–80%) ($p < .001$). A strong correlation was observed between the effects of the different viruses on tumor growth and the activity of the viruses in the inhibition of corneal micropocket angiogenesis. However, three speculations may be considered as a basis for future research. Antiangiogenic activity and antitumor activity of endostatin are dose dependent, but recent experiments reveal a U-shaped curve analogous to interferon-α and TGF-β[485a,485b] in which administration of low doses of endostatin optimally inhibits tumor growth but higher doses do not. A second speculation is that endostatin may aggregate at very high serum levels or that its folding may be effected. A third speculation is that serum plasmin levels may be increased by certain viruses or by high viral titers. Other authors subsequently have reported failure of endostatin gene transfer to significantly inhibit a murine leukemia when endostatin was transduced into hematopoietic stem cells and serum endostatin levels of 300 ng/mL were reached or to inhibit metastases from a fibrosarcoma when serum endostatin levels of up to 700 ng/mL were obtained.[483,484] Of interest is that these authors previously reported, in collaboration with Folkman and O'Reilly, enhanced antitumor activity with an endostatin-angiostatin fusion protein engineered in hematopoietic stem cells.[484,484a]

Endostatin Signaling Network To determine how the endothelial cell genome and proteome react to endostatin treatment, we used a genome-wide expression profile covering 95% of the human genome and phosphorylation analysis on antibody arrays. Briefly, we generated the Human Unigene Chip II containing 74,834 elements, which represents one of the largest gene sets interrogated in array-based gene expression studies to date. Alteration in gene expression was analyzed after 4-hour treatment of human microvascular endothelial cells with 200 ng/mL of human recombinant endostatin (*Pichia pastoris,* endotoxin-free EntreMed/Calbiochem). Using 12 reusable chips, more than 1,800,000 gene expression measurements in total were performed on endostatin-treated endothelium and compared with control samples of untreated endothelium from two different human subjects. The identities of 50,000 gene clusters (spotted DNA clones) have been sequence verified. Averaged ratios of more than 2.0 were considered up-regulated, whereas averaged ratios of less than 0.5 were considered down-regulated. By these criteria, 4,457 Unigene clusters were more than twofold up-regulated and 429 of these were more than fivefold up-regulated. In contrast, 4,814 Unigene clusters were down-regulated by 50% (ratio 0.5) and 421 of these were down-regulated by 80% (ratio 0.2).

Overexpressed genes during endostatin treatment included apoptosis genes, cardiovascular and stress response genes (eg, heat shock), and genes associated with angiogenesis inhibition. Underexpressed genes during endostatin treatment included gene families associated with cancer and angiogenesis induction (the angiogenic switch), as well as transcripts encoding cytokines, cytokine receptors, cellular adhesion molecules, G proteins, G protein–coupled receptors, and transcription factors.

Endostatin down-regulated expression of HIF-1α by 2.5-fold. Under hypoxic conditions, such as in tumor cells in the center of a tumor, where vessels are compressed by high tissue pressure, HIF-lα expression is normally increased and leads to increased expression of VEGF.[365,427] Endostatin also down-regulated many upstream activators of HIF-lα, including c-jun/Fos, Ets, and epidermal growth factor receptor. On the other side, HIF-1α normally helps trigger a coordinated angiogenic response by inducing the expression of genes involved in blood vessel growth, including VEGF and its receptors, VEGFR-2 and neuropilin, as well as nitric oxide synthase and cyclooxygenase 2.

Endostatin also down-regulated the Id transcription factors. These genes are proangiogenic, and deletion of three alleles of Id1 and Id3 results in healthy mice that cannot mount an angiogenic response to implanted tumor cells.[80,81] The $\alpha_V\beta_3$-integrin or its associated metalloproteinase MMP-2 was highly down-regulated in the stunted blood vessels of the residual microscopic tumor mass of Id1(+/–)Id3(–/–) mice. Endostatin substantially down-regulated MMP-2 and $\alpha_V\beta_3$-integrin. In addition to this transcriptional regulation, direct inhibitory effects of endostatin MMP-2 have been reported.[425] Furthermore, Id1 regulates angiogenesis through transcriptional repression of TSP-1.[528] Therefore, endostatin, by down-regulating Id1, up-regulates expression of TSP-1, a powerful angiogenesis inhibitor on its own. Taken together, these pathways provide a general signaling through which endostatin can down-regulate MMP-2 and $\alpha_V\beta_3$-integrin and up-regulate TSP, all events that would result in suppression of the angiogenic response.

Ephrin signaling is down-regulated by endostatin. The ephrin/Eph family was recently shown to participate in the regulation of angiogenesis. Both ephrin B1 and ephrin B2 induce sprouting angiogenesis in vitro to an extent similar to the angiogenic activity of VEGF or angiopoietin 1.[529] Endostatin also down-regulates ephrin A1. Although ephrins generally do not induce endothelial proliferation, ephrin A1, which is up-regulated during capillary tube formation, can promote endothelial cell assembly into a capillary-like tube.[530] We have shown that endostatin inhibits tube formation in vitro.[423]

Endostatin inhibited TNF-α–induced angiogenic signaling by down-regulating the TNF-α receptor. Additionally, nuclear factor (NF)-κB (NF of a κ light chain gene enhancer in B cells) was down-regulated by endostatin. Endostatin inactivation of NF-κB was demonstrated by four different assays, including immunochemistry. It is thought that activation of NF-κB by TNF-α ionizing radiation or chemotherapeutic agents protects cells from apoptosis.[532,533] Therefore, endostatin inhibition of NF-κB in these settings should enhance apoptosis of endothelial cells. An alternative mechanism by which endostatin may mediate endothelial cell arrest and apoptosis is by its down-regulation of activator protein 1 (AP-1). AP-1 consisting of c-Fos and c-Jun normally prevents apoptosis. Of interest is that the promoter regions of VEGF, VEGFR-2, and HIF-1α contain several AP-1 binding elements. These networks define a potential network of targets by which endostatin may exert its antiangiogenic effect. STAT1 and STAT3 (signal transducers and activators of transcription factors) were down-regulated twofold in endothelial cells treated by endostatin. STATs up-regulate genes that encode inhibitors of apoptosis (Bcl family), inducers of angiogenesis (VEGF), and cell-cycle regulators (cyclins D1 and D2 and c-myc).[534] After endostatin treatment of endothelial cells, most of the genes downstream of STAT were strongly down-regulated. These include the apoptosis inhibitor Bcl-2 and the cell-cycle regulators cyclins D1 and D2 and c-myc.

Thrombin receptors (PAR-1 and PAR-2) were also significantly down-regulated by endostatin. Several factors contribute to the proangiogenic activity of thrombin. Thrombin is a potent stimulus for release of VEGF by transcriptional regulation activation of HIF-1α.[535] Thrombin also up-regulates expression of VEGF receptors on endothelial cells.[536] In a positive loop, VEGF accelerates thrombin generation, another proangiogenic event.[537] This loop has implications for cancer patients. The majority of cancer deaths are directly attributable to thrombosis or bleeding. Another link between angiogenesis and thrombin is that cleaved or latent conformations of antithrombin III potently inhibit angiogenesis.[70] We found that endostatin significantly up-regulates antithrombin III. The enzymatic degradation of antithrombin III (58 kDa) to the antiangiogenic form (53 kDa) appears to be by tumor-generated enzymes.[70,512] This observation emphasizes that endostatin down-regulates proangiogenic genes and simultaneously up-regulates genes that lead to inhibition of angiogenesis.

Endostatin directly down-regulates Ets-1 in endothelial cells in a time-dependent manner and decreases the mRNA level of most of the Ets-1 target genes, such as MMP-1 and β_3-integrin. Ets positively regulates angiogenesis by inducing several target genes, including uPA, MMP-1, MMP-3, MMP-9, and β_3-integrin. The elimination of the Ets-1 activity by a dominant negative molecule inhibits angiogenesis in vivo.[538–542] A striking finding is that several pathways thought to be distinct in fact intercommunicate to bring about a focused antiangiogenic response in the tumor bed, directly as a result of endostatin treatment. It is not clear whether many of the small molecular angiogenesis inhibitors produce such a focused antiangiogenic response at the genetic level as endostatin does.

Clinical Implications of Endostatin Several interesting characteristics of endostatin make it advantageous for clinical use in cancer patients. First, it is not toxic.[267] At this writing, endostatin is in phase I and II clinical trials, and, to date, it has been used in not more than approximately 120 patients. However, all centers report that there are virtually no side effects, even in patients who have been on endostatin injected daily subcutaneously without interruption for up to 3.5 years (Patients who receive the subcutaneous preparation of endostatin take their own injections each day at home, such as insulin.

Endostatin does not delay wound healing in patients or in animals.[486] We have confirmed that wound healing in mice is not delayed by endostatin doses sufficient to inhibit growth of tumors in the same animal (J. Marler et al, unpublished data).

Endostatin has no effect on pregnancy in mice. Pregnant mice treated with tumor-regressing doses of endostatin deliver normal babies, even if the mothers bear a tumor that is then inhibited by the endostatin (R. D'Amato et al, unpublished data).

Serum endostatin levels are significantly elevated in Down syndrome patients.[492] Endostatin serum levels in normal individuals range from 4 to 40 ng/mL (20.3 ± 11.5, mean ± SD). For Down syndrome individuals, it is 38.6 ± 20.1, a significant elevation. The collagen XVIII gene is on chromosome 21q22.3. Because Down syndrome is most commonly caused by a duplication of one of the copies of chromosome 21, these individuals have an extra copy of collagen XVIII in which endostatin is a cleavage product. Down syndrome individuals have a low incidence of solid tumors.

A recent study in the United States of 17,987 people with Down syndrome revealed that they have approximately 0.1 the incidence of the control age-matched population for virtually all malignancies except testicular cancer and leukemia.[493] This low incidence of cancer is associated with a large reduction in cancer-associated deaths among Down syndrome patients. It has been proposed that an increase of about one-third of normal endostatin serum levels may represent an effective therapeutic dose to significantly inhibit many solid tumors.[492] When this observation is taken together with endostatin's lack of toxicity, endostatin may someday be used chronically in a preventive mode for patients with a high cancer risk of breast cancer or other tumors.

In a phase I trial, 25 patients who had failed all previous therapy were treated with endostatin.[267] They received a daily intravenous bolus dose of endostatin over a period of 20 minutes. Endostatin was safe and had a linear pharmacokinetic profile up to 599 mg/m^2/d. Tumors regressed in two patients, although not sufficiently to satisfy the criteria for the terms "partial" or "complete" response used for chemotherapy. In one patient with metastatic melanoma, there was prolonged stabilization for 426 days, with a much improved quality of life, and he returned to work.

The limited antitumor effect of bolus dosing in these patients is similar to the weak antitumor effect observed in mice that received bolus dosing.[72] In ongoing phase II trials, patients in Boston are receiving subcutaneous injections of a slow-release preparation of endostatin, which provides a steady-state blood level of endostatin similar to that obtained by continuous intravenous dosing in patients and continuous intraperitoneal pump dosing in mice.[72] In these patients, endostatin is showing more anticancer activity and more prolonged stable disease up to 1 year or more.

Production and Manufacture of Endostatin Recombinant endostatin can be produced in large scale in *E. coli*, *Drosophila* cells, *P. pastoris*, and mammalian cells.[487–491] Current clinical trials in the United States and the Netherlands employ recombinant human endostatin produced in yeast (*P. pastoris*).

Family of Angiogenesis Inhibitors in Matrix Proteins The discovery of endostatin, a specific and potent angiogenesis inhibitor residing as an internal fragment of collagen XVIII, further implicated the potential role of basement membranes in the regulation of angiogenesis. In 1996, three independent lines of evidence led Kalluri and colleagues to launch a new line of investigation into the role of vascular basement membrane in the regulation of angiogenesis: (1) the observation that vascular basement membrane proteins are associated with resting and growth-arrested capillary endothelial cells, whereas proliferating and migrating endothelial cells are under the influence of provisional matrix molecules, such as vitronectin and fibronectin; (2) studies by Madri and by Furcht that suggested that subdomains of type IV collagen exhibit different properties compared with the intact full-length molecule; and (3) the demonstration by Furcht that the NC1 domain can disrupt the assembly of type IV collagen.[498–500,670–673] Kalluri hypothesized that during the inductive phase of angiogenesis involving the degradation of vascular basement membrane, proteolytic degradation fragments of basement membrane are liberated with the potential for positive and negative regulation of capillary endothelial proliferation and migration. Such a potential role for matrix fragments could provide the regulatory balance for an organized formation of new capillaries, especially during development.

A biochemical approach was designed to extract vascular basement membranes and perform degradation with tumor microenvironment–associated enzymes. The isolated vascular basement membrane per se did not reveal any antiangiogenic activity in its solid state. But degradation by various basement membrane–degrading enzymes liberated cryptic domains of collagen molecules from the vascular basement membrane with novel antiangiogenic activity.[500] Interestingly, although these fragments are present in the intact molecules, in this form, they do not exhibit antiangiogenic activity. The initial screen of fragments from the vascular basement membrane identified three antiangiogenic fragments from type IV collagen, known as arrestin, canstatin, and tumstatin. Endostatin was also identified in this collection of basement membrane fragments. The discovery of arrestin, canstatin, tumstatin, and the α_6 chain NC1 domain of type IV collagen was later also independently published by Petitclerc and colleagues.[504]

Arrestin *In Vitro Antiangiogenic Activity* Arrestin (26 kDa) is the NC1 domain fragment of α_1 type IV collagen.[262] Arrestin exhibits antiangiogenic activity in various in vitro and in vivo assays and is found circulating in normal individuals. Recombinant arrestin inhibited the growth of small and large RCC xenografts and prostate carcinoma xenografts in nude mice at doses as low as 4 mg/kg/d intraperitoneally. Syngenic tumors (SCC-PSA1 teratocarcinoma) in 129/Sv mice were significantly reduced by arrestin treatment (1 mg/kg intravenously). The decrease in tumor size was consistent with a decrease in CD31-positive vasculature.[262] In recent studies, the activity of arrestin was further confirmed using different prokaryotic and yeast expression systems.

Mechanism of Action The antiangiogenic and antitumor action of arrestin is potentially mediated by heparan sulfate proteoglycan and $\alpha_1\beta_1$-integrin on proliferating endothelial cells.[262] Two independent studies support the contention that arrestin may function via $\alpha_1\beta_1$-integrin. Senger and colleagues demonstrated that α_1-integrin–neutralizing antibodies can inhibit VEGF-driven angiogenesis without a detectable effect on preexisting vasculature, and VEGF can induce expression of $\alpha_1\beta_1$- and $\alpha_2\beta_1$-integrins.[501] Additionally, Pozzi and colleagues demonstrated that tumors grow more slowly in α_1-integrin null mice when compared with wild-type mice.[502,503] Collectively, all of these studies suggest that arrestin can potentially act as an endogenous inhibitor of $\alpha_1\beta_1$-induced tumor angiogenesis. In a recent study, these observations were tested directly and arrestin was found to compete with type IV collagen binding to $\alpha_1\beta_1$-integrin and inhibit migration, proliferation, and tube formation by proliferating endothelial cells. This activity was dependent on the FAK/cRaf?MEK/ERK1-2/p38 MAPK signaling pathway, without an effect on PI3K/Akt pathway. Furthermore, the action of arrestin depends on $\alpha_1\beta_1$-integrin, and ablation of this integrin in mice makes arrestin nonfunctional. Arrestin also inhibits HIF-1α and VEGF in cultured endothelial cells in an $\alpha_1\beta_1$-integrin–dependent manner.[262a]

Canstatin Canstatin (24 kDa) is the NC1 domain fragment of α_2 type IV collagen.[263] Canstatin exhibits antiangiogenic activity in several in vitro and in vivo assays.[263] Recombinant canstatin inhibits the growth of small and large RCC tumors by four- or threefold with respect to placebo-treated mice. Established human prostate carcinoma (PC-3) in SCID mice or athymic (nu/nu) mice exhibited fractional tumor volumes of about threefold less than placebo-treated mice when treated with 3 mg/kg canstatin. This decrease in tumor size was consistent with a decrease in CD31-positive vasculature.[263] Recent studies using syngeneic mouse Lewis lung tumors (LLC) in C57BL/6 mice and orthotopic MDA-MB 435 breast tumors in nude mice also revealed significant tumor inhibition with recombinant canstatin. The antiangiogenic activity of canstatin was also independently validated subsequently by Petitclerc and colleagues.[504] They demonstrated that recombinant canstatin, tumstatin, and the α_6(IV) NC1 domain can inhibit angiogenesis in a cell adhesion molecule assay. Petitclerc and colleagues also showed that canstatin can bind to $\alpha_v\beta_3$-integrin on endothelial cells.

The mechanism of how canstatin inhibits proliferation and migration of endothelial cells was further investigated. Kamphaus and colleagues investigated the effect of canstatin on ERK activation induced by 20% fetal bovine serum and endothelial mitogens.[263] Canstatin does not act primarily by inhibiting VEGF or bFGF activation of ERK. Instead, canstatin specifically induces apoptosis of endothelial cells with an insignificant effect on nonendothelial cells. Apoptosis of endothelial cells by canstatin is mediated by induction of a steady decrease in FLIP protein (an antiapoptotic protein associated with FAS-mediated apoptosis pathway) levels in the presence of 20% fetal calf serum, bFGF, and VEGF. Interestingly, canstatin did not affect FLIP levels in the absence of growth factors. Panka and colleagues demonstrated that inhibits Akt to induce apoptosis of proliferating endothelial cells. Canstatin's lack of effect on endothelial cells in the absence of growth factors may indicate that only proliferative endothelium is targeted.[262] Recent studies suggested that canstatin binds to $\alpha_v\beta_3$-integrin and $\alpha_3\beta_1$-integrin on proliferating endothelial cells.[504] The importance of $\alpha_v\beta_3$ and $\alpha_3\beta_1$-integrins for the antiangiogenic activity of canstatin is yet to be determined.

Magnon and colleagues argued that canstatin functions act on endothelial cells and tumor cells by inducing mitochondrial damage via the interaction of $\alpha v\beta_3$- and $\alpha v\beta_5$-integrins. Mutagenesis experiments suggest that both N-terminal and C-terminal domains of canstatin may possess antiangiogenic activity. Whether these two fragments bind different integrins and mediate distinct antiangiogenic actions needs further investigation.[263]

Tumstatin Tumstatin (28 kDa) is the NC1 domain fragment of the α_3 collagen molecule and exhibits antiangiogenic activity in both the in vitro and in vivo assays.[71,264,505–507] The antiangiogenic activity has been narrowed down to a 25–amino acid stretch in the middle of the molecule. At equal molar concentrations, the full-length tumstatin exhibits activity similar to that of the 25–amino acid peptide, termed T7 peptide[71,264,505–507] Recombinant tumstatin and T7 peptide exhibit significant inhibition of human tumor xenografts in nude and SCID mice, syngeneic LLC and B16F10 tumors in C57BL/6 mice, the Rip-Tag2 pancreatic cancer model, and orthotopic MDA-MB 435-breast tumor in nude mice at a dosage of 1 mg/kg/d intraperitoneally or intravenously.

Tumstatin (α_3(IV)NC1) binds to endothelial cells via $\alpha_v\beta_3$-integrin and $\alpha_6\beta_1$-integrin.[71,264,505,506] The $\alpha_3\beta_1$-binding activity for tumstatin was also demonstrated by Petitclerc and colleagues.[504] The binding to $\alpha_v\beta_3$ is pivotal for the antiangiogenic activity associated with tumstatin, and the activity is restricted to amino acids 54 to 132 (tumstatin 5) within the 244–amino acid tumstatin using deletion mutagenesis.[71,264,506] Additionally, $\alpha_v\beta_3$ binding to tumstatin is mediated via a mechanism independent of the RGD-containing amino acid sequence and vitronectin/fibronectin binding of proliferating endothelial cells. The antiangiogenic activity of tumstatin can be further localized to a 25–amino acid region within tumstatin 5, and a synthetic peptide representing this region preserves "full" antiangiogenic activity and binds to $\alpha_v\beta_3$-integrin.[71,264,506] Cell biologic experiments demonstrated that the antiangiogenic activity of tumstatin is dependent on $\alpha_v\beta_3$-integrin binding on proliferating endothelial cells.[71,506] These experiments support the notion that through the action of endogenous inhibitors such as tumstatin, $\alpha_v\beta_3$-integrin could also function as a negative regulator of angiogenesis.[71,508–511]

Tumstatin induces apoptosis of proliferating endothelial cells.[507] Maeshima and colleagues demonstrated that tumstatin is an $\alpha_v\beta_3$-integrin–dependent inhibitor of cap-dependent translation mediated through negative regulation of mTOR signaling. In essence, tumstatin is an endothelial cell–specific inhibitor of cap-dependent translation. The mTOR inhibitory property of tumstatin mimics that of rapamycin, except unlike rapamycin, which is pan-specific, tumstatin is specific only for endothelial cells.[507] The action on mTOR is mediated by the FAK-PI3K-Akt pathway downstream of $\alpha_v\beta_3$-integrin. Gene therapy using a tumstatin construct with gemcitabine showed significant efficacy in mouse models. A similar approach of using cancer cells to deliver tumstatin into the tumor microevironment demonstrated a significant reduction in melanoma growth in mice. Caudroy and colleagues elegantly demonstrated that tumstatin is a valuable prognostic indicator for the progression of bronchopulmonary carcinoma.

Endogenous Angiogenesis Inhibitors as Cryptic Tumor Suppressor Proteins With the discovery of angiostatin, endostatin, arrestin, canstatin, and tumstatin, a new paradigm has emerged that puts forward a novel notion that some proteins, such as plasminogen and basement membrane collagens, harbor unique properties that are cryptic and become exposed only on proteolytic degradation. Thus, in their intact form (full length), plasminogen and basement membrane collagen do not exhibit antiangiogenic activity or antitumor activity, but when plasminogen and basement membrane collagens undergo degradation, they now expose or liberate novel cryptic fragments, which possess antiangiogenic activity. How the transition from solid state to soluble state (antiangiogenic) system is regulated is still unknown.

All of these inhibitors are found in the blood of normal individuals. A decrease in the physiologic levels of endostatin, tumstatin, and TSP-1 results in an acceleration of tumor growth. A change in the amino acid sequence of endostatin owing to a polymorphism correlates with an increased susceptibility to prostate cancer. Conversely, an increase in physiologic levels of endostatin results in less propensity for emergence of a solid tumor in Down syndrome patients (owing to an extra copy of type XVIII collagen) (see above).[492] The observation that endostatin is elevated by 1.8-fold in patients with Down syndrome was tested recently using a mouse model. A conditional transgenic mouse was developed to generate just 1.7-fold of endostatin in the systemic circulation. When tumors were placed on these mice, the tumor grew larger by 300%, demonstrating unequivocally that mild elevation in the systemic levels of endostatin can provide significant protection from rapid tumor growth.[512a] In this regard, when mice are deleted in both TSP-1 and tumstatin, the tumors grow much faster when compared with the individual knockouts. These results collectively suggest that the ceiling rate of tumor growth is not determined just by the cancer cells and the genetic defects within them but also by the host-derived endogenous angiogenesis inhibitors (R. Kalluri and J. Folkman, unpublished data).

Collectively, these results argue that angiostatin, endostatin, tumstatin, canstatin, and arrestin may function as cryptic tumor suppressor proteins, offering an additional line of defense against tumor progression by blocking angiogenesis switching.

Antiangiogenic Conformation of Antithrombin III A human small cell lung carcinoma suppressed angiogenesis and tumor growth at remote sites in immunodeficient mice. These cells generated an enzyme in vitro that converted the 58 kDa conformation of circulating antithrombin III to a 53 kDa form of the protein in which the externally configured stressed loop of antithrombin was retracted into the body of the molecule.[70] The 53 kDa "cleaved" form is a specific endothelial inhibitor and a potent angiogenesis inhibitor and has no thrombin binding activity. Antithrombin III has no antiendothelial or antiangiogenic activity. The enzymes that induce this conformational change have not yet been elucidated. Human pancreatic cancer also generates the 53 kDa cleaved antiangiogenic antithrombin.[512]

Tropinin I A novel protein, troponin I, was purified from cartilage during an attempt to find the inhibitors responsible for the avascularity of cartilage.[513] It is a 22 kDa subunit of the troponin complex that, along with tropomyosin, is responsible for the calcium-dependent regulation of striated muscle contraction. It is a specific inhibitor of endothelial cell proliferation and of angiogenesis in the mouse cornea and chick embryo. It inhibits growth of primary tumor and metastases.

Other Angiogenesis Inhibitors That Are Endogenous In addition to the specific angiogenesis inhibitors endostatin, tumstatin, canstatin, and arrestin discussed above, the plasma and tissues contain other endogenous angiogenesis inhibitors that, although not specific, appear to preferentially inhibit endothelial proliferation and/or migration. These inhibitors have quite different structures. The increasing number of endogenous inhibitors of angiogenesis being discovered indicates the existence of a family of molecules that provide physiologic suppression of angiogenesis. An analogy may be drawn to the more than 40 proteins of the clotting system, many of which function to prevent coagulation under normal conditions (see below). Examples of endogenous angiogenesis inhibitors include interferon-β, platelet factor 4, fibronectin fragments, fragments of SPARC, TSP-1, tissue inhibitors of metalloproteinases, certain angiostatic steroids such as tetrahydrocortisol, a nonglucocorticoid, nonmineralocorticoid metabolite of cortisol, and 2-methoxyestradiol, and interleukin-12.[243,246,247,259–261,514–525] TSP also inhibits lumen formation, a rather unique property of an angiogenesis inhibitor.[521] In addition to its cytotoxic properties, mediated by T-cell activation, interleukin-12 also induces the up-regulation of interferon-γ, which itself up-regulates inducible protein 10, reported to be an angiogenesis inhibitor.[526] Certain cryptic antiangiogenic protein fragments are contained within larger proteins of the hemostatic system in addition to angiostatin and the cleaved conformation of antithrombin III. These include an internal fragment (domain 5) of high-molecular-weight kininogen in plasma and the first kringle domain (NK1) or the first two kringle domains (NK2) of HGF, itself a stimulator of angiogenesis in platelets.[527] The hemostatic system, like the extracellular matrix, also appears to store certain angiogenesis inhibitors that may be needed during wound-healing angiogenesis (for a review, see Browder and colleagues[442]).

Synthetic Angiogenesis Inhibitors ***TNP-470*** Takeda neoplastic product 470 (TNP-470) is a synthetic analogue of fumagillin, a compound secreted by the fungus *Aspergillus fumigatus fresenius*, which selectively inhibits methionine aminopeptidase 2, blocks cdk2, and inhibits cdc and phosphorylation of Rb.[59,534,544] Against animal models of human, rabbit, hamster, rat, and mouse tumors, both primary and metastatic, reports from more than 100 laboratories show that TNP-470 has the broadest anticancer spectrum of any known agent.[60] TNP-470 at 30 mg/kg subcutaneously every other day inhibited the growth of human glioblastomas, embryonal rhabdosarcoma, medulloblastoma, meningioma, fibrosarcoma, neurofibrosarcoma, hemangioendothelioma, and gastric, colon, breast, prostate, and esophageal carcinomas, as well as murine Lewis lung carcinoma, melanoma, osteosarcoma, reticulum cell sarcoma, glioma, hepatoma, fibrosarcoma, and mammary, bladder, tongue, and pancreatic cancer, by 50 to 95%, with complete regression in a variety of tumors, especially those of the central nervous system.[603–669]

In early clinical trials with TNP-470 used as a single agent, the best results were that 18% of patients had a 50% regression of tumor. Furthermore, five patients had "complete or dramatic and durable tumor regression, despite having failed all conventional therapy," including patients with carcinoma of the cervix metastatic to the lung, high-grade sarcoma of the kidney, RCC, androgen-independent prostate cancer, and Kaposi's sarcoma.[545–549] TNP-470 also showed promise when used in combination with chemotherapy.[550–552] However, at effective therapeutic doses, some patients have experienced neurocognitive toxicity and minor seizures have been reported. Recently, Satchi-Fainaro,[552a,552b] in the Folkman laboratory, determined that TNP-470 rapidly enters the cerebrospinal fluid. She conjugated TNP-470 to a water-soluble synthetic polymer, (2-hydroxypropyl)methacrylamide (HPMA). Lysosomal enzymes (cathepsin B) in activated endothelial cells cleave the linker between the polymer and the drug, releasing free TNP-470. As a result, TNP-470 does not enter the cerebrospinal fluid, the efficacy of the conjugated HPMA-TNP-470 is significantly greater than free TNP-470 in tumor-bearing animals, and a maximum tolerated dose has not yet been found even at 7 times the previous maximum tolerated dose. The new conjugate HPMA-TNP-470, called Caplostatin,[552b] also potently inhibits vascular permeability induced by VEGF, PAF, and interleukin-2 (pulmonary edema).

Thalidomide In 1994, D'Amato and Folkman reported that the anti-inflammatory drug thalidomide could inhibit angiogenesis induced by bFGF or VEGF in a rabbit cornea micropocket assay.[249] Thalidomide inhibited new blood vessel formation in rabbits and mice independently of its ability to suppress infiltrating host inflammatory cells.[249] Thalidomide reduced the growth of carcinomas in rabbits and Lewis lung carcinoma in mice.[554] In 1999, thalidomide therapy was first used in humans with advanced refractory multiple myeloma based on a suggestion by Folkman to Barlogie.[553] Thirty-two percent of patients treated with thalidomide had a positive response, as assessed by a reduction in the serum levels of myeloma protein and the urine levels of Bence Jones protein.[553] These findings have been confirmed by other studies.[556] Thalidomide is now being tested in numerous clinical trials worldwide for the treatment of a variety of solid tumors and has become one of the most effective drugs for multiple myeloma. It has been approved in Australia for the treatment of multiple myeloma.

Revimide, a more potent analogue of thalidomide, has fewer side effects (ie, less peripheral neuropathy) than thalidomide and is also in clinical trials.

Thalidomide treatment suppresses production of TNF-α, which has been reported to be angiogenic. However, other, more potent inhibitors of TNF-α, such as pentoxifylline or dexamethasone, have little or no activity against corneal angiogenesis.[252] Ibuprofen, which inhibits angiogenesis, actually increases serum levels of TNF-α in mice.[252] Furthermore, TNF-α inhibitors are not effective in animal models of myeloma or in patients. TNF-α suppression therefore does not appear to be a major part of thalidomide's antiangiogenic activity.

Thalidomide does have a direct antiproliferative effect on multiple myeloma cells in vitro, although very high concentrations of thalidomide (up to 100 μM) are required.[556] Nevertheless, this drug might be able to target both cancer cells and vascular endothelial cells. In patients with multiple myeloma, or myelodysplastic syndromes, plasma levels of the proangiogenic proteins VEGF and bFGF were significantly decreased compared with pretreatment levels. This decrease correlated with efficacy of thalidomide therapy.[138]

In the original clinical reports of the antitumor effects of thalidomide against multiple myeloma, decreased microvessel density was not associated with disease remission.[555] This created a question of whether the clinical efficacy of thalidomide was mediated entirely or even partly by its antiangiogenic features.[557] The problem is an assumption that because microvessel density (measured by the method of Weidner and colleagues) can determine cancer prognosis, it should also be useful for determining therapeutic efficacy.[558] Although increased microvessel density in bone marrow is associated with relapse in multiple myeloma or with untreated multiple myeloma in virtually all reports to date, microvessel density has not been an effective measure of therapeutic response in many patients with multiple myeloma. For example, some studies reported that increased microvessel density persists in patients who have undergone a complete response to thalidomide or to stem cell transplantation.[555,559] Microvessel density also remains elevated in patients who have undergone remission after chemotherapy for acute lymphoblastic leukemia.[560] Therefore, microvessel density may not be a useful indicator of efficacy in solid tumors, even though it has continued to be a valid prognostic indicator for predicting future mortality and metastasis.[37,252]

As a substitute for microvessel density, other surrogate markers of efficacy of antiangiogenic therapy are being studied. Circulating bone marrow–derived endothelial cells showed a 10-fold reduction and returned to normal values after thalidomide treatment.[138] Decreased circulating levels of VEGF correlated with thalidomide's therapeutic efficacy in multiple myeloma and other hematologic diseases.[138] However, serum VEGF alone has not been a predictable marker of angiogenesis in other tumors, in part because of the high VEGF content of platelets and because circulating angiogenesis inhibitors are not taken into account.[358]

PRINCIPLES OF ANGIOGENESIS IMPORTANT FOR CLINICAL TRANSLATION **Antiangiogenic Chemotherapy** In some clinical trials, angiogenesis inhibitors are also being administered in combination with conventional chemotherapy. Chemotherapeutic agents have, in fact, been shown to have antiangiogenic properties in animal models, in addition to their ability to induce direct cancer cell death. Paclitaxel, which inhibits microtubule polymerization, inhibits vascular endothelial cell proliferation, motility, and invasiveness in a dose-dependent manner in vitro and tumor angiogenesis in vivo.[562] Secondary effects such as these could contribute to the antitumor efficacy of chemotherapy in vivo and might delay or prevent the acquisition of drug resistance by cancer cells.

Browder and colleagues first proposed that the traditional dose schedule regimen for chemotherapeutic agents cannot, however, provide the sustained blockade of angiogenesis achieved by angiogenesis inhibitors.[563] This could be because chemotherapy is usually administered at the maximum tolerated dose, followed by a treatment-free interval to allow recovery of bone marrow and gastrointestinal tract cells. During the treatment-free interval, microvascular endothelial cells in the tumor bed can resume their proliferation and support tumor regrowth.[563] Browder and colleagues experimented with changing the scheduling and dose of a cytotoxic agent to augment its antiendothelial activity, an approach called "antiangiogenic chemotherapy" (metronomic therapy).

Antiangiogenic chemotherapy was first shown to be effective in tumor-bearing mice.[563] Administration of cyclophosphamide at more frequent intervals at an overall lower dose with a brief treatment-free interval induced sustained apoptosis of endothelial cells in the vascular bed of the tumors and more effectively controlled growth of drug-resistant tumors. This protocol also reduced side effects and avoided bone marrow suppression, These results indicated that the antitumor efficacy of cytotoxic drugs may be improved by changing the schedule and dose to provide optimum cytotoxic targeting of the microvascular endothelial cells in the tumor bed.

These results might also help explain why some patients who receive long-term maintenance or even palliative chemotherapy have stable disease beyond the time that the tumor would have been expected to develop drug resistance. Patients with slow-growing cancers who are on antiangiogenic scheduling of chemotherapy involving continuous-infusion 5-fluorouracil, weekly paclitaxel, or daily oral etoposide have shown an improved outcome despite the fact that in some of these patients, the tumors had already become drug resistant to conventional chemotherapy.[564–571]

Antiangiogenic chemotherapy has also been called metronomic therapy, but the two terms do not have precisely the same meaning. Antiangiogenic chemotherapy signifies that the target of the chemotherapy is microvascular endothelium in the tumor bed.[572] Metronomic therapy indicates that the schedule of administration is at very regular intervals.

Combinations of Antiangiogenic Therapy and Standard Chemotherapy Clinical trials of antiangiogenic chemotherapy are under way at present.[573,574] These trials usually combine very low-dose chemotherapy at frequent intervals with one or more angiogenesis inhibitors. For example, a current clinical trial at the Dana-Farber Cancer Institute, developed by Kieran, combines celecoxib, very low-dose cyclophosphamide, and thalidomide. Every 3 weeks, low-dose etoposide is substituted for cyclophosphamide. In other clinical trials, angiogenesis inhibitors have been added to high-dose conventional chemotherapy. Millar, however, cautioned about possible limitations of combining standard chemotherapy with antiangiogenic therapy or with an oncogene signaling inhibitor that has antiangiogenic activity.[466] Unexpected toxicities may occur or, at the least, lack of increased efficacy. However, we and subsequently others reported that angiogenesis inhibitors can be combined with chemotherapeutic drugs that are administered on an antiangiogenic or metronomic dose and schedule, that is, more frequent than most conventional schedules, and at significantly lower than maximum tolerated doses.[37,563,572,575–577] Administration of chemotherapeutic drugs in this manner is designed to maximize their antiangiogenic activity while reducing the severe and acute toxicities often associated with conventional regimens of maximum tolerated dose.[578] Clinical trials of antiangiogenic chemotherapy (metronomic) are currently under way.[573,574]

Clinical Patterns of Metastasis May Be Governed by Angiogenic Mechanisms Metastases may present at least four common clinical patterns: (1) a primary tumor such as a colon carcinoma is removed, but within a few months, metastases appear; (2) metastases are already present when the primary tumor is first detected; (3) metastases appear first, and the primary tumor remains occult; and (4) the primary tumor is removed (or treated by other therapy), and metastases do not appear until years later (eg, 5–10 years). A fifth and rare pattern is that metastases disappear after removal of the primary tumor (eg, a few cases of RCC). These patterns of metastatic presentation are well recognized, but their biologic basis has been poorly understood.

New experimental evidence suggests that the majority of the presenting patterns of metastases may be dictated by the intensity of angiogenesis in their vascular bed. The essential role that angiogenesis plays in the metastatic cascade can be appreciated by examining animal models that have been developed for each of the common presenting patterns of metastases in cancer patients. These five patterns can be explained by a unifying angiogenic mechanism and will depend mainly on whether a primary tumor generates an angiogenesis inhibitor(s) (eg, angiostatin, endostatin), which circulates and suppresses angiogenesis in remote metastases.[97]

Hematologic Malignancies Are Angiogenic Although solid tumors are known to be angiogenesis dependent, it was assumed until 1993 that leukemias and other hematologic malignancies did not induce angiogenesis to promote their own survival.[579] In 1993, Brunner and colleagues observed that bFGF was expressed by human bone marrow and peripheral blood cells, and the following year, Nguyen and colleagues reported that bFGF was elevated in the urine of newly diagnosed leukemic patients to higher levels than most other malignancies.[170,580] Bone marrow angiogenesis was subsequently found to correlate with multiple myeloma progression and was also observed in the lymph nodes of B-cell non-Hodgkin's lymphoma patients and in bone marrow biopsies from children with newly diagnosed untreated acute lymphoblastic leukemia.[561,581–584] By 1999, cellular levels of another angiogenic protein, VEGF, were reported to predict the outcome of patients with multiple myeloma.[585]Angiogenesis inhibitors might therefore be useful in treating hematologic malignancies. A recent study reported that the retroviral gene transfer of a vector encoding the direct angiogenesis inhibitors angiostatin and endostatin inhibits bone marrow angiogenesis and tumor growth in a mouse model of leukemia.[375] This therapy was shown to directly inhibit endothelial proliferation in vitro but to have no effect on leukemia cell proliferation. Mice inoculated with B-cell, T-cell, or myelogenous leukemias and treated with recombinant endostatin have also been observed to live significantly longer and experience fewer toxic side effects than with conventional chemotherapy (T. Browder, et al, unpublished observation).

Host Angiogenic Response May Be Genetically Controlled A recent finding is that different strains of inbred mice have an approximately 10-fold range of response to a constant dose of angiogenic stimulation (bFGF) in the corneal micropocket assay.[586] Furthermore, the in vitro migratory activity of endothelial cells from aortic rings of selected strains correlates with the in vivo responsiveness. Also, high angiogenesis responders require higher doses of an angiogenesis inhibitor to achieve the same suppression of angiogenesis as a low dose of inhibitor in a low angiogenesis responder. If this early work translates to humans, one can speculate that a low angiogenic host response would decrease the probability of in situ carcinomas switching to the angiogenic phenotype, that tumors that did become angiogenic would grow slowly or be indolent (eg, indolent prostate cancer), and that relatively low doses of angiogenesis inhibitors would be necessary to achieve effective therapy. In contrast, a high angiogenic host response would predict a higher frequency of in situ switching to the angiogenic phenotype and faster-growing tumors, and significantly higher doses of antiangiogenic therapy would be required.

p53 Normally Suppresses Angiogenesis *p53* mutations also allow tumor cells to become resistant to apoptosis under conditions of hypoxia.[587] In mice, *p53* mutations decrease the response of cancer cells to antiangiogenic therapies.[588] Wild-type p53 normally suppresses tumor angiogenesis by up-regulating TSP-1, inducing degradation of HIF-1α, suppressing transcription of VEGF, and down-regulating bFGF-binding protein expression.[75,161,233] The increased neovascularization that occurs following loss of p53 function, however, can be overcome by increasing the dose of antiangiogenic therapy. For example, in mice bearing a mutant *p53*-associated human pancreatic tumor, there was a dose-dependent response to a single angiogenesis inhibitor, varying from 33 to 97% inhibition of tumor growth with tumor regression.[72,589]

It remains to be seen whether this result can be translated to those patients with tumors that possess *p53* mutations. Therefore, in contrast to the maximum tolerated doses of chemotherapy, antiangiogenic therapy dosing may be optimized by titrating against the total angiogenic output of a tumor, analogous to the titration of insulin against blood sugar or warfarin against prothrombin levels. Currently, however, there is no quantitative method for determining the total angiogenic output of a patient's tumor burden, so surrogate markers such as circulating progenitor endothelial cells are being studied.[137]

Slowly Growing Indolent Tumors Rapidly growing tumors are generally more sensitive to conventional cytotoxic chemotherapy than slowly growing indolent tumors. In fact, the most slowly growing tumors (such as neurofibromas and indolent prostate carcinomas) are virtually unresponsive to chemotherapy. It has been assumed by some oncologists that slowly growing tumors would be as unresponsive to antiangiogenic therapy as they are to chemotherapy.[590] However, when two types of human bladder cancers, a rapidly growing highly vascularized tumor and a slowly growing poorly vascularized tumor, were implanted into immunodeficient mice, growth of both tumor types was inhibited by angiogenesis inhibitors. For a given dose of angiogenesis inhibitor, the slower the tumor was growing, the more effective the inhibitor.[590] In carcinogen-treated mice, breast cancers that arose spontaneously and grew very slowly were inhibited and/or regressed by treatment with mouse endostatin.[285] Spontaneously arising carcinomas of the pancreatic beta cells in transgenic mice grew very slowly compared with most transplantable tumors but retained a high degree of sensitivity to angiogenesis inhibitors.[449]

Poorly Vascularized Tumors Another common misconception about antiangiogenic therapy is that it is effective only in highly vascularized tumors. Some cancer patients who have failed conventional therapy lament that their physician told them they were not candidates for antiangiogenic therapy because their tumor was not vascularized. It is sometimes assumed by surgeons that a tumor that appears to be white and avascular (eg, pancreatic cancer) is not a candidate for antiangiogenic therapy. Based on these assumptions, some angiogenesis inhibitor clinical trials currently require a pretreatment biopsy for microvessel density to exclude patients whose tumor microvessel density is too low. Another clinical trial for a new angiogenesis inhibitor is restricted to RCC and other highly vascularized tumors.

There are several flaws in these assumptions. First, virtually any tumor that is large enough to be visible or palpable has already undergone neovascularization to attain that size. Second, the intensity of neovascularization cannot be determined by gross inspection of a tumor. A white neurofibrosarcoma of one or more cubic centimeters may have a microvessel density by microscopy that is similar to the microvessel density of a reddish hepatic carcinoma of a similar size, except in the whitish tumor, the vessels are more compressed. Third, the lower the vascularity of a tumor, the more susceptible it appears to be to antiangiogenic therapy.[590] Highly vascularized tumors may require higher doses of an angiogenesis inhibitor or combinations of angiogenesis inhibitors to achieve a tumor response.

Predicting Efficacy of Antiangiogenic Therapy: Is Microvessel Density Helpful? In 1972, a quantitative method for histologic grading of tumor angiogenesis was developed that correlated the amount of neovascularization with tumor grade in human brain tumors.[591] Additional methods for quantifying the grade of tumor vascularization were developed and followed by the first report of the use of tumor vascularity as a prognostic marker for cutaneous melanoma.[103,592] In 1991, Weidner and colleagues used antiendothelial cell antibodies to identify tumor vasculature and showed that microvessel density was a useful prognostic marker for human breast cancer.[89] Microvessel density measures the relative intensity of angiogenesis in angiogenic clones from one tumor to another. In the past 10 years, microvessel density quantification has become a reproducible prognostic factor for the risk of metastasis. The most plausible explanation for this correlation is that most human tumors contain angiogenic and nonangiogenic cells, both of which enter the circulation, but only the angiogenic cells can form detectable metastases.[2] Although there are a few reports in which microvessel density did not correlate with the risk of metastasis or mortality, this could be due to technical or biologic causes. For example, if a primary tumor that was the source of a biopsy for quantification of microvessel density generated a high level of circulating angiogenesis inhibitor(s), which suppressed the growth of distant metastases, the prognostic value of this test could be negated. For a review of more than 50 publications of microvessel density quantified in more than 8,000 patients as a prognostic indicator of future metastasis or mortality, see Gasparini and Harris.[558,561,593]

Although microvessel density is a useful prognostic marker of metastatic risk, it is not a good indicator of therapeutic efficacy for several reasons. In normal tissues, the degree of vascularization and oxygen/nutrient demand are tightly

Table 11-4 Phase III Clinical Trial Results of Bevacizumab/Chemotherapy Combinations

Tumor Type	Regimen	n	Overall Survival, Mo	HR	PFS, Mo	ORR, %	Additional Toxicities
Colorectal (previously untreated)	IFL + placebo	411	15.6		6.2	34.8	
(Hurwitz et al., 2004)	IFL + BV	402	20.3**	0.66	10.6**	44.8*	Hypertension, GI perforation (1.5%)
Colorectal (previously treated)	FOLFOX4	289	10.7		7.4	9.2	
(Giantonio et al., 2005)	FOLFOX4 + BV	290	12.5*	0.76	5.5**	21.8**	Hypertension, bleeding, neuropathy
	BV	243	10.2		3.5	3.0	Hypertension
NSCLC (previously untreated, non-	PC + placebo	444	10.2		4.5	10	
squamous) (Sandler et al., 2005)	PC + BV	434	12.5*	0.77	6.4**	27**	Hypertension, hemoptysis (fatal in 1.2%)
Breast (previously untreated) (Miller et	Paclitaxel	346	NR		6.1	14.2	
al., 2005b)	Paclitaxel + BV	365	NR	0.67	11.0	28.2**	Hypertension, neuropathy

BV = bevacizumab; FOLFOX4 = fluorouracil, oxaliplatin, leucovorin; GI = gastrointestinal; HR = hazard ratio for overall survival; IFL = irinotecan, fluorouracil, leucovorin; NR = not yet reported; NSCLC = non–small cell lung carcinoma; ORR = overall response rate (partial responses and complete responses); PC = paclitaxel and carboplatin; PFS = progression-free survival.

*$p < .05$ for comparison with control.

**$p < .001$.

coupled. In tumors, however, the degree of vascularization and tumor growth are loosely coupled, or even uncoupled. This may be because in tumor cells, expression of angiogenic factors, such as VEGF, is no longer regulated by oxygen concentration. During tumor regression under antiangiogenic therapy, microvessel density may decrease if capillary dropout exceeds tumor cell dropout (autolysis), increase if tumor cell dropout exceeds capillary dropout, or remain the same if the disappearance of capillaries and the disappearance of tumor cells parallel each other.

Antiangiogenic Activity of Interferon-α: Lessons for Other Angiogenesis Inhibitors Interferon-α has been widely used as an antiviral agent to treat chronic hepatitis but also as a cytotoxic agent to treat certain leukemias and some bladder cancers.[258] The first evidence that interferon-α had antiangiogenic activity was reported in 1980 when it was found to inhibit motility of vascular endothelial cells in vitro in a dose-dependent and reversible manner and was subsequently found to inhibit angiogenesis in vivo.[244,269,270] Experimental studies in mice demonstrated that the antiangiogenic efficacy of interferon-α is optimal at low doses and declines at higher doses.[485a] New blood vessel growth in proliferating hemangiomas has been associated with increased expression of bFGF, and interferon-α has been shown to down-regulate bFGF expression in human cancer cells.[239,240,243,594,595]

The first use of antiangiogenic therapy in a human was in 1988, when pulmonary hemangiomatosis in a 12-year-old boy was successfully treated with low-dose interferon-α therapy (3 million U/m^2).[596,597] Subsequently, infants with life-threatening or sight-threatening hemangiomas were successfully treated with the same low-dose interferon-α.[598–599] Durable complete regressions have been achieved with low-dose interferon-α therapy in patients with solid tumors such as angioblastomas and giant cell tumors, in which tumor angiogenesis was mediated mainly by bFGF.[239–241] Interferon-α at low doses has also been used to successfully treat hemangioendothelioma with or without metastases.[600,602] In a recent report, Kaban and colleagues treated recurrent high-grade giant cell tumors of the maxilla or mandible by simple surgical enucleation to spare nerves and teeth, and after 48 hours, patients received interferon-α, 3 million U/day subcutaneously, for up to 8 months.[241,242] All eight patients had complete and durable regressions without recurrence at follow-up for up to 6 years.

Clinical Signs and Symptoms in Cancer Patients That May Be Based on Angiogenesis Certain clinical signs and symptoms from tumor neovascularization are associated with specific tumor types. For example, retinoblastomas in the posterior eye induce iris neovascularization in the anterior chamber. Certain brain tumors induce angiogenesis in remote areas of the brain. Bone pain in metastatic prostate cancer may be related in part to neovascularization. A problem in the diagnosis of a primary bone tumor is that if the biopsy specimen contains only the neovascular response at the periphery of the tumor, it may be mistaken for granulation tissue or inflammation.

A variety of cancer syndromes, such as inappropriate hormonal activity, hypercoagulation, and cachexia, are secondary to the presence of biologically active peptides released into the circulation from vascularized tumors. Therefore, it might be predicted that an early therapeutic effect of antiangiogenic therapy would be increased appetite, weight gain, and disappearance of certain cancer syndromes. This early therapeutic effect would be most apparent with those angiogenesis inhibitors that had the fewest side effects. The angiogenesis induced by cervical cancer may be observed by colposcopy; the appearance of telangiectasia or "vascular spiders" in a mastectomy scar may herald local recurrence of tumor; color Doppler imaging can demonstrate neovascularization in breast cancer and other tumors; bladder carcinoma is detected by cystoscopy based, in part, on its neovascularization; and mammography often reveals the vascularized rim of a breast tumor.[92,445] In fact, a wide range of radiologic signs of cancer are based on "enhancement" of lesions by radiopaque dyes trapped in the neovasculature of a tumor. Moreover, in some tumors, large central areas cannot be penetrated by radiopaque dyes because of vascular compression, a situation that is unusual in prevascular tumors.

CLINICAL ADVANCES IN THE USE OF ANTIANGIOGENIC THERAPY

The hypothesis that tumor angiogenesis could serve as a target for cancer therapy is now strongly supported by the results of a number of randomized phase III clinical trials across multiple different tumor types (Table 11-4). Bevacizumab, a monoclonal antibody targeting VEGF, is now a standard therapy for metastatic colorectal cancer in combination with 5-fluorouracil–containing chemotherapy.[670] These advances, coupled with our increased understanding of the biologic pathways underlying tumor angiogenesis and the development of improved agents for targeting these pathways, have led to a dramatic increase in the number of clinical trials employing antiangiogenic therapy either alone or in combination with other therapeutic modalities. Currently, the majority of these agents target the VEGF pathway because of its role as a key regulator of tumor angiogenesis. Recent developments in the clinical development of VEGF pathway inhibitors are summarized below.

Therapeutic Approaches to Targeting the VEGF Pathway VEGF is the prototypic member of a family of structurally related, homodimeric growth factors that includes PlGF, VEGF-B, VEGF-C, VEGF-D, and VEGF-E. As described earlier, VEGF family members bind to a family of transmembrane receptor tyrosine kinases that include VEGFR-1 (Flt-1), VEGFR-2 (KDR, Flk-1), and VEGFR-3 (Flt-4) (Figure 11-7). The effects of VEGF on VEGFR- on vascular permeability and endothelial proliferation, migration, and survival are thought to be primarily mediated by VEGFR-2, whereas VEGFR-3 is primarily expressed on lymphatic endothelium.[671,672] Agents targeting the VEGF pathway include monoclonal antibodies that bind the ligand (ie, bevacizumab) or block the receptor (IMC-1121b), as well as small molecule receptor tyrosine kinase inhibitors (RTKIs), such as PTK787, ZD6474, and SU11248. Because of the

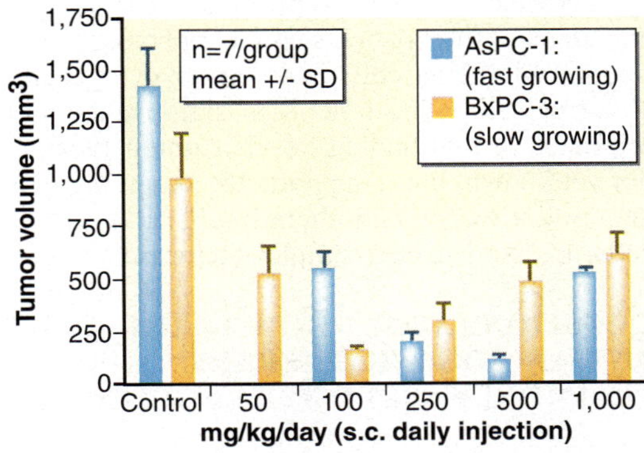

Figure 11-7 Endostatin protein has a biphasic, U-shaped dose-efficacy curve on inhibition of endothelial cell migration and on inhibition of tumor growth. Shown above are human pancreatic cancers in SCID mice. Efficacy is optimal between very low and very high doses depending on the tumor type. [Cancer Research 2005, 65 (23):1-7, in press]

structural similarity of the different receptor tyrosine kinase domains, RTKIs typically inhibit multiple receptors. These profiles of receptor specificity for each inhibitor, as well as their pharmacokinetics and potency for receptor inhibition, are likely to be the key determinants of their clinical activity. Representative agents targeting the VEGF pathway that are currently in clinical testing are listed in Table 11-5.

VEGF Pathway Inhibitors as Anticancer Therapy: Clinical Experience Clinical trials of one of the earliest VEGF pathway inhibitors, bevacizumab, began in 1997. When used as monotherapy for the treatment of advanced solid tumors, the clinical activity of these agents, as judged by objective tumor responses, has generally been low. For example, no partial or complete remissions were observed in 25 patients treated in a phase I trial of bevacizumab.[673] Furthermore, in 243 previously treated patients with colorectal cancer, a 3% objective response rate for bevacizumab monotherapy compared with 9.2% for FOLFOX4 chemotherapy (fluorouracil, oxaliplatin, leucovorin) and 21.8% for the combination. Low response rates have also been observed RTKIs targeting the VEGF pathway, such as SU5416 and ZD6474 when used as monotherapy.[674,675] In the case of SU5416, incomplete inhibition of VEGFR-2 may account in part for the low levels of activity.[676]

One tumor type for which VEGF pathway inhibitors appear to be particularly promising, even when used as monotherapy, is metastatic RCC. These tumors are often marked by inactivation of the VHL gene, leading to VEGF overexpression (reviewed in Rini and Small).[677] In randomized studies, both bevacizumab and Bay 43-9006 have been shown to significantly prolong time to progression compared with placebo controls.[678,679] SU11248 also demonstrated substantial antitumor activity in metastatic RCC, with a 40% objective response rate in phase II testing.[680] Phase III trials are currently in progress to evaluate these drugs either alone or in combination with other targeted or biologic agents.

Combinations of VEGF Pathway Inhibitors and Chemotherapy Because of their generally favorable side-effect profile and the low objective response rates observed when these agents are used as monotherapy, VEGF pathway inhibitors are most often being developed as part of a combination regimen with chemotherapy. Initial results of such combinations were mixed, with one trial in previously treated patients with breast cancer demonstrating an improvement in the objective response rate but no prolongation in overall survival compared with chemotherapy alone.[681]

In 2004, the results of a phase III, randomized, placebo-controlled study were reported comparing standard IFL chemotherapy (irinotecan, fluorouracil, and leucovorin) with or without bevacizumab in patients with previously untreated colorectal cancer.[670] Patients treated with IFL plus bevacizumab had a significantly longer overall survival and progression-free survival, as well as a higher overall response rate (see Table 11-4). This trial provided the definitive evidence that the addition of an angiogenesis inhibitor to chemotherapy could prolong survival, and, based on the results of this trial, bevacizumab received approval from the FDA for use in combination with fluorouracil-containing chemotherapy as first-line treatment for metastatic colorectal cancer.

Preliminary results from three subsequent phase III trials have provided further evidence that the addition of bevacizumab to chemotherapy may provide additional benefit compared with chemotherapy alone (see Table 11-4). In patients with previously untreated non–small cell lung cancer, the addition of bevacizumab to carboplatin and paclitaxel prolonged survival by approximately 2 months compared with treatment with carboplatin and paclitaxel alone.[682] As discussed below, patients with squamous cell histology were excluded from this trial because of a high rate of life-threatening hemoptysis observed in phase II testing of the same regimen. In a trial of previously treated patients with colorectal cancer, patients treated with bevacizumab combined with FOLFOX4 chemotherapy had a prolonged survival compared with those treated with FOLFOX4 alone,[683] although the magnitude of this benefit (1.8 months) appeared to be smaller than that observed in the first-line trial (4.7 months). Finally, in previously untreated patients with metastatic breast cancer, patients receiving bevacizumab in combination with paclitaxel had a longer progression-free survival than those receiving paclitaxel alone. Mature survival data are not yet available for this trial. Taken together, the results of these trials suggest that the benefits of VEGF blockade are not specific to a single tumor type or chemotherapy combination. VEGF pathway inhibitors are now being explored in combination with chemotherapy for virtually every type of solid tumor.

Other agents targeting the VEGF pathway that are being tested in combination with chemotherapy include PTK787 (vatalanib), SU11248 (sunitinib malate), and ZD6474. An interim analysis from a randomized phase III trial comparing FOLFOX4 chemotherapy alone or in combination with PTK787 as first-line therapy for metastatic colorectal cancer showed a nonstatistically significant trend toward improved progression-free survival in the combination arm as judged by central review.[684] Complete results, including overall survival, are not yet available. Preliminary results from a randomized phase II trials suggest that the addition of ZD6474 to docetaxel prolonged progression-free survival compared with docetaxel alone in patients with non–small cell lung carcinoma who progressed after previous chemotherapy.[685] It is not yet known whether RTKIs will provide a benefit similar to that of bevacizumab when used in combination with chemotherapy, although this issue should be addressed by a number of phase III trials currently in progress.

Toxicities Angiogenesis inhibitors have been developed with the hope that they would

Table 11-5 Inhibitors of the VEGF Pathway in Advanced Clinical Development

Agent	Vascular Target	Type	Stage of Development
Agents targeting VEGF ligands			
Bevacizumab	VEGF	Monoclonal antibody	FDA approved (colorectal cancer)
VEGF trap	VEGF, PlGF	VEGF receptor–based fusion protein	Phase I
Agents targeting receptors			
IMC-1121B	VEGFR-2	Monoclonal antibody	Phase I
SU11248 (sunitinib maleate)	VEGFR-1, -2, -3 PDGFR	RTKI (oral)	Phase III
ZD6474	VEGFR-2 EGFR	RTKI (oral)	Phase II
PTK787 (vatalanib)	VEGFR-1, -2 PDGFR	RTKI (oral)	Phase III
Ag-013736	VEGFR-2	RTKI (oral)	Pfizer (Agouron)
BAY 43-9006 (sorafenib tosylate)	VEGFR-2, -3	RTKI (oral)	Phase III
AZD2171	VEGFR-1, -2, -3 PDGFR	RTKI (oral)	Phase II

PDGFR = platelet-derived growth factor receptor; PlGF = placental growth factor; RTKI = receptor tyrosine kinase inhibitor; VEGF = vascular endothelial growth factor; VEGFR = vascular endothelial growth factor receptor.

provide a relatively nontoxic means to slow or prevent tumor growth that could be used over long periods of time, toward the goal of converting cancer into a manageable, chronic condition. Based on the clinical experience to date, it appears that VEGF pathway inhibitors do, in fact, have a generally favorable side-effect profile that is nonoverlapping with chemotherapy. Several toxicities have emerged, however, that appear to be specific to the entire class of agents.

Hypertension The most commonly observed side effect attributable to VEGF pathway inhibitors has been hypertension, which has typically been dose dependent and responsive to medical management. For example, in the randomized phase III trial of bevacizumab combined with chemotherapy for metastatic colorectal carcinoma, grade 3 hypertension was observed in 11% of patients compared with 2.3% in the standard chemotherapy arm.[670] Similar effects have been observed using oral inhibitors of the VEGFR tyrosine kinase such as PTK787.[684] The mechanism for this hypertension remains uncertain but may involve changes in vascular tone mediated by effectors downstream of the VEGF receptor, such as nitric oxide.[685a]

Bleeding and Impaired Wound Healing In a randomized phase II trial of patients with non–small cell lung cancer, 4 cases of fatal hemoptysis were observed in 66 patients treated with bevacizumab, carboplatin, and paclitaxel.[686] This was associated with squamous cell histology, disease location close to major vessels, and tumor necrosis or cavitation. Based on this observation, patients with squamous cell histology, a history of hemoptysis, or brain metastases were excluded from the randomized phase III trial of the same regimen. In this trial, fatal hemoptysis was still observed, albeit at a lower rate: 5 of 434 patients treated in the bevacizumab-containing arm compared with none in the control arm. It is also noteworthy that in patients with colorectal cancer receiving bevacizumab combined with chemotherapy, gastrointestinal perforation occurred in six patients (1.5%), including three with partial or complete tumor responses.[670] A modest impairment in wound healing after major surgery was also observed.[687] Together these results suggest that VEGF blockade may impair normal tissue repair and predispose certain patients to bleeding, particularly at sites of significant tumor regression.

Thromboembolic Events An increased incidence of thromboembolic and cardiovascular events has been observed in some but not all clinical trials of VEGF inhibitors. For example, in a phase I trial of SU5416 combined with gemcitabine and cisplatin, 8 of 19 patients (42%) experienced thromboembolic complications,[688] whereas in phase III trials in colorectal cancer and breast cancer, the incidence was not significantly increased by the addition of bevacizumab to standard chemotherapy. Possible contributing factors include the degree of endothelial disruption caused by a particular regimen,[689] hypercoagulability caused by the tumor itself, and baseline vascular disease. Identifying patients at risk of these complications will be particularly important as newer applications requiring long-term administration of VEGF inhibitors are investigated, for example, as adjuvant therapy or for chemoprevention in high-risk patients.

Potential Mechanisms of Resistance to VEGF Pathway Inhibitors The therapeutic efficacy of conventional chemotherapy for most solid tumors is limited in part by the emergence of drug resistance by rapidly mutating tumor cells. Because antiangiogenic agents are directed against tumor endothelium, which was presumed to be diploid and genetically stable, it was initially thought that tumors may not develop resistance to antiangiogenic therapy as they do to cytotoxic chemotherapy.[690,691] Clinical experience thus far, however, suggests that virtually all tumors do eventually progress despite treatment with a VEGF inhibitor. Recent studies have suggested several potential mechanisms by which tumors may initially have or acquire resistance, or at least decreased sensitivity, to VEGF pathway inhibitors.

Incomplete Target Inhibition Drugs may not be present at sufficiently high concentrations at their targets for a sufficiently long time to cause a sustained inhibition of VEGF receptor signaling and tumor angiogenesis. In trials of the VEGFR inhibitors SU5416 and SU6668, tumor biopsies taken prior to and during treatment revealed that VEGFR phosphorylation was inhibited by less than 50% in all cases, providing a potential explanation for the lack of significant clinical activity observed in these trials.[692] This incomplete target inhibition may be because drugs are not present within the tumor at sufficiently high concentrations, or for prolonged enough periods of time, to effectively inhibit angiogenesis. For other tyrosine kinase inhibitors, such as gefitinib and imatinib, incomplete target inhibition has been shown to result from genetic changes, for example, secondary mutations in epidermal growth factor receptor or BCR-ABL, or epigenetic changes reducing the intracellular concentrations of the inhibitor.[693–695] It is not yet known whether mutations may be present within VEGFR in tumor endothelium.

Bypass of the VEGF Pathway through Expression of Additional Angiogenic Factors Genetic mutations or the activation of pathways such as HIF-1 may lead to the expression of additional angiogenic factors (or the loss of angiogenic inhibitors) by malignant cells in the tumor.[696,697] In turn, these changes may promote the proliferation and survival of tumor endothelial cells even in the presence of VEGF blockade. It has been observed, for example, that advanced-stage breast cancers express a greater number of proangiogenic factors than early-stage cancers do,[698] which may help explain why previously untreated patients with metastatic breast cancer appeared to have a greater benefit from the addition of bevacizumab to standard chemotherapy than previously treated patients.[681,699]

Genetic Alterations within Tumor Endothelium The assumption that tumor endothelium are normal diploid cells and therefore presumably genetically stable has been challenged by the recent observations from murine studies[700] and biopsies from patients with lymphoma[701] that tumor endothelial cells may harbor cytogenetic abnormalities. The functional significance and relevance of this finding to other tumor types is not yet known, but it supports the mounting evidence that tumor endothelial cells, like tumor cells, are likely to be a complex therapeutic target.

QUESTIONS ABOUT HOW TO USE ANTIANGIOGENIC THERAPY COMMONLY ASKED BY CLINICIANS

As the pace of translation of angiogenesis research to clinical application has increased over the past 5 years, clinicians are learning how to use the new modality of antiangiogenic therapy. Some of the questions that they most commonly asked are discussed below:

Can antiangiogenic therapy be administered on a dose and schedule similar to conventional chemotherapy?

There is a fundamental difference between these two modalities: their cellular targets. Chemotherapy is designed to target the cancer cell. Antiangiogenic therapy is designed to target the microvascular endothelial cell in a tumor bed. Chemotherapy is administered as maximum tolerated dose with long off-therapy intervals of 2 to 3 weeks to rescue bone marrow and gastrointestinal mucosa. In contrast, the goal of optimal antiangiogenic therapy is to achieve nearly continuous exposure of vascular endothelium to the angiogenesis inhibitor. The rationale is that vascular endothelial cells in a tumor bed are marinated continuously in angiogenic stimulators such as VEGF and bFGF. This stimulation of endothelial proliferation and migration must be counteracted by the almost continuous presence of angiogenesis inhibitors in the plasma. The 18- to 20-day half-life of bevacizumab (Avastin) accounts in part for its efficacy. Where the overall objective of chemotherapy is maximum tolerated dose, the objective of antiangiogenic therapy is titration of the inhibitor against angiogenic stimulators elaborated by the tumor cell. The two modalities are not mutually exclusive and may be used together.

Can tumors develop resistance to angiogenesis inhibitors as occurs with cytotoxic chemotherapy?

Because endothelial cells are genetically stable, there is less risk of development of the "acquired drug resistance" observed with chemotherapy. For the same reason, bone marrow cells, which are as genetically stable as endothelial cells, rarely develop resistance to cytotoxic chemotherapy. However, after a patient has been treated for months or for more than a year with an angiogenesis inhibitor that blocks the production of a single angiogenic protein, such as VEGF, or its receptor, redundant angiogenic proteins may be expressed by mutant tumor cells. Although approximately 60% of human cancers express VEGF, other angiogenic proteins can be expressed either at the origination of a tumor or later in its life. If a tumor progresses during antiangiogenic therapy, it may be prudent to add another angiogenesis inhibitor or inhibitors or low-dose antiangiogenic chemotherapy (metronomic chemotherapy), instead of discontinuing the original angiogenesis inhibitor. This differs completely from the practice of discontinuing chemotherapy because of tumor progression during therapy.

In mouse studies and in biopsies of patients with lymphoma, it has been shown that endothelial cells in a tumor bed may harbor cytogenetic abnormalities. The functional significance and relevance of this finding to other tumor types is not yet known. Bielenberg and Klagsbrun reported that in mice bearing human tumors, endothelial cells in the tumor vascular bed develop cytogenetic abnormalities. This has been interpreted by some (but not by the authors) to mean that tumor-associated endothelial cells will eventually develop drug resistance similar to tumor cells. However, chromosomal abnormalities in endothelial cells, some of which may have arisen from endothelial phagocytosis of apoptotic bodies of dying tumor cells, may not confer acquired resistance to angiogenesis inhibitors.

Supporting evidence for this statement is that all of the tumors reported by Bielenberg and Klagsbrun have been significantly inhibited by antiangiogenic therapy and some have been eradicated.[700] Drug resistance has not emerged and tumor recurrence has not been observed, even when treatment of human tumors in mice has been carried out for 150 days followed by 150 days of observation off therapy.

Does antiangiogenic therapy increase hypoxia in a tumor and therefore preclude the use of ionizing radiation together with antiangiogenic therapy?

In fact, the initial stages of antiangiogenic therapy increase oxygen delivery to a tumor because vascular leakage decreases and intratumoral tissue pressure is decreased. As antiangiogenic therapy continues, and capillary dropout occurs, tumor cell death matches endothelial cell loss and the efficacy of ionizing radiation actually increases. Furthermore, certain angiogenesis inhibitors suppress expression of HIF-1α and thus prevent the tumor from a compensatory response to hypoxia. These include endostatin, rapamycin, and 2-methoxyestradiol.

Does antiangiogenic therapy reduce blood flow in a tumor and therefore preclude delivery of chemotherapy or other therapies to the tumor?

In fact, the opposite is true. Antiangiogenic therapy increases blood flow and the delivery of chemotherapy to a tumor because of the drop in intratumoral pressure that occurs when vascular permeability of tumor vessels is reduced, a phenomenon also called vessel normalization.

Are slowly growing tumors more refractory to antiangiogenic therapy than rapidly growing tumors?

This is a common misperception based on the analogy that rapidly growing tumors are more responsive to cytotoxic chemotherapy than are slowly growing tumors. Beecken, in the Folkman laboratory, showed the opposite for antiangiogenic therapy of human tumors in mice. The slower the growth of these tumors, the more effective was their inhibition by antiangiogenic therapy. More rapidly growing tumors required higher doses of angiogenesis inhibitors to achieve the same tumor response.

Is a poorly vascularized tumor refractory to antiangiogenic therapy?

Some patients have been told by their oncologist that their tumor would probably not respond to an angiogenesis inhibitor because the tumor is poorly vascularized. The opposite is true. Tumors with a low microvessel density are often easier to treat with an angiogenesis inhibitor because they are producing their own angiogenesis inhibitor(s). Furthermore, gross examination of a tumor even at the operating table does not reveal the extent of its neovascularization. A pancreatic carcinoma is often a white hard mass, but at the microscopic level, it is highly neovascularized.

What is the difference between antiangiogenic therapy and antivascular therapy?

Antivascular therapy, for example, with combretastatin, causes rapid occlusion of tumor vessels (hours), for example, by desquamation of endothelial cells and subsequent thrombosis. This leads to rapid onset of hypoxia, and tumors can undergo massive central necrosis within a few days. Blood flow is rapidly decreased. A compensatory response by surviving tumor cells at the periphery of the tumor is to generate increased HIF-1α and increased expression of VEGF. Therefore, angiogenesis may appear at the periphery of the tumor.

Do some tumors outgrow their blood supply?

Tumors are so critically dependent on new blood supply that if neovascularization is completely prevented, human tumors in mice remain dormant at ~1 mm^3, despite a continuing high rate of tumor cell proliferation balanced by a high rate of tumor cell apoptosis.

The same is true of spontaneous tumors in mice. The misperception that tumors can outgrow their blood supply. Even in zebra fish treated with a nontoxic angiogenesis inhibitor, when the tail fin is transected, it regrows, but only to ~1 mm beyond where the blood vessels have stopped growing (J. Chan, personal communication). This oxygen diffusion limit is similar for tumor cells and for nontumor cells. A Wilms' tumor of the kidney can enter the vena cava and grow in the lumen all the way to the heart but only because it induces a new blood supply, which elongates as the tumor grows. The common misperception that tumors can outgrow their blood supply is based mainly on angiograms of human tumors (ie, renal carcinoma), in which a large necrotic center is surrounded by a thin rim of vascularized tumor. But this pattern is due to compression of vessels previously induced by the tumor. Tumors may compress their blood supply but do not outgrow it.

Do angiogenesis inhibitors have to cross the blood brain barrier to treat a brain tumor?

The angiogenesis inhibitor TNP-470, a synthetic analogue of fumagillin, has a molecular weight of 401 Da, and its polymeric conjugate TNP-470-HPMA (Caplostatin) is 30,000 Da. The low-molecular-weight inhibitor crosses the blood-brain barrier (as proved in mice by mass spectroscopy), but the large-molecular-weight inhibitor does not. Both, however, cause equivalent inhibition of orthotopic human brain tumors in mice. Both selectively inhibit only endothelial proliferation and migration. The larger molecular inhibitor is effective even though it remains mainly inside blood vessels.

FUTURE DIRECTIONS

A long-term goal of antiangiogenic therapy is to be able to treat cancer with a much reduced risk of toxicity and drug resistance. As toxicity and drug resistance are gradually reduced, it may become possible to convert cancer to a chronic manageable disease, such as diabetes. It may eventually become possible to liberate the management of cancer from dependency on knowing the anatomic location.

A starting point toward these ambitious goals could be the use of cancer therapy of relatively low toxicity (including antiangiogenic therapy), guided by specific and sensitive biomarkers in blood or urine. Thus, it might become possible to prevent recurrent colon or breast cancer from ever becoming clinically symptomatic after their initial surgical removal. For individuals at high risk of developing clinically detectable cancer, such as women with the mutated breast cancer gene, it may become possible in the future to avoid bilateral mastectomy and ovariectomy by treating a biomarker with long-term antiangiogenic therapy. An experimental study of spontaneous carcinogen-induced breast cancer in rats revealed that endostatin prevented the onset of breast cancer and prolonged survival compared with untreated controls.[449] High-grade giant cell tumors have been treated with antiangiogenic interferon-α guided by a urinary biomarker, bFGF, which was also employed to show no evidence of disease after therapy was discontinued.[299,338] Calcitonin is the best example of a very specific and sensitive biomarker that could be used to guide antiangiogenic therapy of a medullary carcinoma of the thyroid in the years following surgical removal to prevent its recurrence.

When antibiotics were first introduced in the 1940s, they liberated the treatment of infection from dependency on knowing the anatomic location. The cholesterol-lowering statins are now having a similar effect on the treatment of atherosclerosis.

At this writing, 28 endogenous angiogenesis inhibitors are known to circulate in the blood or to be stored in platelets or in the extracellular matrix. As small molecules are discovered that can elevate these inhibitors, perhaps by only a small percentage, in the future, it may become feasible to develop a new pharmaceutical field in which nontoxic small molecules that are orally available are employed to raise the level of endogenous angiogenesis inhibitors. Individuals with Down syndrome are protected from many cancers, possibly in part owing to their 1.6-fold elevation of circulating endostatin. Doxycycline elevates TSP-1 in vivo) (R. Kalluri, unpublished data).

Finally, it is also possible that, in the future, foods that have high levels of antiangiogenic substances may be studied in clinical trials for prevention of cancer or its recurrence.

REFERENCES

1. Hanahan D, Weinberg RA. The hallmarks of cancer. Cell 2000;100:57–70.
2. Achilles E-G, Fernandez A, Allred EN, et al. Heterogeneity of angiogenic activity in a human liposarcoma: a proposed mechanism for 'no take' of human tumors in mice. J Natl Cancer Inst 2001;93:1075–81.
2a. Folkman J, Kalluri R. Cancer without disease. Nature 2004;427:787.
3. Hudlická O. Growth of capillaries in skeletal and cardiac muscle. Circ Res 1982;50:451–61.
4. Hoppeler H, Kayar SR. Capillarity and oxidative capacity of muscles. News Physiol Sci 1988;3:113–6.
5. Adair TH, Gay WJ, Montani J-P. Growth regulation of the vascular system: evidence for a metabolic hypothesis. Am J Physiol 1990;259:R393–404.
6. Ausprunk DH, Folkman J. Migration and proliferation of endothelial cells in preformed and newly formed blood vessels during tumor angiogenesis. Microvasc Res 1977;15:53–65.
7. Klagsbrun M, Moses M. Molecular angiogenesis. Chem Biol 1999;6:R217–24.
8. Sholley MM, Ferguson GP, Seibel HR, et al. Mechanisms of neovascularization: vascular sprouting can occur without proliferation of endothelial cells. Lab Invest 1984;51:624–34.
9. Folkman J, Brem H. Angiogenesis and inflammation. In: Gallin JI, Goldstein IM, Snyderman R, editors. Inflammation: basic principles and clinical correlates. 2nd ed. New York: Raven Press; 1992. p. 821–39.
10. Folkman J. Angiogenesis in arthritis. In: Smolen J, Lipsky P, editors. Targeted therapies in rheumatology. London: Martin Dunitz; 2002. [In press]
11. Warren BA. The vascular morphology of tumors. In: Peterson H-I, editor. Tumor blood circulation: angiogenesis, vascular morphology and blood flow of experimental human tumors. Florida: CRC Press; 1979. p. 1–47.
12. Coman DR, Sheldon WF. The significance of hyperemia around tumor implants. Am J Pathol 1946;22:821–31.
13. Ide AG, Baker NH, Warren SL. Vascularization of the Brown-Pearce rabbit epithelioma transplant as seen in the transparent ear chamber. AJR Am J Roentgenol 1939;42:891–9.
14. Algire GH, Legallais FY. Growth rate of transplanted tumors in relation to latent period and host vascular reaction. Cancer Res 1947;7:724.
15. Algire GH, Chalkely HW, Legallais FY, Park H. Vascular reactions of normal and malignant tumors in vivo: I. Vascular reactions of mice to wounds and to normal and neoplastic transplants. J Natl Cancer Inst 1945;6:73–85.
16. Day ED. Vascular relationships of tumor and host. Prog Exp Tumor Res 1964;4:57–97.
17. Folkman J. Toward an understanding of angiogenesis: search and discovery. Perspect Biol Med 1985;29:10–36.
18. Folkman J. Tumor angiogenesis: therapeutic implications. N Engl J Med 1971;285:1182–6.
19. Folkman J, Long DM, Becker FF. Growth and metastasis of tumor in organ culture. Cancer 1963;16:453–67.
20. Folkman J, Cole P, Zimmerman S. Tumor behavior in isolated perfused organs: in vitro growth and metastases of biopsy material in rabbit thyroid and canine intestinal segment. Ann Surg 1966;164:491–502.
21. Folkman J. Anti-angiogenesis: new concept for therapy of solid tumors. Ann Surg 1972;175:408–16.
22. Folkman J. The vascularization of tumors. Sci Am 1976;234:58–73.
23. Folkman J, Gimbrone MA Jr. Perfusion of the thyroid. In: Diczfalusy E, editor. Karolinska Symposia on Research Methods in Reproduction Endocrinology, 4th Symposium: Perfusion Techniques. Stockholm: Karolinska Institute; 1971. p. 237–48.
24. Folkman J. The intestine as an organ culture. In: Burdette WJ, editor. Carcinoma of the colon and antecedent epithelium. Springfield (IL): CC Thomas; 1970. p. 113–27.
25. Gimbrone MA Jr, Cotran RS, Folkman J. Endothelial regeneration and turnover. Studies with human endothelial cell cultures. Series Haematol 1973;6:453–5.
26. Jaffe EA, Nachman RL, Becker CG, Minick CR. Culture of human endothelial cells derived from umbilical veins: identification by morphologic and immunologic criteria. J Clin Invest 1972;52:2745–56.
27. Folkman J, Haudenschild CC, Zetter BR. Long-term culture of capillary endothelial cells. Proc Natl Acad Sci U S A 1979;76:5217–21.
28. Taylor S, Folkman J. Protamine is an inhibitor of angiogenesis. Nature 1982;297:307–12.
29. Shing Y, Folkman J, Sullivan R, et al. Heparin affinity: purification of a tumor-derived capillary endothelial cell growth factor. Science 1984;223:1296–8.
30. Folkman J. Antiangiogenesis. In: DeVita VT Jr, Hellman S, Rosenberg SA, editors. Biologic therapy of cancer. Philadelphia: Lippincott; 1991. p. 743–53.
31. Folkman J, Merler E, Abernathy C, Williams G. Isolation of a tumor factor responsible for angiogenesis. J Exp Med 1971;133:275–88.
32. Folkman J. Angiogenesis. In: Jaffe EA, editor. Biology of endothelial cells. Boston (MA): Nijhoff; 1984. p. 412–28.
33. Klagsbrun M, Knighton D, Folkman J. Tumor angiogenesis activity in cell grown in tissue culture. Cancer Res 1976;36:110–4.
34. Auerbach R, Arensman R, Kubai L, Folkman J. Tumor-induced angiogenesis: lack of inhibitor by irradiation. Int J Cancer 1975;15:241–5.
35. Folkman J, Cotran RS. Relation of vascular proliferation to tumor growth. Int Rev Exp Pathol 1976;16:207–48.
36. Folkman J. What is the evidence that tumors are angiogenesis dependent? J Natl Cancer Inst 1990;82:4–6.
37. Kerbel R, Folkman J. Clinical translation of angiogenesis inhibitors. Nat Rev Cancer 2002;2:727–39.
38. Folkman J, Hochberg M. Self-regulation of growth in three dimensions. J Exp Med 1973;138:745–53.
39. Adam JA, Maggelakis AA. Diffusion of regulated growth characteristics of a spherical prevascular carcinoma. Bull Math Biol 1990;52:549–82.
40. Sutherland RM. Cell and environment interactions in tumor microregions: the multicell spheroid model. Science 1988;240:177–84.
41. Sutherland RM, McCredie JA, Inch WR. Growth of multicell spheroids in tissue culture as a model of nodular carcinomas. J Natl Cancer Inst 1971;46:113–20.
42. Holmgren L, O'Reilly MS, Folkman J. Dormancy of micrometastases: balanced proliferation and apoptosis in the presence of angiogenesis suppression. Nat Med 1995;1:149–53.
43. Jain RK. Vascular and interstitial barriers to delivery of therapeutic agents in tumors. Cancer Metastasis Rev 1990;9:253–66.
44. Gimbrone MA Jr, Cotran R, Leapman S, Folkman J. Tumor growth and neovascularization: an experimental model using rabbit cornea. J Natl Cancer Inst 1974;52:413–27.
45. Gimbrone MA Jr, Leapman S, Cotran RS, Folkman J. Tumor dormancy in vivo by prevention of neovascularization. J Exp Med 1972;136:261–76.
46. Hanahan D, Folkman J. Patterns and emerging mechanisms of the angiogenic switch during tumorigenesis. Cell 1996;86:353–64.
47. Brem S, Brem H, Folkman J, et al. Prolonged tumor dormancy by prevention of neovascularization in the vitreous. Cancer Res 1976;36:2807–12.
48. Folkman J. Tumor angiogenesis factor. Cancer Res 1974;34:2109–13.
49. Tannock IF. Population kinetics of carcinoma cells, capillary endothelial cells, and fibroblasts in a transplanted mouse mammary tumor. Cancer Res 1970;30:2470–6.
50. Thomlinson R, Gray L. The histological structure of some human lung cancers and the possible implications for radiotherapy. Br J Cancer 1955;9:539–49.
51. Helmlinger G, Yuan F, Dellian M, Jain RK. Interstitial pH and PO2 gradients in solid tumors in vivo: high-resolution measurements reveal a lack of correlation. Nat Med 1997;3:177–82.
52. Knighton D, Ausprunk D, Tapper D, Folkman J. Avascular and vascular phases of tumour growth in the chick embryo. Br J Cancer 1977;35:347–56.
53. Lien W, Ackerman NB. The blood supply of experimental liver metastases. II. A microcirculatory study of normal and tumor vessels of the liver with the use of perfused silicone rubber. Surgery 1970;68:334–40.
54. Folkman J, Watson K, Ingber D, Hanahan D. Induction of angiogenesis during the transition from hyperplasia to neoplasia. Nature 1989;339:58–61.
55. Thompson WD, Shiach KJ, Fraser RA, et al. Tumors acquire their vasculature by vessel incorporation, not vessel ingrowth. J Pathol 1987;151:323–32.
56. Skinner SA, Tutton PJ, O'Brien PE. Microvascular architecture of experimental colon tumors in the rat. Cancer Res 1990;50:2411–7.
57. Holash J, Maisonpierre PC, Compton D, et al. Vessel cooption, regression, and growth in tumors mediated by angiopoietins and VEGF. Science 1999;284:1994–8.
58. Kim ES, Serur A, Huang J, et al. Potent VEGF blockade causes regression of coopted vessels in a model of neuroblastoma. Proc Natl Acad Sci U S A 2002;99:11399–404.
59. Ingber DM, Fujita T, Kishimoto S, et al. Synthetic analogues of fumagillin that inhibit angiogenesis and suppress tumour growth. Nature 1990;348:555–7.
60. Folkman J. Tumor angiogenesis. In: Wells SA Jr, Sharp PA, editors. Accomplishments in cancer research. Philadelphia (PA): JB Lippincott Williams and Wilkins; 1998. p. 32–44.
61. Hori A, Sasada R, Matsutani E, et al. Suppression of solid tumor growth by immuno-neutralizing monoclonal antibody against human basic fibroblast growth factor. Cancer Res 1991;51:6180–4.
62. Kim KJ, Li B, Winer J, et al. Inhibition of vascular endothelial growth factor-induced angiogenesis suppresses tumour growth in vivo. Nature 1993;362:841–4.
63. Plate KH, Breier G, Millauer B, et al. Up-regulation of vascular endothelial growth factor and its cognate receptors in a rat glioma model of tumor angiogenesis. Cancer Res 1993;53:5822–7.
64. Brooks PC, Montgomery AMP, Rosenfeld M, et al. Integrin $\alpha v\beta 3$ antagonists promote tumor regression by inducing apoptosis of angiogenic blood vessels. Cell 1994;79:1157–64.
65. O'Reilly MS, Holmgren L, Shing Y, et al. Angiostatin: a novel angiogenesis inhibitor that mediates the suppression of metastases by a Lewis lung carcinoma. Cell 1994;79:315–28.
66. O'Reilly MS, Holmgren L, Chen C, Folkman J. Angiostatin induces and sustains dormancy of human primary tumors in mice. Nat Med 1996;2:689–92.
67. O'Reilly MS, Boehm T, Shing Y, et al. Endostatin: an endogenous inhibitor of angiogenesis and tumor growth. Cell 1997;88:277–85.
68. O'Reilly MS, Brem H, Folkman J. Treatment of murine hemangioendotheliomas with the angiogenesis inhibitor AGM-1470. J Pediatr Surg 1994;30:325–30.
69. Boehm T, Folkman J, Browder T, O'Reilly MS. Antiangiogenic therapy of experimental cancer does not induce acquired drug resistance. Nature 1997;390:404–7.
70. O'Reilly MS, Pirie-Shepherd S, Lane WS, Folkman J. Antiangiogenic activity of the cleaved conformation of the serpin antithrombin. Science 1999;285:1926–8.
71. Maeshima Y, Manfredi M, Reimer C, et al. Identification of the anti-angiogenic site within vascular basement membrane-derived tumstatin. J Biol Chem 2001;276:15240–8.
71a. Nyberg P, Xie L, Kalluri R. Endogenous inhibitors of angiogenesis. Cancer Res 2005;65:3967–79.
72. Kisker O, Becker CM, Prox D, et al. Continuous administration of endostatin by intraperitoneally implanted osmotic pump improves the efficacy and potency of therapy in a mouse xenograft tumor model. Cancer Res 2001;61:7669–74.
73. Holash J, Davis S, Papadopoulos N, et al. VEGF-Trap; a VEGF blocker with potent antitumor effects. Proc Natl Acad Sci U S A 2002;99:11393–8.
74. Millauer B, Shawver LK, Plate KH, et al. Glioblastoma growth inhibited in vivo by a dominant-negative Flk-1 mutant. Nature 1994;367:576–9.
75. Dameron KM, Volpert OV, Tainsky MA, Bouck N. Control of angiogenesis in fibroblasts by p53 regulation of thrombospondin-1. Science 1994;265:1582–4.
76. Arbiser JL, Moses MA, Fernandez CA, et al. Oncogenic H-ras stimulates tumor angiogenesis by two distinct pathways. Proc Natl Acad Sci U S A 1997;94:861–6.
77. Chin L, Tam A, Pomerantz J, et al. Essential role for oncogenic Ras in tumour maintenance. Nature 1999;400:468–72.
77a. Tang Y, Kim M, Carrasco D, et al. In vivo assessment of RAS-dependent maintenance of tumor angiogenesis by real-time magnetic resonance imaging. Cancer Res 2005;65:8324–30.
77b. Watnick RS, Cheng Y-N, Rangarajan A, et al. Ras modulates Myc activity to repress thrombospondin-1 expression and increase tumor angiogenesis. Cancer Cell 2003;3:219–31.
78. Cao Y, O'Reilly MS, Marshall B, et al. Expression of angiostatin cDNA in a murine fibrosarcoma suppresses primary tumor growth and produces long-term dormancy of metastases. J Clin Invest 1998;101:1055–63.
79. Streit M, Riccardi L, Velasco P, et al. Thrombospondin-2: a potent endogenous inhibitor of tumor growth and angiogenesis. Proc Natl Acad Sci U S A 1999;96:14888–93.
80. Lyden D, Young AZ, Zagzag D, et al. Id1 and Id3 are required for neurogenesis, angiogenesis and vascularization of tumour xenografts. Nature 1999;401:670–7.
81. Lyden D, Hattori K, Dias S, et al. Impaired recruitment of bone-marrow-derived endothelial and hematopoietic precursor cells blocks tumor angiogenesis and growth. Nat Med 2001;7:1194–201.

81a. Sund M, Hamano Y, Sugimoto, et al. Function of endogenous inhibitors of angiogenesis as endothelium-specific suppressors. Proc Natl Acad Sci 2005;102(8):2934–29.

82. Fidler IJ, Gersten DM, Hart IR. The biology of cancer invasion and metastasis. Adv Cancer Res 1978;28:149–250.

83. Nicolson GL. Cancer metastasis. Sci Am 1979;240:66–76.

84. Nicolson GL. Organ specificity of tumor metastasis: role of preferential adhesion, invasion and growth of malignant cells at specific secondary sites. Cancer Metastasis Rev 1988;7:143–88.

85. Watanabe H, Hori A, Seno M, et al. A sensitive enzyme immunoassay for human basic fibroblast growth factor. Biochem Biophys Res Commun 1991;175:229–35.

86. Zetter BR. Angiogenesis and tumor metastasis. Annu Rev Med 1998;49:407–24.

86a. Kang S-Y, Liu NW, Lee JM, et al. Regulation of stromal thrombospondin-1 in metastatic cancer growth. Proc Supplement Amer Assoc Cancer Res, 96th Annual Meeting 2005; LB15 abstract.

87. Netland PA, Zetter BR. Organ-specific adhesion of metastatic tumor cells in vitro. Science 1984;224:1113–5.

88. Boxberger HJ, Paweletz N, Spiess E, Kriehuber R. An in vitro model study of BSp73 rat tumour cell invasion into endothelial monolayer. Anticancer Res 1989;9:1777–86.

89. Weidner N, Semple JP, Welch WR, Folkman J. Tumor angiogenesis correlates with metastasis in invasive breast carcinoma. N Engl J Med 1991;324:1–8.

90. Weinstat-Saslow D, Steeg PS. Angiogenesis and colonization in the tumor metastatic process: basic and applied advances. FASEB J 1994;8:401–7.

91. Liotta LA, Tryggvason K, Garbisa S, et al. Metastatic potential correlates with enzymatic degradation of basement membrane collagen. Nature 1980;284:67–8.

92. Liotta LA, Saidel MG, Kleinerman J. The significance of hematogenous tumor cell clumps in the metastatic process. Cancer Res 1976;36:889–94.

93. Dvorak HF, Nagy JA, Dvorak JT, Dvorak AM. Identification and characterization of the blood vessels of solid tumors that are leaky to circulating macromolecules. Am J Pathol 1988;133:95–109.

94. Kalebic T, Garbisa S, Glaser B, Liotta LA. Basement membrane collagen: degradation by migrating endothelial cells. Science 1983;221:281–3.

95. Moscatelli D, Gross JL, Rifkin DB. Angiogenic factors stimulate plasminogen activator and collagenase production by capillary endothelial cells [abstract]. J Cell Biol 1981;91:201a.

96. Nagy JA, Brown LF, Senger DR, et al. Pathogenesis of tumor stroma generation: a critical role for leaky blood vessels and fibrin deposition. Biochem Biophys Acta 1989;948:305–26.

97. Folkman J. Angiogenesis in cancer, vascular, rheumatoid and other disease. Nat Med 1995;1:27–31.

98. Chambers AF. The metastatic process: basic research and clinical implications. Oncol Res 1999;11:161–8.

99. Udagawa T, Fernandez A, Achilles E-G, et al. Persistence of microscopic human cancers in mice: alterations in the angiogenic balance accompanies loss of tumor dormancy. FASEB J 2002;16:1361–70.

100. Hicks RM, Chowaniec J. Experimental induction, histology, and ultrastructure of hyperplasia and neoplasia of the urinary bladder epithelium. Int Rev Exp Pathol 1978;18:199–280.

101. Sillman F, Boyce J, Fruchter R. The significance of atypical vessels and neovascularization in cervical neoplasia. Am J Obstet Gynecol 1981;139:154–9.

102. Smith-McCune KK, Weidner N. Demonstration and characterization of the angiogenic properties of cervical dysplasia. Cancer Res 1994;54:800–4.

103. Srivastava A, Laidler P, Davies RP, Horfan K. The prognostic significance of tumor vascularity in intermediate-thickness (0.76–4.0 mm thick) skin melanoma. A quantitative histologic study. Am J Pathol 1988;133:419–23.

104. Weidner N, Folkman J, Pozza F, et al. Tumor angiogenesis: a new significant and independent prognostic indicator in early stage breast carcinoma. J Natl Cancer Inst 1992;84:1875–87.

105. Weidner N, Carroll PR, Flax J, et al. Tumor angiogenesis correlates with metastasis in invasive prostate carcinoma. Am J Pathol 1993;143:401–9.

106. Fang J, Shing Y, Wiederschain D, et al. Matrix metalloproteinase-2 (MMP-2) is required for the switch to the angiogenic phenotype in a novel tumor model. Proc Natl Acad Sci U S A 2000. [In press]

107. Carmeliet P, Dor Y, Herbert JM, et al. Role of HIF-1α in hypoxia-mediated apoptosis, cell proliferation and tumor angiogenesis. Nature 1998;394:485–90.

108. Li C-Y, Shan S, Huang Q, et al. Initial stages of tumor cell-induced angiogenesis: evaluation via skin window chambers in rodent models. J Natl Cancer Inst 2000;92:143–7.

109. Folkman J. Incipient angiogenesis. J Natl Cancer Inst 2000;92:94–5.

110. Rak J, Filmus J, Finkenzeller G, et al. Oncogenes as inducers of tumor angiogenesis. Cancer Metastasis Rev 1995;14:263–77.

111. Holash J, Wiegand SJ, Yancopoulos GD. New model of tumor angiogenesis: dynamic balance between vessel regression and growth mediated by angiopoietins and VEGF. Oncogene 1999;18:5356–62.

112. Senger DR, Brown LF, Claffey KP, Dvorak HF. Vascular permeability factor, tumor angiogenesis and stroma generation. Invasion Metastasis 1994;14:385–94.

113. Kadish JL, Butterfield CE, Folkman J. The effect of fibrin on cultured vascular endothelial cells. Tissue Cell 1979;11:99–108.

114. Ziche M, Morbidelli L, Choudhuri R, et al. Nitric oxide synthase lies downstream from vascular endothelial growth factor-induced but not basic fibroblast growth factor-induced angiogenesis. J Clin Invest 1997;99:2625–34.

115. Papapetropoulos A, Garcia-Cardena G, Madri JA, Sessa WC. Nitric oxide contributes to the angiogenic properties of vascular endothelial growth factor in human endothelial cells. J Clin Invest 1997;100:3131–9.

116. Garcia-Cardena G, Folkman J. Is there a role for nitric oxide in tumor angiogenesis? J Natl Cancer Inst 1998;90:560–1.

117. Ingber DE, Folkman J. How does the extracellular matrix control capillary morphogenesis? Cell 1989;58:803–5.

118. Chen CS, Mrksich M, Huan S, et al. Geometric control of cell life and death. Science 1997;276:1425–8.

119. Yuan F, Chen Y, Dellian M, et al. Time-dependent vascular regression and permeability changes in established human tumor xenografts induced by an anti-vascular endothelial growth factor/vascular permeability factor antibody. Proc Natl Acad Sci U S A 1996;93:14765–70.

120. Kandel J, Bossy-Wetzel E, Radvanyi F, et al. Neovascularization is associated with a switch to the export of bFGF in the multistep development of fibrosarcoma. Cell 1991;66:1095–104.

121. Hanahan D, Christofori G, Naik P, Arbeit J. Transgenic mouse models of tumor angiogenesis: the angiogenic switch, its molecular controls, and prospects for preclinical therapeutic models. Eur J Cancer 1996;14:2386–93.

122. McDonald D, Hashizume H, Baluk P, et al. Openings between defective endothelial cells explain tumor vessel leakiness. Am J Pathol 2000;156:1363–80.

123. Asahara T, Murohara T, Sullivan A, et al. Isolation of putative progenitor endothelial cells for angiogenesis. Science 1997;275:964–7.

124. Shi Q, Rafii S, Wu MH-D, et al. Evidence for circulating bone marrow-derived endothelial cells. Blood 1998;92:362–7.

125. Hatzopoulos AK, Folkman J, Vasile E, et al. Isolation and characterization of endothelial progenitor cells from mouse embryos. Development 1998;125:1457–68.

126. Asahara T, Takahashi T, Masuda H, et al. VEGF contributes to postnatal neovascularization by mobilizing bone marrow-derived endothelial progenitor cells. EMBO J 1999;18:3964–72.

127. Murohara T, Ikeda H, Duan J, et al. Transplanted cord blood-derived endothelial precursor cells augment postnatal neovascularization. J Clin Invest 2000;105:1527–36.

128. Rafii S. Circulating endothelial precursors: mystery, reality, and promise. J Clin Invest 2000:105:17–9.

129. Peichev M, Naiyer AJ, Pereira D, et al. Expression of VEGFR-2 and AC133 by circulating human CD34(+) cells identifies a population of functional endothelial precursors. Blood 2000;95:952–8.

130. Gehling UM, Ergun S, Schumacher U, et al. In vitro differentiation of endothelial cells from AC133-positive progenitor cells. Blood 2000;95:3106–12.

131. Hattori K, Dias S, Heissig B, et al. Vascular endothelial growth factor and angiopoietin-1 stimulate postnatal hematopoiesis by recruitment of vasculogenic and hematopoietic stem cells. J Exp Med 2001:193:1004–14.

132. Hattori K, Heissig B, Tashiro K, et al. Plasma elevation of stromal cell-derived factor-1 induces mobilization of mature and immature hematopoietic progenitor and stem cells. Blood 2001;97:3354–60.

133. Hattori K, Hessig B, Wu Y, et al. Placental growth factor reconstitutes hematopoiesis by recruiting VEGFR1(+) stem cells from bone marrow microenvironment. Nat Med 2002;8:841–9.

134. Heissig B, Hattori K, Dias S, et al. Recruitment of stem and progenitor cells from the bone marrow niche requires MMP-9 mediated release of kit-ligand. Cell 2002;109:625–37.

134a. Peters BA, Diaz LA, Polyak K, et al. Contribution of bone marrow-derived endothelial cells to human tumor vasculature. Nat Med 2005;11:261–2.

135. Reyes M, Dudek A, Jahagirdar B, et al. Origin of endothelial progenitors in human postnatal bone marrow. J Clin Invest 2002;109:337–46.

136. Ito H, Rovira II, Bloom ML, et al. Endothelial progenitor cells as putative targets for angiostatin. Cancer Res 1999;59:5875–7.

137. Monestiroli S, Mancuso P, Burlini A, et al. Kinetics and viability of circulating endothelial cells as surrogate angiogenesis marker in an animal model of human lymphoma. Cancer Res 2001;61:4341–4.

138. Bertolini F, Mingrone W, Alietti A, et al. Thalidomide in multiple myeloma, myelodysplastic syndromes and histiocytosis. Analysis of clinical results and of surrogate angiogenesis markers. Ann Oncol 2001;12:987–90.

139. Folkman J. Role of angiogenesis in tumor growth. Semin Cancer Biol 1992;3:65–71.

140. Polverini P, Leibovich S. Induction of neovascularization in vivo and endothelial proliferation in vitro by tumor-associated macrophages. Lab Invest 1984;51:635–42.

141. Bergers G, Brekken R, McMahon J, et al. Matrix metalloproteinase-9 triggers the angiogenic switch during carcinogenesis. Nat Cell Biol 2000;2:737–44.

142. Coussens LM, Tinkle CL, Hanahan D, Werb Z. MMP-9 supplied by bone marrow-derived cells contributes to skin carcinogenesis. Cell 2000;103:481–90.

143. Schulze-Osthoff K, Risau W, Vollmer E, Sorg C. In situ detection of basic fibroblast growth factor by highly specific antibodies. Am J Pathol 1990;137:85–92.

144. Fukumura D, Xavier R, Sugiura T, et al. Tumor induction of VEGF promotor activity in stromal cells. Cell 1998;94:715–25.

145. Luzzi KJ, MacDonald IC, Schmidt EE, et al. Multistep nature of metastatic inefficiency: dormancy of solitary cells after successful extravasation and limited survival of early micrometastases. Am J Pathol 1998;153:865–73.

146. Cameron MD, Schmidt EE, Kerkvliet N, et al. Temporal progression of metastasis in lung: cell survival, dormancy, and location dependence of metastatic inefficiency. Cancer Res 2000;60:2541–6.

147. Folkman J. Angiogenesis and its inhibitors. In: DeVita VT Jr, Hellman S, Rosenberg SA, editors. Important advances in oncology. Philadelphia: JB Lippincott; 1985. p. 42–62.

148. Cockerill GW, Gamble JR, Vadas MA. Angiogenesis: models and modulators. Int Rev Cytol 1995;159:113–60.

149. Murray JC. Angiogenesis protocols. Totowa, New Jersey: Humana Press; 2001.

150. Christofori G. The role of fibroblast growth factors in tumour progression and angiogenesis. In: Bicknell R, Lewis CE, Ferrara N, editors. Tumour angiogenesis. Oxford (UK): Oxford University Press; 1996. p. 201–37.

151. Friesel RE, Maciag T. Molecular mechanisms of angiogenesis: fibroblast growth factor signal. FASEB J 1995;9:919–25.

152. Folkman J, Shing Y. Angiogenesis. J Biol Chem 1992;267:10931–4.

153. Almaric F, Baldin V, Bosc-Bierne I, et al. Nuclear translocation of basic fibroblast growth factor. Ann N Y Acad Sci 1991;638:127–38.

154. Folkman J, Klagsbrun M, Sasse J, et al. A heparin-binding angiogenic protein—basic fibroblast growth factor—is stored within basement membrane. Am J Pathol 1988;130:393–400.

155. Paulus W, Grothe C, Sensenbrenner M, et al. Localization of basic fibroblast growth factor, a mitogen and angiogenic factor, in human-brain tumors. Acta Neuropathol (Berl) 1990;79:418–23.

156. Takahashi JA, Fukumoto M, Igarashi K, et al. Correlation of basic fibroblast growth factor expression levels with the degree of malignancy and vascularity in human gliomas. J Neurosurg 1992;76:792–8.

157. Chodak GW, Hospelhorn V, Judge SM, et al. Increased levels of fibroblast growth factor-like activity in urine of patients with bladder or kidney cancer. Cancer Res 1988;48:2083–8.

158. Vlodavsky I, Bashkin PK, Korner G, et al. Extracellular matrix-resident growth factors and enzymes: relevance to angiogenesis and metastasis. Proc Annu Meet Am Assoc Cancer Res 1990;31:491–3.

159. Czubayko F, Liaudet-Coopman EDE, Aigner A, et al. A secreted FGF-binding protein can serve as the angiogenic switch in human cancer. Nat Med 1997;3:1137–40.

160. Rak J, Kerbel RS. FGF-2 and tumorangiogenesis: back in the limelight. Nat Med 1997;3:1083–4.

161. Sherif ZA, Nakai S, Pirollo KF, et al. Down-modulation of bFGF-binding protein expression following restoration of p53 function. Cancer Gene Ther 2001;8:771–82.
162. Norrby K. Mast cells and angiogenesis. APMIS 2002;110:355–71.
163. Soutter AD, Nguyen M, Watanabe H, Folkman J. Basic fibroblast growth factor secreted by an animal tumor is detectable in urine. Cancer Res 1993;53:5297–9.
164. Klagsbrun M, D'Amore P. Regulators of angiogenesis. Annu Rev Physiol 1991;53:217–39.
165. Yancopoulos GD, Klagsbrun M, Folkman J. Vasculogenesis, angiogenesis and growth factors. Cell 1998;93:661–4.
166. Uemura A, Ogawa M, Hirashima M, et al. Recombinant angiopoietin-1 restores higher-order architecture of growing blood vessels in mice in the absence of mural cells. J Clin Invest 2002;110:1619–28.
167. Melder RJ, Koenig GC, Witwer BP, et al. During angiogenesis, vascular endothelial growth factor and basic fibroblast growth factor regulate natural killer cell adhesion to endothelium. Nat Med 1996;2:992–7.
168. Griffioen AW, Tromp SC, Hillen HF. Angiogenesis modulates the tumour immune response. Int J Exp Pathol 1998;76:363–8.
169. Griffioen AW, Damen CA, Mayo KH, et al. Angiogenesis inhibitors overcome tumor induced endothelial cell anergy. Int J Cancer 1999;80:315–9.
170. Nguyen M, Watanabe H, Budson AE, et al. Elevated levels of an angiogenic peptide, basic fibroblast growth factor, in the urine of patients with a wide spectrum of cancers. J Natl Cancer Inst 1994;86:356–61.
171. Li VW, Folkerth RD, Watanabe H, et al. Microvessel count and cerebrospinal fluid basic fibroblast growth factor in children with brain tumours. Lancet 1994;344:82–6.
172. Nanus DM, Schmitz-Drager BJ, Motzer RJ, et al. Expression of basic fibroblast growth factor in primary human renal tumors: correlation with poor survival. J Natl Cancer Inst 1993;85:1597–9.
173. Lin RY, Argenta PA, Sullivan KM, Adzick NS. Diagnostic and prognostic role of basic fibroblast growth factor in Wilm's tumor patients. Clin Cancer Res 1995;1:327–31.
174. Dvorak HF. Tumors: wounds that do not heal. Similarities between tumor stroma generation and wound healing. N Engl J Med 1986;315:1650–9.
175. Senger DR, Galli SJ, Dvorak AM, et al. Tumor cells secrete a vascular permeability factor that promotes accumulation of ascites fluid. Science 1983;219:983–5.
176. Ferrara N, Henzel WJ. Pituitary follicular cells secrete a novel heparin-binding growth factor specific for vascular endothelial cells. Biochem Biophys Res Commun 1989;161:851–5.
177. Brown LF, Detmar M, Claffey K, et al. Vascular permeability factor/vascular endothelial growth factor: a multifunctional angiogenic cytokine. In: Goldberg ID, Rosen E, editors. Control of angiogenesis. Berlin: Birkhauser Verlag; 1997. p. 233–69.
178. Ferrara N. Vascular endothelial growth factor. Trends Cardiovasc Med 1993;3:244–50.
179. Rosenthal RA, Megyesi JF, Henzel WJ, et al. Conditioned medium from mouse sarcoma 180 cells contains vascular endothelial growth factor. Growth Factors 1990;4:53–9.
180. Bouck N, Stellmach V, Hsu S. How tumors become angiogenic. Adv Cancer Res 1996;69:135–74.
181. Connolly DT. Vascular permeability factor: a unique regulator of blood vessel function. J Cell Biochem 1991;47:219–23.
182. Dvorak HF, Sioussat TM, Brown LF, et al. Distribution of vascular permeability factor (vascular endothelial growth factor) in tumors: concentration in tumor blood vessels. J Exp Med 1991;174:1275–8.
183. Ferrara N, Houck K, Jakeman L, Leung DW. Molecular and biological properties of the vascular endothelial growth factor family of proteins. Endocr Rev 1992;13:18–32.
184. Breier G, Albrecht U, Sterrer S, Risau W. Expression of vascular endothelial growth factor during embryonic angiogenesis and endothelial cell differentiation. Development 1992;114:521–32.
185. Peters KG, De Vries C, Williams LT. VEGF receptor expression during embryogenesis and tissue repair suggests a role in endothelial differentiation and blood vessel growth. Proc Natl Acad Sci U S A 1993;90:8915–9.
186. Gerber HP, Hillan KJ, Ryan AM, et al. VEGF is required for growth and survival in neonatal mice. Development 1999;126:1149–59.
187. Otani N, Minami S, Yamoto M, et al. The vascular endothelial growth factor/fms-like tyrosine kinase system in human ovary during the menstrual cycle and early pregnancy. J Clin Endocrinol Metab 1999;84:3845–51.
188. Brown LF, Berse B, Jackman RW, et al. Increased expression of vascular permeability factor (vascular endothelial growth factor) and its receptors in kidney and bladder carcinomas. Am J Pathol 1993;143:1255–62.
189. Inoue M, Hager JH, Ferrara N, et al. VEGF-A has a critical, nonredundant role in angiogenic switching and pancreatic beta cell carcinogenesis. Cancer Cell 2002;1:193–202.
190. Gerber HP, Kowalski J, Sherman D, et al. Complete inhibition of rhabdomyosarcoma xenografts growth and neovascularization requires blockade of both tumor and host vascular endothelial growth factor. Cancer Res 2000;60:6253–8.
191. De Vries C, Escobedo JA, Ueno H, et al. The fms-like tyrosine kinase, a receptor for vascular endothelial growth factor. Science 1992;255:989–94.
192. Terman BI, Dougher-Vermazen M, Carrion ME, et al. Identification of the KDR tyrosine kinase as a receptor for vascular endothelial cell growth factor. Biochem Biophys Res Commun 1992;187:1579–86.
193. Klagsbrun M, D'Amore P. Vascular endothelial growth factor and its receptors. Cytokine Growth Factor Rev 1996;7:259–70.
194. Neufeld G, Cohen T, Gengrinovitch S, Poltorak Z. Vascular endothelial growth factor (VEGF) and its receptors. FASEB J 1999;13:9–22.
195. Dvorak HF, Nagy JA, Feng D, et al. Vascular permeability factor/vascular endothelial growth factor and the significance of microvascular hyperpermeability in angiogenesis. Curr Top Microbiol Immunol 1999;237:97–132.
196. Ferrara N. VEGF and the quest for tumour angiogenesis factors. Nat Rev Cancer 2002;2:795–803.
197. Ferrara N. Vascular endothelial growth factor: molecular and biological aspects. Curr Top Microbiol Immunol 1999;237:1–30.
198. Korpelainen EI, Alitalo K. Signaling angiogenesis and lymphangiogenesis. Curr Opin Cell Biol 1998;10:159–64.
199. Kaipainen A, Korhonen J, Mustonen T, et al. Expression of the fms-like tyrosine kinase 4 gene becomes restricted to lymphatic endothelium during development. Proc Natl Acad Sci U S A 1995;92:3566–70.
200. Chang L, Kaipainen A, Folkman J. Lymphangiogenesis. New mechanisms. Ann N Y Acad Sci 2002;979:111–9.
201. Soker S, Takashima S, Miao HQ, et al. Neuropilin-1 is expressed by endothelial and tumor cells as an isoform-specific receptor for vascular endothelial growth factor. Cell 1998;92:735–45.
202. Mamluk R, Gechtman Z, Kutcher ME, et al. Neuropilin-1 binds vascular endothelial growth factor 165, placenta growth factor-2, and heparin via its blb2 domain. J Biol Chem 2002;277:24818–25.
203. Plate K, Breier G, Weich HA, Risau W. Vascular endothelial growth factor is a potential tumour angiogenesis factor in human gliomas in vivo. Nature 1992;359:845–8.
204. Shweiki D, Itin A, Soffer D, Keshet E. Vascular endothelial growth factor induced by hypoxia may mediate hypoxia-initiated angiogenesis. Nature 1992;359:843–5.
205. Levy AP, Levy NS, Goldberg MA. Post-transcriptional regulation of vascular endothelial growth factor by hypoxia. J Biol Chem 1996;271:2746–53.
206. Dor Y, Keshet E. Ischemia-driven angiogenesis. Trends Cardiovasc Med 1997;7:289–94.
207. Shima DT, Adamis AP, Ferrara N, et al. Hypoxic induction of endothelial cell growth factors in retinal cells: identification and characterization of vascular endothelial growth factor (VEGF) as the mitogen. Mol Med 1995;1:182–93.
208. Okada F, Rak J, St. Croix B, et al. Impact of oncogenes on tumor angiogenesis: mutant K-ras upregulation of VEGF/VPF is necessary but not sufficient for tumorigenicity of human colorectal carcinoma cells. Proc Natl Acad Sci U S A 1998;95:3609–14.
209. Iliopoulos O, Levy AP, Jiang C, et al. Negative regulation of hypoxia-inducible genes by the von Hippel-Lindau protein. Proc Natl Acad Sci U S A 1996;93:10595–9.
210. Siemeister G, Weindel K, Mohrs K, et al. Reversion of deregulated expression of vascular endothelial growth factor in human renal carcinoma cells by von Hippel-Lindau tumor suppressor protein. Cancer Res 1996;56:2299–301.
211. Gnarra JR, Zhou S, Merrill MJ, et al. Post-transcriptional regulation of vascular endothelial growth factor mRNA by the product of the VHL tumor suppressor gene. Proc Natl Acad Sci U S A 1996;93:10589–94.
212. Ferrara N. Role of vascular endothelial growth factor in regulation of angiogenesis. In: Teicher BA, editor. Antiangiogenic agents in cancer therapy. New Jersey: Humana Press; 1999. p. 119–42.
213. Aiello LP, George DJ, Cahill MT, et al. Rapid and durable recovery of visual function in a patient with von Hippel-Lindau syndrome after systemic therapy with vascular endothelial growth factor receptor inhibitor SU5416. Ophthalmology 2002;109:1745–51.
214. Roberts WG, Palade GE. Neovasculature induced by vascular endothelial growth factor is fenestrated. Cancer Res 1997;57:765–72.
215. van Bruggen N, Thibodeaux H, Palmer JT, et al. VEGF antagonism reduces edema formation and tissue damage after ischemia/reperfusion injury in the mouse brain. J Clin Invest 1999;104:1613–20.
216. Pepper MS, Ferrara N, Orci L, Montesano R. Potent synergism between vascular endothelial growth factor and basic fibroblast growth factor in the induction of angiogenesis in vitro. Biochem Biophys Res Commun 1992;89:824–31.
217. Goto F, Goto K, Weindel K, Folkman J. Synergistic effects of vascular endothelial growth factor and basic fibroblast growth factor on the bovine capillary endothelial cells within collagen gels. Lab Invest 1993;69:508–17.
218. Stavri GT, Zachary IC, Baskerville PA, et al. Basic fibroblast growth factor upregulates the expression of vascular endothelial growth factor in vascular smooth muscle cells. Synergistic interaction with hypoxia. Circulation 1995;92:11–4.
219. Asahara T, Bauters C, Zheng LP, et al. Synergistic effect of vascular endothelial growth factor and basic fibroblast growth factor on angiogenesis in vivo. Circulation 1995;92:II365–71.
220. Houck KA, Leung DW, Rowland AM, et al. Dual regulation of vascular endothelial growth factor bioavailability by genetic and proteolytic mechanisms. J Biol Chem 1992;267:26031–7.
221. Davis S, Aldrich TH, Jones PF, et al. Isolation of angiopoietin-1, a ligand for the TIE2 receptor, by secretion-trap expression cloning. Cell 1996;87:1161–9.
222. Sato TN, Tozawa Y, Deutsch U, et al. Distinct roles of the receptor tyrosine kinases Tie-1 and Tie-2 in blood vessel formation. Nature 1995;376:70–4.
223. Koblizek TI, Weiss C, Yancopoulos GD, et al. Angiopoietin-1 induces sprouting angiogenesis in vitro. Curr Biol 1998;8:529–32.
224. Suri C, McClain J, Thurston G, et al. Increased vascularization in mice overexpressing angiopoietin-1. Science 1998;282:468–71.
225. Maisonpierre PC, Suri C, Jones PF, et al. Angiopoietin-2, a natural antagonist for Tie2 that disrupts in vivo angiogenesis. Science 1997;277:55–60.
226. Folkman J, D'Amore P. Blood vessel formation: what is its molecular basis? Cell 1996;87:1153–5.
227. Thurston G, Suri C, Smith K, et al. Leakage-resistant blood vessels in mice transgenically overexpressing angiopoietin-1. Science 1999;286:2511–4.
228. Rak J, Yu JL, Klement G, Kerbel RS. Oncogenes and angiogenesis: signaling three-dimensional tumor growth. J Invest Dermatol Symp Proc 2000;5:24–33.
229. Kerbel RS, Viloria-Petit A, Okada F, Rak J. Establishing a link between oncogenes and tumor angiogenesis. Mol Med 1998;4:286–95.
230. Rak J, Yu JL, Kerbel RS, Coomber BL. What do oncogenic mutations have to do with angiogenesis/vascular dependence of tumors? Cancer Res 2002;62:1931–4.
231. Petit AM, Rak J, Hung MC, et al. Neutralizing antibodies against epidermal growth factor and ErB-2/neu receptor tyrosine kinases down-regulate vascular endothelial growth factor production by tumor cells in vitro and in vivo: angiogenic implications for signal transduction therapy of solid tumors. Am J Pathol 1997;151:1523–30.
232. Fernandez A, Udagawa T, Schwesinger C, et al. Angiogenic potential of prostate carcinoma cells overexpressing bcl-2. J Natl Cancer Inst 2001;93:208–13.
233. Ravi R, Mookerjee B, Bhujwalla ZM, et al. Regulation of tumor angiogenesis by p53-induced degradation of hypoxia-inducible factor 1α. Genes Dev 2000;14:34–44.
234. Zhang L, Zu D, Hu M, et al. Wild-type p53 suppresses angiogenesis in human leiomyosarcoma and synovial sarcoma by transcriptional suppression of vascular endothelial growth factor expression. Cancer Res 2000;60:3655–61.
235. Izumi Y, Xu L, di Tomaso E, et al. Tumour biology: Herceptin acts as an anti-angiogenic cocktail. Nature 2002;416:279–80.
236. Relf M, LeJeune S, Scott, PA, et al. Expression of the angiogenic factors vascular endothelial cell growth factor, acidic and basic fibroblast growth factor, tumor growth factor β-1, platelet-derived endothelial cell growth factor, placenta growth factor, and pleiotrophin in human primary breast cancer and its relation to angiogenesis. Cancer Res 1997;57:963–9.

237. Viloria-Petit A, Crombet T, Jothy S, et al. Acquired resistance to the antitumor effect of epidermal growth factor receptor-blocking antibodies in vivo: a role for altered tumour angiogenesis. Cancer Res 200l;61:5090–101.
238. Ciardiello F, Caputo R, Bianco R, et al. Inhibition of growth factor production and angiogenesis in human cancer cells by ZD1839 (Iressa), a selective epidermal growth factor receptor tyrosine kinase inhibitor. Clin Cancer Res 2001;7:1459–65.
239. Kaban LB, Mulliken JB, Ezekowitz RA, et al. Antiangiogenic therapy of a recurrent giant cell tumor of the mandible with interferonα-2a. Pediatrics 1999;103:1145–9.
240. Marler JJ, Rubin JB, Trede NS, et al. Successful antiangiogenic therapy of giant cell angioblastoma with interferon alfa 2b: report of 2 cases. Pediatrics 2002;109:1–5.
241. Kaban LB, Troulis MJ, Ebb D, et al. Antiangiogenic therapy with interferon alpha for giant cell lesions of the jaws. J Oral Maxillofac Surg 2002;60:1101–11.
242. Folkman J. Antiangiogenic therapy with interferon alpha for giant cell lesions of the jaws. J Oral Maxillofac Surg 2002;60:1111–3.
243. Singh RK, Gutman M, Bucana CD, et al. Interferon-α and -β down-regulate the expression of basic fibroblast growth factor in human carcinomas. Proc Natl Acad Sci U S A 1995;92:4562–6.
244. Brouty Boye D, Zetter BR. Inhibition of cell motility by interferon. Science 1980;208:516–28.
245. Kerbel RS. Inhibition of tumour angiogenesis as a strategy to circumvent acquired resistance to anticancer therapeutic agents. Bioessays 1991;13:31–6.
246. Stetler-Stevenson WG, Krutzch HC, Liotta LA. Tissue inhibitor of metalloproteinases (TIMP-2). A new member of the metalloproteinases inhibitor family. J Biol Chem 1989;264:17374–8.
247. Moses MA, Sudhalter J, Langer R. Identification of an inhibitor of neovascularization from cartilage. Science 1990;248:1408–10.
248. Kruger EA, Figg WD. TNP-470: an angiogenesis inhibitor in clinical development for cancer. Exp Opin Invest Drugs 2000;9:1383–96.
249. D'Amato RJ, Loughnan MS, Flynn E, Folkman J. Thalidomide is an inhibitor of angiogenesis. Proc Natl Acad Sci U S A 1994;91:4082–5.
250. Udagawa T, Verheul HMW, D'Amato RJ. Thalidomide and analogs. In: Teicher BA, editor. Antiangiogenic agents in cancer therapy. New Jersey: Humana Press; 1999. p. 263–74.
251. Figg WD, Reed E, Green S, Pluda JM. Thalidomide. A prodrug that inhibits angiogenesis. In: Teicher BA, editor. Antiangiogenic agents in cancer therapy. New Jersey: Humana Press; 1999. p. 407–22.
252. Folkman J. Angiogenesis-dependent diseases. Semin Oncol 2001;28:536–42.
253. Hideshima T, Anderson KC. Molecular mechanisms of novel therapeutic approaches for multiple myeloma. Nat Rev Cancer 2002;2:927–37.
254. Crum R, Szabo S, Folkman J. A new class of steroids inhibits angiogenesis in the presence of heparin or a heparin fragment. Science 1985;230:1375–8.
255. D'Amato R, Lin CM, Flynn E, et al. 2-Methoxyestradiol, an endogenous mammalian metabolite, inhibits tubulin polymerization by interacting at the colchicines site. Proc Natl Acad Sci U S A 1994;91:3964–8.
256. Fotsis T, Zhang Y, Pepper MS, et al. The endogenous oestrogen metabolite 2-methoxyestradiol inhibits angiogenesis and suppresses tumour growth. Nature 1994;368:237–9.
257. Williams JI. Squalamine. A new angiostatic steroid. In: Teicher BA, editor. Antiangiogenic agents in cancer therapy. New Jersey: Humana Press; 1999. p. 153–74.
258. Folkman J, Mulliken JB, Ezekowitz RAB. Antiangiogenic therapy of haemangiomas with interferon A. In: Stuart-Harris R, Penny R, editors. The clinical applications of the interferons. London: Chapman & Hall Medical; 1997. p. 255–65.
259. Voest EE, Kenyon BM, O'Reilly MS, et al. Inhibition of angiogenesis in vivo by interleukin 12. J Natl Cancer Inst 1995;87:581–6.
260. Maione TE, Gray GS, Petro J, et al. Inhibition of angiogenesis by recombinant human platelet factor-4 and related peptides. Science 1990;247:77–9.
261. Rastinejad F, Polverini P, Bouck NP. Regulation of the activity of a new inhibitor of angiogenesis by a cancer suppressor gene. Cell 1989;56:345–55.
262. Colorado PC, Torre A, Kamphaus G, et al. Anti-angiogenic cues from vascular basement membrane collagen. Cancer Res 2000;60:2520–6.
262a. Sudhakar A, Nyberg P, Keshamouni VG, et al. Human alpha1 type IV collagen NC1 domain exhibits distinct antiangiogenic activity mediated by alpha1beta1 integrin. J Clin Invest 2005;115(10):2801–10.
263. Kamphaus GD, Colorado PC, Panka DJ, et al. Canstatin, a novel matrix-derived inhibitor of angiogenesis and tumor growth. J Biol Chem 2000:275:1209–15.
264. Maeshima Y, Colorado PC, Torre A, et al. Distinct antitumor properties of a type IV collagen domain derived from basement membrane. J Biol Chem 2000;275: 21340–8.
265. Brooks PC, Silletti S, von Schalscha TL, et al. Disruption of angiogenesis by PEX, a noncatalytic metalloproteinase fragment with integrin binding activity. Cell 1998;92:391–400.
266. Dawson DW, Volpert OV, Gillis P, et al. Pigment epithelium-derived factor: a potent inhibitor of angiogenesis. Science 1999;285:245–8.
267. Eder JP Jr, Supko JG, Clark JW, et al. Phase I clinical trial of recombinant human endostatin administered as a short intravenous infusion repeated daily. J Clin Oncol 2002;18:3772–84.
268. Gengrinovitch S, Greenberg SM, Cohen T, et al. Platelet factor-4 inhibits the mitogen activity of VEGF121 and VEGF165 using several concurrent mechanisms. J Biol Chem 1995;270:15059–65.
269. Sidky YA, Borden EC. Inhibition of angiogenesis by interferons: effects on tumor- and lymphocyte-induced vascular responses. Cancer Res 1987;47:5155–61.
270. Dvorak HF, Gresser I. Microvascular injury in pathogenesis of interferon-induced necrosis of subcutaneous tumors in mice. J Natl Cancer Inst 1989;81:497–502.
271. Bouck N. Tumor angiogenesis: the role of oncogenes and tumor suppressor genes. Cancer Cells 1990;2:179–85.
272. Volpert OV, Stellmach V, Bouck N. The modulation of thrombospondin and other naturally occurring inhibitors of angiogenesis during tumor progression. Br Cancer Res Treat 1995;36:119–26.
273. Rodriguez-Manzaneque JC, Lane TF, Ortega MA, et al. Thrombospondin-1 suppresses spontaneous tumor growth and inhibits activation of matrix metalloproteinase-9 and mobilization of vascular endothelial growth factor. Proc Natl Acad Sci U S A 2001;98:12485–90.
274. Warren BA, Chauvin WJ, Philips J. Blood-borne tumor emboli and their adherence to vessel walls. In: Day SB, Myers WPL, Stansly P, editors. Cancer invasion and metastasis: biomechanisms and therapy. New York: Raven; 1977. p. 185–97.
275. Sugarbaker EV, Thornthwaite J, Ketcham AS. Inhibitory effect of a primary tumor on metastasis. In: Day SB, Myers WPL, Stansly P, editors. Progress in cancer research and therapy. New York: Raven; 1977. p. 227–40.
276. Clark WH Jr, Elder DE, Guerry DIV, et al. Model predicting survival in stage 1 melanoma based on tumor progression. J Natl Cancer Inst 1989;81:1893–904.
277. Woodruff M. The Walter Hubert Lecture. Interaction of cancer and host. Br J Cancer 1982;46:313–22.
278. Southam CM, Brunschwig A. Quantitative studies of autotransplantation of human cancer. Cancer 1961;14:971–8.
279. Koike A, Moore GE, Mendoza CB, Watne AL. Heterologous, homologous, and autologous transplantation of human tumors. Cancer 1963;16:1065–71.
280. Camphausen K, Moses MA, Beecken W-D, et al. Radiation therapy to a primary tumor accelerates metastatic growth in mice. Cancer Res 2001;61:2207–11.
281. Lange PH, Hekmat K, Bosl G, et al. Accelerated growth of testicular cancer after cytoreductive surgery. Cancer 1980;45:1498–506.
282. Marie P, Clunet J. Fréquence des métastases viscérales chez les souris cancéreuses aprés ablation chirurgicale de leur tumeur. Bull Assoc Fr Etude Cancer 1910;3:19–23.
283. Greene HSN, Harvey EK. The inhibitory influence of a transplanted hamster lymphoma on metastasis. Cancer Res 1960;20:1094–103.
284. Milas L, Hunter N, Mason K, Withers HR. Immunological resistance to pulmonary metastases in C3Hf/Bu mice bearing syngeneic fibrosarcoma of different sizes. Cancer Res 1974;34:61–71.
285. Gorelik E, Segal S, Feldman M. Growth of a local tumor exerts a specific inhibitory effect on progression of lung metastases. Int J Cancer 1978;21:617–25.
286. Bonfil RD, Ruggiero RA, Bustuoabad OD, et al. Role of concomitant resistance in the development of murine lung metastases. Int J Cancer 1988;41:415–22.
287. Simpson-Herren L, Sanford AH, Holmquist JP. Effects of surgery on the cell kinetics of residual tumor. Cancer Treat Rep 1976;60:1749–60.
288. Fisher B, Gunduz N, Saffer EA. Influence of the interval between primary tumor removal and chemotherapy on kinetics and growth of metastases. Cancer Res 1983;43:1488–92.
289. Yuhas JM, Pazmino NH. Inhibition of subcutaneously growing line 1 carcinoma due to metastatic spread. Cancer Res 1974;34:2005–10.
290. Ehrlich P, Apolant H. Beobachtungen über maligne Mäusetumoren. Berl Klin Wochenschr 1905;42:871–4.
291. Bashford EF, Murray JA, Cramer W. The natural and induced resistance of mice to the growth of cancer. Proc R Soc Lond Biol Sci 1907;79:164–87.
292. Gershon RK, Carter RL, Kondo K. Concomitant immunity in tumor-bearing hamsters. Nature 1967;213:674–6.
293. Lausch RN, Rapp F. Concomitant immunity in hamsters bearing DMBA-induced tumor transplants. Int J Cancer 1969;4:226–31.
294. Gunduz N, Fisher B, Saffer EA. Effect of surgical removal on the growth and kinetics of residual tumor. Cancer Res 1979;39:3861–5.
295. Gorelik E. Concomitant tumor immunity and the resistance to a second tumor challenge. Adv Cancer Res 1983;39:71–120.
296. Ruggiero RA, Bustuoabad OD, Bonfil RD, et al. "Concomitant immunity" in murine tumors of non-detectable immunogenicity. Br J Cancer 1985;51:37–48.
297. Himmele JC, Rabenhorst B, Werner D. Inhibition of Lewis lung tumor growth and metastasis by Ehrlich ascites tumor growing in the same host. J Cancer Res Clin Oncol 1986;111:160–5.
298. Prehn RT. The inhibition of tumor growth by tumor mass. Cancer Res 1991;51:2–4.
299. Mohr U, Althoff J, Kinzel V, et al. Melanoma regression induced by "chalone": a new tumour inhibiting principle acting in vivo. Nature 1968;220:138–9.
300. DeWys WD. Studies correlating the growth rate of a tumor and its metastases and providing evidence for tumor-related systemic growth-retarding factors. Cancer Res 1972;32:374–9.
301. O'Reilly M, Rosenthal R, Sage EH, et al. The suppression of tumor metastases by a primary tumor. Surg Forum 1993;44:474–6.
302. Stathakis P, Fitzgerald M, Matthias LJ, et al. Generation of angiostatin by reduction and proteolysis of plasmin. Catalysis by a plasmin reductase secreted by cultured cells. J Biol Chem 1997;272:20641–5.
303. Gately S, Twardowski P, Stack MS, et al. Human prostate carcinoma cells express enzymatic activity that converts human plasminogen to the angiogenesis inhibitor, angiostatin. Cancer Res 1996;56:4887–90.
304. Dong Z, Kumar R, Yang X, Fidler IJ. Macrophage-derived metalloelastase is responsible for the generation of angiostatin in Lewis lung carcinoma. Cell 1997;88:801–10.
305. O'Reilly MS, Wiederschain D, Stetler-Stevenson WG, et al. Regulation of angiostatin production by matrix metalloproteinase-2 in a model of concomitant resistance. J Biol Chem 1999;274:29568–71.
306. Lay AJ, Jiang X-M, Kisker O, et al. Phosphoglycerate kinase acts in tumour angiogenesis as a disulphide reductase. Nature 2000;408:869–73.
307. Heidtmann H-H, Nettelbeck DM, Mingels A, et al. Generation of angiostatin-like fragments from plasminogen by prostate-specific antigen. Br J Cancer 1999;81:1269–73.
308. Lu H, Dhanabal M, Volk R, et al. Kringle 5 causes cell cycle arrest and apoptosis of endothelial cells. Biochem Biophys Res Commun 1999;258:668–73.
309. Lucas R, Holmgren L, Garcia I, et al. Multiple forms of angiostatin induce apoptosis in endothelial cells. Blood 1998;92:4730–41.
310. Griscelli F, Li H, Bennaceur-Griscelli A, et al. Angiostatin gene transfer: inhibition of tumor growth in vivo by blockage of endothelial cell proliferation associated with a mitosis arrest. Proc Natl Acad Sci U S A 1998;95:6367–72.
311. Claesson-Welsh L, Welsh M, Ito N, et al. Angiostatin induces endothelial cell apoptosis and activation of focal adhesion kinase independently of the integrin-binding motif RGD. Proc Natl Acad Sci U S A 1998;95:5579–83.
312. Wu Z, O'Reilly MS, Folkman J, Shing Y. Suppression of tumor growth with recombinant murine angiostatin. Biochem Biophys Res Commun 1997;236:651–4.
313. Cao Y, Chen A, An SSA, et al. Kringle 5 of plasminogen is a novel inhibitor of endothelial cell growth. J Biol Chem 1997;272:22924–8.
314. Ji WR, Castellino FJ, Chang Y, et al. Characterization of kringle domains of angiostatin as antagonists of endothe-

lial cell migration, an important process in angiogenesis. FASEB J 1998;12:1731–8.
315. Ji WR, Barrientos LG, Llinas M, et al. Selective inhibition by kringle 5 of human plasminogen on endothelial cell migration, an important process in angiogenesis. Biochem Biophys Res Commun 1998;247:414–9.
316. Barendsz-Janson AF, Griffioen AW, Muller AD, et al. In vitro tumor angiogenesis assays: plasminogen lysine binding site 1 inhibits in vitro tumor-induced angiogenesis. J Vasc Res 1998;35:109–14.
317. Parsons-Wingerter P, Lwai B, Yang MC, et al. A novel assay of angiogenesis in the quail chorioallantoic membrane: stimulation by bFGF and inhibition by angiostatin according to fractal dimension and grid intersection. Microvasc Res 1998;55:201–14.
318. Cornelius LA, Nehring LC, Harding E, et al. Matrix metalloproteinases generate angiostatin: effects on neovascularization. J Immunol 1998;161:6845–52.
319. Falcone DJ, Khan KM, Layne T, Fernandes L. Macrophage formation of angiostatin during inflammation. A byproduct of the activation of plasminogen. J Biol Chem 1998;273:31480–5.
320. O'Mahony CA, Albo D, Tuszynski GP, Berger DH. Transforming growth factor-β1 inhibits generation of angiostatin by human pancreatic cancer cells. Surgery 1998;124:388–93.
321. O'Mahony CA, Seidel A, Albo D, et al. Angiostatin generation by human pancreatic cancer. J Surg Res 1998;77:55–8.
322. Lijnen HR, Ugwu F, Bini A, Collen D. Generation of an angiostatin-like fragment from plasminogen by stromelysin-1 (MMP-3). Biochemistry 1998;37:4699–702.
323. Patterson BC, Sang QA. Angiostatin-converting enzyme activities of human matrilysin (MMP-7) and gelatinase B/type IV collagenase (MMP-9). J Biol Chem 1997;272:28823–5.
324. Gately S, Twardowski P, Stack MS, et al. The mechanism of cancer-mediated conversion of plasminogen to the angiogenesis inhibitor angiostatin. Proc Natl Acad Sci U S A 1997;94:10868–72.
325. Cao R, Wu HL, Veitonmaki N, et al. Suppression of angiogenesis and tumor growth by the inhibitor K1-5 generated by plasmin-mediated proteolysis. Proc Natl Acad Sci U S A 1999;96:5728–33.
326. Stack S, Gately S, Bafetti LM, et al. Angiostatin inhibits endothelial and melanoma cellular invasion by blocking matrix-enhanced plasminogen activation. Biochem J 1999;340(Pt 1):77–84.
327. Kirsch M, Strasser J, Allende R, et al. Angiostatin suppresses malignant glioma growth in vivo. Cancer Res 1998;58:4654–9.
328. Sim BK, O'Reilly MS, Liang H, et al. A recombinant human angiostatin protein inhibits experimental primary and metastatic cancer. Cancer Res 1997;57:1329–34.
329. Lannutti BJ, Gately ST, Quevedo ME, et al. Human angiostatin inhibits murine hemangioendothelioma tumor growth in vivo. Cancer Res 1997;57:5277–80.
330. Joe YA, Hong YK, Chung DS, et al. Inhibition of human malignant glioma growth in vivo by human recombinant plasminogen kringles 1-3. Int J Cancer 1999;82:694–9.
331. Redlitz A, Daum G, Sage EH. Angiostatin diminishes activation of the mitogen-activated protein kinases ERK-1 and ERK-2 in human dermal microvascular endothelial cells. J Vasc Res 1999;36:28–34.
332. Luo J, Lin J, Paranya G, Bischoff J. Angiostatin upregulates E-selectin in proliferating endothelial cells. Biochem Biophys Res Commun 1998;245:906–11.
333. Tanaka T, Cao Y, Folkman J, Fine HA. Viral vector-targeted anti-angiogenic gene therapy utilizing an angiostatin complementary DNA. Cancer Res 1998;58:3362–9.
334. Moser TL, Stack MS, Asplin I, et al. Angiostatin binds ATP synthase on the surface of human endothelial cells. Proc Natl Acad Sci U S A 1999;96:2811–6.
335. Kost C, Benner K, Stockmann A, et al. Limited plasmin proteolysis of vitronectin. Characterization of the adhesion protein as morpho-regulatory and angiostatin-binding factor. Eur J Biochem 1996;236:682–8.
336. Gorski DH, Mauceri HJ, Salloum RM, et al. Potentiation of the antitumor effect of ionizing radiation by brief concomitant exposures to angiostatin. Cancer Res 1998;58:5686–9.
337. Mauceri HJ, Hanna NN, Beckett MA, et al. Combined effects of angiostatin and ionizing radiation in antitumour therapy. Nature 1998;394:287–91.
338. Tuszynski GP, Sharma MR, Rothman VL, Sharma MC. Angiostatin binds to the tyrosine kinase substrate annexin II through the lysine-binding domain in endothelial cells. Microvasc Res 2002;64:448–62.
339. Felez J, Miles LA, Fabregas P, et al. Characterization of cellular binding sites and interactive regions within reactants required for enhancement of plasminogen activation by tPA on the surface of leukocytic cells. Thromb Haemost 1996;76:577–84.
340. Kassam G, Choi KS, Ghuman J, et al. The role of annexin II tetramer in the activation of plasminogen. J Biol Chem 1998;273:4790–9.
341. Hajjar KA, Jacovina AT, Chacko J. An endothelial cell receptor for plasminogen/tissue plasminogen activator. I. Identity with annexin II. J Biol Chem 1994;269:21191–7.
342. Aitkenhead M, Wang SJ, Nakatsu MN, et al. Identification of endothelial cell genes expressed in an in vitro model of angiogenesis: induction of ESM-1, (beta)ig-h3, and NrCAM. Microvasc Res 2002;63:159–71.
343. Boyko V, Mudrak O, Svetlova M. A major cellular substrate for protein kinases, annexin II, is a DNA-binding protein. FEBS Lett 1994;345:139–42.
344. Chiang Y, Davis RG, Vishwanatha JK. Altered expression of annexin II in human B-cell lymphoma cell lines. Biochim Biophys Acta 1996;1313:295–301.
345. Jiang L, Jha V, Dhanabal M, et al. Intracellular Ca(2+) signaling in endothelial cells by the angiogenesis inhibitors endostatin and angiostatin. Am J Physiol 2001;280:C1140–50.
346. Tarui T, Miles LA, Takada Y. Specific interaction of angiostatin with integrin αvβ3 in endothelial cells. J Biol Chem 2001;276:39562–8.
347. Troyanovsky B, Levchenko T, Mansson G, et al. Angiomotin: an angiostatin binding protein that regulates endothelial cell migration and tube formation. J Cell Biol 2001;152:1247–54.
348. Bratt A, Wilson WJ, Troyanovsky B, et al. Angiomotin belongs to a novel protein family with conserved coiled-coil and PDZ binding domains. Gene 2002;298:69–77.
349. Wajih N, Sande DC. Angiostatin selectively inhibits signaling by hepatocyte growth factor in endothelial and smooth muscle cells. Blood 2002. [In press]
350. Wahl ML, Owen CS, Grant DS. Angiostatin induces intracellular acidosis and anoikis in endothelial cells at a tumor-like low pH. Endothelium 2002;9:205–16.
351. Hajitou A, Grignet C, Devy L, et al. The antitumor effect of endostatin and angiostatin is associated with a down-regulation of vascular endothelial growth factor expression in tumor cell. FASEB J 2002;16:1802–4.
352. Abad MC, Arni RK, Grella DK, et al. The x-ray crystallographic structure of the angiogenesis inhibitor angiostatin. J Mol Biol 2002;318:1009–17.
353. Moses MA, O'Reilly MS. Regulation of angiostatin mobilization by tumor-derived matrix metalloproteinases-2. Methods Mol Med 2003;74:375–90.
354. Apte RS, Niederkorn JY, Mayhew E, Alizadeh H. Angiostatin produced by certain primary uveal melanoma cell lines impedes the development of liver metastases. Arch Ophthalmol 2001;119:1805–9.
355. Verheul HMW, Hoekman K, Luykx-de Bakker S, et al. Platelet: transporter of vascular endothelial growth factor. Clin Cancer Res 1997;3(12 Pt 1):2187–90.
356. Möhle R, Green D, Moore MAS, et al. Constitutive production and thrombin-induced release of vascular endothelial growth factor by human megakaryocytes and platelets. Proc Natl Acad Sci U S A 1997;94:663–8.
357. Verheul HMW, Pinedo HM. Tumour growth: a putative role for platelets? Oncologist 1998;3:ii.
358. Pinedo HM, Verheul HMW, D'Amato RJ, Folkman J. Involvement of platelets in tumour angiogenesis? Lancet 1998;352:1775–7.
359. Verheul HM, Jorna AS, Hoekman K, et al. Vascular endothelial growth factor-stimulated endothelial cells promote adhesion and activation of platelets. Blood 2000;96:4216–21.
360. Indraccolo S, Morini M, Gola E, et al. Effects of angiostatin gene transfer on functional properties and in vivo growth of Kaposi's sarcoma cells. Cancer Res 2001;61:5441–6.
361. Gupta N, Nodzenski E, Khodarev NN, et al. Angiostatin effects on endothelial cells mediated by ceramide and RhoA. EMBO Rep 2001;2:536–40.
362. Tarui T, Majumdar M, Miles LA, et al. Plasmin-induced migration of endothelial cells. A potential target for the anti-angiogenic action of angiostatin. J Biol Chem 2002;277:33564–70.
363. Lay AJ, Jiang XM, Dal E, et al. Plasmin reduction by phosphoglycerate kinase is a thiol-independent process. J Biol Chem 2002;277:9062–8.
364. Abad MC, Geiger J. Crystallization and preliminary x-ray diffraction studies of human angiostatin. Acta Crystallogr D Biol Crystallogr 2002;58(Pt 3):513–4.
365. Indraccolo S, Gola E, Rosato A, et al. Differential effects of angiostatin, endostatin and interferon-α(1) gene transfer on in vivo growth of human breast cancer cells. Gene Ther 2002;9:867–78.
366. Gyorffy S, Palmer K, Gauldie J. Adenoviral vector expressing murine angiostatin inhibits a model of breast cancer metastatic growth in the lungs of mice. Am J Pathol 2001;159:1137–47.
367. Sacco MG, Cato EM, Ceruti R, et al. Systemic gene therapy with anti-angiogenic factors inhibits spontaneous breast tumor growth and metastasis in MMTVneu transgenic mice. Gene Ther 2001;8:67–70.
368. Fukumuri T, Nishitani M, Naroda T, et al. Expression of angiostatin cDNA in a murine renal cell carcinoma suppresses tumor growth in vivo. Urology 2002;59:973–7.
369. Ma HI, Lin SZ, Chiang YH, et al. Intratumoral gene therapy of malignant brain tumor in a rat model with angiostatin delivered by adeno-associated viral (AAV) vector. Gene Ther 2002;9:2–11.
370. Ma HI, Guo P, Li J, et al. Suppression of intracranial human glioma growth after intramuscular administration of an adeno-associated viral vector expressing angiostatin. Cancer Res 2002;62:756–63.
371. Zhang X, Wu J, Fei Z, et al. Angiostatin K(103) gene for treatment of human gliomas: an experimental study. Chin Med J 2000;113:996–1001.
372. Griscelli F, Li H, Cheong C, et al. Combined effects of radiotherapy and angiostatin gene therapy in glioma tumor model. Proc Natl Acad Sci U S A 2000;97:6698–703.
373. Rodolfo M, Cato EM, Soldati S, et al. Growth of human melanoma xenografts is suppressed by systemic angiostatin gene therapy. Cancer Gene Ther 2001;8:491–6.
374. Matsumoto G, Ohmi Y, Shindo J. Angiostatin gene therapy inhibits the growth of murine squamous cell carcinoma in vivo. Oral Oncol 2001;37:368–78.
375. Scappaticci FA, Smith R, Pathak A, et al. Combination angiostatin and endostatin gene transfer induces synergistic antiangiogenic activity in vitro and antitumor efficacy in leukemia and solid tumors in mice. Mol Ther 2001;3:186–96.
376. Hampl M, Tanaka T, Albert PS, et al. Therapeutic effects of viral vector-mediated antiangiogenic gene transfer in malignant ascites. Hum Gene Ther 2001;12:1713–29.
377. Andrawiss M, Maron A, Beltran W, et al. Adeno-mediated gene transfer in canine eyes: a preclinical study for gene therapy of human uveal melanoma. J Gene Med 2001;3:228–39.
378. Shichinohe T, Bochner BH, Mizutani K, et al. Development of lentiviral vectors for antiangiogenic gene delivery. Cancer Gene Ther 2001;8:879–89.
379. Kim JM, Ho SH, Park EJ, et al. Angiostatin gene transfer as an effective treatment strategy in murine collagen-induced arthritis. Arthritis Rheum 2002;46:793–801.
380. Raisler BJ, Berns KI, Grant MI, et al. Adeno-associated virus type-2 expression of pigmented epithelium-derived factor or kringles 1-3 of angiostatin reduce retinal neovascularization. Proc Natl Acad Sci U S A 2002;99:8909–14.
381. Lai CC, Wu WC, Chen SL, et al. Suppression of choroidal neovascularization by adeno-associated virus vector expressing angiostatin. Invest Ophthalmol Vis Sci 2001;42:2401–7.
382. Dabrosin C, Gyorffy S, Margetts P, et al. Therapeutic effect of angiostatin gene transfer in a murine model of endometriosis. Am J Pathol 2002;161:909–18.
383. Mauceri HJ, Seetharam S, Beckett MA, et al. Angiostatin potentiates cyclophosphamide treatment of metastatic disease. Cancer Chemother Pharmacol 2002;50:412–8.
384. Sun X, Kanwar JR, Leung E, et al. Angiostatin enhances B7.1-mediated cancer immunotherapy independently effects on vascular endothelial growth factor expression. Cancer Gene Ther 2001;8:719–27.
385. te Velde EA, Vogten JM, Gebbink MF, et al. Enhanced antitumour efficacy by combining conventional chemotherapy with angiostatin or endostatin in a liver metastasis model. Br J Surg 2002 89:1302–9.
386. Scappaticci FA, Contreras A, Smith R, et al. Statin-AE: a novel angiostatin-endostatin fusion protein with enhanced antiangiogenic and antitumor activity. Angiogenesis 2001;4:263–8.
387. Matsunaga T, Weihrauch DW, Moniz MC, et al. Angiostatin inhibits coronary angiogenesis during impaired production of nitric oxide. Circulation 2002;105:2185–91.

388. Dong Z, Yoneda J, Kumar R, Fidler IJ. Angiostatin-mediated suppression of cancer metastases by primary neoplasms engineered to produce granulocyte/macrophage colony-stimulating factor. J Exp Med 1998;188:755–63.
389. Ambati BK, Joussen AM, Ambati J, et al. Angiostatin inhibits and regresses corneal neovascularization. Arch Ophthalmol 2002;120:1063–8.
390. Hazzard TM, Rohan RM, Molskness TA, et al. Injection of antiangiogenic agents into the macaque preovulatory follicle: disruption of corpus luteum development and function. Endocrine 2002;17:199–206.
391. Drixler TA, Rinks IH, Ritchie ED, et al. Angiostatin inhibits pathological but not physiological retinal angiogenesis. Invest Ophthalmol Vis Sci 2001;42:3325–30.
392. Berns KI, Meneses P, Duvoisin R, et al. Use of recombinant angiostatin to prevent retinal neovascularization. Trans Am Clin Climatol Assoc 2001;112:68–75.
393. Kwon M, Yoon CS, Fitzpatrick S, et al. p22 is a novel plasminogen fragment with antiangiogenic activity. Biochemistry 2001;40:13246–53.
394. Oh SP, Kamagata Y, Muragaki Y, et al. Isolation and sequencing of cDNAs for proteins with multiple domains of Gly-Xaa-Yaa repeats identify a distinct family of collagenous proteins. Proc Natl Acad Sci U S A 1994;91:4229–33.
395. Rehn M, Pihlajaniemi T. Alpha1(XVIII), a collagen chain with frequent interruptions in the collagenous sequence, a distinct tissue distribution, and homology with type XV collagen. Proc Natl Acad Sci U S A 1994;91:4234–8.
396. Carmeliet P, Jain RK. Angiogenesis in cancer and other diseases. Nature 2000;407:249–57.
397. Ortega N, Werb Z. New functional roles for non-collagenous domains of basement membrane collagens. J Cell Sci 2002;115:4201–14.
398. Obeso J, Weber J, Auerbach R. A hemangioendothelioma-derived cell line: its use as a model for the study of endothelial cell biology. Lab Invest 1990;63:259–69.
399. Hohenester E, Sasaki T, Olsen BR, Timpl R. Crystal structure of the angiogenesis inhibitor endostatin at 1.5. A resolution. EMBO J 1998;17:1656–64.
400. Ding Y-H, Javaherian K, Lo K-M, et al. Zinc-dependent dimers observed in crystals of human endostatin. Proc Natl Acad Sci U S A 1998;95:10443–8.
401. Wen W, Moses MA, Wiederschain D, et al. The generation of endostatin is mediated by elastase. Cancer Res 1999;59:6052–6.
402. Felbor U, Dreier L, Bryant RAR, et al. Secreted cathepsin L generates endostatin from collagen XVIII. EMBO J 2000;19:1187–94.
403. Sasaki T, Hohenester E, Timpl R. Structure and function of collagen-derived endostatin inhibitors of angiogenesis. IUBMB Life 2002;53:77–84.
404. Miosge N, Sasaki T, Timpl R. Angiogenesis inhibitor endostatin is a distinct component of elastic fibers in vessel walls. FASEB J 1999;13:1743–50.
404a. Tjin Tham Sjin RM, Satchi-Fainaro R, Birsner AE, et al. A 27-amino-acid synthetic peptide corresponding to the NH2-terminal zinc-binding domain of endostatin is responsible for its antitumor activity. Cancer Res 2005;65:3656–63.
405. Sasaki T, Larsson H, Tisi D, et al. Endostatins derived from collagens XV and XVIII differ in structural and binding properties, tissue distribution and anti-angiogenic activity. J Mol Biol 2000;301:1179–90.
406. Sasaki T, Larsson H, Kreuger J, et al. Structural basis and potential role of heparin/heparan sulfate binding to the angiogenesis inhibitor endostatin. EMBO J 1999;18:6240–8.
407. Kasai S, Nagasawa H, Shimamura M, et al. Design and synthesis of antiangiogenic/heparin-binding arginine dendrimer mimicking the surface of endostatin. Bioorg Med Chem Lett 2002;12:951–4.
408. Boehm T, O'Reilly MS, Keough K, et al. Zinc-binding of endostatin is essential for its antiangiogenic activity. Biochem Biophys Res Commun 1998;252:190–4.
409. Sim BKL, Fogler WE, Zhou XH, et al. Zinc ligand-disrupted recombinant human endostatin: potent inhibition of tumor growth, safety and pharmacokinetic profile. Angiogenesis 1999;3:41–51.
410. Marneros AG, Olsen BR. The role of collagen-derived proteolytic fragments in angiogenesis. Matrix Biol 2001;20:337–45.
411. Ackley BD, Crew JR, Elamaa H, et al. The NC1/endostatin domain of Caenorhabditis elegans type XVIII collagen affects cell migration and axon guidance. J Cell Biol 2001;152:1219–32.
412. Gagnon ML, Bielenberg DR, Gechtman Z, et al. Identification of a natural soluble neuropilin-1 that binds vascular endothelial growth factor: in vivo expression and antitumor activity. Proc Natl Acad Sci U S A 2000;97:2573–8.
413. Miao H-Q, Lee P, Lin H, et al. Neuropilin-1 expression by tumor cells promotes tumor angiogenesis and progression. FASEB J 2000;14:2532–9.
414. Shin D, Garcia-Cardena G, Hayashi S, et al. Expression of ephrinB2 identifies a stable genetic difference between arterial and venous vascular smooth muscle as well as endothelial cells, and marks subsets of microvessels at sites of adult neovascularization. Dev Biol 2001;230:139–50.
415. Wang HU, Chen ZF, Anderson DJ. Molecular distinction and angiogenic interaction between embryonic arteries and veins revealed by ephrin-b2 and its receptor Eph-B4. Cell 1998;93:741–53.
416. Kim YM, Hwang S, Kim YM, et al. Endostatin blocks vascular endothelial growth factor-mediated signaling via direct interaction with KDR/Flk-1. J Biol Chem 2002;277:27872–9.
417. Dixelius J, Larsson H, Sasaki T, et al. Endostatin-induced tyrosine kinase signaling through the Shb adaptor protein regulates endothelial cell apoptosis. Blood 2000;95:3403–11.
418. Chang Z, Choon A, Friedl A. Endostatin binds to blood vessels in situ independent of heparan sulfate and does not compete for fibroblast growth factor-2 binding. Am J Pathol 1999;155:71–6.
419. Seghezzi G, Patel S, Ren CJ, et al. Fibroblast growth factor-2 (FGF-2) induces vascular endothelial growth factor (VEGF) expression in the endothelial cells of forming capillaries: an autocrine mechanism contributing to angiogenesis. J Cell Biol 1998;141:1659–73.
420. Shuster CB, Herman IM. The mechanics of vascular cell motility. Microcirculation 1998;5:239–57.
421. Dixelius J, Cross M, Matsumoto T, et al. Endostatin regulates endothelial cell adhesion and cytoskeletal organization. Cancer Res 2002;62:1944–7.
422. Ergun S, Kilic N, Wurmbach JH, et al. Endostatin inhibits angiogenesis by stabilization of newly formed endothelial tubes. Angiogenesis 2001;4:193–206.
423. Kuo CJ, LaMontagne KR Jr, Garcia-Cardena G, et al. Oligomerization-dependent regulation of motility and morphogenesis by the collagen XVIII NC1/endostatin domain. J Cell Biol 2001;152:1233–46.
424. Wickström S, Veikkola T, Rehn M, et al. Endostatin-induced modulation of plasminogen activation with concomitant loss of focal adhesions and actin stress fibers in cultured human endothelial cells. Cancer Res 2001;61:6511–6.
425. Kim Y-M, Jang J-W, Lee O-H, et al. Endostatin inhibits endothelial and tumor cellular invasion by blocking the activation and catalytic activity of matrix metalloproteinases 2. Cancer Res 2000;60:5410–3.
426. Lee SJ, Jang JW, Kim YM, et al. Endostatin binds to the catalytic domain of matrix metalloproteinase-2. FEBS Lett 2002;519:147–52.
427. Itoh T, Tanioka M, Yoshida H, et al. Reduced angiogenesis and tumor progression in gelatinase a-deficient mice. Cancer Res 1998;58:1048–51.
428. Rehn M, Veikkola T, Kukk-Valdre E, et al. Interaction of endostatin with integrins implicated in angiogenesis. Proc Natl Acad Sci U S A 2001;98:1024–9.
429. MacDonald NJ, Shivers WY, Narum DL, et al. Endostatin binds tropomyosin. A potential modulator of the antitumor activity of endostatin. J Biol Chem 2001;276:25190–6.
430. Karumanchi SA, Jha V, Ramchandran R, et al. Cell surface glypicans are low-affinity endostatin receptors. Mol Cell 2001;7:811–22.
431. Hanai J, Dhanabal M, Karumanchi SA, et al. Endostatin causes G1 arrest of endothelial cells through inhibition of cyclin D1. J Biol Chem 2002;277:16464–9.
432. Dhanabal M, Ramchandran R, Waterman MJF, et al. Endostatin induces endothelial cell apoptosis. J Biol Chem 1999;274:11721–6.
433. Xu R, Yao ZY, Xin L, et al. NC1 domain of human type VIII collagen (alpha 1) inhibits bovine aortic endothelial cell proliferation and causes cell apoptosis. Biochem Biophys Res Commun 2001;289:264–8.
434. Urbich C, Reissner A, Chavakis E, et al. Dephosphorylation of endothelial nitric oxide synthase contributes to the anti-angiogenic effects of endostatin. FASEB J 2002;16:706–8.
435. Morales-Ruiz M, Lee M-J, Zollner S, et al. Sphingosine 1-phosphate activates akt, nitric oxide production, and chemotaxis through a Gi protein/phosphoinositide 3-kinase pathway in endothelial cells. J Biol Chem 2001;276:19672–7.
436. Gallo O, Masini E, Morbidelli L, et al. Role of nitric oxide in angiogenesis and tumor progression in head and neck cancer. J Natl Cancer Inst 1998;90:587–96.
437. Wu P, Yonekura H, Li H, et al. Hypoxia down-regulates endostatin production by human microvascular endothelial cells and pericytes. Biochem Biophys Res Commun 2001;288:1149–54.
438. Sertie AL, Sossi V, Camargo AA, et al. Collagen XVIII, containing an endogenous inhibitor of angiogenesis and tumor growth, plays a critical role in the maintenance of retinal structure and in neural tube closure (Knobloch syndrome). Hum Mol Genet 2000;9:2051–8.
439. Suzuki OT, Sertie AL, Der Kaloustian VM, et al. Molecular analysis of collagen XVIII reveals novel mutations, presence of a third isoform, and possible genetic heterogeneity in Knobloch syndrome. Am J Hum Genet 2002;71:1320-1-9.
440. Fukai N, Eklund L, Marneros AG, et al. Lack of collagen XVIII/endostatin results in eye abnormalities. EMBO J 2002;21:1535–44.
441. Folkman J, Browder T, Palmblad J. Angiogenesis research: guidelines for translation to clinical application. Thromb Haemost 2001;86:23–33.
442. Browder T, Folkman J, Pirie-Shepherd S. The hemostatic system as a regulator of angiogenesis. J Biol Chem 2000;275:1521–4.
443. Ma L, Hollenberg MD, Wallace JL. Thrombin-induced platelet endostatin release is blocked by a proteinase activated receptor-4 (PAR4) antagonist. Br J Pharmacol 2001;134:701–4.
444. Tepper OM, Murayama T, Kearney M, et al. Therapeutic neovascularization as a novel approach to thrombus recanalization and resolution [abstract]. Circulation 2002;106:II-65.
445. Ma L, Elliott SN, Cirino G, et al. Platelets modulate gastric ulcer healing: role of endostatin and vascular endothelial growth factor release. Proc Natl Acad Sci U S A 2001;98:6470–5.
445a. Klement G, Kikuchi L, Kieran M, et al. Early tumor detection using platelet uptake of angiogenesis regulators. In: "American Society of Hematology Annual Meeting" Blood, San Diego, California, 2004.
446. Ma L, del Soldato P, Wallace JL. Divergent effects of new cyclooxygenase inhibitors on gastric ulcer healing: shifting the angiogenic balance. Proc Natl Acad Sci U S A 2002;99:13243–7.
447. Strik HM, Schluesener HJ, Seid K, et al. Localization of endostatin in rat and human gliomas. Cancer 2001;91:10130–9.
448. Black WR, Agner RC. Tumour regression after endostatin therapy. Nature 1998;391:459.
449. Perletti G, Concari P, Giardini R, et al. Antitumor activity of endostatin against carcinogen-induced rat primary mammary tumors. Cancer Res 2000;60:1793–6.
450. Huang X, Wong MK, Zhao Q, et al. Soluble recombinant endostatin purified from *Escherichia coli*: antiangiogenic activity and antitumor effect. Cancer Res 2001;61:478–81.
451. He ZY, Chen ZY, Qiu CP, et al. Cloning, expression and tumor suppression of human endostatin. Sheng Wu Hua Xue Yu Sheng Wu Wu Li Xue Bao 2000;32:333–6.
452. Liu DL, Wen JX, Tong WC, Ben LH. Inhibition of lung adenocarcinoma LA795 in mice by recombinant human endostatin. Di Yi Jun Yi Da Xue Xue Bao 2001;21:917–9.
453. Ye C, Feng C, Wang S, et al. Antiangiogenic and antitumor effects of endostatin of follicular thyroid carcinoma. Endocrinology 2002;143:3522–8.
454. Solaun MS, Mendoza L, De Luca M, et al. Endostatin inhibits murine colon carcinoma sinusoidal-type metastases by preferential targeting of hepatic sinusoidal endothelium. Hepatology 2002;35:1104–16.
455. Iversen PO, Sorensen DR, Benestad HB. Inhibitors of angiogenesis selectively reduce the malignant cell load in rodent models of human myeloid leukemias. Leukemia 2002;16:376–81.
456. Boehle AS, Kurdow R, Schulze M, et al. Human endostatin inhibits growth of human non–small-cell lung cancer in a murine xenotransplant model. Int J Cancer 2001;94:420–8.
457. Kuroiwa M, Ikeda H, Hongo T, et al. Effects of recombinant human endostatin on a human neuroblastoma xenograft. Int J Mol Med 2001;8:391–6.
458. Calvo A, Yokoyama Y, Smith LE, et al. Inhibition of the mammary carcinoma angiogenic switch in C3(1)/SV40

transgenic mice by a mutated form of human endostatin. Int J Cancer 2002;101:224–34.
459. Yokoyama Y, Green JE, Sukhatme VP, Ramakrishnan S. Effect of endostatin on spontaneous tumorigenesis of mammary adenocarcinoma in a transgenic mouse model. Cancer Res 2000;60:4362–5.
460. Bergers G, Javaherian K, Lo KM, et al. Effects of angiogenesis inhibitors on multistage carcinogenesis in mice. Science 1999;284:808–12.
461. Sorensen DR, Read TA, Porwol T, et al. Endostatin reduces vascularization, blood flow, and growth in a rat gliosarcoma. Neurooncology 2002;4:1–8.
461a. Yamaguchi N, Anand-Apte B, Lee M, et al. Endostatin inhibits VEGF-induced endothelial cell migration and tumor growth independently of zinc binding. EMBO J 1999;18:4414–23.
462. Yokoyama Y, Dhanabal M, Griffioen AW, et al. Synergy between angiostatin and endostatin: inhibition of ovarian cancer growth. Cancer Res 2000;60:2190–6.
463. Hanna NN, Seetharam S, Mauceri HJ, et al. Antitumor interaction of short-course endostatin and ionizing radiation. Cancer J 2000;6:287–93.
464. Davidoff AM, Leary MA, Ng CY, et al. Autocrine expression of both endostatin and green fluorescent protein provides a synergistic antitumor effect in a murine neuroblastoma model. Cancer Gene Ther 2001;8:537–45.
465. Sorenson Dr, Leirdal M, Iverson PO, Sioud M. Combination of endostatin and a protein kinase C α DNA enzyme improves the survival of rats with malignant glioma. Neoplasia 2002;4:474–9.
466. Folkman J. Angiogenesis in cancer therapy-endostatin and its mechanisms of action. Exp Cell Res 2005.
467. Feldman AL, Alexander HR, Hewitt SM, et al. Effect of retroviral endostatin gene transfer on subcutaneous and intraperitoneal growth of murine tumors. J Natl Cancer Inst 2001;93:1014–20.
468. Wang X, Liu F, Li X, et al. Inhibitory effect of endostatin mediated by retroviral gene transfer on human liver carcinoma SMMC7721 in vivo. Zhonghua Wai Ke Za Zhi 2002;40:692–5.
469. Cichon T, Jamrozy L, Glogowska J, et al. Electrotransfer of gene encoding endostatin into normal and neoplastic mouse tissues: inhibition of primary tumor growth and metastatic spread. Cancer Gene Ther 2002;9:771–7.
470. Szary J, Szala S. Intra-tumoral administration of naked plasmid DNA encoding mouse endostatin inhibits renal carcinoma growth. Int J Cancer 2001;91:835–9.
471. Yamanaka R, Zullo SA, Ramsey J, et al. Induction of therapeutic antitumor antiangiogenesis by intratumoral injection of genetically engineered endostatin-producing Semliki Forest virus. Cancer Gene Ther 2001;8:796–802.
472. Peroulis I, Jonas N, Saleh M. Antiangiogenic activity of endostatin inhibits C6 glioma growth. Int J Cancer 2002;97:839–45.
473. Read TA, Farhadi M, Bjerkvig R, et al. Intravital microscopy reveals novel antivascular and antitumor effects of endostatin delivered locally by alginate-encapsulated cells. Cancer Res 2001;61:6830–7.
474. Read TA, Sorensen DR, Mahesparan R, et al. Local endostatin treatment of gliomas administered by microencapsulated producer cells. Nat Biotechnol 2001;19:29–34.
475. Joki T, Machluf M, Atala A, et al. Continuous release of endostatin from microencapsulated engineered cells for tumor therapy. Nat Biotechnol 2001;19:35–9.
476. Jin X, Bookstein R, Wills K, et al. Evaluation of endostatin antiangiogenesis gene therapy in vitro and in vivo. Cancer Gene Ther 2001;8:982–9.
477. Ding I, Sun JZ, Fenton B, et al. Intratumoral administration of endostatin plasmid inhibits vascular growth and perfusion in MCa-4 murine mammary carcinomas. Cancer Res 2001;61:526–31.
478. Feldman AL, Restifo NP, Alexander HR, et al. Antiangiogenic gene therapy of cancer utilizing a recombinant adenovirus to elevate systemic endostatin levels in mice. Cancer Res 2000;60:1503–6.
478a. Sauter BV, Martinet O, Zhang WJ, et al. Adenovirus-mediated gene transfer of endostatin in vivo results in high level expression and inhibition of tumor growth and metastases. Proc Natl Acad Sci U S A 2000;97:4802–7.
479. Shi W, Teschendorf C, Muzyczka N, Siemann DW. Adeno-associated virus-mediated gene transfer of endostatin inhibits angiogenesis and tumor growth in vivo. Cancer Gene Ther 2002;9:513–21.
480. Wen XY, Bai Y, Stewart AK. Adenovirus-mediated human endostatin gene delivery demonstrates strain-specific antitumor activity and acute dose-dependent toxicity in mice. Hum Gene Ther 2001;12:347–58.
481. Blezinger P, Wang J, Gondo M, et al. Systemic inhibition of tumor growth and tumor metastases by intramuscular administration of the endostatin gene therapy. Nat Biotechnol 1999;17:343–8.
482. Lefesvre P, Attema J, van Bekkum D. Adenoviral gene transfer of angiostatic ATF-BPTI inhibits tumour growth. BMC Cancer 2002;2:17.
483. Eisterer W, Jiang X, Bachelot T, et al. Unfulfilled promise of endostatin in a gene therapy-xenotransplant model of human acute lymphocytic leukemia. Mol Ther 2002;5:352–9.
484. Pawliuk R, Bachelot T, Zurkiya O, et al. Continuous intravascular secretion of endostatin in mice from transduced hematopoietic stem cells. Mol Ther 2002;5:345–51.
484a. Bachelot T, Pawliuk R, Treilleux I, et al. Retrovirus-mediated gene transfer of an angiostatin-endostatin fusion protein with enhanced anti-tumor properties in vivo [abstract]. Proc Am Assoc Cancer Res 1998;39:271–2.
485. Kuo CJ, Farnebo F, Yu EY, et al. Comparative evaluation of the antitumor activity of antiangiogenic proteins delivered by gene transfer. Proc Natl Acad Sci U S A 2001;98:4605–10.
485a. Slaton JW, Perotte P, Inoue K, et al. Interferon-α-mediated down-regulation of angiogenesis-related genes and therapy of bladder cancer are dependent on optimization of biological dose and schedule. Clin Cancer Res 1999;5:2726–34.
485b. Massague J. TGF-B signaling transduction. Annu Rev Biochem 1998;67:753–91.
486. Berger AC, Feldman AL, Gnant MF, et al. The angiogenesis inhibitor, endostatin, does not affect murine cutaneous wound healing. J Surg Res 2000;91:26–31.
487. Xu R, Du P, Fan JJ, et al. High-level expression and secretion of recombinant mouse endostatin by Escherichia coli. Protein Expr Purif 2002;24:453–9.
488. Park JH, Chang KH, Lee JM, et al. Optimal production and in vitro activity of recombinant endostatin from stably transformed Drosophila melanogaster S2 cells. In Vitro Cell Dev Biol Anim 2001;37:5–9.
489. Trinh L, Noronha SB, Fannon M, Shiloach J. Recovery of mouse endostatin produced by *Pichia pastoris* using expanded bed adsorption. Bioseparation 2000;9:223–30.
490. Xia H, Zhang L, Wen JX, Tong WC. Expression and purification of human endostatin in *Pichia pastoris* and its inhibition on the growth of mouse pulmonary adenocarcinoma cell line LA795. Di Yi Jun Yi Da Xue Xue Bao 2002;22:393–6.
491. Rokstad AM, Holtan S, Strand B, et al. Microencapsulation of cells producing therapeutic proteins: optimizing cell growth and secretion. Cell Transplant 2002;11:313–24.
492. Zorick TS, Mustacchi Z, Bando SY, et al. High serum endostatin levels in Down syndrome: implications for improved treatment and prevention of solid tumours. Eur J Hum Genet 2001;9:811–4.
493. Yang Q, Rasmussen SA, Friedman JM. Mortality associated with Down's syndrome in the USA from 1983 to 1997: a population-based study. Lancet 2002;359:1019–25.
494. Iughetti P, Suzuki O, Godoi PH, et al. A polymorphism in endostatin, an angiogenesis inhibitor, predisposes for the development of prostatic adenocarcinoma. Cancer Res 2001;61:7375–8.
495. Feldman AL, Pak H, Yang JC, et al. Serum endostatin levels are elevated in patients with soft tissue sarcoma. Cancer 2001;91:1525–9.
496. Feldman AL, Alexander HR Jr, Yang JC, et al. Prospective analysis of circulating endostatin levels in patients with renal cell carcinoma. Cancer 2002;95:1637–43.
497. Herbst RS, Hess KR, Tran HT, et al. Phase I study of recombinant human endostatin in patients with advanced solid tumors. J Clin Oncol 2002;20:3792–803.
498. Madri JA. Extracellular matrix modulation of vascular cell behaviour. Transpl Immunol 1997;5:179–83.
499. Furcht LT. Critical factors controlling angiogenesis: cell products, cell matrix, and growth factors. Lab Invest 1986;55:505–9.
500. Kalluri R. Discovery of type IV collagen non-collagenous domains as novel integrin ligands and endogenous inhibitors of angiogenesis. In: Cold Spring Harbor 67th Quantitative Symposium. New York; 2002. [In press]
501. Senger DR, Claffey KP, Benes JE, et al. Angiogenesis promoted by vascular endothelial growth factor: regulation through alpha1beta1 and α2β1-integrins. Proc Natl Acad Sci U S A 1997;94:13612–7.
502. Pozzi A, LeVine WF, Gardner HA. Low plasma levels of matrix metalloproteinase 9 permit increased tumor angiogenesis. Oncogene 2002;21:272–81.
503. Pozzi A, Moberg PE, Miles LA, et al. Elevated matrix metalloprotease and angiostatin levels in integrin alpha 1 knockout mice cause reduced tumor vascularization. Proc Natl Acad Sci U S A 2000;97:2202–27.
504. Petitclerc E, Boutaud A, Prestayko A, et al. New functions for non-collagenous domains of human collagen type IV. Novel integrin ligands inhibiting angiogenesis and tumor growth in vivo. J Biol Chem 2000;275:8051–61.
505. Maeshima Y, Colorado PC, Kalluri R. Two RGD-independent αvβ3-integrin binding sites on tumstatin regulate distinct anti-tumor properties. J Biol Chem 2000;275:23745–50.
506. Maeshima Y, Yerramalla UL, Dhanabal M, et al. Extracellular matrix-derived peptide binds to αvβ3-integrin and inhibits angiogenesis. J Biol Chem 2001;276:31959–68.
507. Maeshima Y, Sudhakar A, Lively JC, et al. Tumstatin, an endothelial cell-specific inhibitor of protein synthesis. Science 2002;295:140–3.
508. Cheresh DA, Stupack DG. Integrin-mediated death: an explanation of the integrin-knockout phenotype? Nat Med 2002;8:193–4.
509. Hynes RO. A reevaluation of integrins as regulators of angiogenesis. Nat Med 2002;8:918–21.
510. Stupack DG, Cheresh DA. ECM remodeling regulates angiogenesis: endothelial integrins look for new ligands. Sci STKE 2002;E7.
511. Stupack DG, Puente XS, Boutsaboualoy S, et al. Apoptosis of adherent cells by recruitment of caspase-8 to unligated integrins. J Cell Biol 2001;155:459–70.
512. Kisker O, Onizuka S, Banyard J, et al. Generation of multiple angiogenesis inhibitors by human pancreatic cancer. Cancer Res 2001;61:7298–304.
512a. Hamano Y, Kalluri R. Tumstatin, the NC1 domain of alpha3 chain of type IV collagen, is an endogenous inhibitor of pathological angiogenesis and suppresses tumor growth. Biochem Biophys Res Commun 2005;333:292–8.
513. Moses MA, Wiederschain D, Wu I, et al. Troponin I is present in human cartilage and inhibits angiogenesis. Proc Natl Acad Sci U S A 1999;96:2645–50.
514. Maione TE, Sharpe RJ. Development of angiogenesis inhibitors for clinical applications. Trends Pharmacol Sci 1990;11:457–61.
515. Homandberg GA, Williams JE, Grant D, et al. Heparin-binding fragments of fibronectin are potent inhibitors of endothelial cell growth. Am J Pathol 1985;120:327–32.
516. Funk SE, Sage EH. Differential effects of SPARC and cationic SPARC peptides on DNA synthesis by endothelial cells and fibroblasts. J Cell Physiol 1993;154:53–63.
517. Good DJ, Polverini PJ, Rastinejad F, et al. A tumor suppressor-dependent inhibitor of angiogenesis is immunologically and functionally indistinguishable from a fragment of thrombospondin. Proc Natl Acad Sci U S A 1990;87:6624–8.
518. Tolsma SS, Volpert OV, Good DJ, et al. Peptides derived from two separate domains of the matrix protein thrombospondin-1 have antiangiogenic activity. J Cell Biol 1993;122:497–511.
519. Murphy-Ullrich JE, Schultz-Cherry S, Hook M. Transforming growth factor-B complexes with thrombospondin. Mol Biol Cell 1992;3:181–8.
520. Sage EH, Bornstein P. Approaches for investigating matrix components produced by endothelial cells: type VIII collagen, SPARC, and thrombospondin. In: Haralson MA, Hassell JR, editors. Extracellular matrix molecules: a practical approach. Oxford: Oxford University Press; 1995. p. 131–60.
521. Tolsma SS, Stack MS, Bouck N. Lumen formation and other angiogenic activities of cultured capillary endothelial cells are inhibited by thrombospondin-1. Microvasc Res 1997;54:13–26.
522. Liotta LA, Steeg PS, Stetler-Stevenson WG. Cancer metastasis and angiogenesis: an imbalance of positive and negative regulation. Cell 1991;64:327–36.
523. Spurbeck WW, Ng CY, Strom TS, et al. Enforced expression of tissue inhibitor of matrix metalloproteinases-3 affects functional capillary morphogenesis and inhibits tumor growth in a murine tumor model. Blood 2002;100:3361–8.
524. Chang C, Werb Z. The many faces of metalloproteases: cell growth, invasion, angiogenesis and metastasis. Trends Cell Biol 2001;11:S37–43.
525. Fassina G, Ferrari N, Brigati C, et al. Tissue inhibitors of metalloproteases: regulation and biological activities. Clin Exp Metastasis 2000;18:111–20.
526. Angiolillo AL, Sgadari C, Taub DD, et al. Human interferon-inducible protein 10 is a potent inhibitor of angiogenesis in vivo. J Exp Med 1995;182:155–62.
527. Colman RW, Pixley RA, Najamunnisa S, et al. Binding of high molecular weight kininogen to human endothelial cells is mediated via a site within domains 2 and 3 of the urokinase receptor. J Clin Invest 1997;100:1481–7.

528. Volpert OV, Pili R, Sidker HA, et al. Id1 regulates angiogenesis through transcriptional repression of thrombospondin-1. Cancer Cell 2002;2:473–83.
529. Brantley DM, Cheng N, Thompson EJ, et al. Soluble Eph A receptors inhibit tumor angiogenesis and progression in vivo. Oncogene 2002;21:7011–26.
530. Sarma V, Wolf FW, Marks RM, et al. Cloning of a novel tumor necrosis factor-α-inducible primary response gene that is differentially expressed in development and capillary tube-like formation in vitro. J Immunol 1992;148:3303–12.
531. Daniel TO, Stein E, Cerretti DP, et al. ELK and LERK-2 in developing kidney and microvascular endothelial assembly. Kidney Int 1996;57:S73–81.
532. Wang CY, Mayo MW, Baldwin AS Jr. TNF- and cancer therapy-induced apoptosis: potentiation by inhibition of NF-kappaB. Science 1996;274:784–7.
533. Beg AA, Baltimore D. An essential role for NF-kappaB in preventing TNF-α-induced cell death. Science 1996;274:782–4.
534. Buettner R, Mora LB, Jove R. Activated STAT signaling in human tumors provides novel molecular targets for therapeutic intervention. Clin Cancer Res 2002;8:945–54.
535. Carmeliet P. Biomedicine. Clotting factors build blood vessels. Science 2001;293:1602–4.
536. Tsopanoglou NE, Maragoudakis ME. On the mechanism of thrombin-induced angiogenesis. Potentiation of vascular endothelial growth factor activity on endothelial cells by up-regulation of its receptors. J Biol Chem 1999;274:23969–76.
537. Zucker S, Mirza H, Conner CE, et al. Vascular endothelial growth factor induces tissue factor and matrix metalloproteinases production in endothelial cells: conversion of prothrombin to thrombin results in progelatinase A activation and cell proliferation. Int J Cancer 1998;75:780–6.
538. Sharrocks AD. The ETS-domain transcription factor family. Nat Rev Mol Cell Biol 2001;2:827–37.
539. Chen Z, Fisher RJ, Riggs CW, et al. Inhibition of vascular endothelial growth factor-induced endothelial cell migration by ETS1 antisense oligonucleotides. Cancer Res 1997;57:2013–9.
540. Nakano T, Abe M, Tanaka K, et al. Angiogenesis inhibition by transdominant mutant Ets-1. J Cell Physiol 2000;184:255–62.
541. Oda N, Abe M, Sato Y. ETS-1 converts endothelial cells to the angiogenic phenotype by inducing the expression of matrix metalloproteinases and integrin beta 3. J Cell Physiol 1999;178:121–32.
542. Iwasaka C, Tanaka K, Abe M, Sato Y. Ets-1 regulates angiogenesis by inducing the expression of urokinase-type plasminogen activator and matrix metalloproteinases-1 and the migration of vascular endothelial cells. J Cell Physiol 1996;269:522–31.
543. Griffith ED, Su Z, Turk BE, et al. Methionine aminopeptidase (type 2) is the common target for angiogenesis inhibitors AGM-1470 and ovalicin. Chem Biol 1997;4:461–71.
544. Sin N, Meng L, Want MQW, et al. The anti-angiogenic agent fumagillin covalently binds and inhibits the methionine aminopeptidase, MetAP-2. Proc Natl Acad Sci U S A 1997;94:6099–103.
545. Kudelka AP, Verschraegen CF, Loyer E. Complete remission of metastatic cervical cancer with the angiogenesis inhibitor TNP-470. N Engl J Med 1998;338:991–2.
546. Bhargava P, Marshall JL, Rizvi N, et al. A phase I and pharmacokinetic study of TNP-470 administered weekly to patients with advanced cancer. Clin Cancer Res 1999;5:1989–95.
547. Chien M, Astumian M, Stadler WM. Normal human urothelial cell (HUC) response to H2O2: senescence-like growth arrest without p16INK4A expression [abstract]. Proc Am Assoc Cancer Res 1998;39:257.
548. Zukiwiski A, Gutterman J, Bui C, et al. Phase I trial of the angiogenesis inhibitor TNP-470 (AGM-1470) in patients (Pts) with androgen independent prostate cancer (AIPCa). Proc Am Soc Clin Oncol 1994;13:A795.
549. Dezube BJ, Von Roenn JH, Holden-Wiltse J, et al. Fumagillin analog in the treatment of Kaposi's sarcoma: a phase I AIDS clinical trial group study. AIDS clinical trial group no. 215 team. J Clin Oncol 1998;16:1444–9.
550. Herbst RS, Madden TL, Tran HT, et al. Safety and pharmacokinetic effects of TNP-470, an angiogenesis inhibitor, combined with paclitaxel in patients with solid tumors: evidence for activity in non–small-cell lung cancer. J Clin Oncol 2002;20:4440–7.
551. Kim ES, Herbst RS. Angiogenesis inhibitors in lung cancer. Curr Oncol Rep 2002;4:325–33.
552. Settles B, Stevenson A, Wilson K, et al. Down-regulation of cell adhesion molecules LFA-1 and ICAM-1 after in vitro treatment with the anti-TNF-α agent thalidomide. Cell Mol Biol 2001;47:1105–14.
552a. Satchi-Fainaro R, Mamluk R, Wang L, et al. Inhibition of vessel permeability by TNP-470 and its polymer conjugate, caplostatin. Cancer Cell 2005;7:251–61.
552b. Satchi-Fainaro R, Puder M, Davies JW, et al. Targeting angiogenesis with a conjugate of HPMA copolymer and TNP-470. Nat Med 2004;10:255–61.
553. Singhal S, Mehta J, Desikan R, et al. Antitumour activity of thalidomide in refractory multiple myeloma. N Engl Med 1999;341:1565–71.
554. Verheul HMW, Panigrahy D, Yuan J, D'Amato RJ. Combination oral anti-angiogenic therapy with thalidomide and sulindac inhibits tumour growth in rabbits. Br J Cancer 1999;79:114–8.
555. Bauditz J, Wedel S, Lochs H. Thalidomide reduces tumour necrosis factor-α and interleukin 12 production in patients with chronic active Crohn's disease. Gut 2002;50:196–200.
556. D'Amato RJ, Lentzsch S, Anderson KC, Rogers MS. Mechanism of action of thalidomide and 3-aminothalidomide in multiple myeloma. Semin Oncol 2001;28:597–601.
557. Raje N, Anderson K. Thalidomide—a revival story. N Engl J Med 1999;341:1606–9.
558. Hlatky L, Hahnfeldt P, Folkman J. Clinical application of antiangiogenic therapy: microvessel density, what it does and doesn't tell us. J Natl Cancer Inst 2002;94:883–93.
559. Rajkumar SV, Fonseca R, Witzig TE, et al. Bone marrow angiogenesis in patients achieving complete response after stem cell transplantation for multiple myeloma. Leukemia 1999;13:469–72.
560. Perez-Atayde AR, Sallan SE, Tedrow U, et al. Spectrum of tumor angiogenesis in the bone marrow of children with acute lymphoblastic leukemia. Am J Pathol 1997;150:815–21.
561. Folkman J. Tumour angiogenesis. In: Holland JF, Frei E III, Bast RC Jr, et al, editors. Cancer medicine. 5th ed. Hamilton (ON): BC Decker; 2000. p. 132–52.
562. Belotti, D, Vergani V, Drudis T, et al. The microtubule-affecting drug paclitaxel has anti-angiogenic activity. Clin Cancer Res 1996;2:1843–9.
563. Browder T, Butterfield CE, Kraling BM, et al. Anti-angiogenic scheduling of chemotherapy improves efficacy against experimental drug-resistant cancer. Cancer Res 2000;60:1878–86.
564. Meta-analysis Group in Cancer. Efficacy of intravenous continuous infusion of fluorouracil compared with bolus administration in advanced colorectal cancer. J Clin Oncol 1998;16:301–8.
565. Gabra H, Cameron DA, Lee LE, et al. Weekly doxorubicin and continuous infusional 5-fluorouracil for advanced breast cancer. Br J Cancer 1996;74:2008–12.
566. Hansen RM, Ryan L, Anderson T, et al. Phase III study of bolus versus infusion fluorouracil with or without cisplatin in advanced colorectal cancer. J Natl Cancer Inst 1996;88:668–74.
567. Abu-Rustum NR, Aghahanian C, Barakat RR, et al. Salvage weekly paclitaxel in recurrent ovarian cancer. Semin Oncol 1997;24(5 Suppl 15):S15-62–7.
568. Loffler TM, Freund W, Lipke J, Hausamen TU. Schedule- and dose-intensified paclitaxel as weekly 1-hour infusion in pretreated solid tumours: results of a phase I/II trial. Semin Oncol 1996;23(6 Suppl 16):32–4.
569. Kakolyris S, Samonis G, Koukourakis M, et al. Treatment of non-small-cell lung cancer with prolonged oral etoposide. Am J Clin Oncol 1998;21:505–8.
570. Chamberlain MC. Recurrent supratentorial malignant gliomas in children. Long-term salvage therapy with oral etoposide. Arch Neurol 1997;54:554–8.
571. Neskovic-Konstantinovic ZB, Bosnjak SM, Radulovic SS, Mitrovic LB. Daily oral etoposide in metastatic breast cancer. Anticancer Drugs 1996;7:543–7.
572. Hanahan D, Bergers G, Bergsland E. Less is more, regularly: metronomic dosing of cytotoxic drugs can target tumour angiogenesis in mice. J Clin Invest 2000;105:1045–7.
573. Colleoni M, Rocca A, Sandri MT, et al. Low-dose oral methotrexate and clophosphamide in metastatic breast cancer: antitumor activity and correlation with vascular endothelial growth factor levels. Ann Oncol 2002;13:73–80.
574. Kerbel RS, Klement G, Pritchard KI, Kamen B. Continuous low-dose anti-angiogenic/metronomic chemotherapy: from the research laboratory into the oncology clinic. Ann Oncol 2002;13:12–5.
575. Klement G, Baruchel S, Rak J, et al. Continuous low-dose therapy with vinblastine and VEGF receptor-2 antibody induces sustained tumour regression without overt toxicity. J Clin Invest 2000;105:R15–24.
576. Bello L, Carrabba G, Giussani C, et al. Low-dose chemotherapy combined with an antiangiogenic drug reduces human glioma growth in vivo. Cancer Res 2001;61:7501–6.
577. Kerbel RS, Folkman J. Reply [letter]. Nat Rev Cancer 2003. [In press]
578. Gately S, Kerbel R. Antiangiogenic scheduling of lower dose cancer chemotherapy. Cancer J 2002;7:427–36.
579. Folkman J. Regulation of angiogenesis. Blood 1993;82 Suppl 1:60.
580. Brunner G, Nguyen H, Gabrilove J, et al. Basic fibroblast growth factor expression in human bone marrow and peripheral blood cells. Blood 1993;81:631–8.
581. Vacca A, Ribatti D, Roncali L, et al. Bone marrow angiogenesis and progression in multiple myeloma. Br J Haematol 1994;87:503–8.
582. Ribatti D, Vacca A, Nico B, et al. Bone marrow angiogenesis and mast cell density increase simultaneously with progression of human multiple myeloma. Br J Cancer 1999;79:451–5.
583. Vacca A, Ribatti D, Presta M, et al. Bone marrow neovascularization, plasma cell angiogenic potential, and matrix metalloproteinase-2 secretion, parallel progression of human multiple myeloma. Blood 1999;93:3064–73.
584. Vacca A, Ribatti D, Roncali L, Dammacco F. Angiogenesis B cell lymphoproliferative diseases. Biological and clinical studies. Leuk Lymphoma 1995;20:27–38.
585. Rak J, Mitsuhashi Y, Bayko L, et al. Mutant ras oncogenes upregulate VEGF/VPF expression: implications for induction and inhibition of tumor angiogenesis. Cancer Res 1995;55:4575–80.
586. Rohan RM, Fernandez A, Udagawa T, et al. Genetic heterogeneity of angiogenesis in mice. FASEB J 2000;14:871–6.
587. Soengas MS, Capodieci P, Polsky D, et al. Inactivation of the apoptosis effector Apaf-1 in malignant melanoma. Nature 2001;409:207–11.
588. Yu, JL, Rak J, Carmeliet P, Coomber BL. Heterogenous vascular dependence of tumour populations. Am J Pathol 2001;58:1325–34.
589. Furuwatari C, Yagi A, Yamagami O, et al. A comprehensive system to explore p53 mutations. Am J Clin Pathol 1998;110:368–73.
590. Beecken W-DC, Fernandez S, Jouddrn SM, et al. Effect of antiangiogenic therapy on slowly growing, poorly vascularized tumours in mice. J Natl Cancer Inst 2001;93:382–7.
591. Brem S, Cotran R, Folkman J. Tumor angiogenesis: a quantitative method for histologic grading. J Natl Cancer Inst 1972;48:347–56.
592. Mlynek ML, van Beunigen D, Leder LD, Streffer C. Measurement of the grade of vascularization in histological tumour tissue sections. Br J Cancer 1985;52:945–8.
593. Gasparini G, Harris AL. Prognostic significance of tumor vascularity. In: Teicher BA, editor. Antiangiogenic agents in cancer therapy. New Jersey: Humana Press; 1999. p. 317–39.
594. Takahashi K, Mulliken JB, Kozakewich HPW, et al. Cellular markers that distinguish the phases of hemangioma during infancy and childhood. J Clin Invest 1994;93:2357–64.
595. Bielenberg DR, Bucana CD, Sanchez R, et al. Progressive growth of infantile cutaneous hemangiomas is directly correlated with hyperplasia and angiogenesis of adjacent epidermis and inversely correlated with expression of the endogenous angiogenesis inhibitor, IFN-β. Int J Oncol 1999;14:401–8.
596. White C, Sondheimer HM, Crouch EC, et al. Treatment of pulmonary hemangiomatosis with recombinant interferon alfa-2a. N Engl J Med 1989;320:1197–200.
597. Folkman J. Successful treatment of an angiogenic disease. N Engl J Med 1989;320:1211–2.
598. Ezekowitz RA, Mulliken JB, Folkman J. Interferon α 2A therapy for "life-threatening" hemangiomas in infancy. N Engl J Med 1992;326:1456–63.
598a. N Engl J Med 1994;330:300.
598b. N Engl J Med 1995;333:595–6.
599. Mulliken JB, Boon LM, Takahashi K, et al. Pharmacologic therapy for endangering hemangiomas. Curr Opin Dermatol 1995;2:109–13.
600. Palmieri G, Montella L, Martignetti A, Bianco AR. Interferon-α-2b at low doses as long-term anti-angiogenic treatment of a metastatic intracranial hemangioendothelioma: a case report. Oncol Rep 2000;7:145–9.
601. Deb G, Donfrancesco A, Ilari I, et al. Hemangioendotheliomas: successful therapy with interferon-α. A study in association with the Italian Pediatric Haematology/Oncology Society (AIEOP). Med Pediatr Oncol 2002;38:118–9.
602. Losso JN. Preventing degenerative diseases by anti-angiogenic functional foods. Food Technol 2002;56:78–88.

603. Kanai T, Konno H, Tanaka T, et al. Effect of angiogenesis inhibitor TNP-470 on the progression of human gastric cancer xenotransplanted into nude mice. Int J Cancer 1997;71:838–41.
604. Kalebic T, Tsokos M, Helman LJ. Suppression of rhabdomyosarcoma growth by fumagillin analog TNP-470. Int J Cancer 1996;68:596–9.
605. Yanase T, Tamura M, Fujita K, et al. Inhibitory effect of angiogenesis inhibitor TNP-470 on tumor growth and metastasis of human cell lines in vitro and in vivo. Cancer Res 1993;53:2566–70.
606. Konno H, Tanaka T, Kanai T, et al. Efficacy of an angiogenesis inhibitor, TNP-470, in xenotransplanted human colorectal cancer with high metastatic potential. Cancer 1996;77:1736–40.
607. Yazaki T, Takamiya Y, Costello PC, et al. Inhibition of angiogenesis and growth of human non-malignant and malignant meningiomas by TNP-470. J Neurooncol 1995;23:23–9.
608. Isobe N, Uozumi T, Kurisu K, et al. Experimental studies of the antitumor effect of TNP-470 on malignant brain tumors. Antitumor effect of TNP-470 on a human medulloblastoma xenograft line. Neuropediatrics 1996;27:136–42.
609. Yamaoka M, Yamamoto T, Ikeyama S, et al. Angiogenesis inhibitor TNP-470 (AGM-1470) potently inhibits the tumor growth of hormone-independent human breast and prostate carcinoma cell lines. Cancer Res 1993;53:5233–6.
610. Taki T, Ohnishi T, Arita N, et al. Anti-proliferative effects of TNP-470 on human malignant glioma in vivo: potent inhibition of tumor angiogenesis. J Neurooncol 1994;19:251–8.
611. McLeskey SW, Zhang L, Trock BJ, et al. Effects of AGM-1470 and pentosan polysulphate on tumorigenicity and metastasis of FGF-transfected MCF-7 cells. Br J Cancer 1996;73:1053–62.
612. Takamiya Y, Brem H, Ojeifo J, et al. AGM-1470 inhibits the growth of human glioblastoma cells in vitro and in vivo. Neurosurgery 1994;34:869–75.
613. Kragh M, Spang-Thomsen M, Kristjansen PE. Time until initiation of tumor growth is an effective measure of the anti-angiogenic effect of TNP-470 on human glioblastoma in nude mice. Oncol Rep 1999;6:759–62.
614. Singh Y, Shikata N, Kiyozuka Y, et al. Inhibition of tumor growth and metastasis by angiogenesis inhibitor TNP-470 on breast cancer cell lines in vitro and in vivo. Breast Cancer Res Treat 1997;45:15–27.
615. Takamiya Y, Friedlander RM, Brem H, et al. Inhibition of angiogenesis and growth of human nerve-sheath tumors by AGM-1470. J Neurosurg 1993;78:470–6.
616. Arbiser JL, Panigrathy D, Klauber N, et al. The antiangiogenic agents TNP-470 and 2-methoxyestradiol inhibit the growth of angiosarcoma in mice. J Am Acad Dermatol 1999;40:925–9.
617. Katzenstein HM, Rademaker AW, Senger C, et al. Effectiveness of the angiogenesis inhibitor TNP-470 in reducing the growth of human neuroblastoma in nude mice inversely correlates with tumor burden. Clin Cancer Res 1999;5:4273–8.
618. Qian CN, Min HQ, Lin HL, et al. Anti-tumor effect of angiogenesis inhibitor TNP-470 on the human nasopharyngeal carcinoma cell line NPC/HK1. Oncology 1999;57:36–41.
619. Beecken WD, Fernandez A, Panigrahy D, et al. Efficacy of antiangiogenic therapy with TNP-470 in superficial and invasive bladder cancer models in mice. Urology 2000;56:521–6.
620. Shusterman S, Grupp SA, Maris JM. Inhibition of tumor growth in a human neuroblastoma xenograft model with TNP-470. Med Pediatr Oncol 2000;35:673–6.
621. Takei H, Lee ES, Cisneros A, et al. Effects of angiogenesis inhibitor TNP-470 on tamoxifen-stimulated MCF-7 breast tumors in nude mice. Cancer Lett 2000;155:129–35.
622. Hotz HG, Reber HA, Hotz B, et al. Angiogenesis inhibitor TNP-470 reduces human pancreatic cancer growth. J Gastrointest Surg 2001;5:131–8.
623. Kato H, Ishikura H, Kawarada Y, et al. Anti-angiogenic treatment for peritoneal dissemination of pancreas adenocarcinoma: a study using TNP-470. Jpn J Cancer Res 2001;92:67–73.
624. Katzenstein HM, Salwen HR, Nguyen NN, et al. Antiangiogenic therapy inhibits human neuroblastoma growth. Med Pediatr Oncol 2001;36:190–3.
625. Kawano T, Yanoma S, Nishimura G, et al. The inhibitory effects of TNP470 on tumour growth of head and neck carcinoma cell producing interleukin-8. J Laryngol Otol 2001;115:802–7.
626. Rooks V, Beecken WD, Iordanescu I, et al. Sonographic evaluation of orthotopic bladder tumors in mice treated with TNP-470, an angiogenic inhibitor. Acad Radiol 2001;8:121–7.
627. Nagabuchi E, VanderKolk WE, Une Y, et al. TNP-470 antiangiogenic therapy for advanced murine neuroblastoma. J Pediatr Surg 1997;32:287–3.
628. Marcus D, Kim S, Brem H. The effect of an antiangiogenic compound (AGM-1470) on transgenic murine retinoblastoma [abstract]. Invest Ophthalmol Vis Sci 1993;34:226.
629. Brem H, Gresser I, Grosfeld J, et al. The combination of antiangiogenic agents to inhibit primary tumor growth and metastasis. J Pediatr Surg 1993;28:1253–7.
630. Brem H, Gotto F, Budson A. Minimal drug resistance after prolonged antiangiogenic therapy with AGM-1470. Surg Forum 1994;45:674–7.
631. Murata R, Nishimura Y, Hiraoka M. An antiangiogenic agent (TNP-470) inhibited reoxygenation during fractionated radiotherapy of murine mammary carcinoma. Int J Radiat Oncol Biol Phys 1997;37:1107–13.
632. Brem H, Folkman J. Analysis of experimental antiangiogenic therapy. J Pediatr Surg 1993;28:445–51.
633. Morita T, Shinohara N, Tokue A. Antitumour effect of a synthetic analogue of fumagillin on murine renal carcinoma. Br J Urol 1994;74:416–21.
634. Yamamoto T, Sudo K, Fujita T. Significant inhibition of endothelial cell growth in tumor vasculature by an angiogenesis inhibitor, TNP-470 (AGM-1470). Anticancer Res 1994;14:1–3.
635. Yatsunami J, Tsuruta N, Fukuno Y, et al. Inhibitory effects of roxithromycin on tumor angiogenesis, growth and metastasis of mouse B16 melanoma cells. Clin Exp Metastasis 1999;17:119–24.
636. Ma G, Masuzawa M, Hamada Y, et al. Treatment of murine angiosarcoma with etoposide, TNP-470 and prednisolone. J Dermatol Sci 2000;24:126–33.
637. Yoshizawa J, Mizuno R, Yoshida T, et al. Inhibitory effect of TNP-470 on hepatic metastasis of mouse neuroblastoma. J Surg Res 2000;93:82–7.
638. Yanai S, Okada H, Misaki M, et al. Antitumor activity of a medium-chain triglyceride solution of the angiogenesis inhibitor TNP-470 (AGM-1470) when administered via the hepatic artery to rats bearing Walker 256 carcinosarcoma in the liver. J Pharmacol Exp Ther 1994;271:1267–73.
639. Egawa S, Tsutsumi M, Konishi Y, et al. The role of angiogenesis in the tumor growth of Syrian hamster pancreatic cancer cell line HPD-NR. Gastroenterology 1995;108:1526–33.
640. Futami H, Iseki H, Egawa S, et al. Inhibition of lymphatic metastasis in a syngeneic rat fibrosarcoma model by an angiogenesis inhibitor, AGM-1470. Invasion Metastasis 1996;16:73–82.
641. Morishita T, Mii Y, Miyauchi Y, et al. Efficacy of the angiogenesis inhibitor O-(chloroacetyl-carbamoyl)fumagillol (AGM-1470) on osteosarcoma growth and lung metastasis in rats. Jpn J Clin Oncol 1995;25:25–31.
642. Yanai S, Okada H, Saito K, et al. Antitumor effect of arterial administration of a medium-chain triglyceride solution of an angiogenesis inhibitor, TNP-470, in rabbits bearing VX-2 carcinoma. Pharm Res 1995;12:653–7.
643. Kamei S, Okada H, Inoue Y, et al. Antitumor effects of angiogenesis inhibitor TNP-470 in rabbits bearing VX-2 carcinoma by arterial administration of microspheres and oil solution. J Pharmacol Exp Ther 1993;264:469–74.
644. Osawa S, Terashima Y, Kimura G, et al. Antitumour effects of the angiogenesis inhibitor AGM-1470 on rat urinary bladder tumours induced by N-butyl-N-(4-hydroxybutyl) nitrosamine. BJU Int 1999;83:123–8.
645. Landuyt W, Theys J, Nuyts S, et al. Effect of TNP-470 (AGM-1470) on the growth of rat rhabdomyosarcoma tumors of different sizes. Cancer Invest 2001;19:35–40.
646. Brem H, Ingber D, Blood C. Suppression of tumor metastasis by angiogenesis inhibition. Surg Forum 1991;42:439–41.
647. Schoof DD, Obando JA, Cusack JC Jr, et al. The influence of angiogenesis inhibitor AGM-1470 on immune system status and tumor growth in vitro. Int J Cancer 1993;55:630–5.
648. Teicher BA, Holden SA, Ara G, et al. Potentiation of cytotoxic cancer therapies by TNP-470 alone and with other anti-angiogenic agents. Int J Cancer 1994;57:920–5.
649. Kato T, Sato K, Kakinuma H, et al. Enhanced suppression of tumor growth by combination of angiogenesis inhibitor O-(chloroacetyl-carbamoyl)fumagillol (TNP-470) and cytotoxic agents in mice. Cancer Res 1994;54:5143–7.
650. Ahmed MH, Konno H, Nahar L, et al. The angiogenesis inhibitor TNP-470 (AGM-1470) improves long-term survival of rats with liver metastasis. J Surg Res 1996;64:35–41.
651. Konno H. Antitumor effect of the angiogenesis inhibitor TNP-470 on human digestive organ malignancy. Cancer Chemother Pharmacol 1999;43 Suppl:S85–9.
652. Mysliwski A, Bigda J, Koszalka P, et al. Synergistic effect of the angiogenesis inhibitor TNP-470 and tumor necrosis factor (TNF) on Bomirski Ab melanoma in hamsters. Anticancer Res 2000;20:4643–47.
653. Mysliwski A, Szmit E, Szatkowski D, et al. Suppression of growth of Bomirski Ab melanoma and its metastasis in hamsters by angiogenesis inhibitor TNP-470. Anticancer Res 1998;18:441–3.
654. Xia JL, Yang BH, Tang ZY, et al. Inhibitory effect of the angiogenesis inhibitor TNP-470 on tumor growth and metastasis in nude mice bearing human hepatocellular carcinoma. J Cancer Res Clin Oncol 1997;123:383–7.
655. Tanaka H, Taniguchi H, Mugitani T, et al. Angiogenesis inhibitor TNP-470 prevents implanted liver metastases after partial hepatectomy in an experimental model without impairing wound healing. Br J Surg 1996;83:1444–7.
656. Matsumoto K, Ninomiya Y, Inoue M, et al. Intra-tumor injection of an angiogenesis inhibitor, TNP-470, in rabbits bearing VX2 carcinoma of the tongue. Int J Oral Maxillofac Surg 1999;28:118–24.
657. Fujioka T, Hasegawa M, Ogiu K, et al. Antitumor effects of angiogenesis inhibitor O-(chloroacetyl-carbamoyl) fumagillol (TNP-470) against murine renal cell carcinoma. J Urol 1996;155:1775–8.
658. Konno H, Tanaka T, Matsuda I, et al. Comparison of the inhibitory effect of the angiogenesis inhibitor, TNP-470, and mitomycin C on the growth and liver metastasis of human colon cancer. Int J Cancer 1995;61:268–71.
659. Tanaka T, Konno H, Matsuda I, et al. Prevention of hepatic metastasis of human colon cancer by angiogenesis inhibitor TNP-470. Cancer Res 1995;55:836–9.
660. Mori S, Ueda T, Kuratsu S, et al. Suppression of pulmonary metastasis by angiogenesis inhibitor TNP-470 in murine osteosarcoma. Int J Cancer 1995;61:148–52.
661. Shishido T, Yasoshima T, Denno R, et al. Inhibition of liver metastasis of human gastric carcinoma by angiogenesis inhibitor TNP-470. Jpn J Cancer Res 1996;87:958–62.
662. Morishita T, Miyauchi Y, Mii Y, et al. Delay in administration of CDDP until completion of AGM-1470 treatment enhances antimetastatic and antitumor effects. Clin Exp Metastasis 1999;17:15–8.
663. Gervaz P, Scholl B, Padrun V, et al. Growth inhibition of liver metastases by the anti-angiogenic drug TNP-470. Liver 2000;20:108–13.
664. Oda H, Ogata Y, Shirouzu K. The effect of angiogenesis inhibitor TNP-470 against postoperative lung metastasis following removal of orthotopic transplanted human colon cancer: an experimental study. Kurume Med J 2001;48:285–93.
665. Saito N, Mitsuhashi M, Hayashi T, et al. Inhibition of hepatic metastasis in mice treated with cell-binding domain of human fibronectin and angiogenesis inhibitor TNP-470. Int J Clin Oncol 2001;6:215–20.
666. Offodile R, Walton T, Lee M, et al. Regression of metastatic breast cancer in a patient treated with the anti-angiogenic drug TNP-470. Tumori 1999;85:51–3.
667. Stadler WM, Kuzel T, Shapiro C, et al. Multi-institutional study of the angiogenesis inhibitor TNP-470 in metastatic renal carcinoma. J Clin Oncol 1999;17:2541–5.
668. Moore JD, Dezube BJ, Gill P, et al. Phase I dose escalation pharmacokinetics of O-chloroacetylcarbamoyl) fumagillol (TNP-470) and its metabolites in AIDS patients with Kaposi's sarcoma. Cancer Chemother Pharmacol 2000;46:173–9.
669. Kudelka AP, Levy T, Verschraegen CF, et al. A phase I study of TNP-470 administered to patients with advanced squamous cell cancer of the cervix. Clin Cancer Res 1997;3:1501–5.
670. Hurwitz H, Fehrenbacher L, Novotny W, et al. Bevacizumab plus irinotecan, fluorouracil, and leucovorin for metastatic colorectal cancer. N Engl J Med 2004;350:2335–42.
671. Hicklin DJ, Ellis LM. Role of the vascular endothelial growth factor pathway in tumor growth and angiogenesis. J Clin Oncol 2005;23:1011–27.
672. Matsumoto T, Claesson-Welsh L. VEGF receptor signal transduction. Sci STKE 2001;RE21.
673. Gordon MS, Margolin K, Talpaz M, et al. Phase I safety and pharmacokinetic study of recombinant human anti-vascular endothelial growth factor in patients with advanced cancer. J Clin Oncol 2001;19:843–50.
674. Holden SN, Eckhardt SG, Basser R, et al. Clinical evaluation of ZD6474, an orally active inhibitor of VEGF and EGF receptor signaling, in patients with solid, malignant tumors. Ann Oncol 2005;16:1391–7.
675. Stopeck A, Sheldon M, Vahedian M, et al. Results of a phase I dose-escalating study of the antiangiogenic agent, SU5416, in patients with advanced malignancies. PG - 2798-805. Clin Cancer Res 2002;8:2798–805.

676. Heymach JV, Desai J, Manola J, et al. Phase II study of the anti-angiogenic agent SU5416 in patients with advanced soft tissue sarcomas. Clin Cancer Res 2004;10:5732–40.
677. Rini BI, Small EJ. Biology and clinical development of vascular endothelial growth factor-targeted therapy in renal cell carcinoma. J Clin Oncol 2005;23:1028–43.
678. Escudier B, Szczylik C, Eisen T, et al. Randomized phase III trial of the Raf kinase and VEGFR inhibitor sorafenib (BAY 43-9006) in patients with advanced renal cell carcinoma (RCC) [abstract]. J Clin Oncol 2005;23.
679. Yang JC, Haworth L, Sherry RM, et al. A randomized trial of bevacizumab, an anti-vascular endothelial growth factor antibody, for metastatic renal cancer. N Engl J Med 2003;349:427–34.
680. Motzer RJ, Rini BI, Michaelson MD, et al. Phase 2 trials of SU11248 show antitumor activity in second-line therapy for patients with metastatic renal cell carcinoma (RCC) [abstract]. J Clin Oncol 2005;23.
681. Miller KD, Chap LI, Holmes FA, et al. Randomized phase III trial of capecitabine compared with bevacizumab plus capecitabine in patients with previously treated metastatic breast cancer. J Clin Oncol 2005;23:792–9.
682. Sandler AB, Gray R, Brahmer J, et al. Randomized phase II/III trial of paclitaxel (P) plus carboplatin (C) with or without bevacizumab (NSC # 704865) in patients with advanced non-squamous non-small cell lung cancer (NSCLC): an Eastern Cooperative Oncology Group (ECOG) Trial - E4599 [abstract]. J Clin Oncol 2005;23.
683. Giantonio BJ, Catalano PJ, Meropol NJ, et al. High-dose bevacizumab in combination with FOLFOX4 improves survival in patients with previously treated advanced colorectal cancer: results from the Eastern Cooperative Oncology Group (ECOG) study E3200 [abstract]. J Clin Oncol 2005;23.
684. Hecht JR, Trarbach T, Jaeger E, et al. A randomized, double-blind, placebo-controlled, phase III study in patients (Pts) with metastatic adenocarcinoma of the colon or rectum receiving first-line chemotherapy with oxaliplatin/5-fluorouracil/leucovorin and PTK787/ZK 222584 or placebo (CONFIRM-1) [abstract]. J Clin Oncol 2005;23.
685. Heymach J, Johnson B, Rowbottom J, et al. A randomized, placebo-controlled phase II trial of ZD6474 plus docetaxel in patients with NSCLC [abstract]. Proc Am Soc Clin Oncol 2005;24:3023.
685a. Fukumura D, Gohongi T, Kadambi A, et al. Predominant role of endothelial nitric oxide synthase in vascular endothelial growth factor-induced angiogenesis and vascular permeability. Proc Natl Acad Sci U S A 2001;98:2604–9.
686. Johnson DH, Fehrenbacher L, Novotny WF, et al. Randomized phase II trial comparing bevacizumab plus carboplatin and paclitaxel with carboplatin and paclitaxel alone in previously untreated locally advanced or metastatic non-small-cell lung cancer. J Clin Oncol 2004;22:2184–91.
687. Scappaticci FA, Fehrenbacher L, Cartwright T, et al. Surgical wound healing complications in metastatic colorectal cancer patients treated with bevacizumab. J Surg Oncol 2005;91:173–80.
688. Kuenen BC, Rosen L, Smit EF, et al. Dose-finding and pharmacokinetic study of cisplatin, gemcitabine, and SU5416 in patients with solid tumors. J Clin Oncol 2002;20:1657–67.
689. Kuenen BC, Levi M, Meijers JC, et al. Potential role of platelets in endothelial damage observed during treatment with cisplatin, gemcitabine, and the angiogenesis inhibitor SU5416. J Clin Oncol 2003;21:2192–8.
690. Boehm T, Folkman J, Browder T, O'Reilly MS. Antiangiogenic therapy of experimental cancer does not induce acquired drug resistance. Nature 1997;390:404–7.
691. Kerbel RS, Yu J, Tran J, et al. Possible mechanisms of acquired resistance to anti-angiogenic drugs: implications for the use of combination therapy approaches. Cancer Metastasis Rev 2001;20:79–86.
692. Davis DW, Takamori R, Raut CP, et al. Pharmacodynamic analysis of target inhibition and endothelial cell death in tumors treated with the vascular endothelial growth factor receptor antagonists SU5416 or SU6668. Clin Cancer Res 2005;11:678–89.
693. Gorre ME, Mohammed M, Ellwood K, et al. Clinical resistance to STI-571 cancer therapy caused by BCR-ABL gene mutation or amplification. Science 2001;293:876–80.
694. Gorre ME, Sawyers CL. Molecular mechanisms of resistance to STI571 in chronic myeloid leukemia. Curr Opin Hematol 2002;9:303–7.
695. Kobayashi S, Boggon TJ, Dayaram T, et al. EGFR mutation and resistance of non-small-cell lung cancer to gefitinib. N Engl J Med 2005;352:786–92.
696. Semenza GL. Targeting HIF-1 for cancer therapy. Nat Rev Cancer 2003;3:721–32.
697. Yamakawa M, Liu LX, Date T, et al. Hypoxia-inducible factor-1 mediates activation of cultured vascular endothelial cells by inducing multiple angiogenic factors. Circ Res 2003;93:664–73.
698. Relf M, LeJeune S, Scott PA, et al. Expression of the angiogenic factors vascular endothelial cell growth factor, acidic and basic fibroblast growth factor, tumor growth factor beta-1, platelet-derived endothelial cell growth factor, placenta growth factor, and pleiotrophin in human primary breast cancer and its relation to angiogenesis. Cancer Res 1997;57:963–9.
699. Miller KD, Wang M, Gralow J, et al. E2100: a randomized phase III trial of paclitaxel versus paclitaxel plus bevacizumab as first-line therapy for locally recurrent or metastatic breast cancer. Proc Am Soc Clin Oncol 2005;23.
700. Hida K, Hida Y, Amin DN, et al. Tumor-associated endothelial cells with cytogenetic abnormalities. Cancer Res 2004;64:8249–55.
701. Streubel B, Chott A, Huber D, et al. Lymphoma-specific genetic aberrations in microvascular endothelial cells in B-cell lymphomas. N Engl J Med 2004;351:250–9.

Section 2

CANCER IMMUNOLOGY

12a

Tumor Antigens

Michael A. Morse, MD

Tumor antigens are protein, peptide, or carbohydrate molecules that, when expressed or presented by tumors, act as a signal for immune effectors (T cells and antibodies) to recognize them as different from normal tissues. Antibodies directly recognize three-dimensional molecular patterns, typically present on surface-expressed proteins, although it is possible to engineer antibody fragments that can bind to intracellular proteins, so-called intrabodies.[1] T cells recognize their epitopes when presented in the context of major histocompatibility complex (MHC) molecules on the cell surface. CD8$^+$ cytolytic T-lymphocyte (CTL) receptors recognize 8 to 10 amino acid–long peptides presented within the peptide binding cleft of MHC class I (human leukocyte antigen [HLA]-A, -B, -C) (Figure 12a-1), whereas CD4$^+$ T helper cell receptors recognize longer peptide fragments (12–18 amino acids) within MHC class II (HLA-DR, -DP, -DQ). These peptides are derived from larger proteins produced by tumors and therefore can originate from any protein, whether nuclear, cytoplasmic, lysosomal, surface expressed, or secreted. For a peptide to be presented in MHC class I molecules, its originating protein is degraded by cytoplasmic proteasomes and the resulting peptides are transported into the lumen of the endoplasmic reticulum via the transporters associated with antigen processing (TAP1 and TAP2).[2] The peptides are complexed with newly synthesized MHC class I molecules and β_2-microglobulin, and the entire complex is then transported to the cell surface. How well a peptide will bind to an MHC molecule depends on whether the peptide sequence results in a structure that allows it to fit within the peptide binding groove of the MHC molecule. Also, certain amino acids in specific locations in the peptide (called anchor motifs) enhance the affinity of the peptide for the MHC molecule.[3–7] Peptides presented in MHC class II molecules generally originate exogenously and are endocytosed and degraded within endosomes that fuse with other vesicles containing MHC molecules, allowing any peptides with an acceptable sequence to bind within the cleft of the MHC class II molecule.[2] This complex is then transported to the cell surface. There is considerable promiscuity in the MHC class II binding of some of these peptides.[8] For example, PADRE (Pan DR epitope) binds to many different MHC class II molecules.

Recently, it has been noted that different patterns of class I restricted peptides may be generated from the same protein depending on whether the processing occurs in the proteasome or the immunoproteasome.[9] The immunoproteasome results from the exchange of several proteasome subunits with other subunits in response to interferon-γ. Its importance is demonstrated by the fact that tumors lacking immunoproteosomes are ignored by CTLs, which should otherwise recognize antigens expressed by these tumors.[10] Tumor antigens may be derived from genetic material not typically expressed in normal tissues; for example, they may be encoded by genes usually silenced in adult tissues or may be mutated genes (eg, mutated *TP53*) or new sequences created by translocations (eg, *bcr-abl* in chronic myelogenous leukemia), introns, pseudogenes, or antisense strands.[11–18] Also, it is not always the case that the T-cell epitope is derived from a linear sequence within the full-length protein. T-cell epitopes may be generated by splicing aberrations, cryptic open reading frames, or post-translational modification.[19] For example, an alternative open reading frame of the human macrophage colony-stimulating factor gene is independently translated and codes for an antigenic peptide recognized by tumor-infiltrating CD8$^+$ T lymphocytes in renal cell carcinoma.[20] A

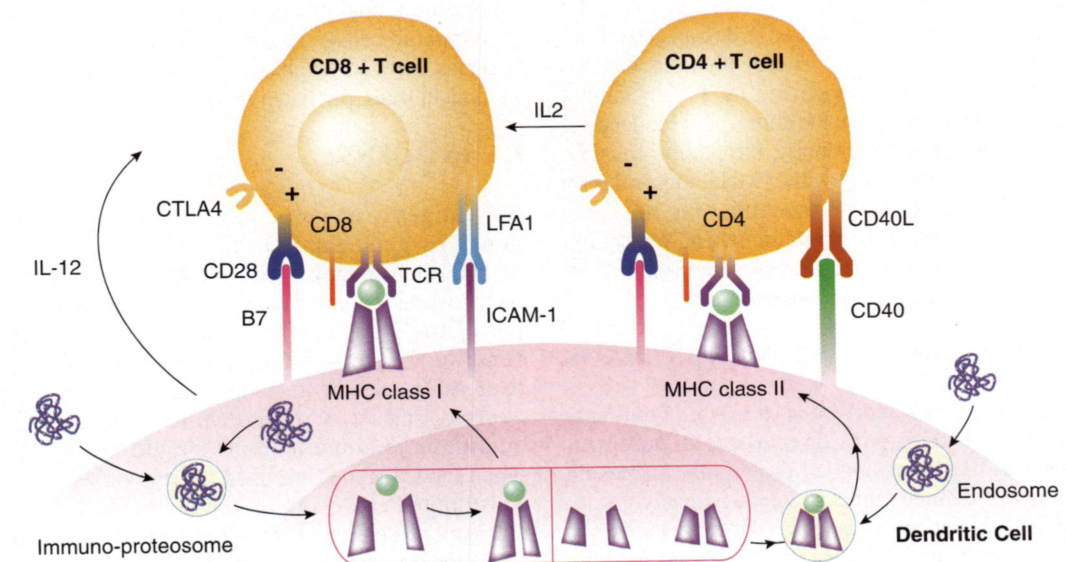

Figure 12a-1 CD8$^+$ cytolytic T-lymphocyte (CTL) receptors recognize 8 to 10 amino acid–long peptides presented within the peptide binding cleft of major histocompatibility complex (MHC) class I (human leukocyte antigen [HLA]-A, -B, -C).

Table 12a-1 Examples of Defined Tumor-Associated Antigens in Cancer Vaccine Clinical Trials and Expression in Major Cancers

Gene	Breast	CRC	Lung	Melanoma	Prostate	Head and Neck	HCC	Bladder	Ovarian
Cancer-Testis									
MAGE-1	12–31	39	10			43	19–75		
MAGE-2		16				38			
MAGE-3	24–27	5	40			44–62	24		
MAGE-5						24			
MAGE-6		3	50	72		48		50	
MAGE-A4	22	16	13			57	5		57
MAGE-12			26–62%	26–62%		26–62%		26–62%	
LAGE-1	15.7		15–50	25–50	25–50	25–50		14–48	21
GAGE-1/2							38		
PAGE					+				
XAGE-1/2	+								
NY-ESO-1	10–40	0-	20–30	45	3–14	6	0	20–30	9–43
SCP-1	33	2–38	12				29		
SSX-1,2,4	23	27	35	43		75	38–72		50
Differentiation antigens									
Gp100				77					
Melan-A/Mart-1				83					
Tyrosinase				100					
NY-BR-1	80								
Mutated proteins									
p53	28	53	55		4–35	13–35	67	38–73	38–70
K-ras	<5	30–60	25	0	+	8		4	25
N-ras				33%					
H-ras								12–18	
Overexpressed antigens									
HER2	30	11	4–29	5	0–16	29	8	58	7–20
MUC-1	>80	45–90	+		17				>80
PSMA					56				
Oncofetal antigens									
CEA	20–60	>95	50–70%			13		0–40	+[1]
AFP							50–70		

+ = expressed but data unavailable on percentage of the time it is expressed.

[1]Mucinous ovarian cancers.[125–137]

CRC = colorectal cancer; HCC = hepatocellular carcinoma.

splicing variant of survivin (survivin 2B) that retains a portion of intron 2 encodes an immunogenic peptide in the context of HLA-A24.[21] Hanada and colleagues described a 9–amino acid FGF-5 peptide generated by protein splicing that could be recognized by T cells cloned from lymphocytes infiltrating a renal cell carcinoma.[22] This type of splicing had not been previously reported in humans. Another unusual antigen was discovered to be translated from an antisense transcript.[23] These situations demonstrate that peptides recognized by T cells cannot always be predicted from the amino acid sequence of the antigen. Most importantly, the protein must be processed and presented within MHC molecules on the cell surface. Some proteins may not have epitopes that fit efficiently within MHC molecules, and some may not reach the processing machinery or may be degraded before presentation.[24]

CLASSIFICATION OF TUMOR ANTIGENS

Excellent reviews and Web sites (<http://www.cancerimmunity.org/peptidedatabase/differentiation.htm>) have catalogued the rapidly increasing number of defined tumor antigens, typically grouping them as cancer-testis (CT) (normally expressed only by testis and placenta but expressed in some cancers), oncofetal (expressed during fetal development and in cancers but not in normal adult tissues), melanoma differentiation antigens, viral (expressed by virally induced tumors), broadly expressed or overexpressed (expressed at higher levels or in a manner recognizable to the immune system by cancers compared with normal tissues), and unique, including those that are lineage restricted, mutated, post-translationally altered, and idiotypic (the unique immunoglobulin or T-cell receptor expressed by lymphoid cells).[3] Examples of tumor-associated antigens, with an emphasis on those being targeted in clinical trials, are listed in Table 12a-1.

CT ANTIGENS

CT antigens (or germ cell antigens), with 44 genes or gene families now identified, were named because they were thought to be expressed only in tumors, spermatocytes, and spermatogonia of the testis and the placenta, where their function is poorly understood. Such limited expression and the fact that the testis does not express class I or II molecules suggest that autoimmune complications should be limited when the CT genes are used for immunization.[25] This limited expression is due to the fact that CT antigens are encoded by genes, usually silent in adult tissues, but reactivated in tumors.[26] This reactivation may occur by hypomethylation of the CpG island in the CT gene promoter.[27] This has led to suggestions that greater expression of these antigens could be achieved by use of demethylating agents, such as 5-aza-2'-deoxycytidine.[28]

The list of CT antigens includes the MAGE, BAGE, and GAGE families; NY-ESO-1/LAGE/CAMEL; SAGE (serial analysis of gene expression); CAGE; SSX-2; TRAG-3; and CT9 and CT10 (see Scanlan and colleagues[29] for a complete list). They are widely expressed such that one or more of these antigens has been identified in colorectal, breast, bladder, lung, head and neck, esophageal, hepatocellular, and prostate carcinomas and melanoma, myeloma, cholangiocarcinoma, and sarcoma.[30–39] Melanoma and bladder non–small cell lung cancer tend to express more than half of the described CT genes, whereas breast and prostate cancers express more than 30% of the CT genes, and a minority of renal and colon cancers express CT genes. Importantly, class I and II epitopes have been identified for the majority of these antigens, although not all are reproducibly immunogenic in vivo.[40]

As a prototypical example of the CT antigens, the human MAGE (hMAGE) genes are related by sharing the MAGE homology domain. The MAGE subfamilies have been subclassified as type I and II MAGE genes.[41] The type I MAGE genes, including the acidic hMAGE-A, -B, and -C, are more restricted to tumor and germ cells, whereas the type II genes, including the genes MAGE-D, -E, -F, -I, -J, -K, and -L2 and necdin, are broadly expressed by both tumor cells and normal tissues. The numerous class I and II epitopes described for the MAGE antigens have been useful for clinical trials, including strategies to target MAGE-A1, -A3, -A4, -A10, and -3DPO4.[42–44] Although these epitopes are generally restricted to one MAGE molecule, an interesting recent observation has been that of a heteroclitic peptide (p248V9) that corresponds to two HLA-A *0201–restricted, cross-recognized epitopes, derived from MAGE-A2, -A3, -A4, -A6, -A10, -A12 (p248G9), and -A1 (p248D9).[43] CTLs specific for this peptide could kill tumor cells expressing all of these MAGE-A proteins.

Clinical studies of vaccines, including MAGE antigens in the form of peptide or dendritic cells loaded with peptides, have demonstrated the induction of MAGE-specific immune responses and occasional clinical responses.[45–48]

The other commonly targeted CT antigen has been NY-ESO-1, for which the following HLA-A2 epitopes have been identified: NY-ESO-$1_{157-167}$, NY-ESO-$1_{157-165}$, and NY-ESO-$1_{155-163}$, although NY-ESO-$1_{157-165}$ may be the naturally processed antigen.[49] A novel observation for NY-ESO-1 has been that of an HLA-A31–restricted epitope that is derived from translation of an alternative open reading frame of the NY-ESO-1 transcript.[50] Notably, NY-ESO-1 is particularly immunogenic, such that half of the patients with NY-ESO-1–expressing tumors possess spontaneously occurring T-cell and antibody responses to this antigen.[51] Vaccination of melanoma patients with NY-ESO-1 peptides has been demonstrated to cause clinical regressions of tumor- and antigen-specific CTL responses.[52]

DIFFERENTIATION ANTIGENS Differentiation antigens, expressed early in the development of normal tissues, are reexpressed in tumors. The antigens have been described in melanomas and melanocytes (tyrosinase, glycoprotein [gp]100, TRP-1, and MART-1/Melan-A) and in epithelial tumors, including Epcam and prostate-specific antigen (PSA), and the oncofetal antigens, such as carcinoembryonic antigen (CEA) (found in colorectal, breast, and lung cancers) and glypican 3 (found in hepatocellular carcinoma). Other than the melanoma antigens associated with melanin biosynthesis, the function of most of the other differentiation antigens is poorly understood. Nonetheless, their relative overexpression in tumors suggests that they can serve as targets of immunotherapies with a reduced but not completely eliminated risk of autoimmunity.

The CEA family includes CEA, CEA cell adhesion molecule (CEACAM) 1, CEA cell adhesion molecule 6, meconium antigen, and Tex.[53] CEA is normally expressed during oncofetal development but is overexpressed in virtually 100% of colorectal cancers, 70% of non–small cell lung cancers, and approximately 50% of breast cancers.[53] Low-level expression is observed in colorectal epithelium, and CEACAM is found on granulocytes and endothelium, where it exhibits angiogenic activity.[54] A number of $CD8^+$ T-cell epitopes that can be recognized in the context of A2, A3, and A24 and $CD4^+$ T cell epitopes that can be recognized in the context of HLA-DR1 and HLA-DR4 have been described, and these epitopes can be used as immunogens to activate T-cell responses against CEA.[55–57] Furthermore, tumors have been found to express many of these epitopes within their MHC molecules.[57] The best-described epitope is the HLA-A2–restricted epitope called CAP-1 and its modified peptide CAP1(6D), which displays enhanced recognition by the T-cell receptor.[58] CEA has been a frequent target of cancer vaccines in the form of peptides, full-length protein, messenger ribonucleic acid–loaded dendritic cells, plasmid deoxyribonucleic acid (DNA), and viral vectors. We and others recently reported that immune responses specific for CEA develop in cancer patients immunized with viral vectors encoding CEA, dendritic cells infected with these vectors, peptide-loaded dendritic cells, and anti-idiotype antibodies mimicking CEA.[59–62] As an alternative strategy, anti-idiotypic antibodies that mimic CEA (from the perspective of the immune system) have also been tested as a vaccine designed to elicit anti-CEA immunity in the setting of advanced colorectal cancer.[63,64]

The family of melanocyte differentiation antigens (Melan-A/MART-1, TRP-1 and -2, gp100, and tyrosinase) is expressed by melanomas and normal skin melanocytes and pigmented retinal epithelial cells. The most extensively studied epitopes are the two native immunodominant HLA-A2–restricted MART-1_{26-35} and MART-1_{27-35} peptides, which have been reported to induce a CTL response in vitro and in vivo.[65,66] Because the magnitude of the response to these epitopes is relatively low, possibly owing to the low affinity of binding to MHC class I, their immunogenicity has been augmented by substituting one or two amino acids.[67–69] The MART-1_{26-35} A27L peptide analogue (ELAGIGILTV), in which the parental immunodominant peptide (MART-1_{26-35}) is modified by replacing the alanine with leucine (A27L), demonstrated better immunogenicity in vitro and in vivo than did the parental sequence (EAAGIGILTV).[68,70] Other approaches to enhancement of immunogenicity have included lipoconjugation.[71] Peptides restricted by HLA-B*3501 and -B45 have also been described. HLA-DP–restricted (class II) epitopes of MART-1 have been demonstrated to activate specific immune responses in patients with melanoma.[72] Studies using MART-1 epitopes with incomplete Freund's adjuvant, interleukin-12, or autologous dendritic cells in patients with high risk or metastatic demonstrated peptide-specific delayed-type hypersensitivity and $CD8^+$ T-cell responses, which correlated with relapse-free survival.[73,74]

Regarding gp100, the immunogenicity of the native HLA-A2–restricted immunodominant epitope of gp100 (gp100 [209-217]) has been enhanced by a substitution of methionine for threonine at position 2 to yield gp100(209-2M). Vaccines based on this modified epitope have been demonstrated to activate specific CTL responses, although clinical responses have been less commonly reported.[75–78] Peptides restricted by HLA-A3, -A24, and -B*3501 have also been described.

The human tyrosinase gene codes for two distinct HLA-A2–restricted epitopes, one of which differs from the gene-encoded sequence as a result of post-translational modification of amino acid residue 370 (asparagine to aspartic acid) and is called $\text{tyrosinase}_{368-376}$ (370D). Peptides restricted by HLA-A1, -A24, -B44, and -B*3501 have also been described. Recent clinical trials of tyrosinase peptides, along with granulocyte-macrophage colony-stimulating factor (GM-CSF) or tyrosinase encoded within viral vectors, have demonstrated the development of delayed-type hypersensitivity and T-cell responses.[79]

BROADLY EXPRESSED ANTIGENS

Some antigens are expressed across many different malignancies (AFP, HER2/neu, MUC-1, WT-1, prostate-specific membrane antigen) or are expressed so broadly that they could be considered "universal antigens" (livin, survivin, hTERT). Many of these antigens are also expressed by normal tissues, but differences in the level or location of expression provide the distinguishing feature between the tumor and normal tissue. Telomerase (hTERT), a reverse transcriptase that stabilizes the ends of chromosomes, can be recognized by $CD8^+$ T cells from cancer patients.[80] Two HLA-A2–restricted peptides derived from hTERT, ^{540}ILAKFLHWL^{548} and ^{865}RLVDDFLLV^{873}, are expressed by human breast, colon, prostate, and melanoma cell lines and can be recognized by peptide-specific CTLs.[81] Because of concern that high-affinity T cells against hTERT, a self-antigen, might be deleted in humans, they modified a lower-affinity peptide and demonstrated that this peptide (pY572) could activate CTLs with the capacity to recognize the wild-type peptide from the blood of five of eight patients with prostate cancer. Importantly, these CTLs did not lyse $CD34^+$ hematopoietic cells, which typically express hTERT.

Survivin, a member of the inhibitor of apoptosis protein family, is expressed during fetal development but becomes undetectable in normal adult tissues. Survivin and its splicing variant, survivin 2B, having been identified by immunohistochemistry in a substantial fraction of breast, colon, squamous cell, lung, and gastric cancers and melanoma. An HLA-A24–restricted antigenic peptide, survivin 2B80-88 (AYACNTSTL), is recognized by the CD8(+)CTLs of cancer patients.[82,83] Clinical trials immunizing patients against survivin have demonstrated induction of antigen-specific T cells without obvious autoimmunity.[84,85]

MUC1, derived from epithelial mucin, is a highly glycosylated, cell surface–expressed type I glycoprotein. Although mucins are expressed by

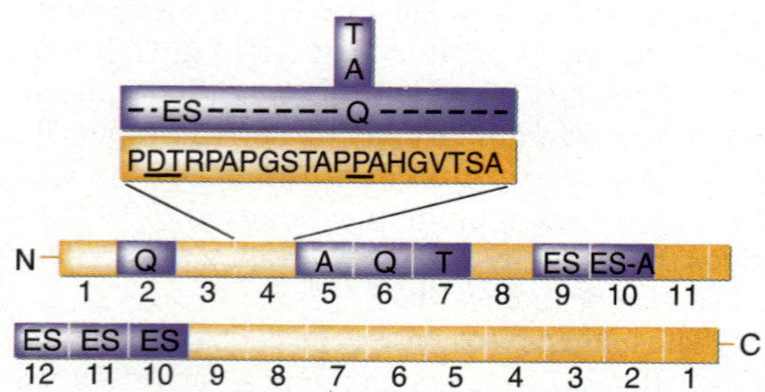

Figure 12a-2 Tandem-repeat structure of the MUC1 tumor antigen. The MUC1 is a unique tumor antigen and contains a protein backbone that is composed of more than 20 homologous repeats of a core sequence PDTRPAPG-STAPPAHGVTSA (ie, single amino acid designations). Each repeat may include some variation, as indicated. For instance, repeat 2 at the amino (*N*-) terminus contains a P→Q change at position 13 of the core sequence. Both CD4+ and CD8+ T cell epitopes as well as antibody binding sites have been identified within the MUC1 sequence, making this an important immune target in the setting of epithelial tumors.

many normal cells, they are expressed aberrantly in breast, ovarian, lung, and colon cancers and hematologic malignancies (myeloma, acute myelogenous leukemia, and some lymphomas).[86] MUC-1 is unique in the expression of an extracellular domain, with a variable number of tandem repeats of 20 amino acids (Figure 12a-2).[87] Interestingly, these tandem repeats can be recognized directly by $CD8^+$ T cells independent of MHC molecules,[88] although peptide epitopes of MUC-1 may also be presented within MHC class I molecules.[89–90] Antibody responses to MUC-1 have also been detected in patients.[91] In addition, sialyl-Tn, a carbohydrate epitope associated with MUC1, has been the target of the cancer vaccine Theratope.[92] The availability of epitopes and the overexpression of MUC1 in many malignancies have made MUC1 a broadly applicable target for cancer vaccination strategies.[93] These have included peptide vaccines,[94] dendritic cells loaded with peptides or viral vectors,[95] and, recently, pox vectors encoding MUC-1,[96] including PANVAC-VF, which is being tested in a phase III study for the treatment of metastatic pancreatic cancer. Another approach has been to conjugate a MUC1 peptide to mannan (polymannose) so that the MUC1 is targeted to mannose receptors on antigen-presenting cells.[97] Immunization with this vaccine led to CTL and antibody responses in some patients.

HER2/neu, a member of the human epidermal growth factor receptor family, is expressed on the surface of breast and ovarian cancers and at a low frequency in lung, pancreatic, and colon cancers. Although best known as the target of the monoclonal antibody trastuzumab (Herceptin), it contains a number of epitopes recognized by T cells that have been extensively studied by Disis and colleagues at the University of Washington.[98] A high rate of 92% of patients vaccinated with their peptide vaccine plus GM-CSF developed T-cell proliferation to HER2/neu peptides. This group has also reported antibody responses to the same vaccine, and, interestingly, these antibody responses inhibit function of the HER2 molecule as well.[99]

PSA, used for monitoring prostate cancer, is also expressed by some breast, ovarian, and salivary gland neoplasms. Antigen-specific T-cell responses have been generated against PSA epitopes.[100,101] Other prostatic antigens of interest as cancer vaccine targets include prostate-specific membrane antigen[102] and prostatic acid phosphatase, which has been the target of Dendreon's dendritic cell vaccine, which has demonstrated activity in patients with hormone-refractory prostate cancer.[103]

UNIQUE ANTIGENS: MUTATED ANTIGENS

Unique antigens are attractive because patients might not be as tolerant to them as they would be to a self-, widely expressed antigen. One way for an antigen to be restricted to tumors is if it is created by a mutation in a protein found in the malignant clone only. For example, many colon, pancreatic, and lung cancers harbor point mutations in the K-*ras* gene at codon 12, where the normal Gly residue is substituted with a Val, Asp, or Cys residue. Ras is an important molecule in the signaling of the epidermal growth factor receptor pathway, and oncogenic mutations cause uncontrolled stimulation of this pathway, resulting in proliferation, migration, and antiapoptotic activities in the tumor cell. Peptides from oncogenic K-*ras* have been shown to be processed and presented in the context of MHC class I in tumor cells in mice and humans.[104,105] Recent clinical trials demonstrated the immunogenicity of these peptide epitopes in humans.[106–108] Mutated *TP53* has also been identified as a potential immunotherapy target. Mutated *TP53,* in addition to losing its tumor-suppressive functions, often accumulates, thus making it an even better target for immune effectors.[109] Induction of CTL activity against *TP53* epitopes, whether derived from wild-type or mutant *TP53*, has been reported in a number of in vitro studies.[110–116] Human clinical trials have demonstrated the induction of T-cell responses specific for *TP53* epitopes following immunization.[107] This study also demonstrated the complexity of using mutated antigens because only 14% of the screened patients were found to be eligible and lack of a suitable mutation was a common reason. Another complexity is that mutated epitopes such as *TP53* may not be processed and presented efficiently by the proteasome.[117]

The genetic instability that can occur in some types of tumors, such as hereditary nonpolyposis colon cancer, caused by defects in mismatch repair genes and the MSI-positive phenotype, can lead to novel protein epitopes. For example, Saeterdal and colleagues described a peptide, SLVRLSS-CVPVALMSAMTTSSSQ, representing a common frameshift mutation in transforming growth factor β (TGF-β) RII, that was recognized by T cells from patients with MSI-positive colon cancers.[118] This group also described an HLA-A2–restricted, $CD8^+$ epitope (RLSSCVPVA) resulting from a common frameshift mutation in TGF-βRII.[119] A CTL clone generated against this peptide was able to kill an HLA-A2–positive colon cancer cell line with mutated TGF-βRII.

Fusion molecules created by translocations of chromosomes give rise to a unique epitope spanning the fusion region (eg, FVEHDDESPGL, an HLA-A2–restricted peptide derived from the BCR-abl fusion in CML).[120] Other epitopes may be found exclusively in one of the partners to the translocation, but because the aberrant molecule is overexpressed, the peptide epitope is also overexpressed. A number of HLA class II–restricted epitopes of BCR-abl have been described as well.[121]

UNIQUE ANTIGENS: IDIOTYPE

Hematologic malignancies that develop from B and T cells (leukemias, lymphomas, and myelomas) express unique B- (immunoglobulin) and T-cell receptors that are unique because they are derived from a single, abnormal clone. The B-cell idiotype has been either purified from the peripheral blood and used as part of a vaccine or the unique portions of the immunoglobulin are identified and cloned so that they may be used as templates for producing vaccines targeting these unique sequences.[122] An initial study immunizing patients who were in remission from low-grade follicular lymphoma with autologous Id conjugated to KLH reported that the majority of patients had Id-specific humoral and/or cellular immune responses.[122] In their follow-up study, 41 patients received a series of injections with vaccines consisting of Id protein conjugated to KLH, and nearly half mounted anti-Id immune responses to the vaccine.[123] A subsequent study demonstrated that an Id-KLH conjugate could activate $CD8^+$ T-cell responses and antibodies in patients in remission from their lymphoma.[124]

SUMMARY AND OTHER CONSIDERATIONS IN CHOOSING TUMOR ANTIGENS

The rapidly expanding list of tumor antigens, driven in part by new techniques for discovery, such as SAGE and Phage display, has provided more options for targeting tumors with immunotherapeutic strategies. The remainder of the subchapters address in more detail how effector cells recognize tumor antigens, how tumor-based immunosuppression may inhibit the response to tumor antigens, how antigens may have been used as part of cancer vaccines, and how to measure immune responses against these tumor antigens. Also, some of the tumor antigens are also measured in the bloodstream as a marker of disease activity (such as CEA).

REFERENCES

1. Lobato MN, Rabbitts TH. Intracellular antibodies as specific reagents for functional ablation: future therapeutic molecules. Curr Mol Med 2004;4:519–28.
2. Lehner PJ, Cresswell P. Processing and delivery of peptides presented by MHC class I molecules. Curr Opin Immunol 1996;8:59–67.
3. Novellino L, Castelli C, Parmiani G. A listing of human tumor antigens recognized by T cells: March 2004 update. Cancer Immunol Immunother 2005;54:187–207.

4. Falk K, Rotzschke O, Stevanovics S, et al. Allele-specific motifs revealed by sequencing of self-peptides eluted from MHC molecules. Nature 1991;351:290–6.
5. Engelhard VH. Structure of peptides associated with class I and class II MHC molecules. Annu Rev Immunol 1994;12:181–207.
6. Sette A, Vitiello A, Reherman B, et al. The relationship between class I binding affinity and immunogenicity of potential cytotoxic T cell epitopes. J Immunol 1994;153:5586–92.
7. van der Burg SH, Visseren MJ, Brandt RM, et al. Immunogenicity of peptides bound to MHC class I molecules depends on the MHC-peptide complex stability. J Immunol 1996;156:3308–14.
8. Neumann F, Wagner C, Kubuschok B, et al. Identification of an antigenic peptide derived from the cancer-testis antigen NY-ESO-1 binding to a broad range of HLA-DR subtypes. Cancer Immunol Immunother 2004;53:589–99.
9. Morel S, Levy F, Burlet–Schiltz O, et al. Processing of some antigens by the standard proteasome but not by the immunoproteasome results in poor presentation by dendritic cells. Immunity 2000;12:107–17.
10. Meidenbauer N, Zippelius A, Pittet MJ, et al. High frequency of functionally active Melan-A-specific T cells in a patient with progressive immunoproteasome-deficient melanoma. Cancer Res 2004;64:6319–26.
11. Wolfel T, Hauer M, Schneider J, et al. A p16INK4a-insensitive CDK4 mutant targeted by cytolytic T lymphocytes in a human melanoma. Science 1995;269:1281–4.
12. Robbins PF, El-Gamil M, Li YF, et al. A mutated beta catenin gene encodes a melanoma-specific antigen recognized by tumor infiltrating lymphocytes. J Exp Med 1996;83:1185–92.
13. Mandruzzato S, Brasseur F, Andry G, et al. A CASP-8 mutation recognized by cytolytic T lymphocytes on a human head and neck carcinoma. J Exp Med 1997;186:785–93.
14. Coulie PG, Lehmann F, Lethe B, et al. A mutated intron sequence codes for an antigenic peptide recognized by cytolytic T lymphocytes on a human melanoma. Proc Natl Acad Sci U S A 1995;92:7976–80.
15. Guilloux Y, Lucas S, Brichard VG, et al. A peptide recognized by human cytolytic T lymphocytes on HLA-A2 melanomas is encoded by an intron sequence of the N-acetylglucosaminyltransferase V gene. J Exp Med 1996;183:1173–83.
16. Aarnoudse CA, van den Doel PB, Heemskerk B, et al. Interleukin-2-induced, melanoma-specific T cells recognize CAMEL, an unexpected product of LAGE-1. Int J Cancer 1999;82:442–8.
17. Moreau-Aubry A, Le Guiner S, Labarriere N, et al. A processed pseudogene codes for a new antigen recognized by a CD8(+) T cell clone on melanoma. J Exp Med 2000;191:1617–24.
18. Wang RF, Wang X, Rosenberg SA. Identification of a novel major histocompatibility complex class II-restricted tumor antigen resulting from a chromosomal rearrangement recognized by CD4+ T cells. J Exp Med 1999;189:1659–68.
19. Schirmbeck R, Riedl P, Fissolo N, et al. Translation from cryptic reading frames of DNA vaccines generates an extended repertoire of immunogenic, MHC class I-restricted epitopes. J Immunol 2005;174:4647–56.
20. Probst-Kepper M, Stroobant V, Kridel R, et al. An alternative open reading frame of the human macrophage colony-stimulating factor gene is independently translated and codes for an antigenic peptide of 14 amino acids recognized by tumor-infiltrating CD8 T lymphocytes, J Exp Med 2001;193:1189–98.
21. Hirohashi Y, Torigoe T, Maeda A, et al. An HLA-A24-restricted cytotoxic T lymphocyte epitope of a tumor-associated protein, survivin. Clin Cancer Res 2002;8:1731–9.
22. Hanada K, Yewdell JW, Yang JC. Immune recognition of a human renal cancer antigen through post-translational protein splicing. Nature 2004;427:252–6.
23. Van Den Eynde BJ, Gaugler B, Probst-Kepper M, et al. A new antigen recognized by cytolytic T lymphocytes on a human kidney tumor results fromreverse strand transcription. J Exp Med 1999;190:1793–800.
24. Valmori D, Gileadi U, Servis C, et al. Modulation of proteasomal activity required for the generation of a cytotoxic T lymphocyte-defined peptide derived from the tumor antigen MAGE-3. J Exp Med 1999;189:895–906.
25. Uyttenhove C, Godfraind C, Lethe B, et al. The expression of mouse gene P1A in testis does not prevent safe induction of cytolytic T cells against a P1A-encoded tumor antigen. Int J Cancer 1997;70:349–56.
26. De Smet C, Lurquin C, Lethe B, et al. DNA methylation is the primary silencing mechanism for a set of germ line and tumor-specific genes with a CpG-rich promoter. Mol Cell Biol 1999;19:7327.
27. Lim JH, Kim SP, Gabrielson E, et al. Activation of human cancer/testis antigen gene, XAGE-1, in tumor cells is correlated with CpG island hypomethylation. Int J Cancer 2005;116:200–6.
28. Sigalotti L, Fratta E, Coral S, et al. Intratumor heterogeneity of cancer/testis antigens expression in human cutaneous melanoma is methylation-regulated and functionally reverted by 5-aza-2'-deoxycytidine. Cancer Res 2004;64:9167–71.
29. Scanlan MJ, Simpson AJ, Old LJ. The cancer/testis genes: review, standardization, and commentary. Cancer Immun 2004;4:1.
30. Mashino K, Sadanaga N, Tanaka F, et al. Expression of multiple cancer-testis antigen genes in gastrointestinal and breast carcinomas. Br J Cancer 2001;85:713–20.
31. Jungbluth AA, Ely S, Diliberto M, et al. The cancer-testis antigens CT7 (MAGE-C1) and MAGE-A3/6 are commonly expressed in multiple myeloma and correlate with plasma cell proliferation. Blood 2005;106:167–74
32. Melloni G, Ferreri AJ, Russo V, et al. Prognostic significance of cancer-testis gene expression in resected non-small cell lung cancer patients. Oncol Rep 2004;12:145–51.
33. Li M, Yuan YH, Han Y, et al. Expression profile of cancer-testis genes in 121 human colorectal cancer tissue and adjacent normal tissue. Clin Cancer Res 2005;11:1809–14.
34. Bolli M, Schultz-Thater E, Zajac P, et al. NY-ESO-1/LAGE-1 coexpression with MAGE-A cancer/testis antigens: a tissue microarray study. Int J Cancer 2005;115:960–6.
35. Ries J, Schultze-Mosgau S, Neukam F, et al. Investigation of the expression of melanoma antigen-encoding genes (MAGE-A1 to -A6) in oral squamous cell carcinomas to determine potential targets for gene-based cancer immunotherapy. Int J Oncol 2005;26:817–24.
36. Segal NH, Blachere NE, Guevara-Patino JA, et al. Identification of cancer-testis genes expressed by melanoma and soft tissue sarcoma using bioinformatics. Cancer Immun 2005;5:2.
37. Utsunomiya T, Inoue H, Tanaka H, et al. Expression of cancer-testis antigen (CTA) genes in intrahepatic cholangiocarcinoma. Ann Surg Oncol 2004;11:934–40.
38. Zhao L, Mou DC, Leng XS, et al. Expression of cancer-testis antigens in hepatocellular carcinoma. World J Gastroenterol 2004;10:2034–8.
39. Li M, Yuan YH, Han Y, et al. Expression profile of cancer-testis genes in 121 human colorectal cancer tissue and adjacent normal tissue. Clin Cancer Res 2005;11:1809–14.
40. Chianese-Bullock KA, Pressley J, Garbee C, et al. MAGE-A1-, MAGE-A10-, and gp100-derived peptides are immunogenic when combined with granulocyte-macrophage colony-stimulating factor and montanide ISA-51 adjuvant and administered as part of a multipeptide vaccine for melanoma. J Immunol 2005;17:3080–6.
41. Barker PA, Salehi A. The MAGE proteins: emerging roles in cell cycle progression, apoptosis, and neurogenetic disease. J Neurosci Res 2002;67:705–12.
42. Atanackovic D, Altorki NK, Stockert E, et al. Vaccine-induced CD4+ T cell responses to MAGE-3 protein in lung cancer patients. J Immunol 2004;172:3289–96.
43. Graff-Dubois S, Faure O, Gross DA, et al. Generation of CTL recognizing an HLA-A*0201-restricted epitope shared by MAGE-A1, -A2, -A3, -A4, -A6, -A10, and -A12 tumor antigens: implication in a broad-spectrum tumor immunotherapy. J Immunol 2002;169:575–80.
44. Thompson LW, Brinckerhoff L, Slingluff CL Jr. Vaccination for melanoma. Curr Oncol Rep 2000;2:292–9.
45. Marchand M, Brasseur F, van der Bruggen P, et al. Perspectives for immunization of HLA-A1 patients carrying a malignant melanoma expressing gene MAGE-1. Dermatology 1993;186:278–80.
46. Marchand M, van Baren N, Weynants P, et al. Tumor regressions observed in patients with metastatic melanoma treated with an antigenic peptide encoded by gene MAGE-3 and presented by HLA-A1. Int J Cancer 1999;80:219–30.
47. Nestle FO, Alijagic S, Gilliet M, et al. Vaccination of melanoma patients with peptide- or tumor lysate-pulsed dendritic cells. Nat Med 1998;4:328–32.
48. Thurner B, Haendle I, Roder C, et al. Vaccination with Mage-3A1 peptide-pulsed mature, monocyte-derived dendritic cells expands specific cytotoxic T cells and induces regression of some metastases in advanced stage IV melanoma. J Exp Med 1999;190:1669–78.
49. Jager E, Chen YT, Drijfhout JW, et al. Simultaneous humoral and cellular immune response against cancer-testis antigen NY-ESO-1: definition of human histocompatibility leukocyte antigen (HLA)-A2-binding peptide epitopes. J Exp Med 1998;187:265–70.
50. Wang RF, Johnston SL, Zeng G, et al. A breast and melanoma-shared tumor antigen: T cell responses to antigenic peptides translated from different open reading frames. J Immunol 1998;161:598–3606.
51. Jager E, Nagata Y, Gnjatic S, et al. Monitoring CD8 T cell responses to NY-ESO-1. Correlation of humoral and cellular immune responses. Proc Natl Acad Sci U S A 2000;97:4760–15.
52. Jager E, Gnjatic S, Nagata Y, et al. Induction of primary NY-ESO-1 immunity. CD8+ T lymphocyte and anti-body responses in peptide-vaccinated patients with NY-ESO-1+ cancers. Proc Natl Acad Sci U S A 2000;97:12198–203.
53. Thomson J, Grunert F, Ziemerman W, et al. CEA gene family. Molecular biology and clinical perspective. J Clin Lab Anal 1991;5:344–66.
54. Kilic N, Oliveira-Ferrer L, Wurmbach JH, et al. Pro-angiogenic signaling by the endothelial presence of CEACAM1. J Biol Chem 2005;280:2361–9.
55. Campi G, Crosti M, Consogno G, et al. CD4(+) T cells from healthy subjects and colon cancer patients recognize a carcinoembryonic antigen-specific immunodominant epitope. Cancer Res 2003;63:8481–6.
56. Ullenhag GJ, Fagerberg J, Strigard K, et al. Functional HLA-DR T cell epitopes of CEA identified in patients with colorectal carcinoma immunized with the recombinant protein CEA. Cancer Immunol Immunother 2004;53:331–7.
57. Berinstein L. Carcinoembryonic antigen as a target for therapeutic anticancer vaccines: a review. J Clin Oncol 2002;20:2197–207.
58. Zaremba S, Barzaga E, Zhu M, et al. Identification of an enhancer agonist cytotoxic T lymphocyte peptide from human carcinoembryonic antigen. Cancer Res 1997;57:4570–7.
59. Marshall L, Gulley JL, Arlen PM, et al. Phase I study of sequential vaccinations with fowlpox-CEA(6D)-TRICOM alone and sequentially with vaccinia-CEA(6D)-TRICOM, with and without granulocyte-macrophage colony-stimulating factor, in patients with carcinoembryonic antigen-expressing carcinomas. J Clin Oncol 2005;23:720–31.
60. Liu KJ, Wang CC, Chen LT, et al. Generation of carcinoembryonic antigen (CEA)-specific T-cell responses in HLA-A*0201 and HLA-A*2402 late-stage colorectal cancer patients after vaccination with dendritic cells loaded with CEA peptides. Clin Cancer Res 2004;10:2645–51.
61. Foon KA, John WJ, Chakraborty M, et al. Clinical and immune responses in resected colon cancer patients treated with anti-idiotype monoclonal antibody vaccine that mimics the carcinoembryonic antigen. J Clin Oncol 1999;17:2889–5.
62. Morse MA, Clay TM, Hobeika AC, et al. Phase I study of immunization with dendritic cells modified with fowlpox encoding carcinoembryonic antigen and costimulatory molecules, Clin Cancer Res 2005;11:3017–24.
63. Bhattachary–Chatterjee M, Nath Barul R, Chatterjee SK, et al. Counterpoint. Cancer vaccines—single-epitope anti-idiotype vaccine versus multiple-epitope antigen vaccine. Cancer Immunol Immunother 2000;49:133–41.
64. Foon KA, John WJ, Chakraborty M, et al. Clinical and immune responses in advanced colorectal cancer patients treated with anti-idiotype monoclonal antibody vaccine that mimics the carcinoembryonic antigen. Clin Cancer Res 1997;3:1267–76.
65. Salio M, Shepherd D, Dunbar PR, et al. Mature dendritic cells prime functionally superior Melan-A-specific CD8+ lymphocytes as compared with nonprofessional APC. J Immunol 2001;167:1188–97.
66. Nestle FO, Alijac S, Gilliet M, et al. Vaccination of melanoma patients with peptide or tumor lysate-pulsed dendritic cells. Nat Med 1998;4:328–32.
67. Romero P, Gervois N, Schneider J, et al. Cytolytic T lymphocyte recognition of the immunodominant HLA-A*0201 restricted Melan-A/MART-1 antigenic peptide in melanoma. J Immunol 1997;158:2366–74.
68. Valmori D, Fonteneau JF, Lizana C, et al. Enhanced generation of specific tumor-reactive CTL in vitro by selected Melan-A/MART-1 immunodominant peptide analogues. J Immunol 1998;160:1750–8.
69. Guichard G, Zerbib A, Le Gal FA, et al. Melanoma peptide MART-1(27-35) analogues with enhanced binding capacity to the human class I histocompatibility molecule HLA-A2 by introduction of a beta-amino acid resi-

due: implications for recognition by tumor-infiltrating lymphocytes. J Med Chem 2000;43:3803–8.
70. Men Y, Miconnet I, Valmori D, et al. Assessment of immunogenicity of human Melan-A peptide analogues in HLA-A*0201/Kb transgenic mice. J Immunol 1999;162:3566–73.
71. Le Gal FA, Prevost–Blondel A, Lengagne R, et al. Lipopeptide-based melanoma cancer vaccine induced a strong MART-27-35-cytotoxic T lymphocyte response in a preclinical study. Int J Cancer 2002;98:221–7.
72. Wong R, Lau R, Chang J, et al. Immune responses to a class II helper peptide epitope in patients with stage III/IV resected melanoma. Clin Cancer Res 2004;10:5004–13.
73. Wang F, Bade E, Kuniyoshi C, et al. Phase I trial of a MART-1 peptide vaccine with incomplete Freund's adjuvant for resected high-risk melanoma. Clin Cancer Res 1999;5:2756–65.
74. Ranieri E, Kierstead LS, Zarour H, et al. Dendritic cell/peptide cancer vaccines: clinical responsiveness and epitope spreading. Immunol Inv 2000;29:121–5.
75. Slingluff CL Jr, Yamshchikov G, Neese P, et al. Phase I trial of a melanoma vaccine with gp100 (280-288) peptide and tetanus helper peptide in adjuvant. Immunologic and clinical outcomes. Clin Cancer Res 2001;7:3012–24.
76. Clay TM, Custer MC, McKee MD, et al. Changes in the fine specificity of gp100(209-217)-reactive T cells in patients following vaccination with a peptide modified at an HLA-A2.1 anchor residue. J Immunol 1999;162:1749–55.
77. Phan GQ, Touloukian CE, Yang JC, et al. Immunization of patients with metastatic melanoma using both class I- and class II-restricted peptides from melanoma-associated antigens. Immunotherapy 2003;26:349–56.
78. Atzpodien J, Fluck M, Reitz M. Individualized synthetic peptide vaccines with GM-CSF in locally advanced melanoma patients. Cancer Biother Radiopharm 2004;19:758–63.
79. Scheibenbogen C, Schmittel A, Keilholz U, et al. Phase II trial of vaccination with tyrosinase peptides and granulocyte-macrophage colony-stimulating factor in patients with metastatic melanoma. J Immunother 2000;23:275–81.
80. Su Z, Dannull J, Yang BK, et al. Telomerase mRNA-transfected dendritic cells stimulate antigen-specific CD8+ and CD4+ T cell responses in patients with metastatic prostate cancer. J Immunol 2005;174:3798–807.
81. Zanetti M, Hernandez X, Langlade-Demoyen P. Telomerase reverse transcriptase as target for anti-tumor T cell responses in humans. Springer Semin Immunopathol 2005;27:87–104.
82. Idenoue S, Hirohashi Y, Torigoe T, et al. A potent immunogenic general cancer vaccine that targets survivin, an inhibitor of apoptosis proteins. Clin Cancer Res 2005;11:1474–82.
83. Schmidt SM, Schag K, Muller MR, et al. Survivin is a shared tumor-associated antigen expressed in a broad variety of malignancies and recognized by specific cytotoxic T cells. Blood 2003;102:571–6.
84. Otto K, Andersen MH, Eggert A, et. al. Lack of toxicity of therapy-induced T cell responses against the universal tumour antigen survivin. Vaccine 2005;23:884–9.
85. Tsuruma T, Hata F, Torigoe T. Phase I clinical study of anti-apoptosis protein, survivin-derived peptide vaccine therapy for patients with advanced or recurrent colorectal cancer. J Transl Med 2004;2:19.
86. Gendler SJ, Spicer AP. Epithelial mucin genes. Annu Rev Physiol 1995;57:607–34.
87. Gendler S, Taylor-Papadimitriou J, Duhig T, et al. Highly immunogenic region of a human polymorphic epithelial mucin expressed by carcinomas is made up of tandem repeats. J Biol Chem 1988;263:12820–3.
88. Takahashi T, Makiguchi Y, Hinoda Y, et al. Expression of MUC1 on myeloma cells and induction of HLA-unrestricted CTL against MUC1 from a multiple myeloma patient. J Immunol 1994;153:2102–9.
89. Brossart P, Heinrich KS, Stuhler G, et al. Identification of HLA-A2-restricted T-cell epitopes derived from the MUC1 tumor antigen for broadly applicable vaccine therapies. Blood 1999;93:4309–17.
90. Apostolopoulos V, Karanikas V, Haurum JS, et al. Induction of HLA-A2-restricted CTLs to the mucin 1 human breast cancer antigen. J Immunol 1997;159:5211–8.
91. Kotera Y, Fontenot JD, Pecher G, et al. Humoral immunity against a tandem repeat epitope of human mucin MUC-1 in sera from breast, pancreatic and colon cancer patients. Cancer Res 1994;54:2856–60.
92. Holmberg LA, Sandmaier BM. Vaccination with Theratope (STn-KLH) as treatment for breast cancer. Exp Rev Vaccines 2004;3:655–63.
93. Finn OJ, Jerome KR, Henderson RA, et al. MUC-1 epithelial tumor mucin-based immunity and cancer vaccines. Immunol Rev 1995;145:61–89.
94. North S, Butts C. Vaccination with BLP25 liposome vaccine to treat non-small cell lung and prostate cancers. Exp Rev Vaccines 2005;4:249–57.
95. Trevor KT, Hersh EM, Brailey J, et al. Transduction of human dendritic cells with a recombinant modified vaccinia Ankara virus encoding MUC1 and IL-2. Cancer Immunol Immunother 2001;50:397–407.
96. Rochlitz C, Figlin R, Squiban P, et al. Phase I immunotherapy with a modified vaccinia virus (MVA) expressing human MUC1 as antigen-specific immunotherapy in patients with MUC1-positive advanced cancer. J Gene Med 2003;5:690–9.
97. Karanikas V, Hwang LA, Pearson J, et al. Antibody and T cell responses of patients with adenocarcinoma immunized with mannan-MUC1 fusion protein. J Clin Invest 1997;100:2783–92.
98. Disis ML, Gooley TA, Rinn K, et al. Generation of T-cell immunity to the HER-2/neu protein after active immunization with HER-2/neu peptide-based vaccines. J Clin Oncol 2002;20:2624–32.
99. Montgomery RB, Makary E, Schiffman K, et al. Endogenous anti-HER2 antibodies block HER2 phosphorylation and signaling through extracellular signal-regulated kinase. Cancer Res 2005;65:650–6.
100. Correale P, Walmsly K, Nieroda C, et al. In vitro generation of human cytotoxic T lymphocytes specific for peptides derived from prostate-specific antigen. J Natl Cancer Inst 1997;89:293–9.
101. Correale P, Walmsley K, Zaremba S, et al. Generation of human cytolytic T lymphocyte lines directed against prostate-specific antigen (PSA) employing a PSA oligoepitope peptide. J Immunol 1998;161:3186–94.
102. Tyoa BA, Simmons VA, Radge H, et al. Evaluation of phase I/II clinical trials in prostate cancer with dendritic cells and PSMA peptides. Prostate 1998;36:39–44.
103. Small EJ, Rini B, Higano C, et al. A randomized, placebo-controlled phase III trial of APC8015 in patients with androgen-independent prostate cancer (AiPCa) [abstract]. Proc Am Soc Clin Oncol 2003;22:382.
104. Abrams SI, Hand PH, Tsang KY, et al. Mutant ras epitopes as targets for cancer vaccines. Semin Oncol 1996;23:118–34.
105. Bristol JA, Schlom J, Abrams SI. Development of a murine mutant Ras CD8+ CTL peptide epitope variant that possesses enhanced MHC class I binding and immunogenic properties. J Immunol 1998;160:2433–41.
106. Gjertsen MK, Bjorheim J, Saeterdal I, et al. Cytotoxic CD4+ and CD8+ T lymphocytes, generated by mutant p21-ras (12Val) peptide vaccination of a patient, recognize 12Val-dependent nested epitopes present within the vaccine peptide and kill autologous tumour cells carrying this mutation. Int J Cancer 1997;72:784–90.
107. Carbone DP, Ciernik IF, Kelley MJ, et al. Immunization with mutant p53- and K-ras-derived peptides in cancer patients: immune response and clinical outcome. J Clin Oncol 2005 Jun 27; Epub ahead of print.
108. Gjertsen MK, Buanes T, Rosseland AR, et al. Intradermal ras peptide vaccination with granulocyte-macrophage colony-stimulating factor as adjuvant: clinical and immunological responses in patients with pancreatic adenocarcinoma. Int J Cancer 2001;92:441–50.
109. Gnjatic S, Cai Z, Viguier M, et al. Accumulation of the p53 protein allows recognition by human CTL of a wild-type p53 epitope presented by breast carcinomas and melanomas. J Immunol 1998;160:328–33.
110. Chikamatsu K, Nakano K, Storkus WJ, et al. Generation of anti-p53 cytotoxic T lymphocytes from human peripheral blood using autologous dendritic cells. Clin Cancer Res 1999;5:1281–8.
111. Houbiers JGA, Nijman HW, Drijfhout JW, et al. In vitro induction of human cytotoxic T lymphocyte responses against peptides of mutant and wild-type p53. Eur J Immunol 1993;23:2072–7.
112. Yanuck M, Carbone DP, Pendleton CD, et al. A mutant p53 tumor suppressor protein is a target for peptide-induced CD8+ cytotoxic T-cells. Cancer Res 1993;53:3257–61.
113. Barfoed AM, Petersen TR, Kirkin AF, et al. Cytotoxic T-lymphocyte clones, established by stimulation with the HLA-A2 binding p5365-73 wild type peptide loaded on dendritic cells in vitro, specifically recognize and lyse HLA-A2 tumour cells over expressing the p53 protein. Scand J Immunol 2000;51:128–33.
114. Eura M, Chikamatsu K, Katsura F, et al. A wild type-sequence p53 peptide presented by HLA-A24 induces cytotoxic T lymphocytes that recognize squamous cell carcinomas of the head and neck. Clin Cancer Res 2000;6:979–86.
115. McArdle SEB, Rees RC, Mulcahy KA, et al. Induction of human cytotoxic T lymphocytes that preferentially recognize tumour cells bearing a conformational p53 mutant. Cancer Immunol Immunother 2000;49:417–25.
116. Keogh E, Fikes J, Southwood S, et al. Identification of new epitopes from four different tumor-associated antigens: recognition of naturally processed epitopes correlates with HLA-A*0201-binding affinity. J Immunol 2001;167:787–96.
117. Theobald M, Ruppert TU, Kuckelkorn UJ, et al. The sequence alteration associated with a mutational hotspot in p53 protects cells from lysis by cytotoxic T lymphocytes specific for a flanking peptide epitope. J Exp Med 1998;188:1017–28.
118. Saeterdal I, Bjorheim J, Lislerud K, et al. Frameshift-mutation-derived peptides as tumor-specific antigens in inherited and spontaneous colorectal cancer. Proc Natl Acad Sci U S A 2001;98:13255–60.
119. Saeterdal I, Gjertsen MK, Straten P, et al. A TGF betaRII frameshift-mutation-derived CTL epitope recognized by HLA-A2-restricted CD8+ T cells. Cancer Immunol Immunother 2001;50:469–76.
120. Wagner WM, Ouyang Q, Pawelec G. The abl/bcr gene product as a novel leukemia-specific antigen: peptides spanning the fusion region of abl/bcr can be recognized by both CD4+ and CD8+ T lymphocytes. Cancer Immunol Immunother 2003;52:89.
121. ten Bosch GJ, Kessler JH, Joosten AM, et al. A BCR-ABL oncoprotein p210b2a2 fusion region sequence is recognized by HLA-DR2a restricted cytotoxic T lymphocytes and presented by HLA-DR matched cells transfected with an Ii(b2a2) construct. Blood 1999;94:1038.
122. Kwak L, Campbell MJ, Czerwinski DK, et al. Induction of immune responses in patients with B-cell lymphoma against the surface-immunoglobulin idiotype expressed by their tumors. N Engl J Med 1992;327:1209–15.
123. Hsu FJ, Caspar CB, Czerwinski D, et al. Tumor-specific idiotype vaccines in the treatment of patients with B-cell lymphoma: long-term results of a clinical trial. Blood 1997;89:3129–35.
124. Bendandi M, Gocke CD, Kobrin CB, et al. Complete molecular remissions induced by patient-specific vaccination plus granulocyte-monocyte colony-stimulating factor against lymphoma. Nat Med 1999;5:1171–7.
125. Bei R, Budillon A, Masuelli L, et al. Frequent overexpression of multiple ErbB receptors by head and neck squamous cell carcinoma contrasts with rare antibody immunity in patients. J Pathol 2004;204:317–25.
126. Brinkmann U, Vasmatzis G, Lee B, et al. *PAGE-1*, an X chromosome-linked *GAGE*-like gene that is expressed in normal and neoplastic prostate, testis, and uterus. Proc Natl Acad Sci U S A 1998;95:10757–62.
127. Cormier JN, Abati A, Fetsch P, et al. Comparative analysis of the in vivo expression of tyrosinase, MART-1/Melan-A, and gp100 in metastatic melanoma lesions: implications for immunotherapy. J Immunother 1998;21:27–31.
128. Junker K, Stachetzki U, Rademacher D, et al. HER2/neu expression and amplification in non-small cell lung cancer prior to and after neoadjuvant therapy. Lung Cancer 2005;48:59–67.
129. Kienstra MA, Neel HB, Strome SE, Roche P. Identification of NY-ESO-1, MAGE-1, and MAGE-3 in head and neck squamous cell carcinoma. Head Neck 2003;25:457–63.
130. Li M, Yuan YH, Han Y, et al. Expression profile of cancer-testis genes in 121 human colorectal cancer tissue and adjacent normal tissue. Clin Cancer Res 2005;11:1809–14.
131. Ries J, Schultze-Mosgau S, Neukam F, et al. Investigation of the expression of melanoma antigen-encoding genes (MAGE-A1 to -A6) in oral squamous cell carcinomas to determine potential targets for gene-based cancer immunotherapy. Int J Oncol 2005;26:817–24.
132. Luo G, Huang S, Xie X, et al. Expression of cancer-testis genes in human hepatocellular carcinomas. Cancer Immun 2002;2:11.
133. Semczuk A, Postawski K, Przadka D, et al. K-ras gene point mutations and p21ras immunostaining in human ovarian tumors. Eur J Gynaecol Oncol 2004;25:484–8.
134. Tureci O, Chen YT, Sahin U, et al. Expression of SSX genes in human tumors. Int J Cancer 1998;77:19–23.
135. Van Der Bruggen P, Zhang Y, Chaux P, et al. Tumor-specific shared antigenic peptides recognized by human T cells. Immunol Rev 2002;188:51–64.
136. Zellweger T, Ninck C, Bloch M, et al. Expression patterns of potential therapeutic targets in prostate cancer. Int J Cancer 2005;113:619–28.
137. Zhao L, Mou DC, Leng XS, et al. Expression of cancer-testis antigens in hepatocellular carcinoma. World J Gastroenterol 2004;10:2034–8.

12b

Cancer Biomarkers

Stephen Chui, MD

The transformation of normal cells into malignant tissue is characterized by progressive gene mutations, alterations in gene transcription and translation, and changes in protein structure and function.[1,2] Such changes in normal cellular function can often be detected and monitored directly in the tissue of interest (via biopsy) and/or in surrogate specimens (eg, bodily fluids such as blood, urine, sputum, and cerebrospinal fluid). Identifying and measuring biomarkers of malignant growth and transformation potentially have important applications in early detection and diagnosis of cancer, classifying the disease, determining the prognosis, and monitoring disease progression, recurrence, or response to therapy.

The term *tumor marker* has traditionally referred to a detectable tumor-associated protein or antigen occurring exclusively or more commonly in association with cancer cells compared with the normal tissue of origin. Most serum tumor markers and many tissue tumor markers have been identified with immunologic techniques that use antisera or monoclonal antibodies prepared in other species immunized with human cancer tissue. More recently, technological advances in high-throughput biomarker analysis (proteomic pattern diagnostics, gene expression profiling) have led to the separation of different populations with respect to outcomes of interest according to groups (signatures) of biologic traits.

BIOMARKER APPLICATIONS

By definition, a biomarker is a property of a cancer associated with a clinical or biologic outcome. A risk marker conveys the earliest evidence of the probability of developing cancer in subjects who are currently without evidence of disease. Inherited genetic abnormalities are the most extensively studied risk markers, such as *BRCA1/2* mutations in breast and ovarian carcinoma, and adenomatous polyposis coli and mismatch repair gene mutations, such as *hMSH2*, *hMLH1*, *hPMS2*, *HMSH3*, and *hMSH6* in colon cancer. The presence of a risk marker indicates that cancer is more likely to occur within a defined time period in subjects with the marker compared with the general population.

Conversely, cancer screening markers distinguish asymptomatic individuals at sufficiently high risk of cancer to justify the use of additional studies to identify previously undetected malignant disease. Screening markers attempt to detect malignant and premalignant disorders at an early stage such that clinical interventions can be effective. Since screening marker tests are intended for use in asymptomatic populations and the proportion of affected persons is likely to be small, an efficacious screening marker exhibits both high sensitivity and high specificity for malignancy. Such a screening marker would therefore be unlikely to miss a case of disease (a sensitivity issue) or lead to false-positive results in individuals without the disease (a specificity issue). Ultimately, the broad applicability of a cancer early detection marker is contingent on improvements in long-term outcomes within a population. Screening mammography for breast cancer, the Papanicolaou (PAP) cell cytology test for cervical cancer, and fecal occult blood testing for colorectal cancer have all been demonstrated to reduce cancer-specific mortality when applied to the general population.[1] On the other hand, considerable uncertainty exists regarding the quantitative cancer-related mortality impact of measuring of serum cancer antigen (CA) 125 as a screening test for ovarian carcinoma and carcinoembryonic antigen (CEA) for gastrointestinal malignancies and performing chest radiography and/or chest computed tomography for lung cancer.

Diagnostic Markers Because of a lack of sensitivity and specificity, measurement of serum tumor markers is rarely of use in the early diagnosis of cancer. Histopathologic analysis of primary tumor tissue continues to remain the "gold standard" for the diagnosis of malignancy. However, tumor markers can still provide important information to aid in (1) distinguishing between benign and malignant disease, (2) identifying the primary site in malignancy of an unclear primary origin, and (3) clarifying issues or distinguishing tumor subtypes in difficult or rare cases that conventional histopathology cannot further classify.[1]

Prognostic Markers Prognostic markers are used to predict the outcome (eg, relapse-free survival, overall survival, time to disease progression) of disease. Traditionally, clinical and histopathologic parameters (eg, tumor size, grade, lymph node status) have been used to assess the prognosis of solid tumors.[1] However, the variability of clinical outcomes within groups of patients classified using these standard schema underscores the limitations of current staging classifications to predict the behavior of tumors over time. Molecular analyses of tumor or serum specimens have the potential to describe and/or reflect on the biologic functions of a particular cancer. The ongoing inclusion of molecular classification markers to prognostic models may help to more accurately define the patient outcomes beyond those subgroups defined by traditional criteria.[1]

Therapy Selection and Response Markers Therapy selection and response markers predict in advance the likelihood of a patient responding to (and therefore benefiting from) a specific therapy. For instance, determination of estrogen receptor (ER) and progesterone receptor (PR) status is useful to predict the response of breast cancers to hormone therapy: up to 70% of ER- and PR-positive advanced breast tumors respond to hormone therapies, whereas less than 5% of ER- and PR-negative tumors respond. ER and PR status also serves as an important breast cancer prognostic marker, with longer disease-free survival and overall survival observed among patients with ER-positive tumors compared with those with ER-negative tumors.[2] Elevated expression levels of HER2 (c-erbB-2), as measured by immunohistochemical staining and/or fluorescence in situ hybridization (FISH) of the *HER2* gene, also predict increased responsiveness of breast tumors to anthracycline chemotherapy versus cyclophosphamide, 4-fluorouracil, and methotrexate[2,3] suggest responsiveness to the anti-HER2 monoclonal antibody trastuzumab[2] and may predict the increased responsiveness of ER-positive tumors to aromatase inhibitor hormone therapy compared with tamoxifen.[2] These observations have led the American Society of Clinical Oncology (ASCO) Panel on Breast Cancer Markers to recommend that ER/PR status and HER2 expression levels be determined for all primary breast cancers at the time of diagnosis.[2]

Interestingly, the efficacy of many novel "targeted therapies" has often not been clearly demonstrated to depend on levels of target expression by the tumor; for example, regardless of levels of epidermal growth factor receptor (EGFR) expression by tumor (as determined by immunohistochemical staining), the EGFR tyrosine kinase inhibitor erlotinib has been shown to prolong survival in advanced non–small cell lung cancer patients after failure of at least one chemotherapeutic regimen, although trends were seen for increased effects of erlotinib on EGFR-positive and -unknown cancers.[2] Ultimately, genotypic analysis may eventually prove to be the superior predictor of therapeutic response to targeted agents: *KIT* and *PDGFRA* mutations in gastrointestinal stromal tumor appear to correlate closely with clinical outcomes in response to imatinib treatment,[2] and mutations in the tyrosine kinase domain of EGFR may predict responsiveness to gefitinib therapy in lung cancer.[2,3]

Recurrence and Metastasis Markers Tumor markers are commonly measured by clinicians in the follow-up and monitoring of patients with previously diagnosed and treated malignancies.

Table 12b-1 Individual Tumor Markers and Their Applications

Primary Malignancy	Tumor Marker	Tumor Marker Characteristics	Tumor Marker Application	References
Testicular germ cell tumors (choriocarcinoma, embryonal carcinoma, teratocarcinoma)	α-fetoprotein	67 kDa plasma protein present in human embryonic serum	Diagnostic Prognostic Therapeutic monitoring	J Clin Oncol 1997;15:594
	hCG	45kDa α/β heterodimeric glycoprotein synthesized by trophoblastic cells of the placenta	Diagnostic Prognostic Therapeutic monitoring	J Clin Oncol 1997;15:594
Hepatocellular carcinoma	α-fetoprotein	67 kDa plasma protein present in human embryonic serum	Diagnostic Therapeutic monitoring	J Hepatol. 2005;43:310
Lung carcinoma	Ki67	Proliferation marker: Polyclonal antibody to Ki67 antigen in the granular components of the nucleolus during late G_1, S, G_2 and M phases.	Prognostic? Prognostic?	Lung Cancer 2001;33:S17–34. Nucleic Acids Res 1997;25:151
	p53 mutation	Tumor suppressor gene: Transcriptional activator involved in growth arrest, DNA repair and apoptosis.	Prognostic?	Clin Can Res 1997;10:1831
	p21 mutation	Mapped to chromosome 17	Prognostic?	N Engl J Med 1990;323:561
	K-ras mutation	Cyclin-dependent kinase inhibitor controlled by p53	Diagnostic?	J Clin Oncol 1988;6:1685.
	hnRNP A2/B1 overexpression	Member of the small GTPase superfamily	Diagnostic?	Cancer Res 1996;56:2285
	Hypermethylation of CpG sequences	Expression evaluated by IHC of sputum epithelial cells PCR analysis of sputum DNA samples		

hCG = human chronic gonadotrophin; IHC = immunohistochemistry; PCR = polymerase chain reaction.

Serum immunoassay markers frequently screened include CA 27.29 (the protein core antigen of the MUC1 glycoprotein detected by the B27.29 monoclonal antibody) for breast cancer, CEA for colorectal cancer, CA 125 for ovarian cancer, and prostate-specific antigen (PSA) for prostate cancer. However, it is important to recognize that the routine use of recurrence markers depends on demonstrating that early detection and diagnosis would result in the provision of effective therapies that would ultimately improve significant health outcomes (eg, overall survival, disease-free survival, quality of life, lesser toxicity, and cost-effectiveness). Data are insufficient to demonstrate clinical benefit for the standard use of CA 27.29 and CEA to detect and/or diagnose breast and colorectal cancer recurrence.[13] Similarly, there are major challenges to the use and interpretation of serial PSA and CA 125 data to monitor for the recurrence or progression of prostate cancer and ovarian cancer, respectively; it should be noted that all of these diseases may progress without an increase in the levels of biochemical markers.[18,19] Conversely, detection of rising serum levels of alpha-fetoprotein and/or β-human chorionic gonadotropin (HCG) can frequently identify patients with recurrent testicular carcinoma, allowing early interventions with effective and frequently curative salvage treatment regimens.[20]

Although most current serum tumor markers may have limited usefulness in screening for disease recurrence after primary therapy, they frequently do have valuable utility in monitoring treatment efficacy in patients. In the absence of other simple tests to document the response, quantification of serum tumor markers may suggest progression or regression of disease. Ideally, such markers would be combined with radiologic or other measurable parameters to confirm the response.[13]

Ideal Cancer Biomarker The definition of an ideal cancer biomarker depends on its application and scientific and/or clinical utility. Nonetheless, an exemplary biomarker would possess the following characteristics: (1) specific expression by malignant and/or premalignant tissue; (2) production by all patients with a specific malignancy; (3) present early in the disease (before clinical evidence of cancer); (4) able to quantitatively reflect tumor volume, behavior, and/or disease progression and thus distinguish tumor growth versus tumor regression owing to effective therapy; and (5) a standardized, reproducible, and validated quantitative assay. Optimally, this test could be performed on (6) surrogate biologic specimens that can be obtained safely and noninvasively and would have (7) a very low false-positive rate and a low false-negative rate (ie, high sensitivity and very high disease specificity). To date, no cancer biomarker has been developed that satisfies all of these criteria.

SERUM IMMUNOASSAY MARKERS

Because of the low prevalence of cancer in the general population and the limited sensitivity for early cancer and specificity for malignancy of individual serum tumor markers, these tests have been generally found to be of little value in screening for cancer in healthy subjects. As prognostic indicators, biochemical markers may provide useful information independent of traditional pathohistologic groupings (Table 12b-1).

Germ Cell Tumors: Gestational Trophoblastic Disease and Testicular Germ Cell Cancer HCG is synthesized nearly exclusively by the trophoblastic cells of the placenta.[21] In patients with choriocarcinoma arising from villous trophoblasts, serum HCG levels exhibit characteristics approaching the ideal tumor marker: HCG levels are elevated in nearly all patients with choriocarcinoma, the levels are extremely sensitive to small changes in tumor burden, and effective systemic therapy is readily available to treat the disease once it has been identified.[22,23] Correspondingly, persistently elevated levels of HCG identify trophoblastic disease patients who are unlikely to achieve complete remission or long-term survival.[24]

Serum levels of HCG and alpha-fetoprotein are also key to the diagnosis, prognosis, and therapeutic monitoring of patients with testicular germ cell tumors (including choriocarcinoma, embryonal carcinoma, and teratocarcinoma), as well as ovarian germ cell tumors. These markers are both sensitive and specific markers for nonseminomatous germ cell testicular tumors. The relatively short half-lives of both HCG and alpha-fetoprotein allow rapid and accurate assessment of tumor burden in response to therapy, helping to guide the administration of appropriate treatment.[4] A multicenter study of over 5,000 testicular carcinoma patients with metastatic disease demonstrated that pretreatment HCG and alpha-fetoprotein levels were independent prognostic factors and has led to incorporation of pretreatment marker levels into the International Germ Cell Cancer Collaborative Group prognostic classification system.[24]

Breast Carcinoma The most important molecular diagnostic and prognostic breast cancer markers are the levels of tumor expression of ER and PR, as well as overexpression of HER2 (c-erb-B2). Expression of ER and/or PR not only helps stratify patients to receive endocrine therapies, it also appears to indicate better-prognosis tumors independent of endocrine-based interventions.[8] Despite these observations, there is, somewhat surprisingly, no standard laboratory methodology to evaluate breast cancer hormone receptor status. Conversely, HER2 overexpression in breast tumors is associated with a worse prognosis. Measurement of HER2 overexpression, generally by FISH analysis, is essential to select patients to receive anti-HER2–based therapies (such as the anti-HER2 monoclonal antibody trastuzumab) and perhaps adds value in predicting the response to anthracycline chemotherapy and endocrine therapies, although the latter remains controversial.[25,26]

Immunoassays using monoclonal antibodies to the CA 15.3 and CA 27.29 protein core antigens of the MUC1 glycoprotein have found widespread use for monitoring of metastatic breast cancer and evaluation of therapeutic response to systemic treatment.[27,28] Nonetheless, the diagnostic value of CA 15.3 and CA 27.29 monitoring for the early detection of recurrent breast cancer remains unproven, with no increases in survival demonstrated despite increased lead time in the detection of recurrence.[29]

The development of technologies capable of capturing and enumerating circulating tumor cells has led to their testing as predictive and therapy response markers. The US Food and Drug Administration–approved Immunicon platform relies on antibody-coated ferrous nanoparticles to isolate individual cells from patient samples, avoiding the high degree of cell loss associated with manual enrichment methods and cytospin slide preparation. In a prospective multicenter trial of 177 patients with untreated metastatic breast cancer, the detection of greater than five circulating tumor cells at baseline was associated with shorter progression-free survival and shorter overall survival. After patients started systemic therapy, finding more than five circulating tumor cells was also associated with worse prognosis, suggesting that circulating tumor cell numbers may help identify patients receiving futile therapy.[30] Along the same lines, quantitation of circulating endothelial cells using similar technologies has led to suggestions that this methodology may be useful to monitor angiogenic activity in response to antiangiogenesis therapy or as a marker of global tumor burden.[31]

Colorectal Carcinoma Serum CEA testing is the most frequently used clinical marker in colorectal cancer patients. Although typically associated with colorectal cancer, elevated serum levels can also be seen in a multitude of other epithelial malignancies, including breast, bladder, cervix, endometrium, gallbladder, stomach, liver, lung, pancreas, ovary, nasopharynx, and thyroid cancers. Furthermore, CEA levels can be elevated in a number of benign conditions, including breast disease, pulmonary emphysema, and inflammatory bowel disease. Owing to a lack of specificity, CEA screening is not recommended as a screening or early diagnostic marker for asymptomatic populations.[13,32] The prognostic use of serum CEA assays is in monitoring colorectal cancer patients after the primary surgical resection of tumor. At least two large clinical studies indicate that rising CEA levels are indicative of recurrence in 81% and 86% of patients, respectively, and provide approximately 5 months of lead time in diagnosis.[33–35] The 2000 update of the clinical practice guidelines of the ASCO references two studies that show that CEA was the most cost-effective approach to detecting potentially curative recurrent disease.[36,37] However, studies are inconclusive and/or contradictory in demonstrating cancer cures attributable to CEA monitoring, leading to ongoing debate as to whether the substantial cost and emotional stress associated with this intervention are worthwhile in the clinical setting.[38–41]

Lung Carcinoma There is a great need to develop effective screening methods for lung cancer owing to the high prevalence of disease and the worse prognosis associated with increasing disease stage at diagnosis.[42] TNM staging remains the most significant prognostic parameter in lung cancer, although numerous cytologic and molecular markers have been shown to be significantly and independently associated with prognosis, including microvessel density as a measure of angiogenesis, decreased levels of apoptosis, Ki-67 immunohistochemistry as a marker of proliferation, cell-cycle checkpoint control mutations, oncogenes, and signal transduction pathway receptor expression.[43,44] *TP53* gene mutations are the most common genetic abnormality in lung cancer,[45,46] although the association of mutated *TP53* and other molecular abnormalities (*P21* gene mutations, mutations in K-*ras*, alterations in RB–cyclin D1 and cyclin E–p16 pathways) with altered prognosis is inconsistent and remains controversial.[43,44,47] Currently, there are no well-established molecular prognostic markers in lung cancer consistently associated with patient survival or response to therapy, although active research continues into the development of early detection, diagnostic, and prognostic markers for this disease.

Ovarian Carcinoma Serum immunoassay for levels of the CA 125 glycoprotein antigen is the best established screening and diagnostic marker for ovarian carcinoma. Initial studies suggested that elevated CA 125 levels were seen in 83% of patients with ovarian carcinoma. However, most of these patients had stage III or IV disease at the time of diagnosis.[48] The value of serum CA 125 for detection of early-stage ovarian carcinoma is more limited. Only 50 to 60% of women with stage I malignancy have elevated serum CA 125 levels.[49,50] Further complicating the usefulness of quantifying CA 125 expression is the antigen's association with coelomic epithelium, including pleura, peritoneum, pericardium, and müllerian epithelia. Several nonmalignant conditions are associated with elevated CA 125 levels, including ovarian cysts, pelvic endometriosis, uterine fibroids, pericarditis, bleeding, pregnancy, and inflammatory processes.[51–53] These benign clinical conditions reduce the specificity of CA 125 screening for early ovarian cancer.

Although CA 125 is not an ideal marker for the detection of early ovarian carcinoma, it still has documented value for clinical follow-up during and after therapy.[54] The absolute level and rate of decline of CA 125 after treatment with chemotherapy predict the final clinical response of disease.[55,56] Among patients who relapse with ovarian carcinoma, elevated CA 125 levels at the time of recurrence are associated with a significantly worse prognosis compared with patients with normal levels.[57]

Prostate Carcinoma Serum PSA is the most widely used marker to detect, stage, and monitor prostate cancer.[58] Early reports suggested that PSA determination combined with digital rectal examination was an effective modality for prostate cancer screening and early detection.[59–61] The Surveillance, Epidemiology, and End Results (SEER) Program and Medicare claims data provided evidence that PSA testing was associated with an increased incidence of prostate cancer diagnosis in the 1980s[62] and was accompanied by migration toward diagnosis of early-stage disease.[63] However, despite these epidemiologic observations, there is still significant uncertainty concerning the impact of PSA screening on prostate cancer mortality.[64–66] Evidence is lacking from prospective studies to support the notion that PSA screening is beneficial in reducing mortality from the disease. There are suggestions that screening often detects what may be indolent, nonaggressive prostate cancer. Depending on the lower limit used, up to 20% of men with prostate cancer will have a "normal" PSA. There is also great overlap between benign and malignant disease: only 30% of men with a PSA of 4 to 10 ng/mL will have cancer, and a PSA up to 20 ng/mL is still compatible with benign prostatic hypertrophy. Furthermore, the great variability in the natural history of prostate cancers and morbidity associated with therapies such as radiation or radical prostatectomy without a proven decrease in mortality has led to debate over the value of PSA quantification as a screening test for prostate cancer.[67,68]

VALIDATING CANCER BIOMARKERS IN CLINICAL TRIALS

It is clear that current histopathology-based staging and risk stratification methods suboptimally predict tumor prognosis and/or therapeutic response. Innovative research in cancer biology has suggested potentially useful candidate markers and marker combinations that may eventually help to better optimize and individualize therapy. Unfortunately, there are currently few markers that have been rigorously tested and developed to allow reliable use in clinical practice.

The ultimate value of a tumor marker is its ability to classify different patient or tumor populations with respect to an outcome of interest. Although thousands of articles are published each year describing genetic mutations, molecular signaling variations, and alterations in protein expression associated with various types of cancer, these studies are predominantly retrospective in nature and have often been performed in only small numbers of patients. To develop these novel markers into tools that can be used reliably in the clinical setting, careful testing will need to be performed in large numbers of tumor specimens and compared with normal controls. Prospective incorporation of novel markers into clinical trials will be crucial to defining the sensitivity and specificity of potentially useful candidate assays. Validation of these markers will depend on careful clinical trial design that selects the appropriate patient population and chooses the proper end point.[69] Close cooperation between clinical researchers and cancer biologists will help translate scientific findings and high-throughput technologies into burgeoning clinically based discovery systems that will powerfully advance the understanding and treatment of human malignancy.

GLOBAL PROFILING OF TUMOR MARKERS

The rapid emergence of technologies capable of simultaneously evaluating multiple tumor properties such as gene mutations and alterations in gene transcription and translation, is transforming the experimental approaches and application of tumor markers.

High-throughput methodologies, such as microarray gene expression profiling, proteomic profiling, comparative genomic hybridization analysis, and metabolomics, enable the simultaneous analysis of thousands of tumor characteristics. Comprehensive profiling of tumors and/or patients has significant implications for malignant diagnosis, prognostic classification, and responses of individual malignancies to therapy.

DNA Microarray Profiling Deoxyribonucleic acid (DNA) microarray technologies are the most frequently used genome-wide approach to diagnose cancer or predict outcomes or response to therapy. DNA microarrays consist of oligonucleotide or complementary DNA probes for measuring the expression of hundreds or thousands of genes (in the form of messenger ribonucleic acid) in a single test.[70] Such assays have the capacity to reveal unique and distinguishable gene expression patterns in human tumors, such as breast,[71] bladder,[72] colon,[73] esophagus,[74] kidney,[75] liver,[76] lung,[77] ovarian, [78,79] pancreatic,[80] and prostate[81] carcinomas, as well as lymphomas,[82] leukemia,[83] and melanoma.[84] Global genomics technologies have led to insights into both the molecular etiology of malignancy and tumor marker discovery.[85,87] DNA microarray techniques are being actively investigated to diagnose and stage cancer, predict recurrence, and even evaluate the likelihood of response to therapy.[88,89]

The application of gene profiling assays to breast cancer illustrates the enthusiasm genotypic analysis to predict both the risk of recurrence and the response to therapy. Gene array analysis has led to the identification of a 21-gene recurrence score (Oncotype DX, Genomic Health Inc, Redwood City, CA, USA), which has been reported to exceed standard measures of patient age, tumor size, and tumor grade in predicting patient outcomes. This assay is based on a panel of 16 "cancer genes" and 5 "reference" genes that categorizes patients as being at low, intermediate, or high risk of recurrence. When this assay was applied to tissue samples from 645 node-negative, ER-positive breast cancer patients who had participated in the National Surgical Adjuvant Breast and Bowel Project (NSABP) B-14 Tamoxifen Benefit Study, it was observed that tamoxifen significantly increased the distant recurrence-free survival (the primary end point) in women deemed at intermediate risk of recurrence by the 21-gene score. Patients identified at high risk of recurrence by the recurrence score assay, however, did not benefit from tamoxifen. Similarly, when the 21-gene recurrence score was applied retrospectively to tissue samples from the NSABP B-20 Chemotherapy Benefit Study, which randomized breast cancer patients to receive either tamoxifen alone or tamoxifen plus adjuvant chemotherapy, the assay accurately predicted the response to chemotherapy. The addition of chemotherapy to tamoxifen in the assay's high-risk category of patients reduced the risk of distant recurrence at 10 years from 88 to 60% ($p = .001$), whereas patients identified as low risk did not benefit from additional chemotherapy. This 21-gene score has been reported to have both prognostic value in identifying high- and low-risk breast tumors and also adds predictive value in classifying those who can be expected to benefit, or not, from adjuvant therapies.[90]

Proteomic Pattern Profiling Surface-enhanced laser desorption ionization time of flight (SELDI-TOF) is a type of mass spectrometry that is useful in generating fingerprints of cell lysates and body fluids using on-chip protein fractionation coupled to time-of-flight separation. The resulting proteomic image can then be "read" using bioinformatics tools. SELDI technology has significant advantages over traditional low-throughput proteomics approaches such as two-dimensional polyacrylamide gel electrophoresis in its speed and amount of tissue required for analysis.[91] However, there continues to be a need to address the reproducibility of SELDI-TOF pattern analysis, along with the requirement (similar to all biomarkers) for validation.

The first application of pattern recognition algorithms coupled with high-throughput proteomic diagnostics was described in an experimental model of ovarian cancer detection. Although conventional therapies produce up to a 90% 5-year survival rate for stage I ovarian cancer, early detection of ovarian carcinoma is confounded by its lack of symptomatology.[92] However, a study using a discriminatory low-resolution high-output mass spectral pattern derived from the sera of women with and without a diagnosis of ovarian cancer was reportedly 100% successful in identifying ovarian cancer in a subsequent small test set of 50 patients and also assigned 95% of 66 healthy and benign controls correctly. Interestingly, this model was unable to classify serum from individuals with other types of malignancy, such as prostate cancer, indicating that disease-specific models can be generated.[93] Other investigators, however, have had difficulty in reproducing their analysis from the same primary data.[94,95]

The value of proteomic pattern diagnostics has been tested in other types of cancer as well. Profiling of blood sera has been used to detect and stage breast cancer in retrospective validation experiments with a sensitivity of 93% for malignancy and a specificity of 91% for controls.[96] Several discovery studies have looked at identifying serum proteomic signatures capable of distinguishing prostate cancer from benign prostatic hypertrophy, a frequent clinical diagnostic dilemma currently requiring biopsy to resolve. Patterns have been identified that are able to classify test sets of benign controls from prostate cancer with a sensitivity > 80% and a specificity > 95%.[97–99] Serum proteomic profiling is also being investigated with great interest to help easily distinguish benign pulmonary nodules from lung cancer.[100]

Unique Challenges to Validating Global Tumor Signature Markers Despite these compelling results, it is important to emphasize that the utility of using gene and protein signature profiles to classify cancers into clinically relevant subgroups still requires prospective large-scale validation studies. Multivariable predictive models have the potential to bring about "overfitting errors" when a large number of predictor variables are fit to a small number of subjects; such errors are not reproducible in a new set of data.[101] For instance, the "Amsterdam 70-gene prognostic signature" of breast cancer developed by the Netherlands Cancer Institute/Antoni van Leeuwenhoek Hospital was initially reported to outperform both the National Institutes of Health and St. Gallen clinicopathologic criteria in predicting recurrences and overall survival.[102] However, although external independent validation of the 70-gene signature continued to show predictive capacities, the outcomes were inferior compared with the original series.[103] As well, it is puzzling to note that distinctive predictive marker sets can often be identified from the same samples when different gene expression profiling platforms are used, with significant implications for the future development of diagnostic tests and biomarker discovery.[104] The performance of tumor signature stratification tools in predicting clinical outcomes demands careful validation using rigorous rules of evidence.

Future of Tumor Profiling Traditionally, oncologists have thought of cancers according to their site of origin (ie, breast, prostate, colon). However, knowing the tissue of origin becomes less important than understanding the intracellular pathway(s) that the cancer is exploiting to survive, grow, and avoid apoptosis. Ultimately, all cancer is a genetic disease, and technologies capable of assessing the myriad abnormalities within a malignant cell are essential not only to identify diagnostic and predictive markers but also to optimize drug discovery and therapy optimization. In particular, there is a growing need for markers and/or tumor profiles that help selected patient populations who would be most likely to respond to the novel, specific, molecularly targeted drugs. Individual prognostic and therapeutic response markers that reflect only one aspect of tumor biology are rapidly being superseded by genomic, transcriptional, and proteomic profiling of malignancies and malignant states.

REFERENCES

1. Srinivas PR, Kramer BS, Srivastava S. Trends in biomarker research for cancer detection. Lancet Oncol 2001;2:698–704.
2. Sidransky D. Emerging molecular markers of cancer. Nat Rev Cancer 2002;2:210–9.

3. Mera SL. Screening for cancer and pre-cancer. Br J Biomed Sci 1995;52:120–41.
4. Duffy MJ. Clinical uses of tumor markers: a critical review. Crit Rev Clin Lab Sci 2001;38:225–62.
5. Allred DC, Harvey JM, Berado M, et al. Prognostic and predictive factors in breast cancer by immunohistochemical analysis. Mol Pathol 1998;11:155–68.
6. Duffy MJ. Prognostic and predictive markers in cancer. J Clin Ligand Assay 1999;22:231–9.
7. McQuire WL. Steroid hormone receptors in breast cancer treatment strategy. Recent Prog Horm Res 1980;36:135–56.
8. Anderson et al. Tumor variants by hormone receptor expression in white patients with node-negative breast cancer from the Surveillance, Epidemiology and End Results database. J Clin Oncol 2001;19:18
9. Paik S, et al. erbB-2 and response to doxorubicin in patients with axillary lymph node positive, hormone receptor-negative breast cancer. J Natl Cancer Inst 1998;90:1361–70.
10. Paik S, et al. NSABP B-15. J Natl Cancer Inst 2000;92:1991–8.
11. Pegram M, Paulett G, Slamon DJ. HER-2/neu as a predictive marker of response to breast cancer therapy. Breast Cancer Res Treat 1998;52:65–77.
12. Ellis MJ, Coop A, Singh B et al. Letrozole is more effective neoadjuvant therapy than tamoxifen for ErbB-1 and/or ErbB-2-positive, estrogen receptor-positive primary breast cancer: evidence from a phase III trial. J Clin Oncol 2001;19:3808–16.
13. Bast RC Jr, Ravdin P, Hayes DF, et al. 2000 UPDATE of recommendations for the use of tumor markers in breast and colorectal cancer: clinical practice guidelines of the American Society of Clinical Oncology. J Clin Oncol 2001;19:1865–78.
14. Shepherd FA, Pereira J, Ciuleanu TE, et al. A randomized placebo-controlled trial of erlotinib in patients with advanced non-small cell lung cancer (NSCLC) following failure of 1st line or 2nd line chemotherapy. A National Cancer Institute of Canada Clinical Trials Group (NCIC CTG) trial. J Clin Oncol 2004;22(14 Suppl):7022.
15. Heinrich MC, Shoemaker JS, Corless CL, et al. Correlation of target kinase genotype with clinical activity of imatinib mesylate (IM) in patients with metastatic GI stromal tumors (GISTs) expressing KIT (KIT+) [abstract]. Proc Am Soc Clin Oncol 2005.
16. Paez et al. EGFR mutations in lung cancer: correlation with clinical response to gefitinib therapy. Science 2004;304:1497–500.
17. Lynch et al. Activating mutations in the epidermal growth factor receptor underlying responsiveness of non-small-cell lung cancer to gefitinib. N Engl J Med 2004;350:2129–39.
18. Kerbrat P, Lhommé C, Fervers B, et al. Standards, options and recommendations: ovarian cancer. Electron J Oncol 2001;1:32–42.
19. Scher HI. Management of prostate cancer after prostatectomy: treating the patient not the PSA. JAMA 1999;281:1642–5.
20. Segal R, Lukka H, Klotz LH, et al, Genitourinary Cancer Disease Site Group, Cancer Care Ontario Practice Guidelines Initiative. Surveillance programs for early stage non-seminomatous testicular cancer: a practice guideline. Can J Urol 2001;8:1184–92.
21. Pierce JG, Parson TF. Glycoprotein hormones. Structure and function. Annu Rev Biochem 1981;50:465–95.
22. Alfthan H, Stenman UH. Pathophysiological importance of various molecular forms of human choriogonadotropin. Mol Cell Endocrinol 1996;125:107–20.
23. Fisher PM, Hancock BW. Gestational trophoblastic disease and their treatment. Cancer Treat Rev 1997;23:1–16.
24. International Germ Cell Cancer Collaborative Group. International germ cell consensus classification. A prognostic factor-based staging system for metastatic germ cell cancers. J Clin Oncol 1997;15:594–603.
25. Cooke T, Reeves J, Lanigan A, et al. HER2 as a prognostic and predictive marker for breast cancer. Ann Oncol 2001;12:S23–8.
26. Yamauchi H, Stearns V, Hayes DF. When is a tumor marker ready for prime time? A case study of c-erbB-2 as a predictive factor in breast cancer. J Clin Oncol 2001;19:2334–56.
27. Stearns V, Yamauchi H, Hayes DF. Circulating tumor markers in breast cancer. Accepted utilities and novel prospects. Breast Cancer Res Treat 1998;52:239–59.
28. Cheung KL, Graves CRL, Robertson JFL. Tumour marker measurements in the diagnosis and monitoring of breast cancer. Cancer Treat Rev 2000;26:91–102.
29. Chan DW, Beveridge RA, Muss H, et al. Use of Truquant BR radioimmunoassay for early detection of breast cancer recurrence in patients with stage II and stage III disease. J Clin Oncol 1997;15:2322–8.
30. Cristofanilli M, Budd GT, Ellis MJ, et al. Circulating tumor cells, disease progression, and survival in metastatic breast cancer. N Engl J Med 2004;351:781–91.
31. Rugo HS, Dickler MN, Scott JH, et al. Circulating endothelial cells: a measure for angiogenesis inhibition [abstract]? Breast Cancer Res Treat 2004;88 Suppl 1:S142.
32. Stevens DP, Mackay IR, Cullen KJ, et al. Carcinoembryonic antigen in an unselected elderly population. A four-year follow-up. Br J Cancer 1975;32:147–52.
33. Wanebo HJ, Llaneras M, Martin T, et al. Prospective monitoring trial for carcinoma of colon and rectum after surgical resection. Surg Gynecol Obstet 1989;169:479–87.
34. Berman JM, Cheung R, Weinberg DS. Surveillance after colorectal cancer resection. Lancet 2000;355:395–9.
35. Minton JP, Hoehn JL, Gerber DM. Results of a 400 patients CEA second-look colorectal cancer study. Cancer 1985;55:1284–90.
36. Graham RA, Wang S, Catalano PJ, et al. Postsurgical surveillance of colon cancer: preliminary cost analysis of physician examination, carcinoembryonic antigen testing, chest x-ray, and colonoscopy. Ann Surg 1998;228:59–63.
37. Castells A, Bessa X, Daniels M, et al. Value of postoperative surveillance after radical surgery for colorectal cancer. Dis Colon Rectum 1998;41:714–24.
38. Moertel CG, Fleming TR, Macdonald JS, et al. An evaluation of the carcinoembryonic antigen (CEA) test for monitoring patients with resected colon cancer. JAMA 1993;270.
39. Chau I, Allen MJ, Cunningham D, et al. The value of routine serum carcino-embryonic antigen measurement and computed tomography in the surveillance of patients after adjuvant chemotherapy for colorectal cancer. J Clin Oncol 2004;22:1420–9.
40. Duffy MJ. Carcinoembryonic antigen as a marker for colorectal cancer. Is it clinically useful? Clin Chem 2001;47:624–30.
41. Seregni E, Ferrari L, Martinetti A, et al. Diagnostic and prognostic tumor markers in the gastrointestinal tract. Semin Surg Oncol 2001;20:147–66.
42. Mountain CT. Revision in the international system for staging of lung cancer. Chest 1997;111:1710–7.
43. Junker K. Prognostic factors in stage I/II non-small cell lung cancer. Lung Cancer 2001;33:S17–24.
44. Niklinski J, Niklinska W, Laudanski J, et al. Prognostic molecular markers in non-small cell lung cancer. Lung Cancer 2001;34:S53–8.
45. Hainaut P, Soussi T, Shomer B, et al. Database of p53 gene somatic mutations in human tumors and cell lines. Updated compilation and future prospects. Nucleic Acids Res 1997;25:151–7.
46. Hussain SP, Hollstein MH, Harris CC. p53 tumor suppressor gene. At the crossroads of molecular carcinogenesis, molecular epidemiology, and human risk assessment. Ann N Y Acad Sci 2000;919:79–85.
47. Flaman JM, Frebourg T, Moreau V, et al. A simple p53 functional assay for screening cell lines, blood, and tumors. Proc Natl Acad Sci U S A 1995;92:3963–7.
48. Bast RC, Klug TL, St John E, et al. A radioimmunoassay using a monoclonal antibody to monitor the course of epithelial ovarian cancer. N Engl J Med 1983;309:169–71.
49. Jacobs I, Davies AP, Bridges J, et al. Prevalence screening for ovarian cancer in postmenopausal women by CA 125 measurement and ultrasonography. BMJ 1993;306:1030–3.
50. Jacobs IJ, Skates S, Davies AP, et al. Risk of diagnosis of ovarian cancer after raised serum CA-125 concentration. A prospective cohort study. BMJ 1996;313:1355–8.
51. Bast RC Jr, Xu FJ, Yu YH, et al. CA 125. The past and the future. Int J Biol Markers 1998;13:179–87.
52. Grover S, Quinn MA, Weidemann P, et al. Factors influencing serum CA 125 levels in normal women. Obstet Gynecol 1992;79:511–4.
53. Zeimet AG, Offner FA, Mullerholzner E, et al. Peritoneum and tissues of the female reproductive tract as physiological sources of CA-125. Tumour Biol 1998;19:275–82.
54. Bast RC, Klug TL, Schaetz IE, et al. Monitoring human ovarian carcinoma with a combination of CA 125, CA 19.9, and carcinoembryonic antigen. Am J Obstet Gynecol 1984;149:553–9.
55. van der Burg MEL, Lammes FB, van Putten WLJ, et al. Ovarian cancer. The prognostic value of the serum half-life of CA 125 during induction chemotherapy. Gynecol Oncol 1988;30:307–12.
56. Yedema CA, Kenemans P, Voorhorst F, et al. CA 125 half-life in ovarian cancer. A multivariate survival analysis. Br J Cancer 1993;67:1361–7.
57. Makar AP, Kristensen G, Bormer OP, et al. Is serum CA 125 at the time of relapse a prognostic indicator for further survival prognosis in patients with ovarian cancer? Gynecol Oncol 1993;49:3–7.
58. Partin AQ, Oesterling JE. The clinical usefulness of prostate specific antigen. Update 1994. J Urol 1994;152:13–68.
59. Cooner WH, Mosley BR, Rutherford CL Jr, et al. Prostate cancer detection in a clinical urological practice by ultrasonography, digital rectal examination and prostate specific antigen. J Urol 1990;143:1146–52.
60. Brawer MK, Chetner MP, Beatie J, et al. Screening for prostate carcinoma with prostate specific antigen. J Urol 1992;147:841–5.
61. Labrie F, Dupont A, Suburu R, et al. Serum prostate specific antigen as pre-screening test for prostate cancer. J Urol 1992;147:846–51.
62. Potosky AL, Miller BA, Albertsen PC, et al. The role of increasing detection in the rising incidence of prostate cancer. JAMA 1995;273:548–52.
63. Perrotti M, Rabbani F, Farkas A, et al. Trends in poorly differentiated prostate cancer 1973 to 1994. Observations from the Surveillance, Epidemiology and End Results database. J Urol 1998;160:81–5.
64. Neal DE, Leung HY, Powell PH, et al. Unanswered questions in screening for prostate cancer. Eur J Cancer 2000;36:1316–21.
65. Potosky AL, Feuer EJ, Levin DL. Impact of screening on incidence and mortality of prostate cancer in the United States. Epidemiol Rev 2001;23:181–6.
66. Perron L, Moore L, Bairati I. PSA screening and prostate cancer mortality. Can Med Assoc J 2002;166:586–91.
67. Graversen PH, Nielsen KT, Gasser TC, et al. Radical prostatectomy versus expectant primary treatment in stages I and II prostatic cancer. A fifteen-year follow-up. Urology 1990;36:493–8.
68. Johansson JE, Holmberg L, Johansson S, et al. Fifteen-year survival in prostate cancer. A prospective, population-based study in Sweden [published erratum appears in JAMA 1997;278:206]. JAMA 1997;277:467–71.
69. Sargent DJ, Conley BA, Allegra C, Collette L. Clinical trial designs for predictive marker validation in cancer treatment trials. J Clin Oncol 2005;23:2020–7.
70. Pusztai L, Ayers M, Stec J, Hortobagyi GN. Clinical applications of cDNA microarrays in oncology. Oncologist 2003;8:252–8.
71. Perou CM, Sorlie T, Eisen MB, et al. Molecular portraits of human breast tumours. Nature 2000;406:747–52.
72. Dyrskjot L, Kruhoffer M, Thykjaer T, et al. Gene expression in the urinary bladder: a common carcinoma in situ gene expression signature exists disregarding histopathological classification. Cancer Res 2004;64:4040–8.
73. Notterman DA, Alon U, Sierk AJ, et al. Transcriptional gene expression profiles of colorectal adenoma, adenocarcinoma, and normal tissue examined by oligonucleotide arrays. Cancer Res 2001;61:3124–30.
74. Kan T, Shimada Y, Sato F, et al. Prediction of lymph node metastasis with use of artificial neural networks based on gene expression profiles in esophageal squamous cell carcinoma. Ann Surg Oncol 2004;11:1070–8.
75. Yang XJ, Tan MH, Kim HL, et al. A molecular classification of papillary renal cell carcinoma. Cancer Res 2005;65:5628–37.
76. Liu K, Lei XZ, Zhao LS, et al. Tissue microarray for high-throughput analysis of gene expression profiles in hepatocellular carcinoma. World J Gastroenterol 2005;11:1369–72.
77. Talbot SG, Estilo C, Maghami E, et al. Gene expression profiling allows distinction between primary and metastatic squamous cell carcinomas in the lung. Cancer Res 2005;65:3063–71.
78. Sawiris GP, Sherman-Baust CA, Becker KG, et al. Development of a highly specialized cDNA array for the study and diagnosis of epithelial ovarian cancer. Cancer Res 2002;62:2923–8.
79. Mok SC, Chao J, Skates S, et al. Prostasin, a potential serum marker for ovarian cancer. Identification through microarray technology. J Natl Cancer Inst 2001;93:1458–64.
80. Heidenblad M, Lindgren D, Veltman JA, et al. Microarray analyses reveal strong influence of DNA copy number alterations on the transcriptional patterns in pancreatic cancer: implications for the interpretation of genomic amplifications. Oncogene 2005;24:1794–801.
81. Halvorsen OJ, Oyan AM, Bo TH, et al. Gene expression profiles in prostate cancer: association with patient subgroups and tumour differentiation. Int J Oncol 2005;26:329–36.
82. Zu Y, Steinberg SM, Campo E, et al. Validation of tissue microarray immunohistochemistry staining and interpre-

tation in diffuse large B-cell lymphoma. Leuk Lymphoma 2005;46:693–701.
83. Kearney L, Horsley SW. Molecular cytogenetics in haematological malignancy: current technology and future prospects. Chromosoma 2005;:1–9.
84. Mori T, Kim J, Yamano T, et al. Epigenetic up-regulation of C-C chemokine receptor 7 and C-X-C chemokine receptor 4 expression in melanoma cells. Cancer Res 2005;65:1800–7.
85. Velculescu VE, Zhang L, Vogelstein B, et al. Serial analysis of great expression. Science 1995;270:484–7.
86. Zhang L, Zhou W, Velculescu VE, et al. Gene expression profiles in normal and cancer cells. Science 1997;276:1268–72.
87. Alizadeh AA, Ross DT, Perou CM, et al. Towards a novel classification of human malignancies based on gene expression patterns. J Pathol 2001;195:41–52.
88. Su AI, Welsh JB, Sapinoso LM, et al. Molecular classifications of human carcinomas by use of gene expression signatures. Cancer Res 2001;61:7388–93.
89. Ryu B, Jones J, Hollingsworth A, et al. Invasion-specific genes in malignancy. Serial analysis of gene expression comparisons of primary and passaged cancers. Cancer Res 2001;61:1833–8
90. Paik S, Shak S, Tang G, et al. A multigene assay to predict recurrence of tamoxifen-treated, node-negative breast cancer. N Engl J Med 2004;351(27).
91. Wulkuhle JD, Liotta LA, Petricoin EF. Proteomic applications for the early detection of cancer. Nat Rev Can 2003;3:267–75.
92. Menon U, Jacobs IJ. Tumor markers. In: Hoskin WJ, Perez CA, Young RC, editors. Principles and practice of gynecologic oncology. Philadelphia: Lippincott, Williams and Wilkins; 2000. p. 165–82.
93. Petricoin EF, et al. Use of proteomic patterns in serum to identify ovarian cancer. Lancet 2002;359:572–7.
94. Baggerly KA, Morris JS, Coombes KR. Reproducibility of SELDI-TOF protein patterns in serum: comparing datasets from different experiments. Bioinformatics 2004;20:777–85.
95. Baggerly KA, Edmonson SR, Morris JS, Coombes KR. High resolution serum proteomic patterns for cancer detection. Endocr Relat Cancer 2004;11:583–4.
96. Li J, Zhang Z, Rosenzweig J, et al. Proteomics and bioinformatics approaches for identification of serum biomarkers to detect breast cancer. Clin Chem 2002;48:1296–304.
97. Adam BL, et al. Serum fingerprinting coupled with a pattern-matching algorithm distinguishes prostate cancer from benign prostate hyperplasia and healthy men. Cancer Res 2002;62:3609–14.
98. Qu Y, et al. Boosted decision tree analysis of surface-enhanced laser desorption/ionization mass spectral serum profiles discriminates prostate cancer from non-cancer patients. Clin Chem 2002;48:1835–43.
99. Petricoin EF, et al. Serum proteomic patterns for detection of prostate cancer. J Natl Cancer Inst 2002;94:1576–8.
100. Ching CD, Mosca P, Fusaro V, et al. Differentiating benign states from non small cell lung cancer using serum proteomic profiling [abstract]. 2004 FDA Science Forum
101. Ransohoff DF. Rules of evidence for cancer molecular-marker discovery and validation. Nat Rev Cancer 2004;4:309–14.
102. Van de Vijver et al. N Engl J Med 2002
103. Picarrt M, et al. Multi-center external validation study of the Amsterdam 70-gene prognostic signature in node-negative untreated breast cancer—interim report. SABCS 2004
104. Pusztai L, Wang J, Coombes K, et al. Cross platform comparison of multigene predictors of response to neoadjuvant paclitaxel/FAC chemotherapy in breast cancer generated by cDNA arrays and Affymetrix GeneChips [abstract]. Proc Am Soc Clin Oncol 2004.

12c

Effectors of Immunity

Timothy M. Clay, PhD
H. Kim Lyerly, MD
Lauretta Odogwu-Oti, MD
Michael A. Morse, MD

The precise mechanisms of the immune response to cancer are increasingly being uncovered and will assist in the design of new immunotherapeutic approaches, as detailed in this book. In this chapter, we provide an overview of the immune response to cancer as a framework for the detailed discussion of the novel therapeutic approaches to follow. This overview seeks to provide a primer on our current understanding of the immune response to cancer, and we focus on concepts and hypotheses rather than on a detailed history of the experimental evidence that led to these concepts being proposed. The concept of immunosurveillance is discussed elsewhere in this book and is not covered here.

OVERVIEW OF EFFECTORS IN THE HOST IMMUNE RESPONSE

The immune response can be divided into the innate system consisting of cells that do not need to be primed to recognize tumor. Rather, they recognize molecular patterns that "signal danger" (see below). The adaptive system consists of effectors that must be "preactivated," that is, they must have been exposed to the antigen (or a molecular mimic) previously to respond to a new challenge. Principal effector cells in the innate immune response to cancer are natural killer (NK) cells, natural killer T (NKT) cells, and macrophages, whereas the principal effectors of adaptive immunity are T lymphocytes and antibodies produced by B cells. Figure 12c-1 summarizes the major components of the antitumor immune response. The role of each of the major cell types is discussed individually below, but it should be stressed that this is a cooperative effort involving many cell types, and it is the quality of the interaction of these cells with the tumor and with each other that dictates how effective this immune response ultimately is. It should also be underscored that tumors can evolve mechanisms that disrupt immune function, and these are discussed later in this chapter.

Cytotoxic T Lymphocytes Cytotoxic T cells are $CD8^+$ T lymphocytes. At the simplest level, cytotoxic T lymphocytes (CTLs) recognize (via their T-cell receptor [TCR]) tumor-derived peptides presented on the surface of the tumor cells by major histocompatibility complex (MHC) molecules. Enormous TCR diversity generated by gene rearrangements and recombination events during T-cell development provides an extremely diverse "repertoire" of T cells expressing different TCRs, which should permit responses to any and all antigens. Indeed, it has been estimated that 10E15 different TCRs can be generated.[1] However, most tumor-associated antigens recognized by T cells are peptides derived from nonmutated self-proteins, and during T-cell development in the thymus, cells expressing TCR that react with self-proteins above a theoretic affinity "threshold" are deleted (negatively selected) to avoid the potential for autoimmunity. Consequently, the repertoire of T cells expressing TCR that can recognize TAA is generally made up of TCRs with only intermediate or low affinity. What does all of this mean? The pool of T cells that can recognize the TAA is depleted of cells expressing high-affinity TCR, which, in part, explains why even when these T cells are present, the tumor can continue to grow and metastasize. In contrast, the T-cell response to viruses is more potent and often clinically effective. There are T cells expressing high-affinity TCR for viral antigens because these are not self-antigens. The T-cell response to common viruses, such as cytomegalovirus and Epstein-Barr virus, is sufficient to suppress the virus in healthy carriers.

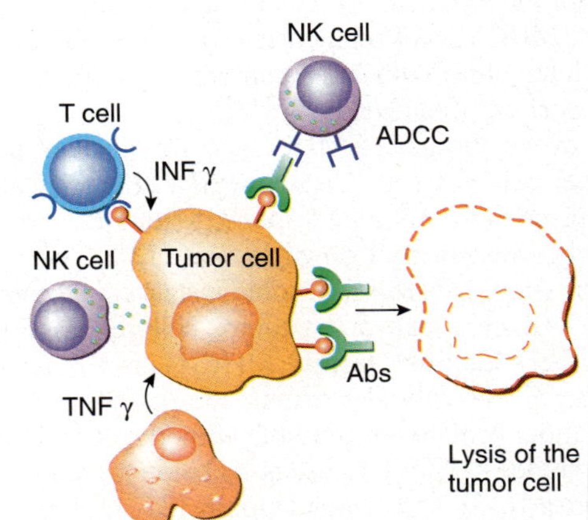

Figure 12c-1 Mechanisms responsible for death of tumor cells co-incubated with immune effector cells or antibodies. T cells, which recognize antigens expressed by the tumor, became activated and produce interferon (IFN) γ and lymphotoxin, which contribute to tumor cell death, as well as other cytokines capable of activating natural killer (NK) cells and macrophages. NK cells release perforin- and granzyme-containing granules. Macrophages release tumor necrosis factor (TNF) γ and other cytokines as well as reactive oxygen intermediates. Antibodies (Abs) to tumor-specific antigens (TSAs) induce arrest of tumor growth or mediate antibody-dependent cellular toxicity (ADCC) by arming effector cells endowed with FcR (NK cells or macrophages).

T-cell recognition of a tumor can lead to activation and proliferation of the T cells and ultimately to direct destruction of the tumor cells by cytotoxic T cells and the support of CTL proliferation by $CD4^+$ T helper (Th) cells (discussed below). However, the context in which antigens are recognized is important. The "two-signal" model of T-cell recognition of antigen indicates that, in addition to TCR engagement by a cognate antigen–MHC complex, the additional interaction of the T cell surface receptor CD28 with CD80 (B7.1) or CD86 (B7.2) on the antigen-presenting cell (APC) is necessary for generation of antigen-specific immune responsiveness. Without this costimulation, antigen-specific T cells enter a state of tolerance and possibly apoptosis. Since tumors will often, through a natural selection process, evolve to lose expression of MHC molecules and key costimulatory molecules to avoid activating CTLs.[2–4]

Other so-called "professional" APCs, namely dendritic cells (DCs), are a key component of CTL responses to tumors (see below). T-cell recognition of tumors also relies on presentation of tumor antigen–derived peptides on the cell surface by MHC molecules. As discussed later, tumors frequently down-regulate expression of MHC molecules and thereby evade recognition by T cells.

Recent studies have further defined the phenotype of T-cell clonotypes based on the definition of so-called naive versus central and effector memory subsets.[5–9] Growing evidence indicates that memory $CD4^+$ and $CD8^+$ T cells comprise at least two functionally distinct subsets: the central memory T cells, which express the chemokine receptor CCR7 and CD62 ligand and home to the T-cell areas of secondary lymphoid organs, and the effector memory T cells, which have lost the expression of CCR7 and have acquired the capacity to migrate to nonlymphoid tissues. Growing evidence suggests that common gamma chain cytokines, interleukin (IL)-2, IL-4, IL-7, and IL-15, play a major role in T-cell homeostasis and may regulate T-cell phenotype. Thus, the naive or memory phenotype of the immune response can be determined and the nature of the T-cell phenotype and can skew the immune response, making it more or less effective at responding to tumors.

T Helper Cells Th cells are $CD4^+$ T lymphocytes that, as the name suggests, provide "help" for other immune cells. Specifically, they secrete cytokines that promote the proliferation and activation of CTLs, B cells, DCs, and other immune cells. They, too, recognize tumor antigen–derived peptides presented by MHC class II molecules via their TCR, and those Th cells that expressed high-affinity TCR for self-TAA are generally considered to be deleted during thymic selection. Again, although tumors can be recognized directly by this mechanism, generally, Th cells are primed by DCs or B cells acting as APCs. Different subsets of Th cells have pronounced differences in their effect on the immune response. Subsets that suppress immune responses or support immune responses, based in part on the cytokines they secrete, have recently been identified and are discussed in greater detail below. An important second signal for B cells has been identified as being provided by CD40 ligand (CD40L), which is expressed on the Th cell surface after activation. At this point, the T-cell surface alone is strongly stimulatory and will activate even naive B cells. The original definition of Th1 versus Th2 T-cell subsets was first made 20 years ago and was based on their distinct cytokine secretion profiles (interferon-γ for Th1 and IL-4 and IL-10 for Th2 cells).[10–13]

Regulatory T Cells A specific group of T cells, suppressor T cells, is thought to be involved in "turning down" the immune response. Like Th cells, suppressor or regulatory T cells, as they are more commonly now called, are stimulated by antigen, but instead of releasing lymphokines that activate B cells (and other cells), suppressor T cells release factors that suppress the B-cell and T-cell responses. Additionally, immunoregulatory T cells can mediate suppression by cell–cell contact, and this suppressive effect is dependent on surface-bound transforming growth factor β on the regulatory T cells.[14]

Although originally proposed by Gershon and Kondo in the 1970s, the concept of suppressor T cells had lapsed into relative obscurity, in part because these cells were so difficult to unequivocally identify.[15] However, recently, Sakaguchi and colleagues were able to identify T regulatory cells (Tregs).[16] These cells are phenotypically identified as $CD4^+CD25^+$ T cells. CD25 and two other subunits (CD122 and CD132) make up the high-affinity IL-2 receptor that is expressed by Tregs. CD25 provides a useful marker for Treg identification because Tregs depend on IL-2 for their survival and function.[17–19]

Unfortunately, CD25 expression has also been found on non-Treg cells, including activated T cells, making the definitive identification of Tregs based on surface phenotypic makers problematic. Other markers, such as GITR and CTLA-4, have also been described on Tregs, but similar to CD25, these markers are often found on activated T cells too.

FoxP3, the forkhead-winged–helix family transcription factor, was originally identified as being responsible for an X-linked recessive inflammatory disease in scurfy mice.[20] FoxP3-deficient mice fail to develop Treg cells, resulting in inflammatory disease. These symptoms can be prevented by adoptive transfer of $CD4^+CD25^+$ Treg cells.[21] Since FoxP3 is crucial for the development and function of Tregs and is not expressed by activated T cells, it is currently the "best" marker for identifying a true $CD4^+$ Treg.[22] Currently, flow cytometric assessment of FoxP3 levels is not reliable, in part because this is a nuclear protein and effective antibodies for intracellular flow cytometry staining are not available, so quantitative reverse transcriptase–polymerase chain reaction is the most informative analysis method for FoxP3 expression.[23]

NK Cells NK cells are a type of lymphocyte that mediates innate immunity against pathogens and tumors. They are identified by their phenotypic expression profile as $CD3^-$, $CD56^+$, and $CD16^+$. They comprise up to 15% of peripheral blood lymphocytes and are found in peripheral tissues, including the liver, peritoneal cavity, and placenta. NK cells use the same killing mechanisms as CTLs (described in detail below) and can secrete cytokines similar to those secreted by CTLs. Unlike B and T cells, NK cells do not express a single, invariant receptor molecule. Instead, they express multiple activating and inhibitory receptors, and, seemingly, the synthesis of these signals determines the functional response of the NK cell. Not all NK cells carry the same group of receptors. Distinct groups of receptors are expressed by different NK cells. Unlike T cells, antigen recognition is not via MHC molecules presenting antigen. In fact, MHC class I molecules can inhibit NK cells by interacting with killer inhibitory receptors on the surface of the NK cells.[24,25]

In the absence of MHC class I molecules, the target cell is lysed. Consequently, NK cells are involved in the immune response to tumors, particularly when tumors down-regulate MHC class I expression. Moreover, in some instances, it seems that NK cells can reject tumor cells expressing NKG2D ligands, despite MHC class I expression.[26,27] NK cells also express the FcγRIII and are a major mediator of antibody-dependent cellular cytotoxicity (ADCC) (discussed below). They also express IL-2R and respond rapidly to IL-2 stimulation, becoming activated, and can reject tumors in mouse models depleted of T cells.

NKT Cells NKT cells are a subset of lymphocytes that express both T-cell and NK-cell markers. They recognize glycolipid antigen in the context of the MHC-like molecule CD1d via their semi-invariant surface TCR. In mice, this is predominantly made up of Vα14 and Vβ11, whereas in humans, most NKT cells express Vα24 and Vβ11 TCR variable region segments.[28,29]

NKT cells are an area of intense study, are thought to play a role in biasing the immune response toward Th1 or Th2 imbalance, and are implicated in immunosurveillance and protection against carcinogenesis; conversely, a regulatory or immunosuppressive subset of NKT cells was also recently reported. NKT cells recognize α-GalCer in the context of the MHC class I–like molecule CD1. Although the number of NKT cells is small, they can produce large amounts of IL-4 or interferon (IFN)-γ, cytokines that promote humoral or cellular immunity, respectively. Recently, a different role has been identified for NKT cells, that of immunosuppressor cells. Studies in mice have demonstrated that NKT cells can mediate suppression of antitumor immunity in vivo, and IL-13 was shown to be the key mediator.[30] More recently, we have shown a similar role for human NKT cells in an in vitro culture system; specifically, the $CD4^+$ subset of NKT cells acts as a regulatory NKT cell, and IL-4 and IL-10 were the key mediators of this suppression.[31]

Macrophages Normal macrophages are phagocytic APCs with a central role in the control of infectious pathogens. A similar role would also be predicted in antitumor immunity, but evidence suggests that, on the contrary, tumor-associated macrophages (TAMs) are immunoinhibitory in function. TAMs mediate immunosuppressive effects through the secretion of prostaglandins, inhibitory cytokines such as IL-10, and the release of reactive oxygen metabolites. Consequently, evidence suggests that increased infiltration by TAMs is inversely correlated with survival in a number of human cancers.[32,33]

B Cells For B cells, tumor antigen recognition occurs via the B-cell receptor (BCR), which is a monospecific immunoglobulin or antibody expressed on the surface of B cells. In a manner analogous to that of the TCR, the BCR locus also permits generation of massive BCR diversity. However, the affinity of the antibodies produced by B cells can undergo a unique process of "affinity maturation" to selectively increase the binding affinity of antibodies.[34] B cells that have been primed by antigen recognition are unable to proliferate and differentiate unless prompted by the action of T-cell lymphokines. Thus, as is true for T cells, the B cell normally receives two stimulating events. First, its antibody receptors bind to the antigen; second, it receives cytokine stimulation from stimulated Th cells. This form of activation is called "T dependent." A few antigens can directly activate B cells. These antigens are free floating in solution and have not been processed in any way. They are usually very large molecules that can bind to numerous antibody receptors on a B cell simultaneously. This multiple binding (crosslinking of BCRs) seems to trigger the B cell into a response without any stimulation from Th cells. Typically, most antigens are first processed by APCs and are then presented to the B cells. These same APCs are also capable of presenting antigen to Th cells. The stimulated Th cells then release lymphokines that act on "primed" B cells, inducing B-cell proliferation and differentiation. Once stimulated, the B cells themselves can function as APCs to recruit even more B and T cells to the inflammatory site. Recognition of antigen results in differentiation of the B cell into a plasma cell, which is essentially an antibody factory that secretes large quantities of that cell's particular antibody. Antibodies patrol the body and tag invaders for destruction by other cells of the immune system. The variety and specificity of antibodies are astounding. There are antibodies specific for the molecules present on virtually every virus and bacterium. However, in cancer, the natural antibody response against tumor cells is weak. Despite this fact, antibodies can be harnessed for effective immunotherapy.

Dendritic Cells The foregoing discussion has not only highlighted many of the cells that play a key role in the immune response to tumors but has also frequently discussed the central role that DCs play in inducing these cells to recognize tumor antigens and become activated to perform their antitumor functions. DCs function to capture, process, and present antigens from dying tumor cells and traffic to draining lymph nodes, where they "prime" CTLs and Th and B cells.[35,36] Thus, DCs are sometimes referred to as the "sentinels" of the immune system. The interplay between NK and NKT cells with DCs is increasingly being revealed, with DCs thus providing a bridge to link innate and adaptive immunity.[37,38] A number of different states of DC maturation have been described, based on surface marker expression and function. So-called "immature" dendritic cells are very efficient at endocytosing antigen and processing the antigenic proteins into short peptides. However, they lack high levels of MHC molecules and costimulatory molecules that are required for optimal T-cell priming. DCs can be "matured" by a variety of agents, including cytokines and other stimuli (eg, bacterial lipopolysaccharide, IFN-γ with CD40L trimer, and Toll-like receptor ligands).[39–42] These "matured" DCs are not as efficient at capturing and processing antigen but have high levels of surface MHC molecules and costimulatory molecules (eg, CD80 [B7.1] or CD86 [B7.2]) and secrete cytokines that stimulate T-cell function (eg, IL-12). Thus, these matured DCs are very potent stimulators of T-cell activation. DCs also act as APCs for B cells and prime B cells. DCs also interact with NK and NKT cells, events that can mediate DC activation and lead to the differentiation of NK and NKT cells. Increasingly, the immune response is being shown to be controlled by a complex network of interactions mediated by cell–cell contact, cytokines, and chemokines and involving the diverse array of cell types. As our understanding of these complex interactions grows, we may develop better methods to harness the immune system to fight cancer. The immune system uses a complex set of "checks and balances" to maintain immune homeostasis, so perturbing one cell type or one interaction may not be sufficient to accomplish the profound changes needed to invoke a potent and long-lived antitumor response to an antigen to which the patient is tolerant. Thus, these basic biology studies elucidating the interplay of all of the elements will shape immunotherapy design.

CELL-MEDIATED KILLING OF TUMOR CELLS

Direct cancer cell lysis is mediated primarily by cytotoxic T cells and NK cells. CTLs and NK cells can kill tumor cells through two different mechanisms: the fas-fas-L pathway and the perforin-granzyme pathway. It was originally believed that the two pathways had separate functions, with Fas-Fas-L being involved in immunity development, activation and elimination of T cells during thymic development and in the periphery, CTL-mediated lysis, activation-induced cell death, regulation of inflammatory responses, and as a costimulatory pathway in T-cell activation. In contrast, the perforin-granzyme pathway was thought to be involved in the immune response to bacterial and viral pathogens. Recent evidence suggests that both pathways can be involved in many of these same areas, so the distinction has become blurred. The mechanism of the Fas-Fas-L (CD95-CD178) pathway was one of the earliest apoptotic signal transduction pathways to be identified. The Fas receptor is a member of the tumor necrosis factor (TNF) receptor family. It is expressed on many tissues, and TNF and other proinflammatory cytokines can increase its expression during inflammation. Fas expression is also increased on activated B and T cells, and it has a role in activation-induced cell death. Fas-Fas-L belongs to the TNF family and is expressed predominantly on activated T cells, macrophages, and neutrophils. However, it has also been detected on various tissues, particularly during inflammation. Fas-mediated apoptosis starts with the binding of a Fas-Fas-L trimer on the effector cell surface to a Fas trimer on the target cell membrane, which results in the formation of the death-inducing signaling complex (DISC) around the cytoplasmic chain of Fas. DISC formation leads to the sequential interaction of Fas with the adaptor protein Fas-associated death-domain protein (FADD) through homologous association of their death domains. Subsequently, a chain of events leads to the eventual apoptosis of the target.

The second pathway used by CTLs and NK cells to kill target cells is the perforin-granzyme pathway. The pore-forming molecule perforin is a crucial effector molecule of cytolysis by CTLs and NK cells. Perforin is a pore-forming molecule that is critical to the cytolytic effector function of CTL and NK cells. It is stored in cytotoxic granules, together with granzymes. On recognition of a target cell, the granules are released, and perforin monomers insert themselves into the target cell membrane and interact to create pores. These perforin pores can cause osmotic lysis of the target cell and allow granzymes to enter the target cell and induce apoptosis through various downstream effector pathways.

ANTIBODY-MEDIATED KILLING OF TUMOR CELLS

Two classic mechanisms of antibody-mediated killing can potentially impact tumors. Human antibodies, especially immunoglobulin (Ig)G1 and IgG3, can direct the killing of tumor cells by ADCC or complement-dependent cytotoxicity. ADCC is triggered by an interaction between the Fc region of an antibody that has bound, through its antigen binding region, to a tumor cell and the Fc receptors (FcRs), particularly FcRI and FcRIII, on immune effector cells such as neutrophils, NK cells, and macrophages. Depending on the type of effector cell involved, the tumor cell is eliminated either by phagocytosis or by lysis. In complement-dependent cytotoxicity, recruitment of the complement component C1q by IgG bound to the tumor cell surface triggers a proteolytic cascade to activate complement. This can potentially lead to the formation of a membrane attack complex that kills the target cell by rupturing its cell membrane. Alternatively, tumor cell–bound C1q can bind to complement receptors, such as C1qR, CR1 (CD35), and CR3 (CD11b/CD18), on effector cells, such as neutrophils, macrophages, and NK cells. This can also trigger cell-mediated tumor cell lysis or phagocytosis, depending on the type of effector cell.

A third means of antibody-induced tumor killing is by the induction of apoptosis, which may occur when antibody crosslinking occurs, antibodies bind to death receptors, or antibodies perturb receptor–ligand interactions and block signals essential for growth or survival.[43,44] For example, apoptosis is at least part of the mechanism of action of rituximab.[45,46]

Recently, evidence has emerged of another antibody-mediated antitumor mechanism that does not involve direct tumor cell killing. Polyclonal antisera generated against the tumor antigen HER2 by peptide vaccination in cancer patients have been shown to block tumor growth by preventing phosphorylation of HER2 on tyrosine Y1248, a residue critical for HER2 signaling through extracellular signal-regulated kinase. These antibodies also suppressed extracellular signal-regulated kinase phosphorylation and inhibited colony formation in soft agar.[47] Thus, anti-HER2 antibodies can effectively suppress HER2 kinase activity and downstream signaling to inhibit the transformed phenotype of HER2-expressing tumor cells.

CYTOKINES IMPORTANT TO THE IMMUNE RESPONSE

A variety of cytokines, both stimulatory and inhibitory to the immune response, are elaborated in the process of immune recognition. Matzinger hypothesized that the process by which the body's defenses recognize and mount immune responses against potential pathogens is initiated through the detection of "danger signals."[48,49] Some of the specific factors that serve as danger signals to the immune system have been discovered and include agents such as TNF-α, CD40L, and IFN-γ. These agents appear to act in part by stimulating the maturation of DCs, particularly in appropriate combinations and temporal sequences.[39,50]

When fully matured, DCs produce cytokines such as IL-12, IL-15, and IL-18, which drive antigen-specific Th1-type immunity. In turn, Th1 responses appear to be important for the generation of antitumor T-cell activity.[51–53]

These cytokines act in part through a direct effect on activated Th cells and stimulate the release of Th1 cytokines, such as IL-2 and IFN-γ.[52] IL-12 also promotes the development of CTLs with a Th1 phenotype (Tc1) and therefore may directly and indirectly enhance the antitumor response to melanoma vaccines.[54] In addition, IL-12 up-regulates class I and II MHC and intercellular adhesion molecule 1 on melanoma cells and therefore may augment the ability of CTLs to recognize and lyse them.[55,56] Overexpression of IL-15 in transgenic mice has shown that this cytokine can enhance both CTL and NK cell function and augments their antitumor effects on melanomas in vivo.[57]

CONCLUSION

Clearly, the immune system has the capacity to attack cancer. However, the immune system, like many biologic systems, is subject to homeostatic mechanisms. Immune homeostasis is the process through which the immune system responds to changes invoked by, for example, viral infection or tumor growth, and seeks to return to equilibrium through a series of positive and negative feedback "loops" that are only just beginning to be defined. The complex interrelationship between DCs, NKT cells, CTLs, Th cells, NK cells, and regulatory T cells; the local cytokine microenvironment; the activation history of these cells; the specific subsets of each cell involved; and the temporal sequence of intercellular interactions all play a part in determining the state of immune responsiveness in a local and body-wide context. Although our understanding of the individual functions of the many cell types and subsets is increasing, we do not yet have a synthesis of how this all interacts as a whole in cancer patients. We do, however, have sufficient insight to design and develop better immunotherapeutic strategies that seek to employ these cells, and as our understanding of the basic immunology underlying the immune response to cancer is extended to a systems biology perspective, we will be able to build on these current approaches.

REFERENCES

1. Davis MM, Bjorkman PJ. T-cell antigen receptor genes and T-cell recognition. Nature 1988;334:395–402.
2. Restifo NP, Marincola FM, Kawakami Y, et al. Loss of functional beta 2-microglobulin in metastatic melanomas from five patients receiving immunotherapy. J Natl Cancer Inst 1996;88:100–8.
3. Khong HT, Restifo NP. Natural selection of tumor variants in the generation of "tumor escape" phenotypes. Nat Immunol 2002;3:999–1005.
4. Chang CC, Campoli M, Restifo NP, et al. Immune selection of hot-spot beta 2-microglobulin gene mutations, HLA-A2 allospecificity loss, and antigen-processing machinery component down-regulation in melanoma cells derived from recurrent metastases following immunotherapy. J Immunol 2005;174:1462–71.
5. Sallusto F, Lenig D, Forster R, et al. Two subsets of memory T lymphocytes with distinct homing potentials and effector functions. Nature 1999;401:708–12.
6. Sallusto F, Langenkamp A, Geginat J, et al. Functional subsets of memory T cells identified by CCR7 expression. Curr Top Microbiol Immunol 2000;251:167–71.
7. Rivino L, Messi M, Jarrossay D, et al. Chemokine receptor expression identifies pre-T helper (Th)1, pre-Th2, and nonpolarized cells among human CD4+ central memory T cells. J Exp Med 2004;200:725–35.
8. Sallusto F, Geginat J, Lanzavecchia A. Central memory and effector memory T cell subsets: function, generation, and maintenance. Annu Rev Immunol 2004;22:745–63.
9. Geginat J, Sallusto F, Lanzavecchia A. Cytokine-driven proliferation and differentiation of human naive, central memory, and effector memory CD4(+) T cells. J Exp Med 2001;194:1711–9.
10. Kim J, Woods A, Becker-Dunn E, et al. Distinct functional phenotypes of cloned Ia-restricted helper T cells. J Exp Med 1985;162:188–201.
11. Mosmann TR, Cherwinski H, Bond MW, et al. Two types of murine helper T cell clone. I. Definition according to profiles of lymphokine activities and secreted proteins. J Immunol 1986;136:2348–57.
12. Stout R, Bottomly K. Antigen-specific activation of effector macrophages by IFN producing (Th1) T cell clones. Failure of IL4 producing (Th2) T cell clones to activate effector function in macrophages. J Immunol 1989;142:760–5.
13. Cher D, Mosmann T. Two types of murine helper T cell clone. II. Delayed type hypersensitivity is mediated by Th1 clones. J Immunol 1987;138:3688–94.
14. Nakamura K, Kitani A, Strober W. Cell contact–dependent immunosuppression by CD4+CD25+ regulatory T cells is mediated by cell surface–bound transforming growth factor . J Exp Med 2001;194:629–44.
15. Gershon RK, Kondo K. Cell interactions in the induction of tolerance: the role of thymic lymphocytes. Immunology 1970;18:723–37.
16. Sakaguchi S, Sakaguchi N, Shimizu J, et al. Immunologic tolerance maintained by CD25+CD4+ regulatory T cells: their common role in controlling autoimmunity, tumor immunity, and transplantation tolerance. Immunol Rev 2001;182:18–32.
17. Almeida AR, Legrand N, Papiernik M, et al. Homeostasis of peripheral CD4+ T cells: IL-2 and IL-2 shape a population of regulatory cells that controls CD4+ T cell numbers. J Immunol 2002;169:4850–60.
18. Klebb G, Autenrieth IB, Haber H, et al. Interleukin-2 is indispensable for development of immunological self-tolerance. Clin Immunol Immunopathol 1996:81:282–6.
19. Malek TR, Bayer AL. Tolerance, not immunity, crucially depends on IL-2. Nat Rev Immunol 2004;4:665–74.
20. Brunkow ME, Jeffery EW, Hjerrild KA, et al. Disruption of a new forkhead/winged-helix protein, scurfin, results in the fatal lymphoproliferative disorder of the scurfy mouse. Nat Genet 2001;27:68–73.
21. Fontenot JD, Gavin MA, Rudensky AY. Foxp3 programs the development and function of CD4+CD25+ regulatory T cells. Nat Immunol 2003;4:330–6.
22. Hori S, Nomura T, Sakaguchi S. Control of regulatory T cell development by the transcription factor Foxp3. Science 2003;299:1057–61.
23. Khattri R, Cox T, Yasayko SA, et al. An essential role for scurfin in CD4+CD25+ T regulatory cells. Nat Immunol 2003;4:337–42.
24. Vales-Gomez M, Reyburn H, Strominger J. Interaction between the human NK receptors and their ligands. Crit Rev Immunol 2000;20:223–44.
25. Makrigiannis AP, Anderson SK. Regulation of natural killer cell function. Cancer Biol Ther 2003;2:610–6.
26. Diefenbach A, Jamieson AM, Liu SD, et al. Ligands for the murine NKG2D receptor: expression by tumor cells and activation of NK cells and macrophages. Nat Immunol 2000;1:119–26.
27. Cerwenka A, et al. Retinoic acid early inducible genes define a ligand family for the activating NKG2D receptor in mice. Immunity 2000;12:721–7.
28. Dellabona P, Padovan E, Casorati M, et al. An invariant $V\alpha 24$-$J\alpha Q/V\beta 11$ T cell receptor is expressed in all individuals by clonally expanded $CD4^-8^-$ T cells. J Exp Med 1994;180:1171–6.
29. Porcelli, S, Yockey CE, Brenner MB, et al. Analysis of T cell antigen receptor (TCR) expression by human peripheral blood $CD4^-8^-$ $\alpha\beta$T cells demonstrates preferential use of several $V\beta$ genes and an invariant TCR α-chain. J Exp Med 1993;178:1–16.
30. Park JM, Terabe M, van den Broeke LT, et al. Unmasking immunosurveillance against a syngeneic colon cancer by elimination of CD4+ NKT regulatory cells and IL-13. Int J Cancer 2005;114:80–7.
31. Osada T, Morse MA, Lyerly HK, Clay TM. Ex vivo expanded human CD4+ regulatory NKT cells suppress expansion of tumor antigen-specific CTL. Int Immunol 2005. [In press]
32. Chen JJ, Lin YC, Yao PL, et al. Tumor-associated macrophages: the double-edged sword in cancer progression. J Clin Oncol 2005;23:953–64.
33. Tsutsui S, Yasuda K, Suzuki K, et al. Macrophage infiltration and its prognostic implications in breast cancer: the relationship with VEGF expression and microvessel density. Oncol Rep 2005;14:425–31.
34. Carsetti R, Rosado MM, Wardmann H. Peripheral development of B cells in mouse and man. Immunol Rev 2004;197:179–91.
35. Banchereau J, Steinman RM. Dendritic cells and the control of immunity. Nature 1998;392:245–52.
36. Mellman I, Steinman RM. Dendritic cells: specialized and regulated antigen processing machines. Cell 2001;106:255–8.
37. Degli-Esposti MA, Smyth MJ, Steinman RM. Some interfaces of dendritic cell biology. APMIS 2003;111:675–97.
38. Degli-Esposti MA, Smyth MJ. Close encounters of different kinds: dendritic cells and NK cells take centre stage. Nat Rev Immunol 2005;5:112–24.
39. Mosca PJ, Hobeika AC, Clay TM, et al. A subset of human monocyte-derived dendritic cells expresses high levels of interleukin-12 in response to combined CD40 ligand and interferon-gamma treatment. Blood 2000;96:3499–504.
40. Mazzoni A, Segal DM. Controlling the Toll road to dendritic cell polarization. J Leukoc Biol 2004;75:721–30.
41. Zou GM, Tam YK. Cytokines in the generation and maturation of dendritic cells: recent advances. Eur Cytokine Netw 2002;13:186–99.
42. Morse MA, Mosca PJ, Clay TM, et al. Dendritic cell maturation in active immunotherapy strategies. Exp Opin Biol Ther 2002;2:35–43.
43. Trauth BC, Klas C, Peters AM, et al. Monoclonal antibody-mediated tumor regression by induction of apoptosis. Science 1989;245:301–5.
44. Ludwig D, Pereira DS, Zhu Z. Monoclonal antibody therapeutics and apoptosis. Oncogene 2003;22:9097–106.
45. Ghetie MA, Bright H, Vitetta ES. Homodimers but not monomers of Rituxan (chimeric anti-CD20) induce apoptosis in human B-lymphoma cells and synergize with a chemotherapeutic agent and an immunotoxin. Blood 2001;97:1392–8.
46. Shan D, Ledbetter JA, Press OW. Apoptosis of malignant human B cells by ligation of CD20 with monoclonal antibodies. Blood 1998;91:1644–52.
47. Montgomery RB, Makary E, Schiffman K, et al. Endogenous anti-HER2 antibodies block HER2 phosphorylation and signaling through extracellular signal-regulated kinase. Cancer Res 2005;65:650–6.
48. Matzinger P. Tolerance, danger, and the extended family. Annu Rev Immunol 1994;12:991–1045.
49. Matzinger P. An innate sense of danger. Semin Immunol 1998;10:399–415.
50. Todryk S, Melcher AA, Hardwick N, et al. Heat shock protein 70 induced during tumor cell killing induces Th1 cytokines and targets immature dendritic cell precursors to enhance antigen uptake. J Immunol 1999;163:1398–408.
51. Avice MN, Demeure CE, Delespesse G, et al. IL-15 promotes IL-12 production by human monocytes via T cell-dependent contact and may contribute to IL-12-mediated IFN-gamma secretion by CD4+ T cells in the absence of TCR ligation. J Immunol 1998;161:3408–15.
52. Barbulescu K, Becker C, Schlaak JF, et al. IL-12 and IL-18 differentially regulate the transcriptional activity of the human IFN-gamma promoter in primary CD4+ T lymphocytes. J Immunol 1998;160:3642–7.
53. O'Donnell MA, Luo Y, Chen X, et al. Role of IL-12 in the induction and potentiation of IFN-gamma in response to bacillus Calmette-Guérin. J Immunol 1999;163:4246–52.
54. Micallef MJ, Darmanin S, Buhagiar JA, et al. Interferon gamma induction in human melanoma cell/allogeneic leukocyte co-cultures is enhanced by interleukin 18 but drug resistant melanoma cells are poorer inducers of IFN-gamma. Int Immunopharmacol 2001;1:295–305.
55. Zitvogel L, Tahara H, Robbins PD, et al. Cancer immunotherapy of established tumors with IL-12. Effective delivery by genetically engineered fibroblasts. J Immunol 1995;155:1393–403.
56. Yue FY, Geertsen R, Hemmi S, et al. IL-12 directly up-regulates the expression of HLA class I, HLA class II and ICAM-1 on human melanoma cells: a mechanism for its antitumor activity? Eur J Immunol 1999;29:1762–73.
57. Yajima T, Nishimura H, Wajjwalku W, et al. Overexpression of interleukin-15 in vivo enhances antitumor activity against MHC class I-negative and -positive malignant melanoma through augmented NK activity and cytotoxic T-cell response. Int J Cancer 2002;99:573–8.

12d

Defects in Antitumor Immunity

Michael A. Morse, MD

The capacity of the immune system to clear diverse infectious organisms has often been suggested as a reason that the immune system should be able to destroy tumors as well. The theory of tumor immunosurveillance states that the immune system continually searches for and eliminates tumor cells by recognizing "differences" with normal cells. This implies that tumors could develop and progress when the immune system fails to recognize or destroy them.[1] This concept was initially controversial because it was observed that athymic nude mice did not necessarily develop tumors with greater frequency than normal mice, and an often discussed issue is whether immunosuppression results in the development of or permits more aggressive behavior by cancers. Certain skin cancers, Kaposi's sarcoma, and lymphoproliferative disorders are more common following solid organ and hematopoietic transplants.[2] This points to the involvement of immunosurveillance in curtailing the actions of oncogenic virus. However, the frequency of noncutaneous, non–virally induced neoplasias, such as carcinomas of the lung, prostate, breast, and colon, is generally not increased among most transplant recipients.[3] Nonetheless, tumors may be more aggressive. In Buell and colleagues' review, transplant patients developed colon cancer at a younger age and had a worse prognosis stage for stage than nontransplant patients.[4] Of course, it is possible that biologically more aggressive tumors develop in transplant patients for reasons other than immunosuppression. For example, dysregulations in the immune response may be associated with the development of some malignancies. Mutations in NOD2, a molecule that interacts with nuclear factor κB and that is associated with Crohn's disease, have been found more often in individuals with nonhereditary and nonpolyposis colon cancers.[5] Nonetheless, reducing immunosuppression does seem to decrease the risk of neoplasms, especially skin cancers.[6] Of course, most animal models of malignancy and most humans with cancer are not systemically immunosuppressed, but it is clear that there is often a failure to activate tumor antigen–specific immune effectors in the cancer-bearing host, and even when they are activated, immune effectors may "ignore" tumors. The reasons for local immunosuppression include both tumor and host factors. Tumors are different from acute infections in that they develop over a prolonged period of time, allowing for long-term interactions with the immune system that result in an altered pattern of immune response. Also, tumors may influence the immune effectors directly through secretion of inhibitory cytokines, by expression of molecules lethal to these effectors, or by "cloaking" themselves to avoid detection. Tumors may also indirectly influence immune effectors by inducing defective antigen-presenting cells or causing activation of T regulatory cells (Tregs) or skewing of T helper (Th) cells toward Th2 responses. The host inflammatory response may also be inhibitory to other immune effects owing to release of proangiogenic molecules and inhibitory cytokines. This immunosuppression within the tumor environment has been elegantly reviewed recently, and we provide an overview.[7]

UNFAVORABLE CYTOKINE MILIEU OF TUMORS

If the immune response to tumors behaved as an acute infection, one would expect the "danger signals" released in the tumor milieu to activate an immune response against the tumor.[8,9] Some of the specific factors that serve as danger signals, such as tumor necrosis factor (TNF)-α, CD40 ligand (CD40L), and interferon (IFN)-γ, act in part by stimulating the maturation of dendritic cells (DCs), particularly in appropriate combinations and temporal sequences.[10,11] When fully matured, DCs produce cytokines, such as interleukin (IL)-12, IL-15, and IL-18, which drive antigen-specific Th1-type immunity. In turn, Th1 responses appear to be important for the generation of antitumor T-cell activity, as described above.[12,13] IL-12 also promotes the development of effector cytotoxic T lymphocytes (CTLs) (called Tc1) and up-regulates class I and II major histocompatibility complex (MHC) and intercellular adhesion molecule 1 on tumor cells and therefore may augment the ability of CTLs to recognize and lyse them.[14,15] Overexpression of IL-15 enhances both CTL and NK cell function and augments their antitumor effects on tumors in vivo.[16] Unfortunately, patients with progressive cancer appear to have a tumor microenvironment in which such danger signals are either absent or masked, and inhibitory factors (eg, IL-10, transforming growth factor [TGF]-β, and prostaglandins) that suppress immune function are increased.[17,18] The effect of TGF-β is complex because it can inhibit tumor growth but also is directly immunosuppressive. Furthermore, it is produced by tumor cells and stromal cells, such as macrophages. TGF-β appears to directly suppress $CD8^+$ effector T cells (and the suppressive effect requires an intact TGF-β receptor II on $CD8^+$ T cells). TGF-β appears to be one of the mediators of the suppressive function of Tregs.[19,20] Indeed, neutralization of TGF-β can enhance the efficacy of antitumor immunizations in animal models.[21] Lee and colleagues reported that TGF-β_1 secreted by tumors impairs natural killer (NK) lytic activity by down-regulating the NK-activating receptor NKG2D. IL-10, produced by Th2 cells and Tregs but also by tumors such as non–small cell lung cancer, pancreatic cancer, and squamous cell carcinomas of the head and neck, impairs DC function and effector T-cell activity and is involved in skewing T-cell helper responses to the Th2 subtype.[22–27] Prostaglandins, particularly PGE_2, generated by cyclooxygenase-2 (COX-2), which is overexpressed in many cancers, suppress T- and B-cell proliferation, inhibit NK cell–mediated cytotoxicity, and inhibit TNF production.[28,29] Prostaglandins also induce the production of IL-10 and enhance regulatory T-cell function.[28,30]

INEFFECTIVE ANTIGEN-PRESENTING CELL FUNCTION INDUCED BY TUMORS

Tumor cells lack the stimulatory molecules needed to activate naive T cells. Therefore, the job of activating T and, subsequently, B cells must be performed by specialized antigen-presenting cells, such as DCs, which acquire antigen released by tumors into their environment. Unfortunately, early in development, tumors may not release enough antigen for uptake and cross-presentation by in situ antigen-presenting cells.[31] Later, the tumor stroma may also prevent effective function of the antigen-presenting machinery by keeping antigen from reaching the DCs. In addition, because DCs, particularly mature DCs, are critical for the induction of antigen-specific immune responses, it is not surprising that the tumor environment is particularly hostile to DC maturation and antigen-presenting functions. For example, immature DCs exposed to tumor cells have significantly lower expression of components of the antigen-presenting machinery (MB1, LMP-2, LMP-7, LMP-10, and endoplasmic reticulum p75) than controls and, consequently, have a decreased ability to present tumor antigens to T cells.[32] Mature DCs tend to be found infrequently within the tumor but are more common in the peritumoral areas.[33] These observations are likely due to high levels of molecular factors that inhibit DC differentiation (vascular endothelial growth factor [VEGF], IL-6, IL-10, TGF-β, macrophage colony-stimulating factor [M-CSF], PGE_2, and COX-2) and low levels of cytokines and other molecules that promote DC differentiation (granulocyte-macrophage colony-stimulating factor [GM-CSF], IL-4).[7,34–38] The tumor and the host macrophages and stromal cells are responsible for these undesirable cytokine profiles. Immature DCs are less capable of stimulating effector T-cell responses and are more likely to cause T-cell unresponsiveness or activate suppressive T cells.[39–41]

Other DC subtypes with suppressive properties accumulate in the tumor microenvironment. Indoleamine 2,3-dioxygenase (IDO)-expressing DCs accumulate in tumors or in regional lymph nodes that drain tumors, likely in response to IL-10, IFN-γ, and regulatory T cells. IDO, by catabolizing tryptophan, which is important for T-cell proliferation, indirectly leads to T-cell death.[42] Plasmacytoid DCs, often called DC2, which home to tumor-infiltrated areas in response to CXCL12, may have immunostimulatory function through their generation of IFN-α but also activate Tregs.[43,44] Immature myeloid cells, identified in mice by expression of CD11b and Gr-1+ but which have no unifying marker in humans and which represent several different cell types in the monocyte or granulocyte pathways, accumulate in response to elevated levels of several cytokines and factors, including VEGF. These cells are capable of suppressing effector T-cell stimulation.[45,46] Finally, myeloid DC (DC1) can be induced within the tumor environment to express molecules such as B7-H1, which cause them to be immunosuppressive. Blocking B7-H1 results in enhanced immunostimulatory capacity of DCs.[47,48]

In addition to the effects on immune recognition of tumors, DCs and other antigen-presenting cells may also have a role in modulating the vascular supply to tumors. Whereas mature DCs generate IL-12, which has antiangiogenic functions, plasmacytoid DCs induce vascularization by producing IL-8.[49] Furthermore Conejo-Garcia and colleagues observed a new DC expressing typical DC and endothelial markers in mice and human ovarian carcinomas.[50] In those tumors expressing β-defensin 29 and elevated levels of VEGF-A, DC precursors were chemoattracted by the β-defensins and then induced by VEGF to form neovasculature. In summary, tumors seem to cause immunosuppressive and proangiogenic antigen-presenting cells to predominate, resulting in a failure of effector T cells to be activated against malignancies and enhancement of mechanisms for tumors to grow and metastasize.

WHEN IMMUNE ACTIVATION IS DANGEROUS TO EFFECTOR T CELLS

Although presentation of tumor antigen to T cells would usually be desirable, the phenomenon of activation-induced cell death (AICD) can occur when previously activated T cells undergo apoptosis following exposure to their cognate antigen.[51,52] Whether AICD occurs is a function of whether the T cells have been preactivated and whether costimulatory molecules are ligated.[53] Resting T cells are relatively resistant to AICD, as are T cells whose CD28 has interacted with the costimulatory molecules CD80 and CD86.[54] Thus, exposure to antigen without costimulatory signals can lead to cell death. This is thought to be mediated by up-regulated expression of surface death ligands and receptors such as Fas/FasL and TNF-related apoptosis-inducing ligand (TRAIL).[55,56] In the absence of costimulatory signals (which cause down-regulation of FasL but are lacking in tumor cells), interactions of Fas on one T cell with FasL on another T cell will lead to AICD. Evidence for AICD has been reported for TIL cells exposed to melanoma, but whether tumor-expressed FasL causes immune evasion in vivo is controversial, although many tumors express FasL.[57–69] It is also important to recognize that activated T cells need not encounter Fas-L directly on tumor cells. Kim and colleagues identified FasL-positive microvesicles in the sera of 21 of 27 head and neck cancer patients.[70] These microvesicles induced activation of the apoptotic pathway via caspase 3 cleavage and also caused a reduction in T-cell receptor (TCR)-ζ chain expression in target lymphocytes. The microvesicle-associated FasL levels also correlated with the extensiveness of the patient's tumor.

DEFECTS IN T-CELL SIGNALING

Defects in the TCR signaling pathways, particularly the loss of the zeta chain portion of the CD3-receptor complex, have been reported in patients with melanoma, renal cell carcinoma, ovarian carcinoma, cervical carcinoma, colon carcinoma, and prostate cancer.[71–76] The zeta chain is an important component of T-cell activation via the TCR and NK cells via the FcγRIII. Defects in signaling ultimately result in lower proliferative responses to antigen, lower cytotoxic function, and lower production of Th1 cytokines. Decreased levels of TCR-ζ expression correlate with prognosis in terms of tumor progression and aggressiveness.[77] The mechanism for zeta chain loss is not clear, but hydrogen peroxide production by tumor-associated macrophages, cleavage by caspases, and granzyme B have all been suggested.[78–80] Finally, some patients may experience defects in the signaling in T cells mediated by nuclear factor κB, which is important for regulating expression of IL-2, TNF, GM-CSF, M-CSF, and IFN-γ.[81,82]

HOW TUMORS WITHSTAND IMMUNE-MEDIATED DESTRUCTION

Although tumor-targeting immune effectors may be stimulated, tumors may be resistant to their cytolytic activities. As Fas/FasL-mediated cytotoxicity is one way that CTLs destroy tumors, Fas-mediated cytotoxicity may be reduced in tumors that down-regulate Fas expression, although the mechanism for this is not well established.[83–85] Similarly, up-regulated inhibitors of Fas-signaling, such as FLIP, protect tumor cells from immune effectors, although up-regulated expression of FLIP has been identified infrequently.[86,87] Inhibitors of granzyme B function, such as PI-9, have been identified in tumors, although their significance is uncertain.[88]

Perhaps most important are the many means that tumors have to escape recognition by immune effects. Tumor cells may down-regulate critical antigen presentation molecules, such as class I MHC, TAP1, and β_2-microglobulin, or fail to express cell-surface costimulatory molecules, such as B7.[89–91] For example, some epithelial tumors, such as breast, prostate, and lung cancer, have been documented to have only low levels of MHC class I molecules or deletion of β_2-microglobulin genes, that is, down-regulation of the antigen-processing machinery.[92,93] Tumors such as melanoma and renal cell carcinoma have been shown to lose β_2-microglobulin.[94–96] Other tumors can down-regulate the expression of particular class I loci or lose the genes for particular class Ia chains. Still other tumors, including small cell carcinoma of the lung, can down-regulate the proteosome component molecules LMP-2 and LMP-7 and TAP1 and TAP2.[97]

REGULATORY T CELL–MEDIATED SUPPRESSION

The immune system seems to be programmed to avoid autoimmunity so that if an immune response becomes activated, regulatory mechanisms must exist to keep it from becoming uncontrolled. In the mid-1980s, Shimizu and colleagues demonstrated that thymically derived CD4 cells that coexpressed the IL-2 receptor alpha chain (CD25), called Tregs, were crucial for control of autoreactive T cells in vivo (Figure 12d-1).[98] These Tregs, now identified by intracellular expression of FOXP3+ (forkhead box P3), inhibit the proliferation of CD25–effector T cells, and it is also believed that these Tregs can inhibit antitumor immune responses.[99] In individuals with ovarian carcinoma, Tregs accumulated in tumors and ascites and were associated with reduced survival.[100] Increased numbers of Tregs have also been demonstrated in the peripheral blood of cancer patients, the tumor-involved lymph nodes of patients with melanoma, and the primary tumor of patients with lung cancer.[101–103] Animal models have demonstrated that Tregs can be activated by immunization.[104] Conversely, Treg cell depletion before immunization results in enhanced tumor antigen–specific T-cell responses.[105–107] Recently, Vieweg and colleagues reported that depletion of Treg prior to immunization of humans with a DC vaccine led to increased antigen-specific T-cell responses.[108] The mechanism of suppression seems to be multifactorial and includes cell–cell contact (via cytotoxic T lymphocyte antigen 4 [CTLA4] or cell-bound TGF-β) or secretion of cytokines, such as TGF-β and IL-10. The CTLA4 expressed by Treg interacts with CD80 and/or CD86 on the surface of DCs to cause a negative signal for T-cell activation. It should also be noted that T cells with inducible regulatory activity, termed Th3, TR1, and $CD8^+$ regulatory cells, have also been described.

CONCLUSIONS

Tumor- and host-related factors result in both diminished effector T-cell activation and impaired

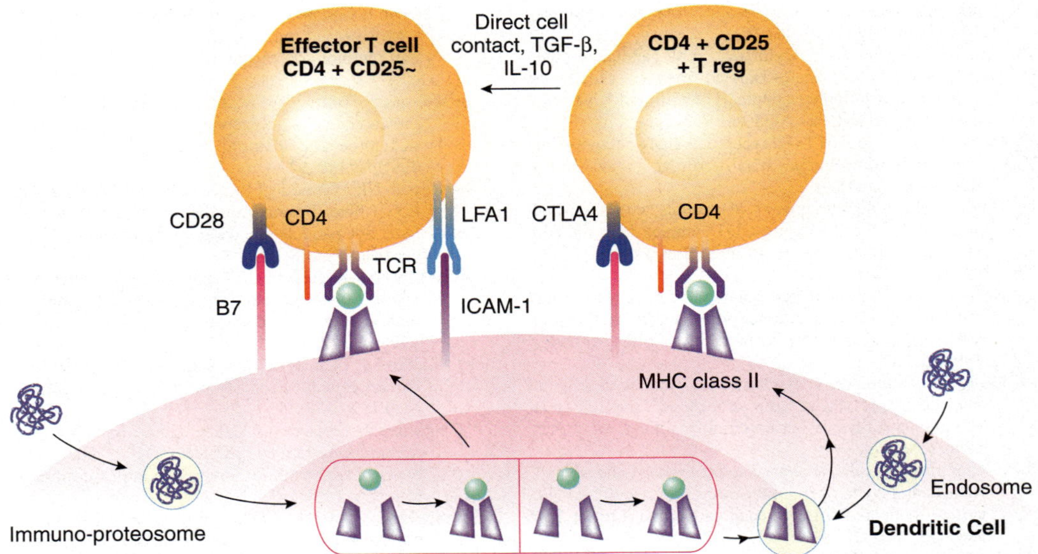

Figure 12d-1 Thymically derived CD4 cells that coexpress the interleukin (IL)-2 receptor alpha chain (CD25), called Tregs, are crucial for control of autoreactive T cells in vivo.

killing capacity of activated T cells in the tumor environment. Efforts to counter the immune dysregulation have included use of exogenously generated DCs (reviewed by Palucka and colleagues[109]) to avoid in situ inhibitory effects on DC function, adjunctive cytokines such as IL-12 to enhance T-cell activation and counteract the inhibitory signals, interferons to up-regulate class I and antigen expression by tumors, and chemotherapy or immune toxins to eliminate regulatory T cells.[110,111] In addition, normal signals that prevent the development of autoimmunity might need to be eliminated to allow an enhanced immune response. For example, CTLA4 expression is not limited to Treg. In fact, effector T cells also express this receptor. When DCs acquire antigen and present it to the TCR, costimulatory molecule engagement is required to activate T-cell proliferation. The positive costimulatory signals are delivered by the binding of CD80 or CD86 on DCs to CD28 on T cells. The engagement of CTLA-4 on effector T cells by these ligands induces cell-cycle arrest and decreased IL-2 production.[112,113] Interestingly, recent data suggest that CD80 binding is not essential for CTLA-4 function.[114] Therefore, CTLA-4 may serve as a general negative signal to T cells and might need to be inhibited if antitumor immune responses are to reach adequate levels of magnitude to destroy tumors. Two drugs in development (MDX-010 and CP-675,206) have demonstrated immunologic activity by inhibiting CTLA4.[115]

REFERENCES

1. Burnet FM. The concept of immunological surveillance. Prog Exp Tumor Res 1970;13:1–27.
2. Ippoliti G, Rinaldi M, Pellegrini C, et al. Incidence of cancer after immunosuppressive treatment for heart transplantation. Crit Rev Oncol Hematol 2005 Jun 22; [Epub ahead of print].
3. Penn I. Cancer complicating organ transplantation. N Engl J Med 1990;323:1767–9.
4. Buell JF, Papaconstantinou HT, Skalow B, et al. De novo colorectal cancer: five-year survival is markedly lower in transplant recipients compared with the general population. Transplant Proc 2005;37:960–1.
5. Kurzawski G, Suchy J, Kladny J, et al. The NOD2 3020insC mutation and the risk of colorectal cancer. Cancer Res 2004;64:1604–6.
6. Otley CC, Maragh SL. Reduction of immunosuppression for transplant-associated skin cancer: rationale and evidence of efficacy. Dermatol Surg 2005;31:163–8.
7. Zou W. Immunosuppressive networks in the tumour environment and their therapeutic relevance. Nat Rev Cancer 2005;5:263–74.
8. Matzinger P. Tolerance, danger, and the extended family. Annu Rev Immunol 1994;12:991–1045.
9. Matzinger P. An innate sense of danger. Semin Immunol 1998;10:399–415.
10. Mosca PJ, Hobeika AC, Clay TM, et al. A subset of human monocyte-derived dendritic cells expresses high levels of interleukin-12 in response to combined CD40 ligand and interferon-gamma treatment. Blood 2000;96:3499–504.
11. Todryk S, Melcher AA, Hardwick N, et al. Heat shock protein 70 induced during tumor cell killing induces Th1 cytokines and targets immature dendritic cell precursors to enhance antigen uptake. J Immunol 1999;163:1398–408.
12. Avice MN, Demeure CE, Delespesse G, et al. IL-15 promotes IL-12 production by human monocytes via T cell-dependent contact and may contribute to IL-12-mediated IFN-gamma secretion by CD4+ T cells in the absence of TCR ligation. J Immunol 1998;161:3408–15.
13. Barbulescu K, Becker C, Schlaak JF, et al. IL-12 and IL-18 differentially regulate the transcriptional activity of the human IFN-gamma promoter in primary CD4+ T lymphocytes. J Immunol 1998;160:3642–7.
14. O'Donnell MA, Luo Y, Chen X, et al. Role of IL-12 in the induction and potentiation of IFN-gamma in response to bacillus Calmette-Guérin. J Immunol 1999;163:4246–52.
15. Yue FY, Geertsen R, Hemmi S, et al. IL-12 directly up-regulates the expression of HLA class I, HLA class II and ICAM-1 on human melanoma cells: a mechanism for its antitumor activity? Eur J Immunol 1999;29:1762–73.
16. Yajima T, Nishimura H, Wajjwalku W, et al. Overexpression of interleukin-15 in vivo enhances antitumor activity against MHC class I-negative and -positive malignant melanoma through augmented NK activity and cytotoxic T-cell response. Int J Cancer 2002;99:573–8.
17. Becker JC, Czerny C, Brocker EB. Maintenance of clonal anergy by endogenously produced IL 10. Int Immunol 1994;6:1605–12.
18. Qin Z, Noffz G, Mohaupt M, Blankenstein T. Interleukin-10 prevents dendritic cell accumulation and vaccination with granulocyte-macrophage colony-stimulating factor gene-modified tumor cells. J Immunol 1997;159:770–6.
19. Chen ML, Pittet MJ, Gorelik L, et al. Regulatory T cells suppress tumor-specific CD8 T cell cytotoxicity through TGF-β signals in vivo. Proc Natl Acad Sci U S A 2005;102:419–24.
20. von Boehmer H. Mechanisms of suppression by suppressor T cells. Nat Immunol 2005;6:338–44.
21. Jia ZC, Zou LY, Ni B, et al. Effective induction of antitumor immunity by immunization with plasmid DNA encoding TRP-2 plus neutralization of TGF-beta. Cancer Immunol Immunother 2005;54:446–52.
22. Lee JC, Lee KM, Kim DW, et al. Elevated TGF-β1 secretion and down-modulation of NKG2D underlies impaired NK cytotoxicity in cancer patients. J Immunol 2004;172:7335–40.
23. Neuner A, Schindel M, Wildenberg U, et al. Cytokine secretion: clinical relevance of immunosuppression in non-small cell lung cancer. Lung Cancer 2001;34 Suppl 2:S79–82.
24. Ebrahimi B, Tucker SL, Li D, et al. Cytokines in pancreatic carcinoma: correlation with phenotypic characteristics and prognosis. Cancer 2004;101:2727–36.
25. Agarwal A, Rani M, Saha GK, et al. Disregulated expression of the Th2 cytokine gene in patients with intraoral squamous cell carcinoma. Immunol Invest 2003;32:17–30.
26. Steinbrink K, Graulich E, Kubsch S, et al. CD4(+) and CD8(+) anergic T cells induced by interleukin 10-treated human dendritic cells display antigen-specific suppressor activity. Blood 2002;99:2468–76.
27. Vicari AP, Trinchieri G. Interleukin-10 in viral diseases and cancer: exiting the labyrinth? Immunol Rev 2004;202:223–36.
28. Harris SG, Padilla J, Koumas L, et al. Prostaglandins as modulators of immunity. Trends Immunol 2002;23:144–50.
29. Pockaj BA, Basu GD, Pathangey LB, et al. Reduced T-cell and dendritic cell function is related to cyclooxygenase-2 overexpression and prostaglandin E2 secretion in patients with breast cancer. Ann Surg Oncol 2004;11:328–39.
30. Sharma S, Yang SC, Zhu L, et al. Tumor cyclooxygenase-2/prostaglandin E2-dependent promotion of FOXP3 expression and CD4+ CD25+ T regulatory cell activities in lung cancer. Cancer Res 2005;65:5211–20.
31. Spiotto MT, Yu P, Rowley DA, et al. Increasing tumor antigen expression overcomes "ignorance" to solid tumors via cross presentation by bone marrow-derived stromal cells. Immunity 2002;17:737–47.
32. Whiteside TL, Stanson J, Shurin MR, et al. Antigen-processing machinery in human dendritic cells: up-regulation by maturation and down-regulation by tumor cells. J Immunol 2004;173:1526–34.
33. Bell D, Chomarat P, Broyles D. In breast carcinoma tissue, immature dendritic cells reside within the tumor, whereas mature dendritic cells are located in peritumoral areas. J Exp Med 1999;190:1417–26.
34. Gabrilovich D, Ishida T, Oyama T, et al. Vascular endothelial growth factor inhibits the development of dendritic cells and dramatically affects the differentiation of multiple hematopoietic lineages in vivo. Blood 1998;92:4150–66.
35. Menetrier-Caux C, Montmain G, Dieu MC, et al. Inhibition of the differentiation of dendritic cells from CD34+ progenitors by tumor cells: role of interleukin-6 and macrophage colony-stimulating factor. Blood 1998;92:4778–91.
36. Shono T, Tofilon PJ, Bruner JM, et al. Cyclooxygenase-2 expression in human gliomas: prognostic significance and molecular correlations. Cancer Res 2001;61:4375–81.
37. Sombroek CC, Stam AG, Masterson AJ, et al. Prostanoids play a major role in the primary tumor-induced inhibition of dendritic cell differentiation. J Immunol 2002;168:4333–43.
38. Yang L, Carbone DP. Tumor-host immune interactions and dendritic cell dysfunction. Adv Cancer Res 2004;92:13–27.
39. Jonuleit H, Schmitt E, Schuler G, et al. Induction of interleukin 10-producing, nonproliferating CD4+ T cells with regulatory properties by repetitive stimulation with allogeneic immature human dendritic cells. J Exp Med 2000;192:1213–22.
40. Dhodapkar MV, Steinman RM, Krasovsky J, et al. Antigen-specific inhibition of effector T cell function in humans after injection of immature dendritic cells. J Exp Med 2001;193:233–8.
41. Hawiger D, Inaba K, Dorsett Y, et al. Dendritic cells induce peripheral T cell unresponsiveness under steady state conditions in vivo. J Exp Med 2001;194:769–79.
42. Mellor AL, Munn DH. IDO expression by dendritic cells: tolerance and tryptophan catabolism. Nat Rev Immunol 2004;4:762–74.
43. Zou W, Machelon V, Coulomb-L'Hermine A, et al. Stromal-derived factor-1 in human tumors recruits and alters the function of plasmacytoid precursor dendritic cells. Nat Med 2001;7:1339–46.
44. Krug A, Veeraswamy R, Pekosz A, et al. Interferon-producing cells fail to induce proliferation of naive T cells but

can promote expansion and T helper 1 differentiation of antigen-experienced unpolarized T cells. J Exp Med 2003;197:899–906.

45. Kusmartsev SA, Li Y, Chen SH. Gr-1+ myeloid cells derived from tumor-bearing mice inhibit primary T cell activation induced through CD3/CD28 costimulation. J Immunol 2000;165:779–85.
46. Almand B, Clark JI, Nikitina E, et al. Increased production of immature myeloid cells in cancer patients: a mechanism of immunosuppression in cancer. J Immunol 2001;166:678–89.
47. Selenko-Gebauer N, Majdic O, Szekeres A, et al. B7-H1 (programmed death-1 ligand) on dendritic cells is involved in the induction and maintenance of T cell anergy. J Immunol 2003;170:3637–44.
48. Curiel TJ, Wei S, Dong H, et al. Blockade of B7-H1 improves myeloid dendritic cell-mediated antitumor immunity. Nat Med 2003;9:562–7.
49. Curiel TJ, Cheng P, Mottram P, et al. Dendritic cell subsets differentially regulate angiogenesis in human ovarian cancer. Cancer Res 2004;64:5535–8.
50. Conejo-Garcia JR, Benencia F, Courreges MC, et al. Tumor-infiltrating dendritic cell precursors recruited by a beta-defensin contribute to vasculogenesis under the influence of VEGF-A. Nat Med 2004;10:950–8.
51. Green DR, Bissonnette RP, Glynn JM, Shi Y. Activation-induced apoptosis in lymphoid systems. Semin Immunol 1992;4:379–88.
52. Kabelitz D, Pohl T, Pechold K. Activation-induced cell death (apoptosis) of mature peripheral T lymphocytes. Immunol Today 1993;14:338–9.
53. Budd RC. Activation-induced cell death. Curr Opin Immunol 2001;13:356–62.
54. Radvanyi L, Shi Y, Vaziri H, et al. CD28 costimulation inhibits TCR-induced apoptosis during a primary T cell response. J Immunol 1996;156:1788–98.
55. Zheng L, Fisher G, Miller RE, et al. Induction of apoptosis in mature T cells by tumour necrosis factor. Nature 1995;377:348–51.
56. Martinez-Lorenzo MJ, Alava MA, Gamen S, et al. Involvement of APO2 ligand/TRAIL in activation-induced death of Jurkat and human peripheral blood T cells. Eur J Immunol 1998;28:2714–25.
57. Zaks TZ, Chappell DB, Rosenberg SA, Restifo NP. Fas-mediated suicide of tumor-reactive T cells following activation by specific tumor. Selective rescue by caspase inhibition. J Immunol 1999;162:3273–9.
58. Radoja S, Saio M, Frey AB. CD8+ tumor-infiltrating lymphocytes are primed for Fas-mediated activation-induced cell death but are not apoptotic in situ. J Immunol 2001;166:6074–83.
59. O'Connell J, Bennett MW, O'Sullivan MG, et al. The Fas counterattack. Fas-mediated T cell killing by colon cancer cells expressing Fas ligand. J Exp Med 1996;184:1075–82.
60. Hahne M, Rimoldi D, Schroter M, et al. Melanoma cell expression of Fas(Apo-1/CD95) ligand. Implications for tumor immune escape. Science 1996;274:1363–6.
61. Shiraki KN, Tsuji T, Shioda K, et al. Expression of Fas ligand in liver metastases of human colonic adenocarcinomas. Proc Natl Acad Sci U S A 1997;94:6420–5.
62. Gastman B, et al. Fas ligand is expressed on human squamous cell carcinomas of the head and neck, and it promotes apoptosis of T lymphocytes. Cancer Res 1999;59:5356–64.
63. Rabinowich H, et al. Lymphocyte apoptosis induced by Fas ligand-expressing ovarian carcinoma cells. Implications for altered expression of T cell receptor in tumor-associated lymphocytes. J Clin Invest 1998;101:2579–88.
64. Koyama S, et al. Fas receptor counterattack against tumor-infiltrating lymphocytes in vivo as a mechanism of immune escape in gastric carcinoma. J Cancer Res Clin Oncol 2001;127:20–6.
65. Bennett M, et al. The Fas counterattack in vivo. Apoptotic depletion of tumor-infiltrating lymphocytes associated with Fas ligand expression by human esophageal carcinoma. J Immunol 1998;160:5669–75.
66. Strand S, et al. Lymphocyte apoptosis induced by CD95 (APO-1/Fas) ligand-expressing tumor cells—a mechanism of immune evasion? Nat Med 1996;2:1361–6.
67. Niehans GA, et al. Human lung carcinomas express Fas ligand. Cancer Res 1997;57:1007–12.
68. Shibakita M, et al. Prognostic significance of Fas and Fas ligand expressions in human esophageal cancer. Clin Cancer Res 1999;5:2464–9.
69. Zietz C, Rumpler U, Sturzl M, Lohrs U. Inverse relation of Fas-ligand and tumor-infiltrating lymphocytes in angiosarcoma. Indications of apoptotic tumor counterattack. Am J Pathol 2001;159:963–70.
70. Kim JW, Wieckowski E, Taylor DD, et al. Fas ligand-positive membranous vesicles isolated from sera of patients with oral cancer induce apoptosis of activated T lymphocytes. Clin Cancer Res 2005;11:1010–20.
71. Finke JH, et al. Loss of T-cell receptor z chain and p56^{lck} in T-cell infiltrating human renal cell carcinoma. Cancer Res 1993;53:5613–6.
72. Gunji Y, et al. High frequency of patients with abnormal assembly of T cell receptor-CD3 complex in peripheral blood T lymphocytes. Jpn J Cancer Res 1994;85:1189–92.
73. Healy C, et al. Impaired expression and function of signal transducing zeta chains in peripheral T cells and natural killer cells in patients with prostate cancer. Cytometry 1998;32:109–19.
74. Lai P, et al. Alteration in expression and function of signal transducing proteins in tumor-associated T and NK cells in patients with ovarian carcinoma. Clin Cancer Res 1996;2:161–73.
75. Nakagomi H, et al. Decreased expression of the signal-transducing z chains in tumor-infiltrating T cell and NK cells of patients with colorectal carcinoma. Cancer Res 1993;53:5610–2.
76. Dworacki G, et al. Decreased zeta chain expression and apoptosis in CD3+ peripheral blood T lymphocytes of patients with melanoma. Clin Cancer Res 2001;7:S947–57.
77. Zea AH, et al. Alterations in T cell receptor and signal transduction molecules in melanoma patients. Clin Cancer Res 1995;1:1327–35.
78. Schmielau J, Finn OJ. Activated granulocytes and granulocyte-derived hydrogen peroxide are the underlying mechanism of suppression of T-cell function in advanced cancer patients. Cancer Res 2001;61:4756–60.
79. Otsuji M, Kimura Y, Aoe T, et al. Oxidative stress by tumor-derived macrophages suppresses the expression of CD3 zeta chain of T-cell receptor complex and antigen-specific T-cell responses. Proc Natl Acad Sci U S A 1996;93:13119–24.
80. Wieckowski E, Wang GQ, Gastman BR, et al. Granzyme B-mediated degradation of T cell receptor zeta chain. Cancer Res 2002;62:4884–9.
81. Li X, Liu J, Park JK, et al. T cells from renal cell carcinoma patients exhibit an abnormal pattern of kappa B-specific DNA-binding activity. A preliminary report. Cancer Res 1994;54:5424–9.
82. Ling W, et al. Impaired activation of NFkappaB in T cells from a subset of renal cell carcinoma patients is mediated by inhibition of phosphorylation and degradation of the inhibitor, IkappaBalpha. Blood 1998;92:1334–41.
83. Nambu Y, Hughes SJ, Rehemtulla A, et al. Lack of cell surface Fas/APO-1 expression in pulmonary adenocarcinomas. J Clin Invest 1998;101:1102–10.
84. Gratas C, Tohma Y, Barnas C, et al. Up-regulation of Fas (APO-1/CD95) ligand and down-regulation of Fas expression in human esophageal cancer. Cancer Res 1998;58:2057–62.
85. Radfar S, Davrinche C, Hollande E. Serial in vivo loss and in vitro gain of Fas expression and function in human cancerous pancreatic duct cells. Int J Cancer 2005;115:214–23.
86. French LE, Tschopp J. Defective death receptor signaling as a cause of tumor immune escape. Semin Cancer Biol 2002;12:51–5.
87. Medema JP, de Jong J, van Hall T, et al. Immune escape of tumors in vivo by expression of cellular FLICE-inhibitory protein. J Exp Med 1999;190:1033–8.
88. Bladergroen BA, Strik MC, Bovenschen N, et al. Expression of the granzyme B inhibitor, protease inhibitor 9, by tumor cells in patients with non-Hodgkin and Hodgkin lymphoma. A novel protective mechanism for tumor cells to circumvent the immune system? Blood 2002;99:232–7.
89. Marincola FM, Jaffee EM, Hicklin DJ, et al. Escape of human solid tumors from T-cell recognition: molecular mechanisms and functional significance. Adv Immunol 2000;74:181–273.
90. Bubenik J. Tumor MHC class I downregulation and immunotherapy. Oncol Rep 2003;10:2005–8.
91. Dissemond J, Gotte P, Mors J, et al. Association of TAP1 downregulation in human primary melanoma lesions with lack of spontaneous regression. Melanoma Res 2003;13:253–8.
92. Jordanova ES, Riemersma SA, Philippo K, et al. Beta2-microglobulin aberrations in diffuse large B cell lymphoma of the testis and the central nervous system. Int J Cancer 2003;103:393–8.
93. Esteban F, Concha A, Delgado M, et al. Lack of MHC class I antigens and tumour aggressiveness of the squamous cell carcinoma of the larynx. Br J Cancer 1990;62:1047–51.
94. Ferrone S, Marincola FM. Loss of HLA class I antigens by melanoma cells: molecular mechanisms, functional significance and clinical relevance. Immunol Today 1995;16:487–94.
95. Restifo NP, Marincola FM, Kawakami Y, et al. Loss of functional beta 2-microglobulin in metastatic melanomas from five patients receiving immunotherapy. J Natl Cancer Inst 1996;88:100.
96. Jakobsen MK, Restifo NP, Cohen PA, et al. Defective major histocompatibility complex class I expression in a sarcomatoid renal cell carcinoma cell line. J Immunother 1995;17:222.
97. Restifo NP, Esquivel F, Kawakami Y, et al. Identification of human cancers deficient in antigen processing. J Exp Med 1993;177:265.
98. Shimizu J, Yamazaki S, Sakaguchi S. Induction of tumor immunity by removing $CD25^+CD4^+$ T cells: a common basis between tumor immunity and autoimmunity. J Immunol 1999;163:5211–8.
99. Shevach EM. CD4+ CD25+ suppressor T cells: more questions than answers. Nat Rev Immunol 2002;2:389–400.
100. Curiel TJ, Coukos G, Zou L, et al. Specific recruitment of regulatory T cells in ovarian carcinoma fosters immune privilege and predicts reduced survival. Nat Med 2004;10:942–9.
101. Wolf AM, Wolf D, Steurer M, et al. Increase of regulatory T cells in the peripheral blood of cancer patients. Clin Cancer Res 2003;9:606–12.
102. Viguier M, Lemaitre F, Verola O, et al. Foxp3 expressing CD4+CD25(high) regulatory T cells are overrepresented in human metastatic melanoma lymph nodes and inhibit the function of infiltrating T cells. J Immunol 2004;173:1444–53.
103. Woo EY, Yeh H, Chu CS, et al. Cutting edge: regulatory T cells from lung cancer patients directly inhibit autologous T cell proliferation. J Immunol 2002;168:4272–6.
104. Hussain SF, Paterson Y. CD4+CD25+ regulatory T cells that secrete TGFbeta and IL-10 are preferentially induced by a vaccine vector. J Immunother 2004;27:339–46.
105. Casares N, Arribillaga L, Sarobe P, et al. CD4+/CD25+ regulatory cells inhibit activation of tumor primed CD4+ T cells with IFN-gamma-dependent antiangiogenic activity, as well as long-lasting tumor immunity elicited by peptide vaccination. J Immunol 2003;171:5931–9.
106. Nagai H, Horikawa T, Hara I, et al. In vivo elimination of CD25+ regulatory T cells leads to tumor rejection of B16F10 melanoma, when combined with interleukin-12 gene transfer. Exp Dermatol 2004;13:613–20.
107. Turk MJ, Guevara-Patino JA, Rizzuto GA, et al. Concomitant tumor immunity to a poorly immunogenic melanoma is prevented by regulatory T cells. J Exp Med 2004;200:771–82.
108. Vieweg J, Su Z, Dannull J. Enhancement of antitumor immunity following depletion of $CD4^+CD25^+$ regulatory T cells [abstract]. J. Clin Oncol 2004;22 14 Suppl:2506.
109. Palucka AK, Laupeze B, Aspord C, et al. Immunotherapy via dendritic cells. Adv Exp Med Biol 2005;560:105–14.
110. Gajewski TF. Integrating IL-12 into therapeutic cancer vaccines. Cancer Chemother Biol Response Modif 2002;20:343–9.
111. Yang I, Kremen TJ, Giovannone AJ, et al. Modulation of major histocompatibility complex class I molecules and major histocompatibility complex-bound immunogenic peptides induced by interferon-alpha and interferon-gamma treatment of human glioblastoma multiforme. J Neurosurg 2004;100:310–9.
112. Chambers CA, Kuhns MS, Egen JG, et al. CTLA-4-mediated inhibition in regulation of T cell responses: mechanisms and manipulation in tumor immunotherapy. Annu Rev Immunol 2001;19:565–94.
113. Doyle AM, Mullen AC, Villarino AV, et al. Induction of cytotoxic T lymphocyte antigen 4 (CTLA 4) restricts clonal expansion of helper T cells. J Exp Med 2001;194:893–902.
114. Chikuma S, Abbas AK, Bluestone JA. B7-independent inhibition of T cells by CTLA-4. J Immunol 2005;175:177–81.
115. Hodi FS, Mihm MC, Soiffer RJ, et al. Biologic activity of cytotoxic T lymphocyte-associated antigen 4 antibody blockade in previously vaccinated metastatic melanoma and ovarian carcinoma patients. Proc Natl Acad Sci U S A 2003;100:4712–7.

12e

Monitoring the Immune Response to Cancer Vaccines

Amy C. Hobeika, PhD
Timothy M. Clay, PhD
H. Kim Lyerly, MD
Michael A. Morse, MD

The quantification of antigen-specific immune responses has become increasingly relevant to the clinical evaluation of cancer immunotherapy strategies.[1,2] Although the primary goal of anticancer immunotherapy is to improve patient outcome, the traditional end points used for evaluation require both extensive resources and long-term follow-up. Early identification of biologic activity may provide a way to prioritize agents for further clinical evaluation. In addition, biologic markers relevant to a specific therapy may be a more direct indicator of immune efficacy. The immune response to tumor-specific antigens can be detected by several highly sensitive immunologic assays. Although effectors such as monocytes, natural killer cells, and antibodies have been shown to have potentially important roles in antitumor immunity, the T-cell response is generally believed to be central to antitumor immune responses. $CD8^+$ cytotoxic T lymphocytes (CTLs) act to cause cytolysis of tumor cells based on the presentation of tumor peptides on the surface of the cells, whereas $CD4^+$ helper T cells are involved in CTL generation. As a result, T cell–based assays have become a significant part of patient analysis in immunotherapy-based clinical trials and in understanding protective immunity.

Assays for measuring T-cell responses traditionally relied on labor-intensive methods that involved in vitro manipulation of bulk populations of cells to expand T-cell levels to a number that was measurable. Unfortunately, these assays made it difficult to compare results between studies and are nonquantitative. More recent advances in T-cell biology have resulted in the development of techniques that possess common desirable characteristics. Although these in vitro T-cell assays also provide distinct advantages over one another, the qualities that make these assays beneficial for clinical studies include the following: they can be performed directly from patient blood or peripheral blood mononuclear cells (PBMCs) without previous manipulation; they are highly sensitive, specific, reliable, and reproducible; they require relatively small quantities of cells; and they are simple and rapid to perform.

PROLIFERATION

The standard proliferation assay involves long-term antigen stimulation of bulk PBMC populations where responding T cells are typically detected by measuring the synthesis of new deoxyribonucleic acid (DNA) using [3H]-thymidine incorporation. A stimulation index can then be calculated by dividing the number of counts per minute for the specimen when exposed to antigen by the counts per minute for the specimen without antigen (unstimulated control). Because it is relatively easy to perform and requires a low number of cells, the proliferation assay has frequently been used in clinical trials of immunotherapy.[3–8] However, although this assay can provide some useful qualitative data and give a general idea of the T-cell activity, it has several drawbacks. Traditional proliferation assays are not truly quantitative in that they reflect the overall amount of proliferation in a culture but do not differentiate between a few cells with high levels of proliferation and large numbers of cells with low levels of proliferation. Additionally, proliferation assays often do not indicate which cell type is responding or detect responses to weak antigens, such as tumor-associated antigens or peptides. It may be due to these issues that this assay has not been convincingly correlated to clinical outcome.[3,5]

Recently, flow cytometry–based assays have been developed that overcome several of the disadvantages posed by the traditional [3H]-thymidine incorporation. Bromodeoxyuridine (BrdU), a thymidine analogue, incorporates into newly synthesized DNA in a manner similar to that of [3H]-thymidine. The cells containing BrdU can then be detected using anti-BrdU fluorescent antibodies.[9] A second method for measuring proliferation by flow cytometry involves the dye carboxyfluorescein succinimidyl ester (CFSE), which binds cellular proteins. Once bound, this stable compound is equally divided among daughter cells, making it possible to count the number of cell divisions based on the twofold reduction in fluorescent intensity.[10,11] Both of these assays allow for identification of individual cells responding to antigen stimulation, resulting in the detection of antigen-specific T cells at a much lower frequency than that of traditional proliferation assays. Moreover, because analysis is performed by flow cytometry, phenotypic details, including effector/memory markers, can be correlated to the responding cells along with functional characteristics using intracellular cytokine staining. One advantage of CFSE when compared with BrdU staining is the requirement for fixation of the cells prior to analysis with BrdU so that further manipulation of the cells is not possible. In contrast, CFSE cells can remain viable and be used for further functional studies. Although these more recent versions of the proliferation assay still require long-term (greater than 24–48 hours) culture, making bystander effects more likely, they offer much more versatility than previous proliferation assays.

PEPTIDE–MAJOR HISTOCOMPATIBILITY COMPLEX MULTIMERS

Peptide–major histocompatibility complex (MHC) multimers were initially described by Altman and colleagues, who showed that by forming a tetrameric complex of peptide-MHC class I, the avidity of the MHC-peptide molecule was increased enough to sufficiently bind $CD8^+$ T cells.[12] These tetrameric complexes are formed by adding biotin groups to recombinant MHC molecules and using avidin to combine four MHC-peptide-biotin monomers together into one complex. Using these stable, fluorescently labeled peptide-MHC tetramers, antigen-specific CTLs can be measured directly from whole blood and cell cultures (Figure 12e-1). The intensity of the staining of $CD8^+$ cells with tetramer appears to correlate strongly with T-cell avidity for the antigen[13]; however, tetramer-positive cells occasionally fail to kill targets expressing the specific epitope.[14] Several studies have demonstrated the ability of peptide-MHC tetramers to quantitate $CD8^+$ T cells specific for tumor antigens or control antigens used in immunotherapy protocols.[15–17] For viral antigens such as cytomegalovirus and Epstein-Barr virus, tetramers have been reported to stain between 0.2 and 2.5% of circulating $CD8^+$ cells.[18–21]

The advantages of peptide-MHC tetramer staining are obvious. They provide reliable, stable, and quantitative data on antigen-specific $CD8^+$ T cells. Tetramers are also practical in that they are easy and quick to use and are commercially available. Similar to other flow-based assays, multiparameter analysis allows for additional phenotypic and functional analysis. Further, tetramers can be used to isolate highly specific and high-avidity $CD8^+$ CTLs, which can be used for various other studies. Dunbar and col-

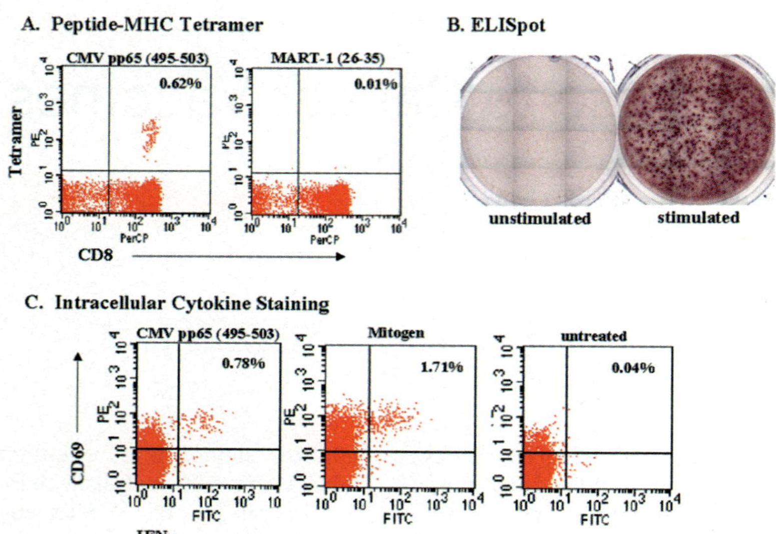

Figure 12e-1 Immune monitoring assays. **A,** Examples of results from a tetramer assay. The CD8+ T cells with T cell receptors that can recognize the antigen CMV in a CMV seropositive individual are depicted. The MART-1 tetramer serves as a control in this individual without evidence of melanoma. **B,** Example of results from an ELISPOT assay showing the spots detected at the site of cells releasing interferon gamma in response to antigen. **C,** Example of results of cytokine flow cytometry showing the CD69+ (i.e., activated) T cells secreting interferon-gamma in response to CMV antigen.

leagues used peptide-MHC tetramers to allow the selection of antigen-specific T cells from peripheral blood or lymph nodes by cell sorting.[22] These selected T cells were cloned for further analysis and were found to respond to specific antigen by cytokine production. Unfortunately, peptide-MHC tetramers also have a number of limitations. Although tetramers can be combined with intracellular cytokine staining to look at functional properties, tetramers themselves provide only phenotypic information and do not indicate whether tetramer-positive cells are also functional. And because the peptide of interest must be synthesized and loaded into the MHC molecule prior to tetramerization, it can be used only to detect immune responses to known antigens. MHC binding peptide epitopes are not always defined for a particular disease, and not all peptides make stable complexes. In addition, each peptide-MHC combination represents only one epitope, possibly giving limited information on the total response to a whole antigen.

The technology behind peptide-MHC multimers is continuing to evolve. Class II MHC tetramers to measure antigen-specific CD4+ T cells are becoming more common and reliable. With an increase in the number of fluorochromes and multicolor flow cytometry, tetramers for multiple peptide epitopes can be analyzed simultaneously along with more in-depth phenotypic analysis. Reversible MHC multimers have recently been developed to aid in techniques such as adoptive transfer.[23] These structures overcome the potential problem of the tetramer binding causing stimulation of the T cell and resulting in subsequent apoptosis or anergy by allowing disassembly of the multimer complexes back into monomer once bound to the T cell. Advances such as these and the increasing optimization of these methods continue to make peptide-MHC multimers an important core technique for monitoring the immune system.

ELISPOT

Cytokine secretion by T cells in response to antigen may be detected by measuring either bulk cytokine production using an enzyme-linked immunosorbent assay (ELISA) or enumerating individual cytokine-producing T cells with an ELISpot assay. Although an ELISA can detect cytokines produced within a cell culture, it does not provide information concerning the specific number of cells responding to stimulation. For this reason, the ELISpot is the preferred method when determining the total number of cells responding to a particular antigen (see Figure 12e-1).

The ELISpot assay consists of six basic steps similar to the ELISA: coating of the microtiter plate with purified cytokine antibody, blocking of the plate to prevent nonspecific absorption of proteins, incubating the cytokine-secreting T cells with antigen, lysing the cells with detergent, adding a labeled secondary antibody, and detecting the antibody-cytokine complex.[24] The final step is typically an enzyme-substrate reaction producing a colored product that can be visualized as a spot or footprint. Each spot represents a single cytokine-producing cell that can be quantitated visually, microscopically, or by using a computerized plate reader. The antigen-specific T-cell precursor frequency is determined by dividing the number of spots or cytokine-secreting cells by the number of cells seeded per well. The ELISpot has been shown to accurately detect the number of antigen-specific T cells by experiments in which known quantities of antigen-specific T cells were added to bulk PBMC preparations.[25]

In addition to being highly sensitive, reliable, and specific, ELISpot assays are also desirable because they can be used for large-scale studies. The computerized plate readers designed for reading ELISpots use digital cameras that can be "trained" for automated reading of plates, allowing for high-throughput data analysis. Other modifications for this assay include a dual-color method that would allow for evaluating two different cytokines at the same time (each cytokine producing a different colored spot or footprint).[26] Although this assay provides more detailed information about cytokine secretion in response to antigen compared with ELISAs, it still does not provide direct phenotypic data on the cells responding.

INTRACELLULAR CYTOKINE ASSAYS

It is also possible to monitor human immune responses by characterizing the cytokine secretion patterns of T cells by flow cytometry, often referred to as cytokine flow cytometry or intracellular cytokine assays (see Figure 12e-1). These assays can be performed on cells from peripheral blood, lymph nodes, or tissue culture. Most methods involve a short period (4–6 hours) of in vitro stimulation of cells with the antigen or mitogen of interest. All or part of this stimulation is done in the presence of a protein secretion inhibitor such as brefeldin A to aid in the detection of the cytokines being expressed.[27] After the stimulation period, cells can be stained for surface markers such as CD4, CD8, and the T-cell activation marker CD69. The cells are then fixed with paraformaldehyde or a similar agent and are permeabilized using a nonionic detergent such as saponin.[28,29] Once permeablized, the intracellular cytokines can be identified for using cytokine-specific antibodies (eg, interferon [IFN]-γ, tumor necrosis factor α, or interleukin-2). The results are read using multicolor flow cytometry.

The ability to combine surface markers to cytokine secretion makes this a valuable assay for determining single-cell cytokine production. With quality cytokine-specific antibodies, this assay is highly sensitive at detecting rare T-cell events. The short-term stimulation gives it an advantage over other assays because it avoids problems commonly associated with longer-term T-cell cultures (eg, proliferation and media changes), and being able to perform it directly on whole blood reduces overall assay time and results in fewer cell manipulations. This assay compares favorably with both peptide-MHC tetramer (and can be combined with tetramer staining) and ELISpot assays,[18,30] and intracellular IFN-γ has been positively correlated to CMV-specific CTL activity measured using a traditional chromium 51 release assay.[31] There are two major drawbacks to intracellular cytokine staining. It can be technically demanding, although, with adequate experience, it is reliably reproducible. In addition, the fixation of the cells to permeabilize them means that they are no longer viable for further manipulations, such as T-cell cloning.

REFERENCES

1. Morse MA, Clay TM, Hobeika AC, et al. Monitoring cellular immune responses to cancer immunotherapy. Curr Opin Mol Ther 2001;3:45–52.
2. Clay TM, Hobeika AC, Mosca PJ, et al. Assays for monitoring cellular immune responses to active immunotherapy of cancer. Clin Cancer Res 2001;7:1127–35.

3. Schreiber S, Kampgen E, Wagner E, et al. Immunotherapy of metastatic malignant melanoma by a vaccine consisting of autologous interleukin 2-transfected cancer cells: outcome of a phase I study. Hum Gene Ther 1999;10:983–93.
4. Salgaller ML, Lodge PA, McLean JG, et al. Report of immune monitoring of prostate cancer patients undergoing T-cell therapy using dendritic cells pulsed with HLA-A2-specific peptides from prostate-specific membrane antigen (PSMA). Prostate 1998;35:144–51.
5. Khleif SN, Abrams SI, Hamilton JM, et al. A phase I vaccine trial with peptides reflecting ras oncogene mutations of solid tumors. J Immunother 1999;22:155–65.
6. Rucker R, Bresler HS, Heffelfinger M, et al. Low-dose monoclonal antibody CC49 administered sequentially with granulocyte-macrophage colony-stimulating factor in patients with metastatic colorectal cancer. J Immunother 1999;22:80–4.
7. Sandmaier BM, Oparin DV, Holmberg LA, et al. Evidence of a cellular immune response against sialyl-Tn in breast and ovarian cancer patients after high-dose chemotherapy, stem cell rescue, and immunization with Theratope STn-KLH cancer vaccine. J Immunother 1999;22:54–66.
8. Disis ML, Grabstein KH, Sleath PR, Cheever MA. Generation of immunity to the HER-2/neu oncogenic protein in patients with breast and ovarian cancer using a peptide-based vaccine. Clin Cancer Res 1999;5:1289–97.
9. Bonhoeffer S, Mohri H, Ho D, Perelson AS. Quantification of cell turnover kinetics using 5-bromo-2'-deoxyuridine. J Immunol 2000;164:5049–54.
10. Lyons AB. Analysing cell division in vivo and in vitro using flow cytometric measurement of CFSE dye dilution. J Immunol Methods 2000;243:147–54.
11. Fulcher D, Wong S. Carboxyfluorescein succinimidyl ester-based proliferative assays for assessment of T cell function in the diagnostic laboratory. Immunol Cell Biol 1999;77:559–64.
12. Altman JD, Moss PA, Goulder PJ, et al. Phenotypic analysis of antigen-specific T lymphocytes. Science 1996;274:94–6.
13. Yee C, Savage PA, Lee PP, et al. Isolation of high avidity melanoma-reactive CTL from heterogeneous populations using peptide-MHC tetramers. J Immunol 1999;162:2227–34.
14. Mackensen A, Veelken H, Lahn M, et al. Induction of tumor-specific cytotoxic T lymphocytes by immunization with autologous tumor cells and interleukin-2 gene transfected fibroblasts. J Mol Med 1997;75:290–6.
15. Lee KH, Wang E, Nielsen MB, et al. Increased vaccine-specific T cell frequency after peptide-based vaccination correlates with increased susceptibility to in vitro stimulation but does not lead to tumor regression. J Immunol 1999;163:6292–300.
16. Romero P, Dunbar PR, Valmori D, et al. Ex vivo staining of metastatic lymph nodes by class I major histocompatibility complex tetramers reveals high numbers of antigen-experienced tumor-specific cytolytic T lymphocytes. J Exp Med 1998;188:1641–50.
17. Dhodapkar MV, Steinman RM, Sapp M, et al. Rapid generation of broad T-cell immunity in humans after a single injection of mature dendritic cells. J Clin Invest 1999;104:173–80.
18. Hobeika AC, Morse MA, Osada T, et al. Enumerating antigen-specific T-cell responses in peripheral blood: a comparison of peptide MHC tetramer, ELISpot, and intracellular cytokine analysis. J Immunother 2005;28:63–72.
19. Burrows SR, Kienzle N, Winterhalter A, et al. Peptide-MHC class I tetrameric complexes display exquisite ligand specificity. J Immunol 2000;165:6229–34.
20. Kuzushima K, Hayashi N, Kudoh A, et al. Tetramer-assisted identification and characterization of epitopes recognized by HLA A*2402-restricted Epstein-Barr virus-specific CD8+ T cells. Blood 2003;101:1460–8.
21. Ouyang Q, Wagner WM, Walter S, et al. An age-related increase in the number of CD8+ T cells carrying receptors for an immunodominant Epstein-Barr virus (EBV) epitope is counteracted by a decreased frequency of their antigen-specific responsiveness. Mech Ageing Dev 2003;124:477–85.
22. Dunbar PR, Ogg GS, Chen J, et al. Direct isolation, phenotyping and cloning of low-frequency antigen-specific cytotoxic T lymphocytes from peripheral blood. Curr Biol 1998;8:413–6.
23. Knabel M, Franz TJ, Schiemann M, et al. Reversible MHC multimer staining for functional isolation of T-cell populations and effective adoptive transfer. Nat Med 2002;8:631–7.
24. Czerkinsky C, Andersson G, Ekre HP, et al. Reverse ELISPOT assay for clonal analysis of cytokine production. I. Enumeration of gamma-interferon-secreting cells. J Immunol Methods 1988;110:29–36.
25. Schmittel A, Keilholz U, Scheibenbogen C. Evaluation of the interferon-gamma ELISPOT-assay for quantification of peptide specific T lymphocytes from peripheral blood. J Immunol Methods 1997;210:167–74.
26. Okamoto Y, Abe T, Niwa T, et al. Development of a dual color enzyme-linked immunospot assay for simultaneous detection of murine T helper type 1- and T helper type 2-cells. Immunopharmacology 1998;39:107–16.
27. Chardin P, McCormick F. Brefeldin A. The advantage of being uncompetitive. Cell 1999;97:153–5.
28. Jung T, Schauer U, Heusser C, et al. Detection of intracellular cytokines by flow cytometry. J Immunol Methods 1993;159:197–207.
29. Prussin C, Metcalfe DD. Detection of intracytoplasmic cytokine using flow cytometry and directly conjugated anti-cytokine antibodies. J Immunol Methods 1995;188:117–28.
30. He XS, Rehermann B, Boisvert J, et al. Direct functional analysis of epitope-specific CD8+ T cells in peripheral blood. Viral Immunol 2001;14:59–69.
31. Ghanekar SA, Nomura LE, Suni MA, et al. Gamma interferon expression in CD8(+) T cells is a marker for circulating cytotoxic T lymphocytes that recognize an HLA A2-restricted epitope of human cytomegalovirus phosphoprotein pp65. Clin Diagn Lab Immunol 2001;8:628–31.

Section 3

CANCER ETIOLOGY

13

Genetic Predisposition to Cancer

Marcia S. Brose, MD, PhD
Thomas C. Smyrk, MD
Henry T. Lynch, MD

The way we think about heredity and cancer underwent a sea change during the twentieth century. When familial adenomatous polyposis (FAP) was described over 100 years ago,[1,2] hereditary cancer syndromes were thought to be very rare. Seventy years ago, a case-control study showed that a positive family history for cancer of the stomach or colon meant a three-fold increased risk for those cancers in family members.[3] In the 1960s, family studies suggested an autosomal dominant mode of genetic transmission for certain clusters of carcinoma of breast, ovary, and colon,[4] a notion that was seriously questioned by many and categorically rejected by some. In the 1980s, the gene for FAP was linked to 5q,[5] then mapped to 5q21,[6,7] ushering in the molecular era in cancer research. The transformation was completed during the 1990s as molecular geneticists made links between mutations and cancers of diverse anatomic sites. There are now more than 40 germline mutations known to be responsible for cancer susceptibility, and it seems that the genetic basis for yet another cancer syndrome is revealed monthly.

The human genome has been mapped, making it almost certain that more cancer susceptibility genes will be found.[8] But the brave new world of molecular biology still must have clinicians in it. Cancer geneticists will not be able to match a subset of our 30,000 to 50,000 genes to hereditary disorders without good, descriptive family studies. Unfortunately, it is rare to pick up a medical chart and find useful information about the family history of cancer.[9,10] A clinician armed with knowledge about the general features of inherited cancer syndromes (Table 13-1) and a willingness to ask about family history constitutes a tremendously effective screen for hereditary cancer.

The estimated number of new cases of cancer diagnosed in the United States during 2005 is 1,372,900.[11] If 5 to 10% of those cases have a primary hereditary etiology (a conservative estimate), then something like 100,000 cancers each year will be attributable to genetic factors. Molecular genetics promises unprecedented power to control or prevent those cancers by testing unaffected members of families whose histories suggest a hereditary syndrome. An individual carrying a cancer-causing germline mutation can be enrolled in surveillance and management programs tailored to the natural history of a particular hereditary disorder, whereas those lacking the mutation can revert to general population cancer screening guidelines.

This rough magic is not without difficulties and drawbacks. Genetic counseling is mandatory, both before and after testing is undertaken. Almost none of the screening and surveillance measures counseled in this chapter have been evaluated in controlled studies; such studies will need to be undertaken where feasible. Ethical and medicolegal dilemmas are sure to arise as patients and their physicians confront privacy and insurability issues. Nevertheless, the translation of genetic knowledge to clinical practice should yield a significant reduction in cancer morbidity and mortality.

Table 13-1 General Features of Hereditary Cancer Syndromes

Same or linked forms of cancer in two or more close relatives
Earlier than usual cancer onset in one or more relatives
Bilateral cancer in paired organs
Multiple primary tumors in the same individual
Specific constellation of tumors are part of known cancer syndrome
Evidence of autosomal dominant transmission of cancer susceptibility

GENETIC BASIS OF CANCER SYNDROMES

Breast-Ovarian Cancer Syndrome **Overview.** In the United States, one woman in eight will develop breast cancer in her lifetime, but some families will be affected at even higher rates. The hereditary breast–ovarian cancer syndrome is characterized by the clustering of breast cancer alone, or breast and ovarian cancer in a single family. Historically, the hereditary breast–ovarian cancer (HBOC) syndrome was recognized in families with an autosomal dominant mode of genetic transmission in the early 1970s.[12,13]

Familial breast cancer accounts for 5 to 10% of all breast cancer, and a substantial number of these cases can be linked to mutations in the genes *BRCA1* or *BRCA2*.[14,15] Familial cases of ovarian cancer comprise up to 8% of all ovarian cancer, and recent reports suggest that most if not all of these may be accounted for by mutations in *BRCA1* or *BRCA2*.[16] *BRCA1* was first linked to chromosome 17q21[17,18] and subsequently isolated in 1994.[19] The existence of breast cancer families without associated mutations in *BRCA1* led to the discovery of a second breast cancer susceptibility gene, *BRCA2*, on chromosome 13q12.[20,21] The scientific and clinical impact of the discovery of these two genes will be discussed below.

***BRCA1* and *BRCA2*: Gene Structure and Function** *BRCA1* and *BRCA2* encode large proteins of 1863 and 3350 amino acids, respectively. They are both complex genes made up of more than 20 exons. Neither gene bears significant homology with other known genes, with the exception of the BRCT domain in the C-terminus of *BRCA1*, a domain found in more than 40 other genes associated with response to DNA damage.[22] It is clear that both *BRCA1* and *BRCA2* are important components of the pathway that protects cells from the effects of DNA damage (reviewed by Venkitaraman[23]). The majority of mutations identified thus far lead to protein truncation, and it is believed that cancer then develops when the second copy is lost. Therefore, it is thought that *BRCA1* and *BRCA2* behave like classic tumor suppressor genes, with the loss of one copy predisposing the carrier to the development of the characteristic cancers of this classic cancer syndrome.

Several lines of investigation have implicated *BRCA1* and *BRCA2* in DNA damage response pathways. An association between *BRCA1* and p53 and the subsequent enhancement of p53 activity incriminates *BRCA1* in p21-mediated cell cycle arrest following DNA damage.[24] In addition, *BRCA1* has been shown to form complexes with both *BRCA2*[25] and Rad51,[26] the human homologue of the *E. coli* gene *RecA,* which is essential to normal recombination and genome stability. Colocalization of *BRCA1*, *BRCA2,* and Rad51 in "nuclear dot" structures is seen to disappear following treatment of cells with DNA-damaging agents that cause double-stranded chromosome breaks.[27] In addition, mouse embryonic stem cells that are homozygous for *BRCA1* null and *BRCA2* truncations are hypersensitive to ionizing radiation and other forms of oxidative damage.[28] The complex network of interactions connecting *BRCA1* and *BRCA2* to cell cycle checkpoints and homologous DNA damage repair has been recently reviewed.[29]

BRCA1 may also play a role in transcription regulation, cell cycle control, and development.[30] Both *BRCA1* and *BRCA2* are nuclear proteins.[31–34] *BRCA1* has been shown to associate with the RNA polymerase holoenzyme[35] and bind CREB,[36] implicating it in transcriptional regulation. *BRCA1* protein levels also have been shown to be altered by variations in hormone levels.[37] During the cell cycle, *BRCA1* and *BRCA2* mRNA levels have been found to increase from low levels at the start of G_1 to maximum levels at the G_1/S transition in parallel to cyclin A levels. Phosphorylation of *BRCA1* also occurs in a cell cycle-dependent manner, suggesting that it may play a role in the G_1/S checkpoint control.[38] Mice with homozygous deletion of *BRCA1* or *BRCA2* die as embryos, revealing a key role for *BRCA1* and *BRCA2* in development.[39–41] However, mice homozygous for a partial deletion of *BRCA2* are viable but show growth retardation and the development of thymic lymphomas.[42,43] Homozygous deletion of *BRCA1* in mouse mammary tissue has been found to lead to the development of tumors.[44]

Clinical Aspects of *BRCA1* and *BRCA2* It is estimated that a family history of breast cancer in the general population confers a 1.7 relative risk of developing the disease.[45–47] The majority of these families will not have a mutation in *BRCA1* or *BRCA2*. However, in a woman who develops breast cancer prior to the age of 40, the chance that she carries a mutation in *BRCA1* may be as high as 10%, or even 20% if she is Ashkenazi Jewish.[15,48–50] This may not be true for *BRCA2,* which may be associated with a slightly older age of diagnosis.[51]

The transmission of the heritable susceptibility to these cancers follows an autosomal dominant pattern. It is estimated that carriers have a 50 to 85% chance of developing breast cancer by the age of 70 and a 16 to 60% risk of developing ovarian cancer.[52,53] Initial reports of a higher than background incidence of prostate cancer have not been confirmed, but there is evidence from several studies of *BRCA1* mutation carriers for an increased risk of colon cancer (RR 2), pancreatic cancer (RR 2-3), gastric cancer (RR 3-7), and fallopian tube cancer (RR 50-100).[54,55] *BRCA2* mutations are associated with an increased incidence of male breast cancer (RR 50-100),[56] as well as an increased risk of prostate cancer (RR 5), pancreatic cancer (RR 4), gall bladder and bile duct cancer (RR 5), stomach cancer (RR 3), and malignant melanoma (RR 3).[57]

Of the women seen in American cancer risk evaluation clinics, *BRCA1* accounts for up to 20 to 30% of breast-ovarian cancer families, whereas *BRCA2* accounts for 10 to 20%. Multiple less penetrant cancer genes that may occur at a higher frequency likely account for the rest of inherited breast cancer risk in families with multiple cases of breast cancer not attributable to *BRCA1* or *BRCA2*.[58,59]

Together, *BRCA1* and *BRCA2* account for most, if not all, familial ovarian cancer.[16] The prevalence of certain *BRCA1* and *BRCA2* mutations is occasionally higher than expected due to the increased transmission of a few mutations ("founder effect") in several subpopulations. Characteristic founder mutations for *BRCA1* and *BRCA2* have been identified in families of Ashkenazi Jewish descent and in Iceland, Finland, Hungary, Russia, France, Holland, Belgium, Sweden, Denmark, and Norway. Most of what we know about *BRCA1* and *BRCA2* has come from studies of whites in the United States and Europe. Significantly less is known about the rates of *BRCA1* and *BRCA2* mutations in families from other ethnic or racial backgrounds.

BRCA1-associated tumors are more likely to be aneuploid, have a high S-phase component,[60] be high grade,[61,62] and be estrogen and progesterone receptor negative.[63] Whether these characteristics result in poorer survival has been difficult to study due to multiple confounding variables, although some studies suggest that this may be the case.[64,65] Evidence from the Breast Cancer Linkage Consortium revealed that unlike *BRCA1*, *BRCA2* tumors are largely indistinguishable from sporadic tumors in their mitotic rate or degree of polymorphism.[60]

Risk Evaluation and Screening The first and most important step in any cancer risk evaluation program is the recording of an accurate history and cancer pedigree. Where possible, it is recommended that all cancers be confirmed by documentation from a hospital record. This is especially true in the case of ovarian cancer, which may be mistaken for stomach or liver cancer as the information is passed through the family. The pedigree helps in identifying the type of cancers and the transmission pattern. Once an accurate pedigree is attained, recommendations can be made regarding the advisability of increased cancer surveillance and DNA testing.

There are several useful models that assist the provider in the evaluation of a patient's risk for the development of breast cancer.[66] These models are based on documented breast cancer risk factors. Other models are available that estimate the probability that the pattern of cancers in a family is the result of a mutation in *BRCA1* or *BRCA2*. These models take into account, to varying degrees, the number, age at diagnosis, and relationship of others in the family who have had breast or ovarian cancer. Although every model has its strengths and weaknesses, knowledge of the appropriate use of different models can help give a range of probabilities that the patient may carry a mutation in one of the two known susceptibility genes.[66]

Due to the expense and difficulty in testing for mutations in *BRCA1* and *BRCA2*, an effort is made to target the testing to the mutations that are felt to be likely in that individual where possible. For example, families of Ashkenazi Jewish descent can be screened relatively quickly and inexpensively first for the three founder mutations, 185delAG, 5382insC in *BRCA1,* and 6174delT in *BRCA2*. These three mutations are thought to account for more than 90% of mutations in this population.[53,67] Where possible, testing is performed on an individual who has been affected with breast or ovarian cancer, thereby increasing the chance that if a genetic alteration exists, it will be identified. Once a mutation is identified in a family, testing of that one mutation can be carried out in the other high-risk individuals. The exception to this approach is in the Ashkenazi Jewish population, where the risk of having more than one founder mutation is sufficient to always warrant screening for all three. In a family where no mutation has been identified, a negative result on testing is uninformative, whereas a negative test on an individual from a family with a known mutation defines the woman's chance of acquiring breast cancer as that of the general population.

For those who desire genetic testing, adequate genetic counseling is required prior to and following the acquisition of any testing results. Once testing has been obtained, those with positive test results have many treatment options available to them including various screening methods, chemoprevention, and prophylactic surgery. Ideally, screening by frequent clinical breast exams, yearly mammography, ultrasound and MRI will identify most breast cancer at stage I or II disease. New evidence that MRI is a more sensitive tool than breast exams, mammography or ultrasound for screening of *BRCA1* mutation carriers has recently been reported,[68] although the impact on mortality is unknown. Chemoprevention with tamoxifen has been shown to reduce the risk of breast cancer in *BRCA1/2* mutation carriers by 50%,[69] although at the price of increased risk of cardiovascular effects and endometrial cancer. Whether newer antiestrogens, raloxifen and anastrazole, currently under study, will be more successful chemopreventive agents remains to be determined (see recent review by Cuzick and colleagues[70]).

Some patients may desire to undergo prophylactic oophorectomy or mastectomy. Unlike breast cancer, ovarian cancer screening has not been shown to be effective, and prophylactic bilateral oophorectomy is the procedure of choice, and has been shown to reduce ovarian cancer risk in mutation carriers by 95%.[71]

In addition, bilateral oophorectomy reduces breast cancer risk by almost 50%.[71] However, because the risk of ovarian cancer increases in the late forties and early fifties, women may wait until after childbearing is complete before choosing to undergo the surgery.

Rebbeck and colleagues,[72] in their update of the efficacy of bilateral prophylactic mastectomy for breast cancer risk reduction in women with *BRCA1* and *BRCA2* mutations, note that research in this area is limited despite the clinical use of this risk-management strategy. Their study estimated the degree of breast cancer risk reduction after surgery in women who carry these mutations. The results showed that breast cancer was diagnosed in 2 (1.9%) of 105 women who had bilateral prophylactic mastectomy and in 184 (48.7%) of 378 matched controls who did not have the procedure, "...with a mean follow-up of 6.4 years. Bilateral prophylactic mastectomy reduced the risk of breast cancer by approximately 95% in women with prior or concurrent bilateral prophylactic oophorectomy and by approximately 90% in women with intact ovaries." They concluded that, overall, bilateral prophylactic mastectomy reduced the risk of breast cancer in women with *BRCA1/2* mutations by approximately 90%.

Despite the decrease in risk, the role of lumpectomy in the presence of a BRCA mutation remains unclear. In the setting of a *BRCA1* or *BRCA2* mutation, Robson and colleagues[73] suggest that the significant risks of contralateral breast cancer and late metachronous ipsilateral breast cancer, "...may prompt the serious consideration of bilateral mastectomy as a preventive measure." However, limited data are available on whether this decrease in breast cancer risk translates into increased survival when compared to multi-modality surveillance of mutation carriers.

Breast Cancer Susceptibility Genes other than *BRCA1/BRCA2* de Jong and colleagues[74] have provided an extensive review focusing on genes other than the high-penetrance *BRCA1/BRCA2* mutations that are involved in breast cancer susceptibility, including the discovery of 13 polymorphisms in 10 genes that are either associated with breast cancer susceptibility or that are in strong linkage disequilibrium with breast cancer causing variants. They discuss recent data that assume that hypermethylation of the promotor region of a gene can also be one of the "hits" acquired in malignant neoplastic development due to silencing of the gene. Germline mutations in other genes of interest found to predispose to breast cancer include the *TP53* gene in the Li-Fraumeni syndrome; the *ATM* gene in ataxia telangiectasia; the *PTEN* gene in Cowden syndrome; and the *LKB1* gene in Peutz-Jeghers syndrome. Polymorphisms in *HRAS1*, *GSTM1*, *GSTP1*, *CYP1B1* (codon 119), *CYP2D6*, *CYP19*, and *VDR* (*Apa*I and poly-A) were also implicated. The group also described finding decreased breast cancer risks in women homozygous for the variant allele for the intron 3, exon 4, and intron 6 polymorphisms in the *TP53* gene, the *Xba*I polymorphism in the *ER* gene, and the PROGINS polymorphism in the *PR* gene. The authors suggest that carriers of these polymorphisms may represent a subpopulation wherein prevention strategies in the future may be applied less intensively than for the general population. Little is known of how the combinations of such polymorphisms might affect breast cancer risk.

The *CHEK2**1100delC variant is an example of a novel lower penetrance allele associated with increased breast cancer risk. The *CHEK2**1100delC variant predisposes to breast cancer in multiple-case families wherein *BRCA1* and *BRCA2* have been excluded. de Bock and colleagues[75] have shown in a large case-control study that harboring the *CHEK2**1100delC mutation increases breast cancer risk albeit to a lesser degree than *BRCA1* and *BRCA2*. How this information should be incorporated into clinical practice is not yet clear, but the authors suggest that "...intensive surveillance, and possibly preventive measures should be considered for newly diagnosed breast cancer cases carrying the *CHEK2**1100delC variant."

Cybulski and colleagues[76] have also recently examined the *CHEK2* gene, which has been associated with a predisposition to breast and prostate cancer in North America and Europe. It is noteworthy that this CHEK2 protein participates in the DNA damage response involving multiple cell types and thereby becomes a good candidate for a multisite cancer susceptibility gene. These investigators identified three founder alleles to be present in Poland, two of which resulted in truncated CHEK2 protein, whereas the remainder is a missense substitution of an isoleucine for a threonine. The majority of common cancer anatomic sites associated with protein-truncating alleles included cancers of the thyroid (odds ratio [OR] 4.9; $p = .0006$), breast (OR 2.2; $p = .02$), and prostate (OR 2.2; $p = .04$). In addition, the missense variant I157T was associated with an increased risk of breast cancer (OR 1.4; $p = .02$), colon cancer (OR 2.0; $p = .001$), kidney cancer (OR 2.1; $p = .0006$), prostate cancer (OR 1.7; $p = .002$), and thyroid cancer (OR 1.9; $p = .04$). Therefore, the range of cancers associated with mutations of the *CHEK2* gene may far exceed breast cancer alone.

Summary With the identification of *BRCA1* and *BRCA2*, we have been able to directly impact the care of people who come from families with mutations in these genes. With the further characterization of additional cancer-prone genes, we hope to gain further insights into the mechanisms that underlie the development of these cancers and their potential for cancer prevention and cure. The cloning of the human genome and the identification of additional risk-associated genes, continues to expand the clinical management of individuals with a strong history of breast and ovarian cancer.[77] Thus, the role of genetic counseling by individuals who specialize in cancer risk assessment will continue to grow in importance. Similarly, an increased understanding of the function of these genes may have significant implications for the treatment of these tumors in the future.[78]

Colorectal Carcinoma **Overview** Approximately 145,300 new cases of colorectal cancer (CRC) will be diagnosed in the United States during 2005.[11] Known hereditary syndromes will account for at least 10% of those, and it is likely that more subtle susceptibility factors contribute to the pathogenesis of many more. A large prospective study[79] recently confirmed what more than a dozen retrospective studies had asserted, that a family history of CRC confers increased risk of the disease. In 1985, analysis of a large colon cancer-prone Utah kindred pointed to the existence of a partially penetrant gene, inherited in an autosomal dominant fashion.[80] The missense mutation in the *APC* gene described by Laken and colleagues (I1307K)[81] is an example of such a mutation. Other low-penetrance mutations may prove to be important contributors to colon cancer risk and are discussed elsewhere in this chapter. This section will review four inherited syndromes featuring increased risk for colon cancer: familial adenomatous polyposis, hereditary nonpolyposis colorectal cancer (Lynch syndrome), familial juvenile polyposis, and Peutz-Jeghers syndrome (PJS).

Familial Adenomatous Polyposis Bulow[82] cites an 1861 clinical patient report by Luschka[83] that may have been FAP. The first definitive report of a patient with multiple colonic polyposis was published in 1881 by Sklifasowski.[84] The first familial example was that of a brother and sister with FAP reported by Cripps[1] in 1882. Additional cases of CRC in patients with FAP were reported by Smith in 1887.[2] The histologic changes from adenoma to adenocarcinoma were first described by Handford.[85] Lockhart-Mummery[86] was the first to report that the relevant hereditary factor in this disease is not the cancer *per se*, but rather the presence of multiple adenomas, which have a tendency to undergo malignant transformation. This sentinel report, emanating from the histories of three FAP families, formed the basis for the now renowned St. Mark's Hospital Polyposis Registry in London, England.

FAP is inherited in an autosomal dominant pattern. The incidence is 1 in 6,000 to 1 in 13,000; Powell and colleagues estimated that more than 50,000 families in the United States could benefit from genetic counseling for this disorder.[87] Affected individuals carry germline mutations of the *APC* gene on chromosome 5q21-q22.[6,7,88–90] About one-third of FAP patients have no family history and probably represent new mutations. Many mutations of *APC* have been described;

80% of them are truncating. There is some correlation between the position of the truncating mutation and phenotype (discussed below).

APC is a large gene, with 15 exons encoding a 2843 residue protein. The gene product participates in several functions, including differentiation, proliferation, apoptosis, adhesion, migration, and chromosomal segregation.[91] First, *APC* may negatively regulate the Wnt-1 signaling pathway by binding to β-catenin.[92,93] Mutated APC product, unable to bind, allows cytoplasmic and nuclear accumulation of β-catenin, with persistent activation of downstream transcription and growth factors. APC protein also colocalizes with the microtubule cytoskeleton, leading to speculation that *APC* is involved in cell migration and cell adhesion.[94] Finally, *APC* might be involved in cell cycle regulation.[95]

Affected individuals have multiple colonic adenomas and, if untreated, will inevitably develop CRC. Adenomas arise in the mid to late teens; 95% of mutation carriers have adenomas by age 35. More than 90% of FAP patients develop duodenal adenomas, but carcinoma supervenes in only about 5%. Gastric polyposis is seen in at least 50% of affected patients; most of the polyps are fundic gland polyps, but gastric adenomas do occur. Although fundic gland polyps are considered to be benign, there are reports of dysplasia in fundic gland polyps and reports of carcinoma arising adjacent to, or in continuity with, fundic gland polyps.[96] Abraham and colleagues[97] have shown that FAP-associated fundic gland polyps often have sporadic *APC* alterations that sporadic fundic gland polyps lack, suggesting that the polyps arising in the hereditary setting are neoplastic. Gastric carcinoma risk, however, is not appreciably elevated in Western FAP patients. In contrast, Japanese and Korean families with FAP have a three- to four-fold excess risk for gastric carcinoma.[98]

Extra-intestinal manifestations of FAP include desmoid tumor, hepatoblastoma, thyroid carcinoma, medulloblastoma, and a litany of benign lesions: sebaceous or epidermoid cysts, lipomas, osteomas, supernumerary teeth, congenital hypertrophy of retinal pigment epithelium, and juvenile nasopharyngeal angiofibromas. Brain tumors, particularly medulloblastomas, are a feature of the Turcot's variant of FAP.[99]

The attenuated variant of FAP (AFAP) presents a particularly difficult diagnostic challenge.[100–102] Adenomas can be sparse (one or two in some patients, dozens in others) and are often right-sided. The adenomas appear at a later age (35–40 years) than in classic FAP, as do colon carcinomas (55 years). Upper gastrointestinal manifestations (fundic gland polyps and duodenal adenomas) are seen with the same frequency as in classic FAP. The first AFAP families to be described had mutations near the proximal end of the *APC* gene; the phenotype has since been seen in families with mutations at the extreme distal end as well.

Genetic testing is available for FAP. If a mutation is found in an affected family member, other at-risk family members can easily be tested for the mutations. Genetic testing is not recommended for children less than 10 years old. If no mutation is found in an affected family member, the test is considered uninformative; a negative result in that setting does not rule out FAP.

Two recent studies compared the phenotype of FAP families with and without documented mutations. Moisio and colleagues[103] identified 38 different germline mutations in *APC* in 47 of 65 (72%) Finnish FAP kindreds. Families without detectable *APC* mutations differed from mutation positive families by having an older mean age of polyposis diagnosis (38.6 years [48 individuals] vs 30.0 years [140 individuals]; p = .001) and a lower proportion of kindreds with extracolonic disease (6/18 v 5/47; p = .04). Heinimann and colleagues[104] studied 36 FAP families, 72% of which were positive for the *APC* germline mutation. The mean age at diagnosis of colonic adenomas was 35.2 years in *APC*-positive families versus 45.3 years in *APC*-negative families. Gastric polyps were found in 14 patients, all of whom were *APC* positive. Finally, patients who were *APC* negative showed a lower number of colonic adenomas at diagnosis and fewer extracolonic manifestations. These authors concluded that patients from FAP families who lacked *APC* germline mutations presented with a notably milder disease phenotype when compared to the *APC*-positive families. Randomized, controlled trials demonstrating the efficacy of screening and management regimens have not been performed and are not likely to be. Nevertheless, the following recommendations are generally agreed upon: affected or at-risk individuals should have annual flexible sigmoidoscopy beginning by age 12. If the family history suggests AFAP, then colonoscopy is required (because the adenomas are more proximal), but can begin later (age 20). Prophylactic colectomy should be considered once multiple adenomas have appeared. However, it may be that prophylactic colectomy can be postponed in AFAP when management by polypectomy is possible; we are following several mutation carriers who develop one or two new adenomas every year but who have not developed carcinoma. Endoscopic surveillance of the rectum and anus should be continued after colectomy. A baseline upper endoscopy is advisable by age 20, with follow-up examinations every two to three years unless symptoms occur. Annual thyroid palpation is suggested, and children at risk for FAP should have serum α-fetoprotein testing every 6 months until 6 years of age in the interest of early detection of hepatoblastoma.

When duodenal adenomas are discovered, they should be removed endoscopically if feasible. Often, however, the adenomas are too numerous to remove; in that case, annual surveillance with biopsy of grossly suspicious lesions is a prudent course. It is hoped that chemoprevention will help control duodenal adenomas, but results thus far have not been encouraging (reviewed by Hawk and colleagues[105]).

Desmoid tumors can be a difficult management problem. These locally aggressive soft-tissue tumors typically arise in the abdominal wall or bowel mesentery. Relentless recurrences are the rule.[106,107] The difficulty of surgical cure, complete with the fact that surgery may initiate the pathogenesis of desmoids, has led to the recommendation that only symptomatic desmoid tumors should be surgically resected.[108] Desmoid tumors may occur in excess in certain FAP families.[107,109,110]

I1307K Ashkenazi Mutation First described by Laken and colleagues,[81] the I1307K mutation/polymorphism is carried by approximately 6% of Ashkenazi Jews and a lower proportion of other Jews; it has not been seen in non-Jews.[81,111,112] Carriers have an approximately two-fold risk of colorectal cancer compared with non-carriers.[81] Rozen and colleagues[113] studied the I1307K APC gene variant in 718 Israeli Jews wherein "....I1307K occurred in 6.2% Ashkenazi participants, in 1.5% of non-Ashkenazi control participants (p = 0.02) and in 10% of Ashkenazim with *familial* neoplasia (relative risk 1.73 [not significant when compared with controls]; 95% confidence interval, 0.7-3.2). Colorectal neoplasia was detected in carriers at a younger age (p <0.05) without excess risk for multiple colorectal neoplasia or non-colorectal neoplasia. I1307K attributable risk for colorectal neoplasia was 0.5–0.6%. Compared with non-carriers, both Ashkenazi and non-Ashkenazi I1307K carriers had similar flanking polymorphic markers (p <0.01)".

The conclusion from this study was that this low penetrant genetic variant poses an approximate 1.7 relative risk for neoplasia in mutation carriers who have familial CRC and that it appears to be clinically equivalent to "...obtaining a family history of sporadic colorectal neoplasia and promoting early screening. I1307K is a founder genetic variant in Jews of different ethnic origin, namely Ashkenazim, but it explains only partially their higher instance of colorectal carcinoma."

Familial Juvenile Polyposis Sporadic juvenile polyps are relatively common (one autopsy study of patients under 21 years reported a prevalence of 1%).[114] Usually solitary, the polyps are innocuous and do not confer increased risk for cancer of the colon.[115] The discovery of multiple juvenile polyps in a patient without a family history of polyposis can create a diagnostic dilemma. The clinical diagnosis of juvenile polyposis (JP) requires histologic confirmation of a juvenile polyp, plus the presence of any of the following: more than 5 juvenile polyps in the colorectum, juvenile polyps elsewhere in the gastrointestinal tract, or a family history of polyposis. Even when there are multiple juvenile polyps and a family history of polyposis, the diagnosis of juvenile polyposis must be made with care, because Cowden syndrome and Bannayan-Riley-Ruvalcaba syndrome have similar polyps but a very different spectrum of associated lesions.[116]

Three variants of JP have been described: a rare, usually fatal juvenile polyposis of infancy with diarrhea, protein-losing enteropathy, and alopecia; juvenile polyps of the colorectum; and generalized juvenile polyposis. (The division between the latter two may be an artifact of variable penetrance, as both the colorectal and gener-

Table 13-2 Hamartomatous Polyposis Syndromes

Syndrome	Phenotype	Mutations
Peutz-Jeghers	Perioral pigmentations, pigmentations of fingers, upper and lower GI hamartomatous lesions, small bowel and pancreas cancer, colorectal cancer and sex cord tumors with annular tubules (SCTAT) of the ovary	*LKBI/STK11* gene[440]
Familial juvenile polyposis	GI hamartomatous polyps, increased risk of GI malignancy (stomach, colorectum), diagnosis made only when features classic for other syndromes are not present.	*SMAD4/DPC4* gene[119] *BMPRIA* gene[120] *PTEN* gene[441]
Cowden syndrome	Colonic hamartomatous polyps but firm association with colorectal cancer yet to be identified, benign and malignant neoplasms of the thyroid, breast, uterus, and skin (multiple trichilemmomas).	*PTEN/MMAC1/DEP1*[283,293] (Finding a germline *PTEN* mutation is molecular evidence for the Cowden syndrome, but absence of an identifiable *PTEN* mutation is non-diagnostic.)
Bannayan-Ruvalcaba-Riley	Microcephaly, fibromatosis, hamartomatous polyposis, hemangiomas, speckled penis; colorectal cancer has not been identified.	*PTEN*

alized forms have been described in one kindred. Extraintestinal anomalies, although not common, have been reported in association with juvenile polyps; these include hydrocephalus, thyroglossal duct cyst, tetralogy of Fallot, coarctation of the aorta, idiopathic hypertrophic subaortic stenosis, and malrotation of the gut.

The inheritance pattern is autosomal dominant. A gene for JP has been mapped to a locus on chromosome 18q21.[117] The gene encodes a component of the TGFβ signaling pathway *MAD4*.[118,119] Mutations in *MADH4* account for about 20% of JP cases. A second gene, bone morphogenetic protein receptor 1A (*BMPR1A*), has been implicated in another 20% of JP.[120] *BMPR1A* is a member of the TGFβ superfamily, and is part of the pathway mediated by MADH4 signaling.

Juvenile polyps may be found in the colorectum (98%), stomach (14%), duodenum (2%), and jejunum and ileum (7%).[121,122] Although the polyps are considered benign, JP patients are at increased risk for CRC. The cumulative lifetime risk was estimated by Järvinen to be 50%,[123] an estimate that compares remarkably well to a report from the University of Iowa describing a large JP kindred in which 16 of 29 (55%) affected individuals developed gastrointestinal cancer.[124] Eleven members of the Iowa kindred had colon cancer and six had gastric cancer.

Affected individuals need regular endoscopic surveillance. Scott-Conner and colleagues[122] recommend upper and lower gastrointestinal endoscopy beginning at age 15 and continuing every 3 years as long as no lesions are detected. If a family carries a *MADH4* or *BMPR1A* mutation, at-risk individuals can be tested to determine whether surveillance is needed. Small numbers of polyps can be managed by polypectomy; in these cases, endoscopy should be repeated yearly until the patient is free of polyps. If there are multiple polyps in the colon, subtotal colectomy is recommended if the rectum can be cleared endoscopically; otherwise, total colectomy is a consideration. For young children with large numbers of polyps, regular colonoscopy with removal of the largest polyps is an option as a temporizing measure until puberty has been attained. Multiple gastric polyps, particularly if dysplasia is present, should prompt consideration of gastrectomy.

Children with large numbers of polyps present a difficult management problem. Colectomy is the prudent choice, but we believe regular colonoscopy with removal of the largest polyps until the patient attains puberty is also an option.[124]

Peutz-Jeghers Syndrome PJS is inherited in an autosomal dominant pattern and has been mapped to a locus on chromosome 19p13.3.[125,126] The gene responsible for the syndrome encodes a serine threonine kinase, STK11 (also known as LKB1).[125] Abnormal (ie, inactive) forms of this kinase may lead to defective control of cellular growth and differentiation. Not all PJS families can be linked to 19p13.3, leading to speculation that there is a second locus for the syndrome.[127,128] The incidence of PJS is unknown; it is thought to be about one-tenth as common as FAP.[80]

The diagnosis of PJS requires histologic confirmation of a hamartomatous, Peutz-Jeghers-type polyp. Because such polyps can be seen in individuals who do not have PJS, clinical diagnosis also requires at least two of the following: small bowel polyposis, family history of PJS; or pigmented macules of buccal mucosa, lips, fingers, and toes.[129] Genetic testing for the syndrome is being developed.[130]

Peutz-Jeghers polyps have been found in the entire gastrointestinal tract. The small bowel is the site affected most often, but stomach and colon are involved as well; esophageal polyps are rare. The polyps are almost always multiple but tend to number in the dozens rather than the hundreds. Peutz-Jeghers polyps have also been described in respiratory mucosa and the urinary tract. One member of the Dutch family originally studied by Peutz suffered from severe nasal polyposis and eventually developed a nasal carcinoma.[131]

PJS carries an increased risk for malignancy. Giardiello and colleagues[129] found a relative risk for cancer 18 times that of the general population in 31 PJS patients. Malignancies involved pancreas (4), breast (2), stomach (2), colon (2), lung (2), and endometrium (1). Spigelman and colleagues[132] reported that 72 retrospectively studied PJS patients were 13 times more likely than the general population to develop a malignancy. The tumors involved colon, stomach, small intestine, ovary, fallopian tube, thyroid, and lung. Investigators from the Mayo Clinic[133] found a relative risk for cancer of 9.9 in 34 PJS patients, with cancers of the colon (7), breast (6), lung (3), and cervix (2) predominating. The Mayo Clinic group found a particularly high incidence of breast and gynecologic cancers, contributing to a relative cancer risk of 18.5 in women, compared to 6.2 in men.

The Dutch family originally described by Peutz has been updated, and the findings further demonstrate that PJS is not a benign condition.[131] Of 22 affected individuals, seven developed carcinoma (3 colon, 1 stomach, 1 gastrointestinal not otherwise specified, 1 breast, and 1 nasal cavity). All patients with malignancy were dead of their disease before the age of 50 years.

Nearly every female PJS patient will have ovarian involvement by sex cord tumor with annular tubules (SCTAT). The tumors are bilateral in at least two-thirds of cases (in contrast to SCTAT in the sporadic setting, which is almost always unilateral). An unusual form of cervical cancer, minimal deviation adenocarcinoma (adenoma malignum), is also characteristic of PJS. This rare tumor accounts for 1 to 3% of all cervical adenocarcinoma but, in one series, affected 4 of 27 women with PJS.[134]

The surveillance protocol advocated by the St. Mark's Polyposis Registry[135] includes yearly hemoglobin and yearly ultrasound of the pelvis in females and of the pancreas in all patients. Testicular ultrasound should also be done in males with feminizing features. Biannual upper and lower endoscopy with small-bowel radiograph are recommended. Regular mammography and cervical smear are critical surveillance measures. Tomlinson and Houlston[136] suggest that upper endoscopy, colonoscopy, and small-bowel radiograph begin in the second decade and that mammography begin at age 25.

The gastrointestinal polyps may be associated with bleeding, obstruction, or intussusception. Conservative removal (snare polypectomy) is favored over segmental resection of bowel to avoid development of a short bowel syndrome.

Differentiating among juvenile polyposis syndrome (JPS), Cowden syndrome, Bannayan-Ruvalcaba-Riley (BRR) syndrome, and PJS can be difficult.[116] Table 13-2 outlines the genetic and clinical features of the hamartomatous polyposes.

Hereditary Nonpolyposis Colorectal Cancer (Lynch Syndrome) The history of hereditary nonpolyposis colorectal cancer (HNPCC) dates to an observation of Aldred Warthin, pathologist at the University of Michigan School of Medicine.[137] He became deeply moved when his seamstress, in 1895, told him that she would likely die of cancer of the colon, stomach, or her female organs, because of the enormous proclivity to these cancers in her family. Unfortunately, just as she had told Warthin, she died at a young age of metastatic endometrial carcinoma. Warthin listened intently, developed her pedigree, and along with other similar cancer prone families published this work in 1913.[138] He updated the family in 1925.[139] The seamstress's family has since been known as Family G.

Lynch and colleagues[4] described the natural history and genetics of two large Midwestern kindreds (Families N and M) in 1966. The clinical genetic features in these families were similar to those of Family G.[4] Dr. A. James French, Warthin's successor as chairman of pathology at the University of Michigan, heard about Lynch's research on Families N and M,[4] and recalled that Warthin, his predecessor, had discovered a similar family (Family G) in 1895. Lynch was then invited by French to take custody of all the detailed documents and pathology specimens which the meticulous Warthin had investigated, catalogued, and published over a span of more than 30 years.[138,139] Family G was then updated and published in 1971.[140] This material is discussed in a more detailed review of the history of HNPCC.[141] Through the use of conversion technology,[142]an *MSH2* mutation was identified in Family G in the year 2000.

Hereditary nonpolyposis colorectal cancer (HNPCC) is inherited in an autosomal dominant pattern. A germline mutation in one of the genes responsible for DNA mismatch repair (MMR) can be demonstrated in the 40 to 60% of families meeting clinical criteria for HNPCC. The incidence has not been definitely established, but a large-scale molecular screening study from Finland indicates that HNPCC accounts for about 2% of the CRC burden in that country.[143] Other estimates of its frequency range much higher.[144,145]

Mutations in six different MMR genes have been identified in HNPCC patients[146,147]: *MLH1*,[148] located on chromosome 3p21.3; *MSH2*[149,150] and *MSH6*,[151] both located on 2p21; *PMS2*,[152] located on 7p22; *MLH3*,[153,154] located on 14q24.3; and possibly *PMS1*,[152] located on 2q31-q33. However, only 40 to 60% of HNPCC patients harbor identifiable germline mutations, most common of which are *MSH2* and *MLH1* mutations.[155] Approximately 90% of the identified HNPCC mutations involve *MLH1* or *MSH2*, whereas mutations in the *MSH6* gene account for approximately 10%. *MSH6* mutations appear to predispose to an atypical form of HNPCC characterized by an excess of endometrial cancer and a deficit of CRC [156] These findings therefore suggest that other genes, including modifier genes, may be of etiologic importance in HNPCC; differing mutation types, environmental factors, and/or chance could also explain the etiology of those 40 to 60% of HNPCC families in which no known cancer-causative germline mutations have to date been identified.[144,147]

All cells of affected individuals carry a nonfunctioning allele of a DNA MMR gene; if the wild-type allele is lost or inactivated, the cell can no longer repair DNA mismatches that inevitably arise during DNA replication. Cells with defective DNA MMR accumulate mutations at a very high rate (as much as 1,000 times that of normal cells). Because DNA mismatches are more likely to occur in DNA microsatellites (areas with multiple repeats of one nucleotide or one pair of nucleotides), defective DNA MMR leads to the phenomenon of microsatellite instability, in which the progeny of the defective cells have varying lengths of a given microsatellite.

The predilection of DNA mismatches for mono- and dinucleotide repeats plays a deciding role in the genetic mutations contributing to carcinogenesis. Nearly all colon cancers with microsatellite instability have mutations in the transforming growth factor β type II receptor (*TGFβIIR*) and *BAX* genes, and those mutations are located in repeating sequences. Mutation of *TGFβIIR* leads to escape from the growth inhibitory effects of TGFβ, whereas mutation of *BAX* interferes with its pro-apoptotic effect. Thus, carcinogenesis in colon cancers with microsatellite instability may involve mutations in critical genes different from those involved in other colon cancers (such as *APC*, *K-ras*, *TP53*).

Individuals carrying germline mutations of *MLH1* or *MSH2* have a lifetime risk for CRC on the order of 80%.[157] The cancers tend to arise proximal to the splenic flexure (70%). The average age at diagnosis is 45 years. Multiple synchronous and metachronous colon cancers are a feature of the syndrome, with 30% of patients developing a second colon cancer within 10 years if a limited operation (right hemicolectomy or segmental resection) is done for the initial cancer. Even when total abdominal colectomy is performed, the rectum is still at risk; Rodriguez-Bigas and colleagues[158] reported that 12% of HNPCC patients had rectal cancer within 12 years after colectomy.

The colon cancers arising via the microsatellite instability pathway, whether hereditary or sporadic, often have clinicopathologic clues to their molecular pathogenesis. Such tumors are usually located proximal to the splenic flexure, and may have mucinous or signet ring cell morphology.[159] Medullary carcinoma, a subtype recently recognized in the World Health Organization classification, is found almost exclusively in tumors with microsatellite instability (MSI-H).[160] There is commonly a host lymphoid response, either in the form of lymphoid aggregates at the edge of the tumor or lymphocytes infiltrating the tumor. The latter have been found to be the single best marker of MSI-status.[161] Jass has developed an algorithm for identifying MSI-H colon cancer.[159]

When one suspects that a tumor has microsatellite instability, immunohistochemical stains for the protein product of the DNA MMR genes *MLH1* and *MSH2* can be a useful confirmatory tool. For example, Marcus and colleagues found that 37 of 38 neoplasms known to be microsatellite instability high (MSI-H) (by PCR analysis) demonstrated the absence of MLH1 or MSH2 expression, and 34 of 34 microsatellite stable (MSS) tumors had intact staining.[162] There are, however, important differences between hereditary and sporadic MSI-H cancers that must be understood. Essentially all sporadic MSI-H colon cancers are the result of hypermethylation of the *MLH1* promotor site. In this situation, no protein is produced and immunohistochemical stains are negative. In the hereditary setting, one allele carries a germline mutation; when the second allele is lost or inactivated, it is possible that the mutant allele will produce a truncated or otherwise altered protein that stains normally but functions abnormally, thus resulting in a falsely normal immunohistochemical stain. Salahshor and colleagues,[163] for example, described intact staining for MLH1 in 2 of 15 MSI-H cancers from patients with known mutations of *MLH1*. In a large series of unselected cases, Lindor and colleagues[164] found that 27 of 818 tumors with intact staining of MLH1 and MSH2 were MSI-H. The authors concluded that immunohistochemistry is a specific (100%) and sensitive (92.3%) screening tool, but that some MSI-H tumors will be missed if only immunohistochemistry is performed. We believe the same general rule applies to testing in the hereditary setting, but would emphasize the possibility of falsely normal staining, if clinical features suggest HNPCC, negative immunohistochemistry should not be taken as definitively ruling out the syndrome.

Jones and colleagues[165] note that a common G-to-C polymorphism at codon 72 in the *TP53* gene has been found to be associated with an increased risk for carcinoma of the lung, nasopharynx, oral cavity, prostate, and breast cancer. These authors suggested that this mutation may also be a marker for genetic susceptibility in CRC and therein they investigated this *TP53* polymorphism and age of onset in Lynch syndrome. Their findings disclosed that Lynch syndrome patients who were heterozygous for this polymorphism developed their CRC 13 years earlier than Lynch syndrome patients who were homozygous for the wild-type allele. They, therefore, concluded that, "combining knowledge of an individual's *TP53* genotype with information on other genetic and environmental risk factors may improve risk estimates and help to identify individuals who are genetically susceptible to developing HNPCC at an earlier age."

Extracolonic Cancers Extracolonic cancers are common in HNPCC.[166] Endometrial carcinoma heads the list; women with HNPCC have a 20 to 60% lifetime risk.[157,167] There is also increased risk for carcinoma of the stomach, ovary, renal pelvis and ureter, small bowel, hepatobiliary tract, and pancreas. Glioblastoma multiforme is seen in some HNPCC families. (Families with colon cancer and brain tumors described under the eponym "Turcot's syndrome" have included FAP families with medulloblastoma and HNPCC families with glioblastoma.[99]) Muir-Torre syndrome (benign and malignant sebaceous skin tumors in combination with colon cancer and other internal malignancies) has been shown by mutational analysis to be a variant of HNPCC.[168] Although the relative risk for breast cancer is not increased in HNPCC, breast cancers arising in HNPCC demonstrate microsatellite instability,[169] suggesting that breast cancer is a tumor integral to HNPCC in some families, albeit with lower penetrance.

Unusual Tumors Molecular pathogenesis of tumors outside the usual Lynch syndrome spectrum remain controversial.

Broaddus and colleagues[170] described two young *MSH2* mutation carriers, one age 34 who developed an adrenal cortical carcinoma, and the second a 39-year-old woman who had a diagnosis of anaplastic carcinoma of the thyroid, tumors that are not usually associated with the Lynch syndrome. Both of these patients were members of families that fulfilled Amsterdam criteria. The adrenal tumor and the thyroid tumor each showed complete loss of immunohistochemical expression for MSH2 protein. Furthermore, neither of these tumors was found to be MSI-H based upon microsatellite instability analysis in accord with the National Institute panel of five microsatellite markers.

Other rare tumors in Lynch syndrome include a report[171] of a malignant fibrous histiocytoma arising in a patient with a germline *MSH2* mutation and a positive family history. A male with a germline *MLH1* mutation and a positive family history developed infiltrating ductal carcinoma of the breast 30 years after early-onset CRC. The breast tumor had MSI positivity—BAT-26 and BAT-40. Wild-type *MLH1* allele was lost in the breast tumor tissue compared to normal tissue and was related to the underlying germline mutation of *MLH1*.[172] Berends and colleagues[173] reported a female with an *MSH2* germline mutation, ovarian cancer, and three metachronous CRCs; she was also found to have an adrenal cortical carcinoma. It is of interest that the original proband in Family N[4] manifested adrenal cortical carcinoma.

Broaddus and colleagues[170] have also discussed the molecular pathogenesis of tumors outside the usual tumor spectrum of the Lynch syndrome and note that this issue remains controversial. The question pertains to whether these tumors are related to defects in DNA mismatch repair (MMR), or whether they have arisen independently of this MMR defect.

Prevalence of a Large Genomic Deletion Encompassing Exons 1-6 of the *MSH2* Gene The cancer susceptibility in Lynch syndrome affecteds is believed to be caused by malfunction of the post-replication mismatch repair germline mutations. Therein, more than 400 different pathogenic mutations have been registered in the International Database of Mutations in HNPCC Kindreds (available at <http://www.nfdht.nl>). Whereas detection of mutations is usually performed by sequencing, we report that one class of mutations, namely large structural rearrangements such as large deletions, is difficult to detect by that method. They can be readily identified by Southern hybridization,[174] multiplex ligation-dependent probe amplification,[175] after conversion to haploidy,[142,176] and by PCR, as reviewed by Lynch and colleagues[177] and Wagner and colleagues[178] who identified this deletion, referred to as the American Founder Mutation, and considered it to be the most common mismatch repair gene mutation responsible for the syndrome in the United States. Lynch and colleagues[177] updated these findings based on the study of 566 family members of 9 probands which have been identified to be at risk and counseled, and therein 137 of these have been tested with 61 showing carriage of the founder mutation. Three families have been found genealogically to descend from a German immigrant family that arrived and first settled in Pennsylvania in the early 1700s. This group has tracked movements of branches of the family from Pennsylvania, through North Carolina, Alabama, Kentucky, Missouri, Iowa, Nebraska, Utah, Texas, and California, and documented carriers of the mutation who have been diagnosed in 14 states. Furthermore, the deletion was not found among 417 European and Australian families with HNPCC. This study is being expanded, wherein current estimates indicate that as many as 16,000 descendants from this original cohort are at increased risk for carriage of this *MSH2*del1-6 mutation (Henry T. Lynch, unpublished data, 2004).

***BRAF* Mutation** Domingo and colleagues[179] note that recently the oncogenic V600E hotspot mutation within *BRAF*, a kinase-encoding gene from the RAS/RAF/MAPK pathway, was found to be associated with sporadic MSI-H CRC. These authors analyzed the *BRAF*-V600E hotspot mutation and identified same "...in 40% (82/206) of the sporadic MSI-H tumours analyzed but in none of the 111 tested HNPCC tumours or in the 45 cases showing abnormal MSH2 immunostaining." They concluded that detection of the V600E mutation in an MSI-H CRC tumor is used against the presence of a germline mutation in either *MLH1* or *MSH2*. Hence, screening for MMR genes will not be necessary in those patients who are positive for the V600E when there is no other significant evidence suggesting an MMR-associated Lynch syndrome mutation. Therefore, the testing of the *BRAF* hotspot, "...is a reliable, fast, and low cost strategy that simplifies genetic testing for HNPCC."

Tobacco Use in Lynch Syndrome To our knowledge, the first study documenting the role of an environmental factor modulating the phenotype of Lynch syndrome was reported by Watson and colleagues,[180] who analyzed germline mutation carriers from the Creighton University Lynch syndrome database in order to ascertain whether tobacco or alcohol use was associated with CRC risk. Findings disclosed that tobacco users had a higher incidence of CRC than non-users, reflected in a hazard ratio of 1.43 ($p < .04$). *MLH1* carriers (vs *MSH2* carriers) and males (vs females) were at statistically significant increased risk of tobacco-associated CRC. However, Cox proportional hazards modeling failed to demonstrate a significant correlation between CRC risk and increased pack-years of use. Cox proportional hazards modeling also failed to show a significant association between alcohol use and CRC risk ($p > .40$). Furthermore, tobacco use and a tobacco use × alcohol use interaction term in the model showed no significant association between alcohol use or the interaction term and CRC risk. It was, therefore, concluded that tobacco use, *MLH1* mutation carriers (as opposed to *MSH2*) and a male sex were significantly associated with an increased risk of CRC (hazard ratios 1.43, 2.07, and 1.58 respectively). Alcohol use did not alter CRC risk. These findings support the need for smoking cessation as an integral part of Lynch syndrome management.

Pedigree Assessment and Lynch Syndrome The diagnosis of HNPCC is based on pedigree assessment. Still widely used are the Amsterdam criteria (Table 13-3),[181] which helped standardize reporting of HNPCC but had limitations as a case-finding tool, notably the failure to acknowledge any contribution from extracolonic cancer. The importance of extracolonic cancer was demonstrated by Wijnen and colleagues,[182] who found three independent variables predictive of germline mutations in *MSH2* or *MLH1*: fulfillment of the Amsterdam criteria, the presence of endometrial cancer in the kindred, and early age at diagnosis of colon cancer. New criteria (Amsterdam II) developed by the International Collaborative Group on HNPCC[183] are listed in Table 13-3, as are the Bethesda Guidelines, which have more recently been shown to be useful.[184,185] Finally, a more detailed algorithmic approach to diagnosis of Lynch syndrome has recently been advocated.[186]

Gene testing is available on a clinical basis but is costly and not as sensitive as testing for FAP. Remember that several genes need to be considered (clinical testing is currently limited to *MLH1* and *MSH2*). Hundreds of different mutations have been described,[147] and although many of them are predicted to be truncating mutations (the easiest to detect), the prevalence of truncating mutations is less than in FAP. Also, it appears that one-third of all pathogenic *MSH2* mutations, at least in the Dutch population, show deletion of almost all of one *MSH2* allele.[174] These large deletions are difficult to detect by the usual screening and sequencing techniques.

Because of the early age of CRC onset in HNPCC and its penchant for the proximal colon, full colonoscopy should be initiated by age 20 to 25 in germline mutation carriers and those at risk based on pedigree analysis. Colonoscopy should be performed at least every year, given the problem of accelerated carcinogenesis of CRC in HNPCC.[144,187] We prefer every other year in high-risk patients who have not had DNA testing and annually in patients with HNPCC germline mutations or who are obligate gene mutation carriers by their position in the pedigree.

CRC Prevention: Colonoscopy Screening Järvinen and colleagues[188] showed the benefit of colonoscopic screening in HNPCC through a controlled clinical trial extending over 15 years.[188] The incidence of CRC was compared in

Table 13-3 Amsterdam I and Amsterdam II Criteria, and Bethesda Guidelines

Amsterdam I criteria[181]:

At least 3 relatives with histologically verified colorectal cancer:

1. One is a first-degree relative of the other two;
2. At least two successive generations affected;
3. At least one of the relatives with colorectal cancer diagnosed at < 50 yrs of age;
4. Familial adenomatous polyposis has been excluded.

Amsterdam II criteria[183]:

At least 3 relatives with an hereditary nonpolyposis colorectal cancer-associated cancer (colorectal cancer, endometrial, stomach, ovary, ureter/renal pelvis, brain, small bowel, hepatobiliary tract, and skin [sebaceous tumors]):

1. One is a first-degree relative of the other two;
2. At least two successive generations affected;
3. At least one of the hereditary nonpolyposis colorectal cancer-associated cancers should be diagnosed at < 50 yrs of age;
4. Familial adenomatous polyposis should be excluded in any colorectal cancer cases;
5. Tumors should be verified whenever possible.

Bethesda Guidelines for testing of colorectal tumors for microsatellite instability[184]:

1. Colorectal cancer diagnosed in a patient who is less than 50 years of age.
2. Presence of synchronous or metachronous colorectal, or other HNPCC-associated tumors,* regardless of age.
3. Colorectal cancer with the MSI-H† histology‡ diagnosed in a patient who is less than 60 years of age.§
4. Colorectal cancer or HNPCC-associated tumor* diagnosed under age 50 years in at least one first-degree relative.‖
5. Colorectal cancer or HNPCC-associated tumor* diagnosed at any age in two first- or second-degree relatives.‖

*Hereditary nonpolyposis colorectal cancer (HNPCC)-associated tumors include colorectal, endometrial, stomach, ovarian, pancreas, ureter or renal pelvis, biliary tract, and brain (usually glioblastoma as seen in Turcot syndrome) tumors, sebaceous gland adenomas and keratoacanthomas in Muir-Torre syndrome, and carcinoma of the small bowel.

†MSI-H = microsatellite instability-high in tumors refers to changes in two or more of the five National Cancer Institute-recommended panels of microsatellite markers.

‡Presence of tumor infiltrating lymphocytes, Crohn disease-like lymphocytic reaction, mucinous/signet-ring differentiation, or medullary growth pattern.

§There was no consensus among the Workshop participants on whether to include the age criteria in guideline 3 above; participants voted to keep less than 60 years of age in the guidelines.

‖Criteria 4 and 5 have been reworded to clarify the Revised Bethesda Guidelines.

two cohorts of at-risk members of 22 HNPCC families. CRC developed in eight screened subjects (6%), compared with 19 controls (16%; $p = .014$). The CRC rate was reduced by 62%. All CRCs in the screened group were local, causing no deaths, compared with nine deaths caused by CRC in the controls. It was concluded that CRC screening at three-year intervals more than cuts in half the risk of CRC, prevents CRC deaths, and decreases overall mortality by about 65% in HNPCC families. The relatively high incidence of CRC even in the screened subjects (albeit without deaths) argues for shorter screening intervals, for example, 1 year. In addition, Vasen and colleagues[189] discovered five interval cancers in HNPCC patients within 3½ years following a normal colonoscopy.

In reviewing this subject, Church[190] suggests that interval CRCs develop from normal epithelium within 3 years or from adenomas that were missed. It is important to realize that colonoscopy "miss" rates are as high as 29% for polyps < 5 mm in diameter.[191] Patients should be advised that colonoscopy is not a perfect screening procedure, and the option of prophylactic colectomy should be discussed.[192,193]

Surgical Measures Subtotal colectomy as a prophylactic measure among HNPCC patients remains controversial, but patients who carry germline mutations should be offered this option as an alternative to lifetime colonoscopic surveillance. Genetic counseling must be provided so that patients can be in a better position to evaluate the various management strategies. Church[193] and Lynch[192] both suggest that prophylactic surgery should be an option for patients likely to show reduced compliance for colonoscopy.

Syngal and colleagues[194] examined the life expectancy and quality-adjusted life expectancy benefits resulting from endoscopic surveillance and prophylactic colectomy among carriers of germline mutations for HNPCC. Both risk-reduction programs showed large gains in life expectancy for mutation carriers, with benefits of 13.5 years for surveillance and 15.6 years for prophylactic proctocolectomy at 25 years of age, compared with no intervention. The benefits of prophylactic colectomy decreased with increasing age.

Gynecologic Screening and Surgical Management Women at risk for HNPCC should have annual screening for endometrial cancer beginning at age 25 to 35 years. Endometrial aspiration and transvaginal ultrasound are advised for screening. Prophylactic hysterectomy and oophorectomy can be considered when childbearing is completed.

Those with hematuria should have annual ultrasound and urinalysis with cytologic examination. This screening should begin at age 30. Periodic upper endoscopy should be performed in families with gastric cancer, and those of oriental origin.

Genotype-Phenotype Heterogeneity HNPCC, not unlike other autosomal dominantly inherited disorders, is noteworthy for genotypic and phenotypic heterogeneity.[144,156,195] *MSH2* mutations may predispose to the more severe phenotypic cancer phenomenon in HNPCC, inclusive of an excess of extracolonic cancer compared to its *MSH1* counterpart. This was investigated by Vasen and colleagues[196] in a study that included 138 families with HNPCC wherein mutations were identified in 79 families (34 with *MLH1*, 40 with *MSH2*, 5 with *MSH6*). These investigators found that the lifetime risk for developing cancer at any anatomic site was significantly higher for *MSH2* mutation carriers as opposed to *MLH1* mutation carriers ($p < .01$). With respect to specific anatomic sites, findings disclosed that, "...The risk of developing colorectal or endometrial cancer was higher in *MSH2* mutation carriers than in *MLH1* mutation carriers, but the difference was not significant ($p = .13$ and $p = .057$, respectively). *MSH2* mutation carriers were found to have a significantly higher risk of developing cancer of the urinary tract ($p < .05$). The risk of developing cancer of the ovaries, stomach and brain was also higher in the *MSH2* mutation carriers than in the *MLH1* mutation carriers, but the difference was not statistically significant." These findings are highly important. In addition, the observation of a significantly higher risk of developing cancer of the urinary tract in those who were carriers of the *MSH2* mutation is equally pertinent.

Hendriks and colleagues[197] performed mutation analysis on 20 families with a germline mutation in *MSH6* wherein they compared the cancer risks between *MSH6* and *MLH1*/*MSH2* mutation carriers. They identified a total of 146 *MSH6* mutation carriers, among whom the cumulative risk for CRC was 69% and only 30% for women. Endometrial carcinoma was present in 71% of the women by age 70. Considering all HNPCC-related tumors, they were significantly lower in *MSH6* compared to *MLH1* or *MSH2* mutation carriers ($p = .002$). Among females with *MSH6* mutations, the risk of CRC was significantly lower ($p = .0049$) and the risk for endometrial cancer significantly higher ($p = .02$) than in *MLH1* and *MSH2* mutation carriers.

Childhood Cancer and MMR Menko and colleagues[198] note that *PMS1*, *PMS2*, *MLH3*, and *EXO1* mutations, while not fully clarified as high-penetrance HNPCC genes, may, nevertheless, apparently play a very small role[199–201] cited by Menko. Although childhood and hematological cancers are not generally considered as part of the HNPCC tumor spectrum, Menko and colleagues note that there has been recent evidence of homozygous mutations in the MMR genes *MLH1*, *MSH2*, and *PMS2* in children with hematological malignancies, solid tumors, and, surprisingly, clinical signs (multiple *café au lait spots*) of neurofibromatosis type 1[202–209] cited by Menko and colleagues. Given this background, Menko and colleagues described a child with multiple *café au lait* spots in association with an oligodendroglioma at age 10, followed by rectal carcinoma at age 12. These lesions were ascribed to a homozygous *MSH6* mutation with predicted pathogenic effects. This child was the youngest of a sibship of four of consanguineous, healthy parents. He died at age 12 of complications of the oligodendroglioma. Importantly, he lacked axillary freckling, neurofibromas, or Lisch noduli. His siblings, two sisters and a brother, were normal. There was an unconfirmed history of CRC in the proband's maternal grandfather, which was diagnosed at age 47.

Molecular testing showed the rectal cancer to be MSI-H phenotype (BAT25, BAT26, and D5S346), while the brain tumor was MSI-stable. Immunohistochemical staining for MLH1 and MSH2 expression was normal in the rectal cancer, whereas MSH6 expression was absent. However, in the brain tumor, MSH6-positive cells were identified. A screening test for Fanconi anemia was negative and no germline *NF1* gene defect was present.

Given that the patient reported by Menko and colleagues[198] was homozygous for an *MSH6* mutation, it is, therefore, noteworthy that heterozygous carriers of the *MSH6* germline mutation show a characteristic phenotype of adult-onset CRC and endometrial cancer.[156] However, Menko and colleagues note that homozygosity for the *MSH6* defect, "...Apparently leads to the clinical picture of *café au lait* spots and childhood malignancies..."

Menko and colleagues conclude that, next to *MLH1*, *MSH2*, and *PMS2*, *MSH6* is also involved in the clinical syndrome of childhood tumors and *café au lait* spots, a fact that has been confirmed by a recent report of this syndrome in siblings with homozygous *MSH6* frameshift mutation,[210] which appears to confirm this association. Menko and colleagues also note that the finding in the brain versus the rectal tumor may indicate that biallelic MMR gene defects are associated with various pathways of carcinogenesis.

In their literature review, Menko and colleagues note that Trimbath and colleagues[206] have also reviewed the subject of *café au lait* spots, childhood colorectal neoplasia, and recessive inheritance in past reports of neurofibromatosis and Turcot syndrome.[206]

Nakagawa and colleagues[211] note that mutations in the *PMS2* gene are rare in the etiology of Lynch syndrome. They provide evidence from five published cases that suggested that, contrary to the Knudson principle, *PMS2* mutations cause HNPCC or Turcot's syndrome only when they are biallelic in the germ line or abnormally expressed. Research continues dealing with the clinical and molecular genetic features of the Lynch syndrome.[145]

Li-Fraumeni Syndrome Li-Fraumeni syndrome (LFS) is inherited as an autosomal dominant.[212,213] Its incidence is unknown. Mutations in the *TP53* gene on chromosome 17p31 are found in about 70% of classical LFS families,[214,215] but *TP53* has been ruled out in some classic families,[216] suggesting that this syndrome is genetically heterogeneous. Genetic testing for *TP53* mutations is available.

The tumor spectrum in LFS was characterized by Lynch and colleagues[217] with the acronym SBLA (Sarcoma, Breast cancer, brain tumors, Leukemia, lymphoma, laryngeal carcinoma, lung cancer, and Adrenal cortical carcinoma). Melanoma, germ cell tumor, pancreatic, gastric, and prostatic carcinomas have also been described in LFS. The clinical diagnosis requires one patient with sarcoma under age 45, a first-degree relative with any type of cancer under age 45, and a third affected family member with sarcoma (any age) or other cancer (less than 45 years old). However, its extensive genotypic and phenotypic heterogeneity must be considered when evaluating suspect families.[218]

The risk of developing noncutaneous malignancy is 50% by age 30 and 90% by age 70. Hisada and colleagues[219] studied the incidence of second and third primary cancers in members of 24 LFS kindreds. The cumulative probability of a second primary cancer was 57% at 30 years after the first cancer diagnosis. Sarcomas and carcinoma of the breast accounted for 46 of the 72 cancers identified.[218] Brain tumors may show an extraordinarily high frequency in certain families.[218]

Annual physical examinations with blood cell counts are advised for LFS patients. Careful attention should be given to sites known to be at risk in LFS. Annual mammography, clinical breast examination, and frequent breast self-examination starting at age 25, are particularly important. Recent interest has focused upon the role of MRI, particularly in young patients with dense breasts.

Malignant Melanoma Inherited risk factors are thought to account for approximately 5 to 10% of melanoma, but gene and mutation frequencies are unknown. Melanoma syndromes have been described as dysplastic nevus syndrome,[220] also known as the familial atypical multiple mole-malignant melanoma syndrome (FAMMM),[221] occasionally, pancreatic carcinoma, and melanoma-astrocytoma syndrome.[222] Three putative melanoma-susceptibility genes have been nominated. The first was *CMM1*, which was mapped to chromosome 1p36. However, no candidate gene at this locus has been identified. A second susceptibility locus was mapped to 9p21; the culprit gene is *CDKN2* (*p16*).[223–225] Finally, germline mutations in the *CDK4* gene on chromosome 12q14 have been documented in rare melanoma-prone families.

Hereditary predisposition to melanoma should be suspected in a patient with findings of invasive melanoma in at least two first-degree relatives and/or multiple atypical nevi in the patient.[221] Early age at melanoma diagnosis and multiple primary melanomas are typical of melanoma-prone families. Although not all melanoma kindreds have dysplastic nevi, 10 to 100 nevi on the upper trunk and limbs, with variability in mole size, shape, and color, are characteristic of many *CDKN2* mutation carriers. Histologically, such nevi show the architectural and cytologic atypia of a dysplastic nevus.

The FAMMM syndrome, as mentioned, is associated with pancreatic cancer.[225] Bergman and colleagues[226] found that the risk for pancreatic cancer in these families is elevated by a factor of 13.4. Astrocytomas and sarcomas occur to excess in some melanoma families.[225] Lynch and colleagues,[225] in a study of Creighton University's familial pancreatic cancer resource composed of 159 families, identified 19 (12%) that showed the FAMMM cutaneous phenotypes. In eight of these families with FAMMM-pancreatic carcinoma (FAMMM-PC), the *CDKN2A* germline mutation was identified. One of the patients with the *CDKN2A* mutation had a sarcoma at age 23 and expired from this disease. Her father had classical FAMMM phenotypic features and manifested a sarcoma, esophageal carcinoma, two malignant melanoma primaries, and died of metastatic cancer. Findings from this study support the existence of the FAMMM-pancreatic cancer (FAMMM-PC) syndrome due to the *CDKN2A* germline mutation.[225]

Various mutations of *CDKN2* have been described. In Dutch melanoma kindreds, a 19-bp deletion has been implicated.[227] Whelan and colleagues[228] linked melanoma/pancreatic cancer predisposition to a missense mutation (Gly93Trp).

Genetic testing for mutations in *CDKN2* is available clinically, but its use is limited by debate over how to use the results.[225,229,230] Four healthy carriers of *CDKN2* mutations, all children of parents who died of pancreatic carcinoma, are being followed (Henry T. Lynch, unpublished data, 2004). Regular endoscopic ultrasound (EUS) of the pancreas is ongoing. However, the risks and benefits of EUS have not been established. Study of pancreatic juice for biomarker association is underway in families from the Creighton University resource that show the FAMMM in association with pancreatic cancer and the *CDKN2A* mutation.

Individuals in melanoma-prone kindreds should perform monthly skin self-examination, possibly with the assistance of a spouse or significant other. Comprehensive dermatologic evaluation by a knowledgeable dermatologist should be done semi-annually. Any suspicious lesions should be excised. Sunburn should be avoided, and use of ultraviolet A/B-blocking sunscreens is encouraged.

Multiple Endocrine Neoplasia **Multiple Endocrine Neoplasia Type 1** Multiple endocrine neoplasia type 1 (MEN1) is a rare autosomal dominant disorder associated with several endocrine tumors that cause as much harm by the hormones they oversecrete as by their malignant potential. The tumors most commonly seen include parathyroid adenomas (90%), gastrinomas (40%), insulinomas (10%) and other gastrointestinal endocrine tumors, as well as prolactinomas (20%) and other tumors in the anterior pituitary. A diagnosis of MEN1 is made with two of the three primary classes of tumors in an individual, with familial MEN1 diagnosed with one case and at least one first-degree relative with one of the three component tumor types (reviewed by Brandi and colleagues[231]). Also seen in this syndrome are carcinoids, lipomas, and angiofibromas. MEN1 was first recognized as a familial disorder by Werner[232] (for review see Marx[233]).

MEN1 often presents as primary hyperparathyroidism and less commonly as Zollinger-Ellison syndrome (ZES), insulinoma, or a pituitary tumor. The majority of those affected will have hyperparathyroidism, with 50% experiencing symptoms by the age of 25.[234] As is the case with other familial cancer syndromes, the presentation may be multifocal, as opposed to the solitary tumors found in most sporadic cases. Management of these tumors can be difficult due to the nature of the hormones they secrete. In addition, these tumors are often small, multiple, and difficult to remove surgically.

The *MEN1* gene was discovered by positional cloning following its localization on chromosome 11q13.[235,236] MEN1 encodes menin, a protein that has been shown to inhibit growth of ras-transformed fibroblasts.[237] More recently it has been shown that inactivation of menin by antisense RNA antagonizes TGF-β-mediated cell growth inhibition, implicating this pathway in menin-related tumor suppression.[238] The majority of mutations documented at this time led to early termination of the protein product, suggesting that it is a classic tumor suppressor gene.[236] Recent evidence now suggests that menin binds DNA, regulates cell proliferation,[239] and induces apoptosis,[240] whereas additional cellular functions continue to be elucidated.

It is now expected that most, if not all, families with MEN1 will carry mutations in this gene. Clinical DNA testing exists and can save an individual from a MEN1 family from periodic biochemical testing of serum calcium, parathyroid hormone, and prolactin, which otherwise is begun as an adolescent. However, genetic testing of individuals at this young age is controversial as it is not clear that parathyroidectomy in childhood is indicated. The fact that biochemical testing is readily available, and often less expensive than mutational analysis of *MEN1,* makes the role of clinical DNA testing uncertain at present. As we learn more about the *MEN1* gene, and can develop effective treatment strategies based on the knowledge of carrier status, DNA testing may take on a more important role.

Multiple Endocrine Neoplasia Type 2 MEN2 families are predisposed to develop the triad of medullary thyroid carcinoma (MTC), pheochromocytoma (PTC), and parathyroid hyperplasia with hyperparathyroidism (HPT) (for review, see Machens and colleagues[241]). MEN2A, which encompasses the majority of the cases, usually presents with MTC, which has been documented in infancy and is the major source of mortality in MEN2. MEN2B families have very early onset, aggressive MTC, as well as HPT and characteristic developmental abnormalities involving hyperplasia of the autonomic nerves of the intestines and characteristic facies due to the disorganized growth of axons on the lips, conjunctiva, and oral mucosa.

Familial medullary thyroid carcinoma (FMTC), the third manifestation of MEN2, consists of families in which only MTC is present. The MTC in FMTC is often later in onset and has a better prognosis than in MEN2A and MEN2B.

MEN2 is caused by mutations in *RET*.[242,243] The role of *RET* in human cancers has recently been reviewed.[244] *RET* is located on chromosome 10q11.2, has 21 exons, and encodes a transmembrane receptor tyrosine kinase. Unlike all other known familial cancer syndrome genes, *RET* is a proto-oncogene. Mutations that increase RET activity lead to the subsequent development of cancer and somatic overgrowth and those that inactivate RET cause Hirschsprung disease (HD), a congenital absence of sympathetic neurons in the distal colon and rectum resulting in severe bowel dysfunction.[245] Unlike most other familial cancer syndromes, MEN2 has a very strong genotype-phenotype association. Ninety-eight percent of MEN2A and 85% of FMTC families have missense mutations altering a cysteine residue in the extracellular juxtamembrane cysteine-rich region (exons 10 and 11), whereas a few FMTC families have missense mutations in the intracellular tyrosine kinase domain encoded by exon 13. Ninety-five percent of MEN2B families have a single mutation, M918T (exon 16), also in the intracellular tyrosine kinase domain (reviewed by Eng[246]).

Prior to the availability of clinical DNA testing for *RET* mutations, biochemical screening and imaging of individuals at risk for this syndrome would begin at the age of 4 or 5 and continue into early adulthood. However, as it is now known that 95% of MEN2A and MEN2B, and 85% of FMTC families had documented mutations in *RET*,[247,248] genetic testing is more accurate and has replaced biochemical screening in the diagnosis and management of MEN2. DNA testing for the few common mutations known to be associated with MEN2 can exclude germline *RET* mutations in > 99% of those at risk and patients with sporadic MTC.[249] In a family with a known mutation, DNA testing is 100% accurate and can save a non-carrier from unnecessary and uncomfortable biochemical screening. Due to the high mortality and very early onset of MTC in MEN2, prophylactic thyroidectomy in all mutation carriers should be performed by age 5 years in MEN2A and no later than age 6 months in MEN2B on the basis of positive DNA testing alone.[231,250]

NEUROFIBROMATOSIS **Neurofibromatosis Type 1** Neurofibromatosis type 1 (NF1) is inherited in an autosomal dominant pattern. The disease incidence is 1 in 3,000, with one-third to one-half of cases representing new mutations. The implicated gene (*NF1*) is a large gene (59 exons) located on chromosome 17q11.2. Many different mutations of *NF1* have been reported; most (70 to 80%) are truncating mutations. A protein truncation test is available for clinical genetic testing.

Clinical diagnosis of NF1 requires two or more of the following: (1) *café au lait* spots, (2) two neurofibromas or one plexiform neurofibroma, (3) multiple axillary or inguinal freckles, (4) sphenoid wing dysplasia or congenital bowing or thinning of long bone cortex, (5) bilateral optic nerve gliomas, (6) two or more iris hamartomas, (7) a first-degree relative with NF1 by these criteria.[251] In addition to the lesions listed above, mutation carriers are at risk for neurofibrosarcoma (3–15% of affected individuals), pheochromocytoma, duodenal carcinoid, neuroblastoma, ependymoma, rhabdomyosarcoma, and Wilms' tumor (WT). Children with NF1 are at increased risk for juvenile myelomonocytic leukemia (juvenile chronic myelogenous leukemia) and the monosomy 7 syndrome, a childhood myelodysplasia.

The *NF1* gene encodes a guanosine triphosphatase-activating protein known as neurofibromin. The gene product negatively regulates signals transduced by ras proteins. Side and colleagues[252] note that NF1 apparently "...functions as a tumor-suppressor gene in immature myeloid cells but inactivation of both NF1 alleles has not been demonstrated in leukemic cells from patients with neurofibromatosis type 1."

There are few screening recommendations for patients with NF1. Blood pressure should be monitored twice a year (pheochromocytoma). Neurologic symptoms (headaches, hearing loss, visual change) should be sought and investigated.

Neurofibromatosis Type 2 NF2 is also autosomal dominant. Disease incidence is 1 in 35,000, with about one-half of cases representing new mutations. The *NF2* gene is on chromosome 22q12.2. Genetic testing is available clinically.

The consensus criteria for NF2 require either (1) bilateral VIIIth nerve masses or (2) a first-degree relative with NF2 in a patient with one of the following: unilateral VIIIth nerve mass, a plexiform neurofibroma, two or more neurofibromas, two or more gliomas, two or more meningiomas, posterior subcapsular cataract at a young age, imaging evidence of an intracranial or a spinal cord tumor.[251]

Patients are at risk for central nervous system (CNS) tumors, the most common of which are vestibular schwannomas, schwannomas at other sites, meningiomas, and ependymomas. Although these tumors are often benign and slow growing, their location within the CNS may lead to intracranial and intraspinal involvement with a high rate of morbidity and mortality. Affected individuals also typically develop hearing loss (often bilateral), imbalance, tinnitus, facial weakness and headache, and posterior capsular lens opacities. The average age at onset is in the mid twenties.[253]

NF2 patients may be clinically subdivided into a severe type and a mild subtype, a classification that is based on the age at onset of symptoms, the number and type of tumors developing, and the duration of disease.[254] The severe type is termed the Wishart form of the disease, which is usually manifested prior to 25 years of age. These patients rarely survive past 50 years of age. Those with the mild subtype, referred to as Gardner subtype, present with symptoms usually later in life (after 25 years of age), develop a lesser number of more slow-growing tumors, have only bilateral vestibular schwannomas, and generally survive beyond the fifth decade. Ruttledge and colleagues[254] suggest that the majority of familial occurrences of NF2 involve only one form of the disease (ie,

Wishart type or Gardner subtype), but they note that Kanter and colleagues[255] have shown that some families will manifest both extremes with intermediate cases occurring within these families.

Baser and colleagues[256] evaluated genotype-phenotype correlations for a variety of non-VIII nerve tumors in 406 patients from the population-based United Kingdom *NF2* registry. Findings disclosed statistically significant genotype-phenotype correlations for intracranial meningiomas, spinal tumors, and peripheral nerve tumors. Individuals with constitutional *NF2* missense mutations, splice-site mutations, large deletions, or somatic mosaicism "...had significantly fewer tumors than did people with constitutional nonsense or frameshift *NF2* mutations. In addition, there were significant intrafamilial correlations for intracranial meningiomas and spinal tumors, after adjustment for the type of constitutional *NF2* mutation. The type of constitutional *NF2* mutation is an important determinant of the number of NF2-associated intracranial meningiomas, spinal tumors, and peripheral nerve tumors."

Annual neurologic examination, to include audiologic and ophthalmologic tests, is advised.

RETINOBLASTOMA Retinoblastoma is the most common intraocular cancer in children. Its incidence is between 1 of 13,500 and 1 of 25,000 live births, affecting males and females equally. Most (90%) retinoblastomas are diagnosed before 3 years of age; bilateral tumors tend to be diagnosed at an earlier age than unilateral ones (12 months vs 18 months).

Only 10% of affected patients have a family history of retinoblastoma, but hereditary retinoblastoma is autosomal dominant, with 90% penetrance. Many apparently sporadic cases represent new germline mutations of the gene (*RB*), which is on chromosome 13q14. The gene product is a negative regulator of cell growth. Dephosphorylated RB controls the cell cycle at the restriction point between G_1 and S phase, and inhibits a variety of transcription factors. Cells lacking RB function proceed unchecked through the cell cycle. All patients with bilateral retinoblastoma (40 to 50%) are considered to carry germline mutations of *RB*. Approximately 20% of unilaterally affected individuals also harbor a germline mutation.

Genetic testing is available and is cost effective. Noorani and colleagues[257] compared molecular and conventional screening of retinoblastoma relatives. The cost of conventional screening was $31,430 (US) for a prototype family with seven at-risk relatives. This involved three clinic examinations and eight examinations under anesthesia over the first 3 years of life for each relative. The molecular strategy (a search for *RB1* germline mutation in the proband and the testing of relatives for that mutation), coupled with clinical follow-up similar to conventional strategy for relatives with the mutation, gave an expected cost of $8,674 (US).

Small retinoblastomas can be treated by cryosurgery, photocoagulation, or radiation therapy. Larger tumors usually require enucleation, emphasizing the importance of early detection.

Second malignant tumors (nonocular) are seen in hereditary retinoblastoma. The incidence has been reported as 4.4% at 10 years, 18.3% at 20 years, and 26.1% at 30 years.[258] Radiation therapy for retinoblastoma contributes to this risk but does not account for all of it. Osteosarcoma and melanoma are the most common second tumors, but brain tumors, sarcomas, leukemias, lymphomas, and pinealoblastoma have been reported.[259] Screening for second tumors is difficult because of the multiple possible sites of involvement.

NEVOID BASAL CELL CARCINOMA SYNDROME (GORLIN'S SYNDROME) The nevoid basal cell carcinoma syndrome (NBCCS) is a rare disorder featuring the early onset of multiple basal cell carcinomas. An enormous number of additional features comprise the phenotype and have been used to enumerate major and minor diagnostic criteria (see below). There is marked variation in clinical expression within and between families, but Wicking and colleagues[260] find no convincing evidence of nonpenetrance. The inheritance pattern is autosomal dominant. Wicking and colleagues[260] estimate the new mutation rate to be at least 14% when they include those families wherein both parents had been examined clinically and radiologically and where paternity was confirmed. However, these authors call attention to the work of Shanley and colleagues[261] who indicated that the new mutation rate might be as high as 81% when all patients with unremarkable family histories were defined.

The gene is *PTCH* on chromosome 9q22.3, a human homolog of the *Drosophila* segment polarity gene *patched*.[260,262,263] Genetic testing is available.[260]

The diagnosis of NBCCS can be established on the basis of two major criteria or one major and two minor criteria.[264] Major criteria are (1) multiple (> 2) basal cell carcinoma, one basal cell carcinoma diagnosed at < 30 years, or > 10 basal cell nevi; (2) any odontogenic keratocyst (proven on histology) or polyostotic bone cyst; (3) palmar or plantar pits (≥ 3); (4) ectopic calcification: lamellar or early (< 20 years) falx calcification; and (5) family history of NBCCS. Minor criteria are (1) congenital skeletal anomaly: bifid, fused, splayed, or missing rib or bifid, wedged, or fused vertebra; (2) occipitofrontal head circumference > 97th percentile, with frontal bossing; (3) cardiac or ovarian fibroma; (4) medulloblastoma; (5) lymphomesenteric cysts; and (6) congenital malformation: cleft lip or palate, polydactyly, eye anomaly (cataract, coloboma, microphthalmia).

Because affected individuals develop multiple basal cell carcinomas by age 20, regular dermatologic screening is advised, with early excision of tumors. Clinicians should be aware that about 5% of patients with NBCCS will develop a medulloblastoma during the first few years of life.[264]

VON HIPPEL-LINDAU DISEASE Von Hippel-Lindau (VHL) disease is inherited as autosomal dominant. Disease incidence is 1 in 36,000. The *VHL* gene is on chromosome 3p25-p26. The gene encodes a protein involved in the transduction of growth signals. Hundreds of different mutations have been described, including missense, nonsense, and deletion mutations. Genetic testing (mutation analysis and linkage analysis) is clinically available.

VHL disease is characterized by multiple cysts in kidney, liver, and pancreas, retinal and cerebellar hemangioblastoma, and increased risk for renal cell carcinoma and pheochromocytoma. Angiomas and cysts of the spleen are occasionally described. Retinal angiomas may also occur, usually in young adulthood, and may produce visual loss. Renal cell carcinoma can occur alone or with pheochromocytoma; occasionally, pheochromocytoma occurs alone. Because pheochromocytoma is an integral lesion in other hereditary syndromes (MEN 2 and NF-1), genetic testing for *VHL* and *RET* mutations has been advocated for patients with familial, multiple, or early-onset pheochromocytoma.[265] Renal cell carcinoma occurs in as many as 75% of affected individuals, with an average age at diagnosis of 40 to 45 years. Pancreatic neoplasms (cystadenocarcinoma, islet cell tumor) cluster in certain families.

Kaelin discusses the *von Hippel-Lindau* tumor suppressor gene (*VHL*) on chromosome 3p25 and how, in its mutated or silenced form, it contributes to > 50% of sporadic clear cell renal cell carcinomas. The *VHL* germline mutations indicate risk for VHL. This disease is characterized by "...an increased risk of blood vessel tumors (hemangioblastomas) and renal cell carcinomas. In this setting, *VHL* inactivation gives risk to premalignant renal cysts. Additional genetic alterations are presumably required for conversion of these cysts to renal cell carcinomas."[266]

Affected individuals are advised to have annual neurologic and ophthalmologic examination; annual red blood cell count (renal cysts and cerebellar hemangioblastoma can produce erythropoietin); regular imaging of CNS, kidneys and pancreas; and annual chemical screening for pheochromocytoma.[267]

WILMS' TUMOR The principal gene for WT (*WT1*) is located at chromosome 11p13. There is a second predisposition locus (WT2) at 11p15.5. A third locus is proposed (WT3) but has not been localized. The *WT1* gene encodes a protein that suppresses transcription downstream from epidermal growth factor receptor 1 and insulin-like growth factor II. Clinical genetic testing is not yet available.

WT affects 1 in 10,000 children. Only 1% of those affected have inherited a germline mutation from a parent. Another 10 to 30% have new germline mutations of *WT1*. *WT1*-related syndromes may present as unilateral or bilateral WT only, WAGR syndrome (Wilms' tumor-aniridia-genitourinary anomalies-retardation), or Drash syndrome (childhood renal failure secondary to mesangial sclerosis). Hemizygosity for *WT1* is associated with developmental anomalies of the genitourinary tract. Aniridia associates with WT because the gene mutated in aniridia is adjacent to *WT1*; thus, aniridia is rare in the general population (1 in 70,000), but WT occurs in 1 of 70 children with aniridia.

WT is also seen in association with Beckwith-Wiedemann syndrome. The WT2 locus on 11p15 appears to be involved in the genetic events responsible for Beckwith-Wiedemann, but the precise gene has not been identified. The disorder features hemihypertrophy, enlarged organs, prominent eyes, and neonatal hypoglycemia. Affected individuals are at risk for hepatoblastoma, adrenocortical carcinoma, and gonadoblastoma in addition to WT.

Hartley and colleagues[268] note that approximately 20% of second primary tumors that develop in WT survivors are leukemias and that they have an atypical distribution, with myeloid leukemias predominating. The cytotoxic therapy for WT may be responsible for some of the myeloid neoplasms, but some of the cases may represent an underlying predisposition to development of a second primary cancer. It is noteworthy that both WT and leukemia/lymphoma occur in NF-1. WT is also an uncommon component of the Li-Fraumeni syndrome.

Although the coexistence of WT and leukemia/lymphoma in families may be uncommon, families of this type may provide important models for elucidating the expression of *WT1* and other genes that may be associated with WT in hematologic forms of cancer. Hartley and colleagues[268] suggest that "Expression and interaction of these genes with other tumor-suppressor genes may have widespread implications for development of second malignancies in certain survivors of WT and of specific tumors in close relatives who may be carriers of germline mutations."[268]

CANCER-ASSOCIATED GENODERMATOSES

Rees[269] indicates that humans show a > 100-fold variation in their sensitivity to the deleterious effects of ultraviolet radiation, wherein the principal determinants are melanin pigmentation as well as differences in skin inflammation and repair processes. Therein, there is a high heritability for pigmentation. Furthermore, susceptibility to cutaneous cancer, which is a key marker of sun sensitivity, appears to be less heritable. Rees indicates that, despite a large number of murine coat-color mutations, there exists only one gene in humans, namely the melanocortin 1 receptor (*MC1R*), and therein it is known to account for substantial variation in skin cancer incidence as well as in skin and hair color. It is, therefore, of interest that, "...Most persons with red hair are homozygous for the alleles of the *MC1R* gene that show varying degrees of diminished function. More than 65 human *MC1R* alleles with nonsynonomous changes have been identified, and current evidence suggests that many of them vary in their physiological activity, such that a graded series of responses can be achieved on the basis of (1) dosage effects (of one or two alleles) and (2) individual differences in the pharmacological profile in response to ligand." This author concludes that this single locus which has been identified within a Mendelian framework, "...can contribute significantly to human pigmentary variation."

Ataxia-Telangiectasia Ataxia-telangiectasia (A-T) is inherited as an autosomal recessive disorder. The frequency of gene mutations in the general population is around 1.4%,[270] and disease incidence is 1 in 30,000 to 1 in 100,000. Cerebellar ataxia is present in all patients, becoming evident as the child learns to walk. The ataxia is truncal at first but gradually comes to include ataxia of gait, intention tremor, dystonia, slurred speech, and apraxia of eye movements. Oculocutaneous telangiectasia begins in late childhood. Other cutaneous signs are vitiligo, *café au lait* spots, and premature graying of the hair. Cellular and humoral immune deficiency is common, probably accounting for frequent sinopulmonary infections. Endocrine dysfunction (glucose intolerance, hypogonadism) is seen in half of affected individuals. A-T patients are unusually sensitive to ionizing radiation, and conventional radiation therapy regimens can be fatal.

The A-T gene is located on chromosome 11q22-23[271,272] and is designated *ATM*.[273] A-T variants (Nijmegen breakage syndrome and Berlin breakage syndrome) are both linked to 8q21, indicating that they are not allelic with A-T. Most reported A-T mutations result in truncated protein. There are several hundred mutations, with very few spontaneously recurring *ATM* mutations, making population screening difficult.[274] Radio-resistant DNA synthesis is the best diagnostic test for A-T. The test is available from a few reference laboratories.

Approximately 15% of A-T patients will die of cancer, with non-Hodgkin's lymphoma, leukemia, and gastric cancer predominating. Medulloblastoma and glioma have also been described in A-T patients. McConville and colleagues[275] describe 14 families with *ATM* mutations and a less severe phenotype and suggest that cancer predisposition may be variable among families. This heterogeneity could result from the position of the *ATM* mutation or the type of mutation involved (eg, missense vs large deletion).

Heterozygotes are at increased risk for breast cancer. Swift and colleagues[276] reported a 6.8-fold increased risk in such patients. Athma and colleagues[270] found increased risk for breast cancer in both younger women (2.9 relative risk) and in women older than age 60 (6.4 relative risk). The authors estimate that 6.6% of breast cancers in the United States occur in women who are A-T heterozygotes. We believe that heterozygous women should begin breast cancer screening at age 30, with regular self-examination and yearly mammograms.

Bloom Syndrome Bloom syndrome (BS) is a rare (about 170 known cases), autosomal recessive disease that occurs more frequently among Ashkenazi Jews. The *BLM* gene is on chromosome 15q26.1. Multiple mutations are possible; the predominant mutation is referred to as "blm," which is a 6-bp deletion, and 7-bp insertion at nucleotide position 2281 in the *BLM* cDNA.[277] Founder mutations have been described in Ashkenazi Jews.[277] BS somatic cells are hypermutable, with markedly elevated chromosome breakage and sister chromatid exchange.

Affected individuals present with short stature, sun-sensitive facial erythema, malar hypoplasia, nasal prominence, small mandible, and dolichocephalic skull.[278] There is immunodeficiency, manifested by bronchitis and bronchiectasis. The hypermutable DNA is responsible for increased frequency of malignancy, with leukemia and lymphoma predominating in younger patients and carcinomas of larynx, lung, esophagus, colon, breast, and cervix seen in adults. The carcinomas arise about 20 years earlier than expected for the general population.[279]

Gruber and colleagues[280] found that Ashkenazi Jews with CRC were more than twice as likely to be heterozygous for the *BLM* mutation than Ashkenazi Jewish controls without CRC (OR = 2.45; 95% CI 1.3-4.8; $p = .0065$). In contrast, the Israeli Ashkenazi Jewish population controls showed an absence of *BLM* carriers, thereby decreasing the likelihood that the results could be biased. Their data were supported by findings in a recent mouse model[281] of Bloom syndrome, which tested the effect of Blm haploinsufficiency and the risk of cancer in mutation carriers. Mice that were heterozygous for a *BLM* mutation developed twice the number of intestinal tumors when crossed with mice carrying a mutation of the *APC* tumor suppressor gene.[281] Gruber and colleagues[280] concluded that, "...Our data similarly show that carriers of a *BLM* mutation have an increased risk for CRC. Possible mechanisms of carcinogenesis include (i) haploinsufficiency, in which a half dose of *BLM* gene product is insufficient for full *BLM* function in the maintenance of genomic integrity, giving rise to an increased mutation rate in the heterozygous cell, and (ii) loss of the normal *BLM* allele in a colonic stem cell, giving rise to a cell clone with the same hypermutability as the Bloom syndrome cell. Whichever the mechanism, our data confirm the importance of genomic instability as a critical element in the pathogenesis of cancer."[280]

Cowden Syndrome and the Multiple Hamartoma Syndromes Cowden syndrome (CS) is an autosomal, dominantly inherited, rare disorder that was the first of the multiple hamartoma syndromes to lend itself to genetic characterization. This syndrome has shared overlapping presentations with Bannayan-Riley-Ruvalcaba syndrome (BRR) and the juvenile polyposis syndrome (JPS). Of greatest interest to the practicing oncologist is the fact that CS patients carry a 25 to 50% lifetime risk of breast cancer and a 3 to 10% lifetime risk of thyroid cancer (for review see Eng[239]; Pilarski and Eng[282]). Unlike CS, BRR does not carry an increased risk of cancer but is now known to be caused by mutations in the same gene, *PTEN*.[283,284]

CS is associated with multiple hamartoma, including gastrointestinal hamartomatous polyps and benign and malignant neoplasms of the breast, thyroid, uterus, and skin. It is also associated with facial trichilemmomas, acral keratosis, and verrucoid or papillomatous papules in virtually all cases. CS is associated with CNS defects in 40% of cases.[285] Cerebellar dysplastic gangliocytoma, also known as Lhermitte-Duclos disease (LDD), is now established as part of the clinical spectrum of CS.[286] Although 90% of CS patients demonstrate symptoms by the age of 20, only 10% exhibit symptoms prior to age 10.[287]

In 1996, CS was mapped to the locus 10q22-23,[287] a region frequently deleted in thyroid tumors.[288] Somatic mutations spanning this region were also commonly found in glioblastoma, breast cancers (in association with CS), and advanced prostate cancer.[289] In 1997, *PTEN* was isolated and identified as the gene responsible for CS. *PTEN* consists of 9 exons spanning 100 kb of DNA.[283,289–291] PTEN is a major lipid 3-phosphatase, which signals down the PI3 kinase/AKT pro-apoptotic pathway. Furthermore, PTEN is a protein phosphatase, with the ability to dephosphorylate both serine and threonine residues. The protein-phosphatase activity has also been shown to regulate cell-survival pathways, such as the mitogen-activated kinase (MAPK) pathway. Although it is well established that PTEN's lipid-phosphatase activity, via the PI3K/AKT pathway, mediates growth suppression, there is accumulating evidence that the protein-phosphatase/MAPK pathway is equally important in the mediation of growth arrest and other crucial cellular functions.[292] All genetic and biochemical studies indicate that *PTEN* acts as a classic tumor-suppressor gene.

In 1996, the International Cowden Syndrome Consortium created a set of major and minor criteria to aid in the diagnosis of Cowden syndrome. Using these criteria to identify 37 CS families and 7 BRR families, 81% of patients had a *PTEN* mutation.[293] Mutations were scattered throughout the gene, but a mutation "hotspot" in exon 5 accounted for 43% of the mutations found in the region encoding the protein tyrosine phosphatase. When mutations in exons 7 and 8, which encode potential phosphorylation sites, were included, the mutation rate increased to 77%.[294] Novel mutations have recently been reported involving larger gene deletions and mutations in the promoter region explaining the presence of disease in patients who were mutation negative.[295]

PTEN screening of BRR families revealed that approximately 60% had mutations for this gene.[239] However, only 10% of JPS patients were *PTEN* mutation carriers, and many of those already showed signs of CS or subsequently developed them. Thus JPS is thought to be a variant of CS with incomplete expressivity.[116] The clinical significance of this association is that patients with JPS and a mutation in *PTEN* may benefit from enhanced screening of the breast, thyroid, skin, and uterus. Finally, when patients with symptoms suggestive of CS but not fulfilling the CS criteria ("CS-like syndromes") were screened for mutations in *PTEN*, only 1 in 64 (2%) of patients carried mutations,[294] supporting the strict use of the International Cowden Consortium criteria for CS.

Attempts to correlate the *PTEN* genotype and phenotype have been limited by small sample size. *PTEN* mutations are associated with LDD in some families,[283,296] but are not clustered in a specific region of the gene. It has been shown recently that as many as 83% of sporadic LDD harbor germline mutations in *PTEN*, supporting a role for *PTEN* testing in these individuals.[297] A trend for greater organ site involvement (5 versus 4 or fewer sites) has been associated with mutations in the protein tyrosine phosphorylase core region; however, larger sample sizes are needed to verify these results.[293] A screen of 177 breast cancer patients with a family history of breast cancer but negative for *BRCA1* and *BRCA2* failed to show *PTEN* coding mutations.[298] Therefore, there appears to be no increased risk of breast cancer in the absence of the other manifestations of CS, and the screening of these patients for *PTEN* in this instance is unwarranted.

Identification of a *PTEN* mutation in a patient is diagnostic for either CS or BRR, but a negative mutation screen is nondiagnostic.[116] *PTEN* carriers should be screened for thyroid and breast cancers starting in their twenties or 5 years earlier than the youngest relative who developed disease. Future work will likely focus on the variable phenotype of *PTEN* mutations and the altered activity of the P13 kinase/AKT pro-apoptotic pathway that may provide potential targets for novel therapies in the future.

Fanconi Anemia Fanconi anemia (FA) is inherited as an autosomal recessive disorder. There are five complementation groups: FA-A at 16q24.3, FA-B (unmapped), FA-C at 9q22.3, FA-D at 3p26-p22, and FA-E (unmapped). The carrier frequency is higher in Ashkenazi Jews (1 in 100), and a founder mutation of FA-C has been described in that population.[299] The cells of homozygotes have chromosomal instability that can be demonstrated as enhancement of chromosome breakage in a mitomycin C chromosome stress test.[300]

Progressive pancytopenia is the principal feature of FA, presenting as anemia, bleeding, and easy bruising in children. Multiple congenital abnormalities are seen in roughly two-thirds of FA patients; these include hyperpigmentation of the skin, *café au lait* spots, skeletal deformities, renal malformations, microphthalmia, ear anomalies and deafness, congenital heart disease, and hypogonadism.

FA patients are at risk for myelodysplastic syndromes and leukemia, usually acute myelogenous leukemia. Hepatocellular carcinoma has been described in about 5% of patients, possibly secondary to anabolic steroid therapy for anemia. Squamous carcinomas of the upper aerodigestive tract, cervix, vulva, and anus can also complicate the course of FA. The FA-A locus on 16q24.3 is an area that often shows loss of heterozygosity in breast cancer. Cleton-Jansen and colleagues[301] have shown that the *FA-A* gene is not the culprit gene in breast cancer, concluding that "Another tumour suppressor gene in this chromosomal region remains to be identified."

Werner Syndrome Werner syndrome (WS) is inherited as autosomal recessive. The incidence is estimated at 1 in 50,000 to 1 in 100,000. Its phenotype is characterized by premature aging, with growth arrest at puberty, cataracts occurring in the second and third decades, premature atherosclerosis, and adult-onset diabetes. The average life span is 47 years.

The WS locus, WRN, maps to chromosomal region 8p12.[302–307] The gene encodes a DNA helicase of 1432 amino acid residues. Bennett and colleagues[302] note that the helicase consensus domain region of WRN has sequence homology with the bacterial RecQ family of helicases, including BLM, the BS gene product.[308] Bennett and colleagues[302] identified MMR in fibroblastoid cells but not in lymphoblastoid cells, a finding that is consistent "...with the possibility that WRN protein could have a cell type- and/or tissue-specific role in mismatch repair. Alternatively, a mutation in *WRN* could predispose cells to mutations in other genes required for mismatch repair activity, at least one of which could be an unknown gene."[302]

Malignant neoplasms associated with WS include sarcoma, melanoma, and carcinoma.[309] Organs at risk for carcinoma include thyroid, stomach, liver, breast, and bile duct. Melanomas may arise in unusual locations, such as the nasal cavity.

Risks and benefits of cancer screening in this syndrome have not been established, but regular melanoma surveillance seems reasonable.

Xeroderma Pigmentosum Xeroderma pigmentosum (XP), mentioned earlier, is inherited as autosomal recessive. The incidence is 1 in 1,000,000 in the United States but 1 in 40,000 in Japan. XP is genetically heterogeneous, with causative loci mapped to 9q34.1 (XP-A), 2q21 (XP-B), 3p25.1 (XP-C), 19q13.2 (XP-D), 11p12-p11 (XP-E), 16p13.2-p13.1 (XP-F), and 13q32-q33 (XP-G). All of the culprit genes play roles in excision repair of DNA pyrimidine dimers induced by ultraviolet light. Mutation analysis is not available as a clinical test.

Affected individuals show an extraordinary hypersensitivity to sun exposure, manifested by childhood onset of photosensitivity, freckling, and irregular pigmentation. Kraemer and colleagues[310] indicate that the frequencies for malignant melanoma and epithelial cancers (squamous and basal cell carcinoma) are respectively 2,000- and 4,800-fold higher in XP patients than their occurrence in the general population of the United States. The median age of the initial cancer in XP is about 8 years, which is close to a half-century earlier than its occurrence in the general population of the United States. Lanza and colleagues[311] note that XP lacks the marked spontaneous chromosomal instability that characterizes other hereditary disorders that show hypersensitivity to mutations with the predisposition to neoplasia, inclusive of AT, FA, and BS. Cellular hypersensitivity to ultraviolet radiation is the hallmark of XP. Laboratory testing for XP is available from reference laboratories.

XP patients are at increased risk for noncutaneous malignancies as well. Brain tumors, leukemias, and carcinomas of lung and stomach have been described. Cultured cells from XP patients are hypersensitive to DNA-binding carcinogens in cigarette smoke and charbroiled food. Neurologic abnormalities are described in 20% of XP patients, and genetic evidence suggests overlap between XP and Cockayne's syndrome (dwarfism with microcephaly, progressive neurologic degeneration, and photosensitivity).[312]

Affected individuals must avoid exposure to carcinogenic effects of sunlight.[313] Assiduous protection from sunlight must begin in infancy, with wide-brimmed hats, long sleeves, and outdoor activities limited to after sunset. Regular examination of skin and eyes, with early excision of lesions, is mandatory. Avoidance of cigarette smoke and grilled food is probably advisable.[314]

Table 13-4 Genetic Syndromes with Inherited Predisposition to Pancreatic Cancer

Familial Syndrome[a]	Gene (Locus)	Relative Risk	Frequency[b]	References
Peutz-Jeghers syndrome	*STK11* / *LKB1* (19p13.3)	132	4%	125,126,440,442-444
Familial pancreatitis	*Cationic trypsinogen* (7q35)	50–60	unknown	445-447
Familial pancreatic cancer syndrome	unknown (4q32-34)	18–57	unknown	320,448
FAMMM syndrome	$p16^{INK4a}$ / *MTS1* (9p21)	13–22	98%	449-452
Hereditary breast-ovarian cancer syndrome	BRCA2 (13q12)	10	7%	453-455
Familial adenomatous polyposis	*APC* (5q21)	5	40%	7,456-460
HNPCC[c]	*hMSH2* (2p22-21) *hMLH1* (3p21.3)	unknown	4–11%	461-463
Ataxia telangiectasia	*ATM* (11q22-23)	unknown	unknown	464,465

[a]All of the above syndromes are inherited in an autosomal dominant fashion, except ataxia telangiectasia, which is an autosomal recessive disorder.

[b]Frequency refers to the frequency of genetic mutation found in sporadically occurring pancreatic carcinomas.

[c]HNPCC: hereditary nonpolyposis colorectal cancer, also known as cancer family syndrome or Lynch syndrome II. HNPCC is typically caused by germline mutations in DNA mismatch repair genes including *hMSH2*, *hMLH1*, *hPMS2*, and *hMSH6*. *hMSH2* and *hMLH1* mutations account for half to two-thirds of HNPCC. The frequency refers to a defect in any one of the five DNA mismatch repair genes causing HNPCC. (Table reproduced by permission from Yee NS et al. Cancer Biol Ther 2003;2:38–47.)

OTHER CANCERS WITH FAMILIAL CLUSTERINGS

Familial Pancreatic Cancer Anecdotal case reports and epidemiologic studies have suggested that pancreatic cancer clusters in some families. Although chance aggregations or a common environmental exposure could account for some familial clusters, evidence for a genetic basis continues to accumulate. Ghadirian and colleagues[315] performed a population-based case-control study in Quebec, Canada and found that 7.8% of pancreatic cancer patients reported a positive family history of pancreatic cancer, compared to 0.6% of controls. Falk and colleagues[316] studied pancreatic cancer in Louisiana and found similar results, as evidenced by an increased risk for pancreatic cancer among persons reporting any cancer in a close relative (OR = 1.86; 95% confidence interval [CI] = 1.42–2.44). The highest risk was seen in those with a history of pancreatic cancer in a close relative (OR = 5.25; 95% CI = 2.08–13.21).

The National Familial Pancreas Tumor Registry at Johns Hopkins is based upon at least two first-degree relatives who have pancreatic cancer.[317] Analysis of these families indicates that even second-degree relatives of affected patients are at increased risk for pancreatic cancer.

When a familial aggregation of pancreatic cancer is recognized, a variety of hereditary cancer disorders needs to be considered. These include HNPCC (*MSH2*, *MLH1*), PJS, FAMMM, familial breast cancer (*BRCA2*), and hereditary pancreatitis.[225] (All of these conditions are discussed elsewhere in this chapter.)

Hereditary pancreatitis is characterized by recurrent episodes of severe chronic pancreatitis. Affected individuals are at risk for pancreatic pseudocysts, pancreatic exocrine failure, diabetes mellitus, and pancreatic cancer. A gene for hereditary pancreatitis has been mapped to chromosome 7q35.[318] This gene encodes a cationic trypsinogen that, when mutated, fails to inactivate trypsin, resulting in autodigestion of the pancreas. Presumably, chronic epithelial injury and regeneration increase the risk for pancreatic cancer.

Even when known hereditary syndromes are excluded, familial aggregations of pancreatic cancer remain. The inheritance pattern in these families appears to be autosomal dominant.

Surveillance of high-risk patients is evolving. Brentnall and colleagues[319] used endoscopic ultrasound, endoscopic retrograde cholangiopancreatography (ERCP), spiral computed tomography, and serum carcinoembryonic antigen and CA19-9 analysis to follow 14 patients from three pancreatic cancer kindreds. Seven patients underwent pancreatectomy on the basis of abnormalities on ultrasonography and ERCP. All seven had histologic dysplasia in the resected specimen; there were no occult carcinomas.

Given the known heterogeneity in pancreatic cancer, it is likely that many differing cancer susceptibility loci will ultimately be identified. For example, Eberle and colleagues[320] have identified a susceptibility locus that maps to chromosome 4q32-34, in an autosomal dominantly inherited pancreatic cancer family. In the case of *BRCA2*, which predisposes to the hereditary breast-ovarian cancer syndrome, Murphy and colleagues[321] found that *BRCA2* mutations significantly increase the risk of pancreatic cancer in individuals with these mutations. Indeed, these investigators indicate that *BRCA2* mutations pose the most common inherited genetic alteration to date that has been identified in familial pancreatic cancer.

van der Heijden and colleagues[322] describe the Fanconi anemia pathway in pancreatic cancer (PC) cells wherein biallelic *BRCA2* mutations that can cause Fanconi anemia are present in approximately 7% of PCs. Attention was given to recent findings that several sequence changes in *FANCC* and *FANCG* occur in PC. Therein, they note that functional defects in the Fanconi pathway can give rise to multiple hypersensitivity to interstrand crosslinking agents such as mitomycin C. Importantly, once the functional implications of these mutations in the Fanconi pathway are more fully comprehended, it may then be possible to initiate clinical trials for the treatment of PC with crosslinking pharmaceutical agents of Fanconi-defective cancers. This research is in full accord with recent developments of targeted chemotherapeutics, wherein the targeting of specific genetic defects in cancer has been taking place. One such example is imatinib which has been shown to be of significant therapeutic promise in patients with chronic myelogenous leukemia[323,324] and in gastrointestinal stromal tumor (GIST).[325–328]

van der Heijden and colleagues[322] note that FA-defective cell lines of CAPAN1, PL11, and Hs766T are all hypersensitive to mitomycin C when compared to other PC cell lines. These authors call attention to their previous studies[329] as an explanation of anecdotal observations wherein a subset of PCs were highly sensitive to mitomycin-containing regimens. Therein, they suggest that, "...pancreatic cancers might be genetically tested for defects in the pathways that repair interstrand crosslinks, such as the FA pathway. Patients with a defect in one of the repair pathways could then be treated rationally with crosslinking agents, possibly at a much lower dose than is customary."

In dealing with a disease as deadly as PC, one must constantly search for new agents that may hold promise. Clearly, this work of van der Heijden and colleagues[322] must be pursued to the fullest possible extent, given their extremely provocative basic science results. The heterogeneity of hereditary pancreatic cancer is demonstrated in Table 13-4.

Familial Gastric Cancer Gastric cancer has many similarities to esophageal carcinoma in that its incidence shows marked geographic variation.

For example, its incidence is exceedingly high in Japan (160/100,000 per year) with high rates also noted in Finland and Chile. In contrast, its incidence is low in the United Kingdom (10/100,000 per year) as well as in the United States, where rates have been declining in these latter areas during the past several decades.

There are two types of gastric adenocarcinoma which can be distinguished histopathologically: (1) intestinal type; (2) diffuse type. Molecular pathology supports the theory that those differences emerge through specific genetic pathways for the two tumor types.[330] The *intestinal* type shows components of glandular or intestinal architecture and tubular structures. The *diffuse* type shows non-coherent, single cells, often with signet-ring cell morphology, and it frequently presents as linitis plastica. Separation of gastric cancer into intestinal and diffuse types is exceedingly useful genetically and epidemiologically.

The intestinal type shows a greater frequency than its diffuse counterpart. In general, the intestinal type is more commonly related to environmental exposures; these include diet (salted fish and meat, and smoked foods), smoking, alcohol, and infection with *Helicobacter pylori*. Indeed, there may be a genetic-environmental interaction in the etiology of gastric carcinoma and *H. pylori* susceptibility.[331–333] El-Omar and colleagues[334] have shown that eradication of *H. pylori* infection leads to resolution of the gastric inflammation and resolution of hypochlorhydria and atrophy in about half of the patients. Importantly, will eradication of *H. pylori* be effective in hereditary forms of gastric cancer?

In contrast, the diffuse type has a low but relatively stable incidence in most parts of the world. In general, it is related to host factors (discussed subsequently).

Familial Risk Factors It is estimated that between 5 and 10% of gastric cancer involves familial clustering. Familial risk for gastric carcinoma was investigated by Hemminki and Jiang[335] employing the nationwide Swedish Family Cancer Database that comprises 10.2 million individuals, with over 34,000 gastric carcinomas. This is the largest study on familial gastric cancer published to date. Standardized incidence rates (SIRs) were 1.31 (95% CI, 0.97–1.70) and 1.47 (1.08–1.92) when a parent presented with gastric cancer or gastric adenocarcinoma respectively. Risk was 1.59 (1.10–2.16) in offspring whose diagnosis was at an age greater than 50 years. Sibling risk for gastric cancer was 3.16 and 5.75 when diagnosed earlier than age 50. Population-attributable proportion of gastric cancer was 0.45%. These authors concluded that environmental factors, possibly *H. pylori* infections, provided the main explanation for familial clustering of gastric cancer. The population-attributable proportion of familial gastric cancer was much lower than that cited in the literature.

Palli and colleagues[336] studied 1,016 patients with gastric cancer and 1,623 population-based controls. Their study was adjusted for potential confounders including diet. Their results showed an increased risk for gastric cancer among those with the following relatives affected: sibling (OR = 2.6); parent (OR = 1.7 [mother affected, OR = 2.3; father affected, OR = 1.3]); two or more siblings (OR = 8.5); both parents (OR = 3.0).

Hereditary Gastric Carcinoma Perhaps the most celebrated family with gastric cancer is that of Napoleon Bonaparte (Figure 13-1). Lying near death on St. Helena in 1821, 52-year-old Napoleon Bonaparte was heard to murmur "Pylorus... My father's pylorus."[337] His father had died of gastric cancer, as had his father's father, his brother, and three sisters. An autopsy showed that Napoleon, too, succumbed to cancer of the stomach (Figure 13-2).

The differential diagnosis of hereditary gastric cancer includes its integral involvement in HNPCC (Lynch syndrome),[338] Park and colleagues[339] have found that after endometrial cancer, gastric cancer is the second most common extracolonic cancer in cases of HNPCC in Korea, an endemic area for gastric cancer, where the relative risk (RR) for gastric cancer is known to be increased four-fold in individuals with HNPCC. FAP, Li-Fraumeni syndrome, and Peutz-Jeghers syndrome are other examples (Figure 13-3).

Hereditary Diffuse Gastric Cancer (HDGC) Hereditary diffuse gastric cancer (HDGC) is a distinctive syndrome, a subset of which are due to the *E-cadherin* gene mutation. Lobular carcinoma of the breast may be an integral lesion in the *E-cadherin* mutation affecteds. HDGC is an autosomal dominantly inherited syndrome. Germline mutations in the *E-cadherin* (*CDH1*) gene were first identified by Guilford and colleagues in three Maori kindreds.[340] Its penetrance is 70 to 80%. The average age of onset of HDGC is about 37 years.

Clinical criteria for defining HDGC families include the following: (1) two or more documented cases in first/second degree relatives, at least one diagnosed at less than age 50 years; (2) Three or more documented diffuse gastric cancers in first/second degree relatives independent of age of onset. Twenty-five to 50% of families meeting these criteria have identifiable germline mutations involving the *E-cadherin* gene. Other families may have unidentified mutations or yet-to-be-defined genes that contribute to HDGC.

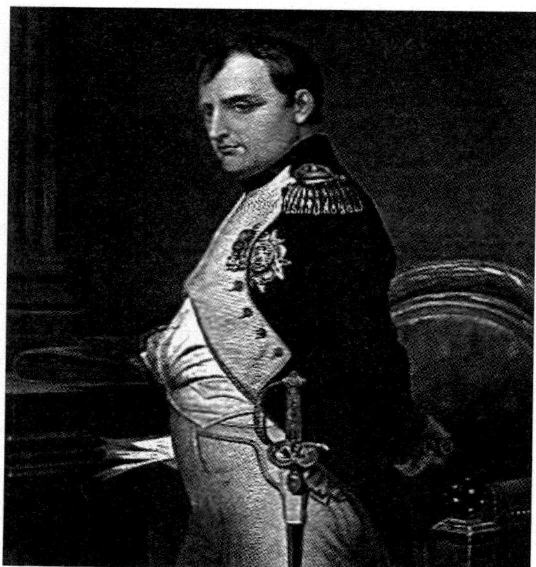

Figure 13-1 Portrait of Napoleon Bonaparte.

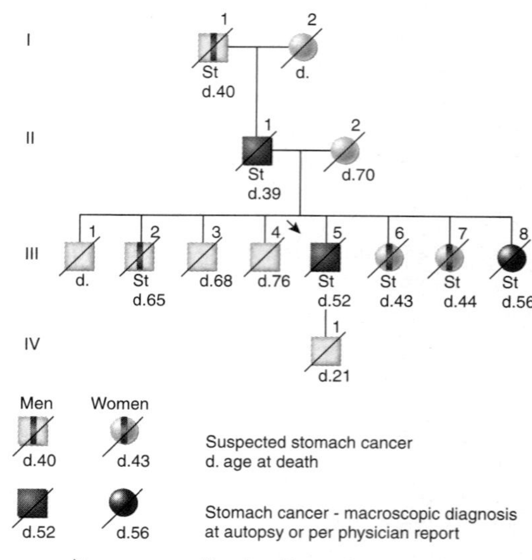

Figure 13-2 Reconstructed pedigree of Napoleon Bonaparte.

Screening Screening for diffuse gastric carcinoma includes endoscopy, endoscopic ultrasound of the stomach, and multiple gastric biopsies. However, this has been exceedingly unproductive in terms of identifying early (and potentially curable) cancer in HDGC in patients with *E-cadherin* mutations. Early diagnosis is clearly the best chance for curative resection, but it is a formidable task. Initial symptoms may be those of advanced disease and they are often nonspecific. When first diagnosed, most cases are locally advanced where over two-thirds present with lymph node involvement. Survival is poor when the disease has advanced beyond the mucosa or submucosa. Lesions tend not to form a grossly visible exophytic mass; rather, they spread submucosally. Emerging new screening technologies include color or fluorescent stains to aid in endoscopic detection. Endoscopic ultrasound is mainly used to stage a previously diagnostic tumor, but it may be useful in identifying early diffuse type gastric cancer.

Prophylactic Surgery Lewis and colleagues,[341] reported their findings on prophylactic gastrectomy in six asymptomatic members of two HDGC families (two males and four females), ages 22, 27, 28, 35, 39, and 40, all of whom were positive for *E-cadherin* mutations. Each of these individuals, when subjected to a research protocol of microscopic sectioning at the time of prophylactic total gastrectomy, had microscopic foci of cancer often at multiple sites, with overlying normal gastric mucosa.

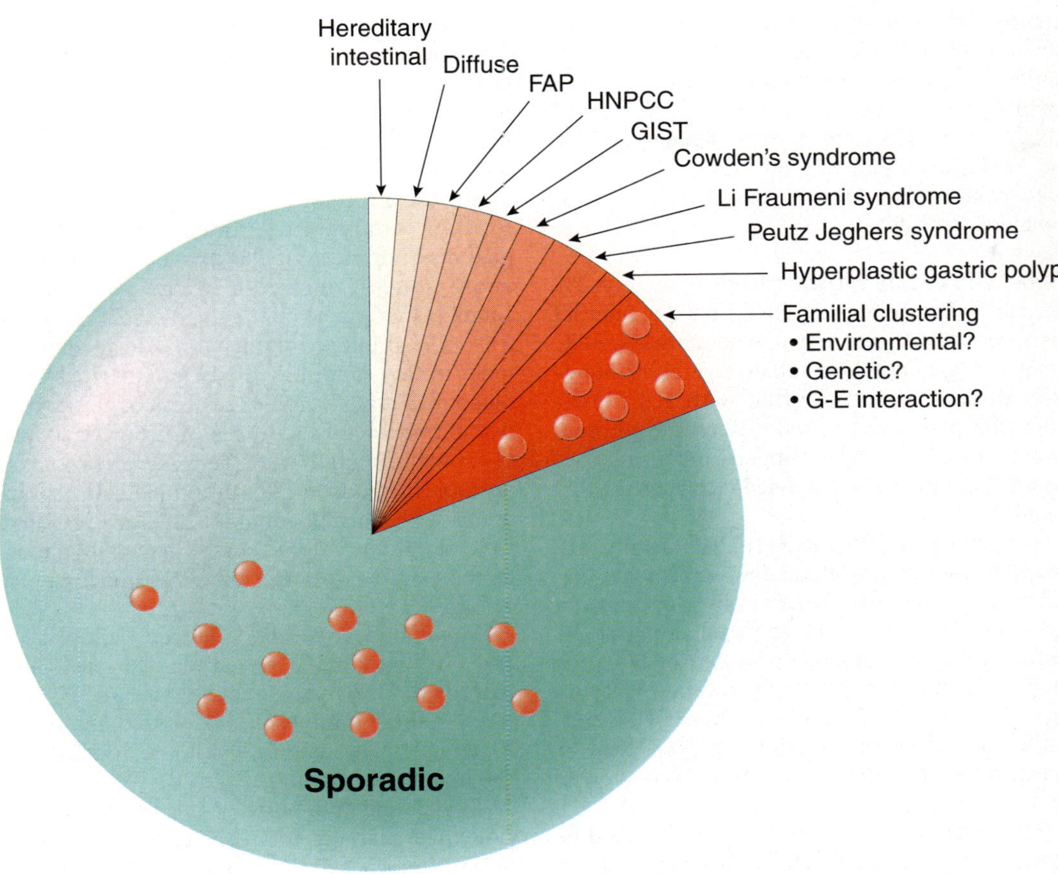

Figure 13-3 Circle graph showing proportions of gastric cancer types.

Huntsman and colleagues[342] and Chun and colleagues[343] have discussed the potential efficacy of surgical prophylaxis. They note that the decision for prophylactic gastrectomy must consider the 2 to 4% risk of mortality and nearly 100% long-term morbidity (chronic diarrhea, dumping syndrome, and weight loss). Ten percent show post-operative complications including infection, myocardial infarction, or leak. Combined results of prophylactic gastrectomy in ten asymptomatic *E-cadherin* mutation carriers in three HDGC families showed that despite negative endoscopic examinations and biopsies, all ten were found to have pathologic evidence for early gastric cancer. Thus, even with intensive endoscopic examinations and random gastric biopsies, this screening approach may be inadequate for early diagnosis and prevention of gastric cancer in HDGC families.

Given the dismal screening results, prophylactic surgery should be presented as a viable option for *E-cadherin* mutation carriers with positive family histories of diffuse gastric cancer. Although the morbidity of this operation may be higher than that for other genetic diseases, it must be realized that the alternative is a mortality risk of over 80% at a young age.[341] For those not desiring prophylactic gastrectomy, we recommend that there be frequent (q 6–12 months) and highly detailed endoscopic mucosal examination with multiple biopsies of even the most subtle of lesions.

Genetic Counseling and Gastric Cancer Lynch and colleagues[344] performed mutation-based genetic counseling in an HDGC family that harbored the *E-cadherin* mutation. A family information service (FIS) was performed,[345] during which 24 family members were thoroughly educated about the clinical and genetic features of HDGC. After giving individual signed consent, they were tested for the E-cadherin mutation, of which 9 were found to be positive and 15 negative. Three of the *E-cadherin* mutation positives were affected and are deceased due to diffuse gastric carcinoma.

None of the 19 patients counseled wanted their results sent to their physicians once they recognized the potential for insurance discrimination. None had undergone endoscopic ultrasound. Three who were positive for the *E-cadherin* mutation expressed strong interest in prophylactic gastrectomy, and one of these has recently undergone prophylactic total gastrectomy and was found to be negative for metastatic disease.

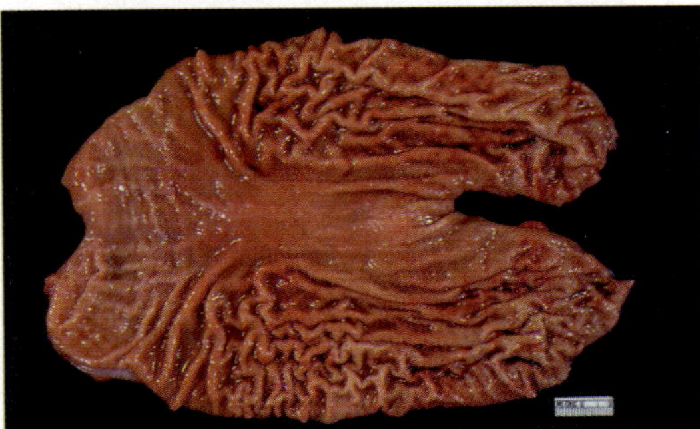

Figure 13-4 Photograph of grossly normal appearing stomach from *E-cadherin* mutation carrier.

During the genetic counseling process, this individual was advised about the importance of undergoing total prophylactic gastrectomy. He realized that he was positive for the *E-cadherin* germline mutation. He was told about the fact that many patients who had undergone prophylactic total gastrectomy had evidence of microscopic metastatic disease in the surgical specimen. He eventually accepted the need for this and underwent the procedure. The examination of the entire stomach (Figure 13-4) revealed three foci of intramucosal signet-cell carcinoma, each < 0.5 mm in dimension (Figure 13-5). There was no evidence of lymph node involvement or distal metastatic spread (TCS, unpublished data).

In conclusion, surveillance, even with intensive endoscopic examinations and random gastric biopsies, may be inadequate for the early diagnosis and prevention of diffuse gastric cancer in HDGC families, hence justifying consideration of prophylactic surgery, particularly among *E-cadherin* mutation carriers. The genetic counselor must discuss the option for prophylactic gastrectomy. Clearly, there is a need for a multidisciplinary group of clinicians, geneticists, and genetic counselors to educate and support the family member in order to enable him or her to make decisions about diagnostic and management options for the future.

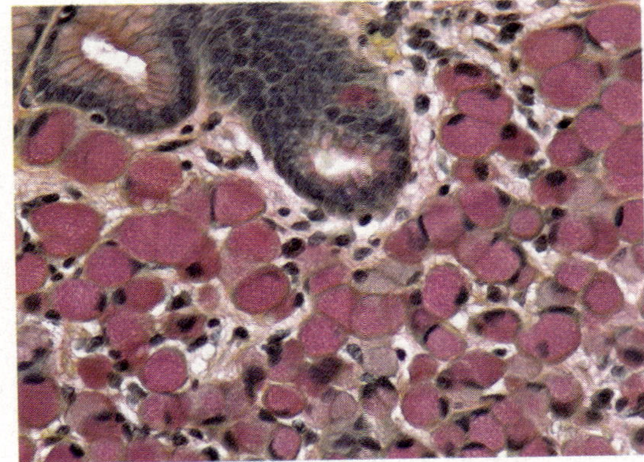

Figure 13-5 Micrograph showing diffuse gastric cancer with signet cell features in *E-cadherin* mutation carrier.

FAP and Gastric Cancer Gastric cancer occurs in excess in patients with FAP, particularly in Japanese FAP families. However, this was not the case in studies of non-Asian patients with FAP in the Johns Hopkins registry[346] in whom there was not an increased relative risk for gastric cancer. Similar results were reported by Jagelman and colleagues,[347] who found gastric cancer in 7 of 1,255 patients with FAP, compared to 10 patients with periampullary carcinoma and 29 with carcinoma elsewhere in the duodenum.

Hyperplastic Polyps A predisposition to gastric cancer may be inherited with a tendency to form hyperplastic polyps. Carneiro and colleagues[348] described a large pedigree characterized by autosomal dominantly inherited predisposition to gastric polyposis coupled with a high incidence of gastric carcinoma. Two of the gastric carcinomas were of the diffuse type and one of these appeared to have originated from hyperplastic polyps. Hyperplastic polyps were found in five of seven family members without carcinoma of the stomach. The remaining two individuals had marked fobeolar hyperplasia. Chronic atrophic gastritis (CAG) with complete intestinal metaplasia was observed in three of the patients. It was concluded that, "Fobeolar hyperplasia/hyperplastic polyps may play a key role in the development of diffuse carcinomas in this inherited polyposis confined to the stomach with the hyperplastic phenotype."[348]

Gastrointestinal Stromal Tumor, St1571 (Glivec) Hirota and colleagues[349] studied a family with multiple gastrointestinal stromal tumor (GIST), which harbored a new type of germline mutation of the *KIT* gene observed at Asp-820 in tyrosine kinase (TK) II domain. These authors indicate that mutations in the TK II domain have been identified in mast cell and germ cell tumors, but heretofore had not been found in GIST tumors. Thus, their family represents the first recorded case of GISTs with TK II known mutations. Furthermore, they note that, "...Because interleukin 3-dependent Ba/F3 murine lymphoid cells transfected with the mutant KIT complementary DNA grew autonomously without any growth factors and formed tumors in nude mice, the mutation was considered to be gain-of-function type."

Nishida and colleagues[350] note that in the first reported case of familial GISTs there was a germline mutation at the juxtamembrane domain of the *KIT* gene. They note, however, that following the original report of Hirota and colleagues,[349] several additional familial GIST cases were described.[351-354] Furthermore, four of these five GIST families manifested the KIT mutation at the juxtamembrane domain,[350–253,354] whereas the remaining family carried the mutation at the TK I domain.[352]

Until recently, there has not been any effective treatment for unresectable metastatic GIST tumor, a lesion which has been invariably fatal. For example, Joensuu and colleagues[328] described a patient with metastatic GIST treated with intensive doxorubicin-based chemotherapy without response. However, ST1571 (Glivec) was started and dramatically reduced metastases. The patient had a complete response within 1 month of the start of ST1571, as evidenced by negative findings on PET and MRI. Toxicity of ST1571 was minimal (mild dyspepsia and slightly increased frequency of bowel movements).

Renal Cell Carcinoma Approximately 2% of renal cell carcinomas (RCC) have a familial basis. As with cancers of many other organs, RCC is not a single entity, but rather several histologically distinct patterns, often with a different molecular pathogenesis and different syndromic associations.[355,356] Von Hippel-Lindau disease, the most common, is discussed elsewhere in this chapter.

Hereditary papillary RCC (HPRC1) is characterized by multiple, bilateral, low-grade renal carcinomas.[357] The gene (*MET*) is on chromosome 7q33.1-34. It is a proto-oncogene encoding a cell-surface receptor for hepatocyte growth factor (HGF). Normal signaling by the receptor tyrosine kinase requires the presence of the HGF ligand. Activating missense mutations in *MET* lead to constitutive signaling, with activation of downstream pathways.

Extrarenal neoplasms have been described in families with papillary renal cell carcinoma.[358] These include carcinomas of the stomach, rectum, breast, lung, pancreas, and bile duct. It is not clear whether these associations are significant.

Penetrance appears to be low (as low as 30% for some mutations). Subclinical disease is often discovered when gene carriers undergo renal imaging. Annual renal imaging beginning at age 30 years is recommended. Familial papillary RCC has also been described in association with papillary carcinoma of the thyroid.[359] That report, describing one kindred, mapped susceptibility to chromosome 1q21.

Hereditary leiomyomatosis and renal cell cancer (HLRCC) is inherited as an autosomal dominant disorder which involves smooth-muscle tumors of the skin and uterus and/or renal cancer. The disorder has been mapped to chromosome 1q42.3-43. Toro and colleagues[360] investigated the role of the *fumarate hydratase* (*FH*) gene in HLRCC. They found *FH* mutations in 31 families; 20 different mutations were identified, 18 of which were novel. Eighty-one patients (47 women and 34 men) had cutaneous leiomyomas. Ninety-eight percent (46/47) of women with cutaneous leiomyomas also had uterine leiomyomas. The authors identified 13 individuals in 5 families with unilateral and solitary renal tumors, whereas 7 individuals from 4 families had papillary type II renal cell carcinoma, and an additional individual manifested a collecting duct carcinoma of the kidney.

Tomlinson and colleagues[361] confirmed the association of uterine leiomyomata as being common tumors in this syndrome that also predisposes to multiple fibroids, cutaneous leiomyomata, and renal cell carcinoma.

Chromosome 3 translocations have been associated with risk for clear cell RCC.[362] Early studies suggested a susceptibility gene at 3p14, possibly involving the FHIT tumor suppressor gene. Subsequently, a variety of chromosome 3 breakpoints have been described, all contained within the pericentromeric regions of 3p and 3q. Further, analysis of tumors from affected patients show loss of the derived chromosome and a somatic mutation of the von Hippel-Lindau (*VHL*) gene on the retained chromosome 3.[363] The proposed model for cancer development in this condition is: (1) an inherited chromosome 3 translocation; (2) loss of the derivative chromosome (with loss of the VHL locus); (3) somatic mutation of the VHL allele on the normal chromosome 3. Individuals from kindreds with chromosome 3 translocations and RCC should be offered surveillance recommendations similar to those for von Hippel Lindau syndrome.

Familial clear cell RCC independent of VHL and chromosome 3 translocations has been described.[364] Because more than half of RCC cases in these families are diagnosed before age 50, annual renal imaging should be offered to at-risk relatives beginning at age 20.

Skates and Iliopoulos[365] discuss the role of molecular markers for renal cell carcinoma in several known hereditary disorders that predispose to this cancer. Therein, they discuss several defined germline mutations in tumor suppressor genes or oncogenes that predispose to the predisposition for renal cell carcinoma. They note, for example, that patients with inactivating mutations in the *Birt-Hogg-Dubé* tumor suppressor gene have a risk of developing oncocytic/chromophobe kidney tumors.[366]

Tuberous sclerosis predisposes to the development of renal tumors. Angiomyolipoma is the most common renal manifestation, but multifocal, bilateral RCC in young patients has been described.[367]

Familial Prostate Cancer Interest in familial prostate cancer risk dates back nearly a half-century to the report by Morganti and colleagues[368] describing an 11-fold increased risk for carcinoma of the prostate in first-degree relatives of index cases compared to age-matched controls. Later, Woolf[369] showed a three-fold increased risk for relatives of affected individuals, and in 1982 Cannon and colleagues[370] concluded that prostate cancer had a stronger familial aggregation in a Utah Mormon genealogic database than breast or colorectal carcinoma. More recent epidemiologic studies confirm these findings and indicate that risk is related to the number of family members affected and the age of the proband at diagnosis.[371]

Segregation analysis has suggested that a highly penetrant autosomal dominant mutant gene could account for 9% of all prostate cancers and 40% of those diagnosed before age 55.[372] Some candidate genes have been identified, the significance of which is unknown at this time. Risks and benefits of surveillance are unproven, but regular screening by serum prostate specific antigen and regular digital rectal examination are reasonable. In high-risk families, screening should begin before age 50. The role of transrectal ultrasound and random prostate biopsies is yet to be evaluated.

Prostate Cancer Genetics The search for the role of heredity in prostate cancer (PC) during the current five-year period showed an exponential increase and has been addressed in no fewer than 112 papers in English (*MEDLINE* search results).[373] Difficulty in identifying genes that predispose to PC is likely due to late age of diagnosis, heterogeneity of the disease, phenocopies (individuals with sporadic forms of the disease interspersed with hereditary cases) in high-risk pedigrees, and genetic complexity.[373,374]

Identification of Novel Prostate Cancer Susceptibility Loci Performing a genome-wide linkage scan for PC susceptibility genes in their study of 36 Jewish families, Friedrichsen and colleagues showed significant linkage to peak at 7q11-21,[373] whereas a genome-wide scan by Tavtigian and colleagues[374] of large, high-risk pedigrees from Utah has provided evidence for linkage to a locus on chromosome 17p. Positional cloning and mutation screening within the defined 17p interval, identified a gene, namely ELAC2, harboring mutations (including a frameshift and a non-conservative missense change) that segregated with PC in two pedigrees.

Xu[375] studied 772 hereditary PC families from the International Consortium for Prostate Cancer Genetics. Xu found that the PC-susceptibility gene linked to 1q24-25 was identified in a defined subset of PC families. However, they accounted for only a relatively small proportion of all families, appearing to play a more prominent role in a subset of families wherein several members were affected at an early age and wherein male-to-male disease transmission was present. A candidate gene in the region, *RNASEL*, on chromosome 1q25, was recently identified as a candidate gene for hereditary PC by Wang and colleagues[376] in association with an increased risk of familial, but not sporadic, PC. However, these results were not confirmed in a large case-control study from Sweden arguing against a significant role for *RNASEL*[377] in PC and suggesting that another gene in the region is behind the increased risk. The HPC1 locus on chromosome 1q24-q25 was identified by linkage analysis of 91 families with three or more affected first-degree relatives.[378,379] In contrast, the search for linkage at chromosome 1q42.2-43 was negative in one study.[380] A putative PC susceptibility gene has been mapped to Xq27-28,[381] a finding that correlates with suggestions of an X-linked mode of inheritance for prostate cancer susceptibility.[382]

Prostate Cancer Risk Associated with Known Cancer Genes *CHEK2*, the upstream regulator of *TP53*, may also contribute to prostate cancer risk,[383] implicating the DNA-damage-signaling pathway in the development of PC. This observation was confirmed when two truncating mutations of *CHEK2* were shown to confer moderate risk of PC.[384]

The Breast Cancer Linkage Consortium found that male carriers of *BRCA2* mutations are at increased risk of PC (OR 4.78; 95% CI, 1.87–12.25; $p = .001$), whereas risk of *BRCA1* mutation carriers was not significantly increased. Prostate tumors with frequent genetic aberrations have been observed in the chromosomal region 12p12-13 harboring *CDKN1B*.[385] Segregation in families with PC was primarily contributed by affected offspring whose age at diagnosis was < 65 years. *E-cadherin* (*CDH1*) has also been associated with prostate carcinogenesis,[386] with the -160 single nucleotide polymorphism acting as a low-penetrant PC susceptibility gene that could explain a proportion of familial PC. Taken together, these findings suggest that germline mutations of *CHEK2*, *BRCA2*, *CDKN1B*, and *CDH1* may play a role in PC susceptibility.

Prostate Cancer in Lynch Syndrome Soravia and colleagues[387] suggest that prostate cancer may be an integral lesion in the Lynch syndrome. They report a family wherein the proband had three metachronous adenocarcinomas of the colon and rectum at ages 54, 57, and 60, and presented with an adenocarcinoma of the prostate at age 61. These investigators performed immunohistochemical (IHC) staining of colonic, rectal, and prostatic tumor tissues and therein found a lack of expression of *MSH2* and *MSH6*. Microsatellite instability (MSI) was evidenced in the rectal, colonic, and prostatic tumors. Since the family fit the Amsterdam criteria for the Lynch syndrome, molecular genetic studies were initiated following the proband's son's manifestation of colorectal cancer at age 35. "...Southern blotting analysis of genomic DNA led to identification of a novel genomic deletion encompassing exon 5 of the MSH2 gene..." These authors indicate that, to the best of their knowledge, this represents the first report wherein MSI and IHC analysis of the prostate adenocarcinoma clearly linked its cause to the germline MMR mutation. They also note that there have been occasional reports[388,389] of prostate carcinoma in Lynch syndrome kindreds and, therefore, appropriately suggest that prostate cancer be included in the Lynch syndrome tumor spectrum.

HNPCC or the Lynch syndrome, as discussed previously, shows a significant increased risk for carcinoma of the ureter and renal pelvis, but to date not the urinary bladder. A statistically significant risk ($p < .001$) for these lesions was found in patients with the Muir-Torre syndrome (MTS) (a variation of HNPCC manifesting sebaceous adenomas, sebaceous carcinomas, and multiple keratoacanthomas) as opposed to HNPCC patients who lacked MTS cutaneous features.

This demonstrates the importance of inquiring into the presence of cancers of all anatomic sites when investigating any patient's family cancer history. In addition, multi-case families, particularly when extended, with pathology verification of cancer, are ideal candidates for formal linkage analysis in the search for genetic susceptibility loci. Such efforts will be of value to molecular geneticists in the search for germline mutations that may predispose to urologic cancer as well as to other cancer types.

Lung Cancer Lung cancer, more than any other solid tumor, is readily identified with an environmental cause, namely, tobacco exposure. Some non-tobacco–related familial clusters have been associated with an earlier age of diagnosis but no genetic loci that might explain these cases have been identified.

In an effort to determine whether a genetic predisposition may exist, Lynch and colleagues[390] evaluated cancer risk in the relatives of 254 consecutively ascertained probands with histologically verified lung cancer and in relatives of 231 probands with other smoking-associated cancers. There was no strong evidence for increased risk of lung cancer in relatives, but there was a significant increased risk for cancers of all anatomic sites among the relatives of lung cancer probands ($p < .001$). Conversely, there were no significant excesses of cancer at all anatomic sites in relatives of probands with other smoking-associated carcinomas. The observed increased risk for cancer at all anatomic sites in the relatives of lung cancer probands could result from an underlying hereditary susceptibility to cancer in general in these families.

Although no familial lung cancer syndrome has been identified, lung cancer presents a model for how the genetics of toxin metabolism may lead to cancer predisposition. Susceptibility to lung cancer may in part be attributable to inter-individual variability in metabolic activation or detoxification of tobacco carcinogens. The glutathione S-transferase M1 (GSTM1) genetic polymorphism has been extensively studied in this context. A recent meta-analysis of the results of 43 case-control studies including > 18,000 individuals identified a slight excess risk of lung cancer in association with the GSTM1 null genotype (odds ratio 1.2).[391] However, a pooled analysis of 9500 subjects involved in 21 case-control studies from the International Collaborative Study on Genetic Susceptibility to Environmental Carcinogens (GSEC) data set performed to assess the role of GSTM1 genotype as a modifier of the effect of smoking on lung cancer risk revealed no evidence of increased risk of lung cancer among carriers of the GSTM1 null genotype (age-, gender- and center-adjusted). In addition, there was no evidence of interaction between GSTM1 genotype and either smoking status or cumulative tobacco consumption.[391] A number of additional studies searching for associations between lung cancer and common genetic polymorphisms have been performed, but like the family studies, no convincing evidence for low penetrance susceptibility genes has emerged from this line of investigation either.

Still, millions of people smoke each year, but not all will develop lung cancer. Tobacco-associated lung cancer has been observed to cluster in some families, prompting further study on genetic determinants of toxin metabolism (for review see Hecht[392] and Bennett and colleagues[393]). Interestingly, mouse models of toxin-related lung cancers have led to the identification of a susceptibility gene in that system.[394] This gene, known as *Pas-1*, has been mapped to the mouse chromosome 6.[395] Identification of homologues to *Pas-1* in humans may eventually lead to breakthroughs in our understanding of the pathogenesis of lung cancer and its genetic determinants.

Familial Neuroblastoma Neuroblastoma is a common tumor of childhood, with almost all cases occurring prior to the age of 10.[396] Heritable predisposition for the development of the disease has been observed but, to date, no susceptibility genes have been isolated.[397] Several chromosomal regions are potential sites for a neuroblastoma susceptibility gene, including 17q, 1p, 11q, and 14q. Chromosome 1p deletions have been reported in as many as 80% of near-diploid neuroblastomas that have been karyotyped, making this a particularly promising locus.[398] These deletions on chromosome 1 have variable proximal break points, but a region of consistent deletion has been mapped to sub-bands of 1p36, possibly marking the location of a tumor suppressor gene important in malignant transformation or progression of neuroblastoma. Further support for this locus comes from the study of a sib pair with neuroblastoma. A1p36 deletion was identified in both tumors through use of double-color fluorescence in situ hybridization, and neither tumor showed evidence of *MYCN* amplification, another common genetic alteration in neuroblastoma. Haplotype analysis showed that the siblings inherited the same paternal 1p36→pter chromosome region in both tumors. However, the maternal 1p region was deleted. These data suggest that the siblings inherited a predisposition to neuroblastoma in the paternal 1p36 region and that tumors developed as a consequence of somatic loss of the maternal 1p36 allele.

Despite the difficulties of identifying a neuroblastoma susceptibility gene, there is convincing evidence that hereditary predisposition to neuroblastoma segregates as an autosomal dominant Mendelian trait. Thus, efforts to identify a susceptibility locus have continued. The most recent progress was reported by Maris and colleagues,[399] who performed linkage analysis on ten families' multiple neuroblastomas and identified a locus at 16p12-13 consistent with linkage (lod = 3.46). Informative recombinants defined a large (26 cM) not yet amenable to candidate gene mutation screening. However, subchromosomal deletions were identified in 5/12 familial (42%) and 55/259 nonfamilial (21%) neuroblastomas at the same locus, narrowing the interval to approximately 13 cM. These data suggest that a gene for hereditary neuroblastoma is located at 16p12-p13 and that inactivation of this gene may contribute to the pathogenesis of sporadic neuroblastomas.[400]

Hematologic Malignancy Most studies dealing with familial aggregations of hematologic neoplasms have lacked adequately matched controls and have focused on the same hematologic malignancy that was present in the proband. In an attempt to address this issue, Shpilberg and colleagues[401] investigated the familial aggregation

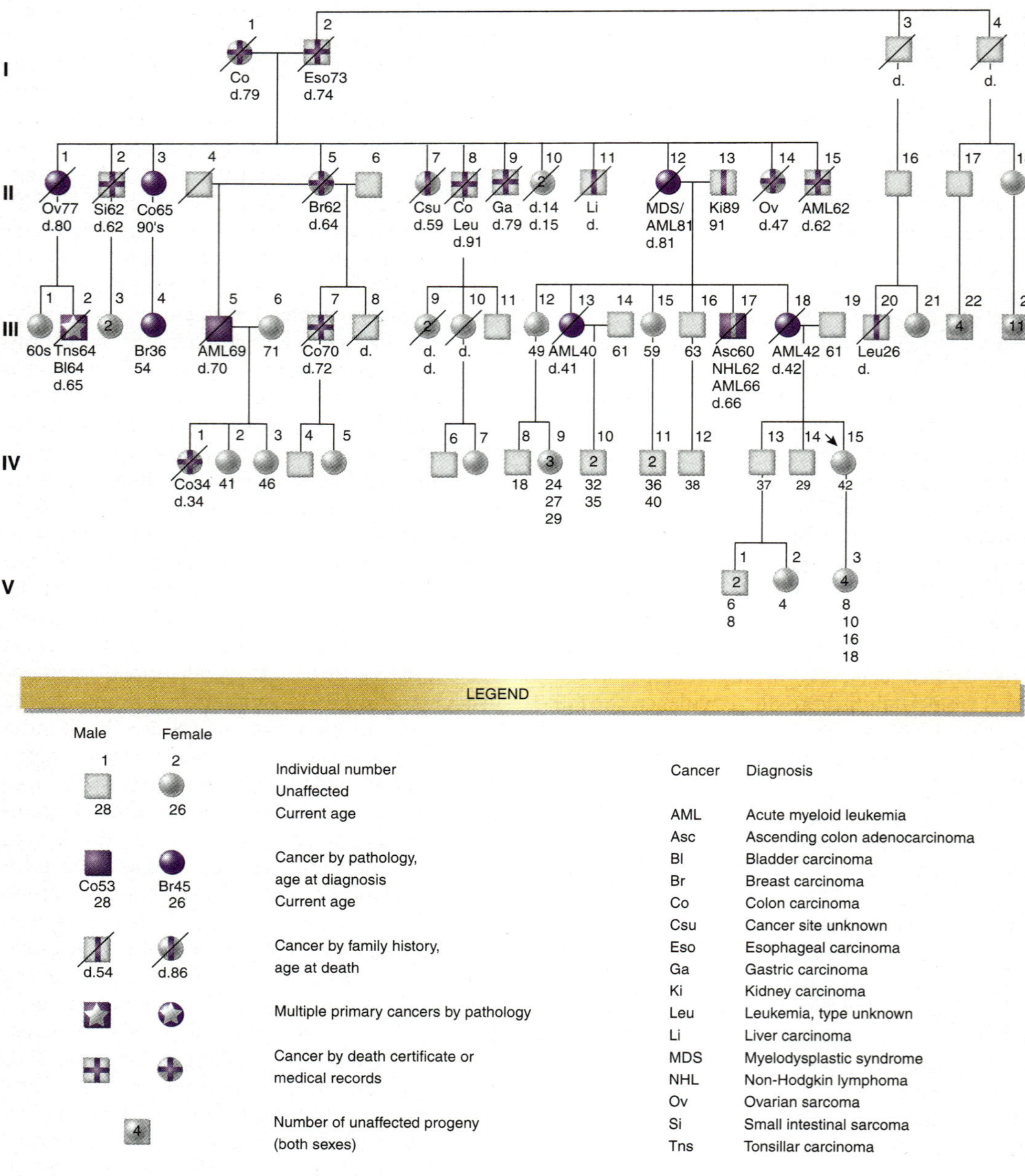

Figure 13-6 Pedigree for hematologic and solid tumor prone family manifesting acute myelogenous leukemia. (Lynch HT, et al. Family with acute myelogenous leukemia, breast, ovarian, and gastrointestinal cancer. Cancer Genet Cytogenet 2002;137:8–14.)

of hematologic cancers in 4,061 family members of 189 patients with a variety of hematologic neoplasms. They compared their findings with control groups of 955 relatives of 36 patients with nonmalignant hematologic disorders and 508 relatives of 33 patients with type II diabetes mellitus. They found that the majority of hematologic cancers among family members differed from those of the probands. Specifically, "The odds ratio for haematological neoplasms among relatives of the index cases adjusted for age, sex, ethnicity, number of relatives in the family, and degree of familial linkage in the study group versus the two control groups was 3.62 (95% confidence interval, 1.44-9.07, $p < .01$)." These findings lend support to the idea of a genetic predisposition to cancer in a subset of patients, with diverse familial clustering of the hematologic neoplasms. Therefore, they suggest that the familial aggregation of hematologic cancer is not necessarily disease specific, which is consistent with an abnormality in the pluripotent hematopoietic stem cell.[401] Alternatively, more differentiated hematologic cells of different types may be susceptible to genetic damage in some families.

Families prone to hematologic malignancies have received a paucity of attention when compared to families with solid tumors. Conversely, hematologic malignancies have had more extensive cytogenetic investigation.[402]

Acute Myelogenous Leukemia We have studied a family[403] with acute myelogenous leukemia (AML) (Figure 13-6) wherein many clues were present that appear to link the presumptive genetic susceptibility of solid tumors to hemato-

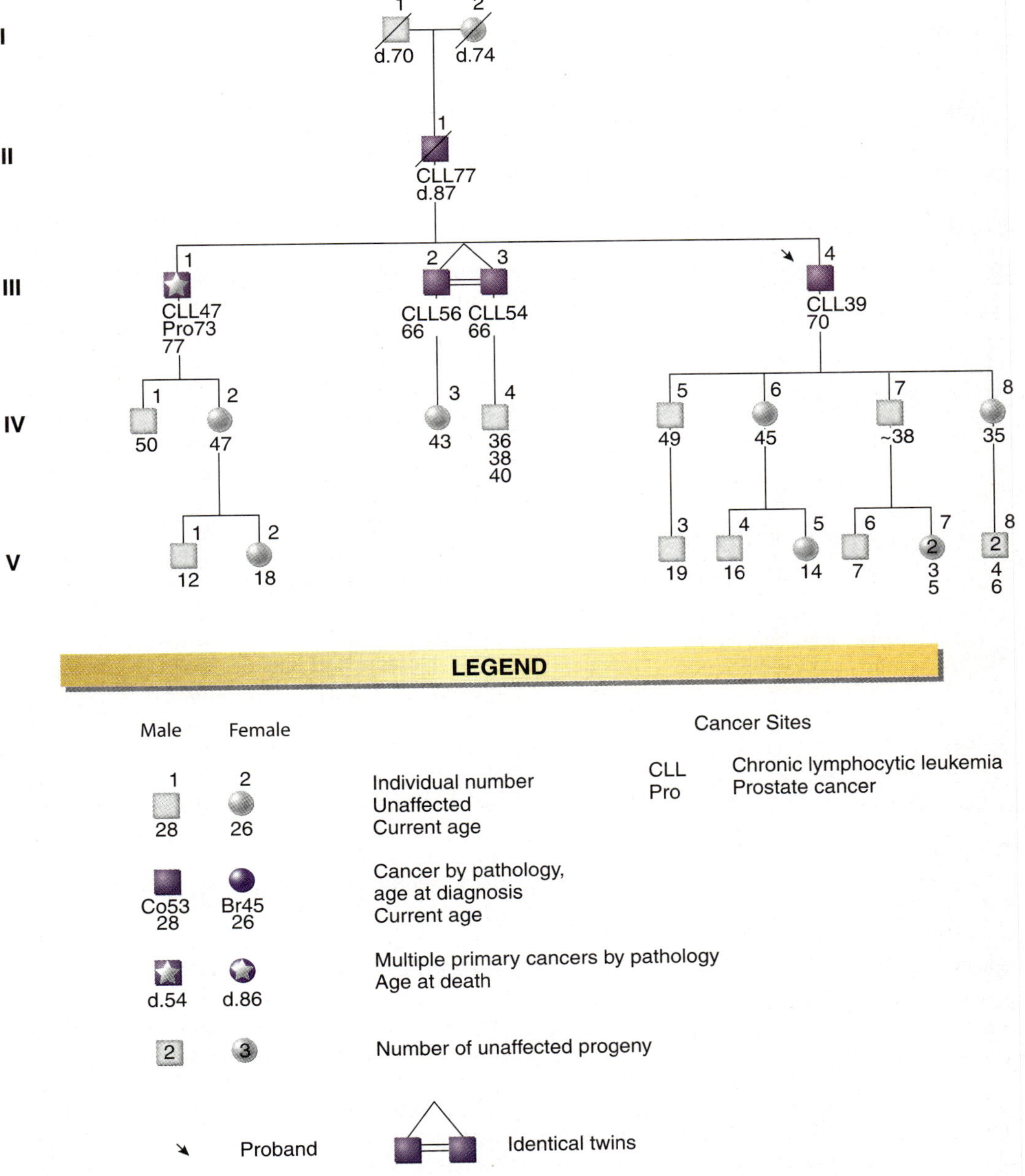

Figure 13-7 Pedigree of a family in which the father and all four children are chronic lymphocytic leukemia (CLL)-affected, findings consistent with an autosomal dominantly-inherited predisposition to CLL. (Lynch HT, et al. Hereditary chronic lymphocytic leukemia: an extended family study and literature review. Am J Med Genet 2002;115:113–117.)

logic cancer in this family. Review of the pedigree shows several examples of key individuals with solid tumors having progeny with hematologic cancer and, conversely, patients with hematologic cancer having progeny with solid tumors. The pedigree appears to be consistent with an autosomal dominant predisposition to both hematologic and solid tumors. In the absence of a hereditary cancer disorder such as the Li-Fraumeni syndrome, these findings appear to be unique, as the hematologic cancers are predominantly AML. There are no premonitory stigmata that may associate this susceptibility to AML.

Chronic Lymphocytic Leukemia We present a family[404] with hereditary chronic lymphocytic leukemia (CLL) (Figure 13-7). Note that the pedigree shows CLL in a father (II-1) and all four of his children (III-1, III-2, III-3, III-4). (Finding a male-to-male transmission excluded X-linked inheritance.) This finding is consistent with an autosomal dominant mode of genetic transmission for susceptibility to CLL. The occurrence of CLL in identical twins in this sibship adds to the likelihood of a primary hereditary etiology. Therefore, hereditary factors appear to be a major contributing causal factor in a subset of CLL cases.[405–407] CLL has also been reported in association with breast cancer.[408]

Yuille and colleagues[409], employing family history questionnaires on 268 CLL-affected individuals, found that a family history of lymphoproliferative disorder (LPD) in a first-degree relative was present in 33 (12%) of those responding to the survey, whereas 15 (6%) reported CLL in a first-degree relative. The largest number of CLL affecteds found in any one of their families was three patients. In their literature survey of CLL families, they identified 81 familial reports of which "…64 were two-case families. Thirty-eight contained an affected sibling, and 16 contained an affected parent and affected offspring. Six pairs of monozygotic twins have been reported. In two of these cases, a first-degree relative was also affected. In five of the families with two or more cases of CLL, other relatives were affected… The largest CLL family reported to date is a six-case family comprising three affected siblings and three affected cousins."[410] Yuille and colleagues[409] suggest that there is an approximate 30-fold increase in risk for CLL in relatives of CLL affecteds.

To date, there has not been any evidence of predisposition genes identified specifically for CLL. However, hematologic cancers inclusive of CLL have been identified in a litany of Mendelian inherited hematologic cancer-prone disorders, particularly such chromosomal breakage syndromes as Bloom's syndrome, Fanconi's aplastic anemia, and ataxia telangiectasia.[411]

Multiple Myeloma The etiology of multiple myeloma (MM) remains obscure, although there are reports of familial clustering that suggest a host susceptibility factor which may act in concert with environmental effects. Lynch and colleagues[412] reported a family with MM (Figure 13-8). Their extended MM family comprised a sibship of 7, wherein 3 patients showed histologically verified MM, whereas two had a monoclonal gammopathy of unknown significance (MGUS). Other tumors in the family included acute lymphocytic leukemia, malignant melanoma, and prostate cancer. Their review of the literature clearly indicates that a subset of familial MM may also include other hematologic cancers as well as solid tumors. More recently, Lynch and colleagues[413] have emphasized the genotypic/phenotypic heterogeneity of MM by describing 39 MM-prone families, with some of the families showing cases of plasma cell dyscrasias, differing hematological malignancies, and/or solid tumors.

Shoenfeld and colleagues,[414] in their review, identified 36 reports of familial MM and added one family of their own. Interestingly, the patients did not show any significant clinical differences from those with nonfamilial myeloma when considering gender, age, distribution of monoclonal proteins, clinical and laboratory data, and prognosis. They did observe an increased incidence of immunoglobulin abnormalities in healthy relatives of the patients manifesting MM.

Horwitz and colleagues[415] described a family wherein multiple myeloma was present in three siblings, two of whom had a history of a monoclonal gammopathy. Their literature review disclosed 38 pairs of siblings with plasma cell disorders, whereas eight families showed a third affected sibling and four families had a fourth affected relative, thereby suggesting that some cases of multiple myeloma may have an hereditary basis. They sug-

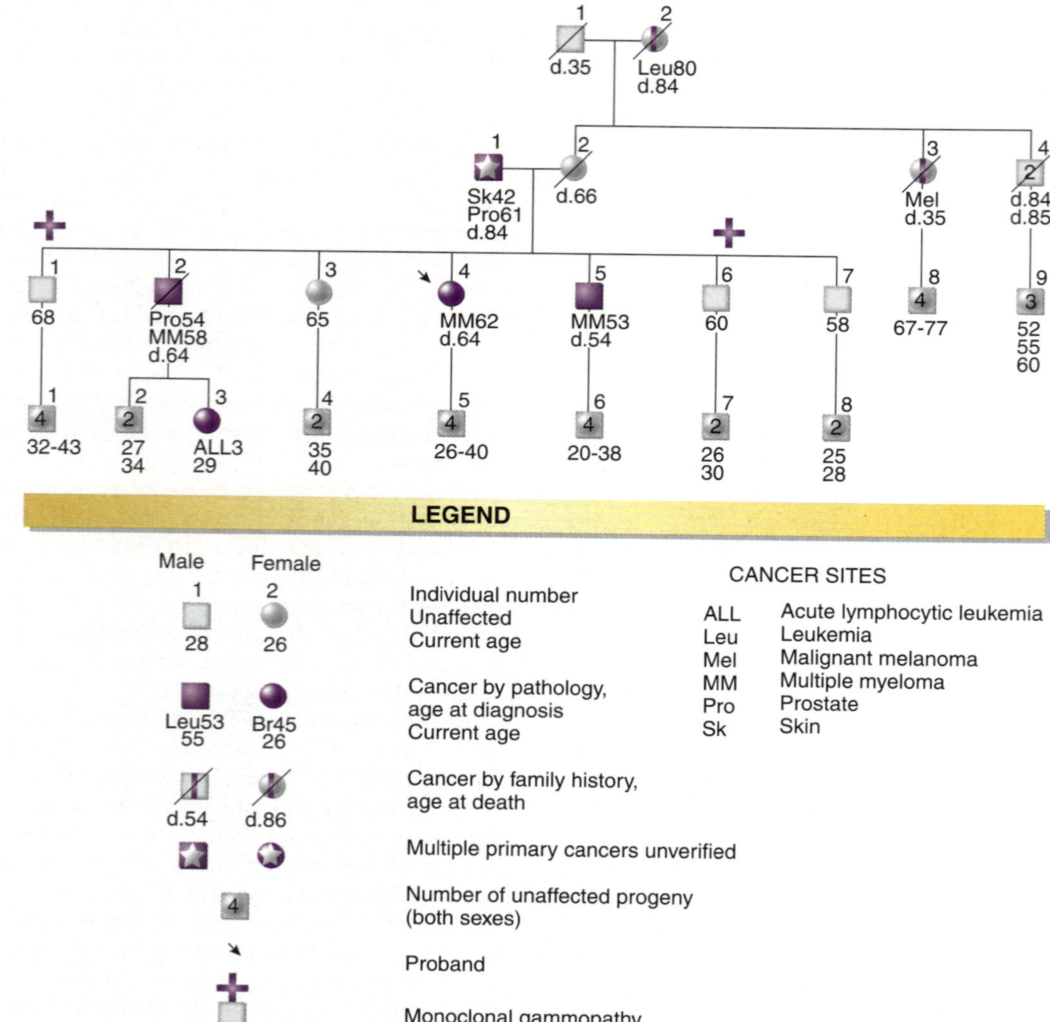

Figure 13-8 Pedigree of multiple myeloma (MM) family with a sibship of seven, showing three siblings with verified MM and two siblings with monoclonal gammopathy of unknown significance. (Lynch HT, et al. Familial multiple myeloma: a family study and review of the literature. J Natl Cancer Inst 2001;93:1479–83.)

gested that other family members may be at increased risk for developing the disease. These authors also noted in their review of the literature that only two other families had three siblings with MM, but they state that, "…five other sibships had combinations of myeloma and monoclonal gammopathy, and two had three siblings with monoclonal gammopathies only. Furthermore, another close relative was affected [with MM] in four of these families. Since approximately 3% of the elderly have benign [monoclonal] gammopathies,[416] the presence of several individuals with such an abnormality in a single family might not be unusual. On the other hand, frank myeloma in three siblings should be very rare."

Bizzaro and Pasini[417] studied a family in which five siblings had a monoclonal gammopathy. MGUS was diagnosed in two of these individuals, following which a family study showed that one sister had died from multiple myeloma, and four of the seven living siblings were discovered to have MGUS.

Hodgkin's Disease and Non-Hodgkin's Lymphoma Research dealing with the genetics of Hodgkin's disease (HD) and non-Hodgkin's lymphoma (NHL) is limited.[418] When considering leukemia or lymphoma in relatives with hematologic malignancies, case-control studies have shown an approximate 3.62-fold risk for these disorders.[401] An approximate 9-fold increased risk for HD among first-degree relatives of HD affecteds has been described, but there was no evidence of an increased risk in NHL.[419]

Ferraris and colleagues[420] estimate that approximately 4.5% of all cases of HD are familial. These authors suggest that shared environmental factors might be important, inclusive of Epstein-Barr virus and other viral agents, which may be acting in concert with genetic determinants to explain the familial aggregation of HD. Mack and colleagues[421] described high concordance for HD in monozygotic twins as compared with dizygotic twins, suggesting a role for genetic factors in the pathogenesis of HD.

X-Linked Lymphoproliferative Syndrome Sullivan[422] has reviewed the history of X-linked lymphoproliferative syndrome (XLP), also known as Duncan's disease. Purtilo and colleagues, some 30 years ago, performed an autopsy on an 8½-year-old male who died following infectious mononucleosis (IM). This was the third male sibling in the family to have died following a bout of IM. This led to their seminal publication in 1975, which described X-linked recessive combined variable immunodeficiency.[423] More than 80 families have now been reported to the XLP syndrome registry established by Purtilo and colleagues.[424]

XLP is characterized by an enormous sensitivity to Epstein-Barr virus (EBV). The phenotype features severe or fatal IM, acquired hypogammaglobulinemia, and malignant lymphoma. Sullivan[422] lists the following phenotypic features: (1) life-threatening EBV infection (58% with a mortality of 96%); (2) immunodeficiency in 31% with a mortality of 45%; (3) lymphoma or Hodgkin's disease in 30% with a mortality of 69%; and (4) aplastic anemia in 3% with a 50% mortality. Most of the lymphomas are extranodal non-Hodgkin's lymphomas, with distal small bowel the site at highest risk.

Genetic linkage studies have localized the XLP locus to the long arm of the X chromosome in Xq24-q25. Coffey and colleagues[425] identified a gene termed *SH2D1A* "…that is mutated in XLP patients and encodes a novel protein composed of a single SH2 domain. *SH2D1A* is expressed in many tissues involved in the immune system. The identification of *SH2D1A* will allow the determination of its mechanism of action as a possible regulator of the EBV-induced immune response." EBV infection in susceptible infants is initially asymptomatic, but by adolescence or early adulthood, IM will occur with 100% mortality by the age of 40.

CLINICAL TRANSLATION

Overview Figure 13-9 shows our recommendations for evaluating and testing individuals suspected of having a hereditary CRC syndrome, as a model example. Family history and physical examination is used to tentatively classify an index patient as sporadic, familial, or hereditary. Family histories are updated regularly, sometimes resulting in reclassification of risk status. Screening and genetic testing options depend on the specific syndrome under consideration. Worth re-emphasizing here is the potential power of such testing when a cancer susceptibility mutation can be identified and at-risk family members can be tested. Individuals who are positive for the mutation can enter surveillance and management programs tailored to the natural history of the particular syndrome involved. In some circumstances, prophylactic surgery may be an option. Individuals lacking the mutation can follow general population screening guidelines. Whether positive or negative, patients in this situation require compassionate genetic counseling.[426] For more thoughts on the importance of family history, and information regarding the National Health Institute's family history project, see Guttmacher and colleagues.[427]

It is important to be aware of factors that might obfuscate pedigree interpretation. These include incomplete gene penetrance in key relatives, early death prior to phenotype expression,

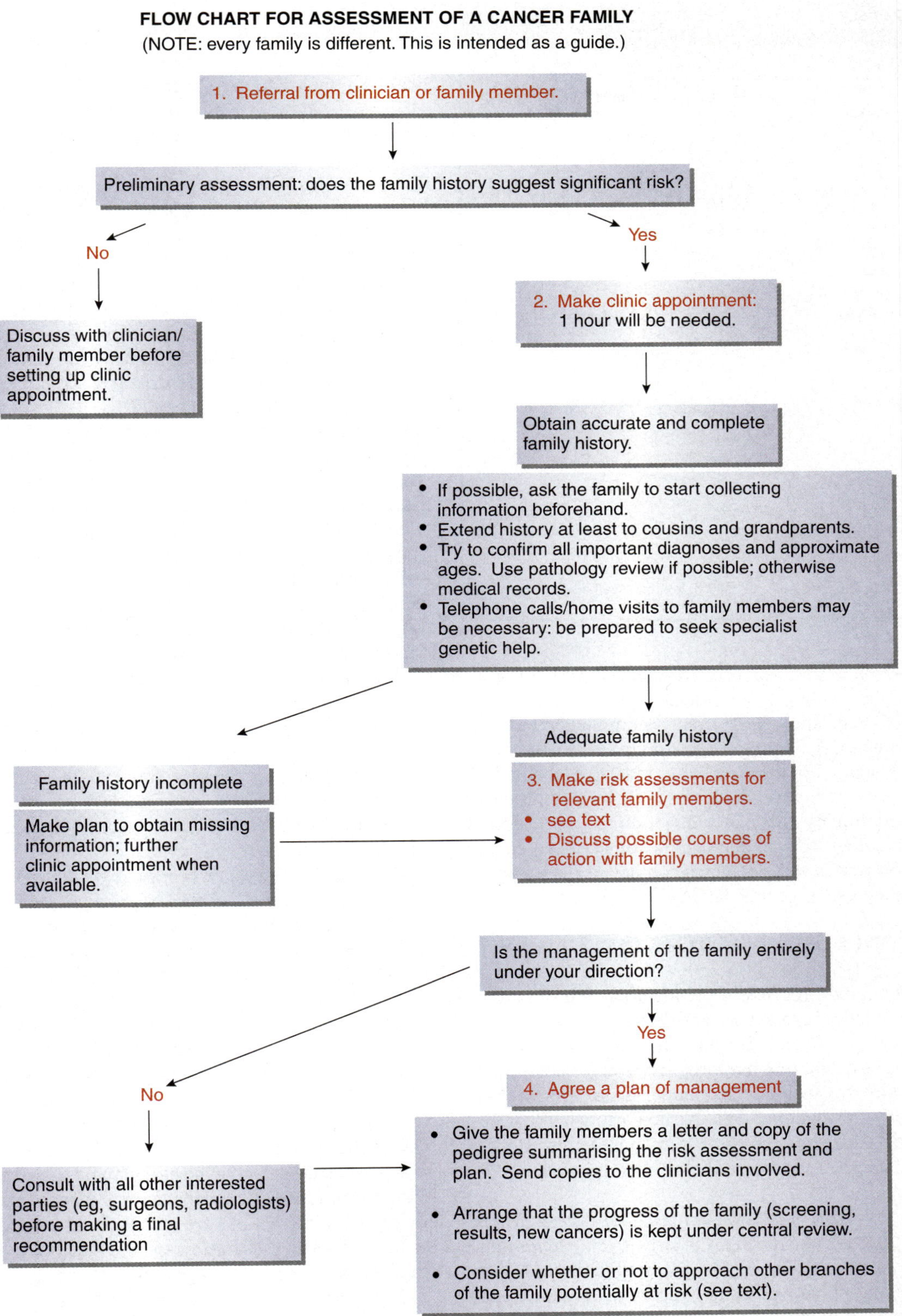

Figure 13-9 Algorithm depicting the process for the study and genetic counseling of families being observed by the Creighton Cancer Genetic Research Team. (Reproduced with permission from Lynch HT, et al. Cancer 1999;86:2449–56.) FIS = Family Information Session; ACS = American Cancer Society.

incomplete family history, false paternity, cancer occurrences that may be sporadic, limited patient and/or physician cooperation, records lost or destroyed, and small family size.

We recommend comprehensive education of all at-risk patients as part of genetic counseling. Detailed coverage of the genetics and natural history of the particular hereditary cancer syndrome, as well as the advantages and disadvantages of DNA testing, can be provided in a large group family information session (FIS).[345] Key relatives in the geographic catchment area may attend the FIS at a designated time so that they can be provided with this educational experience. Alternatively, genetic counseling can be offered as a series of appointments with a genetic counselor and medical team. Informed consent for genetic testing is an extremely complex and important issue in genetic testing and must be obtained with care through a detailed discussion with each participant (see Table 13-5 for essential components). Before blood is collected for DNA testing, patients must be advised of the potential for fear, anxiety, apprehension, and intrafamily strife, as well as insurance and employer discrimination. When a cancer-causing germline mutation is identified, additional genetic counseling on an individual basis at the time of disclosure of these results is required.

Table 13-5 Content of Informed Consent for Genetic Testing

Purpose of the test: if testing is part of a research study, the purpose, aims, and design of the research study
Practical aspects of the testing, including cost, turnaround time, documentation of results
Predictive value of a positive, negative, or indeterminate result and corresponding cancer risk information
Options for cancer risk management in the setting of a positive, negative, or indeterminate result
Possible psychological implications of testing
Individualized assessment of insurance and employment discrimination risks
Alternatives to genetic testing, including the possibility of delaying decision making

We subscribe to the updated guidelines proposed by the American Society of Clinical Oncology,[428] which state that predisposition testing should be offered only when (1) there is a strong family history of cancer, (2) the test can be adequately interpreted, (3) the results will influence medical management of the patient or family members, and (4) laboratories are committed to the validation of testing methodologies. Table 13-6 details hereditary cancer syndromes for which clinical genetic testing is currently available.

Our experience with an HNPCC (Lynch syndrome) family with the *MSH2* mutation illustrates some of the issues that arise during genetic testing.[429] Whether positive or negative for the *MSH2* germline mutation, patients reported considerable emotional stress. Their main concerns centered on reproductive issues, potential transmission of the deleterious gene to their progeny, and discrimination by insurance companies and/or employers. More than one-half of those patients who were found to harbor the *MSH2* mutation considered the option of prophylactic subtotal colectomy. At-risk family members sought genetic risk assessment primarily for benefit to their children and, secondarily, for their own personal health concerns. The patients who were positive for the culprit *MSH2* germline mutation had many concerns about their lifetime cancer destiny.

Medicolegal Issues The prodigious advancement in knowledge about genetic risk, natural history, recommended available surveillance and management, DNA testing, and the need for genetic counseling are affecting decisions in the

Table 13-6 Hereditary Cancer Syndromes for which Clinical Genetic Testing Is Available

Cancer Syndrome	Associated Cancers and Other Features	Gene(s)	Mode of Inheritance
Breast-ovarian cancer syndrome	Early-onset breast cancer Ovarian cancer Prostate cancer Male breast cancer	*BRCA1* *BRCA2*	Autosomal dominant
Hereditary nonpolyposis colorectal cancer	Early onset colon cancer Endometrial cancer Stomach cancer Ovarian cancer Other genitourinary cancers Absence of polyposis	*MLH1* *MSH2* *MSH6*	Autosomal dominant
Familial adenomatous polyposis	Polyposis (> 100 colon polyps) Early-onset colon cancer Desmoid tumors Epidermoid tumors	*APC*	Autosomal dominant
Li-Fraumeni syndrome	Early-onset breast cancer Childhood sarcoma Brain cancer Leukemia Adrenocortical cancer	*TP53*	Autosomal dominant
von Hippel-Lindau syndrome	Renal cell cancer Hemangioblastomas of cerebellum brain stem, spine Retinal angioma Pheochromocytoma	*VHL*	Autosomal dominant

court system. One recent case was adjudicated in favor of a patient with the hereditary breast-ovarian cancer syndrome who followed the recommendations of her gynecologic oncologist and a cancer geneticist to undergo prophylactic oophorectomy, but whose insurance company failed to reimburse for this procedure. Her petition for reimbursement was denied at the district court level, but the Nebraska Supreme Court rendered a favorable decision on her part, ordering the insurance company to provide reimbursement for this indicated procedure.[430]

Standard-of-care concerns apply to physicians as well. In the *Safer* case,[431] a diagnosis of FAP was established in the father of the litigant at age 35. The patient later died. The surviving spouse claimed that although the surgeon discussed her husband's diagnosis, treatment, and cancer management, he failed to disclose the genetic risk for FAP, even though the hereditary nature of FAP was known. The patient's children, then ages 10 and 17, were not advised to seek early colon surveillance. Subsequently, one of the children, at age 36, experienced lower abdominal pain and underwent surgery and extensive chemotherapy for CRC arising in FAP. A claim of negligence was filed against the estate of the surgeon, alleging (1) that he had a duty to warn those known to be at risk of avoidable harm from a genetically transmissible condition existing in his patient, (2) that the physician's duty did extend to members of the immediate family of his patient, and (3) that he had breached these duties.[270] The suit was won by the plaintiff in 1996. Similar cases are likely to become more common as advances in molecular genetics outstrip the ability of physicians to stay current in a very complex field. The physician must not only obtain a sufficiently detailed family history; he or she must also be able to suggest appropriate surveillance and management for the affected family. Finally, genetic testing is not indicated in all heritable cancer syndromes, and current recommendations will continually change as knowledge in the field advances. For these reasons, updated guidelines[428] have been published and will be periodically updated by the American Society of Clinical Oncology for genetic testing for heritable cancer syndromes, to help educate clinicians in the appropriate use of genetic testing.

CONCLUSIONS/FUTURE DIRECTIONS

The rapid progress in the identification of hereditary cancer syndromes and their molecular genetic etiology during the past decade suggests very strongly that research progress in this new millennium will yield an astounding mass of new clinically translational data, particularly when considering the extant heterogeneity in these disorders.

Here are some predictions for the future:

1. *More high-prevalence, low-penetrance mutations will be found that contribute to familial clustering of cancer.* We predict that more highly penetrant, as well as low–penetrance gene mutations, will be identified and will contribute to what we now construe as familial clustering of cancer. Laken and colleagues,[81] as noted earlier, reported a low-penetrance mutation within the *APC* gene. A T-to-A transversion of nucleotide 3920 was identified, resulting in a substitution of lysine for isoleucine at codon 1307 (I1307K). This mutation was found in 6.1% of the 766 Ashkenazi Jewish patients, but none of 243 non-Ashkenazim had the mutation.

Laken and colleagues[81] then examined 211 Ashkenazim with CRC and found that 10.4% of them harbored the I1307K mutation. The authors also observed the mutation more commonly (28%) in Ashkenazim with CRC and a first- or second-degree relative with CRC and/or adenomatous polyps than in Ashkenazim with CRC and an unknown or negative family history. They estimated that carrying this mutation resulted in a doubling of CRC risk over the patient's lifetime. The mutation itself is not pathogenic, but the T-to-A transversion creates a poly-A tract at higher risk for subsequent mutations.

Tomlinson and colleagues[432] subsequently identified a novel susceptibility gene mapped to chromosome 15q14-q22 in an Ashkenazi family with dominantly inherited predisposition to colorectal adenomas and carcinomas. The authors refer to this previously undescribed susceptibility gene on chromosome 15q as *CRAC1* (colorectal adenoma and carcinoma). Interestingly, there were two cases of pancreatic cancer in the family with the suggestion that this could also be part of the phenotype attributable to mutations in the gene. Of further interest is the fact that the family fulfills the Amsterdam criteria for HNPCC but differs in that several of the patients have more colonic adenomas than expected. Genetic linkage analysis excluded germline mutations in *MSH2*, *MLH1*, *PSM1*, *PMS2*, and *MSH6*.

Varley and colleagues[433] suggest that certain *TP53* alleles confer low-penetrance predisposition to the development of cancer. They found a narrow spectrum of *TP53* mutations in children with adrenocortical tumors; some of the mutations had been inherited and some of the families in question had other cancers. No family met criteria for Li-Fraumeni syndrome.

2. *The role of modifier genes will be more fully explored and clarified.* Complex genetic and environmental interactions almost certainly influence phenotypic expression in hereditary syndromes. In the Min mouse, inheritance of the Mom1 locus decreases the size and number of intestinal polyps.[434] In human populations, Moisio and colleagues[435] have shown that genetic polymorphisms in carcinogen metabolism might modify phenotype in HNPCC. They found that in patients carrying germline mutations of *MLH1*, a particular N-acetyltransferase 1 allele was associated with younger patient age at diagnosis and tumor location in the distal colon. As mechanisms for genotype-environment interactions are elucidated, there will be more opportunities for therapeutic intervention, which leads to our next suggestion.

3. *The ability to modulate the effects of deleterious mutations through chemoprevention will continue to grow.* Quite a large body of literature exists on chemoprevention in colon cancer (reviewed by Hawk and colleagues[105]), most of it pertaining to cyclooxygenase inhibitors. Tamoxifen, an anti-estrogen, has been shown to have activity as a chemopreventive agent for breast cancer in patients with DCIS and those with a high risk of breast cancer. Additional indications are currently under study. Many pharmacologic agents under development or currently in trials will undoubtedly aid our ability to inhibit or reverse the process of carcinogenesis.[436]

4. *Microarray technology will make genetic testing more widely available and less expensive.* The newly developed cDNA microarray analysis provides new methodology for cancer genetic research. Bennicelli and Barr[437] have studied the implications of microarray techniques with respect to the biology of sarcomas. Specifically, these authors have shown how relevant knowledge with respect to a better comprehension of sarcoma biology can be obtained through comparative genomic hybridization and microarray techniques. They showed how these powerful technologies "...will facilitate the rapid acquisition of data that provide insight into the molecular genetic and biologic basis of sarcomas."

Finally, these microarray techniques should advance our cause significantly in terms of ferreting out differences between hereditary forms of cancer such as colon, breast, ovary, and endometrium, in the respective hereditary cancer syndromes, and their sporadic counterparts. For example, Kurian and colleagues[438] note that this "...mini-revolution is sweeping the world of science and medicine. DNA chip or microarray technology will have a more profound impact than other recent major advances, including DNA sequencing and the polymerase chain reaction (PCR)."

5. *Gene therapy will become a reality.* We will have the ability to alter cellular function or structure at the molecular level by replacing lost or defective genes or adding genes known to produce beneficial proteins. Everything from inborn errors of metabolism to atherosclerosis to cancer should be amenable to treatment with molecular techniques. For example, phase I clinical trials show that *TP53* replacement therapy induces tumor regression in lung cancer patients.[439] Patients known to carry mutations in cancer-susceptibility genes should be ideal candidates for molecular intervention.

In the next decade, molecular and genetic approaches will likely take center stage in the prevention, diagnosis, and treatment of cancer. Valuable information on the science and ethics of this expanding field is increasingly available and regularly updated for clinicians, health care providers, and the public by major organizations such as the National Institutes of Health (<http://www.genetests.org/>). It will be essential that physicians remain well informed so that they may successfully harness the power of these approaches to the benefit of the patients who seek their assistance.

REFERENCES

1. Cripps WH. Two cases of disseminated polyps of the rectum. Trans Pathol Soc London 1882;33:165–8.
2. Smith T. Three cases of multiple polypi of the lower bowel occurring in one family. St Bartholomew's Hosp Rep 1887;23:225–9.
3. Macklin MT. Inheritance of cancer of stomach and large intestine in man. J Natl Cancer Inst 1960;24:551–71.
4. Lynch HT, Shaw MW, Magnuson CW, et al. Hereditary factors in cancer: study of two large Midwestern kindreds. Arch Intern Med 1966;117:206–12.
5. Herrera L, Kakati S, Gibas L, et al. Brief clinical report: Gardner's syndrome in a man with an interstitial deletion of 5q. Am J Med Genet 1986;25:473–6.
6. Leppert M, Dobbs M, Scambler P, et al. The gene for familial polyposis coli maps to the long arm of chromosome 5. Science 1987;238:1411–3.
7. Kinzler KW, Nilbert MC, Su L-K, et al. Identification of FAP locus genes from chromosome 5q21. Science 1991;253:661–5.
8. Collins FS. Shattuck Lecture—Medical and societal consequences of the Human Genome Project. N Engl J Med 1999;341:28–37.
9. David KL, Steiner-Grossman P. The potential use of tumor registry data in the recognition and prevention of hereditary and familial cancer. NY State J Med 1991;91:150–2.
10. Lynch HT. Cancer and the family history trail. NY State J Med 1991;91:145–7.
11. Jemal A, Murray T, Ward E, et al. Cancer statistics, 2005. CA Cancer J Clin 2005;55:10–30.
12. Lynch HT, Krush AJ, Lemon HM, et al. Tumor variation in families with breast cancer. JAMA 1972;222:1631–5.
13. Lynch HT, Krush AJ. Carcinoma of the breast and ovary in three families. Surg Gynecol Obstet 1971;133:644–8.
14. Ford D, Easton DF, Stratton M, et al. Genetic heterogeneity and penetrance analysis of the BRCA1 and BRCA2 genes in breast cancer families. Am J Hum Genet 1998;62:676–89.
15. Couch FJ, DeShano ML, Blackwood MA, et al. *BRCA1* mutations in women attending clinics that evaluate the risk of breast cancer. N Engl J Med 1997;336:1409–15.
16. Gayther SA, Russell P, Harrington P, et al. The contribution of germline BRCA1 and BRCA2 mutations to familial ovarian cancer: no evidence for other ovarian cancer susceptibility genes. Am J Hum Genet 1999;65:1021–9.
17. Hall JM, Lee MK, Newman B, et al. Linkage of early-onset breast cancer to chromosome 17q21. Science 1990;250:1684–9.
18. Narod SA, Feunteun J, Lynch HT, et al. Familial breast-ovarian cancer locus on chromosome 17q12-q23. Lancet 1991;388:82–3.
19. Miki Y, Swensen J, Shattuck-Eidens D, et al. A strong candidate for the breast and ovarian cancer susceptibility gene BRCA1. Science 1994;266:66–71.
20. Wooster R, Bignell G, Lancaster J, et al. Identification of the breast cancer susceptibility gene BRCA2. Nature 1995;378:789–92.
21. Tavtigian SV, Simard J, Rommens J, et al. The complete BRCA2 gene and mutations in chromosome 13q-linked kindreds. Nat Genet 1996;12:333–7.
22. Wu LC, Wang ZW, Tsan JT, et al. Identification of a RING protein that can interact in vivo with the BRCA1 gene product. Nature Genet 1996;14:430–40.
23. Venkitaraman AR. Cancer susceptibility and the functions of BRCA1 and BRCA2. Cell 2002;108:171–82.
24. Somasundaram K, Zhang H, Zeng YX, et al. Arrest of the cell cycle by the tumour-suppressor BRCA1 requires the CDK-inhibitor P21WAF1/CiP1. Nature 1997;389:187–90.
25. Chen J, Silver DP, Walpita D, et al. Stable interaction between the products of the BRCA1 and BRCA2 tumor. Molecular Cell 1998;2:317–28.
26. Scully R, Chen J, Plug A, et al. Association of *BRCA1* with Rad51 in mitotic and meiotic cells. Cell 1997;88:265–75.
27. Scully R, Chen J, Ochs RL, et al. Dynamic changes of BRCA1 subnuclear location and phosphorylation state are initiated by DNA damage. Cell 1997;90:425–35.
28. Gowen LC, Avrutskaya AV, Latour AM, et al. BRCA1 required for transcription-coupled repair of oxidative DNA damage. Science 1998;281:1009–12.
29. Venkitaraman AR. Tracing the network connecting BRCA and Fanconi anemia proteins. Nature Reviews Cancer 2004;4:266–76.
30. Deng C-X, Wang R-H. Roles of BRCA1 in DNA damage repair: a link between development and cancer. Hum Mol Genet 2003;12(Spec No 1):R113–23.
31. Chen Y, Chen C-F, Riley DF, et al. Aberrant subcellular localization of BRCA1 in breast cancer. Science 1995;270:789–91.
32. Sully R, Ganesan S, Brown M, et al. Location of BRCA1 in human breast and ovarian cancer cells. Science 1996;272:123–6.
33. Thakur S, Zhang HB, Peng Y, et al. Localization of BRCA1 and a splice variant identifies the nuclear localization signal. Mol Cell Biol 1997;17:444–52.
34. Wilson CA, Payton MN, Elliott GS, et al. Differential subcellular localization, expression and biological toxicity of BRCA1 and the splice variant BRCA1-delta11b. Oncogene 1997;14:1–16.
35. Scully R, Anderson SF, Chao DM, et al. BRCA1 is a component of the RNA polymerase II holoenzyme. Proc Natl Acad Sci USA 1997;94:5605–10.
36. Cui JQ, Shao N, Chai Y, et al. BRCA1 splice variants BRCA1a and BRCA1b associate with CBP co-activator. Oncology Reports 1998;5:591–95.
37. Gudas JM, Nguyen H, Li T, et al. Hormone-dependent regulation of BRCA1 in human breast cancer cells. Cancer Res 1995;55:4561–5.
38. Chen Y, Farmer AA, Chen CF, et al. BRCA1 is a 220-kDa nuclear phosphoprotein that is expressed and phosphorylated in a cell cycle-dependent manner. Cancer Res 1996;56:3168–72.
39. Gowen LC, Johnson BL, Latour AM, et al. Brca1 deficiency results in early embryonic lethality characterized by neuroepithelial abnormalities. Nat Genet 1996;12:191–4.
40. Hakem R, de la Pompa JL, Sirard C, et al. The tumor suppressor gene Brca1 is required for embryonic cellular proliferation in the mouse. Cell 1996;85:1009–23.
41. Liu CY, Fleskin-Nikitin A, Li S, et al. Inactivation of the mouse Brca1 gene leads to failure in the morphogenesis of the egg cylinder in early postimplantation development. Genes Dev 1996;10:1835–43.
42. Connor F, Bertwistle D, Mee PJ, et al. Tumorigenesis and a DNA repair defect in mice with a truncating *Brca2* mutation. Nat Genet 1997;17:423–30.
43. Friedman LS, Thistlethwaite FC, Patel KJ, et al. Thymic lymphomas in mice with a truncating mutation in Brca2. Cancer Res 1998;58:1338–43.
44. Xu X, Wagner K-U, Larson D, et al. Conditional mutation of *Brca1* in mammary epithelial cells results in blunted ductal morphogenesis and tumour formation. Nat Genet 1999;22:37-43.
45. Lubin JH, Burns PE, Blot WJ, et al. Risk factors for breast cancer in women in northern Alberta, Canada, as related to age at diagnosis. J Natl Cancer Inst 1982;68:211–7.
46. Bain C, Speizer FE, Rosner B, et al. Family history of breast cancer as a risk indicator for the disease. Am J Epidemiol 1980;111:301–8.
47. Adami HO, Hansen J, Jung B, et al. Characteristics of familial breast cancer in Sweden: absence of relation to age and unilateral versus bilateral disease. Cancer 1981;48:1688–95.
48. FitzGerald MG, MacDonald DJ, Krainer M, et al. Germ-line BRCA1 mutations in Jewish and non-Jewish women with early onset breast cancer. N Engl J Med 1996;334:143–9.
49. Malone KE, Daling JR, Thompson JD, et al. *BRCA1* mutations and breast cancer in the general population: analyses in women before age 35 years and in women before age 45 years with first-degree family history. JAMA 1998;279:922–9.
50. Warner E, Foulkes W, Goodwin P, et al. Prevalence and penetrance of *BRCA1* and *BRCA2* gene mutations in unselected Ashkenazi Jewish women with breast cancer. J Natl Cancer Inst 1999;91:1241–7.
51. Krainer M, Silva-Arrieta S, FitzGerald MG, et al. Differential contributions of *BRCA1* and *BRCA2* to early-onset breast cancer. N Engl J Med 1997;336:1416–21.
52. Easton DF, Steele L, Fields P, et al. Cancer risks in two large breast cancer families linked to BRCA2 on chromosome 13q12-13. Am J Hum Genet 1997;61:120–8.
53. Struewing JP, Hartge P, Wacholder S, et al. The risk of cancer associated with specific mutations of BRCA1 and BRCA2 among Ashkenazi Jews. N Engl J Med 1997;336:1401–8.
54. Brose MS, Rebbeck TR, Calzone KA, et al. Cancer risk estimates for BRCA1 mutation carriers identified in a risk evaluation program. J Natl Cancer Inst 2002;94:1365–72.
55. Thompson D, Easton DF, The Breast Cancer Linkage Consortium. Cancer incidence in BRCA1 mutation carriers. J Natl Cancer Inst 2002;94:1358–65.
56. Couch FJ, Farid LM, DeShano ML, et al. BRCA2 germline mutations in male breast cancer cases and breast cancer families. Nat Genet 1996;13:123–5.
57. Breast Cancer Linkage Consortium. Cancer risks in BRCA2 mutation carriers. J Natl Cancer Inst 1999;91:1310–6.
58. Chenevix-Tranch G, Spurdle AB, Gatei M, et al. Dominant negative ATM mutations in breast cancer families. J Natl Cancer Inst 2002;94:205–15.
59. Dong C, Hemminki K. Modification of cancer risks in off-spring by sibling and parental cancers from 2,112,616 nuclear families. Int J Cancer 2001;92:144–50.
60. Breast Cancer Linkage Consortium. Pathology of familial breast cancer: differences between breast cancers in carriers of *BRCA1* or *BRCA2* mutations and sporadic cases. Lancet 1997;349:1505–10.
61. Marcus JN, Watson P, Page DL, et al. Hereditary breast cancer: pathobiology, prognosis, and BRCA1 and BRCA2 gene linkage. Cancer 1996;77:697–709.

62. Eisinger F, Stoppa-Lyonnet D, Longy M, et al. Germ line mutation at BRCA1 affects the histoprognostic grade in hereditary breast cancer. Cancer Res 1996;56:471–4.
63. Karp SE, Tonin PN, Begin LR, et al. Influence of BRCA1 mutations on nuclear grade and estrogen receptor status of breast carcinoma in Ashkenazi Jewish women. Cancer 1997;80:435–41.
64. Verhoog LC, Brekelmans CTM, Seynaeve C, et al. Survival and tumour characteristics of breast-cancer patients with germline mutations of *BRCA1*. Lancet 1998;351:316–21.
65. Jóhannsson OT, Ranstam J, Borg Å, et al. Survival of *BRCA1* breast and ovarian cancer patients: a population-based study from southern Sweden. J Clin Oncol 1998;16:397–404.
66. Domchek SM, Eisen A, Calzone K, et al. Application of breast cancer risk prediction models in clinical practice. J Clin Oncol 2003;21:593–601.
67. Tonin P, Weber B, Offit K, et al. Frequency of recurrent *BRCA1* and *BRCA2* mutations in Ashkenazi Jewish breast cancer families. Nat Med 1996;2:1179–83.
68. Warner E, Plewes DB, Hill KA, et al. Surveillance of BRCA1 and BRCA2 mutation carriers with magnetic resonance imaging, ultrasound, mammography, and clinical breast examination. JAMA 2004;292:1317–25.
69. Narod SA, Brunet J-S, Ghadirian P, et al. Tamoxifen and risk of contralateral breast cancer in *BRCA1* and *BRCA2* mutation carriers: a case-control study. Lancet 2000;356:1876–81.
70. Cuzick J, Powles T, Veronesi U, et al. Overview of the main outcomes in breast-cancer prevention trials. Lancet 2003;361:296–300.
71. Rebbeck TR, Lynch HT, Neuhausen SL, et al. Prophylactic oophorectomy in carriers of *BRCA1* or *BRCA2* mutations. N Engl J Med 2002;346:1616–22.
72. Rebbeck TR, Friebel T, Lynch HT, et al. Bilateral prophylactic mastectomy reduces breast cancer risk in BRCA1 and BRCA2 mutation carriers: The PROSE Study Group. J Clin Oncol 2004;22:1055–62.
73. Robson M, Svahn T, McCormick B, et al. Appropriateness of breast-conserving treatment of breast carcinoma in women with germline mutations in *BRCA1* or *BRCA2*: a clinic-based series. Cancer 2005;103:44–51.
74. de Jong MM, Nolte IM, te Meerman GJ, et al. Genes other than *BRCA1* and *BRCA2* involved in breast cancer susceptibility. J Med Genet 2002;39:225–42.
75. de Bock GH, Schutte M, Krol-Warmerdam EMM, et al. Tumour characteristics and prognosis of breast cancer patients carrying the germline *CHEK2**1100delC variant. J Med Genet 2004;41:731–5.
76. Cybulski C, Górski B, Huzarski T, et al. *CHEK2* is a multiorgan cancer susceptibility gene. Am J Hum Genet 2004;75:1131–5.
77. Hodgson SV, Morrison PJ, Irving M. Breast cancer genetics: unsolved questions and open perspectives in an expanding clinical practice. Am J Med Genet (Semin Med Genet) 2004;129:56–64.
78. Kennedy RD, Quinn JE, Mullan PB, et al. The role of BRCA1 in the cellular response to chemotherapy. J Natl Cancer Inst 2004;96:1659–68.
79. Fuchs C, Giovannucci E, Colditz G, et al. A prospective study of family history and the risk of colorectal cancer. N Engl J Med 1994;331:1669–74.
80. Burt RW, Bishop DT, Cannon LA, et al. Dominant inheritance of adenomatous colonic polyps and colorectal cancer. N Engl J Med 1985;312:1540–4.
81. Laken SJ, Petersen GM, Gruber SB, et al. Familial colorectal cancer in Ashkenazim due to a hypermutable tract in *APC*. Nat Genet 1997;17:79–83.
82. Bulow S. Familial polyposis coli. Dan Med Bull 1987;34:1–15.
83. Luschka H. Ueber polypose Vegetationen der gesammten Dickdarmschleimhaut. Arch Path Anat Phys Klin Med 1861;20:133–42.
84. Sklifosovski NV. Polyadenoma tractus intestinalis. Vrach 1881;2:55–7.
85. Handford H. Disseminated polypi of the large intestine becoming malignant: strictures (malignant adenoma) of the rectum and of the splenic flexure of the colon; secondary growths in the liver. Trans Path Soc London 1890;41:133–7.
86. Lockhart-Mummery P. Cancer and heredity. Lancet 1925;i:427–9.
87. Powell SM, Petersen GM, Krush AJ, et al. Molecular diagnosis of familial adenomatous polyposis. N Engl J Med 1993;329:1982–7.
88. Bodmer WF, Bailey CJ, Bodmer J, et al. Localization of the gene for familial adenomatous polyposis on chromosome 5. Nature 1987;328:614–6.
89. Nishisho I, Nakamura Y, Miyoshi Y, et al. Mutations of chromosome 5q21 genes in FAP and colorectal cancer patients. Science 1991;253:665–9.
90. Powell SM, Zilz N, Beazer-Barclay Y, et al. APC mutations occur early during colorectal tumorigenesis. Nature 1992;359:235–7.
91. van Es JH, Giles RH, Clevers HC. The many faces of the tumor suppressor gene APC. Exp Cell Res 2001;264:126–34.
92. Munemitsu S, Souza B, Albert I, et al. Regulation of intracellular β-catenin levels by the adenomatous polyposis coli (APC) tumor suppressor protein. Proc Natl Acad Sci USA 1995;92:3046–50.
93. Rubinfeld B, Albert I, Profiri E, et al. Binding of GSK-β with APC/β-catenin complex and regulation of complex assembly. Science 1996;272:1023–6.
94. Smith KJ, Levy DB, Maupin P, et al. Wild-type but not mutant APC associates with the microtubule cytoskeleton. Cancer Res 1994;54:3672–5.
95. Baeg G, Matsumine A, Kuroda T, et al. The tumour suppressor gene product APC blocks cell cycle progression from g0/GI to S phase. EMBO J 1995;14:5618–25.
96. Zwick A, Munir M, Ryan CK, et al. Gastric adenocarcinoma and dysplasia in fundic gland polyps of a patient with attenuated adenomatous polyposis coli. Gastroenterology 1997;113:659–63.
97. Abraham SC, Nobukawa B, Giardiello FM, et al. Fundic gland polyps in familial adenomatous polyposis: neoplasms with frequent somatic adenomatous polyposis coli gene alterations. Am J Pathol 2000;157:747–54.
98. Wallace MH, Phillips RKS. Upper gastrointestinal disease in patients with familial adenomatous polyposis. Br J Surg 1998;85:742–50.
99. Hamilton SR, Liu B, Parsons RE, et al. The molecular basis of Turcot's syndrome. N Engl J Med 1995;332:839–47.
100. Spirio L, Otterud B, Stauffer D, et al. Linkage of a variant or attenuated form of adenomatous polyposis coli to the adenomatous polyposis coli (APC) locus. Am J Hum Genet 1992;51:92–100.
101. Spirio L, Olschwang S, Groden J, et al. Alleles of the APC gene: an attenuated form of familial polyposis. Cell 1993;75:951–7.
102. Lynch HT, Smyrk T, McGinn T, et al. Attenuated familial adenomatous polyposis (AFAP): a phenotypically and genotypically distinctive variant of FAP. Cancer 1995;76:2427–33.
103. Moisio A-L, Järvinen H, Peltomäki P. Genetic and clinical characterisation of familial adenomatous polyposis: a population based study. Gut 2002;50:845–50.
104. Heinimann K, Müllhaupt B, Weber W, et al. Phenotypic differences in familial adenomatous polyposis based on APC gene mutation status. Gut 1998;43:675–9.
105. Hawk E, Lubet R, Limburg P. Chemoprevention in hereditary colorectal cancer syndromes. Cancer 1999;86:2551–63.
106. Lynch HT, Fitzgibbons R Jr., Chong S, et al. Use of doxorubicin and dacarbazine for the management of unresectable intra-abdominal desmoid tumors in Gardner's syndrome. Dis Colon Rectum 1994;37:260–7.
107. Lynch HT, Fitzgibbons R Jr. Surgery, desmoid tumors and familial adenomatous polyposis: case report and literature review. Am J Gastroenterol 1996;91:2598–601.
108. Rodriguez-Bigas MA, Mahoney MC, Karakousis CP, et al. Desmoid tumors in patients with familial adenomatous polyposis. Cancer 1994;74:1270–4.
109. Lynch HT. Desmoid tumors: genotype-phenotype differences in familial adenomatous polyposis—a nosological dilemma. Am J Hum Genet 1996;59:1184–5.
110. Lynch HT, Thorson AG, McComb RD, et al. Familial adenomatous polyposis and extracolonic cancer. Dig Dis Sci 2001;46:2325–32.
111. Prior TW, Chadwick RB, Papp AC, et al. The I1307K polymorphism of the *APC* gene in colorectal cancer. Gastroenterology 1999;116:58–63.
112. Rozen P, Shomrat R, Strul H, et al. Prevalence of the I1307K *APC* gene variant in Israeli Jews of differing ethnic origin and risk for colorectal cancer. Gastroenterology 1999;116:54–7.
113. Rozen P, Naiman T, Strul H, et al. Clinical and screening implications of the I1307K adenomatous polyposis coli gene variant in Israeli Ashkenzi Jews with familial colorectal neoplasia: evidence for a founder effect. Cancer 2002;94:2561–8.
114. Helwig EB. Adenomas of the large intestine in children. Am J Dis Child 1946;72:289–95.
115. Nugent KP, Talbot IC, Hodgson SV, et al. Solitary juvenile polyps: not a marker for subsequent malignancy. Gastroenterology 1993;105:698–700.
116. Eng C, Ji H. Molecular classification of the inherited hamartoma polyposis syndromes: clearing the muddied waters. Am J Hum Genet 1998;62:1020–2.
117. Howe JR, Ringold JC, Summers RW, et al. A gene for familial juvenile polyposis maps to chromosome 18q21.1. Am J Hum Genet 1998;62:1129–36.
118. Howe JR, Ringold JC, Hughes JH, et al. Direct genetic testing for *Smad4* mutations in patients at risk for juvenile polyposis. Surgery 1999;126:162–70.
119. Howe JR, Roth S, Ringold JC, et al. Mutations in the SMAD4/DPC4 gene in juvenile polyposis. Science 1998;280:1086–8.
120. Howe JR, Bair JL, Sayed MG, et al. Germline mutations of the gene encoding bone morphogenetic protein receptor 1A in juvenile polyposis. Nat Genet 2001;28:184–7.
121. Desai DC, Neal KF, Talbot IC, et al. Juvenile polyposis. Br J Surg 1995;82:14–7.
122. Scott-Conner CEH, Hausmann M, Hall TJ, et al. Familial juvenile polyposis: patterns of recurrence and implications for surgical management. J Am Coll Surg 1995;181:407–13.
123. Järvinen HJ. Juvenile gastrointestinal polyposis. Prob Clin Surg 1993;10:749–57.
124. Howe JR, Mitros FA, Summers RW. The risk of gastrointestinal carcinoma in familial juvenile polyposis. Ann Surg Oncol 1998;5:751–6.
125. Jenne DE, Reimann H, Nezu J, et al. Peutz-Jeghers syndrome is caused by mutations in a novel serine threonine kinase. Nat Genet 1998;18:38–44.
126. Hemminki A, Tomlinson I, Markie D, et al. Localization of a susceptibility locus for Peutz-Jeghers syndrome to 19p using comparative genomic hybridization and targeted linkage analysis. Nature Genet 1997;15:87–90.
127. Olschwang S, Markie D, Seal S, et al. Peutz-Jeghers disease: most, but not all, families are compatible with linkage to 19p13.3. J Med Genet 1998;35:42–4.
128. Mehenni H, Blouin J-L, Radhakrishna U, et al. Peutz-Jeghers syndrome: confirmation of linkage to chromosome 19p13.3 and identification of a potential second locus, on 19q13.4. Am J Hum Genet 1997;61:1327–34.
129. Giardiello FM, Welsh SB, Hamilton SR, et al. Increased risk of cancer in the Peutz-Jeghers syndrome. N Engl J Med 1987;316:1511–4.
130. Wang Z-J, Churchman M, Avizienyte E, et al. Germline mutations of the LKB1 (STK11) gene in Peutz-Jeghers patients. J Med Genet 1999;36:365–8.
131. Westerman AM, Entius MM, de Baar E, et al. Peutz-Jeghers syndrome: 78-year follow-up of the original family. Lancet 1999;353:1211–5.
132. Spigelman AD, Murray V, Phillips RKS. Cancer and the Peutz-Jeghers syndrome. Gut 1989;30:1588–90.
133. Boardman LA, Thibodeau SN, Schaid DJ, et al. Increased risk for cancer in patients with the Peutz-Jeghers syndrome. Ann Intern Med 1998;128:896–9.
134. Young RH, Welch WR, Dickersin GR, et al. Ovarian sex cord tumor with annular tubules. Review of 74 cases including 27 with Peutz-Jeghers syndrome and four with adenoma malignum of the cervix. Cancer 1982;50:1384–402.
135. Spigelman AD, Arese P, Phillips RKS. Polyposis: the Peutz-Jeghers syndrome. Br J Surg 1995;82:1311–4.
136. Tomlinson IP, Houlston RS. Peutz-Jeghers syndrome. J Med Genet 1997;34:1007–11.
137. Thorson A, Knezetic JA, Lynch HT. A century of progress in hereditary nonpolyposis colorectal cancer (Lynch syndrome). Dis Colon Rectum 1999;42:1–9.
138. Warthin AS. Heredity with reference to carcinoma as shown by the study of the cases examined in the pathological laboratory of the University of Michigan, 1895–1913. Arch Intern Med 1913;12:546–55.
139. Warthin AS. The further study of a cancer family. J Cancer Res 1925;9:279–86.
140. Lynch HT, Krush AJ. Cancer family "G" revisited: 1895–1970. Cancer 1971;27:1505–11.
141. Lynch HT, Smyrk T, Lynch JF. Molecular genetics and clinical-pathology features of hereditary nonpolyposis colorectal carcinoma (Lynch syndrome): historical journey from pedigree anecdote to molecular genetic confirmation. Oncology 1998;55:103–8.
142. Yan H, Papadopoulos N, Marra G, et al. Conversion of diploidy to haploidy: individuals susceptible to multigene disorders may now be spotted more easily. Nature 2000;403:723–4.
143. Aaltonen LA, Salovaara R, Kristo P, et al. Incidence of hereditary nonpolyposis colorectal cancer and the feasibility of molecular screening for the disease. N Engl J Med 1998;338:1481–7.

144. Lynch HT, de la Chapelle A. Genetic susceptibility to non-polyposis colorectal cancer. J Med Genet 1999;36:801–18.
145. Lynch HT, de la Chapelle A. Genomic medicine: hereditary colorectal cancer. N Engl J Med 2003;348:919–32.
146. Marra G, Boland CR. Hereditary nonpolyposis colorectal cancer: the syndrome, the genes, and historical perspectives. J Natl Cancer Inst 1995;87:1114–25.
147. Peltomäki P, Vasen HFA, International Collaborative Group on Hereditary Nonpolyposis Colorectal Cancer. Mutations predisposing to hereditary nonpolyposis colorectal cancer: database and results of a collaborative study. Gastroenterology 1997;113:1146–58.
148. Bronner CE, Baker SM, Morrison PT, et al. Mutation in the DNA mismatch repair gene homologue hMLH1 is associated with hereditary nonpolyposis colon cancer. Nature 1994;368:258–61.
149. Fishel R, Lescoe MK, Rao MRS, et al. The human mutator gene homolog MSH2 and its association with hereditary nonpolyposis colon cancer. Cell 1993;75:1027–38.
150. Leach FS, Nicolaides NC, Papadopoulos N, et al. Mutations of a mutS homolog in hereditary nonpolyposis colorectal cancer. Cell 1993;75:1215–25.
151. Miyaki M, Konishi M, Tanaka K, et al. Germline mutation of *MSH6* as the cause of hereditary nonpolyposis colorectal cancer. Nat Genet 1997;17:271–2.
152. Nicolaides NC, Papadopoulos N, Liu B, et al. Mutations of two PMS homologues in hereditary nonpolyposis colon cancer. Nature 1994;371:75–80.
153. Batra S, Valdimarsdottir H, McGovern M, et al. Awareness of genetic testing for colorectal cancer predisposition among specialists in gastroenterology. Am J Gastroenterol 2002;97:729–33.
154. Lipkin SM, Wang V, Jacoby R, et al. *MLH3*: a DNA mismatch repair gene associated with mammalian microsatellite instability. Nat Genet 2000;24:27–34.
155. de la Chapelle A. Microsatellite instability phenotype of tumors: genotyping or immunohistochemistry? The jury is still out. J Clin Oncol 2002;20:897–9.
156. Wijnen J, de Leeuw W, Vasen H, et al. Familial endometrial cancer in female carriers of *MSH6* germline mutations. Nat Genet 1999;23:142–4.
157. Vasen HFA, Wijnen JT, Menko FH, et al. Cancer risk in families with hereditary nonpolyposis colorectal cancer diagnosed by mutation analysis. Gastroenterology 1996;110:1020–7.
158. Rodriguez-Bigas MA, Vasen HFA, Pekka-Mecklin J, et al. Rectal cancer risk in hereditary nonpolyposis colorectal cancer after abdominal colectomy. Ann Surg 1997;225:202–7.
159. Jass JR, Do K-A, Simms LA, et al. Morphology of sporadic colorectal cancer with DNA replication errors. Gut 1998;42:673–9.
160. Hamilton SR, Aaltonen LA (eds). Tumours of the Digestive System. Lyon: IARC Press, 2000.
161. Smyrk TC, Watson P, Kaul K, et al. Tumor-infiltrating lymphocytes are a marker for microsatellite instability in colorectal cancer. Cancer 2001;91:2417–22.
162. Marcus V, Madlensky L, Gryfe R, et al. Immunohistochemistry for hMLH1 and hMSH2: A practical test for DNA mismatch repair-deficient tumors. Am J Surg Pathol 1999;23:1248–55.
163. Salahshor S, Koeble K, Rubio C, et al. Microsatellite instability and hMLH1 and hMSH2 expression analysis in familial and sporadic colorectal cancer. Lab Invest 2001;81:535–41.
164. Lindor NM, Burgart LJ, Leontovich O, et al. Immunohistochemistry versus microsatellite instability testing in phenotyping colorectal tumors. J Clin Oncol 2002;20:1043–8.
165. Jones JS, Chi X, Gu X, et al. *p53* polymorphism and age of onset of hereditary nonpolyposis colorectal cancer in a Caucasian population. Clin Cancer Res 2004;10:5845–9.
166. Watson P, Lynch HT. Extracolonic cancer in hereditary nonpolyposis colorectal cancer. Cancer 1993;71:677–85.
167. Dunlop MG, Farrington SM, Carothers AD, et al. Cancer risk associated with germline DNA mismatch repair gene mutations. Hum Mol Genet 1997;6:105–10.
168. Lynch HT, Fusaro RM. Muir-Torre syndrome: heterogeneity, natural history, diagnosis, and management. Prob Gen Surg 1993;10:1–14.
169. Risinger JI, Barrett JC, Watson P, et al. Molecular genetic evidence of the occurrence of breast cancer as an integral tumor in patients with the hereditary nonpolyposis colorectal cancer syndrome. Cancer 1996;77:1836–43.
170. Broaddus RR, Lynch PM, Lu KH, et al. Unusual tumors associated with the hereditary nonpolyposis colorectal cancer syndrome. Mod Pathol 2004;17:981–9.
171. Sijmons R, Hofstra R, Hollema H, et al. Inclusion of malignant fibrous histiocytoma in the tumour spectrum associated with hereditary non-polyposis colorectal cancer. Genes Chromosomes Cancer 2000;29:353–5.
172. Boyd J, Rhei E, Federici MG, et al. Male breast cancer in the hereditary nonpolyposis colorectal cancer syndrome. Breast Cancer Res Treat 1999;53:87–91.
173. Berends MJ, Cats A, Hollema H, et al. Adrenocortical adenocarcinoma in an MSH2 carrier: coincidence or causal relation? Hum Pathol 2000;31:1522–7.
174. Wijnen J, van der Klift H, Vasen H, et al. *MSH2* genomic deletions are a frequent cause of HNPCC. Nat Genet 1998;20:326–8.
175. Schouten JP, McElgunn CJ, Waaijer R, et al. Relative quantification of 40 nucleic acid sequences by multiplex ligation-dependent probe amplification. Nucleic Acids Res 2002;30:57e.
176. Nakagawa H, Yan H, Lockman J, et al. Allele separation facilitates interpretation of potential splicing alterations and genomic rearrangements. Cancer Res 2002;62:4579–82.
177. Lynch HT, Coronel SM, Okimoto R, et al. A founder mutation of the *MSH2* gene and hereditary nonpolyposis colorectal cancer in the United States. JAMA 2004;291:718–24.
178. Wagner A, Barrows A, Wijnen JT, et al. Molecular analysis of hereditary nonpolyposis colorectal cancer in the United States: high mutation detection rate among clinically selected families and characterization of an American founder genomic deletion of the *MSH2* gene. Am J Hum Genet 2003;72:1088–100.
179. Domingo E, Laiho P, Ollikainen M, et al. BRAF screening as a low-cost effective strategy for simplifying HNPCC genetic testing. J Med Genet 2004;41:664–8.
180. Watson P, Ashwathnarayan R, Lynch HT, et al. Tobacco use and increased colorectal cancer risk in patients with hereditary nonpolyposis colorectal cancer (Lynch syndrome). Arch Intern Med 2004;164:2429–31.
181. Vasen HFA, Mecklin J-P, Meera Khan P, et al. The International Collaborative Group on Hereditary Nonpolyposis Colorectal Cancer (ICG-HNPCC). Dis Colon Rectum 1991;34:424–5.
182. Wijnen JT, Vasen HFA, Khan PM, et al. Clinical findings with implications for genetic testing in families with clustering of colorectal cancer. N Engl J Med 1998;339:511–8.
183. Vasen HFA, Watson P, Mecklin J-P, et al. New clinical criteria for hereditary nonpolyposis colorectal cancer (HNPCC, Lynch syndrome) proposed by the International Collaborative Group on HNPCC. Gastroenterology 1999;116:1453–6.
184. Laghi L, Bianchi P, Roncalli M, et al. Revised Bethesda guidelines for hereditary nonpolyposis colorectal cancer (Lynch syndrome) and microsatellite instability. J Natl Cancer Inst 2004;96:1402–3.
185. Umar A, Boland CR, Terdiman JP, et al. Revised Bethesda Guidelines for hereditary nonpolyposis colorectal cancer (Lynch syndrome) and microsatellite instability. J Natl Cancer Inst 2004;96:261–8.
186. Lipton LR, Johnson V, Cummings C, et al. Refining the Amsterdam Criteria and Bethesda Guidelines: testing algorithms for the prediction of mismatch repair mutation status in the familial cancer clinic. J Clin Oncol 2004;22:4934–43.
187. Jass JR, Stewart SM. Evolution of hereditary non-polyposis colorectal cancer. Gut 1992;33:783–6.
188. Järvinen HJ, Aarnio M, Mustonen H, et al. Controlled 15-year trial on screening for colorectal cancer in families with hereditary nonpolyposis colorectal cancer. Gastroenterology 2000;118:829–34.
189. Vasen HFA, Nagengast FM, Khan PM. Interval cancers in hereditary non-polyposis colorectal cancer (Lynch syndrome). Lancet 1995;345:1183–4.
190. Church J. Hereditary colon cancers can be tiny: a cautionary case report of the results of colonoscopic surveillance. Am J Gastroenterol 1998;93:2289–90.
191. Rex DK, Cutler CS, Lemmel GT, et al. Colonoscopic miss rates of adenomas determined by back-to-back colonoscopies. Gastroenterology 1997;112:24–8.
192. Lynch HT. Is there a role for prophylactic subtotal colectomy among hereditary nonpolyposis colorectal cancer germline mutation carriers? Dis Colon Rectum 1996;39:109–10.
193. Church JM. Prophylactic colectomy in patients with hereditary nonpolyposis colorectal cancer. Ann Med 1996;28:479–82.
194. Syngal S, Weeks JC, Schrag D, et al. Benefits of colonoscopic surveillance and prophylactic colectomy in patients with hereditary nonpolyposis colorectal cancer mutations. Ann Intern Med 1998;129:787–96.
195. Nicolaides NC, Littman SJ, Modrich P, et al. A naturally occurring hPMS2 mutation can confer a dominant negative mutator phenotype. Mol Cell Biol 1998;18:1635–41.
196. Vasen HFA, Stormorken A, Menko FH, et al. *MSH2* mutation carriers are at higher risk of cancer than *MLH1* mutation carriers: a study of hereditary nonpolyposis colorectal cancer families. J Clin Oncol 2001;19:4074–80.
197. Hendriks YMC, Wagner A, Morreau H, et al. Cancer risk in hereditary nonpolyposis colorectal cancer due to *MSH6* mutations: impact on counseling and surveillance. Gastroenterology 2004;127:17–25.
198. Menko FH, Kaspers GL, Meijer GA, et al. A homozygous *MSH6* mutation in a child with café au lait spots, oligodendroglioma and rectal cancer. Fam Cancer 2004;3:123–7.
199. Liu T, Yan H, Kuismanen S, et al. The role of *hPMS1* and *hPMS2* in predisposing to colorectal cancer. Cancer Res 2001;61:7798–802.
200. Liu HX, Zhou XL, Werelius B, et al. The role of hMLH3 in familial colorectal cancer. Cancer Res 2003;63:1894–9.
201. Jagmohan-Changur S, Poikonen T, Vilkki S, et al. EXO1 variants occur commonly in normal population: evidence against a role in hereditary nonpolyposis colorectal cancer. Cancer Res 2003;63:154–8.
202. Wang Q, Lasset C, Desseigne F, et al. Neurofibromatosis and early onset of cancers in *hMLH1*-deficient children. Cancer Res 1999;59:294–7.
203. Ricciardone MD, Özçelik T, Cevher B, et al. Human *MLH1* deficiency predisposes to hematological malignancy and neurofibromatosis type I. Cancer Res 1999;59:290–3.
204. de Rosa M, Fasano C, Panariello L, et al. Evidence for a recessive inheritance of Turcot's syndrome caused by compound heterozygous mutations within the PMS2 gene. Oncogene 2000;19:1719–23.
205. Vilkki S, Tsao-J-L., Loukola A, et al. Extensive somatic microsatellite mutations in normal human tissue. Cancer Res 2001;61:4541–4.
206. Trimbath JD, Petersen GM, Erdman SH, et al. Café au lait spots and early onset colorectal neoplasia: a variant of HNPCC? Fam Cancer 2001;1:101–5.
207. Whiteside D, McLeod R, Graham G, et al. A homozygous germ-line mutation in the human MSH2 gene predisposes to hematological malignancy and multiple café-au-lait spots. Cancer Res 2002;62:359–62.
208. Bougeard G, Charbonnier F, Moerman A, et al. Early-onset brain tumor and lymphoma in *MSH2*-deficient children. Am J Hum Genet 2003;72:213–6.
209. Gallinger S, Aronson M, Shayan K, et al. Gastrointestinal cancers and neurofibromatosis Type 1 features in children with a germline homozygous *MLH1* mutation. Gastroenterology 2004;126:576–85.
210. Hegde MR, Blazo MA, Chin LH, et al. A novel homozygous mutation in the MSH6 gene in a Turcot syndrome family characterized by pediatric glioblastoma multiforme, lymphoma, colorectal cancer and neurofibromatosis. Am J Hum Genet 2003;73(Suppl 5):391
211. Nakagawa H, Lockman JC, Frankel WL, et al. Mismatch repair gene *PMS2*: disease-causing germline mutations are frequent in patients whose tumors stain negative for PMS2 protein, but paralogous genes obscure mutation detection and interpretation. Cancer Res 2004;64:4721–7.
212. Li FP, Fraumeni JF. Soft-tissue sarcomas, breast cancer, and other neoplasms: a familial syndrome? Ann Intern Med 1969;71:747–52.
213. Li FP, Fraumeni JF. Familial breast cancer, soft-tissue sarcomas, and other neoplasms. Ann Intern Med 1975;83:833–4.
214. Malkin D, Li FP, Stron LC, et al. Germ line p53 mutations in a familial syndrome of breast cancer, sarcomas and other neoplasms. Science 1990;250:1233–8.
215. Malkin D, Jolly KW, Barbier N, et al. Germline mutations of the p53 tumor-suppressor gene in children and young adults with second malignant neoplasms. N Engl J Med 1992;326:1309–15.
216. Evans SC, Mims B, McMasters KM, et al. Exclusion of a *p53* germline mutation in a classic Li-Fraumeni syndrome family. Hum Genet 1998;102:681–6.
217. Lynch HT, Mulcahy GM, Harris RE, et al. Genetic and pathologic findings in a kindred with hereditary sarcoma, breast cancer, brain tumors, leukemia, lung, laryngeal, and adrenal cortical carcinoma. Cancer 1978;41:2055–64.
218. Lynch HT, McComb RD, Osborn NK, et al. Predominance of brain tumors in an extended Li-Fraumeni (SBLA) kindred, including a case of Sturge-Weber syndrome. Cancer 2000;88:433–9.

219. Hisada M, Garber JE, Fung CY, et al. Multiple primary cancers in families with Li-Fraumeni syndrome. J Natl Cancer Inst 1998;90:606–11.
220. Greene MH, Clark WH, Tucker MA, et al. Acquired precursors of the cutaneous malignant melanoma: the familial dysplastic nevus syndrome. N Engl J Med 1985;312:91–7.
221. Lynch HT, Fusaro RM, Albano WA, et al. Phenotypic variation in the familial atypical multiple mole- melanoma syndrome (FAMMM). J Med Genet 1983;20:25–9.
222. Kaufman DK, Kimmel DW, Parisi JE, et al. A familial syndrome with cutaneous malignant melanoma and cerebral astrocytoma. Neurology 1993;43:1728–31.
223. Gruis NA, van der Velden PA, Sandkuijl LA, et al. Homozygotes for CDKN2 (p16) germline mutation in Dutch familial melanoma kindreds. Nat Genet 1995;10:351–3.
224. Ranade K, Hussussian CJ, Sikorski RS, et al. Mutations associated with familial melanoma impair p16INK4 function. Nat Genet 1995;10:114–6.
225. Lynch HT, Brand RE, Hogg D, et al. Phenotypic variation in eight extended *CDKN2A* germline mutation familial atypical multiple mole melanoma-pancreatic carcinoma-prone families: the familial atypical multiple mole melanoma-pancreatic carcinoma syndrome. Cancer 2002;94:84–96.
226. Bergman W, Watson P, de Jong J, et al. Systemic cancer and the FAMMM syndrome. Br J Cancer 1990;61:932–6.
227. Gruis NA, Sandkuijl LA, van der Velden PA, et al. CDKN2 explains part of the clinical phenotype in Dutch familial atypical multiple-mole melanoma (FAMMM) syndrome families. Melanoma Res 1995;5:169–77.
228. Whelan AJ, Bartsch D, Goodfellow PJ. Brief report: a familial syndrome of pancreatic cancer and melanoma with a mutation in the *CDKN2* tumor-suppressor gene. N Engl J Med 1995;333:975–7.
229. Bergman W, Gruis N. Familial melanoma and pancreatic cancer. N Engl J Med 1996;334:471–2.
230. Whelan AJ, Bartsch D, Goodfellow PJ. Familial melanoma and pancreatic cancer. N Engl J Med 1996;334:472.
231. Brandi ML, Gagel RF, Angeli A, et al. Guidelines foir diagnosis and therapy of MEN type 1 and type 2. J Clin Endocrinol Metab 2001;86:5658–71.
232. Wermer P. Genetic aspects of adenomatosis of endocrine glands. Am J Med 1954;16:363–71.
233. Marx S. Multiple endocrine neoplasia type 1. In: Vogelstein B, Kinzler KW, editors. The Genetic Basis of Human Cancer. New York: McGraw-Hill; 1998. p. 489–506.
234. Skogseid B, Eriksson B, Lundqvist G, et al. Multiple endocrine neoplasia type 1: a 10-year prospective screening. J Clin Endocrinol Metab 1991;73:281–7.
235. Larsson C, Skogseid B, Oberg K, et al. Multiple endocrine neoplasia type 1 gene maps to chromosome 11 and is lost in insulinoma. Nature 1988;332:85–7.
236. Chandrasekharappa SC, Guru SC, Manickam P, et al. Positional cloning of the gene for multiple endocrine neoplasia-type 1. Science 1997;276:404–7.
237. Kim YS, Burns AL, Goldsmith PK, et al. Stable overexpression of MEN1 suppresses tumorigenicity of RAS. Oncogene 1999;18:5936–42.
238. Kaji H, Canaff L, Lebrun JJ, Goltzman D, Hendy GN. Inactivation of menin, a Smad3-interacting protein, blocks transforming growth factor type beta signaling. Proc Natl Acad Sci USA 2001;98:3837–42.
239. Eng C. PTEN: one gene, many syndromes. Hum Mutat 2003;22:183–98.
240. Schnepp RW, Mao H, Sykes SM, et al. Menin induces apoptosis in murine embryonic fibroblasts. J Biol Chem 2004;279:10685–91.
241. Machens A, Ukkat J, Brauckhoff M, et al. Advances in the management of hereditary medullary thyroid cancer. J Intern Med 2005;257:50–9.
242. Mulligan LM, Kwok JBJ, Healey CS, et al. Germ-line mutations of the RET proto-oncogene in multiple endocrine neoplasia type 2A. Nature 1993;363:458–60.
243. Hofstra RM, Landsvater RM, Ceccherini I, et al. A mutation in the RET proto-oncogene associated with multiple endocrine neoplasia type 2B and sporadic medullary thyroid carcinoma. Nature 1994;367:375–6.
244. Santoro M, Carlomagno F, Melillo RM, et al. Dysfunction of the RET receptor in human cancer. Cellular & Molecular Life Sciences 2004;61:2954–64.
245. Romeo G, Ronchetto P, Luo Y, et al. Point mutations affecting the tyrosine kinase domain of the RET proto-oncogene in Hirschsprung's disease. Nature 1994;367:377–8.
246. Eng C. RET proto-oncogene in the development of human cancer. J Clin Oncol 1999;17:380–93.
247. Mulligan LM, Marsh DJ, Robinson BG, et al. Genotype-phenotype correlation in multiple endocrine neoplasia type 2: report of the International RET Mutation Consortium. J Intern Med 1995;238:343–6.
248. Eng C, Clayton D, Schuffenecker I, et al. The relationship between specific *RET* proto-oncogene mutations and disease phenotype in multiple endocrine neoplasia type 2: International *RET* Mutation Consortium analysis. JAMA 1996;276:1575–9.
249. Ponder BA, Ponder MA, Coffey R, et al. Risk estimation and screening in families of patients with medullary thyroid carcinoma. Lancet 1999;1:397–401.
250. Wells SA Jr, Chi DD, Toshima K, et al. Predictive DNA testing and prophylactic thyroidectomy in patients at risk for multiple endocrine neoplasia type 2A. Ann Surg 1994;220:237–50.
251. National Institutes of Health Consensus Development Conference. Neurofibromatosis: conference statement. Arch Neurol 1988;45:575–8.
252. Side L, Taylor B, Cayouette M, et al. Homozygous inactivation of the *NF1* gene in bone marrow cells from children with neurofibromatosis type 1 and malignant myeloid disorders. N Engl J Med 1997;336:1713–20.
253. Evans DG, Huson SM, Donnai D, et al. A clinical study of type 2 neurofibromatosis. Q J Med 1992;84:603–18.
254. Ruttledge MH, Andermann AA, Phelan CM, et al. Type of mutation in the neurofibromatosis type 2 gene (NF2) frequently determines severity of disease. Am J Hum Genet 1996;59:331–42.
255. Kanter WR, Eldridge R, Fabricant R, et al. Central neurofibromatosis with bilateral acoustic neuroma: genetic, clinical, and biochemical distinctions from peripheral neurofibromatosis. Neurology 1980;30:851–9.
256. Baser ME, Kuramoto L, Joe H, et al. Genotype-phenotype correlations for nervous system tumors in neurofibromatosis 2: a population-based study. Am J Hum Genet 2004;75:231–9.
257. Noorani HZ, Khan HN, Gallie BL, et al. Cost comparison of molecular versus conventional screening of relatives at risk for retinoblastoma. Am J Hum Genet 1996;59:301–7.
258. Roarty JD, McLean IW, Zimmerman LE. Incidence of second neoplasm in patients with bilateral retinoblastoma. Ophthalmology 1988;95:1583–7.
259. Moll AC, Imhof SM, Bouter LM, et al. Second primary tumors in patients with retinoblastoma: a review of the literature. Ophthalmic Genet 1997;18:27–34.
260. Wicking C, Gillies S, Smyth I, et al. De novo mutations of the *patched* gene in nevoid basal cell carcinoma syndrome help to define the clinical phenotype. Am J Med Genet 1997;73:304–7.
261. Shanley S, Ratcliffe J, Hockey A, et al. Nevoid basal cell carcinoma syndrome: review of 118 affected individuals. Am J Med Genet 1994;50:282–90.
262. Hahn H, Wicking C, Zaphiropoulos PG, et al. Mutations of the human homolog of Drosophila patched in the nevoid basal cell carcinoma syndrome. Cell 1996;85:841–51.
263. Johnson RL, Rothman AI, Xie J, et al. Human homolog of patched, a candidate gene for the basal cell nevus syndrome. Science 1996;272:1668–71.
264. Cowan R, Hoban P, Kelsey A, et al. The gene for the naevoid basal cell carcinoma syndrome acts as a tumour-suppressor gene in medulloblastoma. Br J Cancer 1997;76:141–5.
265. Crossey PA, Eng C, Ginalska-Malinowska M, et al. Molecular genetic diagnosis of von Hippel-Lindau disease in familial phaeochromocytoma. J Med Genet 1995;32:885–6.
266. Kaelin WG, Jr. The von Hippel-Lindau tumor suppressor gene and kidney cancer. Clin Cancer Res 2004;10:6290s–95s.
267. Lindor NM, Greene MH, Mayo Familial Cancer Program. The concise handbook of family cancer syndromes. J Natl Cancer Inst 1998;90:1039–71.
268. Hartley AL, Birch JM, Harris M, et al. Leukemia, lymphoma, and related disorders in families of children diagnosed with Wilms' tumor. Cancer Genet Cytogenet 1994;77:129–33.
269. Rees JL. The genetics of sun sensitivity in humans. Am J Hum Genet 2004;75:739–51.
270. Athma P, Rappaport R, Swift M. Molecular genotyping shows that ataxia-telangiectasia heterozygotes are predisposed to breast cancer. Cancer Genet Cytogenet 1996;92:130–4.
271. Gatti RA, Berkel I, Boder E, et al. Localization of an ataxia-telangiectasia gene to chromosome 11q22-23. Nature 1988;366:577–80.
272. Lange E, Borresen A-L, Chen X, et al. Localization of an ataxia-telangiectasia gene to a ~500-kb interval on chromosome 11q23.1: linkage analysis of 176 families in an international consortium. Am J Hum Genet 1995;57:112–9.
273. Savitsky K, Bar-Shira A, Gilad S, et al. A single ataxia telangiectasia gene with a product similar to PI-3 kinase. Science 1995;268:1749–53.
274. Telatar M, Teraoka S, Wang Z, et al. Ataxia-telangiectasia: identification and detection of founder-effect mutations in the ATM gene in ethnic populations. Am J Hum Genet 1998;62:86–97.
275. McConville CM, Stankovic T, Byrd PJ, et al. Mutations associated with variant phenotypes in ataxia-telangiectasia. Am J Hum Genet 1996;59:320–30.
276. Swift M, Morrell D, Massey RB, et al. Incidence of cancer in 161 families affected by ataxia-telangiectasia. N Engl J Med 1991;325:1831–6.
277. Ellis NA, Ciocci S, Proytcheva M, et al. The Ashkenazic Jewish Bloom syndrome mutation *blm*Ash is present in non-Jewish Americans of Spanish ancestry. Am J Hum Genet 1998;63:1685–93.
278. German J, Ellis NA. Bloom syndrome. In: Vogelstein B, Kinzler KW, editors. The Genetic Basis of Human Cancer. New York: McGraw-Hill; 1998. p. 301–15.
279. German J. Bloom syndrome: A mendelian prototype of somatic mutational disease. Medicine 1993;72:393–406.
280. Gruber SB, Ellis NA, Rennert G, et al. *BLM* heterozygosity and the risk of colorectal cancer. Science 2002;297:2013.
281. Goss KH, Risinger MA, Kordich JJ, et al. Enhanced tumor formation in mice heterozygous for *Blm* mutation. Science 2002;297:2051–3.
282. Pilarski R, Eng C. Will the real Cowden syndrome please stand up (again)? Expanding mutational and clinical spectra of the *PTEN* hamartoma tumour syndrome. J Med Genet 2004;41:323–6.
283. Liaw D, Marsh DJ, Li J, et al. Germline mutations of the *PTEN* gene in Cowden disease, an inherited breast and thyroid cancer syndrome. Nat Genet 1997;16:64–7.
284. Marsh DJ, Dahia PLM, Zheng Z, et al. Germline mutations in PTEN are present in Bannayan-Zonana syndrome. Nat Genet 1997;16:333–4.
285. Eng C, Parsons R. Cowden syndrome. In: Vogelstein B, Kinzler KW, editors. The Genetic Basis of Human Cancer. New York: McGraw-Hill; 1998. p. 516–26.
286. Eng C, Murday V, Seal S, et al. Cowden syndrome and Lhermitte-Duclos disease in a family: a single genetic syndrome with pleiotrophy? J Med Genet 1994;31:458–61.
287. Nelen MR, Padberg GW, Peeters EAJ, et al. Localization of the gene for Cowden disease to chromosome 10q22-23. Nat Genet 1996;13:114–6.
288. Marsh DJ, Zheng Z, Zedenius J, et al. Differential loss of heterozygosity in the region of the Cowden locus within 10q22-23 in follicular thyroid adenomas and carcinomas. Cancer Res 1997;57:500–3.
289. Li J, Yen C, Liaw D, et al. *PTEN*, a putative protein tyrosine phosphatase gene mutated in human brain, breast, and prostate cancer. Science 1997;275:1943–7.
290. Li DM, Sun H. TEP1, encoded by a candidate tumor suppressor locus, is a novel protein tyrosine phosphatase regulated by transforming growth factor beta. Cancer Res 1997;57:2124–9.
291. Steck PA, Pershouse MA, Jasser SA, et al. Identification of a candidate tumour suppressor gene MMAC1 at chromosome 10q21.3 that is mutated in multiple advanced cancers. Nat Genet 1997;15:356–62.
292. Waite KA, Eng C. Protean *PTEN*: form and function. Am J Hum Genet 2002;70:829–44.
293. Marsh DJ, Coulon V, Lunetta KL, et al. Mutation spectrum and genotype-phenotype analyses in Cowden disease and Bannayan-Zonana syndrome, two hamartoma syndromes with germline PTEN mutation. Hum Mol Genet 1998;7:507–15.
294. Marsh DJ, Dahia PLM, Caron S, et al. Germline PTEN mutations in Cowden syndrome-like families. J Med Genet 1998;35:881–5.
295. Zhou XP, Waite KA, Pilarski R, et al. Germline PTEN promoter mutations and deletions in Cowden/Bannayan-Riley-Ruvalcaba syndrome result in aberrant PTEN protein and dysregulation of the phosphoinositol-3-kinase/Akt pathway. Am J Hum Genet 2003;73:404–11.
296. Nelen MR, van Stavernen WC, Peeters EA, et al. Germline mutations in the PTEN/MMAC1 gene in patients with Cowden disease. Hum Mol Genet 1997;6:1383–7.
297. Zhou XP, Marsh DJ, Morrison CD, et al. Germline inactivation of PTEN and dysregulation of the phosphoinositol-3-kinase/Akt pathway cause human Lhermitte-Duclos disease in adults. Am J Hum Genet 2003;73:1191–8.

298. Carroll BT, Couch FJ, Rebbeck TR, et al. Polymorphisms in PTEN in breast cancer families. J Med Genet 1999;36:94–6.
299. Whitney MA, Saito H, Jakobs PM, et al. A common mutation in the FACC gene causes Fanconi anaemia in Ashkenazi Jews. Nat Genet 1993;4:202–5.
300. Kuffel DG, Lindor NM, Litzow MR, et al. Mitomycin C chromosome stress test to identify hypersensitivity to bifunctional alkylating agents in patients with Fanconi anemia or aplastic anemia. Mayo Clin Proc 1997;72:579–80.
301. Cleton-Jansen A-M, Moerland EW, Pronk JC, et al. Mutation analysis of the Fanconi anaemia A gene in breast tumours with loss of heterozygosity at 16q24.3. Br J Cancer 1999;79:1049–52.
302. Bennett SE, Umar A, Oshima J, et al. Mismatch repair in extracts of Werner syndrome cell lines. Cancer Res 1997;57:2956–60.
303. Goto M, Rubenstein M, Weber J, et al. Genetic linkage of Werner's syndrome to five markers on chromosome 8. Nature (Lond) 1992;355:735–8.
304. Schellenberg GD, Martin GM, Wijsman EM, et al. Homozygosity mapping and Werner's syndrome. Lancet 1992;339:1002.
305. Thomas W, Rubenstein M, Goto M, et al. A genetic analysis of the Werner syndrome region on human chromosome 8p. Genomics 1993;16:685–90.
306. Oshima J, Yu C, Boehnke M, et al. Integrated mapping analysis of the Werner syndrome region of chromosome 8. Genomics 1994;23:100–13.
307. Oshima J, Yu C-E, Puissan C, et al. Homozygous and compound heterozygous mutations at the Werner locus. Hum Mol Genet 1996;5:1909–13.
308. Ellis NA, Groden J, Ye T-Z, et al. The Bloom's syndrome gene product is homologous to RecQ helicases. Cell 1995;83:655–66.
309. Goto M, Miller RW, Ishikawa Y, et al. Excess of rare cancers in Werner syndrome (adult progeria). Cancer Epidemiol Biomarkers Prev 1996;5:239–46.
310. Kraemer KH, Lee MM, Scotto J. Xeroderma pigmentosum: cutaneous, ocular, and neurologic abnormalities in 830 published cases. Arch Dermatol 1987;123:241–50.
311. Lanza A, Lagomarsini P, Casati A, et al. Chromosomal fragility in the cancer-prone disease xeroderma pigmentosum preferentially involves bands relevant for cutaneous carcinogenesis. Int J Cancer (Pred Oncol) 1997;74:654–63.
312. Cleaver J, Kraemer K. Xeroderma pigmentosum and Cockayne syndrome. In: Scriver CR, Beaudet AL, Sly WS, et al, editors. The Metabolic and Molecular Bases of Inherited Disease, 7 ed. New York: McGraw-Hill; 1995. p. 4393–419.
313. Lynch HT, Frichot BCI, Lynch JF. Cancer control in xeroderma pigmentosum. Arch Dermatol 1977;113:193–5.
314. Lynch HT, Frichot BCI, Fisher J, et al. Spontaneous regression of metastatic malignant melanoma in 2 sibs with xeroderma pigmentosum. J Med Genet 1978;15:357–62.
315. Ghadirian P, Boyle P, Simard A, et al. Reported family aggregation of pancreatic cancer within a population-based case-control study in the Francophone community in Montreal, Canada. Int J Pancreatol 1991;10:183–96.
316. Falk RT, Pickle LW, Fontham ET, et al. Life-style risk factors for pancreatic cancer in Louisiana: a case-control study. Am J Epidemiol 1988;128:324–36.
317. Hruban RH, Petersen GM, Goggins M, et al. Familial pancreatic cancer. Ann Oncol 1999;10(suppl 4):S69–S73.
318. Whitcomb DC, Preston RA, Aston CE, et al. A gene for hereditary pancreatitis maps to chromosome 7q35. Gastroenterology 1996;110:1975–80.
319. Brentnall TA, Bronner MP, Byrd DR, et al. Early diagnosis and treatment of pancreatic dysplasia in patients with a family history of pancreatic cancer. Ann Intern Med 1999;131:247–55.
320. Eberle MA, Pfützer R, Pogue-Geile KL, et al. A new susceptibility locus for autosomal dominant pancreatic cancer maps to chromosome 4q32-34. Am J Hum Genet 2002;70:1044–8.
321. Murphy KM, Brune KA, Griffin C, et al. Evaluation of candidate genes *MAP2K4*, *MADH4*, *ACVR1B*, and *BRCA2* in familial pancreatic cancer: deleterious *BRCA2* mutations in 17%. Cancer Res 2002;62:3789–93.
322. van der Heijden MS, Brody JR, Gallmeier E, et al. Functional defects in the Fanconi anemia pathway in pancreatic cancer cells. Am J Pathol 2004;165:651–7.
323. Druker BJ, Talpaz M, Resta DJ, et al. Efficacy and safety of a specific inhibitor of the BCR-ABL tyrosine kinase in chronic myeloid leukemia. N Engl J Med 2001;344:1031–7.
324. Druker BJ, Sawyers CL, Kantarjian H, et al. Activity of a specific inhibitor of the BCR-ABL tyrosine kinase in the blast crisis of chronic myeloid leukemia and acute lymphoblastic leukemia with the Philadelphia chromosome. N Engl J Med 2001;344:1038–42.
325. DeMatteo RP, Heinrich MC, El-Rifai WM, et al. Clinical management of gastrointestinal stromal tumors: before and after STI-571. Hum Pathol 2002;33:466–77.
326. Demetri GD, von Mehren M, Blanke CD, et al. Efficacy and safety of imatinib mesylate in advanced gastrointestinal stromal tumors. N Engl J Med 2002;347:472–80.
327. Tamborini E, Bonadiman L, Greco A, et al. A new mutation in the KIT ATP pocket causes acquired resistance to imatinib in a gastrointestinal stromal tumor. Gastroenterology 2004;127:294–9.
328. Joensuu H, Roberts PJ, Sarlomo-Rikala M, et al. Effect of the tyrosine kinase inhibitor STI571 in a patient with a metastatic gastrointestinal stromal tumor. N Engl J Med 2001;344:1052–6.
329. Kern SE, Hruban RH, Hidalgo M, et al. An introduction to pancreatic adenocarcinoma genetics, pathology and therapy. Cancer Biol Ther 2002;1:607–13.
330. Werner M, Becker KF, Keller G, et al. Gastric adenocarcinoma: pathomorphology and molecular pathology. J Cancer Res Clin Oncol 2001;127:207–16.
331. Straus EW, Patel H, Chang J, et al. *H. pylori* infection and genotyping in patients undergoing upper endoscopy at inner city hospitals. Dig Dis Sci 2002;47:1575–81.
332. El-Omar EM, Chow W-H, Rabkin CS. Gastric cancer and *H. pylori*: Host genetics open the way. Gastroenterology 2001;121:1002–13.
333. Sepulveda AR, Peterson LE, Shelton J, et al. Predicting the risk of gastric cancer using H. pylori gastritis patterns associated with family history of gastric cancer. [abstract] Am J Hum Genet 2000;67(4,suppl 2):14.
334. El-Omar EM, Oien K, Murray LS, et al. Increased prevalence of precancerous changes in relatives of gastric cancer patients: critical role of *H. pylori*. Gastroenterology 2000;118:22–30.
335. Hemminki K, Jiang Y. Familial and second gastric carcinomas: a nationwide epidemiologic study from Sweden. Cancer 2002;94:1157–65.
336. Palli D, Galli M, Caporaso NE, et al. Family history and risk of stomach cancer in Italy. Cancer Epidemiol Biomarkers Prev 1994;3:15–8.
337. Sokoloff B. Predisposition to cancer in the Bonaparte family. Am J Surg 1938;40:673–8.
338. Aarnio M, Salovaara R, Aaltonen LA, et al. Features of gastric cancer in hereditary non-polyposis colorectal cancer syndrome. Int J Cancer (Pred Oncol) 1997;74:551–5.
339. Park YJ, Shin K-H, Park J-G. Risk of gastric cancer in hereditary nonpolyposis colorectal cancer in Korea. Clin Cancer Res 2000;6:2994–8.
340. Guilford P, Hopkins J, Harraway J, et al. *E-cadherin* germline mutations in familial gastric cancer. Nature 1998;392:402–5.
341. Lewis FR, Mellinger JD, Hayashi A, et al. Prophylactic total gastrectomy for familial gastric cancer: therapy based on gene mutation analysis. Surgery 2001;130:612–7.
342. Huntsman DG, Carneiro F, Lewis FR, et al. Early gastric cancer in young, asymptomatic carriers of germ-line *E-cadherin* mutations. N Engl J Med 2001;344:1904–9.
343. Chun YS, Lindor NM, Smyrk TC, et al. Germline *E-cadherin* gene mutations: is prophylactic total gastrectomy indicated? Cancer 2001;92:181–7.
344. Lynch HT, Grady W, Lynch JF, et al. *E-cadherin* mutation-based genetic counseling and hereditary diffuse gastric carcinoma. Cancer Genet Cytogenet 2000;122:1–6.
345. Lynch HT. Family Information Service and hereditary cancer. Cancer 2001;91:625–8.
346. Offerhaus GJ, Giardiello FM, Krush AJ, et al. The risk of upper gastrointestinal cancer in familial adenomatous polyposis. Gastroenterology 1992;102:1980–2.
347. Jagelman DG, DeCosse JJ, Bussey HJR, et al. Upper gastrointestinal cancer in familial polyposis coli. Lancet 1988;i:1149–51.
348. Carneiro F, David L, Seruca R, et al. Hyperplastic polyposis and diffuse carcinoma of the stomach. A study of a family. Cancer 1993;72:323–9.
349. Hirota S, Nishida T, Isozaki K, et al. Familial gastrointestinal stromal tumors associated with dysphagia and novel type germline mutation of KIT gene. Gastroenterology 2002;122:1493–9.
350. Nishida T, Hirota S, Taniguchi M, et al. Familial gastrointestinal stromal tumours with germline mutation of the KIT gene. Nat Genet 1998;19:323–4.
351. Hirota S, Okazaki T, Kitamura Y, et al. Cause of familial and multiple gastrointestinal autonomic nerve tumors with hyperplasia of interstitial cells of Cajal is germline mutation of the *c-kit* gene. Am J Surg Pathol 2000;24:326–7.
352. Isozaki K, Terris B, Belghiti J, et al. Germline-activating mutation in the kinase domain of *KIT* gene in familial gastrointestinal stromal tumors. Am J Pathol 2000;157:1581–5.
353. Maeyama H, Hidaka E, Ota H, et al. Familial gastrointestinal stromal tumor with hyperpigmentation: association with a germline mutation of the *c-kit* gene. Gastroenterology 2001;120:210–5.
354. Beghini A, Tibiletti MG, Roversi G, et al. Germline mutation in the juxtamembrane domain of the kit gene in a family with gastrointestinal stromal tumors and urticaria pigmentosa. Cancer 2001;92:657–62.
355. Linehan WM, Vasselli J, Srinivasan R, et al. Genetic basis of cancer of the kidney: disease-specific approaches to therapy. Clin Cancer Res 2004;10:6282s–9s.
356. Zbar B, Linehan WM. Detection and diagnosis of hereditary and familial renal carcinoma. Kidney Cancer Journal 2004;2:7–14.
357. Schmidt L, Duh FM, Chen F, et al. Germline and somatic mutations in the tyrosine kinase domain of the MET proto-oncogene in papillary renal carcinomas. Nat Genet 1997;16:68–73.
358. Zbar B, Glenn G, Lubensky I, et al. Hereditary papillary renal cell carcinoma: clinical studies in 10 families. J Urol 1995;153:907–12.
359. Malchoff CD, Sarfarazi M, Tendler B, et al. Papillary thyroid carcinoma associated with papillary renal neoplasia: genetic linkage analysis of a distinct heritable tumor syndrome. J Clin Endocrinol Metab 2000;85:1758–64.
360. Toro JR, Nickerson ML, Wei M-H, et al. Mutations in the *fumarate hydratase* gene cause hereditary leiomyomatosis and renal cell cancer in families in North America. Am J Hum Genet 2003;73:95–106.
361. Tomlinson IP, Alam NA, Rowan AJ, et al. Germline mutations in *FH* predispose to dominantly inherited uterine fibroids, skin leiomyomata and papillary renal cell cancer. Nat Genet 2002;30:406–10.
362. Cohen AJ, Li FP, Berg S, et al. Hereditary renal carcinoma associated with a chromosomal translocation. N Engl J Med 1979;301:592–5.
363. Bodmer D, Eleveid MJ, Ligtenberg MJL, et al. An alternative route for multistep tumorigenesis in a novel case of hereditary renal cell cancer and a t(2:3)(q35:q21) chromosome translocation. Am J Hum Genet 1998;62:1475–83.
364. The BT, Giraud S, Sari NF. Familial non-VHL, non-papillary clear-cell renal cancer. Lancet 1997;349:848–9.
365. Skates S, Iliopoulos O. Molecular markers for early detection of renal carcinoma: investigative approach. Clin Cancer Res 2004;10:6296s–301s.
366. Nickerson ML, Warren MB, Toro JR, et al. Mutations in a novel gene lead to kidney tumors, lung wall defects, and benign tumors of the hair follicle in patients with the Birt-Hogg-Dube syndrome. Cancer Cell 2002;2:157–64.
367. Bjornsson J, Short MP, Kwiatkowski DJ, et al. Tuberous sclerosis-associated renal cell carcinoma: clinical, pathologic and genetic features. Am J Pathol 1996;149:1201–8.
368. Morganti G, Gianferrari L, Cresseri A, et al. Recherches clinicostatistiques et genetiques sur les neoplasies de la prostate. Acta Genet Med Gemellol (Roma) 1956;6:304–5.
369. Woolf CM. An investigation of familial aspects of carcinoma of the prostate. Cancer 1960;13:739–44.
370. Cannon L, Bishop DT, Skolnick M, et al. Genetic epidemiology of prostate cancer in the Utah Mormon genealogy. Cancer Surv 1982;1:47–69.
371. Grönberg H, Wiklund F, Damber J-E. Age specific risks of familial prostate carcinoma: a basis for screening recommendations in high risk populations. Cancer 1999;86:477–83.
372. Carter BS, Beaty TH, Steinberg GD, et al. Mendelian inheritance of familial prostate cancer. Proc Natl Acad Sci U S A 1992;89:3367–71.
373. Friedrichsen DM, Stanford JL, Isaacs SD, et al. Identification of a prostate cancer susceptibility locus on chromosome 7q11-21 in Jewish families. Proc Natl Acad Sci U S A 2004;101:1939–44.
374. Tavtigian SV, Simard J, Teng DHF, et al. A candidate prostate cancer susceptibility gene at chromosome 17p. Nat Genet 2001;27:172–80.
375. Xu J, the International Consortium for Prostate Cancer Genetics. Combined analysis of hereditary prostate cancer linkage to *1q24-25*: results from 772 hereditary prostate cancer families from the International Consortium

for Prostate Cancer Genetics. Am J Hum Genet 2000;66:945–57.
376. Wang L, McDonnell SK, Elkins DA, et al. Analysis of the RNASEL gene in familial and sporadic prostate cancer. Am J Hum Genet 2002;71:116–23.
377. Wiklund F, Jonsson B-A, Brookes AJ, et al. Genetic analysis of the *RANSEL* gene in hereditary, familial, and sporadic prostate cancer. Clin Cancer Res 2004;10:7150–6.
378. Smith JR, Freije D, Carpten JD, et al. A genome wide search reveals a major susceptibility locus for prostate cancer on chromosome 1. Science 1996;274:1371–3.
379. Cooney KA, McCarthy JD, Lange E, et al. Prostate cancer susceptibility locus on chromosome 1q: a confirmatory study. J Natl Cancer Inst 1997;89:955–9.
380. Singh RK. No evidence of linkage to chromosome 1q42.2-43 in 131 prostate cancer families from the ACTANE Consortium. Br J Cancer 2002;83:1654–8.
381. Xu J, Schleutker J, Matikainen M, et al. Evidence for a prostate cancer susceptibility locus on the X chromosome. Nat Genet 1998;20:175–9.
382. Monroe KR, Yu MC, Kolonel LN, et al. Evidence of an X-linked or recessive genetic component to prostate cancer risk. Nat Med 1995;1:827–9.
383. Dong X, Wang L, Taniguchi K, et al. Mutations in *CHEK2* associated with prostate cancer risk. Am J Hum Genet 2003;72:270-80.
384. Cybulski C, Huzarski T, Górski B, et al. A novel founder CHEK2mutation is associated with increased prostate cancer risk. Cancer Res 2004;64:2677–9.
385. Chang B-I, Zheng SL, Isaacs SD, et al. A polymorphism in the CDKN1B gene is associated with increased risk of hereditary prostate cancer. Cancer Res 2004;64:1997–9.
386. Jonsson B-A, Adami H-O, Hägglund M, et al. -160C/A polymorphism in the *E-cadherin* gene promoter and risk of hereditary, familial and sporadic prostate cancer. Int J Cancer 2004;109:348–52.
387. Soravia C, van der Klift H, Brundler MA, et al. Prostate cancer is part of the hereditary non-polyposis colorectal cancer (HNPCC) tumor spectrum. Am J Med Genet 2003;121A:159–62.
388. Bapat BV, Madlensky L, Temple LK, et al. Family history characteristics, tumor microsatellite instability and germline MSH2 and MLH1 mutations in hereditary colorectal cancer. Hum Genet 1999;104:167–76.
389. Scott RJ, McPhillips M, Meldrum CJ, et al. Hereditary non-polyposis colorectal cancer in 95 families: differences and similarities between mutation-positive and mutation-negative kindreds. Am J Hum Genet 2001;68:118–27.
390. Lynch HT, Kimberling WJ, Markvicka SE, et al. Genetics and smoking-associated cancers. A study of 485 families. Cancer 1986;57:1640–6.
391. Benhamou S, Lee WJ, Alexandrie AK, et al. Meta- and pooled analyses of the effects of glutathione S-transferase M1 polymorphisms and smoking on lung cancer risk. Carcinogenesis 2002;23:1343–50.
392. Hecht SS. Tobacco smoke carcinogens and lung cancer. J Natl Cancer Inst 1999;91:1194–210.
393. Bennett WP, Hussain SP, Vahakangas KH, et al. Molecular epidemiology of human cancer risk: gene-environment. J Pathol 1999;187:8–18.
394. Dragani TA, Manenti G, Pierotti MA. Genetics of murine lung tumors. Adv Cancer Res 1995;67:83–112.
395. Gariboldi M, Manenti G, Canzian F, et al. A major susceptibility locus to murine lung. Nat Genet 1993;3:132–6.
396. Grovas A, Fremgen A, Rauck A, et al. The National Cancer Data Base report on patterns of childhood cancers in the United States. Cancer 1997;80:2321–32.
397. Tonini GP, Longo L, Coco S, et al. Familial neuroblastoma: a complex heritable disease. Cancer Lett 2003;197:41–5.
398. Brodeur GM. Clinical and biological aspects of neuroblastoma. In: Vogelstein B, Kinzler KW, editors. The Genetic Basis of Human Cancer. New York: McGraw-Hill; 1998. p. 691–711.
399. Maris JM, Matthay KK. Molecular biology of neuroblastoma. J Clin Oncol 1999;17:2264–79.
400. Weiss MJ, Guo C, Shusterman S, et al. Localization of a hereditary neuroblastoma predisposition gene to 16p12-p13. Med Pediatr Oncol 2000;35:526–30.
401. Shpilberg O, Modan M, Modan B, et al. Familial aggregation of haematological neoplasms: a controlled study. Br J Haematol 1994;87:75–80.
402. Sandberg AA. The Chromosomes in Human Cancer and Leukemia, 2nd ed. New York: Elsevier Science Publishing Co., 1990.
403. Lynch HT, Weisenburger DD, Quinn-Laquer B, et al. Family with acute myelogenous leukemia, breast, ovarian, and gastrointestinal cancer. Cancer Genet Cytogenet 2002;137:8–14.
404. Lynch HT, Weisenburger DD, Quinn-Laquer B, et al. Hereditary chronic lymphocytic leukemia: an extended family study and literature review. Am J Med Genet 2002;115:113–7.
405. Shah AR, Maeda K, Deegan MJ, et al. A clinicopathologic study of familial chronic lymphocytic leukemia. Am J Clin Pathol 1992;97:184–8.
406. Fernhout F, Dinkelaar RB, Hagemeijer A, et al. Four aged siblings with B cell chronic lymphocytic leukemia. Leukemia 1997;11:2060–5.
407. Cartwright RA, Bernard SM, Bird CC, et al. Chronic lymphocytic leukaemia: Case control epidemiological study in Yorkshire. Br J Cancer 1987;56:79–82.
408. Linet MS, Van Natta ML, Brookmeyer R, et al. Familial cancer history and chronic lymphocytic leukemia: a case-control study. Am J Epidemiol 1989;130:655–64.
409. Yuille MR, Matutes E, Marossy A, et al. Familial chronic lymphocytic leukaemia: a survey and review of published studies. Br J Haematol 2000;109:794–9.
410. McPhedran P, Heath CW, Lee J. Patterns of familial leukemia: 10 cases of leukemia in two inter-related families. Cancer 1969;24:403–7.
411. Stankovic T, Weber P, Stewart G, et al. Inactivation of ataxia telangiectasia mutated gene in B-cell chronic lymphocytic leukaemia. Lancet 1999;353:26–9.
412. Lynch HT, Sanger WG, Pirruccello S, et al. Familial multiple myeloma: a family study and review of the literature. J Natl Cancer Inst 2001;93:1479–83.
413. Lynch HT, Watson P, Tarantolo S, et al. Phenotypic heterogeneity in multiple myeloma families. J Clin Oncol 2005;23:685–93.
414. Shoenfeld Y, Berliner S, Shaklai M, et al. Familial multiple myeloma. A review of thirty-seven families. Postgrad Med J 1982;58:12–6.
415. Horwitz LJ, Levy RN, Rosner F. Multiple myeloma in three siblings. Arch Intern Med 1985;145:1449–50.
416. Kyle RA, Greipp PR. Idiopathic Bence Jones proteinuria: long-term follow-up in seven patients. N Engl J Med 1984;310:564–7.
417. Bizzaro N, Pasini P. Familial occurrence of multiple myeloma and monoclonal gammopathy of undetermined significance in 5 siblings. Haematologica 1990;75:58–63.
418. Lynch HT, Marcus JN, Lynch JF. Genetics of Hodgkin's and non-Hodgkin's lymphoma: a review. Cancer Invest 1992;10:247–56.
419. Haim N, Cohen Y, Robinson E. Malignant lymphoma in first-degree blood relatives. Cancer 1982;49:2197–200.
420. Ferraris AM, Racchi O, Rapezzi D, et al. Familial Hodgkin's disease: a disease of young adulthood? Ann Hematol 1997;74:131–4.
421. Mack TM, Cozen W, Shibata DK, et al. Concordance for Hodgkin's disease in identical twins suggesting genetic susceptibility to the young-adult form of the disease. N Engl J Med 1995;332:413—8.
422. Sullivan JL. The abnormal gene in X-linked lymphoproliferative syndrome. Curr Opin Immunol 1999;11:431–4.
423. Purtilo DT, Cassel CK, Yank JPS, et al. X-linked recessive progressive combined variable immunodeficiency (Duncan's Disease). Lancet 1975;i:935–40.
424. Hamilton JK, Paquin LA, Sullivan JL, et al. X-linked lymphoproliferative syndrome registry report. J Pediatr 1980;96:669–73.
425. Coffey AJ, Brooksbank RA, Brandau O, et al. Host response to EBV infection in X-linked lymphoproliferative disease results from mutations in an SH2-domain encoding gene. Nat Genet 1998;20:129–35.
426. Lynch HT. Dynamic Genetics Counseling for Clinicians.Springfield, Illinois: CC Thomas, 1969.
427. Guttmacher AE, Collins FS, Carmona RH. The family history—more important than ever. N Engl J Med 2004;351:2333–6.
428. American Society of Clinical Oncology. American Society of Clinical Oncology policy statement update: genetic testing for cancer susceptibility. J Clin Oncol 2003;21:2397–406.
429. Lynch HT, Lemon S, Smyrk T, et al. Genetic counseling in hereditary nonpolyposis colorectal cancer: an extended family with MSH2 mutation. Am J Gastroenterol 1996;91:2489–93.
430. Lynch HT, Severin MJ, Mooney MJ, et al. Insurance adjudication favoring prophylactic surgery in hereditary breast-ovarian cancer syndrome. Gynecol Oncol 1995;57:23–6.
431. Safer v. Estate of Pack, 677 A.2d 1188 (1996).
432. Tomlinson I, Rahman N, Frayling I, et al. Inherited susceptibility to colorectal adenomas and carcinomas: evidence for a new predisposition gene on 15q14-q22. Gastroenterology 1999;116:789–95.
433. Varley JM, McGown G, Thorncroft M, et al. Are there low-penetrance TP53 alleles? Evidence from childhood adrenocortical tumors. Am J Hum Genet 1999;65:995–1006.
434. Dietrich WF, Lander ES, Smith JS, et al. Genetic identification of Mom-1, a major modifier locus affecting Min-induced intestinal neoplasia in the mouse. Cell 1993;75:631–9.
435. Moisio A, Sistonen P, Mecklin J-P, et al. Genetic polymorphisms in carcinogen metabolism and their association to hereditary nonpolyposis colon cancer. Gastroenterology 1998;115:1387–94.
436. Bagchi D, Preuss HG (eds.). Phytopharmaceuticals in Cancer Chemoprevention. New York: CRC Press, 2005.
437. Bennicelli JL, Barr FG. Genetics and the biologic basis of sarcomas. Curr Opin Oncol 1999;11:267–74.
438. Kurian KM, Watson CJ, Wyllie AH. DNA chip technology. J Pathol 1999;187:267–71.
439. Roth JA, Swisher SG, Meyn RE. p53 tumor suppressor gene therapy for cancer. Oncology 1999;13:148–54.
440. Hemminki A, Markie D, Tomlinson I, et al. A serine/threonine kinase gene defective in Peutz-Jeghers syndrome. Nature 1998;391:184–7.
441. Lynch ED, Ostermeyer EA, Lee MK, et al. Inherited mutations in PTEN that are associated with breast cancer, Cowden disease, and juvenile polyposis. Am J Hum Genet 1997;61:1254–60.
442. Giardiello FM, Brensinger JD, Tersmette AC, et al. Very high risk of cancer in familial Peutz-Jeghers syndrome. Gastroenterology 2000;119:1447–53.
443. Su GH, Hruban RH, Bova GS, et al. Germline and somatic mutations of the *STK11/LKB1* Peutz-Jeghers gene in pancreatic and biliary cancers. Am J Pathol 1999;154:1835–40.
444. Sato N, Rosty C, Jansen M, et al. Peutz-Jeghers gene inactivation in intraductal papillary-mucinous neoplasms of the pancreas. Am J Pathol 2001;159:2017–22.
445. Lowenfels AB, Maisonneuve P, Cavallini G, et al. Pancreatitis and the risk of pancreatic cancer. N Engl J Med 1993;328:1433–7.
446. Whitcomb DC, Gorry MC, Preston RA, et al. Hereditary pancreatitis is caused by a mutation in the cationic trypsinogen gene. Nat Genet 1996;14:141–5.
447. Lowenfels AB, Maisonneuve P, Whitcomb DC, et al. Risk factors for cancer in hereditary pancreatitis. Med Clin North Am 2000;84:565–73.
448. Tersmette AC, Petersen GM, Offerhaus GJA, et al. Increased risk of incident pancreatic cancer among first-degree relatives of patients with familial pancreatic cancer. Clin Cancer Res 2001;7:738–44.
449. Lynch HT, Fusaro RM. Pancreatic cancer and the familial atypical multiple mole melanoma (FAMMM) syndrome. Pancreas 1991;6:127–31.
450. Goldstein AM, Fraser MC, Struewing JP, et al. Increased risk of pancreatic cancer in melanoma-prone kindreds with $p16^{INK4}$ mutations. N Engl J Med 1995;333:970–4.
451. Caldas C, Hahn SA, da Costa LT, et al. Frequent somatic mutations and homozygous deletions of the p16 (*MTS1*) gene in pancreatic adenocarcinoma. Nat Genet 1994;8:27–32.
452. Schutte M, Hruban RH, Geradts J, et al. Abrogation of the Rb/p16 tumor suppressive pathway in virtually all pancreatic carcinomas. Cancer Res 1997;57:3126–30.
453. Wooster R, Neuhausen SL, Mangion J, et al. Localization of a breast cancer susceptibility gene, BRCA2, to chromosome 13q12-13. Science 1994;265:2088–90.
454. Tulinius H, Olafsdottir GH, Sigvaldason H, et al. Neoplastic diseases in families of breast cancer patients. J Med Genet 1994;31:618–21.
455. Goggins M, Schutte M, Lu J, et al. Germline *BRCA2* gene mutations in patients with apparently sporadic pancreatic carcinomas. Cancer Res 1996;56:5360–4.
456. Lynch HT, Smyrk T, Kern SE, et al. Familial pancreatic cancer: a review. Sem Oncol 1996;23:251–75.
457. Groden J, Thliveris A, Samowitz W, et al. Identification and characterization of the familial adenomatous polyposis coli gene. Cell 1991;66:589–600.
458. Giardiello FM, Offerhaus GJ, Lee DH, et al. Increased risk of thyroid and pancreatic carcinoma in familial adenomatous polyposis. Gut 1993;34:1394–6.
459. Horii A, Nakatsuru S, Miyoshi Y, et al. Frequent somatic mutations of the APC gene in human pancreatic cancer. Cancer Res 1992;52:6696–8.
460. Yashima K, Nakamori S, Murakami Y, et al. Mutations of the adenomatous polyposis coli gene in the mutation cluster region: comparison of human pancreatic and colorectal cancers. Int J Cancer 1994;59:43–7.

461. Lynch HT, Voorhees GJ, Lanspa SJ, et al. Pancreatic carcinoma and hereditary nonpolyposis colorectal cancer: a family study. Br J Cancer 1985;52:271–3.
462. Jacob S, Praz F. DNA mismatch repair defects: role in colorectal carcinogenesis. Biochimie 2002;84:27–47.
463. Goggins M, Offerhaus GJA, Hilgers W, et al. Pancreatic adenocarcinomas with DNA replication errors (RER$^+$) are associated with wild-type *K-ras* and characteristic histopathology: poor differentiation, a syncytial growth pattern, and pushing borders suggest RER$^+$. Am J Pathol 1998;152:1501–7.
464. Lynch HT, Brand RE, Deters CA, et al. Hereditary pancreatic cancer. Pancreatology 2001;1:466–71.
465. Swift M, Sholman L, Perry M, et al. Malignant neoplasms in the families of patients with ataxia telangiectasia. Cancer Res 1976;36:209–15.

14

Chemical Carcinogenesis

Ainsley Weston, PhD
Curtis C. Harris, MD

Human chemical carcinogenesis is a multistage process that results from exposures, usually in the form of complex chemical mixtures, often encountered in the environment or through our lifestyle and diet (Table 14-1).[1–4] A prime example is tobacco smoke, which can cause cancers at multiple sites including the lung, the bladder, and the head and neck.[5–7] Although most chemical carcinogens do not react directly with intracellular components, they are activated to carcinogenic and mutagenic electrophiles by metabolic processes evolutionarily designed to rid the body of toxins and to modify endogenous compounds. Electrophilic chemical species are naturally attracted to nucleophiles like deoxyribonucleic acid (DNA) and protein, and through covalent bonding to DNA genetic damage results. Once internalized, carcinogens are subject to competing processes of metabolic activation and detoxification, although some chemical species can act directly. There is considerable variation among the human population in these competing metabolic processes, as well as the capacity for repair of DNA damage and cellular growth control. This is the basis for interindividual variation in cancer risk, and is a reflection of gene–environment interactions, which embodies the concept that heritable traits modify the effects of chemical carcinogen exposure.[8] Such variations in constitutive metabolism and DNA repair contribute to the relative susceptibility of individual members of the population to chemical exposures. For example, only 10% of tobacco smokers develop lung cancer, albeit that tobacco use accounts for other fatal conditions, including emphysema, chronic obstructive pulmonary disease, stroke, and heart disease. Within the conceptual framework of multistage carcinogenesis, the primary genetic change that results from a chemical–DNA interaction is termed *tumor initiation.*[9,10] Thus, initiated cells are irreversibly altered and are at a greater risk of malignant conversion than are normal cells. The epigenetic effects of tumor promoters facilitate the clonal expansion of the initiated cells.[10] Selective, clonal growth advantage causes a focus of preneoplastic cells to form. These cells are more vulnerable to tumorigenesis because they now present a larger, more rapidly proliferating, target population for the further action of chemical carcinogens, oncogenic viruses, and other cofactors. Additional genetic changes continue to accumulate. The activation of oncogenes, and the inactivation of tumor suppressor and DNA-repair genes, leads to genomic instability or the so called *mutator phenotype* and an acceleration in the genetic changes taking place.[11,12] This scenario is followed by malignant conversion, tumor progression, and metastasis. The underlying molecular mechanisms that govern chemical carcinogenesis are becoming increasingly understood, and the insights generated are assisting in the development of better methods to investigate human cancer risk and susceptibility.[13] The results of such studies are intended to mold strategies for prevention and intervention. Moreover, insights into the normal operations of so called *gatekeeper* genes,[14] like the tumor suppressor *TP53*, have provided an opportunity to develop new, targeted, therapeutic approaches.[15]

MULTISTAGE CARCINOGENESIS

Carcinogenesis can be divided conceptually into four steps: tumor initiation, tumor promotion, malignant conversion, and tumor progression (Figure 14-1). The distinction between initiation and promotion was recognized through studies involving both viruses and chemical carcinogens.[9,16] This distinction was formally defined in a murine skin carcinogenesis model in which mice were treated topically with a single dose of a polycyclic aromatic hydrocarbon (ie, initiator), followed by repeated topical doses of croton oil (ie, promoter),[9] and this model has been expanded to a range of other rodent tissues, including bladder, colon, esophagus, liver, lung, mammary gland, stomach, and trachea.[17] During the last 50 years, the sequence of events comprising chemical carcinogenesis has been systematically dissected and the paradigm increasingly refined, and both similarities and differences between rodent and human carcinogenesis have been identified.[18,19] Carcinogenesis requires the malignant conversion of benign hyperplastic cells to a malignant state, and invasion and metastasis are manifestations of further genetic and epigenetic changes.[20–22] The study of this process in humans is necessarily indirect and uses information from lifestyle or occupational exposures to chemical carcinogens. Measures of age-dependent cancer incidence have shown, however, that the rate of tumor development is proportional to the sixth power of time, suggesting that at least four to six independent steps are necessary.[23] Partial scheduling of specific genetic events in this process has been possible for some cancers. Exam-

Table 14-1 Selected Examples of Human Chemical Carcinogenesis

Organ System (Specific Pathology)	Chemical Carcinogen	Cocarcinogen
Lung	Metals: As, Be, Cd, Cr, Ni	—
	BCME	—
(Small cell and squamous cell)	Tobacco smoke	Asbestos
	Diesel exhaust	—
Pleural mesothelium	Asbestos	—
Oral cavity	Smokeless tobacco	—
	Betel quid	Slaked lime [$Ca(OH)_2$]
Esophagus	Tobacco smoke	Alcohol
Nasal sinuses	Snuff	Powdered glass
	Isopropyl alcohol	—
Skin (scrotum)	Cutting oil	—
	Coal soot*	—
Liver (angiosarcoma)	Aflatoxin B_1	HBV, HCB
	Vinyl chloride	Alcohol
Bladder	Aromatic amines (eg, 4-ABP and benzidine)	—
	Aromatic amines from tobacco smoke†	—
ALL	Benzene	—
Lymphatic and hemapoietic malignancies	Ethylene oxide	—

4-ABP = 4-aminobiphenyl; ALL = acute lymphoblastic leukemia; BCME = bischloromethyl ether; HBV = hepatitis B virus; HCV = hepatitis C virus.

*Early report of occupational chemical carcinogenesis from 225 years ago.[1]

†Strong circumstantial evidence.[150]

A comprehensive treatise on the evaluation of the carcinogenic risk of chemicals to humans can be found in the ongoing International Agency for Research on Cancer monograph program initiated in 1971.[4]

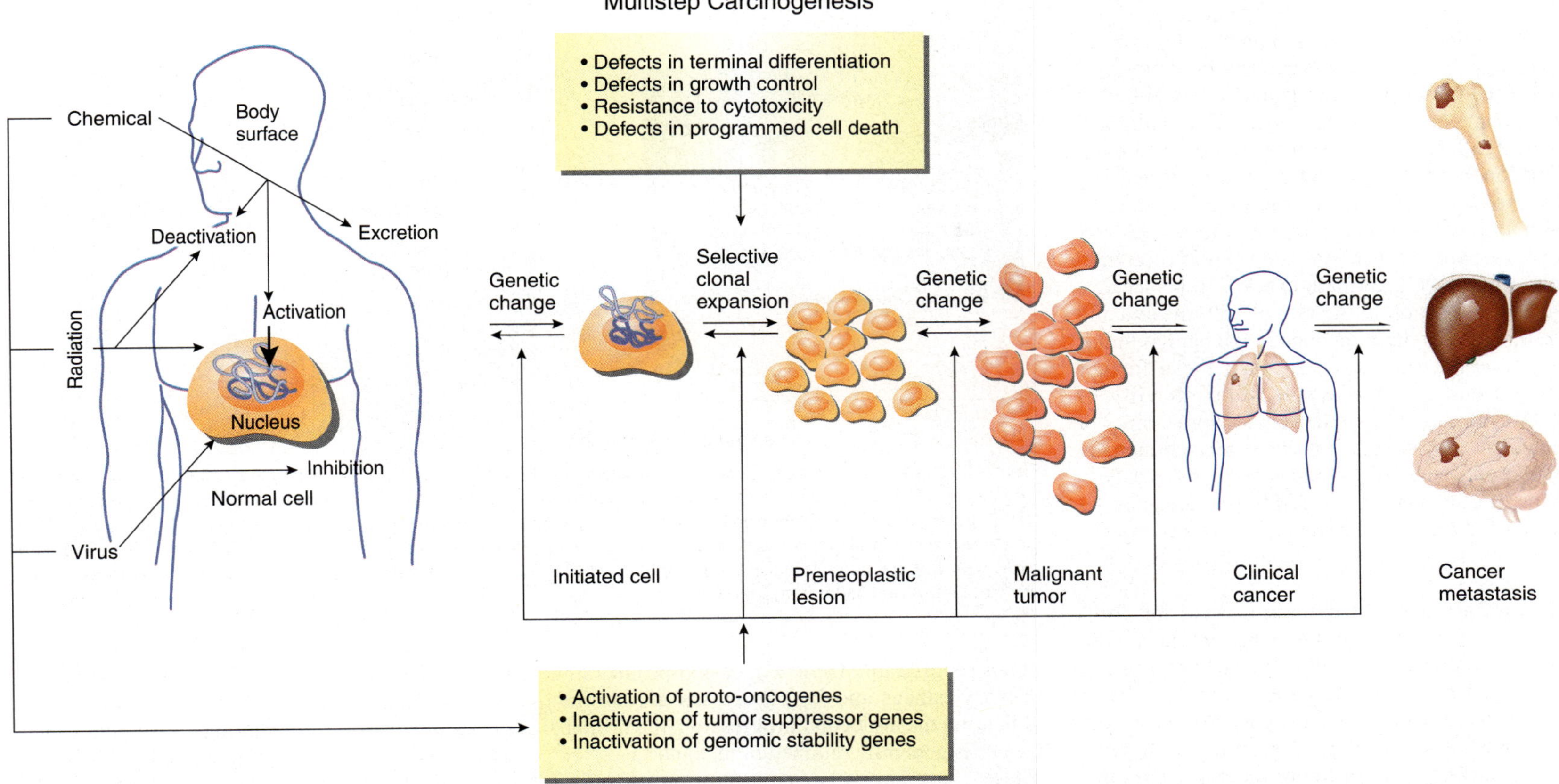

Figure 14-1 Multistage chemical carcinogenesis can be conceptually divided into four stages: tumor initiation, tumor promotion, malignant conversion, and tumor progression. The activation of proto-oncogenes and inactivation of tumor suppressor genes are mutational events that result from covalent damage to DNA caused by chemical exposures. The accumulation of mutations, and not necessarily the order in which they occur, constitutes multistage carcinogenesis.[26,99]

ples of sequential genetic and epigenetic changes that occur with the highest probability are those found in the development of lung cancer[24,25] and colon cancer.[26]

Tumor Initiation The early concept of tumor initiation indicated that the initial changes in chemical carcinogenesis are irreversible genetic damage. However, recent data from molecular studies of preneoplastic human lung and colon tissues implicate epigenetic changes as an early event in carcinogenesis. DNA methylation of promoter regions of genes can transcriptionally silence tumor suppressor genes.[22] For mutations to accumulate, they must arise in cells that proliferate and survive the lifetime of the organism. A chemical carcinogen causes a genetic error by modifying the molecular structure of DNA that can lead to a mutation during DNA synthesis. Most often, this is brought about by forming an adduct between the chemical carcinogen or one of its functional groups and a nucleotide in DNA[17] (the process by which this occurs for the major classes of chemical carcinogens is discussed in detail under "Carcinogen Metabolism"). In general, a positive correlation is found between the amount of carcinogen–DNA adducts that can be detected in animal models and the number of tumors that develop.[27–29] Thus, tumors rarely develop in tissues that do not form carcinogen–DNA adducts. Carcinogen–DNA adduct formation is central to theories of chemical carcinogenesis, and it may be a necessary, but not a sufficient, prerequisite for tumor initiation (the concept of so called nongenotoxic carcinogens is also explored under "Carcinogen Metabolism"). DNA adduct formation that causes either the activation of a proto-oncogene or the inactivation of a tumor suppressor gene can be categorized as a tumor-initiating event (see "Tumor Progression," "Oncogenes and Tumor Suppressor Genes" in this chapter).

Tumor Promotion Tumor promotion comprises the selective clonal expansion of initiated cells. Because the accumulation rate of mutations is proportional to the rate of cell division, or at least the rate at which stem cells are replaced, clonal expansion of initiated cells, produces a larger population of cells that are at risk of further genetic changes and malignant conversion.[20,25,26] Tumor promoters are generally nonmutagenic, are not carcinogenic alone, and often (but not always) are able to mediate their biologic effects without metabolic activation. These agents are characterized by their ability to reduce the latency period for tumor formation after exposure of a tissue to a tumor initiator, or to increase the number of tumors formed in that tissue. In addition, they induce tumor formation in conjunction with a dose of an initiator that is too low to be carcinogenic alone. Croton oil (isolated from *Croton tiglium* seeds) is used widely as a tumor promoter in murine skin carcinogenesis, and the mechanism of action for its most potent constituent, 12-*O*-tetradecanoylphorbol-13-acetate, which occurs via protein kinase C activation, is arguably the best understood among tumor promoters.[30] Chemicals or agents capable of both tumor initiation and promotion are known as complete carcinogens, eg, benzo[*a*]pyrene and 4-aminobiphenyl. Identification of new tumor promoters in animal models has accelerated with the sophisticated development of model systems designed to assay for tumor promotion. Furthermore, ligand binding properties can be determined in recombinant protein kinase C isozymes that are expressed in cell cultures.[31] Chemicals, complex mixtures of chemicals, or other agents that have been shown to have tumor-promoting properties include dioxin, benzoyl peroxide, macrocyclic lactones, bromomethylbenzanthracene, anthralin, phenol, saccharin, tryptophan, dichlorodiphenyltrichloroethane (DDT), phenobarbital, cigarette-smoke condensate, polychlorinated biphenyls (PCBs), teleocidins, cyclamates, estrogens and other hormones, bile acids, ultraviolet light, wounding, abrasion, and other chronic irritation (ie, saline lavage).[17] In addition, protein kinase C is activated and cellular diacylglycerol elevated in laboratory animals maintained on high-fat diets.[32,33]

Malignant Conversion Malignant conversion is the transformation of a preneoplastic cell into one that expresses the malignant phenotype. This process requires further genetic changes. The total dose of a tumor promoter is less significant than frequently repeated administrations, and if the tumor promoter is discontinued before malignant conversion has occurred, premalignant or benign lesions may regress. Tumor promotion contributes to the process of carcinogenesis by the expansion of a population of initiated cells, with a growth advantage, that will then be at risk for malignant conversion. Conversion of a fraction of these cells to malignancy will be accelerated in proportion to the rate of cell division and the quantity of dividing cells in the benign tumor or preneoplastic lesion. In part, these further genetic changes may result from infidelity of DNA synthesis.[34] The relatively low probability of malignant conversion can be increased substantially by the exposure of preneoplastic cells to DNA-damaging agents,[17,35] and this process may be mediated through the activation of proto-oncogenes and inactivation of tumor suppressor genes.

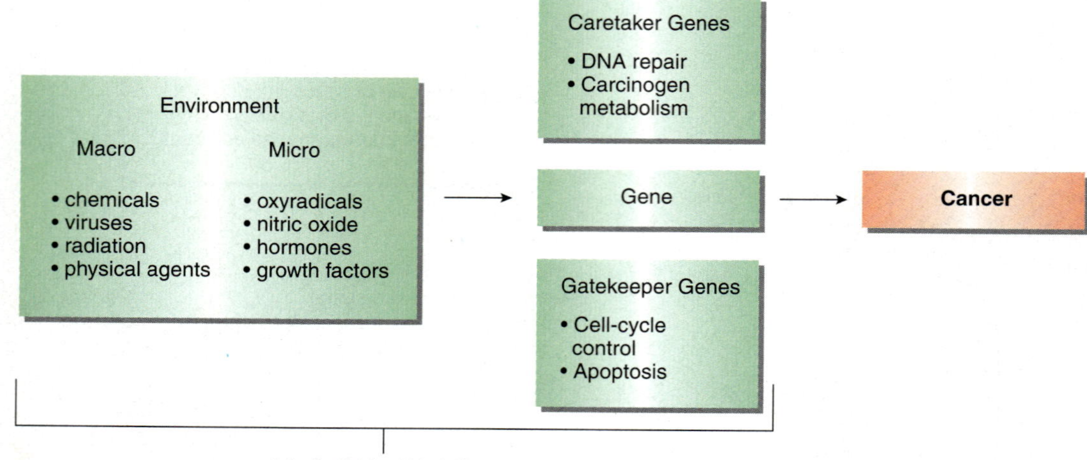

Figure 14-2 The concept of gene–environment interaction is multifaceted: (1) environmental chemicals are altered by the products of metabolic genes; (2) environmental chemicals disrupt the expression (induce or inhibit) of carcinogen metabolizing genes; and (3) environmental exposures cause changes (mutations) in cancer-related genes. The cancer-related genes have been classified as gatekeeper (eg, *APC*) and caretaker genes (eg, *MSH1* and *MLH1*). The interaction of these genes with external and internal environmental agents can lead to the derangement of regulatory pathways that maintain genetic stability and cellular proliferation.

Tumor Progression Tumor progression comprises the expression of the malignant phenotype and the tendency of malignant cells to acquire more aggressive characteristics over time. Also, metastasis may involve the ability of tumor cells to secrete proteases that allow invasion beyond the immediate primary tumor location. A prominent characteristic of the malignant phenotype is the propensity for genomic instability and uncontrolled growth.[36] During this process, further genetic and epigenetic changes can occur, again including the activation of proto-oncogenes and the functional loss of tumor suppressor genes. Frequently, proto-oncogenes are activated by two major mechanisms: in the case of the *ras* gene family, point mutations are found in highly specific regions of the gene (ie, the twelfth, thirteenth, fifty-ninth, or sixty-first codons), and members of the *myc*, *raf*, *HER2*, and *jun* multigene families can be overexpressed, sometimes involving amplification of chromosomal segments containing these genes. Some genes are overexpressed if they are translocated and become juxtaposed to a powerful promoter (eg, the relationship of *bcl-2* and immunoglobulin heavy chain gene promoter regions in B-cell malignancies; see also Philadelphia chromosome, under "Clonal Evolution"). Loss of function of tumor suppressor genes usually occurs in a bimodal fashion, and most frequently involves point mutations in one allele and loss of the second allele by a deletion, recombinational event, or chromosomal nondisjunction. These phenomena confer to the cells a growth advantage as well as the capacity for regional invasion, and ultimately, distant metastatic spread. Despite evidence for an apparent scheduling of certain mutational events, it is the accumulation of these mutations, and not the order or the stage of tumorigenesis in which they occur, that appears to be the determining factor.[24–26] Recent evidence from microarray expression analysis of human cancers supports an alternative, and not mutually exclusive, mode of tumor progression. Gene expression profiles of a primary cancer and its metastases are similar, indicating the molecular progression of a primary cancer is generally retained in its metastases.[37,38] These results have clinical implications in molecular diagnosis of primary cancers and therapeutic strategies.

GENE-ENVIRONMENT INTERACTIONS AND INTERINDIVIDUAL VARIATION

A cornerstone of human chemical carcinogenesis is the concept of gene-environment interactions (Figure 14-2).[8] Potential interindividual susceptibility to chemical carcinogenesis may well be defined by genetic variations in the host elements of this compound system. Functional polymorphisms in human proteins that have, or may have, a role in chemical carcinogenesis include enzymes that metabolize (ie, activate and detoxify) xenobiotic substances, enzymes that repair DNA damage, cell surface receptors that activate the phosphorylation cascade and cell cycle control genes (ie, oncogenes and tumor suppressor genes that are elements of the signal transduction cascade).

Caretaker and Gatekeeper Genes Gatekeeper and caretaker genes are characterized by their control of net cellular proliferation or maintenance of genomic integrity, respectively.[15,39] Examples of gatekeeper genes include *APC* and β-*catenin* in colon epithelial cells, *Rb* in retinal epithelial cells, *NF1* in Schwann cells, and *VHL* in kidney cells. The most prominent example of a gatekeeper is the *APC* gene in colorectal cancer. An alteration in *APC* may lead to a derangement of the cellular proliferation pathway, which is necessary for maintaining a constant cell population. However, this function of *APC* has a high specificity for colonic epithelial cells, but is lacking in most other organs. In murine as well as human colon cancer, *APC* mutation occurs early in carcinogenesis.[40–42] Although other genes such as *K-ras* and *TP53* play significant roles in the later stages of colorectal carcinogenesis, *APC* mutation, and the less-common β-*catenin* mutations, are essential events in neoplastic initiation (for a review, see Kinzler KW and Vogelstein B[39]). If this concept of a gatekeeper pathway holds true for the initiation of neoplasia in general, then the identification of other gatekeeper genes can be anticipated.

Unlike gatekeeper genes, caretaker genes generally maintain genomic stability and are not involved directly in neoplastic initiation. Genetic instability caused by mutations in caretaker genes enhances the probability of mutation in other genes, including those in the gatekeeper pathway. Mismatch DNA-repair genes, such as *MSH2* and *MLH1*, are caretaker genes, and abnormalities in these genes enhance genomic instability and increase the risk of human colon cancer. Based on this knowledge of human colon carcinogenesis, animal models have been developed.[43–45] Similar in vivo, as well as in vitro models, should be developed for carcinogenesis in other tissues. Breast cancer-susceptibility genes, *BRCA1* and *BRCA2*, are also included in the list of caretaker genes.[14] The same report suggested that an individual who inherits a mutated caretaker gene is at a lower risk of cancer as compared with an individual who inherits a mutated gatekeeper gene. This difference is attributed to the finding that three or more additional somatic mutations are required to initiate neoplasia in the caretaker pathway, versus only one additional somatic mutation that is required to initiate neoplasia in the gatekeeper pathway. The analysis of potentially preneoplastic lesions for mutations in gatekeeper and caretaker genes could provide short-term and less-expensive pathobiologic end points for hazard identification and molecular epidemiologic studies.

When chemicals or xenobiotics encounter biologic systems, they become altered by metabolic processes. This is an initial facet of gene–environment interaction. The interindividual variation in carcinogen metabolism and macromolecular adduct formation arising from such processes was recognized 25 to 30 years ago.[46] The cytochrome P450 (CYP) multigene family is largely responsible for the metabolic activation and detoxication of many different chemical carcinogens in the human environment.[47] Cytochrome P450s are Phase I enzymes that act by adding an atom of oxygen onto the substrate; they are induced by polycyclic aromatic hydrocarbons and chlorinated hydrocarbons.[48] Phase II enzymes act on oxidized substrates and also contribute to xenobiotic metabolism. Some Phase II enzymes are methyltransferases; acetyltransferases; glutathione transferases; uridine 5'-diphosphoglucuronosyl transferases; sulfotransferases; nicotinamide adenine dinucleotide (NAD)- and nicotinamide adenine dinucleotide phosphate (NADP)-dependent alcohol dehydrogenases; aldehyde; and steroid dehydrogenases; quinone reductases; NADPH diaphorase; azo reductases; aldoketoreductases; transaminases; esterases; and hydrolases. The pathways of activation and detoxification are often competitive, providing yet further potential for individual differences in propensity for carcinogen metabolism to DNA damaging species.

This scenario is further complicated by a second facet of gene–environment interaction that leads to enzyme induction or inhibition. In this case, environmental exposures alter gene expression, and genes responsible for carcinogen metabolism can be upregulated or repressed by certain chemical exposures.

A third facet of gene–environment interaction occurs when the chemical alters gene structure. Once a procarcinogen is metabolically activated to an ultimate carcinogenic form, it can bind covalently to cellular macromolecules, including DNA. This DNA damage can be repaired by several mechanisms.[49,50] Differences in rates and fidelity of DNA repair potentially influence the extent of carcinogen adduct formation (ie, biologically effective dose) and, consequently, the total amount of genetic damage. The consequences of polymorphisms in genes controlling the cell cycle (serine/threonine kinases, transcription factors, cyclins, cyclin-dependent kinase inhibitors, and cell surface receptors) are much less clear. However, molecular epidemiologic evidence suggests that certain common variants of these types of genes have a role in susceptibility to chemical carcinogenesis.[51,52] The evaluation of polymorphisms as potential biomarkers of susceptibility in the human population is discussed under "Implications for Molecular Epidemiology, Risk Assessment, and Cancer Prevention."

CARCINOGEN METABOLISM

The first chemically identified carcinogens were the polycyclic aromatic hydrocarbons (PAHs).[7,53,54]

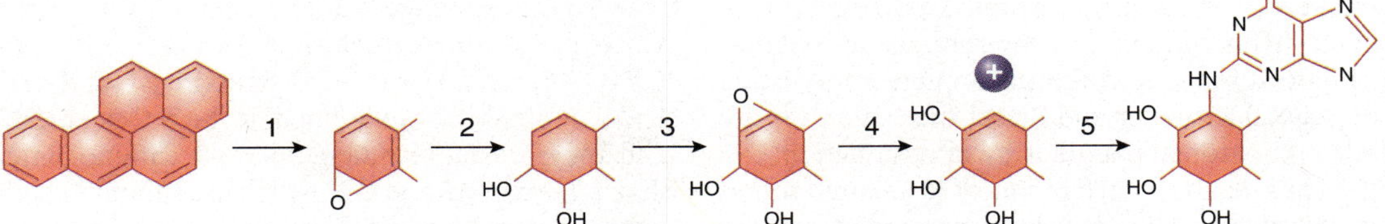

Figure 14-3 Metabolic activation of benzol[*a*]pyrene. (1) Cytochrome P450 (CYP1A1) catalyses initial epoxidation across the 1 - 2, 2 - 3, 4 - 5, 7 - 8 (shown), 9 - 10 and 11 - 12 positions. (2) With the exception of the 1 - 2 and 2 - 3 oxides that convert to phenols, epoxide hydrolase may catalyze the formation of dihydrodiols. (3) Benzo[*a*]pyrene-7, 8-dihydrodiol is further metabolized at the olefinic double bond by cytochrome P450 (CYP1B1 and CYP3A4) to form a vicinal diol-epoxide (r7, t8-dihydroxy-c9, 10 epoxy-7,8,9,10-tetrahydroxybenz[*a*]pyrene). (4) The highly unstable arene ring opens spontaneously to form a carbocation. (5) This electrophic species forms a covalent bond between the 10 position of the hydrocarbon and the exocyclic amino group of deoxyguanosine.

They are composed of variable numbers of fused benzene rings that form from incomplete combustion of fossil fuels and vegetable matter (including tobacco), and they are common environmental contaminants. The PAHs are chemically inert, and require metabolism to exert their biologic effects.[55,56] This is a multistep process, it involves the following: initial epoxidation (cytochrome P450, CYP1A1 is an inducible isoform), hydration of the epoxide (epoxide hydrolase), and subsequent epoxidation across the olefinic bond (CYP1B1; CYP3A4) (Figure 14-3). The result is the ultimate carcinogenic metabolite, a diolepoxide.[57,58] The biology of CYP1A1 metabolism has been elucidated providing a molecular basis for inducibility and interindividual variation,[46,59,60] and variations in cytochrome levels among humans have been documented.[61]

The arene ring of benzo[*a*]pyrene-7,8-diol 9,10-oxide opens spontaneously at the 10 position, giving a highly reactive carbonium ion that can form a covalent addition product (ie, adduct) with cellular macromolecules, including DNA. Several DNA-adducts can be formed, the most abundant being at the exocyclic amino group of deoxyguanosine ([7R]-N^2-[10-{7β,8α,9α-trihydroxy-7,8,9,10-tetrahydro-benz[*a*]pyrene}yl] - deoxyguanosine; BPdG) (Figure 14-4). An alternative pathway of PAH activation, through a mechanism of one electron oxidation, has also been postulated.[62] When benzo[*a*]pyrene is activated by this route, the resulting radical cation is formed at the *meso* position or L-region.[58] The reactive cation forms DNA adducts at the C8 of guanine (BP-6-C8Gua and BP-6-C8dGua), the N7 of guanine (BP-6- N7Gua), and the N7 of adenine (BP-6-N7Ade) (see Figure 14-4). These adducts place strain on the *N*-glycosyl link to the helical backbone and depurination results. Firm evidence for the exfoliation of these adducts in urine was provided recently for exposure scenarios that included coal and tobacco smoke.[63]

Aromatic amines are another class of chemical carcinogens found in cigarette smoke, diesel exhaust, industrial environments and certain cooked foods. The compound, 4-aminobiphenyl, is thought to be responsible for bladder cancer

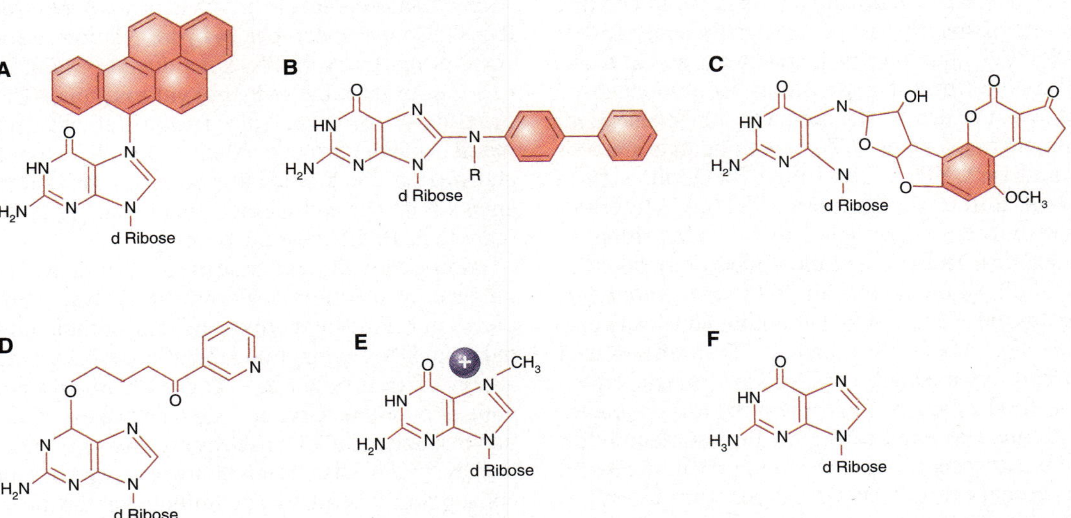

Figure 14-4 Examples of carcinogen–DNA adducts: **A,** N7(benzo[*a*]pyren-6-yl)guanine; **B,** *N*-(deoxyguanosin-8-yl)-{acetyl}aminobiphenyl (when R= H the adduct is not acetylated [R can also be an acetyl group]); **C,** 8,9-dihydro-8-(N5-formyl- 2', 5', 6'-triamino-4'-oxo-N5-pyrimidyl)-9-hydroxy-aflatoxin B1; **D,** O6-[4-Oxo-4(3-pyridyl)butyl]guanine, a mutagenic lesion formed by the metabolism of the tobacco-specific nitrosamine, NNK[73,74]; **E,** N7-methyldeoxyguanosine; and **F,** 3-methyladenosine. Adducts **E,** and **F,** can also result as the small alkyl products of NNK metabolism.[73,74]

among tobacco smokers and rubber industry workers.[64] In addition, nitrated polycyclic aromatic hydrocarbons are environmental contaminants resulting from the incomplete combustion of vegetable matter and diesel fuel, and they are related to aromatic amines by nitroreduction.

The metabolic activation of aromatic amines is complex.[65] They can be converted to an aromatic amide that is catalyzed by an acetyl coenzyme A-dependent acetylation. The acetylation phenotype varies among the population. Persons with the rapid acetylator phenotype are at a higher risk of colon cancer, whereas, those who are slow acetylators are at risk of bladder cancer.[66] This latter association may result from the fact that activation of aromatic amines by *N*-oxidation is a competing pathway for aromatic amine metabolism. Also, the *N*-hydroxylation products when protonated (by acid conditions in the urinary bladder) form reactive electrophiles that bind covalently with DNA or proteins to produce macromolecular damage.

An initial activation step for both aromatic amines and amides is *N*-oxidation by CYP1A2. *CYP1A2* is inducible by phenobarbital, and because it is also responsible for the 3-demethylation of 1,3,7-trimethylxanthine (ie, caffeine), *CYP1A2* phenotype can be determined using this as a probe drug.[67] The reactions of *N*-hydroxyarylamines with DNA appear to be acid catalyzed, but they can be further activated by either an acetyl coenzyme A-dependent O-acetylase or a 3'-phosphoadenosine-5'phosphosulfate-dependent O-sulfotransferase. The *N*-arylhydroxamic acids arise from the acetylation of *N*-hydroxyarylamines or *N*-hydroxylation of aromatic amides; they are not electrophilic and require further activation. The predominant pathway for this occurs through the acetyltransferase-catalyzed rearrangement to a reactive *N*-acetoxyarylamine. Sulfotransferase catalysis forms *N*-sulphonyloxy arylamides. This complex pathway results in two major adduct types, amides (ie, acetylated) and amines (ie, nonacetylated).

The heterocyclic amines form while cooking food, primarily from the pyrolysis (>150°C [302°F]) of amino acids, creatinine, and glucose. They have been recognized as food mutagens,[68] shown to form DNA adducts and cause liver tumors in primates.[69] These compounds are activated by CYP1A2, and their metabolites form DNA adducts in humans.[70] The *N*-hydroxy metabolites of 3-amino-1-methyl-5*H*pyrido[4,3-b]indole (Trp-P-1), 2-amino-6-methyldipyrido[1,2-a:39,29-d]imidazole (Glu-P-1), and 2-amino-3-methyl-imidazo- [4,5-f]quinoline (IQ) can react directly with DNA. Enzymic O-esterification of *N*-hydroxy metabolites plays a key role in activating food mutagens, and the *N*-hydroxy metabolites are also good substrates for transacetylases. This suggests a possible etiologic role for these chemicals in colorectal cancer with the rapid acetylator phenotype.

Aflatoxins (B1, B2, G1, and G2) are metabolites of *Aspergillus flavus* that contaminate cereals, grain, and nuts. A positive correlation exists between dietary aflatoxin exposure and the incidence of liver cancer in developing countries, where grain spoilage is high. Aflatoxins are activated by several cytochrome P450s (CYP2A3; CYP2A6; CYP3A4).[47,71] Aflatoxin B1 and G1 have an olefinic double bond at the 8,9-position, and they are more mutagenic and carcinogenic than aflatoxin B2 and G2, which are saturated and have an ethylenic bond at this position. This implies that the olefinic 8,9-bond is the activation site. Further support for this mechanism comes from studies of DNA-adducts and the prevalence of *TP53* mutations in liver cancer. In people with liver cancer from parts of China and Africa, where food spoilage caused by molds is high, G:C to T:A transversions in codon 249 are frequent.[72] This phenomenon is consistent with metabolic activation of aflatoxin B1 and the formation of depurinating carcinogen–deoxyguanosine adducts.

Carcinogenic *N*-nitrosamines are ubiquitous environmental contaminants and can be found in food, alcoholic beverages, cosmetics, cutting oils, hydraulic fluid, rubber, and tobacco.[73] Tobacco-specific *N*-nitrosamines, such as 4-(methylnitrosoamino)-1-(3-pyridyl)-1-butanone, are carcinogenic in a wide range of animal species. Unlike exposure to many other carcinogens associated with tobacco use, exposure to tobacco-specific *N*-nitrosamines does not require pyrolysis, therefore they may account for the carcinogenic nature of snuff and chewing tobacco.[74] The tobacco-specific nitrosamines are not symmetric so both small alkyl-adducts and large bulky adducts can be formed; for example, 4-(methylnitrosoamino)-1-(3-pyridyl)-1-butanone metabolism gives rise to either a positively charged pyridyl-oxobutyl ion or a positively charged methyl ion, both of which are able to alkylate DNA.[73,74] Endogenous nitrosation forms nitrosamines when an amine reacts with nitrate alone or nitrite in the presence of acid. Thus, nitrite (used in curing meats) and L-cysteine, in the presence of acetaldehyde (a metabolite of alcohol), form *N*-nitrosothiazolidine-4-carboxylic acid. *N*-nitrosodimethylamine undergoes α-hydroxylation, catalyzed primarily by the alcohol inducible *CYP2E1*, to form an unstable α-hydroxynitrosamine. The breakdown products are formaldehyde and methyl diazohydroxide. Methyl diazohydroxide and related compounds are powerful alkylating agents that can add a small functional group at more than 10 different DNA sites.

Non-genotoxic carcinogens may function at the level of the microenvironment by dysregulation of hormones and growth factors, or indirectly inducing DNA damage and mutations through the action of free radicals.[75] These chemicals are none or poorly reactive and are resistant to activation through metabolism. They are also characterized by their persistence in biological systems and consequently tend to accumulate in the food chain. However, they have the ability to stimulate oxyradical formation. There are at least three mechanisms by which this may occur: in the case of persistent organochlorine species, interaction with the Ah receptor could lead to cytochrome P450 induction, similar to PAHs, and associated oxyradical formation; or interaction with other receptors, like IFN-γ, would stimulate elements of the primary immune response and again generate oxyradicals; agents like asbestos would promote oxyradical formation through interaction with ferrous metal and Fenton chemistry. Oxyradicals generated by any one of these mechanisms can then damage DNA. Some of the so called "nongenotoxic" carcinogens might more appropriately be considered to be "oxyradical triggers." Indeed, chronic inflammatory states, which involve oxyradical formation, can also be cancer risk factors.[76]

DNA DAMAGE AND REPAIR

The chemical structure of DNA can be altered by a carcinogen in several ways: the formation of bulky aromatic-type adducts, alkylation (generally small adducts), oxidation, dimerization, and deamination. In addition, double- and single- strand breaks can occur. Chemical carcinogens can cause epigenetic changes, such as altering the DNA methylation status that leads to the silencing of specific gene expression.[77] A complex pattern of carcinogen–DNA adducts likely results from exposure to tobacco smoke, because of the mixture of different chemical carcinogens present.[78]

r7, t8-dihydroxy-c9, 10 epoxy-7,8,9,10-tetrahydroxybenzo[*a*]pyrene (benzo[*a*]pyrene-7,8-diol 9,10-epoxide, BPDE) reacts with the exocyclic (N2) amino group of deoxyguanosine and resides within the minor groove of the double helix; it is typical of polycyclic aromatic hydrocarbons (see Figures 14-3 and 14-4). This adduct, BPdG, appears to be the most common, persistent adduct of benzo[*a*]pyrene in mammalian systems, but others are possible. Some metabolites bind covalently with deoxyadenosine, and proapurinic adducts form through one electron oxidation (see Figure 14-4). This type of adduct, BPdG and others, is thought to induce *ras* gene mutations, which are common in tobacco-smoking-related lung cancers.[29,63,79,80] Aromatic amine adducts are more complex, because they have both acetylated and nonacetylated metabolic intermediates, and they form covalent bonds at the C8, N2, and sometimes O6 positions of deoxyguanosine as well as deoxyadenosine. The major adducts, however, are C8-deoxyguanosine adducts, which reside predominantly in the major groove of the DNA double helix (see Figure 14-4).[65]

Aflatoxin B1 and G1 activation occurs through hydroxylation of the olefinic 8,9-position and adducts are formed at the N7-position of deoxyguanosine. They are relatively unstable and have a half-life of approximately 50 h at neutral pH; depurination products have been detected in rat and human urine.[81] The aflatoxin B1-N7-deoxyguanosine adduct also can undergo ring opening to yield two pyrimidine adducts; alternately, aflatoxin B1-8,9-dihydrodiol could result. This latter possibility could restore the DNA molecular structure if hydrolysis of the original adduct occurs, but a potentially promutagenic lesion would result if the 8,9-dihydrodiol results from degradation of open-ring adduct forms.[82]

DNA alkylation can occur at many sites either following the metabolic activation of certain *N*-nitrosamines, or directly by the action of the *N*-alkylureas (*N*-methyl-*N*-nitrosourea) or the *N*-nitrosoguanidines. The protonated alkyl-functional groups that become available to form lesions in DNA generally attack the following nucleophilic centers: adenine (N1, N3, and N7), cytosine (N3), guanine (N2, O6, and N7), and thymine (O2, N3, and O4). Some of these lesions are known to be repaired (O6-methyldeoxyguanosine), while others are not (N7-methyldeoxyguanosine).[73,74] Furthermore, O6-methyldeoxyguanosine is a promutagenic lesion, whereas N7-methyldeoxyguanosine is not.

Oxyradical damage can form thymine glycol or 8-hydroxydeoxyguanosine adducts. Exposure to organic peroxides (catechol, hydroquinone, and 4-nitroquinoline-*N*-oxide) leads to oxyradical damage; however, oxyradicals and hydrogen peroxide can be generated in lipid peroxidation and the catalytic cycling of some enzymes.[83] Tobacco smoke is also a source of oxyradicals, and by inducing an inflammatory response, tobacco smoke can contribute to diseases such as asthma and chronic heart disease, as well as cancer.[76] Also, certain drugs and plasticizers can stimulate cells to produce peroxisomes.[84] In addition, increased oxyradical formation is mediated through protein kinase C when inflammatory cells are exposed to tumor promoters like phorbol esters.[85]

Another potentially mutagenic cause of DNA damage is the deamination of DNA-methylated cytosine residues. 5-Methylcytosine comprises approximately 3% of deoxynucleotides. In this case, deamination at a CpG dinucleotide gives rise to a TpG mismatch. Repair of this lesion most often restores the CpG; however, repair may cause a mutation (TpA).[86] Deamination of cytosine also can generate a C to T transition if uracil glycosylation and G-T mismatch repair are inefficient. Oxyradicals can enhance the deamination rate, so the activity of inducible nitric oxide synthase and production of high concentrations of nitric oxide could contribute to DNA damage by this mechanism.[87]

Maintenance of genome integrity requires abrogation of DNA damage, and diminished DNA-repair capacity is associated with carcinogenesis, birth defects, premature aging, and foreshortened life-span. DNA-repair enzymes act at DNA-damage sites caused by chemical carcinogens, and six major mechanisms are known: direct DNA repair, nucleotide excision repair, base excision repair, nonhomologous end joining (doublestrand break repair), mismatch repair, and homologous recombination (postreplication repair).[50,88]

In the presence of nonlethal DNA damage, cell-cycle progression is postponed for repair mechanisms. This highly coordinated process involves multiple genes. A DNA-damage recognition sensor triggers a signal transduction cascade and downstream factors direct G1 and G2 arrest in concert with the proteins operationally responsible for the repair process. Although there are at least six discrete repair mechanisms, within five of them there are numerous multiprotein complexes comprising all the machinery necessary to accomplish the step-by-step repair function.

Generically, DNA repair requires damage recognition, damage removal or excision, resynthesis or patch synthesis, and ligation. Recent advances have led to the cloning of more than 130 human genes involved in five of these DNA-repair pathways. A list of these genes and their specific functions was published elsewhere.[89] These genes are responsible for the fidelity of DNA repair, and when they are defective the mutation rate increases. This is the mutator phenotype.[34] Mutations in at least 30 DNA-repair-associated genes have been linked to increased cancer susceptibility or premature aging (Table 14-2).[89] Moreover, the role of common polymorphisms in some of these genes are associated with increased susceptibility in a gene–environment interaction scenario (this is discussed under "Implications for Molecular Epidemiology, Risk Assessment, and Cancer Prevention"). Indeed, molecular epidemiologic evidence suggests that tobacco-smoking-related lung cancer is associated with a polymorphism in the nucleotide excision repair gene, *XPC (ERCC2)*.[90]

Direct DNA repair is effected by DNA alkyltransferases. These enzymes catalyze translocation of the alkyl moiety from an alkylated base (eg, O^6-methyldeoxyguanosine) to a cysteine residue at their active site in the absence of DNA strand scission. Thus, one molecule of the enzyme is capable of repairing one DNA alkyl lesion, in a suicide mechanism. The inactivation of this mechanism by promoter hypermethylation is associated with *K-ras* G to A mutations in colon cancer.[91]

In DNA nucleotide excision repair, lesion recognition, preincision, incision, gap-filling, and ligation are required, and the so-called excinuclease complex comprises 16 or more different proteins. Large distortions caused by bulky DNA adducts (eg, BPDE-dG and 4ABP-dC) are recognized (*XPA*) and removed by endonucleases (*XPF*, *XPG*, *FEN*). A patch is then constructed (*pol* Δ, *pol* ε) and the free ends are ligated.

Base excision repair also removes a DNA segment containing an adduct, however, small adducts (eg, 3-methyladenine) are generally the target so that there is overlap with direct repair. The adduct is removed by a glycosylase (*hOgg1*, *UDG*), an apurinic endonuclease (*APE1* or *HAP1*) degrades a few bases on the damaged strand, and a patch is synthesized (*pol* β) and ligated (DNA ligases: I, II, IIIα, IIIβ, and IV).

DNA mismatches occasionally occur, because excision repair processes incorporate unmodified or conventional, but noncomplementary, Watson–Crick bases opposite each other in the DNA helix. Transition mispairs (G-T or A-C) are repaired by the mismatch repair process more efficiently than transversion mispairs (G-G, A-A, G-A, C-C, C-T, and T-T). The mechanism for correcting mispairings is similar to that for nucleotide excision repair and resynthesis described earlier, but it generally involves the excision of large pieces of the DNA containing mispairings. Because the mismatch recognition protein is required to bind simultaneously to the mismatch and an unmethylated adenine in a GATC recognition sequence, it removes the whole intervening DNA sequence. The parental template strand is then used by the polymerase to fill the gap.

Double-strand DNA breaks can occur from exposure to ionizing radiation and oxidation. Consequences of double-strand DNA breaks are the inhibition of replication and transcription, and loss of heterozygosity. Double-strand DNA break repair occurs through homologous recombination, where the joining of the free ends is mediated by a DNA-protein kinase in a process that also protects the ends from nucleolytic attack. The free ends of the DNA then undergo ligation by DNA ligase IV. Genes known to code for DNA-repair enzymes that participate in this process include *XRCC4, XRCC5, XRCC6, XRCC7, HRAD51B, HRAD52, RPA*, and *ATM*.[87]

Postreplication repair is a damage-tolerance mechanism and it occurs in response to DNA replication on a damaged template. The DNA polymerase stops at the replication fork when DNA damage is detected on the parental strand. Alternately, the polymerase proceeds past the lesion, leaving a gap in the newly synthesized strand. The gap is filled in one of two ways: either by recombination of the homologous parent strand with the daughter strand in a process that is mediated by a helical nucleoprotein (RAD51); or when a single nucleotide gap remains, mammalian DNA polymerases insert an adenine residue. Consequently, this mechanism may lead to recombinational events as well as base-mispairing.

Persistent non-repaired DNA damage blocks the replication machinery. Cells have evolved translesion synthesis (TLS) DNA polymerases to bypass these blocks.[92,93] Most of these TLS polymerases belong to the recently discovered Y-family, have much lower stringency than replicative polymerases and thus are error prone. An increased mutation frequency is an evolutionary trade-off for cellular survival.

MUTATOR PHENOTYPE

Cancer cells contain substantial numbers of genetic abnormalities when compared with normal cells. These abnormalities range from gross changes such as nondiploid number of chromosomes, ie, aneuploidy, and translocations or rearrangements of chromosomes, to much smaller changes in the DNA sequence including deletions, insertions, and single nucleotide substitutions. Therefore, carcinogenesis involves *errors* in (1) chromosomal segregation; (2) repair of DNA damage induced by either endogenous free radicals or environmental carcinogens; and (3) DNA replication. Loeb originally formulated the concept of the mutator phenotype in 1974[94] to account for the high numbers of mutations in cancer cells when compared to the rarity of mutations in normal cells. Recent advances in the molecular analysis of carcinogenesis in human cells and animal

Table 14-2 Examples of Disease Susceptibility and Disease Syndromes Associated with Mutations in DNA-Repair Genes

Gene	Function	Pathology or Cancer
Cancer Susceptibility		
MMR[a]		
MLH1	Damage recognition	HNPCC2[b], glioma
MLH2	DNA binding	HNPCC1, ovarian cancer
MSH3	—	Endometrial cancer
MSH6	Sliding clamp	Endometrial cancer, HNPCC1
PMS1	Damage recognition	HNPCC3
PMS2	Repair initiation	HNPCC4, glioblastoma
NER		
BRCA-1	Directs *p53* transcription towards DNA-repair pathways	Breast cancer, ovarian cancer
RB1	Cell-cycle restriction	Retinoblastoma, breast cancer, and progression osteosarcoma
DSB		
BRCA-2	Regulation of RAD51	Breast cancer, pancreatic cancer
HR		
RAD54	Helicase	Colon cancer, breast cancer, NHL
Other		
TP53 (DSB, NER, HR)	Cell-cycle control; exonuclease; apoptosis; DNA binding	Colon cancer, common somatic defect in human cancer in general; inherited in Li-Fraumeni syndrome and some breast cancers
hOgg1 (Various)	Glycosylase	Cancer susceptibility
Xeroderma pigmentosum (XP)		
NER		
XPD	DNA Helicase	Skin and neurologic, but later onset than XPA
XPB	DNA Helicase	Skin lesions
XPG	Endonuclease	Acute sun sensitivity, mild symptoms; late skin cancer
XPC (and BER)	Exonuclease	Mental retardation; skin sensitivity; microcephaly
DDB1 and DDB2	Binds specific DNA damage	XPE—Mild skin sensitivity
XPA	Damage sensor	XPA—Skin and neurologic problems: the most severe XP
XPC	Damage sensor	XPC—Skin, tongue, and lip cancer
XPE	Damage sensor	XPE—Neurologically normal
PRR		
POLH	Polymerase	XPV—Mild to severe skin sensitivity; neurologically normal
Other syndromes		
NER		
Cockaynes		
CSB	ATPase	Cutaneous, ocular, neurologic, and somatic abnormalities; short stature, progressive deafness, mental retardation, neurologic degeneration, early death; sometimes presents together with XPB
Juberg-Marsidi		
ATRX	Putative helicase	Thalassemia/mental retardation
SB		
Nijmegen		
NBS1	Nibrin, cell-cycle regulation	Microencephaly; mental retardation; immunodeficiency; growth retardation; radiation sensitivity; predisposition to malignancy
Ataxia-telangiectasia		
ATM	Phosphorylation	Neurologic deficiencies, manifest by inability to coordinate muscle actions; skin and corneal telangiectases. Leukemia, lymphoma, and other malignancies (breast cancer?)
MRE11 (Ataxia-like)	Exonuclease	DNA damage sensitivity; genomic instability; telomere shortening; aberrant meiosis; severe combined immunodeficiency
PRKDC	Ser/Thr kinase	SCID
Bloom's		
BLM	DNA Helicase	High rate of spontaneous lymphatic and other malignancy; high rate SCE[c]
Fanconi anemia		
FANCA-G	Protein control	Multiple congenital malformations; chromosome breaks; pancytopenia. Telomere shortening
Werner		
WRN	DNA Helicase/Exonuclease	Premature senility, short stature, exonuclease rapidly progressing cataracts, loss of connective tissue and muscle, premature arteriosclerosis, increase risk of malignancy
RecQ4	DNA Helicase	Osteosarcoma; premature aging.

[a] Repair mechanisms: BER = base excision; DSB = double strand break; HR = homologous recombination; MMR = mismatch; NER = nucleotide excision; PRR = postreplication; SB = strand break.
[b] Diseases: HNPCC = hereditary nonpolyposis colon cancer; NHL = non-Hodgkin lymphoma.
[c] Other abbreviations: SCE = sister chromatid exchange; SCID = severe combined immunodeficiency.

models have refined the mutator phenotype[12] concept that is also linked to the clonal selection theory proposed by Nowell (Figure 14-5).[95]

The fidelity of DNA replication, and the partitioning of equal numbers of chromosomes to the daughter cells, is remarkably accurate in dividing normal cells. Whereas, the maintenance of the species will tolerate few mutations in germ cells, somatic cells may tolerate many more mutations that cause cancer and other life-shortening diseases. Although rare in the human population, inherited mutations in specific genes that are responsible for rare cancer-prone diseases are consistent with the mutator phenotype concept and indicate examples of functional classes of

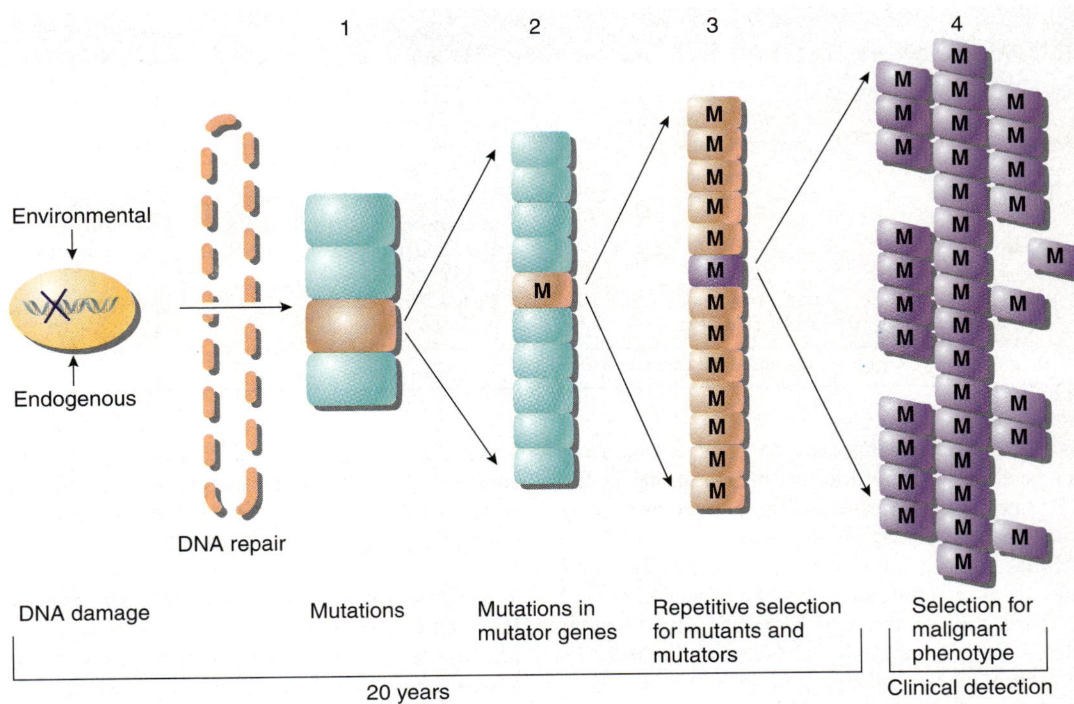

Figure 14-5 Mutation accumulation during tumor progression. (1) Random mutations result when DNA damage exceeds the cell's capacity for error-free DNA repair. (2) These random mutations can result in clonal expansion and mutations in mutator genes (M). (3) Repetitive rounds of selection for mutants yield coselection mutants in mutator genes. (4) From this population of mutant cancer cells, there is selection for cells that escape the host's regulatory mechanisms for the control of cell replication, invasion, and metastasis. (Modified and reproduced with permission from Loeb.[12])

genes that, when mutated, increase the probability of cancer.

Examples of cancer syndromes include those with defective nucleotide excision repair (eg, xeroderma pigmentosum), or mismatch DNA repair (eg, hereditary nonpolyposis colorectal cancer syndrome). Germline mutations in DNA helicases also cause the cancer-prone Bloom and Werner syndromes. Other functional classes of genes required for maintaining genomic stability, that when mutated, may be responsible for the mutator phenotype, include the very genes involved in DNA replication, deoxynucleotide metabolism, cell cycle checkpoints, and mitosis (see Table 14-2). The *TP53* tumor suppressor gene is frequently mutated in human cancer,[96–98] and is involved in DNA repair and recombination, cell cycle checkpoints, and apoptosis.[99] Thus, *TP53* may be an important target gene for a mutator phenotype.

CLONAL EVOLUTION

Clonal evolution in human tumors is complex, because there is evidence that a single progenitor cell gives rise to all the cells in the tumor, as well as evidence for a hierarchical system of stem cells. Both systems likely exist. In tobacco-related cancer of the lung, metachronous bilateral masses have, in some cases, a similar genetic background, whereas in other cases, they are dissimilar.[100,101] In addition, adenosquamous lung carcinomas are most frequently composed of a unique genetic profile, although a small percentage present variability.[102] Together, these findings suggest that multifocal masses may exist where different foci have a common initiated cell as well as multifocal masses where each focus has its own clonal origin.

Cancers of the head and neck are frequently tobacco related and many patients develop metachronous tumors, thus these cancers provide another tumor type in which to approach the question of clonality. Comparative molecular analysis found some paired tumors, arising in the same field, shared a common origin. These findings indicate that a single progenitor cell can replicate, expand, and populate contiguous regions in the process of clonal expansion.[26,103] However, the zonal limits of clonal expansion have not yet been adequately determined.[104,105]

Further evidence for clonality in tumors comes from studies of loss of heterozygosity, where allelic loss invariably affects the same chromosome.[106] Even more convincing is differential methylation in female cancer patients. Inactivation of the X chromosome (by methylation) during embryogenesis is random, so polyclonal female tissues develop with an approximately equal complement of inactivated maternal and paternal X chromosomes. In monoclonal tissues, the same inactive X chromosome should be present in all of the cells. By use of methylation-sensitive restriction enzymes virtually all colorectal tumors in females were found to be monoclonal.[107] Genetic studies have found at least 95% of human tumors to be monoclonal in origin.

In chronic myelogenous leukemia, the early disease phase is characterized by the Philadelphia chromosome, a single reciprocal translocation, t(9;22). The formation of a hybrid gene of *c-abl* with the breakpoint cluster region (*BCR*) activates the proto-oncogene through its in-frame insertion. The resulting gene product has elevated tyrosine kinase activity. The later stages of chronic myeloid leukemia are typified by overgrowth of one or more subclones that have additional karyotypic alterations.[108]

ONCOGENES AND TUMOR SUPPRESSOR GENES

Chronic exposures to carcinogens, accumulation of mutations, development of the mutator phenotype, and clonal selection during several decades result in cancer. Although the phenotypic traits of individual cancers are highly variable, commonly acquired capabilities include limitless replicative potential, self-sufficiency in growth signals, insensitivity to antigrowth signals, evading apoptosis, tissue invasion, sustained angiogenesis, and metastasis.[109] These phenotypic traits reflect a complex molecular circuitry of biochemical pathways and protein machines within cancer cells.[19]

The genes encoding the proteins within the cancer-associated molecular circuitry are of many functional classes and, historically, have been conceptually divided into oncogenes and tumor suppressor genes. Detailed descriptions of oncogenes and tumor suppressor genes are found in Chapters 4 to 7. The *ras* oncogene and the *TP53* tumor suppressor gene will be used as examples of molecular targets of chemical carcinogens.

Activated *ras* genes predominate as the family of oncogenes to be isolated from solid tumors that are induced by chemicals in laboratory animals. Members of the *ras* gene family code for proteins of molecular weight 21,000 (p21); these proteins are membrane bound, have GTPase activity, and form complexes with other proteins. The *ras* genes code for small G-proteins (guanine nucleotide binding) that exert a powerful proliferative response through the signal transduction cascade. The first direct evidence of proto-oncogene activation by a chemical carcinogen was obtained from in vitro studies.[110] A wild-type recombinant clone of the human *Ha-ras* gene (pEC) was modified with benzo[*a*]pyrene-diolepoxide. The treated plasmid was then used to transfect murine NIH-3T3 cells, with the result that the transformed cell foci contained the same point mutations (in either codon 12 or 61) known to exist in activated *ras* genes isolated from human tumors including the bladder (pEJ). In animal models of chemical carcinogenesis and surveys of different types of human tumors that arise from a variety of environmental exposures, *ras* mutations have been found.[31,99,111] For example, tobacco smoke can mutate *K-ras* during the molecular pathogenesis of human lung adenocarcinoma.[80] In rodents, polycyclic aromatic hydrocarbons (3-methylcholanthrene, 7,12-dimethylbenz[*a*]anthracene and benzo[*a*]pyrene) have been used repeatedly to produce both benign tumors and malignant carcinomas. A large proportion of these premalignant and malignant lesions have mutations in either the twelfth or sixty-first codons. Similarly, treatment of rats with either 7,12-dimethylbenz[*a*]anthracene or *N*-methyl-*N*-nitrosourea resulted in the development of mammary carcinomas containing *ras* codon 12 or 61 mutations. These types of mutations also have been observed in mouse skin after initiation with 7,12-dimethylbenz[*a*]anthracene and tumor promotion with 12-*O*-tetradecanoylphorbol-13-acetate. Mutations in *ras* have been found in mouse liver after treatment with vinyl carbamate, hydroxydehydroestragole, or *N*-hydroxy-2-acetylaminofluorene. The same point mutations have been found in murine thymic lymphomas after treatment with *N*-methyl-*N*-nitrosourea or γ-radiation, and in other rodent skin models after treatment with methylmethanesulfonate, α-propiolactone, dimethylcarbamyl chloride, or *N*-methyl-*N*9-nitro-*N*-nitrosoguanidine.

These data indicate that chemical carcinogens may produce site-specific mutations based, in part, on nucleoside selectivity of the ultimate carcinogen. Persistence of a specific mutation, however, also depends on the amino acid substitution in that the function of the mutant protein is altered to confer on the cell a selective clonal growth advantage. The types of mutations that are found in chemically activated *ras* genes cause conformational changes that alter protein binding (GTPase Activating Protein) in such a way that the *ras*-MAP kinase pathway is permanently activated. Data support the hypothesis that *ras* activation is associated with malignant conversion as well as tumor initiation. Transfection of activated *ras* genes into benign papillomas that did not contain a constitutively activated *ras* gene, caused malignant progression.[111] These and other results implicate *ras* mutations in chemical carcinogenesis. Similarly, malignant transformation occurred when immortalized human bronchial epithelial cells were transfected with an activated *ras* gene.[112,113] *Ki-ras* gene mutations are also one of many changes that can arise either early or late in the development of colorectal carcinoma.[106] These findings indicate that the accumulation of mutations, and not necessarily the order in which they occur, contributes to multistage carcinogenesis. Furthermore, the stage of carcinogenesis in which each mutation occurs is not necessarily fixed. In the model for human colorectal carcinoma, *ras* mutations most often occur during malignant conversion, but can be an early event (ie, tumor initiation), but in the rodent skin models, *ras* mutations appear to be primarily a tumor-initiating event. These differences may reflect the type of exposure, both in terms of chemical class and chronic versus acute exposure, or they may be a function of tissue type.

The *TP53* tumor suppressor gene is central in the response pathway to cellular stress.[106] For example, DNA damage caused by chemical carcinogens activates the p53 tumor suppressor protein by post-translational modification to transduce signals to "guard the genome"[114] by engaging cell cycle checkpoints and enhancing DNA repair, and as a fail-safe mechanism, to cause replicative senescence or apoptotic death. Mutations in the *TP53* gene or inactivation of its encoded protein by viral oncoproteins generally lead to a loss of these cellular defense functions. Not surprisingly, *TP53* mutations are common in human cancer.[96–98,115]

Table 14-3 Mutational Spectra of *TP53* in Human Cancers*

Carcinogen Exposure	Neoplasm	Mutation
Aflatoxin B1	Hepatocellular carcinoma	Codon 249 (AGG 6 AGT)
Sunlight	Skin carcinoma	Dipyrimidine mutations (CC 6 TT) on nontranscribed DNA strand
Tobacco smoke	Lung carcinoma	G:C 6 T:A mutations on nontranscribed DNA strand (frequently codons: 157, 248 and 273)
Tobacco and alcohol	Carcinoma of the head and neck	Increased frequency p53 mutations (especially codons 157 and 248)
Radon	Lung carcinoma	Codon 249 (AGG 6 ATG)
Vinyl chloride	Hepatic angiosarcoma	A:T 6 T:A transversions

*For reviews see Greenblatt, Hollstein, Hussain, and Harris.[72, 96, 120, 146]

Molecular analysis of *TP53* can give clues to the environmental etiology of cancer (Table 14-3). It is implicit from the preceding text (see "DNA Damage and Repair") that the covalent binding of activated carcinogens to DNA is not random. Therefore, the formation of a particular DNA lesion to some extent may be deduced from the resulting mutation. A dramatic example of this phenomenon is the previously mentioned *TP53* codon 249 mutation, which is detected in almost all aflatoxin-related hepatocellular carcinomas.[97,116] The striking nature of this association could arise by two distinct mechanisms. First, the third base in codon 249 (AGG) may be unusually susceptible to activated aflatoxin B1 mutations. As discussed earlier, aflatoxin B1-8,9-oxide causes a promutagenic lesion by covalently binding to the N7 position of deoxyguanosine. Alternately, cells bearing the codon 249 lesion may have an important selective growth advantage. Evidence that a combination of these factors is responsible has been presented as well.[116] Another prominent example where circumstantial evidence points to specific molecular events is that of *TP53* mutations indicative of pyrimidine dimer formation in ultraviolet light related skin cancers.[117] In the case of tobacco smoking and lung cancer, G:C to T:A transversions indicate the formation of adducts from activated bulky carcinogens (eg, polycyclic aromatic hydrocarbons).[72,96,118]

Assessment of Causation by the Bradford–Hill Criteria Results obtained from molecular epidemiologic studies can be used for the assessment of causation. Using the "weight of the evidence" principle, Bradford-Hill proposed criteria in the assessment of cancer causation, including strength of association (consistency, specificity, and temporality) and biologic plausibility.[119] These criteria can be applied for the analysis of data obtained in molecular epidemiologic studies.[120] Cigarette smoking has been established as a major risk factor for the incidence of lung cancer (Table 14-4). Codons 157, 248, and 273 of *TP53* are designated as mutational hotspots in lung cancer. The majority of mutations found at these codons are G to T transversions. Furthermore, besides lung cancer, codon 157 also constitutes one of the hotspots for G to T transversions in breast, and head and neck cancers. In smoking-associated lung cancer, the occurrence of G to T transversions has been linked to the presence of benzo[*a*]pyrene in cigarette smoke. Interestingly, codon 157 (GTC to TTC) mutations are not found in lung cancer from never smokers.[96–98] A dose-dependent increase in *TP53* G to T transversion mutations

Table 14-4 Assessment of Causation by the Bradford-Hill Criteria*

Hypothesis:
The chemical carcinogen, benzo[α]pyrene, in tobacco smoke can cause *TP53* hotspot mutations at codons 157, 248, and 273 in human lung carcinogenesis.

Strength of association	Biologic plausibility
Consistency: Cigarette smoking or exposure to coal smoke are associated with a dose-response increase in *TP53* mutations (G to T transversions in human lung cancer).	Tobacco smoke and benzo[α]pyrene are mutagens. Benzo[α]pyrene is metabolically activated and forms benzo[α]pyrene diol-epoxide-DNA adducts in human bronchus *in vitro* (75-fold interindividual variation).
Specificity: Codon 157 (GTC 6 TTC) mutations are uncommon in other types of cancer, including in lung cancer from never smokers.	Benzo[α]pyrene diol-exposide binds to Gs in codons 157, 248, and 273, which are *TP53* mutational hotspots. Benzo[α]pyrene exposure to human cells in vitro produces codon 248 (CGG ≥ CTG) *TP53* mutations.
Temporality: *TP53* mutations can be found in bronchial dysplasia.	Cigarette smoke condensates or benzo[α]pyrene can neoplastically transform human bronchial epithelial cells in the laboratory.

*For reviews see Hill, and DeMarini.[119,151]

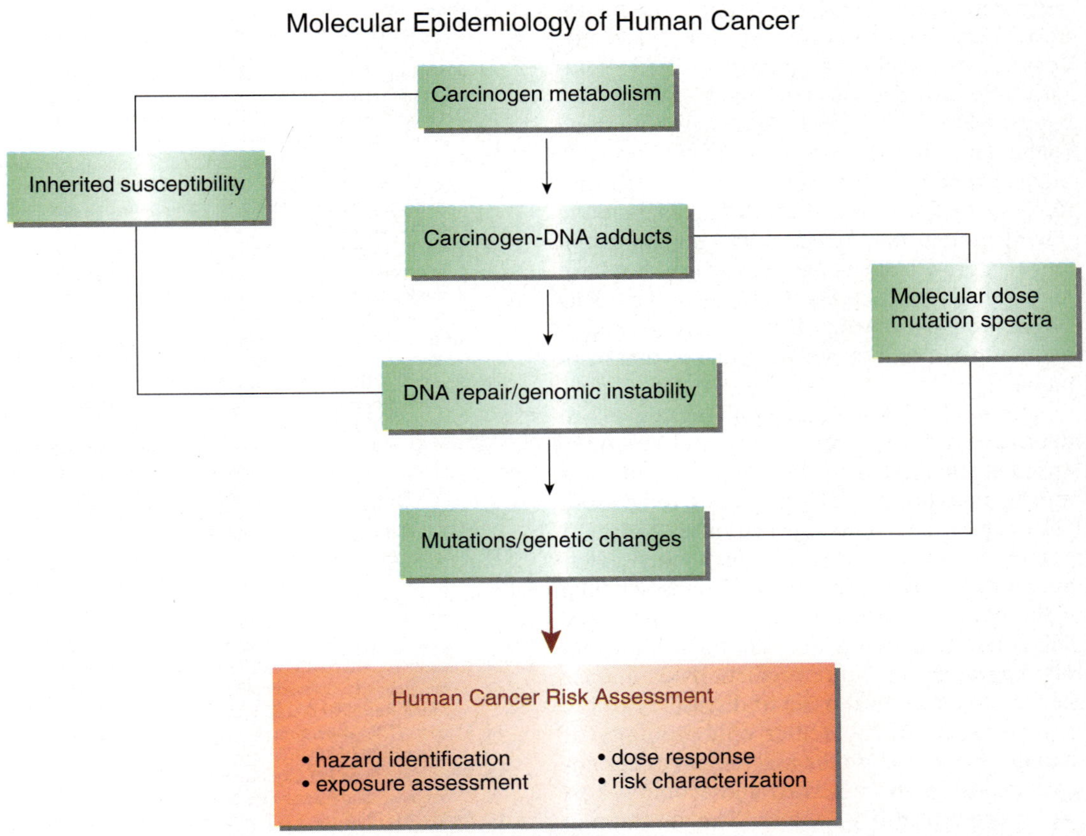

Figure 14-6 Facets of molecular epidemiology that investigate gene–environment interactions. Once internalized, chemical carcinogens are metabolized to reactive species that cause DNA damage (carcinogen DNA adducts). The innate ability to repair DNA damage may reduce or ablate the overall damage burden. Alternately, genetic changes (mutations, clastogenesis) may occur. Carcinogen metabolism and DNA repair are categorizable genetic traits (host factors). DNA adducts (molecular dose) and mutational spectra are measures of exposure. Information from assays designed to investigate host factors and measure exposure can be used for human cancer risk assessment.

with cigarette smoking has been reported in lung cancer.[121] Benzo[α]pyrene diol-epoxide, the metabolically activated form of benzo[*a*]pyrene, has been shown to bind to guanosine residues in codons 157, 248, and 273, which are mutational hotspots in lung cancer.[122] Also, cigarette smoke condensate or benzo[*a*]pyrene neoplastically transforms in vitro human bronchial epithelial cells.[123] In general, molecular and epidemiologic data provide only circumstantial evidence for causation. Bradford-Hill criteria provide a framework for the logical consideration of converging lines of evidence in cancer etiology.

IMPLICATIONS FOR MOLECULAR EPIDEMIOLOGY, RISK ASSESSMENT, AND CANCER PREVENTION

Molecular epidemiology (use of biochemical and molecular biological methods to buttress epidemiological studies) has resulted from the confluence of several disciplines.[124] It encompasses the detection of carcinogen–macromolecular adducts (DNA as a direct genotoxic measure and protein as a surrogate), normal DNA sequence variants (heritable variations), and mutations in target genes (somatic changes). Therefore, these investigations use epidemiologic methods to investigate all aspects of gene–environment interactions and risk assessment in human populations (Figure 14-6).

The biologically effective dose of a chemical carcinogen is governed by the amount that reaches a target tissue in a form that becomes activated to a chemical species capable of causing DNA lesions.[125] Humans are most commonly exposed to complex mixtures of chemicals. Human carcinogen dosimetry at the molecular level requires sensitive and specific methods for carcinogen-macromolecular adduct quantitation. The low levels of adducts that are present in human DNA samples challenge the detection limits of conventional assay systems, and complex mixtures of adducted materials confound simple assay systems.

The most commonly used methods for carcinogen–DNA dosimetry in humans are ^{32}P-nucleotide postlabeling, immunoassays, fluorescence spectroscopy, electrochemical conductance, liquid chromatography/electrospray ionization/tandem mass spectrometry (LC/ESI/MS/MS), and gas chromatography/mass spectroscopy (GC/MS). Each of these techniques currently has its own advantages and limitations, and within the framework of epidemiologic surveys, multiple corroborative end-point analyses seem to provide the most useful information. These methodologies, their application, and their limitations are reviewed extensively elsewhere.[3,29]

For exposure to tobacco smoke, GC/MS has provided a tool to measure aromatic amine protein adducts such as 4-aminobiphenyl hemoglobin. These studies have shown a dose–response relationship between the extent of smoking, type of tobacco used, and the adduct levels.[126] Similarly, tobacco-specific nitrosamine globin adducts have been used to monitor the dose in smokers and snuff dippers. A corroborative approach to the measurement of benzo[*a*]pyrene–DNA adducts has been used in the monitoring of both tobacco and coal smoke exposure. In this study, both GC/MS and fluorescence line-narrowing spectroscopy were used to detect adducts exfoliated in urine.[63,127]

In the case of aflatoxin B1, levels of adducts exfoliated in human urine were measured by GC/MS. 8,9-dihydro-8-(N5-formyl- 2', 5', 6'-triamino-4'-oxo-N5-pyrimidyl)-9-hydroxy-aflatoxin B1 (aflatoxin–N7 guanine) adducts correlated with environmental exposure and disease outcome. Similarly, aflatoxin–albumin adducts provided a corroborative surrogate. Both of these markers were also correlated with 6-hydroxycortisol levels, indicating a role for CYP3A4 in aflatoxin B1 activation. Particularly, the presence of aflatoxin–N7 guanine adducts in urine was associated with liver cancer.[128,129] Based on these findings, a randomized clinical trial of the *interceptor molecule*, chlorophyllin (Derifil), was performed. The test drug or placebo was taken three times daily and urinary AFB1-N7-Gua was monitored by GC/MS. After 12 weeks, adduct levels were > 100% higher among 90 persons taking the placebo than those ($n = 90$) taking chlorophyllin.[81]

Interindividual variation in cancer susceptibility, and, consequently, meaningful human cancer risk assessment, involve determination of inherited host factors as well as exposure assessment. Metabolic polymorphisms have been determined by the use of indicator drugs (eg, caffeine, debrisoquine, dextromethorphan, dapsone, and isoniazid), however, these assays are being replaced by direct genetic assays.[61,67,130] This approach has allowed the investigation of diverse host factors for which indicator drugs were not available, and it has been applied to a wide variety of cancers, including lung, head, and neck.[131,132] Thus, genetic indicators of propensity for carcinogen activation and detoxification, DNA-repair capacity, and cell-cycle control are all features of molecular epidemiologic studies that are complementary to adduct studies because of the implications for a biologically effective dose after exposure.[3]

Cytochrome P450 polymorphisms, involved in carcinogen activation, and glutathione-*S* transferases, uridine diphosphate (UDP) glucuronosyltransferases, sulfotransferases, and *N*-acyltransferases, involved in both carcinogen activation and detoxification, could explain variations in cancer susceptibility among the human population. Evidence that absent protection of a functionally intact *GSTM1* gene correlates with an increased risk of tobacco-related lung cancer.[133,134] Similarly, UDP glucuronosyltransferases (eg, *UGT1A1, UGT1A9, UGT2B7*) have been implicated in cancers of the head and neck. Persons inheriting reduced activity variants of *NAT1* and *NAT2* genes, resulting in the slow acetylator phenotype, are at a greater risk of aromatic amine-induced bladder cancer. This may include persons exposed through tobacco smoke inhalation.[66] Even though the inducible form of arylhydrocarbon hydroxylase (AHH) (*CYP1A1* and *CYP1A2*) has long been suspected of increasing cancer susceptibility in PAH-exposed persons, molecular epidemiologic studies remain inconclusive. Studies of *CYP2D6* metabolizer status and tobacco smoke-related lung cancer are similarly confusing.[8] However, analysis of multiple traits, for example, *CYP1A1* and *GSTM1*, in the same population may help to resolve these issues. Currently, there is a need for improved epidemiologic study design that integrates DNA adduct measures with indicators of metabolic capacity.[135–137]

Many DNA-repair genes have been described recently, and a growing number of polymorphisms have been identified for which molecular epidemiologic studies have provided evidence that genetic variation in these attributes can be a human cancer risk factor.[90,91,138,139] Typically, these types of molecular epidemiological studies initially focus on high exposure groups such as workers, patients taking therapeutic drugs and tobacco smokers. Several polymorphisms in DNA repair genes have now been implicated in tobacco related neoplasams.[140]

The components of cell-cycle control comprise genes that code for cell membrane receptors, intermediate messengers, and transcription factors. Polymorphisms in a number of these genes have been implicated in various cancers, notably: *TP53, p73, BRCA-1, BRCA-2* and *CCND1*.[141–144] However, there is overlap. This is because many of these genes, like *BRCA-1* and *TP53*, are integral components of the DNA repair system. Indeed they constitute a system of genome surveillance that alerts cells of damage status.

Molecular characterization of tumors, that is, molecular profiling, is an important tool that has both etiologic and clinical application. Molecular profiling is a rapidly advancing area that is being propelled by DNA and protein microarray research.[37,38,145] During chemical carcinogenesis, the genome becomes altered and mutations accumulate. These mutations become evident in genes responsible for growth control and cellular homeostasis (including proto-oncogenes, tumor suppressor genes, and some DNA-repair genes), because corruption of these functions is part of carcinogenesis. In respect to chemical carcinogenesis, the most studied genes are Kirsten *ras (Kras)* and *TP53*. *Kras* is mutated in approximately 30% of lung adenocarcinomas, and may prove to be an indicator of prognosis or a guide to treatment.[80] The *TP53* tumor suppressor gene is mutated in most types of human cancers and it is the most commonly mutated gene yet known (eg, mutations in *TP53* are found in approximately 50% of lung cancers). Unlike *ras* gene mutations that are found in highly specific regions (codons 12, 13, 59, and 61), *TP53* mutations occur more widely. This is presumably because a positive growth advantage is conveyed only with specific *ras* mutations and the loss of *TP53* tumor suppressor function can occur with less specificity. However, for some malignancies, *TP53* mutations have provided clues to cancer etiology (see Table 14-3).[119,146] *TP53* is further distinguished from other genetic lesions in that several possible mutant phenotypes can exist. Mutations may simply lead to the absence of *TP53*, an inactive mutant protein may exist, or the mutant might convey a growth advantage. Several studies have investigated *TP53* expression, and even though its role in prognosis has not been clearly defined, it may be that it will provide a guide to treatment options.[147,148]

The goal of molecular epidemiology is to identify risk factors for disease and outcome. Variation among humans in carcinogen biodistribution, metabolism, DNA adduct formation, DNA repair, and potential responses to tumor promoters have important implications in determining cancer risk. An increased understanding of the molecular basis of these differences and their connection with critical steps in carcinogenesis may assist in future predictions of disease risk before the clinical onset of disease.

The facets of molecular epidemiology of human cancer risk are the assessment of carcinogen exposure and inherited and acquired host cancer-susceptibility factors. The interaction between these facets determines cancer risk. When combined with carcinogen bioassays in laboratory animals and classic epidemiology, molecular epidemiology can contribute to the four critical aspects of cancer risk assessment: (1) hazard identification, (2) dose–response assessment, (3) exposure assessment, and (4) risk characterization. Important bioethical considerations accompany the identification of high-risk individuals; these include autonomy, privacy, justice, and equity. Benefits of the knowledge of risk for an individual may be offset by specific concerns relating to that individual's responsibility to family members and psychosocial anxiety regarding the genetic testing of children. Therefore, the uncertainty of current individual risk assessments and the limited availability of genetic counseling services dictate caution. In addition, it is widely held that genetic testing should be restricted to those situations that are amenable to preventative or therapeutic intervention.[149]

ACKNOWLEDGMENTS

We thank Glory Johnson, Karen MacPherson, and Dorothea Dudek for editorial assistance. We also thank Drs. Mark Toraason and Steven H. Reynolds for thoughtful suggestions.

REFERENCES

1. Pott P. Chirurgical observations relative to the cancer of the scrotum. In: Hawes L, Clark W, Collins R, editors. London, 1775.
2. Johnson BL. A review of health-based comparative risk assessments in the United States. Rev Environ Health 2000;15:273–87.
3. Poirier MC, Santella RM, Weston A. Carcinogen macromolecular adducts and their measurement. Carcinogenesis 2000;21:353–9.
4. International Agency for Research on Cancer. IARC monographs on the evaluation of carcinogenic risks to humans. Overall evaluation of carcinogenicity. Monographs volumes 1 to 76. Lyon: IARC;1971–2000.
5. Peto R, Darby S, Deo H, et al. Smoking, smoking cessation, and lung cancer in the UK since 1950: combination of national statistics with two case-control studies. BMJ 2000;321:323–9.
6. Vineis P, Marinelli D, Autrup H, et al. Current smoking, occupation, *N*-acetyltransferase-2 and bladder cancer: a pooled analysis of genotype-based studies. Cancer Epidemiol Biomarkers Prev 2001;10:1249–52.
7. Luch A. Nature and nurture—lessons from chemical carcinogenesis. Nature Rev Cancer 2005;5:113–25.
8. Shields PG, Harris CC. Cancer risk and low-penetrance susceptibility genes in gene-environment interactions. J Clin Oncol 2000;18:2309–15.
9. Berenblum I, Shubik P. A new quantitative approach to the study of the stages of chemical carcinogenesis in the mouse skin. Br J Cancer 1947;1:383–91.
10. Yuspa SH. Overview of carcinogenesis: past, present and future. Carcinogenesis 2000;21:341–4.
11. Jackson AL, Loeb LA. The contribution of endogenous sources of DNA damage to the multiple mutations in cancer. Mutat Res 2001;477:7–21.
12. Loeb LA, Loeb KR, Anderson JP. Multiple mutations and cancer. Proc Natl Acad Sci U S A 2003;100:776–81.
13. Hussain SP, Harris CC. Molecular epidemiology and carcinogenesis: endogenous and exogenous carcinogens. Mutat Res 2000;462:311–22.
14. Kinzler KW, Vogelstein B. Gatekeepers and caretakers. Nature 1997;386:761–3.
15. Woods YL, Lane DP. Exploiting the p53 pathway for cancer diagnosis and therapy. Hematol J 2003;4:233–47.
16. Reddy AL, Fialkow PJ. Papillomas induced by initiation-promotion differ from those induced by carcinogen alone. Nature 1983;304:69–71.
17. Yuspa SH, Poirier MC. Chemical carcinogenesis: from animal models to molecular models in one decade. Adv Cancer Res 1988;50:25–70.
18. Balmain A, Harris CC. Carcinogenesis in mouse and human cells: parallels and paradoxes. Carcinogenesis 2000;21:371–7.
19. Hahn WC, Weinberg RA. Modelling the molecular circuitry of cancer. Nature Rev Cancer 2002;2:331–41.
20. Cairns J. Mutation selection and the natural history of cancer. Nature 1975;255:197–200.
21. Balmain A. Cancer genetics: from Boveri and Mendel to microarrays. Nature Rev Cancer 2001;1:77–82.
22. Jones PA, Baylin SB. The fundamental role of epigenetic events in cancer. Nat Rev Genet 2002;3:415–28.
23. Peto R, Roe FJ, Lee PN, et al. Cancer and ageing in mice and men. Br J Cancer 1975;32:411–26.
24. Russo AL, Thiagalingam A, Pan H, et al. Differential DNA hypermethylation of critical genes mediates the stage specific tobacco smoke-induced neoplastic progression of lung cancer. Clin Cancer Res 2005;11:2466–70.
25. Yokota J, Kohno T. Molecular footprints of human lung cancer progression. Cancer Sci 2004;95:197–204.
26. Vogelstein B, Fearon ER, Hamilton SR, et al. Genetic alterations during colorectal-tumor development. N Engl J Med 1988;319:525–32.
27. Neumann HG. Role of extent and persistence of DNA modifications in chemical carcinogenesis by aromatic amines. Recent Results Cancer Res 1983;84:77–89.
28. Poirier MC, Beland FA. DNA adduct measurements and tumor incidence during chronic carcinogen exposure in animal models: implications for DNA adduct-based human cancer risk assessment. Chem Res Toxicol 1992;5:749–55.
29. Poirier MC. Chemical-induced DNA damage and human cancer risk Nature Rev Cancer 2004;4:630–7.
30. Verma AK, Boutwell RK. Effects of dose and duration of treatment with the tumor-promoting agent, 12-O-tetradecanoylphorbol-13-acetate on mouse skin carcinogenesis. Carcinogenesis 1980;1:271–6.
31. Yuspa SH, Dlugosz AA, Denning MF, Glick AB. Multistage carcinogenesis in the skin. J Investigative Dermatol Symp Proc 1996;1:147–50.
32. Birt DF, Kris ES, Choe M, Pelling JC. Dietary energy and fat effects on tumor promotion. Cancer Res 1992;52:2035s–9s.
33. Choe M, Kris ES, Luthra R, et al. Protein kinase C is activated and diacylglycerol is elevated in epidermal cells

from Sencar mice fed high fat diets. J Nutr 1992;122:2322–9.
34. Loeb LA, Cheng KC. Errors in DNA synthesis: a source of spontaneous mutations. Mutat Res 1990;238:297–304.
35. Wogan GN, Hecht SS, Felton JS, et al. Environmental and chemical carcinogenesis. Sem Cancer Biol 2004;14:473–486.
36. Lengauer C, Kinzler KW, Vogelstein B. Genetic instabilities in human cancers. Nature 1998;396:643–9.
37. Perou CM, Sorlie T, Eisen MB, et al. Molecular portraits of human breast tumors. Nature 2000;406:747–52.
38. Ye QH, Qin LX, Forgues M, et al. Predicting hepatitis B virus-positive metastatic hepatocellular carcinomas using gene expression profiling and supervised machine learning. Nat Med 2003;9:416–23.
39. Kinzler KW, Vogelstein B. Lessons from hereditary colorectal cancer. Cell 1996;87:159–70.
40. Levy DB, Smith KJ, Beazer-Barclay Y, et al. Inactivation of both APC alleles in human and mouse tumors. Cancer Res 1994;54:5953–8.
41. Jen J, Powell SM, Papadopoulos N, et al. Molecular determinants of dysplasia in colorectal lesions. Cancer Res 1994;54:5523–6.
42. Luongo C, Moser AR, Gledhill S, Dove WF. Loss of Apc+ in intestinal adenomas from Min mice. Cancer Res 1994;54:5947–52.
43. Prolla TA, Abuin A, Bradley A. DNA mismatch repair deficient mice in cancer research. Semin Cancer Biol 1996;7:241–7.
44. de Wind N, Dekker M, Berns A, et al. Inactivation of the mouse Msh2 gene results in mismatch repair deficiency, methylation tolerance, hyperrecombination, and predisposition to cancer. Cell 1995;82:321–30.
45. Reitmair AH, Schmits R, Ewel A, et al. MSH2-deficient mice are viable and susceptible to lymphoid tumours. Nat Genet 1995;11:64–70.
46. Harris CC. Interindividual variation in human chemical carcinogenesis: implications for risk assessment. In: Moolgavkar SH, editor. Scientific issues in quantitative risk assessment. Berlin: Springer Verlag 1990. p. 235–51.
47. Guengerich FP. Metabolism of chemical carcinogens. Carcinogenesis 2000;21:345–51.
48. Gonzalez FJ. The role of carcinogen-metabolizing enzyme polymorphisms in cancer susceptibility. Reprod Toxicol 1997;11:397–412.
49. Friedberg EC. How nucleotide excision repair protects against cancer. Nature Rev Cancer 2001;1:22–33.
50. Poirier MC, Weston A. DNA Damage, DNA repair and mutagenesis. In: Bertino J, editor. Encyclopedia of cancer. Vol 2. 2nd ed. San Diego: Elsevier Science; 2002. p. 641–9.
51. Keshava C, Frye BL, Wolff MS, et al. Waf-1 (p21) and p53 polymorphisms in breast cancer. Cancer Epidemiol Biomarkers Prev 2002;11:127–30.
52. Weston A, Godbold JH. Polymorphisms of H-ras-1 and p53 in breast cancer and lung cancer: a meta-analysis. Environ Health Perspect 1997;105 Suppl 4:919–26.
53. Phillips DH. Fifty years of benzo(*a*)pyrene. Nature 1983;303:468–72.
54. Kennaway E. The identification of a carcinogenic compound in coal-tar. Br Med J 1955;2:749–52.
55. Guengerich FP. Metabolism of chemical carcinogens. Carcinogenesis 2000;21:345–51.
56. Miller JA. Carcinogenesis by chemicals: an overview—GHA Clowes memorial lecture. Cancer Res 1970;30:559–76.
57. Sims P, Grover PL, Swaisland A, et al. Metabolic activation of benzo(*a*)pyrene proceeds by a diol-epoxide. Nature 1974;252:326–8.
58. Cooper CS, Grover PL, Sims P. The metabolism and activation of benzo[*a*]pyrene. In: Bridges JW, Chasseaud L, editors. Progress in drug metabolism. New York: Wiley; 1983. p. 295–396.
59. Carrier F, Chang CY, Duh JL, et al. Interaction of the regulatory domains of the murine Cyp1a1 gene with two DNA-binding proteins in addition to the Ah receptor and the Ah receptor nuclear translocator (ARNT). Biochem Pharmacol 1994;48:1767–78.
60. Hayashi S, Watanabe J, Nakachi K, et al. Interindividual difference in expression of human Ah receptor and related P450 genes. Carcinogenesis 1994;15:801–6.
61. Nebert DW, Russell DW. Clinical importance of the cytochromes P450. Lancet. 2002;360:1155–62.
62. Stack DE, Cremonesi P, Hanson A, et al. Radical cations of benzo[*a*]pyrene and 6-substituted derivatives: reaction with nucleophiles and DNA. Xenobiotica 1995;25:755–60.
63. Casale GP, Singhal M, Bhattacharya S, et al. Detection and quantification of depurinated benzo[*a*]pyrene-adducted DNA bases in the urine of cigarette smokers and women exposed to household coal smoke. Chem Res Toxicol 2001;14:192–201.
64. Poirier MC, Beland FA. Aromatic amine DNA adduct formation in chronically exposed mice: considerations for human comparison. Mutat Res 1997;376:177–84.
65. Beland FA, Poirier MC. DNA adducts and carcinogenesis. In: Sirica AE, editor. The pathobiology of neoplasia. New York: Plenum; 1989. p. 57–80.
66. Hein DW, Doll MA, Fretland AJ, et al. Molecular genetics and epidemiology of the NAT1 and NAT2 acetylation polymorphisms. Cancer Epidemiol Biomarkers Prev 2000;9:29–42.
67. Butler MA, Iwasaki M, Guengerich FP, Kadlubar FF. Human cytochrome P-450PA (P-450IA2), the phenacetin O-deethylase, is primarily responsible for the hepatic 3-demethylation of caffeine and N-oxidation of carcinogenic arylamines. Proc Natl Acad Sci U S A 1989;86:7696–700.
68. Felton JS, Malfatti MA, Knize MG, et al. Health risks of heterocyclic amines. Mutat Res 1997;376:37–41.
69. Adamson RH. Induction of hepatocellular carcinoma in nonhuman primates by chemical carcinogens. Cancer Detect Prev 1989;14:215–9.
70. Garner RC, Lightfoot TJ, Cupid BC, et al. Comparative biotransformation studies of MeIQx and PhIP in animal models and humans. Cancer Lett 1999;143:161–5.
71. Guengerich FP, Johnson WW, Shimada T, et al. Activation and detoxication of aflatoxin B1. Mutat Res 1998; 402:121–8.
72. Greenblatt MS, Bennett WP, Hollstein M, Harris CC. Mutations in the p53 tumor suppressor gene: clues to cancer etiology and molecular pathogenesis. Cancer Res 1994;54:4855–78.
73. Hecht SS. Approaches to cancer prevention based on an understanding of *N*-nitrosamine carcinogenesis. Proc Soc Exp Biol Med 1997;216:181–91.
74. Hecht SS. Tobacco smoke carcinogens and lung cancer. J Natl Cancer Inst 1999;91:1194–210.
75. Abdollahi M, Ranjbar A, Shadnia S, Nikfar S, Rezaiee A. Pesticides and oxidative stress: a review. Med Sci Monit. 2004;10:141–7.
76. Hussain SP, Hofseth LJ, Harris CC. Radical causes of cancer. Nat Rev Cancer. 2003 ;3:276–85.
77. Singal R, Ginder GD. DNA methylation. Blood 1999;93:4059–70.
78. Schoket B, Papp G, Levay K, et al. Impact of metabolic genotypes on levels of biomarkers of genotoxic exposure. Mutat Res 2001;482:57-69.
79. Salgia R, Skarin AT. Molecular abnormalities in lung cancer. J Clin Oncol 1998;16:1207–17.
80. Rodenhuis S, Slebos RJ. Clinical significance of ras oncogene activation in human lung cancer. Cancer Res 1992;52:2665s–9s.
81. Egner PA, Wang JB, Zhu YR, et al. Chlorophyllin intervention reduces aflatoxin–DNA adducts in individuals at high risk for liver cancer. Proc Natl Acad Sci U S A 2001;98:14601–6.
82. Hertzog PJ, Smith JR, Garner RC. Characterisation of the imidazole ring-opened forms of trans-8,9-dihydro-8,9-dihydro-8-(7-guanyl)9-hydroxy aflatoxin B1. Carcinogenesis 1982;3:723–5.
83. Poulsen HE, Prieme H, Loft S. Role of oxidative DNA damage in cancer initiation and promotion. Eur J Cancer Prev 1998;7:9–16.
84. Reddy JK, Lalwani ND. Carcinogenesis by hepatic peroxisome proliferators: evaluation of the risk of hypolipidemic drugs and industrial plasticizers to humans. CRC Crit Rev Toxicol 1984;12:1–58.
85. Floyd RA, Watson JJ, Harris J, West M, Wong PK. Formation of 8-hydroxydeoxyguanosine, hydroxyl free radical adduct of DNA in granulocytes exposed to the tumor promoter, tetradecanoylphorbol acetate. Biochem Biophys Res Commun 1986;137:841–6.
86. Sved J, Bird A. The expected equilibrium of the CpG dinucleotide in vertebrate genomes under a mutation model. Proc Natl Acad Sci U S A 1990;87:4692–6.
87. Wachsman JT. DNA methylation and the association between genetic and epigenetic changes: relation to carcinogenesis. Mutat Res 1997;375:1–8.
88. Yu Z, Chen J, Ford BN, et al. Human DNA repair systems: an overview. Environ Mol Mutagen 1999;33:3–20.
89. Ronen A, Glickman BW. Human DNA repair genes. Environ Mol Mutagen 2001;37:241–83.
90. Zhou W, Liu G, Miller DP, et al. Gene–environment interaction for the ERCC2 polymorphisms and cumulative cigarette smoking exposure in lung cancer. Cancer Res 2002;62:1377–81.
91. Esteller M, Toyota M, Sanchez-Cespedes M, et al. Inactivation of the DNA repair gene O6-methylguanine-DNA methyltransferase by promoter hypermethylation is associated with G to A mutations in K-ras in colorectal tumorigenesis. Cancer Res 2000;60:2368–71.
92. Lehmann AR. Replication of damaged DNA by translesion synthesis in human cells. FEBS Lett 2005;579:873–6.
93. Ohmori H, Friedberg EC, Fuchs RP, et al. The Y-family of DNA polymerases. Mol Cell. 2001;8:7–8.
94. Loeb LA. Endogenous carcinogenesis: molecular oncology into the twenty-first century—presidential address. Cancer Res 1989;49:5489–96.
95. Nowell PC. The clonal evolution of tumor cell populations. Science 1976;194:23–8.
96. Hollstein M, Hergenhahn M, Yang Q, et al. New approaches to understanding p53 gene tumor mutation spectra. Mutat Res. 1999;431:199–209.
97. Greenblatt MS, Feitelson MA, Zhu M, et al. Integrity of p53 in hepatitis B x antigen-positive and -negative hepatocellular carcinomas. Cancer Res 1997;57:426–32.
98. Olivier M, Eeles R, Hollstein M, et al. The IARC TP53 database: new online mutation analysis and recommendations to users. Hum Mutat 2002;19:607–14.
99. Vogelstein B, Kinzler KW. Cancer genes and the pathways they control. Nat Med 2004;10:789–99.
100. Huang J, Behrens C, Wistuba II, et al. Clonality of combined tumors. Arch Pathol Lab Med 2002;126:437–41.
101. Shin SW, Breathnach OS, Linnoila RI, et al. Genetic changes in contralateral bronchioloalveolar carcinomas of the lung. Oncology 2001;60:81–7.
102. Niho S, Yokose T, Kodama T, et al. Clonal analysis of adenosquamous carcinoma of the lung. Jpn J Cancer Res 1999;90:1244–7.
103. Califano J, Leong PL, Koch WM, et al. Second esophageal tumors in patients with head and neck squamous cell carcinoma: an assessment of clonal relationships. Clin Cancer Res 1999;5:1862–7.
104. van Oijen MG, Leppers VD, Straat FG, et al. The origins of multiple squamous cell carcinomas in the aerodigestive tract. Cancer 2000;88:884–93.
105. Shimizu S, Yatabe Y, Koshikawa T, et al. High frequency of clonally related tumors in cases of multiple synchronous lung cancers as revealed by molecular diagnosis. Clin Cancer Res 2000;6:3994–9.
106. Fearon ER, Vogelstein B. A genetic model for colorectal tumorigenesis. Cell 1990;61:759–67.
107. Vogelstein B, Fearon ER, Hamilton SR, et al. Clonal analysis using recombinant DNA probes from the X-chromosome. Cancer Res 1987;47:4806–13.
108. Cortes J, O'Dwyer ME. Clonal evolution in chronic myelogenous leukemia. Hematol Oncol Clin North Am 2004;18:671-84.
109. Hanahan D, Weinberg RA. The hallmarks of cancer. Cell 2000;100:57–70.
110. Marshall CJ, Vousden KH, Phillips DH. Activation of c-Ha-ras-1 proto-oncogene by in vitro modification with a chemical carcinogen, benzo(*a*)pyrene diol-epoxide. Nature 1984;310:586–9.
111. Harper JR, Roop DR, Yuspa SH. Transfection of the EJ rasHa gene into keratinocytes derived from carcinogen-induced mouse papillomas causes malignant progression. Mol Cell Biol 1986;6:3144–9.
112. Amstad P, Reddel RR, Pfeifer A, et al. Neoplastic transformation of a human bronchial epithelial cell line by a recombinant retrovirus encoding viral harvey *ras*. Mol Carcinog 1988;1:151–60.
113. Reddel RR, Ke Y, Kaighn ME, et al. Human bronchial epithelial cells neoplastically transformed by *v-Ki-ras:* altered response to inducers of terminal squamous differentiation. Oncogene Res 1988;3:401–8.
114. Lane DP. Cancer. p53, guardian of the genome. Nature 1992;358:15–6.
115. Nigro JM, Baker SJ, Preisinger AC, et al. Mutations in the p53 gene occur in diverse human tumor types. Nature 1989;342:705–8.
116. Ponchel F, Puisieux A, Tabone E, et al. Hepatocarcinoma-specific mutant p53-249ser induces mitotic activity but has no effect on transforming growth factor beta 1-mediated apoptosis. Cancer Res 1994;54:2064–8.
117. Brash DE, Rudolph JA, Simon JA, et al. A role for sunlight in skin cancer: UV-induced p53 mutations in squamous cell carcinoma. Proc Natl Acad Sci U S A 1991;88:10124–8.
118. Hainaut P, Pfeifer GP. Patterns of p53 G->T transversions in lung cancers reflect the primary mutagenic signature of

DNA-damage by tobacco smoke. Carcinogenesis 2001;22:367–74.
119. Hill AB. The environment and disease: association or causation. Proc Roy Soc Med 1965;58:295–300.
120. Hussain SP, Harris CC. Molecular epidemiology of human cancer: contribution of mutation spectra studies of tumor suppressor genes. Cancer Res 1998;58:4023–37.
121. Takeshima Y, Seyama T, Bennett WP, et al. p53 mutations in lung cancers from non-smoking atomic-bomb survivors. Lancet 1993;342:1520–1.
122. Denissenko MF, Pao A, Tang M, Pfeifer GP. Preferential formation of benzo[*a*]pyrene adducts at lung cancer mutational hotspots in P53. Science 1996;274:430–2.
123. Klein-Szanto AJ, Iizasa T, Momiki S, et al. A tobacco-specific *N*-nitrosamine or cigarette smoke condensate causes neoplastic transformation of xenotransplanted human bronchial epithelial cells. Proc Natl Acad Sci U S A 1992;89:6693–7.
124. McMichael AJ. Invited commentary—"molecular epidemiology": new pathway or new travelling companion? Am J Epidemiol 1994;140:1-11.
125. Perera FP, Santella R. Carcinogenesis. In: Schulte P, Perera FP, editors. Molecular epidemiology: principles and practices. New York: Academic Press; 1993. p. 277–300.
126. Skipper PL, Peng X, Soohoo CK, Tannenbaum SR. Protein adducts as biomarkers of human carcinogen exposure. Drug Metab Rev 1994;26:111–24.
127. Duhachek SD, Kenseth JR, Casale GP, et al. Monoclonal antibody—gold biosensor chips for detection of depurinating carcinogen—DNA adducts by fluorescence line-narrowing spectroscopy. Anal Chem 2000;72:3709–16.
128. Groopman JD, Kensler TW. The light at the end of the tunnel for chemical-specific biomarkers: daylight or head-light? Carcinogenesis 1999;20:1–11.
129. Kensler TW, Egner PA, Wang JB, et al. Chemoprevention of hepatocellular carcinoma in aflatoxin endemic areas. Gastroenterology 2004;127:S310–8.
130. Romkes M, Buch SC. Genotyping technologies: application to biotransformation enzyme genetic polymorphism screening. Methods Mol Biol 2005;291:399–414.
131. Nair U, Bartsch H. Metabolic polymorphisms as susceptibility markers for lung and oral cavity cancer. IARC Sci Publ 2001;154:271–90.
132. Bouchardy C, Benhamou S, Jourenkova N, et al. Metabolic genetic polymorphisms and susceptibility to lung cancer. Lung Cancer 2001;32:109–12.
133. Wormhoudt LW, Commandeur JN, Vermeulen NP. Genetic polymorphisms of human *N*-acetyltransferase, cytochrome P450, glutathione-S-transferase, and epoxide hydrolase enzymes: relevance to xenobiotic metabolism and toxicity. Crit Rev Toxicol 1999;29:59–124.
134. Miller DP, Liu G, De Vivo I, et al. Combinations of the variant genotypes of GSTP1, GSTM1, and p53 are associated with an increased lung cancer risk. Cancer Res 2002;62:2819–23.
135. Hengstler JG, Arand M, Herrero ME, Oesch F. Polymorphisms of *N*-acetyltransferases, glutathione-*S*-transferases, microsomal epoxide hydrolase and sulfotransferases: influence on cancer susceptibility. Recent Results Cancer Res 1998;154:47–85.
136. Geisler SA, Olshan AF. GSTM1, GSTT1, and the risk of squamous cell carcinoma of the head and neck: a mini-HuGE review. Am J Epidemiol 2001;154:95–105.
137. Bock KW, Gschaidmeier H, Heel H, et al. Functions and transcriptional regulation of PAH-inducible human UDP-glucuronosyltransferases. Drug Metab Rev 1999;31:411–22.
138. Benhamou S, Sarasin A. ERCC2 /XPD gene polymorphisms and lung cancer: a HuGE review. Am J Epidemiol 2005;161:1–14.
139. Benhamou S, Sarasin A. ERCC2/XPD gene polymorphisms and cancer risk. Mutagenesis 2002;17:463–9.
140. Neumann AS, Sturgis EM, Wei Q. Nucleotide excision repair as a marker for susceptibility to tobacco-related cancers: a review of molecular epidemiological studies. Mol Carcinog 2005;42:65–92.
141. Li G, Wang LE, Chamberlain RM, et al. p73 G4C14-to-A4T14 polymorphism and risk of lung cancer. Cancer Res 2004;64:6863–6.
142. Wu X, Zhao H, Amos CI, et al. p53 Genotypes and haplotypes associated with lung cancer susceptibility and ethnicity. J Natl Cancer Inst 2002;94:681–90.
143. Zhang YJ, Chen SY, Chen CJ, Santella RM. Polymorphisms in cyclin D1 gene and hepatocellular carcinoma. Mol Carcinog 2002;33:125–9.
144. Furberg AH, Ambrosone CB. Molecular epidemiology, biomarkers and cancer prevention. Trends Mol Med 2001;7:517–21.
145. Shih W, Chetty R, Tsao MS. Expression profiling by microarrays in colorectal cancer. Oncol Rep 2005;13:517–24.
146. Harris CC. The 1995 Walter Hubert lecture—molecular epidemiology of human cancer: insights from the mutational analysis of the p53 tumor suppressor gene. Br J Cancer 1996;73:261–9.
147. Cutilli T, Papola F, Di Emidio P, Corbacelli A. p53 tumor suppressor protein and H-RAS oncogene in maxillofacial tumors: immunohistochemical and genetic investigation, induction chemotherapy response and prognosis evaluation. J Chemother 1998;10:411–7.
148. Kandioler-Eckersberger D, Kappel S, Mittlbock M, et al. The TP53 genotype but not immunohistochemical result is predictive of response to cisplatin-based neoadjuvant therapy in stage III non-small cell lung cancer. J Thorac Cardiovasc Surg 1999;117:744–50.
149. Kodish ED. Testing children for cancer genes: the rule of earliest onset. J Pediatr 1999;135:390–5.
150. Poirier MC, Beland FA. Aromatic amine DNA adduct formation in chronically exposed mice: considerations for human comparison. Mutat Res 1997;376:177–84.
151. DeMarini DM, Landi S, Tian D, et al. Lung tumor KRAS and TP53 mutations in nonsmokers reflect exposure to PAH-rich coal combustion emissions. Cancer Res 2001;61:6679–81.

15

Hormones and the Etiology of Cancer

Leslie Bernstein, PhD
C. Leigh Pearce, PhD
Ronald K. Ross, MD
Brian E. Henderson, MD

Substantial and convincing bodies of experimental, clinical, and epidemiologic evidence indicate that hormones play a major role in the etiology of several human cancers. The concept that hormones can increase the incidence of neoplasia was first proposed by Bittner[1] on the basis of experimental studies of estrogens and mammary cancer in mice. This theory has been refined into epidemiologic hypotheses related to cancers of the breast, endometrium, prostate, ovary, thyroid, bone, and testis.[2,3] The underlying mechanism proposed for all of these cancers is that neoplasia is the consequence of prolonged hormonal stimulation of the particular target organ, the normal growth and function of which is controlled by one or more steroid or polypeptide hormones. Evidence is mounting to show that the amount of hormone to which a tissue is effectively exposed is under strong genetic control.[4] Therefore, although external factors such as diet or exogenous hormone use may modify hormone profiles, the current evidence supports a multigenic model of cancer susceptibility, where sequence variants in genes encoding proteins involved in steroid–hormone biosynthesis, metabolism or intracellular signaling and transport, and deoxyribonucleic acid (DNA) binding, repair, and transactivation are also important determinants of individual cancer risk.[4,5]

The major carcinogenic consequence of this hormonal exposure at the end organ is cellular proliferation. The emergence of a malignant phenotype depends on a series of somatic mutations that occur during cell division, but the entire sequence of genes involved in progression from normal cell to a particular malignant phenotype is not known (Figure 15-1). Candidate genes include those in the endocrine and growth factor pathways,[4–6] as well as DNA repair genes, tumor-suppressor genes, and oncogenes.[7,8] Germline mutations have been described in two such tumor-suppressor genes, *BRCA1* and *BRCA2*, which are associated with susceptibility to breast cancer in certain kindreds.[9,10] Germline mutations in *TP53* are also associated in certain kindreds with an increased risk of breast cancer.[11] However, mutations in these genes do not appear to be involved in the majority of sporadic breast cancer. The *HER2/neu* oncogene is overexpressed in advanced breast cancer, is associated with poor prognosis, and probably represents one critical event in the latter part of breast cancer progression.[12]

Neoplasia of hormone-responsive tissues currently accounts for more than 35% of all newly diagnosed male and almost 50% of all newly diagnosed female cancers in the United States. Given that endogenous hormones apparently affect the risk of these cancers and their overall frequency, concern exists about the effects on cancer risk if the same or closely related hormones are administered for therapeutic purposes (eg, as contraceptives, as hormone replacement therapy, or for the prevention of miscarriage).[13] This chapter focuses on breast, endometrial, and ovarian cancers among women and prostate cancer among men and provides a review of the epidemiologic and endocrinologic evidence for the role of hormones in cancer development. It also reviews the current status of the relationship between exogenous hormones and risk of cancers of the breast, endometrium, and ovary. Other less common cancers, cervical cancer, clear cell vaginal adenocarcinoma, thyroid cancer, testicular cancer, and osteosarcoma, appear to have a hormonal basis as well, but these have not been reviewed here.

BREAST CANCER

Breast cancer is the most common cancer in women and is estimated to have accounted for 211,240 new cancer diagnoses and 40,410 deaths in 2005.[14] A perceptible decline in breast cancer mortality has occurred since 1992,[15,16] most likely the result of therapy with tamoxifen and other newer forms of chemotherapy, including therapy that targets *HER2/neu*.[17] Available evidence regarding the hormonal etiology of breast cancer is most consistent with the hypothesis that estrogen is the primary stimulant for breast cell proliferation.[2,3] The simultaneous presence of progesterone further increases the rate of prolifer-

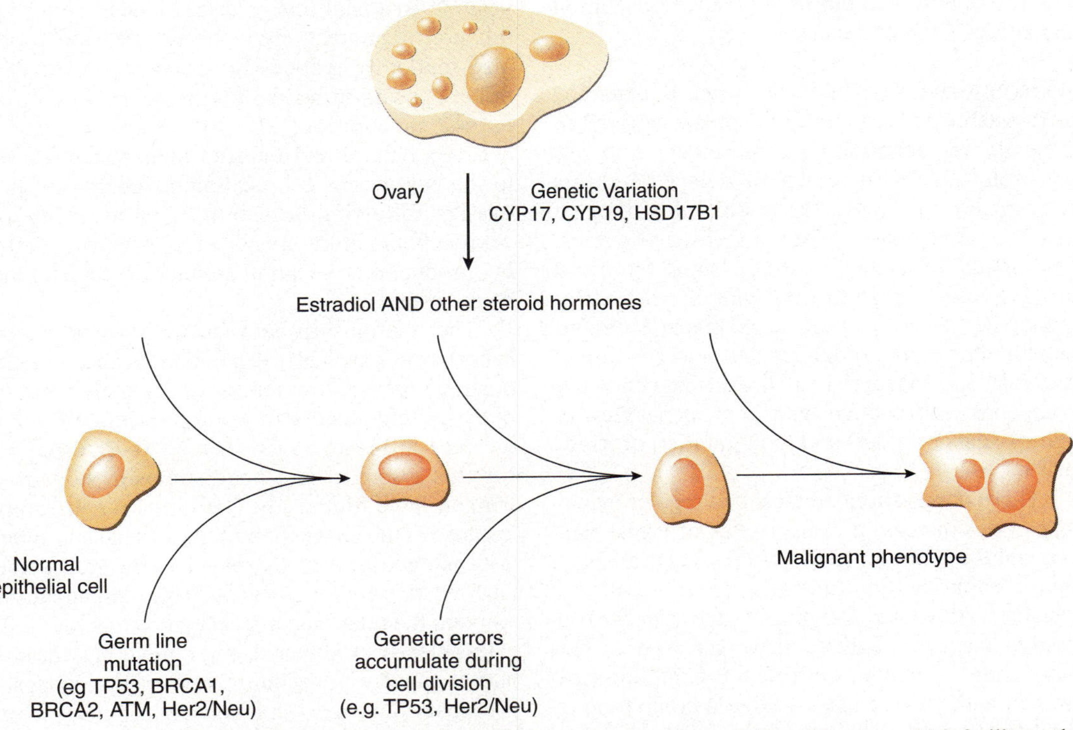

Figure 15-1 Estradiol and other steroid hormones (eg, progesterone) drive breast cell proliferation, which facilitates the accumulation of random DNA copying errors in critical genes on the pathway to a malignant phenotype. Germline mutations in relevant tumor-suppressor genes accelerate the transformation to the malignant phenotype.

Table 15-1 A Summary of Established Hormonal Risk and Protective Factors for Breast Cancer

Risk Factors (increased exposure to estrogen and/or progesterone)
Early menarche
Obesity (postmenopausal women)
Hormone replacement therapy
Protective Factors (reduced exposure to estrogen and/or progesterone)
Lactation
Early age at full-term pregnancy
Physical activity (exercise)

ation.[18] This latter conclusion is based largely on the fact that breast mitotic activity peaks during the luteal phase of the menstrual cycle[19] and is consistent with the increasing number of publications demonstrating that added progestins substantially augment the increased risk of breast cancer from estrogen therapy.[20–24]

The most consistently documented, hormonally related risk factors for breast cancer are early age at menarche, late age at menopause, late age at first full-term pregnancy, and weight (Table 15-1). The age incidence curve for breast cancer emphasizes the importance of ovulation in determining risk.[13] Cases first occur during early adulthood, and the rate of increase in incidence then rises sharply with age until the time of menopause, when it slows dramatically. The rate of increase in the postmenopausal period is approximately one-sixth the rate of increase in the premenopausal period. This age incidence curve appears, then, to be shaped in a major way by the effects of ovarian activity. Therefore, it is critical to understand the determinants, both genetic and environmental, of the onset, regularity, and cessation of ovulation in order to continue to develop effective prevention modalities for breast cancer.

Reproductive Factors Early age at menarche is an established risk factor for breast cancer.[3] In general, risk decreases approximately 5 to 6% for each year that menarche is delayed and this relationship may be further modified by the age at onset of regular ovulatory menstrual cycles. In a study of young women, Henderson and colleagues[25] reported that women with early menarche (ie, age 12 years or younger) and rapid establishment of regular cycles had an almost fourfold increased risk of breast cancer when compared with women with later menarche (ie, age 13 years or older) and long duration of irregular cycles.

These observations suggest that regular ovulatory cycles increase a woman's risk of breast cancer, and they support results from an earlier study that compared circulating hormone levels in daughters of women with breast cancer with those in age-matched daughters of women who do not have breast cancer (controls).[26] Daughters of women with breast cancer, who as a group have at least twice the breast cancer risk of the general population, have higher levels of circulating estrogen and progesterone than daughters of controls.

Although menarche and the onset of ovulation are to some extent genetically determined,[27] it is also critical to establish behaviors that may alter the cumulative number of lifetime ovulatory menstrual cycles. Strenuous physical activity may delay menarche. Adolescent girls who engage in regular ballet dancing, swimming, or running experience a considerable delay in the onset of menses.[28] For example, in one study, ballet dancers had a mean age at menarche of 15.4 years, as compared with 12.5 years for controls. Moderate physical activity during adolescence can lead to anovular menstrual cycles. Girls who engaged in regular, moderate physical activity (averaging at least 600 Kcal of energy expended per week during a 9-month school year) were 2.9 times more likely to be anovular than were girls who engaged in lesser amounts of physical activity.[29] Bernstein and colleagues have reported that lifetime patterns of leisure-time exercise activity significantly impact the risk of breast cancer in both young women (< 40 years of age)[30] and older, postmenopausal women (55–64 years of age).[31] Evidence continues to accumulate in support of a protective effect of physical activity on breast cancer risk with risk reductions observed in both case control and cohort studies, although studies do vary according to the subgroups of women who benefit the most.[32,33]

In the same way that early onset of menarche and regular ovulation equate with a greater cumulative lifetime exposure to estrogen and risk of breast cancer, late occurrence of menopause and extended exposure to ovulatory cycles at the end of menstrual life also increase risk. The breast cancer risk of women whose natural menopause occurs before age 45 years is one-half that of women whose menopause occurs after age 55 years.[34] Artificial menopause, induced either by bilateral oophorectomy or by pelvic irradiation, also markedly reduces breast cancer risk; this effect appears to be slightly greater than that of natural menopause. This difference in impact between natural and induced menopause relates to the continuing, but declining, function of the ovaries following cessation of menses among women with natural menopause and the continuing production of a small amount of testosterone by the ovaries.

The relationship between weight and breast cancer risk is critically dependent on age. Among postmenopausal women, a 10 kg increment in body weight results in an approximately 80% increase in breast cancer risk.[35] An explanation for this effect is that heavier postmenopausal women have higher circulating estrogen levels because of the conversion of the adrenal androgen androstenedione to estrone by the aromatase enzyme present in body fat. In premenopausal women, the relationship between weight and risk is less clearly established, but, if anything, the situation appears to be the reverse of that in postmenopausal women (ie, high weight appears to be associated with reduced risk).[36] This may result from the reduced frequency of ovulatory menstrual cycles associated with high body weight.

Assuming ovarian activity affects breast cancer risk, case control and cohort studies of breast cancer should find higher levels of circulating estradiol among breast cancer patients than among healthy women. Bernstein and colleagues[37] described the results of two concurrent case control studies of premenopausal women in the United States (Los Angeles) and China (Shanghai). Overall, breast cancer patients had 14% higher serum estradiol concentrations, with a case-to-control excess of 17% in Chinese women and 11% in white American women. Los Angeles control women had 21% greater estradiol concentrations than did Shanghai control women, and adjustment for body weight only accounted for 25% of this difference. The results from a pooled analysis of nine prospective studies of endogenous hormones and postmenopausal breast cancer risk provide strong evidence that high estradiol concentrations are predictive of breast cancer risk;[38] women in the highest quintile of exposure have twice the risk of breast cancer as those who are in the lowest exposure quintile. Considering free estradiol, the bioavailable fraction that circulates in blood, women in the highest quintile of exposure have more than 2.5 times the risk of breast cancer as those in the lowest quintile.

Age at First Birth An early age at first birth (ie, before age 20 years) protects against breast cancer, reducing a woman's risk by about 50% relative to nulliparous women. Full-term pregnancies at later ages add smaller increments of protection.[39] Women who have a very late first full-term pregnancy actually are at a higher risk of breast cancer than are nulliparous women. This paradoxical effect of a late first full-term pregnancy has been repeatedly confirmed by epidemiologic studies. Furthermore, a recent full-term pregnancy increases risk. Among women giving birth during the previous 3 years, breast cancer risk is nearly three times higher than that of women of the same age, parity, and age at first birth whose most recent birth occurred at least 10 years earlier.

On the basis of these results, it appears that a first pregnancy confers two contradictory effects on risk of breast cancer: a short-term increase in risk, followed in the long term by a substantial reduction in risk.[40] This apparent paradox has a physiologic explanation based on patterns of estrogen as well as prolactin secretion and metabolism during pregnancy. During the first trimester, the level of bioavailable estradiol rapidly rises, an effect that is more apparent during the first than in subsequent pregnancies.[41] Thus, in terms of estrogen exposure to the breast, the net effect during this early part of pregnancy is an increased risk that is equivalent to the exposure from several ovulatory cycles over a relatively short period of time. In the long run, however, this negative effect of early pregnancy on risk of breast cancer can be overridden by two beneficial hormonal consequences of completing the pregnancy. It has been reported that prolactin levels are substantially lower in parous compared with nulliparous women.[42,43] Prolactin, a polypeptide hormone, regulates lactation and appears to enhance estrogen effects on breast tissue. In addition, parous women have been reported to have lower levels of bioavailable estradiol than their nulliparous counterparts.[44] At a molecular level, it is likely that the hormonal changes during pregnancy induce irreversible differentiation and apoptosis in some cells that have already accumulated one or more of the relevant somatic mutations necessary for breast cancer development.

Evidence is fairly convincing that lactation reduces the risk of breast cancer among premenopausal women,[45–47] but is less consistent for postmenopausal women.[46,48] In two publications, Enger and colleagues showed substantial breast cancer risk reductions for parous premenopausal and postmenopausal women who breast-fed for more than 15 months (35% reduction for premenopausal women and 30% reduction for postmenopausal women relative to similar women who never lactated).[45,48] The reason some studies may have not observed protective effects of lactation could be due to the small proportion of women with sufficient lactation experience. Among premenopausal and postmenopausal women in Shanghai, who had extensive lactation histories, a strong dose-response effect of decreasing breast cancer risk with increasing breast-feeding duration was observed.[49] Variations in the time when supplementary feedings are introduced to the infant as well as the frequency and duration of each breast-feeding episode may also contribute to the inconsistent findings. Lactation would be expected to reduce breast cancer risk by reducing the cumulative number of ovulatory menstrual cycles a woman experiences because breast-feeding results in a substantial delay in reestablishing ovulation following a completed pregnancy.

Diet Much attention has been focused on dietary differences, particularly fat consumption, to explain both the international pattern of breast cancer occurrence and changes in rates of breast cancer following migration to high-risk, usually Western nations from low-risk countries.[50] International breast cancer mortality rates correlate highly with per capita consumption of fat in the diet (correlation coefficient, $r = .93$). When international breast cancer incidence rates rather than mortality rates are considered, the magnitude of the correlation coefficient is still very high ($r = .84$).[50] As implied previously, nutrition likely influences breast cancer occurrence by modifying age at menarche and body weight, but the correlation of fat consumption with international breast cancer mortality remains highly significant, even after statistical adjustment for those factors.

Many case control studies of fat consumption and breast cancer have found only small differences between cases and controls, generally no larger than the differences in total caloric consumption. Similarly, most of the cohort studies that have used food-frequency questionnaires to study the relationship with either total fat, saturated fat, or vegetable fat have found little or no difference in breast cancer risk over a wide range of fat uptake.[51,52]

High-fiber diets may protect against breast cancer, perhaps because fiber reduces the intestinal reabsorption of estrogens excreted via the biliary system.[53] Assessment of fiber intake in epidemiologic studies has been problematic because of a paucity of data on the fiber content of individual foods and disagreement about the most appropriate methods of biochemical analysis to determine the different types of fiber.

Several investigations have been undertaken to demonstrate a reduction in serum estrogen levels following dietary interventions that reduce fat or increase fiber intake.[54] A recent meta-analysis of these studies demonstrated a 7.4% average reduction in estradiol levels of premenopausal women and a 23% reduction in postmenopausal women following trials of reduced dietary fat intake.[54] This analysis could not distinguish between a direct dietary effect on hormone levels and an indirect effect that was due to disruption of ovulatory cycles in premenopausal women; nevertheless, whatever the mechanism, such a reduction in estradiol levels is potentially very important.

Exogenous Hormones Hormone therapy and oral contraceptives are the exogenous counterparts to endogenous hormonal exposures experienced by women and, therefore, are of concern as potential contributors to breast cancer risk.

Oral Contraceptives The relationship of oral contraceptive use to breast cancer risk has been the topic of many review articles. A combined analysis of 54 studies that included more than 150,000 women has provided many important answers about the risk of breast cancer among users of combination oral contraceptives, that is, oral contraceptives that provide estrogen and progestin in combination in a single pill.[55] This analysis indicates that a modest increased risk of breast cancer is observed among current (relative risk [RR] = 1.24) and recent (RR = 1.16) combination oral contraceptive users. Age at first combination oral contraceptive use modifies the association with recent use. For recent users, the risks are highest for those who began combination oral contraceptive use before the age of 20 years. However, total duration of combination oral contraceptive use was not associated with increased risk of breast cancer, once recency of use was taken into account.

The pooled analysis compiled studies that mainly focused on younger women, since most of these studies were conducted at a time when oral contraceptive users had not achieved their perimenopausal and postmenopausal years. The Women's Contraceptive and Reproductive Experiences (Women's CARE) Study, a population-based case control study conducted in 5 geographic regions of the United States,[56] involved more than 4,500 newly diagnosed breast cancer patients and more than 4,500 control subjects who were between the ages of 35 and 64 years. It was specifically designed to assess the impact of oral contraceptives among women who were no longer using oral contraceptives. Relatively few participants in the Women's CARE Study were current oral contraceptive users; many of the women had stopped use at least 20 years earlier. No significant associations were observed between duration of use, estrogen dose of the formulation, age at first use, interval since last use, or use in relation to timing of pregnancy and breast cancer risk. Further, results for younger women (35–44 years) were similar to those for older women (45–64 years), who were more likely to have used earlier formulations but were less likely to have recently used oral contraceptives.

An announcement of a recent International Agency for Research on Cancer review of the existing literature on combination oral contraceptives and breast cancer risk has been published, although the complete analysis is not yet available; this review concludes that breast cancer risk is slightly increased in current or recent oral contraceptive users and that this increase in risk disappears 10 years after oral contraceptive use has ceased.[57]

Hormone Therapy Hormone therapy has evolved over time. Originally designed to reduce the symptoms of menopause, hormone therapy gained popularity because of its efficacy in reducing the risk of osteoporosis and its purported benefits in reducing the risk of heart disease. Initially formulated as estrogen therapy, the number of women using hormone therapy increased through the mid-1970s, when concerns were raised about the carcinogenic potential of estrogen therapy on the endometrium. In the 1980s, cyclic estrogen-progestin regimens became widely recommended and prescribed to eliminate the increase in endometrial cancer associated with estrogen-alone therapy. Initially, these were prescribed as sequential regimens with estrogen given during the first 15 to 20 days of a 28-day cycle followed by 5 to 10 days when both estrogen and progestin were given. More recently, continuous combined regimens have gained favor because they reduce menstrual-like bleeding episodes and because of their ease of administration.

Most studies that have included sufficiently large numbers of women who have used estrogen therapy for extended periods of time (eg, for more than 10 years) indicate a modest increase in breast cancer risk among exposed women, with risk increasing approximately 3% per year of use.[58] Among studies conducted in the United States, where the use of conjugated equine estrogens is the norm, early estimates were that breast cancer risk increased about 2.2% per year of use of a standard dosage regimen (0.625 mg/day).

The Collaborative Group on Hormonal Factors in Breast Cancer pooled data from 51 epidemiologic studies and more than 160,000 women to assess the impact of hormone therapy on breast cancer risk.[59] Where information was available regarding type of hormone preparation used, 80% of women in these studies had used mostly estrogen-only therapy, and 12% of women had used combination hormone therapy. This study showed that

A. Cancers localized to breast

Duration of use and time since last use	Cases/Controls	RR(FSE)*
Never-user	2717/23568	1.00 (0.033)
Last use < 5 years before diagnosis		
Duration < 1 year	99/860	1.09 (0.159)
Duration 1–4 years	288/2037	1.32 (0.110)
Duration 5–9 years	192/1279	1.67 (0.155)
Duration > 10 years	196/1147	1.42 (0.146)
Last use > 5 years before diagnosis		
Duration < 1 year	109/890	1.12 (0.151)
Duration 1–4 years	174/1256	1.13 (0.117)
Duration > 5 years	97/607	1.23 (0.173)

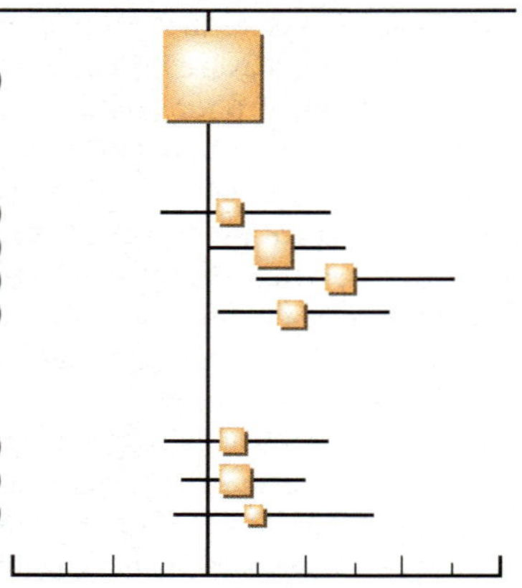

RR and 99% FCI* (axis: 0 0.5 1.0 1.5 2.0 2.5)

B. Cancers spread beyond breast

Duration of use and time since last use	Cases/Controls	RR(FSE)*
Never-user	2101/23568	1.00 (0.039)
Last use < 5 years before diagnosis		
Duration < 1 year	58/860	0.68 (0.146)
Duration 1–4 years	184/2037	0.90 (0.108)
Duration 5–9 years	119/1279	1.04 (0.141)
Duration > 10 years	130/1147	1.25 (0.164)
Last use > 5 years before diagnosis		
Duration < 1 year	68/890	1.01 (0.171)
Duration 1–4 years	108/1256	1.08 (0.143)
Duration > 5 years	47/607	0.88 (0.189)

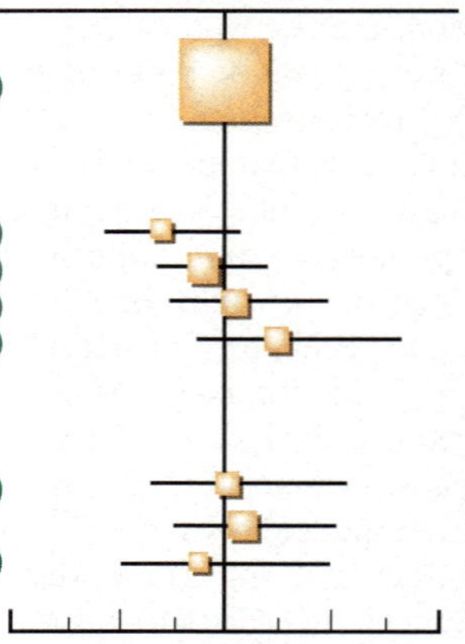

RR and 99% FCI* (axis: 0 0.5 1.0 1.5 2.0)

Figure 15-2 Relative risk of breast cancer by duration and time since last use of hormone therapy according to extent of tumor spread relative to never-users, stratified by study, age at diagnosis, time since menopause, body mass index, parity, and the age of a woman when her first child was born. "Last use within 5 years before diagnosis" includes current users. *Floated standard errors (FTE) and confidence intervals (FCI) calculated from floated variance for each category.

hormone therapy (primarily estrogen therapy) increased breast cancer risk with RRs of 1.09, 1.15, and 1.14, comparing ever users to never users in cohort studies, population-based case control studies, and hospital-based case control studies, respectively. Risk was substantially elevated among women who had used hormone therapy for at least 15 years (RR = 1.58). Risk increased by 2.3% ($p = .0002$) for each year of use among women who had used hormone therapy within 5 years of diagnosis or an equivalent reference date (Figure 15-2). However, women who stopped hormone therapy use 5 or more years earlier had only a modest, nonsignificant increase in risk, regardless of duration of use.

Consistent with these estimates are the results from the Million Women Study, conducted in the United Kingdom, which recruited a cohort of women aged 50 to 64 years who had undergone routine mammography.[60] In this study, incidence of breast cancer was significantly greater among current users of estrogen therapy than among women who had never used hormones (RR = 1.30, 95% Confidence Interval [CI] = 1.22–1.38). Risk increased with increasing duration of use among these current estrogen therapy users, with 5 to 9 years of use associated with an RR of 1.32 and 10 or more years of use associated with an RR of 1.37.

The Women's Health Initiative randomized trial compared an estrogen-alone regimen to placebo among women 50 to 79 years of age who had previously had a hysterectomy and assessed the impact of a combined estrogen plus progestin regimen versus placebo among women 50 to 79 years of age who had an intact uterus. The estrogen-alone regimen consisted of 0.625 mg per day of conjugated equine estrogen,[61] and the combined regimen consisted of 0.625 mg per day of conjugated equine estrogen and 2.5 mg per day of medroxyprogesterone acetate.[23] The results for the estrogen therapy study were somewhat surprising in that, after an average follow-up of 6.8 years, the RR of breast cancer was not elevated (RR = 0.77, 95% CI = 0.59–1.01).[61]

For combined hormone therapy, the Women's Health Initiative assessed only the continuous combined regimen. Three population-based observational studies, published in 1999 and 2000, showed that a combined regimen conferred a greater risk of breast cancer than did an estrogen-alone regimen.[20,21,62] For example, Ross and colleagues found that the increment in risk of each 5 years of use was nearly four times greater for combined hormone therapy users than for estrogen therapy users.[21] Results from the Women's Health Initiative trial arm comparing a continuous combined hormone regimen with placebo provided a risk estimate that was similar to those from these prior studies (RR = 1.24, 95% CI = 1.01–1.54).[23]

Lee and colleagues[24] conducted a meta-analysis of the results of studies that have evaluated the impact of combined hormone therapy on breast cancer risk, separating results for use of sequential (cyclic) combined regimens from those for use of continuous combined regimens and including results from the Collaborative Group on Hormonal Factors in Breast Cancer[59] and the Women's Health Initiative.[23] Overall, users of a combined regimen had substantially elevated risk, with risk increasing 7.6% per year of use.[24] Not all studies provided data on progestin schedule. Those that did showed a small difference in risk between sequential and continuous combined regimens (increase in breast cancer risk per year of use of 8.9% and 10.3%, respectively). Notably, results from Scandinavian studies showed that continuous regimens had a greater impact on risk than sequential regimens. This difference was not as apparent among studies from the United States or the Million Women Study. In the United States, the total dose of progestin is similar in continuous combined compared with sequential regimens, whereas in Scandinavia, continuous combined regimens provide a substantially higher dose of progestin. Thus, evidence is quite strong that the progestin component of combined regimens adds substantially to any increase in breast cancer risk conferred by estrogen alone and that differences in results between the United States and Scandinavia are likely due to differences in the progestin dose administered.

ENDOMETRIAL CANCER

Among the hormone-related cancers, etiologically the best understood is endometrial cancer. All the major demographic characteristics of the disease, as well as the major nondemographic risk factors, are explicable on the basis of cumulative exposure of the endometrium to that fraction of estrogen that is unopposed by the modifying influences of progesterone.[2,3]

Mitotic Activity in the Endometrium Key and Pike summarized the existing data on endometrial mitotic activity during normal menstrual cycles.[63] Mitotic rates are low during days 1 to 4 of the cycle, then increase rapidly and remain stable thereafter until day 19, after which rates essentially drop to zero for the remainder of the cycle. There appears to be a lag period of about 4 days before the full stimulatory effects of unopposed estrogen or the modifying influence of progesterone on endometrial mitotic activity are fully apparent.

The cellular basis for the antiestrogenic activity of progestogens on the endometrium is well understood.[2] Progestogens reduce the concentration of estradiol receptors and increase the activity of the 17-β-hydroxysteroid dehydrogenase type II enzyme, which converts estradiol to estrone,[64,65] a biologically less-potent estrogen because of its lower affinity for cellular estrogen receptors. Luteal phase progesterone causes endometrial cells to differentiate to a secretory

Table 15-2 A Summary of Established Hormonal Risk and Protective Factors for Endometrial Cancer

Risk Factors (increased exposure to "unopposed" estrogen)
Estrogen replacement therapy
Obesity
Sequential oral contraceptives
Late menopause
Protective Factors (decreased exposure to "unopposed" estrogen)
Pregnancy
Combination oral contraceptives

state, and progestogen withdrawal leads to cyclic sloughing of endometrial tissue.

On the basis of the concept that frequency of mitotic activity is the primary determinant of endometrial cancer risk and that such activity is controlled by cumulative exposure to unopposed estrogens, one can readily predict the most important risk factors for this disease (Table 15-2). Pregnancies and oral contraceptives, which expose the endometrium to constant high levels of both estrogen and progestogen, should protect against endometrial cancer development. Estrogen therapy and obesity should increase the risk. All of these predicted effects have been repeatedly well documented in epidemiologic studies.[2]

Estrogen Therapy Hormone therapy in the form of unopposed estrogen therapy gained widespread popularity in the United States during the 1960s and 1970s.[66] Concomitant with this increasing usage, incidence rates of endometrial cancer in postmenopausal women also increased rapidly, especially on the West Coast, where use of estrogen therapy was particularly common.[67] By 1975, the results of epidemiologic case control studies, demonstrating a strong overall association between estrogen therapy and risk of endometrial cancer, were being published.[68,69] Literally dozens of studies have now documented a high relative increase in the risk of endometrial cancer following estrogen therapy. Risk is strongly related both to dose and duration of use, but high relative increments in risk follow even moderate doses taken for moderately long periods of time. Women who use estrogen therapy for 5 years or longer have approximately a 3.5-fold increase in risk compared with that of women who have never used such therapy (Figure 15-3A).[13]

Although use of estrogen clearly increases the incidence of aggressive endometrial cancer, the overall mortality from endometrial cancer among affected users somewhat paradoxically is much lower than among nonusers who develop endometrial cancer.[70] In fact, such women have little reduction in life span when compared with healthy women of the same age. The reasons for this are not completely known, but this phenomenon likely can be explained by the increased medical surveillance among estrogen users. Women who use estrogen therapy tend to be closely monitored because the drug frequently induces vaginal bleeding. Part of the favorable survival experience may also result from patients with estrogen-induced benign hyperplasia being misdiagnosed as having endometrial cancer. Although past users of estrogen therapy have a risk of endometrial cancer that is intermediate between that for current users of comparable duration and lifetime nonusers, risk in such women remains substantially elevated over baseline even after many years without treatment.[71]

As noted above, the newer regimens of hormone therapy typically follow one of two patterns. They either provide a sequence of estrogen and estrogen plus progestin like that of sequential oral contraceptives, or estrogen and progestin are given together daily throughout the cycle. The sequential regimen attempts to reproduce the hormonal pattern of the normal menstrual cycle, albeit at lower levels, of both estrogen and progestogen. One, therefore, might predict that this method of hormone therapy administration would only partially offset the increased risk of endometrial cancer that is associated with unopposed estrogen therapy. Pike and colleagues showed that if progestins are added for less than 10 days per month, the risk is only slightly reduced.[72] However, regimens that include progestins for more than 10 days in a month, or where progestins are given continuously with estrogen, do not increase risk of endometrial cancer.[72]

Some of the most recent data on this issue come from the Million Women Study conducted in Great Britain, which included 716,738 postmenopausal women without prior cancer or hysterectomy who were recruited between 1996 and 2001.[73] Relative to women who had never used any hormonal therapy, endometrial cancer risk was substantially lower among women who had used continuous combined therapy as their most recent hormone therapy with an RR of 0.71 (95% CI = 0.56–0.90). For women using cyclic combined hormone therapy, however, risk did not differ from that of nonusers (RR = 1.05, 95% CI = 0.92–1.22). The number of cases among women taking estrogen-alone therapy was small, as this has rarely been given to women with an intact uterus since the mid-to-late 1970s. Among women on estrogen-alone therapy, the RR of endometrial cancer was substantially lower than prior studies had observed (RR = 1.45, 95% CI = 1.02–2.06). As expected, based on the fact that obesity increases endometrial cancer risk through an estrogen pathway causing endometrial proliferation,[63,74] the impact of combined therapy was greatest among obese women, and the impact of estrogen-alone therapy was greatest among nonobese women.

In reporting results of the Million Women Study, the authors also provided an extensive assessment of the literature on the impact of combined hormone therapy on endometrial cancer risk, calculating a summary estimate of RR comparing users to nonusers of continuous combined therapy and cyclic combined therapy across studies with published data and including their own study.[73] Overall, they estimated that the RR for continuous combined hormone therapy across all studies was 0.88 (95% CI = 0.75–1.03) compared with never users. This estimate, however, was based on relatively few cases, with only 265 cases identified across 6 studies, including the Women's Health Initiative.[75] In the meta-analysis included in the Million Women Study publication,[73] the estimated RR of endometrial cancer associated

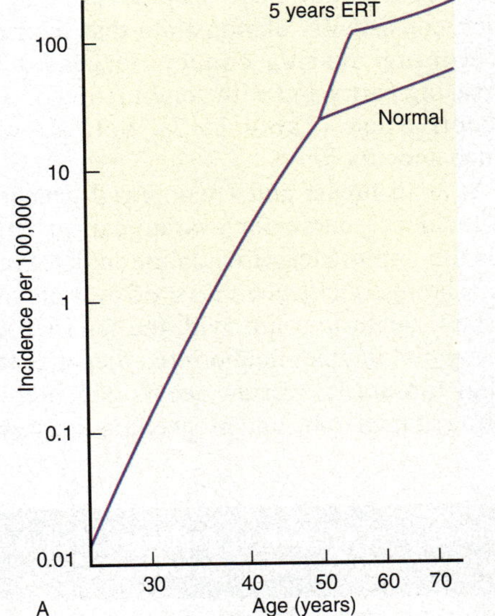

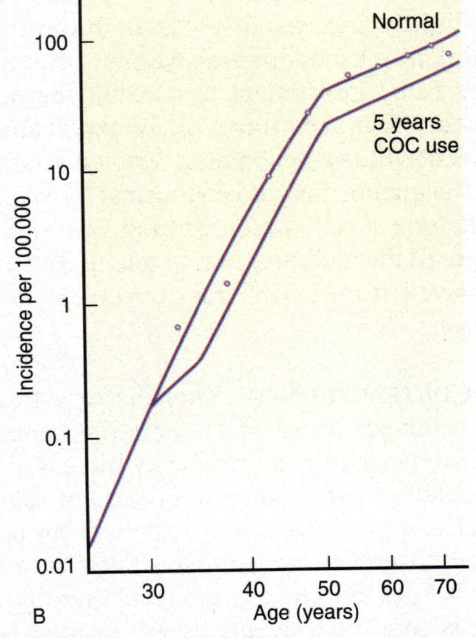

Figure 15-3 Age-specific incidence rates for cancers of the endometrium in women using estrogen therapy (ERT) **(A)** and combination oral contraceptives (COCs) **(B)** for 5 years. Data are from the UK Birmingham Cancer Registry for the years 1968 to 1972. These data largely avoid problems arising from the high hysterectomy and oophorectomy rates in the United States, which artificially distort the age-incidence curves. *Dots* = actual incidence data; *solid lines marked "normal"* = mathematic models predicting these rates from the major known risk factors for these cancers.[13]

with use of cyclic combined hormone therapy was 1.14 (95% CI = 1.01–1.28). This estimate was based on a total of 456 cases, which were included in 6 studies, 4 of which overlap with the studies of continuous combined therapy. Overall, it appears that regimens in which estrogen and progestin are taken daily together (continuous combined hormone therapy) provide a slight protection against endometrial cancer relative to the risk among women who had never used any hormonal regimen, whereas cyclic use of progestins results in a risk of endometrial cancer that is slightly higher than that of women who had never used hormone therapy.

Tamoxifen, an antiestrogen to the breast, acts as an estrogen agonist in the endometrium, and the risk of endometrial cancer is elevated by tamoxifen in a fashion analogous to that of estrogen therapy.[76] Furthermore, the increase in risk is greater among women who previously used estrogen therapy and among those with high body mass.[76] The molecular basis of this agonist effect on the endometrium as opposed to the antagonist activity of tamoxifen on the breast, however, is not totally understood.

Body Weight High body weight leads to increased risk of endometrial cancer at all ages. Studies of postmenopausal women show at least a doubling of risk of endometrial cancer between thin and heavy women.[77,78] Adipose tissue is rich in an aromatase enzyme system that converts androstenedione to estrone. In turn, estrone can be converted directly to estradiol. In addition, protein binding of estrogens in blood is lower in obese women, so the amount of bioavailable estradiol in such women is higher than would be expected from the peripheral conversion of androstenedione to estrone alone.

The explanation for the substantially increased risk of endometrial cancer with obesity in premenopausal women is less obvious.[78] Although obesity does appear to be associated with slightly increased levels of bioavailable estradiol in premenopausal women, this alone appears to be insufficient to account for such a profound effect. The more likely explanation is that obesity in premenopausal women is associated with amenorrhea and subnormal luteal phase progesterone levels, thus resulting in prolonged exposure of the endometrium to unopposed estrogen derived from peripheral conversion in adipose tissue.[79]

Oral Contraceptives The role of estrogens as the principal cause of endometrial cancer is further supported by the markedly increased risk after a relatively short-duration of use of sequential oral contraceptives, which deliver an unopposed estrogen during most of the monthly cycle.[78,80] As potent as estrogen therapy and sequential oral contraceptives are in modifying the risk of endometrial cancer, these effects can be mitigated by the simultaneous administration of progestogens. A series of case control and cohort studies has consistently demonstrated that combined oral contraceptives, which deliver estrogen and progestogen simultaneously during each day of use, decrease the risk of endometrial cancer by 11.7% per year of use (see Figure 15-3B).[13] Use of unopposed estrogen therapy for at least 3 years following discontinuation of oral contraceptive use may counter the reduction in risk observed for oral contraceptive use.[81]

Parity The other major, established risk factor for endometrial cancer, low parity, also is readily explained by the unopposed estrogen hypothesis.[77] The highest risk of endometrial cancer occurs in either married or unmarried nulliparous women, and an incremental decrease in risk occurs with each increment in parity. Nulliparous women have a risk of endometrial cancer that is three to five times that of women with parity of greater than three. This effect is expected as no endometrial mitotic activity occurs during pregnancy because of persistently high progesterone levels.

OVARIAN CANCER

The epidemiology of epithelial ovarian cancer, like breast and endometrial cancer, is well studied. However, the hormonal basis for ovarian cancer appears to differ from that of other hormone-induced cancers in that one of the most important ovarian epithelial cell mitogens is a gonadotropin, follicle-stimulating hormone. The stimulus for cell division in ovarian cancer etiology is not only hormonal, but also a secondary effect following ovulation.[2] In this case, it has been proposed that the epithelial cells within the ovary or covering the ovarian surface are the cells of origin of ovarian cancer. These cells replicate during or after each ovulation; thus, any respite from ovulation would be protective against ovarian cancer. This hypothesis is supported by a large body of epidemiologic data, which consistently demonstrate that the risk of developing ovarian cancer decreases with increasing parity and with combination oral contraceptive use (Table 15-3), both of which induce anovulation.

As with breast and endometrial cancer, the age-incidence curve for ovarian cancer emphasizes the importance of ovulation in determining risk. The age-incidence curve of ovarian cancer can be brought into line with the familiar linear log–log plot of other nonhormone-dependent epithelial tumors if ovarian age is considered as starting at menarche and proceeding at a reduced rate (approximately 30% of normal) during periods of anovulation, including the postmenopausal period.[13]

Table 15-3 A Summary of Established Hormonal Risk and Protective Factors for Ovarian Cancer

Risk Factors (increased number of ovulations)
Late menopause
Protective Factors (decreased number of ovulations)
Pregnancy
Oral contraceptives

Parity Parity has been consistently identified as a protective factor. Compared with parous women, nulliparous women have at least 50% greater risk of ovarian cancer.[82,83] Each pregnancy confers additional protection, whether full-term or incomplete.[84] Considerable attention has been focused on the possible link between fertility drugs and ovarian cancer risk. A recent pooled analysis suggests that the biologic basis of the infertility, rather than the drugs, is responsible for these apparent associations.[85]

Oral Contraceptives Epidemiologic studies have consistently demonstrated that oral contraceptive use decreases the risk of ovarian cancer in a duration-dependent manner analogous to the protective effect on endometrial cancer risk.[86] A review and meta-analysis of 20 epidemiologic studies of ovarian cancer showed that risk of ovarian cancer was 36% lower among women who had used oral contraceptives and that, relative to nonusers, the risk among users decreased approximately 10 to 12% after one year of use and 50% after 5 years of use.[87] The reduction in ovarian cancer risk with oral contraceptive use appears to be long lasting, with reductions in risk persisting for at least 20 to 25 years.[88,89]

Casagrande and colleagues suggested that because the protection afforded by pregnancies and by oral contraceptive use appears to act through a common mechanism, periods of pregnancy and oral contraceptive use could be combined into a single measure of "protected time."[90] They demonstrated that the risk of ovarian cancer clearly decreased as protected time increased. Other epidemiologic studies have confirmed this observation.[91] Other hormonal mechanisms that would impact ovarian cancer risk have been proposed, particularly in relation to oral contraceptives. A study of female macaque monkeys has shown that progestins used in oral contraceptives induce apoptosis in the ovarian epithelium, which should therefore protect against ovarian cancer.[92]

Hormone Therapy The epidemiologic evidence regarding hormone therapy and ovarian cancer risk is equivocal despite the rapidly growing literature on the topic. Early studies did not show an increase in risk associated with estrogen therapy.[93,94]

The results of recent studies are also not consistent. Analyses of the Breast Cancer Detection Demonstration Project, a cohort study that followed women between 1979 and 1998, showed an increased risk of ovarian cancer associated with ever having used estrogen therapy (RR = 1.6, 95% CI = 1.2–2.0) and approximately a 7% increase in risk observed per year of use.[95] No increase in risk was observed for women who used only combined hormone therapy regimens

(RR = 1.1, 95% CI = 0.64–1.7), although the number of cases in this exposure group was small. Similar results for estrogen users were observed in a cohort study of ovarian cancer mortality conducted by the American Cancer Society (Cancer Prevention Study II).[96] Based on 14 years of follow-up and 944 ovarian cancer deaths, the RR of dying from ovarian cancer was 1.51 (95% CI = 1.16–1.96) among women using estrogen therapy at baseline; however, among former users at baseline (when the cohort was formed), risk was not significantly increased (RR = 1.16, 95% CI = 0.99–1.37). Nevertheless, among both current and former users of estrogen therapy, the risk of dying from ovarian cancer increased with increasing duration of use. In contrast to the results from these two studies, Sit and colleagues report no increase in ovarian cancer risk in association with estrogen therapy or with combined hormone therapy in their population-based case control study conducted between 1994 and 1998.[97] Finally, a Danish case control study of ovarian cancer assessed the impact of hormone therapy overall, combining all therapies, but separating out the cumulative increase in risk of ovarian cancer associated with each gram of estrogen intake and of progestin intake.[98] Restricting analysis to women with an intact uterus, they found that each gram of estrogen was associated with a 5.6% increase in risk of ovarian cancer (95% CI = 0.3%–11.2%), whereas cumulative progestin dose did not affect ovarian cancer risk.

Pike and colleagues[99] have conducted a meta-analysis of estrogen therapy in relation to ovarian cancer risk based on 10 studies, including several of the recent studies cited above,[95–97] as well as their own study, which found a nonstatistically significant increase in risk.[100] They report that, across studies, ovarian cancer risk was significantly increased by approximately 24% with 5 years of use of estrogen therapy.[99] For combined hormone therapy, ovarian cancer risk was increased 13% with 5 years of use; however, this result was not statistically significant. They caution that some of the increase in ovarian cancer risk observed with use of estrogen therapy may be a diagnostic bias since, in their own study, risk was elevated solely among women with localized disease.

The Women's Health Initiative has published results on ovarian cancer from the trial of continuous combined estrogen plus progestin therapy versus placebo.[75] During 5.6 years of follow-up, 32 cases of invasive ovarian cancer were diagnosed. Continuous combined therapy was associated with an increase in risk, although the result was not statistically significant (RR = 1.58, 95% CI = 0.77–3.24).

Thus, when we compare results for hormone therapy and ovarian cancer risk to those for oral contraceptive use and ovarian cancer risk, we find that hormone therapy does not offer the protection that is observed with oral contraceptive use. Estrogen therapy alone appears to increase the risk of ovarian cancer; whether combined regimens affect risk is still unsettled.

PROSTATE CANCER

Prostate cancer is the most frequently diagnosed cancer in American men, with an estimated 232,090 cases expected in 2005. It is also the second leading cause of cancer deaths in males, exceeded only by lung cancer, with approximately 30,000 deaths from prostate cancer occurring annually.[14] The prostate is an androgen-regulated organ with androgens considered as the major stimulus for cell division in prostatic epithelium.[5,101] Thus androgens are strong candidates as major contributors to prostatic carcinogenesis. Until recently, only indirect evidence supported a causal role for androgens in prostate cancer development. Results from the Prostate Cancer Prevention Trial (PCPT), using an agent that reduces androgen action in the prostate, provided the first direct evidence in support of an important androgen role in this process.[102] Assessing the role of androgens in prostate cancer development has been difficult, in part because of a lack of easily measurable hormonal events in men as exist in women (eg, menarche, menopause, reproductive experiences). Furthermore, use of exogenous androgens in men is relatively uncommon.

The epidemiology of prostate cancer is dominated by three observations: (1) the profound international and racial/ethnic variation in incidence and mortality, historically reported to be as much as 80-fold between the extremes of high-risk (African Americans) and low-risk (native Japanese and Chinese) populations;[103] (2) the occurrence of occult, subclinical prostate cancer at a relatively comparable prevalence across populations;[104] and (3) the strong relationship between prostate cancer incidence and aging.[5] Prostate cancer is extremely rare before age 50 years, but it is still the most common cancer of American men, in large part because the rate of increase in prostate cancer incidence with aging is greater than for any other cancer.

Some of the indirect evidence for a role of androgens in prostate cancer development has come from comparisons of hormonal profiles of healthy men from racial/ethnic groups at high, intermediate, and low risk of prostate cancer. Asian men, although showing no evidence of low circulating testosterone levels relative to whites and African Americans at any age, have substantially reduced levels of androstanediol glucuronide.[105,106] This hormone reflects 5α-reductase activity (5α-reductase is the prostatic enzyme that bioactivates testosterone to dihydrotestosterone, the most biologically potent human androgen). Based on these results and the presumptive role of androgens in prostate cell proliferation, Ross and colleagues proposed that a 5α-reductase inhibitor might be an effective chemopreventive agent for prostate cancer.[105]

Several additional indirect lines of evidence point to a role of androgens in prostate cancer pathogenesis. Androgens are required for prostate cancer development or progression in most animal models of prostatic adenocarcinoma.[107] Prostate cancer has never been reported to occur in eunuchs or in men with genetically determined decreased 5α-reductase activity, groups with very low androgen activity and highly underdeveloped prostates.[5] Prostate cancers, at least early in their course, are almost uniformly androgen dependent, and androgen ablation therapy has been the mainstay for treating early metastatic prostate cancer for many decades. Somewhat more direct evidence for a role of androgens in prostate carcinogenesis comes from a well-designed prospective study, the Physicians Health Study, which demonstrated that healthy men in the highest quartile of circulating testosterone levels have 2.6 times the likelihood of subsequently developing prostate cancer compared with men in the lowest quartile.[108]

The most convincing evidence for a role of androgens in prostate cancer development comes from the PCPT.[102] In the PCPT, 18,882 healthy men aged 55 years and older, with normal range PSAs, were randomized to receive 5 mg daily of finasteride, a 5α-reductase inhibitor, or placebo. After 7 years, all men were scheduled for an end-of-trial prostate biopsy. Prostate cancer incidence in the treatment arm was reduced approximately 25%. However, paradoxically, there was a statistically significant 25% *increase* in high-grade prostate cancer incidence in the therapeutic arm. These disparate findings have created substantial controversy regarding the role of 5α-reductase inhibitors in prostate cancer prevention in healthy men, as well as substantial disagreement regarding the underlying cause of these curious results. It has been argued, for example, that this finding represents an artifact of disruptive morphological changes induced by finasteride in the prostate, or that the increased risk of high-grade prostate cancer is the result of detection bias owing to finasteride-induced reduction in prostate volume.[109] On the other hand, others have argued that these results are more foreboding with a clear biological basis; for example, Ross and colleagues consider that high-grade prostate cancer precursor cells, possibly with androgen receptor alterations (amplification, gene mutations) thrive in an androgen-depleted environment, that prostate cancer cells with somatic mutations of the 5α-reductase type II gene respond differently to an inhibitor than those without such changes, and that finasteride, by virtue of increased intraprostatic levels of testosterone, selectively stimulates prostate cancer precursor lesions.[110] Understanding the true nature of these results will have enormous public health implications.

GENETIC DETERMINANTS

Familial Risk A family history of breast cancer is associated with an increased risk of the disease.[4] This is particularly apparent when the family history includes a woman who was affected at an early age or had bilateral disease. Whereas a two- to threefold increase in the risk of the disease has been observed in first-degree relatives of women with breast cancer overall, a ninefold increase in risk has been found in the first-degree relatives of premenopausal women with bilateral breast cancer. Very high risks (ie, fivefold or greater) also have been found in women with more than one first-degree relative with breast cancer. Similarly, population-based case control studies have described a two- to threefold increased risk of ovarian cancer in first-degree relatives of ovarian cancer patients.[111,112] Heritability estimates for both breast and ovarian cancer are approximately 25%.[113] The impact of family history on endometrial cancer risk is less clear. Some studies have shown an association between family history and risk of this cancer,[114–117] but this finding has not been consistent.[118] Also, unlike breast and ovarian cancer, heritability estimates from twin studies do not suggest a strong genetic component for endometrial cancer.[113]

Prostate cancer is also a highly familial disease. Men with a first-degree relative with prostate cancer have approximately a two- to threefold increase in risk compared with men with no such history, and this increase is observed across different racial/ethnic groups.[119] As with breast cancer, risk is elevated further when multiple first-degree relatives are affected or when affected relatives are diagnosed at relatively young ages.[120] This strong familial risk has led to the development of several prostate cancer family registries searching for a single locus, high penetrance gene responsible for this familial risk. When linkage analyses have identified a series of possible candidate loci, confirmatory studies in other populations generally have been either nonsupportive or inconclusive.[121]

Genes Significant efforts have been directed toward identifying major genes influencing risk of breast and ovarian cancer using high-risk families. Extraordinary success has been achieved using this approach to identify the highly penetrant, major disease-causing genes, *BRCA1* and *BRCA2*. Yet, mutations in *BRCA1* and *BRCA2* explain less than 10% of the breast[122–124] or ovarian cancer cases.[125] Although *BRCA1* and *BRCA2* are quite important to carriers, a large gap exists in understanding the genetic etiology of breast and ovarian cancer in the general population. All of these observations combined with the epidemiology described above are consistent with a multifactorial etiology for each of these cancers, with hormonal, genetic, and environmental factors playing a role. Most likely, the common forms of breast, ovarian, and endometrial cancers are complex genetic diseases with locus and allelic heterogeneity.

Such complex traits are marked by minor susceptibility genes associated with modest increases in risk, but high population-attributable risk, because the risk allele may be quite common in the population. These types of genes, such as those involved in reproductive endocrinology, may act alone or in combination with common variants of other genes and environmental factors to increase the risk of breast, ovarian, or endometrial cancer. Ultimately common variants in several such genes involved in the biology of the breast, ovary, or endometrium could give rise to a "polygenic" etiology of cancer.

Table 15-4 Candidate Genes and Pathways Relevant to Breast, Ovarian, and Endometrial Cancer Risk

Pathway	Genes
Gonadotropin Signaling	GNRH1, GNRHR, CGA, FSHB, LHB, FSHR, LHCGR, INHA, INHBA, INHBB, ACVR1, ACVR2
Sex Steroid Hormone Biosynthesis	CYP11, CYP17, HSD3B1, HSD3B2, CYP19, HSD17B1, HSD17B2, HSD17B3, STAR
Glucocorticoid Synthesis	CRH, CRHR1/2, POMC (ACTH), MC2R (ACTHR), CYP21, CYP11B
Endogenous/Exogenous Hormone Metabolism	AKR1C1, AKR1C2, AKR1C3, AKR1C4, COMT, CYP1A1, CYP1A2, CYP3A4, CYP3A5, CYP1B1, CYP21, HSD3B1, HSD3B2, HSD17B1, HSD17B2, SRD5A1, SRD5A2, SULT1A1, UGT1A
Hormone Transport/Action	ESR1, ESR2, PGR, SHBG
Growth Hormone/Insulin-like Growth Factor Signaling Axis	GH1, GHR, GHRH, GHRHR, IGF1, IGF2, IGF1R, IGF2R, IGFALS, IGFBP1, IGFBP2, IGFBP3, IGFBP4, IGFBP5, IGFBP6, POU1F1, SST, SSTR1, SSTR2, SSTR3, SSTR4, SSTR5

Exactly which genes and variants are associated with these cancers is unknown, but candidate genes can be selected based on an understanding of the epidemiology, biology, and etiology of the cancer. Table 15-4 shows one potential list of candidate genes and their related pathways. These genes may harbor risk variants for breast, ovarian, or endometrial cancer. For example, one of the most extensively studied genes in all three of these female hormone-related cancers is the progesterone receptor gene (*PGR*). Two variants have been studied in a number of studies. The first is an ALU insertion that is in perfectly correlated with several coding region single nucleotide polymorphisms (SNPs), including two that alter the encoded amino acid (nonsynonymous SNPs).[126–128] The complex is known as PROGINS. The nonsynonymous SNP in exon four (V660L) was recently reported to have a functional consequence on the receptor, but follow-up studies are needed to confirm this report.[129]

Of those studies that could be evaluated in this manner, all but two[130,131] have found that PROGINS is protective against breast cancer among women who carry two copies of the mutant allele.[127,132–134] However, if one summarizes these data using a formal meta-analytic approach, the result indicates a level of heterogeneity of risk estimates across the published studies that is nearly statistically significant (p for heterogeneity = 0.06), suggesting that the finding of a protective effect against breast cancer may not be robust. Conversely, PROGINS has been associated with an increased risk of ovarian cancer among individuals who carry two copies of the mutant allele in most,[127,135–139] but not all studies.[140,141] Pearce and colleagues recently showed that, after a complete characterization of the underlying genetic diversity of the *PGR*, it was not PROGINS that was associated with increased risk of ovarian cancer, but rather a second variant, rs608995.[127] After taking rs608995 into account, PROGINS was not associated with the risk of ovarian cancer in their population-based case control study. This finding is intriguing, but difficult to reconcile with a functional role of the V660L PROGINS complex. This variant has also been explored with regard to risk of endometrial cancer, and a nonsignificant protective effect was observed.[128] Paradoxically, Pijnenborg and colleagues reported that among endometrial cancer cases, those who carry PROGINS are more likely to relapse.[142]

A second variant in the *PGR*, +331G/A , has been studied in all three of these hormone-related female cancers. +331G/A has also been reported to have a functional consequence on the transcription of the receptor.[128] Initially, it was reported that the variant allele was associated with an increased risk of breast cancer;[143] however, two subsequent studies failed to confirm this association.[127,144] One study has shown an association between this variant and an increased endometrial cancer risk,[128] but this finding remains to be confirmed. The findings with regard to ovarian cancer illustrate the importance of large studies and collaborative efforts. The +331G/A *PGR* promoter polymorphism appears to be associated with a modest decrease in risk of endometrioid and clear cell subtypes of ovarian cancer after stratification by histological type of ovarian cancer.[145] Combining data on these two subtypes through meta-analysis using results from three published studies,[141,145] and unpublished data from a fourth study,[127] indicates a strong protective effect of the A allele (meta-analysis odds ratio = 0.56, 95% CI 0.37–0.83). Yet, individually, only one[145] of the four studies[127,141,145] achieved even borderline statistical significance.

As described above using *PGR* as an example, the genetic association literature is extremely inconsistent. Thus, the interpretation of any individual study is difficult. Even when one examines the full complement of available data, the results are often not clear. Lohmueller and colleagues,[146] as well as Ioannidis and colleagues,[147] have estimated that approximately 75% of published association studies are false positives. The difficulty in replicating these association studies has served to underscore the importance of good study design, large samples sizes, and careful interpretation. After a decade of difficult-to-interpret studies, many journals and investigators have realized the importance of collaboration and replication. The National Cancer Institute's Breast and Prostate Cohort Consortium was formed so that robust results could be obtained for many of the key genes and pathways listed in Table 15-4. Similarly, the Breast Cancer Association Consortium and the Ovarian Cancer Association Consortium have been formed in an effort to provide definitive results for the role of genetic variants in the etiology of these cancers. In addition, more comprehensive approaches to studying the role of genetic variation in cancer risk are now in place (see Pearce et al.,[127] for example) so that fully targeting candidate gene regions is now possible and will likely soon become the standard. Whole genome association scans are also being initiated, and the challenges and benefits associated with this approach will likely be understood and resolved over the next several years.[148]

The relationship between genetic control of androgen biosynthesis and metabolic pathways and prostate cancer risk is just now beginning to be understood. A number of years ago Ross and colleagues published a description of a polygenic model of prostate cancer development related to genetic control of androgen pathways to the prostate.[5] Although both genetic control of androgen biosynthesis outside the prostate and transport of androgens to the prostate are of interest, most research to date has centered around androgen signaling within prostatic epithelial cells, especially with regard to (1) the androgen receptor (*AR*) gene encoding the androgen receptor, which is responsible both for androgen transport within prostate cells and for transactivation of genes with androgen response elements in their promoter region, and (2) the steroid 5α-reductase type II (*SRD5A2*) gene, which encodes the type 2 5α-reductase enzyme responsible for metabolic activation of testosterone to dihydrotestosterone in prostatic cells, although other candidate genes in this pathway have also been studied.

Coetzee and Ross proposed that a polymorphic CAG repeat in exon 1 of the androgen receptor gene might predict androgen receptor transactivation activity and, therefore, prostate cancer risk,[149] and later offered some epidemiologic support for this hypothesis.[150] A missense substitution polymorphism in the *SRD5A2* gene has also been linked to prostate cancer risk, but this result has not been easily reproduced.[151] As with female hormone-related cancers, much work still needs to be done in a more systematic pathway driven approach to fully identify the possible contribution of the candidate genes and prostate cancer risk.

CONCLUSION

As our understanding of the relationship between epidemiologic risk factors and the circulating levels of the relevant hormones grows, avenues for primary prevention are becoming apparent. The control of obesity has obvious implications for both endometrial cancer and postmenopausal breast cancer. More information on the relationship between childhood diet and physical activity and the onset of puberty, in conjunction with the hormonal physiology of adolescence and young adulthood may provide increasing avenues for preventing breast, ovarian, and endometrial cancer in women. A large hormonal chemoprevention trial for breast cancer using the antiestrogen drug tamoxifen has already proven successful, and an additional national trial using an alternative selective estrogen receptor modulator, raloxifene, without the same estrogen agonist effects on the endometrium, is underway. In the future, aromatase inhibitors, which are effective in breast cancer therapy, may prove to be effective in breast cancer prevention. Hormonal chemoprevention of ovarian and endometrial cancer is already occurring in the population as a whole through the widespread use of combination oral contraceptives, and of endometrial cancer with use of continuous combined hormone therapy. A national trial to prevent prostate cancer through use of finasteride, a 5α-reductase inhibitor, has been completed and provides convincing evidence for the role of androgens in the development of this disease. A growing knowledge of the mutations and polymorphisms in genes causing increased risk of these cancers should lead to better definition of individual susceptibility. It should then be possible to focus intervention strategies on the higher-risk subgroups of the population.

REFERENCES

1. Bittner JJ. The causes and control of mammary cancer in mice. Harvey Lect 1947;42:221–46.
2. Henderson BE, Ross RK, Bernstein L. Estrogens as a cause of human cancer: the Richard and Hinda Rosenthal Foundation award lecture. Cancer Res 1988;48:246–53.
3. Henderson BE, Ross RK, Pike MC, Casagrande JT. Endogenous hormones as a major factor in human cancer. Cancer Res 1982;42:3232–9.
4. Henderson BE, Feigelson HS. Hormonal carcinogenesis. Carcinogenesis 2000;21:427–33.
5. Ross RK, Pike MC, Coetzee GA, et al. Androgen metabolism and prostate cancer: establishing a model of genetic susceptibility. Cancer Res 1998;58:4497–504.
6. Chan JM, Stampfer MJ, Giovannucci E, et al. Plasma insulin-like growth factor-I and prostate cancer risk: a prospective study. Science 1998;279:563–6.
7. Sager R. Tumor suppressor genes: the puzzle and the promise. Science 1989;246:1406–12.
8. Stanbridge EJ. Identifying tumor suppressor genes in human colorectal cancer. Science 1990;247:12–3.
9. Miki Y, Swensen J, Shattuck-Eidens D, et al. A strong candidate for the breast and ovarian cancer susceptibility gene BRCA1. Science 1994;266:66–71.
10. Wooster R, Bignell G, Lancaster J, et al. Identification of the breast cancer susceptibility gene BRCA2. Nature 1995;378:789–92.
11. Malkin D, Li FP, Strong LC, et al. Germ line p53 mutations in a familial syndrome of breast cancer, sarcomas, and other neoplasms. Science 1990;250:1233–8.
12. Slamon DJ, Clark GM, Wong SG, et al. Human breast cancer: correlation of relapse and survival with amplification of the HER-2/neu oncogene. Science 1987;235:177–82.
13. Henderson BE, Ross RK, Pike MC. Hormonal chemoprevention of cancer in women. Science 1993;259:633–8.
14. American Cancer Society. Cancer facts and figures 2005. Atlanta (GA): American Cancer Society; 2005.
15. Ries L, Eisner M, Kosary C, et al, editors. SEER cancer statistics review, 1975–2002. National Cancer Institute; based on November 2004 SEER data submission posted to the SEER Web site 2005. Available at: http://seer.cancer.gov/csr/1975_2002/ (accessed August 18, 2005).
16. McKean-Cowdin R, Feigelson HS, Ross RK, et al. Declining cancer rates in the 1990s. J Clin Oncol 2000;18:2258–68.
17. Slamon DJ, Leyland-Jones B, Shak S, et al. Use of chemotherapy plus a monoclonal antibody against HER2 for metastatic breast cancer that overexpresses HER2. N Engl J Med 2001;344:783–92.
18. Key TJ, Pike MC. The role of oestrogens and progestagens in the epidemiology and prevention of breast cancer. Eur J Cancer Clin Oncol 1988;24:29–43.
19. Ferguson DJ, Anderson TJ. Morphological evaluation of cell turnover in relation to the menstrual cycle in the "resting" human breast. Br J Cancer 1981;44:177–81.
20. Magnusson C, Baron JA, Correia N, et al. Breast-cancer risk following long-term oestrogen- and oestrogen-progestin-replacement therapy. Int J Cancer 1999;81:339–44.
21. Ross RK, Paganini-Hill A, Wan PC, Pike MC. Effect of hormone replacement therapy on breast cancer risk: estrogen versus estrogen plus progestin. J Natl Cancer Inst 2000;92:328–32.
22. Rossouw JE, Anderson GL, Prentice RL, et al. Risks and benefits of estrogen plus progestin in healthy postmenopausal women: principal results from the Women's Health Initiative randomized trial. JAMA 2002;288:321–33.
23. Chlebowski RT, Hendrix SL, Langer RD, et al. Influence of estrogen plus progestin on breast cancer and mammography in healthy postmenopausal women: the Women's Health Initiative Randomized Trial. JAMA 2003;289:3243–53.
24. Lee SA, Ross RK, Pike MC. An overview of menopausal estrogen-progestin hormone therapy and breast cancer risk. Br J Cancer 2005;92:2049–58.
25. Henderson BE, Pike MC, Casagrande JT. Breast cancer and the oestrogen window hypothesis. Lancet 1981;2:363–4.
26. Henderson BE, Gerkins V, Rosario I, et al. Elevated serum levels of estrogen and prolactin in daughters of patients with breast cancer. N Engl J Med 1975;293:790–5.
27. Kaprio J, Rimpela A, Winter T, et al. Common genetic influences on BMI and age at menarche. Hum Biol 1995;67:739–53.
28. Frisch RE, Gotz-Welbergen AV, McArthur JW, et al. Delayed menarche and amenorrhea of college athletes in relation to age of onset of training. JAMA 1981;246:1559–63.
29. Bernstein L, Ross RK, Lobo RA, et al. The effects of moderate physical activity on menstrual cycle patterns in adolescence: implications for breast cancer prevention. Br J Cancer 1987;55:681–5.
30. Bernstein L, Henderson BE, Hanisch R, et al. Physical exercise and reduced risk of breast cancer in young women. J Natl Cancer Inst 1994;86:1403–8.
31. Carpenter CL, Ross RK, Paganini-Hill A, Bernstein L. Lifetime exercise activity and breast cancer risk among postmenopausal women. Br J Cancer 1999;80:1852–8.
32. McTiernan A, Kooperberg C, White E, et al. Recreational physical activity and the risk of breast cancer in postmenopausal women: the Women's Health Initiative Cohort Study. JAMA 2003;290:1331–6.
33. Vainio H, Bianchini F. IARC handbooks on cancer prevention: weight control and physical activity. Vol 6. Lyon, France: International Agency for Research on Cancer; 2002.
34. Trichopoulos D, MacMahon B, Cole P. Menopause and breast cancer risk. J Natl Cancer Inst 1972;48:605–13.
35. de Waard F, Baanders-van Halewijn EA. A prospective study in general practice on breast-cancer risk in postmenopausal women. Int J Cancer 1974;14:153–60.
36. Willett WC, Browne ML, Bain C, et al. Relative weight and risk of breast cancer among premenopausal women. Am J Epidemiol 1985;122:731–40.
37. Bernstein L, Yuan JM, Ross RK, et al. Serum hormone levels in pre-menopausal Chinese women in Shanghai and white women in Los Angeles: results from two breast cancer case-control studies. Cancer Causes Control 1990;1:51–8.
38. Key T, Appleby P, Barnes I, Reeves G. Endogenous Hormones and Breast Cancer Collaborative Group. Endogenous sex hormones and breast cancer in postmenopausal women: reanalysis of nine prospective studies. J Natl Cancer Inst 2002;94:606–16.
39. MacMahon B, Cole P, Lin TM, et al. Age at first birth and breast cancer risk. Bull World Health Organ 1970;43:209–21.
40. Liu Q, Wuu J, Lambe M, et al. Transient increase in breast cancer risk after giving birth: postpartum period with the highest risk (Sweden). Cancer Causes Control 2002;13:299–305.
41. Bernstein L, Depue RH, Ross RK, et al. Higher maternal levels of free estradiol in first compared to second pregnancy: early gestational differences. J Natl Cancer Inst 1986;76:1035–9.

42. Musey VC, Collins DC, Musey PI, et al. Long-term effect of a first pregnancy on the secretion of prolactin. N Engl J Med 1987;316:229–34.
43. Yu MC, Gerkins VR, Henderson BE, et al. Elevated levels of prolactin in nulliparous women. Br J Cancer 1981;43:826–31.
44. Bernstein L, Pike MC, Ross RK, et al. Estrogen and sex hormone-binding globulin levels in nulliparous and parous women. J Natl Cancer Inst 1985;74:741–5.
45. Enger SM, Ross RK, Henderson BE, Bernstein L. Breastfeeding history, pregnancy experience and risk of breast cancer. Br J Cancer 1997;76:118–23.
46. Newcomb PA, Storer BE, Longnecker MP, et al. Lactation and a reduced risk of premenopausal breast cancer. N Engl J Med 1994;330:81–6.
47. Ursin G, Bernstein L, Wang Y, et al. Reproductive factors and risk of breast carcinoma in a study of white and African-American women. Cancer 2004;101:353–62.
48. Enger SM, Ross RK, Paganini-Hill A, Bernstein L. Breastfeeding experience and breast cancer risk among postmenopausal women. Cancer Epidemiol Biomark Prev 1998;7:365–9.
49. Yuan JM, Yu MC, Ross RK, et al. Risk factors for breast cancer in Chinese women in Shanghai. Cancer Res 1988;48:1949–53.
50. Armstrong B, Doll R. Environmental factors and cancer incidence and mortality in different countries, with special reference to dietary practices. Int J Cancer 1975;15:617–31.
51. Willett WC, Stampfer MJ, Colditz GA, et al. Dietary fat and the risk of breast cancer. N Engl J Med 1987;316:22–8.
52. Holmes MD, Hunter DJ, Colditz GA, et al. Association of dietary intake of fat and fatty acids with risk of breast cancer. JAMA 1999;281:914–20.
53. Cohen LA, Kendall ME, Zang E, et al. Modulation of N-nitrosomethylurea-induced mammary tumor promotion by dietary fiber and fat. J Natl Cancer Inst 1991;83:496–501.
54. Wu AH, Pike MC, Stram DO. Meta-analysis: dietary fat intake, serum estrogen levels, and the risk of breast cancer. J Natl Cancer Inst 1999;91:529–34.
55. Collaborative Group on Hormonal Factors in Breast Cancer. Breast cancer and hormonal contraceptives: collaborative reanalysis of individual data on 53,297 women with breast cancer and 100,239 women without breast cancer from 54 epidemiological studies. Lancet 1996;347:1713–27.
56. Marchbanks PA, McDonald JA, Wilson HG, et al. Oral contraceptives and the risk of breast cancer. N Engl J Med 2002;346:2025–32.
57. Cogliano V, Grosse Y, Baan R, et al. Carcinogenicity of combined oestrogen-progestagen contraceptives and menopausal treatment. Lancet Oncol 2005;6:552–3.
58. Pike MC, Bernstein L, Spicer DV. The relationship of exogenous hormones to breast cancer risk. In: Niederhuber JE, editor. Current therapy in oncology. St. Louis (MO): Mosby; 1993. p. 292–303.
59. Collaborative Group on Hormonal Factors in Breast Cancer. Breast cancer and hormone replacement therapy: collaborative reanalysis of data from 51 epidemiological studies of 52,705 women with breast cancer and 108,411 women without breast cancer. Lancet 1997;350:1047–59.
60. Beral V, Million Women Study Collaborators. Breast cancer and hormone-replacement therapy in the Million Women Study. Lancet 2003;362:419–27.
61. Anderson Gl, Limacher M, Assaf AR, et al. Effects of conjugated equine estrogen in postmenopausal women with hysterectomy: the Women's Health Initiative randomized controlled trial. JAMA 2004;291:1701–12.
62. Schairer C, Lubin JH, Triosi R, et al. Menopausal estrogen and estrogen-progestin replacement therapy and breast cancer risk. JAMA 2000;283:485–91.
63. Key TJ, Pike MC. The dose-effect relationship between 'unopposed' oestrogens and endometrial mitotic rate: its central role in explaining and predicting endometrial cancer risk. Br J Cancer 1988;57:205–12.
64. Wu L, Einstein M, Geissler WM, et al. Expression cloning and characterization of human 17 beta-hydroxysteroid dehydrogenase type 2, a microsomal enzyme possessing 20 alpha-hydroxysteroid dehydrogenase activity. J Biol Chem 1993;268:12964–9.
65. Miettinen MM, Mustonen MV, Poutanen MH, et al. Human 17 beta-hydroxysteroid dehydrogenase type 1 and type 2 isoenzymes have opposite activities in cultured cells and characteristic cell- and tissue-specific expression. Biochem J 1996;314:839–45.
66. Kennedy DL, Baum C, Forbes MB. Noncontraceptive estrogens and progestins: use patterns over time. Obstet Gynecol 1985;65:441–6.
67. Austin DF, Roe KM. Increase in cancer of the corpus uteri in the San Francisco-Oakland standard metropolitan statistical area, 1960–75. J Natl Cancer Inst 1979;62:13–6.
68. Mack TM, Pike MC, Henderson BE, et al. Estrogens and endometrial cancer in a retirement community. N Engl J Med 1976;294:1262–7.
69. Ziel HK, Finkle WD. Increased risk of endometrial carcinoma among users of conjugated estrogens. N Engl J Med 1975;293:1167–70.
70. Chu J, Schweid AI, Weiss NS. Survival among women with endometrial cancer: a comparison of estrogen users and nonusers. Am J Obstet Gynecol 1982;143:569–73.
71. Paganini-Hill A, Ross RK, Henderson BE. Endometrial cancer and patterns of use of oestrogen replacement therapy: a cohort study. Br J Cancer 1989;59:445–7.
72. Pike MC, Peters RK, Cozen W, et al. Estrogen-progestin replacement therapy and endometrial cancer. J Natl Cancer Inst 1997;89:1110–6.
73. Million Women Study Collaborators. Endometrial cancer and hormone-replacement therapy in the Million Women Study. Lancet 2005;365:1543–51.
74. Zeleniuch-Jacquotte A, Akhmedkhanov A, Kato I, et al. Postmenopausal endogenous oestrogens and risk of endometrial cancer: results from a prospective study. Br J Cancer 2001;84:975–81.
75. Anderson GL, Judd HL, Kaunitz AM, et al. Effect of estrogen plus progestin on gynecologic cancers and associated diagnostic procedures: the Women's Health Initiative randomized trial. JAMA 2003;290:1739–48.
76. Bernstein L, Deapen D, Cerhan JR, et al. Tamoxifen therapy for breast cancer and endometrial cancer risk. J Natl Cancer Inst 1999;91:1654–62.
77. Elwood JM, Cole P, Rothman KJ, Kaplan SD. Epidemiology of endometrial cancer. J Natl Cancer Inst 1977;59:1055–60.
78. Henderson BE, Casagrande JT, Pike MC, et al. The epidemiology of endometrial cancer in young women. Br J Cancer 1983;47:749–56.
79. Rogers J, Mitchell GW Jr. The relation of obesity to menstrual disturbances. N Engl J Med 1952;247:53–5.
80. Centers for Disease Control and the National Institute of Child Health and Human Development. Combination oral contraceptive use and the risk of endometrial cancer. The Cancer and Steroid Hormone Study. JAMA 1987;257:796–800.
81. Voigt LF, Deng Q, Weiss NS. Recency, duration and progestin content of oral contraceptives in relation to the incidence of endometrial cancer (Washington, USA). Cancer Causes Control 1994;5:227–33.
82. Wu ML, Whittemore AS, Paffenbarger RS Jr, et al. Personal and environmental characteristics related to epithelial ovarian cancer. I. Reproductive and menstrual events and oral contraceptive use. Am J Epidemiol 1988;128:1216–27.
83. Weiss N. Ovary. In: Schottenfeld D, Fraumeni JF, editors. Cancer epidemiology and prevention. Philadelphia: WB Saunders; 1982. p. 871–80.
84. Newhouse ML, Pearson RM, Fullerton JM, et al. A case control study of carcinoma of the ovary. Br J Prev Soc Med 1977;31:148–53.
85. Ness RB, Cramer DW, Goodman MT, et al. Infertility, fertility drugs, and ovarian cancer: a pooled analysis of case-control studies. Am J Epidemiol 2002;155:217–24.
86. Whittemore AS, Harris R, Itnyre J. Characteristics relating to ovarian cancer risk: collaborative analysis of 12 US case-control studies. II. Invasive epithelial ovarian cancers in white women. Collaborative Ovarian Cancer Group. Am J Epidemiol 1992;136:1184–203.
87. Hankinson SE, Colditz GA, Hunter DJ, et al. A quantitative assessment of oral contraceptive use and risk of ovarian cancer. Obstet Gynecol 1992;80:708–14.
88. Ness RB, Grisso JA, Klapper J, et al. Risk of ovarian cancer in relation to estrogen and progestin dose and use characteristics of oral contraceptives. SHARE Study Group. Steroid Hormones and Reproductions. Am J Epidemiol 2000;152:233–41.
89. Riman T, Dickman PW, Nilsson S, et al. Risk factors for invasive epithelial ovarian cancer: results from a Swedish case-control study. Am J Epidemiol 2002;156:363–73.
90. Casagrande JT, Louie EW, Pike MC, et al. "Incessant ovulation" and ovarian cancer. Lancet 1979;2:170–3.
91. Franceschi S, La Vecchia C, Helmrich SP, et al. Risk factors for epithelial ovarian cancer in Italy. Am J Epidemiol 1982;115:714–9.
92. Rodriguez GC, Walmer DK, Cline M, et al. Effect of progestin on the ovarian epithelium of macaques: cancer prevention through apoptosis? J Soc Gynecol Invest 1998;5:271–6.
93. Whittemore AS, Harris R, Itnyre J. Characteristics relating to ovarian cancer risk: collaborative analysis of 12 US case-control studies. II. Invasive epithelial ovarian cancers in white women. Collaborative Ovarian Cancer Group. Am J Epidemiol 1992;136:1184–203.
94. Coughlin SS, Giustozzi AG, Smith SJ, Lee NC. A meta-analysis of estrogen replacement therapy and risk of epithelial ovarian cancer. J Clin Epidemiol 2000;53:367–75.
95. Lacey JV Jr, Mink PJ, Lubin JH, et al. Menopausal hormone replacement therapy and risk of ovarian cancer. JAMA 2002;288:334–41.
96. Rodriguez C, Patel AV, Calle EE, et al. Estrogen replacement therapy and ovarian cancer mortality in a large prospective study of US women. JAMA 2001;285:1460–5.
97. Sit ASY, Modugno F, Weissfeld JL, et al. Hormone replacement therapy formulations and risk of epithelial ovarian carcinoma. Gynecol Oncol 2002;86:118–23.
98. Glud E, Kjaer SK, Thomsen BL, et al. Hormone therapy and the impact of estrogen intake on the risk of ovarian cancer. Arch Intern Med 2004;164:2253–9.
99. Pike MC, Pearce CL, Wu AH. Prevention of cancers of the breast, endometrium and ovary. Oncogene 2004;23:6379–91.
100. Pike MC, Pearce CL, Peters R, et al. Hormonal factors and the risk of invasive ovarian cancer: a population-based case-control study. Fertil Steril 2004;82:186–95.
101. Coffey DS. Physiological control of prostatic growth: an overview. In: Coffey DS, Isaacs JT, editors. Prostate cancer. Vol 48. Geneva: UICC Technical Report Series; 1979. p. 4–15.
102. Thompson IM, Goodman PJ, Tangen CM, et al. The influence of finasteride on the development of prostate cancer. N Engl J Med 2003;349:215–24.
103. Ross RK, Schottenfeld D. Prostate cancer. In: Schottenfeld D, Fraumeni JF, editors. Cancer epidemiology and prevention. New York: Oxford University Press; 1996. p. 1180–206.
104. Yatani R, Chigusa I, Akazaki K, et al. Geographic pathology of latent prostatic carcinoma. Int J Cancer 1982;29:611–6.
105. Ross RK, Bernstein L, Lobo RA, et al. 5-alpha-reductase activity and risk of prostate cancer among Japanese and US white and black males. Lancet 1992;339:887–9.
106. Lookingbill DP, Demers LM, Wang C, et al. Clinical and biochemical parameters of androgen action in normal healthy Caucasian versus Chinese subjects. J Clin Endocrinol Metab 1991;72:1242–8.
107. Noble RL. The development of prostatic adenocarcinoma in Nb rats following prolonged sex hormone administration. Cancer Res 1977;37:1929–33.
108. Gann PH, Hennekens CH, Ma J, et al. Prospective study of sex hormone levels and risk of prostate cancer. J Natl Cancer Inst 1996;88:1118–26.
109. Mellon JK. The finasteride prostate cancer prevention trial (PCPT)—what have we learned? Eur J Cancer 2005. [In press]
110. Ross RK, Skinner E, Cote RJ. Prevention of prostate cancer with finasteride. N Engl J Med 2003;349:1569–72.
111. Godard B, Foulkes WD, Provencher D, et al. Risk factors for familial and sporadic ovarian cancer among French Canadians: a case-control study. Am J Obstet Gynecol 1998;179:403–10.
112. Stratton JF, Pharoah P, Smith SK, et al. A systematic review and meta-analysis of family history and risk of ovarian cancer. Br J Obstet Gynaecol 1998;105:493–9.
113. Lichtenstein P, Holm NV, Verkasalo PK, et al. Environmental and heritable factors in the causation of cancer—analyses of cohorts of twins from Sweden, Denmark, and Finland. N Engl J Med 2000;343:78–85.
114. Hemminki K, Bermejo JL, Granstrom C. Endometrial cancer: population attributable risks from reproductive, familial and socioeconomic factors. Eur J Cancer 2005. [In press]
115. Parslov M, Lidegaard O, Klintorp S, et al. Risk factors among young women with endometrial cancer: a Danish case-control study. Am J Obstet Gynecol 2000;182:23–9.
116. Gruber SB, Thompson WD. A population-based study of endometrial cancer and familial risk in younger women. Cancer and Steroid Hormone Study Group. Cancer Epidemiol Biomarkers Prev 1996;5:411–7.
117. Parazzini F, La Vecchia C, Moroni S, et al. Family history and the risk of endometrial cancer. Int J Cancer 1994;59:460–2.
118. Olson JE, Sellers TA, Anderson KE, Folsom AR. Does a family history of cancer increase the risk for postmenopausal endometrial carcinoma? A prospective cohort study and a nested case-control family study of older women. Cancer 1999;85:2444–9.

119. Monroe KR, Yu MC, Kolonel LN, et al. Evidence of an X-linked or recessive genetic component to prostate cancer risk. Nature Med 1995;1:827–9.
120. Carter BS, Beaty TH, Steinberg GD, et al. Mendelian inheritance of familial prostate cancer. Proc Natl Acad Sci U S A 1992;89:3367–71.
121. Chung B-L, Turner AR, Isaacs WB, Xu J. Hereditary prostate cancer: the search for major genes and the role of genes involved in androgen action. In: Henderson BE, Ponder B, Ross RK, editors. Hormones, genes and cancer. New York: Oxford University Press; 2003. p. 316–30.
122. Malone KE, Daling JR, Thompson JD, et al. BRCA1 mutations and breast cancer in the general population: analyses in women before age 35 years and in women before age 45 years with first-degree family history. JAMA 1998;279:922–9.
123. Newman B, Mu H, Butler LM, et al. Frequency of breast cancer attributable to BRCA1 in a population-based series of American women. JAMA 1998;279:915–21.
124. McClain MR, Palomaki GE, Nathanson KL, Haddow JE. Adjusting the estimated proportion of breast cancer cases associated with BRCA1 and BRCA2 mutations: public health implications. Genet Med 2005;7:28–33.
125. Risch HA, McLaughlin JR, Cole DE, et al. Prevalence and penetrance of germline BRCA1 and BRCA2 mutations in a population series of 649 women with ovarian cancer. Am J Hum Genet 2001;68:700–10.
126. Rowe SM, Coughlan SJ, McKenna NJ, et al. Ovarian carcinoma-associated TaqI restriction fragment length polymorphism in intron G of the progesterone receptor gene is due to an Alu sequence insertion. Cancer Res 1995;55:2743–5.
127. Pearce CL, Hirschhorn JN, Wu AH, et al. Clarifying the PROGINS allele association in ovarian and breast cancer risk: a haplotype-based analysis. J Natl Cancer Inst 2005;97:51–9.
128. De Vivo I, Huggins GS, Hankinson SE, et al. A functional polymorphism in the promoter of the progesterone receptor gene associated with endometrial cancer risk. Proc Natl Acad Sci U S A 2002;99:12263–8.
129. Agoulnik IU, Tong XW, Fischer DC, et al. A germline variation in the progesterone receptor gene increases transcriptional activity and may modify ovarian cancer risk. J Clin Endocrinol Metab 2004;89:6340–7.
130. Spurdle AB, Hopper JL, Chen X, et al. The progesterone receptor exon 4 Val660Leu G/T polymorphism and risk of breast cancer in Australian women. Cancer Epidemiol Biomarkers Prev 2002;11:439–43.
131. Fabjani G, Tong D, Czerwenka K, et al. Human progesterone receptor gene polymorphism PROGINS and risk for breast cancer in Austrian women. Breast Cancer Res Treat 2002;72:131–7.
132. Dunning AM, Healey CS, Pharoah PD, et al. A systematic review of genetic polymorphisms and breast cancer risk. Cancer Epidemiol Biomarkers Prev 1999;8:843–54.
133. Wang-Gohrke S, Chang-Claude J, Becher H, et al. Progesterone receptor gene polymorphism is associated with decreased risk for breast cancer by age 50. Cancer Res 2000;60:2348–50.
134. Donaldson CJ, Crapanzano JP, Watson JC, et al. PROGINS Alu insertion and human genomic diversity. Mutat Res 2002;501:137–41.
135. McKenna NJ, Kieback DG, Carney DN, et al. A germline TaqI restriction fragment length polymorphism in the progesterone receptor gene in ovarian carcinoma. Br J Cancer 1995;71:451–5.
136. Manolitsas TP, Englefield P, Eccles DM, Campbell IG. No association of a 306-bp insertion polymorphism in the progesterone receptor gene with ovarian and breast cancer. Br J Cancer 1997;75:1398–9.
137. Lancaster JM, Berchuck A, Carney ME, et al. Progesterone receptor gene polymorphism and risk for breast and ovarian cancer. Br J Cancer 1998;78:277.
138. Spurdle AB, Webb PM, Purdie DM, et al. No significant association between progesterone receptor exon 4 Val660Leu G/T polymorphism and risk of ovarian cancer. Carcinogenesis 2001;22:717–21.
139. Tong D, Fabjani G, Heinze G, et al. Analysis of the human progesterone receptor gene polymorphism progins in Austrian ovarian carcinoma patients. Int J Cancer 2001;95:394–7.
140. Lancaster JM, Wenham RM, Halabi S, et al. No relationship between ovarian cancer risk and progesterone receptor gene polymorphism in a population-based, case-control study in North Carolina. Cancer Epidemiol Biomarkers Prev 2003;12:226–7.
141. Terry KL, De Vivo I, Titus-Ernstoff L, et al. Genetic variation in the progesterone receptor gene and ovarian cancer risk. Am J Epidemiol 2005;161:442–51.
142. Pijnenborg JM, Romano A, Dam-de Veen GC, et al. Aberrations in the progesterone receptor gene and the risk of recurrent endometrial carcinoma. J Pathol 2005;205:597–605.
143. De Vivo I, Hankinson SE, Colditz GA, Hunter DJ. A functional polymorphism in the progesterone receptor gene is associated with an increase in breast cancer risk. Cancer Res 2003;63:5236–8.
144. Feigelson HS, Rodriguez C, Jacobs EJ, et al. No association between the progesterone receptor gene +331G/A polymorphism and breast cancer. Cancer Epidemiol Biomarkers Prev 2004;13:1084–5.
145. Berchuck A, Schildkraut JM, Wenham RM, et al. Progesterone receptor promoter +331A polymorphism is associated with a reduced risk of endometrioid and clear cell ovarian cancers. Cancer Epidemiol Biomarkers Prev 2004;13:2141–7.
146. Lohmueller KE, Pearce CL, Pike M, et al. Meta-analysis of genetic association studies supports a contribution of common variants to susceptibility to common disease. Nat Genet 2003;33:177–82.
147. Ioannidis JP, Ntzani EE, Trikalinos TA, Contopoulos-Ioannidis DG. Replication validity of genetic association studies. Nat Genet 2001;29:306–9.
148. Hirschhorn JN, Daly MJ. Genome-wide association studies for common diseases and complex traits. Nat Rev Genet 2005;6:95–108.
149. Coetzee GA, Ross RK. Re: prostate cancer and the androgen receptor. J Natl Cancer Inst 1994;86:872–3.
150. Ingles SA, Ross RK, Yu MC, et al. Association of prostate cancer risk with genetic polymorphisms in vitamin D receptor and androgen receptor. J Natl Cancer Inst 1997;89:166–70.
151. Makridakis NM, Ross RK, Pike MC, et al. Association of mis-sense substitution in SRD5A2 gene with prostate cancer in African-American and Hispanic men in Los Angeles, USA. Lancet 1999;354:975–8.

16

Ionizing Radiation

John B. Little, MD
David J. Grdina, PhD

The hazards of exposure to ionizing radiation were recognized shortly after Roentgen's discovery of the x-ray in 1895. Acute skin reactions were observed in many individuals working with early x-ray generators, and by 1902, the first radiation-induced cancer was reported arising in an ulcerated area of the skin. Within a few years, a large number of such skin cancers were observed, and the first report of leukemia in five radiation workers appeared in 1911.[1] Many experimental and epidemiologic studies have since confirmed the oncogenic effects of radiation.

A number of characteristics specific to ionizing radiation differentiate it from chemical toxic agents or other physical carcinogens. Notable among these is its ability to penetrate cells and to deposit energy within them in a random fashion, unaffected by the usual cellular barriers presented to chemical agents. All cells in the body are thus susceptible to damage by ionizing radiation; the amount of damage incurred will be related to the physical parameters that determine the radiation dose received by the particular cells or tissue.

This chapter briefly reviews the principal cellular effects of radiation, as well as what is known about cellular and molecular mechanisms for radiation carcinogenesis and pharmacologic countermeasures that can mitigate against these processes. The term *carcinogenesis* is used in its broad sense to include the development of all types of malignant neoplasms. Human risk estimates, derived primarily from epidemiologic studies following relatively high-dose radiation exposures, are also presented. However, few reliable human data are available on its oncogenic effects in the dose range below 10 to 20 cGy.

DEVELOPMENT OF RADIATION INJURY

Figure 16-1 is a representation of the interaction of ionizing radiation with biologic tissues and the subsequent development of radiation injury. Such radiation is of two major types: electromagnetic waves or ionizing particles. In either case, interaction with orbital electrons results in ionizations and excitations. The initial deposition of energy in irradiated cells thus occurs in the form of ionized and excited atoms or molecules distributed at random throughout the cells. The ionizations cause most of the chemical changes in the vicinity of the event; this energy may be subsequently transferred through a chain of chemical reactions, finally producing irreversible damage to critical molecules of biologic importance to the cell. It appears that most of the energy that goes into producing excited molecules yields relatively few chemical reactions and is eventually dissipated in the form of heat.

The ionizing event involves the ejection of an orbital electron from a molecule, producing a positively charged or "ionized" molecule. These molecules are highly unstable and rapidly undergo chemical change. This change results in the production of free radicals; these are atoms or molecules containing unpaired electrons. These free radicals are extremely reactive and may lead to permanent damage of the affected molecule, or the energy may be transferred to another molecule. Most of the energy deposited within a cell results in the production of aqueous free radicals because approximately 80% of the cell is water. Chemical damage may be repaired before it is irreversible by the recombination of radicals and dissipation of the associated energy, or it may be modified by agents such as molecular oxygen or sulfhydryl compounds, a class of drugs extensively studied for development as radioprotectors.

As the initial ionizing events are similar for all types of radiation, their biologic effects are also qualitatively similar. However, densely ionizing radiations such as alpha particles produce more biologic damage per unit of energy absorbed. The relative biologic effectiveness (RBE) of different types of radiation relative to x-rays is thus related to their linear energy transfer (LET), a measure of the density of the ionizations produced along the radiation track. The initial critical biologic change is thought to be damage to deoxyribonucleic acid (DNA) molecules in the cell. The time required for the entire chain of physical and chemical events, as shown in Figure 16-1, from the initial interaction until the production of DNA damage is on the order of a microsecond or less. The subsequent development of biochemical and physiologic changes, however, may take hours to days, whereas the induction of cancer may take many years.

PRINCIPAL CELLULAR AND TISSUE EFFECTS OF RADIATION

Cell Killing Radiation can kill cells by two distinct mechanisms. The first is apoptosis, which is also called programmed cell death or interphase death.[2–4] Cells undergoing apoptosis as an immediate consequence of radiation damage usually die in interphase within a few hours of irradiation, irrespective of and without intervening mitosis. They share distinct morphologic changes, including loss of normal nuclear structure and degradation of DNA, which can be demonstrated by a classic pattern of "laddering" on DNA blots. It has long been known that apoptotic cell death can be induced by exposure to relatively low doses of radiation in a few cell types, including small lymphocytes, type A spermatogonia, and oocytes.[2] However, apoptosis may also be a significant cause of death in a broader variety of cell types exposed to higher radiation doses, particularly those of hematopoietic or lymphoid origin.

Early investigations have suggested that radiation-induced apoptosis is dependent on the functional activity of the *TP53* gene, but it soon became evident that *TP53*-independent pathways may also be involved, such as that mediated by the Bcl-2/BAX family,[5] all of which converge on the activation of proteases called caspases.[6] It has been proposed that *TP53*-dependent apoptosis may involve the transcriptional induction of redox-related genes with the formation of reactive oxygen species, leading to cell death by oxidative stress.[7] DNA damage is thought to be important in triggering the apoptotic response.[8,9] However, there is also evidence of the role of membrane damage and signaling pathways outside the nucleus that involve tyrosine kinases, especially ceramide in the apoptotic process.[10] Apoptosis may serve as a protective mechanism for the elimination of heavily DNA-damaged and thus potentially mutated cells from an irradiated population.

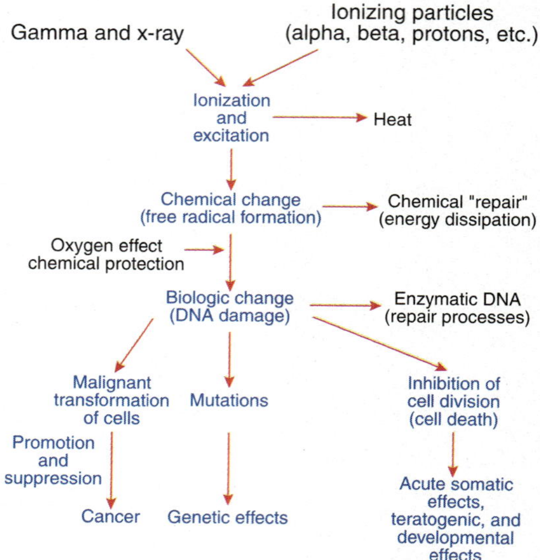

Figure 16-1 Development of radiation injury.

Another potential mechanism for removing heavily damaged cells from an irradiated population is the induction of an irreversible G_1/S arrest.[11] This is observed, for example, following irradiation of human diploid fibroblasts, which are very resistant to apoptosis. The fraction of cells irreversibly blocked in G_1/S is reduced if the cells are allowed to repair potentially lethal damage prior to assaying for survival.[11] This arrest is *TP53* and *ATM* dependent[12–14]; no arrest occurs following irradiation of *ATM* homozygotic cells[11] or of *TP53*$^{-/-}$ cells from patients with Li-Fraumeni syndrome.[12] The activation of the *TP53-p21* pathway by radiation damage in some human tumor cells also suppresses the progression of G_1 cells into the DNA synthetic (S) phase of the cell cycle, as well as enhancing apoptotic cell death.[15,16] Interestingly, overexpression of the c-*myc* oncogene can attenuate this effect in irradiated cells.[17] It has been hypothesized that the absence of a G_1 arrest is responsible for the genetic instability that occurs in irradiated cells lacking normal *TP53* function; cells with extensive genetic damage will progress through the cell cycle and continue proliferation rather than become arrested in G_1 and undergo apoptotic cell death or become senescent. However, the G_1 arrest is only one aspect of a complex cellular response to DNA damage.

The second mechanism for cell killing is radiation-induced reproductive failure. Radiation in sufficient doses can inhibit mitosis, that is, the cell's ability to divide and proliferate indefinitely. The inhibition of cellular proliferation is the mechanism by which radiation kills most mammalian cells. The nature and kinetics of the cytotoxic effects of radiation have been reviewed elsewhere.[2,12] As radiation kills cells by inhibiting their ability to divide, its effects in human beings occur primarily in tissues with high cell turnover or renewal rates characterized by a large amount of proliferative activity. These include tissues such as the bone marrow and the mucosal lining of the stomach and small intestine. Symptoms of acute exposure to whole-body irradiation in human beings are usually observed only following doses of 100 cGy or greater, whereas significant cell killing in vitro can be detected with doses as low as 10 cGy.

Another important somatic effect related to cell killing arises from irradiation of the developing embryo and fetus.[18,19] Whereas irradiation of experimental animals with doses on the order of 200 to 400 cGy during the first trimester of pregnancy has led to a variety of congenital anomalies in the offspring, no such effects were found in large populations of mice exposed to doses below 25 cGy.[18] Moreover, no increase in the frequency of congenital anomalies has been observed in human beings, even following relatively high radiation doses.

Recent epidemiologic studies on the atomic bomb survivors of Hiroshima and Nagasaki focused on mental retardation and other measures of intelligence, such as test scores and school performance.[19] These are presumably more sensitive indicators of radiation effects owing to cell depletion among the neuroblasts during development. Neuroblasts comprise by far the largest population of cells in the early fetus and continue proliferating until the fifth or sixth month of pregnancy. The number of children with such disorders in the atomic bomb survivor study is small, and the mean values for all end points are not significantly different from those in controls for the dose groups below 50 to 100 cGy. The Committee on the Biologic Effects of Ionizing Radiations of the National Research Council (BEIR V Committee) concluded that for mental retardation, the best documented of the developmental abnormalities, the prevalence appeared to increase with dose in a linear manner for individuals irradiated between 8 and 15 weeks, the most sensitive time period after conception.[20] However, the data do not exclude a threshold in the range of 20 to 40 cGy and, indeed, best fit a threshold dose-response relationship with a lower bound of 12 to 20 cGy.[20] On the assumption of a linear, nonthreshold relationship, however, the magnitude of the risk would be approximately a 4% chance of occurrence per 10 cGy for exposure at 8 to 15 weeks of gestational age, with less risk occurring for exposure at other ages.

Mutagenesis The mutagenic effects of ionizing radiation were first described by Herman Muller, in 1927, in his classic experiments with the fruit fly *Drosophila*. Subsequent experiments showed the dose-response relationship for such mutations to be a linear function of exposure over a wide range of radiation doses from as low as 10 to as high as 1,000 cGy. Studies of the induction of single-gene mutations in human cells have been limited to several genetic loci. Of particular note is the X-chromosomal gene for hypoxanthine-guanine phosphoribosyltransferase, first recognized through its human germinal mutations and then extensively studied as a useful reporter gene for somatic mutations in vitro and in vivo in animals and humans.[21,22] The results of most of these studies also suggest that the induction of mutations in human cells is a linear function of dose with doses as low as 10 cGy, and perhaps as low as 1 cGy, and that the dose-rate effect appears to be relatively small.[23,24] DNA structural analyses show that the majority of radiation-induced mutations in human cells result from large-scale genetic events involving loss of the entire active gene and often extending to other loci on the same chromosome.[25]

The major potential consequence of radiation-induced mutations in human populations is heritable genetic effects resulting from mutations induced in germinal cells. Such effects have been examined in several different animal systems.[20,26] For high–dose-rate exposure, the induced mutation rate per gamete generally falls in the range of 10^{-4} to 10^{-5}/cGy. The rates per locus are in the range of 10^{-7} to 10^{-8}/cGy. Protraction of exposure appears to decrease the mutation rate in rodent systems by a factor of 2 or greater. When all of the experimental data for the various genetic end points are considered, the genetic doubling dose (radiation dose necessary to double the spontaneous mutation rate) for low–dose-rate exposure appears to be in the range of 100 cGy. Although significant heritable genetic effects of radiation have not yet been demonstrated in human populations, a doubling dose of 100 cGy is not inconsistent with the absence of a statistically significant increase in hereditary disease among the children of atomic bomb survivors.[27] Indeed, 100 cGy represents approximately the lower 95% confidence interval for the human doubling dose calculated from the atomic bomb survivor data.[20]

Chromosomal Aberrations Radiation can induce two types of chromosomal aberrations in mammalian cells. The first have been termed "unstable" aberrations in that they are usually lethal to dividing cells. They include such changes as dicentrics, ring chromosomes, large deletions, and fragments. These types of aberrations do not allow the equal distribution of genetic material into daughter cells; in many cases, the frequency of such aberrations correlates well with the cytotoxic effects of radiation.

The second type has been termed "stable" aberrations. These include changes such as small deletions, reciprocal translocations, and aneuploidy changes that do not preclude the cell from dividing and proliferating. Figure 16-2 shows a karyotype of a human cell showing a stable aberration. Radiation-induced reciprocal translocations such as have occurred in this cell may be passed on through many generations of cell replication and emerge in clonal cell populations.[28,29]

It is well known that such deletions and translocations can result in gene mutations. It is tempting to speculate that they may play a more fundamental role in the process of radiation carcinogenesis. Typically, cancer cells are aneuploid and contain multiple stable chromosomal aberrations. In a number of cases, specific chromosomal abnormalities are associated with specific tumor types. In some instances, such as the chromosome 8:14 translocation in Burkitt's lymphoma, the chromosomal change results in the activation of a specific oncogene. In others, such as the chromosome 13q14 deletion found in retinoblastoma (RB), tumor development has been ascribed to loss or inactivation of the *RB* tumor suppressor gene. Although radiation-induced cancers show multiple unbalanced chromosomal rearrangements, few show such specific translocations as would be associated with the activation of specific oncogenes or known tumor suppressor genes.[30]

Neoplastic Transformation In Vitro An important cellular effect of radiation is neoplastic transformation, or the conversion of a normal cell to one with the phenotype of a cancer cell, including the ability to form an invasive, malignant tumor on reinjection into syngeneic hosts. Most human cancers have been shown to be clonal in origin. That is, all of the cells within a tumor are descendants of a single cell that has undergone

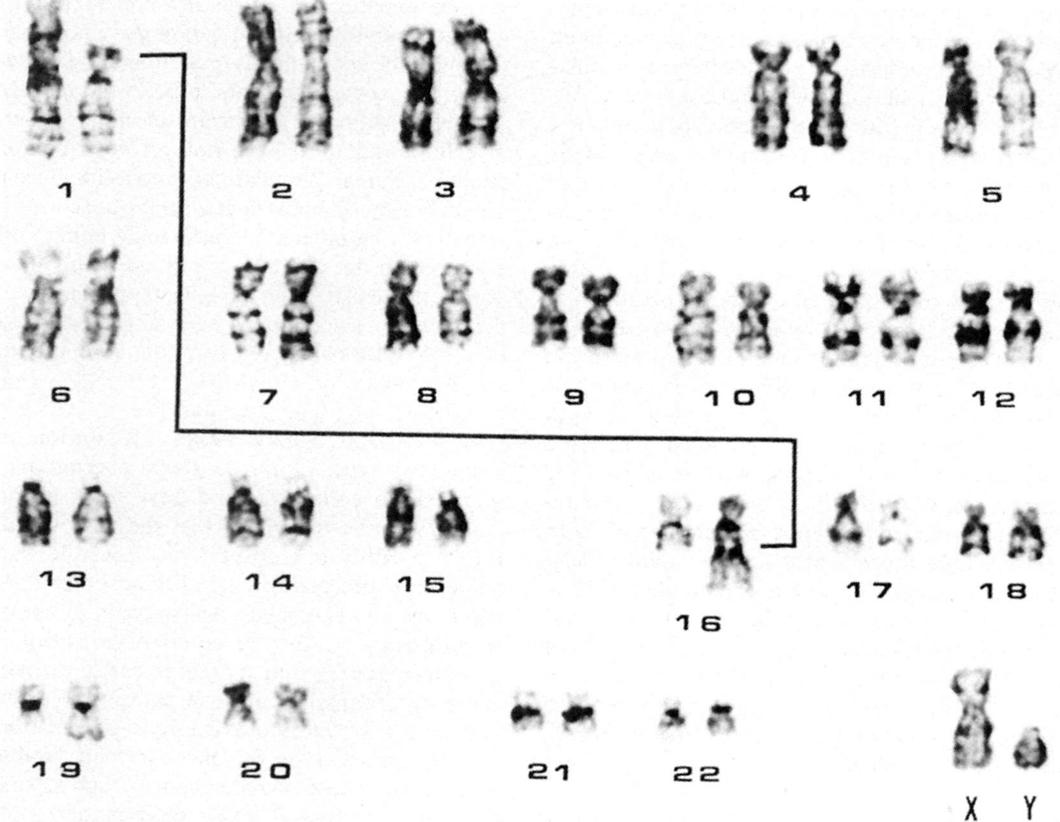

Figure 16-2 Karyotype of normal human diploid fibroblast showing stable chromosomal rearrangement (1:16 translocation) induced by radiation. The irradiated cells were serially subcultivated for 3 months (approximately 20 cell generations) before this cell was analyzed.

the process of neoplastic transformation. The transformation of one or more normal cells in a tissue in vivo is presumed to represent the earliest step in the overall process of carcinogenesis. Whether such a transformed cell can successfully give rise to an invasive, malignant tumor depends on a number of tissue and systemic factors. Although a number of different in vitro transformation systems involving various species and cell types are under investigation, those that generate reliable quantitative data have been restricted to rodent cells, and in none of these is the entire process of malignant transformation measured.[31,32] Rather, surrogate features of transformation are assayed, such as changes in colony morphology, focus formation, or growth under anchorage-independent conditions.

Studies of cellular and animal models for radiation carcinogenesis indicate that it is a progressive, multistep process by which normal cells acquire the various phenotypic characteristics of cancer cells.[33] There appear to be three major independent stages in the malignant transformation of cells in vitro: the development of morphologic changes, cellular immortality, and tumorigenicity.[31] Morphologic changes are many and varied, including the development of abnormalities in cytology, growth pattern, and the control of cell proliferation. Immortalization occurs frequently in rodent cells but extremely rarely in human cells, either spontaneously or as a result of treatment with radiation or chemical carcinogens. It can be induced, however, by transfection of human diploid cells with certain oncogenes and/or genes associated with tumor viruses such as the SV40 T antigen or the E6/E7 genes of human papillomavirus 16 and have been associated with the production of telomerase. Immortalization may thus be an important rate-limiting step in human cell transformation and perhaps in human carcinogenesis in vivo.[31] Tumorigenicity also appears to be an independent phenotype that generally occurs only in previously immortalized cells. A subpopulation of such immortal cells may undergo additional genomic rearrangements that give them a selective growth advantage in vivo perhaps related to factors present in the host animal.[34]

Incubation of cells with various agents either immediately preceding or following exposure or during the 4- to 6-week postirradiation expression period for transformation can markedly modify the ultimate yield of transformed cells.[35–37] The phosphorothioate drug amifostine and its methylated analog were both effective in protecting C3H/10T½ cells against the transforming effects of either low LET gamma rays or fission spectrum neutrons.[35,36] In contrast, the phorbol ester compound 12-0-tetradecanoyl-phorbol-13-acetate (TPA) acts as a potent promoter of x-ray transformation if applied repeatedly beginning either immediately after irradiation or several weeks later. In addition to amifostine, a number of additional drugs have been demonstrated to protect against radiation-induced transformation. These include selenium, retinoids, carotenoids, and ascorbic acid, as well as certain protease inhibitors that have shown promise as chemopreventive agents in vivo.[38–40] Transformation can also be modulated by hormones, growth factors, and anti-inflammatory agents.[38]

It has thus become evident that a number of noncarcinogenic secondary factors can markedly modulate the frequency of radiation-induced transformation. Because transformation can be markedly enhanced, suppressed, or completely inhibited by such factors, they may become the controlling ones in the overall process of transformation of cells exposed to radiation. In many cases, the effects of such agents in vitro have been predictive of those observed in experimental animal systems. It therefore seems likely that secondary factors may be of importance in human radiation carcinogenesis, although there are few epidemiologic data to support this contention.

Radiation-Induced Genomic Instability
This term refers to a phenomenon observed in a number of different cellular systems whereby radiation exposure appears to induce a type of transmissible genetic instability in individual cells that is transmitted to their progeny, leading to a persistent enhancement in the rate at which genetic changes arise in the descendants of the irradiated cell after many generations of replication. The occurrence of such a process could enhance the probability that a single cell lineage would acquire the multiple sequential and interacting gene mutations necessary to convert a normal cell to a full malignant cell. It would also imply that radiation could act at any point in this carcinogenic process. This phenomenon has been termed a nontargeted effect of radiation because genetic damage occurs in cells that in themselves received no direct radiation exposure. The end points studied include malignant transformation, specific gene mutations, and chromosomal aberrations. Typically, this phenomenon is studied by examining the occurrence of such genetic effects in clonal populations derived from single cells surviving radiation exposure.[40] Figure 16-3 shows this schematically.

Early evidence for the existence of such a phenomenon was derived from an examination of the kinetics of radiation-induced malignant transformation of cells in vitro.[41,42] These results suggested that transformed foci did not arise from a single, radiation-damaged cell. Rather, radiation appeared to induce a type of instability in 20 to 30% of the irradiated cell population; this instability enhanced the probability of the occurrence of a second, neoplastic transforming event. This finding is in contradistinction to the classic theories of carcinogenesis in which the initiating event is thought to be rare and likely mutagenic in nature. This second event was a rare one, however, occurring with the frequency of approximately 10^{-6} and involved in the actual transformation of one or more of the progeny of the original irradiated cells after many rounds of cell division. This second transforming event

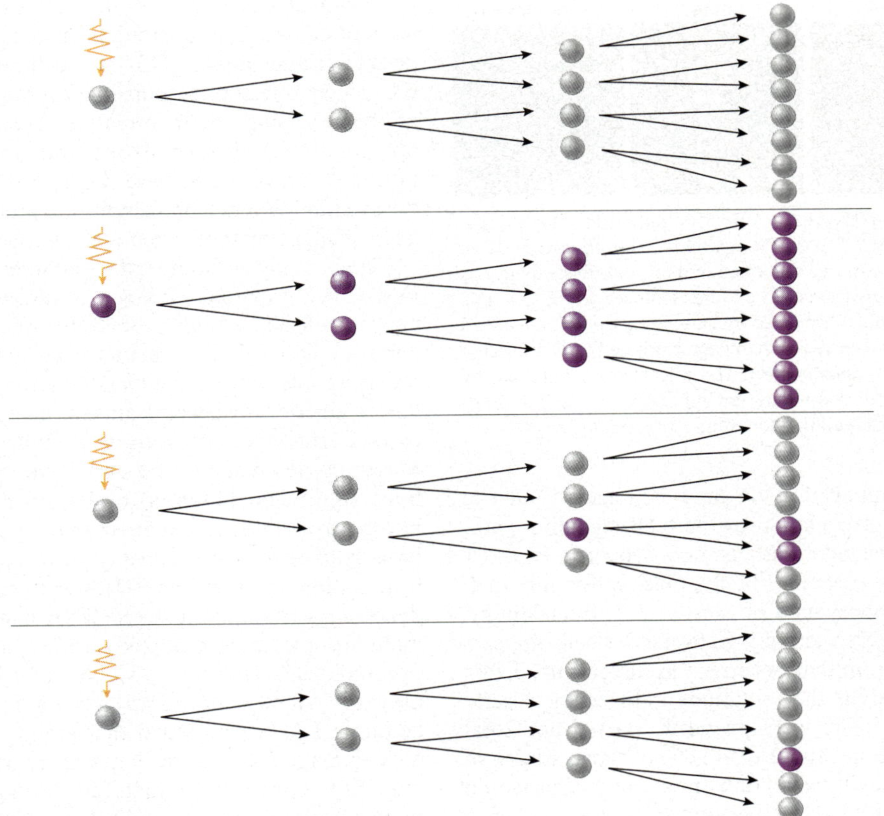

Figure 16-3 Schematic of radiation-induced mutagenesis. *Open circles* represent normal wild-type cells, while *closed circles* represent mutated cells. B is an example of a cell directly mutated by radiation exposure; the mutation is transmitted to all of its progeny. However, most of the cells in the irradiated population will retain the wild-type phenotype (A). C and D are examples of mutations arising as a result of radiation-induced genomic instability. The irradiated cell and its immediate progeny are wild type, but the frequency with which mutations arise amongst the more distant descendants of the irradiated cell is elevated.

occurred with the constant frequency per cell per generation and had the characteristics of a mutagenic event.[43] Thus, neoplastically transformed foci did not appear to arise from the original irradiated cell but rather from one or more of its progeny.

This phenomenon was subsequently demonstrated in a number of experiment systems for various genetic end points.[44–47] In terms of mutagenesis, approximately 10% of clonal populations derived from single cells surviving radiation exposure showed a significant elevation in the frequency of spontaneously arising mutations compared with clonal populations derived from nonirradiated cells.[48,49] This increased mutation rate persisted for approximately 30 to 50 generations postirradiation. The molecular structural spectrum of these late-arising mutants resembles those of spontaneous mutations in that the majority of them are point mutations,[49,50] whereas direct x-ray–induced mutations primarily involve deletions. An enhancement of both minisatellite[51] and microsatellite[52] instability has also been observed in the progeny of irradiated cells selected for mutations at the thymidine kinase locus.

An enhanced frequency of nonclonal chromosomal aberrations was first reported in clonal descendants of mouse hematopoietic stem cells 12 to 14 generations after exposure to alpha radiation.[53] Persistent radiation-induced chromosomal instability has since been shown to occur in a number of other cellular systems.[54–57] Transmission of such chromosomal instability has also been shown to occur in vivo,[58,59] but susceptibility to radiation-induced chromosomal instability differed significantly among different strains of mice.[60,61] Finally, a persistent increase in the rate of cell death has been shown to occur in cell populations many generations after radiation exposure.[62–64] Delayed reproductive failure has been linked to chromosomal instability[65] and malignant transformation,[66,67] and evidence has been presented to suggest that DNA is at least one of the critical targets in the initiation of this phenomenon.[68] It has been proposed that oxidative stress, perhaps consequent to enhanced, *TP53*-independent apoptosis, may contribute to the perpetuation of the instability phenotype in these populations.[65,67,69]

A recent novel phenomenon has been identified and coined *the delayed radioprotective effect*. The delayed radioprotective effect is manifested by an enhanced resistance to ionizing radiation hours to days following exposure of cells to thiol-containing drugs, such as *N*-acetylcysteine and captopril, which have the ability to elevate intracellular antioxidant enzymes, such as manganese superoxide dismutase (MnSOD).[70,71] The underlying mechanism of action responsible for this effect is the activation of the redox-sensitive nuclear transcription factor κB (NF-κB) by thiol-reducing agents, which subsequently results in the elevated transcription of MnSOD. The resulting 10- to 20-fold elevation of intracellular MnSOD facilitates the prevention and removal of radiation-induced oxidative damage and can enhance survival of cells by 10 to 30%. The ability to elevate and maintain prolonged enhanced intracellular antioxidant levels through this mechanism may therefore facilitate the prevention of the genomic instability phenotype if persistent oxidative stress is indeed a causative factor.

Of importance in terms of radiation carcinogenesis and potential chemoprevention strategies are the emerging observations indicating that persistent oxidative stress and genomic instability occur in vivo and may be related to the induction of cancer. The transmission of radiation-induced chromosomal instability in vivo has been demonstrated in several distinct experimental models,[58,59,72] and evidence has been presented to suggest that instability induced in x-irradiated mouse hematopoietic stem cells may be related to the occurrence of the nonspecific genetic damage found in radiation-induced leukemias in these mice.[73] Sensitivity to mammary tumor induction was found not only to be strain specific but to correlate with the strain specificity for the induction of chromosomal instability in mammary epithelial cells irradiated in vivo.[72] These were related to reduced expression of the DNA repair enzymes DNA-PKcs[74] and a high frequency of telomere fusions.[75] This mouse model thus relates radiation-induced genomic instability to a defect in DNA repair and associates it with an enhanced susceptibility to radiation-induced cancer.

It is thus well established that radiation can induce a type of instability in cells that enhances the probability of the occurrence of multiple genetic events in surviving cell populations, sometimes after many generations of replication. Thus, rather than inducing an “initiating” mutation, radiation may play a more general role in the process of carcinogenesis. If this is the case, the initiating event would not be directly related to the tumor itself, but one that enhances the probability that the required mutations would arise in a given cell lineage. Radiation could thus act at any state in tumor development. However, the precise mechanisms for this phenomenon, including how it is initiated and maintained, remain to be elucidated. Various tightly regulated cellular processes may be disrupted by radiation, leading to a chaotic state that perturbs the normal regulatory and signaling pathways, thus disrupting cellular homeostasis, a state from which the cell never completely recovers.[68] It is tempting to speculate that the various factors known to modulate malignant transformation in vitro may act on this process. Interestingly, this concept is consistent with the emerging findings in human populations that suggest that some types of radiation-induced cancer may follow a relative risk model (see below), that is, a given dose of radiation increases the rate of occurrence of cancer at all follow-up times rather than inducing a specific cohort of new tumors.

Bystander Effects in Irradiated Cell Populations It has long been thought that the cell nucleus is the target for the important biologic effects of radiation; these effects occur in the irradiated cell as a direct result of DNA damage that has not been correctly restored by enzymatic repair processes. However, recent evidence shows that targeted cytoplasmic radiation is significantly mutagenic.[76] Moreover, it has become evident that damage signals may be transmitted from irradiated to nonirradiated cells in the population, leading to the occurrence of biologic effects in cells that received no radiation exposure.[77] This phenomenon has been termed the "bystander" effect of radiation; it could be of considerable importance in the carcinogenic effects of very low doses of densely ionizing radiation, such as alpha particles released by radon. Only a small fraction of a person's bronchial epithelial cells, the presumed target for lung cancer, will actually be hit by an alpha particle from residential radon exposure during an exposed person's lifetime.

The experimental model used to study this effect has generally involved the exposure of monolayer cultures of cells to very low fluences of alpha particles, fluences whereby a very small fraction of the cell population will actually be hit by a particle. In the initial study, an enhanced frequency of sister chromatid exchanges was observed in 20 to 40% of cells exposed to fluences by which only 1:1,000 to 1:100 cells were traversed by an alpha particle.[78] Evidence has been presented that this effect involves the secretion of cytokines or other factors by irradiated cells that leads to an up-regulation of oxidative metabolism in bystander cells.[79,80] There is also evidence that incubation with conditioned medium from irradiated cells has cytotoxic effects on nonirradiated cells, which may be related to the release of a factor(s) into the medium, including reactive oxygen species.[81] These findings are reminiscent of the reports that clastogenic activity can be isolated from the plasma of radiation-exposed people.[82]

Of particular note is the observation that an enhanced frequency of specific gene mutations,[83,84] as well as chromosomal aberrations,[85] occurs in bystander cells in populations exposed to very low fluences of alpha particles. As a result, the induced mutation frequency per alpha particle track increases at low fluences at which bystander and directly irradiated cells are at risk of the induction of mutations. This leads to hyperlinearity of the dose-response curve in the low-dose region.

Changes in gene expression also occur in bystander cells in monolayer cultures; the expression levels of tp53, p21[Waf1], CDC2, cyclin B1, and rad51 were significantly modulated in nonirradiated cells in confluent human diploid cell populations exposed to very low fluences of alpha particles.[86] As seen in Figure 16-4, clusters of cells showed enhanced expression of p21[Waf1] as determined by in situ immunofluorescence staining techniques, although only approximately 1 to 2% of the cell nuclei were actually traversed by an alpha particle. This phenomenon involved cell-to-cell communication via gap junctions.[87] Evidence that the up-regulation of the tp53 signaling pathway in bystander cells is a consequence of DNA damage is supported by the observation that tp53 was phosphorylated on serine 15.[87] Interestingly, however, DNA damage in bystander cells appears to differ from that occurring in directly irradiated cells; whereas the mutations induced in directly irradiated cells were primarily partial and total gene deletions, more than 90% of those arising in bystander cells were point mutations.[88] This would be consistent with the evidence that oxidative metabolism is up-regulated in bystander cells[79,80] and has led to the hypothesis that the point mutations are a result of oxidative base damage occurring in bystander cells.[88] The activation of mitogen-activated protein kinase (MAPK) proteins and their downstream effectors in bystander cells[80] is of particular interest in terms of the preliminary evidence that membrane signaling is involved in the bystander effect in monolayer cultures.[89]

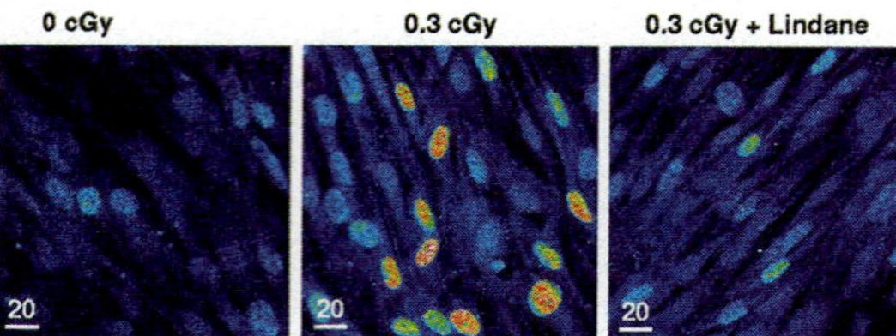

Figure 16-4 Bystander effect of radiation. The expression of p21[Waf1] was determined in individual cells in monolayer cultures of human diploid fibroblasts by in situ immunofluorescence. In cultures exposed to 0.3 cGy (<1 to 2% of nuclei traversed by an alpha particle), enhanced expression occurred in many nonirradiated cells occurring in clusters (*center panel*). The effect was suppressed by incubation with lindane, an inhibitor of gap junction-mediated intercellular communication (*right panel*).

The results of these studies of bystander effects indicate clearly that damage signals can be transmitted from irradiated to nonirradiated cells. In confluent monolayer cultures, this phenomenon involves gap junction–mediated cell-to-cell communication and appears to involve both the induction of reactive oxygen species and the activation of extranuclear signal transduction pathways. Some evidence suggests that regulation of the tp53 damage-response pathway may be central to this phenomenon. These findings could potentially be of considerable significance in terms of residential radon exposure, in which the mutagenic and carcinogenic effects could be greater than those predicted on the basis only of those bronchial epithelial cells actually traversed by an alpha particle.

MOLECULAR MECHANISMS

DNA Damage and Genetic Changes It is well accepted that DNA damage is central to the biologic effects of ionizing radiation. The production of this damage by ionization, resulting specifically in the efficient induction of DNA strand breaks, differentiates ionizing radiation from most other physical and chemical carcinogens. Although ionizing radiation can produce a broad spectrum of DNA lesions, including damage to nucleotide bases, unrepaired or misrepaired DNA double-strand breaks (DSBs) are thought to be the principal lesions responsible for the induction of genetic changes in mammalian cells, including chromosomal abnormalities and gene mutations.[90,91] In contrast, base damage is generally the predominant mechanism for the production of such changes by most chemical carcinogens.

Track analysis studies of x-ray interactions in DNA have provided evidence of clustered damage, which has a high probability of producing complex DSBs.[90] This results from the fact that radiation interactions are usually associated with the production of several closely associated ion pairs. Certain types of DNA base damage, such as 8-hydroxydeoxyguanosine and thymine glycols, have significant potential biologic importance, but the available data suggest that such isolated base damage by itself probably plays a minor role in radiation mutagenesis.[91] However, recent evidence suggests that clustered DNA damage may include abasic sites, oxidized purines, or oxidized pyrimidines.[92] This study, which employed a new method of measuring clustered lesions in genomic DNA, concluded that among all complex damage induced by ionizing radiation, the majority represented clustered damage rather than simple DSBs. The DNA repair proteins Ku70 and Ku80 appear to mediate the repair of such damage.[93] The increased efficiency of DNA breaks induced by high LET radiation appears to result primarily from their greater complexity.[94] Substantial yields of DSBs may also result from secondary electrons with energies well below the ionizing threshold.[95]

Cells possess a complex set of signaling pathways for recognizing such DNA damage and initiating its repair, which are only recently becoming better understood. The *ATM* gene is one of the prime sensors of DNA damage, which activates by phosphorylation a variety of proteins involved in cell cycle control and DNA repair. Two mechanistically distinct pathways that function in complementary ways are involved in the repair of DSBs: nonhomologous end joining (NHEJ), which requires little sequence homology between the DNA ends and is thus error prone, and homologous recombination (HR), which uses extensive homology and is generally error free.[96] NHEJ involves a complex of proteins, including Ku70, Ku80, the DNA-PK catalytic subunit DNA-PKcs, XRCC4, and ligase IV. The NBS1/MRE11/RAD50 complex[97] is also involved in the nucleolytic processing stages of NHEJ; this complex also contributes to HR. HR also involves a complex of proteins, notably RAD51 and other factors in the RAD50 epistasis group.[98] Strong links have been established between recombinational repair and the breast cancer susceptibility proteins BRCA1 and BRCA2,[99–101] as well as the Fanconi's anemia family of proteins.[102] Thus, the metabolic repair of radiation-induced DNA strand breaks involves a large complex of proteins, many of which are associated with clinical syndromes of radiosensitivity and cancer susceptibility.

Unrepaired or misrepaired DSBs lead primarily to large-scale genetic changes that are frequently manifested by chromosomal aberrations. However, the search for genetic changes associated specifically with radiation exposure has proven very disappointing. There is no evidence of site specificity for mutations induced by radiation. The spectrum of molecular-structural changes associated with direct radiation-induced mutations involves primarily partial and total gene deletions, thus differing from that for spontaneous mutations in which point mutations predominate. However, there appears to be no site specificity for DNA breakpoints that lead to deletions, and, similarly, sequence analyses of radiation-induced point mutations have generally shown no site specificity.[103] Furthermore, no genetic alterations unique to radiation have as yet been found in radiation-induced tumors.

Tumor Suppressor Genes It is known that unbalanced translocations can lead to deletions. Because certain cancers that are known to be induced by radiation (such as some types of leukemia and sarcoma) are specifically those in which deletions occur, it has been proposed that the most likely mutational event in the initiation of radiation carcinogenesis involves loss of heterozygosity (LOH) of a tumor suppressor gene.[30] One specific example of this phenomenon is the *RB* tumor suppressor gene located on chromosome 13q14. The hypersensitivity of RB patients to the induction of secondary cancers following radiotherapy, primarily osteosarcomas in the treatment field, is presumably the result of radiation-induced LOH of the *RB* gene.[104] However, RB is a rare disorder, and there are few other examples from animal or human carcinogenesis to support the attractive hypothesis that the induction of LOH at tumor suppressor loci is a general phenomenon in the initiation of radiation carcinogenesis.

Much interest has centered around the *TP53* gene because it appears to play an important role in cell cycle control, radiosensitivity, the development of genetic instability leading to cell transformation, and perhaps in the response of human tumors to radiation or chemotherapy. *TP53* mutations have been found in a wide spectrum of human cancers[105] and in mouse skin tumors induced by ionizing radiation.[106] Mutations of *TP53* have also been associated with lung cancer induced in underground miners by alpha radiation.[107] Although some strains of knockout mice, either hemizygous or homozygous for the *TP53* gene, are more susceptible to radiation-induced tumors,[108] LOH at this locus may not be the initiating event.[109] Indeed, there is increasing evidence that *TP53* mutations may arise late in the development of tumors.[110,111] LOH for *TP53* mutation in knockout mice may also be a secondary event.[109] It is of interest in this context that the expression of *TP53* mutations also appears to occur late in the process of radiation-induced malignant transformation, during the growth of the visible transformed foci,[112] consistent with the findings in some human tumors.[110]

Another area of interest is the role of *TP53* in the control of cellular radiosensitivity because it has been proposed that *TP53* status may be a determinant in the therapeutic responsiveness of certain types of human tumors.[113,114] The absence of normal *TP53* function is associated with enhanced resistance of human diploid fibroblasts to radiation-induced reproductive failure.[12,115] A similar effect has been described in hematopoietic cell lineages in transgenic mice.[116] For cell types that readily undergo apoptosis, such as those of hematopoietic origin, the lack of an apoptotic response in *TP53*-deficient cells renders them more resistant to radiation. The role of *TP53* status in the radiosensitivity of cells derived from human solid tumors, however, remains unclear[117–119] and may depend on tumor type.

Oncogenes Although the involvement of various oncogenes in experimental and human carcinogenesis is well established, no data have emerged from animal models to suggest a general role for oncogene activation in radiation-induced cancer. Activation of members of the *RAS* family has been reported in a small fraction of certain mouse lymphomas,[120,121] and amplification and rearrangement of c-*myc* were found in a small percentage of radiation-induced murine osteosarcomas.[122] Radiation-induced skin papillomas in Car-S mice were notable in their lack of *HRAS* mutations compared with papillomas induced by a chemical carcinogen or TPA.[123] However, these scattered results have not been proven to form a consistent pattern of oncogene activation in radiation carcinogenesis. One special case is the activation of the *RET* oncogene, which has been associated with susceptibility to the induction of papillary carcinoma by radiation in children.[124]

EXPERIMENTAL RADIATION-INDUCED CARCINOGENESIS

General Characteristics of Radiation Carcinogenesis Ionizing radiation has been called a "universal carcinogen" in that it will induce cancer in most tissues of most species at all ages, including the fetus. It is one of the few definitely established carcinogens in human beings and perhaps the only one for which firm dose-response data in human populations are available. It is, however, a relatively weak carcinogen and mutagen. The cancers induced by radiation are of the same histologic types as occur naturally, but the distribution of types may differ. For example, a higher percentage of small cell carcinomas of the lung occur as a result of exposure to alpha radiation in uranium miners; radiation generally induces follicular and papillary carcinomas of the thyroid rather than anaplastic and medullary carcinomas; and chronic lymphocytic leukemia is apparently not induced by radiation, whereas other common types of leukemia are. There is a distinct latency period between exposure to radiation and the clinical appearance of a tumor.

Dose-Response Relationships It has generally been accepted that radiation carcinogenesis is a stochastic process, that is, the probability of the occurrence of the effect increases with dose with no threshold, but the severity of the effect is not influenced by dose. This is in contradistinction to a nonstochastic or deterministic effect, for which both the probability and the severity of the effect vary with dose. There is no clear experimental evidence to suggest that the grade of malignancy, including its invasive or metastatic properties, is a function of dose; radiation-induced cancer appears to be an all-or-none effect. Stochastic effects are those that may arise from damage to a few cells or even a single cell. If this is the case, any dose, no matter how small, carries with it the finite probability of producing the effect. Studies of radiation-induced carcinogenesis in experimental animals and human populations have been designed to test this hypothesis because most environmental exposures are in the low-dose range. Unfortunately, it is very difficult to obtain statistically significant data in either human or animal studies at doses below 10 to 20 cGy of low LET radiation.

Many earlier studies of the effects of radiation in small animals involved its life-shortening properties. Although this effect was originally ascribed to "radiation-induced aging," in which the natural causes of death were accelerated by radiation, a critical examination of this phenomenon by use of techniques such as serial sacrifice experiments and life table analyses has shown that practically all of the life-shortening effect of radiation in experimental animals can be accounted for by the induction of cancer, except perhaps in the high, sublethal dose range.[125,126] Thus, the dose-response relationship for life shortening in animals should reflect that for cancer deaths from all types of radiation-induced tumors in that species. Figure 16-5 shows such a dose-response curve.[127] A generally linear response has been observed for life shortening in a number of different studies.

The dose-response relationships for the induction of cancers in specific tissues of small animals vary with site, sex, and species.[128–130] For low LET radiation, the frequency of induced cancers generally rises with dose in the range of 0 to 300 cGy. In some cases, tumor incidence levels

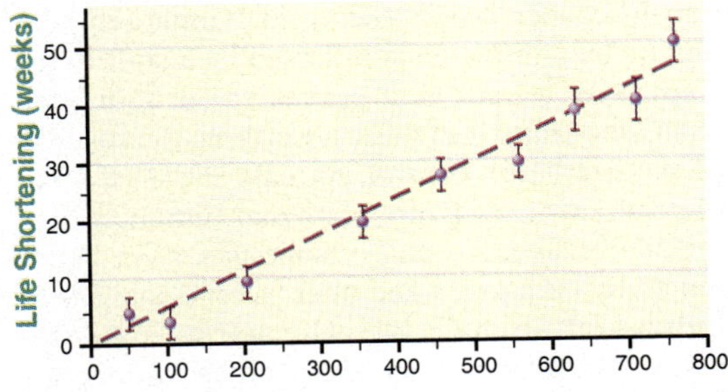

Figure 16-5 Life-shortening in mice as a function of the dose of ionizing radiation. The shortening of life span is ascribed to early death owing to induced cancers. (Reproduced with permission from Lindop P and Rotblat J.[127])

off at higher doses and may even decline. This phenomenon is thought to reflect cell killing. The carcinogenic effect of low LET radiation in rodents is usually reduced with protraction of exposure. In the dose range up to 200 to 300 cGy, the dose-response curves for individual tumor types vary but generally assume a linear-quadratic to near-linear relationship.

For high LET radiation, the rise in cancer incidence with dose is much steeper. The dose-response curves are approximately linear within the range of 0 to 20 cGy, although in some cases they bend over, reaching a plateau at higher doses.[128,131] In contradistinction to low LET radiation, significant increases in cancer and life shortening can be observed after doses as low as 10 cGy of neutrons, alpha particles, or heavy ions.[128,131,132] RBE values in the range of 3 to 15 have been estimated for the carcinogenic effects of these radiations at low doses. There is usually no dose-rate effect for high LET radiation exposure. However, an outstanding example is the induction of mouse mammary tumors by low doses of fast neutrons, in which protraction of exposure appears to increase the carcinogenic effect by a factor of 2 to 3 at doses of 2.5 to 10 cGy.[131]

Modifying Factors As in the case of neoplastic transformation, radiation-induced carcinogenesis in experimental animals can also be modulated by noncarcinogenic secondary factors. Postirradiation treatment with the tumor promoter TPA is known to enhance ultraviolet light–induced mouse skin cancer; a similar phenomenon has been shown for the induction of malignant squamous cell carcinoma of the skin of mice by ionizing radiation.[133]

The induction of carcinogenesis in experimental animals can also be suppressed by treatment with certain agents that are known to inhibit radiation-induced transformation in vitro. An example of this includes amifostine, which is the only drug currently approved for clinical use as a radioprotector by the US Food and Drug Administration.[134] As described by the Kaplan-Meier plots in Figure 16-6, inoculation of B6CF1 hybrid mice with a single dose of 400 mg/kg of amifostine 30 minutes prior to whole-body irradiation with 2 Gy of low LET radiation significantly protected against carcinogenesis in both male and female animals. As discussed earlier, the reduction in cancer deaths owing to lymphoreticular tumors by amifostine is reflected by a shift in the Kaplan-Meier survival curves for drug-treated irradiated animals to those describing the survival of nonirradiated control animals.[135–137] Causes of death owing to lymphoreticular tumors, which included leukemias and lymphomas, were determined by both gross and microscopic analysis of individual animals by veterinarian pathologists.[135] Likewise, certain protease inhibitors have also been shown to suppress the induction of cancer in several different tumor systems.[39] It is well known that the hormonal environment is important in certain radiation-induced rodent cancers, particularly ovarian and mammary tumors. These and other observations again emphasize the importance of noncarcinogenic secondary factors in experimental radiation carcinogenesis. However, the extent to which such factors are important in radiation-induced cancer in human populations is not clear.

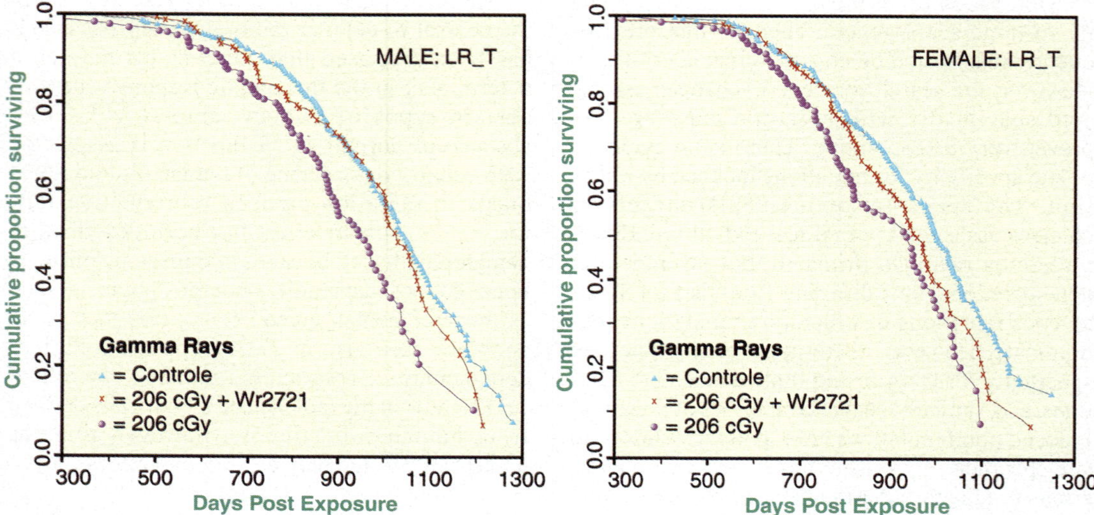

Figure 16-6. Survival curves resulting from lymphoreticular cancers (LR-T), as determined by histopathological analysis of tissues taken from deceased animals that had been irradiated (206 cGy) either with or without amifostine. LR-T includes histiocytic leukemia and lymphoma, lymphocytic-lymphoblastic leukemia and lymphoma, myelogenous leukemia, undifferentiated leukemia and lymphoma, and mixed histiocytic leukemia and lymphoma.

Genetic Susceptibility to Radiation-Induced Cancer The discovery that mutations in a number of specific genes are associated with an enhanced predisposition to single or multiple cancer types has stimulated renewed interest in the potential role of genetic susceptibility in the carcinogenic effects of radiation.[138,139] However, the known genes are highly penetrant and code for rare hereditary disorders. Should a significant fraction of the population be genetically predisposed to radiation-induced cancer, perhaps from mutations in more common but weakly penetrant genes, this fact could be of considerable importance in the development of protection standards.[140]

Although there is little evidence at present to suggest that such genetic factors are involved in most human cancers, they do appear to play a role in these rare hereditary disorders, which may serve as models for radiation-genetic interactions. For example, patients with hereditary retinoblastoma whose somatic cells are heterozygous for the *RB* gene are at markedly increased risk of the development of radiation-induced bone sarcomas,[104] whereas patients with the nevoid basal cell carcinoma syndrome are at high risk of the development of basal cell cancers in irradiated areas. Radiation has also been associated with an enhanced incidence of early-onset breast cancer, although the hereditary nature of radiation-induced breast cancer and its relationship to the breast cancer susceptibility genes *BRCA1 and BRCA2* remain to be clarified. Interestingly, transgenic mice heterozygous for either the *TP53*[108] or *ATM*[141] tumor suppressor genes also show an increased sensitivity to radiation-induced cancer; *ATM* and *TP53* heterozygosity is associated, respectively, with the human cancer–prone disorders ataxia-telangiectasia and Li-Fraumeni syndrome. It is not clear the extent to which more common, low-penetrance susceptibility genes may play a role in genetic predisposition to radiation-induced cancer.[138,140]

HUMAN EPIDEMIOLOGIC STUDIES

There is now a large body of data on radiation-induced cancer derived from epidemiologic studies in irradiated human populations, and it is primarily on the basis of these data that risk estimates are derived. These data are reviewed and analyzed in detail in the latest reports from the BEIR V Committee[20] and the United Nations Scientific Committee on the Effects of Atomic Radiation (UNSCEAR 2000).[142] They are derived primarily from two sources: the long-term follow-up of survivors of the nuclear bombings of Hiroshima and Nagasaki[143] and populations exposed to medical x-rays.[144–146] Information is also available from certain occupational exposures, particularly from individuals with pulmonary and skeletal exposure to alpha radiation. The results of these studies have yielded significant dose-response data for the induction of cancer in at least five tissue sites. Such dose-response data are extremely important in ascribing radiation as the causal agent for the increased incidence of cancer, as well as for estimating the risks associated with a given exposure. Unfortunately, however, the epidemiologic studies yielding useful dose-response data generally involve relatively high-dose exposures (> 10 cGy). Thus, risk estimates in the low-dose range must be derived from an extrapolation from the high-dose data. The shape of the dose-response relationship becomes of critical importance in making such extrapolations.

The observed dose-response curves from the human epidemiologic studies appear to be either linear or linear-quadratic in form (ie, a linear component at low doses with a quadratic component at higher doses); although a threshold (dose below which there is no effect) cannot be formally excluded at very low doses.[147,148] A linear curve implies a constant risk per cGy at all doses, whereas the linear-quadratic model implies a smaller risk per cGy in the low-dose range. The assumption of a linear model simplifies the extrapolation from high to low doses and the corresponding estimation of risks. Furthermore, it is a conservative technique, that is, if anything, it would overestimate rather than underestimate the potential risk. There is no evidence of a proportionally greater effect at low doses, except possibly for very low fluences of alpha particles if a bystander effect occurs in vivo.

A final parameter of importance in determining the hazards of a given dose of radiation is the choice of risk models. For many years, risks were estimated on the basis of an absolute risk model. This model assumed that a specific number of excess cancers was induced by a given radiation dose. Radiation-induced cancers occurred in addition to the natural incidence. Thus, the increased risk could be expressed as the number of excess cancer cases (or cancer deaths) per 10^6 exposed people per year per centigray (the rate per year) or as the total number of excess cancers per 10^6 exposed people per centigray (the total risk or lifetime yield of cancers to be expected from a given radiation dose). The absolute risk model generally assumes a linear dose-response relationship, although, with certain corrections, it can be applied to a linear-quadratic relationship. Because the radiation exposure in Hiroshima included a small fraction of neutrons, the doses in the atomic bomb survivor studies are expressed in sieverts (Sv) rather than grays, a term that takes into account the RBE of neutrons. For our purposes, however, we can consider that 1 Sv equals approximately 1 Gy.

An analysis of the recent data from the atomic bomb survivors suggests that some types of radiation-induced cancer more likely follow a relative risk model.[20,143] This is also true for several different tumor types in mice.[125] The relative risk model implies that radiation increases the natural incidence of cancer at all ages by a dose-dependent factor. Because the excess cancer risk is proportional to the natural incidence, radiation-induced cancers would occur primarily at the times when natural tumors arose, independent of the age at irradiation. Thus, the largest cohort of radiation-induced cancers would occur in older individuals. The relative risk model appears to fit the epidemiologic data for several solid tumors, although it does not appear to be valid for leukemia or bone and lung cancers. In general, the risk estimates derived from the studies involving medical exposures are similar to those of the atomic bomb survivors[146,149,150]; differences in the case of high-dose radiation therapy exposures can be ascribed to cell killing and the effect of dose fractionation.[145] A significantly reduced effect with fractionation for high-dose exposure was observed for lung cancer.[151] This was not the case for breast cancer, although a reduced effect was associated with low–dose-rate protracted exposure.[150]

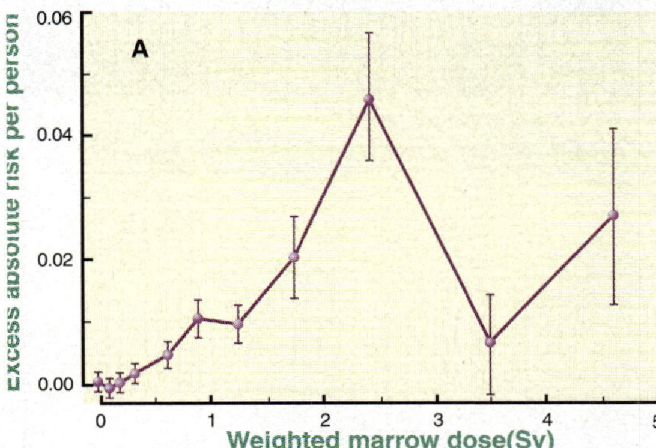

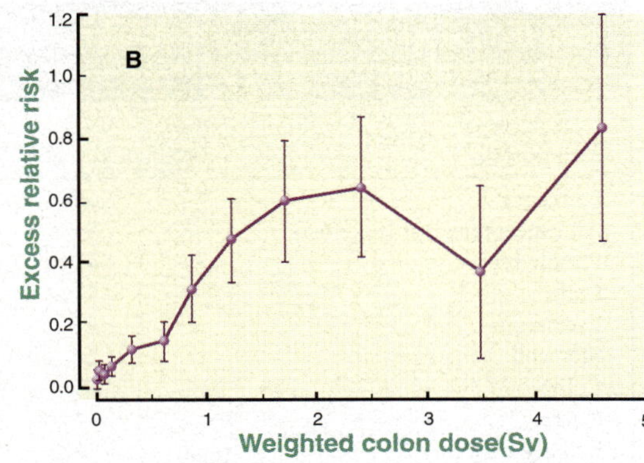

Figure 16-7 Dose-response curves for the induction of cancer in human populations receiving uniform whole-body radiation exposure, derived from epidemiologic data from the atomic bomb survivors of Hiroshima and Nagasaki. **A,** Leukemia. There is a statistically significant upward curvature in the dose range 0.3 Sv and a statistically significant departure from this in the higher dose range. **B,** All cancers except leukemia. There is no statistically significant nonlinearity in the range 0.3 Sv, but the leveling off in the higher dose range is marginally significant. (Reproduced with permission from Pierce et al.[143])

Leukemia At one time, leukemia was thought to be the major radiation-induced cancer to arise from whole-body exposure. We now know the two reasons for this assumption: the spontaneous occurrence of leukemia is low; thus, radiation-induced cases are more readily recognizable; and the latency period in human beings is very short relative to other types of cancer; thus leukemias are recognized earlier. Excess leukemias begin appearing within 2 years after acute radiation exposure, reach a peak incidence within 10 years, and then fall off steadily. This is in contradistinction to other cancers for which the minimum latency period is generally 10 to 15 years, and the appearance of new radiation-induced tumors increases up to 50 years or longer after irradiation. The major sources of data for the induction of leukemia are from the 86,500 members of the life span study of the atomic bomb survivors from whom DS86 (1986) dose estimates are available[143] and from a study of approximately 14,000 patients in the United Kingdom who were treated with radiation for ankylosing spondylitis of the spine.[152]

Figure 16-7A shows the dose-response relationship for the induction of leukemia in the atomic bomb survivors, based on the DS86 dosimetry measurements of organ-absorbed dose. A new dosimetry system, DS02, was recently implemented to replace the DS86. The changes in dose estimates were smaller than what was anticipated, with the primary systematic change being an increase of about 10% in gamma-ray estimates for both Hiroshima and Nagasaki. For both solid cancer and leukemia, estimated age-time patterns and sex difference are virtually unchanged by the dosimetry revision.[153] The data are best described by a linear-quadratic dose-response model in the dose range of 0 to 3 Sv. On the basis of these data,[143] the relative risk at 1 Sv (approximately 100 cGy) is 5.62, and the absolute risk is estimated to be 2.61 excess cancer deaths/10^4 persons exposed/yr/Sv. This latter figure is approximately fourfold higher than that estimated from the data for the British ankylosing spondylitis patients. This may be ascribed to the younger age of the atomic bomb survivors at the time of irradiation and the fact that they received a single acute whole-body exposure.[20] Children appear to be twice as sensitive as adults to the leukemogenic effects of radiation. Studies of in utero exposures to medical x-rays suggest that the unborn child may be as much as 10 times more sensitive than adults to the induction of leukemia following in utero irradiation,[154,155] although no difference was found in the leukemia risk between exposure in utero or during the first 5 years of life among the atomic bomb survivors.[156]

Radiation-induced leukemia in human populations differs in several characteristics from solid tumors. These include the unusually short latency period, high relative risk (Table 16-1), and the fact that the epidemiologic data best fit a linear-quadratic dose-response relationship. This may be related to the nature of the hematopoietic system, which contains less stroma than do most tissues. Therefore, there may be fewer constraints on cell proliferation, in essence allowing a few transformed cells to grow rapidly and be detected earlier as a clinical cancer.

Other Tumors Figure 16-7B shows the dose-response relationship for all cancers except leukemia; the data are best described by a linear model in the dose range of 0 to 3 Sv. Table 16-1 shows the various risk estimates for all types of cancer in which mortality was significantly increased among the atomic bomb survivors. These data are based on approximately 86,500 subjects, of which 50,000 were exposed to greater than 0.005 Sv (0.5 cGy). The most recent estimates indicate that, thus far, there have been about 100 excess leukemias and 440 other cancer deaths attributable to radiation exposure.[144] There have been a total of about 9,300 cancer deaths overall; thus, approximately 6% of all cancer deaths in the population exposed to > 0.005 Sv are associated with

Table 16-1 Summary Measures of Radiation Dose Response for Mortality at Statistically Significant Tissue Sites in Atomic Bomb Survivors of Hiroshima and Nagasaki

Site of Cancer	Relative Risk per Sv*	Excess Deaths (n/10^4/ persons exposed/yr/Sv)	Attributable Risk, %†
Leukemia	5.62	2.61	54
All cancers (except leukemia)	1.53	10.60	7.2
Female breast	2.41	1.48	25
Lung	1.53	1.67	10
Esophagus	1.53	0.42	11
Stomach	1.24	2.11	4.6
Colon	1.65	0.73	12
Ovary	1.94	0.61	15
Urinary tract	1.80	0.48	13
Multiple myeloma	2.15	0.17	17

*Includes both sexes, all ages at exposure, 1950 to 1990 data. Estimates based on weighted organ dose measurements. Adapted from Pierce DA et al.[143]

†Percentage of all cancers observed that can be attributed to the radiation exposure.

radiation, although the overall mortality rate is not significantly increased. As can be seen in Table 16-1, the relative risk at 1 Sv is considerably lower for all other cancer types than it is for leukemia. The excess of cancer deaths/10^4 persons exposed/yr/Sv is approximately 13 for all cancers, including leukemia, ranging from 0.17 to 2.11 in individual tissues.

In addition to breast and lung cancers and leukemia, dose-response data from human epidemiologic studies are available for two other sites not shown in the atomic bomb survivor data in Table 16-1: thyroid and bone cancers. The incidence of bone cancer was not significantly elevated in the atomic bomb survivor studies; the relative and absolute risks are low for the induction of this type of cancer by low LET radiation. The dose-response data have come from studies of persons with elevated body burdens of alpha-emitting radium isotopes as a result of occupational or medical exposures.

Thyroid cancer, on the other hand, is very efficiently induced by low LET radiation in children. Adults are quite resistant. Dose-response relationships are derived from populations receiving therapeutic irradiation, either for an enlarged thymus gland or tinea capitis. Relative risk estimates for the development of thyroid cancer have ranged from 7 to 69 among various age groups, ethnic origins, and studies.[20] However, cancer death rates are not significantly elevated in these populations because radiation apparently induces only papillary- and follicular-type tumors, most of which are curable and tend to progress slowly. Studies of populations exposed from the Chernobyl reactor accident also indicate a significant increase in the incidence of thyroid cancers in children, presumably from radioactive iodine released as a consequence of the accident.[142,157] However, there has been no clear evidence of an increase in overall cancer incidence or mortality, including leukemia in the exposed population, or of any other public health impact aside from the psychological one.[142] On the other hand, increased cancer death rates at several different sites are appearing among the workers at the Mayak Nuclear Weapons facility in the former Soviet Union.[158]

In addition to the results from the atomic bomb survivors, dose-response data are available for breast cancer from several medically exposed populations.[149,150] The results of these studies are generally consistent in terms of risk estimates. Taken as a whole, however, several other interesting findings have emerged. Radiation-induced breast cancers are similar in histopathologic types and age distribution to those arising spontaneously. Women younger than 20 years of age at exposure are at a higher relative risk than adults, similar to the observations for leukemia. As in the case of thyroid cancer, the development of breast cancer is profoundly dependent on hormonal status. Finally, protraction of exposure does not appear to reduce the risk of radiation-induced breast cancer, except for very low dose rates.[150]

Additional epidemiologic studies are also available for the induction of lung cancer.[20] Of particular interest among the underground uranium mine workers in the Colorado plateau has been an apparent multiplicative interaction with cigarette smoking. This observation is consistent with certain experimental findings on alpha radiation–induced lung cancer. However, statistically significant evidence for a more than additive effect between smoking and low LET radiation on lung cancer has not been observed in other epidemiologic studies. This important question needs further investigation.

Finally, it is of passing note that data are now emerging from the studies of the atomic bomb survivors indicating an increase in noncancer mortality among the irradiated survivors.[159] Increasing trends are observed for disorders of the circulatory, digestive, and respiratory systems with doses > 0.5 Sv. The data suggest that 0.8% of noncancer deaths may be associated with the radiation exposure.[159]

Radiation-Induced Secondary Tumors An increase in secondary tumors in the treatment field has now been observed in patients treated for several different types of cancer by radiation therapy, often in conjunction with chemotherapy. In some cases, the incidence of radiation-associated secondary tumors appears to be proportional to dose at the treatment portal, although some epidemiologic data suggest that for leukemia in particular, the tumor incidence may decline at high doses, owing to killing of the target cells. The extent to which genetic factors may play a general role in susceptibility to treatment-induced secondary tumors in cancer patients is unclear. Radiation alone used in conventional treatment regimens may not be a very potent inducer of secondary tumors. This prediction arises from the localized nature of the exposure during clinical radiotherapy, in which the dose to normal tissues is minimized, and from the fact that ionizing radiation tends to be cytotoxic rather than mutagenic. The high radiation doses employed may thus kill potentially transformed cells in the treatment field. Exceptions may be the treatment of Hodgkin's disease, in which lower radiation doses are delivered to a relatively large volume of tissue, and in the use of intensity-modulated radiation therapy (IMRT). IMRT involves the use of more fields with a larger normal tissue volume exposed to lower doses.[160] It has been estimated that IMRT is likely to almost double the incidence of second malignancies compared with conventional radiotherapy from about 1 to 1.75% for patients surviving 10 years.[161] The risk may be even higher for pediatric patients.

Low-Dose Exposures Sufficient data are now available from the atomic bomb survivors to allow an analysis of those survivors who received less than 0.5 Sv; these data are providing preliminary estimates of risk for doses as low as 5 to 10 cGy.[148] They indicate a statistically significant risk in this range consistent with a linear dose-response relationship, with an upper confidence limit on any possible threshold of 6 cGy. A number of epidemiologic studies over the past two decades, however, have purported to show a carcinogenic effect of environmental radiation exposures in the dose range well below 10 cGy. The populations involved are varied but include military personnel exposed during nuclear bomb testing, workers in various nuclear and weapons facilities, and members of the general population living near nuclear facilities or exposed to fallout.

Several reports have analyzed various low-dose epidemiologic studies.[162–164] On the basis of the relative and absolute risk estimates shown in Table 16-1, a significant increase in radiation-associated cancer incidence in populations of these sizes exposed to doses in the range of 10 cGy or less would imply a markedly enhanced sensitivity at low doses, that is, the dose-response curve should show marked hyperlinearity with the excess cancer incidence rising rapidly at very low doses. There are no experimental data to support such a phenomenon; indeed, careful analysis of nearly all of these low-dose studies indicates no significant increase in the incidence of all cancers or of cancers at specific sites. Analyses of a large number of radiation workers from the United Kingdom[165] and Canada[166] indicate that the risk estimates for leukemia and all cancers were consistent with an extrapolation from the atomic bomb survivor data, providing no evidence of an unexpected increase in sensitivity at low doses such as to suggest that the current radiation protection standards might be appreciably in error.

There has also been considerable concern about the risk of lung cancer from exposure to naturally occurring radon in the air of homes and workplaces. The results of several recent epidemiologic studies, however, have been conflicting. For example, a clear association between radon exposure and lung cancer was identified in studies in Sweden and the United Kingdom, whereas equally rigorous investigations in Canada, China, and Missouri found no evidence of excess risk. When a meta-analysis of eight case-control studies was carried out, a positive trend was found consistent with projections of the high-dose data from radon-exposed underground miners.[167] Most radon-induced cancers are expected to occur in cigarette smokers. Overall, however, the carcinogenic risks of residential radon appear to be small,[168] probably of the magnitude of that attributable to passive smoking.[169]

Because the carcinogenic effects of radiation are apparently so small at these low doses, it appears unlikely that they will ever be defined by epidemiologic studies alone. This will likely require a better understanding of the basic mechanisms of radiation carcinogenesis, including the role of factors such as bystander effects, induced genomic instability, and the adaptive response to protracted radiation exposure. In the meantime, risk estimations must be made by extrapolation from the epidemiologic studies at higher doses.

RISK ASSESSMENT

Table 16-2 shows the lifetime excess cancer risk estimates following exposure to 1 cGy as determined by the BEIR V Committee.[20] These estimates were derived from a composite of the epidemiologic data from the atomic bomb survivors and various medical x-ray exposures. They were derived by use of the relative risk model, on the assumption of a linear-quadratic dose-response relationship for leukemia and a straight linear relationship for other tumors. In addition, characteristics such as the latency period, age at exposure, time after exposure, and interaction effects were taken into consideration.

The risk estimates shown in Table 16-2 are for the mean of all ages at exposure. For children younger than 20 years of age, excess cancer mortality per centigray is about 50% higher than the mean for all tumors, whereas it is much lower at ages greater than 65 years. The leukemia risk, on the other hand, rises quite steeply in middle and old age, in which the risk is nearly four times that of young adults and twice that of children.[20] The lifetime excess deaths from all cancers, including leukemia for acute radiation exposure, as shown in Table 16-2, are approximately $800/10^6$ exposed people/cGy. The recent UNSCEAR report estimated that the yield may be 20 to 40% higher on an individual basis[142]; this represents an approximately 1:1,000 (0.1%) effect per centigray. For example, a person receiving 10 cGy acute whole-body exposure would have a 1% chance of developing a lethal cancer during his or her lifetime as a result of this radiation exposure, whereas the chances of dying of cancer unrelated to radiation exposure are approximately 18%. This risk would be lower for low–dose-rate, protracted exposure (see Table 16-2). It should be emphasized, however, that these risks are for uniform whole-body irradiation. Of concern, however, is the rapidly increasing frequency of pediatric patients undergoing computed tomography (CT) diagnostic procedures. Whole-body CT scans, depending on the machine used, can deliver doses in excess of 10 cGy.[170] The estimated lifetime cancer mortality risk attributed, for example, to radiation exposure of a small child is an order of magnitude higher than that for an adult.[171] If the current trend continues, pediatric CT will result in a significantly increased lifetime risk over adult CT owing to both the increased dose per milliampere-second and the increased lifetime risk per unit dose used.

Often the perception of risk, rather than the actual risk itself, is particularly important in the promotion and regulation of health and safety.[172] For example, members of the League of Women Voters and a group of college students were asked to order their perception of the risk of fatality for 30 activities and technologies. Both placed nuclear power in the first position, ahead of smoking, ingestion of alcoholic beverages, and riding in motor vehicles. The risk experts ranked smoking and motor vehicle accidents first (there are about 50,000 motor vehicle deaths in the United States each year, at least 50% of them involving alcohol or drug use), whereas they ranked nuclear power twentieth, in the same range as the ingestion of food coloring and the use of home appliances.

It is of interest to compare the risk of death from various activities associated with everyday living.[173,174] Table 16-3 shows such a comparison. In general, it turns out that the risk from radiation exposure is relatively small when compared with other risks associated with everyday living. Similarly, a comparison of occupational hazards shows that the risks to radiation workers are much lower than those associated with many other occupations. In this context, it is of interest to note the estimation that more than 430,000 excess deaths each year are associated with cigarette smoking in the United States.[172] On the assumption that 40% of the population smokes, such an excess death rate would be comparable with that resulting from approximately 350 cGy of uniform whole-body radiation exposure.

Of concern to the clinical oncologist, however, is the increasingly apparent risk of inducing a secondary malignant tumor as a result of the successful treatment of cancer by high doses of radiation, often in conjunction with chemotherapy. This will, of course, depend on the particular tissue sites included in the radiation field. One could then derive rough risk estimates for radiation alone on the basis of the type of information shown in Table 16-1. The information in Table 16-1, however, was derived from presumably normal people in the general population exposed to tens to hundreds rather than thousands of centigray. As discussed earlier, a number of factors might determine susceptibility to secondary tumors in cancer patients treated with high doses of radiation. Cell killing is one of them; patients treated with radiation for carcinoma of the cervix have not shown an increased incidence of leukemia, presumably because the bone marrow cells in the radiation field are killed by the high radiation doses. On the other hand, a risk factor would be the irradiation of large tissue volumes, as in the treatment of disorders such as Hodgkin's disease; genetic factors would be another. It is well known, for example, that RB patients are at very high risk of developing secondary tumors in the irradiated field. The extent to which genetic hypersusceptibility may be important in some of the more common cancers remains to be determined.

Table 16-2 Lifetime Excess Cancer Risk Estimates for Whole-Body Radiation Exposure to 1.0 cGy

	Cancer Deaths per 10^6 Persons Exposed (excess per cGy)		
Type of Cancer	Acute Exposure*	Protracted Exposure†	Expectation*
Leukemia	95	48	6,850
Nonleukemias	695	347	176,450
All cancers	790	395	183,300

*Estimates from the BEIR V Committee report.[20] See the text for a discussion of these estimates. Normal expectation is the number of cancer deaths (lifetime risk) expected to occur in the general population of 10^6 people.

†Derived from acute exposure data by applying a dose-rate effectiveness factor of 2.

Table 16-3 Risks of Death from Various Activities*

Activity	Risk of Death (per million/yr)
Being a person age 55 years (all causes)	10,000
Smoking a pack of cigarettes daily (all causes)	3,500
Rock climbing for 2 h (accident)	500
Canoeing for 20 h (drowning)	200
Motorcycling for 1,000 miles (accident)	200
Traveling 1,500 miles by car (accident)	40
Being a pedestrian (accident)	40
Working 1 wk as a firefighter (accident)	15
Working 1 wk in agriculture (accident)	10
Fishing (drowning)	10
Eating (choking on aspirated food)	8
Skiing for 10 h (accident)	8
Working 1 mo in a typical factory (accident)	5
Traveling 5,000 miles by air (accident)	5
Having a chest radiograph (radiation-induced cancer)	1
Visiting Denver for 2 mo (cancer from cosmic rays)	1
Living in the vicinity of a nuclear power plant (radiation-induced cancer)	< 0.1

*Estimates derived from various sources.

In most cases, it would seem that a benefit-risk estimation would be positive, that is, the benefit of treatment would outweigh the risk of developing secondary tumors. However, information concerning the relative carcinogenicity of various combinations of radiation and chemotherapeutic agents is now becoming available, and it appears that certain combinations may be more carcinogenic than others. Clearly, additional knowledge is needed to devise effective treatment regimens that might minimize their carcinogenic effects, and thus the risk of developing secondary treatment-induced tumors, while producing an optimal therapeutic gain.

ACKNOWLEDGMENTS

We acknowledge the support of Research Grant FG02-98ER62685 from the US Department of Energy (to J.B.L.), Center Grant ES-00002 from the US National Institutes of Health (to J.B.L.), and National Institutes of Health, National Cancer Institute Grants RO1 CA37435 (to D.J.G.) and RO1 CA99005 (to D.J.G.).

REFERENCES

1. Upton AC. Historical perspectives on radiation carcinogenesis: In: Upton AC, Albert RE, Burns FJ, Shore RE, editors. Radiation carcinogenesis. New York: Elsevier; 1986. p. 1–10.
2. Little JB. Cellular effects of ionizing radiation. I & II. N Engl J Med 1968;278:308–15, 369–76.
3. Williams JR, Little JB, Shipley WU. Association of mammalian cell death with a specific endonucleolytic degradation of DNA. Nature 1974;252:754–5.
4. Geske FJ, Gerschenson LE. The biology of apoptosis. Hum Pathol 2001;32:1029–38.
5. Adams JM, Cory S. The Bcl-2 protein family: arbiters of cell survival. Science 1998;281:1322–6.
6. Thornberry NA, Lazebnik Y. Caspases: enemies within. Science 1998;281:1312–6.
7. Polyak K, Xia Y, Zweier JL, et al. A model for p53-induced apoptosis. Nature 1997;389:300–5.
8. Radford IR. DNA lesion complexity and induction of apoptosis by ionizing radiation. Int J Radiat Biol 2002;78:457–66.
9. Woo RA, Jack MT, Xu Y, et al. DNA damage-induced apoptosis requires the DNA-dependent protein kinase, and is mediated by the latent population of p53. EMBO J 2002;21:3000–8.
10. Watters D. Molecular mechanisms of ionizing radiation-induced apoptosis. Immunol Cell Biol 1999;77:263–71.
11. Little JB, Nagasawa H. Effect of confluent holding on potentially lethal damage repair, cell cycle progression, and chromosomal aberrations in human normal and ataxia-telangiectasia fibroblasts. Radiat Res 1985;101:81–93.
12. Little JB. Failla Memorial Lecture. Changing views of cellular radiosensitivity. Radiat Res 1994;140:299–311.
13. Di Leonardo A, Linke SP, Clarkin K, Wahl GM. DNA damage triggers a prolonged p53-dependent G1 arrest and long-term induction of Cip1 in normal human fibroblasts. Genes Dev 1994;8:2540–51.
14. Jack MT, Woo RA, Hirao A, et al. Chk2 is dispensable for p53-mediated G1 arrest but is required for a latent p53-mediated apoptotic response. Proc Natl Acad Sci U S A 2002;21:3000–8.
15. Kuerbitz SJ, Plunkett BS, Walsh WV, Kastan MB. Wild-type p53 is a cell cycle checkpoint determinant following irradiation. Proc Natl Acad Sci U S A 1992;89:7491–5.
16. Li CY, Nagasawa H, Dahlberg WK, Little JB. Diminished capacity for p53 in mediating a radiation-induced G1 arrest in established human tumor cell lines. Oncogene 1995;11:1885–92.
17. Sheen JH, Dickson RB. Overexpression of c-Myc alters G(1)/S arrest following ionizing radiation. Mol Cell Biol 2002;22:1819–33.
18. Brent RL. Radiation teratogenesis. Teratology 1980;21:281–98.
19. Miller RW. Effects of prenatal exposure to ionizing radiation. Health Phys 1990;59:57–61.
20. National Research Council Committee on the Effects of Ionizing Radiation. Health effects of exposure to low levels of ionizing radiation (BEIR V). Washington (DC): National Academy Press; 1990.
21. Albertini RJ. Validated biomarker responses influence medical surveillance of individuals exposed to genotoxic agents. Radiat Prot Dosimetry 2001;97:47–54.
22. Albertini RJ. Mechanistic insights from biomarker studies: somatic mutations and rodent/human comparisons following exposure to a potential carcinogen. IARC Sci Publ 2004;157:153–77.
23. Grosovsky AJ, Little JB. Evidence for linear response for the induction of mutations in human cells by x-ray exposures below 10 rads. Proc Natl Acad Sci U S A 1985;82:2092–5.
24. Kraemer SM, Waldren CA. Chromosomal mutations and chromosome loss measured in a new human-hamster hybrid cell line, ALC: studies with Colcemid, ultraviolet irradiation, and ^{137}Cs gamma-rays. Mutat Res 1997;379:151–66.
25. Li CY, Yandell DW, Little JB. Molecular mechanisms of spontaneous and induced loss of heterozygosity in human cells in vitro. Somat Cell Mol Genet 1992;18:77–87.
26. Sankaranarayanan K. Estimation of the hereditary risks of exposure to ionizing radiation: history, current status, and emerging perspectives. Health Phys 2001;80:363–9.
27. Abrahamson S. Risk estimates: past, present, and future. Health Phys 1990;59:99–102.
28. Kano Y, Little JB. Mechanisms of human cell neoplastic transformation: x-ray–induced abnormal clone formation in long-term cultures of human diploid fibroblasts. Cancer Res 1985;45:2550–5.
29. Kano Y, Little JB. Persistence of x-ray–induced chromosomal rearrangements in long-term cultures of human diploid fibroblasts. Cancer Res 1984;44:3706–11.
30. Dutrillaux B. Ionizing radiation induced malignancies in man. Radioprotection 1997;32:C431–40.
31. Cox R, Little JB. Oncogenic cell transformation in vitro. In: Nygaard OF, Sinclair WK, Lett JT, editors. Advances in radiation biology. Vol 15. New York: Academic Press; 1992. p. 137–58.
32. Little JB. The relevance of cell transformation to carcinogenesis in vivo. In: Baverstock KF, Strather JW, editors. Low dose radiation—biological basis of risk assessment. London: Taylor and Francis; 1989. p. 439–45.
33. Cox R. The multi-step nature of carcinogenesis and the implications for risk analysis. Int J Radiat Biol 1998;73:373–6.
34. Paquette B, Little JB. In vivo enhancement of genomic instability in minisatellite sequences of mouse C3H/10T1/2 cells transformed in vitro by x-rays. Cancer Res 1994;54:3173–8.
35. Hill CK, Nagy B, Peraino C, Grdina DJ. 2-[(Aminopropyl)amino]ethanethiol (WR1065) is anti-neoplastic and anti-mutagenic when given during ^{60}Co gamma-ray irradiation. Carcinogenesis 1986;7:665–8.
36. Balcer-Kubiczek EK, Harrison GH, Hill CK, Blakely WF. Effects of WR-1065 and WR-151326 on survival and neoplastic transformation in C3H/10T∫ cells exposed to TRIGA or JANUS fission neutrons. Int J Radiat Biol 1993;63:37–46.
37. Little JB. Low-dose radiation effects: interactions and synergism. Health Phys 1990;59:49–55.
38. Chan GL, Little JB. Neoplastic transformation in vitro. In: Upton AC, Albert RE, Burns FJ, Shore RE, editors. Radiation carcinogenesis. New York: Elsevier; 1986. p. 107–36.
39. Kennedy AR. Anticarcinogenic activity of protease inhibitors. In: Troll W, Kennedy AR, editors. Protease inhibitors as cancer chemopreventive agents. New York: Plenum Press; 1993. p. 9–91.
40. Little JB. Radiation carcinogenesis. Carcinogenesis 2000;21:397–404.
41. Kennedy AR, Fox M, Murphy G, Little JB. Relationship between x-ray exposure and malignant transformation in C3H10T1/2 cells. Proc Natl Acad Sci U S A 1980;77:7262–6.
42. Kennedy AR, Little JB. Evidence that a second event in x-ray–induced oncogenic transformation in vitro occurs during cellular proliferation. Radiat Res 1984;99:228–48.
43. Kennedy AR, Cairns J, Little JB. Timing of the steps in transformation of C3H 10T1/2 cells by x-irradiation. Nature 1984;307:85–6.
44. Morgan WF, Day JP, Kaplan MI, et al. Genomic instability induced by ionizing radiation. Radiat Res 1996;146:247–58.
45. Little JB. Radiation-induced genomic instability. Int J Radiat Biol 1998;74:663–71.
46. Baverstock K. Radiation-induced genomic instability: a paradigm-breaking phenomenon and its relevance to environmentally induced cancer. Mutat Res 2000;454:89–109.
47. Romney CA, Paulauskis JD, Nagasawa H, Little JB. Multiple manifestations of x-ray–induced genomic instability in Chinese hamster ovary (CHO) cells. Mol Carcinog 2001;32:118–27.
48. Chang WP, Little JB. Persistently elevated frequency of spontaneous mutations in progeny of CHO clones surviving X-irradiation: association with delayed reproductive death phenotype. Mutat Res 1992;270:191–9.
49. Little JB, Nagasawa H, Pfenning T, Vetrovs H. Radiation-induced genomic instability: delayed mutagenic and cytogenetic effects of x rays and alpha particles. Radiat Res 1997;148:299–307.
50. Grosovsky AJ, Parks KK, Giver CR, Nelson SL. Clonal analysis of delayed karyotypic abnormalities and gene mutations in radiation-induced genetic instability. Mol Cell Biol 1996;16:6252–62.
51. Li CY, Yandell DW, Little JB. Evidence for coincident mutations in human lymphoblast clones selected for functional loss of a thymidine kinase gene. Mol Carcinog 1992;5:270–7.
52. Romney CA, Paulauskis JD, Little JB. X-ray induction of microsatellite instability at autosomal loci in human lymphoblastoid WTK1 cells. Mutat Res 2001;478:97–106.
53. Kadhim MA, Macdonald DA, Goodhead DT, et al. Transmission of chromosomal instability after plutonium alpha-particle irradiation. Nature 1992;355:738–40.
54. Sabatier L, Dutrillaux B, Martin MB. Chromosomal instability. Nature 1992;357:548.
55. Holmberg K, Falt S, Johansson A, Lambert B. Clonal chromosome aberrations and genomic instability in x-irradiated human T-lymphocyte cultures. Mutat Res 1993;286:321–30.
56. Marder BA, Morgan WF. Delayed chromosomal instability induced by DNA damage. Mol Cell Biol 1993;13:6667–77.
57. Kadhim MA, Lorimore SA, Townsend KM, et al. Radiation-induced genomic instability: delayed cytogenetic aberrations and apoptosis in primary human bone marrow cells. Int J Radiat Biol 1995;67:287–93.
58. Pampfer S, Streffer C. Increased chromosome aberration levels in cells from mouse fetuses after zygote x-irradiation. Int J Radiat Biol 1989;55:85–92.
59. Watson GE, Lorimore SA, Wright EG. Long-term in vivo transmission of alpha-particle-induced chromosomal instability in murine haemopoietic cells. Int J Radiat Biol 1996;69:175–82.
60. Watson GE, Lorimore SA, Clutton SM, et al. Genetic factors influencing alpha-particle-induced chromosomal instability. Int J Radiat Biol 1997;71:497–503.
61. Ponnaiya B, Cornforth MN, Ullrich RL. Radiation-induced chromosomal instability in BALB/c and C57BL/6 mice: the difference is as clear as black and white. Radiat Res 1997;147:121–5.
62. Seymour CB, Mothersill C, Alper T. High yields of lethal mutations in somatic mammalian cells that survive ionizing radiation. Int J Radiat Biol Relat Stud Phys Chem Med 1986;50:167–79.
63. Chang WP, Little JB. Delayed reproductive death in x-irradiated Chinese hamster ovary cells. Int J Radiat Biol 1991;60:483–96.
64. Belyakov OV, Prise KM, Trott KR, Michael BD. Delayed lethality, apoptosis and micronucleus formation in human fibroblasts irradiated with x-rays or alpha-particles. Int J Radiat Biol 1999;75:985–93.
65. Limoli CL, Hartmann A, Shephard L, et al. Apoptosis, reproductive failure, and oxidative stress in Chinese hamster ovary cells with compromised genomic integrity. Cancer Res 1998;58:3712–8.
66. Lewis DA, Mayhugh BM, Qin Y, et al. Production of delayed death and neoplastic transformation in CGL1 cells by radiation-induced bystander effects. Radiat Res 2001;156:251–8.
67. Redpath JL, Gutierrez M. Kinetics of induction of reactive oxygen species during the post-irradiation expression of neoplastic transformation in vitro. Int J Radiat Biol 2001;77:1081–5.
68. Limoli CL, Corcoran JJ, Milligan JR, et al. Critical target and dose and dose-rate responses for the induction of

chromosomal instability by ionizing radiation. Radiat Res 1999;151:677–85.
69. Limoli CL, Kaplan MI, Giedzinski E, Morgan WF. Attenuation of radiation-induced genomic instability by free radical scavengers and cellular proliferation. Free Radic Biol Med 2001;31:10–9.
70. Murley JS, Kataoka Y, Weydert CJ, et al. Delayed cytoprotection after enhancement of *Sod2* (*MnSOD*) gene expression in SA-NH mouse sarcoma cells exposed to WR-1065, the active metabolite of amifostine. Radiat Res 2002;158:101–9.
71. Murley JS, Kataoka Y, Cao D, et al. Delayed radioprotection by NFκB-mediated induction of Sod2 (MnSOD) in SA-NH tumor cells after exposure to clinically used thiol-containing drugs. Radiat Res 2004;162:536–46.
72. Ullrich RL, Davis CM. Radiation-induced cytogenetic instability in vivo. Radiat Res 1999;152:170–3.
73. MacDonald D, Boulton E, Pocock D, et al. Evidence of genetic instability in 3 Gy X-ray-induced mouse leukaemias and 3 Gy X-irradiated haemopoietic stem cells. Int J Radiat Biol 2001;77:1023–31.
74. Okayasu R, Suetomi K, Yu Y, et al. A deficiency in DNA repair and DNA-PKcs expression in the radiosensitive BALB/c mouse. Cancer Res 2000;60:4342–5.
75. Gilley D, Tanaka H, Hande MP, et al. DNA-PKcs is critical for telomere capping. Proc Natl Acad Sci U S A 2001;98:15084–8.
76. Wu LJ, Randers-Pehrson G, Xu A, et al. Targeted cytoplasmic irradiation with alpha particles induces mutations in mammalian cells. Proc Natl Acad Sci U S A 1999;96:4959–64.
77. Little JB. Genomic instability and bystander effects: a historical perspective. Oncogene 2003;22:6978–87.
78. Nagasawa H, Little JB. Induction of sister chromatid exchanges by extremely low doses of alpha-particles. Cancer Res 1992;52:6394–6.
79. Narayanan PK, Goodwin EH, Lehnert BE. Alpha particles initiate biological production of superoxide anions and hydrogen peroxide in human cells. Cancer Res 1997;57:3963–71.
80. Azzam E, de Toledo SM, Little JB. Oxidative metabolism modulates signal transduction and micronucleus formation in bystander cells from alpha-particle-irradiated normal human fibroblast cultures. Cancer Res 2002;62:5436–42.
81. Mothersill C, Seymour CB. Cell–cell contact during gamma irradiation is not required to induce a bystander effect in normal human keratinocytes: evidence for release during irradiation of a signal controlling survival into the medium. Radiat Res 1998;149:256–62.
82. Emerit I, Quastel M, Goldsmith J, et al. Clastogenic factors in the plasma of children exposed at Chernobyl. Mutat Res 1997;373:47–54.
83. Nagasawa H, Little JB. Unexpected sensitivity to the induction of mutations by very low doses of alpha-particle radiation: evidence for a bystander effect. Radiat Res 1999;152:552–7.
84. Zhou H, Suzuki M, Randers-Pehrson G, et al. Radiation risk to low fluences of alpha particles may be greater than we thought. Proc Natl Acad Sci U S A 2001;98:14410–5.
85. Little JB, Nagasawa H, Li GC, Chen DJ. Involvement of the nonhomologous end joining DNA repair pathway in the bystander effect for chromosomal aberrations. Radiat Res 2003;59:262–7.
86. Azzam EI, de Toledo SM, Gooding T, Little JB. Intercellular communication is involved in the bystander regulation of gene expression in human cells exposed to very low fluences of alpha particles. Radiat Res 1998;150:497–504.
87. Azzam EI, de Toledo SM, Little JB. Direct evidence for the participation of gap junction-mediated intercellular communication in the transmission of damage signals from alpha-particle irradiated to nonirradiated cells. Proc Natl Acad Sci U S A 2001;98:473–8.
88. Huo L, Nagasawa H, Little JB. HPRT mutants induced in bystander cells by very low fluences of alpha particles result primarily from point mutations. Radiat Res 2001;156:521–5.
89. Nagasawa H, Cremesti A, Kolesnick R, et al. Involvement of membrane signaling in the bystander effect in irradiated cells. Cancer Res 2002;62:2531–4.
90. Goodhead DT. Initial events in the cellular effects of ionizing radiations: clustered damage in DNA. Int J Radiat Biol 1994;65:7–17.
91. Ward JF. Radiation mutagenesis: the initial DNA lesions responsible. Radiat Res 1995;142:362–8.
92. Sutherland BM, Bennett P, Sutherland J, Laval J. Clustered DNA damages induced by x-rays in human cells. Radiat Res 2002;157:611–66.
93. Hashimoto M, Donald CD, Yannone SM, et al. A possible role of Ku in mediating sequential repair of closely opposed lesions. J Biol Chem 2001;276:12827–31.
94. Nikjoo H, Uehara S, Wilson WE, et al. Track structure in radiation biology: theory and applications. Int J Radiat Biol 1998;73:355–64.
95. Boudaiffa B, Cloutier P, Hunting D, et al. Resonant formation of DNA strand breaks by low-energy (3 to 20 eV) electrons. Science 2000;287:1658–60.
96. Jackson SP. Sensing and repairing DNA double-strand breaks. Carcinogenesis 2002;23:687–96.
97. Carney JP, Maser RS, Olivares H, et al. The hMre11/hRad50 protein complex and Nijmegen breakage syndrome: linkage of double-strand break repair to the cellular DNA damage response. Cell 1998;93:477–86.
98. Sonoda E, Takata M, Yamashita YM, et al. Homologous DNA recombination in vertebrate cells. Proc Natl Acad Sci U S A 2001;98:8388–94.
99. Moynahan ME, Chiu JW, Koller BH, Jasin M. Brca1 controls homology-directed DNA repair. Mol Cell 1999;4:511–8.
100. Moynahan ME, Pierce AJ, Jasin M. BRCA2 is required for homology-directed repair of chromosomal breaks. Mol Cell 2001;7:263–72.
101. Xia F, Taghian DG, DeFrank JS, et al. Deficiency of human BRCA2 leads to impaired homologous recombination but maintains normal nonhomologous end joining. Proc Natl Acad Sci U S A 2001;98:8644–9.
102. Taniguchi T, Garcia-Higuera I, Xu B, et al. Convergence of the Fanconi anemia and ataxia telangiectasia signaling pathways. Cell 2002;109:459–72.
103. Grosovsky AJ, de Boer JG, de Jong PJ, et al. Base substitutions, frameshifts, and small deletions constitute ionizing radiation-induced point mutations in mammalian cells. Proc Natl Acad Sci U S A 1988;85:185–8.
104. Wong FL, Boice JD Jr, Abramson DH, et al. Cancer incidence after retinoblastoma. Radiation dose and sarcoma risk. JAMA 1997;278:1262–7.
105. Greenblatt MS, Bennett WP, Hollstein M, Harris CC. Mutations in the p53 tumor suppressor gene: clues to cancer etiology and molecular pathogenesis. Cancer Res 1994;54:4855–78.
106. Ootsuyama A, Makino H, Nagao M, et al. Frequent p53 mutation in mouse tumors induced by repeated beta-irradiation. Mol Carcinog 1994;11:236–42.
107. Hollstein M, Bartsch H, Wesch H, et al. p53 gene mutation analysis in tumors of patients exposed to alpha-particles. Carcinogenesis 1997;18:511–6.
108. Kemp CJ, Wheldon T, Balmain A. p53-deficient mice are extremely susceptible to radiation-induced tumorigenesis. Nat Genet 1994;8:66–9.
109. Bouffler SD, Kemp CJ, Balmain A, Cox R. Spontaneous and ionizing radiation-induced chromosomal abnormalities in p53-deficient mice. Cancer Res 1995;55:3883–9.
110. Offner S, Schmaus W, Witter K, et al. p53 gene mutations are not required for early dissemination of cancer cells. Proc Natl Acad Sci U S A 1999;96:6942–6.
111. Greenblatt MS, Hollstein M, Harris CC. Mutations in the p53 tumor suppressor gene: clues to cancer etiology and molecular pathogenesis. Cancer Res 1994;54:4855–78.
112. Syljuasen RG, Krolewski B, Little JB. Molecular events in radiation transformation. Radiat Res 2001;155:215–21.
113. Lowe SW, Bodis S, McClatchey A, et al. p53 status and the efficacy of cancer therapy in vivo. Science 1994;266:807–10.
114. Taubert H, Meye A, Wurl P. Prognosis is correlated with p53 mutation type for soft tissue sarcoma patients. Cancer Res 1996;56:4134–6.
115. Tsang NM, Nagasawa H, Li C, Little JB. Abrogation of p53 function by transfection of HPV16 E6 gene enhances the resistance of human diploid fibroblasts to ionizing radiation. Oncogene 1995;10:2403–8.
116. Lee JM, Bernstein A. p53 mutations increase resistance to ionizing radiation. Proc Natl Acad Sci U S A 1993;90:5742–6.
117. Brachman DG, Beckett M, Graves D, et al. p53 mutation does not correlate with radiosensitivity in 24 head and neck cancer cell lines. Cancer Res 1993;53:3667–9.
118. McIlwrath AJ, Vasey PA, Ross GM, Brown R. Cell cycle arrests and radiosensitivity of human tumor cell lines: dependence on wild-type p53 for radiosensitivity. Cancer Res 1994;54:3718–22.
119. Suardet L, Li C, Little JB. Radio-induced modulation of transforming growth factor beta1 sensitivity in a p53 wild-type human colorectal-cancer cell line. Int J Cancer 1996;68:126–31.
120. Newcomb EW, Steinberg JJ, Pellicer A. ras oncogenes and phenotypic staging in N-methylnitrosourea– and gamma-irradiation–induced thymic lymphomas in C57BL/6J mice. Cancer Res 1988;48:5514–21.
121. Sloan SR, Newcomb EW, Pellicer A. Neutron radiation can activate K-ras via a point mutation in codon 146 and induces a different spectrum of ras mutations than does gamma radiation. Mol Cell Biol 1990;10:405–8.
122. Sturm SA, Strauss PG, Adolph S, et al. Amplification and rearrangement of c-myc in radiation-induced murine osteosarcomas. Cancer Res 1990;50:4146–53.
123. Pazzaglia S, Mancuso M, Rebessi S, et al. The genetic control of chemically and radiation-induced skin tumorigenesis: a study with carcinogenesis-susceptible and carcinogenesis-resistant mice. Radiat Res 2002;158:78–83.
124. Smida J, Salassidis K, Hieber L, et al. Distinct frequency of ret rearrangements in papillary thyroid carcinomas of children and adults from Belarus. Int J Cancer 1999;80:32–8.
125. Storer JB, Mitchell TJ, Fry RJ. Extrapolation of the relative risk of radiogenic neoplasms across mouse strains and to man. Radiat Res 1988;114:331–53.
126. Thomson JF, Grahn D. Life shortening in mice exposed to fission neutrons and gamma rays. VII. Effects of 60 once-weekly exposures. Radiat Res 1988;115:347–60.
127. Lindop P, Rotblat J. Long-term effects of a single whole-body exposure of mice to ionizing radiations I. Life-shortening. Proc R Soc Lond B 1961;154:332.
128. Fry R, Storer, JB. External radiation carcinogenesis. In: Lett J, editor. Advances in radiation biology. Vol 13. New York: Academic Press; 1987. p. 31–90.
129. Ullrich RL, Storer JB. Influence of gamma irradiation on the development of neoplastic disease in mice. I. Reticular tissue tumors. Radiat Res 1979;80:303–16.
130. Ullrich RL, Storer JB. Influence of gamma irradiation on the development of neoplastic disease in mice. II. Solid tumors. Radiat Res 1979;80:317–24.
131. Ullrich RL. Tumor induction in BALB/c mice after fractionated or protracted exposures to fission-spectrum neutrons. Radiat Res 1984;97:587–97.
132. Little JB, Kennedy AR, McGandy RB. Lung cancer induced in hamsters by low doses of alpha radiation from polonium-210. Science 1975;188:737–8.
133. Bowden GT, Jaffe D, Andrews K. Biological and molecular aspects of radiation carcinogenesis in mouse skin. Radiat Res 1990;121:235–41.
134. Grdina DJ, Murley JS, Kataoka Y. Radioprotectants: current status and new directions. Oncology 2002;63:2–10.
135. Grdina DJ, Carnes BA, Grahn D, Sigdestad CP. Protection against late effects of radiation by *S*-2-(3-aminopropylamino)-ethylphosphorothioic acid. Cancer Res 1991;51:4125–30.
136. Carnes BA, Grdina DJ. In vivo protection by the aminothiol WR-2721 against neutron-induced carcinogenesis. Int J Radiat Biol 1992;61:567–76.
137. Grdina DJ, Carnes BA, Nagy B. Protection by WR-2721 and WR-151327 against late effects of gamma rays and neutrons. Adv Space Res 1992;12:257–63.
138. Sankaranarayanan K, Chakraborty R. Impact of cancer predisposition and radiosensitivity on the population risk of radiation-induced cancers. Radiat Res 2001;156:648–56.
139. Valentin J, editor. Genetic susceptibility to cancer. Annals of the International Commission on Radiological Protection, ICRP publications 79. Tarrytown (NY): Permagon Press; 1999.
140. Baria K, Warren C, Eden OB, et al. Chromosomal radiosensitivity in young cancer patients: possible evidence of genetic predisposition. Int J Radiat Biol 2002;78:341–6.
141. Barlow C, Eckhaus MA, Schaffer AA, Wynshaw-Boris A. ATM haploinsufficiency results in increased sensitivity to sublethal doses of ionizing radiation in mice. Nat Genet 1999;21:359–60.
142. United Nations Scientific Committee on the Effects of Atomic Radiation. Report to the General Assembly with scientific annexes: volume II: effects. New York: United Nations Press; 2000.
143. Pierce DA, Shimizu Y, Preston DL, et al. Studies of the mortality of atomic bomb survivors. Report 12, part I. Cancer: 1950–1990. Radiat Res 1996;146:1–27.
144. Amy Berrington de González AB, Darby S. Risk of cancer from diagnostic x-rays: estimates for the UK and 14 other countries. Lancet 2004;363:345–51.
145. Little MP. Comparison of the risks of cancer incidence and mortality following radiation therapy for benign and malignant disease with the cancer risks observed in the Japanese A-bomb survivors. Int J Radiat Biol 2001;77:431–64.
146. Little MP, Weiss HA, Boice JD Jr, et al. Risks of leukemia in Japanese atomic bomb survivors, in women treated for

cervical cancer, and in patients treated for ankylosing spondylitis. Radiat Res 1999;152:280–92.
147. Hoel D, Li P. Threshold models in radiation carcinogenesis. Health Phys 1998;75:241–50.
148. Pierce DA, Preston DL. Radiation-related cancer risks at low doses among atomic bomb survivors. Radiat Res 2000;154:178–86.
149. Little MP, Boice JD Jr. Comparison of breast cancer incidence in the Massachusetts tuberculosis fluoroscopy cohort and in the Japanese atomic bomb survivors. Radiat Res 1999;151:218–24.
150. Preston DL, Mattsson A, Holmberg E, et al. Radiation effects on breast cancer risk: a pooled analysis of eight cohorts. Radiat Res 2002;158:220–35.
151. Howe GR. Lung cancer mortality between 1950 and 1987 after exposure to fractionated moderate-dose-rate ionizing radiation in the Canadian fluoroscopy cohort study and a comparison with lung cancer mortality in the atomic bomb survivors study. Radiat Res 1995;142:295–304.
152. Weiss HA, Darby SC, Fearn T, Doll R. Leukemia mortality after x-ray treatment for ankylosing spondylitis. Radiat Res 1995;142:1–11.
153. Preston DL, Pierce DA, Shimizu Y, et al. Effect of recent changes in atomic bomb survivor dosimetry on cancer mortality risk estimates. Radiat Res 2004;162:377–89.
154. Boice JD Jr, Miller RW. Childhood and adult cancer after intrauterine exposure to ionizing radiation. Teratology 1999;59:227–33.
155. Doll R, Wakeford R. Risk of childhood cancer from fetal irradiation. Br J Radiol 1997;70:130–9.
156. Delongchamp RR, Mabuchi K, Yoshimoto Y, Preston DL. Cancer mortality among atomic bomb survivors exposed in utero or as young children, October 1950–May 1992. Radiat Res 1997;147:385–95.
157. Astakhova LN, Anspaugh LR, Beebe GW, et al. Chernobyl-related thyroid cancer in children of Belarus: a case-control study. Radiat Res 1998;150:349–56.
158. Shilnikova NS, Preston DL, Ron E, et al. Cancer mortality risk among workers at the Mayak Nuclear Clinic. Radiat Res 2003;159:787–98.
159. Shimizu Y, Pierce DA, Preston DL, Mabuchi K. Studies of the mortality of atomic bomb survivors. Report 12, part II. Noncancer mortality: 1950–1990. Radiat Res 1999;152:374–89.
160. Goffman TE, Glatstein E. Intensity-modulated radiation therapy. Radiat Res 2002;158:115–7.
161. Hall EJ, Wuu C-S. Radiation-induced second cancers: the impact of 3D-CRT and IMRT. Int J Radiat Oncol Biol Phys 2003;56:83–8.
162. Gilbert ES, Omohundro E, Buchanan JA, Holter NA. Mortality of workers at the Hanford site: 1945–1986. Health Phys 1993;64:577–90.
163. Modan B. Low-dose radiation carcinogenesis—issues and interpretation: the 1993 G. William Morgan Lecture. Health Phys 1993;65:475–80.
164. Bruske-Hohlfeld I, Scherb H, Bauchinger M, et al. A cluster of childhood leukaemias near two neighbouring nuclear installations in northern Germany: prevalence of chromosomal aberrations in peripheral blood lymphocytes. Int J Radiat Biol 2001;77:111–6.
165. Muirhead CR, Goodill AA, Haylock RG, et al. Occupational radiation exposure and mortality: second analysis of the National Registry for Radiation Workers. J Radiol Prot 1999;19:3–26.
166. Ashmore JP, Krewski D, Zielinski JM, et al. First analysis of mortality and occupational radiation exposure based on the National Dose Registry of Canada. Am J Epidemiol 1998;148:564–74.
167. Lubin JH, Boice JD Jr. Lung cancer risk from residential radon: meta-analysis of eight epidemiologic studies. J Natl Cancer Inst 1997;89:49–57.
168. National Research Council Committee on the Effects of Ionizing Radiation. Health effects of exposure to radon (BEIR VI). Washington (DC): National Academy Press; 1999.
169. Alavanja MC, Brownson RC, Lubin JH, et al. Residential radon exposure and lung cancer among nonsmoking women. J Natl Cancer Inst 1994;86:1829–37.
170. Parry RA, Glaze SA, Archer BR. The AAPM/RSNA physics tutorial for residents. Radiographics 1999;19:1289-302.
171. Brenner DJ, Elliston CD, Hall EJ, Berdon WE. Estimated risks of radiation-induced fatal cancer from pediatric CT. AJR Am J Roentgenol 2001;176:289–96.
172. Slovic P, Layman M, Kraus N, et al. Perceived risk, stigma, and potential economic impacts of a high-level nuclear waste repository in Nevada. Risk Anal 1991;11:683–96.
173. Centers for Disease Control and Prevention. Cigarette smoking-attributable mortality and years of potential life lost—United States, 1984. MMWR Morb Mortal Wkly Rep 1997;46:444–50.
174. Wilson R, Crouch EA. Risk assessment and comparisons: an introduction. Science 1987;236:267–70.

17

Ultraviolet Radiation Carcinogenesis

James E. Cleaver, PhD
David L. Mitchell, PhD

Mad dogs and Englishmen go out in the mid-day sun.

—Noel Coward

HISTORICAL PERSPECTIVE

Skin cancers occur in uniquely accessible sites and are caused by well-defined environmental agents; consequently, their formation illustrates numerous salient features of carcinogenesis. Skin tumors in humans account for about 30% of all new cancers reported annually.[1,2] Epidemiologic and laboratory studies provide evidence of a direct causal role of sunlight exposure in the induction of cancer,[3,4] and the high rate of skin carcinogenesis is a direct result of the high dose rate from the ultraviolet (UV) light component. Both basal cell carcinoma (BCC) and squamous cell carcinoma (SCC) are found on sun-exposed parts of the body (eg, the face and trunk in men, the face and legs in women), and their incidence is correlated with cumulative sunlight exposure. Tumor incidence and mortality increase with decreasing latitude, corresponding to exposure; skin cancers are less frequent in dark-skinned populations than in lighter-skinned peoples; and tumor incidence increases with occupational exposure, such as in ranchers and fishermen.[5,6] Melanoma, although also associated with sunlight exposure, shows a weaker dependence on total exposure to sunlight and a distribution over the body that is not correlated to exposed areas but is more closely related to intermittent exposures and sunburn in childhood.[7] There may be solar-dependent and -independent pathways for melanoma.

Exposure to direct sunlight in the mid-US latitudes results in the accumulation of a mean lethal dose to unprotected human cells within approximately 30 minutes.[8] The only other human carcinogen that even approaches these exposure levels would be cigarette smoke in very heavy smokers. Variations in individual susceptibility are also clearly observed in skin carcinogenesis. Human skin can be classified into types I to IV, ranging from individuals who always burn and never tan to those who tan but never burn; skin cancer susceptibility varies accordingly.[9] But the most dramatic examples of variations in human susceptibility occur in certain human genetic disorders, especially xeroderma pigmentosum (XP), Cockayne's syndrome (CS), trichothiodystrophy (TTD), basal cell nevus syndrome (BCNS), the porphyrias, and phenylketonuria.[10] Other disorders associated with acquired sun sensitivity include polymorphous light eruption, actinic reticuloid and prurigo, solar urticaria, lupus erythematosus, and Darier's disease, as well as medication and immunologic status. Sunlight exposure also has a major immunosuppressive effect, leading to loss of antigen-presenting Langerhans' cells and the appearance of dyskeratotic keratinocytes (apoptotic sunburn cells) in the upper epidermis, together with the erythemal sunburn response associated with vasodilation caused by a release of prostaglandin.[11] Immunosuppression in organ transplantation and patients with human immunodeficiency virus (HIV) also increases skin cancer incidence.[12]

EPIDEMIOLOGY

Skin Cancer Frequency and Age at Onset

The UV component of sunlight is the major environmental agent that precipitates the clinical symptoms of skin carcinogenesis. This is well established for SCC and BCC but still controversial for melanoma.[13–15] Nonmelanoma skin cancers are by far the most common cancers that occur in the United States each year,[2,16] comprising 30 to 40% of all cancers, and have been increasing steadily for a century.[17,18] As a consequence, there is a wealth of human epidemiologic data on skin cancer risks that are associated with geographic locations, skin type, and various photosensitizing, enhancing, and protective applications.[4,5,18–22] There is also a possibility of greater risk when the exposure is received during childhood and adolescence.[4,23] Nonmelanoma skin cancer is therefore one of the few malignancies for which there is clear evidence of the identification of the initiating agent. The relationship of melanoma to sun exposure and the possible action spectrum are less clear[13] but may be related to acute burns rather than accumulated dose.[4] Neonatal sunburn in mice can induce melanoma but not exposures later in life.[15]

The importance of deoxyribonucleic acid (DNA) as a chromophore for the shorter wavelengths is illustrated by the autosomal recessive disease XP. In this disease, a failure in one cellular protective mechanism, DNA repair, is associated with a major increase in the rate of onset of SCC, BCC, and melanoma.[10] Median onset for skin cancer in the general US population occurs at 50 to 60 years of age; in XP patients, carcinogenesis is accelerated and median onset is within the first decade (Figure 17-1). This early onset is a direct consequence of sunlight-induced changes in DNA of skin cells. An appreciation of the significance of these changes requires describing the

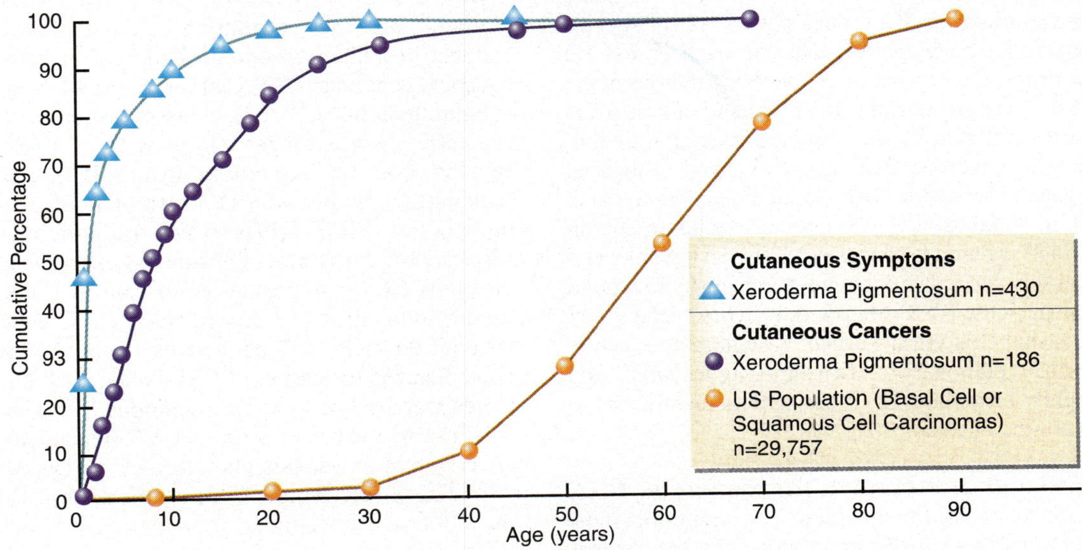

Figure 17-1 Age at onset of xeroderma pigmentosum symptoms. Age at onset of cutaneous symptoms (generally sun sensitivity or pigmentation) was reported for 430 patients. Age at first skin cancer was reported for 186 patients and is compared with age distribution for 29,757 patients with basal cell carcinoma or squamous cell carcinoma in the US general population. (Reproduced with permission from Kraemer KH et al.[120])

photochemical responses of DNA, mechanisms of DNA repair, and their mutagenic and carcinogenic consequences.

Sunlight Spectrum and Wavelengths Responsible for Skin Cancer Ultraviolet radiation (UVR) is divided into three wavelength ranges on the basis of differences in photochemistry and biologic importance. Ultraviolet A (UVA) (320–400 nm) is photocarcinogenic and involved in photoaging but is weakly absorbed in DNA and protein. The relevant chromophores may therefore involve reactive oxygen species (ROS), which secondarily cause damage to DNA.[24] Ultraviolet B (UVB) (290–320 nm) overlaps the upper end of the DNA and protein absorption spectra and is the range mainly responsible for skin cancer through direct photochemical damage to DNA. Ultraviolet C (UVC) (240–290 nm) is not present in ambient sunlight but is readily produced by low-pressure mercury sterilizing lamps. The peak wavelength of mercury excitation (254 nm) coincides with the peak of DNA absorption (260 nm), and this wavelength has been of major importance in experimental studies. Absorption of UVR by stratospheric ozone greatly attenuates these wavelengths so that negligible radiation shorter than 300 nm reaches the earth's surface. Hence, although UVA and UVB light constitute a minute portion of the emitted solar wavelengths (10^{-9}), they are primarily responsible for the sun's pathologic effects.

Physical shielding of the critical cells of the skin is achieved by melanin pigment and keratin layers; intracellular defenses depend on repair of DNA damage, antioxidant enzymes (eg, superoxide dismutase, glutathione reductase), endogenous free radical quenchers, and inducible detoxifying enzymes and biochemical systems.[24] Melanin has multiple functions that can be either harmful or beneficial to the organism.[25] On the one hand, it can be photoprotective, acting as a weak natural sunscreen and scavenger of active chemical species produced by solar UVR. On the other hand, melanin can itself produce active radical species that can damage DNA and has the capacity to bind to drugs in ways that can either benefit or harm the cell.[26] The beneficial role of melanin in humans is best illustrated by the observed reduction in skin cancers, such as BCC and SCC, and protection against sunburn in dark-skinned peoples. In black skin, melanosomes, the cellular compartments in which melanin is sequestered, are oval, single, and densely packed with melanin and clustered around the nucleus. UVR is blocked from the nucleus, and free radicals are absorbed. In contrast, in white skin, melanosomes are round, aggregated, and lightly melanotic. UVR can bypass the clusters to enter the nucleus.

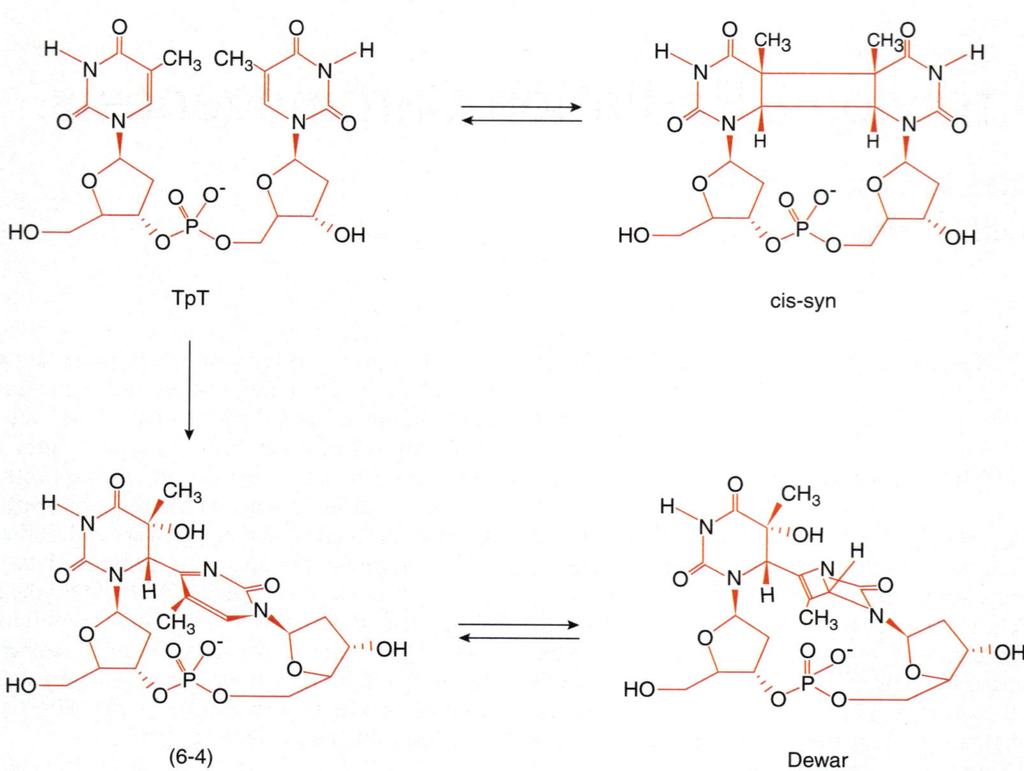

Figure 17-2 Photochemical reactions in a dipyrimidine deoxyribonucleic acid (DNA) sequence leading to the formation of cyclobutane pyrimidine dimers (TpT1, TpT2) or a [6-4] pyrimidine dimer (TpT4) and its photolytic derivative, the Dewar pyrimidone (TpT3). Adapted from Taylor JS and Cohrs MP.[38]

Sunlight-Induced Photoproducts in DNA Action spectra for squamous cell carcinoma indicate that DNA is the target molecule; the absorption spectrum of DNA correlates well with lethality, mutation, and photoproduct formation.[27–31] The energy absorbed by DNA produces molecular changes, some of which involve single bases, whereas others result in interactions between adjacent and nonadjacent bases and still others between DNA and proteins. The relative proportion of DNA photoproducts varies across the UV spectrum.

Dimerizations between adjacent pyrimidines are the most prevalent photoreactions resulting from direct absorption of UVR by DNA. The two major photoproducts are the cyclobutane pyrimidine dimer (CPD) and, at about 25% the frequency, the [6-4] pyrimidine dimer ([6-4]PD) (Figure 17-2). The distribution of these photoproducts in human chromatin depends on base sequence, secondary DNA structure, and DNA-protein interactions.[31–33] Because cytosine more efficiently absorbs longer wavelengths of UVR than thymine, CPDs containing this base are formed more readily after UVB irradiation.[34] In conjunction with [6-4]PDs, which are preferentially induced at thymine-cytosine dipyrimidines, cytosine CPDs may play a major role in UVB (solar) mutagenesis.[35] Recent data show that methylation at PyrCG sequences in the *TP53* gene enhances formation of CPDs and [6-4]PDs at sites that are hot spots for mutations.[36,37] The [6-4]PD can further undergo a UVB-dependent conversion to its valence photoisomer, the Dewar pyrimidinone (see Figure 17-2).[38] In addition to the major photoproducts, other less common lesions can form, including purine-purine and purine-pyrimidine photoadducts, photohydrations, and photo-oxidations.[39] Because the total yield of these photoproducts is only 3 to 4% of the yield of CPDs, their biologic role is considered minimal; however, their importance as premutagenic lesions in specific sites cannot be excluded.

UVA primarily produces damage indirectly through ROS, which, in turn, react with DNA to form base damage, strand breaks, and DNA-protein crosslinks. The importance of these photoproducts is not known, but evidence is accumulating to suggest that UVA may be an important pathogenic component of sunlight. Significant levels of cell killing and mutation induction have been observed in human epidermal cells after irradiation with UVA.[27,29] These data are consistent with earlier studies that suggested that the lethal effects of UVA are not mediated by CPD damage[40,41] and that free radical scavengers can mitigate cytotoxicity.[42] The biologic importance of UVA is perhaps best illustrated by the demonstration that it causes significant levels of tumorigenesis in hairless mice.[43] Recent evidence suggests that UVA may also induce significant levels of CPDs in human cells by some photosensitized triplet energy transfer mechanism and that these lesions should be taken into account to fully understand the biologic effects of UVA.[44]

GENETIC FACTORS IN SKIN CARCINOGENESIS

Excision of UV Photoproducts The idea that DNA damage is an essential component of photocarcinogenesis arose from the discovery that cells from patients suffering from XP are deficient in DNA repair.[45] Since these initial studies, the molecular basis of XP and related diseases has in large part been resolved and the basic mechanism and appropriate genes cloned and characterized.[10,46]

Nucleotide excision repair (NER) is the most important repair process concerned with UV damage. Two major pathways of NER are known: transcription coupled repair (TCR) and global genome repair (GGR). These NER pathways remove pyrimidine dimers and large chemical adducts in DNA and replace the damaged site with a newly synthesized polynucleotide patch approximately 29 bases in length (Figure 17-3).[47,48] TCR removes damage more rapidly from the transcribed strands of transcriptionally active genes, whereas GGR acts more slowly on nontranscribed regions[49] and is regulated by *TP53* through control of XPC and XPE (p48) expression.[50]

NER requires a temporary relaxation of nucleosomal structure such that damaged regions are more accessible to exogenous nucleases. The continuous excision and resynthesis of DNA are associated with a very low net frequency of DNA strand breaks, no more than about 1 in 2×10^8 Da of DNA. Only about 1% of the CPDs produced in DNA are therefore being excised at any instant, but it takes only minutes to complete repair of an individual lesion. Excision therefore sets up a dynamic balance between strand breakage and rejoining and is rate limited by the enzymes involved in the early steps of repair.

Excision repair is a heterogeneous process both between species and within the genome. There is considerable difference between CPDs and [6-4]PDs in their rates of excision from the overall genome of rodent and human fibroblasts and skin,[51] even though the basic mechanisms and patch sizes are essentially the same.[52] [6-4]PDs are the more rapidly excised, 50% being removed from human and rodent cells in 2 to 6 hours. CPDs are much more slowly removed; half are removed from human cell DNA in 12 to 24 hours,[53,54] but negligible amounts are removed from rodent DNA for even longer times. The excision of CPDs may be partly delayed because the strong affinity of the excision system for [6-4]PDs initially sequesters available enzymes. There are also large variations in CPD excision between human subjects.[54] The different rates of excision may reflect the fact that [6-4]PDs are considerably more distortive in DNA and are preferentially located in internucleosomal regions of DNA, which can lead to differences in the binding constant between the damage recognition proteins and the DNA. CPDs are distributed more randomly but with a 10Å periodicity in the DNA wrapped around nucleosomes owing to a preference for formation of dimers on the side of DNA opposite the DNA-protein contact surface.[55,56]

Additional variation in CPD repair occurs on an individual gene basis according to transcriptional activity.[57] An increased excision rate in active genes (TCR) may also occur for [6-4]PDs, but this is less easily resolved against the greater

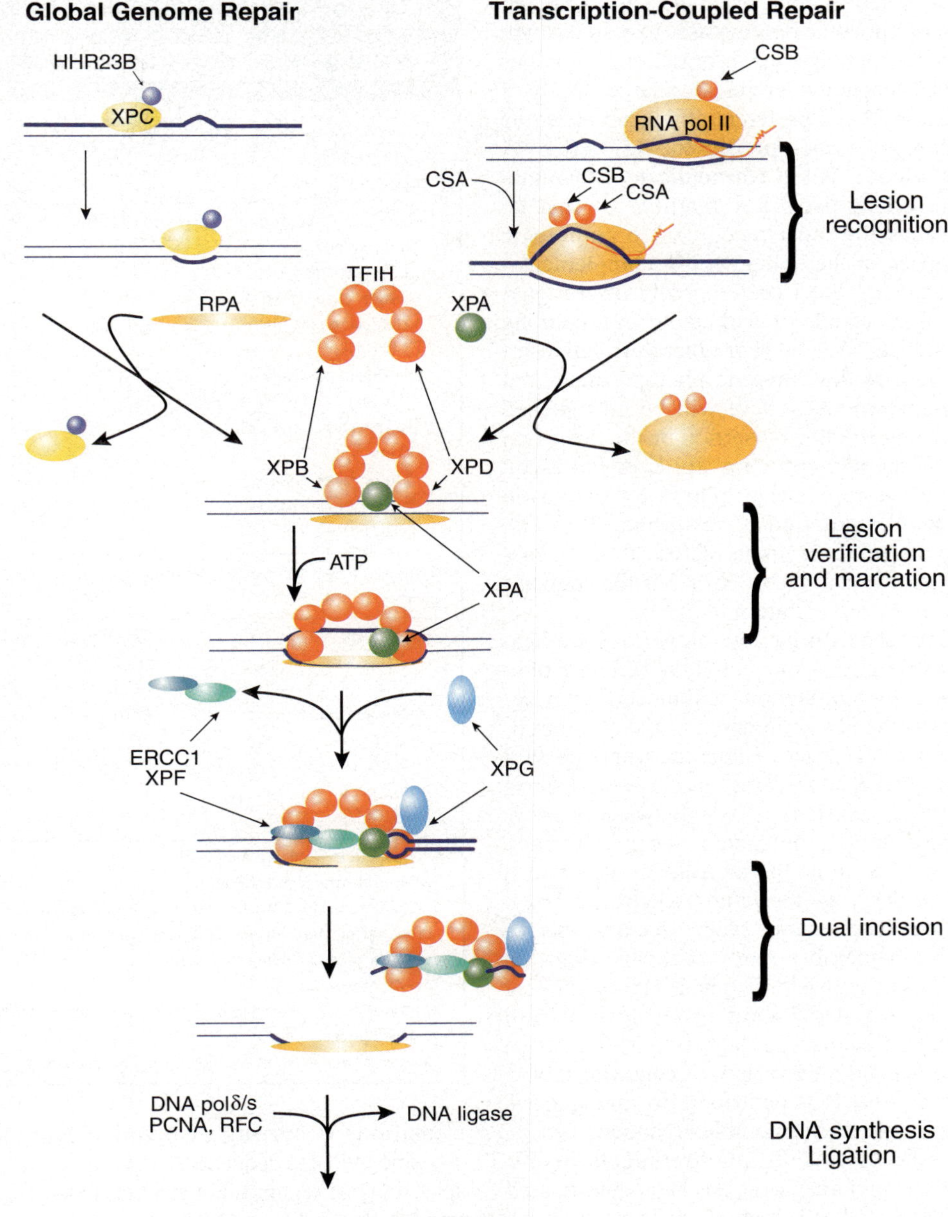

Figure 17-3 Biochemical steps for nucleotide excision repair of cyclobutane pyrimidine dimer (CPDs). Initial recognition of damage involves the XPC and E gene products, followed by XPA and RPA, which bind to photoproducts and download the helicases XPB and D for local unwinding. Excision occurs when ultraviolet-specific endonucleases (XPF/ERCC1 and XPG) make incisions on the 5' and 3' sides. Excision and subsequent polymerization release a 29-base oligonucleotide containing the CPD.

overall rate of excision of these photoproducts in the genome as a whole. The differences in excision from active versus inactive genes occur because a basal transcription factor, TFIIH, and two gene products, Cockayne syndrome A and B (CSA and CSB), regulate basal transcription and bypass of damage by ribonucleic acid (RNA) polymerase II.[58,59] A detailed study of the promoter and first exons of the *PGKI* gene has indicated that excision is slow in regions of promoter binding but increases immediately after the transcription start site.[60] Many of the genes that regulate TCR are associated with the human disorders XP, CS, and TTD, as well as other disorders. Two of the helicases in TFIIH correspond to the *XPB* and *XPD* genes, and others are known to play a role from their analogs in the yeast transcription factor b.[61] TCR also involves the CS genes *CSA* and *CSB*, *XPG*,[62] the mismatch repair gene *MLH2*,[63] and the breast cancer susceptibility gene *BRCA1*.[64]

Mutagenicity of UV Photoproducts and Low-Fidelity DNA Polymerases Most photoproducts act as blocks to the replicative class B polymerases Pol A, D, and E. Depending on their structures, they can, however, be bypassed during DNA replication to different degrees by damage-specific class Y DNA polymerases.[46,65,66] The class Y polymerases Pol H, I, and K have low fidelity owing to expanded active sites.[67] Pol H and I are paralogs, both being closely related to the yeast yRad30 gene product. The expanded active sites allow the polymerases to read through noninformative sequence information. Pol H has the greatest capacity to replicate a large variety of DNA lesions[68] and preferentially inserts adenine in the nascent strand opposite the lesion (the "A rule").[69] Hence, Pol H can replicate a thymine-containing CPD with low fidelity,[70,71] and its absence has the most recognizable pathologic consequence in the human XP-V complementation group.[72,73] Pol I preferentially inserts guanines and is capable of replicating C-containing photoproducts.[74,75] Pol H or I therefore can insert bases opposite dipyrimidine photoproducts, but the 3' complementary base will be mismatched either by an erroneous insertion or the distortion caused by the photoproduct. Pol K or Pol Z can complete the replicative bypass by extension from the mismatched 3' terminus.[76–78] The absence of Pol H results in increased mutagenesis,[79,80] but the absence of Pol Z has the converse effect of reducing mutation rates.[81]

This mechanism has two important implications regarding the mutagenicity of different photoproducts. First, mutations will most often occur where cytosine is a component of the photoproduct because insertion of adenine opposite thymine is a correct and nonmutagenic event. Hence, most CPDs, because they form between two thymine bases, are not mutagenic. Second, the more distortive a lesion is, the more likely it is that it will block DNA synthesis and result in a lethal rather than a mutagenic event. Because the [6-4]PD is considerably more distortive than the CPD (ie, it causes a 47° as opposed to a 7° helical bend), it is more likely to be lethal than mutagenic. Because damage bypass and base insertion depend on a variety of conditions, both CPDs and [6-4] PDs contribute to mutagenesis and tumorigenesis in a complex manner.

The role of specific photoproducts in UV mutagenesis in human cells has been investigated with the use of shuttle vectors. In these systems, UV-irradiated simian virus SV40-based plasmids are transfected into human cells, where they are replicated by the host. The plasmids are subsequently recovered, amplified in bacteria, and analyzed for mutation induction by DNA sequencing. Sites of mutations can then be compared with sites of photoproduct induction in the target sequence. The results of these studies are similar to those obtained in *Escherichia coli*: sites of transition mutations correlated with sites of increased [6-4]PD induction (Table 17-1).[82–84] In particular, sites and frequencies of mutation hot spots in the *lacI* gene transfected into human cells were identical to those determined in *E. coli*.[85] In a shuttle vector system in which photoproduct induction and sites of mutation were examined in the *supF* gene, transfection into SV40-transformed human fibroblasts and monkey kidney cells indicated a similar correlation.[86] In the *supF* gene inserted into the mouse L cell chromosome[87] and in the endogenous *APRT* gene of Chinese hamster ovary cells,[88] most of the mutations consisted of cytosine-to-thymine transitions occurring at thymine-cytosine and cytosine-cytosine sequences. Owing to the strand specificity of repair, there is a bias between mutations in the coding and the noncoding strands of expressed genes that differs according to the NER capacity of the cells.[89,90]

Table 17-1 Ultraviolet C–Induced Mutations Observed in Shuttle Vector pZ189 Replicated in Xeroderma Pigmentosum or Normal Human Cells

Mutations	Number of Plasmids with Base Changes, n (%)*	
	XP	Normal
Independent plasmids sequenced[†]	61 (100)	89 (100)
Point mutations		
Single base substitution	47[‡] (77)	48 (53)
Tandem base substitutions[§]	12 (20)	16 (18)
Multiple base substitutions[‖]	1[‡] (2)	24 (28)
Base insertions and deletions		
Single base insertion	0	2
Single or tandem base deletions	1	3
Types of single or tandem base substitutions and number of changes		
Transitions	67[‡] (94)	61 (75)
GC to AT	66[‡] (93)	59 (73)
AT to GC	1 (1)	2 (2)
Transversions	4[‡] (6)	20 (25)
GC to TA	0[‡]	8 (10)
GC to CG	1 (1)	5 (6)
AT to TA	3 (4)	6 (8)
AT to CG	0	1 (1)

Modified from Bredberg A et al.[145]
XP = xeroderma pigmentosum.
*50 to 300 J/m^2 for XP cells, 100 to 5,000 J/m^2 for normal cells.
†From separate transfections or different mutations in the same transfection, including all experiments.
‡$p < .01$ versus normal.
§Two base substitutions 0 to 2 bases apart or 3 adjacent base substitutions.
‖At least 2 base substitutions more than 3 bases apart.

Because CPDs and [6-4]PDs can both form at sequences shown to be mutation hot spots in shuttle vectors, the identity of the mutagenic lesion has been tested by photoreactivation of the *supF* sequence in plasmids before transfection.[91,92] Enzymatic photoreversal of CPDs reduced the mutation frequency in normal cells by 75% and in XP group A cells by 90%. Because cotransfection of monkey cells with a mixture of unirradiated *supF* plasmid and irradiated plasmid without the *supF* gene did not generate mutations, the role of an SOS-like system, as observed in *E. coli*, did not appear to be responsible for the results.[92] These results are not consistent with the model developed in *E. coli* and suggest that [6-4]PDs may be less mutagenic in human cells. A subsequent analysis using photoreactivation suggested that CPDs occurring at dipyrimidine sites containing at least one cytosine base were the predominant mutagenic lesions induced in human cells and that [6-4]PDs at these sites accounted for only about 10% of the mutations.[91] However, this same study indicated that the frequencies of both CPDs and [6-4]PPs at individual dipyrimidine sites did not correlate with mutation frequency, suggesting that although UV-induced lesions are required for mutagenesis, mutation hot spots are determined by other factors.

A comparison of photoproduct yields, rates of repair, and mutations in the *PGKI* and *TP53* genes, however, has shown that regions of high UV-induced mutation can be caused by either or both high photoproduct yield and low repair.[60,93–95] A combination of initial yields and rates of repair that leave a high net persistent load of photoproducts in a particular site appears to be directly related to the mutational yield. Using ligation-mediated polymerase chain reaction (LMPCR), which allows precise location of damaged bases, the photoproduct distribution in exons 1 and 2 of three *ras* proto-oncogenes was mapped and no correlation between photoproduct frequency and mutation induction in codon 12 of H-*ras* and K-*ras* was found.[96] Further studies with LMPCR showed that the rate of excision repair of CPDs at specific nucleotides in the promoter and exon 1 of the *PGK1* gene varied 15-fold with much reduced repair at transcription factor binding sites.[60] DNA repair at individual nucleotides in the *TP53* tumor suppressor gene was highly variable and sequence dependent, with slow repair observed at seven of eight of the positions associated with mutations.[93] UV-induced mutations in the *TP53* gene are a probable step in the formation of SCC[97,98] and may arise at DNA repair "cold spots" rather than photoproduct "hot spots."

Genetic Disorders of DNA Repair That Affect UV Sensitivity The study of human sunlight-sensitive disorders and the selection of UV-sensitive hamster and mouse cells in culture has identified a series of genetic loci that control the response of mammalian skin to damage (Table 17-2). These loci are all characterized by significant increases in sensitivity to UVC or UVB radiation and include the disorders XP (eight complementation groups),[10] CS (two groups),[99,100] TTD (three groups),[101,102] and BCNS.[103] These disorders are not mutually exclusive because CS overlaps with XP groups B, D, and G and TTD overlaps with groups B and D (see Table 17-2). Many of these genes have also been defined in cell cultures as ERCC 1 to 12 (excision repair cross complementing).[104] Most of these disorders represent recessive mutations associated with a series of genes that regulate human cell DNA repair. Mutations in individual genes have pleiotropic effects on cellular sensitivity to UV light and DNA repair and are associated with a range of clinical syndromes involving skin, nervous system, and immunologic changes.

Mechanism of NER Pyrimidine dimers are repaired by a complex multistep process, which

Table 17-2 Complementation Groups in Xeroderma Pigmentosum and Ultraviolet-Sensitive Chinese Hamster Ovary Cells

Group	Human Chromosome Location	Central Nervous System Repair Disorders	Relative DNA Repair, %
Xeroderma pigmentosum			
A	9q34.1	Yes	2–5
B (Cockayne's syndrome, TTD, and ERCC3)*†	2q21	Yes	3–7
C	3q25	No	5–20
D (Cockayne's syndrome, TTD, and ERCC2)*†	19q13.2	Yes	25–50
E	11p11-12	No	50
F	16q13.1	No	18
G (Cockayne's syndrome)	13q32.3	Yes	< 2
Variant Chinese hamster ovary cells (ERCC)‡	6p21	No	100
1	19q13.2	—	Low
2 (XPD)	19q13.2	—	Intermediate
3 (XPB)	2q21	—	Intermediate
4 (XPF)	16q13.1	—	Low
5 (XPG)	13q 32.3	—	Intermediate

DNA = deoxyribonucleic acid; ERCC = excision repair cross complementing; TTD = trichothiodystrophy.

*Patients also exhibit symptoms commonly associated with Cockayne's syndrome: dwarfism, cutaneous features, and mental retardation. Group B and ERCC3 represent the same complementation group as do group D and ERCC2, F and ERCC4, and G and ERCC5.

†Some patients also have symptoms of TTD.

‡Genes in the ERCC series are found in human and rodent cells and were first identified through selection of ultraviolet-sensitive hamster cells. ERCC1 does not correspond to any xeroderma pigmentosum group, but the corresponding human genes are identified for others. Relative repair in the ERCC series is classified approximately on the basis of relative sensitivity to DNA damage. I am grateful to L. H. Thompson for providing this summary of gene locations and group assignments. Further details can be found on the Web sites <http://xpmutations.org> and <http://www.cgal.icnet.uk/DNA_Repair_Genes.html>.

involves many interacting gene products. In part, it is the need for interacting proteins in repair that gives rise to complex overlapping symptoms in some patients with mutations in these genes. The repair process, in principle, involves removal of a 27 to 29 nt oligonucleotide containing the photoproduct by precisely positioned cleavages, 5 nt on the 3' side of the photoproduct and 24 nt on the 5' side.[105] Once this oligonucleotide is removed, the resulting gap is filled in by the combined action of DNA Pol D, proliferating cell nuclear antigen (PCNA), single-strand binding protein, and ligase I.[47] These processes involve sequential steps of photoproduct recognition, assembly of the excision complex, displacement of the excised fragment, and polymerization of the replacement patch.

The specific binding and association of several proteins are involved in photoproduct recognition. Recognition may occur owing to distortions and single-strandedness in DNA from photoproducts, or the photoproducts could swing out of the DNA helix into a pocket in the protein, as occurs in some other DNA repair enzymes.[106] The XPC-hHR23B complex[107,108] is the earliest damage detector to initiate NER in nontranscribed DNA, acting before the XPA protein, and serves to stabilize XPA binding to the damaged site with a high affinity for the [6-4]PD.[109,110] The XPC protein may be required for transient nucleosome unfolding during NER.[111] This complex is specifically involved in GGR but not TCR, where the arrest of RNA polymerase II at a damaged base may function in its place. Stable association of TFIIH with DNA lesions is dependent on the integrity of XPA and XPC proteins. In addition to the XPA and XPC proteins, the XPE protein has similar binding characteristics but plays a much less prominent role. Two subunits that copurify are associated with XPE, a p48 protein that carries mutations from XPE patients, and a p127 protein, and these may be involved in the repair of less accessible lesions in nontranscribed DNA.[112] The p48 subunit is inducible by tp53 in human cells but is not in rodent cells owing to mutation or methylation of the tp53 response elements in the promoters.[113] Hence, rodent cells fail to repair CPDs in nontranscribed DNA. There is a strong dependence of p48 messenger RNA levels on basal tp53 expression that may provide a link between tp53 and NER.[114]

NER operates by assembly of individual factors at sites of DNA damage rather than by preassembly of holocomplexes.[115] The core protein factors include the XPA-RPA dimer, the six- to nine-subunit TFIIH, the XPC-hHR23B complex, the XPG nuclease, and the ERCC1-XPF nuclease.[47] After assembly, the XPC-hHR23B complex dissociates, the XPG protein cuts 3' to the lesion, and the ERCC1-XPF heterodimer cuts 5' to the CPD. The nuclease complex plus the 29 to 30 nt single-strand fragment is released by the action of transcription factor TFIIH, which contains both 3' to 5' (XPB) and 5' to 3' (XPD) helicases. The XPG protein is also required for TCR of oxidative damage and is a cofactor for thymine glycol glycosylase (nth protein).[62] At least one component of TFIIH, XPB, interacts with tp53 and initiates a signal cascade leading to apoptosis in damaged cells.[116] The whole NER process requires about 100 nt of DNA along which to operate in vitro.[105] PCNA, which is required for repair synthesis, also interacts with GADD45, a damage-inducible protein, which stimulates excision repair in vitro, although its in vivo function is not known.[117] Several components of excision repair, especially the genes *ERCC1*[118,119] and *HR23B*,[108] have rarely been found among clinically recognized syndromes. Inactivation of the *ERCC1* gene produces UV-sensitive cells and causes lethal liver failure in mice,[118] and one neonatal lethal mutation in *ERCC1* has been reported in a human patient. The complexity of these diseases comes not only from the specific role that gene products play in repair but also from other roles as transcription factors, ubiquitylation cofactors, and components of signaling cascades.

XERODERMA PIGMENTOSUM

XP is a rare autosomal recessive disease that occurs at a frequency of about 1 in 250,000 in the United States.[10] Affected patients (homozygotes) have sun sensitivity, resulting in progressive degenerative changes of sun-exposed portions of the skin and eyes, often leading to neoplasia. Some XP patients have, in addition, progressive neurologic degeneration. Obligate heterozygotes (parents) are generally asymptomatic. The median age at onset is 1 to 2 years of age, with skin rapidly taking on the appearance of that seen in individuals with many years of sun exposure. Pigmentation is patchy, and skin shows atrophy and telangiectasia, with development of BCC and SCC. The frequency of cancers is about 2,000 times that seen in the general population under 20 years of age, with an approximate 30-year reduction in life span.[120]

Cells from patients with XP excise pyrimidine dimers at reduced rates of 0 to 90% of normal, except for the variant group, which has near-normal rates.[121] The reductions are similar in all tissues thus far investigated, including skin in vivo, peripheral lymphocytes, fibroblasts, liver cell cultures, and tumor cells. There are seven complementation groups among patients who are deficient in excision repair, and an eighth, the XP variant, has a defect in the low-fidelity polymerase Pol H (see Table 17-2).

Compared with normal cells, cells from XP groups A and D are very sensitive to the lethal effects of UV light and are unable to excise the CPD and the [6-4]PD. XP group A cells also have a reduced capacity to repair the Dewar pyrimidinone, an important lesion induced with increased efficiency by UVB light.[35,51,122]

Group C is one of the largest groups and is often referred to as the common or classic form of XP. The patients show only skin disorders, which vary considerably in severity, depending on the climate. Tumors of the tongue have been observed in several patients. Cells have low but heterogeneous levels of excision repair (10–20% of normal) and are less sensitive to killing by UV light and chemical carcinogens than cells in groups A, B, D, and G. One characteristic of repair unique to this group is that the reduced repair is confined to nontranscribed regions of the genome.[123] These cells insert repair patches into the transcriptionally active regions of their genome at normal rates, corresponding to [6-4]PP and CPD excision.[123] This raises the dilemma that high rates of cell killing, somatic mutation, and cancer from UV light in XP group C are associated with repair deficiencies in the nontranscribed regions of the genome. This, in turn, suggests that activating rather than silencing mutations may be important or that mutations arise from unrepaired lesions in the nontranscribed strand of active genes. Alternatively, global repair deficiencies may cause an overall increase in genomic instability, leading to chromosomal aberrations.

Group E is a rare group that exhibits mild symptoms and residual levels of repair that are between 50 and 100% of normal and lack a DNA-binding protein, p48, which is associated with a larger protein, p127.[124] XPE patients carry mutations in the *P48* gene,[125] but some apparently XPE patients who had normal *P48* were found to be members of other groups that had been misassigned.[126] The role of this protein is still unclear, but it is dependent on tp53 and involved in repair of nontranscribed regions of DNA.[112,114,125]

XP variant cells have normal excision repair but lack a DNA low-fidelity class Y DNA polymerase hRAD30A (Pol H), which is required for accurate replication of pyrimidine dimers.[72,73] In its absence, XP variant cells are very susceptible to UV-induced mutagenesis[79] and exhibit essentially the same symptoms as other XP patients. Carcinogenesis from UV damage in XP patients arises therefore from the loss of either NER capacity or Pol H; both lead to an increase in the amount of persistent DNA damage that becomes the substrate for error generation (mutations, gene rearrangements, deletions, and genomic instability).

COCKAYNE'S SYNDROME

CS is an autosomal recessive disease characterized by cachectic dwarfism, retinal abnormalities, microcephaly, deafness, neural defects, and retardation of growth and development after birth. Carcinomas of the skin as a result of hyperphotosensitivity are not seen in patients with CS, setting this disease apart from XP. CSB knockout mice, however, are sensitive to UVB carcinogenesis.[127]

CS patients are distributed unevenly within the complementation groups, with significantly more group A than B patients.[99] Three patients from two families are known from an XP complementation group B that also shows CS symptoms.[128] CS symptoms have also been reported in a few XP-B, XP-D, and XP-G patients. The UV sensitivity of most CS cells lies in a narrow range, with a dose for 37% survival (D_{37}) about half of normal, and in the same range as that of XP-C cells. Characteristic cellular changes in CS include a failure of DNA and RNA synthesis to recover to normal levels after UV irradiation.[100] The excision of DNA photoproducts from total genomic DNA of CS cells is normal, but repair of transcriptionally active genes is reduced.[129] The CS gene products are involved in coupling excision repair to transcription, but their precise function is not yet clear. They may be involved in the ubiquitination and degradation of stalled RNA Pol II at damaged sites.

CS and XP group C therefore make an interesting contrast. CS cells repair transcriptionally inactive genes, whereas XP-C cells repair only transcriptionally active genes that represent less than 1 to 2% of the whole genome. But whereas XP-C shows elevated carcinogenesis, CS does not, indicating that defective global repair is required for carcinogenesis. The defect in CS cells therefore involves too small a total amount of the genome to trigger genomic instability that is carcinogenic. Mice with defects in XP or CS genes, however, both show elevated carcinogenesis,[130] which raises questions of the different roles of NER in humans and mouse strains.

TRICHOTHIODYSTROPHY

TTD is a rare autosomal recessive disorder characterized by sulfur-deficient brittle hair and ichthyosis. Hair shafts split longitudinally into small fibers, and this brittleness is associated with levels of cysteine or cystine in hair proteins that are 15 to 50% of those in normal individuals. Patients also show physical and mental retardation of varying severity and often have an unusual facial appearance, with protruding ears and a receding chin. Mental abilities range from low normal to severe retardation.[101] Several categories of the disease can be recognized on the basis of UV sensitivity and DNA repair.[102,131] The most severe cases have repair deficiencies and complementation properties that place them in XP groups B and D.[102]

In a detailed analysis of mutations in the *XPD* gene, those that gave rise to XP symptoms corresponded to missense mutations in the DNA helicase motifs of the gene, whereas those that gave rise to TTD were missense mutations in the RNA helicase motifs and the C-terminal end of the protein.[132] Some TTD cases do not have mutations in *XPB* or *XPD* and are due to mutations in a small 8 kDa component of TFIIH that appears to regulate the overall level of the transcription factor.[133] Most cases of TTD therefore affect the function of TFIIH in gene transcription, and the symptoms of this disease indicate a role for this factor in development and hair growth.

CARCINOGENESIS

Carcinogenesis often appears to proceed by a multistep process, the first being an initiation event with subsequent promotional events that can often occur much later. One view of carcinogenesis correlates initiation with the induction of a small number of somatic mutations in a few critical genes and promotion with further alterations in gene expression, copy number, and karyotype. Carcinogenesis appears to involve a process that destabilizes the genome, with resulting variations in the activity of a large number of genes that change and develop over time. Genes that are mutated or destabilized include those for cell cycle regulation, checkpoint and damage response, detoxifying carcinogenic chemicals, DNA repair, and some 50 or more dominantly acting proto-oncogenes activated by mutation, deletion, translocation, or amplification, and tumor suppressor genes, whose loss may contribute to the development of cancer.[134,135]

The comparison between cancer-prone XP patients and CS patients who do not develop cancer is quite revealing. These comparisons suggest that deficiencies affecting DNA repair or replication that involve the whole genome (eg, XP-C, XP-V) predispose patients to cancer; defects that affect repair only of expressed genes (*CSA, CSB*) predispose patients to neurodegeneration and developmental disorders. Deficiencies in both kinds of repair, however, increase mutagenesis, implying that additional genomic instability owing to global deficiencies is necessary for cancer.

Skin cancers include at least three categories of tumor type: SCC, BCC, and melanoma. These have distinct origins, molecular changes and etiology, and eventual outcomes, and each has characteristic genetic and solar components to their development. SCCs and BCCs appear to originate from different locations in the skin and melanoma from the pigment cells. The initial damage produced by solar UVB to the skin is eliminated either by repair or by proliferation and exfoliation from the skin's surface. Some cells in the skin also die by apoptosis following exposure ("sunburn cells"), resulting in the elimination of damaged cells. Stem cells for the epithelium are thought to reside in the bulge region of the hair follicles,[136] but there are also secondary stem cells at the base of each column of epidermal transit, amplifying cells in the epidermal proliferative units.[137] Whether SCCs and BCCs come from different stem cells is currently unknown. A very low frequency of quiescent cells has been observed to retain DNA damage for long periods, seemingly without repair or proliferation.[138] The carcinogen-retaining cells may be stem cells or damaged cells with the potential to become mutants once stimulated to proliferate.

The progression of molecular changes involved in SCC appears to be initiated by inactivating mutations in *TP53* that result in expanding clones in the sun-exposed areas of the skin that are initially confined within the proliferating units.[139] These clones can be very frequent and can break out of the confines of the columnar structure of the proliferative units after chronic UVB irradiation.[139] Over 90% of SCCs are reported to have *TP53* mutations that are characteristic of UV exposure, being in dipyrimidine sequences with notable frequencies of CC to TT changes.[97,98,140] Loss of *TP53* functions can also increase genomic instability during DNA replication when subjected to further UV irradiation.[141,142] Several investigations have also identified activating mutations in the H-*ras* and N-*ras* oncogenes at codon 61 from solar UV exposure.[143–145] However, although over 75% of UV-induced mutations are generally C to T transitions at TC or CC CPD photoproduct sites, the H-*ras* and N-*ras* activation occurred in tumors at a TT site and are transversions not previously identified in model culture systems.[146]

Subsequent to the expansion of *TP53* mutant clones, additional factors come into play with other alterations in gene expression and copy number that have not yet been fully explored. Changes have been observed, for example, in epidermal growth factor, *ras*, nuclear factor κB, JNK2, presenilin, and MMP9, as well as various chromosomal regions identified by allelotyping that control tumor initiation and papilloma to carcinoma conversion.[147–149] There may be an important role for the immune system in SCC formation because immune suppression in organ transplantation patients enhances SCC formation, and the gamma-delta T cells negatively regulate tumor formation.[150] Suppression of DNA repair by the cytokine interleukin-12 may also play a role in immunosuppressed individuals.[151]

BCCs are exemplified by the hereditary disease BCNS. The defect in BCNS appears to be in the human homologue of the *Drosophila* gene *PATCHED* (*PTC*). The gene is involved in embryonic patterning, as well as determining the fate of multiple structures in the developing embryo. Both somatic mutations in sporadic BCCs and single allele mutations in patients with BCNS have provided strong evidence that this tumor suppressor is important in BCC tumorigenesis.[152,153]

The patched protein (PTC) is a transmembrane receptor and with the coreceptor membrane protein smoothened (SMO) regulates signal transduction by the extracellular protein hedgehog (Hh) that binds to PTC.[154] PTC represses the pathway by inhibiting signaling by SMO.[155,156] SMO is released from PTC repression if (1) Hh binds to PTC, (2) PTC is mutationally inactivated, or (3) SMO mutation impedes PTC-SMO protein interaction.[157] Once released from PTC repression, SMO signaling activates transcription factor Gli, which, in turn, up-regulates expression of *PTC* itself and of a variety of other genes depending on tissue, organism, and stage of development. Mutations in *SMO* have been identified in BCCs, and in these tumors, as in BCCs with *PTC* mutations, in situ studies detected increased *PTC* transcript in BCCs compared with overlying epidermis and stroma.[158,159] Thus, increased *PTC* message levels correlate with decreased PTC protein function. More than 50% of BCCs and 90% of SCCs also contain mutations in *TP53* with a specific signature induced by UV light, and many other gene amplifications and deletions have been detected.[160]

Melanoma occurs in a hereditary form among approximately 5 to 12% of all patients.[161] Although this is clinically and histologically indistinguishable from nonfamilial melanoma, there are differences in the age of diagnosis, lesion thickness, and frequency of multiple lesions.[162–164] Significant differences occur in the genetic changes in melanomas according to whether the sites are exposed to chronic (face and hands) or intermittent (trunk and legs) sun damage or are not exposed at all (palms and soles).[165] Melanomas that are not driven by high levels of sun exposure involve a series of mutations, deletions, and amplifications (copy number changes) along the mitogen-activated protein (MAP) kinase pathway.[161,166–171] This pathway involves N-*ras*, *BRAF*, *p16*, the pair of *cyclin D1* and *CDK4*, and *PTEN*. Copy number changes of *cyclin D1* and *CDK4* are mutually exclusive, as are mutations in *ras* and *BRAF*. *PTEN*, being a negative regulator on a parallel *ras*-activated pathway, can occur along with mutations in the *BRAF* arm but is retained in melanomas on chronically sun-exposed skin.

BRAF, a cytoplasmic serine-threonine kinase regulated by *ras*, is mutated in a large fraction of melanoma on unexposed skin.[172] BRAF has been successfully targeted by a small molecule inhibitor in clinical trials in combination with chemotherapy and may become the first line of treatment for certain classes of melanoma.[173] The role of sun damage in chronically exposed regions remains to be fully explored, but melanomas in these regions have fewer mutations and fewer copy number changes.

PREVENTION

Nearly all organisms have behaviors or natural features that lower exposure of DNA to solar UVR and reduce the amount of photodamage. Human behaviors include wearing clothes, hats, sunglasses, and sunscreens and general occupational and recreational lifestyles. Other human behaviors can put individuals at greater risk of skin cancer. Over the past few years, the growth in the cosmetic skin-tanning industry has been considered a major contributor to increased skin cancer frequencies, including melanoma.[174] To reduce the risk of skin cancer, the cosmetic tanning industry uses lamps that emit primarily UVA and are thus considered "safe." Recent data showing CPD induction by UVA call this strategy into question.[44] Along similar lines, sunscreen manufacturers have relied primarily on UVB-blocking strategies based on the idea that UVA does not play a significant role in skin cancer. Both of these strategies are questionable because evidence from the *Xiphophorus* fish melanoma model suggests that UVA may be more effective than UVB in melanoma formation,[175] although this is not supported by recent evidence in mice.[14] The use of UVB sunscreens may even increase melanoma risk by extending exposure to UVA.[176]

In addition to photoprotection, strategies for removing potentially harmful DNA damage within a short time after UV exposure have been researched. One such "morning after" cream contains the bacterial DNA repair enzyme T4 endonuclease V packaged in engineered delivery vehicles that can traverse the stratum corneum, reach cell nuclei in the skin, and repair UV-induced CPDs.[177] This strategy has been shown to enhance DNA repair and reduce cell killing, mutagenesis, and immunosuppression. Similar applications using photolyase are apparently more effective than T4 endonuclease in repairing CPDs from normal human skin cells in vivo.[178] A more controversial therapeutic approach involves the use of thymidine dinucleotides and oligonucleotides that mimic telomeres to stimulate excision repair, decrease UV-induced mutations, and reduce photocarcinogenesis in mice.[179] These and other xenogenic agents delivered to the epidermis in liposomes may have broad applications as active ingredients in modern skin care products.

REFERENCES

1. Scotto J, Fears TR, Fraumeni JF. Incidence of nonmelanoma skin cancer in the United States. Washington, DC, US Department of Health and Human Services; 1983. NIH Publication No.: 83–2433.
2. Scotto J, Fraumeni JF Jr. Skin (other than melanoma). In: Schottenfeld D, Fraumeni JR Jr, editors. Cancer epidemiology and prevention. Philadelphia: W.B. Saunders; 1982. p. 996–1011.
3. Fitzpatrick TB, Sober AJ. Sunlight and skin cancer. N Engl J Med 1985;313:818–20.
4. Armstrong BK, Kricker A. The epidemiology of UV induced skin cancer. J Photochem Photobiol B 2001;63:8–18.
5. Jablonski NG, Chaplin G. The evolution of human skin coloration. J Hum Evol 2000;39:57–106.
6. Grossman L, Wei Q. DNA repair and epidemiology of basal cell carcinoma. Clin Chem 1995;41(Pt 2):1854–63.
7. Armstrong BK. Epidemiology of malignant melanoma: intermittent or total accumulated exposure to the sun? J Dermatol Surg Oncol 1988;14:835–49.
8. Trosko JE, Krause D, Isoun M. Sunlight-induced cyclobutane pyrimidine dimers in human cells in vitro. Nature 1970;228:358–9.
9. Vitaliano PP, Urbach F. The relative importance of risk factors in nonmelanoma skin cancer. Arch Dermatol 1980;116:454–6.
10. Bootsma D, Kraemer KH, Cleaver JE, Hoeijmakers JHJ. Nucleotide excision repair syndromes: xeroderma pigmentosum, Cockayne syndrome, and trichothiodystrophy. In: Vogelstein B, Kinzler KW, editors. The genetic basis of human cancer. New York, NY, McGraw-Hill; 1998. p. 245–74.
11. Kripke ML. Immunological effects of ultraviolet radiation. J Dermatol 1991;18:429–33.
12. London NJ, Farmery SM, Will EJ, et al. Risk of neoplasia in renal transplant patients. Lancet 1995;346:403–6.
13. Kraemer KH, Lee MM, Andrews AD, Lambert WC. The role of sunlight and DNA repair in melanoma and nonmelanoma skin cancer. The xeroderma pigmentosum paradigm. Arch Dermatol 1994;130:1018–21.
14. De Fabo EC, Noonan FP, Fears T, Merlino G. Ultraviolet B but not ultraviolet A radiation initiates melanoma. Cancer Res 2004;64:6372–6.
15. Noonan FP, Recio JA, Takayama H, et al. Neonatal sunburn and melanoma in mice. Nature 2001;413:271–2.
16. Serrano H, Scotto J, Shornick G, et al. Incidence of nonmelanoma skin cancer in New Hampshire and Vermont. J Am Acad Dermatol 1991;24:574–9.
17. Boring CC, Squire TS, Tong T. Cancer statistics 1993. Cancer J Clin 1993;43:7–26.
18. Gallagher RP, Ma D, McLean DI, et al. Trends in basal cell carcinoma, squamous carcinoma and melanoma of the skin from 1973 through 1987. J Am Acad Dermatol 1990;23:413–21.
19. Davies RE, Forbes PD, Urbach F. Effects of chemicals on photobiologic reactions of the skin. Basic Life Sci 1990;53:127–35.
20. Robinson JK, Rademaker AW. Relative importance of prior basal cell carcinomas, containing sun exposure and circulating T lymphocytes on the development of basal cell carcinoma. J Invest Dermatol 1992;99:227–31.
21. Marks R, Staples M, Giles GG. Trends in non-melanomic skin cancer treated in Australia: the second national survey. Int J Cancer 1993;53:585–90.
22. Thompson SC. Reduction of solar keratoses by regular sunscreen use. N Engl J Med 1993;3291:1147–51.
23. Marks R, Jolley D, Lectas S, Foley P. The role of childhood exposure to sunlight in the development of solar kera-

toses and non-melanocytic skin cancer. Med J Aust 1990;152:62–5.

24. Tyrrell RM, Keyse SM. New trends in photobiology: the interaction of UVA radiation with cultured cells. J Photochem Photobiol B 1990;4:349–61.
25. Hill HZ, Li W, Xin P, Mitchell DL. Melanin: a two-edged sword? Pigment Cell Res 1997;10:158–61.
26. Takeuchi S, Zhang W, Wakamatsu K, et al. Melanin acts as a potent UVB photosensitizer to cause an atypical mode of cell death in murine skin. Proc Natl Acad Sci U S A 2004;101:15076–81.
27. Jones CA, Huberman E, Cunningham ML, Peak MJ. Mutagenesis and cytotoxicity in human epithelial cells by far- and near-ultraviolet radiations: action spectra. Radiat Res 1987;110:244–54.
28. Niggli HJ, Cerutti PA. Cyclobutane-type pyrimidine photodimer formation and excision in human skin fibroblasts after irradiation with 313-nm ultraviolet light. Biochemistry 1983;22:1390–5.
29. Tyrrell RM, Pidoux M. Action spectra for human skin cells: estimates of the relative cytotoxicity of the middle ultraviolet, near ultraviolet, and violet regions of sunlight on epidermal keratinocytes. Cancer Res 1987;47:1825–9.
30. Pfeiffer GP, Drouin R, Riggs AD, Homquist GP. In vivo mapping of a DNA adduct at nucleotide resolution: detection of pyrimidine [6-4] pyrimidone photoproducts by ligation-mediated polymerase chain reaction. Proc Natl Acad Sci U S A 1991;88:1374–8.
31. Pfeiffer GP, Drouin R, Riggs AD, Holmquist GP. Binding of transcription factors creates hotspots for UV photoproducts. Mol Cell Biol 1992;12:1798–804.
32. Mitchell DL, Jen J, Cleaver JE. Relative induction of cyclobutane dimers and cytosine photohydrates in DNA irradiated in vitro and in vivo with ultraviolet C and ultraviolet B light. Photochem Photobiol 1991;54:741–6.
33. Mitchell DL, Jen J, Cleaver JE. Sequence specificity of cyclobutane pyrimidine dimers in DNA treated with solar (ultraviolet B) radiation. Nucleic Acids Res 1992;20:225–9.
34. Ellison MJ, Childs JD. Pyrimidine CPDs induced in *Escherichia coli* DNA by ultraviolet radiation present in sunlight. Photochem Photobiol 1981;34:465–9.
35. Mitchell DL, Cleaver JE. Photochemical alterations of cytosine account for most biological effects after ultraviolet irradiation. Trends Photochem Photobiol 1990;1:107–19.
36. Tommasi S, Denissenko MF, Pfeifer GP. Sunlight induces pyrimidine dimers preferentially at 5-methylcytosine bases. Cancer Res 1997;57:4727–30.
37. Mitchell DL. Effects of cytosine methylation on pyrimidine dimer formation in DNA. Photochem Photobiol 2000;71:162–5.
38. Taylor JS, Cohrs MP. DNA, light. and Dewar pyrimidinones: the structure and significance of TpT3. J Am Chem Soc 1987;109:2834–5.
39. Cadet J, Vigney P. The photochemistry of nucleic acids. In: Morrison H, editor. Bioorganic photochemistry: photochemistry and the nucleic acids. New York: John Wiley and Sons; 1990. p. 1–273.
40. Smith PJ, Paterson MC. Abnormal responses to mid-ultraviolet light of cultured fibroblasts from patients with disorders featuring sunlight sensitivity. Cancer Res 1981;41:511–8.
41. Elkind MM, Han A, Chiang-Liu C-M. “Sunlight”-induced mammalian cell killing: a comparative study of ultraviolet and near-ultraviolet inactivation. Photochem Photobiol 1978;27:709–15.
42. Tyrrell RM, Pidoux M. Endogenous glutathione protects human skin fibroblasts against the cytotoxic action of UVB, UVA and near-visible radiations. Photochem Photobiol 1986;44:561–4.
43. Sterenborg HJCM, van der Leun JC. Tumorigenesis by a long wavelength UV-A source. Photochem Photobiol 1990;51:325–30.
44. Courdavault S, Baudouin C, Charveron M, et al. Larger yield of cyclobutane dimers than 8-oxo-7,8-dihydroguanine in the DNA of UVA-irradiated human skin cells. Mutat Res 2004;556:135–42.
45. Cleaver JE. Defective repair replication in xeroderma pigmentosum. Nature 1968;218:652–6.
46. Cleaver JE. Stopping DNA replication in its tracks. Science 1999;285:212–3.
47. Sancar A. Mechanisms of DNA excision repair. Science 1994;266:1954–6.
48. Sancar A, Sancar GB. DNA repair enzymes. Annu Rev Biochem 1988;57:29–67.
49. Hanawalt PC. Transcription-coupled repair and human disease. Science 1994;266:1957–8.
50. Ford JM, Hanawalt PC. Expression of wild-type p53 is required for efficient global genomic nucleotide excision repair in UV-irradiated human fibroblasts. J Biol Chem 1997;272:28073–80.
51. Mitchell DL, Nairn RS. The biology of the (6-4) photoproduct. Photochem Photobiol 1989;49:805–19.
52. Cleaver JE, Jen J, Charles WC, Mitchell DL. Cyclobutane dimers and [6-4] photoproducts are mended with the same patch sizes in human cells. Photochem Photobiol 1991;54:393–402.
53. Cleaver JE. DNA damage and repair in normal, xeroderma pigmentosum, and XP revertant cells analyzed by gel electrophoresis: excision of cyclobutane dimers from the whole genome is not necessary for cell survival. Carcinogenesis 1989;10:1691–6.
54. Freeman SE. Variations in excision repair of UVB-induced pyrimidine CPDs in DNA of human skin in situ. J Invest Dermatol 1988;90:814–7.
55. Gold JM, Smerdon MJ. UV induced [6-4] photoproducts are distributed differently than cyclobutane dimers in nucleosomes. Photochem Photobiol 1990;51:411–7.
56. Mitchell DL, Nguyen TD, Cleaver JE. Nonrandom induction of pyrimidine-pyrimidone [6-4] photoproducts in ultraviolet-irradiated human chromatin. J Biol Chem 1990;265:5353–60.
57. Mellon I, Bohr VM, Hanawalt PC. Preferential repair of an active gene in human cells. Proc Natl Acad Sci U S A 1986;83:8878–82.
58. Schaeffer L, Roy R, Humbert S, et al. DNA repair helicase: a component of BTF2 (TFIIH) basic transcription factor. Science 1993;260:58–63.
59. Licht CL, Stevnser T, Bohr VA. Cockayne syndrome group B cellular and biochemical functions. Am J Hum Genet 2003;73:1217–39.
60. Gao S, Drouin R, Holmquist GP. DNA repair rates mapped along the human PGK-1 gene at nucleotide resolution. Science 1994;263:1438–40.
61. Bootsma D, Hoeijmakers HJ. The molecular basis of nucleotide excision repair syndromes. Mutat Res 1994;307:15–23.
62. Cooper PK, Nouspikel T, Clarkson SG, Leadon SA. Defective transcription coupled repair of oxidative base damage in Cockayne syndrome patients from XP group G. Science 1997;275:990–3.
63. Leadon SA, Avrutskaya AV. Requirement for DNA mismatch repair proteins in the transcription-coupled repair of thymine glycols in *Saccharomyces cerevisiae*. Mutat Res 1998;407:177–87.
64. Gowen LC, Avrutskaya AV, Latour AM, et al. BRCA1 required for transcription-coupled repair of oxidative damage. Science 1998;281:1009–12.
65. Burgers PM, Koonin EV, Bruford E, et al. Eukaryotic DNA polymerases: proposal for a revised nomenclature. J Biol Chem 2001;276:43487–90.
66. Ohmori H, Friedberg EC, Fuchs RPP, et al. The Y-family of DNA polymerases. Mol Cell 2001;8:7–8.
67. Trincao J, Johnson RE, Escalante CR, et al. Structure of the catalytic core of *S. cerevisiae* DNA polymerase h: implications for translesion synthesis. Mol Cell 2001;8:417–26.
68. Johnson RE, Washington MT, Prakash S, Prakash L. Fidelity of human DNA polymerase η. J Biol Chem 2000;275:7447–50.
69. Tessman I In: Bukhari A, Ljungquist E, editors. Abstracts of the Bacteriophage Meeting. Cold Spring Harbor (NY): Cold Spring Harbor Laboratory Press; 1976. p. 87.
70. Johnson RE, Prakash S, Prakash L. Efficient bypass of a thymine-thymine dimer by yeast DNA polymerase eta. Science 1999;283:1001–4.
71. McCulloch SD, Kokoska RJ, Masutani C, et al. Preferential cis-syn thymine dimer bypass by DNA polymerase eta occurs with biased fidelity. Nature 2004;428:97–100.
72. Johnson RE, Kondratick CM, Prakash S, Prakash L. hRAD30 mutations in the variant form of xeroderma pigmentosum. Science 1999;264:263–5.
73. Masutani C, Kusumoto R, Yamada A, et al. The XPV (xeroderma pigmentosum variant) gene encodes human DNA polymerase η. Nature 1999;399:700–4.
74. Tissier A, Frank EG, McDonald JP, et al. Misinsertion and bypass of thymine-thymine dimers by human DNA polymerase iota. EMBO J 2000;19:5259–66.
75. Tissier A, McDonald JP, Frank EG, Woodgate R. Pol iota, a remarkable error-prone human DNA polymerase. Genes Dev 2000;14:1642–50.
76. Woodgate R. Evolution of the two-step model for UV-mutagenesis. Mutat Res 2001;485:83–92.
77. Washington MT, Johnson RE, Prakash L, Prakash S. Human DINB1-encoded DNA polymerase κ is a promiscuous extender of mispaired promer termini. Proc Natl Acad Sci U S A 2002;99:1910–4.
78. Johnson RE, Washington MT, Haracska L, et al. Eukaryotic polymerases i and z act sequentially to bypass DNA lesions. Nature 2000;406:1015–9.
79. Wang YC, Maher VM, McCormick JJ. Xeroderma pigmentosum variant cells are less likely than normal cells to incorporate dAMP opposite photoproducts during replication of UV-irradiated plasmids. Proc Natl Acad Sci U S A 1991;88:7810–4.
80. Wang YC, Maher VM, Mitchell DL, McCormick JJ. Evidence from mutation spectra that the UV hypermutability of xeroderma pigmentosum variant cells reflects abnormal error-prone replication on a template containing photoproducts. Mol Cell Biol 1993;13:4276–83.
81. Gibbs PE, McGregor WG, Maher VM, et al. A human homolog of the *Saccharomyces cerevisiae* REV3 gene, which encodes the catalytic subunit of DNA polymerase zeta. Proc Natl Acad Sci U S A 1998;95:6876–80.
82. Brash DE, Haseltine WA. UV-induced mutation hotspots occur at DNA damage hotspots. Nature 1982;298:189–92.
83. Wood RD, Skopek TR, Hutchinson F. Changes in DNA base sequence induced by targeted mutagenesis of lambda phage by ultraviolet light. J Mol Biol 1984;173:273–91.
84. Tang M-S, Hrncir J, Mitchell D, et al. The relative cytotoxicity and mutagenicity of cyclobutane pyrimidine dimers and [6-4] photoproducts in *Escherichia coli* cells. Mutat Res 1986;161:9–17.
85. Lebkowski JS, Clancy S, Miller JH, Calos MP. The lacI shuttle: rapid analysis of the mutagenic specificity of ultraviolet light in human cells. Proc Natl Acad Sci U S A 1985;82:8606–10.
86. Hauser J, Seidman MM, Sidur K, Dixon K. Sequence specificity of point mutations induced during passage of a UV-irradiated shuttle vector plasmid in monkey cells. Mol Cell Biol 1986;6:277–85.
87. Glazer PM, Sarkar SN, Summers WC. Detection and analysis of UV-induced mutations in mammalian cell DNA using a lambda phage shuttle vector. Proc Natl Acad Sci U S A 1986;83:1041–4.
88. Drobetsky EA, Grosovsky AJ, Glickman BW. The specificity of UV-induced mutations at an endogenous locus in mammalian cells. Proc Natl Acad Sci U S A 1987;84:9103–7.
89. Kress S, Sutter C, Strickland PT, et al. Carcinogen-specific mutational pattern in the p53 gene in ultraviolet B radiation-induced squamous cell carcinomas of mouse skin. Cancer Res 1992;52:6400–3.
90. Dumaz N, Drougard C, Sarasin A, Daya-Grosjean L. Specific UV-induced mutation spectrum in the p53 gene of skin tumors from DNA-repair-deficient xeroderma pigmentosum patients. Proc Natl Acad Sci U S A 1993;90:10519–33.
91. Brash DE, Seetharam S, Kraemer KH, et al. Photoproduct frequency is not the major determinant of UV base substitution hot spots or cold spots in human cells. Proc Natl Acad Sci U S A 1987;84:3782–6.
92. Protic-Sabljic M, Tuteja N, Munson PJ, et al. UV light-induced cyclobutane pyrimidine dimers are mutagenic in mammalian cells. Mol Cell Biol 1986;6:3349–56.
93. Tornaletti S, Pfeiffer GP. Slow repair of pyrimidine dimers at p53 mutation hotspots in skin cancer. Science 1994;263:1436–8.
94. Tornaletti S, Rozek D, Pfeifer GP. The distribution of UV photoproducts along the human p53 gene and its relation to mutations in skin cancer. Oncogene 1993;8:2051–7.
95. Tornaletti S, Rozek D, Pfeifer GP. Mapping of UV photoproducts along the human p53 gene. Ann N Y Acad Sci 1994;726:324–6.
96. Tormanen VT, Pfeifer GP. Mapping of UV photoproducts within ras proto-oncogenes in UV irradiated cells: correlation with mutations in human skin cancer. Oncogene 1992;7:1729–36.
97. Ziegler A, Jonason AS, Leffell DJ, et al. Sunburn and p53 in the onset of skin cancer. Nature 1994;372:773–6.
98. Brash DE, Rudolph JA, Simon JA, et al. A role for sunlight in skin cancer: UV-induced p53 mutations in squamous cell carcinoma. Proc Natl Acad Sci U S A 1991;88:10124–8.
99. Lehmann AR. Three complementation groups in Cockayne syndrome. Mutat Res 1982;106:347–56.
100. Lehmann AR, Kirk-Bell S, Mayne L. Abnormal kinetics of DNA synthesis in ultraviolet light-irradiated cells from patients with Cockayne syndrome. Cancer Res 1979;39:4237–41.
101. Lehmann AR, Arlett CF, Broughton BC, et al. Trichothiodystrophy, a human DNA repair disorder with heteroge-

neity in the cellular response to ultraviolet light. Cancer Res 1988;48:6090–6.
102. Broughton BC, Lehmann AR, Harcourt SA, et al. Relationship between pyrimidine dimers, 6-4 photoproducts, repair synthesis and cell survival: studies using cells from patients with trichothiodystrophy. Mutat Res 1990;235:33–40.
103. Gorlin RJ, Goltz RW. Multiple nevoid basal-cell epithelioma, jaw cysts and bifid rib: a syndrome. N Engl J Med 1960;262:908–12.
104. Busch D, Greiner C, Lewis K, et al. Summary of complementation groups of UV- sensitive CHO cell mutants isolated by large-scale screening. Mutagenesis 1989;4:349–54.
105. Huang JC, Sancar A. Determination of minimum substrate size for human excinuclease. J Biol Chem 1994;269:19034–44.
106. Mol CD, Arvai AS, Sanderson RJ, et al. Crystal structure of human uracil-DNA glycosylase in complex with a protein inhibitor: protein mimicry of DNA. Cell 1995;82:701–8.
107. Shivji MK, Eker AP, Wood RD. DNA repair defect in xeroderma pigmentosum group C and complementing factor from HeLa cells. J Biol Chem 1994;269:22749–57.
108. Masutani C, Sugasawa K, Yanagisawa J, et al. Purification and cloning of a nucleotide excision repair complex involving the xeroderma pigmentosum group C protein and a human homologue of yeast RAD23. EMBO J 1994;13:1831–43.
109. Sugasawa K, Ng JMY, Masutani C, et al. Xeroderma pigmentosum group C protein complex is the initiator of global nucleotide excision repair. Mol Cell 1998;2:223–32.
110. Wood RD. DNA damage recognition during nucleotide excision repair in mammalian cells. Biochimie 1999;81:39–44.
111. Baxter BK, Smerdon MJ. Nucleosome unfolding during DNA repair in normal and xeroderma pigmentosum (group C) human cells. J Biol Chem 1998;273:17517–24.
112. Hwang BJ, Toering S, Francke U, Chu G. p48 activates a UV-damaged-DNA binding factor and is defective in xeroderma pigmentosum group E cells that lack binding activity. Mol Cell Biol 1998;18:4391–9.
113. Tang J, Chu G. Xeroderma pigmentosum complementation group E and UV-damaged DNA-binding protein. DNA Repair 2002;1:601–16.
114. Hwang BJ, Ford JM, Hanawalt PC, Chu G. Expression of the p48 xeroderma pigmentosum gene is p53-dependent and is involved in global genome repair. Proc Natl Acad Sci U S A 1999;96:424–8.
115. Houtsmuller AB, Rademakers S, Nigg AL, et al. Action of DNA repair endonuclease ERCC1/XPF in living cells. Science 1999;284:958–61.
116. Greenblatt MS, Bennett WP, Hollstein M, Harris CC. Mutations in the p53 tumor suppressor gene: clues to cancer etiology and molecular pathogenesis. Cancer Res 1994;54:4855–78.
117. Smith ML, Chen I-T, Zhan Q, et al. Interaction of the p53-regulated protein gadd 45 with proliferating cell nuclear antigen. Science 1994;266:1376–80.
118. McWhir J, Selfridge J, Harrison DJ, et al. Mice with DNA repair gene (ERCC-1) deficiency have elevated levels of p53, liver nuclear abnormalities and die before weaning. Nat Genet 1993;5:217–24.
119. van Duin M, van den Tol J, Warmerdam P, et al. Evolution and mutagenesis of the mammalian excision repair gene ERCC1. Nucleic Acids Res 1988;16:5305–22.
120. Kraemer KH, Lee MM, Scotto J. Xeroderma pigmentosum: cutaneous, ocular and neurological abnormalities in 830 published cases. Arch Dermatol 1987;123:241–50.
121. Zelle B, Lohman PH. Repair of UV-endonuclease-susceptible sites in the 7 complementation groups of xeroderma pigmentosum A through G. Mutat Res 1979;62:363–8.
122. Mitchell DL. The induction and repair of lesions produced by the photolysis of [6-4] photoproducts in normal and UV-hypersensitive human cells. Mutat Res 1988;194:227–37.
123. Venema J, Hoffen AV, Karcagi V, et al. Xeroderma pigmentosum complementation group C cells remove pyrimidine dimers selectively from the transcribed strand of active genes. Mol Cell Biol 1991;11:4128–34.
124. Patterson M, Chu G. Evidence that xeroderma pigmentosum cells from complementation group E are deficient in a homolog of yeast photolyase. Mol Cell Biol 1989;9:5105–12.
125. Itoh T, Nichols A, Linn S. Abnomal regulation of DBB2 gene expression in xeroderma pigmentosum group E strains. Oncogene 2001;20:7041–50.
126. Itoh T, Linn S, Ono T, Yamaizumi M. Reinvestigation of the classification of five cell strains of xeroderma pigmentosum group E with reclassification of three of them. J Invest Dermatol 2000;114:1022–9.
127. Friedberg EC, Meira LB, Cheo DL. Database of mouse strains carrying targeted mutations in genes affecting cellular responses to DNA damage. Version 2. Mutat Res 1998;407:217–26.
128. Weeda G, Ham RCAV, Vermeulen W, et al. A presumed helicase encoded by ERCC-3 is involved in the human repair disorders xeroderma pigmentosum and Cockayne's syndrome. Cell 1990;62:777–91.
129. Venema J, Mullenders JH, Natarajan AT, et al. The genetic defect in Cockayne syndrome is associated with a defect in repair of UV-induced DNA damage in transcriptionally active DNA. Proc Natl Acad Sci U S A 1990;87:4707–11.
130. Berg RJ, Rebel H, van der Horst GT, et al. Impact of global genome repair versus transcription-coupled repair on ultraviolet carcinogenesis in hairless mice. Cancer Res 2000;60:2858–63.
131. Weber CA, Salazar EP, Stewart SA, Thompson LH. ERCC2: cDNA cloning and molecular characterization of a human nucleotide excision repair gene with high homology to yeast RAD3. EMBO J 1990;9:1437–47.
132. Itin PH, Sarasin A, Pittelkow MR. Trichothiodystrophy: update on the sulfur-deficient brittle hair syndromes. J Am Acad Dermatol 2001;44:891–920.
133. Giglia-Mari G, Coin F, Ranish JA, et al. A new, tenth subunit of TFIIH is responsible for the DNA repair syndrome trichothiodystrophy group A. Nat Genet 2004;36:714–9.
134. Stanbridge EJ. Identifying tumor suppressor genes in human colorectal cancer. Science 1990;247:12–3.
135. Vogelstein B, Fearon ER, Kern SE, et al. Allelotype of colorectal carcinomas. Science 1989;244:207–11.
136. Rochat A, Kobayashi K, Barrandon Y. Location of stem cells of human hair follicles by clonal analysis. Cell 1994;76:1063–73.
137. Potten CS. The epidermal proliferative unit: the possible role of the central basal cell. Cell Tissue Kinet 1974;7:77–88.
138. Morris RJ, Fisher SM, Slaga TJ. Evidence that a slowly cycling subpopulation of adult murine epidermal cells retains carcinogen. Cancer Res 1986;46:3061–6.
139. Zhang W, Remenyik E, Zelterman D, et al. Escaping the stem cell compartment: sustained UVB exposure allows p53-mutant keratinocytes to colonize adjacent epidermal proliferating units without incurring additional mutations. Proc Natl Acad Sci U S A 2001;98:13948–53.
140. Nataraj AJ, Trent JC, Ananthaswamy HN. p53 gene mutations and photocarcinogenesis. Photochem Photobiol 1995;62:165–77.
141. Limoli CL, Giedzinski E, Bonner WM, Cleaver JE. UV-induced replication arrest in the xeroderma pigmentosum variant leads to double strand breaks, g-H2Ax formation, and Mre11 relocalization. Proc Natl Acad Sci U S A 2002;99:233–8.
142. Bertrand P, Saintigny Y, Lopez BS. p53's double life: transactivation-independent repression of homologous recombination. Trends Genet 2004;202:235–43.
143. Ananthaswamy HN, Price JE, Goldberg LH, Bales ES. Detection and identification of activated oncogenes in human skin cancers occurring on sun-exposed body sites. Cancer Res 1988;48:3341–6.
144. Keijzer W, Mulder MP, Langeveld JC, et al. Establishment and characterization of a melanoma cell line from a xeroderma pigmentosum patient: activation of N-ras at a potential pyrimidine CPD site. Cancer Res 1989;49:1229–35.
145. Suarez HG, Daya-Grosjean L, Schlaifer D, et al. Activated oncogenes in human skin tumors from a repair-deficient syndrome, xeroderma pigmentosum. Cancer Res 1989;49:1223–8.
146. Bredberg A, Kraemer KH, Seidman MM. Restricted ultraviolet mutational spectrum in a shuttle vector propagated in xeroderma pigmentosum cells. Proc Natl Acad Sci U S A 1986;83:8273–7.
147. Yuspa SH. The pathogenesis of squamous cell cancer: lessons learned from studies of skin carcinogenesis. J Dermatol Sci 1998;17:1–7.
148. Mock BA, Lowry DT, Rehman I, et al. Multigenic control of skin tumor susceptibility in SENCARA/Pt mice. Carcinogenesis 1998;19:1109–15.
149. Nagase H, Mao JH, de Kooning JP, et al. Epistatic interactions between skin tumor modifier loci in interspecific (spretus/musculus) backcross mice. Cancer Res 2001;61:1305–8.
150. Girardi M, Oppenheim DE, Steele CR, et al. Regulation of cutaneous malignancy by gamma delta T cells. Science 2001;294:605–9.
151. Schwarz A, Stander S, Berneburg M, et al. Interleukin-12 suppresses ultraviolet radiation-induced apoptosis by inducing DNA repair. Nat Cell Biol 2002;4:26–31.
152. Johnson RL, Rothman AL, Xie J, et al. Human homolog of patched, a candidate gene for the basal cell nevus syndrome. Science 1996;272:1668–71.
153. Hahn H, Wicking C, Zaphiropoulous PG, et al. Mutations of the human homolog of Drosophila patched in the nevoid basal cell carcinoma syndrome. Cell 1996;85:841–51.
154. Toftgard R. Hedgehog signalling in cancer. Cell Mol Life Sci 2000;57:1720–31.
155. Marigo V, Davey RA, Zuo Y, et al. Biochemical evidence that patched is the hedgehog receptor. Nature 1996;384:176–9.
156. Stone DM, Hynes M, Armanini M, et al. The tumour-suppressor gene patched encodes a candidate receptor for sonic hedgehog. Nature 1996;384:129–34.
157. Xie J, Murone M, Gu Q, et al. Activating SMOOTHENED mutations in sporadic basal cell carcinoma. Nature 1998;391:90–2.
158. Gailani MR, Bale AE. Developmental genes and cancer: role of patched in basal cell carcinoma of the skin. J Natl Cancer Inst 1997;89:1103–9.
159. Reifenberger J, Wolter M, Weber RG, et al. Missense mutations in SMOH in sporadic basal cell carcinomas of the skin and primitive neuroectodermal tumors of the central nervous system. Cancer Res 1998;58:1798–803.
160. Ashton KJ, Weinstein SR, Maguire DJ, Griffiths LR. Molecular cytogenetic analysis of basal cell carcinoma DNA using comparative genomic hybridization. J Invest Dermatol 2001;117:683–6.
161. Goldstein AM, Tucker MA. Genetic epidemiology of cutaneous melanoma: a global perspective. Arch Dermatol 2001;137:1493–6.
162. Barnhill RL, Roush GC, Titus-Ernstoff L, et al. Comparison of nonfamilial and familial melanoma. Dermatology 1992;184:2–7.
163. Kopf AW, Hellman LJ, Rogers GS, et al. Familial malignant melanoma. JAMA 1986;256:1915–9.
164. Aitken JF, Duffy DL, Green A, et al. Heterogeneity of melanoma risk in families of melanoma patients. Am J Epidemiol 1994;140:961–73.
165. Whiteman DC, Watt P, Purdie DM, et al. Melanocytic nevi, solar keratoses, and divergent pathways to cutaneous melanoma. J Natl Cancer Inst 2003;95:806–12.
166. Kamb A, Shattuck-Eidens D, Eeles R, et al. Analysis of the p16 gene (CDKN2) as a candidate for the chromosome 9p melanoma susceptibility locus. Nat Genet 1994;8:23–6.
167. Nobori T, Miura K, Wu DJ, et al. Deletions of the cyclin-dependent kinase-4 inhibitor gene in multiple human cancers. Nature 1994;368:753–6.
168. Bastian B, LeBoit PE, Hamm H, et al. Chromosomal gains and losses in primary cutaneous melanomas detected by comparative genome hybridization. Cancer Res 1998;58:2170–5.
169. Bastian BC, Wesselmann U, Pinkel D, Leboit PE. Molecular cytogenetic analysis of Spitz nevi shows clear differences to melanoma. J Invest Dermatol 1999;113:1065–9.
170. Bastian BC, LeBoit PE, Pinkel D. Mutations and copy number increases of HRAS in Spitz nevi with distinctive histopathologic features. Am J Pathol 2000;157:967–72.
171. Pollock PM, Trent JM. The genetics of cutaneous melanoma. Clin Lab Med 2000;20:667–90.
172. Davies H, Bignell GR, Cox C, et al. Mutations of the BRAF gene in human cancer. Nature 2002;417:949–54.
173. Flaherty K. New molecular targets in melanoma. Curr Opin Oncol 2004;16:150–4.
174. Diffey BL. A quantitative estimate of melanoma mortality from ultraviolet A sunbed use in the U.K. Br J Dermatol 2003;149:578–91.
175. Setlow RB, Grist E, Thompson K, Woodhead AD. Wavelengths effective in induction of malignant melanoma. Proc Natl Acad Sci U S A 1993;90:6666–70.
176. Moloney FJ, Collins S, Murphy GM. Sunscreens: safety, efficacy and appropriate use. Am J Clin Dermatol 2002;3:185–91.
177. Yarosh DB. Enhanced DNA repair of cyclobutane pyrimidine dimers changes the biological response to UV-B radiation. Mutat Res 2002;509:221–6.
178. Stege H. Effect of xenogenic repair enzymes on photoimmunology and photocarcinogenesis. J Photochem Photobiol B 2001;65:105–8.
179. Goukassian DA, Helms E, van Steeg, H, et al. Topical DNA oligonucleotide therapy reduces UV-induced mutations and photocarcinogenesis in hairless mice. Proc Natl Acad Sci U S A 2004;101:3933–8.

18

Inflammation, Trauma, and Physical Agents in Cancer

Michael A. Gallo, PhD
Joseph Aisner, MD

Of the many needs in cancer research, the identification of putative human carcinogens and their inactivation or removal from society is an important priority for prevention of future cancer risks.[1]

Carcinogenesis is a complex, multistep process that results in cancer formation. Physical carcinogens are hypothesized to cause cancer by genetic and epigenetic mechanisms that induce initiation through derivative biochemical reactions 1999.[2] Nonspecific, localized inflammation, and subsequent proliferation result in spontaneous (perhaps ROS-induced) mutations that are then fixed.[3] Further proliferation results in clonal expansion of the mutated gene(s) into cancer (Figure 18-1). This hypothesis is supported by the findings that fiber length and diameter are critical factors in the carcinogenicity of fibrous materials[4,5] and the shape and size of solids such as Bakelite determine the carcinogenic potential. The overarching hypothesis, which is supported by a rich literature, is that solids are chemically inert. However, some solids break down in tissues, hence, there may well be a chemical toxicity involved in some physical carcinogen-induced tumors. Reports that implantation of fragmented carcinogenic solids diminishes or ablates the carcinogenic potential of the material raises intriguing questions regarding the chemical nature of the materials. In the experimental setting, the implanted solids are well-defined materials; this is not the case in the environmental and occupational setting. Particulates in the environment may well be carriers of other carcinogens.

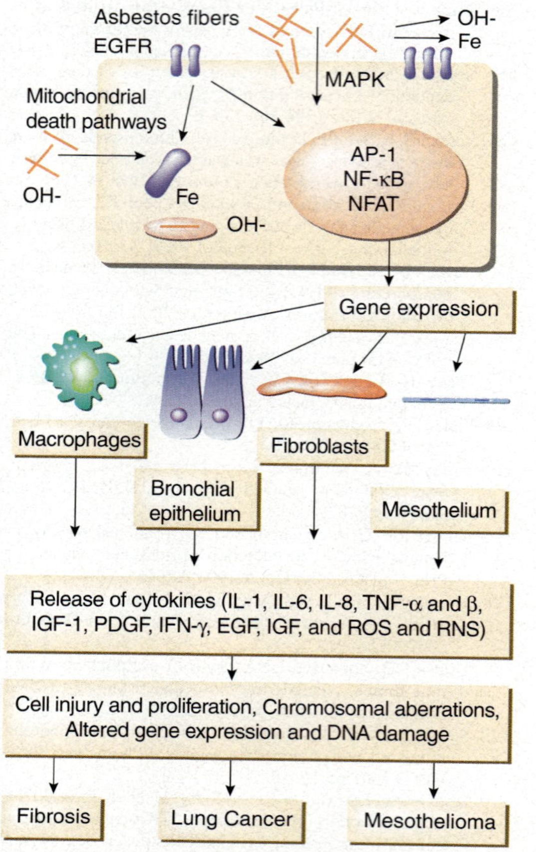

Figure 18-1 Role of oxidants in asbestos-related cell signaling, injury, and disease.

Inflammation is a hallmark of cancers that was reported by Virchow in the mid-nineteenth century.[6] The Virchow hypothesis that cancers originating at the sites of chronic inflammation resulted from cell proliferation is as apt today as it was in the 1860s. Our understanding of the inflammatory process, regardless of the etiologic agent, clearly leads to the elucidation of potential mechanism of many cancers. Importantly, these cancers should be ultimately preventable. Infections and the accompanying inflammation play major roles in 10 to 15% of human cancers.[7] The inflammatory process results in rapid proliferation of cells that aid in wound healing. Proliferating cells may "fix" a mutation in a stochastic manner or the DNA from the proliferating cells may sustain DNA damage from reactive oxygen species generated by leukocytes attracted to the inflamed site by cytokines and chemokines.[8] Generally, inflammation is a limited process. If inflammation persists, as with a non-degradable foreign body, a severe burn or a chronic infection, the risk of tumor initiation and promotion increases markedly. Figure 18-2 depicts the role of chronic inflammation in the development of neoplastic disease. Excellent reviews have been recently published on the role of inflammation and cancer.[6,9,10] Briefly, macrophages respond to chemokines released at the site of the inflammation or wound to enhance healing. Tumor necrosis factor alpha (TNF-α) and transforming growth factor (TGF)-β1 play key roles in healing and carcinogenesis. In addition, macrophages also produce factors that stimulate angiogenesis and breakdown of extracellular matrix. Negus and colleagues, refer to this paradox as the "macrophage balance" hypothesis.[11] The loss of growth control results in the attraction of multiple factors that enhance carcinogenesis.

A large body of literature exists demonstrating the role of inflammation, whether induced by infectious agents, trauma, or foreign bodies, in cancers. Tables 18-1 and 18-2 present a brief survey of agents and processes that are associated with neoplasia. The role of p53 in inflammatory disease related cancer has become very apparent in recent years. This cell cycle regulatory protein is a tumor suppressor and plays a key role in apoptosis, DNA repair, and cancer. Loss of control of p53 (mutated p53) is found in several cancers related to oxidative stress.[12–16] Indeed, p53 mutations have been reported in rheumatoid arthritis synovium clusters as a result of inflammatory mediator induced oxidative stress.[17] This response is analogous to the role of mutated p53 in the pathogenesis of colon cancer, and skin cancer as a result of UV damage.[18] Farrow and Evers hypothesized that inflammation and inflammatory mediators are key factors in the onset of pancreatic cancer and may be the major mediator in other solid tumors such as colon and skin, which are correlated with inflammatory bowel disease, and tumors at burn sites, respectively.[10] Multiple hypotheses exist regarding the mechanisms by which inflammatory mediators affect carcinogenesis, but the most widely accepted is that of the mediators inducing oxidative stress, which in turn alters DNA and releases growth control of the rapidly proliferating cells. Questions exist as to whether the effects are initiated in epithelial cells or in the stromal cells ("landscaper theory" of Kinzler and Vogelstein[19]), but the role of reactive oxygen species

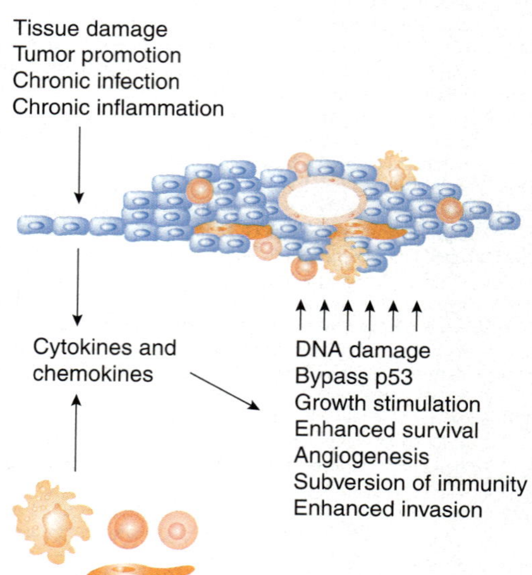

Figure 18-2 Stimulated cytokines and chemokines that contribute to development of malignant disease.

Table 18-1 Chronic Inflammatory Conditions Associated with Neoplasms

Pathologic Condition	Associated Neoplasms(s)	Etiologic Agent
Asbestos silicosis	Mesothelioma, lung carcinoma	Asbestos fibers, silica particles
Bronchitis	Lung carcinoma	Silica, asbestos, smoking (nitrosamines, peroxides)
Cystitis, bladder inflammation	Bladder carcinoma	Chronic indwelling, urinary catheters
Gingivitis, lichen planus	Oral squamous cell carcinoma	
Inflammatory bowel disease, Crohn's disease, chronic ulcerative colitis	Colorectal carcinoma	
Lichen sclerosus	Vulvar squamous cell carcinoma	
Chronic pancreatitis, hereditary pancreatitis	Pancreatic carcinoma	Alcoholism, mutation in trypsinogen gene on Ch. 7
Reflux esophagitis, Barrett's esophagus	Esophageal carcinoma	Gastric acids
Sialadenitis	Salivary gland carcinoma	
Sjögren syndrome, Hashimoto's thyroiditis	MALT lymphoma	
Skin inflammation	Melanoma	Ultraviolet light
Cancers associated with infectious agents		
Opisthorchis, cholangitis	Cholangiosarcoma, colon carcinoma	Liver flukes (*Opisthorchis viverrini* bile acids)
Chronic cholecystitis	Gallbladder cancer	Bacteria, gallbladder stones
Gastritis/ulcers	Gastric adenocarcinoma, MALT	*Helicobacter pylori*
Hepatitis	Hepatocellular carcinoma	Hepatitis B and/or C virus
Mononucleosis	B-cell non-Hodgkin's lymphoma, Burkitt's lymphoma	Epstein-Barr virus
AIDS	Non-Hodgkin's lymphoma, squamous cell carcinomas, Kaposi's sarcoma	Human immunodeficiency virus, human herpesvirus type 8
Osteomyelitis	Skin carcinoma in draining sinuses	Bacterial infection
Pelvic inflammatory disease, chronic cervicitis	Ovarian carcinoma, cervical/anal carcinoma	Gonorrhoeae chlamydia, human papillomavirus
Chronic cystitis	Bladder, liver, rectal carcinoma, follicular lymphoma of the spleen	Schistosomiasis

Modified from refs 29, 67.
MALT = mucosa-associated lymphoid tissue.

(ROS) is prevalent (Figure 18-3). The actions of cytokines and chemokines are presented schematically in Figure 18-4. Vicari and Caux, in an excellent review entitled "Chemokines in Cancer," describe chemokines as a large family[45–50] of structurally related cysteine-containing proteins that bind to G protein-coupled receptors. The role of chemokines is to direct leukocyte trafficking and regulate processes of tumor growth, invasion, and metastasis.[20]

Hence, inflammation is the cornerstone for cancers that are associated with bacterial, viral, and parasitic infections; solid materials such as asbestos, wood dusts and implanted devices; wound healing, and radiation.

Trauma as a causative agent in cancer is not well documented. There is no question that some types of physical injury are associated with specific cancers, but direct causation is difficult to ascertain. Blunt trauma results in localized concentrations of inflammatory mediators, and localized chronic inflammation is associated with cancers.[21] A search of the current literature revealed a few case reports of blunt trauma and tumors. These include reports of a benign lacrimal gland pleotrophic adenoma,[22] synovial sarcoma following a soccer injury,[23] and local lymphomas following blunt trauma to the scalp.[24] Marjolin's ulcers, deep ulcers in old scars, have been reported to develop into squamous cell carcinoma that metastasize, and one might argue that basal cell carcinoma following sunburn is a trauma rather than a radiation-induced tumor. Several authors have reported skin cancers from old deep-burn scars. These thick dense scars usually give rise to squamous cell carcinomas several decades after the initial injury.[25] Bone trauma is estimated to be directly causative of a small percentage of osteosarcoma, whereas some sarcomas develop at the site of healed fractures.[25] Oral cancer has been associated with bad dentures and/or malformed or jagged teeth. These oral cancers are clearly the result of chronic inflammation of the cavity. Skin tumors apparently induced by scarring at points of extreme local heat have been reported in Kashmir and Japan where people use metal or stone warmers close to the skin for prolonged periods.[26,27]

Physical carcinogens represent a broad class of seemingly unrelated agents including alpha and beta particles, gamma radiation, electromagnetic fields, sunlight, extreme temperatures, blunt trauma, solid materials, and gel/plastic materials. The importance of this broad classification is that for the solid and gel type agents it is the shape and size of the material rather than the release of their chemical constituents that is the carcinogenic stimulus. Anecdotal reports of tumors in and around embedded bullets and other munitions have been reported since the late nineteenth century. IARC reported on these agents and cases of sarcomas associated with surgical implants.[28]

Solid carcinogens have been reported in the experimental literature for several decades. Turner reported that implanted Bakelite disks

Table 18-2 Inflammatory Conditions and Their Related Malignancies

Malignancy	Inflammatory Stimulus/Condition
Bladder	Schistosomiasis
Cervical	Papillomavirus
Ovarian	Pelvic inflammatory disease/ taic/tissue remodeling
Gastric	*H. pylori* induced gastritis
MALT lymphoma	*H. pylori*
Esophageal	Barrett's metaplasia
Colorectal	Inflammatory bowel disease
Hepatocellular	Hepatitis virus (B and C)
Bronchial	Silica, asbestos, cigarette smoke
Mesothelioma	Asbestos
Kaposi's sarcoma	Human herpesvirus type 8

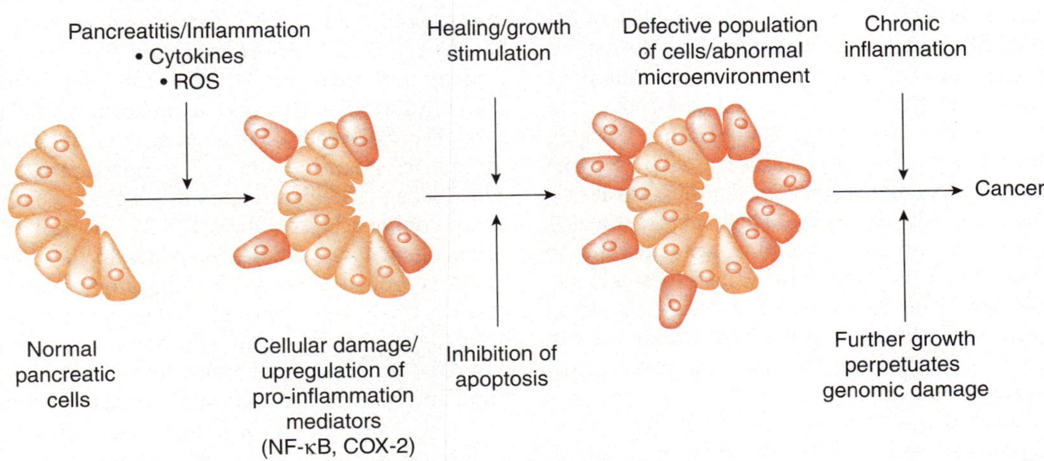

Figure 18-3 Pancreatic cancer: inflammation and the landscaper theory.

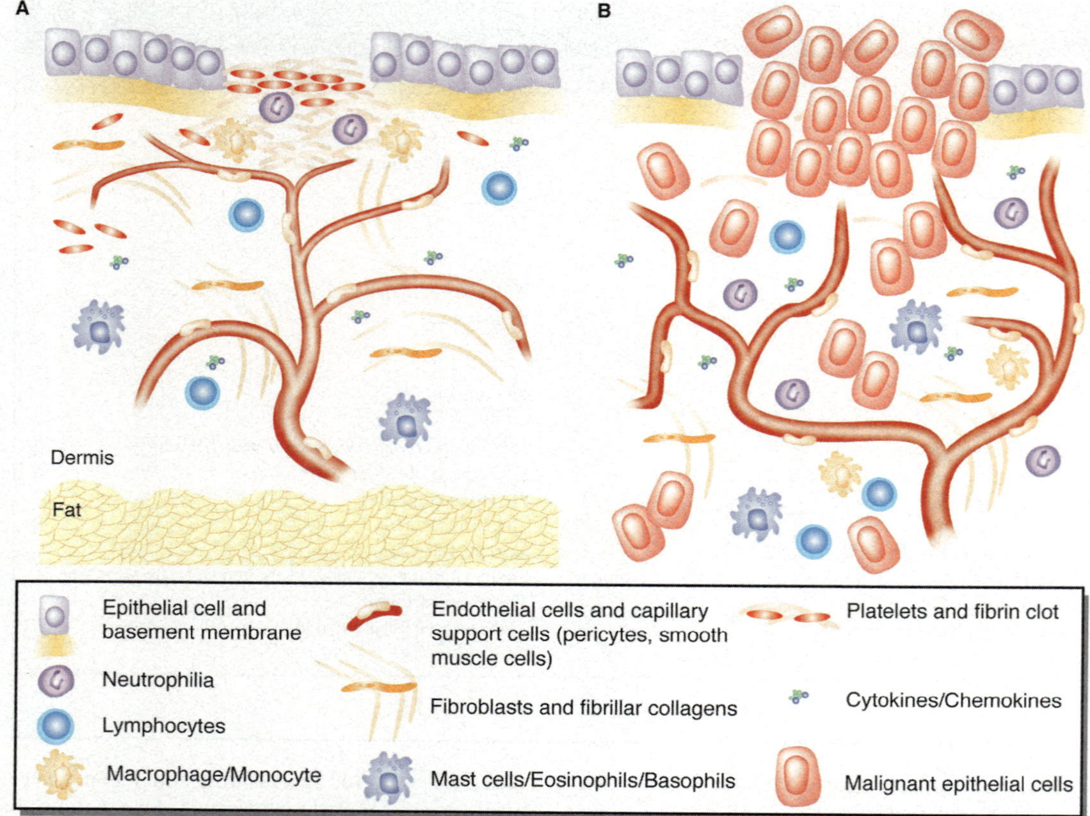

Figure 18-4 Wound healing versus invasive tumor growth.

Table 18-3 Hard and Soft Materials, of Different Shape and Dimension, Found to be Carcinogenic when Implanted in Rodents

Metals
Gold
Platinum
Silver
Steel
Tantalum
Nickel
Metallic alloys
Vitallium (chromium, cobalt, molybdenum)
Water-insoluble polymers
Hydrocarbon polymers (synthetic)
Polyethylene (Polythene)
Polymethylmethacrylate (Lucite)
Polyvinylbenzol (Polystyrol)
Cross-linked polyvinyl alcohol (Ivalon)
Polyester condensate of terephthalate and ethylene glycol (Dacron)
Phenol-formaldehyde condensate (Bakelite)
Halogenated-hydrocarbon polymers (synthetic)
Polyvinyl chloride (PVC, Igelit, Vestolit, Vinnol)
Polyvinylidene chloride (Saran)
Polyfluor(chlor)-olefine (Teflon)
Polymethylmethacrylate chloride (Pliofilm)
Copolymer of vinyl chloride and acrylonitrile (Vinyon N, Dynel)
Aminized hydrocarbon polymers (polyamides) (synthetic)
Polyhexamethylene diamine adipanide (nylon)
Poly-e-Caprolactam, polyurethane (Perlon)
Hydrocarbon polymers (semisynthetic and natural)
Processed latex gum (rubber)
Processed polyglucose (cellulose) (cellophane)
Processed cellulose (linen, parchment paper)
Natural organic materials (silk, keratin, ivory)
Silicon polymers (synthetic)
Processed polydimethylsiloxanes (silicone rubber) (Silastic)
Mixture of different siloxanes (silicone gel for prostheses)

induced local fibrosarcoma in rats,[29] and Oppenheimer and colleagues, reported the carcinogenicity of implanted plastic and metals in rodents.[30–32] The laboratory of Maltoni published a series of studies on the carcinogenic activity of implanted polymeric substances used clinically.[33–35] These are classic studies that defined the carcinogenic potential of these physical agents based on size, shape and placement of the implants. Table 18-3 from Soffritti and colleauges,[36] in *Cancer Medicine e.6* is presented here to accentuate the large number of physical agents shown to be carcinogens in experimental animals. Interestingly, it is not the mass but the shape and size of particular materials that renders them carcinogenic in the rodent models.[34]

By far the most well-studied class of solid agents is fibers in all forms. Asbestos, "the magic mineral," is perhaps the most widely studied of the natural fibers. It was used worldwide in insulation, the automotive, truck, rail, textile, and shipping industries, as well as in paints and sheetrocks. It is safe to say that this mineral is ubiquitous. Workers in the asbestos handling facilities, as well as workers in the above fields and their families, are at risk of asbestos induced disease. There are six silicates classified as asbestos: actinolite, amosite, anthophyllite, tremolite, crocidolite (blue asbestos), and chrysotile (white asbestos) all of which can cause asbestosis.[37] Chrysotile is the most widely used at a rate of several million tons per year, followed by amosite and crocidolite.

Asbestos was first associated with lung cancer by Lynch and Smith in 1935,[38] and the induction of mesothelioma was first reported by Wagner and colleagues in 1960.[39] The overall carcinogenic potential of asbestos has now been reported in clinical, epidemiologic, and experimental settings. Mesothelioma (pleural and peritoneal) is the most widely accepted tumor caused by asbestos. Lung cancer associated with asbestosis is primarily seen in patients with a long history of tobacco smoking. A remarkable synergism exists between tobacco use and asbestos exposure in lung cancer.[40–42] In addition, there are several reports of mesothelioma and pleural plaques in family members of asbestos workers, and community members in asbestos-producing areas.[43]

In cell culture studies asbestos has been shown to activate proto-oncogenes (AP-1) and ERK1/2 pathways in pulmonary epithelial cells and mesothelial cells, and that glutathione-controlled status plays a key role activation.[44–45] Excellent reviews of the cellular actions of asbestos are published in the *International Journal of Biochemistry and Cell Biology*, and *Free Radical Biology and Medicine*.[46–47] The role of p53 and p53-regulated pathways in mesothelioma is strongly supported by studies in mice where a loss of heterozygosity at the p53 tumor-suppressor gene locus markedly affected the carcinogenicity of crocidolite asbestos fibers.[48,49] The overall role of oncogenes and suppressor genes in mesothelioma is well established in laboratory studies, whereas SV40 T-antigen and viral sequences have been reported in up to 80% of human mesothelioma tissues.[50] A recent case-control study identified the presence of SV40, speculated to be from oral polio vaccine, as a major risk factor for malignant mesothelioma in asbestos-exposed individuals.[51]

Man-made mineral fibers (MMMF) and silica are suspect carcinogens. The proposed mechanism of action of these fibers is similar to that of asbestos. Silica is listed as a Group 1 carcinogen by IARC whereas MMMF are listed as Group 2B (suggestive but inconclusive). Recent reviews of the epidemiology of MMMF strongly suggest carcinogenicity of several insulation fibers but the confounding factor in these studies is concurrent exposure to asbestos.[52,53] A multi-site, multi-factor case-control study reported a dose and time-response showing that wood dust, cotton dust, and synthetic fibers increased the odds ratio (OR) for lung and stomach cancer (OR 1.5) for exposure to wood dust, non-Hodgkin lymphoma for exposure to cotton dust (OR 1.9) and bladder cancer for exposure to synthetic fibers (OR 1.8). The question that remains to be answered is whether the man-made fibers and dusts act by mechanisms similar to asbestos or is there a direct carcinogenic action of some or all of these materials.[54]

Particulate air pollution presents a special case in physical carcinogenesis. Particulate matter (PM) is a term used to describe the general mixture of solid particulates and liquid droplets in the air, and is usually described as particles 2.5 to 10 μm (PM_{10}) and particles less than 2.5 μm

($PM_{2.5}$). PM is the result of fixed and mobile sources such as power plants, diesel exhaust from automobiles, buses and trucks, industrial plants, and wood burning stoves. Auto emissions and emissions from small, less efficient gasoline engines also contribute to this pool of pollution. The difference between these particles and those from crystalline sources (asbestos and silicates) is that the PM is a carrier for other potential carcinogens such as polyaromatic hydrocarbons (PAHs), dioxins, heavy metals, and other inherently toxic chemicals. Fine particles less than $PM_{2.5}$ result from combustion and are also formed by chemical reactions in the atmosphere. PM can accumulate in the lung and respiratory tract. The finer the particle the deeper into the lung it can settle, and create inflammatory reactions that can possibly lead to cancer. Several studies have shown positive correlation between PM and lung cancer and recent animal studies reported lung cancer and lymphoma in F344 SPF rats after long-term exposure to diesel fuel.[55–59]

Several laboratories are currently studying diesel exhaust and fine particles for their carcinogenic potential. Of great concern are the ultrafine (0.1 to < 2.5 μm) particles that can readily cross membranes and distribute to and accumulate in other organs of the body. The size distribution of several exhaust streams contains these ultrafine particles, many of which have the same chemical characteristics as the PMs.

The advent and wide use of nanoparticles in drugs, clothing, furniture, personal care products, and paints/pigments bears watching. These particles enter cells, cross the blood brain barrier, and accumulate in lysosomes and macrophages throughout the body. Little toxicology and/or carcinogenicity work on nanoparticles has been published to date, despite the broad worldwide use of these materials. What have we learned?

Gel implants, introduced in the 1960s, became widespread through the end of the century. It is estimated that approximately two million women received silicone breast implants, either post breast cancer surgery (approximately 20%) or for cosmetic breast augmentation.[60,61] Other than the focus on connective tissue diseases, little attention has been paid to the potential long-term effects, including cancer. A few animal studies have shown that silicone implants can induce tumors in rats: fibrosarcomas after subcutaneous implantation, and plasmocytomas of the peritoneum after implantation in the peritoneal cavity.[62,63] The epidemiology studies are mixed. Some show associations whereas others do not. There are provocative epidemiologic findings, though not universally accepted, suggesting that silicone breast implants might reduce breast cancer.[64–71] The possible mechanism of this phenomenon is unknown.

Brinton and colleagues, carried out a large retrospective cohort study of 13,488 patients who received cosmetic breast implants. The average follow-up was 12 years. The standardized incidence ration (SIR) for all tumors was 1.21 (1.1–1.4). The greatest relative risks (RR) were for brain (RR = 2.83) and respiratory (RR = 2.40). However, there was no overall increased risk for implant patients, relative risk (RR) was 1.00 (0.8–1.2). The excesses in brain and respiratory cancers raise interesting questions, but plausible mechanisms are lacking. The overall conclusion is that silicone breast implants do not initiate or promote breast cancer, and probably do not induce tumors in other organs.[72]

Electromagnetic fields (EMF) of low frequency have been studied in several laboratories and have been the subject of many epidemiology studies. EMF are created whenever electricity is generated, transmitted, or used. EMF are made up of electric and magnetic fields and the magnetic flux density is measured in microtesla (μT). One μT is equal to 1 m Gauss and the EMF are proportional to the current generated.[73] The primary EMF are generated at 60 cycles per second or 60 Hertz (60 Hz), which is powerline frequency. However, humans can be exposed to EMF from frequencies ranging from 3 to 3,000 Hz.[74]

Several long-term bioassays in rodents exposed to EMF have been conducted. All studies reported no increase in carcinogenesis. The most extensive study was carried out by the National Toxicology Program in 1,000 F344 rats and 1,000 B6C3F1 mice exposed to doses up to 1,000 μT, 18.5 hours/day for 2 years.[75] Mandeville and colleagues, reported no excess cancers in female F344/N rats exposed up to 2,000 μT (60 Hz) for 20 hours/day for two years.[76] A smaller study at higher EMF (0.5, and 5mT) in F344 was also negative.[77] Seventeen tumor promotion studies have been carried out using chemical carcinogens (DMBA and/or MNU) in combination with EMF. The results are varied. Ten are reported as negative (no promotion of carcinogenicity), seven are positive. These studies are reviewed in Portier and Wolfe.[73] A large body of epidemiologic data have been summarized by the National Institute of Environmental Health Sciences that show conflicting results across exposure levels and even across a single tumor type. The studies that suggest a carcinogenic effect of EMF were conducted primarily on occupationally exposed power line or power station workers. Residential level exposures have routinely been shown to be negative.

Cell phone usage has increased exponentially over the past decade. The hypothesis that cell phone usage increases risk of brain tumors is very controversial and there are studies that support both sides of the argument. Moulder and colleagues, conclude "the existing evidence for a causal relationship between RF radiation from cell phones and cancer is found to be weak and nonexistent."[78] This conclusion is supported by the comments of Elwood that "the epidemiological results fall short... that RF emissions are a cause of human cancer."[79] However, Hardell and colleagues concluded, in a case control study of 1,617 patients with brain tumors, that cell phone use was associated with tumor formation. Ipsilateral use of all phones use gave an increased odds ratio (OR) of 1.8 for astrocytomas. The authors speculated that there may be a tumor promoter effect from cell phone use.[80] Hansson and colleagues, reported that two Swedish epidemiologic studies have shown an association between brain tumors and the use of analog phones.[81] Studies in the United States and Finland have been inconclusive in the relationship between cell phone use as a carcinogen. The controversy continues.

SUMMARY

Cancer associated with physical carcinogens is a preventable disease. The goal of elucidating the carcinogenic potential of physical agents (old and new), and preventing human exposure to these materials is noble and must be pursued.

Physical carcinogens are a serious public health concern. Particulates from insulation, power plants, or mobile sources are ubiquitous. The advent of nanoparticles brings new challenges to researchers and clinicians alike in identifying potential risks. There is also an open question as to the role of smoke micro-particulates in tobacco smoke induced cancers. The new implantation techniques in dentistry and medicine raise concern regarding metal fragments and metal–tissue interactions. The controversies surrounding EMF and RF (cell phones) are still in the fore and must be resolved by laboratory and epidemiology studies. The weak link in the epidemiology studies of all physical carcinogens (proven and potential) is accurate and precise exposure assessment.

REFERENCES

1. Mossman BT, Klein G, Hausen H. Modern criteria to determine the etiology of human carcinogens. Semin Cancer Biol 2004;14:449–52.
2. Kamp DW, Weitzman SA. The molecular basis of asbestos induced lung injury. Thorax 1999;54:638–52.
3. Kane AB. Asbestos bodies: clues to the mechanism of asbestos toxicity. Hum Pathol 2003; 34:735–6.
4. IARC Working Group on the Evaluation of Carcinogenic Risks to Humans: asbestos. Suppl. 1987;7:106–16.
5. Infante P, Schuman L, Dement J, Huff J. Fibrous glass and cancer. Am J Ind Med 1994;26:559–84.
6. Balkwill F, Mantovani A. Inflammation and cancer: back to Virchow? Lancet 2001;357:539–45.
7. Parkin DM, Pisani P, Munoz N, et al, editors. Infections and Human Cancers. Cold Spring Harbor (NY): Cold Spring Harbor Laboratory Press; 1999.
8. Rossi D, Zlotnik A. The biology of chemokines and their receptors. Annu Rev Immunol 2000;18:217–42.
9. Coussens LM, Werb Z. Inflammation and cancer. Nature 2002;420:860–7.
10. Farrow B, Evers BM. Inflammation and the development of pancreatic cancer. Surg Oncol 2002; 10:153–69.
11. Negus RPK, Stamp GWQ, Hadley J, Balkwill FR. Quantitative assessment of the leukocyte infiltrates in ovarian cancer and its relationship to the expression of C-C chemokines. Am J Pathol 1997;150:1723–34.
12. Hollstein M, Sidransky D, Vogelstein B, Harris CC. P53 mutations in human cancers. Science 1991;253:49–53.
13. Levine AJ, Mamand HJ, Finlay CA. The p53 tumour suppressor gene. Nature 1991;351:453–6.
14. Hussain SP, Amstad P, Raja K, et al. Increased p53 mutation load in noncancerous colon tissue from ulcerative colitis: a cancer prone chronic inflammatory disease. Cancer Res 2000;60:3333–7.
15. Jonason AS, Kunals S, Price GJ et al. Frequent clones of p53-mutated keratinocytes in normal human skin. Proc Natl Acad Sci U S A 1996;93:14025–9.
16. Firestein GS, Escheverri F, Yeo M, et al. Somatic mutations in the p53 tumor suppressor gene in rheumatoid arthritis

synovium. Proc Natl Acad Sci U S A 1997;94:10895–900.
17. Yamanishi Y, Boyle DL, Rosengren S, et al. Regional analysis of p53 mutations in rheumatoid arthritis synovium. PNAS 2002;99:10025–30.
18. Levine A. p53, the cellular gatekeeper for growth and division. Cell 1997;88:323–31.
19. Kinzler KW, Vogelstein B. Landscaping the cancer terrain. Science 1998;280:1036–7.
20. Vicari AP, Caux C. Chemokines in cancer. Cytokine Growth Factor Rev 2002;13:143–54.
21. Perl M, Gebhard F, Knoferl MW, et al. The pattern of preformed cytokines in tissues frequently affected by blunt trauma. Shock 2003;19:299–304.
22. Hsu HC. Posttraumatic benign pleomorphic adenoma of the lacrimal gland. Ophthalmologica. 2001;215:235–7.
23. Engel C, Kelm J, Olinger A. Blunt trauma in soccer. The initial manifestation of synovial sarcoma. Zentralbl Chir 2001;126:68–71.
24. Morioka T, Tashima T, Nishio S, et al. Malignant lymphoma of the scalp at the site of a previous blunt trauma: report of two cases. Surg Neurol 1994;42:117–20.
25. Shiffman MA. Can trauma cause or accelerate the growth of cancer. The Forensic Examiner 2004;6–11.
26. Hoffman FL. Cancer in India, Persia and Ceylon, Sankhya. Ind J Statist 1936;2(Part 3):281.
27. Laycock HT. The "Kang Cancer" of West China. Brit Med J 1954;1:982.
28. IARC Monographs on the Evaluation of Carcinogenic Risks to Humans. Surgical implants and other foreign bodies. 1999; Vol.74. Lyon, France.
29. Turner FC. Sarcomas at sites of subcutaneous implanted Bakelite disks in rats. J. Natl Can Inst 1941;2:81.
30. Oppenheimer BS, Oppenheimer ET, Stout AP, Danishefsky I. Malignant tumors resulting from embedding plastics in rodents. Science1953;118:305.
31. Oppenheimer BS, Oppenheimer ET, Danishefsky I, et al. Further studies of polymers as carcinogenic agents in animals. Cancer Res 1955;15:333.
32. Oppenheimer BS, Oppenheimer ET, Danishefsky I, Stout AP. Carcinogenic effects of metals in rodents. Cancer Res 1956;16:439.
33. Maltoni C, Santi I, DelGaudio A. Sarcogenesi del tessuto sottocutaneo nel ratto impianto di dischi di Teflon: sequenza delle modificazioni locali. Il Cancro 1964;17:4.
34. Maltoni C, Sinibaldi C, Morisi, L. Carcinogenicity of vitallium. Long-term bioassays on Sprague-Dawley rats and Swiss mice by subcutaneous implantation. Acta Oncol 1980;1:11.
35. Maltoni C, Sinibaldi C. Carcinogenicity of acrylic resins (polymethyl methacrylate) used in dentistry. Long-term bioassays on Sprague-Dawley rats by subcutaneous implantation. Acta Oncol 1982;3:13.
36. Soffritti M, Minardi, F, Maltoni, C. Physical carcinogens In: Bast RC, Kufe DW, Pollock RE, et al, editors. Cancer medicine 6th ed. Hamilton (ON): BC Decker Inc; 2002. p.314–20.
37. Landrigan PJ, Soffritti M. Collegium Ramazzini Call for an international ban on asbestos. Am J Ind Med 2005;47:471–4.
38. Lynch KM, Smith WA. Pulmonary asbestosis: Carcinoma of the lung in asbestos silicosis. Am J Cancer 1935;24:56–64.
39. Wagner JC, Sleggs CA, Marchand P. Diffuse pleural mesothelioma and asbestos exposure in the North West Cape Province. Br J Ind Med 1960;17:260–71.
40. Hammond E, Selikoff I, Seidman H. Asbestos exposure, cigarette smoking and death rates. Ann NY Acad Sci 1979;330:473–90.
41. Lee CS, Cooper WA. Asbestos exposure and lung cancer. Pathology 2004;36:513–4.
42. Roggli VL. Carcinoma of the lung. In: Roggli VL, Oury TD, Sporn TA, editors. Pathology of asbestos-associated diseases New York: Springer; 2004. p. 193–216.
43. Magnani C, Ivaldi C, Botta M, Terracini B. Pleural malignant mesothelioma and environmental asbestos exposure in Casale Monferrato, Piedmont. Preliminary analysis of a case-control study. Med Lav 1997;88:302.
44. Shukla A, Flanders T, Lounsbury KM, Mossman BT. The γ-glutamylcysteine synthetase and glutathione regulate asbestos-induced expression of activator protein-1 family members and activity. Cancer Res 2004;64:7780–6.
45. Yuan Z, Taatjes DJ, Mossman BT, Heintz NH. The duration of nuclear extracellular signal-regulated kinase 1 and 2 signaling during cell cycle re-entry distinguishes proliferation from apoptosis in response to asbestos. Cancer Res 2004;64:6530–6.
46. Shukla A, Ramos-Nino M, Mossman B. Cell signaling and transcription factor activation by asbestos in lung injury and disease. Int J Biochem Cell Bio 2003;35:1198–1209.
47. Shukla A, Gulumian M, Hei TK, et al. Multiple roles of oxidants in the pathogenesis of asbestos-induced diseases. Free Radic Biol Med 2003;34:1117–29.
48. Marsella JM, Liu BL, Vaslet CA, Kane AB. Susceptibility of p53-deficient mice to induction of mesothelioma by crocidolite asbestos fibers. Environ Health Perspect 1987;105(Suppl.5):1069–72.
49. Vaslet CA, Messier NJ, Kane AB. Accelerated progression of asbestos-induced mesotheliomas in heterozygous p53 +/- mice. Toxicol Sci 2002;68:331–8.
50. Carbone M, Fisher S, Powers A, et al. New molecular and epidemiological issues in mesothelioma. Role of SV40. J Cell Physiol 1999;180:167–72.
51. Cristaudo A, Foddis R, Vivaldi A, et al. SV40 enhances the risk of malignant mesothelioma among people exposed to asbestos: a molecular epidemiologic case-controlled study. Cancer Res 2005; 65:3049–52.
52. Steenland K, Stayner L. Silica, asbestos, manmade mineral fibers, and cancer. Cancer Causes Control 1997;8:491–503.
53. Pohlabein H, Jockel KH, Bruske-Hohlfeld I, et al. Lung cancer and exposure to man-made vitreous fibers: results from a pooled case-control study in Germany. Am J Indl Med 2000;37:469–77.
54. Siemiatycki J, Richardson L, Gerin M, et al. Association between several sites of cancer and nine organic dusts: results from an hypothesis-generating case-control study in Montreal, 1979–1983. Am J Epidemiol 1986;123:235–49.
55. Beeson WL, Abbey DE, Knutsen SF. Long-term concentration of ambient air pollutants and incident lung cancer in California adults: results from the AHSMOG study. Environ Health Perspect 1998;106:813.
56. Dockery DW, et al. An association between air pollution and mortality in six US cities. N Engl J Med 1993;329:1753.
57. Pope CA III, et al. Particulate air pollution as a predictor of mortality in a prospective study of US adults. Am J Respir Crit Care Med 1995;151:669.
58. Pope CA III, Burnett RT, Thun MJ, et al. Lung cancer, cardiopulmonary mortality and long-term exposure to fine particulate air pollution. JAMA 2002;287:1132.
59. Pott F, Dungworth DL, Heinrich U, et al. Lung tumours in rats after intratracheal instillation of dusts. Ann Occup Hyg 1994;38:357.
60. Bright RA, Jeng LL, Moore RM Jr. National survey of self-reported breast implants: 1998 estimates. Long-Term Effects Med Implants 1993;3:81–9.
61. Cook RR, DeLongchamp RR, Woodbury MA, et al. The prevalence of women with breast implants in the United States 1989. J Clin Epidemiol 1995;48:519–26.
62. Food and Drug Administration. Analysis of Dow-Corning data regarding carcinogenicity of silicone gels. Washington, DC: US Government Printing Office.
63. Potter M, Morrison S, Weiner F, et al. Induction of plasmacytomas with silicon gel in genetically susceptible strains of mice. J Natl Cancer Inst 1994;86:1058.
64. Berkel H, Birdsell DC, Jenkins H. Breast augmentation: a risk factor for breast cancer? N Engl J Med 1992;326:1649–53.
65. Brinton LA, Malone KE, Coates RJ, et al. Breast enlargement and reduction: results from a breast cancer case-control study. Plas Reconstr Surg 1996;97:269–75.
66. Deapen DM, Bernstein L, Brody GS. Are breast implants anticarcinogenic? A 14-year follow-up of the Los Angeles study. Plas Reconstr Surg 1997;97:1346–53.
67. Glasser JW, Lee NC, Wingo PA. Does breast augmentation increase the risk of breast cancer? In: Proceedings of the EIS 38th Annual Conference. 1989 April 3–7; Atlanta, GA:CDC; 1989.
68. McLaughlin JF, Nyren O, Blot WJ, et al. Cancer risk among women with cosmetic breast implants. A population-based cohort study in Sweden. J Natl Cancer Inst 1998;90:156–8.
69. Malone KE, Stanford JL, Daling JR, Voight LF. Implants and breast cancer. Lancet 1992;339:1365.
70. Friis S, McLaughlin JK, Mellemkjaer L, et al. Breast implants and cancer risk in Denmark. Int J Cancer 1997;71:956–8.
71. Brinton LA, Lubin JH, Burich, MC, et al. Breast cancer following augmentation mammoplasty. Cancer Causes Control 2000;11:819–27.
72. Brinton LA, Lubin JH, Burich MC, et al. Cancer risks at sites other than the breast following augmentation mammoplasty. Ann Epidemiol 2001;11:248–56.
73. Portier CJ, Wolfe MS. Assessment of Health Effects from Exposure to Power-line Frequency Electric and Magnetic Fields. Working Group Report. National Institute of Environmental Health Sciences. 1998; Available at: www.niehs.nih.gov/emfrapid/home/htm (accessed).
74. Poole C, Ozonoff D. Magnetic fields and childhood cancers. An investigation of dose response analyses. IEEE Engineer Med Biol 1996;15,41–9.
75. NTP. Toxicology and carcinogenesis studies of 60 Hz magnetic fields in F344/N rats and B6C3F1 mice (whole body exposure). NIEHS, NTP, North Carolina; 1998.
76. Mandeville R, Franco E, Sidrac-Ghali S, et al. Evaluation of the potential carcinogenicity of 60 Hz linear sinusoidal continuous-wave magnetic fields in F344 rats. FASEB J 1997;11:1127–36.
77. Yasui M, Kikuchi T, Ogawa M et al. Carcinogenicity test of 50 Hz sinusoidal magnetic fields in rats. Bioelectromagnetics 1997;18:531–40.
78. Moulder JE, Erdreich LS, Malyapa RS, et al. Cell phones and cancer: What is the evidence for a connection. Radiation Res 1999;151:513–31.
79. Elwood JM. Epidemiological studies of radio frequency exposures and human cancer. Bioelectromagnetics 2004;25:235.
80. Hardell L, Mild FH, Carlberg M. Further aspects on cellular and cordless telephones and brain tumors. Int J Oncol 2003;22:399–407.
81. Hansson MK, Hardell L, Kundi M, Mattsson MO. Mobile telephones and cancer: is there really no evidence of an association [review]. Int J Mol Med 2003;12:67–72.

19

Tumor Viruses

Robert C. Gallo, MD
Marvin S. Reitz Jr, PhD

Retroviruses are enveloped viruses that contain a diploid ribonucleic acid (RNA) genome and are defined by the presence of reverse transcriptase (RT), a deoxyribonucleic acid (DNA) polymerase that transcribes RNA into DNA, which is then inserted into the host cell chromosome. These processes often lead to the capture and alteration of genetic material and the transfer of information between cells, with neoplastic transformation of the infected cell being an occasional outcome of infection. Retroviruses are also associated with immunodeficiencies and neurologic diseases, although infection is often asymptomatic. Retroviruses can also enter the germ line and be present as part of the genetic complement of all members of a species. These viruses are called endogenous retroviruses.

Retroviruses were discovered early in the twentieth century. Ellerman and Bang showed the transmission of leukemia in chickens by a cell-free filtrate,[1] and Rous was able to transmit sarcomas in chickens by a similar means.[2] These findings were extended to mammals by Bittner in the case of breast tumors in mice[3] and by Gross for murine leukemias.[4] Gross recognized the importance of inoculating newborn mice for the development of leukemia, and, in many respects, his work heralded the beginning of modern studies of retroviruses. Jarrett and colleagues showed that a similar virus was responsible for leukemia in cats, which was the first demonstration of naturally transmitted leukemia in an outbred species.[5] Theilen and colleagues, Wolfe and colleagues, and Kawakami and colleagues first showed that retroviruses could cause leukemia in primates, specifically in gibbon apes and new world monkeys.[6–8] Biologic assays for these viruses were in use from the 1950s, but a more fundamental understanding of their life cycle was considerably advanced in the early 1970s by the discovery that they contained RT.[9,10] This provided a far simpler and quicker assay for retroviruses, as well as a sensitive and relatively simple tool for their general detection. Another important finding in the 1970s was that some retroviruses (eg, Rous sarcoma virus [RSV]) contained genes for cell transformation and tumorigenesis (called oncogenes) that represented captured cellular genes (proto-oncogenes).[11] This realization led to the identification of dozens of similar genes and to an appreciation of their roles in cell growth and neoplastic transformation.

Despite this work and the interest it engendered, it was widely believed during the 1970s that retroviruses did not play a role in human disease and that they were likely not even present in the human population. Several discoveries made it clear that this was not the case. First, human T-cell leukemia virus type I (HTLV-I), the first infectious human retrovirus, was discovered by Gallo and colleagues and was shown to be a unique virus.[12–15] HTLV-I was soon established as the etiologic agent of adult T-cell leukemia (ATL), a type of leukemia endemic to various locales, including southern Japan and the Caribbean.[16–20] This was quickly followed by the discovery of HTLV-II,[21] a related virus that (although widespread) has not been compellingly associated with any disease.

Several years later, an epidemic of immunodeficiency and malignancies appeared within gay communities, especially in the United States. The first member of another group of human retroviruses was isolated from people with this disease,[22] and when it became possible to culture the virus on a large scale,[23] it was proven to be the etiologic agent of the new disease, called acquired immune deficiency syndrome (AIDS).[24,25] The virus, now called human immunodeficiency virus type 1 (HIV-1), has become established over much of the world, as has AIDS itself, and HIV-1 represents a current global medical and economic catastrophe. As with HTLV-I, a related virus, HIV-2, was discovered.[26] As with HTLV-II and -I, HIV-2 appears to be far less pathogenic than HIV-1.[27]

This chapter summarizes important aspects of the classification and replication cycle of retroviruses and considers some of the pathogenic mechanisms of retroviruses. We also consider endogenous retroviruses and the development of retroviral vectors for gene delivery and therapy.

CLASSIFICATION

The Retroviridae are a large family of viruses that are composed of a core structure surrounded by an envelope that contains a lipid bilayer. The core or capsid contains proteins specified by the *gag* and *pol* genes (Figure 19-1). The former are primarily structural and enclose the products of the latter, which are enzymatic and include RT and a viral protease that processes the Gag proteins. The capsid also encloses two copies of the single-stranded genomic RNA. The area between the capsid and the lipid envelope bilayer is occupied by another Gag protein called the matrix protein (MA). The lipid membrane contains the viral glycoproteins, including a transmembrane protein (TM) and a large surface protein (SU). The entire virion, or extracellular viral particle, is 100 nm in diameter.

Retroviruses have been classified using a variety of criteria.[28] They were originally categorized according to their biologic effects. The subfamilies included oncoviruses, which cause leukemias or other malignancies in their hosts; lentiviruses, or "slow" viruses, which cause slow degenerative diseases in their hosts; and spumaviruses, or foamy viruses, which produce a "foamy" cytopathic effect in infected cultures. The subfamilies have been divided further based on their genomic structures (Table 19-1). They have been historically classified on the basis of the morphology of budding and mature virions in electron micrographs (Table 19-2). As mentioned above, they can also be classified as exogenous or endogenous depending on whether they are transmitted by infection or within the germ line of a species.

STRUCTURE

The simplest retroviruses contain three major genes, *gag*, *pol*, and *env*, all of which are contained in the virion. The genomic RNA, which is generally about 8,000 to 9,000 nucleotides long, contains repeat regions at both ends, called the R region. The DNA form of the genome integrated in the host cell genome contains the R region and other regulatory sequences in structures called the long terminal repeat (LTR) (see Figure 19-1). Retroviruses often become replication defective by loss of large regions of their genomes, which are often replaced by oncogenes derived from the host cell. We now describe the genome and proteins of replication-competent retroviruses.

LONG TERMINAL REPEAT

The viral LTR provides important functions in the viral replication cycle. The LTR is required for integration of the genome into host cell DNA, and elements within the LTR regulate viral RNA expression. The LTR consists of three areas, the U3, R, and U5 regions (Figure 19-2). The U5 region is adjacent to the binding site of the primer for DNA synthesis, which is a cellular transfer ribonucleic acid (tRNA).[29,30] The U5 is the first region to be reverse transcribed as synthesis proceeds left to right. The R region is synthesized next, at which point, the RT must jump to the 3' R

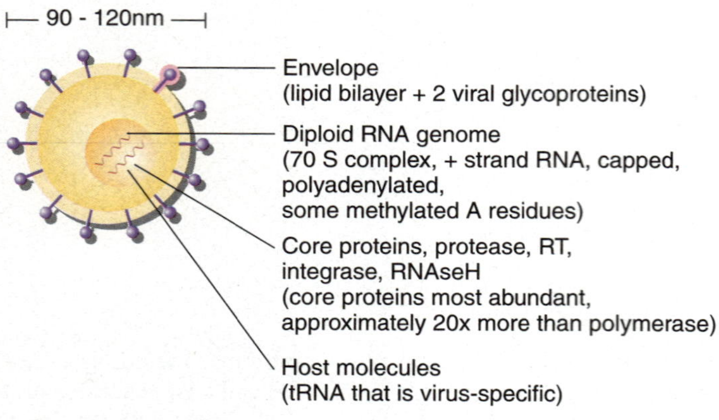

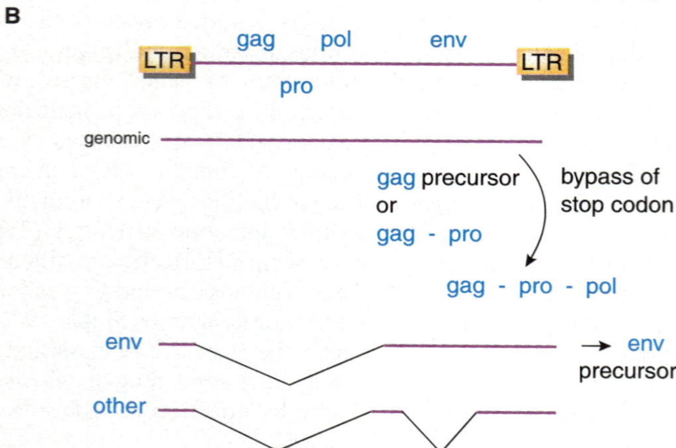

Figure 19-1 **A,** Structure of typical retrovirus virion. **B,** Structure of typical retroviral genome. All replication-competent retroviruses generate a full-length genomic ribonucleic acid (RNA) that encodes the gag and pol products and a singly spliced RNA that encodes the env product. Some retroviruses also generate smaller multiply spliced messages. env = envelope; gag = core proteins; pol = polymerase; pro = protease.

region, where the newly synthesized R complementary deoxyribonucleic acid (cDNA) hydrogen bonds (hybridizes). Synthesis proceeds through U3 right to left (see Figure 19-2). Reverse transcription results in synthesis of a double-stranded DNA with U3, R, and U5 regions at both ends. This DNA is integrated into host cell DNA. After integration, RNA transcription initiates in the 5' LTR and terminates in the 3' LTR.

The U3 region contains promoter regions for the cellular RNA polymerase II and includes canonical CCAT and TATAA boxes (see Figure 19-2).[31,32] These drive RNA transcription, which initiates at the CAP site[33] at the junction of U3 and R. Further to the 3' end, the U3 region contains sequences called enhancers that respond to host cell transcriptional regulatory factors and help regulate levels of viral RNA expression. Examples include NF-κB binding sites in the HIV LTR,[34,35] cyclic adenosine monophosphate–responsive element (CRE) binding sites in the HTLV-I U3,[36] and glucocorticoid receptor binding sites in the U3 of the Maloney mammary tumor virus (MMTV).[37] The types of enhancers that are contained in a viral LTR help determine in what kind of cell the virus can replicate. The R region also has a transcriptional termination-RNA polyadenylation signal (AATAAA) that functions in the 3' LTR. The promoter in the 3' LTR does not function in the presence of the 5' LTR but can become active if the upstream LTR is deleted.

Table 19-1 Retrovirus Groups

Oncornaviruses
Avian leukosis-sarcoma viruses (ALSV)
Avian reticuloendotheliosis virus
Mammalian leukemia and sarcoma viruses (mouse/cat type C viruses)
Mouse mammary tumor virus
Primate type D viruses (Mason-Pfizer monkey virus/simian AIDS virus)
Human T-cell leukemia virus/bovine leukemia virus/simian T-cell leukemia virus
Lentiviruses (including immunodeficiency viruses)
Spumaviruses

Leader Sequence The leader sequence is the RNA sequence located between the 3' end of the 5' LTR and the initiation codon of the *gag* gene. This stretch of RNA contains three important regions. One is the primer binding site, to which (as mentioned above) a cellular tRNA hydrogen bonds and serves as the primer for first-strand cDNA (minus-strand cDNA) synthesis. A second feature of the leader sequence is a splice donor, which is used for generating all spliced subgenomic messenger ribonucleic acids (mRNAs). These spliced mRNAs code for all viral proteins except those from *gag* and *pol*. The third feature of the leader sequence is a packaging signal by which Gag proteins recognize genomic RNA and incorporate it into functional virion cores.[38]

Table 19-2 Retrovirus Morphology

A-type particles
Intracellular core formation and budding
Intracisternal A-type particles (IAP) are products of endogenous proviruses
Noninfectious
B-type particles (MMTV)
Core formation occurs in the cytoplasm
After budding at the plasma membrane, maturation to an eccentric core occurs
Prominent surface spikes
C-type particles
Most oncornaviruses
Initially form electron-dense patches at the plasma membrane
Budding at plasma membrane
Maturation of core to yield centrally located cores
Spikes may or may not be prominent
D-type particles
Mason-Pfizer monkey virus, simian AIDS virus
Intracellular nucleocapsid formation, budding at plasma membrane
Eccentric core
Less prominent spikes
Lentiviruses
Visna-maedi, EIAV, CAEV, SIV, HIV, FIV, BIV
Core formation and budding as for C-type particles
Condensed mature core forms pyramidal shape
Spumaviruses
IAP-like cores

Gag The *gag* gene is always at the 5' end of the central unique (non-LTR) region of the retroviral genome. The Gag proteins are translated from a full-length (unspliced) mRNA as a polyprotein precursor that is processed into three to five mature Gag proteins by the viral protease (one of the proteins encoded by the *pol* gene). The protease (Pro) is translated along with the other *pol* products as extensions of the Gag polyprotein from the same unspliced mRNA by mechanisms that differ from one retroviral group to another.[39–42] The Pol precursor protein is also processed by the viral Pro.

There are three major Gag proteins. These include a nucleic acid binding protein (NC), a small basic protein that is located within the virion capsid and is bound to the genomic RNA. Its positive charge neutralizes the negative charge of the RNA and facilitates RNA packaging and dimerization. The NC also has a zinc finger motif, which is important in RNA binding.[43,44] The motif consists of an arrangement of cysteine and histidine residues present in a specific pattern that facilitates high-affinity binding to RNA and is required for RNA packaging into the virion. The

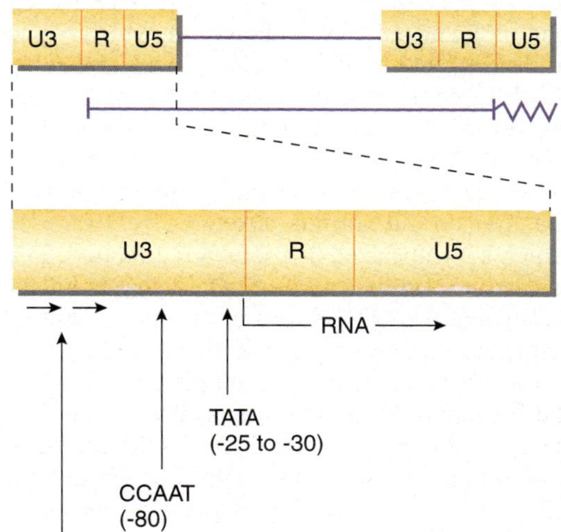

Figure 19-2 Long terminal repeat (LTR) structure. Replication-competent retroviruses contain identical LTRs at the 5' and 3' ends. The U3 portion of the 5' LTR contains all of the enhancer and promoter elements necessary for efficient initiation of transcription of either retroviral or cellular genes. CA = capsid; FeLV = feline leukemia virus; IN = integrase; MA = matrix protein; MMTV = Maloney mammary tumor virus; MuLV = murine leukemia virus; NC = nuclear capsid; PR = protease; RT = reverse transcriptase.

capsid protein (CA) is the major structural protein of the capsid; it forms the shell on the surface of the capsid. The MA is located between the capsid surface and the envelope bilayer. It interacts with the cytoplasmic tail of the TM envelope protein and CA on the capsid surface. Its interaction with the lipid bilayer requires that MA be myristoylated[45,46]; a lack of myristoylation prevents the functional capsid formation.[47]

Pol The *pol* gene is synthesized as an extension of the *gag* gene and encodes enzymatic activities, which include Pro and the viral enzymes required for reverse transcription and integration of viral DNA into the host chromosome. Because viruses require far greater amounts of structural proteins than enzymes, they have had to evolve mechanisms that make synthesis of the *pol* products relatively inefficient. The mechanisms that have been evolved vary among the viruses and are summarized in Figure 19-3. Murine leukemia virus (MuLV) has a stop codon that generally terminates Gag translation. At a low frequency, however, read-through occurs because of suppressor tRNA activity, resulting in a full-length Gag-Pol precursor.[48] Other viruses have semioverlapping reading frames for Pol or Pro and Pol, and synthesis of the extended translational products occurs because slippage at short A-rich regions and the downstream secondary structure of the RNA result in a shift in midtranslation to alternate reading frames.[49–51]

The function of Pro is to cleave the Gag and Gag-Pol polyprotein precursors into the proper mature proteins. As Pro becomes concentrated in nascent virions, it dimerizes and becomes more active. Three different enzymatic activities encoded by *pol* play a role in viral DNA synthesis. These include a DNA polymerase (*RT*), a ribonuclease H (RNaseH) (which removes the template RNA after strand cDNA synthesis), and an integrase (IN), which catalyzes the integration of viral DNA into host cell DNA. The RT and RNaseH are generally contained in a single mature peptide. The three-dimensional structures of the HIV-1 Pro and RT have been solved,[52] and these structures provide a basis for rational design of anti-HIV drugs. HIV IN has an additional function beyond catalysis of integration; it contains a nuclear localization signal, which facilitates transport of the preintegration complex of viral DNA and several viral proteins to the nucleus and helps in infection of nondividing cells.[53]

Envelope The *env* gene encodes a precursor polypeptide containing the signal peptide, which guides the insertion of Env proteins into the cell membrane, the TM, and the outer large SU proteins. The precursor polypeptide, like those for the Gag and Pol proteins, is proteolytically processed, but, in this case, cleavage involves cellular proteases. The Env proteins are translated from a spliced mRNA that uses the cellular splicing machinery, the splice donor upstream of *gag,* and a splice donor upstream from the initiation codon of *env*.[54,55] The TM and SU proteins are organized into a trimer structure on the virion surface that can be visualized by electron microscopy.

The TM protein is generally smaller than the SU protein and penetrates the viral envelope bilayer. The cytoplasmic domain is in contact with the viral MA protein, and the extracellular or ectodomains binds to the SU protein and retains it on the virion surface.[56] Besides its function of retaining and distributing SU, TM plays a role in the fusion of the viral envelope with the target cell membrane during infection.[56] The SU protein is generally heavily glycosylated and is the outermost viral protein.[57] Its major function is to bind to a specific cell-surface protein that serves as the receptor for the virus. Because it is the outermost viral protein, it is the main target of neutralizing antibodies made by the host.[58]

Fusion and entry into the target cell are generally similar to that of other enveloped viruses.[56] After SU binds to the receptor, the envelope proteins undergo conformational changes that result in the insertion of the amino terminus of TM into the target cell membrane and the formation of a six-helix coiled-coil structure in TM.[59,60] These changes promote fusion of the viral envelope with the target cell membrane, which allows viral entry.

Genomic Variation The genomic structure described above is representative of the genomes of the simplest retroviruses; other retroviruses, especially lentiviruses and members of the HTLV group, contain extra genes and have a more complex genomic structure. HIV-1 encodes six regulatory proteins that include a protein that activates viral RNA expression, another that regulates viral RNA splicing patterns, and proteins that interfere with host immune functions. The extra genes result in a more complicated RNA splicing pattern as well, including multiple splicing for many of the regulatory genes. Similarly, HTLV-I (and the related bovine leukemia virus [BLV]) encodes

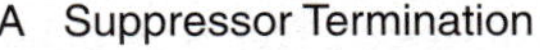

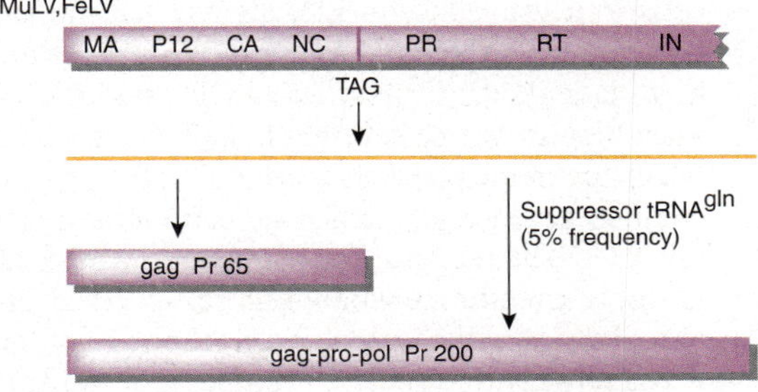

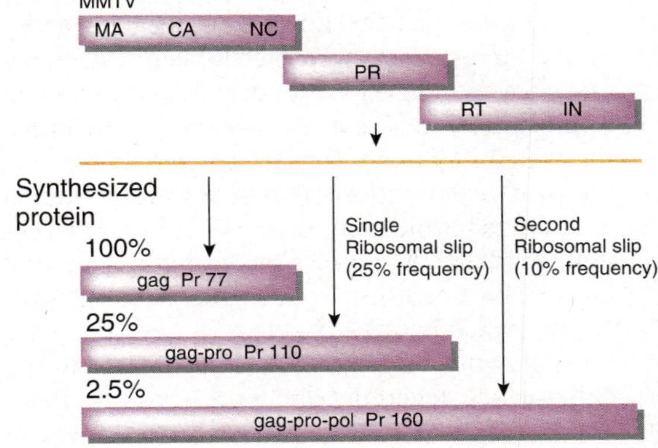

Figure 19-3 Alternative methods different retroviruses use to bypass the gag stop codon to generate the pro-pol products from the full-length genomic transcripts.

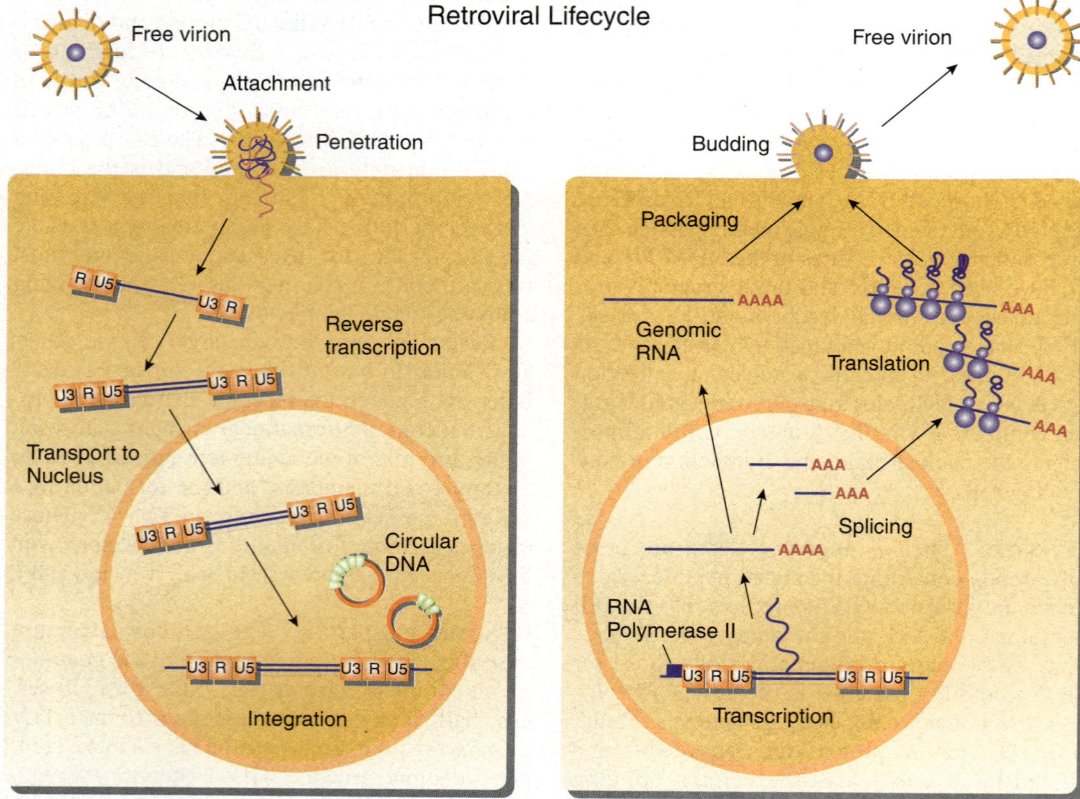

Figure 19-4 Life cycle of retrovirus. Following binding of the retrovirus to its specific cell membrane receptor, the viral and cellular membranes fuse, and the core virion is internalized into the cell. Reverse transcriptase–directed double-stranded retroviral genomic deoxyribonucleic acid (DNA) is then generated, followed by integrase-directed integration into host cell DNA. Retroviral transcripts using host transcriptional machinery then proceed, with the eventual formation of new retroviral virions that bud from the cell surface, allowing a new round of infection to occur.

extra proteins. HTLV-I encodes at least five additional proteins, including (like HIV) a protein that activates viral RNA expression and another that regulates viral RNA splicing patterns. MMTV and the spumaviruses also encode additional proteins, including those that activate viral RNA expression. Other retroviruses, especially those that are acutely transforming (such as the avian and mammalian sarcoma viruses), are generally replication defective and have parts of their genomes deleted and replaced with captured cellular genes that confer transforming capability. These viruses require a replication-competent helper virus for transmission and replication.

REPLICATION CYCLE

The replication cycle includes a number of stages, including entry and the establishment of infection in the target cell, the insertion of viral DNA into the host cell genome (called the provirus), and the synthesis, assembly, and release of virion particles. This process, called horizontal transmission, is summarized in Figure 19-4. In addition, cell replication of a retrovirally infected cell results in replication of the provirus. This is called vertical transmission, and it is the only means of replication for most endogenous viruses, which are present as germline infections.

The first step in infection is the engagement of a specific cell-surface protein by SU on the virion surface. A number of retroviral cell-surface receptors have been identified to date. The first receptor to be identified was the HIV receptor CD4, which is present on the surface of T helper cells.[61] It was subsequently shown that the HIV SU requires a second receptor for functional binding and entry.[62] Following CD4 binding, SU must bind to one of several chemokine receptors, which are in the protein superfamily of G protein–coupled seven-transmembrane serpentine receptors.[62–67] The receptor for one type of MuLV is a multiple membrane–spanning cell-surface protein that normally serves as a transporter protein for cationic amino acids.[68] Another type of MuLV and the gibbon ape leukemia virus (GaLV) use membrane proteins that normally transport inorganic phosphate as their receptors.[69,70] Some members of the avian leukosis virus (ALV) family use a low-density lipoprotein receptor and a tumor necrosis factor receptor for cell attachment and entry.[71,72] MMTV uses a cell-surface protein of unknown function as its receptor.[73] Obviously, the availability of cell-surface receptors limits the kinds of cells a retrovirus is able to enter and, in addition to the elements on the viral LTR that regulate viral RNA expression, provide a second level of host cell restriction. Thus, HIV-1 is generally limited to $CD4^+$ T cells.

Following binding of the SU protein to the cell-surface receptor, the viral envelope fuses with the cell membrane, a process mediated in part by the TM protein. This causes internalization of the naked core of the virion, which begins to disassemble in the cytoplasm. This makes the RT-RNA complex accessible to DNA precursors, and reverse transcription takes place (Figure 19-5). The tRNA hybridized to the primer binding site serves as the initiation point for the synthesis of the first strand (minus strand) of cDNA,[29,30] which is synthesized in a leftward direction. This results in a single strand of cDNA that is known as strong-stop DNA and contains U5 and R sequences.[74] The strong-stop cDNA and RT then jump to the other end of the template RNA, where the R minus-strand cDNA hybridizes to the 3' R region and serves as the primer for the continuation of minus-strand cDNA synthesis through the U3, *env*, *pol*, and *gag*. The RNaseH removes the template RNA except for a nuclease-resistant polypurine tract immediately upstream from the downstream LTR. The residual polypurine tract RNA residue serves as the primer for second-strand (plus-strand) U3-R-U5 DNA synthesis before it is degraded. RNaseH degrades the tRNA primer and the RT jumps again, this time to the other end of the complete minus-strand cDNA. The U3-R-U5 plus-strand cDNA then serves as the primer for the completion of the plus strand, resulting in a double-stranded RNA with complete LTRs at both ends.

After DNA synthesis is completed, it is inserted into the host cell genome by the activity of the viral IN protein, as shown in Figure 19-6. The IN catalyzes cleavage of both viral and host cell DNA. The cleavage of viral DNA eliminates several base pairs from each end of the viral DNA and creates staggered single-stranded ends. The cleavage of host cell DNA also creates staggered ends. These are repaired, resulting in the duplication of four to six base pairs of the host cell DNA at the insertion junctions. The viral DNA is inserted into the cleaved host DNA. The integrated viral DNA is called the provirus. Purified IN has been shown to perform all of these functions in vitro, indicating that no additional cellular proteins are required for integration.[75,76]

The integrated provirus serves as a template for the transcription of viral RNA. Cellular RNA polymerase II, which also transcribes cellular mRNA, is used along with other cellular factors for transcription of viral RNA. The full-length transcript can either serve as viral genomic RNA and become packaged into virions or be used for translation of the Gag and Pol proteins, although the factors that determine this are not clear. RNA splicing, which generates mRNA for all of the other viral proteins, and RNA export from the nucleus to the cytoplasm also rely for the most part on host cellular factors. However, some viruses that have a complex genome and mRNA splicing pattern, such as HTLV and HIV, encode proteins that regulate splicing and actively facilitate nuclear export.[77–79] The Gag and Pol proteins are translated on free ribosomes.[80] The protein at the amino terminus, MA, is myristoylated cotranslationally,[45,46] which directs the Gag and Gag-Pol precursor polypeptides to the inner face of the cell

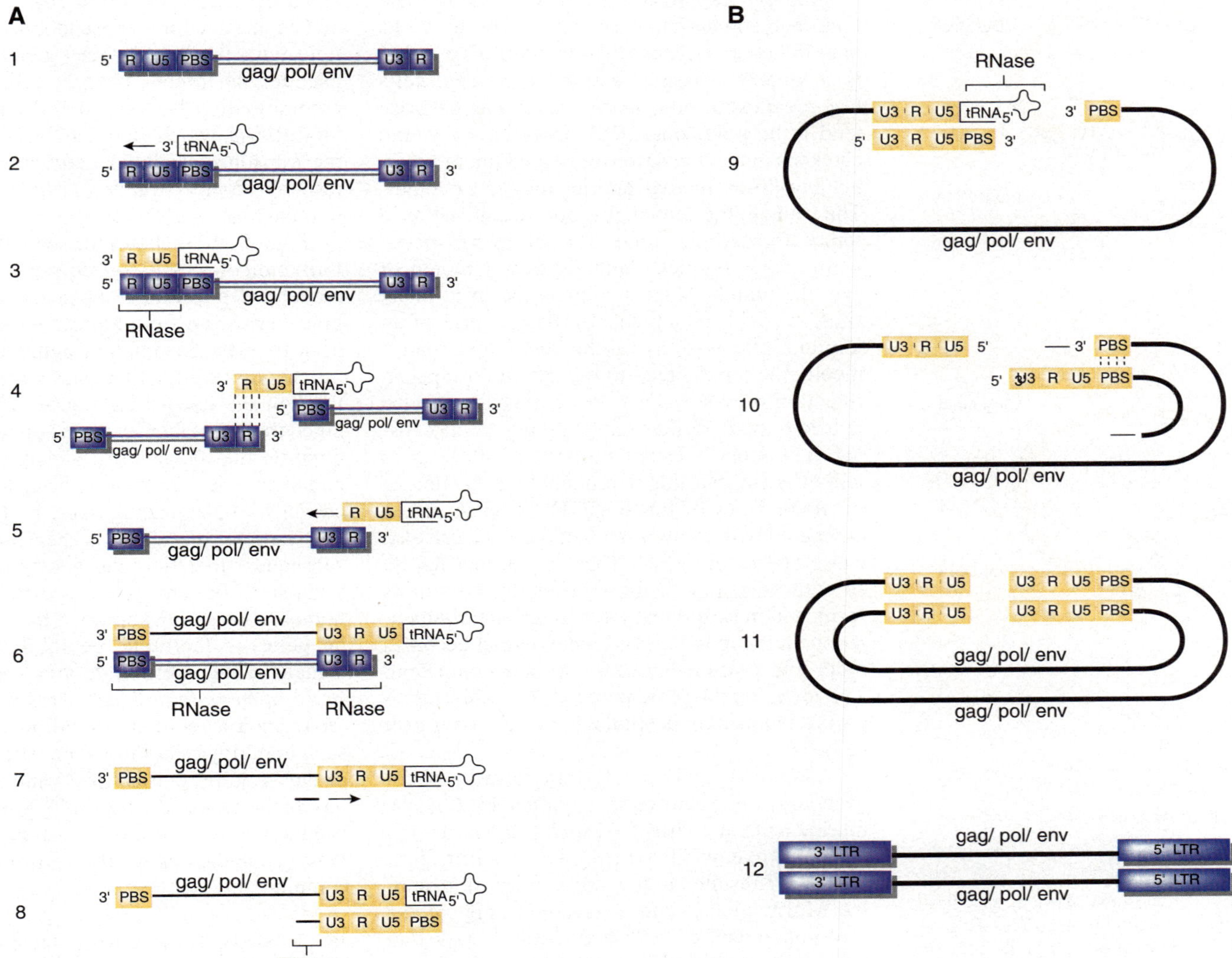

Figure 19-5 Reverse transcription. From a single-stranded ribonucleic acid genomic precursor, reverse transcriptase synthesizes a double-stranded deoxyribonucleic acid (DNA) provirus ready for integration into host cell DNA.

membrane. Here the precursor Gag protein interacts with the packaging signal on the viral RNA to initiate the formation of nascent cores. Cleavage of the Gag and Gag-Pol precursors by the viral protease takes place soon after the virion buds off from the cell surface.[81]

In contrast to Gag and Gag-Pol, Env proteins are synthesized on ribosomes associated with the endoplasmic reticulum.[80] They are glycosylated extensively here and within the Golgi apparatus and are transported to the cell surface, where the signal peptide is removed and cleavage to the mature TM and SU proteins occurs by the action of cellular proteases. The MA protein recognizes the cytoplasmic tail of the TM protein by mechanisms that are not clear and thereby facilitates the assembly of the core with the envelope to form a complete virion.

A few important points with regard to the retroviral replication cycle should be kept in mind. First, proviral formation, which is the product of the integration reaction, results in a stable genetic copy of the virus. This copy is stable; it cannot be removed from the infected cell, and infected cells can and do persist for the life of the host. Furthermore, whenever the cell divides, the provirus is passed on to both daughter cells. As a further consequence, when germline cells are infected, they become part of the genome of subsequent offspring. As a result, 5% or more of the human genome consists of proviruses from past retroviral infections. Integration, however, is not always accurate, and deletions and rearrangements can occur. Integrated proviruses can also occasionally become deleted or rearranged. Reflecting this, most endogenous proviruses are defective and not usually expressed, although expression of some does occur. It is likely, however, that this massive insertion of foreign DNA has had a profound impact on evolutionary processes.

A second important point is that after proviral formation, transcription and translation of viral gene products depend entirely on cellular factors. Thus, a retrovirus generally persists silently in quiescent cells. Activation of infected cells, such as occurs when cells of the immune system are stimulated by antigen or cells are activated by hormones, can activate viral expression, although this is modulated by the suite of transcriptional factor binding sites in the viral LTR. Also, complex retroviruses such as HTLV and HIV encode transcriptional activators that can profoundly affect the activity of the viral RNA polymerase promoter.[82–87]

MECHANISMS OF ONCOGENESIS

Some retroviruses are acutely transforming; they are capable of transforming cells directly. Retroviral induction of neoplasias in vivo in the infected host, however, involves a variety of mechanisms in addition to cell transformation by acutely transforming viruses. These mechanisms are summarized in Figure 19-7.

Oncogene Capture Acutely transforming viruses usually are generated when a cellular proto-oncogene is captured by insertion into the viral genome during viral replication. This process usually causes genetic changes in the proto-oncogene, resulting in an oncogene or a dominant transforming gene. The same process usually also results in a replication-defective virus that requires a helper virus for its replication. The helper virus provides viral proteins to form the

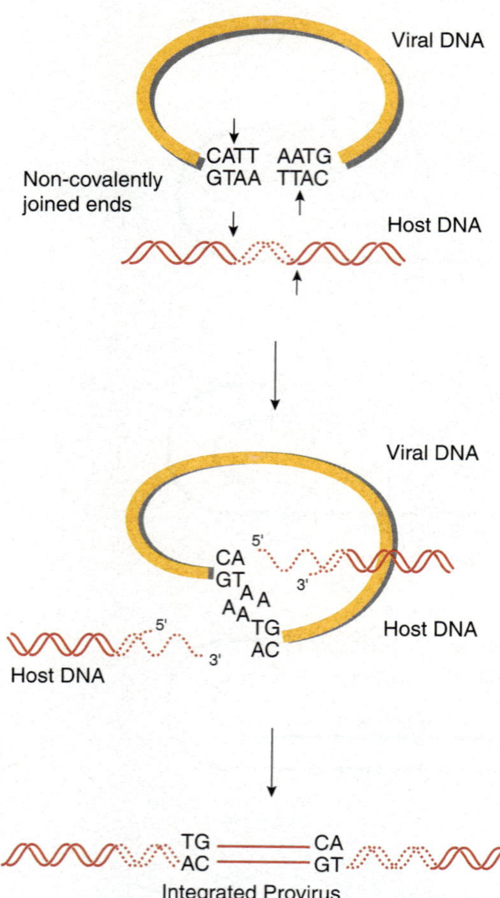

Figure 19-6 Integration. The newly reverse-transcribed double-stranded retroviral deoxyribonucleic acid (DNA) genome and a piece of chromosomal DNA are specifically cleaved by the retroviral integrase protein. This is accompanied by a deletion of two base pairs from the retroviral genome and a duplication of four to six base pairs from the host DNA. Following retroviral genomic insertion into the cleaved host DNA, the DNA is relegated.

virion in which the RNA of the defective virus is packaged. These mixed particles are called pseudotypes.

The first discovered oncogenic virus was RSV, which was shown to be a transmissible agent causing sarcomas in chickens.[2] This was one of the first identified retroviruses. RSV was the first acutely transforming virus of many that was shown to have acquired its oncogenicity by the capture of a cellular gene, in this case, one called *src*.[11] This was made possible in part because RSV, unlike most acutely transforming viruses, is replication competent and does not require a helper virus, thus making it simpler to study. The *src* gene in RSV is inserted as a separate gene immediately 3' of the other viral genes.[38,88] The transforming potential could be assigned to the viral *src* gene (v-*src*) because transformation-defective RSV has mutations specifically in v-*src* and because it confers transforming capability to recombinant viruses that contain it.[89–91] These findings led to the recognition that normal cellular genes, when modified and in the appropriate setting, could cause malignant transformation.

Acutely transforming retroviruses produce tumors in susceptible hosts within days to weeks after infection. Because their transforming ability is so potent, a large fraction of infected cells become transformed; hence, the tumors that arise tend to be polyclonal. RSV infection of young chickens induces a variety of related tumor types, notably fibrosarcomas and histiocytic sarcomas. The younger the animal, the more sensitive it is to tumor formation. Tumor formation can occur within days in chicks younger than 1 month of age; the tumors progress rapidly, occur at many sites, and kill the animal. In the presence of an immune response, as in chickens older than 1 month, the tumors tend to regress and disappear. Injection of v-*src* DNA into chickens can also induce tumors, further implicating v-*src* as causing the tumors.[92] Tumor formation with DNA is less efficient, but this is probably a reflection of the inefficiency of functional DNA uptake when compared with retroviral infection. RSV can also cause tumors in neonate rodents but does not do so with efficiency. Only occasionally do tumors form, and these are restricted to the site of inoculation and tend to regress as the animal becomes older and presumably more immunocompetent. The lower tumorigenic potential probably represents a reduced replication rate of RSV on rodent cells.[93,94]

A more typical acutely transforming oncogene-containing retrovirus is typified by Abelson murine leukemia virus (A-MuLV). Infection of a nude mouse with a replication-competent MuLV[95,96] resulted in the replacement of most of the MuLV genes with a modified copy of the proto-oncogene c-*abl*,[97] a tyrosine kinase that recently became well known because it is the target of the anticancer drug imatinib mesylate (Gleevec). Like most viral oncogenes and their cellular counterparts (summarized in Table 19-3), the *abl* portion of v-*abl* differs genetically from that of c-*abl*. The resultant recombinant virus, A-MuLV, is unable to synthesize any of the viral genes and codes only for a fusion protein containing part of Gag and Abl (v-Abl). The presence of the amino terminal portion of Gag on v-Abl causes it to be myristoylated and transported to the cell membrane, and this is critical for transformation by A-MuLV. The result of the lack of functional viral genes is that A-MuLV is replication defective. It is able to infect and transform target cells only with the assistance of a helper virus. A-MuLV induces B-cell lymphomas in neonate mice, but adult animals are generally resistant to A-MuLV lymphomagenesis.[98]

Several models have been put forth for how cellular sequences are acquired by retroviral genomes; Figure 19-7A summarizes these models. In one scenario, a retrovirus integrates into the host cell genome just upstream from a proto-oncogene.[99] A subsequent deletion removes the 3' portion of the provirus and the 5' portion of the proto-oncogene, fusing the viral genome with cellular sequences and resulting in a reading frame for a fusion protein, generally including part of the *gag* gene. This gene is transcribed under the regulation of the viral LTR, processed, and copackaged into a pseudotype retroviral particle with the helper virus genome. When the pseudotype infects a target cell, RT mediates recombination between the 3' ends of the two viral RNAs, which places a 3' LTR on the end of the transduced cellular gene, which allows the resultant double-stranded DNA to be integrated into the host cell DNA.

Figure 19-7B shows the second model for the formation of acutely transforming viruses. In this model, a replication-competent virus again integrates upstream from a proto-oncogene. On rare occasions, the termination signal in the 3' LTR is not recognized and transcription proceeds through the downstream gene. The large combined transcript then undergoes splicing or recombination that deletes the 3' portion of the viral region and the 5' portion of the cellular region and creates the open reading frame for the viral-proto-oncogene fusion, which is then pseudotyped for subsequent infection and generation of an integratable DNA. This requires that there either be homologous regions between the viral and cellular genes to facilitate recombination or splice signals in the appropriate area for forming the fused open reading frame. This may not be too far-fetched a requirement because examples of such homologies are found between the *pol* gene of the avian retrovirus MC29 and the chicken c-*myc* in the area of the fusion.[100] Such a homology is not obvious in most retroviruses, however, suggesting that the first scenario is probably the more common.

Insertional Activation Most of the retroviruses that cause neoplasms in their hosts are not acutely transforming viruses; they contain the minimum complement of *gag*, *pol*, and *env* genes and are replication competent. Because many of these viruses induce leukemias and are genetically somewhat related, they are collectively referred to as leukemia viruses. Representatives include avian, murine, feline, and gibbon ape leukemia viruses. The kinds of leukemias induced vary with the viral strain; thus, some strains of GaLV are associated with lymphocytic leukemia,[8,101] whereas another strain is associated with myeloid leukemia.[102] Their lack of acutely transforming oncogenes means that they are not competent for direct transformation and do not transform target cells in vitro. The leukemias and other tumors that result from infection of the host are clonal in origin, as is evident from the insertion site of the provirus being identical in all of the neoplastic cells from a given tumor. This reflects the rarity of infection leading to malignant transformation and indicates that infection with the retrovirus preceded (and, by implication, resulted in) transformation. It also suggests that the specific insertion site is important and leads to the concept of insertional mutagenesis. In these kinds of viral neoplasias, the provirus is often found integrated in the vicinity of known cellular proto-oncogenes. The proximity of the viral LTR (or the insertion of the provirus into regulatory regions

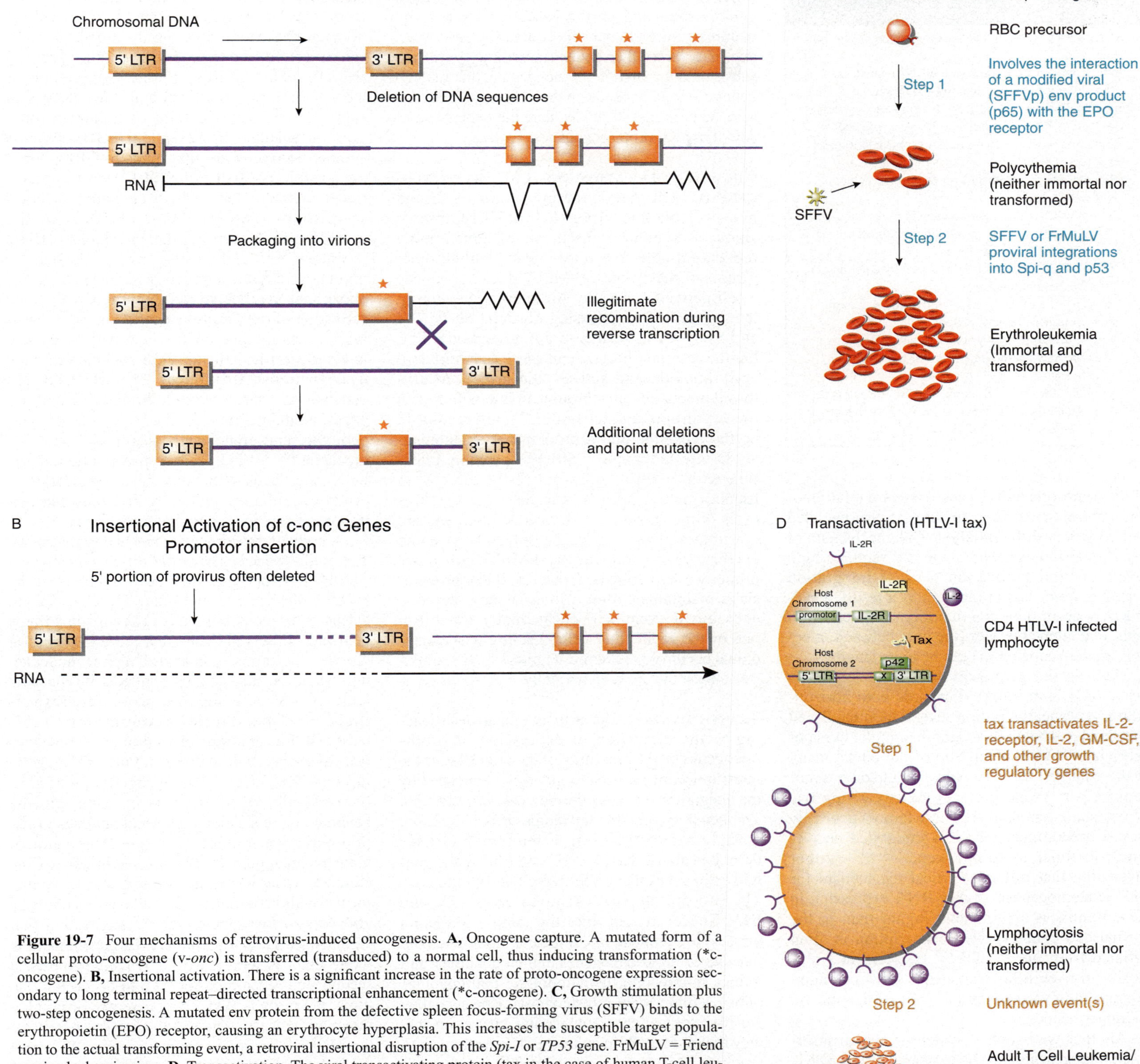

Figure 19-7 Four mechanisms of retrovirus-induced oncogenesis. **A,** Oncogene capture. A mutated form of a cellular proto-oncogene (v-*onc*) is transferred (transduced) to a normal cell, thus inducing transformation (*c-oncogene). **B,** Insertional activation. There is a significant increase in the rate of proto-oncogene expression secondary to long terminal repeat–directed transcriptional enhancement (*c-oncogene). **C,** Growth stimulation plus two-step oncogenesis. A mutated env protein from the defective spleen focus-forming virus (SFFV) binds to the erythropoietin (EPO) receptor, causing an erythrocyte hyperplasia. This increases the susceptible target population to the actual transforming event, a retroviral insertional disruption of the *Spi-I* or *TP53* gene. FrMuLV = Friend murine leukemia virus. **D,** Transactivation. The viral transactivating protein (tax in the case of human T-cell leukemia virus type I) causes expansion of the potential target population through transactivation of growth regulatory genes. Some unknown second event then induces the actual transformation of a clone of these cells.

Table 19-3 Differences Between v-onc and c-onc Genes

Often only a portion of the cellular oncogene is present in v-onc.
v-onc is derived from processed mRNA, which is devoid of introns and flanking sequences.
Loss of cellular control elements (promoters/repressors as well as RNA destabilizers) for some oncogenes (*myc* and *mos*) elevated level of expression in itself may be transforming.
Deletions/rearrangements may affect the structure of the protein itself:
- Loss of C-terminal Tyr-containing region of c-*src* causes loss of phosphorylation-mediated control by host cell kinases.
- v-*erb* B differs from EGF receptor by deletion of the extracellular domain.

v-onc genes are often fused to viral sequences important for transforming function:
- gag-*abl* acquires a myristoylation signal → membrane localization important for transforming activity.
- v-*fms* is the CSF-1 receptor fused to the gag gene product, the latter providing a signal sequence for placement into the cell membrane.

of the proto-oncogene) causes a dysregulation of its expression, leading, in turn, to dysregulated cell growth or differentiation. This mechanism of insertional mutagenesis obviously requires high levels of viral replication because integration occurs more or less at random; as a result, leukemia may occur only in a minority of infected animals, and latency phases (the time between infection and leukemia onset) can be quite lengthy.

ALV is the prototypical simple leukemia virus. ALV is transmitted in birds both horizontally and vertically. Within several months, B-cell lymphoblasts begin to accumulate in the bursa of Fabricius.[103] With involution of the bursa, many of the enlarged follicles regress, but some tumor nodules persist and grow, eventually giving rise to metastatic lymphomas. These tumors generally have a predominant provirus integrated near c-*myc*, a cellular proto-oncogene.[104–106] Further suggesting that this is a critical mechanism for ALV leukemogenesis, c-*myc* RNA expression in these tumors is significantly higher than in the normal cell counterparts. Transcription is often initiated from the 3' LTR,[107] resulting in a chimeric viral-cellular transcript, but continued expression of viral genes and viral replication are no longer needed.

Another well-studied system in which insertional mutagenesis appears to play a critical role is MMTV and murine mammary tumors. As with ALV, MMTV can be transmitted either horizontally or vertically. As with ALV, there is generally a predominant provirus in the mammary tumor cells, with implications similar to those in the case of ALV. Integration was found to occur around but not within a 30 kilobase pair sequence containing the *int-1* proto-oncogene.[108–110] *Int-1* expression generally occurs only in the neural tube of midgestational embryos and in testicular postmeiotic cells, suggesting that inappropriate expression in cells in the breast contributes to tumorigenesis by MMTV. Transgenic mice in which an *int-1* transgene is regulated by the MMTV LTR develop mammary tumors, but this is also the case when any of several other genes (including c-*myc)* are substituted for *int-1*,[111–114] suggesting that tumorigenesis simply depends on the delivery of a breast-specific promoter to dysregulate the expression of any of several proto-oncogenes.

Growth Stimulation and Two-Step Oncogenesis The polycythemic strain of Friend murine leukemia virus (F-MuLV) represents another variation on the theme of transforming replication-defective retroviruses. Unlike other viruses of these types, F-MuLV does not encode a cell-derived oncogene. An internal deletion of the *env* gene encompassing portions of the TM and SU proteins results in a nonfunctional Env, but the resultant protein can serve as a mimic of erythropoietin and activate the growth of erythroid precursor cells through an interaction with the erythropoietin receptor.[115] This results in erythroleukemia and a pronounced splenomegaly in infected mice.[116] Strictly speaking, infection with F-MuLV does not result directly in transformation because the resultant erythrocytes do not form tumors in nude mice and are not immortalized. Thus, the splenomegaly and erythrocytosis induced by FMuLV are more properly a hyperplasia. However, if erythrocytosis is maintained, after a long latency period, a subsequent event will occasionally transform one of the replicating cells, leading to a monoclonal erythroid leukemia. Figure 19-7C summarizes these events schematically.

Transactivation Insertional mutagenesis leading to the activation of expression of proto-oncogenes by the proximity of the viral LTR or the interruption of negative regulatory sequences by the integration event is referred to as *cis*-activation. The genomes of some leukemia viruses are more complex than the simple leukemia viruses described above, such as ALV and MuLV, and contain extra genes that perform regulatory functions. The two prototypical examples are HTLV and BLV. These viruses (like the simple leukemia viruses) are replication competent, do not contain transduced proto-oncogenes in their genomes, and induce monoclonal hematopoietic malignancies only in a minority of infected hosts. However, they are like the acutely transforming viruses in that they transform cells in culture and do not appear to require a specific integration site for oncogenesis (see Figure 19-7D). HTLV is the causative agent for ATL, a monoclonal T-cell lymphoma or leukemia with frequent cutaneous manifestations that is endemic to several areas, including southern Japan and the Caribbean,[16–20] and is also the cause of a neurologic disease resembling multiple sclerosis, called tropical spastic paraparesis or HTLV-associated myelopathy.[117]

HTLV and BLV code for proteins, respectively called Tax[82–84] and p34 Tax,[118] that activate expression by binding to the viral LTR in cooperation with transcription factors. This type of activation by a protein product rather than a DNA regulatory region is called *trans*-activation, and these viral proteins are called transactivators. HTLV-I codes for several other proteins as well, including Rex, a protein that regulates the complex pattern of splicing the mRNAs of HTLV-I.[77,78] Three proteins of unknown function are encoded by HTLVI: p30(II), which is another transactivator that binds to CREB binding protein/p300 (CBP/p300),[119] a transcriptional factor; p12(I), which activates the transcriptional factor NFAT and binds to the cytoplasmic domain of the interleukin (IL)-2 receptor[120,121]; and p13(II), which localizes to mitochondria and interacts with farnesyl pyrophosphate synthetase, an enzyme involved in activation of the proto-oncogene *ras*.[122,123] Most interest has focused on Tax, however, because it is clearly critical to the viral replication cycle through transactivation of the viral LTR and because its transactivation extends to cellular genes, including those for the IL-2 receptor, lymphotoxin, and granulocyte-macrophage stimulating factor.[124–127] The cross-transactivation of cellular genes leads to the idea that dysregulation of growth regulatory genes by Tax may play an important role in its pathogenesis.

A body of experimental evidence suggests that Tax could indeed play a role in leukemogenesis. The HTLV-I provirus in T cells transformed by HTLV-I infection or in leukemic ATL cells often has extensive deletions, but the Tax open reading frame is always preserved. Mice that are transgenic for Tax develop fibrosarcomas or lymphocytic leukemia when the transgene is regulated by the viral LTR or a T cell–specific promoter, respectively.[128,129] Tax directly transforms a rat fibroblast cell line and transforms primary rat embryo cells in cooperation with *ras* in vitro,[130,131] showing that Tax, indeed, has oncogenic properties. Interestingly, when Tax was inserted into the genome of a replication-competent but transformation-defective mutant of herpesvirus saimiri, human hematopoietic cells infected in vitro by the chimeric virus were transformed, and the transformed cells resembled ATL cells in morphology and cell-surface phenotype,[132] suggesting that Tax is indeed important in ATL pathogenesis. It is likely that, as with F-MuLV leukemogenesis, a second step is required for ATL to occur. For one thing, the rarity of ATL as an outcome of HTLV-I infection indicates that a simple infection without the second step is insufficient to cause ATL, and the lack of a common set of integration sites supports the idea that insertional mutagenesis does not play a role. Most tellingly, the leukemic cells do not express viral RNA until after they are put into culture,[133] indicating that, by the time the cells are leukemic, they no longer require viral expression and suggesting that there must be subsequent steps in ATL leukemogenesis.

Recently, a better understanding has begun to emerge about the signaling pathways used by Tax for transactivation and transformation. Tax associates with members of the ATF/CREB family of transcriptional factors,[134–138] and the HTLV-I LTR has three ATF/CREB binding sites. Several cellular genes, such as serum-responsive factor and nuclear factor (NF)-κB/Rel, are transactivated by Tax through the same pathway. Tax also transactivates its LTR, as well as some cellular gene promoters, such as those for IL-2 and the IL-2 receptor, directly through NF-κB.[139–141] This depends on an interaction of Tax and MEKK1, which leads to phosphorylation of the NFκ-B inhibitor Iκ-B. Phosphorylation of Iκ-B targets its removal by ubiquitination and degradation in the proteasome, which unmasks the nuclear localization signal of NFκ-B. This allows it to be transported to the nucleus, where it activates gene expression by binding to NF-kB enhancer elements, which are present in the viral LTR. In addition to contributions to cell transformation from the activation of signaling pathways, Tax also appears to directly affect the cell cycle. Tax can bind to the cell-cycle inhibitor p16/INK4a and interfere with its ability to inhibit the activity of CDK4, a cyclin kinase important for G1–S progression.[142,143] Tax also mediates the phosphorylation of cyclin D3[144] and up-regulates the expression of E2F[145] through ATF/CREB signaling; both of these likely contribute to dysregulation of the cell cycle. Dysregulation of the cell cycle often leads to tp53-mediated apoptosis.[146] It appears that Tax also dysregulates activities of tp53 required for cell-cycle arrest and apoptosis,[147–149] which allows unregulated hyperproliferation and immortalization of cells expressing Tax. Tax appears to inhibit tp53 functions in part by an NF-κB–dependent mechanism and in part by competing with tp53 for binding to CBP/p300. Tax also inhibits MAD1, a protein involved in the G_2/M transition stage of the cell cycle.[150] It is interesting that Tax interferes with the p16/INK4a and tp53 pathways because alteration of these genes or their activities is quite common in naturally occurring cancers.

Retroviruses have also long been associated with immunodeficiency in infected animals, as in the case of FeLV.[151] The best known example of an immunopathogenic virus is, of course, HIV-1, which is the cause of AIDS. Infection with HIV-1 also leads to an increased incidence of several kinds of tumors, most of which are linked to viruses coinfecting HIV-infected individuals. The clearest example is that of human herpesvirus 8 (HHV-8) (also known as Kaposi's sarcoma herpesvirus).[152] HHV-8 is clearly the cause of Kaposi's sarcoma and a B-cell lymphoma called peripheral effusion lymphoma.[153] In the absence of HIV-1 or other immunosuppressive conditions, HHV-8 appears to cause these diseases only rarely. HIV-1 infection raises the risk of these diseases by many orders of magnitude.[154] A greatly elevated incidence of non-Hodgkin's lymphoma (NHL) is also seen in a setting of HIV infection,[154] and at least a substantial portion of these AIDS-NHL cases are associated with Epstein-Barr virus (EBV) infection. Infection with HIV-1 also appears to increase the risk of childhood leiomyosarcomas (associated with EBV), as well as the risks of cervical cancer and hepatocarcinoma. The two latter cancers are associated with human papillomavirus and hepatitis B and C virus infections, respectively. Infection with these viruses tends to be higher in HIV-infected people, but there also appears to be a higher risk of cancer in people who are coinfected with HIV and one of these viruses.

It is also possible that HIV may play a more direct role in tumorigenesis. Mice that are transgenic for Tat, the HIV transactivator protein that is functionally homologous to HTLV-I Tax, develop Kaposi's sarcoma–like lesions.[155] A subset of AIDS-NHL is not associated with EBV, and the reasons for its increased incidence are not clear. Conversely, HTLV-I infection can lead to a loss of function of immune cells in vitro, and immunodeficiency occurs in HTLV-I–infected people, although this may be an epiphenomenon of the associated leukemogenesis.

ENDOGENOUS RETROVIRUSES

Endogenous retroviruses, which are part of the normal genetic complement of species, make up an extremely large fraction (up to 5%) of various mammalian genomes. Many of these appear to have emerged after speciation, based on differences in their type and number among species. Because retroviruses insert at random, and because so many of them are present, it is clear that they have played a profound if unclear role in evolution. It is less clear whether any of them play a role in human cancer or other diseases. First, they are, for the most part, defective because of large deletions, although some have only a few point mutations and a few may be replication competent. A second property of this type of retrovirus is that they are generally not expressed even at the RNA level. This may be because of mutations in the regulatory regions of their LTRs, because of their location in transcriptionally inactive areas of the chromatin, or because of methylation of promoter sequences in the LTR. When endogenous viruses are expressed as RNA, protein, or virions, it is usually in normal placentas or in teratomas, which may reflect the presence of hormone-responsive elements in the LTRs of many endogenous retroviruses. It is possible that integration of endogenous retroviruses may result in recessive mutations. The Hr (hairless) and D (dilute brown) recessive phenotypes in mice are associated with the presence of endogenous retroviruses at the affected loci,[156–158] and reversion of the mutation is associated with proviral deletion, raising the possibility that there may be analogous situations in humans. Indeed, insertion of a GaLV-related provirus upstream from a duplicated pancreatic amylase gene appears to have allowed its expression in saliva[159–161] and may have led to the prevalence of starch-rich foods in the human diet.

One specific endogenous retroviral RNA is highly expressed in the placenta. Its protein product, syncytin, may be important in human placental morphogenesis, and dysregulation of its expression is associated with preeclampsia.[162,163] In general, however, expression or the lack of expression of endogenous retroviral genes has not been associated with human diseases, although the AKR strain of mice develops leukemia by a complex process that involves expression and recombination of endogenous MuLVs.[164–166]

The integration pattern and the content of endogenous retroviruses can differ among members of the same species, suggesting that they are not entirely stable and that many of them are not currently essential to their hosts. Their existence as fixed genetic elements, however, suggests that they were important at one time. Retroviruses that use the same receptor exhibit interference with each other. This is because infection either blocks or down-regulates the cell-surface expression of the receptor, rendering the cell refractory to superinfection. It may be that endogenous retroviruses provided protection by interference against pathogenic retroviruses that no longer exist and are therefore no longer important.

RETROVIRAL VECTORS AND GENE THERAPY

As the understanding of the roles of specific genes in different diseases has evolved, treatment of diseases by gene therapy, or the delivery of desired genes, has become more of a possibility. A primary obstacle is efficient and specific delivery of a gene to the appropriate tissue and cell type. Delivery by transfection of DNA, or introduction into cells in which the membrane has been partially permeabilized by chemicals or an electrical charge, is relatively inefficient, not very specific, and unsuitable for delivery in vivo. Delivery by a gene gun, which shoots DNA on the surface of gold microparticles into skin and muscle, or by direct injection of DNA has resulted in expression of proteins in vivo, but neither is very specific and may be best suited for the delivery of DNA vaccines.

An alternative is to use a recombinant virus to deliver the gene of interest into the appropriate tissue. This method of gene delivery is called transduction. Viruses can be highly tissue specific, and, in principle, transduction appears to represent the best approach to gene delivery. Different viruses have been used for gene delivery, including adenovirus, which has the disadvantages of a lack of persistence and the likelihood of immune responses against viral proteins on repeated administration. Retroviral vectors are perhaps the best studied and most promising transducing vectors.[167–170] They integrate, so they theoretically need to be administered only once. In addition, as seen with the acutely transforming replication-defective retroviruses, the viral genome does not need to be able to code for any viral proteins for the viral genome to be integrated. Their tissue and cell tropisms can be altered by pseudotyping them with different envelope proteins.[171] The only requirements for transduction of the gene of interest are that the vector RNA contains the proper packaging signal and has LTRs at both its ends. The proteins required to form virions are provided by cell lines that express all of the viral proteins from genes that cannot themselves be packaged. When the vector RNA containing the gene of interest is transfected into a packaging cell line, only the vector RNA is packaged into the virion. Because the pseudotyped RNA does not code for viral proteins, the virions are capable only of a single round of infection and integration. This allows the stable expression of the gene of interest in the absence of any of the retroviral proteins, which would be likely to elicit an immune response that would eliminate the genetically altered cells. The majority of retroviral vectors to date are based on the Moloney strain of murine leukemia virus (Mo-MuLV).[167–170] Mo-MuLV vectors efficiently infect a wide variety of cell types, including those of human origin. More recently, retroviral vectors based on lentiviruses have shown promise. They have the advantage of being able to transduce nondividing cells by the same mechanisms that allow lentiviruses to infect resting cells.[172,173]

There are several potential problems with retroviral vectors. One is the possible generation of replication-competent helper viruses during the packaging of the vector, which can occur by homologous recombination. Two approaches have been used to minimize this possibility. One is to place the viral structural genes on different genetic units, so that multiple recombination events must occur before a replication-competent helper virus is generated. A second approach, not mutually exclusive with the first, is to minimize areas of homology among the units expressing the helper virus proteins and the vector by, for example, using heterologous promoters for the helper virus proteins. Another potential problem derives from one of the advantages of retroviral vectors, namely, integration. As mentioned above, insertion in the vicinity of a proto-oncogene could lead to tumorigenesis. Although the risk appears small, it is not zero. This was the apparent reason for three of seven monkeys developing lymphomas in one gene therapy study.[174] This also appears to have been the case in recent gene therapy trials to treat severe combined immunodeficiency. Although the treatment appeared to be effective, two of the patients developed clonal proliferation of T cells in which the retroviral vector was integrated close to the proto-oncogene *LMO2*.[175] Mo-MuLV does not replicate well in human cells, but this is not the case for other potential retroviral vectors. Minimizing integration events by, for example, rigorously excluding the presence of replication-competent helper viruses helps avoid this problem but does not completely eliminate it. Another problem is that expression is not maintained indefinitely; retroviral promoters have a tendency to become inactivated over time. A further limitation is that the genetic capacity of retroviruses is only about 8 to 9 kilobases, which restricts their capability to deliver genes to a single gene or two.

ANTIRETROVIRAL HOST DEFENSES

It has become increasingly evident that host cells have antiretroviral defenses that are distinct from adaptive immunity. One cellular factor called TRIM5 interferes in a species-specific way with a preintegration step in infection by HIV-1 and simian immunodeficiency virus.[176–178] The activity is specific for the viral capsid protein.[177,178] A functionally similar activity in murine cells is called Fv1. APOBEC 3G, a cellular RNA-editing enzyme that deaminates cytosine, also restricts infection with HIV-1 but is blocked by an HIV-1 protein, Vif.[179–181] It was recently shown that APOBEC exists in high- and low-molecular-weight forms.[182] The low-molecular-weight form, which is the active form, predominates in resting T cells, making them less easily infectable by HIV-1.[182] RNA silencing represents a more general antiviral activity; the HIV-1 Tat protein has recently been shown to suppress silencing.[183] It is clear from these examples that the battle between retroviruses and their hosts is an ancient one and involves numerous measures and countermeasures.

CONCLUSIONS

The study of retroviruses has led to much of today's techniques and understanding of molecular biology. This is obviously especially true in the case of cell transformation and tumorigenesis because many retroviruses either cause cancers or, in the case of acutely transforming viruses, capture cellular genes that have the potential to contribute to neoplastic transformation. Retroviruses were the first example of a reversal of the normal order of the flow of genetic information, that is, from RNA to DNA. The identification and elucidation of reverse transcription provided the means for cloning and characterizing mRNA, which greatly facilitated understanding gene expression and function. Studies of the regulation of viral transcription, including transactivation of transcription by viral proteins such as Tat and Tax, have increased knowledge about transcriptional regulation. Much has been learned about RNA splicing from studies of retroviral RNA processing, especially studies of mechanisms of viral proteins that specifically regulate this process (Rex and Rev). Studies of ribosomal slippage and termination suppression, mechanisms used by retroviruses to translate reading frames in transcripts downstream from the first reading frame, have helped elucidate aspects of regulation of translation. We have gained valuable insight on the biochemistry of membranes and membrane fusion from work done on viral entry, and gaining knowledge of the forces involved in viral protein processing and virion assembly has contributed to a better understanding of protein processing and protein–protein interactions. An understanding of how retroviruses package and deliver genetic material holds promise that these viruses will be successfully used to deliver therapeutic genes to appropriate cells and tissues in human diseases. Successful delivery has been achieved in vitro and to some extent in animals in the laboratory, but clinical success in humans is more elusive. However, new generations of vectors currently being studied and developed are bringing us closer to realizing this goal, and it is likely only a matter of time before retroviral viral vectors are used successfully in a clinical setting.

Perhaps one of the most important contributions of retroviral research to human health came in the form of discovery of HTLV-I and HIV-1, two pathogenic human retroviruses. During the 1970s, much of the research carried out with retroviruses came under the aegis of the Virus Cancer Program (VCP) as part of President Nixon's "War on Cancer." The VCP was ended because of a lack of discovery of human cancer viruses and the growing belief that human retroviruses did not exist. Shortly thereafter, however, HTLV-I was discovered and linked to ATL. Although this discovery has not led to better treatment for ATL, it has led to better prevention of infection by, for example, screening blood samples and avoiding transmission by breast-feeding, a common route of infection of babies. Ironically, the most important consequence of the VCP and retroviral research was the relatively rapid discovery and characterization of a virus not directly linked with cancer but with immunodeficiency. HIV-1 was discovered and shown to be the cause of AIDS; a blood test was developed in a relatively short span of time, and therapies based on structural determinations of its RT and protease were developed and are being successfully used. This rapid progress would have been far slower had the means for isolating, culturing, and characterizing retroviruses not already been in place.

REFERENCES

1. Ellerman V, Bang O. Experimentelle Leukemie bei Huhnern. Centralbl Bakteriol Abt 1 (Orig) 1908;46:595–614.
2. Rous P. Transmission of a malignant new growth by means of a cell-free filtrate. J Exp Med 191;13:392–7.
3. Bittner JJ. Some possible effects of nursing on mammary gland tumor incidence. Science 1936;84:164–6.
4. Gross L. "Spontaneous" leukemia developing in C3H mice following inoculation, in infancy, with AK-leukemic extracts, or AK-embryos. Proc Soc Exp Biol Med 1951; 78:36–45.
5. Jarrett W, Martin B, Crichton W, et al. Leukemia in the cat. Transmission experiments with leukemia (lymphosarcoma). Nature 1964;202:566–8.
6. Theilen GH, Gould D, Fowler M, Dungworth DL. C-type virus in tumor tissue of a woolly monkey (*Lagothrix* spp.) with fibrosarcoma. J Natl Cancer Inst 1971;47:881–9.
7. Wolfe LG, Deinhardt F, Theilen GH, et al. Induction of tumors in marmoset monkeys by simian sarcoma virus, type *1* (*Lagothrix*): a preliminary report. J Natl Cancer Inst 1971;47:1115–20.
8. Kawakami TG, Huff SD, Buckley PM, et al. C-type virus associated with gibbon lymphosarcoma. Nat New Biol 1972;235:170–1.
9. Temin HM, Mizutani S. RNA-dependent DNA polymerase in virions of Rous sarcoma virus. Nature 1970;226:1211–3.
10. Baltimore D. RNA-dependent DNA polymerase in virions of RNA tumour viruses. Nature 1970;226:1209–11.
11. Stehelin D, Varmus HE, Bishop JM, Vogt PK. DNA related to the transforming gene(s) of avian sarcoma viruses is present in normal avian DNA. Nature 1976;260:170–3.
12. Poiesz BJ, Ruscetti FW, Gazdar AF, et al. Detection and isolation of type C retrovirus particles from fresh and cultured lymphocytes of a patient with cutaneous T-cell lymphoma. Proc Natl Acad Sci U S A 1980;77:7415–9.
13. Reitz MS, Jr, Poiesz BJ, Ruscetti FW, Gallo RC. Characterization and distribution of nucleic acid sequences of a novel type C retrovirus isolated from neoplastic human T lymphocytes. Proc Natl Acad Sci U S A 1981;78:1887–91.
14. Kalyanaraman VS, Sarngadharan MG, Poiesz B, et al. Immunological properties of a type C retrovirus isolated from

cultured human T-lymphoma cells and comparison to other mammalian retroviruses. J Virol 1981;38:906–15.
15. Poiesz BJ, Ruscetti FW, Reitz MS, et al. Isolation of a new type C retrovirus (HTLV) in primary uncultured cells of a patient with Sézary T-cell leukaemia. Nature 1981;294:268–71.
16. Robert-Guroff M, Ruscetti FW, Posner LE, et al. Detection of the human T cell lymphoma virus p19 in cells of some patients with cutaneous T cell lymphoma and leukemia using a monoclonal antibody. J Exp Med 1981;154:1957–64.
17. Hinuma Y, Nagata K, Hanaoka M, et al. Adult T-cell leukemia: antigen in an ATL cell line and detection of antibodies to the antigen in human sera. Proc Natl Acad Sci U S A 1981;78:6476–80.
18. Catovsky D, Greaves MF, Rose M, et al. Adult T-cell lymphoma–leukaemia in blacks from the West Indies. Lancet 1982;1:639–43.
19. Kalyanaraman VS, Sarngadharan MG, Nakao Y, et al. Natural antibodies to the structural core protein (p24) of the human T-cell leukemia (lymphoma) retrovirus found in sera of leukemia patients in Japan. Proc Natl Acad Sci U S A 1982;79:1653–7.
20. Yoshida M, Miyoshi I, Hinuma Y. Isolation and characterization of retrovirus from cell lines of human adult T-cell leukemia and its implication in the disease. Proc Natl Acad Sci U S A 1982;79:2031–5.
21. Kalyanaraman VS, Sarngadharan MG, Robert-Guroff M, et al. A new subtype of human T-cell leukemia virus (HTLV-II) associated with a T-cell variant of hairy cell leukemia. Science 1982;218:571–3.
22. Barre-Sinoussi F, Chermann JC, Rey F, et al. Isolation of a T-lymphotropic retrovirus from a patient at risk for acquired immune deficiency syndrome (AIDS). Science 1983;220:868–71.
23. Popovic M, Sarngadharan MG, Read E, Gallo RC. Detection, isolation, and continuous production of cytopathic retroviruses (HTLV-III) from patients with AIDS and pre-AIDS. Science 1984;224:497–500.
24. Gallo RC, Salahuddin SZ, Popovic M, et al. Frequent detection and isolation of cytopathic retroviruses (HTLV-III) from patients with AIDS and at risk for AIDS. Science 1984;224:500–3.
25. Sarngadharan MG, Popovic M, Bruch L, et al. Antibodies reactive with human T-lymphotropic retroviruses (HTLV-III) in the serum of patients with AIDS. Science 1984;224:506–8.
26. Clavel F, Guetard D, Brun-Vezinet F, et al. Isolation of a new human retrovirus from West African patients with AIDS. Science 1986;233:343–6.
27. Kanki PJ, M'Boup S, Ricard D, et al. Human T-lymphotropic virus type 4 and the human immunodeficiency virus in West Africa. Science 1987;236:827–31.
28. Teich N. Taxonomy of retroviruses. In: Weiss R, Teich N, Varmus HE, Coffin J, editors. RNA tumor viruses. Cold Spring Harbor (NY): Cold Spring Harbor Laboratory; 1984. p. 509.
29. Dahlberg JE, Sawyer RC, Taylor JM, et al. Transcription of DNA from the 70S RNA of Rous sarcoma virus. I. Identification of a specific 4S RNA which serves as primer. J Virol 1974;13:1126–33.
30. Taylor JM, Illmensee R. Site on the RNA of an avian sarcoma virus at which primer is bound. J Virol 1975;16:553–8.
31. Gannon F, O'Hare K, Perrin F, et al. Organisation and sequences at the 5' end of a cloned complete ovalbumin gene. Nature 1979;278:428–34.
32. Efstratiadis A, Posakony JW, Maniatis T, et al. The structure and evolution of the human beta-globin gene family. Cell 1980;21:653–68.
33. Breathnach R, Chambon P. Organization and expression of eucaryotic split genes coding for proteins. Annu Rev Biochem 1981;50:349–83.
34. Griffin GE, Leung K, Folks TM, et al. Activation of HIV gene expression during monocyte differentiation by induction of NF-kappa B. Nature 1989;339:70–3.
35. Bielinska A, Krasnow S, Nabel GJ. NF-kappa B-mediated activation of the human immunodeficiency virus enhancer: site of transcriptional initiation is independent of the TATA box. J Virol 1989;63:4097–100.
36. Ohtani K, Nakamura M, Saito S, et al. Identification of two distinct elements in the long terminal repeat of HTLV-I responsible for maximum gene expression. EMBO J 1987;6:389–95.
37. Yamamoto KR. Steroid receptor regulated transcription of specific genes and gene networks. Annu Rev Genet 1985;19:209–52.
38. Coffin J. Structure of the retroviral genome. In: Weiss R, Teich N, Varmus HE, Coffin J, editors. RNA tumor viruses. Cold Spring Harbor (NY): Cold Spring Harbor Laboratory; 1984. p. 261.
39. Fan H, Verma IM. Size analysis and relationship of murine leukemia virus-specific mRNAs: evidence for transposition of sequences during synthesis and processing of subgenomic mRNA. J Virol 1978;26:468–78.
40. Pawson T, Harvey R, Smith AE. The size of Rous sarcoma virus mRNAs active in cell-free translation. Nature 1977;268:416–20.
41. Pawson T, Martin GS, Smith AE. Cell-free translation of virion RNA from nondefective and transformation-defective Rous sarcoma viruses. J Virol 1976;19:950–67.
42. von der HK, Duesberg PH. Translation of Rous sarcoma virus RNA in a cell-free system from ascites Krebs II cells. Proc Natl Acad Sci U S A 1975;72:614–8.
43. Schiff LA, Nibert ML, Fields BN. Characterization of a zinc blotting technique: evidence that a retroviral gag protein binds zinc. Proc Natl Acad Sci U S A 1988;85:4195–9.
44. Green LM, Berg JM. A retroviral Cys-Xaa2-Cys-Xaa4-His-Xaa4-Cys peptide binds metal ions: spectroscopic studies and a proposed three-dimensional structure. Proc Natl Acad Sci U S A 1989;86:4047–51.
45. Henderson LE, Krutzsch HC, Oroszlan S. Myristyl amino-terminal acylation of murine retrovirus proteins: an unusual post-translational proteins modification. Proc Natl Acad Sci U S A 1983;80:339–43.
46. Schultz AM, Oroszlan S. In vivo modification of retroviral gag gene-encoded polyproteins by myristic acid. J Virol 1983;46:355–61.
47. Pal R, Reitz MS Jr, Tschachler E, et al. Myristoylation of gag proteins of HIV-1 plays an important role in virus assembly. AIDS Res Hum Retroviruses 1990;6:721–30.
48. Yoshinaka Y, Katoh I, Copeland TD, Oroszlan S. Murine leukemia virus protease is encoded by the gag–pol gene and is synthesized through suppression of an amber termination codon. Proc Natl Acad Sci U S A 1985;82:1618–22.
49. Moore DH, Long CA, Vaidya AB, et al. Mammary tumor viruses. Adv Cancer Res 1979;29:347–418.
50. Jacks T, Townsley K, Varmus HE, Majors J. Two efficient ribosomal frameshifting events are required for synthesis of mouse mammary tumor virus gag-related polyproteins. Proc Natl Acad Sci U S A 1987;84:4298–302.
51. Jacks T, Varmus HE. Expression of the Rous sarcoma virus pol gene by ribosomal frameshifting. Science 1985;230:1237–42.
52. Kohlstaedt LA, Wang J, Friedman JM, et al. Crystal structure at 3.5 A resolution of HIV-1 reverse transcriptase complexed with an inhibitor. Science 1992;256:1783–90.
53. Gallay P, Hope T, Chin D, Trono D. HIV-1 infection of nondividing cells through the recognition of integrase by the importin/karyopherin pathway. Proc Natl Acad Sci U S A 1997;94:9825–30.
54. Weiss SR, Varmus HE, Bishop JM. The size and genetic composition of virus-specific RNAs in the cytoplasm of cells producing avian sarcoma-leukosis viruses. Cell 1977;12:983–92.
55. Mellon P, Duesberg PH. Subgenomic, cellular Rous sarcoma virus RNAs contain oligonucleotides from the 3' half and the 5' terminus of virion RNA. Nature 1977;270:631–4.
56. Kowalski M, Potz J, Basiripour L, et al. Functional regions of the envelope glycoprotein of human immunodeficiency virus type 1. Science 1987;237:1351–5.
57. Marquardt H, Gilden RV, Oroszlan S. Envelope glycoproteins of Rauscher murine leukemia virus: isolation and chemical characterization. Biochemistry 1977;16:710–7.
58. Nowinski RC, Fleissner E, Sarkar NH, Aoki T. Chromatographic separation and antigenic analysis of proteins of the oncornaviruses. II. Mammalian leukemia-sarcoma viruses. J Virol 1972;9:359–66.
59. Rabenstein M, Shin YK. A peptide from the heptad repeat of human immunodeficiency virus gp41 shows both membrane binding and coiled-coil formation. Biochemistry 1995;34:13390–7.
60. Lu M, Blacklow SC, Kim PS. A trimeric structural domain of the HIV-1 transmembrane glycoprotein. Nat Struct Biol 1995;2:1075–82.
61. Dalgleish AG, Beverley PC, Clapham PR, et al. The CD4 (T4) antigen is an essential component of the receptor for the AIDS retrovirus. Nature 1984;312:763–7.
62. Feng Y, Broder CC, Kennedy PE, Berger EA. HIV-1 entry cofactor: functional cDNA cloning of a seven-transmembrane, G protein-coupled receptor. Science 1996;272:872–7.
63. Alkhatib G, Combadiere C, Broder CC, et al. CC CKR5: a RANTES, MIP-1alpha, MIP-1beta receptor as a fusion cofactor for macrophage-tropic HIV-1. Science 1996;272:1955–8.
64. Deng H, Liu R, Ellmeier W, et al. Identification of a major co-receptor for primary isolates of HIV-1. Nature 1996;381:661–6.
65. Dragic T, Litwin V, Allaway GP, et al. HIV-1 entry into CD4+ cells is mediated by the chemokine receptor CCCKR-5. Nature 1996;381:667–73.
66. Choe H, Farzan M, Sun Y, et al. The beta-chemokine receptors CCR3 and CCR5 facilitate infection by primary HIV-1 isolates. Cell 1996;85:1135–48.
67. Doranz BJ, Rucker J, Yi Y, et al. A dual-tropic primary HIV-1 isolate that uses fusin and the beta-chemokine receptors CKR-5, CKR-3, and CKR-2b as fusion cofactors. Cell 1996;85:1149–58.
68. Albritton LM, Tseng L, Scadden D, Cunningham JM. A putative murine ecotropic retrovirus receptor gene encodes a multiple membrane-spanning protein and confers susceptibility to virus infection. Cell 1989;57:659–66.
69. Wilson CA, Eiden MV, Anderson WB, et al. The dual-function hamster receptor for amphotropic murine leukemia virus (MuLV), 10A1 MuLV, and gibbon ape leukemia virus is a phosphate symporter. J Virol 1995;69:534–7.
70. Olah Z, Lehel C, Anderson WB, et al. The cellular receptor for gibbon ape leukemia virus is a novel high affinity sodium-dependent phosphate transporter. J Biol Chem 1994;269:25426–31.
71. Bates P, Young JA, Varmus HE. A receptor for subgroup A Rous sarcoma virus is related to the low-density lipoprotein receptor. Cell 1993;74:1043–51.
72. Brojatsch J, Naughton J, Rolls MM, et al. CAR1, a TNFR-related protein, is a cellular receptor for cytopathic avian leukosis-sarcoma viruses and mediates apoptosis. Cell 1996;87:845–55.
73. Golovkina TV, Dzuris J, van den Hoogen B, et al. A novel membrane protein is a mouse mammary tumor virus receptor. J Virol 1998;72:3066–71.
74. Haseltine WA, Kleid DG, Panet A, et al. Ordered transcription of RNA tumor virus genomes. J Mol Biol 1976;106:109–31.
75. Craigie R, Fujiwara T, Bushman F. The IN protein of Moloney murine leukemia virus processes the viral DNA ends and accomplishes their integration in vitro. Cell 1990;62:829–37.
76. Bushman FD, Fujiwara T, Craigie R. Retroviral DNA integration directed by HIV integration protein in vitro. Science 1990;249:1555–8.
77. Ohta M, Nyunoya H, Tanaka H, et al. Identification of a *cis*-regulatory element involved in accumulation of human T-cell leukemia virus type II genomic mRNA. J Virol 1988;62:4445–51.
78. Seiki M, Inoue J, Hidaka M, Yoshida M. Two *cis*-acting elements responsible for posttranscriptional *trans*-regulation of gene expression of human T-cell leukemia virus type I. Proc Natl Acad Sci U S A 1988;85:7124–8.
79. Feinberg MB, Jarrett RF, Aldovini A, et al. HTLV-III expression and production involve complex regulation at the levels of splicing and translation of viral RNA. Cell 1986;46:807–17.
80. Purchio AF, Jovanovich S, Erikson RL. Sites of synthesis of viral proteins in avian sarcoma virus-infected chicken cells. J Virol 1980;35:629–36.
81. Yoshinaka Y, Luftig RB. Murine leukemia virus morphogenesis: cleavage of P70 in vitro can be accompanied by a shift from a concentrically coiled internal strand ("immature") to a collapsed ("mature") form of the virus core. Proc Natl Acad Sci U S A 1977;74:3446–50.
82. Fujisawa J, Seiki M, Kiyokawa T, Yoshida M. Functional activation of the long terminal repeat of human T-cell leukemia virus type I by a trans-acting factor. Proc Natl Acad Sci U S A 1985;82:2277–81.
83. Felber BK, Paskalis H, Kleinman-Ewing C, et al. The pX protein of HTLV-I is a transcriptional activator of its long terminal repeats. Science 1985;229:675–9.
84. Sodroski J, Rosen C, Goh WC, Haseltine W. A transcriptional activator protein encoded by the x-lor region of the human T-cell leukemia virus. Science 1985;228:1430–4.
85. Arya SK, Guo C, Josephs SF, Wong-Staal F. Trans-activator gene of human T-lymphotropic virus type III (HTLVIII). Science 1985;229:69–73.
86. Sodroski J, Rosen C, Wong-Staal F, et al. Trans-acting transcriptional regulation of human T-cell leukemia virus type III long terminal repeat. Science 1985;227:171–3.
87. Sodroski J, Patarca R, Rosen C, et al. Location of the trans-activating region on the genome of human T-cell lymphotropic virus type III. Science 1985;229:74–7.

88. Vogt PK. Spontaneous segregation of nontransforming viruses from cloned sarcoma viruses. Virology 1971;46:939–46.
89. Martin GS. Rous sarcoma virus: a function required for the maintenance of the transformed state. Nature 1970;227:1021–3.
90. Kawai S, Hanafusa H. The effects of reciprocal changes in temperature on the transformed state of cells infected with a Rous sarcoma virus mutant. Virology 1971;46:470–9.
91. Bader JP. Temperature-dependent transformation of cells infected with a mutant of Bryan Rous sarcoma virus. J Virol 1972;10:267–76.
92. Fung YK, Crittenden LB, Fadly AM, Kung HJ. Tumor induction by direct injection of cloned *v-src* DNA into chickens. Proc Natl Acad Sci U S A 1983;80:353–7.
93. Boettiger D, Love DN, Weiss RA. Virus envelope markers in mammalian tropism of avian RNA tumor viruses. J Virol 1975;15:108–14.
94. Altaner C, Temin HM. Carcinogenesis by RNA sarcoma viruses. XII. A quantitative study of infection of rat cells in vitro by avian sarcoma viruses. Virology 1970;40:118–34.
95. Abelson HT, Rabstein LS. Lymphosarcoma: virus-induced thymic-independent disease in mice. Cancer Res 1970;30:2213–22.
96. Abelson HT, Rabstein LS. Influence of prednisolone on Moloney leukemogenic virus in BALB-c mice. Cancer Res 1970;30:2208–12.
97. Reddy EP, Smith MJ, Srinivasan A. Nucleotide sequence of Abelson murine leukemia virus genome: structural similarity of its transforming gene product to other *onc* gene products with tyrosine-specific kinase activity. Proc Natl Acad Sci U S A 1983;80:3623–7.
98. Scher CD, Siegler R. Direct transformation of 3T3 cells by Abelson murine leukaemia virus. Nature 1975;253:729–31.
99. Varmus HE. Form and function of retroviral proviruses. Science 1982;216:812–20.
100. Walther N, Lurz R, Patschinsky T, et al. Molecular cloning of proviral DNA and structural analysis of the transduced myc oncogene of avian oncovirus CMII. J Virol 1985;54:576–85.
101. Gallo RC, Gallagher RE, Wong-Staal F, et al. Isolation and tissue distribution of type-C virus and viral components from a gibbon ape (*Hylobates lar*) with lymphocytic leukemia. Virology 1978;84:359–73.
102. Kawakami TG, Kollias GV Jr, Holmberg C. Oncogenicity of gibbon type-C myelogenous leukemia virus. Int J Cancer 1980;25:641–6.
103. Cooper MD, Payne LN, Dent PB, et al. Pathogenesis of avian lymphoid leukosis. I. Histogenesis. J Natl Cancer Inst 1968;41:373–8.
104. Hayward WS, Neel BG, Astrin SM. Activation of a cellular *onc* gene by promoter insertion in ALV-induced lymphoid leukosis. Nature 1981;290:475–80.
105. Neel BG, Hayward WS, Robinson HL, et al. Avian leukosis virus-induced tumors have common proviral integration sites and synthesize discrete new RNAs: oncogenesis by promoter insertion. Cell 1981;23:323–34.
106. Fung YK, Fadly AM, Crittenden LB, Kung HJ. On the mechanism of retrovirus-induced avian lymphoid leukosis: deletion and integration of the proviruses. Proc Natl Acad Sci U S A 1981;78:3418–22.
107. Payne GS, Bishop JM, Varmus HE. Multiple arrangements of viral DNA and an activated host oncogene in bursal lymphomas. Nature 1982;295:209–14.
108. van Ooyen A, Kwee V, Nusse R. The nucleotide sequence of the human int-1 mammary oncogene; evolutionary conservation of coding and non-coding sequences. EMBO J 1985;4:2905–9.
109. van Ooyen A, Nusse R. Structure and nucleotide sequence of the putative mammary oncogene *int-1*; proviral insertions leave the protein-encoding domain intact. Cell 1984;39:233–40.
110. Nusse R, Varmus HE. Many tumors induced by the mouse mammary tumor virus contain a provirus integrated in the same region of the host genome. Cell 1982;31:99–109.
111. Stewart TA, Pattengale PK, Leder P. Spontaneous mammary adenocarcinomas in transgenic mice that carry and express MTV/myc fusion genes. Cell 1984;38:627–37.
112. Sinn E, Muller W, Pattengale P, Tepler I, et al. Coexpression of MMTV/v-Ha-ras and MMTV/c-myc genes in transgenic mice: synergistic action of oncogenes in vivo. Cell 1987;49:465–75.
113. Matsui Y, Halter SA, Holt JT, et al. Development of mammary hyperplasia and neoplasia in MMTV-TGF alpha transgenic mice. Cell 1990;61:1147–55.
114. Bouchard L, Lamarre L, Tremblay PJ, Jolicoeur P. Stochastic appearance of mammary tumors in transgenic mice carrying the MMTV/c-neu oncogene. Cell 1989;57:931–6.
115. Li JP, D'Andrea AD, Lodish HF, Baltimore D. Activation of cell growth by binding of Friend spleen focus-forming virus gp55 glycoprotein to the erythropoietin receptor. Nature 1990;343:762–4.
116. Ruscetti SK, Janesch NJ, Chakraborti A, et al. Friend spleen focus-forming virus induces factor independence in an erythropoietin-dependent erythroleukemia cell line. J Virol 1990;64:1057–62.
117. Gessain A, Barin F, Vernant JC, et al. Antibodies to human T-lymphotropic virus type-I in patients with tropical spastic paraparesis. Lancet 1985;2:407–10.
118. Willems L, Chen G, Portetelle D, et al. Structural and functional characterization of mutants of the bovine leukemia virus transactivator protein p34. Virology 1989;171:615–8.
119. Zhang W, Nisbet JW, Bartoe JT, et al. Human T-lymphotropic virus type 1 p30(II) functions as a transcription factor and differentially modulates CREB-responsive promoters. J Virol 2000;74:11270–7.
120. Albrecht B, D'Souza CD, Ding W, et al. Activation of nuclear factor of activated T cells by human T-lymphotropic virus type 1 accessory protein p12(I). J Virol 2002;76:3493–501.
121. Mulloy JC, Crownley RW, Fullen J, et al. The human T-cell leukemia/lymphotropic virus type 1 p12I proteins bind the interleukin-2 receptor beta and gamma (c) chains and affects their expression on the cell surface. J Virol 1996;70:3599–605.
122. D'Agostino DM, Zotti L, Ferro T, et al. The p13II protein of HTLV type 1: comparison with mitochondrial proteins coded by other human viruses. AIDS Res Hum Retroviruses 2000;16:1765–70.
123. Lefebvre L, Vanderplasschen A, Ciminale V, et al. Oncoviral bovine leukemia virus G4 and human T-cell leukemia virus type 1 p13(II) accessory proteins interact with farnesyl pyrophosphate synthetase. J Virol 2002;76:1400–14.
124. Tschachler E, Bohnlein E, Felzmann S, Reitz MS Jr. Human T-lymphotropic virus type I tax regulates the expression of the human lymphotoxin gene. Blood 1993;81:95–100.
125. Miyatake S, Seiki M, Malefijt RD, et al. Activation of T cell-derived lymphokine genes in T cells and fibroblasts: effects of human T cell leukemia virus type I p40x protein and bovine papilloma virus encoded E2 protein. Nucleic Acids Res 1988;16:6547–66.
126. Inoue J, Seiki M, Taniguchi T, et al. Induction of interleukin 2 receptor gene expression by p40x encoded by human T-cell leukemia virus type 1. EMBO J 1986;5:2883–8.
127. Fujii M, Sassone-Corsi P, Verma IM. c-fos promoter trans-activation by the tax1 protein of human T-cell leukemia virus type I. Proc Natl Acad Sci U S A 1988;85:8526–30.
128. Grossman WJ, Kimata JT, Wong FH, et al. Development of leukemia in mice transgenic for the tax gene of human T-cell leukemia virus type I. Proc Natl Acad Sci U S A 1995;92:1057–61.
129. Nerenberg M, Hinrichs SH, Reynolds RK, et al. The tat gene of human T-lymphotropic virus type 1 induces mesenchymal tumors in transgenic mice. Science 1987;237:1324–9.
130. Tanaka A, Takahashi C, Yamaoka S, et al. Oncogenic transformation by the tax gene of human T-cell leukemia virus type I in vitro. Proc Natl Acad Sci U S A 1990;87:1071–5.
131. Pozzatti R, Vogel J, Jay G. The human T-lymphotropic virus type I tax gene can cooperate with the *ras* oncogene to induce neoplastic transformation of cells. Mol Cell Biol 1990;10:413–7.
132. Grassmann R, Dengler C, Muller-Fleckenstein I, et al. Transformation to continuous growth of primary human T lymphocytes by human T-cell leukemia virus type I X-region genes transduced by a herpesvirus saimiri vector. Proc Natl Acad Sci U S A 1989;86:3351–5.
133. Clarke MF, Trainor CD, Mann DL, et al. Methylation of human T-cell leukemia virus proviral DNA and viral RNA expression in short- and long-term cultures of infected cells. Virology 1984;135:97–104.
134. Yin MJ, Gaynor RB. HTLV-1 21 bp repeat sequences facilitate stable association between Tax and CREB to increase CREB binding affinity. J Mol Biol 1996;264:20–31.
135. Suzuki T, Fujisawa JI, Toita M, Yoshida M. The trans-activator tax of human T-cell leukemia virus type 1 (HTLV-1) interacts with cAMP-responsive element (CRE) binding and CRE modulator proteins that bind to the 21-base-pair enhancer of HTLV-1. Proc Natl Acad Sci U S A 1993;90:610–4.
136. Zhao LJ, Giam CZ. Human T-cell lymphotropic virus type I (HTLV-I) transcriptional activator, Tax, enhances CREB binding to HTLV-I 21-base-pair repeats by protein-protein interaction. Proc Natl Acad Sci U S A 1992;89:7070–4.
137. Adya N, Giam CZ. Distinct regions in human T-cell lymphotropic virus type I tax mediate interactions with activator protein CREB and basal transcription factors. J Virol 1995;69:1834–41.
138. Gachon F, Peleraux A, Thebault S, et al. CREB-2, a cellular CRE-dependent transcription repressor, functions in association with Tax as an activator of the human T-cell leukemia virus type 1 promoter. J Virol 1998;72:8332–7.
139. Leung K, Nabel GJ. HTLV-1 transactivator induces interleukin-2 receptor expression through an NF-kappa B-like factor. Nature 1988;333:776–8.
140. Ballard DW, Bohnlein E, Lowenthal JW, et al. HTLV-I tax induces cellular proteins that activate the kappa B element in the IL-2 receptor alpha gene. Science 1988;241:1652–5.
141. Siekevitz M, Josephs SF, Dukovich M, et al. Activation of the HIV-1 LTR by T cell mitogens and the trans-activator protein of HTLV-I. Science 1987;238:1575–8.
142. Low KG, Dorner LF, Fernando DB, et al. Human T-cell leukemia virus type 1 Tax releases cell cycle arrest induced by p16INK4a. J Virol 1997;71:1956–62.
143. Suzuki T, Kitao S, Matsushime H, Yoshida M. HTLV-1 Tax protein interacts with cyclin-dependent kinase inhibitor p16INK4A and counteracts its inhibitory activity towards CDK4. EMBO J 1996;15:1607–14.
144. Neuveut C, Low KG, Maldarelli F, et al. Human T-cell leukemia virus type 1 Tax and cell cycle progression: role of cyclin D-cdk and p110Rb. Mol Cell Biol 1998;18:3620–32.
145. Lemasson I, Thebault S, Sardet C, et al. Activation of E2F-mediated transcription by human T-cell leukemia virus type I Tax protein in a p16(INK4A)-negative T-cell line. J Biol Chem 1998;273:23598–604.
146. Wu X, Levine AJ. p53 and E2F-1 cooperate to mediate apoptosis. Proc Natl Acad Sci U S A 1994;91:3602–6.
147. Pise-Masison CA, Radonovich M, Sakaguchi K, et al. Phosphorylation of p53: a novel pathway for p53 inactivation in human T-cell lymphotropic virus type 1-transformed cells. J Virol 1998;72:6348–55.
148. Akagi T, Ono H, Tsuchida N, Shimotohno K. Aberrant expression and function of p53 in T-cells immortalized by HTLV- I Tax1. FEBS Lett 1997;406:263–6.
149. Mulloy JC, Kislyakova T, Cereseto A, et al. Human T-cell lymphotropic/leukemia virus type 1 Tax abrogates p53-induced cell cycle arrest and apoptosis through its CREB/ATF functional domain. J Virol 1998;72:8852–60.
150. Jin DY, Spencer F, Jeang KT. Human T cell leukemia virus type 1 oncoprotein Tax targets the human mitotic checkpoint protein MAD1. Cell 1998;93:81–91.
151. Hoover EA, Mullins JI, Quackenbush SL, Gasper PW. Experimental transmission and pathogenesis of immunodeficiency syndrome in cats. Blood 1987;70:1880–92.
152. Chang Y, Cesarman E, Pessin MS, et al. Identification of herpesvirus-like DNA sequences in AIDS-associated Kaposi's sarcoma. Science 1994;266:1865–9.
153. Cesarman E, Chang Y, Moore PS, et al. Kaposi's sarcoma-associated herpesvirus-like DNA sequences in AIDS-related body-cavity-based lymphomas. N Engl J Med 1995;332:1186–91.
154. Goedert JJ. The epidemiology of acquired immunodeficiency syndrome malignancies. Semin Oncol 2000;27:390–401.
155. Vogel J, Hinrichs SH, Reynolds RK, et al. The HIV tat gene induces dermal lesions resembling Kaposi's sarcoma in transgenic mice. Nature 1988;335:606–11.
156. Stoye JP, Fenner S, Greenoak GE, et al. Role of endogenous retroviruses as mutagens: the hairless mutation of mice. Cell 1988;54:383–91.
157. Cachon-Gonzalez MB, Fenner S, Coffin JM, et al. Structure and expression of the hairless gene of mice. Proc Natl Acad Sci U S A 1994;91:7717–21.
158. Jenkins NA, Copeland NG, Taylor BA, Lee BK. Dilute(d) coat colour mutation of DBA/2J mice is associated with the site of integration of an ecotropic MuLV genome. Nature 1981;293:370–4.
159. Meisler MH, Ting CN. The remarkable evolutionary history of the human amylase genes. Crit Rev Oral Biol Med 1993;4:503–9.
160. Ting CN, Rosenberg MP, Snow CM, et al. Endogenous retroviral sequences are required for tissue-specific expression of a human salivary amylase gene. Genes Dev 1992;6:1457–65.

161. Samuelson LC, Wiebauer K, Snow CM, Meisler MH. Retroviral and pseudogene insertion sites reveal the lineage of human salivary and pancreatic amylase genes from a single gene during primate evolution. Mol Cell Biol 1990;10:2513–20.

162. Knerr I, Beinder E, Rascher W. Syncytin, a novel human endogenous retroviral gene in human placenta: evidence for its dysregulation in preeclampsia and HELLP syndrome. Am J Obstet Gynecol 2002;186:210–3.

163. Mi S, Lee X, Li X, et al. Syncytin is a captive retroviral envelope protein involved in human placental morphogenesis. Nature 2000;403:785–9.

164. Devare SG, Rapp UR, Todaro GJ, Stephenson JR. Acquisition of oncogenicity by endogenous mouse type C viruses: effects of variations in env and gag genes. J Virol 1978;28:457–65.

165. Chien YH, Verma IM, Shih TY, et al. Heteroduplex analysis of the sequence relations between the RNAs of mink cell focus-inducing and murine leukemia viruses. J Virol 1978;28:352–60.

166. Elder JH, Gautsch JW, Jensen FC, et al. Biochemical evidence that MCF murine leukemia viruses are envelope (env) gene recombinants. Proc Natl Acad Sci U S A 1977;74:4676–80.

167. Hogge DE, Humphries RK. Gene transfer to primary normal and malignant human hemopoietic progenitors using recombinant retroviruses. Blood 1987;69:611–7.

168. Miller AD, Jolly DJ, Friedmann T, Verma IM. A transmissible retrovirus expressing human hypoxanthine phosphoribosyltransferase (HPRT): gene transfer into cells obtained from humans deficient in HPRT. Proc Natl Acad Sci U S A 1983;80:4709–13.

169. Williams DA, Lemischka IR, Nathan DG, Mulligan RC. Introduction of new genetic material into pluripotent haematopoietic stem cells of the mouse. Nature 1984;310:476–80.

170. Mann R, Mulligan RC, Baltimore D. Construction of a retrovirus packaging mutant and its use to produce helper-free defective retrovirus. Cell 1983;33:153–9.

171. Wilson C, Reitz MS, Okayama H, Eiden MV. Formation of infectious hybrid virions with gibbon ape leukemia virus and human T-cell leukemia virus retroviral envelope glycoproteins and the gag and pol proteins of Moloney murine leukemia virus. J Virol 1989;63:2374–8.

172. Follenzi A, Ailles LE, Bakovic S, et al. Gene transfer by lentiviral vectors is limited by nuclear translocation and rescued by HIV-1 pol sequences. Nat Genet 2000;25:217–22.

173. Naldini L, Blomer U, Gallay P, et al. In vivo gene delivery and stable transduction of nondividing cells by a lentiviral vector. Science 1996;272:263–7.

174. Donahue RE, Kessler SW, Bodine D, et al. Helper virus-induced T-cell lymphoma in nonhuman primates after retroviral-mediated gene transfer. J Exp Med 1992;176:1125–35.

175 . Hacein-Bey-Abina S, Von Kalle C, Schmidt M, et al. LMO2-associated clonal T cell proliferation in two patients after gene therapy for SCID-X1. Science 2003;302:415–9.

176. Towers G, Bock M, Martin S, et al. A conserved mechanism of retrovirus restriction in mammals. Proc Natl Acad Sci U S A 2000;97:12295–9.

177. Cowan S, Hatziioannou T, Cunningham T, et al. Cellular inhibitors with Fv1-like activity restrict human and simian immunodeficiency virus tropism. Proc Natl Acad Sci U S A 2002;99:11914–9.

178. Owens CM, Yang PC, Gottlinger H, et al. Human and simian immunodeficiency virus capsid proteins are major viral determinants of early, postentry replication blocks in simian cells. J Virol 2003;77:726–31.

179. Mangeat B, Turelli P, Caron G, et al. Broad antiretroviral defense by human APOBEC3G through lethal editing of nascent reverse transcripts. Nature 2003;424:99–103.

180. Shindo K, Takaori-Kondo A, Kobayashi M, et al. The enzymatic activity of CEM15/Apobec-3G is essential for the regulation of the infectivity of HIV-1 virion but not a sole determinant of its antiviral activity. J Biol Chem 2003; 278:44412–6.

181. Zheng YH, Irwin D, Kurosu T, et al. Human APOBEC3F is another host factor that blocks human immunodeficiency virus type 1 replication. J Virol 2004;78:6073–6.

182. Chiu YL, Soros VB, Kreisberg JF, et al. Cellular APOBEC3G restricts HIV-1 infection in resting CD4+ T cells. Nature 2005;435:108–14.

183. Bennasser Y, Le SY, Benkirane M, Jeang KT. Evidence that HIV-1 encodes an siRNA and a suppressor of RNA silencing. Immunity 2005;22:607–19.

20

Herpesviruses

Jeffrey I. Cohen, MD

Eight herpesviruses have been isolated from humans: Herpes simplex 1, herpes simplex 2, and varicella-zoster virus, which are members of the Alphaherpesvirinae subfamily; cytomegalovirus, human herpesvirus 6, and human herpesvirus 7, which are members of the Betaherpesvirinae subfamily; and Epstein-Barr virus (EBV) and human herpesvirus 8 (HHV-8, Kaposi's sarcoma-associated herpesvirus), which are members of the Gammaherpesvirinae subfamily. Two of these herpesviruses are associated with human tumors. EBV has been detected in lesions from patients with nasopharyngeal carcinoma, Burkitt's lymphoma, Hodgkin's disease, and certain other lymphoid tumors. HHV-8 is associated with Kaposi's sarcoma, primary effusion lymphoma, and Castleman's disease.

Herpesviruses are ubiquitous in nature, and nearly every animal species is infected by at least one herpesvirus. The transforming animal herpesviruses include *Herpesvirus saimiri,* which induces fatal T-cell lymphomas in certain species of monkeys and rabbits and transforms human T cells in vitro, and murine herpesvirus 68, which causes lymphoproliferative lesions in mice. Viruses homologous to EBV and HHV-8 have been identified in macaques.

PROPERITES OF HERPESVIRUSES

Herpesviruses are enveloped virions that contain a deoxyribonucleic acid (DNA) core surrounded by an icosahedral nucleocapsid and a tegument. The viral genome consists of linear, double-stranded DNA varying in size from 120 to 240 kilobase pairs, depending on the virus. The smallest herpesviruses contain approximately 70 unique genes, while the largest contain about 200 genes. Virions contain 30 to 35 structural proteins.

Infection of cells with herpesviruses begins with adsorption and fusion of the virion envelope with the cell membrane. The envelope glycoproteins are important mediators of adsorption and fusion. The viral capsid is released into the cytoplasm and is transported to the nucleus where the linear viral DNA circularizes. In infections that result in production of progeny viruses and lysis of the host cell, immediate-early, early, and subsequently late viral genes are transcribed in the nucleus and their proteins are synthesized in the cytoplasm, while translation of host cell ribonucleic acids (RNAs) is inhibited. Early lytic replication is associated with irreversible cytocidal inhibition of host DNA, RNA, and protein synthesis. Virion DNA is replicated and assembled into nucleocapsids in the nucleus. Nucleocapsids undergo initial envelopment by budding through the inner lamella of the nuclear membrane. Viral proteins and glycoproteins modify the host cell's cytoplasmic membranes. Virions are released by exocytosis or by cytoplasmic de-envelopment and re-envelopment at the plasma membrane.

All herpesviruses have the capacity to establish latent infection as well as to undergo lytic infection. The capacity to establish latent infection in vivo and to reactivate from latency ensures a source of virus to infect previously uninfected individuals. Herpesviruses are ubiquitous in most human populations. Almost all adults latently harbor herpes simplex 1, varicella-zoster virus, human herpesviruses 6 and 7, and EBV. Reactivation in adults results in transmission of virus to infants, children, or young adults, perpetuating nearly uniform adult infection and persistence of the virus over many generations.

ONCOGENIC FEATURES OF HERPESVIRUSES

Several features of herpesvirus replication are important for the maintenance of latency and for oncogenicity. To be oncogenic, herpesviruses must be capable of maintaining their viral genome in the cell, avoid killing the cell, avoid destruction of the cell by the immune system, and activate appropriate cellular growth control regulatory pathways. Because EBV is the best studied of the human herpesviruses, which latently infects cells and has a strong association with human neoplasia, this virus is used to illustrate the principles of herpesvirus infection relevant to oncogenicity.

First, viral DNA must be maintained in the cell. EBV establishes latent infection in B lymphocytes. Because B lymphocytes replicate, the virus must have a way to ensure transmission to cell progeny. The EBV genome is usually maintained in B cells either as a multicopy circular episome in the host cell, or by integrating the viral DNA into the host genome. Episomes are formed by fusion of the direct repeat sequences that are present at both termini of the linear genome present in virions. The Namalwa Burkitt tumor cell line contains a complete copy of the entire EBV genome integrated into the host cell DNA and no additional episomal viral DNA. Analysis of the DNA sequence indicates that the viral genome is integrated into the host DNA at the terminal direct repeat sequence of the virus.

Second, a cell transformed by a virus must avoid immune clearance. To achieve this, a virus can only express a limited number of viral genes. Replication of herpesviruses in cells results in inhibition of host cell protein synthesis and lysis of the host cell. Analysis of the EBV DNA sequence indicates nearly 100 possible gene products; however, latent infection of B cells with EBV results in expression of 12 or fewer genes.[1,2] This limited repertoire of gene products prevents frequent viral replication, with death of the infected cell, and restricts the ability of the immune system to recognize and destroy a cell latently infected with the virus.

Third, specific viral proteins interact with other cell proteins or directly transactivate other cell genes to provide additional functions necessary for immortalization. Proteins encoded by several DNA tumor viruses transactivate expression of cell genes which may be important to initiate or maintain neoplasia. Several EBV proteins interact with cellular proteins to activate transcription of viral and cellular genes or to engage signal transduction pathways in the cell (see below).

EPSTEIN-BARR VIRUS: AN ONCOGENIC HUMAN HERPESVIRUS

Effect on B-Cell Growth In Vitro Infection of primary B cells with EBV in vitro results in transformation of the cells, which can then proliferate indefinitely. B-cell activation antigens, including CD23, are expressed on the surface of the EBV-transformed B cells. The supernatant of EBV-transformed B cells contains a 35-kilodalton (kDa) protein thought to represent a soluble, cleaved form of CD23. CD23 may be a growth factor for B cells and the soluble form of CD23 may have autocrine growth factor activity. EBV infection of Burkitt's lymphoma cells in vitro results in up-regulation of a number of cellular proteins, including CD44, and two G protein-coupled peptide receptors.[3]

Gene Expression in Transformed Lymphocytes Six different EBV nuclear proteins, two membrane proteins, and two nontranslated RNAs are known to be expressed in latently infected B lymphocytes that have been growth transformed by EBV in vitro (Table 20-1). The EBV nuclear proteins EBNA-1, EBNA-2, EBNA-LP, EBNA-3A, EBNA-3B, and EBNA-3C comprise the EBV nuclear antigen complex. EBNA-1 binds to the oriP sequence (origin of viral DNA replication) on EBV DNA and allows the virus genome to be maintained as an episome in transformed B cells.[4] EBNA-1 also transactivates its own expression. EBNA-1 transcripts are initiated from one of four

Table 20-1 Selected EBV Genes and Their Cellular Homologs and Activities

Gene	Expression Class	Cellular Homolog	Activity
EBNA-1	Latent, lytic	None	Episome maintenance, transactivates viral genes, inhibits apoptosis
EBNA-2	Latent	Notch	Transactivates viral and cellular genes, inhibits apoptosis
EBNA-3A,B,C	Latent	None	Regulates EBNA-2 activity, transactivates cellular genes
EBNA-LP	Latent	None	Increases EBNA-2 activity
LMP-1	Latent, lytic	CD40	Transactivates cellular genes, inhibits apoptosis
LMP-2	Latent	None	Prevents EBV reactivation
EBERs	Latent	None	Up-regulate cellular genes
BARF1	Lytic	CSF-1R	Inhibits interferon-α
BCFR1	Lytic	IL-10	Inhibits interferon-γ and IL-12
BHRF1	Lytic	bcl-2	Inhibits apoptosis
BALF1	Lytic	bcl-2	Regulates BHRF1 activity
BZLF1	Lytic	None	Inhibits interferon-γ effects, inhibits function of p53, inhibits TNF-α, initiates lytic infection

different promoters. The Cp and Wp promoters are used to express EBNA-1 in lymphoblastoid cell lines in vitro; the Qp promoter is used in tissues from Burkitt's lymphoma, nasopharyngeal carcinoma, and Hodgkin's disease; and the Fp promoter is used during lytic replication.[5] Transgenic mice expressing EBNA-1 develop B-cell lymphomas.[6] EBNA-1 inhibits its own protein degradation by proteosomes[7] and limits its own translation[8] both of which may reduce its presentation to CD8+ cytotoxic T cells; however, EBNA-1 remains a target for cytotoxic cells.[9,10] EBNA-1 inhibits apoptosis induced by expression of p53.[11]

EBNA-2 is required for B-cell transformation by EBV. EBNA-2 transactivates expression of the EBV genes LMP-1[12] and LMP-2,[13] and the cellular genes CD23, CD21, c-*myc*, and c-*fgr*,[14,15] which encodes a protein tyrosine kinase and is a member of the *src* gene family. EBNA-2 does not bind DNA directly but interacts with several cellular proteins. EBNA-2 is targeted to the LMP-1, LMP-2, Cp EBNA, and CD23 promoters by the GTGGGAA-binding protein Jκ, and thereby activates these promoters.[16] EBNA-2 is a functional homolog of the Notch receptor, which uses Jκ to regulate gene expression during development.[17] EBNA-2 also interacts with the DNA-binding protein PU-1 to transactivate the LMP-1 promoter[18] and with AUF to transactivate the EBNA Cp promoter.[19] The transactivation domain of EBNA-2 is essential for B-lymphocyte transformation.[20] This domain interacts with several transcription factors, including TFIIB and the TATA-binding protein-associated factor TAF40.[21] EBNA-2 inhibits apoptosis mediated by Nur77.[22] EBNA-2 is a major determinant of the type-specific transforming difference between the two naturally occurring types of EBV.

EBNA-LP interacts with and enhances the ability of EBNA-2 to transactivate LMP-1 and LMP-2.[23] Although EBNA-LP binds to the retinoblastoma protein, heat shock proteins, and p53 in vitro,[24] the significance of these interactions is uncertain. Deletion of the carboxy terminus of EBNA-LP markedly reduces the ability of the virus to transform B lymphocytes.[25]

EBNA-3A, EBNA-3B, and EBNA-3C are encoded by three tandem open reading frames. These three proteins are distantly related. The EBNA-3 proteins bind to Jκ preventing it from binding DNA, thereby inhibiting transactivation by EBNA-2.[26] EBNA-3C is a regulator of transcription that up-regulates expression of LMP-1 and CD21. EBNA-3C binds to Nm23-HI, a human metastasis suppressor protein, and inhibits the protein's ability to suppress migration of Burkitt's lymphoma cells.[27] EBNA-3A and EBNA-3C are essential for B-lymphocyte transformation in vitro, while EBNA-3B is dispensable.[28]

Two latent membrane proteins, LMP-1 and LMP-2, are expressed in B cells that have been growth transformed by EBV. Both proteins are present in lipid rafts on the surface of B cells.[29] LMP-1 functions as a transforming oncogene; rodent cells expressing the protein form tumors in nude mice.[30] Expression of LMP-1 in EBV-negative Burkitt's lymphoma cells results in B-cell clumping and increased villous projections. Up-regulation of bcl-2, bfl-1, and A20 by LMP-1 in B cells protects the cells from apoptosis.[31] Expression of LMP-1 in epithelial cells inhibits differentiation of the cells.[32]

LMP-1 interacts with several cellular proteins. LMP-1 is a functional homolog of CD40, a member of the tumor necrosis factor receptor (TNFR) family. The carboxy terminus of LMP-1 interacts with the TNFR-associated factors (TRAFs) 1, 2, 3, and 5, TRADD, RIP, and Janus-activated kinase-3 (JAK3) in vitro.[33-35] LMP-1 functions as a constitutively active form of CD40 resulting in activation of NF-κB, stress-activated protein kinases, signal transducers and activators of transcription (STATs), adhesion molecules, the B7 costimulatory molecule, c-*jun* N-terminal kinase, and B-cell proliferation. LMP-1 can functionally substitute for CD40 in transgenic mice.[36] LMP-1 up-regulates expression of intracellular adhesion molecules, Fas, CD40, and matrix metalloproteinase-9[37] in B cells and epidermal growth factor in epithelial cells.[38]

LMP-1 is essential for transformation of B lymphocytes by EBV.[39] Expression of LMP-1 in the skin of transgenic mice induces epithelial hyperplasia with increased expression of keratin 6.[40] Expression of LMP-1 in lymphocytes of transgenic mice results in the development of B-cell lymphomas; these tumors contain elevated levels of the antiapoptotic proteins Bcl-2 and A20.[41] Analysis of EBV-containing human lymphomas shows that LMP-1 localizes with TRAF-1, TRAF-3, and that activated NF-κB is present, suggesting that these activities may have an important role in oncogenesis.[42]

LMP-2 is dispensable for transformation of B cells,[43] but induces a transforming phenotype in epithelial cells.[44] Two forms of LMP-2 (LMP-2A and LMP-2B), which differ only in their first exon, are expressed in latently infected B cells. LMP-2 prevents lytic reactivation of EBV-infected primary B cells and calcium mobilization in response to activation of the B-cell receptor complex by cross-linking of surface immunoglobulin. LMP-2 is tyrosine phosphorylated and associates with the *src* family and *syk* protein-tyrosine kinases that are coupled to the B-cell receptor complex.[45] Binding of LMP-2 to these proteins results in their constitutive phosphorylation, which inhibits their ability to mediate signaling for virus reactivation.[45,46] B cells from transgenic mice expressing LMP-2 survive even without normal B-cell receptor signaling activity.[47] LMP-2A activates beta-catenin signaling pathways in epithelial cells.[48]

The two EBV-encoded RNAs, EBER-1 and EBER-2, are the most abundant EBV RNAs in latently infected B cells; however, they are not required for latent or lytic EBV infection or cell transformation in vitro.[49] The EBERs up-regulate expression of bcl-2 and IL-10.[50] These RNAs are not polyadenylated and interact with the nuclear antigens La and EAP, ribosome protein L22, the double-stranded RNA-activated protein kinase, and interferon-inducible oligoadenylate synthetase.[51,52]

Epstein-Barr Virus Genes Expressed during Productive Infection Infection of epithelial cells with EBV results in productive infection, with replication of virus and lysis of infected cells. Immediate-early genes encode regulators of virus gene expression, including the BZLF1 and BRLF1 proteins, which act as switches to initiate lytic infection. The BZLF1 protein inhibits TNF-α signaling by reducing expression of the TNF receptor.[53] BZLF1 protein also inhibits the expression of the interferon-γ receptor and the activity of interferon-γ,[54] and inhibits the function of p53.[55] Early genes encode proteins that are involved in viral DNA synthesis, such as the viral DNA polymerase and thymidine kinase. Late genes encode structural proteins of the virus, including the viral capsid antigen and the major envelope glycoprotein gp350.

Three viral genes expressed during productive infection are functional homologs of cellular genes and are important for the survival of EBV-infected B cells. The EBV BCRF-1 protein is homologous to interleukin-10 and has interleukin-10 activity.[56] Recombinant BCRF-1 and BCRF-1 secreted from EBV-infected cells inhibit interferon-γ release from activated human peripheral blood mononuclear cells and secretion of interleukin-12 from macrophages. Because interferon-γ is important for the activity of T cells, expression of BCRF-1 during lytic infection may inhibit the ability of cytotoxic T cells to destroy EBV-infected cells. BCRF-1 protein also acts as a B-cell growth factor.

The EBV BARF-1 protein acts as a soluble receptor for colony stimulating factor 1.[57] BARF-1 inhibits interferon-α secretion by human monocytes. Because interferon-α inhibits outgrowth of EBV-infected B cells in vitro, BARF-1 may act in concert with BCRF-1 to inhibit interferon and promote increased survival of EBV-infected cells.

The EBV BHRF-1 protein is homologous to Bcl-2, a cellular protein that is activated in follicular lymphomas and protects cells from apoptosis. BHRF-1 colocalizes with bcl-2 in the cytoplasm and protects Burkitt's lymphoma cells from apoptosis.[58] EBV BALF-1 is also homologous to bcl-2 and antagonizes the antiapoptotic effect of BHRF-1.[59]

Table 20-2 Diseases Associated with EBV Latent Gene Expression

Disease	EBERs	EBNA-1	EBNA-2	LMP-1	LMP-2
Burkitt's lymphoma	+	+	–	–	–
Nasopharyngeal carcinoma	+	+	–	+	+
Hodgkin's disease	+	+	–	+	+
Peripheral T-cell lymphoma	+	+	–	+	+
Lymphoproliferative disease	+	+	+	+	+

Animal Models Several animal models have been used to study EBV oncogenesis. EBV-infected cell lines produce B-cell tumors when inoculated intracerebrally into nude mice. Inoculation of peripheral blood leukocytes from EBV-seropositive humans into mice with severe combined immunodeficiency results in development of human B-cell lymphomas in the animals. Inoculation of these mice with peripheral blood leukocytes from EBV-seronegative humans results in engraftment of a human immune system, and if these latter mice are subsequently injected with cell-free EBV, the animals develop immunoblastic lymphomas. These B cell tumors express the full complement of EBNA and LMP genes characteristic of latently infected, growth-transformed cell lines.[60] Cotton-top tamarins inoculated with a large dose of cell-free EBV develop multifocal large-cell lymphomas over the ensuing few weeks. These tumors express EBNA-1, EBNA-2, EBNA-LP, and LMP-1[61] and are monoclonal or oligoclonal in origin. Inoculation of Rag2 knockout mice with CD34+ human cord blood cells followed by injection with EBV results in EBV+ B-cell proliferative lesions in the liver and spleen,[62] while inoculation of NOD/SCID mice with human CD34+ cells followed by injection with EBV results in lymphomas that express the EBV latency genes.[63]

Clinical Aspects EBV infection is usually spread by saliva. The virus infects B cells directly or oropharyngeal epithelial cells, and then spreads to subepithelial B cells.[64] During primary infection, up to a few percent of the peripheral blood B lymphocytes are infected with EBV and have the capacity to proliferate indefinitely in vitro. Natural killer (NK) cells, suppressor T cells, and HLA- and EBNA- or LMP-restricted cytotoxic T cells control the latently infected B lymphocytes. T- and B-cell interactions release lymphokines and cytokines, giving rise to many of the clinical manifestations of acute infectious mononucleosis. After recovery, the fraction of B cells latently infected with EBV in the peripheral blood remains at 1 in 10^5 to 1 in 10^6. These lymphocytes are the primary site of EBV persistence and a source of virus for persistent infection of epithelial surfaces.

The B-cell tumors that occur early after EBV infection are usually lymphoproliferative processes in which latent virus infection in B cells is the principal cause of proliferation. Oral hairy leukoplakia may be the epithelial counterpart. In contrast, Burkitt's lymphoma and nasopharyngeal carcinoma occur long after primary EBV infection; although etiologically related to EBV, viral gene expression may not be important to the growth of the clinically evident malignant cells.

Lymphoproliferative Disease EBV is associated with B-cell lymphoproliferative disease in patients with congenital immunodeficiency. X-linked lymphoproliferative syndrome is an inherited immunodeficiency of males who have apparently normal cellular and humoral immune responses before infection with EBV. With EBV infection, most of the patients die of a fatal lymphoproliferative disorder or fulminant hepatitis, but some survive with hypogammaglobulinemia. EBV nuclear antigens have been detected in lesions from these patients. The gene mutated in X-linked lymphoproliferative syndrome has been identified as SAP,[65] also termed SH2D1A or DSHP. SAP encodes an SH2-containing protein that interacts with the signaling lymphocyte-activation molecule (SLAM) on B and T cells, and with 2B4 on NK and T cells.

EBV is also associated with fatal infectious mononucleosis in persons with no known underlying genetic predisposition or in patients with congenital immunodeficiencies, such as severe combined immunodeficiency. EBV lymphoproliferative disease occurs in patients who are immunosuppressed as a result of transplantation or acquired immunodeficiency syndrome (AIDS).[66,67] Risk factors for development of lymphoproliferative disease include EBV-seronegativity prior to transplant, receipt of T-cell depleted bone marrow or antilymphocyte antibody, and concurrent cytomegalovirus disease. Lymphoproliferative lesions are most commonly seen in the lymph nodes, liver, lungs, kidney, bone marrow, or small intestine. Tumors in transplant patients are usually classified as lymphomas or immunoblastic sarcomas; some patients have hyperplastic lesions. The proliferating lymphocytes in these tumors generally do not have chromosomal translocations.

AIDS-related lymphomas may be systemic (nodal or extranodal) lymphomas, primary central nervous system lymphomas, or primary effusion lymphomas. Primary effusion lymphomas often contain EBV in addition to HHV-8. Although most B-cell tumors in transplant recipients and central nervous system lymphomas in AIDS patients contain EBV, about 50% of other lymphomas in AIDS patients contain EBV. Tumors in patients with AIDS are usually either immunoblastic lymphomas or Burkitt's lymphomas; most of the latter have c-*myc* translocations.

Tissues from transplant recipients or AIDS patients with EBV lymphoproliferative disease show expression of EBERs, EBNA-1, EBNA-2, and LMP-1 (Table 20-2). The EBV viral load in the peripheral blood has been used to predict development of disease and to follow patients after therapy. The expression of these EBV genes, which are targets for cytotoxic T cells, has important implications for therapy. Infusion of EBV-specific cytotoxic T cells, nonirradiated donor leukocytes, or HLA-matched allogeneic cytotoxic T cells have been effective in some cases for treatment of EBV lymphoproliferative disease.[68-70] Anti-CD20 antibody (rituximab) has induced remissions in some patients, and has been used in some studies as pre-emptive therapy when EBV viral DNA in the blood is rising in transplant recipients at risk of lymphoproliferative disease,[71] although other studies suggest that pre-emptive therapy may be unnecessary.[72]

Burkitt's Lymphoma Seroepidemiologic studies show a strong association between Burkitt's lymphoma and EBV in Africa. More than 90% of African Burkitt's lymphomas are associated with EBV, whereas only approximately 20% of Burkitt's lymphomas in the United States are associated with the virus. African patients with Burkitt's lymphoma often have high levels of antibody to EBV antigens, and the virus can be recovered from the tissue. Burkitt's lymphoma tissues express EBERs and EBNA-1, but not EBNA-2, EBNA-3, or LMP-1.

Burkitt's lymphomas contain chromosomal translocations that result in c-*myc* dysregulation. The most common chromosomal translocation, t(8;14), places a portion of the c-*myc* oncogene adjacent to an immunoglobulin heavy chain gene. Less common translocations involve the c-*myc* oncogene and the κ or λ immunoglobulin light chain genes t(2;8) and t(8;22), respectively. These translocations result in high constitutive expression of c-*myc*. Dysregulated expression of c-*myc* in EBV-immortalized lymphoblastoid cell lines results in highly transformed cells that form tumors when injected into immunodeficient mice.[73] Transgenic mice that express a mutated human c-*myc* that is derived from a Burkitt's lymphoma and is fused to the Igλ locus develop tumors that have histologic and phenotypic features of Burkitt's lymphomas.[74] Thus, engineering a portion of a Burkitt's lymphoma chromosomal translocation into mice can reconstitute the features of the disease.

EBV-associated endemic Burkitt's lymphoma is thought to develop in steps. First, EBV infection may expand the pool of differentiating and proliferating B cells. Second, chronic holoendemic malaria may cause T-cell suppression and B-cell proliferation. Third, enhanced proliferation of differentiating B cells may favor the chance occurrence of a reciprocal c-*myc* (t[8;14] or t[8;22]) translocation placing c-*myc* partially under the control of immunoglobulin-related transcriptional enhancers, with development of a monoclonal tumor.

Nasopharyngeal Carcinoma The nonkeratinizing nasopharyngeal carcinomas are uniformly associated with EBV. Seroepidemiologic studies indicate that patients with nasopharyngeal carcinoma have high levels of antibodies to EBV antigens. A large prospective study of Taiwanese men showed that those with IgA antibodies to viral capsid antigen (VCA) and anti-EBV deoxyribonuclease (DNAse) antibodies had a markedly increased risk of developing nasopharyngeal carcinoma when compared to those men without these antibodies.[75] These antibodies are useful in screening patients for early detection of nasopharyngeal carcinoma and are prognostic for patients after treatment. Another study showed that quantitating the level of EBV DNA in plasma of patients with advanced nasopharyngeal carcinoma was useful for monitoring patients and predicting outcomes.[76] Nasopharyngeal carcinoma tissue contains EBV genomes in every cell. Biopsy tissue shows expression of EBERs, EBNA-1, LMP-1, and LMP-2. These tumors are monoclonal with regard to EBV infection, indicating that EBV infection precedes malignant cell outgrowth at the cellular level. Unlike Burkitt's lymphoma, the association of EBV with nasopharyngeal carcinoma is uniform and universal.

Hodgkin's Disease Persons with a history of infectious mononucleosis are at a greater risk of developing Hodgkin's disease.[77] Patients with Hodgkin's disease generally have higher titers of antibody to EBV VCA than does the general population. Tissues from approximately 40 to 60% of patients with Hodgkin's disease contain EBV genomes. Cases of Hodgkin's disease in patients with human immunodeficiency virus (HIV) or from developing countries are more likely to contain EBV genomes than persons without HIV or from developed countries.[78] The EBV genome is present in Reed-Sternberg cells and the viral genome is monoclonal. EBV is more often associated with aggressive subtypes (especially mixed cellularity) of Hodgkin's disease. Reed-Sternberg cells from tumors express EBERs, EBNA-1, LMP-1, and LMP-2, but not EBNA-2. Tumors from patients with EBV+ Hodgkin's disease and some from patients with lymphoproliferative disease arise from postgerminal center cells.[2,79] Infusion of cytotoxic T cells generated from 11 patients with relapsed Hodgkin's disease and measurable disease resulted in complete remissions in 2 patients, partial remission in 1 patient, stable disease in 5 patients, and no response in 3 patients.[80]

Other Tumors Associated with Epstein-Barr Virus EBV genomes and EBNA-1, LMP-1, and LMP-2 have been detected in tissues from patients with peripheral T-cell lymphomas; EBNA-2, however, is not present.[81] EBV DNA has also been detected in central nervous system lymphomas from patients with no underlying immunodeficiency, T cells in patients with virus-associated hemophagocytic syndrome, nasal T/NK-cell lymphoma, carcinoma of the palatine tonsil, supraglottic laryngeal carcinoma, and angioimmunoblastic lymphadenopathy. EBV DNA and nuclear antigens have been detected in thymic carcinomas and in lesions from lymphomatoid granulomatosis.

EBV DNA has been found in leiomyosarcomas in AIDS patients,[82] and viral RNA and EBNA-2 have been detected in smooth muscle tumors in organ transplant recipients.[83] EBV DNA, RNA, and EBNA-1 (but not EBNA-2 or LMP-1) were detected in 7% of primary gastric carcinomas, especially in undifferentiated lymphoepithelioma-like carcinomas.

Although some reports suggested that EBV is associated with breast carcinomas, in most of these studies EBV was detected by PCR and viral proteins were found in only a fraction of the tumor cells.[84,85] More recent studies using in situ hybridization and immunochemistry have generally not supported an association of EBV and breast carcinoma.[86,87]

HUMAN HERPESVIRUS 8 AND MALIGNANCIES

In 1994, Chang and colleagues detected sequences of a new human herpesvirus in Kaposi's sarcoma tissues from patients with AIDS.[88] This agent is now termed human herpesvirus 8 (HHV-8) or Kaposi's sarcoma-associated herpesvirus. Sequence analysis indicates that HHV-8, like EBV, is a member of the gammaherpesvirus subfamily. However, while EBV is a lymphocryptovirus (gammaherpesvirus-1), HHV-8 is a Rhadinovirus (gammaherpesvirus-2).

HHV-8 is present in B cells in asymptomatic persons. B-cell lines derived from primary effusion lymphomas maintain HHV-8 in a latent state and can be induced to undergo lytic virus replication by the addition of phorbol ester or butyrate. Foscarnet, ganciclovir, and cidofovir, but not acyclovir, inhibit virus production when these cells are induced to replicate virus.[89]

Infection of dermal microvascular endothelial cells in vitro with HHV-8 results in transformation of the cells with maintenance of long-term infection. The cells become spindle shaped and show loss of contact inhibition with anchorage-independent growth.[90] The cells can be induced to undergo lytic replication with TPA. HHV-8 also transforms bone marrow-derived endothelial cells; however, the virus is present in only a small fraction of the cells and proliferation is likely caused by a paracrine mechanism.[91] Integrin $\alpha_3\beta_1$ is a receptor for the virus in some cells.[92]

VIRAL PROTEINS

HHV-8 encodes a large number of cellular homologs (Table 20-3) that have been grouped into different classes, depending on when they are expressed in primary effusion lymphoma cell lines.[93] Several HHV-8 genes may contribute to its oncogenicity.

Expression of the HHV-8 *K1* gene in rodent fibroblasts results in transformation of the cells.[94] Substitution of the STP oncogene in *Herpesvirus saimiri* with the HHV-8 *K1* gene maintains the transforming activity of *Herpesvirus saimiri* in vitro and in vivo. K1 is a transmembrane protein whose cytoplasmic domain has an immunoreceptor tyrosine-based activation motif (ITAM). The K1 protein induces tyrosine phosphorylation in cells[95] and activates the Akt signaling pathway.[96] Expression of this gene in cells results in constitutive calcium-dependent signal activation in B cells in the absence of exogenous stimuli.[97]

The HHV-8 *K2* gene encodes an interleukin (IL)-6 homolog (vIL-6). IL-6 is a B-cell growth factor and acts as an autocrine growth factor for lymphoid tumors resulting in proliferation.[98] vIL-6 prevents death of IL-6–dependent B9 cells in vitro,[99] promotes hematopoiesis, and induces vascular endothelial growth factor (VEGF) to promote angiogenesis.[100] The K3 and K5 proteins induce rapid endocytosis of MHC class I molecules from the surface of cells.[101] The K5 protein also downregulates ICAM-1 and B7.2, which results in inhibition of NK cell-mediated cytotoxicity.[102]

The HHV-8 *K4*, *K4.1*, and *K6* genes encode three chemokines: the viral macrophage inflammatory proteins (MIP)-II, -III, and -I, respectively. vMIP-I inhibits replication of HIV strains dependent on CCR5.[99] Each of the viral chemokines partially block HIV infection of peripheral blood mononuclear cells and are angiogenic. vMIP-I and vMIP-III are chemokine receptor agonists for CCR8[103] and CCR4,[104] respectively, while vMIP-II is a broad-spectrum chemokine receptor antagonist. vMIP-II is a chemoattractant for eosinophils,[105] binds to both CC and CXC chemokines, and blocks calcium mobilization induced by chemokines.[106]

The HHV-8 *K8* and *ORF50* genes encode the homologs of the EBV BZLF1 and BRLF1 proteins, and transactivate expression of other HHV-8 genes during lytic viral replication. K8 and ORF50 inhibit the activity of p53.[107,108] The HHV-8 K9, K11.1, and K10.5 proteins are referred to as viral interferon regulatory factor (vIRF)-1, -2, and -3, respectively. Each of these proteins inhibits virus-mediated activation of the interferon-α promoter. vIRF1and vIRF3 inhibit p53-mediated apoptosis[109,110] and transform NIH 3T3 cells, which can then induce tumors in nude mice.[111] vIRF3 (also called latency-associated nuclear antigen 2 [LANA2]) protects cells from p53-induced apoptosis.[113,112] HHV-8 ORF45

Table 20-3 Selected HHV-8 Genes and Their Cellular Homologs and Activities

Gene	Expression Class	Cellular Homolog	Activity
K1	II	ITAM motif	Transformation, activates signaling pathways
K2	II	IL-6	B-cell growth factor; angiogenesis; hematopoiesis
K3	III	None	Reduces surface MHC class I
K4	II	MIP-1α	Chemokine receptor antagonist; angiogenesis; chemotaxis
K4.1	II	MIP-1α	Chemokine receptor agonist; angiogenesis; chemotaxis
K5	II	None	Inhibits NK cell activity; reduces surface MHC class I
K6	II	MIP-1α	Chemokine receptor agonist; angiogenesis; chemotaxis
K8	III	None	Inhibits p53
K9	II	IRF	Represses interferon activity; transformation; inhibits p53
K10.5 (LANA-2)	II	IRF	Represses interferon activity; inhibits apoptosis; inhibits p53
K11.1	I	IRF	Represses interferon activity
K12 (Kaposin)	II	None	Transformation
K14	II	OX-2	Induces proinflammatory cytokines
K15 (LAMP)	III	None	Binds TRAFs; inhibits B-cell receptor signaling
ORF4	II	CR2	Complement binding protein
ORF16	II/III	Bcl-2	Inhibits apoptosis
ORF71	I	FLIP	Inhibits apoptosis; activates NF-κB
ORF72	I	Cyclin D	Cell-cycle progression; inhibits Rb
ORF73 (LANA-1)	I	None	Episome maintenance, inhibits p53 and Rb
ORF74	II	GPCR	Angiogenesis; transformation and proliferation

Expression: class I = latent gene, expressed in uninduced primary effusion lymphoma cells, not induced by phorbol ester; class II = expressed in uninduced cells, induced by TPA; class III = lytic gene, expressed only after induction by TPA (includes many structural proteins and DNA replication enzymes). FLIP = FLICE inhibitory protein; GPCR = G protein-coupled receptor; IRF = interferon regulatory factor; ITAM = immunoreceptor tyrosine-based activation motif; MHC= major histocompatibility complex; MIP = macrophage inflammatory protein; NK = natural killer; Rb = retinoblastoma protein; TRAFs = TNFR associated factors.

blocks the activity of IRF7 and inhibits the activation of interferon-α and –β.[113]

The HHV-8 K12 protein, also called kaposin, induces transformation of cells; injection of these transformed cells into nude mice results in highly vascularized sarcomas.[114] The HHV-8 K14 protein, a homolog of the cellular OX2 protein, stimulates monocytes to produce proinflammatory cytokines such as TNF-α, IL-1β, and IL-6.[115] HHV-8 ORF4 protein inhibits the complement system.[116] HHV-8 ORF16 encodes a homolog of the cellular Bcl-2 protein and inhibits bax-induced apoptosis.[117] The ORF71 gene encodes a homolog of cellular FLIP that blocks apoptosis. HHV-8 ORF71 activates NF-κB, promotes tumor growth, and is required for survival of KSHV-infected lymphoma cells.[118–120] HHV-8 ORF72 encodes a cyclin D homolog that binds to and activates cdk6 and stimulates cell-cycle progression in normally quiescent fibroblasts.[121] The viral cyclin protein phosphorylates and thereby inactivates the retinoblastoma tumor-suppressor protein.[122]

HHV-8 ORF73 encodes LANA1 that localizes with viral DNA episomes and tethers them to chromosomes during cell division.[123] Like EBV EBNA-1, HHV-8 LANA1 is required for persistence of the episome in dividing cells and transactivates its own promoter. In addition, LANA1 inhibits the activity of both p53 and the retinoblastoma protein,[124,125] and up-regulates expression and stabilizes β-catenin.[126]

HHV-8 ORF74 encodes a G protein-coupled receptor that is homologous to the cellular IL-8 receptor; unlike the latter protein, however, the HHV-8 receptor is constitutively active and induces cellular proliferation.[127] This protein activates angiogenesis,[128] activates the Akt signaling pathway,[129] and induces lesions that resemble Kaposi's sarcoma in transgenic mice.[130] ORF74 activates NF-κB and c-*jun*-N-terminal kinase, and up-regulates IL-1, IL-8, tumor necrosis factor (TNF), fibroblast growth factor (FGF), and VEGF.

HHV-8 K15 encodes the latency-associated membrane protein (LAMP). HHV-8 K15, like EBV LMP-1, interacts with TRAFs 1, 2, and 3.[131] K15 suppresses tyrosine phosphorylation and intracellular calcium mobilization, inhibiting B-cell–receptor signaling.[132]

CLINICAL ASPECTS

Seroprevalence rates for HHV-8 vary from < 5% in normal blood donors in the United States or United Kingdom to 30 to 35% in HIV-positive homosexual men.[133] Antibody to HHV-8 is more common in African and Mediterranean populations. At least 85% of patients with Kaposi's sarcoma have antibodies to HHV-8.[134] The prevalence of Kaposi's sarcoma is lower in women than in men, and HIV-seropositive women have a much lower incidence of antibody to HHV-8 than do seropositive men. HHV-8 seropositivity in HIV-positive homosexual men is predictive of subsequent development of Kaposi's sarcoma.[135] The virus is not thought to be pathogenic in most healthy individuals and can persist in a latent phase for life; however, in immunocompromised persons, it is strongly associated with Kaposi's sarcoma. Thus, although infection with HHV-8 appears to be required for development of Kaposi's sarcoma, it is probably not sufficient by itself, and other cofactors, such as HIV and impaired cellular immunity, may have important roles. HHV-8 is thought to be sexually transmitted in homosexual men[133] and has been associated with sexual transmission and intravenous drug use in women.[136] In endemic populations (eg, Africa) HHV-8 may be transmitted vertically from mother to child and between siblings. HHV-8 has been transmitted by renal allografts, and kidney transplant recipients have subsequently developed Kaposi's sarcoma in cells of donor origin.[137,138]

Kaposi's Sarcoma HHV-8 has been found in nearly all biopsies of classic Kaposi's sarcoma, African endemic Kaposi's sarcoma, Kaposi's sarcoma in HIV-seronegative transplant recipients and homosexual men, and Kaposi's sarcoma in patients with AIDS.[139] HHV-8 is present in the endothelial and spindle cells of the tumor, but not in normal endothelium.[140] Most of the tumor cells are latently infected with the virus, but 1 to 5% of the spindle cells in HIV-positive Kaposi's sarcoma show lytic HHV-8 infection. LANA1, K12, viral cyclin, ORF71, ORF74, and vMIP-III are expressed in these tissues. Various studies indicate that Kaposi's sarcoma can be polyclonal, oligoclonal, or monoclonal. HHV-8 is also present in the peripheral blood mononuclear cells of approximately 50% of patients with Kaposi's sarcoma, and its presence is predictive of development of the malignancy.[133] HHV-8 has also been detected in the saliva of patients with Kaposi's sarcoma and, infrequently, in semen. Foscarnet and ganciclovir reportedly reduce the frequency of new Kaposi's sarcoma lesions in some, but not all, studies.[141,142] Cidofovir had no effect on treatment of established lesions.[143] In contrast, HIV protease inhibitors have been reported to induce regression of Kaposi's sarcoma lesions.[144]

Primary Effusion Lymphoma HHV-8 has also been found in primary effusion lymphomas in patients with AIDS.[140,145] These body cavity-based lymphomas of B-cell lineage are located in the pleural, peritoneal, or pericardial space and usually contain EBV genomes as well as HHV-8. Some HHV-8–positive lymphomas have been found in patients without AIDS. LANA1, K12, viral cyclin, ORF71, and IRF3 are expressed in these lymphomas; approximately 20% of the cells express vIL-6.

Multicentric Castleman's disease HHV-8 has also been detected in biopsies from some patients with multicentric Castleman's disease, especially in the variant known as the plasma cell type.[140,146] This disease is usually polyclonal and presents as generalized lymphadenopathy, fever, and hypergammaglobulinemia. HHV-8 is detected more frequently in biopsies from HIV-positive patients than in biopsies from those patients without HIV. HHV-8 is present in the immunoblastic B cells of the mantle zone of the lesions. These lesions express multiple proteins including the latency-associated proteins LANA1, ORF71, vIRF1, vIRF3, and vIL-6, and lytic proteins.[147]

Other Diseases HHV-8 is associated with fever, plasmacytosis, and bone marrow failure after kidney and stem cell transplantation.[148] Although initial reports detected HHV-8 sequences in dendritic cells from multiple myeloma and in prostatic carcinomas, other studies have not confirmed these findings.[140] HHV-8 has been detected in lung lesions of patients with primary pulmonary hypertension in some, but not other, studies; these lesions share many of the features of angioproliferative lesions seen in Kaposi's sarcoma.[149] HHV-8 has been found in a variety of other tumors, including angioimmunoblastic lymphadenopathy with dysproteinemia and angiosarcoma, but detection of the virus has been inconsistent among various studies.

ONCOGENIC POTENTIAL OF OTHER HUMAN HERPESVIRUSES

Cytomegalovirus is not oncogenic in humans. Although viral antigen or viral DNA has been demonstrated in some tumors (eg, Kaposi's sarcomas in AIDS patients, colon carcinomas), a similar level of cytomegalovirus antigen or DNA indicative of latent infection has been detected in nontumor tissue from control patients. Similarly, initial seroepidemiologic studies suggested a role for herpes simplex virus 2 in cervical carcinoma, yet there has been no convincing evidence for viral DNA or antigen in these tissues. Finally, although human herpesvirus-6 DNA has been detected in some lymphomas, it is unknown whether the virus is involved in the pathogenesis of these tumors or whether the virus is associated with the non-neoplastic lymphocytes.

REFERENCES

1. Kieff E, Rickinson AB. Epstein-Barr virus and its replication. In: Knipe DM, Howley PM, editors. Fields virology. Philadelphia: Lippincott Williams & Wilkins; 2001. p. 2511–73.
2. Thorley-Lawson DA, Gross A. Persistence of the Epstein-Barr virus and the origins of associated lymphomas. N Engl J Med 2004;350:1328–37.
3. Birkenbach M, Josefsen K, Yalamanchili R, et al. Epstein-Barr virus-induced genes: first lymphocyte-specific G protein-coupled peptide receptors. J Virol 1993;67:2209–20.
4. Yates J, Warren N, Reisman D, Sugden B. A *cis*-acting element from the Epstein-Barr viral genome that permits stable replication of recombinant plasmids in latently infected cells. Proc Natl Acad Sci U S A 1984;81:3806–10.
5. Deacon EM, Pallesen G, Niedobitek G, et al. Epstein-Barr virus and Hodgkin's disease: transcriptional analysis of virus latency in the malignant cells. J Exp Med 1993;177:339–49.
6. Wilson JB, Bell JL, Levine AJ. Expression of Epstein-Barr virus nuclear antigen 1 induces B cell neoplasia in transgenic mice. EMBO J 1996;15:3117–26.
7. Levitskaya J, Shapiro A, Leonchiks A, et al. Inhibition of ubiquitin/proteosome-dependent protein degradation by the Gly-Ala repeat domain of the Epstein-Barr virus nuclear antigen 1. Proc Natl Acad Sci U S A 1997;94:12616–21.
8. Yin Y, Manoury B, Fahraeus R. Self-inhibition of synthesis and antigen presentation by Epstein-Barr virus-encoded EBNA1. Science 2003;301:1371–4.
9. Voo KS, Fu T, Wang HY, et al. Evidence for the presentation of major histocompatibility complex class I-restricted Epstein-Barr virus nuclear antigen 1 peptides to CD8+ T lymphocytes. J Exp Med 2004;199:459–70.
10. Lee SP, Brooks JM, Al-Jarrah H, et al. CD8 T cell recognition of endogenously expressed Epstein-Barr virus nuclear antigen 1. J Exp Med 2004;199:1409–20.
11. Kennedy G, Komano J, Sugden B. Epstein-Barr virus provides a survival factor to Burkitt's lymphomas. Proc Natl Acad Sci U S A 2003;100:14269–74.
12. Wang F, Tsang SF, Kurilla MG, et al. Epstein-Barr virus nuclear antigen 2 transactivates latent membrane protein. J Virol 1990;64:3407–16.
13. Zimber-Strobl U, Kremmer E, Grasser F, et al. The Epstein-Barr virus nuclear antigen 2 interacts with an EBNA2 responsive *cis*-element of the terminal protein 1 gene promoter. EMBO J 1993;12:167–75.
14. Wang F, Gregory C, Sample C, et al. Epstein-Barr virus latent membrane protein (LMP-1) and nuclear proteins 2 and 3C are effectors of phenotypic changes in B lymphocytes: EBNA-2 and LMP-1 cooperatively induce CD23. J Virol 1990;64:2309–18.
15. Knutson JC. The level of c-fgr RNA is increased by EBNA-2, an Epstein-Barr virus gene required for B-cell immortalization. J Virol 1990;64:2530–6.
16. Henkel T, Ling PD, Hayward SD, Peterson MG. Mediation of Epstein-Barr virus EBNA-2 transactivation by recombination signal-binding protein Jkappa. Science 1994;265:92–5.
17. Gordadze AV, Peng R, Tan J, et al. Notch IIC partially replaces EBNA2 function in B cells immortalized by Epstein-Barr virus. J Virol 2001;75:5899–912.
18. Johannsen E, Koh E, Mosialos G, et al. Epstein-Barr virus nuclear protein 2 transactivation of the latent membrane protein 1 promoter is mediated by Jkappa and PU.1. J Virol 1995;69:253–62.
19. Fuentes-Panana EM, Peng R, Brewer G, et al. Regulation of the Epstein-Barr virus C promoter by AUF1 and the cyclic AMP/protein kinase A signaling pathway. J Virol 2000;74:8166–75.
20. Cohen JI. A region of herpes simplex virus VP16 can substitute for a transforming domain of Epstein-Barr virus nuclear protein 2. Proc Natl Acad Sci U S A 1992;89:8030–4.
21. Tong X, Wang F, Thut CJ, Kieff E. The Epstein-Barr virus nuclear protein 2 acidic domain can interact with TFIIB, TAF40, and RPA70 but not with TATA-binding protein. J Virol 1995;69:585–8.
22. Lee JM, Lee KH, Weidner M, et al. Epstein-Barr virus EBNA2 blocks Nur77- mediated apoptosis. Proc Natl Acad Sci U S A 2002;99:11878–83.
23. Peng CW, Xue Y, Zhao B, et al. Direct interactions between Epstein-Barr virus leader protein LP and the EBNA2 cidic domain underlie coordinate transcriptional regulation. Proc Natl Acad Sci U S A 2004;101:1033–8.
24. Szekely L, Selivanova G, Magnusson KP, et al. EBNA-5, an Epstein-Barr virus-encoded nuclear antigen, binds to the retinoblastoma and p53 proteins. Proc Natl Acad Sci U S A 1993;90:5455–9.
25. Mannick JB, Cohen JI, Birkenbach M, et al. The Epstein Barr virus nuclear protein encoded by the leader of the EBNA RNAs is important in B lymphocyte transformation. J Virol 1991;65:6826–37.
26. Robertson ES, Lin J, Kieff E. The amino-terminal domains of Epstein-Barr virus nuclear proteins 3A, 3B, and 3C interact with RBPJkappa. J Virol 1996;70:3068–74.
27. Subramanian C, Cotter MA, Robertson ES. Epstein-Barr virus nuclear protein EBNA-3C interacts with the human metastatic suppressor Nm23-HI: a molecular link to cancer metastasis. Nat Med 2001;7:350–5.
28. Tomkinson B, Robertson E, Kieff E. Epstein-Barr virus nuclear proteins (EBNA) 3A and 3C are essential for B lymphocyte growth transformation. J Virol 1993;67:2014–25.
29. Higuchi M, Izumi KM, Kieff E. Epstein-Barr virus latent-infection membrane proteins are palmitoylated and raft-associated: protein 1 binds to the cytoskeleton and through TNF receptor cytoplasmic factors. Proc Natl Acad Sci U S A 2001;98:4675–80.
30. Wang D, Liebowitz D, Kieff E. An EBV membrane protein expressed in immortalized lymphocytes transforms established rodent cells. Cell 1985;43:831–40.
31. Fries KL, Miller WE, Raab-Traub N. Epstein-Barr virus latent membrane protein 1 blocks p53-mediated apoptosis through the induction of the A20 gene. J Virol 1996;70:8653–9.
32. Dawson CW, Rickinson AB, Young LS. Epstein-Barr virus latent membrane protein inhibits human epithelial cell differentiation. Nature 1990;344:777–80.
33. Devergne O, Hatzivassiliou E, Izumi KM, et al. Association of TRAF1, TRAF2, and TRAF3 with an Epstein-Barr virus LMP1 domain important for B-lymphocyte transformation: role in NF-κB activation. Mol Cell Biol 1996;16:7098–108.
34. Izumi KM, Kieff ED. The Epstein-Barr virus oncogene product latent membrane protein 1 engages the tumor necrosis factor receptor-associated death domain protein to mediate B lymphocyte growth transformation and activate NF-κB. Proc Natl Acad Sci U S A 1997;94:12592–7.
35. Gires O, Kohlhuber F, Kilger E, et al. Latent membrane protein 1 of Epstein-Barr virus interacts with JAK3 and activates STAT proteins. EMBO J 1999;18:3064–73.
36. Uchida J, Yasui T, Takaoka-Shichijo Y, et al. Mimicry of CD40 signals by Epstein-Barr virus LMP-1 in B lymphocyte responses. Science 1999;286:300–3.
37. Yoshizaki T, Sato H, Furukawa M, et al. The expression of matrix metalloproteinase 9 is enhanced by Epstein-Barr virus latent membrane protein 1. Proc Natl Acad Sci U S A 1998;95:3621–6.
38. Miller WE, Cheshire JL, Raab-Traub N. Interaction of tumor necrosis factor receptor-associated factor signaling proteins with the latent membrane protein 1 PXQXT motif is essential for induction of epidermal growth factor receptor expression. Mol Cell Biol 1998;18:2835–44.
39. Kaye KM, Izumi KM, Kieff E. Epstein-Barr virus latent membrane protein 1 is essential for B-lymphocyte growth transformation. Proc Natl Acad Sci U S A 1993;90:9150–4.
40. Wilson JB, Weinberg W, Johnson R, et al. Expression of the BNLF-1 oncogene of Epstein-Barr virus in the skin of transgenic mice induces hyperplasia and aberrant expression of keratin 6. Cell 1990;61:1315–27.
41. Kulwichit W, Edwards RH, Davenport EM, et al. Expression of the Epstein-Barr virus latent membrane protein 1 induces B cell lymphoma in transgenic mice. Proc Natl Acad Sci U S A 1998;95:11963–8.
42. Liebowitz D. Epstein-Barr virus and a cellular signaling pathway in lymphomas from immunosuppressed patients. N Engl J Med 1998;338:1413–21.
43. Longnecker R, Miller CL, Tomkinson B, et al. Deletion of DNA encoding the first five transmembrane domains of Epstein-Barr virus latent membrane proteins 2A and 2B. J Virol 1993;67:5068–74.
44. Scholle F, Bendt KM, Raab-Traub N. Epstein-Barr virus LMP2A transforms epithelial cells, inhibits cell differentiation, and activates Akt. J Virol 2000;74:10681–9.
45. Miller CL, Burkhardt AL, Lee JH, et al. Integral membrane protein 2 of Epstein-Barr virus regulates reactivation from latency through dominant negative effects on protein-tyrosine kinases. Immunity 1995;2:155–66.
46. Miller CL, Lee JH, Kieff, E, Longnecker R. An integral membrane protein (LMP2) blocks reactivation of Epstein-Barr virus from latency following surface immunoglobulin crosslinking. Proc Natl Acad Sci U S A 1994;91:772–6.
47. Caldwell RG. Wilson JB, Anderson SJ, Longnecker R. Epstein-Barr virus LMP2A drives B cell development and survival in the absence of normal B cell receptor signals. Immunity 1998;9:405–11.
48. Morrison JA, Klingelhutz AJ, Raab-Traub N. Epstein-Barr virus latent membrane protein 2A activates beta-catenin signaling in epithelial cells. J Virol 2003 77:12276–84.
49. Swaminathan S, Tomkinson B, Kieff E. Recombinant Epstein-Barr virus with small RNA (EBER) genes deleted transforms lymphocytes and replicates in vitro. Proc Natl Acad Sci U S A 1991;88:1546–50.
50. Kitagawa N, Goto M, Kurozumi K, et al. Epstein-Barr virus-encoded poly(A)(–) RNA supports Burkitt's lymphoma growth through interleukin-10 induction. EMBO J 2000;19:6742–50.
51. Clarke PA, Schwemmle M, Schickinger J, et al. Binding of the Epstein-Barr virus small RNA EBER-1 to double-stranded RNA-activated protein kinase. Nucleic Acids Res 1991;19:243–8.
52. Sharp TV, Raine DA, Gewert DR, et al. Activation of the interferon-inducible (2'–5') oligoadenylate synthetase by the Epstein-Barr virus RNA, EBER-1. Virology 1999;257:303–13.
53. Morrison TE, Mauser A, Klingelhutz A, et al. Epstein-Barr virus immediate-early protein BZLF1 inhibits tumor necrosis factor alpha-induced signaling and apoptosis by downregulating tumor necrosis factor receptor 1. J Virol 2004;78:544–9.
54. Morrison TE, Mauser A, Wong A, et al. Inhibition of interferon-gamma signaling by an Epstein-Barr virus immediate-early protein. Immunity 2001;15:787–99.
55. Mauser A, Saito S, Appella E, et al. The Epstein-Barr virus immediate-early protein BZLF1 regulates p53 function through multiple mechanisms. J Virol 2002;76:12503–12.
56. Hsu D-H, de Waal Malefyt R, Fiorentino DF, et al. Expression of interleukin-10 activity by Epstein-Barr virus protein BCRF1. Science 1990;250:830–2.
57. Cohen JI, Lekstrom K. The Epstein-Barr virus BARF1 protein is dispensable for B cell transformation and inhibits interferon alpha secretion from mononuclear cells. J Virol 1999;73;7627–32.
58. Henderson S, Huen D, Rowe M, et al. Epstein-Barr virus-coded BHRF1 protein, a viral homolog of bcl-2, protects

human B cells from programmed cell death. Proc Natl Acad Sci U S A 1993;90:8479–83.
59. Bellows DS, Howell M, Pearson C, et al. Epstein-Barr virus BALF1 is a bcl-2-like antagonist of the herpesvirus anti-apoptotic bcl-2 proteins. J Virol 2002;76:2469–79.
60. Rowe M, Young LS, Crocker J, et al. Epstein-Barr virus (EBV)-associated lymphoproliferative disease in the SCID mouse model: implications for the pathogenesis of EBV-positive lymphomas in man. J Exp Med 1991;173:147–58.
61. Young LS, Finerty S, Brooks L, et al. Epstein-Barr virus gene expression in malignant lymphomas induced by experimental virus infection of cotton-top tamarins. J Virol 1989;63:1967–74.
62. Traggiai E, Chicha L, Mazzucchelli L, et al. Development of a human adaptive immune system in cord blood cell-transplanted mice. Science 2004;304(5667):104–7.
63. Islas-Ohlmaayer M, Padgett-Thomas A, Domiati-Saad R, et al. Experimental infection of NOD/SCID mice reconstituted with human CD34+ cells with Epstein-Barr virus. J Virol 2004;78:13891–900.
64. Cohen JI. Epstein-Barr virus infection. N Engl J Med 2000;343:481–92.
65. Sayos J, Wu C, Morra N, et al. The X-linked lymphoproliferative-disease gene product SAP regulates signals induced through the co-receptor SLAM. Nature 1998;395:462–9.
66. Cohen JI. Epstein-Barr virus lymphoproliferative disease associated with acquired immunodeficiency. Medicine 1991;70:137–60.
67. Paya CV, Fung JJ, Nalesnik MA, et al. Epstein-Barr virus induced posttransplant lymphoproliferative disorders. Transplantation 1999;68:1517–25.
68. O'Reilly RJ, Small TN, Papadopoulos E, et al. Biology and adoptive cell therapy of Epstein-Barr virus-associated lymphoproliferative disorders in recipients of marrow allografts. Immunol Rev 1997;157:195–216.
69. Rooney CM, Smith CA, Ng YC, et al. Infusion of cytotoxic T cells for the prevention and treatment of Epstein-Barr virus-induced lymphomas in allogeneic transplant recipients. Blood 1998;5:1549–55.
70. Haque T, Wilkie GM, Taylor C, et al. Treatment of Epstein-Barr-virus-positive post-transplantation lymphoproliferative disease with partly HLA-matched allogeneic cytotoxic T cells. Lancet 2002;360:436–42.
71. van Esser JW, Niesters HG, van der Holt B, et al. Prevention of Epstein-Barr virus-lymphoproliferative disease by molecular monitoring and preemptive rituximab in high-risk patients after allogeneic stem cell transplantation. Blood 2002;99:4364–9.
72. Wagner HJ, Cheng YC, Huls MH, et al. Prompt versus preemptive intervention for EBV lymphoproliferative disease. Blood 2004 103:3979–81.
73. Lombardi L, Newcomb EW, Dalla-Favera R. Pathogenesis of Burkitt lymphoma: expression of an activated c-myc oncogene causes the tumorigenic conversion of EBV-infected human B lymphocytes. Cell 1987;49:161–70.
74. Kovalchuk AL, Qi C-F, Torrey TA, et al. Burkitt lymphoma in the mouse. J Exp Med 2000;192:1183–90.
75. Chien Y-C, Chen J-Y, Liu M-Y, et al. Serological markers of Epstein-Barr virus infection and nasopharyngeal carcinoma in Taiwanese men. N Engl J Med 2001;345:1877–82.
76. Lin JC, Wang WY, Chen KY, et al. Quantification of plasma Epstein-Barr virus DNA in patients with advanced nasopharyngeal carcinoma. N Engl J Med 2004;350:2461–70.
77. Hjalgrim H, Askling J, Rostgaard K, et al. Characteristics of Hodgkin's lymphoma after infectious mononucleosis. N Engl J Med 2003;349:1324–32.
78. Glaser SL, Lin RJ, Stewart SL, et al. Epstein-Barr virus associated Hodgkin's disease: epidemiologic characteristics in international data. Int J Cancer 1997;70:375–82.
79. Timms JM, Bell A, Flavell JR, et al. Target cells of Epstein-Barr-virus (EBV)-positive post-transplant lymphoproliferative disease: similarities to EBV-positive Hodgkin's lymphoma. Lancet 2003;361:217–23.
80. Bollard CM, Aguilar L, Straathof KC, et al. Cytotoxic T lymphocyte therapy for Epstein-Barr Virus+ Hodgkin's disease. J Exp Med 2004;200:1623–33.
81. Chen C-L, Sadler RH, Walling DM, et al. Epstein-Barr virus gene expression in EBV-positive peripheral lymphomas. J Virol 1993;67:6303–8.
82. McClain KL, Leach CT, Jensen HB, et al. Association of Epstein-Barr virus with leiomyosarcomas in young people with AIDS. N Engl J Med 1995;332:12–8.
83. Lee ES, Locker J, Nalesnik M, et al. The association of Epstein-Barr virus with smooth-muscle tumors occurring after organ transplantation. N Engl J Med 1995;332:19–25.
84. Labrecque LG, Banres DM, Fentiman IS, et al. Epstein-Barr virus in epithelial cell tumors: a breast cancer study. Cancer Res 1995;55:39–45.
85. Bonnet M, Guinebretiere J-M, Kremmer E, et al. Detection of Epstein-Barr virus in invasive breast cancers. J Natl Cancer Instit 1999;99:1376–81.
86. Chu PG, Chang KL, Chen Y-Y, et al. No significant association of Epstein-Barr virus infection with invasive breast carcinoma. Am J Pathol 2001;159:571–8.
87. Deshpande CG, Badve S, Kidwai N, et al. Lack of expression of the Epstein-Barr virus (EBV) gene products, EBER, EBNA1, LMP1, and LMP2A, in breast cancer cells. Lab Investig 2002;82:1993–99.
88. Chang Y, Cesarman E, Pessin MS, et al. Identification of herpesvirus-like DNA sequences in AIDS-associated Kaposi's sarcoma. Science 1994;266:1865–9.
89. Kedes DH, Ganem D. Sensitivity of Kaposi's sarcoma-associated herpesvirus replication to antiviral drugs. J Clin Invest 1997;99:2082–6.
90. Moses AV, Fish KN, Ruhl R, et al. Long-term infection and transformation of dermal microvascular endothelial cells by human herpesvirus 8. J Virol 1999;73:6892–902.
91. Flore O, Rafii S, Ely S, et al. Transformation of primary human endothelial cells by Kaposi's sarcoma-associated herpesvirus. Nature 1998;394:588–92.
92. Akula SM, Pramod NP, Wang FZ, et al. Integrin alpha3beta1 (CD 49c/29) is a cellular receptor for Kaposi's sarcoma-associated herpesvirus (KSHV/HHV-8) entry into the target cells. Cell 2002;108:407–19.
93. Sarid R, Flore O, Bohenzky RA, et al. Transcription mapping of the Kaposi's sarcoma-associated herpesvirus (human herpesvirus 8) genome in a body cavity-based lymphoma cell line (BC-1). J Virol 1998;72:1005–12.
94. Lee H, Guo J, Li M, et al. Identification of an immunoreceptor tyrosine-based activation motif of K1 transforming protein of Kaposi's sarcoma-associated herpesvirus. Mol Cell Biol 1998;18:5219–28.
95. Lee H, Veazey R, Williams K, et al. Deregulation of cell growth by the K1 gene of Kaposi's sarcoma-associated herpesvirus. Nat Med 1998;4:435–40.
96. Tomlinson CC, Damania B. The K1 protein of Kaposi's sarcoma-associated herpesvirus activates the Akt signaling pathway. J Virol 2004;78:1918–27.
97. Lagunoff M, Majeti R, Weiss A, Ganem D. Deregulated signal transduction by the K1 gene product of Kaposi's sarcoma-associated herpesvirus. Proc Natl Acad Sci U S A 1999;96:5704–9.
98. Chatterjee M, Osborne J, Bestetti G, et al. Viral IL-6-induced cell proliferation and immune evasion of interferon activity. Science 2002;298:1432–5.
99. Moore, PS, Bashoff C, Weiss RA, Chang Y. Molecular mimicry of human cytokine and cytokine response path-way genes by KSHV. Science 1996;274:1739–44.
100. Aoki Y, Jaffe ES, Chang Y, et al. Angiogenesis and hematopoiesis induced by Kaposi's sarcoma-associated herpesvirus-encoded interleukin-6. Blood 1999;93:4034–43.
101. Ishido S, Wang C, Lee B-S. Downregulation of major histocompatibility complex class I molecules by Kaposi's sarcoma-associated herpesvirus K3 and K5 proteins. J Virol 2000;74:5300–9.
102. Ishido S, Cook J-K, Lee-B-S. Inhibition of natural killer cell-mediated cytotoxicity by Kaposi's sarcoma-associated herpesvirus K5 protein. Immunity 2000;13:365–74.
103. Dairaghi DJ, Fan RA, McMaster BE, et al. HHV-8-encoded vMIP-1 selectively engages chemokine receptor CCR8: agonist and antagonist profiles of viral chemokines. J Biol Chem 1999;274:21569–74.
104. Stine JT, Wood C, Hill M, et al. KSHV-encoded CC chemokine vMIP-III is a CCR4 agonist, stimulates angiogenesis, and selectively chemoattracts TH2 cells. Blood 2000;95:1151–7.
105. Bashoff C, Endo Y, Collins PD, et al. Angiogenic and HIV-inhibitory functions of KSHV-encoded chemokines. Science 1997;278:290–4.
106. Kledal TN, Rosenkilde MM, Coulin F, et al. A broad-spectrum chemokine antagonist encoded by Kaposi's sarcoma-associated herpesvirus. Science 1997;277:1656–9.
107. Park J, Seo T, Hwang S. The K-bZIP protein from Kaposi's sarcoma-associated herpesvirus interacts with p53 and represses its transcriptional activity. J Virol 2000;74:11977–82.
108. Gwack Y, Hwang S, Byun H, et al. Kaposi's sarcoma-associated herpesvirus open reading frame 50 represses p53-induced transcriptional activity and apoptosis. J Virol 2001;75:6245–8.
109. Nakamura H, Li M, Jung JU. Inhibition of p53 tumor suppressor by viral interferon regulatory factor. J Virol 2001;75:7572–82.
110. Rivas C, Thlick AE, Parravicini C, et al. Kaposi's sarcoma-associated herpesvirus LANA2 is a B cell specific latent viral protein that inhibits p53. J Virol 2001;75:429–438.
111. Li M, Lee H, Guo J, et al. Kaposi's sarcoma-associated herpesvirus viral interferon regulatory factor. J Virol 1998;72:5433–40.
112. Burysek L, Pitha PM. Latently expressed human herpesvirus 8-encoded interferon regulatory factor 2 inhibits double-stranded RNA-activated protein kinase. J Virol 2001;75:2345–52.
113. Zhu FX, King SM, Smith EJ, et al. A Kaposi's sarcoma-associated herpesviral protein inhibits virus-mediated induction of type I interferon by blocking IRF-7 phosphorylation and nuclear accumulation. Proc Natl Acad Sci USA 2002;99:5573–8.
114. Muralidhar S, Pumferry AM, Hassani M, et al. Identification of kaposin (open reading frame K12) as a human herpesvirus 8 (Kaposi's sarcoma-associated herpesvirus) transforming gene. J Virol 1998;72:4980–8.
115. Chung YH, Means RE, Choi JK, et al. Kaposi's sarcoma-associated herpesvirus OX2 glycoprotein activates myeloid-lineage cells to induce inflammatory cytokine production. J Virol 2002;76:4688–98.
116. Spiller OB, Blackbourn DJ, Mark L, et al. Functional activity of the complement regulator encoded by Kaposi's sarcoma-associated herpesvirus. J Biol Chem. 2003;278:9283–9.
117. Cheng EH-Y, Nicholas J, Bellows DS, et al. A bcl-2 homolog encoded by Kaposi sarcoma-associated virus, human herpesvirus 8, inhibits apoptosis but does not heterodimerize with bax or bak. Proc Natl Acad Sci U S A 1997;94:690–4.
118. Sun Q, Zachariah S, Chaudhary PM. The human herpes virus 8-encoded viral FLICE-inhibitory protein induces cellular transformation via NF-κB activation. J Biol Chem 2003;278:52437–45.
119. Guasparri I, Keller SA, Cesarman E. KSHV vFLIP is essential for the survival of infected lymphoma cells. J Exp Med 2004;199:993–1003.
120. Djerbi M, Screpati V, Catrina AL, et al. The inhibitor of death receptor signaling, FLICE-inhibitory protein defines a new class of tumor progression factors. J Exp Med 1999;190:1025–31.
121. Swanton C, Mann DJ, Fleckenstein B, et al. Herpes viral cyclin/Cdk6 complexes evade inhibition by CDK inhibitor proteins. Nature 1997;390:184–7.
122. Chang Y, Moore PS, Talbot SJ, et al. Cyclin encoded by KS herpesvirus. Nature 1996;382:410.
123. Ballestas ME, Chatis PA, Kaye KM. Efficient persistence of extrachromosomal KSHV DNA mediated by latency-associated nuclear antigen. Science 1999;284:641–4.
124. Friborg J, Kong W, Hottiger MO, et al. p53 inhibition by the LANA protein of KSHV protects against cell death. Nature 1999;402:889–94.
125. Radkov SA, Kellam P, Boshoff C. The latent nuclear antigen of Kaposi sarcoma-associated herpesvirus targets the retinoblastoma-E2F pathway and with the oncogene h-*ras* transforms primary rat cells. Nat Med 2000;6:1121–7.
126. Fujimuro M, Wu FY, ApRhys C, et al. A novel viral mechanism for dysregulation of beta-catenin in Kaposi's sarcoma-associated herpesvirus latency. Nat Med 2003;9:300–6.
127. Arvanitakis L, Geras-Raaka E, Varma A, et al. Human herpesvirus KSHV encodes a constitutively active G-protein–coupled receptor linked to cell proliferation. Nature 1997;385:347–50.
128. Bais C, Santomasso B, Coso O, et al. G-protein–coupled receptor of Kaposi's sarcoma-associated herpesvirus is a viral oncogene and angiogenesis activator. Nature 1998;391:86–9.
129. Sodhi A, Montaner S, Patel V, et al. Akt plays a central role in sarcomagenesis induced by Kaposi's sarcoma herpesvirus-encoded G protein-coupled receptor. Proc Natl Acad Sci U S A 2004;101:4821–6.
130. Yang BT, Chen SC, Leach MW. Transgenic expression of the chemokine receptor encoded by human herpesvirus 8 induces an angioproliferative disease resembling Kaposi's sarcoma. J Exp Med 2000;191:445–54.
131. Glenn M, Rainbow L, Aurade F, et al. Identification of a spliced gene from Kaposi's sarcoma-associated herpesvirus encoding a protein with similarities to latent membrane proteins 1 and 2A of Epstein-Barr virus. J Virol 1999;73:6953–63.
132. Choi J-K, Lee B-S, Shim SN, et al. Identification of the novel K15 gene at the rightmost end of the Kaposi's sarcoma-associated herpesvirus genome. J Virol 2000;74:436–46.
133. Martin JN, Ganem DE, Osmond DH, et al. Sexual transmission and the natural history of human herpesvirus 8 infection. N Engl J Med 1998;338:948–54.

134. Simpson GR, Schulz TF, Whitby D, et al. Prevalence of Kaposi's sarcoma-associated herpesvirus infection measured by antibodies to recombinant capsid protein and latent immunofluorescence antigen. Lancet 1996;348:1133–8.
135. Gao SJ, Kingsley L, Hoover DR, et al. Seroconversion of antibodies to Kaposi's sarcoma-associated herpesvirus related latent nuclear antigens prior to onset of Kaposi's sarcoma. N Engl J Med 1996;335:233–41.
136. Cannon MJ, Dollard SC, Smith DK, et al. Blood-borne and sexual transmission of human herpesvirus 8 in women with or at risk for human immunodeficiency virus infection. N Engl J Med 2001;344:637–743.
137. Regamey N, Tamm M, Wernli M, et al. Transmission of human herpesvirus 8 infection from renal-transplant donors to recipients. N Engl J Med 1998;339:1358–63.
138. Barozzi P, Luppi M, Facchetti F, et al. Post-transplant Kaposi sarcoma originates from the seeding of donor-derived progenitors. Nat Med 2003;9:554–61.
139. Moore PS, Chang Y. Detection of herpesvirus-like DNA sequences in Kaposi's sarcoma in patients with and those without HIV infection. N Engl J Med 1995;332:1181–5.
140. Dupin N, Fisher C, Kellam P, et al. Distribution of human herpesvirus-8 latently infected cells in Kaposi's sarcoma, multicentric Castleman's disease, and primary effusion lymphoma. Proc Natl Acad Sci U S A 1999;96:4546–51.
141. Glesby MJ, Hoover DR, Weng S, et al. Use of antiherpes drugs and the risk of Kaposi's sarcoma: data from the Multicenter AIDS Cohort Study. J Infect Dis 1996;173:1477–80.
142. Martin DF, Kuppermann BD, Wolitz RA, et al. Oral ganciclovir for patients with cytomegalovirus retinitis treated with ganciclovir implant. Roche Ganciclovir Study Group. N Engl J Med 1999;340:1063–70.
143. Little RF, Merced-Galindez F, Staskus K, et al. A pilot study of cidofovir in patients with Kaposi sarcoma. J Infect Dis 2003;187:149–53.
144. Cattelan AM, Calabro ML, Aversa SML, et al. Regression of AIDS-related Kaposi's sarcoma following antiretroviral therapy with protease inhibitors: biological correlates of clinical outcome. Eur J Cancer 1999;35:1809–15.
145. Cesarman E, Chang Y, Moore PS, et al. Kaposi's sarcoma-associated herpesvirus-like DNA sequences in AIDS-related body-cavity-based lymphomas. N Engl J Med 1995;332:1186–91.
146. Soulier J, Grollety L, Oksenhendler E, et al. Kaposi's sarcoma-associated herpesvirus-like DNA sequences in multicentric Castleman's disease. Blood 1995;86:1276–280.
147. Katano H, Sato Y, Kurata T, et al. Expression and localization of human herpesvirus 8-encoded proteins in primary effusion lymphoma, Kaposi's sarcoma, and multicentric Castleman's disease. Virology 2000;269:335–44.
148. Luppi M, Barozzi P, Schultz TF, et al. Bone marrow failure associated with human herpesvirus 8 infection after transplantation. N Engl J Med 2000;323:1378–85.
149. Cool CD, Rai PR, Yeager ME, et al. Expression of human herpesvirus 8 in primary pulmonary hypertension. N Engl J Med 2003;349:1113–22.

Papillomaviruses and Cervical Neoplasia

Christopher P. Crum, MD
Catherine M. McLachlin, MD

The causal relationship between human papillomaviruses (HPVs) and cervical neoplasia is an accepted fact, and this virus has been the focus of strategies designed to elucidate mechanisms of virus-induced tumorigenesis, to improve the diagnosis and screening of uterine cervical neoplasms, and to exploit the host immune response to prevent these diseases. Technological advances have dictated both the tempo and the direction of this research, which began with descriptive and experimental pathology, progressed to molecular biology, and finally involved molecular immunology in efforts to both implicate the virus directly in producing neoplasia and to unravel the mechanisms of host response and prevention with vaccines.

DEFINITIONS, TISSUE SPECIFICITY, AND MECHANISMS OF INFECTION AND TRANSFORMATION

Definitions Genital "infections" are best defined by the presence of clinically or colposcopically identifiable flat or raised lesions that contain papillomaviral deoxyribonucleic acid (DNA), the prototype of which is genital warts. In this instance, infectious virus is likely to be identified within the epithelium (Figure 21-1A). More recently, the term *infection* has been expanded to include HPV-related precancerous lesions, or even cancers, the term being used loosely to denote the presence of viral DNA. However, integrated viral DNA rather than virions is more likely to be identified in advanced lesions (Figure 21-1B).[1] As is detailed subsequently (see "Risk Factors"), HPV DNA may be associated with no visible abnormality; active, clinically, or morphologically conspicuous infection; and advanced neoplasia (Tables 21-1 and 21-2). The hallmark of significant HPV infection is a morphologic transformation of the target tissue. This is not synonymous with the term *transformation* as classically applied to changes in cultured cells produced after introduction of HPV nucleic acids. Rather, it defines the morphologic alterations that can be most consistently associated with the presence of HPV nucleic acids. Depending on host factors and HPV type involved in the infection, it may be defined as a low- or high-grade genital precancer, either of which is distinct from the normal epithelium (see Figures 21-1 and 21-2).

Specificity The squamous epithelium is most susceptible to HPV infections. In particular, squamocolumnar junctions, where basal or reserve cells are undergoing expansion in the form of squamous or columnar cell differentiation (transformation zones), are most vulnerable to the genital papillomaviruses.[2,3] These transformation zones contain multipotent cells that by virtue of their biology or location render them uniquely vulnerable and may be found in the larynx, oropharyngeal mucosa, anus, esophagus, subungual mucosa (nail bed), and conjunctiva. Kreider and colleagues demonstrated that some of these sites are particularly vulnerable to experimental infection with genital viruses.[4] This indicates that the genital HPV types require specific conditions provided by certain locales for infection to occur or characteristics facilitating morphologic transformation once infection has taken place. One component of this equation is the infection of cells that are either undergoing shifts in differentiation or are capable of doing so once infected.[5–7]

Mechanism of Infection Papillomaviruses are epitheliotropic, circular, double-stranded DNA viruses that infect the squamous epithelium. The interval from exposure to the development of a lesion varies from a few weeks to several months and perhaps longer.[8] It is presumed that the virus gains access to the cervix or lower female genital tract through defects in the epithelium that expose the basal epithelial cells to virion particles.[3] In support of this hypothesis are the demonstration of papillomavirus DNA and ribonucleic acids in basal cells and the observation that experimental infection of the

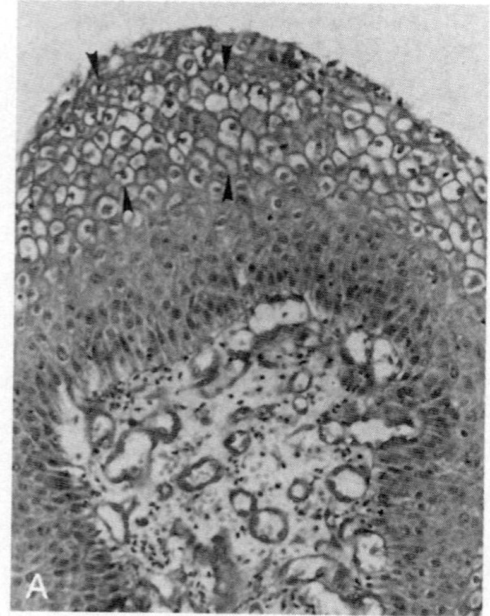
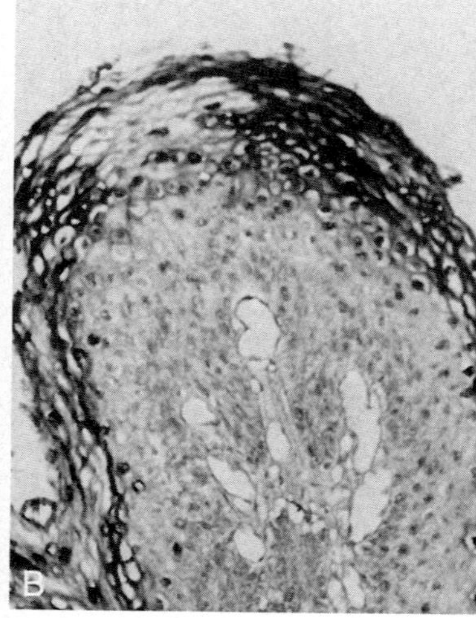
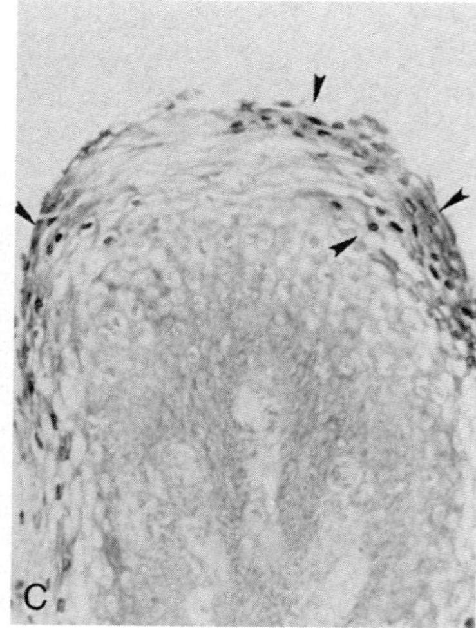

Figure 21-1 Histopathology of a classic human papillomavirus (HPV) infection (condyloma) of the cervix associated with low-risk HPV types (HPV type 6 or 11). **A,** Morphologic features of HPV infection include nuclear atypia in the superficial epithelial cells with prominent cytoplasmic halos (*arrowheads*). The lower cell layers contain minimal cytologic atypia. **B,** Appearance following in situ hybridization with a biotin-labeled mixed deoxyribonucleic acid (DNA) probe containing HPV types 6 and 11 (VIRATYPE, Life Technologies, Gaithersburg, MD). The dark staining in the superficial cell nuclei and cytoplasm represents viral DNA and ribonucleic acid produced during viral replication. **C,** An immunoperoxidase stain for HPV capsid proteins, highlighting several dark-staining nuclei in the superficial epithelium (*arrowheads*).

Table 21-1 Definitions

HPV = Human papillomavirus.
CIN = Cervical intraepithelial neoplasia, synonymous with papillomavirus-related squamous intraepithelial lesions. Low-grade CIN (CIN I) is synonymous with flat or exophytic condyloma and exhibits nuclear atypia, principally in the upper epithelial layers.
High-grade CIN (CIN II or III) is characterized by atypia in all epithelial layers.
HPV-related lesion = Includes HPV infections such as condylomata, but also includes any lesion associated with papillomaviruses, including high-grade CIN and various invasive carcinomas.
Occult or latent HPV = Defined as the presence of HPV DNA in the absence of morphologic evidence of HPV infection (ie, no lesion is present).
High-risk HPV = HPV with documented association with cancer (this is not an assessment of cancer risk and will vary between high-risk HPVs).
Low-risk HPV = HPV with no association with cancer.
VLP = Viral-like particle; pertains to papillomavirion-like particles generated in vitro.

Table 21-2 Genital HPVs and Their Relationship to Disease

HPV(s)	Associated Diseases
16	More than 50% of high-grade CIN and carcinomas (both squamous and adenocarcinoma)
18	10% of squamous carcinomas, 50% of adenocarcinomas and adenocarcinomas in situ, and 90% of neuroendocrine carcinomas
31, 45	5% to 10% of CIN, squamous carcinomas
33, 39, 51, 52, 55, 56, 58, 59, 68	Less than 3% (each) of CIN, squamous carcinomas
6, 11, 40, 42, 53, 54, 57, 66, 84	Low-risk HPVs, essentially never detected in carcinoma
61, 62, 64, 67, 69–72, 81, cp6108, iso39	Insufficient data to ascertain risk

Adapted from Stoler MH et al[15]; Peyton CL et al[29]; and Hughes SA et al.[62]

squamous mucosa by HPV is enhanced by disturbing the epithelial surface (and hence exposing the basal cells) prior to exposure.[9] As the cells containing the viral DNA approach the upper layers of the epithelium, the virus replicates and assembles into virions, which can be detected by electron microscopy or immunohistochemistry (see Figure 21-1).[10] Some of the superficial cells in the infected epithelium characteristically display enlarged, hyperchromatic nuclei, with or without cytoplasmic halos (koilocytotic atypia), and the mature virus usually concentrates in this cell population (see Figure 21-1).[10,11] Uncoupling of cell-cycle control also occurs in these cells, the nuclei of which may express cell-cycle proteins (Ki-67, cyclin E, p16^{ink4}).[12,13] The genital squamous epithelium is the principal site for HPV infection, but infection may occur in other sites, as discussed above. Moreover, HPV nucleic acids have been isolated from neoplasms not clearly derived from squamous-committed epithelial cells, most notably adenocarcinomas and undifferentiated carcinomas (small cell carcinoma).[14,15]

MECHANISMS OF NEOPLASTIC TRANSFORMATION

The mechanism by which HPV infection produces neoplastic transformation has been progressively elucidated and consists of at least four components (Figure 21-3).[3] The first is the direct effects of the viral oncoproteins on the cell cycle, mediated via interactions between E6 and E7 oncoproteins of cancer-associated (high-risk) HPVs and the tp53 and Rb proteins, respectively (see Figure 21-3). A direct influence of these oncoproteins on other cell-cycle regulators, such as cyclin E, has also been demonstrated.[4] Compensatory elevation in expression of the cyclin-dependent kinase inhibitor p16 results from the above disturbances.[13] The second effect is also mediated via viral oncoproteins and consists of abnormalities in centrosome duplication, leading to genomic instability, subsequently reflected in progressive allelic imbalance.[16,17] The latter include alterations in 3p and specific amplifications at 3q25-27.[18,19] The third component is mediated via E6 and consists of telomerase up-regulation and a disruption of normal replicative senescence.[20] These events occur ultimately as a function of expression of viral oncoproteins (E6 and E7). A fourth mechanism is the inactivation of tumor suppressor genes by methylation.[21]

HPV AND HUMAN GENITAL NEOPLASIA

Risk Factors HPV infection is ubiquitous in the young, sexually active population, peaks in the early reproductive years, is often transient, and becomes increasingly less prevalent with increasing age.[22,23] However, persistent infection by the same HPV type is strongly associated with the risk of a current or subsequent cervical neoplasm.[24] At least 30 HPV types are associated with cervical neoplasia, with a broad gradient of risk imposed by these HPV types. Types 6 and 11 are prototypical "low-risk" HPVs associated with genital warts (condylomata).[25,26] In contrast, type 16 is the prototypical "high-risk" HPV, present in more than

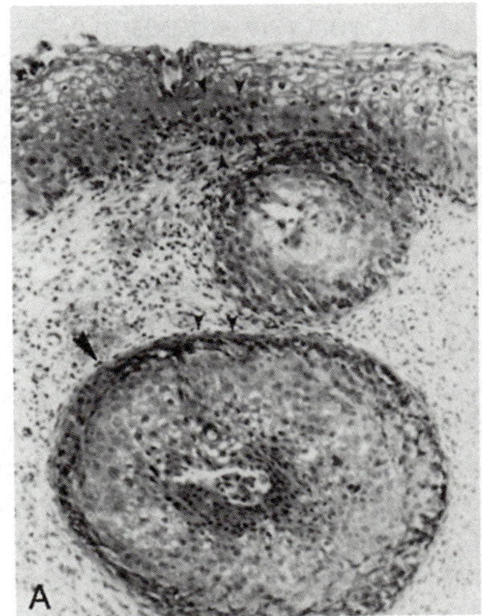

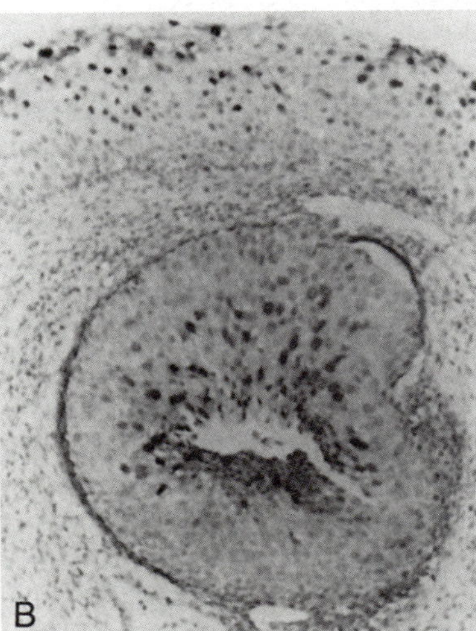

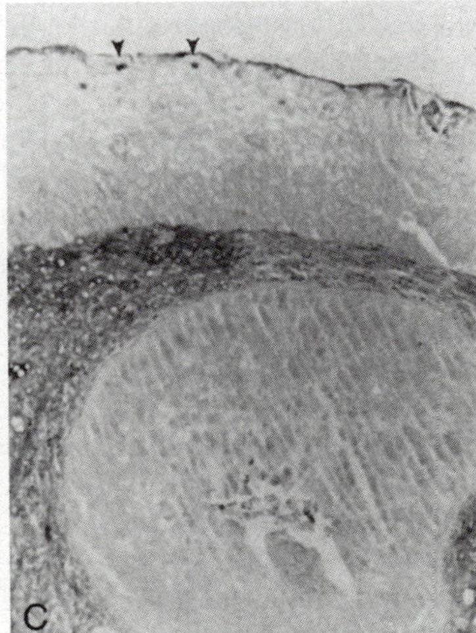

Figure 21-2 Histopathology of cervical intraepithelial neoplasm associated with high-risk human papillomavirus (HPV) types (ie, 16, 31, 33, 35, and so on). **A,** Lesion involving the superficial and crypt (gland) epithelium (*large arrowhead*). Koilocytotic atypia is present (*upper right*), but, in addition, nuclear atypia is conspicuous in the lower cell layers (*small arrows*). **B,** Appearance following in situ hybridization with a mixed probe containing HPV types 31, 33, and 35. Note the similar distribution of staining as in Figure 24-1B. In contrast to Figure 24-1C, capsid proteins are infrequently identified by immunostaining, with rare positive nuclei observed (*arrowheads*).

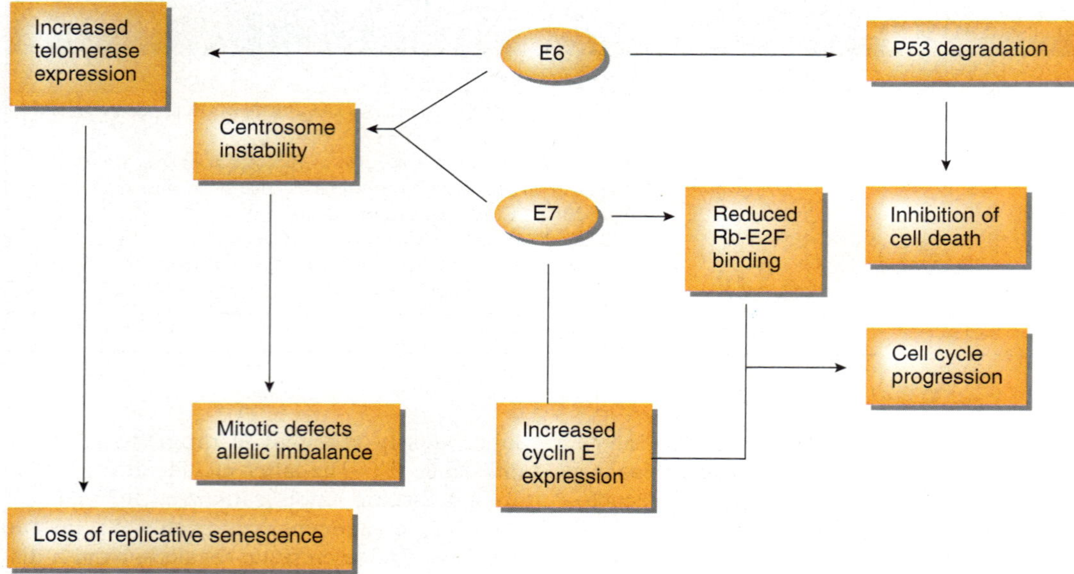

Figure 21-3 Schematic of potential mechanisms of human papillomavirus–related neoplastic transformation.

50% of cervical carcinomas.[27] HPV 18 predominates in glandular and neuroendocrine carcinomas.[14,15,28] However, all of these HPVs may be found in women with normal cytology. A variety of other HPVs are associated with cancer at a lower frequency. Currently, these "intermediate-risk" and the high-risk types are combined into a single category. The presence of any HPV, high or low risk, does not exclude the subsequent emergence of another HPV infection of different risk, meaning that infection with one virus may serve as a surrogate marker for subsequent infection by a high-risk HPV.[8] Predictably, most HPVs detected in women with normal Pap smears have some association with cancer risk, albeit low.[29]

If a woman is found to harbor a high-risk HPV in her genital tract, what is her risk of developing a high-grade squamous intraepithelial lesion (HSIL)? In general, approximately 15% of reproductive-age women will score positive for high-risk HPVs. The risk of HSIL ranges from less than 5% to over 80%, depending on whether the Pap smear is normal, contains a minor or nondiagnostic atypia (atypical squamous cells of undetermined significance [ASCUS]), or is HSIL. Repeated detection of the same HPV type—even in the presence of a normal Pap smear—increases the risk to nearly 20%.[24] There is a strong theoretic basis for assuming that intratypical sequence variants influence outcome following infections by HPV 16.[30] However, the use of this information in patient management awaits greater consistency in study design and outcome and a clearer understanding of the mechanisms influencing the relationship between intratypical variants and the risk of developing high-grade cervical intraepithelial neoplasia (CIN) or cancer.

Human leukocyte antigen (HLA) molecules regulate immune responses to foreign antigens and discrimination of self- from non–self-antigens. In addition, it was recently reported that certain HLA class II haplotypes (linked class II alleles) are positively associated with low- and high-grade squamous intraepithelial lesions or invasive cervical cancer, whereas other class II haplotypes are negatively associated or protective.[31]

It should be emphasized, however, that even though a number of associations between HLA class II types and cervical neoplasia or HPV infection have been identified, the precise mechanisms underlying these associations remain to be clarified.

Young, sexually active women are at greatest risk of HPV infection and preinvasive cervical neoplasia, and this risk drops significantly with increasing age. As many as 39% of adolescents may score positive at a single visit.[22] The index of HPV detection drops further with the approach of menopause, presumably signifying a long-standing and effective immune response to the virus that follows the onset of sexual activity and exposure to HPVs in early life.[22,23]

The risk of anogenital neoplasia or HPV infection in immunosuppressed individuals is well documented, particularly in transplantation patients.[32] Human immune deficiency virus (HIV) infection has been the most intensively studied. The risk of HPV positivity and persistent positivity is increased in women who are HIV positive.[33] Furthermore, persistence was 1.9 (95% confidence interval [CI] 1.5–2.3) times greater if the subject had a CD4 cell count < 200 cells/μL (vs > 500 cells/μL) in one study.[34] The risk of a subsequent squamous intraepithelial lesion is significantly higher in HIV-infected women.[35] The proportion of advanced precursor lesions is not significantly higher, but the risk of lesion persistence is.[34,35] The risk of invasive carcinoma in HIV-infected women is controversial but may be influenced by the level and duration of immunosuppression.[36,37]

Sexual behavior patterns in male consorts also influence the risk of both HPV and other sexually transmitted diseases. Thomas and colleagues linked risk in Thai women with male behavior, specifically unprotected intercourse with prostitutes.[38] Castilla and colleagues found that the prevalence rates of penile HPV between Spain and Columbia explained the differences in cancer rate.[39] Another group showed that monogamous wives of husbands who had sexual relationships both before and during the marriage had a substantial risk of cervical cancer (relative risk 6.9; 95% CI 2.3–20.7]).[40]

Oral contraceptive use modestly increases the risk of cervical neoplasia, possibly by a preferential increase in the risk of glandular neoplasms.[41] There is also an association (independent of HPV) between smoking and cervical neoplasia that shows a dose response.[42] The association between *Chlamydia* infection and cervical neoplasia is controversial.[43]

In summary, a multitude of factors, virus and host related, influence the risk of papillomavirus-related cervical neoplasia before, during, and following exposure and lesion progression.

APPLICATIONS TO CLINICAL MEDICINE

Background The prevention of cervical cancer is based on the Pap smear. Because the majority of cervical cancers are preceded by a cervical precursor (CIN) lesion, often by many years, the detection of these precursors is fundamental to cancer prevention. Precursor lesions are recognized clinically on colposcopy, where precursor lesions can be identified following the application of acetic acid.[44] The use of colposcopy has maximized the targeting of lesions for biopsy, and outpatient removal is the usual approach, including cryotherapy, laser, and, recently, loop electrical excision.[45] The latter procedures target the entire transformation zone, removing the lesion and replacing the process of chronic repair with a brief period of reepithelialization. Recurrence after removal or ablation is linked to either inadequate excision or infection by another HPV following therapy. The former is increased when margins are positive. Infection with new HPV types appears to explain why many "recurrences" following ablation for high-grade precursors are low grade in nature. Reinfection with the same HPV type is uncommon except in immunosuppressed women.

HPV Testing in Management of the Abnormal Pap Smear HPV testing has emerged as a viable management tool for a subset of women with abnormal cervical cytology. Because HPV is so strongly linked to cervical neoplasia and because high-risk HPV types predominate in the cervix, a substantial proportion of women with a cytologic diagnosis of low- or high-grade precancerous changes will score positive. For this reason, HPV testing is of limited value in this population. However, women with nondiagnostic squamous atypias (ASCUS) present a management dilemma in which the clinician must decide between colposcopy or Pap smear follow-up.

HPV testing offers the additional opportunity to triage the patient into colposcopy and follow-up groups by immediately testing the cytologic sample, which is possible with the newer liquid-based technologies. Newer generations of HPV testing, such as the Hybrid Capture II test, are extremely sensitive and will detect more than 95% of women with histologically proven preinvasive disease.[46] If HPV negative, women with ASCUS have a less than 1% risk of high-grade CIN, in contrast to a 20% risk if they are HPV positive.[46] Similar results have been seen with the management of abnormal glandular cells on the smear.[47] Recently, the test has been approved as an adjunct to the Pap smear for screening women over age 30. The basis for this approach lies in the high negative predictive value of both a normal smear and negative HPV assay, which may permit a longer cytology screening interval. This concept is currently being introduced into and tested in the practice setting, but long-term studies are needed to ascertain the safety of extending follow-up intervals to 3 years.[48]

Surrogate Markers of HPV Infections for Diagnosis The laboratory management of early cervical neoplasia is based on criteria derived from prior studies correlating the high-risk prototypes (such as type 16) with high-grade squamous intraepithelial lesions (CIN grades II and III).[49] However, the distinction of a preinvasive lesion from a benign inflammatory process may be difficult and can influence management decisions.

Improving the precision of these diagnoses has been the focus of studies designed to identify biomarkers that may simplify the distinction of HPV-related neoplasia from its mimics. Because HPVs disrupt cell function, it is logical to presume that alterations in host genes may serve as "surrogate markers" for HPV infection. Host genes reported to be up-regulated in cervical neoplasia include telomerase, p16^{ink4}, cyclin E, Ki-67, MN, and others.[12] Some of these, such as Ki-67, cyclin E, and p16^{ink4}, have practical value in triaging histologic abnormalities.[12,13] As the identification and screening of new biomarkers evolve, it is possible that screening of Pap smears, or cervical samples for host gene alterations, will become standard practice. However, whether such markers will exceed the sensitivity and specificity of HPV testing remains to be determined.

Clinical Management Management of HPV-related cervical neoplasms continues to be defined and redefined, in step with the methods used for lesion removal. Most women with low- or high-grade CIN on Pap smear or an atypical smear that is HPV positive will be referred to colposcopic examination. Of those who have a negative examination or a low-grade CIN on biopsy, 10 to 13% will develop a biopsy-proven high-grade CIN within 2 years. Many practitioners will follow patients with low-grade abnormalities and negative colposcopy by repeat cytology in 6 to 12 months, with attention to this risk.

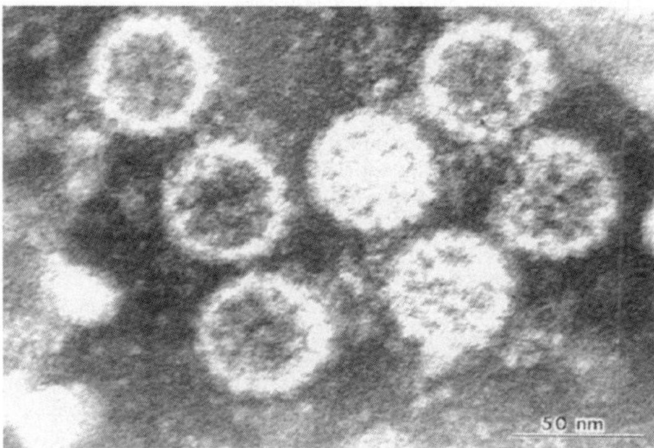

Figure 21-4 Electron micrograph depicting papillomavirus-like particles generated in vitro. Courtesy of Ian Frazer, MD, Princess Alexandra Hospital, Queensland, Australia.

Biopsy-proven high-grade CIN is typically managed by the loop electrical excision procedure or cone biopsy. Thus, the outcome of a given case will be dependent on the application of the histologic criteria for distinguishing low- from high-grade squamous intraepithelial lesions.[50] Long-term follow-up of all women with cervical abnormalities, treated or otherwise, customarily includes Pap smear evaluations but may eventually include periodic HPV testing as well.

Prevention Efforts to elucidate the immune response to HPV have evolved from studies of fusion proteins and linear epitopes to the production in vitro of virus-like particles (VLPs) (Figure 21-4).[51–55] VLPs are produced by expressing the entire late region of papillomaviruses in eukaryotic systems, contain the conformational epitopes operative in generating host immunity, and can be used to study (or generate) host immunity.[56–59] This avenue of investigation was the most promising because it offered the advantage of intact particles that were highly immunogenic. Recent large-scale trials have validated the merits of VLP vaccination, demonstrating high efficacy for both preventing infection and lesions attributed to the HPV type(s) targeted in the vaccine.[60,61] Trials are ongoing that test multivalent vaccines containing not only HPV 16 but also HPVs 18, 6, and 11 (the latter two target genital warts). These trials are expected to prove successful, and if they demonstrate lasting immunity, it is conceivable that these vaccines will be introduced within 5 years and that the next 20 years will witness the beginning of a reduction in the incidence of not only cervical cancer but also penile, anal, oropharyngeal, and other papillomavirus-related diseases in humans.

REFERENCES

1. Cullen AP, Reid R, Campion M, Lorincz AT. Analysis of the physical state of different human papillomavirus DNAs in intraepithelial and invasive cervical neoplasm. J Virol 1991;65:606–12.
2. Richart RM. Cervical intraepithelial neoplasia. In: Sommers SC, editor. Pathology annual. New York: Appleton-Century-Crofts; 1973. p. 301.
3. Munger K, Howley PM. Human papillomavirus immortalization and transformation functions. Virus Res 2002;89:213–28.
4. Kreider JW, Howett MK, Wolfe SA, et al. Morphologic transformation in vivo of human uterine cervix with papillomavirus from condylomata acuminata. Nature 1985;317:639.
5. Kreider JW, Howett MK, Stoler MH, et al. Susceptibility of various human tissues to transformation in vivo with human papillomavirus type II. Int J Cancer 1987;39:459.
6. Quade BJ, Yang A, Wang Y, et al. Expression of the p53 homologue p63 in early cervical neoplasia. Gynecol Oncol 2001;80:24–9.
7. Witkiewicz AK, Hecht JL, Cviko A, et al. Microglandular hyperplasia: a model for the de novo emergence and evolution of endocervical reserve cells. Hum Pathol 2005;36:154–61.
8. Koutsky LA, Holmes KK, Critchlow CW, et al. A cohort study of the risk of cervical intraepithelial neoplasia grade 2 or 3 in relation to papillomavirus infection. N Engl J Med 1992;327:1272–8.
9. Kreider JW, Howett MK, Stoler MH, et al. Susceptibility of various human tissues to transformation in vivo with human papillomavirus type 11. Int J Cancer 1987;39:459–65.
10. Meisels A, Morin C. Human papillomavirus and cancer of the uterine cervix. Gynecol Oncol 1981;12 Suppl:111.
11. Purola E, Savia E. Cytology of gynecologic condyloma acuminatum. Acta Cytol 1977;21:26–31.
12. Keating JT, Cviko A, Riethdorf S, et al. Ki-67, cyclin E, and p16^{INK4} are complementary surrogate biomarkers for human papilloma virus-related cervical neoplasia. Am J Surg Pathol 2001;25:884–91.
13. Sano T, Masuda N, Oyama T, Nakajima T. Overexpression of p16 and p14^{ARF} is associated with human papillomavirus infection in cervical squamous cell carcinoma and dysplasia. Pathol Int 2002;52:375–83.
14. Pirog EC, Kleter B, Olgac S, et al. Prevalence of human papillomavirus DNA in different histological subtypes of cervical adenocarcinoma. Am J Pathol 2000;157:1055–62.
15. Stoler MH, Walker AN, Mills SE. Small cell neuroendocrine carcinoma of the cervix: a human papillomavirus type 18 associated cervix cancer. Lab Invest 1989;60:92A.
16. Duensing S, Duensing A, Crum CP, Munger K. Human papillomavirus type 16 E7 oncoprotein-induced abnormal centrosome synthesis is an early event in the evolving malignant phenotype. Cancer Res 2001;61:2356–60.
17. Duensing S, Lee LY, Duensing A, et al. The human papillomavirus type 16 E6 and E7 oncoproteins cooperate to induce mitotic defects and genomic instability by uncoupling centrosome duplication from the cell division cycle. Proc Natl Acad Sci U S A 2000;97:10002–7.
18. Heselmeyer K, Schrock E, du Manoir S, et al. Gain of chromosome 3q defines the transition from severe dysplasia to invasive carcinoma of the uterine cervix. Proc Natl Acad Sci U S A 1996;93:479–84.
19. Rader JS, Gerhard DS, O'Sullivan MJ, et al. Cervical intraepithelial neoplasia III shows frequent allelic loss in 3p and 6p. Genes Chromosomes Cancer 1998;22:57–65.
20. Klingelhutz AJ, Foster SA, McDougall JK. Telomerase activation by the E6 gene product of human papillomavirus type 16. Nature 1996;380:79–82.
21. Feng Q, Balasubramanian A, Hawes SE, et al. Detection of hypermethylated genes in women with and without cervical neoplasia. J Natl Cancer Inst 2005;97:273–82.
22. Rosenfeld WD, Rose E, Vermund SH, et al. Follow-up evaluation of cervicovaginal human papillomavirus infection in adolescents. J Pediatr 1992;121:307–11.
23. Melkert PW, Hopman E, van den Brule AJ, et al. Prevalence of HPV in cytomorphologically normal cervical smears, as determined by the polymerase chain reaction, is age-dependent. Int J Cancer 1993;53:919–23.
24. Bory JP, Cucherousset J, Lorenzato M, et al. Recurrent human papillomavirus infection detected with the hybrid capture II assay selects women with normal cervical smears at risk for developing high grade cervical lesions: a longitudinal study of 3091 women. Int J Cancer 2002;102:519–25.
25. de Villiers EM, Gissmann L, zur Hausen H. Molecular cloning of viral DNA from human genital warts. J Virol 1981;40:932–5.
26. Gissmann L, Wolnik L, Ikenberg H, et al. Human papillomavirus types 6 and 11 DNA sequences in genital and laryngeal papillomas and in some cervical cancers. Proc Natl Acad Sci U S A 1983;80:560–3.
27. Durst M, Gissman L, Ikenberg H, zur Hausen H. A papillomavirus DNA from a cervical carcinoma and its prevalence in cancer biopsy samples from different geographic regions. Proc Natl Acad Sci U S A 1983;80:3812.
28. Boshart M, Gissman L, Ikenberg H, et al. A new type of papillomavirus DNA, its presence in genital cancer biopsies

and in cell lines derived from cervical cancer. EMBO J 1984;3:1151.
29. Peyton CL, Gravitt PE, Hunt WC, et al. Determinants of genital human papillomavirus detection in a US population. J Infect Dis 2001;183:1554–64.
30. Xi LF, Critchlow CW, Wheeler CM, et al. Risk of anal carcinoma in situ in relation to human papillomavirus type 16 variants. Cancer Res 1998;58:3839–44.
31. Hildesheim A, Wang SS. Host and viral genetics and risk of cervical cancer: a review. Virus Res 2002;89:229–40.
32. Fairley CK, Sheil AG, McNeil JJ, et al. The risk of ano-genital malignancies in dialysis and transplant patients. Clin Nephrol 1994;41:101–5.
33. Ahdieh L, Klein RS, Burk R, et al. Prevalence, incidence, and type-specific persistence of human papillomavirus in human immunodeficiency virus (HIV)-positive and HIV-negative women. J Infect Dis 2001;184:682–90.
34. Ellerbrock TV, Chiasson MA, Bush TJ, et al. Incidence of cervical squamous intraepithelial lesions in HIV-infected women. JAMA 2000;283:1031–7.
35. La Ruche G, Leroy V, Mensah-Ado I, et al. Short-term follow up of cervical squamous intraepithelial lesions associated with HIV and human papillomavirus infections in Africa. Int J STD AIDS 1999;10:363–8.
36. Parkin DM, Wabinga H, Nambooze S, Wabwire-Mangen F. AIDS-related cancers in Africa: maturation of the epidemic in Uganda. AIDS 1999;13:2563–70.
37. Duncan ME, Tibaux G, Pelzer A, et al. A socioeconomic, clinical and serological study in an African city of prostitutes and women still married to their first husband. Soc Sci Med 1994;39:323–33.
38. Thomas DB, Ray RM, Kuypers J, et al. Human papillomaviruses and cervical cancer in Bangkok. III. The role of husbands and commercial sex workers. Am J Epidemiol 2001;153:740–8.
39. Castilla J, Barrio G, de la Fuente L, Belza MJ. Sexual behaviour and condom use in the general population of Spain, 1996. AIDS Care 1998;10:667–76.
40. Agarwal SS, Sehgal A, Sardana S, et al. Role of male behavior in cervical carcinogenesis among women with one lifetime sexual partner. Cancer 1993;72:1666–9.
41. Lacey JV Jr, Brinton LA, Barnes WA, et al. Use of hormone replacement therapy and adenocarcinomas and squamous cell carcinomas of the uterine cervix. Gynecol Oncol 2000;77:149–54.
42. Deacon JM, Evans CD, Yule R, et al. Sexual behaviour and smoking as determinants of cervical HPV infection and of CIN3 among those infected: a case-control study nested within the Manchester cohort. Br J Cancer 2000;83:1565–72.
43. Reesink-Peters N, Ossewaarde JM, Van Der Zee AG, et al. No association of anti-*Chlamydia trachomatis* antibodies and severity of cervical neoplasia. Sex Transm Infect 2001;77:101–2.
44. Richart RM. Current concepts in obstetrics and gynecology: the patient with an abnormal Pap smear—screening techniques and management [review]. N Engl J Med 1980;302:332–4.
45. Ferenczy A. Management of the patient with an abnormal Papanicolaou test. Recent developments. Obstet Gynecol Clin North Am 1993;20:189–202.
46. Solomon D, Schiffman M, Tarone R. Comparison of three management strategies for patients with atypical squamous cells of undetermined significance: baseline results from a randomized trial. J Natl Cancer Inst 2001;93:293–9.
47. Ronnett BM, Manos MM, Ransley JE, et al. Atypical glandular cells of undetermined significance (AGUS): cytopathologic features, histopathologic results, and human papillomavirus DNA detection. Hum Pathol 1999;30:816–25.
48. Hoyer H, Scheungraber C, Kuehne-Heid R, et al. Cumulative 5-year diagnoses of CIN2, CIN3 or cervical cancer after concurrent high-risk HPV and cytology testing in a primary screening setting. Int J Cancer 2005.
49. Crum CP, Mitao M, Levine RU, Silverstein S. Cervical papillomaviruses segregate within morphologically distinct precancerous lesions. J Virol 1985;54:675–81.
50. Wright TC, Ferenczy A, Kurman RJ. Precancerous lesions of the cervix. In: Kurman RJ, editor. Blaustein's pathology of the female genital tract. 4th ed. New York: Springer Verlag; 1994. p. 246–53.
51. Zhou J, Sun XY, Stenzel DJ, Frazer IH. Expression of vaccinia recombinant HPV 16 L1 and L2 ORF proteins in epithelial cells is sufficient for assembly of HPV virion-like particles. Virology 1991;185:251–7.
52. Kirnbauer R, Taub J, Greenstone H, et al. Efficient self-assembly of human papillomavirus type 16 L1 and L1-L2 into virus-like particles. J Virol 1993;67:6929–36.
53. Ghim SJ, Jenson AB, Schlegel R. HPV-1 L1 protein expressed in cos cells displays conformational epitopes found on intact virions. Virology 1992;190:548–52.
54. Hagensee ME, Yaegashi N, Galloway DA. Self-assembly of human papillomavirus type 1 capsids by expression of the L1 protein alone or by coexpression of the L1 and L2 capsid proteins. J Virol 1993;67:315–22.
55. Rose RC, Bonnez W, Reichman RC, Garcea RL. Expression of human papillomavirus type 11 L1 protein in insect cells: in vivo and in vitro assembly of viruslike particles. J Virol 1993;67:1936–44.
56. Zhou J, Sun XY, Stenzel DJ, Frazer IH. Expression of vaccinia recombinant HPV 16 L1 and L2 ORF proteins in epithelial cells is sufficient for assembly of HPV virion-like particles. Virology 1991;185(1):251–7.
57. Kirnbauer R, Booy F, Cheng N, et al. Papillomavirus L1 major capsid protein self-assembles into virus-like particles that are highly immunogenic. Proc Natl Acad Sci U S A 1992;89(24):12180–4.
58. Ghim SJ, Jenson AB, Schlegel R. HPV-1 L1 protein expressed in cos cells displays conformational epitopes found on intact virions. Virology 1992;190(1):548–52.
59. Hagensee ME, Yaegashi N, Galloway DA. Self-assembly of human papillomavirus type 1 capsids by expression of the L1 protein alone or by coexpression of the L1 and L2 capsid proteins. J Virol 1993;67(1):315–22.
60. Koutsky LA, Ault KA, Wheeler CM, et al, Proof of Principle Study Investigators. A controlled trial of a human papillomavirus type 16 vaccine. N Engl J Med 2002;347:1645–51.
61. Harper DM, Franco EL, Wheeler C, et al, GlaxoSmithKline HPV Vaccine Study Group. Efficacy of a bivalent L1 virus-like particle vaccine in prevention of infection with human papillomavirus types 16 and 18 in young women: a randomised controlled trial. Lancet 2004;364:1757–65.
62. Hughes SA, Sun D, Gibson C, et al. Managing atypical squamous cells of undetermined significance (ASCUS): human papillomavirus testing, ASCUS subtyping, or follow-up cytology? Am J Obstet Gynecol 2002;186(3):396–403.

22

Hepatitis Viruses

Max W. Sung, MD

Swan N. Thung, MD

The viral causes of infectious hepatitis were recognized as early as 1885, when an outbreak of jaundice was reported in shipyard workers who had received smallpox vaccination with human lymph.[1] The transmissible agent was subsequently found to be a "filterable" virus. The actual isolation and characterization of hepatitis viruses did not occur until the last quarter of the 20th century. The hepatitis A and B viruses (HAV and HBV) were isolated first, followed by the hepatitis C, D, and E viruses (HCV, HDV, and HEV), and then, more recently, by the hepatitis viruses HGF, HGV (hepatitis G, also called hepatitis GB virus C [GBV-C]), and TTV (transfusion-transmitted virus).

The epidemiologic association of hepatocellular carcinoma (HCC) with hepatitis viruses was first noted with chronic HBV infection in the 1980s. Since then, chronic HCV infection has also been implicated in the pathogenesis of HCC, as well as in that of other cancers such as cholangiocarcinoma and non-Hodgkin's lymphoma. Table 22-1 summarizes the characteristics of hepatitis viruses.

HEPATITIS B VIRUS

HBV is a partially double-stranded deoxyribonucleic acid (DNA) virus packaged with a core protein (HBcAg) and DNA polymerase, and enclosed by envelope proteins (HBsAg).[2] Following receptor-mediated entry into hepatocytes, the virus enters the nucleus, where the viral DNA is frequently

Table 22-1 Hepatitis Viruses

Hepatitis Virus	HAV	HBV	HCV	HDV	HEV
Structure					
Family	Picornaviridae	Hepadnaviridae	Flaviviridae	Deltaviridae	Caliciviridae/togavirus
Size (nm)	28	42	38–50	36	32
Genome	Single-stranded RNA (+) 7.5 kb	Double-stranded DNA 3.2 kb	Single-stranded RNA (+) 9.4 kb	Single-stranded RNA (+) 1.7 kb	Single-stranded RNA (+) 7.8 kb
Envelope proteins	None	Large, middle, major HBsAg	E1, D2	Yes (major HBsAg from HBV)	None
Capsid proteins	VP1, VP2, VP3	HBcAg	NS2, NS3, NS4	Small and large HDAg (p24, 27)	2
Genomic integration	No	Yes	No	No	No
Genotypes	4	5	6 (15 subtypes)	3	3
Serotypes	1	1	?	?	1
Clinical					
Incubation period	30 days	75 days	50 days	75 days	40 days
Transmission	Fecal–oral	Parenteral	Parenteral	Parenteral	Fecal–oral
Tissues infected	Liver	Liver, blood mononuclear cells	Liver, blood mononuclear cells	Liver	Liver
Virus persistence	No	Yes	Yes	Yes	No
Association with HCC	No	Yes	Yes	No	No
Acute hepatitis	Yes	Yes	Yes	Yes	Yes
Chronic hepatitis	No	Yes	Yes	Yes	No
Progression to chronic hepatitis after acute infection	0%	1%–10% adults, 90% neonates	50%–80%	2%–5% co-infection, 70%–90% superinfection	0%
Diagnosis					
Acute	IgM anti-HAV	IgM anti-HBc, HBsAg, HBeAg, HBV DNA	HCV RNA, anti-HCV	IgG anti-HDAg (>1:1,000), HDV RNA	IgM anti-HEV, HEV RNA
Chronic	NA	HBsAg, HBeAg,+ HBV DNA	HCV RNA, anti-HCV	IgG anti-HDAg (>1:1,000)	NA
Past infection	IgG anti-HAV[a]	Anti-HBs, anti-HBc, anti-HBe	Anti-HCV	IgG anti-HDAg (<1:1,000)	IgG anti-HEV
Treatment					
Acute	—	—	—	—	—
Chronic	—	Interferon-α, lamivudine, adefovir, entecavir	Interferon-α, ribavirin	Interferon-α	—
End stage	Transplantation	Transplantation + HBIg	Transplantation	Transplantation	Transplantation
Prevention					
Pre-exposure	HAV vaccine	HBV vaccine	—	HBV vaccine	Sanitation of water supply
Post-exposure	HAV vaccine + Ig	HBV vaccine + HBIg			

DNA = deoxyribonucleic acid; HAV = hepatitis A virus; HBcAg = hepatitis B core antigen; HBeAg = hepatitis B enzyme antigen; HBIg = hepatitis B immunoglobulin; HBsAg = hepatitis B surface antigen; HBV = hepatitis B virus; HCC = hepatocellular carcinoma; HCV = hepatitis C virus; HDAg = hepatitis D antigen; HDV = hepatitis D virus; HEV = hepatitis E virus; Ig = immunoglobulin; IgG = immunoglobulin G; IgM = immunoglobulin M; RNA = ribonucleic acid.

[a]Also post vaccination.

integrated into the host genome. Protein synthesis proceeds from four open reading frames (ORFs): the envelope proteins (large, middle, and major HBsAg) from the pre-S1, pre-S2, and S gene sequences; the e antigen (HBeAg) and HBcAg from the pre-C and C gene sequences; the DNA polymerase protein from the P gene; and the transactivator X protein from the X gene. HBeAg contains peptides from the pre-C gene sequence, which permits the protein to be secreted; in contrast, HBcAg lacks these peptides and remains in the cell. DNA replication proceeds via ribonucleic acid (RNA) intermediates in the nucleus. The virus particles are then assembled in the cytoplasm and released by the hepatocytes. The virus itself is not cytopathic; hepatocyte destruction results from immune-mediated responses to viral antigens, leading to hepatic necrosis and inflammation.

In most adult patients, viral infection is cleared by neutralizing antibodies and cytolytic T lymphocytes.[3] Viral infection persists in up to 10% of adults and 90% of neonates following acute infection. The frequency of viral persistence following acute infection is related to age, sex, and immune deficiency. Persistence occurs in 90% of infants under 1 year of age, 30% of children aged 1 through 5 years, and 10% of adults; in men twice as often as in women; and in immune-deficient individuals, such as those with human immunodeficiency virus (HIV) infection, renal insufficiency requiring hemodialysis, or Down syndrome.[4] Patients exposed to large pools of potentially infected plasma, such as those with hemophilia, are also at risk for chronicity.

Chronically infected patients have positive serum HBV DNA and HBsAg. Serum HBeAg may also be present. Clearance of the virus may occur spontaneously, with seroconversion of HBeAg in 10% and of HBsAg in 1 to 2% of cases per year.[4] Chronically infected patients exhibit a wide range of pathology, from asymptomatic carrier status to mild or severe hepatitis, cirrhosis, or HCC in various combinations.[5,6] It is important to note that in up to 15% of HBsAg carriers, HBeAg seroconversion may be associated with persistent high levels of HBV DNA and with high-grade histologic activity indicative of active viral replication. These patients have been found to acquire a mutation in the pre-C region, which ablates the synthesis of HBeAg.[7]

Hepatitis B virus is transmitted parenterally from infected patients, in whom concentrations in the blood approach 10^{10}/mL (concentrations in body secretions, such as semen and saliva, are only one one-thousandth that in blood).[8] Settings in which HBV may be transmitted include those involving parenteral exposure to infected blood products: transfusions, use of contaminated needles in intravenous drug administrations, sexual intercourse, and perinatal or in utero exposures (mother to infant).[9–12] Infants of HbeAg+ mothers have a 70% chance of infection and a 90% risk of chronic infection.[13] Transmission has also been reported in institutions for the mentally retarded, day care centers, and family environments with close interpersonal contacts.[14,15] The virus has been shown to be quite stable at ambient temperatures, and contamination of surfaces in the homes of chronically infected persons has been documented.[16] The mode of transmission in intrafamilial contacts may be inapparent percutaneous exposure—although oral spread cannot be excluded, because the accidental ingestion of HbsAg+ human serum has been reported to result in HBV infection.

HBV and Hepatocellular Carcinoma Epidemiologic Considerations The evidence for an epidemiologic association between chronic HBV infection and HCC is overwhelming. An estimated 387 million people worldwide are chronic carriers of HBV, and the risk of HCC developing in this population is more than 200 times the risk found in the noninfected population.[17] In low endemic areas, HCC was found in about 0.4% of autopsies; in high endemic areas, where HBV infection is 10 times higher, 20 to 40% of all cancers are HCCs.

In the best prospective study from Taiwan, 22,707 men were tested for HBsAg, with 3,454 positive results (15.2%).[18] In the 7-year follow-up, 116 cases of HCC were diagnosed.[19] All of the men with HCC had previously tested positive for HBsAg, except for 3 who had serologic markers of previous HBV infection. None of the HBsAg– controls developed HCC. HBsAg carriers at especially high risk were those with active infection (HBeAg/HBV DNA+) and those with cirrhosis. In another prospective study of 824 Alaska natives who were HBsAg carriers, the annual incidence for HCC was 387 per 100,000 population, accounting for 57% of cancer-related deaths. In the noncarrier Alaska native population, HCC accounted for 2% of all cancer-related deaths.[20]

These two studies not only indicate an association between HBV and HCC, but also strongly suggest a causal relationship. Carcinogenesis is generally accepted to be a multistep process involving initiation, promotion, and progression. The question arises as to whether, despite this overwhelming epidemiologic evidence, HBV infection alone can be responsible for all of those processes.

Several observations indicate that other agents—alone or in combination with HBV—play a role in the development of HCC. In industrialized and developing countries respectively, 68% and 11% of HCC patients lack the serologic markers of HBV infection. However, these data must be treated cautiously, because they depend on the sensitivities of the assays for serologic markers. Those percentages may change substantially with the use of polymerase chain reaction (PCR), which can detect minimal amounts of HBV DNA in serum or tissue.[21] More compelling evidence for the contribution of other factors to hepatic carcinogenesis are these observations: (1) within one region, the prevalence of HBV infection may be relatively uniform, but HCC is not[22]; (2) HCC is found more frequently in men than in women; and (3) in some endemic areas, variations in HCC rates have been reported according to ethnic group or place of birth.[23]

Besides HBV, other factors in the development of HCC may include other chronic viral hepatitis infections (such as HCV), cirrhosis of any origin, genetic disposition, androgenic–anabolic and oral contraceptive steroids, and immune system function. In addition, alcohol, cigarettes, and aflatoxin have all been implicated as causative agents, as have nonalcoholic steatohepatitis, α1-antitrypsin deficiency, and schistosomiasis.

Aflatoxin exposure from ingestion of contaminated food has been implicated as a cause of HCC. However, most of the correlation studies were performed in high HBV-endemic areas, without taking into account HBV status, and were plagued by inaccurate assessments of aflatoxin exposure. A 1987 study in Swaziland addressed the relationships between aflatoxin exposure, HBV infection, and the incidence of HCC.[24] In that study, HBsAg prevalence varied little from region to region, but aflatoxin exposure varied by as much as a factor of 5. The incidence of HCC also varied by a factor of 5 and correlated well with aflatoxin exposure, suggesting that aflatoxin may act as an independent risk factor. Furthermore, in countries where aflatoxin is highly suspected, cases of HCC have frequent G:C to T:A transversions in codon 249 of the *TP53* gene, providing a molecular epidemiologic signature for this particular mutation.[25] A meta-analysis of 49 published studies found that the mean proportion of HCCs with the codon 249 mutation was positively correlated with aflatoxin exposure ($p = .0001$).[26]

Alcohol consumption and cigarette smoking have also been implicated in the causation of HCC in case control and cohort studies. However, when HBV status was taken into account, alcohol consumption remained a risk factor, but cigarette smoking did not.[27,28] The role of cirrhosis as the causative link was addressed in a cross-sectional study from France that showed that the relative risk for HCC was about twice as great in HBV-associated cirrhosis as in alcoholic cirrhosis.[29] HBV-associated HCC occurs in the absence of cirrhosis in up to 27% of patients (Figure 22-1).[18]

Oral contraceptive use has also been recognized as a risk factor.[30]

Mechanisms of Oncogenicity Application of the technology of molecular biology to HBV infection gave several clues regarding the mecha-

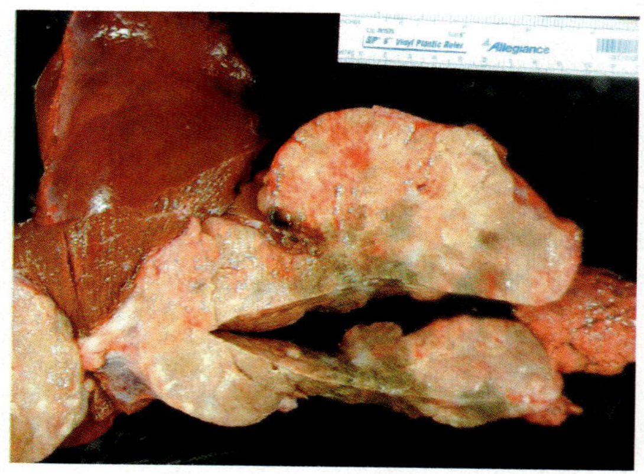

Figure 22-1 Hepatocellular carcinoma in noncirrhotic HBV-infected liver.

nisms by which HBV infection leads to HCC. A uniform mechanism valid for every HCC is still elusive, however. The subsections that follow review the genetic organization of HBV during infection and the possible mechanism or mechanisms by which it can cause HCC.

Integration of HBV DNA The availability of cloned HBV DNA made it possible to detect HBV DNA in HCCs. Epidemiologic studies based on serologic markers were confirmed, because all the HCCs induced by HBV infection contained chromosomally integrated HBV DNA in various forms. The long latency period that elapses between infection and development of HCC makes it very unlikely that the HBV DNA codes form a dominantly acting, classic oncogene. Furthermore, during the latency period, the HBV DNA becomes fragmented and rearranged; thus, neither the inserted HBV DNA sequences nor the chromosomal sites of insertion are uniform in the various HCCs.

Chromosomally integrated HBV DNA may release the growth control of hepatocytes by coding for a factor (similar to the X protein), which activates otherwise dormant genes and proto-oncogenes, or which silences anti-oncogenes; by inserting HBV DNA sequences that can activate and influence the transcription of cellular genes; by causing chronic inflammation with cell death and hepatocyte regeneration and with fibrosis; and by activating the immune system, thereby liberating cytokines at the wrong time in the wrong place. A comprehensive characterization of gene expression profiles of HBV-related HCC and noncancerous liver samples has been reported using 5'-read expressed sequence tag clusters to a complement DNA (cDNA) microarray system containing 12,393 genes.[31] Altered transcription of multiple genes was noted, including many genes involved in cell cycle regulation and biotransformation, but no overriding trends could be identified.

Activation of Oncogenes, Growth Factors, and Receptors Although the DNA sequences of the woodchuck hepatitis virus are not integrated adjacent to the coding sequences of the *myc* gene, rearrangements of the *myc* gene with a 5 to 50 times higher expression were found in several HCCs. The rearrangements found in woodchuck HCCs are similar to those found in human B- and T-cell leukemias, Burkitt lymphoma, and mouse plasmacytoma.[32]

Mutations and activation of the genes belonging to the *ras* family are associated with a wide variety of human cancers. Mutations in the *ras* genes are not regularly found in human HCCs, but activated H-*ras* and K-*ras* genes have been detected in some HCCs.[33,34] In other tissues, high expression of *ras* genes—as well as mutated sequences—is associated with malignant transformation; the role of the *ras* gene in HCCs therefore cannot be overlooked.

Among the growth factors analyzed in HCCs, insulin-like growth factor 2 (*IGF2*), originally called somatomedin A, seems to be involved in the development of HCCs. The *IGF2* RNAs are differentially spliced: the most abundant species found in fetal woodchuck liver represent the predominant species in both precancerous liver nodules and HCCs in the woodchuck. Furthermore, the pattern of *IGF2* RNAs in precancerous liver nodules is similar to that found in fully malignant HCCs. Thus, the activation of *IGF2* transcripts may contribute to the growth of precancerous nodules.[35]

Because the development of carcinomas can be viewed as a disturbance of the signal transducing system, it is intriguing that HBV DNA is sometimes integrated in a frame next to a liver cell sequence that bears a striking homology not only to the v-*erb*-A oncogene, but also to the DNA-binding domains of the human glucocorticoid receptor, estrogen receptor genes, and the retinoic acid receptor. The inappropriate expression of such genes because of HBV DNA integration might be a contributory factor to the development of HCC.

The HBV DNA integration into chromosomal DNA was found to have a relationship to oncogenes, receptors, growth factors, and (in at least one case) a normal protein, cyclin A.[36] Cyclins A and B are well conserved during evolution and play an important role in mitotic division. HBV DNA is inserted into the intron of cyclin A, and this insertion might influence the progression phase of HCCs.

This brief and by no means complete summation of the insertion sites of HBV DNA leads unequivocally to the conclusion that the integration of HBV DNA can be viewed only as guilt by association; the "smoking gun" has yet to be identified.

Tumor Suppressor Genes Several lines of evidence indicate that HBV DNA insertion into chromosomes may be associated with inactivation of a tumor suppressor gene. First, the long latency period that elapses between infection and development of HCC and the fact that not all infections lead to HCC are compatible with the notion, as seen in retinoblastoma, that one allele is altered genetically, and the other is somatically mutated. Indeed, in children with the Beckwith–Wiedemann congenital malformation syndrome, 10% of the cases are associated with mutations on chromosome 11, leading to tumor formation, including hepatoblastoma, Wilms' tumor, rhabdomyosarcoma, and adrenal carcinoma. That chromosome 11 codes for a tumor suppressor gene was shown by Stanbridge and colleagues, who found that the malignant phenotype was repressed when the normal chromosome 11 was present in somatic hybrids between tumorigenic and nontumorigenic cells.[37] The loss of that normal chromosome led to a reversion to the malignant phenotype. (The suppressor gene in retinoblastoma was mapped to chromosome 13.)

In 45% of HCC cases, alleles from chromosome arm 11p are missing, and in 50% of HCCs, alleles from chromosome arm 13q are missing.[38] In addition, HBV DNA integration was mapped to chromosome 11 in many cases. It has also been shown that the *TP53* gene functions as a tumor suppressor, and in many human cancers, including HCC, mutations occur in that gene, with the mutated gene subsequently acting as an oncogene.[25,39] Furthermore, although evidence—albeit circumstantial—for the role of suppressor genes in HCC is furnished by transgenic mice carrying the *TEAD1* gene (TEA domain family member 1) coding for T antigen (SV40 transcriptional enhancer factor), the tumorigenic activity of the SV40 T antigen is associated with its ability to bind to the suppressor gene product. In transgenic mice expressing SV40 T antigen, HCC develops after a long period of hyperplasia.[40] Furthermore, mouse hepatocytes immortalized by T antigen were transfected with a selectable gene and HBV DNA. All of the cells in which HBV replicated displayed malignant growth characteristics and were tumorigenic.

It has been well documented that aflatoxin B1 exposure is associated with a specific mutation at codon 249 in the *TP53* tumor suppressor gene in hepatic tumors.[25] Studies of tumor specimens from patients with HCC have also shown a strong association of codon 249 mutations with HBsAg positivity in the serum and HBV DNA in tumor tissue, suggesting an association of HBV with these mutations.[26,41,42]

Role of HBx Protein The HBx protein coded by the X gene of HBV has transactivating activity on a number of viral and cellular genes that may be involved in the development of HCC.[43] For instance, the HBx protein has been shown to interact with members of the bZip family and to bind and inactivate the *TP53* tumor suppressor protein.[44,45] Its genomic localization is analogous to that of the human T-cell lymphotropic viruses (HTLV-I and -II, and HIV), namely, it is at the 3' end of the linearized genome.

Interestingly, other DNA viruses with oncogenic activity also code for transactivating activity. For example, the T antigen of *TEAD1*, the MS-EA protein of Epstein–Barr virus, the IE protein of herpes simplex, and the *tat* protein of HIV (which, despite being an RNA virus, shares some steps in its replicative cycle with HBV). The sequence coding for the HBx protein is well conserved among the various subtypes of HBV and in the woodchuck and ground squirrel hepatitis viruses. Despite the similar genetic organization of the hepadnaviruses, duck hepatitis virus does not contain the sequences coding for the HBx protein, and infection with that virus does not lead to HCC. In many HCCs, viral DNA is inserted near or within the coding sequences of the HBx protein; thus, it is possible that expression of this protein, or of a fusion protein with cellularly coded genes, plays an important role in the development of HCC.[46]

That specific cellular proteins, in concert with virally coded proteins, are involved in HCC is suggested by the finding that chimpanzees infected with HBV display the classic symptoms and signs of hepatitis as judged morphologically in the liver, and by the appearance in those primates of elevated serum enzymes, together with viral antigens and the corresponding antibodies. In contrast to the human disease, however, HBV infection in the chimpanzee does not lead to HCC. Recent studies with HBx-expressing transgenic mice under authentic promoter control showed a high rate of HCC development (86%).[47]

HBV-Induced Hepatocytic Hyperplasia and Necrosis As a consequence of HBV infection leading to HCC hepatocytic nodules, ground glass–appearing cells (containing HBsAg and displaying hyperplasia, necrotic inflammation, fibrosis, portal inflammation, and, in many cases, cirrhosis) can be detected in the liver. The causal relation between the infection and the liver cell injury has not been elucidated. The evidence that the immune system is involved is only circumstantial.[48]

The availability of vaccines and the production of viral antigens by recombinant DNA technology made it possible to determine that the production of antibodies against HBsAg is T cell–dependent; HBcAg is more immunogenic and elicits antibodies in T cell–dependent and –independent ways.[49,50] HBcAg-specific, functionally competent CD4 helper and CD8 suppressor T cells were detected in chronic infection, but HBsAg-specific T cells were not found.[51] The T-cell clones that were HBcAg-specific were HLA-dr (d-related human leukocyte antigen)–restricted and secreted interleukin-2 (IL-2), interferon-γ, and tumor necrosis factor. For such involvement of the immune system, HBV is obliged to enter the cells of the immune system to present the antigen. There are indications that, albeit rarely, lymphocytes and monocytes are infected with HBV in vivo. Although immune system involvement could adequately explain the cascade of events that lead from infection through inflammation, necrosis, and regeneration, with subsequent genetic changes leading to HCC, the results obtained with transgenic mice indicate that HCC can develop without the contributions of the immune system. Transgenic mice carrying HBV DNA sequences have been produced in several laboratories.[52] The livers of these animals synthesize HBsAg and secrete virus into the serum, but the immune system is tolerant. In one case, a programmed response characterized by inflammation, regenerative hyperplasia, and aneuploidy led to the development of HCC. The incidence of HCC was influenced by sex and age and was directly related to liver cell injury and nonsecreted HBsAg content of the liver cells.

To summarize, several factors, directly or indirectly, alone or in combination, can lead to HCC, but the integration of HBV DNA in one form or another is obligatory in HBV-associated hepatocarcinogenesis.

Primary Prevention **Pre-exposure Prophylaxis** Effective vaccines for prophylaxis against HBV infection were first introduced by Krugman in 1981, using inactivated human HBsAg+ serum. The HBsAg particles were subsequently purified from seropositive human sera and used in the plasma-derived vaccine. Advances in genetic engineering enabled the large-scale production of HBsAg protein product by viral expression vectors coding the S gene in bakers' yeast.[53] More than 90% of patients developed adequate levels of anti-HBs (10 mIU/mL) following a series of three injections at 0, 1, and 6 months; in these subjects, protection from subsequent hepatitis B infection was almost complete.[54] Some patients develop "breakthrough" HBV infection despite protective levels of anti-HBs; one of these subjects was shown to have acquired an infection with an HBsAg mutant virus, in which a mutation in the S gene resulting in an amino acid substitution at position 145 rendered the virus insensitive to the neutralizing antibody raised by conventional HBsAg vaccine.[55,56]

Of vaccinated subjects, 90% retain detectable levels and 80% retain protective levels of anti-HBs 5 years after vaccination.[57] The side effects of vaccination include mild pain at the site of injection and mild temperature elevation. No cases of HIV transmission have been reported with either the plasma-derived or recombinant vaccine. However, 5% of vaccinated subjects develop an inadequate response (between 2.1 and 9.9 mIU/mL), and another 5% produce no anti-HBs. Lack of response may be due to immune suppression, such as in subjects with renal failure or HIV infection; to older age (> 60 years); or to route of injection (intramuscular is superior to subcutaneous or intradermal administration). In 25% of nonresponders or inadequate responders, an additional dose produced adequate levels of anti-HBs; an additional series of three injections produced adequate anti-HBs in 50 to 60%. Co-administration of the vaccine with interferon-α, thymopentin, or IL-2 is being investigated for enhancement of response in the remaining 15 to 25%.

Other vaccines for preventing HBV infection are currently under investigation. HBsAg vaccines incorporating the pre-S2 polypeptide may induce responses in individuals who fail to respond to the conventional vaccine.[58] A monoclonal antibody, 2F10, has been raised that is an "internal image" anti-idiotype antibody capable of mimicking the group-specific "a" determinant of HBsAg. The antibody can generate B- and T-cell responses to HBsAg when injected into mice. A 15-mer peptide from the hypervariable region of 2F10 has been isolated that is capable of generating immune responses similar to those from the intact antibody and that has potential for vaccine development.[59]

Large-scale production of immunogenic protein can be accomplished using insects or worms infected with viral vectors or using transgenic plants.[60] Recombinant HBsAg obtained from transgenic tobacco plants has been shown to elicit B- and T-cell immune responses when injected into mice.[61] Tests in which animals are fed with transgenic potatoes encoding recombinant HBsAg are currently in progress and may offer a more economical program for large-scale vaccination. Vaccine administration can also be facilitated by multiple pressure or scratch techniques using vaccinia virus vectors and by oral administration using adenovirus vectors.[62,63]

Despite the development of safe and effective vaccines for HBV infection, the incidence of hepatitis B in the United States has increased. In contrast, a decrease in HBV infection incidence has been demonstrated following vaccination programs in Taiwan and Switzerland. The failure in the United States may be attributable to inadequate vaccination of high-risk subjects (only 10% were vaccinated) and the fact that 30 to 40% of new HBV cases did not fall into the high-risk category.[64,65] The current recommendation for a universal hepatitis B vaccination program in childhood should result in the vaccination of all subjects and should effectively reduce the incidence of HBV infection.[66] Such an approach has reduced the prevalence rate of HBsAg+ serum by 99% in Alaska and from 9.8% to 0.7% in children 15 years and younger in Taiwan.[67,68]

The effectiveness of HBV vaccination in the primary prevention of chronic HBV infection and HCC has already been demonstrated in pilot vaccination projects. In Taiwan, universal HBV vaccination was initiated with newborns of HBsAg+ mothers in 1984 and was extended to all children by 1989. The average annual incidence of HCC in children has since decreased to 0.36 from 0.70 per 100,000 children (1981–1986 to 1990–1994).[69]

Postexposure Prophylaxis For prevention after HBV exposure, such as after delivery of a neonate from an infected mother, after needlestick puncture from an infected patient, or after sexual intercourse with an infected partner, administration of hepatitis B immunoglobulin (HBIg) followed by HBV vaccination has been more than 90% effective.[70] Vaccination without HBIg produced only 70 to 80% anti-HBs responses.

Blood Donor Screening With the introduction of HBsAg antibody screening in blood donors, the incidence of transfusion-associated hepatitis decreased to 6% from 33% of hepatitis cases over three decades. Since the addition of anti-HCV screening, only 0.3% of hepatitis in the United States is transfusion related.[71]

Secondary Prevention **Screening for HCC** Locally advanced and metastatic HCC usually responds poorly to anticancer treatments. Early HCC is, however, effectively treated by surgical and nonsurgical modalities, with prolonged survival. It is not clear whether lead-time bias might be responsible, in part, for the survival prolongation.

Because of the high prevalence of HBV infection in certain regions of China, a screening program for HCC was instituted for adults over the age of 35 with chronic HBV infection. The screening tests used were serum α-fetoprotein and liver ultrasonography performed every 6 months. The α-fetoprotein has a sensitivity of 70%, given that up to 30% of HCCs do not secrete it. The specificity of α-fetoprotein depends on the threshold level chosen. For levels of more than 1,000 ng/mL, α-fetoprotein is close to 100% specific. For levels of 20 to 200 ng/mL, false positives outnumber true positives. Liver ultrasonography has up to 70% sensitivity for the detection of HCCs less than 2 cm, but has poor specificity. However, the combination of α-fetoprotein and ultrasonography increases both sensitivity and specificity. Of the 1.3 million people screened in the Chinese program, 500 cases of HCC were detected.[68] A similar screening program was reported from Alaska; it screened 1,400 HBsAg carriers and detected 20 cases of HCC.[20,68] A randomized study demonstrating the survival benefit for the screened population as compared with controls has yet to be completed.

Treatment of Chronic HBV Infection For the treatment of chronic HBV infection to be effective, it must eliminate viral replication, resolve hepatic necrotic inflammation, and prevent progression to cirrhosis and HCC. The most effective treatment to date is interferon-α given at a dose of 5 MU daily or 10 MU three times weekly for 12 to 24 weeks. Meta-analysis of 15 randomized controlled trials showed that interferon-α produced seroconversion of HBeAg in 33% of recipients as compared with 12% of untreated controls.[72] Seroconversion of HBsAg occurred in 10% of treated patients as compared with rare instances in controls. Of patients who clear HBeAg, 65% also clear HBsAg at a mean follow-up of 4.3 years. Of patients who clear both HBeAg and HBsAg, 50 to 100% also clear serum HBV DNA, with improvement in hepatic necrotic inflammation and normalization of serum alanine aminotransferase (ALT). It should be noted that some patients might clear HBeAg, but still maintain high serum levels of HBV DNA. These patients, who are HBsAg+ and anti-HBe+, may have acquired mutations in the pre-C sequence that ablated synthesis of HBeAg, but that did not affect viral replication.

Factors predicting a favorable response to interferon-α include high serum ALT, low serum HBV DNA, and active hepatic necrotic inflammation.[73] Patients with normal ALT or high serum HBV DNA rarely respond to interferon. It should be noted that Asian patients who demonstrate predictors favorable to interferon, do not respond as well as Caucasian and African American patients.[74] Patients receiving interferon-α treatment, particularly those with more severe hepatitis, may experience a flare-up of hepatic necrotic inflammation, but will not usually require treatment interruption. Prednisone priming before treatment with interferon-α has been reported in pilot studies to be more effective than interferon-α alone. This approach has not been confirmed in large-scale studies, however, and is not used as standard treatment.[75,76]

Other drugs that have been shown in pilot studies to be effective and tolerated include the second-generation nucleoside analogues famciclovir and lamivudine (3-thiacytidine). These analogues, administered orally, were found to be well tolerated and effective in reducing serum HBV DNA levels and serum aminotransferase levels following a 1-month course of treatment. Unfortunately, patients relapsed rapidly after treatment cessation. Prolonged administration of lamivudine for 1 year has been shown in a randomized trial to produce sustained suppression of serum HBV DNA (44% vs. 16%), HBeAg seroconversion (32% vs. 11%), sustained normalization of serum ALT (41% vs. 7%), and decreased hepatic fibrosis (5% vs. 20%).[77] However, viral resistance in HBV mutants with substitutions in the YMDD motif of the polymerase gene occurred in 38% of patients after 2 years and in 67% of patients after 4 years of lamivudine therapy.[78] But recent studies have shown that newer nucleoside analogues such as adefovir dipivoxil and entecavir can be active against lamivudine-resistant mutants as well as against wild-type HBV.[79,80] Results from randomized trials of adefovir dipivoxil and entecavir showed significant improvement in liver inflammation after 48 weeks of treatment and reduction in hepatic fibrosis in chronic hepatitis B infection.[81,82] HBsAg vaccine was shown in one study to be effective in 3 of 14 patients with chronic HBV infection, with clearance of serum HBV DNA after three injections.[83]

For patients with liver cirrhosis caused by chronic HBV infection, orthotopic liver transplantation may provide a long-term survival benefit. Recurrence of HBV infection, however, occurs at rates of 40% and 50% at 1 and 3 years following transplantation. Recurrence is particularly high in patients with positive serum HBV DNA at the time of surgery: 83% at 3 years post transplantation as compared with 58% at 3 years post transplantation in patients negative for HBeAg and HBV DNA at the time of surgery.[84,85] Long-term therapy with high-dose HBIg post transplantation reduced HBV recurrence to 35% from 75% and increased survival to 82% from 50% at 3 years post transplantation.[85] These studies indicate that patients with HBV-related cirrhosis but with negative HBeAg and HBV DNA may benefit from liver transplantation with HBIg treatment following their surgery.

The effectiveness of interferon-α in the secondary prevention of HCC in patients with chronic HBV infection has been demonstrated. In one study, 101 men with chronic HBV infection were randomized to placebo or interferon-α treatment. Follow-up was between 1.1 and 11.5 years after the end of therapy. HCC was detected in 1 of 67 treated patients as compared with 4 of 34 placebo controls ($p = .013$).[86] In another study, the cumulative occurrence rate of HCC in 313 patients (94 treated with interferon-α, 219 not treated) was assessed at the end of 3, 5, and 10 years. Rates for treated versus untreated patients were 4.5% versus 13.3% at 3 years, 7.0% versus 19.6% at 5 years, and 17.0% versus 30.8% at 10 years ($p = .0124$).[87]

The Role of HDV in HCC HDV ("delta virus") is an RNA virus with envelope proteins that are derived from HBV.[88] HDV infection therefore requires the presence of HBV and can occur concurrently (HDV/HBV coinfection) or in the setting of an established chronic HBV infection (HDV superinfection). Acute HDV/HBV coinfection is self-limiting, with 2 to 5% persisting as chronic HDV infection. However, acute HDV superinfection can persist in 70 to 90% of cases, and progression to cirrhosis is more accelerated than with chronic HBV infection alone.[89]

Acute HDV superinfection generally induces an exacerbation of chronic HBV hepatitis, but may induce fulminant hepatitis in 17% of cases.[90] Diagnosis of acute and chronic HDV infection is made by the presence in serum of immunoglobulin G anti-hepatitis D protein (IgG anti-HDAg) at titers of more than 1:1,000, or of HDAg, or of HDV RNA.[91] Serum IgG anti-HDAg may persist in low titers (< 1:1,000) after resolution of HDV infection.

HDV has not been associated with HCC. Patients with HBV-associated cirrhosis and HCC have a prevalence of chronic HDV infection similar to that of patients with HBV-associated cirrhosis without HCC. Chronic HDV infection, however, may accelerate the development of cirrhosis, thereby increasing the risk for HCC.

Prevention is of particular importance for patients with chronic HBV infection because of the aggressive clinical course of HDV superinfection. Treatment of chronic HDV/HBV infection with interferon-α requires higher doses than does HBV infection alone; moreover, the time to response is longer (4 to 6 months), and the rate of relapse after cessation of treatment (90%) is higher.[92]

Like HBV, HDV is transmitted through parenteral exposure; preventive measures are geared toward safe practices in blood banks, abstinence from intravenous drug use, and vaccination against HBV. No commercial vaccine is currently available for HDV.

HEPATITIS C VIRUS

HCV was first isolated from non-A, non-B infectious plasma in 1989.[93] HCV is a member of the family Flaviviridae, which includes yellow fever virus, dengue viruses, and Japanese encephalitis virus. HCV measures 30 to 60 μm and is an enveloped virus with a single-stranded, linear, positive-sense RNA genome approximately 9.5 kb in length.[94]

The virus contains one large ORF capable of encoding a polyprotein precursor of 3,011 amino acids. Structural proteins are encoded at the 5' end. The 5' noncoding region precedes the large coding sequence and represents the most highly conserved sequence among the various viral isolates.[95] The 5' noncoding region contains a series of three short ORFs. The amino terminal of the transcript is cleaved to produce the core protein, an unglycosylated, basic, 19 to 22 kDa protein (p22). Two putative enveloped glycoproteins of 33 to 35 kDa and 70 to 72 kDa are designated E1 and E2, respectively. The amino terminal of E2 contains a hypervariable region that exhibits significant variation between HCV isolates. Four nonstructural domains follow (NS2 to NS5). The NS2 region is extremely hydrophobic, but its function has not been identified. The NS3 region encodes a 60 kDa protein that contains a viral protease involved in polyprotein processing and a putative helicase enzyme that is probably involved in unwinding the RNA genome for replication. The NS4 region is also extremely hydrophobic and shows 50% sequence homology among the various HCV types. The function of NS4 is not known. The NS5 region encodes a

116 kDa RNA-dependent RNA polymerase that replicates the RNA genome.

Phylogenetic analysis of the NS5 and E1 nucleotide sequences from samples obtained worldwide led to the identification of six major genetic groups and 14 subgroups.[96] Genotypes 1 to 3 are distributed worldwide, accounting for 70 to 80% of HCV infection in Western countries. Genotypes 4 and 5 are distributed primarily in Africa, and genotype 6, in Asia. Response to treatment with interferon-α is poor in patients with genotype 1 HCV infection.[97] Several reports have suggested correlations between these various genotypes and the severity of liver disease, the outcome of interferon treatment, and the development of HCC.[98] In addition, the population of HCV genomes ("quasi-species") shows genetic heterogeneity in infected individuals, which may be the reason that clearing the virus in the host is difficult.

HCV is the most common cause of nonalcoholic liver disease and the leading reason for orthotopic liver transplantation in the United States.[97] Although HCV incidence has declined since 1989 because of blood donor screening, an estimated 38,000 new cases occur annually in the United States.[98] Previously, more than 150,000 individuals were acutely infected with HCV annually.[99] Nearly 4 million people in the United States are currently infected with the virus. The infection is more common in minority populations (3.2% of African Americans and 2.1% of Mexican Americans) than in non-Hispanic white populations (1.5%).

HCV is transmitted through blood and blood products. Risk factors include blood transfusion and intravenous drug use.[89] Sexual and perinatal transmissions are less important routes of transmission. Perinatal transmission occurs more readily when the mother is coinfected with HBV.[98] In approximately 40% of patients with HCV, no recognizable risk factors are present.[99]

The clinical presentation of acute hepatitis C is mild and produces symptoms in only 20% of patients.[100] However, 80% of patients acutely infected with HCV do not clear the virus; they become chronically infected with HCV. Of chronically infected individuals, 20% develop cirrhosis within 20 years, and once the disease is established, they go on to develop HCC at a rate of 1 to 4% per year.[101] Fulminant hepatitis is rare in hepatitis C.

HCV infection is diagnosed with a third-generation enzyme-linked immunosorbent assay (ELISA) for antibodies to HCV. The test incorporates antigens from the nucleocapsid, NS3, NS4, and NS5 regions.[102] It has a sensitivity of 97%, but false positives require confirmation with a third-generation recombinant immunoblotting assay. In patients with negative anti-HCV because of recent acute infection or immunosuppression, direct detection of HCV RNA with reverse transcriptase PCR is required to assess for active infection.[103] Seroconversion of anti-HCV does not occur until the 9th week following acute HCV infection. It should also be noted that patients who successfully clear the virus may remain positive for anti-HCV for many years.[104,105]

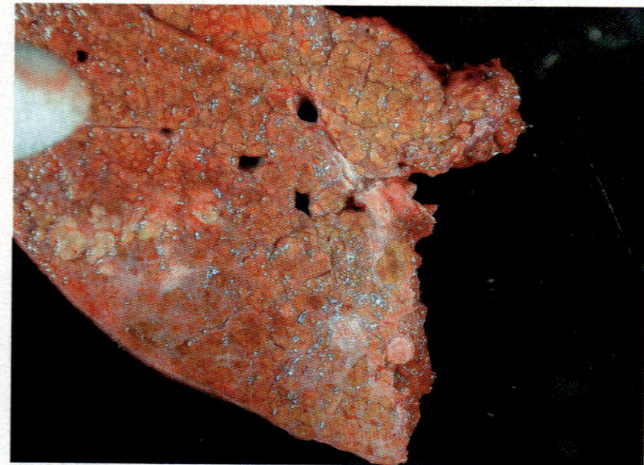

Figure 22-2 Multifocal HCC in HCV cirrhosis.

Quantitative methods, such as the branched DNA signal amplification assay, have been used to identify candidates for interferon therapy, to monitor viral load during the course of chronic infection and antiviral treatment, and, prior to liver transplantation, to predict recurrent infection in the allografts.[106]

HCV and HCC A significant proportion of patients with HCC are infected with HCV.[107–109] Patients with well-documented transfusion-related hepatitis C progressed from acute to chronic hepatitis, to cirrhosis, and finally to HCC after 7 to 23 years (Figure 22-2). Similar observations were made in chimpanzees years after inoculation with serum from a patient with chronic non-A, non-B hepatitis.

The epidemiologic evidence for an association of HCV with HCC is compelling. Case-control studies from Japan, Italy, Spain, South Africa, and Taiwan have shown that the prevalence of anti-HCV positivity in patients with HCC is substantially higher than in control populations. From 60 to 70% of Japanese patients with HCC were seropositive for antibodies to HCV. A similar prevalence was reported in Western Europe. HCV RNA and the viral proteins can be detected in both the tumor and the surrounding cirrhotic nodules of the HCC patients.[110,111] In a prospective study, 246 patients with well-compensated cirrhosis who were positive for anti-HCV by ELISA were followed for 10 years. Of these 246 patients, 56 developed HCC (annual incidence of 2.2%).[112]

The role of HCV in the malignant transformation of hepatocytes is not clear, however. Although 30% of HCCs in HBV carriers developed in the absence of cirrhosis, HCC arising in chronic HCV infection is, with only rare exceptions, associated with cirrhosis.[113–115] Findings suggest an indirect role of HCV in hepatocarcinogenesis, probably through the continuous cell regeneration that results from the chronic microinflammatory process, which predisposes hepatocytes to mutations and malignant transformation.[116–118] Case-control studies have suggested a synergism in the development of HCC of chronic HCV infection with HBV markers and a history of alcohol intake.[119] Recent studies in transgenic mice expressing the HCV core protein have suggested that the core protein may have a more direct role in hepatocarcinogenesis by binding to nuclear factors that regulate growth and by accumulating reactive oxygen species.[120]

It should be noted that an increased risk for non-Hodgkin's lymphoma and cholangiocarcinoma have been demonstrated in epidemiologic studies of patients with chronic HCV infection.[121–123] Intrahepatic B cells in patients with chronic HCV infection have been shown to be infected with HCV, clonally expanded, and activated to secrete IgM molecules, suggesting a role for HCV-induced B-cell expansion resulting in mixed cryoglobulinemia or non-Hodgkin's lymphoma.[124] Several studies have shown an increased risk for cholangiocarcinoma in anti-HCV+ patients.[125,126] The detection of HCV RNA in cholangiocarcinomas further supports the potential role of HCV in the pathogenesis of cholangiocarcinoma.[127,128]

Prevention and Treatment Little is known about either passive or active immunity to HCV. Recent studies have shown that reinfection with HCV following a previous infection is quite common.[129,130] That finding suggests that long-lasting immunity to HCV infection is nonexistent. HCV has the ability to mutate rapidly under immune pressure and to exist simultaneously as a series of related but immunologically distinct variants, any one of which can become the predominant strain when a coexistent strain comes under immune pressure.[131] This coexistence of multiple mutants has been termed "quasi-species." Neutralizing antibodies to HCV have been shown to develop, but they are strain-specific and are ineffective against the emerging strains. Major efforts are under way to develop a vaccine that would bypass these obstacles and provide protective immunity.

Before the discovery of HCV, interferon-α was found to be beneficial in patients with chronic non-A, non-B hepatitis.[132] Subsequent randomized controlled trials for chronic hepatitis using HCV RNA and antibody assays have shown that interferon-α administered for 6 months produced disappearance of serum HCV RNA, normalization of serum aminotransferases, and improvement in hepatic inflammation in up to 50% of treated patients.[133] However, relapses following cessation of treatment were common, with increases in serum HCV RNA, elevation of serum aminotransferases, and increased hepatic inflammation. Sustained responses were seen in 6 to 15% of patients treated with interferon-α. More recently, the combination of interferon-α with ribavirin at a dose of 1,000 to 1,200 mg daily has produced sustained responses in 30 to 40% of patients; this combination is currently the standard treatment for previously nontreated patients.[134] Pegylated interferon-α monotherapy has shown sustained responses in 35 to 40% of cases, similar to combination therapy with ribavirin.[135] A randomized trial of pegylated interferon-α plus ribavirin versus interferon-α plus ribavirin showed resolution of HCV RNA in 54% versus 47% of patients ($p = .01$).[136]

For patients with end-stage liver cirrhosis from chronic HCV infection, orthotopic liver transplantation may prolong survival. Recurrence of HCV infection is close to 100% post transplantation, but unlike recurrent HBV infection, the clinical course is indolent, and liver cirrhosis may not appear until many years after the surgery.[137] In approximately 10% of cases, however, progression of recurrent hepatitis C to liver failure occurs within a few years because of cirrhosis or massive hepatic necrosis. Fibrosing cholestatic hepatitis post transplantation has also been reported.[138,139] Treatment with interferon-α post transplantation showed a 28% response in normalization of ALT and a 100% response in reduction of HCV RNA. HCV RNA invariably returned to the pretreatment level after cessation of treatment, however.[140] In studies before 1989, HBIg administration was shown to reduce HCV seroconversion in transplantation patients[141]; however, HBIg is no longer effective because, in 1990, donor screening for anti-HCV eliminated plasma rich in anti-HCV. Based on these data, a monoclonal antibody directed against HCV has been evaluated in an HCV-infected mouse model and is currently in phase I/II clinical trials in patients with chronic HCV infection and post liver transplantion.[142]

Primary Prevention Prevention of HCV transmission has made great strides since the introduction of HCV screening in 1990 with the first-generation anti-HCV assay. With the refinement of diagnostic assays, the incidence of post-transfusion HCV hepatitis in the United States has been reduced to less than 0.3%. However, posttransfusion HCV hepatitis remains a problem in many parts of the world where donor screening has not been systematic and where contaminated instruments have been used in blood procurement, mass immunization, and surgical or dental procedures. Currently, the major identifiable risk is intravenous drug use with contaminated needles; transmission during sex or birthing is rare. With the lack of an effective HCV vaccine, pre-exposure prophylaxis is not possible. Since the introduction of blood donor screening in 1990, the plasma pools for hepatitis B immunoglobulin and hyperimmunoglobulin are devoid of anti-HCV antibodies and hence not likely to be effective for postexposure prophylaxis.

Secondary Prevention Although interferon-α has been used for the treatment of chronic HCV infection, an international survey also found it to be effective in secondary prevention of HCC. The overall relative HCC risk was three times higher in untreated patients than in interferon-treated anti-HCV+ patients and more than six times higher in untreated versus treated anti-HCV+/anti-HBc– patients.[143] In a report by the International Interferon-α Hepatocellular Carcinoma Study Group, which involves 21 centers, data on HCC occurrence were collected on 637 patients. Of these 637 patients, 281 received interferon, and 356 did not receive it. For anti-HCV+ patients without HBV markers, 29 of 129 untreated patients (20%) and 6 of 116 treated patients (5%) developed HCC.[144]

REFERENCES

1. Zuckerman AJ. The history of viral hepatitis from antiquity to the present. In: Deinhardt F, Deinhardt J, editors. Viral hepatitis: laboratory and clinical science. New York: Marcel Dekker; 1983. p. 3–32.
2. Pugh JC, Bassendine MF. Molecular biology of hepadnavirus replication. Br Med Bull 1990;46:329–53.
3. Hollinger FB, Dienstag JL. Hepatitis viruses. In: Lennette A, Balrus A, Hausler WH Jr, Shadomy HJ, editors. Manual of clinical microbiology. 4th ed. Washington (DC): American Society of Microbiology; 1985. p. 813–35.
4. McMahon BL, Alward WLM, Hall DB, et al. Acute hepatitis B infection. Relation of age to the clinical expression of disease and subsequent development of the carrier state. J Infect Dis 1985;151:599–603.
5. Desmet VJ, Gerber MA, Hoofnagle JH, et al. Classification of chronic hepatitis: diagnosis, grading and staging. Hepatology 1994;19:1513–20.
6. Thung SN, Gerber MA, Popper H. Basic morphologic patterns of viral hepatitis A, B, non-A, non-B, and delta agent in animal and man. In: Chisari PV, editor. Advances in hepatitis research. New York: Masson; 1983. p. 293.
7. Okamoto H, Yotsumoto S, Akahane Y, et al. Hepatitis B viruses with precore region defects prevail in persistently infected hosts along with seroconversion to the antibody against e antigen. J Virol 1990;64:1298–303.
8. Heathcote J, Cameron CH, Dane BS. Hepatitis B antigen in saliva and semen. Lancet 1974;1:71–3.
9. Alter HJ, Holland PV, Purcell RH. The emerging pattern of post-transfusion hepatitis. Am J Med Sci 1975;270:329–34.
10. Centers for Disease Control. Changing patterns of groups at high risk for hepatitis B in the United States. MMWR Morb Mortal Wkly Rep 1988;37:429–32.
11. Szmuness W, Much MI, Prince AM, et al. On the role of sexual behavior in the spread of hepatitis B infection. Ann Intern Med 1975;83:489–95.
12. Gerety RJ, Schweitzer IL. Viral hepatitis type B during pregnancy, the neonatal period, and infancy. J Pediatr 1977;90:368–74.
13. Gerety RJ, Hoofnagle JH, Markenson JA, Barker LF. Exposure to hepatitis B virus and development of the chronic HBAg carrier state in children. J Pediatr 1974;84:661–5.
14. Hadler SC, McFarland L. Hepatitis in day care centers: epidemiology and prevention. Rev Infect Dis 1986;8:548–57.
15. Bernier RH, Sampliner R, Gerety R, et al. Hepatitis B infection in households of chronic carriers of hepatitis B surface antigen: factors associated with prevalence of infection. Am J Epidemiol 1980;116:199–211.
16. Bond WW, Favero MS, Petersen NJ, et al. Survival and hepatitis B virus after drying and storage for one week. Lancet 1981;1:550–1.
17. Szmuness W. Hepatocellular carcinoma and the hepatitis B virus: evidence for a causal association. Prog Med Virol 1978;24:40–69.
18. Beasley RP, Hwang LY, Lin CC, Chien CS. Hepatocellular carcinoma and hepatitis B virus. A prospective study of 22,707 men in Taiwan. Lancet 1981;2:1129–33.
19. Beasley RP. Hepatitis B virus. The major etiology of hepatocellular carcinoma. Cancer 1988;61:1842–56.
20. McMahon BJ, Alberts SR, Wainwright RB, et al. Hepatitis B sequelae. Prospective study in 1400 hepatitis B surface antigen–positive Alaska native carriers. Arch Intern Med 1990;150:1051–4.
21. Kaneko S, Miller RH, Feinstone SM, et al. Detection of serum hepatitis B virus DNA in patients with chronic hepatitis using the polymerase chain reaction assay. Proc Natl Acad Sci U S A 1989;86:312–6.
22. Van Rensburg SJ, Cook-Mozafarri P, van Schalkwyk DJ, et al. Hepatocellular carcinoma and dietary aflatoxin in Mozambique and Transkei. Br J Cancer 1985;51:713–26.
23. Lee HP, Day NE, Shanmugaratnam K. Trends in cancer incidence in Singapore, 1968–1982. IARC Scientific Publications, No. 91. Lyon (France): International Agency for Research on Cancer; 1988.
24. Peers F, Bosch X, Kaldor J, et al. Aflatoxin exposure, hepatitis B virus infection and liver cancer in Swaziland. Int J Cancer 1987;39:545–53.
25. Hsu IC, Metcalf RA, Sun T, et al. Mutational hotspot in the *p53* gene in human hepatocellular carcinomas. Nature 1991;350:427–8.
26. Stern MC, Umbach DM, Yu MC, et al. Hepatitis B, aflatoxin B_1, and *p53* codon 249 mutation in hepatocellular carcinomas from Guangxi, People's Republic of China, and a meta-analysis of existing studies. Cancer Epidemiol Biomarkers Prev 2001;10:617–25.
27. Oshima A, Tsukuma H, Hiyama T, et al. Follow-up study of HBs Ag-positive blood donors with special reference to effect of drinking and smoking on development of liver cancer. Int J Cancer 1984;34:775–9.
28. Trichopoulos D, Day NE, Kaklamani E, et al. Hepatitis B virus, tobacco smoking, and ethanol consumption in the etiology of hepatocellular carcinoma. Int J Cancer 1987;39:45–9.
29. Hadengue A, N'Dri N, Benhamou JP. Relative risk of hepatocellular carcinoma in HBsAg positive vs alcoholic cirrhosis. A cross-sectional study. Liver 1990;10:147–51.
30. Neuberger J, Forman D, Doll R, Williams R. Oral contraceptives and hepatocellular carcinoma. Br Med J (Clin Res Ed) 1986;292:1355–7.
31. Xu XR, Huang J, Xu ZG, et al. Insight into hepatocellular carcinogenesis at transcriptome level by comparing gene expression profiles of hepatocellular carcinoma with those of corresponding noncancerous liver. Proc Natl Acad Sci U S A 2001;98:150–94.
32. Moroy T, Marchio A, Etiemble J, et al. Rearrangement and enhanced expression of c-*myc* in hepatocellular carcinoma of hepatitis virus infected woodchucks. Nature 1986;324:276–9.
33. Ochiya T, Fujiyama A, Fukushige S, et al. Molecular cloning of an oncogene from a human hepatocellular carcinoma. Proc Natl Acad Sci U S A 1986;83:4993–7.
34. Takada S, Koike K. Activated N-*ras* gene was found in human hepatoma tissue but only in a small fraction of the tumor cells. Oncogene 1989;4:189–93.
35. Yang DY, Rogler CE. Analysis of insulin-like growth factor II (IGF-II) expression in neoplastic nodules and hepatocellular carcinomas of woodchucks utilizing in situ hybridization and immunocytochemistry. Carcinogenesis 1991;12:1893–901.
36. Wang J, Chenivesse X, Henglein B, Brechot C. Hepatitis B virus integration in a cyclin A gene in a hepatocellular carcinoma. Nature 1990;343:555–7.
37. Stanbridge EJ, Flandermeyer RR, Daniels DW, Nelson-Rees WA. Specific chromosome loss associated with the expression of tumorigenicity in human cell hybrids. Somat Cell Genet 1981;7:699–712.
38. Wang HP, Rogler CE. Deletions in human chromosome arms 11p and 13q in primary hepatocellular carcinomas. Cytogenet Cell Genet 1988;48:72–8.
39. Bressac B, Kew M, Wands J, Ozturk M. Selective G to T mutations of *p53* gene in hepatocellular carcinoma from southern Africa. Nature 1991;350:429–31.
40. Held WA, Mullins JJ, Kuhn NJ, et al. T antigen expression and tumorigenesis in transgenic mice containing a mouse major urinary protein/SV40 T antigen hybrid gene. EMBO J 1989;8:183–91.
41. Lunn RM, Zhang YJ, Wang LY, et al. *p53* Mutations, chronic hepatitis B virus infection, and aflatoxin exposure in hepatocellular carcinoma in Taiwan. Cancer Res 1997;57:3471–7.
42. Wang SK, Wang ZZ, Lu XL, et al. The presence of HBV genomic DNA in tumor tissue correlates with *p53* aberrations in human hepatocellular carcinoma in Qidong, China. Cancer Genet Cytogenet 1999;113:191–2.
43. Colgrove R, Simon G, Ganem D. Transcriptional activation of homologous and heterologous genes by the hepatitis B virus X gene product in cells permissive for viral replication. J Virol 1989;63:4019–26.
44. Feitelson MA. Hepatitis B X antigen and *p53* in the development of hepatocellular carcinoma. J Hepatobiliary Pancreat Surg 1998;5:367–74.
45. Andrisani OM, Barnabas S. The transcriptional function of the hepatitis B virus X protein and its role in hepatocarcinogenesis. Int J Oncol 1999;15:373–9.
46. Wollersheim M, Debelka U, Hofschneider PH. A transactivating function encoded in the hepatitis B virus X gene is conserved in the integrated state. Oncogene 1988;3:545–52.
47. Yu DY, Moon HB, Son JK, et al. Incidence of hepatocellular carcinoma in transgenic mice expressing the hepatitis B virus X-protein. J Hepatol 1999;31:123–32.
48. Eggink HG, Houthoff HJ, Huitema S, et al. Cellular and humoral immune reactions in chronic active liver disease. I. Lymphocyte subsets in liver biopsies of patients with untreated idiopathic autoimmune hepatitis, chronic active hepatitis B and primary biliary cirrhosis. Clin Exp Immunol 1982;50:17–24.

49. Milich DR. Genetic and molecular basis for T- and B-cell recognition of hepatitis B viral antigens. Immunol Rev 1987;99:71–103.
50. Milich DR, McLachlan A, Moriarty A, Thornton GB. Immune response to hepatitis B virus core antigen (HBcAg): localization of T cell recognition sites within HBcAg/HBeAg. J Immunol 1987;139:1223–31.
51. Ferrari C, Penna A, Giuberti T, et al. Intrahepatic, nucleocapsid antigen-specific T cells in chronic active hepatitis B. J Immunol 1987;139:2050–8.
52. Chisari FV, Klopchin K, Moriyama T, et al. Molecular pathogenesis of hepatocellular carcinoma in hepatitis B virus transgenic mice. Cell 1989;59:1145–56.
53. McAleer WJ, Buynak EB, Maigetter RZ, et al. Human hepatitis B vaccine from recombinant yeast. Nature 1984;307:178–80.
54. McLean AA, Hilleman MR, McAleer WJ, Buynak EB. Summary of worldwide experience with H-B-Vax (B, MSD). J Infect 1983;7(Suppl 1):95–104.
55. Carman WF, Zanetti AR, Karayiannis P, et al. Vaccine-induced escape mutant of hepatitis B virus. Lancet 1990;336:325–9.
56. Waters JA, Kennedy M, Voet P, et al. Loss of the common "a" determinant of hepatitis B surface antigen by a vaccine-induced escape mutant. J Clin Invest 1992;90:2543–7.
57. Hadler SC, Francis DP, Maynard JE, et al. Long-term immunogenicity and efficacy of hepatitis B vaccine in homosexual men. N Engl J Med 1986;315:209–14.
58. Neurath AR, Kent SBH, Strick N, et al. Genetic restriction of immune responsiveness to synthetic peptides corresponding to sequences in the pre-S region of the hepatitis B virus (HBV) envelope gene. J Med Virol 1985;17:119–25.
59. Pride MW, Shi H, Anchin JM, et al. Molecular mimicry of hepatitis B surface antigen by an anti-idiotype-derived synthetic peptide. Proc Natl Acad Sci U S A 1992;89:11900–4.
60. Mason HS, Lam DM, Arntzen CJ. Expression of hepatitis B surface antigen in transgenic plants. Proc Natl Acad Sci U S A 1992;89:11745–9.
61. Thanavala Y, Yang YF, Lyons P, et al. Immunogenicity of transgenic plant–derived hepatitis B surface antigen. Proc Natl Acad Sci U S A 1995;92:3358–61.
62. Rutgers T, Hauser P, De Wilde M. Potential future recombinant vaccines. In: Ellis RW, editor. Hepatitis B vaccines in clinical practice. New York: Marcel Dekker; 1993. p. 383–407.
63. Lubeck MD, Davis AR, Chegavata M, et al. Immunogenicity and efficacy testing in chimpanzees of an oral hepatitis B vaccine based on live recombinant adenovirus. Proc Natl Acad Sci U S A 1989;86:6763–7.
64. Williams WW, Hickson MA, Kane MA, et al. Immunization policies and vaccine coverage among adults. The risk for missed opportunities. Ann Intern Med 1988;108:616–25.
65. Alter MJ, Hadler SC, Margolis HS, et al. The changing epidemiology of hepatitis B in the United States. Need for alternative vaccination strategies. JAMA 1990;263:1218–22.
66. Hepatitis B virus: a comprehensive strategy for eliminating transmission in the United States through universal childhood vaccination. Recommendations of the Immunization Practices Advisory Committee (ACIP). MMWR Recomm Rep 1991;40(RR-13):1–25.
67. Harpaz R, McMahon BJ, Margolis HS, et al. Elimination of new chronic hepatitis B virus infections: results of the Alaska immunization program. J Infect Dis 2000;181:413–8.
68. Ni YH, Chang MH, Huang LM, et al. Hepatitis B virus infection in children and adolescents in a hyperendemic area. Fifteen years after mass hepatitis B vaccination. Ann Intern Med 2001;135:796–800.
69. Chang MH, Chen CJ, Lai MS, et al. Universal hepatitis B vaccination in Taiwan and the incidence of hepatocellular carcinoma in children. N Engl J Med 1997;336:1855–9.
70. Stevens CE, Taylor PE, Tong MJ, et al. Yeast-recombinant hepatitis B vaccine. Efficacy with hepatitis B immune globulin in prevention of perinatal hepatitis B virus transmission. JAMA 1987;257:2612–6.
71. Alter HJ, Houghton M. Clinical Medical Research Award. Hepatitis C virus and eliminating post-transfusion hepatitis. Nat Med 2000;6:1082–6.
72. Wong DKH, Cheung AM, O'Rourke K, et al. Effect of α-interferon treatment in patients with hepatitis B e antigen–positive chronic hepatitis B. Ann Intern Med 1993;119:312–23.
73. Brook MG, Karayiannis P, Thomas HC. Which patients with chronic hepatitis B virus infection will respond to α-interferon therapy? A statistical analysis of predictive factors. Hepatology 1989;10:761–3.
74. Lok AS, Wu PC, Lai CL, et al. A controlled trial of interferon with or without prednisone priming for chronic hepatitis B. Gastroenterology 1992;102:2091–7.
75. Perrillo RP, Schiff ER, Davis GL, et al. A randomized, controlled trial of interferon alfa-2b alone and after prednisone withdrawal for the treatment of chronic hepatitis B. The Hepatitis Interventional Therapy Group. N Engl J Med 1990;323:295–301.
76. Reichen J, Bianchi L, Frei PC, et al. Efficacy of steroid withdrawal and low-dose interferon treatment in chronic active hepatitis B. Results of a randomized multicenter trial. Swiss Association for the Study of the Liver. J Hepatol 1994;20:168–74.
77. Dienstag JL, Schiff ER, Wright TL, et al. Lamivudine as initial treatment for chronic hepatitis B in the United States. N Engl J Med 1999;341:1256–63.
78. Liaw RF. Impact of YMDD mutations during lamivudine therapy in patients with chronic hepatitis B. Antivir Chem Chemother 2001;12(Suppl 1):67–71.
79. Yang H, Westland CE, Delaney W 4th, et al. Resistance surveillance in chronic hepatitis B patients treated with adefovir dipivoxil for up to 60 weeks. Hepatology 2002;36:464–73.
80. Levine S, Hernandez D, Yamanaka G, et al. Efficacies of entecavir against lamivudine-resistant hepatitis B virus replication and recombinant polymerases in vitro. Antimicrob Agents Chemother 2002;46:2525–32.
81. Gilson RJ, Chopra KB, Newell AM, et al. A placebo-controlled phase I/II study of adefovir dipivoxil in patients with chronic hepatitis B virus infection. J Viral Hepat 1999;6:387–95.
82. Chang TT, Hadziyannis S, Cianciara J, et al. Sustained viral load and ALT reduction following 48 weeks of entecavir treatment in subjects with chronic hepatitis B who have failed lamivudine [abstract]. Hepatology 2002;36(4 Pt 2):300A.
83. Pol S, Driss F, Carnot F, et al. Efficacite d'une immunotherapie par vaccination contre le virus de l'hepatite B sur la multiplication virale B. CR Acad Sci III 1993;316:688–91.
84. Todo S, Demetris AJ, Van Thiel DH, et al. Orthotopic liver transplantation for patients with hepatitis B virus–related liver disease. Hepatology 1991;13:619–26.
85. Samuel D, Muller R, Alexander G, et al. Liver transplantation in European patients with the hepatitis B surface antigen. N Engl J Med 1993;329:1942–7.
86. Lin SM, Sheen IS, Chien RN, et al. Long-term beneficial effect of interferon therapy in patients with chronic hepatitis B virus infection. Hepatology 1999;29:971–5.
87. Ikeda K, Saitoh S, Suzuki Y, et al. Interferon decreases hepatocellular carcinogenesis in patients with cirrhosis caused by the hepatitis B virus: a pilot study. Cancer 1998;82:827–35.
88. Wang KS, Choo QL, Weiner AJ, et al. Structure, sequence and expression of the hepatitis delta viral genome. Nature 1986;323:508–14.
89. Smedile A, Rizzetto M, Gerin JL. Advances in hepatitis D virus biology and disease. Prog Liver Dis 1994;12:157–75.
90. Buti M, Esteban R, Jardi R, et al. Clinical and serological outcome of acute delta infection. J Hepatol 1987;5:59–64.
91. Di Bisceglie A, Negro F. Diagnosis of hepatitis delta virus infection. Hepatology 1989;10:1014–6.
92. Farci P, Mandas A, Coiana A, et al. Treatment of chronic hepatitis D with interferon alfa-2a. N Engl J Med 1994;330:88–94.
93. Choo QL, Kuo G, Weiner AJ, et al. Isolation of cDNA clone derived from a blood-borne non-A, non-B viral hepatitis genome. Science 1989;244:359–62.
94. Kato N, Hijikata M, Ootsuyama Y, et al. Molecular cloning of the human hepatitis C virus genome from Japanese patients with non-A, non-B hepatitis. Proc Natl Acad Sci U S A 1990;87:9524–8.
95. Han JH, Shyamala V, Richman KH, et al. Characterization of the terminal regions of hepatitis C viral RNA: identification of conserved sequences in the 5' untranslated region and poly(A) tails at the 3' end. Proc Natl Acad Sci U S A 1991;88:1711–5.
96. Bukh J, Purcell RH, Miller RH. At least 12 genotypes of hepatitis C virus predicted by sequence analysis of the putative E1 gene of isolates collected worldwide. Proc Natl Acad Sci U S A 1993;90:8234–8.
97. Alter MJ. Epidemiology of hepatitis C in the West. Semin Liver Dis 1995;15:5–14.
98. Thaler MM, Park CK, Landers DV, et al. Vertical transmission of hepatitis C virus. Lancet 1991;338:17–8.
99. Alter MJ, Margolis HS, Krawczynski K, et al. The natural history of community-acquired hepatitis C in the United States. N Engl J Med 1992;327:1899–905.
100. Hoofnagle JH. Hepatitis C: the clinical spectrum of disease. Hepatology 1997;26(3 Suppl 1):15S–20S.
101. Alter HJ, Seeff LB. Recovery, persistence, and sequelae in HCV infection. A perspective on long-term outcome. In: Stramer SL, editor. Blood safety in the new millennium. Bethesda (MD): American Association of Blood Banks; 2001. p. 123–66.
102. Barrera J, Francis B, Ercilla G, et al. Improved detection of anti-HCV in post-transfusion hepatitis by a third-generation ELISA. Vox Sang 1995;68:15–8.
103. Garson JA, Ring C, Tuke P, Tedder RS. Enhanced detection by PCR of hepatitis C virus RNA. Lancet 1990;336:878–9.
104. Gretch D, Lee W, Corex L. Use of aminotransferase, hepatitis C antibody, and hepatitis C polymerase chain reaction RNA assays to establish the diagnosis of hepatitis C virus infection in a diagnostic virology laboratory. J Clin Microbiol 1992;30:2145–9.
105. Takaki A, Wiese M, Maertens G, et al. Cellular immune responses persist and humoral responses decrease two decades after recovery from a single-source outbreak of hepatitis C. Nat Med 2000;6:578–82.
106. Iino S, Komata M, Kumada H, et al. Quantification of HCV RNA by branched DNA probe assay. J Med Pharm Sci 1993;2:327.
107. Nalpas B, Driss F, Pol S, et al. Association between HCV and HBV infection in hepatocellular carcinoma and alcoholic liver disease. J Hepatol 1991;12:70–4.
108. Saito I, Miyamura T, Ohbayashi A, et al. Hepatitis C virus infection is associated with the development of hepatocellular carcinoma. Proc Natl Acad Sci U S A 1990;87:6547–9.
109. Gerber MA. Relation of hepatitis C virus to hepatocellular carcinoma. J Hepatol 1993;17:108–11.
110. Gerber MA, Shieh YS, Shim KS, et al. Detection of replicative hepatitis C virus sequences in hepatocellular carcinoma. Am J Pathol 1992;141:1271–7.
111. Haruna Y, Hayashi N, Kamada T, et al. Expression of hepatitis C virus in hepatocellular carcinoma. Cancer 1994;73:2253–8.
112. Colombo M. The role of hepatitis C virus in hepatocellular carcinoma. Recent Results Cancer Res 1998;154:337–44.
113. Kew MC, Popper H. Relationship between hepatocellular carcinoma and cirrhosis. Semin Liver Dis 1984;4:136–46.
114. Levrero M, Tagger A, Balsano C, et al. Antibodies to hepatitis C virus in patients with hepatocellular carcinoma. J Hepatol 1991;12:60–3.
115. Furuya K, Nakamura M, Yamamoto Y, et al. Macroregenerative nodule of the liver. A clinicopathologic study of 345 autopsy cases of chronic liver disease. Cancer 1988;61:99–105.
116. Theise ND, Lapook JD, Thung SN. A macroregenerative nodule containing multiple foci of hepatocellular carcinoma in a non-cirrhotic liver. Hepatology 1993;17:993–6.
117. Theise ND, Schwartz M, Miller C, Thung SN. Macroregenerative nodules and hepatocellular carcinoma in 44 sequential adult liver explants with cirrhosis. Hepatology 1992;16:949–55.
118. Tarao K, Ohkawa S, Shimizu A, et al. Significance of hepatocellular proliferation in the development of hepatocellular carcinoma from anti-hepatitis C virus–positive cirrhotic patients. Cancer 1994;73:1149–54.
119. Tagger A, Donato F, Ribero ML, et al. Case-control study on hepatitis C virus (HCV) as a risk factor for hepatocellular carcinoma: the role of HCV genotypes and the synergism with hepatitis B virus and alcohol. Brescia HCC Study. Int J Cancer 1999;81:695–9.
120. Koike K, Moriya K, Kimura S. Role of hepatitis C virus in the development of hepatocellular carcinoma: transgenic approach to viral hepatocarcinogenesis. J Gastroenterol Hepatol 2002;17:394–400.
121. Dammacco F, Gatti P, Sansonno D. Hepatitis C virus infection, mixed cryoglobulinemia, and non-Hodgkin's lymphoma: an emerging picture. Leuk Lymphoma 1998;31:463–76.
122. Shaib Y, El-Serag HB. The epidemiology of cholangiocarcinoma. Semin Liver Dis 2004;24:115–25.
123. Donato F, Gelatti U, Tagger A, et al. Intrahepatic cholangiocarcinoma and hepatitis C and B virus infection, alcohol intake, and hepatolithiasis: a case-control study in Italy. Cancer Causes Control 2001;12:959–64.
124. Franzin F, Efremov DG, Pozzato G, et al. Clonal B-cell expansion in peripheral blood of HCV-infected patients. Br J Haematol 1995;90:548–52.

125. Shaib YH, El-Serag HB, Davila JA, et al. Risk factors of intrahepatic cholangiocarcinoma in the United States: a case-control study. Gastroenterology 2005;128:620–6.
126. Kobayashi M, Ikeda K, Saitoh S, et al. Incidence of primary cholangiocellular carcinoma of the liver in Japanese patients with hepatitis C virus–related cirrhosis. Cancer 2000;88:2471–7.
127. Yin F, Chen B. Detection of hepatitis C virus RNA sequences in hepatic portal cholangiocarcinoma tissue by reverse transcription polymerase chain reaction. Chin Med J (Engl) 1998;111:1068–70.
128. Lu H, Ye MQ, Thung SN, et al. Detection of hepatitis C virus RNA sequences in cholangiocarcinomas in Chinese and American patients. Chin Med J (Engl) 2000;113:1138–41.
129. McOmish F, Chan SW, Dow BC, et al. Detection of three types of hepatitis C virus in blood donors: investigation of type-specific differences in serologic reactivity and rate of alanine aminotransferase abnormalities. Transfusion 1993;33:7–13.
130. Farci P, Alter HJ, Govindarajan S, et al. Lack of protective immunity against reinfection with hepatitis C virus. Science 1992;258:135–40.
131. Ogata NR, Alter HJ, Miller RH, Purcell RH. Nucleotide sequence and mutation rate of the H strain of hepatitis C virus. Proc Natl Acad Sci U S A 1991;88:3392–6.
132. Hoofnagle JH, Mullen KD, Jones DB, et al. Treatment of chronic non-A non-B hepatitis with recombinant human α interferon. N Engl J Med 1986;315:1575–8.
133. Davis GL, Balart LA, Schiff ER, et al. Treatment of chronic hepatitis C with recombinant interferon alfa. A multicenter randomized, controlled trial. N Engl J Med 1989;321:1501–6.
134. Poynard T, Marcellin P, Lee SS, et al. Randomised trial of interferon α2b plus ribavirin for 48 weeks or for 24 weeks versus interferon α2b plus placebo for 48 weeks for treatment of chronic infection with hepatitis C virus. International Hepatitis Interventional Therapy Group (IHIT). Lancet 1998;352:1426–32.
135. Zeuzem S, Feinman SV, Rasenack J, et al. Peginterferon alfa-2a in patients with chronic hepatitis C. N Engl J Med 2000;343:1666–72.
136. Manns MP, McHutchison JG, Gordon SC, et al. Peginterferon alfa-2b plus ribavirin compared with interferon alfa-2b plus ribavirin for initial treatment of chronic hepatitis C: a randomized trial. Lancet 2001;358:958–65.
137. Wright TL, Donegan E, Hsu HH, et al. Recurrent and acquired hepatitis C viral infection in liver transplant recipients. Gastroenterology 1992;103:317–22.
138. Kim-Schluger L, Sheiner P, Thung SN, et al. Severe recurrent cholestatic hepatitis following orthotopic liver transplantation. Hepatology 1996;23:971–6.
139. Sheiner PA, Kim-Schluger L, Emre S, et al. Retransplantation for recurrent hepatitis C. Liver Transplant Surg 1997;3:130–6.
140. Wright TL, Combs C, Kim M, et al. Interferon-α therapy for hepatitis C virus infection after liver transplantation. Hepatology 1994;20(4 Pt 1):773–9.
141. Feray C, Gigou M, Didier S, et al. Incidence of hepatitis C in patients receiving different preparations of hepatitis B immunoglobulins after liver transplantation. Ann Intern Med 1998;128:810–6.
142. Ilan E, Arazi J, Nussbaum O, et al. The hepatitis C virus (HCV)-Trimera mouse: a model for evaluation of agents against HCV. J Infect Dis 2002;185:153–61.
143. Bonino F, Oliveri F, Colombatto P, Brunetto MR. Impact of interferon-α therapy on the development of hepatocellular carcinoma in patients with liver cirrhosis: results of an international survey. J Viral Hepat 1997;4(Suppl 2):79–82.
144. International Interferon-a Hepatocellular Carcinoma Study Group. Effect of interferon-α on progression of cirrhosis to hepatocellular carcinoma: a retrospective cohort study. Lancet 1998;351:1535–9.

Parasites

Piero Mustacchi, MD, ScD
Anne G. Kasmar, MD, MSc

The intensity of parasitic infection frequently correlates with its prevalence.[1] Thus, when relatively uncommon neoplasms are noted with undue frequency in countries with a high prevalence of parasitic diseases, the question of the role of parasites arises. In this respect, the two most intriguing examples are probably the relationships of schistosomiasis to bladder cancer and that of malaria to Burkitt's lymphoma. Classic references have been presented before.[2]

SCHISTOSOMIASIS AND CANCER OF THE BLADDER

Epidemiologic Aspects The data associating schistosomiasis (frequently called bilharzia in Africa) and neoplasia are overwhelming, but explanations for this association remain speculative.[3,4] Data published so far have been retrospective and, therefore, have yielded only relative frequencies, with their well-known inherent limitations.

Geography In Africa, squamous cell carcinoma of the bladder is greatly over-represented among the fellaheen of Egypt and the Africans of Mozambique, Zimbabwe, and Zambia (formerly Rhodesia), all countries where *Schistosoma haematobium* is endemic. An age-standardized mortality rate for bladder cancer of 10.8 per 100,000 males places Egypt at the top of the list of the 54 countries providing data for the 1987 WHO database.[5] Observations made in Ghana and Tanzania[6] suggest an association, however, and none emerges from Tanzania, Uganda, or French-speaking West Africa, where *Schistosoma haematobium* is endemic but bladder cancer apparently is rare.

No prospective study measuring the risk of developing bladder cancer in infected and uninfected persons is yet available. Although differences in relative frequencies may reflect differences in risk, the interplay of other factors, such as geopolitical variations in case finding, can result in spurious differences and erroneous associations. If the postulated association is correct, one of several conditions must obtain: the worm (1) produces a carcinogen, (2) carries a virus, or (3) is cocarcinogenic to some other insult. In this case, there are many unanswered questions regarding geographic differences in vesical cancer observed where schistosomiasis is endemic. These range from whether there is geographic uniformity in the host's reaction to infection to whether other environmental variables (such as the bright food coloring used in the candy popular in the Nile delta) interact and are additionally responsible for vesical neoplasia.

Age and Sex Egyptian data from the Alexandria Cancer Registry disclose a five-fold sex-linked disparity in the annual age-adjusted incidence rate of bladder cancer: 19.2 per 10^5 males and 3.6 per 10^5 females.[5] Bilharzial (ie, schistosomal) bladder cancer attacks men preferentially and seems to be especially common in those with HLA-B16 and Cw2 antigens.[7] In Egyptian hospital series, the mean age of patients is 41 years, about 5 years younger than that of patients with nonbilharzial bladder cancer,[5,8] and the sex ratio ranges from 5:1 to 9:1. Possibly reflecting the lower frequency of schistosomal infestation prevalent in the early 1990s (as compared with the 1960s), mean patient age increased from 47 ± 13.6 to 53 ± 12.2 years.[9] In Ghana, 5 of 13 males with bladder cancer came to autopsy before age 36 years.[10] In Mozambique, too, bilharzial bladder cancer occurs earlier in life, but the sex ratio (M/F 1.75:1) is not as striking as in Egypt.[11] Whether this difference from Egypt reflects a greater susceptibility of females in Mozambique, a reduced risk in males, or simply a vagary resulting from under-reporting remains unresolved.

Urban/Rural Distribution In Egypt, additional support for an association with bilharzial infection can be found in the relative paucity of bladder cancer cases (10 among 33 cancers) reported from hospitals serving the nonparasitized Italian and Greek residents of metropolitan Cairo, compared with the large number observed in hospitals attending Egyptian peasants (45 among 74 cancers).[7,9] In Egypt, clinical history of urinary schistosomiasis is associated with increased bladder cancer risk: this explains some 16% of the bladder cancer cases.[12]

Frequency and Severity of Infection The association of bladder cancer with schistosomal infection seems to become stronger with longer-standing and more severe infection.[8] In the Nile delta, *Schistosoma* ova in the urine correlate with bladder status: cytologically benign epithelium, squamous metaplasia, benign tumors, and, finally, cancer.

The severity of infection tends to rise sharply with opportunities for exposure. In Egypt, it is directly related to the extent of perennial irrigation through canals, which creates a constant risk of reinfection, and inversely related to control measures and availability of safe and effective therapy. In Ghana, where different agricultural conditions prevail, schistosomiasis is essentially a prepubertal disease, and only a small proportion of the population is infested, as compared with the extent in Egypt. Comparative studies in these two countries indicate a rather clear and direct relationship between parasitic infection with *S. haematobium* and frequency of bladder cancer.[10] Thus, the peculiar agricultural setting of the Nile valley singles out this region for a dose–response relationship not encountered in other parts of Africa.

Variability in Diagnostic Criteria of Schistosomiasis Many reports of schistosomal bladder cancer fail to define the diagnostic criteria for infection. Ruling out a diagnosis of schistosomiasis because of the absence of ova in the centrifuged urine specimen would be unrealistic in many cases of contracted bladder due to bilharzial fibrosis, in which the dense scar tissue precludes shedding of ova from the submucosa. Conversely, sound epidemiologic practices require that when evidence of infestation in ova-negative bilharzial patients is sought by rectal scrapings or radiographic studies, the same diagnostic refinements be used in every member of the group studied.

One study conducted in the Nile delta concluded that only 11% of the men and 3% of the women could be considered infected, on the basis of presence of *Schistosomal* ova in the initial urinalysis. On the basis of this diagnostic criterion, only a suggestive association of infection and cancer of the bladder was demonstrated ($p = .04$). By expanding the criteria for diagnosis of schistosomiasis to include the presence of ova in any centrifuged urine sample, and other evidence of infection obtained by endoscopic or radiologic procedures, the prevalence of infection was increased three-fold. After correcting for age, sex, and residence, the relative risk of developing bladder cancer among the bilharzial patients was double that in the comparison population group. By adopting the expanded definition of schistosomiasis, the probability that the association of infection and cancer occurred by chance was much lower ($p = .002$).[10]

Geographic Variability in Schistosomal Virulence Within East Africa, a coastal strain of *S. haematobium* is more virulent than that at Lake Victoria, where infested bladders do not show severe changes.

When *Schistosoma mansoni* is considered, the Brazilian and Puerto Rican strains are the most virulent, as measured by the production of liver disease in infested mice. Under the same experimental conditions, the Egyptian strain caused the least liver damage and the Tanzanian strain produced the fewest eggs.[13] Variability in *S. mansoni* virulence has been cited to explain the high frequency of liver cancer in Mozambique but not in Egypt, even though schistosomal liver cirrhosis is common in both countries. This type of explanation is, at best, tentative because other, as yet undetected, environmental carcinogenic hazards can be at work.

Progression of Bilharzial Bladder Cancer (BBC) Although traditionally considered a disease of slow growth rate with a tendency to recur locally rather than to metastasize, BBC often shows a high proliferative index and a low rate of apoptosis. An over-representation of the protein encoded by the *MDM2* gene found in the majority of the studied cases, may account for the frequent inactivation of the *TP53* control pathway observed in BBC, thereby underlining the accumulation of DNA damage and the aggressive clinical course of BBC.[14]

Monosomy9 may be an early chromosomal change in the urothelium of the bilharzial infected bladder, and a predictor of incipient carcinoma in patients with bilharzial cystitis.[15]

Role of Urinary Infection Although the causative role of schistosomiasis is now accepted, various associated factors have been proposed in the induction of BBC [16] especially infection with the liberation of N-nitroso compounds.[16] In Egypt, but not in Mozambique, bladder calculi and incrustations of vesical ulcers are frequent complications of schistosomal infection. The experimental work linking some nitroso products of bacterial metabolism to carcinogenesis may perhaps reinvigorate the old carcinogenic hypothesis of the early Egyptian workers who implicated "alkaline urine." In fact, the urinary excretion of nitrite and N-nitroso compounds is increased in patients with *S. haematobium* infection.[17] The prevalence of urinary nitrites found in symptomatic active bilharzial cystitis increases in patients who also have schistosomal bladder cancer.[18,19] In noncancerous bladders, infection with *S. haematobium* increases significantly the ability of the vesical bacterial flora to reduce nitrates to the nitrite precursors of N-nitroso compounds.[20]

Compared to controls, schistosome-infested patients have a three-fold higher urinary nitrate and the proposition that this is due to the ability of their inflammatory cells to synthesize nitric oxide, seems plausible.[21,22] The endogenous production of nitric oxide and alkylation of DNA by N-nitroso compounds formed by reaction of nitrite with urinary secondary amines, could account for the significant excess of transitions at CpG dinucleotides in the *TP53* gene in BBC as compared with the non-bilharzial counterpart.[23] Moreover, inactivation of *TP53* could be responsible for the conversion of a low grade tumor to an invasive one.[24,25] The detection of multiple *TP53* mutations in invasive BBC of the squamous cell variety is suggestive of the involvement of a carcinogenic agent with maintenance of preferential activation of the H-*ras* gene.[26] On the other hand, in bladder cancer, the presence or absence of schistosomal ova does not seem to affect the expression of CD44.[27]

Urinary tract infection has been associated with increased chromosomal breakage in the urothelium. The frequency of micronuclei is reduced significantly after antihelminthic treatment.[28] Urothelial carcinogenesis in the presence of schistosomiasis seems to proceed along different pathways from those linked to cigarette smoking, which appears to have a significant impact on mutation of the *TP53* gene with A:T to G:C transitions, that are not observed in bilharzial bladder cancer.[29] The latter also displays $p16^{INK4}$ alterations more frequently than other bladder tumors.[30]

Carbohydrate antigen 19-9 (CA 19-9) seems to be elevated only in transitional cell carcinoma of the schistosomal bladder, but not in the other histologic varieties.[31]

Apoptosis in Schistosomal Bladder Cancer Certain genes, such as Bcl-2, contribute to oncogenesis by suppressing apoptosis. In the presence of schistosomiasis Bcl-2 was significantly expressed in squamous cell bladder cancer as compared with the transitional cell cancer[32] but this was not confirmed in another study.[33]

Pathology of Benign and Preneoplastic Schistosomal Bladder Lesions An intense, delayed-sensitivity reaction is elicited by viable *Schistosoma* eggs plugging the vesical venules leading to tubercules, nodules, or polyps. In bilharzial cystitis, the papilloma, covered as it is by one or two layers of flattened cells, which merge with the transitional epithelium at its base, is essentially a granuloma and not a precancerous lesion. With recurrent inflammation and fibrosis, some transitional epithelial cells become sequestered in the vesical submucosa and acquire a globular arrangement around a central cavity. When they open into the bladder cavity, the cystic formations become pseudoglandular. These structures, as part of cystitis glandularis, are at times precancerous; an adenocarcinoma may arise from the columnar epithelium, into which their lining has differentiated.

In patients with schistosomiasis, squamous metaplasia is frequently encountered because it is a common concomitant of chronic inflammation. This type of metaplasia is a nearly consistent precursor of bladder cancer, and for this reason, leukoplakia acquires clinical importance as a precancerous condition.

Site of Origin In patients in Western countries, bladder cancer frequently arises in the trigone; in patients in Egypt, it usually develops in areas remote from the ureters, mostly in the anterior and posterior bladder walls. This peculiarity tends to strengthen its association with schistosomal infection because the scanty or altogether absent submucosal tissue of the trigone discourages significant deposition of ova (Table 23-1).

Table 23-1 Anatomic Distribution of Vesical Cancer in Egypt and the United States

Site	Egypt (%)	United States (%)
Trigone	3	21
Lateral wall	34	47
Anterior wall	22	8
Posterior wall	30	18
Vault	11	6

Histologic Classification Table 23-2 contrasts the over-representation of squamous cell carcinoma of the bladder in countries like Egypt, Kuwait, Mozambique, South Africa (Bantu population),[34] and Zimbabwe, where the association with schistosomiasis is considered important, with the Ugandan and white South African experiences where the reverse applies.

Within the same country, squamous cell carcinoma of the bladder is markedly over-represented only in areas where schistosomiasis is endemic.[35,36] Moreover, the more intense the infection, the greater is the proportion of squamous cell cancers with a reciprocal decrease in the frequency of transitional cell neoplasms (Figure 23-1).[37] Adenocarcinoma of the bilharzial bladder is particularly aggressive: this may be explained by its proneness to develop gross chromosomal aberrations combined with high cell proliferation.[38]

A rare, though distinct, variant of squamous cell cancer is verrucous carcinoma of the bilharzial bladder (Figure 23-2). Despite reports to the contrary, a large proportion develop into invasive squamous cell carcinoma, with which they share the same adverse prognosis.[39]

Experimental Data Half a century ago, papillomatous hyperplasia of the vesical wall was observed in African sooty monkeys within 3 months of infection with *S. haematobium*. More recently, carcinoma of the bladder was diagnosed in a baboon killed 26 weeks after infection.[40] In a number of nonhuman primates, infection with *S. haematobium* resulted in epithelial proliferation, squamous metaplasia, and transitional cell carcinoma of the urinary bladder.[41] The American opossum has also been found experimentally suitable for infection with *S. haematobium*.[42] These experimental observations are important because eggs of *S. haematobium*, lyophilized worms, and urine from bilharzia patients have not been found to be carcinogenic to mice.[43,44] Furthermore, *Schistosoma* ova, alone or in the presence of 3-methylcholanthrene, lacked urothelial topical carcinogenicity or cocarcinogenicity in mice.[45] However, 2-acetyl-aminofluorene appears to promote malignant and benign bladder neoplasms of mice infested with schistosomes more often than does either agent alone.[46] Similarly, N-methyl-N-nitrosourea and *S. haematobium* caused bladder tumors in 5 of 16 hamsters, whereas no oncogenic effect was seen with either alone. Three *S. haematobium* infected

Table 23-2 Histologic Distribution of Bladder Cancer in Africa

Type	Egypt	Kuwait	East Africa	South Africa Bantus	South Africa Whites	Uganda	Zimbabwe
Squamous	232	100	58	16	11	26	207
Transitional	134	23	28	2	0	31	63
Anaplastic	2	1	13	4	129	7	7
Adenocarcinoma	20	4	0	1	0	5	20
Total	388	128	99	23	140	69	297

baboons treated with N-butyl-N-butazolnitrosamine all developed extensive bladder cancer.[47]

Cancer development was thought to have been accelerated by schistosomal infection, presumably acting as a late-stage cocarcinogen by virtue of its direct proliferative effect on the urothelium.[48] Similarly, an increased incidence of hepatoma has been described after administration of carcinogen to mice infested with *S. mansoni*.[43] This occurs even though the toxic morphologic alterations occurring in the liver are fewer than those observed in noninfected mice exposed to the same hepatocarcinogen.[49]

Helminthic Infestations and Viruses In one study, human papilloma virus was not detected in 25 cases of BBC.[50] Another study [51] found the virus in 23 out of 40 cases. In 1 of 4 capuchin monkeys, C-type virus particles were found in a papillary carcinoma induced by *S. haematobium* that had not been present earlier in the normal bladder tissue. In mice infected with *S. mansoni*, the parasitic disease may enhance the acute effect of hepatitis virus, but no evidence has been found as yet that the chronic cirrhosis-like picture results from this.[52]

Metabolic Observations during Schistosomiasis Increased urinary excretion of free 3-hydroxykynurenine, 3-hydroxyanthranilic acid, and 2-amino-3-hydroxyacetophenone has been documented in some patients with bladder cancer. These ortho-aminophenol derivatives of tryptophan are generally excreted as conjugates of sulfuric acid or glucuronic acid. They are related to the carcinogenic metabolites of β-naphthylamine and are themselves carcinogenic to mice.

The relative resistance of the trigone to schistosomal bladder cancer would make less tenable an etiologic hypothesis predicated on the topical action of an endogenous urinary carcinogen, were it not for the increased activity of urinary β-glucuronidase in vesical infections, including schistosomiasis. Under these circumstances the enzymatic release of the active carcinogen from its glucuronide could well become a significant biologic factor that determines the anatomic localization of the neoplasm. In the study of bilharzial cancer, the metabolism of tryptophan along the formylkynurenine pathway leading to nicotinic acid has elicited considerable interest.[53] The justification for this interest originally stemmed from industrial oncology; however, epidemiologic support is also derived from the high prevalence of classic pellagra that used to be observed in Egypt but not in other parts of Africa where squamous bladder cancer is infrequently reported despite endemic schistosomiasis. In pellagra, exaggeration of the pathway from tryptophan to nicotinic acid occurs, producing larger amounts of tryptophan intermediates along the formylkynurenine pathway.

Our understanding of the role played by *Schistosoma* infection in disturbed tryptophan metabolism is complicated by geographic variations of dietary habits. In fact, serotonin metabolites such as 5-hydroxyindoleacetic acid, which are excreted in large amounts by plantain-eating Africans, are low in Africans on other diets.[54,55] Similar differences attributable to dietary habits have been found between bilharzial patients in Mozambique and in South Africa. Egyptian peasants are not plantain-eaters but subsist mostly on beans, lentils, and rice. Those with bilharzial cancer metabolize tryptophan in a manner reminiscent of the pattern seen in many patients with spontaneous bladder cancer, with increased excretion of 3-hydroxyanthranilic acid, anthranilic acid, 5-hydroxyindoleacetic acid, and kynurenine. The excretion of these metabolites is enhanced by a loading dose of tryptophan.

Schistosomiasis should not be considered the only causal factor in the associated excretion of abnormal tryptophan metabolites because, with or without cancer, vesical schistosomiasis is almost universally accompanied by urinary tract infection. The bacterial flora may, thus, contribute to a spurious accumulation of some metabolites of tryptophan. Moreover, untreated pellagra is associated with increased urinary excretion of anthranilic acid, acetylkynurenine, and 5-hydroxyindoleacetic acid.

Potentially carcinogenic metabolites of tryptophan, which may be the true oncogenic agent in the presence of bilharzial bladder inflammation, are principally determined by hepatic metabolic patterns. Factors that bear on this are coincident infestation of the liver by *S. mansoni*, pyridoxine deficiency, and chronic protein starvation. In the presence of advanced abnormalities in any of these factors, lesser amounts of potential carcinogenic metabolites might be formed owing to lack of hepatic enzymes or cofactors. No mutagens were detected by the Ames test in the urine of patients suffering from bilharzial bladder cancer [56] or in soluble extracts of eggs and adult *Schistosoma japonicum* worms.[57] A weak promoting activity was noted for *S. japonicum* soluble egg antigen, which resulted in the recovery of Epstein-Barr virus (EBV) from cultured human lymphoid cells that harbored the viral genome.[57]

The hepatic drug-metabolizing capacity of mice infected with *S. mansoni* is markedly reduced.[58] The mutagen inactivating potential of *S. japonicum*-infected mouse liver is similarly reduced.[59] This results in longer persistence of the mutagen in the animal body.[60] It seems likely that the carcinogen dose is a determining factor in the aggressiveness of a bladder tumor, and that a low-grade carcinoma can be converted into a high-

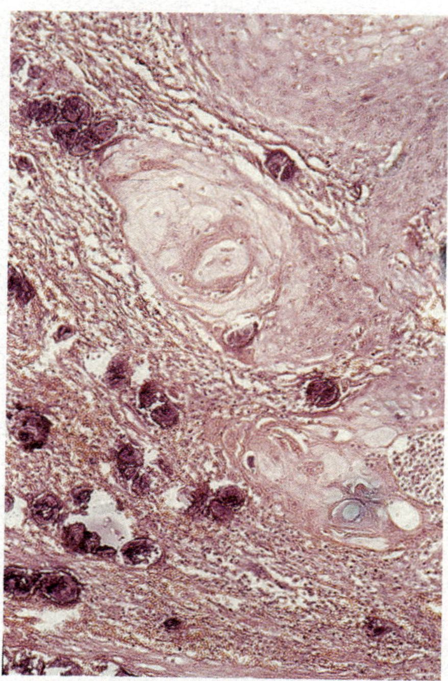

Figure 23-1 Bilharzial bladder cancer. Infiltrating well-differentiated squamous cell carcinoma with adjacent calcified *S. hematobium* eggs. (H & E × 100). (Courtesy of Drs M. R. Mahran and M. El-Baz, Mansoura University, Egypt).

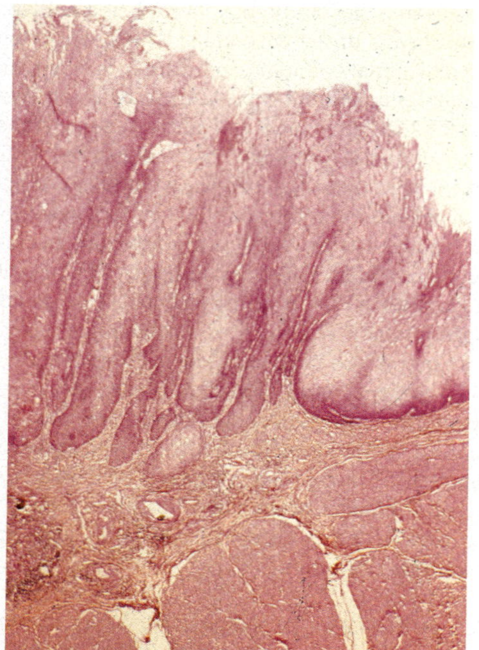

Figure 23-2 Verrucous carcinoma (noninvasive) of bladder with superficial filamentous elongated surface projections. (H & E × 40). (Courtesy of Drs M. R. Mahran and M. El-Baz, Mansoura University, Egypt.)

grade one if exposed continuously to low doses of N-nitroso compounds.[61] This would explain, at least in part, the over-representation of deeply invasive squamous cell cancers in the bilharzial urinary bladder.[61] The significant excess of transitions at C_pG dinucleotides in the *TP53* gene in bilharzial bladder cancer has been attributed to the endogenous production of nitric oxide provoked by the inflammatory response to schistosomal ova.[62]

A study of the frequency of mutant active *ras* oncogenes in bilharzial bladder cancer concluded that it was not higher than in nonbilharzial cancer.[63] In view of its isolation from direct exposure to putative carcinogens present in the urine, a defunctionalized bilharzial bladder might seem an unlikely site for the development of neoplastic changes. Nonetheless, adenocarcinoma has been reported in a defunctionalized bladder showing extensive metaplasia.[64] Quantitative estimates of infection with *S. haematobium* have shown, however, that its overall severity is unlikely to be the sole factor in the pathogenesis of endemic vesical cancer.[65]

SCHISTOSOMIASIS AND CANCER OF OTHER SITES

Large Intestine Although acknowledging the frequency of benign schistosomal polyposis, Egyptian data tend to discount any association of *S. mansoni* or *S. haematobium* with cancer of the large intestine. On the other hand, in Asia, intestinal infestation with *S. japonicum* is considered a significant contributory factor to the development of cancer of the colon and rectum. *S. japonicum* lays a very large number of eggs (2,000 per day per pair of worms) while *S. mansoni*'s eggs are considerably fewer and, thus, cause fewer pathologic problems.[66]

In one report from China, where in endemic areas the prevalence of schistosomiasis may reach 44 per 100,000 persons, 48% of colectomy specimens for colorectal carcinoma obtained from 1951 to 1974 were associated with *S. japonicum* infestation. Associated inflammatory changes, pseudopolyps, and transitional mucosal changes of schistosomal granulomatous disease progressing to mucosal atypia and to carcinoma were reminiscent of bowel carcinoma in patients with ulcerative colitis, save for the ova deposited in all layers of the bowel.[67] Nonetheless, 92% of cancers were well differentiated, compared with 69% in the group without schistosomiasis. An ecologic study of 49 Chinese rural counties indicates that both schistosomal infestation and dietary factors contribute to the remarkable geographic variation of colon cancer in China.[68]

In Shanghai, patients with intestinal schistosomiasis and cancer of the large intestine are, on average, 6 years younger than patients with spontaneous intestinal cancer.[69,70] However, Chinese patients whose history of schistosomiasis entailed an elevated relative risk (RR) of rectal cancer (RR 8.3; CI 3.1 to 22.6) did not show a parallel increase in their RR for cancer of the colon.[71]

Compared to controls, Chinese patients with schistosomal rectal cancer showed a higher proportion of base-pair substitutions at CpG nucleotides and a higher frequency of arginine missense mutations, conceivably the result of genotoxic agents produced endogenously through the course of schistosomiasis japonica.[72]

The Breast In Egyptian hospital material, the male-to-female breast cancer ratio is substantially greater than in the West. If corroborated by incidence studies, this observation would be a valuable epidemiologic observation worthy of further investigation. Hyperestrogenism secondary to bilharzial liver fibrosis has been invoked as one possible cause.

The Liver Conflicting observations on the association of schistosomiasis and hepatic cancer are difficult to reconcile without further data. In Egypt[5] and Mozambique,[11] bilharzial liver cirrhosis is very common; carcinoma of the liver, however, is prevalent only in Mozambique, where it is the most common cancer among males. The association of cirrhosis from *S. japonicum* with hepatoma has been reported only infrequently and appears, thus, not to be causal.

In Japan, liver cancer correlated highly with three factors: HBsAg (OR = 10.0), history of schistosomiasis (OR = 9.5), daily intake of alcohol (OR = 3.2), concurrent viral hepatitis, with the combination of hazards acting multiplicatively or at least synergistically.[73–77] In experimental animals, infection with *S. japonicum*, alone[78] or in combination with N-2-fluorenyl acetamide, induced or accelerated the occurrence of liver tumors.[79] Disturbing are the reports of decreased response to hepatitis B vaccine among children of mothers with schistosomiasis, since the vaccine protects against hepatocellular carcinoma and may diminish the severity of liver disease in patients with schistosomiasis.[80] The relationship between schistosomiasis and hepatocellular carcinoma is confounded by co-infection with hepatitis B virus [81–83] However remnants of schistosomal eggs were found in the severe granulomatous reaction present within a well-differentiated hepatocellular carcinoma that had developed in a hepatitis B and C seronegative chimpanzee.[84]

Lymphoma Eight cases of solitary follicular lymphoma of the spleen were found among 863 spleens removed from patients with hepatosplenic schistosomiasis. The rarity of an isolated tumor at this site and of this type suggests a causal link, possibly mediated by cycles of follicular hyperplasia and involution occurring in the spleen in the course of advanced schistosomiasis.[85]In a Nigerian series, lymphoreticular tumors were over-represented in infected individuals (16%) as compared with uninfested ones.[86]

Other Organs Immunohistochemically confirmed invasive squamous cell carcinoma of the prostate was diagnosed in two prostatic schistosomiasis patients coming from a population where prostatic cancer is uncommon[87] and male breast cancer strikingly high. This suggests that in schistosomiasis, impaired liver detoxication mechanisms may result in increased estrogen and diminished androgen levels [88] Co-existent schistosomiasis and prostatic carcinoma have been reported in unusually young patients.[89] On the other hand, the Egyptian cases indicate no relationship between bilharziasis and cancer of the lungs, pancreas, prostate, seminal vesicles, urethra, vulva, vagina, cervix uteri, body of the uterus, or ovaries.[5] As would be expected, surgical or autopsy material in countries with high schistosomal endemicity from time to time shows the presence of *Schistosoma* ova in various tissues, including cancerous ones. The literature contains a number of isolated reports of such coincidences. Moreover, in areas where infestation is endemic, schistosomal tissue reaction may be so intense and proliferative as to be mistaken clinically for cancer of the large intestine[90] or the cervix.[91]

Evaluation of Carginogenicity of Schistosomiasis According to accepted international criteria, infection with *S. haematobium* is carcinogenic to humans (group 1); infection with *S. mansoni* is not classifiable as to its carcinogenicity to humans (group 3); infection with *S. japonicum* is possibly carcinogenic to humans (group 2B).[92]

EAST ASIAN DISTOMIASIS

Liver and Pancreas *Clonorchis sinensis* is endemic in parts of Japan, Korea, and China; a similar species, *Opisthorchis viverrini*, causes distomiasis in Thailand. Liver fluke infections have been associated with multi-focal intrahepatic bile duct adenocarcinoma in those areas of Asia where distomiasis is endemic: Thailand, where 70 to 90% of the population of the northeast part of the country are infected with *O. viverrini*, has the highest recorded incidence of cholangiocarcinoma in the world. Similarly in Korea, where infestation with *C. sinensis* is very prevalent, cholangiocarcinoma accounts for more than 20% of liver cancers.[93] In Indonesia, Taipei, and Taiwan, where distomiasis is considered uncommon, cholangiocarcinoma is infrequent. Imported cases of distomiasis are seen in the United States where up to 26% of Southeast Asian immigrants have active liver fluke infection.[94] Since the parasite can live up to 30 years, it represents a long-term hazard to infected persons.[95]

Human infection results from eating raw or undercooked parasitized freshwater fish. In humans, the ingested parasites excyst in the duodenum and ascend the bile ducts and canaliculi, where they mature, causing biliary epithelial hyperplasia and fibrosis. Similarities between the histopathologic responses in infected humans and experimental animals have been documented, including the development of cholangiocarcinoma in dogs and cats experimentally infected with *Clonorchis*. Hamsters administered dimethylnitrosamine for 10 weeks after infection with *Opisthorchis* developed mucin-secreting cholangiocarcinomas, whereas noninfected animal controls failed to develop tumors. This observation, as well as other observations,[96] are in keeping with experimental evidence pointing to infection as a promoter.[97] In the Far East, nitrosamines are commonly found in such traditional Chinese preserved foods as salted fish, dried shrimp, and sausage.[98] Precursors of nitroso compounds have been identified in the body fluid of men infested with *O. viverrini*.[99] Pancreatic ducts may also be infected with *C. sinensis*; this frequently results in squamous metaplasia and mucous gland hyperplasia. In one instance in the United States, an immigrant with *C. sinensis* in the common bile duct developed a well-differentiated ductal adenocarcinoma of the pancreas.[100]

Evaluation of Carcinogenicity of Distomiasis Infection with *O. viverrini* is carcinogenic to humans (group 1); infection with *O. felineus* is not classifiable as to its carcinogenicity to humans (group 3); infection with *C. sinensis* is probably carcinogenic to humans (group 2A).[101]

MALARIA

The geographic distribution of Burkitt's lymphoma in the classic malarial belt initially suggested the possible role of an arthropod vector in oncogenesis. This fits with the notion that the risk for this lymphoma declines with increasing westernization and effective malaria eradication.[102,103] The possibility that drugs taken for malaria prophylaxis could have contributed to the development of Burkitt's lymphoma [104,105] was considered unlikely because no increase (and indeed a decrease) in endemic Burkitt's lymphoma (eBL) was observed in the Malagasy Republic[106] and in Imesi, West Africa,[107] where intensive antimalarial prophylaxis was practiced; moreover, cases occur [108] among persons not receiving malaria prophylaxis.

More significant are the epidemiologic observations that have linked eBL to the combined effect of malaria and infection with the EBV.[109] Endemic BL is only found in areas where malaria is holoendemic or hyperendemic; within these areas, it is absent in malaria-free pockets, such as urban centers. Within endemic areas, the peak incidence of eBL follows closely the incidence of severe *Plasmodium falciparum* malaria, and malarial prophylaxis reduces the incidence of the lymphoma.[106,107]

Vigorous cellular and serologic responses occur during malarial infection.[110] This renders plausible the argument that persistent reticuloendothelial stimulation experienced among malarial populations conditions the EBV-infected African patient to develop a neoplasm rather than a self-limited disease, such as infectious mononucleosis.[111] This view finds support in the observation that each one of the erythrocytic, exoerythrocytic, and sexual forms of the parasite is structurally differentiated and probably contains a multitude of biologically active antigenic constituents.[112,113] In this respect, it is interesting to note that in endemic malarial areas, the distribution of hyper-reactive malarial splenomegaly parallels the distribution of eBL, and that the peak age incidence of eBL follows closely the peak age incidence of severe *P. falciparum* malaria.[109]

In situ hybridization for the detection of EBER-1 and EBER-2 RNA, has demonstrated that acute infection with malaria leads to colonization of lymph nodes by virus-infected lymphoblasts in 60% of the cases.[114]

One way of explaining the observation that the malaria patient harboring a multitude of parasite-derived antigens becomes a host susceptible to eBL is the suggestion that malaria patients produce so many nonspecific and "useless" antibodies that they are unable to recognize and respond to the threat posed by a small clone of malignant lymphoid cells.[115] This view is supported by experimental data. In mice, antigenic stimulation and immune suppression often result in an increased incidence of lymphomas. Mice repeatedly injected with *Plasmodium berghei* sometimes develop malignant lymphoma that is morphologically similar to Burkitt's lymphoma and sometimes develop persistent antigenic stimulation without significant tumorigenesis.[116–118] Lymphomas are frequently induced by Moloney leukemogenic virus in mice infected with *P. berghei* but rarely occur in mice given either plasmodium or virus alone.[119] Acute malaria, which increases B-cell proliferation, also impairs EBV-specific T-cell responses.[102,120] This results in a larger pool of EBV-infected cells with increased likelihood for chromosomal translocation and lymphomagenesis.[121] In children, the risk of developing Burkitt's lymphoma is related to antibody titers against EBV capsid antigens.[122] The clinical manifestations probably are promoted by other environmental factor(s), such as holoendemic malaria [123] and phorbol exposure.[124]

Of considerable interest are studies on the frequency of sickle-cell trait in eBL patients and controls. Persons with sickle trait are not protected from being bitten by mosquitoes or from malarial infection, but they are protected against the lethal effect of overwhelming *P. falciparum* malaria in early childhood and from the intense reticuloendothelial stimulation that sometimes progresses to hyper-reactive malarial splenomegaly.[125] Sickle cells exposed to low oxygen tension do not support the growth of parasites in vitro. A similar phenomenon may explain why children with the sickle-cell trait have a lower *P. falciparum* parasitemia. As a result, a lower mortality rate, lower IgM levels, and reduced lymphoproliferation (as measured by spleen size) are found among individuals with hemoglobin AS genotype. However, most studies attempting to relate eBL to AS hemoglobinopathy have failed to reach statistical significance.[120] Other hemoglobinopathies, such as hereditary ovalocytosis, also protect against malaria. If eBL turns out to be underrepresented in populations where both ovalocytosis and malaria are prevalent, as in Papua, New Guinea,[126]such information would provide strong supporting evidence for malaria as a cofactor in the genesis of eBL.[120] In this event, the observation that in Uganda malarial endemicity also correlates with non–Burkitt's non–Hodgkin lymphoma, would acquire added significance.[127]

The small differences in titers of malarial antibodies observed in Burkitt's lymphoma patients and controls [128] were attributed to the fact that many in the experimental group had received several courses of antimalarial drugs, which may have lowered the level of malaria-specific antibodies.[110] A probable role of malaria emerges also from the following considerations. African children with eBL develop autoantibodies, the elevated titers of which show no linear correlation with EBV titers for viral capsid antigen (VCA) or Epstein-Barr nuclear antigen (EBNA),[129] suggesting that a factor independent of EBV causes an immunologic imbalance and autoantibody production. The notion that this could be due to malaria is supported by the observation that Caucasians suffering from acute *P. falciparum* malaria develop autoantibodies,[130,131] and that experiments in vitro demonstrated that normal human lymphocytes can produce autoantibodies as a response to malarial antigens.[132]

In the genesis of eBL, regardless of whether malaria is considered the initiator and EBV the promoter or vice versa, neither hypothesis accounts for the fact that in vitro infection of B cells with EBV and stimulation with malaria antigens has yet to produce a cell that carries the chromosomal tumorigenic translocations found in both sporadic and endemic BL.[122] Overexpression of *c-myc* appears to be central to the pathogenesis of Burkitt's and atypical Burkitt's lymphoma. Although *c-myc* translocation occurs in all cases of Burkitt's lymphoma, differences are seen in the translocation patterns in the endemic and sporadic varieties of the disease. Typically, sporadic Burkitt's lymphoma has translocations involving sequences within or immediately 5' to *myc* on chromosome 8 and sequences within or near the immunoglobulin heavy chain S region on chromosome 14. In contrast, endemic Burkitt's lymphoma tends to be characterized by a translocation involving sequences on chromosome 8 further upstream from *myc* and sequences within or near the JH region on chromosome 14.[133] Thus, it seems likely that other unidentified factors (genetic, nutritional, or environmental) play a significant role in tumorigenesis.

AMERICAN BURKITT'S LYMPHOMA

By the early 1970s, approximately 100 cases of Burkitt's lymphoma had been confirmed by the American Burkitt's Lymphoma Registry.[134] Space-time clustering is suggested by the American data.[135,136] Although malaria is associated with Burkitt's lymphoma in Africa, the relative rarity of the tumor in relation to the holoendemic nature of malaria indicates that a combination of genetic factors plus specific environmental factors may be operative. Host and environmental factors other than malaria are probably important in North American cases.[134]

CANCER IN ANIMALS

Observations made by Fibiger [137] on gastric cancer in rats infested with a nematode are now all but discredited. A question that remains to be evaluated is whether the nematode helped localize some unidentified carcinogens in the diet, similar to the induction of sarcomas at the site of subcutaneous injection of sodium chloride in rats being fed 3-methylcholanthrene.

Sarcoma is an almost inevitable complication of infection of the liver or the subcutaneous tissues of rats with *Cysticercus fasciolaris*, the larval form of the common tapeworm of the cat, *Taenia taeniaformis*. Washed, ground-up *C. fasciolaris* produced peritoneal sarcomas in half the injected rats, the proportion reaching 91% if the animals were genetically related to the parasitized host. The active agent appears to be associated with the calcium carbonate corpuscles of the parasite, but the mechanism is not clear.[138] Although not directly implicated in vesical carcinogenesis, there is suggestive evidence that infestation with another nematode, *Trichosomoides crassicauda*, increases the incidence of tumors in the bladders of rats receiving 2-acetylaminofluorine.[139]

Another nematode, *Spirocerca lupi*, has been associated with the development of esophageal sarcoma in dogs. Here the reported association seems to be described only in the southern United States, thereby adding a possible geographic dimension to the problem.

Some neoplastic responses to parasitic infestation are a kind of cecidiosis and may represent the end of a hypothesized evolutionary sequence by which parasite secretions stimulate the host to form protective structures (cecidia) that benefit the parasite.

REFERENCES

1. Jordan P. Egg output on bilharziasis in relation to epidemiology, pathology, treatment and control. In: Mostofi FK, editor. Bilharziasis. Berlin, Germany: Springer-Verlag; 1967.
2. Mustacchi P. Parasites. In: Holland JF, Frei E III, Bast RC Jr, et al., editors. Cancer medicine, 4th ed. Baltimore, MD: Williams & Wilkins; 1996.
3. Cheever AW. Schistosomiasis and neoplasia. J Natl Cancer Inst 1978;61:13.
4. Gentile JM. Schistosome related cancers: a possible role for genotoxins. Exp Mutagen 1985;7:775.
5. Bedwani R, El-Khwsky F, La Vecchia C, et al. Descriptive epidemiology of bladder cancer in Egypt. Int J Cancer 1993; 55:351.
6. Kitinya JN, Lauren PA, Eshleman LJ et al. The incidence of squamous and transitional cell carcinomas of the urinary bladder in northern Tanzania in areas of high and low levels of endemic *Schistosoma haematobium* infection. Trans R Soc Trop Med Hyg 1986;80:935–9.
7. Wishahi M, El-Baz HG, Shaker ZA. Association between HLA-A, B, C and DR antigens and clinical manifestations of *Schistosoma haematobium* in the bladder. Eur Urol 1989;16:138.
8. Aboul Nasr A, Gazyerli M, Fawz RM, El-Sibal L. Epidemiology and pathology of cancer of the bladder in Egypt. Acta Unio Int Contra Cancrum 1962;18:528.
9. Koraitim MM, Metwalli NE, Atta MA, El-Sadr AA. Changing age-incidence and pathological types of Schistosoma-associated bladder carcinoma. J Urol 1995:154:1714.
10. Mustacchi P, Shimkin MB. Cancer of the bladder and infestation with *Schistosomiasis haematobium*. J Natl Cancer Inst 1958;20:825.
11. Prates MD, Gillman J. Carcinoma of the urinary bladder in the Portuguese East African with special reference to bilharzial cystitis and preneoplastic lesions. South Afr J Med Sci 1959;24:13.
12. Bedawi R, Renganathan E, El-Khwsky F, et al. Schistosomiasis and the risk of bladder cancer in Alexandria, Egypt. Brit J cancer 1998;77:1186.
13. Warren KS. A comparison of Puerto Rican, Brazilian, Egyptian, and Tanzanian strains of *Schistosoma mansoni* in mice: penetration of cercariae, maturation of schistosomas and production of liver disease. Trans R Soc Trop Med Hyg 1967;61:795.
14. Osman I, Scher H, Zhang ZF, et al. Expression of Cyclin D1, but not cyclins E and A, is related to progression in bilharzial bladder cancer. Clin Cancer Res 1997;3:2247.
15. Ghaleb AH, Pizzolo JG, Melamed MR. Aberrations of chromosomes 9 and 17 in bilharzial bladder cancer as detected by fluorescence *in situ* hybridization. Am J Clin Path 1996;106:234.
16. Badawi AF, Mostafa MH, Probert A, O'Connor PJ. Role of schistosomiasis in human bladder cancer: evidence of association, aetiological factors and basic mechanisms of carcinogenesis. Eur J Cancer Prev 1995;4:45.
17. Tricker AR, Mostafa HH, Spiegelhalder P, Preussman P. Urinary nitrite and nitroso compounds in bladder cancer patients with schistosomiasis (bilharziasis). IARC Sci Publ 1991;105:178.
18. El-Aaser AA, El-Merzabani MM, El-Bolkain Ibrahim AS. A study on the etiological factors of bilharzial bladder cancer in Egypt. 5-urinary nitrites in a rural population. Tumori 1980;66:400.
19. Tricker AR, Mostafa MH, Spiegelhalder B, Preussman R. Urinary excretion of nitrate, nitrite and N-nitroso compounds in Schistosomiasis and bilharzias bladder cancer patients. Carcinogenesis 1989;10:547–52.
20. Hicks RM, Ismail MM, Walters CL, et al. Association of bacteriuria and urinary nitrosamine formation with *Schistosoma haematobium* infection in the Qalyub area of Egypt. Trans R Soc Trop Med Hyg 1982;76:519.
21. Abdel Mohsen MA, Hassan AAM, El-Sewedy SM, et al. Biomonitoring of N-nitroso compounds, nitrite and nitrate in the urine of Egyptian bladder cancer patients with or without *Schistosoma haematobium* infection. Int J Cancer 1999;82:789.
22. Badawi AF. Nitrate, nitrite and *N*-nitroso compounds in human bladder cancer associated with schistosomiasis. Int J Cancer 2000;85:598.
23. Warren W, Biggs PJ, El-Baz M et al. Mutations in the *p53* gene in schistosomal bladder cancer: a study of 92 tumors from Egyptian patients and a comparison between mutational spectra from schistosomal and non-schistosomal urothelial tumors. Carcinogenesis 1995;16:1181.
24. Badawi AA. Molecular and genetic events in schistosomiasis-associated human bladder cancer: role of oncogenes and tumor suppressor genes. Cancer Letters 1996;105:123.
25. Osman I, Scher HI, Zhang ZF, et al. Alterations affecting the p53 control pathway in Bilharzial-related bladder cancer. Clin Cancer Res 1997;3:531.
26. Ramchurren N, Cooper K, Summerhayes. Molecular events underlying schistosomiasis-related bladder cancer. Int J Cancer 1995;62:237.
27. Gadalla HA, Kamel NA, Badary FA, Elanany FG. Expression of CD44 protein in bilharzial and non-bilharziala bladder cancers. BJU Int 2004;93:151–5.
28. Anwar WA, Rosin, MP. Reduction in chromosomal damage in schistosomiasis patients after treatment with praziquantel. Mutat Res 1993;298:17.
29. Habuchi T, Takahashi R, Yamada H, et al. Influence of cigarette smoking and schistosomiasis on p53 gene mutation in urothelial cancer. Cancer Res 1993;53:3795.
30. Tamimi Y, Bringuier PP, Smit F, et al. Homozygous deletions of p16^{INK4} occur frequently in bilharziasis-associated bladder cancer. Int J Cancer 1996;68:183.
31. Fouad M, Khallaf E. CA 19-19 in carcinoma of the bilharzial bladder. J R Coll Surg Edinb 1994;39:246–8.
32. Swellam M, Abd-Elmaksoud N, Halim MH, et al. Incidence of Bcl-2 expression in bladder cancer: relation to schistosomiasis. Clin Biochem 2004;37:798–802.
33. Badr KM, Nolen JD, Derose PB, Cohen C. Muscle invasive schistosomal squamous cell carcinoma of the urinary bladder: frequency and prognostic significance of p53, BCL-2, HER2/neu and proliferation (MIB-1). Hum Path 2004;35:184–9.
34. Higginson J, Oettle AG. Cancer of the bladder in the South African Bantu. Acta Unio Inter Contra Cancrum 1962;18:580.
35. Kitinya JN, Lauren PA, Eshleman LJ, et al. The incidence of squamous and transitional cell carcinomas of the urinary bladder in northern Tanzania in areas of high and low levels of endemic *Schistosoma haematobium* infection. Trans R Soc Trop Med Hyg 1986;80:935.
36. Thomas JE, Nassett MT, Sigola LB, Taylor P. Relationship between bladder cancer incidence, *Schistosoma haematobium* infection, and geographical region in Zimbabwe. Trans R Soc Trop Med Hyg 1990;84:551.
37. Lucas SB. Squamous cell carcinoma of the bladder and schistosomiasis. East Afr Med J 1982;59:345.
38. Shabaan AA, Elbaz AE, Tribukait B. Primary nonurachal adenocarcinoma in the bilharzial urinary bladder: deoxyribonucleic acid flow cytometric and morphologic characterization in 93 cases. Urology 1998;51:469.
39. Mahran MR, El-Baz M. Verrucous carcinoma of the bilharzial bladder. Scand J Urol Nephrol 1993;27:189.
40. Gillman J, Prats MD. Histologic types and histogenesis of bladder cancer in the Portuguese East African with special reference to bilharzial cystitis. Acta Unio Inter Contra Cancrum 1952;18:560.
41. Kuntz RE, Cheever AW, Myers BJ. Proliferative epithelial lesions of the urinary bladder of nonhuman primates infested with *Schistosoma haematobium*. J Natl Cancer Inst 1972;48:223.
42. Kuntz RW, Myers BJ, Moore JA, Huang TC. Parasitologic aspects of *Schistosoma haematobium* (Iran) infections in the American opossum (*Didelphis marsupialis*) Int J Parasitol 1975;5:21.
43. El-Ghaffar YA. Failure to induce bladder cancer in mice. Bladder implantation with paraffin wax pellets of lyophilized urine from bilharzial patients. Cancer 1966;19:1225.
44. Shimkin MB, Mustacchi PO, Cram EB, Wright WH. Lack of carcinogenicity of lyophilized *Schistosoma* in mice. J Natl Cancer Inst 1955:16:47.
45. Al-Hussaini M, McDonald, DF. Lack of urothelial topical tumorigenicity and cotumorigenicity of *Schistosoma* ova in mice. Cancer Res 1967;27:228.
46. Hashem M, Boutros K. The influence of bilharzial infection on the carcinogenesis of the mouse bladder. An experimental study. J Egyptian Med Assoc 1961;44:598.
47. Hicks RM, James C, Webbe G, Nelson GS. *Schistosoma haematobium* and bladder cancer. Trans Roy Soc Trop Med Hyg 1977;71:288.
48. Hicks RM. The canopic worm: role of bilharziasis in the aetiology of human bladder cancer. J Roy Soc Med 1983;76:16.
49. Liu LB, Domingo EO, Stenger RJ, et al. An ultrastructural study of the toxic and carcinogenic effects of 2-amino-5-azotoluene on the livers of schistosome-infected and uninfected mice. Cancer Res 1969;29:837.
50. Cooper K, Haffajee Z, Taylor L. Human papillomavirus and schistosomiasis associated bladder cancer. Mol Path 1997;50:145.
51. Khaled HM, Raafata A, Mokhtar N, et al. Human papilloma virus infection and overexpression of p53 protein in bilharzial bladder cancer. Tumori 2001;87:256–61.
52. Warren KS, Rosenthal MS, Domingo EO. Mouse hepatitis virus (MHV3) infection in chronic murine *Schistosomiasis mansoni*. Bull NY Acad Med 1969;45:211.
53. Mousa AH, Abdel Wahab AFO, Mousa W, et al. Tryptophan metabolism in hepatosplenic bilharziasis. Trans R Soc Trop Med Hyg 1967;61:640.
54. Fripp PH. Bilharziasis and bladder cancer. Br J Cancer 1965;19:292.
55. Trout GE, Gillman J, Prates MD. Bilharzial cystitis and the urinary excretion of tryptophan metabolites in the Portuguese East African. Acta Unio Int Contra Cancrum 1962;18:575.
56. Everson RB, Gad-el-Mawla NM, Attia MA, et al. Analysis of human urine for mutagens associated with carcinoma of the bilharzial bladder by the Ames *Salmonella* plate assay. Interpretation employing quantitation of viable lawn bacteria. Cancer 1983;51:371.
57. Ishii A, Matsuoka H, Aji T, et al. Evaluation of the mutagenicity and the tumor promoting activity of parasite extract: *Schistosoma japonicum* infection and *Clonorchis sinensis*. Mutat Res 1989;224:229.
58. Cha YN, Edwards R. Effects of *Schistosoma mansoni* infection on the hepatic drug-metabolizing capacity of mice. J Pharmacol Exper Ther 1976;199:432.
59. Matsuoka H, Aji T, Ishii A, et al. Reduced levels of mutagen processing potential in the *Schistosoma japonicum*-infected mouse liver. Mutat Res 1989;227:153.
60. Aji T, Matsuoka H, Ishii A, et al. Retention of a mutagen, 3 amino-1-methyl-5 H-pyrido[4,3,6] indole (Trp P2) in the liver of mice infected with *S. japonicum*. Mutat Res 1994;305:265.
61. Badawi AF, Mostafa MH, O'Connor PJ. Involvement of alkylating agents in schistosome-associated bladder cancer: the possible basic mechanisms of induction. Cancer Lett 1992;63:171.

62. Warren W, Biggs PJ, El-Baz M, et al. Mutations in the p53 gene in schistosomal bladder cancer: a study of 92 tumors from Egyptian patients and a comparison between mutational spectra from schistosomal and non-schistosomal urothelial tumors. Carcinogenesis 1995;16:1181–9.
63. Fujita J, Nakayama H, Onoue H, et al. Frequency of active ras oncogenes in human bladder cancers associated with schistosomiasis. Jpn J Cancer Res (Gann) 1987;78:915.
64. Elem B, Alam SZ. Total intestinal metaplasia with focal adenocarcinoma in a *Schistosoma*-infested defunctioned urinary bladder. Brit J Urol 1984;56:331.
65. Elem B, Purohit R. Carcinoma of the urinary bladder in Zambia. A quantitative estimation of *Schistosoma haematobium* infection. Brit J Urol 1983;55:275.
66. Ishii A, Matsuoka H, Aji T, et al. Parasite infection and cancer with special emphasis on *Schistosoma japonicum* infections (Trematoda). A review. Mutat Res 1994;305:273.
67. Chen MC, Chuang CY, Chang PY, Hu TC. Evolution of colorectal cancer in schistosomiasis. Cancer 1980;46:1661.
68. Guo W, Zheng W, Li JY, et al. Correlation of colon cancer mortality with dietary factors, serum markers and schistosomiasis in China. Nutr Cancer 1993;20:13.
69. Huan-Wen T, Yueh-Ying Y. A pathologic study of intestinal schistosomiasis associated with cancer. Chinese Med J 1958;77:244.
70. Ming-Chai C, Shan-Chi CW. Acute colonic obstruction in *Schistosoma japonica*. A clinical study of 40 cases 14 associated with carcinoma. Chinese Med J 1957;75:517.
71. Xu Z, Su DL. *Schistosoma japonicum* and colorectal cancer: an epidemiologic study in the People's Republic of China. Inter J Cancer 1984;34:315.
72. Zhang R, Takahashi S, Orita S et al. *p53* gene mutations in rectal cancer associated with schistosomiasis japonica in Chinese patients. Cancer Letters 1998;131:215.
73. Inaba Y, Maruchi N, Matsuda M, et al. A case-control study on liver cancer with special emphasis on the possible aetiological role of schistosomiasis. Int J Epidemiol 1984;13:408.
74. Kojiro M, Kakizoe S, Yano H, et al. Hepatocellular carcinoma and *Schistosomiasis japonica*. A clinicopathologic study of 59 autopsy cases of hepatocellular carcinoma associated with chronic schistosomiasis japonica. Acta Pathol Jpn 1986;36:525.
75. Iida F, Iida R, Kamijo H et al. Chronic Japanese schistosomiasis and hepatocellular carcinoma: ten years of follow-up in Yamanashi prefecture, Japan. Bull WHO 1999;77:573.
76. Takemura Y, Kikuchi S, Inaba Y. Epidemiologic study of the relationship between schistosomiasis due to *Schistosoma japonicum* and liver cancer/cirrhosis. Am J Trop Med Hyg 1998;59:551.
77. Badawi AA, Michael MS. Risk factors for hepatocellular carcinoma in Egypt: the role of hepatitis-B viral infection and schistosomiasis. Anticancer Res 1999;19:4563.
78. Amano T, Oshima T. Hepatoma formation in ddY mice with chronic schistosomiasis japonica. Jpn J Cancer Res (Gann) 1988;79:173.
79. Miyasato M. Experimental study on the influence of *Schistosoma japonicum* infection on carcinogenesis of mouse liver treated with N-2-fluorenyl acetamide (2-FAA) Jpn J Parasitol 1984;33:41.
80. WHO Expert Committee on the Control of Schistosomiasis. Public health impact of schistosomiasis: disease and mortality. Bull WHO 1993;71:657.
81. Li ZJ, Luo DD, Dai JZ, Zheng LL, et al. Immunohistochemical detection of HBsAg and HbcAg in the liver of patients with schistosomiasis japonica complicated by hepatocellular carcinoma. J Tongji Med Univ 1991;11:141–4.
82. Itoshima T, Fedail SS, Suliman I et al. Hepatitis B virus markers in patients with schistosomiasis, liver cirrhosis and hepatocellular carcinoma in Khartoum, Sudan. Acta Med Okayama 1989;43:241–4.
83. Hassan MM, Zaghloul AS, El-Serag HB et al. The role of hepatitis C in hepatocellular carcinoma: a case control study among Egyptian patients. J Clin Gastroenterol 2001;33:123–6.
84. Abe K, Kagei N, Teramura Y, Ejima H. Hepatocellular carcinoma associated with chronic *Schistosoma mansoni* infection in a chimpanzee. J Med Primatol 1993;33:237–9.
85. Andrade ZA, Abreeu WN. Follicular lymphoma of the spleen with hepatosplenic *Schistosomiasis mansoni*. Am J Trop Med Hyg 1971;20:237.
86. Edington GM, von Lichtenberg F, Nwabuebo I, et al. Pathologic effects of schistosomiasis in Ibadan, western state of Nigeria, I. Incidence and intensity of infection; distribution and severity of lesions. Am J Trop Med 1970;19:982.
87. Al Adnani, MS. Schistosomiasis, metaplasia and squamous cell carcinoma of the prostate: histogenesis of the squamous cells determined by localization of specific markers. Neoplasma 1985;32:613.
88. Sherif M, Ibrahim AS, El-Aaser AA. Prostatic carcinoma in Egypt: epidemiology and etiology. Scand J Urol Nephrol (Suppl) 1980;55:25-s6.
89. Cohen RJ, Edgaar SG, Cooper K. Schistosomiasis and prostate cancer. Pathology 1995;27:115.
90. Mustacchi PO, El-Sibai I. Advanced schistosomal proctitis simulating clinically cancer of the rectum. Gastroenterology 1951;19:137.
91. Schwartz DA. Carcinoma of the uterine cervix and schistosomiasis in West Africa. Gynecol Oncol 1984;19:365.
92. IARC Monographs on the evaluation of carcinogenic risks to humans. Vol. 61. Lyon: IARC; 1994. p.100.
93. Shin H-R, Lee C-U, Park H-J et al. Hepatitis B and C virus, *Chlonorchis sinensis* for the risk of liver cancer: a case-control study in Pusan, Korea. Int J Epidem 1996;25:933.
94. Schwartz DA. Cholangiocarcinoma associated with liver fluke infection: a preventable source of morbidity in Asian immigrants. Am J Gastroentrol 1986;81:76–9.
95. Sun T, ed. Clonorchiasis and opisthorchiasis. In: Pathology and clinical features of parasitic diseases, Vol. 5. New York, NY: Masson Monogr Diagn Path 1982. p. 243.
96. Thamavit W, Pairojkul C, Tiwawech D et al. Strong promoting effect of *Opisthorchis viverrini* infection on dimethylnitrosamine-initiated hamster liver. Cancer Letters 1994;78:121.
97. Thamavit W, Tiwawech D, Moore MA, et al. Equivocal evidence of complete carcinogenicity after repeated infection of Syrian hamsters with *Opisthorchis viverrini*. Toxicol Pathol 1996; 24: 493–7.
98. Schwartz DA. Cholangiocarcinoma associated with liver fluke infection: a preventable source of morbidity in Asian immigrants. Am J Gastroenterol 1986;81:76.
99. Haswell-Elkins MR, Satama S, Tsuda M, et al. Liver fluke infection and cholangiocarcinoma: model of endogenous nitric oxide and extragastric nitrosation in human carcinogenesis. Mutat Res 1994;305:241–52.
100. Colquhoun BPD. Adenocarcinoma of the pancreas associated with *C. sinensis* infection. Can Med Assoc J 1987;136:153.
101. IARC Monographs on the evaluation of carcinogenic risks to humans, Vol. 61. Lyon: IARC; 1994. p.162.
102. Cook-Mozaffari P, Newton R, Beral V, Burkitt DP. The geographical distribution of Kaposi's sarcoma and of lymphomas in Africa before the AIDS epidemic. Brit J Cancer1998;78:1521.
103. Ojesina AI, Akang EE, Ojemakinde KO. Decline in the frequency of Burkitt's lymphoma relative to other childhood malignancies in Ibadan, Nigeria. Ann Trop Paediatr 2002;22:159–63.
104. Sadoff L. Aetiology of Burkitt's lymphoma. Lancet 1972;2:1414.
105. Sadoff L. Antimalarial drugs and Burkitt's lymphoma. Lancet 1973;2:1262.
106. Bruce-Chwatt LJ. Antimalarial drugs and Burkitt's lymphoma. Lancet 1974;1:223.
107. McGucken RB. Antimalarial drugs and Burkitt's lymphoma. Lancet 1974;1:68.
108. Aghai E, Hulu N, Virag I, et al. Childhood non-Hodgkin's lymphoma—a study of 17 cases in Israel. Cancer 1974;33:1411.
109. Facer CA, Playfair JHL. Malaria, Epstein-Barr virus and the genesis of the lymphomas. Adv Cancer Res 1989;53:33.
110. Riley EM, Hviid L, Theander TG. Malaria. In: Kierszenbaum F, editor. Parasitic infections and the immune system. San Diego: Academic Press; 1994. p. 119–43.
111. O'Connor GT. Persistent immunologic stimulation as a factor in oncogenesis with special reference to Burkitt's tumor. Am J Med 1970;48:279.
112. Jayawardena AN. In: Mansfield JM, ed. Parasitic diseases, Vol. I. Immunology. New York, NY: Marcel Dekker; 1981. p. 88–163.
113. Neva FA, Sheagren JN, Shulman NR, Canfield CJ. Malaria: host-defense mechanisms and complications. Ann Intern Med 1970;73:295.
114. Facer C, Khan G. Detection of EBV RNA (EBER-1 and EBER-2) in malaria lymph nodes by in situ hybridization. Microbiol Immunol 1997;41:891–4.
115. Warrens AE. Burkitt's lymphoma and disordered immunoglobulin response. Lancet 1974;1:742.
116. Evans AS. Clinical syndromes associated with EB virus infection. Adv Intern Med 1972;18:77.
117. Kreger G, O'Conor GT. Epidemiologic and immunologic considerations on the pathogenesis of Burkitt's tumor. Recent Results Cancer Res 19712;32:211.
118. Sizaret P, O'Conor GT, Beaumont R, Laval M. Serum protein patterns in mice following primary and challenge infection with *Plasmodium berghei*. Z Tropenmed Parasitol 1971;22:260.
119. Weddeburn N. Effect of concurrent malarial infection on development of virus-induced lymphoma in Balb/c mice. Lancet 1970;2:1114.
120. Whittle HC, Brown J, Marsh K, et al. T-cell control of Epstein-Barr virus-infected B-cells is lost during *P. falciparum* malaria. Nature 1984;312:449.
121. Magrath I. The pathogenesis of Burkitt's lymphoma. Adv Cancer Res 1990;55:145.
122. De-The G, Geser A, Day NE, et al. Epidemiological evidence for causal relationship between Epstein-Barr virus and Burkitt's lymphoma from Ugandan prospective study. Nature 1978;274:756.
123. Epstein MA, Achong BG. The Epstein-Barr virus. Berlin, Germany: Springer Verlag; 1979.
124. Van den Bosch C, Griffin BE, Kazembe P, et al. Are plant factors a missing link in the evolution of endemic Burkitt's lymphoma? Br J Cancer 1993;68:1232.
125. Morrow RH, Sever JL, Henderson BE. Antibody levels to infectious agents other than Epstein-Barr virus in Burkitt's lymphoma patients. Cancer Res 1974;34:1212.
126. Castelino D, Saul A, Myler P, et al. Ovalocytosis in Papua New Guinea—dominantly inherited resistance to malaria. Southeast Asian J Trop Med Public Health 1981;12:549.
127. Schmauz R, Mugerwa JW, Wright DH. The distribution of non-Burkitt, non-Hodgkin's lymphoma in Uganda in relation to malarial endemicity. Int J Cancer 1990;46:650.
128. Morrow RH. Epidemiological evidence for role of falciparum malaria. In: Burkitt's lymphoma: a human cancer model. Lenoir G, O'Conor G, Olweny C, editors. Lyon: IARC Science Publication No.60; 1985. p. 177–85.
129. Vainio E, Lenoir GM, Franklin RM. Autoantibodies in three populations of Burkitt's lymphoma patients. Clin Exp Immunol 1983;54:387.
130. Daniel-Ribeiro CT, de Roquefeuil S, Druilhe P, et al. Abnormal anti-single stranded (ss) DNA activity in sera from *Plasmodium falciparum* infected individuals. Trans R Soc Trop Med Hyg 1983;78:742.
131. Mortazavi-Milan SM, Stiele HE, Holborow EJ. Antibody to intermediate filaments of the cytoskeletons in the sera of patients with acute malaria. Clin Exper Immunol 1983;55:177.
132. Kataaha PK, Hacer CA, Holborow EJ. Stimulation of autoantibodies production in normal blood lymphocytes by malaria culture supernatants. Parasite Immunol 1984;6:481.
133. Bishop PC, Rao K, Wilson WH. Burkitt's lymphoma: molecular pathogenesis and treatment. Cancer Invest 2000;18:574.
134. Levine PH, Cho BR. Burkitt's lymphoma: clinical features of North American cases. Cancer Res 1974;34:1219.
135. Levine PH, Sandler SG, Komp DM, et al. Simultaneous occurrence of "American Burkitt's lymphoma" in neighbors. N Engl J Med 1973;288:562.
136. Patton LL, McMillan CW, Webster WP. American Burkitt's lymphoma: a 10-year review and case study. Oral Surg Oral Med Oral Pathol 1990;69:307.
137. Fibiger J. Untersuchung fiber eine Nematode (Spiroptera sp.n.) und deren F_higkeitt, papillomatose und karzinomatose Geschwulstbildungen in Magen der Ratte hervorzurufen. Z Krebsforsch 1913;13:217.
138. Dunning WF, Curtis MR. Multiple peritoneal sarcoma in rats from intraperitoneal injection of washed ground *Taenia* larvae. Cancer Res 1946;6:668.
139. Chapman WH. The incidence of a nematode, *Trichosomoides crassicauda*, in the bladder of laboratory rats: treatment with nitrofurantoin and preliminary report of their influence on urinary calculi and experimental tumors. J Invest Urol 1964;2:52.

Section 4

CANCER EPIDEMIOLOGY, PREVENTION, AND SCREENING

24

Cancer Epidemiology

Michael J. Thun, MD, MS
Ahmedin Jemal, DVM, PhD

The magnitude of the human and economic costs of cancer in the United States is enormous. Based on current incidence rates and the age structure of the population, approximately one of every two men and one in three women in the United States will be diagnosed with an invasive cancer during their lifetime.[1] Malignant diseases afflict two out of every three families. The annual cost of cancer is estimated to be $189.8 billion–69.4 billion (US) for direct medical costs, $16.9 billion (US) for lost productivity, and $103.5 billion for indirect mortality costs.[2]

This chapter describes the use of epidemiologic methods to monitor patterns of cancer occurrence and to identify factors that may increase or decrease the risk of cancer. By definition, epidemiologic studies examine the occurrence and determinants of disease in populations rather than in individual patients. This chapter describes the measures used to characterize disease occurrence in epidemiologic studies, the role of surveillance and descriptive epidemiology to monitor temporal trends, geographic patterns, and disparities, and the approaches used in analytic epidemiology to identify etiologic factors that influence cancer occurrence or progression.

MEASURES OF DISEASE OCCURRENCE

The primary measures of cancer occurrence are incidence or death rates, usually expressed per 100,000 persons per year. Incidence rates represent the number of newly diagnosed cases that occur each year in a population of specified size. Mortality rates represent the corresponding number of deaths, also generally expressed per 100,000 person years of observation. It is essential that rates be expressed based on a common person-time denominator if comparisons are to be made across populations of varying size and length of observation.[3]

Another measure of cancer occurrence, more familiar to the public, is the total number of newly diagnosed cancers or deaths that occur in a given year in a specified geographic area. Information on the count of cancer cases or deaths can be useful in determining health services needs for a region. However, numerator data alone do not allow valid comparisons of risk across populations that differ in size, duration of follow-up, or age. Thus, the number of cases or deaths in a given geographic area does not in itself communicate the average risk of individuals in the population.

Age and Age-Adjustment A fundamental characteristic of many cancers is that incidence and death rates increase exponentially with age during adulthood. The increase in the age-specific incidence rate of all cancers combined is so large that about 76% of all invasive cancers occur among the approximately 19% of the United States population 55 years of age or older.[1] Figure 24-1 shows that the death rate from all cancers combined increases progressively after age ten, and that the incidence rate increases with age except among persons age 85 and above. The decrease in cancer incidence rates in the oldest age group is probably an artifact of less complete diagnosis in the elderly and lower lung cancer incidence in the generations that preceded the peak of cigarette smoking in the United States, because the downturn has occurred at progressively later ages over time, and occurs at different ages according to race and sex.

Rather than characterize all of the age-specific rates shown in Figure 24-1, vital statistics data and epidemiologic studies often present a single age-adjusted or age-standardized rate to compare cancer occurrence across populations with a different age composition. Age standardization serves a dual purpose: it summarizes the age-specific rates into a single number, and eliminates age differences between the populations by assigning them all a "standard" age distribution.[4] Age-specific rates are multiplied times the number of people within the corresponding five-year age group in a "standard" population. The products, or number of cases expected in each age group in the standard population, are then summed across all age groups and divided by the total number of people in the population to yield the age-standardized rate. The issue of age-standardization is particularly relevant now, because, beginning with 1999 mortality and incidence data, United States cancer statistics are standardized to the year 2000 population estimates rather than to the 1970 United States age distribution.[5] The implications of this for the age-adjusted rates and temporal trends in the rates are discussed below.

CANCER SURVEILLANCE

Descriptive epidemiologic studies measure the occurrence of cancer and other health-related factors in relation to person (eg, age, sex, race, social class, behavioral factors etc), place, and time. This section describes the systems that collect and report data on cancer incidence and mortality. It also discusses current patterns and trends in cancer occurrence, counts, individual lifetime probability of developing various cancers, and disparities in cancer occurrence and survival across subgroups of the population.

Date Collection and Reporting Population-based statistics on cancer incidence and mortality are collected under several systems. Mortality data have been available nationally for most of the United States since 1930.[6] Causes of death are

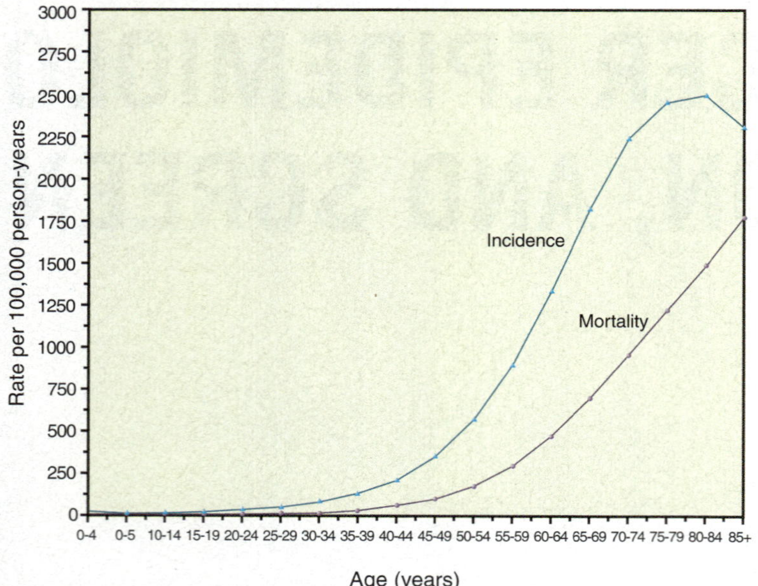

Figure 24-1 Age-specific incidence and mortality rates from all cancers combined, United States, 1997–2001.

reported on death certificates filed in the states. From these, the underlying cause of death is determined[7,8] using criteria specified by the World Health Organization (WHO). Beginning with 1999, cancer deaths have been coded according to the tenth revision of the International Classification of Diseases (ICD-10).[5]

Cancer incidence has been monitored since 1973 by the Surveillance, Epidemiology, and End Results (SEER) program of the National Cancer Institute (NCI).[1] Temporal trends in incidence can be evaluated since 1973 for approximately 10% of the population of the United States. Through subsequent expansions, the SEER program now encompasses 26% of the United States population. Incidence and survival data from SEER and mortality data from the National Center for Health Statistics are published annually in the SEER Cancer Statistics Review, 1973 to 1998, and are available on the Internet at <www-seer.ims.nci.nih.gov>.

Many states not covered by SEER began cancer incidence registries during the 1980s. The system of state registries has been enhanced by the North American Association of Central Cancer Registries (NAACCR)[9,10] and by the National Program of Cancer Registries (NPCR), administered by the Centers for Disease Control and Prevention (CDC).[11] By 2004, 45 states, the District of Columbia, Puerto Rico, the Virgin Islands, and Palau were receiving appropriations from CDC to support their cancer registries.[9] State-specific cancer incidence and mortality data are available on the Internet at <http://statecancerprofiles.cancer.gov/>. Incidence data for the combined SEER and NPCR registries are published annually.[10]

Many hospital registries also tabulate data on cancer care provided in their facility.[10–14] Hospital registries are not population–based; yet they provide much of the primary data for state and other population-based registries. Hospitals that participate in the Approvals Program of the American College of Surgeons (ACoS) receive an annual report from the National Cancer Data Base (NCDB) that allows them to compare the cancer care statistics from their facility with those of other approved hospitals. The types and frequencies of cancers treated at a particular hospital may not be representative of the population as a whole. However, NCDB is currently the only registry that provides feedback regarding cancer care at the hospital level.

International statistics on cancer occurrence are compiled by the International Agency for Research on Cancer (IARC), part of the World Health Organization (WHO). Nationwide incidence data are available from a few countries. More commonly, incidence data are collected in regional registries.[15] Where cancer incidence data are not available, the IARC uses age-, gender-, and cancer site-specific mortality statistics to estimate incidence. International data are available in both tabular[16,17] and map form through the IARC Globocan Web site available at <www.dep.iarc.fr>. Mortality statistics reported to IARC derive mainly from the WHO mortality database.[17]

Age-Adjusted Incidence and Death Rates Table 24-1 shows the average age-adjusted incidence and death rates from various cancers in the United States during the period 1997 to 2001. The death rates represent the entire United States; the incidence rates cover 11 SEER registries.[1] The rates in Table 24-1 are standardized to the age distribution of the United States population in the year 2000[1] and can be compared validly to any other rates that are age-adjusted to the same standard population. They cannot be compared to many international statistics, however, since vital statistics published by IARC are standardized to the world population which is based

Table 24-1 Average Annual Age-Adjusted Incidence and Death Rates[a] for Selected Cancer Sites, United States, All Races by Sex, 1997–2001

	Incidence Rates		Death Rates	
Cancer Sites	Males	Females	Males	Females
All sites	554.3	414.4	251.1	166.7
Brain	7.2	4.9	5.6	3.8
Breast	1.2	135.2	0.3	27.0
Colon and rectum	63.4	46.4	25.3	17.7
Corpus and uterus, NOS	—	24.5	—	4.1
Esophagus	7.7	2.0	7.7	1.8
Hodgkin's disease	3.0	2.4	0.6	0.4
Kidney and renal pelvis	15.7	7.8	6.1	2.8
Larynx	6.7	1.4	2.6	0.5
Leukemias	15.9	9.4	10.2	5.9
Liver and intrahepatic bile duct	9.1	3.5	6.7	2.9
Lung and bronchus	79.1	49.1	77.9	40.8
Melanomas of the skin	21.4	13.8	3.9	1.8
Multiple myeloma	6.9	4.6	4.7	3.2
Non-Hodgkin's lymphomas	23.3	15.7	10.5	6.9
Oral cavity and pharynx	15.7	6.4	4.3	1.6
Ovary	—	13.9	—	8.9
Pancreas	12.6	9.7	12.2	9.2
Prostate	172.3	—	31.5	—
Stomach	12.6	6.1	6.6	3.3
Testis	5.2	—	0.3	—
Thyroid	3.8	10.4	0.4	0.5
Urinary bladder	36.1	9.1	7.6	2.3
Uterine cervix	—	9.3	—	2.9
Uterine corpus	—	24.0	—	4.1

[a]Rates are per 100,000 and are age-adjusted to the 2000 US standard population.
Data source: Surveillance, Epidemiology, and End Results Program, 12 Registries, NCI, 2004.

Table 24-2 Cancer Incidence and Death Rates, 2001, United States: Age-Adjusted to the 1970 and 2000 US Standard Population

Cancer Site	Sex	Incidence Rates			Mortality Rates		
		1970	2000	% Change	1970	2000	% Change
All malignant cancers	Male	448.7	537.3	19.8	189.4	243.5	28.5
	Female	337.4	402.0	19.1	130.9	164.1	25.4
Colon and rectum	Male	47.8	59.5	24.5	18.5	24.2	30.9
	Female	34.7	44.1	27.0	12.8	17.0	33.3
Lung and bronchus	Male	60.7	73.6	21.2	60.8	75.1	23.4
	Female	39.1	46.4	18.8	33.9	40.9	20.9
Breast	Female	112.6	132.1	17.3	21.1	25.9	23.1
Prostate	Male	147.4	171.4	16.3	19.2	29.1	51.3

on the international age distribution in approximately 1960.[16–18]

Table 24-2 illustrates the effect of standardizing 2001 incidence and death rates to the year 2000 instead of the 1970 age standard. The age-adjusted rates for all cancers combined and for the four most common cancers are 15 to 50% higher when adjusted to the year 2000 standard, even though the age-specific rates are identical in these calculations. Although it is periodically necessary to update the age-standard to reflect the contemporary age structure of the population, this change should not be misinterpreted as a true increase in cancer occurrence. Rather, it acknowledges that the aging and growth of the United States population increase the actual number of cancer cases and cancer occurrence rates, because of the increase in cancer risk with aging.

Estimated Number of Cases and Deaths from Cancer Other widely cited indices of cancer occurrence are the estimates of new cases and deaths, published annually by the American Cancer Society (ACS).[19] Table 24-3 shows the estimated number of new cases and deaths predicted by ACS to occur in 2002. The estimates of new cases are based on data from the SEER program, projected onto census information about the size and age-structure of the United States population.[20] The estimated number of deaths is based on the actual number of cancer deaths recorded annually in the United States from 1979 until the most recent year for which data are available, projected forward to the current year. The value of the ACS projections is that they are current, readily understood by the public, and reasonably accurate when compared to the actual counts of cancer deaths, tabulated several years later. However, they represent projections rather than actual measurements. Because they estimate the absolute number of cancer cases and deaths rather than the rates shown in Figure 24-1, they increase with growth of the population and aging, even when age-specific rates remain constant.

Figures 24-2 and 24-3 show the ten most common incident and fatal cancers, respectively, among United States' men and women, ranked according to the percentage each contributes to all cancers. The percentages are based on the ACS estimates for 2002.[19] Cancer of the lung and bronchus is the most common cancer site causing death in both sexes, whereas prostate cancer (in men) and breast cancer (in women) are the leading incident cancers. Four cancers (lung and bronchus, breast, prostate, and colon and rectum) make up slightly over half of all incident invasive cancers and deaths in both sexes.[19]

Age affects the types of cancer that occur, as well as their frequency. Table 24-4 shows the ranking of the most common fatal cancers at different ages in males and females.[19] Up to age 19, the five most common fatal cancers in both sexes include leukemia, brain and other nervous system (ONS), bones and joints, endocrine system, and soft tissues. In women age 20 to 39 and 40 to 59 years, breast cancer is the most common fatal cancer. At age 60 and above, the four most common fatal cancers are lung and bronchus, female breast, prostate, and colon and rectum.

Because the age-standardized death rates from heart disease have been decreasing more rapidly in the United States than the age-standardized death rate from cancer, cancer has become the most common cause of death among persons 40 to 74 years of age.[19] If the current trends in the age-standardized death rates from cancer and heart disease continue, cancer will become the most common cause of death in the overall population in the year 2018.

Individual Risk of Cancer Individuals frequently ask about their personal risk of developing cancer by a certain age or over a specific time period. Table 24-5 illustrates the probabilities (and odds) of developing or dying from invasive cancer within certain age ranges, based on average incidence rates in the United States between 1999 and 2001.[19] It is important to note that these probabilities are based on population averages and may either over- or underestimate the risk for an individual. Personal factors that can cause an individual's risk to be greater or less than the national average include genetic susceptibility, lifestyle behaviors such as smoking, and competing causes of death. The average lifetime probability of developing cancer also increases with the longevity of the population. Nevertheless, the probabilities shown in Table 24-5 illustrate the average individual's risk of developing an invasive cancer at various ages.

One measure of disease frequency that is rarely used for cancer is prevalence, or the percentage of people alive during a particular time period, who have ever been diagnosed with cancer. Prevalence is generally expressed as a rate per 100,000 people. In reality, it reflects a combination of the incidence rate and survival, and is not an actual measure of disease occurrence. Prevalence imperfectly reflects the continuing burden of cancer in a population, because there is no reliable way to distinguish between people who have been disease free for some specified period following cancer treatment and those who struggle with active disease.[21]

Validity of Cancer Surveillance Data The quality of routinely collected medical information varies over time and across countries. Consequently, data quality can influence apparent temporal trends and international differences. Information on deaths from cancer derives from causes of death reported on death certificates that are coded systematically to indicate the probable underlying cause of death. Death registration is a statutory requirement in many countries. The accuracy of death certificate data depends upon the disease under study (rapidly fatal diseases are more accurately recorded), the person completing the certificate (attending physician vs coroner), and the age of the patient (diagnoses are often less well documented in the elderly).[22] Despite the many well documented limitations of death certificates,[23] valid temporal comparisons of mortality rates have been possible in most developed countries in populations under age 75 since the 1960s.[24] Validation studies within SEER have found over 90% agreement between the clinical diagnosis and the underlying cause of death for 17 cancer sites that represent over two-thirds of cancers in the United States.[25,26] Major cancers such as lung, breast, prostate, pancreas, and ovary are included in this group. Other sites, such as cancers of the colon or rectum, can also be reliably classified from death certificates. when selected sites are combined but not when separate. Although issues of data quality are fundamentally important, routinely collected data can be informative in both descriptive and analytic studies if appropriate consideration is given to data quality in relation to the cancer and research question of interest.

Temporal Trends in Cancer Occurrence in the United States Cancer incidence and mortality rates continue to change over time in the United States. The largest increase occurred in the age-adjusted death rates from cancer of the lung and bronchus in men between 1930 and 1991 (Figure 24-4).[27] This increase was followed by a decline in lung cancer death rates in men from 1992 to 2001. Lung cancer death rates did not increase sharply in American women until after 1960, 30 years after the steep rise in men, because of the later uptake of cigarette smoking by American women than men. The age-adjusted death rates from lung cancer have now begun to level off in American women (Figure 24-5), and are anticipated to show a steady decline. The gender differences in these temporal trends in lung

Table 24-3 Estimated Number of New Cancer Cases and Deaths by Sex for All Sites, United States, 2005*

	Estimated New Cases			Estimated New Deaths		
	Both Sexes	Male	Female	Both Sexes	Male	Female
All sites	1,372,910	710,040	662,870	570,280	295,280	275,000
Oral cavity and pharynx	29,370	19,100	10,270	7,320	4,910	2,410
Tongue	7,660	5,050	2,610	1,730	1,120	610
Mouth	10,070	5,370	4,700	1,890	1,100	790
Pharynx	8,590	6,520	2,070	2,130	1,490	640
Other oral cavity	3,050	2,160	890	1,570	1,200	370
Digestive system	253,500	134,370	119,130	136,060	75,020	61,040
Esophagus	14,520	11,220	3,300	13,570	10,530	3,040
Stomach	21,860	13,510	8,350	11,550	6,770	4,780
Small intestine	5,420	2,840	2,580	1,070	580	490
Colon†	104,950	48,290	56,660	56,290	28,540	27,750
Rectum	40,340	23,530	16,810	—	—	—
Anus, anal canal, and anorectum	3,990	1,750	2,240	620	230	390
Liver and intrahepatic bile duct	17,550	12,130	5,420	15,420	10,330	5,090
Gallbladder and other biliary	7,480	3,330	4,150	3,340	1,270	2,070
Pancreas	32,180	16,100	16,080	31,800	15,820	15,980
Other digestive organs	5,210	1,670	3,540	2,400	950	1,450
Respiratory system	184,800	102,420	82,380	168,140	93,990	74,150
Larynx	9,880	7,920	1,960	3,770	2,960	810
Lung and bronchus	172,570	93,010	79,560	163,510	90,490	73,020
Other respiratory organs	2,350	1,490	860	860	540	320
Bones and joints	2,570	1,480	1,090	1,210	670	540
Soft tissue (including heart)	9,420	5,530	3,890	3,490	1,910	1,580
Skin (excluding basal and squamous)	66,000	37,580	28,420	10,590	6,920	3,670
Melanoma-skin	59,580	33,580	26,000	7,770	4,910	2,860
Other nonepithelial skin	6,420	4,000	2,420	2,820	2,010	810
Breast	212,930	1,690	211,240	40,870	460	40,410
Genital system	321,050	241,570	79,480	59,920	31,010	28,910
Uterine cervix	10,370	—	10,370	3,710	—	3,710
Uterine corpus	40,880	—	40,880	7,310	—	7,310
Ovary	22,225	—	22,220	16,210	—	16,210
Vulva	3,870	—	3,870	870	—	870
Vagina and other genital, female	2,140	—	2,140	810	—	810
Prostate	232,090	232,090	—	30,350	30,350	—
Testis	8,010	8,010	—	390	390	—
Penis and other genital, male	1,470	1,470	—	270	270	—
Urinary system	101,880	71,090	30,790	26,590	17,420	9,170
Urinary bladder	63,210	47,010	16,200	13,180	8,970	4,210
Kidney and renal pelvis	36,160	22,490	13,670	12,660	8,020	4,640
Ureter and other urinary organs	2,510	1,590	920	750	430	320
Eye and orbit	2,120	1,090	1,030	230	110	120
Brain and other nervous system	18,500	10,620	7,880	12,760	7,280	5,480
Endocrine system	27,650	7,550	20,100	2,370	1,080	1,290
Thyroid	25,690	6,500	19,190	1,490	630	860
Other endocrine	1,960	1,050	910	880	450	430
Lymphoma	63,740	33,050	30,690	20,610	10,930	9,680
Hodgkin's disease	7,350	3,980	3,370	1,410	780	630
Non-Hodgkin's lymphoma	56,390	29,070	27,320	19,200	10,150	9,050
Multiple myeloma	15,980	8,600	7,380	11,300	5,660	5,640
Leukemia	34,810	19,640	15,170	22,570	12,540	10,030
Acute lymphocytic leukemia	3,970	2,180	1,790	1,490	850	640
Chronic lymphocytic leukemia	9,730	5,780	3,950	4,600	2,520	2,080
Acute myeloid leukemia	11,960	6,530	5,430	9,000	5,040	3,960
Chronic myeloid leukemia	4,600	2,640	1,960	850	430	420
Other leukemia‡	4,550	2,510	2,040	6,630	3,700	2,930
Other and unspecified primary sites	28,590	14,660	13,930	46,250	25,370	20,880

*Rounded to the nearest 10; excludes basal and squamous cell skin cancers and in situ carcinomas except urinary bladder.

About 58,490 carcinoma in situ of the breast and 46,170 melanoma in situ will be newly diagnosed in 2005.

† Estimated deaths for colon and rectum cancers are combined.

‡ More deaths than cases suggests lack of specificity in recording underlying causes of death on death certificates.

American Cancer Society, Surveillance Research, 2005. Data source: Estimates of new cases are based on incidence rates from 1979 to 2001, National Cancer Institute's Surveillance, Epidemiology and End Results Program, nine oldest registries. Estimates of deaths are based on data from US mortality public use data tapes, 1969 to 2002. National Center for Health Statistics, Center for Disease Control and Prevention; 2004.

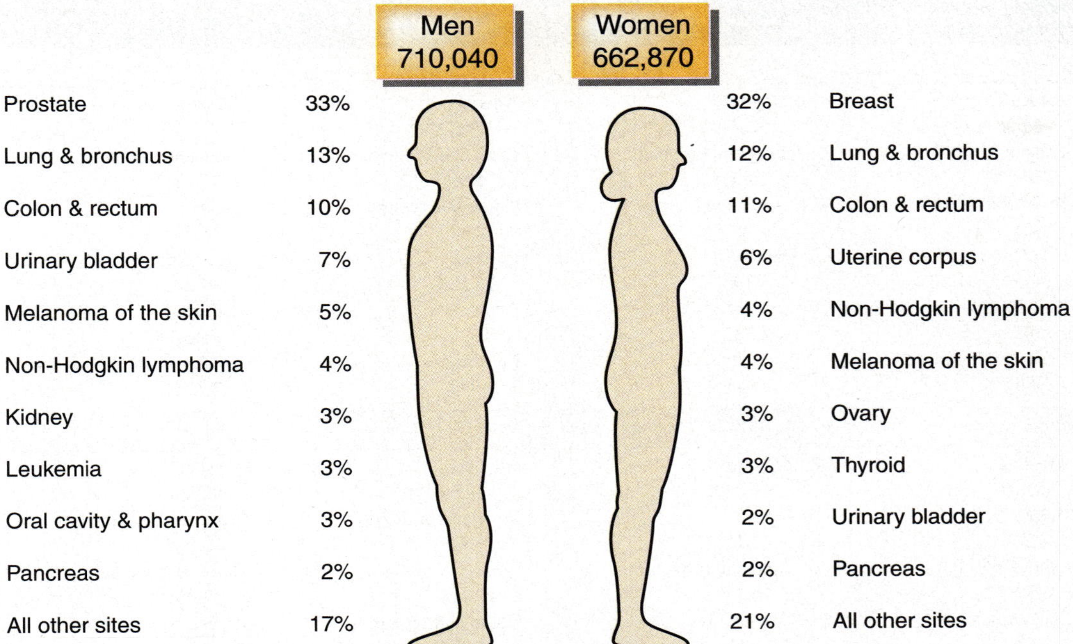

Figure 24-2 Estimated percentage of new cancer cases for 10 leading sites by sex, United States, 2005. *Excludes basal and squamous cell skin cancers and in situ carcinomas except urinary bladder. Source: American Cancer Society, Cancer facts and figures, 2005.

cancer closely parallel sex-specific changes in smoking. They provide a remarkable record of how tobacco smoking has affected lung cancer mortality and incidence in the United States.

Two other large changes in cancer death rates since 1930 involve the decline in stomach cancer death rates in both sexes, and the decrease in uterine (cervix and corpus combined) death rates in women. The decrease in stomach cancer is largely attributed to the introduction of refrigeration (with reduced use of salted and smoked foods and increased availability of fresh vegetables and fruit), and perhaps to improved living conditions that decreased chronic infection with helicobacter in childhood.[28] The decrease in the cervical cancer death rate is partly (but not entirely) attributable to early detection by PAP testing. The decline in death rates from cancer of the uterine cervix and corpus began well before 1945,[19] when the PAP test began to be introduced, and prior to widespread usage of PAP testing in the 1970s. It is unclear to what extent changes in surgical practice, nutrition, personal hygiene, or reproductive factors may also have contributed.

Temporal trends in the incidence of specific cancers, monitored in nine NCI SEER registries, are shown in Figure 24-6.[19] In men, the large increase in diagnoses of prostate cancer between 1989 and 1992 dominates the incidence trends in other cancer. This reflects the widespread introduction of screening for prostate specific antigen (PSA) in the late 1980s.[29] The prostate malignancies diagnosed by PSA represent real prostate cancer, but the apparent temporal increase is exaggerated by improved detection of tumors that would previously have gone undiagnosed. The shift toward earlier and more complete diagnosis of prostrate cancer has had a much greater impact on prostate cancer incidence (see Figure 24-6) than mortality (see Figure 24-4).

When all cancers in men and women are combined (Figure 24-7), the age-adjusted rate peaked in 1992 for cancer incidence and in 1991 for mortality. Both incidence and death rates subsequently decreased each year through 1996. If 1992 rates are used as a common baseline, the average annual decrease from 1992 through 2001 was 1.0% for mortality and 0.7% for incidence.[30] Much of the decline in cancer incidence was contributed by the large fall in prostate cancer incidence (see Figure 24-6), several years after the introduction of PSA testing,[29] although sustained reductions in the lung cancer incidence in men and colorectal cancer in both sexes also contributed.

The temporal trend in cancer death rates for all sites combined is substantially different in men from that in women (Figure 24-8). Whereas the combined death rate from all cases in men increased over most of 1930 to 1991, the rate in women has not changed markedly since the 1960s. This is because the decrease in death rates from cancers of the stomach, uterus, and colorectum has largely offset the increase in lung cancer mortality in women but not in men.

Whereas the death rate from all cancers combined decreased from 1991 to 2001, the total number of cancer deaths continued to increase, albeit more slowly than in earlier years (Figure 24-9). As mentioned, the decrease in the death rates did not completely offset the aging and growth of the population. Future trends in the number of cases and deaths from cancer will continue to be influenced by aging of the "baby-boomer" generation for several decades. The demographic trends make it difficult to reduce the total number of cancer cases and deaths. It is therefore important to distinguish between trends in age-adjusted occurrence rates and trends in the number of people affected when discussing "progress" against cancer.

Variations Across Socioeconomic, Ethnic, and Racial Groups The impact of socioeconomic status on cancer occurrence and survival is usually examined indirectly, through comparisons of racial and ethnic groups. Many analyses

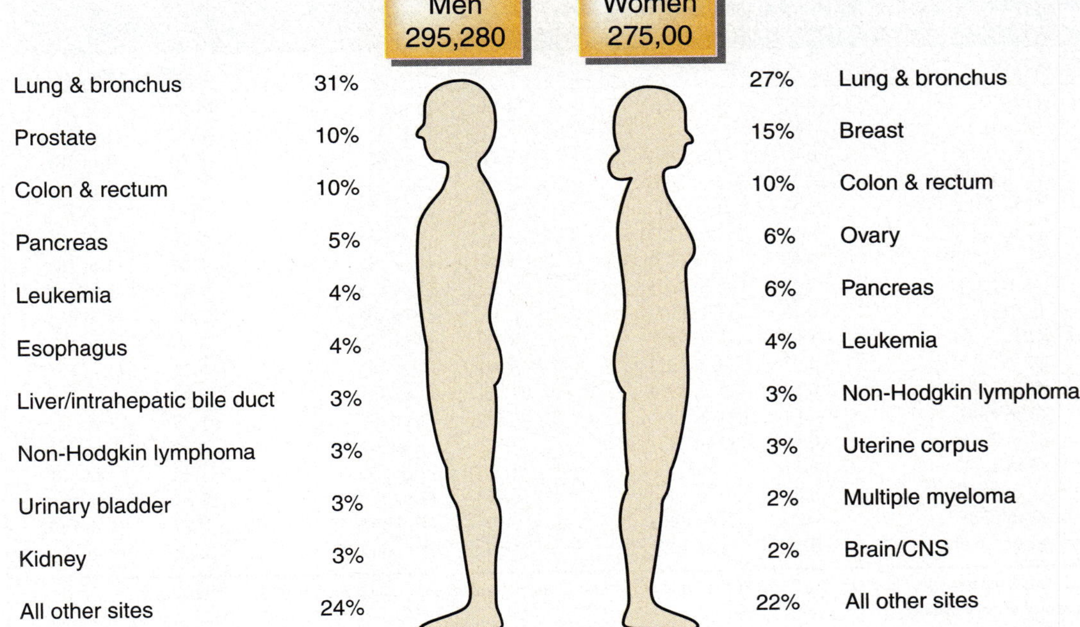

Figure 24-3 Estimated percentage of cancer deaths for 10 leading sites by sex, United States, 2005. *Excludes basal and squamous cell skin cancers and in situ carcinomas except urinary bladder. Source: American Cancer Society, Cancer facts and figures, 2005.

Table 24-4 Reported Deaths for the Five Leading Cancer Sites by Gender and Age, United States, 2002

Males	< 20	20–39	40–59	60–79	> 80
All sites 288,768	All sites 1,282	All sites 4,626	All sites 52,489	All sites 156,527	All sites 73,839
Lung and bronchus 90,121	Leukemia 382	Leukemia 599	Lung and bronchus 16,044	Lung and bronchus 55,996	Lung and bronchus 17,681
Prostate 30,446	Brain and ONS 327	Brain and ONS 516	Colon and rectum 5,257	Colon and rectum 14,973	Prostate 15,795
Colon and rectum 28,472	Endocrine 104	Colon and rectum 413	Pancreas 3,195	Prostate 13,539	Colon and rectum 7,820
Pancreas 14,877	Bones and joints 96	Non-Hodgkin's lymphoma 401	Liver and bile duct 2,733	Pancreas 8,312	Leukemia 3,409
Non-Hodgkin's lymphoma 12,058	Soft Tissue 82	Lung and bronchus 394	Esophagus 2,470	Leukemia 5,919	Urinary bladder 3,331
Females	**< 20**	**20–39**	**40–59**	**60–79**	**> 80**
All sites 268,503	All sites 989	All sites 5,403	All sites 49,570	All sites 129,699	All sites 82,840
Lung and bronchus 67,509	Leukemia 296	Breast 1,331	Breast 12,115	Lung and bronchus 39,943	Lung and bronchus 16,064
Breast 41,514	Brain and ONS 244	Uterine cervix 499	Lung and bronchus 11,129	Breast 17,218	Colon and rectum 12,030
Colon and rectum 28,132	Endocrine 88	Leukemia 433	Colon and rectum 3,857	Colon and rectum 11,904	Breast 10,849
Pancreas 15,387	Bones and joints 83	Lung and bronchus 370	Ovary 3,285	Pancreas 7,869	Pancreas 5,436
Ovary 14,682	Soft Tissue 71	Brain and ONS 349	Pancreas 1,999	Ovary 7,349	Non-Hodgkin's lymphoma 4,029

Note: "All Sites" excludes in situ carcinomas except urinary bladder.
ONS = other nervous system.
Source: US mortality public use data tape 2002. National Center for Health Statistics, Centers for Disease Control and Prevention; 2004.

show that African-Americans experience disproportionately high cancer rates, but few studies have separated the impact of poverty and its attendant risk factors from genetic differences associated with race.[31]

Table 24-6 shows that incidence and death rates from all cancers combined and from the four most common cancers were generally higher in African Americans than other racial and ethnic groups during the years 1997 to 2001.[1] The one exception to this was breast cancer incidence in women, where the rate was highest in whites. Among men, the incidence of all invasive cancers combined (per 100,000) was 598 in African Americans, 480 in whites, 327 in Hispanics, 326 in Asian/Pacific islanders, and 178 in American Indians. The high incidence in African American men involves cancers of the prostate, and lung and bronchus (shown in Table 24-6) as well as oropharynx, larynx, esophagus, pancreas and multiple myeloma (not shown in Table 24-6). The cancer incidence rate in African Americans has decreased from 1992 to 2001, as it has in other racial and ethnic groups.[1]

Table 24-5 Probability of Developing Invasive Cancers Within Selected Age Intervals by Gender, United States, 1999-2001*

		Birth to 39 (%)	40 to 59 (%)	60 to 79 (%)	Birth to Death (%)
All sites†	Male	1.41 (1 in 71)	8.52 (1 in 12)	34.63 (1 in 3)	45.59 (1 in 2)
	Female	1.97 (1 in 51)	9.1 (1 in 11)	22.51 (1 in 4)	38.18 (1 in 3)
Bladder‡	Male	0.02 (1 in 4,262)	0.41 (1 in 243)	2.41 (1 in 41)	3.56 (1 in 28)
	Female	0.01 (1 in 8,876)	0.12 (1 in 804)	0.65 (1 in 153)	1.13 (1 in 88)
Breast	Female	0.48 (1 in 207)	4.18 (1 in 24)	7.49 (1 in 13)	13.39 (1 in 7)
Colon and rectum	Male	0.07 (1 in 1,484)	0.9 (1 in 111)	3.96 (1 in 25)	5.90 (1 in 17)
	Female	0.06 (1 in 1,586)	0.69 (1 in 145)	3.04 (1 in 33)	5.54 (1 in 18)
Leukemia	Male	0.15 (1 in 659)	0.22 (1 in 461)	0.85 (1 in 118)	1.47 (1 in 68)
	Female	0.13 (1 in 799)	0.14 (1 in 697)	0.48 (1 in 206)	1.04 (1 in 96)
Lung and bronchus	Male	0.03 (1 in 3,164)	1.06 (1 in 95)	5.75 (1 in 17)	7.63 (1 in 13)
	Female	0.03 (1 in 2,977)	0.81 (1 in 123)	3.91 (1 in 26)	5.71 (1 in 18)
Melanoma	Male	0.13 (1 in 795)	0.51 (1 in 195)	1.08 (1 in 93)	1.89 (1 in 53)
	Female	0.21 (1 in 484)	0.4 (1 in 248)	0.53 (1 in 190)	1.28 (1 in 78)
Non-Hodgkin's lymphoma	Male	0.14 (1 in 724)	0.46 (1 in 217)	1.32 (1 in 76)	2.18 (1 in 46)
	Female	0.09 (1 in 1,147)	0.31 1 in 328)	1.00 (1 in 100)	1.80 (1 in 56)
Prostate	Male	0.01 (1 in 9,879)	2.58 (1 in 39)	14.76 (1 in 7)	17.81 (1 in 6)
Uterine cervix	Female	0.16 (1 in 636)	0.29 (1 in 340)	0.27 (1 in 368)	0.77 (1 in 130)
Uterine corpus	Female	0.06 (1 in 1,632)	0.72 (1 in 139)	1.57 (1 in 64)	2.62 (1 in 38)

*For those free of cancer at beginning of age interval. Based on cancer cases diagnosed during 1999-2001. The "1 in" statistic and the inverse of the percentage may not be equivalent due to rounding.
†All sites exclude basal and squamous cell skin cancers and in situ cancers except urinary bladder.
‡Includes invasive and in situ cancer cases.
Data source: DEVCAN Software, Version 5.2, Surveillance, Epidemiology, and End Results Program, Division of Cancer Control and Population Sciences, National Cancer Institute; 2004.

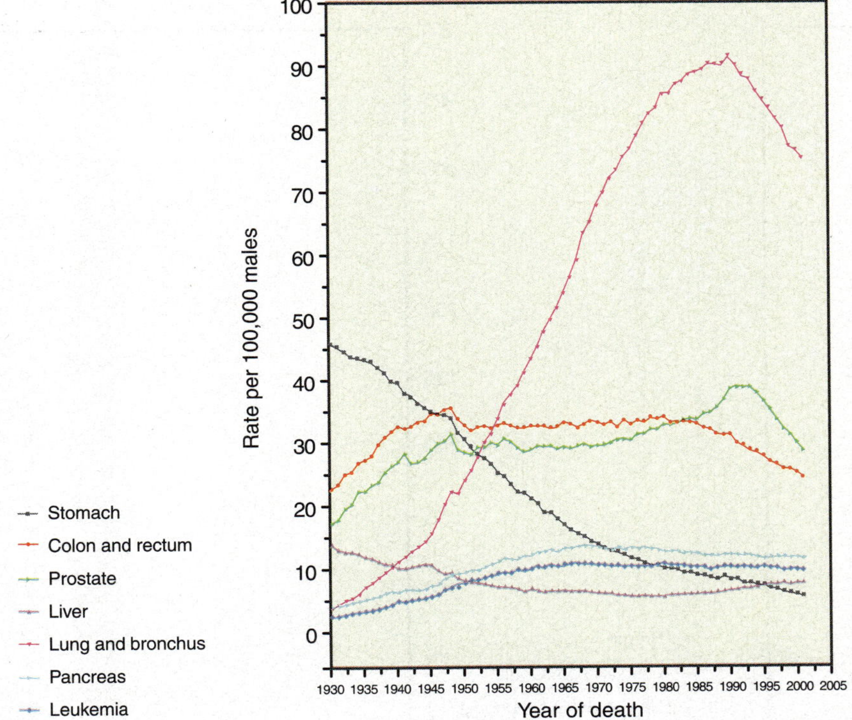

Figure 24-4 Age-adjusted cancer death rates among males for selected cancer types, United States, 1930 to 2001. *Rates are per 100,000 population per year and are age-adjusted to the 2000 US standard population. Note: Due to changes in ICD coding, numerator information has changed over time. Rates for cancers of the liver, lung and bronchus, and colon and rectum are affected by these changes. American Cancer Society, Surveillance Research, 2005. Data source: US mortality public use data tapes, 1960 to 2001, US mortality volumes, 1930 to 1959. National Center for Health Statistics, Centers for Disease Control and Prevention; 2004.

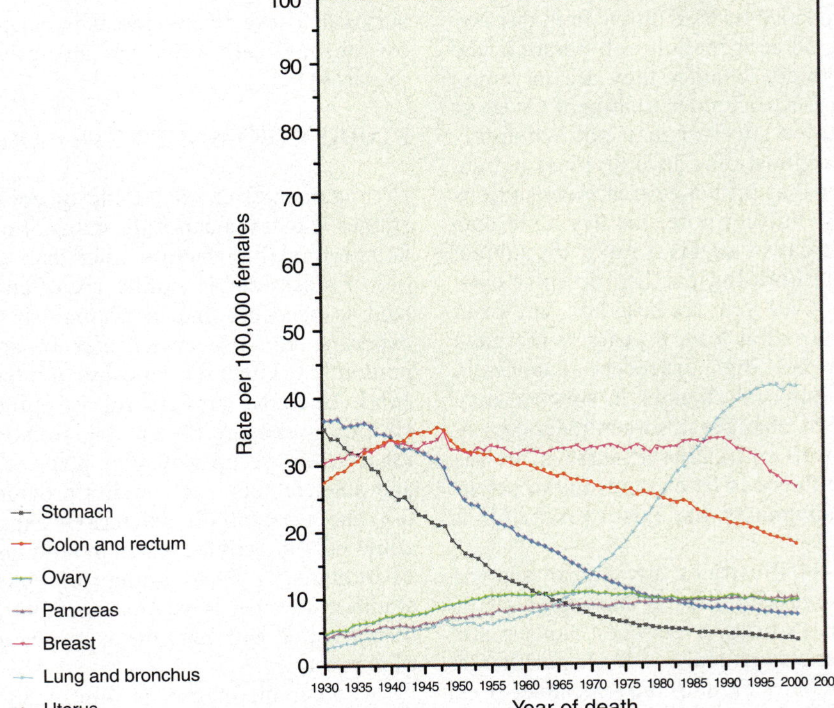

Figure 24-5 Age-adjusted cancer death rates among females for selected cancer types, United States, 1930 to 2001. *Rates are per 100,000 population per year and are age-adjusted to the 2000 US standard population. Note: Due to changes in ICD coding, numerator information has changed over time. Rates for cancers of the uterus, lung and bronchus, and colon and rectum are affected by these changes. *Uterus cancer death rates are for uterine cervix and uterine corpus combined. American Cancer Society, Surveillance Research, 2005. Data source: US mortality public use data tapes, 1960 to 2001, US mortality volumes, 1930 to 1959. National Center for Health Statistics, Centers for Disease Control and Prevention; 2004.

Table 24-7 shows the findings of one study that measured cancer incidence by race within strata of income and educational attainment, markers of socioeconomic status.[31] Within comparable strata of education and income, African Americans age 25 and above have similar or lower incidence of all cancers combined than did white Americans. The implication of this study is that many of the disparities in cancer incidence associated with race may be caused by factors associated with poverty rather than by genetic correlates of race. Lower socioeconomic status limits educational attainment, reduces access to medical screening, and is often associated with greater exposure to tobacco, heavy alcohol consumption, poor nutrition, physical inactivity, overweight, and other risk factors.[32] It should be noted that the incidence rates in Table 24-7 are age-standardized to the 1970 United States population and thus cannot be compared to the race- and ethnicity-specific incidence rates in Table 24-6.

Cancer is frequently diagnosed at a later stage among persons of lower income and educational status, contributing to poorer survival.[33,34] This is reflected in Figure 24-10, where the percentage of cancers diagnosed at a localized stage (confined to the organ of origin) was lower for many cancer sites among African Americans than whites between 1995 and 2000.[35] The difference in stage is largest for cancers of the female breast and uterine cervix and corpus. Lower use of mammography contributes to the racial disparity in stage at diagnosis for breast cancer.[36] The stage difference is more difficult to explain for cervical cancer, however, because the use of PAP testing is actually higher in African American than in white women.[36] PAP testing is underutilized in postmenopausal women of all races. It may be that the lack of PAP testing in older African American women contributes particularly to their higher death rates from cervical cancer.

Other ethnic groups in the United States also have distinctive cancer patterns.[32,37] Relative to whites, age-adjusted incidence and mortality rates among Mexican-Americans (Hispanics) are higher for gallbladder, stomach, and cervical cancers; American Indian men and women have lower incidence rates of most cancers other than gallbladder, stomach, and cervix; Japanese Americans have higher rates of stomach and liver cancer; Chinese Americans have higher rates of nasopharyngeal, liver, and stomach cancer; Native Hawaiians have higher death rates from esophagus, liver, pancreas, lung, breast, and cervical cancer; Filipino-Americans have lower risk of most cancers other than stomach, liver, oral cavity, and esophagus. Many of these ethnic differences are known to reflect differences in tobacco use, dietary habits, infectious exposures, or medical care. For example, the high rate of stomach cancer among recent migrants from Latin America, Asia, and parts of Africa correlates with their higher prevalence of chronic helicobacter infection in childhood, greater dietary consumption of salted and smoked preserved

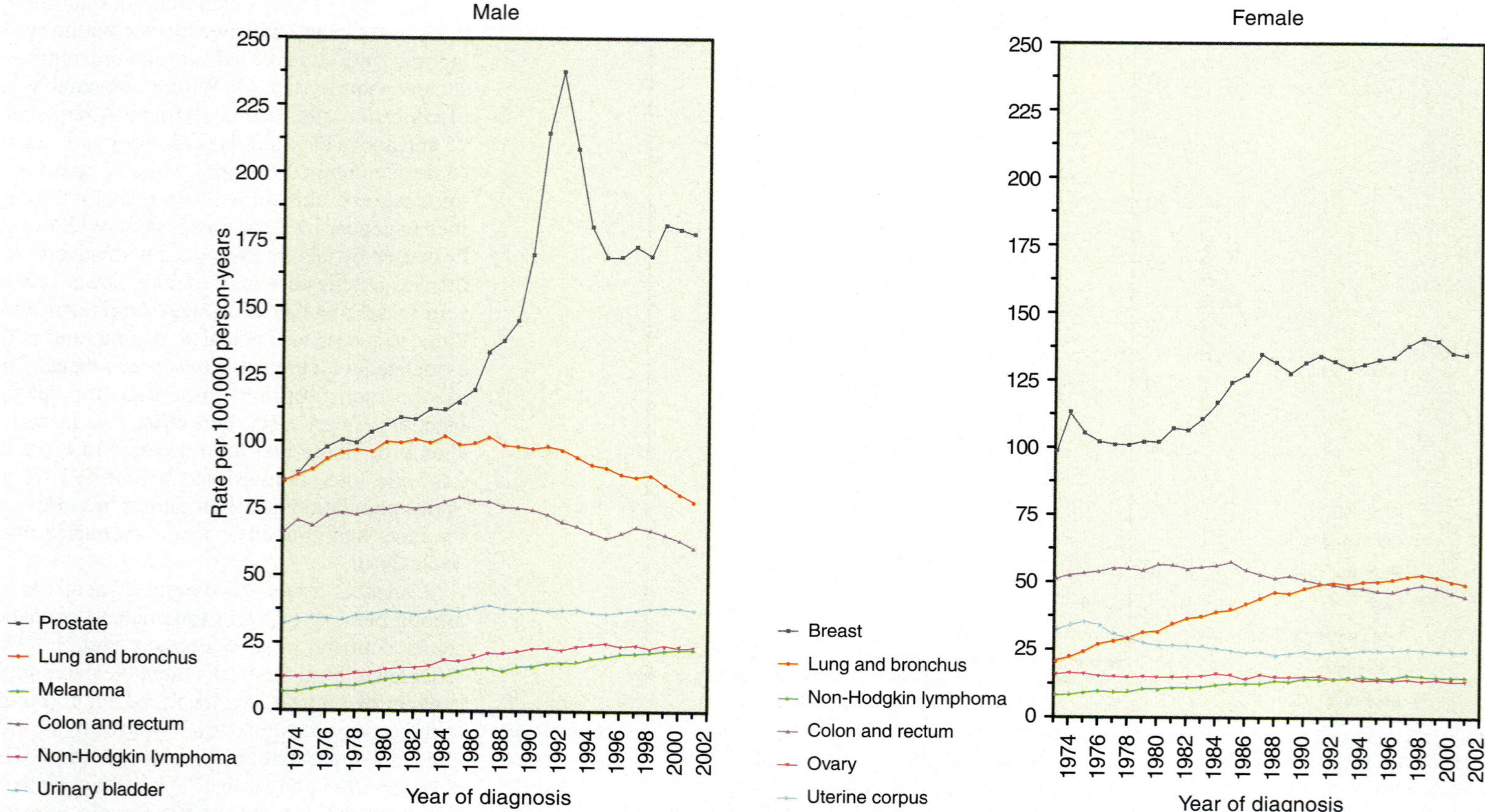

Figure 24-6 Age-adjusted cancer incidence rates for males and females by site, United States, 1973 to 2001. *Rates are per 100,000 population per year and are age-adjusted to the 2000 US standard population. American Cancer Society, Surveillance Research, 2005. Data source: NCI, Surveillance, Epidemiology, and End Results Program, 1973–2001, Division of Cancer Control and Population Sciences, National Cancer Institute; 2004.

food, and lower consumption of fresh fruits and vegetables. Similarly, ethnic groups with increased liver cancer usually have higher prevalence of infection with chronic hepatitis B, or less commonly C virus. The incidence of cervical cancer reflects exposure to human papilloma virus 16, especially when sexual activity begins at an early age with multiple partners, whereas the death rate from cervical cancer varies according to the utilization of PAP testing and early diagnosis and treatment.

SURVIVAL OF PATIENTS WITH CANCER

The survival of patients with cancer is monitored by the National Cancer Institute SEER registries in the United States.[1] Relative survival is determined by following-up cancer patients over a series of one-year intervals and then comparing the percentage of these patients who remain alive to the corresponding percentage in the general population of similar age, race, and sex.[38,39] A relative survival of 100 percent means that the same percentage of cancer patients survived as in the general population. A relative survival greater than 100 indicates better survival among the cancer patients than in the general population, whereas a relative survival less than 100 signifies the opposite.

Five-year relative survival differs from disease-free survival, since it includes all persons who have not yet died, whether they are in remission, disease free, or under treatment. Average five-year relative survival may not accurately predict the prognosis for an individual patient due to factors that influence treatment options and longevity. Furthermore, the available data on five-year relative survival rates are subject to certain methodological limitations: estimates from a given year are based on data from patients diagnosed at least 8 years in the past, and may not reflect the most recent advances in treatment[30]; temporal changes in survival may be influenced by changes in screening and early detection as well as treatment; survival trends may also be influenced by changes in the extent of disease at diagnosis that exist even within a given stage.

Figure 24-11 illustrates that 5-year relative survival is generally shorter among African Americans than whites, even when cancers are diagnosed at the same stage.[32,34] Disparities in survival are seen for eight of the ten cancer sites shown, and are largest in absolute terms for cancers of the female breast, uterine cervix and corpus, colon and rectum, and prostate. Racial differences in survival probably reflect lower access to medical care and poor nutrition as well as other unidentified factors that may affect survival. These discrepancies in cancer survival by race and ethnicity are an active area of research.

STUDIES OF CANCER ETIOLOGY

A fundamental characteristic of epidemiologic studies is that the exposure status of participants is determined by factors other than randomization. Epidemiologic studies are often characterized as observational to distinguish them from experimental studies where subjects are assigned randomly to either the exposure of interest or placebo. Because participants in epidemiologic studies make their own decisions regarding tobacco use, occupation, diet, place of residence, and other factors, such studies provide information about potentially deleterious exposures that could not ethically be tested in randomized trials of humans. A disadvantage of observational studies, however, is that extraneous factors may be correlated with both the exposure and disease of interest.

Another distinction is often made between descriptive and analytic epidemiologic studies.[4] Descriptive studies usually characterize risk factor prevalence and/or disease occurrence based on aggregate data on the entire population. These studies identify personal characteristics, geographic locations, and time periods

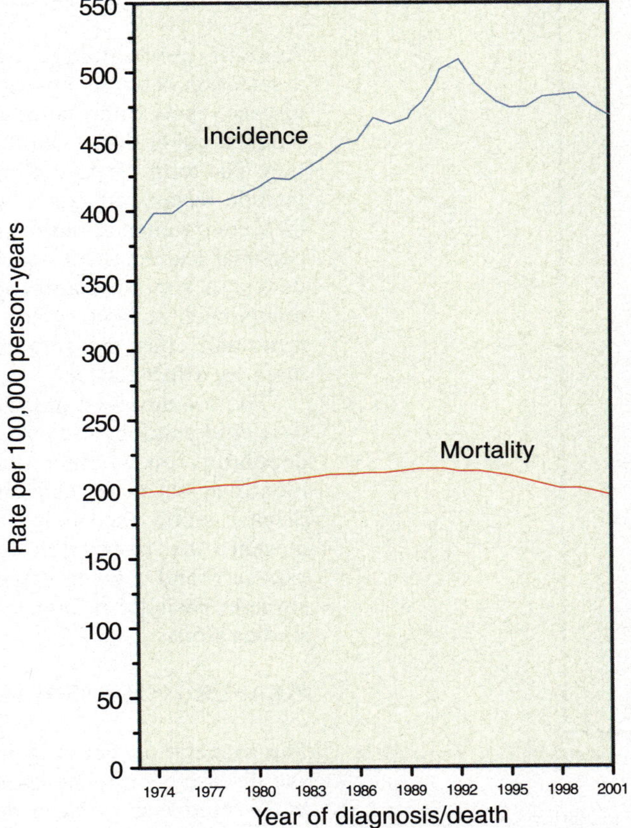

Figure 24-7 Age-adjusted cancer incidence and mortality rates for males and females for all sites combined, United States, 1973 to 2001. *Rates are per 100,000 population per year and are age-adjusted to the 2000 US standard population. American Cancer Society, Surveillance Research, 2005. Data source: NCI, Surveillance, Epidemiology, and End Results Program, 1973–2001, Division of Cancer Control and Population Sciences, National Cancer Institute, 2004. US mortality public use data tapes, 1960 to 2001, US mortality volumes, 1930 to 1959. National Center for Health Statistics, Centers for Disease Control and Prevention; 2004.

associated with unusually high or low risk of cancer, thereby generating hypotheses that can be tested elsewhere. Special caution is warranted in interpreting ecological studies that use aggregate statistics on populations to imply that a particular factor as causal. In contrast, analytic studies measure the exposure and disease status of individuals rather than aggregate statistics on the overall population. Analytic studies are more able to test prespecified (a priori) hypotheses by measuring the association between individual exposure and subsequent disease.

DESCRIPTIVE STUDIES

The huge geographic and temporal variation in many types of cancer provides strong evidence that cancer is not an intrinsic consequence of life, but is affected by lifestyle and environmental factors in addition to inherited genes. Doll and Peto, in 1981, compared the cumulative incidence (percent of people affected) by various cancers in countries with the highest and lowest risk around the world.[40] Table 24-8 shows the range of cumulative incidence that they observed in 1976. Also shown is the ratio of the highest to the lowest cumulative incidence in the age range 35 to 64 years, a range intended to reduce the reporting error in poorer countries. From the data in Table 24-8 and other lines of evidence, Doll and Peto inferred that approximately 75 to 80% of cancer deaths occurring in the United States in 1970 could theoretically be avoided.

Much of the enormous geographic and temporal variation in cancer rates is real rather than an artifact of incomplete registration of cases and deaths in economically developing countries. Some of the ranges shown in Table 24-8 have narrowed over time, yet high rates of cancer of the stomach persist in Japan, China, and parts of South America, nasopharyngeal cancer in southern China, colon cancer in Eastern Europe, Denmark and New Zealand, cervical cancer in parts of South and Central America and Africa, liver cancer in much of Asia and sub-Saharan Africa, and melanoma in Australia.

The Doll and Peto analysis is descriptive only in that it uses routinely collected data on cancer incidence and mortality to demonstrate the large variation in cancer risk across countries.[40] It does not make inferences about why a particular cancer is common or uncommon in a certain region based on the descriptive data alone; rather, it considers all of the information available from analytic studies, clinical medicine, and basic research in estimating the fraction of cancers attributable to smoking, nutrition, alcohol consumption, and other factors.[40] Validity in epidemiologic studies depends partly upon the conclusions being drawn as well as on the quality of the underlying data.

Studies in migrants who move from low to high, or high to low risk areas support the idea that many cancers are largely avoidable.[41] The change in cancer occurrence is seen more quickly after migration for some cancers than others. For instance, the low incidence of colon cancer seen in Japan rises substantially in the first generation of Japanese who migrate to Hawaii or to the continental United States. In contrast, the low rate of breast cancer among women in Japan who migrate to the United States continues to rise into the second generation after migration. Ultimately, breast cancer incidence among Japanese American women rises to equal or exceed the rate among American white women.[4]

Time trends within countries also illustrate the importance of exogenous, as well as genetic, factors on cancer occurrence. Figure 24-12 shows the increase in death rates from colon, and to a lesser extent breast cancer, in Japan between 1955 and 1985.[42] Major changes in diet and other factors occurred in Japan after World War II. Figure 24-12 also shows the temporal increase in fat intake, based on per capita estimates of the total amount of fat in foods reportedly consumed in Japan during these years. These data alone do not establish that fat consumption caused the increase in death rates from colon and breast cancer. Certain other factors not shown in Figure 24-12 may also have contributed to the increase. These include increased consumption of total calories or meat, diminished consumption of fresh fruit and vegetables, and reduced physical activity. However, the temporal trends in Japan clearly show that mortality from breast and colorectal cancer is affected by external factors as well as by genetic inheritance.

Another example of how ecological studies have contributed to nutritional epidemiology is the correlation between per capita consumption (or disappearance) of various foods in selected countries and national cancer rates. Figure 24-13 shows the strong correlation (0.89) between per capita consumption of red meat in the late 1960s and the incidence of colorectal cancer in women.[43] These correlation studies do not measure the behavior or disease experience of individuals, nor can they separate other unmeasured risk factors such as physical inactivity, caloric intake, or abdominal obesity from the measured correlation with red meat consumption. Nevertheless, these ecological studies generate hypotheses that can be tested in other research including analytic epidemiologic studies as well as basic and clinical research.

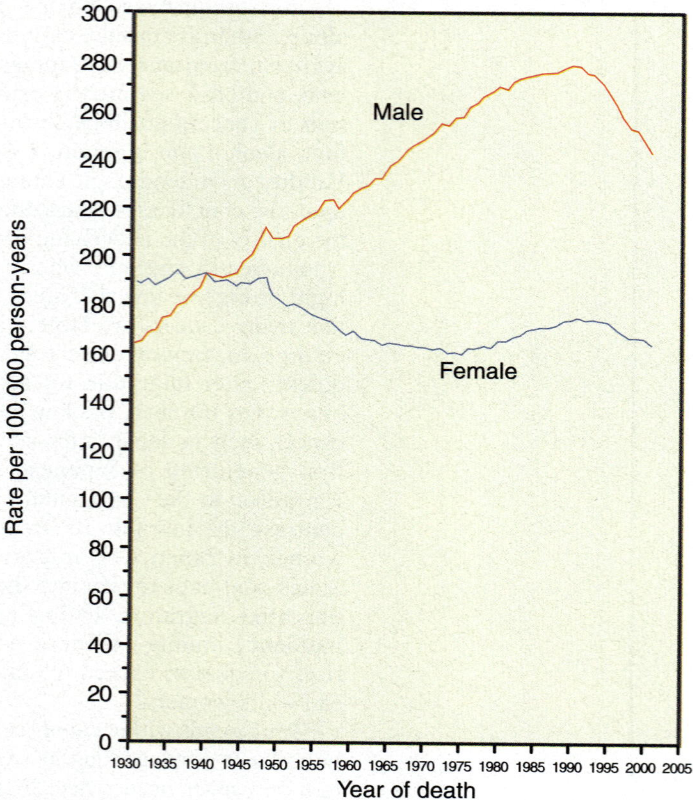

Figure 24-8 Cancer death rates, all sites combined, all races, by sex, United States, 1930 to 2001. *Age–adjusted to the 2000 US population. Data source: US mortality public use data tapes, 1960 to 2001, US mortality volumes, 1930 to 1959. National Center for Health Statistics, Centers for Disease Control and Prevention; 2004.

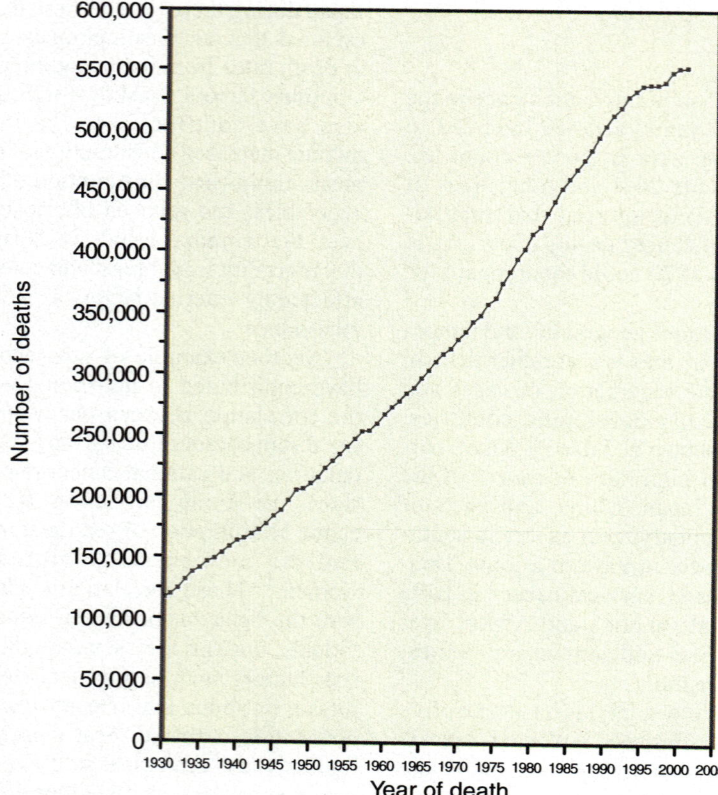

Figure 24-9 Number of cancer deaths, all sites combined, all races, men and women combined, United States, 1930 to 2001. Data source: US mortality public use data tapes, 1960 to 2001, US mortality volumes, 1930 to 1959. National Center for Health Statistics, Centers for Disease Control and Prevention; 2004.

ANALYTIC EPIDEMIOLOGY

Analytic epidemiologic studies measure the association between a particular exposure and a disease, using information collected from individuals, rather than from the aggregate population. The term "exposure" is defined broadly to include behavioral factors such as smoking or diet, environmental pollutants such as asbestos, personal characteristics such as obesity or tendency to sunburn, anthropometric measurements such as body mass index, and genetic traits and other measurable biological factors that may affect cancer.

The two most common study designs in analytic epidemiology are cohort and case-control, depending on whether the subjects are first identified based on characteristics other than disease status (see below). Both approaches measure the association between a particular exposure and a given disease; both provide a stronger basis for inference than do descriptive studies alone.

MEASURES OF ASSOCIATION

The association between individual exposure and disease occurrence is most often expressed as the relative risk (RR or rate ratio) in a cohort study or odds ratio (OR) in a case-control study.[4] For example, a cohort study could measure the association between human papilloma virus (HPV) infection and cervical cancer by determining the incidence of cervical cancer among a defined group of women in a health maintenance organization who do or do not have chronic HPV infection. The increase associated with HPV infection could be expressed as the RR, or the incidence rate among infected women divided by the incidence among the uninfected women. Alternatively, the association could also be estimated from a case control study of women with cervical cancer, by comparing HPV infection among cases with the prevalence among non-cases or controls.

Both the RR and the OR characterize the association between the exposure and disease in relative terms. Both measures reflect the frequency of disease occurrence among exposed subjects as a multiple of the rate among unexposed persons. A second, less commonly used measure of association, however, is the absolute change in risk associated with exposure. This can be estimated in cohort but not usually in case-control studies. The absolute risk (or rate difference, RD) equals the rate among the exposed persons minus the rate in the unexposed. In our specific example of cervical cancer and HPV infection, the RD would reflect the absolute magnitude of the increase in cervical cancer incidence associated with HPV infection. The RD is informative because it describes the absolute impact of the exposure on disease occurrence better than does the RR. This absolute impact is dependent on the background risk of disease in unexposed persons as well as upon

Table 24-6 Average Annual Incidence and Mortality Rates* for Selected Cancer Sites by Race and Ethnicity, United States, 1997-2001

Incidence	White	African American	Asian/Pacific Islander	American Indian/ Alaskan Native	Hispanic†
All sites					
Male	556.5	689.2	385.9	263.2	419.8
Female	429.8	400.1	302.8	222.5	309.9
Breast (female)	141.7	119.9	96.8	54.2	89.6
Colon and rectum					
Male	63.1	72.9	56.3	38.3	49.6
Female	45.9	56.5	38.6	32.7	32.5
Lung and bronchus					
Male	77.9	117.2	60.5	46.0	45.2
Female	51.3	54.5	28.5	23.4	23.9
Prostate	167.4	271.3	100.7	51.2	140.0
Stomach					
Males	10.8	18.8	21.9	15.7	17.8
Females	5.0	9.9	12.4	8.9	10.0
Liver and bile duct					
Males	7.2	11.8	21.1	8.3	13.5
Females	2.9	3.9	7.7	4.8	5.8
Cervix uteri	8.9	11.8	9.5	6.0	16.2
Mortality	**White**	**African American**	**Asian/Pacific Islander**	**American Indian/ Alaskan Native**	**Hispanic†**
All sites					
Male	245.5	347.3	151.2	167.0	174.0
Female	165.5	196.5	100.5	113.4	111.6
Breast (female)	26.4	35.4	12.6	13.6	17.3
Colon and rectum					
Male	24.8	34.3	15.8	17.1	18.0
Female	17.1	24.5	10.8	11.7	11.6
Lung and bronchus					
Male	76.6	104.1	40.2	49.8	39.6
Female	41.6	39.9	19.2	26.6	14.9
Prostate	28.8	70.4	13.0	20.2	23.5
Stomach					
Males	5.8	13.3	11.9	7.3	9.7
Females	2.8	6.3	7.0	4.1	5.3
Liver and bile duct					
Males	6.1	9.3	15.6	8.3	10.6
Females	2.7	3.8	6.6	4.3	5.1
Cervix uteri	2.6	5.6	2.8	2.8	3.6

*Rates are per 100,000 and are age-adjusted to the 2000 US standard population.
†Hispanics are not mutually exclusive from Whites, African Americans, Asian/Pacific Islanders, or American Indian/Alaskan Natives.
Note: Incidence data are from the 12 SEER areas; mortality data are from all states except data for Hispanics; data for Hispanics include deaths that occurred in all states except Connecticut, Louisiana, New Hampshire, and Oklahoma.
Source: Surveillance, Epidemiology and Results Program, 1973–2001, Bethesda, MD: Division of Cancer Control and Population Sciences, National Cancer Institute; 2004.
Mortality derived from data originating from the National Center for Health Statistics, Centers for Disease Control and Prevention; 2004.

Table 24-7 Incidence Rates* by Race, Income, and Educational Level, Ages 25 and Over, in San Francisco, Oakland, Detroit and Atlanta, 1978 to 1982

	White	African American
Educational level		
< 12 years of school	385.9	383
High school graduate	352.6	324.4
Some college	342.1	339.8
College graduate	338.3	270.6
Total	350.5	328.7
Income level (annual)		
Less than $15,000	403.2	371.7
$15,000–$24,999	352.7	341.9
$25,000–$29,999	348.1	285.8
$30,000 and over	336.8	326.6
Total	349.3	323.4

*Rates are per 100,000 and are age-adjusted to the 1970 US standard population.[33]

the RR. If the disease is rare, an exposure with RR = 10 will affect relatively few people. In contrast, if the disease is common, an exposure with RR = 1.5 would have a very large absolute impact on the population. The RD is less commonly measured in epidemiologic studies than is the RR, partly because it is only obtainable from cohort studies, and partly because it is more variable across different populations than is the RR.

Another measure of association is attributable risk, used to estimate the fraction or burden of disease in the population caused by the exposure of interest. This may be expressed as either the percentage of disease caused by the exposure among exposed persons, or the corresponding percentage in the overall population, which includes both exposed and unexposed persons. In either case, estimates of attributable risk are based on the assumption that an association is causally related to the exposure of interest, rather than merely reflecting chance or correlated factors that have not been controlled for.

Cohort Studies Epidemiologic studies of various populations, or cohorts have contributed much to our understanding of how tobacco, radiation, and other occupational and environmental factors can increase cancer risk, and more recently, how nutritional and genetic factors may modify this risk. Two central characteristics of cohort studies are (1) participants are selected because of some common characteristic that precedes the disease being studied and are then followed forward for some specified time period (unlike case-control studies), and (2) participants are not randomly assigned to their exposure status by the researchers (unlike randomized clinical trials).

In some cohort studies, the population is defined based on records pertaining to the particular exposure being studied. This is true in many occupational and environmental cohort studies such as the Atomic Bomb Survivors Study, the Underground Uranium Miners Study, and studies of asbestos-exposed workers.[44] In these, the historical records from workplaces and other places with unusually high-level exposures are used to define the cohort and to estimate the degree of exposure. The health or vital status of the cohort is then followed forward for some specified time period, during which disease occurrence is measured.

Alternatively, cohorts may be defined by some common attribute that makes them easier to identify and to follow. Examples of these are the British Doctor's Study, the Harvard Nurses' Health and Health Professionals Studies, and the several large cohorts assembled by the American Cancer Society through its network of volunteers. Although some of these cohorts are defined by occupation, the exposures of interest are usually lifestyle factors such as smoking, nutritional patterns, or other factors that are common in the general population. Information is collected by questionnaire at the time of enrollment and periodically thereafter. Exposures of interest can also be measured in blood specimens or other tissues that were collected before the advent of disease and then stored.

All cohort studies are prospective in the sense that subjects are classified as "exposed" or "unexposed," and then followed-up over time to assess disease occurrence. This temporal sequence

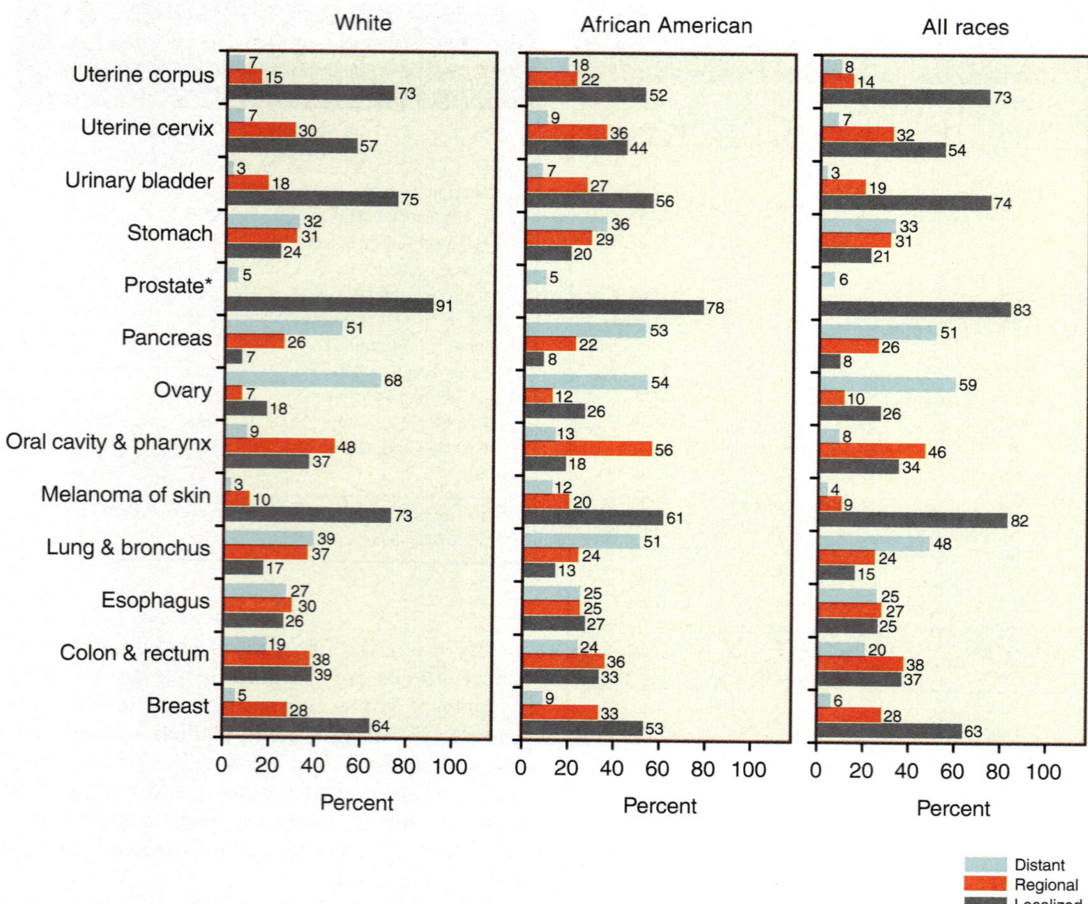

Figure 24-10 Percent distribution of cancer cases by race and stage at diagnosis, United States 1995–2000. *The rate for localized stage represents localized and regional stages combined. Note: Staging according to Surveillance, Epidemiology, and End Results (SEER) historic stage categories rather than the American Joint Committee on Cancer (AJCC) staging system. For each site and race, stage categories do not total 100% because sufficient information is not available to assign a stage to all cancer cases. Source: Ries LAG, Eisner MP, Kosary CL, et al.

exists whether the observation period begins in the distant past and extends towards the present, as in many historical cohort studies, or begins in the present and extends forward into the future. The ability of cohort studies to document exposure status before the occurrence of disease is an important strength, because it avoids the possibility that factors resulting from the disease itself may alter the reporting or measurement of exposure.[25]

Other important strengths of cohort studies, besides their logical temporal progression from exposure to disease, are their ability to study uncommon exposures (eg, unusual occupational and environmental exposures), and to measure the actual rates of disease occurrence and absolute measures of risk. Their disadvantages are that they are expensive to initiate, not well suited to studying rare diseases, and require considerable effort to ensure that, at most, only a small percentage of subjects are lost to follow-up. Ensuring adequate follow-up is an important concern for the validity of cohort studies.

Occupationally exposed workers have unfortunately served as the sentinel for many of the recognized industrial carcinogens, especially in workplaces where prolonged, heavy exposure caused unusual clusters of rare cancers.[45] Examples are the historical epidemics of scrotal cancer in former chimney sweeps,[46] bladder cancer in aniline dye workers,[47] osteosarcoma of the jaw in radium watch dial painters,[48] angiosarcoma of the liver in chemical workers exposed to vinyl chloride monomer,[49] and mesothelioma among asbestos-exposed workers.[44] In many of the early occupational studies, the association between very high exposure levels and a particular disease was strong and could be recognized simply through clinical observation. More recently, systematic epidemiologic studies have been used to estimate the dose-response relationship at lower levels of exposure, or to assess whether smaller increases also occurred in more common cancers. For example, the association between lung cancer and employment in poorly ventilated underground uranium mines has been known for over a century. Efforts to quantify the dose-response relationship between lower exposures to radon and lung cancer continue to have important implications for the general population with domestic exposure to radon gas seeping into cellars. Occupational studies are most informative when records exist to quantify exposure, where there is a substantial range in the intensity and duration of exposure, and where the workforce is large.

A more recent development in large prospective cohort studies, at least with respect to cancer, is their potential to measure biological markers in blood, urine, and other tissues, and to relate this to subsequent disease occurrence. Some markers, such as the measurements of aflatoxin metabolites in urine,[50] or cotinine in the serum or urine of persons exposed to second-hand smoke,[51] provide a more accurate measure of current internal exposure than could be obtained from questionnaires alone. In some cases, laboratory measurements based on stored serum, urine, or DNA provide the only reliable data on exposure. Biological specimens are essential in determining the presence or absence of serum antigens to hepatitis B or C, the concentrations of serum estrone among post-menopausal women not taking hormone replacement, and the profile of specific genetic polymorphisms that may modify an individual's susceptibility to a particular carcinogen. Biological specimens are usually collected on all willing members of the cohort, processed, and stored long term in liquid nitrogen. When a sufficient number of cases of a particular cancer have accrued during follow-up, the specimens are then analyzed on the cases, as well as on a sample of controls.

An example of how measurements of hormones, growth factors, nutrients etc. in blood can be informative about cancer is the recent study by Chan and colleagues of insulin-like growth factor-1 (IGF-1) in relation to prostate cancer in the Physician's Health Study.[52] This analysis found a strong positive association between IGF-1 in plasma collected from men and their subsequent development of prostate cancer. Plasma samples had been collected and stored on nearly 15,000 of the 22,000 male physicians who participated in this study. The fact that these blood samples preceded the diagnosis of prostate cancer, and that prostate specific antigen (PSA) levels were also measured on the stored specimens circumvented concern that prevalent prostate cancer might have affected the concentrations of IGF-1.

CASE-CONTROL STUDIES

Subjects in case-control studies are selected based on whether they have (cases) or have not (controls) been diagnosed with the specific disease under study. Cases and controls may then be interviewed about past and ongoing exposures, and the proportion of cases with a particular exposure is compared to that of the controls to determine if there is an association between the exposure and the disease.[4,22]

The preferred approach in a case-control study is that cases and controls are drawn from the same population. Ideally, cases are identified from population-based cancer registry rather than

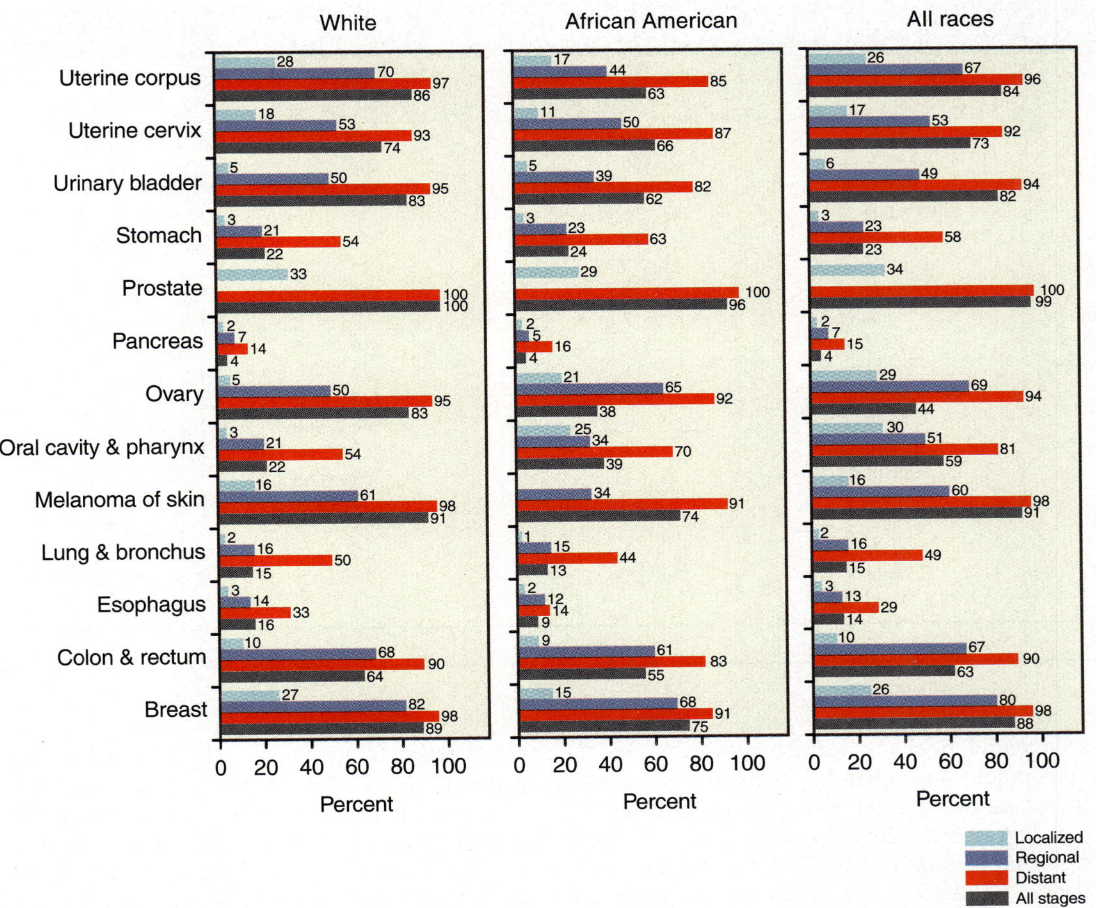

Figure 24-11 Five-year relative survival from various cancers, by race and stage at diagnosis, United States 1995–2000. Note: Staging according to Surveillance, Epidemiology, and End Results (SEER) historic stage categories rather than the American Joint Committee on Cancer (AJCC) staging system. Source: Ries LAG, Eisner MP, Kosary CL, et al.

a hospital, and controls are identified from the general population from which the cases arose. To the extent possible, cases should represent a single disease rather than a mixture of diseases with possibly diverse etiologies.

Advantages of case control over cohort studies are that they are efficient for studying rare diseases, quicker and less expensive than cohort studies to initiate, and because of their smaller size, better able to collect detailed information on a wide variety of exposures of interest. Their disadvantages are that, because subjects are aware of their disease status, case-control studies are more susceptible to biased reporting of exposures. For instance the case-control approach is not well suited to studying the relationship between alcohol consumption and oropharyngeal cancer, since cases might report their alcohol consumption more honestly than the controls (reporting bias), and controls who drink heavily may be unwilling to participate in the study (selection bias). The former results in differential misclassification of exposure, meaning that the exposure information is systematically flawed to over- or to underestimate the differences in exposure between cases and controls. In this case, the association between drinking and oropharyngeal cancer may be exaggerated by both the reporting and selection bias.

Case-control studies are highly efficient in studying uncommon cancers such as brain cancer. The sample size can be much smaller, because only the cases and a sample of controls are studied, rather than the entire base population from which the cases arose. Case-control studies can also be situated in populations that broaden the range of the exposure of interest. For example, Whittemore and colleagues studied the relation of diet and physical activity to colorectal cancer among Chinese in North America and in China.[53] By including cases and controls from China as well as North America, this study took advantage of the far greater range in dietary fat and protein consumption between these two regions, compared to the range within each region. The odds ratio (and 95 percent confidence intervals) between consumption of saturated fat and colorectal cancer among Chinese men in North America was OR = 2.1 (1.6–2.7), similar to that among women in North America. However, among men in China the odds ratio associated with saturated fat was smaller: OR = 1.2 (0.84–1.7), as it was in women. By demonstrating a stronger association between saturated fat and colorectal cancer in North America than in China, the study adds to the aggregate evidence that fat consumption is correlated with and may contribute to the high incidence of colorectal cancer in the United States.

WHAT CONSTITUTES "PROOF" IN EPIDEMIOLOGICAL STUDIES?

There has been vigorous philosophic and scientific debate over what constitutes "proof" when epidemiologic and other evidence is evaluated with respect to policy. Cohort and case control studies are, in principle, less definitive than are randomized clinical trials because they cannot control completely for unmeasured or incompletely measured risk factors that may be associated with both the exposure and disease of interest. However, the information from observational studies is often considered sufficient for public health action if chance, bias, or confounding can be reasonably excluded as alternative explanations for the findings.

Reliance on observational data as a basis for policy is inevitable in situations where randomized trials are unethical or unfeasible. The criteria frequently used to make a judgment of causation were first proposed in the 1964 Surgeon General's report on Smoking and Health,[54] subsequently expanded by Sir Austin Bradford Hill,[55] and later incorporated by organizations such as the International Agency for Research on Cancer (IARC).[56]

The inference that an association is causal is supported when

1. the association is strong (higher relative risks being more likely to indicate cause);
2. risk increases or decreases with exposure in a dose-response gradient;
3. consistent findings are seen in multiple studies with different investigators, different study populations, and designs;
4. the exposure (cause) precedes the disease;
5. it appears biologically plausible that the exposure could cause the disease;
6. the association is specific between the exposure and a single disease; and
7. the epidemiologic findings fit coherently with information from other types of research and other epidemiologic studies.

Certain of these criteria are considered more necessary than others. For example, an association that is reproducible in multiple epidemiologic studies and is consistent with other experimental and clinical research is far more credible than an association that meets only the criteria of specificity—one exposure causing one disease. In fact, the overwhelming evidence linking tobacco smoking with multiple types of cancer is strengthened, rather than diminished by the large number of cancers that it causes. In general, no

Table 24-8 Range of Cumulative Incidence* for Common Cancers Among Males and (for Certain Cancers) Among Females

Site of Origin of Cancer	High Incidence Area	Sex	Cumulative Incidence, % in High Incidence Area	Ratio of Highest Rate to Lowest Rate	Low Incidence Area
Skin (chiefly nonmelanoma)	Australia, Queensland	Male	>20	>200	India, Bombay
Esophagus	Iran, northeast section	Male	20	300	Nigeria
Lung and bronchus	England	Male	11	35	Nigeria
Stomach	Japan	Male	11	25	Uganda
Cervix, uteri	Columbia	Female	10	15	Israel: Jewish
Prostate	United States, blacks	Male	9	40	Japan
Liver	Mozambique	Male	8	100	England
Breast	Canada, British Columbia	Female	7	7	Israel: non-Jewish
Colon	United States, Connecticut	Male	3	10	Nigeria
Corpus uteri	United States, California	Female	3	30	Japan
Buccal cavity	India, Bombay	Male	2	25	Denmark
Rectum	Denmark	Male	2	20	Nigeria
Bladder	United States, Connecticut	Male	2	6	Japan
Ovary	Denmark	Female	2	6	Japan
Nasopharynx	Singapore: Chinese	Male	2	40	England
Pancreas	New Zealand: Maori	Male	2	8	India, Bombay
Larynx	Brazil, Sao Paulo	Male	2	10	Japan
Pharynx	India, Bombay	Male	2	20	Denmark
Penis	Parts of Uganda	Male	1	300	Israel: Jewish

*Based on rates adjusted to the world standard population.

single criterion from the above list should be considered necessary or sufficient to consider an exposure causally related to a disease.

IARC CLASSIFICATION OF CARCINOGENS

Because it would be impossible for individual clinicians or even governments to evaluate the many substances suspected of carcinogenicity, IARC has established a formal process that systematically evaluates known and suspected carcinogens.[56] The evaluations are done by international working groups of experts who meet, ensure that all relevant and appropriate data have been collected, prepare accurate summaries of the data, and classify the evidence into one of four categories (1) "Sufficient evidence" of carcinogenicity in humans [signifying that, in the opinion of the working group, a causal relationship has been established between the agent and human cancer in studies in which chance, bias and confounding can be excluded with reasonable confidence] (2) "Limited evidence" of carcinogenicity [the agent has been associated with increased risk of human cancer, but that chance, bias and confounding cannot be ruled out with reasonable confidence] (3) "Inadequate evidence" of carcinogenicity [available studies are of insufficient quality, consistency, or statistical power to permit a conclusion regarding the carcinogenicity of the agent, or no data on carcinogenicity in humans were available], and (4) "Evidence suggesting lack of carcinogenic activity" [several adequate studies of use or exposure are mutually consistent in not showing an increased risk for specified cancer sites, conditions and levels of exposure]. A complete list of the IARC monograph classification of agents, mixtures, and other substances is available on the Internet at <www.iarc.fr>.

The same IARC Web site lists the various iatrogenic exposures that have been linked to cancer. These include diagnostic and therapeutic exposure to ionizing radiation, cancer treatment with alkylating agents such as melphalan, cyclophosphamide, busulfan and mechlorethamine, immunosuppression (which increases risk of non-Hodgkin's lymphoma and B-immunoblastic sarcomas), hormone medications (such as diethylstilbestrol, unopposed estrogen, and androgens), and antibiotics such as chloramphenicol.

SUMMARY

Population research contributes to our understanding of cancer at many levels. Certain fundamental concepts such as individual risk, survival, and population attributable risk are measurable only in populations, not individuals. In cancer surveillance, epidemiologic methods are used to measure cancer incidence, mortality, and survival, to identify high-risk subgroups, and to

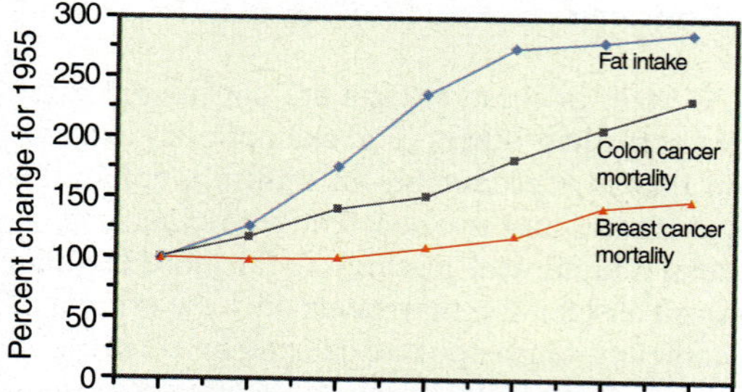

Figure 24-12 Time trends in per capita consumption of fat and death rates from colon and breast cancer in Japan, 1955–1985. Reprinted with permission.

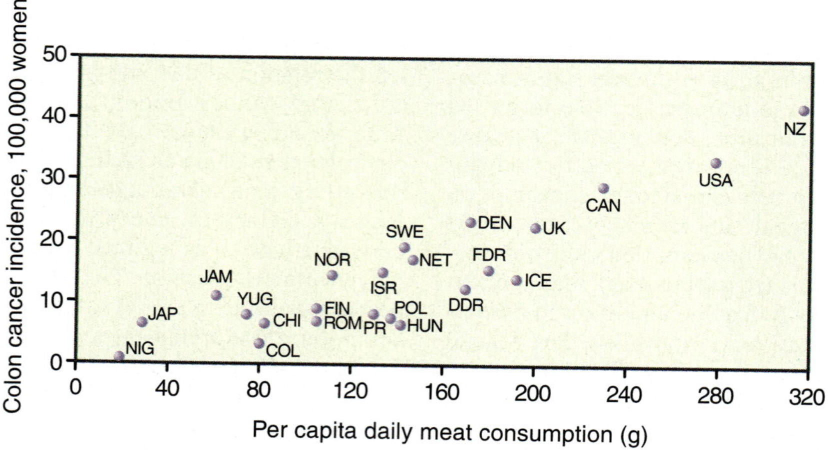

Figure 24-13 Correlation between per capita meat consumption and incidence of colon cancer in women. Reproduced with permission.

monitor progress (or lack of progress) against the disease. In etiologic research, epidemiologic studies have been crucial in identifying and characterizing the carcinogenicity of tobacco, radiation, and many other occupational, environmental, and infectious agents. Epidemiologic studies often provide conclusive information on effective strategies to prevent disease many decades before the precise causal mechanism is identified.

REFERENCES

1. Ries L, Eisner M, Kosary C, et al. SEER cancer statistics review, 1975–2002. Bethesda, Maryland: National Cancer Institute; 2005.
2. National Institutes of Health. Disease statistics. Fact book, fiscal year 2003. Bethesda, Maryland: National Institute of Health, National Heart, Lung and Blood Institute; 2003. p. 53.
3. Rothman K, Greenland S. Measures of disease frequency. In: Rothman K, Greenland S, editors. Modern epidemiology. Philadelphia, PA: Lippincott-Raven; 1998. p. 53.
4. Hennekens C, Buring J. Epidemiology in medicine. Boston: Little, Brown; 1987. p. 66–73.
5. Anderson R, Minino A, Hoyert D, Rosenberg H. Comparability of cause of death between ICD-9 and ICD-10: preliminary estimates. National Vital Stat Reports 2001;49:1–32.
6. Wingo PA, Cardinez CJ, Landis SH, et al. Long-term trends in cancer mortality in the United States, 1930–1998. Cancer 2003;97:3133–275.
7. National Center for Health Statistics. Vital statistics of the United States, 1930, 1931, ...1959, Vol. 2. Mortality, parts A and B. Hyattsville, MD: Public Health Service; 1988.
8. National Center for Health Statistics. Vital statistics of the United States, 1950–2001, Volume II. Mortality, parts A and B. Washington, DC: Public Health Service; 2005.
9. Centers for Disease Control and Prevention. Cancer Registries: the Foundation for Cancer Prevention and Control, Vol. 2005. Centers for Disease Control and Prevention; 2005. Available at: http://www.cdc.gov/cancer/npcr/awards.htm (accessed June 15, 2005).
10. U.S. Cancer Statistics Working Group. United States cancer statistics: 2001 incidence and mortality. Atlanta, GA: Department of Health and Human Services, Centers for Disease Control and Prevention, and National Cancer Institute; 2004.
11. MMWR. State cancer registries: status of authorizing legislation and enabling regulations-United States. MMWR Morb Mortal Wkly Rep 1994;43:71–5.
12. Menck H, Smart C, editors. Central cancer registries: design management, and use. Switzerland: Hargood Academic Publishers; 1994.
13. Jensen O, Parkin D, Maclennan R, et al. Cancer registration: principles and methods. Lyon, France: IARC Scientific Publications; 1991.
14. American College of Surgeons. Standards of the Commission on Cancer, Vol II, registry operations and data standards (ROADS). Chicago, IL: American College of Surgeons; 1996.
15. Ferlay J, Black R, Whelan S. CIVII: Cancer incidence in five continents, Vol VII. Lyon, France: IARC CancerBase No. 2, 1997.
16. Parkin D, Whelan S, Ferlay J, et al, editors. Cancer incidence in five continents, Vol. VII. Vol. 143. Lyon, France: IARC Scientific Publication; 1997. p. 1028–9.
17. World Health Organization. World health statistics annual, 1996. Geneva: World Health Organization, 1998.
18. Waterhouse J, Muir C, Correa P, Powell J, editors. Cancer incidence in five continents, Vol. III. Lyon, France: IARC Scientific Publications; 1976.
19. Jemal A, Murray T, Ward E, et al. Cancer statistics, 2005. CA Cancer J Clin 2005;55:10–30.
20. Tiwari RC, Ghosh K, Jemal A, et al. A new method of predicting US and state-level cancer mortality counts for the current calendar year. CA Cancer J Clin 2004;54:30–40.
21. Wingo P, Parkin D, Eyre H. Measuring the occurrence of cancer: impact and statistics. Chapter 1. In: Lenhard R, Brady L, Osteen R, Gansler T, editors. Clinical oncology, 3rd ed. Atlanta, Georgia: American Cancer Society; 2001.
22. Kelsey J, Thompson W, Evans A. Methods on observational epidemiology. New York: Oxford University Press; 1986.
23. Messite J, Stellman S. Accuracy of death certificate completion. JAMA 1996;275:794–6.
24. Doll R, Muir C, Fraumeni J. Introduction. In: Sidebottom E, editor. Trends in cancer incidence and mortality, Vol. 19/20. Plainview: Cold Spring Harbor Laboratory Press; 1994. p. 1–4.
25. Percy C, Miller B, Ries L. Effect of changes in cancer classification and the accuracy of cancer death certificates on trends in cancer mortality. Ann NY Acad Sci 1990;609:87–98.
26. Percy C, Stanek E, Gloeckler L. Accuracy of cancer death certificates and its effect on cancer mortality statistics. Nat Cancer Inst Monogr 1982;59:467–75.
27. Thun M, Henley S, Calle E. Tobacco use and cancer: an epidemiologic perspective for geneticists. Oncogene 2002;21:7307–25.
28. Nomura A. Stomach cancer. In: Schottenfeld D, Fraumeni J, editors. Cancer epidemiology and prevention. New York: Oxford University Press; 1996. p. 707–24.
29. Gann P. Interpreting recent trends in prostate cancer incidence and mortality. Epidemiology 1997;8:117–9.
30. Jemal A, Clegg LX, Ward E, et al. Annual report to the nation on the status of cancer, 1975–2001, with a special feature regarding survival. Cancer 2004;101:3–27.
31. Baquet C, Horm J, Gibbs T, Greenwald P. Socioeconomic factors and cancer incidence among blacks and whites. J Natl Cancer Inst 1999;83:551–7.
32. American Cancer Society. Cancer facts & figures 2003, Special section on cancer disparities. Atlanta, Georgia: American Cancer Society, Inc; 2004.
33. Singh G, Miller B, Hankey BF, Edwards BK. Area socioeconomic variations in U.S. cancer incidence, mortality, stage, treatment, and survival. NCI Cancer Surveillance Monograph Series, number 4. Vol. NIH Publication No. 03-5417. Bethesda, MD: National Cancer Institute; 2003.
34. Howard J, Hankey B, Greenberg R, et al. A collaborative study of differences in the survival rates of black patients and white patients with cancer. Cancer 1992;69:2349–60.
35. American Cancer Society. Cancer facts and figures for African Americans 2005–2006. Atlanta, Georgia: American Cancer Society; 2005.
36. Breen N, Wagener D, Brown M, et al. Progress in cancer screening over a decade: results of cancer screening from the 1987, 1992, and 1998 National Health Interview Surveys. J Natl Cancer Instit 2001;93:1704–13.
37. Miller B, Kolonel L, Bernstein L, et al, editors. Racial/ethnic patterns of cancer in the United States 1988–1992. NIH Pub. No. 96-4104, Bethesda, MD: National Cancer Institution; 1996.
38. Wingo P, Gloeckler-Ries L, Parker S, Heath C. Long-term cancer patient survival in the United States. Cancer Epidemiol Biomarkers Prev 1998;7:271–82.
39. Ederer F, Axtell L, Cutler S. The relative survival rate: a statistical methodology. Nat Cancer Inst Monogr 1961;6:101–21.
40. Doll R, Peto R. The causes of cancer: Quantitative estimates of avoidable risks of cancer in the United States today. J Natl Cancer Inst 1981;66:1191–308.
41. Thomas D, Kargas M. Migrant studies. In: Schottenfeld D, Fraumeni J, editors. Cancer epidemiology and prevention. New York: Oxford University Press; 1996. p. 236–66.
42. Willett W. The search for the cause of breast and colon cancer. Nature 1989;338:389–93.
43. Armstrong B, Doll R. Environmental factors and cancer incidence and mortality in different countries, with special reference to dietary practices. Int J Cancer 1975;15:617–31.
44. Monson R. Occupation. In: Schottenfeld D, Fraumeni J, editors. Cancer epidemiology and prevention, 2nd ed. New York: Oxford University Press; 1996. p. 313–405.
45. Checkoway H, Pearce N, Kreibel D. Research methods in occupational epidemiology, (2nd edition). Oxford, U.K.: Oxford University Press; 2004. p. 384.
46. Pott P. Cancer scroti. Chirurgical observations. London: Hawes, Clarke, Collins; 1775. p. 63–8.
47. Case R, Pearson J. Tumors of the urinary bladder in workmen engaged in the manufacture and use of certain dyestuff intermediates in the British chemical industry. Part II. Further consideration of the role of aniline and of the manufacture of auramine and magenta (fuchsine) as possible causative agents. Br J Indust Med 1954;11:213–6.
48. Martland H, Humphries R. Osteogenic sarcoma in dial painters using luminous paint. Arch Pathol 1929;7:406–17.
49. Creech JJ, Johnson M. Angiosarcoma of liver in the manufacture of polyvinyl chloride. J Occup Med 1974;16:150–1.
50. Qian G, Ross R, Yu M, et al. A follow-up study of urinary markers of aflatoxin exposure and liver cancer risk in Shanghai, People's Republic of China. Cancer Epidemiol Biomarkers Prev 1994;3:3–10.
51. Pirkle J, Flegal K, Bernert J, et al. Exposure of the US population to environmental tobacco smoke. JAMA 1996;275:1233–40.
52. Chan J, Stampfer M, et al. Plasma insulin-like growth factor-1 and prostate cancer risk: a prospective study. Science 1998;279:563–6.
53. Whittemore A, Wu-Williams A, Lee M, et al. Diet physical activity and colorectal cancer among Chinese in North America and China. J Natl Cancer Inst 1990;82:915–26.
54. U.S. Public Health Service. Smoking and health. Report of the Advisory Committee to the Surgeon General of the Public Health Service: PHS Publication No. 1103, U.S. Department of Health, Education, and Welfare, Public Health Service, Centers for Disease Control; 1964.
55. Hill A. The environment and disease: association or causation? Proc R Soc Med 1965;58:295–300.
56. IARC. IARC Monographs on the evaluation of the carcinogenic risk of chemicals to humans: chemicals, industrial processes and industries associated with cancer in humans. Vol. 1-29. Lyon: International Agency for Research on Cancer; 1982.

Prevention of Tobacco-Related Cancers

Paul F. Engstrom, MD
Margie L. Clapper, PhD
Robert A. Schnoll, PhD

Tobacco smoke consists of more than 4,000 chemical compounds and approximately 60 known carcinogens. Half of these compounds occur naturally in the green tobacco leaf, whereas the remainder are generated when tobacco is burned. The complex mixture of chemicals in tobacco smoke includes carbon monoxide, hydrogen cyanide, benzene, formaldehyde, nicotine, phenol, polycyclic aromatic hydrocarbons (PAHs), and tobacco-specific nitrosamines (TSNAs). Although the chemical composition of mainstream and sidestream smoke is similar, the concentration of many constituents is higher in sidestream or "passive" smoke.

Nicotine, the second most abundant constituent of tobacco smoke, is present in both mainstream and sidestream smoke and is rapidly absorbed by the alveoli of the lungs. Subsequent release of dopamine via activation of cholinergic receptors in the brain and modulation of hormones such as epinephrine and cortisol is believed to lead to nicotine dependence. The effect of polymorphisms in the dopamine transporter (*SLC6A3*) and dopamine D2 receptor (*DRD2*) genes on smoking initiation and nicotine dependence remains controversial and is a subject of intense investigation.[1]

CARCINOGENIC AND GENOTOXIC EFFECTS OF TOBACCO CONSTITUENTS

Efforts to study the carcinogenic effects of cigarette smoke in animal models have been met with limited success owing to the inability of most animals to inhale as deeply as humans. The results from recent studies in A/J mice, which spontaneously develop lung adenomas and adenocarcinomas and additional lung neoplasms on carcinogen exposure, have confirmed that environmental (sidestream) tobacco smoke is, indeed, a lung carcinogen.[2] Furthermore, the highest lung tumor multiplicity and incidence were observed in animals that were allowed to recover in filtered air for 4 months following a 5-month exposure (6 hours per day, 5 days per week) to mainstream and sidestream cigarette smoke, a smoking history similar to that of a former smoker.

The potent ability of metabolically activated PAHs (ie, benzo[*a*]pyrene) and TSNAs [specifically 4-(methylnitrosamino)-l-(3-pyridyl)-l-butanone (NNK)] to induce pulmonary tumors in rodents at doses similar to those experienced during a lifetime of smoking has been attributed to their potential to form bulky deoxynucleic acid (DNA) adducts.[3] Although chemical carcinogens prefer to bind to guanine, the specific position within this base is dependent on the chemical properties of the carcinogen. For example, aromatic amines prefer to bind to the C8 position, whereas PAHs bind preferentially to the N2 position of guanine. Smoke-induced DNA adducts are present in many tissues from smokers, including lung, bronchus, larynx, kidney, bladder, esophagus, liver, aorta, and placenta.[4] Adduct levels correlate with the amount smoked and the duration of exposure,[5] and decrease in a time-dependent manner following smoking cessation.

If left unrepaired, smoke-induced DNA adducts can cause mutations in oncogenes and tumor suppressor genes, thus conferring a preneoplastic phenotype. (For a review, see Sekido and colleagues.[6]) The most frequent alteration is mutation of *TP*53 (usually G-T transversion), which is present in greater than 75% of small cell lung carcinomas and approximately 50% of non–small cell lung carcinomas (NSCLCs). Mutant *TP53* has also been detected in exfoliated cells (sputum, bronchial lavage or brushings) from chronic smokers[7] and thus may serve as an early biomarker of lung cancer risk. K-*ras* mutations (primarily G-T transversions) are detected at a much lower frequency (20 to 30% for lung adenocarcinomas and 15 to 20% for all NSCLCs). Mutation of *TP53* and K-*ras* is frequently found at the surgical margin in presumed "non-neoplastic" lung tissue.[8]

Gene inactivation via promoter hypermethylation has been established as a mechanism by which lung tumors can arise independent of K-*ras* mutation. More than 30 genes involved in cell cycle control, differentiation and signaling, invasion, and apoptosis have been identified, which are silenced transcriptionally in lung cancers. (For a review, see Belinsky.[9]) For example, hypermethylation of *p16* and death-associated protein kinase (*DAPK*) is a frequent event in non–small cell lung cancers[10] and in the bronchial brush specimens of former smokers, especially those with a previous history of cancer.[11] Strong support for *p16* promoter hypermethylation as an early predictive marker of lung cancer risk is provided by the detection of hypermethylation in exfoliated cells from chronic smokers without clinical evidence of disease[7] and in the sputum of 100% of patients with squamous cell lung carcinoma up to 3 years prior to clinical diagnosis.[12] Methylation of the adenomatous polyposis coli (*APC*) gene, the putative gatekeeper of colorectal cancer, was present in 96% of primary lung cancer tissues and 47% of the serum and/or plasma samples from the same individuals.[13]

GENETIC VARIATION IN CANCER SUSCEPTIBILITY

DNA Repair Capacity The rate at which adducts are removed from DNA is dictated by the activity of DNA repair enzymes. A recent meta-analysis of two specific polymorphisms in the nucleotide excision repair gene xeroderma pigmentosum complementary group D (*XPD*) indicates that these variants confer a high risk of developing lung cancer.[14] A polymorphism in the x-ray cross-complementing group 1 (*XRCC1*) gene, a coordinator of base excision repair, may also be a predictor of the risk of squamous cell carcinoma of the lung, but only in individuals with less than 40 pack-years of smoking.[15] Likewise, the adjusted odds ratios for lung cancer risk associated with two polymorphisms in the excision repair complementing group 2 (*ERCC2*) gene correlate inversely with pack-year history.[16] Although single polymorphisms in the DNA repair genes *XPA*, *XPD*, *XRCC1*, and *XRCC3* confer only a moderate risk of lung cancer, the risk increases considerably when combinations of variant alleles are considered.[17]

Detoxification Enzyme Activity Several enzyme systems involved in the metabolism and detoxification of carcinogenic smoke constituents exhibit genetic polymorphisms that have been associated with differential susceptibility for cancer. Epidemiologic and clinical data continue to suggest that polymorphisms in select phase I (carcinogen activating) and II (carcinogen inactivating) detoxification enzymes may serve as biomarkers of increased risk of smoking-related cancers.

Cytochrome P-450 2D6 Cytochrome P-450 2D6 (CYP2D6) is a phase I enzyme responsible for converting the tobacco-specific nitrosamine NNK to highly reactive metabolites.[18] Identification of numerous polymorphisms in this gene has led to the classification of individuals as either recessive poor metabolizers (PMs) (approximately 9%) or homozygous or heterozygous dominant extensive metabolizers (EMs).[19] Initial studies demonstrated that individuals who exhibited the EM phenotype were at increased risk of lung cancer compared with PMs.[20] In contrast, more recent meta-analyses indicate that the association between the CYP2D6 polymorphism and susceptibility for lung cancer is not persuasive.[21,22] The results from DNA-based assays continue to remain equivocal, and the lung cancer risk for light and heavy smokers with the PM genotype does not differ significantly.[23] However, nicotine metabolism may be altered in smokers who are CYP2D6 ultrarapid metabolizers.[24] An association between the EM phenotype and increased risk of bladder and cervical cancer has been suggested.[25,26]

Cytochrome P-450 1A1 Cytochrome P-450 1A1 (CYP1A1) is a phase I inducible microsomal enzyme that oxygenates carcinogenic PAHs such as benzo[*a*]pyrene to facilitate their ultimate detoxification and excretion. (For a review, see Whitlock.[27]) CYP1A1 is expressed at a low level in the lung of nonsmokers and can be induced 100-fold in smokers. Recent analyses of human lung tissue suggest that induction occurs, in part, via demethylation of the CYP1A1 promoter by tobacco smoke.[28] Nicotine was identified recently as a potent and rapid inducer of pulmonary CYP1A1, suggesting its ability to accelerate the metabolism of carcinogens in cigarette smoke.[29] High inducibility of aryl hydrocarbon hydroxylase, the product of the *CYP1A1* gene, in selected individuals has been attributed to polymorphisms in the gene[30] and correlated with high DNA adduct levels.[31]

The potential contribution of polymorphisms in the *CYP1A1* gene to increased risk of lung cancer remains equivocal and an area of intense investigation. Comprehensive analysis of data pooled from 11 studies indicates that a polymorphism in exon 7 of the *CYP1A1* gene may confer an increased risk of squamous cell carcinoma of the lung, especially in nonsmokers and women.[32] Independent analysis of results pooled from 14 case-control studies yielded an odds ratio of 4.85 for the risk of lung adenocarcinoma in white nonsmokers carrying an Ile-Val polymorphism in *CYP1A1*.[33] Investigations in Japanese populations have confirmed the association of an MspI restriction fragment length polymorphism in the 3' noncoding region of *CYP1A1* with increased lung cancer risk.[34] However, a meta-analysis of published case-control studies yielded little support for variation in the *CYP1A1* gene (MspI or Ile-Val polymorphisms) as a determinant of lung cancer risk in whites.[35] Evaluation of smoking data from the Nurses' Health Study suggested that females with the MspI polymorphism who start smoking before age 18 may be at increased risk of breast cancer.[36]

Cytochrome P-450 2E1 The phase I enzyme cytochrome P-450 2E1 (CYP2E1) catalyzes the oxidation and DNA adduct formation of benzene, nitrosamines, and other carcinogens.[37] A polymorphism in the *CYP2E1* gene has been associated with lung cancer in Japanese populations.[38] However, this association has not been replicated in whites. The CYP2E1 polymorphism, when combined with polymorphisms in either the *CYP2D6* or *GSTM1* gene, has been strongly associated with lung cancer risk, producing odds ratios of 14.0 and 6.0, respectively.[39]

***N*-Acetyltransferase 2** Although *N*-acetyltransferase 2 (NAT2) is classified as a phase II enzyme, its ability to both inactivate aromatic amines and activate specific arylamine metabolites in cigarette smoke has been suggested.[40] Corresponding acetylation rates (slow vs rapid) are controlled by a single gene. Slow acetylation is an autosomal recessive trait that occurs in approximately 50 to 60% of Western populations. Slow acetylators are less efficient in detoxifying arylamines (potent bladder carcinogens)[41] and possess higher levels of tobacco-related arylamine hemoglobin adducts than rapid acetylators, with adduct levels increasing with the number of cigarettes smoked per day.[42] In contrast to bladder cancer, in which slow acetylation correlates with increased risk,[43,44] phenotypic and genotypic analyses of lung cancer patients have produced conflicting results, with the majority failing to reveal an association between acetylator status and cancer risk.[45,46] One explanation for these inconsistencies is the recently identified, statistically significant interaction between *NAT2* genotype and pack-year history of smoking.[47] The NAT2 rapid acetylator genotype was found to confer a decreased risk of lung cancer among nonsmokers but an increased lung cancer risk in heavy smokers. Likewise, the additive risk of lung cancer faced by those carrying the *NAT2* genotype in combination with a polymorphism in microsomal epoxide hydrolase is dependent on cumulative smoke exposure. An association between risk for postmenopausal breast cancer and the slow acetylator genotype has also been established with respect to smoking dose.[48]

Glutathione *S*-Transferase M1 The glutathione *S*-transferases (GSTs) are a family of enzymes that catalyze the conjugation of PAHs and other toxic intermediates with glutathione. The resulting conjugate is more water soluble and more readily excreted from the body. The gene encoding the M1 isozyme is deleted in approximately 50% of the general population. This polymorphic expression, when combined with the ability of M1 to inactivate highly reactive epoxides, such as benzo[*a*]pyrene-4,5-oxide, has prompted a detailed investigation of the role of the null genotype in determining individual susceptibility to a variety of cancers. Several studies have suggested an association between the GSTM1 null genotype and increased risk of various smoking-related cancers. A meta-analysis of the relationship between GSTM1 status and lung cancer risk in 12 case-control studies classified the GSTM1 null genotype as a moderate risk factor for all histologic subtypes of lung cancer (odds ratio = 1.4).[49] The unavailability of standardized data on smoking history prohibited analysis of this variable. The results from a recent case-control study suggest that black smokers with the null genotype are at a very high risk of developing lung cancer (odds ratio = 8.2) compared with black nonsmokers with the wild-type genotype.[50] The trend between increasing risk and greater pack-year history of smoking was highly significant. Furthermore, GSTM1 null women who live with husbands who are heavy smokers (a smoking history of ≥ 40 pack-years) are at a significantly increased risk of developing lung cancer compared with females who are GSTM1 null and exposed to low-dose environmental tobacco smoke (ETS) (husbands with a history of ≤ 40 pack-years).[51]

Although the GSTM1 null genotype confers only a modest risk of lung cancer, individuals who carry both the GSTM1 null genotype and a second high-risk polymorphism appear to be at a significantly increased risk of developing lung cancer. In most instances, individuals with the combined genotype metabolically activate carcinogens at a fast rate while being less efficient in providing cellular protection from the resulting reactive intermediates. This association has been well established for the combined mutant CYP1A1/GSTM1 null genotype[52,53] and confirmed by biochemical data, which indicate that K-*ras* mutations are sixfold more likely to be present in lung tumors from smokers who carry both the variant CYP1A1 and GSTM1 null genotypes compared with those who possess the corresponding wild-type alleles.[54] Likewise, high DNA adduct levels are observed in smokers who are slow acetylators for NAT and lack the *GSTM1* gene,[55,56] whereas adduct levels are low in smokers who are fast acetylators for NAT and *GSTM1* positive.[56] Other polymorphisms that confer a high risk of lung cancer when combined with the GSTM1 null genotype include microsomal epoxide hydrolase His113/His139 (homozygous),[57] CYP2E1 wild type,[58] and GSTP1 Val.[59]

Gender In 1987, lung cancer surpassed breast cancer as the leading cause of cancer-related death in women. Several biologic rationales for the increased susceptibility of females for lung cancer have been suggested. First, sex differences in the metabolism of nicotine and other tobacco smoke constituents have been proposed. Female lung cancer patients have a significantly higher level of pulmonary DNA adducts compared with men, despite a smaller smoking history.[60] The frequency of the CYP1A1 (NcoI) polymorphism is significantly greater among female lung cancer patients than controls.[53] Findings from an independent study indicate that CYP1A1 expression is significantly elevated within the lungs of female smokers compared with male smokers.[31] Second, growth stimulatory effects, specifically gastrin-releasing peptide receptor expression, are more common among females (smokers and nonsmokers) than males.[61] Lastly, exogenous and endogenous estrogens appear to contribute to the development of lung adenocarcinoma in women. Early age at menopause (< 40 years) is associated with a reduced risk of adenocarcinoma of the lung, whereas use of estrogen therapy confers a higher risk.[62] Recent discovery of the potent ability of tobacco smoke to induce the expression of CYP1B1, a phase I enzyme involved in both the activation of procarcinogens in smoke and the hydroxylation of 17β-estradiol to reactive catechol estrogens, has provided new insight into the role of estrogens in lung tumorigenesis.[63]

APPROACHES TO SMOKING CESSATION

Assessment of the last 2 years of nicotine addiction treatment research gives reason for disappointment and optimism. On the one hand, since our last review of this literature,[64] the US adult rate of tobacco use has decreased modestly, from 22.8% in 2001 to 22.1% in 2003.[65,66] The national objective set by Healthy People 2010 of reducing the population rate of smoking to < 12% will not be attained. On the other hand, the spread of municipal bans on smoking in public places, quit lines, and the development of new pharmacotherapies suggest that substantial reductions in the prevalence of smoking are on the horizon. Further, the release of the surgeon general's report *The Health Consequences of Smoking*[67] and national action plans for nicotine addiction treatment[68] provide blueprints for the ascertainment of national health objectives. In the following paragraphs, we review recent developments in nicotine addiction treatment and discuss several important topics in this field, such as prevention and harm reduction.

Table 25-1 Guide to the Evaluation and Management of Smokers for Physicians

Step 1 (Ask). Evaluate the smoking history of every patient.
Institute official policy concerning the mandatory assessment of tobacco use status (ie, is patient a current smoker, a former smoker, or a nonsmoker?)
Include assessment of tobacco use status as part of the collection of vital signs
Ensure that the tobacco use status of each patient is included in the patient's medical records in a way that is easily detected by the entire health care team (eg, smoking status stickers)
Step 2 (Advise). Convey concise, forthright, and individualized quitting advice to all smokers.
Indicate that the patient should quit (not just cut down) immediately and that you will be helping him or her achieve this goal
Express to the patient that quitting smoking is crucial to ensure present and future health
Associate current smoking with present health problems if applicable and emphasize the economic, health (eg, impact of smoking on fetus), and social impact of smoking (eg, effects of second-hand smoke on family members)
Involve all clinic staff in encouraging the patient to quit by reinforcing cessation messages
Step 3 (Assess). Evaluate the patient's readiness to quit.
Assess patient's readiness to change and willingness to make a quit attempt
Assess patient's interest in behavioral and pharmacologic smoking cessation treatments
Provide referral to patients interested in participating in formal cessation programs
Consider patient's age, ethnicity, gender, and particular health-related risks
For patients in the precontemplation stage, provide motivational messages (eg, identify acute [eg, shortness of breath], long-term [eg, cancer, heart attacks], and environmental [eg, increased risk of cancer and other health problems among family members] adverse health effects of smoking for patient and review benefits of smoking cessation [eg, improved health, improved self-esteem, cessation of worry about effects of second-hand smoke])
Step 4 (Assist). Provide direct smoking cessation assistance to the patient.
Formulate quit plan: set quit date within 2 weeks; have patient solicit encouragement and support from family; remove smoking cues from the environment (eg, cigarettes, ashtrays)
Encourage the use of nicotine replacement therapy (NRT) (ie, the patch or the gum) or bupropion (Zyban)
Provide quitting advice: total abstinence is the goal; encourage family members who smoke to quit
Provide problem-solving (ie, identify situations that increase the chance of smoking, such as being with other smokers, stress, negative mood, and drinking alcohol) and coping skills (ie, avoid tempting situations, stress management using positive self-talk or exercise) training and clinician support (ie, confidence in patient's ability to quit, discuss feelings about quitting, express willingness to help, and listen to patient's fears about quitting)
Provide self-help educational material tailored to individual's ethnicity, gender, and age
Step 5 (Arrange). Schedule follow-up contact to review cessation progress.
Plan follow-up contacts within 1 week of quit date and within the first month of cessation (eg, telephone or postcard reminders, in-person visits)
Reward successes and reinforce cessation advice if a relapse occurs; review use of NRT; if relapse occurred, review patient's thoughts about why it happened and how to avoid relapse in the future, including the need for more intensive behavioral therapies

Adapted from Fiore MC et al.[69]

Smoking Cessation Interventions The implementation of nicotine addiction treatment should be guided by clinical practice guidelines, which are based on the accumulated literature on smoking cessation interventions.[69] To summarize, the guidelines indicate that (1) brief tobacco cessation interventions of 3 to 5 minutes can be effective; (2) there is a dose-response relationship between the intensity and duration of behavioral smoking cessation interventions and their effectiveness; (3) there are five "first-line" pharmacotherapies that increase quit rates; (4) clinicians and health care programs must ensure that all smokers are identified and provided with appropriate treatment; and (5) insurance plans should reimburse patients and physicians for the provision of nicotine addiction treatments. The provision of smoking cessation treatment should be tailored to the smoker's characteristics, such as the individual's readiness to change or ethnic or cultural barriers. In addition, the most effective approach to smoking treatment involves the combination of behavioral and pharmacologic treatment.[69] The effects of these treatments are independent and additive. Here we review the current literature on various smoking interventions. We urge readers to consider evaluating these interventions both in terms of the abstinence rate yielded and the proportion of smokers that the interventions reach (ie, the impact value).[70]

Self-Help Methods Although the use of booklets or pamphlets for guiding smokers in the process of cessation is popular and seen as a component of a formal cessation program, their efficacy as a stand-alone therapy is limited.[69] Recent meta-analytic studies of cessation self-help guides concluded that this approach does not increase quit rates when added to other forms of smoking cessation treatment[71] or compared with other intervention approaches.[72] However, there is evidence that efficacy can be enhanced when telephone counseling is included as an adjunct to self-help[73] or when the content of self-help material is tailored to characteristics of the smoker that are related to the ability to quit, such as motivation.[74]

Quit Lines Telephone lines are becoming more available for smoking cessation treatment and are endorsed by the Subcommittee on Cessation of the Intra-agency Committee on Smoking and Health in their national action plan for tobacco cessation.[68] Quit lines are cost effective and can reach many smokers with personally relevant and empirically based interventions.[75] In one study, the addition of counseling via a quit line to computer-generated quit advice increased short-term cessation to 21% versus the quit advice alone (12%).[76] Zhu and colleagues found that smokers receiving counseling sessions through the California Smokers' Helpline showed a quit rate at 3 months of 23.7% versus 16.5% among smokers in a control condition.[77] Research is needed to assess the long-term efficacy of quit lines, the specific components of quit lines that promote cessation, and the feasibility of integrating quit lines with pharmacotherapy.

Behavioral Counseling Successful smoking intervention requires behavioral counseling with a trained counselor.[72] Although heterogeneity among studies makes identifying specific elements responsible for cessation difficult,[78] meta-analytic studies conclude that the following components of behavioral smoking interventions are critical for successful cessation: (1) problem-solving training, including techniques to avoid relapse and manage stress (eg, identifying events or internal states that trigger smoking and learning to deal with these in novel ways); (2) intratreatment social support, such as encouragement, understanding, and concern (eg, help the smoker to develop confidence); and (3) extratreatment social support from friends and family (eg, training smokers to enlist the help of friends and family). Because a relatively small proportion of smokers use this treatment approach (ie, about 6%),[79] identifying methods to encourage smokers to enroll in formal cessation counseling programs is a priority.

Physician-Based Interventions With 80% of smokers seeing a physician annually, physician-delivered interventions represent a cost-effective way to disseminate cessation messages and services to many smokers.[80] This approach may be especially effective because smokers perceive physicians as a valuable, credible, and reliable source of health information and generally adhere to their advice.[81] Thus, public health agencies have tried to urge physicians to implement smoking interventions by providing treatment guidelines and training manuals in the context of the "5 A's" model shown in Table 25-1.[69] Studies indicate that spending 5 minutes discussing cessation with patients can yield quit rates of 10%.[69,82] Next to trained behavioral counselors, physicians are the most effective providers of cessation treatment.[72] Unfortunately, most physicians do not take advantage of this opportunity to provide cessation advice and assistance,[83] perhaps because they are not adequately trained to do so or do not have the time.[84] Although recent evidence suggests that the rate of physician use of the 5 A's model approach is increasing,[85] additional research is needed to identify ways in which implementation of this model can be improved. One recent study, which trained health care providers in the model (not just physicians), serves as an excellent example of this initiative.[86] A meta-analysis of nurse-based interventions for smoking indicates that such interventions yield an odds ratio of 1.47 compared with controls.[87] In addition, a review article indicates that pharmacists should be considered possible advocates of nicotine addiction treatment.

Pharmacologic Interventions There are currently six approved pharmacotherapies for smoking cessation treatment, of which five are forms of nicotine replacement therapy (NRT) and bupropion, a non-nicotine medication originally designed to treat depression.[88] In addition, several new medications are in the process of being evaluated.[88] Pharmacotherapies are regarded as an essential component of nicotine addiction treatment, yielding quit rates that are close to twice those found compared with placebo or behavioral counseling only.[72,89] Although use of pharmacotherapies has increased substantially over the past several years, these medications remain underused.[88] Further, the following important clinical research issues remain largely unexplored: (1) the relative efficacy of pharmacotherapies, (2) the impact of long-term pharmacotherapy use, and (3) the effectiveness and safety of pharmacotherapies for light smokers, adolescents, and pregnant women who smoke.

Nicotine Replacement Therapies The delivery mechanisms for NRT can be via gum, a transdermal patch, nasal spray, an inhaler, and a lozenge, and several of these are available in varying dosages over the counter to enable matching of the NRT with the level of smoking. NRTs are designed to address the physiologic elements of nicotine addiction and assist with cessation by ameliorating the symptoms of withdrawal and craving. A recent meta-analytic review indicated that NRTs can almost double the probability for successful cessation versus placebo or no NRT, with odds ratios ranging from 1.66 (for gum) to 2.35 (for the inhaler).[89] Certain NRTs, namely, the nasal spray, inhaler, and gum, have unfavorable side-effect profiles; therefore, adherence to these NRT forms is lower relative to the patch.[90] Including more than one NRT may improve cessation rates compared with single NRTs, but very little is known about the relative effectiveness of NRTs or how the effectiveness of NRTs can be enhanced by tailoring their use to specific characteristics among smokers.[89] Because NRT forms differ in terms of whether they provide acute versus steady nicotine replacement, characteristics such as the regularity of smoking and desire for control over nicotine dosing may be factors that moderate the relative response to forms of NRTs.[91] Thus, future study is needed to examine ways to enhance NRT use and efficacy.

Bupropion Several antidepressant drugs have been examined as treatments for nicotine addiction, including moclobemide (Manerix), fluoxetine (Prozac), and nortriptyline (Pamelor), but only bupropion (Zyban) is approved by the US Food and Drug Administration and recommended as a first-line medication for smoking cessation. Close to 20 studies have assessed the efficacy of bupropion, showing that the medication yields an abstinence rate of about 30% versus placebo[92] and outperforms NRT.[93] Bupropion is thought to help smokers quit by affecting the noradrenergic system and enhancing concentrations of dopamine and by serving as an antagonist for nicotinic acetylcholine receptors.[94] Despite bupropion's relative efficacy, there remains a need for new drug discovery because the large majority of smokers taking bupropion eventually relapse.

Other Pharmacotherapies Several anxiolytic agents have been assessed for nicotine addiction, including diazepam, mepromate, metoprolol, and oxprenolol, but preliminary data suggest that these medications are not effective.[95] Other studies have assessed the use of buspirone for smoking cessation; however, the findings have been inconsistent.[96,97] Naltrexone, an opioid antagonist, has also been studied, but its efficacy was comparable to that of placebo, and sedation was a common adverse side effect.[98] In contrast, two other medications are showing promising results for nicotine addiction treatment. Varenicline is a nicotine agonist currently under investigation in phase III trials by Pfizer. Although independent studies have not been conducted, industry data indicate that varenicline is outperforming placebo and bupropion in terms of short-term abstinence rates.[88] Finally, in light of data indicating that the cannabinoid CB_1 receptor may influence nicotine addiction,[99] there has been growing interest in rimonobant, a selective cannabinoid 1 receptor antagonist. Studies show that this drug can reduce nicotine self-administration,[100] can alter behavior maintained by nicotine-associated cues in the absence of nicotine,[101] and can double quit rates versus a placebo.[102] These two medications may indeed become useful pharmacotherapies for nicotine addiction in the coming years.

Tailoring Smoking Cessation Interventions for Special Populations Although clinical practice may not always adhere to this principle, most researchers acknowledge that, to be effective, nicotine addiction treatment must be tailored to the unique characteristics of the smoker, whether these are demographic, psychological, or related to the smoker's health status. For instance, behavioral smoking cessation interventions are more effective when they consider (1) the smoker's motivation level according to the transtheoretical (TT) model, (2) unique cultural beliefs or attitudes that impede successful cessation among a specific ethnic group, (3) unique beliefs and attitudes that impede successful cessation among adolescents, and (4) unique beliefs and emotions that impede cessation among hospitalized smokers.

Stage of Change The TT model can guide the implementation of nicotine addiction treatment because it considers the smoker's motivation to quit in selecting specific elements of a behavioral cessation treatment. In short, the TT model characterizes smokers in terms of their motivation to quit and then uses specific psychological techniques for different stages (eg, precontemplators receive consciousness raising, whereas those in preparation receive reinforcement strategies). Although some research has not supported hypotheses of the TT model,[103] there are ample data indicating that TT model–tailored approaches outperform generic approaches. Borland and colleagues found that use of computer-generated TT model–tailored cessation material enhanced quit rates compared with standard print material (20% vs 12%),[76] and Lawrence and colleagues reported that a TT model–tailored cessation intervention with pregnant women enhanced cessation rates compared with standard care.[104] As such, there is adequate empiric support for the tailoring of cessation content and strategies to the smoker's level of motivation to quit.

Minority Smokers Assessing recent trends in smoking prevalence rates across ethnic groups underscores the need for targeted cessation programs for blacks. Among white and Hispanic high school students, smoking rates from 1991 to 2003 decreased from 31 to 25% and from 25.3 to 18.4%, respectively, but the rate for blacks increased from 12.6 to 15.1%.[105] Blacks exhibit higher rates of cardiovascular disease and cancer morbidity and mortality versus whites.[106,107] Unfortunately, there have been few treatment efficacy studies for blacks, and many of those published manifest methodologic shortcomings, such as a lack of randomization and biochemical verification.[108] Behavioral counseling interventions that employed content tailored to be culturally relevant have been more effective.[104] The one pharmacotherapy trial with blacks found that bupropion significantly increased rates of cessation versus placebo.[109] As future intervention studies with blacks are planned, the following issues should be considered. First, blacks experience more stress than whites (eg, poverty, crime, unemployment, discrimination), which increases psychological stress reactions, such as engaging in unhealthful behaviors such as smoking.[110] Blacks who experience more stress are more likely to start smoking as adolescents and are more likely to be smokers as adults.[111] Second, blacks are less knowledgeable about the adverse health effects of smoking than are whites, believe that quitting would be too difficult given their stressful lives, and believe that smoking is a critical method for coping with stress.[108] Third, blacks are more likely to smoke mentholated cigarettes, which are more addictive,[112] and they smoke fewer cigarettes than whites but exhibit higher nicotine intake and slower nicotine metabolism.[113] This latter finding suggests that blacks may respond more favorably to NRTs that have steady (eg, patch) versus acute (eg, spray, lozenge) forms of administration. Lastly, greater religious affiliation and spirituality have been linked to a lower probability of smoking among blacks,[114] and blacks with greater social support are more likely to successfully quit smoking in treatment studies.[115] Thus, interventions for blacks must address stressors, attitudes about stress, and unique smoking and physiologic patterns.

Women Smokers Although the rates of lung cancer morbidity have plateaued and the rates of lung cancer mortality have been steadily decreasing for men, the lung cancer morbidity and mortality rates among women have been increasing.[116] Even when controlling for smoking history and other key risk factors, women are more susceptible to developing lung cancer than men, perhaps because of unique molecular changes that occur more frequently in women, such as *TP53* mutations, or because of estrogen signaling.[116] Nevertheless, whereas the rate of tobacco use among men has decreased by 50% since 1960, the rate among women has decreased only by 25%.[117] Further, cancers that are either exclusive to women (eg, cervical) or occur almost exclusively among women (ie, breast) have been linked to tobacco use, and women who smoke are at risk of experiencing adverse effects during pregnancy if they continue to smoke while pregnant.[118] The reasons why women have not shown the same decrease in smoking as men include aggressive marketing directed toward young girls that emphasize the weight control benefits of smoking.[119] Indeed, postcessation weight gain is a salient barrier to cessation among women.[120] In addition, depression, which is more prevalent among women,[121] may be an important barrier to cessation.[122] Medications such as rimonobant, which can yield weight loss and possibly treat nicotine addiction, may be especially effective for women. In addition, further study is needed to examine the potential for women to show greater responsiveness to antidepressant medications such as bupropion. Lastly, in light of relatively discouraging results from behavioral smoking cessation trials with pregnant women, recent efforts have been directed toward examining pharmacotherapy for pregnant women who continue to smoke. The negative reproductive effects from smoking (eg, birth defects, spontaneous abortions, cardiovascular disorders) are thought to be largely attributable to the various toxins, such as lead and carbon monoxide, in cigarettes rather than from nicotine per se.[123] To date, two NRTs (the gum and the patch) have been shown to be safe and effective for promoting cessation from tobacco use among pregnant women.[118] Further, although additional studies of the safety and efficacy of bupropion for smoking cessation among women are needed, a small randomized controlled study found that bupropion yielded a quit rate of 45% versus 10% for placebo in this population of smokers.[124]

Adolescents Cessation programs must be directed toward adolescents because the vast majority of adult smokers begin to smoke during adolescence. As such, assisting adolescents to quit smoking before tobacco use becomes an ingrained addiction can lower the adult smoking rate. The past few years have shown that there is, perhaps, reason for optimism. The latest Youth Risk Behavior Surveillance results indicate that the prevalence of current cigarette use among high school students has decreased from 27.5% in 1991 to 21.9% in 2003, and gains have been seen across both genders and across most ethnic and racial groups.[125] Even so, adolescents are still in need of smoking cessation interventions. Interventions for youth smoking must include a variety of approaches, including community-based measures such as counteradvertising (eg, "The Truth Campaign"), penalties (eg, penalties for being caught smoking, such as school suspension, denial of a driver's license, monetary fines, and mandated cessation programs), smoking bans, restricted sales, and taxation. However, formal cessation programs are also needed, and a recent review indicates that school-based programs can double quit rates when compared with usual care.[126] Long-term follow-up of smoking outcomes is rare in adolescent smoking cessation studies, and relapse rates are high. As such, additional trials are needed to evaluate more intensive and more innovative smoking cessation treatments for adolescents, including the use of pharmacotherapy. Two trials indicated that NRT was not effective for adolescents,[126] and a recent study found that bupropion and the patch were equally poor at maintaining long-term abstinence among adolescents.[127] As interventions with this population move forward, researchers should consider that adolescents are less interested in quitting smoking than adults, believing instead that they will quit when they are older and without formal assistance.[128] In addition, because psychological (eg, depression, health values, motivation to quit), social (eg, peer support), familial (eg, parental approval or parental smoking status), smoking-related (eg, addiction), and societal (eg, access to cigarettes) factors predict cessation, comprehensive programs involving behavioral counseling, peer education, NRT, and community restrictions are likely to be most successful. Finally, considering the benefits of physician-based tobacco treatments for adults, pediatricians are logical agents for providing cessation counseling to adolescents, and such an approach should be the focus of future research.[81]

Cancer Patients About one-third of cancer patients who were smokers before diagnosis continue to smoke during treatment, and many who quit return to smoking post-treatment.[129] Because continued patient smoking reduces the duration of survival, heightens the risk of disease recurrence and a second primary tumor, reduces treatment efficacy, and causes pulmonary embolisms, venous thrombosis, and mucositis,[129] it is imperative that smoking cessation treatment be made available in the oncologic setting. Relatively few studies, however, have tested smoking interventions for cancer patients, and many of those that have been conducted have suffered from methodologic shortcomings, such as a small sample size. A recent study examined the use of the 5 A's model at cancer treatment facilities but did not find a significant reduction in patient smoking. A second study, which assessed a tailored behavioral counseling cessation program, also yielded null results.[130] The high rate of barriers to cessation, such as depression and fatalistic beliefs,[131] suggests that patients require more intensive interventions, including tailored behavioral counseling and pharmacotherapy, a treatment approach that is currently under investigation as a multisite randomized clinical trial.[132]

ENVIRONMENTAL TOBACCO SMOKE Exposure to ETS is causally linked to cancer,[133] heart disease,[134] asthma, acute lower and upper respiratory illnesses, middle ear disease, reduced lung function, and impaired lung development.[135] Children and adolescents and employees at work sites without bans on public tobacco use (eg, blue-collar and service workers) are especially vulnerable to the adverse health impact of ETS exposure. An estimated half of all children in the United States may be exposed to ETS,[136] and many industries around the country, such as restaurants and casinos, still permit tobacco use in public areas. Serum cotinine among children exposed to parental tobacco use can be detected,[137] as are tobacco-specific lung carcinogens, such as NNK and NNAL (4-(methylnitrosamino)-1-(3-pyridyl)-1-butanol) among casino patrons.[138] Because the primary source of ETS exposure among children and adolescents is parental tobacco use, smoking cessation interventions must be provided to parents, and pediatricians may be a useful source of intervention because most infants are seen by these physicians on a regular basis. In a recent review, Klerman concluded that interventions directed to assist parents to quit smoking have been effective, even if they are of minimal intensity.[137] Common elements of successful interventions are motivational interviewing (ie, counseling that is nonjudgmental and focuses on resolving ambivalence about behavior change) and problem-solving skills integrated within health care clinics, follow-up telephone booster sessions, and the provision of self-help manuals.[136] However, outside the context of formal studies, health care workers, especially pediatricians, do not typically provide cessation treatment to parents.[139] Constraints on the amount of time that physicians have, limited training, a lack of third-party reimbursement for cessation services, and negative beliefs about the provision of cessation treatment (eg, parents do not want to hear about smoking cessation) are all factors that moderate physician behavior.[140] Finally, interventions in the workplace to reduce ETS exposure must include bans on public smoking and the provision of formal cessation assistance. There is little question that bans on public tobacco use lower

ETS exposure[141] and reduce smoking rates.[142] In addition, a review of workplace smoking cessation treatments indicates that significant reductions in smoking rates are found when formal behavioral counseling and/or NRT are provided.[143] A recent study also indicated that the provision of personalized risk assessment feedback to smokers can play a role in reducing workplace smoking rates.[144]

Genetics of Tobacco Addiction The variability in people's susceptibility to tobacco initiation and ability to quit suggests that genetic polymorphisms, individually or in combination, may explain some of these behaviors.[145] Several genetic pathways have been proposed to explain the genetic influence on smoking and cessation behavior, including genes responsible for metabolizing nicotine (eg, *CYP2A6*) and regulating physiologic reward, such as dopaminergic and serotoninergic genes.[145] This literature is dominated by case-control studies, has rarely considered gene-gene or gene-environment (eg, personality or depression) interactions, and has been limited by methodologic shortcomings, such as low statistical power and population stratification bias. Understanding the genetic basis of nicotine addiction is a complex process, which poses a unique brand of conceptual and methodologic issues.[129] As studies in this pioneering area of research move forward, there is a growing promise that understanding the genetic correlates of nicotine addiction can lead to innovative personalized methods for treating[146] and preventing the development of nicotine addiction.[147]

Smoking Initiation Researchers have assessed polymorphisms on dopamine receptor gene *DRD2*, dopamine transporter gene (*DAT VNTR*), serotonin transporter gene (*5HTT LPR*), and the cytochrome P-450 2A6 gene (*CYP2A6*). Polymorphisms in the *DRD2* gene may be linked to smoking initiation in that the Taq1A polymorphism is marginally associated with an increased probability of being a smoker in pooled analyses.[145] In contrast, pooled analyses of studies on polymorphisms in *DAT VNTR*, *5HTT LPR*, and *CYP2A6* indicate that polymorphisms in these genes are not predictive of smoking initiation.[145]

Persistent Smoking and Smoking Cessation Meta-analyses of pooled data indicate that polymorphisms in *DRD2*, *DAT VNTR*, *5HTT LPR*, and *CYP2A6* genes are not associated with persistent smoking.[145] With regard to smoking cessation, pooled analyses indicate that polymorphisms in the *DRD2* and *DAT VNTR* genes are not associated with the ability to quit smoking, but effects have been detected for polymorphisms in *5HTT LPR* and in *CYP2A6* genes.[145] In particular, the short allele of the *5HTT LPR* gene is associated with a lower probability of successful smoking cessation, whereas the reduced-activity polymorphism of the *CYP2A6* gene is associated with a greater likelihood of successful smoking cessation.

New Genes The findings from recent trials of rimonobant, a CB_1 receptor antagonist, indicate that the cannabinoid CB_1 receptor may influence nicotine addiction. Animal studies that compare CB_1 knockout mice with wild-type littermates show that this receptor can influence the acute effects of and motivational processes underlying nicotine, such as locomotor behavior, antinociceptive effects, and the rewarding effects of nicotine as measured by conditioned place preference. Variants in the CB_1 receptor may influence susceptibility to nicotine addiction and the ability to quit smoking. A study by Zhang and colleagues found that the TAG haplotype (TAG; rs806379 [hCV1652584], rs1535255 [hCV8943758], and rs2023239 [hCV11600616]) was related to polysubstance addiction in European Americans, blacks, and a Japanese sample.[99] Interestingly, the TAG haplotype is related to a reduction in CB_1 messenger ribonucleic acid, which has implications for dopaminergic function, thereby suggesting that the CB_1 receptor may represent a reward pathway for addictive substances, including nicotine. Future studies are planned to elucidate the effect of this gene on nicotine addiction.

Prevention of Tobacco Use The most effective way to reduce the rate of tobacco-related morbidity and mortality is to prevent smoking initiation. Because nearly all smokers begin to use tobacco when they are under the age of 18 years, tobacco prevention efforts must be directed toward children and adolescents. A comprehensive approach to tobacco prevention must consider the range of factors that determine smoking initiation. A recent review outlines the multidimensional framework for smoking initiation among adolescents, highlighting the following as risk factors: low socioeconomic status, weight concern (among girls), conduct disorder (among boys), genetic polymorphisms, tolerance for nicotine, attention deficits, depression, peer influence, parental exposure, tobacco advertising, and low cost of cigarettes.[148] Specific factors play a greater influence at specific time points in the trajectory from experimentation to regular use. For instance, experimentation is more likely if the child is exposed to peer encouragement, has poor parental monitoring or little disapproval, is exposed to commercial advertising for tobacco use, and exhibits a curiosity about the consequences of tobacco use. In contrast, a high tolerance for nicotine or genetic polymorphisms that lower endogenous dopamine concentrations may play a greater role in determining the progression from experimentation to regular use. In recognizing the psychological and social factors that underlie the risk of initiating tobacco use, tobacco prevention initiatives have been either school-based education and counseling programs or community-based projects.

School-Based Programs These programs are based on the assumption that addressing psychological and social influences that promote tobacco use will effectively inoculate children and adolescents from starting to smoke. These programs adopt either a social influences model or the related, yet more intensive and comprehensive, social competence enhancement (or life skills training) approach. The former teaches students about the role that social factors (eg, peer influence) play in determining their risk of tobacco use, works with students to develop norms that discourage tobacco use, and instructs students in skills to resist negative social influences. The latter approach focuses on intensive instruction in personal self-management and social competency skills (eg, refusing pressure to try cigarettes). In a recent review of these programs, 15 of 25 studies reported significant 2-year reductions in smoking rates of 9 to 14.2%[149] in schools that implemented such prevention programs compared with control schools. It should be noted, however, that these gains may not be maintained over a longer follow-up duration, as shown in a large examination of a social influence prevention program that included a 12-year follow-up assessment.[150] As such, a critical priority for the field of tobacco control is the development and evaluation of innovative school-based tobacco prevention programs that address other risk factors (beyond psychological and social) through the integration of community-wide initiatives.

Community-Based Programs Mass media education (eg, billboards and television commercials) and legislative policy (ie, restricting advertising and access, raising taxes, and instituting bans) can influence individual behavior and societal norms concerning tobacco use.[151] Tobacco advertising promotes adolescent smoking, and the tobacco industry has maintained a long-standing and aggressive marketing program designed to encourage youth to initiate tobacco use.[152] For instance, prior to the Joe Camel advertising campaign, the market share for Camel cigarettes among those aged 12 to 17 years was less than 1%, but it increased to 13% after 5 years.[153] Despite the Master Settlement Agreement's restrictions on tobacco marketing, the tobacco industry spent $694 million to promote its product in 2000, an increase of 87% since 1996.[154] Fortunately, countermarketing efforts can effectively prevent youth tobacco use, especially when they are combined with more intensive school-based programs.[155] Persuasive data come from Florida's evaluation of The Truth Campaign, which portrayed youth confronting the tobacco industry in humorous yet confrontational ways. The campaign yielded an 18% reduction in smoking among middle school students and an 8% reduction in smoking among high school students after 1 year, and 40% and 18% reductions, respectively, after year 2, reductions that exceeded national declines,[156] were independent of tax increases[157] and were maintained after 4 years.[158] Similar mass media counteradvertising campaigns in California, Minnesota, Massachusetts, and Oregon yielded significant reductions in youth smoking rates as well.[155] Elements common to these programs related to effectiveness are the use of an antismoking brand, underscoring tobacco industry manipulation, the deglamorization of smoking, the use of messages that elicit strong emotional responses, the delineation of the short- and long-term health effects of smoking, and the dispelling of smoking myths.[155]

Several legislative policies are critical for effective tobacco prevention. Restricting youth access to tobacco products through enforcement of laws preventing tobacco sales to those under age 18 years (eg, "It's the Law") lowers sales of cigarettes to minors; however, the effectiveness of this approach is dependent on implementation of penalties to nonadherent vendors.[159] In addition, tobacco sales are affected by price increases,[160] to which youth are especially sensitive. Data indicate that a 10% increase in the cost of cigarettes would reduce the prevalence of smoking by close to 7% and a $2 per pack increase in cigarettes would prevent approximately 6 million children from initiating tobacco use.[68] Lastly, perhaps the most encouraging development in the area of tobacco control has been the steady growth in public smoking bans. Comprehensive bans on smoking in indoor public spaces yield a 10% reduction in the prevalence of smoking[161] and reduce respirable suspended particles, a marker for ETS exposure, by 84%.[161] Further, a fascinating study by Sargent and colleagues illustrated the health benefits of public smoking bans.[162] The rates of hospital admissions for myocardial infarction (MI) in Helena, Montana, during a comprehensive ban on public and workplace smoking and then after the ban was lifted were examined. The rates of MI admissions were significantly reduced, from an average of 40 admissions per year in years when the ban was not in place to 24 per year during the ban. There was no change in MI admission rates in areas outside Helena, where such a ban was not enacted. Although confirmation of these findings is needed, these data suggest that bans on indoor public tobacco use can translate into measurable health benefits. Importantly, the implementation of clean indoor air legislation does not diminish revenues in restaurants and bars[163] or in recreational venues, such as bingo halls or other charity-run gaming facilities.[164]

REFERENCES

1. Lerman C, Patterson F, Berrettini W. Treating tobacco dependence: state of the science and new directions. J Clin Oncol 2005;23:311–23.
2. Bogen KT, Witschi H. Lung tumors in A/J mice exposed to environmental tobacco smoke: estimated potency and implied human risk. Carcinogenesis 2002;23:511–9.
3. Hoffmann D, Hecht SS. Advances in tobacco carcinogenesis. In: Cooper CS, Grover PL, editors. Handbook of experimental pharmacology. Vol 94. Berlin: Springer-Verlag; 1990. p. 511–9
4. Beach AC, Gupta RC. Human biomonitoring and the ^{32}P-postlabeling assay. Carcinogenesis 1992;13:1053–74.
5. Phillips DH, Hewer A, Martin CN, et al. Correlation of DNA adduct levels in human lung with cigarette smoking. Nature 1988;336:26–9.
6. Sekido Y, Fong KM, Minna JD. Molecular genetics of lung cancer. Annu Rev Med 2003;54:73–87.
7. Kersting M, Friedl C, Kraus A, et al. Differential frequencies of *p16^{INK4a}* promoter hypermethylation, *p53* mutation, and K-*ras* mutation in exfoliative material mark the development of lung cancer in symptomatic chronic smokers. J Clin Oncol 2000;18:3221–9.
8. Jassem J, Jassem E, Jakobkiewicz-Banecka J, et al. *P53* and K-*ras* mutations are frequent events in microscopically negative surgical margins from patients with nonsmall cell lung carcinoma. Cancer 2004;100:1951–60.
9. Belinsky SA. Silencing of genes by promoter hypermethylation: key event in rodent and human lung cancer. Carcinogenesis [In press]
10. Zochbauer-Muller S, Fong KM, Virmani AK, et al. Aberrant promoter methylation of multiple genes in non-small cell lung cancers. Cancer Res 2001;61:249–55.
11. Soria JC, Rodriguez M, Liu DD, et al. Aberrant promoter methylation of multiple genes in bronchial brush samples from former cigarette smokers. Cancer Res 2002;62:351–5.
12. Palmisano WA, Divine KK, Saccomanno G, et al. Predicting lung cancer by detecting aberrant promoter methylation in sputum. Cancer Res 2000;60:5954–8.
13. Usadel H, Brabender J, Danenberg KD, et al. Quantitative adenomatous polyposis coli promoter methylation analysis in tumor tissue, serum, and plasma DNA of patients with lung cancer. Cancer Res 2002;62:371–5.
14. Hu Z, Wei Q, Wang X, Shen H. DNA repair gene XPD polymorphism and lung cancer risk: a meta-analysis. Lung Cancer 2004;46:1–10.
15. Park JY, Lee SY, Jeon HS, et al. Polymorphism of the DNA repair gene XRCC1 and risk of primary lung cancer. Cancer Epidemiol Biomarkers Prev 2002;11:23–7.
16. Zhou W, Liu G, Miller DP, et al. Gene-environment interaction for the ERCC2 polymorphisms and cumulative cigarette smoking exposure in lung cancer. Cancer Res 2002;62:1377–81.
17. Popanda O, Schattenberg T, Phong CT, et al. Specific combinations of DNA repair gene variants and increased risk for non-small cell lung cancer. Carcinogenesis 2004;25:2433–41.
18. Crespi CI, Penman BW, Gelboin HV, Gonzales FJ. A tobacco smoke-derived nitrosamine, 4-(methylnitrosamino)-1-(3-pyridyl)-1 butanone, is activated by multiple human cytochrome P450s including the polymorphic human cytochrome P4502D6. Carcinogenesis 1991;12:1197–201.
19. Evans DAP, Mahgoub A, Sloan TP, et al. A family and population study of the genetic polymorphism of debrisoquine oxidation in a white British population. J Med Genet 1980;17:102–5.
20. Ayesh R, Idle JR, Ritchie JC, et al. Metabolic oxidation phenotypes as markers for susceptibility to lung cancer. Nature 1984;312:169–70.
21. Christensen PM, Gotzsche PC, Brosen K. The sparteine/debrisoquine (CYP2D6) oxidation polymorphism and the risk of lung cancer: a meta-analysis. Eur J Clin Pharmacol 1997;51:389–93.
22. Rostami-Hodjegan A, Lennard MS, Woods HF, Tucker GT. Meta-analysis of studies of the CYP2D6 polymorphism in relation to lung cancer and Parkinson's disease. Pharmacogenetics 1998;8:227–38.
23. Laforest L, Wikman H, Benhamou S, et al. CYP2D6 gene polymorphism in Caucasian smokers: lung cancer susceptibility and phenotype-genotype relationships. Eur J Cancer 2000;36:1825–32.
24. Saarikoski ST, Sata F, Husgafvel-Pursiainen K, et al. CYP2D6 ultrarapid metabolizer genotype as a potential modifier of smoking behaviour. Pharmacogenetics 2000;10:5–10.
25. Kaisary A, Smith P, Jaczq E, et al. Genetic predisposition to bladder cancer: ability to hydroxylate debrisoquine and mephenytoin as risk factors. Cancer Res 1987;47:5488–93.
26. Warwick AP, Redman CWE, Jones PW, et al. Progression of cervical intraepithelial neoplasia to cervical cancer: interactions of cytochrome P450 CYP2D6 EM and glutathione *S*-transferase GSTM1 null genotypes and cigarette smoking. Br J Cancer 1994;70:704–8.
27. Whitlock JP. Induction of cytochrome P4501A1. Annu Rev Pharmacol Toxicol 1999;39:103–25.
28. Anttila S, Hakkola J, Tuominen P, et al. Methylation of cytochrome P4501A1 promoter in the lung is associated with tobacco smoking. Cancer Res 2003;63:8623–8.
29. Iba MM, Scholl H, Fung J, et al. Induction of pulmonary CYP1A1 by nicotine. Xenobiotica 1998;28:827–43.
30. Nakachi K, Imai K, Hayashi S-I, Kawajiri K. Polymorphisms of the CYP1A1 and glutathione S-transferase genes associated with susceptibility to lung cancer in relation to cigarette dose in a Japanese population. Cancer Res 1993;53:2994–9.
31. Mollerup S, Ryberg D, Hewer A, et al. Sex differences in lung CYP1A1 expression and DNA adduct levels among lung cancer patients. Cancer Res 1999;59:3317–20.
32. Le Marchand L, Guo C, Benhamou S, et al. Pooled analysis of the CYP1A1 exon 7 polymorphism and lung cancer (United States). Cancer Causes Control 2003;14:339–46.
33. Hung RJ, Boffetta P, Brockmoller J, et al. CYP1A1 and GSTM1 genetic polymorphisms and lung cancer risk in Caucasian non-smokers: a pooled analysis. Carcinogenesis 2003;24:875–82.
34. Kawajiri K, Nakachi K, Imai K, et al. Identification of genetically high risk individuals to lung cancer by DNA polymorphisms of the cytochrome P4501A1 gene. FEBS Lett 1990;263:131–3.
35. Houlston RS. CYP1A1 polymorphisms and lung cancer risk: a meta-analysis. Pharmacogenetics 2000;10:105–14.
36. Ishibe N, Hankinson SE, Colditz GA, et al. Cigarette smoking, cytochrome *P450 1A1* polymorphisms, and breast cancer risk in the Nurses' Health Study. Cancer Res 1998;58:667–71.
37. Kato S, Shields PG, Caporaso NE, et al. Cytochrome P450IIE1 genetic polymorphisms, racial variation, and lung cancer risk. Cancer Res 1992;52:6712–5.
38. Uematsu F, Ikawa S, Kikuchi H, et al. Restriction fragment length polymorphism of the human CYP2E1 (cytochrome P450IIE1) gene and susceptibility to lung cancer: possible relevance to low smoking exposure. Pharmacogenetics 1994;4:58–63.
39. El-Zein R, Zwischenberger JB, Wood TG, et al. Combined genetic polymorphism and risk for development of lung cancer. Mutat Res 1997;381:189–200.
40. Lang NP, Kadlubar FF. Aromatic and heterocyclic amine metabolism and phenotyping in humans. Prog Clin Biol Res 1991;372:33–47.
41. Mommsen S, Aagaard J. Susceptibility in urinary bladder cancer: acetyltransferase phenotypes and related risk factors. Cancer Lett 1986;32:199–205.
42. Vineis P. Epidemiological models of carcinogenesis: the example of bladder cancer. Cancer Epidemiol Biomarkers Prev 1992;1:149–53.
43. Hein DW. Acetylator genotype and arylamine-induced carcinogenesis. Biochim Biophys Acta 1988;948:37–66.
44. Vineis P, Marinelli D, Autrup H, et al. Current smoking, occupation, N-acetyltransferase-2 and bladder cancer: a pooled analysis of genotype-based studies. Cancer Epidemiol Biomarkers Prev 2001;10:1249–52.
45. Cascorbi I, Brockmöller J, Mrozikiewicz PM, et al. Homozygous rapid arylamine N-acetyltransferase (NAT2) genotype as a susceptibility factor for lung cancer. Cancer Res 1996;56:3961–6.
46. Bouchardy C, Mitrunen K, Wikman H, et al. N-Acetyltransferase NAT1 and NAT2 genotypes and lung cancer risk. Pharmacogenetics 1998;8:291–8.
47. Zhou W, Liu G, Thurston SW, et al. Genetic polymorphisms in N-acetyltransferase-2 and microsomal epoxide hydrolase, cumulative cigarette smoking, and lung cancer. Cancer Epidemiol Biomarkers Prev 2002;11:15–21.
48. Ambrosone CB, Freudenheim JL, Graham S, et al. Cigarette smoking, N-acetyltransferase 2 genetic polymorphisms, and breast cancer risk. JAMA 1996;276:1494–501.
49. McWilliams JE, Sanderson BJS, Harris EL, et al. Glutathione S-transferase M1 (GSTM1) deficiency and lung cancer risk. Cancer Epidemiol Biomarkers Prev 1995;4:589–94.
50. Ford JG, Li Y, O'Sullivan MM, et al. Glutathione S-transferase M1 polymorphism and lung cancer risk in African-Americans. Carcinogenesis 2000;21:1971–5.
51. Kiyohara C, Wakai K, Mikami H, et al. Risk modification by CYP1A1 and GSTM1 polymorphisms in the association of environmental tobacco smoke and lung cancer: a case-control study in Japanese nonsmoking women. Int J Cancer 2003;107:139–44.
52. Alexandrie AK, Sundberg MI, Seidegard J, et al. Genetic susceptibility to lung cancer with special emphasis on CYP1A1 and GSTM1: a study on host factors in relation to age at onset, gender and histological cancer types. Carcinogenesis 1994;15:1785–90.
53. Dresler C, Fratelli C, Babb J, et al. Gender differences in genetic susceptibility to lung cancer. Lung Cancer 2000;30:153–60.
54. Noda N, Matsuzoe D, Konno T, et al. Risk for K-ras gene mutations in smoking-induced lung cancer is associated with cytochrome P4501A1 and glutathione S-transferase micro1 polymorphisms. Oncol Rep 2004;12:773–9.
55. Hou SM, Falt S, Yang K, et al. Differential interactions between GSTM1 and NAT2 genotypes on aromatic DNA adduct level and HPRT mutant frequency in lung cancer patients and population controls. Cancer Epidemiol Biomarkers Prev 2001;10:133–40.
56. Godschalk RW, Dallinga JW, Wikman H, et al. Modulation of DNA and protein adducts in smokers by genetic polymorphisms in GSTM1, GSTT1, NAT1 and NAT2. Pharmacogenetics 2001;11:389–98.

57. Habalova V, Salagovic J, Kalina I, Stubna J. Combined analysis of polymorphisms in glutathione S-transferase M1 and microsomal epoxide hydrolase in lung cancer patients. Neoplasma 2004;51:352–7.
58. Wang J, Deng Y, Li L, et al. Association of GSTM1, CYP1A1 and CYP2E1 genetic polymorphisms with susceptibility to lung adenocarcinoma: a case-control study in Chinese population. Cancer Sci 2003;94:448–52.
59. Wang J, Deng Y, Cheng J, et al. GST genetic polymorphisms and lung adenocarcinoma susceptibility in a Chinese population. Cancer Lett 2003;201:185–93.
60. Ryberg D, Hewer A, Phillips DH, Haugen A. Different susceptibility to smoking-induced DNA damage among male and female lung cancer patients. Cancer Res 1994;54:5801–3.
61. Shriver SP, Bourdeau HA, Gubish CT, et al. Sex-specific expression of gastrin-releasing peptide receptor: relationship to smoking history and risk of lung cancer. J Natl Cancer Inst 2000;92:24–33.
62. Taioli E, Wynder EL. Endocrine factors and adenocarcinoma of the lung in women. [letter]. J Natl Cancer Inst 1994;86:869–70.
63. Meireles SI, Verma B, Stoyanova R, et al. Modulation of gene expression in murine lung tissue by tobacco smoke exposure. Proc Am Assoc Cancer Res 2004;45:352.
64. Engstrom PF, Clapper M, Schnoll RA. Prevention of tobacco-related cancers. In: Kufe DW, Pollack RE, Weichselbaum RR, et al, editors. Cancer medicine. 6th ed. Hamilton (ON): BC Decker; 2003. p. 383–96.
65. Centers for Disease Control and Prevention. Cigarette smoking among adults—United States. MMWR Morb Mortal Wkly Rep 2004;53:427–31.
66. Centers for Disease Control and Prevention. State-specific prevalence of current cigarette smoking among adults—United States. MMWR Morb Mortal Wkly Rep 2004;53:1035–7.
67. US Department of Health and Human Services. The health consequences of smoking: a report of the surgeon general. Atlanta: US Department of Health and Human Services, CDC, National Center for Chronic Disease Prevention and Health Promotion, Office on Smoking and Health; 2004.
68. Fiore MC, Croyle RT, Curry SJ, et al. Preventing 3 million premature deaths and helping 5 million smokers quit: a national action plan for tobacco cessation. Am J Public Health 2004;94:205–10.
69. Fiore MC, Bailey WC, Cohen SJ, et al. Treating tobacco use and dependence. In: Clinical practice guideline. Rockville (MD): US Department of Health and Human Services, Public Health Service; 2000.
70. Abrams DB, Orleans CT, Niaura R, et al. Integrating individual and public health perspectives for treatment of tobacco dependence under managed care: a combined stepped-care and matching model. Ann Behav Med 1996;18:290–304.
71. Lancaster T, Stead LF. Self-help interventions for smoking cessation. Cochrane Database Syst Rev 2000;CD001118.
72. Mojica WA, Suttorp MJ, Sherman SE, et al. Smoking-cessation interventions by type of provider: a meta-analysis. Am J Prev Med 2004;26:391–401.
73. Curry SJ. Bridging the clinical and public health perspectives in tobacco treatment research: scenes from a tobacco treatment research care. Cancer Epidemiol Biomarkers Prev 2001;10:281–5.
74. Prochaska JO, Velicer WF, Fava JL, et al. Evaluating a population-based recruitment approach and a stage-based expert system intervention for smoking cessation. Addict Behav 2001;26:583–602.
75. Ossip-Klein DJ, McIntosh S. Quitlines in North America: evidence base and applications. Am J Med Sci 2003;326:201–5.
76. Borland R, Balmford J, Segan C, et al. The effectiveness of personalized smoking cessation strategies for callers to a quitline service. Addiction 2003;98:837–46.
77. Zhu SH, Anderson CM, Tedeschi GJ, et al. Evidence of real-world effectiveness of a telephone quitline for smokers. N Engl J Med 2002;347:1087–93.
78. Piasecki TM, Baker TB. Any further progress in smoking cessation treatment? Nicotine Tob Res 2001;3:311–23.
79. Pierce JP, Gilpin EA, Emery SL, et al. Tobacco control in California: who's winning the war? An evaluation of the Tobacco Control Program 1989-1996. La Jolla (CA): University of California, San Diego; 1998.
80. Kottke TE. Observing the delivery of smoking-cessation interventions. Am J Prev Med 1998;14:71–2.
81. Stein RJ, Haddock CK, O'Byrne KK, et al. The pediatrician's role in reducing tobacco exposure in children. Pediatrics 2000;106:1–17.
82. Silagy C, Stead LF. Physician advice for smoking cessation. Cochrane Database Syst Rev 2001;CD000165.
83. Doescher MP, Saver BG. Physicians' advice to quit smoking. The glass remains half empty. J Fam Pract 2000;49:543–7.
84. Thorndike AN, Rigotti NA, Stafford RS, Singer DE. National patterns in the treatment of smokers by physicians. JAMA 1998;279:604–8.
85. National Committee for Quality Assurance. The state of managed care quality. 1999. Available at http://www.ncqa.org/communications/some/SO4C2004.pdf. Accessed 17 August 2005.
86. Katz DA, Muehlenbruch DR, Brown RL, et al. Effectiveness of implementing the agency for healthcare research and quality smoking cessation clinical practice guideline: a randomized, controlled trial. J Natl Cancer Inst 2004;96:594–603.
87. Rice VH, Stead LF. Nursing interventions for smoking cessation. Cochrane Database Syst Rev 2004;CD001188.
88. Foulds J, Burke M, Steinberg M, et al. Advances in pharmacotherapy for tobacco dependence. Exp Opin Emerg Drugs 2004;9:39–53.
89. Silagy C, Lancaster T, Stead L, et al. Nicotine replacement therapy for smoking cessation. Cochrane Database Syst Rev 2004;CD000146.
90. Hajek P, West R, Foulds J, et al. Randomized comparative trial of nicotine polacrilex, a transdermal patch, nasal spray, and an inhaler. Arch Intern Med 1999;159:2033–8.
91. Houtsmuller EJ, Henningfield JE, Stitzer ML. Subjective effects of the nicotine lozenge: assessment of abuse liability. Psychopharmacology (Berl) 2003;167:20–7.
92. Hughes JR, Shiffman S, Callas P, Zhang J. A meta-analysis of the efficacy of over-the-counter nicotine replacement. Tob Control 2003;12:21–7.
93. Jorenby DE, Leischow SJ, Nides MA, et al. A controlled trial of sustained-release bupropion, a nicotine patch, or both for smoking cessation. N Engl J Med 1999;340:685–91.
94. George TP, O'Malley SS. Current pharmacological treatments for nicotine dependence. Trends Pharmacol Sci 2004;25:42–8
95. Hughes JR, Stead LF, Lancaster T. Antidepressants for smoking cessation. Cochrane Database Syst Rev 2000;CD000031.
96. Cinciripini PM, Lapitsky L, Seay S, et al. A placebo-controlled evaluation of the effects of buspirone on smoking cessation: differences between high- and low-anxiety smoke. J Clin Psychopharmacol 1995;15:182–91.
97. Farid P, Abate MA. Buspirone use for smoking cessation. Ann Pharmacother 1998;32:1362–4.
98. David S, Lancaster T, Stead LF. Opioid antagonists for smoking cessation. Cochrane Database Syst Rev 2001;CD003086.
99. Zhang PW, Ishiguro H, Ohtsuki T, et al. Human cannabinoid receptor 1: 5' exons, candidate regulatory regions, polymorphisms, haplotypes and association with polysubstance abuse. Mol Psychiatry 2004;9:916–31.
100. Cohen C, Perrault G, Voltz C, et al. SR141716, a central cannabinoid (CB(1)) receptor antagonist, blocks the motivational and dopamine-releasing effects of nicotine in rats. Behav Pharmacol 2002;13:451–63.
101. Cohen C, Perrault G, Griebel G, et al. Nicotine-associated cues maintain nicotine-seeking behavior in rats several weeks after nicotine withdrawal: reversal by the cannabinoid (CB(1)) receptor antagonist, rimonabant (SR141716). Neuropsychopharmacology 2005;30:145-55.
102. Anthenelli RM, Despres JP. Effects of rimonabant in the reduction of major cardiovascular risk factors. Results from the STRATUS-US Trial (Smoking Cessation in Smokers Motivated to Quit). Presented at the American College of Cardiology 53rd Annual Scientific Session; 2004; New Orleans, LA.
103. Sutton S. Back to the drawing board? A review of applications of the transtheoretical model to substance use. Addiction 2001;96:175–86.
104. Lawrence T, Aveyard P, Evans O, Cheng KK. A cluster randomised controlled trial of smoking cessation in pregnant women comparing interventions based on the transtheoretical (stages of change) model to standard care. Tob Control 2003;12:168–77.
105. Centers for Disease Control and Prevention. Indoor air quality in hospitality venues before and after implementation of a clean indoor air law. MMWR Morb Mortal Wkly Rep 2004;53:1038–41.
106. Centers for Disease Control and Prevention. Self-reported heart disease and stroke among adults with and without diabetes—United States, 1999-2001. MMWR Morb Mortal Wkly Rep 2003;52:1065–70.
107. Jemal A, Tiwari RC, Murray T, et al. Cancer statistics. CA Cancer J Clin 2004;54:8–29.
108. Mazas CA, Wetter DW. Smoking cessation interventions among African Americans: research needs. Cancer Control 2003;10:87–9.
109. Ahluwalia JS, Harris KJ, Catley D, et al. Sustained-release bupropion for smoking cessation in African Americans: a randomized controlled trial. JAMA 2002;288:468–74.
110. Taylor SE. Health psychology. 5th ed. Boston: McGraw Hill; 2003.
111. Landrine H, Klonoff EA. Racial discrimination and cigarette smoking among blacks: findings from two studies. Ethn Dis 2000;10:195–202.
112. Garten S, Falkner RV. Role of mentholated cigarettes in increased nicotine dependence and greater risk of tobacco-attributable disease. Prev Med 2004;38:793–8.
113. Perez-Stable EJ, Herrera B, Jacob P, Benowitz NL. Nicotine metabolism and intake in black and white smokers. JAMA 1998;280:152–6.
114. Airhihenbuwa CO, Kumanyika SK, TenHave TR, Morssink CB. Cultural identity and health lifestyles among African Americans: a new direction for health intervention research? Ethn Dis 2000;10:148–64.
115. Nollen NL, Catley D, Davies G, et al. Religiosity, social support, and smoking cessation among urban African American smokers. Addict Behav [In press]
116. Patel JD, Bach PB, Kris MG. Lung cancer in US women: a contemporary epidemic. JAMA 2004;291:1763–8.
117. Giovino GA. Epidemiology of tobacco use in the United States. Oncogene 2002;21:7326–40.
118. Oncken CA, Kranzler HR. Pharmacotherapies to enhance smoking cessation during pregnancy. Drug Alcohol Rev 2003;22:191–202.
119. US Department of Health and Human Services. Women and smoking: a report of the surgeon general. Washington (DC): US Department of Health and Human Services, Public Health Service, Office of the Surgeon General; 2001.
120. Filozof C, Fernandez Pinilla MC, Fernandez-Cruz A. Smoking cessation and weight gain. Obes Rev 2004;5:95–103.
121. Weissman MM, Bland RC, Canino GJ, et al. Cross-national epidemiology of major depression and bipolar disorder. JAMA 1996;276:293–9.
122. Hitsman B, Borrelli B, McChargue DE, et al. History of depression and smoking cessation outcome: a meta-analysis. J Consult Clin Psychol 2003;71:657–63.
123. Dempsey DA, Benowitz NL. Risks and benefits of nicotine to aid smoking cessation in pregnancy. Drug Saf 2001;24:277–322.
124. Chan B, Einarson A, Koren G. Effectiveness of bupropion for smoking cessation during pregnancy. J Addict Dis 2005;24:19–23.
125. Centers for Disease Control and Prevention. Youth Risk Behavior Surveillance—United States, 2003. MMWR Morb Mortal Wkly Rep 2004;53:1–100.
126. Garrison MM, Christakis DA, Ebel BE, et al. Smoking cessation interventions for adolescents: a systematic review. Am J Prev Med 2003;25:363–7.
127. Killen JD, Robinson TN, Ammerman S, et al. Randomized clinical trial of the efficacy of bupropion combined with nicotine patch in the treatment of adolescent smokers. J Consult Clin Psychol 2004;72:729–35.
128. Balch GI, Tworek C, Barker DC, et al. Opportunities for youth smoking cessation: findings from a national focus group study. Nicotine Tob Res 2004;6:9–17.
129. Schnoll RA, Zhang B, Rue M, et al. Brief physician-initiated quit smoking strategies for clinical oncology settings: a trial coordinated by the Eastern Cooperative Oncology Group. J Clin Oncol 2003;21:355–65.
130. Schnoll R, Rothman RL, Wielt DB, et al. A randomized pilot study of cognitive-behavioral therapy vs. basic health education for smoking cessation among cancer patients. Ann Behav Med [In press]
131. Schnoll RA, Malstrom M, James C, et al. Correlates of tobacco use among smokers and recent quitters diagnosed with cancer. Patient Educ Couns 2002;46:137–45.
132. Schnoll RA, Lazev AB, Sobel M, et al. Preliminary results from a randomized trial of bupropion for smoking cessation among cancer patients. Paper presented at the 11th Annual Meeting of the Society for Research on Nicotine and Tobacco; 2005; Prague, The Czech Republic.
133. Sasco AJ, Secretan MB, Straif K. Tobacco smoking and cancer: a brief review of recent epidemiological evidence. Lung Cancer 2004;45 Suppl 2:3–9.
134. Leone A, Giannini, D, Bellotto C, Balbarini A. Passive smoking and coronary heart disease. Curr Vasc Pharmacol 2004;2:175–82.

135. Environmental Protection Agency. Health effects of exposure to environmental tobacco smoke. Tob Control 1997;6:346–53.
136. Gehrman CA, Hovell MF. Protecting children from environmental tobacco smoke (ETS) exposure: a critical review. Nicotine Tob Res 2003;5:289–301.
137. Klerman L. Protecting children: reducing their environmental tobacco smoke exposure. Nicotine Tob Res 2004;6 Suppl 2:39–53.
138. Anderson KE, Kliris J, Murphy L, et al. Metabolites of a tobacco-specific lung carcinogen in nonsmoking casino patrons. Cancer Epidemiol Biomarkers Prev 2003;12:1544–6.
139. Tanski SE, Klein JD, Winickoff JP, et al. Tobacco counseling at well-child and tobacco-influenced illness visits: opportunities for improvement. Pediatrics 2003;111:E162–7.
140. Zapka JG, Fletcher K, Pbert L, et al. The perceptions and practices of pediatricians: tobacco intervention. Pediatrics 1999;103:e65.
141. Siegel M, Albers AB, Cheng DM, et al. Effect of local restaurant smoking regulations on environmental tobacco smoke exposure among youth. Am J Public Health 2004;94:321–5.
142. Brownson RC, Hopkins DP, Wakefield MA. Effects of smoking restrictions in the workplace. Annu Rev Public Health 2002;23:333–48.
143. Moher M, Hey K, Lancaster T. Workplace interventions for smoking cessation. Cochrane Database Syst Rev 2003;CD003440.
144. Schnoll RA, Miller SM, Wang H, et al. Change in smoking behavior at the worksite following a cancer risk feedback intervention: a pilot study. Am J Health Behav 2005;29:215–27.
145. Munafo M, Clark T, Johnstone E, et al. The genetic basis for smoking behavior: a systematic review and meta-analysis. Nicotine Tob Res 2004;6:583–97.
146. Walton R, Johnstone E, Munafo M, et al. Genetic clues to the molecular basis of tobacco addiction and progress towards personalized therapy. Trends Mol Med 2001;7:70–6.
147. Swan GE. Implications of the genetic epidemiology for the prevention of tobacco use. Nicotine Tob Res 1999;1 Suppl 1:49–56.
148. Turner L, Mermelstein R, Flay B. Individual and contextual influences on adolescent smoking. Ann N Y Acad Sci 2004;1021:175–97.
149. Skara S, Sussman S. A review of 25 long-term adolescent tobacco and other drug use prevention program evaluations. Prev Med 2003;37:451–74.
150. Peterson AV, Kealey KA, Mann SL, et al. Hutchinson Smoking Prevention Project: long-term randomized trial in school-based tobacco use prevention—results on smoking. J Natl Cancer Inst 2000;92:1979–91.
151. Sowden A, Arblaster L, Stead L. Community interventions for preventing smoking in young people. Cochrane Database Syst Rev 2003;CD001291.
152. Pierce JP, Gilpin EA, Choi WS. Sharing the blame: smoking experimentation and future smoking-attributable mortality due to Joe Camel and Marlboro advertising and promotions. Tob Control 1999;8:37–44.
153. Arnett JJ, Terhanian G. Adolescents' responses to cigarette advertisements: links between exposure, liking, and the appeal of smoking. Tob Control 1998;7:129–33.
154. Federal Trade Commission. Report to Congress for 2000 pursuant to the federal cigarette labeling and advertising act. Washington (DC): Federal Trade Commission; 2002.
155. Farrelly MC, Niederdeppe J, Yarsevich J. Youth tobacco prevention mass media campaigns: past, present, and future directions. Tob Control 2003;12:i35–47.
156. Sly DF, Heald GR, Ray S. The Florida "truth" anti-tobacco media evaluation: design, first year results, and implications for planning future state media evaluation. Tob Control 2001;10:9–15.
157. Farrelly MC, Healton CG, Davis KC, et al. Getting to the truth: evaluating national tobacco countermarketing campaigns. Am J Public Health 2002;92:901–7.
158. Niederdeppe J, Farrelly MC, Haviland ML. Confirming "truth": more evidence of a successful tobacco countermarketing campaign in Florida. Am J Public Health 2004;94:255–7.
159. Lantz PM, Jacobson PD, Warner KE, et al. Investing in youth tobacco control: a review of smoking prevention and control strategies. Tob Control 2000;9:47–63.
160. Tauras JA. Public policy and smoking cessation among young adults in the United States. Health Policy 2004;68:321–32.
161. Levy DT, Friend KB. The effects of clean indoor air laws: what do we know and what do we need to know? Health Educ Res 2003;18:592–609.
162. Sargent RP, Shepard RM, Glantz SA. Reduced incidence of admissions for myocardial infarction associated with public smoking ban: before and after study. BMJ 2004;328:977–80.
163. Centers for Disease Control and Prevention. Impact of a smoking ban on restaurant and bar revenues—El Paso, Texas, 2002. MMWR Morb Mortal Wkly Rep 2004;53:150–2.
164. Glantz SA, Wilson-Loots R. No association of smoke-free ordinances with profits from bingo and charitable games in Massachusetts. Tob Control 2003;12:411–3.

26

Nutrition in the Etiology and Prevention of Cancer

Steven K. Clinton, MD, PhD
Edward L. Giovannucci, MD, ScD, DPH
Elizabeth C. Miller, MS, RD, LD

Over the last two centuries, improvements in food production, processing, storage, and distribution have led to major changes in diet composition within the economically developed nations. During this period, life expectancy also dramatically increased in these countries because of a combination of factors, including public health measures, improved occupational safety, and major reductions in nutrient deficiency syndromes. As the population has aged, there has been a shift in the major causes of morbidity and mortality toward chronic diseases such as cancer and cardiovascular disease. These changes are associated with an increasingly overweight and sedentary population. Although nutritional deficiencies still plague subpopulations in developed nations such as the poor, the aged, alcoholics, and the chronically ill, we now recognize that the affluent diet contributes to the pathogenesis of chronic diseases that afflict the vast majority of the population. Efforts to understand the etiologies of various cancers have led to epidemiologic and laboratory studies that strongly implicate certain dietary patterns and specific nutrients. In recent years, the inter-relationships between diet, nutrition, and cancer have expanded to encompass support of patients undergoing therapy and during survivorship.

It is important to establish a conceptual framework for organizing data regarding diet, nutrition, and cancer that will help readers provide guidance to the public and patients. Organizations such as the National Cancer Institute, the American Cancer Society, and the American Institute for Cancer Research have published recommendations defining achievable dietary and nutritional goals for the entire population that may help reduce the overall cancer burden through primary prevention (Table 26-1). Some individuals, particularly those deemed to be at higher risk of specific types of cancer as a result of environmental exposures, family history, or the presence of premalignant conditions are increasingly interested in the unique dietary and lifestyle interventions that may be tailored to lower their chances of developing cancer. Patients actively undergoing cancer therapy represent another group profoundly interested in the role of dietary and nutritional factors to enhance the efficacy of treatment while reducing the frequency and severity of side effects. Finally, as cancers are detected earlier and treatment interventions become more successful, the number of cancer survivors is increasing rapidly. Those completing cancer therapy are seeking information regarding diet and lifestyle interventions that will lower their risk of recurrence (secondary prevention) and reduce the severity of long-term complications of their cancer treatment, including therapy-related second malignancies and long-term organ dysfunction. Thus, those involved in cancer therapy and management of long-term health are increasingly being asked to provide evidence-based guidance in an area where scientific studies are few, and purveyors of alternative diet or nutrient-based interventions are allowed to market products in the absence of scientific data regarding efficacy and safety. We briefly review each of these categories of intervention and provide information that will assist in counseling individuals and groups interested in dietary and nutritional interventions. We believe this is a useful framework because it is likely that dietary variables may have unique effects during the prediagnostic phase, after diagnosis and during therapy, and following effective treatment.

The vast majority of research conducted in the field of diet, nutrition, and cancer focuses on etiology and prevention. Thus, this chapter emphasizes the public health model and focuses on the interventions that may reduce the overall cancer burden of large populations. We then consider the evidence for the prevention of cancers involving specific organs. Rather than detailing the complex, often incomplete, and occasionally contradictory literature concerning the role of diet in the etiology of specific cancers, this chapter provides a general guide with an emphasis on the major emerging concepts in the area. We conclude with a brief overview of the role of diet and nutrition to enhance therapy and survivorship.

METHODOLOGIC ISSUES IN DIET, NUTRITION, AND CANCER STUDIES

It is valuable to briefly consider how dietary recommendations are established. The unbiased detection and quantification of risks that are associated with variations in diet and nutrient intake would ideally be achieved through randomized, prospective trials. Unfortunately, the enormous costs of long-term nutrition studies and the scientific difficulties in controlling or measuring nutrient intake, limit their feasibility. Current nutritional guidelines for disease prevention are therefore based on the integration of information derived from a variety of different epidemiologic approaches and laboratory investigations. Thus, most guidelines are provided by committees convened by organizations such as the National Cancer Institute, the American Cancer Society, the American Institute of Cancer Research /World Cancer Research Fund, and the World Health Organization, among others.[1–4] The evidence derived from epidemiologic studies, clinical investigations, and laboratory studies are reviewed and discussed by expert committees relative to criteria of causality. Causality is defined as a specific occurrence or outcome that is consistently preceded by a known set of circumstances or conditions. In nutritional sciences, clear representations of causality have been the demonstration of single-nutrient deficiency syndromes and their complete reversal by exposure to the nutrient. For example, the lack of fruits and vegetables in the diet leads to scurvy, which is readily reversed by vitamin C. Unfortunately, relationships between diet and cancer are much more complex than simple deficiency syndromes. To establish causality, conclusions about the occurrence of an event and its etiologic factor are based on several established criteria. These criteria have evolved over many years and include consistency, strength of association, biologic gradient, temporality, specificity, biologic plausibility, biologic mechanism, coherence, and experimental evidence.[5] Precisely quantitating risk has been difficult because the etiologies of most cancers are multifactorial and poorly understood. Human cancers show striking variations based on factors such as age, sex, race, socioeconomic status, and genetics as well as many occupational and lifestyle variables. The potential for complex interactions between these factors and diet is enormous, and this emphasizes the difficulties in demonstrating causal associations with the same clarity as is demonstrable for high-risk environmental exposures, such as cigarette smoking.

Assessment of the Human Diet Nutritional epidemiology poses some unique obstacles, in that food is a universal exposure, which is in stark contrast to many cancer-causing environmental exposures, such as cigarette smoke. Table 26-2 details the strengths and limitations of various types of study designs used in nutrition research.

Table 26-1 Public Health Guidelines for Disease Prevention

	American Institute of Cancer Research[2]	American Heart Association[17]	United States Department of Agriculture[12]	American Cancer Society[1]
Body weight	Avoid being underweight or overweight and limit weight gain during adulthood to less than 5 kg (11 pounds).	Balance the number of calories you eat with the number you use each day.	Maintain body weight in a healthy range, balance calories from foods and beverages with calories expended.	Choose foods that maintain a healthful weight. Maintain a healthful weight throughout life. Lose weight if you are currently overweight or obese.
Physical activity	If occupational activity is low or moderate, take an hour's brisk walk or similar exercise daily, and also exercise vigorously for a total of at least one hour a week.	Maintain a level of physical activity that keeps you fit and matches the number of calories you eat.	Engage in regular physical activity and reduce sedentary activities to promote health, psychological well-being, and a healthy body weight	Adults: engage in moderate activity of ≥ 30 minutes, at least 5 days per week. Children and Teens: ≥ 60 minutes per day of moderate-to-vigorous activity, at least 5 days per week.
Plant-based diet	Choose predominantly plant-based diets rich in a variety of vegetables and fruits, pulses (legumes), and minimally processed starchy staple foods.			Eat a variety of healthful foods, with an emphasis on plant sources.
Vegetable & fruit	Eat 15 to 30 ounces or five or more portions a day of a variety of vegetables and fruits, all year round.	Eat a variety of fruits and vegetables. Choose 5 or more servings per day.	Consume a sufficient amount of fruits and vegetables while staying within energy needs. Choose a variety of fruits and vegetables each day.	Eat 5 or more servings of a variety of fruits and vegetables each day.
Breads, grains, & cereals	Eat 20–30 ounces or more than seven portions a day of a variety of cereals, grains, pulses (legumes), roots, tubers, and plantains.	Eat a variety of grain products, including whole grains. Choose 6 or more servings per day	Consume 3 or more ounce-equivalents of whole-grain products per day, with the rest of the recommended grains coming from enriched or whole grain products.	Choose whole grains in preference to processed (refined) grains and sugars.
Animal products	If eaten at all, limit intake of red meat to less than 3 ounces daily. It is preferable to choose fish, poultry, or meat from non-domesticated animals in place of red meat.	Include fat-free and low fat milk products, fish, legumes (beans), skinless poultry, and lean meats.		Limit consumption of red meats, especially those high in fat, and processed meats.
Dietary fat	Limit consumption of fatty foods, particularly those of animal origin. Choose modest amounts of appropriate vegetable oils.	Limit foods high in saturated fat, trans fat and /or cholesterol. Choose fats with 2 grams or less saturated fat per serving, such as liquid and tub margarine, canola oil, and olive oil.	Keep total fat intake between 20 and 35% of calories, with most fats coming from sources of polyunsaturated and monounsaturated fatty acids, such as fish, nuts, and vegetable oils.	Limit your intake of high-fat foods, particularly from animal sources. Choose foods low in fat.
Processed foods & refined sugar	Prefer minimally processed foods. Limit consumption of refined sugar.	Limit your intake of foods high in calories or low in nutrition, including foods like soft drinks and candy that have a lot of sugars.	Choose and prepare foods and beverages with few added sugars or caloric sweeteners.	
Salt & sodium	Limit consumption of salted foods and use of cooking and table salt. Use herbs and spices to season foods.	Eat less than 6 grams of salt per day (2,400 milligrams of sodium).	Consume less than 2,300 mg (approximately 1 tsp of salt) of sodium per day. Choose and prepare foods with little salt.	
Alcohol	Alcohol consumption is not recommended. If consumed at all, limit alcoholic drinks to less than two drinks a day for men and one for women.	Have no more than one alcoholic drink per day if you are a woman and not more than two if you are a man.	Those who choose to drink alcoholic beverages should do so sensibly and in moderation defined as one drink/day for women and up to two drinks/day for men	If you drink alcoholic beverages, limit consumption
Food storage	Do not eat food which, as a result of prolonged storage, is liable to contamination. Use refrigeration and other appropriate methods to preserve perishable food as purchased and at home.		Chill (refrigerate) perishable food promptly and defrost foods properly.	
Food preparation	Do not eat charred foods. For meat and fish eaters, avoid burning of meat juices. Consume the following only occasionally: meat and fish grilled (broiled) in direct flame; cured, and smoked meats		Clean hands, food contact surfaces, and fruits and vegetables. Meat and poultry should not be washed or rinsed. Separate raw, cooked, and ready-to-eat foods.	
Food additives	When levels of additives, contaminants and other residues are properly regulated, their presence in food and drink is not known to be harmful. However, unregulated or improper use can be a health hazard, and this applies particularly in economically developing countries.			
Tobacco	Do not smoke or chew tobacco			
Miscellaneous	For those who follow the above recommendations, dietary supplements are probably unnecessary, and possibly unhelpful, for reducing cancer risk		Consume a variety of nutrient-dense foods and beverages within and among the basic food groups.	Increase access to healthful foods in schools, worksites, and communities

Table 26-2 Types of Studies Used to Assess Diet and Disease Relationships

Study Type	Methods	Strengths	Limitations
Ecologic/correlational studies	The unit of observation is a population defined by a discriminator location (Japan v. United States, northern v. southern latitudes). Mortality or incidence among groups is compared with estimates of nutrient or food intake.	Large differences in cancer incidence and dietary patterns are often identified and hypotheses can be generated.	There are often many diet and lifestyle differences between populations, therefore correlations between disease incidence and dietary factors are confounded by known or unknown variables. Cancer incidence data and diet patterns may not be similarly quantitated among nations.
Case-control studies	Individuals experiencing a disease are identified and a similar group of matched subjects without the disease are identified. Information about past diet and nutrients is obtained from both the cases and controls for comparison.	Studies can be conducted over a relatively short period of time.	Selection bias can occur if a non-representative control group is selected. Recall bias can occur when subjects with a disease alter their perceptions and recall of past dietary habits. This often occurs when participants are familiar with a particular diet/disease hypothesis.
Prospective/cohort studies	A study population is identified and diet patterns assessed. The population is followed over time for disease outcome and changes in exposure to dietary risk factors.	Dietary intake can be monitored periodically over time. Diet assessment does not rely on long-term memory and is less affected by recall bias. Biochemical measures can be obtained periodically.	Long periods of time may be necessary for a disease to be diagnosed, therefore cohort studies often require many years of follow-up. A large number of subjects are required to compensate for subjects who drop out, are lost to follow-up, and the possibility that the frequency of the outcome of interest is low. Long term, large prospective studies are expensive.
Randomized controlled trials	Individuals are screened and a proper target population is identified, based on specific characteristics, and randomized to a control arm (standard of care) or an intervention arm. The subjects are followed for disease outcome or other biomarkers.	Especially useful for testing compounds (vitamins and minerals) that can be incorporated into pills or capsules and provided in a double-blind fashion over a period of years.	Difficult to implement for many nutrition and cancer hypotheses (weight loss, exercise, dietary fat, fiber, fruits and vegetables) because trials of dietary change cannot be blinded. Manipulation of single dietary components in large-scale intervention studies is difficult because foods are complex and contain many compounds. Compliance with food changes may be difficult to determine. Randomized, controlled trials can take a long time to complete and can be very expensive.

The critical limiting feature of most human studies is the imprecision of quantifying nutrient intake. Estimating the usual intake of foods or nutrients as well as accounting for intraindividual variation over time is a critical area of research.[6–8] An estimate of human nutrient intake is derived from a two-step process. First, interviews, questionnaires, or food diaries must determine the amounts and types of foods that are consumed.[9] This information can then be used to calculate nutrient intake if an accurate database has been established that quantifies the amount of each nutrient contained in the foods that are consumed by the population under investigation. Each step can be associated with significant error and contributes to the challenges in defining nutrient and cancer associations. The human diet is a complex array of foods that exhibits significant day-to-day and seasonal variations. The complexity of diet also differs widely among populations, cultures, and geographic areas. This often requires the development of different assessment methods for each population or subgroup. Future progress will depend, in part, on identifying biomarkers of nutrient exposure. Development of valid and reliable biomarkers of nutrient intake offers the promise of improved precision in epidemiologic studies because of reduced misclassification of participants according to intake estimates [10]

Laboratory Models The effects of nutrients and their interactions on carcinogenesis can be rigorously tested in animal models. Although the information derived from animal models must be extrapolated to humans with caution, it does provide important evidence for the biologic plausibility of relationships suggested by epidemiologic studies. The nutrient requirements of most laboratory animals have been precisely defined, and purified ingredients can be used to formulate diets for cancer studies. The rapid emergence of new animal models based on transgenic and knockout technology has provided new opportunities to examine interactions between specific genetic targets and dietary variables.[11]

PUBLIC HEALTH GUIDELINES FOR CANCER PREVENTION

We begin this section with a synthesis of public health dietary guidelines for cancer prevention published by several organizations including the American Cancer Society (ACS), American Institute of Cancer Research (AICR)/World Cancer Research Fund (WCRF), and the National Cancer Institute (NCI), The American Heart Association (AHA) and the American Diabetes Association (ADA).[1,2,4,12] The public health approach is a preventive strategy to decrease the overall disease incidence by reducing the adverse dietary habits of the entire population. Implementation of dietary recommendations requires cooperation among the media, food industry, nutritional scientists, public health personnel, medical practitioners, educators, and government agencies.[2,13] To achieve success, dietary recommendations must be clear as well as feasible and have minimal risk, low cost to society, and the potential to benefit many people.[2,13] Past efforts have been successful in the area of nutrition. For example, iron fortification of cereals benefits a large number of children and adult women, although risk is limited to a small number of individuals with hemochromatosis. Although much remains to be learned before the impact of the proposed recommendations on health can be precisely quantified, most experts agree that a number of dietary recommendations can be made with a reasonable degree of certainty, with the likelihood of minimal risk, and the potential for significant public health benefits.[2,3,13–15] The decision to formulate recommendations must take into account several factors, including strength of the evidence, potential benefits to society if the disease could be prevented, likelihood and severity of an adverse effect, and the feasibility of reducing exposure to the risk factor. In addition, economic issues, relative to the food and agricultural industry, are factors that may influence the decisions of committees to define nutritional guidelines. Table 26-1 summarizes current population-based dietary recommendations that together may lower the risk of chronic diseases, including cancer.[2,13,15–17]

Public Health Guidelines for Nutrition and Cancer Prevention: ***Maintain a Healthful Weight*** Increasingly, studies are documenting that obesity is a risk factor for human cancer.[18] Women with a body mass index (BMI) of greater than 25 kg/m^2, and men with a BMI greater than 27 kg/m^2 should make weight loss a priority. Weight loss of just 5 to 10% is associated with improved health and can reduce the incidence or severity of several diseases. Weight loss is best achieved by reducing total calorie consumption and increasing calorie expenditure to create a negative energy balance resulting in a modest, but consistent weight loss over time. Maximum weight loss of 1 to 2 pounds per week is appropriate for most people. Rapid weight loss achieved through fad diets does not encourage individuals to establish healthy eating patterns and weight loss is typically not maintained with these regimens. Regardless of adult weight, minimizing weight gain during adulthood is an important way to reduce cancer risk.[1,2,4,18]

Consume Five to Nine Servings of Fruits and Vegetables Each Day and a Variety of Whole Grains and Cereals It is estimated that widespread compliance with this recommendation could reduce cancer incidence by 20% (AICR). Several hundred studies have examined the relationships between fruit and vegetable intake and cancer risk.[2,14,16,19] The vast majority suggests a significant protective effect of a plant-based diet relative to cancer risk at many sites. Fruits and vegetables not only contain a diverse array of vitamins, minerals, fiber and phytochemicals, but they are lower in calories and fat than most other foods. A variety of fruits and vegetables should be included at every meal. Additionally, emphasis should be placed on consumption of whole-grain breads, cereals, and pastas that provide fiber, B vitamins, and a variety of phytochemicals. Consumption of refined carbohydrates should be limited. Foods rich in refined carbohydrate include cookies, pastries, candy, soda pop, and white bread. These foods contribute to a calorie-rich diet and are essentially devoid of nutrients.

Consume a Low-Fat Diet The role of dietary fat in cancer risk remains controversial and a convincing role for dietary fat, independent of other factors in human cancer, remains to be definitively demonstrated. Defining the contribution of dietary fat, and the different types of fat, in the etiology of many cancers, especially those of the breast, colon, pancreas, endometrium, and prostate, is an active area of investigation.[1,2,4,13,14,20] A significant reduction in fat can be achieved through the consumption of foods such as fruits, vegetables, and whole grains. The relationship between diets high in fat, especially saturated fat, and cardiovascular disease is well established. Most organizations recommend reducing total fat intake to 30% or less of total energy intake, with saturated fats representing less than 10% of total calories and dietary cholesterol limited to less than 300 mg/d.

For People Who Enjoy Red Meat, Moderate Portion Sizes Are Advisable Choose fresh meats more often than highly processed meats. Consumption of three ounces of red meat (beef, lamb, and pork) per day probably does not significantly contribute to overall cancer risk of a population, especially if meat does not displace consumption of fruits, vegetables, and whole grains. Choosing a variety of meats, including fresh chicken, fish, and turkey, is reasonable. Although relationships remain uncertain, diets rich in processed meat are associated with risk of several cancers, and thus should be consumed in moderation.[2] Meat that is cooked at very high temperatures, grilled, and charred favors the formation of certain types of chemical carcinogens and should be consumed in moderation.[2]

Participate in Physical Activity Daily and Moderate-to-Vigorous Intensity Exercise Several Days Each Week The energy expenditure associated with physical activity is a critical component of maintaining a healthy body weight and preventing adult weight gain associated with risk of several types of cancer.[1,2,4] A combination of daily physical activity and regular bouts of moderate-to-vigorous intensity exercise has been shown in many studies to reduce cancer risk independent of weight and diet.[21,22] Physical activity should be incorporated into activities of daily living in combination with regular moderate-to-vigorous intensity exercise on most days of the week.

Alcohol, If Consumed At All, Should Be Limited The risks and potential benefits of modest alcohol consumption remain a subject of debate. Although the health effects of specific types of alcoholic beverages is an active area of research, chronic consumption of alcohol is strongly associated with cancers of the oropharynx, larynx, and esophagus.[2,13] Tobacco smoking acts synergistically with alcohol in the pathogenesis of these cancers. Alcoholic beverages probably contribute to liver cancer, and may have a role in gastric, pancreatic, and colon cancers.[2] Even a moderate amount of daily alcohol consumption may slightly, but significantly, increase the risk of breast cancer.[23] Because there is some evidence that alcohol in moderation may reduce the risk of heart disease, individuals need to consider their personal health history when deciding whether or not to consume alcohol. For those who choose to drink, alcohol intake should be limited to one drink per day for women and two drinks per day for men.

Dietary Supplements Are Probably Unnecessary in the Context of a Healthy Diet An increasing proportion of the American population consumes some type of self-prescribed nutritional supplement on a regular basis. The public perceives nutrient supplements and alternative medications as an important form of self-therapy for the prevention and treatment of many ailments, including cancer.[1,2,4] Multivitamin and mineral supplements are usually inexpensive, easy to consume, relatively free of side effects when taken at the dosages approximating the recommended dietary allowance (RDA), and can be obtained without a prescription. There has been very little evidence in support of routine dietary supplements for population-wide cancer prevention. Although it is clear that Americans can achieve adequate nutrient intake by consuming a diet based on the above recommendations, a standard multivitamin/mineral supplement providing the recommended dietary allowance may be beneficial to some and entails minimal risk. Increasingly, supplements are being aggressively marketed that contain high concentrations of specific nutrients combined with other components such as herbals, extracts, and concentrates. Consumers should be aware that regulations regarding implied health claims and requirements for demonstrating safety and efficacy are minimal and the buyer should maintain skepticism and caution.

SUMMARY OF RESEARCH EFFORTS FOCUSING ON SPECIFIC CANCERS

It is unlikely that any food, nutrient, or dietary pattern will influence all cancers uniformly.[1,2,4] Thus, in reviewing the relationships between nutrition and cancer risk, it is important to examine the data for each tissue or organ separately. It is clear that research will continue to improve our ability to identify individuals at high risk of specific cancers based on genetic tests, family history, exposure to carcinogenic agents, and the presence of premalignant conditions. The future goal is to provide tailored dietary recommendations and chemopreventive strategies for individuals at risk. Additional research will define unique preventive strategies for various cancers. The following is a brief summary of the current understanding of relationships between diet, nutrition, and the risk of specific cancers.

Colon and Rectum Colorectal cancer is the second leading cause of cancer death in the United States, with 5% of the population predicted to develop cancer of the large bowel by the age of 75 years.[1,2,4] Genetic factors and premalignant conditions are being characterized that will define high-risk groups for chemoprevention and diet intervention studies that show promise in preclinical testing. The international variation in colorectal cancer is large (Figure 26-1), and although diagnostic differences may account for some of the international variation, it is unlikely to account for the greater than tenfold variations that are observed between nations.[2] The lower rates in Japan suggest that cultural and lifestyle variables rather than industrialization are the critical factors.[2,24,25] Dramatic increases in incidence among Japanese and Chinese migrants to the United States[26] clearly indi-

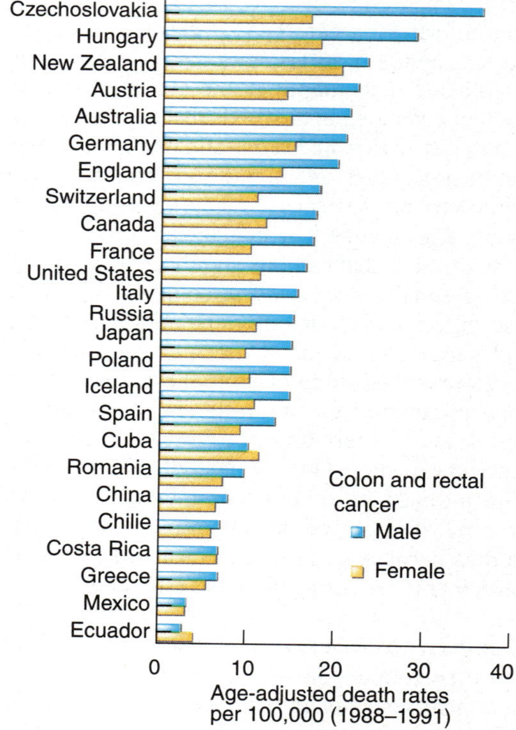

Figure 26-1 Age-adjusted death rates per 100,000 population from colon and rectal cancer in selected countries. (Adapted from Boring CC, Squires TS, Tong T, Montgomery S. Cancer Statistics, 1994. CA Cancer J Clin 1994;44:7.)

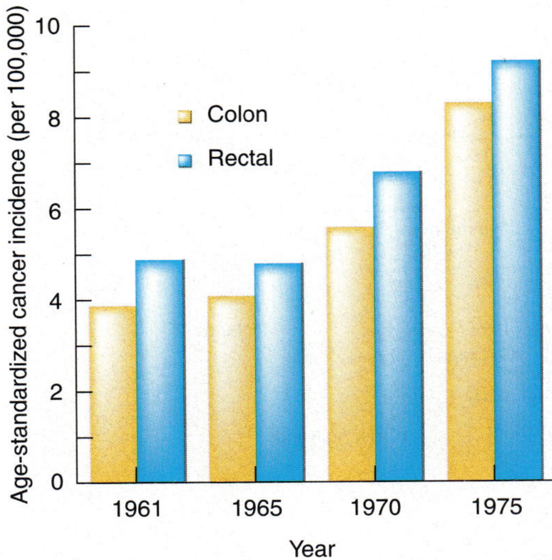

Figure 26-2 Age-standardized colon and rectal cancer incidence per 100,000 men in Japan from 1960 through 1977.

cate that international variations primarily result from environmental influences rather than genetic background.[27,28] Examination of time trends in colorectal cancer incidence, particularly in Japan since the 1940s, strongly suggests major contributions from lifestyle factors associated with westernization of their culture (Figure 26-2).[1,2,27,29]

Energy Balance and Physical Activity Energy intake, metabolic efficiency, physical activity, and various measures of body size or obesity are intimately interrelated. It is difficult to quantitate or ascertain the role of each component in colon cancer risk without considering them as a group. An inverse association between physical activity and risk of colon cancer has been consistently reported.[1,2,21,26,30–33] Several studies have found an association between BMI and elevated risk of colon cancer in men, although this relationship is weaker among women.[28,34–37] These associations between obesity and inactivity with risk of colon cancer have been observed in several countries (United States, China, Sweden, and Japan), among men and women, and for both occupational and recreational activities. Obesity is also directly associated with risk of colon adenoma.[38] Some evidence suggests that height (perhaps a proxy of the net energy intake during childhood and adolescence) also is related to a higher risk of colon cancer.[39–41] Studies in rodent models of colon carcinogenesis have reported enhanced tumorigenesis with greater *ad libitum* intake[42] and reduced risk with restricted intake.[43] Overall, the evidence is convincing that physical activity and appropriate energy balance will decrease risk of colon cancer.[44]

Dietary Lipid and Meats The relationship between total fat intake, fat saturation, or different sources of fat and risk of colon cancer remains an active area of research, but definitive conclusions are not yet possible.[1,2] Food consumption data from geographically defined populations show striking correlations between estimated fat intake, especially saturated fat, and colorectal cancer incidence.[45–47] Many [1,2,26,48–50] but not all studies report a positive association between dietary fat and risk of colon cancer. Most of these studies also show a direct association between total energy intake and risk of colon cancer, which is not surprising, given the high correlation between fat and energy intake. A population-based case-control study suggests that dietary fat accounts for 60% of colorectal cancer risk among Chinese migrants to the United States (Figure 26-3). The relative risk of a high-fat diet, however, depends on the level of physical activity and on gender. Other cohort studies report that fat from red meats rather than total fat, may increase colon cancer risk,[35,49,51,52] whereas a recent study suggested that regular consumption of red meat for at least ten years significantly increases risk of colon cancer.[53] Thus, moderation in lipids and meats should be considered for those at risk of colorectal cancer.

Fruits, Vegetables, and Fiber Diets rich in plant products, particularly grains and vegetables, are often associated with a lower risk of colon cancer and many have postulated that the fiber content is a major mediating factor.[1,2,13,21,45,49,50,54-57] The chemistry of dietary fiber is exceptionally complex, and unfortunately, the quantitative and qualitative assessment of fiber intake in human studies is very difficult. However, the majority of studies suggest a diet rich in diverse fiber-containing foods may be beneficial. A meta-analysis of case-control studies of colon cancer found a combined odds ratio (OR) of 0.58 between the highest and lowest quintiles on the basis of fiber intake but an even stronger OR of 0.48 on the basis of vegetable consumption.[57] The European Prospective Investigation into Cancer (EPIC) study also found a 40% reduction in colon cancer risk for the highest quintile versus the lowest quintile of dietary fiber intake in over 500,000 individuals.[58] A few intervention trials using very specific sources of dietary fiber have been undertaken thus far, the results are equivocal.[59–62]

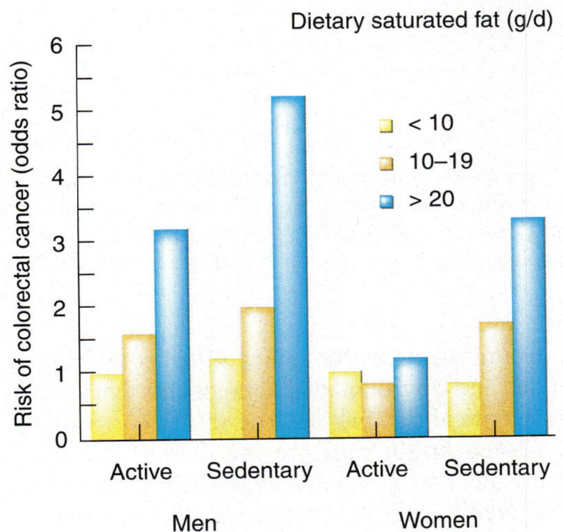

Figure 26-3 The risk of colorectal cancer in Chinese migrants to the United States according to dietary fat intake and level of physical activity. (Reproduced with permission from Whittemore AS, Wu-Williams AH, Lee M, et al., Diet, physical activity and colorectal cancer among Chinese in North America and China. J Natl Cancer Inst, 1990;82:915–26.)

Alcohol and Folate A positive association between alcohol intake and risk of colon cancer [1,2]is consistent among many ecologic, cohort, and population-based case-control studies.[1,2,29,63] Alcohol is also related to higher risk of colorectal adenoma.[1,2,64,65] Overall, the effects seem to be related more to total alcohol intake rather than to the source of alcohol.[1,2] Studies suggest that the elevated risk associated with alcohol occur predominantly in the rectum or distal colon.[52] Recent studies indicate that high intakes of folate or methionine, both of which are crucial for normal methyl group metabolism and, particularly, deoxyribonucleic acid (DNA) methylation, appears to mitigate the influence of alcohol. The risk of colorectal adenoma and cancer was elevated in individuals with high intakes of alcohol and low intakes of methionine and folate.[66,67] This suggests that alcohol, which has a well-known adverse effect on methyl group metabolism, increases the risk of colorectal cancer via this mechanism.

Carcinogens and Cooking Methods Variations in food preparation may lead to a different pattern or concentration of pyrolysis products in food. A number of mutagenic pyrolysis products are produced during cooking, and several have been found to be carcinogenic in laboratory animals, even if very few have been found to be specific for the colon.[1,2,68] Heterocyclic amines are one class of potent carcinogens formed during the cooking of meat, particularly under conditions of high temperature for prolonged periods of time.[69] Well-done grilled red meat was recently associated with the risk of colorectal adenomas.[69] Other investigations have focused on the production of mutagens within the digestive tract as a result of bacterial metabolism.[68] Human feces contain substances that are mutagenic in bacterial test systems,[68] and correlational studies indicate that fecal mutagenicity is greater in populations that are at high risk for colorectal cancer.[70] Human subjects fed a high-risk diet rich in protein, fat, energy, and animal products showed greater concentrations of fecal mutagens than did those fed a low-risk diet.[71]

In summary, increased risk of colorectal cancer is strongly associated with a physically inactive lifestyle, and an affluent dietary pattern, which is rich in high-fat foods (especially from animal products) and low in fruits, whole grain products, and, vegetables.[1,2,4] The individual contributions of alcohol, energy intake, folate, methionine, meats, and specific fiber components require further investigation.[1,2,4] The potential interactions among these components and other factors contributing to risk, such as exercise and genetics, are numerous. At present, it is prudent to consider the combined impact of the total diet and physical activity when making recommendations for colon cancer prevention rather than focusing on a single factor.

BREAST CANCER

Cancer of the breast is most common in the affluent nations of North America and Western Europe, and much less common in many parts of Asia and Africa,[1,2] and like colorectal cancer, we observe that migrants from low-risk nations show increasing risk after moving to a high-risk nation,[1,2,13,27,46,54] particularly in succeeding generations. This observation suggests that nutritional or other environmental factors active during youth and adolescence may have a long-term and major impact on subsequent risk of breast cancer.[1,2,4] The risk of breast cancer is influenced by multiple factors that are difficult to modify, however a number of dietary and nutritional factors characteristic of an affluent culture have been proposed to enhance risk of breast cancer and are briefly summarized.[1,2,13,44,46,54,72,73]

Energy Balance, Weight, and Obesity The role of energy intake as a stimulator of mammary carcinogenesis has been well established by rodent studies using diet or energy restriction,[74,75] or by regression analysis of *ad libitum* feeding.[42,76] Higher body weight or BMI in women is associated with greater risk;[2,77] furthermore, adult weight gain is associated independently of body weight with enhanced risk of postmenopausal breast cancer.[78,79] Overall, higher levels of adult physical activity seem to be associated with a modest protection against breast cancer risk and the protective effect may also be independent of BMI or weight gain as an adult.[80,81] However, the precise relationships between energy intake, energy expenditure, anthropometrics, and risk of breast cancer must be examined for different critical periods in a woman's life cycle. The effects of these factors may vary during adolescence, the reproductive years, and the postmenopausal period.

Dietary Fat The controversy concerning the contribution of dietary fat to risk of breast cancer can best be appreciated through examination of the representative data presented in Figure 26-4. Geographic studies show strong correlations between national rates of breast cancer and the estimated per capita fat consumption.[82,83] There are wide international variations in breast cancer rates as well as per capita fat consumption or the percentage of calories derived from fat. Breast cancer rates have been observed to increase significantly in populations migrating from low-risk areas, such as Japan, where diets were traditionally low in fat, to high-risk areas, such as the United States, where populations consume diets rich in fat.[27,54] Time-trend studies also support a dietary fat and breast cancer association. Within Japan, estimates of per capita daily fat intake have risen over the decades following World War II. During this period, breast cancer mortality increased in Japan by more than 30%. Correlation does not prove cause and effect, and many investigators argue that fat intake may be an

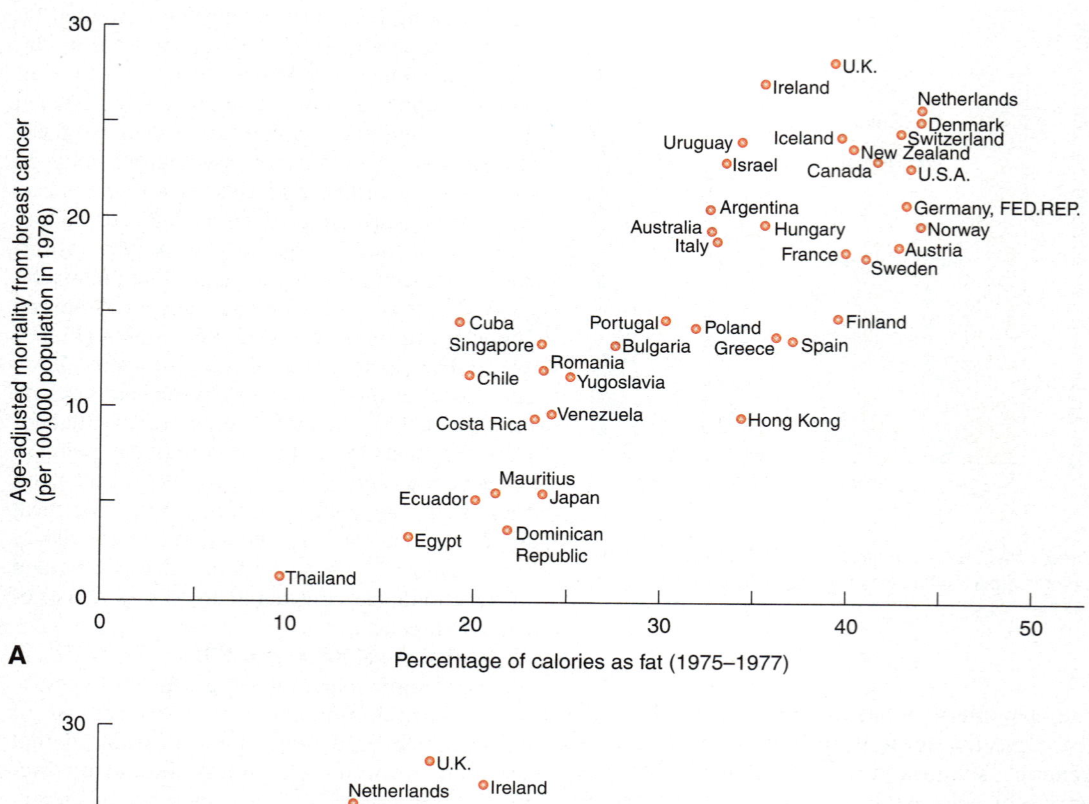

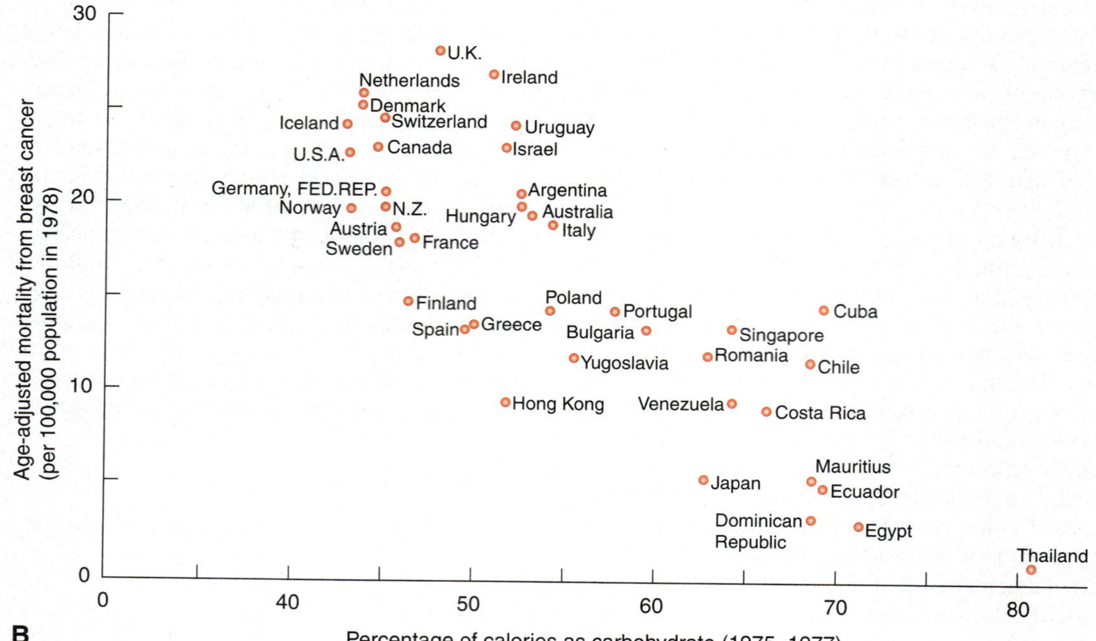

Figure 26-4 International correlation of **A,** estimated dietary fat intake (percentage of calories as fat) and **B,** estimated carbohydrate intake (percentage of calories as carbohydrate) and age-adjusted breast cancer mortality. (Reproduced with permission from Carroll KK. Carbohydrate and cancer. In: Alfin-Slater RB, Kritchevsky D, editors. In human nutrition. A comprehensive treatise. Vol 7. Cancer and nutrition. New York: Plenum; 1991. p.97.)

indicator of some other unidentified combination of diet and environmental components that are the truly critical risk factors. The strong correlations observed might indicate the overall effect of many dietary factors that change simultaneously. The relationship between fat intake and risk of breast cancer has been examined in many case-control studies with inconsistent results.[2,84] Prospective cohort studies have not provided compelling evidence for the high dietary fat/breast cancer association.[1,2,48] In the largest cohort study, the Nurses' Health Study,[85] there was no significant relationship between a low fat diet or specific types of fat and breast cancer risk. Although the epidemiologic data have not provided definitive results concerning dietary fat and breast cancer, accumulated evidence from more than 100 animal studies using chemical carcinogens, hormones, irradiation, or viruses to induce breast cancer indicate that as a single variable, fat enhances mammary carcinogenesis (Figure 26-5).[2,42,76,86] Overall, the possibility that achievable reductions in fat intake during adulthood will cause an appreciable reduction in breast cancer risk remains uncertain; several intervention trials are ongoing to evaluate low fat

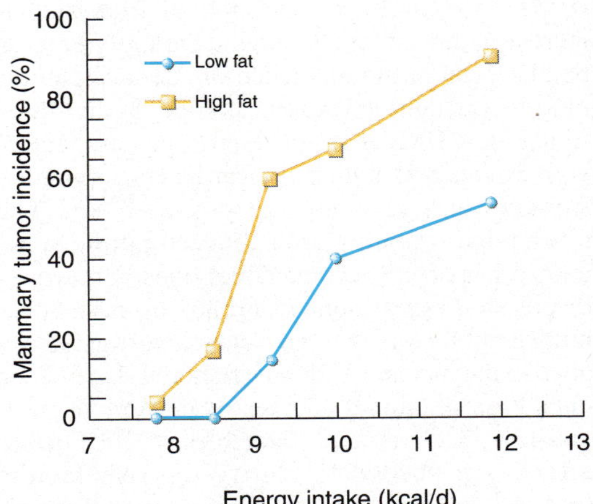

Figure 26-5 The effects of low-and high-fat diets at different levels of caloric intake on spontaneous mammary tumorigenesis in C3H female mice. (Adapted from Tannenbaum A. The dependence of tumor formation on the composition of the calorie-restricted diet as well as on the degree of restriction. Cancer Res 1945;5:616–25.)

dietary patterns on breast cancer risk. For example, the WINS Trial, a secondary prevention study, recently reported a significant 24% reduction in breast cancer recurrence after a median follow-up of 5 years in women assigned to a low fat (average = 33 ± 17 grams per day) dietary pattern compared to controls consuming a higher fat diet (average = 51 ± 24 grams per day) calories from fat.[87]

Alcohol Use Recent reviews of the accumulated evidence concerning alcohol intake and risk of breast cancer suggest a positive association.[1,2,88–90] The relative risk (RR) from the consumption of one typical serving of beer, wine, or liquor (approximately 12 g of ethanol) per day is estimated to be 1.4, whereas three drinks per day approximately doubles the risk. A recent meta-analysis that pooled studies from Canada, The Netherlands, Sweden, and the United States found a linear relationship between breast cancer risk and each 10 g increase in daily alcohol consumption.[23]

Other Dietary Factors Overall, plant-based diets rich in vegetables, fruits and grains may contribute to an overall dietary pattern associated with a decrease in the risk of breast cancer,[1,2] but a specific role for selected fruits and vegetables has not been observed.[91,92] There are no consistent relationships for the consumption of specific vitamins or minerals and breast cancer risk, and recommendations regarding supplement use for prevention remain to be defined.[2] Other bioactive compounds found in the diet, such as soy isoflavones, lignins, and fiber, may play a role in breast cancer, but evidence remains insufficient for recommendations.[1,2,4] In summary, the most well-established recommendations for breast cancer prevention are to consume a plant-based dietary pattern, engage in vigorous physical activity on a regular basis, avoid or limit intake of alcoholic beverages, and minimize lifetime weight gain through physical activity and energy restriction.

Prostate Cancer Cancer of the prostate is one of the most frequently diagnosed malignancies in American men, and it is especially common among the African American population.[2,93,94] Prostate cancer is a disease of aging men and the international distribution of prostate cancer is similar to that of colon and breast cancer; therefore, it correlates with affluent dietary patterns.[2,93] Relationships between diet and prostate cancer are not clearly defined and specific recommendations to prevent the disease remain speculative. A role for weight gain, energy balance, and activity is suggested by some human studies and clearly demonstrated in rodent studies.[2,18,93,95–97] International and intra-country correlational studies suggest associations between prostate cancer mortality and the per capita intake of total fat.[2,93] Similarly, several analytic epidemiologic studies and case control studies have reported associations between total fat or the consumption of high-fat foods and prostate cancer,[2,93] particularly saturated fats from animal products.[2,93,95,96,98,99]

Several studies suggest that the antioxidant nutrients, vitamin E and selenium, may influence prostate cancer risk. The most provocative data is derived from a randomized intervention trial with vitamin E conducted in Finland among men at high risk of lung cancer.[100] A significantly lower risk of prostate cancer was noted among men randomized to vitamin E supplementation.[100] The possible role of selenium in the prevention of prostate cancer has been hypothesized on the basis of an ongoing chemoprevention study designed to examine the effects of supplemental selenium on recurrence of skin cancer in populations of geographic areas having low soil selenium. Selenium supplementation did not influence the risk of skin cancer, although supplementation was associated with a nonsignificant reduction in all-cause mortality and a statistically significant reduction in total cancer mortality and risk of prostate cancer.[101] A protective effect was also suggested by a study reporting that low concentrations of toenail selenium are related to a greater risk of prostate cancer.[102] Additional studies designed to further investigate the hypothesis that vitamin E and selenium can prevent prostate cancer are ongoing including the largest prostate cancer chemoprevention trial to date, the Selenium and Vitamin E Chemoprevention Trial (SELECT), which began randomizing 33,000 men in the fall of 2001.

The overall consumption of fruits and vegetables has not shown a consistent reduction in risk of prostate cancer.[2,93] However, a reduced risk of prostate cancer associated with the consumption of tomatoes and processed tomato products has been observed in the prospectively evaluated Health Professional's Follow-up Study.[103–106] On the basis of these findings, it has been hypothesized that the carotenoid lycopene may account for some of the anticancer properties of tomato products although other compounds found in tomato foods may also be important.[107–110] Lycopene is the potent antioxidant carotenoid providing the red color to tomato products and is hypothesized to have anticancer properties.[93] Blood lycopene concentrations obtained prior to diagnosis are inversely related to the risk of prostate cancer.[111,112] However, it is premature to conclude that lycopene mediates a protective effect against prostate cancer or that lycopene is the only component of tomato products that may contribute to the association.

The possibility that calcium, phosphorus, and vitamin D are interacting components of a complex network of dietary and endocrine factors modulating prostate cancer risk is under investigation.[113] Several studies suggest that men consuming diets rich in calcium, either from foods or supplements, experience an increased risk of prostate cancer.[113,114] Prostate cells express vitamin D receptors and exposure to a ligand tends to induce differentiation pathways. Although uncertain at present, these findings warrant additional investigation.

In summary, epidemiologic studies and a limited number of laboratory investigations suggest a role for diet in prostate cancer. Rates of prostate cancer are higher in nations consuming an affluent dietary pattern and sedentary lifestyle, although the contributions of specific components, such as fat and energy intake, are not well defined. The possibility that selenium, vitamin E, calcium, vitamin D, tomatoes, soy, and other dietary factors influence the risk of prostate cancer are being actively investigated.

Lung Cancer Lung cancer is currently the most common worldwide malignancy and the leading cause of cancer-related death.[2] Cigarette smoking accounts for the vast majority of cases and incidence rates continue to climb in parallel with the globalization of cigarette manufacturing, marketing, and advertising.[2,115] Certain occupational exposures, such as to asbestos or radiation, may act synergistically with cigarette smoking to increase the risk.[115] Compared with the role of tobacco, the potential contribution of diet and nutrition is relatively trivial. However, the inverse relationship between the greater intake of fruits and vegetables and lower risk of lung cancer has been a frequent finding in human nutritional epidemiology.[2,116,117] Many hypothesized that β-carotene found in fruits and vegetables or vitamin A derived from cleavage of β-carotene may be the critical active agents in these foods.[2,118] However, two randomized controlled intervention trials in high-risk population found no reduction, and perhaps an increase, in the incidence of lung cancer among male smokers after several years of supplementation with β-carotene at 20 or 30 mg/d.[119] These reports emphasize that protective benefits of diets rich in fruits and vegetables probably involve many interacting components and will not be reproduced by providing a single agent. A number of other nutrients including vitamin E, selenium, vitamin C, fat, soy, and retinoids are undergoing continuing evaluation regarding a protective role against lung cancer[2,120]; however, their roles remain uncertain. Overall, elimination of cigarette smoking and occupational risk factors will have the greatest impact on decreasing the incidence of lung cancer. Among high-risk individuals, the frequent consumption of a diverse array of fruits, vegetables and other plant foods may provide some degree of protection against lung cancer.

Oral Cavity, Larynx, and Oropharynx Cancers Like lung cancer, cancers of the oral cavity and the larynx are strongly related to the use of tobacco products.[1,2,4] Case-control studies completed over several decades have documented associations between the consumption of alcoholic beverages and cancers of these tissues. A dose–response relationship of alcohol and oral cancer, independent of tobacco usage, has been observed in a number of studies (Figure 26-6).[121] Additional evidence is derived from studies of populations, such as alcoholics, who exhibit increased risk, and Seventh-Day Adventists and Mormons in the United States, who abstain from alcohol and have a much lower risk.[122,123] It is of interest that feeding pure alcohol as part of a nutritionally sound diet does not produce oral cancers in experimental animals. The extent that this represents biochemical differences between man and rodents, the lack of a direct carcinogenic effect of ethanol, the presence of carcinogens in alcoholic beverages consumed by man, the passive inhalation of ambient tobacco smoke in the places where ethanol is consumed, or the importance of other interacting carcinogens and nutritional deficits must be further evaluated. Both epidemiologic and laboratory studies provide convincing evidence supporting a protective role for diets rich in fruits and vegetables.[2,34] In addition, clinical and laboratory investigation has suggested that vitamin A and analogues or metabolites, as well as certain carotenoids, may serve as inhibitors of carcinogenesis in the oral and respiratory epithelia. In summary, tobacco products are major contributors to cancers of the mouth and pharynx, especially in conjunction with the consumption of alcoholic beverages.[2] Further efforts to better define the role of vitamin A, synthetic retinoids, and other phytochemicals as possible chemopreventive agents for high-risk groups is warranted.

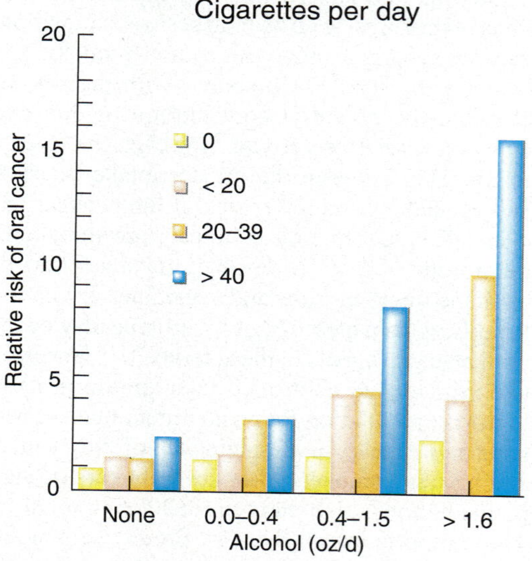

Figure 26-6 The interactions between alcohol intake and cigarette smoking on the relative risk of oral cancer. (Adapted from Rothman K, Keller A. The effect of joint exposure to alcohol and tobacco on risk of cancer of the mouth and pharynx. J Chron Dis 1972;25:711–16.)

Esophageal Cancer Squamous cell cancer of the esophagus is the eighth most common cancer worldwide and varies several-hundred-fold between nations and between geographic regions within nations.[2] The incidence is particularly high in an area extending from the southern border of the Caspian Sea in Iran across central Asia to China. The incidence of esophageal cancer in the United States is comparatively low. In most developed nations, correlational analyses and case-control studies indicate that the major risk factors are ethanol and cigarette smoking.[2,13,54] Risk increases in proportion to the amount of alcohol consumed.[2,124] A number of studies show an alcohol dose–response relationship after controlling for cigarette smoking, although the two factors may show a significant additive effect.[2] Increasing consumption of alcohol generally is associated with the marginal intake of many nutrients, which is thought to predispose individuals to greater risk. For example, alcohol may interact with folate, vitamin B_{12}, and methyl group metabolism to modulate risk.[125] A number of studies suggest an inverse relationship between risk of esophageal cancer and the consumption of fresh fruits and vegetables.[2,116,126] In certain parts of Asia where alcohol consumption does not explain the high risk for esophageal cancer, there may be a relationship between esophageal cancer and the indigenous diet which is low in fresh fruits, vegetables, and animal products, and the estimated intakes of vitamin A, vitamin C, riboflavin, zinc, and several trace elements, such as molybdenum, frequently are cited as being low as well.[2,127,128] In summary, cigarette smoking and alcohol consumption are the most important etiologic factors in affluent nations. The possibility that marginal intakes of one or more nutrients may contribute to risk in affluent populations has been suggested but not firmly established. The most important protective dietary intervention is the frequent consumption of fruits and vegetables.[2]

Adenocarcinoma of the Esophagus and Gastric Cardia The incidence of adenocarcinoma of the distal esophagus and gastric cardia have been increasing rapidly over the last two decades in the United States and Western Europe.[129,130] Among white men, adenocarcinoma of the distal esophagus has increased more than 350% since the mid-1970s.[131] Current or past cigarette smoking may be one of the contributing factors.[131,132] However, one of the most consistent observations has been a positive association between risk and body mass index (BMI).[129] As the prevalence of obesity has increased in the United States, a parallel trend can be observed in the incidence of adenocarcinoma of the esophagus and gastric cardia.[130] One study found that BMI was more strongly associated with esophageal and gastric cardia cancer in nonsmokers and younger age groups.[133,134] The mechanism remains under investigation; however, it has been speculated that obesity may predispose to gastroesophageal reflux disease. Other nutritional factors that have been investigated relative to the increased adenocarcinoma risk include diets high in animal sources of fat, low in fiber, and low in fruits and vegetables.[135,136] Further efforts are needed to clarify the risk factors responsible for the dramatic increase in the incidence of adenocarcinoma of the esophagus and to devise effective intervention strategies.

Stomach Cancer Gastric cancer is the second most common cancer worldwide.[137] The incidence varies dramatically among countries and is highest in parts of Asia (eg, Japan) and South America. A dramatic decrease in the incidence of stomach cancer in many affluent nations has been documented over the last century. In the United States, the current rate is among the lowest in the world, whereas in 1930, gastric cancer was the most frequently diagnosed malignancy in Americans.[66] In recent years, investigators have identified a divergent incidence pattern for cancers of the gastric cardia and distal stomach, which suggests different etiologies. Adenocarcinomas of the cardia are typically grouped etiologically with those arising from the metaplastic distal esophagus showing a similar histology and may share risk factors.

The efforts to identify the causes of stomach cancer have proceeded in several major directions: (1) the protective role of diets rich in fruit and vegetables; (2) the benefits of vitamin C; (3) the protective effects of modern food processing and storage, thereby reducing spoilage and the use of salt-curing, pickling, and nitrates for preservation;[2,132,138,139] (4) the role of *Helicobacter pylori* infection and interactions with dietary factors;[138–140] (5) identification of natural carcinogens or precursors such as nitrates, found in foods; (6) the production of carcinogens during grilling or barbecuing of meats; and (7) the synthesis of carcinogens from dietary precursors in the stomach. These concepts are briefly reviewed.

Populations consuming abundant quantities of fresh fruits and vegetables experience a significantly lower risk of stomach cancer and efforts to identify components of these foods that have protective properties are underway.[2,116,141] The potentially active ingredients include, provitamin A carotenoids, tocopherols, vitamin C, and other bioactive phytochemicals.[2,142] The data regarding a protective effect for vitamin C have been more thoroughly investigated with the majority of case-control studies, cohort studies, or investigations of plasma ascorbic acid suggesting benefits for vitamin C.[2] However, intervention studies with vitamin C supplements have not yet demonstrated chemopreventive activity. Epidemiologic studies have consistently identified an increased risk associated with greater consumption of salt, which is used in many cultures as a preservative of dried meats and pickled vegetables.[2] Heating meats to high temperatures produces polycyclic aromatic hydrocarbons and other carcinogens found in high quantities in grilled, charbroiled, and smoke-cured meats.[143] For example, the quantity of polycyclic aromatic hydrocarbons in a large, well-done charbroiled steak is equivalent to that found in the smoke of 600 cigarettes.[143] Subpopulations at high risk for gastric cancer in Iceland, Hungary, and Latvia were found to have greater exposure to polycyclic aromatic hydrocarbons in smoked meats.[144] Continuing efforts are directed toward the identification of dietary factors that may accentuate the endogenous production of mutagens such as nitrosamines found in food or produced in the stomach from precursors.[1,2,54] Many nitrosamines are stomach carcinogens in experimental animals, and several studies have suggested an association between increased levels of nitrate in the diet or drinking water and risk of gastric cancer.[54,138]

Liver Cancer Primary hepatocellular carcinoma is very rare in the United States and Northern Europe. In contrast, it is one of the most frequent types of cancer in the developing nations of sub-Saharan Africa and Asia, and is now ranked as the third most common cancer worldwide.[2] Hepatitis B and C infections appear to be the major etiologic factors in many high-risk areas, where the carrier state imparts an RR of approximately 200-fold.[145] Contamination of foods with carcinogenic fungal products, such as certain aflatoxins, also may contribute to risk in some populations.[13,54,146] Aflatoxins are found in geographic areas where food processing and storage are not optimal. Groups with high aflatoxin exposure often have high rates of hepatitis B infection, parasitic infections, and nutritional deficiencies, which may interact to determine risk. In low-risk nations, the regular and high consumption of alcohol is an important dietary factor in the pathogenesis of liver cancer.[1,2,45,96,124,147] The data also suggest that other cofactors may act in an additive or synergistic fashion.[148] It has been hypothesized that liver cancer primarily occurs in those whose cumulative experiences with ethanol, viral hepatitis, and toxin exposure lead to cirrhosis. The cellular and molecular events that are associated with cirrhosis and formation of regenerative nodules that may participate in the initiation and progression to cancer are under investigation.

Pancreatic Cancer Pancreatic cancer is frequently detected at an advanced stage and thus is highly lethal. Cigarette smoking has been firmly established as one etiologic factor.[1,2,4] The RR of smoking at least a pack per day is approximately four-fold, compared with that of nonsmokers.[2] A rapid reduction in risk over the first 2 years associated with quitting smoking could potentially eliminate 25% of deaths from pancreatic cancer.[149] Descriptive studies have suggested associations between an increased risk for pancreatic cancer and a number of components that are characteristic of the affluent diet, such as meat, fat, protein, eggs, milk, and alcohol.[2,13,45,54,150] In contrast, the majority of epidemiologic studies suggest that the frequent consumption of fruits and vegetables may reduce the risk of pancreatic cancer.[2,116] Excess energy intake, low physical activity, and obesity are positively associated with pancreatic cancer risk,[151] and are supported by animal models where dietary restriction produces acinar cell atrophy, reduces DNA synthesis,[152] and inhibits experimental pancreatic carcinogenesis.[153] Furthermore, a diet high in glycemic load may increase risk of pancreatic cancer, particularly in those with elevated body mass index or with low physical activity.[154] The evidence is most consistent with the conclusion that coffee has little contribution to the risk of pancreatic cancer.[2]

Endometrial Cancer In general, endometrial cancer shows an international distribution similar to that of other cancers of affluence, such as breast, colon, and prostate cancers. Evidence for association between endometrial cancer and excess energy intake and obesity continues to accumulate.[1,2,18,54,96] The role of fruits and vegetables in decreasing the risk of endometrial cancer is supported by data from some studies.[2,155] At the present time, the most appropriate guidance is to avoid obesity through reduced energy consumption and regular physical exercise coupled with a diet rich in fruits, vegetables, and grains.

Ovarian Cancer There are considerable international and geographic variations in the incidence and mortality rates of ovarian cancer. The disease is more common in nations exhibiting Western culture, especially among the higher socioeconomic groups.[1,2,54] Although some of the geographic variation may result from reproductive variables, there are suggestive relationships to dietary components.[13,54,156] At present, no conclusive role for dietary components in the pathogenesis of ovarian cancer has been established, but additional studies are needed, particularly in conjunction with known risk factors of low parity and specific inherited genetic abnormalities.[2]

Bladder Cancer Bladder cancer is more frequent in industrialized nations, especially among smokers and those in urban areas and of lower socioeconomic status.[2,45,116,157,158] The majority of epidemiologic and case-control studies support the hypothesis that the frequent consumption of fruits and vegetables will reduce risk.[2,116,157,159] A diet rich in cruciferous vegetables such as broccoli, but not other classes of fruits and vegetables, has been associated with a significantly reduced bladder cancer risk in both smokers and nonsmokers among 47,000 men enrolled in the Health Professional's Follow-Up Study (HPFS).[159] The role of fluid intake in bladder cancer risk has frequently been proposed.[2,160] The prospective evaluation of fluid intake found a significant inverse association between total daily fluid intake and bladder cancer risk, with no evidence for a benefit or risk from specific sources of fluid.[160] Laboratory studies have found that the nonnutritive sweeteners cyclamates and saccharine may be weak initiators or promoters of bladder carcinogenesis in rodents, but their contribution to human cancer probably is very small.[2,13,54] Although some studies suggest an association between coffee consumption and bladder cancer most of the investigations do not support a meaningful relationship.[2,13]

CURRENT RESEARCH

Specific Foods, Nutrients, and Dietary Components Frequently Associated with Cancer Prevention Many people at risk of cancer focus their attention on specific foods or nutrients in part because of the extensive marketing of products and publicity generated by the popular press. This tendency is facilitated by the news media when science reporters publicize results of single studies or preliminary findings, often confusing readers with contradictory and conflicting results. The following section briefly summarizes data regarding selected food components or nutrients and might assist the medical practitioner in responding to specific inquiries from individuals.

Vitamins **Vitamin A** Vitamin A is essential for the normal growth and development of epithelial tissues. Vitamin A deficiency is common in many parts of the developing world, but is extremely rare in Americans. Vitamin A is provided in the diet as retinol and its esters, primarily from milk and organ meats, and as β-carotene and a few other provitamin A carotenoids in yellow and leafy green vegetables. A protective effect of consuming foods rich in vitamin A has been hypothesized for several types of cancer [1,2,13,54,116,161] at this time, however, there is no clear evidence that vitamin A supplementation will decrease the risk of cancer in populations or individuals consuming a healthy diet. Although many studies in laboratory models indicate that vitamin A deficiency increases the susceptibility of tissues to chemical carcinogenesis, these observations do not support the concept that a lower risk will be observed by excessive supplementation in persons with adequate vitamin A status. The use of vitamin A and synthetic retinoids as pharmacologic agents in chemoprevention trials to determine their efficacy in specific high-risk populations is an important area of translational research.[162]

Vitamin D In contrast to many nutrients, comparatively little effort has focused on the role of vitamin D in human cancer,[13,161] but several studies suggest a relationship between lower vitamin D intake and colon cancer.[13,95,163] Cancer cells derived from many human tumors express the receptor for 1,25-dihydroxy vitamin D3 and respond to this agent in vitro, but the pathophysiologic significance in human cancer remains to be determined.[161] There are vitamin D analogues in development that do not have hypercalcemic effects, but which continue to interact with receptors on many cancer cells. These compounds may lead to the development of novel chemopreventive or therapeutic agents.

Vitamin E Vitamin E is a family of eight compounds that are collectively referred to as *tocopherols*. Vegetable oil, eggs, and whole grains are the major sources of dietary vitamin E. The antioxidant and free radical scavenger properties of vitamin E suggest a possible role as an antineoplastic vitamin;[161] however, few rodent or epidemiologic studies provide strong evidence to support the consumption of vitamin E supplements to prevent cancer.[164] Additional studies focusing on cancers of the lung, cervix, and prostate are particularly worthy of additional investigation. An NCI funded national effort evaluating the ability of selenium or vitamin E to prevent prostate cancer is underway and should help to elucidate the role of vitamin E in prostate cancer prevention.

Vitamin C Vitamin C, which includes ascorbic acid and dehydroascorbic acid, functions as a water-soluble antioxidant and a component of several enzymatic reactions in intermediary metabolism. Citrus fruits, leafy vegetables, tomatoes, and potatoes are rich sources of vitamin C. Despite the large volume of publications in the last decade, very little evidence supports a critical role of vitamin C in the etiology of most human cancers.[13,54,161] Supplement studies, although few in number, have failed to show a reduced risk of cancer.[165] Some provocative evidence concerns the ability of vitamin C to inhibit the formation of carcinogenic nitrosamines, which ultimately may reduce the incidence of cancers that are thought to be associated with nitrosamines, such as gastric cancer. At present, there is no evidence to suggest that consumption of vitamin C supplements at levels higher than can be achieved in a well-balanced diet containing ample fresh fruits and vegetables is useful in the prevention or treatment of human cancer.[2]

Folate Folate is an essential water-soluble B vitamin required for the normal metabolism of amino acids, methyl groups, and nucleotides and found in many vegetables, fruits, beans, and whole grains, and folic acid is found in fortified grain products in the United States.[166] Folate plays a role in the methylation of DNA, which may be critical for the normal regulation of gene expression and tissue differentiation. Epidemiologic and laboratory studies are beginning to accumulate evidence suggesting that insufficient folate may relate to the risk of several malignancies, particularly colon cancer.[2,14,99,167] Unlike many other nutrients, mild to moderate folate deficiency is relatively prevalent in the American population because of the consumption of a highly refined diet with poor intake of fruits and vegetables.

MINERALS **Calcium** Calcium is hypothesized to reduce the risk of colon cancer, but enhance the risk of prostate cancer. For example, a prospective, cohort study in the United States found that those who develop colon cancer had a significantly lower intake of calcium and vitamin D. Calcium supplementation of 1.2 g/d reduced the proliferative rate of colonic cells in patients who are considered to be at an increased risk of colon cancer.[168] Some laboratory studies report that calcium reduces the loss of superficial epithelial cells and the proliferation of basal crypt cells.[169] Several clinical trials to determine the effects of calcium supplementation on polyp formation are currently ongoing with initial reports suggesting a modest benefit. Conversely, calcium from dietary sources and from supplements has been demonstrated in at least two prospective studies to increase the risk of prostate cancer,[113,114] particularly cancers with more aggressive characteristics. At this time, it is appropriate to target calcium intake at RDA levels from a variety of food sources. The RDA is currently 1,000 mg/d for those ages 19 to 50 years and 1,200 mg/d for people older than age 50 years.

Selenium Selenium is a mineral required in the diet at very small concentrations with an RDA of 55 micrograms per day for both men and women. Grains, cereals, seafood, and meat are good sources of selenium. Selenium is an essential constituent of glutathione peroxidase, and it participates in the destruction of hydrogen peroxide and organic hydroperoxides, using reducing equivalents from glutathione. Selenium, thus, participates in cellular and tissue defense against oxidative damage. A major obstacle for epidemiologic studies is that estimates of dietary selenium intake are unreliable, especially in the developed nations where foods are extensively processed and shipped for long distances, because the selenium content of food is very sensitive to soil concentrations. An inverse association between the selenium levels in forage crops from different geographic areas or tissue selenium and mortality rates from certain cancers has been suggested.[2,13,101,102,170] A landmark human intervention trial reported that selenium supplements might reduce the risk of lung, colon, and prostate cancer.[101] However, larger randomized controlled trials are required to confirm and expand upon these findings. Overall, individuals choosing to consume a selenium supplement should be advised to consume the requirement of 55 μg per day and not more than 400 μg per day because there is a narrow margin between safe and potentially toxic dosages.

FOODS AND FOOD COMPONENTS **Soy Products** People living in countries such as Japan and China where soy foods are consumed regularly have a much lower risk of cancers of the breast, colon, and prostate than do people living in the United States where soy foods are not commonly consumed. However, many other variables in addition to soy probably contribute to the geographic variations. Soy foods contain several components, including soy protein, isoflavones, lignins, and saponins, which have been investigated for their anticancer effects in laboratory models.[171,172] Although many studies are currently underway, there is no convincing evidence that suggests the use of soy supplements, soy extracts, pure soy concentrates, or other soy components currently marketed, will significantly impact human cancer risk. Some concerns have been raised about the risks and benefits for soy consumption relative to breast or endometrial cancer. Several soy isoflavones have a chemical structure similar to estrogen and may bind to the estrogen receptor and act as weak estrogen. It is plausible that high amounts of phytoestrogens may actually increase cell proliferation, although this remains controversial. At this time it is probably prudent for women at high risk of breast cancer to avoid concentrated isoflavone supplements, but it is unlikely that moderate amounts of soy foods as part of a plant-based diet will increase cancer risk.[173]

β-Carotene Foods rich in β-carotene, such as many fruits and vegetables, are associated with a lower risk of cancer. However, recent intervention trials with β-carotene clearly question the validity of the hypothesis that the benefits of a plant-based diet can be produced through β-carotene supplements. Two large intervention studies of β-carotene demonstrated a higher risk of lung cancer in smokers.[119,174] Although β-carotene is a potential antioxidant and source of vitamin A, supplements should be discouraged for cancer prevention and dietary sources should be encouraged.

Lycopene and Other Carotenoids The bright red color of tomato products is caused by the nonprovitamin carotenoid lycopene. Interest in lycopene has emerged because many studies demonstrate that the consumption of tomato products is associated with a lower risk of several cancers, particularly prostate cancer.[105,106,108] However, at the present time it is prudent to consume tomato products as a source of lycopene and other phytochemicals rather than assume that the benefits will be achieved from the lycopene enriched extracts currently being aggressively marketed.

Omega-3 Fatty Acids, Fish Oil, and Olive Oil Diets rich in total fat have a high caloric density and contribute to excess energy intake and obesity. Thus, most healthy dietary patterns are lower in total fat than the current American pattern. However, the types of lipids may also have an impact on cancer. Fish is a rich source of omega-3 fatty acids that can influence cell biology through a number of mechanisms including modulation in the production of bioactive lipids such as prostaglandins and leukotrienes. Animal models suggest some benefits for cancers of the prostate and breast.[175] Olive oil has generated interest because of its lack of association with cancers in studies where total lipids, saturated fats, and other measures of lipid intake demonstrate positive associations. Like other lipids, olive oil contributes to caloric intake and risk of obesity, but can be used in certain recipes to replace other types of lipid that may have a greater association with cancer and cardiovascular disease. Overall, very little definitive data is available regarding lipid sources and human cancer risk and specific recommendations are not possible at this time.

Food Irradiation Americans are increasingly concerned about contamination of food by disease-causing microorganisms. Exposure of foods to irradiation is an effective means of sterilization and increasing the shelf life of foods. Contrary to misperceptions by much of the public, the food does not become a source of radiation, and the changes in the food appear to be minimal with no evidence that cancer risk is a concern.

Organic and Natural Foods Government regulators will continue to evaluate information and provide updated standards and recommendations to consumers regarding expectations when the term "organic" is used in food labeling. In general, the term refers to foods grown without the use of synthesized pesticides or herbicides, and has been expanded to include nongenetically manipulated foods. At the present time, there are no studies demonstrating that consuming organic foods will substantially lower cancer risk when compared to the same foods produced by standard farming practices.[1,2]

Pesticides, Herbicides, and Environmental Contaminants in Food Residues of pesticides and herbicides are found in low concentrations in fruits and vegetables. Overall, studies have not clearly defined cancer risks associated with exposure to these compounds at low concentrations and the preponderance of data supports the recommendation that fruits and vegetables should be consumed at greater concentrations. Additional concerns relate to the accumulation of some environmental toxins in meats, including fish, but without clear evidence of a cancer risk. Certainly, exposures to high concentrations of these compounds through industrial and agricultural exposures are associated with toxicity and concerns about cancer risk. Overall, regulatory agencies must continue to monitor agents and ensure safety at expected exposure levels.[1,2,4]

Artificial Sweeteners (Aspartame and Saccharin) Artificial sweeteners are the basis of many low-calorie foods currently marketed. No links between aspartame and cancer have been identified. Saccharin has been shown to slightly enhance the risk of bladder cancer in rodent studies when provided in concentrations that would greatly exceed that consumed by humans. Human epidemiologic studies have not identified saccharin consumption as a risk factor for human cancer.[1,2]

Sugar Highly refined simple sugars provide calories but without the nutrients associated with whole foods. Diets containing large amounts of simple sugars are frequently nutrient poor and might also contribute to promoting obesity and hormonal changes that could potentially increase cancer risk. However, sugars per se are not carcinogens, and a diet with a modest amount of sweets should not be a concern in the context of a healthy dietary pattern.[1,2]

Tea Investigations of green and black teas are currently underway to determine whether these products may have anticancer properties in humans to support data derived from laboratory studies. Thus far, tea has not been shown to lower the risk of any human cancer, but important studies are under way.[1,2]

SURVIVORSHIP: DIET AND NUTRITIONAL GUIDANCE DURING AND FOLLOWING CANCER TREATMENT

Although the focus of this chapter is diet and nutrition in the etiology and prevention of cancer, we briefly introduce the emerging field of diet and nutrition during cancer survivorship. "Survivorship" is now accepted as beginning at the time of cancer diagnosis and continuing throughout the life of the individual. Diet and nutrition may have a role in several components of cancer survivorship, including (1) enhancing the benefits of treatment and reducing the frequency or severity of acute treatment related toxicities; (2) promoting recovery during the immediate post-treatment phase; (3) support of patients suffering from cancer cachexia and during terminal phases of incurable or advanced cancers; and (4) promoting long-term survivorship by reducing the chance of recurrent disease, secondary prevention of cancer, and reducing the frequency and severity of late-complications of therapy and enhancing overall health and longevity. At current rates, more than 1.2 million Americans are diagnosed with cancer each year and more than 9 million are categorized as survivors. The need for scientifically based recommendations is now acute and has not keep pace with the desire of patients or survivors to obtain information on diet and nutrition. The American Cancer Society recently published a review of the field summarizing the state of research, providing guidelines for communicating with survivors.[176]

Diet and nutrition represents, for many cancer patients, an opportunity to counteract the profound sense of loss of control that accompanies cancer treatment. Quality of life is improved when patients feel that they are active participants in the course of their care. Unfortunately, scientific evidence to help a patient choose optimal diet and nutritional information is insufficient in most areas. Cancer survivors are faced with a bewildering array of sources of dietary information ranging from well-intended family and friends, to alternative health care providers, and those marketing products or selling publications touting dietary approaches. Coupled with the limited training and knowledge of nutrition by many health care providers, such as physicians and nurses, a survivor is frequently confused or easily misled. Although definitive and detailed guidelines are not possible at the present, the following provides a framework for communicating with patients and directing future survivorship research.

Active Treatment Phase Cancer treatment often includes surgery, radiation, chemotherapy, or biologic treatments, as well as combinations of approaches as multimodality interventions are established for a greater number of clinical scenarios. The key to guiding a patient undergoing therapy is to individualize the nutritional support. The care team should monitor individual needs through assessment of body weight, lean body mass, and the presence of eating or digestive impairments. Treatments for some cancers may compromise nutritional status caused by impairment of food intake, digestion, absorption, and metabolism of nutrients. For example, loss of appetite, nausea, vomiting, altered taste and smell perception, constipation, and diarrhea may transiently occur. Individually tailored interventions to nutritionally support a patient during these periods will enhance quality of life. In some patients, maintaining adequate energy intake is an obstacle and specific commercially prepared and tested nutritional products can easily be incorporated into a diet plan. Early referrals of patients at high risk for nutritional complications to trained nutritionists, particularly registered dietitians, can prevent the development of more severe malnutrition that may limit the ability of the medical team to provide the optimal treatment intensity.[176]

The use of nutritional supplements during therapy is controversial and few studies have been conducted to provide detailed guidance. For example, vitamin supplements with high dosages of antioxidants (vitamins C or E, selenium, etc) during chemotherapy or radiation therapy are considered by some clinicians to potentially reduce the efficacy of treatments that may depend on oxidative stress in the cancer cell as the mechanism of action. However, others suggest that antioxidant supplements may provide a benefit to patients by limiting damage to normal tissues such as bone marrow. In general, it is prudent for clinicians to advise patients undergoing chemotherapy or radiation therapy to limit antioxidants to levels that do not exceed the RDAs for specific nutrients and avoid other products that contain herbals or extracts enriched in antioxidant components. Folic acid is one nutrient where large dosages exceeding the RDA could influence the outcome of chemotherapy with agents such as methotrexate or 5-flurouracil (5-FU) that target metabolic pathways involving folate. Daily supplements containing folate above the RDA should be discouraged for these patients.[176]

Recovery Following Treatment The days and weeks following completion of intensive treatment are points in the cancer care continuum where many patients explore dietary and nutritional interventions to enhance survivorship. During this period, the frequency of contacts with health care providers lessens and the patient is concerned about the efficacy of treatment and recovery from therapy. Diet and physical activity should be a component of the treatment plan with the goal of restoring muscle mass and functional status. Health care providers must continue to question patients regarding supplements and alternative medical treatments and provide counseling as needed. Continuing individualized nutritional evaluation will identify those with more serious long-term nutritional complications of therapy, such as dysphagia, malabsorption, and bowel changes common in those treated for cancers of the oral pharynx, esophagus, stomach, pancreas, bowel, and others. A focus on energy balance and ensuring adequate intake of essential nutrients is critical. For example, gastric surgery or resection of the terminal ileum may lead to a vitamin B_{12} deficiency unless parenteral administration is initiated.[176]

Advanced Cancer In general, progressive cancer is associated with a loss of appetite, and if a patient does not succumb quickly to a complication of the disease or comorbid condition, progressive weight loss and other features of malnutrition will become evident. Unfortunately, many families and caretakers have the impression that reversal of the nutritional deficits will significantly prolong life. In reality, the failure to control the growth of the cancer, rather than malnutrition, is the critical issue. Frequently, the patient and caregivers experience conflict based on loss of appetite and food consumption. The medical team should be alert and identify conflicts centering on food, help establish understanding, and provide guidance to families. In the setting of advanced disease, dietary and nutritional interventions can contribute to a sense of well being and quality of life. Dietitians and the medial team can assist the patient in altering food choices and eating patterns and help maintain nutritional status in the setting of advanced disease often complicated by pain control issues and the resulting constipation caused by side effects of narcotic analgesics. Some medications can be coupled with limited physical activity to enhance appetite and improve bowel function. In some cases, additional nutritional support may be indicated.[176]

PREVENTION OF CANCER RECURRENCE AND LONG-TERM COMPLICATION OF THERAPY

The patient who achieves a complete remission from cancer is concerned about the reappearance of the primary cancer. In addition, survivors of certain cancers are at greater risk of second primaries, for example, survivors of oral or lung cancer may experience an approximately 10% chance of a second tobacco-related primary cancer yearly. Many cancer survivors are also at risk for cancers of other sites, often related to treatment, for example, secondary leukemia in cured testis cancer patients following treatment with etoposide based chemotherapy or secondary breast cancer in survivors of adolescent lymphoma treated with mediastinal radiation. Very little research has been undertaken to establish optimal dietary patterns to prevent recurrent disease or second primaries at the same or different sites. In general, most experts will focus on the dietary recommendations summarized at the beginning of this chapter and by various groups for the prevention of cancer.[1, 2,176]

As the population of cancer survivors expands, and physicians continue to monitor them over longer periods, long-term complications of treatments that are potential targets of dietary interventions are becoming apparent. For example, premature menopause in women treated with chemotherapy for breast cancer may contribute to accelerated osteoporosis[177] that may require alterations in dietary calcium and physical activity. Mediastinal radiation in young adults and children may contribute to premature coronary atherosclerosis. Medical caregivers should emphasize early interventions with dietary and exercise patterns that will maintain healthy blood cholesterol and triglyceride profiles. Although very little research concerning diet and nutrition has thus far been accumulated to provide clear guidance to cancer survivors, we anticipate that future efforts in this area will expand rapidly as a result of patient demands and the response of the National Institutes of Health through their support of survivorship issues.

REFERENCES

1. Byers T, Nestle M, McTiernan A, et al. American Cancer Society guidelines on nutrition and physical activity for cancer prevention: reducing the risk of cancer with healthy food choices and physical activity. CA Cancer J Clin 2002;52:92–119.
2. World Cancer Research Fund. Food, nutrition and the prevention of cancer: a global perspective. Washington, D.C.: American Institute for Cancer Research; 1997.
3. World Health Organization. Diet Nutrition and the prevention of chronic diseases. Geneva, Switzerland: WHO; 1990.
4. Eyre H, Kahn R, Robertson RM. Preventing cancer, cardiovascular disease, and diabetes. A common agenda for the American Cancer Society, the American Diabetes Association, and the American Heart Association. Stroke 2004;35:1999–2010.
5. Weed DL, Greenwald P, Kramer BS, editors. Cancer prevention and control. New York: Marcel Dekker, Inc.; 1995.
6. Medlin C, Skinner JD. Individual dietary intake methodology: a 50-year review of progress. J Am Diet Assoc 1988;88:137.
7. Block G. A review of validations of dietary assessment methods. Am J Epidemiol 1982;115:492–505.
8. Willett W. Nutritional epidemiology. 2nd Ed. New York: Oxford University Press; 1998.
9. Barett-Connor E. Nutrition epidemiology: how do we know what they ate? Am J Clin Nutr 1991;54(1 Suppl): 182–7.
10. Colditz GA, Willet WC. Epidemiologic approaches to the study of diet and cancer. In: Alfin-Slater RB, Kritchevsky D, editors. Human nutrition: a comprehensive treatise. Vol 7. New York: Plenum; 1991:51.
11. Patel AC, Nunez NP, Perkins SN, et al. Effects of energy balance on cancer in genetically altered mice. J Nutr 2004;134(12 Suppl):3394–8.
12. U.S. Department of Health and Human Services and U.S. Department of Agriculture. Dietary guidelines for Americans. Washington, DC: US Government Printing Office; 2005.
13. National Academy of Sciences Committee on Diet and Health Food and Nutrition Board. Diet and health: implications for reducing risk of chronic disease. Rockville, MD: Academy Press; 1989.
14. Willett WC. Goals for nutrition in the year 2000. *CA* Cancer J Clin 1999;49:331–52.
15. National Academy of Sciences National Research Council. Nutrient requirements of laboratory animals. Vol 10. Washington, DC: National Academy Press; 1978.
16. American Cancer Society. Nutrition and cancer cause and prevention. New York: American Cancer Society; 1984.
17. Krauss R, Eckel R, Howard B. AHA dietary guidelines revision 2000: a statement for healthcare professionals from the Nutrition Committee of the American Heart Association. Circulation 2000;102:2284–99.
18. Calle EE, Rodriguez C, Walker-Thurmond K, Thun MJ. Overweight, obesity, and mortality from cancer in a prospectively studied cohort of U.S. adults. N Engl J Med 2003;348:1625–38.
19. Dorgan JF, Sowell A, Swanson CA, et al. Relationships of serum carotenoids, retinol, alpha-tocopherol, and selenium with breast cancer risk: results from a prospective study in Columbia, Missouri (United States). Cancer Causes Control 1998;9:89–97.
20. Nagai M, Hashimoto T, Yanagawa H, et al. Relationship of diet to the incidence of esophageal and stomach cancer in Japan. Nutrition & Cancer 1982;3:257–68.
21. Slattery ML, Caan BJ, Potter JD, et al. Dietary energy sources and colon cancer risk. Am J Epidemiol 1997;145:199–210.
22. Sesso H, Paffenbarger RJ, Lee I. Physical activity and breast cancer risk in the College Alumni Health Study (United States). Cancer Causes Control 1998;9:433–9.
23. Smith-Warner SA, Spiegelman D, Yaun SS, et al. Alcohol and breast cancer in women: a pooled analysis of cohort studies. JAMA 1998;279:535–40.
24. Jensen OM, MacLennan R, Wahrendorf J. Diet, bowel function, fecal characteristics, and large bowel cancer in Denmark and Finland. Nutr Cancer 1982;4:5–19.
25. Ward JM, Anjo T, Ohannesian L, et al. Inactivity of fecapentaene-12 as a rodent carcinogen or tumor initiator. Cancer Lett 1988;42:49–59.
26. Whittemore AS, Wu-Williams AH, Lee M, et al. Diet, physical activity, and colorectal cancer among Chinese in North America and China. J Natl Cancer Inst 1990;82:915–26.
27. Haenszel W. Cancer mortality among the foreign-born in the United States. J Natl Cancer Inst 1961;26:37.
28. McMichael AJ, McCall MG, Hartshorne JM, Woodings TL. Patterns of gastro-intestinal cancer in European migrants to Australia: the role of dietary change. Int J Cancer 1980;25:431–7.
29. Hirayama T. Association between alcohol consumption and cancer of the sigmoid colon: observations from a Japanese cohort study. Lancet 1989;2:725–7.
30. Albanes D, Blair A, Taylor PR. Physical activity and risk of cancer in the NHANES I population. Am J Public Health 1989;79:744–50.
31. Ballard-Barbash R, Schatzkin A, Albanes D, et al. Physical activity and risk of large bowel cancer in the Framingham Study. Cancer Res 1990;50:3610–3.
32. Lee IM, Paffenbarger RS Jr, Hsieh C. Physical activity and risk of developing colorectal cancer among college alumni. J Natl Cancer Inst 1991;83:1324–9.
33. Martinez ME, Giovannucci E, Spiegelman D, et al. Leisure-time physical activity, body size, and colon cancer in women. Nurses' Health Study Research Group. J Natl Cancer Inst 1997;89:948–55.
34. Must A, Jacques PF, Dallal GE, et al. Long-term morbidity and mortality of overweight adolescents. A follow-up of the Harvard Growth Study of 1922 to 1935. N Engl J Med 1992;327:1350–5.
35. Bostick RM, Potter JD, Kushi LH, et al. Sugar, meat, and fat intake, and non-dietary risk factors for colon cancer incidence in Iowa women. Cancer Causes Control 1994;5:38–52.
36. Lee IM, Paffenbarger RS Jr. Quetelet's index and risk of colon cancer in college alumni. J Natl Cancer Inst 1992;84:1326–31.
37. Phillips RL, Snowdon DA. Dietary relationships with fatal colorectal cancer among Seventh-Day Adventists. J Natl Cancer Inst 1985;74:307–17.
38. Giovannucci E, Ascherio A, Rimm EB, et al. Physical activity, obesity, and risk for colon cancer and adenoma in men. Ann Intern Med 1995;122:327–34.
39. Chute CG, Willett WC, Colditz GA, et al. A prospective study of body mass, height, and smoking on the risk of colorectal cancer in women. Cancer Causes Control 1991;2:117–24.
40. Albanes D, Jones DY, Schatzkin A, et al. Adult stature and risk of cancer. Cancer Res 1988;48:1658–62.
41. Albanes D, Taylor PR. International differences in body height and weight and their relationship to cancer incidence. Nutr Cancer 1990;14:69–77.
42. Clinton SK, Imrey PB, Alster JM, et al. The combined effects of dietary protein and fat on 7,12-dimethylbenz [a] anthracene-induced breast cancer in rats. J Nutr 1984;114:1213–23.
43. Klurfeld DM, Weber MM, Kritchevsky D. Inhibition of chemically induced mammary and colon tumor promotion by caloric restriction in rats fed increased dietary fat. Cancer Res 1987;47:2759–62.
44. Colditz GA, Cannuscio CC, Frazier AL. Physical activity and reduced risk of colon cancer: implications for prevention. Cancer Causes Control 1997;8:649–67.
45. Armstrong B, Doll R. Environmental factors and cancer incidence and mortality in different countries, with

special reference to dietary practices. Int J Cancer 1975;15:617–31.
46. Carroll KK, Khor HT. Dietary fat in relation to tumorigenesis. Prog Biochem Pharmacol 1975;10:308–53.
47. Rose DP, Boyar AP, Wynder EL. International comparisons of mortality rates for cancer of the breast, ovary, prostate, and colon, and per capita food consumption. Cancer. 1986;58:2363–71.
48. Willett WC, Hunter DJ, Stampfer MJ, et al. Dietary fat and fiber in relation to risk of breast cancer. An 8-year follow-up. JAMA 1992;268:2037–44.
49. Giovannucci E, Rimm EB, Stampfer MJ, et al. Intake of fat, meat, and fiber in relation to risk of colon cancer in men. Cancer Res 1994;54:2390–7.
50. Lyon JL, Mahoney AW, West DW, et al. Energy intake: its relationship to colon cancer risk. J Natl Cancer Inst 1987;78:853–61.
51. Goldbohm RA, van den Brandt PA, van 't Veer P, et al. A prospective cohort study on the relation between meat consumption and the risk of colon cancer. Cancer Res 1994;54:718–23.
52. Willett WC, Stampfer MJ, Colditz GA, et al. Relation of meat, fat, and fiber intake to the risk of colon cancer in a prospective study among women. N Engl J Med 1990;323:1664–72.
53. Chao A, Thun MJ, Connell CJ, et al. Meat consumption and risk of colorectal cancer. JAMA 2005;293:172–82.
54. National Academy of Sciences Committee on Diet Nutrition and Cancer. Diet, nutrition and cancer. Washington, DC: National Academy Press; 1982.
55. Jensen OM. The epidemiology of large bowel cancer. In: Reddy BS, Cohen LA, editors. Diet, nutrition, and cancer: a critical evaluation. Vol I: Macronutrients and cancer. Boca Raton: CRC;1986. p. 27.
56. Giovannucci E, Stampfer MJ, Colditz G, et al. Relationship of diet to risk of colorectal adenoma in men. J Natl Cancer Inst 1992;84:91–8.
57. Trock B, Lanza E, Greenwald P. Dietary fiber, vegetables, and colon cancer: critical review and meta-analyses of the epidemiologic evidence. J Natl Cancer Inst 1990;82:650–61.
58. Bingham SA, Day NE, Luben R, et al. Dietary fibre in food and protection against colorectal cancer in the European Prospective Investigation into Cancer and Nutrition (EPIC): an observational study. Lancet 2003;361:1496–1501.
59. Macrae F. Wheat bran fiber and development of adenomatous polyps: evidence from randomized, controlled clinical trials. Am J Med 1999;106(1A):38–42.
60. Alberts DS, Einspahr J, Rees-McGee S. Effects of dietary wheat bran fiber on rectal epithelial cell proliferation in patients with resection for colorectal cancers. J Natl Cancer Inst 1990;82:1280.
61. Alberts DS, Einspahr J, Ritenbaugh C, et al. The effect of wheat bran fiber and calcium supplementation on rectal mucosal proliferation rates in patients with resected adenomatous colorectal polyps. Cancer Epidemiol Biomarkers Prev 1997;6:161–9.
62. Alberts DS, Martinez ME, Roe DJ, et al. Lack of effect of a high-fiber cereal supplement on the recurrence of colorectal adenomas. Phoenix Colon Cancer Prevention Physicians' Network. N Engl J Med 2000;342:1156–62.
63. Freudenheim JL, Graham S, Marshall JR, et al. Lifetime alcohol intake and risk of rectal cancer in western New York. Nutr Cancer 1990;13:101–9.
64. Kono S, Ikeda N, Yanai F, et al. Alcoholic beverages and adenomatous polyps of the sigmoid colon: a study of male self-defense officials in Japan. International Journal of Epidemiology 1990;19:848–52.
65. Kikendall JW, Bowen PE, Burgess MB, et al. Cigarettes and alcohol as independent risk factors for colonic adenomas. Gastroenterology 1989;97:660–4.
66. Giovannucci E, Rimm EB, Stampfer MJ, et al. Folate, methionine, and alcohol intake and risk of colorectal adenoma. J Natl Cancer Inst 1993;85:875–84.
67. Giovannucci E, Rimm EB, Ascherio A, et al. Alcohol, low-methionine—low-folate diets, and risk of colon cancer in men. J Natl Cancer Inst 1995;87:265–73.
68. Bruce WR. Recent hypotheses for the origin of colon cancer. Cancer Res 1987;47:4237–42.
69. Sinha R, Rothman N. Role of well-done, grilled red meat, heterocyclic amines (HCAs) in the etiology of human cancer. Cancer Letters 1999;143:189–94.
70. Mower HF, Ichinotsubo D, Wang LW, et al. Fecal mutagens in two Japanese populations with different colon cancer risks. Cancer Res 1982;42:1164–9.
71. Kuhnlein HV, Kuhnlein U, Bell PA. The effect of short-term dietary modification on human fecal mutagenic activity. Mutation Res 1983;113:1–12.
72. Goodwin PJ, Boyd NF. Critical appraisal of the evidence that dietary fat intake is related to breast cancer risk in humans. J Natl Cancer Inst 1987;79:473–85.
73. Hirohata T, Nomura AM, Hankin JH, Kolonel LN, Lee J. An epidemiologic study on the association between diet and breast cancer. J Natl Cancer Inst 1987;78:595–600.
74. Gillette C, Zhu Z, Westerlind K, et al. Energy availability and mammary carcinogenesis: effects of calorie restriction and exercise. Carcinogenesis 1997;18:1183–8.
75. Tannenbaum A. The dependence of tumor formation on the composition of the calorie-restricted diet as well as on the degree of restriction. Cancer Res 1945;5:616.
76. Clinton SK, Alster JM, Imrey PB, et al. Effects of dietary protein, fat and energy intake during an initiation phase study of 7,12-dimethylbenz [a] anthracene-induced breast cancer in rats. J Nutr 1986;116:2290–302.
77. Albanes D. Caloric intake, body weight and cancer. A review. Nutr Cancer 1987;9:199.
78. Huang Z, Hankinson S, Colditz G, et al. Dual effects of weight and weight gain on breast cancer risk. JAMA 1997;278:1407–11.
79. Ziegler RG, Hoover RN, Nomura AM, et al. Relative weight, weight change, height, and breast cancer risk in Asian-American women. Journal of the National Cancer Institute 1996;88:650–60.
80. Breslow RA, Ballard-Barbash R, Munoz K, Graubard BI. Long-term recreational physical activity and breast cancer in the National Health and Nutrition Examination Survey I epidemiologic follow-up study. Cancer Epidemiol Biomarkers Prev 2001;10:805–8.
81. Rockhill B, Willett WC, Hunter DJ, et al. A prospective study of recreational physical activity and breast cancer risk. Arch Intern Med 1999;159:2290–6.
82. Carroll KK. Dietary polyunsaturated fat versus saturated fat in relation to mammary carcinogenesis. J Natl Cancer Inst 1979;62:1009–12.
83. Prentice R, Kakar F, Hursting S, et al. Aspects of the rational for the Women's Health Trial. J Natl Cancer Inst 1988;80:802–14.
84. Boyd N, Martin L, Noffel M, et al. A meta-analysis of dietary fat and breast cancer risk. Br J Cancer 1993;68:627–36.
85. Holmes M, Hunter D, Colditz G, et al. Association of dietary intake of fat and fatty acids with risk of breast cancer. JAMA 1999;281:914–20.
86. Clinton S, Alster J, Imrey P, et al. The combined effects of dietary protein and fat intake during the promotion phase of 7,12-dimethylbenz[α]anthracene-induced breast cancer in rats. J Nutr 1988;118:1577–85.
87. Chlebowski RT, Blackburn GL, Elashoff C, et al. Dietary fat reduction in postmenopausal women with primary breast cancer: phase III Women's Intervention Nutrition Study (WINS) ASCO conference proceedings abstract. J Clin Oncol 2005;23(16S):3.
88. Garland M, Hunter D, Colditz G, et al. Alcohol consumption in relation to breast cancer risk in a cohort of United States women 25–42 years of age. Cancer Epidemiol Biomarkers Prev 1999;8:1017–21.
89. Willett W, Stampfer M, Colditz G, et al. Moderate alcohol consumption and the risk of breast cancer. N Engl J Med 1987;316:1174–80.
90. Longnecker M, Berlin J, Orza M, Chalmers T. A meta-analysis of alcohol consumption in relation to risk of breast cancer. JAMA 1988;260:652–6.
91. Smith-Warner S, Spiegelman D, Yaun S, et al. Intake of fruits and vegetables and risk of breast cancer: a pooled analysis of cohort studies. JAMA 2001;285:769–76.
92. van Gils CH, Peeters PH, Bueno-de-Mesquita HB, et al. Consumption of vegetables and fruits and risk of breast cancer. JAMA 2005;293:183–93.
93. Clinton SK, Giovannucci E. Diet, nutrition, and prostate cancer. Annu Rev Nutr 1998;18:413–40.
94. Ross RK, Shimizu H, Paganini-Hill A, et al. Case-control studies of prostate cancer in blacks and whites in southern California. J Natl Cancer Inst1987;78:869–74.
95. Kolonel LN, Yoshizawa CN, Hankin JH. Diet and prostatic cancer: a case-control study in Hawaii. Am J Epidemiol 1988;127:999–1012.
96. Mukherjee P, Sotnikov AV, Mangian HJ, et al. Energy intake and prostate tumor growth, angiogenesis, and vascular endothelial growth factor expression. J Natl Cancer Inst 1999;91:512–23.
97. Nilsen TI, Vatten LJ. Anthropometry and prostate cancer risk: a prospective study of 22,248 Norwegian men. Cancer Causes Control 1999;10:269–75.
98. Le Marchand L, Kolonel LN, Wilkens LR, et al. Animal fat consumption and prostate cancer: a prospective study in Hawaii. Epidemiology 1994;5:276–82.
99. Giovannucci E, Rimm EB, Colditz GA, et al. A prospective study of dietary fat and risk of prostate cancer. J Natl Cancer Inst 1993;85:1571–9.
100. Heinonen OP, Albanes D, Virtamo J, et al. Prostate cancer and supplementation with alpha-tocopherol and beta-carotene: incidence and mortality in a controlled trial. J Natl Cancer Inst 1998;90:440–6.
101. Clark LC, Combs GF Jr, Turnbull BW, et al. Effects of selenium supplementation for cancer prevention in patients with carcinoma of the skin. A randomized controlled trial. Nutritional Prevention of Cancer Study Group. JAMA 1996;276:1957–63.
102. Yoshizawa K, Willett WC, Morris SJ, et al. Study of prediagnostic selenium level in toenails and the risk of advanced prostate cancer. J Natl Cancer Inst 1998;90:1219–24.
103. Giovannucci E, Ascherio A, Rimm EB, et al. Intake of carotenoids and retinol in relation to risk of prostate cancer. J Natl Cancer Inst 1995;87:1767–76.
104. Giovannucci E, Rimm E, Liu Y, et al. A prospective study of tomato products, lycopene, and prostate cancer risk. J Natl Cancer Inst 2002;94:391–8.
105. Hadley C, Miller E, Schwartz S, Clinton S. Tomatoes, lycopene, and prostate cancer: progress and promise. Exp Biol Med 2002;227:869–80.
106. Miller E, Hadley C, Schwartz S, et al. Lycopene, tomato products, and prostate cancer prevention. Have we established causality? Pure Appl Chem 2002;74:1435–41.
107. Clinton SK. Lycopene: chemistry, biology, and implications for human health and disease. Nutr Rev 1998;56:35–51.
108. Giovannucci E. Tomatoes, tomato-based products, lycopene, and cancer: review of the epidemiologic literature. J Natl Cancer Inst 1999;91:317–31.
109. Boileau TW-M, Liao Z, Kim S, et al. Prostate carcinogenesis in n-methyl-n-nitrosourea (NMU)-testosterone-treated rats fed tomato powder, lycopene, or energy-restricted diets. J Natl Cancer Inst 2003;95(21)1578-1586.
110. Clinton SK, Emenhiser C, Schwartz SJ, et al. cis-trans lycopene isomers, carotenoids, and retinol in the human prostate. Cancer Epidemiol Biomarkers Prev 1996;5:823–33.
111. Gann PH, Ma J, Giovannucci E, et al. Lower prostate cancer risk in men with elevated plasma lycopene levels: results of a prospective analysis. Cancer Res 1999;59:1225–30.
112. Wu K, Erdman JW Jr, Schwartz SJ, et al. Plasma and dietary carotenoids, and the risk of prostate cancer: a nested case-control study. Cancer Epidemiol Biomarkers Prev 2004;13:260–9.
113. Giovannucci E, Rimm EB, Wolk A, et al. Calcium and fructose intake in relation to risk of prostate cancer. Cancer Res 1998;58:442–7.
114. Chan J, Stampfer M, Ma J, et al. Dairy products, calcium, and prostate cancer risk in the Physicians' Health Study. Am J Clin Nutr 2001;74:549–54.
115. Department of Health Education and Welfare D. Smoking and Health: a report of the Surgeon General. Vol DHEW Pugl. No. (PHS) 79-50066. Rockville, MD: Office on Smoking and Health, Office of the Assistant Secretary for Health, Public Health Service, US Department of Health Education and Welfare; 1979:1164.
116. Block G, Patterson B, Subar A. Fruit, vegetables, and cancer prevention: a review of the epidemiological evidence. Nutr Cancer 1992;18:1–29.
117. Steinmetz KA, Potter JD, Folsom AR. Vegetables, fruit, and lung cancer in the Iowa Women's Health Study. Cancer Res 1993;53:536–43.
118. Menkes M, Comstock G, Vuilleumier J, et al. Serum beta-carotene, vitamins A and E, selenium, and the risk of lung cancer. N Engl J Med 1986;315:1250–4.
119. Omenn GS, Goodman GE, Thornquist MD, et al. Risk factors for lung cancer and for intervention effects in CARET, the Beta-Carotene and Retinol Efficacy Trial. J Natl Cancer Inst 1996;88:1550–9.
120. Bandera EV, Freudenheim JL, Marshall JR, et al. Diet and alcohol consumption and lung cancer risk in the New York State Cohort (United States). Cancer Causes Control 1997;8:828–40.
121. Burch JD, Howe GR, Miller AB, Semenciw R. Tobacco, alcohol, asbestos, and nickel in the etiology of cancer of the larynx: a case-control study. J Natl Cancer Inst 1981;67:1219–24.
122. DeLint J, Levinson T. Mortality among patients treated for alcoholism: a 5-year follow-up. Can Med Assoc J 1975;113:385.
123. Lyon J, Klauber M, Gardner J, Smart C. Cancer incidence in Mormons and non-Mormons in Utah 1966-1970. N Engl J Med 1976;294:129.
124. Tuyns AJ. Alcohol et Cancer. Lyons, France: International Agency for Research on Cancer; 1978.

125. Jaskiewicz K, Marasas WF, Lazarus C, et al. Association of esophageal cytological abnormalities with vitamin and lipotrope deficiencies in populations at risk for esophageal cancer. Anticancer Res 1988;8:711–5.
126. Graham S, Marshall J, Haughey B, et al. Nutritional epidemiology of cancer of the esophagus. Am J Epidemiol 1990;131:454–67.
127. van Rensburg SJ. Epidemiologic and dietary evidence for a specific nutritional predisposition to esophageal cancer. J Natl Cancer Inst 1981;67:243.
128. Cook-Mozaffari PJ, Azordegan F, Day NE, et al. Oesophageal cancer studies in the Caspian Littoral of Iran: results of a case-control study. Br J Cancer 1979;39:293–309.
129. Vaughan TL, Davis S, Kristal A, Thomas DB. Obesity, alcohol, and tobacco as risk factors for cancers of the esophagus and gastric cardia: adenocarcinoma versus squamous cell carcinoma. Cancer Epidemiol Biomarkers Prev 1995;4:85.
130. Blot WJ, McLaughlin JK. The changing epidemiology of esophageal cancer. Sem Oncology 1999;26(5 Suppl 15):2–8.
131. Devesa SS, Blot WJ, Fraumeni JF Jr. Changing patterns in the incidence of esophageal and gastric carcinoma in the United States. Cancer 1998;83:2049.
132. Gammon MD, Schoenberg JB, Ahsan H, et al. Tobacco, alcohol, and socioeconomic status and adenocarcinomas of the esophagus and gastric cardia. J Natl Cancer Inst 1997;89:1277.
133. Chow WH, Blot WJ, Vaughan TL. Body mass index and risk of adenocarcinomas of the esophagus and gastric cardia. J Natl Cancer Inst 1998;90:150.
134. Mayne S, Nararro S. Diet, obesity and reflux in the etiology of adenocarcinomas of the esophagus and gastric cardia in humans. J Nutr 2002;132(11 Suppl):3467–70.
135. Brown LM, Swanson CA, Gridley G. Adenocarcinoma of the esophagus: role of obesity and diet. J Natl Cancer Inst 1995;87:104.
136. Chen H, Ward M, Graubard B, et al. Dietary patterns and adenocarcinoma of the esophagus and distal stomach. Am J Clin Nutr 2002;75:137–44.
137. Boring CC, Squires TS, Tong T, Montgomery S. Cancer statistics, 1994. CA Cancer J Clin 1994;44:7–26.
138. Correa P, Cuello C, Fajardo LF, et al. Diet and gastric cancer: nutrition survey in a high-risk area. J Natl Cancer Inst 1983;70:673–8.
139. Fox JG, Dangler CA, Taylor NS, et al. High-salt diet induces gastric epithelial hyperplasia and parietal cell loss, and enhances *Helicobacter pylori* colonization in C57BL/6 mice. Cancer Res 1999;59:4823–8.
140. Parsonnet J, Friedman G, Vandersteen D, et al. *Helicobacter pylori* infection and the risk of gastric carcinoma. N Engl J Med 1991;325:1127.
141. Terry P, Nyren O, Yuen J. Protective effects of fruits and vegetables on stomach cancer in a cohort of Swedish twins. Int J Cancer 1998;76:35.
142. Lu SH, Ohshima H, Fu HM, et al. Urinary excretion of N-nitrosamino acids and nitrate by inhabitants of high- and low-risk areas for esophageal cancer in Northern China: endogenous formation of nitrosoproline and its inhibition by vitamin C. Cancer Res 1986;46:1485–91.
143. Lijinsky W, Shubik P. Benzo[α]pyrene and other polynuclear hydrocarbons in charcoal-broiled meat. Science 1964:53.
144. Dungal N. The special problem of stomach cancer in Iceland with particular reference to dietary factors. JAMA 1961;176:789.
145. Beasley RP, Hwang LY, Lin CC, Chien CS. Hepatocellular carcinoma and hepatitis B virus. A prospective study of 22 707 men in Taiwan. Lancet 1981;2:1129–33.
146. Wogan GN. Dietary factors and special epidemiological situations of liver cancer in Thailand and Africa. Cancer Res 1975;35:3499.
147. Austin H, Delzell E, Grufferman S, et al. A case-control study of hepatocellular carcinoma and the hepatitis B virus, cigarette smoking, and alcohol consumption. Cancer Res 1986;46:962–6.
148. Yu MC, Mack T, Hanisch R, et al. Hepatitis, alcohol consumption, cigarette smoking, and hepatocellular carcinoma in Los Angeles. Cancer Res 1983;43:6077–9.
149. Fuchs C, Colditz G, Stampfer M, et al. A prospective study of cigarette smoking and the risk of pancreatic cancer. Arch Intern Med 1996;156:2255–60.
150. Longnecker DS, Morgan RGH. Diet and cancer of the pancreas: epidemiological and experimental evidence. In: Reddy BS, Cohen LA, editors. Diet, nutrition, and cancer: a critical evaluation. Vol I: Macronutrients and cancer. Boca Raton: CRC; 1986. p. 11.
151. Michaud D, Giovannucci E, Willett W, et al. Physical activity, obesity, height, and the risk of pancreatic cancer. JAMA 2001;286:921–9.
152. Nevalainen TJ, Janigan DT. Degeneration of mouse pancreatic acinar cells during fasting. Virchows Arch B Cell Pathol 1974;15:107–18.
153. Roebuck BD, Yager JD Jr, Longnecker DS. Dietary modulation of azaserine-induced pancreatic carcinogenesis in the rat. Cancer Res 1981;41:888–93.
154. Michaud D, Liu S, Giovannucci E, et al. Dietary sugar, glycemic load, and pancreatic cancer risk in a prospective study. J Natl Cancer Inst 2002;94:1293–1300.
155. Littman A, Beresford S, White E. The association of dietary fat and plant foods with endometrial cancer. Cancer Causes Control 2001;12:691–702.
156. Kushi LH, Mink PJ, Folsom AR, et al. Prospective study of diet and ovarian cancer. Am J Epidemiol 1999;149:21–31.
157. Clinton SK, Michaud, D., Giovannucci, E. Nutrition and bladder cancer. In: Heber D, Blackburn GL, Go VLW, editors. Nutritional oncology. San Diego, CA: Academic Press; 1997. p. 463.
158. Michaud D, Clinton S, Rimm E, et al. Risk of bladder cancer by geographic region in a U.S. cohort of male health professionals. Epidemiology 2001;12:719–26.
159. Michaud DS, Spiegelman D, Clinton SK, et al. Fruit and vegetable intake and incidence of bladder cancer in a male prospective cohort. J Natl Cancer Inst 1999;91:605–13.
160. Michaud DS, Spiegelman D, Clinton SK, et al. Fluid intake and the risk of bladder cancer in men. N Engl J Med 1999;340:1390–7.
161. Merrill AH, Foltz AT, McCormick DB. Vitamins and cancer. In: Alfin-Slater RB, Kritchevsky D, editors. Human nutrition: a comprehensive treatise. Vol 7. New York: Plenum; 1992. p. 262.
162. Greenwald P, Nixon D, Malone W, et al. Concepts in cancer chemoprevention research. Cancer 1990;65:1483–90.
163. McCullough ML, Giovannucci EL. Diet and cancer prevention. Oncogene 2004;23:6349–64.
164. Lonn E, Bosch J, Yusuf S, et al. Effects of long-term vitamin E supplementation on cardiovascular events and cancer: a randomized controlled trial. JAMA 2005;293:1338–47.
165. Watkins M, Erickson J, Thun M, et al. Multivitamin use and mortality in a large prospective study. Am J Epidemiol 2000;152:149–62.
166. U.S. Food and Drug Administration. Folic acid fortification fact sheet. Washington, DC: Office of Public Affairs; 1996.
167. Freudenheim JL, Graham S, Marshall JR, et al. Folate intake and carcinogenesis of the colon and rectum. Int J Epidemiol 1991;20:368–74.
168. Lipkin M. Calcium modulation of intermediate biomarkers in the gastrointestinal tract. In: Lipkin M, Kelloff G., Newmark H, editors. Calcium, vitamin D and cancer. Boca Raton, FL: CRC; 1991.
169. Caderni G, Stuart EW, Bruce WR. Dietary factors affecting the proliferation of epithelial cells in the mouse colon. Nutr Cancer 1988;11:147–53.
170. Clark LC. The epidemiology of selenium and cancer. Fed Proc 1985;44:2584–9.
171. Zhou J, Gugger E, Tanaka T, et al. Soybean phytochemicals inhibit the growth of transplantable human prostate carcinoma and tumor angiogenesis in mice. J Nutr 1999;129:1628–35.
172. Zhou J, Mukherjee P, Gugger E, et al. Inhibition of murine bladder tumorigenesis by soy isoflavones via alterations in the cell cycle, apoptosis, and angiogenesis. Cancer Res 1998;58:5231–8.
173. Messina M, Loprinzi C. Soy for breast cancer survivors: a critical review of the literature. J Nutr 2001;131(11 Suppl):3095S–108.
174. The Alpha-Tocopherol Beta-Carotene Cancer Prevention Study Group. The effect of vitamin E and beta carotene on the incidence of lung cancer and other cancers in male smokers. N Engl J Med 1994;330:1029–35.
175. Rose D, Connolly J. Effects of dietary omega-3 fatty acids on human breast cancer growth and metastases in nude mice. J Natl Cancer Inst 1993;85:1743–7.
176. Brown JK, Byers T, Doyle C, et al. Nutrition and physical activity during and after cancer treatment: An American Cancer Society guide for informed choices. CA Cancer J Clin 2003;53(5):268–91.
177. Shapiro C, Manola J, Leboff M. Ovarian failure after adjuvant chemotherapy is associated with rapid bone loss in women with early-stage breast cancer. J Clin Oncol 2001;19:3306–11.

27

Chemoprevention of Cancer

Michael B. Sporn, MD
Scott M. Lippman, MD

There are two general approaches to the problem of control of cancer. The classic approach, followed for more than a hundred years, has been to deal with the disease once it becomes symptomatic in its terminal stages, which are characterized by clinical symptoms or laboratory findings related to the phenomenon of invasiveness or metastasis. Invasion and metastasis have long been considered the "true" hallmarks of cancer. Once patients have been diagnosed with "cancer," as defined by the above criteria, they have then been treated with the various modalities of surgery, radiation therapy, chemotherapy, immunotherapy, or other treatments directed at the eradication of detectable lesions. Despite some spectacular successes in the treatment of relatively rare cancers, this approach has not yet led to a significant decrease in cancer mortality resulting from the common forms of many metastatic epithelial cancers, such as carcinoma of the lung, breast, colon, prostate, pancreas, and other sites.[1]

An alternative approach to the problem of cancer control is one that attempts, first, to provide new understanding of the fundamental nature of the chronic disease process that eventually leads to invasive and metastatic carcinoma, and second, to develop new pharmacologic agents that arrest or reverse this chronic disease process in its earliest stages, well before it reaches its terminal invasive and metastatic phase.[2,3] This alternative approach is known as chemoprevention.[2,4] It is based on the concept that the very term "cancer," widely used by clinicians, laboratory scientists, and laypersons alike, is a misnomer because it is inadequate to describe the pathogenesis of the disease process as it actually occurs in the patient. The term cancer denotes a static circumstance, whereas the disease, in reality, is an evolving chronic molecular and cellular process—carcinogenesis. By focusing on end-stage invasive and metastatic disease, we lose the opportunity to intervene in the disease process at earlier stages, when it may be more amenable to the use of pharmacologic agents for its prevention. Since 20 years or more may elapse between the original mutagenic initiation of the carcinogenic process and the subsequent development of invasive or metastatic cells,[5,6] there is a long window of opportunity in which to use preventive agents. Indeed, since there is only a stochastic probability that an early stage of carcinogenesis will progress to a later one, the intrinsic biology of the carcinogenic process suggests that preventive agents can be developed and successfully used.[5,6] Perhaps the most significant aspect of carcinogenesis is that most people do *not* develop invasive and metastatic carcinoma, despite endogenous and exogenous mutational burdens and often significant preinvasive neoplastic lesions in various epithelia. Most heavy smokers do *not* develop lung cancer.

The natural history of the disease process of carcinogenesis thus convincingly indicates that there are intrinsic biologic mechanisms that protect the organism against the development of clones of malignant cells.[7,8] It would therefore seem reasonable to use these mechanisms to design strategies for prevention of cancer. It is paradoxical that the phenomenon that not all dysplastic, preinvasive lesions progress to invasiveness has been used as an argument against the clinical use of chemopreventive agents, with the false premise that since a patient may not yet have an invasive lesion (does not yet have "cancer"), the patient is therefore "healthy."[9] In this regard, the oncology community lags far behind the cardiovascular community in recognizing and accepting the importance of early precursor lesions as antecedents of clinically symptomatic and life-threatening disease. In cardiovascular medicine, it is well accepted that precursor lesions, such as fatty streaking and arterial plaques, have an important causal relationship to the end-stage clinical outcomes of myocardial infarction and stroke.[10] Great advances have been made in the development of new drugs that can lower cholesterol levels and that have had a major impact on lowering mortality from cardiovascular disease.[11] Moreover, the fact that not all arterial precursor lesions progress to a thrombotic or embolic state has not been used as an argument against interventive chemoprevention, and it is generally accepted that patients with extensive precursor lesions in their arterial tree may be at high risk of serious, life-threatening events. There is widespread acceptance of the concepts that patients with such lesions are *not* healthy from a cardiovascular perspective, even though they may not be symptomatic, and that it is appropriate to use pharmacologic agents to prevent further progression of early arterial lesions.

Rather than dismissing precursor lesions of invasive cancer as biologically insignificant on the grounds that not all of these lesions progress to invasiveness, the oncology community should attempt to understand the intrinsic mechanisms in epithelia that prevent progression of these lesions, and then design new pharmacologic agents that could enhance the activity of such mechanisms. These concepts provide the basis for the ultimate use of chemoprevention to control cancer death rates.

AGENTS FOR CHEMOPREVENTION AND THEIR MECHANISM OF ACTION

Types of Chemopreventive Agents In the broadest sense, agents for chemoprevention of cancer fall into two principal categories:[4] (1) those that prevent the mutagenic initiation of the carcinogenic process ("blocking" agents) and (2) those that prevent the further promotion or progression of lesions that have already been established ("suppressing" agents). Since mutation continues as part of the entire chronic process of carcinogenesis, the distinction between the two categories, at least in the dimension of time, is artifactual. However useful the concept of two-stage carcinogenesis (initiation followed by promotion) was in the past to describe relatively simple experimental systems in laboratory rodents, it can no longer be accepted as a valid model for the process of carcinogenesis in human subjects, in whom mutation and continued initiation of molecular lesions play an ongoing role throughout the rest of the individual's life span. Extensive information is now available on the ability of cells, such as neutrophils and macrophages, to generate potent agents, such as superoxide, hydrogen peroxide, hydroxyl radical, and nitric oxide, all of which can damage deoxyribonucleic acid (DNA). It is now clear that endogenous metabolism as well as exposure to exogenous agents can have major influences on the process of carcinogenesis.[12]

In this chapter, we discuss both types of agents, since both have found clinical application. Although various dietary constituents, such as ascorbic acid, β-carotene, folic acid, and α-tocopherol (vitamin E), have been the subject of many clinical trials to prevent cancer (reviewed in the last part of this chapter), for the most part, the results with vitamins and other nutrients have been disappointing. It should be clear by now that if chemoprevention is truly to have a practical impact on the control of cancer, it will be necessary to develop a fundamentally pharmacologic approach to the problem. In the face of the intense mutagenic pressure that drives the process of carcinogenesis, it will be necessary to use agents that either are potent antimutagens or can significantly alter patterns of gene expression.

Retinoids The molecules that have been most intensively studied for chemoprevention of carcinogenesis are the retinoids, which are defined as natural and synthetic analogues of retinol (vitamin A).[2,13] More than a thousand such molecules have been made by synthetic chemistry,[14] and as knowledge of the receptors that mediate their mechanism of action increases, so also does the number of new agents that are ligands for these receptors. Of particular importance to retinoid studies has been the unification of molecular and cell biology that occurred with the discovery of the steroid receptor superfamily.[15,16] This has been a major advance in the attempt to develop new agents for the chemoprevention of carcinogenesis, since it is now apparent that the intracellular receptors for the retinoids, vitamin D, and thyroid hormone—as well as those for the classic steroids such as estrogens, progestogens, androgens, and glucocorticoids—all belong to a superfamily involved in the selective regulation of transcription of specific genes that control cell differentiation and proliferation.[15–17] Studies on the mechanism of action of the above ligands with their respective receptors now provide the basis for rational design, development, and testing of new agents for the chemoprevention of carcinogenesis.

The impact of this new knowledge has been especially important in studies of retinoids. Many years ago, Wolbach and Howe demonstrated that the normal function of retinoids was essential for the proper regulation of the differentiation and proliferation of all the epithelia that are the common sites of carcinogenesis in men and women.[18] They clearly recognized that during retinoid deficiency there was a failure of stem cells to mature into appropriate differentiated cells; this was accompanied by enhanced cellular proliferation, with the formation of lesions resembling those found in malignant or premalignant tissues. It is now known that retinoids are required to maintain normal differentiation and proliferation of almost all cells, including nonepithelial cells of mesenchymal origin, during both embryogenesis and adult life.[19]

Further advances related to the chemoprevention of carcinogenesis came from organ culture and cell culture studies. It was shown that retinoids could reverse the premalignant lesions induced in mouse prostate organ cultures by carcinogenic hydrocarbons such as 3-methylcholanthrene[20] and that retinoids could act directly on cells previously treated with such carcinogens to suppress the appearance of the malignant phenotype.[21] The latter cell culture studies were particularly important because they emphasized that the continuing presence of the retinoid was essential for the suppression of malignancy; removal of the retinoids from the cultures allowed the expression of the transformed state in cells that had previously been exposed to carcinogen. This phenomenon of a continued requirement for a retinoid to suppress carcinogenesis has also been seen repeatedly in many studies in intact animals and undoubtedly is clinically relevant. However, there are also some situations in which retinoids can alter the differentiation of invasive neoplastic cells and induce terminal differentiation. The most striking example of this phenomenon is the induction of terminal differentiation in many types of teratocarcinoma and leukemia cells, of both animal and human origin.[22–24]

Several synthetic retinoids have been successfully used in a large number of studies for the prevention of carcinogenesis in experimental animals. Among those that have potential for clinical application are the following: all-*trans*-retinoic acid (tretinoin), 4-hydroxyphenyl all-*trans*-retinoic acid amide (fenretinide), 13-*cis*-retinoic acid (isotretinoin), and 9-*cis*-retinoic acid and its derivatives. There are six known retinoic acid receptors (RAR) that mediate the actions of these retinoids. The first receptors to be cloned, RAR-α, RAR-β, and RAR-γ, bind all-*trans*-retinoic acid and 9-*cis*-retinoic acid with high affinity,[25,26] but bind neither fenretinide nor 13-*cis*-retinoic acid. These latter two retinoids are presumably prodrugs; the isomerization of 13-*cis*- to all-*trans*-retinoic acid occurs readily. However, the enzymatic hydrolysis of fenretinide to the free acid has yet to be shown, either in cell culture or in vivo.

More recently, three new retinoid receptors, known as RXR-α, RXR-β, and RXR-γ, have been cloned;[27] these retinoid X receptors (RXRs) bind only 9-*cis*-retinoic acid[25,26] and do not bind any of the other three retinoids just mentioned above. However, since all-*trans*-retinoic acid can be metabolized to the 9-*cis* derivative, it is ultimately a potential ligand for the RXRs in vivo. The importance of the RXRs is emphasized by their ability to form heterodimers with many other members of the steroid receptor superfamily, including RARs, the vitamin D receptor, and the thyroid hormone receptor. RXRs and their ligands are thus permissive systems that can modulate the activity of other ligands and receptors in the steroid receptor superfamily. With the recent demonstration that terpenoid molecules other than 9-*cis*-retinoic acid can act as ligands for RXRs, the functional domain of this system now appears to be even broader than anticipated. Ligands that are specific for binding only to RXRs are known as "rexinoids."

There is an extensive literature on the use of retinoids to arrest or reverse the process of carcinogenesis and to prevent the development of invasive carcinoma in experimental animals.[28] Of particular importance are the many studies that have shown the efficacy of retinoids when they are administered after animals have been treated with a carcinogen; this experimental design is highly relevant to human populations. Significant activity has been shown for all-*trans*-retinoic acid, 13-*cis*-retinoic acid, 9-*cis*-retinoic acid,[29] fenretinide, and many other retinoids, as reviewed by Moon and colleagues.[28] The epithelial sites studied include breast, skin, lung, bladder, pancreas, liver, oropharynx, esophagus, stomach, and prostate. In addition to efficacy as single agents, retinoids have been particularly effective when used in combination with other preventive agents, especially tamoxifen.

Tamoxifen Tamoxifen is a nonsteroidal triphenylethylene derivative that binds to the estrogen receptor.[30] It has both estrogenic and antiestrogenic actions, depending on the target tissue. It is strongly antiestrogenic on mammary epithelium, hence its use in both the prevention and treatment of breast cancer, and it is proestrogenic on uterine epithelium, hence the current controversy regarding its safety in cancer prevention,[9] especially since an increased incidence of endometrial carcinoma has been found in women treated chronically with tamoxifen.[30] It is therefore inappropriate to refer to tamoxifen simply as an antiestrogen. The term selective estrogen receptor modulator (SERM) is more appropriate.

Tamoxifen was originally screened in a drug development program oriented toward discovering new contraceptive agents. Although it was effective in rats, it was not a useful drug for control of fertility in women, and it was not until the early 1970s that it was shown to be useful for clinical palliation of advanced breast cancer. Subsequently, animal studies performed in rats, using both dimethylbenzanthracene (DMBA) and nitrosomethylurea as carcinogens, showed that tamoxifen was highly effective in preventing the development of experimental breast cancer;[31,32] these results have also been confirmed in the mouse model in which murine mammary tumor virus is the carcinogen.

The mechanism of action of tamoxifen is complex. Clearly, its principal mechanism of action is mediated by its binding to the estrogen receptor and the blocking of the proliferative actions of estrogen on mammary epithelium. One suggested mechanism for this antiproliferative action is the induction by tamoxifen of the synthesis of the cytokine transforming growth factor-β (TGF-β), which acts as a negative autocrine regulatory molecule.[33] However, it has also been shown that tamoxifen can induce synthesis of TGF-β in estrogen receptor-negative cells, such as fetal fibroblasts.[34] Moreover, immunohistochemical studies have shown that tamoxifen induces the synthesis of TGF-β in the stromal (mesenchymal) compartment of breast cancers, suggesting a paracrine as well as autocrine mechanism of action, independent of an interaction with the estrogen receptor.[35] Reports of some clinical efficacy of tamoxifen in the treatment of women with estrogen receptor-negative breast carcinomas would appear to be in accord with these mechanistic conclusions,[36] although these findings are controversial. Other studies that are in accord with these observations are the findings that tamoxifen can lower the circulating levels of insulin-like growth factor I (IGF-I) in breast cancer patients.[37,38] IGF-I is a potent mitogen for breast cancer cells and may act by endocrine, paracrine, and autocrine routes to stimulate their growth. This agent has undergone large-scale phase III testing for breast cancer prevention, which is discussed later in this chapter under "Chemoprevention Trials," "Breast."

Raloxifene Although the risks are actually quite small, there is major concern about the safety of the use of tamoxifen as a chemopreventive agent for the prophylaxis of breast cancer because of its estrogenic effect on uterine epithelium and the attendant increased risk of development of uterine cancer. Thus, there has been a search for new agents that would resemble tamoxifen in their overall mechanism of action, but would be inhibitory to the growth of uterine epithelium. One such molecule is raloxifene, the chemical structure of which is totally different from that of tamoxifen; tamoxifen is a triphenylethylene derivative, but raloxifene is a benzothiophene. Like tamoxifen, raloxifene binds to the estrogen receptor and has both estrogenic and antiestrogenic actions; it is another estrogen-response modifier. It has been shown to have both therapeutic and preventive activity on breast tumors induced in rats by chemical carcinogens.[32] Most notably, in contrast to tamoxifen, raloxifene does not act as an estrogen agonist in the uterus and does not stimulate the growth of uterine epithelium in ovariectomized rats.[39] However, raloxifene is strongly estrogenic in its positive actions on bone and serum lipids; it is a potent agent for prevention of bone loss in the ovariectomized rat.[39] Because of this unusual spectrum of pharmacologic activity, raloxifene is an attractive agent for the prevention of bone loss in osteoporotic, postmenopausal women, which is its primary therapeutic application at present. Raloxifene has been shown to prevent ER-positive breast cancer in women who have used this agent as treatment for osteoporosis and is undergoing clinical testing for breast cancer prevention in a phase III trial called the Study of Tamoxifen and Raloxifene (STAR), which is discussed later in this chapter under "Chemoprevention Trials," "Breast."

Deltanoids (Vitamin D and Its Synthetic Analogues) Another important ligand of the steroid receptor superfamily is 1,25-dihydroxycholecalciferol (1,25-DHCC), the active metabolite of dietary vitamin D. 1,25-DHCC has potent actions in controlling the expression of many genes and can induce differentiation in many tumor cells, particularly those of myeloid lineage.[40,41] However, because of its marked hypercalcemic activity, it is not a suitable agent for clinical chemoprevention. A large number of synthetic analogues of 1,25-DHCC have been made, with the goal of increasing differentiative activity and decreasing calcemic actions;[42] we have suggested the term "deltanoids," analogous to "retinoids," for the entire family of natural and synthetic molecules related to 1,25-DHCC.[43] Many of the new analogues are markedly less calcemic and more active in inducing differentiation, and some have been shown to be active in the prevention of breast cancer in animal experiments.[43,44] The clinical potential for the use of these agents is still unrealized.

Finasteride Prostate carcinogenesis in both experimental animals and humans is driven by androgen, in much the same way that mammary carcinogenesis is driven by estrogen. The testosterone metabolite 5α-dihydrotestosterone (DHT) has higher binding affinity for the androgen receptor than testosterone and is believed to play a critical role in the development of the prostate gland. DHT is formed from testosterone by the action of the enzyme 5α-reductase, and several androgen analogues have been developed as antagonists of this enzyme. One of these analogues, finasteride, is now in widespread use to treat benign prostatic hyperplasia (BPH)[45] and has been tested in a large-scale phase III trial called the Prostate Cancer Prevention Trial (PCPT), which is discussed later in this chapter under "Chemoprevention Trials," "Prostate."

Difluoromethylornithine Agents that can suppress cell proliferation are obvious candidates for chemoprevention if they have sufficient selectivity. One such molecule is difluoromethylornithine (DFMO), a potent irreversible inhibitor of the enzyme ornithine decarboxylase, which catalyzes the formation of putrescine, a polyamine involved in DNA synthesis.[46] There is a very extensive literature on the use of DFMO to prevent carcinogenesis in animal models of colon, bladder, breast, liver, skin, and stomach cancer.[47] The National Cancer Institute (NCI) has conducted extensive preclinical and clinical toxicologic evaluations of this drug, and further clinical trials are in progress.

Nonsteroidal Anti-Inflammatory Drugs A large number of nonsteroidal anti-inflammatory drugs (NSAIDs) have shown potent chemopreventive activity in many test systems. Among the NSAIDs that have been studied at length are aspirin, ibuprofen, sulindac, and piroxicam. All of these molecules are cyclooxygenase inhibitors that block prostaglandin synthesis, and they are in widespread clinical use for the chronic treatment of various inflammatory diseases, most notably osteoarthritis or rheumatoid arthritis. There is therefore an abundance of information about the safe dosage for their long-term administration that would be required for a chemoprevention trial. All of these inhibitors of prostaglandin synthesis have been shown to be active in a multiplicity of animal models for the suppression of carcinogenesis, with particular efficacy in preventing experimental colon carcinogenesis. Most recently, attention has been focused on selective cyclooxygenase-2 (COX-2) inhibitors, such as rofecoxib (Vioxx) or celecoxib (Celebrex), since these have the potential to prevent cancer with fewer undesirable side effects than classic NSAIDs.[48] Based on these results, a number of clinical trials have been conducted or are underway. Clinical data from a colorectal polyp prevention trial show that the selective COX-2 inhibitor rofecoxib at 25 mg per day for 18 months is associated with an increased number of cardiovascular events (acute myocardial infarction and stroke), and this agent has been voluntarily withdrawn from the world market. Although limited clinical data indicate an increase in cardiovascular events with celecoxib, there are other clinical data indicating no increase in these events, and celecoxib continues to be marketed worldwide. The clinical NSAID prevention trials are discussed in greater detail later in this chapter under "Chemoprevention Trials," "Colon and Rectum."

***N*-Acetylcysteine and Oltipraz** Glutathione in its reduced form (GSH) is a critical molecule in the chemical deactivation of many carcinogens. Since glutathione itself is not a practical agent for chemoprevention, a great deal of effort has been devoted to the development of exogenous agents that would elevate intracellular GSH levels. This principle, termed electrophile counterattack,[49] has been the basis of extensive investigation. *N*-acetylcysteine and oltipraz are two of the most important such molecules that act by this mechanism. These agents can block the mutagenic activity of a variety of carcinogens by preventing their binding to DNA, either directly or indirectly; a substantial decrease in DNA adducts has been seen if either *N*-acetylcysteine or oltipraz is given to animals when they are treated with carcinogens such as aflatoxin, benzo[*a*]pyrene, or acetylaminofluorene.[50,51] Both agents are active in animal test systems for the prevention of cancer, and both are in clinical trial.

CHEMOPREVENTION TRIALS

Numerous randomized controlled trials (RCTs) of chemoprevention in many sites have been reported to date (Table 27-1). Chemoprevention entered the realm of standard clinical practice, when, following unblinding of the Breast Cancer Prevention Trial (BCPT) in 1998, the Food and Drug Administration (FDA) approved tamoxifen for breast-cancer risk reduction in high-risk women. The second and only other FDA-approved agent in a chemoprevention setting is celecoxib, which was approved in 1999 for helping in the control of familial adenomatous polyposis (FAP). Several other RCTs also show promise for helping to introduce other chemopreventive agents into standard practice in certain settings.[52,53]

HEAD AND NECK **Oral Premalignancy** Oral leukoplakia is a premalignant lesion that manifests with a white patch unclassifiable as any other disorder.[54] Current management ranges from observation to excision (discussed in detail in Chapter 79, "Neoplasms of the Head and Neck"), depending on the location, extent, and histology of the lesion. Chemoprevention may become standard systemic therapy in certain cases, such as those involving aneuploidy (further discussed below) or extensive multiple lesions.[55]

Oral leukoplakia is an excellent model system for clinical testing of chemopreventive agents with potential activity throughout the aerodigestive tract. This lesion is related to tobacco use and associated with squamous cell carcinoma. It is easily monitored clinically, cytologically, and histologically and is related to carcinogenesis in other aerodigestive tract sites.[54,55] The oral leukoplakia system has been used for clinical laboratory translational studies of agent effects on histopathologic and other intermediate end-point biomarkers of carcinogenesis.[55–57]

Systemic retinoid, β-carotene, vitamin E, and selenium intervention have been used in nonrandomized chemoprevention trials in oral leukoplakia.[52,54,58] Only the retinoids have had their

Table 27-1 Randomized Chemopreventional Trials

Author (Year)	Study Setting/Endpoint	Design	Number	Intervention	Primary Outcome
Head and Neck					
Hong et al (1986)[59]	Oral leukoplakia	Phase II	44	Isotretinoin (1–2 mg/kg/d)	Positive
Stitch et al (1986)[62]	Oral leukoplakia	Phase II	65	Vit A (200,000 IU/wk)	Positive
Han et al (1990)[63]	Oral leukoplakia	Phase II	61	Retinamide (40 mg/d)	Positive
Lippman et al (1993)[60]	Oral leukoplakia	Phase II	70	Isotretinoin (0.5 mg/kg/d)	Positive
Chiesa et al (1993)[64]	Oral leukoplakia	Phase II	80	Fenretinide (200 mg/d)	Positive
Epstein et al (1994)[65]	Oral leukoplakia	Phase II	22	Topical bleomycin (1%)	Positive
Hong et al (1990)[75]	Prior SCC	Phase III	103	Isotretinoin (100 $mg/m^2/d$)	Positive (SPT)
Bolla et al (1994)[80]	Prior SCC	Phase III	316	Etretinate (50, 25 mg/d)	Negative
Lung					
Heimburger et al (1988)[85]	Metaplasia	Phase II	73	Vit B_{12} (500 μg/d); Folic acid (10 mg/d)	Positive
Arnold et al (1992)[82]	Metaplasia	Phase II	150	Etretinate (25 mg/d)	Negative
van Poppel et al (1992)[86]	Micronuclei	Phase II	114	βC (20 mg/d)	Positive
Lee et al (1994)[83]	Metaplasia	Phase II	87	Isotretinoin (1 mg/kg/d)	Negative
van Poppel et al (1995)[87]	8-oxodG	Phase II	122	βC (20 mg/d)	Negative
McLarty et al (1995)[88]	Metaplasia	Phase II	755	βC (50 mg/d); Vit A (25,000 IU qod)	Negative
Kurie et al (2000)[84]	Metaplasia	Phase II	70	Fenretinide (200 mg/d)	Negative
Kurie et al (2002)[89]	Metaplasia, RAR-β	Phase II	177	9*c*RA (100 mg/d); isotretinoin (1 mg/kg) + Vit E (1,200 IU)	Positive (9*c*RA)
Lam et al (2002)[90]	Dysplasia	Phase II	101	Anethole dithiolethione (75 mg/d)	Positive
ATBC Cancer Prevention Study (1994)[91]	Lung cancer	Phase III (2 × 2 factorial)	29,133	βC (20 mg/d); Vit E (50 mg/d)	Negative
Omenn et al (CARET) (1996)[95]	Lung cancer	Phase III	18,314	βC (30 mg/d); Vit A (25,000 IU/d)	Negative
Pastorino et al (1993)[96]	Prior NSCLC	Phase III	307	Vit A (300,000 IU/d)	Positive (SPT)
van Zandwijk et al (2000)[97]	Prior HNC, NSCLC	Phase III (2 × 2 factorial)	2,592	Vit A (300,000/150,000 IU/d); NAC (600 mg/d)	Negative
Lippman et al (2001)[98]	Prior NSCLC	Phase III	1,166	Isotretinoin (30 mg/d)	Negative
Colon					
Bussey et al (1982)[123]	FAP	Phase II	36	Vit C (3 g/d)	Positive (polyp)
McKeown-Eyssen et al (1988)[124]	Adenoma	Phase II	137	Vits C (400 mg/d), E (400 mg/d)	Negative
DeCosse et al (1989)[125]	FAP	Phase II	58	Vits C (4 g/d), E (400 mg/d); Fiber (22.5 g/d)	Positive (polyp)
Gregoire et al (1989)[117]	Prior cancer	Phase II	30	Calcium (1,200 mg/d)	Negative (LI)
Stern et al (1990)[116]	Prior FAP	Phase II	31	Calcium (1,200 mg/d)	Negative (LI)
Labayle et al (1991)[114]	FAP	Phase II	10	Sulindac (300 mg/d)	Positive (polyps)
Kikendall et al (1991)[122]	Adenoma	Phase II	257	βC (15 mg/d)	Negative
Barsoum et al (1992)[118]	Adenoma	Phase II	14	Calcium (1.25 g/d)	Positive (LI)
Wargovich et al (1992)[115]	Adenoma	Phase II	20	Calcium (2,000 mg/d)	Positive (LI)
Paganelli et al (1992)[128]	Adenoma	Phase II	41	Vits A (30,000 IU/d), E (70 mg/d), C (1 g/d)	Negative (LI)
Alberts et al (1992)[127]	Adenoma	Phase II	100	WBF (2.0 or 13.5 g/d); Calcium (250 or 1,500 mg/d)	Negative (LI)
Giardiello et al (1993)[99]	FAP	Phase II	22	Sulindac (300 mg/d)	Positive (polyps)
MacLennan et al (1995)[126]	Adenoma	Phase II	395	Fat (< 25% of calories); WBF (11 g/d); βC (20 mg/d)	Negative (polyps)
Bostick et al (1993)[119]	Adenoma	Phase II	21	Calcium (1,200 mg/d)	Negative (LI)
Roncucci et al (1993)[129]	Adenoma	Phase II	209	Vits A (30,000 IU/d), C (1 g/d), E (70 mg/d); Lactulose (20 g/d)	Positive
Greenberg et al (1994)[130]	Adenoma	Phase II	751	βC (25 mg/d); Vits E (400 mg/d), C (1 g/d)	Negative
Cats et al (1995)[120]	HNPCC	Phase II	30	Calcium (1,500 mg/d)	Negative (LI)
Baron et al (1995)[104]	Adenoma	Phase II	333	Calcium (3,000 mg/d)	Negative (LI)
Baron et al (1999)[121]	Adenoma	Phase II	913	Calcium (3,000 mg/d)	Positive
Schatzkin et al (2000)[110]	Adenoma	Phase II	1,905	Low fat (20% of total calories), High fiber (18 g/1000 kcal); Fruits and vegetables (3.5 servings/1000 kcal)	Negative
Alberts et al (2000)[111]	Adenoma	Phase II	1,303	High fiber (13.5 g/d)	Negative
Steinbach et al (2000)[100]	FAP	Phase II	77	Celecoxib (800 mg/d)	Positive
Baron et al (2002)[103]	Adenoma	Phase II	1,121	Aspirin (80 mg/d)	Positive
Giardiello et al (2002)[102]	FAP	Phase II	41	Sulindac (150 mg/d, 300 mg/d)	Negative
Skin					
Moriarty et al (1982)[132]	AK	Phase II	50	Etretinate (75 mg/d)	Positive
Watson (1986)[133]	AK	Phase II	15	Etretinate (75 mg/d)	Positive
Kligman & Thorne (1991)[131]	AK	Phase II	527	Topical tretinoin (0.05%)	Negative
Kligman & Thorne (1991)[131]	AK	Phase II	455	Topical tretinoin (0.10%)	Positive
Yarosh et al (2001)[141]	Xeroderma pigmentosum	Phase II	30	Topical T4 endonuclease V (1%)	Positive
Levine et al (1997)[139]	Prior BCC/SCC	Phase III	524	Isotretinoin (5-10 mg/d); Vit A (25,000 IU/d)	Negative
Greenberg et al (1990)[136]	Prior BCC/SCC	Phase III	1,805	βC (50 mg/d)	Negative
Tangrea et al (1992)[137]	Prior BCC	Phase III	981	Isotretinoin (10 mg/d)	Negative
Moon et al (1997)[138]	AK	Phase III	2,298	Vit A (25,000 IU/d)	Positive
Bouwes Bavinck et al (1995)[135]	Renal transplant	Phase III	38	Acitretin (30 mg/d)	Positive
Clark et al (1996)[140]	Prior BCC/SCC	Phase III	1,312	Selenium (200 μg/d)	Negative
Breast					
Fisher et al (1998)[142]	High risk/BC	Phase III	13,388	Tamoxifen (20 mg/d)	Positive
Veronesi et al (1998)[146]	BC	Phase III	5,408	Tamoxifen (20 mg/d)	Negative
Powles et al (1998)[147]	High risk/BC	Phase III	2,471	Tamoxifen (20 mg/d)	Negative
Fisher et al (1999)[144]	DCIS/BC	Phase III	1,804	Tamoxifen (20 mg/d)	Positive
Veronesi et al (1999)[151]	CBC	Phase III	2,972	Fenretinide (200 mg/d)	Negative

(Continued)

Table 27-1 Randomized Chemopreventional Trials *(Continued)*

Author (Year)	Study Setting/Endpoint	Design	Number	Intervention	Primary Outcome
Esophagus/Stomach					
Munoz et al (1985)[158]	Geographic risk	Phase II	610	Vit A (50,000 IU/wk); Riboflavin (200 mg/wk); Zinc (50 mg/wk)	Negative
Zaridze et al (1993)[161]	Geographic risk	Phase II	532	Riboflavin (80 mg/wk); Vits A 100,000 IU/wk), E (80 mg/wk); βC (40 mg/d)	Negative
Blot et al (1993)[164]	Geographic risk	Phase III	29,584	Multiple vitamins/minerals	Negative
Li et al (1993)[165]	Geographic risk	Phase III	3,318	Multiple vitamins/minerals	Negative
Buiatti et al (1994)[166]	Geographic risk	Phase II	222	Bismuth (120 mg qid); Amoxicillin (500 mg qid)	Negative (*H. pylori*)
Bladder					
Alfthan et al (1983)[168]	SBT	Phase II	32	Etretinate (25–50 mg/d)	Positive
Pederson et al (1984)[169]	SBT	Phase II	73	Etretinate (50 mg/d)	Negative
Studer et al (1984)[170]	SBT	Phase II	86	Etretinate (25–50 mg/d)	Positive
Lamm et al (1994)[171]	SBT	Phase II	65	Megadose vitamins	Positive
Cervix					
Byrne et al (1986)[173]	CIN 2, 3	Phase II	26	HLI (0.8×10^6 IU/wk)	Negative
Yliskoski et al (1990)[174]	CIN 1, 2	Phase II	20	HLI (9×10^6 IU/d)	Negative
Frost et al (1990)[175]	CIN 2	Phase II	10	IFN-α2b (4×10^6 IU/wk)	Negative
Dunham et al (1990)[176]	CIN 1-3	Phase II	14	IFN-α2b (6×10^6 IU/wk)	Negative
de Vet et al (1991)[179]	CIN 1-3	Phase II	278	βC (10 mg/d)	Negative
Butterworth et al (1992)[177]	CIN 1, 2	Phase II	235	Folic acid (10 mg/d)	Negative
Meyskens et al (1994)[180]	CIN 2, 3	Phase II	301	Topical tretinoin (0.372%)	Positive (CIN 2)
Childers et al (1995)[178]	CIN 1, 2	Phase II	331	Folic acid (5 mg/d)	Negative
Follen et al (2001)[181]	CIN 2, 3	Phase II	39	Fenretinide (200 mg/d)	Negative
Keefe et al (2001)[182]	CIN 2, 3	Phase II	103	βC (30 mg/d)	Negative
All Cancer					
Hennekens et al (1996)[185]	Healthy men	Phase III	22,071	βC (50 mg qod)	Negative
Lee et al (1999)[186]	Healthy women	Phase III	39,876	βC (50 mg qod)	Negative

Adapted and updated from Table 2 of Lippman SM et al.[52]

ATBC = Alpha-Tocopherol, Beta-Carotene; AK = actinic keratosis; BC = breast cancer; BCC = basal cell carcinoma; CARET = β-Carotene and Retinol Efficacy Trial; CBC = contralateral breast cancer; βC = beta-carotene; CIN = cervical intraepithelial neoplasia (CIN 1, mild dysplasia; CIN 2, moderate dysplasia; CIN 3, severe dysplasia); 9cRA = 9-*cis*-retinoic acid; DCIS = ductal carcinoma in situ; FAP = familial adenomatous polyposis; HLI = human leukocyte interferon; HNPCC = hereditary nonpolyposis colon cancer; *H. pylori* = *Helicobacter pylori*; IFN = interferon; kcal = kilocalories; LI = labeling index; NAC = *N*-acetylcysteine; NSCLC = non–small cell lung carcinoma; 8-oxodG = 8-oxo-7,8-dihydro-2'-deoxyguanosine; RAR-β = retinoic acid receptor-β; SBT = superficial bladder tumors; SCC = squamous cell carcinoma; SPT = second primary tumors; Vit = vitamin; WBF = wheat bran fiber.

preliminary activity confirmed in randomized trials.[59–64] In the only other randomized drug intervention trial, significant activity was reported with topical bleomycin.[65] Although interesting, the potential value of this local approach is limited by its inability to treat the diffuse aerodigestive epithelial field at risk.

Five randomized retinoid trials in oral premalignancy have been reported. The first of these, reported in 1986, was a short-term, placebo-controlled, double-blind study of high-dose isotretinoin.[59] For 3 months, 44 subjects received either 1 to 2 mg/kg/d of isotretinoin or placebo. Major clinical responses occurred in 67% (16 of 24) of isotretinoin recipients and in 10% (2 of 20) of placebo recipients ($p = .0002$). Histologic major responses (reversal of atypia) occurred in 54% (13 of 24) of isotretinoin recipients and 10% (2 of 20) of placebo recipients ($p = .01$). Although isotretinoin was active, over half of responders had recurrences of or developed new lesions within 3 months of stopping it. Also, the high-dose isotretinoin regimen was unacceptably toxic for long-term use.

A second randomized trial was conducted to solve the toxicity and relapse problems encountered in the first.[60,61] In an induction phase, 70 patients received high-dose isotretinoin therapy (1.5 mg/kg/d for 3 months). In a subsequent maintenance phase, stable and responding patients were randomized to 9 months of low-dose isotretinoin (0.5 mg/kg/d) or β-carotene (30 mg/d). Fifty-three subjects qualified for full evaluation. Treatment failure (disease progression or new lesion development) during or after maintenance therapy was 8% (2 of 24) and 55% (16 of 29) in the isotretinoin and β-carotene groups, respectively ($p < .001$). The toxic effects of low-dose isotretinoin therapy were generally mild, although significantly greater than those of β-carotene. The maintenance isotretinoin dose produced tolerable and reversible mucocutaneous dryness and hypertriglyceridemia.

The three other randomized trials reported significant retinoid activity in oral premalignancy. Natural vitamin A had significant activity in a 6-month placebo-controlled trial in 54 Asian betel nut chewers.[62] The synthetic retinamide, *N*-4-(hydroxycarbophenyl) retinamide had significant activity in a 4-month placebo-controlled trial.[63] A maintenance trial tested fenretinide (versus no treatment) in preventing relapse or new lesion development after complete laser resection of premalignant oral lesions.[64] Interim results on 137 randomized patients who received no treatment or fenretinide at a dose of 200 mg/d for 52 weeks and with 1-year follow-up indicate a significantly lower failure rate in the retinoid arm. There were 11 treatment failures (9 recurrences, 2 new premalignant oral lesions, 0 cancers) in the fenretinide arm and 21 treatment failures (8 recurrences, 12 new lesions, and 1 cancer) in the no-treatment control arm.[64]

Adjunctive laboratory studies of retinoic acid receptors, *p53* and loss of heterozygosity (LOH) have been integrated into recent clinical retinoid trials in oral premalignancy. Earlier in vitro and in vivo studies show that expression of the RAR-β messenger ribonucleic acid (mRNA) is sequentially lost with carcinogenic progression to dysplasia and cancer in the head and neck, and that RAR-β expression can be upregulated by retinoic acid in vitro in cancer cell lines. In a prospective isotretinoin trial, RAR-β mRNA was detected via in situ hybridization with antisense RNA in only 21 (40%) of 52 premalignant oral lesions ($p = .003$).[66] RAR-β mRNA expression increased significantly in response to high-dose isotretinoin (from 40 to 90%, $p < .001$), in direct association with clinical response ($p = .04$). These translational data conform with strong preclinical data indicating that RAR-β is the nuclear receptor most highly regulated by retinoids.

Studies of *p53* are another major area of translational research within head and neck cancer chemoprevention trials. Frequent alterations of the *p53* gene and its protein product occur in head and neck cancer and in adjacent normal-appearing and premalignant tissue.[55] A prospective study revealed a lack of *p53* modulation by isotretinoin, and a significant correlation between lesion resistance to isotretinoin and levels of *p53* accumulation ($p = .006$).[67] Promising results in advanced oral intraepithelial neoplasia (IEN) have been achieved by *p53* targeting. ONYX-015 is a replication-competent adenovirus that selectively replicates in and causes lysis of cells with deficient *p53* activity. A complete regression of dysplasia occurred in 7 of 19 advanced oral IEN patients who were taking ONYX-015.[68]

The molecular markers aneuploidy and LOH (at 3p and 9p) have been documented in oral premalignant lesions, providing evidence of genetic instability and clonal expansion in preinvasive head and neck lesions, and found to be significant predictors of cancer development in this setting.[69,70] Complete resection (no dysplasia at the margins) does not prevent oral cancer, which is frequently aggressive, in patients with aneuploid dysplastic leukoplakia.[70] Complete resection also did not statistically significantly reduce oral cancer in patients with molecular high-risk lesions defined by LOH patterns, unless the completeness was confirmed molecularly,[71] illustrating the importance of molecular confirmation of complete resection in this setting. The roles of optimal surgical margin width and molecularly confirmed complete resection in reducing cancer risk in high-risk LOH settings should be examined further. Topical supravital toluidine blue staining may be helpful in identifying oral IEN with molecularly marked high cancer risk and in guiding surgical margin widths since this staining recently was found to be associated with the presence of LOH in dysplastic, minimally dysplastic, or nondysplastic oral IEN.[72,73] LOH also has been used to monitor molecular response to chemoprevention.[69]

Prevention of Second Primary Tumors Compelling factors support the testing of retinoids in the adjuvant setting of second primary tumor prevention after definitive therapy of primary head and neck cancer.[52–55] Oral premalignancy, which is linked to second primary tumor development through field carcinogenesis and other shared etiologic and biologic features, responds to retinoids. Second primary tumors occur in a diffuse pattern throughout the aerodigestive tract and bladder, making them beyond the control of local therapies. Second primary tumors are a major cause of death following "cure" of head and neck cancer and are the leading cancer-related cause of death after resection of early-stage disease. Second primary tumors develop at a constant rate of approximately 6% per year.[52,54]

The first phase III adjuvant trial to prevent these second primary tumors involved high-dose isotretinoin.[74] Following definitive local therapy of primary head and neck tumors, 103 patients received either isotretinoin (100 mg/m^2/d) or placebo for 1 year. This isotretinoin regimen was intolerable, and protocol doses were reduced to 50 mg/m^2/d after the first 44 enrolled patients. At a median follow-up of 32 months for all patients, the rate of second primary tumors was significantly lower in the retinoid group (4%) than in the placebo group (24%) ($p = .005$). The retinoid, however, had no significant effect on disease recurrence, disease-free survival, or overall survival.

A follow-up analysis of this trial after a median of 55 months was recently reported.[75] Isotretinoin's protective effect against all second primary tumors had decreased since the 32-month follow-up but remained statistically significant ($p = .04$). In the subset of only tobacco-related second primary tumors, the retinoid's protective effect remained at a similar level of statistical significance ($p = .008$). Reversible retinoid effects in all second primary tumors and other carcinogenic settings are the norm. The strong long-term retinoid effect, without treatment, against these tobacco-related second primary tumors is unprecedented.

Stringent prospective methods employed to effect surgical salvage of second primary tumor patients, most of whom came from the placebo group, may have masked the retinoid's ability to improve survival. The study population included a large percentage of patients with stages III and IV disease, who frequently experience early treatment failure and death from primary disease recurrence. Therefore, this trial could not indicate whether isotretinoin can improve survival in patients with early-stage disease.

Isotretinoin's significant activity in this initial second primary tumor prevention trial led to an NCI intergroup phase III trial of isotretinoin that was designed to prevent second primary tumors associated with stages I and II head and neck cancer.[76] This trial's design called for low-dose isotretinoin to solve the toxicity problems encountered in the first trial. Low-dose isotretinoin was given for 3 years to prevent second primary tumors in over 1,000 patients with definitively treated early-stage head and neck cancer. The lower dose was better tolerated than was the high-dose isotretinoin regimen but had no effect on second primary tumors, recurrence, or survival.[77] The survival rate in former smokers was significantly better than in current smokers, providing the first definitive proof of a benefit of smoking cessation in this setting. A high-dose bioadjuvant regimen of isotretinoin combined with interferon-alpha and vitamin E substantially reduced recurrence and second primary tumors associated with locally advanced head and neck cancer in a phase-II trial.[78] These results led to an ongoing phase III adjuvant trial (coordinated by the Eastern Cooperative Oncology Group) of this regimen in locally advanced disease.

Investigators in France assessed the efficacy of the synthetic retinoid etretinate in preventing second primary tumors following definitive therapy of stage I-III squamous cell carcinomas of the oral cavity and oral pharynx.[79] By random assignment, patients received either etretinate or placebo at doses of 50 mg/d for 1 month, followed by 25 mg/d for 2 years. Second primary tumor rates in the two study arms did not differ significantly. Interpretation of this trial was clouded by insufficient details on study compliance and second primary tumor diagnostic criteria; however, certain valuable data were reported. The French trial confirmed earlier prospective data on the high rate of second primary tumors associated with head and neck cancer. After 41 months' median follow-up, 24% of placebo recipients had developed second primary tumors. Also, data from this trial support the field carcinogenesis theory concerning aerodigestive tract cancers: approximately 80% of second primary tumors developed in the head and neck, lungs, or esophagus.

The Lung Premalignancy Premalignant conditions of the lung have been the arena for several clinical and translational chemoprevention trials.[55,81] Four randomized trials of retinoids in smokers with metaplasia have been reported.[82–90] The first of these trials was a placebo-controlled trial of etretinate for the reversal of metaplasia appearing in sputum samples.[82] Therapy lasted 6 months. Metaplasia was reversed in the sputum of 32% of etretinate subjects and 30% of placebo subjects. The second trial was a placebo-controlled trial of isotretinoin.[83] This trial evaluated metaplasia in bronchial biopsy specimens. By random assignment, 87 subjects received either placebo or isotretinoin for 6 months. Both study groups experienced a substantial reduction in metaplasia index: 54% in the isotretinoin arm and 60% in the placebo arm. Smoking cessation was closely correlated with a significant reduction in the metaplasia index. A more recent study involved fenretinide.[84] This study's overall design (except for the drug) and negative primary result were similar to those of the earlier isotretinoin study.[83] Despite the generally negative data (see Table 27-1), encouraging phase IIb data have emerged from recent studies of 9-*cis*-retinoic acid[89] and anethole dithiolthione,[90] especially in former smokers.

Prevention of Primary Lung Cancer The NCI-sponsored Alpha-Tocopherol, Beta-Carotene (ATBC) Cancer Prevention Study was a phase III trial of α-tocopherol and β-carotene to prevent primary lung cancer. The ATBC study involved 29,133 male smokers between 50 and 69 years of age who had smoked an average of one pack of cigarettes a day for approximately 36 years.[91] This trial's 2×2 factorial design called for α-tocopherol (50 mg/d) and β-carotene (20 mg/d) to be given in a randomized, double-blind, placebo-controlled fashion. The factorial design allowed the study scientists to assess the individual effects of each agent. Significant increases in lung cancer incidence (18% increase, $p = .01$) and total mortality (8%, $p = .02$) occurred in the β-carotene-treated subjects after 6.1 years' median follow-up. α-Tocopherol had no significant impact on the lung cancer mortality rate, and there was no evidence of an interaction between α-tocopherol and β-carotene. The β-carotene results from this large-scale phase III trial are consistent with experimental lung carcinogenesis studies.[92,93] These laboratory data and definitive clinical results contradict the epidemiologic data on β-carotene and underscore the need to confirm data of this type[53] before public health recommendations are made. The α-tocopherol group had a long-term nonsignificant trend of reduced lung cancer incidence and a significant positive secondary analysis in prostate cancer, a 32% decrease in incidence and 41% decrease in mortality.[94]

The Beta-Carotene and Retinol Efficacy Trial (CARET) is the other major NCI phase III lung cancer chemoprevention trial. This trial tested the combination of β-carotene (30 mg/d) plus retinyl palmitate (25,000 IU/d) in 17,000 smokers and asbestos workers.[95] It confirmed the major finding of the ATBC study with its primary finding that the β-carotene combination increased lung cancer risk in this high-risk population. There was no evidence from either the ATBC study or the CARET that β-carotene increased lung cancer risk in nonsmokers, former, or moderate (less than one pack a day) smokers.

Prevention of Second Primary Tumors Second primary tumors in lung cancer are related to those associated with head and neck cancer through etiology, region, and biology. An adjuvant trial of the natural vitamin A ester retinyl palmitate achieved a significant reduction in lung second primary tumors.[96] Patients were randomly assigned to receive either 300,000 IU of retinyl palmitate daily (150 patients) or no treatment (157 patients) for 12 months following complete resection of stage I non–small cell lung cancer. Compliance was over 80%, and toxic effects were minimal. At a median follow-up of 46 months, second primary tumors occurred in 29 (8%) of control patients and in 18 (12%) of retinyl palmitate recipients. Thirteen patients in the retinoid group and 25 in the control group developed tobacco-related second primary tumors, whose development time was significantly shorter in the control arm than in the retinoid arm (p = .045). Recurrence and disease-free and overall survival rates were not significantly different between the retinoid and placebo groups.

These encouraging results with second primary tumors and retinoid activity in related carcinogenic systems led to two large-scale phase III retinoid trials in the setting of second primary tumor prevention; one was in Europe and the other in the United States. The European trial, called the European Study on Chemoprevention with Vitamin A and *N*-Acetylcysteine (EUROSCAN),[97] was an open-label multicenter trial of 2 years of retinyl palmitate and *N*-acetyl-L-cysteine (NAC) in a 2 × 2 factorial design. Its aim was to prevent second primary tumors following definitive therapy of early-stage head and neck cancer (larynx Tis, T1–3, N0–1; oral cavity T1–2, N0–1) and non–small cell lung cancer (pT1–2, N0–1, and T3 N0). Involving 2,592 patients, EUROSCAN found that retinyl palmitate and/or NAC produced no improvement in event-free survival, survival, or incidence of second primary tumors. The U.S. multicenter phase III Lung Intergroup Trial (LIT) (NCI I 91–0001) involved low-dose isotretinoin to prevent second primary tumors after definitive therapy of stage I non–small cell lung cancer.[98] Although LIT results were neutral overall, a provocative secondary finding of a drug interaction with smoking status was reported. Lung-cancer recurrence and mortality were potentially increased in current smokers and decreased in nonsmokers.

Colon and Rectum Colorectal trial designs have primarily employed the intermediate end points of adenomatous polyp development and response and hyperproliferation markers. Several NSAIDs, calcium salts, fiber, and vitamin micronutrient combinations in the prevention of colon cancer have been studied.[52,53,99–126] NSAIDs' ability to inhibit colon carcinogenesis was suggested by preclinical and epidemiologic studies[52,53] and is an active area of mechanism research.[113]

Sulindac and celecoxib can effectively treat (but not prevent) adenomas in FAP.[99–102] High-dose celecoxib (800 mg/d) reduced large-bowel polyposis by 28%[91] and duodenal polyposis, which is difficult to resect, by 14%[101] (versus placebo). The risk of sporadic adenomas was reduced by calcium (1,200 mg/d) 15% overall[104] and even more in later-stage disease[103,105] (versus placebo).

Three recent large RCTs have tested the efficacy of aspirin in preventing sporadic adenomas, showing significant reductions in recurrent adenomas among patients treated for one or more years. Sandler and colleagues[106] randomized 635 colorectal cancer survivors to aspirin (325 mg/d) versus placebo. The aspirin group had a significant reduction in the number of patients with incident adenomas and a significant delay in the time to the first adenoma after a median follow-up of 12.8 months. Baron and colleagues[107] randomized 1,121 patients with prior adenomas to aspirin (81 or 325 mg/d) versus placebo and reported a reduction in the adenoma risk in the low-dose aspirin group, especially in the risk of advanced adenomas (41% risk reduction). Interim results from another trial evaluating aspirin's effects against incident adenomas show preventive effects after 1 year in 272 randomized patients with prior adenomas.[108] An RCT of another NSAID, rofecoxib, led to the drug's withdrawal from the world market because of preliminary data indicating a significant association with serious heart events; subsequent preliminary data from the same trial showed that rofecoxib also was producing a significant reduction (versus placebo) in sporadic adenomas.[109] Preliminary data from one of three ongoing RCTs of celecoxib have raised safety concerns for celecoxib with respect to cardiovascular events; celecoxib continues to be marketed worldwide, and the safety concerns are under continuing review.

Recent cancer epidemiology trials have established a link between dietary factors and cancer prevention. This link led to RCTs of low-fat, high-fiber and high-fruit-and-vegetable diets in patients with sporadic adenomas.[110–112] Although the clinical trials did not result in reduced short-term adenoma rates, the randomized epidemiologic studies still underscore the evolution of cancer epidemiology in designing better cancer-prevention studies.

Trials of vitamins alone in relation to the colon have achieved largely negative results (see Table 27-1). The largest randomized trial of β-carotene or combined vitamins C and E given in a placebo-controlled, 2 × 2 factorial fashion was recently reported.[130] Lasting 4 years, this study included 864 patients having at least one adenoma within 3 months of study entry, and excluded patients with familial polyposis or a history of colorectal cancer. Neither β-carotene nor the vitamin combination was active.

The Skin Chemoprevention trials in reversing premalignant skin lesions and in preventing skin cancer have been conducted. Topical application of the retinoid tretinoin has exhibited dose-related activity against actinic keratosis in nonrandomized and randomized trials.[131] Systemic retinoid therapy has achieved significant activity against actinic keratosis in two placebo-controlled trials.[132,133] Topical formulations of eflornithine, colchicines, or 5-FU have produced significant activity in suppressing or regressing actinic keratosis. Aminolevulinic acid HCl with photodynamic therapy and sodium diclofenac recently received FDA approvals for treating actinic keratosis.

The NCI has sponsored a series of small trials of isotretinoin that achieved reductions in skin tumor incidence. One of these trials was conducted in five xeroderma pigmentosum patients at extremely high risk of developing nonmelanoma skin cancer.[134] This trial achieved a significant reduction in the number of skin cancers during the 2 years of high-dose isotretinoin (2 mg/kg/d) treatment (p = .02). Subsequent studies from these investigators have shown that this chemopreventive effect was dose related. The beneficial effect of this approach was lost after cessation of treatment. A randomized placebo-controlled trial tested the retinoid acitretin in 38 renal transplant recipients.[135] This study showed significant reductions in premalignant lesions and skin cancers. The chemopreventive effects were reversible after the 6-month retinoid intervention.

Several large-scale, long-term phase III chemoprevention trials have been conducted in subjects at much lower risk of developing skin cancer.[136–140] Only one of these trials was positive. In this trial, retinol (25,000 IU/d) significantly reduced the incidence of primary squamous cell (but not basal cell) skin cancer in patients with actinic keratosis.[138] The other trials, all negative, involved β-carotene, retinol, very low-dose isotretinoin and selenium in patients with previous skin cancers. The study of selenium (200 μg/d in brewer's yeast) was negative in its primary end point of preventing squamous cell and basal cell carcinomas of the skin in 1,312 patients having histories of nonmelanoma skin cancer and living in low-selenium-intake regions of the United States.[140] This trial, however, produced provocative secondary findings of significant positive selenium effects on prostate, lung, and colon cancer incidence and of total cancer incidence and mortality, which were attenuated in the longer term as shown by an analysis at the end of the blinded treatment period.

A recent novel randomized trial of a topical DNA-repair enzyme in xeroderma pigmentosum resulted in a reduction in the rates of actinic keratosis and basal cell carcinoma.[141]

The Breast Based on highly significant positive results of the Breast Cancer Prevention Trial

(BCPT), tamoxifen became the first chemopreventive agent to earn FDA approval. Conducted by the National Surgical Adjuvant Breast and Bowel Project (NSABP), the BCPT compared tamoxifen with placebo in preventing breast cancer in 13,388 women at high risk of this disease.[142] The major high-risk eligibility criteria were age > 60 years old and history of lobular carcinoma in situ (LCIS), or women from 35 to 59 years old with 5-year breast cancer risk of 1.66% based on the Gail model. The actual overall average, 5-year baseline, breast cancer risk was 3.2%.

At a median follow-up of 55 months, primary invasive breast cancer findings for the tamoxifen and placebo groups were 89 versus 175 respectively for a 49% relative reduction ($p < .00001$). The relative breast cancer risk reduction was similar for all age and risk groups and was limited to estrogen receptor-positive tumors. Relative risk reductions of invasive breast cancer were 56% and 86% for women with a history of LCIS and atypical hyperplasia respectively. Tamoxifen achieved a 50% reduction (35 versus 69 cases) in noninvasive breast cancers. Tamoxifen nonsignificantly reduced overall and breast cancer mortality.

Beneficial secondary findings included 19% fewer fractures in the tamoxifen group. Secondary adverse findings associated with tamoxifen were increased endometrial cancers, vascular events and cataracts. Neutral secondary findings included coronary heart disease and depression of mental function.

Although the BCPT successfully completed testing its primary hypothesis, it also raised several key unresolved issues, such as effects on mortality, optimal tamoxifen duration, generalizability of results, and the issue of prevention versus treatment.

The FDA recently approved tamoxifen for breast cancer risk reduction in high-risk women.[53] The FDA recommendation is 20 mg/d for 5 years for high-risk women and warns of tamoxifen-associated risks. The FDA also approved and recommended tamoxifen for reducing the incidence of contralateral breast cancers, based on consistent secondary adjuvant data.[143]

Adverse tamoxifen effects make this agent's use a complex, highly individualized decision. In general, an improved tamoxifen risk-to-benefit ratio applies in (1) higher breast cancer risk at any age, (2) any breast cancer risk at lower age, and (3) hysterectomy at any breast cancer risk of women > 50 years old.

The NSABP B-24 study tested 5 years of tamoxifen (20 mg/d) versus placebo as adjuvant therapy after resection and radiation in 1,804 patients with ductal carcinoma in situ.[144] At 74 months median follow-up, 5-year incidences of all breast cancer events (invasive and noninvasive) were 8.2% and 13.4% in the tamoxifen and placebo groups respectively, representing a 43% relative risk reduction ($p = .0009$). The cumulative incidence at 5 years of all invasive breast cancer events in the tamoxifen group was 4.1% versus 7.2% in the placebo group ($p = .004$).

The current NSABP prevention trial is the Study of Tamoxifen and Raloxifene (STAR). Secondary analyses from osteoporosis trials provided the strong rationale supporting raloxifene in the STAR,[143,145] which continues to be in the treatment and follow-up phase after successfully completing its accrual of approximately 19,000 randomized women.

Two smaller European (Italian and British) tamoxifen breast cancer prevention trials, however, were negative.[146,147] The major way both trials differed from the BCPT was in having much lower study powers. With 13,388 women and 368 breast cancer events, the BCPT had about two times the sample size and three times the number of events of both European trials combined. Each trial also had individual differences from the BCPT. The key British trial differences were a population of younger age, stronger family history, and concurrent use of hormone replacement therapy (26%). The key Italian trial differences were a relatively low-risk population and poor compliance.

The International Breast Cancer Intervention Study (IBIS-I) trial randomized 7,410 women and showed a 32% reduction in breast cancer risk with tamoxifen.[148] The positive results in this and the BCPT (the two stronger RCTs in this setting) were limited to estrogen receptor-positive cancers.

Based largely on results of the Anastrozole, Tamoxifen Alone or in Combination (ATAC) trial, there is great interest in aromatase inhibitors for breast cancer prevention in postmenopausal women. Involving 9,366 patients, ATAC found that the aromatase inhibitor anastrozole was more effective than was tamoxifen in reducing recurrence and contralateral breast cancer.[149] Anastrozole produced fewer vascular and endometrial events but more musculoskeletal events and fractures than did tamoxifen. These adjuvant ATAC data have led to IBIS RCTs of anastrozole versus placebo in high-risk postmenopausal women and versus tamoxifen in resected ductal carcinoma in situ.[150] The NSABP is planning a new RCT to compare the winner from STAR with an aromatase inhibitor in high-risk women. Despite the enthusiasm for raloxifene and aromatase inhibitors, tamoxifen remains the only proven and FDA-approved agent for preventing breast cancer in high risk women. Agents under development to prevent estrogen receptor-negative breast cancer include RXR-selective retinoids, and inhibitors of COX-2 and epidermal growth factor receptor.

The retinoid fenretinide has exhibited potent chemopreventive activity in breast carcinogenesis models and a favorable clinical toxicity profile. These data led to a large-scale, placebo-controlled Italian trial of fenretinide to prevent contralateral breast cancer (second primary tumors) in approximately 3,000 women who had previously undergone resection for early-stage, node-negative breast cancer.[151] Contralateral breast cancers in this setting occur at a rate of approximately 0.8% per year. The intervention will last 5 years and consists of 200 mg/d of fenretinide, with monthly 3-day drug holidays to avoid ocular toxicity (reduced night vision) associated with fenretinide-induced reductions in plasma retinol levels. There was no significant overall effect of fenretinide in preventing contralateral breast cancer, but a trend toward benefit in premenopausal (but not postmenopausal) women.

The Prostate Prostate cancer mortality has declined in the United States in recent years (SEER Cancer Statistics Review 1975–2000) but remains the most common visceral malignancy in U.S. men.[1] It is estimated that 230,110 new cases of and 29,900 deaths (the second leading cause of cancer death) from prostate cancer will occur in the U.S. in 2004, and 380,000 new cases are predicted to occur annually by 2025. The lifetime risks of developing and dying from prostate cancer are 17.6% and 2.8% respectively for white U.S. men and 20.6% and 4.7% respectively for African-American men,[152] the highest such risks in the world. Earlier detection with widespread prostate-specific antigen (PSA) screening and advances in prostate cancer surgery and radiation therapy have not prevented frequent morbidity and treatment complications in the men treated for localized disease.[153,154] Prostate carcinogenesis is an androgen-driven process, and a large-scale RCT, the Prostate Cancer Prevention Trial (PCPT), tested finasteride (5 mg/d), which inhibits 5-alpha-reductase from converting testosterone into the more potent androgen dihydrotestosterone, versus placebo for seven years in 18,882 men 55 years of age or older who had normal digital rectal exam (DRE) and PSA. Finasteride reduced the 7-year prostate cancer prevalence by 24.8%[155] but also increased high-grade disease—6.4% (finasteride) versus 5.1% (placebo). PCPT analyses also indicated a high risk of prostate cancer, including high-grade disease, among men with normal PSA levels.[156] The biology behind the provocative clinical results of the PCPT will be studied intensively in translational studies based on the PCPT's invaluable repository of biological specimens and correlative patient data. Another very large RCT, the Selenium and Vitamin E Cancer Prevention Trial (SELECT), is ongoing (although accrual has been completed) and evaluating selenium versus vitamin E versus combined selenium and vitamin E versus placebo in over 35,000 men whose eligibility requirements included a normal DRE and PSA and an age of 55 years or older (except African-American men, who were eligible at age 50 years or older). The rationale for SELECT is based largely on secondary findings from the two large RCTs, the ATBC and Nutritional Prevention of Cancer studies.[157]

Esophagus and Stomach In the United States, esophageal carcinoma is strongly associated with tobacco and alcohol abuse. Causes of this cancer in other parts of the world, such as China, however, appear to include nutritional deficiencies and exposure to carcinogens, such as *N*-nitroso compounds.

Several large placebo-controlled chemoprevention trials against esophageal or gastric carcinogenesis have been conducted. Subjects for most of these trials came from geographic regions with established high risks of esophageal or gastric cancers. Four trials were of multiple natural compounds. The applicability of the findings in developing countries to esophageal cancer in the United States and other developed countries with different epidemiologic risk profiles is not clear.

The first placebo-controlled, randomized trial to reverse esophageal squamous carcinogenesis was conducted in Huixian, China.[158] This trial was based on several factors, including epidemiologic and endoscopic studies in high-risk geographic areas. Subjects received a combination of retinol, riboflavin, and zinc for 13.5 months. The intervention achieved no overall reduction in the occurrence of premalignant lesions. Two subset analyses revealed that (1) micronuclei frequency in the esophagus, but not in the oral cavity, decreased significantly in association with the chemopreventive regimen[159] and (2) increased plasma micronutrient levels (primarily retinol) were associated with a reduction in dysplastic lesions, regardless of treatment arm.[160] This trial also illustrated an issue of concern to many investigators studying vitamins, minerals, and micronutrients. Plasma micronutrient levels in the Huixian trial increased substantially in about 50% of placebo recipients. Evidently these control subjects obtained readily available trial compounds via their diet or in over-the-counter preparations of vitamins and minerals. Poor study compliance, either in the form of drop-ins or dropouts, can greatly reduce the statistical power of a randomized trial.

The second phase IIb trial was conducted in Uzbekistan. Retinol, β-carotene, and vitamin E with or without riboflavin were given in a factorial design to high-risk subjects with oral leukoplakia and/or chronic esophagitis.[161] As in the Huixian study, none of the vitamin regimens had a significant effect on esophageal premalignancy.

An RCT in Linxian, China, tested celecoxib (200 mg/bid) and selenomethionine (200 μg/qd) in a 2 × 2 factorial design for effects on moderate or mild esophageal squamous dysplasia. Celecoxib did not improve either moderate or mild dysplasia. Selenomethionine did not improve moderate dysplasia but did improve mild dysplasia ($p = .02$).[162] There also have been trials in the prevention of esophageal adenocarcinoma, which has the fastest rising incidence of all cancers in western countries.[163] The adenocarcinoma precursor, Barrett's esophagus, has been studied intensively. In 2003, the United States FDA approved a photosensitizing porphyrin mixture (Photofrin) in conjunction with photodynamic therapy (PDT) for the ablation of high-grade dysplasia in patients with Barrett's esophagus who cannot or choose not to undergo esophagectomy. This approval was based on a multicenter RCT involving 138 patients randomized to Photofrin PDT plus omeprazole and 70 patients randomized to omeprazole alone (<http://www.fda.gov/cder/foi/label/2003/20451s012_photofrin_lbl.pdf>). Follow-up ranged from 2 to 3.6 years and showed that a complete and sustained eradication of high-grade dysplasia occurred in 77% of the patients treated with combination therapy versus in 39% of the patients treated with omeprazole alone ($p < .0001$). This chemopreventive approach involves intravenous injection of Photofrin, which is activated 40 to 50 hours later by endoscopically applied red light for a maximum of three treatment courses.

Two NCI placebo-controlled phase III trials of multiple vitamins and minerals were conducted in the high-risk area of Linxian, China. One trial employed a complex modified factorial design to test four different vitamin-mineral combinations given to 29,584 subjects for 5 years at doses of one to two times the US recommended daily allowance (RDA).[164] The combination of β-carotene, α-tocopherol, and selenium was associated with 4% and 21% reductions in the esophageal cancer and gastric cancer mortality rates respectively. The gastric cancer mortality reduction was significant ($p < .05$). In the other phase III trial, only higher risk subjects with esophageal dysplasia received either 26 vitamins and minerals (including β-carotene, α-tocopherol, and selenium, at two to three times the US RDA) or placebo in a two-arm design.[165] This intervention was associated with two nonsignificant changes: an 18% increase in mortality from gastric cancer and a 16% reduction in mortality from esophageal cancer. Interpretation of these two contrasting studies is made difficult by the many different interventions and end points.

A placebo-controlled study of 220 subjects from Venezuela reported no significant effect of bismuth and amoxicillin on *Helicobacter pylori* eradication rates.[166] The bacterium *H. pylori* has been implicated in the etiology of gastric carcinogenesis.

The Bladder In vivo animal model, in vitro, and epidemiologic studies have shown that retinoids are active against bladder carcinogenesis.[167] The retinoid etretinate has been tested in three randomized clinical trials in patients following resection of superficial bladder tumors.[168–170] Two of these trials employed prolonged low-dose etretinate, which appeared to be effective.[144,170] Results of the two positive trials require confirmation, however, because of these trials' limited patient numbers and follow-up. A fourth randomized trial compared a multivitamin preparation at RDA levels alone or supplemented with 40,000 IU retinol, 100 mg pyridoxine, 2,000 mg ascorbic acid, 400 IU of α-tocopherol, and 90 mg zinc. The estimated 5-year tumor recurrence rate was 91% in the RDA arm versus 41% in the megadose arm ($p = .0014$).[171]

Fenretinide is a leading candidate for new trials in bladder cancer chemoprevention. This retinoid has a high therapeutic index against rodent bladder carcinogenesis and has produced encouraging clinical results in a phase IIa trial.[172] Other promising agents entering clinical trials include COX-2 inhibitors and DFMO.[53]

The Cervix The characteristic multistep histologic evolution of cervical carcinogenesis, the well-documented rates of progression and spontaneous regression within each histopathologic grade (cervical intraepithelial neoplasia [CIN] 1, 2, and 3), and ease in monitoring make cervical carcinogenesis an excellent human model for studying chemoprevention agents.

Cervical dysplasia has been studied in over 10 randomized trials,[173–182] including negative trials of locally applied interferon, folic acid and β-carotene. Only one of these trials was positive, and it involved the retinoid tretinoin.[180] The positive, randomized tretinoin trial used an intermittent schedule of locally applied tretinoin in 301 subjects—141 with biopsy-proved moderate (CIN 2) cervical dysplasia and 160 with severe (CIN 3) dysplasia.[180] Compared with placebo, tretinoin had significant activity in moderate dysplasia: complete regression rates of 43% versus 27% respectively ($p = .04$). It had no activity in severe dysplasia. A subsequent RCT of topical tretinoin for a shorter duration was negative.[183]

The major risk factor for cervical cancer is a human papilloma virus (HPV) infection, usually HPV-16. An HPV-16 virus-like particle vaccine was tested recently in an RCT involving 2,392 young women. The vaccine produced a marked reduction in the incidence of both HPV-16 infection and HPV-16-associated CIN.[184]

Overall Cancer Two important large US trials have tested the ability of β-carotene to reduce overall cancer incidence. The Physicians' Health Study was a 12-year test of β-carotene effects on overall cancer incidence.[185] β-Carotene produced no significant differences in overall incidence of cancer (including lung cancer). Only 11% of this population were current smokers. Similar β-carotene results of the Women's Health Study were reported.[186]

CONCLUSIONS

The clinical maturation of cancer chemoprevention is illustrated by the FDA's approval of several agents to prevent cancer or to treat or prevent IEN. Celecoxib, diclofenac, Photofrin (in conjunction with PDT), and tamoxifen (in three distinct breast cancer prevention settings) are more recent additions to a growing list of FDA-approved agents for cancer prevention, which includes hepatitis B vaccine, bacillus Calmette-Guerin, valrubicin, masoprocol, 5-fluorouracil, and aminolaevulinic acid (with PDT). The preventive efficacies of aspirin, calcium, and finasteride also have been established in definitive RCTs. Recent translational studies, such as the study of tamoxifen activity in *BRCA2*-positive women[187] and of retinoic acid activity in patients with the *GG* genotype of the *cyclin D1* gene,[188] suggest the broad potential of pharmacogenetics for advancing cancer chemoprevention. New directions for preventive drug development include the convergent development of molecular-targeted drugs for cancer prevention and cancer therapy.[189] Prevention drug development is beginning to converge with therapy drug development at the level of early-phase clinical testing, aided by important advances in our molecular understanding of neoplasia, cancer risk and prognosis, and mechanisms of new, less toxic, and more cytostatic, molecular-targeted drugs. This new direction will depend on technological advances, such as in molecular imaging, to achieve its promise in reducing the burden of major cancers.

REFERENCES

1. Jemal A, Murray T, Ward E, et al. Cancer statistics 2005. CA Cancer J Clin 2005;55:10–30.
2. Sporn MB, Dunlop NM, Newton DL, Smith JM. Prevention of chemical carcinogenesis by vitamin A and its synthetic analogues (retinoids). Fed Proc 1976;35:1332–8.
3. Sporn MB. Carcinogenesis and cancer: different perspectives on the same disease. Cancer Res 1991;51:6215–8.
4. Wattenberg LW. Chemoprevention of cancer. Cancer Res 1985;45:1–8.
5. Symposium on early lesions and the development of epithelial cancer. Cancer Res 1976;36:2475–706.
6. Boone CW, Kelloff GJ, Steele VE. Natural history of intraepithelial neoplasia in humans with implications for cancer chemoprevention strategy. Cancer Res 1992;52:1651–9.
7. Sporn MB, Suh N. Chemoprevention: an essential approach to control cancer. Nature Rev Cancer 2002;2:537–43.
8. Kelloff GJ. Perspectives on cancer chemoprevention research and drug development. Adv Cancer Res 1999;78:199–334.
9. Fugh-Berman A, Epstein S. Tamoxifen: disease prevention or disease substitution? Lancet 1992;340:1143–5.
10. Ross R. The pathogenesis of atherosclerosis: a perspective for the 1990s. Nature 1993;362:801–9.
11. Manson JE, Tosteson H, Ridker PM, et al. The primary prevention of myocardial infarction. N Engl J Med 1992;326:1406–16.
12. Ames BN, Shigenaga MK, Hagen TM. Oxidants, antioxidants, and the degenerative diseases of aging. Proc Natl Acad Sci U S A 1993;90:7915–22.
13. Sporn MB, Roberts AB, Goodman DS, editors. The retinoids. 2nd ed. New York: Raven Press; 1994.
14. Dawson MI, Hobbs PD. The synthetic chemistry of retinoids. In: Sporn MB, Roberts AB, Goodman DS, editors. The retinoids. 2nd ed. New York: Raven Press; 1994. p. 5–178.
15. Green S, Chambon P. A superfamily of potentially oncogenic hormone receptors. Nature 1986;324:615–7.
16. Evans RM. The steroid and thyroid hormone receptor superfamily. Science 1988;240:889–95.
17. O'Malley B. The steroid receptor superfamily: more excitement predicted for the future. Mol Endocrinol 1990;4:363–9.
18. Wolbach SB, Howe PR. Tissue changes following deprivation of fat soluble A vitamin. J Exp Med 1925;42:753–77.
19. Sporn MB, Roberts AB. Role of retinoids in differentiation and carcinogenesis. Cancer Res 1983;43:3034–40.
20. Lasnitzki I. The influence of A hypervitaminosis on the effect of 20-methylcholanthrene on mouse prostate glands grown in vitro. Br J Cancer 1955;9:434–41.
21. Merriman RL, Bertram JS. Reversible inhibition by retinoids of 3-methylcholanthrene-induced neoplastic transformation in C3H/10T1/2 CL8 cells. Cancer Res 1979;39:1661–6.
22. Strickland S, Mahdavi V. The induction of differentiation in teratocarcinoma stem cells by retinoic acid. Cell 1978;15:393–403.
23. Breitman TR, Selonick SE, Collins SJ. Induction of differentiation of the human promyelocytic leukemia cell line (HL-60) by retinoic acid. Proc Natl Acad Sci U S A 1980;77:2936–40.
24. Gudas LJ, Sporn MB, Roberts AB. Cellular biology and biochemistry of the retinoids. In: Sporn MB, Roberts AB, Goodman DS, editors. The retinoids. 2nd ed. New York: Raven Press; 1994. p. 443–520.
25. Allegretto EA, McClurg MR, Lazarchik SB, et al. Transactivation properties of retinoic acid and retinoid X receptors in mammalian cells and yeast. J Biol Chem 1993;268:26625–33.
26. Allenby G, Janoch R, Kazmer S, et al. Binding of 9-cis-retinoic acid and all-trans-retinoic acid to retinoic acid receptors α, β, and γ. J Biol Chem 1994;269:16689–95.
27. Mangelsdorf DJ, Umesono K, Evans RM. The retinoid receptors. In: Sporn MB, Roberts AB, Goodman DS, editors. The retinoids. 2nd ed. New York: Raven Press; 1994. p. 319–49.
28. Moon RC, Mehta RG, Rao KV. Retinoids and cancer in experimental animals. In: Sporn MB, Roberts AB, Goodman DS, editors. The retinoids. 2nd ed. New York: Raven Press; 1994. p. 573–96.
29. Anzano MA, Byers SW, Smith JM, et al. Prevention of breast cancer in the rat with 9-cis-retinoic acid as a single agent and in combination with tamoxifen. Cancer Res 1994;54:4614–7.
30. Jordan VC, editor. Long-term tamoxifen treatment for breast cancer. Madison (WI): University of Wisconsin Press; 1994. p. 289.
31. Jordan VC, Allen KE, Dix CJ. Pharmacology of tamoxifen in laboratory animals. Cancer Treat Rep 1980;64:745–9.
32. Gottardis MM, Jordan VC. Antitumor actions of keoxifene and tamoxifen in the N-nitrosomethylurea-induced rat mammary carcinoma model. Cancer Res 1987;47:4020–4.
33. Knabbe C, Lippman ME, Wakefield LM, et al. Evidence that TGF-β is a hormonally regulated negative growth factor in human breast cancer cells. Cell 1987;48:417–28.
34. Colletta AA, Wakefield LM, Howell LM, et al. Antioestrogens induce the secretion of active TGF-β from human fetal fibroblasts. Br J Cancer 1990;62:405–9.
35. Butta A, MacLennan K, Flanders KC, et al. Induction of transforming growth factor β1 in human breast cancer in vivo following tamoxifen treatment. Cancer Res 1992;52:4261–4.
36. Nolvadex Adjuvant Trial Organization. Controlled trial of tamoxifen as a single adjuvant agent in the management of early breast cancer. Br J Cancer 1988;57:608–11.
37. Colletti RB, Roberts JD, Devlin JT, Copeland KC. Effect of tamoxifen on plasma insulin-like growth factor I in patients with breast cancer. Cancer Res 1989;49:1882–4.
38. Pollak MJ, Costantino C, Polychronakos C, et al. Effect of tamoxifen on serum insulin-like growth factor I levels in stage I breast cancer patients. J Natl Cancer Inst 1990;82:1693–7.
39. Black LJ, Sato M, Rowley ER, et al. Raloxifene (LY139481 HCI) prevents bone loss and reduces serum cholesterol without causing uterine hypertrophy in ovariectomized rats. J Clin Invest 1994;93:63–9.
40. Lowe KE, Maiyar AC, Norman AW. Vitamin D–mediated gene expression. Crit Rev Eukaryot Gene Expr 1992;2:65–109.
41. Studzinski GP, McLane JA, Uskokovic MR. Signalling pathways for vitamin D-induced differentiation: implications for therapy of proliferative and neoplastic diseases. Crit Rev Eukaryot Gene Expr 1993;3:279–312.
42. Ikekawa N, Ishizuka S. Molecular structure and biological activity of vitamin D metabolites and their analogues. In: Bol M, Daux WL, editors. Molecular structure and biological activity of steroids. Boca Raton (FL): CRC Press; 1992. p. 293–316.
43. Anzano MA, Smith JM, Uskokovic MR, et al. 1α,25-dihydroxy-16-ene-23-yne-26,27-hexafluorocholecalciferol (Ro24-5531), a new deltanoid (vitamin D analogue) for prevention of breast cancer in the rat. Cancer Res 1994;54:1653–6.
44. Guyton KZ, Kensler TW, Posner GH. Cancer chemoprevention using natural vitamin D and synthetic analogs. Annu Rev Pharmacol Toxicol 2001;41:421–42.
45. Stoner E. The clinical effects of a 5α-reductase inhibitor, finasteride, on benign prostatic hyperplasia. The Finasteride Study Group. J Urol 1992;147:1298–302.
46. Pegg AE. Polyamine metabolism and its importance in neoplastic growth and as a target for chemotherapy. Cancer Res 1988;48:759–74.
47. Ratko TA, Detrisac CJ, Rao KV, et al. Interspecies analysis of the chemopreventive efficacy of dietary α-difluoromethylornithine. Anticancer Res 1990;10:67–72.
48. Gupta RA, DuBois RN. Colorectal cancer prevention and treatment by inhibition of cyclooxygenase-2. Nature Rev Cancer 2001;1:11–21.
49. Prestera T, Zhang Y, Spencer SR, et al. The electrophile counterattack response: protection against neoplasia and toxicity. Adv Enzyme Regul 1993;33:281–96.
50. DeFlora S, Izzotti A, D'Agostini F, et al. Chemopreventive properties of *N*-acetylcysteine and other thiols. In: Wattenberg L, Lipkin M, Boone CW, Kelloff GJ, editors. Cancer chemoprevention. Boca Raton (FL): CRC Press; 1992. p. 183–94.
51. Kensler TW, Egner PA, Trush MA, et al. Mechanisms of protection against aflatoxin tumorigenicity in rats fed 5-(2-pyrazinyl)-4-methyl-1,2-dithiol-3-thione (oltipraz) and related 1,2-dithiol-3-thiones and 1,2-dithiol-3-ones. Cancer Res 1987;47:4271–7.
52. Lippman SM, Benner SE, Hong WK. Cancer chemoprevention. J Clin Oncol 1994;12:851–73.
53. Lippman SM, Lee JJ, Sabichi AL. Cancer chemoprevention: progress and promise. J Natl Cancer Inst 1998;90:1514–28.
54. Vokes EE, Weichselbaum RR, Lippman SM, et al. Head and neck cancer. N Engl J Med 1993;328:184–94.
55. Hong WK, Lippman SM, Hittelman WN, et al. Retinoid chemoprevention of aerodigestive cancer: from basic research to the clinic. Clin Cancer Res 1995;1:677–86.
56. Papadimitrakopoulou V, Izzo J, Lippman SM, et al. Frequent inactivation of $p16^{INK4a}$ in oral premalignant lesions. Oncogene 1997;14:1799–803.
57. Lippman SM, Lee JS, Lotan R, et al. Biomarkers as intermediate end points in chemoprevention trials. J Natl Cancer Inst 1990;82:555–60.
58. Benner SE, Winn RJ, Lippman SM, et al. Regression of oral leukoplakia with α-tocopherol: a community clinical oncology program chemoprevention study. J Natl Cancer Inst 1993;85:44–7.
59. Hong WK, Endicott J, Itri LM, et al. 13-cis-retinoic acid in the treatment of oral leukoplakia. N Engl J Med 1986;315:1501–5.
60. Lippman SM, Batsakis JG, Toth BB, et al. Comparison of low-dose isotretinoin with β-carotene to prevent oral carcinogenesis. N Engl J Med 1993;328:15–20.
61. Papadimitrakopoulou VA, Hong WK, Lee JS, et al. Low-dose isotretinoin versus β-carotene to prevent oral carcinogenesis: long-term follow-up. J Natl Cancer Inst 1997;89:257–8.
62. Stich HF, Hornby AP, Mathew B, et al. Response of oral leukoplakias to the administration of vitamin A. Cancer Lett 1988;40:93–101.
63. Han J, Lu Y, Sun Z, et al. Evaluation of N-4-(hydroxycarbophenyl) retinamide as a cancer prevention agent and as a cancer chemotherapeutic agent. In Vivo 1990;4:153–60.
64. Chiesa F, Tradati N, Marazza M, et al. Fenretinide (4-HPR) in chemoprevention of oral leukoplakia. J Cell Biochem 1993;17F:255–61.
65. Epstein JB, Wong FLW, Millner A, Le ND. Topical bleomycin treatment of oral leukoplakia: a randomized double-blind clinical trial. Head Neck 1994;16:539–44.
66. Lotan R, Xu X-C, Lippman SM, et al. Suppression of retinoic acid receptor β in premalignant oral lesions and its upregulation by isotretinoin. N Engl J Med 1995;332:1405–10.
67. Lippman SM, Shin DM, Lee JJ, et al. p53 and retinoid chemoprevention of oral carcinogenesis. Cancer Res 1995;55:16–9.
68. Rudin CM, Cohen EE, Papadimitrakopoulou VA, et al. An attenuated adenovirus, ONYX-015, as mouthwash therapy for premalignant oral dysplasia. J Clin Oncol 2003;21:4546–52.
69. Lippman SM, Hong WK. Molecular markers of the risk of oral cancer. N Engl J Med 2001;344:1323–6
70. Sudbø J, Lippman SM, Lee JJ, et al. The influence of resection and aneuploidy on mortality in oral leukoplakia. N Engl J Med 2004;350:1405–13.
71. Zhang L, Poh CF, Lam WL, et al. Impact of localized treatment in reducing risk of progression of low-grade oral dysplasia: molecular evidence of incomplete resection. Oral Oncol 2001;37:505–12.
72. Guo Z, Yamaguchi K, Sanchez-Cespedes M, et al: Allelic losses in OraTest-directed biopsies of patients with prior upper aerodigestive tract malignancy. Clin Cancer Res 2001;7:1963–8.
73. Epstein JB, Zhang L, Poh C, et al. Increased allelic loss in toluidine blue-positive oral premalignant lesions. Oral Surg Oral Med Oral Pathol Oral Radiol Endod 2003;95:45–50.
74. Lippman SM, Sudbo J, Hong WK. Oral cancer prevention and the evolution of molecular-targeted drug development. J Clin Oncol 2005;23:346–56.
75. Hong WK, Lippman SM, Itri LM, et al. Prevention of second primary tumors with isotretinoin in squamous-cell carcinoma of the head and neck. N Engl J Med 1990;323:795–801.
76. Benner SE, Pajak TF, Lippman SM, et al. Prevention of second primary tumors with isotretinoin in squamous cell carcinoma of the head and neck: long term follow-up. J Natl Cancer Inst 1994;86:140–1.
77. Khuri FR, Kim ES, Lee JJ, et al. The impact of smoking status, disease stage, and index tumor site on second primary tumor incidence and tumor recurrence in the head

and neck retinoid chemoprevention trial. Cancer Epidemiol Biomarkers Prev 2001;10:823–9.

78. Khuri F, Lee JJ, Lippman SM, et al. Isotretinoin effects on head and neck cancer recurrence and second primary tumors. Proc Annu Meet Am Soc Clin Oncol 2003;22:90 (359).
79. Shin DM, Khuri FR, Murphy B, et al. Combined interferon-α, 13-cis-retinoic acid and α-tocopherol in locally advanced head and neck squamous cell carcinoma: novel bioadjuvant phase II trial. J Clin Oncol 2001;19:3010–7.
80. Bolla M, Lefur R, Ton Van J, et al. Prevention of second primary tumours with etretinate in squamous cell carcinoma of the oral cavity and oropharynx: results of a multicentric double-blind randomized study. Eur J Cancer 1994;30A:767–72.
81. Mao L, Lee JS, Kurie JM, et al. Clonal genetic alterations in the lungs of current and former smokers. J Natl Cancer Inst 1997;89:857–62.
82. Arnold AM, Browman GP, Levine MN, et al. The effect of the synthetic retinoid etretinate on sputum cytology: results from a randomized trial. Br J Cancer 1992;65:737–43.
83. Lee JS, Lippman SM, Benner SE, et al. A randomized placebo-controlled trial of isotretinoin in chemoprevention of bronchial squamous metaplasia. J Clin Oncol 1994;12:937–45.
84. Kurie JM, Lee JS, Khuri FR, et al. N(4-hydroxyphenyl) retinamide in the chemoprevention of squamous metaplasia and dysplasia of the bronchial epithelium. Clin Cancer Res 2000;6:2973–9.
85. Heimburger DC, Alexander B, Birch R, et al. Improvement in bronchial squamous metaplasia in smokers treated with folate and vitamin B_{12}: report of a preliminary randomized, double-blind intervention trial. JAMA 1988;259:1525–30.
86. van Poppel G, Kok FJ, Hermus RJJ. Beta-carotene supplementation in smokers reduces the frequency of micronuclei in sputum. Br J Cancer 1992;66:1164–8.
87. van Poppel G, Poulsen H, Loft S, Verhagen H. No influence of β-carotene on oxidative DNA damage in male smokers. J Natl Cancer Inst 1995;87:310–1.
88. McLarty JW, Holiday DB, Girard WM, et al. β-Carotene, vitamin A, and lung cancer chemoprevention: results of an intermediate endpoint study. Am J Clin Nutr 1995;62(6 Suppl):1431S–8S.
89. Kurie JM, Lotan R, Lee JJ, et al. Randomized, placebo-controlled trial of 9-*cis* retinoic acid (9cRA) versus 13-*cis* retinoic acid (13cRA) plus alpha-tocopherol (AT) in the reversal of biomarkers of bronchial preneoplasia in former smokers. Proc Amer Soc Clinical Oncol 2002;21:295a.
90. Lam S, MacAulay C, le Riche JC, et al. A randomized phase IIb trial of anethole dithiolethione in smokers with bronchial dysplasia. J Natl Cancer Inst 2002;94:1001–9.
91. The Alpha-Tocopherol, Beta-Carotene Cancer Prevention Study Group. The effect of vitamin E and beta-carotene on the incidence of lung cancer and other cancers in male smokers. N Engl J Med 1994;330:1029–35.
92. Wang X-D, Liu C, Bronson RT, et al. Retinoid signaling and activator protein-1 expression in ferrets given β-carotene supplements and exposed to tobacco smoke. J Natl Cancer Inst 1999;91:60–6.
93. Paolini M, Cantelli-Forti G, Perocco P, et al. Co-carcinogenic effect of β-carotene. Nature 1999;398:760–1.
94. Heinonen OP, Albanes D, Virtamo J, et al. Prostate cancer and supplementation with alpha-tocopherol and beta-carotene: incidence and mortality in a controlled trial. J Natl Cancer Inst 1998;90:440–6.
95. Omenn GS, Goodman GE, Thornquist MD, et al. Effects of a combination of beta carotene and vitamin A on lung cancer and cardiovascular disease. N Engl J Med 1996;334:1150–5.
96. Pastorino U, Infante M, Maioli M, et al. Adjuvant treatment of stage I lung cancer with high-dose vitamin A. J Clin Oncol 1993;11:1216–22.
97. van Zandwijk N, Dalesio O, Pastorino U, et al (For the European Organization for Research and Treatment of Cancer Head and Neck and Lung Cancer Cooperative Groups). EUROSCAN, a randomized trial of vitamin A and *N*-acetylcysteine in patients with head and neck cancer or lung cancer. J Natl Cancer Inst 2000;92:977–86.
98. Lippman SM, Lee JJ, Karp DD, et al. Randomized phase III intergroup trial of isotretinoin to prevent second primary tumors in stage I non-small-cell lung cancer. J Natl Cancer Inst 2001;93:605–18.
99. Giardiello FM, Hamilton SR, Krush AJ, et al. Treatment of colonic and rectal adenomas with sulindac in familial adenomatous polyposis. N Engl J Med 1993;328:1313–6.
100. Steinbach G, Lynch PM, Phillips RK, et al. The effect of celecoxib, a cyclooxygenase-2 inhibitor, in familial adenomatous polyposis. N Engl J Med 2000;342:1946–52.
101. Phillips RK, Wallace MH, Lynch PM, et al. A randomised, double blind, placebo controlled study of celecoxib, a selective cyclooxygenase 2 inhibitor, on duodenal polyposis in familial adenomatous polyposis. Gut 2002;50:857–60.
102. Giardiello FM, Yang VW, Hylind LM, et al. Primary chemoprevention of familial adenomatous polyposis with sulindac. N Engl J Med 2002;346:1054–9.
103. Baron JA, Cole BF, Mott LA. Aspirin chemoprevention of colorectal adenomas. Proc Am Assoc Cancer Res 2002;43:669.
104. Baron JA, Tosteson TD, Wargovich MJ, et al. Calcium supplementation and rectal mucosal proliferation: a randomized controlled trial. J Natl Cancer Inst 1995;87:1303–7.
105. Wallace K, Baron JA, Cole BF, et al. Calcium carbonate chemoprevention in the large bowel: effects on hyperplastic polyps, tubular adenomas, and more advanced lesions. Proc Am Assoc Cancer Res 2002;43:163–4.
106. Sandler RS, Halabi S, Baron JA, et al. A randomized trial of aspirin to prevent colorectal adenomas in patients with previous colorectal cancer. N Engl J Med 2003;348:883–90.
107. Baron JA, Cole BF, Sandler RS, et al. A randomized trial of aspirin to prevent colorectal adenomas. N Engl J Med 2003;348:891–9.
108. Benamouzig R, Deyra J, Martin A, et al. Daily soluble aspirin and prevention of colorectal adenoma recurrence: one-year results of the APACC trial. Gastroenterology 2003;125:328–36.
109. Bresalier RS, Sandler RS, Quan H, et al. Cardiovascular events associated with rofecoxib in a colorectal adenoma chemoprevention trial. N Engl J Med 2005;352:1092–102.
110. Schatzkin A, Lanza E, Corle D, et al. Lack of effect of a low-fat, high-fiber diet on the recurrence of colorectal adenomas. N Engl J Med 2000;342:1149–55.
111. Alberts DS, Martinez ME, Roe DJ, et al. Lack of effect of a high-fiber cereal supplement on the recurrence of colorectal adenomas. N Engl J Med 2000;342:1156–62.
112. Levin B. Dietary intake and recurrence of colorectal adenoma. Lancet 2000;356:1286–7.
113. Hwang DH, Fung V, Dannenberg AJ. National Cancer Institute workshop on chemopreventive properties of nonsteroidal anti-inflammatory drugs: role of COX-dependent and independent mechanisms. Neoplasia 2002;4:1–7.
114. Labayle D, Fischer D, Vielh P, et al. Sulindac causes regression of rectal polyps in familial adenomatous polyposis. Gastroenterology 1991;101:635–9.
115. Wargovich MJ, Isbell G, Shabot M, et al. Calcium supplementation decreases rectal epithelial cell proliferation in subjects with sporadic adenoma. Gastroenterology 1992;103:92–7.
116. Stern HS, Gregorie RC, Koshtan H. Long-term effects of dietary calcium on risk markers for colon cancer in patients with familial polyposis. Surgery 1990;108:528–33.
117. Gregoire RC, Stern HS, Yeung KS, et al. Effect of calcium supplementation on mucosal cell proliferation in high risk patients for colon cancer. Gut 1989;30:376–82.
118. Barsoum GH, Hendrickse C, Winslet MC, et al. Reduction of mucosal crypt cell proliferation in patients with colorectal adenomatous polyps by dietary calcium supplementation. Br J Surg 1992;79:581–3.
119. Bostick RM, Potter JD, Fosdick L, et al. Calcium and colorectal epithelial cell proliferation: a preliminary randomized, double-blinded, placebo-controlled clinical trial. J Natl Cancer Inst 1993;85:132–41.
120. Cats A, Kleibeuker JH, van der Meer R, et al. Randomized, double-blind, placebo-controlled intervention study with supplemental calcium in families with hereditary nonpolyposis colorectal cancer. J Natl Cancer Inst 1995;87:598–603.
121. Baron JA, Beach M, Mandel JS, et al. Calcium supplements for the prevention of colorectal adenomas. N Engl J Med 1999;340:101–7.
122. Kikendall JW, Mobarhan S, Nelson R, et al. Oral beta carotene does not reduce the recurrence of colorectal adenomas [abstract]. Am J Gastroenterol 1991;36:1356.
123. Bussey HJR, DeCosse JJ, Deschner EE, et al. A randomized trial of ascorbic acid in polyposis coli. Cancer 1982;50:1434–9.
124. McKeown-Eyssen G, Holloway C, Jazmaji V, et al. A randomized trial of vitamins C and E in the prevention of recurrence of colorectal polyps. Cancer Res 1988;48:4701–5.
125. DeCosse JJ, Miller HH, Lesser ML. Effect of wheat fiber and vitamins C and E on rectal polyps in patients with familial adenomatous polyposis. J Natl Cancer Inst 1989;81:1290–7.
126. MacLennan R, Macrae F, Bain C, et al. Randomized trial of intake of fat, fiber, and beta carotene to prevent colorectal adenomas. J Natl Cancer Inst 1995;87:1760–6.
127. Alberts D, Rees-McGee S, Einspahr J, et al. Double-blind, placebo controlled study of wheat bran fiber (WBF) vs. calcium carbonate (CALC) in patients with resected adenomatous polyps. Proc Am Assoc Cancer Res 1992;33:207.
128. Paganelli GM, Biasco G, Brandi G, et al. Effect of vitamins A, C, and E supplementation on rectal cell proliferation in patients with colorectal adenomas. J Natl Cancer Inst 1992;84:47–51.
129. Roncucci L, Donato PD, Carati L, et al. Antioxidant vitamins or lactulose for the prevention of the recurrence of colorectal adenomas. Dis Colon Rectum 1993;36:227–34.
130. Greenberg ER, Baron JA, Tosteson TD, et al. A clinical trial of antioxidant vitamins to prevent colorectal adenoma. N Engl J Med 1994;331:141–7.
131. Kligman AM, Thorne EG. Topical therapy of actinic keratosis with tretinoin. In: Marks, R, editor. Retinoids in cutaneous malignancy. Cambridge (MA): Blackwell Scientific Publications; 1991. p. 66–73.
132. Moriarity M, Dunn J, Darragh A, et al. Etretinate in treatment of actinic keratosis: a double blind crossover study. Lancet 1982;1:364–5.
133. Watson AB. Preventative effect of etretinate therapy on multiple actinic keratoses. Cancer Detect Prev 1986;9:161–5.
134. Kraemer KH, DiGiovanna JJ, Moshell AN, et al. Prevention of skin cancer in xeroderma pigmentosum with the use of oral isotretinoin. N Engl J Med 1988;318:1633–7.
135. Bouwes Bavinck JN, Tiben LM, Van Der Woude FJ, et al. Prevention of skin cancer and reduction of keratotic skin lesions during acitretin therapy in renal transplant recipients: a double-blind, placebo-controlled study. J Clin Oncol 1995;13:1933–8.
136. Greenberg ER, Baron JA, Stukel TA, et al. A clinical trial of β-carotene to prevent basal-cell and squamous-cell cancers of the skin. N Engl J Med 1990;323:789–95.
137. Tangrea JA, Edwards BK, Taylor PR, et al. Long-term therapy with low-dose isotretinoin for prevention of basal cell carcinoma: a multicenter clinical trial. J Natl Cancer Inst 1992;84:328–32.
138. Moon TE, Levine N, Cartmel B, et al. Effect of retinol in preventing squamous cell skin cancer in moderate-risk subjects: a randomized, double-blind, controlled trial. Cancer Epidemiol Biomarkers Prev 1997;6:949–56.
139. Levine N, Moon TE, Cartmel B, et al. Trial of retinol and isotretinoin in skin cancer prevention: a randomized, double-blind, controlled trial. Southwest Skin Cancer Prevention Study Group. Cancer Epidemiol Biomarkers Prev 1997;6:957–61.
140. Clark LC, Combs GF Jr, Turnbull BW, et al. Effects of selenium supplementation for cancer prevention in patients with carcinoma of the skin. JAMA 1996;276:1957–63.
141. Yarosh D, Klein J, O'Connor A, et al. Effect of topically applied T4 endonuclease V in liposomes on skin cancer in xeroderma pigmentosum: a randomised study. Lancet 2001;357:926–9.
142. Fisher B, Costantino JP, Wickerham DL, et al. Tamoxifen for prevention of breast cancer: report of the national surgical adjuvant breast and bowel project P-1 study. J Natl Cancer Inst 1998;90:1371–88.
143. Lippman SM, Brown PH. Tamoxifen prevention of breast cancer: an instance of the fingerpost. J Natl Cancer Inst 1999;91:1809–19.
144. Fisher B, Dignam J, Wolmark N, et al. Tamoxifen in treatment of intraductal breast cancer: national surgical adjuvant breast and bowel project B-24 randomised controlled trial. Lancet 1999;353:1993–2000.
145. Cummings SR, Eckert S, Krueger KA, et al. The effect of raloxifene on risk of breast cancer in postmenopausal women: results from the MORE randomized trial. JAMA 1999;281:2189–97.
146. Veronesi U, Maisonneuve P, Costa A, et al. Prevention of breast cancer with tamoxifen: preliminary findings from the Italian randomised trial among hysterectomised women. Lancet 1998;352:93–7.
147. Powles T, Eeles R, Ashley S, et al. Interim analysis of the incidence of breast cancer in the Royal Marsden Hospital tamoxifen randomised chemoprevention trial. Lancet 1998;352:98–101.

148. Cuzick J,.Forbes J, Edwards R, et al.. First results from the International Breast Cancer Intervention Study (IBIS-I): a randomised prevention trial. Lancet 2002;360:817–24.
149. Baum M, Buzdar A, Cuzick J, et al. Anastrozole alone or in combination with tamoxifen versus tamoxifen alone for adjuvant treatment of postmenopausal women with early-stage breast cancer: results of the ATAC (Arimidex, Tamoxifen Alone or in Combination) trial efficacy and safety update analyses. Cancer 2003;98:1802–10.
150. Cuzick J. Aromatase inhibitors in prevention—data from the ATAC (Arimidex, Tamoxifen Alone or in Combination) trial and the design of IBIS-II (the second International Breast Cancer Intervention Study). Recent Results Cancer Res 2003;163:96–103 [discussion 264–6].
151. Veronesi U, De Palo G, Marubini E, et al. Randomized trial of fenretinide to prevent second breast malignancy in women with early breast cancer. J Natl Cancer Inst 1999;91:1847–56.
152. Ries LAG, Elsner MP, Kosary CL, et al, editors. SEER Cancer Statistics Review, 1975–2001, http://seer.cancer.gov/csr/1975_2001/ (accessed December 2, 2004).
153. Stanford JL, Feng Z, Hamilton AS, et al. Urinary and sexual function after radical prostatectomy for clinically localized prostate cancer: the Prostate Cancer Outcomes Study. JAMA 2000;283:354–60.
154. Potosky AL, Legler J, Albertsen PC, et al. Health outcomes after prostatectomy or radiotherapy for prostate cancer: results from the Prostate Cancer Outcomes Study. J Natl Cancer Inst 2000;92:1582–92.
155. Thompson IM, Goodman PJ, Tangen CM, et al. The influence of finasteride on the development of prostate cancer. N Engl J Med 2003;347:215–24.
156. Thompson IM, Pauler DK, Goodman PJ, et al. Prevalence of prostate cancer among men with a prostate-specific antigen level < or =4.0 ng per milliliter. N Engl J Med 2004;350:2239–46.
157. Lippman SM, Goodman PJ, Klein EA, et al. Designing the selenium and vitamin E cancer prevention trial (SELECT). J Natl Cancer Inst 2005;97:94–102.
158. Munoz N, Bang LJ, Day NE, et al. No effect of riboflavin, retinol, and zinc on prevalence of precancerous lesions of oesophagus: randomized double-blind intervention study in high-risk population of China. Lancet 1985;2:111–4.
159. Munoz N, Hayashi M, Bang LJ, et al. Effect of riboflavin, retinol and zinc on micronuclei of buccal mucosa and of the esophagus: a randomized double-blind intervention study in China. J Natl Cancer Inst 1987;79:687–91.
160. Wahrendorf J, Munoz N, Jian-Bang L, et al. Blood, retinol and zinc riboflavin status in relation to precancerous lesions of the esophagus: findings from a vitamin intervention trial in the People's Republic of China. Cancer Res 1988:48:2280–3.
161. Zaridze D, Evstifeeva T, Boyle P. Chemoprevention of oral leukoplakia and chronic esophagitis in an area of high incidence of oral and esophageal cancer. Ann Epidemiol 1993;3:225–34.
162. Limburg P, Wei W, Ahnen D, et al. Chemoprevention of esophageal squamous cancer: randomized placebo-controlled trial in a high-risk population. Gastroenterology 2002;122:A71.
163. Kelty CJ, Marcus SL, Ackroyd R. Photodynamic therapy for Barrett's esophagus: a review. Dis Esophagus 2002;15:137–44.
164. Blot WJ, Li JY, Taylor PR, et al. Linxian nutrition intervention trials: supplementation with specific vitamin/mineral combinations, cancer incidence, and disease-specific mortality in the general population. J Natl Cancer Inst 1993;85:1483–92.
165. Li J-Y, Taylor PR, Li B, et al. Linxian nutrition intervention trials: multiple vitamin/mineral supplementation, cancer incidence, and disease-specific mortality among adults with esophageal dysplasia. J Natl Cancer Inst 1993;85:1492–8.
166. Buiatti E, Munoz N, Vivas J, Cano E, et al. Difficulty in eradicating *Helicobacter pylori* in a population at high risk of stomach cancer in Venezuela. Cancer Causes Control 1994;5:249–54.
167. Sporn MB, Squire RA, Brown CC, et al. 13-*cis*-retinoic acid inhibition of bladder carcinogenesis in the rat. Science 1977;195:487–9.
168. Alfthan O, Tarkkanen J, Grohn P, et al. Tigason (etretinate) in prevention of recurrence of superficial bladder tumors. Eur Urol 1983;9:6–9.
169. Pederson H, Wolf H, Jensen SK, et al. Administration of a retinoid as prophylaxis of recurrent noninvasive bladder tumors. Scand J Urol Nephrol 1984;18:121–3.
170. Studer UE, Biedermann C, Chollet D, et al. Prevention of recurrent superficial bladder tumors by oral etretinate: preliminary results of a randomized, double-blind, multicenter trial in Switzerland. J Urol 1984;131:1469–72.
171. Lamm DL, Riggs DR, Shrivers JS, et al. Megadose vitamins in bladder cancer: a double-blind clinical trial. J Urol 1994;151:21–6.
172. Decensi A, Bruno S, Costantini M, et al. Phase IIa study of fenretinide in superficial bladder cancer, using DNA flow cytometry as an intermediate end point. J Natl Cancer Inst 1994;86:138–41.
173. Byrne MA, Moller BR, Taylor-Robinson D, et al. The effect of interferon on human papillomaviruses associated with cervical intraepithelial neoplasia. Br J Obstet Gynaecol 1986;93:1136–44.
174. Yliskoski M, Cantell K, Syrjanen K, et al. Topical treatment with human leukocyte interferon of HPV 16 infections associated with cervical and vaginal intraepithelial neoplasias. Gynecol Oncol 1990;36:353–7.
175. Frost L, Skajaa K, Hvidman LE, et al. No effect of intralesional injection of interferon on moderate cervical intraepithelial neoplasia. Br J Obstet Gynaecol 1990;97:626–30.
176. Dunham AM, McCartney JC, McCance DJ, et al. Effect of perilesional injection of alpha-interferon on cervical intraepithelial neoplasia and associated human papillomavirus infection. J R Soc Med 1990;83:490–2.
177. Butterworth CE, Hatch KD, Soong S-J, et al. Oral folic acid supplementation for cervical dysplasia: a clinical intervention trial. Am J Obstet Gynecol 1992;166:803–9.
178. Childers JM, Chu J, Voigt LF, et al. Chemoprevention of cervical cancer with folic acid: a phase III Southwest Oncology Group intergroup study. Cancer Epidemiol Biomarkers Prev 1995;4:155–9.
179. de Vet HCW, Knipschild PG, Willebrand D, et al. The effect of beta-carotene on the regression and progression of cervical dysplasia: a clinical experiment. J Clin Epidemiol 1991;44:273–83.
180. Meyskens FL, Surwit E, Moon TE, et al. Enhancement of regression of cervical intraepithelial neoplasia II (moderate dysplasia) with topically applied all-trans-retinoic acid: a randomized trial. J Natl Cancer Inst 1994; 86:539–43.
181. Follen M, Atkinson EN, Schottenfeld D, et al. A randomized clinical trial of 4-hydroxyphenylretinamide for high-grade squamous intraepithelial lesions of the cervix. Clin Cancer Res 2001;7:3356–65.
182. Keefe KA, Schell MJ, Brewer C, et al. A randomized, double blind, phase III trial using oral beta-carotene supplementation for women with high-grade cervical intraepithelial neoplasia. Cancer Epidemiol Biomarkers Prev 2001;10:1029–35.
183. Ruffin MT, Bailey JM, Normolle DP, et al. Topical all-trans retinoic acid in high grade squamous intraepithelial lesions. Proc Am Assoc Cancer Res 2003;44:1301, abstract 5677.
184. Koutsky LA, Ault KA, Wheeler CM, et al. A controlled trial of a human papillomavirus type 16 vaccine. N Engl J Med 2002;347:1645–51.
185. Hennekens CH, Burning JE, Manson JE, et al. Lack of effect of long-term supplementation with beta carotene on the incidence of malignant neoplasms and cardiovascular disease. N Engl J Med 1996;334:1145–9.
186. Lee I-M, Cook NR, Manson JE, et al. Beta carotene supplementation and incidence of cancer and cardiovascular disease: the Women's Health Study. J Natl Cancer Inst 1999;91:2102–6.
187. King MC, Wieand S, Hale K, et al. Tamoxifen and breast cancer incidence among women with inherited mutations in BRCA1 and BRCA2: National Surgical Adjuvant Breast and Bowel Project (NSABP-P1) Breast Cancer Prevention Trial. JAMA 2001;286:2251–6.
188. Izzo JG, Papadimitrakopoulou VA, Liu DD, et al. Cyclin D1 genotype, response to biochemoprevention, and progression rate to upper aerodigestive tract cancer. J Natl Cancer Inst 2003;95:198–205.
189. Abbruzzese JL, Lippman SM. The convergence of cancer prevention and therapy in early-phase clinical drug development. Cancer Cell 2004;6:321–6.

28

Cancer Screening and Early Detection

Robert A. Smith, PhD
Stephen W. Duffy, MSc
Harmon J. Eyre, MD

Cancer screening and early detection have major importance in the survival of patients with some cancers. A feature common to most of the more prevalent cancers, that is, cancers of the skin, breast, cervix, endometrium, ovary, testis, colon and rectum, prostate, and lung, is that stage at diagnosis is the primary determinant of prognosis, and prognosis generally is better and treatment more successful if the disease is detected while still localized. Secondary prevention of cancer is distinguished from primary prevention in that it is an intervention focused on (1) detecting and treating early invasive disease, and thus preventing death from cancer; or (2) altering the natural history of the disease by identifying precursor lesions known to be predictive of eventual malignancy and treating them, thus preventing progression to invasive disease.

KEY CRITERIA IN THE DECISION TO SCREEN

The observation that a particular cancer has more favorable survival if diagnosed at an early stage is important, but only one element in the decision matrix used to determine whether or not to offer cancer screening to an asymptomatic population.[1,2] In general, the following criteria should be met:[3]

1. The disease should be an important health problem, as measured by morbidity, mortality, and other measures of disease burden.
2. The disease should have a detectable preclinical phase.
3. Treatment of disease detected before the onset of clinical symptoms should offer benefits compared with treatment after the onset of symptoms.
4. The screening test should meet acceptable levels of accuracy and cost.
5. The screening test and follow-up requirements should be acceptable to individuals at risk and to their health care providers.

These criteria are important considerations prior to any decision to offer screening to a healthy population. However, although each criterion is important, there are no measurable thresholds to guide decision making; thus, the decision matrix requires considering the criteria collectively.[4,5] For example, a disease may not be an important cause of mortality but may account for significant morbidity. A high false-positive rate may be acceptable when screening for cancers at some organ sites but not at others owing to the costs (financial, or harms to individuals) associated with diagnostic testing after an abnormal screening examination. A screening test may not meet the criteria very well, but the disease may be of great concern to the population at risk and the test will therefore be acceptable despite limitations. Values, in addition to scientific evidence, play a role in policy decisions about screening.[5]

Disease Burden The International Agency for Research on Cancer estimates that in 2002 there were 10.9 million new cases of cancer and 6.9 million deaths, excluding basal and squamous cell cancers of the skin and in situ cervix, breast, or melanoma lesions.[6] Lung cancer (1.35 million) is the most common cancer, followed by breast cancer (1.15 million), colorectal cancer (1 million), and stomach cancer (.93 million). Lung cancer also is the most common cause of death from cancer (1.18 million deaths), followed by stomach cancer (700,000 deaths), liver cancer (598,000 deaths), and colorectal cancer (529,000). There is considerable international variation in the incidence of these and other cancers, although the world's regions tend to be more similar than different owing to common environmental exposures and lifestyles.

Characteristics of the Disease If a disease is judged to be an important health problem, additional disease-specific criteria must be met to justify screening. These include the natural history of the disease, the nature of the disease latency period, and the degree to which treatment before the onset of clinically apparent disease truly improves prognosis compared with that achieved with later treatment.

Screening recommendations typically represent an interplay between the age at which to begin screening and a screening interval, so that there will be both a sufficient prevalence of detectable occult disease to justify screening large numbers of healthy individuals, and an interval that is likely to detect most cancers at an early stage in a population adherent with screening recommendations. Most cancers have a long preclinical phase, which technically begins following the first reproduction of malignant cells. At a point late in the preclinical phase, a tumor may become detectable by a screening test before the onset of symptoms, hence the "detectable" period in the preclinical phase. The detectable preclinical phase (DPCP), also known as the "sojourn time," is the estimated duration of time in which an occult tumor can be detected with a screening test before the onset of symptoms.[7] For screening to be successful, the sojourn time should be sufficiently long to insure that periodic screening provides the opportunity to detect most disease in the target population before the onset of symptoms. If the sojourn time is short, then the necessary screening interval may be so short that screening is impractical. Conversely, if the sojourn time is long, then screening too frequently will waste health care resources. The screening interval should always be shorter than the estimated mean duration of the sojourn time. When a screening interval equals or exceeds the mean sojourn time, there will be a higher rate of interval cancers (cancers that arise and present with clinical manifestations between regularly scheduled screens), and thus, poorer prognosis in that subset of the incident cases. The interrelationship between the sojourn time and the lead time is shown in Figure 28-1.

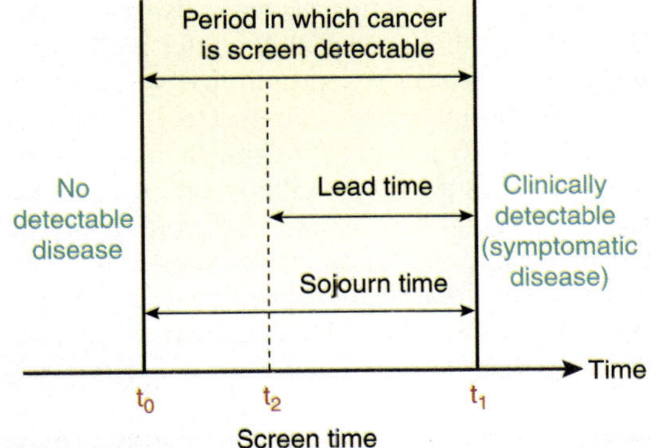

Figure 28-1 The natural history of cancer. In this figure, t1-t0 is the duration of the preclinical screen-detectable period, known as the "sojourn time"; t1-t2 is the amount of time by which the diagnosis is advanced by screening, known as the "lead time." The sojourn time is often assumed to have an exponential distribution, which confers exactly the same distribution on the lead time. Under this model the expected lead time of a screen-detected case is equal to the mean sojourn time (MST)

Treatment of screen-detected cancers should offer advantages compared with treatment of disease that presents with symptoms. These advantages may be measured by any single outcome or combination of outcomes: lower mortality, lower morbidity, and/or improved quality of life. However, it is important not to equate detection of occult disease with better outcomes, since this may not always be the case, and the magnitude of the benefit may not be sufficient to warrant screening the population.[8]

IS THE SCREENING TEST EFFECTIVE?

The ultimate determinant of whether a screening test is effective in public health terms is whether its routine use leads to a reduction in mortality or morbidity. In terms of its diagnostic effect (which is a necessary condition for its effectiveness), the primary measures are sensitivity (S), specificity (Sp), positive predictive values (PPV), and negative predictive value (NPV).

Sensitivity and Specificity The sensitivity is the probability that the test will have a positive result when applied to a person who truly has the disease. The specificity is the probability of a negative result when applied to a person who does not have the disease. The conventional formulas for calculating sensitivity and specificity are shown in Table 28-1. These are intuitively reasonable definitions, and they have obvious practical applications: A sensitive test will tend to catch disease cases and an insensitive test will miss them, possibly leading to false reassurance and actual delay in diagnosis; a specific test will tend only to catch disease cases, whereas a nonspecific test will raise suspicion of disease in normal subjects, leading to unnecessary further diagnostic investigations and possibly treatments.

Clearly then, high sensitivity and high specificity are desirable features. However, in general, they tend to be negatively correlated. For example, consider a blood test that we class as positive if the value of a continuous assay exceeds a certain cutoff. A high cutoff will confer high specificity and low sensitivity, and vice versa. Other complications include cost-effectiveness of detection. MRI is more sensitive than mammography, but has poorer specificity, and thus, much higher financial and human costs.[9] It should be borne in mind that there is a difference between screening and diagnosis. A positive screening test is not generally a definitive diagnosis of any condition; rather,, it merely indicates whether or not further diagnostic work-up is necessary (thus, the ubiquitous use of the term "false positive" for recalled subjects who are finally diagnosed normal is arguably misleading). Therefore, it is unreasonable to expect 100% sensitivity or specificity. In screening for cancer, one would prefer to avoid further diagnostic work-up in more than 10% of truly disease-negative subjects, and if at all possible one would not want to miss more than 10% of disease-positive subjects. These are arbitrary figures, but are reasonable.

Table 28-1 Measures of Screening Performance

	Disease Status	
Screening Test Results	Yes	No
Positive	a	b
Negative	c	d

Sensitivity = a/(a + c); specificity = d/(b + d); positive predictive value (PPV) = a/(a + b); negative predictive value (NPV) c/(c + d)

Finally, we should not confuse test sensitivity with program sensitivity. The latter is the proportion of cases arising in people attending a screening program that are actually detected as a result of screening (as opposed to cases arising symptomatically between screens). Program sensitivity is a function of test sensitivity, the duration of sojourn time, and the time interval between screens.

Positive and Negative Predictive Values The positive predictive value is the probability that a subject with a positive screening result actually has the disease. For example, in mammography, it is not unusual to recall 5% of subjects screened for further investigation and to finally diagnose only 0.5% of screened subjects with cancer. In this case, the PPV is 10%. This figure seems low, superficially, but generally is acceptable to screened populations.[10] The benefit of early detection for the 5 women per thousand with breast cancer is considered to outweigh the temporary inconvenience and anxiety for the 45 women per thousand with a positive test who do not have cancer. The complement of positive predictive value is the proportion of screen positive subjects who do not have disease. This should not be confused with overdiagnosis (see next section).

The NPV is the probability that a subject screened negative is truly free of disease and is in some sense a quantification of the reassurance value of a negative test. It is arguably more important to have a high NPV, as this will mean that few disease subjects are missed and potentially have diagnosis and treatment delayed.

Overdiagnosis In the context of screening, overdiagnosis is the diagnosis through screening of disease that would never have given rise to clinical symptoms during the lifetime of the case. Overdiagnosis is commonly applied to circumstances that, although quite disparate, result in the same lack of benefit from early detection. First is the theoretical possibility of diagnosis of lesions that have no biological propensity to progress. This clearly happens in the case of screen-detected premalignant lesions of the uterine cervix and large bowel, and possibly in cancers of the prostate. The issue is controversial in the case of mammography, as there are some in situ lesions with dubious potential for progression. These lesions are, however, likely to be a minority of ductal carcinoma in situ (DCIS) cases.[11] The second circumstance pertains to the early diagnosis and treatment of a cancer that would not have produced symptoms before a patient died from some other cause. This kind of overdiagnosis is of greatest concern when screening is offered to individuals who have very limited longevity because of life-limiting comorbid conditions, with little possibility of benefiting from any preventive health measure.

Whether the risks of overdiagnosis and the harm to the patient as a result are outweighed by the benefits is a matter of judgment. For breast and cervical cancer, willingness of subjects to participate despite the likelihood of some overdiagnosis, albeit not fully quantified, suggests that for these cancers, the risks are outweighed by the benefits.

All the above issues are discussed in the sections on specific cancers below.

Cost-Effectiveness The cost of screening extends far beyond the cost of the screening test. There are costs associated with diagnostic evaluations and the cost of treatment of screen-detected disease that may never have become clinically apparent. For these reasons, decisions about screening should be made only after careful consideration of whether the implementation of a screening test meets well-defined criteria related not only to disease burden, benefit of early detection, test performance, and acceptability to the population, but also costs. Put another way, does the potential exist for a favorable balance between the benefits of screening and the limitations and costs of screening?

There are two basic models for the evaluation of costs and outcomes: cost-benefit analysis (CBA) and cost-effectiveness analysis (CEA). In CBA, benefits are expressed in monetary terms, whereas benefits in CEA are expressed as health outcomes.[12] Benefits in CBA may be based on a human capital model, in which case a life is assigned a monetary value, or alternatively, individuals are given an opportunity to establish what the benefit is worth to them. However, assigning a dollar value to health is inherently both difficult and arbitrary.[12] Nevertheless, if costs exceed benefits, the intervention is judged to be not cost-beneficial and therefore not justified. In contrast, cost-effectiveness studies in medicine are focused on the unit or net cost of achieving a particular health-related outcome.[13] In cancer screening, cost-effectiveness can be expressed in terms of the cost to detect one cancer, prevent one death, add a year of life, or add a quality-adjusted year of life. At the most basic level, the most appropriate and intuitive estimate of the cost-effectiveness of cancer screening is an estimate of the marginal cost per year of life saved (MCYLS). The marginal costs of screening are the costs incurred by implementing a screening program minus the costs of case detection and management without screening. The marginal effectiveness is the years of life expected and gained in the screened group minus the years of life expected in the group not undergoing screening. The MCYLS is the fraction of the marginal costs of screening divided by the marginal effectiveness. In general, if a screening test achieves a benchmark of less than $40,000 (US) per MCYLS, costs are judged to be within acceptable limits of cost-effectiveness.[12] This conventional benchmark, which has been applied for several decades, has never been adjusted for inflation.

Acceptability to Individuals at Risk and Health Care Providers No matter how effective a screening test may be, its potential to reduce disease burden is highly dependent on adherence with recommended screening intervals and follow-up procedures. Low participation in cancer screening among both providers (low rate of referral) and the public (low and irregular attendance) can be due to low awareness, low perceptions of individual risk, high costs, low access, and aversion to the test, learning test results, and follow-up. Probably the single most important factor related to screening participation, apart from having health insurance, is a recommendation from an individual's health care provider.[14]

METHODOLOGIC ISSUES IN THE EVALUATION OF EARLY-DETECTION PROGRAMS

The issue of whether or not a screening intervention is effective may appear superficially to be a simple matter. Theoretically, one only need observe whether persons live longer or have a lesser risk of dying from the disease in question as a result of application of a screening test. Case reports or anecdotal evidence of good outcomes following cancer detection in asymptomatic persons should not, however, be trusted as evidence of screening effectiveness. Evaluations of screening tests done outside the context of a rigorous research design are subject to many biases that may (and usually do) invalidate the conclusions being drawn. Included among these complicating factors are lead-time and length biases, subject self-selection, and overdiagnosis.

Known Biases in the Evaluation of Screening Programs **Lead-Time Bias** As described earlier, the interval between the moment an occult condition can be detected and the moment that condition would have become known by patient awareness of signs or symptoms is known as the lead time. Unless lead time is accounted for, comparisons of survival rates in screened and unscreened populations will be misleading. There always is a bias toward better survival rates in the screened group because the length of the lead time moves the point at which survival begins to be measured forward. Thus, it is possible that earlier detection only moves forward the time of a patient's diagnosis, without moving back the time of death (Figure 28-2). If lead-time bias is present, screen-detected cancers appear to have better survival, but in fact, death occurs at the same point it would have without screening. It is traditional to think of lead time as a disadvantage, but it is only so in terms of complicating the process of data analysis. In clinical terms, it is the essential benefit of screening. A screening test that does not advance the time of diagnosis will not improve the prognosis.

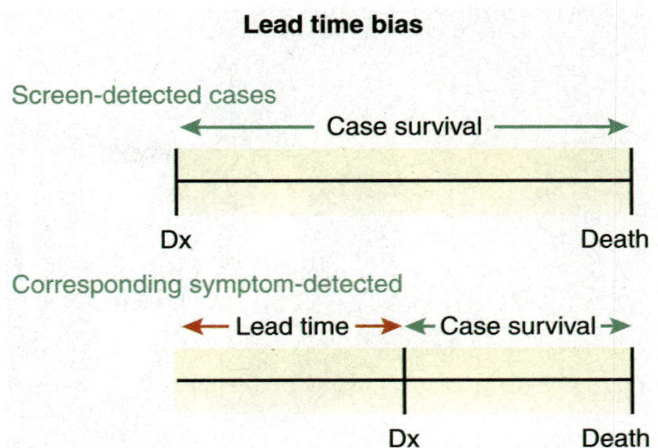

Figure 28-2 Lead time bias. In this figure, Dx is the time of diagnosis. Note that the screen-detected cases and the cases diagnosed with symptoms each die at the same time, but the survival time looks greater in the screen-detected case because of lead time bias. Adapted from www.3.cancer.gov/prevention/lss/vaslides.html

Length Bias Because of variations in tumor growth rates and other biologic characteristics, more of the cancers with long preclinical phases will be detected when a population is screened. A tumor with a longer preclinical phase may also be a more indolent and less-threatening lesion. This bias toward detection of less-threatening cancers is "length bias" (Figure 28-3). This form of potential bias complicates the interpretation of outcome differences between cancers detected by screening and those found outside the screening program because the cancers most likely to escape detection may be the very cancers that have the greatest likelihood of causing death.

Overdiagnosis Overdiagnosis is an extreme example of length bias. Because early-detection intervention is more likely than symptom recognition to yield lesions that might never become clinically significant cancers, survival statistics for screening detected cancers may be inflated. The occurrence of overdiagnosis may be suspected if an imbalance between the incidence rate in a screening program and the expected incidence rate in the absence of screening persists in a cohort after an extended period of follow-up.

Patient Self-Selection Individuals who elect to receive early detection tests may be different from those who do not in ways that could affect their survival or recovery from disease. For example, users of early-detection services may be more health conscious, more likely to control risk factors such as smoking or diet, more alert to the signs and symptoms of disease, more adherent to treatment, or generally healthier.

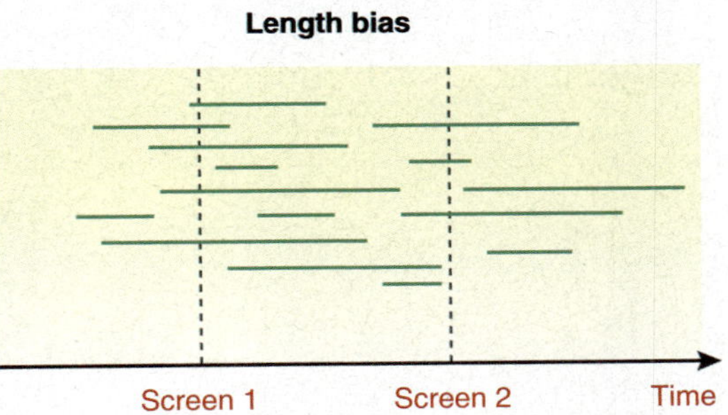

Figure 28-3 Length bias. In this figure, the horizontal lines represent the sojourn times of individual tumors detected in a screening program. The two screening examinations detect 6 out of 8 long sojourn time tumors, but only 2 out of 6 short sojourn time tumors.

Research Designs for Screening Evaluation Researchers use several different approaches to study cancer-screening effectiveness, including descriptive studies, case-control studies, and randomized controlled trials. Each of these strategies has certain strengths and weaknesses. Some methods are more powerful than others, but no single approach can provide all the answers needed for the evaluation of screening efficacy. Assessing the effectiveness of a screening intervention almost always requires combining evidence from multiple sources based on different research methodologies.

Descriptive Studies Uncontrolled studies based on the experience of individual physicians, hospitals, and nonpopulation-based registries can yield important information about screening. Indeed, the first evidence that screening may contribute to disease control often is reported from descriptive studies, as is evidence about the performance parameters of detection tests, such as sensitivity, specificity, and positive predictive values. Descriptive studies, however, do not establish efficacy because of the absence of an appropriate control group and the influence of the potential biases described previously.

Case-Control Studies Retrospective case-control studies can provide additional evidence on screening effectiveness. The advantage of this approach is that it is a low-cost strategy that may provide evidence more quickly than prospective studies when the screening procedure is already in clinical use.[15] Although mortality reduction can be an end point measured in these studies, case-control studies are subject to bias and confounding from uncontrolled factors.

Randomized Clinical Trials The most rigorous assessment of screening is by randomized clinical trials (RCT) that measure cancer-specific mortality reduction as the primary end point. As a qualification to this, in a trial of cervical screening, where the object is to prevent invasive cervical cancer from occurring, a valid end point would be incidence of the disease. In an RCT, the distorting effects of self-selection are bypassed through random assignment to either an experimental group invited to receive screening or an uninvited group. The mortality end point is not subject to the effects of lead-time or length bias, or overdiagnosis. An RCT of screening evaluates the effect of an invitation to screening rather than screening per se, that is, end results are based on comparisons between invited and uninvited groups rather than screened and unscreened groups. The distinction is important since noncompliance to the invitation to screening in the experimental group, and contamination in the control group (ie, participation in screening outside of the trial), have an effect on the magnitude of the observed outcome. Although RCTs are the most desirable study design from a methodological perspective, the large sample sizes required, their expense, and their long duration have tended to limit the number of RCTs of screening that have been conducted.

All-cause mortality rather than disease-specific mortality has been proposed as a preferable end point in RCTs on the basis of possible biases in assignment of cause of death in experimental and control groups in a trial.[16] Cause of death committees need to, and usually do, build safeguards into the death ascertainment process so that these biases are avoided, or, at the least, minimized. These safeguards include blinded review and a consensus process that referees disputes between multiple reviewers. Thus, although some level of misallocation may occur, there is little evidence that the rate of error approaches a level that would measurably bias end results.[17] It has been shown that in breast cancer screening, breast cancer mortality is an appropriate and reliable end point, and that all-cause mortality is inefficient and of little if any value.[18] This is also likely to be the case in evaluation of screening for other cancers.

BREAST CANCER

Disease Burden In the United States in 2005, the American Cancer Society (ACS) estimates that 211,240 women will be diagnosed with invasive breast cancer, and an additional 58,490 women will be diagnosed with ductal carcinoma in situ (DCIS).[19] Approximately 40,410 women are expected to die from breast cancer in 2005.[19] Breast cancer is uncommon in men. In 2005, the ACS estimated that there would be 1,690 new cases of male breast cancer and 460 deaths, less than 1% of the annual incidence and mortality among women. The most recent 5-year survival rate for breast cancer cases diagnosed in 1992 is 85%.[20] When calculated by extent of disease at diagnosis, survival is much improved if breast cancer is diagnosed while still localized (98%) and is progressively poorer for regional (81%) and distant disease (26%).[21]

Screening and Diagnostic Methods The most effective screening test for the early detection of breast cancer is mammography. Guidelines for early breast cancer detection emphasize an age-related combination of breast self-examination (BSE), clinical breast examination (CBE), and mammography as a complete program of surveillance. After age 40 years, the principal roles of BSE and CBE are to identify masses that were not detected on mammography owing to test limitations, rapid tumor growth, or human error. Increasingly, magnetic resonance imaging (MRI) and ultrasound are being added to mammography for women who are at very high risk of breast cancer at a younger age, since each of these techniques offers unique advantages for imaging the dense breast.

Mammography Mammography is an x-ray examination of the breasts to detect abnormalities that may be breast cancer (Figures 28-4 through 28-6). Modern mammography is done on dedicated imaging equipment designed to produce a high-quality image of the breast at a minimum x-ray dose. Average breast dose per view has been reduced from several centigrays (rads) to 1 to 2 milliGray (0.1–0.2 rads) per view.[22] Image quality and interpretive skills have also been improved through early efforts by the American College of Radiology's Mammography Accreditation Program (ACRMAP), and subsequently, the passage of the Mammography Quality Standards Act (MQSA) of 1992, which requires a facility to meet a broad range of technical and personnel standards in order to be certified by the US Food and Drug Administration (FDA).[23] Until recently, breast cancer screening was limited to dedicated x-ray equipment that produced images on x-ray film. The introduction of new, full-field digital units that capture the image electronically with solid state detectors instead of film is a new competing technology that may offer significant advantages over conventional film-screen units. A large prospective study comparing screen film mammography with digital mammography completed enrollment in 2004.[24]

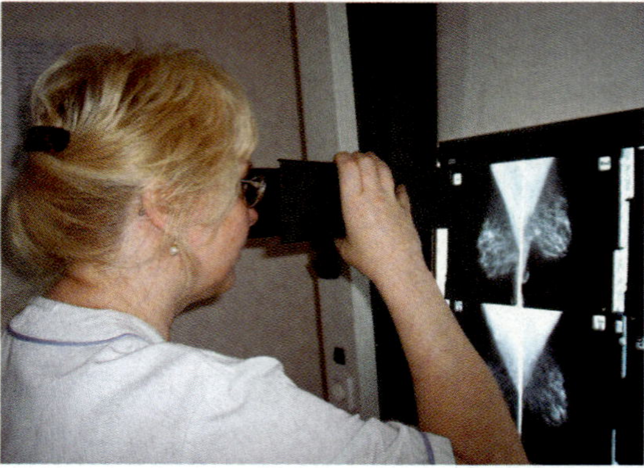

Figure 28-4 Dr. Nadja Lindhe seen screening asymptomatic women using a multiviewer, Department of Mammography, Central Hospital, Falun Sweden. Courtesy of Dr. Laszlo Tabar.

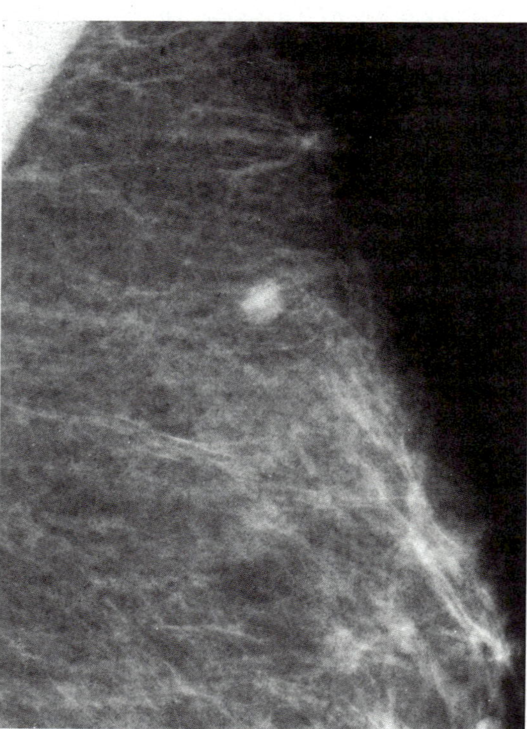

Figure 28-5 Medio-lateral oblique projection of the left breast of a 66-year-old asymptomatic woman. In the axillary portion of the breast a < 10 mm solitary circular lesion is seen. Courtesy of Dr. Laszlo Tabar.

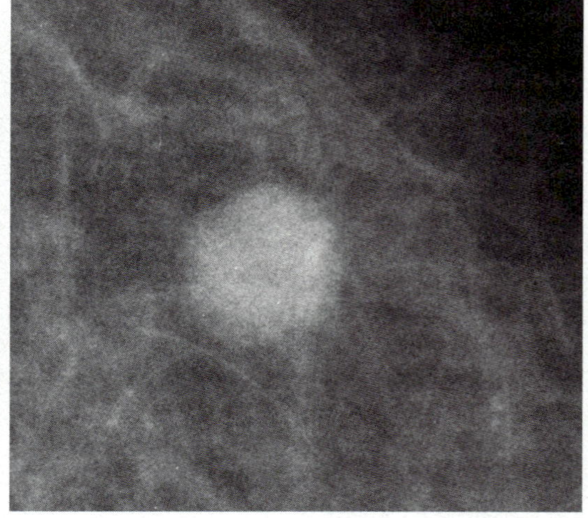

Figure 28-6 Microfocus magnification image of the circular abnormality in Figure 28-5 shows an ill-defined, solitary, mammographically malignant lesion, later confirmed to be an invasive ductal carcinoma. Courtesy of Dr. Laszlo Tabar.

A screening examination involves two views of each breast: a craniocaudal (CC) view and a mediolateral oblique (MLO) view. Prior to taking the x-ray, a radiology technologist positions a woman's breast in a compression device. Although breast compression results in some discomfort, it should not be painful. Adequate compression contributes to image quality by evening the thickness of the breast, separating breast tissues that may obscure a lesion, permitting even penetration, preventing motion blur, improving contrast (by decreasing radiation scatter), and reducing radiation dose to the breast. After the examination, a radiologist examines the films for abnormalities. The rate of abnormal interpretations is generally higher for first screening examinations, but overall, the average range of initial abnormal interpretations is 5 to 10%.[25] In most instances, abnormalities are resolved through additional diagnostic mammography imaging with special views, or by ultrasonography. Abnormalities that cannot be resolved with additional imaging (including ultrasonography) generally will proceed to biopsy with fine needle aspiration, ultrasonographically or radiographically directed core needle biopsy, or surgical excision.

The sensitivity and specificity of mammography fall within acceptable parameters and vary somewhat by age, with sensitivity, specificity, and PPV improving in successive age groups of women. Historically, discussions of mammographic sensitivity and specificity have been influenced by the debate over the value of screening women under age 50 (discussed below), leading to the misleading conclusion that sensitivity, specificity, and PPV were uniform for postmenopausal women and measurably poorer in premenopausal women.[26,27] However, sensitivity measures available from the trials also are influenced by the screening interval, especially for women under age 50. More recent data examining sensitivity, specificity, and PPV by age have shown that there is a continuum of improvement with increasing age, and that performance in adjacent decades of life is more similar than different.[28–31]

No other cancer screening test has been studied as extensively as mammography. There have been eight randomized trials published to date. The most recently published results of these are shown in Figure 28-7. This indicates a 20% reduction in breast cancer mortality with invitation to screening. The International Agency for Research on Cancer's in-depth review concluded that the benefits of actually receiving screening were higher, of the order of a 35% breast cancer mortality reduction.[32]

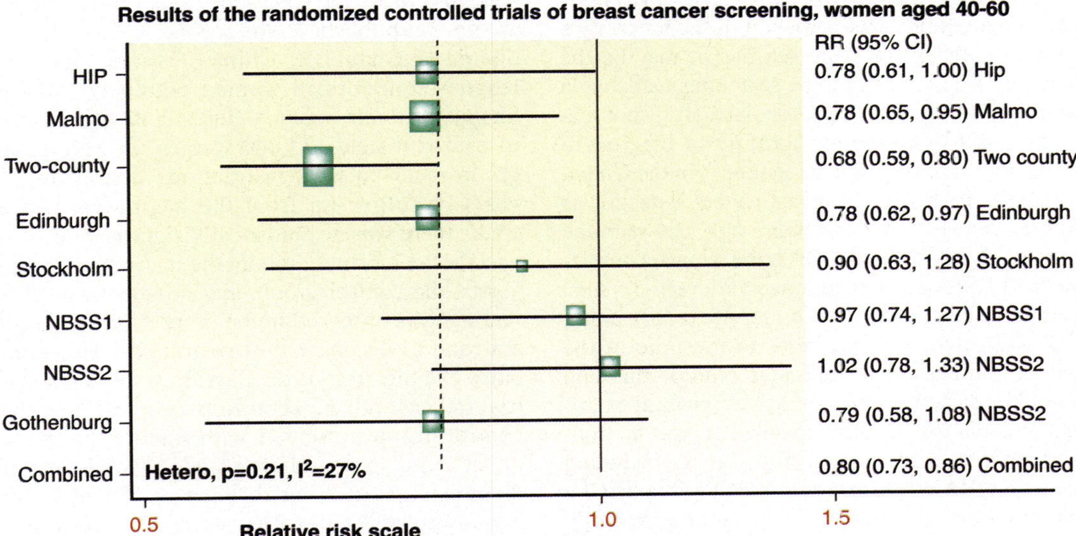

Figure 28-7 Results of randomized controlled trials of breast cancer screening, women aged 40–69.

During the past two decades, the issue of breast cancer screening with mammography among women under age 50 has dominated deliberations about breast cancer screening and has been a source of persistent debate in the United States and in Europe.[26,33–37] Although many leading medical organizations in the United States endorsed breast cancer screening for women aged 40 to 49 years, some equally prominent organizations did not. For the most part, the dispute over screening policy for women under age 50 was based on the lack of clear evidence from the world's trials that mammography screening for women aged 40 to 49 years was effective.

Prior to 1997, two trials (the Health Insurance Plan of Greater New York trial and the Swedish Two-County trial) had shown a statistically significant reduction in breast cancer mortality among women aged 50 years and older, but no statistically significant reduction in deaths from an individual trial had been observed for women aged 40 to 49 years.[38,39] More recent analyses of trial data have provided important insights about screening in different age groups of women and have helped explain why early trial results were less favorable results in premenopausal women.[40,41] In the individual trials, a mortality benefit begins to appear relatively early (at about 5 years) for women aged 50 and over at randomization, whereas it occurs much later for women ages 40 to 49 at randomization. With accumulating years of follow-up in the 40- to 49-years group, the relative risk (RR) of mortality steadily improves. Recent analysis of the Two-County data provides a clinically intuitive explanation for the delay in benefit observed in women under age 50, based on the interrelationship between tumor histology, sojourn time, and age.[40,42] As described earlier, the mean breast cancer sojourn time (ie, potential lead time) is shorter (1.7 years) in women under age 50 compared with women over age 50 (≥ 3.3 years).[43] Because the majority of the world's trials screened women aged 40 to 49 at randomization at an interval of 24 months, faster tumor growth rates in women in their forties meant that these women were less likely to benefit from mammography when it was offered every 2 years compared with women aged 50 and older. Whereas a 2-year interval was equally effective in both age groups for grade 2, medullary, and invasive lobular tumors, and was effective in reducing deaths among grade 3 tumors diagnosed in women aged 50 and older; it was not effective for grade 3 tumors diagnosed in women aged 40 to 49. The results from the Gothenburg trial, which screened women aged 39 to 49 at 18-month intervals, show that the timing of the benefit, which appears at 6 to 8 years, is similar to that observed for women aged 50 and over.[44] In the Gothenburg trial, which screened women aged 40 to 49 every 18 months and showed a 44% reduction in breast cancer mortality, the proportional interval cancer incidence was 18% in the first 12 months after a negative screen and increased to more than 50% in the period of 12 to 18 months.[44] Data from service screening programs also support these conclusions.[45] Based on findings related to faster tumor growth rates, most organizations that recommend screening for women in their forties emphasize the advantage of screening annually.

Evaluation of Mammography Service Screening Programs Whereas the RCTs of breast cancer screening had clearly demonstrated the benefit of early breast cancer detection, the establishment of routine screening with mammography as health policy, that is, "service screening," posed new questions. Is mammography less or more effective outside of the experimental setting, especially since screening standards, protocols, and technology have improved? Answering this question is not so straightforward. In 1999, Sjönell and Stahle reported that the assumption that mammography was beneficial was illusionary, since widespread screening with mammography in Sweden had apparently little impact on breast cancer mortality.[46] However, Sjönell and Stahle failed to correctly identify the years when Swedish counties introduced screening, failed to account for the time it takes to introduce screening into a population, failed to consider that different counties would have different screening take-up rates, and finally, failed to distinguish between screened and unscreened cohorts in their mortality analysis. In the case of breast cancer, in any 10-year period after the introduction of screening, usually more than 50% of the breast cancer deaths will occur in women diagnosed before the introduction of screening, a group that clearly could not have benefited from the intervention.[47] Ideally, the analysis of service screening should be able to isolate screened and unscreened cohorts, and to classify women on the basis of whether or not they were invited to screening, attended screening (screen-detected and interval cancers), and whether or not they were nonattenders (not invited, or refusers). With these data, as well as information on access to screening, breast cancer mortality can be estimated for women who actually attend screening and for the population as a whole, the latter simulating a classic intention-to-treat analysis. Differences in mortality over time will be attributable to screening, improvements in therapy, and increased awareness, although distinguishing between screening and nonscreening factors is complex and can be only indirectly estimated.

Investigators from Sweden have been able to classify breast cancer cases before and after the introduction to screening on the basis of exposure to screening.[45,47,48] These studies typically show around a 30% reduction in breast cancer mortality associated with the policy of offering screening, and a 40% or higher reduction with individual exposure to screening. The studies incorporate control for the various biases and estimation of the changes in mortality from other changes in addition to screening. The data demonstrate that organized screening with high rates of attendance in a setting that achieves a high degree of programmatic quality assurance can achieve breast cancer mortality reductions equal to or greater than observed in the randomized trials.

Physical Examinations CBE and BSE CBE involves physical palpation of the breast by a trained clinician. In some settings, it may be the only method of breast cancer screening available to women.[49] In other settings, regular CBE is not recommended once mammography is offered to women for breast cancer screening.[50] In the United States, its role in early breast cancer detection is defined primarily by a woman's age. Between the ages of 20 and 40 years, CBE is the clinical complement to BSE and is recommended every 3 years. Beginning at age 40, CBE commonly is done annually, and often near and prior to the time of the annual mammogram. Technique is important and should be systematic. A competent physical examination includes palpation in small segments, from the nipple to the periphery of the breast, including the axilla. Various techniques exist to organize the examination, and personal preference probably should be the deciding factor.[51]

There have been no randomized trials of the efficacy of CBE as a single screening modality. CBE has been included in some randomized trials of mammography, but any estimation of the sensitivity of CBE in these early studies must be interpreted in the historical context of the sensitivity of mammography at that time. The fact that some trials have examined the combined modality of mammography and CBE and the observation that a small percentage of palpable masses are not seen on mammography have led to guidelines that include routine CBE, ideally near to and prior to the occasion of mammography, as part of the screening regimen, to increase sensitivity.[52] However, in a setting of high-quality mammography, and high adherence with regular mammography, routine CBE contributes very little to the detection of breast cancer.[53] Of course, if a patient has a palpable mass, then she is no longer asymptomatic and screening mammography is inappropriate.

BSE has obvious appeal as a screening test because it is simple and convenient, has no apparent financial cost to participants, is noninvasive, and is intended to lead to earlier awareness of the presence of breast cancer symptoms. However, recommendations for BSE have been controversial because of a lack of definitive evidence for its efficacy and concerns about harms, including (1) the possibility that BSE promotion distracts from the importance of mammography, (2) false reassurance, (3) heightened anxiety about breast cancer, (4) anxiety during the examination, and (5) false positives.[54] Results from two RCTs of BSE are now available, and neither has demonstrated a reduction in mortality in a group trained to do BSE compared with a group receiving usual care. The first RCT of BSE was conducted in St. Petersburg and Moscow in 1985, with results published only from the St. Petersburg arm.[55] The results from St. Petersburg show no difference in mortality between the BSE instruction group and the control group, and also no difference in tumor size or stage between the two groups, although compliance with BSE was low, and women in both the experimental group and control group were also receiving CBE.[56] Results from Moscow are not yet published. The second RCT was conducted in Shanghai, China. Thomas and colleagues randomized women employed by the Shagnhai Textile Industry Bureau into two groups of approximately 133,000 women, in which one group received BSE instruction.[57] At 10 to 11 years of follow-up from the beginning of the study, there was no statistically significant difference in the mortality rate in the instruction group versus the control group, and no significant difference was observed in the proportion of Tis (in situ) and T1 lesions in the two groups.[58] However, close examination of the data from the Shanghai trial indicated that a significant proportion of the control group presented with tumors that were under 2 cm (45%) and not advanced at the time of diagnosis, suggesting that the combination of high awareness and access to health care in this region meant there was uncertain potential to improve on tumor characteristics at diagnosis through the initiation of BSE. In addition, the study group had nonsignificant reductions of around 10% in node positive tumors and tumors at T2 stage or worse.

BSE and CBE potentially offer some advantage for the detection of palpable masses in women who have not reached an age when mammography is recommended, or to detect cancers missed by mammography or faster growing tumors among women in an age group in which mammography is recommended. However, the unique advantage of systematic physical exams is unclear in an age group or population compared with self-detection during normal activities in a population that has gained heightened awareness of breast cancer symptoms and the importance of prompt reporting of new breast changes. Although heightened awareness is key, it also is unclear whether that can be achieved through educational messages alone, or whether BSE instruction and periodic CBE reinforce heightened awareness, which likewise may be true for women undergoing regular mammography as well.[59] Because prognosis is very strongly influenced by tumor size, women should be continually educated about the importance of reporting any new breast symptom to a health care professional.

New Technology Among the unique challenges to breast cancer screening is surveillance in high-risk groups. Women who are known or suspected to be at elevated risk because of mutations on breast cancer susceptibility genes of known penetrance are at significantly elevated risk of breast cancer at an earlier age, a period when greater breast density poses a challenge to conventional mammography. Recently, there have been several reports comparing the effectiveness of clinical breast exam, ultrasound, mammography, and magnetic resonance imaging in high-risk women. Kriege and colleagues reported findings from a Netherlands study comparing the efficacy of CBE, mammography, and MRI in a group of 1,909 women at high risk.[60] Study participants had a cumulative lifetime breast cancer risk of 15% or more, and 358 were carriers of germ-line mutations of known susceptibility to breast cancer. Women were screened every 6 months with CBE, and yearly with mammography and MRI. Kriege and colleagues reported significantly superior sensitivity of MRI (79.5%) in the detection of invasive breast cancer compared with mammography (33.3%) and CBE (17.9%). Further, MRI was superior to mammography in finding tumors smaller than 1 cm (43.2% vs 14%) and was associated with a higher rate of detection of localized breast cancer (52.4% vs 21.4%). In a similar study, Warner and colleagues compared the sensitivity and specificity of mammography, ultrasound, MRI, and CBE in a group of 236 Canadian women aged 25 to 65 years with known *BRCA1* or *BRCA2* mutations.[61] CBE was conducted twice yearly, that is, on the day of the imaging examination, and then at the 6 month interval. All imaging examinations were conducted annually and interpreted independently. The investigators estimated sensitivity and specificity for each of the 4 modalities, and then compared the sensitivity of all 4 screening tests combined with conventional breast cancer screening, that is, mammography and CBE alone. Of the 22 cancers detected, 77% were detected by MRI compared with only 36% by mammography, 33% by ultrasound, and 9% by CBE. In both studies, MRI was less specific than mammography. Both studies showed that multimodal testing was superior to using any one test alone. In particular, Warner and colleagues showed that all four screening modalities combined had a sensitivity of 95% compared with 45% for mammography and CBE alone.[61] These reports and others have strengthened the evidence supporting the value of MRI for the detection of breast cancer in younger, high-risk women, a group for which screen film mammography is less sensitive.

Screening Recommendations Screening guidelines for breast cancer generally are based on age-specific recommendations for periodic testing, and may include periodic regimens of BSE, CBE by a trained health professional, and mammography (Table 28-2). The ACS no longer recommends that women conduct monthly BSE, although the guidelines do stress that women may elect to do BSE regularly, irregularly, or not at all, but what is most important for all women is to be educated about the importance of heightened vigilance about new breast symptoms.[62] The ACS recommends CBE every 3 years between ages 20 and 39, and annually thereafter. CBE should take place prior to mammography, because if a mass is present, it can be brought to the attention of the radiologist, and a diagnostic evaluation can be considered. If CBE follows mammography and a mass that was not seen on the mammogram is detected, then the patient would need to return for additional directed imaging. CBE before mammography avoids potential waste of resources. Beginning at age 40, women should have annual mammography and CBE.[62] Guidelines from the American Medical Association and the American College of Radiology are equivalent to ACS recommendations.[63,64] In 2002, the United States Preventive Services Task Force (USPSTF) upgraded their

Table 28-2 Recommendations for Early Detection of Cancer in Average-Risk Asymptomatic Individuals

Cancer Site	Population	Test or Procedure	Frequency
Cervix[a]	Women, 3 years after 1st vaginal intercourse; no later than age 21	Pap test and pelvic examination	< age 30: Annual testing with conventional Pap tests or every two years using liquid-based Pap tests. ≥ age 30: After three normal test results in a row, screening every 2–3 years with cervical cytology (conventional or liquid-based Pap test) alone, or every three years with an HPV DNA test plus cervical cytology ≥ age70: women who have had 3+ normal Pap tests and no abnormal Pap tests within 10 years Women who have had a total hysterectomy for benign reasons may choose to stop screening
Breast[b]	Women age 20+	Clinical breast exam (CBE)	Every 3 years on the occasion of a periodic checkup, age 20–39; annual, age 40+[c]
		Mammography	Annual, age 40+
Colorectal[d]	Men and women age 50+	Fecal occult blood test (FOBT)	Annual, age 50+
		Fecal immunochemical test (FIT)	Annual, age 50+
		Flexible sigmoidoscopy (FSIG)	Every 5 years, starting at age 50
		FOBT or FIT, and FSIG	Annual FOBT or FIT, and FSIG every 5 years starting at age 50
		Colonoscopy	Every 10 years starting at age 50
		Double contrast barium enema	Every 5 years, starting at age 50
Prostate[e]	Men age 50+	Digital rectal examination (DRE) and prostate-specific antigen test (PSA)	For those who seek regular testing, annual DRE and PSA starting at age 50

[a]Both the American College of Obstetricians and Gynecologists (ACOG) and USPSTF recommend the same algorithm for initiation of screening, and the screening interval. ACOG recommends annual pelvic exam after age 30; USPSTF recommends discontinuing screening at age 65.
[b]The American Cancer Society (ACS), American College of Radiology (ACR), and American Medical Association (AMA) endorse the guidelines shown. The United States Preventive Services Task Force (USPSTF) recommends mammography every 1–2 years for women aged 40 and older.
[c]Beginning at age 40, annual CBE should be done prior to mammography.
[d]The ACS, ACR, American College of Gastroenterology, American Gastroenterological Association, American Society of Colon and Rectal Surgeons, American Society for Gastrointestinal Endoscopy, Crohn's and Colitis Foundation of America, Oncology Nursing Society, and Society of American Gastrointestinal Endoscopic Surgeons have endorsed these guidelines for average risk adults. The USPSTF also recommends screening for colorectal cancer beginning at age 50 with each of the tests listed above, but does not specify the periodicity of testing.
[e]No organization recommends that average-risk men undergo routine testing for prostate cancer. Rather, the ACS, AMA, USPSTF, the American Academy of Family Physicians, the American College of Physicians-American Society of Internal Medicine, and the American Urologic Association recommend that clinicians (1) discuss the potential benefits and possible harms of PSA screening; (2) consider patient preferences; and (3) individualize the decision to test.

breast cancer screening guidelines to recommend that women aged 40 years and older should receive mammography every 1 to 2 years with or without clinical breast examination.[65]

There is no upper age limit to ACS breast cancer screening guidelines as long as a woman is in good health. Women at significantly higher risk of breast cancer should talk with their health care providers about initiating screening earlier, and potentially with multimodal screening as noted above.[62]

COLORECTAL CANCER

Disease Burden In the United States, colorectal cancer is the third most common cancer diagnosed among men and women and the third leading cause of cancer mortality. In 2005, it was estimated that 145,290 men and women will be diagnosed with colorectal cancer and 54,290 will die from this disease.[19] Five-year survival is 90% if the disease is diagnosed while still localized (ie, confined to the wall of the bowel), but only 68% for regional disease (ie, disease with lymph node involvement), and 10% if there are distant metastases.[21]

Screening and Diagnostic Methods The goal of screening for colorectal cancer is both the detection of early-stage adenocarcinomas and the detection and removal of adenomatous polyps, which are accepted as being potential precursors for colorectal cancer. Reduction in colorectal cancer morbidity and mortality through screening is achieved through a combination of (1) a more favorable stage at diagnosis of occult disease and (2) disease prevention resulting from the removal of precursor lesions.

Polyps are common in adults over age 50. Since the majority of polyps will not develop into adenocarcinoma, histology and size determine their clinical importance as precursor lesions.[66–68] The most common and clinically important polyps are adenomatous polyps, which represent about one-half to two-thirds of all colorectal polyps and are associated with the greatest risk of colorectal cancer (Figures 28-8 and 28-9). Other polyps, which include incidental hyperplastic polyps and mucosal tags, are not believed to have clinical significance in the development of colorectal cancer. The evidence for the importance of colorectal polyps in the development of colorectal cancer is largely indirect, but is nonetheless convincing. First, adenomatous polyps and adenocarcinomas in the colon and rectum have a similar anatomic distribution, and the average age at which polyps begin to appear in adults precedes the age-incidence distribution of colorectal cancer,[69] with conventional estimates of about 10 years for the time required for an adenomatous polyp < 1 cm to become an invasive lesion.[70] Second, there is a strong association between polyp size and the grade of dysplasia, with higher-grade dysplasias more commonly observed in large polyps.[66] Third, epidemiologic evidence has shown higher risks of colorectal cancer after 14 years among individuals who had large polyps removed from the rectum or sigmoid colon and subsequently received no follow-up testing.[71] Fourth, individuals with familial adenomatous polyposis (FAP) have a nearly 100% probability of developing colorectal cancer and will experience earlier onset and extensive distribution of polyps throughout the colon and rectum.[72] Fifth, epidemiologic evidence has shown a lower incidence of colorectal cancer among individuals who have had large adenomatous polyps removed compared with the general population.[73,74] As will be seen below, the protection offered by screening and removal of adenomatous polyps extends only to the area of the bowel that has been examined.

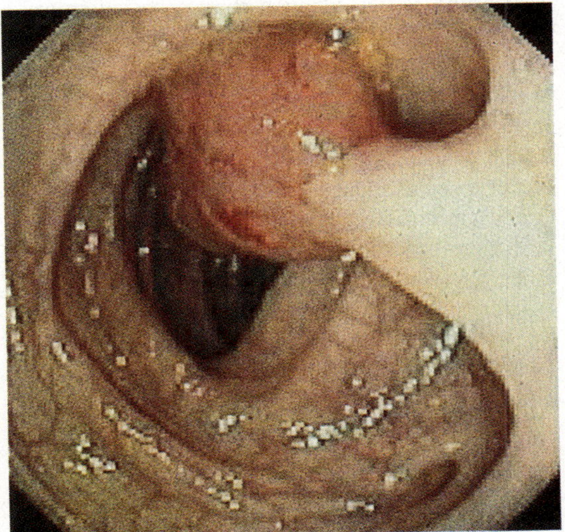

Figure 28-8 Malignant pedunculated polyp without invasion of the stalk.

There are a number of screening methods for colorectal cancer, and they fall into two general categories: stool tests, which include testing for occult blood or exfoliated DNA, and structural exams, which include flexible sigmoidoscopy, colonoscopy, CT colonography (both 2D and 3D), and double contrast barium enema. These tests may be used alone or in combination (to improve sensitivity, or in some instances, to

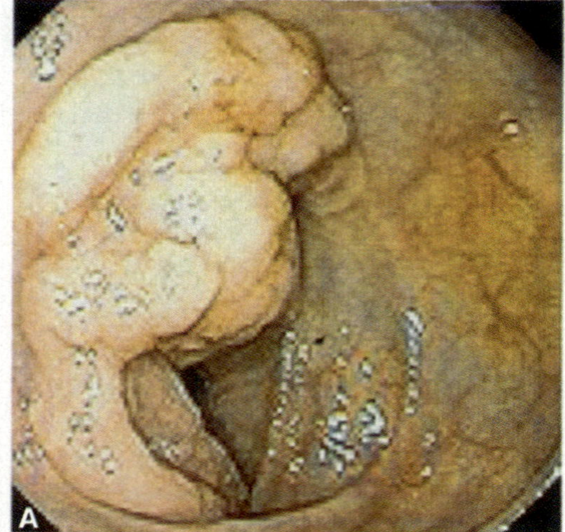

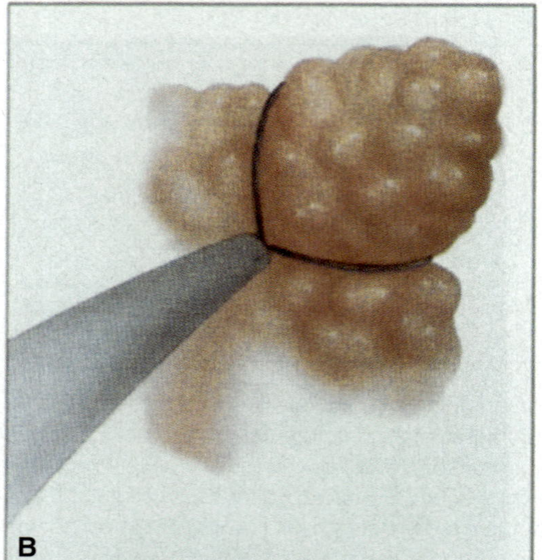

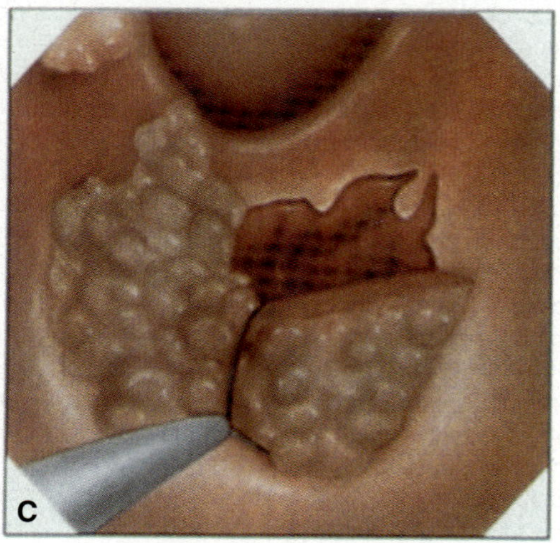

Figure 28-9 Piecemeal polypectomy of a sessile polyp. **A,** Colonoscopic view of a large sessile villous adenoma. **B,** Snare resection of a portion of the sessile polyp. **C,** Piecemeal removal of a sessile polyp.

ensure a complete examination). Screening tests for colorectal cancer vary in terms of the degree of underlying evidence supporting their use, potential efficacy, cost-effectiveness, and acceptability among patients. Nevertheless, any one of these alternatives, applied in a program of regular surveillance, has the potential to reduce deaths from colorectal cancer.

Stool Tests (*g*FOBT, *i*FOBT, and Stool DNA Tests) Stool blood tests are conventionally known as fecal occult blood tests (FOBT) because they aim to discover the presence of occult blood in stool, which may derive from colorectal cancer or larger (> 2 cm) polyps. Because small polyps do not tend to bleed, and bleeding from cancers or large polyps may be intermittent, the proper use of stool blood tests requires serial specimens (2 or 3) during the occasion of testing, as well as annual testing.[75–77] The most common stool blood tests (*g*FOBT) in use today are guaiac-based tests, followed by immunochemical tests (*i*FOBT). Guaiac-based tests detect blood in the stool through the pseudoperoxidase activity of heme or hemoglobin, while the immunochemical tests react to human hemoglobin. Guaiac-based tests can be processed in the physician's office, whereas the immunochemical tests are processed in a laboratory. Rehydration of *g*FOBT specimens improves sensitivity but remains controversial because it also increases the rate of false positives. A positive *g*FOBT or *i*FOBT is the basis for a diagnostic work-up to examine the entire colon with colonoscopy in order to rule out the presence of advanced neoplasia.

Because DNA mutations associated with colorectal cancer are relatively well understood, and because colorectal polyps and malignancies exfoliate cells into the lumen, it is possible to examine the stool for an array of mutations. Early clinical studies in small numbers of patients with a multitarget DNA-based stool assay approach suggested high sensitivity and specificity for both colorectal cancer and premalignant adenomatous polyps.[78] More recent investigations in larger populations have shown lower sensitivity (52%) for cancer than early studies (with similar specificity), but considerably better sensitivity for one-time testing compared with *g*FOBT.[79] Although stool DNA testing is a promising technology and is likely to undergo further refinement, there is not consensus that it is an acceptable screening test for average-risk adults.[80,81]

The observation that cancers detected through stool blood testing (*g*FOBT) had more favorable stages and better survival than cases diagnosed with symptoms led to prospective trials in Europe and the United States evaluating the efficacy of FOBT in reducing deaths from colorectal cancer. In the Minnesota trial, 46,551 asymptomatic participants aged 50 to 80 were randomly assigned to one of three groups: a group that would receive an annual invitation to screening, a group that would receive an invitation to biennial screening, and a control group that would receive usual care.[82] Participants with a positive *g*FOBT received a total colon examination with colonoscopy. After 14 years of follow-up, the 13-year cumulative mortality in the group offered annual screening was 5.33 per 1,000, compared with 8.33 per 1,000 in the biennially screened group and 8.83 in the usual-care (control) group. Annual screening was associated with a statistically significant 33% reduction in deaths from colorectal cancer compared with usual care. The reduction in deaths associated with biennial screening compared with usual care was not statistically significant at the time of initial follow-up. Similar results with 2 yearly *g*FOBT have been observed in two other trials.[83,84] In a subsequent analysis of Minnesota trial data with 18 years of follow-up, Mandel and colleagues also observed a 20% reduction in incidence in the group invited to annual screening, and an 18% reduction in incidence in the group invited to biennial screening, likely attributable to detection and removal of advanced neoplasia.[85]

The sensitivity and specificity of a *g*FOBT can be influenced by the type of *g*FOBT (performance characteristics vary), whether or not the specimen is rehydrated (ie, adding a drop of water to the slide window before processing), and by variations in interpretation, specimen collection, number of samples collected per test, screening interval, and other factors.[86] The reported sensitivity of a single FOBT varies considerably, from less than 50% to approximately 90%.[86] In a recent report by Lieberman and Weiss, the sensitivity of a single, 3-panel *g*FOBT for cancer or high-grade dysplasia was 35.6%, and 23.9% for all advanced neoplasia, reinforcing the importance of annual testing to achieve the program sensitivity observed in the randomized controlled trials.[87]

The performance of *g*FOBT is highly dependent on following a recommended protocol.[76,86,88] Although dietary restrictions have been recommended to reduce the rate of false positives, recent data suggest that dietary restrictions do not influence the false positivity rate in nonrehydrated tests, and they may reduce the compliance rate with testing.[89,90] Specimens should be collected over a 3-day period from successive bowel movements, with two samples placed on each test card. Once three samples have been collected, FOBT cards should be returned according to the provider's instructions, and the test should be processed without rehydration to reduce the rate of false positives. Annual testing following this regimen is required in order to achieve the program sensitivity observed in the randomized controlled trials.

Recent data provide reason to be concerned that the quality of *g*FOBT testing in the United States is seriously deficient, and provide a good example of the importance of strict adherence to recommended procedures for screening. In the recent comparison of stool DNA testing with *g*FOBT, Imperiale and colleagues observed that one-time *g*FOBT testing using the take-home method was only 13% sensitive for cancer, with poorer performance, in part, attributable to in-office processing of test results. Further, in the same study of veteran males reported earlier, Collins and colleagues compared the performance of a single sample, in-office *g*FOBT following digital rectal examination (DRE). Keeping in mind that the sensitivity for advanced neoplasia of one-time *g*FOBT when done properly is very low, the sensitivity for advanced neoplasia with the in-office procedure was only 4.9%.[91] The observation that one-third of primary care physicians reported that this was the only method of stool blood testing that they conducted, and that an additional 41% reported using both the in-office and take-home methods, suggests that millions of *g*FOBTs done each year are literally worthless, and provides at least indirect evidence for one reason that colorectal cancer mortality hasn't dropped more despite the volume of stool blood testing.[92,93] Many physicians have difficulty bypassing the opportunity to do FOBT with stool acquired during DRE, having little confidence that the patient will complete the preferred at-home protocol, but it is clear from the evidence that this kind of testing for fecal occult blood not only is wasteful of time and resources, but a negative result also provides false reassurance. Although convenient and common,[92] a one-sample *g*FOBT for colorectal cancer screening with stool collected during a digital rectal examination (DRE) is not recommended.[76,93] Additional data from Nadel and colleagues reveal further problems with stool blood testing, specifically that follow-up of positive *g*FOBTs commonly is inappropriate.[92] Nearly 1 in 3 physicians surveyed reported repeating the *g*FOBT if the first test was positive, and a higher percentage reported follow-up with flexible sigmoidoscopy rather than colonoscopy. One third of adults in the National Health Interview Survey who reported having had a positive FOBT reported that they received no follow-up.[92] A positive stool test should be followed with a colonoscopy.

Flexible Sigmoidoscopy Sigmoidoscopy is a relatively simple procedure that requires minimal preparation prior to the examination.[94] Sigmoidoscopes used in screening may be rigid (25 cm) or flexible (35 or 60 cm) although the most common sigmoidoscope in use is flexible and about 60 cm in length, allowing for examination of somewhat less than half of the colon (Figure 28-10). Operator visualization is achieved through either fiberscope or videoscope. Patient preparation involves a saline laxative enema 1 to 2 hours before the examination, and the test is generally performed without sedation. Prior to beginning flexible sigmoidoscopy (FSIG), the examiner should perform a DRE.[95] A skilled examiner can complete the examination in less than 10 minutes. If the test is positive, the patient is generally referred for colonoscopy. Biopsy during sigmoidoscopy can be done, but is rare outside of specialty settings for two reasons: First, the presence of polyps in the distal bowel signals an elevated risk of polyps or cancer in the proximal bowel, and the patient may be referred for colonoscopy; second, biopsy with electrocautery poses the risk of explosion of ignited hydrogen or methane in the incompletely prepared bowel. For patient safety and greater test sensitivity, total colon examination is generally postponed until a full bowel preparation can be done prior to colonoscopy.[77]

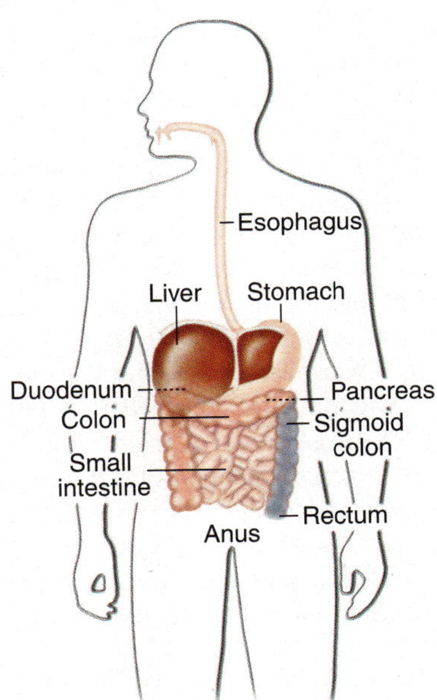

Figure 28-10 Reach of flexible sigmoidoscopy (shaded area) in screening for colorectal cancer and adenomatous polyps. (Source: Centers for Disease Control and Prevention.)

At present, there are several ongoing randomized trials of FSIG underway,[96] and thus, current evidence for the efficacy of FSIG derives from case-control investigations. Selby and colleagues compared the screening histories of patients who died from colorectal cancer with those of controls matched for age and sex.[97] Evaluation of patient records revealed that a history of rigid sigmoidoscopy was associated with 59% fewer deaths from colorectal cancer lesions in the region of the bowel within reach of the sigmoidoscope. Consistent with this interpretation was the finding that there was no protective effect from sigmoidoscopy for death due to cancers that developed in the proximal colon, that is, that part of the colon outside the reach of the instrument. Newcomb and colleagues observed a 79% reduction in colorectal cancer mortality in patients who had a history of one or more sigmoidoscopies compared with patients who had never had a sigmoidoscopy, and in subsequent analysis they observed a long-term protective effect against incidence in the distal bowel.[98,99]

Combined Stool Blood Testing and FSIG The combination of annual FOBT (either guaiac or immunochemical tests) and FSIG every 5 years is superior to either FOBT or FSIG alone insofar as the two examinations together constitute a quasi-total colon examination. FOBT provides for some surveillance in the proximal colon (outside of the reach of FSIG), and FSIG in the distal colon has higher sensitivity and specificity than FOBT and provides an opportunity to visualize cancer and polyps. Clearly, the advantage of adding FSIG to FOBT is far greater than the addition of FOBT to FSIG. The combination of FOBT and sigmoidoscopy was evaluated in a controlled trial that randomized asymptomatic individuals aged 40 and older into a group that would receive annual screening with rigid sigmoidoscopy and FOBT or with rigid sigmoidoscopy alone. After 5 to 11 years of follow-up, the investigators observed fewer colorectal cancer deaths in the group receiving annual FOBT and sigmoidoscopy compared with the group receiving sigmoidoscopy alone (0.36 versus 0.63 per 1,000; p = .53).[100] More recently, a simulation of combined FOBT and flexible sigmoidoscopy (based on findings from colonoscopy) suggested that the combined exam would achieve 76% sensitivity for advanced neoplasia.[87]

Barium Enema Barium enema is an x-ray examination of the bowel that derives contrast from barium (a single-contrast study) or the combination of barium and instilled air (a double-contrast study). Double-contrast barium enema (DCBE) is more sensitive than the single-contrast study for both malignancies and polyps. Because the addition of air into the colon can cause some discomfort, the single-contrast study may be used for patients who the physician anticipates would tolerate DCBE poorly. Bowel preparation for DCBE is similar to that required for colonoscopy since residual stool can mask lesions or lead to false positives. Prior to the examination, a flexible tube is inserted into the rectum to introduce barium into the bowel. Fluoroscopic examination monitors the progress of the barium through the bowel (patients may be required to roll and assume various positions to insure bowel cavities will be coated with barium). Once the bowel is completely coated, x-rays are taken. If the patient has a positive test, the next step is a colonoscopy. The evidence for the efficacy of DCBE is largely indirect, based on the performance of DCBE in detecting small malignant lesions and polyps and on the known benefits of early detection and polypectomy for reducing mortality from colorectal cancer. Winawer and colleagues reported comparative results of DCBE and colonoscopy for 580 patients enrolled in the National Polyp Study who underwent surveillance following diagnosis of adenomatous polyps.[101] The proportion of examinations in which adenomatous polyps identified by colonoscopy also being detected by DCBE was significantly influenced by the size of the lesion, with DCBE sensitivity increasing with the size of the lesion. Although DCBE identified some lesions missed by colonoscopy, the number was comparatively much smaller. The authors concluded colonoscopy was a more effective method of surveillance than DCBE in patients who have undergone colonoscopic polypectomy. Among all currently recommended screening tests, DCBE is the least used. In a recent study of colorectal cancer screening among Medicare beneficiaries between 1979 and 1999, the median rate for DCBE was only 2.2%.[102]

Colonoscopy Like DCBE, colonoscopy is a total colon examination (Figure 28-11) and requires thorough bowel preparation. The modern colonoscope is capable of examining the entire bowel, with the examination terminating at the cecum. The instrument generally is far more complex than a sigmoidoscope since it must be capable of air insufflation, irrigation, suction, and the passage of biopsy forceps and polypectomy snares.[103] Like sigmoidoscopes, the tip of the instrument is equipped with a small video camera and light to provide high-resolution visualization of the wall of the bowel. Patients generally go on a liquid diet one or more days before the examination, followed by either ingestion of oral lavage solutions or saline laxatives to stimulate bowel movements until the

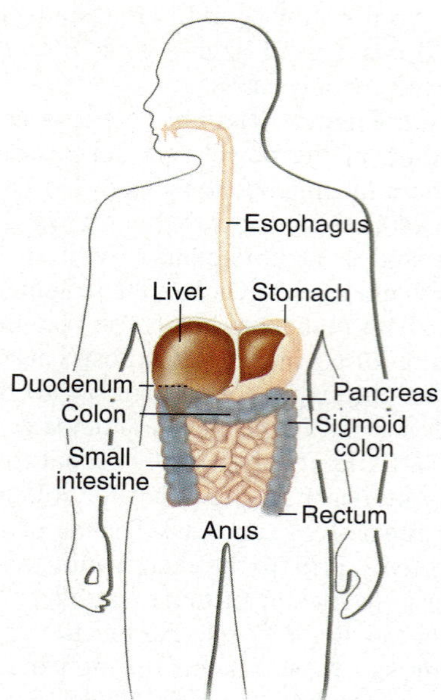

Figure 28-11 Reach of colonoscopy (shaded area) in screening for colorectal cancer and adenomatous polyps. (Source: U.S. Centers for Disease Control and Prevention.)

bowel is clean. Proper bowel preparation is a critical element in the accuracy and cost-effectiveness of screening with colonoscopy.[104] It is common for the patient to receive a mild sedative prior to the procedure, but it is not essential for those who tolerate the procedure with only mild discomfort.[105] Colonoscopy is commonly done in a hospital, but can also be done in an outpatient setting. The examination is more complex than sigmoidoscopy, with higher risk of complications, mostly because of the effects of sedation, biopsy, or polypectomy.[106] A skilled operator can complete an uncomplicated examination in approximately 30 minutes.[107]

Colonoscopy has a unique advantage among all screening tests for colorectal cancer in that direct visualization of the entire bowel is possible, and clinically significant adenomas can be identified and removed during the examination. Evidence for the effectiveness of colonoscopy is indirect in that no large trials with mortality end points have been conducted to evaluate the efficacy of screening. However, as with DCBE, the high sensitivity of the test to detect advanced neoplasia and to identify and remove high-risk adenomatous polyps has been regarded as sufficient for colonoscopy to be included among recommended screening tests. In the large majority of screening procedures (over 90%), the cecum can be visualized; when colonoscopy is incomplete, the examination may be repeated, or a total colon examination may be achieved with DCBE, or CT colonography.[77] In a case-control study of 32,702 veterans, patients who had undergone colonoscopy with polypectomy were significantly less likely to develop colorectal cancer (odds ratio, 0.48; 95% CI, 0.35–0.66).[108] In the Telemark Polyp Study, 400 asymptomatic men and women aged 50 to 59 and 399 controls were randomly selected from the Telemark, Norway population registries. The experimental group was offered flexible sigmoidoscopy, and participants with detected polyps received colonoscopy with polypectomy and two subsequent rounds of colonoscopy. After 13 years of follow-up, the relative risk of colorectal cancer in the group receiving colonoscopy and polypectomy was 0.2 (95% CI, 0.03–0.95, $p = .02$).[74]

CT Colonography The use of computed tomography for colorectal cancer screening, that is, CT colonography or virtual colonoscopy, is an imaging procedure that uses computer programming to combine multiple helical CT scans in order to create two- or three-dimensional images of the interior of the colon. These images can be rotated for different views and even combined for a complete, "virtual" view of the colon that can be viewed in a manner that simulates the insertion and withdrawal of a colonoscope. The term "virtual colonoscopy" was coined in the mid-1990s by researchers at Wake Forest University who described this procedure as simulating conventional colonoscopy.[109] Evaluation studies of CT colonography have typically used study designs that first performed the CT exam, which was then followed by optical colonoscopy, with the examiner blinded to the results of the CT exam. Although early results with 2D imaging were disappointing, more recent back-to-back evaluations of CT colonography using faster scanners, updated 3D luminal displays, and oral stool tagging with digital subtraction have demonstrated sensitivities for large adenomas equivalent to colonoscopy.[110] Sensitivity is lower for lesions ≤ 6 mm, although these lesions are regarded as clinically insignificant and raise questions as to whether there is actual value in test sensitivity for lesions that pose no real threat in the near term. Although these results were produced in an expert setting, meta-analysis suggests a wider range of sensitivities consistent with both the introduction of a new technology and different, unstandardized approaches to technique.[111] A collaborative American College of Radiology Imaging Network/NCI trial comparing virtual colonoscopy with optical colonoscopy is presently under way.

Screening Recommendations Most organizations recommend that average-risk adults should be regularly screened for colorectal cancer beginning at age 50, although there are differences in recommended options for regular surveillance. As shown in Table 28-2 recommendations for average-risk individuals include five options for regular surveillance beginning at age 50, including annual FOBT (guaiac or immunochemical, flexible sigmoidoscopy every 5 years; annual FOBT and flexible sigmoidoscopy every five years after initial screening with both tests; total colon examination (TCE) with double-contrast barium enema every 5 years; or TCE with colonoscopy every 10 years. Neither stool DNA testing nor virtual colonoscopy is included in current guidelines. Annual DRE is no longer recommended because of low sensitivity, but DRE should be done prior to FSIG or colonoscopy. Although there is strong consensus about colorectal cancer screening among U.S. organizations that issue guidelines, the USPSTF does not specify an interval for testing.[76,77,80,112] Guidelines for higher-risk individuals are also shown in Table 28-3. Higher-risk individuals include those with a family history of adenomatous polyps or colorectal cancer, a family history of familial adenomatous polyposis (FAP), a family history of hereditary nonpolyposis colorectal cancer (HNPCC), or a personal history of inflammatory bowel disease.[76,77] In general, colorectal cancer screening guidelines for higher-risk individuals recommend earlier onset of surveillance and more thorough examinations of the colon.

CERVICAL CANCER

Disease Burden In 2005, an estimated 10,370 new cases of invasive cervical cancer will to be diagnosed among women in the United States, and 3,710 deaths from cervical cancer were expected.[19] The decline in cervical cancer mortality has been dramatic in U.S. women, declining more than 70% between 1930 and 1980. Similar declines in incidence have been observed as well. In the recent period, rates declined by 4.6% per year between 1975 and 1981, declined at a much smaller annual rate (–1.1%) between 1981 and 1997, and then have declined at a greater annual rate (–4.8%) between 1997 and 2002.[21] Age-adjusted incidence rates per 100,000 women are higher among African American women (10.3) compared with white women (6.8), as are age-adjusted mortality rates (5.0 vs 2.3), and the magnitude of these differences has been declining over time. Five-year survival is very good for women diagnosed with localized disease (92.2%), but declines considerably for disease diagnosed regionally (54.7%) and with distant metastasis (16.5%).[21]

The relatively small incidence rate compared with other cancers and the long-term downward trend in incidence and mortality is a measure of the success of the Papanicolaou test, developed by Dr. George Nicolas Papanicolaou in the 1920s (Figure 28-12), at detecting precursor lesions, that is, cervical intraepithelial neoplasia (CIN).[113] Rates of treatable precursor lesions are considerably higher. Although there is no system for surveillance of precursor lesions, a recent report from the Centers for Disease Control and Prevention's (CDC) National Breast and Cervical Cancer Early Detection Program (NBCCEDP) summarizing findings from a broad spectrum of program participants throughout the United States showed an overall abnormality rate of 3.8% and a ratio of CIN III/carcinoma in situ (CIS) to invasive disease of 9:1 and a ratio of CIN II or worse to invasive disease of 18.5:1.[114]

Screening and Diagnostic Methods It is generally accepted that screening for cancer of the cervix, specifically precancerous lesions, is effective in reducing both the incidence and mortality from cervical cancer. Cervical cancer is

Table 28-3 Guidelines for Screening and Surveillance for Early Detection of Colorectal Polyps and Cancer for Individuals at Greater Than Average Risk

Risk Category and Description	Recommendation	Age to Begin	Screening Interval and Recommendation
Moderate risk			
People with single, small (< 1 cm) adenomatous polyps	Colonoscopy	At the initial polyp diagnosis	TCE within 3 years after initial polyp removal; if normal, follow recommendations for average-risk individuals
People with large (≥ 1 cm) or multiple adenomatous polyps of any size	Colonoscopy	At time of initial polyp diagnosis	TCE within 3 years after initial polyp removal; if normal TCE every 5 years
Personal history of curative-intent resection of colorectal cancer	TCE	Within 1 year after resection	If normal, TCE in 3 years; If second TCE is normal, TCE in 5 years
Colorectal cancer or adenomatous polyps, in first-degree relative younger than age 60 or in 2 or more first-degree relatives of any ages	TCE	40 years, or 10 years before the youngest case in the family, whichever is earlier	Every 5 years
Colorectal cancer in other relatives (not first-degree)	Follow recommendations for age-risk individuals		
High risk			
Family history of FAP	Early surveillance with endoscopy, counseling to consider genetic testing, and referral for specialty care	Puberty	If genetic test is positive or polyposis is confirmed, consider colectomy; otherwise, continue endoscopy every 1–2 years
Family history of HNPCC	Colonoscopy and counseling to consider genetic testing	21 years	If untested, or if genetic test is positive, colonoscopy every 2 years until age 40; after age 40, colonoscopy every year
Inflammatory bowel disease	Colonoscopy with biopsies for dysplasia	8 years after the start of pancolitis; 12–15 years after the start of left-sided colitis	Colonoscopy every 1–2 years

FAP = familial adenomatous polyposis; HNPCC = hereditary nonpolyposis colorectal cancer; TCE = total colon examination.

[a]Digital rectal examination (DRE) should be done at the time of each sigmoidoscopy, colonoscopy, or DCBE.

[b]TCE includes either colonoscopy or DCBE. Flexible sigmoidoscopy should be added to DCBE in those instances when the rectosigmoid colon is not well visualized; DCBE should be added to the examination in those instances when the entire colon can not be visualized by colonoscopy.

[c]FOBT and flexible sigmoidoscopy should begin at age 50; repeat FOBT annually, and flexible sigmoidoscopy every 5 years.

Adapted from American College of Physicians.[88]

characterized by a long sojourn time, with potentially cancerous lesions progressing through a succession of identifiable stages prior to invasive disease. If precursor lesions are detected prior to the point of progression to invasive disease, a variety of treatment options are available and the disease is almost certainly curable, and the progression to invasive disease preventable. Age-specific incidence data previously available from NCI's Surveillance, Epidemiology, and End Results (SEER) program and from cross-sectional studies of small geographic areas or clinic populations are consistent with the following observations: (1) the prevalence of precursor dysplastic lesions is greater among younger women compared with older women; (2) a significant proportion of premalignant lesions will regress, especially in younger women; (3) carcinoma in situ (CIN) of the cervix peaks in the midthirties; and (4) the incidence of invasive disease peaks in the midforties, remaining relatively constant among white women and continuing to rise among African American women.[21,115,116]

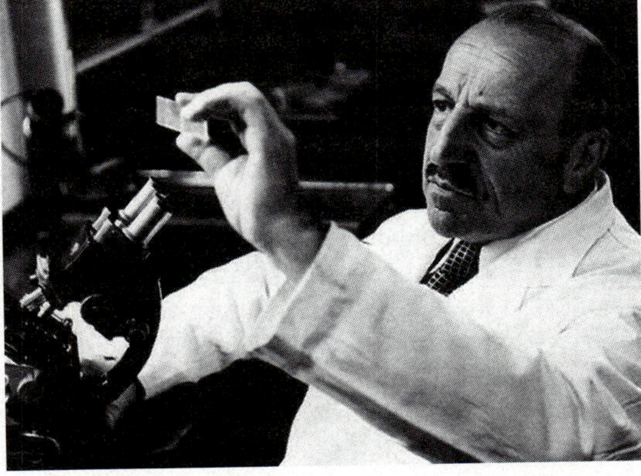

Figure 28-12 Dr. George Nicolas Papanicolaou (1883–1962) is credited with the development of the Pap test. (Reprinted with permission from the Telsa Memorial Society of New York.)

Although there has never been a randomized trial of the efficacy of screening for cancer of the cervix, it has been observed that cytologic screening was an accepted part of medical care among both women and providers before the randomized trial with a mortality end point had become the standard by which the efficacy of a screening test is evaluated.[2] Even so, the logic of cytologic screening has always measured up well against criteria applied to the value of a screening test. Screening with the Pap smear is comparatively inexpensive and is widely accepted by both the public and providers. Perhaps the most widely cited evidence for the contribution of cytologic screening to the reduction in cervical cancer mortality is the long-term decline in the death rate from cervical cancer in the United States coincident with the introduction of the Pap smear, although it has been noted that death rates had begun to decline prior to widespread use of the test, perhaps owing to other factors such as an increase in the hysterectomy rate and trends in the underlying epidemiology of disease.[117] However, there can be little argument that cytologic screening has primarily influenced the long-term trend. Scientific evidence for the efficacy of cervical cytology in reducing the incidence of invasive disease and mortality exists in nonexperimental studies, specifically, observational studies and case-control studies. The best examples of observational studies are the evaluations of cervical cancer mortality rates in five Nordic countries before and after the introduction of screening programs.[118–122] Comparing mortality rates before and after the introduction of cytologic screening between two time periods (1963 to 1967 and 1978 to 1982), mortality reductions between 8 and 73% were observed. Factors underlying this wide range of mortality reductions are also consistent with a screening effect. In Norway, where participation rates were lowest, mortality remained comparatively unchanged, whereas in Iceland, which organized an aggressive screening program that had high rates of participation, the mortality reduction (73%) was greatest among the five countries.[118,120,122] More recent investigations of population trends in the United Kingdom and the Republic of Ireland show similar associations with the organization and intensity of screening as was observed in the Nordic countries. Mortality in England, Wales, and Scotland has declined for over 30 years, with an accelerating rate since reorganization of the screening program in the 1980s, whereas in the Irish Republic, which has no screening program, mortality rates have been increasing at an average annual rate of 1.5% each year since 1978.[123] Numerous examples of case-control studies also show a benefit from cervical cancer screening, typically examining the screening histories of women diagnosed with invasive disease compared with matched controls.[124,125] Today, cervical cancer screening research focuses more on effectiveness and cost-effectiveness of various screening than on issues of efficacy.

The Pap test is the most widely used cancer-screening test in the world. At the most basic level, the Pap test involves the collection of exfoliating epithelial cells from the cervical squamocolumnar junction, or transformation zone. Both the ectocervix and endocervix should be sampled. Various collection tools (spatula, cotton swab, Cytobrush, Cervix brush, Cytopick, etc.) are available for specimen collection. Boon and colleagues evaluated various approaches to specimen collection and found that the combination of spatula and Cytobrush, or the Cytopick, had the best performance as measured by presence of endocervical cells. They also concluded that the spatula alone or the combination of spatula and cotton swab gave poor performance and were not recommended.[126] The two samples should be applied to one side of a glass slide and quickly fixed (usually with a spray fixative) to prevent air-drying. The slide is then examined under a microscope by a cytotechnologist.

Although the Pap test is simple to conduct, its accuracy is greatly dependent on achieving a high level of quality in specimen collection, slide preparation, and microscopic examination and interpretation. Even under the best of circumstances, the Pap smear has a significant error rate.[127] Sampling error is estimated to account for about two-thirds of false-negative tests whereas errors in interpretation account for the remaining third.[128] A technology assessment of cervical cytology by the Duke University Center for Clinical Health Policy Research conducted for the Agency for Health Care Policy and Research (AHCPR) concluded that conventional Pap smear screening had specificity of 98%, but sensitivity of only 51%.[128] Sensitivity is lower when the threshold of a positive test is higher, that is, in the case of a high-grade squamous intraepithelial lesion (HSIL) versus a low-grade squamous intraepithelial lesion (LSIL) or atypical cells of undetermined significance (ASCUS).

In an effort to improve the accuracy and cost-effectiveness of the Pap smear, several new screening technologies have evolved, with each taking a somewhat different approach to resolving some of the shortcomings—mainly sampling error and detection error—of the conventional Pap smear. Liquid-based cytology uses similar specimen collection techniques to the conventional Pap smear, but instead of placing the sample on a glass slide, the sample is suspended in a fixative solution, after which it is dispersed, filtered, and then distributed on a glass slide in a monolayer. Accuracy is increased because there are fewer artifacts (blood, mucus, etc.) and because cells are not overlapping (Figure 28-13). The test has been shown to have higher sensitivity, especially in populations with a lower prevalence of cytologic abnormalities, although, like the Pap smear sensitivity, still is dependent on collecting an adequate sample.[128–130] Computer aided diagnosis applies neural-network technology to identify false negatives among the pool of Pap smears interpreted as normal. A computerized algorithm is applied to identify slides that are likely to contain abnormal cells, suspicious areas are targeted, and a cytotechnologist then decides whether the slide should be further reviewed. Each of these technologies has greater sensitivity than the Pap smear, but each also is a more expensive screening test. A comparative review of these new technologies concluded that their application was more cost-effective when incorporated into protocols of less frequent screening, and that cost-effectiveness was higher in populations with higher disease prevalence.[131] With annual screening, they offer little added advantage to life expectancy over the conventional Pap smear.

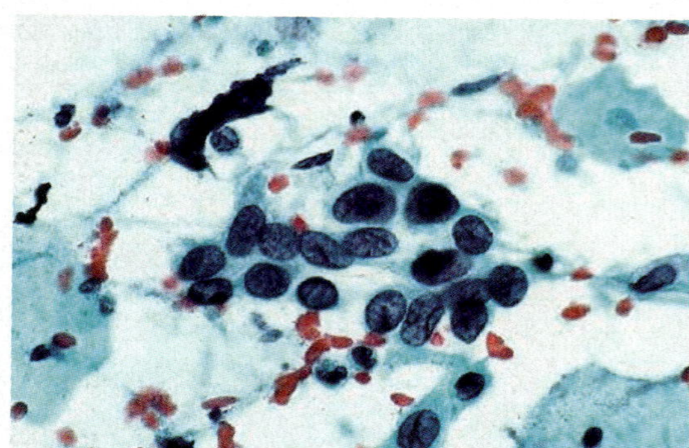

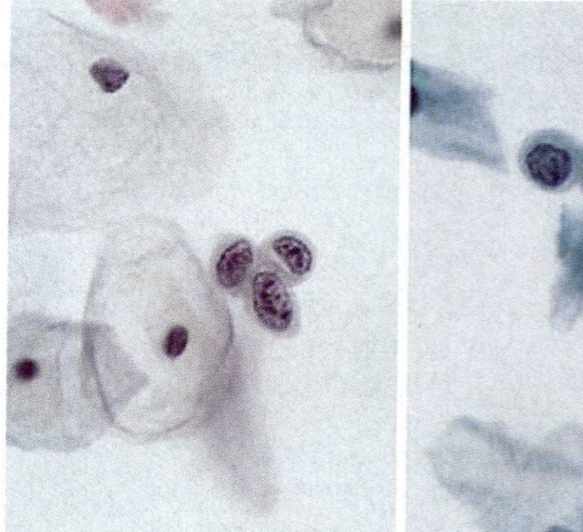

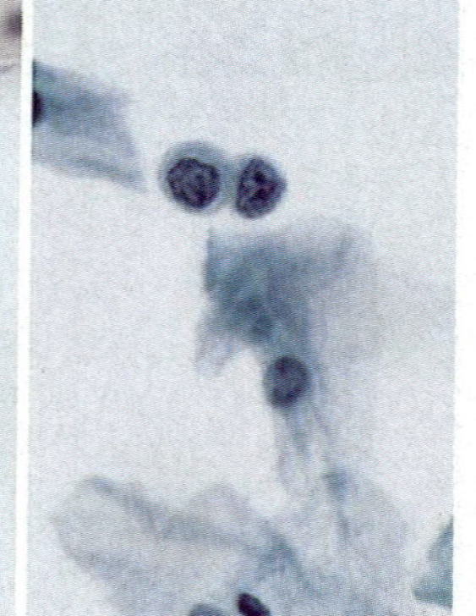

Figure 28-13 Examples of conventional cervical cytology (*left*) and liquid based cytology (*right*), interpreted as a high-grade squamous intraepithelial lesion (HSIL). (Source: U.S. Centers for Disease Control and Prevention.)

Because of the strong association between infection with particular subtypes of human papillomavirus (HPV) and cervical cancer, HPV testing is increasingly finding application for surveillance and risk stratification, specifically as a strategy for risk assignment in order to distinguish a high-risk group for more aggressive surveillance, primary screening, triaging women with low-grade Pap-smear abnormalities (atypical cells of undetermined significance [ASCUS], atypical glandular cells of undetermined significance [AGUS], or low-grade squamous intraepithelial lesion [LSIL]), or for follow-up of women with confirmed CIN.[132–135] Current testing for HPV DNA is done with the hybrid capture test, which is the only test that has been approved by the FDA for commercial use. However, the hybrid capture test determines only the presence of HPV and not the specific subtypes of HPV infection, which requires polymerase chain reaction (PCR) techniques.[136] The value and the potential for HPV testing rest on the strong evidence that infection with particular subtypes of HPV—in particular, HPV type 16 and 18—probably is a necessary, not just sufficient, etiologic factor in nearly all cervical neoplasia.[137] At this time, HPV testing does appear to have value for triaging women with ASCUS and AGUS, specifically with regard to greater cost-effectiveness related to the management of the mildly abnormal Pap smear, although formal recommendations will await the completion of ongoing studies. Still, there is growing evidence that HPV testing may represent a less resource-intense strategy for women at demonstrated lower risk, as well as a more sensitive surveillance strategy when combined with cytology for women at elevated risk.[138–140] On the other hand, HPV testing as a basis for defining a low-risk group that needs less surveillance, or a high-risk group that needs more intensive surveillance, is not so straightforward for several reasons. First, HPV infection may be active, latent, or transient; thus, the potential for misclassification at testing is high. Second (and even more problematic for a program of risk assessment with cross-population screening), exposure opportunities vary in individuals over time. Apart from the fact that a person may test negative because the infection is latent or the viral load low, they may also acquire an infection in the period after testing.[141] Third, since HPV infection is common in adults who have had more than one sexual partner, and since most individuals with HPV infection do not develop cervical cancer, public health education would face an enormous challenge to avoid stigma associated with testing positive for a sexually acquired infection. However, it is likely that the accumulation of additional evidence as well as a growing awareness in the public of the role of HPV in cervical cancer etiology will lead to the use of HPV information in testing and triaging, not only for screening and surveillance in specific groups, but also monitoring vaccine effectiveness.[142]

After years of evolution in cytologic classification systems for Pap smear results, the NCI sponsored a meeting in 1988 to develop a new system, widely adopted, and revised twice since that time, to both standardize cytologic nomenclature and address shortcomings in the various systems in use. These shortcomings included uneven cytologic/histologic correlation, low reliability, and confusion in the communication with referring physicians, by both the use of different systems and the inconsistent use of nomenclature within a system. This new system, known as the Bethesda System, was intended to provide "a uniform format for cytopathology reports that is intended to communicate clinically relevant information using standardized terminology."[143] The current Bethesda System is shown in Table 28-4.[144]

Screening Recommendations The ACS updated guidelines for cervical cancer screening in 2002 (see Table 28-2).[145] According to the

Table 28-4 Bethesda System 2001

Specimen Type	Indicate Conventional Smear (Pap Smear) vs Liquid-Based vs Other
Specimen Adequacy	
Satisfactory for evaluation	Describe presence or absence of endocervical/transformation zone component and any other quality indicators, eg, partially obscuring blood, inflammation, etc
Unsatisfactory for evaluation	Specimen rejected/not processed (specify reason), or Specimen processed and examined, but unsatisfactory for evaluation of epithelial abnormality because of (specify reason)
General Categorization (optional)	Negative for Intraepithelial Lesion or Malignancy Epithelial Cell Abnormality: See Interpretation/Result (specify "squamous" or "glandular" as appropriate) Other: See Interpretation/Result (eg, endometrial cells in a woman > 40 years of age)
Automated Review	If Case Examined by Automated Device, Specify Device and Result
Ancillary Testing	Provide a brief description of the test methods and report the result so that it is easily understood by the clinician.
Interpretation/Result	
Negative for Intraepithelial Lesion or Malignancy	When there is no cellular evidence of neoplasia, state this in the General Categorization above and/or in the Interpretation/Result section of the report, whether or not there are organisms or other non-neoplastic findings)
Organisms	*Trichomonas vaginalis* Fungal organisms morphologically consistent with *Candida* spp Shift in flora suggestive of bacterial vaginosis Bacteria morphologically consistent with *Actinomyces* spp. Cellular changes consistent with Herpes simplex virus
Other Non-neoplastic Findings (Optional to report; list not inclusive)	Reactive cellular changes associated with inflammation (includes typical repair) radiation intrauterine contraceptive device (IUD) Glandular cells status post hysterectomy Atrophy
Other	Endometrial cells (in a woman ≥ 40 years of age) (Specify if "negative for squamous intraepithelial lesion")
Epithelial Cell Abnormalities	
Squamous Cell	Atypical squamous cells of undetermined significance (ASC-US) cannot exclude HSIL (ASC-H) Low grade squamous intraepithelial lesion (LSIL) encompassing: HPV/mild dysplasia/CIN 1 High grade squamous intraepithelial lesion (HSIL) encompassing: moderate and severe dysplasia, CIS/CIN 2 and CIN 3 with features suspicious for invasion (if invasion is suspected) Squamous cell carcinoma
Glandular Cell	Atypical endocervical cells (NOS or specify in comments) endometrial cells (NOS or specify in comments) glandular cells (NOS or specify in comments) Atypical endocervical cells, favor neoplastic glandular cells, favor neoplastic Endocervical adenocarcinoma in situ Adenocarcinoma endocervical endometrial extrauterine not otherwise specified
Other Malignant Neoplasms	Specify
Educational Notes and Suggestions (Optional)	Suggestions should be concise and consistent with clinical follow-up guidelines published by professional organizations (references to relevant publications may be included).

Adapted from Solomon D, et al.[144]

ACS, cervical cancer screening should begin approximately 3 years after the onset of vaginal intercourse, but no later than 21 years of age. Cervical screening should be performed annually with conventional cervical cytology smears, or every 2 years using liquid-based cytology, until age 30, after which screening with the Pap test may continue every 2 to 3 years for those women who have had three consecutive, technically satisfactory normal/negative cytology results. Alternatively, for women aged 30 and over for whom less frequent screening is appropriate, cervical screening may be performed every 3 years using conventional or liquid-based cytology combined with a test for DNA from high-risk HPV types. Frequency of combined cytology and HPV DNA testing should not be more often than every 3 years. In 2004, a consensus conference of leading agencies further addressed the issue of HPV testing and endorsed adding HPV DNA testing to cervical cytology for women 30 years and older, including guidance for women who test positive for high-risk HPV subtypes, but are negative on cytology, to have the tests repeated in 6 to 12 months rather than being referred immediately for colposcopy, and if either test is subsequently positive, colposcopy should be performed.[140] Women who are age 70 and older with an intact cervix and who have had (1) three or more documented, consecutive, technically satisfactory normal/negative cervical cytology tests; and (2) no abnormal/positive cytology tests within the 10-year period prior to age 70, may elect to cease cervical cancer screening. Women over the age of 70 should discuss their need for cervical cancer screening with a health care professional and make an informed decision about continuing screening based on the potential benefits, harms, and limitations of screening. Recommendations for cervical cancer screening from the USPSTF are similar. ACS guidelines also address screening recommendations for women a history of in utero exposure to diethylstilbestrol (DES), women who are immunocompromised (including HIV+), and women with a history of subtotal or total hysterectomy.

Historically, screening guidelines in the United States have recommended more aggressive surveillance than in those in Europe, with the organizations in the United States endorsing earlier ages to begin testing, more frequent testing, and not specifying an age to stop screening. Although the new recommendations still endorse more aggressive screening than many European countries, they specify a more rational, cost-effective approach than earlier guidelines. Still, it is apparent that many U.S. clinicians are hesitant to embrace less frequent cervical cancer screening,[146] despite good evidence that overscreening is wasteful of resources and contributes to potential harms.[146–148]

PROSTATE CANCER

Disease Burden Adenocarcinoma of the prostate is the most common cancer (excluding skin cancer) diagnosed in American men and a significant public health problem. An estimated 232,090 new cases of prostate cancer will be diagnosed in the United States in 2005 and an estimated 30,350 men in the United States will die of this disease.[19] The incidence of prostate cancer is particularly high in African American men, who have roughly twice the incidence as white men.[21] African American men with newly diagnosed prostate cancer have been shown to have higher PSA values than white men, after adjustment for age at diagnosis and for grade and clinical stages of cancer.[149] Also, even within clinical stage categories at diagnosis, African American men have significantly greater cancer volumes. The explanation for these race-related differences is unclear.

Prostate cancer is sometimes observed to be a disease a man is more likely to die "with" than "because of," and competing causes of death are important, owing to the older average age at prostate cancer diagnosis. In fact, however, prostate cancer is the usual cause of death for men with advanced disease. It is exceeded only by lung cancer as a cause of cancer death, accounting for about 10% of all male cancer deaths.[19] Prognosis is good if the diagnosis is made when the cancer is still localized to the prostate; but nearly one-third of prostate cancers are diagnosed after the tumor has spread locally, and in 1 of 10 cases, the disease has distant metastases at diagnosis. The 5-year survival rate for men with advanced prostate cancer is only 34%.[21]

Screening and Diagnostic Methods The principal methods that have been evaluated as early prostate cancer detection tools are the digital rectal examination (DRE), the prostate-specific antigen (PSA) blood test, and transrectal ultrasonography (TRUS).

DRE Palpable asymmetry of the prostate gland and, particularly, hard nodular areas sometimes indicate presence of prostate cancer. Jacobsen and colleagues conducted a population-based case-control study on all men who died of prostate cancer in Olmsted County from 1976 to 1991.[150] They found case subjects were half as likely as control subjects to have had any DRE in the 10 years before diagnosis. The investigators concluded that if their findings could be replicated, screening DREs might prevent as many as 50 to 70% of the deaths due to prostate cancer. In a more recent case-control study, Weinmann and colleagues observed that DRE was associated with a statistically significant 35% reduced risk of death from prostate cancer in white men, and a nonsignificant 14% reduction in African American men.[151] Two other case-control studies observed a smaller, although nonsignificant, protective effect.[152,153] However, in both cases these studies were small, and in aggregate, these investigations are suggestive of a modest reduction in deaths from prostate cancer associated with DRE.

The principal limitations of DRE are that the majority of palpable cancers that are not early cancers and many clinically important cancers are located in regions of the gland that are inaccessible to digital palpation. Although it has poor sensitivity, the DRE often is recommended as one component of prostate cancer screening because it may detect cancers missed by other tests, it is a low-cost procedure, and it has value in evaluating other prostate abnormalities such as benign prostatic hyperplasia.[154]

PSA PSA became widely used for screening and diagnosis following its commercial introduction as a test for monitoring prostate cancer patients. This pattern of use resulted in a marked increase in prostate cancer incidence rates in the United States in the late 1980s. This trend peaked in 1992, and subsequently declined, revealing a classic pattern of rise and decline in incidence consistent with the detection of a sizable prevalence of occult disease that without screening would potentially have been detected in subsequent years. Over the remainder of the decade, the incidence rate rose to "catch up" with the earlier incidence trend.

The principal strengths of the PSA test are its sensitivity, reasonable cost, and high patient acceptance. The principal drawback of the test is its imperfect specificity, owing to the fact that common conditions such as benign prostatic hyperplasia and prostatitis can cause borderline or markedly abnormal test results. These false-positive results can lead to expensive further diagnostic evaluation and unwarranted patient anxiety. Conversely, the high sensitivity of the test may result in considerable overdiagnosis, with small indolent cancers that might require no treatment, or less aggressive cancers that would not become life threatening in an older male before death from other causes occurred, being gathered in the same net as the aggressive, potentially life-threatening cancers. Current diagnostic algorithms are imperfect for distinguishing among these prognostic groups with complete confidence. Although it is common to equate slow progression with overdiagnosis, a Swedish study with a 21-year follow-up of men with early-stage disease who were initially untreated showed a significant decrease in disease-free survival after 15 years, with prostate cancer mortality increasing from 15 per 1,000 person years in the first 15 years of follow-up to 44 per 1,000 person years after 15 years.[155] These findings provide further support for current guidelines that stress that expected longevity is an important consideration in decisions about both testing for early detection and therapy.

Another major concern about the utility of PSA is the lack of a dependable cutoff level. The PSA has been criticized for the lack of a good balance between sensitivity and specificity, and the fact that the conventional cutoff level (4 ng/mL) does not detect all prostate cancers. In fact, prostate cancer may be present even with very low levels of PSA. Recent results from the Prostate Cancer Prevention Trial showed that sensitivity measurably increased with successively lower PSA cutoff values and for higher grade disease, but that with each increment in sensitivity, specificity significantly declined.[156] These findings add to the evidence indicating that PSA levels lower than 4 ng/mL can not be assumed to be normal and that the patient and physician will need to consider a number of factors in order to decide about further evaluation.

Evidence supporting the effectiveness of PSA testing alone or in combination with DRE and TRUS is available from several sources. Early comparative studies showed that prostate cancer detection in asymptomatic men could be increased by PSA and related testing.[157,158] In addition, it was demonstrated that the stage distribution of screen-detected cancers was much more favorable than that which occurred in the general, unscreened population. The American Cancer Society National Prostate Cancer Detection Project showed that after 5 years of annual testing by PSA, DRE, and TRUS, 92% of cancers detected were localized to the prostate, compared with 66% in a contemporaneous national database covering men the same age.[159]

Population mortality trends may reflect on the effectiveness of prostate cancer screening. Etzioni and colleagues have argued that decreases in mortality reported within the first decade after the onset of widespread PSA testing are unlikely to be due to PSA testing, given the long natural history of prostate cancer.[160] However, a decline in prostate cancer mortality could be due to the increased interest in early detection of prostate cancer with DRE that began prior to the PSA era, as manifested by earlier stage at diagnosis and by increasing surgery rates for localized prostate cancer in the decade prior to the onset of widespread PSA testing. Another possible explanation for the decline in prostate cancer mortality is that there has been a shift in the tendency to classify prostate cancer as the underlying cause of death.[161] Alternatively, Tarone and colleagues have argued that stage-specific survival rates suggest that the rapid decrease in mortality preceded a large increase in incidence of high-grade lesions diagnosed before metastasis.[162] Thus, rather than viewing the mortality trend in the context of the estimated average lead time gained, it is reasonable to view the reduction in the incidence rate of advanced disease as predictive of a subsequent reduction in prostate cancer mortality rates.[162]

Results also are available from a natural experiment comparing prostate cancer mortality trends in the Federal State of Tyrol, Austria, where PSA testing had been made freely available, with the rest of the country, which did not have a screening program. After the introduction of the program, a significant shift toward a more favorable stage at diagnosis was observed in Tyrol compared with the rest of Austria, followed by a much greater and statistically significant decline in the prostate cancer mortality rate.[163] More recent updates of the Tyrol experience show continued downstaging of disease and continued reduction in expected mortality.[164]

Two large randomized trials of prostate cancer screening are also underway. The European Randomized Study of Screening for Prostate Cancer (ERSPC) is being conducted in seven European countries, and the U.S. National Cancer Institute (NCI) Prostate, Lung, Colorectal, and Ovarian Cancer Trial (PLCO) is studying multimodality screening in men and women at 10 locations in the United States.[165,166] The ERSPC and PLCO trials have entered into collaboration with the common goal of "sound and efficient evaluation of the screening programs."[167] The collaboration also provides an opportunity to increase statistical power and carry out subgroup analysis that might not be possible in a smaller study. Study investigators estimate that definitive results should be available from 2005 to 2008.[167]

One of the questions related to prostate cancer screening is whether treatment is necessary and effective in early prostate cancer. In a study in Sweden, symptomatic men with localized prostate cancer (UICC stage T1b, T1c, or T2) were randomized to receive either radical prostatectomy or watchful waiting.[168] After an average 6.2 years of follow-up, there was a statistically significant difference in the rate of distant metastases (relative hazard 0.63, 95% CI, 0.41–0.96) and disease-specific mortality (relative hazard 0.50, 95% CI, 0.27–0.91) in the group randomized to radical treatment compared with the group randomized to watchful waiting. In an accompanying editorial, Walsh[169] applauded the results and claimed that they were the first concrete evidence to answer Whitmore's often cited and fundamental question, "Is cure necessary in those in whom it may be possible, and is cure possible in those in whom it is necessary?"[170] However, Walsh also noted that although these results answered a fundamental question about the whether or not treatment reduced prostate cancer mortality, men still will be well served by careful consideration of treatment options based on tumor characteristics and expected longevity.[169]

Transrectal Ultrasonography (TRUS) TRUS uses a small rectal probe placed against the prostate gland to image the entire gland. Areas of the gland with differing morphology often yield different images. Unfortunately, cancer has no unique and reliably assessed ultrasonographic signature, and TRUS has been shown to have poor specificity when employed as the sole screening modality. It does, however, play a very important role in the early detection process. It is a means of accurately measuring gland dimensions and calculating total gland volume. This information is useful in evaluating borderline elevations in PSA using PSA density (PSAD). More importantly, TRUS is the means for directing needle biopsies of the prostate gland for diagnostic purposes.

Screening Recommendations Over the years there has been considerable confusion about general recommendations related to prostate cancer screening in men at average and higher risk. This confusion has arisen because of different wording in guidelines that distinguish between recommendations for population-based screening versus individualized decisions about testing for early detection. Further, in some cases advice has been vague with respect to the physician's responsibility to either initiate conversations about testing or simply be prepared to discuss testing if the patient inquires about whether or not testing is appropriate. Finally, it also is the case that a considerable volume of testing may take place in response to generalized symptoms related to voiding, etc., which increase in prevalence with increasing age. Although inferential evidence suggests a benefit from testing for early detection, the general state of evidence is insufficient to recommend for or against screening for prostate cancer with PSA and DRE, or to determine if benefits outweigh harms.[171] Thus, the American Cancer Society, The American Academy of Family Physicians, the American College of Physicians-American Society of Internal Medicine, the American Medical Association, and the American Urologic Association recommend that for men age 50 and older and men at higher risk of prostate cancer, clinicians (1) discuss with patients the potential benefits and possible harms of PSA screening, (2) consider patient preferences, and (3) individualize the decision to screen (see Table 28-2).[76,172–174]

Both the ACS and the American Urologic Association provide some additional guidance to help clinicians and men make informed decisions. Men at high risk, including men of African descent (specifically, sub-Saharan African descent) and men with a first-degree relative diagnosed at a younger age should begin testing at age 45. Men at even higher risk of prostate cancer owing to multiple first-degree relatives diagnosed with prostate cancer at an early age could begin testing at age 40.[175] Persons with a strong family history of prostate cancer have increased risk of death from the disease, and screening individuals with inheritable risk may yield greater benefit compared with the general population.[176,177] Discovery of genetic markers of prostate cancer risk may further refine the targeting of populations that may benefit most from screening interventions.[178] When genetic tests become available, it will be important to address which individuals are most suited for testing and how they are to be identified. In each instance, subsequent testing would depend on initial PSA results. In addition, these recommendations do not bypass the general recommendation related to informing patients about the potential benefits and possible harms of PSA screening as well as considering patient preferences.

Although no upper age limit has been established over which PSA testing is not recommended, there is some evidence that men with less than a 10-year life expectancy are unlikely to gain years of life from early detection, because of the long natural history of untreated localized prostate cancer and competing causes of death.[155,179] Thus, a significant proportion of men over the age of 70 are reaching an age when further PSA testing may not be beneficial in terms of life extension and treatment may result in a net decrease in the quality of life. Algorithms for estimating life expectancy and the likelihood of benefiting from preventive care have been proposed by Walter and Covinsky.[180] The implications from their estimates of projected longevity by age in the context of comorbidity indicate that chronological age is a poor stand alone measure for making determinations about whether or not an individual may benefit from cancer screening.

Despite the fact that we do not yet know the exact cause or causes for the observed differences in prostate cancer in African American men, special efforts at screening are justified to lessen the disparity. Starting testing at younger ages in African American men may be reasonable in an attempt to catch tumors earlier when they are smaller. Different investigators have proposed age- and race-adjusted PSA values for cancer detection, with lower PSA cutoff levels for African American men.[181,182] There are limited data, however, on the effectiveness of these targeting strategies.

LUNG CANCER

Disease Burden Lung cancer is the second most common cancer and the leading cause of death from cancer among both men and women in the United States. In 2005, 172,570 new cases of lung cancer and 163,510 deaths were predicted.[19] Lung cancer is relatively uncommon before age 50, with rates increasing rapidly after age 50. Overall, lung cancer has a very poor prognosis. The most recent 5-year survival statistics show only 15% of cases surviving 5 years, with nearly 65% of patients succumbing within a year of diagnosis.[21] Five-year survival is measurably better (49%) when the disease is diagnosed while still localized, but only 16% of cases are diagnosed without regional disease or distant metastases.[21] The majority of lung cancers develop in individuals with a history of cigarette smoking. Risk of lung cancer declines with cessation at any age compared with individuals who continue smoking, but the decline is greater among those who cease smoking at an early age.[183]

Screening and Diagnostic Methods The available technologies for detecting occult lung cancer include imaging modalities and cytologic and molecular evaluations of lung sputum. Chest x-ray has some, although likely limited, potential as a screening tool, especially in comparison with new imaging technologies that achieve higher resolution (Figure 28-14). With conventional chest radiography, two images are normally taken: a posterior-anterior view and a lateral view. The sensitivity of

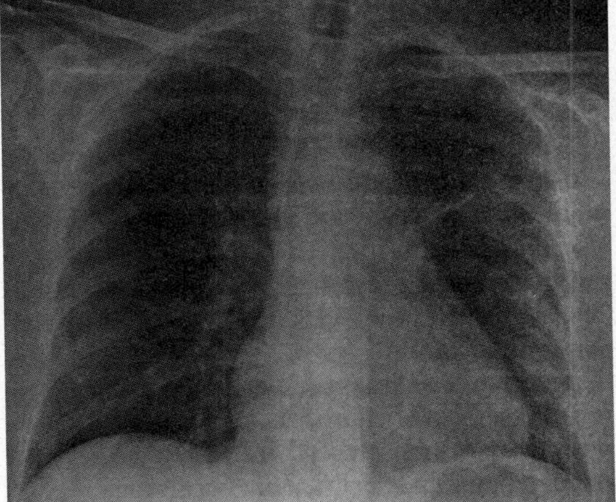

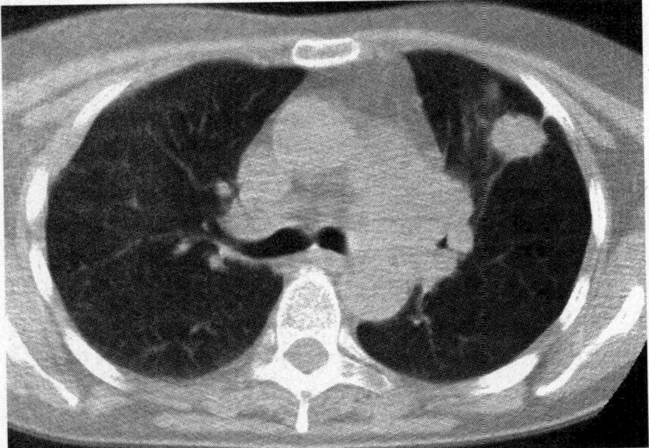

Figure 28-14 **(L)** Chest radiograph shows a 2 cm left upper lobe cancer. This is the median size of tumors detected in the Mayo Lung Project screening study that was initiated in 1971. **(R)** CT scan of the same left upper lobe cancer. (Images courtesy of David Yankelevitz, M.D., Department of Radiology, New York-Presbyterian Hospital-Weill Cornell Medical Center, New York, NY.)

chest radiographs is dependent on the size and location of the lesion, the quality assurance factors related to image quality, and the skill of the interpreting physician.[184] Failure to detect lesions at a favorable, or even larger, size can occur because the lesions can be obscured by the mediastinum and other aspects of chest structure, or as commonly occurs, because of errors in perception on the part of the interpreter.[185] To date, trials of lung cancer screening with chest radiography have not shown sufficient evidence to conclude that chest radiography is an effective screening tool,[186] although because of study limitations its potential still is being evaluated in a large U.S. trial and compared with spiral CT in another more recently initiated prospective randomized trial.[187,188]

Low-dose computed tomography (CT)—that is, spiral or helical CT—produces multiple images of the lung conventionally in 5 mm multiplanar slices that can produce a three-dimensional display of the lung (Figure 28-15).[189] Low-dose CT is more sensitive than chest radiography in the detection of small pulmonary nodules, is commonly used in diagnostic studies, and is regarded as having the greatest potential for early detection of lung malignancies.[190,191] Owing to the higher resolution and the ability to image nodules under 1 cm in size, a high proportion of individuals undergoing screening will require short-term follow-up, which has led to concerted efforts to develop protocols for triaging those cases with clear malignant potential for further evaluation.[192] Sputum cytology was believed to have potential for the early detection of lung cancer, but it showed little added advantage over chest radiography in the NCI cooperative trials and was not associated with any reduction in deaths from lung cancer. However, further attempts to identify molecular markers from sputum associated with elevated risk or malignancy, as well as the application of autofluorescence bronchoscopy and positron emission tomography (PET) are potentially valuable new directions in the early detection of lung cancer.[193]

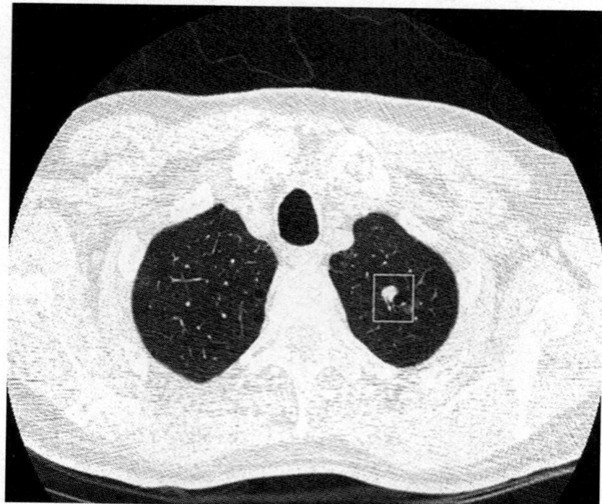

Figure 28-15 CT screen detected 7 mm left upper lobe cancer. This is the median size for cancers detected with CT screening. (Images courtesy of David Yankelevitz, M.D., Department of Radiology, New York-Presbyterian Hospital-Weill Cornell Medical Center, New York, NY.)

In the 1970s and 1980s, four prospective trials of lung cancer screening were carried out using combinations of chest radiography and sputum cytology.[194–198] None of these studies showed a significant reduction in lung cancer mortality associated in the experimental groups, although some results were suggestive of a survival benefit.[199,200] Although results of prospective trials were disappointing in the presence of such significant disease burden, these trials also were methodologically limited at inception in their ability to demonstrate a benefit from screening. Although none of the studies showed fewer deaths in the experimental group compared with the control group, none of the studies compared disease outcome in a group offered screening with a group not invited to screening. In each of the trials, there was an element of early detection intervention in the control group. Further, chest radiography alone and in combination with sputum cytology improved the stage of diagnosis and was associated with more favorable survival, which has also been observed in case-finding series. In spite of limitations in study design and paradoxical findings in RCTs and case-finding series, for many years it has been widely accepted that lung cancer screening is not effective, whereas, recent reevaluation of the trial data has led to the conclusion that there is insufficient evidence to recommend for or against lung cancer screening.[201,202]

Newer technology for the early detection of lung cancer appears to be more promising than conventional chest radiography. The Early Lung Cancer Action Project (ELCAP) is designed to evaluate screening with low-radiation-dose CT.[203] In a report of the baseline experience with 1,000 volunteers aged 60 and over with a smoking history of at least 10 pack-years (eg, a pack year = one pack per day for a year) and who would be acceptable candidates for thoracic surgery, low-dose CT significantly outperformed conventional chest radiography in the detection of small pulmonary nodules. Low-dose CT identified 233 participants with noncalcified nodules and 27 malignancies, of which 26 were resectable and 23 were stage 1 disease. In contrast, conventional chest radiography identified 68 noncalcified nodules, of which 7 were malignant and 4 were stage 1. Work-up of positive CT results was based on the size of the nodule and change observed on repeat screening. Based on the average tumor size in the ELCAP study, the authors project a 5-year survival of 80% for cases diagnosed using low-dose CT.[203] Based on growing evidence that spiral CT may truly provide for a successful early detection strategy, the NCI launched the National Lung Screening Trial (NLST) in September 2002.[188,204] The trial has enrolled 50,000 current and former smokers aged 55 to 74 who were randomized to an experimental group who will be invited to receive annual spiral CT, or a control group that will be invited to receive annual chest radiography. Study participants are scheduled to undergo three rounds of annual screening.[188] A number of trials also are underway in Europe.[205]

Screening Recommendations At this time, no organization recommends routine screening for lung cancer among the general adult population or among individuals who are at higher risk because of tobacco or occupational exposures.[76,201] The ACS recently revised its narrative related to testing for early lung cancer detection. However, today a growing number of institutions and facilities are promoting CT screening to asymptomatic individuals at risk of lung cancer, and some have argued that the current evidence is sufficient to promote screening to individuals at significant risk of lung cancer.[206] With greater interest in spiral CT testing among health care providers and individuals at higher risk, the ACS determined that updated guidance about early lung cancer detection was appropriate. Further, given the high rate of positive results that occur with CT screening for lung cancer and the complexity of the algorithm for working up small nodules,[207] there is reason to be concerned about broad dissemination of lung screening outside of experienced, multispecialty settings and prior to validation of this new technology.[76] The ACS recommends that, to the extent possible, individuals at risk of lung cancer owing to current or prior smoking history, history of significant exposure to second-hand smoke, or occupational history be aware of their continuing lung cancer risk. Those who seek testing for early lung cancer detection should be informed about what is currently known about the benefits, limitations, and risks associated with conventional and emerging early detection technologies, as well as the associated diagnostic procedures and treatment. Given the complexity of diagnostic and follow-up algorithms associated with early lung cancer testing, the ACS discourages testing in a setting that is not linked to multidisciplinary specialty groups for diagnosis and follow-up. Individuals who choose to undergo testing should have access to testing and follow-up that meets state-of-the-art standards, with informed decision making at every step of an ongoing process. Individuals interested in early detection also should be encouraged to participate in trials. The route to testing should be through an individual's primary care physician. The referring physician can assist patients to understand their risks and reach informed decisions about testing and provide support if early detection tests are positive. If an individual seeks testing and does not have a referral from a primary care provider, the radiologist who provides testing is obliged to provide information about benefits, risks and limitations of testing as described above, and must become the individual's physician of record until proper alternative care arrangements can be made. Individuals who are current smokers also should be informed that the more immediate preventive health priority is the elimination of tobacco use altogether, since smoking cessation offers the surest route at this time to reducing the risk of premature mortality from lung cancer.[183]

TESTICULAR CANCER

Disease Burden An estimated 8,010 new cases of testicular cancer will be diagnosed and 390 men will die of the disease in the United

States in 2005.[19] Testicular cancer accounts for approximately 1% of all cancers in men and is four times more common among white men than African American men. The majority of testicular cancers are diagnosed at a localized stage. Recent advances in the treatment of testicular cancer have made it possible to cure most cases of the disease even when it is diagnosed at an advanced stage. As a result, testicular cancer mortality in the United States has fallen 60% in recent years without much change in the distribution of disease stage at diagnosis.[21]

Screening and Diagnostic Methods Testicular cancer is generally detected through patient self-detection and physician palpation. There are no tests available to detect testicular cancer at an asymptomatic stage. Suspicious masses may be further evaluated through ultrasonography and biopsy.

There have been no randomized trials of the efficacy of testicular examination, either by a physician or by individuals. However, detecting testicular cancer at an early stage has advantages in that survival is somewhat better, but the greater advantage would be a reduction in the likelihood of undergoing toxic treatment or major surgery. Still, no organization recommends either routine testicular self-exam or examination of the testicles for lumps or nodules or any change in the size, shape, or consistency of the testes.[208] What is likely to offer greater advantage is health education to promote the seeking of medical care promptly, since patient delay after becoming aware of a testicular abnormality has been associated with poorer survival.[209] Khadra and Oakeshott investigated the degree to which a sample of men aged 18 to 50 in London were aware of testicular cancer and practiced testicular self-examination (TSE).[210] Although approximately 90% of men reported that they had heard of testicular cancer, only 1 in 4 knew the age range most commonly affected, and only about 22% of respondents reported practicing monthly TSE. Similar findings have been reported by Ward and colleagues.[211]

The issue of regular TSE by asymptomatic men is somewhat controversial. Self-palpation of the testes is simple and low cost, but has low specificity and predictive value, and performance of periodic self-examination is infrequent even by men educated about the technique.[212,213] Since self-examinations or clinical examinations result in additional encounters with physicians to have suspicious findings evaluated, of which nearly all will be determined to not be cancer, false alarms do burden the health care system and can be costly. Geczi and colleagues recently evaluated the impact of a 3-year program of public education about testicular cancer, TSE, and the importance of responding promptly to symptoms.[214] Based on the low yield of cancers detected and the high false positive rate, the investigators concluded that the evidence did not justify screening programs for young men, and instead, efforts should focus on increased awareness for the population at risk and health care professionals that typically see men in the commonly affected age group.

Screening Recommendations No organization recommends routine screening for testicular cancer in average-risk men. The American Academy of Family Physicians recommends palpation of the testicles for men aged 13 to 39 who fall into a higher-risk group because of a history of cryptorchidism, orchiopexy, or testicular atrophy.[215] The USPSTF recommends against routine screening for testicular cancer in asymptomatic adolescent and adult males.[208]

ENDOMETRIAL CANCER

Disease Burden Cancer of the endometrium is the most common cancer of the female reproductive organs in the United States. In 2005, 40,880 new cases of endometrial cancer will be diagnosed in the United States, and 7,310 women will die from the disease.[19] Prognosis is very much associated with stage at diagnosis. From 1992 to 1998, the 5-year relative survival rate for localized disease among United States white women was 96%, 63% for regional disease, and 26% for distant disease.[21] African American women have poorer survival at each stage of disease and are more likely to be diagnosed with late-stage endometrial cancer.[21]

Screening and Diagnostic Methods Endometrial cancer may be detected through a variety of means; however, the efficacy of screening for endometrial cancer has never been evaluated in a large prospective randomized trial. The Pap test may fortuitously identify endometrial abnormalities, but it is too insensitive to be used as a screening technique for detection of endometrial cancer.[216] Today, the endometrial biopsy is the most common technique used to obtain endometrial tissue, and evaluation of endometrial histology has been the gold standard of determining the status of the endometrium.[217] More recently, interest in screening for endometrial cancer with endometrial biopsy and transvaginal ultrasonography (TVU) has been stimulated because of increased risk of endometrial cancer in women at elevated risk of breast cancer who are taking tamoxifen for chemoprevention.[218] However, two recent studies of screening asymptomatic women for endometrial cancer with endometrial biopsy and transvaginal ultrasound reported disappointing results,[219,220] and each report harms associated with diagnostic assessments, including unnecessary biopsies and in some cases uterine perforations. Recently, the ACS updated screening recommendations for endometrial cancer and concluded that a risk-based approach was reasonable only for women at high risk of endometrial cancer.[76] The population defined as at high risk of endometrial cancer includes women known to carry HNPCC-associated mutations, women who appear to have a substantial likelihood of being a mutation carrier based on the presence of known mutation carriers in the family, and women from families with an autosomal dominant predisposition to colon cancer in the absence of genetic testing results.[221]

Screening Recommendations At the time of menopause, all women should be informed about the risks and symptoms of endometrial cancer and strongly encouraged to report any unexpected bleeding or spotting to their physician. However, there is no evidence to support screening asymptomatic women, and some evidence against screening.[76] Women with or at risk of HNPCC should be offered endometrial screening annually beginning at age 35. Owing to the absence of strong scientific evidence supporting the value of this recommendation, informed decision making following a discussion of options, including benefits, risks, and limitations of testing, is appropriate.[76]

OVARIAN CANCER

Disease Burden Ovarian cancer is the fifth most common cancer and the fifth leading cause of cancer death among women in the United States. An estimated 22,220 new cases of ovarian cancer were predicted to be diagnosed in 2005, and about 16,210 deaths are expected.[19] Ovarian cancer has the highest mortality rate of all gynecologic cancers and it accounts for 6% of all cancer deaths in women. About 45% of all ovarian cancer patients survive 5 years after diagnosis, but prognosis for survival is largely dependent on the extent of disease at diagnosis. Women diagnosed with local disease experience a 94% 5-year survival rate and women with distant disease have only a 29% 5-year survival. Unfortunately, only 19% of women present with localized disease at diagnosis.[21]

Screening and Diagnostic Methods Potential screening tests for ovarian cancer include vaginal ultrasound, CA-125 antigen as a tumor marker, and bioinformatic analysis of proteomic patterns. The sensitivity and specificity of pelvic examination for the detection of ovarian cancer are imprecisely defined but certainly poor, and thus cannot be regarded as a screening method.

Ultrasonography Abdominal ultrasonography has been used in ovarian cancer screening with poor results, owing to low specificity.[222] Transvaginal ultrasonography, however, is capable of detecting small ovarian masses and may distinguish some benign masses from some malignant adnexal masses. Even this more proximal examination, however, still only poorly predicts which masses are cancers and which are due to benign diseases of the ovary. Color Doppler ultrasonography is a technique that may further improve the specificity of the transvaginal ultrasonography, but current data are insufficient to suggest that this or any other imaging modality is useful as a screening tool in average-risk asymptomatic women. Nevertheless, with these limitations in mind, transvaginal ultrasonography may be appropriate for women with a high risk of ovarian cancer, as noted above.

CA-125 The most extensively studied ovarian cancer serum marker is CA-125. CA-125 is a tumor-associated antigen, and its main use is for surveillance in women who have already had surgery to remove an epithelial ovarian cancer.[223]

This marker manifests an increased level in many women with ovarian cancer, but noncancerous diseases of the ovaries can also increase the blood levels of CA-125.[224] Additionally, only half of early ovarian cancers produce enough CA-125 to cause a positive test. It is clearly a powerful serum marker, although the exact algorithm for its use is still in evolution. Although CA-125 arguably is not accurate enough for use in the general population, as with transvaginal ultrasonography, it has been recommended for women at high risk of disease.[225]

Proteomic Patterns Investigators have applied intensive pattern recognition algorithms to identify a key subset of peptides that discriminates ovarian cancer cases from control subjects. After this algorithm was developed in "training" data, it was applied to the analysis of serum samples from 116 patients whose ovarian cancer status was unknown to the investigators. They correctly identified all 50 patients with ovary cancer including 18 with localized disease yielding a sensitivity of 100%. Specificity was 95%, having correctly classified 63 of 66 noncancer subjects. Although encouraging, the suitability of this approach for general screening of women at risk has not yet been studied, and, as is often the case, results achieved in select clinical series have yet to be duplicated in asymptomatic women.[226] In fact, a move to market a commercial test in 2003 was delayed by the FDA because of concerns about reliability and reproducibility, and as of 2005, the expectation that there soon would be screening for ovarian cancer based on proteomic patterns is yet unrealized.[227,228]

Much of the evidence concerning the effectiveness of ovarian cancer screening has come from nonrandomized cohort studies. In one study, five cancers were diagnosed among over 5,000 self-referred asymptomatic women who underwent periodic screening by abdominal ultrasonography.[229] Transvaginal ultrasonography was used in a study of 3,220 asymptomatic postmenopausal women, and this yielded only two early ovarian cancers.[230] A case-control study of CA-125 using stored sera reported a specificity of 100% for the most commonly used cutoff level, but sensitivity was only 57%.[231] Einhorn and colleagues studied CA-125 in a single screening of 5,550 women.[232] Only six cancers were detected, two of which were advanced at diagnosis. Jabobs and colleagues studied CA-125 and transabdominal ultrasonography in 22,000 women.[233] Three hundred forty-five women had elevated CA-125. Of 19 cancers detected, 11 were associated with elevated CA-125, indicating a sensitivity of 57%. Trials are currently under way to test an algorithm that measures CA-125 velocity to predict risk of ovarian cancer.[234]

Screening Recommendations Although ovarian cancer clearly meets disease burden criteria in terms of suitability as a target for screening interventions, there are no screening interventions with sufficient sensitivity and specificity for use in the general population at risk of ovarian cancer. Neither the ACS nor the USPSTF recommend ovarian cancer screening in average-risk women, and, in fact, the USPSTF specifically recommends against screening for ovarian cancer in average-risk women.[235] In 1994, a National Institutes of Health Consensus Panel concluded that all women should have a comprehensive family history taken, and that women with two or more first-degree relatives should be offered counseling about their ovarian cancer risk by a gynecologic oncologist (or other specialist qualified to evaluate family history and discuss hereditary cancer risks), since these women have a 3% chance of being positive for an ovarian cancer hereditary syndrome. Women with a known hereditary ovarian cancer syndrome, including breast-ovarian cancer syndrome, site-specific ovarian cancer syndrome, and HNPCC, should receive annual rectovaginal pelvic examinations, CA-125 determinations, and transvaginal ultrasonography until childbearing is completed or at least until age 35, at which time prophylactic bilateral oophorectomy is recommended.[225] Although women with these hereditary syndromes are estimated to represent only 0.05% of the female population, they have a 40% estimated lifetime risk of ovarian cancer.

MELANOMA AND NONMELANOMA SKIN CANCER

Disease Burden Melanoma and nonmelanoma skin cancers together are the most common cancers, accounting for nearly half of all malignancies. More than one million cases of nonmelanoma skin cancer are diagnosed each year, and in 2005 it is estimated that 59,580 melanoma cases will be diagnosed.[19] Melanoma accounts for only about 4% of the skin cancer cases, but causes the majority of skin cancer deaths. In 2005 it is estimated that there will be 2,820 deaths from nonmelanoma skin cancer and 7,700 deaths from melanoma skin cancer in the United States.[19] Five-year survival is very good when melanoma is diagnosed while still localized (98.3%), and poor (16%) when distant metastases are present.[21]

Screening and Diagnostic Methods The principal aim of skin examinations is early identification of melanoma because of the greater life-threatening potential of this disease. Identification of nonmelanoma skin cancer and precursor lesions is an additional potential benefit that may be achieved by total skin examination. Skin cancer screening involves a 2- to 3-minute visual inspection of the patient's entire body, including the scalp, hands, and feet. It also may involve questions to the patient regarding sun exposure, sun protection, and family history. A total examination of the skin is preferable to examining only the sunlight-exposed areas of the body because skin cancers often occur at anatomic sites that are not directly exposed to sources of risk. One study reported sensitivity of 93.3%, specificity of 97.8%, positive predictive value of 54%, and negative predictive value of 99.8% when dermatologists did the screening.[236]

There is insufficient evidence to establish whether a decrease in mortality occurs with routine examination of the skin.[237] No randomized clinical trial has evaluated the effectiveness of periodic screening on reducing melanoma mortality, although a large trial in Queensland, Australia, has completed the pilot phase and is presently underway.[238] Evidence relevant to skin cancer screening recommendations is based primarily on results from community-wide screenings, case-control studies, and observational studies. Studies of high-risk populations report that patients routinely screened by dermatologists have mean tumor thicknesses of detected malignant melanoma that are thinner than that of historical or population-based controls.[239] The American Academy of Dermatology program of skin cancer screening has examined over 600,000 people of various risk categories since 1985. In addition to the detection of over 35,000 nonmelanoma skin cancers, melanomas diagnosed by screening were more likely than historical controls to have lesions smaller than 1.5 mm.[240] The effectiveness of skin cancer screening may be increased if targeted to high-risk persons such as white patients older than age 20 with atypical mole syndrome or congenital melanocytic nevi, patients with specific phenotypic traits, or patients with a history of nonmelanoma skin cancer.[241]

Screening Recommendations The ACS recommends skin examination during the occasion of a periodic preventive health examination.[242] The American College of Preventive Medicine recommends periodic total cutaneous examinations for targeted populations at high risk of malignant melanoma.[243] High-risk groups include those with the following traits or conditions: white race, fair complexion, presence of pigmented lesions (dysplastic or atypical nevus), several large nondysplastic nevi, many small nevi, moderate freckling, or familial dysplastic nevus syndrome.[244,245] Although recommending alertness to skin abnormalities, particularly in high-risk individuals, the USPSTF concluded that the evidence was insufficient to recommend for or against routine screening for skin cancer using a total-body skin examination for the early detection of cutaneous melanoma, basal cell cancer, or squamous cell skin cancer.[246]

ORAL CANCER

Disease Burden An estimated 29,370 new cases of oral cancer were expected to be diagnosed in the United States in 2005, and 7,320 deaths are expected.[19] The disease is more common in men compared with women, and it occurs more frequently in African Americans compared with whites. Incidence increases steadily with age until about age 65, when the rate levels off. Oral cancers diagnosed while still localized have 82% 5-year survival, but only approximately one-third of oral cancers are diagnosed at a localized stage.[21]

Screening and Diagnostic Methods Oral cancer occurs in a region of the body that is generally accessible to physical examination by the patient, the dentist, and the physician. Screening can be made more efficient by inspecting the high-risk sites where 90% of all squamous cell cancers arise: the floor of the mouth, the ventrolateral aspect of the tongue, and the soft-palate complex.[247] Leukoplakia and erythroplastic lesions are the earliest and most serious signs of squamous cell carcinoma. An inspection of the oral cavity should be part of every physical examination in a dentist or physician's office.[248] Symptoms include sores on the lip or the mouth, oral bleeding, persistent white or red patches in the mouth or on the gums, oral swelling and/or pain, sore throat, and difficulty swallowing. There is now significant evidence that visual inspection for oral premalignancies significantly reduces mortality from oral cancer in a high-risk population.[249]

Screening Recommendations At this time, no organization recommends routine screening for oral cancer, although the ACS recommends that on the occasion of a routine physical examination the oral cavity should be examined.[242] Insofar as oral cancer is easily detected and often curable in its early stages, recent evidence demonstrating the efficacy of screening for oral cancer will likely lead to renewed efforts to identify cost-effective strategies to identify an appropriate population for routine surveillance.

CONCLUSION

In the near term, the greatest potential for reducing deaths from cancer is through early detection. The adoption of healthier lifestyles, as well as risk identification and modification via genomics and proteomics, is believed to offer even greater potential in the long run, but at this time that potential is uncertain. However, it also is the case that the fullest benefit of applied early-detection strategies remains unfulfilled in the United States because of inequalities in access to screening, uneven quality of screening, and because screening is poorly integrated into routine health care.[250,251] Screening under opportunistic conditions rather than through a system is inefficient at both the individual and population levels;[252] moreover, without a system, there is no readiness to implement any new early-detection technology that could improve disease control. A comprehensive system of early detection potentially not only leads to high levels of participation, but also insures that all the elements of a program of early detection and intervention are highly competent, interrelated, and interdependent. A system has the potential not only to increase quality, but also to reduce the volume of small errors that contribute to incremental erosion of efficiency, as well as the volume of gross failures that result in death when mortality is avoidable. Although there are many practical barriers that must be overcome to establish true population-based screening programs, a system of organized screening holds the greatest potential to realize the benefits of reducing the incidence rate of advanced cancers, and subsequently avoiding premature mortality.

REFERENCES

1. Cole P, Morrison AS. Basic issues in cancer screening. In: Miller AB, editor. Screening in cancer. Geneva: International Union Against Cancer; 1978. p. 7.
2. Morrison A. Screening in chronic disease. New York: Oxford University Press; 1992.
3. Wilson JMG, Junger G. Principles and practice of screening for disease. Geneva, Switzerland: World Health Organization; 1968.
4. Smith RA. Screening fundamentals. Monogr Natl Cancer Inst 1997;22:15–22.
5. Shapiro S. Screening for secondary prevention of disease. In: Armenian HK, Shapiro S, editors. Epidemiology and health services. New York: Oxford University Press; 1998. p. 183–206.
6. Parkin DM, Bray F, Ferlay J, Pisani P. Global cancer statistics, 2002. CA Cancer J Clin 2005;55:74–108.
7. Duffy SW, Chen HH, Tabar L, Day NE. Estimation of mean sojourn time in breast cancer screening using a Markov chain model of both entry to and exit from the preclinical detectable phase. Stat Med 1995;14:1531–43.
8. Miller AB. Fundamental issues in screening for cancer. In: Schottenfeld D, Fraumeni JF, editors. Cancer epidemiology and prevention. 2nd ed. New York: Oxford University Press; 1996. p. 1433–52.
9. Lehman CD, Schnall MD, Kuhl CK, Harms SE. Report of the Working Groups on Breast MRI: report of the High-Risk Screening Group. Breast J 2004;10 Suppl 2:S9–12.
10. Schwartz LM, Woloshin S, Sox HC, et al. US women's attitudes to false positive mammography results and detection of ductal carcinoma in situ: cross sectional survey. BMJ 2000;320:1635–40.
11. Yen MF, Tabar L, Vitak B, et al. Quantifying the potential problem of overdiagnosis of ductal carcinoma in situ in breast cancer screening. Eur J Cancer 2003;39:1746–54.
12. Garber AM, Weinstein MC, Torrance GW, Kamlet MS. Theoretical foundations of cost-effectiveness analysis. In: Gold MR, Siegel JE, Russell LB, Weinstein MC, editors. Cost-effectiveness in health and medicine. New York: Oxford University Press; 1996. p. 25–53.
13. Eisenberg JM. Clinical economics. A guide to the economic analysis of clinical practices. JAMA 1989;262:2879–86.
14. Ruffin MT, Gorenflo DW, Woodman B. Predictors of screening for breast, cervical, colorectal, and prostatic cancer among community-based primary care practices. J Am Board Fam Pract 2000;13:1–10.
15. Cronin KA, Weed DL, Connor RJ, Prorok PC. Case-control studies of cancer screening: theory and practice. J Natl Cancer Inst 1998;90:498–504.
16. Black WC, Haggstrom DA, Welch HG. All-cause mortality in randomized trials of cancer screening. J Natl Cancer Inst 2002;94:167–73.
17. Nystrom L, Andersson I, Bjurstam N, et al. Long-term effects of mammography screening: updated overview of the Swedish randomised trials. Lancet 2002;359:909–19.
18. Tabar L, Duffy SW, Yen M-F, et al. All-cause mortality among breast cancer patients in a screening trial: support for breast cancer mortality as an end point. J Med Screen 2002;9:1–4.
19. Jemal A, Murray T, Ward E, et al. Cancer statistics, 2005. CA Cancer J Clin 2005;55:10–30.
20. Ries L, Eisner M, Kosary C, et al. SEER Cancer Statistics Review, 1973–1999. Bethesda (MD): National Cancer Institute; 2002.
21. Ries L, Eisner M, Kosary C, et al. SEER Cancer Statistics Review, 1975–2002. Bethesda (MD): National Cancer Institute; 2005.
22. Hendrick RE. Quality control in mammography: the American College of Radiology's Mammography Screening Accreditation Program. Curr Opin Radiol 1989;1:203–11.
23. Destouet JM, Bassett LW, Yaffe MJ, et al. The ACR's Mammography Accreditation Program: ten years of experience since MQSA. J Am Coll Radiol 2005;2:585–94.
24. Pisano ED, Gatsonis CA, Yaffe MJ, et al. American College of Radiology Imaging Network Digital Mammographic Imaging Screening Trial: objectives and methodology. Radiology 2005;236:404–12.
25. Joy JE, Penhoet EE, Petitti DB. Saving women's lives: strategies for improving breast cancer detection and diagnosis. Washington, DC: The National Academies Press; 2005.
26. Fletcher SW, Black W, Harris R, et al. Report of the International Workshop on Screening for Breast Cancer [comments]. J Natl Cancer Inst 1993;85:1644–56.
27. Kerlikowske K, Grady D, Barclay J, et al. Effect of age, breast density, and family history on the sensitivity of first screening mammography [comments]. JAMA 1996;276:33–8.
28. Sickles EA. Breast cancer screening outcomes in women ages 40–49: clinical experience with service screening using modern mammography. J Natl Cancer Inst Monogr 1997;22:99–104.
29. May DS, Lee NC, Nadel MR, et al. The National Breast and Cervical Cancer Early Detection Program: report on the first 4 years of mammography provided to medically underserved women [comments]. AJR Am J Roentgenol 1998;170:97–104.
30. Smith RA. Breast cancer screening among women younger than age 50: a current assessment of the issues. CA Cancer J Clin 2000;50:312–36.
31. Broeders MJ, Verbeek AL, Straatman H, et al. Repeated mammographic screening reduces breast cancer mortality along the continuum of age. J Med Screen 2002;9:163–7.
32. IARC Working Group on the Evaluation of Cancer-Preventive Strategies. Breast cancer screening. Lyon: IARC Press; 2002.
33. Bailar JC. Mammography before age 50 years? [editorial]. JAMA 1988;259:1548–9.
34. Eckhardt S, Badellino F, Murphy GP. UICC meeting on breast-cancer screening in pre-menopausal women in developed countries. Geneva, 29 September–1 October 1993. Int J Cancer 1994;56:1–5.
35. Forrest AP, Alexander FE. A question that will not go away: at what age should mammographic screening begin? [editorial; comment]. J Natl Cancer Inst 1995;87:1195–7.
36. National Institutes of Health Consensus Development Panel. National Institutes of Health Consensus Development Conference Statement: breast cancer screening for women ages 40–49, January 21–23, 1997. J Natl Cancer Inst 1997;89:1015–26.
37. Berry DA. The utility of mammography for women aged 40 to 50 years (Con). In: De Vita VT, Hellman S, Rosenberg SA, editors. Progress in Oncology, 2002. Boston: Jones and Bartlett Publishers; 2003. p. 346–72.
38. Shapiro S, Venet W, Strax P, et al. Ten- to fourteen-year effect of screening on breast cancer mortality. J Natl Cancer Inst 1982;69:349–55.
39. Tabar L, Fagerberg CJ, Gad A, et al. Reduction in mortality from breast cancer after mass screening with mammography. Randomised trial from the Breast Cancer Screening Working Group of the Swedish National Board of Health and Welfare. Lancet 1985;1:829–32.
40. Swedish Cancer Society and the Swedish National Board of Health and Welfare. Breast-cancer screening with mammography in women aged 40–49 years. Int J Cancer 1996;68:693–9.
41. Tabar L, Chen HH, Fagerberg G, et al. Recent results from the Swedish Two-County Trial: the effects of age, histologic type, and mode of detection on the efficacy of breast cancer screening. J Natl Cancer Inst Monogr 1997;22:43–7.
42. Tabar L, Duffy SW, Vitak B, et al. The natural history of breast carcinoma: what have we learned from screening? Cancer 1999;86:449–62.
43. Duffy SW, Day NE, Tabar L, et al. Markov models of breast tumor progression: some age-specific results. J Natl Cancer Inst Monogr 1997;22:93–7.
44. Bjurstam N, Bjorneld L, Duffy SW, et al. The Gothenburg breast screening trial: first results on mortality, incidence, and mode of detection for women ages 39–49 years at randomization [comments]. Cancer 1997;80:2091–9.
45. Tabar L, Yen MF, Vitak B, et al. Mammography service screening and mortality in breast cancer patients: 20-year follow-up before and after introduction of screening. Lancet 2003;361:1405–10.
46. Sjonell G, Stahle L. [Mammographic screening does not reduce breast cancer mortality]. Lakartidningen 1999;96:904–5, 908–13.
47. Duffy S, Tabar L, Chen HH, et al. The impact of organized mammographic service screening on breast cancer mortality in seven Swedish counties. Cancer 2002;95:458–69.
48. Tabar L, Vitak B, Tony HH, et al. Beyond randomized controlled trials: organized mammographic screening substantially reduces breast carcinoma mortality. Cancer 2001;91:1724–31.
49. Pinotti JA, Barros AC, Hegg R, Zeferino LC. Breast cancer control programme in developing countries. Eur J Gynaecol Oncol 1993;14:355–62.
50. Ballard-Barbash R, Klabunde C, Paci E, et al. Breast cancer screening in 21 countries: delivery of services, notification of results and outcomes ascertainment. Eur J Cancer Prev 1999;8:417–26.
51. Saslow D, Hannan J, Osuch J, et al. Clinical breast examination: practical recommendations for optimizing performance and reporting. CA Cancer J Clin 2004;54:327–44.

52. Feig SA, Shaber GS, Schwartz GF, et al. Thermography, mammography, and clinical examination in breast cancer screening. Review of 16,000 studies. Radiology 1977;122:123–7.
53. Bobo JK, Lee NC, Thames SF. Findings from 752,081 clinical breast examinations reported to a national screening program from 1995 through 1998. J Natl Cancer Inst 2000;92:971–6.
54. Baxter N. Preventive health care, 2001 update: should women be routinely taught breast self-examination to screen for breast cancer? CMAJ 2001;164:1837–46.
55. Semiglazov VF, Moiseyenko VM, Bavli JL, et al. The role of breast self-examination in early breast cancer detection (results of the 5-years USSR/WHO randomized study in Leningrad). Eur J Epidemiol 1992;8:498–502.
56. Semiglazov VF, Moiseenko VM, Manikhas AG, et al. [Interim results of a prospective randomized study of self-examination for early detection of breast cancer (Russia/St. Petersburg/WHO)]. Vopr Onkol 1999;45:265–71.
57. Thomas DB, Gao DL, Self SG, et al. Randomized trial of breast self-examination in Shanghai: methodology and preliminary results [comments]. J Natl Cancer Inst 1997;89:355–65.
58. Thomas DB, Gao DL, Ray RM, et al. Randomized trial of breast self-examination in Shanghai: final results. J Natl Cancer Inst 2002;94:1445–57.
59. Smith R. Commentary: breast self examination: do we really know what we think we know? BMJ-USA 2003;3:168–9.
60. Kriege M, Brekelmans CT, Boetes C, et al. Efficacy of MRI and mammography for breast-cancer screening in women with a familial or genetic predisposition. N Engl J Med 2004;351:427–37.
61. Warner E, Plewes DB, Hill KA, et al. Surveillance of BRCA1 and BRCA2 mutation carriers with magnetic resonance imaging, ultrasound, mammography, and clinical breast examination. JAMA 2004;292:1317–25.
62. Smith RA, Saslow D, Sawyer KA, et al. American Cancer Society guidelines for breast cancer screening: update 2003. CA Cancer J Clin 2003;53:141–69.
63. Short MP, Nielsen NH, Young DC, et al. Mammography screening for asymptomatic women: report of the Council on Scientific Affairs. Chicago: American Medical Association; 1999.
64. Feig SA, D'Orsi CJ, Hendrick RE, et al. American College of Radiology guidelines for breast cancer screening. AJR Am J Roentgenol 1998;171:29–33.
65. U.S. Preventive Services Task Force. Summaries for patients. Screening for breast cancer: recommendations from the U.S. Preventive Services Task Force. Ann Intern Med 2002;137(5 Pt 1):I47.
66. O'Brien M, Winawer S, Zauber A, et al. The National Polyp Study. Patient and polyp characteristics associated with high-grade dysplasia in colorectal adenomas. Gastroenterology 1990;98:371–9.
67. Giacosa A, Frascio F, Munizzi F. Epidemiology of colorectal polyps. Tech Coloproctol 2004;8 Suppl 2:s243–7.
68. Bond JH. Colon polyps and cancer. Endoscopy 2003;35:27–35.
69. Stryker S, Wolff B, Culp C, et al. Natural history of untreated colonic polyps. Gastroenterology 1987;93:1009–13.
70. Winawer SJ, Fletcher RH, Miller L, et al. Colorectal cancer screening: clinical guidelines and rationale [comments] [published errata appear in Gastroenterology 1997;112:1060 and 1998;114:625]. Gastroenterology 1997;112:594–642.
71. Atkin WS, Morson BC, Cuzick J. Long-term risk of colorectal cancer after excision of rectosigmoid adenomas [comments]. N Engl J Med 1992;326:658–62.
72. Rustgi A. Hereditary gastrointestinal polyposis and nonpolyposis syndromes. N Engl J Med 1994;331:1694–702.
73. Winawer SJ, Zauber AG, Ho MN, et al. Prevention of colorectal cancer by colonoscopic polypectomy. The National Polyp Study Workgroup [comments]. N Engl J Med 1993;329:1977–81.
74. Thiis-Evensen E, Hoff GS, Sauar J, et al. Population-based surveillance by colonoscopy: effect on the incidence of colorectal cancer. Telemark Polyp Study I. Scand J Gastroenterol 1999;34:414–20.
75. Young G, St. John J. Selecting an occult blood test for use as a screening tool for large bowel cancer. Front Gastrointest Res 1991;18:135–56.
76. Smith RA, von Eschenbach AC, Wender R, et al. American Cancer Society guidelines for the early detection of cancer: update of early detection guidelines for prostate, colorectal, and endometrial cancers. Also: update 2001—testing for early lung cancer detection. CA Cancer J Clin 2001;51:38–75; quiz 77–80.
77. Winawer S, Fletcher R, Rex D, et al. Colorectal cancer screening and surveillance: clinical guidelines and rationale—update based on new evidence. Gastroenterology 2003;124:544–60.
78. Ahlquist DA, Skoletsky JE, Boynton KA, et al. Colorectal cancer screening by detection of altered human DNA in stool: feasibility of a multitarget assay panel. Gastroenterology 2000;119:1219–27.
79. Imperiale TF, Ransohoff DF, Itzkowitz SH, et al. Fecal DNA versus fecal occult blood for colorectal-cancer screening in an average-risk population. N Engl J Med 2004;351:2704–14.
80. Levin B, Brooks D, Smith RA, Stone A. Emerging technologies in screening for colorectal cancer: CT colonography, immunochemical fecal occult blood tests, and stool screening using molecular markers. CA Cancer J Clin 2003;53:44–55.
81. Ouyang DL, Chen JJ, Getzenberg RH, Schoen RE. Noninvasive testing for colorectal cancer: a review. Am J Gastroenterol 2005;100:1393–403.
82. Mandel JS, Bond JH, Church TR, et al. Reducing mortality from colorectal cancer by screening for fecal occult blood. Minnesota Colon Cancer Control Study [published erratum appears in N Engl J Med 1993;329:672] [comments]. N Engl J Med 1993;328:1365–71.
83. Hardcastle JD, Thomas WM, Chamberlain J, et al. Randomised, controlled trial of faecal occult blood screening for colorectal cancer. Results for first 107,349 subjects. Lancet 1989;1:1160–4.
84. Kronborg O, Fenger C, Olsen J, et al. Randomised study of screening for colorectal cancer with faecal-occult- blood test [comments]. Lancet 1996;348:1467–71.
85. Mandel JS, Church TR, Bond JH, et al. The effect of fecal occult-blood screening on the incidence of colorectal cancer. N Engl J Med 2000;343:1603–7.
86. Ransohoff DF, Lang CA. Screening for colorectal cancer with the fecal occult blood test: a background paper. American College of Physicians [comments]. Ann Intern Med 1997;126:811–22.
87. Lieberman DA, Weiss DG. One-time screening for colorectal cancer with combined fecal occult-blood testing and examination of the distal colon. N Engl J Med 2001;345:555–60.
88. American College of Physicians. Suggested technique for fecal occult blood testing and interpretation in colorectal cancer screening. Ann Intern Med 1997;126:808–10.
89. Cole SR, Young GP. Effect of dietary restriction on participation in faecal occult blood test screening for colorectal cancer. Med J Aust 2001;175:195–8.
90. Pignone M, Campbell MK, Carr C, Phillips C. Meta-analysis of dietary restriction during fecal occult blood testing. Eff Clin Pract 2001;4:150–6.
91. Collins JF, Lieberman DA, Durbin TE, Weiss DG. Accuracy of screening for fecal occult blood on a single stool sample obtained by digital rectal examination: a comparison with recommended sampling practice. Ann Intern Med 2005;142:81–5.
92. Nadel MR, Shapiro JA, Klabunde CN, et al. A national survey of primary care physicians' methods for screening for fecal occult blood. Ann Intern Med 2005;142:86–94.
93. Sox HC. Office-based testing for fecal occult blood: do only in case of emergency. Ann Intern Med 2005;142:146–8.
94. Levin TR, Palitz AM. Flexible sigmoidoscopy: an important screening option for average-risk individuals. Gastrointest Endosc Clin N Am 2002;12:23–40, vi.
95. Byers T, Levin B, Rothenberger D, et al. American Cancer Society guidelines for screening and surveillance for early detection of colorectal polyps and cancer: update 1997. CA Cancer J Clin 1997;47:154–60.
96. Weissfeld JL, Schoen RE, Pinsky PF, et al. Flexible sigmoidoscopy in the PLCO cancer screening trial: results from the baseline screening examination of a randomized trial. J Natl Cancer Inst 2005;97:989–97.
97. Selby JV, Friedman GD, Quesenberry CPJ, Weiss NS. A case-control study of screening sigmoidoscopy and mortality from colorectal cancer [comments]. N Engl J Med 1992;326:653–7.
98. Newcomb PA, Norfleet RG, Storer BE, et al. Screening sigmoidoscopy and colorectal cancer mortality [comments]. J Natl Cancer Inst 1992;84:1572–5.
99. Newcomb PA, Storer BE, Morimoto LM, et al. Long-term efficacy of sigmoidoscopy in the reduction of colorectal cancer incidence. J Natl Cancer Inst 2003;95:622–5.
100. Winawer SJ, Flehinger BJ, Schottenfeld D, Miller DG. Screening for colorectal cancer with fecal occult blood testing and sigmoidoscopy [comments]. J Natl Cancer Inst 1993;85:1311–8.
101. Winawer SJ, Stewart ET, Zauber AG, et al. A comparison of colonoscopy and double-contrast barium enema for surveillance after polypectomy. National Polyp Study Work Group [comments]. N Engl J Med 2000;342:1766–72.
102. Cooper GS, Koroukian SM. Geographic variation among Medicare beneficiaries in the use of colorectal carcinoma screening procedures. Am J Gastroenterol 2004;99:1544–50.
103. Waye JD. Colonoscopy [comments]. CA Cancer J Clin 1992;42:350–65.
104. Rex DK, Imperiale TF, Latinovich DR, Bratcher LL. Impact of bowel preparation on efficiency and cost of colonoscopy. Am J Gastroenterol 2002;97:1696–700.
105. Takahashi Y, Tanaka H, Kinjo M, Sakumoto K. Sedation-free colonoscopy. Dis Colon Rectum 2005;48:855–9.
106. Cobb WS, Heniford BT, Sigmon LB, et al. Colonoscopic perforations: incidence, management, and outcomes. Am Surg 2004;70:750–8.
107. Rex DK, Bond JH, Winawer S, et al. Quality in the technical performance of colonoscopy and the continuous quality improvement process for colonoscopy: recommendations of the U.S. Multi-Society Task Force on Colorectal Cancer. Am J Gastroenterol 2002;97:1296–308.
108. Muller AD, Sonnenberg A. Prevention of colorectal cancer by flexible endoscopy and polypectomy. A case-control study of 32,702 veterans [comments]. Ann Intern Med 1995;123:904–10.
109. Vining DJ. Virtual endoscopy: is it reality? Radiology 1996;200:30–1.
110. Pickhardt PJ, Choi JR, Hwang I, et al. Computed tomographic virtual colonoscopy to screen for colorectal neoplasia in asymptomatic adults. N Engl J Med 2003;349:2191–200.
111. Mulhall BP, Veerappan GR, Jackson JL. Meta-analysis: computed tomographic colonography. Ann Intern Med 2005;142:635–50.
112. U.S. Preventive Services Task Force. Screening for colorectal cancer: recommendation and rationale. Ann Intern Med 2002;137:129–31.
113. Koss LG. The Papanicolaou test for cervical cancer detection. A triumph and a tragedy [comments]. JAMA 1989;261:737–43.
114. Lawson H, Lee N, Thames S, et al. Cervical cancer screening among low-income women: results of a national screening program, 1991–1995. Obstet Gynecol 1998;92:745–52.
115. Celentano DD, deLissovoy G. Assessment of cervical cancer screening and follow-up programs. Atlanta: Centers for Disease Control; 1990.
116. Moscicki AB, Shiboski S, Hills NK, et al. Regression of low-grade squamous intra-epithelial lesions in young women. Lancet 2004;364:1678–83.
117. Gardner JW, Lyon JL. Efficacy of cervical cytologic screening in the control of cervical cancer. Prev Med 1977;6:487–99.
118. Laara E, Day NE, Hakama M. Trends in mortality from cervical cancer in the Nordic countries: association with organised screening programmes. Lancet 1987;1:1247–9.
119. Hakama M, Magnus K, Petterson F, et al. Effect of organized screening on the risk of cervical cancer in the Nordic countries. In: Miller AB, Chamberlain J, Day NE, et al, editors. Cancer screening. Cambridge: Cambridge University Press; 1991. p. 153–62.
120. Johannesson G, Geirsson G, Day N. The effect of mass screening in Iceland, 1965–74, on the incidence and mortality of cervical carcinoma. Int J Cancer 1978;21:418–25.
121. Hakama M. Effect of population screening for carcinoma of the uterine cervix in Finland. Maturitas 1985;7:3–10.
122. Magnus K, Langmark F, Andersen A. Mass screening for cervical cancer in Ostfold county of Norway 1959–77. Int J Cancer 1987;39:311–6.
123. Comber H, Gavin A. Recent trends in cervical cancer mortality in Britain and Ireland: the case for population-based cervical cancer screening. Br J Cancer 2004;91:1902–4.
124. Olesen F. A case-control study of cervical cytology before diagnosis of cervical cancer in Denmark. Int J Epidemiol 1988;17:501–8.
125. Macgregor JE, Campbell MK, Mann EM, Swanson KY. Screening for cervical intraepithelial neoplasia in north east Scotland shows fall in incidence and mortality from invasive cancer with concomitant rise in preinvasive disease. BMJ 1994;308:1407–11.
126. Boon ME, de Graaff Guilloud JC, Rietveld WJ. Analysis of five sampling methods for the preparation of cervical smears. Acta Cytol 1989;33:843–8.
127. Shingleton HM, Patrick RL, Johnston WW, Smith RA. The current status of the Papanicolaou smear. CA Cancer J Clin 1995;45:305–20.

128. McCrory DC, Matchar DB, Bastian L, et al. Evaluation of cervical cytology Agency for Health Care Policy and Research evidence report. Rockville (MD): 1999. p. 1–418.
129. Hutchinson ML, Zahniser DJ, Sherman ME, et al. Utility of liquid-based cytology for cervical carcinoma screening: results of a population-based study conducted in a region of Costa Rica with a high incidence of cervical carcinoma. Cancer 1999;87:48–55.
130. Guo M, Hu L, Martin L, et al. Accuracy of liquid-based Pap tests: comparison of concurrent liquid-based tests and cervical biopsies on 782 women with previously abnormal Pap smears. Acta Cytol 2005;49:132–8.
131. Brown AD, Garber AM. Cost-effectiveness of 3 methods to enhance the sensitivity of Papanicolaou testing. JAMA 1999;281:347–53.
132. van Muyden RC, ter Harmsel BW, Smedts FM, et al. Detection and typing of human papillomavirus in cervical carcinomas in Russian women: a prognostic study. Cancer 1999;85:2011–6.
133. Kim JJ, Wright TC, Goldie SJ. Cost-effectiveness of human papillomavirus DNA testing in the United Kingdom, The Netherlands, France, and Italy. J Natl Cancer Inst 2005;97:888–95.
134. Sasieni P, Cuzick J. Could HPV testing become the sole primary cervical screening test? J Med Screen 2002;9:49–51.
135. Cuzick J. HPV testing in cervical screening. Pharmacoepidemiol Drug Safety 2001;10:33–6.
136. Jenkins D, Sherlaw-Johnson C, Gallivan S. Assessing the role of HPV testing in cervical cancer screening. Papilloma Report 1998;9:89–101.
137. Franco EL, Rohan TE, Villa LL. Epidemiologic evidence and human papillomavirus infection as a necessary cause of cervical cancer. J Natl Cancer Inst 1999;91:506–11.
138. Cuzick J, Szarewski A, Cubie H, et al. Management of women who test positive for high-risk types of human papillomavirus: the HART study. Lancet 2003;362:1871–6.
139. Sherman ME, Lorincz AT, Scott DR, et al. Baseline cytology, human papillomavirus testing, and risk for cervical neoplasia: a 10-year cohort analysis. J Natl Cancer Inst 2003;95:46–52.
140. Wright TC Jr, Schiffman M, Solomon D, et al. Interim guidance for the use of human papillomavirus DNA testing as an adjunct to cervical cytology for screening. Obstet Gynecol 2004;103:304–9.
141. Bosch FX, Manos MM, Munoz N, et al. Prevalence of human papillomavirus in cervical cancer: a worldwide perspective. International biological study on cervical cancer (IBSCC) Study Group [comments]. J Natl Cancer Inst 1995;87:796–802.
142. Munoz N, Bosch FX, Castellsague X, et al. Against which human papillomavirus types shall we vaccinate and screen? The international perspective. Int J Cancer 2004;111:278–85.
143. Broder S. Rapid communication—the Bethesda system for reporting cervical/vaginal cytologic diagnoses—report of the 1991 Bethesda workshop. JAMA 1992;267:1892.
144. Solomon D, Davey D, Kurman R, et al. The 2001 Bethesda System: terminology for reporting results of cervical cytology. JAMA 2002;287:2114–9.
145. Saslow D, Runowicz C, Solomon D, et al. American Cancer Society guideline for the early detection of cervical neoplasia and cancer. CA Cancer J Clin 2002;52:342–62.
146. Saint M, Gildengorin G, Sawaya GF. Current cervical neoplasia screening practices of obstetrician/gynecologists in the US. Am J Obstet Gynecol 2005;192:414–21.
147. Sawaya GF. Papanicolaou testing: when does more become less? Am J Med 2005;118:159–60.
148. Sawaya GF, McConnell KJ, Kulasingam SL, et al. Risk of cervical cancer associated with extending the interval between cervical-cancer screenings. N Engl J Med 2003;349:1501–9.
149. Moul JW, Sesterhenn IA, Connelly RR, et al. Prostate-specific antigen values at the time of prostate cancer diagnosis in African-American men. JAMA 1995;274:1277–81.
150. Jacobsen SJ, Bergstralh EJ, Katusic SK, et al. Screening digital rectal examination and prostate cancer mortality: a population-based case-control study [comments]. Urology 1998;52:173–9.
151. Weinmann S, Richert-Boe KE, Van Den Eeden SK, et al. Screening by prostate-specific antigen and digital rectal examination in relation to prostate cancer mortality: a case-control study. Epidemiology 2005;16:367–76.
152. Friedman GD, Hiatt RA, Quesenberry CP Jr, Selby JV. Case-control study of screening for prostatic cancer by digital rectal examinations [comments]. Lancet 1991;337:1526–9.
153. Richert-Boe KE, Humphrey LL, Glass AG, Weiss NS. Screening digital rectal examination and prostate cancer mortality: a case-control study. J Med Screen 1998;5:99–103.
154. Basler JW, Thompson IM. Lest we abandon digital rectal examination as a screening test for prostate cancer [editorial; comment]. J Natl Cancer Inst 1998;90:1761–3.
155. Johansson JE, Andren O, Andersson SO, et al. Natural history of early, localized prostate cancer. JAMA 2004;291:2713–9.
156. Thompson IM, Ankerst DP, Chi C, et al. Operating characteristics of prostate-specific antigen in men with an initial PSA level of 3.0 ng/ml or lower. JAMA 2005;294:66–70.
157. Mettlin C, Lee F, Drago J, Murphy GP. The American Cancer Society National Prostate Cancer Detection Project. Findings on the detection of early prostate cancer in 2425 men. Cancer 1991;67:2949–58.
158. Catalona WJ, Smith DS, Ratliff TL, et al. Measurement of prostate-specific antigen in serum as a screening test for prostate cancer [published erratum appears in N Engl J Med 1991;325:1324] [comments]. N Engl J Med 1991;324:1156–61.
159. Mettlin C. The American Cancer Society National Prostate Cancer Detection Project and national patterns of prostate cancer detection and treatment [published erratum appears in CA Cancer J Clin 1997;47:325]. CA Cancer J Clin 1997;47:265–72.
160. Etzioni R, Legler JM, Feuer EJ, et al. Cancer surveillance series: interpreting trends in prostate cancer—part III: quantifying the link between population prostate-specific antigen testing and recent declines in prostate cancer mortality. J Natl Cancer Inst 1999;91:1033–9.
161. Feuer EJ, Merrill RM, Hankey BF. Cancer surveillance series: interpreting trends in prostate cancer—part II: cause of death misclassification and the recent rise and fall in prostate cancer mortality. J Natl Cancer Inst 1999;91:1025–32.
162. Tarone RE, Chu KC, Brawley OW. Implications of stage-specific survival rates in assessing recent declines in prostate cancer mortality rates. Epidemiology 2000;11:167–70.
163. Bartsch G, Horninger W, Klocker H, et al. Prostate cancer mortality after introduction of prostate-specific antigen mass screening in the Federal State of Tyrol, Austria. Urology 2001;58:417–24.
164. Horninger W, Berger A, Pelzer A, Screening for prostate cancer: updated experience from the Tyrol study. Can J Urol 2005;12 Suppl 1:7–13.
165. Standaert B, Denis L. The European Randomized Study of Screening for Prostate Cancer: an update. Cancer 1997;80:1830–4.
166. Gohagan J, Prorok P, Kramer B. The prostate, lung, colorectal and ovarian cancer screening trial of the National Cancer Institute. Cancer 1995;75:1869–73.
167. de Koning HJ, Auvinen A, Berenguer Sanchez A, et al. Large-scale randomized prostate cancer screening trials: program performances in the European Randomized Screening for Prostate Cancer trial and the Prostate, Lung, Colorectal and Ovary cancer trial. Int J Cancer 2002;97:237–44.
168. Holmberg L, Bill-Axelson A, Helgesen F, et al. A randomized trial comparing radical prostatectomy with watchful waiting in early prostate cancer. N Engl J Med 2002;347:781–9.
169. Walsh PC. Surgery and the reduction of mortality from prostate cancer. N Engl J Med 2002;347:839–40.
170. Whitmore WF Jr. Natural history of low-stage prostatic cancer and the impact of early detection. Urol Clin North Am 1990;17:689–97.
171. Screening for prostate cancer: recommendation and rationale. Ann Intern Med 2002;137:915–6.
172. American Academy of Family Physicians. Periodic health examinations: summary of AAFP policy and recommendations & age charts: AAFP; 2002.
173. American College of Physicians. Screening for prostate cancer. Ann Intern Med 1997;126:480–4.
174. American Medical Association. Report 9 of the Council on Scientific Affairs (A-00). Screening and early detection of prostate cancer. AMA; 2001.
175. Negri E, Pelucchi C, Talamini R, et al. Family history of cancer and the risk of prostate cancer and benign prostatic hyperplasia. Int J Cancer 2005;114:648–52.
176. Rodriguez C, Calle EE, Miracle-McMahill HL, et al. Family history and risk of fatal prostate cancer. Epidemiology 1997;8:653–7.
177. Carter HB, Pearson JD, Metter EJ, et al. Longitudinal evaluation of prostate-specific antigen levels in men with and without prostate disease [comments]. JAMA 1992;267:2215–20.
178. Thompson I, Leach RJ, Pollock BH, Naylor SL. Prostate cancer and prostate-specific antigen: the more we know, the less we understand. J Natl Cancer Inst 2003;95:1027–8.
179. Pearson J, Landis P, Fozard J, Carter H. When is PSA testing no longer necessary? J Urol 1998;157:178.
180. Walter LC, Covinsky KE. Cancer screening in elderly patients: a framework for individualized decision making. JAMA 2001;285:2750–6.
181. Presti JC Jr, Hovey R, Bhargava V, et al. Prospective evaluation of prostate specific antigen and prostate specific antigen density in the detection of carcinoma of the prostate: ethnic variations [comments]. J Urol 1997;157:907–12.
182. Morgan TO, Jacobsen SJ, McCarthy WF, et al. Age-specific reference ranges for prostate-specific antigen in black men [comments]. N Engl J Med 1996;335:304–10.
183. Peto R, Darby S, Deo H, et al. Smoking, smoking cessation, and lung cancer in the UK since 1950: combination of national statistics with two case-control studies [comments]. BMJ 2000;321:323–9.
184. Black WC. Lung cancer. In: Kramer BS, Gohagan JK, Prorok PC, editors. Cancer screening: theory and practice. New York: Marcel Dekker; 1999. p. 327–77.
185. Muhm JR, Miller WE, Fontana RS, et al. Lung cancer detected during a screening program using four-month chest radiographs. Radiology 1983;148:609–15.
186. Humphrey LL, Teutsch S, Johnson M. Lung cancer screening with sputum cytologic examination, chest radiography, and computed tomography: an update for the U.S. Preventive Services Task Force. Ann Intern Med 2004;140:740–53.
187. Kramer BS, Gohagan J, Prorok PC, Smart C. A National Cancer Institute sponsored screening trial for prostatic, lung, colorectal, and ovarian cancers. Cancer 1993;71(2 Suppl):589–93.
188. Ford LG, Minasian LM, McCaskill-Stevens W, et al. Prevention and early detection clinical trials: opportunities for primary care providers and their patients. CA Cancer J Clin 2003;53:82–101.
189. Mulshine JL. New developments in lung cancer screening. J Clin Oncol 2005;23:3198–202.
190. Smith IE. Screening for lung cancer: time to think positive [comment]. Lancet 1999;354:86–7.
191. Henschke CI. Computed tomography screening for lung cancer: principles and results. Clin Cancer Res 2005;11:4984s–7s.
192. Henschke CI, Yankelevitz DF, Naidich DP, et al. CT screening for lung cancer: suspiciousness of nodules according to size on baseline scans. Radiology 2004;231:164–8.
193. Rossi A, Maione P, Colantuoni G, et al. Screening for lung cancer: new horizons? Crit Rev Oncol Hematol 2005.
194. Fontana RS, Sanderson DR, Woolner LB, et al. Screening for lung cancer. A critique of the Mayo Lung Project. Cancer 1991;67(4 Suppl):1155–64.
195. Berlin NI. Overview of the NCI cooperative early lung cancer detection program. International Conference on Prevention and Early Diagnosis of Lung Cancer, Varese, Italy; 1998.
196. Frost JK, Ball WC Jr, Levin ML, et al. Early lung cancer detection: results of the initial (prevalence) radiologic and cytologic screening in the Johns Hopkins study. Am Rev Respir Dis 1984;130:549–54.
197. Kubik A, Polak J. Lung cancer detection. Results of a randomized prospective study in Czechoslovakia. Cancer 1986;57:2427–37.
198. Melamed MR, Flehinger BJ, Zaman MB, et al. Screening for early lung cancer. Results of the Memorial Sloan-Kettering study in New York. Chest 1984;86:44–53.
199. Fontana RS. The Mayo Lung Project: a perspective. Cancer 2000;89(11 Suppl):2352–5.
200. Kubik A, Haerting J. Survival and mortality in a randomized study of lung cancer detection. Neoplasma 1990;37:467–75.
201. U.S. Preventive Services Task Force. Lung cancer screening: recommendation statement. Ann Intern Med 2004;140:738–9.
202. Strauss G, Dominioni L. Varese meeting report. Lung Cancer 1999;23:171–2.
203. Henschke CI, McCauley DI, Yankelevitz DF, et al. Early Lung Cancer Action Project: overall design and findings from baseline screening [comments]. Lancet 1999;354:99–105.
204. Gohagan JK, Marcus PM, Fagerstrom RM, et al. Final results of the Lung Screening Study, a randomized feasibility study of spiral CT versus chest X-ray screening for lung cancer. Lung Cancer 2005;47:9–15.

205. Hirsch FR, Bunn PA Jr, Dmitrovsky E, et al. IV international conference on prevention and early detection of lung cancer, Reykjavik, Iceland, August 9–12, 2001. Lung Cancer 2002;37:325–44.
206. Strauss GM, Dominioni L, Jett JR, et al. Como international conference position statement: lung cancer screening for early diagnosis 5 years after the 1998 Varese conference. Chest 2005;127:1146–51.
207. Henschke CI, Naidich DP, Yankelevitz DF, et al. Early lung cancer action project: initial findings on repeat screenings. Cancer 2001;92:153–9.
208. U.S. Preventive Services Task Force. Screening for testicular cancer: recommendation statement: Agency for Healthcare Research and Quality(AHRQ); 2002.
209. Moul JW, Paulson DF, Dodge RK, Walther PJ. Delay in diagnosis and survival in testicular cancer: impact of effective therapy and changes during 18 years. J Urol 1990;143:520–3.
210. Khadra A, Oakeshott P. Pilot study of testicular cancer awareness and testicular self-examination in men attending two South London general practices. Fam Pract 2002;19:294–6.
211. Ward KD, Vander Weg MW, Read MC, et al. Testicular cancer awareness and self-examination among adolescent males in a community-based youth organization. Prev Med 2005;41:386–98.
212. Sheley JP, Kinchen EW, Morgan DH, Gordon DF. Limited impact of testicular self-examination promotion. J Community Health 1991;16:117–24.
213. Buetow SA. Testicular cancer: to screen or not to screen? [comments]. J Med Screen 1996;3:3–6.
214. Geczi L, Gomez F, Horvath Z, et al. Three-year results of the first educational and early detection program for testicular cancer in Hungary. Oncology 2001;60:228–34.
215. American Academy of Family Physicians. Age charts for the periodic health examination. Kansas City: American Academy of Family Physicians; 1994.
216. Burk JR, Lehman HF, Wolf FS. Inadequacy of Papanicolaou smears in the detection of endometrial cancer. N Engl J Med 1974;291:191–2.
217. Walker JL, Nunez ER. Endometrial cancer. In: Kramer BS, Gohagan JK, Prorok PC, editors. Cancer screening: theory and practice. New York: Marcel Dekker; 1999. p. 531–66.
218. van Leeuwen FE, Benraadt J, Coebergh JW, et al. Risk of endometrial cancer after tamoxifen treatment of breast cancer [comments]. Lancet 1994;343:448–52.
219. Barakat RR, Gilewski TA, Almadrones L, et al. Effect of adjuvant tamoxifen on the endometrium in women with breast cancer: a prospective study using office endometrial biopsy [In process citation]. J Clin Oncol 2000;18:3459–63.
220. Gerber B, Krause A, Muller H, et al. Effects of adjuvant tamoxifen on the endometrium in postmenopausal women with breast cancer: a prospective long-term study using transvaginal ultrasound [In Process Citation]. J Clin Oncol 2000;18:3464–70.
221. Burke W, Daly M, Garber J, et al. Recommendations for follow-up care of individuals with an inherited predisposition to cancer. II. BRCA1 and BRCA2. Cancer Genetics Studies Consortium [comments]. JAMA 1997;277:997–1003.
222. Jacobs IJ, Menon U. Progress and challenges in screening for early detection of ovarian cancer. Mol Cell Proteomics 2004;3:355–66.
223. Duffy MJ. Evidence for the clinical use of tumour markers. Ann Clin Biochem 2004;41(Pt 5):370–7.
224. Moss EL, Hollingworth J, Reynolds TM. The role of CA125 in clinical practice. J Clin Pathol 2005;58:308–12.
225. National Institutes of Health consensus Development Conference Statement. Ovarian cancer: screening treatment, and followup. NIH Consensus Statement 1994. Bethesda: National Institutes of Health 1994:1–30.
226. Petricoin EF, Ardekani AM, Hitt BA, et al. Use of proteomic patterns in serum to identify ovarian cancer. Lancet 2002;359:572–7.
227. Baggerly KA, Morris JS, Edmonson SR, Coombes KR. Signal in noise: evaluating reported reproducibility of serum proteomic tests for ovarian cancer. J Natl Cancer Inst 2005;97:307–9.
228. Ransohoff DF. Lessons from controversy: ovarian cancer screening and serum proteomics. J Natl Cancer Inst 2005;97:315–9.
229. Campbell S, Bhan V, Royston P, et al. Transabdominal ultrasound screening for early ovarian cancer [comments]. BMJ 1989;299:1363–7.
230. DePriest PD, van Nagell JR Jr, Gallion HH, et al. Ovarian cancer screening in asymptomatic postmenopausal women. Gynecol Oncol 1993;51:205–9.
231. Helzlsouer KJ, Bush TL, Alberg AJ, et al. Prospective study of serum CA-125 levels as markers of ovarian cancer [comments]. JAMA 1993;269:1123–6.
232. Einhorn N, Sjovall K, Knapp RC, et al. Prospective evaluation of serum CA 125 levels for early detection of ovarian cancer. Obstet Gynecol 1992;80:14–8.
233. Jacobs I, Davies AP, Bridges J, et al. Prevalence screening for ovarian cancer in postmenopausal women by CA 125 measurement and ultrasonography [comments]. BMJ 1993;306:1030–4.
234. Skates SJ, Xu FJ, Yu YH, et al. Toward an optimal algorithm for ovarian cancer screening with longitudinal tumor markers. Cancer 1995;76(10 Suppl):2004–10.
235. Screening for ovarian cancer: recommendation statement. Ann Fam Med 2004;2:260–2.
236. Rampen FH, Casparie-van Velsen JI, van Huystee BE, et al. False-negative findings in skin cancer and melanoma screening. J Am Acad Dermatol 1995;33:59–63.
237. Helfand M, Mahon SM, Eden KB, et al. Screening for skin cancer. Am J Prev Med 2001;20(3 Suppl):47–58.
238. Aitken JF, Elwood JM, Lowe JB, et al. A randomised trial of population screening for melanoma. J Med Screen 2002;9:33–7.
239. Tiersten AD, Grin CM, Kopf AW, et al. Prospective follow-up for malignant melanoma in patients with atypical-mole (dysplastic-nevus) syndrome. J Dermatol Surg Oncol 1991;17:44–8.
240. Geller AC, Zhang Z, Sober AJ, et al. The first 15 years of the American Academy of Dermatology skin cancer screening programs: 1985–1999. J Am Acad Dermatol 2003;48:34–41.
241. Swetter SM, Waddell BL, Vazquez MD, Khosravi VS. Increased effectiveness of targeted skin cancer screening in the Veterans Affairs population of Northern California. Prev Med 2003;36:164–71.
242. Smith RA, Cokkinides V, Eyre HJ. American Cancer Society guidelines for the early detection of cancer, 2003. CA Cancer J Clin 2003;53:27–43.
243. Ferrini R, Woolf SH. American College of Preventive Medicine practice policy. Screening for prostate cancer in American men. Am J Prev Med 1998;15:81–4.
244. Tucker MA, Halpern A, Holly EA, et al. Clinically recognized dysplastic nevi. A central risk factor for cutaneous melanoma [comments]. JAMA 1997;277:1439–44.
245. McDonald CJ. American Cancer Society perspective on the American College of Preventive Medicine's policy statements on skin cancer prevention and screening [comment]. CA Cancer J Clin 1998;48:229–31.
246. U.S. Preventive Services Task Force. Screening for skin cancer: recommendations and rationale. Am J Prev Med 2001;20(3 Suppl):44–6.
247. Mashberg A, Samit A. Early diagnosis of asymptomatic oral and oropharyngeal squamous cancers. CA Cancer J Clin 1995;45:328–51.
248. Smart CR. Screening for cancer of the aerodigestive tract. Cancer 1993;72(3 Suppl):1061–5.
249. Sankaranarayanan R, Ramadas K, Thomas G, et al. Effect of screening on oral cancer mortality in Kerala, India: a cluster-randomised controlled trial. Lancet 2005;365:1927–33.
250. Meissner HI, Smith RA, Rimer BK, et al. Promoting cancer screening: learning from experience. Cancer 2004;101(5 Suppl):1107–17.
251. Smith RA, Wender RC. Cancer screening and the periodic health examination. Cancer 2004;100:1553–7.
252. Miles A, Cockburn J, Smith RA, Wardle J. A perspective from countries using organized screening programs. Cancer 2004;101(5 Suppl):1201–13.

Section 5

CLINICAL TRIALS AND OUTCOMES ASSESSMENT

29

Statistical Innovations in Cancer Research

Donald A. Berry, PhD

Statistics chapters in medical volumes are usually introductions to traditional statistical concepts. This chapter is different. Its goal is to introduce researchers and clinicians to innovations in the design and analysis of cancer experiments, especially clinical trials. One reason for this tack is that numerous good biostatistics texts are available to readers. Another is that in the modern world of Internet search engines such as Google (Google Inc, Mountain View, CA), the curious reader can find out as much as desired about any particular statistical method.

The principal goals of the innovations presented in this chapter are to (1) use information from clinical trials more efficiently in drawing conclusions about treatment effects, (2) use patient resources more efficiently whereas treating patients who participate in clinical trials as effectively as possible, and (3) identify better drugs and therapeutic strategies more rapidly, moving them more quickly through the development process. The underlying premise is to exploit all available evidence, placing information gleaned from an ongoing clinical trial into the context of what is already known. The innovations considered are intuitively appealing, but some are controversial. Some innovations are being used in actual clinical trials, whereas others are still being developed and evaluated for such use.

This chapter addresses two types of innovations. One is a natural extension of the traditional practice of statistics. The other type represents a sea change and is based on a Bayesian statistical philosophy. Because not all readers will be familiar with the Bayesian approach, it is described and related to the more familiar frequentist approach. Readers who are familiar with Bayesian ideas may wish to skip "Bayesian Updating" below. An important distinction between the two approaches is one of attitude. The Bayesian approach is tailored to on-line learning (as data accrue), and the frequentist approach is tied to particular experiments and to the experiment's design; however, there is substantial overlap. Much of this chapter's development of clinical trial design employs the Bayesian approach as a tool for finding designs that tend to treat patients in the clinical trial more effectively, and that identify better drugs more rapidly. But the frequentist properties (such as false-positive rate and power) of the design thus derived can be found, usually by simulation. Ensuring that a design has pre-specified frequentist properties means that the design is frequentist and that the Bayesian approach served as a tool for finding a good frequentist design.

In the early days of clinical trials, designs could not be very complicated. For example, if the treatment assigned to the next patient were to depend on the currently available results of the patients previously treated in the trial, it would be difficult to evaluate the trial's false-positive rate. Such a calculation may be impossible using standard mathematical methods. But in the modern era, the availability of high-speed computers and sophisticated computational methods makes such calculations routine. For example, modern computers can be used to simulate trials with even the most complicated of designs and evaluate design properties such as power and false-positive rate. All that is required is that the design be specified prospectively.

PRELIMINARIES

The basis of all experimentation is comparison. Evaluating an experimental therapy in a clinical trial requires information about the outcomes of these patients had they received some other therapy. The best way to address this issue is to randomize patients to the experimental therapy and to some comparison therapy. Although there are ways to learn without randomizing, there are limitations to approaches that do not employ randomization. And randomization does not require equal assignment probabilities to the therapeutic strategies, or "arms," being compared. Unbalanced randomization is possible, as is randomization that is adaptive in the sense that assignment probabilities depend on the accumulating data in the trial. (The latter possibility is a principal focus of this chapter.)

Most clinical trials are conducted in accord with a protocol. The traditional goal is science and not the effective treatment of patients in the trial.[1] Protocols may refer to the retrospective or sporadic collection of data, but they are usually prospective. A prospective protocol lays out how the trial is to be conducted, including how patients will be assigned to therapy, and when the trial will end. Deviations from a protocol may make scientific inferences from the trial difficult or impossible (although they may be necessary to avoid exposing participants to unnecessary risks).

BAYESIAN APPROACH

This section is not essential for reading the remainder of this chapter. But the material covered will help readers understand some of the approaches and attitudes. The goals of this section are to show how Bayesian learning takes place and how the Bayesian approach relates to the more traditional frequentist approach. This introduction is necessarily superficial. Philosophical issues, in particular, are barely touched upon. Further reading includes a comprehensive but elementary introduction to Bayesian ideas and methods,[2] a discussion of their role in medical research,[3] and an elegant and useful text describing more advanced Bayesian methods.[4]

Bayesian Updating The defining characteristic of any statistical approach is how it deals with uncertainty. In the Bayesian approach, uncertainty is measured by probability. Any event that has an unknown occurrence has a probability. The frequentist approach uses probabilities as well, but in a more restricted fashion, as will be seen in the next section. Examples of probabilities in the

Bayesian approach that do not have frequentist counterparts include the following: the probability that the drug is effective, the probability that a certain patient will respond to a particular chemotherapy, and the probability that the future results in the trial will show a statistically significant benefit for a particular therapy.

The Bayesian paradigm is one of learning. As information becomes available one updates one's knowledge about the unknown aspects of the process that is producing the information. The fundamental tool for learning under uncertainty is Bayes' rule. Bayes' rule relates inverse probabilities. An example that will be familiar to many readers is finding the positive predictive value (PPV) of a diagnostic test: In view of a positive test result, what is the probability that the individual being tested has the disease in question? The inverse probability is that of a positive test given the presence of the disease, which is called the test's *sensitivity*. PPV also depends on the test's *specificity*, which is the probability of a negative test, given that the individual does not have the disease. And PPV depends on the prevalence of disease in the population. In applying Bayes' rule to statistical inference, the analog of PPV is the "posterior probability" that a hypothesis is true given the experimental results. The analog of disease prevalence is the "prior probability" that the hypothesis is true.

Consider an overly simplified numerical example, one with only two possible response rates (r): $r = 0.75$ and $r = 0.50$. If you are accustomed to thinking about PPV for diagnostic tests, consider one of these to be that the "patient has the disease" and the other to be that the "patient does not have the disease." The question is this: Is r equal to 0.75 or 0.50? Before any experimentation these two possibilities are regarded to be equally likely: $P(r = 0.75) = P(r = 0.50) = 1/2$.

The focus of the Bayesian approach is learning. Probabilities are calculated as new information becomes available, and is taken to be "given." Statisticians have a notation that facilitates thinking about and calculating probabilities as new information accrues. They use vertical bars to separate the event of interest from data or parameters that are regarded to be known (or taken to be given): $P(A|B)$ is read "probability of A given B." Write R for tumor response and N for non-response. Using this notation, for example, $P(R|r = 0.75) = 0.75$. More interesting is the probability of $r = 0.75$ given a tumor response: $P(r=0.75|R)$. These two expressions are the inverses of each other, with the roles of the event of interest and the event being assumed. Bayes' rule is the relationship between these two expressions. Namely, that the updated (posterior) probability of $r = 0.75$ is as follows:

$$P(r = 0.75|R) = P(R|r = 0.75)P(r = 0.75)/P(R).$$

The denominator on the right-hand side follows from the law of total probability:

$$\begin{aligned} P(R) &= P(R|r = 0.75)P(r = 0.75) + P(R|r = 0.50)P(r = 0.50) \\ &= (0.75)(1/2) + (0.5)(1/2) = 5/8. \end{aligned}$$

That is, $P(R)$ is the average of the two response rates under consideration, 0.75 and 0.50, where the average is with respect to the corresponding prior probabilities—half each in this example. Substituting the numerical values into Bayes' rule, the posterior probability of $r = 0.75$ is as follows:

$$P(r = 0.75|R) = (0.75)(1/2)/(5/8) = 3/5.$$

Therefore, the new evidence boosts the probability of $r = 0.75$ from 1/2 (or 50%) to 60%. And since total probability is 100%, the evidence in a single response lowers the probability of $r = 0.50$ from 50 to 40%. (For further explanation and examples, see Chapter 5 of *Statistics: A Bayesian Perspective*.[2])

Consider a second independent observation. The probabilities of the two values of r prior to this second observation are posterior to the first observation. If the second observation is also a response, then a second application of Bayes' rule applies to give $P(r = 0.75|R, R) = 9/13 = 69\%$, which is a further increase from the previous values of 50 and 60%. On the other hand, if the second observation is a non-response then $P(r = 0.75|R, N) = 3/7 = 43\%$, a decrease from 60%. This process can go on indefinitely, updating either after each observation or all at once on the basis of whatever evidence happens to be available. The current probabilities of the various possible values of response rate r can be found at any time. These probabilities depend on the original prior probability and on the intervening data. This process of updating and on-line learning is an important advantage of the Bayesian approach to designing clinical trials.

The above example considered only two possible values of r. More realistically, the response rate r may be any number between 0 and 1. The left-hand panel in Figure 29-1A shows a constant or flat curve that is a candidate prior distribution. The flat curve indicates that the probability is spread equally over this range of values of r. This might be termed an "open-minded prior distribution" because the posterior distribution depends almost entirely on the evidence from the experiment at hand. After a single tumor response, Bayesian updating serves to change the probability distribution to the one shown in the right-hand panel of Figure 29-1A—that is, the right-hand panel is the posterior distribution after observing R when the prior distribution is the one shown in the left-hand panel. The shift in the distribution to larger values of r corresponds to the intuitive notion that larger response rates become more likely after observing R. Bayes' rule quantifies this intuition.

There are many candidate prior distributions other than the first one shown in Figure 29-1A. Three other prior/posterior pairs are shown in Figures 29-1B, -1C, and -1D. The right-hand panel within each pair is the posterior distribution after observing R when the prior distribution is that shown in the left-hand panel. Moreover, the left-hand curves in Figures 29-1B, -1C, and -1D

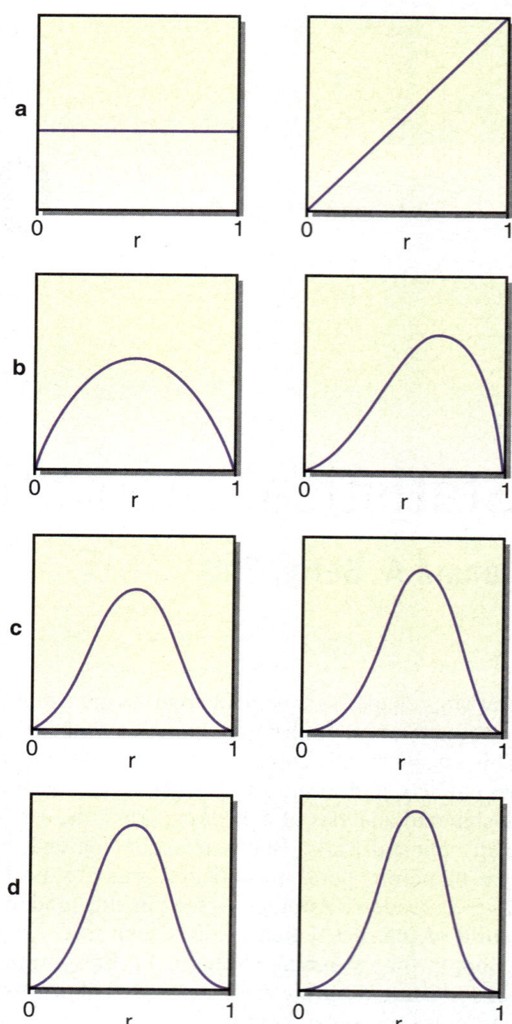

Figure 29-1 Prior distributions of response rate r. The left-hand panel in each pair is the prior distribution of response rate r. The right-hand panel is the posterior distribution of r after having observed a response in a single patient. The (predictive) probability of a response for each left-hand panel is 0.500, increasing in the right-hand panels to 0.667, 0.600, 0.571, 0.556 in cases "a" through "d," respectively. Changes are greater and learning is more rapid when the prior distribution reflects greater uncertainty.

are themselves posterior distributions for the right-hand curves in Figures 29-1A, -1B, and -1C, respectively, but when the observation is an N. Intuitively, after a non-response the concentration of probabilities shifts to smaller values of r. Mathematically, observing R means to multiply the current distribution by r (the response rate) and renormalize it so that the area under the curve is 1. Similarly, observing an N means to multiply by $(1-r)$, the rate of non-response.

An implication is that moving left to right and top to bottom in Figure 29-1 corresponds to starting with the prior distribution in the left-hand panel of Figure 29-1A and observing RNRNRNR. The eight curves shown in Figure 29-1 are proportional to the following respective functional forms: 1, r, $r(1-r)$, $r^2(1-r)$, $r^2(1-r)^2$, $r^3(1-r)^2$, $r^3(1-r)^3$, $r^4(1-r)^3$. Each observation of response increases the exponent of r by 1 and each observed N increases the exponent of (1–r) by 1. As is evident in the figure, additional observations lead to narrower distributions. As the number of observations increases, the distribution tends to concentrate about a single point, which is the "true" value of r, the response rate that is producing the observations.

The principal message of this section is not the numerical calculation defining the updated distribution, but the fact that updated distributions can be found using the Bayesian approach at any time during a clinical trial.

PRIOR PROBABILITIES Bayesian updating requires a starting point: a prior distribution of the various parameters. In the example, one must have a probability distribution for response rate r in advance of or separate from the experiment in question. This prior distribution may be subjectively assessed or based explicitly on the results of previous experiments. In some settings, such as some regulatory scenarios, an appropriate default distribution is non-informative or open-minded[2] in the sense that all possible values of the parameters are assigned the same prior probabilities. The left-hand panel of Figure 29-1A is an example.

Non-informative or flat prior distributions limit the benefits of taking a Bayesian approach if they ignore information that is available from outside the experiment. However, the benefit of employing Bayesian updating may be substantial even if one starts with a flat distribution that does not reflect anyone's assessment of the prior information. Flat prior distributions serve some important roles. One role is that it may be helpful to distinguish the evidence in the data in the experiment under consideration from that present before the experiment. Another is that the Bayesian conclusions that arise from using flat priors are often the same as the corresponding frequentist conclusions.

Prior distributions are usually based on historical data. Suppose that a similar drug (or the same drug in a possibly different patient population) gave a response rate of 50% in 20 patients: 10 responders and 10 non-responders. The corresponding likelihood of response rate r (see "Frequentist/Bayesian Comparison" below) is $r^{10}(1-r)^{10}$. Given that there may be differences between the historical setting and that of the current trial, it would not be reasonable to use this as a prior distribution for r, but it would be appropriate to somehow exploit this relevant information. One possibility (another will be described in "Hazards over Time") is to discount the historical evidence as it applies to the context of the current trial. For example, weighing an historical observation as having the information equivalent of 30% that of a current observation would mean using a prior distribution proportional to $r^3(1-r)^3$. This is the distribution shown in Figure 29-1D, left-hand panel.

ROBUSTNESS PRINCIPLE

In the presence of enough data, essentially all observers will have similar posterior distributions. This is the robustness principle. An implication is that the particular prior distribution assumed does not matter much when the sample size is moderate or large. As an example, consider the eight distributions shown in Figure 29-1 and think of each of them in turn as being the prior distribution of a different person. Parameter r is the response rate to a particular drug. Suppose that 40 patients are treated in a trial and 20 of them respond. Applying the robustness principle, the eight people in question will come to very nearly the same conclusion about the drug's response rate. The eight posterior distributions are shown in Figure 29-2. The curves are nearly superimposed. The eight 95% probability intervals will also be very similar. The data outweighs any of the prior distributions shown in Figure 29-1.

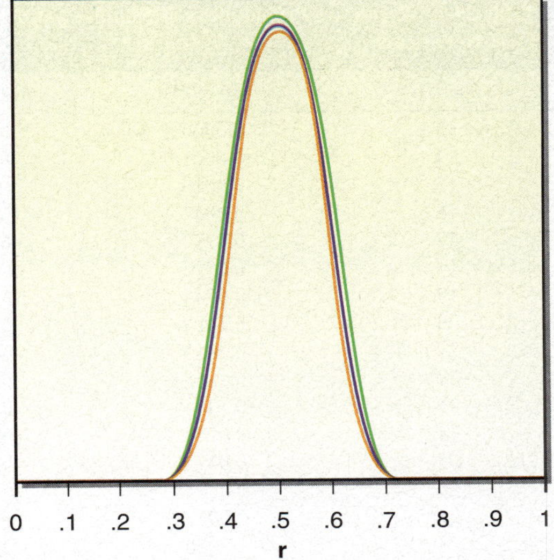

Figure 29-2 Posterior distributions for response rate r based on an experiment with 20 responses and 20 failures. The eight prior distributions considered are the eight distributions shown in Figure 29-1. Except for proportionality constants these are 1, r, $r(1-r)$, $r^2(1-r)$, $r^2(1-r)^2$, $r^3(1-r)^2$, $r^3(1-r)^3$, and $r^4(1-r)^3$. The corresponding posterior distributions are proportional to $r^{20}(1-r)^{20}$, $r^{21}(1-r)^{20}$, $r^{21}(1-r)^{21}$, $r^{22}(1-r)^{21}$, $r^{22}(1-r)^{22}$, $r^{23}(1-r)^{22}$, $r^{23}(1-r)^{23}$, and $r^{24}(1-r)^{23}$. These eight posterior distributions are very similar, demonstrating the robustness principle.

If two prior distributions are markedly different, then the robustness principle still applies, but it could take a good deal of data to bring two disparate distributions close together.

FREQUENTIST/BAYESIAN COMPARISON In the frequentist approach, hypotheses and parameters do not have probabilities. Rather, probability assignments apply only to data, with particular values assumed for any unknown parameters in calculating these probabilities. For example, the ubiquitous p-value is the probability of data as or more extreme than the observed data assuming that the null hypothesis is true. In symbols:

Frequentist p-value: $P(\text{observed or more extreme data}|H0)$

Bayesian posterior probability: $P(H0|\text{observed data})$

It is easy to confuse these two concepts. A p-value is commonly interpreted as the probability of no effect, and 1 minus the p-value as the probability of an effect. This interpretation is wrong. This is trying to have a Bayesian posterior probability without a prior probability, which is impossible.

There are two important differences between a frequentist p-value and a Bayesian posterior probability. One is the inversion of the conditions: what is assumed in the former has a probability in the latter. The second difference is that p-values include the probabilities of results other than those observed in the experiment.

As an example, consider a single-arm phase II trial for testing $H0$: $r = 0.5$ versus $H1$: $r = 0.75$. Assuming a type I error rate $\alpha = 5\%$, a sample size of $n = 33$ gives 90% power. Suppose the final results are 22 responses of 33 patients. The (frequentist) one-sided p-value is the probability of 22 *or more* responses of the 33 patients assuming the null hypothesis, $H0$: $r = 0.5$. Under this assumption the probability of observing 22, 23, 24, ... responses is 0.0225+0.0108+0.0045+ ... = 0.0401. Since this p-value is less than 5%, observing 22 responses is said to be "statistically significant."

The Bayesian measure is the posterior probability of the hypothesis that $r = 0.75$ (which is one minus the probability of $r = 0.5$) given 22 responses out of 33 trials. (As indicated above, the Bayesian calculation depends only on the probability of the data actually observed, 22 responses of 33, whereas the frequentist calculation also includes probabilities of 23, 24, etc, responses.) Using Bayes' rule:

$$P(H1|22\text{ of }33) = P(22\text{ of }33|H1)P(H1)/P(22\text{ of }33)$$

As above, the denominator follows from the law of total probability:

$$\begin{aligned} P(22\text{ of }33) &= P(22\text{ of }33|H1)P(H1) + P(22\text{ of }33|H0)P(H0) \\ &= (0.0823)(0.5) + (0.0225)(0.5) \\ &= 0.0524 \end{aligned}$$

So

$$P(H1|22\text{ of }33) = (0.0823)(0.5)/0.0524 = 0.785$$
$$P(H0|22\text{ of }33) = (0.0225)(0.5)/0.0524 = 0.215$$

The above calculation considers just two hypotheses, $r = 0.5$ and $r = 0.75$. In considering other values of r, Bayes' rule weighs them by $P(22\text{ of }33|r)$, which is called the *likelihood function* of r. The likelihood function is pictured in Figure 29-3. It indicates the degree of support for response rate r provided by the observed data. Values of r having the same likelihood are equally supported by the data. Only relative likelihoods matter. For example, conclusions about $r = 0.5$ versus 0.75 depend only on the ratio of their likelihoods, 0.0823 and 0.0225, values that are highlighted in Figure 29-3. Since 0.0823/0.0225 = 3.66, the data lend 3.66 times as much support to $r = 0.75$ as they do to $r = 0.5$.

The conclusions of the two approaches are different conceptually and numerically. In the frequentist approach the results are statistically sig-

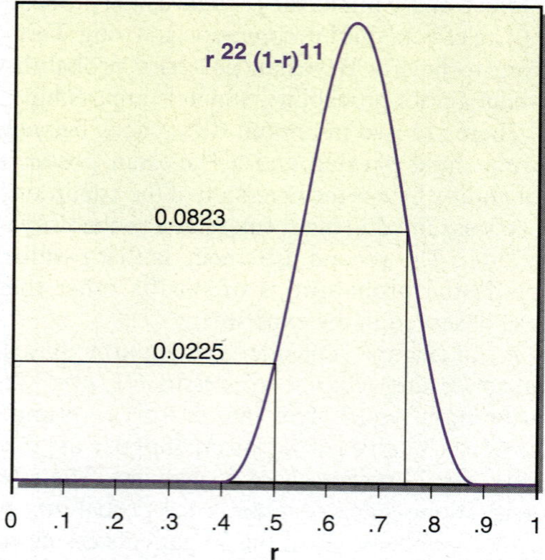

Figure 29-3 Likelihood of r for 22 responses out of 33 observations. The likelihood is $P(22 \text{ of } 33|r)$, which is proportional to $r^{22}(1-r)$.[11] The likelihoods at $r = 0.5$ and 0.75 are highlighted. These values are used in the calculational example in the text.

Table 29-1 Predictive Probabilities of Number S of Responses after 33 Patients given 13 Responses in the First 16 Patients

S (of 33)	$P(S\|r = 0.5)$	$P(S\|r = 0.75)$	$P(S)$	$P(H1)$
13	0.0000	0.0000	0.0000	0.0002
14	0.0001	0.0000	0.0000	0.0006
15	0.0010	0.0000	0.0000	0.0017
16	0.0052	0.0000	0.0002	0.0050
17	0.0182	0.0000	0.0007	0.0148
18	0.0472	0.0001	0.0019	0.0432
19	0.0944	0.0005	0.0042	0.1192
20	0.1484	0.0025	0.0082	0.2887
21	0.1855	0.0093	0.0162	0.5491
22	0.1855	0.0279	0.0341	0.7851
23	0.1484	0.0668	0.0701	0.9164
24	0.0944	0.1276	0.1263	0.9705
25	0.0472	0.1914	0.1857	0.9900
26	0.0181	0.2209	0.2129	0.9966
27	0.0052	0.1893	0.1820	0.9989
28	0.0010	0.1136	0.1091	0.9996
29	0.0001	0.0426	0.0409	0.9999
30	0.0000	0.0075	0.0072	1.0000

Columns $P(S|r = 0.5)$ and $P(S|r = 0.75)$ assume the indicated value of r in calculating the probability. Column $P(S)$ is the weighted average of the two previous columns, where the respective weights are 0.039 and 0.961. The last column gives $P(H1)$, the probability of $H1$ (r = 0.75), given S responses after 33 patients. The shaded cells are described in the text.

nificant, with p-value = .0401. Some researchers interpret statistical significance as meaning that $H0$ is unlikely to be true. That is not what it means. The Bayesian posterior probability of $H0$ addresses this question. This probability is 0.215. Although smaller than the prior probability of 0.50 because the data point somewhat more strongly to $H1$ than to $H0$, it is 5 times as large as the p-value.

Interval estimates also have different interpretations in the two approaches. In the Bayesian approach, one can find the probability that a parameter lies in any given interval. In the frequentist approach, confidence intervals have a long-run frequency interpretation for fixed and given parameters. So it is not correct to say that the probability is 95% that the parameter in question is in a 95% confidence interval. Despite the different interpretations, there is a point of agreement between the two approaches. Namely, if the prior distribution is flat (such as the left-hand panel of Figure 29-1A) then the Bayesian posterior probability of a confidence interval is essentially the same as the frequentist level of confidence. For example, if the prior distribution is flat then the Bayesian posterior probability that a parameter lies in its 95% confidence interval is in fact 95%. For prior distributions that are not flat the posterior probability of a 95% confidence interval may be greater than or less than 95%. If the historical data upon which the prior distribution is based are consistent with those from the current experiment, then the posterior probability that the parameter is in the 95% confidence interval will be greater than 95%. If the historical data are different from those in the current experiment, then the probability of the 95% confidence interval will typically be less than 95%.

PREDICTIVE PROBABILITIES

The ability to calculate the probabilities of future results is important for designing trials and for monitoring trials. The Bayesian approach allows for calculating such probabilities without assuming any particular hypothesis. For a specified experimental design, one can find the conditional probabilities of the future data for each parameter value and average them with respect to the current probabilities of the various parameter values. Predictive probabilities will be exploited extensively in this chapter.

Consider the 33-patient trial described above. Suppose that the first 16 patients have been treated, with 13 responses and three nonresponses. What will be the results after the data from the full complement of 33 patients are available? The number of responses will be between 13 and 30, but it is possible to say more. In particular, it seems most unlikely that there will be no responses in the next 17 patients after having seen 13 in the first 16 patients. And it is.

It might seem reasonable to use an estimate of r (such as the current rate, $13/16 = 0.81$) and calculate the probabilities of the results of the next 17 patients assuming this value of r, but this would be wrong. Such a calculation incorporates the uncertainty in the future data for the given r but it fails to incorporate uncertainty in r. Bayesian predictive probabilities incorporate both types of uncertainty. Table 29-1 shows the results assuming just two values of r, 0.5 and 0.75. The first column (the leftmost column) lists the possible numbers (S) of responses after 33 patients. The second and third columns show the probabilities of the possible values of S for these two values of r. The corresponding probabilities without conditioning on r are shown in the fourth column. This is a weighted average of the second and third columns. The weights are the respective probabilities of the two values of r conditional on having observed 13 responses in the first 16 patients: 0.039 for r = 0.5 and 0.961 for r = 0.75. The fourth column evinces greater variability (greater standard deviation) than either of the previous two columns. Typically, including when all values of r between 0 and 1 are considered (that is, all values have positive probability), predictive probabilities reflect greater uncertainty about future results than when conditioning on a particular value of r. (The rightmost column of Table 29-1 will be discussed in the next section.)

For convenience in this example, equal prior probabilities are assumed: $P(H1) = P(H0) = 0.5$. Although there is no vertical bar "|" in these expressions, these probabilities can depend on other available evidence, such as the results of earlier clinical and preclinical trials. There may be additional information from biological assessments, such as when considering targeted therapies. These overall conditions are taken to be understood in setting down $P(H0)$ and $P(H1)$.

Bayesian versus Frequentist Interim Analyses There are numerous commonalties and a few differences between the Bayesian and frequentist approaches. This section addresses a principal difference. In the Bayesian approach, one makes an observation and updates the probabilities of the various hypotheses. This simple process implies a degree of flexibility that is difficult to mimic in the frequentist approach.

Consider the trial design described above, with $n = 33$ patients and testing $H0$: $r = 0.5$ versus $H1$: $r = 0.75$. Observing 22 or more responses will be sufficient to reject $H0$ in favor of $H1$. However, assigning 33 patients to an experimental therapy without assessing the interim results is ethically problematic and would likely be questioned by institutional review boards. If the results are conclusive (either positive, strongly suggesting $r > 0.5$, or negative, suggesting $r \leq 0.5$) part of the way through the trial, then the trial should be stopped. Suppose, for example, that after treating 16 patients, one finds that 13 respond and three do not. From a Bayesian perspective, the updated probability of $H1$ is 96.1% (assuming prior probability $P(H0) = 0.5$).

Whether this probability is "conclusive" is not clear. The decision as to whether to continue a trial is complicated. It depends on the consequences of the trial given the current results and also given future results. In the Bayesian approach, the consequences of future results can be weighed by their predictive probabilities. For example, suppose the impact of the trial depends on whether the posterior probability of $H1$ is > 95% when the data from the full complement of 33 patients becomes available. Then one can calculate the predictive probability of this event. The rightmost column in Table 29-1 shows the posterior probability of $H1$ assuming S responses of 33 patients. The shaded values are those having $P(H1|S/16) > 95\%$. To achieve > 95% posterior probability requires at least 24 responses in the 33 patients. The predictive probability of this event is the sum of the predictive probabilities for $S \geq 24$ (the fourth column in Table 29-1), which is 0.8642. Although the current probability of $H1$ is > 95%, this characteristic will be lost with probability $1 - 0.8642 = 0.1358$. That this has moderate probability indicates the tentative nature of the current conclusion. The possibility that the current conclusion is moderately likely to change can be factored into the decision to continue the trial.

Alternatively, and mixing Bayesian and frequentist concepts, if the impact of the trial depends on achieving (one-sided) statistical significance then the Bayesian predictive probability of this event means adding the probabilities of 22 and 23 responses to 0.8642, the total being 0.9684.

If the predictive probability that the current conclusion will be maintained is sufficiently high then one may reasonably decide to stop a trial. This is true for both claims of futility and superiority. The possibility of stopping a trial early on the basis of predictive probability should be stated explicitly in the trial's protocol.

The focus of the frequentist perspective is the type I error rate, α. This is the probability of rejecting $H0$ when $H0$ is true, which depends on the trial design. For a fixed sample size of 33 patients, the calculation is straightforward. Rejecting $H0$ for ≥ 22 responses means $\alpha = 0.0401$ (see the previous section). The calculation becomes more complicated when there is a possibility of stopping the trial early. In the example, if the trial is stopped and $H0$ is rejected if there are 13 or more responses in the first 16 patients then α is increased because there is additional opportunity for rejecting $H0$. Assuming $r = 0.5$, the probability of rejecting $H0$ is now 0.0712. (The possibility that r is different from its null value plays no role in calculating the type I error rate.) Because this is greater than 0.05, the convention is to modify the stopping and rejection criteria to reduce α to about 0.05. For example, rejecting only if there are 14 responses or more out of 16 patients treated, or if there are 23 or more responses after 33 patients are treated, gives an overall type I error rate of 0.0326.

It follows that it is more difficult to draw a conclusion of statistical significance when there are interim analyses. The reason is that the type I error rates are calculated assuming that a particular hypothesis (the null hypothesis of no effect) is true. In a sense, an investigator is penalized for interim analyses in the frequentist approach. There are no such penalties for interim analyses in a Bayesian perspective. The reason is that Bayesian probabilities do not condition on any particular hypothesis.

Although it is not a Bayesian quantity, the type I error rate of any Bayesian design, however complicated, can be evaluated. If the design has interim analyses, then such a calculation incorporates appropriate penalties. This calculation is straightforward in a simple example such as that given above. In more complicated settings it can require Monte Carlo simulations. To find α via simulation in the above example, toss a fair coin 16 times. Make a tick mark if 13 or more "heads" result, and stop tossing. Otherwise, toss the coin an additional 17 times and make a tick mark if the total number of heads is 22 or more. Repeat the process thousands of times. (Program a computer to do the tossing!) Estimate α to be the number of tick marks divided by the number of times the process was simulated. Assuming that the random number generator is working properly, the proportion with tick marks will be about 7%.

ANALYSIS ISSUES

The purpose of this section is to consider two types of analysis issues. The first is an extension of the previous section. The second is unrelated to the first and deals with a particular aspect of survival analysis.

Hierarchical Modeling: Synthesizing Information When analyzing data from a clinical trial, other information is usually available about the treatment under consideration. This section deals with a method called hierarchical modeling. One of its uses is synthesizing information from different sources. The method applies in many settings, including meta-analysis and incorporating historical information. A hierarchical model is a random-effects model. In a meta-analysis, for example, one level of the experimental unit is the patient (within a trial) and the second level is the trial itself. Hierarchical models also apply for design issues such as combining results across diseases or disease subtypes and for such seemingly disparate issues as cluster randomization. Design issues for hierarchical modeling will be considered in the next section.

Reconsider the phase II trial discussed above, where 21 of 33 patients responded. The one-sided p-value is 0.08 for the null hypothesis $H0$: $r = 0.50$, and so the results are not statistically significant at the 5% level. Now consider an earlier phase I trial using the same treatment in which 15 of 20 patients responded. This information seems relevant, even if the population being treated might have been somewhat different and the trial might have been conducted at a different institution. But it is not obvious how to incorporate the information into an analysis. The frequentist approach is experiment-specific, which requires imagining that the two trials are part of some larger experiment. If one assumes that the entire set of data resulted from a single trial involving 53 patients with 36 responses, then from a frequentist perspective this would lead to a p-value of 0.0063, which is highly statistically significant. But this conclusion is wrong because the assumption is wrong, and it is not clear how to make it right.

Any Bayesian analysis that assumes that the same response rate applies in both trials would be similarly flawed. Response rate r may be reasonably expected to vary from one trial to another. Two response rates may be different even if the eligibility criteria in the two trials are the same. For one thing the eligibility criteria may be applied differently. But even if the patients accrued are apparently similar, there are differences in the use of concomitant therapy and variations in the ability to assess clinical and laboratory variables. A way to repair the analysis is to explicitly consider two values of r, say r_1 for the first trial and r_2 for the second.

Recapitulating, there are two extreme assumptions that lead to analyses that are easy to carry out, but wrong. One is to assume that r_1 and r_2 are unrelated and to base any inferences about r_2 on the results of the second trial alone. The other is to assume that $r_1 = r_2$ and combine the results in the two trials.

The two r-values may be the same or different. In a Bayesian hierarchical model, both possibilities are allowed, but neither is assumed. Namely, r_1 and r_2 are regarded as having come from a population of r-values. The population may have little variability (homogeneity) or substantial variability (heterogeneity). The observed response rates give information concerning the extent of heterogeneity, with disparate rates suggesting greater heterogeneity. When the observed rates are similar, the precision of estimates of r_1 and r_2 will be greater than when the observed rates are disparate. In the former case there will be greater "borrowing of strength" across the trials. If it happens that the results of the trials are very different, then there will be little borrowing and the information from any one trial will not apply much beyond that trial.

More generally, there may be any number of related studies or databases that provide supportive information regarding a particular therapeutic effect. The studies may be heterogeneous and may consider different patient populations. The next example is generic, but it is more complicated than the previous example because it includes nine studies.[5] The only commonalty in the studies is that all addressed the efficacy of the same therapy.

The response rates can take on any value between 0 and 1. The number S of responses and sample size n is shown for each study in Table 29-2 and in Figure 29-4. There are nine response rates,

Table 29-2 Numbers of Responses *S*, Sample Size *n*, Observed Response Proportions (Including Its Standard Error) and Adjusted Estimates of Response Rates by Study

Study No.	Responses *S*	Sample Size *n*	Observed Response Proportions (Standard Error)	Bayes Estimate (Standard Deviation)
1	11	16	0.69 (0.116)	0.69 (0.094)
2	20	20	1.00 (0.000)	0.90 (0.064)
3	4	10	0.40 (0.155)	0.53 (0.121)
4	10	19	0.53 (0.115)	0.57 (0.094)
5	5	14	0.36 (0.128)	0.48 (0.109)
6	36	46	0.78 (0.061)	0.77 (0.058)
7	9	10	0.90 (0.095)	0.80 (0.097)
8	7	9	0.78 (0.139)	0.73 (0.110)
9	4	6	0.67 (0.192)	0.68 (0.125)
Totals	106	150	0.71 (0.037)	0.68 (0.064)

The Bayes estimate column is described in the text.

r_1, r_2 up to r_9, one for each study. Each of the nine sample response proportions *S*/*n* is an estimate of the corresponding *r*. There were 106 responses among 150 patients. If all nine of the response rates are assumed to be equal then the posterior distribution of the common response rate *r* (assuming a flat prior distribution) is that shown in Figure 29-4, labeled "pooled analysis."

Even though this pooled analysis is wrong, the overall estimate of 106/150 may be quite reasonable. However, the precision associated with this estimate is too great (equivalently, its standard error is too small). In contrast, the "hierarchical analysis" curve in Figure 29-4 is a Bayesian estimate of the distribution of the response rates in the population of the studies. (This curve is the mean posterior distribution assuming a noninformative prior for the parameters in a particular class of distributions for *r*-values, called *beta distributions*.) As is typical of hierarchical analyses, this curve shows greater variability than does the analogous curve under the assumption of homogeneity.

In a hierarchical analysis, an individual study's *r* has a distribution that depends on the data from that study, but it also depends on the data from the other studies. The rightmost column in Table 29-2 shows the mean of the distribution of each study's response rate. This is also the predictive probability of the response for a future patient in that study. The individual study probabilities are shrunk toward the overall mean. This shrinkage is greater for smaller studies, and for studies with observed proportions further from the overall mean. Hierarchical borrowing is defensible because it does not make the assumption that all studies had the same true response rate, and because the extent of borrowing is determined by the data.

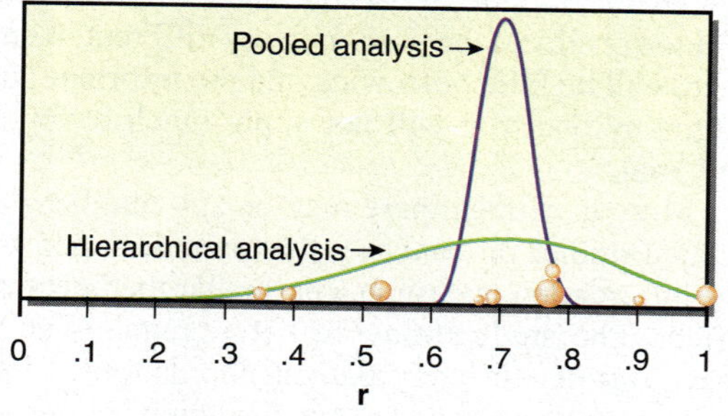

Figure 29-4 Response comparisons. The dot plot on the *r*-axis shows the observed response proportions given in Table 29-2. The areas of the dots are approximately proportional to sample sizes *n*. The pooled analysis curve shows the distribution of response rate *r* assuming no study effect. The hierarchical analysis curve shows the Bayesian estimate of the distribution of response rates allowing for heterogeneity across the various studies.

Figure 29-5 provides a pictorial comparison of the rightmost two columns in Table 29-2, demonstrating shrinkage. The Bayesian estimates are intermediate between simple pooling (complete shrinkage) and each trial standing alone. The amount of shrinkage—including the two extremes mentioned above—depends on the prior distribution of the population of trials. This aspect of the prior distribution should be set in advance, or varied to allow for assessing the sensitivity of the overall conclusion.

Shrinkage is a consequence of hierarchical modeling. The motivation for such modeling is to use the available information appropriately in improving precision or in decreasing the required sample size. Consider study number 1 in Table 29-2. Simply pooling the data from the other eight studies would greatly increase the precision of its estimated response rate. Namely, the standard error would be reduced from 0.116 to 0.037. But in view of the possibility of heterogeneity in the studies, such pooling would not be justified. Borrowing hierarchically also strengthens the conclusion, but not as much. The standard deviation of the Bayes estimate is only about 20% smaller, from 0.116 to 0.094. Although smaller than the reduction with unabashed pooling, this reduction implies that more than 50% savings in sample size is necessary to carry out a clinical trial (in the setting of study number 1 in Table 29-2) with the same precision: $(0.116/0.094)^2 - 1 = 52\%$. For example, to achieve the same standard error in a stand-alone study would require 25 as opposed to 16 patients in study number 1 of Table 29-2.

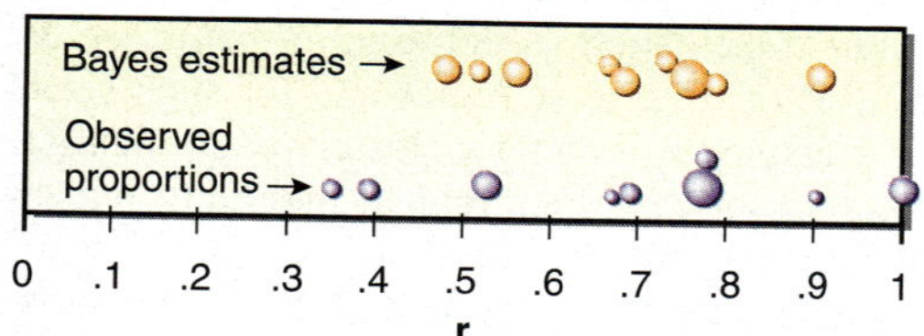

Figure 29-5 Observed response proportions compared to the adjusted response rate estimates. Values are given in the two rightmost columns in Table 29-2. The dot plot on the *r*-axis shows the observed response proportions, just as in Figure 29-4. The Bayes estimates assume a hierarchical model and show shrinkage toward the overall mean.

Patient covariates can be incorporated into a hierarchical analysis, thus adjusting for known differences in the studies but still accounting for unknown effects. In this example and in more complicated hierarchical settings as well,[6] modeling allows for borrowing from other studies and databases. If the results are consistent across studies then the amount of borrowing will be greater. If the results are sufficiently different (after accounting for covariates) then this suggests heterogeneity among the studies and there is little borrowing.

Hierarchical Modeling in Trial Design

There are many settings in which trials can be set up to borrow strength from related, but not necessarily identical, experimental units.

Consider designing a trial for a therapy for a disease that has several subtypes, such as several different histologies that exist for one type of tumor. The response rates will likely differ for the different subtypes. The setting is essentially the same as that of the previous section. Now the focus is the tumor response rate within the individual subtype. These have a distribution, just as in the previous section. Recognizing the possibility of borrowing across subtypes means greater precision for estimating each individual response rate and therefore that the sample size within each subtype can be smaller.

The extent of borrowing depends on the results, just as in the previous section. That means that the savings in terms of sample size cannot be predicted with certainty. However, this is not a problem if the interim results can be monitored. The interim results can be used to determine the precision associated with the estimates of the various response rates. (This is a special case of an adaptive sample size to be described later in this chapter.) If interim results will not be available when the decision to stop the trial must be made, then the uncertainties regarding heterogeneity across subtypes can be assessed at the trial design stage and the sample size chosen accordingly, recognizing that the eventual precisions cannot be predicted perfectly.

Hazards over Time Time-to-event analyses are ubiquitous in cancer research. There are Bayesian analogues of the frequentist survival analyses with which the reader may be familiar. And there are hierarchical Bayesian analogues in which survival curves are allowed to depend on the category of patient or to vary with the study in a meta-analysis. However, the purpose of this section is not to extend the more traditional survival models and analyses to the Bayesian setting, rather, to focus on a narrow and relatively simple aspect of survival analysis, but one that enables greater understanding of cancer and its treatment, by using data from a clinical trial, protocol 8541 of the Cancer and Leukemia Group B (CALGB).[7]

This trial considered three different dose schedules of cyclophosphamide, Adriamycin (doxorubicin), and 5-fluorouracil (CAF) in the treatment of node-positive breast cancer: high, moderate (mod), and low. These are respectively, four cycles of CAF at 600, 60, and 600 mg/m^2, six cycles at 400, 40, 400, and four cycles at 300, 30, 300. The primary endpoint was disease-free survival, which is shown in Figure 29-6 for the three dose-groups using Kaplan-Meier plots. There are no *p*-values provided for the various comparisons (high versus moderate; high versus low) because whether these are statistically significant is not material to the purpose.

Time-to-event curves such as those in Figure 29-6 are standard but they do not tell the whole story regarding any benefit of increasing dose and dose intensity. A clearer picture is contained in hazard plots over time. Hazards are the proportions of events within a particular time period as a fraction of those patients who are at risk at the beginning of the period. For example, suppose the event is recurrence and there are 100 patients in a group that are at risk in the first year. If 10 of these patients experience a recurrence of the disease in the first year, then the first-year hazard is 10%. Going into the second year there are 90 patients at risk. If another 18 experience recurrences in the second year, then the second-year hazard is 18/90 = 20%. When calculating hazards from survival plots such as those in Figure 29-6, one subtracts the current year's survival proportion from the previous year's survival proportion and divides by the previous year's survival proportion. The resulting yearly hazards are shown in Figure 29-7.

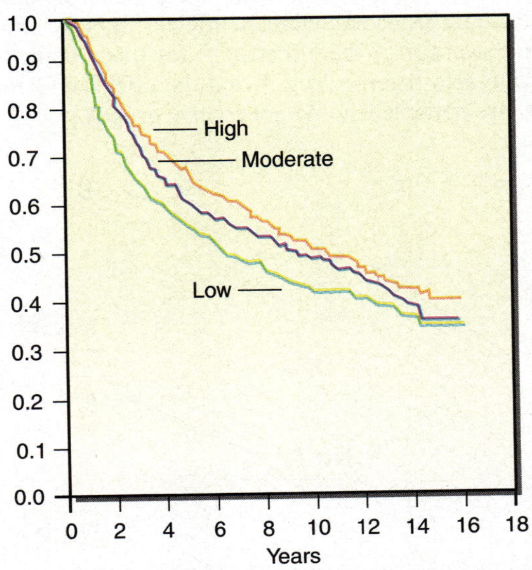

Figure 29-6 Disease-free survival proportions for the three CAF dose groups of CALGB 8541.

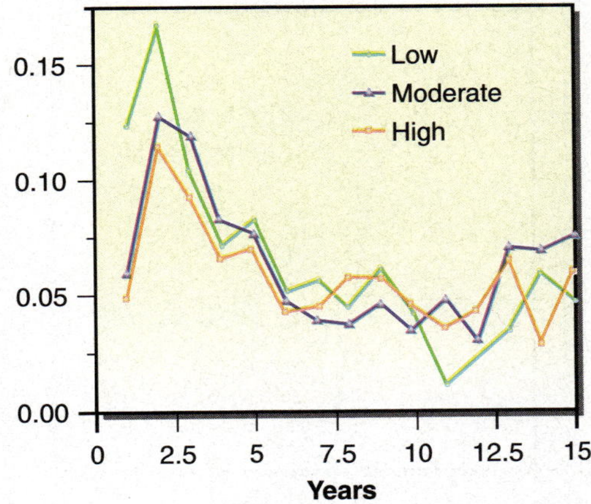

Figure 29-7 Hazards for the three CAF dose groups of CALGB 8541, Derived from Figure 29-6.

A striking observation from Figure 29-7 is that the hazards decrease over time (after the second year) for all three treatment arms. This is a reflection of the heterogeneity of the disease. The most aggressive tumors recur early, giving the high hazards evident in the first few years. Once their tumors have recurred, patients are removed from the at-risk population. The remaining tumors are less aggressive and so they recur at a lower rate.

Regarding a treatment arm effect, the apparent benefit of the high-dose schedule is restricted to the first five years or so. Actually, the hazard for patients on the high-dose schedule is lower than those of the other two arms in each of the first six years. (Although it is not much lower in the last few of these six years, and it is not much lower than the moderate-dose schedule at any time.) This observation is impressive because each year is like a new study, with previous recurrences not counted when starting a new year.

Another observation from Figure 29-7 is that after five years the risks of all three groups converge, with the annual risk of recurrence being approximately 5% in all three groups.

The reduction in hazard of recurrence for the high versus low dose schedules is 14% over the 18 years of follow-up (95% confidence interval: 6–22%). This is an average over these years (weighted over time because of the differences in at-risk sample sizes over time). But because there is no reduction at all in the later years, the overall reduction is being carried by the early years. Restricting to the first three years, the reduction is 24% (13–33%). A benefit of chemotherapy that is restricted to the first few years is typical in breast cancer trials. An implication is that a hazard reduction seen early in a trial, say one with a median of three years of follow-up, will deteriorate over time. This is because the comparison will eventually involve averaging over periods where there is no longer a treatment benefit.

In the later years, the hazards of about 5% are very similar to the annual hazard for patients with node-negative breast cancer. Interestingly, convergence to about 5% applies irrespective of the

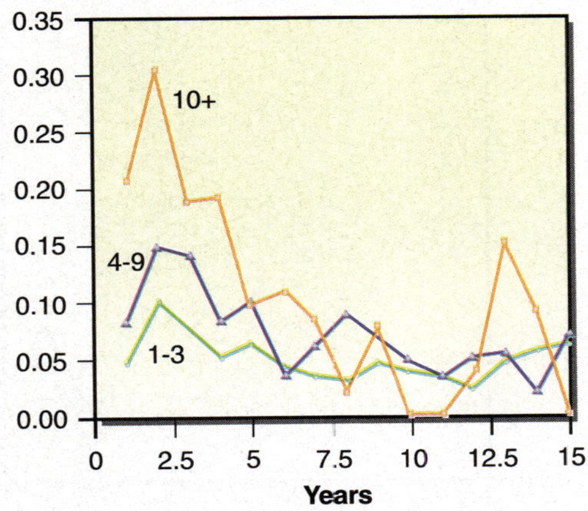

Figure 29-8 Hazards for the three categories of positive lymph nodes (1–3, 4–9, and 10 or more) for CALGB 8541. There are few patients at risk in the later years, especially in the 10+ group, and for two reasons. One is that this was the smallest group to start, with 174 of the 1,550 patients in the trial, and the other is that the disease recurred early for most in this group. The peak at 13 years indicates a point where there were only 24 patients at risk, and 3 of these had disease recurrence in the 13th year.

number of positive lymph nodes. Figure 29-8 shows this effect. It gives hazard plots for three categories of positive nodes: 1 to 3, 4 to 9, and 10 or more (for the three dose groups combined). Early in the trial, patients with 10$^+$ positive nodes have a very high annual recurrence rate of 20 to 30%. However, after five years or so, the annual hazard is about 5% in all three groups. So, a woman with a large number of positive nodes who has not experienced disease recurrence in the first five years or so has the same updated prognosis as a woman with a small number of positive nodes, including no positive nodes. The effects of both the number of positive nodes and dose of CAF have worn off after five years.

An important aspect of CALGB 8541 is the role of tumor HER2/neu expression, and in particular its interaction with the dose of CAF.[8] HER2/neu assessment was carried out for a subset of 992 patients from the original study. Its interaction with dose was shown to be significant in a multivariate proportional hazards model. But the manner of interaction is easiest to understand using hazards. Figure 29-9 shows the effect of dose of CAF separately for patients with HER2/neu–negative (n = 720) and HER2/neu–positive (n = 272) tumors. HER2/neu negative tumors (in the left-hand panel of Figure 29-9) show no dose effect. The entire benefit of the high- over the moderate-dose treatment schedule, and the high- over the low-dose treatment schedule that is observed in these patients is concentrated in those with HER2/neu positive tumors. Moreover, this benefit occurs through a reduction in hazard in each of the first three to four years. Again, each year is a separate study and so each of these years provides a separate confirmation of the overall conclusion. The hazard reduction in the first three years for patients receiving the high-dose treatment schedule, as compared with the other two

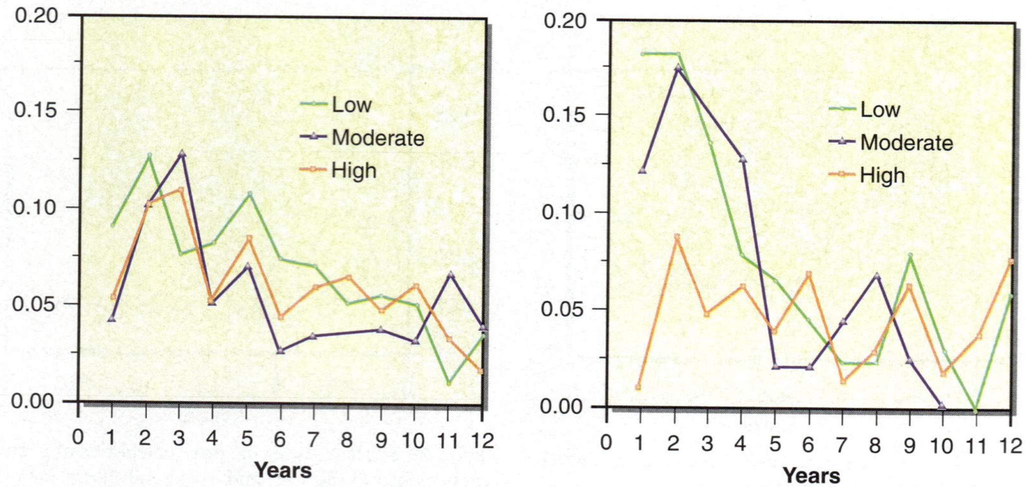

Figure 29-9 Annual disease-free survival hazards for a subset of patients ($n = 992$) in CALGB. The subset consists of patients for whom the expression of HER-2/neu in the patient's tumor was assessed. The left-hand panel represents patients with HER-2/neu–negative tumors and the right-hand panel patients with HER-2/neu–positive tumors.

groups combined, was 65% among patients with HER2/neu–positive tumors. HER2/neu overexpression apparently conveys a poor prognosis for lower doses but not for higher doses—it might even provide a favorable prognosis for patients receiving higher doses.

Many of the conclusions in this section would have been difficult or impossible to make without considering hazards over time.

A final comment regarding hazards relates to the common problem of predicting survival results into the future for patients already accrued to a trial. This differs from the general problem of prediction discussed earlier in "Predictive Probabilities." Consider Figure 29-6. Some of the patients have as little as 10 years of follow-up information. As more follow-up information becomes available, there will be no change in these curves prior to the 10-year time point. But the curves are subject to change beyond 10 years. Because the focus is on patients for whom the tumor has not yet recurred, the way the curves will change depends on the hazards beyond 10 years. The information available about these hazards is shown in Figure 29-7. For predicting when and whether a patient's disease will recur, consider hazards one year at a time, always building on her current year of follow-up. Each incremental hazard prediction depends on the data for the corresponding year.

PRINCIPLES OF STATISTICAL DESIGN: FACTORIAL EXPERIMENTS

Most comparative drug trials in oncology have two treatment arms. Typically, one uses an experimental agent and the other does not. The patients in both arms may receive additional therapy based on the current standard of care for the type and stage of their cancer, and on their prior treatment. They may have surgery and receive concomitant radiation and other chemotherapy, which may include several drugs. If the experimental drug is shown to be sufficiently effective, then it will be incorporated into the standard therapy.

This approach is simple and clean. It is sometimes called KISS: "Keep it simple, stupid." But it has a number of drawbacks. One is that it is not possible to assess the individual contributions of the various components of polychemotherapy that are developed in this way. Another is that the approach provides a mechanism for adding drugs to standard regimens but not for subtracting them. An experimental agent's effectiveness may require all other components of the standard regimen. Adding an experimental drug to a standard regimen, however, may make other components of the regimen unnecessary. In the latter case, there is no way of knowing which components these are.

To some extent this conundrum is inevitable. Studying the possible removal of a component of standard chemotherapy is difficult, and for ethical reasons this is so even if the component has never been proven to contribute to the overall effectiveness of the combination. However, better approaches for developing drugs would alleviate the problem and could lead to more rapid development of better therapies.

At any given time, various experimental agents are being studied by different clinical trial groups, in most cases by adding them to therapy that is standard for the disease in question. One group may be studying drug A and another drug B. If both are shown to be effective it will not be clear which is better and whether the combination of drugs A and B would prove better than, just as good as, or worse than using only one of the drugs.

A fundamental principle of optimal experimental design in statistics is in stark contrast with KISS: Change the various contributing factors in such a way as to learn efficiently about their impact on outcome. This impact may involve interactions between the factors and it is important to learn about such interactions. What is required is to model relationships and exploit the available data to inform the model. From the perspective of optimal design, the KISS principle more appropriately stands for "Keep it simple AND stupid."

An alternative to varying one factor at a time in separate studies is using factorial designs. In the simplest example considered above, patients would be assigned to one of four regimens: A alone, B alone, A and B in combination, and neither. (The last of these does not mean "no therapy" since all patients receive standard therapy.) These four possibilities are shown schematically in Figure 29-10 where "A" means that the patient receives A and "No A" means the patient does not receive A. The factors may be drugs, or other interventions (eg, "A" could be radiation therapy, or surgery before rather than after chemotherapy, or a high dose as opposed to a low dose of a drug). Reading from left to right in Figure 29-10 may not indicate time. The two drugs may be given concurrently or sequentially, A before B or B before A. Indeed, sequential vs. concurrent administration of drugs could be another factor in a factorial design (see Citron and colleagues[9] for example).

An advantage of factorial designs is that they enable estimating the "main effects" of the individual drugs and therefore a single trial answers two (or more) questions. Another advantage is that factorial designs allow for assessing interactions between the factors. For example, comparing the difference between the top two cases in Figure 29-10 with the difference between the bottom two cases addresses whether the effect of B is the same when it is given with drug A as when it is given without drug A. Table 29-3 shows the types of interactions that are possible for the four combinations of drugs A and B considered in Figure 29-10, assuming that the endpoint is response rate. For negative interactions, the effect of the combination is less than the sum of the individual drug effects. For positive interactions, the effect of the combination is greater than the sum of the individual drug effects.

There are no compensating disadvantages to using factorial designs! In particular, the sample size is no greater than for a two-armed design that addresses the effect of just one of the two drugs. Each patient contributes equally to estimating the main effects of both factors. For example, assuming equal sample sizes in the four possible combinations, the estimated main effect of B is the simple average of the effect of B for those patients who also receive drug A and the effect of B for those patients who do not receive drug A.

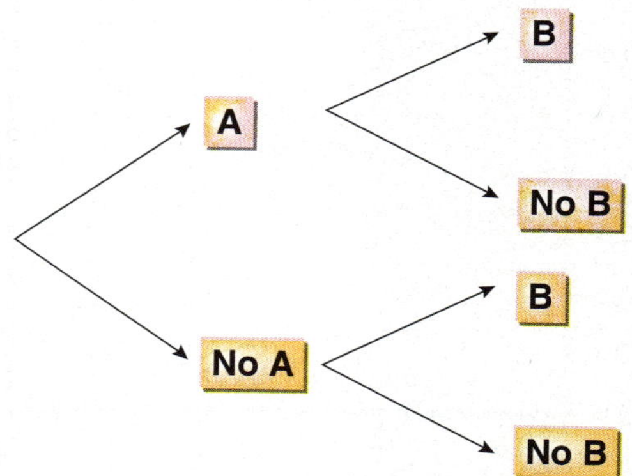

Figure 29-10 A 2×2 factorial design considering drugs A and B and their combination. There are 4 possible treatment combinations.

Table 29-3 Response Rates (%) for the Four Treatment Combinations in a Factorial Design in Which Drugs A and B Are Added to Standard Therapy (Hypothetical Effects)

Treatment Combination	Neither Effective	A Effective B Not	B Effective A Not	Additive Effects	Negative Interaction	Positive Interaction (Example i)	Positive Interaction (Example ii)
A and B	20	30	30	40	30	50	40
A, No B	20	30	20	30	30	30	20
B, No A	20	20	30	30	30	30	20
Neither	20	20	20	20	20	20	20

A limitation of using factorial designs is that some treatment combinations may not be ethically or practically possible. For example, one of the combinations in Figure 29-10 is neither of the two drugs. In some oncology settings it may not be possible to have such a treatment arm. Including only three arms in the trial is better than having only two, but then individual drug effects cannot be assessed and the sample size advantages of the factorial design are lost.

When a two-armed trial is designed to have a particular power, a second factor can be added without increasing the sample size. The power for assessing the interaction between the factors is not as great as for assessing a main effect, but there will be some information about interactions. The sample size can be increased if high power for assessing an interaction is required, but a reasonable and usually a more realistic alternative is to keep the sample size the same and accept modest power for assessing interactions. It may happen that the interaction is strong enough to show statistical significance. Moreover, any interaction that is clinically important is likely to show at least a hint of an interaction in the trial's results and this may lead to a follow-on trial to better quantify the degree of interaction.

Learning about interactions is essential, both clinically and scientifically, and interactions cannot be identified from a single two-armed trial. At best, three separate, two-armed trials would be required, and the likelihood of their being completed is not high. For example, one trial could compare A with No A, a second could compare B with No B, and a third could compare the combination with A alone. There are several disadvantages of this approach relative to factorial designs: (1) The total sample size is three times as large; (2) the third trial may not be possible if both single-agent trials turn out to be effective as single agents; (3) neither drug may be effective on its own but the combination may be effective; and (4) outcomes of clinical trials are heterogeneous, even if they employ the same patient eligibility criteria. Therefore, treatment effects would be confounded with any trial effects. Possibility (3), that only in combination are the two drugs effective, could happen in a variety of ways, one of which is when the two drugs target different but parallel metastatic pathways. In this circumstance (represented in the rightmost column in Table 29-3), both drugs would fail their respective two-armed trials and be abandoned, with the effectiveness of the combination never discovered.

Factorial designs can consider more than two factors and more than two levels per factor. For example, Henderson and colleagues[10] considered three dose schedules of doxorubicin and paclitaxel versus no paclitaxel in node-positive breast cancer using a 3 × 2 factorial design. This trial was noteworthy in answering two important clinical questions: increasing the dose of doxorubicin (in combination with 600 ng/m^2 of cyclophosphamide) from 60 to 75 to 90 ng/m^2 in four q3week cycles did not improve either disease-free or overall survival, and adding four q3-week cycles of paclitaxel (75 ng/m^2) did improve both. Moreover, it answered a third question because there was not a hint of an interaction between the two factors.

Figure 29-11 shows a somewhat more complicated example, a 2 × 2 × 3 factorial design. Now there are three doses of drug C. (An application would be a modification of the aforementioned trial reported by Henderson and colleagues[10] in which cyclophosphamide would have been used at two doses. A could be paclitaxel, B would then be cyclophosphamide, and C would be doxorubicin.) Again, data from every patient contributes to estimating the main effects of A, B, and C separately and so there is no increase in sample size. Estimating three-way interactions have less power than estimating two-way interactions, but the results from the factorial design in Figure 29-11 will contain some information about the three-way interaction of drugs A, B, and C.

Factorial designs apply in both phases II and III. In phase II they are especially relevant in proof-of-concept trials involving multiple investigational agents. Such trials may involve many drugs, and many more possible combinations of the drugs. The number of drugs and their combinations may be so large that a balanced factorial design is not tenable. A modification is to use an adaptive randomization scheme, as discussed in a subsequent section of this chapter. The efficacy and toxicity of the various combinations could be explored using unbalanced assignments, favoring combinations that the accumulating data suggest are promising. If it turns out that one of the drugs is ineffective, whether used with or without the other drugs, it would then be dropped.

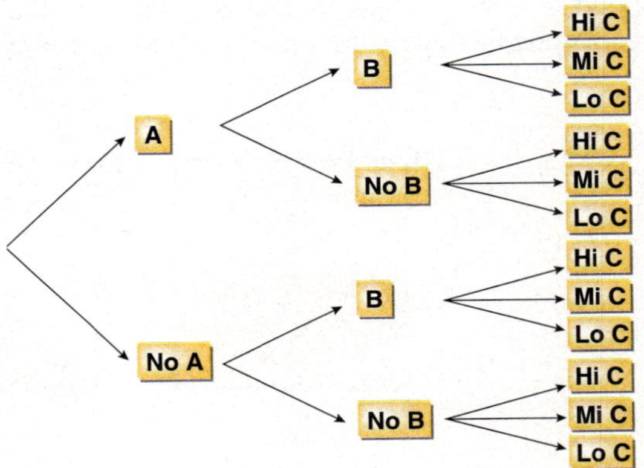

Figure 29-11 A 2×2×3 factorial design considering drugs A and B, Three levels of drug C, and their combinations. There are 12 possible treatment combinations.

In many oncology drug settings, toxicity is as important as efficacy. There are ways to incorporate them both in a factorial design. For example, one can establish the notion of *admissible combinations* based on toxicity. This involves allowing only certain of the full factorial combinations at the start of the trial. As experience accrues about toxicity, other combinations become admissible, or the number of admissible combinations shrinks. The assignment to treatment combinations within the set of admissible combinations can be made either randomly or adaptively based on accumulating information about efficacy (see below).

DECISION ANALYSIS AND CHOOSING SAMPLE SIZE

Clinical practice and clinical research involve making decisions. An example of the latter is choosing the sample size of a clinical trial. It is impossible to precisely predict the result of making a particular decision, but one can list the possible results and associate (predictive) probabilities with each of the possibilities. Also associated with each possible result are the consequences of that result. A list of results, probabilities, and consequences characterizes each decision, and allows for choosing one decision over another.

The consequences of a particular decision are many faceted. Consider the case in which consequences are unidimensional, and numerical. A particular "number" can always be assigned to a consequence, at least in theory. A numerical assignment that indicates the overall worth or benefit of a consequence is called its utility. The decision analytic approach is to average the utilities with respect to the associated predictive probabilities. The resulting average is the utility of the decision in question, and the various possible decisions can be compared on the basis of their utilities. The central role of predictive probabilities in this process makes the Bayesian approach ideally suited for decision making.

The terms decision making, decision analysis, and decision theory are used more or less interchangeably. Many references develop this subject more deeply than is possible to report here.[11–14]

A simple example will help fix the concept. One is offered an opportunity to win a prize that has a utility of 10. The utility of playing for the prize is –1. There are two decisions: play or not play. If one plays, then he will end up with a utility of either 9 or −1. Suppose that the probability of the former is r. (A class of decisions not considered here, performing an experiment to get information about r, is interesting and revealing.) The utility of playing is then $9r - (1-r) = 10r - 1$. The utility of not playing is 0. Playing is optimal if $r > 0.1$.

Averaging utilities to assess taking gambles is well and good. But it is less clear that it is appropriate when outcomes are health states or the results of clinical trials. Moreover, it may be difficult to assess the utilities of such outcomes. However, one must make a decision, and when faced with a list of outcomes and their associated probabilities for each available decision, reducing the lists to a single dimension greatly facilitates choosing among them. In addition, varying the probabilities and utilities assumed allows for assessing the sensitivity of the various aspects of the decision process.

Consider a decision-analytic approach for choosing a sample size in a two-armed clinical trial. The purpose of clinical trials is to learn about competing therapies. The benefit of learning about competing therapies is that it may affect the future treatment of patients having the disease in question. In a decision analysis one can consider delivering good medicine to all patients who have the disease. The utility of any particular design of a clinical trial is its consequent effect on patients who have the disease, including the patients in the trial as well as those outside the trial. This approach contrasts with the stark attitude of the Belmont Report[1] in which the knowledge derived from treating patients in the trial is distinguished from the treatment of patients who present after the trial.

Consider the patients who will benefit from the conclusions of the clinical trials being planned. Call this the "patient horizon" N. Its numerical value depends on the prevalence of the disease and the availability of alternative treatments. The population of patients with primary breast cancer who might benefit from an advance in therapy is very large. But N is small in a rare type of children's cancer. Experimentation has a greater value when N is large, whereas treating the current patients more effectively has a greater value when N is small. Therefore, these two extremes have different sample size implications. However, they are addressed in the same way when choosing sample sizes via power calculations. In the case of a small N, a substantial portion of the patients, perhaps all, may be in the clinical trial and so few if any subsequent patients will get to take advantage of the results obtained in the trial. In the case of a large N, a trial may be too small to enable an informed choice between the two treatments and so the very large number of patients outside the trial may receive inferior therapy. A conclusion of this section is that when the goal is treating as many patients as effectively as possible, the sample sizes of the clinical trials depend greatly on the magnitude of N.

The value of N is not usually precisely known. In particular, N depends on the effectiveness and side effects of both treatments, which are also unknown. However, a consequence of this section is that only the order of magnitude of N should be considered in choosing the sample sizes of clinical trials. Precision in fixing N is not very important. Considering the extremes, diseases or conditions that are very common (large N), call for larger trials than do rare diseases (small N). Moreover, when N is unknown, the results of this section rely on replacing N with its mean. So experts could assess the annual size of the patient population and the potential availability of other therapies over the next several years. Patients presenting in the future could be discounted by the probability that they will be treated using one of the treatments involved in the trial. This gives an expected value of N that can be used in designing the trial.

Table 29-4 Optimal Sample Sizes of a Clinical Trial when the Patient Horizon is N

Patient Horizon, N	1,000,000	100,000	10,000	1,000	100
Single trial sample size	1000	320	100	32	10
Sample size for the first of two trials	170	78	36	17	8

Sample sizes are given with two-digit accuracy. The optimal sample sizes for N = 1,000,000 are for a particular prior distribution of the unknown parameters. The ratios of optimal sample sizes within each row apply for arbitrary prior distributions. For example, if the optimal single-trial sample size for N = 1,000,000 were 2000 then that for N = 100 would be 20.

For convenience, consider dichotomous outcomes: response and non-response. The goal is to treat as many of the N patients as successfully as possible with one of two therapies. The utility of any trial is the number of responses over the patient horizon (including both those in the trial and those beyond). An optimal sample size maximizes the expected number of responses over the patient horizon N. By definition, patients in the horizon are those who present after the trial and who are given the therapy that performed better in the trial.

The optimal trial sample size has an order of magnitude the square root of N.[15] If there are two clinical trials (followed by implementation of the better performing therapy in clinical practice), then the first of the two should have a sample size with an order of magnitude the cube root of N. Table 29-4 considers a setting in which the optimal trial sample size for a common disease with N of about one million turns out to be 1,000. The point of Table 29-4 is to compare this with the corresponding optimal sample sizes for more rare diseases. The table also shows the optimal sample size for the first of two clinical trials. The sample sizes are strikingly different for common versus uncommon diseases.

In a decision analysis one can explicitly consider asymmetry in information concerning the treatment arms under consideration. The allocation proportions should also be asymmetric. As above, continue to assume a two-armed trial with the goal being to effectively treat as many patients in horizon N as possible. Consider the particular forms of prior information about the unknown rates of response that are shown in Figure 29-12. Suppose the response rate for one of the arms, say arm 1, has distribution A and that for the other arm, arm 2, has either distribution A, B, or C.

Consider N = 100 or greater, as indicated in Table 29-5. The table shows the optimal sample sizes for each of the arms. As discussed above, these increase with N in proportion to the square root of N (approximately). Consider the case of N = 1,000 and distribution A for both response rates. The table indicates that 21 patients should be assigned to one of the arms and 20 to the other. In view of symmetry, either arm 1 or arm 2 could get the extra patient. Using this assignment, the resulting response proportion among the 1,000 patients in the horizon is 65%. Increasing either or both sample sizes decreases this response proportion. And decreasing either or both sample sizes decreases this response proportion. To consider the extremes, both not running a clinical trial at all and running a trial entering all 1,000 patients have expected response proportions of 50%.

For the case distribution A versus B in Table 29-5, arm 2 is more promising than arm 1 and so it is assigned to more patients in the trial—about $\sqrt{3} - 1 = 73\%$ more for a large N. For distribution A versus C, the response rate for arm 2 is known to be 0.5. The response rate for arm 1 could be greater than 0.5 or less than 0.5. The trial's pur-

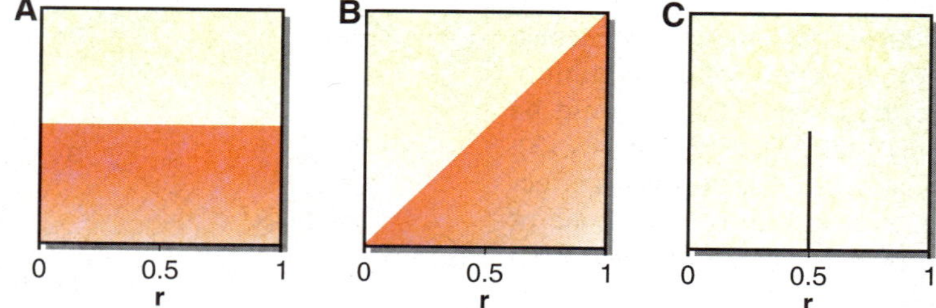

Figure 29-12 Three different prior distributions for r, the rate of response. Under distribution A, r is equally likely to be any value between 0 and 1. The density in B is proportional to r, which means, for example, that r greater than 0.5 is three times as probable as r less than 0.5. (These two distributions are the same as the two in Figure 29-1A.) Under distribution C, all the probability is concentrated on r = 0.5 and so in this case the arm's effectiveness is assumed to be known.

Table 29-5 Optimal Allocations of Sample Size to Arms 1 and 2 in a Two-Armed Clinical Trial plus Response Proportion among the N Patients for That Allocation

Patient	Prior Distributions of Rates from Figure 29-12; Optimal Success Proportion								
Horizon, N	1: A	2: A	Prop	1: A	2: B	Prop	1: A	2: C	Prop
100	6	5	0.63	4	8	0.71	9	0	0.60
1,000	21	20	0.65	16	30	0.74	29	0	0.62
10,000	70	69	0.66	56	98	0.75	99	0	0.62
Large N	$\sqrt{N/2}$	$\sqrt{N/2}$	2/3	$\sqrt{N/3}$	$\sqrt{N}$	3/4	$\sqrt{N}$	0	5/8

For each value of N there are three pairings of prior distributions of the arm 1 and arm 2 response rates considered. The optimal asymptotic (large N) response proportion is the expected value of the maximum of the two response rates, where the expectation is with respect to the prior distribution.

Prop = response proportion.

pose—in addition to treating patients effectively—is to identify whether the arm 1 response rate is greater than or less than 0.5. To achieve this purpose it would be a waste to allocate patients to arm 2 because its response rate is known. Arm 2 is held in reserve and will be used after the trial should it turn out that arm 1's observed response rate is less than 0.5.

This section assumes no interim monitoring. There could be a substantial benefit in response rate achieved if updating is possible during the trial. Such updating could be used to modify the proportions of patients allocated to the two arms, and it could be used to determine when the clinical trial should end. These possibilities and other related modifications are considered in the next section. However, the next section is not explicitly decision analytic, and in particular it does not address maximizing the overall response proportion in choosing a clinical trial design.

ADAPTIVE DESIGNS OF CLINICAL TRIALS

The first step in planning a trial is to assess the available evidence regarding the hypotheses and parameters of interest. In a Bayesian approach, the trial designer addresses the possibility of using this information in a prior distribution or incorporating it in a hierarchical model along with the results of the trial being planned.

At the planning stage it is important to consider the possible state of affairs when the trial is over. One consideration is the set of implications and consequences of each possible result. Another is the predictive probability of each possible result. The previous section presents an approach in which utilities are assessed for the former and weighed with respect to the latter. The present section deals with designs that are more flexible than the ones in the previous section. Although the designs in this section are not based on an explicit consideration of utilities, the goals are efficient learning and effective treatment of patients. For an explicit decision-analytic generalization of some parts of this section, see *Bandit Problems: Sequential Allocation of Experiments*.[16]

Consider a trial having a particular design. Calculating the predictive probabilities of the trial's results is always possible, even for the most complicated of designs (although the most complicated designs require simulations). These calculations allow for finding a variety of the design's attributes, including the probability of achieving a statistically significant benefit of one therapy over another, the expected number of patients in the trial, and the expected number of patients in the trial who successfully respond to their assigned treatment. Comparing the calculations for different designs facilitates choosing one design over another.

Designs of clinical trials are usually static in the sense that the sample size and any prescription for assigning treatment, including for randomization protocols, are fixed in advance. Results observed during the trial are not used to guide its course. There are exceptions. Some phase II cancer trials have two stages, with stopping after the first stage possible if the results are not sufficiently promising. And most phase III protocols specify interim analyses that determine whether the trial should be stopped early for sufficiently strong evidence of a difference between competing treatment arms. However, traditional early stopping criteria are very conservative and so few trials stop early.

The simplicity of trials with static designs makes them solid inferential tools. Their sample sizes tend to be large, at least in comparison with the alternatives to be discussed in this section. And they usually consider two therapeutic strategies, or arms, thus enabling straightforward treatment comparisons. That is not to say that static trials always give clear answers as to whether one arm is better than the other, but only that they usually allow for an unambiguous quantification of the uncertainty regarding whether one arm is better.

Despite their virtues, static trials result in slow and unnecessarily costly drug development. Hundreds of millions of dollars and many years can be expended in developing a single cancer drug, one that may not make it to market. For a company developing a moderate number of drugs (say 20 or more), this circumstance is tolerated because costs are balanced by profits from other drugs. Smaller companies are at the mercy of the prevailing attitudes toward drug development and risk going bankrupt.

The tradition of drug development is one at a time. The number of cancer drugs available for development is increasing exponentially. It is inefficient to focus on a single drug whereas myriad others are sitting on the sidelines waiting to be evaluated. The standard types of errors in drug development are false positives and false negatives. These errors apply to drugs actually being tested. Another kind of error applies to drugs not under investigation: Every such drug is a false neutral. A drug not being developed has no chance of helping anyone. Finite resources limit the ability of the medical establishment to develop therapies. But when resources are limited we should approach their allocation in a more rational way. And what makes sense today may well be different from the ways of the past.

Pharmaceutical companies and medical researchers generally must be able to consider hundreds or thousands of drugs for development at the same time. Static trials inhibit the simultaneous processing of many drugs. And they cannot efficiently address dose-response questions when many drugs are under consideration. Dynamic designs that are integrated with the drug development process are necessary for reasonable progress in medical research.

The focus of this section is a family of designs that are dynamic in the sense that observations made during the trial can affect the subsequent course of the trial. The general class of designs is adaptive or sequential. The focus is clinical trials, but the ideas apply at least as forcefully in the preclinical setting. A main bottleneck of the drug development process occurs at the level of the preclinical animal toxicity/carcinogenicity studies. There are many opportunities for using adaptive designs in the preclinical area that will efficiently identify the best drugs to move forward in trials for humans.

Using an adaptive design means examining the accumulating data periodically, or even continually, with the goal of modifying the trial's design. These modifications depend on what the data show about the unknown hypotheses. Among the modifications possible are stopping early, restricting eligibility criteria, expanding accrual to additional sites, extending accrual beyond the trial's original sample size if its conclusion is still not clear, dropping arms or doses, and adding arms or doses. All of these possibilities are considered in the light of the accumulating information. Adaptive designs also include unbalanced randomization where the degree of imbalance depends on the accumulating data. For example, arms that give more information about the hypothesis in question or that are performing better than other arms can be weighted more heavily.[16]

Adaptation is not limited to the data accumulating in the trial. Information that is reported from other ongoing trials can also be used. This is easier to effect if one takes a Bayesian approach, possibly using hierarchical modeling as described in the previous section.

Adaptive designs are increasingly being used in cancer trials. This is true for trials sponsored by pharmaceutical companies, and more generally. For example, a variety of trials at The University of Texas M. D. Anderson Cancer Center (MDACC) are prospectively adaptive, as described below.

Continuous Reassessment Method (CRM) in Phase I Trials The purpose of phase I cancer trials is to identify the maximum tolerated dose (MTD). The most commonly used phase I designs are variants of the so-called "3 + 3" design. Patients are admitted in groups of three. If none of the three patients experiences toxicity then the dose is increased one level for the next group of three. If two or three of the three patients experience toxicity then the next lower dose is the MTD. If one of the three experiences toxicity then three more patients are added at the same dose level. If two or more of the six patients at that dose experience toxicity then again the next lower dose is the MTD.[17]

This design is adaptive, but its adaptation is very crude. Such a design is likely to assign low doses and to select an MTD that is ineffective. Moreover, such a design ignores important information that is available in the trial. In particular, dose assignments are not based on sufficient statistics.[18] An alternative approach uses Bayesian updating: the continual reassessment method (CRM) of O'Quigley and colleagues.[19] In this method, updating takes place assuming a particular model of the relationship between dose and toxicity (such as the logistic function). The CRM too is adaptive. Each patient is assigned to the dose having the probability of toxicity closest to some predetermined target value. This is the Bayesian posterior probability calculated from the data available up to that point (and so it is based on sufficient statistics).

The CRM more effectively finds the MTD than does the 3 + 3 design. The CRM is the standard design used in phase I trials at MDACC. But it is rather crude and is being improved in a number of ways. One of these ways is based on the fundamental principle that ignoring information is wrong. (A catch, of course, is that taking information into account is work, and it can require modeling.) There is some information that accrues about efficacy in a phase I trial. This information is limited, especially regarding the dose-efficacy relationship. But at a minimum, in proceeding to phase II with a particular dose (usually the MTD), one should use the efficacy information from those patients in phase I who were assigned to that dose. This notion leads to using a phase I/II design that addresses safety and efficacy simultaneously, or one that focuses on efficacy after an initial focus on toxicity. Such an approach is efficient from the perspective of both time and patient resources.

A way in which both 3 + 3 and CRM designs are crude is the need to pause the accrual while waiting for toxicity information.[20,21] Such pauses are inefficient and they cause logistical problems. Trials should be paused or stopped if there are safety concerns, not because the design cannot get out of its own way. In getting information about toxicity (or efficacy), there is seldom a magical dose that the next patient must get. All doses are potentially informative. Rather than stopping, one should use a design that models dose response (toxicity and efficacy) and is able to assign a next dose even though patients previously treated are not yet fully evaluable.

Another way in which both 3 + 3 and CRM designs are crude is the assumption that toxicity is dichotomous. An approach that is better—again because of using all available information—would be to account for the severity of toxicity. Again, it would be better to consider both the severity of toxicity and the efficacy in a phase I/II design.[22] Assigning utilities to the various possible health states would lead to weighing these two conflicting desiderata in a decision analysis.

Adaptive Dose-finding in Phase II Trials In many diseases, the standard phase II dose-finding design is to allocate a fixed number of patients to each of a number of doses in a grid. Such questions are generally of less interest in cancer because of the MTD mentality: administer as much drug as the patient can tolerate. But with the increasing interest in biological agents, dose finding for efficacy is becoming important in cancer research.

After seeing the results of a dose-finding trial, the investigators usually wish they had assigned patients in some other fashion. Perhaps the dose-response curve was shifted more to the left or right than anticipated. If so, then the assignment of a bulk of the patients on one end or the other was wasted. Or perhaps the slope of the dose-response curve is greater than anticipated and the response of patients assigned to the flat regions of the curve would have been more informative if the doses assigned had been in the region where the slope is apparently greatest. Or perhaps the results for the early patients made it clear that the dose-response curve was flat over the entire range and therefore the trial could have stopped earlier. Or perhaps the results of the trial show that the standard deviation of the outcome of interest is greater or less than anticipated and so the trial should have been larger or could have been smaller.

The approach of Berry and colleagues[23] is to proceed sequentially, analyzing the data as it accumulates (see also the approach of Malakoff[24]). There are two stages of the trial, first dose ranging (phase II) and then confirmatory (phase III), if the latter is warranted. The dose-ranging stage continues until a decision is made that the drug is not sufficiently effective to pursue future development or that the optimal dose for the confirmatory phase III trial is sufficiently well known. (Switches to phase III can be effected seamlessly and without stopping accrual, and this is so even if the endpoint of interest is delayed, such as time to progression. See below.) The example trial of Berry and colleagues[23] involves a biological neuroprotective agent for stroke. But the same principles of trial design apply in cancer research. Each patient entering the trial is assigned the dose (one of 16, including a placebo) that maximizes the information about the dose-response relationship, given the results observed so far. This dose could be in the region of the greatest apparent slope, or it could be the placebo or a high dose. But future patients are not assigned to doses in any region where accumulating evidence suggests that the dose-response curve is flat.

In the dose-ranging stage, neither the number of patients assigned to any particular dose nor the total number of patients assigned in this stage are fixed in advance. The dose-ranging sample size will be large when the data suggest that the drug has moderate benefit, when the dose-response curve is gently sloping, or when the standard deviation of the responses is moderately large. It will tend to be small if the drug has substantial benefit, if the drug has no benefit, if the dose-response curve rises over a narrow range of doses, or if the standard deviation of the responses turns out to be small. (In addition, and somewhat nonintuitively, the dose-ranging stage will be small if the standard deviation of the responses is very large. The reason is that a sufficiently large standard deviation means that a very large sample size would be required to demonstrate a beneficial drug effect. The required sample size may be so large that it would be impossible to study the drug and so the trial stops in the dose-ranging phase before substantial resources go down the drain.)

In the stroke trial considered by Berry and colleagues,[23] the ultimate endpoint is an improvement in the stroke scale from baseline to 13 weeks. If the accrual rate is large then the benefit of adaptive assignment can be limited by delays in obtaining the endpoint information. To minimize the effects of delayed information, each patient's stroke scale is assessed weekly between baseline and week 13. Within-patient measurements are correlated, with correlations greater if they are closer together in time. We incorporate a longitudinal model into the analysis of the trial and carry out Bayesian predictions of the ultimate endpoint based on the current patient-specific information, and we update the probability distributions of the treatment effect accordingly.

Adaptive dosing is more effective than is the standard design at identifying the right dose. And it usually identifies the right dose with a smaller sample size than when using fixed dose assignments. Another advantage is that many more doses can be considered in an adaptive design. (Even though some doses will be little used and some may never be used, these cannot be predicted in advance.) An adaptive design therefore has some ability to distinguish responses at adjacent doses and to estimate the nuances of the dose-response curve.

The circumstances of the stroke trial are similar to those in many other types of trials. Finding the right dose is a ubiquitous problem in pharmaceutical development, and it is seldom done well or efficiently. The adaptive nature of the stroke trial would be less advantageous if we had not exploited early endpoints. Cancer, too, is characterized by the availability of information about a patient's performance (local control of the disease, biomarkers, etc.) before reaching the primary endpoint. Finally, the possibility of moving seamlessly into phase III depending on the phase II results exists for many types of drugs. That issue leads naturally to the subject of the next section.

Seamless Phases II and III The convention of categorizing drug development into phases is unfortunate. We proceed from one phase to the next when we think we know something: the MTD from phase I, or that a drug's impact on a phase II endpoint will translate into a benefit in phase III, and at the phase II dose. In the Bayesian approach one never takes a quantity to be perfectly known. Instead, the Bayesian perspective is to carry along uncertainty with whatever knowledge is available. Phases of drug development are arbitrary labels that describe a process that is, or should be, continuous.

One of the consequences of partitioning drug development into phases is that there are delays between phases. For example, there is a pause between phases II and III to set up one or more pivotal studies. As mentioned above in the context of the stroke trial, its design allows for avoiding such a hiatus. At each time point, say weekly, the algorithm that guides the conduct of the trial carries out a decision analysis and recommends either (1) continue the dose-ranging stage of the trial, (2) stop the trial for lack of efficacy (inadequate slope of the dose-response curve or, more accurately, evidence of a positive dose-response that is insufficient to justify continuing the trial), or (3) shift into a confirmatory trial. This shift can be made seamlessly, with no break in the accrual. Indeed, it is even theoretically possible to effect such a shift in a double-blind trial without informing the investigators: they simply continue to randomize doses, but unbeknownst to them, the only two being assigned are the phase III dose and the placebo.

A trial designed at MDACC[25] encompasses both phases II and III. If there is a switch to phase III, this switch is seamless. The anticipated effect of the drug is on local control. We model survival as it depends on local control and as it depends on treatment. (Although the possibility is remote, we allow for the experimental drug to have a beneficial effect on survival that is not mitigated by local control.) So local control is a surrogate endpoint in a way similar to the way early stroke scale assessments are surrogate endpoints in the stroke trial. But the clear focus is on survival as the main endpoint and the utility of the surrogate endpoint must be demonstrated by the results actually observed in the trial. The trial exploits any relationships that exist, but do not assume such relationships. The data in the trial are analyzed frequently and adapted to the accruing evidence.

The seamless aspect is as follows. Initially, only MDACC patients are accrued to the trial. Think of this as phase II. If the accumulating data are sufficiently strong in suggesting that the drug has no effect on local control or survival, then the trial stops. If the data suggest that the drug may have an impact on local control and that this impact translates into a survival benefit, then the trial will be expanded to include other centers and the accrual rate will increase accordingly. During such an expansion, patients continue to accrue at MDACC so that there is no downtime in the local accrual whereas other centers gear up to join the trial. This is efficient use of patient resources because data from the patients who accrued early at MDACC contribute to the eventual inferences about survival. These patients are the most informative of all those enrolled because their follow-up times are the longest.

The trial continues until stopping occurs because (1) continuing would be futile, judged by predictive probabilities, (2) the maximum sample size is reached, or (3) the predictive probability of eventually achieving statistical significance becomes sufficiently large. If the third event occurs, the accrual ceases and the pharmaceutical company prepares a marketing application.

The sample size of a conventional phase III trial with the desired operating characteristics is 900. We take this to be the maximum sample size in the seamless design as well. Actual accrual is very likely to be much less than this maximum sample size, and on average it will be about half as large. On the other hand, incorporating the same number of interim analyses in a conventional design using a conventional type of stopping boundary allows for only a slight decrease in the average sample size. Under any hypothesis, null or alternative, the Bayesian design occasionally leads to a relatively large trial (close to 900 patients). However, a pleasant aspect of the design is that the sample size is large precisely when a large trial is necessary. Conventional trials may well (and sometimes do!) come to their predetermined end with an ambiguous conclusion. In a Bayesian approach one may choose to continue such a trial to resolve the ambiguity, and this option has substantial utility. (Carrying this argument to the maximum sample size, there may be times for which stopping at 900 is ill advised, but for logistical reasons we specified a maximum size.)

Reductions in sample size result from two characteristics of the seamless design described above. First are the frequent analyses to assess the predictive probability of eventual statistical significance. The second is the explicit modeling of the possible relationship between local control and survival. Of the two, the second is more important.

A conventional drug development strategy involves running a phase II trial that addresses the local control, digesting the results, and if the results are positive, starting to develop phase III trials with survival as the primary endpoint. As indicated above, in comparison with such a strategy, a seamless approach can greatly reduce the sample size. In addition, a seamless design minimizes pauses between phases and so the total drug development time is greatly shortened.

Adaptive Allocation The adaptive designs discussed so far are motivated by the desire to learn efficiently and as rapidly as possible. Another kind of adaptive design aims to treat patients in the trial as effectively as possible. These designs use adaptive allocation in which patients are more likely to be assigned to therapies that are performing better. In addition to making clinical trials more attractive to patients and thereby increasing participation in clinical trials, such strategies have the important side benefit of being efficient, and so they result in rapid learning.

More than a dozen trials at MDACC have been designed and are being conducted using adaptive allocation. Our standard approach is to randomize the treatment assignment, but we shift the weights toward better performing arms as the trial proceeds and the results accumulate. Many of these trials have more than two arms. The arms are sometimes distinct therapies, and sometimes they are closely related. An example of the latter is an MDACC trial involving five doses (including 0) of a drug (pentostatin). The goal is to inhibit graft-versus-host-disease (GVHD) in leukemia patients who are receiving bone marrow transplants. The problem is that the drug may inhibit the successful engraftment of the transplant, which is necessary for survival. Such inhibition may be related to dose. We use a combination endpoint: survival at 100 days free of GVHD. The conflict between engraftment and freedom from GVHD means that the dose-response curve may not be monotone. In particular, it may increase for small doses and then decrease. Initially we assign doses in a graduated fashion, climbing the dose ladder slowly. But as doses become admissible, we assign patients to those that have been performing well.

Consider a patient who qualifies for the trial. To decide which pentostatin dose to assign we calculate the current (Bayesian) probabilities that each admissible dose is better than the placebo. This calculation uses all the information from the patients treated to date. We allocate doses randomly, with weights proportional to these probabilities. We consider other allocation algorithms, including assigning in proportion to the powers of these probabilities. The assignments involve some degree of randomization, but all patients are more likely to receive doses that are performing better. Doses that are doing sufficiently poorly become inadmissible in the sense that their assignment weight becomes 0. When and if it is learned that the drug is effective, the trial is stopped. When and if it is learned that the drug is ineffective, then again the trial is stopped. Patients in the trial benefit from data collected in the trial. The explicit goal is to treat patients more effectively, but in addition we learn efficiently. We evaluate each design's frequentist operating characteristics using Monte Carlo simulation, possibly modifying the parameters of the assignment algorithm to achieve desired characteristics.

Process or Trial? Evaluating Many Drugs Simultaneously Using Adaptive Allocation The greatest need for innovation and the greatest room for improving drug development is the process of effectively dealing with the enormous numbers of potential drugs that are available for development. The notion of developing drugs one at a time is part of the pharmaceutical culture. It will change. Companies that are able to screen many drugs simultaneously and effectively will survive and others will not.

Many different drugs should be evaluated in the same preclinical experiment or collection of experiments. Information should be updated frequently or even continually. The extent to which any particular drug is used and the order of drugs used will depend on the available data. Drugs that are apparently more promising will move faster through the preclinical setting. Drugs that give disappointing data will languish. And the sample sizes of patients treated with drugs that have promises and toxicities that are not clear will tend to be large so as to enable resolving uncertainties.

These ideas and imperatives apply as well to drugs' clinical development. As an example, MDACC is building the foundation for a phase II trial for evaluating drugs that is more a process than a trial. The idea is an extension of the adaptive assignment strategies described in the previous section. We start with a number of treatment arms plus a control—possibly a standard therapy. We randomize to the arms and learn about their relative efficacy as the trial proceeds. Arms that perform better get used more often. An arm that performs sufficiently poorly gets dropped. An arm that does well enough graduates to phase III, and if it does sufficiently well it might even replace the control. As more arms become available, they are added to the mix.

The result is that better arms (better treatments) move through quickly and poorer arms get dropped. Patients in the trial are provided with better treatment (when the arms are not equally good). Patients outside the trial get access to better drugs more rapidly.

EXTRAIM ANALYSES A common circumstance is that a clinical trial ends without a clear conclusion. For example, a statistical significance level of 5% in the primary endpoint may be required for drug registration, and the *p*-value may turn out to be 6%. The regulatory agency then suggests that the trial was "under-powered" and that the company should carry out another trial. It would be much more efficient to simply increase the sample size in the present trial. The problem is that the possibility of such an extension increases the type I error rate. The principle is identical to that for interim analyses.

The solution is to build into the design the possibility of continuing the trial depending on the results, and suitably adjusting the significance levels. In contrast to the adjustments for interim analyses, the adjustments for "extra-im" (extraim) analyses are reversed, with much of the overall significance level "spent" at the originally planned sample size. For example, taking equal significance levels at each possible termination point is preferable to O'Brien-Fleming stopping boundaries because the latter are too conservative for extraim analyses. Allowing for extending the trial increases the maximal sample size and the average sample size. But a modest increase in the average sample size (such as 20%) comes with a substantial increase in statistical power (such as 80% increasing to 95%). The reason for this beneficial trade-off is that the trial is extended only when such an extension is worthwhile.

The "penalty" in the significance level can be either partially or fully offset by including futility analyses as part of the design. Namely, the trial would be stopped for sufficiently negative results at preset interim time points. The reason such analyses offset the penalty for extraim analyses is that the null hypothesis is never rejected when the trial stops for futility. Decreasing the opportunity for a type I error also decreases the power of the trial. However, this decrease is usually quite modest and in any case is more than compensated by the increase in power due to the extraim analyses.

The increment in sample size depends on the available data at the time the decision is made to continue the accrual. It also depends on the number of possible extensions. In trials I have designed, I have based each extension on the predictive power. The usual definition of power assumes a particular value of the parameter of interest, say r. Predictive power considers all possible values of r. The data available at the time of the extraim analysis play two roles. First, they count in the final results of the trial. Second, they are used to update the (Bayesian) probability distribution of r. Fix the total sample size n and calculate the power for detecting each possible value of r. Average this power with respect to the probability distribution of r to give the predictive power for sample size n. Extend the accrual by the minimum sample size that gives a total sample size having a pre-specified predictive power. If there is no such value of n, then continuing the accrual may be unwise.

There is an aspect of the above development that may be unrealistic. Namely, it assumes that the endpoints for those patients treated in the trial so far are available at the time of the extraim analysis. Even if the endpoint is tumor response, there is a delay in obtaining this information. There is no need to stop the trial just because some of the endpoint information is unavailable. Rather, these data can be predicted along with those from patients not yet accrued. If there is some early information (biomarkers, performance status, etc) that is correlated with the endpoint of interest then this can be used to inform the prediction. A special and important case is when the endpoint is the time to an event. The fact that a patient has not yet reached an event is useful information in predicting the time to that event. However, if there is no patient-specific early information, then patients treated but not yet assessed for response are treated in the same way as patients not yet treated. (This set of issues is sufficiently important that they deserve being addressed separately. See the next section.)

The above process is complicated. But it can be completely and precisely described. That means it can be simulated. The simulations can be carried out under various assumptions about the parameter of interest. In particular, the false-positive rate can be calculated. If there is a target significance level (such as 5%), then the various inputs into the design (number and type of extraim analyses, number, and type of futility analyses, etc) can be varied until that target is achieved. An advantage of simulations is that each iteration provides data from a fully accrued trial. Therefore it is possible to check any characteristic of interest regarding the trial's design by calculating the proportion of the trials that have that characteristic. Characteristics of interest include the power, the actual sample size, and the probability of extending the accrual.

AUXILIARY VARIABLES, BIOMARKERS, AND BIOLOGICAL AGENTS

The adaptive designs considered in the previous section are based on information on the primary endpoint that accrues during the trial. If the primary endpoint is delayed and the accrual is sufficiently fast, then adaptive methods are of limited value. This section addresses statistical procedures for designs that exploit information that accrues during the trial other than the primary endpoint.

USING AUXILIARY VARIABLES Information that accrues during a trial has a broad interpretation. Suppose that the endpoint is time to progression and a patient has not yet progressed. That is information, and it can be used to update the distributions of whatever parameters are involved.

In addition, information accrues about each patient's circumstances and each patient's condition. Whether the patient's tumor has responded is information, and this is so even if response is not the endpoint of interest. Moreover, time to tumor response can be informative. A patient's performance status can change over time (or not!) and such information is important and the various possibilities can be used prospectively in designing a trial. There are many such variables that might be considered. They are auxiliary variables because they may contain information about the primary endpoint even though they are not themselves endpoints.

The critical issue is how to take advantage of the wealth of information that accrues in a trial. The answer is modeling. A model can relate the early information to the primary endpoint.

There are several benefits of modeling. One benefit was considered in the sections on adaptive dose finding and on seamless phases. Waiting for long-term endpoints may rule out the ability to modify the design of a clinical trial during its course. Using auxiliary variables can make adaptation possible. Another benefit of modeling is that the relationship between the primary endpoint and auxiliary variables may allow for announcing the trial results earlier or for getting earlier regulatory approval of an experimental drug. For example, suppose that survival is the primary endpoint and that modeling its relationship with response was considered explicitly in the design of the trial. Accrual to the trial has ended and all patients have been treated. There is insufficient information to conclude drug benefit on the basis of survival alone. But the drug has a positive impact on tumor response. And it turns out that in both the experimental treatment and control groups there is a clear relationship between response and survival. A model can use this information to conclude a survival benefit.

The distinction between the auxiliary variable and surrogate endpoints is critically important. Surrogate endpoints are those that can substitute for the primary endpoint in the sense that the effect of a treatment on the primary endpoint is wholly explained by its effect on the surrogate endpoint. This is generally too high a hurdle. Auxiliary variables require a correlation and not a substitution. In the above example, tumor response is an auxiliary variable and it is not assumed to be a surrogate for survival. The focus of the definitive analysis is the primary endpoint and not the auxiliary variable. The conclusion of the trial is still that the drug improves survival or not.

A model incorporating early information can be arbitrarily complicated and, in particular, it can contain all the variables discussed above. However, one should tiptoe into model development and consider one auxiliary variable at a time. Especially important is considering the possibility that any relationship between the auxiliary variable and the primary endpoint depends on treatment. Consequently, treatment must be explicitly considered in the equation. If it happens that there is an interaction between the auxiliary variable and treatment, such as that the tumor response is related to survival in the control group but not in the treatment group, then the model automatically discounts the auxiliary variable and relies on survival data alone.

Little is lost by modeling, and potential gains are large, as indicated in the seamless phase II/III trial design presented earlier. Moreover, as indicated previously, the gains and any losses can be assessed by simulation.

A special type of auxiliary variable is a biomarker. Models relating to primary endpoints can be based on longitudinal models that incorporate biomarker information that accrues over time. An example of a longitudinal model is described by Berry and colleagues,[23] in the context of a stroke trial.

Developing Biological Agents Biological agents present special drug development problems. Historically, oncology drug development has dealt primarily with cytotoxic agents. Drug activity has been judged by assessing the tumor growth. An effective biological agent may well have an impact that slows tumor growth rather than killing the tumor. Or it might have little effect on the local tumor's growth but halt the tumor's spread. And it may not be desirable to seek or employ its maximum tolerated dose.

A possible strategy is to include stable disease with partial and complete tumor response as the phase II endpoint. Another is to use time-to-progression as the phase II endpoint. The latter has the drawback that sample sizes and the length of time to trial may increase, but not as much as when skipping phase II entirely. Both strategies may succeed. And both have the advantage that they do not involve a paradigm shift for the oncology research community. But there are better options.

There are two types of biological agents, those with and those without measurable targets (such as specific oncoproteins). I distinguish between these as follows: If there is a target and the drug does not affect the target then the drug cannot be effective. Circumstances are usually more complicated and affecting a particular target may not be a drug's only mechanism. In such a case the drug is in essence a generic biological agent that might affect cancer through a variety of pathways.

Another reason one might view a targeted agent to be generic is when the assessment of the expression of the target is subject to error. An example is trastuzumab, which may well benefit tumors that have normal levels of HER2/neu because laboratory tests are not perfect in assessing expression levels.[26,27]

Whether or not a biological agent has a measurable target, the section "Using Auxiliary Variables" applies. If there is a target, think of it as a biomarker and develop a longitudinal model to relate its level with the primary endpoint, usually the time to progression or the overall survival. If there is no measurable target then identify auxiliary variables (biological and otherwise) that may be correlated with the primary endpoint. Model the possibility of a relationship should one exist. Again, the goal is to learn early and quickly as to whether the drug has a benefit, and by which route that benefit travels.

ACKNOWLEDGMENTS

The author thanks the Cancer and Leukemia Group B for permission to use data from CALGB 8541.

REFERENCES

1. The National Commission for the Protection of Human Subjects of Biomedical and Behavioral Research (US). The Belmont report. Ethical principles and guidelines for the protection of human subjects of research, 1979. Available at: http://ohsr.od.nih.gov/guidelines/belmont.html (accessed July 12, 2005).
2. Berry DA. Statistics: a Bayesian perspective. Belmont (CA): Duxbury Press, 1996.
3. Berry DA. A case for Bayesianism in clinical trials (with discussion). Stat Med 1993;12:1377–1404.
4. Speigelhalter DJ, Abrams KR, Myles JP. Bayesian approaches to clinical trials and health-care evaluation. Chichester, England: Wiley, 2004.
5. DuMouchel W. Bayesian metaanalysis. In: Berry DA, editor. Statistical methodology in the pharmaceutical sciences. New York: Marcel Dekker, 1989, p. 509–29.
6. Thall PF, Wathen JK, Bekele BN, et al. Hierarchical Bayesian approaches to phase II trials in diseases with multiple subtypes. Stat Med 2003;22:763–80.
7. Budman DR, Berry DA, Cirrincione CT, et al. Dose and dose intensity as determinants of outcome in the adjuvant treatment of breast cancer. J Natl Cancer Inst 1998;90:1205–11.
8. Thor A, Berry DA, Budman D, et al. *erb*B-2, p53 and efficacy of adjuvant therapy in lymph node-positive breast cancer. J Natl Cancer Inst 1998;90:1346–60.
9. Citron ML, Berry, DA, Cirrincione C, et al. Randomized trial of dose-dense versus conventionally scheduled and sequential versus concurrent combination chemotherapy as postoperative adjuvant treatment of node-positive primary breast cancer: First report of Intergroup C9741/Cancer and Leukemia Group B Trial 9741. J Clin Oncol 2003;21:1431–39.
10. Henderson IC, Berry DA, Demetri GD, et al. Improved outcomes from adding sequential paclitaxel but not from escalating doxorubicin dose in an adjuvant chemotherapy regimen for patients with node-positive primary breast cancer. J Clin Oncol 2003;21:976–83.
11. Sox HC, Blatt MA, Higgins MC, Marton KI. Medical decision making. Boston: Butterworth and Heinemann, 1988.
12. Clemen RT. Making hard decisions. Boston: PWS-Kent, 1991.
13. Berry DA. Decision analysis and Bayesian methods in clinical trials. In: Thall PF, editor. Recent advances in clinical trial design and analysis. New York: Kluwer Press, 1995, p. 125–54.
14. Lewis RJ, Berry DA. Decision theory. In: Armitage P, Colton T, editors. Encyclopedia of biostatistics. Vol. 2. New York: John Wiley & Sons, 1998, p. 1109–18.
15. Cheng Y, Su F, Berry DA. Choosing sample size for a clinical trial using decision analysis. Biometrika 2003;90:923–36.
16. Berry DA, Fristedt B. Bandit problems: Sequential allocation of experiments. London: Chapman-Hall, 1985.
17. Dixon WJ. The up-and down method for small samples. J Am Stat Assoc 1965;60:967–78.
18. Berry DA, Lindgren BW. Statistics: Theory and methods, 2nd ed. Belmont (CA): Duxbury Press, 1996.
19. O'Quigley J, Pepe M, Fisher L. Continual reassessment method: a practical design for phase I clinical trials in cancer. Biometrics 1990;52:673–84.
20. Thall PF, Lee JJ, Tseng C-H, Estey E. Accrual strategies for phase I trials with delayed patient outcome. Stat Med 1999;18:1155–69.
21. Cheung YK, Chappell R. Sequential designs for phase I clinical trials with late-onset toxicities. Biometrics 2000;56:1177–82.
22. Thall PF, Russell KT. A strategy for dose-finding and safety monitoring based on efficacy and adverse outcomes in phase I/II clinical trials. Biometrics 1998;54:251–64.
23. Berry DA, Mueller P, Grieve AP, et al. Adaptive Bayesian designs for dose-ranging drug trials. In: Gatsonis C, Carlin B, Carriquiry A, editors. Case studies in Bayesian statistics V. New York: Springer-Verlag, 2001, p. 99–181.
24. Malakoff D. Bayes offers a "new" way to make sense of numbers. Science 1999;286:1460–64.
25. Inoue LYT, Thall P, Berry DA. Seamlessly expanding a randomized phase II trial to phase III. Biometrics 2002;58:264–72.
26. Paik S, Bryant J, Tan-Chiu E, et al. Real-world performance of HER2 testing—National Surgical Adjuvant Breast and Bowel Project experience. J Natl Cancer Inst 2002;94:852–54.
27. Roche PC, Suman VJ, Jenkins RB, et al. Concordance between local and central laboratory HER2 testing in the Breast Intergroup Trial N9831. J Natl Cancer Inst 2002;94:855–7.

30

Cancer Outcomes

James A. Talcott, MD, SM

Because the goal of all medical research is to identify therapeutic strategies that improve patient outcomes, in a sense all clinical investigation is outcomes research. However, traditional clinical research views disease primarily from a biological perspective and therefore defines outcomes from that perspective. For example, in most cancer studies tumor shrinkage is measured, because it is a logical surrogate for survival, the definitive outcome, from the biological perspective. Although biological phenomena play a central role in the thinking of outcomes researchers, they view medical care from additional perspectives and, as a result, measure additional outcomes.

"Outcomes research" here refers to a loosely defined group of research objectives and methodologies that complement and expand the biological medical research model by measuring nonbiological outcomes that reflect their view of medical care in additional contexts. Lipscomb and colleagues, in their introduction to the monograph produced by the National Cancer Institute's Cancer Outcomes Measurement Working Group (COMWG), defined outcomes research as "the scientific field devoted to measuring and interpreting the impact of medical conditions and health care on individuals and populations… and describes, interprets, and predicts the impact of various influences, especially (but not exclusively) interventions on 'final' endpoints that matter to decision makers: patients, providers, private payers, government agencies, accrediting organizations and society at large."[1] Like traditional clinical researchers, outcomes researchers are seeking interventions that delay death from disease and neutralize its manifestations, but also those that will preserve or improve patients' quality of life, support their decision-making autonomy, ensure consistent, high-quality medical care, and maximize economic efficiency. To accomplish these goals, they use specialized, usually quantitative techniques and the perspective of social sciences. Asking questions that presume that biological processes are core elements of medical care, but not the only ones, outcomes researchers have adapted the methods of psychologists, sociologists, economists, and biostatisticians, including behavioral models, psychometric measurements, economic analyses, and decision analytical techniques (Table 30-1). When successful, these techniques address issues important to patients that their physicians have undervalued or overlooked, refine the objectives of treatment and incorporate additional perspectives from patients, physicians, payers, and policy makers.

Basic scientists have dramatically improved our understanding of the complex processes that underlie human disease, and translational research has brought new biological insights to bear on treatment. However, the therapeutic innovations made possible by new biological insights into cancer and other diseases bring fresh challenges. It may be especially difficult to identify appropriate indications for biologically powerful interventions, use them efficiently and fully appreciate and manage potentially complex and unexpected consequences. The techniques of outcomes researchers, if successful, allow us to evaluate treatment innovations more comprehensively and refine their use to meet the needs of patients, and of society, more completely.

HISTORY

Because of both historical circumstances and the distinctive natural history of cancer, outcomes research developed largely outside of oncology. Oncologists, like other medical subspecialists, came late to the field, which was developed largely by generalists, particularly in General Internal Medicine. However, the discontinuous natural history of cancer, which renders it less tractable to techniques useful in studying other chronic diseases, was another obstacle for outcomes researchers to overcome.

Low back pain, benign prostatic hyperplasia, degenerative joint disease and most other chronic diseases that outcomes researchers first studied have a relatively straightforward and clinically transparent natural history, a progression that leads to ongoing doctor–patient dialogue. They progress symptomatically and inexorably toward a definitive "fix" that is often a surgical procedure. Although specific diagnostic tests may be necessary to identify the key clinical milestones that trigger or mandate treatment, most patients with these diseases experience progressive illness directly through increasing symptoms, provoking naturally evolving treatment discussions with their doctors.

In contrast, the crucial transitions in cancer's natural history are unobservable and usually clinically silent. Primary cancers and metastases begin as single cellular events that may take years of growth to produce symptoms or tumor masses large enough for medical detection, even when they occur in easily observable sites such as skin. As a result, patients experience the clinical course of cancer as discontinuous: although the cancer has been growing in most cases for years, the initial diagnosis of cancer or the discovery of a metastasis comes "out of the blue," suddenly presenting an asymptomatic patient with a shocking prognosis and often frightening treatment options. Treatments for apparently localized cancers often present a "high stakes" potential for cure that makes toxic, invasive interventions acceptable to patients who feel few if any symptoms from their disease. Methods developed to investigate chronic diseases with less discontinuous natural histories required significant adjustment to encompass the challenging natural history of cancer, which took time. However, despite its later start in cancer medicine, outcomes research is now firmly entrenched.

The impetus for the rapid growth in medical outcomes research arose both from within academia and from larger societal trends. Beginning in the early 1970s, Wennberg and colleagues found striking variations in medical practice patterns in adjacent small geographic areas, corresponding to hospital service areas.[2] Although some of the variation they found could be explained by medical factors, much could not, forcing investigators to consider non-medical explanations, including

Table 30-1 Perspective, Goals, and Outcomes in Clinical Research

Perspective	Goal	Outcome Measured
Traditional (biological)	Define, measure and modify the biological processes that underlie disease	Survival, other biological variables (eg, tumor "response," or shrinkage, blood pressure, cardiac arrhythmias, etc.). Physician-reported information about adverse effects, such as toxicity scales.
Quality of life	Measure the impact of disease and medical interventions on the patient's experience of living.	Patient-reported outcomes, including functional status, "bother," and preferences.
Economics	Define and compare medical interventions' use of economic resources, both absolutely (cost minimization) and in terms of the benefit achieved (cost-benefit analyses).	Marginal costs and changes in quality-adjusted survival (or other indicators of health benefits)
Quality of health care	Identify and correct factors that produce medical harm	Medical error rates

social and economic causes .[3,4] The documentation of practice variation led directly to questions about the quality of medical care: if the use of some procedures and the overall intensity of medical care varied strikingly, which practice patterns were most helpful to patients?[5] From a systems approach, three components of health care could be seen: structure, process, and outcomes. Each aspect of care underwent scrutiny. Structure and process were easier to define and measure than outcomes but could not be evaluated in isolation from them. Meaningful comparisons of the structure and processes of alternative practice patterns required measuring their outcomes, the output of medical care.[6]

At the same time that the extent of practice variation was being appreciated, the rapidly rising costs of health care forced businesses and governments, the largest purchasers of health care, to attend to its economic efficiency. The realization by officials of General Motors in the 1970s that health care was a greater cost component of car making than steel, for example, forced it to examine closely the quality of the health care it was purchasing. Similarly, the United States government, the largest single purchaser of medical care through the Medicare and Medicaid programs, observed that health care costs were the most rapidly increasing segment of expenditures. The awareness of the growing cost of health care prompted the next major step in the development of outcomes research.

Early studies examined the effect of the structure of health care delivery on use and costs. The practice pattern variation documented by Wennberg and colleagues, as well as anecdotal evidence, suggested that a significant proportion of health care utilization was inappropriate and thus wasteful. Varying the payment structure of health care insurance was a potential corrective. Financial disincentives, such as increased health insurance deductibles, it was hoped, could reduce inappropriate use of health care and thus help control costs, at the same time protecting patients from the risk of iatrogenic injury from unnecessary medical interventions. The RAND Health Insurance Study (HIS), a randomized trial, compared health care utilization when care was provided free to patients to that of plans requiring patients make out of pocket patient payments, or deductibles, for their care.[7] It found that requiring patient payments reduced health care expenditures by a third compared to care provided free.[8]

However, the objective of the HIS was not to devise incentives to reduce health care utilization per se, but rather to specifically reduce the use of inappropriate care whose elimination would not compromise patients' health. To assess potential harms, investigators used both process and outcome indicators. Using guidelines for medical appropriateness developed by physician evaluators, the study found that the results of financial disincentives were disappointing: under financial pressure from copayments, patients reduced appropriate and inappropriate use of health care in equal measure.[9] The HIS investigators also undertook the more challenging measurement task of assessing health outcomes. They developed health status measures, including the most widely used survey instrument in medical research, the Medical Outcomes Study Short Form 36-Item Health Survey (SF-36).[10,11] Using these measures, the study found sparse evidence that patient groups who reduced medical care expenditures and utilization because of co-payments had worse health outcomes.[12] These combined results, although ambiguous, ruled out a quick fix to the system by using financial incentives to reduce inappropriate health care use: they found no evidence that patients can distinguish appropriate from inappropriate medical care. The lasting benefit of the HIS, however, was a major advance in the field of medical outcomes measurement.

Other studies of structure, process and outcomes followed this pioneering study. One found that HMOs reduced hospitalization compared to fee-for-service plans without evidence of reduced patient health outcomes.[13] Another used appropriateness criteria to determine whether practice pattern variations could be explained by varying use of inappropriate care, a potential target whose elimination would produce savings without harming patients. Studying several expensive medical procedures, investigators found that although inappropriate use of procedures was common, especially for some procedures with complex and vague indications such as cardiac catheterization, and varied by geographic area, it accounted for only a small part of medically unexplained variation.[14,15] Further work needed to be done.

This line of inquiry led directly to the creation of the Agency for Health Care and Policy Research (AHCPR) in 1989. As stated in the legislation that created it, the new Agency's goal was "to enhance the quality, appropriateness, and effectiveness of health care services, and access to such services, through the establishment of a broad base of scientific research and through the promotion of improvements in clinical practice and in the organization, financing, and delivery of health care services." Although funding a range of research, AHCPR devoted a substantial portion of its research budget to funding a series of Patient Outcomes Research Teams (PORTs), multidisciplinary groups whose task was to address a major clinical problem comprehensively, largely through existing data and methods but also new studies targeting crucial knowledge gaps. Their objective was to identify appropriate treatments that improved patient outcomes and promulgate them through evidence-based guidelines (vs expert opinion-based guidelines, a much inferior alternative highly vulnerable to existing biases). The first group of PORTs addressed chronic conditions other than cancer, such as back pain, cataracts, hip fractures, and diabetes, although some studies of localized prostate cancer were included in the PORT that addressed benign prostatic hyperplasia. The second wave of PORTs 5 years later included additional chronic diseases, more cancer (adding local breast cancer and continuing the prostate cancer PORT) as well as acute disease management (pediatric asthma, pelvic inflammatory disease, infants with diarrhea) and diagnostic technology (right heart catheterization and medical testing before cataract surgery). The policy aspect of the Agency's charge, guidelines, proved troublesome. Guidelines produced by an early PORT for treating back pain discouraged the early use of surgical interventions. Politically well-connected back surgeons led a backlash that accomplished a sustained challenge to Agency funding (and the elimination of the Federal Office for Technology Assessment). In late 1998, the Agency was transformed into the current Agency for Healthcare Research and Quality (AHRQ), which simultaneously removed the troublesome policy component and made explicit the ultimate goal of outcomes research, improving quality of care. During the brief life of AHCPR, however, outcomes research established itself throughout the medical research structure. In oncology, perhaps the clearest indicator of the recognition of outcomes research was the National Cancer Institute's creation and sponsorship of the Cancer Outcomes Measurement Working Group in 2001 to evaluate the state of the science of outcomes measurement and recommend approaches to improve its scientific quality and usefulness.[16]

OUTCOMES METHODS

Study Designs **Randomized Trials** Outcomes researchers use the gold standard clinical research design, randomized trials, but also recognize their limitations. These trials' crucial design element is that investigators assign interventions, through a chance-driven mechanism invisible to enrolling physicians, to patents who meet explicit eligibility criteria. As a result, randomized trials provide a powerful if expensive mechanism for answering a single research question within a single, fairly homogeneous population under controlled circumstances. The research design's power arises both from random assignment, which in sufficiently large studies reliably balances measured and unmeasured prognostic factors, and from reducing other potential sources of clinical variation by tightly controlling patient characteristics and constraining responses to clinical contingencies. The study protocol excludes patients at increased risk of treatment toxicity or of death from comorbid disease before the effects of treatment can be determined. It also dictates treating physicians' treatment options, including diagnostic testing, treatment modifications and other medical interventions. As a result, randomized trials take place in a hothouse environment that often produces results unrepresentative of clinical practice when the intervention is used more widely by physicians in practice with less experience with the experimental therapy and greater clinical discretion. Randomized trials assess the *efficacy* of medical interventions, in contrast to *effectiveness*, the impact of the intervention in real-world conditions. Without the investigators' specialized expertise and the research protocol's constraints on patient selection and clinical practice variations, the results may be less gratifying. To obtain the clearest answer to whether the experimental treatment can work under optimal conditions, the randomized trial releases authority on the question of whether it will work under typical conditions.

A separate problem with randomized trials is more troublesome for the kinds of questions of interest to outcomes researchers. For a patient to be enrolled in a randomized trial, she must accept that no preferred treatment for her problem exists and, by implication, that her doctor cannot help her select the best approach to her disease. This position, *equipoise,* is psychologically difficult for some patients to accept, especially those with life-threatening diseases like cancer. For physicians, deeply committed to the treatments they provide and well aware of how much their patients, especially those with cancer, depend on them for their expertise, arriving at equipoise may be even more difficult than for their patients. As a result, trial enrollment becomes increasingly difficult the more fundamental the aspect of medical care the trial investigates, and progressively easier the more trivial the deviation from current practice the experimental intervention represents. As a result, although important efforts have been made to identify and overcome barriers to completing trials,[17,18] outcomes researchers accept that they cannot rely on randomized trials to study the most important aspects of medical care, while remaining mindful that they remain the most definitive mechanism to document successful innovation. Another consequence of the emotional difficulty that randomization poses, particularly for patients with life-threatening diseases like cancer and perhaps for their physicians as well,[19] is the eager embrace of non-randomized studies with little probability of benefit, such as phase I trials. Patients report they are motivated by the hope of clinical benefit[20] and expect it,[21] despite little objective support for that belief in the consent forms they sign to enter the trial.[22]

Outcomes researchers have had growing influence on the practice of randomized trials. Although the definitive outcome of most randomized cancer trials is either survival or a biological intermediate variable, some recent trials have had patient-reported primary outcomes. Two pivotal trials that led to approval of new drug indications by the US Food and Drug Administration (FDA), which requires demonstration of "clinical benefit," had patient-reported elements in their primary outcomes. The first study found that mitoxantrone palliated prostate cancer patients with painful bone metastases, using a reduction in reported pain without an offsetting increase in narcotic use as the main outcome.[23] The second found that gemcitabine produced clinical benefit in patients with advanced pancreatic cancer, measured by a newly created composite of measurements of pain (analgesic consumption and pain intensity), Karnofsky performance status, and weight. Demonstrating benefit required a sustained improvement lasting at least 4 weeks in at least one parameter without worsening in any other.[24]

Outcomes research has a more fundamental role in cancer research. Because most advanced cancers are not curable by current methods, palliation is the primary therapeutic objective for the great majority of patients treated by medical oncologists. As a result, changes in quality of life are a central measure of the efficacy of treatment, although as a rule any intervention that prolongs symptomatic patients' lives improves their self-reported quality of life, even when the survival benefit is marginal.[25] Definitive measurement of quality of life remains challenging, and currently other more biological outcomes dominate cancer trials. However, as methodological progress addresses these challenges, the role of quality of life outcomes will grow in randomized cancer trials.

Observational Studies Observational research offers practical and cost advantages over randomized trials, but at a methodological cost. Because entering the study does not affect patients' treatments, observational studies accrue them more easily than randomized trials. However, because treating physicians, not study procedures, determine the treatment patients receive, confounding by other factors associated with the treatment is unavoidable, making causal inferences about the effects of treatment difficult. Because observational studies need not use prospectively collected data, enrollment of individual patients is unnecessary if data recorded for other purposes, such as routine medical record keeping, disease registries or even billing, is available for analysis. Observational studies using existing data may include hundreds of thousands of patients, producing extraordinarily powerful studies that produce very precise estimates of outcomes, and they are usually more representative of the typical patient experience, particularly when the population is geographically based, than randomized trial populations consisting of the small proportion of patients willing to enroll in them. The power of observational studies based on large existing databases is so great that trivial clinical differences between groups regularly achieve statistical significance. In large observational studies, issues of potential confounding and bias, not statistical significance, are the main challenges for investigators. The Health Insurance Portability and Accountability Act (HIPAA) has made observational studies more difficult, because variables that identify patients even approximately, including the time of diagnosis, are in general not accessible to investigators without patient consent.[26]

The data in retrospective observational studies are problematic. Because the previous data were recorded for other purposes, the data may have little relevance to the most interesting study hypotheses, sharply limiting both the range of research questions that can be asked, and the alternative explanations for the results that can be explored. Further, the investigators do not control the procedures that ensure the quality of the collected data, resulting in possibly unreliable data. These limitations assign observational studies a secondary role in treatment questions, particularly close calls easily overshadowed by confounding and bias. However, observational studies can make important contributions, especially when large databases are thoughtfully constructed with research purposes in mind, the study explores novel relationships, the effects of interest are large, or randomized trials are unethical, too expensive or persistently unsuccessful.

The major observational study designs are cohort studies and case-control studies. In a cohort study, investigators identify the characteristics and health status of a group of patients at a particular time point and evaluate subsequent outcomes. Previously recorded information can produce a cohort study retrospectively. Administrative data collected for billing purposes, particularly for large, geographically based databases, such as national or regional health care authorities or the Medicare insurance program in the United States, permit massive cohort studies, providing data to determine both entry criteria and outcomes. However, billing databases often may not collect medically relevant data for many research questions, and the data that is collected may be ambiguous.

Potosky and colleagues dramatically increased the value of the Medicare database for cancer research by merging it at the patient level with the National Cancer Institute's Surveillance, Epidemiology and End Results (SEER) database, the population-based cancer registry maintained by the National Cancer Institute that now includes the cancers in about 15% of the US population.[27] The combined SEER-Medicare database has been exploited in scores of retrospective cancer cohort studies that document the relationships of a variety of factors, including sociodemographic characteristics, geographic location, and treatment modalities, with survival. However, because the Medicare database is largely confined to patients aged 65 or older (a constraint not felt in nations with national health services), it has little to say about cancers in younger patients, and the SEER database lacks important information about therapy after the initial treatment. It contains no patient-reported quality of life information. To overcome the last limitation, some investigators have used the Medicare or SEER-Medicare data to identify patients with particular cancer diagnoses and stages or who have undergone particular treatments in order to survey them about quality of life issues.[28] One large study, the Prostate Cancer Outcomes Study (PCOS), used SEER to identify prostate cancer patients within 6 months of diagnosis and surveyed them at regular intervals, most recently at 5 years after diagnosis.[29,30] Among the recent uses of the SEER-Medicare database are studies that examine the relationship between provider procedure or case volume and patient outcomes, or volume-outcome studies,[31–33] demographic characteristics, such as age or race,[34,35] and economic studies.[36,37]

Large prospective cohort studies are costly to perform, but if carefully constructed, can produce a rich yield in both epidemiological and clinical research results. The Nurses Health Study and the Health Professionals Follow-up Study each evaluated tens of thousands of subjects who, because of their medical training, give reliable information about not only their personal experience but also their medical histories, allowing investigators to have greater faith in their reports and spares them the need to document any reported medical events with medical records. Study participants are surveyed regularly, providing new and updated information about risk factors and medical events, newly hypothesized risk factors, and other patient-reported information, such as quality of life items.[38–41] Further, blood specimens from participants allow investigators to examine a broad range of biomarkers.[42–45]

The case-control study is an efficient design for identifying factors associated with uncommon outcomes. Although cancer is a common diagnosis, specific cancer diagnoses and outcomes may be infrequent, especially in smaller populations. In these studies, investigators compare the frequency of risk factors, including interventions, of patients with (cases) and without (controls) the condition of interest from the same population. The ratio of risk factors in the cases and controls is algebraically equivalent to the relative risk associated with the risk factor: the finding that patients with oral cancers have ten times as often used chewing tobacco as those without the diagnosis, for example, is equivalent to a tenfold increased risk of oral cancer from using chewing tobacco. Like cohort studies, case-control studies are limited by the data that has been collected or may be collected by the investigators. Case-control studies that arise from the populations in cohort studies, or nested case-control studies, have been very useful, especially within large cohort studies, for which much of the data of interest have already been collected. Of course, if all the data used in the analyses is prerecorded, eliminating the need for new data collection, their most expensive and time-consuming task, investigators can use all non-cases in the cohort study as controls.

Although case-control studies have made a major contribution to studies of cancer etiology, they have less often been used to assess diagnostic or therapeutic interventions. One innovative approach used clinical information recorded in a health maintenance organization's database to evaluate the efficacy of sigmoidoscopy in preventing colorectal cancer, using patients who died of the disease as cases. In this way, the investigators were able to demonstrate that the risk of death from distal colon or rectal cancer (within the range of the procedure) was reduced by more than half in patients who had undergone the procedure within 10 years.[46] Because the study was observational, causality could not be directly observed, and the authors required ingenuity to address other potential explanations for the statistically strong association, such as the possibility that patients who would undergo the uncomfortable procedure were health-conscious in other ways that could account for their lower colorectal cancer rate. However, a randomized trial addressing the question using the definitive outcome for screening trials, mortality, would have been far more time consuming and costly, requiring thousands of patients and at least 10 years of follow-up. Although studies of relatively inexpensive and simple screening procedures in colorectal cancer have been completed with mortality outcomes,[47–50] studies using complex, expensive procedures like sigmoidoscopy or colonoscopy use intermediate outcomes, such as the diagnosis of cancer or numbers of colonic polyps.[51,52] In principal, cases could be selected for a case-control study based on good or bad functional or quality of life outcomes, instead of typical selection factors such as disease diagnosis or death. However, indicators of quality of life are far less likely to be recorded reliably than cancer mortality or tumor shrinkage.

Modeling Studies Mathematical models are attempts to identify quantitative relationships between outcomes of interest and factors that influence them. Unlike a mathematical model that describes physical phenomena, such as the archetypical equation of Einstein, $e = mc^2$, a mathematical model in medicine is an attempt to sketch a useful description of the medical situation using as few variables as possible. With these tools, the model builder hopes to identify the most important factors in a clinical situation and understand the relationships between them, but she understands that the resultant understanding is approximate. Because a model built in a single *training* population may reflect idiosyncratic or chance relationships that may not apply to other populations, it must be assessed in other *testing* populations to demonstrate its validity. Put another way, all medical models are wrong, but some can be shown to be useful.

Models are used for a variety of purposes, including adjusting for prognostic differences between patient groups in controlled trials, evaluating diagnostic or prognostic tests, and developing clinical decision or prediction rules.[53,54] One such model produced a clinical prediction rule that identified cancer patients with febrile neutropenia at low risk of medical complications after broad-spectrum antibiotic therapy has began,[55] allowing experiments with outpatient management.[56,57] However, in outcomes research the modeling perspective is most prominently featured in the decision analytic approach. The primary research product of decision analysis is a working mathematical model that relates the key factors in a general or clinical population that affect the outcome of interest. These models can be used to select the intervention that on average is best, using currently available options and what is known about them, as well as to test the potential effects of "what if" scenarios that include changed parameters (such as efficacy or cost) of existing options as well as novel interventions or approaches. The outcomes of interest for such models can be straightforward medical outcomes, such as survival, or alternative outcomes more specific to outcomes research, such as quality of life, organ function, or survival adjusted for impaired quality of life, expressed as quality-adjusted life years, or QALYs.

QALYs have received special interest because, if certain assumptions are made, they can be considered a "common currency" through which the consequences of all healthcare interventions can be measured and then compared against alternatives. Each intervention can be assigned an average benefit in QALYs alone or as a cost-effectiveness "price," the ratio of QALYs obtained per unit of cost. Not surprisingly, the results of cost-effectiveness analysis (CEA) are enormously appealing to policy-makers and payers. In theory, CEA allows the universe of potential medical interventions to be compared and ranked, producing "league tables" with the interventions that produce health benefits (QALYs) most efficiently (lowest cost per QALY) at the top and less efficient interventions progressively lower on the list. Using this list, health policy decision makers could simply proceed down the list from the most cost-effective treatments, approving progressively less cost-effective interventions until the available budget for health care is exhausted, with confidence that the process purchases the most health benefit possible with the available funding.

In the most direct attempt to apply this methodology to public policy, the state of Oregon attempted to prioritize services for its Medicaid process, as part of a plan to increase insurance coverage to nearly all residents. Its legislature created the Oregon Health Services Commission and charged it with defining a set of "basic" services that all public and private health insurance must cover. The first pass at ranking services produced alarmingly counterintuitive results, such as ranking orthodontic care above treatment for Hodgkin lymphoma. The resultant reassessment found technical problems, and cost-effectiveness procedures were overridden. Instead, the Commission created categories for services based on types of conditions or the outcomes of treatment, and ranked them by its assessment of their value to society, value to an individual and whether they are essential to health care. Opinions differed strongly on why the cost-effectiveness approach failed. Some argued that a fundamental conflict exists between the purposes of health care and the cost-effectiveness approach.[58] Most, however, found that correctable errors in execution were responsible and that the rational framework of CEA is better than the existing approach.[59–61]

One useful and transparent method for evaluating survival in cancer patients, Time Without Symptoms and Toxicity (TWiST), classifies the life of cancer survivors broadly.[62] Patients spend time experiencing treatment-related toxicity, cancer-related symptoms or without either, or TWiST. Outcomes can be performed comparing the time that patients spend in the high-quality TWiST state,[63] or weights can be applied to the toxicity and symptom states, producing a straightforward approximation of QALYs.[64] Although the TWiST method can be subjected to the same criticisms of other methods that attempt to quantify quality of life decrements, it has a straightforward appeal to clinicians who observe the qualitative differences in patients on treatment, in remission and in relapse.

Quality of Care Studies of quality of care arise from at least two major research streams, studies of medical practice variability and studies of medical injury and its implications for malpractice litigation and patient safety. Each has evolved and interacts with the other.

The studies of medical practice variation by Wennberg and colleagues are described above. They documented variation in medical practice patterns within small geographic areas that could not be explained medically. After establishing their research methodology, which persuasively confirmed both the variation and the absence of explanations for it from medical contingencies or patient preferences, they attempted to identify optimal practice patterns that exclude inefficient or harmful medical care. Using physician experts to define appropriate care and working through medical organizations, they undertook quality improvement campaigns to induce physicians to standardize their care on optimal practice patterns.[65] They also examined patient outcomes to compare practice patterns. Using claims data, they calculated risk-adjusted mortality rates and the frequency of adverse outcomes, such as preoperative mortality or re-operation or other salvage interventions, to determine the settings in which patients did better or worse.[66–68] Most recently, they compared mortality in regions in which health care was more or less expensive. They found that patients in higher-cost regions did not have better outcomes, implying that a substantial portion of medical care expenditures could be eliminated without harming patients.[69,70] This approach has led to studies of the relationship between the volume of procedures performed by providers and patient outcomes, also known as volume-outcomes studies.[32,33,71] This research approach has identified some of the major factors that influence the relationship. Not all surgical procedures show the same strong relationship between volume and outcomes. The effect is strongest for the most complex procedures, such as esophagectomy, compared to less challenging procedures performed in equally ill patients, such as pneumonectomy.[31] Outcomes are related to both hospital and provider volume, indicating that both institutional factors and treating teams influence quality.[72,73] This debate has complex ramifications, because it can be used to support both efforts to identify and remedy contributing factors to quality and restricting procedures to high-volume, regional referral centers.[74]

Another stream of research arose from the debate over malpractice litigation. For some, malpractice lawsuits are a humane, effective means of compensating patients for injury from substandard medical care while discouraging negligent medical practice. For others, they are an irrational, punitive process that so burdens providers financially, especially those who care for patients at high risk, that competent physicians are discouraged from practice, denying patients their services unnecessarily. The Harvard Malpractice study, reported in 1991, examined medical records in New York state using explicit criteria to determine how often medical care harmed hospitalized patients. They screened patients' charts for indicators of adverse events, occurrences that injured patients or prolonged their hospitalization, and then determined their relationship to medical error, negligence and subsequent disability. They found that adverse events occurred in over 3% of hospital admissions, 30% caused permanent injury or death, and negligence was responsible in about one third of cases. Malpractice cases were filed in less than 5% of patients who experienced an adverse event caused by negligence, and no negligence was found in most cases that were filed. The results had profound implications for both the effectiveness of the medical malpractice process and for the safety of hospitalized patients.[75–77] They, along with a series of high-visibility mishaps, primarily in cancer care, led directly to the Institute of Medicine report decrying the prevalence of medical error in the United States[78] and dramatically expanded efforts to reduce medical error, including the redirection of the Agency for Health Care Policy and Research to explicitly include quality of care in its research mission under its new name, the Agency for Healthcare Research and Quality.

These studies represent only a small part of an area of research whose importance has been increasingly recognized.

OUTCOMES, OR ENDPOINTS The starting point of any study is choosing the outcome of interest. For good reason, survival is the "gold standard" outcome for all medical researchers, including outcomes researchers: it is important and unambiguous. However, more traditional medical researchers focus on "biological" disease-specific markers, such as tumor shrinkage in oncology. Such endpoints interest outcomes researchers largely to the extent that they are surrogate indicators of prolonged survival or improved or deferred symptoms. However, outcomes researchers use other endpoints crafted to answer other questions. We have described the main research designs of outcomes researchers. We now discuss the endpoints used in these analyses.

Quality of Life Disease and its treatment may affect both the length and the quality of life. Quality of life is daunting to define, much less measure. The goal of medical researchers is to measure the contribution of health to quality of life, or health-related quality of life (HRQOL). Because of cancer's devastating potential and, in some cases, the possibility of cure, patients and physicians are willing to accept toxicity from treatments that would be unacceptable for less frightening diagnoses. Therefore, quality of life assessment in oncology extends beyond the effects of cancer to the effects from its treatment. Cancer, like other serious illnesses, may have additional non-medical consequences that affect quality of life, such as out-of-pocket costs or difficulties obtaining or continuing work or medical insurance. Depending on the clinical situation or research objective, researchers may define HRQOL differently. The patient's perspective may differ from that of the investigators. For example, researchers to their surprise have found that, despite well-documented, large increases of urinary incontinence and erectile dysfunction, men report little if any decline in their HRQOL a year after treatment for early prostate cancer.[79,80] Although these results could be explained if the survey instruments were too poorly designed to detect the HRQOL consequences or if impotence or incontinence simply do not affect quality of life, some patients may simply consider only the cancer, not the effects of its treatment, to be health-related. For patients with prostate cancer, which causes no specific symptoms, they may feel they have nothing to report, regardless of the impact of their treatment on their quality of life.

Investigators take two approaches to measuring quality of life. One approach attempts to identify and measure the physical consequences of disease and its treatment, including symptoms and dysfunction. The alternative approach attempts to identify the global impact of disease and treatment on the patient's experience, referred to as utility or preference assessment. Each approach has different uses, strengths and weakness, although attempts to link them with varying success have been described.[81,82] Measuring specific areas of dysfunction provide useful descriptions of patient states, but the results do not permit the investigator to report an overall conclusion about the summed effects, or global utility, of the health state in question. Measurement of global utility permits straightforward adjustment of survival to account for decreased quality of life, creating a "universal currency" unit that includes both the length and the quality of survival, the quality-adjusted life-year, or QALY.

To assume that interventions will produce a particular yield in QALYs, even on average, requires several assumptions: that it is possible to measure how much a potential change in health status would affect patients' overall assessment of their health-related quality of life, that the relationship between the health state and the self-assessed quality of life remains constant over time, and that all elements in the postulated health state can be assessed in combination or separately and then combined mathematically. The validity of each assumption can be questioned.

Determining how much to adjust quality of life for an impaired health state requires that patients express their preferences such that investigators can quantify them. Several ingenious instruments have been developed to accomplish that, but each can be challenging for patients, especially if they are uncomfortable with numbers. The approach with the firmest theoretical underpinnings is the standard reference gamble (SRG). In it patients report the point at which they are indifferent to staying in the impaired health state or a theoretical gamble with 2 outcomes, death or "perfect health," with progressively more or less attractive odds. For example, a patient who reports he would be unable to speak because of a laryngectomy to treat a pharyngeal cancer[83] or accepting a gamble in which perfect health is three times more likely than death (odds 3:1) indicates that his quality adjustment for living without a larynx is .75: for him life without a larynx is 75% as good as being in perfect health. Not surprisingly, many people are unable to produce consistent, meaningful responses when challenged with the standard reference gamble. Other approaches, such as the time-trade-off (TTO), in which patients are asked how many years of life in an impaired health state they would be willing to trade for 10 years in perfect health, or simply a global assessment, in which patients are asked how they would rate the impaired health state on a scale of 100, where 0 is death and 100 perfect health, represent less daunting mental tasks but are still very demanding to many patients uncomfortable with quantitative expression, a state often referred to as innumeracy, by analogy with illiteracy,[84] and the alternatives are also less theoretically valid than the SRG. This measurement problem remains vexing despite the resourcefulness of thoughtful investigators mindful of the great potential usefulness of QALYs.

The other assumptions are also subject to challenge. Although decision analysis assumes stable preferences, patients adapt to poor health and reduced function; observers are often surprised how highly disabled patients rate the quality of their lives despite being burdened with disabilities that healthier persons might think to be nearly intolerable. It is impossible to obtain direct assessments of all possible health states, because the potential permutations of organ dysfunction and other disease symptoms are nearly limitless. Therefore some mechanical procedure is necessary for scoring combinations of health states, be it additive (arithmetic), synergistic (multiplicative) or some combination. Arriving at a generally applicable formula for measuring complex health states is difficult. One can imagine that, for example, sudden-onset dysfunction that might be highly distressing to an otherwise healthy young individual, resulting in sharply decreased self assessed quality of life, might seem relatively insignificant to a patient with the lowered health expectations of older age or a more profound disability that renders the new dysfunction trivial by comparison or moot. For example, amputation to excise an osteosarcoma, even if curative, would profoundly alter the life of an adolescent, whereas an older adult forced by chronic respiratory failure to exclusively wheelchair mobility might find an amputation due to chronic diabetic vascular insufficiency no hindrance and perhaps even an improvement over managing the complications of the condition. The problem of adaptation does not disappear if one gives up on measuring preferences to measure dysfunction instead. Because the individual response to disability varies, investigators distinguish dysfunction from the response to dysfunction, called bother, or distress.

Even if incompletely persuasive methodologically, decision-analytic models offer a mechanism for examining the structure of a clinical problem, producing both the optimal decision on average situation under typical circumstances or in a specific situation of particular interest, but also identifying the factors with the greatest impact on the outcome. As a result, the exercise can illuminate whether adequate information on key factors is available to make authoritative decisions about the appropriate clinical strategy. A jarring result can shine a light on inadequately examined assumptions. A cost-effectiveness analysis (CEA) examined the use of prophylactic intravenous immunoglobulins (IVIG) to prevent infectious complications of chronic lymphocytic leukemia. Despite a well-designed trial demonstrating the clinical efficacy of IVIG in this setting, the model's calculations found that under any plausible assumption, the cost-effectiveness of the therapy was over $1 million per QALY.[85]

Costs Measuring economic efficiency has long been a goal of outcomes research. In part because the major economic inputs in health care, specialized, highly skilled labor and complex technology, are difficult to monetarize, but also because of the highly regulated structure and complex payment schemes, the economic aspects of health care are difficult to study. The standard units of expenditure, costs, are not measured but calculated, based on ratios between what is billed, charges, and true economic costs. Medicare requires that each hospital report department-specific cost to charge ratios. Charges are determined through negotiations, which are in turn dependent on bargaining power. The largest purchasers, usually health care plans, negotiate the lowest charges, and those with the least power, such as individual uninsured patients in the United States, have the highest charges. A third category is the record of actual economic activity, charges paid, but is rarely the economic outcome of interest. Accepted procedures for economic analyses have also been published.[86–89]

As noted above, a common use of cost data in medicine is to arrive at a common measure of value for medical maneuvers, the cost-effectiveness ratio in quality-adjusted life years, of QALYs. With such a "price," it is possible to rank the medical "efficiency" of various components of health care. The most straightforward use of cost-effectiveness analysis would be to rank potential interventions in a *league table* from the most to the least efficient (ie, from the lowest to the highest cost-effectiveness ratio), accepting all the interventions until the total expenditures exhaust the health care budget and rejecting the rest. That approach, in which each medical procedure is pitted against all others, has been rare in the United States. The most visible attempt, the Oregon Medicaid reform attempt, which failed, is described above. Far more common is analysis that asks only whether a procedure has an acceptably low cost-effectiveness ratio, either that of renal dialysis, a procedure to which the United States government made an early commitment to fund, or a range, often calibrated to dialysis, of $30,000 to $70,000 US per QALY. In this approach, *all* interventions meeting the threshold are recommended for acceptance by payers. Given the economic implications, many such analyses are performed by advocates of the intervention, often with a financial stake, who use studies with the most favorable results in their central analysis, or bad case, whether or not they are representative.

However, there is a further problem. Each additional procedure, whether or not it meets a cost-effectiveness criterion, adds to total health care expenditures. Only if each additional intervention is balanced by eliminating a less cost-effective intervention with the same total cost does this approach make medical care more efficient. If not, new technology adds to the total cost of health care. The latter situation holds today, accounting for the rapid increases in health care expenditures,[90] and the cost of cancer care is rising faster than any other area in medicine. It is easy to break a budget with cost-effective care. Controlling costs must be approached with the global budget in mind, not the absolute acceptance or rejection of individual interventions.

Measures of Quality As noted above, the quality of care in medical care can be measured at three levels: structure, process, and outcomes, and each has been subject to analysis and evaluation by investigators. The quality field is in its early years, but some approaches deserve mention. In this brief discussion, I omit references to the highly valuable quality improvement movement, a direct descendant of the approach that has been so successful in improving the safety of industries like commercial aviation.

Studies of structure have attempted to identify optimal institutional characteristics, such as for-profit versus nonprofit, teaching versus non-teaching, and referral centers versus community institutions.[91] Although these distinctions sometimes yield useful insights, the categories overlap and contain divergent institutions within them. Perhaps the most fertile current approach examines volume-outcome relationships. For most procedures, especially the most complex, providers and institutions that perform the most procedures have better outcomes, however assessed. Why the advantage occurs is not always evident, although one can imagine that staff experience, supporting structures, and specialized expertise might contribute. However, decisive factors may surprise. For example, much of the success of high-volume centers treating myocardial infarction has been attributed to more consistent prescription of beta-blockers on discharge.

Process is relatively easy to study, because procedures and many other interventions are regularly recorded for billing purposes. The highest quality providers would be most expected to consistently use the best practice patterns. However, defining them requires reference to a standard. One approach developed by the RAND Corporation polls expert panels iteratively to rate candidate process and outcome indicators of quality care in terms of validity and feasibility. The approach brings to bear substantial weight of clinical expertise with the opportunity to interact, exploring and testing the rationales of advocates. However, the process gives great sway to individual prejudices and idiosyncrasies. The larger difficulty with expert opinion-based results is that they tend to codify the currently accepted biases within the field.[74]

The alternative to guidelines based on expert opinion is evidence-based guidelines. Such guidelines are based on formal procedures to evaluate existing evidence, conform to strict methodological guidelines and clearly indicate the strength of the conclusions and the supporting evidence.[92] Despite increasing support for the development of evidence-based guidelines from the Cochran Collaborative, medical authorities under financial pressure to choose between competing, high-cost interventions, and, more recently as part of its research mission, from ARHQ, the process is time-consuming and can be performed successfully only when high-quality evidence is available. As a result, the process should generally be limited to settings in which the results are likely to be most useful: when practice variation is great, the clinical or economic implications are the most substantial and adequate evidence is available. Attention must also be paid to the dissemination of guidelines. Presentations that obscure the key findings or present them so densely that the target audience is repelled are unlikely to influence practice. The American Society of Clinical Oncology has produced a long series of useful guidelines for the practice of oncology.[93,94]

Once guidelines are established, measuring compliance with them provides useful process indicators of quality. The value of such studies lies in determining not only the frequency of compliance with indicators but also the factors that depress it. Such studies find clinical factors, such as severity of illness and overriding contraindications, and structural factors, such as inadequate information systems support and other barriers, account for discrepancies more than the resistance of clinicians.[95]

The ultimate endpoint for judging quality is patient outcomes. Because death (but not cause-specific mortality) is recorded reliably and its importance as a goal of therapy is unquestioned, many investigators have compared death rates to evaluate quality. When comparative trials are randomized, such comparisons produce unambiguous conclusions, because patients can be presumed to be similar clinically. However, for observational comparisons, adjustment for potential confounders is necessary. This process, risk adjustment, has proven the major barrier to accepting the results of quality comparisons based on patient mortality rates. Complicated patients are routinely referred to specialized centers, producing the belief that their patients have poorer prognoses that adjustment procedures cannot fully capture. Analyses that compare regions, not hospitals, sidestep that concern most successfully.[69,96] Other outcomes, more ambiguous and less well documented than mortality, are vexed by the risk-adjustment problem at least as much.

REFERENCES

1. Lipscomb J, Gotay C, Snyder C. Introduction to Outcomes Assessment in Cancer. Measures, Methods and Applications. In: Lipscomb J, Gotay C, Snyder C, editors. Outcomes Assessment in Cancer. Measures, Methods and Applications. Cambridge: Cambridge University Press; 2005. p. 1–13.
2. Wennberg J, Gittelsohn A. Small area variations in health care delivery. Science 1973;182:1102–8.
3. Wennberg JE. Factors governing utilization of hospital services. Hosp Pract 1979;14:115–21, 126–7.
4. Wennberg JE, Fowler FJ, Jr. A test of consumer contribution to small area variations in health care delivery. J Maine Med Assoc 1977;68:275–9.
5. Wennberg JE, Freeman JL, Culp WJ. Are hospital services rationed in New Haven or over-utilised in Boston? Lancet 1987;1:1185–9.
6. Wennberg JE, Bunker JP, Barnes B. The need for assessing the outcome of common medical practices. Annu Rev Public Health 1980;1:277–95.
7. Newhouse JP. A summary of the Rand Health Insurance Study. Ann N Y Acad Sci 1982;387:111–4.
8. Newhouse JP, Manning WG, Morris CN, et al. Some interim results from a controlled trial of cost sharing in health insurance. N Engl J Med 1981;305:1501–7.
9. Siu AL, Sonnenberg FA, Manning WG, et al. Inappropriate use of hospitals in a randomized trial of health insurance plans. N Engl J Med 1986;315:1259–66.
10. Kisch AI, Torrens PR. Health status assessment in the health insurance study. Inquiry 1974;11:40–52.
11. Brook RH, Ware JE, Jr, Davies-Avery A, et al. Conceptualization and measurement of health for adults in the Health Insurance Study: Overview. Santa Monica, Calif.: Rand; 1979.
12. Ware JE, Jr, Brook RH, Rogers WH, et al. Comparison of health outcomes at a health maintenance organisation with those of fee-for-service care. Lancet 1986;1:1017–22.
13. Sloss EM, Keeler EB, Brook RH, et al. Effect of a health maintenance organization on physiologic health. Results from a randomized trial. Ann Intern Med 1987;106:130–8.
14. Chassin MR, Kosecoff J, Park RE, et al. Does inappropriate use explain geographic variations in the use of health care services? A study of three procedures. JAMA 1987;258:2533–7.
15. Leape LL, Park RE, Solomon DH, et al. Does inappropriate use explain small-area variations in the use of health care services? JAMA 1990;263:669–72.
16. Lipscomb J, Gotay C, Snyder C. Outcomes Assessment in Cancer. Measures, Methods and Applications. Cambridge: Cambridge University Press; 2005.
17. Donovan J, Mills N, Smith M, et al. Quality improvement report: Improving design and conduct of randomised trials by embedding them in qualitative research: ProtecT (prostate testing for cancer and treatment) study. Commentary: presenting unbiased information to patients can be difficult. BMJ 2002;325:766–70.
18. George SL. Reducing patient eligibility criteria in cancer clinical trials. J Clin Oncol 1996;14:1364–70.
19. Joffe S, Cook EF, Cleary PD, et al. Quality of informed consent in cancer clinical trials: a cross-sectional survey. Lancet 2001;358:1772–7.
20. Daugherty C, Ratain MJ, Grochowski E, et al. Perceptions of cancer patients and their physicians involved in phase I trials. J Clin Oncol 1995;13:1062–72.
21. Cheng JD, Hitt J, Koczwara B, et al. Impact of quality of life on patient expectations regarding phase I clinical trials. J Clin Oncol 2000;18:421–8.
22. Horng S, Emanuel EJ, Wilfond B, et al. Descriptions of benefits and risks in consent forms for phase 1 oncology trials. N Engl J Med 2002;347:2134–40.
23. Tannock IF, Osoba D, Stockler MR, et al. Chemotherapy with mitoxantrone plus prednisone or prednisone alone for symptomatic hormone-resistant prostate cancer: a Canadian randomized trial with palliative end points. J Clin Oncol 1996;14:1756–64.
24. Burris HA 3rd, Moore MJ, Andersen J, et al. Improvements in survival and clinical benefit with gemcitabine as first-line therapy for patients with advanced pancreas cancer: a randomized trial. J Clin Oncol 1997;15:2403–13.
25. Helsing M, Bergman B, Thaning L, Hero U. Quality of life and survival in patients with advanced non-small cell lung cancer receiving supportive care plus chemotherapy with carboplatin and etoposide or supportive care only. A multicentre randomised phase III trial. Joint Lung Cancer Study Group. Eur J Cancer 1998;34:1036–44.
26. O'Herrin JK, Fost N, Kudsk KA. Health Insurance Portability Accountability Act (HIPAA) regulations: effect on medical record research. Ann Surg 2004;239:772–6; discussion 776–8.
27. Potosky AL, Riley GF, Lubitz JD, et al. Potential for cancer related health services research using a linked Medicare-tumor registry database. Med Care 1993;31:732–48.
28. Fowler FJ Jr, Barry MJ, Lu-Yao G, et al. Patient-reported complications and follow-up treatment after radical prostatectomy. The National Medicare Experience: 1988–1990 (updated June 1993). Urology 1993;42:622–9.
29. Potosky AL, Harlan LC, Stanford JL, et al. Prostate cancer practice patterns and quality of life: the Prostate Cancer Outcomes Study. J Natl Cancer Inst 1999;91:1719–24.
30. Potosky AL, Davis WW, Hoffman RM, et al. Five-year outcomes after prostatectomy or radiotherapy for prostate cancer: the prostate cancer outcomes study. J Natl Cancer Inst 2004;96:1358–67.
31. Begg CB, Cramer LD, Hoskins WJ, Brennan MF. Impact of hospital volume on operative mortality for major cancer surgery. JAMA 1998;280:1747–51.
32. Schrag D, Cramer LD, Bach PB, et al. Influence of hospital procedure volume on outcomes following surgery for colon cancer. JAMA 2000;284:3028–35.
33. Bach PB, Cramer LD, Schrag D, et al. The influence of hospital volume on survival after resection for lung cancer. N Engl J Med 2001;345:181–8.
34. Godley PA, Clark JA, Gellantly DD, et al. Race and prostate cancer: attitudes toward diagnosis and treatment among newly diagnosed patients. Proc Annu Meet Am Soc Clin Oncol 2004;23:A6056.
35. Sundararajan V, Hershman D, Grann VR, et al. Variations in the use of chemotherapy for elderly patients with advanced ovarian cancer: a population-based study. J Clin Oncol 2002;20:173–8.
36. Ramsey SD, Berry K, Etzioni R. Lifetime cancer-attributable cost of care for long term survivors of colorectal cancer. Am J Gastroenterol 2002;97:440–5.
37. Brown ML, Riley GF, Potosky AL, Etzioni RD. Obtaining long-term disease specific costs of care: application to Medicare enrollees diagnosed with colorectal cancer. Med Care 1999;37:1249–59.
38. Collins MM, Meigs JB, Barry MJ, et al. Prevalence and correlates of prostatitis in the health professionals follow-up study cohort. J Urol 2002;167:1363–6.
39. Laden F, Neas LM, Tolbert PE, et al. Electric blanket use and breast cancer in the Nurses' Health Study. Am J Epidemiol 2000;152:41–9.
40. Schernhammer ES, Laden F, Speizer FE, et al. Night-shift work and risk of colorectal cancer in the nurses' health study. J Natl Cancer Inst 2003;95:825–8.
41. Bacon CG, Giovannucci E, Testa M, et al. The association of treatment-related symptoms with quality-of-life outcomes for localized prostate carcinoma patients. Cancer 2002;94:862–71.
42. Ishibe N, Hankinson SE, Colditz GA, et al. Cigarette smoking, cytochrome P450 1A1 polymorphisms, and breast cancer risk in the Nurses' Health Study. Cancer Res 1998;58:667–71.
43. Giovannucci E, Pollak M, Platz EA, et al. Insulin-like growth factor I (IGF-I), IGF-binding protein-3 and the risk of colorectal adenoma and cancer in the Nurses' Health Study. Growth Horm IGF Res 2000;10 Suppl A:30–1.
44. Tranah GJ, Giovannucci E, Ma J, et al. Epoxide hydrolase polymorphisms, cigarette smoking and risk of colorectal adenoma in the Nurses' Health Study and the Health Professionals Follow-up Study. Carcinogenesis 2004;25:1211–8.
45. Giovannucci E, Stampfer MJ, Krithivas K, et al. The CAG repeat within the androgen receptor gene and its relationship to prostate cancer. Proc Natl Acad Sci U S A 1997;94:3320–3.
46. Selby JV, Friedman GD, Quesenberry CPJ, Weiss NS. A case-control study of screening sigmoidoscopy and mortality from colorectal cancer 'see comments. N Engl J Med 1992;326:653–7.
47. Mandel JS, Bond JH, Church TR, et al. Reducing mortality from colorectal cancer by screening for fecal occult blood. N Engl J Med 1993;328:1365–71.
48. Mandel JS, Church TR, Ederer F, Bond JH. Colorectal cancer mortality: effectiveness of biennial screening for fecal occult blood. J Natl Cancer Inst 1999;91:434–7.
49. Hardcastle JD, Chamberlain JO, Robinson MH et al. Randomised controlled trial of faecal-occult-blood screening for colorectal cancer. Lancet 1996;348:1472–7.

50. Scholefield JH, Moss S, Sufi F, et al. Effect of faecal occult blood screening on mortality from colorectal cancer: results from a randomised controlled trial. Gut 2002;50:840–4.
51. Thiis-Evensen E, Hoff GS, Sauar J, et al. Population-based surveillance by colonoscopy: effect on the incidence of colorectal cancer. Telemark Polyp Study I. Scand J Gastroenterol 1999;34:414–20.
52. Winawer SJ, Zauber AG, Ho MN, et al. Prevention of colorectal cancer by colonoscopic polypectomy. The National Polyp Study Workgroup. N Engl J Med 1993;329:1977–81.
53. Wasson JH, Sox HC, Neff RK, Goldman L. Clinical prediction rules. Applications and methodological standards. N Engl J Med 1985;313:793–9.
54. Talcott JA, Finberg R, Mayer RJ, Goldman L. The medical course of cancer patients with fever and neutropenia. Clinical identification of a low-risk subgroup at presentation. Arch Intern Med 1988;148:2561–8.
55. Talcott JA, Siegel RD, Finberg R, Goldman L. Risk assessment in cancer patients with fever and neutropenia: a prospective, two-center validation of a prediction rule. J Clin Oncol 1992;10:316–22.
56. Talcott JA, Whalen A, Clark J, et al. Home antibiotic therapy for low-risk cancer patients with fever and neutropenia: a pilot study of 30 patients based on a validated prediction rule. J Clin Oncol 1994;12:107–14.
57. Rubenstein EB, Rolston K, Benjamin RS, et al. Outpatient treatment of febrile episodes in low-risk neutropenic patients with cancer. Cancer 1993;71:3640–6.
58. Hadorn DC. Setting health care priorities in Oregon. Cost-effectiveness meets the rule of rescue. JAMA 1991;265:2218–25.
59. Dixon J, Welch HG. Priority setting: lessons from Oregon. Lancet 1991;337:891–4.
60. Eddy DM. Oregon's methods. Did cost-effectiveness analysis fail? JAMA 1991;266:2135–41.
61. Fisher ES, Welch HG, Wennberg JE. Prioritizing Oregon's hospital resources. An example based on variations in discretionary medical utilization. JAMA 1992;267:1925–31.
62. Gelber RD, Gelman RS, Goldhirsch A. A quality-of-life-oriented endpoint for comparing therapies. Biometrics 1989;45:781–95.
63. Gelber RD, Goldhirsch A, Cavalli F. Quality-of-life-adjusted evaluation of adjuvant therapies for operable breast cancer. The International Breast Cancer Study Group. Ann Intern Med 1991;114:621–8.
64. Gelber RD, Goldhirsch A, Cole BF, et al. A quality-adjusted time without symptoms or toxicity (Q-TWiST) analysis of adjuvant radiation therapy and chemotherapy for resectable rectal cancer. J Natl Cancer Inst 1996;88:1039–45.
65. Wennberg JE, Blowers L, Parker R, Gittelsohn AM. Changes in tonsillectomy rates associated with feedback and review. Pediatrics 1977;59:821–6.
66. Wennberg JE, Roos N, Sola L, et al. Use of claims data systems to evaluate health care outcomes. Mortality and reoperation following prostatectomy. JAMA 1987;257:933–6.
67. Wennberg JE, Freeman JL, Shelton RM, Bubolz TA. Hospital use and mortality among Medicare beneficiaries in Boston and New Haven. N Engl J Med 1989;321:1168–73.
68. Lu-Yao GL, Potosky AL, Albertsen PC, et al. Follow-up prostate cancer treatments after radical prostatectomy: a population-based study. J Natl Cancer Inst 1996;88:166–73.
69. Fisher ES, Wennberg DE, Stukel TA, et al. The implications of regional variations in Medicare spending. Part 1: the content, quality, and accessibility of care. Ann Intern Med 2003;138:273–87.
70. Fisher ES, Wennberg DE, Stukel TA, et al. The implications of regional variations in Medicare spending. Part 2: health outcomes and satisfaction with care. Ann Intern Med 2003;138:288–98.
71. Begg CB, Riedel ER, Bach PB, et al. Variations in morbidity after radical prostatectomy. N Engl J Med 2002;346:1138–44.
72. Schrag D, Panageas KS, Riedel E, et al. Hospital and surgeon procedure volume as predictors of outcome following rectal cancer resection. Ann Surg 2002;236:583–92.
73. Hu JC, Gold KF, Pashos CL, et al. Role of surgeon volume in radical prostatectomy outcomes. J Clin Oncol 2003;21:401–5.
74. Talcott JA. Quality of care in prostate cancer: important to start and too important to stop here. J Clin Oncol 2003;21:1902–3.
75. Brennan TA, Leape LL, Laird NM, et al. Incidence of adverse events and negligence in hospitalized patients. Results of the Harvard Medical Practice Study I. N Engl J Med 1991;324:370–6.
76. Leape LL, Brennan TA, Laird N, et al. The nature of adverse events in hospitalized patients. Results of the Harvard Medical Practice Study II. N Engl J Med 1991;324:377–84.
77. Localio AR, Lawthers AG, Brennan TA, et al. Relation between malpractice claims and adverse events due to negligence. Results of the Harvard Medical Practice Study III. N Engl J Med 1991;325:245–51.
78. Kohn DB, Kantoff PW, Eglitis MA, et al. Retroviral-mediated gene transfer into mammalian cells. Blood Cells 1987;13:285–98.
79. Clark JA, Rieker P, Propert KJ, Talcott JA. Changes in quality of life following treatment for early prostate cancer. Urology 1999;53:161–8.
80. Litwin MS, McGuigan KA, Shpall AI, Dhanani N. Recovery of health related quality of life in the year after radical prostatectomy: early experience. J Urol 1999;161:515–9.
81. Torrance GW, Furlong W, Feeny D, Boyle M. Multi-attribute preference functions. Health Utilities Index. Pharmacoeconomics 1995;7:503–20.
82. Furlong WJ, Feeny DH, Torrance GW, Barr RD. The Health Utilities Index (HUI) system for assessing health-related quality of life in clinical studies. Ann Med 2001;33:375–84.
83. McNeil BJ, Weichselbaum R, Pauker SG. Speech and survival: tradeoffs between quality and quantity of life in laryngeal cancer. N Engl J Med 1981;305:982–7.
84. Gigerenzer G, Edwards A. Simple tools for understanding risks: from innumeracy to insight. BMJ 2003;327:741–4.
85. Weeks JC, Tierney MR, Weinstein MC. Cost effectiveness of prophylactic intravenous immune globulin in chronic lymphocytic leukemia. N Engl J Med 1991;325:81–6.
86. Russell LB, Gold MR, Siegel JE, et al. The role of cost-effectiveness analysis in health and medicine. Panel on Cost-Effectiveness in Health and Medicine JAMA 1996;276:1172–7.
87. Siegel JE, Weinstein MC, Russell LB, Gold MR. Recommendations for reporting cost-effectiveness analyses. Panel on Cost-Effectiveness in Health and Medicine JAMA 1996;276:1339–41.
88. Weinstein MC, Siegel JE, Gold MR, et al. Recommendations of the Panel on Cost-effectiveness in Health and Medicine. JAMA 1996;276:1253–8.
89. Gold MR, Siegel JE, Russell LB, Weinstien MC, editors. Cost Effectiveness in Health and Medicine. New York: Oxford University Press; 1996.
90. Bodenheimer T. High and rising health care costs. Part 1: seeking an explanation. Ann Intern Med 2005;142:847–54.
91. Stern RS, Juhn PI, Gertler PJ, Epstein AM. A comparison of length of stay and costs for health maintenance organization and fee-for-service patients. Arch Intern Med 1989;149:1185–8.
92. Field MJ, Lohr KN. Guidelines for clinical practice: From development to use. Washington, DC: National Academy Press; 1992.
93. American Society of Clinical Oncology. Recommendations for the use of hematopoietic colony-stimulating factors: evidence-based, clinical practice guidelines. J Clin Oncol 1994;12:2471–508.
94. Loblaw DA, Mendelson DS, Talcott JA, et al. American Society of Clinical Oncology recommendations for the initial hormonal management of androgen-sensitive metastatic, recurrent, or progressive prostate cancer. J Clin Oncol 2004;22:2927–41.
95. Ellrodt AG, Conner L, Riedinger M, Weingarten S. Measuring and improving physician compliance with clinical practice guidelines. A controlled interventional trial Ann Intern Med 1995;122:277–82.
96. Cowper PA, DeLong ER, Peterson ED, et al. Geographic variation in resource use for coronary artery bypass surgery. IHD Port Investigators. Med Care 1997;35:320–33.

Part III

Principles of Cancer Diagnosis

Section 6

CANCER PATHOLOGY

31

Principles of Cancer Pathology

James L. Connolly, MD
Jeffrey D. Goldsmith, MD
Helen H. Wang, MD, DrPH
Janina A. Longtine, MD
Ann M. Dvorak, MD
Harold F. Dvorak, MD

Pathologists are physicians who are concerned primarily with the study of disease in all its aspects: that is, causation, diagnosis, pathogenesis, mechanisms, natural history, anatomic and biochemical features, progression, and prognosis. In many respects, therefore, pathologists are "doctors' doctors"—consultants with specialized knowledge that can be helpful to the clinician who is caring directly for the patient. Nowhere in medicine is this adage more true than in the care of patients with cancer.

Pathologists engage in several types of activity: *anatomic pathology,* which includes surgical pathology, cytology, and autopsy pathology; *clinical pathology,* also known as laboratory medicine—that is, the direction of clinical laboratories; and *experimental pathology,* or basic investigations of the pathogenesis of disease. However, these distinctions have become increasingly blurred as advances in technology such as immunohistochemistry, flow cytometry, and molecular biologic approaches to cancer diagnosis have moved from the research laboratory into the clinic.

This chapter reviews the basic principles of pathology as they apply to neoplastic disease. The goal is to provide oncologists with a better understanding of what pathologists do; how they arrive at diagnoses; what tools, especially modern ones, they have at their disposal; and how the oncologist can interact most productively with the pathologist to achieve the greatest benefit for the patient.

TUMOR STRUCTURE AND TUMOR STROMA GENERATION

Tumor Structure What is a tumor?

Although physicians know very well what they mean when they use the term "tumor", the question is not a simple one to answer in a concise and comprehensive manner. The word "tumor" is of Latin origin; it means "swelling." But not all swellings are tumors in the modern sense of the term (eg, the swellings of inflammation and repair). The distinguished pathologist Wallace H. Clark[1] has offered an excellent definition, paraphrased as follows: a tumor (fully evolved) is a population of abnormal cells characterized by temporally unrestricted growth and the ability to grow in at least three different tissue compartments—the original compartment; the mesenchyme of the primary site (tumor invasion); and a distant mesenchyme (tumor metastasis). Clark's definition usefully emphasizes the progressive nature of tumor growth; the common (though not exclusive) origin of tumors as benign growths; their gradual acquisition of autonomy; and, at some stage, their ability to grow in new tissues distant from their site of origin—that is, to metastasize.

Although some tumors (eg, leukemias, ascites tumors) grow as cell suspensions, most tumors grow as solid masses of tissue. Solid tumors have a distinct structure that mimics that of normal tissues[2–4] and that comprises two distinct but interdependent compartments: the parenchyma (neoplastic cells) and the stroma that the neoplastic cells induce and in which they are dispersed. In many tumors, including those of epithelial cell origin, a basal lamina separates clumps of tumor cells from stroma. However, the basal lamina is often incomplete, especially at points of tumor invasion.

All tumors have stroma and require stroma for nutritional support and for removal of waste products. In the case of leukemias, blood plasma serves as stroma, although an additional stromal response, angiogenesis, may develop in the bone marrow.[5] When tumors grow in body cavities, a plasma exudate (eg, ascites) provides stroma.[6,7] In solid tumors, stroma includes connective tissue, blood vessels, and, very often, inflammatory cells, all of which are interposed between the malignant cells and normal host tissues. In all tumors, stroma is largely a product of the host and is induced as the result of tumor cell–host interactions. Solid tumors, regardless of their type or cellular origin, require stroma if they are to grow beyond a minimal size of 1 to 2 mm.[8] The stroma of solid tumors may also limit the influx of inflammatory cells or the egress of tumor cells ("invasion"). Stroma, therefore, at once provides a lifeline that is necessary for tumor growth and imposes a barrier that inhibits and may regulate interchange of fluids, gases, and cells.

The singular importance of new blood vessel formation to tumor survival and growth has rightly led to an emphasis on tumor angiogenesis; however, that emphasis has been accompanied by an unfortunate tendency to undervalue other tumor stromal components. Blood vessels are only one component of tumor stroma. In fact, in many

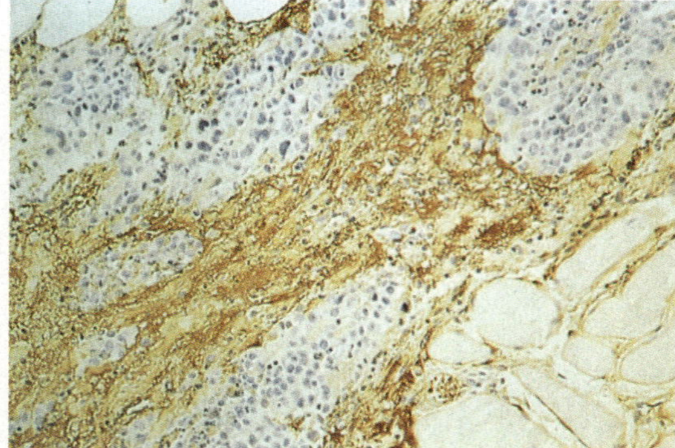

Figure 31-1 Immunoperoxidase staining reaction of line 10 guinea pig undifferentiated bile duct carcinoma exposed to a monoclonal antibody specific for fibrin (supplied by Dr. Gary Matsueda). Tumor comprises nests of malignant cells interspersed in a stroma that stains heavily for fibrin. Immunoperoxidase stain; ×50 original magnification.

tumors, interstitial connective tissue comprises the bulk of stroma, and blood vessels are only a minor component of the stromal mass.

For the most part, tumor stroma is formed of elements that are derived from the circulating blood and from adjacent host connective tissues.[9,10] Plasma components include water and plasma proteins, together with various types and numbers of inflammatory cells. Almost any element found in normal connective tissue may be represented in tumor stroma, including even bone and cartilage. Generally speaking, the major components of tumor stroma include, in addition to new blood vessels, leaked plasma and plasma proteins, proteoglycans and glycosaminoglycans, interstitial collagens (primarily types I and III), fibrin (Figure 31-1), fibronectin, and cells of two general types: normal connective tissue cells such as fibroblasts, and inflammatory cells that are derived from the blood.[9,10]

Although all tumor stroma contain the same basic building blocks, pathologists have long recognized that tumors differ markedly from each other in stromal content. Sometimes the differences are primarily quantitative. At one extreme are desmoplastic tumors, such as many carcinomas of the breast, stomach, and pancreas, in which as much as 90% or more of the total tumor mass consists of stroma. At the other extreme are tumors such as medullary and lobular carcinomas of the breast and many lymphomas, in which only minimal stroma is deposited. In other cases, differences in stromal content among various tumors are largely qualitative. For example, some carcinomas of the breast provoke the deposition of abundant elastic tissue and collagen; others (eg, medullary carcinoma of the breast) induce an extensive lymphocytic infiltrate and little else in the way of stroma. Even within a single tumor, there may be significant variations in stromal composition from one area to another. Stromal heterogeneity should not be surprising in view of the well-recognized heterogeneity of the parenchymal cells present within individual tumors.

Tumor Stroma Generation **Steps in the Process** Studies of transplantable tumors have yielded important information concerning the pathogenesis of tumor stroma generation (Figures 31-2 and 31-3).[3,4,9,11] Among the earliest steps in the process is local vascular hyperpermeability to circulating macromolecules. Increased vascular permeability is attributable to vascular permeability factor/vascular endothelial growth factor (VPF/VEGF, VEGF-A), a multifunctional cytokine that is synthesized and secreted by most animal and human tumors.[11–14]

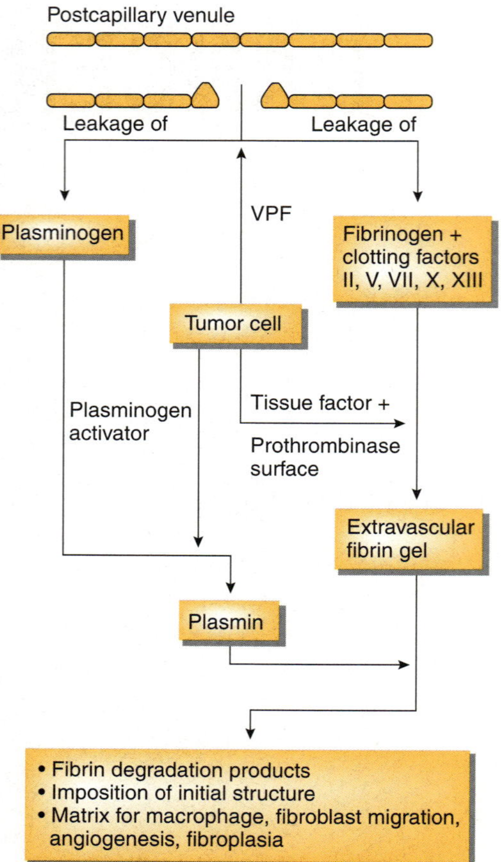

Figure 31-2 Schematic diagram of tumor stroma generation.

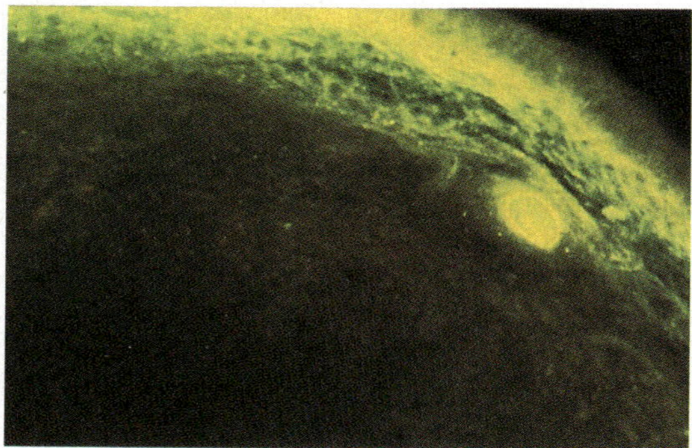

Figure 31-3 Lewis lung carcinoma growing in flank of a syngeneic C57Bl/6 mouse that had received a macromolecular tracer, 70 kDa fluoresceinated dextran, 15 minutes previously. Bright-staining apple-green fluorescence forming a rim around the tumor represents extensive extravasation of tracer into surrounding normal connective tissue from leaky blood vessels at the tumor–host interface. The tumor itself is virtually unstained, appearing as a "black hole," because tracer at its periphery diffuses poorly into tumor. Fluorescence microscopy; magnification ×15.

Among other activities, VEGF-A renders the microvasculature hyperpermeable to plasma and plasma proteins with a potency some 50,000 times that of histamine. It ranks among the most powerful vascular permeabilizing substances known (see Figures 31-2 and 31-3).[7,11–14] When injected into skin or other normal tissues, VEGF-A, like mediators of inflammation such as histamine, provokes the extravasation of a protein-rich plasma exudate. As with histamine, the primary target of VEGF-A action is postcapillary venules and small veins whose lining endothelial cells express the two VEGF-A tyrosine kinase receptors VEGFR-1 (*FLT1*) and VEGFR-2 (*KDR*).

An important and almost immediate consequence of VEGF-A action is leakage of plasma proteins, including fibrinogen and other clotting factors. Vascular hyperpermeability and extravasation of plasma proteins lead to activation of the coagulation system by a tissue factor–mediated mechanism.[15] As a result, extravasated plasma fibrinogen is rapidly clotted to form an extravascular gel of cross-linked fibrin (see Figures 31-1 and 31-2).

Extravascular fibrin deposits are important because they dramatically alter the local microenvironment, transforming the erstwhile inert extravascular matrix of normal adult tissues into a proangiogenic provisional matrix that favors and apparently stimulates inward migration of host mesenchymal cells.[11,14] Indeed, fibrin implanted in animals without tumor cells induces the invasion of new blood vessels and fibroblasts, resulting in a vascularized connective tissue that is not dissimilar in appearance or composition to tumor stroma. Other plasma proteins (eg, plasma fibronectin), as well as locally synthesized structural proteins (eg, cellular fibronectins, tenascin), hyaluronan, and proteoglycans (eg, chondroitin sulfate–rich proteoglycan and decorin) also contribute to this new tissue.[9,11,14]

The fibrin gel deposited by tumors is modulated by proteases (see Figures 31-1 and 31-2) and gradually replaced by an ingrowth of fibroblasts and new blood vessels that give rise to loose connective tissue similar to the "granulation tissue" of healing wounds.[4] After an additional period of time, the granulation tissue is further transformed into the poorly vascularized, densely collagenous scar-like connective tissue characteristic of tumor desmoplasia. Simultaneously, of course, other tumor cells have broken away from the original tumor site and have begun to recapitulate at nearby sites—particularly at the tumor's growing edge—the same sequence of events: increased vascular permeability and new fibrin deposition. Thus, at any one time, growing desmoplastic tumors consist of older, generally more centrally placed portions, comprising tumor cells that are encased in poorly vascularized, dense collagenous stroma, and a more active, newer, fibrin-rich peripheral zone that interfaces with the surrounding host tissue.

Critical Role of VEGF-A in Stroma Formation At this point, something more needs to be said about VEGF-A because of its central role in tumor angiogenesis and stroma generation. (For detailed accounts, see recent reviews[11–13].)

VEGF-A is expressed in several different isoforms as the result of alternative splicing of a single, highly conserved gene. VEGF-A is the founding member of a family of proteins whose members include placenta growth factor and VEGF-B, -C, -D, and -E.[12] At present, much more is known about VEGF-A than about other, more recently discovered family members. In addition to its potent function as an effecter of vascular hyperpermeability, VEGF-A has other actions that make important contributions to angiogenesis and stroma generation. Thus, VEGF-A stimulates endothelial cell division and migration. It also induces endothelial cells to express increased amounts of tissue factor, urokinase, tissue plasminogen activator, and matrix metalloproteases.[11–13] Collectively, those endothelial cell products induce clotting and initiate fibrinolysis and degradation of collagen and other elements of pre-existing matrix—all-important steps in angiogenesis and stroma generation.

A number of factors serve to regulate VEGF-A expression in tumor cells. VEGF-A expression is greatly stimulated by tissue hypoxia and, perhaps independently, by low tissue pH, conditions that are commonly present in the tumor microenvironment.[11–13] However, it would be a mistake to think that hypoxia is the only factor responsible for VEGF-A overexpression by tumor cells. Many tumor cells make substantial amounts of VEGF-A under normoxic or even hyperoxic conditions. Other factors that induce overexpression include cytokines (eg, epidermal growth factor, basic fibroblast growth factor), certain hormones (eg, thyroglobulin), and, perhaps of more general interest, various oncogenes (eg, *src*, *ras*) and tumor suppressor genes including the von Hippel–Lindau protein.[11–13]

Relationship of Tumor Stroma Generation to Wound Healing and Other Examples of Pathologic and Physiologic Angiogenesis and Stroma Generation The events of stroma generation in transplantable tumors closely mimic those of normal wound healing.[4,16] As occurs in tumors, VEGF-A expression is strikingly upregulated in healing wounds[16] and in various analogous pathologic and physiologic processes that involve new blood-vessel and stroma formation, including rheumatoid arthritis, psoriasis, delayed hypersensitivity, diabetic retinopathy, and corpus luteum formation.[11] In all of these processes, the initial event is a local increase in vascular permeability, followed in turn by extravascular clotting, fibrin deposition, and infiltration of new blood vessels and connective tissue cells, leading to the development of granulation tissue and finally of dense, fibrous connective tissue (termed "desmoplasia" in tumors and scars or "fibroplasia" in the other entities). It would seem, therefore, that tumors have preempted and subverted, for their own purposes, a fundamental host mechanism, the wound healing response, as the means to acquire the stroma they need to grow and spread.[4]

Of course, some differences exist. Platelets, which play several critical roles in wound healing, seem not to participate to any great extent in tumor stroma generation; however, many platelet functions can be subsumed by tumor cells, which express similar or analogous cytokines and growth factors. Tumors differ from healing wounds in another important respect. At wound sites, overexpression of VEGF-A and consequent vascular hyperpermeability are limited to a period of a few days, presumably until oxygen tension has returned to normal.[16] By contrast, VEGF-A expression and vascular hyperpermeability are not limited in tumors; they persist indefinitely. Thus, tumors in some sense behave as wounds that do not heal.[4]

The analogy between wound healing and tumor stroma generation may be taken one step further. Except in lower vertebrates that are capable of regenerating normal tissues, wound healing does not recapitulate ontogeny but, instead, replaces injured parenchyma and stroma with connective tissue whose functional capacities fall well short of the original normal tissue. In the same manner, the stroma of a malignant tumor is generally a disorganized and poorly supportive parody of normal connective tissue. The vascular supply is often marginal. Tumor blood vessels are structurally and functionally abnormal, unevenly spaced, and often unequal to the task of supporting the growth and even the life of rapidly metabolizing tumor cells.[10,17] The result is irregular blood flow in leaky blood vessels, uneven perfusion, shifting zones of anoxia, low pH, and, commonly, necrosis and apoptosis.[10,18] In fact, the presence of necrosis is sometimes helpful to the pathologist in distinguishing malignant tumors from their benign counterparts and from certain non-neoplastic processes.

Stroma Generation in Autochthonous Human Tumors Detailed interventional studies of the type required to elucidate the pathogenesis of tumor stroma generation in animal tumors are not ethically feasible in humans. Nonetheless, there is good reason to believe that similar mechanisms are involved in human malignancy. First, VEGF-A is overexpressed at both the messenger ribonucleic acid (mRNA) level and the protein level in most primary and metastatic human tumors that have been studied. These include carcinomas arising in the gastrointestinal tract, pancreas, stomach, breast, ovary, kidney, and bladder, and glioblastomas.[11,13] Second, the specific, high-affinity receptors for VEGF-A are both also overexpressed in the microvascular endothelial cells that supply those tumors. Finally, many human tumors exhibit evidence of vascular hyperpermeability to plasma proteins, including spillage of fibrinogen with deposition of cross-linked extravascular fibrin as observed in animal tumors[4,13]. Taken together, this is strong evidence that the pathogenesis of stroma formation in human tumors closely follows that in animal tumors, although allowance must be made for species differences and for the generally slower growth rate of autochthonous human tumors.

ROLE OF THE SURGICAL PATHOLOGIST IN THE DIAGNOSIS AND MANAGEMENT OF CANCER PATIENTS

Surgical pathologists have the definitive role in tumor diagnosis. No matter how high the index of clinical suspicion, a diagnosis of cancer is neither conclusively established nor safely assumed in the absence of a tissue diagnosis. With few exceptions, definitive therapy for cancer should not be undertaken in the absence of a tissue diagnosis. Policies supporting this practice are written into the bylaws of most hospitals and are regularly monitored by hospital tissue committees and by accrediting agencies.

The surgical pathologist has the task to provide an accurate, specific, and sufficiently comprehensive diagnosis to enable the clinician to develop an optimal plan of treatment and, to the extent possible, to estimate prognosis. Not many years ago, the simple designation "benign" or "malignant" provided the clinician with all of the information necessary to provide appropriate care for the patient. This is no longer the case. Cancer is not a single disease. Tumors come in more than 300 distinct varieties, each with a characteristic biology. Moreover, tumors have a historical course of development and progression; in an individual patient, they may be first recognized at any stage along that course.

The tremendous advances in all fields of oncology require a great deal of additional information. In fact, to permit the most appropriate classification for research, prognosis, and therapeutic intervention, nearly every case requires a fuller understanding of the patient's particular tumor. Details of the type and origin of the tumor, its differentiation and level of invasion, the numbers of lymph nodes with and without metastatic tumor, the presence or absence of hormone receptors, the activity of specific enzymes, ploidy, frequency of mitosis, and percentage of cells in the S-phase may all be relevant in the pathologic assessment of neoplasia. For example, molecular pathology, using nucleic acid probes with or without amplification by the polymerase chain reaction to detect expression of specific tumor genes or gene mutations, is rapidly becoming standard practice and promises an increasingly important role for pathology in the clinical management of cancer patients.

Surgical pathologists deal primarily with structure. Careful gross examination of excised tissue with the naked eye is followed by a more detailed examination of tissue sections in the compound light microscope. Intraoperative examination may make use of frozen tissue sections, but in most instances, pathologists rely on the better preservation of structure afforded by permanent tissue sections stained with hematoxylin and eosin (H&E) and occasionally other dyes. Histochemistry, immunohistochemistry, and electron microscopy are helpful or necessary supplements for diagnosis in 10 to 15% of solid tumors.

Surgical pathologists collaborate closely with cytopathologists in diagnoses involving exfoliated cells or needle aspirates, and with clinical pathologists, who make use of other techniques, such as culture for microorganisms, flow cytometry, and specialized laboratory tests of a biochemical, immunologic, or molecular nature. For most of these supplementary studies, the specimen must be specially processed while it is still fresh—that is, prior to tissue fixation. The surgical pathologist is responsible to coordinate these various activities and to synthesize the resulting information into a comprehensive diagnosis that is maximally informative to the clinician caring for the patient.

Methods for Obtaining Specimens Tissue may be obtained in a number of ways. Each method has its appropriate place and uses, depending on the clinical circumstances. Sampling body fluids for exfoliated cells or scraping or brushing to obtain cells are rapid, efficient, and low-risk techniques. Those methods, and the related technique of fine-needle aspiration (FNA) biopsy, are discussed in greater detail later in this chapter.

For obvious reasons, those approaches do not always reveal the primary tumor site or the extent of disease. Cutting-needle biopsies, core-needle biopsies, and drill biopsies obtain tissue cores for histologic examination or for special studies that permit evaluation of architectural structure. Incisional biopsy (along with FNA) is often the method of choice for lesions that are inoperable or too large for ready excision, or when excision could lead to functional or cosmetic impairment. Excisional biopsy is often favored because it provides generous amounts of tissue for diagnosis and may itself afford sufficient surgical therapy for some tumors—for example, small- to medium-sized breast cancers.

Biopsy interpretation has many potential pitfalls. These include inadequate tissue sampling and artifacts induced by the procedure itself, such as thermal damage caused by an electrocautery or laser. Benign findings do *not* exclude the possibility that a tumor or other significant pathologic condition is present but was not included in the tissue submitted for examination. The clinician must be prepared to perform a second, often more extensive, procedure if the first does not yield sufficient diagnostic information.

Gross Handling of Specimens The pathologist must regard a biopsy as the definitive surgical specimen and must therefore properly triage each biopsy, particularly excisional biopsies. To approach triage appropriately, the pathologist must be informed about the patient's clinical history, the differential diagnosis, relevant laboratory results, gross tissue examination, and frozen section findings, if any. Individually or together, these factors dictate whether special studies are required. Often, tissue arrives in the pathology laboratory in formalin or another fixative. If a specimen has been so treated, it is already too late to perform many special studies (eg, microbiologic cultures, certain types of immunohistochemistry, flow cytometry, and optimal electron microscopy) that may prove to be critical for diagnosis. To avoid the need for repeat biopsy, the surgeon should consult the pathologist in advance. Frequently, the goal of biopsy is to determine whether a lesion is benign or malignant, with the expectation of performing additional surgery if the lesion proves malignant. In this case, supplementary tests may properly be deferred to the subsequent, more definitive surgery, at which time larger amounts of tissue become available for analysis.

Specimens should be marked with clips, sutures, or ink to provide anatomic orientation, and the method of marking should be described in the pathology submission sheet. The gross specimen should also be described with regard to its appearance and characteristics, taking care to measure in three dimensions the size of the specimen and, if visible, the lesion itself and the distances between the lesion edges and the excision (resection) margins. Excision margins should be identified and marked with ink before any dissection, thus permitting accurate measurement of these distances under microscopy. Depending on the type of specimen and the clinical circumstances, margins can be evaluated by analysis of frozen sections. All lymph nodes associated with a cancer specimen need to be dissected out, described (including location), and processed for histology.

Certain biopsies require still more careful examination—for example, breast biopsies, in which no lesion may be visible to the naked eye. Breast specimens with calcification also often require specimen radiography. Ideally, therefore, a radiograph of the intact specimen should be obtained, then the margins should be inked, the specimen "breadloafed," and radiographs taken of each slice. Sections should then be coded, individually processed for histology, and correlated with the corresponding radiographs.[19,20]

Preparation of Microscopy Sections Microscopy requires that tissues be cut with a microtome into thin sections that can be stained with dyes such as H&E, toluidine blue, and other stains for specific tissue components such as mucus, glycogen, cytoplasmic granules, collagen, bacteria, and fungi. The sectioning methods most commonly used are frozen sections and paraffin-embedded (permanent) sections.

Frozen sections can be prepared rapidly (within minutes) during the course of surgery while the patient is still under anesthesia. They are therefore of the greatest practical value when an immediate answer is required for an important clinical question. Frozen sections are useful for determining whether a lesion is a neoplasm and, if so, whether it is benign or malignant. They can provide information about the extent of regional tumor metastases that may govern decisions concerning further surgery (eg, mediastinal lymph node involvement in primary carcinoma of the lung, peripancreatic lymph node involvement in carcinoma of the pancreas). Following definitive cancer surgery, they allow the pathologist to determine whether the resection margins—for example, those of skin, gut, or pulmonary lesions—are adequate. If resection margins are inadequate, additional tissue can be removed immediately, without the need for a subsequent operation. Perhaps the most common current use of frozen sections is to determine, while the specimen is still fresh, the appropriate additional work-up necessary for this particular tissue. For example, if the metastatic tumor found in a lymph node is recognized as a poorly differentiated carcinoma, special fixation and electron microscopy may be required for proper diagnosis. On the other hand, if the tumor is a lymphoma, an entirely different set of studies may be required, such as those for cell-surface antigen markers and gene rearrangement.

Some tumors, such as those arising in the soft tissues or breast, are best evaluated in permanent sections. In contrast to frozen sections, permanent sections are prepared from tissues that have been fixed, dehydrated, and embedded in paraffin wax as a supporting medium before sectioning. Although they require more time for preparation (generally 12 to 24 hours), permanent sections offer a number of important advantages over frozen sections. Permanent sections are generally thinner (typically 5 μm) and, because freezing artifacts are avoided, are of better overall quality, permitting greater certainty of interpretation. Certain tissues, such as those containing fat or bone, cut poorly as frozen sections but may be satisfactorily studied in permanent sections. As a general rule, if insufficient tissue is available for both frozen and permanent sections, only permanent sections should be prepared. Although the opinions just expressed certainly represent a majority view, some excellent pathology departments routinely diagnose tumors on the basis of frozen sections and prepare permanent sections primarily for archival purposes.

Microscopy Interpretation of Tissue Sections In cases of suspected cancer, the first task of the surgical pathologist is to decide whether a neoplasm is present. As noted earlier, the word "tumor" is Latin for "swelling," and various types of "swelling" can masquerade as neoplasms. These include inflammatory lesions, repair, hypertrophy, hyperplasia (eg, keloids), choristomas (ectopic rests), and hamartomas (masses of mature cells that are appropriate to a given site but are arranged in a disorganized fashion as the result of aberrant differentiation). The initial distinction is often easily made. For example, hyperplastic polyps of the colon, nasal polyps, and skin tags are not likely to be confused with true neoplasms. Sometimes, however, the task is less straightforward.

Not infrequently, tumors generate an extensive inflammatory response. It is not unusual, for example, in endoscopic biopsies of gastric carcinomas, to find only after a prolonged search rare individual cancer cells "buried" in an extensive inflammatory cell infiltrate. Healing ulcerations of the gastrointestinal or cervical mucosa may sometimes closely resemble the carcinomas or pre-malignant lesions that arise in those tissues (eg, squamous intraepithelial lesions, low or high grade). Finally, atypical hyperplasia can be very difficult to distinguish from in situ carcinoma and, even when no

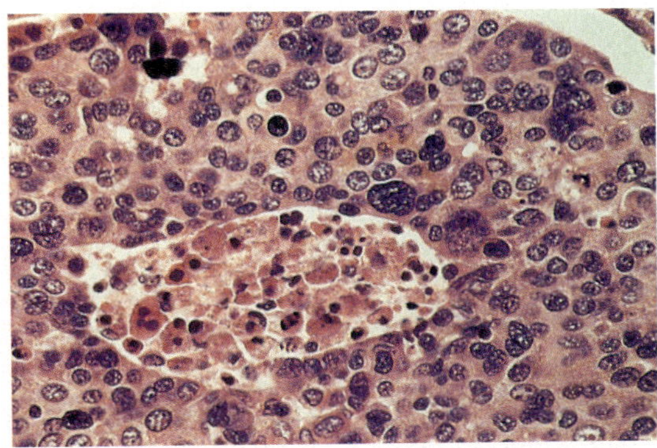

Figure 31-4 Undifferentiated carcinoma of lung. The tumor is composed of irregularly arranged pleomorphic tumor cells with large nuclei and prominent nucleoli. A central necrotic zone, typical of this type of tumor, is present. There is little stroma. Hematoxylin and eosin stain; ×100 original magnification.

evidence of tumor is found, may represent an important diagnostic finding. For example, patients whose breast biopsies show atypical hyperplasia have a four- to five-fold increased risk of developing breast cancer at a later time.[21]

Having decided, on the basis of criteria such as cellular abnormalities or invasion, that a neoplasm is present (see below), the pathologist's next task is to classify it. A number of classification schemes are possible, but the most important is based on the tumor's histogenetic or cytogenetic origin. The combination of histogenetic and cytogenetic classification is often supplemented by other useful descriptors such as those provided by the tumor's gross or microscopic appearance (eg, polypoid, papillomatous), by the degree of cellular differentiation (eg, well or poorly differentiated; Figure 31-4), and, perhaps most importantly, by the expected biologic behavior (benign or malignant).

Broadly speaking, tumors of epithelial cell origin are termed adenomas or papillomas when benign and carcinomas when malignant. Carcinomas account for approximately 80% of all malignant tumors. Their classification is often further qualified on the basis of the type of epithelium present: for example, glandular (adenocarcinoma, Figure 31-5), squamous (squamous cell carcinoma, Figure 31-6), urothelial cell (urothelial cell carcinoma). Addition of the suffix "–oma" to the cell of origin also describes benign tumors of mesenchymal origin (eg, lipomas, fibromas). Malignant tumors of mesenchymal origin are called sarcomas (eg, liposarcomas, fibrosarcomas).

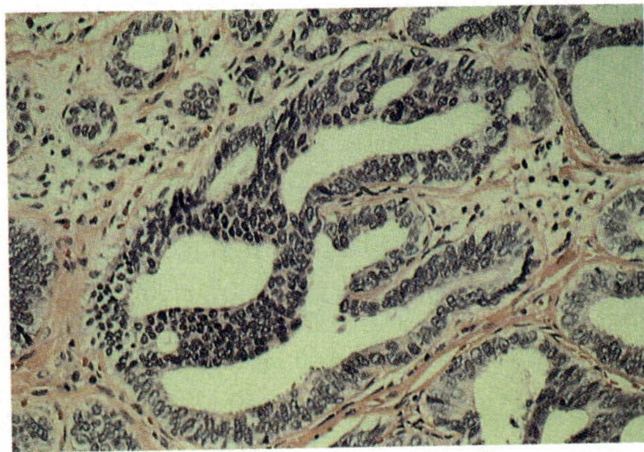

Figure 31-5 Adenocarcinoma of the breast. The tumor is arranged in the form of fairly well-differentiated glands separated by a fibrous connective tissue stroma. Moderate numbers of inflammatory cells, mostly lymphocytes, are present in the stroma. Hematoxylin and eosin stain; ×65 original magnification.

Most tumors consist of a single type of neoplastic cell. However, a few tumors contain neoplastic cells of more than one type—for example, Wilms' tumors. Even rarer are tumors that contain neoplastic cells deriving from more than a single germ layer—for example, teratomas (dermoid cysts). Certain tumors have long been identified with trivial names that do not follow any well-ordered classification scheme. Examples include seminomas (for carcinomas of testicular epithelial cell origin), hypernephromas (for renal cell carcinomas), and melanomas (for melanocarcinomas; Figure 31-7). Other tumors, because of prolonged usage, continue to bear eponyms (eg, Hodgkin's disease, Kaposi's sarcoma).

The pathologist must carry classification further still. Even within a single organ and within a single type of epithelium, several different tumor types may arise, each with its own special characteristics, prognosis, and response to therapy. In the breast, for example, the two most common types of malignant tumor are infiltrating ductal carcinoma (sometimes designated as carcinoma "not otherwise specified"), which accounts for approximately 80% of infiltrating breast cancers, and infiltrating lobular carcinomas, which account for about an additional 9% of breast cancers. Those two tumors, together accounting for nearly 90% of breast cancers, have similar prognoses that are less favorable than the prognoses of the other, less common types of breast carcinoma (ie, tubular, mucinous or colloid, medullary, papillary, and adenoid cystic carcinomas).[22]

One of the most important distinctions that the surgical pathologist can make is the distinction between tumors that are benign and those that are malignant. In general, benign tumors share certain properties. The neoplastic cells that make up the tumor are usually well differentiated, closely resembling the corresponding cells of normal tissue. Benign tumors tend to expand uniformly in all directions unless impeded by surrounding structures. For example, compression by the bony skull often causes meningiomas to take on a flattened appearance. As expansile masses, benign tumors cause compression atrophy of surrounding normal tissues. As a result, a thin rim of fibrous connective tissue can form around the tumor. This enveloping connective tissue rim may serve as a "capsule" that renders benign tumors discrete, readily palpable, and easily movable. However, not all benign tumors have capsules. Some examples are leiomyomas of the uterus, hemangiomas, and adenomatous polyps of the large intestine.

Malignant tumors, or cancers, are characterized primarily by the abnormality of their neoplastic cells. These cellular abnormalities are of two general types, those involving intercellular relationships and those affecting individual neoplastic cells. With regard to intercellular relationships, malignant tumors commonly exhibit increased cell numbers and altered orientation of both neoplastic cells and stroma that may be best described as "helter-skelter" or disorganized. For example, carcinomas of the skin may comprise squamous cells that differentiate and mature fairly normally; however, the cells are commonly organized into nests, in which the least differentiated cells are situated peripherally, and the most differentiated cells are positioned centrally, where they form keratin pearls. Further, these tumor cell nests are surrounded by disorganized stroma. Disturbed intercellular arrangements such as these are of great help to the pathologist reading a tissue section; much of tumor diagnosis depends on the pathologist's ability to recognize altered microscopic tissue patterns.

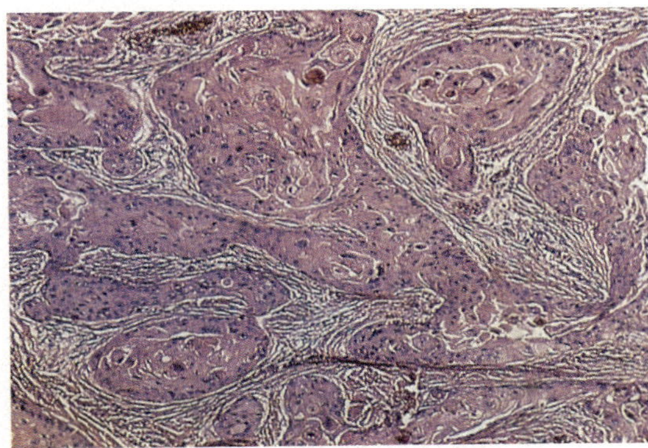

Figure 31-6 Squamous cell carcinoma of the skin of the face. Tumor consists of an island of well-differentiated squamous epithelium separated by fibrous connective-tissue stroma. Note that the epithelium forms "keratin pearls." Hematoxylin and eosin stain; ×60 original magnification.

Abnormalities of individual neoplastic cells may also be helpful in diagnosis, particularly increased numbers of mitoses and cytologic features relating to the state of tumor-cell differentiation. Cytologic features of malignancy include altered polarity, tumor-cell enlargement, increased ratio of nuclear to cytoplasmic area (may approach 1:1 instead of the normal 1:4 or 1:6, although exceptions exist), pleomorphism (variation in size and shape) of tumor cells and their nuclei, clumping of nuclear chromatin and distribution of chromatin along the nuclear mem-

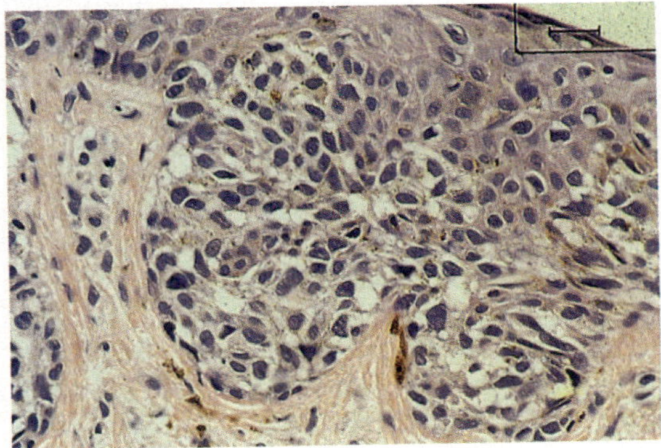

Figure 31-7 Malignant melanoma arising in skin. Tumor is composed of large, irregular cells with large nuclei, prominent nucleoli, and abundant, clear cytoplasm, peppered with dots and larger accumulations of melanin pigment. Hematoxylin and eosin stain; ×100 original magnification.

brane, enlarged nucleoli, atypical or bizarre mitoses (eg, tripolar), and tumor giant cells with one or more nuclei. However, some malignant tumors are well differentiated—so well differentiated, in fact, that their malignant cells cannot be distinguished from those of benign tumors or even from normal cells by any available diagnostic method. In such instances, the recognition of abnormal cellular relationships becomes especially important for correct diagnosis.

Anaplasia (from the Greek "to form backwards") is a term that describes the degree of tumor cell differentiation or, more correctly, the lack thereof. Although well entrenched, the term is an unfortunate one. It implies that tumors arise from mature, differentiated cells by a process of de-differentiation (ie, differentiation in reverse). Few pathologists hold that view today. Mammalian cells, once differentiated, generally lack the ability to reverse that process. Also, strong and growing evidence is providing support for the alternative explanation—namely, that tumors arise from populations of undifferentiated "stem" or "reserve" cells that are present in many, perhaps in all, organs capable of cell renewal.[23–27]

Stem cells constitute a minority cell population that lacks differentiation markers, making them difficult to identify. However, positive recognition of stem cells has been achieved in several organs—for example, bone marrow, epidermis, liver, and gastrointestinal tract mucosa.[28] Stem cells have a high capacity for cell proliferation but, unless stimulated, may divide infrequently. Stem cells alone have the capacity to regenerate normal tissues and, by extension, tumor-cell populations. Oncologists have become increasingly aware that stem cells may be the critically important target of cancer therapy. Destruction of differentiated tumor cells, without the simultaneous killing of tumor stem cells, will not lead to permanent tumor eradication.

Malignant tumors invariably lack a capsule. Instead, they extend crab-like projections into the surrounding host tissues without respect for normal anatomic boundaries. This behavior is called "invasion." Malignant tumor cells often invade lymphatics and veins and are transported by lymph or blood flow to distant sites, opening the possibility of metastasis. Invasion is not a property confined to malignant tumor cells; placental trophoblasts, inflammatory cells, and many proliferations in fetal life also have the capacity to invade tissues. To be considered malignant, a tumor need not be invasive at the time of removal; it may have been "caught" before it had time to invade, or it may not yet have progressed to the point of acquiring the capacity to invade. Epithelial tumors that have not extended through the underlying basement membrane at the time of diagnosis but that exhibit all other properties of malignancy are described as "in situ carcinomas" and can almost certainly be cured by complete excision.[29]

Ancillary Staining and Analytic Methods Immunohistochemistry is the most commonly employed ancillary technique in surgical pathology (see "Role of the Immunohistochemist" later in this chapter), but special stains also aid in differential diagnosis and classification of tumors. Examples include the Van Gieson stain or the Masson trichrome method for distinguishing collagen and muscle, the Weigert stain for elastic tissue, silver stains for reticulin fibers, and special stains for mucins, amyloid, lipids, myelin, and glycogen—all substances whose identification may aid in the diagnosis of one type of tumor or another. In other instances, enzyme histochemistry may be essential for defining cell lineage, as in certain types of leukemia. Examples include chloroacetate esterase or endogenous peroxidase staining for cells of myelomonocytic lineage and alpha naphthyl butyrate esterase (called "nonspecific" esterase) staining for monocytes and macrophages.

Other techniques that may occasionally aid the surgical pathologist in tumor diagnosis are specimen radiography (for localizing and analyzing crystalline material such as calcium in breast biopsies) and morphometry.

Excision Margins An important concern is the adequacy of tumor excision. Depending on the tissue, a decision about adequacy can be made from either frozen or permanent sections. If the tumor forms a discrete mass and the margins of the specimen are clearly recognizable, determination of excision margins is usually straightforward. Examples of tumors whose excision is likely to give clearly defined margins include those arising in the gastrointestinal tract, lung, and skin. The margins of tumors arising in soft tissues (eg, many sarcomas and breast carcinomas) and diffusely infiltrating tumors (eg, infiltrating lobular carcinoma of the breast, signet ring tumors of the gastrointestinal tract, and nerve-invading tumors such as adenoid cystic carcinomas of the salivary glands, gliomas, and glioblastomas) may be much more difficult to define. In at least certain histologic patterns of breast carcinoma, factors such as the extent of intraductal growth must be considered when evaluating resection margins.[30,31] In patients treated with excision and radiotherapy for invasive breast cancer, the evaluation of excision margins in the context of an extensive intraductal component provides more prognostic information than does the evaluation of margins alone.[32]

Tumor Grading, Staging, and Prognosis Pathologists are often called on to grade tumors or to participate in their staging so as to estimate tumor prognosis. Tumor staging (eg, the well-known tumor, nodes, metastasis [TNM] system) has proven to be of great value in estimating prognosis.

Staging tries to measure the extent of spread of a cancer within a patient. It uses parameters such as tumor size, lymph node involvement, and the presence of other metastases. Clearly, objective determinations made by the pathologist on resected tumor specimens have a critical impact on accurate tumor staging.

With rare exceptions, such as papillary carcinoma of the thyroid, the single most important

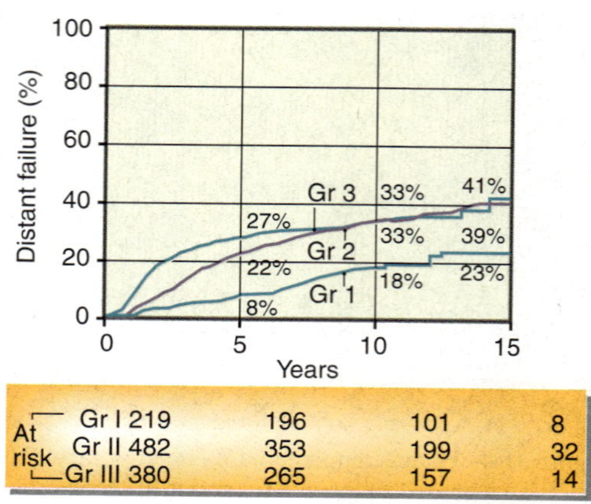

Figure 31-8 Actuarial rates of distant failure for 1,081 patients with invasive breast cancer related to histologic grade of tumor. Grading was performed using Elston's modification of the Bloom and Richardson grading system, which takes into consideration architectural pattern, nuclear grade, and mitotic activity (J. Connolly and S. Schnitt, unpublished data).

risk factor in determining tumor prognosis is the presence of metastases to regional lymph nodes. Therefore, the pathologist must search diligently to find, examine, and prepare histologic sections from all lymph nodes included in resected tissue.

"Tumor grading" has traditionally referred to a pathologist's judgment as to a tumor's degree of differentiation and growth rate, often on a scale of I to III, where III represents the least differentiated, fastest dividing tumors (ie, the tumors presumed to have the worst prognosis). Formal grading systems have improved in recent years with stricter standardization of criteria (Figure 31-8).[33]

Tumor grading does, however, have shortcomings. Each type of tumor requires a different scale, and scoring is subjective and not always reproducible. Also, tumors are typically heterogeneous; areas that vary significantly in differentiation and mitotic activity exist side by side, with the attendant risk of sampling error. Because prognosis is invariably linked to the most malignant portions of a tumor, it follows that, for accurate diagnosis and grading, sufficient tissue and microscopic sections must be sampled to find the most malignant areas. Moreover, a regular (though not invariant) feature of malignant tumors is progression,[34,35] the property by which tumors become more and more malignant over time. Tumor progression is thought to result from genomic instability[36] that leads to specific mutations of oncogenes or loss of tumor suppressor genes; from other genetic alterations, such as gene amplification; and from epigenetic changes that result in altered patterns of gene expression. Overt carcinogens, environmental promoters, and local factors such as hypoxia and nutrient deprivation, may all contribute to those changes and therefore to tumor progression. Finally, the correlation between histologic appearance and biologic behavior is seldom perfect.

Pathologists are continuously on the lookout for more useful tumor-specific features that may be important independent predictors of tumor prognosis. For example, carcinomas of the prostate are now usefully graded on the basis of tissue architecture and neoplastic cell pattern.[37] A variety of criteria, including nuclear differentiation, degree of gland or tubule formation, and mitotic activity, have been usefully combined to grade breast carcinomas.[33,38,39] Carcinoma of the breast illustrates other tumor-specific factors that affect prognosis and will now be discussed in greater detail, as an important example.

Factors Important in Predicting Risk for Local Recurrence or Distant Metastases in Patients with Invasive Breast Cancer

Separate consideration must be given to the risks of local recurrence of cancer in the breast and of distant metastases. The factors that affect each type of spread are not identical.

Local Recurrence In patients with infiltrating ductal carcinoma treated with breast-conserving surgery and radiation therapy, the factors predictive of local recurrence are not clearly related to known factors that predict for the development of distant metastasis. A large study on patients with clinical stage I or II infiltrating carcinomas of the breast made that point.[40] Treatment consisted of complete surgical excision of the primary tumor (without margin evaluation by microscopy), followed by radiation therapy totaling at least 60 Gy to the primary site. Of 34 separate tumor characteristics that were subjected to multivariate analysis, the only factor that was found to be associated with an increased risk of local breast recurrence was the presence of an extensive intraductal component (EIC-positive).

EIC positivity was identified in two distinct groups of tumors: (1) tumors which were predominantly ductal carcinomas in situ with areas of focal invasion; and (2) primarily invasive tumors in which (a) the ducts and lobules were not obliterated, (b) virtually all preserved ducts were involved by ductal carcinoma in situ, and (c) tumors in which ductal carcinoma in situ was present adjacent to the invasive tumor.[41] Of all study cases, 28% fell into the EIC-positive group, and 26% of those patients developed local tumor recurrence, compared with only 7% of patients with EIC-negative tumors (p = .001).[41] A number of other investigators have confirmed the finding that the presence of EIC is associated with a higher risk for breast cancer recurrence after local excision and radiation therapy.[42,43]

There seem to be two likely explanations for the increased risk of local recurrence in patients with EIC-positive tumors. One is that the residual tumor in this group of patients is less radiosensitive than that in patients with EIC-negative tumors. The second is that the subclinical residual tumor burden following excision is consistently larger in EIC-positive than in EIC-negative patients and may have been too large to have been eradicated by the cosmetically acceptable doses of radiation therapy that were delivered. Although both explanations are possible, the residual tumor burden has been found to be consistently larger in EIC-positive than in EIC-negative patients.[30]

EIC positivity is currently used to determine the extent of surgical excision. Patients with EIC-positive tumors frequently require a larger excision than patients with EIC-negative tumors. Some patients with EIC-positive tumors may require a mastectomy to obtain adequate margins. Patients with EIC-positive tumors with negative margins may be adequately treated with local excision "lumpectomy" and radiation therapy.[32]

Distant Metastases As is the case with many other tumors, the single most important predictor of systemic spread of breast cancer is involvement of the regional lymph nodes. Unless treated, most patients with involved axillary lymph nodes will ultimately die from metastatic spread of their disease. The greater the number of involved axillary lymph nodes, the greater the likelihood that tumor cells have spread elsewhere in the body to indeterminate locations only to become clinically manifest at a later time. Thus, in one large series, 87% of the patients with ≥ 13 involved axillary lymph nodes developed metastatic spread within 10 years, but only 20% of node-negative patients did so.[44]

Complete axillary dissection is becoming less common, especially with the advent of sentinel lymph node mapping. Radioactive isotopes or blue dye, or both, are injected either at the tumor site or into the overlying skin some time prior to the axillary exploration. At the time of surgery, only the "hot" or "blue" lymph nodes are removed. Immunocytochemistry is commonly performed on those nodes to identify tumor cells, but that procedure is not recommended by the College of American Pathologists at this time.[45] The reason is that a fairly large percentage of patients with ductal carcinoma in situ have positive nodes by immunocytochemistry, but have a less than 1% chance of developing distant metastases. In addition, the significance of micrometastases (2 mm or less in size in a single node) has not as yet been clearly demonstrated.

Given the important prognostic significance of positive lymph nodes and recent evidence that patient survival improves with adjuvant therapy, criteria are now urgently needed for identifying the 20 to 30% of lymph node–negative patients who will nonetheless develop metastatic disease after primary breast treatment. Factors worthy of consideration include the degree of tumor differentiation and the mitotic index as discussed earlier in this chapter. In addition, other more specific factors may play a role. One likely candidate is the capacity of tumor cells to find their way into vascular spaces, such as lymphatics or small blood vessels.[46–49]

Newer Criteria for Assessing Breast Carcinomas Several scoring systems have been used to grade breast cancers. Generally speaking, most include the degree of nuclear differentiation and the degree to which the tumor is able to form glands. An attempt is also made to estimate tumor growth rate by measuring mitotic activity. Using such criteria, the survival rates in one series of node-negative patients with grades 1 through 3 tumors varied from 86 to 64% at 5 years, and from 49 through 25% at 15 years.[50]

One approach for assessing tumor differentiation involves the use of flow cytometry. Tumors with normal diploid or tetraploid deoxyribonucleic acid (DNA) content have been repeatedly shown to have a better prognosis than aneuploid tumors do.[51–53] However, not all workers agree with this conclusion as it applies to node-negative patients.[54,55]

Tumor growth rate can be measured in a number of ways, including standard counts of mitotic figures per 10 high-power fields, the percentage of cells in the S-phase as determined by flow cytometry, and the ^{3}H thymidine labeling index.[51–53] In a large study of DNA ploidy and S-phase fraction in lymph node–negative patients with breast cancer, no correlation was found between S-phase fraction and survival among patients with aneuploid tumors.[51] The aneuploid tumors constituted two-thirds of cases studied. Among diploid tumors, however, the S-phase fraction was highly predictive of recurrence.[51]

One of the most intensively studied and widely used measures of breast cancer evaluation is tumor expression of estrogen receptor (ER) and progesterone receptor (PR). Those measures are, in fact, the only ones for which standardized quality control is currently available. Most studies have shown that lymph node–negative patients with ER-positive tumors have a significantly better disease-free survival and, in some cases, better overall survival than patients whose tumors are ER-negative.[56] The difference between the survival rates of patients with ER-positive tumors and ER-negative tumors decreases with time, and some studies have suggested that the survival curves will eventually merge.[57] Taken together, these observations suggest that tumors expressing estrogen and progesterone receptors tend to proliferate more slowly than tumors lacking such receptors. Thus, ER measurements may not represent an independent prognostic factor per se, but may instead provide yet another method of assessing tumor growth rate or differentiation. The true value in determining the ER status of a tumor is to predict which patients may benefit from adjuvant hormonal chemotherapy. Patients whose tumors are ER-positive are often treated with pharmaceutical agents that bind to the estrogen receptor and block endogenous estrogen binding. In postmenopausal patients, use of aromatase inhibitors that reduce estrogen production may provide an alternative adjuvant therapy.

Another criterion for assessing breast cancer prognosis—measurement of microvascular density—has come into prominence recently. As noted earlier, tumors must induce new blood vessels if they are to grow beyond minimal size. Therefore, intratumor microvascularity, taken as a measure of tumor angiogenesis, might be expected to provide a useful index of tumor aggressiveness. Investigating that possibility, Weidner and colleagues[58] performed counts of blood vessel frequency on breast cancer tissue sections. After immunostaining sections with anti–factor VIII–related antigen to ensure detection of all microvessels, they found that, as with other tumor properties such as mitotic index, individual breast cancers were heterogeneous with respect to microvessel density. They therefore selected zones that exhibited the highest blood vessel density ("hot spots") and found that hot spots in cancers of patients with metastases had mean vessel counts of 101 ± 49 per 200× field, significantly higher than the 45 ± 21 value for patients without metastases. Multivariate analysis of the data revealed that intratumor microvascular density provided an independent prognostic indicator of lymph node metastasis and of both relapse-free and overall patient survival. Most follow-up studies have confirmed those findings in breast[59] and in other tumors such as head and neck,[60] lung,[61,62] and prostate.[63]

Unfortunately, measurements of tumor microvascular density are laborious and subject to interobserver variability. For those reasons, the technique is unlikely to be used routinely outside of research settings. Nonetheless, the studies by Weidner and colleagues emphasize the importance of angiogenesis in human tumor biology, and they support the principle that angiogenesis may be a worthy target in biologic approaches to breast cancer therapy.

A somewhat different approach has been to correlate prognosis with the type of blood vessels that tumors generate. Only in the last few years have attempts been made to classify tumor blood vessels into their several distinct types.[10,64,65] Recently gathered evidence correlates tumors that generate one particular type of blood vessel, the so-called glomeruloid bodies or glomeruloid microvascular proliferations, with poor prognosis.[66,67]

Many studies are now in progress attempting to identify other factors that may predict for risk in node-negative patients. These include evaluation of Ki-67,[59] epidermal growth factor receptors,[68–70] insulin-like growth factors,[71,72] transforming growth factor,[73,74] cathepsin D,[75] and various oncogenes and their products. A recent review of prognostic factors in breast cancer cataloged and evaluated them.[45]

Oncologists have long sought therapeutic agents that would spare normal tissue and specifically target tumor cells. The use of antiestrogenic agents in ER–positive breast cancers has long been an established practice. A newer approach has been to target the *HER2/neu* antigen, which is overexpressed in certain breast and ovarian cancers. The antigen is targeted by a therapeutic agent, trastuzumab (Herceptin), consisting of a humanized monoclonal antibody that binds to the *HER2/neu* protein.[76] Initial clinical trials have demonstrated that trastuzumab specifically targets tumor cells and has a significant impact on patient survival.[77]

In the past, pathologists and oncologists have sought markers that predict tumor prognosis. We are now entering an era in which it will be more important to identify markers that help to predict the response to new and different therapeutic modalities.

Surgical Pathologist's Report Findings should be presented comprehensively, in terms that are understandable to both the pathologist and the clinicians caring for the patient. The report should provide enough information so that the clinicians can follow the thought processes of the pathologist, much as if they were viewing the case with the pathologist at a double-headed microscope. The report should contain all the information to which the pathologist has access (ie, tumor size, grade, and nodal status) that is necessary to stage a patient with cancer. That information varies with tumor origin, type, and staging system employed. The report should include the results of all specialized tests performed, their interpretation, and the synthesis and coordination of all clinically useful information available to the pathologist that may be of aid in diagnosis and management.

A helpful method to standardize the reporting of malignancies has been the introduction of synoptic reporting. The Association of Directors of Anatomic Pathology and The College of American Pathologists Cancer Committee have both produced synoptic reporting guidelines that are available on their Web sites.

Finally, reports should be issued in a timely manner. Failure to report results promptly may delay patient care (thus uselessly adding to the cost of medical care), lead to error and confusion, and at the very least prolong anxiety in patients who are often already distraught.

ROLE OF THE CYTOPATHOLOGIST

Cytology is used for both screening and diagnosis of lesions that may represent cancer or its precursors. Specific benefits include cost-effectiveness, rapid turnaround time, and diagnosis with minimal patient risk. Because cytology specimens usually consist of a very small quantity of cells or tissue fragments, optimal techniques for sample collection and slide preparation alike are crucial. Moreover, as in all areas of pathology, cytologic diagnosis should never be made "in a vacuum." Pertinent clinical data and communication between the cytopathologist and the clinician are essential and will facilitate rapid, accurate, and definitive cytologic diagnoses.

Methods for Obtaining Specimens The methods of obtaining cells for microscopy fall into two categories. In the first, a medium that contains naturally exfoliated cells (eg, urine, sputum, body cavity fluids) is obtained. In the second, cells of interest for examination are obtained using an instrument, such as a brush or a needle with a syringe.

Preparation of Cytologic Specimens for Microscopy The preparation of a cytologic specimen depends on the type of specimen. When cells are collected using an instrument, the cells can be either rinsed into a preservative solution or simply spread directly onto slides.[78–80] When the cells are collected in a medium, natural or artificial, the specimen needs to be processed to separate the medium from the cells. Possibilities include centrifugation, cytocentrifugation, filtering, or processing through a machine, such as a ThinPrep processor[81] or a PrepStain system.[82]

The optimal final product for every type of preparation is a slide holding a thin layer of evenly dispersed cells. Cells thinly spread on a slide dry out very easily; slides therefore need to be immediately fixed (using either 95% ethanol or a commercially available spray fixative) and then stained with Papanicolaou or H&E stain. Alternatively, slides allowed to air dry can be stained with a Romanowsky-type stain.

Microscopy Interpretation of Cytologic Specimens In contrast to surgical pathologists, cytopathologists deal primarily with cells without regard to stroma. Although some architectural features are maintained in cytology specimens, many are lost in the process of specimen collection and preparation. Therefore, cytopathologists rely mainly on the cytologic features of malignancy and on residual structural features such as cohesion versus dyshesion to determine the benign or malignant nature of the lesion.

Cytopathologists usually report their result in one of four categories: "positive," "suspicious," "atypical," or "negative."[83–85] A "positive" diagnosis indicates sufficient confidence in the malignant nature of the lesion that the pathologist is prepared to have the patient undergo definitive treatment such as surgical resection or chemotherapy based on the cytologic diagnosis alone.

Where doubt exists, the report should be less definitive and should fall into the "suspicious" category. Other diagnostic tests, such as a repeat cytology sample or a surgical biopsy, should be performed to determine with certainty the nature of the lesion before the patient undergoes definitive therapy. Occasionally, other evidence of malignancy, such as clinical and radiologic findings, is so strong that clinicians feel confident in implementing definitive therapy with a "suspicious" diagnosis. That must be a decision of the responsible clinician.

When cellular abnormalities whose clinical significance is not known are present, the report should be placed in the "atypical" category. Other diagnostic tests may be in order, depending on the clinical situation. Definitive therapy should never be initiated solely on the basis of atypia.

A "negative" cytology result means that no abnormal cells were found in the sample examined. All parties concerned must realize that a "negative" finding does not necessarily indicate absence of malignancy in the patient. False negative cytology results are often the result of sampling error. Laboratory error may produce both false negative and false positive results.

Exfoliative Cytology Exfoliative cytology involves microscopic examination of cells exfoliated from the respiratory (sputum), urinary (urine), or female genital tracts. The use of the Papanicolaou (Pap) smear to screen for cervical cancer and its precursors in the general asymptomatic population has been instrumental in dramatically lowering the mortality rate from cervical cancer over the last four decades.[86–88]

A problem inherent in all screening tests is the need to balance sensitivity and specificity.[88] Lowering the threshold for a diagnosis of atypia means that fewer cases of neoplasia will be missed. However, the trade-off is that more patients without neoplastic disease will receive additional, expensive studies such as colposcopy to rule out the presence of cancer or its precursors. The importance of proper sample collection and preparation needs to be emphasized. Failure to fix samples immediately, to create a thin-enough smear, or to ensure the absence of significant amounts of blood may all result in specimens that are inadequate or suboptimal for diagnosis. Putting the sampled materials into a preservative medium and using a machine to make slides with a thin layer of cells can obviate most of the above pitfalls; however, the cost of preparation is significantly increased.[81,82]

Since human papillomavirus (HPV) was shown to be a necessary, though not sufficient, cause of cervical neoplasia,[89] testing for high-risk (oncogenic) types of HPV has now been added to the screening program for cervical neoplasia. Testing for high-risk HPV had initially been used to triage women with equivocal cytology results (ie, atypical squamous cells of undetermined significance [ASC-US]).[90] Recently, the US Food and Drug Administration approved the use of the "high-risk" panel of Hybrid Capture 2 HPV DNA Test (HC2, which detects HPV types 16, 18, 31, 33, 35, 39, 45, 51, 52, 56, 58, 59, and 68) as an adjunct to cervical cytology screening in women aged 30 years or older.[91] In fact, for women in that age group, a strategy that uses HPV testing in combination with cytology for primary screening at 3-year intervals provides a greater reduction in cancer risk (91.9%) and is less costly (lifetime cost of $1,647 US) than is annual conventional cytology (89.5% reduction, with lifetime cost of $2,457 US).[92] Women who are negative both for cytology and for HPV can be screened every three years. Those whose cytology diagnosis is more serious than ASC-US, and those whose cytology diagnosis is ASC-US with positive HPV, should be immediately referred for colposcopy. Those who have negative cytology and positive HPV results should undergo both tests again at 6 to 12 months. Those whose cytology shows ASC-US, but negative HPV results, may repeat cytology at 12 months.

Cytologic examinations of sputum and urine are not currently used to screen the general population, but are instead used to detect cancers in high-risk patients who either have had exposures that increase their risk of developing cancers or already have symptoms that may be caused by cancers in the lung or urinary bladder.[93,94] Similarly, patients with an increased risk of esophageal adenocarcinoma or squamous cell carcinoma can be surveyed by non-endoscopic sampling with balloon or encapsulated samplers.[95–97] A breast duct lavage technique has been proposed to detect cellular atypia for risk stratification in women at high risk for breast cancer.[98,99] For patients with symptoms or other clinical evidence of disease, more invasive procedures—such as bronchoscopy, cystoscopy, upper gastrointestinal endoscopy, colposcopy, and fine-needle aspirations or excisional biopsies—are called for if a diagnosis cannot be made on exfoliative cytology.

Endoscopic Cytology In areas amenable to endoscopy, such as the bronchial tree and the gastrointestinal and urinary tracts, cytologic specimens obtained with brushing and washing techniques aimed at grossly identifiable lesions may serve a diagnostic function. Paired cytology and biopsy can improve the likelihood of diagnosing malignancy in a single procedure.[100,101] Because brush samples cover a wide area, they provide greater diagnostic sensitivity than biopsies, particularly in the case of early lesions that are not grossly obvious. However, endoscopic biopsies generally provide more information, particularly in determinations of tumor type and presence of invasion. Endoscopic FNA, either with the flexible needle used for injecting esophageal varices (sclerotherapy needle) or with a transbronchial aspiration needle, may make it possible to obtain samples from lesions lying deep to necrotic debris or to normal mucosa.[102] This technique is further enhanced by adding ultrasound guidance.[103] Endoscopic ultrasound-guided FNAs have enabled endoscopists to reach further than was possible with biopsy forceps. They can now sample mural lesions and even lesions adjacent to the gastrointestinal tract, such as lymph nodes and pancreas.[104–106]

Cytology of Body Cavity and Cerebrospinal Fluids Fluids are removed from body cavities not only for the purpose of therapy (eg, to relieve pressure on vital organs), but also for diagnosis. With the exception of mesotheliomas, the presence of tumor cells in body cavities (Figure 31-9) implies metastasis. Determining the site of the primary tumor is usually difficult, if not impossible; but certain morphologic clues may occasionally allow the cytopathologist to suggest a site of origin. If the cytology is consistent with the clinical findings and results from other studies, a positive cytologic diagnosis can lead directly to treatment. Current cytologic specimens should always be compared to previous cytologic or histologic specimens, if available.

Reactive mesothelial cells share certain characteristics with carcinoma cells, and the parallels should be considered in the differential diagnosis. Panels of immunocytochemical stains may prove useful (see "Role of the Immunohistochemist"). Sometimes (eg, in the case of mesotheliomas) tumor growth may be confined to the surfaces lining body cavities, without significant exfoliation of malignant cells. Under those circumstances, a biopsy of the cavity wall is required to establish the diagnosis. An alternative approach for future investigation may be to analyze tumor cell–free effusions for secreted products of malignant cells or other tumor-cell markers. One successful, though preliminary, application of this approach is the finding of high levels of the angiogenic factor VPF/VEGF (VEGF-A) in effusions by immunoassay.[107]

Aspiration Cytology The earliest work on aspiration cytology was reported from Memorial Hospital in New York in the 1930s.[108] Subsequently, the impetus for this technique shifted to Europe and was not "rediscovered" in the United States until the 1970s.[109]

Cytopathologists, surgeons, and other clinicians can successfully perform an aspiration of a palpable lesion. In the case of non-palpable lesions, a radiologist or clinician performs the aspiration under computed tomography, ultrasound, or fluoroscopic guidance. Deep aspiration procedures of this kind are expensive, time-consuming, and invasive. For those reasons, it is desirable that a cytotechnologist or cytopathologist attend the procedure to ensure specimen adequacy and optimal slide preparation. A further advantage of having experienced personnel on hand is effective triage of material for special studies such as immunocytochemistry (Figure 31-10), electron microscopy, flow cytometry, and tissue culture.

Definitive aspiration cytology diagnoses, rendered by an experienced cytopathologist, can pro-

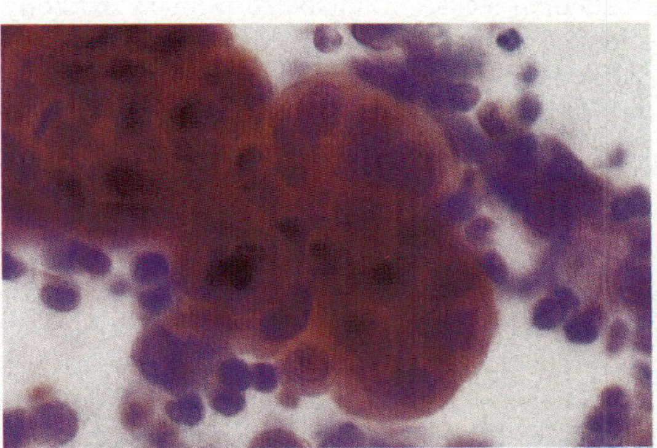

Figure 31-9 Ovarian papillary serous adenocarcinoma in ascitic fluid. Cells are present in three-dimensional clusters with nuclear molding and irregular hyperchromatic nuclei. Papanicolaou stain; ×250 original magnification.

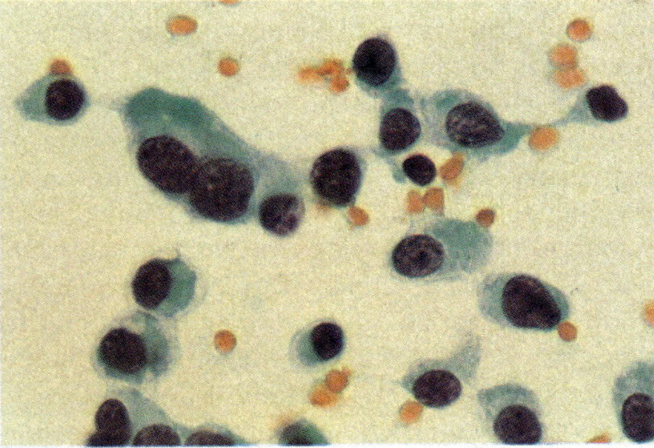

Figure 31-10 Metastatic neuroendocrine tumor as seen in a fine-needle aspiration biopsy of liver. Note eccentric nuclei with "salt and pepper" chromatin and abundant granular cytoplasm. Immunocytochemical stains confirmed the diagnosis. Papanicolaou stain; ×250 original magnification.

vide the basis for definitive therapy. However, such diagnoses need to be viewed in the context of all other laboratory studies and clinical findings. Specific problems and pitfalls are associated with aspirations of various sites.

The Thyroid FNA biopsy is the first test used in most patients with a solitary thyroid nodule. The technique is safe and inexpensive and leads to a better selection of patients for surgery than does any other test.[110] FNA permits the accurate diagnosis of papillary, medullary, and anaplastic carcinomas; it is less useful in the diagnosis of follicular nodules. Certain cytologic features help to distinguish between the various types of follicular lesions,[111] but a definitive diagnosis is not possible by FNA. In that situation, FNA serves only to distinguish patients needing immediate surgery for thyroid disease from those who may be safely followed with or without hormonal suppression. However, even that limited information can eliminate many unnecessary surgeries.[112]

The Breast In the hands of an experienced cytopathologist, the diagnostic specificity of breast aspiration is very high, and a positive diagnosis may safely lead to mastectomy or other definitive treatment.[85,113] Of course, atypical and suspicious cases require further workup. FNA of the breast may also be performed on nonpalpable lesions under the guidance of conventional or stereotactic mammography or ultrasonography.[114–116]

As compared with core biopsy, breast cytology presents certain inherent problems. These include inability to distinguish infiltrating from in situ carcinoma and difficulty in rendering a specific benign diagnosis.[117,118] However, the needles used in FNA cost much less than core needles do, and they are more readily tolerated by patients. Most labs continue to show an increase in FNA of the breast, especially for palpable lesions, but that increase is much less than the increase in core biopsies of the breast.[119] Furthermore, there seems to be a tendency for clinicians to use FNA for lesions that are clinically benign and core biopsies for lesions that are clinically worrisome.[120]

Lungs Aspiration cytology of the lungs may lead to diagnosis of both primary and metastatic tumors and of non-neoplastic lesions such as tuberculosis and fungal infections.[121] As in the case of histologic lung-tissue sections, distinguishing primary from metastatic carcinoma is not always possible.

The Abdomen Aspiration cytology is particularly useful in pretreatment diagnosis of malignancies in the liver, pancreas, kidney, and retroperitoneum.[122] A diagnosis of metastatic tumor or lymphoma spares the patient major surgery and provides a basis for definitive therapy. Poorly differentiated tumors may be difficult to type, but the use of adjunct techniques is often helpful in establishing a definitive diagnosis.

Lymph Nodes Some pathologists question the role of aspiration cytology in the diagnosis of lymph node lesions.[123] FNA can provide useful information to obviate the need for surgery in cases of suspected metastatic carcinoma or melanoma from a known primary to palpable lymph nodes. FNA can also help to identify infections. Lymph node aspirates may provide a diagnosis and classification of lymphoproliferative disorders, especially when used in conjunction with flow cytometry or another immunophenotyping technique.[124,125] If, on FNA, a lymphoproliferative lesion is suspected without a definitive diagnosis, the patient can proceed to have an excisional biopsy for final diagnosis.

APPLICATION OF ANCILLARY STUDIES ON CYTOLOGIC MATERIALS Nearly all ancillary studies, such as those involving immunocytochemistry, electron microscopy, flow cytometry, and molecular biology, can be applied to cytologic materials (see "Role of the Immunohistochemist," next, for details).

Few of the diagnostic tests introduced into medicine have actually lowered the cost of high-quality patient care. Cytopathology is one of them. It offers the advantages of low morbidity, rapid turnaround time, and outstanding cost effectiveness. The problems in cytology should not detract from its usefulness. All procedures have limitations, and the oncologist needs to be informed alike about the benefits and the pitfalls of this technique.

ROLE OF THE IMMUNOHISTOCHEMIST

Immunohistochemistry has become an important adjunct in the evaluation of human neoplasms. A detailed discussion of the technical aspects of immunohistochemistry is beyond the scope of this chapter, but the interested reader can consult several review articles and monographs.[126–131] The commercial availability of a broad range of reagents, including prediluted reagents in kit form, has made it possible for high-quality immunohistochemistry to be performed in most pathology laboratories. The most commonly employed immunohistochemical techniques are those in which enzymes, such as horseradish peroxidase or alkaline phosphatase, are used in conjunction with specific antibodies to provide color reactions at sites of antigen–antibody interactions. Variations of the avidin–biotin complex (ABC) technique are the most widely used in current practice.

The ABC procedure generally requires four sequential steps: an unlabeled primary antibody directed against the antigen of interest, a biotin-labeled anti-immunoglobulin secondary antibody, preformed avidin–biotin peroxidase complexes, and finally a chromogenic substrate (typically diaminobenzidine), which is enzymatically converted by the peroxidase moiety to a colored signal. One variation of the ABC method employs streptavidin, which has greater sensitivity than avidin and exhibits less nonspecific binding.[126]

It should be noted that the sensitivity of any immunohistochemical procedure is, in large part, related to the reagents and detailed procedures employed. As a consequence, comparing the results of immunohistochemical studies from different institutions that employ different reagents and methods is difficult. Almost any type of pathology specimen may be suitable for immunohistochemical staining, including fresh-frozen tissue, fixed tissue, and cytologic preparations. Unfortunately, however, not all antigens are equally well preserved after these various treatments, and the approach taken for immunohistochemical staining must depend on the antigen or antigens of interest. For example, although many cytoplasmic antigens are detectable in fixed, paraffin-embedded tissue, others, such as many cell surface–associated antigens, are destroyed or masked by common fixatives. They may be demonstrable only in fresh-frozen tissue or in cytologic preparations. Antigen retrieval methods, such as pretreatment with proteolytic enzymes or heating (using a microwave oven, steamer, pressure cooker, or autoclave), may permit the identification of otherwise undemonstrable antigens in fixed, paraffin-embedded tissue sections.[132,133] Finally, not all fixatives are equivalent with regard to antigen preservation. Although cross-linking fixatives, such as formaldehyde, are often suitable, they are suboptimal for detecting certain antigens of diagnostic importance, such as those located on intermediate filaments, which are best demonstrated in fresh-frozen or alcohol-fixed tissue.[128,134,135]

APPLICATIONS Immunohistochemistry has widespread applicability in the evaluation of human tumors. Some of the more common applications are listed in Table 31-1 and are discussed below.

Categorizing "Undifferentiated" Malignant Tumors Not infrequently, a pathologist examining routine H&E-stained paraffin sections recognizes the presence of a malignant tumor but is unable to characterize the tumor further. This is understandable. Histologically undifferentiated tumors often lack visually recognizable characteristics that would permit more accurate classification. Yet further classification is often important in making clinical decisions about appropriate therapy and prognosis. Immunohistochemistry may be helpful in such situations (Figure 31-11).

But before performing immunohistochemistry, the pathologist must first develop a differential diagnosis, and that diagnosis will depend on the tumor's histologic appearance, anatomic location, radiologic characteristics, and the patient's clinical history. Only then is the pathologist in a

Table 31-1 Common Applications of Immunohistochemistry in the Evaluation of Human Tumors

1. Categorization of "undifferentiated" malignant tumors
2. Determination of site of origin of metastatic tumors
3. Subclassification of tumors in various organ systems and tissue compartments (e.g., central nervous system tumors, germ cell tumors, sarcomas)
4. Distinction between carcinomas and malignant mesotheliomas
5. Categorization of leukemias and lymphomas
6. Detection of antigens of potential prognostic or therapeutic importance
   a. Estrogen and progesterone receptors
   b. Oncogene and tumor suppressor gene products
   c. Markers of proliferative activity

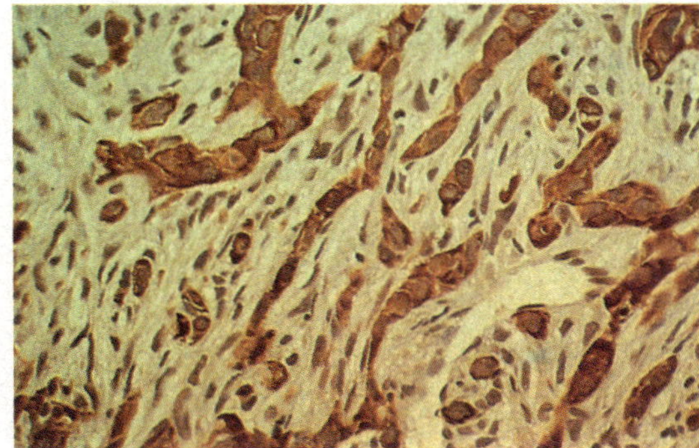

Figure 31-11 Immunoperoxidase staining of a monoclonal antibody specific for keratin in a poorly differentiated squamous cell carcinoma of skin. The "spindle cell" form of the tumor mimics tumors of connective-tissue origin, and its true nature can often be determined only by immunohistochemistry. Immunoperoxidase stain; ×100 original magnification.

position to select antibodies that will permit a more definitive diagnosis.

The common problem of an undifferentiated tumor composed of large cells with an epithelioid appearance will serve as an example. The differential diagnosis in such cases typically includes undifferentiated carcinoma, lymphoma, and malignant melanoma. Distinction among these tumor types can often be made using a panel of antibodies as illustrated in Table 31-2. Unfortunately, this table represents an ideal result that is not always achieved in practice. Some carcinomas show staining for vimentin or S100 protein, some melanomas show immunoreactivity for keratin, and some neoplasms other than melanomas express HMB-45.[135–140] Such results emphasize the need to use a panel of antibodies, rather than a single antibody, in evaluating tumors.

Determining Site of Origin of Metastatic Tumors On routine microscopy examination, tumors may be classifiable with regard to general histologic type (eg, adenocarcinoma, squamous cell carcinoma). However, the site of origin may not be reliably determined using histologic cues alone. It would be highly desirable to have available antibodies specific for tumors arising in various sites. At present, however, very few organ- or tissue-specific antigens have been identified, thus limiting the ability of immunohistochemistry to resolve such problems in every instance.

Table 31-3 lists a number of useful antigens. It should be noted that antigens specific for some of the more common tumors—such as carcinomas of the colon, endometrium, and pancreas—are not currently available. Furthermore, some of the antigens listed in Table 31-3 have now been demonstrated in neoplasms other than those for which they were initially thought to be "specific." For example, the melanoma-associated antigen detected by one widely used antibody (HMB-45) has been found in some nonmelanocytic tumors.[137] A more recent approach for the subclassification of metastatic carcinomas exploits differences in the cytokeratin profiles of tumors from different primary sites.[141]

Subclassifying Tumors in Various Organ Systems In some organs and tissue compartments, overlapping features may make it difficult to subclassify certain tumors solely on histologic grounds. Some of the distinctions are, at present, only of academic interest; for example, determining whether a high-grade sarcoma shows neural, myogenous, or fibrous differentiation. Other distinctions have therapeutic and prognostic significance.

For example, in some cases, distinguishing with certainty an anaplastic seminoma from an embryonal carcinoma of the testis may be difficult or impossible by routine microscopy examination. Such a distinction has both therapeutic and prognostic implications. However, immunostaining for the intermediate filament keratin is often useful in such a case, because seminomas are typically keratin-negative, and embryonal carcinomas are usually keratin-positive.[142,143] Similar situations are encountered in other organ systems and tissue compartments.

Table 31-2 Idealized Immunohistochemical Evaluation of the "Undifferentiated" Malignant Tumor[a]

Antibody to	Tumor Type		
	Carcinoma	Lymphoma	Melanoma
Keratin	+	–	–
Epithelial membrane antigen	+	–	–
Vimentin	–	+ or –	+
Leukocyte common antigen	–	+	–
S100 protein	–	–	+
HMB-45	–	–	+

[a]In which the differential diagnosis includes carcinoma, lymphoma, and melanoma (see text).

Table 31-3 Antigens with Highly Restricted Specificity

Antigen	Tumor Specificity
Factor VIII–related antigen	Vascular tumors
Gross cystic disease fluid protein	Breast carcinomas; cutaneous tumors with protein apocrine differentiation
HMB-45	Melanoma, renal angiomyolipoma
Muscle-specific actin	Smooth muscle and skeletal muscle tumors
Myoglobin	Skeletal muscle tumors
Prostate-specific antigen	Prostatic carcinomas
Thyroglobulin	Thyroid follicular cell tumors

Table 31-4 Immunohistochemical Distinction between Metastatic Adenocarcinoma and Malignant Mesothelioma Involving the Pleura or Peritoneum

	Adenocarcinoma	Mesothelioma
Keratin	+	+
Vimentin	+ or –	+ or –
Carcinoembryonic antigen	+ or –	–
Leu-M1	+ or –	–
B72.3	+ or –	–
Ber-EP4	+ or–	–
Calretinin	–	+

Distinguishing between Carcinomas and Malignant Mesotheliomas A common problem encountered by the surgical pathologist is making the distinction between metastatic adenocarcinoma and malignant mesothelioma involving the pleura or peritoneum.[144–148] Immunohistochemical staining using a panel of antibodies is often useful in making this distinction (Table 31-4).

Categorizing Leukemias and Lymphomas One of the most common uses for immunohistochemistry is the correct diagnosis and classification of leukemias and lymphomas. A detailed discussion of this subject is beyond the scope of this chapter, but the interested reader can consult recent articles and reviews.[149–152] In brief, immunohistochemistry is a useful adjunct to morphology and histochemistry in making the distinction between acute leukemias of the lymphoid and myeloid types and in distinguishing hairy-cell leukemia from other types of leukemic infiltrates in the bone marrow and at other sites. In addition, the technique is useful for subclassifying non–Hodgkin's lymphomas and Hodgkin's disease and in distinguishing the two conditions in problematic cases.

Detecting Antigens of Potential Prognostic or Therapeutic Significance Immunohistochemistry can be used to detect a variety of antigens of possible prognostic and therapeutic importance, including estrogen and progesterone receptors in breast cancers, protein products of oncogenes (such as *HER2/neu* in breast cancers), antigens associated with tumor cell proliferation such as Ki-67 and the P-glycoprotein product of the multiple drug resistance (*MDR*) gene.[153–161]

Ki-67 is of particular interest.[162] It is a nuclear antigen present in all proliferating cells; that is, it is present in the G1, S, G2, and M phases of the cell cycle, but absent in G0 cells. Therefore, by staining for Ki-67, it is possible to measure the tumor growth fraction directly, simply, and in a manner more readily applicable to clinical specimens than are the ^{3}H–thymidine radiolabeling methods. Ki-67 staining also yields results that are more reproducible than those obtained by counting mitotic figures. Recently, a number of antibodies that identify the Ki-67 antigen in formalin-fixed, paraffin-embedded tissue sections became available.[163]

Recognizing Invasive Carcinoma Using Myoepithelial Markers The distinction between invasive adenocarcinoma and its histologic mimics can be extremely difficult in core biopsies of the prostate, the test of choice for the diagnosis of prostatic adenocarcinoma. Accurate diagnosis of invasive carcinoma in these small biopsies is extremely important because of the profound clinical and therapeutic consequences. The observation that benign lesions arising from glandular structures such as the prostate are invested with a layer of non-neoplastic myoepithelial cells has been exploited since the discovery of antibodies that are relatively specific for myoepithelial differentiation (eg, p63, calponin, and cytokeratin 903). The presence of myoepithelial cells surrounding nests of cells, as detected by immunohistochemistry, effectively excludes a diagnosis of invasive carcinoma;[164] lack of such an investment strongly suggests invasive carcinoma (Figure 31-12). These immunohistochemical markers of myoepithelial differentiation are also used extensively in the diagnosis of mammary carcinoma, in which markers such as p63 are useful for distinguishing in situ mammary carcinoma from the invasive form.

Limitations An appreciation of the limitations of immunohistochemistry in tumor diagnosis is as important as an understanding of its many useful applications. Potential limitations in the immunohistochemical evaluation of solid tumors can be broadly characterized as technical and interpretive.

Technical Limitations Because demonstration of various types of antigens by immunostaining requires appropriate tissue preparation, advance planning for immunohistochemistry is essential so that the specimen may be handled appropriately. For example, if, on clinical grounds or at intraoperative examination (ie, frozen section or tissue imprint), an excised lymph node shows features suspicious for a lymphoma, a portion of the specimen might be snap-frozen to permit reliable demonstration of lymphocyte surface markers, because some of those markers are not well demonstrated in fixed, paraffin-embedded tissue. In cases of suspected carcinoma in which demonstration of intermediate filament proteins is likely to be important, fixation of a portion of the tumor in an alcohol-based fixative may be advisable. As in any laboratory procedure, the use of appropriate positive and negative controls is mandatory in immunohistochemistry. Controls serve as a check on the technical adequacy of the procedure. If the appropriate controls are omitted or are suboptimal, the results of immunostaining must be viewed with caution.

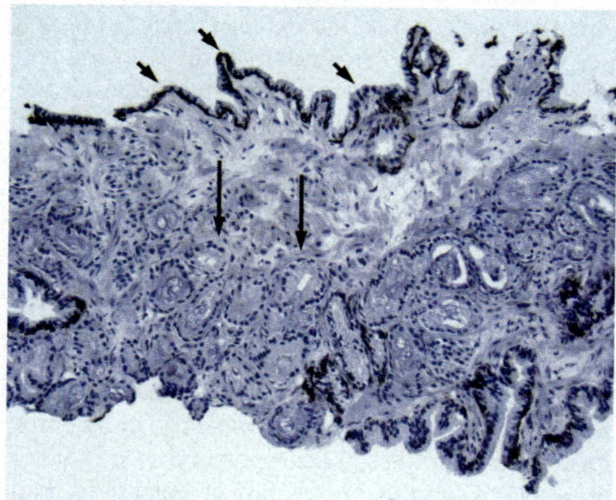

Figure 31-12 Immunoperoxidase staining for cytokeratin 903, a marker specific for prostatic myoepithelial cells. The absence of a rim of myoepithelial cells (*long arrows*) in the center of the photomicrograph confirms the presence of invasive adenocarcinoma. Note the surrounding benign glands (*short arrows*) that show expression of cytokeratin 903, which denotes the presence of myoepithelial cells, and, thus, the benign nature of these glands. Hematoxylin counterstain. Original magnification, 200×. Photograph courtesy of Dr. Elizabeth Genega.

Interpretive Limitations Correct interpretation of immunohistochemical stains performed on tumor specimens depends not only on the technical adequacy of the procedure, but also on interpretive factors. In most cases, a panel of antibodies is more useful than a single antibody. The antibodies that make up the panel must be selected thoughtfully, on the basis of a carefully prepared differential diagnosis. A haphazard approach to immunostaining is strongly discouraged, because it will only serve to compound diagnostic confusion.

Accurate interpretation of staining also requires familiarity with the sensitivity and specificity of the antibodies in question. Negative reactions are more difficult to interpret than positive reactions are. Even with the use of other controls, it is difficult to be certain that a reaction is a true negative unless the section in question stains positively for a complementary antigen. For example, in the analysis of an undifferentiated malignant tumor in which the differential diagnosis includes lymphoma and carcinoma, a negative reaction for keratin (the intermediate filament characteristic of many carcinomas) does not by itself rule out the possibility of carcinoma. However, if a negative keratin stain is accompanied by positive staining for the leukocyte common antigen (a marker present in most lymphomas), the likelihood of lymphoma is greatly enhanced. Some antibodies are of great diagnostic value in terms of both sensitivity and specificity—the antibodies to prostate-specific antigen, for example. Others are of limited diagnostic value even when used as part of a panel—antibodies to the intermediate filament vimentin, for example.

Pathologists who use immunohistochemistry must be experienced and aware of the limitations of the methodology, which is evolving at a rapid pace. An antigenic profile suitable today for diagnosing a particular type of tumor may tomorrow be shown to be suboptimal or less specific than was originally thought. Immunohistochemistry is a valuable tool for aiding in the diagnosis of difficult-to-identify tumors. However, it is only an adjunct to diagnosis, and the results must be interpreted in the context of other findings, particularly routine histologic sections and the clinical setting.

ROLE OF THE ELECTRON MICROSCOPIST

Although it makes use of radically different technology, electron microscopy (EM) seeks the same type of information as that gleaned from immunohistochemistry—that is, detection of differentiated organelles ("markers" in the case of immunohistochemistry) that permit more accurate tumor identification and classification. EM is not useful in determining whether individual cells are malignant or benign. However, it is a powerful tool for recognizing subcellular structures not detectable under light microscopy. The presence of particular structures under EM permits confident identification of cells—for example, whether they are of epithelial or melanocyte origin.

Although advances in immunohistochemistry have somewhat reduced the need for EM in tumor diagnosis, they have by no means eliminated the need altogether. EM remains a powerful but generally underutilized approach to tumor diagnosis.[165–168] Moreover, validation of new immunohistochemical reagents is often best accomplished by ultrastructural study of replicate tissue samples.

Technical Considerations Appropriate tissue handling, fixation, and processing are of even greater importance in EM than in immunohistochemistry.[169] Advance planning and consultation between the clinician, the surgical pathologist, and the electron microscopist are therefore important. In many cases, having a pathologist or knowledgeable technician in the operating room or at the bedside at the time of biopsy is advantageous. Tissue can then be fixed immediately and trimmed appropriately.

Tissue must be cut into small pieces because chemical fixatives penetrate slowly (taking minutes to hours), and the electron microscope glaringly exposes artifacts in poorly fixed tissues that are not detectable at the lower resolution afforded by light microscopy. In at least one dimension, the tissue must be no thicker than 1 mm. To achieve that small size, further trimming may be necessary after a brief preliminary fixation. Mixtures of glutaraldehyde and paraformaldehyde provide optimal fixation.[169] Vials of fixative can be frozen beforehand and thawed immediately before use, thereby avoiding the time-consuming need to prepare fresh fixative for each case. Tissues fixed in formalin or in other "routine" fixatives designed for light microscopy give inadequate tissue preservation for electron microscopy. Once tissues are fixed inappropriately, they generally cannot be recovered for adequate EM, and repeat biopsy becomes the best option. Peripheral blood, bone marrow, and cell-containing fluids (eg, pleural effusions, and spinal or synovial fluid) are handled somewhat differently from samples of solid tissue.[169]

Applications The great strength of EM lies in its exquisite resolution, which permits recognition of intracellular structures, organelles, or products that are undetectable under light microscopy.

EM is often helpful in the diagnosis of "undifferentiated" malignant tumors and in determining the origin of metastatic tumors of unknown primary site (Figures 31-13 and 31-14). The recognition of cytoplasmic premelanosomes within tumor

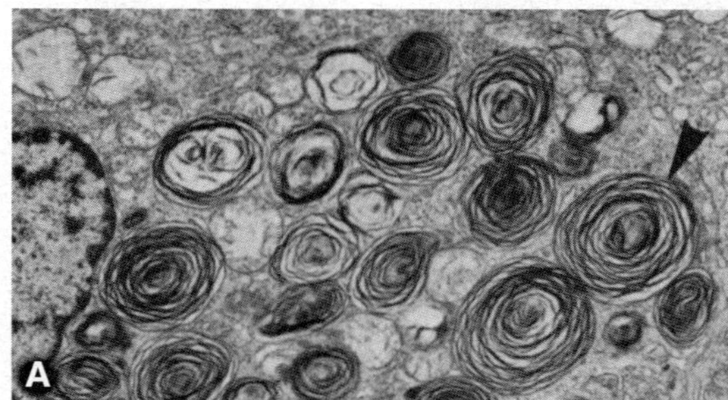

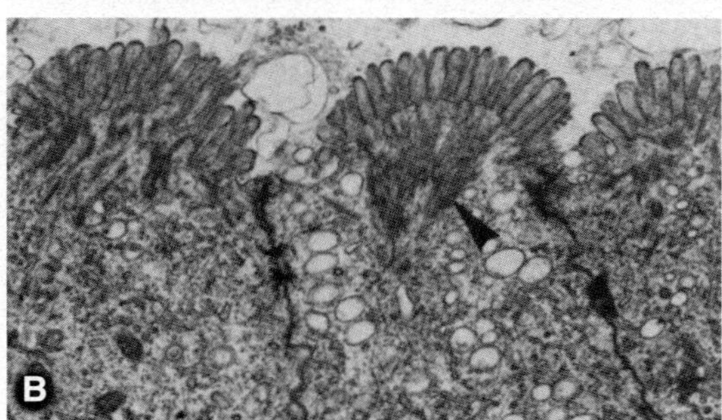

Figure 31-13 **A,** Electron micrograph from a lung mass shows typical surfactant-containing lamellar bodies ("surfactant bodies" [*arrowhead*]) that fill the cytoplasm of a tumor cell, allowing the specific diagnosis of primary alveolar cell carcinoma of the lung to be made. ×12,500 original magnification. **B,** Electron micrograph from a lung mass shows apical cytoplasm of three tumor cells at high magnification. Note the short, blunt, surface microvilli and the dense terminal web (*arrowhead*) of cytoskeletal filaments that traverse the apical cytoplasm to enter individual microvilli. The tumor cells are joined by epithelial junctions and contain numerous apical cytoplasmic vesicles. The identification of the differentiated organelle, the terminal web, allows the specific diagnosis of metastatic adenocarcinoma of gut absorptive epithelial cell origin to be made. ×19,000 original magnification.

cells permits amelanotic malignant melanomas to be distinguished from the undifferentiated carcinomas and lymphomas with which they can be confused. Other ultrastructural features whose recognition may permit definitive diagnosis are the cytoplasmic granules characteristic of carcinoid tumors, the norepinephrine- and epinephrine-containing granules found in pheochromocytomas, the "terminal webs" characteristic of primary gastrointestinal carcinomas of absorptive epithelial cell origin,[170] the lamellar (surfactant) bodies found only in type II pneumocytes (and therefore diagnostic of alveolar cell carcinomas of the lung,)[171] the tonofilaments and desmosomes found in mesothelial cells and squamous cells, and the cytoplasmic glycogen aggregates and calligraphic nucleoli typical of germinomas. The presence of intercellular junctions permits the distinction of carcinomas from lymphomas, even if the carcinoma's primary site cannot be determined.

EM is also helpful in subclassifying tumors, an exercise that may have important therapeutic implications. The use of ultrastructural cytochemistry for endogenous peroxidase may allow the important distinction of acute myeloblastic leukemia from acute lymphoblastic leukemia. Histiocytosis X may be diagnosed by identification of Birbeck bodies characteristic of Langerhans cells. EM may also permit accurate diagnosis of lysosomal storage diseases and of bacterial, fungal, and viral infections.

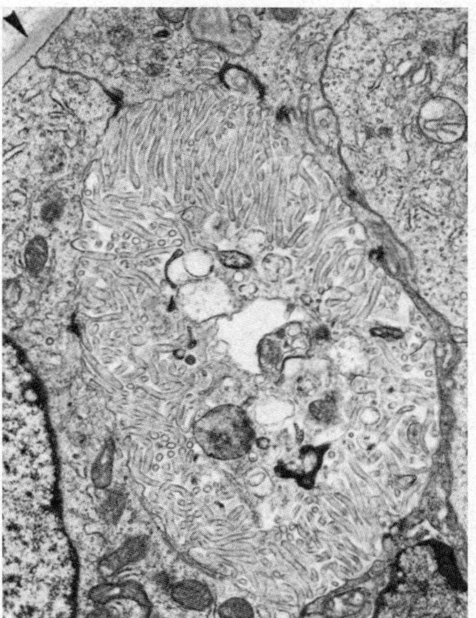

Figure 31-14 High-magnification electron micrograph of pleural tumor shows three typical features of mesothelial cells: (1) numerous elongated, thick surface microvilli that (2) do not display evidence of terminal web differentiation, and (3) desmosomes that connect individual cells surrounding the extracellular acinar space and basal lamina (*arrowhead*). Another feature diagnostic of mesothelial cells—dense bundles of tonofilaments—is not seen in this high-magnification image. In concert, these four ultrastructural findings allow an ultrastructural diagnosis of mesothelioma to be made in the presence of light microscopy evidence of a malignant tumor proliferation of the pleura. ×22,000 original magnification.

Finally, EM is important in identifying the histogenesis of newly recognized neoplasms. A recent example (Figure 31-15) is the recognition that certain spindle cell tumors of the gastrointestinal tract, previously thought to be of smooth muscle origin, in fact arise from autonomic neurons (gastrointestinal tract autonomic nerve tumors).[170]

Limitations As in immunohistochemistry, the limitations of EM are both technical and interpretive. Technical limitations such as improper tissue handling and delayed or inappropriate fixation or processing have already been alluded to. Another limitation is sampling error, which is attributable to the very small size of the specimen that can be studied on an EM grid. Expense is also a limitation. Whereas the availability of commercial reagents, defined protocols, and relatively simple interpretation have permitted immunohistochemistry to be established in almost any hospital pathology laboratory, the same cannot be said for diagnostic EM. The costly electron microscope, the fairly elaborate support equipment, and the need for experienced technical and professional personnel have limited the application of this methodology to large tertiary-care centers, mostly at academic institutions. Of particular importance is the need for a pathologist who is well trained in both surgical pathology and EM. Asking a basic science-oriented electron microscopist or an EM technician to take a few pictures of a tumor specimen is a prescription for error or futility.

ROLE OF THE CLINICAL PATHOLOGIST

The role of the clinical pathologist or "laboratorian" is obvious and familiar to the oncologist and requires only brief mention here. Clinical pathologists are interested in measurements of body fluids that lead to the early detection and monitoring of cancer. The field of tumor antigens and tumor markers has generated a great deal of interest, and some of those antigens and markers are discussed elsewhere in this volume. At least in theory, tumor-specific antigens circulating in the plasma could be useful in tumor diagnosis and prognosis, assessment of tumor burden, prediction of recurrence, and guidance for treatment.

Properties of an ideal tumor marker include great sensitivity, specificity, and accuracy in reflecting total tumor burden. A tumor marker should also be prognostic of outcome and predictive of tumor recurrence. Unfortunately, none of the tumor markers discovered to date fulfills all of those criteria. In fact, none is uniquely produced by tumor cells. Normal cells of one sort or another make all of the tumor markers thus far recognized, and plasma or serum levels in tumor patients differ only quantitatively, not qualitatively, from those in normal control subjects or in patients with other diseases. Recently, a new concept has emerged—namely, that cancer may be diagnosed by testing a panel of serum proteins using proteomic methods, even when these proteins have not been identified.[172,173] This approach, though not as yet ready for routine use, merits further exploration.

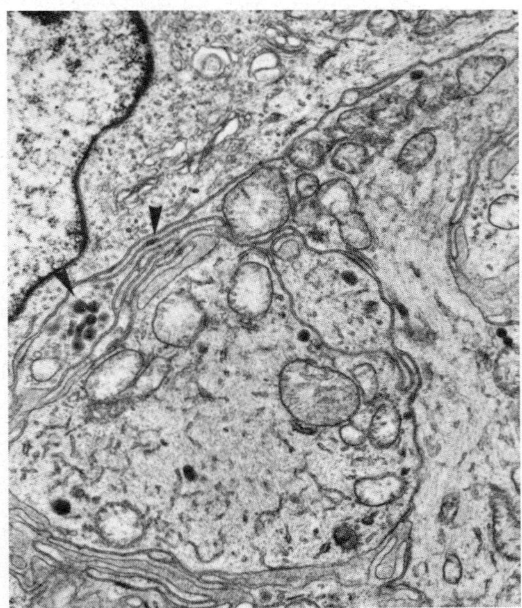

Figure 31-15 This high-magnification electron micrograph of a gastric tumor shows tumor cells diagnostic for the newly delineated entity gastrointestinal autonomic nerve tumor. The elongated tumor cells are neurites, which contain numerous mitochondria and neurofilaments. Small numbers of dense core granules are present in larger cell processes adjacent to tumor plasma membranes and in Golgi areas (not shown). The number of dense core granules increases in smaller axons with synaptic connections to adjacent neurites (*arrowheads*). Basal lamina is absent from these cells, thus ruling out an origin from Schwann cells. ×19,000 original magnification.

However, the role of the clinical pathologist has recently expanded into other areas of oncology. Particularly important is the molecular biologic diagnosis of tumors—for example, T-cell lymphomas—by detection of gene rearrangements.[174,175] Demonstration of such rearrangements may be especially important as a supplement to the work of the surgical pathologist and the immunohistochemist in distinguishing "clonal" (and therefore presumably malignant) lesions from benign but highly reactive lymph nodes. The clinical laboratory is exhibiting increasing interest in the assessment of solid tumor clonality as a way to understand tumorigenesis and to help in diagnosis and estimation of prognosis. In recent years, the cytogenetics laboratory has enjoyed a renaissance of activity in defining consistent chromosome abnormalities in a growing list of leukemias, lymphomas, and solid tumors. At present, specific chromosomal abnormalities are of greatest clinical importance in only a few tumors, primarily lymphomas and leukemias[176,177] (for example, in acute and chronic myeloid leukemia and in acute lymphocytic leukemia); however, it is now clear that nonrandom chromosomal changes are to be found in a variety of solid tumors, and cytogenetic information is likely to become increasingly useful in defining tumor progression and prognosis.[24,48,178–180]

In a similar vein, interest in the use of flow cytometric analysis of tumor cell suspensions for determination of tumor ploidy and the fraction of replicating cells has been increasing in recent years. Early results indicate that such information is useful in defining the prognosis of renal, breast, and certain other types of tumors.[24,51,52,54,181]

ROLE OF THE MOLECULAR PATHOLOGIST

The molecular pathologist practices at the interface of anatomic and clinical pathology, using the principles, theories, and techniques of molecular biology to make or confirm diagnoses of cancer, to provide more specific classification of cancer, and to provide prognostic or therapeutic information.

Somatic mutations (ie, mutations that occur during the lifetime of an individual in tissue outside of the germline) are central to the development of cancer.[182] Neoplastic progression is characterized by a succession of mutations in critical genes. These mutations may be gene deletions, duplications, point mutations, or chromosomal translocations, in any combination, in the DNA of the tumor cells. The mutations affect regulation of the cell cycle, cellular differentiation, apoptosis, and cell–cell and cell–matrix interactions. They are associated with altered gene expression.

Different neoplasms have different combinations of genetic alterations, and those differences can be exploited in the laboratory for diagnostic, prognostic, or therapeutic purposes. Some genetic alterations are required for the development of specific tumor types. Those alterations are therefore discrete, objective indicators of the associated neoplasm. The best examples are the chromosomal translocations seen in some leukemias, lymphomas, and soft-tissue tumors (Table 31-5). Other genetic alterations, such as *TP53* missense mutations that inactivate the protein's normal role in cell cycle control, seem to be common to many malignancies.[183] Still other genetic changes are seen in subsets of neoplasms—for example, the amplification of the *HER2/neu* gene that is present in 10 to 30% of breast carcinomas and that provides both prognostic information and targeted therapeutic options with trastuzumab.[184] HPV genotyping has proved to be a useful adjunct tool in the diagnosis of precancerous cervical dysplasias.[185]

Table 31-5 Recurrent Chromosomal Translocations in Human Neoplasia

Malignancy	Chromosomal Translocations	Genes Involved
Acute myelogenous leukemia	t(8;21)(q22;q22)	*RUNX1/RUNX1T1*
	inv(16)(p13;q22)	*CBFB/MYH11*
	t(15;17)(q22;q21)	*PML/RARA*
	t(9;11)(p21-22;q23)	*MLL/MLLT3*
Acute lymphoblastic leukemia	t(12;21)(p12;q22)	*ETV6/RUNX1*
	t(9;22)(q34;q11)	*BCR/ABL*
	t(1;19)(q23;p13)	*TCF3/PBX1*
	t(4;11)(q21;q23)	*MLL*/AF4
Chronic myelogenous leukemia	t(9;22)(q34;q11)	*BCR/ABL*
Follicular lymphoma	t(14;18)(q32;q21)	*IGH@/BCL2*
Chondrosarcoma, myxoid	t(9;22)(q22;q12)	*TEC/ETS1*
Clear cell sarcoma (MMSP)	t(12;22)(q13;q12)	*ATF1/ETS1*
Ewing's sarcoma/PNET	t(11;22)(q24;q12)	*FLI1/EWSR1*
	t(21;22)(q22;q12)	*ERG/EWSR1*
Liposarcoma, myxoid	t(12;16)(q13;p11)	*DDIT3/FUS*
Rhabdomyosarcoma, alveolar	t(2;13)(q35-37;q14)	*PAX3/FOXO1A*
	t(1;13)(p36;q14)	*PAX7/FOXO1A*
Synovial sarcoma	t(X;18)(p11,q11)	*SSX1/SYT1*
		SSX2/SYT1

MMSP = malignant melanoma of the soft parts; PNET = peripheral neuroectodermal tumor.

Many cancer-related molecular pathology tests focus on genetic alterations that are markers of specific tumor types. The new World Health Organization classification of leukemias characterizes leukemia subtypes by specific chromosomal translocations.[186] For example, the Philadelphia chromosome, t(9;22)(q34;q11), juxtaposes the 5' portion of the *BCR* gene to the 3' portion of the *ABL* gene, creating a new chimeric *BCR-ABL* gene that is the sine qua non for chronic myelogenous leukemia (CML). The chromosomal breakpoints occur within the introns (non-coding regions) of the genes so that the exons (coding regions) remain intact and can be transcribed into mRNA and translated into a unique 210 kDa fusion protein that is an activated tyrosine kinase. It is this fusion protein that is oncogenic for hematopoietic cells and present in all cases of CML. The molecular pathologist can look for this specific marker of disease in a variety of ways, including complete cytogenetic analysis, fluorescence in situ hybridization on metaphase spreads or intact interphase nuclei, Southern blot hybridization on tumor DNA, reverse-transcriptase polymerase chain reaction (RT-PCR) on tumor mRNA, or Western blot on tumor protein. The most commonly used methods are karyotype, fluorescence in situ hybridization, and RT-PCR. All of these technologies are labor-intensive and costly, which has limited their application. However, higher throughput technologies such as real-time RT-PCR have made more routine applications realistic.[187] RT-PCR assays have the added advantage of being sensitive as well as specific. As few as 1 abnormal cell in 100,000 can be detected, making the technique useful for following minimal residual disease post therapy.

Molecular pathology assays are central not only to the accurate subclassification of neoplasms, but also to treatment guidance, especially with targeted therapies, such as those employing small-molecule inhibitors. Imatinib mesylate, a tyrosine kinase inhibitor, blocks the tyrosine kinase activity of *BCR-ABL* and inhibits the proliferation of CML tumor cells. Most patients experience a significant hematologic and cytogenetic remission. Real-time RT-PCR assays offer a sensitive quantitative assessment of minimal residual disease by determining the amount of chimeric *BCR-ABL* mRNA expression relative to the expression of a control gene. Serial monitoring over time documents the kinetics of the leukemic clone, providing prognostic information and allowing for therapeutic intervention. Patients with a 3-log reduction in *BCR-ABL* transcripts compared to baseline have a significantly better progression-free survival than those who have a lesser response.[188] Rising levels of *BCR-ABL* can indicate the emergence of a clone resistant to imatinib, triggering a screen for mutational analysis.[189]

Clinical resistance to imatinib is associated primarily with mutations in the kinase domain of *BCR-ABL*. The mutations lead to amino acid substitutions and conformational changes in the imatinib binding site. Different mutations predict different clinical outcomes and require different therapeutic strategies, from dose escalation to combined therapy to transplantation.[189] Second generation *ABL* kinase inhibitors that are active in imatinib-resistant *BCR-ABL* mutants have been discovered and are being investigated in clinical trials.[190]

The interplay of the molecular pathologist and targeted therapy is not limited to hematologic malignancies. Clinical trials of gefitinib, a drug that binds to the ATP cleft of the tyrosine kinase domain of epidermal growth factor receptor (*EGFR*), showed that 10% of nonsmall cell lung carcinomas that overexpressed *EGFR* responded clinically.[191,192] Clinical response is correlated with the presence of specific heterozygous, gain of function, in-frame deletion mutations or point mutations associated with amino acid substitutions in the *EGFR* kinase domain.[193,194] Microdissection of relatively pure populations of nonsmall cell lung carcinoma from frozen tissue or paraffin-embedded sections, followed by DNA isolation and sequence analysis of the exons containing the clustered mutations, identifies the patients who are likely to respond to gefitinib or similar targeted drugs.

As the molecular basis of neoplastic transformation and progression for various cancers becomes clearer, more applications will become incorporated into the diagnostic laboratory. Recently, microarray technology has been successfully employed to stratify neoplasms by disease outcome. Pathologists will play a central role in determining the best way to incorporate these new biologic markers and technologies into the diagnostic laboratory. For example, chronic lymphocytic leukemia (CLL) is a heterogeneous disorder. It may follow an indolent course with no need for therapy or, alternatively, a rapidly progressive course that is resistant to treatment. Somatic mutation analysis of the immunoglobulin heavy chain gene variable region (mutated vs. unmutated) stratifies these two clinical groups, but requires expensive and time-consuming sequencing techniques that are unlikely to be universally available.[195,196] Gene-expression profiling of CLL has shown differences in the expression patterns of several hundred genes.[197,198] The expression of one of these genes, *ZAP70* (a member of the Syk family of tyrosine kinases that normally plays a role in T cell receptor signaling, natural killer cell activation, and early B cell development), has emerged as a potential surrogate marker for risk stratification of CLL.[199] *ZAP70* expression can be analyzed by real-time PCR, flow cytometry, or immunoperoxidase staining. Pathologists will have to determine the most informative and cost-effective technique.

The chemotherapeutic agents used to treat cancer often have narrow therapeutic indexes with an inherent risk of toxicity. Pharmacogenetics—the study of the role of genetic inheritance in individual variation in drug response and toxicity—will affect the practice of oncology.[200] For example, thiopurine *S*-methyltransferase (*TPMT*) is a cytosolic enzyme that catalyzes the *S*-methylation of the cytotoxic thiopurine drugs, including 6-thioguanine and 6-mercaptopurine. Genetic polymorphisms in *TPMT* lead to variable in vivo activity of the enzyme. In the white population, 89% have high enzyme activity, 11% have intermediate activity, and 1 in 300 have undetectable activity. The latter are at risk of severe, and potentially fatal, myelosuppression after standard-dose thiopurine therapy.[201] Patients can be screened by phenotypic or genotypic assays to identify those who require a reduced dosage.

ROLE OF THE AUTOPSY PATHOLOGIST

Autopsies do not receive the respect they were at one time accorded, and the autopsy rate has declined precipitously throughout the United States from approximately 90% of hospital deaths in some teaching hospitals in the late 1960s to the current average rate of approximately 5%.[202] One widely voiced but erroneous reason for this change in attitude and practice is the belief that autopsies no longer yield much in the way of useful information. They are considered to have been preempted by new technologies, such as magnetic resonance imaging and other pathologic and biochemical tests performed on the patient during life.

In a series of cases from 1986 to 1995, clinically undiagnosed or misdiagnosed malignancies were found in 44% of autopsies—a rate similar to that reported in studies from 1923 and 1972. Among the undiagnosed cancers, 57% were felt to be directly related to the patient's death.[203] A recent paper indicates that, at a contemporary US institution, an autopsy could yield a major error rate of 8.4 to 24.4% and a class I error rate of 4.1 to 6.7%.[204]

Another concern is clinicians' fear of malpractice suits resulting from new findings revealed at autopsy that had not been diagnosed during life. Still another is the fact that the Joint Commission for the Accreditation of Health Care Organizations has greatly reduced its emphasis on the hospital autopsy rate for accreditation purposes.

Psychological factors may also play a negative role. Because of the significant side effects that accompany the longer survivals achieved with modern cancer therapy, the family of the deceased may feel that the patient had "suffered enough." Also, the autopsy serves as a symbol of failure, reminding the clinician that a cure could not be effected. Finally, there is a negative economic incentive for performing autopsies. Neither the pathologist, the hospital, nor the oncologist is reimbursed the cost in time, effort, and materials involved in performing an autopsy or in persuading a reluctant family to permit an autopsy.

Despite those objections, autopsy continues to have an important role in patient care. In fact, advances in technology have done little to change the incidence of unexpected, clinically significant findings at autopsy. In our experience, it is most unusual for an unexpected autopsy finding to lead to litigation, and if an egregious error in patient management has occurred, is it not the responsibility of the medical profession to discover this?

Autopsy has an important role in evaluating the care of the cancer patient who has succumbed to the illness. The autopsy will obviously not offer direct benefit to the dead patient, but it may be essential for supporting or refuting clinical impressions, determining the extent of residual disease and the adequacy of therapy, evaluating new therapies, identifying the ultimate and proximate causes of death, and revealing unexpected findings that affected patient care. As a means of advancing knowledge, clinicians should regard an autopsy as the final contribution that they and the deceased patient can make to an understanding of disease. The usefulness of an autopsy is greatly enhanced when the clinician takes the time to address with the pathologist specific questions that need to be answered at postmortem examination.

SUMMARY AND CONCLUSIONS

Perhaps the most important theme of this chapter has been its emphasis on the role of the pathologist as a member of the medical team caring for the patient with cancer. The importance of close communication between the oncologist, surgeon, radiotherapist, other clinicians, and the pathologist cannot be overemphasized. Patient care will be optimized if the pathologist is consulted in advance of procedures designed to obtain tissue samples for definitive diagnosis. Just a single opportunity may exist to obtain tissue that will make a complete diagnosis possible, and it will be unfortunate if that opportunity is lost because portions of the specimen are not appropriately triaged for immunohistochemistry, electron microscopy, flow cytometry, culture, or other special procedures. Implementation of a high level of communication and cooperation between pathologists and clinicians has led to important contributions in the treatment and care of patients with malignant melanoma and breast cancer, among other examples. Those examples should serve as useful models for the study of other types of cancers.

REFERENCES

1. Clark WH. Tumour progression and the nature of cancer. Br J Cancer 1991;64:631–44.
2. Cotran RS, Kumar V, Collins T, editors. Robbins pathologic basis of disease. 6th ed. Philadelphia: WB Saunders Company; 1999.
3. Dvorak HF, Nagy JA, Dvorak AM. Structure of solid tumors and their vasculature: implications for therapy with monoclonal antibodies. Cancer Cells 1991;3:77–85.
4. Dvorak HF. Tumors: wounds that do not heal. Similarities between tumor stroma generation and wound healing. N Engl J Med 1986;315:1650–9.
5. Dickson DJ, Shami PJ. Angiogenesis in acute and chronic leukemias. Leuk Lymphoma 2001;42:847–53.
6. Nagy JA, Masse EM, Herzberg KT, et al. Pathogenesis of ascites tumor growth: vascular permeability factor, vascular hyperpermeability, and ascites fluid accumulation. Cancer Res 1995;55:360–8.
7. Senger DR, Galli SJ, Dvorak AM, et al. Tumor cells secrete a vascular permeability factor that promotes accumulation of ascites fluid. Science 1983;219:983–5.
8. Folkman J, Shing Y. Angiogenesis. J Biol Chem 1992;267:10931–4.
9. Yeo TK, Dvorak HF. Tumor stroma. In: Colvin R, Bhan A, McCluskey R, editors. Diagnostic immunopathology. 2nd ed. New York: Raven Press; 1995. p. 685–97.
10. Dvorak HF. Rous-Whipple Award Lecture. How tumors make bad blood vessels and stroma. Am J Pathol 2003;162:1747–57.
11. Brown LF, Detmar M, Claffey K, et al. Vascular permeability factor/vascular endothelial growth factor: a multifunctional angiogenic cytokine. EXS 1997;79:233–69.
12. Claesson-Welsh L. Vascular growth factors and angiogenesis. Berlin: Springer-Verlag; 1999.
13. Dvorak HF. Vascular permeability factor/vascular endothelial growth factor: a critical cytokine in tumor angiogenesis and a potential target for diagnosis and therapy. J Clin Oncol 2002;20:4368–80.
14. Dvorak HF, Nagy JA, Feng D, et al. Vascular permeability factor/vascular endothelial growth factor and the significance of microvascular hyperpermeability in angiogenesis. Curr Top Microbiol Immunol 1999;237:97–132.

15. Dvorak HF, Senger DR, Dvorak AM, et al. Regulation of extravascular coagulation by microvascular permeability. Science 1985;227:1059–61.
16. Brown LF, Yeo KT, Berse B, et al. Expression of vascular permeability factor (vascular endothelial growth factor) by epidermal keratinocytes during wound healing. J Exp Med 1992;176:1375–9.
17. Vaupel P, Kallinowski F, Okunieff P. Blood flow, oxygen and nutrient supply, and metabolic microenvironment of human tumors: a review. Cancer Res 1989;49:6449–65.
18. Tannock IF, Rotin D. Acid pH in tumors and its potential for therapeutic exploitation. Cancer Res 1989;49:4373–84.
19. Connolly JL, Schnitt SJ. Evaluation of breast biopsy specimens in patients considered for treatment by conservative surgery and radiation therapy for early breast cancer. Pathol Annu 1988;23:1–23.
20. Owings D, Hann L, Schnitt SJ. How thoroughly should needle localization breast biopsies be sampled for microscopic examination? A prospective mammographic–pathologic correlative study. Am J Surg Pathol 1990;14:578–83.
21. Dupont WD, Page DL. Risk factors for breast cancer in women with proliferative breast disease. N Engl J Med 1985;312:146–51.
22. McDivitt RW, Stewart FW, Berg JW. Tumors of the breast. Bethesda, MD: Armed Forces Institute of Pathology; 1968.
23. Pierce GB. The cancer cell and its control by the embryo. Rous-Whipple Award Lecture. Am J Pathol 1983;113:117–24.
24. Tannock IF, Hill RP, editors. The basic science of oncology. 2nd ed. New York: McGraw-Hill, Inc.; 1992.
25. Knudson AG. Stem cell regulation, tissue ontogeny, and oncogenic events. Semin Cancer Biol 1992;3:99–106.
26. Beachy PA, Karhadkar SS, Berman DM. Tissue repair and stem cell renewal in carcinogenesis. Nature 2004;432:324–31.
27. Reya T, Morrison SJ, Clarke MF, Weissman IL. Stem cells, cancer, and cancer stem cells. Nature 2001;414:105–11.
28. Reid LM. Stem cell biology, hormone/matrix synergies and liver differentiation. Curr Opin Cell Biol 1990;2:121–30.
29. Schnitt SJ, Silen W, Sadowsky NL, et al. Ductal carcinoma in situ (intraductal carcinoma) of the breast. N Engl J Med 1988;318:898–903.
30. Holland R, Connolly JL, Gelman R, et al. The presence of an extensive intraductal component (EIC) following a limited excision correlates with prominent residual disease in the remainder of the breast. J Clin Oncol 1990;8:113–8.
31. Schnitt SJ, Connolly JL, Khettry U, et al. Pathologic findings on re-excision of the primary site in breast cancer patients considered for treatment by primary radiation therapy. Cancer 1987;59:675–81.
32. Gage I, Schnitt SJ, Nixon AJ, et al. Pathologic margin involvement and the risk of recurrence in patients treated with breast-conserving therapy. Cancer 1996;78:1921–8.
33. Elston CW. The assessment of histological differentiation in breast cancer. Aust N Z J Surg 1984;54:11–5.
34. Foulds L. The experimental study of tumor progression: a review. Cancer Res 1954;14:327–39.
35. Hill RP. Tumor progression: potential role of unstable genomic changes. Cancer Metastasis Rev 1990;9:137–47.
36. Nowell PC. Mechanisms of tumor progression. Cancer Res 1986;46:2203–7.
37. Gleason DF. Histologic grade, clinical stage, and patient age in prostate cancer. NCI Monogr 1988;7:15–8.
38. Bloom HJG, Richardson WW. Histological grading and prognosis in breast cancer. Br J Cancer 1957;11:359–77.
39. Scharf ERW, Hadley RS. Prognosis in carcinoma of the breast. Lancet 1938;2:582–3.
40. Schnitt SJ, Connolly JL, Harris JR, et al. Pathologic predictors of early local recurrence in stage I and II breast cancer treated by primary radiation therapy. Cancer 1984;53:1049–57.
41. Connolly JL, Boyages J, Nixon AJ, et al. Predictors of breast recurrence after conservative surgery and radiation therapy for invasive breast cancer. Mod Pathol 1998;11:134–9.
42. Jacquemier J, Kurtz J, Amalric R, et al. An assessment of extensive intraductal component as a risk factor for local recurrence after breast-conserving therapy. Br J Cancer 1990;61:873–6.
43. Peterse JL, van Dongen JA, Bartelink H. Recurrence of breast carcinoma after breast conserving treatment. Eur J Surg Oncol 1988;14:123–6.
44. Fisher ER, Sass R, Fisher B. Pathologic findings from the National Surgical Adjuvant Project for Breast Cancers (protocol no. 4). X. Discriminants for tenth year treatment failure. Cancer 1984;53(Suppl):712–23.
45. Fitgibbons PL, Page DL, Weaver D. Prognostic factors in breast cancer. Arch Pathol Lab Med 2000;124:966–78.
46. Epstein AH, Connolly JL, Gelman R, et al. The predictors of distant relapse following conservative surgery and radiotherapy for early breast cancer are similar to those following mastectomy. Int J Radiat Oncol Biol Phys 1989;17:755–60.
47. Lee AK, DeLellis RA, Wolfe HJ. Intramammary lymphatic invasion in breast carcinomas. Evaluation using ABH isoantigens as endothelial markers. Am J Surg Pathol 1986;10:589–94.
48. Rosen PP, Groshen S. Factors influencing survival and prognosis in early breast carcinoma (T1N0M0–T1N1M0). Assessment of 644 patients with median follow-up of 18 years. Surg Clin North Am 1990;70:937–62.
49. Toikkanen S, Joensuu H, Klemi P. Nuclear DNA content as a prognostic factor in T1–2N0 breast cancer. Am J Clin Pathol 1990;93:471–9.
50. Elston CW, Ellis IO. Pathological prognostic factors in breast cancer. I. The value of histological grade in breast cancer: experience from a large study with long-term follow-up. Histopathology 1991;19:403–10.
51. Clark GM, Dressler LG, Owens MA, et al. Prediction of relapse or survival in patients with node-negative breast cancer by DNA flow cytometry. N Engl J Med 1989;320:627–33.
52. Fallenius AG, Franzen SA, Auer GU. Predictive value of nuclear DNA content in breast cancer in relation to clinical morphologic factors. A retrospective study of 227 consecutive cases. Cancer 1988;62:521–30.
53. von Rosen A, Rutqvist LE, Carstensen J, et al. Prognostic value of nuclear DNA content in breast cancer in relation to tumor size, nodal status, and estrogen receptor content. Breast Cancer Res Treat 1989;13:23–32.
54. Muss HB, Kute TE, Case LD, et al. The relation of flow cytometry to clinical and biologic characteristics in women with node negative primary breast cancer. Cancer 1989;64:1894–900.
55. Powles TJ, Hardy JR, Ashley SE, et al. Chemoprevention of breast cancer. Breast Cancer Res Treat 1989;14:23–31.
56. Fisher B, Redmond C, Fisher ER, Caplan R. Relative worth of estrogen or progesterone receptor and pathologic characteristics of differentiation as indicators of prognosis in node negative breast cancer patients: Findings from National Surgical Adjuvant Breast and Bowel Project Protocol B-06. J Clin Oncol 1988;6:1076–87.
57. Boyages J, Recht A, Connolly J, et al. Factors associated with local recurrence as a first site of failure following the conservative treatment of early breast cancer. Recent Results Cancer Res 1989;115:92–102.
58. Weidner N, Folkman J, Pozza F, et al. Tumor angiogenesis: a new significant and independent prognostic indicator in early-stage breast carcinoma. J Natl Cancer Inst 1992;84:1875–87.
59. Gasparini G, Dal Fior S, Pozza F, Bevilacqua P. Correlation of growth fraction by Ki-67 immunohistochemistry with histologic factors and hormone receptors in operable breast carcinoma. Breast Cancer Res Treat 1989;14:329–36.
60. Gasparini G, Weidner N, Maluta S, et al. Intratumoral microvessel density and *p53* protein: correlation with metastasis in head-and-neck squamous-cell carcinoma. Int J Cancer 1993;55:739–44.
61. Yamazaki K, Abe S, Takekawa H, et al. Tumor angiogenesis in human lung adenocarcinoma. Cancer 1994;74:2245–50.
62. Macchiarini P, Fontanini G, Hardin MJ, et al. Relation of neovascularisation to metastasis of non-small-cell lung cancer. Lancet 1992;340:145–6.
63. Wakui S, Furusato M, Itoh T, et al. Tumour angiogenesis in prostatic carcinoma with and without bone marrow metastasis: a morphometric study. J Pathol 1992;168:257–62.
64. Pettersson A, Nagy JA, Brown LF, et al. Heterogeneity of the angiogenic response induced in different normal adult tissues by vascular permeability factor/vascular endothelial growth factor. Lab Invest 2000;80:99–115.
65. Sundberg C, Nagy JA, Brown LF, et al. Glomeruloid microvascular proliferation follows adenoviral vascular permeability factor/vascular endothelial growth factor-164 gene delivery. Am J Pathol 2001;158:1145–60.
66. Goffin JR, Straume O, Chappuis PO, et al. Glomeruloid microvascular proliferation is associated with *p53* expression, germline *BRCA1* mutations and an adverse outcome following breast cancer. Br J Cancer 2003;89:1031–4.
67. Straume O, Chappuis PO, Salvesen HB, et al. Prognostic importance of glomeruloid microvascular proliferation indicates an aggressive angiogenic phenotype in human cancers. Cancer Res 2002;62:6808–11.
68. Fox SB, Smith K, Hollyer J, et al. The epidermal growth factor receptor as a prognostic marker: results of 370 patients and review of 3009 patients. Breast Cancer Res Treat 1994;29:41–9.
69. Perez R, Pascual M, Macias A, Lage A. Epidermal growth factor receptors in human breast cancer. Breast Cancer Res Treat 1984;4:189–93.
70. Sainsbury JR, Farndon JR, Needham GK, et al. Epidermal-growth-factor receptor status as predictor of early recurrence of and death from breast cancer. Lancet 1987;1:1398–402.
71. Bonneterre J, Peyrat JP, Beuscart R, et al. Prognostic significance of IGF1 receptors (IGF1-R) in human breast cancer. Breast Cancer Res Treat 1989;14:166.
72. Klijn JG, Portengen H, van Putten WL, et al. The prognostic value of receptors for somatostatin (SS-R), insulin-like growth factor-1 (IGF-1-R) and epidermal growth factor (EGF-R) in human breast cancer [abstract]. Proc Am Soc Clin Oncol 1989;8:A78.
73. Barrett-Lee P, Travers M, Luqmani Y, Coombes RC. Transcripts for transforming growth factors in human breast cancer: Clinical correlates. Br J Cancer 1990;61:612–7.
74. Watson P, Barrett J, Pantazis C, Guthrie T. Color video analysis of transforming growth factor alpha expression in female breast cancer [abstract]. Proc Am Soc Clin Oncol 1988;7:A138.
75. Tandon AK, Clark GM, Chamness GC, et al. Cathepsin D and prognosis in breast cancer. N Engl J Med 1990;322:297–302.
76. Carter P, Presta L, Gorman CM, et al. Humanization of an anti-*p185HER2* antibody for human cancer therapy. Proc Natl Acad Sci U S A 1992;89:4285–9.
77. Pegram MD, Lipton A, Hayes DF, et al. Phase II study of receptor-enhanced chemosensitivity using recombinant humanized anti-*p185HER2/neu* monoclonal antibody plus cisplatin in patients with *HER2/neu*-overexpressing metastatic breast cancer refractory to chemotherapy treatment. J Clin Oncol 1998;16:2659–71.
78. Crystal BS, Wang HH, Ducatman BS. Comparison of different preparation techniques for fine needle aspiration specimens. A semiquantitative and statistical analysis. Acta Cytol 1993;37:24–8.
79. Ducatman BS, Hogan CL, Wang HH. A triage system for processing fine needle aspiration cytology specimens. Acta Cytol 1989;33:797–9.
80. Wang HH, Sovie S, Trawinski G, et al. ThinPrep processing of endoscopic brushing specimens. Am J Clin Pathol 1996;105:163–7.
81. Linder J, Zahniser D. ThinPrep Papanicolaou testing to reduce false-negative cervical cytology. Arch Pathol Lab Med 1998;122:139–44.
82. Bishop JW, Bigner SH, Colgan TJ, et al. Multicenter masked evaluation of AutoCyte Prep thin layers with matched conventional smears. Including initial biopsy results. Acta Cytol 1998;42:189–97.
83. The uniform approach to breast fine-needle aspiration biopsy. National Cancer Institute Fine-Needle Aspiration of Breast Workshop Subcommittees. Diagn Cytopathol 1997;16:295–311.
84. Page DL, Johnson JE, Dupont WD. Probabilistic approach to the reporting of fine-needle aspiration cytology of the breast. Cancer 1997;81:6–9.
85. Wang HH, Ducatman BS. Fine needle aspiration of the breast. A probabilistic approach to diagnosis of carcinoma. Acta Cytol 1998;42:285–9.
86. Craemer DW. The role of cervical cytology in the declining morbidity and mortality of cervical cancer. Cancer 1974;34:2018–27.
87. Miller AB, Lindsay J, Hill GB. Mortality from cancer of the uterus in Canada and its relationship to screening for cancer of the cervix. Int J Cancer 1976;17:602–12.
88. Wang HH, Ducatman BS. Introduction. In: Wang HH, Ducatman BS, editors. The Pap smear: controversies in practice. New York: Arnold Publishers; 2002. p. 1-11.
89. Walboomers JM, Jacobs MV, Manos MM, et al. Human papillomavirus is a necessary cause of invasive cervical cancer worldwide. J Pathol 1999;189:12–9.
90. Wright TC Jr, Cox JT, Massad LS, et al. 2001 Consensus guidelines for the management of women with cervical cytological abnormalities. JAMA 2002;287:2120–9.
91. Wright TC Jr, Schiffman M, Solomon D, et al. Interim guidance for the use of human papillomavirus DNA testing as an adjunct to cervical cytology for screening. Obstet Gynecol 2004;103:304–9.

92. Goldie SJ, Kim JJ, Wright TC. Cost-effectiveness of human papillomavirus DNA testing for cervical cancer screening in women aged 30 years or more. Obstet Gynecol 2004;103:619–31.
93. Brown FM. Urine cytology. It is still the gold standard for screening? Urol Clin North Am 2000;27:25–37.
94. Patz EF Jr, Goodman PC, Bepler G. Screening for lung cancer. N Engl J Med 2000;343:1627–33.
95. Falk GW, Chittajallu R, Goldblum JR, et al. Surveillance of patients with Barrett's esophagus for dysplasia and cancer with balloon cytology [see comments]. Gastroenterology 1997;112:1787–97.
96. Leoni-Parvex S, Mihaescu A, Pellanda A,. Esophageal cytology in the follow-up of patients with treated upper aerodigestive tract malignancies. Cancer 2000;90:10–6.
97. Tsang TK, Hidvegi D, Horth K, Ostrow JD. Reliability of balloon-mesh cytology in detecting esophageal carcinoma in a population of US veterans. Cancer 1987;59:556–9.
98. Dooley WC, Ljung BM, Veronesi U, et al. Ductal lavage for detection of cellular atypia in women at high risk for breast cancer. J Natl Cancer Inst 2001;93:1624–32.
99. O'Shaughnessy JA, Ljung BM, Dooley WC, et al. Ductal lavage and the clinical management of women at high risk for breast carcinoma. Cancer 2002;94:292–8.
100. Geisinger KR. Endoscopic biopsies and cytologic brushings of the esophagus are diagnostically complementary. Am J Clin Pathol 1995;103:295–9.
101. Wang HH, Jonasson JG, Ducatman BS. Brushing cytology of the upper gastrointestinal tract. Obsolete or not? Acta Cytol 1991;35:195–8.
102. Layfield LJ, Reichman A, Weinstein WM. Endoscopically directed fine needle aspiration biopsy of gastric and esophageal lesions. Acta Cytol 1992;36:69–74.
103. Wiersema MJ, Wiersema LM, Khusro Q, et al. Combined endosonography and fine-needle aspiration cytology in the evaluation of gastrointestinal lesions. Gastrointest Endosc 1994;40:199–206.
104. Agarwal B, Abu-Hamda E, Molke KL, et al. Endoscopic ultrasound-guided fine needle aspiration and multidetector spiral CT in the diagnosis of pancreatic cancer. Am J Gastroenterol 2004;99:844–50.
105. Hernandez LV, Mishra G, George S, Bhutani MS. A descriptive analysis of EUS-FNA for mediastinal lymphadenopathy: an emphasis on clinical impact and false negative results. Am J Gastroenterol 2004;99:249–54.
106. Jhala NC, Jhala DN, Chhieng DC, et al. Endoscopic ultrasound-guided fine-needle aspiration. A cytopathologist's perspective. Am J Clin Pathol 2003;120:351–67.
107. Yeo KT, Wang HH, Nagy JA, et al. Vascular permeability factor (vascular endothelial growth factor) in guinea pig and human tumor and inflammatory effusions. Cancer Res 1993;53:2912–8.
108. Martin HE, Ellis EB. Biopsy by needle puncture and aspiration. Ann Surg 1930;92:169–81.
109. Linsk JA. Aspiration cytology in Sweden: the Karolinska Group. Diagn Cytopathol 1985;1:332–5.
110. Mazzaferri EL. Management of a solitary thyroid nodule. N Engl J Med 1993;328:553–9.
111. Tulecke MA, Wang HH. ThinPrep for cytologic evaluation of follicular thyroid lesions: correlation with histologic findings. Diagn Cytopathol 2004;30:7–13.
112. Hamberger B, Gharib H, Melton LJ 3rd, et al. Fine-needle aspiration biopsy of thyroid nodules. Impact on thyroid practice and cost of care. Am J Med 1982;73:381–4.
113. Frable WJ. Needle aspiration of the breast. Cancer 1984;53(Suppl):671–6.
114. Azavedo E, Svane G, Auer G. Stereotactic fine-needle biopsy in 2594 mammographically detected non-palpable lesions. Lancet 1989;1:1033–6.
115. Hann L, Ducatman BS, Wang HH, et al. Nonpalpable breast lesions: evaluation by means of fine-needle aspiration cytology. Radiology 1989;171:373–6.
116. Lofgren M, Andersson I, Bondeson L, Lindholm K. X-ray guided fine-needle aspiration for the cytologic diagnosis of nonpalpable breast lesions. Cancer 1988;61:1032–7.
117. Berner A, Davidson B, Sigstad E, Risberg B. Fine-needle aspiration cytology vs. core biopsy in the diagnosis of breast lesions. Diagn Cytopathol 2003;29:344–8.
118. Sun W, Li A, Abreo F, et al. Comparison of fine-needle aspiration cytology and core biopsy for diagnosis of breast cancer. Diagn Cytopathol 2001;24:421–5.
119. Tabbara SO, Frost AR, Stoler MH, et al. Changing trends in breast fine-needle aspiration: results of the Papanicolaou Society of Cytopathology Survey. Diagn Cytopathol 2000;22:126–30.
120. Xie HB, Salhadar A, Haara A, et al. How stereotactic core-needle biopsy affected breast fine-needle aspiration utilization: an 11-year institutional review. Diagn Cytopathol 2004;31:106–10.
121. Tao LC. Lung, pleura, and mediastinum. In: Kline TS, editor. Guides to clinical aspiration biopsy. New York: Igaku-Shoin; 1988. p. 1.
122. Cafferty LL, Katz RL, Ordonez NG, et al. Fine needle aspiration diagnosis of intraabdominal and retroperitoneal lymphomas by a morphologic and immunocytochemical approach. Cancer 1990;65:72–7.
123. Hehn ST, Grogan TM, Miller TP. Utility of fine-needle aspiration as a diagnostic technique in lymphoma. J Clin Oncol 2004;22:3046–52.
124. Dong HY, Harris NL, Preffer FI, Pitman MB. Fine-needle aspiration biopsy in the diagnosis and classification of primary and recurrent lymphoma: a retrospective analysis of the utility of cytomorphology and flow cytometry. Mod Pathol 2001;14:472–81.
125. Meda BA, Buss DH, Woodruff RD, et al. Diagnosis and subclassification of primary and recurrent lymphoma. The usefulness and limitations of combined fine-needle aspiration cytomorphology and flow cytometry. Am J Clin Pathol 2000;113:688–99.
126. Dabbs DJ. Diagnostic immunohistochemistry. Philadelphia: Churchill Livingstone; 2002.
127. Hsu SM, Raine L, Fanger H. A comparative study of the peroxidase–antiperoxidase method and an avidin–biotin complex method for studying polypeptide hormones with radioimmunoassay antibodies. Am J Clin Pathol 1981;75:734–8.
128. Nagle RB. Intermediate filaments. Efficacy in surgical pathology diagnosis. Am J Clin Pathol 1989;91(Suppl 1):S14–8.
129. Sheibani K, Tubbs RR. Enzyme immunohistochemistry: technical aspects. Semin Diagn Pathol 1984;1:235–50.
130. Sternberger LA. Immunocytochemistry. 3rd ed. New York: John Wiley & Sons; 1986.
131. Taylor CR. Immunomicroscopy: a diagnostic tool for the surgical pathologist. Philadelphia: WB Saunders; 1986.
132. Cattoretti G, Suurmeijer AJH. Antigen unmasking on formalin-fixed paraffin-embedded tissues using microwaves: a review. Adv Anat Pathol 1995;2:2–9.
133. Miller RT, Swanson PE, Wick MR. Fixation and epitope retrieval in diagnostic immunohistochemistry: a concise review with practical considerations. Appl Immunohistochem Mol Morphol 2000;8:228–35.
134. Battifora H, Kopinski M. The influence of protease digestion and duration of fixation on the immunostaining of keratins. A comparison of formalin and ethanol fixation. J Histochem Cytochem 1986;34:1095–100.
135. Pinkus GS, Kurtin PJ. Epithelial membrane antigen—a diagnostic discriminant in surgical pathology: immunohistochemical profile in epithelial, mesenchymal, and hematopoietic neoplasms using paraffin sections and monoclonal antibodies. Hum Pathol 1985;16:929–40.
136. Azumi N, Battifora H. The distribution of vimentin and keratin in epithelial and nonepithelial neoplasms. A comprehensive immunohistochemical study on formalin- and alcohol-fixed tumors. Am J Clin Pathol 1987;88:286–96.
137. Bacchi CE, Bonetti F, Pea M, Martignoni G, Gown A. HMB-45: a review. Appl Immunohistochem 1996;4:73–85.
138. Drier JK, Swanson PE, Cherwitz DL, Wick MR. S100 protein immunoreactivity in poorly differentiated carcinomas. Immunohistochemical comparison with malignant melanoma. Arch Pathol Lab Med 1987;111:447–52.
139. Gould VE. The coexpression of distinct classes of intermediate filaments in human neoplasms. Arch Pathol Lab Med 1985;109:984–5.
140. Zarbo RJ, Gown AM, Nagle RB, et al. Anomalous cytokeratin expression in malignant melanoma: One- and two-dimensional Western blot analysis and immunohistochemical survey of 100 melanomas. Mod Pathol 1990;3:494–501.
141. Wang NP, Zee S, Zarbo RJ. Coordinate expression of cytokeratins 7 and 20 defines unique subsets of carcinomas. Appl Immunohistochem Mol Morphol 1995;3:99–107.
142. Battifora H, Sheibani K, Tubbs RR, et al. Antikeratin antibodies in tumor diagnosis. Distinction between seminoma and embryonal carcinoma. Cancer 1984;54:843–8.
143. Miettinen M, Virtanen I, Talerman A. Intermediate filament proteins in human testis and testicular germ-cell tumors. Am J Pathol 1985;120:402–10.
144. Carella R, Deleonardi G, D'Errico A, et al. Immunohistochemical panels for differentiating epithelial malignant mesothelioma from lung adenocarcinoma: a study with logistic regression analysis. Am J Surg Pathol 2001;25:43–50.
145. Ordonez NG. The immunohistochemical diagnosis of mesothelioma. Differentiation of mesothelioma and lung adenocarcinoma. Am J Surg Pathol 1989;13:276–91.
146. Otis CN, Carter D, Cole S, Battifora H. Immunohistochemical evaluation of pleural mesothelioma and pulmonary adenocarcinoma. A bi-institutional study of 47 cases. Am J Surg Pathol 1987;11:445–56.
147. Sheibani K. Immunopathology of malignant mesothelioma. Hum Pathol 1994;25:219–20.
148. Wick MR, Loy T, Mills SE, et al. Malignant epithelioid pleural mesothelioma versus peripheral pulmonary adenocarcinoma: a histochemical, ultrastructural, and immunohistologic study of 103 cases. Hum Pathol 1990;21:759–66.
149. Falini B, Mason DY. Proteins encoded by genes involved in chromosomal alterations in lymphoma and leukemia: clinical value of their detection by immunocytochemistry. Blood 2002;99:409–26.
150. Gocke CD. Non-Hodgkin's lymphoma. In: Dabbs DJ, editor. Diagnostic immunohistochemistry. New York: Churchill Livingstone; 2002. p. 113–34.
151. Kadin ME. Hodgkin's lymphoma. In: Dabbs DJ, editor. Diagnostic immunohistochemistry. New York: Churchill Livingstone; 2002. p. 135–46.
152. Oertel J, Huhn D. Immunocytochemical methods in haematology and oncology. J Cancer Res Clin Oncol 2000;126:425–40.
153. McClelland RA, Berger U, Miller LS, et al. Immunocytochemical assay for estrogen receptor: relationship to outcome of therapy in patients with advanced breast cancer. Cancer Res 1986;46(Suppl):4241s–3s.
154. Battifora H. Immunocytochemistry of hormone receptors in routinely processed tissues. The new gold standard. Appl Immunohistochem 1994;2:143–6.
155. Garcia RL, Coltrera MD, Gown AM. Analysis of proliferative grade using anti-PCNA/cyclin monoclonal antibodies in fixed, embedded tissues. Comparison with flow cytometric analysis. Am J Pathol 1989;134:733–9.
156. Gerdes J, Lelle RJ, Pickartz H, et al. Growth fractions in breast cancers determined in situ with monoclonal antibody Ki-67. J Clin Pathol 1986;39:977–80.
157. Pertschuk LP, Feldman JG, Eisenberg KB, et al. Immunocytochemical detection of progesterone receptor in breast cancer with monoclonal antibody. Relation to biochemical assay, disease-free survival, and clinical endocrine response. Cancer 1988;62:342–9.
158. Ross JS, Fletcher JA. The *HER2/neu* oncoprotein in breast cancer: prognostic factor, predictive factor and target for therapy. Oncologist 1998;3:237–52.
159. Slamon DJ, Godolphin W, Jones LA, et al. Studies of the *HER-2/neu* proto-oncogene in human breast and ovarian cancer. Science 1989;244:707–12.
160. van de Vijver MJ, Peterse JL, Mooi WJ, et al. *neu*-Protein overexpression in breast cancer. Association with comedo-type ductal carcinoma in situ and limited prognostic value in stage II breast cancer. N Engl J Med 1988;319:1239–45.
161. Weinstein RS, Kuszak JR, Kluskens LF, Coon JS. P-Glycoproteins in pathology: the multidrug resistance gene family in humans. Hum Pathol 1990;21:34–48.
162. Gerdes J. Ki-67 and other proliferation markers useful for immunohistological diagnostic and prognostic evaluations in human malignancies. Semin Cancer Biol 1990;1:199–206.
163. Mauri FA, Girlando S, Dalla Palma P, et al. Ki-67 antibodies (Ki-S5, MIB-1, and Ki-67) in breast carcinomas. A brief quantitative comparison. Appl Immunohistochem Mol Morphol 1994;2:171–6.
164. Hedrick L, Epstein JI. Use of keratin 903 as an adjunct in the diagnosis of prostate carcinoma. Am J Surg Pathol 1989;13:389–96.
165. Dvorak HF, Brown LF, Detmar M, Dvorak AM. Vascular permeability factor/vascular endothelial growth factor, microvascular hyperpermeability, and angiogenesis. Am J Pathol 1995;146:1029–39.
166. Dvorak HF, Nagy JA, Berse B, et al. Vascular permeability factor, fibrin, and the pathogenesis of tumor stroma formation. Ann N Y Acad Sci 1992;667:101–11.
167. Ghadially FN. Diagnostic electron microscopy of tumours. London: Butterworths; 1980.
168. Henderson DW, Papadimitriou JM. Ultrastructural appearances of tumours. A diagnostic atlas. Edinburgh: Churchill Livingstone; 1982.
169. Dvorak AM. Monograph—Procedural guide to specimen handling for the ultrastructural pathology service laboratory. J Electron Microsc Tech 1987;6:255–301.
170. Dvorak AM. Gut autonomic nerve (GAN) tumors. In: Watanabe S, Wolff M, Sommers SC, editors. Digestive

disease pathology. Philadelphia: Field and Wood Medical Publishers, Inc.; 1989. p. 49–66.
171. Dvorak AM, Monahan-Earley RA. Neurological findings and loss of consciousness in a previously well forty seven year old woman: alveolar cell carcinoma of the lung, metastatic to the brain. Norelco Report 1985;32:29–36.
172. Alexe G, Alexe S, Liotta LA, et al. Ovarian cancer detection by logical analysis of proteomic data. Proteomics 2004;4:766–83.
173. Carr KM, Rosenblatt K, Petricoin EF, Liotta LA. Genomic and proteomic approaches for studying human cancer: prospects for true patient-tailored therapy. Hum Genomics 2004;1:134–40.
174. Kadin ME, Said J. T-cell lymphomas and leukemias of post-thymic differentiation. Clin Lab Med 1988;8:135–50.
175. Weiss LM, Hu E, Wood GS, et al. Clonal rearrangements of T-cell receptor genes in mycosis fungoides and dermatopathic lymphadenopathy. N Engl J Med 1985;313:539–44.
176. Kurzrock R, Gutterman JU, Talpaz M. The molecular genetics of Philadelphia chromosome–positive leukemias. N Engl J Med 1988;319:990–8.
177. Nowell PC, Croce CM. Chromosomal approaches to oncogenes and oncogenesis. FASEB J 1988;2:3054–60.
178. Vogelstein B, Fearon ER, Hamilton SR, et al. Genetic alterations during colorectal-tumor development. N Engl J Med 1988;319:525–32.
179. Rabbitts TH. Chromosomal translocations in human cancer. Nature 1994;372:143–9.
180. Nowell PC. Cytogenetic approaches to human cancer genes. FASEB J 1994;8:408–13.
181. el-Naggar AK, Batsakis JG, Teague K, et al. Acridine orange flow cytometric analysis of renal cell carcinoma. Clinicopathologic implications of RNA content. Am J Pathol 1990;137:275–80.
182. Vogelstein B, Kinzler K, editors. The genetic basis of human cancers. 2nd ed. New York: McGraw-Hill; 2002.
183. Hahn WC, Weinberg RA. Rules for making human tumor cells. N Engl J Med 2002;347:1593–603.
184. Ross JS, Fletcher JA. *HER-2/neu* (*c-erb-B2*) gene and protein in breast cancer. Am J Clin Pathol 1999;112(Suppl 1):S53–67.
185. Saslow D, Runowicz CD, Solomon D, et al. American Cancer Society guideline for the early detection of cervical neoplasia and cancer. CA Cancer J Clin 2002;52:342–62.
186. Jaffe ES, Harris NL, Stein H, Vardiman J, editors. World Health Organization classification of tumors, pathology and genetics of tumors of haematopoietic and lymphoid tissues. Lyon, France: IARC Press; 2001.
187. Gabert J, Beillard E, van der Velden VH, et al. Standardization and quality control studies of "real-time" quantitative reverse transcriptase polymerase chain reaction of fusion gene transcripts for residual disease detection in leukemia—a Europe Against Cancer program. Leukemia 2003;17:2318–57.
188. Hughes TP, Kaeda J, Branford S, et al. Frequency of major molecular responses to imatinib or interferon alfa plus cytarabine in newly diagnosed chronic myeloid leukemia. N Engl J Med 2003;349:1423–32.
189. Branford S, Rudzki Z, Parkinson I, et al. Real-time quantitative PCR analysis can be used as a primary screen to identify patients with CML treated with imatinib who have BCR-ABL kinase domain mutations. Blood 2004;104:2926–32.
190. Shah NP, Tran C, Lee FY, et al. Overriding imatinib resistance with a novel ABL kinase inhibitor. Science 2004;305:399–401.
191. Fukuoka M, Yano S, Giaccone G, et al. Multi-institutional randomized phase II trial of gefitinib for previously treated patients with advanced non-small-cell lung cancer (The IDEAL 1 Trial) [corrected]. J Clin Oncol 2003;21(12):2237-46.
192. Kris MG, Natale RB, Herbst RS, et al. Efficacy of gefitinib, an inhibitor of the epidermal growth factor receptor tyrosine kinase, in symptomatic patients with non-small cell lung cancer: a randomized trial. JAMA 2003;290:2149–58.
193. Lynch TJ, Bell DW, Sordella R, et al. Activating mutations in the epidermal growth factor receptor underlying responsiveness of non-small-cell lung cancer to gefitinib. N Engl J Med 2004;350:2129–39.
194. Paez JG, Janne PA, Lee JC, et al. *EGFR* mutations in lung cancer: correlation with clinical response to gefitinib therapy. Science 2004;304:1497–500.
195. Damle RN, Wasil T, Fais F, et al. Ig V gene mutation status and CD38 expression as novel prognostic indicators in chronic lymphocytic leukemia. Blood 1999;94:1840–7.
196. Hamblin TJ, Davis Z, Gardiner A, et al. Unmutated Ig V(H) genes are associated with a more aggressive form of chronic lymphocytic leukemia. Blood 1999;94:1848–54.
197. Klein U, Tu Y, Stolovitzky GA, et al. Gene expression profiling of B cell chronic lymphocytic leukemia reveals a homogeneous phenotype related to memory B cells. J Exp Med 2001;194:1625–38.
198. Rosenwald A, Alizadeh AA, Widhopf G, et al. Relation of gene expression phenotype to immunoglobulin mutation genotype in B cell chronic lymphocytic leukemia. J Exp Med 2001;194:1639–47.
199. Wiestner A, Rosenwald A, Barry TS, et al. *ZAP-70* expression identifies a chronic lymphocytic leukemia subtype with unmutated immunoglobulin genes, inferior clinical outcome, and distinct gene expression profile. Blood 2003;101:4944–51.
200. Weinshilboum R. Inheritance and drug response. N Engl J Med 2003;348:529–37.
201. Goetz MP, Ames MM, Weinshilboum RM. Primer on medical genomics. Part XII: Pharmacogenomics—general principles with cancer as a model. Mayo Clin Proc 2004;79:376–84.
202. Burton EC, Phillips RS, Covinsky KE, et al. The relation of autopsy rate to physicians' beliefs and recommendations regarding autopsy. Am J Med 2004;117:255–61.
203. Burton EC, Troxclair DA, Newman WP 3rd. Autopsy diagnoses of malignant neoplasms: how often are clinical diagnoses incorrect? JAMA 1998;280:1245–8.
204. Shojania KG, Burton EC, McDonald KM, Goldman L. Changes in rates of autopsy-detected diagnostic errors over time: a systematic review. JAMA 2003;289:2849–56.

Section 7

IMAGING

32

Principles of Imaging

Edward F. Patz Jr., MD

Ever since the discovery of the x-ray more than 100 years ago, imaging has become an essential diagnostic tool in every aspect of clinical medicine. Noninvasive studies provide clinicians with information invaluable in designing optimal patient management strategies. As technology improves and our basic understanding of cancer grows, the capabilities and indications of imaging studies in the practice of oncology will continue to evolve.

Conventional radiologic studies rely on anatomic and morphologic features in suggesting a diagnosis, Such studies have provided an important dimension to the understanding of tumors, and they continue to be the mainstay of most radiology departments. Plain films in particular are easy to perform, deliver a low dose of radiation, are relatively inexpensive, and still provide a tremendous amount of diagnostic information. In oncology, cross-sectional imaging studies including computed tomography (CT), magnetic resonance (MR) imaging, and nuclear medicine scans have also become a standard part of the diagnostic evaluation. As the resolution of multidetector CT improves, the addition of multiplanar reconstruction to anatomic information will lead to imaging unsurpassed by any other modality.

The type and frequency of examination depend on the tumor and the clinical situation. Imaging studies are currently used in a number of scenarios when cancer is a concern. These scenarios include screening the asymptomatic individual, complementing the clinical work-up of a symptomatic patient, and following the progression of disease. Each scenario has a set of unique issues, particularly when applied to the cancer patient. But before any imaging study is requested, it is imperative to understand the type of abnormality suspected, whether the contemplated test can provide the necessary information, and—just as importantly—what can and will be done with the resulting information to change the course of the disease.

Although conventional imaging studies provide invaluable diagnostic information, cancer needs to be recognized as a disease of the genes. Thus, imaging studies that extend beyond traditional anatomic description to elucidate the fundamental biology of the disease would be enormously useful for patient management. This new direction toward molecular imaging is essential to address many of the basic diagnostic issues in oncology.

The genesis of molecular imaging came in the 1990s, with the use of positron emission tomography (PET) imaging and the glucose analog ^{18}F 2-fluoro-2-deoxy-D-glucose (FDG).[1] PET imaging has been used to differentiate benign from malignant lesions, to stage tumors, and to predict recurrent disease.[2] Over the last several years, FDG-PET imaging has become one of the most important tools used to evaluate cancer patients. PET has provided a new model and direction for tumor imaging—one that goes beyond the traditional anatomic and morphologic description to provide biochemical, metabolic, and molecular information.[3–11]

Clearly, as more is learned about cancer, additional tools will be developed for the diagnostic armamentarium. Radiology has just begun to integrate some of the basic properties of tumors into imaging strategies. As the move toward molecular imaging continues, the development of new targets, techniques, and tumor-specific imaging ligands (probes) should provide more accurate diagnostic information.[12–15] Improvements in lesion characterization and prognosis will then hopefully translate into a more rationale-based therapeutic approach with better outcomes.

Although the technology is undergoing a dramatic expansion, it is incumbent upon the radiologic community to carefully study the new imaging techniques to determine if they are truly useful and cost effective. The ability to create ever more spectacular images does not necessarily improve clinical management and outcomes. Hypothesis-driven, evidence-based studies are essential if the radiologic community is to truly have an effect on patient care. Because imaging is a fundamental part of diagnostic evaluation, understanding the utility of particular tests will guide an efficient patient evaluation.

This section's collection of chapters provides an overview of imaging principles, with a focus on the cancer patient. Imaging plays a central role in clinical management, and the information presented here provides general guidelines for using radiologic studies in everyday practice.

REFERENCES

1. Mankoff DA, Bellon JR. Positron-emission tomographic imaging of cancer: glucose metabolism and beyond. Semin Radiat Oncol 2001;11:16–27.
2. Rohren EM, Turkington TG, Coleman RE. Clinical applications of PET in oncology. Radiology 2004;231:305–32.
3. Delbeke D. Oncological applications of FDG PET imaging: brain tumors, colorectal cancer, lymphoma and melanoma. J Nucl Med 1999;40:591–603.
4. He Q, Xu RZ, Shkarin P, et al. Magnetic resonance spectroscopic imaging of tumor metabolic markers for cancer diagnosis, metabolic phenotyping, and characterization of tumor microenvironment. Dis Markers 2003–2004;19(2–3):69–94.
5. Perkins AC, Frier M. Radionuclide imaging in drug development. Curr Pharm Des 2004;10:2907–21.
6. Laruelle M, Slifstein M, Huang Y. Relationships between radiotracer properties and image quality in molecular imaging of the brain with positron emission tomography. Mol Imaging Biol 2003;5:363–75.
7. Acton PD, Kung HF. Small animal imaging with high resolution single photon emission tomography. Nucl Med Biol 2003;30:889–95.
8. Shah K, Jacobs A, Breakefield XO, Weissleder R. Molecular imaging of gene therapy for cancer. Gene Ther 2004;11:1175–87.
9. Sokolov K, Aaron J, Hsu B, et al. Optical systems for in vivo molecular imaging of cancer. Technol Cancer Res Treat 2003;2:491–504.
10. Choy G, Choyke P, Libutti SK. Current advances in molecular imaging: noninvasive in vivo bioluminescent and fluorescent optical imaging in cancer research. Mol Imaging 2003;2:303–12.
11. Blasberg RG. Molecular imaging and cancer. Molr Cancer Ther 2003;2:335–43.
12. Tsien RY. Imagining imaging's future. Nat Rev Mol Cell Biol 2003;(Suppl):SS16–21.
13. Herschman HR. Molecular imaging: looking at problems, seeing solutions. Science 2003;302:605–8.
14. Gillies RJ. In vivo molecular imaging. J Cell Biochem Suppl 2002;39:231–8.
15. Campa MJ, Serlin SB, Patz EF Jr. Development of novel tumor imaging agents using phage-display combinatorial peptide libraries. Acad Radiol 2002;9:927–32.

32a

Imaging Cancer of Unknown Primary Site

Kitt Shaffer, MD, PhD

Imaging and management of patients with metastatic disease without a known primary site are difficult and often frustrating for both clinicians and patients. Approximately 3% to 5% of new diagnoses of cancer are classified as cancer of unknown primary (CUP), and approximately 60% of these are of adenocarcinoma histology.[1,2] Overall median survival of patients with CUP is only about 4 months,[3] but certain subsets of patients may have much longer survival. It can be important to diagnose the primary site in some patients because a small percentage of tumors may have relatively specific treatment—for example, hormonally dependent tumors or germ-cell tumors. However, it is also important to spare the majority of patients for whom no specific treatment is likely to be effective from unnecessarily costly and cumbersome work-ups. Localization of the primary tumor may occasionally allow local control to be established, with a reduction in symptoms as a result of continued growth of the primary lesion and a decreased risk of additional metastatic lesions.

In an autopsy study of 375 patients who died soon after organ transplantation, 3% had occult malignancies including thyroid carcinoma, small-bowel carcinoid, lung cancer, laryngeal cancer, renal cell carcinoma, and seminoma.[4] In a study of 1,000 patients with CUP at M.D. Anderson Cancer Center, median survival was 11 months. Patients with fewer metastatic sites did slightly better, as did those with histology other than adenocarcinoma.[5] Patients with disease limited to nodal sites probably do slightly better overall than those with visceral sites of disease.[6] Despite extensive imaging work-ups, the primary site in patients with metastatic unknown primary tumor is found in fewer than 25% of cases.

Unfortunately, because the majority of CUP cases are adenocarcinomas, they may be very difficult to discriminate histologically (Figure 32a-1). Newer pathology methods, including immunohistochemistry and genetic analyses, may help in some of these cases and are likely to have an even greater role in future. Certain specific imaging strategies—such as breast magnetic resonance imaging (MRI) to search for occult breast primary in patients with axillary nodes—may be used, but immunohistochemistry—for example, analysis of cytokeratins or thyroid transcription factors—may be more helpful than random CT scanning.[7] Newer imaging methods such as positron emission tomography (PET) and MRI may also offer more specific diagnoses in some cases. In a series of 11 cases of CUP, PET localized the primary site (mostly lung cancer) in just under half.[8] With PET, the potential exists to substitute a single imaging modality for multiple imaging methods (Figure 32a-2). Therefore, although PET is a relatively expensive procedure, it may be more cost-effective than the combination of multiple plain films, CT scanning, ultrasonography, and nuclear medicine examinations.[9]

In analyzing the patient with CUP, it is important to determine the location of the metastases and any suggestive imaging features that may allow a tailored search for the likeliest primary site. Most metastatic disease in cancer patients is detected at a time when the primary tumor has already declared itself, usually through symptoms such as flank pain or hematuria in renal cell carcinoma, obstruction and bleeding in gastrointestinal (GI) tumors, or persistent infection and respiratory symptoms in lung cancer. In the setting of CUP, the primary lesion is asymptomatic. CUP patients therefore show a slight preponderance of the more clinically silent yet overall more rare tumors such as cholangiocarcinoma or pancreatic carcinoma, because these tumors are more likely to grow undetected long enough for metastases to develop. However, the commonest overall causes of CUP are the commonest tumors: those of breast, lung, prostate, and GI tract. It is also important to consider tumors with a tendency to spread widely while the primary lesion is still quite small—for example, some lung cancers, melanoma, and breast tumors.

Comparisons between clinical research studies of CUP are particularly difficult, because new diagnostic modalities are continually being pursued, and last year's CUP may be more easily diagnosed with this year's new imaging and histology methods. Even among contemporaneous studies, the particular imaging and histology methods used may vary widely from study to study. Some studies include all patients who had CUP at initial presentation; others may exclude patients who reach a specific diagnosis as a consequence of a tailored and often extensive additional work-up. Patients who die soon after initial presentation with aggressive tumors are less likely to be diagnosed in terms of a primary site. Patients with advanced disease causing significant morbidity at diagnosis may be less likely to undergo further detailed diagnostic work-up to try to find a primary site. Specific imaging work-ups vary widely from institution to institution. All of these factors limit the ability to generalize about CUP across clinical studies.

The site and pattern of metastatic disease may sometimes both suggest a specific primary site. One of the commonest presentations for CUP is metastasis to neck nodes. Although squamous cell histology is often reported, suggesting a head-and-neck primary site, other sources must also be considered—for example, uterine, cervical, or lung primary tumors. Neck-node metastases without known primary site constitute approximately 10% of cases of CUP, with approximately 75% ultimately proven to originate from a head-and-neck tumor. In a study of 75 patients presenting with cervical nodal metastases, thorough imaging and clinical exam revealed the head-and-neck primary site in approximately 40% of patients.[10]Results of PET scanning for neck nodes are still controversial. In cervical nodal metastases from unknown primary site, PET found an occult head-and-neck primary in 5% to 25% of cases in which CT, MRI, and clinical exam failed to localize a primary. Ipsilateral tonsillectomy, a standard method for detection of occult primary tumors, was positive in approximately 25% of cases.[11] But, in another study of 13 patients with squamous cell carcinoma metastases in cervical lymph nodes, only one primary site was correctly identified using PET, as compared with six false-positive sites.[12] Clearly, larger studies are needed to determine the most appropriate role for PET in this clinical situation.

In another study of PET in patients with metastases outside of neck nodes, a primary was located in about 25% of cases.[13] The addition of

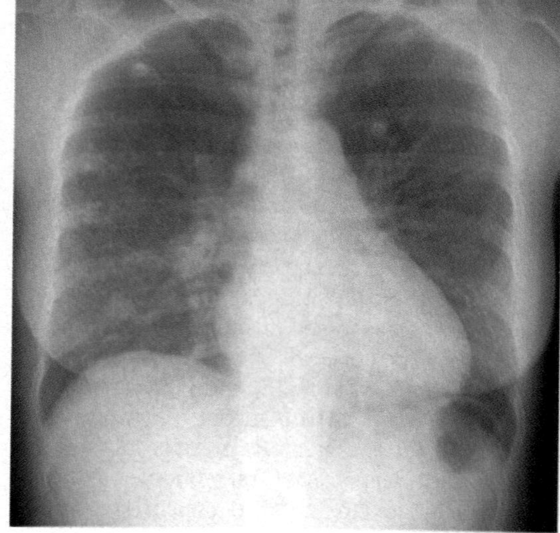

Figure 32a-1 Frontal chest film of a 42-year-old female who presented with shortness of breath. Diffuse reticular abnormalities are present in both lungs, with a suggestion of discrete nodules and hilar adenopathy. At attempted bronchoscopy, the patient developed acute respiratory decompensation and died. Bronchial washings revealed adenocarcinoma. The likely primary sites would include breast, lung, and gastrointestinal tract.

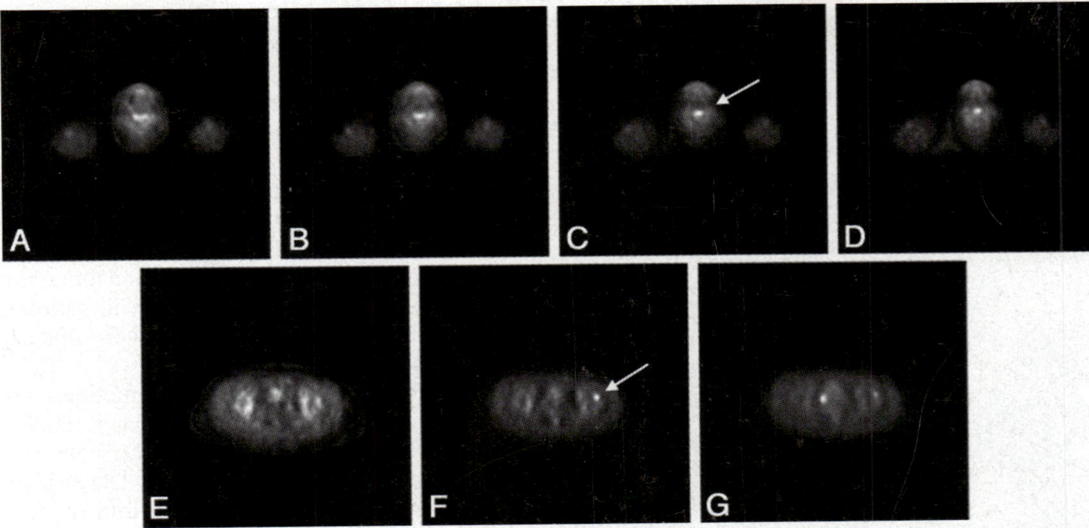

Figure 32a-2 Positron emission tomography in a 49-year-old female who presented with a bilateral neck adenopathy, pathologically squamous cell carcinoma. Images **A** to **D** are of the neck region, showing focal uptake in the hypopharynx and base of tongue (*arrow*). At endoscopy, squamous cell carcinoma was found in the base of the tongue. Images **E** to **G** are of the pelvis; they show a metastatic lesion to the left hip (*arrow*).

CT in fused PET/CT imaging (Figure 32a-3) may increase detection rates to 33%.[14] PET was used to locate a primary site in a series of 53 cases of metastatic disease and no known primary despite extensive conventional diagnostic work-up. Most cases presented with cervical adenopathy containing metastatic foci. PET found a primary site in approximately 50% of the cases, of which approximately 40% originated in lung, approximately 30% originated in a head-and-neck site, and one case each originated at occult breast and GI sites. False-positive sites were also seen in the tonsils in several patients.[15]

For adenocarcinoma metastatic to cervical nodes, the list of possible sources must include breast, renal cell,[16] and GI primaries, as well as lung. Follicular thyroid carcinomas in particular may be small and clinically occult, yet capable of yielding symptomatic metastases to cervical nodes and other sites: one case report described a solitary metastasis to the right petrous apex presenting as trigeminal neurinoma.[17] PET can be helpful in the detection of metastatic disease from the thyroid, which may be otherwise occult.[18] Papillary thyroid metastases to neck nodes can occasionally be cystic, which may help in suggesting the primary site.[19]

Another common presentation of CUP is axillary nodal metastatic disease. Occult breast cancer presents as axillary metastases in approximately 1% of operable cases. In a study of 6,000 cases of breast cancer, 20 patients presented with axillary metastases, but normal physical exam and mammography—that is, less than 1% would have been termed CUP, at least initially.[20] In 40 cases of axillary metastases with negative mammography and clinical exam, breast MRI identified the primary site in 28 cases (70%).[21,22] In a study of 22 women with axillary metastases and normal physical exam and mammography, MRI detected the breast primary site in 19 women (86%).[23]

Pleural metastases are not an uncommon presentation for CUP (Figure 32a-4), occurring in 12% of patients in one study of chemical pleurodesis of malignant effusions.[24] Analysis of pleural fluid for carcinoembryonic antigen (CEA) or cancer antigen 125 (CA125) may help to determine the most likely site of origin. Elevated CEA is most consistent with lung, breast, or mucinous GI tract origin; elevated CA125 is more suggestive of ovarian, fallopian tube, or endometrial carcinoma.[25] In one study of ovarian carcinoma, survival was actually better for patients who initially presented as CUP with either pleural metastases or supraclavicular metastases than for patients presenting with intra-abdominal spread. It was proposed that the CUP patients were in better physical condition at the time of diagnosis and that they could withstand more aggressive chemotherapy, which accounted for their slightly longer survival.[26]

The utility of mammography as a routine part of a CUP work-up is questionable. In a study of 31 women with metastatic disease in which breast

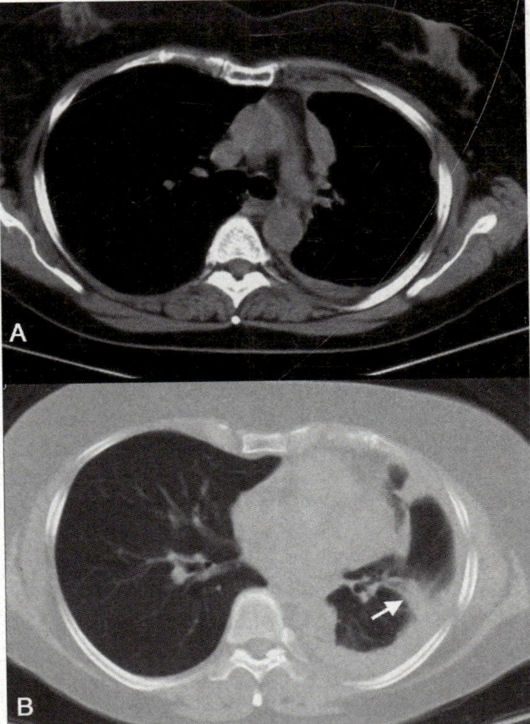

Figure 32a-4 Computed tomography images from a study in a 59-year-old female with left chest pain. Diffuse left pleural thickening is evident extending both medially and laterally as well as into the major fissure (*arrow*). No other abnormalities were seen, and the patient's mammogram was normal. Likely primary sites include breast, lung, and ovaries. Image **A** is displayed with soft-tissue windows; **B** is displayed with lung windows.

Figure 32a-3 Positron emission tomography (PET)/computed tomography (CT) and fusion images from a 60-year-old male with carcinoma of unknown primary. The combination of PET and CT can reduce false positive results and may increase the detection rate of the primary tumor to 33% from 25%. In this case, images showed diffuse visceral metastases in liver as well as in pelvic nodes and bones, but did not reveal the primary site.

cancer was considered as a possible diagnosis, the sites of metastases were lung (45%), nodes (19%) and abdomen (16%). After further work-up, a primary site was eventually determined in almost 90% of cases, with lung (45%), breast (16%), and ovary (16%) being the most common. In only one case did mammography correctly identify a breast primary. Mammography yielded false-positive results in three cases, and false-negative results in five more.[27] Most breast cancer that is metastatic at diagnosis has a clinically evident primary site. In patients who show no symptoms suggestive of a breast primary, mammography is probably of limited value. Breast MRI may, in many cases, be more revealing because it is better able to detect a small lesion in the midst of breast parenchyma.[22]

Metastasis to the central nervous system (CNS) is another common presentation of CUP. In a study of patients with CNS metastases and no primary site known at presentation or after routine initial staging, survival was better for single than for multiple lesions, and was best for those who underwent resection of a single lesion followed by radiation.[28] During follow-up, the primary site became evident in 82% of patients; it was most commonly in lung (78%). In a retrospective study of 181 patients presenting with solitary brain metastasis, about half had no known primary site. About half of those patients still had no primary site identified after further work-up, and in 5%, no primary site was found even at autopsy. The common primary sites in this study included lung carcinoma, melanoma, and prostate carcinoma.[29] When the brain is involved in metastatic disease of unknown primary, it is rarely an isolated site. In a series of 220 patients with brain metastases from unknown site, only 39 patients (18%) had brain metastases alone. Most of the metastases were adenocarcinomas, and about one-third of cases ultimately had a primary site identified, most often in lung.[30]

Skin and soft-tissue metastases are a relatively rare presentation of CUP. Metastatic melanoma to skin from an unknown primary site may sometimes represent atypical cutaneous or subcutaneous origin of the tumor. Based on a review of survival data in this situation, metastatic melanoma should have a 5-year survival of only approximately 10%; yet, in a study of 11 cases, an 8-year survival of 83% was actually observed, suggesting that at least some of the cases were not metastatic disease, but rather atypical histologic presentation of a primary cutaneous or subcutaneous site.[31] Solitary soft-tissue metastasis is not a common site for CUP, and it is sometimes initially mistaken for primary sarcoma. In a review of 11 cases of soft-tissue metastases without known primary, 9 cases (82%) were ultimately found to be caused by lung cancer, with colon cancer found in one case.[32]

Metastasis to bone is common in malignancies of many types, and may be the first manifestation of CUP in some cases. Skeletal metastases can lead to significant morbidity caused by pain and pathologic fracture. In a series of patients seen over a 6-year period at an orthopedic hospital, bone metastasis from CUP was found in approximately 30% of all cases of bony metastasis. The primary site was determined before death in 88% of cases and at autopsy in 4%, with 8% remaining unknown. Primary sites included lung cancer (approximately 40%), prostate cancer (approximately 20%), breast cancer (approximately 8%), and hepatocellular carcinoma (approximately 8%), with isolated cases of pancreatic and renal cell carcinoma.[33]

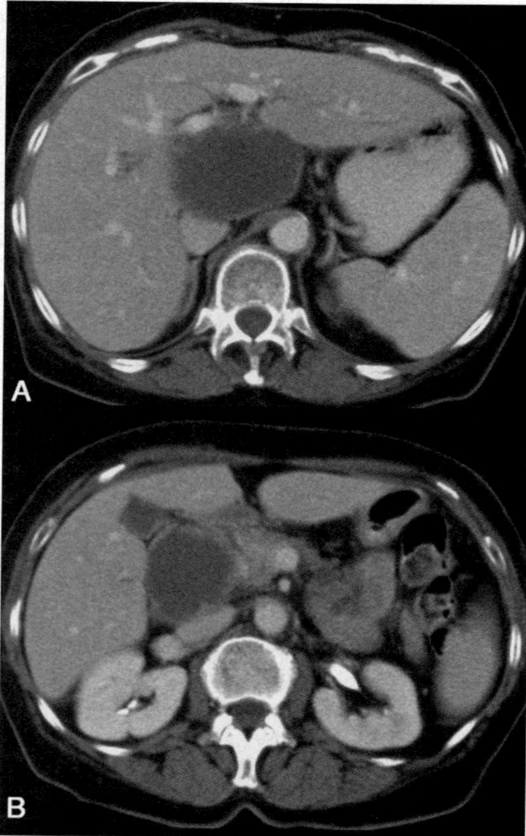

Figure 32a-5 Computed tomography (CT) images from a study in a 47-year-old female who presented with a left axillary node. At biopsy, this node contained squamous cell carcinoma. The CT scan was done as part of a search for a primary site. The unsuspected large necrotic mass in the porta hepatis displaces portal vessels forward **(A)** and also displaces the pancreatic head toward the midline **(B)**. On a later study, the uterus was noted to be enlarged, with central low attenuation suggestive of a cervical primary.

The liver is another common presenting site for CUP. New immunohistochemical methods for detecting specific cytokeratins can help to discriminate certain common tumor sites yielding metastatic disease to the liver: these include biliary, colon, rectum, and pancreas.[34] Certain specific histologic features may suggest more specific sites, such as invasive lobular breast carcinoma or carcinoma of GI origin in the case of signet ring morphology. Squamous histology may suggest cervical or head-and-neck origin (Figure 32a-5). Even carcinoid tumors, which most typically present with localizing symptoms that suggest the primary site, can occasionally be very indolent and may present as CUP.[35]

Adrenal masses are common and may represent benign adenomas or metastatic disease from unknown primary site. Of all patients presenting with suspected metastatic disease of unknown primary site, the adrenal is involved in approximately 6% of cases. As a solitary site, the adrenal is rather rare (<1%). In most such cases, the adrenal masses are large or bilateral and are therefore unlikely to be mistaken for adenomas.[36] In a study of fine-needle aspiration of adrenal masses ranging in size from 3 cm to 12 cm in patients without known malignancy, 6% were unsuspected metastases.[37]

Thromboembolic events can sometimes be the first indication of occult malignancy. Trousseau first described the connection between venous thrombosis and malignancy. The risk of cancer is increased by between threefold and 20-fold in patients presenting with venous thromboembolism without a known precipitating cause.[38] Deep venous thrombosis of an upper extremity is more worrisome as a sign of occult malignancy than is thrombosis of a lower extremity. Among patients with lower extremity deep venous thrombosis, the rate of diagnosis of cancer in the following 12 months was approximately 10%; in patients with upper-extremity thrombosis, it was almost 25%. Common underlying cancers included lymphoma, lung cancer, colon, or prostate.[39] In the setting of CUP with thromboembolic complications, those cancers are the most likely primary tumors to be considered.

The management of CUP can be a frustrating and unrewarding experience for patients and their caregivers. Despite an exhaustive work-up, the primary site is found in less than 25% of CUP cases.[7] Although most CUP patients have a rapid downhill course, a significant subset of up to 10% may have relatively long survival.[1] Remembering that empiric therapy is in some cases equally effective regardless of the actual primary site, it may sometimes be best to limit work-ups or to tailor them to specific clinical situations. Some generalizations may help in the determination. Tumors presenting as metastases without known primary are likely in two settings: tumors that metastasize while small, and tumors arising in clinically silent areas. In the first group are lung carcinoma, breast carcinoma, and melanoma. In the second group are melanoma, cholangiocarcinoma, pancreatic carcinoma, and, occasionally, carcinoid tumors. The advent of PET scanning may have a significant impact on CUP in the future, because the technology allows the entire body to be surveyed in a single study, which may greatly simplify the search for a primary site in some cases.

REFERENCES

1. Brigden ML, Murray N. Improving survival in metastatic carcinoma of unknown origin. Postgrad Med 1999;105:63–4,67–74.
2. Hammar SP. Metastatic adenocarcinoma of unknown primary origin. Hum Pathol 1998;29:1393–402.
3. Hillen HF. Unknown primary tumours. Postgrad Med J 2000;76:690–3.

4. Torbenson MS, Wang J, Nichols L, et al. Occult nonhematopoietic malignancies present at autopsy in solid organ transplant patients who died within 100 days. Transplantation 2001;71:64–9.
5. Hess KR, Abbruzzese MC, Lenzi R, et al. Classification and regression tree analysis of 1000 consecutive patients with unknown primary carcinoma. Clin Cancer Res 1999;5:3403–10.
6. Chorost MI, Lee MC, Yeoh CB, et al. Unknown primary. J Surg Oncol 2004;87:191–203.
7. Varadhachary GR, Abbruzzese JL, Lenzi R. Diagnostic strategies for unknown primary cancer. Cancer 2004;100:1776–85.
8. Lassen U, Daugaard G, Eigtved A, et al. ^{18}F–FDG whole body positron emission tomography (PET) in patients with unknown primary tumours (UPT). Eur J Cancer 1999;35:1076–82.
9. Marom EM, Erasmus JJ, Patz EF. Lung cancer and positron emission tomography with fluorodeoxyglucose. Lung Cancer 2000;28:187–202.
10. Weber A, Schmoz S, Bootz F. CUP (carcinoma of unknown primary) syndrome in head and neck: clinic, diagnostic, and therapy. Onkologie 2001;24:38–43.
11. Nieder C, Gregoire V, Ang KK. Cervical lymph node metastases from occult squamous cell carcinoma: cut down a tree to get an apple? Int J Radiat Oncol Biol Phys 2001;50:727–33.
12. Greven KM, Keyes JW Jr, Williams DW 3rd, et al. Occult primary tumors of the head and neck: lack of benefit from positron emission tomography imaging with 2-^{18}F-fluoro-2-deoxy-D-glucose. Cancer 1999;86:114–8.
13. Joshi U, van der Hoeven JJ, Comans EF, et al. In search of an unknown primary tumour presenting with extracervical metastases: the diagnostic performance of FDG–PET. Br J Radiol 2004;77:1000–6.
14. Gutzeit A, Antoch G, Kuhl H, et al. Unknown primary tumors: detection with dual-modality PET/CT—initial experience. Radiology 2004;234:227–34.
15. Bohuslavizki KH, Klutmann S, Kroger S, et al. FDG PET detection of unknown primary tumors. J Nucl Med 2000;41:816–22.
16. Dal Cin P, Sciot R, De Wever I, et al. Diagnosis of primary renal cell carcinoma in a left supraclavicular lymph node by chromosome analysis. J Urol 1996;156:171–2.
17. Kachhara R, Nair S, Radhakrishnan VV, et al. Solitary metastasis from occult follicular carcinoma of the thyroid mimicking trigeminal neurinoma—case report. Neurol Med Chir (Tokyo) 2001;41:360–3.
18. Stevens KJ, Smith SL, Denley H, et al. Is mammography of value in women with disseminated cancer of unknown origin? Clin Oncol (R Coll Radiol) 1999;11:90–2.
19. Lloyd MS, Nash AG. “Occult” breast cancer. Ann R Coll Surg Engl 2001;83:420–4.
20. Ruda R, Borgognone M, Benech F, et al. Brain metastases from unknown primary tumour: a prospective study. J Neurol 2001;248:394–8.
21. Dede F, Ajoedi ND, Ansari SM, et al. Metastatic thyroid cancer occurring as an unknown primary lesion: the role of ^{18}F FDG positron emission tomography. Clin Nucl Med 2001;26:396–9.
22. North JH Jr. Occult thyroid carcinoma manifested as a cystic neck mass. South Med J 1997;90:1027–8.
23. Foroudi F, Tiver KW. Occult breast carcinoma presenting as axillary metastases. Int J Radiat Ocol Biol Phys 2000;47:143–7.
24. Olson JA Jr, Morris EA, Van Zee KJ, et al. Magnetic resonance imaging facilitates breast conservation for occult breast cancer. Ann Surg Oncol 2000;7:411–5.
25. Orel SG, Weinstein SP, Schnall MD, et al. Breast MR imaging in patients with axillary node metastases and unknown primary malignancy. Radiology 1999;212:543–9.
26. Martinez-Moragon E, Aparicio J, Sanchis J, et al. Malignant pleural effusion: prognostic factors for survival and response to chemical pleurodesis in a series of 120 cases. Respiration 1998;65:108–13.
27. Pinto MM, Bernstein LH, Rudolph RA, et al. Diagnostic efficiency of carcinoembryonic antigen and CA125 in the cytological evaluation of effusions. Arch Pathol Lab Med 1992;116:626–31.
28. Zang RY, Zhang ZY, Cai SM, et al. Epithelial ovarian cancer presenting initially with extraabdominal or intrahepatic metastases: a preliminary report of 25 cases and literature review. Am J Clin Oncol 2000;23:416–9.
29. Giordana MT, Cordera S, Boghi A. Cerebral metastases as first symptom of cancer: a clinico-pathologic study. J Neurooncol 2000;50:265–73.
30. Nguyen LN, Maor MH, Oswald MJ. Brain metastases as the only manifestation of an undetected primary tumor. Cancer 1998;83:2181–4.
31. Bowen GM, Chang AE, Lowe L, et al. Solitary melanoma confined to the dermal and/or subcutaneous tissue: evidence for revisiting the staging classification. Arch Dermatol 2000;136:1397–9.
32. Glockner JF, White LM, Sundaram M, McDonald DJ. Unsuspected metastases presenting as solitary soft tissue lesions: a fourteen-year review. Skeletal Radiol 2000;29:270–4.
33. Katagiri H, Takahashi M, Inagaki J, et al. Determining the site of the primary cancer in patients with skeletal metastasis of unknown origin: a retrospective study. Cancer 1999;86:533–7.
34. Tot T. Adenocarcinomas metastatic to the liver: the value of cytokeratins 20 and 7 in the search for unknown primary tumors. Cancer 1999;85:171–7.
35. Mahmood T, Mudad R. Carcinoid syndrome with unknown primary: a case report. Am J Clin Oncol 1999;22:384–6.
36. Lee JE, Evans DB, Hickey RC, et al. Unknown primary cancer presenting as an adrenal mass: frequency and implications for diagnostic evaluation of adrenal incidentalomas. Surgery 1998;124:1115–22.
37. Lumachi F, Borsato S, Brandes AA, et al. Fine-needle aspiration cytology of adrenal masses in noncancer patients: clinicoradiologic and histologic correlations in functioning and nonfunctioning tumors. Cancer 2001;93:323–9.
38. Otten HM, Prins MH. Venous thromboembolism and occult malignancy. Thromb Res 2001;102:V187–94.
39. Girolami A, Prandoni P, Zanon E, et al. Venous thromboses of upper limbs are more frequently associated with occult cancer as compared with those of lower limbs. Blood Coagul Fibrinolysis 1999;10:455–7.

32b

Imaging Neoplasms of the Central Nervous System, Head, and Neck

Christopher J. Hurt, MD

Norman J. Beauchamp Jr, MD, MHS

Neuroradiologic imaging plays a central role in the diagnosis and treatment of tumors of the central nervous system (CNS) and of the head and neck. A number of imaging modalities are available, including computed tomography (CT), magnetic resonance imaging (MRI), nuclear medicine, and angiography. Deciding which of these imaging options to rely on can be daunting, but a reasonable generalization is that, for initial characterization, MRI is the modality of choice intracranially and within the spinal canal, and that CT and MRI are the modalities of choice extracranially. Both modalities enable exquisite detection of tumors by exploiting biophysical differences between pathology and normal tissue.

Once the lesion is detected, the ability to localize it to a given anatomic region is perhaps the most important step in narrowing the list of differential diagnostic possibilities. For example, if a lesion can be identified as being in the cerebellopontine angle, a differential list of three tumors (acoustic schwannoma, meningioma, and epidermoid) would include the correct diagnosis more than 90% of the time. Increased specificity is occasionally possible based on the unique imaging characteristics of a given lesion.

Besides an understanding of the capabilities of imaging approaches, an awareness of their limitations is also essential. Such an awareness helps to ensure detection of lesions when present and to avoid false-positive interpretations (for example, mistaking an artifact for a lesion). A comprehensive look at artifacts is beyond the scope of this review, but a few of the more common limitations are presented. For example, patient motion universally compromises the detection of pathology because of blurring of anatomic information. Other limitations are more modality-specific. MRI is uniquely sensitive to motion *within* the patient—for example, blood flow and cerebrospinal fluid (CSF) flow have the potential to generate pseudo-lesions. In the presence of highly dense material—bone or calcium, for instance—the x-rays used in CT become "hardened." The result can be obscuration of detail adjacent to bone or appearance of pseudo-lesions attributable to dark and bright lines.

In this chapter, then, the approach to discussing neoplasms will be location focused, considering the CNS first and the head and neck second. The primary emphasis will be MRI and CT evaluation. When the use of additional imaging techniques is valuable in diagnosis, that fact will be specifically mentioned.

CENTRAL NERVOUS SYSTEM

Just as each CNS tumor possesses unique clinical, macroscopic, histopathologic, and molecular features, each tumor also possesses its own radiologic features. Albeit generally not pathognomonic, a coupling of the information on location and patient age to radiographic appearance can often be highly suggestive of a histologic diagnosis.

Obviously, imaging assists in tumor grading by delineating invasion, infiltration, and necrosis. These features are characterized by CT as the presence of nonanatomic structures and areas of abnormal density. MRI uses a series of pulse sequences that are differentially targeted to define anatomy (T1-weighted [T1W] images), breakdown of the blood–brain barrier (T1W images following administration of intravenous contrast), and the extent of tumor and edema (T2-weighted [T2W] images and T1W images following administration of intravenous contrast) to interrogate for disease. Staging is not as widely used for CNS tumors. However, neuroimaging can reveal subarachnoid space (SAS) and rare extra-CNS spread, and can determine requisite resection coverage. Notably, despite the fact that contrast enhancement margins are often viewed to represent tumor extent, malignant cells can be present beyond enhancing regions or even beyond areas of abnormal intensity on MR images.

As stated in the introduction, lesion localization is often more telling in regard to the differential diagnostic possibilities. Localization begins by classifying the lesion as intra- or extra-axial. Manifestations suggesting the former are cortical thickening, extensive vasogenic edema, sharp margins with dural surfaces, containment of all lesion margins within brain parenchyma, and absence of overlying contrast enhancement of the leptomeninges (ie, leptomeningeal [LM] enhancement) or bone infiltration. Extra-axial processes typically demonstrate obtuse parenchymal margins, cortical buckling, linear dural enhancement adjacent to the tumor (also called "dural tail"), overlying bone infiltration or reaction, lesion-margin SAS dilatation, and cranial nerve (CN) or LM contrast enhancement. In addition, cytotoxic and vasogenic edema would be absent. (Vasogenic edema is associated with intra-axial neoplasms and is characterized by hypodensity on CT or hyperintensity on T2W MRI that involves white matter, but that spares gray matter.)

The remainder of the CNS section highlights useful characteristics of individual tumors first in the brain and second in the spinal cord.

The Brain Meningioma is by far the most common intracranial extra-axial neoplasm. On CT, 60% of lesions are hyperdense to brain. On MRI, lesions tend to be hypo- to isointense to cortex on T1W MR images (T1WI) and iso- to hyperintense to cortex on T2W MR images (T2WI), although signals can vary because of vascularity, calcifications, cystic foci, or intrinsic mottling or speckling. Most meningiomas enhance markedly on both CT and MRI with contrast. CT with contrast probably provides better demonstration of the broad-based dural margin and confirmation of the extra-axial location.

Differentiation from peripherally located lymphoma or other lesions with prominent enhancement can occasionally be challenging. Stippled or solid calcification is seen in approximately 20% of lesions.[1] MRI can miss some calcified meningiomas that are detected by CT. Nonetheless, without contrast, some meningiomas can also go unnoticed on CT.

Dural tails are characteristic, being present in 72% of lesions; they represent enhancement along tumor margins affecting the pachymeninges. However, studies disagree as to whether dural tails are tumor or benign reactive tissue. Dural tails can also, on rare occasions, be seen with gliomas, acoustic schwannomas, and metastases. In addition, MRI has shown enhancing dural thickening, which proved to represent tumoral extension within and around the dura.

In 20 to 46% of cases, meningiomas yield bone lysis or sclerosis, usually representing reaction, although occasionally indicating invasion. Indeed, meningiomas can exhibit aggressive features such as necrosis, fatty or cystic degeneration, parenchymal or osseous infiltration, and vasogenic edema. Nonetheless, growth is typically progressive, causing mass effect.

Angiographically, a tumor blush can be seen. This blush is a manifestation of neovascularity within the lesion.

In addition to evaluating tumor size and location, and presence of blood–brain barrier breakdown, MRI can also evaluate tumor metabolism. This technique is called MR spectroscopy. Although a comprehensive review of metabolites is beyond the scope of this chapter, certain patterns of metabolites can help to differentiate higher-grade from lower-grade tumor, glial from non-glial tumors, and tumors from abscess. Spectroscopic features are not unique for meningiomas, but significant *N*-acetylaspartate (NAA) and creatine (CR) reductions, with elevated choline (CHO) peaks, may be seen.

Schwannoma represents the second most common extra-axial mass, characteristically located in the internal auditory canal (IAC) or cerebellar pontine angle (CPA), where it accounts for 75 to 90% of lesions. Overall, schwannomas account for 7 to 8% of intracranial neoplasms.

MRI with contrast is the best way to screen patients suspected of acoustic schwannoma originating from CN VIII. The technique shows greater sensitivity than CT, especially for residual and recurrent cases. Schwannomas are typically proximal to the very dense, and thus CT-limiting, petrous bone. Schwannomas tend to be slightly iso- to hypointense on T2WI and, like meningiomas, isointense to gray matter on T1WI. Nonetheless, schwannomas rarely exhibit dural tails, and they tend to exuberantly enhance to a greater degree than meningiomas do. Such enhancement is homogeneous in 70% of cases. Vestibular schwannomas may also exhibit cystic or hemorrhagic degeneration and edema; however, bony reaction is exceedingly uncommon. A lesion entering and expanding the IAC favors schwannoma over meningioma; a flat dural-based lesion or non-expanded IAC favors meningioma.

After meningiomas and epidermoids, schwannomas of CN V or VII represent the next most common CPA mass. Location and growth pattern differentiate these lesions from CN VIII schwannomas. Epidermoids typically arise in the CPA (suprasellar cistern, peripineal region, or prepontine cistern), where they represent 3 to 6% of tumors. Tumor edges tend to be scalloped, corresponding to infiltration, commonly into the brainstem. MRI provides excellent characterization of epidermoids. These lesions have signal characteristics similar to CSF on T1W and T2W sequences and do not enhance. Similarly, on CT, the lesion is hypodense (water-like density). As a result, before advanced MRI imaging sequences were introduced, these lesions were difficult to differentiate from CSF-filled arachnoid cysts. However, two newer MRI sequences—fluid attenuation inversion recovery (FLAIR) and diffusion-weighted imaging (DWI)—enable differentiation of epidermoids from arachnoid cysts.[2] On these sequences, the signal within the epidermoid is heterogeneous and does not follow CSF in signal intensity (SI). MR spectroscopy can also be useful. Spectroscopically, epidermoids exhibit lactate peaks. Arachnoid and porencephalic cysts show no peaks, and cystic astrocytomas peak for NAA, CHO, CR, and occasionally lactate.[3]

In the pineal region, pineal germ cell and pineal cell tumors, peripineal masses, and pineal cysts can be seen. Once localized to the pineal region, the differential diagnosis can be further narrowed by understanding the relative tumor-type frequency by patient age and imaging appearance. A rough rule of thumb is that two-thirds of pineal-region tumors are germ cell tumors, and two-thirds of the germ cell tumors are germinomas.

The "typical" germinoma markedly and homogeneously enhances. On CT, more than 50% of germinomas are hyperdense to normal brain, and the remainder exhibit isodensity. On MRI, these lesions are iso- to hypointense on T1WI and T2WI. Typically, lesions are found to engulf a densely calcified pineal gland. In that setting, a "most likely" diagnosis of germinoma can be made from an imaging perspective. However, the lesions are not always homogeneous; cystic degeneration is seen in 33%. Lastly, CSF tumor spread can occur in up to 50% of pineal-region germinomas. Response to radiation therapy is also a defining characteristic of germinomas; tumor disappears as soon as 2 weeks after therapy. Notably, the "non-typical" appearance of cystic degeneration typically predicts poor radiotherapy (RT) outcome.

Other germ cell tumors observed in the region are teratomas, choriocarcinomas, endodermal sinus tumors, and embryonal cell tumors. These cancers can be further differentiated based on signal characteristics. The presence of imaging characteristics consistent with fat (hypodense on CT; hyperintense on T1W) is a hallmark of teratomas. Imaging characteristics consistent with hemorrhage suggest choriocarcinoma, a lesion that hemorrhages at a high rate, where other lesions in this region rarely do.

Serology can be used to distinguish a number of lesions in this region. Indeed, for pineal-region tumors, biochemical tumor markers are (besides patient age) probably more important factors in determining tumor type than MRI appearance is.

In terms of pineal cell tumors, pineoblastomas are often also considered to belong to the class of primitive neuroectodermal tumors (PNETs), which is discussed below. Pineoblastomas are typically slightly hyperdense on CT and markedly enhance and have low SI on T2WI and FLAIR. Calcification is more common with pineal cell tumors than with pineal germinomas. SAS can be seen with pineoblastomas, but only rarely with pineocytomas. The former can engulf or "explode" normal pineal calcification; the latter can cystically degenerate, resembling a complex benign congenital pineal cyst.

Suspected lesions in the sellar region are best evaluated by MRI due to the proximity of the dense base of the skull and the technique's ability to image in multiple planes, which facilitates anatomic localization and definition of the tumor's relationship to adjacent structures—useful in delineating tumor origin. Pituitary adenomas are common lesions in this location. They are differentiated into macro- and microadenomas. Macroadenomas are 1 cm or larger in size and arise within or engulf the normal pituitary gland. They can enlarge the pituitary fossa, depressing the sellar floor or ascending into the suprasellar cistern via the diaphragma sella. Microadenomas (<1 cm) can be more challenging to diagnose. They do not yield bony aberrations, presenting as mere intraglandular abnormal density or signal intensity. Macroadenomas have a propensity to hemorrhage because of their marginal blood supply, giving high SI on T1WI. Tumors of both sizes typically enhance less than the surrounding gland. Cavernous sinus invasion is a typical harbinger of high hormone levels and complex surgery.

A lesion that can have a very similar appearance is a large sellar-region meningioma. Blood vessel involvement can be a useful differentiator: whereas pituitary adenomas, like meningiomas, can encircle the internal cerebellar artery in the parasella, adenomas tend not to narrow vessel lumens. Craniopharyngiomas can mimic pituitary tumors when located in the suprasellar region. However, in the suprasella, macroadenoma extension represents the most common lesion. Also, craniopharyngiomas typically exhibit cysts or frequent calcification, or both. Such cysts can give high SI on non-contrast T1WI, a finding that would be very atypical for a meningioma.

Other regional neoplasms include germ cell tumors and hypothalamic or chiasmatic astrocytomas. Of note, 28% of suprasellar germinomas exhibit cystic degeneration and CSF seeding. It is important to remember that masses other than true neoplasms—for example, basilar tip aneurysm and granulomatous disease such as sarcoid, can give a similar appearance in this region. Correlation with clinical evaluation is therefore imperative.

Overall, 86% of choroid plexus papillomas (CPP) are seen in children younger than 5 years. They account for 42% of brain tumors in children younger than 2 months, 3% of all intracranial pediatric tumors, and 0.5% of all intracranial neoplasms. Notably, 80% occur at the glomus of the lateral ventricles in children.[4] Characteristic frond-like growth and avid enhancement are notable. Hydrocephalus is also typical, attributable to CSF overproduction, outlet obstruction, or arachnoidal adhesions from tumor-associated proteinaceous material or blood. Thus, in a pediatric patient, identifying an isolated enhancing lesion in the atrium of the lateral ventricle with associated ventricular dilatation would support a "most likely" diagnosis of CPP, regardless of density or other MRI signal characteristics.[5]

In adults, CPPs are found in the fourth ventricle rather than the lateral ventricles, again reinforcing the importance of age and location in constructing an appropriate differential diagnosis. Moreover, a glomus-region tumor in an adult would more likely be a meningioma. In adults, metastases, lymphoma, and astrocytoma must also be considered as possibilities for masses in the region.

Ependymomas arise from ventricular ependyma and typically account for 6% of gliomas. Location is usually the posterior fossa, in association with the fourth ventricle. Growth is characteristic, expanding the foramina of Luschka and Magendie, filling the fourth ventricle, and even growing out the ventricular foramina. Further, ependymomas typically calcify in 40 to 50% of children; medulloblastomas do not. Stippled calcification can assume a hyperdense CT appearance, but noncalcified regions are usually hypo- to isodense to brain. Cysts can occur (15%), as can hemorrhage (10%). The mixture of calcium, hemorrhage, and cysts yields a heterogeneous picture on T2WI; T1WI typically reveals a lesion hypointense with cortex. Enhancement is typically mild and heterogeneous. SAS seeding occurs with a high incidence. Lastly, up to 20% of lesions are located in the supratentorial parenchyma, where they can exhibit ring enhancement with central necrosis, thus resembling high-grade astrocytomas. In differentiating ependymoma from medulloblastoma, the other common pediatric tumor of the fourth ventricular region, medulloblastomas narrow the fourth ventricle, do not grow out of the ventricular foramina, and do not calcify.

Subependymomas are rare benign ventricular lesions that are typically located in the lateral recesses of the fourth ventricle or in the lateral ventricles along the septum pellucidum. SI and density are similar to those of gray matter, and calcification is highly unlikely. To differentiate these tumors from adult CPPs or ependymomas, note that, when located in the fourth ventricle, subependymomas almost never enhance. (Enhancement is more typical in supratentorial subependymomas.) Mass effect can be seen, but edema does not occur.

Central neurocytoma is the accepted name for the formerly misnamed intraventricular oligodendroglioma. Neurocytomas are benign lesions characteristically located along the septum pellucidum; they commonly precipitate hydrocephalus. The lesions frequently exhibit calcification and variable enhancement, thus yielding a heterogeneous MRI appearance. The lesion can be misdiagnosed as an intraventricular oligodendroglioma because of a similarity in imaging characteristics. Rare intraparenchymal lesions have been reported. In fact, a distinction between oligodendroglioma and neurocytoma is not possible radiologically; electron microscopy and immunohistology are required. Nonetheless, making the distinction is critical, because neurocytomas may not require RT. In general, purely intraventricular oligodendrogliomas are very atypical; in the absence of infiltration into the extraventricular region, a diagnosis of neurocytoma should be favored.

Subependymal giant-cell astrocytoma (SEGA) can also be seen as a mostly intraventricular, sharply defined, frequently calcified, strongly enhancing mass at the foramen of Monro. SEGA is commonly associated with tuberous sclerosis; should subependymal nodules or cortical tubers be present as well, the diagnosis is fairly conclusive.

Other entities to consider in the ventricles or along the septum pellucidum are metastasis, and germinomas. Hemangiocytomas, lipomas, dermoids, and SAS seeding from primary CNS lesions, lymphoma, leukemia, or non-CNS primary malignancies can all occur as extra-axial masses. Dermoids may also rupture, yielding SAS seeding as well.

Astrocytomas are intra-axial lesions—that is, subpial and extraventricular. For determining lesion subtype and grade, patient age, presence of necrosis, vascularity, and margin characteristics are particularly important. Glioblastoma multiforme (GBM), which represents 50 to 60% of gliomas, most often presents as a single lesion in the frontal, parietal, and temporal lobes, although true multicentricity is noted in 2.3% of cases. With MRI, GBM exhibits prominent SI heterogeneity on T2WI, with high SI regions centrally, rims that are less hyperintense to isointense, and surrounding finger-like areas of high SI. GBM is typified by irregular infiltrative margins, poor demarcation, impressive edema exerting mass effect, necrosis, and hypervascularity seen as flow voids or as high perfusion on contrast-enhanced cerebral blood volume (CBV) studies. Lesion hemorrhage has been found to correlate with histologic grade.

A challenge with glial tumors is to differentiate tumor extent from edema. Specifically, on T2W sequences, edema is hyperintense, as is most of the tumor itself. Fortunately, whereas low-grade glial tumors may not enhance, GBMs characteristically enhance. This contrast enhancement can be used to better demarcate the extent of the tumor. Abscess must be ruled out when considering GBM. Clinical history may make the case clear, but DWI can prove useful, because a pyogenic abscess is bright, whereas cysts and necrosis are dark.[6] Similarly, the corpus callosum is an extremely tightly packed white-matter fiber tract and is largely resistant to edema. Hyperintensity in the corpus callosum in the setting of an intra-axial tumor is more consistent with tumor infiltration.

An enhancing non-necrotic infiltrative lesion suggests anaplastic astrocytoma. These lesions tend to elicit edema, exert mass effect, and exhibit hemorrhagic—and occasionally cystic—portions. A non-enhancing or non-edematous lesion with relatively homogeneous high SI involvement of both gray and white matter on T2WI suggests a low-grade astrocytoma.

Enhancement, necrosis, and edema are not always a defining characteristic of tumor aggressiveness. For example, gliomatosis cerebri (GC) may not enhance. Indeed, necrosis and edema can also be absent in GC, which can be multilobar, can involve and enlarge deep gray-matter structures, and can extend to the brainstem and cervical cord. Grossly, structures appear normal in shape, leading to a normal CT appearance, but MRI reveals abnormal SI on long TR scans. In this instance, it is the extensive area of infiltration that should facilitate making the diagnosis.

Similarly, a number of intra-axial lesions that enhance have a characteristically benign course. These include cerebellar pilocytic astrocytomas, pleomorphic xanthoastrocytomas, hemangioblastomas, and gangliogliomas.

Pilocytic astrocytoma of the cerebellum, most often seen as a cyst with a mural nodule, is unusual as a benign astrocytoma in that it enhances, albeit to an unpredictable extent. Moreover, spectroscopically, a lactate doublet is typically seen, which normally is only seen with high-grade lesions. Furthermore, high metabolic activity is seen with positron emission tomography (PET). Anaplastic transformation can occur, and growth can be infiltrative. The lesions that infiltrate the brainstem are typically fibrillary (a histologic type accounting for 15% of cerebellar astrocytomas) and exhibit a more aggressive appearance than the pilocytic variety. MRI is best to evaluate such lesions, because of the beam-hardening artifact of the petrous bones that plagues CT in the posterior fossa. Relative to cortex, the lesions are typically iso- to hypointense on T1WI and hyperintense on T2WI. In the absence of enhancement, long-TR MRI is needed to fully delineate the high SI mass.[7] Perfusion-weighted imaging (PWI), with maps of relative CBV (rCBV), has been used to assess tumor grade, revealing a direct correlation—that is, rCBV in GBM is 3 to 5 times greater than in low-grade astrocytomas. The rCBV also appears to correlate with histologic vascularity.

Spectroscopically, high-grade astrocytomas typically exhibit increased lactate and lipid peaks. Reduced NAA and elevated CHO are seen, yielding a characteristically high CHO:NAA ratio for high-grade lesions. A CHO:CR > 1 also typifies tumor. Characteristic lactate:H_2O ratios exist for all three major astrocytoma groups, and a typical CHO:H_2O ratio exists for low-grade astrocytomas. Cysts in low-grade lesions have also been found to accumulate lactate.

Gangliogliomas account for approximately 2% of gliomas; 64 to 80% of those occur in patients under 30 years of age. Lesions are typically well circumscribed and located in the brain periphery, especially the gray matter of temporal lobes. Among these legions, 38 to 50% are cystic; 50% exhibit faint enhancement; and 33% show calcification. Presentation as a cyst with an enhancing mural nodule can be seen. Because of slow growth, bony remodeling can be seen, but aggressive transformation and LM and SAS spread have been reported. MRI and CT can only suggest higher grade with the presence of edema; PET and ^{201}Tl single-photon emission computed tomography (SPECT) appear to be useful for this distinction, with lower activity seen in lower-grade lesions. In the peripheral temporal lobes, a pleomorphic xanthoastrocytoma (PXA) could be entertained as a potential lesion. PXAs expand gray and white matter, variably enhance, and remodel bone because of their slow growth. Cysts with enhancing mural nodules can be seen with PXA, as can an infiltrative appearance.

Oligodendrogliomas account for 4 to 8% of gliomas. Classic appearance is a sharply demarcated lesion in the frontal or temporal lobe that fails to elicit any edematous response.[8] Calvarial erosion can be seen because of a peripheral location and a slow growth pattern. Calcification occurs in 40 to 80% of cases; but, despite the greater frequency of calcification relative to calcification in astrocytoma, the higher prevalence of the astrocytoma renders a calcified mass more likely to be astrocytoma than oligodendroglioma. The calcification character of oligodendroglioma is chunky; that of astrocytoma tends to be stippled. Cystic and hemorrhagic degeneration can be seen, yielding varying SI. Lesions typically appear iso- to hypodense on CT. On MRI, they exhibit low SI on T1WI and abnormally high SI on T2WI. Enhancement is mild and poorly defined in 50% of cases, although higher-grade lesions appear to enhance more often on CT. Mixed astrocytomatous histology is seen in 33 to 50% of lesions, but these heterogeneous lesions tend to be better defined than pure astrocytomas are. Spectroscopically, NAA is typically attenuated, and lactate tends to be absent.

PNET encompasses tumors such as medulloblastoma, ependymoblastoma, pineoblastoma, and primary cerebral neuroblastoma. Histology is typically hypercellular, yielding lesions iso- to hypointense with gray matter on T2WI and hypointense to cortex on T1WI. Lesions enhance, but less so than do pilocytic astrocytomas or GBM. Location and a patient age below 10 years tend to suggest the diagnosis. Indeed, PNET together with cerebellar astrocytoma, ependymoma, and brainstem glioma accounts for 95% of pediatric posterior fossa tumors. MRI with contrast greatly helps in distinguishing these lesions.

Medulloblastoma is the classic and most common PNET, and thus one of the most common pediatric posterior fossa tumors: 33% of tumors in this region and 50% of cerebellar tumors are medulloblastomas. On CT, lesions typically appear hyperdense, although up to 70% of cases in children may exhibit an atypical appearance. Edema is not always present. Calcification has been reported at rates of 10 to 21%. Cyst formation has been found to occur at rates of 10 to 20% in children and 59 to 82% in adults. Hemorrhage has also been noted. At presentation, 15 to 50% of children have SAS seeding; thus, primary imaging with contrast-enhanced MRI should be performed of the entire CNS axis. High recurrence rates of 25% in children younger than 2 years and 80% in children younger than 10 years are found. Older age groups account for 20% of medulloblastomas, a proportion that represents 6% of gliomas. Lesions in the older age range often simulate posterior fossa extra-axial lesions; however, a well-demarcated hemispheric lesion, mildly to moderately enhancing, located on the cerebellar surface suggests medulloblastoma as a possibility. Spectroscopically, medulloblastomas have NAA:CHO and CR:CHO ratios that tend to run lower than the same ratios in astrocytomas. In all pediatric posterior fossa tumors, ^{201}Tl SPECT appears to offer an overall sensitivity greater than 75% and a 90% specificity for detection.

Dysembryoplastic neuroepithelial tumors (DNETs) are hypodense on CT, hypointense on T1WI, and hyperintense on T2WI. They typically reside in the temporal lobe. Cortical infiltration can be seen as cortical thickening. Cystic degeneration is seen in more than 80% of cases; however, enhancement and edema are both inconsistent findings.[9] Calcification and bony remodeling can also be seen. Ipsilateral temporal lobe atrophy with poor gray–white matter definition has been noted. That said, most DNETs involve subcortical white matter; however, lesions can be confined to gray matter. Aggressiveness also varies, with some lesions resembling PXAs or gangliogliomas.

Desmoplastic infantile ganglioglioma occurs in children younger than 2 years and is usually found as lesions with a meningeal base in the frontal or parietal lobes. Cystic change with enhancing peripheral rims is nearly invariable, although calcified rims can also be seen. Calcification and hemorrhage occur less often than in PNET; edema is variably present. Desmoplasia results in a low SI rim on T2WI.

Hemangioblastoma represents the most common primary neoplasm of the adult posterior fossa. It is seen as a cystic cerebellar mass with a mural nodule in 55 to 65% of cases. Although mural nodules enhance, cyst walls do not. Patient age permits the distinction from the similar-appearing pilocytic astrocytoma. Mural-nodule flow voids, which correspond to lesion vascularity, permit the same distinction. Angiographically, dense nodule enhancement is seen, with a single, dilated, tortuous arterial feeder and multiple dilated veins. Vasculature can appear displaced because of cysts. Non-cystic lesions can be seen in 40% of cerebellar lesions and in nearly all spinal cord and medulla lesions. Multiplicity strongly suggests von Hippel–Lindau (VHL) disease. Overall, 25% of patients with hemangioblastoma have VHL.[10] Cerebellar involvement is also suggestive of VHL, because 66 to 88% of VHL patients show lesions in this area. Interestingly, 40% of all hemangioblastoma patients exhibit polycythemia because of increased erythropoietin production.

CNS lymphoma is often best suggested by clinical scenario, than by particular imaging findings. Indeed, SAS lymphoma can be unapparent on imaging. Nonetheless, CNS lymphoma is classically hyperdense on CT, with strong, homogeneous enhancement in approximately 90% of cases. However, non-enhancing lesions, and even transiently vanishing lesions after steroid therapy, have been reported. Typical MRI appearance, relative to gray matter, is slightly low SI on T1WI and slightly high SI on PDWI and T2WI. Edema can be variable, but is often severe, with marked mass effect. Growth across the corpus callosum has been seen in 38% of cases. Lesions are multiple in more than 50% of cases, with either intra- or extra-axial involvement, including calvarial, LM, or pachymeningeal. That percentage further increases in patients with acquired immunodeficiency syndrome (AIDS).

AIDS CNS lymphoma can have an atypical appearance, with lesions that are hypodense, necrotic, and peripherally enhancing, rendering distinction from GBM or toxoplasmosis challenging. Nonetheless, CNS lymphoma is thallium-avid, which toxoplasmosis is not, allowing differentiation of these two lesions. Moreover, in one series, 50% of AIDS CNS lymphoma cases had a periventricular lesion, while only 3% of toxoplasmosis occupied this location. In another series, ventricular encasement and subependymal spread were seen in 38% of AIDS CNS lymphoma patients. In addition, in one series examining AIDS CNS lymphoma, 82% of lesions were less than 2 cm in size, often multiple in number, and frequently located in the temporal lobes and basal ganglia. The same series found that, in non-AIDS CNS lymphoma, 75% of lesions were greater than 2 cm in size, primarily solitary, and located deep in the parietal lobes.[11] Spectroscopically, all CNS lymphomas tend to exhibit increased CHO and decreased CR and NAA, plus marked lipid elevation.

Metastatic lesions to the CNS can present as intra- or extra-axial in location, with lung and breast carcinoma proving to be the most frequent primary for either location. Other primaries that classically metastasize to the CNS are melanoma, and renal cell and gastrointestinal carcinoma. Calvarial deposits can appear lytic, blastic, or mixed. Typically, intra-axial metastases lodge at the gray–white junction because of decreasing vasculature caliber. Moreover, based on vascular flow dynamics, 80% of lesions deposit in terminal branches of the cerebellar artery, and 20% deposit in terminal branches of the vertebrobasilar system. Lesions are usually well defined, yield severe vasogenic edema that exerts mass effect, and are occasionally necrotic. Metastases essentially always enhance; contrast improves metastatic lesion detection and distinction from edema. Multiplicity strongly suggests the diagnosis, although 50% of metastases are singular deposits; indeed, 20% of solitary intra-axial masses are metastases. The clinical scenario often offers the best differentiation from CNS primary malignancy, although the fact that metastatic lesions do not exhibit growth across the corpus callosum provides another method of distinction.

Hemorrhage is classically synonymous with choriocarcinoma, melanoma, and renal cell and thyroid carcinoma, but the higher prevalence of lung and breast cancer means that these latter two malignancies prove to be the most common hemorrhagic metastatic lesions. Hemorrhage can render the typical hypodense appearance hyperdense on CT. Calcification can commonly be seen with metastatic mucinous adenocarcinoma, osteosarcoma, and chondrosarcoma. Increased cellularity, as with small cell, renal cell, and certain intestinal carcinomas, can yield an SI similar to that of gray matter. Melanin content in melanoma appears hyperintense on T1WI and dark on T2WI because of paramagnetic effects.[12] Hemorrhage or lack of melanin results in mixed SI patterns.

Metastases can account for LM, dural, SAS, subependymal, and intraventricular masses, and for nerve-root masses on CNs exiting to the extracranium. In the latter scenario, lymphoma and inflammatory entities must also be entertained as a possible diagnosis. Spectroscopically, metastatic lesions show attenuated NAA and CR–

phosphocreatine peaks, and prominent lipid and lactate, with correlation of larger lesions with lower CHO and greater lipid and lactate.

Evaluating CNS tumors post-surgery is challenging and deserves special mention. Residual tumor can be considered when continued enhancement is seen within the resection site less than 2 days after surgery, provided that preoperative enhancement occurred. Nonetheless, distinction from surgical blood products can be difficult. Without preoperative enhancement, differentiation from postoperative edema can be impossible, rendering growth the only indication of residual tumor. Postoperative granulation tissue enhances after 2 days and can persist for months. Postoperative intraparenchymal or pial enhancement beyond 1 year is abnormal, but nearly all cases exhibit postoperative dural enhancement for up to decades. Absent, mild, focal, or diffuse enhancement is considered normal; nodular dural, pial, or ependymal enhancement is suggestive of recurrent local tumor, LM metastasis, or blooming infection.

Post-RT patients also deserve particular consideration because of the challenge of differentiating residual and recurrent tumor from radionecrosis, given their indistinguishable enhancement patterns. Radionecrosis evolution appears to correlate with total RT dose, fractional dose size, number of fractions, total delivery time, volume treated, patient age, and survival time.

Post-RT manifestations are divided into early (during, or within weeks of, RT) and delayed (more than 4 months post-RT) types. The former type proves transient, appearing as white-matter high SI on T2WI and FLAIR because of imposed edema. Delayed effects are more common and are further subclassified as early (months post-RT) and late (months to years post-RT). The latter is most common, seen in 5 to 15% of irradiated patients. Early delayed injury is also transient, but late delayed effects are often irreversible and either focal or diffuse, affecting white more than gray matter. Within 2 years, 70% of focal delayed, late post-RT findings become manifest.

Focal radiation injury usually appears in the primary tumor site and can hemorrhage focally in the absence of necrosis. Lesions typically exhibit enhancement, edema, hypodensity on CT, and high SI on T2WI, thus mimicking glioma or metastasis. PET might prove useful in suggesting the diagnosis, because, relative to normal brain, tumor exhibits increased activity on ^{18}F fluorodeoxyglucose or ^{11}C-labeled deoxyglucose PET; radionecrosis has decreased activity. Nonetheless, hypometabolic gliomas must be considered. Moreover, correlation between PET and recurrent tumor is poor with intensive RT. The distinction can be made with 85% accuracy, and even higher rates can be achieved with high-grade tumors. PWI might also have utility, because, in contrast to neoplasm, radionecrosis yields decreased rCBV.

Diffuse late injury is typically located in the periventricular region or posterior centrum semiovale and appears as marked demyelination—that is, white-matter decreased density and increased SI on T2WI and proton density–weighted imaging (PDWI). The rate of severe white matter lesions increases with age, volume irradiated, dose, and survival time.[13] Post-RT telangiectasias and cavernomas have also been reported, seen as single or multiple sites of hemosiderin deposition (ie, low SI on T2WI and GEI, with no surrounding edema). RT-induced tumors have been reported and are most often meningiomas and gliomas. Spectroscopically, CHO and CR are attenuated with radionecrosis, and lipid can be elevated.

In the future, preoperative brain tumor evaluation may include genetic screening, because numerous genetic aberrancies have been associated with specific brain tumor lines. For example, 90% of all astrocytomas exhibit inactivation of the *p16* and *RB* (chromosome 13q) genes, which help to control *E2F1* transcription factor, a regulator of the G1 cell cycle. With the advent of molecular imaging, protocols may attempt to use imaging drugs or viruses to image such known suspect genes.

Spinal Cord Spinal cord neoplasms are intramedullary, intradural extramedullary, and extradural in location, each location possessing a particular differential. Overall, spinal cord neoplasms are uncommon, totaling 4 to 10% of all CNS tumors.

MRI with post-contrast images is crucial to the evaluation of suspected lesions in all locations. Neoplasms tend to enhance, to focally or diffusely enlarge the cord, and to give high SI on proton-density imaging (PDI) and T2WI. On CT, neoplasms are characterized by posterior element involvement, partial or absent pre-vertebral soft-tissue swelling, and osteoblastic alterations. Primary and metastatic lesions are both seen. Of the former, astrocytoma and ependymoma are the most common neoplasms; they are impossible to differentiate with imaging.

Astrocytomas represent 40% of cord tumors, typically occur in the cervicothoracic region, usually occupy the full cord diameter, and are occasionally exophytic. Cysts can be seen as low SI on T1WI and PDWI. Enhancement is the norm, but is uneven and less than that seen with ependymomas. Ependymomas represent 50 to 60% of cord tumors in the third to fifth decades of life. They tend to be more focal and well circumscribed, and they occupy the central cord. Central cyst formation with non-enhancing walls can be seen. On T1WI, ependymomas are isointense to cord and exhibit high, heterogeneous SI on T2WI. Hemorrhage is often seen, yielding low SI T2WI rims from the hemosiderin. Location is generally the cervicothoracic region.[14]

Hemangioblastomas can occur in the spinal cord, especially in the cervicothoracic region. Intramedullary metastases typically enlarge the cord, evoke edema, and enhance. Intramedullary or LM metastases are seen in 3% of patients with metastatic disease. On MRI, LM metastases are seen as enhancing nodules that yield an irregular cord margin, although the entire SAS can enhance, and tumor deposits can be present on nerve roots. Pial metastases can give linear cord surface enhancement. On T1WI, CSF can appear abnormally low in SI, giving decreased cord–CSF definition. A parameningeal mass is potentially a presentation of leukemia (chloroma) or a mode of lymphomatous spread, growing through intervertebral foramina.

In terms of extramedullary intradural neoplasms, meningiomas represent 25% of spinal canal neoplasms, with 80% occurring in the thoracic area. Lesions are usually singular, although multiple lesions have been reported. Meningiomas tend to enhance, and on T1WI, they are iso- to hypointense, with heterogeneous texture. Cord compression, calcification, dural tails, and widened neural foramina can be seen. However, widened neural foramina are more common with schwannomas, which are usually solitary, commonly occur in the sensory nerve root sheath, and often exhibit hemorrhage, thrombosis, sinusoidal dilation, and cystic or fatty degeneration. Schwannomas can be purely intradural (two-thirds), partially intra- and extradural (one-sixth), or purely extradural (one-sixth). In contrast, neurofibromas are often multiple and rarely exhibit hemorrhage, vascular aberrations, or fatty change. Schwannomas and neurofibromas both have low SI on T1WI and high SI on T2WI; both enhance; and, when hemorrhagic, both become iso- to hyperintense on T1WI and hypointense on PDI and T2WI. Although bone erosion can occur, calcification is unusual for schwannomas and neurofibromas as compared with meningiomas.

HEAD AND NECK

In contrast to other body locations, evaluation of a mass in the head and neck aerodigestive system focuses less on differential diagnosis and histologic differentiation and more on assessing the most effective therapeutic intervention. In more than 90% of cases, mucosal mass histology is squamous cell carcinoma (SCC). The imaging features of SCC are non-specific on both CT and MRI, such that an adenocarcinoma cannot be distinguished from a SCC. Nonetheless, given the preponderance of SCC, such distinction is rendered moot, and SCC is assumed to be the histologic type, especially given that therapeutic issues are similar regardless of particular histology.

In general, SCC exhibits intermediate SI on post-contrast T1WI and T2WI, plus mild enhancement. On CT, the density is similar to that of muscle, with faint mass enhancement. With both imaging modalities, necrosis can be seen in large masses and in SCC-associated lymphadenopathy. One caveat for head-and-neck imaging is that superficial lesions are still best evaluated by endoscopy; indeed, imaging can fail to detect aberrancies in such locations. In addition, post therapy, especially post RT, recurrences present special challenges to accurate interpretation.

Therapeutic options for SCC include surgery, RT, brachytherapy, and chemotherapy, alone or in various combinations. Certain tumor imaging features, such as cartilage invasion, help to determine which therapy to implement. Accordingly, knowledge of each therapeutic modality's indications and contraindications, which are established based on particular imaging findings, is critical to appropriate imaging interpretation. By adequately describing tumor extent *and* pertinent areas devoid of tumor, clinicians can reach the best-informed treatment decision. Many such decisions are contingent on the site of tumor origin. Moreover, origin site also makes either MRI or CT ideal for diagnostic evaluation. Consequently, the subsections that follow consider specific neoplasm origin sites.

The Nasopharynx MRI is the preferred modality for evaluating patients with nasopharyngeal carcinoma (NPC). Given that surgery is not a primary treatment modality for this tumor site, the most important factors in NPC evaluation are extent of skull base and intracranial involvement.

MRI with contrast appears to be most useful for delineating the 31 to 48% propensity for infiltration along the skull base foramina and nerve roots. In addition, bony skull base involvement appears to be better evaluated with MRI than CT: low SI tumor is seen to replace high SI bone marrow on T1WI. Perineural spread, especially to the pterygopalatine fossa via the maxillary division of CN V, is best visualized with fat-suppressed, contrast-enhanced axial and coronal MRI.

Multiplanar scanning is critical for NPC evaluation because the tumor growth pattern often traverses a superoinferior direction. Multidetector CT with coronal and sagittal reconstructions might represent a reasonable substitute for direct multiplanar MRI. Nonetheless, subtle infiltration of tensor and levator veli palatini musculature is best evaluated with the greater soft-tissue resolution of MRI. Note that 45% of NPCs exhibit retropharyngeal spread and that 80% demonstrate nodal spread.

NPC is T-staged based on the presence of infiltration of the nasal cavity, orbits, and other surrounding cavities and structures. The thin walls of these cavities are better depicted with CT; however, MRI is superior for distinction between neoplasm and obstructed sinus secretions or inflammatory disease. Generally, neoplasm exhibits intermediate SI and solid contrast enhancement; inflammatory disease is bright on T2WI, with typical peripheral mucosal enhancement patterns. Recent studies suggest that tumor volume may better predict radiochemotherapy outcomes than T-staging does.

Sinonasal Cavity For the best evaluation of sinonasal cavity carcinoma (SNC), combined MRI and CT are required. The reasons are the same as those earlier specified for NPC invasion. MRI with contrast best detects perineural invasion along the maxillary division of CN V, which is seen as neural enlargement with enhancement.[15] SNC meningeal infiltration is also best evaluated with contrast-enhanced MRI, wherein dural enhancement greater than 5 mm in thickness, focal dural nodularity, and pial enhancement are suggestive of neoplastic infiltration. In contrast, thin, linear dural enhancement typically represents a reactive phenomenon to adjacent tumor. Obviously, meningeal disease and infiltration into the intracranial compartment require not only head-and-neck, but also craniofacial surgery.

Because tumors often obstruct the ostia of sinuses, inflammatory disease is typically seen superimposed on neoplasm. The two can be differentiated 95% of the time by the intermediate SI of SNC on T2WI. Benign inflammation tends to be hyperintense. Inflammatory manifestations run the gamut from mere obstructed secretions to mucoceles with sinus enlargement. Chronic sinusitis represents a known risk factor for SNC. In addition, inverted papilloma, a benign neoplasm, has a 6 to 27% coincidental rate of SCC.

The bony destruction that characterizes SNC in up to 80% of cases can be distinguished from that of benign etiologies better on thin-section CT than on MRI.[16] Malignancies tend to completely destroy bony walls, exhibiting marginal irregularity; polyps, mucoceles, and other benign inflammatory conditions usually remodel, thin, and expand bone. Such findings also hold true at the anterior cranial fossa, where benign lesions such as sinonasal polyposis and inverted papilloma can elicit a bony appearance that suggests infiltration more aggressive than is histologically present.

Oral Cavity Oral-cavity carcinoma (OCC) can be evaluated equally well with CT and MRI. Overall, the accuracy of CT staging is 81 to 94%. The shortcomings—for example, inability to evaluate periosteum, and difficulty in distinguishing inflammation and neoplastic bone infiltration—apply in both modalities.

One of the most critical factors in therapeutic decision-making for OCC is the degree of involvement of the mandible or maxilla. With periosteal involvement, most surgeons resect a periosteal margin to ensure complete tumor removal. If the cortex is focally involved without marrow infiltration, a segmental resection of a mandibular portion can be performed with primary closure using plates. With bone-marrow infiltration or extensive cortical involvement, a segmental resection of the mandible with wide margins is likely required, which obviously necessitates bone grafting for the surgical defect.

Unfortunately, imaging cannot detect periosteal involvement; however, the periosteum can be biopsied. Extensive preparation is a requisite for permanent sections; mandibular cortex and marrow cannot be intraoperatively biopsied for frozen sections. Consequently, surgeons rely on preoperative evaluation to determine whether to remove mandibular segments. Furthermore, bone biopsies in the exposed, non-sterile environment of the mouth can lead to secondary osteomyelitis. CT best demonstrates bony erosion. Other findings that suggest neoplastic mandibular infiltration include abnormal bone-marrow density, pathologic fracture, and aggressive periosteal reaction. In nearly all instances, neoplastic erosion is lytic; however, sclerotic margins can be present, especially with prior RT. Bone erosion contraindicates wide local excision, necessitating resection with either a partial mandibulectomy or maxillectomy; the amount of bone erosion also influences the type of surgical resection. MRI best demonstrates soft-tissue infiltration of the dark SI of mandibular or maxillary cortex; replacement of bright marrow by intermediate SI tumor on T1WI; and contrast enhancement in bone or contrast enhancement of nerves traversing the mandible, especially the inferior alveolar nerve. Observance on either CT or MRI of simultaneous tumor on both sides of the mandible implies infiltration.

Evaluation of the mandible or maxilla proves difficult when dental amalgam lies adjacent to suspected neoplasm. In such cases, CT metallic spray artifact and MRI susceptibility artifact can result in obscuration of tumor margin. Additionally, tumor at tooth roots (eg, alveolar ridge malignancies) is difficult to evaluate because of subtle infiltration, frequent association with carious odontogenic disease infiltrating bone, and frequent extraction of the offending tooth, leading to bony reactive changes. It is also important to note that osteoradionecrosis, radiation fibrosis, and osteomyelitis secondary to dental caries can simulate neoplastic infiltration.

Besides mandible and maxilla, the other element particularly scrutinized during OCC evaluation is infiltration of the retromolar triangle region, with subsequent complex spread patterns, such as to the pterygopalatine fossa or pterygomandibular raphe. Bilateral tongue infiltration across the midline is also of therapeutic consideration, because a total glossectomy proves essential for surgical cure in such scenarios. In most instances, patients elect an RT–chemotherapy combination, with consequent tracheostomy because of lack of airway protection, rather than undergo total glossectomy. Floor-of-mouth neoplasm often leads to obstruction or infiltration of submandibular gland ducts. Ductal enlargement with sialadenitis—seen as abnormal submandibular gland enlargement, enhancement, density, or SI—can be observed with OCC. Metachronous and synchronous OCC are seen 40% of the time, and nodal spread is apparent 30% of the time, at presentation.

The Oropharynx In oropharyngeal carcinoma (OPC), the overall staging accuracies of CT and MRI are 96% and 70 to 86% respectively. Most OPC involves the base of the tongue or tonsils. The tonsils are an especially frequent site of SCC and often are associated with bilateral lymphadenopathy. Tonsillar carcinoma can also spread to the soft palate, nasopharynx, parapharyngeal tissue, and (occasionally) the base of the tongue, subsequently infiltrating into the mandible when advanced. Overall, OPC nodal spread is seen in 65% of OPC patients at presentation.

Obviously, the same issues concerning the mandible require consideration in evaluating OPC.

Moreover, because of associated lymphadenopathy and the earlier-described issues concerning total glossectomy, bilaterality also remains a very important aspect for OPC. OPC is also prone to infiltrate pre-epiglottic fat, a quadrangular area best seen on sagittal images. CT and MRI sensitivities for pre-epiglottic invasion are both 100%; specificities are 93% and 84 to 90% respectively. MRI accuracy for pre-epiglottic fat infiltration has been reported to be 90%. Because fat is very bright on T1WI, low-SI tumor infiltrating pre-epiglottic fat from the vallecula or tongue base can be appreciated with relative ease on MRI. Pre-epiglottic fat infiltration implies supraglottic larynx involvement and, accordingly, often requires a horizontal or limited supraglottic laryngectomy. Extension into the epiglottis or epiglottic petiole also requires laryngeal surgery in addition to attention to the oropharyngeal process. The extent of pre-epiglottic fat infiltration can influence the possibility for voice-conserving surgery.

The Larynx A number of manuscripts have demonstrated that the volume of laryngeal SCC (LC) predicts the success or failure of primary RT. For instance, one study found that, for treatment with RT alone, a supraglottic tumor volume less than 6 cm^3 had an 89% likelihood of local control, while a tumor volume greater than 6 cm^3 had only a 52% chance of primary site control.[17] Accordingly, measuring the LC dimensions or using a tumor volumetric algorithm or definition is important. For CT, 1 mm-thick sections through the lesion typically afford the most accurate volumetric measurement. LC volume predicts not only the potential for RT to cure the lesion, but also prognosis.

Because tumors that cross glottic boundaries portend worse prognoses, the supero-inferior LC location relative to the supraglottis, glottis, and subglottis remains an important concern. That location is best appreciated on coronal T1WI, although reconstructive coronal imaging might represent an adequate alternative. The supero-inferior LC extent also determines the surgical technique implemented for tumor extraction. Tumors limited to the supraglottis—that is, those with no exolaryngeal or transglottic spread—that exhibit no cartilage invasion and only limited pre-epiglottic fat infiltration can be treated with a standard supraglottic laryngectomy, whereby the resection plane lies in the laryngeal ventricle. Supraglottic tumors with glottic involvement limited to the true vocal cord, with only minimal thyroid cartilage invasion and no arytenoid cartilage infiltration, can be treated with a voice-sparing supracricoid laryngectomy. Tumors with extension greater than 5 mm; with more than minimal thyroid, cricoid, or arytenoid cartilage infiltration; or with bulky supraglottic disease require total laryngectomy.

In nearly all institutions, LC cartilaginous invasion remains a contraindication to RT, because of concomitant radionecrosis predisposition. RT seldom cures tumors with cartilaginous invasion, even with only early invasion. Accordingly, detection of thyroid, arytenoid, or cricoid cartilage invasion is critical in LC evaluation. Although overall TNM staging accuracy appears better for CT than for MRI (ie, 73 to 95% versus 85%), the cumulative impression is that MRI is more sensitive than CT for detection of laryngeal cartilage invasion. CT, although less sensitive, possesses more specificity than MRI. On MRI, cartilage invasion is seen as replacement of either low-SI cartilage with higher SI tissue on T2WI, or high-SI T1 marrow with low-SI tissue, plus cartilaginous enhancement on post-contrast T1WI. MRI false-positive cases are likely secondary to inflammatory cartilaginous change induced by adjacent tumor. On CT, cartilaginous lysis, erosion, and circumferential tumor must be identified; whether sclerosis should also be included in that list remains debatable. Nonetheless, one study found that glottic tumor volumes of more than 3.5 cm^3, with no or only single laryngeal cartilage sclerosis, had a 90% chance of local control with RT alone.[18] A tumor volume of less than 3.5 cm^3 with sclerosis of two laryngeal cartilages, or of more than 3.5 cm^3 with no or single cartilage sclerosis, had a 40 to 50% rate of control. A tumor volume greater than 3.5 cm^3, with combined sclerosis of ipsilateral arytenoid and adjacent cricoid cartilage had a less than 20% rate of control. In up to 50% of cases, inflammatory change attributable to proximal tumor might also account for sclerotic cartilage seen on CT that fails to prove positive for tumor.

Periglottic spread into fat deep to laryngeal mucosa is another area in which MRI is more sensitive than CT, leading to better overall tumor delineation. Although no relationship exists between pre-epiglottic space involvement and local control, the likelihood of maintaining a functional larynx after RT is significantly higher with tumors invading less than 25% of the pre-epiglottic space than with more extensive tumors.

LYMPHADENOPATHY

Neck-node palpation is widely accepted as an insufficient examination, with sensitivities and specificities in approximately the 60 to 70% range. CT, MRI, and ultrasonography for lymph node (LN) assessment all have their proponents, and sensitivities and specificities for LN examination in the N0 neck vary widely. Generally, CT or MRI finds 40 to 60% of occult metastases in an N0 neck, with 25 to 35% proving to be false positives. Because the consensus appears to be to treat a neck with a 20% or greater risk for occult metastases, early detection of metastatic disease clearly becomes essential. The most recent Radiology Diagnostic Oncology Group study of LN assessment revealed that CT might be more reliable and accurate than MRI for predicting LN neoplastic invasion.[19] Even so, the ability of CT to exclude LN neoplastic infiltration was poor, reaching a negative predictive value of only 90%, with a criterion of 5 mm for the maximum transverse LN diameter; the associated positive predictive value was 44%. MRI was unable to obtain a 90% negative predictive value by any size criterion. Yousem and colleagues later demonstrated that central LN necrosis and extracapsular spread was better demonstrated with CT than with MRI, with accuracies of 90% and 78% respectively.[20]

The general consensus appears to be that CT best demonstrates LN necrosis, which represents a reliable criterion for metastatic disease. But, regardless of modality in this situation, contrast is required, as is excellent fat suppression in the case of MRI. Unfortunately, imaging does not detect extracapsular spread, which has been pathologically documented to be relatively high once LNs are larger than 2 cm—that is, 53% for LNs 2 cm to 3 cm and 74% for LNs larger than 3 cm, as compared with 23% for LNs smaller than 1 cm.

More institutions are using PET to identify pathologic lymphadenopathy, both before and after therapy—especially because PET has been reported to yield results superior to CT and MRI for detection of LNs harboring metastatic disease. Combining CT with PET allows accurate localization and more exact definition of disease extent.

PET, with or without CT, has also proved valuable in detecting carcinomas with unknown primary origin. In instances in which a neoplasm-laden LN is identified and conventional imaging, endoscopy, and clinical evaluation have failed to detect a primary tumor, PET can elucidate 25 to 50% of primary malignancies. Often the lesions reside in the nasopharynx, a tonsil, the pyriform sinus apex, or the tongue base. However, certain upper thoracic and breast carcinomas can account for lesions in such situations. The extent to which PET should be used for primary evaluation of all head and neck SCCs remains to be determined. Currently, PET is primarily used for detection of residual recurrent disease after surgery, RT, or chemotherapy.

For routine LN evaluation, most institutions suspect pathology for LNs with a maximum transverse diameter in excess of 10 mm, although 6 to 7 mm has been recommended. Using a 10 mm criterion, coupled with the presence of central nodal necrosis or rounded LN morphology, imaging can achieve an overall accuracy of approximately 75% for identifying neoplastic LNs. Nonetheless, microscopic LN infiltration remains a shortcoming of head-and-neck imaging, proving to be present in 20 to 30% of cases despite negative results on imaging.

EXTRAMUCOSAL MASSES

Extramucosal head-and-neck spaces are grossly partitioned into masticator, parotid, carotid, parapharyngeal, retropharyngeal, and prevertebral spaces. For evaluation of masses in such territories, MRI is generally preferred because of its superior soft-tissue discrimination, lack of ionizing radiation, and more-acceptable contrast-agent risk profile. Moreover, the multiplanar capability of MRI proves useful for evaluating lesions in such regions.

In 80% of cases, extramucosal head-and-neck inflammatory lesions and benign neoplasms are hyperintense on T2WI, and malignancies are intermediate to dark. Exceptions include benign processes such as chronic sialadenitises; Warthin tumors; fungal disease; microbacterial infections; fibromatous lesions; some schwannomas; approximately 30% of parathyroid adenomas; chronic sinusitis, with secretions of greater than 25% protein concentration; and chronically inspissated sinonasal secretions—all of which can be hypointense to intermediate in SI on T2WI.[21] Similarly, certain malignancies such as lymphoma, adenoid cystic carcinoma, low-grade mucoepidermoid carcinoma, synovial sarcoma, and rhabdomyosarcoma can be relatively bright on T2WI.

Using MRI, specific histologic diagnosis of extramucosal space lesions can be made, including such hypervascular lesions as juvenile angiofibromas, hemangiomas, and paragangliomas, which may show flow voids suggestive of their highly vascular nature. Head-and-neck cystic lesions such as branchial cleft, thyroglossal duct, dermoid cyst, ranula, and lymphangioma can also be reasonably easy to detect and characterize based on location and density or SI characteristics. Similarly, lipomas and other fat-containing lesions suggestive of a benign etiology can be readily detected by MRI and CT.

Sarcomas of the head and neck can exhibit variable, heterogeneous density, SI, and enhancement characteristics. Necrosis can be present in such lesions, rendering specific characterization difficult. Chondroid and osseous lesions are better distinguished with CT than with MRI, but combination of the two to examine tumor cartilage caps might help to distinguish benign from malignant lesions.[22]

CONCLUSION

Imaging plays an integral role in the team approach to managing patients suffering from CNS and head-and-neck malignancies. Essential information regarding staging and tumor extent is gained, and that information affects surgical approach, contraindicates particular treatment modalities, and permits monitoring for treatment outcome and recurrence. The future is apt to bring many more developments and innovations in radiology to further improve care for CNS and head-and-neck cancer patients.

REFERENCES

1. Grossman RI, Yousem DM. Neuroradiology: the requisites. 2nd ed. St. Louis, MO: Mosby; 2003.
2. Gao PY, Osborn AG, Smirniotopoulos JG, et al. Radiologic–pathologic correlation. Epidermoid tumor of the cerebellopontine angle. AJNR Am J Neuroradiol 1992;13:863–72.
3. Chang KH, Song IC, Kim SH, et al. In vivo single-voxel proton MR spectroscopy in intracranial cystic masses. AJNR Am J Neuroradiol 1998;19:401–5.
4. Anderson DR, Falcone S, Bruce JH, et al. Radiologic–pathologic correlation. Congenital choroid plexus papillomas. AJNR Am J Neuroradiol 1995;16:2072–6.
5. Wang Z, Sutton LN, Cnaan A, et al. Proton MR spectroscopy of pediatric cerebellar tumors. AJNR Am J Neuroradiol 1995;16:1821–33.
6. Kim YJ, Chang KH, Song IC, et al. Brain abscess and necrotic or cystic brain tumor. Discrimination with signal intensity on diffusion-weighted MR imaging. AJR Am J Roentgenol 1998;171:1487–90.
7. Kane AG, Robles HA, Smirniotopoulos JG, et al. Radiologic–pathologic correlation. Diffuse pontine astrocytoma. AJNR Am J Neuroradiol 1993;14:941–5.
8. Lee YY, Van Tassel P. Intracranial oligodendrogliomas. Imaging findings in 35 untreated cases. AJR Am J Roentgenol 1989b;152:361–9.
9. Ostertun B, Wolf HK, Campos MG, et al. Dysembryoplastic neuroepithelial tumors. MR and CT evaluation. AJNR Am J Neuroradiol 1996;17:419–30.
10. Ho VB, Smirniotopoulos JG, Murphy FM, et al. Radiologic–pathologic correlation. Hemangioblastoma. AJNR Am J Neuroradiol 1992;13:1343–52.
11. Dina TS. Primary central nervous system lymphoma versus toxoplasmosis in AIDS. Radiology 1991;179:823–8.
12. Atlas SW, Braffman BH, LoBrutto R, et al. Human malignant melanomas with varying degrees of melanin content in nude mice. MR imaging, histopathology, and electron paramagnetic resonance. J Comput Assist Tomogr 1990;14:547–54.
13. Tsuruda JS, Kortman KE, Bradley WG, et al. Radiation effects on cerebral white matter. MR evaluation. AJR Am J Roentgenol 1987;149:165–71.
14. McCormick PC, Torres R, Post KD, et al. Intramedullary ependymoma of the spinal cord. J Neurosurg 1990;72:523–32.
15. Curtin HD, Williams R, Johnson J. CT of perineural tumor extension. Pterygopalatine fossa. AJR Am J Roentgenol 1985;144:163–9.
16. Hudgins PA. Sinonasal imaging. Neuroimaging Clin N Am 1996;6:319–31.
17. Mancuso AA, Mukherji SK, Mendenhall WM, et al. Value of pre-treatment CT as a predictor of outcome in supraglottic cancer treated with radiation therapy alone [abstract]. Radiology 1994;193P:262.
18. Pameijer FA, Mancuso AA, Mendenhall WM, et al. Can pretreatment computed tomography predict local control in T3 squamous cell carcinoma of the glottic larynx treated with definitive radiotherapy? Int J Radiat Oncol Biol Phys 1997;37:1011–21.
19. Curtin HD, Ishwaran H, Mancuso AA, et al. Comparison of CT and MR imaging in staging of neck metastases. Radiology 1998;207:123–30.
20. Yousem DM, Som PM, Hackney DB, et al. Central nodal necrosis and extracapsular neoplastic spread in cervical lymph nodes. MR imaging versus CT. Radiology 1992;182:753–9.
21. Dillon WP, Som PM, Fullerton GD. Hypointense MR signal in chronically inspissated sinonasal secretions. Radiology 1990;174:73–8.
22. Russell EJ, Levy JM, Breit R, et al. Osteocartilaginous tumors in the parapharyngeal space arising from bone exostoses. AJNR Am J Neuroradiol 1990;11:993–7.

Imaging Neoplasms of the Thorax

Jeremy J. Erasmus, MD
Mylene T. Truong, MD
H. Page McAdams, MD

Thoracic imaging is important in the management of patients with lung cancer, mediastinal neoplasms, and malignant pleural mesothelioma. In these patients, imaging is used to determine the anatomic extent of disease and appropriate therapeutic management. This chapter reviews the use of conventional anatomic imaging and newer thoracic imaging techniques such as positron emission tomography (PET) in staging, assessing treatment response, and monitoring for tumor recurrence after treatment of lung cancer, mediastinal neoplasms, and malignant pleural mesothelioma.

LUNG CANCER

STAGING **Nonsmall-Cell Lung Cancer** Because most patients with lung cancer have advanced disease at presentation, diagnosis is usually not difficult. However, treatment and prognosis, which both depend on the anatomic extent of disease, can be more difficult to determine. Comprehensive patient evaluation, including imaging, is usually performed to define disease extent in patients with nonsmall-cell lung cancer (NSCLC).

The International System for Staging Lung Cancer describes the anatomic extent of disease in a traditional TNM system that enables a standardized description of NSCLC in terms of the primary tumor (T), lymph nodes (N), and metastases (M).[1] The primary tumor is described according to its size, location, and extent of local invasion. Computed tomography (CT) is more accurate than chest radiographs in assessing these parameters, and CT is typically used to evaluate patients after initial diagnosis. More recently, use of whole-body PET imaging with [^{18}F] fluoro-2-deoxy-D-glucose (FDG-PET) has been increasing in NSCLC staging.[2–5] Currently, FDG-PET imaging is usually combined with CT, because the relatively poor spatial resolution of PET imaging limits its utility in the evaluation of the primary tumor and in the determination of the precise anatomic location of regions of increased focal FDG uptake. Integrated CT-PET scanners that can acquire co-registered, spatially matched functional and morphologic data overcome the limitations inherent in both modalities when used separately. In fact, staging of NSCLC has been reported to be more accurate with integrated CT-PET than with the use of visual correlation of PET and CT images acquired separately.[2,6]

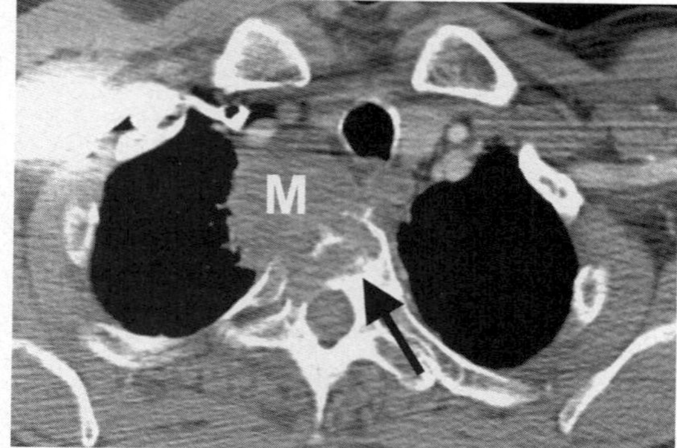

Figure 32c-1 Nonsmall-cell lung cancer and vertebral body invasion. Computed tomograph of chest shows mass (M) in the right upper lobe with destruction (*black arrow*) of the adjacent vertebral body.

In terms of the primary tumor, CT and magnetic resonance imaging (MRI) are both useful in confirming gross chest wall (Figure 32c-1) or mediastinal invasion, but are inaccurate in differentiating between anatomic contiguity and subtle invasion.[7–10] MRI can be a useful adjunct to CT in showing the extent of great vessel, pericardial, or cardiac involvement, particularly if there is a contraindication to the intravenous administration of iodinated contrast. Additionally, because of its superior soft-tissue contrast resolution and multiplanar ability, MRI is particularly useful in the evaluation of patients with superior sulcus tumors (Figure 32c-2).[11–13]

The presence of nodal metastases and their location are important in determining management and prognosis for patients with NSCLC.[1,14] Size is the only criterion used to diagnose nodal metastases, with nodes greater than 10 mm in the short-axis diameter considered abnormal.[15] Chest radiographs are not sensitive or specific in evaluating nodal metastases (Figure 32c-3). CT and MRI are better in this regard, but because enlarged nodes can be hyperplastic and small nodes can contain metastases, the accuracy of CT and MRI in the detection of metastases to hilar and mediastinal nodes is not optimal.[11,16,17] FDG-PET imaging can be used to improve the detection of nodal metastases (Figure 32c-4).[18–20] In this regard, integrated CT-PET, as compared with CT and with CT and PET interpreted separately, has the highest accuracy of regional lymph node staging (sensitivity: 89%; specificity: 94%; positive predictive value: 89%; negative predictive value: 94%; accuracy: 93%).[6] Current recommendations state that FDG-PET imaging should be performed in patients with no CT findings of nodal metastatic disease to corroborate the CT findings when no distant metastasis (M0) are found or to redirect nodal sampling by identifying an otherwise undetected site of metastasis.

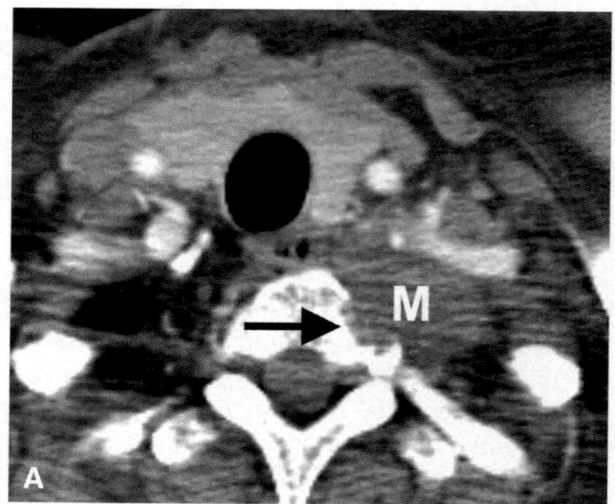

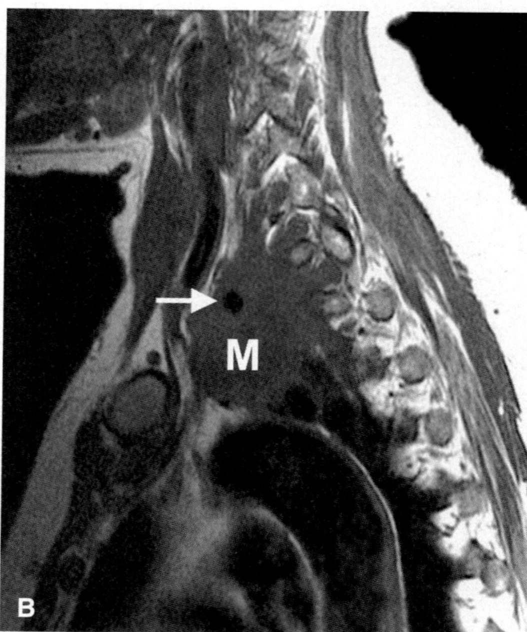

Figure 32c-2 Superior sulcus tumor with invasion of the chest wall and brachial plexus. **A,** Computed tomograph of chest shows mass (M) in the apex of the left hemithorax with focal destruction (*black arrow*) of the adjacent vertebral body. **B,** Sagittal T_1-weighted magnetic resonance image shows mass in the apex of the left hemithorax with encasement of the left subclavian artery (*white arrow*) and C8, T1, and T2 roots of the brachial plexus. Note that the tumor extends to the intervertebral neural foramina.

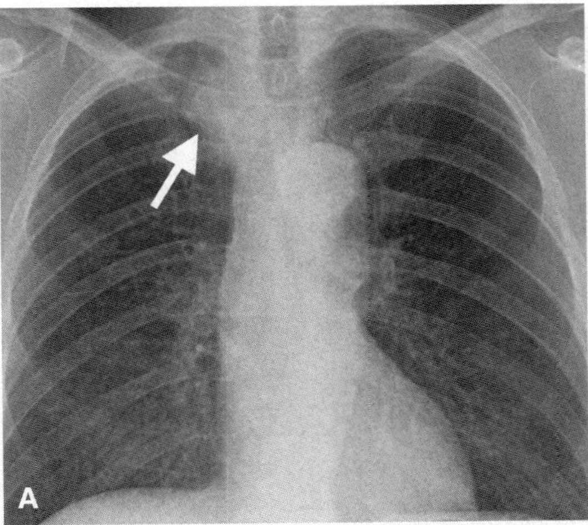

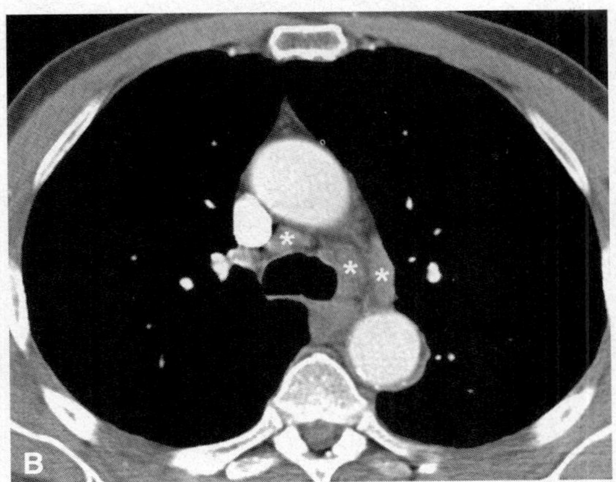

Figure 32c-3 Nonsmall-cell lung cancer with nodal metastases. **A,** Posteroanterior chest radiograph shows poorly marginated mass (*arrow*) in the right upper lobe. Hilar and mediastinal contours are normal without findings of adenopathy. **B,** Computed tomograph of chest shows 12- to 18-mm paratracheal and aortopulmonary window nodes (*asterisks*). Mediastinoscopy confirmed metastatic disease.

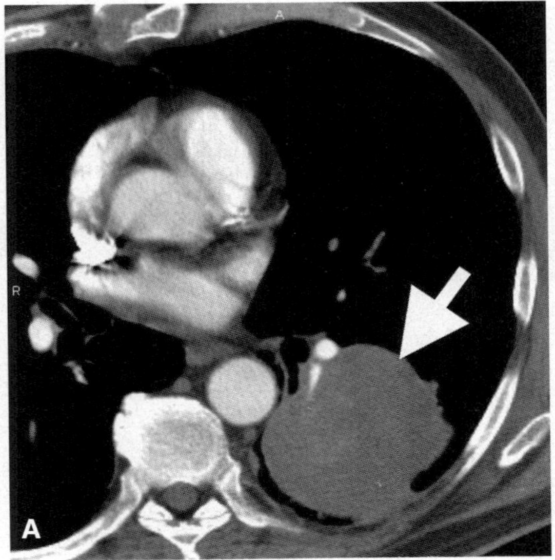

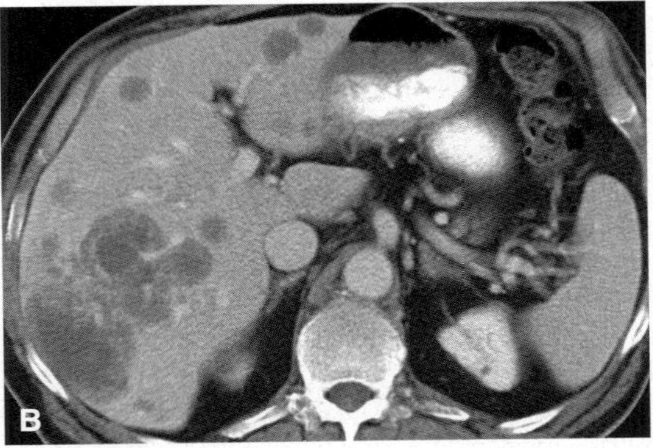

Figure 32c-5 Nonsmall-cell lung cancer and liver metastases. **A,** Computed tomograph of chest shows mass (*arrow*) in left lower lobe. **B,** Computed tomograph of the abdomen reveals numerous low-attenuation lesions within the liver, with peripheral contrast enhancement. Biochemical parameters of liver function were normal. Biopsy confirmed metastatic disease.

Although patients with NSCLC commonly have metastases to the adrenal glands, kidneys, liver, brain, bones, and lymph nodes at presentation, the role of imaging in the detection of these metastases is not clearly defined. Because the combination of normal findings from a clinical examination and laboratory tests has a negative predictive value greater than 95% for extrathoracic metastatic disease, it has been suggested that routine radiologic evaluation for occult extrathoracic metastasis may not be required.[21,22] However, routine imaging of the abdomen is still performed in most patients with NSCLC because clinical and laboratory findings are unreliable in the detection of adrenal, renal, hepatic, and abdominal nodal metastases (Figure 32c-5). In this regard, CT is the primary modality used to diagnose and characterize intra-abdominal lesions, and a confident diagnosis of benignity or malignancy is frequently possible. For instance, if an adrenal mass contains fat or has an attenuation value of less than 10 Hounsfield units (HU) on a noncontrast CT scan, the mass can be considered benign without the need for FDG-PET imaging, MRI, or biopsy.[23,24] Routine CT or MRI of the central nervous system has also been advocated, because up to 18% of patients with NSCLC have brain metastases at presentation.[25] However, brain metastases are usually associated with neurologic signs and symptoms, and if the patient is asymptomatic, imaging of the brain is frequently not performed.[21,26] Similarly, imaging rarely reveals occult skeletal metastases, and therefore bone radiographs, ^{99m}Tc-labeled methylene diphosphonate bone scintigraphy, and MRI are usually performed only if the patient has focal bone pain or an elevated alkaline phosphatase level.[21,27,28]

Because staging of NSCLC performed on the basis of symptoms, laboratory findings, and conventional radiologic imaging can be inaccurate, whole-body imaging with FDG-PET is being used to improve the accuracy of staging (Figure 32c-6). FDG-PET has a higher sensitivity and specificity than does CT in detecting metastases to the adrenal glands, bones, and extrathoracic lymph nodes. Whole-body PET imaging stages intra- and extrathoracic disease in a single study and detects occult extrathoracic metastases in up to 24% of patients selected for curative resection.[4,5,29] It is important to note that the incidence of detection of occult metastases has been reported to increase as the T and N staging descriptors increase (ie, 7.5% in early-stage disease to 24% in advanced disease).[30] In this regard, a recent randomized controlled trial of the role of PET in early-stage lung cancer (more than 90% of patients with T1–2N0) showed that dis-

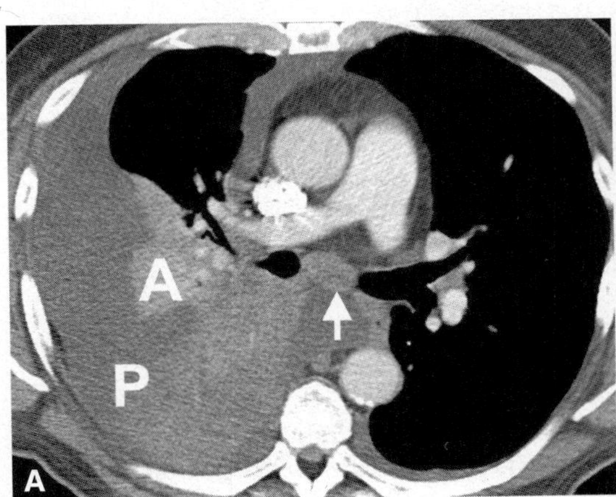

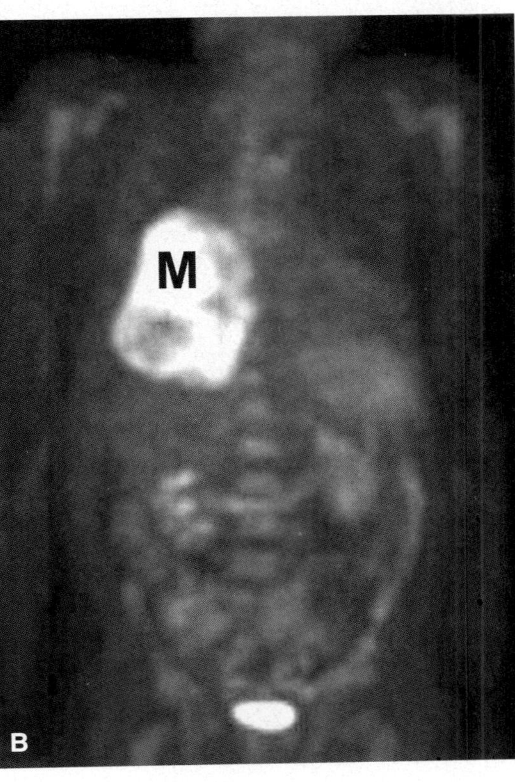

Figure 32c-4 Nonsmall-cell lung cancer and intrathoracic adenopathy. **A,** Computed tomograph of chest shows complex pleuroparenchymal abnormality in the right hemithorax caused by pleural effusion (P), atelectasis (A), obstructive consolidation, and mass. Note the enlarged subcarinal lymph node (*arrow*). **B,** Whole-body coronal positron emission tomography with ^{18}F fluoro-2-deoxy-D-glucose (FDG) shows increased FDG uptake within the mass (M) and adjacent lung. Note absence of hypermetabolism in the region of enlarged subcarinal adenopathy consistent with reactive hyperplasia.

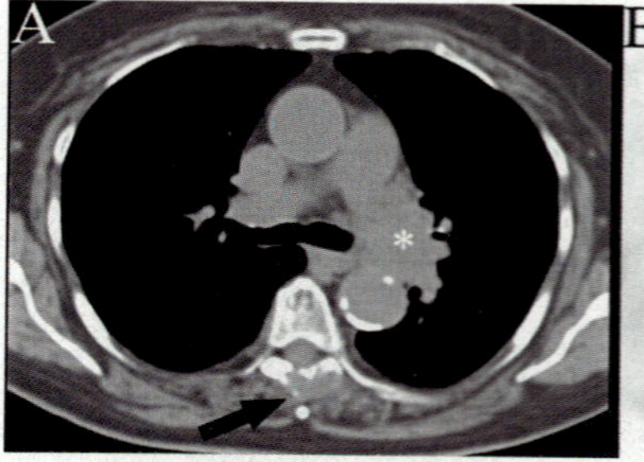

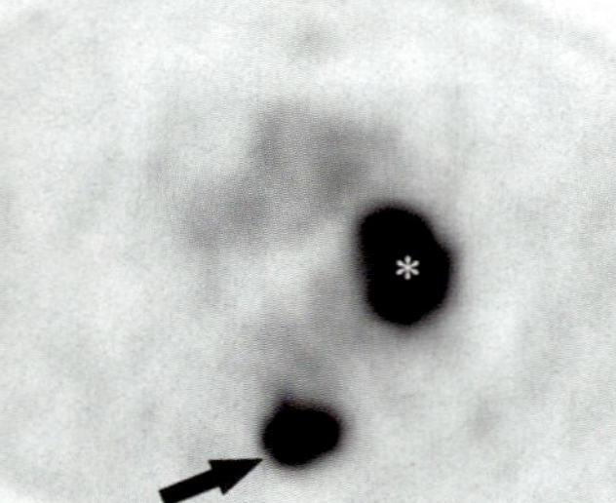

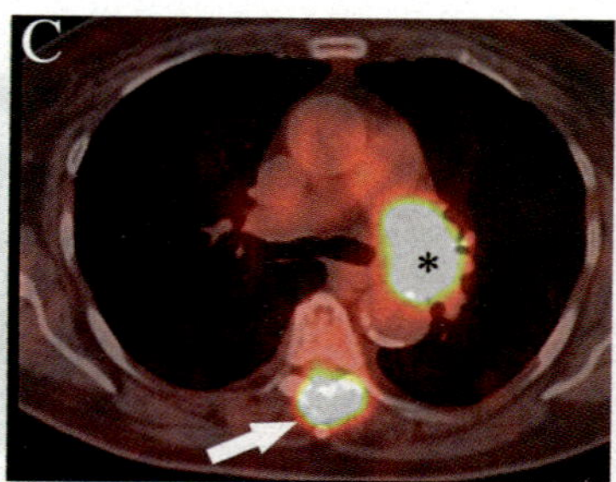

Figure 32c-6 Nonsmall-cell lung cancer in a patient being assessed for surgical resection. **A,** Axial computed tomography (CT) , **B,** positron emission tomography (PET), and **C,** integrated CT-PET show diffuse uptake of ^{18}F fluoro-2-deoxy-D-glucose (FDG) in primary lung malignancy (*asterisks*) and in lytic thoracic vertebral lesion (*arrows*). Patient was asymptomatic. Aspiration biopsy was positive for metastasis.

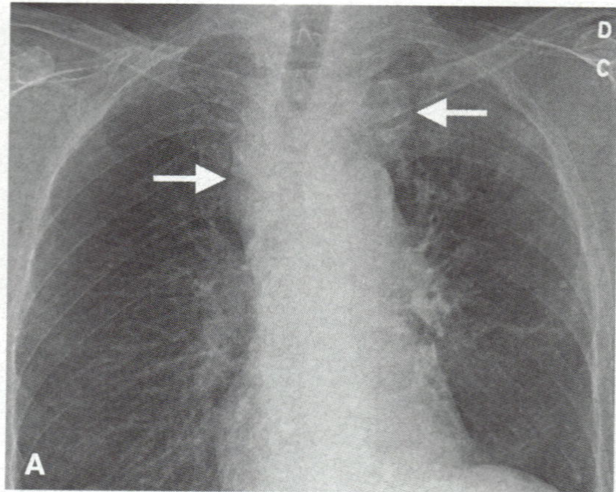

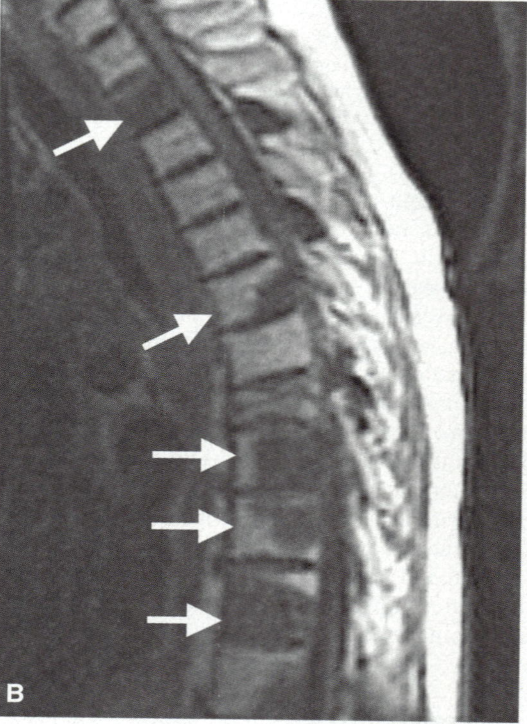

Figure 32c-7 Extensive small-cell lung cancer manifesting as intrathoracic adenopathy and bone metastases. **A,** Posteroanterior chest radiograph shows mediastinal contour abnormality (*arrows*). Computed tomograph (not shown) confirmed mediastinal adenopathy. **B,** Sagittal T_1-weighted magnetic resonance image of the thoracic spine shows decreased signal in numerous vertebral bodies (*arrows*) consistent with metastases.

tant metastases were rarely detected (< 2.5%), although PET improved the accuracy of staging and led to more stage-specific therapy.[31] Two studies with a higher proportion of more advanced lung cancers considered resectable by standard clinical staging showed that PET imaging prevented nontherapeutic surgery in 1 in 5 patients.[4,5]

Small-Cell Lung Cancer Small-cell lung cancer (SCLC) is generally staged as limited disease (malignancy confined to a hemithorax and regional lymph nodes) or extensive disease (malignancy with noncontiguous metastases to the contralateral lung or distant metastases).[32] Most patients with SCLC have extensive disease at presentation. Common sites of metastatic disease include liver, bones, bone marrow, brain, and retroperitoneal lymph nodes (Figure 32c-7).[33]

No consensus has emerged regarding the imaging studies and invasive procedures that should be performed in a staging evaluation of SCLC, but evaluation for extrathoracic metastatic disease is usually directed at the common sites of metastases. SCLC differs from NSCLC in that central nervous system metastases are common at presentation,[32,34] and, because most of the patients are asymptomatic, CT or MRI of the brain is often routinely performed.[35] Similarly, routine CT or MRI of the abdomen is performed because metastases to the liver and abdominal nodes are common at presentation, and the patients are often asymptomatic.[32,34] Although patients with SCLC who have bone and bone marrow metastases are also often asymptomatic and frequently have normal blood alkaline phosphatase levels, isolated bone and bone marrow metastases are uncommon.[32,34,36,37] Consequently, ^{99m}Tc-labeled methylene diphosphonate bone scintigraphy and MRI are usually performed only if the patient has other findings of extensive disease. Whole-body FDG-PET imaging has been suggested to possibly be useful in improving and simplifying the staging of SCLC.[38]

Assessing Treatment Response The antitumor effect of a treatment in patients with solid tumors can be determined by clinical or biochemical evaluation (or both), by surgical pathologic restaging, or by serial measurements of tumor size on radiologic images. Tumors are usually measured on chest radiographs or CT images; treatment response, largely decided using a single measurement of the largest tumor diameter, is determined using uniform criteria known as the Response Evaluation Criteria in Solid Tumors (RECIST).[39] Because marked inconsistency can exist in the measurement of lung lesions from radiographs and CT images, the suggestion has been made that measurement of tumor volume may allow an earlier and more accurate assessment of tumor response.[40–42] The accurate assessment of treatment response is further complicated by the recent development of treatment regimens in which the antitumor effect is cytostatic and a reduction in tumor size as a manifestation of treatment response is unlikely. Accurate determination of response may thus require functional and molecular techniques that assess metabolism, growth kinetics, angiogenesis growth factors, tumor cell markers, and in vivo genetic and gene expression alterations.[43] In this regard, PET is a clinically available method that is sensitive and specific for studying molecular interactions in vivo. FDG uptake, increased in most malignant tumors, can be measured using PET, and such measurement may provide an early and sensitive assessment of the antitumor effect of anticancer chemotherapy.[44–46] This early prediction of tumor response during first-line chemotherapy would allow patients with nonresponding tumors to receive second-line or alternative treatment early in the course of therapy. In a recent study evaluating the ability of FDG-PET to predict response to chemotherapy in patients with advanced NSCLC, the reduction of metabolic activity after one cycle of chemotherapy correlated closely with final outcome of therapy.[46] Furthermore, PET may have an important role in guiding patient care after surgery or radiation therapy, because it is more accurate than conventional studies in detecting recurrent tumor.[47,48]

MEDIASTINAL MASSES

Mediastinal tumors comprise a diverse group of abnormalities including congenital, inflammatory, and neoplastic lesions. To assist in diagnosis and management, these masses are usually imaged with CT or MRI, and are described according to the site of origin and location in the mediastinum. Although CT provides the requisite information in most patients with mediastinal abnormalities, MRI, because of its multiplanar capability, is especially useful in the evaluation of the diaphragm and anatomically complex regions such as the aortopulmonary window. Contrast resolution with MRI is superior to that with CT, and thus MRI can be useful in delineating mediastinal anatomy and demonstrating vascular structures without contrast enhancement (Figure 32c-8). MRI is also the preferred modality for evaluating neurogenic tumors within the mediastinum because it may simultaneously assess (1) intraspinal extension, (2) spinal-

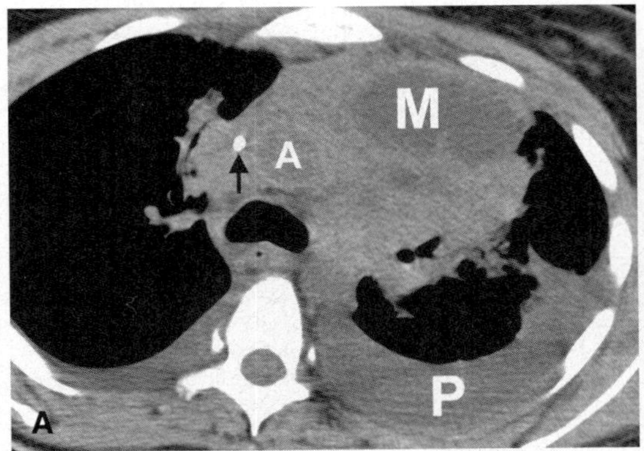

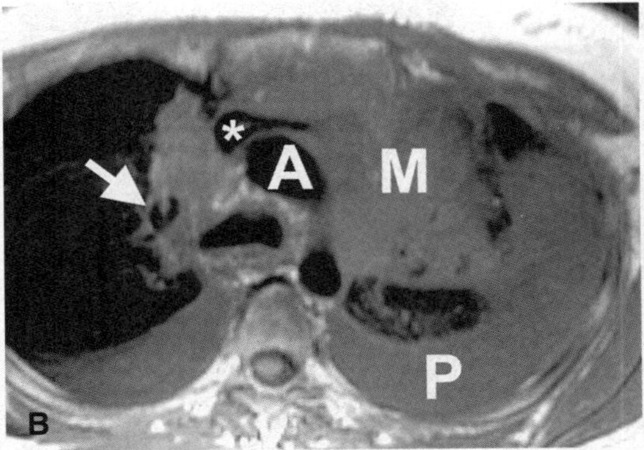

Figure 32c-8 Hodgkin's lymphoma in a patient with clinical findings suggestive of obstruction of the superior vena cava (SVC). Patient was allergic to iodinated contrast. **A,** Noncontrast computed tomograph shows diffuse heterogeneous anterior mediastinal mass (M) and bilateral pleural effusions (P). Note central venous catheter in SVC (*arrow*) and poor visualization of SVC and aorta (A). **B,** Axial T_1-weighted magnetic resonance image shows anterior mediastinal mass with intermediate signal intensity and flow within compressed left brachiocephalic vein (*asterisk*) and SVC (*arrow*). More distal images (not shown) showed patency of markedly narrowed SVC.

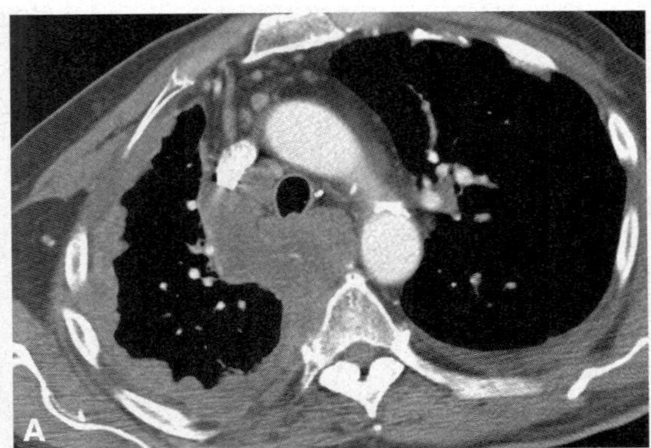

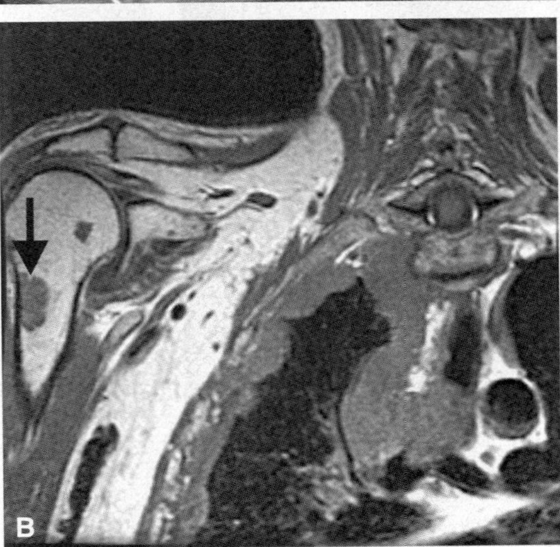

Figure 32c-10 Malignant pleural mesothelioma manifesting as diffuse pleural mass. **A,** Computed tomograph of chest shows lobular pleural mass encasing the right hemithorax. **B,** Coronal T_1-weighted magnetic resonance image shows diffuse pleural mass and reveals metastases in the right humerus (*arrow*).

cord abnormalities, (3) longitudinal extent of tumor, and (4) extradural extension.

CT and MRI are particularly useful in showing local soft-tissue and vascular invasion and early dissemination to regional lymph nodes in tumors such as thymomas and thymic carcinomas (Figure 32c-9). Also, because of the varying composition of soft tissue, fat, calcium, and hemorrhage in teratomas, CT and MRI can occasionally differentiate these tumors from thymomas and lymphomas.[49,50] CT is also usually used as the primary staging modality in patients with suspected mediastinal lymphoma. Because FDG-PET has high sensitivity and specificity in detecting lymphoma and because it provides complementary staging information, it is being increasingly used for the initial staging of lymphoma; when available, it has replaced ^{67}Ga citrate single photon emission computed tomography.[51–55] Additionally, FDG-PET has high diagnostic accuracy in the early prediction of response to chemotherapy, is useful in restaging lymphoma after initial treatment, and helps in the detection of early relapse after completion of therapy.[56–60] Residual masses after chemotherapy or radiation therapy are common, and distinction of a fibrotic mass from persistent or recurrent tumor can be difficult by CT imaging. In these cases, FDG-PET is useful in detecting persistent disease in residual masses and in predicting relapse of lymphoma.[61]

MALIGNANT PLEURAL MESOTHELIOMA

Because accurate anatomic staging is becoming important in determining the selection of patients for potentially curative resection, radiologic evaluation is an essential component in the appropriate management of patients with malignant pleural mesothelioma (MPM).[62,63] Chest radiographic abnormalities suggestive of MPM (unilateral pleural effusion with or without a lobular or multifocal pleural mass) are usually further evaluated with CT to assess the extent of local chest wall and mediastinal invasion and the presence of nodal and lung metastases. In patients with potentially resectable disease, MRI can be performed to further examine the local extent of tumor (Figure 32c-10).

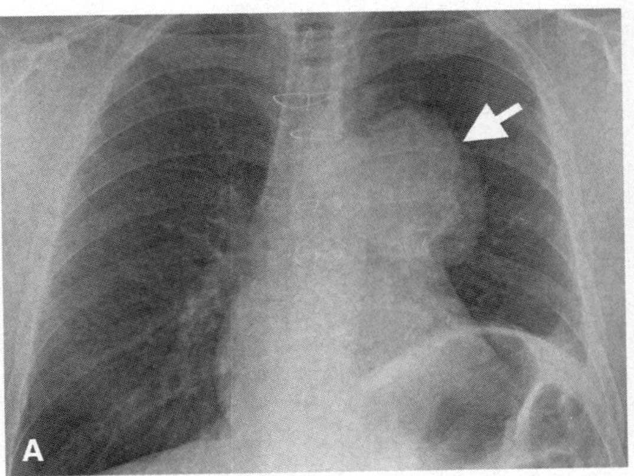

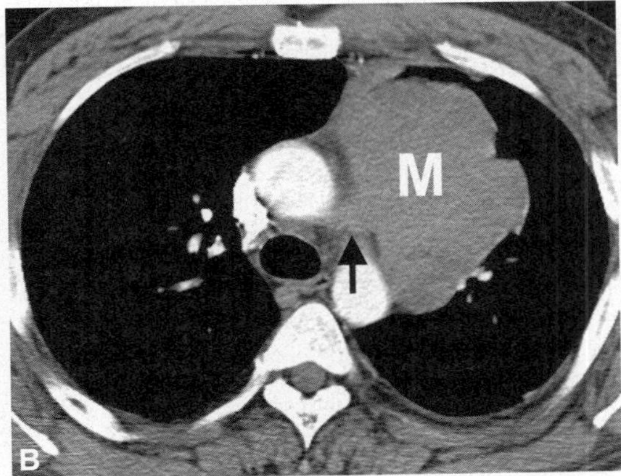

Figure 32c-9 Invasive thymoma manifesting as a mediastinal mass. **A,** Posteroanterior chest radiograph shows left mediastinal mass (*arrow*). Note elevation of left hemidiaphragm caused by paralysis secondary to phrenic nerve involvement. **B,** Chest computed tomograph reveals large lobular mediastinal mass (M) with extension into the aortopulmonary window (*arrow*).

In a recent study, MRI and CT were found to be of nearly equivalent diagnostic accuracy in the staging assessment of patients with MPM.[64] However, MRI was more accurate than CT in assessing invasion of the diaphragm and limited focal chest wall invasion. Accordingly, initial imaging evaluation of patients with MPM is usually performed using CT. In patients considered surgical candidates who have questionable areas of local tumor extension on CT, MRI may provide additional information before extrapleural pneumonectomy (EPP) is attempted. FDG-PET imaging has been used to evaluate MPM and may aid in the preoperative evaluation of patients being considered for EPP.[65,66] Although the role of FDG-PET in the staging of MPM has not been fully elucidated, in our experience, integrated CT-PET imaging improves accuracy of MPM staging and is important in determining the appropriate therapy in patients being considered for EPP.[67] In this regard, CT-PET is particularly useful in detecting unsuspected extrathoracic metastases (Figure 32c-11).

CONCLUSION

Conventional anatomic imaging (chest radiographs, CT, MRI) is an integral component in the

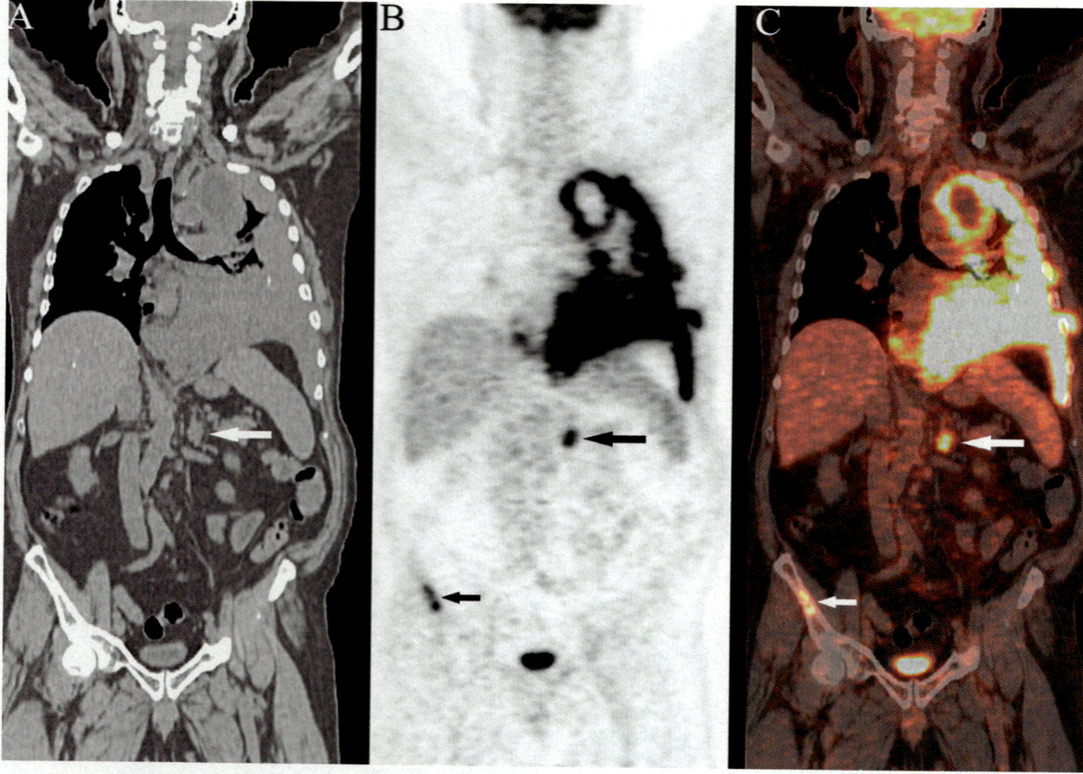

Figure 32c-11 Malignant pleural mesothelioma in a patient being evaluated for extrapleural pneumonectomy. **A,** Coronal computed tomography (CT), **B,** positron emission tomography (PET), and **C,** integrated CT-PET show diffuse uptake of ^{18}F fluoro-2-deoxy-D-glucose in primary left pleural tumor and focal areas of increased uptake in the left adrenal mass (*long arrows*) and pelvis localized to right iliac bone (*short arrows*). These occult metastases were not detected on conventional staging evaluation.

evaluation and management of patients with thoracic neoplasms. Radiologic imaging is useful for (1) improving the accuracy of clinical staging of lung cancer and malignant pleural mesothelioma, (2) assessing the anatomic extent and presence of local invasion of mediastinal neoplasms, and (3) determining therapeutic response. PET complements conventional radiologic assessment of thoracic neoplasms and improves the accuracy of staging and determination of therapeutic response.

REFERENCES

1. Mountain CF. Revisions in the international system for staging lung cancer. Chest 1997;111:1710–7.
2. Lardinois D, Weder W, Hany TF, et al. Staging of non-small-cell lung cancer with integrated positron-emission tomography and computed tomography. N Engl J Med 2003;348:2500–7.
3. Verhagen AF, Bootsma GP, Tjan-Heijnen VC, et al. FDG-PET in staging lung cancer: how does it change the algorithm? Lung Cancer 2004;44:175–81.
4. Reed CE, Harpole DH, Posther KE, et al. Results of the American College of Surgeons Oncology Group Z0050 trial: the utility of positron emission tomography in staging potentially operable non-small cell lung cancer. J Thorac Cardiovasc Surg 2003;126:1943–51.
5. van Tinteren H, Hoekstra OS, Smit EF, et al. Effectiveness of positron emission tomography in the preoperative assessment of patients with suspected non-small-cell lung cancer: the PLUS multicentre randomised trial. Lancet 2002;359:1388–93.
6. Antoch G, Stattaus J, Nemat AT, et al. Non-small cell lung cancer: dual-modality PET/CT in preoperative staging. Radiology 2003;229:526–33.
7. Ratto GB, Piacenza G, Frola C, et al. Chest wall involvement by lung cancer: computed tomographic detection and results of operation. Ann Thorac Surg 1991;51:182–8.
8. Yokoi K, Mori K, Miyazawa N, et al. Tumor invasion of the chest wall and mediastinum in lung cancer: evaluation with pneumothorax. Radiology 1991;181:147–52.
9. Martini N, Heelan R, Westcott J, et al. Comparative merits of conventional, computed tomographic, and magnetic resonance imaging in assessing mediastinal involvement in surgically confirmed lung carcinoma. J Thorac Cardiovasc Surg 1985;90:639–48.
10. McLoud TC. CT of bronchogenic carcinoma: indeterminate mediastinal invasion. Radiology 1989;173:15–6.
11. Webb WR, Gatsonis C, Zerhouni EA, et al. CT and MR imaging in staging non-small cell bronchogenic carcinoma: report of the Radiologic Diagnostic Oncology Group. Radiology 1991;178:705–13.
12. Webb WR, Sostman HD. MR imaging of thoracic disease: clinical uses. Radiology 1992;182:621–30.
13. McLoud TC, Filion RB, Edelman RR, et al. MR imaging of superior sulcus carcinoma. J Comput Assist Tomogr 1989;13:233–39.
14. Mountain CF, Dresler CM. Regional lymph node classification for lung cancer staging. Chest 1997;111:1718–23.
15. Glazer GM, Gross BH, Quint LE, et al. Normal mediastinal lymph nodes: number and size according to American Thoracic Society Mapping. AJR Am J Roentgenol 1985;144:261–5.
16. McLoud TC, Bourgouin PM, Greenberg RW, et al. Bronchogenic carcinoma: analysis of staging in the mediastinum with CT by correlative lymph node mapping and sampling. Radiology 1992;182:319–23.
17. Shimoyama K, Murata K, Takahashi M, et al. Pulmonary hilar lymph node metastases from lung cancer: evaluation based on morphology at thin-section, incremental, dynamic CT. Radiology 1997;203:187–95.
18. Dwamena BA, Sonnad SS, Angobaldo JO, Wahl RL. Metastases from non-small cell lung cancer: mediastinal staging in the 1990s: meta-analytic comparison of PET and CT. Radiology 1999;213:530–6.
19. Vansteenkiste JF, Stroobants SG, De Leyn PR, et al. Lymph node staging in non-small-cell lung cancer with FDG-PET scan: a prospective study on 690 lymph node stations from 68 patients. J Clin Oncol 1998;16:2142–9.
20. von Haag DW, Follette DM, Roberts PF, et al. Advantages of positron emission tomography over computed tomography in mediastinal staging of non-small cell lung cancer. J Surg Res 2002;103:160–4.
21. Silvestri GA, Littenberg B, Colice GL. The clinical evaluation for detecting metastatic lung cancer. A meta-analysis. Am J Respir Crit Care Med 1995;152:225–30.
22. Tanaka K, Kubota K, Kodama T, et al. Extrathoracic staging is not necessary for non-small-cell lung cancer with clinical stage T1–2 N0. Ann Thorac Surg 1999;68:1039–42.
23. Boland GW, Lee MJ, Gazelle GS, et al. Characterization of adrenal masses using unenhanced CT: an analysis of the CT literature. AJR Am J Roentgenol 1998;171:201–4.
24. Mayo-Smith WW, Boland GW, Noto RB, et al. State-of-the-art adrenal imaging. Radiographics 2001;21:995–1012.
25. Hooper RG, Tenholder MF, Underwood GH, et al. Computed tomographic scanning of the brain in initial staging of bronchogenic carcinoma. Chest 1984;85:774–6.
26. Colice GL, Birkmeyer JD, Black WC, et al. Cost-effectiveness of head CT in patients with lung cancer without clinical evidence of metastases. Chest 1995;108:1264–71.
27. Michel F, Soler M, Imhof E, Perruchoud AP. Initial staging of non-small cell lung cancer: value of routine radioisotope bone scanning. Thorax 1991;46:469–73.
28. Salvatierra A, Baamonde C, Llamas JM, et al. Extrathoracic staging of bronchogenic carcinoma. Chest 1990;97:1052–58.
29. Pieterman RM, van Putten JW, Meuzelaar JJ, et al. Preoperative staging of non-small-cell lung cancer with positron-emission tomography. N Engl J Med 2000;343:254–61.
30. MacManus MP, Hicks RJ, Matthews JP, et al. High rate of detection of unsuspected distant metastases by PET in apparent stage III non-small-cell lung cancer: implications for radical radiation therapy. Int J Radiat Oncol Biol Phys 2001;50:287–93.
31. Viney RC, Boyer MJ, King MT, et al. Randomized controlled trial of the role of positron emission tomography in the management of stage I and II non-small-cell lung cancer. J Clin Oncol 2004;22:2357–62.
32. Darling GE. Staging of the patient with small cell lung cancer. Chest Surg Clin N Am 1997;7:81–94.
33. Jelinek JS, Redmond J, Perry JJ, et al. Small cell lung cancer: staging with MR imaging. Radiology 1990;177:837–42.
34. Abrams J, Doyle LA, Aisner J. Staging prognostic factors, and special considerations in small cell lung cancer. Semin Oncol 1988;15:261–77.
35. van de Pol M, van Oosterhout AGM, Wilmink JT, et al. MRI in detection of brain metastases at initial staging of small-cell lung cancer. Neuroradiology 1996;38:207–10.
36. Stahel RA, Mabry M, Skarin AT, et al. Detection of bone marrow metastasis in small-cell lung cancer by monoclonal antibody. J Clin Oncol 1985;3:455–61.
37. Stahel RA, Ginsberg R, Havemann K, et al. Staging and prognostic factors in small cell lung cancer: a consensus report. Lung Cancer 1989;5:119–26.
38. Schumacher T, Brink I, Mix M, et al. FDG-PET imaging for the staging and follow-up of small cell lung cancer. Eur J Nucl Med 2001;28:483–8.
39. Therasse P, Arbuck SG, Eisenhauer EA, et al. New guidelines to evaluate the response to treatment in solid tumors. European Organization for Research and Treatment of Cancer, National Cancer Institute of the United States, National Cancer Institute of Canada. J Natl Cancer Inst 2000;92:205–16.
40. Yankelevitz DF, Gupta R, Zhao B, et al. Small pulmonary nodules: evaluation with repeat CT—preliminary experience. Radiology 1999;212:561–6.
41. Werner-Wasik M, Xiao Y, Pequignot E, et al. Assessment of lung cancer response after nonoperative therapy: tumor diameter, bidimensional product, and volume. A serial CT scan-based study. Int J Radiat Oncol Biol Phys 2001;51:56–61.
42. Erasmus JJ, Gladish GW, Broemeling L, et al. Interobserver and intraobserver variability in measurement of non-small-cell carcinoma lung lesions: implications for assessment of tumor response. J Clin Oncol 2003;21:2574–82.
43. Weissleder R. Molecular imaging: exploring the next frontier. Radiology 1999;212:609–14.
44. Young H, Baum R, Cremerius U, et al. Measurement of clinical and subclinical tumour response using [^{18}F]-fluorodeoxyglucose and positron emission tomography: review and 1999 EORTC recommendations. European Organization for Research and Treatment of Cancer (EORTC) PET Study Group. Eur J Cancer 1999;35:1773–82.
45. Weber WA, Schwaiger M, Avril N. Quantitative assessment of tumor metabolism using FDG-PET imaging. Nucl Med Biol 2000;27:683–7.
46. Weber WA, Petersen V, Schmidt B, et al. Positron emission tomography in non-small-cell lung cancer: prediction of

response to chemotherapy by quantitative assessment of glucose use. J Clin Oncol 2003;21:2651–7.

47. Bury T, Corhay JL, Duysinx B, et al. Value of FDG-PET in detecting residual or recurrent nonsmall cell lung cancer. Eur Respir J 1999;14:1376–80.
48. Patz EF, Lowe VJ, Hoffman JM, et al. Persistent or recurrent bronchogenic carcinoma: detection with PET and 2-[^{18}F]-2-deoxy-D-glucose. Radiology 1994;191:379–82.
49. Moeller KH, Rosado-de-Christenson ML, Templeton PA. Mediastinal mature teratoma: imaging features. AJR Am J Roentgenol 1997;169:985–90.
50. Brown LR, Aughenbaugh GL. Masses of the anterior mediastinum: CT and MR imaging. AJR Am J Roentgenol 1991;157:1171–80.
51. Friedberg JW, Fischman A, Neuberg D, et al. FDG-PET is superior to gallium scintigraphy in staging and more sensitive in the follow-up of patients with de novo Hodgkin lymphoma: a blinded comparison. Leuk Lymphoma 2004;45:85–92.
52. Wirth A, Seymour JF, Hicks RJ, et al. Fluorine-18 fluorodeoxyglucose positron emission tomography, gallium-67 scintigraphy, and conventional staging for Hodgkin's disease and non-Hodgkin's lymphoma. Am J Med 2002;112:262–8.
53. Bangerter M, Moog F, Buchmann I, et al. Whole-body 2-[^{18}F]-fluoro-2-deoxy-D-glucose positron emission tomography (FDG-PET) for accurate staging of Hodgkin's disease. Ann Oncol 1998;9:1117–22.
54. Kostakoglu L, Leonard JP, Kuji I, et al. Comparison of fluorine-18 fluorodeoxyglucose positron emission tomography and Ga-67 scintigraphy in evaluation of lymphoma. Cancer 2002;94:879–88.
55. Yamamoto F, Tsukamoto E, Nakada K, et al. ^{18}F-FDG PET is superior to ^{67}Ga SPECT in the staging of non-Hodgkin's lymphoma. Ann Nucl Med 2004;18:519–26.
56. Spaepen K, Stroobants S, Dupont P, et al. Early restaging positron emission tomography with ^{18}F-fluorodeoxyglucose predicts outcome in patients with aggressive non-Hodgkin's lymphoma. Ann Oncol 2002;13:1356–63.
57. Spaepen K, Stroobants S, Dupont P, et al. Prognostic value of positron emission tomography (PET) with fluorine-18 fluorodeoxyglucose ([^{18}F]FDG) after first-line chemotherapy in non-Hodgkin's lymphoma: is [^{18}F]FDG-PET a valid alternative to conventional diagnostic methods? J Clin Oncol 2001;19:414–9.
58. Jerusalem G, Beguin Y, Fassotte MF, et al. Early detection of relapse by whole-body positron emission tomography in the follow-up of patients with Hodgkin's disease. Ann Oncol 2003;14:123–30.
59. Guay C, Lepine M, Verreault J, et al. Prognostic value of PET using ^{18}F-FDG in Hodgkin's disease for posttreatment evaluation. J Nucl Med 2003;44:1225–31.
60. Kostakoglu L, Coleman M, Leonard JP, et al. PET predicts prognosis after 1 cycle of chemotherapy in aggressive lymphoma and Hodgkin's disease. J Nucl Med 2002;43:1018–27.
61. Naumann R, Vaic A, Beuthien-Baumann B, et al. Prognostic value of positron emission tomography in the evaluation of post-treatment residual mass in patients with Hodgkin's disease and non-Hodgkin's lymphoma. Br J Haematol 2001;115:793–800.
62. Greene F, Page DL, Fleming ID, et al., editors. Pleural mesothelioma. In: American Joint Committee on Cancer (AJCC) cancer staging manual. 6th ed. New York: Springer-Verlag; 2002. p. 179–84.
63. Patz EF Jr, Rusch VW, Heelan R. The proposed new international TNM staging system for malignant pleural mesothelioma: application to imaging. AJR Am J Roentgenol 1996;166:323–7.
64. Heelan RT, Rusch VW, Begg CB, et al. Staging of malignant pleural mesothelioma: comparison of CT and MR imaging. AJR Am J Roentgenol 1999;172:1039–47.
65. Schneider DB, Clary-Macy C, Challa S, et al. Positron emission tomography with ^{18}F-fluorodeoxyglucose in the staging and preoperative evaluation of malignant pleural mesothelioma. J Thorac Cardiovasc Surg 2000;120:128–33.
66. Flores RM, Akhurst T, Gonen M, et al. Positron emission tomography defines metastatic disease but not locoregional disease in patients with malignant pleural mesothelioma. J Thorac Cardiovasc Surg 2003;126:11–6.
67. Truong MT, Erasmus JJ, Marom EM, Munden RF. Imaging evaluation in the diagnosis and staging of malignant pleural mesothelioma. Semin Roentgenol 2004;39:386–96.

32d

Imaging Neoplasms of the Abdomen and Pelvis

Haesun Choi, MD
Harmeet Kaur, MD
Evelyne M. Loyer, MD
Paul M. Silverman, MD

Technologic innovations in computed tomography (CT), magnetic resonance imaging (MRI), and ultrasonography have greatly improved our ability to diagnose abdominopelvic neoplasms and to monitor treatment efficacy. Although plain films and air-contrast techniques remain fundamental to the imaging armamentarium, they have largely been supplanted by cross-sectional imaging. Endoscopic ultrasonography, functional MRI, and positron emission tomography (PET) are new approaches whose roles are increasing in scope. The choice of technique is determined by the organ being studied, the suspected pathology, the patient's clinical condition, and the experience of the radiologist and endoscopist.

Conventional ultrasonography is often the initial screening examination, but it has a limited role in the diagnosis and staging of abdominopelvic neoplasms. However, endoscopic and transvaginal ultrasonography have respectively become important adjuncts in the evaluation of gastrointestinal (GI) and pancreatic malignancies and of gynecologic malignancies.

CT has become the primary diagnostic modality used in oncologic radiology. The development of multislice CT (MSCT) has dramatically improved the examination speed, enabling the imaging of very thin slices and multiple phases of contrast administration.[1] Thus, the role of CT has expanded to the point that relatively invasive studies—such as CT arteriography, CT arterial portography, and certain vascular studies—can now be replaced by noninvasive evaluations with MSCT. GI and intravenous (IV) contrast administration is required in most cases, assuming that the patient has normal renal function and no history of allergy to iodine. IV contrast should be given through a needle of adequate bore, using an injector to achieve an injection rate of 3 to 5 mL/s depending on the specific CT protocol. With contrast injection at those rates, helical (spiral) CT can acquire multiphasic images of an organ or mass that can help to characterize the disease and to more easily define its stage. In some cases, three-dimensional (3D) reconstructions can help radiologists to more confidently stage neoplastic disease (Figure 32d-1). Three-dimensional CT imaging also provides a roadmap to guide surgical intervention.[2,3]

MRI is generally used as a second-line imaging technique because of its cost and relatively limited availability, but it may be the primary imaging modality used in patients allergic to iodine. In such cases, gadolinium-enhanced MRI may be performed. However, implanted cardiac pacemakers and certain intracerebral aneurysmal clips are absolute contraindications for MRI. In evaluations of the liver, MRI is mainly a problem-solving modality for lesions that are difficult to characterize by CT. Technical advances in both software and hardware have allowed enhanced triphasic acquisition within a single breath hold, similar to multiphasic CT. An important differentiating feature between the two modalities lies in the cell-specific contrast agent—iron oxide particulates—uniquely available for MRI. The iron oxide particulates are taken up by reticular endothelial cells and, in liver imaging, maximize lesion detectability on MRI and, more importantly, increase the specificity at the same time.[4,5] Magnetic resonance cholangiopancreatography (MRCP) has emerged as a noninvasive alternative to endoscopic retrograde cholangiopancreatography (ERCP). MRCP has been particularly useful in patients in whom ERCP has failed or the Whipple procedure has been performed.[6]

MRI is superior to CT when high soft-tissue contrast or direct multiplanar images are needed, as in the evaluation of large abdominal masses. In the case of soft-tissue tumors involving the extremities, MRI is widely accepted as the superior examination. In the pelvis, MRI is used to assess rectal tumors and gynecologic malignancies. The application of phased-array or endorectal coils improves the signal-to-noise ratio, leading to improved resolution for evaluating cervical, uterine, and prostate cancers. MR angiography (MRA) can also be readily performed in conjunction with MRI and plays an important part in local staging of renal and pancreatic carcinomas.

PET has been increasingly used in oncology. PET is a metabolic imaging technique that uses a radiolabeled glucose analog, ^{18}F fluorodeoxyglucose (FDG). The FDG is metabolized by the cells but, unlike glucose, remains trapped there after phosphorylation. FDG-PET imaging relies on the increased glycolytic rate and higher uptake of radiolabeled glucose in malignant cells than in normal cells. On FDG-PET, the glucose metabolic activity can be quantitated.

Although the role of FDG-PET is still being defined and its value is not equal for all malignancies, many of its clinical applications have already affected patient management. Increased accuracy in staging is seen with esophageal carcinoma, melanoma, and lymphoma, with an immediate impact on therapeutic decisions.[7] In lymphoma in the restaging setting, the distinction between scar tissue and true residual tumor is quicker and more reliable with FDG-PET than with conventional assessment. In addition, a high negative predictive value of PET for progression after treatment has been reported.[8] GI stromal tumor (GIST) is a rare tumor whose avidity for FDG is very high. PET is highly sensitive in the detection of tumor nodules and the assessment of treatment response in GIST.[9] The value of PET in other abdominal and pelvic tumors such as liver metastasis, GI carcinomas, and gynecologic and urinary malignancies has not yet been clearly established. Evaluation of hepatic, renal, and prostate tumors is impaired by the high physiologic concentration of FDG in those organs.[7]

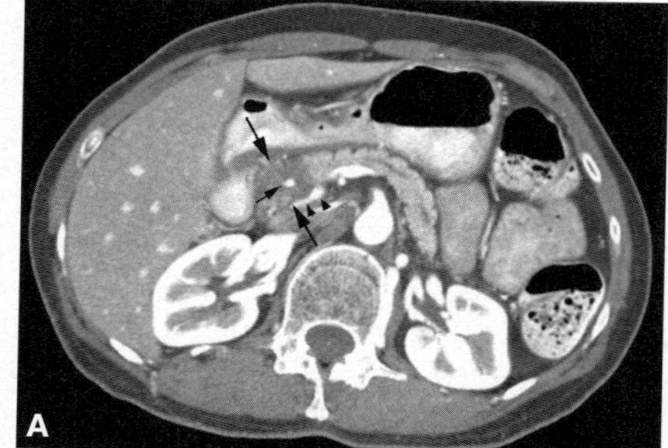

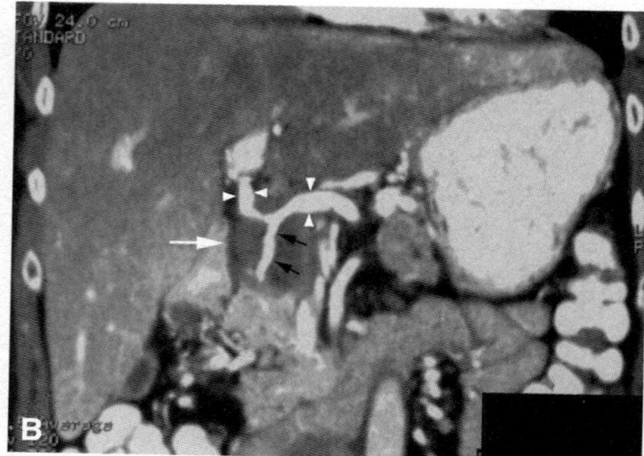

Figure 32d-1 Pancreatic adenocarcinoma. **A,** A contrast-enhanced computed tomography image during the pancreatic phase demonstrates a hypodense mass (*large arrows*) in the head of the pancreas, completely encasing the hepatoduodenal artery (*small arrow*) and compressing the main portal vein (*arrowheads*). **B,** A reconstructed coronal image depicts the mass (*large arrow*), which involves not only the hepatoduodenal artery (*small arrows*), but also the common hepatic artery and celiac trunk (*arrowheads*).

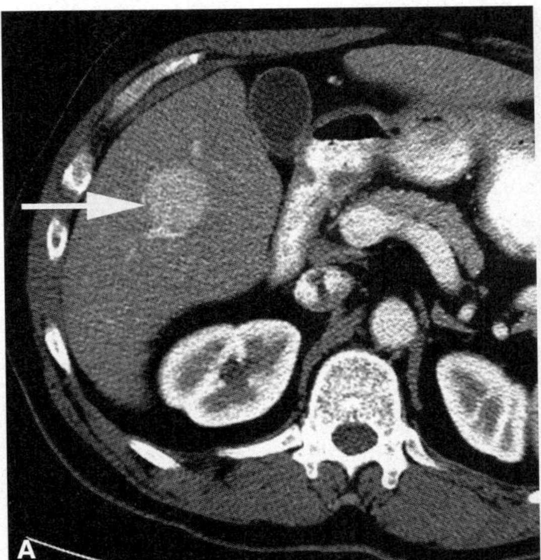

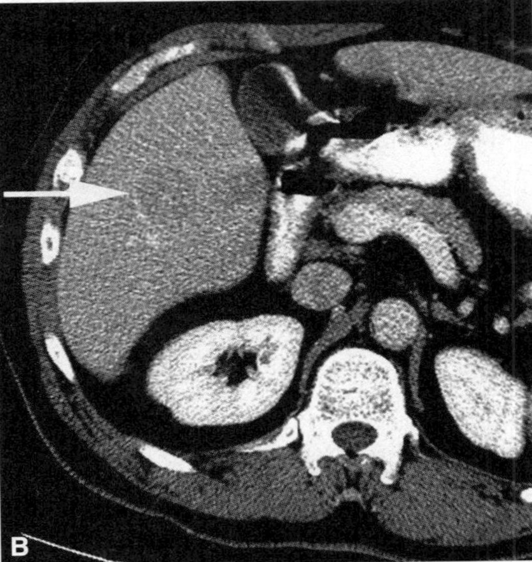

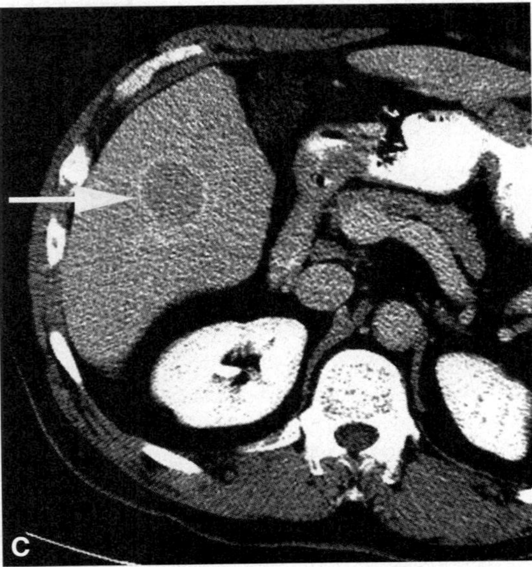

Figure 32d-2 Hepatocellular carcinoma. **A,** An early arterial phase image of enhanced computed tomography (CT) demonstrates a well-defined enhancing mass (*arrow*) in the right lobe of the liver. **B, C,** The mass becomes invisible (isodense to the liver parenchyma, *arrow*) on the late arterial phase image **B** and hypodense (*arrow*) on a portal venous phase image **C** of the enhanced CT, leaving the rim hyperdense. This is typical of hepatocellular carcinoma.

The sections that follow consider the role of each of the various imaging modalities in specific regions of the abdomen and pelvis, highlighting the benefits and limitations in each case.

THE GASTROINTESTINAL TRACT

Detection of GI tumors relies primarily on luminal contrast techniques and endoscopy. Both techniques are used to assess the mucosa of the upper GI tract and colon. Air-contrast barium studies of the esophagus, stomach, and colon require technical skill and an optimized approach to be diagnostic. Patients must fast before undergoing studies of the upper GI tract, and the colon must be thoroughly emptied before a barium enema.[10] With proper preparation, subtle mucosal abnormalities representing early neoplasms can be detected.[11,12] CT colonography has a sensitivity of 81% for the detection of colon polyps larger than 1 cm in diameter.[13] One study found CT colonography, or "virtual colonoscopy," to be a sensitive method for the detection of clinically relevant polyps and adenomas; however, multicenter trials are needed to confirm this early result.[14]

Endoscopy, because it allows both direct visualization of a mucosal tumor and the ability to obtain tissue for biopsy, tends to supersede air-contrast barium studies. Colonoscopy has been advocated as the screening modality for colon cancer, but the optimal screening program is now being debated because of recent technologic developments in MSCT and CT colonography.[15] Endoscopic ultrasonography is an adjunctive study used for local staging because of its ability to evaluate the depth of tumor penetration through the wall (T stage) in the esophagus, stomach, and rectum, with an accuracy of 85% and a sensitivity of 67% to 97%.[16] It also has the capability to detect nodal spread, although with less accuracy.

Small-bowel tumors are, for the time being, not accessible to endoscopy. For them, evaluation is performed using a barium examination, with graded compression of the opacified loops. This study requires the patient to drink a significant volume of contrast material. Depending on individual transit time, the duration of the examination can exceed 2 hours. Small-bowel enteroclysis is another, more sensitive technique for detecting abnormalities of the small bowel. Unfortunately, it involves invasive intubation of the proximal jejunum and infusion of barium alone or barium and methylcellulose for a double-contrast effect. Successful application of the technique also is highly dependent on the expertise of the radiologists and technologists. Multiple images of the distended loops are obtained. Although the distention aids in the detection of abnormalities, this benefit must be weighed against the patient's discomfort from the nasojejunal intubation.[17,18]

Although CT sometimes can visualize mural and extramural involvement, the technique has not been used for tumor detection mainly because controlling bowel distention and appropriate opacification so as to assess the mucosa is difficult. However, CT colonography combining the air-contrast enema technique and helical CT may have utility as a screening tool.[14] Stromal tumors and lymphoma, which tend to grow exophytically, are more readily demonstrated on CT. Small-bowel tumors (such as carcinoid tumors) may be diagnosed on CT by detection of mesenteric involvement in addition to local and distant metastatic disease.[19] CT is the best modality to stage these tumors. Locally, the extent of a mass can be assessed grossly for extension into the peritoneal fat or to adjacent organs. Nodal, peritoneal, and hepatic metastases are also best assessed with CT.[20–22] As described earlier, endoscopic ultrasonography is used to define the T stage of the tumor.

The role of MRI in GI tumors is very limited, except for tumors in the rectum. For rectal tumors, MRI has shown superior capability in local staging at the time of diagnosis and in monitoring the disease after treatment.[23]

THE LIVER

Radiographic evaluation of liver disease relies on ultrasonography, CT, and MRI.[24] These techniques enable detection, and often characterization, of focal and diffuse hepatic processes. Ultrasonography is inexpensive and readily available, but its value compared with single-slice helical CT (SSCT), MSCT, and MRI is limited by its lower sensitivity and specificity. Recent advances in Doppler technique and ultrasonography contrast material can aid in the characterization of hepatic lesions. Intraoperative ultrasonography is widely used before hepatic resection because of its high sensitivity.[25]

The initial evaluation of primary and metastatic liver tumors is usually done with CT, although MRI is also appropriate and relies on similar morphologic and vascular criteria, as well as signal characteristics on T_2-weighted images. With the introduction of helical CT, biphasic acquisition has become a standard method for evaluating and characterizing primary hepatic neoplasms because it provides morphologic and physiologic information. The pattern of enhancement defined with the multiphasic technique provides key information for diagnosis.[26] Hypervascular tumors have a rapid and brief uptake of contrast; cholangiocarcinoma and adenocarcinoma in general have a less intense, more delayed, and persistent contrast uptake (Figures 32d-2 and 32d-3).[27] Specific patterns of enhancement have also been defined for hemangioma and, to a lesser extent, focal nodular hyperplasia (FNH).[26,28,29] The multiphasic technique is used for the evaluation of hypervascular tumors, primary hepatocellular carcinoma (HCC) and metastasis (neuroendocrine, carcinoid, and choriocarcinoma), because it improves lesion detection. Paulson and colleagues evaluated metastases from carcinoid tumor and found that one third of the lesions were most conspicuous on the arterial phase and one sixth were seen only on the arterial phase.[30] Similarly, additional tumor nodules are seen on the arterial phase in patients with HCC.[31]

In contrast, hypovascular tumors (such as metastases from lung and GI neoplasms) require imaging in the hepatic venous phase (HVP) only. A sensitivity of 85.1% was achieved with helical

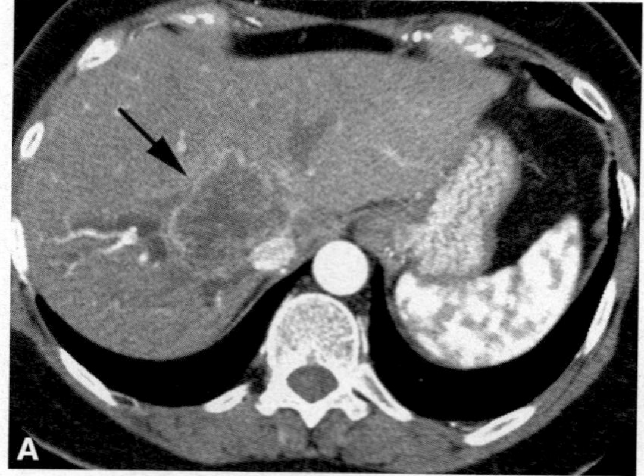

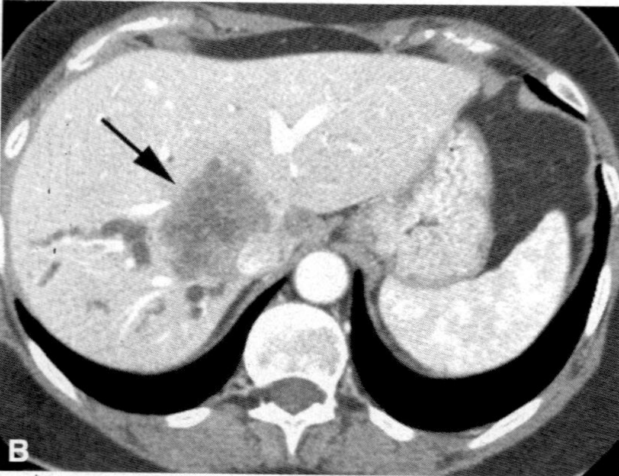

Figure 32d-3 Cholangiocarcinoma. **A,** A contrast-enhanced computed tomography (CT) image obtained during the late arterial phase shows a hypodense mass (*arrow*) in the right lobe of the liver. **B,** A contrast-enhanced CT image obtained during the portal venous phase shows the mass (*arrow*) enhancing.

CT in the detection of hepatic metastases from colorectal carcinoma.[32]

Despite a recent dramatic improvement in the detection of hypervascular tumors by helical CT, in transplant populations the sensitivity of the technique remains suboptimal for screening the cirrhotic liver for malignant hepatic nodules.[33,34] Current MSCT permits shortening the scan time of the entire liver to 10 seconds or less, and it is possible to conduct a multiphasic study in which the liver is scanned in the hepatic arterial phase, late arterial phase, and HVP.[35] Recent data on the use of the double arterial phase protocol indicates that this technique has a higher sensitivity than helical CT; however, an accurate estimate of sensitivity would require correlation with results in an explanted liver.[36] Distinguishing between dysplastic nodules and small HCC is difficult. Equally difficult is the characterization of a small enhancing focus that may be caused by a benign or nontumor source.[33,37] Lesion characterization also remains a problem for very small, subcentimeter lesions, which are being detected with increased frequency.[38]

As a first-line oncologic imaging approach, MRI is used mainly as a problem-solving modality or in patients who are allergic to iodine. The dynamic imaging capabilities of both CT and MRI are critical to their utility. Focal areas of fatty infiltration can easily be differentiated from a mass lesion using in- and out-of-phase sequences. Hypervascular metastasis and benign hypervascular neoplasms such as FNH and adenoma can be differentiated on MRI by using a liver-specific contrast in addition to traditional gadolinium compound. For example, FNH is typically highly vascular in the early arterial phase on Gd-enhanced MRI (as on enhanced CT); it is also enhanced by liver-specific contrast, while metastasis is not. Liver-specific contrast also maximizes lesion detectability and is often used before metastasis resection. MRI can be particularly useful in the event of discrepant clinical and CT findings and in monitoring recurrent tumors. CT or ultrasonography is generally employed to guide needle biopsies of liver lesions; physical characteristics of the lesion itself (accessibility, visualization, etc), equipment availability, and radiologist expertise will dictate the modality that is chosen.

THE BILIARY DUCT

Ultrasonography, CT, and MRI are all used in the examination of a jaundiced patient.[24] Conventional transabdominal ultrasonography can easily identify bile duct obstruction as the origin for the jaundice—and the level of the obstruction—but it may not be able to determine its cause, often because of gaseous interpositions. Endoscopic ultrasonography is used to explore the distal common bile duct and the pancreatic head.

CT is currently the primary imaging modality used to identify the cause of bile duct obstruction. SSCT and MSCT can produce thin sections from the level of the porta hepatis to the pancreatic head, displaying the extrahepatic bile ducts and pancreas. Using either technique, the site of obstruction can be defined and assessed for the presence of stones, soft-tissue mass arising from the biliary tree or pancreas, or extrinsic involvement by adenopathy or adjacent neoplasm. In general, the cause of the obstruction can be classified into one or more of these categories, although differentiation between a benign inflammatory process and a malignant obstruction is not always possible before surgical exploration.

Cholangiocarcinoma, involving the hilum of the liver, and gallbladder carcinoma are often large at the time of diagnosis because symptoms are often lacking in the early stage of the disease. Tumors arising in the common hepatic duct and common bile duct tend to be small and are more difficult to detect. A biliary stent placed to relieve the jaundice may limit the quality of the imaging studies by creating artifacts attributable to the stent itself or to an inflammatory process occurring following stent placement. Ideally, diagnostic CT should be done before stent placement. Helical CT allows detection of small tumors limited to subtle wall thickening. These tumors are usually hypovascular, although papillary tumors or tumors with neuroendocrine differentiation are hypervascular and best seen during the arterial phase. On CT, assessment of the extent of the tumor along the biliary tree; detection of involvement of the adjacent organs, portal vein, and hepatic artery; and detection of distant metastasis are possible, but with variable accuracy.[39,40]

THE PANCREAS

Detection of small pancreatic tumors with CT is primarily based on the difference in enhancement between tumor and normal parenchyma. Most ductal adenocarcinomas enhance less than the surrounding normal parenchyma does. Additional findings show a focal change in texture or an abrupt change in the caliber of the pancreatic or bile duct. When a dedicated technique is used, tumors as small as 5 mm can be detected.[41]

Accurate definition of the relationship of the tumor with the superior mesenteric artery, celiac axis, and superior mesenteric portal venous confluence and detection of extrapancreatic disease will determine whether the tumor is potentially resectable. (See Figure 32d-1.) The accuracy of CT in predicting unresectability is well established.[42]

If a diagnosis is not achieved with CT, then MRCP or cholangiography (such as ERCP or percutaneous transhepatic cholangiography) is used to define the obstruction. Cholangiography also allows brushing for cytologic evaluation. Endoscopic ultrasonography (EUS) is used to explore distal duct obstructions and the ampullary region of the pancreas. At the same setting, EUS-guided biopsy can provide a cytologic diagnosis of a mass.[43]

Fast and ultrafast dynamic MRI using paramagnetic contrast agents and the fat-suppression technique have improved the ability of MRI to image the pancreas.[44,45] Although some studies suggest that helical CT is superior to MRI in staging and detection of pancreatic cancer,[46] another study found that MRI can detect more small tumors than CT can.[47]

KIDNEYS AND ADRENAL GLAND

In cancer patients with adrenal lesions, the most common diagnostic dilemma is distinguishing adrenal adenoma from metastasis. A distinction can be made using either noncontrast CT or chemical-shift MRI (Figure 32d-4). Both techniques rely on detection of characteristic intracellular lipids in adenomas. In noncontrast CT, detection of a low-attenuation-value mass provides a reliable means of discriminating benign adenoma from metastatic disease; a threshold value of 10 Hounsfield units (HU) has a sensitivity of 71% and a specificity of 98%.[48] This result is comparable to those obtained with chemical-shift MRI. In the identification of lipid-poor adenomas, delayed contrast-enhanced CT is more valuable. Threshold attenuation values of 30 to 40 HU or a percentage of enhancement washout of 60% at 15 minutes are equally efficacious. In a study combining noncontrast and delayed contrast-enhanced CT, 96% of adenomas were characterized correctly.[49] The most common primary tumor of the adrenal gland is adrenal carcinoma, which characteristically presents as large heterogeneous masses with areas of necrosis.

In the radiologic characterization of renal masses, the objective is to distinguish solid malignant lesions that require surgical intervention from benign conditions (complex cysts,

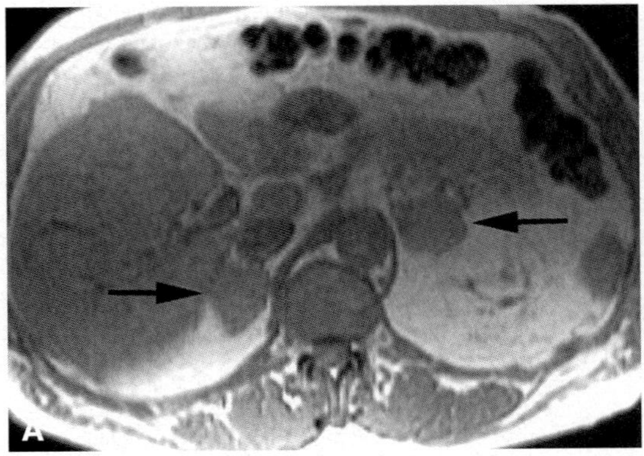
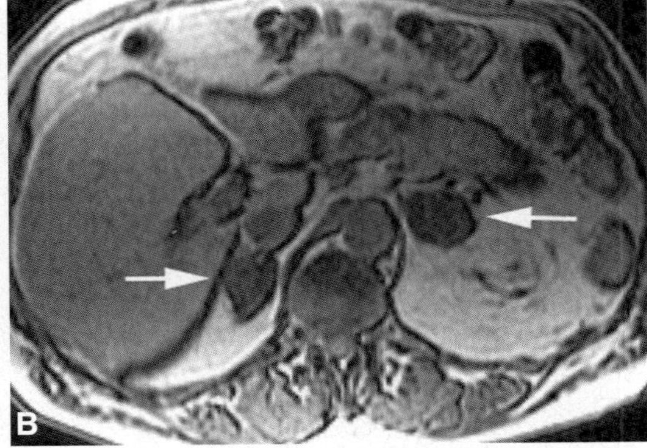

Figure 32d-4 Adrenal adenoma. **A,** An axial in-phase magnetic resonance (MR) image shows homogenous, bilateral adrenal masses (*arrows*). **B,** An axial out-of-phase MR image shows a significant decrease in the signal intensity of the masses (*arrows*).

abscesses, pseudotumors, and angiomyolipomas). Ultrasonography is excellent at identifying and characterizing simple cysts. The limitations are large body habitus and lesion size, because only 25% of masses between 10 and 15 mm are detected by ultrasonography.[50] Thin-section CT can correctly characterize most lesions greater than 1 cm in size. Enhancement indicates vascularity and favors a malignant process. MRI is comparable to CT in evaluating renal masses and can be used in case of adverse reaction to contrast or compromised renal function. CT and MRI are both used in the staging of renal cell carcinoma. The multiplanar capability of MRI assists in determining the relationship of large renal cell tumors to adjacent structures. Transitional cell carcinoma of the upper and lower urinary tract is best diagnosed by intravenous pyelography or retrograde pyelography; CT and MRI are used primarily in staging.

THE FEMALE REPRODUCTIVE TRACT

Ultrasonography is usually the initial imaging modality in the evaluation of adnexal masses. The combination of gray-scale imaging, color Doppler, and duplex Doppler is highly accurate in the detection and characterization of ovarian masses.[51] MRI can be used to identify the site origin and to characterize certain ovarian masses, such as dermoid tumors with a fat element, and hemorrhagic cysts and masses that are indeterminate on ultrasonography. Once the diagnosis is made, CT is the primary imaging modality in staging and monitoring ovarian cancers. Peritoneal carcinomatosis is best identified on CT. When the tumor is large (which is often the case in ovarian cancers), MRI plays an important role in surgical planning.

MRI is superior to CT and ultrasonography in the staging of cervical and endometrial cancer. The excellent soft-tissue resolution of the technique enables definition of uterine and cervical zonal anatomy. When supplemented by the use of dynamic contrast scanning, MRI is highly accurate in the detection of small tumors and in the evaluation of the depth of stromal and myometrial invasion. Cervical tumors can be identified accurately in 91% of invasive lesions (Figure 32d-5).[52] MRI provides the most accurate means for noninvasive pretreatment evaluation of tumor size, parametrial invasion, and depth of stromal invasion—criteria that are important prognostic determinants in cervical cancer. In endometrial cancer, tumor grade and depth of myometrial invasion are the most important prognostic factors. MRI provides the most accurate means for preoperative assessment of depth of myometrial invasion.[53] CT and MRI have comparable accuracies in the evaluation of nodal involvement, because both techniques rely on nodal size and shape as the criteria for the presence of metastasis. Lymphangiography permits evaluation of nodal architecture, but is invasive. Helical CT, MRI, and lymphangiography are comparable in the detection of nodal metastasis.[54] The use of PET in nodal disease has the potential to improve sensitivity and specificity over other modalities; however, its utility is limited in nodes less than 1 cm in diameter.[55] CT is the most efficient and widely used screening modality in the follow-up of ovarian, cervical, and uterine cancers. However, MRI is superior in the evaluation of locally recurrent disease within the pelvis and should be used routinely in the follow-up of cervical cancer.

THE PROSTATE

Transrectal ultrasonography (TRUS) is currently an initial imaging modality used in patients with suspected prostate carcinoma. The role of ultrasonography in staging prostate cancer is still limited. One advantage of TRUS is that it provides access for the biopsy of suspicious masses for definitive diagnosis. MRI is at least as sensitive as, and perhaps more sensitive than, ultrasonography in detecting the tumors. It is probably the most accurate imaging modality in T3 and T4 staging (eg, extracapsular extension or seminal vesicle involvement), but it does not allow biopsy.[56,57] A pelvic phased-array or endorectal coil should be used to optimize the diagnostic and staging accuracy of MRI. Also, following biopsy, it is advisable to postpone MRI at least 6 to 8 weeks. The advantage of MRI over TRUS is the former's ability to evaluate pelvic lymph nodes and bones simultaneously.

Either CT or MRI can be used to evaluate retroperitoneal and pelvic lymphadenopathy and distant metastasis; however, CT is the primary imaging modality used because of its wider availability. Either CT or MRI can detect bone metastasis, but a bone scan is the most sensitive modality available to evaluate bone disease.

Imaging has a limited role in monitoring prostate carcinoma after treatment. Posttreatment clinical surveillance uses serial serum PSA measurements. Bone scan and CT are the primary screening modalities for suspected recurrent disease with possible metastasis. In monitoring locally advanced disease or a suspected local recurrence, MRI (endorectal) is superior to CT. Imaging of the prostate is continuously evolving. PET has not yet been proven useful in detecting prostate carcinomas; however, magnetic resonance spectroscopy, based on the high choline levels in prostate carcinoma tissue, is under

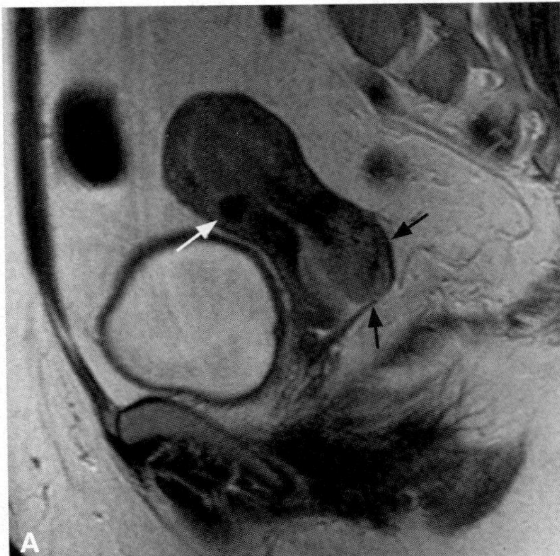
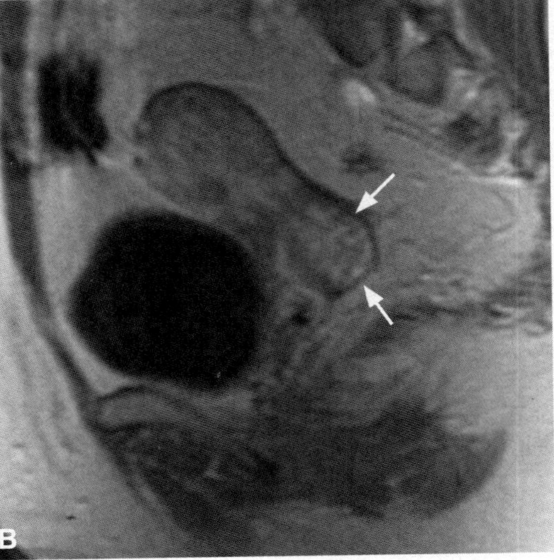

Figure 32d-5 Cervical carcinoma. **A,** A sagittal T_2-weighted magnetic resonance (MR) image demonstrates a hyperintense cervical mass (*black arrows*) extending into the posterior lip. A small leiomyoma (*white arrow*) is also noted at the anterior wall of the uterus. **B,** A dynamic sagittal T_1-weighted MR image shows the mass (*arrows*) enhancing, in contrast to the nonenhancing stroma.

extensive clinical investigation, with promising results.[58] The technique may contribute to identifying patients with clinically significant prostate carcinoma. It may also aid in monitoring local disease and in detecting local recurrence following external beam radiation or hormonal therapy.

CONCLUSION

In summary, CT, MRI, and ultrasonography are the major fundamental imaging modalities used in the diagnosis and staging of abdominopelvic neoplasms. Recent technologic advances in MSCT have brought that technique to the forefront of oncologic imaging.

REFERENCES

1. Ji H, McTavish JD, Mortele KJ, et al. Hepatic imaging with multidetector CT. Radiographics 2001;21(Spec No):S71–80.
2. Smith PA, Ratner LE, Lynch FC, et al. Role of CT angiography in the preoperative evaluation for laparoscopic nephrectomy. Radiographics 1998;18:589–601.
3. Takahashi S, Murakami T, Takamura M, et al. Multi-detector row helical CT angiography of hepatic vessels: depiction with dual-arterial phase acquisition during single breath hold. Radiology 2002;222:81–8.
4. Bartolozzi C, Lencioni R, Donati F, Cioni D. Abdominal MR: liver and pancreas. Eur Radiol 1999;9:1496–512.
5. Beavers KL, Semelka RC. MRI evaluation of the liver. Semin Liver Dis 2001;21:161–77.
6. Fulcher AS, Turner MA. Magnetic resonance pancreatography (MRP). Crit Rev Diagn Imaging 1999;40:285–322.
7. Rohren EM, Turkington TG, Coleman RE. Clinical application of PET in oncology. Radiology 2004;231:305–32.
8. Spaepen K, Stroobants S, Dupont P, et al. Early restaging positron emission tomography with ^{18}F-fluorodeoxyglucose predicts outcome in patients with aggressive non-Hodgkin's lymphoma. Ann Oncol 2002;13:1356–63.
9. Stroobants S, Goeminne J, Seegers M, et al. ^{18}FDG-positron emission tomography for the early prediction of response in advanced soft tissue sarcoma treated with imatinib mesylate (Glivec®). Eur J Cancer 2003;39:2012–20.
10. Laufer I, Kressel HY. Principles of double-contrast diagnosis. In: Laufer I, Levine MS, editors. Double-contrast gastrointestinal radiology. 2nd ed. Philadelphia: W.B. Saunders; 1992. p. 9–54.
11. Laufer I. Assessment of the accuracy of double-contrast gastroduodenal radiology. Gastroenterology 1976;71:874–8.
12. Laufer I, Smith NC, Mullens JE. The radiological demonstration of colorectal polyps undetected by endoscopy. Gastroenterology 1976;70:167–70.
13. Steine S, Stordahl A, Lunde OC, et al. Double-contrast barium enema versus colonoscopy in the diagnosis of neoplastic disorders: aspects of decision-making in general practice. Fam Pract 1993;10:288–91.
14. Yee J, Akerkar GA, Hung RK, et al. Colorectal neoplasia: performance characteristics of CT colonography for detection in 300 patients. Radiology 2001;219:685–92.
15. Levine MS, Glick SN, Rubesin SE, Laufe I. Double-contrast barium enema examination and colorectal cancer: a plea for radiologic screening. Radiology 2002;222:313–5.
16. Montgomery RC, Ridge JA. Radiologic staging of gastrointestinal cancer. Semin Surg Oncol 1998;15:143–50.
17. Maglinte DD, Lappas JC, Kelvin FM, et al. Small bowel radiography: how, when, and why? Radiology 1987;163:297–305.
18. Ha HK, Shin JH, Rha SE, et al. Modified small-bowel follow-through: use of methylcellulose to improve bowel transradiance and prepare barium suspension. Radiology 1999;211:197–201.
19. Buckley JA Fishman EK. CT evaluation of small bowel neoplasms: spectrum of disease. Radiographics 1998;18:379–92.
20. Charnsangavej C. New imaging modalities for follow-up of colorectal carcinoma. Cancer 1993;71:4236–40.
21. Charnsangavej C, DuBrow RA, Varma DG, et al. CT of the mesocolon. Part 2. Pathologic considerations. Radiographics 1993;13:1309–22.
22. Granfield CA, Charnsangavej C, Dubrow RA, et al. Regional lymph node metastases in carcinoma of the left side of the colon and rectum: CT demonstration. AJR Am J Roentgenol 1992;159:757–61.
23. Brown G, Richards CJ, Newcombe RG, et al. Rectal carcinoma: thin-section MR imaging for staging in 28 patients. Radiology 1999;211:215–22.
24. Charnsangavej C, Loyer EM, Iyer RB, et al. Tumors of the liver, bile duct, and pancreas. Curr Probl Diagn Radiol 2000;29:69–107.
25. Machi J. Intraoperative and laparoscopic ultrasound. Surg Oncol Clin North Am 1999;8:205–26.
26. Nino-Murcia M, Olcott EW, Jeffrey RB Jr, et al. Focal liver lesions: pattern-based classification scheme for enhancement at arterial phase CT. Radiology 2000;215:746–51.
27. Loyer EM, Chin H, DuBrow RA, et al. Hepatocellular carcinoma and intrahepatic peripheral cholangiocarcinoma: enhancement patterns with quadruple phase helical CT—a comparative study. Radiology 1999;212:866–75.
28. Buetow PC, Pantongrag-Brown L, Buck JL, et al. Focal nodular hyperplasia of the liver: radiologic–pathologic correlation. Radiographics 1996;16:369–88.
29. Yamashita Y, Hatanaka Y, Yamamoto H, et al. Differential diagnosis of focal liver lesions: role of spin-echo and contrast-enhanced dynamic MR imaging. Radiology 1994;193:59–65.
30. Paulson EK, McDermott VG, Keogan MT, et al. Carcinoid metastases to the liver: role of triple-phase helical CT. Radiology 1998;206:143–50.
31. Oliver JH 3rd, Baron RL, Federle MP, Rockette HE Jr. Detecting hepatocellular carcinoma: value of unenhanced or arterial phase CT imaging or both used in conjunction with conventional portal venous phase contrast-enhanced CT imaging. AJR Am J Roentgenol 1996;167:71–7.
32. Valls C, Andia E, Sanchez A, et al. Hepatic metastases from colorectal cancer: preoperative detection and assessment of resectability with helical CT. Radiology 2001;218:55–60.
33. Baron RL Peterson MS. From the RSNA refresher courses: screening the cirrhotic liver for hepatocellular carcinoma with CT and MR imaging: opportunities and pitfalls. Radiographics 2001;21:S117–32.
34. Peterson MS, Baron RL, Marsh JW Jr, et al. Pretransplantation surveillance for possible hepatocellular carcinoma in patients with cirrhosis: epidemiology and CT-based tumor detection rate in 430 cases with surgical pathologic correlation. Radiology 2000;217:743–9.
35. Foley WD, Mallisee TA, Hohenwalter MD, et al. Multiphase hepatic CT with a multirow detector CT scanner. AJR Am J Roentgenol 2000;175:679–85.
36. Murakami T, Kim T, Takamura M, et al. Hypervascular hepatocellular carcinoma: detection with double arterial phase multi-detector row helical CT. Radiology 2001;218:763–7.
37. Dodd GD 3rd, Baron RL, Oliver JH 3rd, Federle MP. Spectrum of imaging findings of the liver in end-stage cirrhosis: part II, focal abnormalities. AJR Am J Roentgenol 1999;173:1185–92.
38. Schwartz LH, Gandras EJ, Colangelo SM, et al. Prevalence and importance of small hepatic lesions found at CT in patients with cancer. Radiology 1999;210:71–4.
39. Tillich M, Mischinger HJ, Preisegger KH, et al. Multiphasic helical CT in diagnosis and staging of hilar cholangiocarcinoma. AJR Am J Roentgenol 1998;171:651–8.
40. Feydy A, Vilgrain V, Denys A, et al. Helical CT assessment in hilar cholangiocarcinoma: correlation with surgical and pathologic findings. AJR Am J Roentgenol 1999;172:73–7.
41. McNulty NJ, Francis IR, Platt JF, et al. Multi-detector row helical CT of the pancreas: effect of contrast-enhanced multiphasic imaging on enhancement of the pancreas, peripancreatic vasculature, and pancreatic adenocarcinoma. Radiology 2001;220:97–102.
42. Legmann P, Vignaux O, Dousset B, et al. Pancreatic tumors: comparison of dual-phase helical CT and endoscopic sonography. AJR Am J Roentgenol 1998;170:1315–22.
43. Wiersema MJ. Endoscopic ultrasonography. J Gastrointest Surg 2002;6:129–32.
44. Murakami K, Nawano S, Moriyama N, Onuma Y. Usefulness of magnetic resonance imaging with dynamic contrast enhancement and fat suppression in detecting a pancreatic tumor. Jpn J Clin Oncol 1998;28:107–11.
45. Takehara Y. Fast MR imaging for evaluating the pancreaticobiliary system. Eur J Radiol 1999;29:211–32.
46. Freeny PC. Pancreatic carcinoma: imaging update 2001. Dig Dis 2001;19:37–46.
47. Irie H, Honda H, Kaneko K, et al. Comparison of helical CT and MR imaging in detecting and staging small pancreatic adenocarcinoma. Abdom Imaging 1997;22:429–33.
48. Boland GW, Lee MJ, Gazelle GS, et al. Characterization of adrenal masses using unenhanced CT: an analysis of the CT literature. AJR Am J Roentgenol 1998;171:201–4.
49. Caoili EM, Korobkin M, Francis IR, et al. Adrenal masses: characterization with combined unenhanced and delayed enhanced CT. Radiology 2002;222:629–33.
50. Jamis-Dow CA, Choyke PL, Jennings SB, et al. Small (≤3-cm) renal masses: detection with CT versus US and pathologic correlation. Radiology 1996;198:785–8.
51. Funt SA, Hann LE. Detection and characterization of adnexal masses. Radiol Clin North Am 2002;40:591–608.
52. Hricak H, Lacey CG, Sandles LG, et al. Invasive cervical carcinoma: comparison of MR imaging and surgical findings. Radiology 1988;166:623–31.
53. Frei KA, Kinkel K. Staging endometrial cancer: role of magnetic resonance imaging. J Magn Reson Imaging 2001;13:850–5.
54. Scheidler J, Hricak H, Yu KK, et al. Radiological evaluation of lymph node metastases in patients with cervical cancer. A meta-analysis. JAMA 1997;278:1096–101.
55. Narayan K, Hicks RJ, Jobling T, et al. A comparison of MRI and PET scanning in surgically staged loco-regionally advanced cervical cancer: potential impact on treatment. Int J Gynecol Cancer 2001;11:263–71.
56. Bartolozzi C, Crocetti L, Menchi I, et al. Endorectal magnetic resonance imaging in local staging of prostate carcinoma. Abdom Imaging 2001;26:111–22.
57. Presti JC Jr, Hricak H, Narayan PA, et al. Local staging of prostatic carcinoma: comparison of transrectal sonography and endorectal MR imaging. AJR Am J Roentgenol 1996;166:103–8.
58. Koutcher JA, Zakian K, Hricak H. Magnetic resonance spectroscopic studies of the prostate. Mol Urol 2000;4:143–52; discussion 153.

32e

Imaging of Musculoskeletal Neoplasms

R. Lee Cothran, MD
Clyde A. Helms, MD

Primary musculoskeletal neoplasms are relatively uncommon as compared with malignancies of other organ systems. Musculoskeletal involvement of malignancy is more often a result of metastatic disease from neoplasms of nonmusculoskeletal origins. These metastatic lesions are the ones most commonly evaluated by imaging. However, with the advent of computed tomography (CT), magnetic resonance (MR), and positron emission tomography (PET) imaging and advances in technique and equipment for percutaneous interventions, radiographic examination has become a critical component of the preoperative work-up of almost all instances of primary musculoskeletal malignancy.

Radiographs ("plain films") continue to be the mainstay of the primary evaluation of osseous neoplasms. It is from the radiograph that the abnormality is initially characterized. The lesion is determined to be either "aggressive" or "nonaggressive" based on its radiographic appearance. It is important that the foregoing terminology not be misinterpreted such that "aggressive" is considered equivalent to "malignant," because this is not always the case. The same is true for nonaggressive lesions. Although nonaggressive lesions are often benign, some malignant bone lesions—metastatic disease or myeloma, for example—may have a deceptively nonaggressive appearance on radiographs. Regardless, the radiograph is the starting point for an initial assessment of primary osseous lesions and for determination of the differential diagnosis.

After this initial evaluation is performed, cross-sectional imaging may be used to further define the anatomic detail of a lesion:

- Is there a soft-tissue component?
- If so, what is the extent of the soft-tissue component?
- What is the relationship to neurovascular structures?
- What anatomic compartments are involved?
- What is the extent of marrow involvement, and in special instances, are "skip lesions" present?

The answers to these questions can be gleaned from cross-sectional imaging and may help to narrow the differential diagnosis obtained from the radiograph, but they should not be used in isolation to generate a differential diagnosis. The primary importance of cross-sectional evaluation is treatment planning.

Primary neoplasms of the soft tissues of the musculoskeletal system may not be visible on radiographs. They often present as palpable masses or as pain or mass effect on adjacent structures. It remains important to obtain radiographs for an initial assessment of adjacent osseous involvement and for determining the presence or extent of mineralization within the mass. On radiographs, certain details may be visualized that are more difficult to visualize with cross-sectional imaging; the clues provided can be important in developing a differential diagnosis. However, because many soft-tissue musculoskeletal neoplasms have no adjacent osseous involvement or mineralization, cross-sectional imaging plays a somewhat greater role in developing a differential diagnosis for them than for primary osseous lesions.

Cross-sectional imaging is occasionally diagnostic, as in the pathognomonic appearance of benign lipomas (Figure 32e-1) or in cases in which the number or distribution of the masses is diagnostic, such as in neurofibromatosis (Figure 32e-2). However, in many soft-tissue masses, imaging characteristics are not diagnostic of the tumor type, and a differential diagnosis can be based only on probabilities. Such a differential diagnosis takes into account the signal characteristics of the mass, the anatomic location of the mass, the age of the patient, and the clinical presentation, among other factors. In some instances, cross-sectional imaging will not even determine whether a lesion is benign or malignant; but, even in those cases, it will provide valuable information about the extent of the lesion and its anatomic relationships. That information will be important in the eventual sampling of the lesion and in subsequent therapy.[1]

The appearance of musculoskeletal masses on MR imaging (MRI) is relatively nonspecific in many instances, because most tumors have similar signal characteristics: high T2 signal, and low or intermediate T1 signal (Figure 32e-3). However, for some tumors, MRI may provide a diagnosis—or at least a very limited differential—based on signal characteristics, location, and distribution. Tumors in which MRI may provide a definitive diagnosis include benign lipomas,[2] pigmented villonodular synovitis, most hemangiomas (Figure 32e-4), and many neural tumors. Plantar fibromatosis (Figure 32e-5), Morton neuromas, accessory muscles, and myxomas are all masses that may be easily diagnosed with MRI. Some masses have characteristics that may narrow the differential diagnosis considerably—for example, fluid–fluid levels in aneurysmal bone cysts and telangiectatic osteosarcomas. MRI can also be very useful in differentiating an enchondroma from a chondrosarcoma by evaluating for the presence of a soft-tissue mass, which is almost never present in an enchondroma.[3]

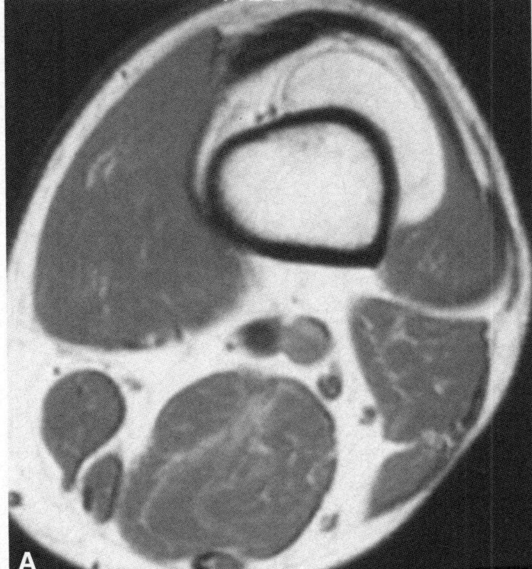

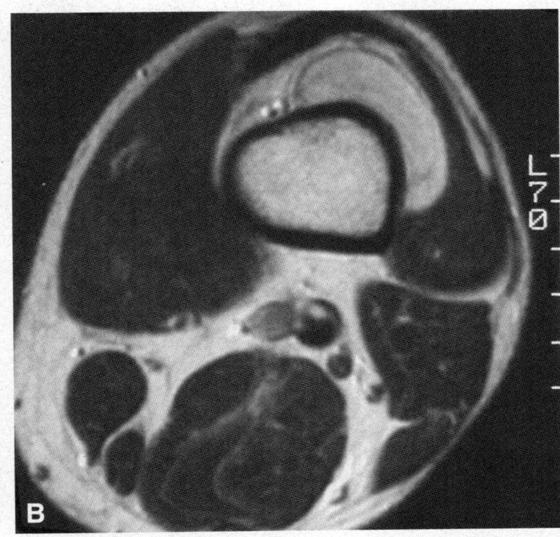

Figure 32e-1 **A,** T1-weighted and **B,** T2-weighted (without fat suppression) axial magnetic resonance images through the distal thigh reveal a high T1-, high T2-signal mass anterior to the distal femur consistent with a benign lipoma. Note how the signal characteristics match those of subcutaneous fat on both sequences.

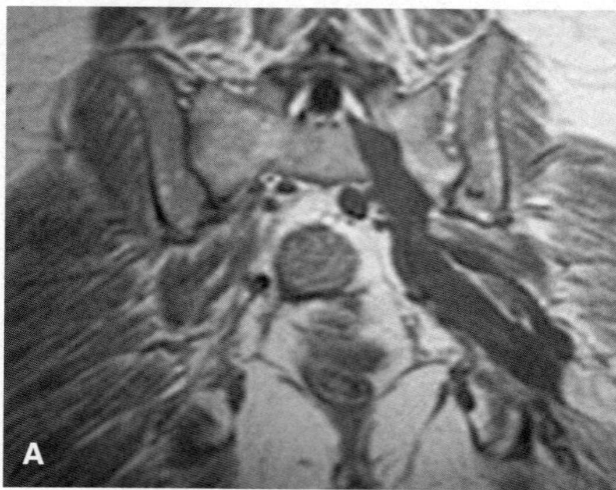

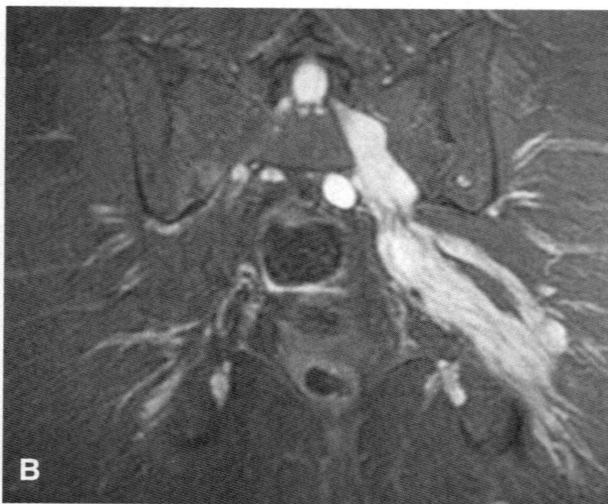

Figure 32e-2 **A,** T1-weighted and **B,** T2-weighted, fat-suppressed coronal magnetic resonance (MR) images through the sacrum reveal low-to-intermediate T1-signal, high T2-signal masses extending along the path of the sacral nerve roots and proximal sciatic nerve consistent with neurogenic tumors—in this case, neurofibromas. MR imaging permits a confident diagnosis based on distribution of the masses.

Given the primary purposes of cross-sectional imaging—to determine anatomic extent and to delineate relationships to adjacent tissues and compartments—MRI, even though it may not provide a definitive diagnosis in all cases, is of primary importance in the evaluation of musculoskeletal neoplasms. This importance reflects the superior ability of MRI, as compared with CT, to distinguish tissue types and to evaluate soft-tissue edema and marrow abnormality. CT has application in occasional cases in which characterization of mineralization is important. (MRI is not as helpful in characterizing mineralization because of many factors, including the artifact caused by the paramagnetic effect of calcium.) CT also has proven quite useful as a guide for percutaneous biopsy.[4] Ultrasonography is primarily useful as a guidance modality for percutaneous biopsy in select cases. It is also occasionally used to provide information on the solid or cystic nature of a known mass or to evaluate for flow within a lesion,[5] but it is not a primary diagnostic modality for musculoskeletal neoplasms. PET imaging currently has limited application in musculoskeletal neoplasms; it is primarily used for identification of distant soft-tissue metastases, although some research suggests that quantitative analysis of glucose metabolism might help to differentiate benign from malignant primary bone lesions.[6,7] However, quantitative analysis of glucose metabolism is not standard practice. The standardized uptake value (SUV)—widely used in other malignancies—shows considerable overlap in the case of benign and malignant musculoskeletal lesions.[8]

Dynamic contrast-enhanced MRI of musculoskeletal masses has been described as a potential tool for establishing a more accurate diagnosis.[9] The pattern and degree of delayed enhancement and the patterns of dynamic enhancement reportedly have potential utility in the characterization of masses.[10] However, the utility of contrast enhancement for musculoskeletal neoplasms is relatively limited in practice. The primary utility occurs in those few cases in which a very bright T2 lesion needs to be classified as solid or cystic. A solid lesion will exhibit at least a small degree of enhancement throughout the mass; a cystic or fluid-filled lesion will enhance only peripherally. Because of the reduced ability of CT imaging to distinguish subtle tissue differences, intravenous contrast administration may have an increased role in CT evaluation of musculoskeletal malignancies in geographic locations where MRI is not easily accessible.

Once a lesion has been identified and characterized, a biopsy or a resection of the lesion for histologic evaluation is often necessary so that a more specific diagnosis can be made before definitive therapy is delivered. Percutaneous sampling of musculoskeletal neoplasms has become increasingly important in these pretreatment evaluations. As the tools for performing such biopsies have improved, and as the experience level with the techniques has improved, percutaneous sampling has become an alternative to open biopsy in many cases.[11] Larger-gauge needles with acquisition of tissue cores are necessary for characterizing most lesions, but experienced pathologists may be able to make an accurate diagnosis of some neoplasms based on smaller-gauge fine-needle aspiration.[12]

Many musculoskeletal masses are palpable and therefore may be percutaneously sampled by an experienced physician without the need for imaging guidance. In cases that require imaging assistance, CT scanning provides excellent visualization of a path for needle placement. Although fluoroscopic guidance may be used for biopsies, the greater delineation of anatomic structures and the improved ability to evaluate for soft-tissue components of osseous masses and for thinning of the cortex make CT imaging the modality of choice in many, if not most, cases. The advantages potentially reduce the required number of needle placements, allow better visualization of structures that are to be avoided, and therefore theoretically reduce the complication rate and improve the biopsy yield. MRI may be used as a guide for percutaneous sampling, but special non-ferromagnetic sampling equipment and, often, an open MR scanner or an otherwise modified imaging system are required. As a result, percutaneous sampling of musculoskeletal masses may be more time-consuming. Ultrasonography may also be used as a guidance modality for sampling soft-tissue masses, but it is of limited utility in predominantly osseous lesions.

Regardless of the modality used to guide percutaneous sampling, it is critical that the physician performing the biopsy be in communication with the surgeon in charge of the definitive therapy. In many instances, the compartmental anatomy of a lesion is vital to the surgeon's eventual approach.[13,14] Surgical therapy in many sarcomas can be radically altered because of a need to resect the biopsy tract after compartments not involved by tumor are contaminated by passing a needle through them on the biopsy approach. In some cases, a lack of communication between the

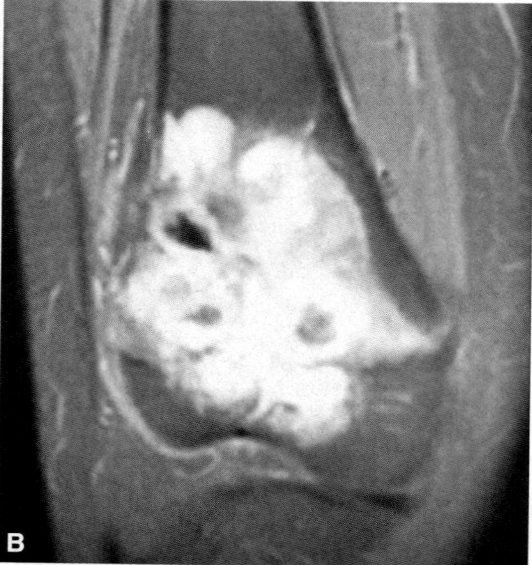

Figure 32e-3 **A,** T1-weighted and **B,** T2-weighted, fat-suppressed coronal magnetic resonance images of an osteosarcoma in the distal femur. These signal characteristics are common in malignant and benign tumors; consequently, the signal alone is not diagnostic.

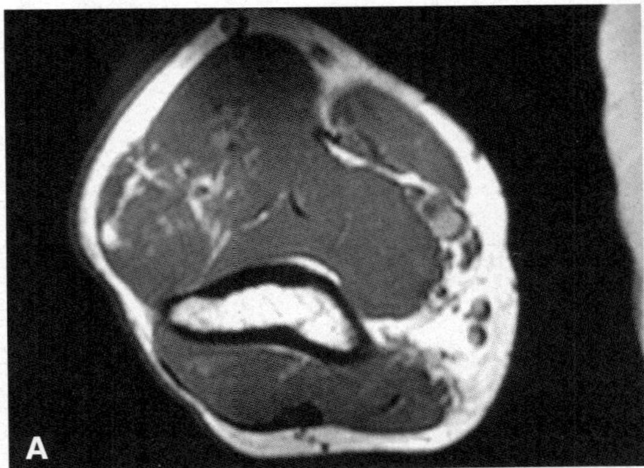

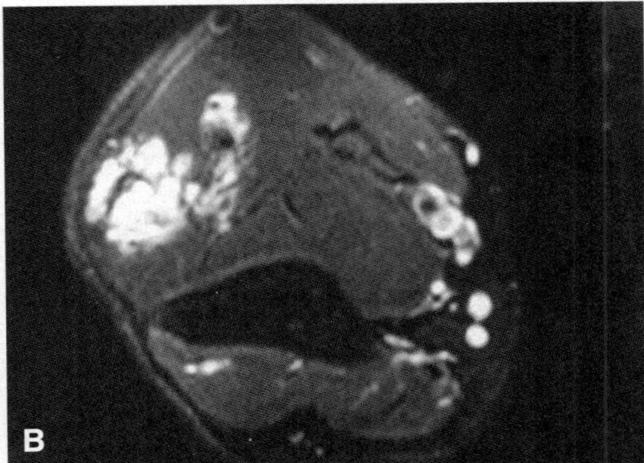

Figure 32e-4 **A,** T1-weighted and **B,** T2-weighted, fat-suppressed axial magnetic resonance images through the upper arm reveal a lobulated mass with interdigitating fat signal and extension through fascial planes. These characteristics are diagnostic of a soft-tissue hemangioma.

physician performing the biopsy and the surgeon may even result in an amputation having to be performed when a limb-sparing procedure might otherwise have been an option.

Involvement of the pathologist in the discussion concerning a lesion to be percutaneously sampled is also critical. Interpretation of the histology of musculoskeletal neoplasms is best performed by a pathologist with particular experience in musculoskeletal oncology. The differences between malignant and benign histology may be subtle and can depend on characteristics of the lesion that cannot be obtained from a gross or microscopic sample alone. Histologic characteristics or patterns that would be interpreted as benign in one anatomic location may be interpreted as more ominous or aggressive in another. The radiologic assessment can therefore play a critical role in the eventual histologic diagnosis. Ultimately, a cooperative effort between the radiologist, the surgeon, the pathologist, and the oncologist is optimal for a complete assessment and development of a treatment plan.

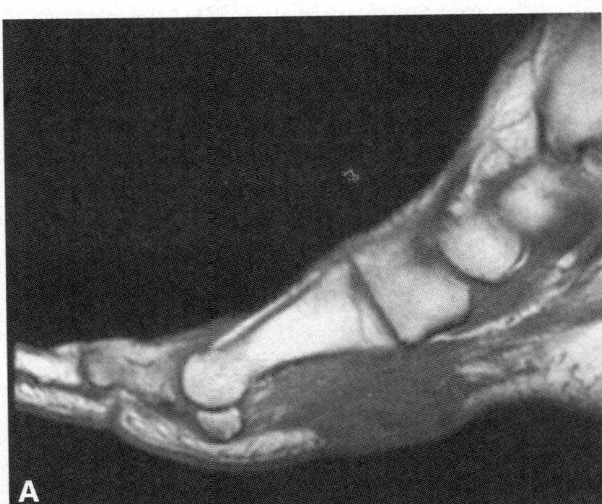

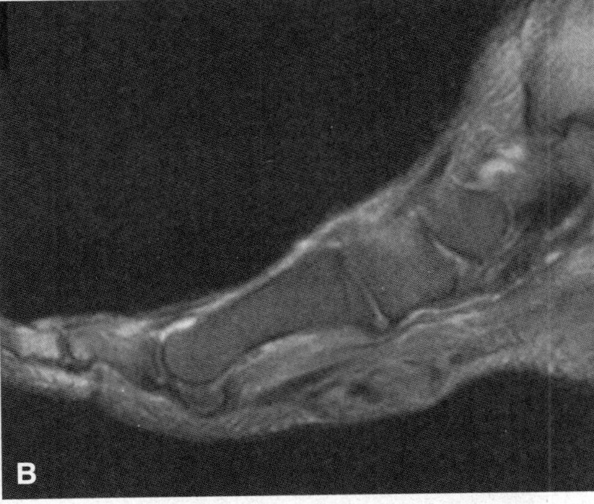

Figure 32e-5 **A,** T1-weighted and **B,** T2-weighted, fat-suppressed sagittal images of the foot reveal low-T1-, low-T2-signal mass in the plantar aspect of the foot. This combination of signal characteristics and location is diagnostic of plantar fibromatosis.

In summary, imaging evaluation of musculoskeletal neoplasms has become a critical part of developing a treatment plan. Imaging has also provided an avenue for characterizing and even sampling lesions before institution of definitive therapy, thus reducing the risk of biopsy in many patients and providing a greater degree of information about the anatomy and extent of a tumor than has been available in the past. As a result, unnecessary interventions can be avoided and a much more focused therapeutic plan can be established for patients in whom further intervention is required.

REFERENCES

1. Berquist T, Ehman R, King B, et al. Value of MR imaging in differentiating benign from malignant soft tissue masses: study of 95 lesions. AJR Am J Roentgenol 1990;155:1251–5.
2. Gaskin CM, Helms CA. Lipomas, lipoma variants, and well-differentiated liposarcomas (atypical lipomas): results of MRI evaluations of 126 consecutive fatty masses. AJR Am J Roentgenol 2004;182:733–9.
3. Murphy MD, Flemming DJ, et al. Enchondroma versus chondrosarcoma in the appendicular skeleton—differentiating features. Radiographics 1998;18:1213–37.
4. Edeiken B, deSantos LA. Percutaneous needle biopsy of the irradiated skeleton. Radiology 1983;146:653–5.
5. Park KS, Choi BI, Won HJ, et al. Intratumoral vascularity of experimentally induced VX2 carcinoma: comparison of color Doppler sonography, power Doppler sonography, and microangiography. Invest Radiol 1998;33:39–44.
6. Dimitrakopoulou-Strauss A, Strauss LG, Schwarzbach M, et al. Dynamic PET ^{18}F-FDG studies in patients with primary and recurrent soft-tissue sarcomas: impact on diagnosis and correlation with grading. J Nucl Med 2001;42:713–20.
7. Wu H, Dimitrakopoulou-Strauss A, Heichel TO, et al. Quantitative evaluation of skeletal tumours with dynamic FDG PET: SUV in comparison to Patlak analysis. Eur J Nucl Med 2001;28:704–10.
8. Aoki J, Watanabe H, Shinizaki T, et al. FDG PET of primary benign and malignant bone tumors: standardized uptake value in 52 lesions. Radiology 2001;219:774–7.
9. Versraete KL, Van der Woude HJ, Hogendoorn PCW, et al. Dynamic contrast-enhanced MR imaging of musculoskeletal tumors: basic principles and clinical applications. J Magn Reson Imaging 1996;6:311–21.
10. Geirnaerdt MJA, Hogendoorn PCW, Bloem JL, et al. Cartilaginous tumors: fast contrast-enhanced MR imaging. Radiology 2000;214:539–46.
11. Leffler SG, Chew FS. CT-guided percutaneous biopsy of sclerotic bone lesions: diagnostic yield and accuracy. AJR Am J Roentgenol 1999;172:1389–92.
12. Ward WG, Kilpatrick S. Fine-needle aspiration biopsy of primary bone tumors. Clin Orthop Relat Res 2000;373:80–7.
13. Anderson MW, Temple HT, Dussault RG, et al. Compartmental anatomy: relevance to staging and biopsy of musculoskeletal tumors. AJR Am J Roentgenol 1999;173:1663–71.
14. Toomayan GA, Robertson F, Major NM. Lower extremity compartmental anatomy: clinical relevance to radiologists. Skeletal Radiol 2005;34:307–13.

32f

Imaging the Breast

Lawrence W. Bassett, MD, FACR
Olegario Jay Lara, DO

Today, breast imaging encompasses numerous technologies. Mammography is the primary screening and diagnostic tool. Ultrasonography is the major adjunctive technology. Image-guided biopsies have become the preferred method for tissue diagnosis. In addition, magnetic resonance imaging (MRI) and radionuclide imaging are under investigation as additional adjunctive tools for diagnostic breast evaluation.

TYPES OF MAMMOGRAPHY

There are two basic types of mammographic examinations: screening and diagnostic. "Screening mammography" refers to examination of an asymptomatic woman to detect clinically occult breast cancer.[1] The screening examination includes two views of the breast, sometimes called the "standard views": a mediolateral oblique view and a craniocaudal view.[2] Controversies over the exact statistical benefit from screening mammography continue, but a recent review of the current literature by the U.S. Institute of Medicine recommended mammography as the most effective screening tool for breast cancer detection.[3] In addition, a recent report of screening in seven Swedish counties encompassing approximately 33% of the population of Sweden showed a 40 to 45% reduction in breast carcinoma mortality among women actually screened.[4] That study indicated that most of the reduction in breast carcinoma mortality noted in recent years resulted primarily from screening.

"Diagnostic mammography," also called "consultative" or "problem-solving" mammography, is performed when clinical findings such as a palpable lump or an abnormal screening mammogram require additional study.[5] Diagnostic mammography may entail additional views of the breast such as spot compression and magnification, a correlative clinical examination, and ultrasonography. With some exceptions, a radiologist should be present during the performance of a diagnostic mammography study.

Diagnostic mammography should also be performed when a biopsy is being considered for a palpable lump in a woman older than 30 years of age. Diagnostic mammography before biopsy of a palpable mass is intended to define the nature of the clinical abnormality and to find any other (unexpected) lesions, including multifocal carcinomas or intraductal extension of an invasive carcinoma. To correlate the clinical with the imaging findings, a radiopaque marker ("BB") should be placed over any area of clinical concern before the diagnostic mammogram is performed.

STANDARDIZED MAMMOGRAPHY REPORTING

The American College of Radiology (ACR) Breast Imaging Reporting and Data System (BI-RADS) mammography report should include the reason or reasons for the examination, the tissue composition of the breast, a description of the findings using the standardized lexicon, and a final assessment with a management recommendation.[6]

Breast-Tissue Composition The overall density of a patient's breast tissue helps to determine the sensitivity of mammography. The standardized mammography report therefore includes a statement about the overall composition of the breast in terms of the relative amounts of fatty and dense tissue. Because breast cancers are radiodense (eg, white on mammograms), radiolucent fat (dark gray-to-black on mammograms) provides an excellent background in which to see cancers. On the other hand, dense fibroglandular tissue can obscure small cancers.

Breast composition can be characterized as one of four types: (1) the breast is almost entirely fat (< 25% glandular, Figure 32f-1A); (2) there are scattered islands of fibroglandular tissue (approximately 25 to 50% glandular); (3) the breast tissue is heterogeneously dense (approximately 51 to 75% glandular), which may lower the sensitivity of mammography; and (4) the breast tissue is extremely dense (> 75% glandular), which will lower the sensitivity of mammography (Figure 32f-1B).

Findings The standard lexicon descriptors for reporting abnormal findings on mammograms indicate the likelihood of malignancy. Masses and calcifications are the most common findings, and their radiographic presentation is an important clue to their cause.

Overall Impression and Assessment Category The standardized report concludes with one of seven assessment categories, indicating the likelihood of malignancy and the recommendations for management (Table 32f-1). Category 0 (incomplete, needs additional imaging evalua-

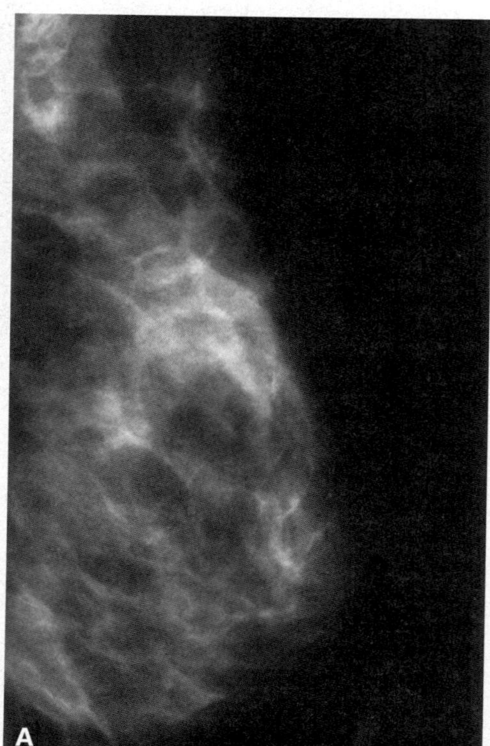

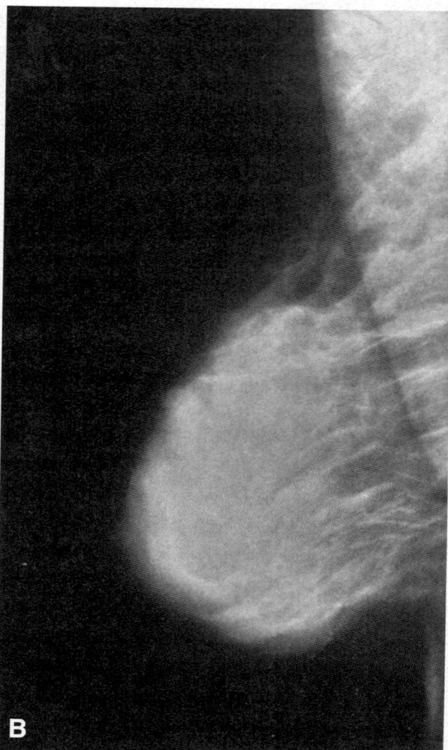

Figure 32f-1 Varying breast tissue composition: **A,** Primarily fatty breast, with scattered islands of fibroglandular tissue. Mammography has high sensitivity in this type of breast. **B,** Extremely dense breast. The sensitivity of mammography is limited because of the dense tissue, which could obscure a carcinoma.

Table 32f-1 American College of Radiology Mammography Assessment Categories

Category	Assessment	Description
0	Incomplete assessment	Additional imaging or prior mammograms, or both, are needed for comparison.
1	Negative	There is nothing to comment on. Routine screening recommended.
2	Benign finding	A definitely benign finding described. Routine screening recommended.
3	Probably benign finding	Very high probability of being benign; <2% risk of malignancy. Short-term follow-up recommended to establish stability.
4	Suspicious abnormality	Not characteristic, but has reasonable probability of being malignant. Biopsy should be considered.
5	Highly suggestive of malignancy	These lesions have a high probability (≥ 95%) of being cancer. Appropriate action should be taken.
6	Known, biopsy-proven malignancy	This category is reserved for lesions identified on the imaging study with biopsy proof of malignancy before definitive therapy. Appropriate action should be taken.

tion) is used for a screening examination in which a definitive recommendation cannot be made until more information is obtained. Once additional work-up has been completed, a final assessment is assigned. The *Mammography Quality Standards Act* (MQSA) requires that the assessment category be included in the mammography report.[7]

THE MAMMOGRAM WITH NORMAL FINDINGS

The mammographic appearance of the normal breast varies (see Figure 32f-1). Because younger women usually have more fibroglandular tissue, their breasts tend to be more "dense." However, the variation in normal breast density patterns of younger and older women is great. An increase in breast density has been reported in postmenopausal women in conjunction with exogenous hormone replacement.

THE MAMMOGRAM WITH ABNORMAL FINDINGS

Masses The features that most significantly indicate whether a mass is benign or malignant are its shape and margins (Figure 32f-2).

Figure 32f-2 Terminology used to describe masses.

The shape can be round, oval, lobular, or irregular. Circumscribed oval and round masses are usually benign. An irregular shape suggests a greater likelihood of malignancy.

The margins can be described as circumscribed, microlobulated, obscured (partially hidden by adjacent tissue), indistinct (ill-defined), or spiculated (characterized by lines radiating from the mass). The likelihood of malignancy with a circumscribed mass is very low, but additional work-up may be necessary to verify that the margins are completely circumscribed. Typical examples of benign circumscribed masses are cysts (Figure 32f-3) and fibroadenomas (Figure 32f-4). Ultrasonography can determine whether a circumscribed mass is cystic or solid. If the mass is a simple cyst, no further work-up is necessary. If the mass is solid, the shape and margins should be evaluated carefully, possibly with magnification mammography. Unless previous mammograms establish it as a new finding, a solitary, completely circumscribed, nonpalpable, solid mass is often managed by 6-month follow-up examination to establish that the mass is stable (not growing).[8] If the mass is stable, continued mammographic surveillance is recommended for at least 2 years. If a circumscribed mass is directly adjacent to fibroglandular tissue of similar density, the margins of the mass may be obscured, and spot compression is used to show the margins of the mass more completely.

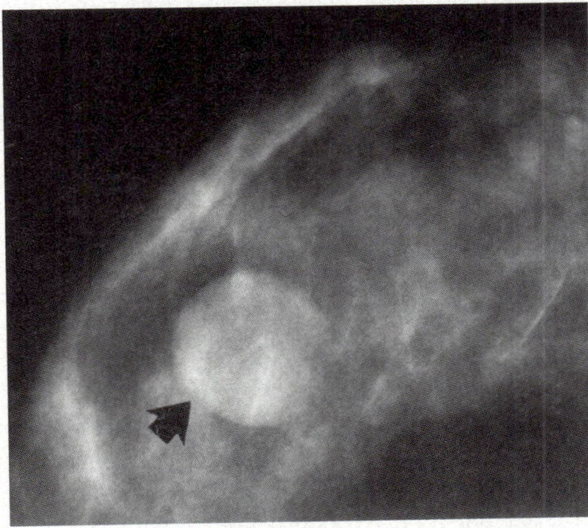

Figure 32f-3 Cyst: Mediolateral oblique mammogram shows a round, circumscribed mass (*arrow*) in the subareolar area. Ultrasonography revealed a simple cyst.

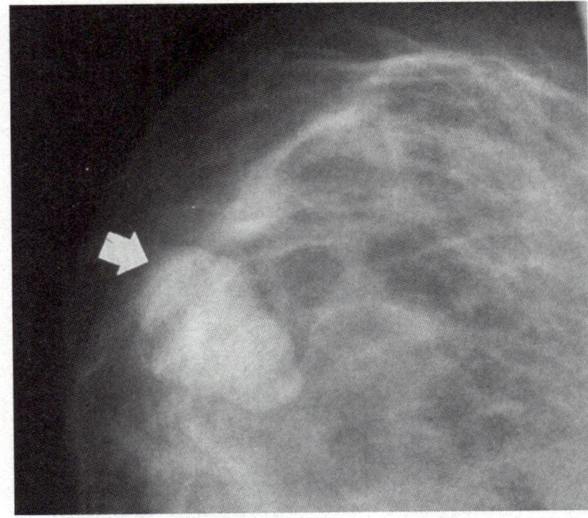

Figure 32f-4 Fibroadenoma: Mediolateral mammogram shows a lobular, circumscribed mass (*arrow*). Biopsy revealed fibroadenoma.

Masses with irregular shapes and indistinct or spiculated margins have a higher likelihood of being malignant. Indistinct margins (Figure 32f-5) generally raise suspicion of malignancy, and spiculated margins (Figure 32f-6) are highly suggestive of malignancy. Nonetheless, a small number of cancers may exhibit a round shape and relatively circumscribed margins.

The density of a mass can be designated as low, intermediate (see Figures 32f-3 and 32f-4), or high (see Figure 32f-5) by comparing it with an area of

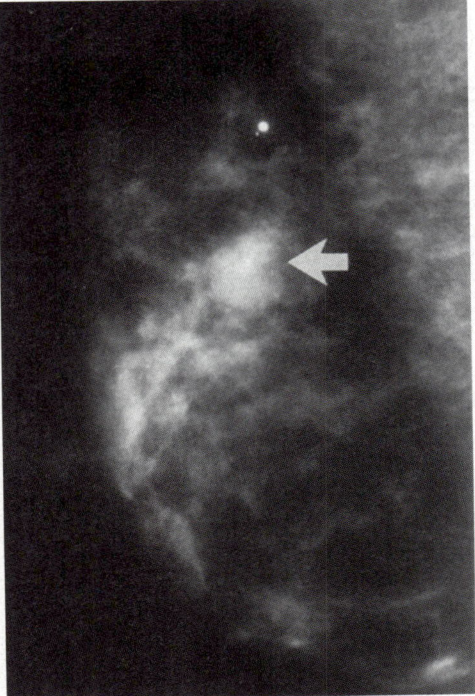

Figure 32f-5 Invasive ductal carcinoma: Close-up of mammogram shows a mass (*arrow*) with an irregular shape and ill-defined margins.

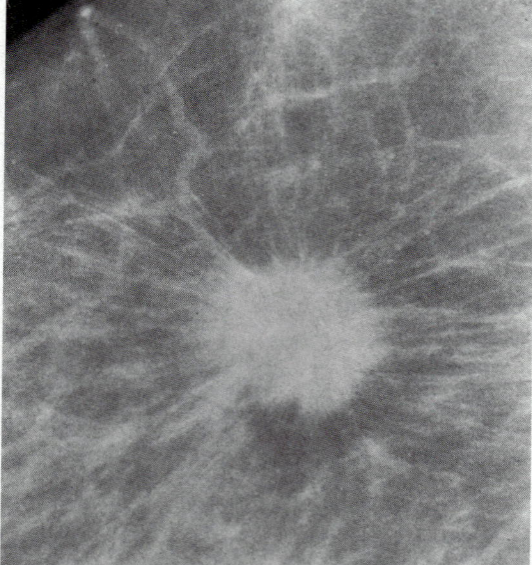

Figure 32f-6 Invasive ductal carcinoma: Close-up of mammogram shows a mass with irregular shape and spiculated margins.

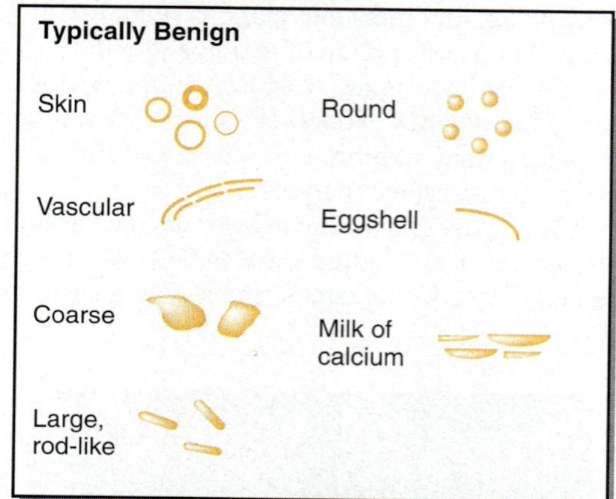

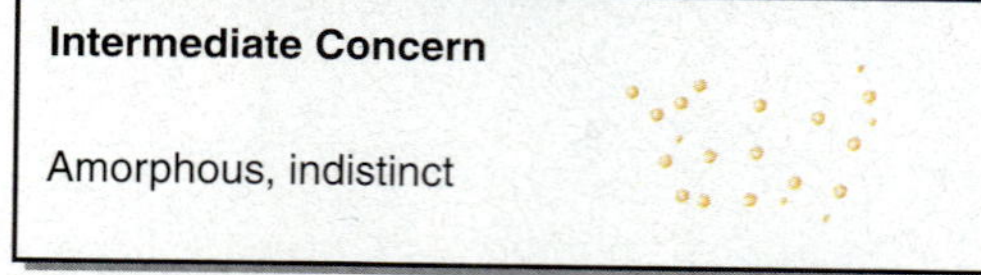

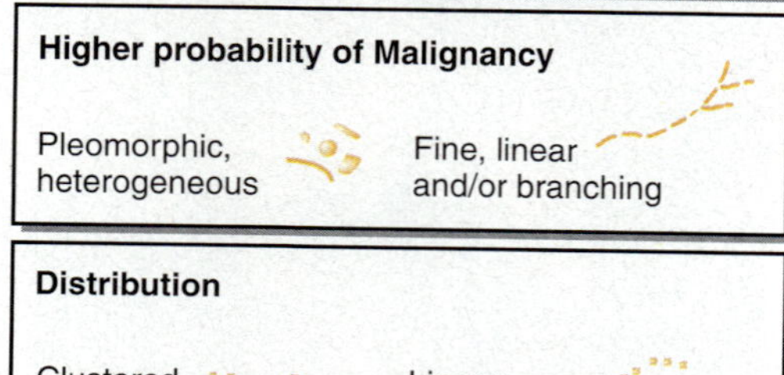

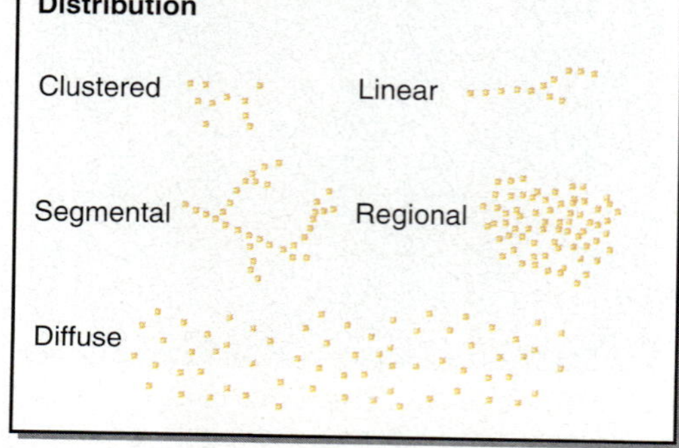

Figure 32f-7 Terminology used to describe calcifications.

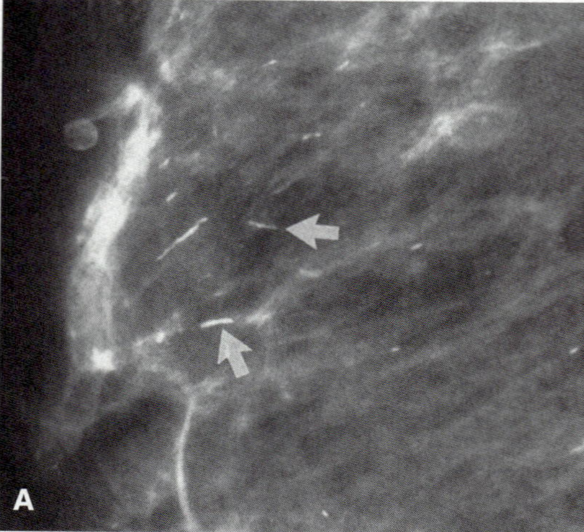

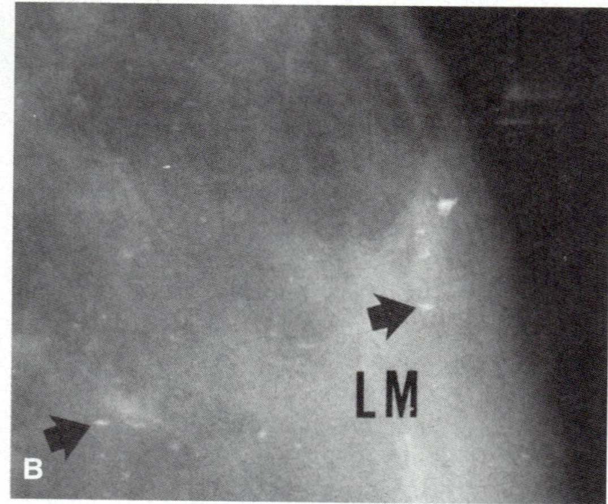

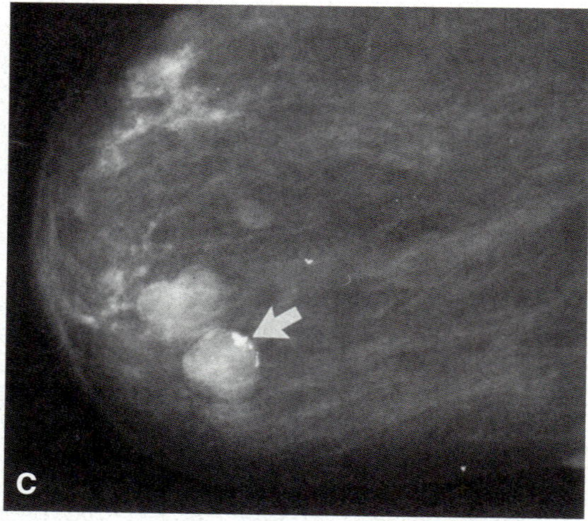

Figure 32f-8 Typically benign calcifications: **A,** Rod-like calcifications (*arrows*) of benign secretory disease (duct ectasia). **B,** Ninety-degree lateral mammograms reveal calcifications (*arrows*) that layer at the bottom of fluid-filled microcysts. These are sometimes called "milk of calcium" or "teacup calcifications" (analogous to tea leaves that settle to the bottom of a cup). **C,** Coarse calcification (*arrow*) on the rim of a fibroadenoma.

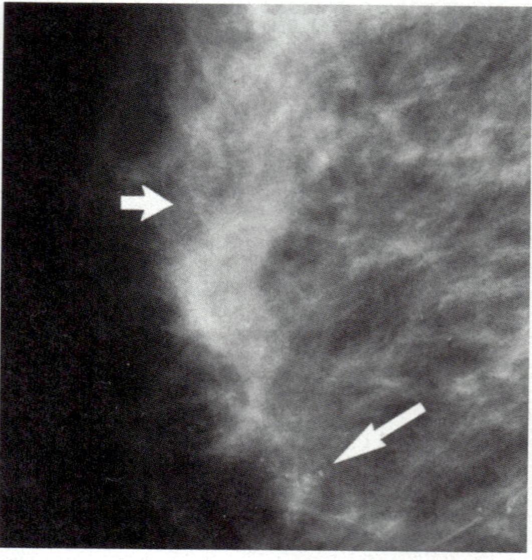

Figure 32f-9 Barely visible intermediate (amorphous, indistinct) calcifications (*arrows*).

normal breast tissue on the mammogram. Benign masses tend to be lower in density than carcinomas are, but density is frequently not a reliable sign.[9]

CALCIFICATIONS In the BI-RADS lexicon, calcifications are categorized as typically benign, intermediate-concern, or higher probability of malignancy (Figure 32f-7).

"Typically benign" calcifications include skin, vascular, coarse, large rod-like, round, eggshell, and milk-of-calcium types (Figure 32f-8). Many calcifications are so typical of a benign lesion that additional work-up is unnecessary. However, if any doubt exists, magnification mammography should be performed.

"Intermediate-concern" calcifications are tiny, amorphous, or indistinct (Figure 32f-9).

"Higher probability of malignancy" calcifications can be pleomorphic, heterogeneous, or fine, linear, and branching (casting) in any combination (Figure 32f-10). Malignant calcifications may occur with or without an associated mass.[10] Calcifications are often the only evidence of an intraductal carcinoma or ductal carcinoma in situ (DCIS).[11]

Calcifications can also be characterized by their distribution: the terms "grouped" or "clustered" calcifications refer to groups of more than five within a small tissue volume (< 2 cm^3); they can be benign or malignant (Figure 32f-10A). Fine, linear, branching calcifications arranged in a line that may have small branch points (Figure 32f-10B) is a distribution that raises suspicion of malignancy. Segmental calcifications (Figure 32f-11) that are distributed in a duct and its branches also suggest malignancy. Regional calcifications occupy a larger volume of breast tissue and can be associated with either benign or malignant conditions. Diffuse or scattered calcifications are distributed randomly through the breast and are almost always benign.

INDIRECT SIGNS OF MALIGNANCY Other indirect or subtle signs that may suggest malignancy include a neodensity, architectural distortion, or asymmetry.[12] Identifying these subtle signs may require careful comparison with previous examinations. Any new or evolving density that is identified by comparison with previous mammograms should lead to further evaluation. Ultrasonogra-

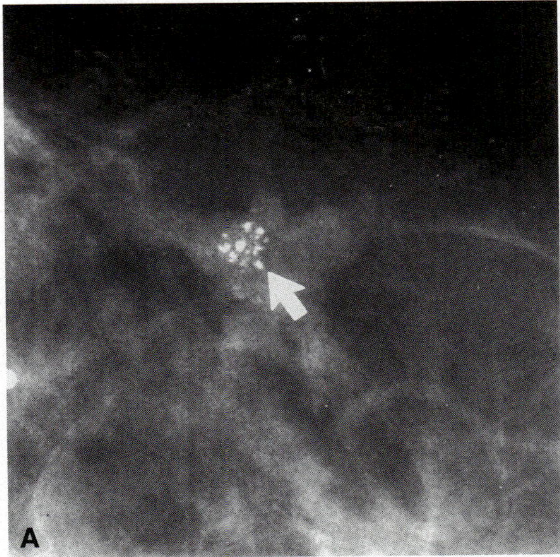

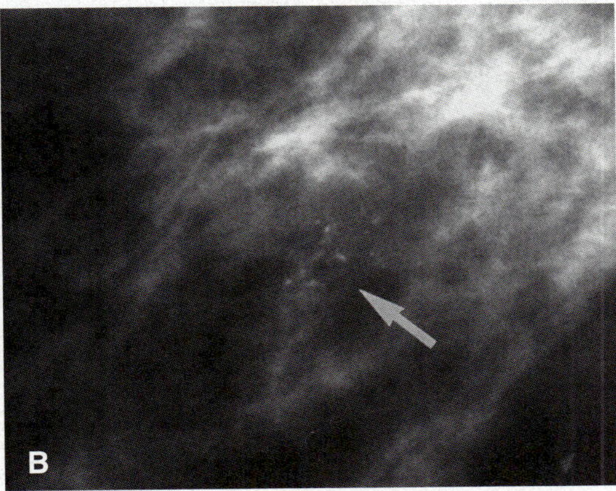

Figure 32f-10 Calcifications with higher probability of malignancy: **A,** This cluster manifests pleomorphic calcifications (*arrows*) of varying size and shape. Biopsy revealed intraductal cribriform carcinoma. **B,** Fine, linear, branching calcifications (*arrow*) are highly suggestive of intraductal carcinoma. Biopsy revealed comedocarcinoma with calcification of necrotic debris in the center of tumor-filled duct.

phy may be indicated if the neodensity has features suggestive of a cyst.

Architectural distortion is the appearance on a mammogram of spicules without an associated mass (Figure 32f-12). The differential diagnosis includes scarring from previous surgery, radial scar, and carcinoma.

Asymmetric breast tissue is one of the most difficult findings to evaluate. The breasts tend to be relatively symmetric in their distribution of fibroglandular tissue. Minor asymmetry between the two breasts is a common variant, but a new or prominent asymmetry warrants further investigation. Further work-up should include a correlative clinical breast examination, additional mammographic views, and ultrasonography. When asymmetry is associated with architectural distortion, calcifications, or an underlying mass, the probability of malignancy is greater, and a biopsy should be considered.

MAMMOGRAPHY FOR PREOPERATIVE PLANNING

Mammography before biopsy of a palpable abnormality is useful for excluding bilateral or multifocal lesions, but not for evaluating ipsilateral axillary nodes. Although normal-sized or enlarged axillary nodes can be visualized in the mediolateral oblique views, no mammographic criteria effectively exclude nodal involvement.[13] Consequently, histologic assessment of the nodes remains essential to staging invasive carcinomas.

MAMMOGRAPHY OF THE POSTSURGICAL BREAST

Postsurgical changes on mammograms may include skin thickening or retraction, architectural distortion, asymmetry, calcification, and fat necrosis.[14] Any of these changes can mimic a carcinoma. Knowledge of the sites of previous breast surgery or biopsy is therefore important when interpreting mammograms. When patients have undergone breast-conservation surgery, knowledge of the location of the lumpectomy scar and comparison of the current study with a baseline postsurgical study are particularly important. In general, a scar should decrease in size over time.

Breast-conservation therapy for extensive intraductal carcinoma manifested by calcifications (see Figure 32f-11) entails special management protocols before and after surgery (Figure 32f-13). Multiple localization needles ("bracketing") may be required preoperatively to guide excision of malignant calcifications. Specimen radiography is useful to show that the calcifications are in the specimen. If calcifications extend to the margins of the specimen, re-excision can be performed before wound closure. Before radiotherapy is started, magnification mammography should also be performed directly over the surgical site to rule out residual malignant calcifications—even if the inked margins were clear histologically. If calcifications are still present, local re-excision or a mastectomy may be considered.[15]

ULTRASONOGRAPHY

The normal breast exhibits some typical features on ultrasonography (Figure 32f-14). Sonographic images depict the skin as double parallel lines, below which is a layer consisting of hypo-

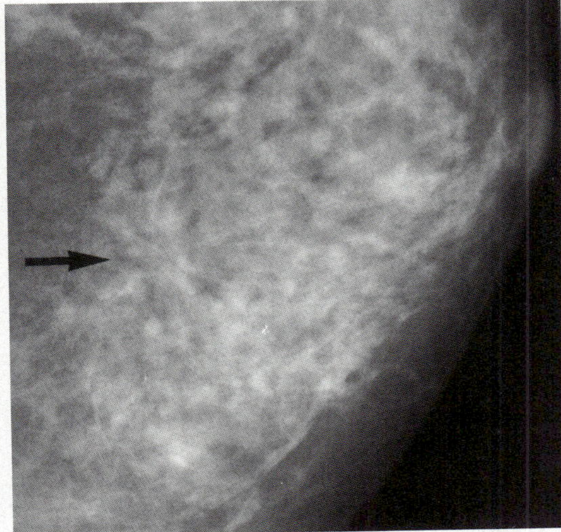

Figure 32f-11 Segmental distribution of the fine, linear, branching calcifications (*arrows*) of intraductal comedocarcinoma.

Figure 32f-12 Invasive carcinoma presenting as a subtle architectural distortion. Biopsy revealed an 8 mm invasive ductal carcinoma.

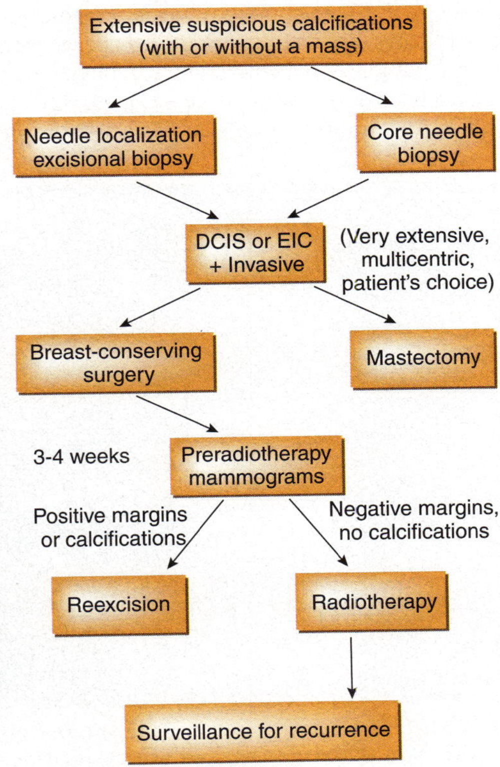

Figure 32f-13 Protocol for managing extensive suspicious calcifications.

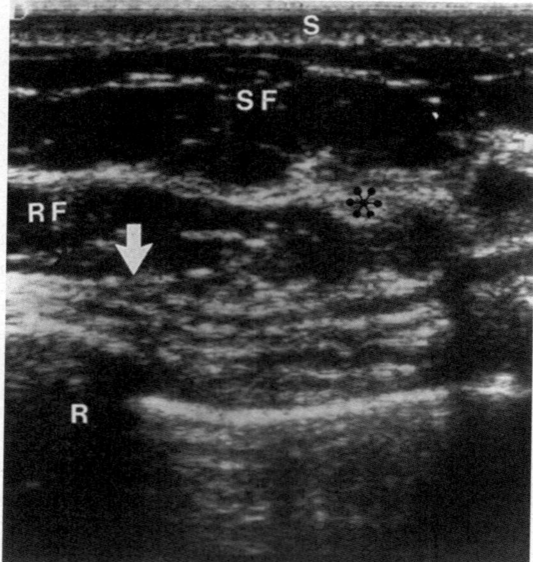

Figure 32f-14 Ultrasonography of the normal breast: The skin (S) lies between two bright echogenic lines on the surface of the breast. The subcutaneous fat (SF) is hypoechoic. The fibroglandular tissue (*) is relatively echogenic. Retroglandular fat (RF) is also present. The ultrasonographic appearance will vary according to the relative proportions of fat and fibroglandular tissue. Arrows = anterior boundary of pectoral muscle; R = rib.

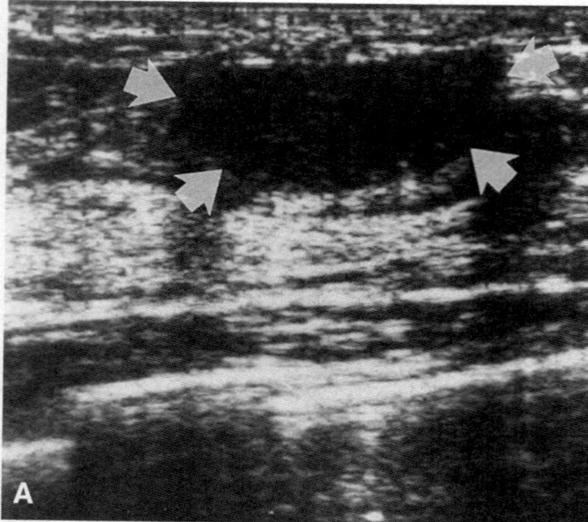

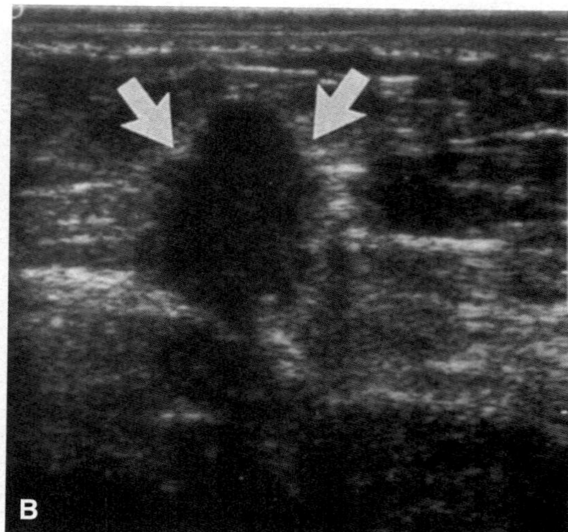

Figure 32f-16 Ultrasonography features typical of benign and malignant masses: **A,** This benign fibroadenoma (*arrows*) is characterized by an oval shape, wider-than-tall dimensions, and circumscribed margins. **B,** This carcinoma (*arrows*) has an ill-defined irregular shape, taller-than-wide dimensions, low-level heterogeneous internal echoes, and ill-defined margins.

echoic lobules of subcutaneous fat. Fibroglandular tissue in the breast is more echogenic than fat. Hypoechoic fat may also be visible deep to the glandular tissue and adjacent to the pectoral muscle, which lies at the base of the breast, overlying the ribs and chest wall.

The role of ultrasonography in breast imaging continues to evolve. The traditional role of ultrasonography is to differentiate cysts from solid masses.[16–18] Characteristic ultrasonographic features of a cyst are its round or oval shape, circumscribed margins, anechoic interior, and enhanced distal echoes posterior to the cyst (Figure 32f-15). Continuing improvements in ultrasonography equipment have led to the identification of additional features that may help to differentiate benign from malignant solid masses.[19] These additional features include the shape, margins, and echogenicity of a breast mass (Figure 32f-16). It remains to be seen whether these signs are reliable enough to avoid the need for biopsy of solid masses that have "benign" ultrasonographic features.

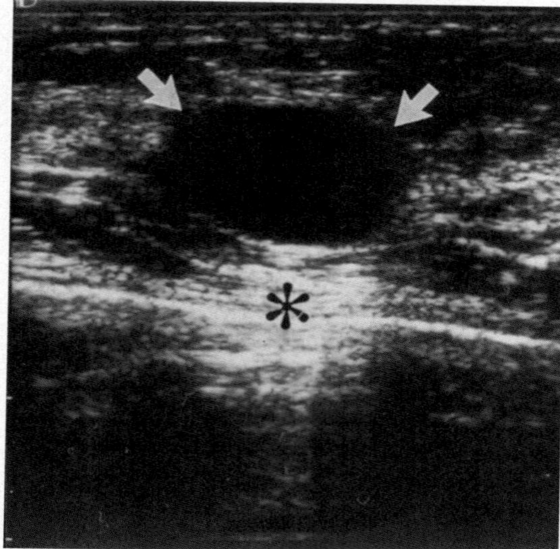

Figure 32f-15 Sonogram of a cyst: The cyst (*arrow*) is characterized by an oval or round shape, circumscribed margins, absence of internal echoes (anechoic interior), clearly defined posterior wall, and enhancement of distal echoes (*).

Although ultrasonography has not yet been proven effective for breast cancer screening, evidence is growing that the technology can be useful in identifying multifocal carcinoma in the dense breast.[20] Ultrasonography also plays an important role in guiding interventional procedures such as fine-needle aspiration biopsy, core-needle biopsy, and prebiopsy needle localization of breast masses or calcifications.[21,22]

IMAGING-GUIDED NEEDLE BIOPSY OF THE BREAST

The positive predictive value of breast biopsies that have been prompted by mammographic abnormalities—that is, the number of cancers detected divided by the number of biopsies done—has been reported to be in the range of 10 to 40%,[23] with a desirable range being 25 to 40%.[1] Concerns about the positive predictive value of imaging studies relate to the cost and morbidity of biopsies that are performed for what later prove to be benign conditions. Some reports suggest that the costs of such biopsies may exceed the costs of screening.[24]

As an alternative to open-breast biopsy, percutaneous needle biopsy results in lower costs, less morbidity, no breast scarring, and no changes in subsequent mammograms. In Europe, fine-needle aspiration cytology (FNAC) has largely replaced excisional biopsy, thus reducing the overall costs of mammographic screening.[25] In the United States, barriers to wider acceptance of FNAC for nonpalpable breast abnormalities have included inadequate numbers of skilled cytopathologists, variability in the reported accuracy, high rates of insufficient samples, and the current medicolegal environment.[26] Even when adequate specimens are obtained, a definitive diagnosis is not always possible. For example, FNAC cannot differentiate infiltrating carcinoma from in situ carcinoma. However, when properly performed and interpreted by an experienced cytologist, FNAC can be a useful tool in identifying benign masses such as fibroadenoma.

In recent years, core needle biopsy (CNB) of the breast has been widely adopted in the United States as a substitute for excisional biopsy.[27] Compared with FNAC, CNB can offer a more specific diagnosis, greater accuracy, and fewer inadequate specimens, without the requirement for specially trained cytopathologists. Stereotactic mammography equipment can be used to guide CNB for the evaluation of calcifications and masses that have been identified only on mammography. Stereotactically guided core needle biopsies are performed with an automated 14-gauge core biopsy gun or a vacuum-assisted directional biopsy device with a 14- or 11-gauge needle. Ultrasonography is also commonly used to guide needle biopsies.[28]

Imaging–pathology correlation is essential after a needle biopsy has been performed.[29] If the results of an imaging study and a needle biopsy are discordant, an excisional biopsy is indicated. Furthermore, because of the possibility of sampling error, some needle biopsy pathology results necessitate an excisional biopsy to rule out coexistent carcinoma. Cases of atypical ductal hyperplasia diagnosed at needle biopsy are generally agreed to require excisional biopsy.[30] The need for excisional biopsy for other pathologies, such as lobular carcinoma in situ, atypical lobular hyperplasia, radial scar, and papilloma remains controversial.

OTHER BREAST IMAGING MODALITIES

Digital Mammography With digital mammography, an image of the breast is recorded electronically rather than on film. The acquired digital image can be stored in computer memory and printed later as a film or displayed and interpreted on a high-definition monitor. The potential advantages of digital mammography include the ability to post-process images and emphasize areas of interest, to transmit images for remote consultations or interpretations ("teleradiology"), and to employ computer-aided detection.[31] Digital mammography may eventually reduce other problems associated with conventional film–screen mammography, such as film library space and lost films. Digital images can also be viewed on diagnostic workstations within seconds.

Digital mammography reduces the time necessary for mammography-guided procedures, such as stereotactic CNB and prebiopsy needle localization. Current disadvantages of digital mammography include the high cost of the equipment (two to three times that of conventional mammography), limitations in viewing-station technology, and difficulty of making comparisons with previous conventional images.

MRI of the Breast MRI has been used successfully to evaluate silicone breast implants for intracapsular or extracapsular rupture.[32] Initially though, MRI was not reliable for detection or diagnosis of breast cancer.[33] However, the use of intravenous contrast agents has made MRI highly sensitive for breast cancer detection.[34–37] Nonetheless, high cost and low specificity continue to limit the use of MRI as a screening tool. Another problem is that MRI cannot reliably identify intermediate- and low-grade ductal carcinoma in situ. Nevertheless, contrast-enhanced MRI of the breast appears to have several potential roles: (1) determining the size and extent of known invasive cancers; (2) identifying multicentric lesions; (3) evaluating the ipsilateral breast of a woman with axillary metastases and unknown primary; and (4) identifying a recurrent carcinoma in a conservatively treated breast. Multicenter clinical trials are currently underway to determine the exact roles of MRI in breast cancer management (Figure 32f-17).

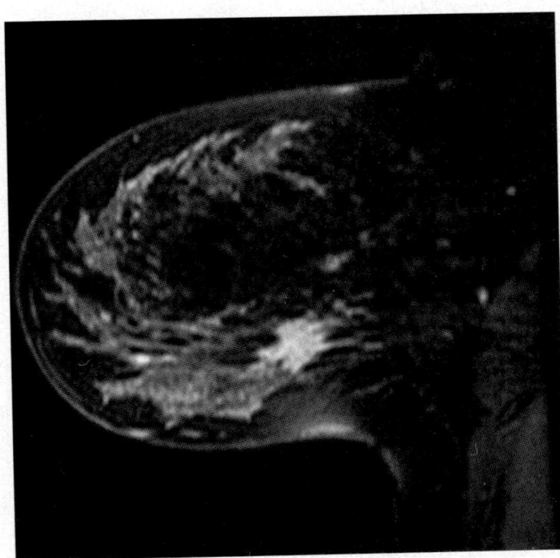

Figure 32f-17 Enhancing spiculated mass demonstrated on a sagittal MRI image.

Radionuclide Imaging Focal radionuclide uptake in breast cancers has been identified with positron emission tomography (PET) after the injection of ^{18}F-fluorodeoxy-D-glucose (FDG).[38] This labeled compound may also accumulate in abnormal axillary nodes.

PET imaging requires additional research to determine its sensitivity and specificity in breast cancer detection. Nonetheless, PET scanning is a useful tool for detecting metastatic disease in patients with stage II or greater disease.

In clinical practice, nuclear scans with ^{99m}Tc sulfur colloid have shown early promise for the identification of sentinel nodes before surgery.[39–41] The labeled compound is injected near a biopsy-proven breast cancer. The injected material tracks along potential routes of tumor spread in the lymphatic vessels. At subsequent surgery, sentinel nodes (which drain the primary cancer site) are identified with a handheld radionuclide probe, and the nodes are removed and evaluated histologically. If the sentinel node is negative for tumor, axillary node dissection and its potential complications may be avoided.

REFERENCES

1. Agency for Health Care Policy and Research (AHCPR [US]), Quality Determinants of Mammography Guideline Panel. Quality determinants of mammography. Clinical practice guideline No. 13. AHCPR Publication No. 95-0632. Rockville (MD): Dept. of Health and Human Services (US), Public Health Service, AHCPR; 1994.
2. American College of Radiology (ACR). Standards for the performance of screening mammography [adopted by the ACR Council 1990, revised 1994]. In: ACR digest of official actions. Reston (VA): ACR; 1994.
3. Institute of Medicine (US), Committee on Technologies for the Early Detection of Breast Cancer. Mammography and beyond—developing technologies for the early detection of breast cancer. Washington (DC): National Academy Press; 2001. Available at: http://www.iom.edu/report.asp?id=5456 (accessed July 24, 2002).
4. Duffy SW, Tabar L, Chen H, et al. The impact of organized mammography service screening on breast carcinoma mortality in seven Swedish counties. Cancer 2002;95:458–69.
5. American College of Radiology (ACR). Standards for the performance of diagnostic mammography and problem-solving breast evaluation [adopted by the ACR Council 1994]. In: ACR digest of official actions. Reston (VA): ACR; 1994.
6. American College of Radiology (ACR). ACR BI-RADS—mammography. In: ACR breast imaging reporting and data system, breast imaging atlas. 4th ed. Reston (VA): ACR; 2003.
7. Food and Drug Administration (US), Center for Devices and Radiological Health. Writing the mammography report. Mammography Matters 1998;5(4):10.
8. Sickles EA. Management of probably benign breast lesions. Radiol Clin North Am 1995;33:1123–30.
9. Jackson VP, Dines KA, Bassett LW, et al. Diagnostic importance of radiographic density of noncalcified breast masses: analysis of 91 lesions. AJR Am J Roentgenol 1991;157:25–8.
10. Egan RL, McSweeney MB, Sewell CW. Intramammary calcifications without an associated mass in benign and malignant diseases. Radiology 1980;137:1–7.
11. Stomper PC, Connelly JL, Meyer JE, Harris JR. Clinically occult ductal carcinoma in situ detected with mammography: analysis of 100 cases with radiologic–pathologic correlation. Radiology 1989;172:235–41.
12. Sickles EA. Mammographic features of 300 consecutive nonpalpable breast cancers. AJR Am J Roentgenol 1986;146:661–3.
13. Kalisher L, Chu AM, Peyster RG. Clinicopathological correlations of xeroradiography in determining involvement of metastatic axillary nodes in female breast cancer. Radiology 1976;121:333–5.
14. Mendelson EB. Evaluation of the postoperative breast. Radiol Clin North Am 1992;30:107–38.
15. Stomper PC, Margolin FR. Ductal carcinoma in situ: the mammographer's perspective. AJR Am J Roentgenol 1994;162:585–91.
16. Sickles EA, Filly RA, Callen PW. Breast cancer detection with ultrasonography and mammography: comparison using state-of-the-art equipment. AJR Am J Roentgenol 1983;140:843–5.
17. Kopans DB, Meyer JE, Lindfords KK. Whole-breast US imaging: 4-year follow-up. Radiology 1985;157:505–7.
18. Bassett LW, Kimme-Smith C, Sutherland LK, et al. Automated and hand-held breast US: effect on patient management. Radiology 1987;165:103–8.
19. Stavros AT, Thickman D, Rapp CL, et al. Solid breast nodules: use of sonography to distinguish between benign and malignant lesions. Radiology 1995;196:123–34.
20. Berg WA, Gilbreath PL. Multicentric and multifocal cancer: whole-breast US in preoperative evaluation. Radiology 2000;214:59–66.
21. Fornage BD, Coan JD, David CL. Ultrasound-guided needle biopsy of the breast and other interventional procedures. Radiol Clin North Am 1992;30:167–85.
22. Jackson VP. The current role of ultrasonography in breast imaging. Radiol Clin North Am 1995;33:1161–70.
23. Bassett LW, Liu TH, Giuliano AE, Gold RH. The prevalence of carcinoma in palpable vs impalpable mammographically detected lesions. AJR Am J Roentgenol 1991;157:21–4.
24. Cyrlak D. Induced costs of low-cost screening mammography. Radiology 1988;168:661–3.
25. Azevado E, Svane G, Aver G. Stereotactic fine-needle biopsy in 2594 mammographically detected nonpalpable lesions. Lancet 1989;1:1033–6.
26. Jackson VP, Bassett LW. Stereotactic fine-needle aspiration biopsy for nonpalpable breast lesions. AJR Am J Roentgenol 1990;154:1196–7.
27. Parker SH, Lovin JD, Jobe WE, et al. Nonpalpable breast lesions: stereotactic automated large-core biopsies. Radiology 1991;180:403–7.
28. Parker SH, Jobe WE, Dennis MA, et al. US-guided automated large core breast biopsy. Radiology 1993;187:507–11.
29. Bassett LW, Winchester DP, Caplan RB, et al. Stereotactic breast CNB: report of the Joint Task Force of the ACR, ACS, COAP. CA Cancer J Clin 1997;47:171–90.
30. Jackman RJ, Nowels KW, Shepard MJ, et al. Stereotaxic large-core needle biopsy of 450 nonpalpable breast lesions with surgical correlation in lesions with cancer or atypical hyperplasia. Radiology 1994;193:91–5.
31. Shtern F. Digital mammography and related technologies: a perspective from the National Cancer Institute. Radiology 1992;183:629–30.
32. Gorczyca DP, Sinha S, Ahn CY, et al. Silicone breast implants in vivo: MR imaging. Radiology 1992;185:407–10.
33. El Yousef SJ, O'Connell DM, Duchesneau RH, et al. Benign and malignant breast disease: magnetic resonance and radiofrequency pulse sequences. AJR Am J Roentgenol 1985;145:1–8.
34. Harms SE, Flamig DP, Evans WP, et al. MR imaging of the breast: current status and future potential. AJR Am J Roentgenol 1994;163:1039–47.
35. Heywang SH, Wolf A, Pruss E, et al. MR imaging of the breast with Gd-DTPA: use and limitations. Radiology 1989;171:95–103.
36. Heywang-Kobrunner SH, Schlegel A, Beck R, et al. Contrast-enhanced MRI of the breast after limited surgery and radiation therapy. J Comput Assist Tomogr 1993;17:891–900.
37. Orel SG, Schnall MD, LiVolsi VA, Troupin RH. Suspicious breast lesions: MR imaging with radiographic–pathologic correlation. Radiology 1994;190:485–93.
38. Wahl RL. Current status of PET in breast cancer imaging, staging and therapy. Semin Roentgenol 2001;3:250–60.
39. Winchester DJ, Sener SF, Winchester DP, et al. Sentinel lymphadenectomy for breast cancer: experience with 180 consecutive patients: efficacy of filtered technetium 99m sulphur colloid with overnight migration time. J Am Coll Surg 1999;188:597–603.
40. Krag DN, Harlow S, Weaver D, Ashikaga T. Radiolabeled sentinel node biopsy: collaborative trial with the National Cancer Institute. World J Surg 2001;25:823–8.
41. Veronesi U, Paganelli G, Viale G, et al. Sentinel lymph node biopsy and axillary dissection in breast cancer: results in a large series. J Natl Cancer Inst 1999;91:302–3.

Radionuclide Imaging in Cancer Medicine

R. Edward Coleman, MD

The discipline of nuclear medicine consists of radionuclide imaging and radionuclide therapy with the number of patients having radionuclide imaging studies being much greater than those who have radionuclide therapy. The use of radionuclide imaging and therapeutic procedures is increasing because they have an important role in the management of patients with cancer.

Radionuclide imaging is the most commonly performed procedure in molecular imaging. Nuclear medicine has been performing molecular imaging since the first radionuclide studies that were performed with I-131 sodium iodide for diagnosing and treating thyroid cancer.

To perform radionuclide imaging, a radioactive material (radiopharmaceutical) is administered and the radiation emitted by the radiopharmaceutical detected by sensitive radiation detectors located outside of the patient being studied. Radiopharmaceuticals that provide more sensitive and specific detection of cancers are being developed, and the methods of detecting the radiation are improving.

Radiopharmaceuticals consist of a radionuclide and a molecule that determines the localization. For I-131 sodium iodide, the radionuclide and the molecule are the same. For technetium-99m (Tc-99m) methylene diphosphonate (MDP), the radionuclide is Tc-99m and the molecule that determines the distribution is MDP. Radiochemists are continuing to improve the ways for radiolabeling new molecules that are developed by basic scientists in molecular biology and pharmacology laboratories.

Radionuclide imaging is commonly separated into single photon imaging and positron imaging. The devices used for imaging the single photon-emitting radionuclides are different than those for imaging positron-emitting radionuclides. Single photon radionuclides emit gamma rays in the energy range of approximately 75 to 360 KeV. These radionuclides include Tc-99m, I-131, Tl-201, In-111, Ga-67, etc. Devices known as gamma cameras detect these radionuclides, and these devices can perform regional imaging, whole-body imaging, and single photon emission computed tomography (SPECT) imaging.[1]

Positron-emitting radionuclides such as F-18, C-11, N-13, and O-15 emit a positive electron from the nucleus.[1,2] The positive electron travels a short distance through tissue and interacts with a free or loosely bound negative electron. The positive electron and negative electron annihilate each other, and their mass is converted to energy. This energy consists of two photons, each of 511 KeV, which are given off in opposite directions. The simultaneous detection of the two photons by detectors placed around the body provides a line of response. By obtaining multiple lines of response, the distribution of radioactivity in the body can then be determined. Positron emission tomography (PET) is able to more accurately correct for scatter of the radiation in the body and absorption of the radiation by the body than SPECT imaging. Furthermore, PET provides higher resolution lesion detection than SPECT imaging.

A major advance that is occurring in radionuclide imaging is the combination of gamma camera and computed tomography (CT) scanners and the combination of PET and CT scanners.[2] The radionuclide images provide excellent information concerning the biology of a process, but very little, if any, anatomic information. By combining the high resolution anatomic information from CT imaging and the biologic information from SPECT and PET imaging, greater diagnostic information is available. Furthermore, the CT scan can provide information concerning the attenuation of the photons in the body, and this attenuation can be corrected for more accurate radionuclide imaging.

This chapter will divide radionuclide imaging into the single photon techniques and PET. Radionuclide probe detectors are being increasingly used for the intraoperative localization of radioactivity for such studies as lymphoscintigraphy for the identification of sentinel lymph nodes, but this will not be discussed in this chapter.

SINGLE PHOTON TECHNIQUES

Gamma camera imaging is available at every major hospital in the United States. Radiopharmaceuticals are available from central radiopharmacies, which provide the requested radiopharmaceutical on a unit dose basis. Thus, the hospital or outpatient imaging center does not need to compound the radiopharmaceutical on site, but can purchase it in a form that is ready to be administered. The central radiopharmacies are able to provide all the radiopharmaceuticals used in imaging.

In this section, the studies that are performed using single photon-emitting radionuclides in cancer imaging will be addressed.

Bone Scanning Radionuclide bone imaging is one of the most commonly performed procedures in nuclear medicine (Figure 32g-1). The bone scan has been used for more than 40 years to evaluate patients with suspected metastatic bone disease, primary bone tumors, and primary soft tissue tumors.[3–5] Bone scintigraphy with Tc-99m MDP is very sensitive for detecting bone disease, it is widely available, and it is safe. The radiation dose that the patient receives is comparable to that of conventional radiographic procedures. Because the whole body is included in the imaging, it is an excellent method for evaluating patients with suspected metastatic disease that can occur throughout the skeleton. Abnormal areas of accumulation are seen related to osteoblastic activity. Purely lytic lesions such as multiple myeloma may be missed on the bone scan.

The bone scan can detect an abnormality prior to the radiograph becoming abnormal. Bone scans are quite sensitive for the detection of metastatic disease, but the specificity is lower than the sensitivity. Any process involving bone will result in increased bone turnover and an abnormality on the bone scan. Thus, inflammatory, traumatic, and metabolic abnormalities will result in increased areas of localization on the bone scan. Plain radiographs are frequently needed to correlate with the bone scan to determine the cause of the abnormality on the bone scan. For some lesions, such as sacral abnormalities, CT scanning is particularly helpful for correlation. For other lesions, MRI correlation may be helpful.[5]

Certain primary cancers, such as breast cancer, lung cancer, and prostate cancer, commonly spread to the bone. However, not every patient with these cancers needs a bone scan. The true positive yield in stage 1 and stage 2 breast cancer is very low (< 3%). Thus, these patients should have preoperative scans only when they are symptomatic or have laboratory values worrisome for metastatic disease. The use of prostate-specific antigen (PSA) has helped to clarify the role of bone scanning in the initial evaluation of patients with prostate cancer.[3] Several studies have now shown that bone scanning is not indicated in patients with newly diagnosed prostate cancer if the serum PSA levels are in the lower range of abnormal (10–20 mg/mL) and if they do not have bone pain suggestive of metastatic disease.

Gallium Scintigraphy Ga-67 citrate scintigraphy has been proven to be useful in the management of lymphoma: staging the extent of the disease, determining the response to therapy, detecting relapse or progression of disease, and predicting outcome.[6–8] Gallium scintigraphy has

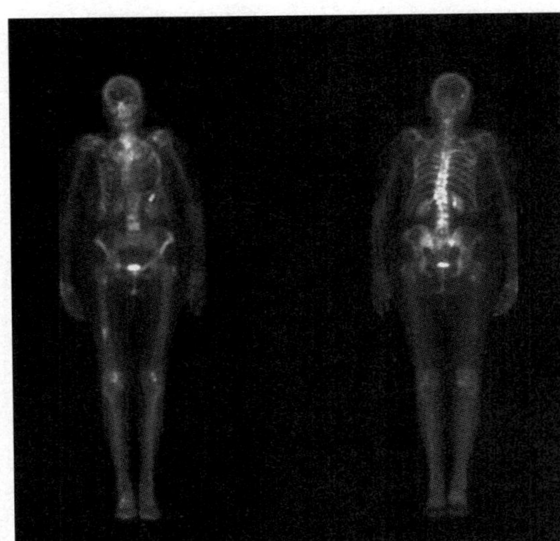

Figure 32g-1 Whole-body Tc-99m MDP bone scan revealing widespread metastatic disease.

been used in other cancers such as melanoma, hepatocellular carcinoma, sarcoma, and lung cancer, but the utility in the cancers other than lymphoma is extremely limited. The primary use of gallium scintigraphy in Hodgkin's and non-Hodgkin's lymphoma has been to evaluate the response to treatment in assessing a residual mass after therapy. Gallium scintigraphy is able to assess the response based on the observation that gallium is a tumor viability agent. Several studies have demonstrated that patients who had positive scans at the end of treatment either died or had tumor progression, whereas most patients with negative scans after treatment achieved complete remission.

Although gallium scintigraphy has been the standard for assessing therapeutic response in lymphoma in many institutions for many years, FDG-PET imaging is now being shown to be superior to gallium scintigraphy, and PET imaging has replaced gallium imaging in most institutions.[7,8]

Thallium-201 and Tc-99m MIBI Tl-201 was originally described as a myocardial perfusion and viability agent and has shown some effectiveness in oncology.[9] Technetium-99m methoxy-isobutyl isonitrile (Tc-99m MIBI) is now replacing Tl-201 scintigraphy in many nuclear cardiology applications and is being increasingly used in oncologic imaging.

Thallium-201 chloride behaves similarly to potassium chloride in most biologic systems. Tumors concentrate potassium ions and thallium ions in a similar manner. Tc-99m MIBI is a lipophilic cation greatly influenced by the negative charges on mitochondria and appears to concentrate related to the increased mitochondrial density in tumors. The washout of MIBI from tumor cells has been observed to be related to the multidrug-resistant P-glycoprotein system that has MIBI as a substrate.[10,11] The rapid clearance of MIBI from tumor cells may be a marker of multidrug resistance. Thallium and MIBI have been evaluated in several tumors and they have gained limited use in some tumors.[10–15] Brain tumors, bone and soft tissue sarcomas, lung cancers, thyroid cancer, and breast cancer accumulate these tracers. However, only in breast cancer has MIBI gained significant use.[12–14] MIBI breast studies appear to be useful to patients at high risk who have mammograms that are difficult to interpret. For example, women with dense breasts or who have architectural distortion and are at high risk of having malignant lesions may benefit from MIBI imaging.

Monoclonal Antibody Imaging The concept of radiolabeling a monoclonal antibody that reacts with a tumor antigen appears very appealing as a "magic bullet." The development of monoclonal antibodies for imaging cancer has been very difficult. The only monoclonal antibody imaging that is performed in many patients is ProstaScint imaging.[16,17] The other antibodies approved by the Food and Drug Administration have not proven to have adequate sensitivity and specificity to be of use. The clinical study with ProstaScint has not shown great accuracy, but the studies provide information that is not available from other techniques. For example, in the presurgical staging of prostate cancer, ProstaScint has a sensitivity of 63% for detecting lymph node metastasis at the time of surgery. Bone scans have been demonstrated to be more sensitive than ProstaScint imaging for detection of osseous metastases. The imaging of ProstaScint is not easy. The antibody is labeled with indium-111, and SPECT and planar imaging are performed 3 to 5 days after injection. Performing the SPECT scans on a SPECT/CT device improves the anatomic information for correlation with the ProstaScint images.

Somatostatin Receptor Scintigraphy and MIBG Somatostatin receptors have been identified on cells of neuroendocrine origin as well as other cells such as lymphocytes.[18,19] Somatostatin receptor scintigraphy has been performed using Octreoscan. A high sensitivity for neuroendocrine tumors such as gastrinoma, glucagonoma, paraganglioma, pheochromocytoma, and carcinoid tumors has been demonstrated.[19] Furthermore, a high sensitivity has been shown in nonsmall-cell lung cancer and meningioma, with other tumors such as breast cancer, lymphoma, and astrocytoma demonstrating uptake of the radiopharmaceutical. Octreoscan is frequently used in imaging neuroendocrine tumors.

Metaiodobenzylguanidine (MIBG) labeled with 123 or I-131 is very sensitive for the detection of pheochromocytomas, carcinoid tumors, and neuroblastomas[20,21] (Figure 32g-2). The accuracy of MIBG and Octreoscan is not different in the detection of neuroendocrine tumors. In institutions that are using I-131 MIBG for treating neuroendocrine tumors, MIBG has been the preferred imaging agent.[22,23] Methods of labeling Octreoscan with a therapeutic radionuclide are under development, but are not available at this time.[19,24]

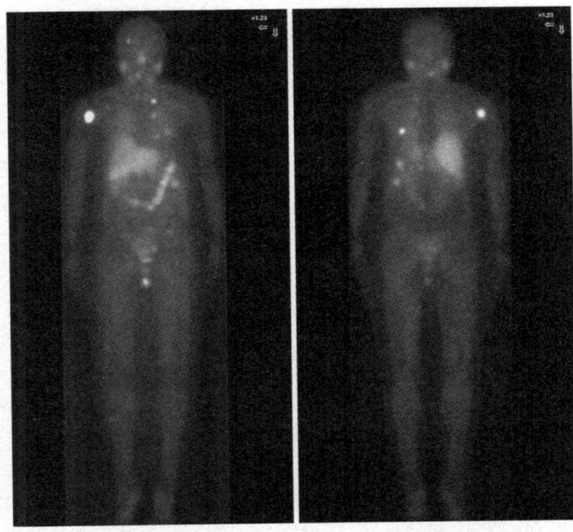

Figure 32g-2 I-131 metaiodobenzylguanidine (MIBG) whole-body bone scan in a patient with metastatic pheochromocytoma demonstrating multiple MIBG-avid metastases.

POSITRON EMISSION TOMOGRAPHY (PET)

The use of PET imaging is rapidly increasing in the United States. The radiopharmaceutical used for oncologic PET imaging is fluorine-18 2-fluoro-2-deoxyglucose (FDG). FDG behaves very similarly to glucose. Both FDG and glucose are transported across the cell membrane by glucose transporter proteins, and both are phosphorylated. Once phosphorylated, the FDG-6-phosphate is not further metabolized in most tissues. However, in the liver, because of the high concentration of phosphatase enzymes, the FDG-phosphate can be dephosphorylated and is transported out of the cell.

Malignant cells have an increased glycolytic rate. FDG is concentrated in malignant cells more than in normal tissue.

For a clinical PET study, the FDG is administered to the patient after a 4-hour fast. Approximately 1 hour after injection of the FDG, the patient is placed in the PET scanner for the imaging. The imaging procedure takes approximately 30 minutes for the whole-body study.

Medicare first started paying for FDG-PET scans in 1998. In late 2002, Medicare was paying for diagnosis, staging, and restaging of lung cancer, colorectal cancer, melanoma, lymphoma, head and neck cancer, and esophageal cancer. In addition, staging and restaging of breast cancer and monitoring the effect of therapy on breast cancer was reimbursed. Other third party payers generally have policies similar to Medicare for coverage of PET imaging.

Lung Cancer The most common use of FDG-PET imaging is in diagnosis, staging, and restaging of lung cancer.[25] PET is very accurate in the characterization of lung nodules that are indeterminate on a CT scan (Figure 32g-3). A meta-analysis

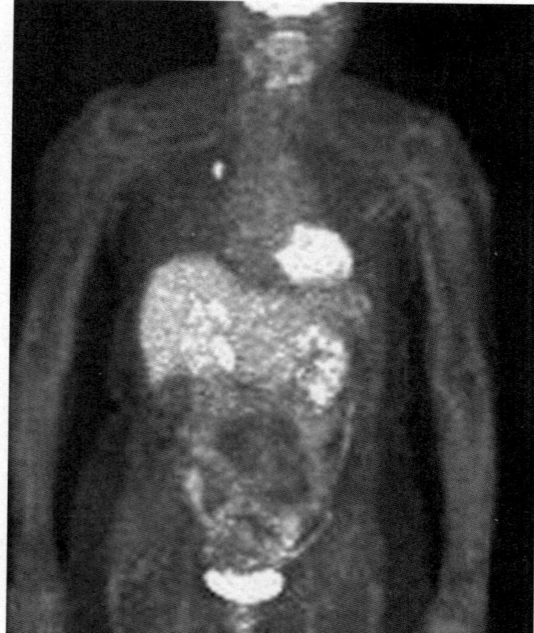

Figure 32g-3 Patient who has a solitary pulmonary nodule that is indeterminate on CT scan and abnormal on whole-body F-18 2-fluoro-2-deoxyglucose positron emission tomography (FDG-PET). Subsequent surgery documented nonsmall-cell lung cancer.

of 1,174 focal pulmonary lesions found that PET operates at sensitivity of 96.8% and a specificity of 77.8%.[26] False positive nodules generally relate to granulomatous inflammatory processes.

PET has been demonstrated to be more accurate than CT in staging the mediastinum. In patients who have had conventional imaging for evaluation of metastatic disease, PET will identify previously undetected metastatic disease in 10 to 15% of patients (Figure 32g-4). PET has also been demonstrated to be very accurate in monitoring the effects of treatment.

Colorectal Carcinoma PET is not frequently used for the diagnosis and initial staging of patients with colorectal cancer. It is used in the initial staging of high-risk patients for whom surgery could be avoided if metastasis could be identified.[27]

FDG-PET in colorectal cancer patients is primarily used for the detection of recurrent or metastatic disease. PET has been shown to be more accurate than CT for staging recurrent cancer. The sensitivity of FDG-PET imaging is lower for mucinous adenocarcinoma than nonmucinous adenocarcinoma. PET is useful in evaluating patients who have a history of colorectal cancer, rising CEA, and negative CT. Approximately 70% of these patients will have the cause of the rising CEA detected on the FDG-PET scan.

Malignant Melanoma PET imaging does not replace lymphoscintigraphy in identification of regional nodal disease. Patients with intermediate- or high-risk tumors benefit from having a PET scan because of the prevalence of regional or distant disease at presentation in these patients.[28] In several studies, PET has been shown to be more sensitive

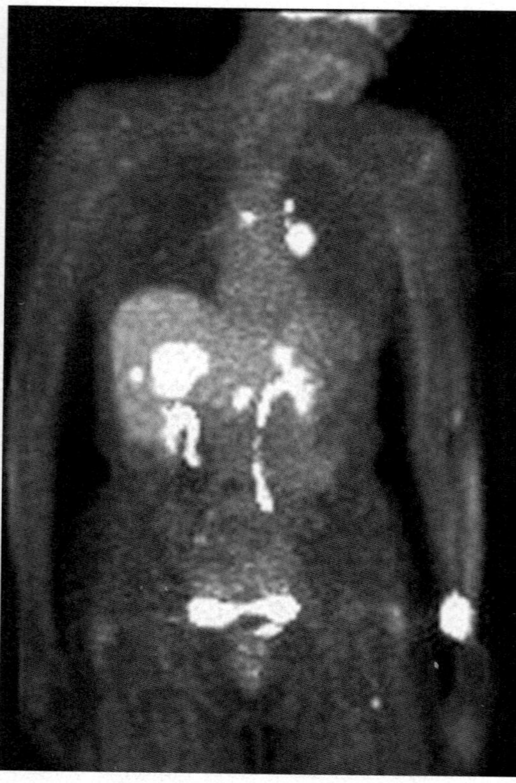

Figure 32g-4 Whole-body F-18 2-fluoro-2-deoxyglucose positron emission tomography (FDG-PET) scan in a patient who has a primary lung cancer with hilar, liver, and bone metastases.

than conventional imaging in staging metastatic melanoma. In some institutions, PET is being used as a surveillance procedure in high-risk patients. In patients with recurrent tumor, FDG-PET can identify the distribution of tumor in those patients. Unsuspected distant metastases are identified in approximately 15% of patients, which changes the patient from surgical to nonsurgical therapy.

Lymphoma PET is used in lymphoma for pretreatment staging, post-treatment detection of residual disease, prediction of treatment effect, and diagnosis of recurrent tumor.[28] FDG-PET is very accurate in staging Hodgkin's disease and high-grade non-Hodgkin's lymphoma. FDG-PET is more accurate in staging patients than gallium or CT scanning.[7,8]

Many studies have demonstrated the ability of FDG-PET to differentiate viable tumor from fibrosis in a residual post-treatment mass. PET has been demonstrated to be superior to gallium scintigraphy in making this differentiation. Even early during the course of therapy, FDG-PET imaging can predict eventual treatment response. FDG-PET has been demonstrated to provide prognostic information at the completion of a course of therapy.

Head and Neck Cancer PET imaging has been demonstrated to be useful in identifying the head and neck primary cancer in 20 to 40% of patients who present with metastatic squamous cell cancer in a neck lymph node even after a negative clinical examination and CT.[29] PET does not provide any advantage over CT in primary tumor staging. The primary advantage of PET imaging is evaluation of therapy when fibrosis, edema, and loss of tissue planes may confound the ability to evaluate tumor response by physical examination or anatomic imaging. PET is superior to the other modalities in identifying recurrence of head and neck cancer after treatment.

Esophageal Cancer PET imaging is rarely used for the diagnosis of esophageal cancer.[29] Endoscopic ultrasound has been found to be more accurate than PET and/or CT scanning in detection of paraesophageal lymph nodes, but PET is more accurate in the detection of distant disease. PET is also used in evaluating response to therapy of the esophageal cancer and assessing recurrent esophageal cancer after therapy.

Breast Cancer FDG-PET at this time does not play a role in diagnosis of breast cancer,[30] nor is it accurate enough to replace lymphoscintigraphy in the evaluation of axillary lymph nodes. FDG-PET is accurate in staging breast cancer and detection of metastatic disease. Furthermore, PET can predict early during a course of therapy whether the patient will respond to the therapy or not.

CONCLUSION

Radionuclide imaging in cancer medicine consists of standard imaging techniques and new methods. PET imaging is having an increasingly important role in diagnosing, staging, and restaging many cancer patients. New radiopharmaceuticals will be available that will improve our ability to diagnose and stage cancer.

REFERENCES

1. Coleman RE. SPECT and PET in cancer imaging. Cancer 1991;67:1261–70.
2. Rohren EM, Turkington TG, Coleman RE. Clinical applications of PET in oncology. Radiology 2004;231:305–32.
3. Kosuda S, Yoshimura I, Aizawa T, et al. Can initial prostate specific antigen determinations eliminate the need for bone scans in patients with newly diagnosed prostate carcinoma? A multicenter retrospective study in Japan. Cancer 2002;94:964–72.
4. Hamaoka T, Madewell JE, Podoloff DA, et al. Bone imaging in metastatic breast cancer. J Clin Oncol 2004;22:2942–53.
5. Taoka T, Mayr NA, Lee HJ, et al. Factors influencing visualization of vertebral metastases on MR imaging versus bone scintigraphy. AJR Am J Roentgenol 2001;176:1525–30.
6. Israel O, Mor M, Epelbaum R, et al. Clinical pretreatment risk factors and Ga-67 scintigraphy early during treatment for prediction of outcome of patients with aggressive non-Hodgkin lymphoma. Cancer 2002;94:873–8.
7. Kostakoglu L, Goldsmith SJ. Positron emission tomography in lymphoma: comparison with computed tomography and gallium-67 single photon emission computed tomography. Clin Lymphoma 2000;1:67–74.
8. Kostakoglu L, Leonard JP, Kuji I. Comparison of fluorine-18 fluorodeoxyglucose positron emission tomography and Ga-67 scintigraphy in evaluation of lymphoma. Cancer 2002;94:879–88.
9. Yamamoto Y, Nishiyama Y, Toyama Y, et al. Comparison of 201 Tl-with 67 Ga single photon emission tomography in the diagnosis of head and neck cancer recurrence. Nucl Med Commun 2002;23:187–91.
10. Sao A, Shiun SC, Hsu NY, et al. Technetium-99m methoxyisobutylisonitrile chest imaging for small-cell lung cancer. Relationship to chemotherapy response (six courses of combination of cisplatin and etoposide) and p-glyco-

protein or multidrug resistance related protein expression. Ann Oncol 2001;12:1561–6.
11. Luker GD, Flagg TP, Sha Q, et al. MDR1 P-glycoprotein reduces influx of substrates without affecting membrane potential. J Biol Chem 2001;276:49053–60.
12. Leung JW. New modalities in breast imaging: digital mammography, positron emission tomography, and sestamibi scintimammography. Radiol Clin North Am 2002;40:467–82.
13. Kim R, Osaki A, Hirai T, et al. Utility of technetium-99m methoxyisobutyl isonitrile uptake analysis for prediction of the response to chemotherapy in advanced and relapsed breast cancer. Breast Cancer 2002;9:240–7.
14. Bombardieri E, Crippa F, Baio SM, et al. Nuclear medicine advances in breast cancer imaging. Tumori 2001;87:277–87.
15. Yamamoto Y, Nishiyama Y, Fukunaga K, et al. 99mTc-MIBI SPECT in small cell lung cancer patients before chemotherapy and after unresponsive chemotherapy. Ann Nucl Med 2001;15:329–35.
16. Freeman LM, Krynyckyi BR, Li Y, et al. The role of 111In Capromab Pendetide (Prosta-ScintR) immunoscintigraphy in the management of prostate cancer. Q J Nucl Med 2002;46:131–7.
17. Wong TZ, Turkington TG, Polascik TJ, Coleman RE. ProstaScint (capromab pendetide) imaging technique using hybrid gamma camera-CT technology. AJR Am J Roentgenol 2005;184:678–80.
18. Warner RR, O'dorisio TM. Radiolabeled peptides in diagnosis and tumor imaging: clinical overview. Semin Nucl Med 2002;32:79–93.
19. De Gerder WW, Lamberts SW. Somatostatin and somatostatin analogues: diagnostic and therapeutic uses. Curr Opin Oncol 2002;14:53–7.
20. Ohta H. I-123 MIBG scintigraphy. Pheochromocytoma. Ann Nucl Med 2002;16:frontpage, 278.
21. Zuetenhorst JM, Hoefnageli CA, Boot H, et al. Evaluation of 111 In-pentetreotide, 131 I-MIBG and bone scintigraphy in the detection and clinical management of bone metastases in carcinoid disease. Nucl Med Commun 2002;23:735–41.
22. Yanik GA, Levine JE, Matthay KK, et al. Pilot study of iodine-131-metaiodobenzylguanidine in combination with myeloablative chemotherapy and autologous stem-cell support for the treatment of neuroblastoma. J Clin Oncol 2002;20:2142–9.
23. Safford SD, Coleman RE, Gockerman JP, et al. Iodine-131 metaiodobenzylguanidine is an effective treatment for malignant pheochromocytoma and paraganglioma. Surgery 2003;134:956–62.
24. Anthony LB, Woltering EA, Espenan GD, et al. Indium-111-pentetreotide prolongs survival in gastroenteropancreatic malignancies. Semin Nucl Med 2002;32:123–32.
25. Hagge RJ, Coleman RE. Positron emission tomography: lung cancer. Semin Roent 2002;37:110–7.
26. Gould MK, Maclean CC, Kuschner WG, et al. Accuracy of positron emission tomography for diagnosis of pulmonary nodules and mass lesions: a meta-analysis. JAMA 2001;285:914–24.
27. Vitola J, Delbeke D. Positron emission tomography for evaluation of colorectal carcinoma. Semin Roent 2002;37:118–28.
28. Abella-Columna E, Valk PE. Positron emission tomography imaging in melanoma and lymphoma. Semin Roent 2002;37:129–39.
29. Lowe VJ, Stack BC Jr. Esophageal cancer and head and neck cancer. Semin Roent 2002;37:140–50.
30. Dehdashti F, Siegel BA. Evaluation of breast and gynecologic cancers by positron emission tomography. Semin Roent 2002;37:151–68.

33

Interventional Radiology for the Cancer Patient

Marshall E. Hicks, MD
Michael J. Wallace, MD
Sanjay Gupta, MD

By using standard imaging modalities that best define the neoplasm, the interventional radiologist applies minimally invasive percutaneous techniques to establish diagnoses, initiate therapeutic management of the patient with cancer confined to a certain anatomic region, and provide supportive care for cancer patients. These procedures include a variety of approaches: intra-arterial infusion, embolization, and chemoembolization; portal vein occlusion; balloon angioplasty; percutaneous tumor injection; focused ultrasonography, radiofrequency, laser, or cryoablation; biopsy and drainage (gastrostomy, nephrostomy) techniques; repositioning of central venous catheters; placement of long-term venous access devices, stents, and vena cava filters; intravascular foreign body retrieval; and thrombolysis, among others. Both vascular and nonvascular radiologic procedures are performed more rapidly, more efficiently, and more cost-effectively with less morbidity and mortality than their surgical alternatives. Selected components of these responsibilities are described in greater detail in this chapter.

INTRA-ARTERIAL THERAPY

The delivery of therapeutic agents intra-arterially requires selective vascular catheterization, which is accomplished by tailoring the catheter configuration to the vascular anatomy. Coaxial systems with 2- to 3-French (F) catheters delivered through 4- to 6.5-F access catheters have markedly facilitated the technical challenge of intravascular therapy through small vessels (segmental and subsegmental). A nonthrombogenic environment is created by the use of a heparinized saline solution to periodically flush the angiographic catheters and sheaths.

Infusion Therapy The goal of intra-arterial chemotherapy is to deliver high-dose chemotherapy into the artery supplying the neoplasm. Several experimental and clinical studies have shown that a 20 to 30% higher response rate can be achieved. However, the benefits of prolonged survival rates and improved quality of life are not consistently realized, and the patients are rarely cured.[1] These techniques did not gain enthusiastic support and have not been used as frontline therapy in many tumors, but, rather, are employed after failure of other treatments and to test new drug regimens.

Embolization Embolization is the occlusion of the arterial supply to the tumor to create ischemia and tumor necrosis and to arrest growth by the intra-arterial delivery of particulate materials, sclerosing solutions, and substances introduced in a liquid state that eventually solidify. Interruption of a vessel at its origin by an embolus has an effect similar to a surgical ligation. Collateral circulation is available immediately; the more central the occlusion, the more abundant is the collateral circulation that must be pursued and occluded when it supplies the neoplasm. Peripheral (segmental and subsegmental) vascular embolization is best accomplished with coaxial catheters and small particles. Multiple arteries supplying a neoplasm or an organ can be converted to a single source by selective occlusion, allowing the collaterals to redistribute flow.

Typically, at The University of Texas M. D. Anderson Cancer Center, peripheral embolization is accomplished with absorbable gelatin sponge particles and powder (Gelfoam), polyvinyl alcohol foam (PVA, Ivalon) granules, and acrylic copolymer gelatin particles (Embosphere Microspheres). Gelatin sponge segments or stainless steel coils are used for central (larger vessel) occlusion.

The indications for transcatheter embolization of neoplasms are (1) to control bleeding, particularly gastrointestinal hemorrhage, from ulcerated tumors in patients who are not operative candidates; (2) preoperatively, to facilitate surgical resection by decreasing blood loss and operating time or to allow hypertrophy of the nonembolized tissue as in the liver (eg, portal vein embolization); (3) to inhibit tumor growth; (4) to relieve pain by decreasing tumor bulk; and (5) to decrease the release of hormonally active substances by tumor.

The complications of embolization were analyzed by Hemingway and Allison[2] over a 10-year period in 284 patients who underwent 410 embolizations. Minor complications occurred in 16% and serious complications (ischemia, hemorrhage) in 6.6%, with death in 2%. The postembolization syndrome (fever, elevated white blood count [WBC], and discomfort) was encountered in 42.7% of the procedures. The underlying abnormality and vascular bed usually determine the nature of the complication.

Chemoembolization Chemoembolization is the combination of infusion and embolization and/or related therapies. Decreasing arterial flow will create ischemia and increase contact time between the infusate and the tumor cells, which increases tumor cell kill and accelerates tumor necrosis or programmed cell death (apoptosis). Several techniques have been used, including (1) balloon occluded arterial infusion; (2) injection of a chemotherapeutic agent, with or without iodized oil and with embolic particles; (3) arterial infusion after the injection of biodegradable starch microspheres; (4) embolization with liposomes or microcapsules containing cytotoxic drugs; and (5) intravascular or direct injection of sclerosing solutions ± iodized oil, genes, growth factors, or polymer–drug conjugates.

Another theoretical consideration is the concept of "enhanced permeability and retention" (EPR) suggested by Maeda and colleagues.[3] Newly formed tumor vessels are more "leaky" (permeable) than normal and, coupled with a lack of lymphatics in the neoplasm, result in retention of molecules of higher molecular weight (greater than 30,000 Daltons) for a more prolonged period. This may explain, in part, the accumulation of iodized oil or the increase in concentration of polymer conjugates of chemotherapeutic agents in neoplasms.

In Japan, the technique of chemoembolization that has gained wide clinical acceptance since 1983 is the use of embolic material mixed with chemotherapeutic agents and iodized oil delivered into the arterial supply to a neoplasm followed by Gelfoam embolization. The iodized oil (lipiodol/Ethiodol) acts as a contrast medium, an embolic agent, and a vehicle or drug carrier. When injected into the hepatic artery, the iodized oil rapidly enters the portal vein, primarily through the peribiliary plexus, and passes through the sinusoids into the hepatic veins and the general circulation.[4] This results in a dual embolization, that is, the hepatic artery and the portal vein. There is temporary vascular and sinusoidal occlusion and congestion. Removal of lipiodol is accomplished by reestablishment of arterial flow and phagocytosis of the oil by the Kupffer cells. Particulate materials (polylactic acid, Gelfoam, polyvinyl alcohol foam, or Ivalon), even in the sizes of 1 μm and larger, cause hepatic arterial occlusion, necrosis, and fibrosis. The necrotic and fibrotic areas are bypassed by vessels similar to the "capillarized" sinusoids observed in cirrhotic livers of humans. These vessels act as sinusoidal shunts in the embolized areas.[5] Embolization increases fibrosis in an already fibrotic (cirrhotic) liver and should be used with caution in such patients.

Hepatic Neoplasms: Hepatocellular Carcinoma The hepatic blood supply consists of 70 to 80% portal vein and 20 to 30% hepatic arterial flow. The hepatic tumor is nearly completely nourished by the arterial blood supply. This allows more specific treatment to the neoplasms through the hepatic artery, while preserving normal hepatic function.

In the Far East, the annual incidence of hepatocellular carcinoma (HCC) is as high as 150 cases per million, while in Western countries the frequency is markedly less.[6] HCC is the most frequent tumor worldwide, with an estimated one million deaths per year. Currently, surgical removal of the tumor represents the only potentially curative treatment. However, curative resection is only possible in fewer than 10% of patients.[6] Systemic chemotherapy for HCC is disappointing because of the low response rate (20–30%). Hepatic artery embolization and chemoembolization are currently considered frontline treatments, along with ablative therapy, for unresectable HCC that appears confined to the liver.

It is our experience that the type of HCC seen at M. D. Anderson in the United States, and perhaps in institutions in other Western countries, is different from that more commonly treated by interventional radiologists in Japan.[7] Nodular HCC is seen in fewer than 25% of our patients, while in Japan, it comprises approximately 75% of patients. This type of tumor can be approached by ablation, chemoembolization, or the combination of both, but also by surgery with a 2-year survival rate of approximately 50%. However, there are no randomized studies performed in Japan to compare these different techniques in patients with HCC (5 cm in diameter or less) and Childs A or B liver disease.

Preoperative (Neoadjuvant) Chemoembolization Hepatic artery chemoembolization has been recommended preoperatively even for lesions of 5 cm in diameter or less. Harada and colleagues used neoadjuvant chemoembolization preoperatively with lipiodol, doxorubicin, mitomycin C, and Gelfoam in 105 patients to cause tumor necrosis, minimize spillage of viable tumor cells during resection, and destroy microscopic intrahepatic metastases not included in the resected specimen and compared it with no preoperative treatment in 35 patients.[8] They recorded tumor reduction in 61%, with considerable complications in 53% and a surgical delay of 72.9 ± 52.0 days. They concluded that the only clinical indication for the use of preoperative chemoembolization was to reduce tumor bulk in patients who had borderline resectable lesions. The high complication rate and prolonged surgical delay minimized its use.[8–10]

Palliative Chemoembolization In their series of 1,061 patients, including those with large inoperable HCC treated with Gelfoam particles mixed with doxorubicin and mitomycin C, Yamada and colleagues[6] reported survival rates of 51% at 1 year, 28% at 2 years, 13% at 3 years, 8% at 4 years, and at 6% at 5 years. The 1-year, 2-year, and 3-year survival rates increased to 72%, 55%, and 47%, respectively, in 66 patients with tumors smaller than 5 cm in diameter.[6] Nakamura and colleagues demonstrated improved results in their patients who were treated with iodized oil, doxorubicin, and gelatin sponge embolization. The survival rates of their 443 patients were 56.3% at 1 year, 33.3% at 2 years, 18.3% at 3 years, 11.8% at 4 years, and 8.0% at 5 years, slightly but significantly better than the control group of patients who were embolized with Gelfoam and doxorubicin.[11]

Ohishi and colleagues[12] described their experience with more than 500 patients with inoperable HCC with a 4-year survival rate of 20.4%, using anticancer drugs, gelatin sponge, and iodized oil. From the same group, Uchida and colleagues[13] reported a 3-year survival rate of 55% in their series of 99 nodular HCCs (< 5 cm in diameter) treated with subsegmental iodized oil chemoembolization. More recently, they used SMANCS (styrene maleic acid neocarzinostatin) soluble in lipiodol as the chemoembolic agent, followed by Gelfoam. Matsui and colleagues reported that subsegmental chemoembolization with iodized oil and anticancer drugs followed by gelatin sponge particles or a mixture of iodized oil and absolute ethanol in 82 patients with nodular HCC (< 4 cm in diameter, Childs classes A and B) yielded 1-year and 4-year survival rates of 100% and 67%, respectively.[14]

In the study of 38 consecutive patients with HCC, 35% stage I, 62% stage II, and 3% stage III, and 51% with cirrhosis, Solomon and colleagues reported the results of chemoembolization with cisplatin, doxorubicin, mitomycin C, Ethiodol, and polyvinyl alcohol particles.[15] In 7 patients, the lesions became resectable after chemoembolization. Among 25 patients evaluable for morphologic response, 36% had a partial response (PR), 32% had a minor response (MR), and 32% remained stable. No patient had progression of disease while receiving therapy. The cumulative survival was 60% at 1 year, 41% at 2 years, and 16% at 3 years. Two patients developed progressive hepatic failure. The 30-day mortality was 8%. These results compare favorably with the response and survival rates for chemoembolization of advanced HCC from Asia and Europe.[16] Consistently among studies, patients shown to benefit most from chemoembolization for HCC include those with less advanced hepatic disease (ideally Childs-Pugh class A) and less advanced tumor (such as lack of vascular invasion and asymptomatic tumors).

Complications Undoubtedly, with chemoembolization, there is an increased local effect along with an increase in local toxicity. Sakamoto and colleagues reported an incidence of 102 (4.4%) complications in 2,300 chemoembolization procedures for hepatic neoplasms. Of those related to chemoembolic agents, 63 (1.8%) produced injury to the liver, including acute liver failure, liver abscess, intrahepatic biloma formation, liver infarction, and multiple intrahepatic aneurysms. Injury to extrahepatic structures, probably a result of inadvertent chemoembolization of adjacent arteries, occurred in 28 episodes (0.9%), including severe cholecystitis, gallbladder and splenic infarctions, gastrointestinal mucosal lesions (ulcers, especially along the lesser curvature of the stomach), pulmonary embolism or infarction, tumor rupture, and variceal bleeding. In 39 (1.7%), the complications were caused by catheter or guidewire trauma leading to iatrogenic dissection, occlusion, or vascular perforation.[17]

Local Tissue Ablation Image-guided tumor ablation of focal hepatic malignancies can be accomplished by (1) direct intratumoral percutaneous ethanol injection (PEI), hot water or saline, acetic acid, or chemotherapeutic agents that induce tumor cell death; or (2) high-energy radiofrequency (RF), interstitial laser photocoagulation (ILP), microwave, cryotherapy, or high-intensity focused ultrasound (HIFU) that causes coagulation necrosis.[18,19] These procedures can be performed under imaging guidance by interventional radiologists or by surgeons in the operating suite. The procedures performed by the interventional radiologists offer advantages over the conventional surgical approach to the treatment of small hepatic neoplasms in that they are less invasive, less expensive, and can be performed on an outpatient basis using conscious sedation. PEI is well established for the treatment of HCC, but it is much less successful in the treatment of hepatic metastases, where thermal ablation methods are more promising. Multiple studies have demonstrated that these treatments can cause destruction of tumor with low morbidity and mortality, although the best results have been seen with lesions smaller than 5 cm.[18,19] Ebara and colleagues[20] reported a 20-year experience with PEI in lesions less than or equal to 3 cm. The local recurrence rate at 3 years was 10%, with overall 3- and 5-year survival rates of 81% and 60%, respectively. Shiina and Niwa[21] combined PEI and iodized oil chemoembolization with survival rates of 79% for 1 year and 38% for 5 years.

Livraghi and colleagues compared RF ablation versus PEI in the treatment of small HCC (3 cm diameter). Complete necrosis was achieved in 47 of 52 tumors (90%) in 1.2 sessions per tumor with RF and 48 of 60 tumors (80%) in 4.8 sessions per tumor with PEI. One major (hemothorax) and four minor complications (bleeding, hemobilia, pleural effusion, and cholecystitis) occurred with RF, while there were none with ethanol.[19] Lencioni and colleagues reported treatment of HCC with either RF ablation or PEI in a randomized series of 102 patients with hepatic cirrhosis. Although there was no overall difference in 1- and 2-year survival, there was a significant difference in 1- and 2-year local recurrence-free survival in patients treated with RF ablation (98% vs 83% and 96% vs 62%, respectively). The study was limited to patients with either a single 5 cm diameter or smaller HCC or patients with a maximum of three HCCs of 3 cm diameter or less.[22] However, up to 25% of the lesions in Ebara's study[20] with PEI could not have been treated by radiofrequency ablation because of anatomic considerations, emphasizing that there is still a role for PEI in small tumors despite results that, overall, favor radiofrequency ablation. Thermal ablation for hepatic metastases from colorectal cancer has also been reported to improve survival. Median survival time was increased to 39 months from 21 to 25 months (reported natural history) in a study reported by Gillams and Lees.[23]

Randomized Studies As summarized in the French and American literature, three randomized studies of groups of patients[24–26] with unresectable HCC without severe liver cirrhosis were treated with iodized oil chemoembolization with epidoxorubicin or doxorubicin and/or cisplatin and Gelfoam particles or powder. This approach definitely reduced tumor growth but often caused liver damage and/or failure, which required increased hospitalization and was definitely more expensive.[9] These groups were randomized against supportive therapy with no chemoembolization; there was no significant improvement in survival. Undoubtedly, the patient selection criteria employed in these randomized studies differed from those in Japan, where the tumors are more frequently nodular, encapsulated, hypervascular, and positive for hepatitis B or C antibodies. In Japan, selection of patients for chemoembolization is done earlier in the course of the disease because of their aggressive screening program, which may account for the better results achieved.

Two randomized studies have reported more favorable results with chemoembolization compared with bland embolization and/or conservative therapy. Llovet and colleagues reported survival probabilities at 1 and 2 years of 75% and 50% for embolization alone, 82% and 63% for chemoembolization (doxorubicin and Gelfoam), and 63% and 27% for control, respectively.[27] The study was stopped early because of the proven survival benefit. This study included patients with unresectable HCC, but without severe liver disease. Only 12% of the patients enrolled were included in the final analysis.[27] Another study by Lo and colleagues demonstrated a benefit in survival for patients with unresectable HCC treated with chemoembolization (lipiodol, cisplatin, and Gelfoam) compared with a control group treated with symptomatic therapy only.[28] Survival in the chemoembolization group was 57% at 1 year, 31% at 2 years, and 26% at 3 years, compared with 32%, 11%, and 3%, respectively, in the control group.

Transarterial Brachytherapy Internal radiation by transhepatic arterial delivery of yttrium-90 microspheres has been reported by Geschwind and colleagues as a promising form of therapy for HCC.[29] Yttrium-90 is a beta emitter with high energy emission and a short half-life. The concept of delivery is similar to chemoembolization with selective distribution of the beta-emitting microparticles to vascular tumor beds. Thus, a relatively high amount of radiation can be "selectively" delivered to the tumor, theoretically reducing the potential for organ toxicity, which is a limitation of external beam therapy. In a study of 80 patients classified as Okuda stage I ($n = 54$) and stage II ($n = 26$) treated with yttrium-90 microspheres, median survival duration and 1-year survival rates were 628 days and 63%, and 384 days and 51%, respectively.[29]

Portal Vein Embolization (PVE) Successful resection of the liver depends on the volume and normal function of the residual hepatic parenchyma. Portal vein branch ligation, stenosis, or occlusion results in atrophy of the affected lobe or segment and global hypertrophy of the remainder of the liver because of hepatocyte growth factors (hematopoietin A [HGF], insulin, glucagon).[30] HCC is most frequently accompanied by cirrhosis, whereas metastases from other primary neoplasms are usually scattered through otherwise normal liver. Preoperative PVE can be accomplished by percutaneous transhepatic approach in preparation for hepatectomy, when there is too little hepatic parenchyma to permit safe resection.[31] After percutaneous transhepatic occlusion of a lobar or segmental branch of the portal vein, de Baere and colleagues reported adequate hypertrophy (after 30 days) of the future remnant liver (FLR) of 90% ± 52% after cyanoacrylate and iodized oil injection.[32] Modified polyvinyl acetate, fibrin glue with lipiodol, Gelfoam, and thrombin, or absolute ethanol itself, have been used for portal vein embolization. A combination of particles and embolization coils are used at M. D. Anderson. PVE is performed if the FLR was estimated to be less than 25% of the total liver volume. For embolizations performed prior to extended right hepatectomy, extension of the preoperative embolization to segment IV is required in many patients. The range of reported mean absolute FLR increase is 46 to 70%, depending on the particle type used for embolization. PVE results in hepatocyte apoptosis, so the postembolization syndrome associated with transarterial embolization and necrosis does not occur. Fulminant liver insufficiency (post-PVE or postresection) also did not occur in a report of 44 patients treated with PVE at M. D. Anderson.[31]

In an attempt to facilitate the procedure, Kan and Wallace[33] demonstrated in animals that segmental atrophy and diffuse hypertrophy of the residual normal liver could be accomplished by chemoembolization of a lobar or segmental branch of the hepatic artery with a 3:1 or 4:1 ratio of Ethiodol to absolute ethanol mixture in pigs and rats, respectively. Hepatic artery embolization with Ethiodol gains rapid access to the portal vein, primarily through the peribiliary plexus; lipiodol with ethanol is, therefore, a dual embolization of the hepatic artery and portal vein. Cheng and colleagues treated 200 patients with HCC by Ethiodol/ethanol (3:1) injection into the segmental hepatic artery supplying the HCC.[34] Twenty patients were subsequently subjected to segmental or lobar hepatectomy after 6 weeks. All biochemical tests reverted to normal within 2 weeks. Preoperatively, six patients were estimated to have insufficient liver volume to withstand resection, but the liver subsequently hypertrophied to permit resection. In seven patients, there was complete necrosis of the HCC. All patients survived without major associated complications, and the 1-year survival was 95%. They reported that transarterial Ethiodol/ethanol administration was a safe and efficacious method for the treatment of HCC. It effectively decreased tumor size, caused hepatic hypertrophy, improved liver function, and allowed a wider range of patients to undergo hepatectomy with a better survival rate.[34]

HEPATIC METASTASES **Colorectal Metastases** Currently, the treatment of colorectal cancer to the liver is reserved for metastatic disease confined to the liver.[35] Although there is no proven survival benefit, there is an increase in local response rate when compared with systemic chemotherapy alone. There are also palliative benefits for symptomatic patients.[36,37] Pajkos and colleagues treated 41 patients with metastatic colorectal carcinoma to the liver with chemoembolization consisting of Adriamycin (doxorubicin) (50 mg), mitomycin C (8 mg), cisplatin (50 mg) or carboplatin (150 mg), lipiodol (10 mL), and starch microspheres every 6 weeks, as well as systemic 5-fluorouracil (5-FU) (425 mg/m^2) and leucovorin 20 mg/m^2 for 5 days every 28 days. The response rate was 68%, with a median survival time of 15 months.[38] Combination therapies are also being advocated in order to offer more patients palliative or survival benefits. Vogl and colleagues reported a mean reduction of tumor size of 35% in metastatic liver lesions treated with transarterial chemoembolization.[39] All patients in the study initially had unresectable disease that was also too large for treatment with percutaneous laser induced thermotherapy (LITT) alone. After chemoembolization, 50% of the patients had sufficient decrease in tumor bulk to allow treatment with LITT. Median survival in the group with combined therapy was 26 months.

Neuroendocrine Metastases Hepatic artery embolization is indicated for patients with multiple, nonresectable, hormonally active tumors. The goal of treatment is to reduce tumor bulk and hormone secretion. The 5-year postembolization survival range is 50 to 60%, with symptomatic and biochemical response ranges of 40 to 80% and 50 to 60%, respectively.[40] Moertel and colleagues chronicled their 10-year experience in 111 patients with neuroendocrine hepatic metastases, usually hypervascular, receiving vascular occlusion therapy by a variety of methods.[41] Seventy-one patients also received subsequent alternating chemotherapy regimens (dacarbazine + doxorubicin, alternating with streptozotocin + 5-FU). Objective regression rates of 60% with vascular occlusion alone and 80% with sequential therapy of vascular occlusion and chemotherapy were observed. A median survival time of 37 months was experienced by patients with islet cell carcinoma and 49 months by those with carcinoid hepatic metastases. Repeated embolizations were preferred.

At M. D. Anderson, the best results for metastatic disease of the liver treated with hepatic artery embolization with Ivalon or Gelfoam segments/powder have been observed in patients with metastatic neuroendocrine tumors to the liver. Sequential and periodic embolization is required for effective palliation. Gupta and colleagues have reported on 81 patients with carcinoid syndrome who were treated with either bland embolization (n = 50) or chemoembolization (n = 31).[42] Imaging was available in 69 patients for evaluation of a response. Of these patients, a partial response occurred in 46 patients (67%), minimal response in 6 patients (8.7%), stable disease in 11 (16%), and progression of tumor in 6 (8.7%). The median response duration was 17 months in patients with a partial response. A reduction of tumor-related symptoms occurred in 63%, with a median progression-free survival of 19 months, and a median overall survival time of 31 months.[42] These 69 patients with carcinoid tumor were compared with 54 patients who had islet cell tumor with metastases to the liver in a subsequent study by Gupta and colleagues.[43] Patients with carcinoid tumor benefited from a higher response rate and a longer progression-free survival (67% vs 35% and 23 months vs 16 months, respectively). Although chemoembolization did not prove to be beneficial for survival in patients with carcinoid tumor compared with bland embolization, it did result in improved overall survival and improved response (32 months vs 18 months and 50% vs 25%, respectively) in patients treated for islet cell tumor.

Other Hepatic Metastases Other types of hepatic metastases that are treated by chemoembolization at M. D. Anderson are metastatic ocular melanoma, metastatic leiomyosarcoma, and, on occasion, metastatic breast carcinoma and metastatic hypernephroma. For metastatic ocular melanoma, chemoembolization with cisplatin and Ivalon produced a response rate of 46% and a median survival period of 11 months.[44] The longest survival was 5 years from the initial chemoembolization. In the past, these patients lived for 2 to 6 months from presentation with hepatic metastases. Additional studies have been reported using hepatic arterial infusion of carboplatin-based chemotherapy or fotemustine with response rates of 38% and 40%, respectively.[44] Hepatic artery immunoembolization has also been reported with variable responses.[44] Patients with metastatic leiomyosarcoma to the liver were treated at M. D. Anderson with chemoembolization every 4 weeks, with cisplatin (150 mg) and Ivalon, 150 to 250 μm (150 mg), followed by vinblastine infusion (10 mg/m^2) of 2 hours into vessels that had undergone chemoembolization.[45] The response rate was 70% and lasted 4 to 19 months (median 9 months). Usually, a response greater than a PR was observed. This compared well with the response rate of 15% obtained after systemic therapy with ifosfamide with doxorubicin. It should be noted that these are not common tumors and that most are treated on protocol studies. The more common types of hepatic metastases from colorectal carcinoma and carcinoma of the breast are generally treated by systemic or intra-arterial chemotherapy. Our approach to chemoembolization of hepatic metastases is similar to that of hepatocellular carcinoma, that is, a hypervascular tumor is more likely to benefit from the treatment than a hypovascular tumor. The goal of treatment, whether it is to provide symptomatic relief or to prolong survival, must be considered against the risk of complications.

Genitourinary Neoplasms **Renal Carcinoma** Renal artery embolization for carcinoma is sometimes performed preoperatively to decrease operative blood loss in patients with extensive local tumor. One recent study has shown a survival benefit to preoperative embolization, although previous studies have not demonstrated this advantage.[46] Embolization of renal carcinoma is also performed for palliative relief of symptoms in patients with extensive local tumor, or as a cytoreductive measure when the patients are not candidates for surgery because of their general medical status.[47] Sequential renal artery embolization that preserves as much renal parenchyma and function as possible has also been used in the management of congestive heart failure caused by arteriovenous shunting through the renal carcinoma, and for hypertension, hypercalcemia, polycythemia, and hemorrhage caused by the renal neoplasm. Selective segmental embolization is especially necessary and effective in patients with an elevated serum creatinine level or a neoplasm in a solitary kidney. Embolization should be done, preserving at least 50% of the kidney to maintain adequate function. Percutaneous radiofrequency ablation has also been reported for the treatment of renal cell carcinoma, especially in patients who are not eligible for surgery because of comorbidities, or as a nephron-sparing alternative to surgery.[48] Ahrar and colleagues from M. D. Anderson describe their experience with 29 patients with 30 renal tumors who underwent percutaneous RF ablation.[49] A total of 88 overlapping ablations were performed in 34 sessions on the 30 tumors. Technical success was achieved in all cases. Follow-up imaging was available in 26 patients. Twenty-four of these 26 patients were treated for eradication of primary tumor, and imaging showed complete ablation in 23 of 24 patients (96%). Mean and median follow-up were 10 months and 7 months, respectively. Two patients were treated with RF ablation for gross hematuria. Both remain asymptomatic at last follow-up of 6 and 27 months for each. Four patients had major complications, including gross hematuria and urinary obstruction in three patients. All were successfully treated. One patient had persistent weakness of the anterior abdominal wall. None of the patients in the study had a significant degradation of renal function following treatment.

BIOPSY

Percutaneous biopsy has been the most cost-effective contribution to the diagnosis and management of the patient with cancer. Almost all tissues, including the myocardium, are accessible to percutaneous biopsy. A variety of needles (11–25 gauge) as well as biopsy forceps are efficient in obtaining representative specimens. Biopsy guns are available to automate the procedure. However, a negative biopsy does not exclude malignancy and may merely be an error in sampling. Most biopsies of lesions in adults are scheduled electively on an outpatient basis. Prothrombin time and platelet counts are determined, and any correctable coagulopathies are remedied. Intravenous sedation and local analgesics are usually adequate, while general anesthesia is reserved for children. After the biopsy, the patient is observed for approximately 1 to 3 hours before discharge from the department.

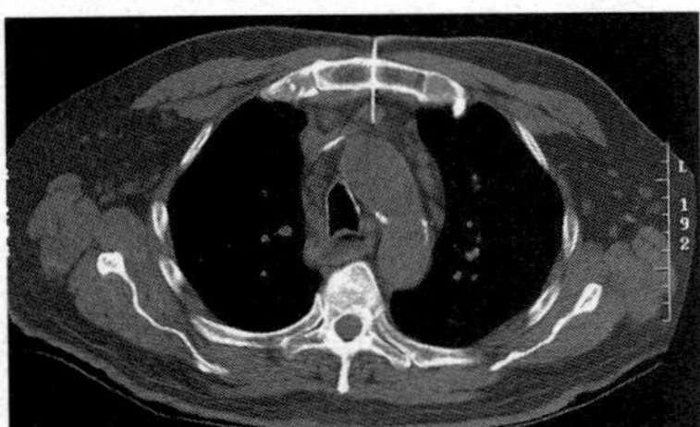

Figure 33-1 Biopsy of a mediastinal lymph node in a 45-year-old male with lymphoma. An 18 gauge guide needle was placed transsternally and samples were obtained through the 18 gauge needle with a 22 gauge needle.

The Thorax Guidance by fluoroscopy or computed tomography (CT) is usually adequate for biopsy of the lung or mediastinum (Figure 33-1).[50] The reported accuracy of percutaneous transthoracic needle biopsy of patients with lung cancer and pulmonary metastases is 90 to 98%,[51] while the diagnostic yield for local pulmonary infection in immunocompromised patients is 73%.[52] Positive cytology is disclosed in 72% of attempted biopsies of mediastinal masses, with a 9% incidence of complications.[53] Serious complications of lung and mediastinal biopsies include systemic air embolization, hemorrhage, pericardial tamponade, seeding of malignant cells into the needle track, lung torsion, and empyema. These are rare and should not alter the indications for biopsy. Pneumothorax is the most frequent complication (5–61%) done under fluoroscopic guidance. CT guidance may be associated with a higher frequency probably because it requires more time and the average size of the lesion is smaller. The reported incidence with CT guidance is 22 to 45%. In the study described by Cox and colleagues, smaller lesions (< 2 cm), biopsied under CT guidance and the presence of emphysema strongly correlated with the occurrence of pneumothorax, 42% with CT versus 21% with fluoroscopically guided biopsy.[54]

The Abdomen Guided by fluoroscopy, ultrasonography, CT, and magnetic resonance imaging (MRI), 84 to 95% of biopsies yielded adequate diagnostic material for cytologic analysis. When a 20- to 23-gauge needle is used, biopsies of the liver, pancreas, kidney, adrenal, spleen, and ovary, among other organs, are performed with a sensitivity of 86.6%, a specificity of 98.6%, and an accuracy of 90%. The overall complication rate in another study of 63,180 biopsies was 0.16%. Seeding of malignant cells along the needle tract was 0.05%.[55–57]

Lymph Nodes Metastatic lymphadenopathy from carcinoma can be detected with a high degree of accuracy (83–95%) by fine-needle aspiration (FNA) directed by fluoroscopy of lymph nodes that are opacified on lymphography, CT, or ultrasonography. At M. D. Anderson, the accuracy of needle biopsy of lymph nodes involved by lymphoma is now 80% with the help of immunocytochemical cell markers, deoxyribonucleic acid (DNA) flow cytometry, cytogenetics, molecular studies, and cytospin and cell block techniques for cytology.[58]

Musculoskeletal Biopsy The diagnostic accuracy of percutaneous skeletal biopsy is 80% (range, 50–94%).[59] At M. D. Anderson, the overall diagnostic accuracy of 78.6% was reported in a series of 178 patients with primary skeletal tumors who underwent percutaneous needle biopsy. The procedure was more accurate for malignant neoplasms (83%) than benign tumors (64.2%).[60] The frequency of positive bacterial cultures has been low for biopsies performed in patients with unsuspected infectious diseases.

INTRATUMORAL GENE THERAPY

Intratumoral injection of adenoviral or retroviral wild-type TP53 constructs in animal models results in tumor regression in a variety of different tumors, including nonsmall-cell lung cancer (NSCLC), leukemia, glioblastoma, and breast, liver, ovarian, colon, kidney, and prostate cancers. Roth and Cristiano demonstrated the safety and feasibility of using a retroviral wild-type TP53 (wt-TP53) in patients with advanced NSCLC.[61] Tumors regressed in 3 of 7 evaluable patients after bronchoscopic or CT-guided intratumoral injection of retroviral wt-TP53. In addition, Swisher and Roth administered adenovirus vector containing wt-TP53 complementary DNA (Ad-TP53) to 28 patients with NSCLC.[62] Patients received up to six intratumoral injections, at monthly intervals, of Ad-TP53 by percutaneous fine-needle injection (23 patients) or bronchoscopy (5 patients). Apoptosis was demonstrated in post-treatment biopsy specimens from 11 patients. Vector-related toxicity was minimal, despite 84 courses in 28 patients. Therapeutic activity in 25 patients available for follow-up included PR in 2 patients (8%), and disease stabilization (2–14 months) in 16 patients (64%). Repeated intratumoral injections of Ad-TP53 appear to be well tolerated, resulting in transgene expression of wt-TP53, and were seen to mediate antitumor activity in a subset of patients with advanced NSCLC. A phase II trial by Swisher and colleagues was designed to assess the locoregional efficacy of Ad-TP53 and radiotherapy in patients with nonmetastatic NSCLC. The 1-year overall survival rate was 45.5%, with most failures because of metastatic disease progression, and not local failure. Twelve of 19 biopsied patients (63%) showed no active tumor 3 months after completion of therapy.[63]

MECHANICAL DEVICES

Vena Cava Filters Cancer patients, especially those with hypercoagulability, experience an increased incidence of thrombophlebitis and pulmonary embolism. The percutaneous placement of a vena cava filter is the optimal therapeutic approach for patients with pulmonary embolism who have a contraindication to anticoagulation or who develop recurrent emboli despite adequate anticoagulation. There are numerous filters currently in use, including the Greenfield filter (Boston Scientific Vascular, Watertown, MA), the Bird's Nest filter (Cook, Bloomington, IN), the Simon Nitinol filter (Nitinol Medical Technologies, Woburn, MA), the Vena Tech filter (Vena Tech, Evanston, IL), the TrapEase filter (Cordis Europa NV, the Netherlands), and the Gunther Retrievable filter (William Cook Europe, Bjaeverskov, Denmark). In ex vivo tests, Kasmouris and colleagues demonstrated that the Bird's Nest filter and the Simon Nitinol filter were the most efficient,[64] while Hammer and colleagues concluded that the Bird's Nest filter had the highest clot-trapping capacity.[65]

The stainless steel Greenfield filter, the reference standard since 1972, is now delivered via a 12-F catheter placed through a 14-F sheath. The success rate of percutaneous placement was 99%; it was placed via the right femoral vein in 70% and via the left femoral or internal jugular vein in the remainder. At 30 days, there was a 3% incidence of recurrent pulmonary embolism and 98% caval patency. Incomplete opening was seen in 2% and insertion site hematoma in 1%.[66] The Bird's Nest filter also requires a 12-F insertion system through a 14-F sheath. The clinical incidence of recurrent pulmonary embolism was 2% and the caval patency rate was 97%.[67] It is certain that the patency rate over time for all filters is considerably lower if tested by inferior venacavography. Extensive collateral venous circulation can occur without signs or symptoms. The Simon Nitinol filter, the TrapEase filter, and a newer version of the Vena Tech filter are all designed to be delivered through a sheath that is ≤ 9-F. The advantages are decreased risk of puncture site hemorrhage and increased flexibility (so that the devices can be placed via nonstandard access routes, such as a contralateral vessel). In addition, these three filters all offer MR compatibility.

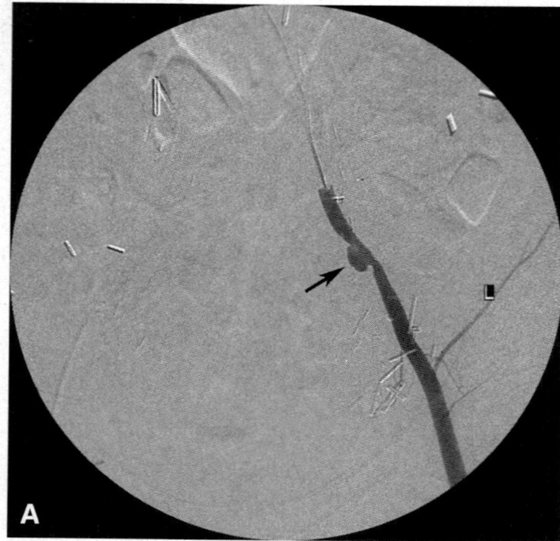

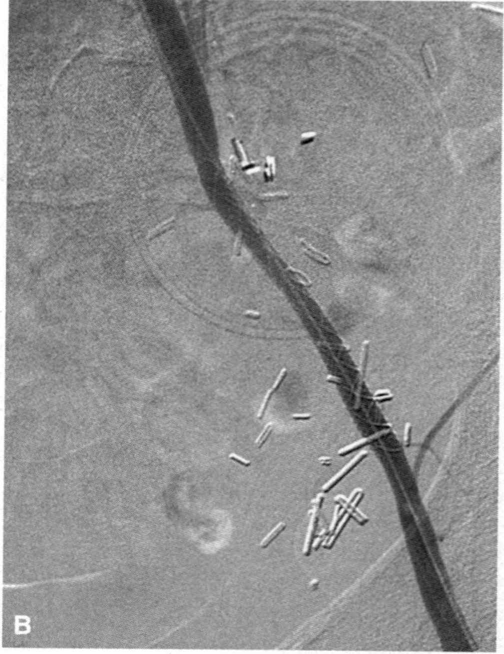

Figure 33-2 A 47-year-old female treated with a covered stent (Wallgraft) for an iliac artery pseudoaneurysm as a complication of treatment of cervical cancer. An iliac artery-ureteral fistula was suspected because of intermittent, significant hematuria and the triad of previous pelvic surgery, previous pelvic radiation, and a chronic ureteral endoprosthesis. **A**, A left external iliac artery pseudoaneurysm (*arrow*) was identified during a selective digital subtraction angiogram that was the presumed site of the ureteral-iliac artery fistula resulting in intermittent hematuria. **B**, The patient was treated with an intra-arterial metallic stent covered with PET excluding the pseudoaneurysm. No recurrent hemorrhage occurred.

Wallace and colleagues reported on the experience of vena cava filter placement in 308 patients with venous thromboembolic disease and malignancy at M. D. Anderson.[68] Median survival was 145 days and 207 days for patients with solid and liquid tumors, respectively. Patients with metastatic or disseminated disease were 3.7 times as likely to die as those with local disease, and patients with deep venous thrombosis (DVT) and a history of hemorrhage were twice as likely to die as those with DVT and no history of hemorrhage. Major complications included pulmonary emboli ($n = 4$), new caval thrombus ($n = 14$), retroperitoneal hemorrhage ($n = 2$), and maldeployed filters ($n = 2$).

Metallic Stents Metallic stents, bare and covered, were developed to restore or preserve the luminal patency and to cover gaps and fistulas of tubular structures—vena cavae, arteries, biliary ducts, tracheobronchial tree, and the gastrointestinal tract—caused by malignant neoplasms or the complications of therapy (Figure 33-2). These devices are usually delivered by fluoroscopic and/or endoscopic guidance. Metal stents (stainless steel, nitinol [nickel/titanium], and Elgiloy [cobalt/chromium]) have major advantages over plastic tubes in that they can be introduced in a compressed form in a small delivery system with more flexibility and versatility and can be self-or custom-expanded by balloon catheters. The internal working diameter of metal stents may be much greater than that of plastic stents and provide greater relief of obstruction. Metallic stents, however, are much more expensive and, in most cases, are not retrievable once placed. Pron and colleagues summarized the experience with nonvascular stents in more than 109 series involving 4,753 patients, including only six randomized trials in the biliary ducts and the esophagus. In both these sites, metallic stents were superior to plastic for palliation of obstructive signs and symptoms on the basis of longer and better patency and lower reintervention costs.[69]

The metallic stents, bare or covered, employed in the management of the oncologic patient include the self-expandable Gianturco "Z" stent (Cook Inc., Bloomington, IN), Wallstent Wallgraft and Strecker or Ultraflex (Boston Scientific Vascular, Watertown, MA), EndoCoil (InStent Inc., Eden Prairie, MN), Viabahn (W.L. Gore and Associates, Inc., Flagstaff, AZ), and the balloon-assisted Palmaz stent (Johnson & Johnson; Cordis Interventional Systems, Warren, NJ). The "Z" stent or zig-zag configuration has the greatest radial expansile force, comprising the least metal, but is the most rigid. This stent will continue to expand over time until it reaches its resting diameter. With installation, a minimum of two bodies for stability and adequate fixation should be used with a diameter of 20% greater than the normal diameter of the stenotic tubular structure to be dilated. The "Z" stent is available with and without barbs to limit migration. The Wallstent is also self-expandable and made of stainless steel with a criss-cross construction with a tantalum core to increase its radiopacity. The Wallstent I is a two-layer stainless steel mesh with a polyurethane coating (Permalume) between the wires. It is the most flexible and adapts well to almost all contours and is especially appropriate for tortuous vessels or curved bronchi and biliary ducts. The Wallstent does foreshorten by 20% when deployed. The Palmaz stent is derived from an etched stainless steel cylinder with a diamond contour when expanded and is rigid, requiring balloon assistance to distend it to the necessary diameter. The Palmaz stent has excellent radial force, but will not expand beyond the limits of the specific balloon size inflated. It is most effective in short segmental stenoses. Other stents are slight modifications of those described.

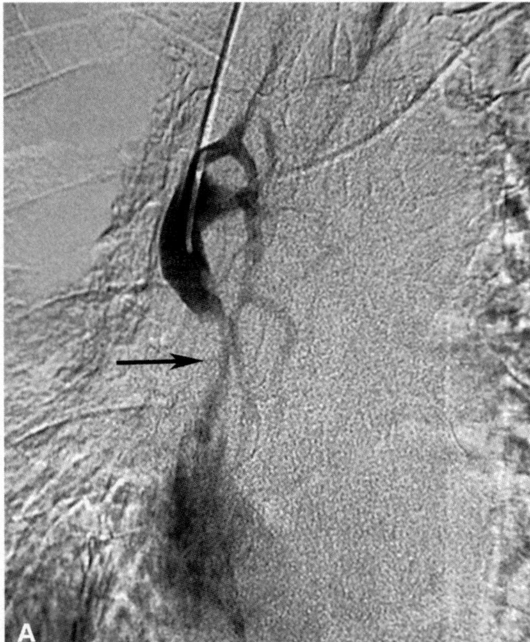

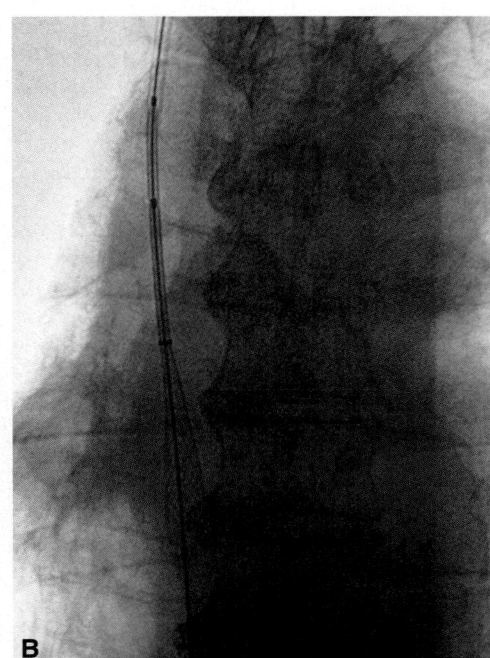

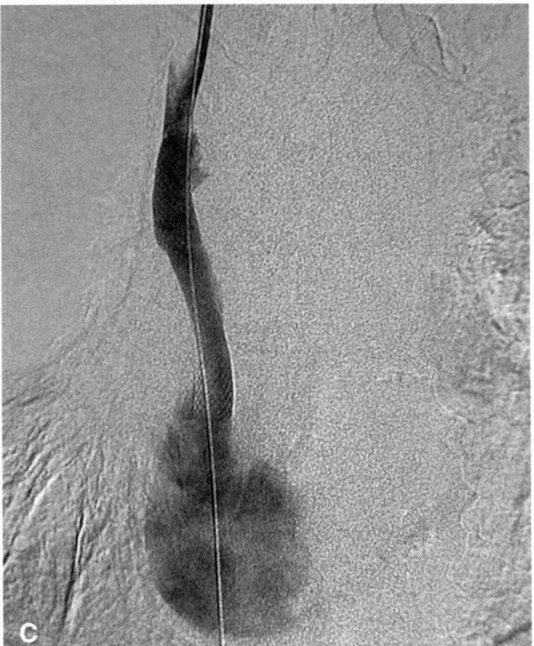

Figure 33-3 A 43-year-old male with lymphoma and superior vena cava (SVC) syndrome. **A**, Superior vena cavagraphy demonstrated severe narrowing (*arrow*) of the SVC with collateral veins. **B**, Deployment of the self-expanding Wallstent. **C**, Following placement of a Wallstent, the SVC is widely patent. The patient experienced complete symptomatic relief.

VENOUS STENOSIS Vena cava syndrome is most frequently the result of intrinsic or extrinsic malignant disease (74–95%). Primary neoplasms, by their extension and localization and secondary malignancies, especially as they affect mediastinal, retroperitoneal, and pelvic lymph nodes, will create stenosis and obstruction by extrinsic compression. The complications of radiation therapy and chemotherapy include mediastinal fibrosis and thrombophlebitis, especially because of toxic irritation of chemotherapeutic agents or faulty placement of the central venous catheter.[70]

Superior vena cava syndrome (SVC) symptoms have been grouped into four classes: (1) central nervous system (CNS) related: headache, blurred vision, and cognitive dysfunction; (2) laryngopharyngeal edema, producing dyspnea and hoarseness; (3) nasal or facial edema; and (4) other signs of venous congestion and dilatation.[71] In addition to the stenosis or obstruction, there is frequently thrombosis complicating the mediastinal compression or intraluminal invasion by the tumor. Parish and colleagues reported the average survival time after the diagnosis of malignant SVC obstruction to be 7 months.[72] Results of the treatment of venous stenosis using either the Gianturco "Z" stent or the Wallstent are similar, with the Gianturco "Z" preferred in the straight vessels and the superior or inferior vena cava, and the Wallstent in the more tortuous brachiocephalic or pelvic vessels. These stents can effectively palliate symptoms with malignant vena cava stenosis in 68 to 80% of patients.[70] Intraluminal thrombus or thrombophlebitis may be approached by mechanical or pharmaceutical thrombolysis followed by stenting.[71] Depending on the etiology, a "Z" stent may be preferred, especially if increased radial force is necessary or desirable. The patient is usually immediately aware of a relief of the symptoms of congestion once the stent has permitted adequate flow (Figure 33-3). Systemic anticoagulation is maintained, if flow is impaired.

ESOPHAGEAL STENTS Effective palliation of dysphagia is the main therapeutic goal of the interventional radiologist. Surgery has high morbidity and mortality as well as a high rate of recurrent dysphagia. Radiation therapy and/or chemotherapy provide relief of dysphagia in approximately 40% of patients, but may take 4 to 6 weeks to be effective. Laser therapy is highly effective in the treatment of malignant dysphagia; however, this therapy must be repeated about every 4 weeks, and it is ineffective on extrinsic compression of the esophagus.

Indications for esophageal stent placement are (1) contraindications to surgery or irradiation; (2) recurrent dysphagia after initial successful radiation, chemotherapy, or surgery; (3) circumferential stenosis or malignant stricture of the upper esophagus larger than 6 cm; (4) rapidly growing tumors; (5) extraluminal compression by neoplasm or adenopathy; (6) tracheoesophageal fistula; and (7) esophageal leak. Contraindications to esophageal stent placement include (1) cancer located less than 2 cm from the upper esophageal sphincter, (2) extremely limited life expectancy, and (3) lack of patient motivation. The relative contraindications include (1) total luminal obstruction, (2) noncircumferential tumor stenoses prohibiting anchoring of the stent, (3) angulated lesions leading to horizontal positioning of the stent, and (4) excessively bleeding or necrotic lesion.[69,73–75]

Insertion of self-expanding covered (polyurethane, silicone, latex) metallic endoprostheses for the palliation of malignant esophageal obstruction is an effective therapy that can be carried out with relative ease. Successful palliation of symptoms can be expected in more than 95% of cases. The average survival after stent placement was 24 weeks. Complication necessitating further intervention occurred in 10%. Placement of metallic esophageal endoprostheses is substantially better than endoscopic laser therapy for palliation of dysphagia in patients with inoperable esophageal carcinoma. The use of bare or covered metallic stents provides equal palliation in patients with dysphagia.[73–75]

Stomach and Proximal Small Bowel Self-expandable metallic prostheses (Wallstent, Gianturco "Z" stent, Ultraflex Nitinol Mesh stent, and EndoCoil stent) have been deployed to palliate patients with malignant stenoses of the stomach and proximal small bowel. Such prostheses will relieve intrinsic and extrinsic obstructive disease caused by primary neoplasms of the stomach (especially an outlet obstruction), duodenum, biliary tract, and proximal jejunum and secondary compression from a carcinoma of the pancreas, lymph node metastases, and peritoneal implants, with symptoms of early satiety, nausea, vomiting, and weight loss. Recurrent disease after successful treatment will also present with similar complaints. Access to the obstructive process may be by surgical, endoscopic, or an interventional radiologic approach.[69,74,76,77] Operative morbidity and mortality maybe as high as 25%, justifying the search for other alternatives.

The interventional radiologic management may be by the peroral or nasal catheter or the direct percutaneous transgastric technique facilitated by fluoroscopic guidance. The most frequent stent employed for gastric outlet and proximal small bowel obstruction has been the bare Wallstent. These uncovered stents have increased flexibility and decreased migration, but do have the potential for tumor ingrowth, which is less likely with covered stents.[69,76] Patients who have previously undergone a surgical procedure develop strictures related to local recurrence at or near the surgical anastomosis. The distorted anatomy may limit the use of a stent. Adequate evaluation for multiple strictures is important because this may also preclude placement. Although the numbers of such patients treated are small, the success rate has been rewarding.[74]

Colon Stents The incidence of obstruction in patients with colon carcinoma is approximately 30%. The placement of a metal stent may alleviate acute symptoms and allow appropriate preoperative management and evaluation for subsequent elective resection. In the event of disseminated carcinomatosis, a metallic stent may serve to palliate the patient's disease.[69,74,78,79]

A variety of bare or covered stents are available; the Wallstent is most frequently employed. DeGregorio and colleagues studied 126 consecutive patients with large bowel obstruction from colon carcinoma treated by covered Wallstent prostheses.[78] The obstruction was relieved by stenting in 91%. Eighty-one (70%) patients went on to bowel preparation and primary resection, while 34 (30%) had palliative stenting with a mean survival of 6.8 months. Eleven patients (9%) required colostomy for persistent obstruction. Complications occurred in 12% and included self-limited bleeding, stent migration, and symptomatic erosion and perforation. Canon and colleagues cautioned against balloon dilatation to facilitate stenting because of the risk of perforation of a friable tumor.[80] Binkert and colleagues noted that there was a significant cost saving of 28.8% in patients who underwent preoperative stent placement for malignant stenosis as palliation or in preparation for definitive reaction.[81]

Biliary Stents Pancreatic carcinoma, cholangiocarcinoma, and ampullary carcinoma are the primary neoplasms to produce intrinsic biliary obstruction, while extrinsic compression is the result of lymphadenopathy, hepatocellular carcinoma, or hepatic metastasis.[69,77,82–84] The first description of percutaneous biliary drainage in the United States appeared in 1965, when a percutaneously introduced catheter was placed in the obstructed biliary duct for up to 5 days.[83,85] Nonsurgical palliation of malignant biliary obstruction, accomplished either endoscopically or percutaneously, is now a well-established modality. The methods used include drainage by external or internal/external percutaneous biliary catheter or by biliary endoprosthesis.[77,82,83]

The aim of palliative therapy is to provide relief of jaundice and pruritus as well as associated cholangitis, and, most importantly, to prepare patients for anticancer therapy. Neither the endoscopic nor the percutaneous approach has an advantage with regard to influencing survival, and the choice of technique is often a team decision, based on the available local expertise (Figure 33-4). Internal drainage by the endoscopist is preferable because of the inconvenience of an external catheter, pain of the tube entry site, bile leakage around the catheter, and sepsis from skin organisms. If possible, most patients should be treated with an endoprosthesis, a metallic stent rather than plastic catheters.[69]

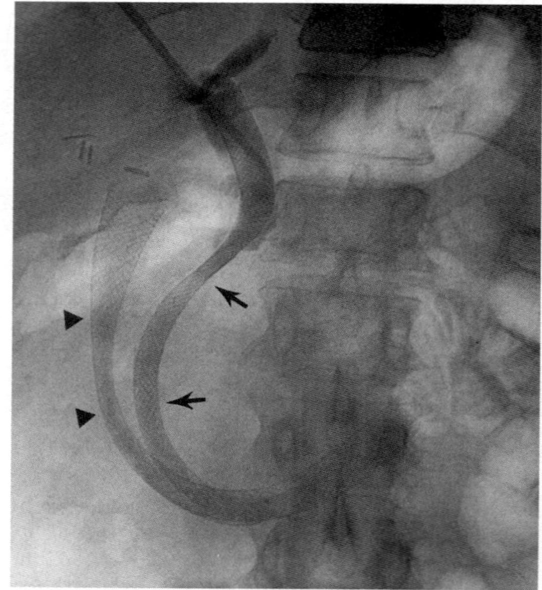

Figure 33-4 Patient with pancreatic cancer and a combined duodenal and biliary obstruction is managed by placement of metallic stents into the duodenum (*arrowheads*) and the common bile duct (*arrows*). The duodenal stent was placed endoscopically, and the biliary Wallstent was placed percutaneously because of the inability to cannulate the bile duct endoscopically. An external percutaneous biliary drainage catheter has been used to inject the biliary Wallstent at the time of placement to confirm patency.

Speer and colleagues described 70 patients with malignant biliary obstruction who were randomized to undergo drainage by either the percutaneous method (33 patients) or endoscopic stenting (37 patients).[84] The success rate of endoscopic stents relieving jaundice (81% vs 61% for the percutaneous method) and the complication rate (19% vs 67%) were significantly different in favor of the endoscopic approach. In addition, the 30-day mortality in the two groups (15% vs 33%) also favored patients who were palliated endoscopically. For patients who cannot be managed by internal drainage because of repeated occlusion, conversion to internal/external drainage may provide effective long-term palliation.[83] Various types of metallic endoprosthesis, both bare and covered, are commercially available for use in the biliary tree and have been described previously.

Cholangitis, hemorrhage, and bile leakage are the most common complications of endoprosthesis placement. There is a lower incidence of cholangitis in patients treated with a metallic endoprosthesis compared with a plastic endoprosthesis. Plastic stents are more prone to migrate (3–6% of cases). Metallic stents may be dislodged by balloon dilation immediately following deployment, but long-term spontaneous migration is negligible. In addition, loss of electrolytes and fluids, as well as pH imbalance may occur with external, but not internal, drainage. Stent occlusion remains a significant problem. The advent of expandable metallic stents, placed either endoscopically or transhepatically, has reduced the rate of occlusion of the stent, although occlusion secondary to tumor ingrowth or overgrowth remains a problem. Prospective randomized studies comparing endoscopically placed expandable metallic stents versus their plastic counterparts have shown an increased patency rate for metallic stents. However, even covered stents are subject to ingrowth, although somewhat delayed.[72,82,83,85]

Transjugular Intrahepatic Portosystemic Shunts The formation of a transjugular intrahepatic portosystemic shunt (TIPS), by placing a metallic stent between the hepatic and portal venous systems, is an accepted means of decreasing the sequelae associated with portal hypertension.[86] Indications include gastrointestinal variceal bleeding, ascites, portal gastropathy, hepatic hydrothorax, grade 4 varices (prophylactic) prior to myelosuppressive therapy, and Budd-Chiari syndrome. Cancer patients with hepatic disease may be candidates for this procedure. Wallace and colleagues, have reported 38 patients with malignancy and hepatic disease treated by TIPS placement at M. D. Anderson for the indications above.[87] Technical success was 97%. The mean portosystemic gradient decreased from 18.5 mm Hg to 7.5 mm Hg. Recurrent variceal hemorrhage occurred in only 1 of 19 patients (5%), and ascites/hydrothorax resolved or was significantly improved in 9 of 12 patients (75%). (Figure 33-5) The Achilles heel of TIPS has been the frequent occurrence of intimal hyperplasia and occlusion of the stent, with primary 1-year patency rates reported at 25 to 66%.[88] Development of covered stents to prevent stenosis has shown dramatic promise, with two studies demonstrating identical 1-year primary patency of 84%.[89,90]

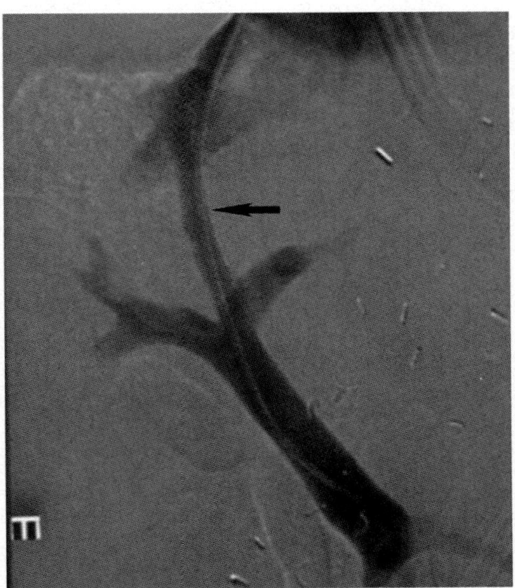

Figure 33-5 A communication between the right hepatic vein and the portal vein was formed by performance of a transjugular intrahepatic portosystemic shunt (*arrow*) in this 56-year-old male with cirrhosis and variceal bleeding.

REFERENCES

1. Charnsangavej C, Wallace S. Interventional radiologic techniques in the diagnosis and treatment of hepatobiliary malignancy. In: Wanebo H, editor. Surgery for gastrointestinal cancer: a multidisciplinary approach. PA: Lippincott-Raven; 1997. p.597–606.
2. Hemingway AP, Allison DJ. Complications of embolization: analysis of 410 procedures. Radiology 1988;166:669–72.
3. Maeda H, Seymour LW, Miyamoto Y. Conjugates of anticancer agents and polymers: advantages of macromolecular therapeutics in vivo. Bioconjug Chem 1992;3:351–62.
4. Kan Z. Dynamic study of iodized oil in the liver and blood supply to hepatic tumors. Acta Radiol 1996;37 Suppl 408:1–25.
5. Tancredi T, McCuskey PA, Kan Z, Wallace S. Changes in rat liver microcirculation after experimental hepatic arterial embolization: comparison of different embolic agents. Radiology 1999;211:177–81.
6. Yamada R, Kishi K, Sato M, et al. Transcatheter arterial chemoembolization (TACE) in the treatment of unresectable liver cancer. World J Surg 1995;19:795–800.
7. Yamashita Y, Takahashi M, Baba Y, et al. Hepatocellular carcinoma with or without cirrhosis: a comparison of CT and angiographic presentations in the United States and Japan. Abdom Imaging 1993;18:168–75.
8. Harada T, Matsuo K, Inoue T, et al. Is preoperative hepatic arterial chemoembolization safe and effective for hepatocellular carcinoma? Ann Surg 1996;224:4–9.
9. Lehnert T, Herforth C. Chemoembolization for hepatocellular carcinoma: what, when and for whom. Ann Surg 1996;224:1–3.
10. Uchida M, Kohno H, Kubota H, et al. Role of preoperative transcatheter arterial oily chemoembolization for resectable hepatocellular carcinoma. World J Surg 1996;20:326–31.
11. Nakamura H, Mitani T, Murakami T, et al. Five-year survival after transcatheter chemoembolization for hepatocellular carcinoma. Cancer Chemother Pharmacol 1994;33:S89–92.
12. Ohishi H, Yoshimura H, Uchida H, et al. Transcatheter arterial embolization using iodized oil (lipiodol) mixed with an anticancer drug for the treatment of hepatocellular carcinoma. Cancer Chemother Pharmacol 1989;23:S33–6.
13. Uchida H, Ohishi H, Matsuo N, et al. Transcatheter hepatic segmental arterial embolization using lipiodol mixed with an anticancer drug and Gelfoam particles for hepatocellular carcinoma. J Cardiovasc Interv Radiol 1990;13:140–5.
14. Matsui O, Kadoya M, Yoshikawa J, et al. Small hepatocellular carcinoma: treatment with subsegmental transcatheter arterial embolization. Radiology 1993;188:79–83.
15. Solomon B, Soulen MC, Baum RA, et al. Chemoembolization of hepatocellular carcinoma with cisplatin, doxorubicin, mitomycin-C, Ethiodol and polyvinyl alcohol: prospective evaluation of response and survival in a U.S. population. J Vasc Interv Radiol 1999;10:793–8.
16. Llovet JM. Updated treatment approach to hepatocellular carcinoma. J Gastroenterol 2005;40:225–35.
17. Sakamoto I, Aso N, Nagaoki K, et al. Complications associated with transcatheter arterial embolization for hepatic tumors. Radiographics 1998;18:605–19.
18. Goldberg SN, Livraguhi T. Solbiati L, Gazella GS. In situ ablation of focal hepatic neoplasms. In: Gazelle GS, Saini S, Mueller PR, editors. Hepatobiliary and pancreatic radiology: imaging and intervention. New York, NY: Thieme;1998. p.470–502.
19. Livraghi T, Goldberg SN, Lazzaroni S, et al. Small hepatocellular carcinoma: treatment with radio-frequency ablation versus ethanol injection. Radiology 1999;210:655–61.
20. Ebara M, Okabe S, Kita K, et al. Percutaneous ethanol injection for small hepatocellular carcinoma: therapeutic efficacy based on a 20-year observation. J Hepatol 2005;43:458–64.
21. Shiina S, Niwa Y. Percutaneous ethanol injection therapy in the treatment of liver neoplasms. In: Cope C, editor. Current techniques in interventional radiology. Philadelphia: Current Medicine; 1994. p.3.1–3.18.
22. Lencioni R, Allgaier H, Cioni D, et al. Small hepatocellular carcinoma in cirrhosis: randomized comparison of radiofrequency thermal ablation versus percutaneous ethanol injection. Radiology; 2003;228:235–40.
23. Gillams AR, Lees WR. Survival after percutaneous, image-guided, thermal ablation of hepatic metastases from colorectal cancer. Dis Colon Rectum 2000;43:656–61.
24. Groupe D'Etude et de Traitement du Carcinome Hepatocellulaire. A comparison of lipiodol chemoembolization and conservative treatment for unresectable hepatocellular carcinoma. N Engl J Med 1995;332:1256–61.
25. Madden MV, Krige JEJ, Bailey S, et al. Randomized trial of targeted chemotherapy with lipiodol and 5-epidoxorubicin compared with symptomatic treatment for hepatoma. Gut 1993;34:1598–600.
26. Pelletier G, Roche A, Ink O, et al. A randomized trial of hepatic arterial chemoembolization in patients with unresectable hepatocellular carcinoma. J Hepatol 1990;11:181–4.
27. Llovet JM, Real MI, Montana X, et al. Arterial embolisation or chemoembolisation versus symptomatic treatment in patients with resectable hepatocellular carcinoma: a randomised controlled trial. Lancet 2002;359:1734–9.
28. Lo C-M, Ngan H, Tso W-K, et al. Randomized controlled trial of transarterial lipiodol chemoembolization for unresectable hepatocellular carcinoma. Hepatology 2002;35:1164–71.
29. Geschwind JF, Salem R, Carr BI, et al. Yttrium-90 microspheres for the treatment of hepatocellular carcinoma. Gastroenterology 2004;127(5 Suppl 1):S194–205.
30. Ueno S, Aikou T, Tanabe G, et al. Exogenous hepatocyte growth factor markedly stimulates liver regeneration following portal branch ligation in dogs. Cancer Chemother Pharmacol 1996;91:763–71.
31. Madoff DM, Abdalla EK, Gupta S, et al. Transhepatic ipsilateral right portal vein embolization extended to segment IV: improving hypertrophy and resection outcomes with spherical particles and coils. J Vasc Interv Radiol 2005;16:215–25.
32. de Baere T, Roche A, Elias D, et al. Preoperative portal vein embolization for extension of hepatectomy indications. Hepatology 1996;24:1386–91.
33. Kan Z, Wallace S. Transcatheter liver lobar ablation: an experimental trial in an animal model. Eur Radiol 1997;7:1071–5.
34. Cheng YF, Kan Z, Chen CL, Lee TY. The efficacy and safety of preoperative lobar or segmental ablation via transarterial administration of Ethiodol and ethanol mixture in the treatment of hepatocellular carcinoma: a clinical study. World J Surg 2000;24:844–50.
35. Lian-Xin L, Wei-Hui Z, Hong-Chi J. Current treatment for liver metastases from colorectal cancer. World J Gastroenterol 2003;9:193–200.
36. Pentecost MJ, Teitelbaum GP, Katz M, Daniels JR. Chemoembolization in hepatic malignancy. Semin Interv Radiol 1992;9:28–36.
37. Lang E, Brown CL. Colorectal metastases to the liver: selective chemoembolization. Radiology 1993;189:417–22.
38. Pajkos G, Szentpétery L, Kristo K, Izsó J. Combined treatment of colorectal cancer liver metastases: intrahepatic chemoembolization and systemic chemotherapy. Orv Hetil 1998;139:1013–7.
39. Vogl T, Mack, M, Balzer J, et al. Liver metastases: neoadjuvant downsizing with transarterial chemoembolozation before laser induced thermotherapy. Radiology 2003;229:457–64.
40. Ramage JK, Davies AHG, Ardill, J, et al. Guidelines for the management of gastroenteropancreatic neuroendocrine (including carcinoid) tumors. Gut 2005;54:1–16.
41. Moertel CG, Johnson CM, McKusick MA, et al. The management of patient with advanced carcinoid tumors and islet cell carcinoma. Ann Intern Med 1994;120:302–9.
42. Gupta S, Yao J, Ahrar K, et al. Hepatic arterial embolization and chemoembolization for the treatment of patients with metastatic carcinoid tumors: the M. D. Anderson experience. Cancer J 2003;9:261–7.
43. Gupta S, Johnson M, Murthy, et al. Hepatic arterial embolization and chemoembolization for the treatment of patients with metastatic neuroendocrine tumors. Cancer 2005. [In press]
44. Feldman E, Pingpank J, Alexander H. Regional treatment options for patients with ocular melanoma metastatic to the liver. Ann Surg Oncol 2004;11:290–7.
45. Mavligit GM, Zukwiski AA, Ellis LM, et al. Gastrointestinal leiomyosarcoma metastatic to the liver. Durable tumor regression by hepatic chemoembolization infusion with cisplatin and vinblastine. Cancer 1995;75:2083–8.
46. Zielinski H, Szmigielski S, Petrovich Z. Comparison of preoperative embolization followed by radical nephrectomy with radical nephrectomy alone for renal cell carcinoma. Am J Clin Oncol 2002;23:6–12.
47. Campbell S, Flanigan R, and Clark J. Nephrectomy in metastatic renal cell carcinoma. Curr Treat Options Oncol 2003;4:363–72.
48. Gervais D, Arellano R, Mueller P. Percutaneous radiofrequency ablation of renal cell carcinoma. Eur Radiol 2005;12:960–7.

49. Ahrar K, Matin S, Wood C, et al. Percutaneous radiofrequency ablation of renal tumors: technique, complications, and outcomes. J Vasc Interv Radiol 2005;16:670–88.
50. Gupta S, Wallace MJ, Morello FA Jr, et al. CT-guided percutaneous needle biopsy of intrathoracic lesions by the transsternal approach: experience in 37 patients. Radiology 2002;222:57–62.
51. Westcott JL. Lung biopsy. In: Dondelinger RF, Rossi P, Kurdziel JC, Wallace S, editors. Interventional radiology. Stuttgart, Germany: Georg Thieme Verlag; 1990. p.9–17.
52. Castellino R, Blank N. Etiologic diagnosis of focal pulmonary infection in immunocompromised patients by fluoroscopically guided percutaneous needle aspiration. Radiology 1979;133:563–7.
53. Rosenberger A, Adler OB. Mediastinal biopsy. In: Dondelinger RF, Rossi P, Kurdziel JC, Wallace S, editors. Interventional radiology. Stuttgart, Germany: George Thieme Verlag; 1990. p.18–26.
54. Cox JE, Chiles C, McManus CM, et al. Transthoracic needle aspiration biopsy: variables that affect risk of pneumothorax. Radiology 1999;212:165–8.
55. Smith EH. Complications of percutaneous abdominal fine-needle biopsy [review]. Radiology 1991;178:253–8.
56. Stewart CJ, Coldewey J, Stewart IS. Comparison of fine needle aspiration cytology and needle core biopsy in the diagnosis of radiologically detected abdominal lesions. J Clin Pathol 2002;55:93–7.
57. Charboneau J, Reading C, Welch T. CT and sonographically guided needle biopsy: current techniques and new innovations. Am J Radiol 1990;154:1–10.
58. Carrasco CH, Richli WR, Lawrence D, et al. Fine needle aspiration biopsy of lymphoma. Radiol Clin North Am 1990;28:879–83.
59. Carrasco CH, Charnsangavej C, Richli WR, Wallace S. Bone biopsy. In: Dondelinger RF, Rossi P, Kurdziel JC, Wallace S, editors. Interventional radiology. Stuttgart, Germany: Georg Thieme Verlag; 1990. p.58–63.
60. Ayala AG, Zornoza J. Primary bone tumors: percutaneous needle biopsy: radiologic-pathologic study of 222 biopsies. Radiology 1983;149:675–9.
61. Roth JA, Cristiano RJ. Gene therapy for cancer: what have we done and where are we going? J Natl Cancer Inst 1997;89:21–39.
62. Swisher SG, Roth JA. p53 gene therapy for lung cancer. Curr Oncol Rep 2002;4:334–40.
63. Swisher SG, Roth JA, Komaki R J, et al. Induction of p53-regulated genes and tumor regression in lung cancer patients after intratumoral delivery of adenovirus p53 (INGN 201) and radiation therapy. Clin Cancer Res 2003;9:93–101.
64. Kasmouris AA, Williams AC, Delichatsios MA, Athanasoulis CA. Inferior vena cava filters: in vitro comparison of clot capture and flow dynamics. Radiology 1988;166:361–6.
65. Hammer FD, Rousseau HP, Joffre FG, et al. In vitro evaluation of vena cava filters. J Vasc Interv Radiol 1994;5:869–76.
66. Cho KJ, Proctor MC, Greenfield LJ. Efficacy and problems associated with inferior vena cava filters. In: Cope C, editor. Current techniques in interventional radiology, 2nd ed. Philadelphia: Current Medicine; 1994. p.8.1–8.3.
67. Roehm JOF, Johnsrude IS, Barth MH, Gianturco C. The Bird's Nest filter inferior vena cava filter: progress report. Radiology 1988;168:745–9.
68. Wallace M, Jean J, Gupta S, et al. Use of inferior vena caval filters and survival in patients with malignancy. Cancer 2004;101:1902–7.
69. Pron G, Common A, Simons M, Ho CS. Interventional radiology and use of metal stents in nonvascular clinical practice: a systemic overview. Semin Cardiovasc Interv Radiol 1999;10:613–28.
70. Charnsangavej C, Carrasco CH, Wallace S, Gianturco C. Self-expanding endovascular prostheses in the treatment of venous stenoses. In: Cope C, editor. Current techniques in interventional radiology, 2nd ed. Philadelphia: Current Medicine; 1994. p.10.1–10.10.
71. Kee ST, Kinoshita L, Razavi MK, et al. Superior vena cava syndrome: treatment with catheters directed thrombolysis and endovascular stent placement. Radiology 1998;206:187–93.
72. Parish JM, Marschke RF, Dines DE, Lee RE. Etiologic considerations in superior vena cava syndrome. Mayo Clin Proc 1981;56:407–13.
73. Cwikiel W, Tranberg K-G, Cwikiel M, Lillo-Gil R. Malignant dysphagia: palliation with esophageal stents—long term results in 100 patients. Radiology 1998;207:513–8.
74. Maxin M, Absher D, Pong E. The role of metal stents in the management of gastrointestinal obstructive disease. Appl Radiol 1999;(Suppl):26–32.
75. Raijman I, Siddique I, Ajani J, Lynch P. Palliation of malignant dysphagia and fistulae with coated expandable metal stents: experience with 101 patients. Gastroint Endosc 1998;48:172–9.
76. de Baere T, Harry G, Ducreux M, et al. Self-expanding metallic stents as palliative treatment of malignant gastroduodenal stenosis. AJR Am J Roentgenol 1997;169:1079–83.
77. Feretis C, Benakis P, Dimopoulos C, et al. Duodenal obstruction caused by pancreatic head carcinoma: palliation with self-expandable endoprostheses. Gastroint Endosc 1997;46:161–5.
78. DeGregorio MA, Mainar A, DiAgostino H, et al. Transanal metallic stents for malignant colonic obstruction: experience in 126 patients. J Vasc Interv Radiol 1999;10 Suppl 2:219.
79. Mainar A, Tejero E, Maynar M, et al. Colorectal obstruction: treatment with metallic stents. Radiology 1996;198:761–4.
80. Canon CL, Baron TH, Morgan DE, et al. Treatment of colonic obstruction with expandable metal stents: radiologic features. AJR Am J Roentgenol 1997;168:199–205.
81. Binkert CA, Ledermann H, Jost R, et al. Acute colonic obstruction: clinical aspects and cost-effectiveness of preoperative and palliative treatment with self-expanding metallic stents—a preliminary report. Radiology 1998;206:199–204.
82. Morgan RA, Adam A. Percutaneous management of biliary obstruction. In: Gazelle GS, Saini S, Mueller PR, editors. Hepatobiliary and pancreatic radiology: imaging and intervention. New York: Thieme; 1998. p.677–709.
83. Raijman I, Wallace S, Ajani J. The Shapiro article reviewed. Malignant biliary obstruction: nonoperative and palliative techniques by Marcelle Shapiro. Oncology 1995;9:499–503.
84. Speer ERG, Cotton PBS, Russell RCA, et al. Randomized trial of endoscopic versus percutaneous stent insertion in malignant obstructive jaundice. Lancet 1987;2:57–62.
85. Dodd GD, Greening RR, Wallace S. The radiologic diagnosis of cancer. In: Nealon T, editor. Management of patients with cancer, 3rd ed. Philadelphia: W.B. Saunders; 1965. p.72–113.
86. Barton RE, Rosch J, Saxon RR, et al. TIPS: short- and long-term results: a survey of 1750 patients. Sem Interv Radiol 1995;12:364–7.
87. Wallace M, Madoff D, Ahrar K, Warneke C. Transjugular intrahepatic portosystemic shunts: experience in the oncology setting. Cancer 2004;101:337–45.
88. Saxon RR, Ross PL, Mendel-Hartvig J, et al. Transjugular intrahepatic portosystemic shunt patency and the importance of stenosis location in the development of recurrent symptoms. Radiology 1998;207:683–93.
89. Rossi P, Salvatori F, Fanelli F, et al. Polytetrafluoroethylene-covered nitinol stent-graft for transjugular intrahepatic portosystemic shunt creation: 3-year experience. Radiology 2004;231:820–30.
90. Charon J, Alaeddin F, Pimpalwar S, et al. Results of a retrospective multicenter trial of the Viatorr expanded polytetrafluoroethylene-covered stent-graft for transjugular intrahepatic portosystemic shunt creation. J Vasc Interv Radiol 2004;15:1219–30.

Part IV

Principles of Therapeutic Modalities

Section 8

SURGICAL ONCOLOGY

34

Principles of Surgical Oncology

Raphael E. Pollock, MD, PhD, FACS
Donald L. Morton, MD, FACS

Surgery is the oldest modality of cancer therapy and still forms the mainstay of treatment in solid tumors. It remains a paradigm that more patients are cured by surgery when it is used as a single treatment in comparison with any other individual form of cancer therapy. Even in the contemporary multimodality cancer therapy milieu, it is the rare solid-tumor patient whose care does not include a surgical component. To be maximally effective, the cancer surgeon must function as a member of the oncology team and is frequently the first oncology specialist that a patient will consult. The cancer surgeon is commonly charged with the responsibility to establish a tissue diagnosis for a suspicious lesion; this may require an operative procedure or an image-directed or other biopsy approach. The cancer surgeon will usually bear the responsibility for communicating the biopsy findings to the patient, completing the procedures needed to stage the cancer, and initiating subsequent interaction between the patient and other members of the multimodality oncology team. Because of these responsibilities, it is most often the cancer surgeon who initially explains to the patient the sequence and rationale of the various treatment components that will be used to manage the specific malignancy. To be maximally effective, the cancer surgeon must therefore be aware of the different therapeutic options, the natural history of a given malignancy, and how these factors will be integrated into a well-conceived and appropriate multimodality treatment algorithm. It is also usually the cancer surgeon's responsibility to provide initial information about prognosis and to make decisions about follow-up care and surveillance to detect tumor recurrence. In these regards, the cancer surgeon is unlike almost any other surgical specialist in that the commitment to a given patient is for both the acute and the long-term components of the patient's disease process.

Over the years, the practice of surgical oncology has come full circle. Originally, surgeons attempted to treat cancer conservatively by removing only the gross lesion. Unfortunately, this led to extremely high rates of local recurrence and subsequent patient mortality. In the late nineteenth century, surgeons began to undertake complete en bloc resections and amputations to treat patients with malignant lesions. These techniques yielded improved results, but the procedures were ablative and mutilating. With the advent of complementary and effective treatment modalities, notably radiation therapy in the 1920s and chemotherapy after the 1940s, the orientation of surgical resection is once again becoming conservative.

Adjuvant chemotherapy, alone or in combination with radiation therapy, has improved disease-free survival and prolonged quality life for patients who have been rendered free of gross disease by surgery but who still have a high likelihood of recurrence as a consequence of microscopic residual metastases. Randomized clinical trials have demonstrated the benefit of adjuvant chemotherapy in a variety of tumors, including breast cancer, colon cancer, osteogenic sarcoma, testicular cancer, ovarian cancer, and certain lung cancers. In some cancers (eg, sarcoma), the benefit of adjuvant therapy is modest; however, in other tumor systems, such as testicular and bone cancer, it has resulted in two- and threefold improved overall survival rates.

Surgery is most effective in the treatment of localized primary tumor and associated regional lymphatics. This is accomplished by en bloc surgical procedures that attempt to encompass gross and microscopic tumor in all contiguous and adjacent anatomic locations. Intuitively, it appears logical that surgery should have little role in disease management once a neoplasm has spread from the primary location to a distant site. However, prolonged survival is possible following the surgical resection of some metastases in the lung, liver, or brain. For example, a 5-year survival rate up to 40% can be anticipated after surgical resection of solitary colorectal metastasis in the liver.

Surgery operates by zero-order kinetics, in which 100% of excised cells are killed. In contrast, chemotherapy and radiation therapy operate by first-order kinetics, and only a fraction of tumor cells are killed by each treatment. These zero- and first-order processes are complementary. Surgical resection reduces the tumor burden, which hopefully increases the efficacy of nonsurgical adjuvant therapies intended to eliminate microscopic residual disease, thereby decreasing the risk of recurrence.

During the past two decades, major improvements in both operative technique and the use of combined modality therapy have significantly reduced the morbidity and mortality associated with the surgical treatment of solid neoplasms. For example, breast-preserving surgery has become an alternative to mastectomy in patients with breast carcinoma, limb salvage is often possible in patients with bone and soft-tissue sarcomas, and sexual potency/urinary continence can frequently be preserved for patients with prostate cancer. Because surgery is increasingly combined with other treatment modalities, it is essential that most patients with solid neoplasms have their treatment planned by a multidisciplinary team, which includes radiation and medical oncologists as well as surgical oncologists. To retain a primary role in the management of the cancer patient, the successful surgical oncologist must be able to coordinate and integrate the efforts of the entire oncologic team.

HISTORICAL CONSIDERATIONS

Oncology (from the Greek words *onkos*, meaning mass or tumor, and *logos*, meaning study) is the study of neoplastic diseases. Early authors suggested that certain families, races, and working classes were predisposed to neoplastic transformations. In 1862, Edwin Smith, an American Egyptologist, discovered the apparently earliest recordings of the surgical treatment of cancer.[1] Written in Egypt circa 1600 BC, this treatise was based on teachings possibly dating back to 3000 BC. The Egyptian author advised surgeons to contend with tumors that might be cured by surgery but not to treat those lesions that might be fatal.

Hippocrates (460–375 BC) was the first to describe the clinical symptoms associated with cancer. He advised against treating terminal patients, who would enjoy a better quality of life without surgical intervention.[2] He also coined the terms *carcinoma* (crab legs tumor) and *sarcoma* (fleshy mass). In the second century AD, Galen published his classification of tumors, describing cancer as a systemic disease caused by an excess of black bile.[3] Galen cautioned that as a systemic disease, cancer was not amenable to cure by surgery, which was often promptly followed by patient death. This strong admonition against surgery persisted for more than 1,500 years until eighteenth-century pathologists discovered that cancer often grew locally before spreading to other anatomic sites. Prior to the advent of safe general anesthetics, surgery was used primarily to manage trauma or severe infectious problems such as abscess drainage. In that era, cancer surgery consisted primarily of amputation or cauterization of surface tumors of the trunk or extremities. Patients were usually unwilling to submit to the pain of tumor surgery, when there was little likelihood of improved survival.

During the eighteenth and nineteenth centuries, advances in anatomic pathology led to an increase in autopsies, which, in turn, resulted in a better understanding of human physiology. The early work of Morgagni, Le Dran, and Da Salva established that there was an initial period of local tumor growth prior to distant dissemination. This led to the understanding that not all tumors were systemic, and that certain lesions cause death solely by local invasive growth. Percival Pott (1714–1788) was the first to describe a specific etiologic factor associated with cancer development. In 1775, Pott demonstrated a high incidence of cancer of the scrotum in chimney sweeps who had reached puberty and recommended wide local resection for cure. In 1829, the French Surgeon Joseph Recamier (1774–1852) first described the complicated process of tumor dissemination. The first recorded elective tumor resection was performed in 1809 by Ephraim McDowell, an American surgeon. He successfully removed a 22-pound ovarian tumor from a patient, who subsequently survived 30 years. McDowell's work, which included 12 more ovarian resections, stimulated greater interest in elective surgery for cancer patients.

Surgeons were initially hindered by the extreme discomfort that patients experienced during surgical procedures, as well as the lack of agents that could reduce the incidence of infection. Crawford Long (1815–1878) was the first to use ether for general anesthesia in 1842, but it was the reported work of John Collins Warren (1778–1856) and William T.G. Morton (1819–1868) that brought the potential of anesthesia to public attention. The surgical procedure in Warren's first published account of ether anesthesia (1846) was the elective removal of a tongue carcinoma for which submaxillary gland resection and partial glossectomy were performed. Warren was also responsible for the first American-authored textbook of tumor surgery, *Surgical Observations on Tumors*, published in 1838. Joseph Lister (1827–1912) was the first to report the successful use of antisepsis during elective surgery. In 1867, Lister applied Pasteur's concept that bacteria caused infection, when he introduced the use of carbolic acid as an antiseptic agent in conjunction with heat sterilization of surgical instruments. Lister is also credited with the introduction of absorbable ligatures, as well as the placement of drainage tubes to control secretions and dead space in surgical wounds. Robert Wood Johnson developed the individual sterile dressing pack in 1876, which also remarkably improved postoperative wound-contamination problems.

Even with the advent of antisepsis and general anesthesia, surgical oncology in the second half of the nineteenth and early twentieth centuries was still associated with high patient mortality rates. Cancer was rarely diagnosed in the early stages; consequently, few patients were considered candidates for curative surgery. Those surgeons who did attempt surgical excision of malignant lesions were hindered by rudimentary anesthesia, which was also independently associated with high patient mortality. Antibiotics were not yet available, and surgical instruments were crude. The importance of the microscope to evaluate frozen tissues for surgical margins was not yet appreciated, and surgeons had great faith in their own unaided gross visual assessment of the tumor perimeter. However, several important developments in this era led to rapid advancements in surgical oncology. Emphasizing meticulous surgical technique, gentle tissue handling, and applications of listerian principles, pioneers such as Albert Theodore Billroth (first gastrectomy, laryngectomy, and esophagectomy), William Stewart Halsted (en bloc resection, radical mastectomy), as well as many other more contemporary surgeons defined and advanced the boundaries of surgical oncology, as summarized in Table 34-1.[2,3]

Table 34-1 Landmark Advances in Surgical Oncology

Year	Event	Surgeon
1775	Etiologic basis of cancer	Percival Pott
1809	Elective oophorectomy	Ephraim McDowell
1829	Metastatic process	Joseph Recamier
1846	Ether as anesthesia	John Collins Warren
1867	Carbolic acid as antisepsis	Joseph Lister
1873	Laryngectomy	Albert Theodore Billroth
1878	Resection of rectal tumor	Richard von Volkman
1880	Esophagectomy	Albert Theodore Billroth
1881	Gastrectomy	Albert Theodore Billroth
1890	Radical mastectomy	William Stewart Halsted
1896	Oophorectomy for breast cancer	G.T. Beatson
1904	Radical prostatectomy	Hugh H. Young
1906	Radical hysterectomy	Ernest Wertheim
1908	Abdominoperineal resection	W. Ernest Miles
1909	Thyroid surgery (Nobel Prize)	Theodore Emil Kocher
1910	Craniotomy	Harvey Cushing
1912	Cordotomy for the treatment of pain	E. Martin
1913	Thoracic esophagectomy	Franz Torek
1927	Resection of pulmonary metastases	George Divis
1933	Pneumonectomy	Evarts Graham
1935	Pancreaticoduodenectomy	Allen O. Whipple
1945	Adrenalectomy for prostate cancer	Charles B. Huggins
1957	Isolated limb perfusion	Oliver Creech
1958	Organization of National Adjuvant Breast and Bowel Project (NSABP) to conduct prospective randomized trials	Bernard Fisher
1965	Hormonal therapy of cancer	Charles Huggins
1971	Free tissue transfer with microvascular anastomosis	Harry Buncke

Ongoing innovations to advance effective surgical primary tumor control have improved surgical outcomes and quality of life. Advances in microvascular surgery now permit the free transfer of complex autologous tissues, such as free jejunal grafts to reconstitute the upper aerodigestive system or osteomyocutaneous flaps to reconstruct extremities and other mobile body parts such as the jaw. Automatic stapling devices, as well as endoscopic instrumentation coupled with high-resolution fiberoptics, have remarkably advanced intra-abdominal, thoracic, and pelvic tumor surgery, resulting in less-morbid procedures that require significantly less patient recuperation time and effort (Figure 34-1). Enhanced biomedical monitoring and the emergence of critical care medicine have made it possible to safely undertake increasingly complicated surgical procedures. A more sophisticated awareness of the patterns of tumor progression has made possible less-invasive surgical approaches. Examples include sentinel node biopsy as a replacement for

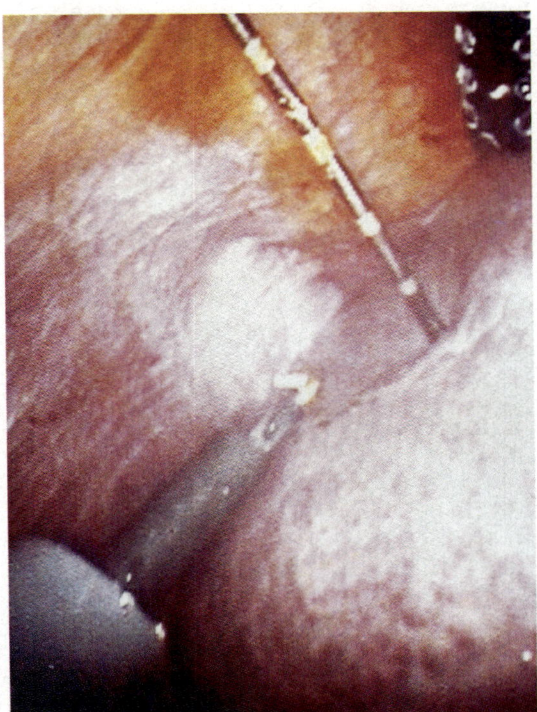

Figure 34-1 Laparoscopic ultrasound of dome of liver with cutting needle biopsy prior to resection of hepatic colorectal metastases. Note ultrasound unit in left lower foreground, percutaneously placed biopsy needle in the liver, and diaphragm in the background. Courtesy of Nicolas Vauthey, MD, Department of Surgical Oncology, University of Texas M.D. Anderson Cancer Center.

formal lymphadenectomy in early-stage melanoma and breast carcinoma, and the introduction of radiofrequency ablation with ultrasonography guidance, which has markedly enhanced surgical cancer control of multifocal liver disease while minimizing patient morbidity.

THE CONTEMPORARY ROLE OF SURGICAL ONCOLOGY

Surgical oncologists are surgeons who devote most of their time to the study and treatment of malignant neoplastic disease. They must possess the necessary knowledge, skills, and clinical experience to perform both the standard as well as extraordinary surgical procedures required for patients with cancer. Surgical oncologists must be able to diagnose tumors accurately and to differentiate aggressive neoplastic lesions from benign reactive processes. In addition, surgical oncologists should have a firm understanding of radiation oncology, medical oncology, and hematology. They must also be capable of organizing interdisciplinary studies of cancer. Surgical oncologists should also be trained in pathology, because they will be called on to excise appropriate tumor samples for pathologists and make decisions about adequacy of surgical margins. Surgical oncologists have a shared role with medical oncologists as the "primary care physicians" of cancer treatment. Almost all cancer patients will initially be managed by one of these two specialists who will bear the ultimate responsibility for coordinating appropriate multimodality care for the individual patient.

Not surprisingly, given the complexity of contemporary multidisciplinary approaches to the cancer patient, free-standing cancer centers have developed facilities to provide the needed planning expertise, clinical care, patient support services, and access points to clinical trials. Cancer center professional staff share the exclusive goal of eradicating neoplastic disease. Comprehensive cancer centers are frequently (but not invariably) affiliated with academic medical institutions and offer the complete spectrum of oncology therapies, clinical trials, rehabilitation, and social services, as well as basic and translational research programs to move new knowledge from the laboratory bench to the patient bedside. In this contemporary oncology milieu, the role of the surgical oncologist has expanded, while the overall impact of noncancer surgical specialists has declined.

Surgical oncology is more of a cognitive than a technical surgical specialty. With the exception of a small cluster of index operations, such as regional pancreatectomy, limb salvage and retroperitoneal sarcoma surgery, isolated limb perfusion, and multisegment liver resection, most of the surgical procedures that are performed by surgical oncologists are similar to those performed by a surgeon not oncologically trained. What frequently differentiates these two types of surgeons is not merely knowledge about *how* to do a specific operation, but an awareness of *how and when* to do that operation; that is, the cognitive knowledge of contemporary multimodality cancer care. A broad knowledge of cancer in its presenting and recurring forms, as well as an awareness of the molecules driving tumor proliferation and dissemination, is an integral part of the special cognitive database of the surgical oncologist.

As part of the larger surgical community, the surgical oncologist is a critical conduit of cancer information to colleagues in general surgery and other surgical specialties. This individual makes academic presentations at large surgical meetings, such as those of the American College of Surgeons or the Society of Surgical Oncology, directs hospital-based tumor boards, and consults on behalf of individual cancer patients. Because of their leading role in the initial diagnosis of cancer, it is not surprising that surgical oncologists are also frequently in leadership roles in cancer prevention and screening programs. Nationally based multimodality clinical trial groups also depend on surgical oncology expertise to help in trial design, establishing the criteria of surgical quality control, educating trial participants regarding standards of surgical care (including indications for procedures), as well as assistance in accurate data collection, analysis, and presentation of trial results.

COMBINED MODALITY THERAPY

Pediatric oncologists pioneered the use of combined modality therapy (radiation in combination with chemotherapy and surgery) as effective management of childhood neoplasms. Control of localized retinoblastoma in children has been dramatically increased by using multimodality therapy. The cure rate for patients with Wilms' tumor is 75%, if surgical therapy is followed by chemotherapy and, in some cases, radiation, an increase of 40% over operation alone. Embryonal rhabdomyosarcoma responds best to combinations of radiation, chemotherapy, and operation. Until recently, the effectiveness of multimodality therapy was only occasionally demonstrable for adult neoplasms. A striking example is the approach to skeletal and soft-tissue sarcomas. Surgical therapy, the accepted method for local management of most skeletal and soft-tissue sarcomas of the extremities, is associated with frequent treatment failure if used alone. In the past, approximately 50% of patients with soft-tissue sarcomas and 80% of those with bone sarcomas eventually succumbed to distant metastases, even after amputation of the extremity bearing the primary tumor. Consequently, multimodality treatment regimens were developed to improve these results. Preoperative chemotherapy with intra-arterial doxorubicin followed by radiation resulted in extensive tumor cell necrosis in as many as 75% of patients.[4] The effectiveness of this preoperative therapy permitted local resection of the sarcoma and salvage of a viable functional extremity. Local recurrence rates were as low as with amputation, and long-term results were functionally and psychologically superior. In addition, there was no decrease in overall or disease-free survival rates. Multimodality therapy is also effective for localized breast cancers. In clinical trials, radiation and minimal surgery were demonstrably as effective as mastectomy in the control of small breast cancers. Survival and local recurrence rates were the same for both groups, and patients treated with multimodality therapy were spared the physical deformity and psychological problems of mastectomy.

In selecting appropriate therapy, surgery and radiation are still the most successful means of treating cancer localized to the primary site and/or regional lymph nodes. Because these forms of therapy exert their effects locoregionally, neither is usually considered curative once the disease has metastasized beyond these sites. However, both methods are frequently useful as palliative treatments, and occasional long-term survival follows surgical resection of single-organ metastases.

An emerging component of the multimodality approach is tumor immunotherapy. The concept of immunostimulation with biologic response modifiers or nonspecific immunomodulators is not new in cancer therapy. Nearly a century ago, William B. Coley developed the basis for nonspecific cancer immunotherapy using mixed bacterial vaccines (Coley toxin). Since then, whole-cell or cell-fragment tumor vaccines have been introduced for active specific immunotherapy of neoplastic disease, and some of these have reached clinical applications maturity. In melanoma, which is the focus of most cancer vaccine research, immunochemotherapy is now used as an adjuvant to surgery for treatment of local and regional neoplastic disease, as well as to prolong the survival of patients with distant metastases. Cytokines such as interferon are being used to modulate the immune response and have proved effective in some diseases, such as chronic myeloid leukemia and hairy-cell leukemia. Use of the colony-stimulating factor (CSF) is invaluable in accelerating hematopoietic recovery from high-dose chemotherapy, as well as a comparison of bone marrow transplantation protocols.

Unlike surgery and radiation therapy, systemic therapies, such as chemotherapy, immunotherapy, and hormonal therapy, are treatments that can kill tumor cells that have already metastasized to distant sites. These systemic modalities have a greater chance of cure in patients with minimal (or even subclinical) tumor burden, as compared with those patients with clinically evident disease. Consequently, surgery and radiation therapy may be useful in decreasing a given patient's tumor burden, thereby maximizing the impact of subsequent systemic approaches.

Whether the goals of therapy should be cure or palliation depends on the stage of a specific cancer. If the cancer is localized without evidence of spread, it may be possible to eradicate the cancer and cure the patient. When the cancer has spread beyond the possibility of cure, the goal is to control symptoms and maintain maximum activity and quality of life for as long as possible (Figure 34-2). Patients are generally judged incurable if they have distant metastases or evidence of extensive local infiltration of critical structures adjacent to tumor. However, some patients are potentially curable even though they have distant metastases. For example, patients with solitary pulmonary, hepatic, or cerebral metastases may still be curable by resection, and patients with widespread choriocarcinoma or ovarian carcinoma metastases may still be cured using chemotherapy. Histologic proof of distant metastases should be obtained before the patient is deemed incurable. Occasionally, an exploratory celiotomy or thoracotomy may be necessary to determine the histology of ambiguous lesions in the lungs or liver. In rare situations, the clinical situation may point so overwhelmingly to distant metastases that the patient may be considered incurable without biopsy. For each anatomic site, there are certain local criteria that place the patient unequivocally in an incurable status, whereas other anatomic constraints may imply a poor prognosis but are not an absolute indication of incurability per se. In equivocal situations where extensive studies fail to demonstrate metastatic or incurable local extension, the patient deserves the benefit of the doubt and should be treated for cure.

The selection of therapeutic modalities depends not only on the type and extent of cancer, but also on the patient's general condition and the presence of any coexisting disease. For example, surgery may be contraindicated in a patient who has had a recent myocardial infarction. A patient with preexisting diabetes will be much more susceptible to the toxic effects of hormonal therapy with corticosteroids. Renal disease may increase the toxicity of some of the chemotherapeutic agents, such as methotrexate or ifosfamide. In addition, acute or chronic infection or bleeding may make any form of cancer therapy dangerous and must be addressed before initiating definitive oncology treatment.

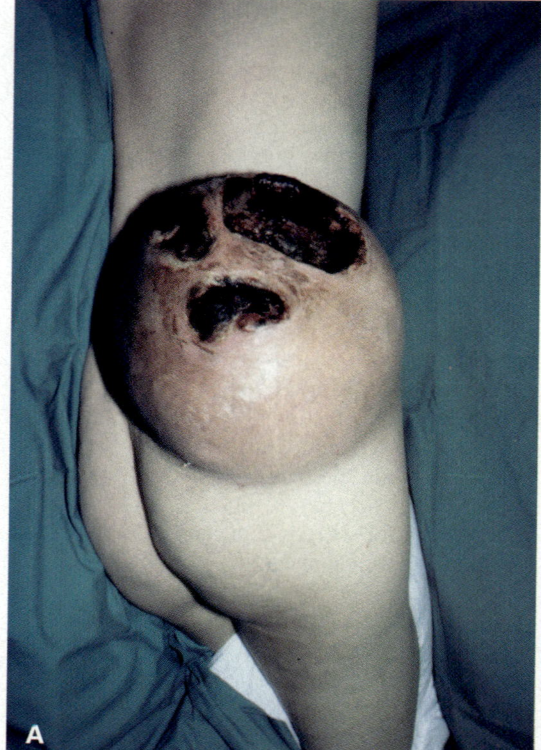

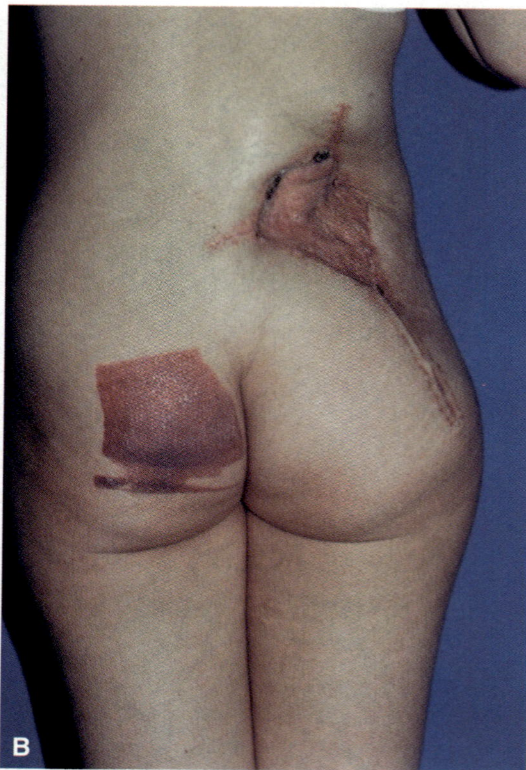

Figure 34-2 Palliative surgery. **A,** A patient with a large fungating tumor occupying the lumbar triangle and superior buttock region. This patient had already developed lung metastases and was suffering from intractable pain. The tumor itself created a socially unacceptable situation and prevented her from interacting with her family. **B,** The same patient several weeks after a negative margin wide local excision with skin graft closure. The patient's pain problem was eliminated, and she was able to fully interact with her family. Systemic therapy for her metastatic disease could be initiated.

The patient's psychologic make-up and life situation also must be considered. A patient who is unable to accept the realities of a given treatment should be offered other treatment options, if possible. Consultation with a psychiatrist experienced in cancer (a psycho-oncologist) may help the patient deal with the reality of the disease and its treatment. This is particularly true for surgical procedures that significantly alter the patient's appearance, such as mastectomy, or those that involve a change of organ function, such as colostomy. Encouraging the patient to talk with others who have successfully undergone and adjusted to the particular operation will be helpful. Experimental forms of therapy should also be avoided in some patients whose potential noncompliance might jeopardize both themselves as well as the clinical trial. For example, patients who are unwilling to tolerate the inconvenience of an intra-arterial catheter (and might therefore remove it themselves) should not undergo treatment that depends on this form of angioaccess.

Extensive staging procedures may indicate that a tumor is localized to a primary site and/or regional lymph nodes, and hence curable by local therapy (surgery and/or radiation). However, approximately 60% of localized malignant tumors ultimately recur, suggesting that many such patients must have had subclinical metastases at the time of initial diagnosis. The probability of cure may be improved if systemic approaches are coupled with local treatment. Chemotherapeutic drugs must be given when the number of tumor cells is low enough to permit their destruction at doses that can be tolerated by the patient. The opportunity for cure is most likely during the early stage of disease or immediately after surgery when the tumor burden has been minimized. Adjuvant chemotherapy has remarkably improved surgical results in some malignancies, primarily because of cytocidal effects on clinically undetectable neoplastic cells outside the operative field. Neoadjuvant or induction chemotherapy that is initiated prior to local and regional treatments also can affect micrometastatic distant disease while significantly cytoreducing the primary tumor. After a course of neoadjuvant chemotherapy, the tumor may be surgically resected with or without concomitant preoperative or postoperative radiotherapy.

Classically, surgery has been first in the sequence of therapies for solid neoplasms, but increasing evidence suggests that it should perhaps be the last. Chemotherapy and radiation therapy both work by first-order kinetics. However, because of tumor cell heterogeneity, it can be anticipated that resistant clones of viable neoplastic cells may persist in the primary tumor after these therapies. Such clonal heterogeneity is more likely in large tumors that are both poorly perfused by chemotherapeutic agents and are also relatively

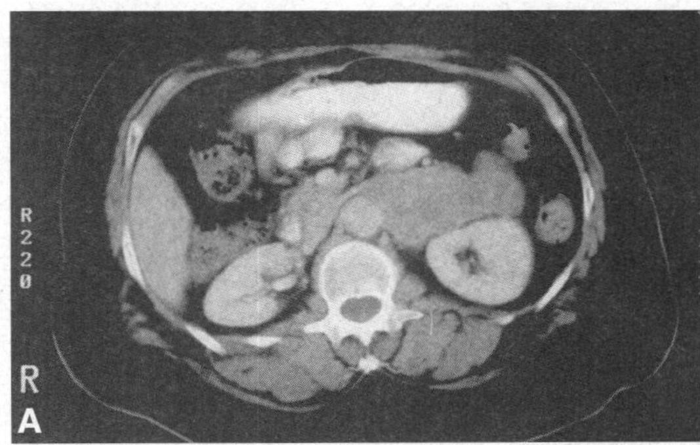

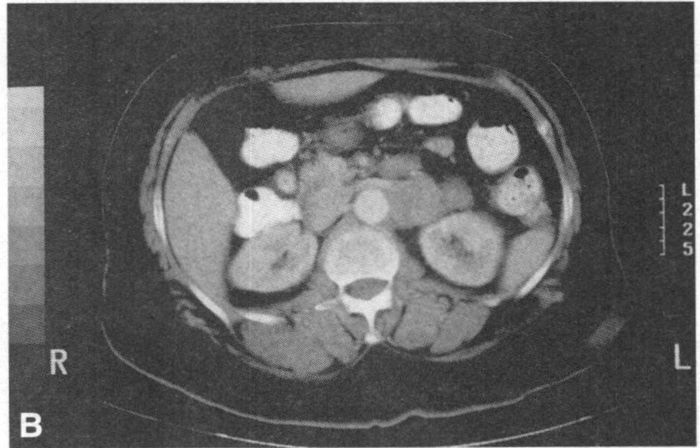

Figure 34-3 Neoadjuvant chemotherapy. A patient with a large perinephric malignant fibrous histiocytoma located in the left side of the abdomen and retroperitoneum. **A,** Before treatment with neoadjuvant chemotherapy. **B,** After four courses of doxorubicin-based multidrug chemotherapy. Note the approximate 50% reduction in overall tumor size. At the time of surgery it was possible to save the left kidney while achieving a negative margin resection. Pathologic analysis demonstrated nearly 100% necrosis of this neoadjuvantly treated tumor.

hypoxic and therefore resistant to radiation therapy. Because surgery works by zero-order kinetics, it effectively removes the local residual primary tumor cells that are resistant to these other modalities. In addition, this sequence of preoperative therapies can cause shrinkage of tumor mass because of the destruction of chemo- and radiosensitive tumor cells (Figure 34-3). The frequent possibility of less-ablative surgery resulting in tissue (and function) preservation is a major dividend of this preoperative cytoreduction by neoadjuvant treatment. There have been promising results from clinical trials that have applied these concepts in bone and soft-tissue sarcomas, locally advanced breast cancer, and other neoplasms.

A growing neoplasm can evade immune attack by producing specific and nonspecific immunosuppression. Specific immunosuppression can be caused by antigens shed from the tumor into the blood. These antigens, which circulate alone or as antigen–antibody complexes, can inhibit the lymphocyte-mediated destruction of tumor cells in vitro and may play a similar role in vivo. Nonspecific or generalized immunosuppression is attributed to humoral factors produced by or in response to the neoplasm. Any therapeutic maneuver that lowers tumor burden may reverse specific and nonspecific immunosuppression, thereby altering the immune balance in favor of the patient. In this respect, cancer surgery may be thought of as immunotherapy in that it effectively removes the immunosuppressive cancer cell mass. Once the tumor mass has been removed, the patient's immune system then may be able to destroy subclinical micrometastases. This premise suggests that local disease should be considered as a manifestation of systemic illness, whether or not the patient has clinically overt metastases. Surgery for apparently localized tumors can thus favorably affect the host–tumor relationship and may even contribute to cure in the patient with subclinical distant metastases.

SURGICAL COMPONENTS OF CANCER MANAGEMENT

Prevention The old adage that an ounce of prevention is worth a pound of cure certainly applies in solid-tumor oncology. As the role of genetic mutations that predispose to subsequent cancer development expands, one can anticipate that prophylactic surgery will be extended to encompass these conditions. In these situations, it is imperative that the surgical oncologist become intimately knowledgeable about the indications, limitations, and ethical considerations regarding genetic counseling, if only because it will be the responsibility of the surgeon to alert other family members at risk and arrange for appropriate testing.

The above emerging indications are being added to an already established role for prophylactic surgery in predisposing conditions such as cryptorchidism associated with subsequent testicular carcinoma, long-standing ulcerative colitis or familial polyposis associated with colon carcinoma, multiple endocrine neoplasia syndromes associated with the development of medullary carcinoma of the thyroid, and oral leukoplakia associated with subsequent development of squamous cell carcinoma. Assessing the risk to benefit ratio of prophylactic surgery is critical but frequently inexact. The future advent of inexpensive and reliable genetic screening technologies, coupled with emerging insights derived from the new field of molecular epidemiology, should bring more definitive understanding of prophylactic surgery benefits in populations at risk.

Biopsy and Diagnosis of Tumors The diagnosis of solid tumors depends on locating and performing a biopsy of the lesion. Biopsy evidence will be used to determine the histology and/or grade of a tumor, which is a prerequisite for planning definitive therapy. Significant therapeutic errors have been made when biopsy confirmation of malignancy was not obtained prior to treatment, as in the radical mastectomies that were performed for nodular fat necrosis. Even when biopsy reports from another hospital are available, the slides of the previous biopsy must be obtained and reviewed prior to the institution of therapy. This is essential because all too often (and particularly in rare neoplasms) an erroneous interpretation may have been made in the initial pathology assessment.

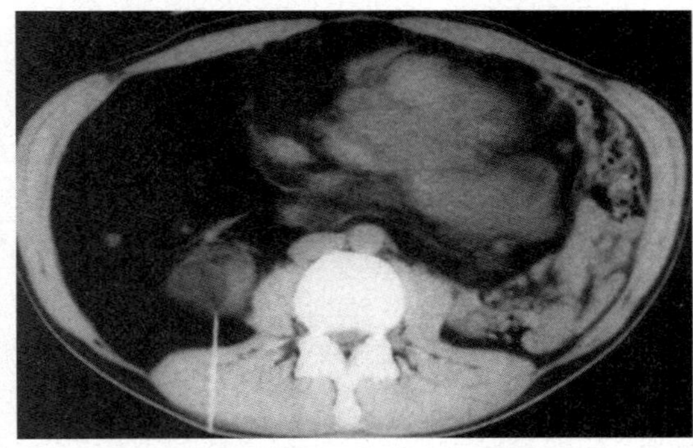

Figure 34-4 Computed tomography (CT) image-directed biopsy. A patient with a large retroperitoneal liposarcoma occupying nearly 75% of the total abdominal and retroperitoneal space. A CT-directed needle biopsy is being performed in an area of suspected liposarcoma dedifferentiation. The posterior approach through the lumbar musculature allowed positive identification of dedifferentiation, which led to initial neoadjuvant therapy prior to an ultimately successful surgical resection.

Biopsy is easiest when the tumor is near the surface or involves an orifice that can be examined with appropriate visualizing instruments, such as the bronchoscope, colonoscope, or cystoscope. Carcinomas of the breast, tongue, or rectum can be seen or palpated and a portion can be excised for definitive diagnosis. In contrast, deep-seated lesions may grow to quite a large size before causing symptoms. Ultrasonography, computed tomography (CT), and magnetic resonance imaging (MRI) are all useful techniques for localizing such lesions at the time of invasive biopsy (Figure 34-4). However, although image-directed needle biopsy may be useful in some patients, exploratory surgery is often required to obtain a definitive biopsy that establishes the exact histologic diagnosis. Fortunately, such procedures can now be frequently performed on an outpatient basis by using minimally invasive technology such as laparoscopic surgical approaches.

Three methods are commonly used to biopsy suspicious lesions: needle biopsy and open incisional or excisional biopsy. Regardless of the method used, the pathologic interpretation of the tumor mass will be valid only if a representative section of tumor is obtained. The surgical oncologist must be aware that a sampling error can occur with needle and incisional biopsies where only small portions of the total tumor mass are submitted for pathologic examination. It is the surgeon's task to provide adequate tissue for diagnosis. Orientation of the specimen, as may be necessary, is also the responsibility of the surgeon. It is axiomatic that adequate tissue can provide the basis for diagnosis by an adequate pathologist, whereas inadequate tissue will be insufficient for diagnosis by an adequate or inadequate pathologist.

Fine-needle aspiration (FNA) is a cytologic technique in which cells are aspirated from a tumor using a needle and syringe. The technique can be performed using image-directed guidance and is particularly helpful in the diagnosis of relatively inaccessible lesions, such as deep visceral tumors. Because the aspirate consists of disaggregated cells rather than intact tissue, diagnosis of malignancy usually depends on detection of abnormal intracellular features, such as nuclear pleomorphism; thus the margin of error is higher than with other biopsy techniques. In addition, because of the lack of intact tumor architecture, FNA cannot distinguish invasive from noninvasive malignancy. Negative results do not rule out malignancy. Depending on the clinical context, such as distinguishing carcinoma in situ from an infiltrating malignancy, other types of biopsy may be more appropriate.

Cutting-core biopsy is the simplest method of histologic (as opposed to cytologic) diagnosis and may be useful for biopsy of subcutaneous masses and muscular masses, as well as some internal organs, such as liver, kidney, and pancreas. The added benefit is that this method is inexpensive and causes minimal disturbance of the surrounding tissue. Cutting-core biopsies are performed with a large-bore needle, such as the Vim Silverman or Tru Cut. This technique retrieves a small piece of intact tumor tissue, which allows the pathologist to study the invasive relationship between cancer cells and the surrounding microenvironment. The danger of implanting tumor cells in a needle track during biopsy is extremely small. This risk can be avoided altogether if the needle track is positioned so that it can be excised en bloc at the time of the definitive surgical procedure. Needle biopsy may be less appropriate if the specimen is small, which increases the likelihood of the needle missing the lesion or the biopsy not being representative of the entire tumor. Consequently, a needle biopsy report that is negative for malignant disease should be viewed with skepticism if it is inconsistent with the clinical presentation and should be followed by incisional or excisional biopsy.

Incisional biopsy for pathologic examination involves removal of a small portion of the tumor mass. It is best performed in circumstances where the incisional wound can be totally excised in continuity with the definitive surgical resection in the event that any tumor cells are spilled at the time of biopsy. Incisional biopsy is indicated for deeper subcutaneous or intramuscular tumor masses when initial needle biopsy fails to establish a diagnosis. Incisional biopsy includes the instrument removal of tumor portions during endoscopic examination of the bronchus, esophagus, rectum, or bladder, and also includes suction or curettage of the endometrium, as well as laparoscopic biopsy.[5]

An incisional biopsy is also appropriate when a tumor is so large that complete local excision would violate wide tissue planes and impair a subsequent wide local resection for curative purposes. If possible, an incisional biopsy should retrieve a deep section of tumor, as well as a margin of normal tissue. Incisional biopsies suffer from the same disadvantages as needle biopsies in that the removed portion may not be representative of the entire tumor. Consequently, a negative biopsy does not preclude the possibility of cancer in the residual mass.

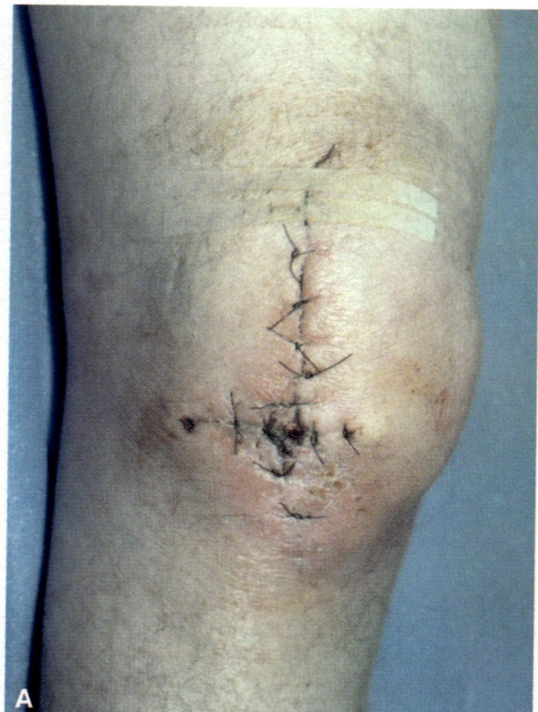

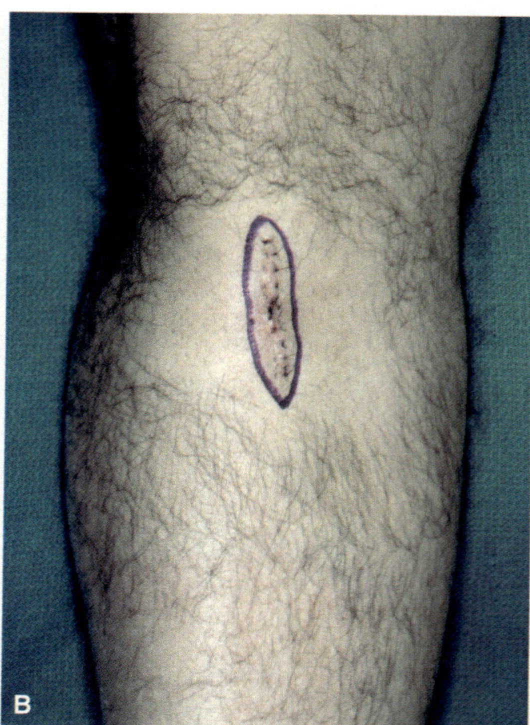

Figure 34-5 Appropriate and inappropriate biopsy incisions. **A,** A patient with a cruciate-shaped biopsy scar overlying the patellar tendon that contained a synovial sarcoma. Note the erythema in this infected incision. This ill-conceived biopsy scar would have required a wide-field soft tissue and osseous composite resection to encompass all of the violated tissue planes. Unfortunately, tumor was *intruded* into the joint space at the time of this biopsy, and this patient ultimately required an above-knee amputation to treat this small, otherwise limb-salvageable sarcoma. **B,** An appropriately oriented incisional biopsy scar in the lower extremity. Note the alignment of the scar parallel with the long axis of the extremity and the meticulous placement of small biopsy wound sutures. The entire scar could be excised at surgery (blue ellipse) with minimal concomitant normal tissue sacrifice.

Excisional biopsy completely removes the local tumor mass. It is used for small, discrete masses that are 2 to 3 cm in diameter, where complete removal will not interfere with a subsequent wider excision that may be required for definitive local control. Excisional biopsy allows the pathologist to examine the entire lesion. However, this method is contraindicated in large tumor masses because the biopsy procedure could scatter tumor cells throughout a large surgical field that would need to be widely and totally encompassed by the ultimate surgical resection. For this reason, excisional biopsy is usually contraindicated for skeletal and soft tissue sarcomas, whereas it is very useful for superficial squamous or basal cell carcinomas or malignant melanomas.

The excisional method is also used for polypoid lesions of the colon, for thyroid and breast nodules, for small skin lesions, and when the pathologist cannot make a definitive diagnosis from tissue removed by incisional biopsy. An unbiopsied lump is also surgically removed when the suspicious character of the lesion, the need for its removal (whatever the diagnosis), and the nonmutilating nature of the operation render such an approach feasible. Examples of such procedures include hemithyroidectomy for thyroid nodules after inconclusive fine-needle aspiration and a right hemicolectomy for a cecal mass that might be either inflammatory or neoplastic. In the latter instance, colonoscopic biopsy is informative only if positive for neoplasm.

Surgeons should always mark the excisional biopsy margins with sutures or metal clips so that if removal is incomplete and further excision is needed the positive margin can be accurately identified in situ. Orientation of biopsy incisions is also extremely important. Ill-conceived incisions can unnecessarily open up additional tissue planes, necessitating subsequent wider radiotherapy fields or more extensive ultimate surgical resections. For example, tumors of the extremities are best biopsied by using incisions that run parallel to the long axis of that limb. This facilitates a definitive en bloc resection that encompasses the biopsy track (Figure 34-5). Biopsy incisions should be closed using meticulous hemostasis because a hematoma can lead to widespread dissemination of tumor cells with contamination of tissue planes. Instruments, gloves, gowns, and drapes should be discarded and replaced with unused substitutes if the definitive surgical resection immediately follows the biopsy procedure.

Lymph nodes should be carefully selected for biopsy. Axillary nodes may be preferable to groin nodes if both are enlarged because of a decreased likelihood of postoperative infection. Other caveats are also noteworthy. For example, lymph node specimens preserved in formaldehyde cannot be analyzed for cytogenetics or flow cytometric immunophenotyping. The laboratory work-up for lymphoma usually requires unfixed sterile tissue. Cervical lymph nodes should not be biopsied until a careful search for a primary tumor has been made using nasopharyngoscopy, esophagoscopy, and bronchoscopy because enlargement of the upper cervical nodes by metastases is usually caused by laryngeal, oropharyngeal, and nasopharyngeal primary neoplasms. In contrast, supraclavicular nodes are more frequently enlarged as a result of metastases from primary tumors of the thoracic or abdominal cavities or breast.

The tumor specimen may be prepared for pathologic examination by either frozen or permanent section. Frozen sections are made at the time of biopsy, and pathologic diagnosis can be obtained within 10 to 20 minutes. Frozen sections are used when the diagnosis is required to assess resectability at the time of major surgery, or to check tumor margins intraoperatively. Frozen-section biopsy-proven carcinomatosis may mandate abandoning a procedure with a curative intent in favor of a palliative approach. Occasionally, mediastinoscopy, laparoscopy (peritoneoscopy), thoracoscopy, exploratory thoracotomy, or even laparotomy is necessary to obtain adequate representative tissue samples for microscopic examination to confirm diagnosis or tumor stage.

Staging Tumor staging is a system used to describe the anatomic extent of a specific malignant process in an individual patient. Staging systems cluster relevant prognostic factors about the primary tumor, such as size, grade, and location, as well as information about dissemination to regional sites, such as lymph nodes or distant metastatic loci. Accurately staging a cancer is absolutely essential in designing an appropriate therapeutic program and advising about prognosis. Without accurate staging, it is impossible to meaningfully compare the results of therapies administered in different centers. New forms of therapy can be appropriately evaluated only by comparing the impact of current therapy of neoplasms of equivalent stage.

The recognized importance of staging has led to a variety of international and national attempts to standardize the staging of the patient with cancer. To date, no single system has been universally accepted. The American Joint Committee on Cancer (AJCC) has recommended a staging system ranging from stage I (small, localized malignancy) to stage IV (distant metastatic spread).[6] Both the AJCC and the Union Internationale Contre Cancer (International Union Against Cancer, UICC) have adopted a shared TNM system that defines a cancer in terms of the primary tumor (T), the presence or absence of nodal metastases (N), and the presence or absence of distant metastases (M). Increasing numerals after the T, such as T1, T2, T3, or T4, indicate lesions of increasing size that are usually associated with a poorer prognosis. The absence of nodal metastasis is designated as N0, the presence of nodal metastasis is N1, and for more extensive nodal involvement, additional numbers may be used. Finally, distant metastases are indicated by adding the numeral 1 following M for metastases, or the numeral 0 signifying their absence. Thus, a small lesion that has neither spread to regional nodes nor metastasized to distant sites would be designated as T1 N0 M0. A larger lesion that involved regional nodes but not distant sites might be identified as T2 N1 M0. A large neoplasm associated with both regional and distant metastases would be designated T3 N1 M1. For some tumor types, such as soft tissue sarcoma, a G for grade of malignancy is added. High-grade tumors are less differentiated and tend to metastasize more readily.

The TNM system has four chronologic classifications. The clinical classification (cTNM or TNM) represents the extent of the disease prior to first definitive treatment, as determined from physical examination, imaging studies, endoscopy, biopsy, surgical exploration, and any other relevant findings. The pathologic classification (pTNM) incorporates the additional information available at the time of surgery or derived from pathologic examination of a completely resected specimen. This is especially useful in planning adjuvant therapy. The retreatment classification (rTNM) is used to stage a cancer that has recurred after a disease-free interval; it includes clinical and/or pathologic evidence of recurrence. Finally, the autopsy classification (aTNM) is based on postmortem examination.

Patterns of Tumor Spread In general, a malignant tumor may spread (1) by infiltrating surrounding tissue, (2) via the lymphatics, (3) by vascular invasion, or (4) by implantation in serous cavities. However, many cancers spread by more than one route, and an orderly course of metastasis is not predictably certain. For example, patients with breast cancer or melanoma can manifest distant metastatic disease in the lungs, liver, or skeleton without ever developing evidence of lymph node metastases. Table 34-2 summarizes the metastatic patterns of various human tumors.

Table 34-2 Patterns of Neoplastic Spread for Common Human Cancers

Neoplasms	Hematogenous	Lymphatic	Local Infiltration (Expressed as Local Recurrence)
Adenocarcinoma			
Breast	4	3	2
Endometrium	1	2	1
Ovary	2	3	4
Stomach	4	4	3
Pancreas	4	4	3
Colon	3	3	1
Kidney	2	2	2
Prostate	3	3	3
Liver	1	1	4
Epidermal carcinoma			
Lung	4	3	2
Oropharynx	1	3	3
Larynx	1	3	2
Cervix	1	4	3
Transitional cell carcinoma			
Bladder	2	3	4
Cutaneous neoplasm			
Squamous cell carcinoma	1	2	1
Melanoma	3	3	2
Basal cell carcinoma	0	0	1
Sarcoma			
Bone	4	1	1
Soft tissue	4	1	3
Brain neoplasm	0	0	4

Does not occur; 0 = < 1%; 1 = 1–5%; 2 = 15–30%; 3 = 30%; 4 = 50%.

Cancer cells may also spread by direct extension through tissue spaces and planes. Some neoplasms, such as soft tissue sarcomas and adenocarcinomas of the stomach or esophagus, may extend for a considerable distance (10–15 cm) along tissue planes beyond the palpable tumor mass. Other neoplasms, such as a basal cell carcinoma of skin, rarely extend for more than a few millimeters beyond the visible margin. Even though most central nervous system (CNS) tumors infrequently metastasize, they may penetrate nearby brain tissue, and their location can cause death by interfering with vital CNS functions.

Tumor cells can readily enter the lymphatics and extend through these channels by permeation or embolization to the lymph nodes. Permeation is the growth of a colony of tumor cells along the course of the lymphatic vessel. This commonly occurs in the skin lymphatics in carcinoma of the breast and in the perineural lymphatics in carcinoma of the prostate. Lymphatic involvement is extremely common in malignant epithelial neoplasms of all types, except basal cell carcinoma of the skin, which metastasizes to regional lymphatics in less than 0.1% of cases, or mesenchymal neoplasms, such as sarcomas, which metastasize to lymph nodes in only 2 to 5% of cases.

Spread along the lymphatics by embolization to regional or distant lymph nodes is of great clinical importance. Tumor cells travel within anastomosing lymphatics and can spread to proximal nodal basins via the collateral lymphatic channels. Lymph node metastases are first confined to the subcapsular space; at this stage, the node is not enlarged and may appear normal to the naked eye. Gradually, the tumor cells permeate the sinusoids and replace the nodal parenchyma. There is little direct spread from node to node, because the nodal capsule is not penetrated until a late stage. However, when an involved lymph node is more than 3 cm in diameter, tumor has usually extended beyond the capsule into the perinodal fat, indicating an ominous prognosis.

Lymph from the abdominal organs and lower extremities drains into the cisterna chyli, and then into the thoracic duct, which finally opens into the left jugular vein. By using this route, tumor cells can pass freely from the lymphatic system into the bloodstream. Oncologists originally believed that solid neoplasms first involved regional lymph nodes and then spread into the bloodstream by drainage into the thoracic duct and then to other parts of the body. An alternative explanation now favored by some oncologists assumes that the presence of cancer cells in regional lymph nodes indicates an unfavorable host–tumor relationship and the concomitant high likelihood of distant (albeit subclinical) metastases. However, this argument is weakened by the 30 to 50% rate of long-term (25–30 year) cure after complete lymphadenectomy for lymph node metastases.

Cancer cells may reach the bloodstream either through the thoracic duct or by direct invasion of blood vessels. Capillaries offer no resistance to tumor cell transgression. Small veins are frequently invaded, whereas thicker-walled arteries are rarely violated. Veins frequently form a plexus extending to the subendothelial regions, which provide a portal of entry through the thin vein wall. When the vascular endothelium is destroyed, a thrombus can form that is quickly invaded by tumor. This combination of thrombus and tumor may detach to form large tumor emboli. Vascular invasion is common in both carcinomas and sarcomas and is associated with a poor prognosis. Some types of neoplasms have a remarkable tendency to grow as a solid column along the course of veins. For example, renal cell carcinoma can grow into the renal vein and up the inferior vena cava extending to the right atrium. In this situation, a spectacular en bloc removal requiring cardiopulmonary bypass may still result in long-term survival or even cure.

Tumor cells occasionally gain entrance to serous cavities by growing through the wall of an organ. Many tumor cells can grow in suspension without a supporting matrix and may widely spread within the peritoneal cavity or attach to serous surfaces. Thus, widespread peritoneal seeding is common with gastrointestinal and ovarian cancers. Similarly, malignant gliomas may spread widely within the CNS via the cerebrospinal fluid.

Although much is known about the routes of tumor spread, the mechanisms underlying this process remain unclear. Some cancers are metastatic at the time of clinical discovery, whereas others of the same type and in the same organ tissue may remain localized for years. Metastases may dominate the presenting clinical picture while the primary tumor remains latent and asymptomatic or even undetectable. For example, cerebral metastases from silent cancers in the bronchus or the breast are often mistaken for primary benign CNS neoplasms.

A surgical oncology resection is designed to remove the primary neoplasm and the usual contiguous lymphatic and vascular routes of tumor spread with the intent to ablate every cancer cell in the body. According to this view of surgical therapy, cure is achieved by the mechanical removal of all cancer cells. However, cancer cells are frequently found in operative wound washings or in the drainage from postoperative wounds. In that many of these patients never develop recurrent cancer, host immune defenses must be effective in destroying any tumor cells missed at the time of resection.[5,7] Similarly, the demonstrably viable tumor cells that are frequently found in the blood or lymphatics of cancer patients seldom lead to metastatic implants.

Prolonged remission is also evidence of effective immune defenses. Rapidly progressive cancer sometimes recurs 10 or more years after successful treatment of the primary tumor. During the preceding long period of clinical remission, the growth of tumor cells has presumably been inhibited by host defenses. Host immune mechanisms may also have a role in the salvage of patients undergoing resection of metastases in distant organs, such as the lung or liver. It is likely that these patients have other subclinical metastases, which presumably are destroyed by host immune mechanisms in that subset of postresection patients who subsequently become disease-free long-term survivors.

Preoperative Preparation The preoperative patient is frequently in relatively poor physical condition. This is because many malignant tumors have toxic effects on the host that are disproportionate to the size of the lesion. Patients may have a poor nutritional status because of interference with normal alimentary function, as is often encountered with cancers of the mouth, pharynx, esophagus, intestinal tract, and appended glandular organs, such as the pancreas. Pain may contribute to anorexia and consequent severe electrolyte disorder. Every effort should be made to correct nutritional deficiencies, restore depleted blood volume, and correct hypoproteinemia prior to extensive surgical procedures. Total parenteral nutrition (TPN) can be used to prepare the malnourished patient for a major operation, although reconstitution is a slow process, and TPN may chiefly serve to interrupt further deterioration by restoring positive nitrogen balance. Surgical morbidity and mortality following extensive cancer operations will predictably be problematic if critical physiologic and biochemical deficiencies are not corrected in advance.

Table 34-3 American Society of Anesthesiologists: Physical Status Classification

Class	Description
P-1	A normal healthy patient
P-2	A patient with mild systemic disease
P-3	A patient with severe systemic disease
P-4	A patient with severe systemic disease that is a constant threat to life
P-5	A moribund patient who is not expected to survive without the operation
P-6	A declared brain-dead patient whose organs are being removed for donor purposes

Modified from Saklad M. Grading of patients for surgical procedures. Anesthesiology 1941;2:281.

Determining the risk inherent in a given operation is a complicated and inexact assessment based on a number of factors. The physical status of the patient, including cardiopulmonary reserve, comorbid conditions, debility inherent to a specific operation, hepatic and renal function, and the intent of surgical procedure (curative versus palliative) are all pertinent to this assessment. The technical complexity of an operation, the type of anesthetic used, and the relative experience of the involved health care personnel can all impact on the complications of a procedure. Various schema for risk assessment, such as the five-level physical status classification of the American Society of Anesthesiologists (Table 34-3) and the Eastern Cooperative Oncology Group five-step performance scale (Table 34-4) may be useful in assessing the appropriateness of a given operation for a specific patient.

Operative mortality is defined as mortality that occurs within 30 days of an operative procedure. In cancer patients, the underlying disease is a major determinant of operative mortality. Although it is true that comparable operations are usually more morbid in the geriatric age group as compared with other adults, advanced age per se should not disqualify a patient from a potentially curative surgical procedure.

Table 34-4 Eastern Cooperative Oncology Group: Performance Scale and Corresponding Karnofsky Rating

Grade	Description
0	Fully active, able to carry on all predisease activities without restriction (Karnofsky 100)
1	Restricted in physically strenuous activity, but ambulatory and able to carry out work of a light or sedentary nature, for example, light housework/office work (Karnofsky 80–90)
2	Ambulatory and capable of all self-care, but unable to carry out any work activities; up and about more than 50% of waking hours (Karnofsky 60–70)
3	Capable of limited self-care; confined to bed or chair 50% or more of waking hours (Karnofsky 40–50)
4	Completely disabled; cannot carry on any self-care; totally confined to bed or chair (Karnofsky 30 or less)

Because of their high-risk nature, decisions about the indications for palliative surgical procedures are particularly difficult. For example, palliative surgery for extensive metastatic disease or symptomatic intestinal obstruction secondary to carcinomatosis has a 20 to 30% perioperative mortality. In such circumstances, the risk to benefit ratio and ultimate surgical objectives must be defined as clearly as possible and accepted by patient, family, and surgeon.

Operative Considerations Once a decision has been made to proceed with surgical therapy, the operative procedure itself must be carefully planned for the specific surgical patient. It is essential to realize that the best (and often the only) opportunity for cure is with the first resection, at the time of initial tissue plane, lymphatic, and blood vessel potential exposure to tumor cells that may be dislodged within the operative field (see Figure 34-4). A subsequent recurrence may be difficult to distinguish from the normal postsurgical inflammatory reaction and scarring.

When a preliminary biopsy has been performed, the entire operative field should be reprepared after the biopsy incision is closed. The risk of implanting cancer cells into the wound is greatly increased if the tumor is inadvertently entered during an operative procedure with curative intent. Should this happen, the cut surface of the tumor must be electrocauterized and isolated from the remainder of the wound. Only then can the operation continue, preferably through a new plane of dissection that allows a much wider margin around the tumor. Many different cytotoxic preparations, such as sodium hypochlorite solution, nitrogen mustard, and thiotepa, have been used to irrigate the wound following cancer surgery in an effort to sterilize the operative site. None has proven to be effective in decreasing local recurrence rates. Local recurrence is an unfavorable prognostic factor and is usually, although not invariably, associated with systemic disease. For most types of malignancy, the rate of 5-year survival after wide resection of local recurrence is at least 20%. Local recurrence can occur despite every effort to isolate the tumor or to avoid spilling cancer cells into the operative field. For example, malignant cells in local lymphatics may be unrecognized at the time of the initial operation, or blood-borne cells may implant into the fresh wound. Manipulation of the tumor at any time during the surgical procedure can greatly increase the number of cancer cells recovered from the bloodstream. Likewise, it is also important to use an appropriately large incision so as to minimize unnecessary manipulation of the tumor. There are reports of a correlation between the presence of tumor cells in the bloodstream during the operative procedure and local recurrence. This possibility could be secondary to perioperative tumor cell implantation, which, in turn, may be facilitated by immunosuppression induced by surgery and anesthesia.[8]

Types of Cancer Operations Wide local resection with removal of an adequate margin of normal peritumoral tissue may be adequate treatment of low-grade neoplasms that very rarely metastasize to regional nodes or widely infiltrate adjacent tissues. Basal cell carcinomas and mixed tumors of the parotid gland are examples of such tumors. In contrast, neoplasms that spread widely by infiltration into adjacent tissues, such as soft tissue sarcomas and esophageal and gastric carcinomas, must be excised with a wide margin of normal tissue. This wide tissue margin between the line of excision and the tumor mass may also act as a protective barrier against intraoperative tumor cell traversal into severed lymphatics and vessels. Tumor cells may have been implanted in the incision when an incisional biopsy alone had been previously performed. To encompass potentially contaminated tissues, it is extremely important to remove a wide segment of skin and underlying muscle, fat, and fascia beyond the limits of the original incision (Figure 34-6).

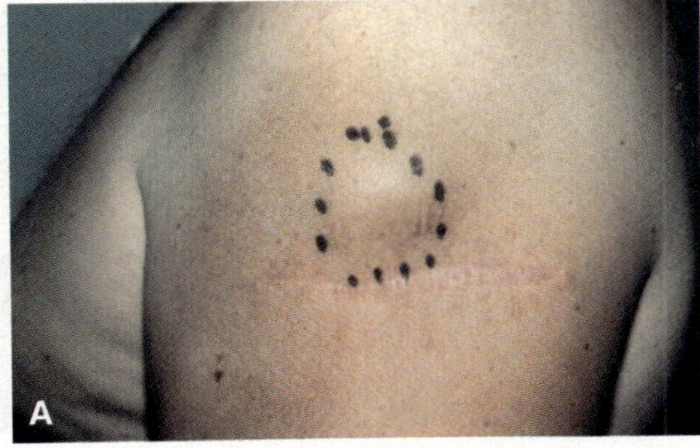

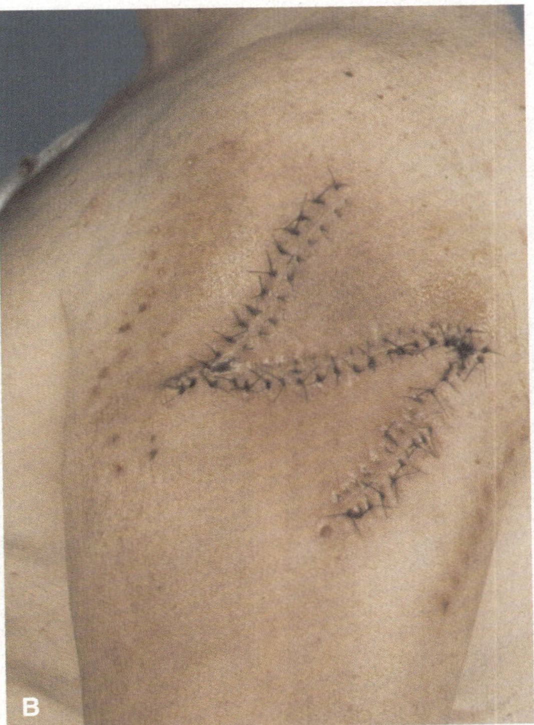

Figure 34-6 Surgical strategies to encompass all potential tissues at risk. **A,** A patient with a recurrent synovial sarcoma previously resected through a transverse scar that lies perpendicular to the long axis of the extremity. The recurrent tumor is enclosed within the black dotted circle. The entire field, including the previous scar, is at risk of harboring tumor cells; therefore, an appropriate surgical strategy must be created to remove tissues at risk. The recurrent nature of this tumor suggests that radiation therapy may be necessary after resection; consequently, avoiding skin grafting or flap reconstruction is important. **B,** A double Z-plasty technique was used to encompass the entire recurrent tumor as well as previous resection scar, thereby avoiding the use of tissue transfer or skin grafting, but necessitating creation of a wide surgical field. It would have been preferable for this patient to have had an initial tumor excision through a scar placed parallel with the long axis of the extremity at the time of the first resection.

Malignant neoplasms are usually not truly encapsulated. The tumor is commonly encased by a pseudocapsule that is composed of a compression zone of normal tissue interspersed with neoplastic cells. This pseudoencapsulation offers a great temptation for simple enucleation in that the tumor may be easily dislodged from its bed. However, this approach must be resisted because microscopic extensions of tumor from the primary through the pseudocapsule will be left behind after simple enucleation, dooming the patient to a local recurrence. Ideally, the surgeon should operate through normal tissues at all times and never encounter or even directly visualize the neoplasm during its removal. Dissection should proceed with meticulous care to avoid tumor cell spillage. Surprising amounts of skin, subcutaneous fat, and muscle can usually be sacrificed with little functional loss. However, tumor involvement of major vessels, nerves, joints, or bones may require sacrifice of these structures. Occasionally, even amputation may be necessary as an initial surgical procedure if a curative result is to be obtained. The extent of operation must be based solely on the extent of resection needed to achieve negative margins and not by plans for subsequent surgical reconstruction. The problem of reconstruction should be approached as a separate surgical procedure. This usually requires the participation of plastic and reconstructive surgeons and other surgical specialists who have been consulted prior to the resection so that an appropriate reconstructive strategy can be articulated (Figure 34-7).

During the operation, enhanced awareness of tumor extent and/or pathologic evaluation of resected margins may indicate that an alteration is needed in the initial operative plan. Decisions regarding the extent of resection are difficult and require experienced judgment. It is usually better to proceed with a potentially curative extirpation of the tumor mass, unless there is unequivocal histologic confirmation that the lesion has extended beyond the boundaries of curative surgical resection.

Many neoplasms metastasize via the lymphatics, and operations have been designed to remove the primary neoplasm and draining regional lymph nodes in continuity with all intervening tissues. Circumstances favor this type of operative approach when the lymph nodes draining the neoplasm lie adjacent to the tumor bed or when there is a single avenue of lymphatic drainage that can be removed without sacrificing vital structures. It is important to avoid cutting across

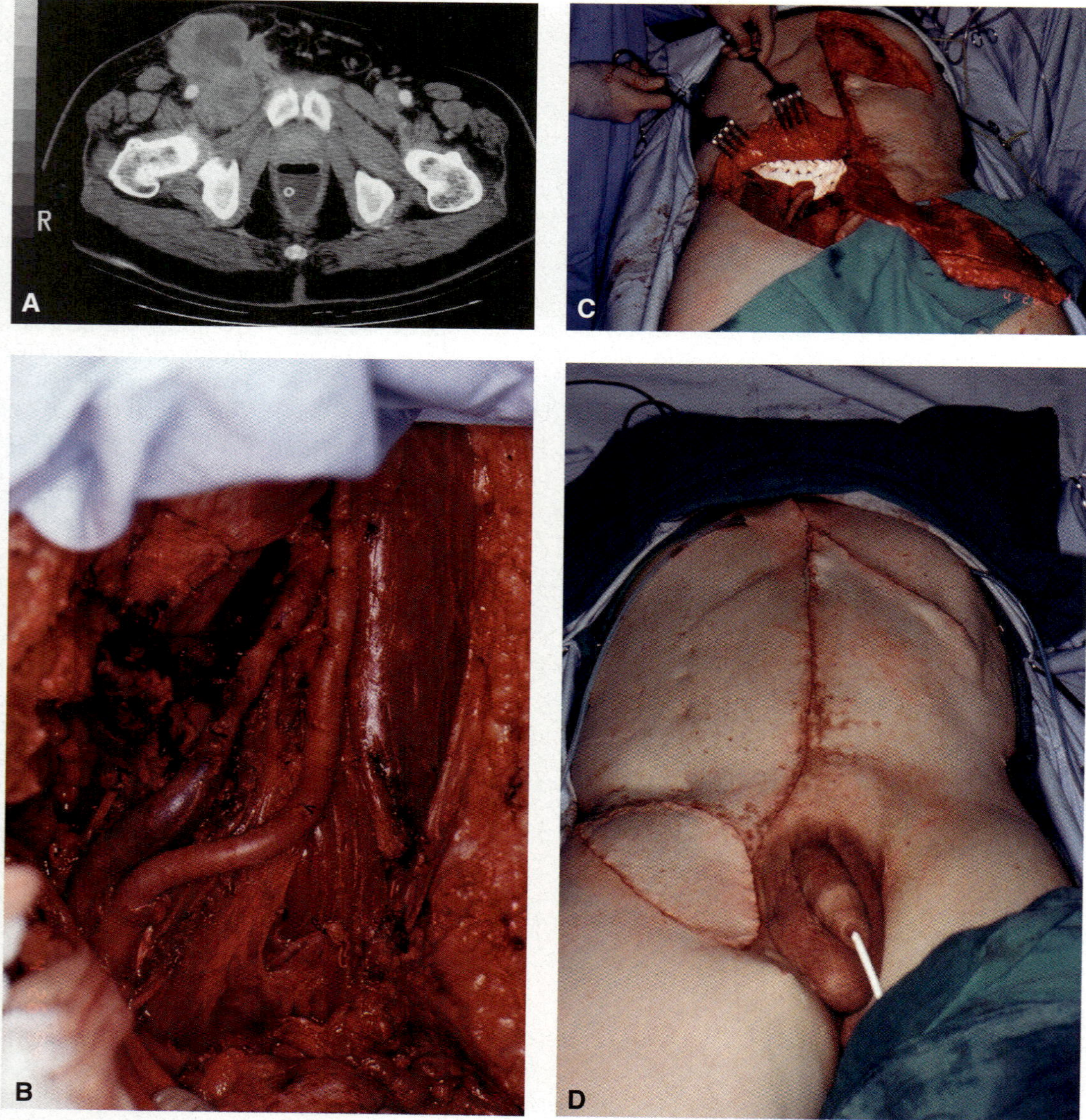

Figure 34-7 The role of reconstructive surgery as a part of the multimodality care of the oncology patient. **A,** A computed tomography scan of patient with multiply recurrent high-grade sarcoma of the proximal thigh, groin, and pelvis referred for radical hemipelvectomy. This patient had never received neoadjuvant chemoradiation; an aggressive course of same was the initial form of therapy for this patient. **B,** The surgical field after tumor resection. Note that all of the soft tissue of the lower abdominal wall, proximal thigh, and groin have been resected, and the iliofemoral vasculature can be seen in the depths of the wound. **C,** Reconstruction of this defect is accomplished by creation of a new inguinal ligament using Gortex mesh (white material). Note that the Gortex mesh can be tailored to accommodate the iliofemoral vasculature, thereby avoiding vessel constriction. A contralateral rectus abdominis musculocutaneous flap based on the intact inferior epigastric vascular system is mobilized and rotated into the surgical defect. **D,** Upon completion of the surgical procedure, the patient is rendered free of disease with an intact and fully functional extremity.

involved lymphatic channels, which markedly increases the possibility of local recurrence.

At the present time, it is generally agreed that en bloc regional lymph node dissection is indicated for clinically demonstrable nodal involvement with metastatic tumor. However, in many cases, the tumor has already spread beyond regional nodes. Although the cure rates following resection in such circumstances may be quite low (20–50%), undue pessimism should not prevent such patients from receiving appropriate surgical treatment. En bloc removal of the involved lymph nodes may offer the only chance for cure and can at least provide significant palliative local control. Regional lymph node involvement should therefore not be viewed as a contraindication to surgery but as a possible indication for adjuvant therapies, such as radiation or chemotherapy.

The routine dissection of regional nodes in close proximity to the primary malignancy is recommended for most cancer types even when these structures are not clinically involved with tumor. This recommendation is based on the high rate of locoregional recurrence following surgical resection when multiple lymph nodes are microscopically involved and the high error rate when palpation alone is used to assess possible lymph node involvement with tumor. Microscopic tumor dissemination to regional lymph nodes can be detected in 20 to 40% of clinically node-negative carcinomas and melanomas.

The validity of elective or prophylactic lymph node dissection has been challenged because it is not clear whether cure rates are improved if subclincally positive lymph nodes are removed before they become clinically palpable. Actively accruing prospective randomized clinical trials are currently addressing this question for many types of neoplasms. Regardless of direct therapeutic benefit, knowledge of regional node tumor status can affect staging and subsequent treatment. In many neoplasms, prognosis depends on the status of the lymph node basin draining the primary tumor. Some breast cancer patients with metastases to regional nodes derive significant survival benefit from adjuvant chemotherapy or hormonal therapy. Some patients with melanomas may become eligible for investigational adjuvant trials only if lymph node metastases can be demonstrated. Finally, a comparison of experimental results from different institutions depends on accurate staging before therapy is initiated.

In addition to questions of timing, the extent of lymph node dissection is also controversial. Sentinel lymphadenectomy is a promising new technique for detection of early nodal disease and is currently under investigation in multicenter trials. Detection of the sentinel node (ie, the first lymph node draining a primary tumor) was introduced by Morton and colleagues for melanoma[9] and is now being applied to breast carcinoma[7] and other neoplasms.[10] Initially, the technique relied on the injection of a vital blue dye at the tumor site and visual tracking of this dye along the lymphatics draining to the nodal basin. Subsequently, sentinel node mapping has been facilitated by adding a radiolabeled isotope to the dye and monitoring its path using a handheld gamma probe.[11,12] Sentinel lymphadenectomy is a low-morbidity procedure that accurately stages the regional lymph nodes and identifies the 60 to 80% of melanoma and breast cancer patients who do not require complete lymphadenectomy.

Advances in surgical technique, anesthesia, and supportive care (blood transfusion, antibiotics, and fluid and electrolyte management) permit more radical, extensive, and lengthy operative procedures. Such procedures offer a chance for a cure that cannot be achieved by other means and are justified in selected situations, if there is no evidence of distant metastases. For example, some slow-growing primary tumors may reach an enormous size and widely infiltrate locally without metastasizing to distant sites. Supraradical operative procedures should be considered for these extensive and nearly inoperable tumors because the occasional patient is cured. However, such operations should be undertaken only by experienced surgeons who can select those patients most likely to benefit. As an example of carefully indicated radical surgery, pelvic exenteration is a well-conceived operation capable of curing patients with radiation-treated recurrent cancer of the cervix and certain well-differentiated and locally extensive adenocarcinomas of the rectum. This operation removes all pelvic organs (bladder, uterus, and rectum) and soft tissues within the pelvis. Bowel function is restored with colostomy. Urinary tract drainage is established by anastomosis of the ureters into a segment of the bowel (ileum or sigmoid colon). The 5-year relapse-free survival is 25% when pelvic exenteration is used to manage these problems. It is also imperative that the surgical oncologist be willing to accept responsibility for helping to optimize the postoperative emotional and psychological rehabilitation of the patient prior to embarking on extensive resections, such as hemipelvectomy, forequarter amputation, mutilating operations for head and neck carcinomas, or total pelvic exenteration.

Surgical resection of selected localized recurrent neoplasms may produce a long period of remission. Surgical procedures are frequently successful in controlling recurrent soft tissue sarcomas, anastomotic recurrences of colon cancer, certain basal and squamous cell carcinomas of skin, and local breast cancer recurrence following segmental mastectomy. However, surgical resection of locally recurrent tumors in patients with synchronous metastatic disease is usually not indicated unless the entire local recurrence can be completely excised and there is also some form of not previously used (yet effective) therapy available to control the metastases.

Historically, routine second-look operations to detect early recurrence of colon cancer were advocated by Gilbertsen and Wangensteen. However, the improvement in outcome after these second-look procedures has not been sufficient to justify their routine use. In contrast, more recent longitudinal follow-up strategies using tumor markers such as carcinoembryonic antigen (CEA) have been more useful in selecting patients likely to benefit from reoperation.

Although logic might suggest that once a neoplasm has metastasized to a distant site, it is no longer curable by surgical resection, experience shows otherwise. The removal of metastatic lesions in the lung, liver, or brain occasionally produces a clinical cure. Resection of disseminated tumor may be indicated in selected patients with slowly growing metastasis, especially if the lesion is solitary. Even multiple metastases may be successfully resected if their growth rate is slow, or if regional or systemic chemotherapies administered before surgery have resulted in disease stabilization or tumor shrinkage. Prior to undertaking resection, an extensive work-up should be performed to rule out metastatic spread to other body sites outside of the proposed operative field.

Some patients with isolated liver metastases may benefit from surgical resection. Resection is recommended for the patient whose primary tumor has been controlled, who has no evidence of extrahepatic metastases, and who has a solitary liver metastasis or metastases located in one hepatic lobe. Although only a minority of patients with colon cancer metastatic to the liver will meet these requirements of operability, approximately 25 to 40% will survive more than 5 years after resection. In certain circumstances, the results for resection of pulmonary metastatic lesions have also been very satisfactory. For example, resection of a solitary or limited pulmonary metastasis for some tumor types, such as osteogenic sarcoma, results in a higher survival rate than resection of primary bronchogenic carcinoma of the lung. Resection of pulmonary metastases may be indicated even when more than one metastatic lesion is present, particularly if the metastases have been demonstrably responsive to systemic or regional therapies prior to surgery, or the tumor has a long doubling time.

Surgical procedures are sometimes indicated to palliate symptoms without attempting to cure the patient, thereby prolonging a useful and comfortable life. A palliative operation may be justified to relieve pain, hemorrhage, obstruction, or infection when it can be done without untoward risk to the patient. Palliative surgery may also be applicable when there are no better nonsurgical means of palliation, or when the procedure will improve the quality of life, even if it does not result in prolonged survival. In contrast, surgery that only prolongs a miserable existence is not of benefit to the patient. Examples of indicated palliative surgical procedures include (1) colostomy, enteroenterostomy, or gastrojejunostomy to relieve obstruction; (2) cordotomy to control pain; (3) cystectomy to control hemorrhagic tumors of the bladder; (4) amputation for intractably painful tumors of the extremities; (5) simple mastectomy for carcinoma of the breast, when the tumor is infected, large, ulcerated, and locally resectable (even in the presence of distant metastases); (6) potentially obstructing colon resection in the presence of hepatic metastases; and (7) destruction of liver metastases by using radiofrequency ablation. Surgery for residual disease is a special application of palliative surgery. In some patients, extensive yet isolated local spread of malignancy precludes gross total resection of all disease. In these patients, cytoreductive surgery may be of benefit provided that (1) other forms of effective treatment are available for use after surgery, and (2) that reduction of tumor bulk will enhance the effectiveness of these postsurgical therapies.

Problems with exsanguinating hemorrhage, perforated viscus, abscess formation, or impending obstruction of a hollow viscus, such as gastrointestinal organs, critical blood vessels, or respiratory structures, are sometimes amenable to emergency surgical intervention. Emergency surgery may also be indicated to decompress tumors that are invading the CNS or that are destroying critical neurologic components by exerting pressure in closed spaces. The cancer patient being evaluated for emergency surgery may be neutropenic or thrombocytopenic as a consequence of recent myelosuppressive chemotherapy. Sometimes a potential catastrophe can be avoided by operating on such patients expectantly just after they have gone through the nadir of their most recent myelosuppressive chemotherapy. Because of the high risks involved, each patient and the patient's family must be made aware of the dangers and benefits of the proposed surgery, as well as of other potentially effective treatments that might be available if the patient survives this emergency operation.

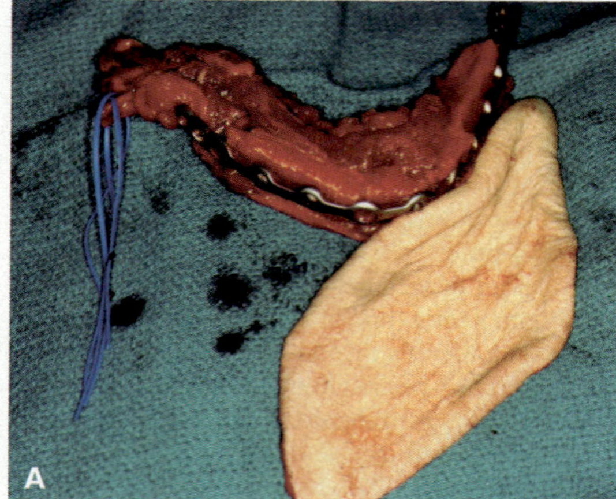

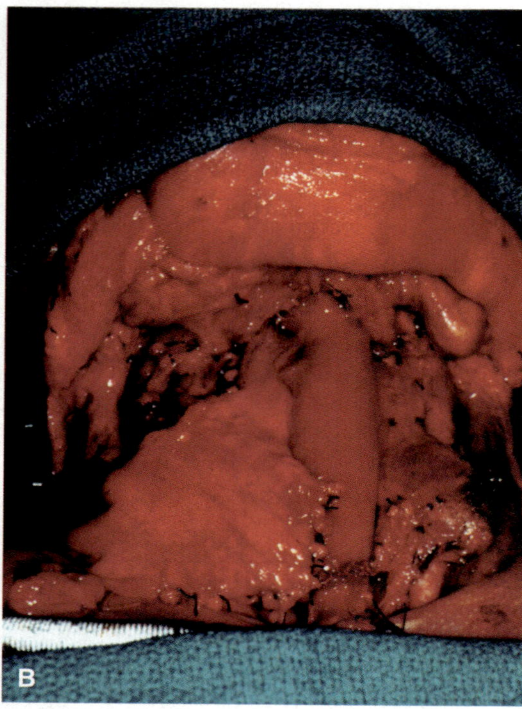

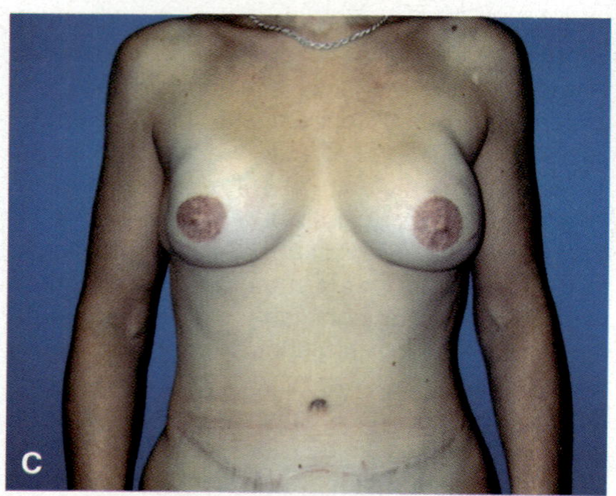

Figure 34-8 Complex contemporary reconstruction approaches. **A,** An osteomyocutaneous composite tissue graft used to reconstruct the mandible. Note the metal plate holding two ribs in proper position to provide a new bony strut, the vascularized overlying full thickness skin, and the vascular pedicle in the upper left corner. **B,** Jejunal free flap after inset to reconstruct the upper aerodigestive tract. **C,** Bilateral modified radical mastectomies reconstructed using free transverse rectus abdominis myocutaneous (TRAM) flaps. Courtesy of Michael Miller, MD, Department of Plastic and Reconstructive Surgery, University of Texas M.D. Anderson Cancer Center.

Reconstructive surgery after tumor resection has remarkably improved the quality of life for many cancer patients. The routine application of microvascular anastomotic techniques has enabled the free transfer of composite grafts containing skin, muscle, and/or bone to surgically created bodily defects. Breast reconstruction after mastectomy, tissue transfers as part of extremity surgery for sarcoma or mandible reconstruction, and aerodigestive reconstruction using jejunal-free grafts (Figure 34-8) are examples of these dramatic improvements in the combined surgical management of complex cancer problems. In the future, applications of the new discipline of tissue engineering will remarkably extend the reconstructive armamentarium. Using these approaches in the future, it may be possible to custom-grow nerve, fat, muscle, bone cartilage, or other body components as replacements for tissues that will need to be resected as part of a composite cancer procedure (Figure 34-9).[13] After resection, the tissue-engineered prostheses will then be implanted, thereby avoiding the constraints of only having dispensable autologous body parts available for reconstructive purposes.

SURGICAL ONCOLOGY IN THE FUTURE

Within the next decade, cancer is predicted to replace cardiovascular disease as the leading cause of death among Americans. Given that there are no more than approximately 30 to 40 surgical oncologists produced yearly in the United States, it is clear that the traditional surgical oncology educational roles in academic medical centers, as well as in the larger health care community, will continue and perhaps come under increasing pressure to expand.

As multimodality care grows in complexity and chemotherapy/radiotherapy move more prominently into the neoadjuvant position, surgical oncologists will have to become increasingly involved in clinical trial design. To be effective in this arena, understanding the natural history of specific malignancies will require an expanded knowledge base about the mutated genes and their cognate proteins that drive solid-tumor proliferation and metastasis. Surgical oncologists will have to become more knowledgeable about these factors, both during training and as a lifelong commitment to self-education.

In light of these changing demographics and increasing pressures for knowledge, it is perhaps unfortunate that the Accreditation Council for Graduate Medical Education (ACGME) has not yet granted formal subspecialty status to surgical oncology. This inaction may temporarily impede the growth of surgical oncology by discouraging some from entering the specialty. This prospect is unfortunate, given the emerging need for an expanded cadre of trained surgical oncologists who will be committed to working with other cancer specialists in developing new combined modality treatment programs.

On the other hand, the recent creation of the Surgical Oncology Advisory Council by the American Board of Surgery points to a change in how surgical oncologists will be trained in the future. It can be anticipated that traditional residency training will be decreased to a shorter 2-year core training program with a 4-year surgical oncology training component to begin after this basic residency core. Board certification would occur at the conclusion of this latter training period and more closely reflect the selected surgical subspecialty, such as surgical oncology. In the contemporary 80-hour work-week era, such an approach will best utilize available clinical training resources while providing increased opportunities for in-depth exposure to multimodality oncology care.

It is also certain that surgical oncologists will be unable (and do not desire) to perform all of the increasing number of cancer resections that will be needed by the United States population in the future. In the final analysis, the most important consideration may be the willingness of surgical oncologists to think innovatively about surgery as part of multimodality care, while preserving, and even improving, the quality of the surgical product that is being offered. Fortunately, many of the most talented surgical trainees being produced in

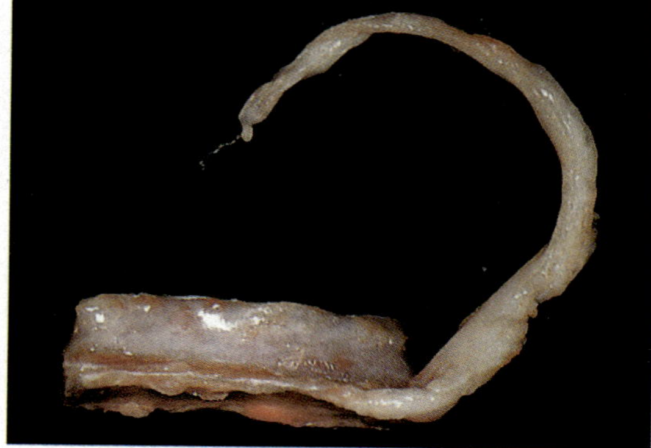

Figure 34-9 Tissue-engineered vascularized osseus graft. This graft was grown in vivo in a biodegradable strut that had been implanted into the rib of a sheep. In the future, such cultured tissues might be useful in reconstructive procedures, thereby avoiding dependency on available and dispensable autologous tissues. Courtesy of Michael Miller, MD, Department of Plastic and Reconstructive Surgery, University of Texas M.D. Anderson Cancer Center.

the United States have embraced this challenge and are gravitating to postresidency surgical oncology fellowship training. Surgical fellowship programs focusing on oncology are now available in nearly all of the surgical specialties. This favorable state of surgical oncology as a "superspecialty" bodes well for the future. Our patients and our medical colleagues expect this of us (and the solid-tumor challenge demands this of us) if we are to work together and succeed in eliminating cancer as the major public health hazard that it currently represents.

The rapid development of telesurgery, aided by the application of surgical robotics, promises to markedly change surgical oncology practice in the future. This rapidly evolving technology will be applied in the contexts of remote surgery, intraoperative expert consultation/assistance, surgical oncology cognitive and technical knowledge dissemination, and will also be used to enhance operative abilities of human surgical oncologists via successful collaboration with operative robots.

Telesurgery Telesurgery has been defined by Eadie and colleagues as "surgery, procedure, or technique performed on an inanimate trainer, animate model, or patient in which the surgeon is not at the immediate site of the model or the patient being operated upon. Visualization and manipulation of the tissues and equipment is performed using electronic devices."[14] The telesurgical approach can be applied to professional education and competence assessment tasks, surgical discussion and consultation among remote conferees, and surgery using "telemanipulation" (the extension of a person's movements to a remote location)[14] and "telepresence" (telemanipulation with added sensory information to make the operator feel that they are present at the remote site).[14] Telesurgery may even be used to provide emergency surgical care even if only a remote surgeon is available. The remote surgeon can interact and also direct all members of the OR team, including nursing and anesthesia personnel, while working with locally positioned surgical assistants of varying surgical expertise.

With the recent advent of broadband technology, digitized patient care information (including real-time data) can be transmitted anywhere, thereby minimizing distance problems in health care delivery. Image capture technology, high-resolution display panels, and improved laparoscopic equipment technology and robotics enable one surgeon to join another physical part of the operating team, even from a distance. The feasibility of this approach was first demonstrated by Marescaux and colleagues in 2001.[15,16] In this initial experience, a patient underwent elective nonemergent laparoscopic cholecystectomy in Strasbourg, France, under the surgical leadership of a surgeon operating from a computer control center in New York City while assisted by other practitioners located in France. The operation was performed without difficulty and in all other regards was quite comparable to the same procedure as would have been performed by a totally on-site surgical team.

This approach has been used for a variety of surgical interventions including herniorrhaphy, cholecystectomy, and thyroidectomy. For example, a recent successful experience in Ontario, Canada, was reported in which expert surgeons located in southern Ontario performed cholecystectomies for more than 20 patients located in northern Ontario.[17] The patients in this series readily accepted this arrangement owing to the convenience of surgery close to home, in their local hospital, with the involvement of their local surgeon who assumed responsibility for postoperative care. The money saved in reduced transportation costs for both patients and surgical specialists may markedly alter the role of surgical oncologists in the future as the trend toward regionalization of complex surgical oncology care into outcome-defined centers of excellence accelerates in tandem with the increasing prevalence and incidence of solid malignancy in the future.

Telesurgery will likewise also have major future impact on the teaching (and certification) of surgical skills. Problems with large numbers of trainees crowded around a small surgical field can be addressed by appropriate camera placement with image capture at close proximity and transmission anywhere in the world to an audience of any size or composition.[16,18] These approaches will maximize the likelihood that dissemination of surgical knowledge is both rapid and global. "Teleproctoring" (ie, the monitoring and evaluation of surgical trainees and practitioners for credentialing and recredentialing) can also be anticipated. This is especially apparent as we move into an era of more frequent recredentialing, where criteria for success will include favorable assessments of intraoperative surgical management skills. Such evaluations could be conducted from afar using panels of experts. In a similar vein, the possibility of remote intraoperative teleconsultation in which consultants might even use robotic arms to conduct critical or challenging portions of operations can likewise be anticipated.[18] The concept that the operating room is the exclusive domain of the surgeon and operating team predictably will change.[16] One can even anticipate an era where patients or their families will demand the use of distant experts, a major alteration in the public perception of best practice standards of surgical care.[16]

Juxtaposed against these remarkable future changes due to the anticipated widespread deployment of telesurgery are daunting concerns about cost; legal liability across jurisdictions or even continents; licensing and credentialing; and regulations, patient confidentiality, and potential problems with patient safety.[14] Loss of communication between remote and local surgeons, telesystem failures, and life threatening issues such as acute intraoperative bleeding or cardiac arrest will mandate change in our concepts of surgical qualifications and accountability—exciting and challenging issues for the future.

Robotic Surgery Surgical robots grew out of an interest in improving laparoscopic approaches to the surgical patient. Current iteration laparoscopic equipment has several drawbacks. These include lack of haptic feedback (force/pressure and texture/tactility), forcing the surgeon to compensate by using visual cues even more extensively.[19] In addition, positioning laparoscopic instruments is counterintuitive for most operators because one must move the instruments in the opposite direction of the desired target to which it is displayed on the monitor (fulcrum effect).[19] This difficulty can compromise hand-eye coordination, particularly in delicate dissections. An additional concern is that the typical laparoscopic prehensile attachment has four degrees of movement, whereas the human hand has seven degrees of movement. Moreover, physiologic tremor is transmitted via laparoscopic instruments, whereas tremor can be eliminated using robots by filtering the visual image presented to the surgeon, thereby decreasing purposeless movements and the postural compromise otherwise needed to reduce normal tremor.[19,20] Likewise, robots can restore normal hand-eye coordination by eliminating the fulcrum effect. Robots have the potential to enhance dexterity by improving accuracy and precision of movement through the operative field while increasing endurance. This is because the operator can assume a braced or sitting position, an ergonomically more comfortable operating stance compared to the customary upright surgical positioning.[20] Robots are also advantageous in another regard: By using binocular attachments or cameras, three-dimensional vision is possible as compared to two-dimensional laparoscopic views.[20] Magnified three-dimensional images can be coupled with a 10:1 or even 100:1 gross movement scaledown.[14] This combination allows extremely precise surgical maneuvers heretofore impossible, such as the therapeutic cannulation of the retinal veins (5 μm diameter) as compared to the current best microvascular sutured anastamoses involving vessels of 50 μm minimum diameter.[14] Other relative potential advantages of surgical robots include the possible future incorporation of diverse sensing devices for color, smell, heat, or other parameters relevant to enhanced surgical efficacy. In addition, the ability of robots to be sterilized, and their resistance to either infectious agents or radiation present important advantages, particularly regarding remote-site surgery.[19]

However, juxtaposed against these many advantages are several important caveats. At this time, robots lack any judgment abilities; they are unable to utilize quantitative information, totally lack haptic capacities, and they are very expensive.[19] Their current physical size is best described as bulky, and there is a lack of compatible other equipment as well as surgical instrumentation.[19] Some of these concerns have already been addressed by effectively integrating safeguards such as manual override options, ability to restrict robotic motions to designated "safe" operating fields, and the safety freeze control feature in which the robotic arm will freeze in place if there is any interruption of electrical power.[14] This latter technology can significantly reduce potential patient injury caused by an uncontrolled and floppy robotic arm in the event of sudden power or control loss.[14] An additional level of control is the already deployed voice-activated robotic arm to achieve optimal (and safe) robotic arm placement.[16] Finally, the amount of force or pressure that robots can apply to tissues in the operative field can also be precisely stipulated so that extremely large or small forces can be controllably exerted.[14]

Robots currently have demonstrated their ability in microvascular surgical applications and other manipulations in very small spaces. In cardiac surgery, robots can be programmed to gate and synchronize visual images to the rate of the beating heart, thereby allowing surgery to be performed on a motionless-appearing heart while avoiding the use of cardioplegia.[14] In oncology applications, robotic surgery has proven useful in radical prostatectomy, esophagectomy, adrenalectomy, nephrectomy, pelvic node dissection, transanal-rectal resection, pediatric laparoscopic surgery and other applications requiring small precise maneuvers in anatomically constrained operative fields.[19]

In the future, it can be anticipated that robots will be coupled with intraoperative imaging technologies such as MRI to better guide the surgeon in identifying normal and pathologic anatomy, thereby enhancing operative dissection.[19] Wireless transmitted direct retinal visual display systems in which a surgical image is projected directly onto the operator's retina are already in prototypic development.[14] Electronic chemical vapor-sensing olfactory systems, coupled with an odor generator at a remote surgeon's control site, could enhance operative realism for the remote surgeon.[14] It can also be anticipated that in the future surgical robots will be more modular, smaller, more robust, more easily assembled/disassembled, and easier to transport.[17] The above advancements certainly will facilitate the role of robotics in telesurgery; as artificial intelligence is more directly applied it can be anticipated that the robot will be better able to collaborate with the human members of the surgical team by becoming aware and even more interactive with the other animate and inanimate surgeons "scrubbed" in an operation! The implications for oncology care is obvious and even daunting, yet if handled with discernment, almost certainly will result in improved surgical outcomes for the many additional patients for whom there will be such needs in the future.

REFERENCES

1. Breasted JH. The Edwin Smith surgical papyrus. Chicago: University of Chicago Press; 1930.
2. Hill GJ II. Historic milestones in cancer surgery. Semin Oncol 1979;6:409–27.
3. Antman KA, Eilber FR, Shiu MH. Soft tissue sarcomas: current trends in diagnosis and management. Curr Prob Cancer 1989;13:339–67.
4. Eilber FC, Rosen G, Eckardt J, et al. Treatment induced pathologic necrosis: a predictor of local recurrence and survival in patients receiving neoadjuvant therapy for high-grade extremity soft tissue sarcoma. J Clin Oncol 2001;19:3203–9.
5. Minnard EA, Conlon KC, Hoos A, et al. Laparoscopic ultrasound enhances standard laparoscopy in the staging of pancreatic cancer. Ann Surg 1998;2:182–7.
6. Greene FL, Balch CM, Page DL, et al, editors. American Joint Committee on Cancer (AJCC) Cancer staging manual. 6th ed. New York: Springer-Verlag; 2002.
7. Giuliano AE, Kirgan DM, Guenther JM, Morton DL. Lymphatic mapping and sentinel lymphadenectomy for breast cancer. Ann Surg 1994;220:391–8.
8. Pollock RE, Lotzova E, Standford SD. Surgical stress impairs natural killer cell programming of tumor for lysis in patients with sarcomas and other solid tumors. Cancer 1992 70:2192–202.
9. Morton DL, Wen D-R, Wong JH, et al. Technical details of intraoperative lymphatic mapping for melanoma. Arch Surg 1992;127:392–9.
10. Levenback C, Burke TW, Gershenson DM, et al. Intraoperative lymphatic mapping for vulvar cancer. Obstet Gynecol 1994;84:163–7.
11. Krag DN, Meijer SJ, Weaver DL, et al. Minimal-access surgery for staging of malignant melanoma. Arch Surg 1995;130:654–8.
12. Van der Veen H, Hoekstra OS, Paul MA, et al. Gamma sentinel node biopsy to select patients with melanoma or lymphadenoma. Br J Surg 1994;81:1769–70.
13. Patrick CW Jr, Mikos AG, McIntire LV. Frontiers in tissue engineering, 1st ed. New York: Pergamon Press; 1998.
14. Eadie LH, Seifalian AM, Davidson BR. Telemedicine in surgery. Br J Surg 2003;90:647–58.
15. Marescaux J, Leroy J, Gogner M, et al. Transatlantic robot-assisted telesurgery. Nature 2001;413:379–80.
16. Merrell R C Telemedicine and telesurgery in the operating room. Bull Am Coll Surg 2005;90:8–13.
17. Anvari M. Robot-assisted remote telepresence surgery. Semin Laparosc Surg 2004;11:123–28.
18. Rafiq A, Moore JA, Zhao X, et al. Digital video capture and synchronous consultation in open surgery. Ann Surg 2004;123:567–73.
19. Lanfranco AR, Castellanos AE, Sesai JP, et al. Robotic surgery: a current perspective. Ann Surg 2004;239:14–21.
20. Marescaux J, Leroy J, Rubino F, et al. Transcontinental robot-assisted remote telesurgery: feasibility and potential applications. Ann Surg 2002;235:487–92.

Section 9
RADIATION ONCOLOGY

35

Principles of Radiation Oncology

Arno J. Mundt, MD
John C. Roeske, PhD
Theodore D. Chung, MD, PhD
Ralph R. Weichselbaum, MD

Radiation oncology is a field devoted to the treatment of benign and malignant diseases with ionizing radiation (IR). The field was born not long after the discovery of x-rays by Wilhelm Roentgen in 1895.[1] Radiation therapy (RT) was soon being used in the treatment of a wide variety of malignant tumors.[2,3] It was also soon recognized, however, that radiation produced adverse effects on normal tissues. In fact, due to the significant cutaneous toxicity associated with the available low-energy machines, RT had limited applicability until the introduction of high-energy (megavoltage) therapy in the 1950s. Only then was it possible to treat deep-seated tumors without excessive toxicity.

Over the past 20 years, tremendous advances have been made in imaging and treatment delivery, allowing for improved targeting and increased sparing of normal tissues. Increased understanding of radiobiology has also provided a means of further reducing the risk of treatment sequelae while increasing the efficacy of treatment. RT currently occupies an important role in the management of benign and malignant diseases throughout the body in both children and adults and offers an effective means of palliation when cure is not possible.

PHYSICAL BASIS OF RADIATION THERAPY

Types of Radiation RT is delivered primarily with high-energy photons (gamma rays and x-rays) and charged particles (electrons). The distinction between gamma rays and x-rays lies in their origin; gamma rays originate from excited and unstable nuclei, whereas x-rays are produced by electron energy transitions within the atom or through the deceleration of high-kinetic energy electrons (bremsstrahlung).[4,5] Gamma rays are typically produced by radioactive sources used in brachytherapy (see below), whereas x-rays are generated by linear accelerators and used in external beam RT. Within a linear accelerator, a narrow beam of electrons is accelerated to nearly the speed of light before striking a tungsten target.[5] As the electrons decelerate, they emit bremsstrahlung radiation (x-rays) with a spectrum ranging from zero to their maximum kinetic energy. Beam quality is often expressed as the highest-energy photons produced in kVp (kilovolts peak) or MV (megavolts). Therapeutic beam energies range from 50 kVp to 25 MV or greater. In this energy range, the relevant interactions of photons with matter include the photoelectric effect, Compton effect, and pair production.[4,5] Compton effect is the predominant interaction for therapeutic beams, whereas for energies below 50 kVp, the photoelectric effect is the most important interaction, and pair production is the primary interaction at energies above 25 MV. As a result of these interactions, electrons are set into motion, causing ionization and excitation of other atoms in the medium. As an x-ray beam passes through matter, its intensity is reduced and can be expressed by the following formula:

$$I(x) = Io e^{-\mu x}$$

where Io is the initial intensity of the photon beam, I (x) is the intensity after traversing a depth x and μ is the material's linear attenuation coefficient. High-energy beams are less attenuated than low-energy beams and thus are used for the irradiation of deep-seated tumors. Radiation intensity from a point source also decreases as the inverse square of the distance from the source, a dependence known as the inverse square law.[4,5]

Unlike a photon beam, a charged particle travels a known range in tissue proportional to its energy. Tissues beyond the range of the charged particle are thus not irradiated. Electrons are the most common therapeutic charged particles and are also produced by a linear accelerator. Instead of striking a tungsten target, the beam passes through a series of filters that broaden and shape it. Charged particles interact with matter through three primary processes: soft collisions (coulomb force interactions with outer shell electrons), hard "knock on" collisions (direct interactions with electrons), and nuclear field interactions.[5] Typically, a 1 MeV electron will undergo 10^5 interactions before losing its energy.[4] Soft collisions account for approximately half the energy transferred to matter. The remaining energy is transferred primarily by the relatively fewer, but more energetic, hard collisions.

Other therapeutic modalities include neutrons[6,7] and protons.[8,9] Neutron beams are generated by bombarding a beryllium target with a cyclotron-accelerated proton beam.[5] Like photons, neutrons are exponentially attenuated. Interactions with tissue include neutron–proton collisions and neutron–nuclei reactions, which set heavy charged particles in motion. Proton beams are also generated by a cyclotron. Unlike neutrons, protons primarily deposit their dose near the end of their range, a phenomenon known as a Bragg peak.[4,5] The Bragg peak can be modified to encompass the tumor without delivering high doses to more distal tissues.[8,9]

Radiation Absorbed Dose The quantification of radiation has evolved over time. In the early twentieth century, units of skin erythema and the roentgen, a measure of ionization produced in air, were used. Today, the accepted unit of measurement is "absorbed dose," which is the energy absorbed per unit mass. Physically, absorbed dose represents the energy deposited by secondary charged particles in the medium. The unit of absorbed dose is the gray (Gy), which is defined as the absorption of 1 joule per kilogram (J/kg).[4,5] One gray is equivalent to 100 centigray (cGy) or 100 rads.

TREATMENT PLANNING AND DELIVERY

External Beam Therapy The goal of treatment planning is to uniformly irradiate a specified target while minimizing the dose to surrounding normal tissues.[10] The spatial distribution of radiation delivered depends on a number of factors including patient anatomy, tissue density, beam energy, and the configuration of radiation portals. Because of the often complex tumor geometry, image-based three-dimensional (3D) planning is essential.[11-14] Both the concepts of treatment planning and the technical considerations related to 3D planning are described below.

Simulation and Target Delineation Simulation involves patient positioning, fabrication of treatment aids, including immobilization devices, and may include the selection of treatment fields.[15] Most patients are simulated in the supine position; however, specific positions are often indicated to minimize the dose delivered to neighboring normal tissues. Breast and lung cancer patients, for example, are simulated with their arms overhead to allow for the use of angled (oblique) beams which do not transverse the arms. Other specialized positions include the "frog leg" position (vulvar cancer) and the "chin tuck" position (pituitary tumors). Immobilization is accomplished with the aid of thermoplastics, foam cradles, bite blocks, and other accessories. The goal of immobilization is to minimize the day-to-day set-up variability caused by patient movement. On a conventional simulator, field borders are chosen under fluoroscopic guidance on the basis of patient anatomy and knowledge of tumor spread. More recently, computed tomography (CT) simulators allow for direct acquisition of CT data with the patient in the treatment position. Selection of beam orientations is performed virtually.

Imaging occupies a central role in RT planning, providing geometric information on external patient contour and tumor size, shape, and location relative to adjacent critical structures.[16,17] For 3D planning, the process begins with the acquisition of a CT scan with the patient immobilized in the treatment position. Three volumes are defined for planning:[18] the gross tumor volume (GTV), the clinical target volume (CTV), and the planning target volume (PTV). The GTV is the tumor visible on the treatment planning images. Regions of microscopic spread define the CTV. The PTV encompasses both the GTV and CTV with an added margin due to the uncertainty in the treatment delivery process. The PTV includes the effects of organ motion and day-to-day setup uncertainty and typically ranges from 3 to 10 mm.[19,20] In addition, surrounding normal tissues are delineated. Dedicated CT simulators are often used in this process. Most of these scanners are capable of both axial (one slice at a time) and spiral scanning techniques. Spiral or helical CT allows data to be acquired while the table and x-ray beam simultaneously translate and rotate, respectively. The spiral mode is preferred due to its faster acquisition time. Multislice CT scanners have recently been adopted in CT simulation allowing for multiple slices to be acquired simultaneously. These scanners use multiple rows of detectors and acquire images faster and with a lower tube heat compared with conventional CT scanners. Multislice scanners are particularly useful for simulation of lung cancer patients since breathing artifacts can be minimized. Moreover, this technology can be used to simulate respiratory-gated treatments.

Although CT is the primary imaging modality for treatment planning, magnetic resonance imaging (MRI) provides important complementary information,[21–23] especially for intracranial and head and neck tumors. Recently, MRI simulators have been introduced into RT clinics. The MRI simulator consists of an open-MRI system, flat table top, and an external laser marking system. MRI simulators have been used to provide better delineation of the prostate for RT treatment planning. However, since this technology is relatively new, its clinical role is not fully defined. Other modalities, such as positron emission tomography (PET) and single photon emission computed tomography (SPECT), also provide complementary information.[24,25] Hybrid scanners, such as the PET/CT scanner have increasingly gained clinical acceptance. These devices provide both anatomical (CT) and functional (PET) imaging. Moreover, because these scans are obtained with the patient in the same position, the PET and CT data share a common coordinate system. Imaging data can also be cross-correlated to transfer regions of interest from one study to another.[26–28]

Treatment Planning Treatment planning is performed interactively on a computer and is used to generate a dose distribution superimposed on CT images. Variables considered in planning include beam energy and modality, number of portals and beam angles, relative beam weights, and beam-modifying devices (wedges, compensators). Beam energy is chosen on the basis of patient anatomy. High-energy photon beams are used for deep-seated tumors; superficial tumors may be treated with orthovoltage-energy photon beams (100–250 kVp) or with electrons. Beam number is determined by a variety of factors including tumor size, shape, and location. Beam modifying devices are used to compensate for variations in external patient anatomy.

A number of tools have been developed that aid in the design and evaluation of a treatment plan.[29–32] Beam's eye view (BEV) allows the visualization of the tumor geometry relative to critical structures from the perspective of the radiation beam.[29] Beam orientations are chosen that encompass the PTV but spare adjacent critical structures. In addition, BEV also permits the design of customized shielding blocks. Quantitative evaluation of treatment plans is performed using dose volume histograms (DVH) and dose surface histograms (DSH).[31,32] DVH represents the volume of a particular organ irradiated as a function of dose. The surface area as a function of dose is represented by DSH and is used in the evaluation of hollow organs. Such quantitative evaluation assists in the selection of the optimal treatment plan. Other treatment planning tools include digitally reconstructed radiographs[30] and volume rendering.[33,34]

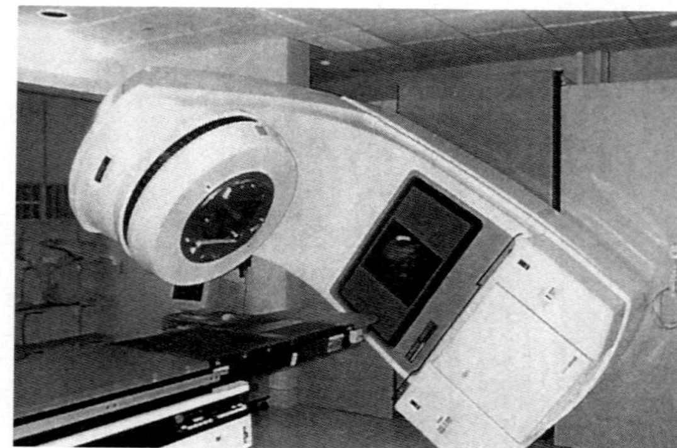

Figure 35-1 A linear accelerator.

Treatment Delivery and Verification Linear accelerators are used to administer external beam RT (Figure 35-1). Most modern accelerators have dual photon energies ranging from 4 to 24 MV, and four to six electron energies (6–22 MeV). Accelerators are equipped with a gantry which rotates through 360°, allowing treatment from any angle. Non-co-planar beams may be delivered through a combination of gantry and treatment table rotations. The beam produced is rectangular in shape. Beam shaping is accomplished with either Cerrobend blocks or a multileaf collimator (MLC). Cerrobend is a low-melting-point alloy which attenuates nearly all of the beam.[5] Custom blocks are designed for each field and are placed manually. MLC, as the name implies, consists of a series of leaves within the machine head, which are typically 0.5 to 1.0 cm in width.[35,36] An MLC increases the efficiency of treatment delivery by obviating the need for changing blocks between fields and offers the capability of delivering intensity-modulated radiation therapy (IMRT) (see below). An alternative treatment delivery approach is helical tomotherapy (Figure 35-2). On the outside, the Tomotherapy unit looks like a CT scanner. However, this device is equipped with a compact linear accelerator. Treatment is delivered as the beam rotates around the patient while the couch moves continuously though the gantry. Simultaneously, a set of binary collimators open and close according the treatment plan.

RT is delivered with the patient placed on the treatment table in a customized immobilization

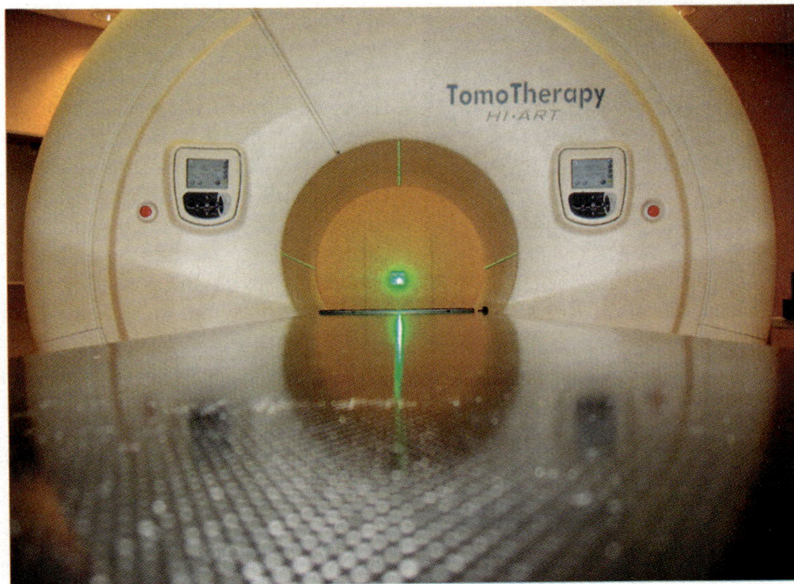

Figure 35-2 A helical tomotherapy unit.

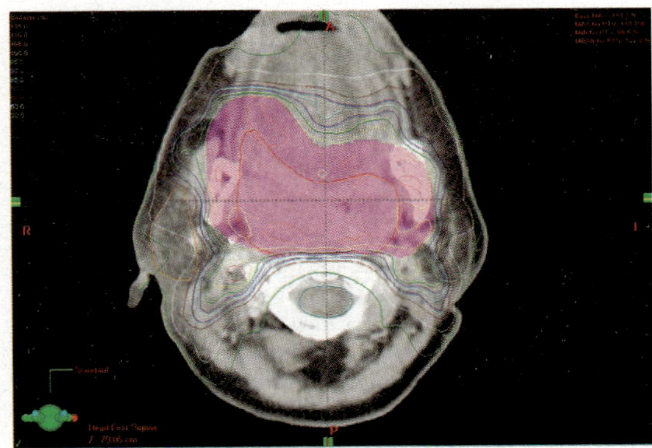

Figure 35-3 An intensity-modulated radiation therapy treatment plan in a patient with head and neck cancer.

device. The patient is positioned so that the center of the PTV is at the isocenter, the center of rotation of all moving parts of the machine (gantry, collimator, and table). On the first day of treatment, set-up films are obtained and compared with those taken at simulation. The positions of anatomic landmarks are evaluated, and patient moves are made as needed. Films are also obtained at each treatment angle, showing both the internal anatomy and the field aperture. In recent years, electronic portal imaging devices (EPIDs) have been introduced.[37,38] EPIDs offer the potential advantages of online verification, as well as the ability to monitor and compensate for patient motion during therapy.[39,40] Image-guided (IG) technologies have taken on an important role in RT. Video, ultrasound and on-board imaging devices allow physicians the unprecedented ability to monitor patient (and tumor) position in three dimensions on a daily basis. As IG technologies mature, daily modification of the treatment planning parameters (known as adaptive radiotherapy) based on the patient position, and the size and location of the tumor, may be possible. Treatment delivery may be aided through a record-and-verify system, a computer program which monitors treatment parameters for each patient.[41,42] Such programs are becoming increasingly integrated into comprehensive information systems with links to the simulator and treatment planning computers.

Intensity-Modulated Radiation Therapy Conventional external beam RT is delivered with beams of uniform intensity. Recent advances, however, have made the use of beams of varying intensity possible. This approach, known as intensity-modulated RT (IMRT), allows the high-dose region to be better *conformed* to the shape of the PTV.[43–46] Better conformality translates to increased sparing of surrounding tissues, thereby allowing the delivery of higher radiation doses to the tumor. The beam intensity patterns used in IMRT are derived using an inverse process[45,46] and delivered using an MLC fitted on a linear accelerator. Beam intensity is varied by computer-controlled movement of the leaves of the MLC into and out of the beam's path. Delivery of IMRT requires accurate patient positioning and immobilization.[15]

Increasing interest is focusing on IMRT. While initially available at only a limited number of academic institutions, the increasing availability of commercial treatment planning systems in recent years has resulted in its widespread use. A survey of practicing radiation oncologists in the United States in 2002 revealed that 32% had adopted IMRT and 95% of the IMRT non-users planned to adopt it within 1 to 3 years.[47] A follow-up survey performed in 2004 noted that the prevalence of IMRT use continued to grow at a rapid rate, with 73.2% of those surveyed stating they had begun using it in their clinics.[48]

IMRT has been shown to be a promising approach in several disease sites. In prostate cancer, IMRT is used to minimize the volume of the bladder and rectum irradiated, allowing higher doses to be delivered to the prostate.[49,50] IMRT has also been used to decrease xerostomia (dry mouth) in head and neck cancer patients by reducing the volume of parotid tissue irradiated.[51,52] IMRT also has shown promise in the treatment of pediatric tumors[53] and gynecologic malignancies.[54,55]

Examples of IMRT Treatment Plans

Head and Neck Figure 35-3 illustrates an axial CT image, with isodose lines superimposed in a patient with head and neck cancer. Note that the high dose isodose lines conform to the shape of the target tissues minimizing dose to the neighboring parotid glands, reducing the risk of chronic xerostomia.

Prostate Figure 35-4 shows an axial slice through the lower pelvis in a patient with early-stage prostate cancer treated with IMRT. The IMRT plan significantly reduces the dose delivered to the bladder and rectum compared with conventional RT planning. Recent attention has also been focused on sparing other normal structures, including the penile bulb, in an attempt to reduce the risk of RT-related impotence.[56]

Gynecology At the University of Chicago, IMRT is used as an alternative to traditional whole pelvic RT in women with gynecologic malignancies.[57] Conventional whole pelvic RT results in the irradiation of significant portions of the small bowel. In contrast, the conformity achieved with IMRT reduces the volume of normal tissues irradiated. An IMRT plan in a patient with endometrial cancer undergoing adjuvant intensity-modulated pelvic RT is shown in Figure 35-5. In women receiving concomitant chemoradiotherapy, an additional normal tissue that can be spared is the pelvic bone marrow within the iliac crests.[58]

Brachytherapy Brachytherapy involves the placement of radioactive sources either within an existing body cavity (eg, the vagina) in close proximity to the tumor (intracavitary) or directly within a tumor (interstitial). Intracavitary brachytherapy is accomplished with the aid of specialized applicators; the best known and most widely used is the Fletcher-Suit applicator for carcinoma of the cervix. A tube-like tandem is inserted into the uterus, and colpostats are positioned against the lateral fornices. Other applicators include Heyman-Simon capsules

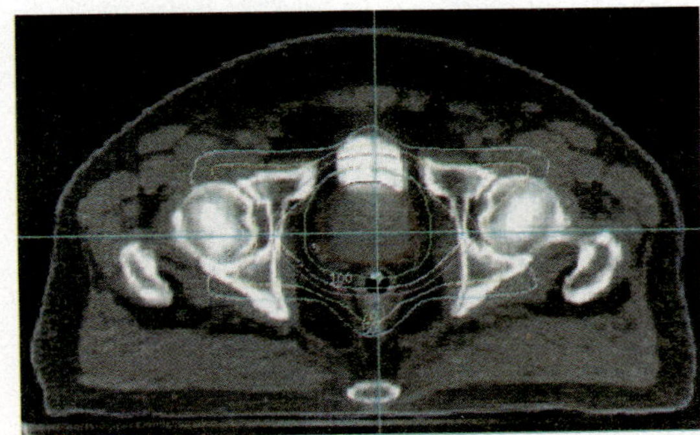

Figure 35-4 Example of an IMRT treatment plan in a patient with early-stage prostate carcinoma. Isodose lines are superimposed on an axial CT image.

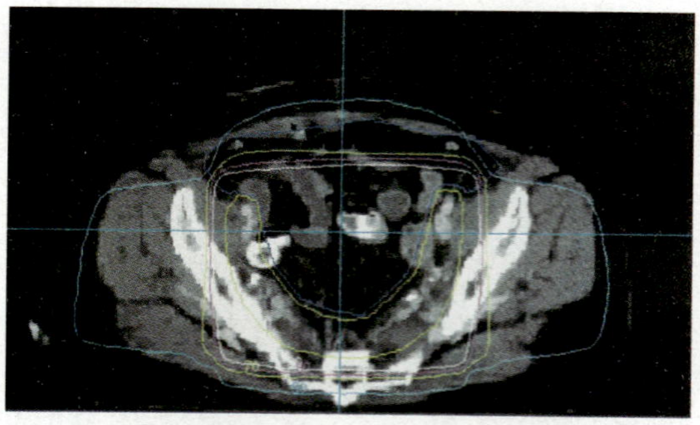

Figure 35-5 Example of an IMRT plan in a patient with early-stage endometrial cancer undergoing adjuvant intensity-modulated pelvic irradiation delivered on a helical tomotherapy machine.

(uterine cancer) and vaginal cylinders (uterine and vaginal tumors). Intracavitary brachytherapy may also be performed by inserting radioactive sources within a nasogastric tube (nasopharynx, esophageal tumors), biliary stents (cholangiocarcinoma), or directly within the lumen of a bronchus (lung cancer). Interstitial brachytherapy involves placing within a tumor hollow needles that can be replaced by flexible plastic catheters. Interstitial brachytherapy in gynecologic tumors uses a variety of treatment aids, for example a Syed template.[59] In head and neck cancer, catheters are typically placed freehand via a submental approach.

At most centers, brachytherapy is currently performed with afterloading techniques that minimize exposure to the staff. Radioactive sources are placed either temporarily or permanently. Brachytherapy was initially instituted with the use of naturally occurring isotopes, such as radium or radon, but with the availability of artificially produced isotopes, it has been practiced more frequently with cesium 137, iridium 198, and iodine 125. Plans are generated by digitizing and reconstructing source positions from plane radiographs. Three-dimensional dose calculations are performed, and the dose is calculated to a limited number of normal tissue points. Recently, CT-guided brachytherapy has been an area of research interest.[60] Examples of intracavitary and interstitial brachytherapy in cervical and prostate cancer are shown in Figures 35-6 and 35-7.

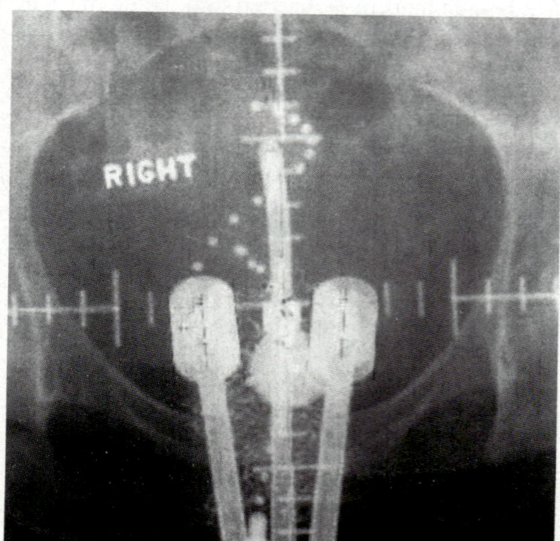

Figure 35-6 Intracavitary brachytherapy in a patient with early-stage cervical cancer.

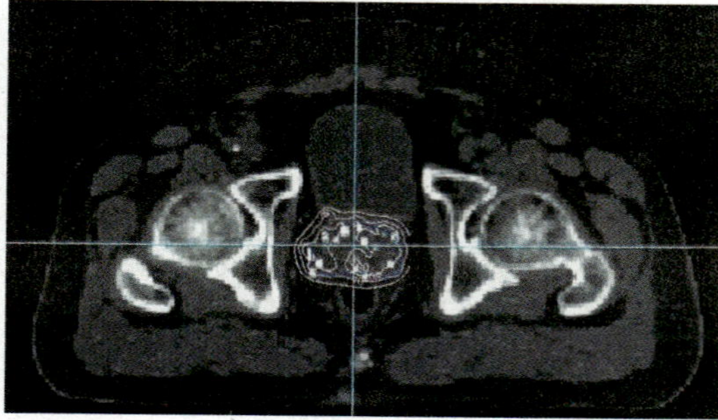

Figure 35-7 Interstitial brachytherapy in a patient with prostate carcinoma.

Brachytherapy has been traditionally delivered over 3 to 4 days as an inpatient procedure at a low dose rate (LDR), for example, 40 to 70 cGy/h. In recent years, high dose rate (HDR) techniques have been introduced using high-activity iridium sources with dose rates exceeding 200 cGy/min. Unlike LDR, HDR is an outpatient procedure requiring only minimal anesthesia. It is particularly appealing to the elderly and patients with multiple medical problems. Promising results have been reported in many sites, including the head and neck,[61] cervix,[62] endometrium,[63] and prostate.[64]

Stereotactic Radiosurgery and Radio-Therapy Stereotactic radiosurgery (SRS) is a technique used to precisely deliver a single, high-dose fraction of external beam radiation to a small, intracranial volume. It was first developed by Leksell in the early 1950s as an alternative to surgery.[65] The technique has since evolved to include heavy charged particles, gamma rays from Co-60 (gamma knife), and megavoltage beams from linear accelerators. The delivery of multiple fractions using the stereotactic process is known as stereotactic radiotherapy (SRT).[66] SRS and SRT have been used to supplement conventional external beam treatment in primary or metastatic brain tumors.[67] SRS is used to treat benign conditions, such as arteriovenous malformations (AVMs),[68] pituitary adenomas,[69] and acoustic neuromas.[70]

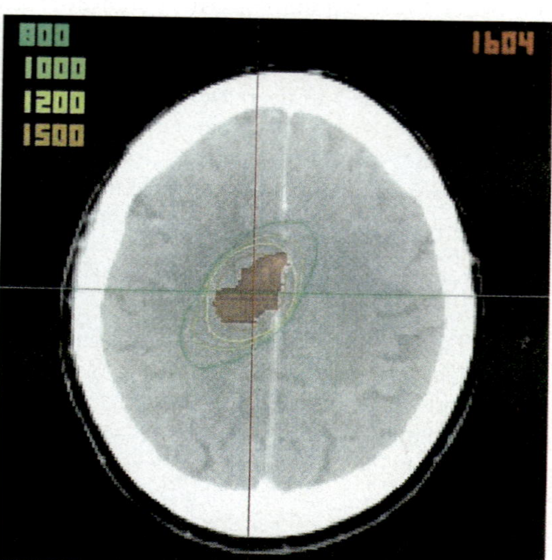

Figure 35-8 Stereotactic radiosurgery treatment plan in a patient with a solitary brain metastasis from a lung primary.

Both SRS and SRT involve the localization of a targeted lesion within a stereotactic frame. The stereotactic frame is either fixed (screwed into the cranium) (SRS) or relocatable (SRT). A stereotactic frame allows positioning of a patient with millimeter accuracy.[71] The goal of SRS/SRT is to conform the dose distribution to the targeted lesion while minimizing the dose to normal, surrounding brain parenchyma. In practice, this is accomplished with the use of multiple non-co-planar arcs. An example of an SRS treatment plan in a patient with a solitary brain metastasis from lung cancer is shown in Figure 35-8. This plan consists of five non-co-planar arcs and was delivered with 6 MV photons on a linear accelerator.

BIOLOGIC BASIS OF RADIATION THERAPY

Cellular Response to Radiation Radiation randomly interacts with molecules within the cell. Although the critical target for cell killing is the deoxyribonucleic acid (DNA),[72] damage to the cellular and nuclear membranes and other organelles may also be important. Radiation deposition results in DNA damage manifested by single- and double-strand breaks (DSBs) in the sugar-phosphate backbone of the DNA molecule. Cross-links between DNA strands and chromosomal proteins also occur. The mechanism of DNA damage differs among the various radiation types. For example, electromagnetic radiation is *indirectly* ionizing via short-lived, hydroxyl free radicals produced primarily by the ionization of cellular H_2O.[73] Protons and other heavy particles are *directly* ionizing and damage DNA directly.[74] Consequently, different types of radiation have varying relative biologic effectiveness (RBE). Directly ionizing radiation (eg, neutrons) has a greater RBE than indirectly ionizing radiation (photons or electrons).[75,76]

Radiation damage is primarily manifested by the loss of cellular reproductive capacity. Lethally irradiated cells are, thus, said to undergo a reproductive death. Consequently, most cell types do not show morphologic evidence of radiation damage until they attempt to divide. Alternatively, some cell types are killed via the induction of apoptosis.[77] A cell that has sustained lethal damage following radiation exposure may undergo one or more divisions prior to metabolic death and loss from the tumor population.

The concept that cell death following radiation exposure may not be manifested until several cell divisions later has clinical relevance, such that tumors associated with very slowly proliferating cancers may persist for months and appear histologically viable. The histologic appearance may clear only after tumor cells have had the opportunity to attempt to divide. Prostate carcinoma, for example, may require up to 24 months after RT prior to obtaining a normal biopsy.[78]

Radiation Survival Analysis Radiation survival can be studied both in vitro and in vivo. In

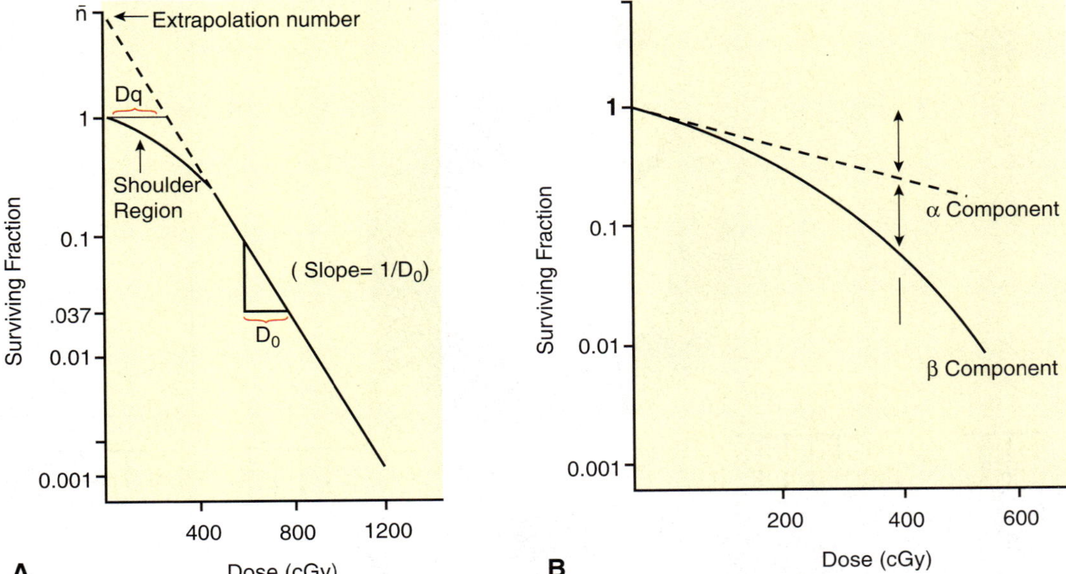

Figure 35-9 Models for survival curve analysis. Experimental data are typically shown as the fraction of cells surviving a dose of radiation plotted on a logarithmic scale, whereas the dosage of radiation is plotted on a linear scale (**A**). When using the multitarget model, the shoulder region is quantified by extrapolation of the exponential portion of the curve to the y-axis intercept. This point is referred to as *n* (extrapolation number), whereas a horizontal line drawn from 100% survival to the extrapolation line is referred to as Dq (or quasi-threshold dose). Slope of the terminal portion of the survival curve is quantified by the term Do, which is the inverse of the slope and designated as the radiosensitivity of the cells or tissue under study (**B**). When using the linear-quadratic models for survival analysis, there are two components for cell killing. The alpha component represents the initial slope, and the beta component represents the terminal slope of the survival curve. The alpha component is proportional to the dose, whereas the beta component is proportional to the square of the dose. The dose at which the alpha and beta components are equal is referred to as the alpha/beta ratio, which, for example, is 400 cGy in **B**.

vitro experiments usually involve irradiating exponentially growing cells to known doses of radiation. Cells are plated, and after 2 to 3 weeks, colonies are stained. The surviving fraction is then calculated by dividing the number of colonies by the plating efficiency of unirradiated cells. A survival curve is then generated by graphing the log of the surviving fraction versus the absorbed dose (Figure 35-9). Typically, survival curves are characterized by an initial shoulder, followed by exponential decrease in the fraction of surviving cells at higher doses.

In vivo models examine both the inherent radiosensitivity of tumor cells and environmental influences, such as hypoxia and host immunity. A model commonly used to study radiation effects is the growth delay assay, which measures the time interval required for a tumor exposed to radiation to regrow to a specified volume (Figure 35-10).[79] An assay that analyzes the dose required to control 50% of tumors is the TCD50 assay, which has been widely employed to study tumors in a variety of experimental systems.[80] The radiobiologic use of transplantable solid tumor systems in experimental animals has been reviewed by Hall.[75] Radiation survival parameters can be assayed for normal tissues in vivo as well as for tumors. For acutely responding tissues, in vivo survival is measured by studying clones of normal tissues regrowing in situ (eg, skin, jejunal crypt cells) or cells transplanted to another site (bone marrow stem cells). To study radiation effects in late-responding tissues, such as the nervous system, functional assays, such as paralysis and death, may be employed.

Models of Radiation Survival Curve Analysis Two empirically derived mathematical models have been used to analyze radiation survival data (see Figure 35-9). In the multitarget model, the reciprocal of the slope of the survival curve is defined as D0, the radiosensitivity of the cell population or tissue under investigation. D0 is the dose required to reduce the surviving fraction to 37% in the exponential portion of the survival curve. The width of the shoulder region is represented by the quantities n or Dq. Dq is the quasi-threshold dose, or the point at which killing becomes exponential.

The linear quadratic model (surviving fraction = eccD-5D2) fits radiation survival data to a continuously bending curve, where D is dose and a and 0 are constants. The linear component, a measure of the initial slope, termed *alpha,* represents single-hit killing kinetics and dominates the radiation response at low doses. The quadratic component of cell killing, termed *beta,* represents multiple-hit killing and causes the curve to bend at higher doses. The ratio of alpha to beta is the dose at which the linear and quadratic components of cell killing are equal. The more linear the response to killing of cells at low radiation dose, the higher the value of alpha, and the greater the radiosensitivity of the cells.[81] Neither model has a firmly established biologic basis and, therefore, both should be viewed as mathematical tools to describe the cellular radiosensitivity.

Molecular Events Following Cellular Exposure to Ionizing Radiation The ultimate fate of the irradiated cell is not only a function of the radiation dose but also influenced by the cell's natural defenses, including the ability to detect the DNA lesions and to repair them with high fidelity. Furthermore, recent advances have revealed DNA is not the only cellular target that influences the radiation response. IR also interacts directly with lipid and protein signaling pathways and modulates gene expression through a

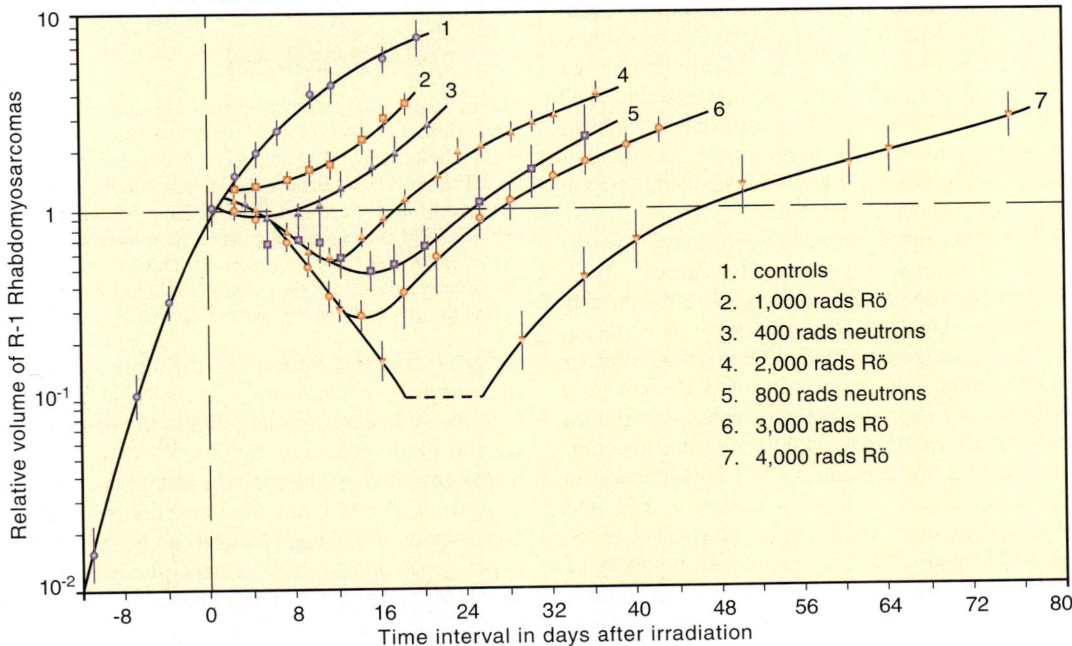

Figure 35-10 Data points represent volume changes observed in tumors in animal models after irradiation. After an initial decrease in the volume size, tumors grow back to the original volume over a time interval referred to as the growth delay. Curve 1 is the growth of an unirradiated control tumor. Curves 2, 4, 6, and 7 represent the growth of tumors irradiated with 1,000, 2,000, 3,000, and 4,000 cGy of photons. Curves 3 and 5 represent the growth of tumors irradiated with 400 and 800 cGy of 152 MeV neutrons. Growth delay is prolonged with increasing dosage and more densely ionizing radiation, such as neutrons. Source: Barendsen and Broerse.[7]

variety of mechanisms including the direct activation of transcription factors. IR-induced activation of these signaling pathways can affect critical processes such as cell-cycle regulation, DNA repair, apoptosis, and tissue repopulation. Figure 35-11 illustrates the current perspective on the interactions between IR-induced DNA damage and cell signaling.

Molecular Sensors and Effectors of Radiation-Induced DNA Damage As shown in Figure 35-11, components of the DNA-dependent protein kinase (DNA-PK) complex are involved in sensing DSBs as well as the repair of these breaks. DNA-PK consists of the 470 kDa cat- 10 alytic serine/threonine kinase (DNA-PKCs) and the 70 and 80 kDa Ku heterodimer.[82–84] Ku binds directly to sites of DSBs,[85,86] and DNA-PKCs is recruited to sites of Ku/DNA complexes where it is activated.[84] The Ataxia Telangiectasia Mutated (ATM) protein is also involved in sensing DNA damage and is related to DNA-PKCs and other members of the phosphatidylinositol (PI) 3-kinase (PIK) family. ATM proteins are involved in cell-cycle regulation, recombination, telomere length control and the multiple steps in the cellular response to DNA damage.[87–89] Investigators have recently revealed that ATM phosphorylates a nuclease, Artemis, and directly affects radiation-induced DNA damage, independently of ATM-dependent cell-cycle checkpoint arrest.[90]AT cells, like DNA-PKCs/Ku-deficient cells, are hypersensitive to IR.[91–93] AT cells that are deficient in ATM or express a nonfunctional mutant protein also exhibit defects in IR-induced growth arrest,[94–96] radioresistant DNA synthesis and chromosome instability.[97,98] Because ATM is one of most widely studied components in the cellular response to DNA damage, it has been placed in the center of this figure. However, numerous other factors, such as the AT and Rad3-related (ATR) protein kinase, are essential for cell-cycle modulation after the induction of other types of DNA damage.[98] The red bars indicate three main cell-cycle checkpoints in late G1, late G2 and S; dashed lines show that the effect is of DSBs;[85,86] DNA-PKCs is recruited to sites of Ku/DNA complexes; and the question mark denotes links between G2 arrest and P53-mediated apoptosis currently under investigation.

The *TP53* tumor suppressor gene plays a pivotal role in the cellular response to IR. Through its C-terminal domain, the P53 protein can bind directly to radiation-damaged DNA and to single-stranded DNA ends, suggesting that P53 can act as a sensor of DNA damage. Exposing cells to DNA damaging agents or to restriction endonucleases that induce DNA breaks results in the stabilization and accumulation of P53 in the nucleus.[94,100] This increase in P53 is associated with transcription of P21 and BAX, leading to the induction of G1 arrest or apoptosis. ATM and CHK2, a mammalian homolog of Cds1/Rad53 that is activated by ATM, phosphorylates P53 and thereby prevents its degradation. DNA-PK interacts with the N-terminal region of P53 and contributes to its sequence-specific DNA binding, transactivation function, and stability.[101–104] Thus, P53 is an effector as well as sensor of DNA damage. c-Abl, a non-receptor tyrosine kinase, associates with P53104, 105 to stabilize and induce its pro-apoptotic functions through a kinase-independent mechanism.[105] c-Abl also interacts with the P53-related protein P73 in the response to IR and other genotoxic agents.[106–108] c-Abl has been implicated in inhibiting the Mdm2 oncoprotein as well.[109] Mdm2 binds the transcriptional activation domain of P53 and blocks its ability to regulate target genes and to exert antiproliferative effects. Mdm2 also promotes the degradation of P53 via the ubiquitination/proteasome pathway. The role of P53 in cell-cycle regulation is discussed below.

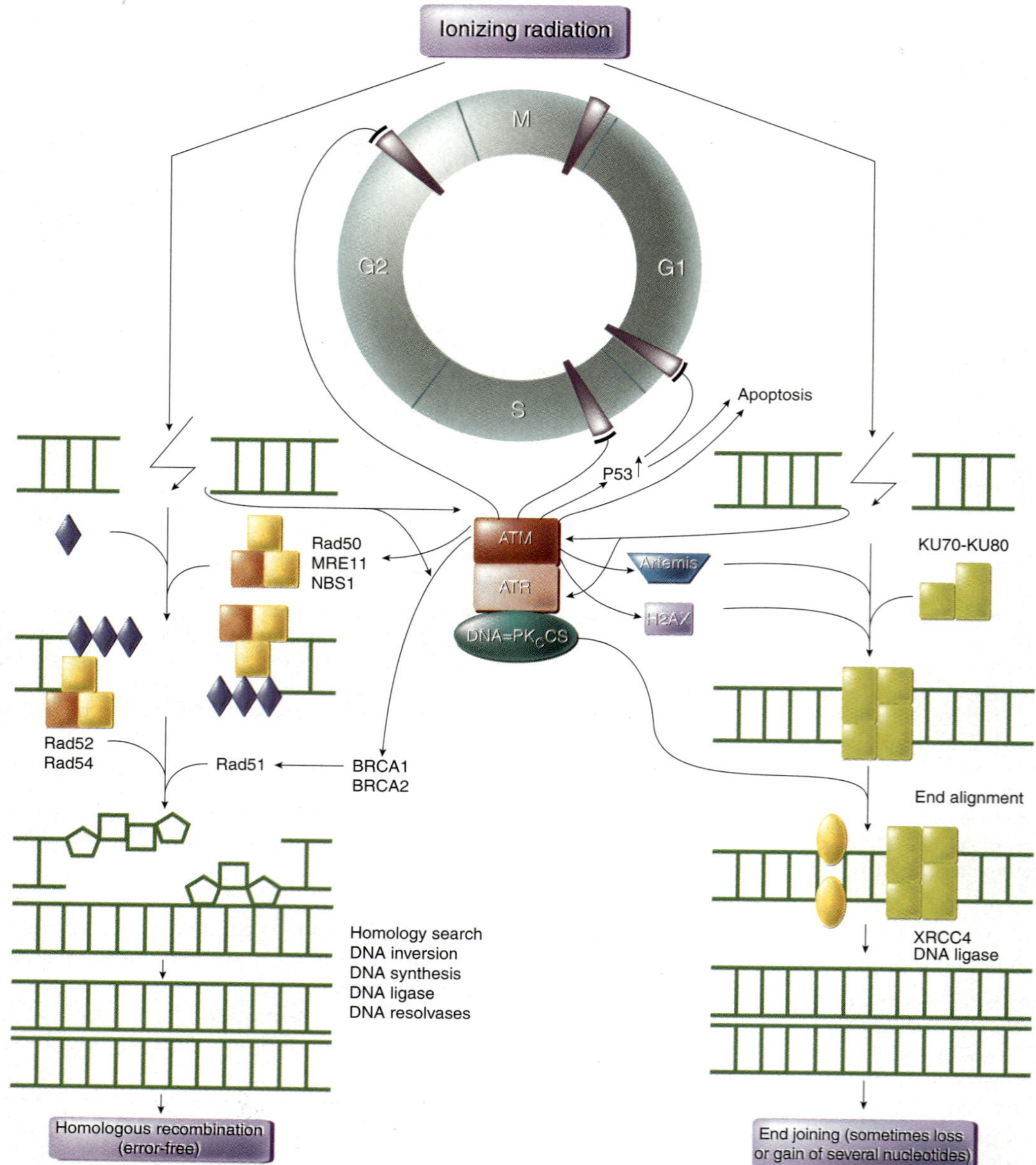

Figure 35-11 The presence of double-strand breaks (DSBs) leads to activation of the ataxia-telangiectasia-mutated (ATM) protein kinase. Targets of ATM phosphorylation include *TP53* and NBS1 and probably the phosphorylated histone variant H2AX. In this way, ATM influences cell-cycle progression and DSB repair, and if the face of overwhelming damage apoptosis. Preclinical studies have shown that delivery of an adenoviral vector expressing an antisense to ATM sensitizes prostate cancer cells to IR treatment.[98] AT patients exhibit pronounced toxicity to radiation, and therefore a cancer therapy strategy to block ATM expression/function requires localization to tumor tissue. Elk-1 and ATF-2.[130] In turn, binding of activated c-*Jun* to the AP-1 site in the c-*Jun* gene promoter contributes to the activation of c-*Jun* transcription in a positive feedback loop. IR-induced activation of the c-*Jun* gene is blocked by the antioxidant *N*-acetyl-L-cysteine (NAC).[131] IR also induces expression of the c*fos* and *jun-B* genes, which encode proteins that associate with c-*Jun*.

The Role of Growth and Stress-Signaling Pathways in the Radiation Response IR-induced activation of signaling pathways can have a variety of consequences, including increased or decreased radiosensitivity, inducing proliferation, differentiation or apoptosis or affecting biologic behavior (eg, invasiveness or metastases). Several of the key pathways that have been explored are summarized.

Ras, Raf, and MAPK Signaling The Ras/Raf signaling pathway mediates growth signals from receptors such as the epidermal growth factor receptor (EGFR), which is a member of the ErbB family. Overexpression of EGFR has been associated with uncontrolled proliferation, anchorage-independent growth, autocrine growth regulation, and increased radioresistance. IR activates the small G-protein Ras, which in turn activates c-Raf, a serine/threonine kinase that interacts with Ras.[110] Activating mutations in the *Ras* oncogene have been associated with radioresistance in certain cell lines.[111] Activation of c-Raf-1 has also been implicated in the development of radioresistance.[112,113] Ras and Raf thus represent potential targets for increasing radiosensitization. For example, farnesyltransferase inhibitors, which block cell membrane attachment and thereby activation of Ras, enhance IR-induced cell death.[114] In addition, down-regulation of Raf expression with anti-sense oligonucleotides sensitizes tumor cells to the cytotoxic effects of radiation.[115] IR-induced Ras activation leads to upregulation of mitogen-activated protein kinase (MAPK).[116,117]

PKC Signaling Protein kinase C (PKC) was the first cytoplasmic serine/threonine kinase found to be activated during the cellular response to IR.[118] IR-induced activation of PKC has been attributed to the generation of phospholipase A2-mediated oxidation products.[119] c-Abl also phosphorylates and activates cytoplasmic PKCs in irradiated cells.[120] IR-induced activation of PKCs is associated with translocation of PKCs to the nucleus.[120] PKC inhibitors block IR-induced activation of the early growth response 1 gene (*EGR-1*) and c-*Jun*.[118] In addition, PKC inhibitors such as calphostin C, PKC 412, and chelyrithine chloride, exhibit greater than additive antitumor effects in animal models when used in combination with IR.[121–123] Radioprotection of b-FGF-treated endothelial cells is also mediated by PKC activation.[124] Selective modulation of PKC could thus represent a strategy to enhance tumor cell killing or normal tissue survival. Inhibitors of the EGFR block IR-induced activation of MAPK,[125] indicating that EGFR, Ras, Raf, and MAPK all lie in the same IR response pathway. A recent phase II trial of a blocking antibody to EGFR has shown substantial improvement in the responses of head and neck tumors to radiotherapy.[126] Agents that target the intracellular tyrosine kinase region include small molecule tyrosine kinase inhibitors (TKIs), which act by interfering with ATP binding to the receptor, and various other compounds that act at substrate-binding regions or downstream components of the signaling pathway.[125] This group of compounds offers several advantages in cancer chemotherapy, including the possibility of inhibiting specific deregulated pathways in cancer cells while having minimal effects on normal cell function. They also have favorable pharmacokinetic and pharmacodynamic properties and low toxicity. Some TKIs, such as the reversible synthetic anilinoquinazoline inhibitor ZD1839 (Iressa), are now undergoing phase II to III clinical trials. A number of preclinical studies confirm Iressa's activity in a broad spectrum of tumor types, both as monotherapy and in combination with commonly used cytotoxic agents. A recent report suggests that the relative expression of ErbB isotypes may alter the potency of these agents. For example, SU11925, a small molecule inhibitor of the tyrosine kinase activity of both EGFR and human EGF-receptor 2 (HER-2), exhibits similar potency against EGFR and HER-2 in vitro; however, higher plasma concentrations of SU11925 are required to inhibit EGFR phosphorylation in vivo in tumors that also express high levels of HER-2 than in tumors that express EGFR alone.[126] This observation suggests that it is more difficult to inhibit EGFR phosphorylation in cells that express high levels of HER-2.

Lyn/c-Abl/SAPK Lyn, a member of the c-Src family of non-receptor protein tyrosine kinases (PTKs), is activated in IR-treated cells[128,129] and is required for induction of the stress-activated protein kinase (SAPK), a member of the mitogen-activated protein kinase (MAPK) family, which is involved in the apoptotic response to genotoxic stress. Lyn inhibits the cyclin-dependent kinase Cdc2 in irradiated cells which is necessary for progression through the premitotic checkpoint[128] and inhibits DNA-PKCs activity.[129] c-Abl activates MEKK-1, and thereby confers activation of the SEK1->SAPK pathway. In this context, SAPK induces the activation of transcription factors including c-*Jun*.

Early Response Genes IR induces expression of the *EGR-1* gene.[132] Transcription of it is conferred by IR-induced activation of serum response (CARG) elements in the EGR-1 promoter.[132] As found for c-*Jun*, treatment with NAC blocks induction of the *EGR-1* gene in the IR response.[133] These findings showed that IR activates the c-*Jun* and *EGR-1* genes by ROS-mediated signaling mechanisms. The finding that IR activates gene transcription provided the experimental basis for the design of gene therapy strategies in which the spatial and temporal control of gene expression are regulated by high-energy x-rays. In this approach, a radio-inducible promoter, such as that from the *EGR-1* gene, is inserted upstream to sequences encoding a therapeutic protein. The CARG elements in the EGR-1 promoter have been used to activate IR-induced transcription of tumor necrosis factor (TNF) or the HSV-1 thymidine kinase (TK).[134–136]

The TNF protein functions as a radiosensitizer and, in high local TNF concentrations, selectively increases the sensitivity of the tumor to IR treatment in the absence of systemic toxicity.[137] Several clinical trials are underway in which the EGR-1/CARG promoter–TNF construct is delivered to tumors in an adenoviral vector and activated by local radiotherapy.

Classic Aspects of DNA Repair in Radiotherapy Irradiated cells that are not lethally damaged may undergo repair of the damage to their DNA. Sublethal damage repair (SLDR) is operationally defined as the enhancement in survival when a dose of radiation is separated over a period of time. SLDR may be represented by the extrapolation number (*n*) of the radiation survival curve when a multitarget survival model is employed.[138-142]

Sublethal damage has been studied in vitro and in vivo. In general, SLDR experiments divide a single dose into two relatively equal doses spaced at variable time intervals. Elkind and colleagues investigated this phenomenon in great detail.[138,143] Figure 35-12 shows results representative of split-dose experiments. An enhancement in survival,

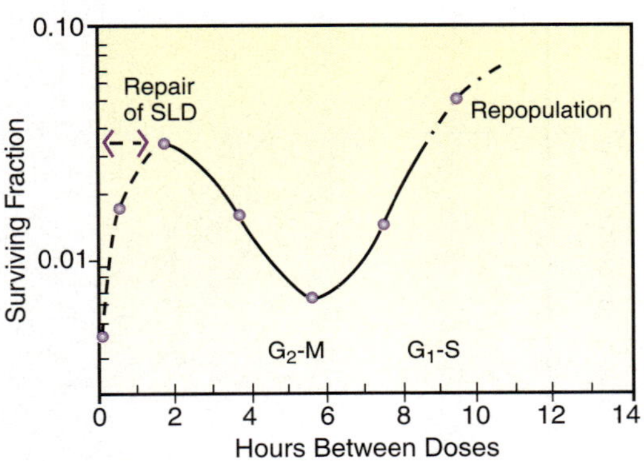

Figure 35-12 The surviving fractions of Chinese hamster cells exposed to two doses of x-rays separated by various time intervals are shown. When the two doses are given together (time between doses = 0 hours), the surviving fraction is equal to that observed after the single larger dose of radiation. As the two doses are separated by time, an enhancement in survival occurs and is interpreted as the repair of sublethal damage (*dashed line*). Subsequent radiation doses result in a reduction in the surviving fraction. This reduction in survival occurs because of more sensitive phases of the cell cycle (G2 and M). Later time points demonstrate increased surviving fractions due to radiation synchronization of cells and their entry into resistant phases of the cell cycle (G1 and S) Source: Elkind.[38,39]

following two doses separated in time, is observed in exponentially growing Chinese hamster cells at 2 hours. This enhancement in survival is due to the rapid repair of SLD and is followed by a subsequent decline in survival at 5 hours and then another increase in survival at 8 hours. This variability in survival is caused by synchronization of the exponentially growing cell populations by the first radiation dose and subsequent treatment with a second dose during the radioresistant S-phase (t = 2 hours) or radiosensitive G2-M phase of the cell cycle (t = 6 hours).[139,141,142]

The concept of SLDR is important during a course of fractionated RT because the shoulder region of the survival curve is recapitulated due to SLDR.[140] Fractionation magnifies the surviving fraction after each treatment to an exponent equal to the number of treatments. Therefore, small differences in survival after each dose may have a great impact on treatment outcome. Most human tumor cell lines studied in vitro have relatively small shoulders;[144,149] however, a large capacity for SLDR has been reported for some human tumor cell lines.[79,145]

The ability of tissues to undergo SLDR has been demonstrated using a variety of normal tissue clonogenic or functional assays.[150–152] The capacity of different cell populations to repair SLD is reflected by the width of the shoulder (or initial slope) of their survival curve. An increase in the total dose required to give the same biologic damage when a single dose (D1) is split into two doses (total dose D2), with a time interval between doses to obtain a single biologic end point, is the capacity of a normal tissue to repair SLD. The difference in the two doses, D2 – D1, is the measure of SLDR by the tissue, provided that the two doses are larger than those that generate the shoulder region of the survival curve.[81,151,153]

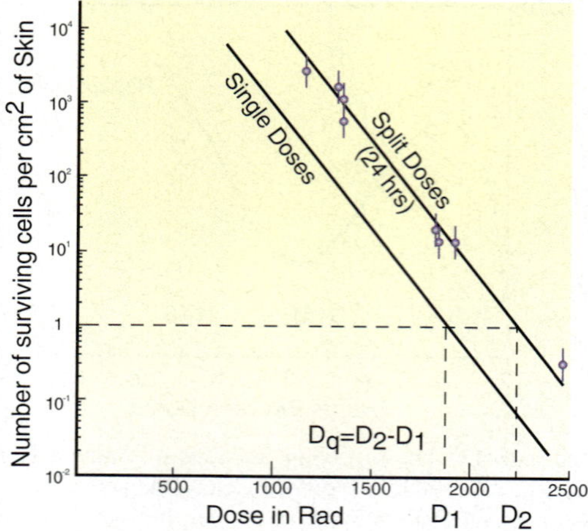

Figure 35-13 Single-dose and two-dose survival curves for epithelial cells. The D0 is 135 cGy. The ordinate is not the surviving fraction, as in survival curves for cells cultured in vitro, but is the number of surviving cells per square centimeter of skin (plating efficiency is obviously not known in vivo). In the two-dose survival curve, the interval between dose fractions is 24 hours. Although the curves are parallel (similar D0), their graphic horizontal separation number (n), may then be calculated from D0 and Dq. Source: Weners.[195,196]

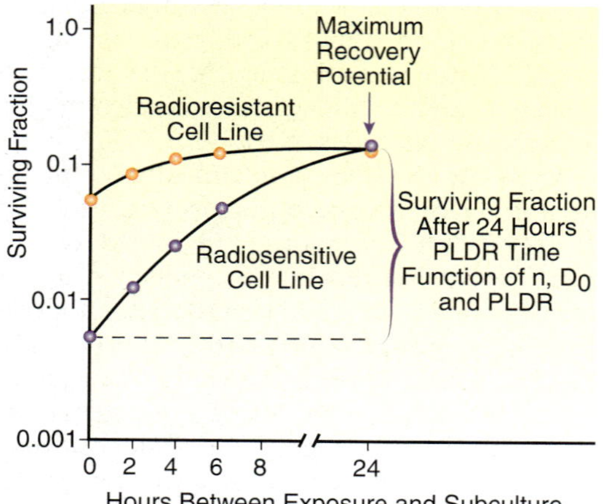

Figure 35-14 Maximum recovery potential (MRP) for radioresistant and radiosensitive cells. Confluent cell lines (noncycling) were irradiated and immediately subcultured, which resulted in an initial surviving fraction (0), which is generally equal to or slightly less than the surviving fraction of exponentially growing cells in tissue culture. However, when these irradiated confluent cells are not subcultured for the indicated time intervals, an enhancement in survival, interpreted as STR repair of potentially lethal damage (PLDR), occurs. The surviving fractions of cells after a 24-hour delay in subculture (maximum recovery potential [MRP]) of confluent cells is dependent on n, D0, and PLDR. The initial surviving fraction of cells at 0 hours is dependent on no and D0 but not on PLDR.

(Figure 35-13), D2 – D1 = Dq. If the D0 is known, then n can be calculated from the equation:

$$\log_e n = Dq/D0$$

Varying environmental conditions can influence cell survival after a dose of x-rays. Thus, damage that is potentially lethal under a given set of conditions may not be lethal if postirradiation conditions are altered.[154,155] The enhancement in survival seen following manipulation of postirradiation conditions is referred to as the repair of potentially lethal damage (PLD). PLD repair (PLDR) has been demonstrated in vitro[156,157] (Figure 35-14). PLDR has also been shown to occur in vivo.[156,158,159] PLDR is reported to be more pronounced in large tumors, presumably because a large proportion of cells are in G1 or G0. PLDR has been described to occur principally in the G1 phase of the cell cycle. Efficient PLDR occurs in a variety of human tumor cell lines in vitro.[160–163] Weichselbaum and colleagues,[163–165] and Guichard and colleagues[166] have suggested that PLDR contributes to radiotherapy failure under certain circumstances.

PLDR and/or SLDR may not be expressed under all conditions in vivo. For example, cells must be genetically competent to repair these types of damages, and the tumor environment may affect the proliferative status of tumor cells.[155,165,167] Also, radiation (or chemotherapy) may induce tumor proliferation, which allows fixation of radiation damage before PLDR or SLDR is complete.[155,167] Therefore, PLDR is likely to be most important in tumor cells of intermediate or high radiosensitivity when cells are quiescent between fractions. The 24-hour PLDR-surviving fraction, following treatment of human tumor cells in plateau-phase culture with a similar dose, is referred to as the maximum recovery potential (MRP).[80] Figure 35-14 shows that although two cell lines have different amounts of initial lethal damage induced by a constant radiation dose (a function of D0 and n), the surviving fraction after a 24-hour delay in subculture (a function of n, D0, PLDR) may be similar.

Molecular Aspects of DNA Repair in the Cellular Response to Ionizing Radiation All eukaryotes have evolved several mechanisms to repair DSBs, which indicate the importance and difficulty of repairing this type of DNA injury. The two main pathways are homologous combination (HR) and nonhomologous end-joining (NHEJ). These two repair modes differ in their requirement for a homologous template DNA and in the fidelity of DSB repair. Whereas HR ensures accurate DSB repair, NHEJ does not. The contributions of these two DSB repair pathways are likely to differ depending on the stage of the cell cycle.[99] However, the pathways are not mutually exclusive because repair events that involve both pathways can be detected. HR is most efficient in the S and G2 phases of the cell cycle because of the availability of sister chromatids as repair templates.[168] In the absence of a sister chromatid, DSB repair in G1 phase could still efficiently occur through NHEJ.

HR can repair DSBs by using the undamaged chromatid as a template, which results in the accurate repair of the DSB. HR is mediated through the RAD52 family of proteins.[169] These proteins include RAD50, RAD51, RAD52, RAD54 and meiotic recombination 11 (MRE11). The initial cellular response to DSBs is mediated through ATM and Nijmegen breakage syndrome 1 (NBS1).[170] Subsequent steps of DSB repair through HR include DNA-end recognition, possibly by RAD52, and nucleolytic processing of the broken ends of DNA into 3'-end single-stranded DNA. This single-stranded DNA is bound by the RAD51 protein which mediates crucial steps in the reaction—the search for a homologous duplex template DNA and the formation of joint molecules between the broken DNA ends and the repair template. Other proteins, including replication protein A (RPA), RAD52, RAD5430 and several RAD51-related proteins (eg, RAD51B, RAD51C, RAD51D, XRCC2, XRCC3, and DMC1),[171] are thought to function as accessory proteins for *RAD51* at various stages of HR. In mammalian cells, RAD51 forms nuclear foci in response to IR and decreased expression of RAD51 confers sensitivity to IR-induced DNA lesions.[172] The later steps of the process include polymerization of nucleotides to restore degraded DNA strands and resolution of the recombination intermediates. Mice with targeted disruption of the *RAD51* gene exhibit an embryonic lethal phenotype.[173] Moreover, the failure to generate RAD51–/– stem cells has indicated that RAD51 is essential for cell viability. RAD51 interacts with *TP53*[174] and *BRCA1*.[175] Although the breast cancer susceptibility proteins BRCA1 and BRCA2 are clearly implicated in HR, their roles are not well understood. Other studies have demonstrated that RAD51 is phosphorylated by c-Abl in IR-treated cells and that this response contributes to the down-regulation of RAD51 activity in ATP-dependent DNA strand exchange reactions.[172] Treatment of cells with IR is also associated with inactivation of RAD51 by caspase-3-mediated proteolytic cleavage.[176]

In contrast to HR, NHEJ uses little or no homology to couple DNA ends. This pathway is not only used to repair DSBs generated by IR or other exogenous DNA-damaging agents, but is also required to process the DSB intermediates that are generated during V(D)J recombination.[177] Several proteins that are involved in NHEJ have been identified. The Ku heterodimer, which consists of Ku70 and Ku80, has a high affinity for DNA ends, which indicates that it has an early role in the NHEJ process. Ku bound to a DNA end attracts the catalytic subunit of the DNA-dependent protein kinase (DNA-PKCs), a 470-kDa polypeptide with a protein kinase domain near its carboxyl terminus.[178] DNA-PKCs can subsequently phosphorylate several cellular target proteins, including P53, the Ku polypeptides and itself. At present, it is unclear which phosphorylation targets of DNA-PKCs are relevant in vivo. A complex that consists of DNA ligase IV and XRCC4 (X-ray-repair-crosscomplementing defective repair in Chinese hamster mutant 4) accomplishes the final ligation step. Cell lines or animals that lack either of the genes encoding these proteins do not carry out V(D)J recombination and are sensitive to ionizing radiation.[179] In addition to the involvement of the RAD50–MRE11-containing complex in HR, genetic experiments with yeast indicate that this complex also has a role in NHEJ.[180]

Although cells deficient in components of the NHEJ and HR pathways are more radiosensitive than their wild-type counterparts, few advances have been made in the development of inhibitors of IR-induced DSB repair. Initial attempts at inhibiting DNA repair in irradiated tumors were associated with increased normal tissue toxicity. A more recent strategy using antisense oligonucleotides to the *RAD51* gene has resulted in enhancement of the effects of radiation on glioma cells in vitro and in animal models.[181] With improvements in the selective delivery of radiotherapy, the spatial targeting of IR-induced DSBs to tumors should theoretically establish inhibition of DNA repair as an attractive therapeutic approach.

Modulation of chromatin structure and function represents another novel strategy for biological targeting. Histone H2AX, a minor histone H2A variant, encodes a conserved Sr-Gln-Glu (SQE) motif in the carboxyl-terminal tail. IR induces phosphorylation of the Ser residue by ATM/ATR family kinases to form foci of H2AX immunoreactivity a DNA double-strand breaks. Weichselbaum and colleagues showed that peptides that mimic the H2AX carboxyl terminus block induction of H2AX foci and enhance cell death in irradiated radioresistant tumor cells.

Cell-Cycle Checkpoints, Integration of Signalling, and DNA Repair It is necessary for one phase of the cell cycle to be completed before initiating events associated with the following phase. Failure to achieve accurate completion of events may lead to genetic instability and/or cell death. Cells have evolved mechanisms to monitor genomic instability associated with DNA damage. The surveillance mechanisms and resulting inhibition of cell-cycle progression are referred to as *checkpoint controls.* For example, a DNA damage checkpoint control communicates information between a DNA lesion and the regulatory components of the cell cycle. Radiation-induced single-strand breaks (SSBs) and DSBs are associated with the initiating signal that activates checkpoint controls. In general, the cell cycle is delayed at one of the checkpoints by inhibiting cyclin-dependent kinases (CDKs) until DNA repair is complete. Following exposure to ionizing radiation, cells arrest at the checkpoints. Cell-cycle regulation in irradiated and nonirradiated cells has recently been reviewed.[182,183]

DNA damage and its effect on cell-cycle progression have been intensively studied in yeast and Xenopus oocyte, as well as in mammalian cells. Studies show that the kinase activity of Cdc2-cyclin B complex is required for the G2-to-M-phase (G2/M) transition in the normal cell cycle and that tyrosine phosphorylation of Cdc2 inhibits its kinase activity.[184] Both inhibition of Cdc2 kinase activity and enhanced phosphorylation of Cdc2 have been observed following DNA damage. The phosphorylation state of Cdc2 is maintained by the kinases Wee1 and Myt1 and by the phosphatase Cdc25.[120, 122, 124,185] Cdc2 is inactivated by phosphorylation of Thr-14 and Tyr-15 in the ATP-binding domain by the Wee1 kinase.[186] Phosphorylation of Tyr-15 is also mediated in part by IR-induced activation of the Lyn tyrosine kinase.[127,128] Although checkpoint regulation of both sides exists, it is thought that regulation of Cdc25 activity is an important factor in the maintenance of G2 arrest after DNA damage. In mammalian cells, two kinases, Chk1 and Cds1 (also known as Chk2), have been identified[119,187,188] and shown to phosphorylate Cdc25C and prevent it from dephosphorylating (Ser-216) and activating Cdc2.[85,119,187–190]

Phosphorylation of Cdc25 facilitates association with the 14-3-3 protein, resulting in its export from the nucleus; however, the mechanism of Chk1 and Cds1 activation following irradiation is not clear. Studies in Chk1-deficient cells have also shown that this kinase is required for initiating G2 arrest[190,192] and is a downstream effector of ATM. The response of Cds1 to DNA damage has been shown to be dependent on the activity of ATM. The ATM-dependent DNA damage checkpoint pathway regulates both the G1-S and G2-M transitions in the response of mammalian cells to IR treatment. The IR-induced arrest at the G1-S DNA damage checkpoint is mediated predominately by P53-dependent induction of P21 expression and thereby inhibition of the Cdk2 kinase.[193]

P53 promotes arrest at the G0/G1 checkpoint. Following radiation exposure, P53 protein levels rise due to post-translational modifications that increase the P53 half-life. This rise is transient and is correlated with the presence of damaged DNA. DNA strand breaks are the most potent inducer of P53 following IR exposure.[181] Cell-cycle arrest is induced by P53 when the protein acts as a transcriptional activator. One of the most important genes induced is $P21^{waf\text{-}cip}$. The interaction of P21 with the cyclin E/CDK2 complex inhibits the progression of cells into the S-phase. P21 also binds directly to proliferating cell nuclear antigen (PCNA). In addition, P53 interacts with MDM2 and GADD45. As described above, MDM2 negatively regulates P53 and likely functions during the recovery phase in the late G1-phase. GADD45 inhibits the progression of cells into the S-phase. A second mechanism of regulating the G1 checkpoint by P53 is mediated by direct binding to proteins such RPA. Bristow and colleagues[194] showed that rat fibroblast clones expressing increasing levels of transfected mutant P53 showed loss of the G1/S checkpoint and increasing levels of radioresistance. The increased survival was not associated with loss of apoptosis, but consistent with observations of improved double-strand break repair.[195] This is not consistent with a "more time for repair" hypothesis for the G1/S checkpoint, because checkpoint abrogation would then be expected to sensitize and not protect. Interestingly, the radiosensitivity of P53 null fibroblasts remained unchanged, indicating a gain of function of mutant P53, possibly due to improved damage sensing via the carboxy terminus of the protein which is known to bind to damaged DNA in a nonsequence-dependent manner.

Pharmacological agents that override the G2/M block often sensitize the cells to IR.[196] The classic inhibitor of the IR-induced G2 arrest response is caffeine. The precise mechanism for the effects of caffeine on G2 arrest is unresolved, although ATM has been proposed as the target.[197] Treatment of irradiated P53-deficient cells with caffeine is associated with activation of Cdc2 and hence mitotic cell death.[198] These findings are in concert with reports which demonstrate that abrogation of the G2 checkpoint results in differential radiosensitization of G1 checkpoint defective cells.[199] Caffeine and its analogues, however, have not proven to be effective radiosensitizers in the clinic, in part because of the toxicities associated with levels required for inhibition of IR-induced G2 arrest. The CHK1 inhibitors, UCN01 and SB-218078, block DNA damage-induced G2 arrest in human cells.[200–202] These findings and the demonstration that UCN01 does not inhibit hCHK2[200,201] have supported lack of involvement of CHK2 in the G2 arrest response. Whereas UCN01 is undergoing clinical evaluation as a radio- and chemosensitizer, other inhibitors of CHK1/2, such as debromohymenialdisine,[203] are under development. It is noteworthy that the concept of caffeine-induced override of G2-M block has been challenged by investigators who suggest this cell-cycle perturbation and enhancement of the induced DNA damage associated with caffeine are attributed to inhibition of DNA repair and or DNA synthesis.[204–206]

Both the initiation and elongation stages of DNA replication (S-phase checkpoint) are inhibited by IR. In budding yeast, the genes that regulate the S-phase checkpoint are RAD17, RAD24, RAD53, and MEC3 and MEC1. The sequence of gene interaction and function in mammalian cells is under investigation. The ATM gene product plays a role in replicon initiation and chain elongation. Both MEC1 and ATM are members of the *PI3K* gene family.

Fractionation Early in the twentieth century, it became apparent that RT was equally efficacious but better tolerated when administered in divided doses,[207] a concept known as *fractionation.* Fractionation spares normal tissues by allowing time for repair and repopulation of normal cells. In addition, fractionation increases tumor cell kill due to reoxygenation and reassortment of tumor cells into sensitive phases of the cell cycle.[208] Conventional fractionation schemes involve a daily fraction of 1.8 to 2 Gy 5 days a week. Total treatment times depend on the total dose prescribed and thus range from 3 to 7 weeks. Various mathematical models have been proposed to equate total dose, time, and fraction size and achieve an isoeffective dose. However, clinical utility of these models remains controversial.

Clinical interest in altered fractionation has been resurrected due to recently reported improved outcomes in patients with advanced head and neck cancer. *Hyperfractionation* is defined as the use of reduced size fractions given twice or more per day such that a greater total dose is delivered by increasing the number of treatments (50–60 vs 30–35) in the same total treatment time. Thus, relatively rapidly dividing cell populations may have a higher proportion of cells in the most sensitive phases of the cell cycle at each treatment. Cells in late-responding normal tissues are slowly proliferating, and therefore, after a few fractions, many surviving cells will be concentrated in the more resistant phases. This strategy has been applied to a variety of tumors, including primary brain tumors[208] and head and neck cancer.[210]

Accelerated fractionation decreases the overall treatment time to diminish clonogenic proliferation between successive doses. Treatment is given 2 to 4 times per day, employing fraction sizes of 1.5 to 2 Gy per treatment with 4 to 6 hour interfraction intervals.[81,211] The total daily dose is thus 3 to 6 Gy and the total dosage is given in 3 to 4 weeks. Although treatment interruptions are often necessary due to acute toxicity,[210] the total treatment time is substantially reduced. *Hypofractionation* is the use of larger than standard daily fractions. This approach is typically used when palliation is the goal. Treatment may involve 4 to 10 Gy fractions delivered weekly or several times a week as opposed to daily.

Modifiers of the Radiation Response The extent of DNA damage following radiation exposure is dependent on several factors. One of the most important is cellular oxygen.[212] Hypoxic cells are considerably less radiosensitive than aerated cells. In fact, anoxic cells require 2 to 3 times the radiation dose to produce an equivalent amount of cell kill as do oxygenated cells. The difference in radiosensitivity between hypoxic and aerated cells is known as the oxygen enhancement ratio (OER). Oxygen is believed to prolong the lifetime of the short-lived free radicals produced by the interaction of x-rays and cellular H_2O. Indirectly ionizing radiation is consequently less efficacious in tumors with significant areas of hypoxia and necrosis. In contrast, damage following exposure to directly ionizing radiation is independent of cellular oxygen levels.[214]

Thomlinson and Gray observed that tumors "outgrow" their vasculature resulting in necrotic areas and suggested that tumor cells adjacent to the anoxic region may be clonogenic but hypoxic.[214, 215] As shown in Figure 35-15, the oxygen tension within the tumor falls with the distance from the capillary producing a hypoxic region. In some experimental tumor systems, reoxygenation of hypoxic tumor cells occurs within 24 hours.[217] A clinical observation that supports the importance of oxygen levels in patients undergoing RT is that severe anemia is associated with worsened local control in a variety of tumors. Several studies have demonstrated improved survival in patients with locally advanced cervical cancer treated with RT when hemoglobin levels were above 11 g as compared with patients with lower hemoglobin levels.[218–220] Anemia has been associated with poorer survival rates following RT in other tumors, including endometrial, bladder, and pharyngeal cancers.[221–223] The importance of cellular oxygen is also demonstrated by improvements in outcome in patients receiving hyperbaric oxygen.[224,225]

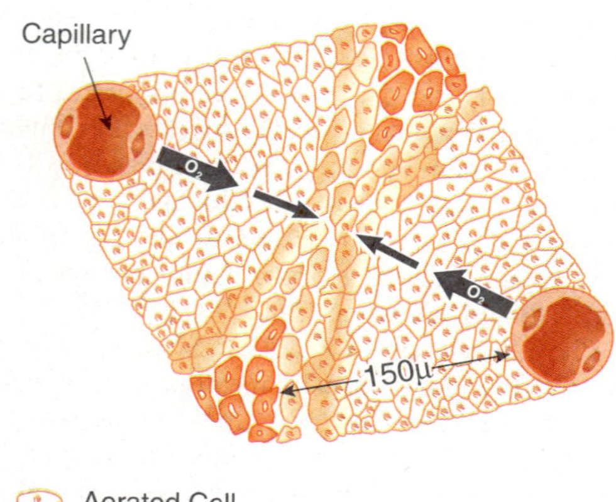

Figure 35-15 Oxygen diffusion through tissue from a capillary resulting in hypoxic cells. Oxygen diffuses an average of 150 Ci from the capillary. Cells beyond this region are anoxic and nonviable. Cells at the periphery of this radius are hypoxic but viable.

Numerous chemicals have been shown to modify the effects of ionizing radiation. An important class of compounds are the hypoxic cell sensitizers, including metronidazole, misonidazole, and etanidazole.[226] These agents mimic oxygen and have been shown in vitro to increase cell kill of hypoxic cells.[227] Clinical experience, however, with these agents has been mixed. Only two prospective trials has demonstrated a benefit to their use in conjunction with RT.[228,229] Toxicity is common, particularly peripheral neuropathy. More promising results with less toxicity have been noted with the newest hypoxic sensitizer nimorazole.[230]

A second class of radiation sensitizers are the thymidine analogues iododeoxyuridine (IUdR) and bromodeoxyuridine (BudR), we had better incorporated. Both are incorporated into DNA in the place of thymidine and render DNA more susceptible to radiation damage. Although several nonrandomized trials have been promising,[232,233] no prospective trial has demonstrated a significant benefit to their use. Of note, both are associated with considerable acute toxicity.

Multiple chemotherapeutic agents sensitize cells to radiation including 5-fluorouracil, actinomycin D, cisplatin, gemcitabine, fludarabine, paclitaxel, doxorubicin, hydroxyurea, mitomycin C, topotecan, and vinorelbine. The mechanism of radiosensitization varies among the different agents. Cisplatin inhibits both SLDR and PLDR.[232] Inhibition of repair may also help explain the radiosensitizing properties of topotecan.[233] Doxorubicin increases cellular oxygen levels by inhibiting mitochondrial and tumor cell respiration.[234] Hydroxyurea is toxic to cells in the S-phase and inhibits entry of cells into the G1- from the S-phase.[235] Mitomycin C is preferentially toxic to hypoxic cells.[236] Paclitaxel synchronizes cells into the G2- and M-phases.[237]

Other drugs act as radioprotectors by protecting normal tissues from radiation damage while reportedly not affecting tumor radiosensitivity. The best known radioprotector is amifostine, a derivative of cysteamine which acts as a free radical scavenger. Following administration, amifostine quickly penetrates into normal tissues, but only slowly into tumors, and thereby results in a preferential protection of normal tissues. Promising results have been reported in head and neck cancer patients undergoing RT.[238] Amifostine has also been used to reduce chemotherapy-related sequelae.[239] Various endogenous biologic response modifiers also act as radio protectors, including interleukin-1 and granulocyte macrophage colony-stimulating factor (GM-CSF);[240,241] neither are classic radioprotectors, since they do not directly scavenge free radicals but, rather, improve bone marrow tolerance compartment.

Growth Factor and Cytokine Induction Following Radiation Exposure Growth and Regeneration Kinetics The percentage of cycling tumor cells is called the growth fraction (GF). In human solid tumors, it is usually a small proportion of the total number of cells. If the GF remains constant with time, the growth rate of the tumor is proportional to the GF. If the GF decreases with time, the rate of the tumor growth slows. Solid tumors usually grow at a slower rate as they enlarge, and so growth is approximated by the Gompertz formula.[81,244] In circumstances of equilibrium in normal tissues, each mitotic division results in the average of only one new cell. Usually, one daughter cell is lost by desquamation or metastasis. By definition, the cell loss factor (CLF) in a steady state is 1. Maximum growth occurs if the CLF is reduced to 0. The only requirement for growth is a reduction from 1.0 in the CLF, that is, an average of < 1 of two daughter cells of a division is lost. A CLF of < 1 is characteristic of regeneration of both normal tissue and malignant growth. Tumor growth is usually characterized by CLFs that are closer to 1 than 0.

An index for the potential regeneration of tumors and normal tissue populations is the proliferative activity of the cell population.[81] One common measurement of tumor growth is the potential doubling time (PDT), which is defined as the time required to double the number of clonogenic cells if the CLF decreases to 0. In this concept, the doubling time is equal to the cell-cycle time. Tumors with a high rate of both cell production and loss have the potential for early and rapid regeneration after irradiation or other cytotoxic treatment. Thus, even though a tumor may exhibit slow pretreatment growth, it may regenerate rapidly. Excessive protraction in the time of radiation fractionation or split-course regimens may give inferior local control results if accelerated proliferation occurs during the period when radiation is not given. Clonal proliferation during tumor regression after irradiation was demonstrated by Hermens and Barendsen, who showed an exponential increase in clonogen number in a rat rhabdomyosarcoma during a time of tumor shrinkage (Figure 35-16).[245] Accelerated repopulation of irradiated tumors and tissues may be associated with the recruitment of quiescent

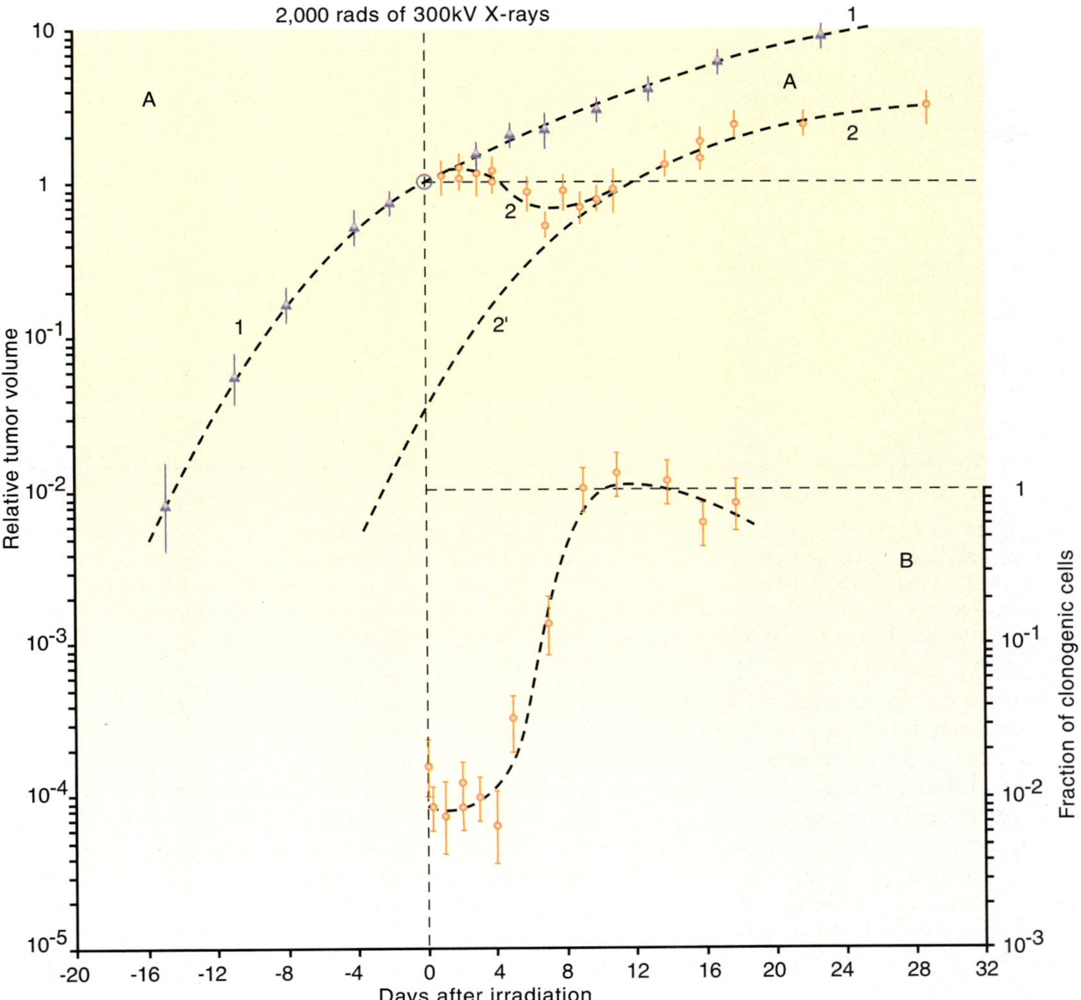

Figure 35-16 Growth curves of rat rhabdosarcoma tumors irradiated in vivo demonstrating accelerated repopulation **(A).** Volume change in the tumor after a single dose of 2,000 cGy. Curve 1 is the growth of an unirradiated tumor. Curve 2 represents regression and regrowth of an irradiated tumor **(B).** Exponential increase in the fractions of clonogenic cells as a function of time after irradiation. Cells were obtained from the tumors irradiated in **A,** and the colony-forming assay was used to determine clonogenic potential. This figure demonstrates that there is an exponential increase in the number of clonogenic cells within 6 to 10 days after irradiating a tumor in vivo and that clonogens can repopulate during tumor regression. Source: Hermens AF and Barendsen GW.[245]

cells into the cell cycle. This effect is associated with radiation-mediated induction of the immediate early genes c-*Jun* and *EGR1*.[246]

Although the induction of genes following DNA damage was well known in bacteria, it was only relatively recently that induction of the transcription of the proinflammatory cytokine *TNF*α gene provided support for the theory that gene activation mediates the mammalian cell response to DNA damage.[247] *TNF*α is transcriptionally induced following irradiation of human tumor cells in vitro[245] and has paracrine and autocrine effects on tumor cell killing and might account for some of the systemic effects of localized RT. bFGF is induced in endothelial cells and mediates protection against apoptosis. The concept of the induction and release of growth factors following IR was initially reported in tumor cells and in normal endothelial cells.[249] Subsequent studies showed that IR induces expression of genes encoding other growth factors, such as the platelet-derived growth factor, interleukin-1[189] and bFGF.[185] IR-induction of TGFO, which is proposed to mediate fibrosis following IR and thereby to mediate some of the late effects of RT on normal tissues. Other cytokines have been also reported to be induced following radiation.[250] Potential applications of these observations is the use of TNFα or other cytokines as potential radioenhancing agents in gene therapy combined with ionizing radiation (see below). It has subsequently been discovered that b-FGF protects some of the lung endothelium from radiation-mediated apoptosis and has potential as a radioprotector.[251] Also, secretion of growth factors and cytokines may be an important step in radiation carcinogenesis in normal cells. Inhibition of molecular mediators of deleterious late radiation effects on normal tissues may increase the therapeutic ratio and presents the possibility of genetic manipulation in clinical radiotherapy.

The recent demonstration of EGFR activation by ionizing radiation makes this receptor and other members of ErbB receptor tyrosine kinase family important targets for radiosensitizing therapeutic interventions.[250] The radiation-induced activation of EGFR results in cytoprotective signaling dominantly involving MAPK and PI3K. The inhibition of EGFR by tyrphostin TK inhibitors or through overexpression of a dominant-negative (DN) EGFR inhibit the radiation-induced cytoprotective response and results in significant radiosensitization of xenograft tumors in mice. The monoclonal antibody, IMC-C225, which blocks the binding of EGF, exhibits antitumor activity in EGFR+ tumors and enhances radiation toxicity in cultured human squamous cell carcinoma; it also increases taxane-, platinum-induced cytotoxicity in non-small cell lung carcinoma xenografts.[253] In A431 head and neck squamous cell xenografts, IMC-C225 administered in conjunction with irradiation yielded a radiation enhancement factor of 3.62, attributable to both tumor necrosis and antiangiogenesis.[252] In phase I pharmacokinetic studies, IMC-C225 has a long half-life, lending itself to convenient weekly administration. The reported toxicity profile of IMC-C225 is limited to allergic and dermatologic reactions. An ongoing phase III international multicenter randomized study in locally advanced squamous cell carcinoma of the head and neck is evaluating therapeutic radiation therapy, either alone or in conjunction with IMC-C225. Preclinical studies have shown that ZD1839, an oral anilinoquinazoline, inhibits the epidermal growth factor receptor-associated TK, and has an additive to synergistic effect in combination with radiation or chemotherapy in colon, head and neck, and non-small cell lung cancers. Phase I clinical trials have shown modest dose-related toxicity, and antitumor activity has been reported in a variety of malignancies including lung cancer.[255]

Induction of Apoptosis The response of eukaryotic cells to IR and other DNA-damaging agents includes the induction of apoptosis. For more than 40 years, radiobiologists have been aware of cells in irradiated specimens that display the features of apoptosis. Despite this knowledge, the role of apoptosis in end points important in radiation therapy is not clear. The current model suggests that tumor cells with apoptotic propensity are more sensitive to radiation. If this hypothesis is confirmed, strategies can be envisioned that may restore apoptotic propensity to radioresistant tumor cells for therapeutic benefit.

Direct evidence for the activation of caspases in the induction of apoptosis comes from studies with peptide inhibitors,[256] the cowpox virus protein CRMA,[257] and the baculovirus protein P35.[258] Overexpression of CRMA inhibits the induction of apoptosis in diverse settings, including activation of the Fas receptor and treatment with TNFα.[259,260] Similarly, the P35 protein functions as an inhibitor of caspases and blocks apoptosis in insect and mammalian cells.[261] The recent finding that IR-induced apoptosis involves activation of a CRMA-insensitive pathway has supported the existence of apoptotic signals that are distinct from those activated by Fas and TNK.[262] In this context, caspase-3 is inhibited by P35 but not CRMA in vitro, and IR-induced activation of caspase-3, like the induction of apoptosis, involves a P35-sensitive, CRMA-insensitive pathway.[262] Whereas caspase-3 is activated by IR, as well as Fas ligand and TNF, these findings are explained by involvement of a CRMA-sensitive caspase in the Fas- and TNF-induced, but not the IR-induced, cascade. IR-induced activation of caspase-3 is associated with the proteolytic cleavage of poly-(ADP-ribose) polymerase (PARP),[263] DNA-PK,[264] protein kinase C8,265,266 and protein kinase C.[267] The activation of caspase 3 and the subsequent substrate cleavage in irradiated cells are regulated by members of the Bc1-2/Bc1-x1 family.[268] Bc1-2 and Bc1-xL block the release of cytochrome *c* from the mitochondria of cells exposed to IR and other agents.[269–271] Whereas cytochrome *c* is not released from the mitochondria of cells induced to undergo apoptosis with Fas ligand,[82] this event upstream to activation of caspase-3[118] and the insensitivity of IR-induced caspase-3 activity to CRMA[262] support distinct apoptotic signals in Fas- and IR-treated cells.

IR-induced apoptosis is mediated at least in part by c-Abl dependent activation of P53 and its homolog, P73.[272] IR also induces translocation of SAPK to mitochondria, interaction of SAPK and Bcl-xL, and thereby release of cytochrome *c*.[273,274] In turn, cytochrome *c* activates caspase-3 and the cleavage of diverse proteins that confer the apoptotic response.[275,276] Bcl-2 and Bcl-xL block IR-induced cytochrome *c* release and apoptosis.[273,277,278] These findings have supported the transduction of DNA damage-induced signals to mitochondria as a determinant of cell fate in the IR response.

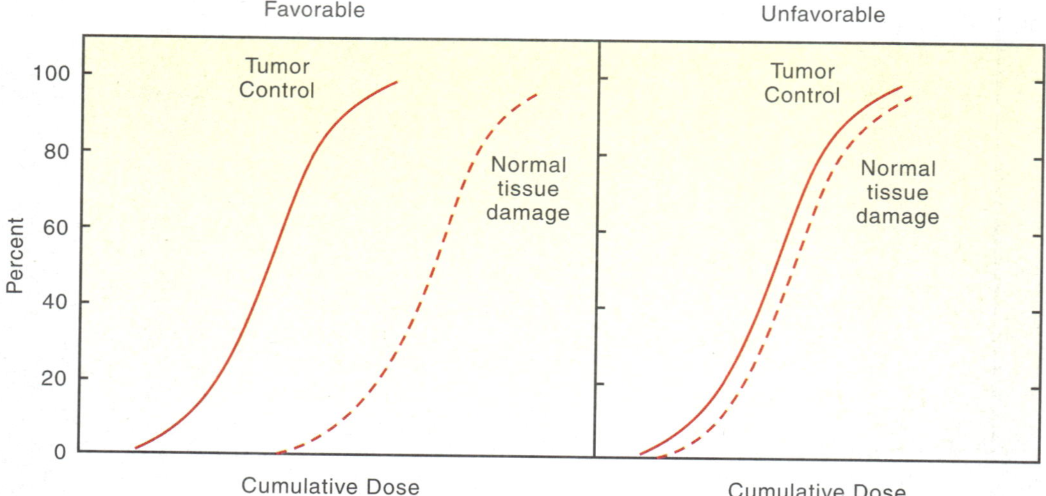

Figure 35-17 Dose control and complication curves in curable and noncurable tumors treated with radiotherapy. The percentages of tumor control and normal tissue damage are sigmoidal. In a radiocurable tumor, such as Hodgkin's disease, the dose required to control a tumor is less than the normal tissue tolerance. This results in a favorable therapeutic ratio. The dosage required to control an unfavorable tumor, such as pancreatic carcinoma, is approximately that of the normal tissue tolerance, resulting in an unfavorable therapeutic ratio. Source: Varian, Palo Alto, California.

Dose Response and the Therapeutic Ratio

Various levels of radiation yield different tumor-control probabilities, depending on the size and anatomic extent of the lesion. The total number of surviving cells is proportional to the initial number and biologic characteristics of clonogenic cells and the total cell kill achieved with a specified dose of radiation. Dose-response relationships for local control of homogeneous tumor groups have been empirically determined. The higher the doses of radiation delivered, the more likely is tumor control (Table 35-1).

The dose of radiation that can be delivered to a tumor is limited by the probability of serious normal tissue complications. Therefore, the choice of a tumor dose is based on the relative probability of tumor control and normal tissue complications. The potential therapeutic gain can be estimated for an average group of patients on the basis of tumor size, histologic type, and the normal tissues that will be included in the treatment fields. Figure 35-17 shows a theoretic dose-response relationship for tumor control and normal tissue complications. The therapeutic ratio is defined as the percentage of tumor cures obtained at a given level of toxicity for normal tissues. Hill suggests that the therapeutic ratio is better defined in a ratio of radiation doses required to produce a given percentage of tumor control and complications.[244] Figure 35-17A depicts a favorable therapeutic ratio and Figure 35-17B depicts an unfavorable therapeutic ratio. The greater the displacement between the two curves (in the favorable situation), the more radiocurable is the tumor.

Table 35-1 Relationship of Tumor Diameter and Dose to Percent Local Control

Dose (5 × 200 cGy/wk)	% Control: Squamous Cell Carcinoma	% Control: Adenocarcinoma
5,000	> 90% microfoci 50% 2–3 cm nodes	> 90% subclinical
6,000	80–90% T1 pharynx and larynx	
7,000	90% 1–3 cm nodes 80% T3–T4 tonsil	90% axillary

Gene Therapy and Radiation Therapy

Experimental RT has been combined with gene therapy in a variety of different strategies. These include the use of a various viral and nonviral vectors to transduce tumor cells with enzymes that convert specific prodrugs to radiosensitizers, cytotoxins and/or immunomodulatory cytokines and other molecules that disrupt signaling pathways. Prodrug converting enzymes include herpes simplex virus (HSV), thymidine kinase and bacterial cytosine deaminase. In another approach, the tumor suppressor gene P53 is employed to modulate radiation-mediated apoptosis in cells that lack P53. Limitations of gene therapy include the lack of transduction of the entire tumor cell population as well as the lack of control of gene expression. In an attempt to compensate for lack of uniform tumor transduction and to achieve spatial and temporal control of gene therapy, Weichselbaum and colleagues delineated a strategy whereby a radiation-inducible promotor is ligated to a therapeutic gene of interest.[279] Radiation-inducible DNA sequences from the EGR-1 promoter were ligated to a DNA encoding TNFα and cloned into a nonreplication competent adenoviral vector. Tumors treated with ionizing radiation and EGR–TNFα regressed more rapidly and to a greater extent than tumors treated with EGR–TNFα or radiation alone. TNFα was induced seven-fold over background levels in the tumor, but not in the blood, thus achieving control over gene expression. This approach to gene therapy overcomes some of the limitations of limited viral transduction by employing a diffusible cytokine. This strategy has been recently evaluated for safety in phase I clinical trials and is currently being tested for efficacy in phase II trials in patients with pancreatic and esophageal cancer.

In another strategy that targets gene therapy by IR, it has been demonstrated that genetically engineered herpes viruses can be induced to proliferate in irradiated tumors. Herpes virus can cause lethal encephalitis and has been modified to be less neurovirulent by one of two strategies. Herpes genes that encode enzymes necessary for viral DNA synthesis or the gamma1 *34.5* gene are deleted. The *34.5* gene prevents host protein syntheses shut-off, which has evolved to defeat HSV proliferation. Advani and colleagues employed a herpes virus (with gamma *34.5* deleted) combined with radiation and demonstrated a superior antitumor effect when compared with radiation or herpes virus alone in a flank model of human gliomas.[280] These findings were extended and confirmed by Bradley and colleagues who employed IR and genetically engineered (GSE) herpes in an intracranial model of glioma and demonstrated a prolongation of survival in animals treated with the combination of herpes and ionizing radiation.[281]

Cytotoxic applications of adenovirus have also been investigated. This virus exerts its control over host cell growth regulation by a complex set of proteins that facilitate viral replication. Adenoviral infection induces cellular p53 protein which is proapoptotic and therefore detrimental to the viral life cycle. The virally encoded E1B protein blocks p53 action, preventing apoptosis and allowing for viral replication to proceed. The ONYX-15 virus is an E1B deleted adenovirus that restricts lytic activity to cells expressing mutant p53. Freytag and colleagues have shown that ONYX-15 virus combined with radiation leads to enhanced tumor cell killing in tumors expressing mutant p53 in vivo.[282] DeWeese and colleagues used a prostate specific antigen selective replication restricted adenovirus in a phase I dose escalation study in patients with locally recurrent prostates cancer. They showed that the highest dose levels of virus administered were associated with a decrease in PSA.[283]

Another strategy that has been used to improve the therapeutic ratio of radiotherapy by gene therapy has been to introduce genes that selectively protect normal tissue. An example of this is the delivery of manganese superoxide dismutase (MSOD) to normal cells to protect against radiation damage. Greenberger and colleagues have studied the delivery of liposome-MnSOD complexes for protecting both normal lung and bladder tissue in mice treated with ionizing radiation.[284] Other investigators have shown that tissue levels of TGF-beta1 can be reduced by soluble TGFbeta type II receptor gene therapy and ameliorated radiation-induced pulmonary injury in rats.[285]

Another gene-based strategy is based on the overexpression of EGFR-CD533. This dominant negative EGFR variant lacks the C-terminal 533 amino acids and forms nonfunctioning heterodimeric complexes with wt EGFR receptors.[286] Schmidt-Ullrich and colleagues have studied the potential therapeutic application of EGFR-CD533 in human tumor xenograft models.[287] These investigators demonstrated that overexpression of EGFR-CD533 in mammary carcinoma cells abrogates the EGFR-mediated cytoprotective response induced by IR and enhances radiosensitivity.[288] They subsequently incorporated EGFR-CD533 into a replication-incompetent adenovirus (Ad) and showed that Ad-EGFR-CD533 delays growth of U-373 MG glioma xenograft tumors and overcomes the enhanced tumorigenic effects of EGFRvIII expression.[289]

Antiangiogenic Therapy Combined with Radiation Therapy Ionizing radiation has been reported to mediate vascular collapse and thrombosis of very small tumor vessels. However, until recently, ionizing radiation was not considered to target the tumor vessels. Tumor endothelial cells arise from host endothelium and are genetically stable, compared with tumor cells, and therefore are less likely to become resistant to DNA-damaging agents. Also one tumor vessel may supply up to 10^6 tumor cells with nutrients, thus amplifying the cytotoxic antitumor effects of IR. Teicher and colleagues conducted investigations combining radiation and synthetic antiangiogenesis compounds and demonstrated an increase in tumor cure and tumor growth delay.[290] In spite of potential toxicities of the antiangiogenesis drugs, these investigators validated the tumor vasculature as a potential target for RT. In concert with these findings, the synthetic angiogenesis inhibitor, TNP-470, has been found to potentiate the effects of radiotherapy in the treatment of human glioblastoma multiforme xenografts in the nude mouse.[291] Other studies have demonstrated that the endogenous angiogenesis inhibitor, angiostatin, enhances radiation-mediated tumor regressions without an increase in toxicity.[292] The potentiation of radiotherapy by angiostatin was observed in several human tumor xenografts, including a human glioma. A brief exposure to angiostatin enhances tumor regression when delivered at the same time as radiation.[293] These findings also showed that a prolonged course of angiostatin is not necessary for optimal therapeutic effects. The demonstration that endostatin similarly potentiates the anti-tumor effects of radiotherapy indicates that the interaction is broadly applicable to angiogenesis inhibitors.[294]

Another strategy has been to potentiate the effectiveness of radiotherapy with agents that function by directly blocking positive regulators of angiogenesis. For example, administration of antibodies against the vascular endothelial growth factor (VEGF) potentiates radiotherapy of murine and human tumor models, including that of a glioma xenograft.[293] In clinical trials, Willet and colleagues demonstrated that anti-VEGF antibody decreases tumor perfusion, vascular volume and microvascular density in rectal cancer patients.[295] Similar findings have been corroborated in other studies using anti-VEGF antibodies or inhibitors (SU5416, SU6668, PTK787) of the VEGF signaling pathway in combination with radiotherapy.[296-300] In addition, COX-2 inhibitors have been reported to enhance the antitumor efficacy of radiotherapy without increasing toxicity.[301-303] These findings collectively demonstrate that inhibition of tumor angiogenesis potentiates the efficacy of radiation therapy.

Recently, investigators have suggested that vascular endothelial cell apoptosis represents a primary lesion in radiation-induced injury, at least in the GI tract. Fuks and colleagues demonstrated that basic FGF increases survival of intestinal crypts and prevents GI syndrome in C57Bl/6 mice.[304] More recently, these authors suggested that microvascular damage regulates tumor cell response to radiation.[305]

Clinical Radiaiton Oncology RT alone is used as curative therapy in a variety of tumor types. Treatment may consist of external beam alone, brachytherapy alone, or a combination of the two. Although combined modality therapy is more common today, definitive RT is still used in early-stage head and neck as well as gynecologic tumors. RT alone is associated with results comparable with that obtained with surgery for tumors of the oral cavity,[306] oropharynx,[307] supraglottic larynx,[308] and glottis.[309] Moreover, definitive RT is often associated with better long-term functional outcome than surgery. Definitive RT was recently compared in a large prospective randomized trial with radical surgery in women with early-stage operable cervical cancer. RT was associated with identical tumor control rates with less long-term sequelae.[310] Another tumor type that may be treated with RT alone is early-stage Hodgkin's disease.[311]

RT alone is also the treatment of choice in elderly patients. A common belief is that the elderly are at higher risk of acute and chronic RT sequelae. However, numerous investigators have demonstrated that age per se is not associated with increased toxicity.[312,313] Instead, comorbidities present in the elderly may increase their risk.[314]

Adjuvant Therapy A more common use of RT is in combination with surgery and/or chemotherapy. When combined with surgery, RT may be given prior to (preoperative), following (postoperative), or during (intraoperative) surgery. Although common in the past, preoperative RT is less used today except in large borderline resectable tumors, for example, rectal cancer[315] and soft tissue sarcomas.[316] In contrast, postoperative RT is used in many tumor sites including tumors of the central nervous system,[317] head and neck,[318] breast,[319] lung,[320] genitourinary,[321] and gastrointestinal tract.[322] In patients with resectable disease, postoperative RT is preferred because it allows treatment to be tailored to the pathology findings, and higher doses are possible; moreover, there is reduced potential for interference in normal wound healing. Indications for postoperative RT include close/positive margins, residual disease, and lymph node involvement. Potential disadvantages of postoperative RT include delaying therapy until wound healing is complete and reduced vascularity of tissues following surgery. Intraoperative RT is the delivery of a single large fraction during surgery with either electrons or low energy photons.[323] This is accomplished with either a dedicated treatment machine in the operating room or by transporting the patient to the RT department during surgery. An important benefit is that normal tissues, for example small bowel, can be displaced out of the treatment field. A disadvantage is that the total treatment is delivered in a single fraction, which obviates the benefit of fractionation. Promising results have been reported in retroperitoneal soft tissue sarcoma.[324] Brachytherapy has also been used at the time of surgery. It is imperative, however, to delay loading for several days to allow for adequate wound healing.[325]

When combined with chemotherapy, chemotherapy may be administered prior to (neoadjuvant), during (concomitant), or following RT (maintenance). Chemoradiotherapy approaches have been shown to improve local control and eradicate micrometastatic disease. Neoadjuvant chemotherapy has been used in a number of sites including early-stage non-Hodgkin's lymphoma[326] and small-cell lung cancer.[327] A potential advantage is that bulky disease sites can be cytoreduced allowing for smaller treatment volumes. However, increasing evidence suggests that concomitant chemoradiotherapy is preferable in a variety of disease sites. Concomitant chemoradiotherapy is used in locally advanced cancer of the lung,[328] head and

Table 35-2 Interaction of Radiotherapy and Chemotherapy

Chemotherapy drug and radiation active against different tumor cell subpopulations based on hypoxia, cell-cycle specificity, and pH
Decreased tumor cell repopulation following fractionated radiation due to effects of chemotherapy
Increased tumor cell recruitment from G0 into a therapy-responsive cell-cycle phase
Increased tumor cell oxygenation following radiation with improved drug or radiation activity
Improved drug delivery with shrinkage of tumor
Early eradication of tumor cells preventing emergence of drug and/or radiation resistance
Eradication of cells resistant to one treatment modality by the other treatment
Cell-cycle synchronization
Inhibition of repair of sublethal radiation damage or inhibition of recovery from potentially lethal radiation damage

neck,[329] esophagus,[330] bladder,[331] and cervix.[332] Possible interactions between chemotherapeutic drugs and radiation are summarized in Table 35-2.

In select sites, all three modalities are combined. A variety of schedules have been used. Examples include neoadjuvant chemotherapy, surgery, and postoperative RT (locally advanced breast cancer)[333] and surgery followed by concomitant postoperative chemoradiotherapy (cancer of the pancreas and rectum).[334,335]

Prophylactic Therapy The most common example is the prophylactic treatment of regional, clinically uninvolved lymph nodes. Prophylactic cranial irradiation (PCI) is used in patients with limited-stage small-cell lung cancer[336] and children with high-risk acute leukemia.[337] Other examples include breast irradiation in men with prostate cancer who receive diethylstilbestrol (DES), whole lung RT in patients with bulky mediastinal Hodgkin's disease, and liver RT in advanced Hodgkin's disease and pancreatic cancer.[338–340]

Palliative Therapy RT is an important means of providing rapid and effective palliation due to local and/or metastatic disease. Osseous metastases secondary to breast, prostate, and other cancers are treated with localized fields and short-course regimens, for example, 30 Gy in 10 fractions. Pain relief is achieved in more than 70% of patients.[341] The optimal fractionation schedule, however, remains unclear. Rapid large fractions, for example, 20 Gy over 5 days, are equivalent to more protracted regimens using smaller daily doses.[342] Such approaches are indicated in patients with symptomatic long-bone sites that are not in close proximity to critical organs. More rapid schedules may be possible. The Radiation Therapy Oncology Group (RTOG) is currently comparing 8 Gy in 1 fraction with 30 Gy in 10 fractions in a randomized trial. Large-field (hemibody) irradiation has been used in patients with widespread bone metastases.[343,344] Promising results have also been reported with intravenous 144Sr344 and samarium.[345]

Whole-brain RT is indicated in patients with cerebral metastases. Treatment is typically delivered over 10 days to a total dose of 30 Gy. As with osseous metastases, controversy exists over the optimal treatment regimen in these patients. Borgelt and colleagues reviewed various regimens ranging from 20 Gy in 5 fractions to 40 Gy in 20 fractions on two randomized trials. No differences were seen in frequency or duration of response. Overall, 50% of patients had significant improvement in neurologic symptoms. However, the less protracted regimens resulted in more rapid overall response rates.[346] Protracted regimens are indicated, however, in patients with controlled primaries and solitary metastases.

Other indications for palliative RT include spinal cord compression,[347] liver metastases,[348] orbital metastases,[349] and carcinomatous meningitis.[350] Palliative RT is also used in symptomatic locally advanced lung[351] and ovarian cancer.[352] Brachytherapy can be used in palliative treatment as well, for example, bronchial,[353] biliary,[354] and esophageal[355] obstructions.

Therapy for Benign Disease RT is used in a wide variety of benign tumors and conditions, such as keloids,[356] hemangiomas,[357] desmoids,[358] and pterygium.[359] Other indications include renal[360] and cardiac[361] transplant rejection, macular degeneration,[362] and heterotopic bone prophylaxis following arthroplasty.[363] While attention has now turned to the use of drug-eluting stents, promising results have been reported in the prevention of re-stenosis in patients undergoing coronary angioplasty.[364]

RADIATION SEQUELAE **Acute Sequelae** Acute radiation sequelae, such as skin desquamation, mucositis, and diarrhea, occur during or immediately following treatment. Such sequelae are believed to be due to the interruption of repopulation of rapidly proliferating tissues.[365] The type of reaction is dependent on the site irradiated. The one exception is fatigue, which occurs in almost all patients. Most acute sequelae are self-limited and respond to pharmacologic management, such as diphenoxylate hydrochloride with atropine sulfate (diarrhea) and viscous lidocaine (esophagitis). It is imperative to control symptoms and avoid prolonged treatment breaks, since treatment protraction has been correlated with worse tumor control in several disease sites.[366–368] Prophylactic medication may also be helpful. Promising results have been reported using sucralfate in patients undergoing thoracic irradiation to decrease the severity of esophagitis.[369,370]

The severity of acute sequelae is dependent on a variety of factors. Two major factors are fraction size and treatment volume. Whenever large treatment volumes are used, it is thus imperative to reduce the daily fraction size to minimize acute sequelae. A commonly held belief is that older patients are at higher risk of acute sequelae. However, recent reports have disputed this belief.[371]

Chronic Sequelae Chronic reactions, such as fibrosis, fistulae, and necrosis, occur months to years following treatment and are due, in part, to damage to slowly proliferating tissues. Other factors, including vascular damage, may also play a part in their development. Chronic reactions, like acute reactions, are dependent on the irradiated site. Chronic reactions, however, are often permanent. Sequelae vary widely in severity, ranging from mild fibrosis to small bowel obstruction, fistulae, and second malignancies. Overall, the risk of a second malignancy following RT is low. The notable exception is osteosarcoma arising in irradiated bones in children treated for retinoblastoma, particularly the hereditary type.[372]

Select chronic radiation sequelae are responsive to medical management, for example, pneumonitis is managed with bronchodilators and, if necessary, a course of corticosteroids. Recent evidence supports the role of angiotensin II receptor antagonist in the treatment and prevention of radiation nephritis.[373] Prophylactic medications may also decrease the risk of select late sequelae. Promising results have been reported with pilocarpine in head and neck cancer to decrease the incidence of xerostomia.[374] Recently, zinc sulfate has been found to reduce the risk of significant taste alterations in patients with head and neck cancer.[375] The most important means of reducing the risk of chronic sequelae, however, is prevention. Strict attention to optimal technique is imperative. Soft tissue sarcoma patients, for example, should never receive treatment to the entire circumference of the extremity in order to reduce the risk of chronic edema. The risk of late sequelae is also reduced by avoiding the use of large daily fractions, since fraction size is a major determinant of late effects.[376,377] As noted earlier, new approaches including 3D CRT, IMRT, and inverse treatment planning should further aid in reducing the risk of late sequelae.

FUTURE DIRECTIONS

Since its first use a century ago, the role of RT in the treatment of cancer has undergone tremendous changes. Its role will continue to change in the coming years. Definitive wide-field irradiation approaches will be replaced with small-volume treatment delivered in conjunction with chemotherapy. In general, combined modality approaches will become more common, particularly organ preservation techniques.[361] RT will be increasingly integrated into high-dose chemotherapy and stem cell programs, providing improved control of bulky and refractory disease sites. Imaging will continue to be more and more important in the planning and delivery of RT.

The twenty-first century will see increased understanding and application of radiobiologic concepts to clinical radiation oncology. Potential strategies include induction of apoptosis, modification of cellular resistance, modulation of cell-cycle regulation, and predictive assays for tumor control. Radiogenetic therapy will be introduced into the clinic. Selected genes linked to radio-inducible promoters whose expression can be regulated by ionizing radiation may improve the therapeutic ratio of RT. These and other approaches will continue to concretize the importance of RT in the treatment of the cancer patient.

REFERENCES

1. Roentgen WC. On a new kind of rays [preliminary communication]. Translation of a paper read before the Physikalische-medicinischen Gesellschaft of Wurzburg on December 28, 1895. Br J Radiol 1931;4:32–6.
2. Coutard H. Roentgentherapy of epitheliomas of the tonsillar region, hypopharynx and larynx from 1920 to 1926. AJR Am J Roentgenol 1932;28:313–32.
3. Paterson RP. The radical x-ray treatment of carcinomata. Br J Radiol 1936;9:671–9.
4. Attix FH. Introduction to radiological physics and radiation dosimetry. New York (NY): John Wiley and Sons Inc; 1986.
5. Khan F. The physics of radiation therapy. 2nd ed. Baltimore (MD): Williams and Wilkins; 1994.
6. Laramore GE. The use of neutrons in cancer therapy: a historical perspective through the modern era. Semin Oncol 1997;24:672–285.
7. Vynckier S, Schmidt R. The physical basis for radiotherapy with neutrons. Rec Res Cancer Res 1998;150:1–30.
8. Bonnett DE. Current developments in proton therapy: a review. Phys Med Biol 1993;38:1371–92.
9. Miller DW. A review of proton beam radiotherapy. Med Phys 1995;22(11 Pt 2):1943–54.
10. Goitein M, Laughlin J, Purdy JA, et al. State-of-the-art of external photon beam treatment planning. Int J Radiat Oncol Biol Phys 1991;21:9–24.
11. Michalski JM, Sur RK, Harms WB, Purdy JA. Three dimensional conformal radiation therapy in pediatric parameningeal rhabdomyosarcomas. Int J Radiat Oncol Biol Phys 1995;33:985–92.
12. Graham MV, Purdy JA, Emami B, et al. Preliminary results of a prospective trial using three dimensional radiotherapy for lung cancer. Int J Radiat Oncol Biol Phys 1995;33:993–1000.
13. Sibley GS, Mundt AJ, Shapiro C, et al. The treatment of stage III non-small cell lung cancer using high dose conformal radiotherapy. Int J Radiat Oncol Biol Phys 1995;33:1001–8.
14. Yang FE, Chen GTY, Ray P, et al. The potential for normal tissue dose reduction with neoadjuvant hormonal therapy in conformal treatment planning for stage C prostate cancer. Int J Radiat Oncol Biol Phys 1995;33:1009–18.
15. Bentel G. Patient positioning and immobilization in radiation oncology. New York (NY): McGraw-Hill; 1999. p.1–38.
16. Austin-Seymour M, Chen GTY, Rosenman J, et al. Tumor and target delineation: current research and future directions. Int J Radiat Oncol Biol Phys 1995;33:1041–52.
17. Kuszyk BS, Ney DR, Fishman EK. The current state of the art in three dimensional imaging. Int J Radiat Oncol Biol Phys 1995;33:1029–1029.
18. ICRU Report 50. Dose specification for reporting external beam therapy with photons and electrons. Washington DC: International Commission on Radiation Units and Measurements; 1993.
19. Van Herk M, Bruce A, Kroes APG, et al. Quantification of organ motion during conformal radiotherapy of the prostate by three dimensional image registration. Int J Radiat Oncol Biol Phys 1995;33:1211–320.
20. Roeske JC, Forman JD, Messina CF, et al. Evaluation of changes in the size and location of the prostate, seminal vesicles, bladder, and rectum during a course of external beam radiation therapy. Int J Radiat Oncol Biol Phys 1995;33:1321–9.
21. Levin DN, Hu X, Tan KK, et al. The brain: integrated three-dimensional display of MR and PET images. Radiology 1989;172:783–9.
22. Kooy H, vanHerk M, Barnes PD, et al. Image fusion for stereotactic radiotherapy and radiosurgery treatment planning. Int J Radiat Oncol Biol Phys 1994;28:1229–34.
23. Hamilton RJ, Sweeney PJ, Pelizzari CA, et al. Functional imaging in treatment planning of brain lesions. Int J Radiat Oncol Biol Phys 1997;21:683–93.
24. Nestle U, Walter K, Schmidt S, et al. 18F-deoxyglucose positron emission tomography (FDG-PET) for the planning of radiotherapy in lung cancer: high impact in patient with atelectasis. Int J Radiat Oncol Biol Phys 1999;44:593–7.
25. Suga K, Kume N, Nishigauchi K, et al. 201Tl SPECT as an indicator for early prediction of therapeutic effects in patients with non-small cell lung cancer. Ann Nucl Med 1998;12:355–62.
26. Pelizzari CA, Chen GTY, Spelbring DA, et al. Accurate three-dimensional registration of CT, PET, and/or MR images of the brain. J Comput Assist Tomogr 1989;13:20–6.
27. Kessler ML, Pitluck S, Petti P, Castro JR. Integration of multimodality imaging data for radiotherapy treatment planning. Int J Radiat Oncol Biol Phys 1991;21:1653–67.
28. Van Herk M, Kooy HM. Automatic three-dimensional correlation of CT-CT, CT-MRI, and CT-SPECT using chamfer matching. Med Phys 1994;21:1163–78.
29. McShan DL, Silverman A, Lanza DM, et al. A computerized three-dimensional treatment planning system utilizing interactive color graphics. Br J Radiol 1979;52:478–81.
30. Sherouse GW, Novins K, Chaney EL. Computation of digitally reconstructed radiographs for use in radiotherapy treatment design. Int J Radiat Oncol Biol Phys 1990;18:651–8.
31. Dryzmala RE, Mohan R, Brewster L, et al. Dose-volume histograms. Int J Radiat Oncol Biol Phys 1991;21:71–8.
32. Yu L, Song Y, Li S-D, et al. A method of analyzing rectal surface area irradiated in prostate conformal radiotherapy. Int J Radiat Oncol Biol Phys 1995;33:1121–6.
33. Drebin RA, Carpenter L, Hanrahan P. Volume rendering. Computer Graphics 1988;22:65–74.
34. Drebin RA, Magid D, Robertson DD, Fishman EK. Fidelity of three-dimensional CT imaging for detecting fracture gaps. J Comput Assist Tomogr 1989;13:487–9.
35. Boyer AL, Ochran TG, Nyerick CE, et al. Clinical dosimetry for the implementation of a multileaf collimator. Med Phys 1992;19:1255–61.
36. Brahme A. Optimization of radiation therapy and the development of multileaf collimation. Int J Radiat Oncol Biol Phys 1993;25:373–5.
37. Meertens H, van Herk M, Bijhold J, Bartelink H. First clinical experience with a newly developed electronic portal imaging device. Int J Radiat Oncol Biol Phys 1990;18:1173–81.
38. Boyer AL, Antonuk L, Fenster A, et al. A review of electronic portal imaging devices (EPIDs). Med Phys 1992;19:1–16.
39. Michalski JM, Wong JW, Gerber RL, et al. The use of in-line image verification to estimate the variation in radiation therapy dose delivery. Int J Radiat Oncol Biol Phys 1993;27:707–16.
40. Dong L, Boyer AL. An image correlation procedure for digitally reconstructed radiographs and electronic portal images. Int J Radiat Oncol Biol Phys 1995;33:1053–60.
41. Fraass BA, McShan DL, Kessler ML, et al. A computer-controlled conformal radiotherapy system. I: overview. Int J Radiat Oncol Biol Phys 1995;33:1139–58.
42. Kessler ML, McShan DL, Fraass BA. A computer-controlled conformal radiotherapy system. III: graphical simulation and monitoring of treatment delivery. Int J Radiat Oncol Biol Phys 1995;33:1173–80.
43. Mohan R, Leibel SA. Intensity modulation of the radiation beam. In: Devita VT, Hellman S, Rosenberg SA, editors. Cancer: principles and practice of oncology. Philadelphia (PA): Lippincott-Raen; 1997.
44. Verhey LJ. Comparison of three-dimensional conformal radiation therapy and intensity-modulated radiation therapy systems. Semin Radiat Oncol 1999;9:78–98.
45. Stein J, Mohan R, Wang XH, et al. Number and orientations of beams in intensity-modulated radiation treatments. Med Phys 1997;24:149–60.
46. Yu C, Symons MJ, Du MN, et al. A method for implementing dynamic photon beam intensity modulation using independent jaws and a multileaf collimator. Phys Med Biol 1995;40:769–87.
47. Mell LK, Roeske JC, Mundt AJ. A survey of intensity-modulated radiation therapy use in the United States. Cancer 2003;98:204–11.
48. Mell LK, Mundt AJ. Survey of IMRT use in the United States – 2004. Presented at the 87th Annual Meeting of the American Radium Society, Barcelona, Spain; April 2005.
49. Teh BS, Amosson CM, Mai WY et al. Intensity modulated radiation therapy (IMRT) in the management of prostate cancer. Cancer Invest 2004;22:913–24.
50. De Meerleer G, Vakaet L, Meersschout S, et al. Intensity-modulated radiotherapy as primary treatment for prostate cancer: acute toxicity in 114 patients. Int J Radiat Oncol Biol Phys 2004;60:777-87.
51. Chao KS, Majhail N, Huang CJ, et al. Intensity-modulated radiation therapy reduces late salivary toxicity without compromising tumor control in patients with oropharyngeal carcinoma: a comparison with conventional techniques. Radiother Oncol 2001;61:275–80.
52. Lee N, Xia P, Fischbein N, et al. Intensity-modulated radiation therapy for head-and-neck cancers: the UCSF experience focusing on target volume definition. Int J Radiat Oncol Biol Phys 2003;57:49–60.
53. Huang E, The BS, Strother DR, et al. Intensity-modulated radiation therapy for pediatric medulloblastoma: early report on the reduction of ototoxicity. Int J Radiat Oncol Biol Phys 2002;52:599–605.
54. Roeske J, Lujan A, Rotmensch J, et al. Intensity-modulated whole pelvic radiation therapy in patients with gynecologic malignancies. Int J Radiat Oncol Biol Phys 2000;48:1613–21.
55. Mundt AJ, Lujan AE, Rotmensch J, et al. Intensity-modulated whole pelvic radiotherapy in women with gynecologic malignancies. Int J Radiat Oncol Biol Phys 2002;52:1330–7.
56. Roach M, Winter K, Michalski JM, et al. Penile bulb dose and impotence after three-dimensional conformal radiotherapy for prostate cancer on RTOG 9406: findings from a prospective, multi-institutional, phase I/II dose-escalation study. Int J Radiat Oncol Biol Phys 2004;60:1351–6.
57. Mundt AJ, Mell LK, Roeske JC. Preliminary analysis of chronic gastrointestinal toxicity in gynecology patients treated with intensity-modulated whole pelvic radiation therapy. Int J Radiat Oncol Biol Phys 2003;56:1354–60.
58. Lujan AE, Mundt AJ, Yamada SD, et al. Intensity modulated radiotherapy as a means of reducing dose to the bone marrow in gynecologic patients receiving whole pelvic radiotherapy. Int J Radiat Oncol Biol Phys 2003;57:516–21.
59. Syed AMN, Puthawala A, Neblett D, et al. Transperineal interstitial/intracavitary "Syed-Neblett" applicator in the treatment of carcinoma of the uterine cervix. Endocuriether Hyperther Oncol 1986;2:1–13.
60. Nag S, Cardenes H, Chang S, et al. Proposed guidelines for image-based intracavitary brachytherapy for cervical carcinoma: report from the Image-Guided Brachytherapy Working Group. Int J Radiat Oncol Biol Phys 2004;60:1160–72.
61. Leung TW, Wong VY, Wong CM, et al. High dose rate brachytherapy for carcinoma of the oral tongue. Int J Radiat Oncol Biol Phys 1997;39:1113–20.
62. Stitt JA, Fowler JF, Thomadsen BR, et al. High dose rate intracavitary brachytherapy for carcinoma of the cervix: the Madison System: I. Clinical and radiobiological considerations. Int J Radiat Oncol Biol Phys 1992;24:335–48.
63. Knocke TH, Kucera H, Weidlinger B, et al. Primary treatment of endometrial carcinoma with high-dose-rate brachytherapy: results of 12 years of experience with 280 patients. Int J Radiat Oncol Biol Phys 1997;37:359–65.
64. Grills IS, Martinez AA, Hollander M, et al. High dose rate brachytherapy as prostate monotherapy reduces toxicity compared to low dose rate palladium seeds. J Urol 2004;171:1098–104.
65. Leksell LT. The stereotactic method and radiosurgery of the brain. Acta Chir Scand 1951;102:316–9.
66. Gill SS, Thomas DGT, Warrington AP, Brada M. Relocatable frame for stereotactic external beam radiotherapy. Int J Radiat Oncol Biol Phys 1991;20:599–603.
67. Sturm V, Kober B, Hover KH, et al. Stereotactic percutaneous single dose irradiation of brain metastases with a linear accelerator. Int J Radiat Oncol Biol Phys 1987;13:279–82.
68. Loeffler JS, Alexander E, Siddon RL, et al. Stereotactic radiosurgery for intracranial arteriovenous malformations using a standard linear accelerator. Int J Radiat Oncol Biol Phys 1989;17:673–7.
69. Mitsumori M, Shrieve DC, Alexander E, et al. Initial clinical results of LINAC-based stereotactic radiosurgery and stereotactic radiotherapy for pituitary adenomas. Int J Radiat Oncol Biol Phys 1998;42:573–80.
70. Kamerer D, Lunsford LD, Miller M. Gamma knife: an alternative treatment for acoustic neuromas. Ann Otol Rhinol Laryngol 1988;97:631–5.
71. Corn BW, Curran WJ, Shrieve DC, Loeffler JS. Stereotactic radiosurgery and radiotherapy: new developments and new directions. Semin Oncol 1998;24:707–14.
72. Dizdaroglu M. Measurement of radiation-induced damage in DNA at the molecular level. Int J Radiat Biol 1992;61:175–9.
73. Ward JF. DNA damage produced by ionizing radiation in mammalian cells: identities, mechanisms of formation, and reparability. Prog Nucleic Acid Res Mol Biol 1988;35:95–8.
74. Phillips MH, Griffin TW. Physics of high-linear energy transfer (LET) particles and protons. In: Perez CA, Brady LW, editors. Principles and practice of radiation oncology. Philadelphia (PA): Lippincott-Raven Publishers; 1997.
75. Griffin TW, Wambersie A, Laramore G, Castro J. International clinical trials in radiation oncology, high LET:

heavy particle trials. Int J Radiat Oncol Biol Phys 1988;14:83–8.
76. Laramore GE, Griffin TW, Maor MH. Mixed beam radiation therapy for carcinoma of the prostate: results of a randomized RTOG trial. Int J Radiat Oncol Biol Phys 1985;11:1621–5.
77. Hellman S, Weichselbaum RR. Radiation oncology and the new biology. Cancer J Sci Am 1995;1:174–9.
78. Cox JD, Kline RW. Prostate biopsies after irradiation for adenocarcinoma. Int J Radiat Oncol Biol Phys 1983;9:229–32.
79. Barranco SC, Rmsdahl NM, Humphrey RM. The radiation response of human malignant melanoma cells grown in vitro. Cancer Res 1971;31:830–3.
80. Weichselbaum RR, Beckett MA. The maximum recovery potential of human tumor cells may predict clinical outcome in radiotherapy. Int J Radiat Oncol Biol Phys 1987;13:709–11.
81. Withers HR. In: Perez CA, Brady LW, editors. Principles and practice of radiation oncology. Philadelphia (PA): JB Lippincott; 1987. p.67–98.
82. Carter T, Vancurova I, Sun I, et al. A DNA-activated protein kinase from HeLa cell Nuclei. Mol Cell Biol 1990;10:6460–71.
83. Jackson SP, MacDonald JJ, Lees-Miller S, et al. GC box binding induces phosphorylation of Spl by a DNA-dependent protein kinase. Cell 1990;63:155–65.
84. Lees-Miller SP, Chen Y, Anderson CW. Human cells contain a DNA-activated protein kinase that phosphorylates simian virus 40 T antigen, mouse P53 and the human Ku autoantigen. Mol Cell Biol 1990;10:6472–81.
85. Boubnov NV, Hall KT, Wills Z, et al. Complementation of the ionizing radiation sensitivity, DNA end binding, and V(D)J recombination defects of double-strand break repair mutants by the p86 Ku autoantigen. Proc Natl Acad Sci U S A 1995;92:890–4.
86. Lees-Miller SP, Godbout R, Chan DW, et al. Absence of p350 subunit of DNA-activated protein kinase from a radiosensitive human cell line. Science 1995;267:1183–5.
87. Lavin MF, Khanna KK, Beamish H, et al. Relationship of the ataxia-telangiectasia protein ATM to phosphoinositide 3-kinase. Trends Biochem 1995;20:382–3.
88. Savitsky K, Bar-Shira A, Gilad S, et al. A single ataxia telangiectasia gene with a product similar to PI-3 kinase. Science 1995;268:1749–53.
89. Zakian VA. ATM-related genes: what do they tell us about functions of the human gene? Cell 1995;82:685–7.
90. Riballo E, Kuhne M, Rief N, et al. A pathway of double-strand break rejoining dependent upon ATM, Artemis, and progeins locating to gamma-H2AX foci. Mol Cell 2004;16:715–24.
91. Chen PC, Lavin MF, Kidson C, Moss D. Identification of ataxia telangiectasia heterozygotes, a cancer prone population. Nature 1978;274:484–6.
92. Paterson MC, Anderson AK, Smith BP, et al. Enhanced radiosensitivity of cultured fibroblasts from ataxia telangiectasia heterozygotes manifested by defective colony-forming ability and reduced DNA repair replication after hypoxic gamma irradiation. Cancer Res 1979;39:3725–34.
93. Taylor AMR, Harnden DG, Arlett CF, et al. Ataxia-telangiectasia: a human mutation with abnormal radiation sensitivity. Nature 1975;258:427–9.
94. Kastan MB, Zhan Q, el-Deiry WS, et al. A mammalian cell cycle checkpoint pathway utilizing P53 and GADD45 is defective in ataxia-telangiectasia. Cell 1992;71:587–97.
95. Khanna KK, Lavin MF. Ionizing radiation and UV induction of P53 protein by different pathways in ataxia-telangiectasia cells. Oncogene 1993;8:3307–12.
96. Khanna KK, Beamish H, Yan J, et al. Nature of G1/S cell cycle checkpoint defect in ataxia-telangiectasia. Oncogene 1995;11:609–18.
97. Hawley RS, Friend S. Strange bedfellows in even stranger places: the role of ATM in meiotic cells, lymphocytes, tumors, and its functional links to P53. Genes Dev 1997;10:2383–8.
98. Guha C, Guha U, Tribius S, et al. Antisense ATM gene therapy: a strategy to increase the radiosensitivity of human tumors. Gene Ther 2000;7:852–8.
99. Zhou BB, Elledge SJ. The DNA damage response: putting checkpoints in perspective. Nature 2000;408:433–9.
100. Lammering G, Hewit T, Hawkins W, et al. Epidermal growth factor receptor as a genetic therapy target for carcinoma cell radiosensitization. J Natl Cancer Inst 2001;93:921–9.
101. Hirao A, Kong YY, Matsuoka S, et al. DNA damage-induced activation of P53 by the checkpoint kinase Chk2. Science 2000;287:1824–7.
102. Shieh SY, Ahn J, Tamai K, et al. The human homologs of checkpoint kinases Chk1 and Cds1 (Chk2) phosphorylate P53 at multiple DNA damage-inducible sites [published erratum appears in Genes Dev 2000 Mar 15;14:750]. Genes Dev 2000;14:289–300.
103. Ko LJ, Prives C. P53: puzzle and paradigm. Genes Dev 1996;10:1054–72.
104. Lees-Miller SP, Sakaguchi K, Ullrich SJ, et al. Human DNA-activated protein kinase phosphorylates serines 15 and 37 in the amino-terminal transactivation domain of human P53. Mol Cell Biol 1992;12:5041–9.
105. Woo RA, McLure KG, Lees-Miller SP, et al. DNA dependent protein kinase acts upstream of P53 in response to DNA damage. Nature 1998;394:700–4.
106. Sionov RV, Moallem E, Berger M, et al. c-Abl neutralizes the inhibitory effect of Mdm2 on P53. J Biol Chem 1999;274:8371–4.
107. Sionov R, Coen S, Goldberg Z, et al. c-Abl regulates P53 levels under normal and stress conditions by preventing its nuclear export and ubiquitination. Mol Cell Biol 2001;5869–78.
108. Gong J, Costanzo A, Yang H. The tyrosine kinase c-Abl regulates p73 in apoptotic response to cisplatin-induced DNA damage. Nature 1999;806–9.
109. Yuan ZM, Huang Y, Whang Y, et al. Role for the c-Abl tyrosine kinase in the growth arrest response to DNA damage. Nature 1996;382:272–4.
110. Sklar MD. The *RAS* oncogene increases the intrinsic resistance of NIH 3T3 cells to ionizing radiation. Science 1988;239:645–7.
111. Bernhard EJ, Stanbridge EJ, Gupta S, et al. Direct evidence for the contribution of activated N-*RAS* and K-*RAS* oncogenes to increased intrinsic radiation resistance in human tumor cell lines. Cancer Res 2000;60:6597–600.
112. Kasid UN, Pfeifer A, Weichselbaum RR, et al. The *RAF* oncogene is associated with a radiation-resistant human laryngeal cancer. Science 1987;237:1039–41.
113. Kasid UN, Pfeifer A, Brennan T, et al. Effect of antisense-craf-1 on tumorigenicity and radiation sensitivity of a human squamous carcinoma. Science 1989;243:1354–6.
114. Bernhard EJ, Kao G, Cox AD, et al. The farnesyltransferase inhibitor FTI-277 radiosensitizes H-ras transformed rat embryo fibroblasts. Cancer Res 1996;56:1727–30.
115. Soldatenkov VA, Dritschilo A, Wang FH, et al. Inhibition of Raf-1 protein kinase by antisense phosphorothioate oligodeoxyribonucleotide is associated with sensitization of human laryngeal squamous carcinoma cells to gamma radiation. Cancer J Sci Am 1997;3:13–20.
116. Stevenson MA, Pollock S, Coleman CN, et al. X-irradiation, phorbolesters, and H2O2 stimulate mitogen-activated protein kinase activity in HIH-3T3 cells through the formation of reactive oxygen intermediates. Cancer Res 1994;54:12–5.
117. Dent P, Reardon DB, Park JS, et al. Radiation-induced release of transforming growth factor alpha activates the epidermal growth factor receptor and mitogen-activated protein kinase pathway in carcinoma cells, leading to increased proliferation and protection from radiation-induced cell death. Mol Biol Cell 1999;10:2493–506.
118. Hallahan D, Sukhatme V, Sherman M, et al. Protein kinase C mediates x-ray inducibility of nuclear signal transducers, EGR-1 and c-Jun. Proc Natl Acad Sci U S A 1991;88:2156–60.
119. Hallahan DE, Virudachalam S, Kuchibhotla J, et al. Membrane-derived second messenger regulates x-ray-mediated tumor necrosis factor alpha gene induction. Proc Natl Acad Sci U S A 1994;91:4897–901
120. Yuan ZM, Utsugisawa T, Ishiko T, et al. Activation of protein kinase CTM by the c-Abl tyrosine kinase in response to ionizing radiation. Oncogene 1998;16:1643–8.
121. Zaugg K, Rocha S, Resch H, et al. Differential P53-dependent mechanism of radiosensitization in vitro and in vivo by the protein kinase C-specific inhibitor PKC412. Cancer Res 2001;61:732–8.
122. Acevedo-Duncan M, Pearlman J, Zachariah B. Sensitivity of human glioma U-373MG cells to radiation and the protein kinase C inhibitor, calphostin C. Cell Prolif 2001;34:31–41.
123. Chmura SJ, Mauceri HJ, Advani S, et al. Decreasing the apoptic threshold of tumor cells through protein kinase C inhibition and sphingomyelinase activation increases tumor killing by ionizing radiation. Cancer Res 1997;57:4340–7.
124. Haimovitz-Friedman A, Kan CC, Ehleiter D, et al. Ionizing radiation acts on cellular membranes to generate ceramide and initiate apoptosis. J Exp Med 1994;180:525–35.
125. Traxler P, Bold G, Buchdunger E, et al. Tyrosine kinase inhibitors: from rational design to clinical trials. Med Res Rev 2001;21:499–512.
126. Christensen JG, Schreck RE, Chan E, et al. High levels of HER-2 expression alter the ability of epidermal growth factor receptor (EGFR) family tyrosine kinase inhibitors to inhibit EGFR phosphorylation in vivo. Clin Cancer Res 2001;7:4230–8.
127. Kharbanda S, Yuan ZM, Rubin E, et al. Activation of the src-like P56/P53lyn tyrosine kinase by ionizing radiation. J Biol Chem 1994;269:20739–43.
128. Kharbanda S, Saleem A, Yuan ZM, et al. Nuclear signaling induced by ionizing radiation involves colocalization of the activated p56/P53lyn tyrosine kinase with P34CDC2. Cancer Res 1996;3617–21.
129. Kumar S, Pandey P, Bharti A, et al. Regulation of DNA-dependent protein kinase by the Lyn tyrosine kinase. J Biol Chem 1998;273:25654–8.
130. Minden A, Karin M. Regulation and function of the JNK subgroup of MAP kinases. Biochimica et Biophysica Acta 1997;1333:F85–104.
131. Datta R, Hallahan D, Kharbanda S, et al. Involvement of reactive oxygen intermediates in the induction of c-Jun gene transcription by ionizing radiation. Biochemistry 1992;31:8300–6.
132. Datta R, Rubin E, Sukhatme V, et al. Ionizing radiation activates transcription of the EGR-1 gene via CARG elements. Proc Natl Acad Sci U S A 1992;89:10149–53.
133. Datta R, Taneja N, Sukhatme V, et al. Reactive oxygen intermediates target CARG sequences to mediate activation of the immediate early transcription factor EGR-1 by ionizing radiation. Proc Natl Acad Sci U S A 1993;90:2419–22.
134. Hallahan D, Mauceri H, Seung L, et al. Spatial and temporal control of gene therapy using ionizing radiation. Nat Med 1995;1:786–91.
135. Marples B, Scott SD, Hendry JH, et al. Development of synthetic promoters for radiation-mediated gene therapy. Gene Therapy 2000;7:511–17.
136. Takahashi M, Fukuda K, Ohata T, et al. Increased expression of inducible and endothelial constitutive nitric oxide synthases in rat colon tumors induced by azoxymethane. Cancer Res 1997;57:1233–7.
137. Mauceri HJ, Hanna NN, Wayne JD, et al. Tumor necrosis factor alpha (TNF-alpha) gene therapy targeted by ionizing radiation selectively damages tumor vasculature. Cancer Res 1996;56:4311–4.
138. Elkind MM. The initial part of the survival curve. Does it predict outcome of fractionated radiotherapy? Radiat Res 1988;114:425–8.
139. Elkind MM, Witmore GF. Radiobiology of cultured mammalian cells. New York (NY): Gordon and Breach; 1967.
140. Elkind MM. Fractionated dose radiotherapy and its relationship to survival curve shapes. Cancer Treat Rev 1976;3:2–6.
141. Elkind MM, Sutton H. Radiation response of mammalian cells grown in culture I. Repair of x-ray damage in surviving Chinese hamster cells. Radiat Res 1960;13;556–60.
142. Elkind MM, Sutton-Gilbert H, Moses WB, et al. Radiation response in cells in culture V. Temperature dependence of the repair of x-ray damage in surviving cells (aerobic and hypoxic). Radiat Res 1965;25:359–63.
143. Elkind MM, Sutton HG. X-ray damage and recovery in mammalian cells in culture. Nature 1959;184:1293–7.
144. Boothman DA, Bouvard I, Hughes EN. Identification and characterization of x-ray induced proteins in human cells. Cancer Res 1989;49:2871–4.
145. Carney DN, Mitchell JB, Kinsella T. In vitro radiation and chemotherapeutic sensitivity of established cell lines in human small cell lung cancer and large cell morphology variants. Cancer Res 1983;43:2806–9.
146. Kelland LR, Bingle L, Edwards S, Steel G. High intrinsic radiosensitivity of a newly established and characterized human embryonal rhabdomyosarcoma cell line. Br J Cancer 1989;59:160–3.
147. Peckman MJ. In: Steele GG, Adams GE, editors. The biological basis of radiotherapy. New York (NY): Elsevier; 1983. p.1–15.
148. Weichselbaum RR, Beckett MA, Vijayakumar S, et al. Radiobiological characterization of head and neck and sarcoma cell lines derived from patients prior to radiotherapy. Int J Radiat Oncol Biol Phys 1990;19:313–7.
149. Weichselbaum RR, Rotmensch J, Ahmed-Swan S, Beckett MA. Radiobiological characterization of 53 human tumor cell lines. Int J Radiat Oncol Biol Phys 1989;16:553–7.
150. Fowler JF. Review: total doses in fractionated radiotherapy. Int J Radiat Oncol Biol Phys 1984;2:103–6.

151. Hall EJ. Radiobiology for the radiologist. Philadelphia (PA): JB Lippincott; 1988. p.17–160.
152. Thames HD, Henry JH. Fractionation in radiotherapy. London, U.K.: Taylor & Francis; 1987.
153. Withers HR. Regeneration of intestinal mucosa after irradiation. Cancer 1971;28:78–83.
154. Phillips RA, Tolmach LJ. Repair of potentially lethal damage in x-irradiated HeLa cells. Radiat Res 1966;29:413–7.
155. Weichselbaum RR, Nove J, Little JB. Deficient recovery from potentially lethal radiation damage in ataxia telangiectasia and xeroderma pigmentosum. Nature 1978;27:261–5.
156. Hahn GM, Bagshaw MA, Evans RG, Gordon LF. Repair of potentially lethal lesions in x-irradiated density inhibited Chinese hamster cells. Radiat Res 1973;55:280–4.
157. Hahn GM, Little JB. Plateau phase cultures of mammalian cells: an in vitro model for human cancer. Curr Top Radiat Res 1972;8:39–43.
158. Little JB, Hahn GM, Friendel E, Tubiana M. Repair of potentially lethal radiation damage in vitro and in vivo. Radiology 1973;106:689–93.
159. Rubin PJ, Coper R, Phillips TL. Radiation biology and radiation oncology syllabus (set RT 1:radiation oncology). Chicago (IL): American College of Radiology; 1975.
160. Kinsella TJ, Mitchell JB, McPherson S, et al. In vitro radiation studies on Ewing's sarcoma cell lines and human bone marrow. Application to the clinical use of total body irradiation. Int J Radiat Oncol Biol Phys 1984;10:1005–11.
161. Puck TT, Marcus PI. Action of x-rays on mammalian cells. J Exp Med 1956;108:553–7.
162. Powers WE, Palmer LA. Biologic basis of preoperative radiation therapy. Am J Roentgenol Radium Ther Nucl Med 1968;102:176–92.
163. Weichselbaum RR, Dahlberg W, Beckett MA, et al. Radiation resistant and repair proficient human tumor cell lines may be associated with radiotherapy failure in head and neck cancer patients. Proc Natl Acad Sci U S A 1986;83:2683–7.
164. Weichselbaum RR, Little JB, Nove J. Response of human osteosarcoma in vitro to irradiation. Evidence for unusual cellular repair activity. Int J Radiat Oncol Biol Phys 1977;31:295–9.
165. Weichselbaum RR, Schmit A, Little JB. Cellular repair factors influencing radiocurability of human malignant tumors. Br J Cancer 1982;45:10–4.
166. Guichard M, Weichselbaum RR, Little JB, Malaise EP. Potential lethal damage as a possible determinant of human tumor radiosensitivity. Radiother Oncol 1984;1:263–7.
167. Weichselbaum RR, Nove J, Little JB. X-ray sensitivity of human tumor cells in vitro. Int J Radiat Oncol Biol Phys 1980;6:437–40.
168. Johnson RD, Jasin M. Sister chromatid gene conversion is a prominent double-strand break repair pathway in mammalian cells. EMBO J 2000;19:3398–407.
169. Jackson SP. Sensing and repairing DNA double-strand breaks. Carcinogenesis 2002;23:687–96.
170. Khanna KK, Jackson SP. DNA double-strand breaks: signaling, repair and the cancer connection. Nat Genet 2001;27:247–54.
171. Wood RD, Mitchell M, Sgouros J, Lindahl T. Human DNA repair genes. Science 2001;291:1284–9.
172. Yuan ZM, Huang Y, Ishiko T, et al. Regulation of Rad51 function by c-Abl in response to DNA damage. J Biol Chem 1998;273:3799–802.
173. Shu Z, Smith S, Wang L, et al. Disruption of muREC2/RAD51L1 in mice results in early embryonic lethality which can be partially rescued in a P53(-/-) background. Mol Cell Biol 1999;8686–93.
174. Sturzbecher HW, Donzelmann B, Henning W, et al. P53 is linked directly to homologous recombination processes via RAD51/RecA protein interaction. EMBO J 1996;15:1992–2002.
175. Bhattacharyya A, Ear US, Koller BH, et al. The breast cancer susceptibility gene BRCA1 is required for subnuclear assembly of RAD51 and survival following treatment with the DNA cross-linking agent cisplatin. J Biol Chem 2000;275:23899–903.
176. Flygare J, Hellgren D, Wennborg A. Caspase-3 mediated cleavage of HSRAD51 at an unconventional site. Eur J Biochem 267;5977–82.
177. Taccioli GE, Rathbun G, Oltz E, et al. Impairment of V(D)J recombination in double-strand break repair mutants. Science 1993;260:207–10.
178. Critchlow SE, Bowater RP, Jackson SP. Mammalian DNA double-strand break repair protein XRCC4 interacts with DNA ligase IV. Curr Biol 1997;7:588–98.
179. Grawunder U, Wilm M, Wu X, et al. Activity of DNA ligase IV stimulated by complex formation with XRCC4 protein in mammalian cells. Nature 1997;388:492–5.
180. Wilson S, Warr N, Taylor DL, Watts FZ. The role of Schizosaccharomyces pombe RAD32, the MRE11 homologue, and other DNA damage response proteins in non-homologous end joining and telomere length maintenance. Nucleic Acids Res 1999;27:2655–61.
181. Ohnishi T, Taki T, Hiraga S, et al. In vitro and in vivo potentiation of radiosensitivity of malignant gliomas by antisense inhibition of the RAD51 gene. Biochem Biophys Res Commun 1998;245:319–24.
182. Taneja N, Davis M, Choy JS, et al. Histone H2AX phosphorylation as a predictor of radiosensitivity and target for radiotherapy. J. Biol Chem 2004;279:2273–80.
183. Iliakis G. Cell cycle regulation in irradiated and non-irradiated cells. Semin Oncol 1997;24:602–15.
184. Poon RY, Chau MS, Yamashita K, Hunter T. The role of CDC2 feedback loop control in the DNA damage checkpoint in mammalian cells. Cancer Res 1997;57:5168–78.
185. Haimovitz-Friedman A, Vlodavsky I, Chaudhuri A, et al. Autocrine effects of fibroblast growth factor in radiation damage repair in endothelial cells. Cancer Res 1991;51:2552–8.
186. Gallardo D, Drazan K, McBride W. Adenovirus-based transfer of wild-type P53 gene increases ovarian tumor radiosensitivity. Cancer Res 1996;56:4891–3.
187. Mundt A, Roeske J, Weichselbaum R. Principles of radiation oncology. In: Bast RC, Kufe DW, Pollock RE, et al, editors. Cancer medicine, 5th ed. Hamilton (ON): BC Decker; 2000. p. 465–78.
188. Ito Y, Pandey P, Sathyanarayana P, et al. Interaction of hematopoietic protein kinase 1 (HPK1) and c-Abl tyrosine kinase in response to genotoxic stress. J Biol Chem 2001;276:25959–69.
189. Woloschak GE, Chang-Liu CM, Jones PS, Jones CA. Modulation of gene expression in Syrian hamster embryo cells following ionizing radiation. Cancer Res 1990;50:339–44.
190. Kharbanda S, Ren R, Pandey P, et al. Activation of the c-Abl tyrosine kinase in the stress response to DNA-damaging agents. Nature 1995;376:785–8.
191. Mueller PR, Coleman TR, Kumagai A, Dunphy WG. Myt1: a membrane associated inhibitory kinase that phosphorylates Cdc2 on both threonine-14 and tyrosine-15. Science 1995;270:86–90.
192. Sanchez Y, Wong C, Thomas RS, et al. Conservation of the Chk1 checkpoint pathway in mammals: Linkage of DNA damage to CDK regulation through CDC25. Science 1997;1497–501.
193. Spitz F, Nguyen D, Skibber J, et al. Adenoviral-mediated wild-type P53 gene expression sensitizes colorectal cancer cells to ionizing radiation. Clin Cancer Res 1996;2:1665–71.
194. Peacock JW, Chung S, Bristow RG, et al. The P53-mediated G1 checkpoint is retained in tumorigenic rat embryo fibroblast clones transformed by the human papillomavirus type 16 E7 gene and EJ-ras. Mol Cell Biol 1995;15:1446–54.
195. Bristow RG, Hu Q, Jang A, et al. Radioresistant MTP53-expressing rat embryo cell transformants exhibit increased DNA-dsb rejoining during exposure to ionizing radiation. Oncogene 1998;16:1789–802.
196. Palayoor ST, Macklis RM, Bump EA, Coleman CN. Modulation of radiation-induced apoptosis and G2/M block in murine T-lymphoma cells. Radiat Res 1995;235–43.
197. Blasina A, de Weyer IV, Laus MC, et al. A human homologue of the checkpoint kinase Cds1 directly inhibits Cdc25 phosphatase. Curr Biol 1999;9:1–10.
198. Abrieu A, Fisher D, Simon MN, et al. MAPK inactivation is required for the G2 to M-phase transition of the first mitotic cell cycle. EMBO J 1997;16:6407–13.
199. Abbott DW, Holt JT. Mitogen-activated protein kinase 2 activation is essential for progression through the G2/M checkpoint arrest in cells exposed to ionizing radiation. J Biol Chem 1999;274:2732–42.
200. Wright JH, Munar E, Jameson DR, et al. Mitogen-activated protein kinase activity is required for the G(2)/M transition of the cell cycle in mammalian fibroblasts. Proc Natl Acad Sci U S A 1999;96:11335–40.
201. New L, Jiang Y, Zhao M, et al. PRAK, a novel protein kinase regulated by the P38 MAP kinase. EMBO J 1998;17:3372–84.
202. Rane MJ, Coxon PY, Powell DW, et al. P38 kinase-dependent MAPKAPK-2 activation functions as 3-phosphoinositide-dependent kinase-2 for Akt in human neutrophils. J Biol Chem 2001;276:3517–23.
203. Kumar S, McDonnell PC, Gum RJ, et al. Novel homologues of CSBP/P38 MAP kinase: activation, substrate specificity and sensitivity to inhibition by pyridinyl imidazoles. Biochem Biophys Res Commun 1997;235:533–8.
204. Deplanque G, Ceraline J, Mah-Becherel MC, et al. Caffeine and the G2/M block override: a concept resulting from a misleading cell kinetic delay, independent of functional P53. Int J Cancer 2001;94:363–9.
205. Deplanque G, Vincent F, Mah-Becherel MC, et al. Caffeine does not cause override of the G2/M block induced by UVc or gamma radiation in normal human skin fibroblasts. Br J Cancer 2000;83:346–53.
206. Yasutake H, Tsuchiya H, Tomita K, et al. Inhibitory effect of caffeine on potentially lethal damage repair in cisplatin-treated human osteosarcoma cells. Anticancer Res 1995;15:831–7.
207. Regaud C, Ferroux R. Discordance des effects de rayons X, d'une part dans le testicule, par le fractionment de la dose. C R Soc Biol 1927;97:431–4.
208. Suit H, Witte R. Radiation dose fractionation and tumor control probability. Radiat Res 1966;29:267–73.
209. Jeremic B, Shibamoto Y, Grujicic D, et al. Hyperfractionated radiation therapy for incompletely resected supratentorial low-grade glioma. A phase II study. Radiother Oncol 1998;49:49–54.
210. Brizel DM, Albers ME, Fisher SR, et al. Hyperfractionated irradiation with or without concurrent chemotherapy for locally advanced head and neck cancer. N Engl J Med 1998;338:1798–804.
211. Wang CC. Cancer of the head and neck. In: Wang CC, editor. Clinical radiation oncology. Littleton (MA): PSG Publishing; 1988. p.120–79.
212. Peters LJ, Brock WA, Travis EL. Radiation biology at clinically relevant fractions. In: Important advances in oncology. Philadelphia (PA): JB Lippincott; 1990. p.65–83.
213. Littbrand B, Revesz L. The effect of oxygen on cellular survival and recovery after radiation. Br J Radiol 1969; 42:914–7.
214. Raju MR, Amols HI, Bain E, et al. A heavy particle comparative study. III. OER and RBE. Br J Radiol 1978;51:712–9.
215. Thomlison H, Gray L. Histological structure of some human lung cancers and the possible implications for radiotherapy. Br J Cancer 1955;9:539–63.
216. Thomlison RH. In: Modern trends in radiotherapy, Vol 1. Deelay TJ, Wood CAP, editors. London, U.K.: Butterworths Scientific Publications; 1967. p. 52–72.
217. Van Putten LM. Tumor reoxygenation during fractionated radiotherapy. Eur J Cancer 1968;4:173–7.
218. Bush RS, Jenkin RDT, Allt WEC, et al. Definitive evidence for hypoxic cells influencing cure in cancer therapy. Br J Cancer 1978;37(Suppl 3):302–7.
219. Evans JC, Bergsio P. The influence of anemia on the results of radiotherapy in carcinoma of the cervix. Radiology 1965;84:709–12.
220. Hierlihy P, Jenkin RDT, Stryker JA. Anemia as a prognostic factor in cancer of the cervix. A preliminary report. J Cancer Med Assoc 1969;100:1100–4.
221. Overgaard J, SandHansen H, Jorgensen K, Hjelm-Hansen M. Primary radiotherapy of larynx and pharynx carcinoma—an analysis of some factors influencing local control and survival. Int J Radiat Oncol Biol Phys 1986;12:515–9.
222. Quilty PM, Duncan W. The influence of hemoglobin level on the regression and long term local control of transitional cell carcinoma of the bladder following photon irradiation. Int J Radiat Oncol Biol Phys 1986;12:1735–8.
223. Rustowski J, Kupsc W. Factors influencing the results of radiotherapy in cases of inoperable endometrial cancer. Gynecol Oncol 1982;14:185–8.
224. Dische S, Anderson PJ, Sealy R, Watson ER. Carcinoma of the cervix-anaemia. Radiotherapy and hyperbaric oxygen. Br J Radiol 1983;56:251–5.
225. Henk JM. Does hyperbaric oxygen have a future in radiation therapy? Int J Radiat Oncol Biol Phys 1981;7:1125–30.
226. Chapman JD. Hypoxic sensitizers: implications for radiation therapy. N Engl J Med 1979;301:1429–32.
227. Coleman CN, Bump EA, Kramer RA. Chemical modifiers of cancer therapy. J Clin Oncol 1988;6:709–11.
228. Lee DJ, Cosmatos D, Marcial V, et al. Results of an RTOG phase III trial (RTOG 85-27) comparing radiotherapy plus etanidazole with radiotherapy alone for locally advanced head and neck carcinoma. Int J Radiat Oncol Biol Phys 1995;32:567–76.
229. Overgaard J, Hansen HS, Andersen AP, et al. Misonidazole combined with split-course radiotherapy in the treatment of invasive carcinoma of the larynx and pharynx: report

from the DAHANCA 2 study. Int J Radiat Oncol Biol Phys 1989;16:1065–8.
230. Overgaard J, Hansen HS, Overgaard M, et al. A randomized double-blind phase III study of nimorazole as a hypoxic radiosensitizer of primary radiotherapy in supraglottic larynx and pharynx carcinoma. Results of the Danish Head and Neck Cancer Study (DAHANCA) Protocol 5-85. Radiother Oncol 1998;42:135–46.
231. Kinsella TJ, Dobson PP, Mitchell JB, et al. The use of halogenated thymidine analogs as clinical radiation sensitizers: rationale, current status, and future prospects: nonhypoxic cell sensitizers. Int J Radiat Oncol Biol Phys 1984;10:1399–406.
232. Phuphanich S, Levin EM, Levin VA. Phase I study of intravenous bromodeoxyuridine used concomitantly with radiation therapy in patients with primary malignant brain tumors. Int J Radiat Oncol Biol Phys 1984;10:1769–72.
233. Chang AE, Kinsella TJ, Rowland TJ, et al. A phase I study of intraarterial iododeoxyuridine in patients with colorectal liver metastases. J Clin Oncol 1989;7:662–9.
234. Dritschillo A, Pizo A, Kellman A, et al. The effect of cis-platinum on the repair of radiation damage in plateau phase Chinese hamster (V-79) cells. Int J Radiat Oncol Biol Phys 1979;5:1345–9.
235. Ng CE, Bussey AM, Raaphorst GP. Inhibition of potentially lethal damage and sublethal damage repair by camptothecin and etoposide in human melanoma cell lines. Int J Radiat Biol 1994;66:49–57.
236. Durand R. Adriamycin: a possible indirect radiosensitizer of hypoxic cells. Radiology 1979;119:217–22.
237. Sinclair WK. The combined effect of hydroxyurea and x-rays on Chinese hamster cells in vitro. Cancer Res 1968;28:198–206.
238. Gran C, Overgaard J. Radiosensitizing and cytotoxic properties of mitomycin-C in a C3H mouse mammary carcinoma in vivo. Int J Radiat Oncol Biol Phys 1991;20:265–9.
239. Geard C, Jones JM, Schiff PB, et al. Taxol and radiation. Monogr Natl Cancer Inst 1993;15:89–94.
240. Buntzel J, Kuttner K, Frohlich D, Glatzel M. Selective cytoprotection with amifostine in concurrent radiochemotherapy for head and neck cancer. Ann Oncol 1998;9:505–9.
241. Nagy B, Dale PJ, Grdina D. Protection against cis-diamminedichloroplatinum cytotoxicity and mutagenicity in V79 cells by 2([aminopropyl]amino)ethanethil. Cancer Res 1986;46:1132–6.
242. Neta R, Oppenheim JJ, Douches SD. Interdependence of the radioprotective effects of human recombinant interleukin 1, alpha tumor necrosis factor, granulocyte macrophage colony stimulating factor. J Immunol 1988;140:108–11.
243. Oppnehiem JJ, Neta R, Tiberghein P, et al. IL-1 enhances survival of lethally irradiated mice treated with allogenic bone marrow cells. Blood 1989;74:2257–61.
244. Patt HM, Tyree EB, Straube RL, et al. Protection against x-irradiation. Science 1949;110:213–5.
245. Hermens AF, Barendsen GW. Changes of cell proliferation characteristics before and after x-irradiation. Eur J Cancer 1969;5:173–7.
246. Jeggo PA, Kemp LM. X-ray sensitive mutants of Chinese hamster ovary cell line: isolation and cross sensitivity to other DNA damaging agents. Mutat Res 1983;112:313–7.
247. Hallahan DE, Spriggs DR, Beckett MA, et al. Increased tumor necrosis factor expression following ionizing radiation exposure. Proc Natl Acad Sci U S A 1989;86:10104–7.
248. Hallahan DE, Spriggs DR, Beckett MA, et al. Increased tumor necrosis alpha mRNA after cellular exposure to ionizing radiation. Proc Natl Acad Sci U S A 1989;86:10104–9.
249. Witte L, Fuks Z, Haimovitz-Friedman A, et al. Effects of radiation on the release of growth factors from cultured bovine, porcine, and human endothelial cells. Cancer Res 1989;49:5066–73.
250. Woloschak GE, Liu GMC, Jones S, Jones C. Modulation of gene expression in Syrian hamster embryo cells following ionizing radiation. Cancer Res 1990;50:339–43.
251. Fuks Z, Alfieri A, Haimovitz-Friedman A, et al. Intravenous basic fibroblast growth factor protects the lung but not mediastinal organs against radiation-induced apoptosis in vivo. Cancer J Sci Am 1995;1:62–5.
252. Schmidt-Ullrich RK, Dent P, Grant S, et al. Signal transduction and cellular radiation responses. Radiat Res 2000;153:245–57.
253. Herbst RS, Langer CJ. Epidermal growth factor receptors as a target for cancer treatment: the emerging role of IMC-C225 in the treatment of lung and head cancers. Semin Oncol 2002;29:27–36.
254. Milas L, Mason K, Hunter N, et al. In vivo enhancement of tumor radioresponse by C225 antiepidermal growth factor receptor antibody. Clin Cancer Res 2000;6:701–8.
255. Raben D, Helfrich BA, Chan D, et al. ZD1839, a selective epidermal growth factor receptor tyrosine kinase inhibitor, alone and in combination with radiation and chemotherapy as a new therapeutic strategy in non-small cell lung cancer. Semin Oncol 2002;29:37–46.
256. Thornberry NA. The caspase family of cysteine proteases. Br Med Bull 1997;53:478–90.
257. Kondo T, Yokokura T, Nagata S. Activation of distinct caspase-like proteases by Fas and reaper in Drosophila cells. Proc Natl Acad Sci U S A 1997;94:11951–6.
258. Bump NJ, Hackett M, Hugunin M, et al. Inhibition of ICE family proteases by baculovirus antiapoptotic protein p35. Science 1995;269:1885–8.
259. Enari M, Hug H, Nagata S. Involvement of an ICE-like protease in Fas-mediated apoptosis. Nature 1995;375:78–81.
260. Cryns VL, Bergeron L, Zhu H, et al. Specific cleavage of alpha-fodrin during Fas- and tumor necrosis factor-induced apoptosis is mediated by an interleukin-1 beta-converting enzyme/Ced-3 protease distinct from the poly(ADP-ribose) polymerase protease. J Biol Chem 1996;271:31277–82.
261. Clem RJ. Baculoviruses and apoptosis: the good, the bad, and the ugly. Cell Death Differ 2001;8:137–43.
262. Datta R, Kojima H, Banach D, et al. Activation of a CRMA-insensitive, P35-sensitive pathway in ionizing radiation-induced apoptosis. J Biol Chem 1997;272:1965–9.
263. Hallan E, Blomhoff HK, Smeland EB, Lomo J. Involvement of ICE (Caspase) family in gamma-radiationinduced apoptosis of normal B lymphocytes. Scand J Immunol 1997;46:601–8.
264. Tong X, Liu B, Dong Y, Sun Z. Cleavage of ATM during radiation-induced apoptosis: caspase-3-like apoptotic protease as a candidate. Int J Radiat Biol 2000;76:1387–95.
265. Chauhan D, Pandey P, Ogata A, et al. Cytochrome c-dependent and independent induction of apoptosis in multiple myeloma cells. J Biol Chem 1997;272:29995–7.
266. Matassa AA, Carpenter L, Biden TJ, et al. PKCdelta is required for mitochondrial-dependent apoptosis in salivary epithelial cells. J Biol Chem 2001;276:29719–28.
267. Frutos S, Moscat J, Diaz-Meco MT. Cleavage of zetaPKC but not lambda/iotaPKC by caspase-3 during UV-induced apoptosis. J Biol Chem 1999;274:10765–70.
268. Salvesen GS, Dixit VM. Caspases: intracellular signaling by proteolysis. Cell 1997;91:443–6.
269. Bossy-Wetzel E, Newmeyer DD, Green DR. Mitochondrial cytochrome c release in apoptosis occurs upstream of DEVD-specific caspase activation and independently of mitochondrial transmembrane depolarization. EMBO J 1998;17:37–49.
270. Burri SH, Kim CN, Fang G, et al. Loop domain deletional mutant of Bcl-xL is as effective as p29Bcl-xL in inhibiting radiation-induced cytosolic accumulation of cytochrome c (cyt c), caspase-3 activity, and apoptosis. Int J Radiat Oncol Biol Phys 1999;43:423–30.
271. Kirsch DG, Doseff A, Chau BN, et al. Caspase-3-dependent cleavage of Bcl-2 promotes release of cytochrome c. J Biol Chem 1999;274:21155–61.
272. Petrini JH. The MRE11 complex and ATM: collaborating to navigate S phase. Curr Opin Cell Biol 2000;12:293–6.
273. Kharbanda S, Saxena S, Yoshida K, et al. Translocation of SAPK/JNK to mitochondria and interaction with BclxL in response to DNA damage. J Biol Chem 2000;275:322–7.
274. Lim DS, Kim ST, Xu B, et al. ATM phosphorylates p95/nbs1 in an S-phase checkpoint pathway. Nature 2000;404:613–7.
275. Gatei M, Young D, Cerosaletti KM, et al. ATM-dependent phosphorylation of nibrin in response to radiation exposure. Nat Genet 2000;25:115–9.
276. Zhao S, Weng YC, Yuan SS, et al. Functional link between ataxia-telangiectasia and Nijmegen breakage syndrome gene products. Nature 2000;405:473–7.
277. Wu X, Ranganathan V, Weisman D, et al. ATM phosphorylation of Nijmegen breakage syndrome protein is required in a DNA damage response. Nature 2000;405:477–82.
278. Baumann P, Benson FE, West SC. Human Rad51 protein promotes ATP-dependent homologous pairing and strand transfer reactions in vitro. Cell 1996;87:757–66.
279. Mauceri HJ, Hanna NN, Beckett MA, et al. Combined effects of angiostatin and ionizing radiation in antitumor therapy. Nature 1998;394:287–92.
280. Advani SJ, Chung SM, Yan SY, et al. Replication-competent, nonneuroinvasive genetically engineered herpes virus is highly effective in the treatment of therapy-resistant experimental human tumors. Cancer Res 1999;59:2055–8.
281. Bradley JD, Kataoka Y, Advani S, et al. Ionizing radiation improves survival in mice bearing intracranial high-grade gliomas injected with genetically modified herpes simplex virus. Clin Cancer Res 1999;5:1517–22.
282. Rogulski KR, Freytag, SO, Zhang, K, et al. In vivo antitumor activity of ONYX-015 is influenced by p53 status and is augmented by radiotherapy. Cancer Res 1193–6.
283. DeWeese TL, van der Poel H, Li S, et al. A phase I trial of CV706, a replication-competent, PSA selective oncolytic adenovirus, for the treatment of locally recurrent prostate cancer following radiation therapy. Cancer Res 2001;61:7464–72.
284. Epperley MW, Guo HL, Jefferson M, et al. Cell phenotype specific kinetics of expression of intratracheally injected manganese superoxide dismutase-plasmid/liposomes (MnSOD-FL) during lung radioprotective gene therapy. Gene Ther 2003;10:163–71.
285. Rabbani ZN, Anscher MS, Zhang X, et al. Soluble TGFbeta type II receptor gene therapy ameliorates acute radiation induced pulmonary injury in rats. Int J. Radiat Oncol Biol Phys 2003;57:563–72.
286. Spivak-Kroizman T, Rotin D, Pincahsi D, et al. Heterodimerization of c-cerbB2 with different epidermal growth factor receptor mutants elicit stimulatory or inhibitory responses. J Biol Chem 1992;267:8056–63.
287. Lammering G, Hewit TH, Valerie K, et al. Anti-erbB receptor strategy as a gene therapeutic intervention to improve radiotherapy in malignant human tumours. Int J Radiat Biol 2003;79:561–8.
288. Contessa JN, Reardon DB, Todd D, et al. The inducible expression of dominant-negative epidermal growth factor receptor-CD533 results in radiosensitization of human mammary carcinoma cells. Clin Cancer Res 1999;5:405–11.
289. Lammering G, Hewit TH, Holmes M et al. Inhibition of the type III epidermal growth factor receptor variant mutant receptor by dominant-negative EGFR-CD533 enhances malignant glioma cell radiosensitivity. Clin Cancer Res 2004;10:6732–43.
290. Kakeji Y, Teicher BA. Preclinical studies of the combination of angiogenic inhibitors with cytotoxic agents. Invest New Drugs 1997;15:39–48.
291. Lund EL, Bastholm L, Kristjansen PE. Therapeutic synergy of TNP-470 and ionizing radiation: effects on tumor growth, vessel morphology, and angiogenesis in human glioblastoma multiforme xenografts. Clin Cancer Res 2000;6:971–8.
292. Mauceri HJ, Hanna NN, Beckett MA, et al. Combined effects of angiostatin and ionizing radiation in antitumour therapy. Nature 1998;394:287–91.
293. Gorski DH, Beckett MA, Jaskowiak NT, et al. Blockage of the vascular endothelial growth factor stress response increases the antitumor effects of ionizing radiation. Cancer Res 1999;59:3374–8.
294. Hanna NN, Seetharam S, Mauceri HJ, et al. Antitumor interaction of short-course endostatin and ionizing radiation. Cancer J 2000;6:287–93.
295. Willet CG, Boucher Y, di Tomaso E, et al. Direct evidence that the VEGF-specific antibody bevacizumab has antivascular effects in human rectal cancer. Nat Med 2004;10:145–7.
296. Lee CG, Heijn M, di Tomaso E, et al. Anti-vascular endothelial growth factor treatment augments tumor radiation response under normoxic or hypoxic conditions. Cancer Res 2000;60:5565–70.
297. Kozin SV, Boucher Y, Hicklin DJ, et al. Vascular endothelial growth factor receptor-2-blocking antibody potentiates radiation-induced long-term control of human tumor xenografts. Cancer Res 2001;61:39–44.
298. Geng L, Donnelly E, McMahon G, et al. Inhibition of vascular endothelial growth factor receptor signaling leads to reversal of tumor resistance to radiotherapy. Cancer Res 2001;61:2413–9.
299. Hess C, Vuong V, Hegyi L, et al. Effect of VEGF receptor inhibitor PTK787/ZK222584 (correction of ZK222548) combined with ionizing radiation on endothelial cells and tumour growth. Br J Cancer 2001;85:2010–6.
300. Ning S, Laird D, Cherrington JM, Knox SJ. The antiangiogenic agents SU5416 and SU6668 increase the antitumor effects of fractionated irradiation. Radiat Res 2002;157:45–51.
301. Dicker AP, Williams TL, Grant DS. Targeting angiogenic processes by combination rofecoxib and ionizing radiation. Am J Clin Oncol 2001;24:438–42.
302. Kishi K, Petersen S, Petersen C, et al. Preferential enhancement of tumor radioresponse by a cyclooxygenase-2 inhibitor. Cancer Res 2000;60:1326–31.

303. Milas L. Cyclooxygenase-2 (COX-2) enzyme inhibitors as potential enhancers of tumor radioresponse. Semin Radiat Oncol 2001;11:290–9.
304. Maj KG, Paris F, Haimovitz-Friedman A, et al. Microvascular function regulates intestinal crypt response to radiation. Cancer Res 2003;63:4338–41.
305. Garcia-Barros M. Paris F, Cordon-Cardo C, et al. Tumor response to radiotherapy regulated by endothelial cell apoptosis. Science 300:1155–9.
306. Million RR. Carcinomas of the oral cavity and oropharynx. Curative treatment with preservation of function. Front Radiat Ther Oncol 1993;27:20–
307. Lee WR, Mendenhall WM, Parsons JT, et al. Carcinoma of the tonsillar region: a multivariate analysis of 243 patients treated with radical radiotherapy. Head Neck 1993;15:283–8.
308. Medenhall WM, Parsons JT, Stringer SP, Cassisi NJ. Radiotherapy for carcinoma of the supraglottis. Otolaryngol Clin North Am 1997;30:145–61.
309. Fein DA, Medenhall WM, Parsons JT, Million RR. T1-2 squamous cell carcinoma of the glottic larynx treated with radiotherapy: a multivariate analysis of variables potentially influencing local control. Int J Radiat Oncol Biol Phys 1993;25:605–11.
310. Landoni F, Maneo A, Colombo A, et al. Randomized study of radical surgery versus radiotherapy for stage IB-IIA cervical cancer. Lancet 1997;350:535–540.
311. Farah R, Ultmann J, Griem M, et al. Extended mantle radiation therapy for pathologic stage I and II Hodgkin's disease. J Clin Oncol 1988;6:1047–52.
312. Pignon T, Gregor A, Schaake-Koning C, et al. Age has no impact on acute and late toxicity of curative thoracic radiotherapy. Radiother Oncol 1998;46:239–48.
313. Mitchell PA, Waggoner S, Rotmensch J, Mundt AJ. Cervical cancer in the elderly treated with radiation therapy. Gynecol Oncol 1998;71:291–8.
314. Roeske JC, Mundt AJ, Halpern H, et al. Late rectal sequelae following definitive radiation therapy for carcinoma of the uterine cervix: a dosimetric analysis. Int J Radiat Oncol Biol Phys 1997;37:351–8.
315. Pahlman L, Glimelius B, Ginman C, et al. Preoperative irradiation of primarily non-resectable adenocarcinoma of the rectum and rectosigmoid. Acta Radiol Oncol 1985;24:35–39.
316. Barkley H, Martin R, Romsdahl M, et al. Treatment of soft tissue sarcomas by preoperative irradiation and conservative surgical resection. Int J Radiat Oncol Biol Phys 1988;14:693–9.
317. Connell PP, Macdonald RL, Mansur DB, et al. Tumor size predicts control of benign meningiomas treated with radiotherapy. Neurosurgery 1999;44:1194–9.
318. Peters LJ, Goepfert H, Ang KK, et al. Evaluation of the dose for postoperative radiation therapy of head and neck cancer: first report of a prospective randomized trial. Int J Radiat Oncol Biol Phys 1993;26:3–11.
319. Heimann R, Powers C, Halpern HJ, et al. Breast preservation in stage I and II carcinoma of the breast: the University of Chicago experience. Cancer 1996;78: 1722–30.
320. Lad T, Lung Cancer Study Group. The benefit of adjuvant treatment for resected locally advanced non-small cell lung cancer. J Clin Oncol 1988;6:9–17.
321. Anscher MS, Prosnitz LR. Postoperative radiotherapy for patients with carcinoma of the prostate undergoing radical prostatectomy with positive margins, seminal vesicle involvement and/or penetration through the capsule. J Urol 1987;138:1407–12.
322. Hoskins RB, Gunderson LL, Dosoretz DE, et al. Adjuvant postoperative radiotherapy in carcinoma of the rectum and rectosigmoid. Cancer 1985;55:61–6.
323. Gunderson LL, Willett CG, Harrison LB, et al. Intraoperative irradiation: current and future status. Semin Oncol 1998;24:715–31.
324. Kinsella TJ, Sindelar WF, Lack E, et al. Preliminary results of a randomized study of adjuvant radiation therapy in resectable adult retroperitoneal soft tissue sarcomas. J Clin Oncol 1988;6:18–25.
325. Shiu M, Turnball A, Nori D, et al. Control of locally advanced extremity soft tissue sarcomas by function saving resection and brachytherapy. Cancer 1984;53:1385–92.
326. Glick J, Kim K, Earle J, et al. An ECOG randomized phase III trial of CHOP vs CHOP + radiotherapy for intermediate grade early stage non-Hodgkin's lymphoma. Proc Am Soc Clin Oncol 1995;14:391–5.
327. Perry M, Eaton W, Propert K. Chemotherapy with or without radiation therapy in limited stage small-cell carcinoma of the lung. N Engl J Med 1987;316:912–8.
328. Schaake-Koning C, Van den Bogaert W, Dalesio O, et al. Effects of concomitant cisplatin and radiotherapy in inoperable non-small cell cancer. N Engl J Med 1992; 326:524–30.
329. Haraf DJ, Stenson K, List M, et al. Continuous infusion paclitaxel, 5-fluorouracil, and hydroxyurea with concomitant radiotherapy in patients with advanced or recurrent head and neck cancer. Semin Oncol 1997;24(Suppl):S2–S68.
330. Herskovic A, Martz K, Al-Sarraf M, et al. Combined chemotherapy and radiotherapy compared with radio-therapy alone in patients with cancer of the esophagus. N Engl J Med 1992;326:1593–8.
331. Shipley WU, Prout JR, Eisenstein AB, et al. Treatment of invasive bladder cancer by cisplatin and irradiation in patients unsuited for surgery: a high success rate in clinical stage T2 tumors in a National Bladder Cancer Group trial. JAMA 1987;258:931–6.
332. Keys HM, Bundy BN, Stehman FB, et al. Cisplatin, radiation, and adjuvant hysterectomy compared with radiation and adjuvant hysterectomy for bulky stage IB cervical carcinoma. N Engl J Med 1999;340:1154–61.
333. Bonadonna G, Veronesi U, Bronhilla T, et al. Primary chemotherapy to avoid mastectomy in tumors with diameters three centimeters or more. J Natl Cancer Inst 1990;82:1539–45.
334. Kalser MH, Ellenberg SS, for Gastrointestinal Tumor Study Group. Pancreatic cancer: adjuvant combined radiation and chemotherapy following curative resection. Arch Surg 1985;120:899–904.
335. Krook JE, Moertel CG, Gunderson LL, et al. Effective surgical adjuvant therapy for high-risk rectal carcinoma. N Engl J Med 1991;324:709–15.
336. Auperian A, Arriagada R, Pignon JP, et al. Prophylactic cranial irradiation for patients with small-cell lung cancer in complete remission. Prophylactic cranial irradiation overview collaborative group. N Engl J Med 1999;341:476–84.
337. Schrappe M, Reiter A, Riehm H. Prophylaxis and treatment of neoplastic meningeosis in childhood acute lymphoblastic leukemia. J Neurooncol 1998;38:159–165.
338. Lee CK, Bloomfield CD, Goldman AI, et al. The therapeutic utility of lung irradiation for Hodgkin's disease patients with large mediastinal masses. Int J Radiat Oncol Biol Phys 1981;7:151–54.
339. Lee CK, Bloomfield CD, Levitt SD. Liver irradiation in stage IIA Hodgkin's disease patients with splenic involvement. Am J Clin Oncol 1984;7:149–157.
340. Komaki R, Wadler S, Peters T, et al. High-dose local irradiation plus prophylactic hepatic irradiation and chemotherapy for inoperable adenocarcinoma of the pancreas. A preliminary report of a multi-institutional trial (Radiation Therapy Oncology Group Protocol 8801). Cancer 1992;69:2807–12.
341. Price P, Hoskin PJ, Easton D. Low dose single fraction radiotherapy in the treatment of metastatic bone pain: a pilot study. Radiother Oncol 1998;12:297–301.
342. Tong C, Gilliack L, Hendrickson FR. The palliation of symptomatic osseous metastases: final results of the study by the Radiation Therapy Oncology Group. Cancer 1982;50:893–6.
343. Salazar OM, Rubin P, Hendrickson FR, et al. Single-dose half-body irradiation for the palliation of multiple bone metastases from solid tumors: a preliminary report. Int J Radiat Oncol Biol Phys 1981;7:773–81.
344. Scher HI, Chung LWK. Bone metastases: improving the therapeutic index. Semin Oncol 1994;21:630–5.
345. Sefarini A, Houston SJ, Resche I, et al. Palliation of pain associated with metastatic b cancer using samarium-153 lexidronam: a double blind placebo controlled clinical trial. J Clin Oncol 1998;16:1574–81.
346. Borgelt BB, Gelber R, Brady LW, et al. The palliation of hepatic metastases: results of the Radiation Therapy Oncology Group pilot study. Int J Radiat Oncol Biol Phys 1981;7:587–91.
347. Findlay GFG. Adverse effects of the management of malignant spinal cord compression. J Neurol Neurosurg Psych 1984;47:761–5.
348. Liebel SA, Pajak TF, Massullo V, et al. A comparison of misonidazole sensitized radiation therapy to radiation therapy alone for the palliation of hepatic metastases: results of the Radiation Therapy Oncology Group prospective trial. Int J Radiat Oncol Biol Phys 1990;13:1057–62.
349. Dobrowsky W. Treatment of choroid metastases. Br J Radiol 1988;61:140–44.
350. Zachariah B, Zachariah SB, Vorghese R, Balducci L. Carcinomatous meningitis: clinical manifestations and management. Int J Clin Pharmacol Ther 1995;33:7–12.
351. Rees GJ, Tevrell CE, Barley VC, Newman HF. Palliative radiotherapy for lung cancer: two versus five fractions. Clin Oncol 1997;9:90–5.
352. Adelson MD, Wharton JT, Delclos L, et al. Palliative radiotherapy for ovarian cancer. Int J Radiat Oncol Biol Phys 1993;13:531–5.
353. Cotter GW, Larscy C, Ellingwood KE, Herbert D. Inoperable endobronchial obstructing lung cancer treated with combined endobronchial and external beam irradiation: a dosimetric analysis. Int J Radiat Oncol Biol Phys 1993;27:531–5.
354. Montemaggi P, Costamagna G, Dobelbower RR, et al. Intraluminal brachytherapy in the treatment of pancreas and bile carcinomas. Int J Radiat Oncol Biol Phys 1995;32:437–41.
355. Taal BG, Aleman BM, Koning CC, Boot H. High dose rate brachytherapy before external beam radiotherapy in inoperable oesophageal cancer. Br J Cancer 1996;74: 1452–57.
356. Kovalic J, Perez C. Radiation therapy following keloidectomy: a 20-year experience. Int J Radiat Oncol Biol Phys 1989;17:77–80.
357. Schild S, Buskirk S, Frick L, Cupps R. Radiotherapy for large symptomatic hemangiomas. Int J Radiat Oncol Biol Phys 1991;21:729–35.
358. Sherman N, Romsdahl M, Evans H, et al. Desmoid tumors: a 20-year radiotherapy experience. Int J Radiat Oncol Biol Phys 1990;19:37–49.
359. Van den Brenck HAA. Results of prophylactic postoperative irradiation in 1300 cases of pterygium. AMJ Am J Roentgenol 1968;103:723–7.
360. Sutherland DER, Ferguson RM, Rynasiewicz JJ, et al. Total lymphoid irradiation versus cyclosporin for retransplantation in recipients at high risk to reject renal allografts. Transplant Proc 1983;15:460–65.
361. Frist WH, Winterland AW, Gerhardt EB, et al. Total lymphoid irradiation in heart transplantation: adjuvant treatment for recurrent rejection. Ann Thorac Surg 1989;48:863–4.
362. Berson AM, Finger PT, Sherr DL, et al. Radiotherapy for age-related macular degeneration: technique and preliminary subjective response. Int J Radiat Oncol Biol Phys 1996;36:861–6.
363. Ritter MA, Vaughn RB. Ectopic ossification after total hip arthroplasty: predisposing factors, frequency and effect on results. J Bone J Surg 1977;59A:345–8.
364. Tierstein PS, Massullo V, Jani S, et al. Catheter-based radiotherapy to inhibit restenosis after coronary stenting. N Engl J Med 1997;336:1697–1703.
365. Stevens KR. The stomach and intestines. In: Moss WT, Cox JD, editors. Radiation oncology, rationale, techniques. St Louis (MO): CV Mosby; 1989. p. 362–408.
366. Perez CA, Grigsby PW, Castro-Vita H, et al. Carcinoma of the uterine cervix. I. Impact of prolongation of overall treatment time and timing of brachytherapy on outcome of radiation therapy. Int J Radiat Oncol Biol Phys 1995;32:1275–99.
367. Skladowski K, Law MG, Maciejewski B, et al. Planned and unplanned gaps in radiotherapy: the importance of gap position and gap duration. Radiother Oncol 1994;30:109–20.
368. Meredith R, Salter M, Kim R, et al. Sucralfate for radiation mucositis: results of a double-blind randomized trial. Int J Radiat Oncol Biol Phys 1997;37:275–9.
369. Smith LM, Donaldson SS, Egbert PR, et al. Aggressive management of second primary tumors in survivors of hereditary retinoblastoma. Int J Radiat Oncol Biol Phys 1989;17:499–505.
370. Moulder JE, Fish BL, Cohen EP. Angiotensin II receptor antagonists in the treatment and prevention of radiation nephropathy. Int J Radiat Oncol Biol Phys 1998;73:415–21.
371. LeVeque FG, Montgomery M, Potter D, et al. A multicenter, randomized, double-blind, placebo-controlled, dose-titration study of oral pilocarpine for treatment of radiation-induced xerostomia in head and neck cancer patients. J Clin Oncol 1993;11:1124–31.
372. Ripamonti C, Zecca E, Brunelli C, et al. A randomized, controlled clinical trial to evaluate the effects of zinc sulfate on cancer patients with taste alterations caused by head and neck irradiation. Cancer 1998;82:1938–45.
373. Withers HR, McBride WH. Biologic basis of radiation therapy. In: Perez CA, Brady LW, editors. Principles and practice of radiation oncology. Philadelphia, PA: Lippincott-Raven; 1997.
374. The Department of Veteran Affairs Laryngeal Cancer Study Group. Induction chemotherapy plus radiation compared

with surgery plus radiation in patients with advanced laryngeal cancer. N Engl J Med 1991;324:1685–90.

375. Mundt AJ, Sibley G, Williams S, et al. Patterns of failure and outcome of complete responders following high-dose chemotherapy and autologous bone marrow trans-plantation for metastatic breast cancer. Int J Radiat Oncol Biol Phys 1994;30:151–60.

376. Mundt AJ, Sibley G, Williams SF, Hallahan DE. Patterns of failure and outcome following high-dose chemotherapy and bone marrow transplantation with involved field radiotherapy for relapsed/refractory Hodgkin's disease. Int J Radiat Oncol Biol Phys 1995;33:261–70.

377. Coleman CN. Beneficial liaisons: radiobiology meets cellular and molecular biology. Radiother Oncol 1993;28:1–15.

35a

Photodynamic Therapy of Cancer

Tayyaba Hasan, PhD
Bernhard Ortel, MD
Nicolas Solban, PhD
Brian W. Pogue, PhD

OVERVIEW

Photodynamic therapy (PDT) is based on the concept that (1) certain photosensitizers can be localized (somewhat preferentially) in neoplastic tissue, and (2) subsequently, these photosensitizers can be activated with the appropriate wavelength (energy) of light to generate active molecular species, such as free radicals and singlet oxygen ($^1O_2$) that are toxic to cells and tissues. PDT is a binary therapy, and a potential advantage of PDT is its inherent dual selectivity. First, selectivity is achieved by an increased concentration of the photosensitizer in target tissue, and second, the irradiation can be limited to a specified volume. Provided that the photosensitizer is nontoxic, only the irradiated areas will be affected, even if the photosensitizer does bind to normal tissues. Selectivity can be further enhanced by binding photosensitizers to molecular delivery systems that have high affinity for target tissue.[1–5] For photoactivation, the wavelength of light is matched to the electronic absorption spectrum of the photosensitizer so that photons are absorbed by the photosensitizer and the desired photochemistry can occur. Except in special situations, where the lesions being treated are very superficial, the range of activating light is typically between 600 and 900 nm. This is because endogenous molecules, in particular hemoglobin, strongly absorb light below 600 nm and therefore capture most of the incoming photons.[6] The net effect would be the impairment of penetration of the activating light through the tissue. The reason for the 900 nm upper limit is that energetics beyond this wavelength are not sufficient to produce $^1O_2$, the activated state of oxygen, perhaps critical for successful PDT.

This chapter provides an overview of the field; excellent reviews and texts on this topic exist.[7–10] In particular, the reader is referred to a recent review by Dougherty and colleagues.[11] A brief introduction to the relevant photochemistry is given in the next section so that the conceptual basis of PDT may be better understood. Although spatial control of illumination, mentioned above, provides specificity of tissue destruction, it can also be a limitation of PDT. Target sites must be accessible to light delivery systems, and issues of light dosimetry need to be addressed.[12–14] In general, the amenability of lasers to fiberoptic coupling makes the task of light delivery to most anatomic sites manageable, although precise dosimetry remains complex and elusive. The effective penetration depth, δ_{eff}, of a given wavelength of light is a function of the optical properties, such as absorption and scatter of the tissue being interrogated. The fluence (light dose) in a tissue is related to the depth, d, as: $e^{-d/\delta_{eff}}$. Typically, the effective penetration depth is about 2 to 3 mm at 630 nm and increases to 5 to 6 mm at longer wavelengths (700–800 nm).[15–17] These values can be altered by altering the biologic interactions and physical characteristics of the photosensitizer; however, the relationships are complex. Factors such as self-shielding and photobleaching (self-destruction of the photosensitizer during the PDT) further complicate precise dosimetry and are discussed further below. In general, photosensitizers with longer absorbing wavelengths and higher molar absorption coefficients at these wavelengths are more effective photodynamic agents.

From a practical point of view, characteristics of the given photosensitizer most relevant to PDT are its concentration, c (measured on a spectrophotometer), and the extinction coefficient, ε, which are related by the relationship: $A = \varepsilon\, c\, l$, where A is the absorption value determined spectrophotometrically, and ε is the molar extinction coefficient and can be viewed as a measure of efficiency with which the molecule absorbs light of a given wavelength. It is a characteristic of the absorbing chemical species at a specified wavelength under defined conditions, such as solution and solid. In the above equation, l is the pathlength of light. (In practical terms, this is the width of the cuvette used for determining the absorption values of the photosensitizing agent.)

BASICS OF LIGHT AND PDT-RELATED PHOTOCHEMISTRY

Light is a form of electromagnetic radiation that covers a wide range of wavelengths, λ. Between electromagnetic radio wavelengths in the meter (m) range to gamma rays with wavelengths around 10^{-11} m, visible light relevant to PDT covers the limited range of 4 to 7×10^{-7} m (400–700 nm). The energy content (E) of light is related to the wavelength of absorption by $E = h\nu = hc/\lambda$, where h is Planck's constant (6.63×10^{-34}Js), v is the frequency, c is the speed of light in vacuum (3.0×10^8 m/s), and λ is the wavelength. When light is absorbed, the energy of the absorbed photons causes the absorbing molecule to be electronically excited. (Other processes, such as scattering and reflection also occur, as discussed below in the dosimetry section.) This excitation energy may be converted into heat (kinetic energy) by the collision of the excited molecule with surrounding molecules by radiationless decay. Alternatively, it may be re-emitted as fluorescence. The electronic energy levels between which transitions occur by absorption of ultraviolet-visible light (λ = 200–700 nm) may be represented by the simplified energy level diagram presented in Figure 35a-1.

With conventional light sources, typical absorption of light by a molecule involves a single photon exciting the molecule to the first excited singlet state S_1. From this energized state the molecule may initiate photochemistry (depending on the chemical structure) or intersystem cross to an electronically different excited state, the first triplet state T_1. From S_1, the excited molecule may also relax back to S_0 by radiation-

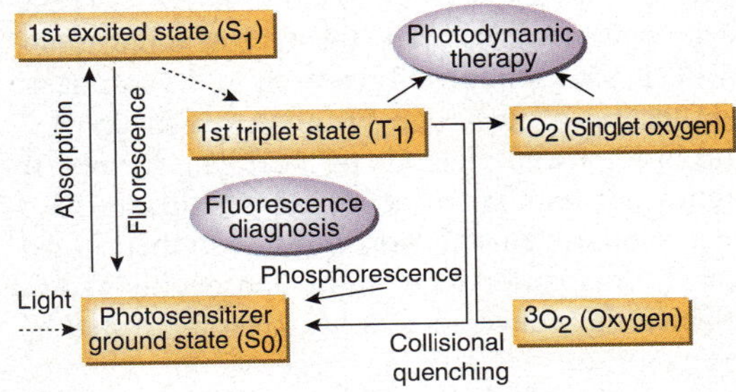

Figure 35a-1 A simplified energy level diagram for the photoexcitation of a photosensitizer (PS). Absorption of a photon results in the excitation of the absorbing molecule from the ground singlet state (S_0), to the first excited singlet state (S_1). Fluorescence, which can be used for diagnostic purposes, comes during de-excitation from S_1, back to the ground state S_0. Alternatively, the first triple state (T_1) is generated after intersystem crossing from S_1. Phosphorescence is emitted when the molecule relaxes back to S_0 from T_1. T_1 can initiate photochemical reactions directly, giving rise to reactive free radicals, or transfer its energy to the ground state oxygen molecules ($^3O_2$) to give rise to excited singlet state oxygen molecules ($^1O_2$). Adapted from Pogue B and Hasan T.[223]

less decay and generate heat or may re-emit radiation as fluorescence, which may be used for diagnostic purposes. In general, T_1 is longer lived and chemically more reactive so that the biologically relevant photochemistry is often mediated by this state. T_1 can initiate photochemical reactions directly, giving rise to reactive free radicals, or transfer its energy to the ground state oxygen molecules ($^3O_2$) to give rise to excited singlet state oxygen molecules $^1O_2$. This excitation to produce $^1O_2$ requires at least 20 kcal/mole, which places limits on the wavelength of absorption of the photosensitizer. If the energetics are appropriate, photo-oxidative reactions may occur by $^1O_2$ mediation. This photodynamic mechanism of cytotoxicity is the generally accepted one for most photosensitizers currently under investigation, although other competing mechanisms exist. T_1 can also potentially relax to S_0 by radiationless decay or by radiative decay as phosphorescence.

Table 35a-1 Selected Non-PF Photosensitizers and Experimental Clinical Studies*

Photosensitizer	Cutaneous Lesions	Early Upper Aerodigestive, Esophagus, Bronchus	Gynecology (Endometrial, Cervical, Vulvar)	Age-Related Macular Degeneration	Other Applications
ALA-PpIX	X	X	X		X
BPD-MA	X		X	X	
Porphycenes	X				
MACE	X				
Tin-etio-purpurin	X		X	X	
mTHPC	X	X	X		
Npe6				X	
Pc4	X				
Lutetium Texaphyrin	X		X		

ALA-PpIX = δ-aminolevulinic acid-induced protoporphyrin IX; BPD-MA = benzoporphyrin derivative monoacid A; MACE = mono-aspartyl chlorin e_6; mTHPC = meta-tetrahydroxyphenyl-chlorin; Npe6 = *N*-aspartyl chlorin e6; Pc4 = a silicon phtalocyanine.

*This list is not meant to be exhaustive; because PDT is rapidly expanding, there are likely to be more applications than listed here.

PHOTOSENSITIZERS

There are a fairly large number of photosensitizers under preclinical development at the present time. No attempt is made in this chapter to cover all these comprehensively. The reader is referred to the many existing reviews.[11,18–21] Only a few photosensitizers that are in advanced stages of clinical development in the United States are discussed.

Anionic Lipophilic Photosensitizers By far, most of the clinical experience in PDT has been with Porfimer sodium (Photofrin, PF), and for a long time, preclinical studies were dominated by investigations using some form of Hematoporphyrin derivative (HPD). Clinical results with PF have been promising, and this photosensitizer has received regulatory approval in a number of countries. However, it is plagued by prolonged cutaneous phototoxicity, which can last up to 4 to 6 weeks. In addition, it is poorly characterized chemically and has relatively low absorption in the wavelength region of therapeutic interest. These factors, plus an increase in the clinical applications of PDT, have stimulated research in the synthesis and testing of new, non-PF photosensitizers[20–23] and in improved methods of localizing them.[23] A significant number of new photosensitizers have been synthesized and show promise in their initial testing. In addition to avoiding nonspecific phototoxicity, their development has been motivated by the possibility of treating larger tumor volumes because of the greater penetration depth of longer wavelengths of light. Therefore, the properties that were aimed for in the development of these sensitizers were improved selectivity, longer wavelengths of light absorption, and increased extinction coefficient (molar absorptivity) at these wavelengths. Currently there may be over 30 photosensitizers in laboratory investigations, all of which are tetrapyrrole compounds. A selected few compounds that are being tested preclinically and clinically are summarized in Table 35a-1.

In general, these newer compounds show somewhat improved selectivity for tumor over normal tissue compared with PF and consequently have reduced associated cutaneous phototoxicity. For some, the pharmacokinetics are reasonably rapid with plasma half-lives that are often biphasic, with values ranging from a few hours to up to a few days. They also have superior photochemical properties in the absorption at longer wavelengths and corresponding extinction coefficients. For example, the chlorins have red-shifted absorption spectra (λ_{max} 650–670 nm), compared with 630 nm for PF[24–26] and extinction coefficients in the 3 to 5×10^4 $M^{-1}cm^{-1}$ range compared with the estimated values of up to 2×10^3 M^{-1} cm^{-1} for PF. Of the newer photosensitizers, the most developed is benzoporphyrin derivative monoacid A (BPD-MA).[27,28] For clinical applications, this molecule is liposomally formulated and has good absorbance at longer wavelengths. BPD-MA has shown encouraging results in the phase I-II clinical studies for the treatment of cutaneous malignancies (both primary and metastatic lesions). However, because of its effectiveness in the obliteration of neovessels, this compound has been successfully implemented by QLT Phototherapeutics and Ciba-Vision as a first-line treatment of age-related macular degeneration (AMD) of the eye.[29–31] This direction was stimulated by a series of preclinical studies,[29] where intraocular tumors implanted in rabbit eyes were used as a model for neovasculature. These studies showed that the very efficient destruction of these tumors could be attributed primarily to the destruction of the tumor neovasculature; the established choroidal vessels remained largely intact. Currently, the use of BPD-MA in the liposomal formulation called verteporfin is used in Visudyne therapy, marketed by Novartis Ophthalmics, for the treatment of classic subfoveal neovascularization (CNV) due to AMD. This treatment was approved in the United States by the FDA in 2001 following promising phase I and II clinical trials demonstrating that the treatment could slow the loss of vision in patients with CNV, pathologic myopia, and ocular histoplasmosis.[32] Currently, Visudyne treatment has been approved in 70 different countries and has rapidly become a major commercial success for PDT treatment, which will likely become approved for other indications in ophthalmology in the near future. At the time of the writing of this chapter, BPD-MA (Visudyne) is commercially available in 70 countries for the treatment of predominantly classic subfoveal CNV caused by AMD. It is also approved in 40 countries, including the European Union, United States, and Canada, for the treatment of subfoveal CNV due to pathologic myopia (severe near-sightedness). In 15 countries, Visudyne is also approved for presumed ocular histoplasmosis or other macular diseases. For the occult form of subfoveal CNV, Visudyne is approved in the European Union and United States. Clinical trials are ongoing to achieve approval for treatment of CNV with chlorin and phthalocyanine-based photosensitizers produced by other companies, perhaps expanding the variety of compounds and mechanisms of action that will be used in AMD therapy.

Cationic Photosensitizers A different group of photosensitizers that merits a brief mention are the cationic photosensitizers. In contrast to the porphyrins, which derive their PDT effect in large part via destruction of the tumor vasculature, cationic photosensitizers are suggested to be cellularly localized molecules and to act at the tumor cell level. It is believed that the basis for their preferential accumulation in tumor tissue is that the electrical potential across the mitochondrial membrane in tumor cells is much steeper than in normal cells.[33] This steep gradient leads to a high accumulation in tumor cells of compounds with a delocalized positive charge. The best developed of the series are the benzophenothiazinium dyes.[34,35] In systematic investigations of these dyes, Cincotta and colleagues showed high cure rates in two animal models of sarcoma, using the cationic photosensitizer 5-ethylamino-9-diethylaminobenzo[a]phenothiazinium chloride activated with 652 nm irradiation.[35] Minimal damage to surrounding and overlying skin tissue was observed, pointing to the selectivity of this compound. Histologic and fluorescein dye exclusion data indicated minimal damage to the irradiated vasculature within and surrounding the tumor. Cellular uptake of these compounds appears to occur rapidly, within seconds. In an attempt to combine vascular and cellular effects, a benzophenothiazinium sensitizer and BPD-MA were used in PDT of EMT-6 tumors in Balb/c mice. The treatment produced a synergistic effect, compared with the single treatments.[36] Using the iodinated form of the cationic photosensitizer, it was shown that the antitumor effect was mediated by both T cells and natural killer (NK) cells, indicating that PDT can elicit antitumor protective immunity.[37] These preclinical studies may be useful in various clinical settings and are currently under development.

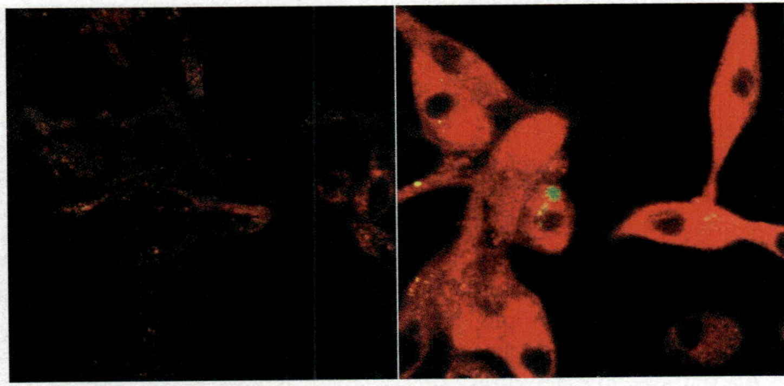

Figure 35a-2 Confocal laser scanning fluorescence micrographs showing increased aminolevulinic acid (ALA)-induced protoporphyrin IX (PpIX) levels with cellular differentiation. Human prostate cancer cell line LNCaP was exposed to 0.3 mM ALA for 4 hours. The red fluorescence stems from PpIX synthesized within the cells. The cells on the left were grown in androgen-free medium. The cells on the right were pretreated for 4 days with the synthetic androgen receptor ligand R1881, which acts as a differentiating agent.

δ-Aminolevulinic Acid-Based PDT Typically, in the application of PDT, presynthesized sensitizers are administered, followed by a delay period that, depending on the photosensitizer, may vary from 30 minutes to 7 days. The rationale for the shorter times is that the photosensitizer is largely in the bloodstream during irradiation so that a shutdown of the tumor vasculature may be achieved. At longer delays, the photosensitizer is expected to be cleared from normal tissues, and there is some preferential retention in tumor tissue; light activation then leads to photocytotoxicity, as already discussed.

Recently, there has been much interest in a different approach to PDT where, instead of a photosensitizer being administered in a synthetic form, a precursor is administered, and the photosensitizer is synthesized in situ in tumors.[38] This is the case with δ-aminolevulinic acid (ALA). ALA is a naturally occurring precursor in the biosynthetic pathway for heme production. The last step in the biosynthetic route involves conversion of protoporphyrin IX (PpIX), a photosensitizing species, to heme (a nonphotosensitizing agent). Under physiologic conditions, cellular heme synthesis is regulated in a negative feedback control of the enzyme ALA synthase by free heme. ALA synthase then becomes the rate-limiting step. When exogenous ALA is added, the control mechanism is bypassed, and downstream metabolites are synthesized in excess. Under these conditions, ferrochelatase, which catalyzes iron insertion into PpIX, becomes the rate-limiting enzyme. Following the addition of exogenous ALA, the low physiologic rate of iron insertion by ferrochelatase is unable to compensate for the excess PpIX that is formed. PpIX, therefore, accumulates in cells and renders them photosensitive.

ALA-based PDT has been used primarily in the treatment of nonmelanoma skin cancers because of the skin's accessibility to light treatment and the availability of a preparation of ALA for topical use.[38,39] In this indication, ALA-based PDT compares well with other forms of PDT and likewise has favorable patient acceptance owing to excellent cosmetic results.[40] Although cutaneous lesions are easily sensitized with topical preparations, other tumor locations need systemic sensitization by ingestion of ALA doses up to 60 mg/kg body weight. For PDT of oral cancer, systemic ALA photosensitization has been successful.[41,42] Patients with Barrett's esophagus, precancerous dysplasia and early esophageal carcinomas are being efficiently treated with oral ALA-based PDT, although the current data suggest that the treatment is most successful in smaller tumor regions.[43–45] In this specific indication, selective PpIX accumulation in the epithelium seems to help prevent strictures that are a complication of PDT with PF.[46,47] Clinical trials are ongoing to improve the overall efficacy of Barrett's treatment, examining variations in drug delivery and light dosimetry to optimize treatment conditions.

In contrast to most tetrapyrrole photosensitizers, ALA-PpIX localizes in cells (where it is synthesized) rather than in the tumor vasculature.[40,48] The effects of exogenous ALA cannot be imitated by administration of presynthesized PpIX.[18] ALA[49] and ALA-PpIX[41] are rapidly cleared from the system, which results in an acceptably short period (< 24 h) of cutaneous photosensitivity. This is viewed as an advantage over some of the other photosensitizers where light protection may be required for several weeks.

Concurrent with clinical studies in humans, there has been much experimental work in cell culture and in animals aimed at understanding the mechanisms of ALA-based PDT, in order to develop strategies for more effective clinical response.[50–52] At present, our knowledge of the mechanisms involved in ALA-based PDT is limited. For example, the reason for preferential ALA uptake and conversion by tumors and dysplastic tissue is not clear. No matter how good the delivery of ALA may be, the formation of PpIX requires the activity of several enzymes, the manipulation of which presents an opportunity to improve PDT. At this point, the relative importance of various enzymes seems dependent on the tumor/tissue type. For example, it has been proposed that some tumors contain lower levels of ferrochelatase, resulting in enhanced ALA-PpIX accumulation. A reduced availability of iron reduces heme formation by ferrochelatase, and iron metabolism has been shown to play a role in ALA-based PDT.[53,54] There is some indication that porphobilinogen deaminase is another important enzyme and is up-regulated under exogenous ALA stimulation.[55]

Proliferating tissues and malignant cells are generally considered more efficient in ALA-PpIX formation,[51] but recently an inverse relationship has been documented in which growth arrest was associated with differentiation.[56] In differentiating (growth-arrested) primary keratinocytes, an increased production of ALA-PpIX was accompanied by an up-regulation of coproporphyrinogen oxidase at the mRNA level,[57] compared with their nondifferentiated (proliferating) counterparts. The increased cellular PpIX content enhanced PDT efficacy. The same increase of ALA-PpIX formation with cellular differentiation was also found in other cellular models of differentiation,[57,58] including a human prostate cancer cell line (LNCaP). In the latter, differentiation was induced with a synthetic androgen receptor ligand, which resulted in an up to 10-fold enhanced ALA-PpIX production and led to enhanced photocytotoxicity. Figure 35a-2 shows a dramatic increase in the PpIX content in differentiated LNCaP cells by confocal scanning fluorescence microscopy after 4 hours of ALA exposure. Quantification showed a more than 10-fold enhancement in the PpIX content of the differentiated LNCaP cells over the undifferentiated ones, along with an increase in PDT responsiveness. These findings suggest a potential for a new combined therapeutic regimen, where induction of differentiation precedes ALA-based PDT and makes tumors more susceptible to photosensitization.

In order to improve the penetration of topically applied ALA and improve selectivity, the development of ALA esters is being investigated. The cells take these up, and esterase hydrolysis yields ALA that enters the heme pathway and induces PpIX production.[59] ALA esters have different molecular properties, which alter pharmacokinetics and bioavailability. The data indicate that the altered properties further improve the diagnostic and therapeutic potential significantly beyond what is achieved with ALA-based PDT.[60,61] The rapid degradation of the ester compounds in the blood limits the penetration to immediately near the site of topical application, thereby limiting PpIX production in surrounding normal tissues and improving the overall tumor to normal tissue selectivity. Several of these esters are in preclinical and clinical investigations.[60–65]

BIOLOGIC MECHANISMS OF PDT

Cellular Mechanisms The cellular mechanisms involved in PDT have been studied extensively, and as with other modalities, these depend on the specific conditions under which they are investigated. These mechanisms have been reviewed,[11,66] and only the more recent developments are discussed below.

In complex environments, such as cells and tissues, the subcellular localization of the photosensitizer is important for effective photochemistry to occur. For electron transfer reactions, an interaction between excited sensitizer and a donor or acceptor molecule is necessary; if these happen to be cellular targets, photobiologic effects occur. Energy transfer reactions involving $^1O_2$ require close proximity of sensitizer and target, since $^1O_2$ can diffuse only about 20 nm in cells because of efficient quenching in biologic environments.[67] Therefore, the cellular structures close to both a high sensitizer and a high oxygen concentration will be preferentially damaged on illumination. Subcellular localization is mainly dependent on the physicochemical properties of the photosensitizer, but may be altered by using specific delivery vehicles (see below) and modifying the status of the cell itself.[57] In a series of studies, Kessel and colleagues[68,69] have shown that sensitizers that localize in mitochondria are very rapid inducers of apoptosis, in contrast to photosensitizers localized in lysosomes and plasma membranes.[68–70] Figure 35a-3 shows the primarily mitochondrial localization of BPD-MA which, on photosensitization, induces apoptosis efficiently (see below). For lysosomal photosensitizers, the mode of cell death is dominated by necrosis, possibly because of the release of lysosomal enzymes and other toxic moieties. There is, however, a possibility of lysosomally localized photosensitizer relocating to mitochondria within the first few seconds of illumination, where they may be considerably more phototoxic.[71]

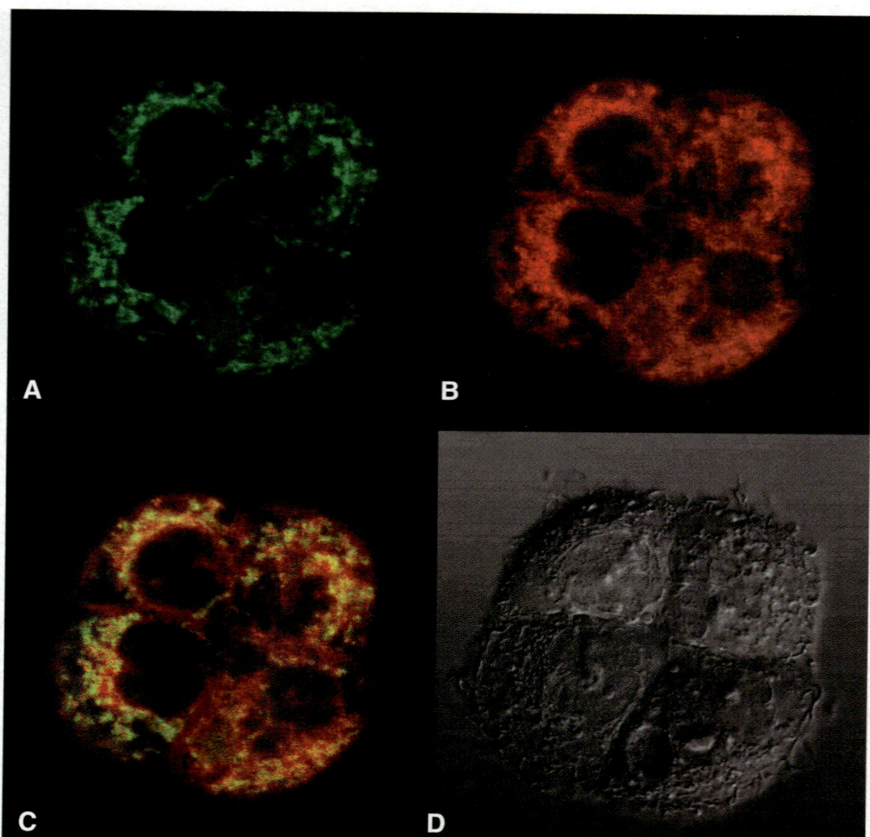

Figure 35a-3 The predominantly mitochondrial localization of the photosensitizer benzoporphyrin derivative monoacid A (BPD-MA) by confocal laser scanning microscopy. OVCAR-3 cells were incubated in 92 nm BPD-MA for 3 hours and 10 nm rhodamine 123, a mitochondrial probe, for 20 minutes. **A,** Green fluorescence of rhodamine 123; **B,** Red BPD-MA fluorescence; **C,** Combination of A+B, where yellow indicates co-localization; **D,** Differential interference contrast transmission image.

Apoptosis induction by photosensitizers primarily localized to the mitochondria is an extremely rapid process.[72] The mechanisms behind this rapid induction have now partly been elucidated and, in general, are consistent with the hypothesis of Liu and colleagues, which proposes the release of cytochrome *c* from mitochondria being a critical signal for the induction of apoptosis.[73] Following PDT with a different photosensitizer, a very early step is the loss of cytochrome *c* into the cytosol.[74–76] In addition, a rapid loss of mitochondrial membrane potential is observed on PDT attributed to the opening of the so-called mitochondrial transition pore.[77] The loss of cytochrome *c* after PDT results in a sharp increase of caspase (cysteine protease acting on aspartic acid) 3 activity via complex formation with 2'-deoxyadenosine 5'-triphosphate (dATP),[75] apoptosis-activating factor-1 (APAF-1), and procaspase 9, and subsequent cleavage of procaspase 9 can activate procaspase 3.[78,79] Caspase 3 is a key player in the induction of apoptosis and involved in the cleavage of a number of proteins,[80] including DNA fragmentation factor (DFF) and poly-ADP-ribose polymerase (PARP), which are involved in the final steps of the apoptotic process. Photodynamic treatment with the photosensitizers Pc4 (a silicon phthalocyanine), BPD-MA, and aluminium phthalocyanine (AlPc) has been shown to induce cleavage of PARP in different cell lines.[72,81,82] In addition, DFF activation was shown after PDT.[74] The very rapid induction of PARP cleavage in thymic lymphoma-resistant to x-rays (LY-R) cells after Pc4-mediated PDT, which is PDT dose dependent and can occur within 10 minutes following illumination.

Another aspect of PDT-induced apoptosis relevant to oncologic applications is that it appears to bypass the usual pathways for apoptotic control. Bcl-2, a protein found in the outer membrane of the mitochondria, is known to be an antiapoptotic. The overexpression of this protein has been associated with chemotherapy and radiation resistance.[83] Consistent with these observations, it was reported that in Chinese hamster ovary (CHO) cells, the presence of Bcl-2 partly protects against apoptosis induction by photodynamic treatment with Pc4.[84] This could be due not only to the known antioxidant effect of Bcl-2, but also due to its ability to interfere with calcium homeostasis, which has been shown to play a role in photodynamically induced cell death.[85] However, it is more likely that Bcl-2 is involved in the inhibition of the cytochrome *c* release after PDT, known to be an important mechanism of modulation of apoptosis by Bcl-2.[86,87] Similarly, it was shown that PDT with BPD-MA was less effective in apoptosis induction in HL-60 cells overexpressing Bcl-2.[88] In these cells the activation of caspase 3 and 6 was also diminished, indicating again their key role in PDT-induced apoptosis. In accordance with these results, it was shown that blocking of Bcl-2 using retrovirus transfection with antisense Bcl-2 increases the sensitivity of MGC803 cells to PDT-induced apoptosis.[89] However, a reversal of the conventional inverse relationship between Bcl-2 expression and apoptosis induction was shown in an interesting study by Kim and colleagues.[90] Using AlPc as sensitizer, an enhanced sensitivity of a Bcl-2-transfected breast cancer cell line was demonstrated. This unexpected result was explained by the simultaneous increase in Bax, a proapoptotic Bcl-2 family member. It was postulated that Bcl-2 might be preferentially damaged by PDT, thereby increasing the Bax:Bcl-2 ratio, which subsequently leads to enhanced apoptosis. These observations are of significance in cancer therapy since, as mentioned above, overexpression of Bcl-2 is often involved in resistance mechanisms against chemotherapeutic agents.[83]

Studies show the involvement of a different signal transduction cascade in growth arrest and apoptosis induced by PDT using Pc4.[91–93] The WAF1/CIP1/p21 protein, which is an inhibitor of cyclin kinases was induced after PDT. This induction, in turn, is believed to lead to the inhibition of cyclin D1 and D2 and their catalytic subunits cyclin-dependent kinase 2 (cdk2) and cdk6. These processes result in an arrest of the cells in the G0/G1 phase of the cell cycle. It was suggested that the increase in WAF1/CIP1/p21 and the subsequent induction of growth arrest was induced by nitric oxide (NO), produced during PDT.[94] In a follow-up study, it was shown that PDT, using Pc4, can cause a hypophosphorylation of retinoblastoma protein (Rb), and decrease free E2F.[92] E2F is a family of transcription factors, which regulate the G1-S transition in the cell cycle, and its inhibition causes arrest of the cells in the G0/G1 phase. This is the final step in the cascade involved in cell-cycle regulation that is affected by PDT. Using cells transfected with the viral protein E6, which abrogates p53 function, Fisher and colleagues showed that PDT with PF caused hypophosphorylation of Rb and subsequent cell-cycle arrest.[95] Growth arrest was independent of the p53 status of the cells, but the apoptotic response was clearly diminished in the cells without functional p53. However, despite the abrogation of the p53-mediated apoptotic pathway, the clonogenic survival following PDT was similar for cells with wild-type p53 or cells with abrogated p53 function. Cells resistant to apoptosis might, therefore, still be sensitive to PDT. Furthermore, a mutation in p53, which occurs in about 50% of human tumors, does not seem to influence its sensitivity to PDT.

Besides the apoptotic pathways described above, other signaling molecules have been implicated in the induction of apoptosis after PDT, such as ceramide formed after activation of sphingomyelinase by PDT.[96,97] In addition, phospholipases A and C have been shown to play a role in PDT-induced apoptosis.[98] The modulating effect of different kinases on the apoptosis induction by PDT is not well understood, but several recent studies have implicated the stress-activated kinases stress-activated protein kinase/Jun N-terminal kinase (SAPK/JNK) and p38/high-osmolarity glycerol response (HOG1) in the control of apoptosis[99,100] as well as the nonreceptor-mediated tyrosine kinase Etk/bmx.[101] Apart from a necrotic or apoptotic response, cells can also undergo a rescue response after PDT, dependent on cell type, photosensitizer, and PDT dose. Several stress proteins involved in cell rescue have been shown to be up-regulated following PDT: heat shock proteins,[76,102,103] glucose-regulated proteins,[104–106] and heme oxygenase.[107] In addition, phospholipase A, prostaglandin E2, and 3'-5'-cyclic adenosine monophosphate (cAMP) were implicated in cellular rescue responses after PDT.[85,108,109]

PDT has also been shown to regulate adhesion molecules,[110] surface receptors such as major histocompatibility complex (MHC) class I and II,[111] and a number of cytokines.[112–114] Cytokine induction by PDT has been shown to be under control of various transcription factors, such as activator protein 1 (AP-1) and nuclear factor kappa B (NFκB).[115] These cellular changes probably play a role in the induction of an immune response after PDT, which is being exploited for developing new therapies.

In Vivo Mechanisms For most sensitizers in clinical and preclinical use, three primary mechanisms of PDT-mediated tumor destruction in vivo have been proposed: cellular, vascular, and immunologic. The relative contribution of each depends, among other factors, on the nature of the photosensitizer and its localization within the tumor tissue, tumor type (vascularity and macrophage content), and the time delay of irradiation after photosensitizer administration (which is one determinant of site of localization, eg, vascular vs parenchymal). The two most investigated mechanisms in vivo are viewed as involving (1) direct tumor cell photoinactivation, and (2) vascular destruction. The third, immunologic, is currently being investigated intensively in many laboratories, and a substantial understanding of this pathway can be anticipated in the near future.[116–118] The PDT response with any photosensitizer involves interplay of all pathways. For example, using in vivo–in vitro analyses, Henderson and Dougherty have shown that the photosensitizer bacteriochlorophyll *a* has a direct cell-kill potential of ~50% at the end of the light treatment and exhibits no vascular shutdown until 3 to 4 hours after the termination of irradiation.[119] On the other hand, with PF, vascular shutdown begins almost immediately after the initiation of light exposure. Direct cell destruction is expected to dominate when the photosensitizer content is high within the tumor cells at the time of light activation. The actual mechanisms of cell death have been discussed above in some detail, and the initial event may be simple organelle damage, such as membrane lipid peroxidation, disruption of lysosomal membrane, loss of mitochondrial membrane potential, and membrane enzyme inhibition.[120] Under the typical protocols, vascular damage is considered the dominant mechanism of tumor death in vivo for most photosensitizers being investigated clinically. Damage is believed to be initiated by release of factors such as eicosanoids, in particular thromboxane,[121] histamines, and tumor necrosis factor-α (TNF-α).[114] Macroscopically, the vascular PDT response is characterized by acute erythema, edema, blanching, and sometimes necrosis. Microscopically, the tumor tissue is characterized by endothelial cell damage,[119,122] platelet aggregation, vasoconstriction, and hemorrhage following PDT.[123] That a clean dissection of the mechanism(s) responsible for PDT-induced tumor destruction is not possible was pointed out in elegant studies.[124,125] radiation-induced fibrosarcoma (RIF) cells in which PDT resistance had been induced in vitro were implanted in mice and subjected to PF-mediated PDT under typical conditions in which a shutdown of the vasculature is generally believed to be the dominant mode of tumor destruction. As the resistance to PDT was induced within the tumor cells, it was expected that in vivo the tumor response to PDT (via vascular shutdown-induced hypoxia) would be similar for the parent and the resistant cell lines.[125] However, the observation was that the resistance to PDT was maintained in vivo, suggesting that direct cytotoxicity was a major component in the tumor photodestruction. As is the case with other modalities, extrapolation of in vitro observations to in vivo mechanisms is not always possible. Quite contradictory observations have been made; for example, although PF-mediated PDT in vivo causes platelet aggregation, photosensitization in vitro leads to an inhibition of platelet aggregation.[126]

It has been shown in some tumor treatments that the modulation of immune effects may play a role in PDT-induced destruction of tumors.[11,114,117,127–134] Nseyo and colleagues have reported high concentrations of interleukin (IL)-1β, IL-2, and TNF-α in the urine of patients treated with PDT for bladder cancer.[127] The reasons for the release of these cytokines and the role they may play in PDT are not well understood. In a study aimed at understanding the mechanisms responsible for PDT-induced potentiation of antitumor immunity, Gollnick and colleagues demonstrated in a balb/c mouse model that PDT delivered to normal and tumor tissue in vivo causes marked changes in the expression of cytokines IL-6 and IL-10, but not TNF-α.[112] IL-6 mRNA and protein were strongly enhanced in the PDT-treated EMT6 tumor. PDT also increased IL-6 mRNA in exposed spleen and skin. The investigators concluded that the general inflammatory response to PDT might be mediated, at least in part, by IL-6. In contrast, IL-10 mRNA in the tumor decreased following PDT, while it was induced in the normal skin of mice exposed to a PDT regime that strongly inhibits the contact hypersensitivity (CHS) response. The coincidence of the kinetics of IL-10 induction with the known kinetics of CHS inhibition observed in these studies suggests that the enhanced IL-10 expression is instrumental in the observed suppression of cell-mediated responses seen following PDT.

In an interesting approach to exploiting immune effects, Steele and colleagues demonstrated that the selective photodestruction of suppressor T cells using monoclonal antibody-HP conjugates resulted in limited increased tumor regression in treated mice, compared with control mice.[128] This enhanced regression was attributed to immune system stimulation after irradiation, leading to the increased killing activity of specific cytotoxic T lymphocytes against target tumor cells. Enhanced NK-cell activity following PDT was also suggested to be operative by possibly lowering the metastatic potential of surviving tumor cells.[129,130] Increased immunity by colony inhibition assays was also demonstrated in mice treated with BPD-MA–mediated PDT.[131] Macrophage involvement (TNF-α production) has been reported and studied by Korbelik and colleagues.[117,133,135] Studies show that tumor-associated macrophages accumulate up to 9 times the PF levels present in tumor cells. This enhanced accumulation is attributed to the association of most porphyrins with low density lipoprotein (LDL).[134] In addition to the direct release from macrophages of factors such as TNF-α that may mediate phototoxicity, an indirect mechanism of macrophage-mediated cytotoxicity in PDT has also been suggested.[136] According to this hypothesis, initial PDT-induced damage to tumor cells forms exposed lipid fragments. These fragments are then recognized as targets by macrophages. This recognition of possibly reparable cells by macrophages and subsequent phagocytosis is then responsible for tumor cell cytotoxicity. The observation of immune response stimulation in tumor treated with PDT has initiated a new hypothesis that PDT-mediated vaccines could be produced more effectively than by other means, and work by Gollnick and colleagues has indicated that this may be true.[118] In addition to the above evidence of immune stimulation, immune suppression has also been reported following PDT with both PF and BPD-MA.[137,138] This observed immune system suppression is being investigated for novel applications, such as organ transplantation and the treatment of autoimmune diseases.

PHOTODYNAMIC THERAPY DOSIMETRY

In principle, photodynamic response is obtained wherever a photosensitizer, oxygen, and light occur simultaneously. Early studies by Bown and colleagues[139] indicated that the presence of photosensitizer and light were of equal importance, and that there existed some level of drug-light reciprocity in the tissue response,[139,140] in that decreasing the drug level by some factor would cause the same loss of effect, equivalent to alternatively decreasing the light delivered by the same factor. This reciprocity is lost in the presence of additional mitigating factors such as photobleaching, oxygen limitation, and excessive photosensitizer concentration leading to self-shielding of the light delivered.[141,142] The extent of the tissue response is modulated by the amounts of both the photosensitizer and the light, and in general, it varies in a dose-dependent manner for both. There appears to be a threshold component for PDT effects to be lethal,[143–146] below which tissue damage is reparable. This threshold value can be different for tumor and normal tissue, as well as vary between photosensitizers and with time after injection,[145] providing an opportunity for added selectivity.[146]

However the drug-light dependence of some photosensitizers is especially complex, such as with ALA-PpIX, where the photosensitizer is produced within the cells after injection of ALA. The maximal production of PpIX is observed at 4 to 6 hours after injection, and there is a complex interaction between optical dose rate and the magnitude of the effect observed. Recent observations have shown that a pretreatment of light followed by a dark interval of 2 hours to allow regeneration of PpIX significantly increases the PDT effect, as measured in normal mouse skin, and variations of this dosimetric regimen will likely become important to maximize the efficacy of the treatment.[147-149] Dose rate effects are thought to be inherently linked to oxygen dependency, as discussed further below.

In Vivo Light Dosimetry Although the significance of accurate light delivery in PDT has been known for decades,[15–17,150,151] many clinical PDT studies have ended without success because of problems with delivering the appropriate amount of light to the tissue[140] or from overdelivery of light causing ulcerations, perforations, or strictures.[152,153] Intracavity irradiation requires the use of specialized delivery probes and monitoring systems,[15,154,155] which allow delivery of light equally to the walls of the tissue, and incorporate integrating sphere effects into the dose calculations. In larger bulk tissues, prediction of the light fluence within the tissue is complicated because it requires accurate estimation of the tissue absorption, scatter and anisotropy parameters, along with analytic or computational means to predict the light fluence. Elaborate methods to measure the interaction parameters have been developed,[156] and relatively simple expressions for diffusion theory prediction of light propagation in tissue-like media have been derived.[143,150] Probes that can be placed on the surface of tissue have been developed by several investigators and companies and perhaps offer the easiest and most reliable method to estimate light dose to the surface of a tissue.[15,157,158] Integrated systems that measure the fluence rate either interstitially or on the surface of the tissues being treated are being implemented in many academic clinical PDT centers, but have not yet been integrated into commercial PDT treatments.[158,159]

In Vivo Photosensitizer Dosimetry Measurement of photosensitizer concentration in tissue has been an issue of significant interest for several decades, with the most accepted method of quantification being biopsy sampling of the tissue and chemical extraction of the compound to be quantified by spectrophotometric assay.[160,161] Throughout this time, there has been interest in using the fluorescent properties of the photosensitizer to directly measure the concentration in vivo, and although useful qualitative case studies have been shown, the data have been largely confounded by variations in tissue optical properties, drug localization, and aggregation variations, all of which can alter the intensity of the fluorescence detected independently of the absolute concentration. More recently, some probes have been developed that allow quantitative measurement of the fluorescence from small fiber systems, which are below the length scale of scattering within tissue, thereby limiting the effect of tissue optical properties.[161,162] Clinical implementation of some elegant fluorescence-based methods currently exist.[163]

Photobleaching of the drug during irradiation has largely been ignored, but has become especially important with the increased use of ALA-PDT, since PpIX appears to have a rapid photobleaching rate.[48,144,147,148,164] Wilson and colleagues have presented the possibility of using photobleaching of the photosensitizer as an indirect measure of the deposited PDT dose in the tissue, since the integrated loss of signal is an indirect measure proportional to the singlet oxygen produced, assuming that singlet oxygen mechanisms are causing the photodegradation. Alternatively, others have suggested the photobleaching degradation products that are optically active could be used to monitor the deposited dose.[165,166] This work continues in search of a good method to quantify deposited dose in tissue.

In Vivo Oxygen Dosimetry With most photosensitizers under investigation, in addition to amounts of photosensitizer and light, PDT efficacy is also oxygen dependent.[167–173] It is generally accepted that the oxygen dependence is based on the requirement to form the active species, singlet oxygen, from interaction of the excited photosensitizer with molecular oxygen dissolved in the tissue. This concept was mostly based on extrapolation from solution chemistry, since the detection of singlet oxygen in vivo has not been possible until very recently.[174–177] Other reactive oxygen species, such as hydroxyl radicals and superoxide anion could also be important active species with some photosensitizers, although this remains to be proven in vitro or in vivo.[178] Under anoxic conditions, the PDT effects of PF are abolished.[179] It should be noted that the relationship between tumor blood flow or oxygen concentration and PDT is not a simple one, as demonstrated in the study by Fingar and colleagues, in which the artificial oxygen carrier Fluosel-DA (20%) did not enhance PDT tumor destruction.[180] Similarly, Iinuma and colleagues demonstrated that in contrast to results from ionizing radiation, pretreatment of animals with nicotinamide, a homogenizer of tumor blood flow and oxygen concentration, did not enhance PDT response.[48] In contrast to these observations, increased respiratory oxygen tension of 100% does enhance PDT efficacy with PF.[181]

An interesting consequence of this oxygen dependence is the effect of the fluence rate (the rate of photon delivery) on PDT efficiency. Within the range of fluence rates for linear photochemistry, there should be no effect of fluence rate on the efficacy of PDT, assuming that there is an overabundance of oxygen available. In a clinical situation, higher subthermal fluence rates have been thought to be favorable because total irradiation time can be shortened. However, as shown in Figure 35a-4 and discussed below, reduced efficacy of tumor destruction[48,170,171,173] has been reported when fluence rates, in the range typically applied in clinical studies (~100–200 mW/cm^2), were used in PDT. This lowered effect has been attributed to oxygen depletion during the irradiation due to oxygen consumption in the photochemical reaction at a rate greater than the rate of reperfusion. In vitro measurements and photochemical calculations confirm that an oxygen limitation to singlet oxygen production should exist in vivo when the available oxygen supply is limited and when the optical fluence rate and photosensitizer concentration in tissue are both high.[182–186]

Depletion of oxygen during photoirradiation has been investigated either by measuring the hypoxic cell fraction in the tumor immediately after PDT[169] or by directly measuring tissue oxygen tension during irradiation, using oxygen electrodes of various types.[172,187–189] The exact changes during PDT remain complex to discern exactly because of the problems of sampling small spatial regions with electrodes, and the fact that the response is highly heterogeneous. Observations have shown both increases and decreases in oxygen tension following PDT,[190,191] indicat-

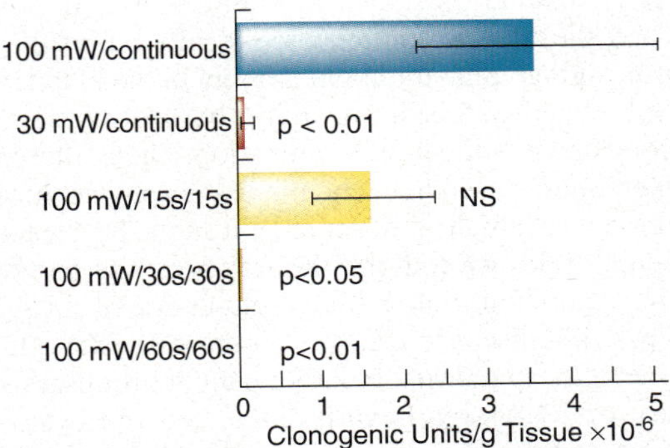

Figure 35a-4 The effect of fluence rate and light fractionation on BPD-mediated photodynamic therapy. Benzoporphyrin derivative monoacid A was administered to rats with nitroblue tetrazolium positive cells (NBT) II tumors implanted into the bladder wall. One hour later, tumors were exposed to a total fluence of 30 J/cm^2 of 690 nm irradiation under the following conditions: 100 mW/cm^2 continuous; 100 mW/cm^2 fractionated 15 s on/15 s off; 100 mW/cm^2 30 s on/30 s off; 100 mW/cm^2 60 s on/60 s off. Tumors were disaggregated 24 hours later and tumor cells were plated for colony formation assay. Colonies (50 cells or more) were counted 9 days later after fixing with methanol and staining with crystal violet. The Wilcoxon rank sum test was used to compare the number of clonogenic cells with data at 100 mW/cm^2 and continuous wave irradiations.

ing high degrees of heterogeneity occur, and the response depends significantly upon the photosensitizer and protocol used.[192] Oxygen depletion during PDT has important practical implications and may be an important limitation of PDT. Tumor tissues are not homogeneous and may contain fractions of hypoxic cells because the induction of neovessels lags tumor growth. In the extreme case, tumor necrosis occurs from lack of nutrients as well as lack of oxygen. It occurs especially in such hypoxic regions that PDT may be less effective because of the limited availability of oxygen.[169,171] Even for the tumor cells located near blood vessels, oxygen might become depleted when high fluence rates are used, consuming oxygen faster than it is replaced from the circulating blood. This problem can be obviated to some extent by using lower fluence rates or fractionated irradiation, as shown in preclinical studies.[52,173,193–197] In studies in an orthotopic rat bladder tumor model, Iinuma and colleagues showed that at the fluence rate of 100 mW/cm^2 and total cumulative light dose of 30 J/cm^2, PDT mediated by BPD-MA was enhanced almost 1,000-fold when a light fractionation regimen (λ = 690 nm) of 60 seconds on and 60 seconds off was used (see Figure 35a-4).[48] At shorter intervals, the enhancement was absent or modest, presumably because oxygen depleted during the initial phase of PDT could not be replenished rapidly enough. Also, for the same fluence (30 J/cm^2), tumor cell cytotoxicity was much enhanced when the fluence rate was 30 mW/cm^2 rather than 100 mW/cm^2. Sitnik and colleagues[172,187] studied the effects of fluence rate on oxygen concentration in a murine RIF tumor model during and after PDT, using 5 mg/kg of PF and fluence rates of 30, 75, or 150 mW/cm^2. Median pO_2 before PDT ranged from 2.9 to 5.2 mm/Hg in the three treatment groups. Within the first minute of illumination, median tumor pO_2 decreased with all fluence rates to values between 0.7 and 1.1 mm/Hg. During prolonged illumination (20–50 J/cm^2), pO_2 recovered at 30 mW/cm^2 fluence rate, but remained low at the 150 mW/cm^2 fluence rate (median pO_2 of 1.7 mm/Hg). There was also a direct correlation between tumor regrowth times and recovery of oxygen levels within the tumor tissues. These preclinical studies appear to suggest that fluence rates lower than those being used currently should produce more efficient clinical PDT response. The problem that has to be addressed, then, is the practicality of treatment times and intervals. Fractionation needs to be accomplished within seconds to minutes and, in contrast to ionizing radiation, is ineffective at longer intervals of hours, possibly because of efficient repair mechanisms following PDT. The key exception to this rule is ALA-PpIX photodynamic therapy where fractionation on the timescale of hours has shown a significant advantage, likely because of the allowing of increased production of PpIX in the intervening time period; however, the exact mechanism of this enhancement is still to be determined.[149]

Recent studies have shown that following PDT with both PF and BPD-MA, tumor oxygenation can rise significantly above pretreatment values.[190,192] This rise can lead to increased radiation sensitivity as demonstrated by Chen and colleagues[198] and could lead to a new application for PDT as a useful adjuvant to radiation therapy of hypoxic tumors.

PHOTODYNAMIC THERAPY WITH TARGETED MOLECULAR DELIVERY SYSTEMS

An important determinant of successful PDT targeting is the localization of the photosensitizer in neoplastic tissue. Although most photosensitizers in their currently used formulations provide adequate selectivity for the limited indications that PDT is used for at this time, the reach and the ease of use would be greatly enhanced if significantly high selective accumulation in tumor tissues could be achieved. The threshold effect discussed above combined with the increased selective localization could minimize the need for precise light dosimetry and concerns of toxicity in complex sites, such as the abdominal cavity. In order to optimize photodynamic action, the idea of drug targeting, as introduced by Ehrlich,[199] has also been applied to PDT. The basic assumption is that molecular delivery systems have an ability to interact selectively with their targets. The rationale for the use of molecular delivery systems for photosensitizers is similar to that for the delivery of chemotherapeutics and toxins. There are, however, two fundamental differences in the requirement in the photon- and the nonphoton-based approaches. First, in conventional therapy, the drug has to be freed to elicit the appropriate biologic response. This is not a prerequisite when macromolecular carrier molecules are used for delivery of photosensitizers in PDT.[33,200,201] Second, in PDT, the requirements for specificity of the delivery molecule are less stringent. This is a consequence of the inherent double selectivity mentioned earlier. As long as the delivery agent has preferential (not necessarily exclusive) affinity for the target tissue, improved selective photodestruction is expected. Therefore, motivations for carrier-mediated PDT are (1) increased concentrations of the photosensitizers at target sites; (2) the possibility of using nontumor-localizing photosensitizers with efficient photochemistry, thus providing a greater repertoire of usable chemicals; and (3) broadening the application of PDT and minimizing the need for precise light dosimetry.

Tumor targeting with antibodies is based on (1) the assumption that new antigens are present on tumor cells, and (2) the ability to obtain specific mAbs that recognize these antigens. Neoplastic transformation is assumed to generate new and specific antigenic components not present in normal tissue. In practice, this is not always true, and mAbs with uniquely high level of specificity for tumor markers are generally nonexistent. Many molecules considered tumor antigens probably represent quantitative differences in glycosylation patterns rather than distinct proteins. Photoimmunoconjugates differ from other immunoconjugates in that in the case of mAb–photosensitizer conjugates, no effector function for the mAb or antibody internalization is required for toxicity because active cytotoxic species can act effectively at the cell membrane level. However, internalized conjugates could be more effective. In cases where drug resistance (eg, via the enhanced P-glycoprotein pump efflux) may be a problem, mAb–photosensitizer conjugates may be expected to be unaffected as long as binding to the cell surface is not seriously impaired. The potential for cytotoxicity of antigen-negative cells because of the diffusivity of free radicals may also be considered an advantage, since tumors generally contain heterogeneous cell populations.

As a recent example of growth factor immunotargeting, Savellano and colleagues have conjugated the photosensitizer BPD to the EGFR Ab C225. Figure 35a-5, which shows specific phototoxicity using this photoimmunoconjugate of A-431, an EGFR-expressing cell line (Figure 35a-5A), while no phototoxicity is observed in NR6, an EGFR-negative cell line (Figure 35a-5B).[202] Another photoimmunoconjugate was used in vivo for the treatment of ovarian cancer in mice.[203] Figure 35a-6 shows an increase in survival of treated mice.

In summary, the existing investigations of mAb–photosensitizer conjugates are promising. Better-characterized and purified conjugates are needed, along with careful pharmacokinetic information in vivo in appropriate animal models. An aspect that is being explored is the use of photosensitizer–immunoconjugates synthesized with antibody fragments, synthetic mAbs and fragments, and single-chain and chimeric antibodies. Such experiments will solve some of the prob-

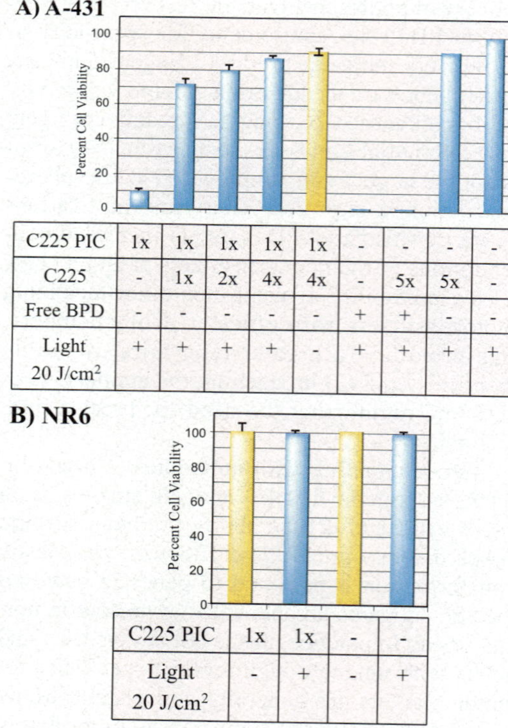

A) A-431

C225 PIC	1x	1x	1x	1x	1x	-	-	-	-
C225	-	1x	2x	4x	4x	-	5x	5x	-
Free BPD	-	-	-	-	-	+	+	-	-
Light 20 J/cm^2	+	+	+	+	-	+	+	+	+

B) NR6

C225 PIC	1x	1x	-	-
Light 20 J/cm^2	-	+	-	+

Figure 35a-5 Phototoxicity experiments. The molar loading ratio of the photoimmune conjugate (PIC) was ~7 benzoporphyrin derivative (BPD)/antibody. Light doses were either 0 J/cm^2 (■) or 20 J/cm^2 (■). **A,** epidermal growth factor receptor (EGFR)-overexpressing A-431 cells were incubated at 37°C for 40 h with C225 PIC (approximately 20 nM antibody content or, equivalently, 140 nM BPD content), either in the absence or in the presence of 1×, 2×, or 4× fold equivalents of unmodified C225 antibody (approximately 20, 40, and 80 nM antibody content, respectively). Control experiments included 140 nM free BPD, 140 nM free BPD + 5× equivalents (100 nM antibody content) of unmodified C225, 5× equivalents of unmodified C225 and media only. **B,** EGFR-negative NR6 cells were incubated at 37°C for 40 h with C225 PIC (approximately 40 nM antibody content or, equivalently, 280 nM BPD content). Percent killing is relative to media only.

lems associated with mAb transport and antispecies response. As a variety of photoimmunoconjugates become available, it will be important to establish the effect of the molecular features of the photoimmunoconjugates on their biologic behavior. Studies have shown that the molecular charge may be critical in establishing the route of delivery for optimal selectivity.[204,205] Similarly, the presence of enzyme-cleavable linkages could further enhance the efficacy of photoimmunoconjugates.

TARGETED OPTICAL IMAGING

The real utility of photoimmunotargeting may lie in its use as a detection modality and therapeutic response monitoring methodology. With this as a focus, Soukos and colleagues have tested an anti-epidermal growth factor receptor (EGFR) MAb coupled to either the near infrared fluorescent dye Cy5.5 for detection or to the photochemically active dye, chlorin (ce_6) for therapy of premalignancy in the hamster cheek pouch carcinogenesis model.[206] Figure 35a-7 shows a representative image from an animal with a papillary tumor measuring 5 mm in diameter. The normal cheek pouch has no visible fluorescence (Figure 35a-7A), whereas the tumor-bearing pouch has a clearly delineated tumor in the fluorescence image (Figure 35a-7B) after systemic injection of anti-EGFR-Cy5.5 MAb conjugate. Furthermore, PDT with the anti-EGFR-ce_6 MAb conjugate showed a significant reduction of EGFR-overexpressing cells compared with non-illuminated areas. These findings suggested that the overexpression of EGFR might be used as a marker for early diagnosis and treatment of oral precancer, since head and neck cancers, including oral cancer and precancer, overexpress EGFR. Targeting the EGFR with antibody-delivered photoactive molecules may destroy the EGFR overexpressing cells, while the normal, low expression levels of EGFR in the healthy tissue do not lead to enough PS concentration in the normal mucosa. Targeted PDT thus will cause the premalignant lesion to regress. The MAb-bound fluorescent dye may also allow the monitoring of the progress of the treatment. These results demonstrate the potential for development of immunotargeted photodiagnosis as a diagnostic tool and as a method of monitoring response to therapy.

Diagnosis Using ALA Although therapeutic indications are expanding, the use of ALA-induced PpIX (ALA-PpIX) has gained much interest in diagnostics.[43] PpIX fluorescence is being developed for the detection of early malignancies, carcinomas in situ, and cancer precursor lesions. By minimally invasive diagnostic procedures, accessible organs, such as the bladder,[207–209] oral cavity,[210,211] lungs,[212] upper and lower gastrointestinal tract,[213,214] and cervix,[215,216] to name a few, are being viewed with optical devices, and ALA-PpIX fluorescence is used to detect suspicious areas for guided biopsy and therapy. In urology, ALA-PpIX is used for the early diagnosis of urothelial dysplasia and carcinoma. An image from a cystoscopic examination of the bladder is shown in Figure 35a-8. In this case, the ALA is administered locally by instillation and remains for about 2 hours in the bladder. Subsequently, the physician first performs cystoscopy under white light illumination. Then, filtered blue light is used to excite the red porphyrin fluorescence, which is observed through the cystoscope. With white light, the lesion can be barely distinguished, while blue light-induced ALA-PpIX fluorescence clearly demonstrates the outline of the neoplasia. In larger patient groups, this use of ALA significantly enhanced the cystoscopic detection of malignant and dysplastic lesions,[208] and in the application of imaging following surgical resection, it has been shown to be a useful "second-look" tool to find remaining dysplastic tissues, thereby significantly reducing the local recurrence rate following surgery.[209]

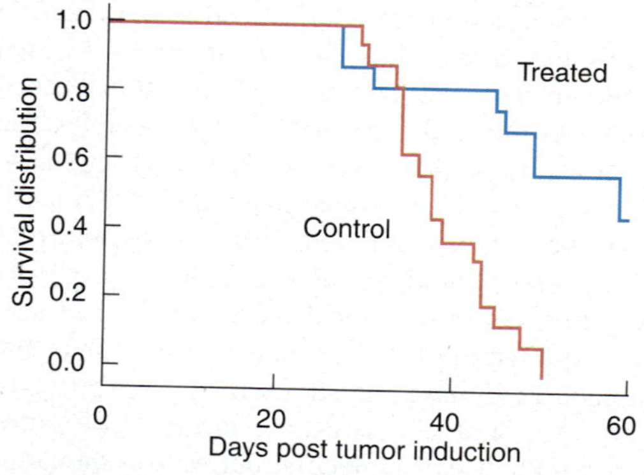

Figure 35a-6 Photoimmunotherapy of ovarian cancer in vivo. Ascites (NIH:OVCAR-3 cells)-bearing mice were treated with the photoimmunoconjugate OC 125 mAb conjugated to chlorin derivative. Twenty-four hours later, mice in the experimental group were treated with a total of 15 J/cm^2 of 656 nm irradiation interperitoneally with a cylindrically diffusing fiber. The photoimmunotherapy was repeated 3 times, 1 week apart, and survival of the treated mice was compared with survival of untreated controls.[203]

Guided Surgery Using ALA ALA-PpIX has been shown to be useful not only for detecting premalignant or malignant tissue, but also for the detection of tumor margins. During surgery for primary brain tumors, the surgical challenge is to remove the malignant tissue as radically as possible, while preserving as much of the healthy brain tissue as possible. The finger-like extensions of these so-called gliomas infiltrate the healthy tissue and thus it is often difficult to distinguish the tumor margins. If the patient ingests ALA prior to surgery, the tumor-associated disruption of the blood-brain barrier results in increased ALA delivery to tumor areas and consequently higher localized PpIX concentrations. Under a modified operating microscope, blue light-induced PpIX fluorescence is then used to guide the targeted resection of the fluorescent malignant tissue with careful sparing of nonfluorescent normal brain. This strategy has been employed successfully in clinical studies and has resulted in prolonged patient survival, which is a sensitive measure of efficient surgery in brain tumors.[217–220] An exciting development in the use of ALA-induced PpIX is the recent approval of hexyl-ALA for diagnosis and guidance imaging of resection in bladder cancer.

PERSPECTIVES

In the past decade PDT has received a number of regulatory approvals worldwide and applications continue to grow. Since the publication of the previous edition of this chapter, PDT with PF was approved by the FDA for the treatment of Barrett's esophagus and is used routinely as a first-line treatment of AMD. The first approval of optical diagnosis in cancer was obtained in Sweden for hexyl-ALA–induced PpIX in the diagnosis and surgical guidance of bladder cancer. In general, all tumors appear to respond to the treatment; however, cure rates are not easily evaluated for a large proportion of the patient population because most of the cancers treated with PDT are refractory to all other treatments.[10,11,221,222] Limitations of light penetration make this therapy most appropriate for small and/or superficial lesions, such as bladder carcinoma in situ, early-

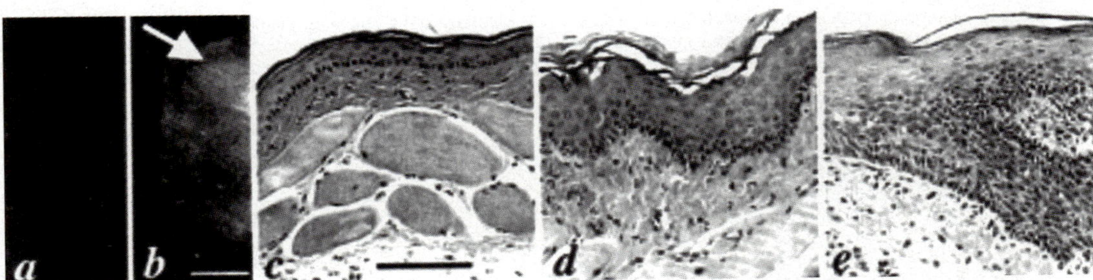

Figure 35a-7 Fluorescence images of normal (**a**) and carcinogen-treated (**b**) hamster cheek pouches, 6 days after the injection of the EGFR-Cy5.5 conjugated (**c**) (bar, 5 mm). An area of increased fluorescence can be seen within the carcinogen-treated cheek pouch (*arrow*). H&E histology shows normal mucosal epithelium for the carcinogen-untreated cheek pouch (**c**) (bar, 100 µm), mild dysplasia for the carcinogen-treated cheek pouch (**d**), and moderate dysplasia for the hot spot (**e**).[206]

stage field cancerization of the oral mucosa, vulvar and early cervical cancers, early lung cancer, Barrett's esophagus, and cancers of the biliary tract. PDT may also have an important role in the purging of tumor cells from bone marrow or peripheral blood. In certain cases where relatively large solid tumors are in locations with delicate surrounding structures, PDT may be used with light administered interstitially using multiple fibers. Examples of such applications are tumors of the brain, prostate, and in specific situations, residual disease in intraperitoneal carcinomatosis, as in ovarian and certain gastrointestinal malignancies. Increasing regulatory approval of this modality for some of the above indications has been encouraging and has stimulated research on new photosensitizers, better methods of localization, and improved resources for light delivery and dosimetry.

Overall, PDT has the potential of being a palliative therapy, a component of combination regimens (eg, with radio-, chemo-, and/or differentiation therapy), or a primary therapy depending on the specific indications. The photosensitizing agents used in PDT all have reasonable fluorescence, and this has spurred much activity in using these molecules for diagnostic purposes and for providing guidance for margins of resection. This aspect of photomedicine is at its infancy and may be expected to grow significantly in the near future with the development of newer technologies. Another interesting aspect of PDT that may be of importance in oncology, and medicine in general, is that PDT is a dynamic process. As photosensitizers travel through different compartments of the tissue, the predominant site of damage (eg, cellular or vascular) could, to some extent, be selected by the choice of the timing of light exposure following photosensitizer administration. This could broaden the scope of application of this modality.

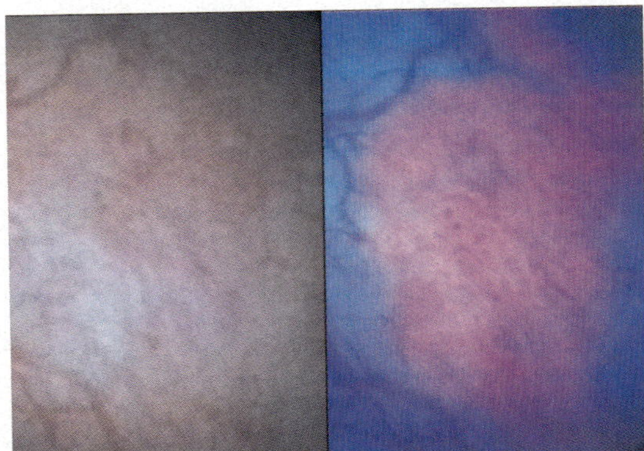

Figure 35a-8 Fluorescence diagnosis of urothelial dysplasia in the bladder clinically. Cystoscopic images of the bladder wall of patients after instillation of 50 mL of a 3% aminolevulinic acid solution for 2 hours for the induction of PpIX formation. The conventional white light image to the left did not show the extent of the neoplastic lesion, which is revealed by the pink PpIX fluorescence under blue illumination of the same view on the right. (Image courtesy of Reinhold Boumgartner, PhD.)

The long-term utility of PDT will be determined from results of well-designed controlled clinical trials, using selectively localized photosensitizers and convenient light sources, such as diode lasers, possibly with built-in light dosimetry components. The increased regulatory approvals of PDT and associated optical detections are exciting developments for cancer research, therapy, and diagnosis.

ACKNOWLEDGMENTS

Support of the authors was provided by National Institutes of Health Grants R01 AR40352 (T.H.), RO1 CA78734 (B.W.P.), PO1 CA84203 (T.H., B.O., B.W.P.), by the Office of Naval Research Contract N00014-94-1-0927 (B.O.), and by the Department of Defense (PC040158) to N.S. during the preparation of this chapter.

REFERENCES

1. van Dongen GA, Visser GW, Vrouenraets MB. Photosensitizer-antibody conjugates for detection and therapy of cancer. Adv Drug Deliv Rev 2004;56:31–52.
2. Vrouenraets MB, Visser GW, Snow GB, van Dongen GA. Basic principles, applications in oncology and improved selectivity of photodynamic therapy. Anticancer Res 2003;23:505–22.
3. Hasan T. Photosensitizer delivery mediated by macromolecular carrier systems. In: Dougherty TJ, Henderson BW, editors. Photodynamic therapy: basic principals and clinical applications. New York: 1992. p. 187–200.
4. Strong L, Yarmush DM and Yarmush ML. Antibody-targeted photolysis. Photophysical, biochemical, and pharmacokinetic properties of antibacterial conjugates. Ann NY Acad Sci 1994;745:297–320.
5. Sharman WM, van Lier JE, Allen CM. Targeted photodynamic therapy via receptor mediated delivery systems. Adv Drug Deliv Rev 2004;56:53–76.
6. Wilson BB, Patterson MS, Flock ST, Moulton JD The optical absorption and scattering properties of tissues in the visible and near-infrared wavelength range. In: Douglas Dall'Acqua M, editor. Light in biology and medicine. Vol. 1. New York: Plenum; 1988. p. 45–52.
7. Dolmans DE, Fukumura D, Jain RK. Photodynamic therapy for cancer. Nat Rev Cancer 2003;3:380–7.
8. Brown SB, Brown EA, Walker I. The present and future role of photodynamic therapy in cancer treatment. Lancet Oncol 2004;5:497–508.
9. Sibata CH, Colussi VC, Oleinick NL, Kinsella TJ. Photodynamic therapy in oncology. Expert Opin Pharmacother 2001;2:917–927.
10. Dougherty TJ, Marcus SL. Photodynamic therapy. Eur J Cancer 1992;28A:1734–42.
11. Dougherty TJ, Gomer CJ, Henderson BW, et al. Photodynamic therapy. J Natl Cancer Inst 1998;90:889–905.
12. Wilson BC. Photodynamic therapy: light delivery and dosage for second-generation photosensitizers. Photosensitizing compounds: their chemistry, biology and clinical use. CIBA Found Symp 1989;146:60–73.
13. Star WM. Light dosimetry in vivo. Phys Med Biol 1997;42:763–87.
14. Grossweiner LI. PDT light dosimetry revisited. J Photochem Photobiol B 1997;38:258–68.
15. Wilson BC, Muller PJ, Yanch JC. Instrumentation and light dosimetry for intra-operative photodynamic therapy (PDT) of malignant brain tumours. Phys Med Biol 1986;31:125–33.
16. Grossweiner LI, Hill JH, Lobraico RV. Photodynamic therapy of head and neck squamous cell carcinoma: optical dosimetry and clinical trial. Photochem Photobiol 1987;46:911–7.
17. Star WM, Marijnissen JP, van Gemert MJ. Light dosimetry in optical phantoms and in tissues: I. Multiple flux and transport theory. Phys Med Biol 1988;33:437–54.
18. Dougherty TJ. Photosensitizers: therapy and detection of malignant tumors. Photochem Photobiol 1987;45:879–89.
19. Detty MR, Gibson SL, Wagner SJ. Current clinical and preclinical photosensitizers for use in photodynamic therapy. J Med Chem 2004;47:3897–915.
20. Gomer CJ. Preclinical examination of first and second generation photosensitizers used in photodynamic therapy. Photochem Photobiol 1991;54:1093–107.
21. Boyle RW, Dolphin D. Structure and biodistribution relationships of photodynamic sensitizers. Photochem Photobiol 1996;64:469–85.
22. Pushpan SK, Venkatraman S, Anand VG, et al. Porphyrins in photodynamic therapy—a search for ideal photosensitizers. Curr Med Chem AntiCanc Agents 2002;2:187–207.
23. Peng Q, Moan J. Correlation of distribution of sulphonated aluminium phthalocyanines with their photodynamic effect in tumour and skin of mice bearing CaD2 mammary carcinoma. Br J Cancer 1995;72:565–74.
24. Alian W, Andersson-Engels S, Svanberg K, Svanberg S. Laser-induced fluorescence studies of meso-tetra(hydroxyphenyl)chlorin in malignant and normal tissues in rats. Br J Cancer 1994;70:880–5.
25. Pogue BW, Redmond RW, Trivedi N, Hasan T. Photophysical properties of tin ethyl etiopurpurin I (SnET2) and tin octaethylbenzochlorin (SnOEBC) in solution and bound to albumin. Photochem Photobiol 1998;68:809–15.
26. Pogue BW, Ortel B, Chen N, et al. A photobiological and photophysical-based study of phototoxicity of two chlorins. Cancer Res 2001;61:717–24.
27. Aveline B, Hasan T, Redmond RW. Photophysical and photosensitizing properties of benzoporphyrin derivative monoacid ring A (BPD-MA). Photochem Photobiol 1994;59:328–35.
28. Aveline BM, Hasan T, Redmond RW. The effects of aggregation, protein binding and cellular incorporation on the photophysical properties of benzoporphyrin derivative monoacid ring A (BPDMA). J Photochem Photobiol B 1995;30:161–9.
29. Schmidt-Erfurth U, Hasan T, Gragoudas E, et al. Vascular targeting in photodynamic occlusion of subretinal vessels. Ophthalmology 1994;101:1953–61.
30. Schmidt-Erfurth U, Miller J, Sickenberg M, et al. Photodynamic therapy of subfoveal choroidal neovascularization: clinical and angiographic examples. Graefes Arch Clin Exp Ophthalmol 1998;236:365–74.
31. Schmidt-Erfurth U, Miller JW, Sickenberg M, et al. Photodynamic therapy with verteporfin for choroidal neovascularization caused by age-related macular degeneration: results of retreatments in a phase 1 and 2 study. Arch Ophthalmol 1999;117:1177–87.
32. Bressler NM. Treatment of age-related macular degeneration with photodynamic therapy (TAP) study group. Pho-

todynamic therapy of subfoveal choroidal neovascularization in age-related macular degeneration with verteporfin: two-year results of 2 randomized clinical trials-tap report 2. Arch Ophthalmol 2001;119:198–207.

33. Oseroff AR, Ohuoha D, Hasan T, et al. Antibody-targeted photolysis: selective photodestruction of human T- cell leukemia cells using monoclonal antibody-chlorin e6 conjugates. Proc Natl Acad Sci U S A 1986;83:8744–8.
34. Cincotta L, Foley JW, Cincotta AH. Novel red absorbing benzo[a]phenoxazinium and benzo[a]phenothiazinium photosensitizers: in vitro evaluation. Photochem Photobiol 1987;46:751–8.
35. Cincotta L, Foley JW, MacEachern T, et al. Novel photodynamic effects of a benzophenothiazine on two different murine sarcomas. Cancer Res 1994;54:1249–58.
36. Cincotta L, Szeto D, Lampros E, et al. Benzophenothiazine and benzoporphyrin derivative combination phototherapy effectively eradicates large murine sarcomas. Photochem Photobiol 1996;63:229–37.
37. Hendrzak-Henion JA, Knisely TL, Cincotta L, et al. Role of the immune system in mediating the antitumor effect of benzophenothiazine photodynamic therapy. Photochem Photobiol 1999;69:575–81.
38. Kennedy JC, Pottier RH. Endogenous protoporphyrin IX, a clinically useful photosensitizer for photodynamic therapy. J Photochem Photobiol B 1992;14:275–92.
39. Gupta AK, Ryder JE. Photodynamic therapy and topical aminolevulinic acid: an overview. Am J Clin Dermatol 2003;4:699–708.
40. Peng Q, Warloe T, Berg K, et al. 5-Aminolevulinic acid-based photodynamic therapy. Clinical research and future challenges. Cancer 1997;79:2282–308.
41. Grant WE, Hopper C, MacRobert AJ, et al. Photodynamic therapy of oral cancer: photosensitisation with systemic aminolaevulinic acid. Lancet 1993;342:147–8.
42. Mustajoki P, Timonen K, Gorchein A, et al. Sustained high plasma 5-aminolaevulinic acid concentration in a volunteer: no porphyric symptoms. Eur J Clin Invest 1992;22:407–11.
43. Kelty CJ, Brown NJ, Reed MW, Ackroyd R. The use of 5-aminolaevulinic acid as a photosensitiser in photodynamic therapy and photodiagnosis. Photochem Photobiol Sci 2002;1:158–68.
44. Barr H, Shepherd NA, Dix A, et al. Eradication of high-grade dysplasia in columnar-lined (Barrett's) oesophagus by photodynamic therapy with endogenously generated protoporphyrin IX. Lancet 1996;348:584–5.
45. Tan WC, Fulljames C, Stone N, et al. Photodynamic therapy using 5-aminolaevulinic acid for oesophageal adenocarcinoma associated with Barrett's metaplasia. J Photochem Photobiol B, Biol 1999;53:75–80.
46. Ell C, Gossner L. Photodynamic therapy. Recent Results Cancer Res 2000;155:175–81.
47. Gossner L, Ell C. Photodynamic therapy of gastric cancer. Gastrointest Endosc Clin N Am 2000;10:461–80.
48. Iinuma S, Schomacker KT, Wagnieres G, et al. In vivo fluence rate and fractionation effects on tumor response and photobleaching in photodynamic therapy with two photosensitizers in an orthotopic rat tumor model. Cancer Res 1999;59:6164–70.
49. Berlin NI, Neuberger A, Scott JJ. The metabolism of d-aminolevulinic acid. 1. Normal pathways, studied with the aid of 15N. Biochem J 1956;64:80–90.
50. Malik Z, Lugaci H. Destruction of erythroleukaemic cells by photoactivation of endogenous porphyrins. Br J Cancer 1987;56:589–95.
51. Iinuma S, Farshi SS, Ortel B, Hasan T. A mechanistic study of cellular photodestruction with 5-aminolaevulinic acid-induced porphyrin [published erratum appears in Br J Cancer 1994 Dec;70(6):1283]. Br J Cancer 1994;70:21–8.
52. Hua Z, Gibson SL, Foster TH, Hilf R. Effectiveness of delta-aminolevulinic acid-induced protoporphyrin as a photosensitizer for photodynamic therapy in vivo. Cancer Res 1995;55:1723–31.
53. Pourzand C, Reelfs O, Kvam E, Tyrrell RM. The iron regulatory protein can determine the effectiveness of 5- aminolevulinic acid in inducing protoporphyrin IX in human primary skin fibroblasts. J Invest Dermatol 1999;112:419–25.
54. Rittenhouse-Diakun K, Van Leengoed H, Morgan J, et al. The role of transferrin receptor (CD71) in photodynamic therapy of activated and malignant lymphocytes using the heme precursor delta-aminolevulinic acid (ALA). Photochem Photobiol 1995;61:523–8.
55. Gibson SL, Cupriks DJ, Havens JJ, et al. A regulatory role for porphobilinogen deaminase (PBGD) in delta-aminolaevulinic acid (delta-ALA)-induced photosensitization? Br J Cancer 1998;77:235–43.
56. Ortel B, Sharlin D, O'Donnell D, et al. Differentiation enhances aminolevulinic acid-dependent photodynamic treatment of LNCaP prostate cancer cells. Br J Cancer 2002;87:1321–7.
57. Ortel B, Chen N, Brissette J, et al. Differentiation-specific increase in ALA-induced protoporphyrin IX accumulation in primary mouse keratinocytes. Br J Cancer 1998;77:1744–51.
58. Li G, Szewczuk MR, Pottier RH, Kennedy JC. Effect of mammalian cell differentiation on response to exogenous 5-aminolevulinic acid. Photochem Photobiol 1999;69:231–5.
59. Gaullier JM, Berg K, Peng Q, et al. Use of 5-aminolevulinic acid esters to improve photodynamic therapy on cells in culture. Cancer Res 1997; 57:1481–6.
60. Xiang W, Weingandt H, Liessmann F, et al. Photodynamic effects induced by aminolevulinic acid esters on human cervical carcinoma cells in culture. Photochem Photobiol 2001;74:617–23.
61. Luksiene Z, Eggen I, Moan J, et al. Evaluation of protoporphyrin IX production, phototoxicity and cell death pathway induced by hexylester of 5-aminolevulinic acid in Reh and HPB-ALL cells. Cancer Lett 2001;169:33–9.
62. Kloek J, Akkermans W, van Beijersbergen H, Henegouwen GM. Derivatives of 5-aminolevulinic acid for photodynamic therapy: enzymatic conversion into protoporphyrin. Photochem Photobiol 1998;67:150–4.
63. Kloek J,van Beijersbergen H. Prodrugs of 5-aminolevulinic acid for photodynamic therapy. Photochem Photobiol 1996;64:994–1000.
64. Lange N, Jichlinski P, Zellweger M, et al. Photodetection of early human bladder cancer based on the fluorescence of 5-aminolaevulinic acid hexylester-induced protoporphyrin IX: a pilot study. Br J Cancer 1999;80:185–93.
65. Uehlinger P, Zellweger M, Wagnieres G, et al. 5-Aminolevulinic acid and its derivatives: physical chemical properties and protoporphyrin IX formation in cultured cells. J Photochem Photobiol B 2000;54:72–80.
66. Oleinick NL, Evans HH. The photobiology of photodynamic therapy: cellular targets and mechanisms. Radiat Res 1998;150:S146–56.
67. Peng Q, Moan J, Nesland JM. Correlation of subcellular and intratumoral photosensitizer localization with ultrastructural features after photodynamic therapy. Ultrastruct Pathol 1996;20:109–29.
68. Kessel D, Luo Y. Mitochondrial photodamage and PDT-induced apoptosis. J Photochem Photobiol B, Biol 1998;42:89–95.
69. Kessel D. The role of subcellular localization in initiation of apoptosis by photodynamic therapy. Photochem Photobiol 1997;65:410–5.
70. Dahle J, Steen HB, Moan J. The mode of cell death induced by photodynamic treatment depends on cell density. Photochem Photobiol 1999;70:363–7.
71. Wood SR, Holroyd JA, Brown SB. The subcellular localization of Zn(II) phthalocyanines and their redistribution on exposure to light. Photochem Photobiol 1997;65:397–402.
72. He J, Whitacre CM, Xue LY, et al. Protease activation and cleavage of poly(ADP-ribose) polymerase: an integral part of apoptosis in response to photodynamic treatment. Cancer Res 1998;58:940–6.
73. Liu X, Kim CN, Yang J, et al. Induction of apoptotic program in cell-free extracts: requirement for dATP and cytochrome c. Cell 1996;86:147–57.
74. Granville DJ, Carthy CM, Jiang H, et al. Rapid cytochrome c release, activation of caspases 3, 6, 7 and 8 followed by Bap31 cleavage in HeLa cells treated with photodynamic therapy. FEBS Lett 1998;437:5–10.
75. Varnes ME, Chiu SM, Xue LY, Oleinick NL. Photodynamic therapy-induced apoptosis in lymphoma cells: translocation of cytochrome c causes inhibition of respiration as well as caspase activation. Biochem Biophys Res Commun 1999;255:673–9.
76. Kessel D, Luo Y. Photodynamic therapy: a mitochondrial inducer of apoptosis. Cell Death Differ 1999;6:28–35.
77. Green DR, Reed JC. Mitochondria and apoptosis. Science 1998;281:1309–12.
78. Thornberry NA, Lazebnik Y. Caspases: enemies within. Science 1998;281:1312–6.
79. Nunez G, Benedict MA, Hu Y, Inohara N. Caspases: the proteases of the apoptotic pathway. Oncogene 1998;17:3237–45.
80. Porter AG, Janicke RU. Emerging roles of caspase-3 in apoptosis. Cell Death Differ 1999;6:99–104.
81. Luo Y, Kessel D. Initiation of apoptosis versus necrosis by photodynamic therapy with chloroaluminum phthalocyanine. Photochem Photobiol 1997;66:479–83.
82. Belzacq AS, Jacotot E, Vieira HL, et al. Apoptosis induction by the photosensitizer verteporfin: identification of mitochondrial adenine nucleotide translocator as a critical target. Cancer Res 2001;61:1260–4.
83. van Brussel JP, Mickisch GH. Circumvention of multidrug resistance in genitourinary tumors. Int J Urol 1998;5:1–15.
84. He J, Agarwal ML, Larkin HE, et al. The induction of partial resistance to photodynamic therapy by the protooncogene BCL-2. Photochem Photobiol 1996;64:845–52.
85. Penning LC, Rasch MH, Ben-Hur E, et al. A role for the transient increase of cytoplasmic free calcium in cell rescue after photodynamic treatment. Biochim Biophys Acta 1992;1107:255–60.
86. Yang J, Liu X, Bhalla K, et al. Prevention of apoptosis by Bcl-2: release of cytochrome c from mitochondria blocked. Science 1997;275:1129–32.
87. Kluck RM, Bossy-Wetzel E, Green DR, Newmeyer DD. The release of cytochrome c from mitochondria: a primary site for Bcl-2 regulation of apoptosis. Science 1997;275:1132–6.
88. Granville DJ, Jiang H, An MT, et al. Bcl-2 overexpression blocks caspase activation and downstream apoptotic events instigated by photodynamic therapy. Br J Cancer 1999;79:95–100.
89. Zhang WG, Ma LP, Wang SW, et al. Antisense bcl-2 retrovirus vector increases the sensitivity of a human gastric adenocarcinoma cell line to photodynamic therapy. Photochem Photobiol 1999;69:582–6.
90. Kim HR, Luo Y, Li G, Kessel D. Enhanced apoptotic response to photodynamic therapy after bcl-2 transfection. Cancer Res 1999;59:3429–32.
91. Whitacre CM, Feyes DK, Satoh T, et al. Photodynamic therapy with the phthalocyanine photosensitizer Pc 4 of SW480 human colon cancer xenografts in athymic mice. Clin Cancer Res 2000;6:2021–7.
92. Ahmad N, Mukhtar H. Mechanism of photodynamic therapy-induced cell death. Methods Enzymol 2000;319:342–58.
93. Colussi VC, Feyes DK, Mulvihill JW, et al. Phthalocyanine 4 (Pc 4) photodynamic therapy of human OVCAR-3 tumor xenografts. Photochem Photobiol 1999;69:236–41.
94. Gupta S, Ahmad N, Mukhtar H. Involvement of nitric oxide during phthalocyanine (Pc4) photodynamic therapy-mediated apoptosis. Cancer Res 1998;58:1785–8.
95. Fisher AM, Ferrario A, Rucker N, et al. Photodynamic therapy sensitivity is not altered in human tumor cells after abrogation of p53 function. Cancer Res 1999;59:331–5.
96. Separovic D, He J, Oleinick NL. Ceramide generation in response to photodynamic treatment of L5178Y mouse lymphoma cells. Cancer Res 1997;57:1717–21.
97. Separovic D, Mann KJ, Oleinick NL. Association of ceramide accumulation with photodynamic treatment-induced cell death. Photochem Photobiol 1998;68:101–9.
98. Agarwal ML, Larkin HE, Zaidi SI, et al. Phospholipase activation triggers apoptosis in photosensitized mouse lymphoma cells. Cancer Res 1993;53:5897–902.
99. Agostinis P, Assefa Z, Vantieghem A, et al. Apoptotic and anti-apoptotic signaling pathways induced by photodynamic therapy with hypericin. Adv Enzyme Regul 2000;40:157–82.
100. Xue L, He J, Oleinick NL. Promotion of photodynamic therapy-induced apoptosis by stress kinases. Cell Death Diff 1999;6:855–64.
101. Xue LY, Qiu Y, He J, et al. Etk/Bmx, a PH-domain containing tyrosine kinase, protects prostate cancer cells from apoptosis induced by photodynamic therapy or thapsigargin. Oncogene 1999;18:3391–8.
102. Xue LY, He J, Oleinick NL. Rapid tyrosine phosphorylation of HS1 in the response of mouse lymphoma L5178Y-R cells to photodynamic treatment sensitized by the phthalocyanine Pc 4. Photochem Photobiol 1997;66:105–13.
103. Gomer CJ, Ryter SW, Ferrario A, et al. Photodynamic therapy-mediated oxidative stress can induce expression of heat shock proteins. Cancer Res 1996;56:2355–60.
104. Gomer CJ, Ferrario A, Rucker N, et al. Glucose regulated protein induction and cellular resistance to oxidative stress mediated by porphyrin photosensitization. Cancer Res 1991;51:6574–9.
105. Morgan J, Whitaker JE, Oseroff AR. GRP78 induction by calcium ionophore potentiates photodynamic therapy using the mitochondrial targeting dye victoria blue BO. Photochem Photobiol 1998;67:155–64.
106. Xue LY, Agarwal ML, Varnes ME. Elevation of GRP-78 and loss of HSP-70 following photodynamic treatment of

V79 cells: sensitization by nigericin. Photochem Photobiol 1995;62:135–43.

107. Gomer CJ, Luna M, Ferrario A, Rucker N. Increased transcription and translation of heme oxygenase in Chinese hamster fibroblasts following photodynamic stress or Photofrin II incubation. Photochem Photobiol 1991;53:275–9.
108. Penning LC, VanSteveninck J, Dubbelman TM. HPD-induced photodynamic changes in intracellular cyclic AMP levels in human bladder transitional carcinoma cells, clone T24. Biochem Biophys Res Commun 1993;194:1084–9.
109. Penning LC, Dubbelman TM. Fundamentals of photodynamic therapy: cellular and biochemical aspects. Anticancer Drugs 1994;5:139–46.
110. Runnels JM, Chen N, Ortel B, et al. BPD-MA-mediated photosensitization in vitro and in vivo: cellular adhesion and beta1 integrin expression in ovarian cancer cells. Br J Cancer 1999;80:946–53.
111. King DE, Jiang H, Simkin GO, et al. Photodynamic alteration of the surface receptor expression pattern of murine splenic dendritic cells. Scand J Immunol 1999;49:184–92.
112. Gollnick SO, Liu X, Owczarczak B, et al. Altered expression of interleukin 6 and interleukin 10 as a result of photodynamic therapy in vivo. Cancer Res 1997; 57:3904–9.
113. Kick G, Messer G, Goetz A, et al. Photodynamic therapy induces expression of interleukin 6 by activation of AP-1 but not NF-kappa B DNA binding. Cancer Res 1995;55:2373–9.
114. Evans S, Matthews W, Perry R, et al. Effect of photodynamic therapy on tumor necrosis factor production by murine macrophages. J Natl Cancer Inst 1990;82:34–9.
115. Piret B, Legrand-Poels S, Sappey C, Piette J. NF-kappa B transcription factor and human immunodeficiency virus type 1 (HIV-1) activation by methylene blue photosensitization. Eur J Biochem 1995;228:447–55.
116. Hunt DW, Chan AH. Influence of photodynamic therapy on immunological aspects of disease—an update. Expert Opin Investig Drugs 2000;9:807–17.
117. Korbelik M, Dougherty GJ. Photodynamic therapy-mediated immune response against subcutaneous mouse tumors. Cancer Res 1999;59:1941–6.
118. Gollnick SO, Vaughan L, Henderson BW. Generation of effective antitumor vaccines using photodynamic therapy. Cancer Res 2002;62:1604–8.
119. Henderson BW, Dougherty TJ. How does photodynamic therapy work? Photochem Photobiol 1992;55:145–57.
120. Dubbelman TMAR. Porphyrin-photosensitized modification of subcellular structures. In: Jori G, Perria C, editors. Photodynamic therapy of tumors and other diseases. Padova, Italy: Libreria Progetto Editore; 1985. p. 93–5.
121. Fingar VH, Wieman TJ, Doak KW. Role of thromboxane and prostacyclin release on photodynamic therapy-induced tumor destruction. Cancer Res 1990;50:2599–603.
122. Schmidt-Erfurth U, Bauman W, Gragoudas E, et al. Photodynamic therapy of experimental choroidal melanoma using lipoprotein-delivered benzoporphyrin. Ophthalmology 1994;101:89–99.
123. Fingar VH, Taber SW, Haydon PS, et al. Vascular damage after photodynamic therapy of solid tumors: a view and comparison of effect in pre-clinical and clinical models at the University of Louisville. In Vivo 2000;14:93–100.
124. Fingar VH, Wieman TJ. Studies on the mechanism of photodynamic therapy induced tumor destruction. In: Dougherty TJ, editor. PDT Mechanisms II. Bellingham (WA): Proc SPIE; 1990. p. 168–77.
125. Adams K, Rainbow AJ, Wilson BC, Singh G. In vivo resistance to photofrin-mediated photodynamic therapy in radiation-induced fibrosarcoma cells resistant to in vitro Photofrin-mediated photodynamic therapy. J Photochem Photobiol B 1999;49:136–41.
126. Henderson BW, Owczarczak B, Sweeney J, Gessner T. Effects of photodynamic treatment of platelets or endothelial cells in vitro on platelet aggregation. Photochem Photobiol 1992;56:513–21.
127. Nseyo UO, Whalen RK, Duncan MR, et al. Urinary cytokines following photodynamic therapy for bladder cancer. A preliminary report. Urology 1990;36:167–71.
128. Steele JK, Liu D, Stammers AT, et al. Suppressor deletion therapy: selective elimination of T suppressor cells in vivo using a hematoporphyrin conjugated monoclonal antibody permits animals to reject syngeneic tumor cells. Cancer Immunol Immunother 1988;26:125–31.
129. Gomer CJ. The effect of localized porphyrin photodynamic therapy on the induction of tumour metastasis. Br J Cancer 1987;56:27–32.
130. Gomer CJ, Ferrario A, Hayashi N, et al. Molecular, cellular, and tissue responses following photodynamic therapy. Lasers Surg Med 1988;8:450–63.
131. Logan PM, Newton J, Richter A, et al. Immunological effects of photodynamic therapy. In: Dougherty TJ, editor. PDT Mechanisms II. Bellingham (WA): Proc SPIE; 1990. p. 153–8.
132. Krosl G, Korbelik M. Potentiation of photodynamic therapy by immunotherapy: the effect of schizophyllan (SPG). Cancer Lett 1994;84:43–9.
133. Korbelik M, Sun J, Posakony JJ. Interaction between photodynamic therapy and BCG immunotherapy responsible for the reduced recurrence of treated mouse tumors. Photochem Photobiol 2001;73:403–9.
134. Hamblin MR, Newman EL. On the mechanism of the tumour-localising effect in photodynamic therapy. J Photochem Photobiol B, Biol 1994;23:3–8.
135. Korbelik M, Krosl G. Photofrin accumulation in malignant and host cell populations of a murine fibrosarcoma. Photochem Photobiol 1995;62:162–8.
136. Korbelik M, Krosl G. Enhanced macrophage cytotoxicity against tumor cells treated with photodynamic therapy. Photochem Photobiol 1994;60:497–502.
137. Lynch DH, Haddad S, King VJ, et al. Systemic immunosuppression induced by photodynamic therapy (PDT) is adoptively transferred by macrophages. Photochem Photobiol 1989;49:453–8.
138. Simkin G, Obochi M, Hunt DWC, et al. Effect of photodynamic therapy using benzoporphyrin derivative on the cutaneous immune response. In: Dougherty TJ, editor. Optical methods for tumor treatment and detection: mechanisms and techniques in PDT IV. Bellingham (WA): Proc SPIE; 1995. p. 23–33.
139. Bown SG, Tralau CJ, Smith PD, et al. Photodynamic therapy with porphyrin and phthalocyanine sensitisation: quantitative studies in normal rat liver. Br J Cancer 1986;54:43–52.
140. Marijnissen JP, Versteeg JA, Star WM, van Putten WL. Tumor and normal tissue response to interstitial photodynamic therapy of the rat R-1 rhabdomyosarcoma. Int J Radiat Oncol Biol Phys 1992;22:963–72.
141. Barr H. The significance of the nature of the photosensitizer for photodynamic therapy: quantitative and biological studies in the colon. Br J Cancer 1990;62:730–5.
142. Moesta KT, Greco WR, Nurse-Finlay SO, et al. Lack of reciprocity in drug and light dose dependence of photodynamic therapy of pancreatic adenocarcinoma in vitro. Cancer Res 1995;55:3078–84.
143. Patterson MS, Wilson BC, Graff R. In vivo tests of the concept of photodynamic threshold dose in normal rat liver photosensitized by aluminum chlorosulphonated phthalocyanine. Photochem Photobiol 1990;51:343–9.
144. Georgakoudi I, Nichols MG, Foster TH. The mechanism of Photofrin photobleaching and its consequences for photodynamic dosimetry. Photochem Photobiol 1997;65:135–44.
145. Farrell TJ, Wilson BC, Patterson MS, Olivo MC. Comparison of the in vivo photodynamic threshold dose for photofrin, mono- and tetrasulfonated aluminum phthalocyanine using a rat liver model. Photochem Photobiol 1998;68:394–9.
146. Lilge L, Wilson BC. Photodynamic therapy of intracranial tissues: a preclinical comparative study of four different photosensitizers. J Clin Laser Med Surg 1998;16:81–91.
147. Robinson DJ, de Bruijn HS, van der Veen N, et al. Fluorescence photobleaching of ALA-induced protoporphyrin IX during photodynamic therapy of normal hairless mouse skin: the effect of light dose and irradiance and the resulting biological effect. Photochem Photobiol 1998;67:140–9.
148. Robinson DJ, de Bruijn HS, van der Veen N, et al. Protoporphyrin IX fluorescence photobleaching during ALA-mediated photodynamic therapy of UVB-induced tumors in hairless mouse skin. Photochem Photobiol 1999;69:61–70.
149. Thissen MR, de Blois MW, Robinson DJ, et al. PpIX fluorescence kinetics and increased skin damage after intracutaneous injection of 5-aminolevulinic acid and repeated illumination. J Invest Dermatol 2002;118:239–45.
150. Grossweiner LI. Optical dosimetry in photodynamic therapy. Lasers Surg Med 1986;6:462–6.
151. Werkhaven J, Harris DM, Krol G, Hill JH. Light dosimetry in animal models: application to photodynamic therapy in otolaryngology. Laryngoscope 1986;96:1058–61.
152. D'Hallewin MA, Baert L. Long-term results of whole bladder wall photodynamic therapy for carcinoma in situ of the bladder. Urology 1995;45:763–7.
153. Panjehpour M, Overholt BF, Haydek JM, Lee SG. Results of photodynamic therapy for ablation of dysplasia and early cancer in Barrett's esophagus and effect of oral steroids on stricture formation. Am J Gastroenterol 2000;95:2177–84.
154. van Staveren HJ, Beek JF, Keijzer M, Star WM. Integrating sphere effect in whole-bladder-wall photodynamic therapy: II. The influence of urine at 458, 488, 514 and 630 nm optical irradiation. Phys Med Biol 1995;40:1307–15.
155. Marijnissen JP, Baas P, Beek JF, et al. Pilot study on light dosimetry for endobronchial photodynamic therapy. Photochem Photobiol 1993;58:92–9.
156. Bays R, Wagnieres G, Robert D, et al. Light dosimetry for photodynamic therapy in the esophagus. Lasers Surg Med 1997;20:290–303.
157. Profio AE, Doiron DR. Dose measurements in photodynamic therapy of cancer. Lasers Surg Med 987;7:1–5.
158. Vulcan TG, Zhu TC, Rodriguez CE, et al. Comparison between isotropic and nonisotropic dosimetry systems during intraperitoneal photodynamic therapy. Lasers Surg Med 2000;26:292–301.
159. Johansson T, Thompson MS, Stenberg M, et al. Feasibility study of a system for combined light dosimetry and interstitial photodynamic treatment of massive tumors. Appl Opt 2002;41:1462–8.
160. Lilge L, O'Carroll C, Wilson BC. A solubilization technique for photosensitizer quantification in ex vivo tissue samples. J Photochem Photobiol B 1997;39:229–35.
161. Lee CC, Pouge BW, Strawbridge RR, et al. Comparison of photosensitizer (AlPcS2) quantification techniques: in situ fluorescence microsampling versus tissue chemical extraction. Photochem Photobiol 2001;74:453–60.
162. Lee CC, Pogue BW, O'Hara JA, et al. Spatial heterogeneity and temporal kinetics of photosensitizer (AlPcS2) concentration in murine tumors RIF-1 and MTG-B. Photochem Photobiol Sci 2003;2:145–50.
163. Glanzmann T, Hadjur C, Zellweger M, et al. Pharmacokinetics of tetra(m-hydroxyphenyl)chlorin in human plasma and individualized light dosimetry in photodynamic therapy. Photochem Photobiol 1998;67:596–602.
164. Moan J. Effect of bleaching of porphyrin sensitizers during photodynamic therapy. Cancer Lett 1986;33:45–53.
165. Konig K, Schneckenburger H, Ruck A, Steiner R. In vivo photoproduct formation during PDT with ALA-induced endogenous porphyrins. J Photochem Photobiol B 1993;18:287–90.
166. Ahram M, Cheong WF, Ward K, Kessel D. Photoproduct formation during irradiation of tissues containing protoporphyrin. J Photochem Photobiol B 1994;26:203–4.
167. Moan J, Sommer S. Oxygen dependence of the photosensitizing effect of hematoporphyrin derivative in NHIK 3025 cells. Cancer Res 1985;45:1608–10.
168. Star WM, Marijnissen HP, van den Berg-Blok AE, et al. Destruction of rat mammary tumor and normal tissue microcirculation by hematoporphyrin derivative photoradiation observed in vivo in sandwich observation chambers. Cancer Res 1986;46:2532–40.
169. Henderson BW, Fingar VH. Oxygen limitation of direct tumor cell kill during photodynamic treatment of a murine tumor model. Photochem Photobiol 1989;49:299–304.
170. Gibson SL, van der Meid KR, Murant RS, Hilf R. Increased efficacy of photodynamic therapy of R3230AC mammary adenocarcinoma by intratumoral injection of Photofrin II. Br J Cancer 1990;61:553–7.
171. Foster TH, Murant RS, Bryant RG, et al. Oxygen consumption and diffusion effects in photodynamic therapy. Radiat Res 1991;126:296–303.
172. Sitnik TM, Hampton JA, Henderson BW. Reduction of tumour oxygenation during and after photodynamic therapy in vivo: effects of fluence rate. Br J Cancer 1998;77:1386–94.
173. Veenhuizen RB, Stewart FA. The importance of fluence rate in photodynamic therapy: is there a parallel with ionizing radiation dose-rate effects? Radiother Oncol 1995;37:131–5.
174. Patterson MS, Madsen SJ, Wilson BC. Experimental tests of the feasibility of singlet oxygen luminescence monitoring in vivo during photodynamic therapy. J Photochem Photobiol B 1990;5:69–84.
175. Georgakoudi I. Singlet oxygen- versus nonsinglet oxygen-mediated mechanisms of sensitizer photobleaching and their effects on photodynamic dosimetry. Photochem Photobiol 1998;67:612–25.

176. Baker A, Kanofsky JR. Quenching of singlet oxygen by biomolecules from L1210 leukemia cells. Photochem Photobiol 1992;55:523–8.
177. Niedre M, Patterson MS, Wilson BC. Direct near-infrared luminescence detection of singlet oxygen generated by photodynamic therapy in cells in vitro and tissues in vivo. Photochem Photobiol 2002;75:382–91.
178. Timmins GS, Davies MJ. An EPR spin trapping study of albumin protein radicals formed by the photodynamic action of haematoporphyrin. J Photochem Photobiol B 1993;21:167–73.
179. Henderson BW. Probing the effects of photodynamic therapy through in vivo-in vitro methods. In: Kessel D, editor. Photodynamic therapy of neoplastic disease. Boca Raton (FL): CRC Press; 1990. p. 169–88.
180. Fingar VH, Mang TS, Henderson BW. Modification of photodynamic therapy-induced hypoxia by fluosol-DA (20%) and carbogen breathing in mice. Cancer Res 1988;48:3350–4.
181. Chen Q, Huang Z, Chen H, et al. Improvement of tumor response by manipulation of tumor oxygenation during photodynamic therapy. Photochem Photobiol 2002;76:197–203.
182. Foster TH, Gao L. Dosimetry in photodynamic therapy: oxygen and the critical importance of capillary density. Radiat Res 1992;130:379–83.
183. Foster TH, Hartley DF, Nichols MG, Hilf R. Fluence rate effects in photodynamic therapy of multicell tumor spheroids. Cancer Res 1993;53:1249–54.
184. Nichols MG, Foster TH. Oxygen diffusion and reaction kinetics in the photodynamic therapy of multicell tumour speroids. Phys Med Biol 1994;39:2161–81.
185. Henning JP, Fournier RL, Hampton JA. A transient mathematical model of oxygen depletion during photodynamic therapy. Radiat Res 1995;142:221–6.
186. Pogue BW, Hasan T. A theoretical study of light fractionation and dose-rate effects in photodynamic therapy. Radiat Res 1997;147:551–9.
187. Sitnik TM, Henderson BW. The effect of fluence rate on tumor and normal tissue responses to photodynamic therapy. Photochem Photobiol 1998;67:462–6.
188. Tromberg BJ, Orenstein A, Kimel S, et al. In vivo tumor oxygen tension measurements for the evaluation of the efficiency of photodynamic therapy. Photochem Photobiol 1990;52:375–85.
189. Tromberg BJ, Kimel S, Orenstein A, et al. Tumor oxygen tension during photodynamic therapy. J Photochem Photobiol B 1990;5:121–6.
190. Henderson BW, Busch TM, Vaughan LA, et al. Photofrin photodynamic therapy can significantly deplete or preserve oxygenation in human basal cell carcinomas during treatment, depending on fluence rate. Cancer Res 2000;60:525–9.
191. Pogue BW, Braun RD, Lanzen JL, et al. Analysis of the heterogeneity of pO2 dynamics during photodynamic therapy with verteporfin. Photochem Photobiol 2001;74:700–6.
192. Pogue BW, O'Hara JA, Goodwin IA, et al. Tumor PO(2) changes during photodynamic therapy depend upon photosensitizer type and time after injection. Comp Biochem Physiol A Mol Integr Physiol 2002;132:177–84.
193. Gibson SL, van der Meid KR, Murant RS, et al. Effects of various photoradiation regimens on the antitumor efficacy of photodynamic therapy for R3230AC mammary carcinomas. Cancer Res 1990;50:7236–41.
194. Gibson SL, Foster TH, Feins RH, et al. Effects of photodynamic therapy on xenografts of human mesothelioma and rat mammary carcinoma in nude mice. Br J Cancer 1994;69:473–81.
195. Gibson SL, Nguyen ML, Foster TH, et al. Efficacy of photodynamic therapy on original and recurrent rat mammary tumors. Photochem Photobiol 1995;61:196–9.
196. Foster TH, Gibson SL, Raubertas RF. Response of Photofrin-sensitised mesothelioma xenografts to photodynamic therapy with 514 nm light. Br J Cancer 1996;73:933–6.
197. van Geel IP, Oppelaar H, Rijken PF, et al. Vascular perfusion and hypoxic areas in RIF-1 tumours after photodynamic therapy. Br J Cancer 1996;73:288–93.
198. Chen B, Pogue BW, Goodwin IA, et al. Blood flow dynamics after photodynamic therapy with verteporfin in the RIF-1 tumor. Radiat Res 2003;160:452–9.
199. Ehrlich P. Collected studies on immunity, New York: Wiley; 1906.
200. Hasan T. Photosensitizer delivery mediated by macromolecular carrier systems. In: Dougherty TJ, Henderson BW, editors. Photodynamic therapy: basic principles and clinical applications. New York: Marcel Dekker; 1992. p. 187–200.
201. Yarmush ML, Thorpe WP, Strong L, et al. Antibody targeted photolysis. Crit Rev Ther Drug Carrier Syst 1993;10:197–252.
202. Savellano MD, Hasan T. Targeting cells that overexpress the epidermal growth factor receptor with PEGylated BPD vertoporfin photosensitizer immunoconjugates. Photochem Photobiol 2003;77:431–9.
203. Goff BA, Blake J, Bamberg MP, Hasan T. Treatment of ovarian cancer with photodynamic therapy and immunoconjugates in a murine ovarian cancer model. Br J Cancer 1996;74:1194–8.
204. Hamblin MR, Miller JL, Hasan T. Effect of charge on the interaction of site-specific photoimmunoconjugates with human ovarian cancer cells. Cancer Res 1996;56:5205–10.
205. Duska LR, Hamblin MR, Bamberg MP, Hasan T. Biodistribution of charged F(ab')2 photoimmunoconjugates in a xenograft model of ovarian cancer. Br J Cancer 1997;75:837–44.
206. Soukos NS, Hamblin MR, Keel S, et al. Epidermal growth factor receptor-targeted immunophotodiagnosis and photoimmunotherapy of oral precancer in vivo. Cancer Res 2001;61:4490–6.
207. Kriegmair M, Baumgartner R,, Knuchel R, et al. Detection of early bladder cancer by 5-aminolevulinic acid induced porphyrin fluorescence. J Urol 1996;155:105–10.
208. Koenig F, McGovern FJ, Larne R, et al. Diagnosis of bladder carcinoma using protoporphyrin IX fluorescence induced by 5-aminolaevulinic acid. BJU Int 1999;83:129–35.
209. Riedl CR, Daniltchenko D, Koenig F, et al. Fluorescence endoscopy with 5-aminolevulinic acid reduces early recurrence rate in superficial bladder cancer. J Urol 2001;165:1121–3.
210. Leunig A, Betz CS, Mehlmann M, et al. Detection of squamous cell carcinoma of the oral cavity by imaging 5-aminolevulinic acid-induced protoporphyrin IX fluorescence. Laryngoscope 2000;110:78–83.
211. Betz CS, Stepp H, Janda P, et al. A comparative study of normal inspection, autofluorescence and 5-ALA-induced PPIX fluorescence for oral cancer diagnosis. Int J Cancer 2002;97:245–52.
212. Baumgartner R, Huber RM, Schulz H, et al. Inhalation of 5-aminolevulinic acid: a new technique for fluorescence detection of early stage lung cancer. J Photochem PhotobiolB 1996;36:169–74.
213. Mayinger B, Horner P, Jordan M, et al. Endoscopic fluorescence spectroscopy in the upper GI tract for the detection of GI cancer: initial experience. Am J Gastroenterol 2001;96:2616–21.
214. Mayinger B, Neidhardt S, Reh H, et al. Fluorescence induced with 5-aminolevulinic acid for the endoscopic detection and follow-up of esophageal lesions. Gastrointest Endosc 2001;54:572–8.
215. Hillemanns P, Weingandt H, Baumgartner R, et al. Photodetection of cervical intraepithelial neoplasia using 5-aminolevulinic acid-induced porphyrin fluorescence. Cancer 2000;88:2275–82.
216. Duska LR, Wimberly J, Deutsch TF, et al. Detection of female lower genital tract dysplasia using orally administered 5-aminolevulinic acid induced protoporphyrin IX: a preliminary study. Gynecol Oncol 2002;85:125–8.
217. Friesen SA, Hjortland GO, Madsen SJ, et al. 5-Aminolevulinic acid-based photodynamic detection and therapy of brain tumors [review]. Int J Oncol 2002;21:577–82.
218. Kaneko S. Intraoperative photodynamic diagnosis of human glioma using ALA induced protoporphyrin IX. No Shinkei Geka 2001;29:1019–31.
219. Stummer W, Stepp H, Moller G, et al. Technical principles for protoporphyrin-IX-fluorescence guided microsurgical resection of malignant glioma tissue. Acta Neurochir 1998;140:995–1000.
220. Stummer W, Stocker S, Novotny A, et al. In vitro and in vivo porphyrin accumulation by C6 glioma cells after exposure to 5-aminolevulinic acid. J Photochem Photobiol B, Biol 1998;45:160–9.
221. Marcus SL. Photodynamic therapy of human cancer. Proc IEEE 1992;80:869–86.
222. McCaughan JS Jr. Photodynamic therapy: a review [In Process Citation]. Drugs Aging 1999;15:49–68.
223. Pogue B, Hasan T. Targeting in photodynamic therapy and photo-imaging. OPN 2003;14:36–43.

Hyperthermia

Mark W. Dewhirst, DVM, PhD
Ellen Jones, MD, PhD
Thaddeus Samulski, PhD
Zeljko Vujaskovic, MD, PhD
Chuan Y. Li, PhD
Leonard Prosnitz, MD

INTRODUCTION

The rationale for use of hyperthermia (HT) as a treatment of cancer rests on several mechanisms. HT is known to cause direct cytotoxicity and also acts as a radiation (RT) and chemosensitizer. In addition, HT improves tumor oxygenation and delivery of novel drug carriers, such as liposomal agents. Recent developments in the field of gene therapy may also establish a role for HT as a strategy for targeted, localized induction of gene therapy using the heat shock promoter.

Despite the strong biological rationale, implementation of HT in the clinic presents significant challenges. The primary hurdle is to heat tumors to defined temperature ranges in a precise and reproducible manner. Ease of clinical application is critically important. Current techniques for measuring temperature are invasive and the definition and calculation of thermal dose have not been well defined. Further improvements in technologies to deliver HT and measure thermal dose remain crucial, although significant progress has been made on these issues over the past 5 years.

Two recently published pivotal trials have demonstrated for the first time that prospective control of thermal dose, when HT is combined with RT, has an impact on tumor response and duration of local tumor control. A third key paper reports that measurement of thermal dose can be achieved using MRI-based noninvasive thermometry methods and that parameters derived from these measurements are prognostically important. Collectively, these trials set the stage for establishing methods for writing a prescription for HT and for controlling thermal dose in real time.

In spite of the technical difficulties in delivering HT, however, there are many published randomized trials of HT in human cancer patients. The majority demonstrated a local control and/or survival advantage with the addition of HT to RT. Thus, even with the limitations of current technology, the promise of HT is emerging from clinical trials.

As the technology improves, the benefits of this form of therapy will only become more visible.

THE BIOLOGY OF HYPERTHERMIA

Definition of Hyperthermia HT means elevation of temperature to a supra-physiological level. For discussions in this chapter, this refers to temperatures between 40° to 45°C. Higher temperatures are used for thermal ablation, but will not be discussed here.

Hyperthermic Cell Killing, the Arrhenius Relationship, and Thermal Isoeffect Dose When cells are heated in vitro, they die exponentially and the rate of killing increases with temperature. The Arrhenius relationship has been used to define the temperature dependence of the rate of cell killing, which can then be used as a method for thermal dosimetry. This is done by plotting the log of the slope (1/Do) of cell survival curves as a function of temperature (Figure 35b-1). Typically, Arrhenius plots have a biphasic curve. The temperature at which the slope changes is referred to as a "breakpoint." Above the breakpoint for nearly all cell types, increase in temperature of 1.0°C doubles the rate of cell killing. The breakpoint for human cells is near 43.5°C, and below the breakpoint the rate of cell killing drops by a factor of 2–4 for each 1.0°C drop in temperature. The change in slope below the breakpoint is due to development of thermotolerance during heating. The slopes of Arrhenius plots derived from in vivo and in vitro studies are virtually identical.[1] Collectively, these data provide a strong rationale for using the Arrhenius relationship as a basis for thermal dosimetry.

The recognition that there is a definable relationship between the rate of cell killing and temperature led Sapareto and Dewey[2] to propose using this relationship to normalize thermal data from HT treatments. The rationale came from observations that time-temperature histories vary from patient to patient and that temperatures within tumors were almost always nonuniform, thereby preventing the goal of reaching a uniform target temperature-time combination for therapy. The formulation takes the following form:

$$\text{CEM } 43°\text{C} = tR^{(43-T)}$$

Where CEM 43°C = cumulative equivalent minutes at 43°C (the temperature suggested for normalization), t = time of treatment, T = average temperature during desired interval of heating and R is a constant. When above the breakpoint, R = 0.5. When below the breakpoint, R = 0.25.

For a complex time-temperature history, the heating profile is broken into short intervals of

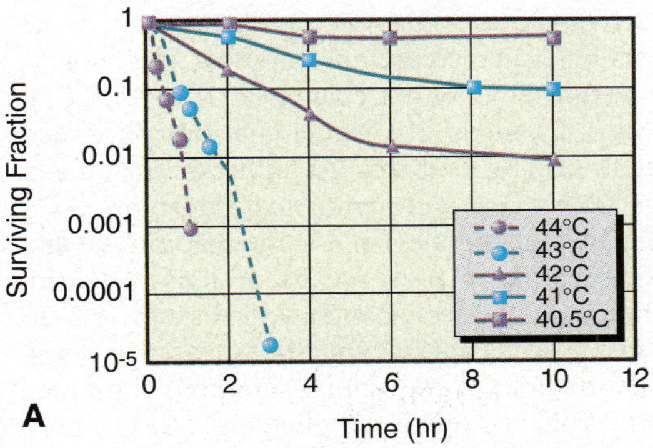

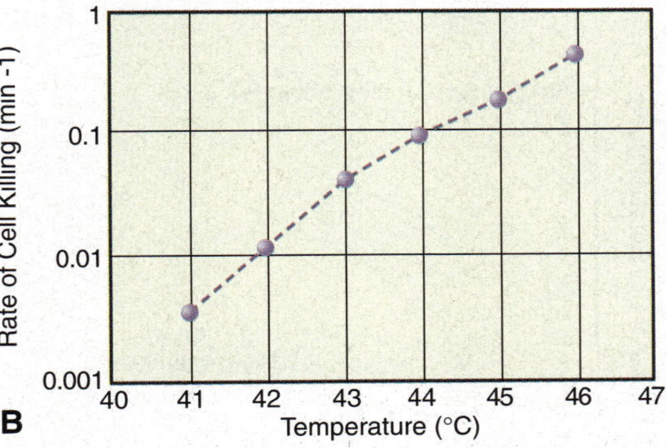

Figure 35b-1 **A,** Cell survival curves for V79 cells, plotted as log of surviving fraction as a function of time of heating at a defined temperature. Data replotted from Raaphorst GP et al.[92] **B,** Arrhenius plot from same data. Note change in slope of Arrhenius plot above and below 43°C.

time "t" length (typically 1–2 min), where the temperature remains relatively constant. CEM 43°C is calculated for each interval and summed to give a final CEM 43°C for the entire HT treatment as follows:

$$\text{CEM } 43°\text{C} = \Sigma t R^{(43\text{-}T_{avg})}$$

The CEM 43°C (thermal isoeffect dose) formulation has been used successfully in clinical trials to retrospectively assess heating efficacy.[3–6] This dosimetry concept has been evaluated prospectively in two recently published phase III trials (see "Clinical Hyperthermia" below for details).[7–9] These trials have been critical for showing that prospective control of thermal dose delivery can affect probability for response and duration of local tumor control.

Modifiers of Thermal Cytotoxicity There are factors that are known to affect the position and slopes of the Arrhenius plot. These factors have potential clinical relevance (Figure 35b-2).

Thermotolerance Thermotolerance is a transient adaptation to thermal stress that renders surviving heated cells more resistant to additional heat stress. It is caused by up-regulation of synthesis of heat shock proteins within cells during and after thermal stress. Thermotolerance tends to shift the Arrhenius plot to the right and downward, indicating that higher temperatures are needed to achieve equivalent rates of cell killing in thermotolerant as compared with nonthermally tolerant cells. Generally thermotolerance is avoided clinically by using 2 to 3 days between HT treatments to allow for its decay.

Acute Acidification Acute acidification will sensitize cells to killing in two ways. The Arrhenius plot is shifted to the left and the breakpoint nearly disappears because thermotolerance induction is inhibited. Methods for achieving acute tumor-specific acidification have been studied extensively in preclinical models and in humans and are discussed in more detail in the section below "Hyperthermia and Physiology."[10–13]

Step Down Heating Step down heating occurs when temperatures rise above the breakpoint and then drop below the breakpoint for the remainder of a treatment.[4] This occurs clinically when power is turned down after heating has started in response to pain or excessively high normal tissue temperatures or when perfusion increases in response to increased temperatures. When step down heating occurs, thermotolerance induction is prevented during that heating session.

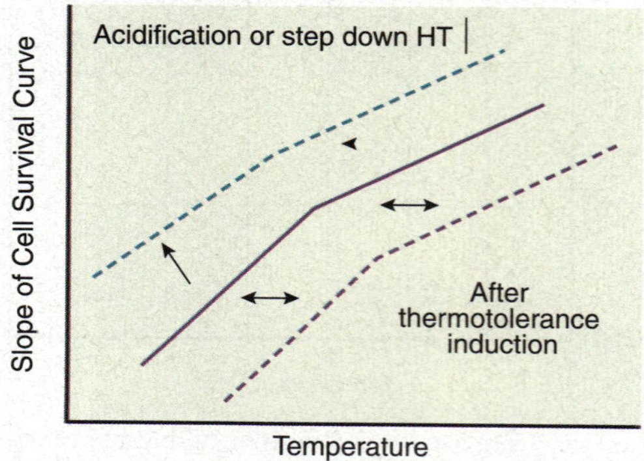

Figure 35b-2 Comparison of the effects of modifiers of the Arrhenius relationship (eg, thermal sensitivity).

MECHANISMS OF HYPERTHERMIC CYTOTOXICITY

Cellular and Tissue Responses to Hyperthermia **Targets for Hyperthermic Cytotoxicity** When cells are exposed to elevated temperatures (≥ 40.0°C), the predominant molecular target appears to be protein.[14] The heat of inactivation for cell killing and thermal damage is similar to the energy needed for protein denaturation (130–170 kcal/mole).[14,15] Additional evidence for proteins as being the primary target for cell killing is the importance of heat shock proteins in protecting thermotolerant cells from thermal damage. One of the primary functions of heat shock proteins is to refold other proteins that have been denatured or damaged.[16] Two modes of death are induced by HT: apoptosis and necrosis.[17,18]

Some cellular organelles are especially important in thermal responses. Modification of cell membrane lipid content or use of membrane active agents, such as alcohols, can sensitize cells to heat killing, but the sensitization is probably related to destabilization of the membrane as it relates to lipid-protein interactions.[19] The cytoskeleton of cells, which control many signal transduction pathways is particularly heat sensitive.[20,21] Enzymes in the respiratory chain are more heat sensitive than enzymes in the glycolytic pathway.[14,22] Finally, the DNA repair process is heat sensitive and this may be one of the mechanisms that leads to heat-induced radio- and chemosensitization.[23,24] Chromosomal aberrations can occur if cells are in S-phase during the time of heating[25,26] or if centrilobar damage occurs.[27]

HYPERTHERMIA AND PHYSIOLOGY

Tumor blood flow and metabolism have important influences on the efficacy of HT and, conversely, the physiologic consequences of HT can influence the efficacy of other treatments that the patient may receive.

Physiologic Response to Hyperthermia As temperatures are increased, the first tissue reaction is an increase in blood flow. The temperature threshold for this change is 41° to 41.5°C in skin.[28] Changes in vascular permeability also occur, leading to edema. At higher thermal doses vascular stasis and hemorrhage develop. As a rough estimate, one can assume that muscle and skin perfusion increase by at least 10-fold, whereas tumor perfusion may increase by 1.5- to 2-fold.[29] Mechanisms underlying vascular stasis may include arteriovenous shunting, thrombus formation, and leukocyte plugging.[30] It is rare to achieve temperatures high enough in the clinic to cause vascular damage, but there are physiologic changes in tumors at lower temperatures that are potentially beneficial (Figure 35b-3).

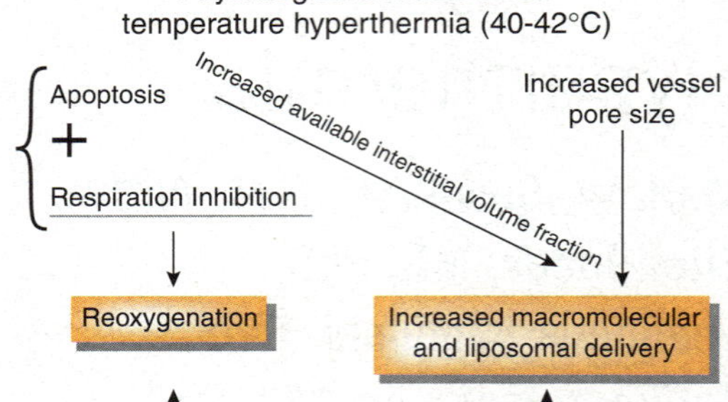

Figure 35b-3 Physiologic and therapeutic benefits to low or mild temperature hyperthermia (eg, 40°–42°C).

Taking Advantage of Physiological Response to Hyperthermia ***Improvement in Macromolecular and Liposomal Drug Delivery*** A liposome is a small lipid vesicle (≈100 nm diameter) that contains water or saline in the center. Drugs can be loaded into liposomes at high concentration. HT has been shown to augment liposomal drug delivery. 100 nm diameter liposomes do not extravasate at normothermia (34°C for mouse skin), but extravasate well at 40° to 42°C[31,32] (Figure 35b-4). HT does not cause liposomal extravasation from normal vessels. When temperature-sensitive liposomes are used, even better antitumor effects can be achieved, particularly using rapid drug release liposomes.[33] It has been recently reported that liposomal extravasation and release can be monitored noninvasively with MRI using a novel $MnSO_4$ doxorubicin-loaded liposome.[34] The mechanism of tumor cell killing with this formulation includes vascular destruction, occurring secondary to high drug concentrations that accumulate around vessels post-HT.[35]

There is no physiologic advantage to using HT to augment delivery of small molecular

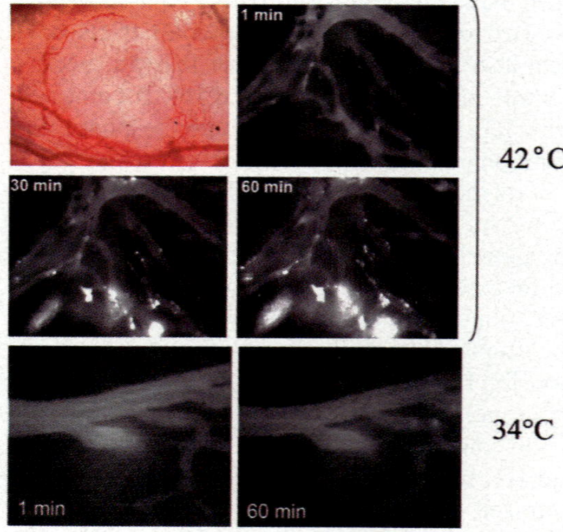

Figure 35b-4 Effect of 42°C hyperthermia (HT) on 100 nm liposomal extravasation from tumor vs normal tissue microvessels. Note that enhancement of extravasation is readily observable when the tumor is heated, whereas there is little extravasation at normothermia. HT does not increase extravasation of liposomes from normal microvessels (data not shown). Data similar to previously published results.[31]

weight drugs (< 1,000 MW), although HT increases cellular drug uptake.[36] In contrast, HT augments transvascular delivery of monoclonal antibodies, for example.[37] Recently, polymeric peptides that can carry drugs or radioisotopes have been designed to undergo inverse phase transition in the typical HT temperature range. When this occurs, these peptides transition from a water-soluble state to form aggregates that accumulate in tumor tissue.[38] The available volume fraction (space between cells and stromal fibers) increases after heating as cells undergo either necrosis or apoptosis.[39] This may increase the space available for macromolecular and liposomal accumulation.

Effects of HT on Tumor Metabolism and Oxygenation Enzymes for aerobic metabolism are more heat sensitive than those involved in anaerobic metabolism.[22] Kelleher and colleagues reported decreases in ATP and increases in lactate concentration occurring concomitantly with reduction in tumor blood flow following HT.[40] These results are consistent with the theory that a reduction in tumor respiration occurs after HT treatment.

A shift toward anaerobic metabolism could decrease oxygen consumption rates, which could lead to improvement in tumor oxygenation. Oleson suggested that some of the benefits of HT in the clinical setting (other than its cytotoxic and radiosensitizing effects) may result from improvements in oxygenation.[41] Results from several studies in rodent tumors and human tumor xenografts indicate improvement in tumor oxygenation resulting from thermal exposures below those that cause vascular damage (eg, 41°–43°C, 60 min).[42,43]

It has been reported that HT improves tumor oxygenation in canine and human tumors.[44–46] In the human studies, failure to reoxygenate after the first HT fraction led to a significantly lower probability to achieve pathologic complete response at the time of surgery[45,46] (Figure 35b-5). Excessively high temperatures can decrease oxygenation, but this is not commonly observed in clinical treatments because such temperatures are difficult to achieve.

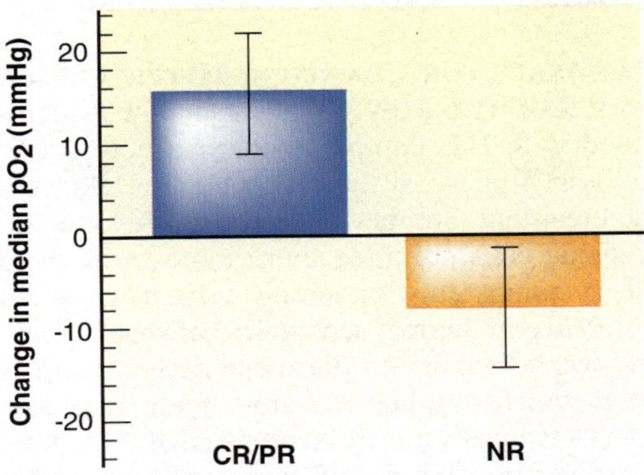

Figure 35b-5 Relationship between change in Eppendorf electrode hypoxic fraction, as measured 24 hour post the first hyperthermia (HT) and clinical response in patients with locally advanced breast cancer. These patients were treated with a combination of Taxol, radiation therapy, and HT. Reoxygenation is clearly associated with those patients who achieved either a complete or partial response. Data reprinted with permission of the author and publisher.[46]

NORMAL TISSUE DAMAGE FROM HYPERTHERMIA

Thermal damage to tissues is dependent on the severity of the injury and the tissue type being heated. Mild damage can merely lead to edema, whereas more severe injury can lead to massive necrosis and organ failure. This subject has been reviewed in detail recently.[47] When significant damage ensues, there is apoptosis, necrosis, inflammatory reaction with edema, focal hemorrhage, and granulocytic infiltrates within a few days following exposure. Chronic changes, seen after a few weeks, include fibrosis, parenchymal necrosis (death of tissue cells), and lymphohistiocytic infiltration. The ranking of thermal sensitivities of tissues does not follow classical principles of cytotoxic agents, dictating that the most sensitive tissues are those with the highest proliferative activity or potential. The most sensitive tissues include brain, the cells of which have almost no proliferative potential, as well as testis, which is highly proliferative. There is no clear ranking by tissue type, either. For example, peripheral nerves are heat resistant, spinal cord is intermediate, and brain is very sensitive.

There is no inherent difference in the thermal sensitivity between tumor and normal tissues. However, the microenvironment of tumors, which is often acidotic and nutritionally deprived, leads to an increase in thermal sensitivity.[48]

PHYSIOLOGIC APPROACHES TO ENHANCE THERMAL CYTOTOXICITY

pH Modification It is well established that an acute reduction in extracellular pH can greatly enhance sensitivity to HT. Cells adapted to grow at low pH are relatively resistant to HT killing as a result of heat shock protein up-regulation.[49] Acute acidification of such cells below their resting pH can lead to catastrophic cell death, because they have little reserve to further increase proton pumping. It is the reduction in intracellular pH that is actually responsible for the increase in cytotoxicity.[11] Induction of hyperglycemia will push tumor cells toward glycolysis, leading to increases in lactic acid production. Selectivity for tumors occurs because of alterations in respiratory pathways and a propensity toward sensitivity to the Crabtree effect.[50,51] The addition of the respiratory inhibitor, MIBG (metaiodobenzylguanidine) can further enhance selective acidification in tumors.[12,52,53] Pharmacologic agents that block the extrusion of hydrogen ions from cells has also been investigated.[13]

The use of hyperglycemia improves response to CT + HT and RT + HT in rodents.[54–56] One human study in a few patients suggested improvement in response with the use of hyperglycemia with RT + HT.[57] However, pH was not measured and the study was not randomized.

Tumor Blood Flow Reduction during HT Will Increase Temperatures A number of vasoactive agents have been shown to reduce tumor blood flow, including those that are normally considered to be vasodilators. The reason for this paradoxical effect in tumors relates to vascular steal that is created by (1) a relative lack of arteriolar input to tumors,[58] (2) pre-existing vasodilation in the few arterioles that tumors have, and (3) the presence of relatively high flow resistance that is exacerbated when blood pressure is reduced, as is frequently encountered with the use of vasodilators.[59,60] Many studies have been conducted in murine models with agents such as hydralazine.[61] Although use of such agents can quite effectively decrease tumor blood flow, they may not be easily implemented clinically because of the risks of inducing hypotension. In humans, reduction in tumor blood flow following hydralazine administration does not occur in the absence of hypotension.[62] Continuous administration of nitroprusside to a dose that decreases mean arterial pressure by 20% has been shown to yield very modest improvement in temperatures in spontaneous canine tumors, which is insufficient to justify clinical development.[63]

Another approach would be to use agents that cause peripheral vasoconstriction, tumor perfusion reduction, and lowered oxygenation, such as nitric oxide synthase inhibitors.[64–66] The nitric oxide synthase inhibitor L-NAME increased temperatures during HT application to muscle of normal beagles.[67] In two older pet dogs with spontaneous soft tissue sarcomas, however, pancreatitis developed post-HT application to the tumor-bearing area. Both animals had comorbid conditions that predisposed them toward developing pancreatitis. There is still merit in this approach in humans, since nitric oxide synthase inhibitors have been used in septic shock,[68] and thus far, pancreatitis has not been reported as a side effect of NO synthase inhibition in humans.

IMMUNOLOGICAL EFFECTS OF HYPERTHERMIA

A basic physiologic response to infection is to increase body temperature to help fight the infectious disease.[69] Many viral and bacterial pathogens are thermally sensitive and elevations in temperature are effective in altering both adaptive and innate immunity. Additionally, the metabolism of all cells is increased at elevated temperature, at least up to temperatures of 40°C.[14] This could accelerate immune reactivity.

HT has been shown to have specific immunological effects that could augment immune reactivity toward tumors, including (1) enhanced lymphocyte trafficking,[70] (2) HT-induced maturation of dendritic cells,[71] and (3) heat shock protein 70 (HSP70) mediated regulation of immune rejection of a variety of syngeneic tumor lines by chaperoning MHC Class I epitopes.[72] HSP70-chaperoned proteins show enhanced ability to stimulate dendritic cells and augment T-cell specific antitumor reactivity.[73]

HT augments the innate immune system as well. Peptide sequences in HSP70 can stimulate NK cell reactivity,[74] up-regulate $\alpha4\beta7$ integrin, which is the lymphocyte homing receptor of high endothelial cells of lymph nodes, and serve as chemokines for trafficking and activation of macrophages, via binding of toll-like receptors.[75] The heat shock protein Gp96 may also play a role in augmenting the adaptive and innate immune systems as well.[76]

HYPERTHERMIA AND METASTASES

Preclinical data are mixed with respect to whether local HT affects metastasis development. Local HT enhanced metastatic rates when the B16 melanoma was grown in the mouse foot pad.[77,78] Two other studies with different tumor models showed either a reduction in metastases following local HT[79] or no effect on the incidence of metastases, relative to controls.[80]

The question is difficult to answer in clinical trials unless the primary therapy has a high probability for local control. In a phase III trial of canine patients with primary malignant melanomas treated with the radiation ± HT, there was no difference in the likelihood for metastasis between the two arms.[81] However, local recurrence was a common event and its onset was frequently followed by appearance of distant metastases. In a phase III randomized trial of human melanomas treated in a similarly designed trial, there was significant improvement in the likelihood for survival when the local tumor was controlled. Since the radiotherapy + HT arm had improved local control, the combination therapy reduced the probability for metastases.[82,83] In a study comparing graded doses of radiation ± HT of canine soft tissue sarcomas, higher normal tissue temperatures surrounding tumor were correlated with lower likelihood for distant metastases.[84]

A large series of patients ($N = 95$) with previously untreated high-grade soft tissue sarcomas provides the most easily interpretable data because the local control rate following preoperative HT + RT was near 90%.[85] Fifty percent of these patients went on to develop distant metastases. This rate is essentially identical to that seen with preoperative RT alone.[86] The conclusion is that with the exception of one preclinical study with B16 melanoma, there is no evidence that local-regional HT causes an increase in metastases.

The results following whole-body HT are more provocative. In a randomized phase II study, dogs with soft tissue sarcomas received RT + local HT or RT + local HT + whole-body HT.[87] The combination of local + whole-body HT + RT did not improve local control over local HT + RT, and it increased the likelihood for distant metastases. In a separate study, alteration in the location of metastases of dogs with primary osteosarcomas was seen following treatment with whole-body HT.[88] It has also been reported that patients who had a fever during or shortly after receiving brachytherapy for carcinoma of the cervix had an increased risk of developing distant metastases.[89]

RADIATION AND HYPERTHERMIA

Rationale for Combining Hyperthermia with Radiotherapy When radiation is combined with HT, complementary effects occur. Cells in S-phase of the cell cycle are relatively radioresistant, but they are most sensitive to HT. Hypoxic cells are three times more resistant to RT, as compared with aerobic cells. There is no difference in thermal sensitivity between aerobic and hypoxic cells. As discussed earlier, there is good evidence in human tumors (soft tissue sarcoma and locally advanced breast) that HT causes reoxygenation, which will further improve radiation response. Finally, HT inhibits the repair of both sublethal and potentially lethal damage by inactivating crucial DNA repair pathways.[90–93]

Factors to Consider when Combining Hyperthermia with Radiotherapy The interaction between RT and HT is described by the "thermal enhancement ratio" or TER, which is defined as the ratio of doses of RT to achieve an isoeffect for RT/(RT + HT). A number of murine studies compared TERs for tumor and normal tissues, and in some cases it was possible to demonstrate therapeutic gain (ie, $TER_{tumor} > TER_{normal\ tissue}$).[94] TERs for late tissue complications in feet and skin of mice were lower than TERs for moist desquamation.[95,96]

TERs for local tumor control have been estimated to be > 1 for several human tumor types.[97] TER values for normal tissue damage have been less than tumor in the same patient populations, suggesting potential for therapeutic gain for RT + HT compared with RT alone. Prospective randomized trials in dogs with spontaneous tumors have also shown evidence for improved local tumor control with RT + HT compared with RT alone,[98–100] with no clinical increase in frequency of clinically relevant late normal tissue complications.

In summary, most available data from preclinical and clinical studies indicate that therapeutic gain is achievable for the combination of HT with RT. HT does not appear to enhance the incidence or severity of late normal tissue complications.

HYPERTHERMIA AND CHEMOTHERAPY

Rationale for Using Hyperthermia with Chemotherapy Many chemotherapeutic agents have been shown to exhibit synergism with HT including cisplatin and related compounds: melphalan, cyclophosphamide, nitrogen mustards, anthracyclines, nitrosoureas, bleomycin, mitomycin C, and hypoxic cell sensitizers.[36] The mechanisms that underlie the synergy may include (1) increased cellular uptake, (2) increased oxygen radical production, and (3) increased DNA damage and inhibition of repair. Hypoxia and pH are also important in the thermochemotherapeutic response.[101–105]

Factors to Consider when Combining Hyperthermia with Chemotherapy **Reversal of Drug Resistance** An important factor in the potential use of HT with many drugs is its ability to reverse, at least partially, drug resistance. Examples of drugs for which this has been shown include cisplatin,[106] melphalan,[107] nitrosoureas,[108] and doxorubicin, when combined with the multiple drug resistance inhibitor, verapamil.[109]

In Vitro Results May Not Predict In Vivo Activity Tubulin binding agents, such as Taxol, show no evidence for interaction in vitro,[110] but studies in combination with radiation therapy in vivo are more encouraging.[111] Generally speaking, most antimetabolites do not interact with HT when given concomitantly.[36] However, it is important to consider issues such as time of drug exposure and temperature, both of which may be important in determining where and when to expect a positive interaction. When 5FU has been given simultaneously with HT, there have been only additive effects.[112] However, 5FU has been shown to interact supra-additively with HT when simulated as continuous infusion. Heating to 39° to 41°C can lead to enhanced conversion to active metabolites, thereby increasing drug cytotoxicity. In addition, continuous infusion protocols with this drug may lead to cell-cycle block in S-phase, a relatively HT-sensitive part of the cell cycle.[113]

Sequencing For most drugs (excluding 5FU and perhaps other antimetabolites), the optimal sequence between heat and drug is to administer them simultaneously or to give the drug immediately before the onset of heating. For platinum-containing drugs, the tissue extraction rate of drug may be increased with HT, further substantiating the rationale for use of this sequence.[114]

Lack of Interaction Etoposide and the vinca alkaloids have failed to show synergistic interaction with HT.[36]

Trimodality Therapies The combination of HT, drugs, and radiation has been evaluated preclinically.[115] Limited, but encouraging pilot human data, based on the combination of the hypoxic cell sensitizer, etanidazole, radiation, and HT have been reported.[116] The combination of 5FU, HT, and radiation therapy has yielded favorable responses in patients with locally advanced colorectal cancer in a phase II study,[117] which has led to the current conduct of a randomized phase III trial of 5FU + radiation ± HT. Similarly, a pilot trial of HT + cisplatin + RT in patients with locally advanced cervix cancer[118] has led to initiation of a phase III multinational multi-institutional phase III trial comparing cisplatin CT + RT with and without HT.

Hyperthermia and Gene Therapy Several investigators have exploited the heat shock response as a means to perform gene therapy. The heat shock promoter is highly inducible and relatively quiescent under normothermic conditions.[119–121] The heat inducibility has been used to minimize therapeutic gene expression in normal tissues by focusing the heat on the tumor bearing region only.[122]

Examples of therapeutic genes that have been investigated include interleukin 12 (as a modulator of immune function and angiogenesis),[123] thy-

Table 35b-1 Summary of Hyperthermia Methods

Class	Method	Power Directed to Tumor Site?	Frequency	Coupling Medium	Invasive Thermometry Requirements	Advantages	Disadvantages
EM				Superficial			
	Magnetic induction	No		Air	Fiber optic or high resistance lead thermistors	Simple to operate	Eddy currents follow path of least resistance; heating pattern is not controllable
	Capacitive RF	Sometimes-use different sized applicators	5 to 30 MHz	Saline	Same as above	Simple to operate	Superficial fat heats; limits use to thin patients
	Microwave waveguide	Yes, by physical placement of waveguide(s) over tumor	433, 915, 2,450 MHz	Water	Same as above	Simple to operate	Limited depth of heating; heating pattern highly dependent on power deposition pattern
EM				Deep			
	Magnetic induction	No		Air	Same as above	Simple to operate	Eddy currents follow path of least resistance; heating pattern is not controllable
	Capacitive RF	Partially by physical location of applicators	5 to 30 MHz	Saline	Same as above	Simple to operate	Superficial fat heats; limits use to thin patients
	Phased RF or microwave arrays	Partially by altering phase and amplitude of power from different antennas	100 to 200 MHz	Water	Same as above	Better focus capability than other EM methods	Technically challenging
Ultrasound				Superficial			
	Planar ultrasound transducers: single or multiple	Yes, mainly by physical placement of transducer(s) over region of tumor	1 to 3 MHz	Degassed water	Metal device preferable (ie, thermocouple or thermistor); avoid plastic	Similar to waveguides	Good coupling to body required; air and bone prohibit penetration and can lead to pain
Ultrasound				Deep			
	Focused transducer array	Yes	0.5 to 2 MHz	Degassed water	Same as above	The most focusable method	Limited size of acoustic window(s); air and bone reflect power

midine kinase conversion of the prodrug ganciclovir to a toxic chemotherapeutic agent,[124–126] other cytokines such as TNFα, and restoration of wild-type *TP53* to induce apoptosis.[127–129] There are potential advantages to be gained through augmentation of immune function by HSP70 as well.[130]

HYPERTHERMIA PHYSICS

HT is usually delivered by exposing tissues to conductive heat sources, or nonionizing radiation, such as electromagnetic (EM) or ultrasound (US) fields. Although these modalities deposit energy in tissue by different physical mechanisms, they have general similarities. They are sensitive to the heterogeneity of tissue properties, geometry of blood flow, and the practical problems of coupling energy into tissue. HT can be administered using either invasive sources or noninvasively using externally applied power. A brief discussion of the noninvasive methods is provided below (Table 35b-1). Further details on all methods are available elsewhere.[131,132]

Electromagnetic Heating When an electric field (E-field) exists in materials of finite electrical conductivity, resistant heating occurs. For all tissue types, the electrical conductivity increases as the EM frequency increases. This implies improved penetration for low frequency or long wavelengths. However, the ability to localize EM energy deposition is dependent on the wavelength. The longer the wavelength, the broader the focus of heating. Thus, there is a fundamental constraint on noninvasive heating by EM techniques that does not allow localized heating at depths greater than 2 to 5 cm. Utilization of EM techniques to achieve deep heating results in regional energy deposition involving substantial volumes of normal tissue.

EM Heating Devices A range of EM heating devices has been developed for external applications of HT. These devices can be separated into two categories: superficial applicators with effective penetration into tissue in the range of 2 to 5 cm, and deep heating devices that have effective penetration > 5 cm. Examples of superficial devices include waveguides and microstrip or patch antennas[133,134] that operate in the microwave band typically at 433, 915, or 2,450 MHz.[131] All of these devices are usually coupled into tissue through a deionized water bolus. This bolus is usually temperature controlled to maintain the skin temperature below 43°C.

In order to heat at depths > 5 cm, one has to use lower EM frequencies in the RF band (5–200 MHz). There are three basic techniques for EM deep heating: magnetic induction, capacitive coupling, and phased array fields.

Magnetic induction heating uses a time varying magnetic field to induce eddy currents in conductive tissue.[131] The magnetic field distribution is not sensitive to tissue type and is consistently predictable. However, the eddy current distribution is governed by paths of least resistance and will be affected by tissue conductivity. One way to more selectively deliver power to tumor with this method is to use ferromagnetic metals, implanted within the tumor volume.[135–137] These metals have often been designed to undergo a Curie point transition, where their magnetic properties change with temperature, thereby providing self-regulated temperature control.

Deep heating using the capacitive technique uses RF fields in the frequency range of 5 to 30 MHz.[131] Ion currents are driven between two or more conductive electrodes. Heating tends to be concentrated at the electrodes, so temperature controlled saline pads or bolus are used to cool the skin and underlying fat.[138] Varying the size of the respective electrodes can shift the current distribution toward the smallest of the electrodes. The thickness of the superficial fat layer is a significant limitation because of resistive heating. Therefore, RF capacitive heating is used almost exclusively in Asia, where patients tend to be thinner.

The third option for noninvasive deep heating is the RF-phased array.[139] These devices consist of an array of RF antennas arranged in a geometric pattern surrounding the body region that is to be heated. The antennas are driven from a common RF source. This allows the RF fields (which are sine waves) from the antennas to add together to form a null or a focus. One can achieve better and deeper power deposition into tissue than by operating the antennas independently. In general the phased array technique has more flexibility for controlling power deposition than magnetic induction and capacitive techniques.

Ultrasound Heating Energy transfer from an acoustic field is associated with viscous friction. Penetration of ultrasound fields decrease with frequency. However, because the wavelength of an ultrasound field is several orders of magnitude smaller than that of EM fields, the problems of applicator size and focusing of ultrasound field energy in deeper tissues are greatly reduced. However, anatomic geometry and tissue heterogeneity (air reflects, bone preferentially absorbs) severely limit the utility of ultrasound. The availability of an adequate "acoustic window" (a path unobstructed by bone or air proximal and distal to the target) is often a problem in clinical applications. The entry window size determines the size and depth of the target volume.

Ultrasound devices are coupled into tissue using a temperature controlled degassed water bolus. Single and multiple transducer plane wave devices have been designed for superficial tumors (2–5 cm) heating, which typically operate in the 1 to 3 MHz range.[140–142] Specialized ultrasound arrays have been developed to facilitate simultaneous application of HT with RT, which will maximize the cytotoxic interactions between these two treatments.[140,141] Deep heating with ultrasound is accomplished by using scanned focused transducers, phased arrays, or multiple scanned focused transducers.[143–145] Ultrasound frequencies for deep heating are in the 0.5 to 2 MHz range.

Measurement of Temperatures During Hyperthermia The most commonly used method currently involves physically placing thermometers into the tumor. Invasive thermometry has many disadvantages: (1) patient discomfort, (2) risk of hemorrhage and/or infection, (3) requirement of physician time and image verification, and (4) limited amount of data obtained makes it difficult to control power or alter treatment. Noninvasive thermometry is under development and if successfully implemented, it will revolutionize the way that hyperthermia is practiced because it will allow for real-time adjustment of heating devices.

Invasive thermometry is done by inserting blind-ended catheters into a tumor and using either ultrasound or CT guidance. Thermometers are then placed inside these catheters. Multipoint devices remain in one fixed position during treatment or single point devices are physically moved inside the catheter during heating. There are guidelines published for how these measurements should be taken.[146–149]

Invasive thermometry provides valuable information about the quality of a treatment. A number of clinical reports have correlated temperature-related parameters to treatment outcome[5,6,150] and two recent phase III trials used prospective control of thermal dose, as measured using noninvasive thermometry to increase tumor response and duration of local control following thermoradiotherapy (see "Clinical Hyperthermia" below for details).[7,8]

Noninvasive Thermometry The limitation of invasive techniques for characterizing temperature distributions has stimulated the development of noninvasive thermometry. MRI is currently the preferred technology, although several other methods have been investigated.[151–157] Several MR parameters are temperature sensitive including the relaxation time T_1, T_2, bulk magnetization, and the proton resonance frequency. The latter has shown to provide the best temperature sensitivity and is most commonly used.[158]

Clinical studies in patients with extremity soft tissue sarcomas have reported resolution of 0.5° to 1°C[150] (Figure 35b-6). Similar accuracy has been reported for pelvic malignancies.[159] There are significant issues to deal with that may limit the usefulness of MR thermometry, however. Drift in MR magnet coils and motion of the patient or parts of the patient, created by factors such as peristalsis, must be corrected. Despite these concerns, a recent clinical report has been published showing that thermal dose parameters, derived from temperatures measured using MRI-based noninvasive thermometry, are correlated with treatment outcome in patients with locally advanced colorectal cancer treated with thermochemoradiotherapy.[159]

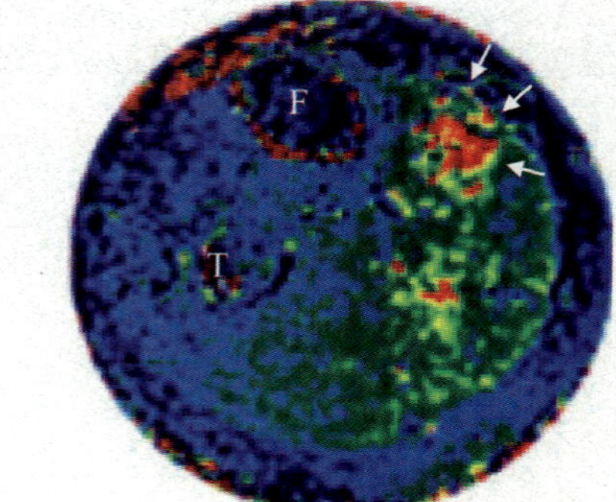

Figure 35b-6 Example of noninvasive thermometry data acquired from a patient with a lower extremity soft tissue sarcoma. The patient was placed inside the MRI and HT was administered using a phased RF array. MR thermal data were obtained during the heating procedure. The measurement was made using phase difference (chemical shift) magnetic resonance imaging. The temperature coefficient of this measurement is approximately 0.01 ppm/°C. The method in human patients has yielded a temperature resolution of 1.0°C, as calibrated against invasive measurements. Location of the tibia (T) and fibula (F) are noted, as well as the tumor site (*arrows*). The tissues inside the 44°, 42°, and 41°C isotherms are red, yellow, and green, respectively. Data replotted from Carter DL et al.[192]

CLINICAL HYPERTHERMIA

General Considerations HT alone has been studied in the treatment of superficial tumors. Although an occasional response is noted, the duration is typically quite short.[160,161] Long-term tumor control has not been described with the use of HT as a sole treatment modality. HT alone remains widely practiced in certain alternative and complementary medicine clinics. Its use, however, is not supported by any peer-reviewed published scientific data.

A large number of phase I/II reports over the last two decades attest to the efficacy of HT + RT. The patients have been primarily those with superficial malignancies (and thus more amenable to heating) but present as a component of generalized disease. The most common clinical presentation has been local recurrence of breast carcinoma. With HT + RT, clinical response rates have doubled from 25 to 35% for RT alone to 50 to 70% with RT + HT.[162] The great majority of patients have had systemic disease as well; thus, survival data and long-term local control have infrequently been reported.

In addition to phase II studies, approximately 20 to 25 phase III trials have now been conducted worldwide with approximately two-thirds published in the English literature. These trials, for the most part, have been positive, lending additional validity to the information obtained from phase II studies.

Overall, HT is well tolerated and does not appear to significantly increase early or late toxicity of radiation.[97–100] The therapeutic ratio is thus improved by the addition of HT to RT. The most common side effect of HT is superficial or subcutaneous tissue burns, generally first or second degree in character and small in volume. Such burns occur in approximately 5% of patients treated in our clinic; characteristically they do not exceed 3 to 4 cm in maximum diameter. Third degree burns are rarely seen—less than 1% of all patients treated. Complications (particularly infections) from the placement of thermometry catheters interstitially within the tumor have also been reported,[163] but are quite infrequent if thermometry catheters are removed following each HT treatment.[164] There are potential medical contraindications to HT, related to the physiological stresses of heating. The latter has sometimes been compared with a moderately intense exercise workout. Guidelines for patient selection for deep hyperthermia have been developed by RTOG.[148]

Published data on the efficacy of local-regional HT + CT is much less frequent. Both animal and human data have recently been reviewed.[162] Particularly encouraging phase II results have been reported for sarcomas[165] and breast carcinoma (J Park et al, personal communication; Duke University Medical Center, unpublished data). Additionally, significant activity is seen when chemotherapy is administered to extremity tumors, via perfusional or infusional methods, where the perfusate is heated.[166,167]

Positive phase II results have also been reported for triple combinations of drug, HT, and radiotherapy. Examples include a phase II trial of 5FU, leucovorin, HT, and radiotherapy for locally advanced rectal cancer[168] and a pilot phase II trial evaluating the combination of cisplatin + RT + HT for locally advanced cervix cancer.[118] No phase III data are as yet reported, but trials are underway for locally advanced rectal carcinoma and cervical carcinoma.

Relationship Between Thermal Dose and Outcome The conduct of clinical trials and clinical practice of HT has been inhibited by difficulties in establishing quantifiable thermal dose parameters that correlate well with outcome in both tumor and normal tissue. As with any therapy, sound dosimetry is required to write a verifiable treatment prescription. Quality assurance standards have been established for treatment set up and invasive thermometry,[146,148,169,170] but a standard system for thermometry data reporting is still not established. A number of parameters have been described, based on simple descriptions of multipoint thermometry such as minimum or average temperature. The tenth percentile of the temperature distribution, which is commonly referred to as the T90 (90% of measured points exceed this value) has often been used. To deal with variations in temperatures and times of heating between patients, clinical data have been converted to thermal dose, defined as cumulative equivalent minutes at 43°C (CEM 43°C) at the minimum, average or T90 temperature point in order to permit comparative analysis.[4]

Many trials have shown positive relationships between such measures of thermal dose and treatment outcome.[4–6,150] In all of these studies, thermal analysis was performed retrospectively. It has been more difficult to demonstrate that prospective control of thermal dose relates to clinical outcome. Two studies compared various numbers of HT fractions, given in combination with fractionated RT,[171,172] using the assumption that more treatments would yield greater cumulative thermal dose. Neither study showed benefit with more HT fractions. This could be due to the fact that there was considerable overlap in thermal doses between arms because temperature is a stronger determinant of thermal dose than time of HT (see Biology section). Thrall and colleagues tested the hypothesis that RT combined with whole-body HT + local HT would yield greater CEM 43°C T90 than local HT alone and superior local control rates in dogs with soft tissue sarcomas.[87] This study failed to show any advantage for whole-body + local HT, even though thermal doses were higher in the whole-body + local HT arm. Induction of thermotolerance during the whole-body HT, which was administered prior to application of local heating may have reduced the overall effect of HT in the combined group.

The first attempt to prospectively control thermal dose, as prescribed by the CEM 43°C T90, was a study of preoperative RT and HT for soft tissue sarcomas. The outcome variable was pathologic complete response (CR) assessed at the time of surgery. Even though the thermal goal was reached in the majority of patients, the projected CR rate was not achieved.[173] A number of explanations are possible, but a major consideration is the limited number of tumor temperatures that were sampled with invasive thermometry and the small number of patients enrolled into the trial. Certain 31-MRS parameters were associated with pathologic outcome in this patient series, suggesting that mitigating features of tumor heterogeneity may have masked the thermal dose effect.[174]

Two additional phase III trials have recently been reported, however, showing that prospective control of thermal dose, when HT is combined with RT, has an effect on tumor response and duration of local control. Details of those trials are discussed below.

Clinical Trials Overview In this section we will focus on the major published phase III trials. These trials have involved a wide variety of disease sites: superficial malignancies and tumors deep within the body, and palliative as well as potentially curative patients. The more important of these trials are summarized in Table 35b-2. Several other important trials are still in progress.

Breast Cancer Chest wall recurrences of breast cancer are well suited for strategies employing HT. They are difficult to control with conventional approaches, even when patients have not been previously treated.

Five separate phase III trials were conducted, which were subsequently combined in an international collaborative study.[175] Patients were randomized to either RT alone or RT with HT. A significant improvement in CR rate was seen for patients receiving HT + RT compared with RT alone, 59% in the former group, 41% in the latter, with an odds ratio of 2.3 (95% CI 1.4–3.8). The greatest effect was observed in patients with recurrent lesions in previously irradiated areas where further irradiation was limited to low doses. Survival advantages were not apparent.

Other Superficial Malignancies A prior study was conducted by the RTOG comparing RT versus RT + HT in superficial measurable tumors (RTOG 8104).[176–178] Three hundred seven patients were enrolled; approximately half had head and neck tumors, one-third breast carcinoma (chest wall recurrences), with the remaining patients having a variety of superficial malignancies. Patients treated with RT + HT had a CR rate of 32% compared with 30% for those receiving RT. Subgroup analysis revealed significant improvements in duration of local control in patients with tumors < 3 cm and in those with breast and/or chest wall recurrences. For lesions > 3 cm there was no difference in outcome. It was postulated that the better outcome in smaller tumors was a consequence of better heating. This trial was characterized by highly variable HT techniques and inadequate thermal dosimetry. These issues led to the development of subsequent RTOG guidelines for performing hyperthermia.[146]

Head and Neck Cancer Two trials demonstrated an advantage to HT + RT. The first study randomized 65 patients to RT alone versus RT + HT.[179] RT doses consisted of 50 Gy in 5 weeks to the primary site and regional lymphatics, followed by an additional 10 to 15 Gy to sites of gross disease in daily fractions of 2 Gy. HT was given twice a week with 72 hours between each session. HT + RT significantly improved response in patients with stage III and IV disease. Patients in stage III receiving RT + HT had a 58% CR compared with 20% in the RT group. Similarly patients with stage IV disease achieved a CR of 38% compared with 7% for those receiving RT alone. There was no benefit for patients with stage I and II disease, with > 90% achieving a CR with either treatment. This trial evaluated both the primary site as well as neck nodes, despite difficulties of effectively heating most primary head and neck tumors.

A second trial restricted evaluation to metastatic cervical lymph nodes in 41 patients with advanced local regional squamous cell carcinoma of the head and neck randomized to treatment with either RT alone or RT + HT.[180,181] The CR rate was 41% for RT alone versus 83% for RT + HT. The 5-year actuarial probability of local control in the neck was 24% for RT alone versus 69% in the combined arm. Five year survival was 0 for RT alone and 53% in the RT + HT group. All of these differences were statistically significant. Two patients in the combined group developed late osteonecrosis of the mandible. Interpretation of normal tissue complications is difficult, however, since the only long-term survivors were in the combined group. Thermal parameters reported in this study included the T_{min}, T_{max}, T90, and cumulative equivalent minutes at 42.5°C. There was no clear relationship between thermal dose received and outcome. Nonetheless, this well-executed and described phase III trial, despite the relatively small number of patients, is an important component of the evidence suggesting the value of hyperthermia.

Table 35b-2 Summary of Key Phase III Clinical Trial Results Comparing Radiotherapy Alone to Radiotherapy Plus Hyperthermia

				Rx Arm							Hyperthermia	End Points		Significance	
Author	Tumor Type/ Location	Type of Trial	n	RT	RT + HT	Total RT Dose (Gy)	Dose/Fx and/ or Dose Rate	No. Fx	Mean Tx Time	No Fx	Thermal Dose Goals or Reported Data	Control Arm (RT)	Treatment Arm (RT + HT)	(p <.05)	Effect of Heating Quality
van der Zee[186]	Pelvic	Multicenter	358	176	182					1/wk up to 5tx (1–4 h post RT)	Target = 60 min after any point in tumor is 42°C Average total HT duration = 90 min	CR 39% @ 3 mo	CR 55% @ 3 mo	Yes	41% of patients received fewer than 5 HT tx because of refusal
												OS 24% @ 3y	OS 30% @ 3y	Yes	
	Rectal		143	71	72	46–50	1.8–2.3 Gy + 10–24 Gy boost		42d (29–81)			LC 26% @ 3y	LC 38% @ 3y	Yes	
												CR 15% @ 3 mo	CR 21% @ 3 mo	No	
												OS 22% @ 3y	OS 13% @ 3y	No	
	Bladder		101	49	52	66–70	2 Gy		48 d (21–127)			LC 8% @ 3y	LC 16% @ 3y	NR	
												CR 51% @ 3 mo	CR 73% @ 3 mo	Yes	
												OS 22% @ 3 y	OS 28% @ 3y	No	
	Cervical		114	56	58	42	1.8–2.0 Gy + brachy-therapy boost	23–28	48 d (35–121)			LC 33% @ 3y	LC 42% @ 3y	No	
												CR 57% @ 3 mo	CR 83% @ 3 mo	Yes	
												OS 27% at 3 y	OS 51% at 3 y	Yes	
												LC 41% @ 3 y	LC 61% @ 3 y	Yes	
Sneed[185]	Glioblastoma (after RT)	Single institution	68	33	35	59.4	1.8 Gy	33	32 d	2Fx (pre-/ post BT)	Median (Range) CEM 43° T90: 14.1 (0–771)	TTP median 33 week	TTP median 33 wk	Yes	8 patients had only 1 HT tx
						60	0.4-0.6 Gy/[125]I		100 hr		Median (range) CEM 43° T50: 74.6 (0.1–4,652)	TTLTP 35 wk	TTLTP 57 wk	Yes	
												OS 15% @ 2 y	OS 31% @ 2 y	Yes	
Emami[182]	Various	Multicenter	173	87	86	Prior dose + study dose < 100 Gy	10 Gy ± 10%/d; (0.4–0.5 Gy/h)		1 d	1 or 2 (Pre ± post-RT)	Goal: T_{min} 43° C for 60 min	Median survival 76 week	Median survival 85 wk		No thermal dose relationship found
												CR 54%	CR 57%	No	Only 1 patient met criteria for "adequate HT treatment"
												PR 24%	PR 14%	No	T90 < 40.5 vs T90 > 40.5 CR 53% vs 68% respectively
												LC at 2 y 37%	LC at 2 y 43%	No	
	Head and neck		75	35	40							OS at 2 y 29%	OS at 2 y 36%	NR	
												CR 52%	CR 62%	No	
	Pelvis		75	37	38							PR 37%	PR 10%	No	
												CR 57%	CR 60%	No	
Vernon1[175]	Breast	Multicenter	306	135	171	29–50 Gy ± boost	1.8–4 Gy	Varied	2–5 wk	1 to 8	Goal: T >42.5° C q 30 min	PR 8%	PR 10%	No	
												CR 41%	CR 59%	Yes	
												Actuarial survival 40% at 2 y	Actuarial survival 40% at 2 y	No	
Overguaard[82]	Melanoma	Multicenter	68	65	63	24–27 Gy	8 or 9 Gy	3	8d	3	Goal: 43°C q 60 min	CR 35% @ 3 mo	CR 62% @ 3 mo	Yes	62% had T_{max} >60 CEM 43°C
			Patients had more than one tumor									LC 28% @ 5 y	LC 46% @ 5 y	Yes	9% reached T_{min} target > 60 CEM 43°C
												RR (RT + HT vs RT alone) CR = 4.01; 2 y local control = 1.73			Local control at 5 y When AvT_{max} > 76 CEM 43°C (n = 27) 54% When Av T_{max} > 1–76 CE 43°C (n = 27) 36%
Sugimachi[184]	Esophagus	Single institution	66	34[a]	32[a]	30 Gy	2 Gy *Patients also received chemo	13	3 wk	6	42.5–44.0°C q 30 min	Downstaging effect of neoadjuvant therapy			NR
												Effective in 44%	Effective in 69%	Yes	
												OS 24% @ 3 y	OS 50% @ 3 y	NR	

(Continued)

Table 35b-2 Summary of Key Phase III Clinical Trial Results Comparing Radiotherapy Alone to Radiotherapy Plus Hyperthermia *(Continued)*

				Rx Arm						Hyperthermia		End Points		Significance	
Author	Tumor Type/ Location	Type of Trial	*n*	RT	RT + HT	Total RT Dose (Gy)	Dose/Fx and/ or Dose Rate	No. Fx	Mean Tx Time	No Fx	Thermal Dose Goals or Reported Data	Control Arm (RT)	Treatment Arm (RT + HT)	(*p* <.05)	Effect of Heating Quality
Valdagni[180]	Head and neck	Single institution	41	23 (19)	21 (17)	64–70 Gy	2.0–2.5 Gy	NR	30 d	2 vs 6 Fx	Goal: T_{min} + 42.5°C q 30 min	CR 37% @ 3 mo	CR 82% @ 3 mo	Yes	CR 86% vs 80% for 2 vs 6 HT doses; no correlation for CR vs thermal parameters
			Multiple nodes in some												
Valdagni[181]	5-y followup on above patients			21/22 nodes	6/18 nodes	"	"	"	"	"	"	Act probe of control 24% at 5 y OS 0% at 5 y	Act probe of control 69% at 5 y OS 53% at 5 y	Yes Yes	
Perez[176]	Head and neck	Multicenter	218	107	111	32 Gy	4 Gy	8			Goal: 42.5°C for 60 min biw; "Good" HT = 45 min @ 42.5°C x 4fx	CR 28%	CR 32%	No	52% patients in RT + HT group rec'd full Rx; few rec'd "good HT"
Perez[177]	Final report on Trial		236	117	119	"	"	"	"	"	"	Overall CR 30%; CR for lesions <3cm 25%	Overall CR 32%; CR for lesions <3cm 52%	No overall and in subgroup	
Datta[179]	Head and neck	Single institution	65	32	33	50 Gy + boost	2.0 Gy/d	25	5 wk	biw	Goal: 20 min @ 42.5°C	CR 31% @ 8 wk Disease-free survival difference	CR 55% @ 8 wk	Yes No overall Yes, in stages III and IV	NR

[a]Patients also received chemotherapy.

Abbreviations: Act probe = act variant probability; BT = brachytherapy; CEM = cumulative equivalent minutes; CR = complete response; DFS = disease-free survival; Fx = radiation therapy fraction; HT = hyperthermia; LC = local control; OS = overall survival; PathCR = pathologic response; PR = partial response; RT radiation therapy; T = temperature; TTP = time to progression; TTLTP = time to local tumor progression; Tx = time of heating.

A trial of interstitial hyperthermia was carried out primarily in head and neck patients by the RTOG.[182] This trial entered 173 patients with persistent or recurrent tumors after prior RT and/or surgery that were amenable to interstitial RT. The lesion site was head and neck in approximately 45% of patients, the pelvis in approximately 40%, with miscellaneous sites accounting for the rest. Patients were randomized to receive interstitial RT alone or combined with interstitial HT. There was no difference in CR rates or 2-year survival. There were major quality assurance issues with this trial. Only 1 patient was considered to have had adequate HT.

Esophagus Two randomized studies demonstrated an advantage to the addition of HT to chemoradiotherapy or CT alone in neoadjuvant treatment of esophagus cancer. In the first study, 53 patients with squamous cell carcinoma of the thoracic esophagus were randomized to preoperative HT + RT + CT (bleomycin), compared with RT + CT alone.[183] HT + CT were given concurrently 1 hour prior to RT in a 3-week regimen with a total RT dose of approximately 32 Gy. Clinical complete responses as well as pathologic responses were significantly improved in the trimodality arm, pathologic CR of 26% combined in the trimodality group versus 8% in the chemoradiotherapy alone group.

In a follow-up study, an additional 40 patients were treated with CT alone (bleomycin and cisplatin) or combined with HT.[184] No RT was given in this trial. Again an improvement in histopathologic response was noted favoring the HT group (19% vs 41%).

Malignant Melanoma A major multicenter trial was carried out in Europe in patients with metastatic melanoma. Seventy patients with 134 metastatic or recurrent malignant melanoma lesions were randomized to receive RT or RT followed by HT.[82] Overall there was a significant benefit for RT + HT, with a 2-year local control of 46% in the combined group compared with 28% RT alone. Quality assurance was similarly an issue in this trial with only 14% of treatments achieving the objective of 43°C for 60 minutes. Despite this, positive benefits were seen.

Glioblastoma Multiforme A University of California in San Francisco study evaluated interstitial HT + brachytherapy RT boost for selected patients with glioblastoma multiforme.[185] Patients whose tumors were implantable following external beam RT and CT were randomized to receive brachytherapy RT alone or combined with HT. One hundred twelve patients were accrued and 79 qualified for brachytherapy and were randomized. The remaining patients were dropped from the protocol because of disease progression. Both time to tumor progression and survival were significantly improved for the HT patients compared with those treated with brachytherapy alone. Two-year survivals were 31 and 15%, respectively. Toxicity appeared to be slightly greater in the HT patients, with 7 grade 3 toxicities reported compared with 1 in the brachytherapy alone group. Extensive thermal dose data

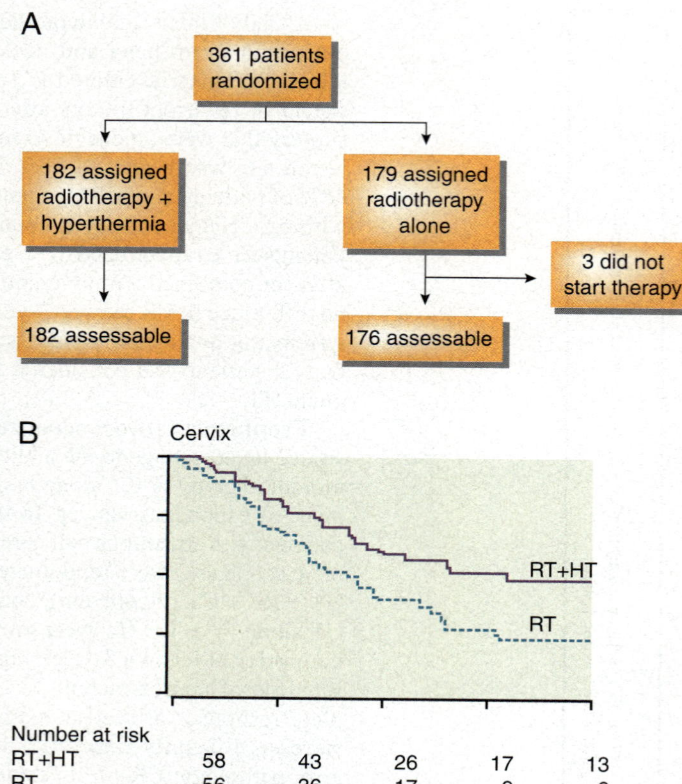

Figure 35b-7 **A,** Clinical trial design. **B,** Overall survival following HT + RT vs RT alone for locally advanced cervix cancer. A distinct survival advantage was seen with the addition of HT ($p = .009$). Rectal and bladder cancer survival were not significantly affected by heat. HT = hyperthermia; RT = radiotherapy. Figure reproduced with the permission of the author and publisher.[186]

were reported. Good heating was achieved in most patients, but no correlation found between thermal dose and response.

Carcinoma of the Cervix Perhaps the most significant phase III trial is that of the Dutch group, which explored the use of RT alone versus RT + HT in patients with locally advanced pelvic tumors.[186] This study randomized 361 patients with previously untreated locally advanced pelvic tumors to receive RT alone or RT + HT. There were approximately equal numbers of patients with rectal, bladder, and cervix carcinoma. No CT was given in this trial. CR rates were 39% after RT alone and 55% after RT + HT ($p = < .001$). Duration of local control was also significantly improved with RT + HT compared with RT alone. Most of the benefit appeared to occur in patients with cervical carcinoma in whom the CR rate following RT + HT was 83% compared with 57% after RT alone. Three-year survival was 27% in the RT alone group of cervix cancer patients, 51% in the RT + HT group ($p = .003$) (Figure 35b-7). HT treatments were given once weekly for a total of five treatments. Generally, thermal goals were not achieved. Detailed thermal dose analyses were not published.

Although the effect of HT in this study was fairly dramatic, it has been criticized for suboptimal therapy in the control arm, namely RT alone as opposed to RT + CT. At the time the trial was initiated in 1990, the role of CT in locally advanced cervix carcinoma was not established. Subsequently, a number of studies published in 1999/2000 have demonstrated a survival advantage for concurrent cisplatin + RT in cervical carcinoma.[187–191] Two new phase III trials have now been initiated comparing CT + RT + HT to CT + RT in the United States and the Netherlands. The control arm in the US trial is CT + RT, whereas in the Netherlands it is RT + HT.

Prospective Control of Thermal Dose Is Related to Superior Outcome Two recently completed phase III trials used extensive invasive thermometry to control the amount of HT delivered, as defined by CEM 43°C at the T90.[7,8] An important aspect of these trials was the requirement that patients were not randomized until it was determined that the tumors were heatable, using preset criteria. This was determined by performing a test HT. If the tumor was deemed heatable during that first HT, then they were randomized to receive either a low or high thermal dose, as accumulated over the course of thermoradiotherapy.

Superficial tumors were the subjects of the human trial. One hundred twenty patients were enrolled and 109 were deemed heatable and were randomized. Those patients who randomized to the low HT dose group received no further HT, but received conventionally fractionated RT, with the total dose being determined by whether or not they had had prior RT. Those patients who were randomized to the high HT group were targeted to receive more than 10 CEM 43°C T90, whereas the low HT dose patients were targeted to 0.5 to 1

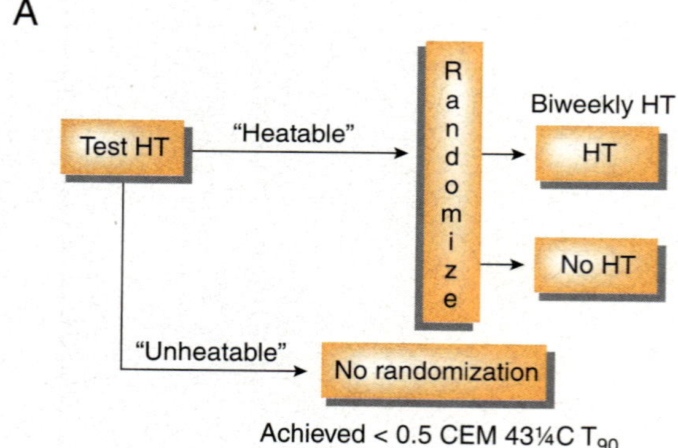

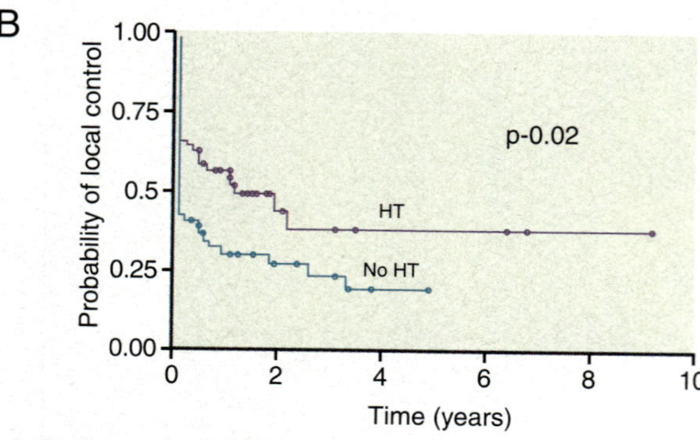

Figure 35b-8 **A,** Clinical trial design. **B,** Duration of local control in patients with superficial tumors treated with a low vs high cumulative thermal dose combined with radiation therapy. The difference in complete response rate was significant as well as duration of local control following administration of a higher cumulative thermal dose. Figure reproduced with permission of the author and publisher.[9]

CEM 43°C T90 from the single HT treatment that they received. The CR rate in the high HT dose arm was 66.1% versus 42.3% in the low HT dose arm, with an odds ratio of 2.7 (p = .02; Figure 35b-8).

The canine trial involved pet dogs with spontaneous soft tissue sarcomas.[8] These animals were treated with conventionally fractionated RT, to a total dose of 52 Gy, combined with either low or high dose HT. This trial was different from the human trial in that animals that were randomized to low HT continued to be administered HT treatments, but the duration of HT was shortened so as to not exceed 2 to 5 CEM 43°C T90 over the entire treatment course. Animals in the high HT dose group were targeted to receive 20 to 50 CEM 43°C T90. The endpoints in this trial were duration of local control, metastasis-free, and overall survival. One hundred twenty-two dogs were accrued into the trial and of these 109 met the criterion of having heatable tumors. The median duration of local control was not significantly different between the two arms, but after adjusting for other variables, such as tumor grade, volume, and institution where treatment was administered, thermal dose was found to be significantly important (p = .023). Other variables found to be important were tumor grade, volume, and HT treatment duration.

Summary of Clinical Trials Results of the published phase III trials above are intriguing. Apart from the two early RTOG trials, they all appear to demonstrate substantial benefits for HT + RT. However, many of the trials were associated with significant design and implementation problems, including relatively small numbers of patients, thermal dosimetry information that was highly variable in nature, thermal goals that were often not achieved, and control arms that may not have represented optimal standard therapy. Despite these difficulties, the generally positive nature of these trials suggest the future of HT is quite promising and that technological advances may well lead the way to even more positive results. The two positive thermal dose escalation trials provide strong rationale for implementing strict thermal dose requirements for future HT trials.

ACKNOWLEDGMENTS

This work was supported by a grant from the NIH/NCI CA42745.

REFERENCES

1. Field SB, Morris CC. The relationship between heating time and temperature: its relevance to clinical hyperthermia. Radiother Oncol 1983;1:179–86.
2. Sapareto SA, Dewey WC. Thermal dose determination in cancer therapy. Int J Radiat Oncol Biol Phys 1984;10:787–800.
3. Dewey WC. Arrhenius relationships from the molecule and cell to the clinic. Int J Hyperthermia 1994;10:457–83.
4. Dewhirst MW. Thermal dosimetry. In: Seegenschmiedt M, Fessenden P, Vernon CC, editors. Thermoradiotherapy and thermochemotherapy. Berlin: Springer-Verlag; 1995. p. 123–8.
5. Seegenschmiedt MH, Martus P, Fietkau R, et al. Multivariate analysis of prognostic parameters using interstitial thermoradiotherapy (IHT-IRT): tumor and treatment variables predict outcome. Int J Radiat Oncol Biol Phys 1994;29:1049–63.
6. Oleson JR, Samulski TV, Leopold KA, et al. Sensitivity of hyperthermia trial outcomes to temperature and time: implications for thermal goals of treatment. Int J Radiat Oncol Biol Phys 1993;25:289–97.
7. Jones EL, Oleson JR, Prosnitz LR, et al. A randomized trial of hyperthermia and radiation for superficial tumors. J Clin Oncol 2005. [In Press]
8. Thrall DE, LaRue S, Yu D, et al. Prospective application of thermal dose is related to duration of local tumor control in canine sarcomas. J Clin Oncol 2005. [In review]
9. Jones E, Oleson, JR, Dewhirst, MW, et al. A randomized trial of hyperthermia and radiation for superficial tumors. J Clinical Oncol 2005. [In press]
10. Leeper DB, Engin K, Thistlethwaite AJ, et al. Human tumor extracellular pH as a function of blood glucose concentration. Int J Radiat Oncol Biol Phys 1994;28:935–43.
11. Wahl ML, Bobyock SB, Leeper DB, et al. Effects of 42 degrees C hyperthermia on intracellular pH in ovarian carcinoma cells during acute or chronic exposure to low extracellular pH. Int J Radiat Oncol Biol Phys 1997;39:205–12.
12. Zhou R, Bansal N, Leeper DB, et al. Intracellular acidification of human melanoma xenografts by the respiratory inhibitor m-iodobenzylguanidine plus hyperglycemia: a 31P magnetic resonance spectroscopy study. Cancer Res 2000;60:3532–6.
13 Zhou R, Bansal N, Leeper DB, et al. Enhancement of hyperglycemia-induced acidification of human melanoma xenografts with inhibitors of respiration and ion transport. Acad Radiol 2001;8:571–82.
14. Lepock JR. Cellular effects of hyperthermia: relevance to the minimum dose for thermal damage. Int J Hyperthermia 2003;19:252–66.
15. Dewey WC, Hopwood LE, Sapareto SA, et al. Cellular responses to combinations of hyperthermia and radiation. Radiology 1977;123:463–74.
16. Morimoto RI, Kroeger PE, Cotto JJ. The transcriptional regulation of heat shock genes: a plethora of heat shock factors and regulatory conditions. Exs 1996;77:139–63.
17. Vidair CA, Dewey WC. Division-associated and division-independent hyperthermic cell death: comparison with other cytotoxic agents. Int J Hyperthermia 1991;7:51–60.
18. Ohnishi K, Ohnishi T. Heat-induced p53-dependent signal transduction and its role in hyperthermic cancer therapy. Int J Hyperthermia 2001; 17:415–27.
19. Raaphorst GP, Hyperthermia. In: Field SB, editor. An introduction to the practical aspects of clinical hyperthermia. London: Taylor and Francis; 1990. p. 10.
20. Coss RA, Linnemans WA. The effects of hyperthermia on the cytoskeleton: a review. Int J Hyperthermia 1996;12:173–96.
21. Liang P, MacRae TH. Molecular chaperones and the cytoskeleton. J Cell Sci 1997;110:1431–40.
22. Streffer C. Metabolic changes during and after hyperthermia. Int J Hyperthermia 1985;1:305–19.
23. Kampinga HH, Dikomey E. Hyperthermic radiosensitization: mode of action and clinical relevance. Int J Radiat Biol 2001;77:399–408.
24. Dewhirst M, Lora-Michiels M, Viglianti B, et al. Carcinogenic effects of hyperthermia. Int J Hyperthermia 2003. [In press]
25. Dewey WC, Miller HH. Effect of temperature on x-ray induced cell lethality and chromosomal aberrations. Int J Radiat Biol Relat Stud Phys Chem Med 1970;18:91–3.
26. Dewey WC, Westra A, Miller HH, et al. Heat-induced lethality and chromosomal damage in synchronized Chinese hamster cells treated with 5-bromodeoxyuridine. Int J Radiat Biol Relat Stud Phys Chem Med 1971;20:505–20.
27. Vidair CA, Doxsey SJ, Dewey WC. Heat shock alters centrosome organization leading to mitotic dysfunction and cell death. J Cell Physiol 1993;154:443–55.
28. Dewhirst MW, Sim D, Gross J, et al. Effects of heating rate on normal and tumor microcirculatory function. In: ASME. Heat and mass transfer in the microcirculation of thermally significant vessels. Anaheim (CA): 1986.
29. Song CW. Effect of local hyperthermia on blood flow and microenvironment: a review. Cancer Res 1984;44:4721s–30s.
30. Reinhold HS. Physiological effects of hyperthermia. Recent results. Cancer Res 1988;107:32–43.
31. Kong G, Braun RD, Dewhirst MW. Hyperthermia enables tumor-specific nanoparticle delivery: effect of particle size. Cancer Res 2000;60:4440–5.
32. Kong G, Braun RD, Dewhirst MW. Characterization of the effect of hyperthermia on nanoparticle extravasation from tumor vasculature. Cancer Res 2001;61:3027–32.
33. Kong G, Anyarambhatla G, Petros WP, et al. Efficacy of liposomes and hyperthermia in a human tumor xenograft model: importance of triggered drug release. Cancer Res 2000;60:6950–7.
34. Viglianti BL, Abraham SA, Michelich CR, et al. In vivo monitoring of tissue pharmacokinetics of liposome/drug using MRI: illustration of targeted delivery. Magn Reson Med 2004;51:1153–62.
35. Chen Q, Tong S, Dewhirst MW, et al. Targeting tumor microvessels using doxorubicin encapsulated in a novel thermosensitive liposome. Mol Cancer Ther 2004;3:1311–7.
36. Dahl O. Interaction of heat and drugs in vitro and in vivo. In: Seegenschmiedt M, Fessenden P, Vernon C, editors. Thermoradiotherapy and thermochemotherapy. Berlin: Springer-Verlag; 1995. p. 103–55.
37. Hauck M, Zalutsky M, Dewhirst MW, Enhancement of radiolabeled monoclonal antibody uptake in tumors with local hyperthermia. In: Torchilin V, editor. Targeted delivery of imaging agents. Boca Raton (FL): CRC Press; 1995. p. 335–61.
38. Meyer DE, Kong GA, Dewhirst MW, et al. Targeting a genetically engineered elastin-like polypeptide to solid tumors by local hyperthermia. Cancer Res 2001;61:1548–54.
39. Krol A, Dewhirst MW, Yuan F. Effects of cell damage and glycosaminoglycan degradation on available extravascular space. Int J. Hyperthermia 2002. [In press]
40. Kelleher DK, Nauth C, Thews O, et al. Localized hypothermia: impact on oxygenation, microregional perfusion, metabolic and bioenergetic status of subcutaneous rat tumours. Br J Cancer 1998;78:56–61.
41. Oleson JR. Hyperthermia from the clinic to the laboratory: a hypothesis. Eugene Robertson Special Lecture. Int J Hyperthermia 1995;11:315–22.
42. Song CW, Park H, Griffin RJ. Improvement of tumor oxygenation by mild hyperthermia. Radiat Res 2001;155:515–28.
43. Vujaskovic Z, Song CW. Physiological mechanisms underlying heat-induced radiosensitization. Int J Hyperthermia 2004;20:163–74.
44. Vujaskovic Z, Poulson JM, Gaskin AA, et al. Temperature-dependent changes in physiologic parameters of spontaneous canine soft tissue sarcomas after combined radiotherapy and hyperthermia treatment. Int J Radiat Oncol Biol Phys 2000;46:179–85.
45. Brizel DM, Scully SP, Harrelson JM, et al. Radiation therapy and hyperthermia improve the oxygenation of human soft tissue sarcomas. Cancer Res 1996;56:5347–50.
46. Jones EL, Prosnitz LR, Dewhirst MW, et al. Thermochemoradiotherapy improves oxygenation in locally advanced breast cancer. Clin Cancer Res 2004;10:4287–93.
47. Dewhirst MW, Viglianti BL, Lora-Michiels M, et al. Basic principles of thermal dosimetry and thermal thresholds for tissue damage from hyperthermia. Int J Hyperthermia 2003;19:267–94.
48. Engin K, Leeper D, Thistlethwaite A, et al. Tumor extracellular pH as a prognostic factor in thermoradiotherapy. Int J Radiat Oncol Biol Phys 1994;29:125–32.
49. Coss RA, Storck CW, Wachsberger PR, et al. Acute extracellular acidification reduces intracellular pH, 42 degrees C-induction of heat shock proteins and clonal survival of human melanoma cells grown at pH 6.7. Int J Hyperthermia 2004;20:93–106.
50. Crabtree H. LXI. Observations on the carbohydrate metabolism of tumours. Biochemical Journal 1929;23:536–45.
51. Newsholme E, Crabtree B, Ardawi M. The role of high rates of glycolysis and glutamine utilization in rapidly dividing cells. Bioscience Reports 1985;5:393–400.
52. Biaglow JE, Manevich Y, Leeper D, et al. MIBG inhibits respiration: potential for radio- and hyperthermic sensitization. Int J Radiat Oncol Biol Phys 1998;42:871–6.
53. Burd R, Lavorgna SN, Daskalakis C, et al. Tumor oxygenation and acidification are increased in melanoma xenografts after exposure to hyperglycemia and meta-iodo-benzylguanidine. Radiat Res 2003;159:328–35.
54. van den Berg AP, van den Berg-Blok AE, Kal HB, et al. A moderate elevation of blood glucose level increases the effectiveness of thermoradiotherapy in a rat tumor model II. Improved tumor control at clinically achievable temperatures. Int J Radiat Oncol Biol Phys 2001;50:793–801.
55. Kozin SV, Zaitsev AV, Yarmonenko SP. Antitumour effect of irradiation followed by hyperglycemia and hyperthermia: the dependence on tumour size and blood flow. Int J Hyperthermia 1996;12:147–56.

56. Mueller-Klieser W, Walenta S, Kelleher DK, et al. Tumour-growth inhibition by induced hyperglycaemia/hyperlact-acidaemia and localized hyperthermia. Int J Hyperthermia 1996;12:501–11.
57. Nagata K, Murata T, Shiga T, et al. Enhancement of thermoradiotherapy by glucose administration for superficial malignant tumours. Int J Hyperthermia 1998;14:157–67.
58. Dewhirst M, Ong E, Rosner G, et al. Arteriolar oxygenation in tumor and subcutaneous arterioles: effects of inspired air oxygen content. Br J Cancer 1996;74:S247–51.
59. Sevick EM, Jain RK. Geometric resistance to blood flow in solid tumors perfused ex vivo: effects of tumor size and perfusion pressure. Cancer Res 1989;49:3506–12.
60. Sevick EM, Jain RK. Viscous resistance to blood flow in solid tumors: effect of hematocrit on intratumor blood viscosity. Cancer Res 1989;49:3513–9.
61. Jirtle RL. Chemical modification of tumour blood flow. Int J Hyperthermia 1988;4:355–71.
62. Dewhirst MW, Prescott DM, Clegg S, et al. The use of hydralazine to manipulate tumour temperatures during hyperthermia. Int J Hyperthermia 1990;6:971–83.
63. Poulson JM, Vujaskovic Z, Gaskin AA, et al. Effect of calcitonin gene related peptide vs sodium nitroprusside to increase temperature in spontaneous canine tumours during local hyperthermia. Int J Hyperthermia 2004;20:477–89.
64. Meyer RE, Shan S, DeAngelo J, et al. Nitric oxide synthase inhibition irreversibly decreases perfusion in the R3230Ac rat mammary adenocarcinoma. Br J Cancer 1995;71:1169–74.
65. Fukumura D, Yuan F, Endo M, et al. Role of nitric oxide in tumor microcirculation. Blood flow, vascular permeability, and leukocyte-endothelial interactions. Am J Pathol 1997;150:713–25.
66. Hahn JS, Braun RD, Dewhirst MW, et al. Stroma-free human hemoglobin A decreases R3230Ac rat mammary adenocarcinoma blood flow and oxygen partial pressure. Radiat Res 1997;147:185–94.
67. Poulson JM, Dewhirst MW, Gaskin AA, et al. Acute pancreatitis associated with administration of a nitric oxide synthase inhibitor in tumor-bearing dogs. In Vivo 2000;14:709–14.
68. Schoonover LL, Stewart AS, Clifton GD. Hemodynamic and cardiovascular effects of nitric oxide modulation in the therapy of septic shock. Pharmacotherapy 2000;20:1184–97.
69. Hanson DF. Fever, temperature, and the immune response. Ann N Y Acad Sci 1997;813:453–64.
70. Ostberg JR, Gellin C, Patel R, et al. Regulatory potential of fever-range whole body hyperthermia on Langerhans cells and lymphocytes in an antigen-dependent cellular immune response. J Immunol 2001;167:2666–70.
71. Manjili MH, Wang XY, Park J, et al. Cancer immunotherapy: stress proteins and hyperthermia. Int J Hyperthermia 2002;18:506–20.
72. Menoret A, Chaillot D, Callahan M, et al. Hsp70, an immunological actor playing with the intracellular self under oxidative stress. Int J. Hyperthermia 2002;18:490–505.
73. Milani V, Noessner E, Ghose S, et al. Heat shock protein 70: role in antigen presentation and immune stimulation. Int J Hyperthermia 2002;18:563–75.
74. Multhoff G. Activation of natural killer cells by heat shock protein 70. Int J Hyperthermia 2002;18:576–85.
75. Asea A, Kraeft SK, Kurt-Jones EA, et al. HSP70 stimulates cytokine production through a CD14-dependant pathway, demonstrating its dual role as a chaperone and cytokine. Nat Med 2000;6:435–42.
76. Hilf N, Singh-Jasuja H, Schild H. The heat shock protein Gp96 links innate and specific immunity. Int J Hyperthermia 2002;18:521–33.
77. Nathanson SD, Cerra RF, Hetzel FW, et al. Changes associated with metastasis in B16-F1 melanoma cells surviving heat. Arch Surg 1990;125:216–9.
78. Nathanson SD, Nelson L, Anaya P, et al. Development of lymph node and pulmonary metastases after local irradiation and hyperthermia of footpad melanomas. Clin Exp Metastasis 1991;9:377–92.
79. Ando K, Urano M, Kenton L, et al. Effect of thermochemotherapy on the development of spontaneous lung metastases. Int J Hyperthermia 1987;3:453–8.
80. Bataille N, Vallancien G, Chopin D. Antitumoral local effect and metastatic risk of focused extracorporeal pyrotherapy on Dunning R-3327 tumors. Eur Urol 1996;29:72–7.
81. Dewhirst MW, Sim DA, Forsyth K, et al. Local control and distant metastases in primary canine malignant melanomas treated with hyperthermia and/or radiotherapy. Int J Hyperthermia 1985;1:219–34.
82. Overgaard J, Gonzalez Gonzalez D, Hulshof MC, et al. Randomised trial of hyperthermia as adjuvant to radiotherapy for recurrent or metastatic malignant melanoma. European Society for Hyperthermic Oncology. Lancet 1995;345:540–3.
83. Overgaard J, Gonzalez Gonzalez D, Hulshof MC, et al. Hyperthermia as an adjuvant to radiation therapy of recurrent or metastatic malignant melanoma. A multicentre randomized trial by the European Society for Hyperthermic Oncology. Int J Hyperthermia 1996;12:3–20.
84. Gillette SM, Dewhirst MW, Gillette EL, et al. Response of canine soft tissue sarcomas to radiation or radiation plus hyperthermia: a randomized phase II study. Int J Hyperthermia 1992;8:309–20.
85. Prosnitz LR, Maguire P, Anderson JM, et al. The treatment of high-grade soft tissue sarcomas with preoperative thermoradiotherapy. Int J Radiat Oncol Biol Phys 1999;45:941–9.
86. Pisters WT, O'Sullivan BO, Demetri GD, Sarcomas of nonosseous tissues. In: Bast RC, et al, editors. Cancer medicine. Hamilton (ON): BC Decker; 2000. p. 1906–30.
87. Thrall DE, Prescott DM, Samulski TV, et al. Radiation plus local hyperthermia versus radiation plus the combination of local and whole-body hyperthermia in canine sarcomas. Int J Radiat Oncol Biol Phys 1996;34:1087–96.
88. Lord PF, Kapp DS, Morrow D. Increased skeletal metastases of spontaneous canine osteosarcoma after fractionated systemic hyperthermia and local X-irradiation. Cancer Res 1981;41:4331–4.
89. Kapp DS, Lawrence R. Temperature elevation during brachytherapy for carcinoma of the uterine cervix: adverse effect on survival and enhancement of distant metastasis. Int J Radiat Oncol Biol Phys 1984;10:2281–92.
90. Mivechi NF, Dewey WC. DNA polymerase alpha and beta activities during the cell cycle and their role in heat radiosensitization in Chinese hamster ovary cells. Radiat Res 1985;103:337–50.
91. Raaphorst GP, Ng CE, Yang DP. Thermal radiosensitization and repair inhibition in human melanoma cells: a comparison of survival and DNA double strand breaks. Int J Hyperthermia 1999;15:17–27.
92. Raaphorst GP, Szekely J, Lobreau A, et al. A comparison of cell killing by heat and/or X-rays in Chinese hamster V79 cells, friend erythroleukemia mouse cells, and human thymocyte MOLT-4 cells. Radiat Res 1983;94:340–9.
93. Raaphorst GP, Yang DP, Ng CE. Effect of protracted mild hyperthermia on polymerase activity in a human melanoma cell line. Int J Hyperthermia 1994;10:827–34.
94. Overgaard J. The effect of sequence and time intervals of combined hyperthermia and radiation treatment. Br J Radiol 1977;50:763–5.
95. Stone HB. Thermal enhancement of radiation-induced leg contracture. Int J Radiat Oncol Biol Phys 1990;18:595–602.
96. Urano M, Kenton LA, Kahn J. The effect of hyperthermia on the early and late appearing mouse foot reactions and on the radiation carcinogenesis: effect on the early and late appearing reactions. Int J Radiat Oncol Biol Phys 1988;15:159–66.
97. Overgaard J. The current and potential role of hyperthermia in radiotherapy. Int J Radiat Oncol Biol Phys 1989;16:535–49.
98. Gillette EL, McChesney SL, Dewhirst MW, et al. Response of canine oral carcinomas to heat and radiation. Int J Radiat Oncol Biol Phys 1987;13:1861–7.
99. Dewhirst MW, Sim DA. The utility of thermal dose as a predictor of tumor and normal tissue responses to combined radiation and hyperthermia. Cancer Res 1984;44:4772s–80s.
100. Denman DL, Legorreta RA, Kier AB, et al. Therapeutic responses of spontaneous canine malignancies to combinations of radiotherapy and hyperthermia. Int J Radiat Oncol Biol Phys 1991;21:415–22.
101. Herman TS, Teicher BA, Jochelson M, et al. Rationale for use of local hyperthermia with radiation therapy and selected anticancer drugs in locally advanced human malignancies. Int J Hyperthermia 1988;4:143–58.
102. Herman TS, Teicher BA, Varshney A, et al. Effect of hypoxia and acidosis on the cytotoxicity of mitoxantrone, bisantrene and amsacrine and their platinum complexes at normal and hyperthermic temperatures. Anticancer Res 1992;12:827–36.
103. Holden SA, Teicher BA, Herman TS. Effect of environmental conditions (pH, oxygenation, and temperature) on misonidazole cytotoxicity and radiosensitization in vitro and in vivo in FSaIIC fibrosarcoma. Int J Radiat Oncol Biol Phys 1991;20:1031–8.
104. Teicher BA, Herman TS, Holden SA. Effect of pH, oxygenation, and temperature on the cytotoxicity and radiosensitization by etanidazole. Int J Radiat Oncol Biol Phys 1991;20:723–31.
105. Teicher BA, Herman TS, Holden SA, et al. Effect of oxygenation, pH and hyperthermia on RSU-1069 in vitro and in vivo with radiation in the FSaIIC murine fibrosarcoma. Cancer Lett 1991;59:109–17.
106. Hettinga JV, Konings AW, Kampinga HH. Reduction of cellular cisplatin resistance by hyperthermia--a review. Int J Hyperthermia 1997;13:439–57.
107. Laskowitz DT, Elion GB, Dewhirst MW, et al. Hyperthermia-induced enhancement of melphalan activity against a melphalan-resistant human rhabdomyosarcoma xenograft. Radiat Res 1992;129:218–23.
108. Da Silva VF, Feeley M, Raaphorst GP. Hyperthermic potentiation of BCNU toxicity in BCNU-resistant human glioma cells. J Neurooncol 1991;11:37–41.
109. Averill DA, Su C. Sensitization to the cytotoxicity of Adriamycin by verapamil and heat in multidrug-resistant Chinese hamster ovary cells. Radiat Res 1999;151:694–702.
110. Leal BZ, Meltz ML, Mohan N, et al. Interaction of hyperthermia with Taxol in human MCF-7 breast adenocarcinoma cells. Int J Hyperthermia 1999;15:225–36.
111. Cividalli A, Cruciani G, Livdi E, et al. Hyperthermia enhances the response of paclitaxel and radiation in a mouse adenocarcinoma. Int J Radiat Oncol Biol Phys 1999;44:407–12.
112. Urano M, Kahn J, Reynolds R. The effect of 5-fluorouracil at elevated temperatures on a spontaneous mouse tumour: Arrhenius analysis and tumour response. Int J Radiat Biol 1991;59:239–49.
113. Kido Y, Kuwano H, Maehara Y, et al. Increased cytotoxicity of low-dose, long-duration exposure to 5-fluorouracil of V-79 cells with hyperthermia. Cancer Chemother Pharmacol 1991;28:251–4.
114. Vaden SL, Page RL, Williams PL, et al. Effect of hyperthermia on cisplatin and carboplatin disposition in the isolated, perfused tumour and skin flap. Int J Hyperthermia 1994;10:563–72.
115. Herman TS, Teicher BA. Sequencing of trimodality therapy [cis- diamminedichloroplatinum(II)/hyperthermia/radiation] as determined by tumor growth delay and tumor cell survival in the FSaIIC fibrosarcoma. Cancer Res 1988;48:2693–7.
116. Bornstein BA, Herman TS, Hansen JL, et al. Pilot study of local hyperthermia, radiation therapy, etanidazole, and cisplatin for advanced superficial tumours. Int J Hyperthermia 1995;11:489–99.
117. Rau B, Wust P, Gellermann J, et al. [Phase II study on preoperative radio-chemo-thermotherapy in locally advanced rectal carcinoma]. Strahlenther Onkol 1998;174:556–65.
118. Jones EL, Samulski TV, Dewhirst MW, et al. A pilot phase II trial of concurrent radiotherapy, chemotherapy, and hyperthermia for locally advanced cervical carcinoma. Cancer 2003;98:277–82.
119. Huang Q, Hu JK, Lohr F, et al. Heat-induced gene expression as a novel targeted cancer gene therapy strategy. Cancer Res 2000;60:3435–9.
120. Borrelli M, Schoenherr D, Wong A, et al. Heat-activated transgene expression from adenovirus vectors infected into human prostate cancer cells. Cancer Res 2001;61:1113–21.
121. Schmidt M, Heimberger T, Gruensfelder P, et al. Inducible promoters for gene therapy of head and neck cancer: an in vitro study. Eur Arch Otorhinolaryngol 2004;261:208–15.
122. Lohr F, Huang Q, Hu K, et al. Systemic vector leakage and transgene expression by intratumorally injected recombinant adenovirus vectors. Clin Cancer Res 2001;7:3625–8.
123. Lohr F, Hu K, Huang Q, et al. Enhancement of radiotherapy by hyperthermia-regulated gene therapy. Int J Radiat Oncol Biol Phys 2000;48:1513–8.
124. Braiden V, Ohtsuru A, Kawashita Y, et al. Eradication of breast cancer xenografts by hyperthermic suicide gene therapy under the control of the heat shock protein promoter. Hum Gene Ther 2000;11:2453–63.
125. Blackburn RV, Galoforo SS, Corry PM, et al. Adenoviral-mediated transfer of a heat-inducible double suicide gene into prostate carcinoma cells. Cancer Res 1998;58:1358–62.
126. Lee YJ, Lee H, Borrelli MJ. Gene transfer into human prostate adenocarcinoma cells with an adenoviral vector: Hyperthermia enhances a double suicide gene expression, cytotoxicity and radiotoxicity. Cancer Gene Ther 2002;9:267–74.
127. Okamoto K, Shinoura N, Egawa N, et al. Adenovirus-mediated transfer of p53 augments hyperthermia-induced apoptosis in U251 glioma cells. Int J Radiat Oncol Biol Phys 2001;50:525–31.

128. Qi V, Weinrib L, Ma N, et al. Adenoviral p53 gene therapy promotes heat-induced apoptosis in a nasopharyngeal carcinoma cell line. Int J Hyperthermia 2001;17:38–47.
129. Tamamoto T, Yoshimura H, Takahashi A, et al. Heat-induced growth inhibition and apoptosis in transplanted human head and neck squamous cell carcinomas with different status of p53. Int J Hyperthermia 2003;19:590–7.
130. Ito A, Matsuoka F, Honda H, et al. Heat shock protein 70 gene therapy combined with hyperthermia using magnetic nanoparticles. Cancer Gene Ther 2003;10:918–25.
131. Hand JaJ, JR. Physical techniques in clinical hyperthermia. New York: John Wiley and Sons; 1986.
132. Cossett JM. Interstitial, endocavitary, and perfusional hyperthermia. Clinical thermology. Berlin: Springer-Verlag; 1990. p. 1.
133. Lee ER, Wilsey TR, Tarczy-Hornoch P, et al. Body conformable 915 MHz microstrip array applicators for large surface area hyperthermia. IEEE Trans Biomed Eng 1992;39:470–83.
134. Samulski TV, Fessenden P, Lee ER, et al. Spiral microstrip hyperthermia applicators: technical design and clinical performance. Int J Radiat Oncol Biol Phys 1990;18:233–42.
135. Brezovich IA, Atkinson WJ, Lilly MB. Local hyperthermia with interstitial techniques. Cancer Res 1984;44:4752s–6s.
136. Brezovich IA, Meredith RF. Practical aspects of ferromagnetic thermoseed hyperthermia. Radiol Clin North Am 1989;27:589–602.
137. Meijer JG, van Wieringen N, Koedooder C, et al. The development of PdNi thermoseeds for interstitial hyperthermia. Med Phys 1995;22:101–4.
138. Rhee JG, Lee CK, Osborn J, et al. Precooling prevents overheating of subcutaneous fat in the use of RF capacitive heating. Int J Radiat Oncol Biol Phys 1991;20:1009–15.
139. Turner PF. Regional hyperthermia with an annular phased array. IEEE Trans Biomed Eng 1984;31:106–14.
140. Moros EG, Straube WL, Klein EE, et al. Simultaneous delivery of electron beam therapy and ultrasound hyperthermia using scanning reflectors: a feasibility study. Int J Radiat Oncol Biol Phys 1995;31:893–904.
141. Moros EG, Straube WL, Myerson RJ. Potential for power deposition conformability using reflected-scanned planar ultrasound. Int J Hyperthermia 1996;12:723–36.
142. Underwood HR, Burdette EC, Ocheltree KB, et al. A multi-element ultrasonic hyperthermia applicator with independent element control. Int J Hyperthermia 1987;3:257–67.
143. Hynynen K, Roemer R, Anhalt D, et al. A scanned, focused, multiple transducer ultrasonic system for localized hyperthermia treatments. Int J Hyperthermia 1987;3:21–35.
144. Tobias J, Hynynen K, Roemer R, et al. An ultrasound window to perform scanned, focused ultrasound hyperthermia treatments of brain tumors. Med Phys 1987;14:228–34.
145. Shimm DS, Hynynen KH, Anhalt DP, et al. Scanned focussed ultrasound hyperthermia: initial clinical results. Int J Radiat Oncol Biol Phys 1988;15:1203–8.
146. Dewhirst MW, Phillips TL, Samulski TV, et al. RTOG quality assurance guidelines for clinical trials using hyperthermia. Int J Radiat Oncol Biol Phys 1990;18:1249–59.
147. Waterman FM, Dewhirst MW, Fessenden P, et al. RTOG quality assurance guidelines for clinical trials using hyperthermia administered by ultrasound. Int J Radiat Oncol Biol Phys 1991;20:1099–107.
148. Sapozink MD, Corry PM, Kapp DS, et al. RTOG quality assurance guidelines for clinical trials using hyperthermia for deep-seated malignancy. Int J Radiat Oncol Biol Phys 1991;20:1109–15.
149. Emami B, Stauffer P, Dewhirst MW, et al. RTOG quality assurance guidelines for interstitial hyperthermia. Int J Radiat Oncol Biol Phys 1991;20:1117–24.
150. Kapp DS, Cox RS. Thermal treatment parameters are most predictive of outcome in patients with single tumor nodules per treatment field in recurrent adenocarcinoma of the breast. Int J Radiat Oncol Biol Phys 1995;33:887–99.
151. Haverman J, Sminia, P, Wondergem, J, et al. Effects of hyperthermia on the central nervous system: what did we learn from animal studies? Int J Hyperthermia 2005. [In press]
152. Arthur R, Straube, WL, Trobaugh, JW, Moros, EG. Noninvasive estimation of hyperthermia temperatures with ultrasound. Int J Hyperthermia 2005. [In press]
153. Denis de Senneville B, Quesson B, Moonen CTW. Magnetic resonance temperature imaging. Int J Hyperthermia 2005. [In press]
154. Gellerman J, Wlodarczyk W, Feussner A, et al. Methods and potentials of magnetic resonance imaging for monitoring radiofrequency hyperthermia in a hybrid system. Int J Hyperthermia 2005. [In press]
155. Kuroda K. Non-invasive MR thermography using water proton chemical shift. Int J Hyperthermia 2005. [In press]
156. Lindner L, Reinl HM, Schlemmer M, et al. Paramagnetic thermosensitive liposomes for MR-thermometry. Int J Hyperthermia 2005. [In press]
157. McDannold N. Quantitative MRI-based temperature mapping based on the proton resonant frequency shift: review of validation studies. Int J Hyperthermia 2005. [In press]
158. Carter DL, MacFall JR, Clegg ST, et al. Magnetic resonance thermometry during hyperthermia for human high-grade sarcoma. Int J Radiat Oncol Biol Phys 1998;40:815–22.
159. Gellerman J, Wlodarczyk, W, Wust, P, et al. Non-invasive magnetic resonance thermography of recurrent rectal carcinoma in a 1.5 Tesla hybrid system. Cancer Res 2005. [In press]
160. Meyer JL. The clinical efficacy of localized hyperthermia. Cancer Res 1984;44:4745s–51s.
161. Dewhirst MW, Connor WG, Sim DA. Preliminary results of a phase III trial of spontaneous animal tumors to heat and/or radiation: early normal tissue response and tumor volume influence on initial response. Int J Radiat Oncol Biol Phys 1982;8:1951–61.
162. Falk MH, Issels RD. Hyperthermia in oncology. Int J Hyperthermia 2001;17:1–18.
163. van der Zee J, Peer-Valstar JN, Rietveld PJ, et al. Practical limitations of interstitial thermometry during deep hyperthermia. Int J Radiat Oncol Biol Phys 1998;40:1205–12.
164. Sneed PK, Dewhirst MW, Samulski T, et al. Should interstitial thermometry be used for deep hyperthermia? Int J Radiat Oncol Biol Phys 1998;40:1015–7.
165. Issels RD, Abdel-Rahman S, Wendtner C, et al. Neoadjuvant chemotherapy combined with regional hyperthermia (RHT) for locally advanced primary or recurrent high-risk adult soft-tissue sarcomas (STS) of adults: long-term results of a phase II study. Eur J Cancer 2001;37:1599–608.
166. Eggermont AM, Brunstein F, Grunhagen D, et al. Regional treatment of metastasis: role of regional perfusion. State of the art isolated limb perfusion for limb salvage. Ann Oncol 2004:15.
167. Thompson JF, Kam PC. Isolated limb infusion for melanoma: a simple but effective alternative to isolated limb perfusion. J Surg Oncol 2004;88:1–3.
168. Rau B, Wust P, Tilly W, et al. Preoperative radiochemotherapy in locally advanced or recurrent rectal cancer: regional radiofrequency hyperthermia correlates with clinical parameters. Int J Radiat Oncol Biol Phys 2000;48:381–91.
169. Hand JW, Lagendijk JJ, Bach Andersen J, et al. Quality assurance guidelines for ESHO protocols. Int J Hyperthermia 1989;5:421–8.
170. Lagendijk JJ, Van Rhoon GC, Hornsleth SN, et al. ESHO quality assurance guidelines for regional hyperthermia. Int J Hyperthermia 1998;14:125–33.
171. Kapp DS, Petersen IA, Cox RS, et al. Two or six hyperthermia treatments as an adjunct to radiation therapy yield similar tumor responses: results of a randomized trial. Int J Radiat Oncol Biol Phys 1990;19:1481–95.
172. Engin K, Tupchong L, Moylan DJ, et al. Randomized trial of one versus two adjuvant hyperthermia treatments per week in patients with superficial tumours. Int J Hyperthermia 1993;9:327–40.
173. Maguire PD, Samulski TV, Prosnitz LR, et al. A phase II trial testing the thermal dose parameter CEM 43 degrees T90 as a predictor of response in soft tissue sarcomas treated with preoperative thermoradiotherapy. Int J Hyperthermia 2001;17:283–90.
174. Dewhirst M, Poulson JM, Yu D, et al. Relation between pO2, 31P magnetic resonance spectroscopy parameters and treatment outcome in patients with high grade soft tissue sarcomas treated with thermoradiotherapy. Int J Radiat Oncol Biol Phys 2005;61:480–491.
175. Vernon CC, Hand JW, Field SB, et al. Radiotherapy with or without hyperthermia in the treatment of superficial localized breast cancer: results from five randomized controlled trials. International Collaborative Hyperthermia Group. Int J Radiat Oncol Biol Phys 1996;35:731–44.
176. Perez CA, Gillespie B, Pajak T, et al. Quality assurance problems in clinical hyperthermia and their impact on therapeutic outcome: a Report by the Radiation Therapy Oncology Group. Int J Radiat Oncol Biol Phys 1989;16:551–8.
177. Perez CA, Pajak T, Emami B, et al. Randomized phase III study comparing irradiation and hyperthermia with irradiation alone in superficial measurable tumors. Final report by the Radiation Therapy Oncology Group. Am J Clin Oncol 1991;14:133–41.
178. Sakaguchi Y, Stephens LC, Makino M, et al. Apoptosis in tumors and normal tissues induced by whole body hyperthermia in rats. Cancer Res 1995;55:5459–64.
179. Datta NR, Bose AK, Kapoor HK, et al. Head and neck cancers: results of thermoradiotherapy versus radiotherapy. Int J Hyperthermia 1990;6:479–86.
180. Valdagni R, Amichetti M. Report of long-term follow-up in a randomized trial comparing radiation therapy and radiation therapy plus hyperthermia to metastatic lymph nodes in stage IV head and neck patients. Int J Radiat Oncol Biol Phys 1994;28:163–9.
181. Valdagni R, Amichetti M, Pani G. Radical radiation alone versus radical radiation plus microwave hyperthermia for N3 (TNM-UICC) neck nodes: a prospective randomized clinical trial. Int J Radiat Oncol Biol Phys 1988;15:13–24.
182. Emami B, Scott C, Perez CA, et al. Phase III study of interstitial thermoradiotherapy compared with interstitial radiotherapy alone in the treatment of recurrent or persistent human tumors. A prospectively controlled randomized study by the Radiation Therapy Group. Int J Radiat Oncol Biol Phys 1996;34:1097–104.
183. Sugimachi K, Kitamura K, Baba K, et al. Hyperthermia combined with chemotherapy and irradiation for patients with carcinoma of the oesophagus—a prospective randomized trial. Int J Hyperthermia 1992;8:289–95.
184. Sugimachi K, Kuwano H, Ide H, et al. Chemotherapy combined with or without hyperthermia for patients with oesophageal carcinoma: a prospective randomized trial. Int J Hyperthermia 1994;10:485–93.
185. Sneed PK, Stauffer PR, McDermott MW, et al. Survival benefit of hyperthermia in a prospective randomized trial of brachytherapy boost +/– hyperthermia for glioblastoma multiforme. Int J Radiat Oncol Biol Phys 1998;40:287–95.
186. van der Zee J, Gonzalez Gonzalez D, van Rhoon GC, et al. Comparison of radiotherapy alone with radiotherapy plus hyperthermia in locally advanced pelvic tumours: a prospective, randomised, multicentre trial. Dutch Deep Hyperthermia Group. Lancet 2000;355:1119–25.
187. Morris M, Eifel PJ, Lu J, et al. Pelvic radiation with concurrent chemotherapy compared with pelvic and para-aortic radiation for high-risk cervical cancer. N Engl J Med 1999;340:1137–43.
188. Keys HM, Bundy BN, Stehman FB, et al. Cisplatin, radiation, and adjuvant hysterectomy compared with radiation and adjuvant hysterectomy for bulky stage IB cervical carcinoma. N Engl J Med 1999;340:1154–61.
189. Peters WA 3rd, Liu PY, Barrett RJ 2nd, et al. Concurrent chemotherapy and pelvic radiation therapy compared with pelvic radiation therapy alone as adjuvant therapy after radical surgery in high-risk early-stage cancer of the cervix. J Clin Oncol 2000;18:1606–13.
190. Rose PG, Bundy BN, Watkins EB, et al. Concurrent cisplatin-based radiotherapy and chemotherapy for locally advanced cervical cancer. N Engl J Med 1999;340:1144–53.
191. Whitney CW, Sause W, Bundy BN, et al. Randomized comparison of fluorouracil plus cisplatin versus hydroxyurea as an adjunct to radiation therapy in stage IIB-IVA carcinoma of the cervix with negative para-aortic lymph nodes: a Gynecologic Oncology Group and Southwest Oncology Group study. J Clin Oncol 1999;17:1339–48.
192. Carter DL, MacFall JR, Clegg ST, et al. Magnetic resonance thermometry during hyperthermia for human high-grade sarcoma. Int J Radiat Oncol Biol Phys 1998;40:815–22.

Section 10
MEDICAL ONCOLOGY

36

Principles of Medical Oncology

William N. Hait, MD, PhD
James F. Holland, MD, ScD (hc)
Emil Frei III, MD
Donald W. Kufe, MD
Robert C. Bast Jr, MD
Waun Ki Hong, MD

Medical oncology evolved from a subspecialty of internal medicine whose hallmark was the ability to diagnose cancer and to safely administer dangerous drugs to the branch of medicine most directly linked to modern molecular biology. A medical oncologist understands the biologic basis of malignant transformation and applies this knowledge to the prevention, early detection, and treatment of cancer patients. An individual with cancer should be viewed in the context of the etiology, pathogenesis, pathology, and biochemistry of the particular neoplastic process and humanistically as a whole person.

Training of medical oncologists originated in cancer institutes, divisions of hematology, and departments of pharmacology. The subspecialty was established as a separate discipline by the American Board of Internal Medicine in 1971.[1] Approximately 8,000 certified internists have been further certified by the Board in the subspecialty of medical oncology. There are over 21,000 members of the American Society of Clinical Oncology, and approximately half of the 24,000 members of the American Association of Cancer Research are physicians. Medical oncologists and hematologists have overlapping interests in neoplastic diseases of the hematopoietic tissues and share historic interests in training subspecialists in both fields. However, because each discipline became more complex, individual training programs are the preferred approach.

In this chapter, we introduce the subspecialty by attempting to define a set of principles that underlie the practice of medical oncology.

PRINCIPLES

Principle n. *an important underlying law or assumption required in a system of thought.*

Certain principles underlie the practice of medical oncology and are listed in Table 36-1. These tenets, not mathematically derived or subject to rigorous validation, should nonetheless serve the purpose of providing both the uninitiated young practitioner and the seasoned veteran with a perspective gleaned from the several vantage points of the authors.

The treatment of cancer is multidisciplinary, requiring consultation with knowledgeable colleagues in related subspecialties. The practice of medical oncology is dependent on highly productive interactions with cognate disciplines, particularly surgical oncology, radiation oncology, radiology, and pathology. Multiple other interactions occur with nursing oncology, psycho-oncology, neuro-oncology, gynecologic oncology, rehabilitation medicine, and, for young patients, pediatric oncology. Infectious diseases are common complications of cancers and their treatments, forming a natural alliance with specialists in infectious diseases. Today, with the gratifying number of long-term survivors, the medical oncologist must work closely with primary care physicians for follow-up surveillance and psychologists and psychiatrists, who may be required to address the existential complexities of survivorship and the sequelae of treatment.

The medical oncologist is often involved in the final decisions concerning management and is frequently the final common pathway through which decisions are implemented. The timing of surgery and radiotherapy, the decision whether to take a curative or a palliative approach, and the decision whether watchful waiting is the appropriate course or whether vigorous action is necessary are often entrusted to the medical oncologist.

Most patients have a relationship with other physicians before being diagnosed with cancer; a family physician or internist who referred the patient to a medical oncologist and other specialists may already have been involved with the patient before the recognition of a neoplastic disease. Medical oncologists must recognize their interest and continuing role in the management of

Table 36-1 Principles of Medical Oncology
The treatment of cancer is multidisciplinary, requiring consultation with knowledgeable colleagues in related subspecialties.
The suspicion of cancer is based on clinical acumen and the diagnosis on examination of tissue.
Prevention is more effective than treatment.
The medical treatment of cancer patients is based on a clear understanding of the mechanism of drug action, the potential for harmful side effects, mechanisms of drug resistance, and the principles of therapeutics.
Early-stage cancers are more curable than late-stage cancers; the first treatment is more effective than the next.
The best treatment is often found through participation in clinical trials.
Cancer surveillance must be based on validated assumptions.
Oncologic care is for life.

patients with multisystem disease and communicate with them effectively. In the absence of such consultants, however, the medical oncologist must also implement all aspects of internal medicine. Elsewhere, this book contains detailed descriptions of various diseases; the modalities used in their treatment; the pharmacologic, immunologic, neurologic, psychological, biochemical, epidemiologic, and molecular biologic aspects of cancers; and the complications that cancers cause. Oncologic emergencies, rehabilitation, and the oncologist's relationship to medical informatics and to government are also presented. Familiarity with these topics constitutes a foundation for medical oncology from which the principles derive.

The suspicion of cancer is based on clinical acumen and the diagnosis on examination of tissue. Oncologists must be highly competent internists to diagnose, exclude, and treat cancer. Many diseases can mimic the signs and symptoms of cancer, but the medical oncologist must not miss a nonmalignant cause. Conversely, the internist and the medical oncologist must remember that cancer, like syphilis in the past, is the "great masquerader" and, thus, must be considered in every differential diagnosis.[2] A medical oncologist must understand the pathophysiology of cancer, the genetic predispositions, and the basic pharmacology that is the bedrock of effective cancer treatment. All cancers are not the same, and all patients with a given type of cancer do not behave in a similar manner.

For complex new syndromes appearing in a patient who once had cancer, such as pulmonary insufficiency, meningoencephalopathy, or inexplicable pain, it is indispensable to establish by objective criteria that cancer is the proximate cause. Cancer patients are not protected from other symptomatic noncancerous diseases, such as pulmonary fibrosis and central nervous system disorders, or painful conditions, such as a herniated disk. No symptom should be attributed to cancer without persuasive evidence. Yet cancer must be suspected every time.

To ascribe a finding to cancer requires histologic proof. Modern medical oncologists will need to both understand the histologic appearance of malignant and premalignant lesions and be able to understand the interpretation of complex profiles of gene transcription and protein translation, as well as chromosomal abnormalities and gene sequences, to properly diagnose and manage their patients. These advances will lead to an even greater number of individuals who know that they are at risk of developing cancer, living with a diagnosis of cancer, or putatively cured of cancer but are concerned about recurrence. It is an exceptional case when a medical oncologist can consider treatment without a histologic diagnosis. Certain oncologic emergencies, such as spinal cord compression or superior vena cava syndrome, were once considered exceptions, but with modern imaging and biopsy techniques, a tissue diagnosis can usually be made rapidly and safely. Cytologic diagnoses may provide sufficient information in the presence of unambiguous clinical syndromes, but cytology of the bronchus, stomach, cervix, and body fluids has produced sufficient numbers of false-positive identifications to show that corroborating evidence is essential. Highly specific biochemical markers may be helpful when clinical and radiologic findings are characteristic and when a major intracavitary (cranial, thoracic, or abdominal) biopsy procedure would constitute an ominously serious event for a particular patient. Even elevation of human chorionic gonadotropin, alpha-fetoprotein, or cancer antigen (CA) 125 or CA 19-9 in the presence of compatible clinical manifestations is rarely sufficient, with the possible exception of relapsing disease. It is always preferable to have histologic evidence whenever possible.

The management of cancer patients requires an understanding of the genetics, biology, and pharmacology of neoplasia and the psychosocial impact of a cancer predisposition or diagnosis on patient and physician. The practice of medical oncology requires wisdom, sensitivity, and resourcefulness. For the patient in whom relatively asymptomatic findings lead to a diagnosis of cancer, it is useful to consider that the day before the discovery, the patient was living with cancer. It is a source of some encouragement to patients to know that a diagnosis of cancer does not lead immediately or inevitably to death. The medical oncologist may be able to stress the long-term evolution of a cancer, the several stages that intervene between the carcinogenic stimulus, genetic mutations, selection of cells with a survival advantage, and the appearance of an autonomous neoplasm. Because this process usually takes years and often decades, it is of value to place the neoplastic process in perspective (vide infra). This is particularly important when a patient is being urged to make an immediate decision regarding surgery, radiation, or chemotherapy. When one considers that, on average, it will take more than 5 years for a malignant cell to undergo the requisite 30 doublings to achieve a 1 cm (1 billion cell) mass required for most diagnoses, an additional week or two to gather information and opinions is unlikely to have a negative impact on the ultimate course of the disease.

Increasingly, individuals are recognized to harbor genetic predispositions to cancer owing to mutations or polymorphisms. The oncologist must combine an understanding of the impact of these changes on the probability of being diagnosed with cancer and weigh the risks and benefits of medical intervention while being sensitive to the emotional impact that this knowledge has on individuals and their families. In some, cancer or the prevention of cancer may become a chronic process requiring ongoing treatment analogous to the management of diabetes or hypertension. Similarly, oncologists must recognize environmental exposures that increase the risk of cancer and attempt intervention to mitigate that risk. An increasing number of patients who might have developed cancer will be at greater risk of dying from other diseases than of dying from cancer.

Table 36-2 Cancers Curable with Chemotherapy
Choriocarcinoma
Acute lymphocytic leukemia of childhood
Burkitt's lymphoma
Hodgkin's disease
Acute promyelocytic leukemia
Large follicular center cell lymphoma
Embryonal carcinoma of testis
Hairy cell leukemia

The medical oncologist must distinguish between a neoplasm in which a chance for cure exists versus one that is currently incurable ("precurable"). Most cancers are curable if detected early, and most cancers are incurable if detected late. Thus, a 1 cm tumor of 1×10^9 cells is often curable, whereas a tumor mass approaching 1×10^{12} cells is usually fatal. Whereas the former is likely to be driven by few genetic mutations, confined to one or two critical pathways, the latter is likely to harbor multiple mutations in several pathways that make successful treatment less likely. The medical oncologist must therefore appreciate the importance of prevention, screening, and early detection and must actively educate colleagues and patients.

Advances in our understanding of cancer biology encourage the belief that one day all cancers will be prevented or cured. It is axiomatic that the day before the first metastatic choriocarcinoma was cured with high-dose methotrexate,[3,4] metastatic cancer, in general, was considered incurable by most observers. Similar considerations apply to every neoplastic disease that is now curable (Table 36-2). Other neoplasms are currently not cured by medicines alone but require participation of surgery or radiotherapy as an intrinsic part of the therapeutic process (Table 36-3).

Patients are often influenced by their present state of subjective well-being. It is the responsibility of an oncologist to recognize the often pernicious behavior of cancer in its potential for recurrence and metastasis. In this context, the medical oncologist

Table 36-3 Cancers Subcurable with Chemotherapy*
With regional therapy
Wilms' tumor
Osteosarcoma
Ewing's sarcoma
Embryonal rhabdomyosarcoma
Adenocarcinoma of breast
Small cell carcinoma of lung
Squamous cell carcinoma of upper aerodigestive tract†
Adenocarcinoma of ovary
Thymoma
Without regional therapy
Acute lymphocytic leukemia of adulthood
Acute myeloid leukemia
Lymphomas, some subsets

*By definition, < 50% curable with chemotherapy alone; cure rates obtained with chemotherapy plus regional therapy are significantly superior to those with regional therapy alone (ie, chemotherapeutic cure of micrometastatic disease only).
†Cure rates < 50% in most series.

must interact directly with the patient and family, as well as with the chart, films, slides, and other critical raw data. It is important to understand how patients make choices so as to present information in a way that does not bias an eventual decision. Additionally, altering behavior of patients and their families is likely to occur.[5] For example, following a "scare" that a lung nodule could have been malignant may be the best time to treat nicotine addiction in the patient and in members of the family. The diagnosis of cancer constitutes a serious emotional burden that may distort ordinary reason. By firsthand intimacy with the diagnosis, the extent of the disease, and the patient's attitudes and infirmities, the medical oncologist can make rational recommendations to the patient and to the other physicians involved.

Explanations of disease, anticipated therapies, protocols in which there is randomization, and unknowns must be tailored to the intellectual and emotional levels of the particular patient. It is never permissible to lie, but it may be prudent not to deposit all of the truth at once on a patient who cannot accept the full details and ramifications of diagnosis and management. "Your patient has no more right to all the truth you know than to all the medicine in your saddlebags" was a humane and ethical tenet advanced by Oliver Wendell Holmes more than a century ago.[6] It is dishonest to twist facts or to deny specific features, such as the existence of metastases. By the same token, it is wrong to deny a patient an opportunity to make final dispositions with respect to self, family, religion, the law, and business by falsely stating that a disease is benign or cured. Families who assert that the patient must not know because the patient could not stand it are usually twice wrong: the patient often knows already or may be more distraught by being excluded from knowing, and the patient ordinarily incorporates the information into his or her life equation indistinguishably from other patients. A reading of Tolstoy's masterful *The Death of Ivan Ilyich* should convince any doubting oncologist about the terror of uncertainty and the value of direct and honest, yet humane, interactions with the patient. When a patient asks, "There is hope, isn't there?" the oncologist can always be positive. Hope is a uniquely human characteristic that sustains the will to continue, and all oncologists and all patients do hope for a better outcome.

The treatment of patients with life-threatening disease can take its toll on providers of care. A sense of frustration can affect anyone who encounters barriers to successful completion of an important task. This is particularly true of intellectual tasks and invisible barriers. When the barrier is a lethal disease about which the oncologist can do little that is effective, the frustration can be all consuming. Oncologists who encounter several instances of recrudescent or refractory disease in a short time (especially if punctuated by the deaths of young or favorite patients, uninterrupted by counterbalancing compensatory successes) may well experience frustration, a sense of inadequacy, and depression. Frequent repetition of this cyclic phenomenon may lead to burnout.

The medical oncologist knows that many of today's cancers are not yet curable. To the extent that the medical oncologist can be involved, actually and conceptually, in the solution to these complex mysteries, the frustration is lessened. Cancer research, whether at the basic or the clinical level, is held in high esteem by our fellow citizens. Group identity, "being one of the team," helps offset the self-deprecation when human tragedies mount despite one's best efforts. The camaraderie of other oncologists helps because they battle the same enemy with the same primitive weapons. Another oncologist can understand the trauma and the distress; it is an encounter on familiar terrain.

The appreciation that the horizon is distant, and that oncologists are all working intently to see beyond it, puts present frustration in a more appropriate perspective. Involvement in the systematized academic pursuit, whether in an academic setting, a medical school outreach, an oncology society, or a local collaborative group, provides the security of collegial support. A sound mind in a sound body implies rest, exercise, nutrition, and enjoyment. To ensure the last, the first three are prerequisites. Avocation and vacation are a portion of good mental health, included in the terms *rest* and *exercise*.

If these stratagems do not help the potentially burnt out oncologist find a new orientation and a more resilient response to the inevitable future traumas, the oncologist may well consider an alternative occupation. Many oncologists have moved honorably to laboratory, administrative, or pharmaceutical positions, where they are insulated from the difficulties of patients' illnesses.

Finally, all oncologists can benefit from the vast array of continuing medical education programs given at academic medical centers, on the World Wide Web, at national meetings such as the American Association for Cancer Research and the American Society of Clinical Oncology, and through textbooks such as *Cancer Medicine*.

Prevention is more effective than treatment. The seminal work of Dr. Bert Vogelstein of John Hopkins Medical School demonstrated that as a normal epithelium transforms through dysplasia, anaplasia, and, eventually, neoplasia, there is a progressive increase in genetic mutations, a process that may take many years.[7] Similarly, as chronic myelogenous leukemia progresses from the chronic phase, through the accelerated phase, to blast crisis, more chromosomal and genetic abnormalities are acquired. Exposure to environmental carcinogens, most commonly through tobacco use owing to nicotine addiction, accelerates the oncogenic process most prominently in the bronchial mucosa. These mutations activate complex signaling pathways that favor cell viability and inactivate pathways that normally balance uncontrolled growth through programmed cell death. Not surprisingly, many of these molecular changes impart resistance to cancer treatment. It follows that the earlier a cancer is diagnosed and treated, the more effective the treatment. Furthermore, the oncogenic process provides substantial time for interventions that could prevent the formation of cancer in susceptible individuals.

Numerous studies now confirm that inhibition of cyclooxygenases within the intestinal epithelium with nonsteroidal anti-inflammatory drugs, including aspirin, naproxen, and ibuprofen, has prevented many cases of colorectal cancer.[8,9] Hepatitis B vaccines have dramatically reduced the incidence of hepatoma, once the eastern world's most common malignancy, by preventing the chronic inflammation and cellular damage produced by chronic hepatitis.[10] Retinoic acid can decrease the appearance of second malignancies in heavy smokers,[11] and tamoxifen can prevent breast cancer in patients at substantial risk.[12] Minor surgical interventions, such as colonic polypectomy[13] and loop electrosurgical procedure for carcinoma in situ of the cervix,[14] can prevent colon and cervical cancer, respectively.

Increasingly, the medical oncologist will be called on to decide whether medical or surgical prevention is indicated in individuals without cancer but for whom cancer is a significant risk. This will require a sophisticated understanding of medical genetics, genomics, and proteomics, which will ultimately extend to subtle genetic abnormalities, such as single nucleotide polymorphisms and circulating biomarkers. In addition, the use of preventive drugs will require long-term monitoring because they will likely be used each day for years. Currently, the medical oncologist is asked to decide who should receive tamoxifen for prevention of breast cancer, retinoids for prevention of head and neck cancer, and oral contraceptives for prevention of ovarian cancer. Medical oncologists frequently advise patients regarding the benefits of prophylactic oophorectomy and mastectomy in patients with *BRCA1* and *BRCA2* mutations. Similarly, oncologists must be aware that the hepatitis B vaccine will prevent hepatoma, and a vaccine being developed against human papillomavirus will prevent many cases of cancer of the uterine cervix.[15] The oncologist must take a leading role in treating addiction to nicotine in all of its manifestations and must educate physicians and the public on the importance of early detection through appropriate screening.

Medical oncologists should counsel patients and families about good nutrition and healthy sexual practices as well as screening tests available for some cancer types. Several chapters of this treatise deal with prevention and early detection, and numerous publications that deal with these topics are available for distribution to patients and families from the National Cancer Institute (NCI) and the American Cancer Society (ACS). The NCI Cancer Information Service (800-4-CANCER) and the ACS National Cancer Information Center (800-ACS-2345) will send available publications free of charge and publish this information on their Web sites (<www.cancer.gov> and <www.cancer.org>, respectively).

The medical treatment of cancer patients is based on a clear understanding of the mechanism of drug action, the potential for harmful side effects, mechanisms of drug resistance, and the principles of therapeutics. For a drug to be effective, it must hit its target, the target must be integral to the viability of cancer cells, and it must be present in the tumor being treated.

The drug–target interaction must disable cancer cells better than normal cells. Modern methods of treatment adhere to these basic principles of cancer pharmacology and are important means by which one can predict a patient's response to treatment.

We have entered the era of "targeted therapies," broadly defined as the selective alteration of molecules that are essential to malignant cell growth. These new medications are likely to be less toxic than traditional cancer chemotherapy drugs that most commonly target deoxyribonucleic acid (DNA) or microtubules. The proper use of the new targeted therapies will require an understanding of the molecular pathways responsible for malignancy in general and possibly in each individual's tumor. Recent examples include imatinib to inhibit the transforming oncogenic protein in chronic-phase chronic myelogenous leukemia (bcr-abl)[16]; gefitinib to effectively treat patients with non–small cell lung cancer by targeting those individuals whose tumors harbor activating mutations in the epidermal growth factor receptor[17]; erlotinib, which was shown to extend survival in patients with non–small cell lung cancer[18]; trastuzumab to treat metastatic breast cancer in patients whose cancers have amplification of the *HER2/neu* oncogene[19]; cetuximab to treat colorectal cancers by targeting the epidermal growth factor receptor[20]; and bevacizumab to treat colorectal cancer by targeting the vascular endothelial growth factor receptor and blocking angiogenesis.[21]

In addition, one must appreciate the importance of drug resistance and recognize it when it occurs. When choosing treatment for recurrent disease, one should consider the likely cross-resistance to several natural products owing to the multidrug resistance phenotype mediated by the adenosine triphosphate binding cassette family transporters (eg, P-glycoprotein, MRPs), the low probability of response to drugs of the same drug class (eg, taxanes), or sequential hormonal therapies when selecting drugs with the same mechanism of action (eg, aromatase inhibitors).

Treatment of cancer patients includes the use of drugs for host support. The effects of the tumor and its products on the structure and function of the patient's normal tissues, as well as the mind and emotions, define an understanding of the disease process and of the patient in whom it takes place. It is not sufficient to order a therapy with the appropriate dose and schedule. There must be a broad understanding of and attention to potential toxicities, which represent the drug's effects on normal tissues. A medical oncologist should understand the interaction of the administered drug with target molecules present in normal tissues and the potential for drug–drug interactions to avoid unnecessary toxicities.

The availability of effective antibiotics and the use of platelet transfusions were intrinsic to early cures of the acute leukemias. Colony-stimulating factors (filgrastim, sargramostim) have significantly altered the prospect of drug-induced granulocytopenia, and recombinant erythropoietin can diminish drug-induced anemia. Means to ameliorate thrombocytopenia other than with platelet transfusions are under intense investigation.

The use of cytokines to collect circulating hematopoietic progenitor (CD34) cells enabled the convenient collection of marrow-repopulating precursors, allowing autologous stem cell transfusions to substitute for autologous marrow transfusion. New antibiotics make granulocytopenia less ominous, and oral prophylaxis with antibiotics and antifungal agents has decreased hospital admissions. These assets allow chemotherapy to be given more safely at the intended dose and schedule without delay or dose reduction.

The availability of highly effective antiemetics makes cancer chemotherapy less dreaded than in the past. The emergence of psycho-oncology as a widely appreciated discipline has also made it possible for patients to strengthen their resolve to undertake approaches aimed at cure or to accept the unlikelihood of cure with greater serenity.

Intravenous medications that may be toxic to the venous wall, and vesicant if extravasated, require the use of central venous access. When venipuncture is difficult because of anatomy or obesity, repeated needle sticks and much time are wasted in attempting peripheral cannulation. Needle phobia is a perverse part of being under treatment; it can be largely obviated by establishing permanent venous access.

Most patients with cancer are over the age of 60 and are receiving treatment for comorbid conditions. Therefore, care must be taken when prescribing treatments that could have dire drug interactions, leading to untoward side effects. No modern physician should be without electronic tools, such as handheld computers, that contain a compendium of drug interactions, drug descriptions, and appropriate methods of monitoring for efficacy and toxicity. A medical oncologist benefits from using an electronic medical record system that saves time and prevents errors through on-line calculation of dosing and electronic ordering. These systems also allow the creation of databases that can be queried for identification of trends and unexpected results (see Chapter 142, "Oncologic Emergencies").

Therapies that are totally appropriate for someone whose disease might be cured by judicious application of surgery, radiotherapy, and/or chemotherapy might be totally inappropriate when applied to someone with widely metastatic disease for whom no known cure exists. Therapy with curative intent may be toxic but of relatively short duration. On the one hand, conservatism aims at saving a life, not avoiding toxicity; on the other hand, treatment for palliative purposes would not ordinarily condone similar risks and iatrogenic effects that diminish the quality of life, even temporarily. The same is true for therapies aimed at cancer prevention because these are often taken by asymptomatic individuals for prolonged periods of time. The recent experiences with high-dose cyclooxygenase II inhibitors over long periods, which caused increased cardiovascular side effects in patients participating in one of two cancer prevention studies, resulted in serious consequences for the pharmaceutical manufacturers.[22]

Certain principles govern the application of therapies, no matter what the disease. These were enunciated more than a half-century ago by Robert F. Loeb, Bard Professor of Medicine at Columbia University's College of Physicians and Surgeons. These simple rules have profundity and nearly universal applicability but must be tempered, however, by an understanding of the neoplastic process.

The first law is if what you are doing is "doing good," keep doing it. It is implicit that a physician measure the effects of any intervention on both the tumor and the host. The lessons learned from the treatment of acute lymphocytic leukemia of childhood are noteworthy. For example, vincristine plus prednisone is an excellent induction treatment, but in 1968, a question was raised: Why not keep administering this highly active induction regimen rather than shifting to antimetabolite management? A cohort of children who were induced into remission by vincristine and prednisone were randomized to continue the induction treatment or shift to the antimetabolite. They rapidly became resistant and relapsed, whereas those who were shifted to the antimetabolite experienced long-term sustained remissions and cures (Cancer and Leukemia Group B, unpublished data). Thus, the first law of therapeutics does not always apply to cancer for which sequential treatment regimens may have special importance. Much of curative oncology relates to the biology of the unseen tumor, for which the current clinical status may not be informative. The first law seems more applicable to clinically recognizable disease.

The second law of therapeutics states that if what you are doing is not "doing good," stop doing it. Most therapeutic regimens have little chance of success if after 8 weeks of treatment they have failed to elicit therapeutic benefit. Indeed, most patients show incipient tumor regression earlier. It is, nonetheless, advantageous to undertake a second month of treatment in most instances because a well-documented early increase in tumor diameter on radiographic examinations or increased pain can, indeed, be followed by tumor regression. If no symptomatic or objective benefit occurs after 2 months, a third month will not likely be beneficial. A few therapies work more slowly, however, and should be considered differently. New therapies that inhibit tumor growth that differentiate cancer cells may cause tumor stasis, however, and require different assessments of effectiveness. Before stopping treatment, corroborating information should be sought by direct measurements, radiography, or biochemical markers. Increased bony uptake of radionuclides can be a sign of bone healing, even of a previously unsuspected lesion, and is not a suitable end point. The appearance of a new metastatic deposit or the continued growth of a previously documented tumor despite chemotherapeutic treatment speaks against continuing that regimen. Always remember that it is not that the patient has failed the therapy but that the therapy has failed the patient.

Hippocrates' admonition, *Primum non nocere* (First do no harm), is also subject to reassessment in oncology.[23] Thus, the second law of therapeutics does not extend to toxic effects unless they are life-threatening or profoundly disabling. With many of the therapeutic agents available today, complete avoidance of toxicity would doom many patients to death from their neoplasm. Some patients can obtain cure, and more can achieve meaningful remission by accepting the transient effect of intensive therapy that kills tumor cells and normal cells alike. The patient almost always recovers, but the less resilient tumor may not. To treat a population of patients at so low a dose that it would avoid toxic harm (ie, lethal jeopardy) to any patient would surely exact a higher price in depriving others of adequate doses to achieve maximum benefit. Curative and subcurative cancer chemotherapy, as we know it today, is often toxic but rarely fatal. Attempts to abrogate toxicity for all by reducing the dose of an established regimen might compromise benefit for the majority.[24,25] Dose adjustment for an individual may be necessary and prudent but must always be considered with respect to other means of mitigating toxicity without dose reduction.

The third law of therapeutics—if you do not know what to do, do nothing—counsels against uninformed action. In many circumstances, a rush to judgment or, worse, a rush to do something, anything, can be disastrous. Aside from oncologic emergencies, there is rarely an occasion when observing the evolution of symptoms and findings or seeking consultation with another individual for a fresh viewpoint is contraindicated because of time pressure. In the presence of pain, one should not delay pain relief, but other therapy may be delayed to build an informed formulation. In the presence of a differential diagnosis that includes diseases other than cancer, particularly infections, one must be certain that delay does not risk mortality or morbidity from the other possible disorders. Thus, the time invested for observation and consultation should not be extravagant.

The fourth law of therapeutics is never make the treatment worse than the disease. This relates to total life equation: the price the oncologist knows the patient may be obliged to pay in present side effects to attain future real effects. Often the patient's vision is foreshortened because today's symptoms caused by drug toxicity can be more severe than the original complaints related to the cancer. The medical oncologist must ascertain the patient's attitude toward quality of life versus duration of life. It is a medical oncologist's responsibility to counsel the patient concerning this weighty topic. It is critical to distinguish therapy with curative intent from a palliative orientation. The proper goal is maximal life at maximal quality. It is a modification of the commentary that one should die young as late as possible. For some patients, the toxic effects of treatment outweigh the value of possible extension of life. This perception is often related directly to age. The treatments imperative for young patients may be inappropriate and unwise for patients in their eighties. Pain and disability from cancer may temper the desirability of certain therapies, which offer only temporary and partial relief. It is not a kindness to defer death only transiently by rescuing a dying patient back to a raft of suffering. Heroic efforts are justified only when a meaningful therapeutic option exists.

It is inappropriate for the medical oncologist to substitute professional judgment for a patient's ardent wishes when the patient strives to accomplish something that is a reasonable therapeutic goal. The medical oncologist must serve as a bastion of reality, however, advising the patient of what is possible and of what is likely. In the course of doing this, the laws of therapeutics and of humanity always include hope.

Early-stage cancers are more curable than late-stage cancers; the first treatment is more effective than the next. Since no method of prevention is likely to be completely effective, medical oncologists must recommend appropriate tests to detect cancer at its earliest possible stage. They include mammography, colonoscopy, occult blood in the feces, digital rectal examination of the prostate, Papanicolaou smears, and examination of the skin and body orifices for signs of premalignancy, such as leukoplakia and dysplastic nevi, and will soon include a variety of validated biomarkers that will identify early cancer or the presence of premalignancies, for example, ductal carcinoma in situ, prostatic intraepithelial neoplasia, colonic polyps, and cervical dysplasia. As described above, progression of cancer leads to the acquisition of mutations or changes in gene expression that select for cell survival over cell death. Many of these changes, such as the expression of the bcl-2 protein, mutation or deletion of the *TP53* tumor suppressor gene, and alterations in topoisomerases, allow tumor cells to exist in harsh environments characterized by hypoxia and a low pH. These same changes produce tumor cells that are increasingly resistant to cancer therapies.

Cancer cells that emerge following initial treatment often represent clones of cells with intrinsic resistance or cells in which the treatment has selected for drug resistance mechanisms. For example, the expression of P-glycoprotein increased several-fold in breast cancers following therapy, and this increase was associated with a markedly increased relative risk of failing to respond to chemotherapy.[26] This reality places a premium on getting it right the first time so that medical oncologists and their team must be certain that they have all of the requisite information at hand to allow the best choice for initial treatment. For example, treating a breast cancer patient without knowledge of the status of estrogen and progesterone receptors and the *HER2/neu* oncogene correctly measured would likely compromise the initial treatment of breast cancer patients. Similarly, embarking on the treatment of acute myelogenous leukemia without full genotyping and phenotyping risks making the wrong choice for initial treatment. Furthermore, resistance to imatinib is associated with both P-glycoprotein and specific mutations in the *BCR:ABL* gene. These changes are becoming defined, and new drugs are being developed to overcome these forms of resistance.

The advantage of treating early-stage patients who, by definition, have a lower body burden of cancer has proved so persuasive that the profession and patients have accepted the technique of postsurgical or adjuvant chemotherapy, acknowledging that this entails treating some if not the majority of patients whose risk of relapse and body burden of cancer are already zero. Adjuvant therapy after surgery has been demonstrated to be curative in several diseases for which surgery alone has low cure rates and chemotherapy alone cannot cure metastatic disease. Breast cancer, Wilms' tumor, and osteosarcoma are the prime examples. In many diseases, there is evidence of prolonged disease-free survival and of longer survival, such as stage II and III breast cancer,[27,28] stage III ovarian cancer,[29] and stage III colon cancer.[30] Recent evidence suggests that transcriptional profiling of breast cancer specimens may help identify patients for whom adjuvant therapy is unnecessary.[31]

Because adjuvant treatment is aimed at micrometastatic disease remote from the primary tumor, exploration of chemotherapy before surgery ("neoadjuvant") has been undertaken in a few types of cancer. In addition to earlier exposure of the micrometastases, this approach has two additional beneficial characteristics. First, regression of the primary lesion predicts that the micrometastases will also likely be sensitive.[32] Failure of the primary neoplasm to regress affords an opportunity to shift chemotherapeutic treatment while there is still a chance of affecting the micrometastases with a new regimen. Second, regression of the primary tumor may make primary surgery unnecessary, allowing curative radiotherapy, as in some head and neck cancers and as shown in a large series of patients with breast cancer.[33] In other instances, surgery after chemotherapy may be technically easier, although not always less radical, because there is no certainty that every cell has been eradicated at the original boundaries. Induction chemotherapy of sarcomas has allowed a major reduction in amputations, however, in favor of limb-sparing surgery. Induction chemotherapy often diminishes mastectomy for large breast cancers in favor of lumpectomy and radiotherapy. Induction or concurrent chemotherapy may also significantly enhance the effectiveness of radiotherapy for other tumors, such as anal carcinoma, thereby decreasing the need for surgery.

Treatment of recurrent disease is too often empiric. The response to these subsequent treatments predictably diminishes over time. For example, a breast cancer patient whose tumor strongly expresses the estrogen and progesterone receptor has a $>50\%$ chance of responding to first-line hormonal therapy, with a likely duration of response of ~18 months.[34] On relapse, that same patient's probability of response to second-line therapy is cut in half, as is the likely duration of response.[35] Similarly, patients with metastatic prostate cancer have a very high initial response to androgen ablation but limited if any meaningful response to further hormonal treatments once they relapse. Precisely why this occurs is an important area of cancer research, and one can anticipate that discoveries in this area will likely improve the treatment of cancer patients in the future.

The best treatment is often found through participation in clinical trials. The most common and lethal cancers, including lung, colon, and breast, are often incurable by approved treatments. Approximately half of all adults diagnosed with cancer succumb to their disease. Relapsed, advanced disease is almost never cured and may not be effectively treated. Furthermore, most approved treatments have significant risks of side effects and produce limited prolongation of life. Yet, despite these facts, most patients receive standard rather than experimental therapies. For many, the best choice of treatment may be available only through clinical trials.

Patients are increasingly involved in decisions regarding the choice of therapy, having been empowered by information widely available through the Internet. Patients with cancer are often apprehensive that they may not receive the best treatment and will challenge us with appropriately tough questions before moving ahead. The medical oncologist can speak with greater authority when a deliberate comparison is being made because the goal of such studies is toward improvement on the standard, not toward finding treatments that are equally good.

A number of ethical issues are abrogated by the certainty that a specific patient's disease is not currently curable. For asymptomatic patients with indolent disease, precurability eliminates the need to rush to treatment. Many problems are initially best approached by masterful observation, particularly where age and comorbidity are factors. Where a rapid course portending symptoms or inquietude prevails, however, therapy is indicated. For metastatic disease for which no cure is known, it is not only ethical but also important that a systematically designed investigation of new treatments through participation in clinical trials be undertaken early in the course of the patient's disease. This allows assessment of a drug's activity before toxicity arises from conventional therapies that might limit dosing. Conventional therapies might also elicit resistance of one or another kind or immune system depression, which might foreclose the opportunity to recognize the activity of the candidate compound.

For diseases with an especially unfavorable outlook and rare therapeutic success, delays in introducing candidate compounds to ensure that they carry little or no risk of toxicity are an unwise investment of resources and time, let alone the patient's short-lived opportunity for possible benefit. The outcome of unsuccessfully treated cancer is more ominous than the hazards of clinical investigation.

Patients should be made aware of clinical trials as part of the initial discussions regarding treatment. Too often patients are not aware of clinical trials and discover this option through friends or the Internet rather than through their physicians. Heavily pretreated patients are usually precluded from phase II and III clinical trials, thereby depriving patients of their choice to receive potentially active drugs. A trial of candidate phase II agents prior to conventional chemotherapy for metastatic breast cancer has been conducted without significant compromise in response to the established regimen.[36] Today, therapies aimed at validated molecular targets may enter the clinic once proof of principle is obtained in cell lines and safety is confirmed in animal models. Although clinical activity was notoriously unpredictable from human xenografts, new mouse models based on manipulation of mouse embryonic stem cells to either knock in or knock out genes to produce tumors that mimic human cancers may be more promising. Major differences in pharmacokinetics exist between mouse and man, and the ultimate test remains the carefully designed, meticulously conducted clinical trial. The testing of new targeted therapies is likely to change how we view early trials of anticancer drugs. For example, the phase I trial of imatinib did not reach a maximum tolerated dose. Rather, the dose was determined based on "maximum biological dose," that is, the dose in which the target enzyme was maximally inhibited.[37] Similarly, dynamic imaging techniques, such as positron emission tomography, predict the responsiveness to imatinib in patients with gastrointestinal stromal tumors well before changes occur in tumor size.[38]

Therefore, until the day arrives when all cancers are preventable or curable, enrollment of patients in clinical trials will be the hallmark of the practice of the best medical oncologists. No cancer is so well treated that an improvement in outcome or therapeutic approach cannot readily be imagined. Thus, research is imperative.

An individual in practice cannot devote the same time and energy to clinical research as one who serves full time on the faculty of a university, research institute, or hospital. However, the private practitioner has an opportunity to participate in clinical trials through cooperative groups or in collaboration with cancer centers; this opportunity should not be wasted. Every oncologist participated in clinical research during his or her training, and the oncologist's office should include the capacity to perform clinical research. It is the responsibility of the medical oncologist to discuss clinical trials with patients in a way that does not bias an ultimate decision.

Participation in clinical research serves to keep the practitioner current and provides the opportunity for patients to receive therapy in a setting in which they may be most comfortable. There is much reason to anticipate that progress would be more rapid if clinical research were accepted as an integral part of the practice of medical oncology, as it is in pediatric oncology. The technology exists in medical informatics for community oncologists to ally themselves with their alma mater or other academic centers to participate in diagnostic, preventive, and therapeutic research trials using the computer, electronic mail, and fax as expedient tools. The NCI has initiated an expanded participation project in which oncologists can access many important research protocols. Abundant resources can be found on the Internet at <www.cancer.gov>. Those oncologists who have so heavy a workload that it prevents their devoting the necessary time to participate in clinical research risk depriving their patients of access to research advances. Sharing the workload with a newly recruited colleague would upgrade the practice. Clinical investigation should serve as the bridge to fundamental science and the excitement generated by the new molecular biologic understanding of the cancer cell.

Cancer surveillance must be based on validated assumptions. Following completion of curative therapy and attainment of a complete remission or following adjuvant therapy, surveillance for early signs of recurrence is based on the logical assumption that the earlier a recurrence is detected, the better the outcome of a therapeutic intervention. Although true in principle, in practice, this is rarely the case. There are several reasons for this illogical result, including the possibilities that surveillance tests are insensitive or nonspecific or that further treatment options are ineffective. Overtesting of patients at low risk of recurrence increases the probability of a false-positive result and the attendant morbidity, psychological or physical, associated with attempting to make a definitive diagnosis. In contrast, undertesting in patients at risk of recurrence of a form of cancer for which effective salvage therapy is available (eg, germ cell tumors, large cell lymphoma, Hodgkin's disease, osteosarcoma, breast cancer) is inexcusable. Thus, the oncologist must be aware of the predictive value of surveillance tests (tumor markers, imaging studies) in the context of specific malignancies and apply them accordingly.

Standards for quantifying diagnostic tests used frequently in surveillance have been adopted in most parts of the world (Système Internationale [SI] units), except the United States. It is impossible to read an international medical journal without being thoroughly familiar with SI units. They are presented in Table 36-4 so that readers can have ready access to a source for translation from the old nomenclature, characteristically American, which pervades this treatise.

Oncologic care is for life. The relationship of a medical oncologist with patients is intimate and should not end once therapies aimed at controlling the spread of cancer are no longer effective. The medical oncologist must be skilled in the principles and practice of palliative care and collaborate actively with specialists in symptom control, for example, neurologists, psychiatrists, and hospice staff. No greater feeling of abandonment can occur than when a patient is abruptly released from care by an oncologist who fails to recognize this lifelong responsibility.

It is, however, also the responsibility of the medical oncologist to address end-of-life planning

Table 36-4 Representative Système International Units for Laboratory Tests of Importance in Oncology

Component	Present Reference Interval	Present Unit	Conversion Factor	Intervals	Unit Symbols
Albumin	4.0–6.0	g/dL	10.0	40–60	g/L
Alpha-fetoprotein, radioimmunoassay	0–20	ng/mL	1.00	0–20	μg/L
Bilirubin					
Total	0.1–1.0	mg/dL	17.10	2–18	μmol/L
Conjugated	0–0.2	mg/dL	17.10	0–4	μmol/L
Calcium	8.8–10.3	mg/dL	0.2495	2.20–2.58	mmol/L
Cholesterol	< 200+	mg/dL	0.02586	< 5.20	mmol/L
Cortisol	4–19	μg/dL	27.59	110–520	nmol/L
Creatinine	0.6–1.2	mg/dL	88.40	50–110	μmol/L
Fibrinogen	200–400	mg/dL	0.01	2.0–4.0	g/L
Glucose	70–110	mg/dL	0.05551	3.9–6.1	mmol/L
Hemoglobin					
Male	14.0–18.0	g/dL	10.0	140–180	g/L
Female	11.5–15.5	g/dL	10.0	115–155	g/L
Immunoglobulins					
IgG	500–1200	mg/dL	0.01	5.00–12.00	g/L
IgA	50–350	mg/dL	0.01	0.50–3.50	g/L
IgM	30–230	mg/dL	0.01	0.30–2.30	g/L
IgD	< 6	mg/dL	10	< 60	mg/L
IgE	20–1,000	ng/mL	1.00	20–1000	μg/L
Iron	80–180	μg/dL	0.1791	14–32	μmol/L
Iron-binding capacity	250–460	μg/dL	0.1791	45–82	μmol/L
Lipoproteins					
Low density (LDL), as cholesterol	50–190	mg/dL	0.02586	1.30–4.90	mmol/L
High density (HDL), as cholesterol	30–70	mg/dL	0.02586	.80–1.80	mmol/L
Magnesium	1.8–3.0	mg/dL	0.4114	0.80–1.20	mmol/L
	1.6–2.4	mEq/L	0.500		
Metanephrines (as normetanephrine)	0–2.0	mg/24 h	5.458	0–11.0	μmol/d
Osmolality	280–300	mOsm/kg	1.00	280–300	nmol/kg
Phosphate (as inorganic P)	2.5–5.0	mg/dL	0.3229	0.80–1.60	mmol/L
Potassium	3.5–5.0	mEq/L	1.00	3.5–5.0	mmol/L
Protein, total	6–8	g/dL	10.0	60–80	g/L
Serotonin	8–21	μg/dL	0.05675	0.45–1.20	μmol/L
Thyroxine, free (T_4)	0.8–2.8	ng/dL	12.87	10–36	pmol/L
Triiodothyronine (T_3)	75–220	ng/dL	0.01536	1.2–3.4	nmol/L
Urate (as uric acid)	2.0–6.0	mg/dL	59.48	120–360	μmol/L
Urea nitrogen	8–18	mg/dL	0.3570	3.0–6.5	mmol/L
Vanillylmandelic acid	< 6.8	mg/24 h	5.046	< 35	μmol/d

with the patient and the family. Advice regarding living wills, power of attorney, and resuscitation falls squarely within the purview of the medical oncologist. This responsibility is highlighted in states that require that do not resuscitate (DNR) orders be written on patient charts prior to death. In the absence of such orders, when a nurse finds a patient apparently dead, she must, by law, initiate emergency calls for resuscitative efforts.

When death comes from cancer as the expected final event of a gradual deterioration of vital forces, resuscitative efforts do not succeed. When we are unable to keep someone alive, the likelihood of bringing him or her back to meaningful life is infinitesimal. Resuscitative efforts should be applied to patients with cancer who were not expected to die because reversible phenomena, such as pulmonary emboli, cardiac arrhythmias, aspiration, and similar events, can provoke unexpected death in a patient with a neoplasm, just as in any other hospitalized or ambulatory patient. It is, however, in the circumstance of gradual decline and predictable disintegration of body functions that resuscitative efforts place great physical and emotional stress on the distraught family as well as on nursing and ancillary personnel, house staff, and attending physicians. Many patients, particularly the elderly and those apprised of the progress of their disease, can discuss the decision not to resuscitate with equanimity and, indeed, with a certain personal satisfaction of avoiding the fruitless anguish that such a procedure entails for the surviving family. Many patients are eager to sign living wills or to appoint a health care proxy if these possibilities are presented to them.

Because of the legal implications involved, where particular religious scruples obtain or where families have emotionally uncontrolled members who cannot accept the anticipated death of a loved one, the medical oncologist should spend considerable time planning for an eventual death. Medical oncologists, through their organizations, should also invest effort to alter laws that place significant administrative burdens on them and their colleagues and that infringe on the appropriate professional practice of medicine. DNR forms are a technique of documentation and constitute further evidence that society has moved medicine onto a new plateau of accountability.

The medical oncologist should make known his or her intentions concerning the advisability of resuscitative efforts for each particular patient in advance to forestall unnecessary trauma to the patient, family, and staff; to forestall litigation; and to settle in advance any serious disagreements with the patient or family. An impasse might occasion a medical oncologist to find a suitable substitute physician if there is irresolvable conflict concerning the plans surrounding an anticipated death.

DNR orders do not imply that there be diminution of oncologic effort to control or palliate the disease before death. However, if good judgment indicates that continued efforts are fruitless and can only inflict suffering, with no prospect of benefit, discontinuation of active therapy should always be accompanied by DNR orders.

SUMMARY

The medical oncologist stands at the crossroads of modern molecular biology and medical practice and often serves as the final common pathway for the application of cancer research to patients. A complex corpus of information is available that expands rapidly, both deeper into the nature of the cancer process and wider into new approaches that provide demonstrated effectiveness in therapy, prevention, or support.

The increasing appreciation that oncogenes and tumor suppressors act through usurpation of normal autocrine and paracrine signaling pathways provides a variety of new targets for therapy. The realization that malignant transformation is a multistep process of accumulation of genetic abnormalities over long periods of time gives impetus for the design of rational preventive strategies and guidance to target patients at highest risk. These pathways have already led to effective targeted therapies that are less toxic than traditional cancer chemotherapy. Thus, the tide of fundamental discovery is washing away many of the unknowns and the flyspeck observations. It is axiomatic that certain cancers can be cured today without knowing the intimate nature of neoplasia. How better the day, perhaps soon upon us, when we know what we are doing!

Clinical accomplishments have similarly been exceptionally productive in the 49 years since the first cancer was cured with drugs.[3] A large assortment of drugs has since been provided. A new array of genetically engineered drugs support host function, and others that are still early in their development are on the way. Imaging technologies will continue to revolutionize the ability to detect, stage, treat, and monitor cancers. Biochemical markers of tumor behavior will provide increasing diagnostic and monitoring capacity and may offer new targets for therapy.

There is probably no cancer in which some progress in diagnosis or therapy has not been achieved in the last decade. Similar achievements for cancer prevention are materializing. Oncologists must assume greater responsibility for health preservation. Much could be accomplished by applying what is already known about lifestyle, diet, and exercise. Medical facts without political action were slow to change the tax on health that tobacco levies. A concerted effort within most states has begun, but a federal role in managing the tobacco plague has been thwarted.

The horizon has never been closer. Although still distant, there are enough promising paths to follow that one of them may prove considerably faster than even reasonable optimism would suppose. The information that serves as our foundation, its rate of accrual, its revelations, and the demonstrated success of translating science to clinical applications augur well for the future of medical oncology and for cancer patients.

REFERENCES

1. Kennedy BJ, Calabresi P, Carbone PP, et al. Training program in medical oncology. Ann Intern Med 1973;78:127–30.
2. Holland J. The diseases that cancer causes. J Chron Dis 1963;16:635.
3. Hertz R, Li MC, Spencer DB. Effect of methotrexate therapy upon choriocarcinoma and chorioadenoma. Proc Soc Exp Biol Med 1956;93:361–6.
4. Holland JF. Methotrexate therapy of metastatic choriocarcinoma. Am J Obstet Gynecol 1958;75:195–9.
5. Mitka M. "Teachable moments" provide a means for physicians to lower alcohol abuse. JAMA 1998;279:1767–8.
6. Holmes O. Medical essays: the young practitioner.
7. Vogelstein B, Fearon ER, Hamilton SR, et al. Genetic alterations during colorectal-tumor development. N Engl J Med 1988;319:525–32.
8. Thun MJ, Namboodiri MM, Heath CW Jr. Aspirin use and reduced risk of fatal colon cancer. N Engl J Med 1991;325:1593–6.
9. Koehne CH, Dubois RN. COX-2 inhibition and colorectal cancer. Semin Oncol 2004;31:12–21.
10. O'Brien TR, Kirk G, Zhang M. Hepatocellular carcinoma: paradigm of preventive oncology. Cancer J 2004;10:67–73.
11. Hong WK, Lippman SM, Itri LM, et al. Prevention of second primary tumors with isotretinoin in squamous-cell carcinoma of the head and neck. N Engl J Med 1990;323:795–801.
12. Fisher B, Costantino JP, Wickerham DL, et al. Tamoxifen for prevention of breast cancer: report of the National Surgical Adjuvant Breast and Bowel Project P-1 Study. J Natl Cancer Inst 1998;90:1371–88.
13. Thiis-Evensen E, Hoff GS, Sauar J, et al. Population-based surveillance by colonoscopy: effect on the incidence of colorectal cancer. Telemark Polyp Study I. Scand J Gastroenterol 1999;34:414–20.
14. Boardman LA, Steinhoff MM, Shackelton R, et al. A randomized trial of the Fischer cone biopsy excisor and loop electrosurgical excision procedure. Obstet Gynecol 2004;104:745–50.
15. Koutsky LA, Ault KA, Wheeler CM, et al. A controlled trial of a human papillomavirus type 16 vaccine. N Engl J Med 2002;347:1645–51.
16. Druker BJ, Talpaz M, Resta DJ, et al. Efficacy and safety of a specific inhibitor of the BCR-ABL tyrosine kinase in chronic myeloid leukemia. N Engl J Med 2001;344:1031–7.
17. Lynch TJ, Bell DW, Sordella R, et al. Activating mutations in the epidermal growth factor receptor underlying responsiveness of non-small-cell lung cancer to gefitinib. N Engl J Med 2004;350:2129–39.
18. US Food and Drug Administration. Available at: www.fda.gov division. 2004.
19. Slamon DJ, Leyland-Jones B, Shak S, et al. Use of chemotherapy plus a monoclonal antibody against HER2 for metastatic breast cancer that overexpresses HER2. N Engl J Med 2001;344:783–92.
20. Cunningham D, Humblet Y, Siena S, et al. Cetuximab monotherapy and cetuximab plus irinotecan in irinotecan-refractory metastatic colorectal cancer. N Engl J Med 2004;351:337–45.
21. Hurwitz H, Fehrenbacher L, Novotny W, et al. Bevacizumab plus irinotecan, fluorouracil, and leucovorin for metastatic colorectal cancer. N Engl J Med 2004;350:2335–42.
22. Masters BA, Kaufman M. Painful withdrawal for makers of Vioxx: pulling of arthritis drug raises questions on marketing, safety risks. Washington Post 2004 ;Sect. A:1, 8.
23. Holland JF. Ethics for a clinical investigator. Non primum non nocere. Am J Med 1979;66:554–5.
24. Frei E III. Combination cancer therapy: presidential address. Cancer Res 1972;32:2593–607.
25. Frei E III, Canellos GP. Dose: a critical factor in cancer chemotherapy. Am J Med 1980;69:585–94.
26. Trock BJ, Leonessa F, Clarke R. Multidrug resistance in breast cancer: a meta-analysis of MDR1/gp170 expression and its possible functional significance. J Natl Cancer Inst 1997;89:917–31.
27. Systemic treatment of early breast cancer by hormonal, cytotoxic, or immune therapy. 133 randomised trials involving 31,000 recurrences and 24,000 deaths among 75,000 women. Early Breast Cancer Trialists' Collaborative Group. Lancet 1992;339:71–85.
28. Perloff M, Norton L, Korzun AH, et al. Postsurgical adjuvant chemotherapy of stage II breast carcinoma with or without crossover to a non-cross-resistant regimen: a Cancer and Leukemia Group B study. J Clin Oncol 1996;14:1589–98.
29. McGuire WP, Hoskins WJ, Brady MF, et al. Cyclophosphamide and cisplatin compared with paclitaxel and cisplatin in patients with stage III and stage IV ovarian cancer. N Engl J Med 1996;334:1–6.
30. Moertel CG, Fleming TR, Macdonald JS, et al. Levamisole and fluorouracil for adjuvant therapy of resected colon carcinoma. N Engl J Med 1990;322:352–8.
31. Paik S, Shak S, Tang G, et al. A multigene assay to predict recurrence of tamoxifen-treated, node-negative breast cancer. N Engl J Med 2004;351:2817–26.
32. Rosen G, Caparros B, Huvos AG, et al. Preoperative chemotherapy for osteogenic sarcoma: selection of postoperative adjuvant chemotherapy based on the response of the primary tumor to preoperative chemotherapy. Cancer 1982;49:1221–30.
33. Jacquillat C, Weil M, Baillet F, et al. Results of neoadjuvant chemotherapy and radiation therapy in the breast-conserving treatment of 250 patients with all stages of infiltrative breast cancer. Cancer 1990;66:119–29.
34. Sawka CA, Pritchard KI, Shelley W, et al. A randomized crossover trial of tamoxifen versus ovarian ablation for metastatic breast cancer in premenopausal women: a report of the National Cancer Institute of Canada Clinical Trials Group (NCIC CTG) trial MA.1. Breast Cancer Res Treat 1997;44:211–5.
35. Robertson JF, Osborne CK, Howell A, et al. Fulvestrant versus anastrozole for the treatment of advanced breast carcinoma in postmenopausal women: a prospective combined analysis of two multicenter trials. Cancer 2003;98:229–38.
36. Costanza ME, Weiss RB, Henderson IC, et al. Safety and efficacy of using a single agent or a phase II agent before instituting standard combination chemotherapy in previously untreated metastatic breast cancer patients: report of a randomized study—Cancer and Leukemia Group B 8642. J Clin Oncol 1999;17:1397–406.
37. Druker BJ, Sawyers CL, Kantarjian H, et al. Activity of a specific inhibitor of the BCR-ABL tyrosine kinase in the blast crisis of chronic myeloid leukemia and acute lymphoblastic leukemia with the Philadelphia chromosome. N Engl J Med 2001;344:1038–42.
38. Demetri GD, von Mehren M, Blanke CD, et al. Efficacy and safety of imatinib mesylate in advanced gastrointestinal stromal tumors. N Engl J Med 2002;347:472–80.

Section 11
CHEMOTHERAPY

37

Cytokinetics

Teresa Ann Gilewski, MD
Larry Norton, MD

Cytokinetics is the study of the kinetics of cellular growth, a fundamental attribute of all multi-cellular life. Because oncology is the study of malignant growth, it is rooted, in a very fundamental sense, in this discipline. All the cardinal features of a cancer—its proclivity to increase in size, to disseminate, and to destroy the function of normal organs—are dependent on the reproduction of its cells. For this reason, growth kinetic concepts pervade clinical thinking in both overt and obscure ways. As evidence, we need only refer to the everyday language of clinicians, which is replete with kinetic terms: indolent growth, rapid growth, slow or no regression ("refractory to therapy"), and brisk regression ("responsive to therapy"). The meanings of these descriptive terms seem intuitive. They are, however, more complex and profound than a superficial familiarity would reveal. Is indolent growth always slow, never to accelerate? Is rapid growth always virulent, never to decelerate? How does the quantification of cellular proliferation relate to macroscopic growth patterns? What are the connections between growth rate and other attributes of cancer? Do the presumed sites of action of anticancer drugs, the disruption of mitosis, associate growth pattern with response to therapy? Is there a difference in this regard between the impact of drugs on cancer cells and on such rapidly proliferating host tissues as hematopoietic progenitors and gastrointestinal mucosa? How does expression profiling, univariate or multivariate as by microarray, of genes related to mitosis, apoptosis, and micromorphology correlate with prognosis, natural history, or response to therapy?

An important development in the past two decades has been the asking of kinetic questions in experimental treatment protocols. Can prognosis be predicted by pretreatment cytokinetic measurements? Does drug resistance emerge rapidly between diagnosis and the first opportunity to initiate chemotherapy? Is prognosis improved by shrinking a tumor mass as rapidly as possible, even before surgical removal? What is the optimal scheduling of non–cross-resistant chemotherapies? What is the relationship between drug dose and the rate of tumor regression? Can we use molecular (based on DNA, mRNA, or protein) information to plan treatment? These and similar issues are important to both the scientist who studies cytokinetics in the laboratory and the health care professional who treats patients and gathers information in the clinic.

The field of cytokinetics actually comprises two intertwined disciplines. The first is the study of cell proliferation. This is of interest not primarily in the biologic sense of examining how cells divide (which is discussed elsewhere in this volume), but in the numeric sense of studying how fast they divide, how many are dividing, and how biologic measurements, such as DNA content per cell and gene expression, relate to these kinetic processes. The second aspect of cytokinetics is growth curve analysis, the description of rates of change of cell number over time in both the unperturbed and perturbed (therapeutic) situation. The two disciplines are closely related, in that the kinetics of cellular proliferation partially determines the kinetics of tumor growth. In addition, both cellular proliferation and tumor growth are now thought to relate to many biologic characteristics of a cancer, including its tendency to invade, metastasize, and respond to drug therapy. Hence, this chapter will consider both of these disciplines, their connections, and their clinical implications.

CELL PROLIFERATION

Mitotic Cycle: Percentage of Labeled Mitoses Curves Mitosis, or cell division, is the basic biologic process that results in an increase in somatic cell numbers over time. The term *growth* applies to the increasing volume of a cellular population and is measured in units of volume (cubic centimeters) or weight (milligrams). Growth is largely the consequence of increasing numbers of cells but also can be influenced by the increasing size of the individual cells, edema, changes in the context of the extracellular matrix, hemorrhage, and infiltration by host cells, such as leukocytes. The term *proliferation* specifically applies to an increase in the number of cells, which is measured as cell number as a function of time. Cells divide by progressing through a sequence of steps that are collectively called the mitotic cycle. Other names for the mitotic cycle are the proliferative cycle, the generation cycle, and the cell cycle.

Classic autoradiographic techniques were first used to divide the cell cycle into four phases.[1,2] The terms for these phases, described below, are still used today, although the method of assessment is now often biochemical or biophysical, not biologic as in the original usage.

The two key events in mitosis are the synthesis of DNA, which occurs mostly in the S-phase or S (for synthesis), and the actual division of the parent cell into two daughters during the M-phase or M (for mitosis). The M-phase is typified micromorphologically by the metaphase plate. The time gap between cell division and DNA synthesis is gap number 1, or G_1. The time gap between DNA synthesis and cell division is gap number 2, or G_2. Although the term *mitosis* is often used to refer to the M-phase, the adjective *mitotic* properly refers to all cells that are engaged in any portion of the whole process of self-replication. This whole process includes the submicroscopic events (G_1, S, G_2) that precede the M-phase, as well as the M-phase itself. This usage has the advantage of distinguishing cells that provide evidence of their intention to divide, from those cells, called G_0 cells, which do not express that intention.

Cell cycle phases are best understood in the context of their means of quantification. The venerable mitotic index, the counting of metaphase figures in histologic slides, is of real scientific value. However, this is very labor intensive, so it has, unfortunately, decreased in popularity.[3] An important variant of the mitotic index, also infrequently applied, is the stathmokinetic technique, in which a mitotic poison is applied prior to counting.[4]

Of all the older techniques, however, the most important, by far, is the thymidine labeling index (TLI).[5] Here viable cells are exposed briefly in vitro to a radiolabeled precursor of DNA. The most common thymidine label is tritium (^3H), but carbon 14 (^{14}C) has also been used. The percentage of tumor cells with autoradiographic grains over their nuclei estimates the fraction of cells that were in S-phase during the period of thymidine exposure. Newer variants use monoclonal antibodies directed against proteins expressed during proliferation (see below) to allow mitotic (ie, cycling) cells to be identified visually.[6–8] In all these techniques, the microanatomy of the specimen is preserved so that the microscopist can actually know that the cell being counted is one of interest.

The highest refinement of the TLI is the percentage of labeled mitoses (PLM) curve. This technique counts, as a function of time after exposure, the number of M-phases that contain radioactive label. This measures the cells currently in M-phase that had been in S-phase during the exposure to radioisotope. The PLM method formerly was used to study human disease, but this application has been prohibited because it requires whole-body exposure to a long-lived radioisotope. In spite of its limitations, the technique has been of fundamental importance in the field of cytokinetics because it directly estimates the durations of phases of the cell cycle. Its theory is illustrated schematically in Figure 37-1. In Figure 37-1A, tritiated thymidine is administered as a pulse to label cells in the S-phase. As time passes (Figure 37-1B), the labeled cells move beyond S and transverse G_2. At this moment, no M-phase cells contain label, so the PLM is zero. Over the next short interval of time (Figure 37-1C), labeled cells enter the M-phase. The PLM goes from zero to 100%, as shown in the graph at the bottom of Figure 37-1. The time elapsed from the pulse labeling to the achievement of 100% PLM is equivalent to the sum of the durations of G_2 and M. The time required for the PLM to drop again to zero is the same as the time required for all the cells labeled during the S-phase to pass through their M-phase. This is the same as the duration of S-phase (Figure 37-1D). If we follow the population through a second generation, the PLM will again rise from 0 to 100% (Figure 37-1E). Figures 37-1C and 37-1E are the same except for a translocation in time, which is equivalent to one full cell cycle.

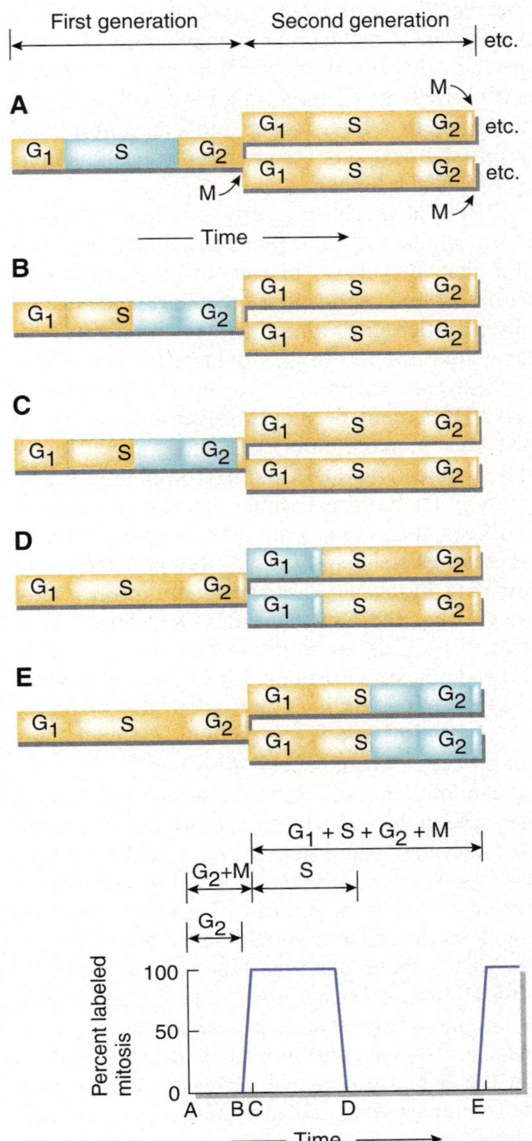

Figure 37-1 The mitotic cycle and percent labeled mitoses curve.

Actual PLM curves would be as sharp and as precise as is this hypothetic example were cycle lengths homogeneous and invariable, but, unfortunately, they are neither. Another complication is that because of the pharmacokinetics of radioisotopes and other technical considerations, it is rare for label ever to be present in all M-phase cells. Thus, sophisticated mathematic methods must be used to estimate phase lengths by model fitting.[9] In spite of these limitations, however, almost everything that we now know concerning cycle dynamics has been learned from the PLM method.

It has been observed in animal models that the labeling index (LI) decreases with increasing tumor size, whether measured in cubic millimeters or milligrams.[10,11] This is thought to be the major cause of the slowing of growth as a tumor (or a normal tissue, for that matter) gets larger. The fact the growth rate is a function of tissue size has major consequences, which are discussed in the discussion of fractal biology below and in the section "New Concepts." The rate of decrease is slower for malignant than benign tissues, as demonstrated by the maintenance of high labeling indexes in large and metastatic cancers, illustrated below using specific examples.

The drop in LI, slow as it is in malignancy, is not irregular. In fact, curve fitting has shown that the logarithm of the LI is linear in the logarithm of the tumor size. This may be related to the histologic architecture of the cancer, which is lost to varying degrees, compared with the tissue of origin. Structure may be quantified as a fractal (or mass) dimension.[12] Less structure (more anaplasia) means that the fractal dimension is close to 3. Total loss of structure (complete anaplasia) would mean that the fractal dimension equals 3. The rate of decline of the LI is directly related to the fractal dimension of the entire tissue, with more anaplastic tissues showing a slower rate of decline than the highly structured normal tissues from which they originated. Total lack of structure (complete anaplasia, which almost never occurs in nature), would be associated with a fractal dimension of 3 and pure exponential growth, with no decline in the LI. The link between fractal dimension and LI might be that the cell number (N) relates to the diameter of the tissue (L) raised to the fractal dimension (D) power, whereas the volume of the tissue (V) is related to L^3. Hence, N/V decreases as V gets larger. If LI were proportional to N/V, as would be the case were the probability of mitosis determined by the concentration of a soluble growth factor produced by the cells, this might explain the relationship between LI and tumor size.[13] Also to be considered, however, is the possibility that the cell loss (or apoptotic) fraction AF might bear a power-function relationship with V. Should LI/V drop at a faster rate than AF/V, the rates of cell production and loss would eventually converge at a plateau value of V. These and related concepts are discussed below in the section on the Gompertzian growth model.

Cell Cycle Phases and DNA Content At its birth, a normal mammalian somatic cell contains a diploid number of chromosomes, and hence diploid (2N) DNA content. Following a successful cell division, the new cell generally experiences a time gap before it begins to engage in measurable DNA synthesis. Some very primitive or embryonic cells enter DNA synthesis immediately, but these are exceptions to the usual pattern. We have termed this gap G_1, but a new cell is properly called G_1 only if it exhibits the biologic intention of entering the S-phase. Should the cell never actually progress to the point of starting DNA synthesis, it would properly be classified as G_0. Because both G_0 and G_1 cells are diploid in DNA content, we avoid the presumption of prescience by considering the two phases together. In performing this grouping, we recognize that the lengths of the G_0-G_1 phases are highly variable, fitting a log-normal probability distribution that is skewed markedly to the right, that is, toward longer times. Because the cells on the far right end of the distribution will never divide within the life span of the host, they are the G_0 cells.

This statistical distinction between G_0 and G_1 has biologic correlates. Between their M- and S-phases, cells prepare to enter the S-phase by progressing through defined stages that are dependent on protein synthesis.[14] These stages are regulated enzymatically by processes partially sensitive to such extracellular influences as growth factors and the supply of nutrients. Cancer cells may be less dependent on these external signals and conditions than are normal cells, which may account for their ability to grow in suspension cultures without extracellular matrix. This ability may be related to the activity of oncogenes or to the deregulation of suppressor genes, such as *TP53* or the retinoblastoma gene. The potency of genes like simian virus 40 large T antigen (*SV40LT*) to transform cells is particularly relevant to this point.[15,16] Recently, it has been observed that normal human cells can be transformed by the insertion of three genes—*SV40LT*, *hTERT* (which encodes the catalytic subunit of telomerase), and an oncogenic *ras*—all of which convey some element of growth factor autonomy.[17]

Cells in G_1 have already progressed beyond several preliminary steps to prepare for the S-phase, whereas G_0 cells need further time to complete early synthetic events so that they can enter the G_1-phase. These differences can be exploited in the laboratory to discriminate G_0 from G_1 cells. G_0 cells tend to be smaller, and have lower RNA and protein contents than do G_1 cells, as well as specific, characteristic messenger RNAs (mRNAs) and proteins.[18–20] For example, the Ki-67 antigen is present in all mitotic cells (G_1, S, G_2, M), but is not found in G_0 cells.[8] Also, G_0 cells do not metabolize the cationic dye rhodamine, which is thought, but has not been proven, to reflect the cells' relatively low mitochondrial activity.[21,22] However, G_0 cells, in spite of their distinctive biologic characteristics, can be stimulated by external influences to proceed through the sequence of events that leads them into the G_1-phase and eventually into the S-phase. This phenomenon is called *recruitment*.

After the M-phase, but before DNA synthesis accelerates, the cell either commits to proliferate by entering the S-phase or stops dividing by differentiating into a nonmitotic cell. The ratio $G_1/(G_0 + G_1)$ at any one time defines the proportion of cells entering their next S-phase. A particular restriction point at the G_1:S interface, now called *Start*, may be regulated by the p34cdc2 protein, which may couple with different cyclin proteins (whose levels vary within the cell cycle) to permit, alternately, a cell's entry into the S- or its entry into the M-phase.[23] Normally, the M-phase cannot take place unless the S-phase has been completed, and the S-phase cannot take place unless the M-phase has been completed. Abnormalities in this system could result in an unblocking of the normal "block to re-replication" which prevents parts of the genome from being replicated more than once during a single S-phase.[24] Such abnormalities are one possible etiology for aberrant levels of DNA per neoplastic cell (see below). Once the cell enters the S-phase, its progression through the rest of the cycle is largely self-regulated.[25] This regulation involves direct controls, in which a step must be completed before the next step commences, as well as indirect feedback loops.[26]

The S-phase, lasting between 12 and 24 hours in mammalian cells, is generally much less variable than the G_0-G_1 phase. Specific regions of chromosomes replicate at specific times, clusters of replication units initiating synchronously, with the whole complex process transpiring in a highly orchestrated manner.[27] During the S-phase, a cell's DNA content should increase from 2N to 4N. A very small number of S_0 cells may actually stop synthesizing DNA before completing the S-phase.[28] Their ultimate fate is unclear, although it is likely that some can resume the S-phase, whereas others are prevented from proceeding by intrinsic blocks in their self-regulation. Cells completing the S-phase enter the second gap, marked by a dramatic diminution in the rate of DNA synthesis. G_2 usually lasts for about 3 hours in mammalian cells, ending when the M phase begins. Rarely, a cell can rest in the G_2-phase and not proceed into actual cell division.[29]

The initiation of the M-phase may depend on the same molecular trigger as Start, but in a complex interplay with different cyclins and other factors, which are beyond the scope of this chapter.[30] The M-phase is composed of several parts. In prophase, the cell assumes the shape of a sphere.[31] The microtubules and microfilaments of the cell's cytoskeleton rearrange, the Golgi apparatus disperses into small vesicles, protein synthesis drops, and the dispersed chromosomes (duplicated during the S-phase) cease metabolic activity and then condense into transportable units.[32] During prometaphase, these units orient themselves linearly toward opposite ends of the cell and move to the midplane to form the metaphase plate. In anaphase, spindle fibers attached to kinetochores on each chromosome guide them toward centrosomes in opposite ends of the cell. In telophase, the nuclei reform, the chromosomes de-condense, and the cell normally divides into two approximately equal halves, one new nucleus per daughter cell. The M-phase is the least variable in length, lasting about 1 hour in most mammalian cells.

The total duration of the cell cycle varies considerably, but the average in human cancer is between 2 and 4 days. This is in marked contrast with the cell cycle in *Drosophila*, which may take minutes, or with that of mammalian embryos, which may take hours. Some normal cells, such as some human neurons, may never divide at all. Cancer is not always a disease of rapid proliferation, but it is always one of persistent proliferation. If a large number of cancer cells are dividing, even if they are dividing with deliberate speed, they will produce many offspring, which, by continuing to divide, will inevitably lead to an abnormal accumulation over time. For a given tissue, malignant or benign, the length of the cell cycle in vivo is fairly constant in spite of variations in the number of cycling cells in that population. However, subtle changes in cycle kinetics have been seen in cancers in laboratory animals that are allowed to grow large and phase lengths can shift significantly as cells are cultured in vitro.[33–35] This is in addition to changes in the LI during tumor growth, discussed above.

Flow Cytometry The variation in cellular DNA content during the proliferative cycle can be exploited analytically by a collection of automated methods called *flow cytometry*. Visual procedures, such as mitotic index, TLI, and static Ki-67 staining, are slow, laborious, and subjective. These negative features may change with technologic advances in assessing cellularity on slides and in the automated counting of visually distinctive cells.[36,37] At present, however, flow methods are the most rapid and quantitative.[38] The major disadvantage of such techniques as flow cytometry, in which the cells being analyzed are not visualized, is that normal stromal cells, normal blood cells, and tumor cells of various types and degrees of oxygenation are all counted together. Another disadvantage is that reliable flow cytometry requires meticulous technique and hence constant attention to quality control. Nevertheless, flow cytometry has become the most widely applied method of cytokinetic assessment in the modern clinic. Hence, it has been the most productive in terms of accumulation of literature.

In fluorescence-activated cell sorting, a suspension of individual cells is automatically counted by being allocated into bins by DNA content, RNA content, cell size, antibody label, or combinations of such factors.[39,40] This can be performed on fresh tissue—leukemias, tumor cells in effusions or ascites, enzymatically dispersed solid tumors—or on cells recovered from paraffin-embedded specimens.[41] Enzymatic methods of dispersing fresh or fixed solid tumor specimens have been shown to produce high single-cell yields, representative of the tissue as a whole, with low degrees of contamination by cellular debris.[42]

Flow cytometry can be used to measure RNA per cell, which, as mentioned above, is helpful in distinguishing G_0 from G_1 cells. Various techniques of tagging cells for the purpose of sorting are being employed. For example, cells can be labeled by the Ki-67 antibody (conjugated to a fluorescent dye).[8] Unfixed, viable cells can be exposed to bromodeoxyuridine, which is incorporated during the S-phase.[43] These cells will then react with an antibromodeoxyuridine antibody tagged with a fluorescent dye, a method that has proven reliable in studies of solid tumors.[44] Bromodeoxyuridine can also be administered intravenously (IV) to patients several hours prior to a biopsy. The tissue so recovered can then be examined for an S-phase label or can be exposed to tritiated thymidine to provide a double label, useful for examining phase durations, particularly in leukemia.[45]

The primary value of flow cytometry for cytokinetics is in its measurement of DNA content.

DNA content is usually assessed by the use of intercalating or base-pair affinity dyes. The standard output of this technique is the DNA flow cytogram, also called a DNA histogram. Standardization of the G_0-G_1 peak for DNA histograms uses diploid cells from the same species as the tissue being studied.[46] Human lymphocytes from normal donors are commonly used for many clinical applications. In the assessment of human breast cancer, for instance, lymphocytes are often obtained from normal lymph nodes removed at the time of primary surgery. The completed histogram graphs the relative proportions of cells with 2N DNA (ie, diploid cells in the G_0-G_1-phase), 4N DNA (ie, tetraploid cells in the G_2-M-phase), and DNA content between 2N and 4N, called the S-phase fraction. Another cytometric term in common use is the proliferative index, the fraction of cells that are in the S-, G_2-, or M-phase.

By measuring DNA content per cell, flow cytometry can also identify cells with abnormal amounts of DNA in the G_0-G_1 peak, termed *aneuploid*. Categories include near diploid (within 10% of 2N), hypodiploid (any value less than 2N), simple hyperdiploid (between 2N and 4N), tetraploid (4N), near-tetraploid (within 10% of 4N), hypertetraploid (greater than 4N), or combinations, called *multiploid*. Each aneuploid G_0-G_1 peak is expected to have a corresponding G_2-M peak with twice as much DNA. The DNA index is the ratio between the fluorescence channel of the malignant G_0–G_1 peak and the normal diploid G_0–G_1-peak; < 0.9 or > 1.1 is often considered abnormal. The S-phase fraction may be impossible to measure in the presence of marked aneuploidy. This is especially true when a diploid G_2–M peak overlaps with an aneuploid S peak. An overview of the literature suggests that ploidy can now be measured in more than 90% of solid tumors, and the S-phase fraction in about 80% of specimens. However, the classification of DNA histograms is not well standardized at present, so interpretations are highly variable, especially when paraffin-embedded, rather than fresh source material, is used.[47]

Mitotic Compartments When a cell divides, the daughters must either remain in a mitotically quiescent state, enter the G_1-phase, or die. There are no other possibilities. Entering the G_1-phase means that the cell has positioned itself to divide again. Such a cell is thereby a member of the proliferative fraction, also called the *growth fraction* or the *growth compartment*.[48] The second possibility is that the cell enters a prolonged G_0-phase (or, rarely, an S_0-phase or an arrested G_2-phase), which means that the cell has joined the nonproliferative or quiescent fraction. Classically, the growth fraction is measured by dividing the LI by the ratio of the durations of the S-phase and the total cycle time.[49]

The S-phase fraction as measured by flow cytometry includes S_0 cells in the quiescent fraction. For this and other technical reasons, the S-phase fraction is usually larger than the TLI. It correlates with, but is not equivalent to, the growth fraction.[50] About 2 to 20% of cells in a typical cancer are in the S-phase at any point in time. Because the S-phase occupies one-quarter to one-half of the cell cycle, the growth fraction is usually 4 to 80%, with an average of less than 20%. Some normal tissues, such as bone marrow and alimentary mucosa, have larger growth fractions and shorter mitotic cycle times than many cancers, even cancers of those tissues.[51,52]

Nonproliferative cells fall into three categories. Some highly differentiated cells are thought to be permanently nonproliferative but might survive for the whole life of the organism. Classical teaching is that many neurons fall into this category, although this issue is still under investigation. However, most terminally differentiated cells, such as the polymorphonuclear leukocyte, have a finite life span. The third type of nonproliferative cell is in an unstable G_0-phase, which means that it may be recruited into the G_1-phase with the proper extracellular signal. Stem cells share with neurons the property of living as long as the organism. But, like unstable G_0 cells, they can periodically, or on demand, produce viable progeny.[53,54] Stem cells are also called *clonogenic cells* because of their capacity for unlimited proliferation. The signal for stem cell recruitment is often from physiologic changes in the environment, such as cell death or cell injury, or extracellular influences, such as by drugs or hormones. An operational definition of stem capacity is the ability to form colonies in soft agar.[29,55] Cell culture experiments have found that from 1% to less than 0.1% of the cells in many common tumors have this property, but this may be an underestimate, because in vitro conditions may be more austere than those occurring naturally in vivo. Yet, even though malignant clonogenic cells are a minority population in a cancer, they are the prime targets of anticancer therapy because they constantly replenish the whole population. If chemotherapy preferentially kills mitotic cells, which is the mitotoxicity hypothesis, the ability of tumor stem cells to remain in the G_0-phase for long periods may be one reason for failure of therapy.[56]

The third possible fate for a cell is death. Cells lost from any phase of the cell cycle are collectively called the cell loss fraction.[57] Cell loss is important because the growth rate is the difference between cell production and cell loss. The common mechanism for cell death is apoptosis, which is under genetic control.[58] Other mechanisms are desquamation and necrosis. Whatever the mechanism, a tumor with much cell loss may appear to be growing slowly, when in fact, the rate of mitosis may be high. A well-known clinical example is basal cell epithelioma of the skin, which grows slowly in spite of showing a large number of metaphase figures.

The significant effect of apoptotic cell loss on growth rate may be illustrated by a hypothetic numeric example. Let us imagine a tumor with a growth fraction of 100%, no cell loss, and a mitotic cycle time of 3 days. This tumor will double in size every 3 days. In this case, the generation time is equal to the doubling time, the time it takes the cell number to double in size. If, however, cells are lost from the tumor at one-half the rate of cell production, a cell loss fraction of 50%, the tumor will double in 6 days rather than in 3 days. As mentioned elsewhere, growth fraction tends to get smaller as a mass increases in size. If the apoptotic fraction stays the same, or gets smaller at a slower rate, a plateau size will eventually be reached where mitosis equals apoptosis. The mathematics of these rate changes would result in the final tissue size, which relates to the degree of malignancy of that tissue. The importance of cell loss, however, goes beyond its impact on growth rate. Each mitotic cycle carries with it a finite probability of mutation.[59] A tumor with a higher cell loss rate takes more mitotic cycles to double in size than a tumor with a lower cell loss rate. Thus, the rate of cell loss, especially the rate of apoptotic, physiologic cell loss, relates directly to the rate of mutations toward biologic properties of clinical importance.

Cytokinetics and Biologic Diversity Since 1980, thousands of studies have been published that have assayed the cytokinetics of clinical cancers. There have been major as well as minor applications. One use has been in the screening of cytologic specimens for malignant cells. This exercise exploits the observation that with few exceptions (noted below), normal cells are diploid, whereas about 70% of clinical cancers are aneuploid. Screening, however, has been of secondary interest. The major use of kinetic measurements has been for correlation with clinical course. The S-phase fraction, the TLI, and aneuploidy have all been evaluated as prognostic factors. The S-phase fraction may be no higher in neoplastic than in some normal tissues. However, within a given histologic type of cancer, both a high S-phase fraction and the presence of aneuploidy are frequently associated with a growth rate that is relatively more rapid, a malignant behavior that is relatively more aggressive, and a therapeutic response that is relatively poorer.

The reasons for the consistent association of aneuploidy with high S-phase fraction are conjectural. One possibility is that aneuploidy is caused by high S-phase activity because it is the consequence of errors in chromosomal construction. The reasoning in this regard is that a high S-phase fraction implies a large number of mitotic cycles per unit of time, which provides more opportunities for erroneous DNA replication. Against this argument is the observation that many normal tissues, such as bone marrow and epithelia, have high S-phase fractions but do not normally become aneuploid. This leaves another possibility: High S-phase fraction is not the cause of aneuploidy but rather the consequence of the chromosomal abnormalities reflected in the aneuploid state. Such abnormalities may be linked with oncogene activation or suppressor gene inactivation. Some clinically benign tumors are aneuploid, so chromosomal abnormalities do not always mean frank cancerous behavior. Yet aneuploidy is clearly a step in tumor progression: DNA errors lead to growth stimulation, high cell turnover results in more opportunities for error, and errors produce increasing genetic aberrancy. The question of how fast mutations accumulate by this process is clinically relevant and will be discussed in the context of growth curve models.

Regardless of the rate of mutations, however, the neoplastic process is so closely related to spontaneous genetic change that tumor progression toward increasing malignancy is regarded as an intrinsic property of cancer.[45,60] The clonal origin of tumors has been described.[61] It has been stated that over 80% of clinical cancers are monoclonal by glucose-6-phosphate dehydrogenase (G6PD) isotype or cytogenetics.[62] Yet clonal evolution as the tumors evolve leads to heterogeneity in morphology, metastatic behavior, biochemistry, ploidy, immunogenicity, steroid and growth factor receptors, and drug sensitivity.[63] Metastases tend to grow faster than do the primary tumors from which they arise.[64,65] There is ample evidence that cytokinetics either underlies or is a direct covariate of tumor progression, that is, the mechanism relating aneuploidy to S-phase fraction also relates tumor progression to S-phase fraction. This will be illustrated in the discussion of clinical correlates of cytokinetics below in the context of the doubling time and the Skipper–Schabel model.

As discussed theoretically above, the third determinant of growth rate, cell loss, is also relevant to the generation of genetic changes. High rates of cell turnover are implicated in carcinogenesis. Elevated levels of thyroid stimulating hormone predispose to thyroid cancer.[66] Chronic thermal injury with compensatory hyperplasia and hyperplasia secondary to solar damage lead to skin cancer.[67,68] Hyperproliferation of the bone marrow in dysmyelopoiesis and in chronic granulocytic leukemia can result in acute leukemia.[69,70] Hyperproliferation of the epithelium, as of the colon in inflammatory bowel disease and polyps, and of the breast in murine models and clinical specimens, is also associated with neoplastic transformation.[71–74] Indeed, chemical carcinogenesis requires a growth promoter.[75] It is possible that the hyperproliferation of cancer cells as a compensatory response to chronic antineoplastic drug treatment may predispose to the development of drug resistance in Hodgkin's lymphoma and gastrointestinal cancer.[76,77]

All the statistical associations among S-phase fraction, ploidy, cell loss fraction, and clinical behavior are of major scientific interest. It must be cautioned, however, that these associations are not always of practical importance, especially when kinetic parameters are highly correlated with more easily measured prognostic factors, such as tumor size. As is seen with any weak prognostic factor, small studies often have false-negative results. Conversely, false-positive reports may arise via data-driven subset analysis. For example, imagine that a population of patients is divisible into those with some arbitrary factor X and those without X, those with Y and those without Y, those with Z and those without Z, and so on. A small study may show that aneuploidy means poor prognosis for patients with Y but good prognosis for patients without Y, whereas both X and Z seem unrelated to ploidy and prognosis. Here the subset allocation (by Y) is chosen because ploidy seems to be useful within the subset, not because there is a biologic reason to suspect that ploidy and Y should be related. In fact, if ploidy carried no prognostic significance whatsoever, there is a real possibility that some other arbitrary division would distinguish the patients merely by chance. This other arbitrary division could be draped in the illusion of biologic tenability, but it would not prove reproducible in prospective confirmatory studies. Hence, purely statistical phenomena such as these should always be kept in mind when reading conflicting data concerning cytokinetics and clinical behavior.

Clinical Cytokinetics: The Example of Breast Cancer Cytokinetic parameters have been evaluated for correlation with pathologic features, prognostic value and prediction of response to therapy in nearly all types of malignant growth.[78] For the purpose of brevity, breast cancer can be used as an example. There are numerous publications regarding the potential role of TLI, S-phase fraction by flow cytometry (SPF) and ploidy.[78,79] Many of the results are conflicting. As of 2000, the American Society of Clinical Oncology (ASCO) guidelines do not recommend routine evaluation of flow cytometric or immunohistochemical analysis of DNA content or S phase to aid in assessment of prognosis or treatment of breast cancer.[80]

The breast cancer literature is filled with reports of putative prognostic factors that correlate, to various degrees, with proliferative measurements. These include c-*erb*B2 (*HER2*/neu), epidermal growth factor receptor (EGFR, HER-1), mutant p53, cathepsin D and other proteases, nm-23, urokinase-type plasminogen activator (uPA) and plasminogen activator inhibitor type-I (PAI-1), and other mutation suppressors.[81–83] HER-2 is a protooncogene, located on chromosome 17q21-22, which is amplified in approximately 30% of primary breast cancers. It encodes a 185 kDa glycoprotein with tyrosine kinase activity that is involved in the transduction of signals for growth. Amplification and over-expression of c-*erb*B2 are observed at all stages of primary breast cancer and in lesions in all metastatic sites. Over-expression of c-*erb*B2 in node-positive patients correlates with high SPF and aneuploidy, but not with TLI.[84–86] Moreover, over-expression or gene amplification of HER2/neu have been found in some studies to be an independent prognostic factor whereas other studies have not confirmed this observation.[80] As of 2000 the ASCO guidelines did not recommend use of HER2/neu in early stage breast cancer to assess prognosis.[80] However, these guidelines do recommend HER2/neu analysis to identify patients for whom trastuzumab (a monoclonal antibody targeted to HER2/neu) or anthracycline based therapy may be of particular benefit.

The *TP53* gene is one of the tumor suppressor genes involved by deletion or inactivation in the development of breast cancer. Wild-type p53 protein arrests cell division at the interface of G_1 and S, binds DNA in a sequence-specific manner, and is a transcriptional activator.[87] Cathepsin D is an estrogen-related protein that acts as a peptide growth factor and may facilitate cancer cell migration and invasion.[88] In 2000 the ASCO panel felt data was insufficient to warrant routine evaluation of p53 or cathepsin D in breast cancer.[80] Insulin-like growth factors and cyclooxygenase-2 (COX-2) and cyclins are other parameters under evaluation to assess breast cancer proliferation.[89–91]

All these data signify that the growth fraction, as estimated by a large number of currently available techniques, is positively correlated with some aggressive manifestations of breast cancer, but not others, and never strongly or consistently. Hence, factors other than growth fraction alone must be important determinants of the malignant behavior of this disease. As discussed in other sections of this chapter, apoptosis—particularly the rate of change of the apoptotic fraction—is clearly a cytokinetic process of great potential in this regard. Numerous ongoing evaluations will aid in the identification of those factors of clinical significance. Recently, gene-expression signature has been found to be a predictor of breast cancer prognosisl.[92] Many of the genes implicated relate to such cytokinetic events as mitosis and apoptosis, whereas others are linked to microanatomy, which obviously underlies the fractal dimension. The further development of this field is anticipated eventually to lead to a strategy by which we may select optimal candidates for specific postoperative adjuvant chemotherapy regimens, including no treatment at all for those with already superb prognoses.

GROWTH CURVE ANALYSIS

That cytokinetic measurements correlate at all with the clinical behavior of cancers supports one of the key underpinning concepts of modern oncology, that cancer is fundamentally a disease of abnormal cellular proliferation. This manifests in two main ways. The first is that cell growth is the reason why cancers grow large and hence destructive. The second is the concept that cell proliferation is intimately associated with the generation of tumor heterogeneity. However, the fact that cytokinetic measures correlate weakly with many aspects of clinical cancer suggests that the whole picture is not yet clear, that some major but not yet obvious pieces of the puzzle are missing. Connecting cytokinetic observations at the cellular level with the analysis of how cell numbers and tumor volumes change over time may be our best method of solving this enigma. Our tool is the *growth curve*, a type of mathematic function that describes increases and decreases in the number of cells at the macroscopic level.

Understanding the totality of the cytokinetic/growth-curve relationship may be important in itself because it may allow us to better understand carcinogenesis in a way that may inform prevention strategies, with cancer prevention our ultimate goal. At present, however, the more immediate issue is that anticancer therapy is largely intended to reverse growth by killing or removing cancer cells. Growth curves not only summarize clinical course, but they also relate to the rate of emergence of mutations toward clinically relevant cellular diversity. Through both these attributes, growth curves are proving to be useful in explaining human cancer and in indicating new directions for therapeutic research. In this section we will review the history of modern growth curve analysis with an emphasis on clinical applications and the most recent implications regarding the molecular bases for cancer and its metastases.

Skipper–Schabel–Wilcox (Log-Kill) Model and the Concept of the "Doubling Time" This model of tumor growth, formulated and popularized by investigators at the Southern Research Institute, is commonly called the log-kill model. It was the original, and is still the preeminent, model of tumor growth and therapeutic regression.[93–95] The model is based on the observation that leukemia L1210 in BDF_1 or DBA mice grows exponentially until it reaches a lethal tumor volume of 10^9 cells (1 cubic centimeter).[96] Ninety percent of the leukemia cells divide every 12 to 13 hours. This percentage is the same for both a tiny tumor and a tumor close to the lethal volume. As a result, the doubling time is always constant: if it takes 11 hours for 100 cells to grow into 200 cells, it will take 11 hours for 10^7 cells to grow into 2 times 10^7 cells. This pattern generalizes for any constant fractional increase: if it takes 40 hours for 10^3 cells to grow into 10^4 cells (an increase by a factor of 10), it will take 40 hours for 10^7 cells to grow into 10^8 cells.

Exponential growth and its associated concept of the doubling time are clinically relevant.[97] Different histologic types of cancer display a great variety of doubling times within the observable range of tumor sizes.[98] The most therapeutically responsive human cancers, such as testicular cancer and choriocarcinoma, tend to have doubling times that are < 1 month long. Less responsive cancers, such as squamous cell cancer of the head and neck, seem to double in about 2 months. The relatively unresponsive cancers, such as colon adenocarcinoma, tend to double every 3 months. Clearly, this clinical observation may relate to the higher chemosensitivity of proliferating cells (see below), that is, if a tumor has a high fraction of dividing cells, it will tend to grow faster and will also tend to be more responsive to drugs that kill dividing cells. Alternatively, tumors with a higher rate of cell loss tend to have a relatively slower growth rate and also a higher rate of mutations toward drug resistance. A combination of factors may be relevant, in that slower growth due to fewer mitoses may impede therapeutic response because of kinetics, whereas slower growth owing to a high rate of apoptosis may impede response due to drug resistance.

An unspoken assumption in these theoretic considerations is that the doubling time remains fixed and thereby accurately summarizes the proliferative behavior of a given tumor for its entire life history. This assumption is almost always incorrect as will be examined in some detail below. Nevertheless, we may use exponential growth to illustrate some important properties of growth, properties that are also relevant to more complex growth patterns. The first is that when an exponentially growing collection of homogeneously sensitive cells is treated with a specific chemotherapy regimen, the fraction of cells killed is always the same, regardless of the initial size of the malignant population. This has been demonstrated in experimental animal cancers that do indeed grow exponentially, L1210 being the major example.[99] If a given dose of a given drug reduces 10^6 cells to 10^5, the same therapy applied against 10^4 cells will result in 10^3 survivors. These two cytoreductions are both examples of a one-log kill, which means a 90% decrease in cell number. The second is that it was shown quite early in the development of experimental medical oncology that for many drugs the log kill increases with increasing dose. Hence, it requires higher drug dosages to eradicate larger inoculum sizes of transplanted tumors.[100] In addition, if two or more drugs are used, the log kills are multiplicative, that is, imagine that a given dose of drug A kills 90% of a population of cells (a one log kill) when administered as a single agent. Imagine as well that were we to treat the same population of cells with a given dose of drug B as a single agent, we would also kill 90%. Then drug B added to therapy with drug A should kill 90% of the 10% of cells left after drug A alone, resulting in a kill of 99% of the cells (a two-log kill). In other words, two one-log kills equal one two-log kill. As a numeric example, if treatment A given alone leaves 10^5 cells out of 10^6, and if treatment B given alone would accomplish the same, the combination A + B (at full doses of each) should be able to reduce 10^6 cells to 10^4. If treatment C is also a one-log kill therapy, A + B + C against 10^6 cells should leave only 10^3 cells. If A + B + C is used to treat 10^3 cells, only 10^0, or one, cell should remain. Thus, if enough drugs at adequate doses were applied against a tumor of sufficiently small size, the number of cells left after treatment should be smaller than one, which means that the tumor is destroyed. This concept, the fundamental concept underlying combination chemotherapy, was first demonstrated to be of major value in the design of early curative approaches to childhood leukemia.[101] Other applications will be discussed below.

When the concept of fractional kill was first applied to the postoperative adjuvant treatment of micrometastases, say from breast cancer, it engendered enormous optimism.[102,103] After all, micrometastases are very small collections of cancer cells. Indeed, very small solid tumors in the laboratory contain a higher percentage of actively dividing cells than do their larger counterparts. It is thought, as mentioned above, that most chemotherapeutic agents preferentially damage mitotic cells. Hence, the fraction of cells killed in a small tumor should actually be even greater than the fraction of cells killed in a histologically identical tumor of larger size. As a consequence, according to the Skipper–Schabel–Wilcox model, if the log-kill estimate is wrong, the error should be in the direction of underestimating the impact of therapy against micrometastases. Putting this all together, tumors of small volume should be easily cured by aggressive combination chemotherapy, even more readily than would be predicted by the model.

Clinical trials, unfortunately, have not entirely confirmed these optimistic predictions. An illustration is the postoperative adjuvant chemotherapy of early-stage breast cancer. After quality surgery very few cells should be left, largely disseminated in multiple micrometastatic sites. By Skipper's model, these should be easily reduced to below the volume of a single cell by appropriate drug therapy.[104] The adjuvant chemotherapy of breast cancer with active agents at conventional doses does indeed reduce the probability of patients developing stage IV disease and does result in improved survival. However, in composite, this effect is relatively modest.[105,106] Is this because the duration of the therapy is not long enough? Assume that a given drug combination causes a one-log kill with each application. Six cycles of that combination should cure tumors of fewer than 10^6 cells. For tumors of exactly 10^6 cells, the six cycles would leave just one cell to regrow. If this were the case, then merely extending the duration of treatment beyond six cycles should kill the remaining cell and thereby increase the cure rate. From a modeling perspective, this same argument generalizes for higher degrees of cell kill and higher tumor cell burdens. Yet, durations of exposure to the same chemotherapeutic regimen longer than 4 to 6 months have not improved results in adjuvant chemotherapy.[106] Hence, the predictions of the model (that cure in this setting should be easy, and that duration of therapy should increase that likelihood) do not match actual observations.

What is wrong? If we accept the basic tenets of the Skipper–Schabel-Wilcox model, the failure of adjuvant chemotherapy to cure all cases of early breast cancer can only be due to cellular biochemical drug resistance. Skipper and colleagues were aware of the divergence between their theory and actual experience and, for this reason, hypothesized that some cells in the tumor must be refractory to the drugs used at the dose levels employed.

When, later in this section, we explore the implications of other models, we will see that it is not always necessary to hypothesize the existence of absolutely refractory cells. Nevertheless, the inclusion of the concept of absolutely resistant cells in the Skipper–Schabel–Wilcox model can account for many observations. According to this reasoning, once all the sensitive cells are eliminated by a certain length of treatment, continuing the same therapy for a longer duration will not give better results. The reason is that all the cells left after that initial course are drug resistant and therefore cannot be killed by further use of the same drugs. It is further assumed that such resistance is acquired during a cancer's growth history (by the occurrence of mutations, a phenomenon called *tumor progression*). If that were the case, the only way to guarantee the absence of resistant cells is to initiate therapy at so small a tumor size that no recalcitrant mutants are as yet present. In L1210, the transplantable mouse leukemia that was used to formulate the Skipper model, drug-resistant cells are rarely found in small aliquots, which would seem to support the above reasoning. If this same reasoning were to apply to human cancer, it would mean that such drug-resistant cells would have to arise spontaneously between the time of the carcinogenic event and the time of the appearance of diagnostically large amounts of tumor. This concept leads to the conclusion that the development of a curative strategy depends entirely on the answers to two questions: when in the course of growth does resistance develop? Can tumors be diagnosed early enough so that we can start treatment when the (small) tumor is still curable?[107]

Delbruck–Luria Model as Applied to Cancer To try to answer these two questions, theoreticians have turned to quantitative models of the emergence of drug resistance. Indeed, the development of such models was one of the first major activities in the field of growth curve analysis. That is because drug resistance, by biochemical mechanisms unknown at that time, was recognized quite early to be important in cancer therapeutics.[108] The original work, however, was not based on the study of cancer cells, but rather some pioneering experiments in bacteriology. In 1943, Luria and Delbruck found that different bacterial cultures developed resistance to bacteriophage infection at random (and hence different) times in their growth histories. In fact, resistance often developed long before exposure to the viruses.[109] Later, when the cultures were exposed to the viruses, the survival of the resistant bacteria could be assessed, thereby measuring the percentage of cells that had randomly acquired resistance. Luria and Delbruck reasoned that those cultures that had experienced a mutation earlier in their histories had had more time to develop a high percentage of resistant bacteria.

A new way of stating this observation is as follows: If a bacterium mutates toward property X with probability x at each mitosis, the probability of the cell not developing property X in one mitosis is $1 - x$. In y mitoses, the probability of no mutations occurring is $(1 - x)^y$. If each mitosis produces two viable cells (no cell loss), it takes $N - 1$ mitoses (over $\log_2 N$ generation times) for one cell to grow into N cells, that is, one mitosis produces two cells, each of these two cells undergoes mitosis (for a cumulative total of three mitoses) to produce four cells, each of these four divides (for a cumulative total of seven mitoses) to produce eight cells, and so on. Hence, the probability of not finding any bacteria with property X in N cells is $\exp[(N - 1) * \ln(1 - x)]$, which is approximately $\exp[-x(N - 1)]$, because x is small. (A numeric example of the application of this formula is given below.)

Within a decade of Delbruck and Luria's original observation regarding bacteria, the same pattern was found by Law to apply to the emergence of methotrexate resistance in L1210 cells.[110] Thus, antimetabolite resistance was reasoned to be a trait acquired spontaneously at random times in the pretreatment growth of this cancer. The more modern view of cancer biology has not diminished enthusiasm for this critically important concept of acquired mutations. Abnormalities of the process regulating the entry of G_1 cells into S could disinhibit replication, producing aberrant levels of DNA per neoplastic cell at each cell division.[111–114] By this mechanism, aneuploidy as well as drug resistance should be a function of the number of mitoses. Cell loss would actually increase the probability of mutations per given cell number, because more cell divisions would have been required to produce that cell number than if no cell loss had occurred. Hence, the worst situation regarding the development of cellular heterogeneity would be a high proliferation rate coupled with a high apoptotic rate, which as we have seen in the previous section is a common occurrence in poor-prognosis cancers.

Goldie–Coldman Model In a qualitative sense, the kinetic observations of Delbruck, Luria, Law, and others were highly influential in the genesis and development of the concept of combination chemotherapy.[115] If tumor cells could acquire resistance to a drug prior to exposure to that drug, then the therapist could be faced with a disease heterogeneous in drug sensitivity even at the time of first diagnosis. Because it is numerically unlikely that any one cell could spontaneously become resistant to many different drugs (particularly if the drugs have different biochemical sites of action), only with combinations of drugs could one hope to eradicate all cells.[116] Because of its influence on the development of combination chemotherapy this concept has been formative of modern medical oncology.

In a quantitative sense, the Delbruck–Luria model was re-applied to human cancer in 1979 by the work of Goldie and Coldman.[117,118] These authors later refined their original model to include multiple sublines with double or higher orders of drug resistance and also the presence of cell loss.[119] Their analysis contended that there is a high probability that mutations arise over a two-log (100-fold) increase in tumor size.

This can be shown by the following calculation (based on the new formulation above): Let us take a tenable mutation rate x of 10^{-6}.[120] Using the expression $\exp[-x(N - 1)]$ that we derived above, the probability of no mutants in 10^5 cells is $\exp[-10^{-6}(10^5 - 1)]$, which equals 0.905. Similarly, the probability of no mutants in 10^7 cells is 0.000045, that is, it is unlikely that 10^5 cells have a drug-resistant mutant, but extremely likely that 10^7 cells have at least one such cell.

In this regard, it should be noted that whereas Goldie and Coldman focused on the property of drug resistance, an even clearer illustration of their concept might be found in the acquisition of metastatic ability. The capacity to metastasize is now established to be a reflection of genetic lability.[121] The approximate volume of 10^7 packed cells is 0.01 cubic centimeter. If tumor cells are mixed with benign host tissue (including stromal cells, fibrosis, extracellular secretions, blood and lymphatic vessels, cellular infiltrate, and fluid-filled space) at a packing ratio of 1:10, 10^7 cancer cells will occupy a volume of 0.1 cubic centimeter. At a packing ratio of 1:100, which is often more realistic, 10^7 cancer cells would be found in a tumor volume of about 1.0 cubic centimeter. This example of scaling relates directly to clinical data. In primary breast cancer, the best predictor of axillary metastases is tumor size. Only 17% of invasive ductal lesions < 1 cm in diameter are metastatic to the axilla, contrasted with 41% of lesions of 2 cm in diameter and 68% of tumors of 5 to 10 cm.[122] For primary breast cancer that does not involve axillary lymph nodes, the probability of eventual metastatic spread increases sharply when the mass in the breast is > 1 cm in diameter.[123] Hence, metastatic ability is conspicuously more common in tumors larger than this critical size. A 1 cm spherical tumor contains a volume of slightly over 0.5 cubic centimeter, which is right in the middle of the range of 0.1 to 1.0 cubic centimeter described above as likely harboring between 10^5 and 10^7 cancer cells.

These calculations fit the model with reassuring precision. However, they cannot be regarded as proof of the model, because other explanations are possible (see "New Concepts" below). Moreover, some very specific predictions of the Goldie–Coldman model have not been confirmed in the clinic, as discussed immediately below. This illustrates the complexity of the biology underlying common tumor growth curves and illustrates that all models are useful, only in that they summarize empiric observations and motivate experiments. Models never explain phenomena: they merely describe phenomena in mathematic language.

The specific, testable predictions of the Goldie–Coldman model regard drug sensitivity. Using the calculations above, the model predicts that a cancer arising from a single, drug-sensitive malignant cell has a 90% chance of being curable at 10^5 cells. Yet, if it has a 90% chance of being curable at that size, it will almost certainly become incurable by the time it grows to 10^7 cells. Thus, tumors larger than 0.1 to 1.0 cubic cm should always be incurable with any single agent. This line of reasoning led these authors to conclude that the best chemotherapeutic strategy was to treat as small a tumor as possible as early as possible. The earliest possible treatment might be perioperative or even preoperative. They also concluded that once treatment is started, as many effective drugs as possible should be applied as soon as possible. This strategy, according to the model, is needed to prevent cells that are already resistant to one drug from mutating to resist others.

These recommendations are intuitive, conforming to established empiric principles of combination chemotherapy.[124] They differ from classic principles, only in that they concentrate on the emergence of resistance during treatment, as contrasted with the other possibility that resistance is already present at the start of treatment. Most uniquely, these recommendations imply that if several drugs cannot be used simultaneously at good therapeutic levels (because of overlapping toxicity or competitive interference), they should be used in a strict alternating sequence.

The recommendation for strict alternation is based on several assumptions. All are based on the principle of *symmetry*. Imagine that a tumor has two types of cells, type A and type B. The A-cells are sensitive only to therapy A, whereas the B-cells are sensitive only to therapy B. Symmetry means that A-cells are as sensitive to therapy A as B-cells are sensitive to therapy B. The second assumption is that the rate of mutation toward biochemical resistance is also symmetrical. This means that the A-cells mutate toward resistance to A at the same rate as the B-cells mutate to resistance to B. The third assumption is that the growth patterns and growth rates of the two types of cells are equivalent.[125] Critical appraisal of the various assumptions and conclusions of the Goldie–Coldman model has raised several interesting points. It would be informative to examine these in some detail, not only to illuminate this one hypothesis but also to show the relevance of growth curve analysis to clinical problems.

The first, and most basic, assumption that we must question concerns the notion that all chemotherapeutic failure is rooted in absolute drug resistance. This is a widely held assumption, but it is not above criticism. In fact, evidence to the contrary is found easily in clinical experience. For example, lymphomas and acute leukemias frequently respond to chemotherapy when they relapse from a complete remission induced by the same chemotherapy. Patients with Hodgkin's disease who achieve complete remission with combination chemotherapy and who relapse ≥ 18 months later have an excellent chance of attaining complete remission again when the same chemotherapy is reapplied.[126] A similar situation is found in the treatment of breast adenocarcinoma. Stage IV (recurrent, metastatic disease) frequently responds to chemotherapy that had worked previously but been discontinued. Various illustrations of this phenomenon have been documented in the literature. For example, the Cancer and Leukemia Group B (CALGB) treated patients with advanced breast cancer with cyclophosphamide, Adriamycin (doxorubicin), and 5-fluorouracil (CAF), with or without tamoxifen.[127] Although none of these patients had prior chemotherapy for their advanced disease, some had had prior adjuvant chemotherapy. All parameters of disease sensitivity to treatment—the response rate, response duration, and overall survival—were unaffected by patients' past histories of adjuvant chemotherapy. Similarly, patients on trials at the National Cancer Institute in Milan who developed stage IV breast cancer after adjuvant cyclophosphamide, methotrexate, and 5-fluorouracil (CMF) responded as well to CMF for advanced disease as those who previously had been randomized to be treated with radical mastectomy alone.[128] From these observations we may safely conclude that breast cancers that regrow after exposure to adjuvant CMF are not universally resistant to CMF.[129] We have more recently observed that patients experiencing recurrence of stage IV disease after the failure of high-dose chemotherapy (autologous bone marrow transplantation [ABMT]) can benefit in terms of tumor response to the reapplication of conventional doses of chemotherapy drugs. Hence, all chemotherapeutic failure cannot be attributed to permanent drug resistance. It is possible that some cancers escape cure because a temporary absolute drug resistance develops that then reverses over time. It is also possible, however, that at least some cancers can escape cure by the use of drugs, even though some of their cells are not absolutely resistant to these drugs. This important possibility will be developed further as we consider growth models other than simple, symmetric exponential growth.

Another prediction from the Goldie–Coldman model that is interesting to examine is that tumors > 1.0 cubic centimeter (10^7 cells at a packing ratio of 1:100, 10^9 cells at maximum density packing) cannot be cured with single drugs. Two rapidly growing cancers, gestational choriocarcinoma and Burkitt lymphoma, both with dense packing of their cancer cells, have been cured with single drugs.[130] Cures are achieved even when therapy is initiated at tumor sizes much larger than 1.0 cubic centimeter. Childhood acute lymphoblastic leukemias, other pediatric cancers, adult lymphomas, and germ cell tumors of greater than 10^{10} cells are frequently cured with two-drug and three-drug regimens. Hence, contradicting the model, the size of 10^7 cells does not always mean incurability.

For the purposes of planning chemotherapy schedules, the Goldie–Coldman model speculates that mutations develop rapidly during the treatable portion of a cancer's growth history. This may seem tenable, because in our previous discussion of cell proliferation, we established that genetic liability is a key attribute of neoplasia. Yet, clinical observations hint at a deeper level of complexity.

As a starting example, let us examine metastatic ability as a measure of the rate of mutations. A primary breast cancer left untreated to grow in the breast, as was standard practice in the nineteenth century, always became metastatic.[131] Yet at 30 years of follow-up after radical mastectomy (with no adjuvant chemotherapy), more than 30% of patients are alive and free of disease.[132,133] The mortality rate drops gradually from about 10% per year in the first year to about 2% per year by year 25, but a plateau is reached after 30 years, with a rate of mortality indistinguishable from that of the general population.[134–136] Hence, whereas most, if not all, breast cancers can become metastatic if left alone long enough, and many have already done so by the time of initial presentation, some have not. This speaks against the universal, rapid development of mutations.

Let us consider another situation, the case of a primary cancer that is diagnosed in the breast before it has developed metastatic ability. If the cancer cells in the breast are not completely removed or destroyed, will the residual cells mutate rapidly to produce metastatic clones? A protocol of the NSABP considered this question.[137] Some patients with primary disease were treated by lumpectomy without radiotherapy. The local relapse rate was significant, indicating that residual tumor was left unchecked. Yet, such patients did not have a higher metastatic rate (measured by the survival rate) than patients treated adequately de novo by lumpectomy plus immediate radiotherapy or by mastectomy.

This latter result is surprising, because some metastases from residual cancer should be expected even if that residual disease did not progress in its ability to release metastatic clones. Longer follow-up of this trial might eventually reveal a higher rate of distant metastases. However, the absence at 12 years of a major negative survival impact of local recurrence indicates that tumor can remain in a breast, grow in the breast, and yet not develop metastatic cells at a very high rate. If metastases develop, therefore, the odds are high that they have already done so before the time of first clinical presentation.

Because this view was first expounded in the first edition of this textbook, more recent evidence concerning radiotherapy to the chest wall after mastectomy has become available. These data may be regarded as confirmatory. Several papers have shown that for patients with a high probability of local recurrence the use of such radiotherapy decreases the chances of local and (the key point) distant recurrence.[138–140] Yet the differences are small, and are not apparent for many years after primary therapy. At high rates of mutations the local residual disease would be expected to produce metastatic clones universally: hence, the rate of mutations cannot be very high. For further discussion of the practical and natural philosophical implications of these results, the reader is referred to a paper by Hellman.[141]

In a similar vein, the Goldie–Coldman model concludes that for chemotherapy to be effective it must be started as soon as possible after diagnosis. To restate the rationale: the hypothesized rapid mutation rates would otherwise produce cells that would be resistant to all treatments. Here as well, however, contradictory evidence is well known. For example, in a pioneering trial in the treatment of acute leukemia, the response to an antimetabolite (A) was the same whether that drug was used first or sequentially after the use of a different antimetabolite (B).[142] Had mutations toward the drug A occurred rapidly during treatment with drug B, we should not have expected these results. Another two examples are found in the treatment of breast cancer. In a randomized trial, the International (Ludwig) Breast Cancer Study Group found that it was equally effective to give node-positive breast cancer patients either 7 months of chemotherapy starting within 36 hours of surgery or 6 months of chemotherapy starting about 4 weeks later.[143] Again, rapid mutation rates should have impeded response after the delay, but this did not occur. A very important result was obtained in a trial of high-dose chemotherapy (with autologous hematopoietic stem cell rescue, ABMT) for metastatic breast cancer.[144] Here patients in complete remission from conventionally dosed chemotherapy were randomized to receive high dose therapy and ABMT immediately or were followed in an unmaintained remission. Those 90% who relapsed from the unmaintained remission were then treated identically with ABMT. The duration of disease control and survival from the time of ABMT was the same in both arms of the trial. (Incidentally, this translated to an overall improved median duration of disease control and survival for the patients receiving delayed ABMT. This is partially because the 10% of patients who remained disease free for more than 5 years from the conventional therapy without ABMT raised the whole curve. It is also because the delayed ABMT patients had an overall duration of disease control that was the sum of that which they experienced from the conventional therapy and from the ABMT.) Had mutations toward resistance to chemotherapy occurred rapidly during the unmaintained remission, the delayed-ABMT arm should have done worse. A trial in stage B nonseminomatous testicular cancer provides yet another example.[145] This trial randomized patients after retroperitoneal lymph node dissection either to two cycles of cisplatin combination chemotherapy or to observation. At a median follow-up of 4 years, 6% of patients randomized to adjuvant chemotherapy relapsed, compared with 49% of patients randomized to observation. Yet, because the response of relapsing cases to subsequent chemotherapy was excellent, there was no significant survival difference between the two approaches. Hence, this is evidence that most testicular carcinomas retained their chemosensitivity in spite of a prolonged period of unperturbed growth. We may conclude, therefore, that leukemia cells, and breast and testicular cancer cells that are residual after surgery, can grow unperturbed and yet not develop drug-resistant mutants at a fast rate.

There are other challenges to the validity of the Goldie–Coldman model. The model concludes that adjuvant treatment must be instituted as early as possible in the growth history of a cancer to be effective. Yet several pilot studies and one major multi-institutional trial failed to find an advantage to preoperative chemotherapy for primary breast cancer.[146,147] The model also concludes that if drugs are used postoperatively, they have to be used as soon as possible after surgery to be effective. Hence, Goldie–Coldman recommends that all drugs in an adjuvant regimen be introduced immediately, lest their biologic impact be dampened by mutations toward drug resistance. This hypothesis was questioned in a trial by the CALGB that gave node-positive primary breast cancer patients 8 months of an adjuvant CMF (plus vincristine and prednisone) regimen.[148,149] The CMFVP was followed by either more CMFVP or by 6 months of vinblastine, Adriamycin (doxorubicin), thiotepa, and Halotestin (VATH). Patients receiving the crossover therapy had a significantly improved disease-free survival, especially those with four or more involved axillary nodes. In a similar vein, it is of note that a trial in Milan found no advantage to doxorubicin following CMF for patients with one to three involved nodes, that is, the crossover effect was not seen in patients with lower risk of relapse.[150] This differs from the results of a pivotal trial using paclitaxel in the adjuvant setting, which is discussed below. The point is that for many patients, dominant resistance to VATH did not develop during the 8 months of CMFVP treatment in those cells escaping CMFVP. This result, therefore, does not confirm the Goldie–Coldman hypothesis. The implications of the CALGB's results in patients with higher degrees of nodal involvement, including the issues of simultaneous versus sequential therapies, dose scheduling, and optimal duration, are discussed in more detail below.

The assertion most singularly identified with the Goldie–Coldman model is the recommendation for alternating chemotherapy sequences. To repeat: they say that it is so important to give drugs as early as possible that if one cannot deliver a true simultaneous combination using all the drugs, one should alternate sequences rather than use the drugs in sequential blocks. Has this strategy demonstrated unequivocal advantages? Numerous attempts to improve the prognosis of patients with small-cell lung cancer (SCLC) by alternating chemotherapy sequences have resulted in little or no benefit.[151] Another relevant trial concerns the treatment of diffuse aggressive non-Hodgkin's lymphoma. The National Cancer Institute (NCI) found no advantage to a ProMACE-MOPP hybrid, which delivered eight drugs during each monthly cycle, over a treatment plan delivering a full course of repeated cycles of ProMACE (prednisone, methotrexate, Adriamycin [doxorubicin], cyclophosphamide, etoposide), which was then followed by cycles of MOPP (mechlorethamine, vincristine, procarbazine, prednisone).[152]

The Goldie–Coldman principle was also examined in the context of advanced Hodgkin's disease, where MOPP was compared with MOPP alternating with Adriamycin (doxorubicin), bleomycin, vinblastine, and dacarbazine (ABVD). ABVD is an effective first-line therapy for Hodgkin's disease and is also an effective salvage regimen for patients who are refractory to MOPP.[153,154] Among chemotherapy-naive patients, MOPP-ABVD was found to be superior to MOPP, with regard to complete remission rate, freedom from progression, and survival.[155,156] These results suggested that there might be some advantage to the "all drugs early" idea. However, the CALGB found that the complete remission rate and failure-free survival with MOPP-ABVD, although better than with MOPP alone, was not different from that with ABVD alone.[157] Indeed, the superiority of MOPP-ABVD and ABVD over MOPP may have been due to differences in dose received, because only about 40% of MOPP patients received full doses of the cytotoxic agents by the third cycle, whereas these percentages were greater than 70% on ABVD and on MOPP-ABVD. At comparable levels of received dose, there were no clear advantages to the alternation of MOPP and ABVD over ABVD alone. Similarly, the NCI found no advantage to MOPP alternating with lomustine, Adriamycin (doxorubicin), bleomycin, and streptozocin over MOPP alone.[158] An American intergroup trial has found that a hybrid of MOPP-ABVD was superior in complete remission duration, failure-free survival, and overall survival to MOPP followed by ABVD.[159] As with MOPP-ABVD in the CALGB trial, however, it is possible that this result may be explained by dose differences, that is, patients treated with the hybrid regimen received higher doses because of the necessity to modify for toxicity the doses of MOPP in the regimen that delivered MOPP followed by ABVD. It is also possible that the earlier introduction of doxorubicin in the hybrid might have been advantageous because such an approach could diminish the adverse impact of the emergence of multi-drug resistance. These points are discussed below in the context of the Norton–Simon model.

Lessons learned in the treatment of the lymphomas have extended to the treatment of breast cancer, that is, alternating cycles that have not resulted in a dosage difference have not proved advantageous. For example, the VATH regimen is active against tumors relapsing from or failing to respond to CMF, and thereby meets the non–cross-resistance requirements of the Goldie–Coldman model.[160] Yet, in patients with advanced disease, the CALGB found no advantage to CMFVP alternating with VATH over CAF or VATH alone.[161] A direct comparison of alternating and sequential chemotherapy in the adjuvant chemotherapy of breast cancer was conducted in Milan. This group had previously generated historically controlled data that suggested a benefit from a sequential approach, the rationale for which is discussed below.[162,163] In the more recent study, female patients with stage II breast cancer involving four or more axillary lymph nodes were randomized between two arms.[164] Arm I prescribed four 3-week courses of A (Adriamycin [doxorubicin]), followed by eight 3-week courses of intravenous C (CMF), symbolized as AAAACCCCCCCC. Arm II stipulated the use of two courses of intravenous CMF alternated with one course of doxorubicin four times for a total of 12 courses, symbolized as CCACCACCACCA. The total amounts of doxorubicin and CMF in both arms were equal. Yet the patients who received arm I had a higher disease-free survival and a higher overall survival than those on arm II. With total dose controlled, alternating courses of chemotherapy were found to be inferior to a crossover therapy plan. These preliminary results have been confirmed by long-term follow-up analysis.[165]

The sequential application of drugs has proved to be a useful strategy in the treatment of leukemias. In adult acute myelogenous leukemia, a high rate of complete remission is obtained with cytarabine plus anthracyclines, but the duration of the responses is short. Postremission maintenance therapy has been shown by the CALGB to be relatively ineffective when given at low doses.[166] Moreover, a trial showed that 32 months of postremission therapy were not superior to 8 months of the same therapy, similar to the failure of longer courses of adjuvant chemotherapy to improve results achieved by 4 to 6 months of such treatment in breast cancer.[106,167] A randomized trial was recently reported that studied 596 patients out of 1,088 who had achieved complete remission with induction chemotherapy.[168] This trial was designed to question the effectiveness of intensive postremission chemotherapy, exploiting the steep dose-response curve for cytarabine.[169] The study found that the high-dose regimen was the best of three different dose schedules of cytarabine. Indeed, the best results were comparable with those reported in similar patients undergoing allogeneic BMT during first remission.[168,170] The Children's Cancer Group (CCG) has reported that intensive induction, followed sequentially by intensive consolidation and later intensification, was superior to other strategies in the treatment of childhood acute lymphoblastic leukemia.[171] These observations have major practical and theoretic implications, as they suggest that strategies other than those advocated by the Goldie-Coldman hypothesis may have more significant clinical impact.

The foregoing detailed examination of the Goldie–Coldman model is provided not only to provide discussion points regarding this particular concept but also to illustrate the relevance of growth curve analysis to treatment design. The Goldie–Coldman model is mathematically sensible and may well be applicable to some aspects of cancer biology. The model is also of major historic importance in that its publication in the mid-1980s rekindled interest in the quantitative development of drug resistance. These two points are valid even though several of the model's major predictions have not been sustained by clinical data. Yet, we are left with an enigma: how can a model that is so reasonable and seemingly so well grounded in kinetic dogma (log-kill) fail to generate a successful clinical strategy? One reason for a discrepancy between tenable theory and empiric results is the invalidity of underlying assumptions. An assumption of particular consequence in this regard, one that merits re-evaluation in face of the negative data reviewed above, concerns the concept of absolute drug resistance.

Implications of Relative Drug Resistance The Goldie–Coldman model is very centered on the idea of absolute drug resistance. Yet, it is now well established that much drug resistance is relative rather than absolute.[172] A cell that is absolutely resistant cannot be killed with any pharmacologic dose level of the agent. Relative drug resistance, on the other hand, depends on the dose level employed. In terms of the Skipper–Schabel-Wilcox model, one tumor may experience a log kill of two (99% reduction in cell number) when it is exposed to a certain dose and duration of treatment. Another, more resistant, tumor may experience a log kill of one (90% shrinkage) when it is treated with exactly the same therapy. However, if the dose intensity of chemotherapy against the relatively resistant tumor is increased, the log kill can increase as well.[173,174]

Clinically, even two-fold increases in dose level can sometimes have profound effects on the curative impact of chemotherapy.[172] Yet, this is not always seen with all drugs, nor in all diseases.[175] In retrospective analyses of the adjuvant chemotherapy of operable breast cancer and of the chemotherapy of advanced lymphoma, a high dose seems to be a key beneficial variable.[176–178] Yet, even here, the validity of conclusions based on retrospective data has been questioned.[179,180] In randomized trials in childhood acute lymphoblastic leukemia, adult germ cell tumors, advanced breast cancer, and breast cancer in the adjuvant setting, the higher-dose regimen has proven superior.[181–185] Yet, results do not indicate a strictly rising dose-response relationship. For example, doses of cyclophosphamide over 600 mg/m^2 do not improve results in the adjuvant chemotherapy of breast cancer,[185] nor do doses of doxorubicin over 60 mg/m^2.[186]

How do we explain this complicated relationship between dose and effect? From a kinetic viewpoint, the importance of dose is defensible. In many animal experiments, the log kill will be greater for the regimen with a higher dose intensity.[187] But dose intensity is a concept that requires careful definition. Intensity is not just the total amount of drug received, nor is it just the amount of drug received per unit of time; rather, it is a mathematic combination of both. Dose intensity is actually a combination of dose escalation (raising the dose level, the number of milligrams per squared meter) and dose density (increasing the amount of drug per unit of time, usually by shortening the total duration of treatment, while keeping the total amount of drug constant). If regimen I gives X amount of drug over Y days, and if regimen II gives $2X$ amount of drug over Y days, then regimen II is clearly more dose intensive. Regimen III, giving X amount of drug over $Y/2$ days, is also more intensive than regimen I. Although the dose rate of drug delivery of regimen III ($2X/Y$ drug per day) is equivalent to regimen II, regimen II delivers more total drug and thus may be superior to regimen III in clinical efficacy. Hence, dose intensity alone may not account for clinical superiority. Yet, sometimes, once a certain minimal total dose is achieved, further increases in total dose are unimportant. For example, a number of trials have shown that durations of adjuvant chemotherapy for a particular regimen longer than 4 to 6 months do not improve clinical results in operable breast cancer.[188–191] Therefore, once the minimal total dose is determined empirically and adhered to, dose intensity should be an important determinant of cell kill.

The shape of the relationship between cell-killing capacity and dose is not totally clear for any drug, but for some agents, some data suggest a strictly proportional relationship, up to a point. We may use as an example the randomized trial by the CALGB that treated node-positive breast cancer patients by one of three plans of CAF adjuvant treatment (cyclophosphamide, Adriamycin [doxorubicin], 5-fluorouracil).[184] (Further studies on dose levels greater than those employed in this trial are discussed in the next section.) Let Z equal a certain total cumulative dose of chemotherapy: the three regimens gave either $2Z$ over 4 months (plan I), $2Z$ over 6 months (plan II), or Z over 4 months (plan III). Plan I was superior to plan III in reducing the rate of recurrence, but no difference between plan I and plan II has as yet been reported, except for a subset of patients.[192] Hence, the total anticancer influence of each of these regimens seems to be strictly proportional to the total dose administered. For plan I, it was $2Z$, the sum of $2Z$ over the first 4 months plus zero for the 2 additional months. Plan II also gave $2Z$ but over the entire 6 months. Plan III delivered half as much total anticancer influence, the sum of Z over the first 4 months, then zero for the remaining 2 months. A proportional dose-response relationship would predict that plan III should be inferior to both plan I and plan II, which was observed. One qualifier in this argument is that if CAF chemotherapy cures some patients, then plan I might eventually prove to be superior to plan II. This is because the cancer cell killing accomplished at 4 months from $2Z$ given over 4 months should be greater than the cell killing measured at 4 or at 6 months from $2Z$ given over 6 months. For some patients given $2Z$ over 4 months, the log kill might be enough to preclude disease re-growth. This might explain the superiority of plan I in patients with HER2–overexpressing tumors.[192] That such tumors may be especially sensitive to higher dose levels of doxorubicin is now suggested by the results of several corroborating studies.[193,194]

The global conclusion of this analysis is that clinical treatment failure may be the consequence of insufficient dose intensity (ie, $2Z$ over 6 months when it could have been given over 4 months). A tumor may relapse because some of its cells, relatively but not absolutely insensitive to the agents applied, are not exposed to enough drug to be eradicated. This is analogous to a bacterial infection relapsing because an insufficient dose intensity of an antibiotic is applied, even though the microorganisms are sensitive in vitro. In both infection and neoplasia, however, prolonged or repeated episodes of low-dose therapy can give rise to absolute resistance by the selection of biochemically resistant cells.

If insufficient dose intensity is a major cause of failure to cure, then it is possible that increased dose intensity itself can improve clinical results.[195,196] This statement is phrased as a possibility rather than as a certainty because it is highly dependent on the host tolerance to the chemotherapy and also on the shape (degree of steepness and nonlinearity) of the dose-response curve for each agent for each disease. It also depends on the shape of the curve of tumor volume regression, which is considered in the next paragraphs.

Gompertzian Model and Fractal Geometry The log-kill model originated from, and is expressed in terms of, exponential growth. How realistic is this pattern of growth for human cancer? Only some tumors in some special situations seem to follow this pattern. Nodular pulmonary metastases and, much less commonly, measurable lesions in other sites do seem to follow exponential growth during periods of observation that are short in relation to the total life histories of the tumors.[197–199] Doubling times, ranging from 1 week to 1 year, with a median of 1 to 3 months, correlate with histologic type, growth fraction, and cell loss fraction. Yet, many, if not all, human cancers do not grow exponentially because they do not have constant doubling times.[200–202]

In 1825, Benjamin Gompertz described the nonexponential growth pattern that has received the most attention by cytokineticists.[203] It differs from exponential growth in several important ways. In exponential growth, the fixed doubling time means that the growth rate relative to tumor size always remains constant. In Gompertzian growth, however, the doubling time increases steadily as the tumor grows larger. Figure 37-2 illustrates a typical breast cancer (the specifics of this tumor's Gompertzian growth are detailed below). Between 10^2 cells and clinical appreciation at 10^{10} cells, the shape of the growth curve on the semilogarithmic plot deflects downward. An exponential curve would appear as a straight line. The progressive respective slowing of Gompertzian growth may be more the result of decreased cell production than of increased cell loss in larger tumors, that is, the fraction of dividing cells seems to decrease as the tumor gets larger, possibly in proportion to the ratio of tumor cells over total tumor volume, which decreases as volume increases as a consequence of fractal geometry.[204] Failure to appreciate the existence of Gompertzian growth can lead to certain errors. For example, the false assumption of exponential growth would suggest that the tumor's doubling time when below the level of clinical appreciation is the same as that which is clinically observed. That doubling time would be unrealistically slow.[205] The assumption of exponentiality has led to some unrealistic estimates of the time from carcinogenesis to the appearance of clinical disease, that is, estimates that are too long.

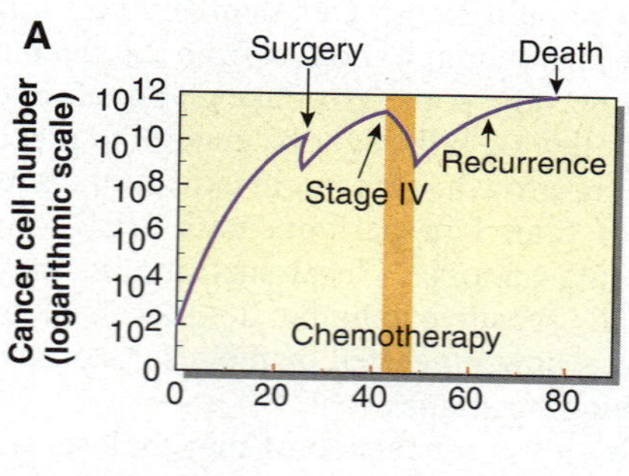

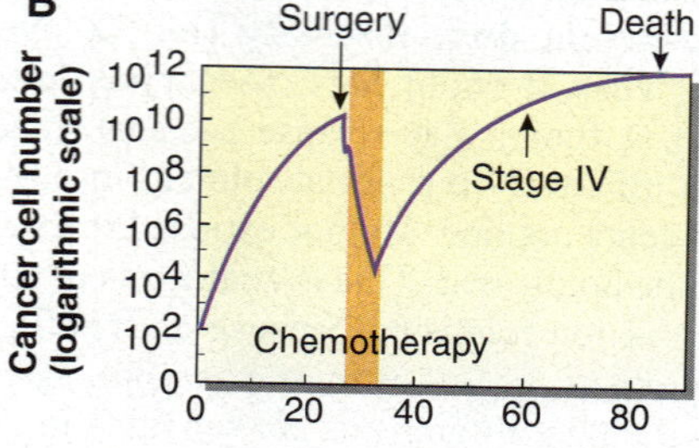

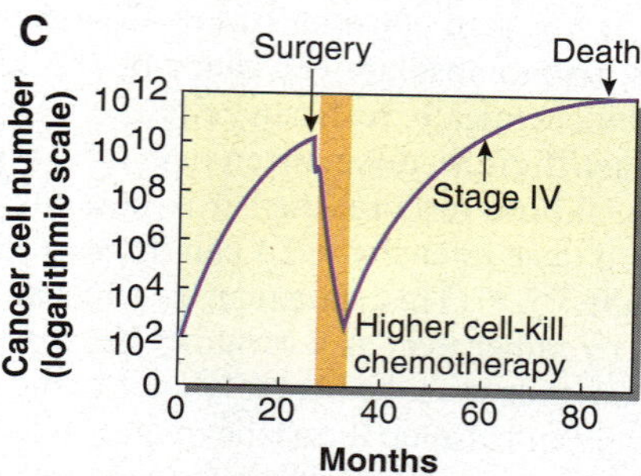

Figure 37-2 Gompertzian model of breast cancer growth.

The biologic basis for Gompertzian growth is still unclear. An old, now unpopular, concept is that a solid tumor "outgrows" its supply of nutrients and so cannot sustain unimpeded exponential growth. This has been challenged by evidence that large tumors, with relatively slow growth rates, usually have adequate vascularity. Indeed, that may be why they are large tumors: they can induce the blood vessels (neovascularization) that allow them to grow to large size.[206] A new concept concerns the relation between the cancer cell and its local environment, which includes other like cancer cells.[207] Most cancers are composed of repeating elements—such as branching tree patterns or multiple nodules—that are self-similar over various scales of size. Such patterns are called fractals. The dimension of a fractal is called its mass dimension: a mass dimension of 3 means that the structure is solid and regular (like densely packed sand), a mass dimension of 2 means that the cells are arranged in a sheet. The average mean mass dimension for a normal tissue is about 2.7, which means that the number of cells is proportional to the length of the tissue raised to the 2.7 power.[208–213] The volume of the tissue is proportional to the length raised to the power of 3.0. Therefore, a fractal geometric pattern means that the number of cells is proportional to the tumor volume raised to a power ≤ 1, that power being a function of the mass dimension, say 2.7/3.0 in the above example.

Cancers tend to have mass dimensions of greater than 2.7, but they vary widely, with the more malignant tumors having mass dimensions closer to 3.0. Smaller mass dimensions produce lower power constants and, therefore, low ratios of number of cells per volume of tumor. Such tumors, with relatively few cells per microscopic field, tend to be more benign, whereas cancers with higher mass dimensions (more cancer cells and little intervening stroma) tend to be more malignant. It has been shown that masses growing in a manner that preserves the power relationship between cell number and volume follow a Gompertzian curve. For example, let N, the total number of cells in a mass, be proportional to the average radius of the mass raised to a fractal dimension d less than 3. If the number of mitotic cells in N is proportional to the radius raised to a fractal dimension less than D, the growth fraction (mitotic/total cell numbers) would decrease as N becomes larger. Similarly, the apoptotic-necrotic death fraction, also being fractal, would also decline, but at a different rate. At the inception of growth cell production must exceed cell death. But if over time the death fraction declines at a slower rate than the mitotic fraction, the gap between the two rates would narrow and Gompertzian-like growth would result.

In such Gompertzian-like growth the rate of deviation from exponentiality is functionally related to the power constants: values of the mitotic fractal close to 3 give more aggressive growth, and smaller values, balanced against cell loss, give Gompertzian curves that may plateau at a relatively benign size, as in ductal carcinoma in situ of the breast.[207] An interesting aspect of this thesis is that a precancerous mass can suddenly become recognizable as malignant with just a small additional increment in the mitotic power constant over a certain threshold. Because the power constant reflects the mass dimension, tissues with widely varying mass dimensions can be benign, but once the power constant is close to a critical degree (probably greater than 2.85–2.90), a further small change toward increased mass dimension could describe malignant transformation.

The molecular bases of the power constants that define Gompertzian growth are an active topic of study, but several hypotheses concern autocrine and paracrine growth factor loops, which might also determine invasion and metastases.[207] That is, if the cells are responding to a concentration of growth factors and if that concentration is proportional to the number of cells divided by their total volume, this would be enough to explain Gompertzian growth. Clearly, rates of apoptosis, which, like rates of mitosis, vary as a function of tissue size, relate to these phenomena as well, including sensitivity to ambient soluble factors. That so many of the genes implicated in malignant transformation affect mitosis, apoptosis, and microanatomy (measured by the fractal dimension), such as adhesion molecules, provides a potential bridge between modern cytokinetics and the molecular biology of cancer. This is further discussed under "New Concepts" below.

Some of the important characteristics and implications of Gompertzian growth are illustrated in the next paragraphs.[214]

Speer–Retsky Model In the nineteenth century, breast cancer was often managed from diagnosis to death without surgery or any other effective treatment.[131] Speer, Retsky, and colleagues used survival histories for such patients, plus the growth histories of mammographic shadows, and data for disease-free survival following mastectomy, to fit a model in which tumors grow in randomly increasing steps of Gompertzian plateaus.[215–217] This work is interesting because it demonstrates that growth curves that deviate far from exponentiality can fit clinical data. However, the validity of the model has been challenged on several counts. First, it is questionable whether the temporary plateaus that are predicted by the model are ever actually observed.[179] Second, the Speer–Retsky model predicts that to maximize the efficacy of postsurgical adjuvant chemotherapy, it should be applied intermittently over a prolonged duration so as to coincide with the presumed growth spurts. This approach, however, proved ineffective in a clinical trial.[218] Third, the same clinical data as used by Speer and Retsky can be fitted more parsimoniously, and with greater accuracy, by a family of simple Gompertzian curves.[214] A family of exponential curves could also be fitted to these data; however, the model that would result could not account for both disease-free survival and overall survival because the time from relapse to death would be too short. The curve used in Figure 37-2 is the median curve from the family of simple Gompertzian curves mentioned above.[214] Note that it takes just 3 months for the tumor to increase by two logs from 10^2 to 10^4. Yet, it takes 5 months for 10^9 cells to grow just one log to 10^{10}. This is a realistic example of increasing doubling time with increasing tumor volume.

Norton–Simon Model The Skipper–Schabel–Wilcox model is so meaningful because it conceptualizes both tumor growth (in the limited case this is exponential) and tumor regression (in the exponential case it is log-kill) in response to chemotherapy. We have already discussed the profound implications of the positive association between the rate of tumor regression and the dose intensity of chemotherapy. Experimental and clinical data also indicate that the rate of tumor regression is positively related to the growth rate of the unperturbed tumor just prior to treatment.[219,220] This important observation is corroborated by experimental data: the logarithm of the surviving fraction of an experimental neoplasm is negatively correlated with the logarithm of the tumor size at the time of treatment.[221]

This log–log relationship extends the Skipper–Schabel-Wilcox model. In exponential growth, the growth rate is always proportional to tumor size. If a tumor at size X is growing at rate Y, the same tumor at size $2X$ would grow at rate $2Y$. On a logarithmic scale, these growth rates would appear to be the same because the rate of growth per tumor size (Y/X) is the same in both cases. A rate of regression proportional to growth rate is, therefore, also proportional to tumor size, which results in a constant proportional (or "log") kill, that is, imagine that a tumor at size X shrinks at rate Z to achieve a size $X/2$ in 1 week (a change in size by the proportion of one half). The same tumor at size $2X$, if treated with the same chemotherapy, would shrink at rate $2Z$ to achieve size X in 1 week (also a change by the proportion of one-half). The absolute volume shrinkage would be $X/2$ in the first case and X in the second case, but the proportional change would be one-half in both cases (X to $X/2$; $2X$ to X). The distinction between the Skipper–Schabel–Wilcox model and the Norton–Simon model is that in Gompertzian growth, unlike exponential growth, the growth rate of the unperturbed tumor is always changing, that is, if a tumor at size X grows at rate Y, the same tumor at size $2X$ would grow at a rate less than $2Y$.

In Figure 37-2, a realistic numeric example illustrates the implications of Gompertzian regression. In Figure 37-2A the tumor is observed to grow to clinical diagnosis at 10^{10} cells (about 10 cubic centimeters of packed tumor cells or about 100 cubic centimeters at a packing ratio of 1:10). Let us assume for the purposes of this illustration that 90% of the tumor is in the breast and axillary lymph nodes, and about 10% of the cells are scattered in various micrometastatic sites. The mass in the breast itself would be about 5 cm in diameter. If this mass and the axillary contents are removed completely (or destroyed completely with radiotherapy), the total body's burden of tumor is reduced to the 10^9 metastatic cells. Because the 10^9 cancer cells are spread throughout the body, they are invisible to our diagnostic tests. No adjuvant therapy is given. The tumor grows for 13.5 months until it reaches about 10^{11} cells in total number, which is large enough for detection as metastases. At this time, chemotherapy is employed, reducing the total cell number to about 10^9 (a two-log kill). A period of remission is experienced but the tumor eventually relapses, leading to death at 10^{12} cells.

Figure 37-2B graphs the same tumor, but here the same chemotherapy is applied in the adjuvant setting at a total tumor size of 10^9 cells. The relative rate of growth (the slope of the curve on this semilogarithmic plot) is faster for the tumor at 10^9 cells than it would be for the same tumor at 10^{11} cells. This is clear from inspection of Figure 37-2A. According to the Norton–Simon model, the relative rate of regression of the 10^9-cell tumor will be faster as well, even though the dose and schedule of chemotherapy are identical. Figure 37-2B shows that the chemotherapy that had caused a two-log kill of 10^{11} cells causes instead a five-log kill of 10^9 cells. The 10^4 cells that result re-grow to relapse as stage IV disease at 10^{11} cells and to kill the patient at 10^{12} cells. Comparison of Figures 37-2A and 37-2B demonstrates a remarkable result. The time from surgery to stage IV is clearly longer when adjuvant chemotherapy is applied. However, the time from surgery to death is identical! The greater fractional kill in the adjuvant setting is counterbalanced by a faster fractional regrowth. This may explain why the adjuvant chemotherapy of breast cancer has less impact on overall survival (a function of eventual tumor body burden) than on disease-free survival. It may also explain why the survival duration of patients with stage IV breast cancer has remained fairly stable in recent decades in spite of more aggressive approaches to management.[222–224]

What if another chemotherapy plan, more aggressive but still subcurative, is used in the adjuvant setting against the 10^9 cells? This is illustrated in Figure 37-2C. If 10^2 cells are left instead of 10^4, it will take only 3.5 months longer for the tumor to reach 10^{12}, because the growth from 10^2 cells to 10^4 cells is very rapid. Hence, adjuvant therapies can differ greatly in log kill, with only a slight effect on eventual clinical results measured years later. This slight impact could easily be lost in the "noise" caused by random fluctuations, especially in clinical data sets of small size.

The pessimistic side of this observation is that much more aggressive chemotherapy may produce little real clinical benefit. Short-course very high-dose chemotherapy with hematopoietic stem cell rescue has been employed in an effort to eradicate all breast cancer cells in the adjuvant setting. The results of randomized trials in this regard are largely negative. At a landmark annual meeting of the American Society of Clinical Oncology in 1999, several studies of the short-course high-dose approach were presented, all negative except for one (Bezwoda) which was later retracted over issues of data veracity.[225–227] The largest American trial coordinated for the Intergroup by the CALGB shows no effect on survival after long term follow-up.[226]

The optimistic side of this analysis is that if the model holds, current adjuvant chemotherapies for breast cancer are actually bringing us much closer to total cellular eradication than we might otherwise be led to suspect. It is possible that the use of multiple cycles of effective therapy might be enough to bring some patients beyond the threshold of disease eradication.[228] Even with drug-sensitive diseases, such as bacterial infections responsive to antibiotics, more than one cycle is almost always necessary for cure. Further studies of multi-cycle high-dose regimens have completed accrual, and some preliminary results are expected soon. Of course, it is not known if dose escalation is obligatory for the success of adequately planned multi-cycle regimens because other considerations, such as dose density, might prove to be more potent as a therapeutic manipulation.

The basic concept is that patient survival can be improved to a significant degree only when tumor cell populations are actually eradicated or when their regrowth is otherwise meaningfully impeded. In our previous discussion of cellular proliferation, we concluded that heterogeneity in drug sensitivity is a characteristic of neoplasia. How can tumor cell eradication be accomplished in a heterogeneous cancer? The answer may lie in the application of kinetic principles. Gompertzian regression means that slower-growing collections of tumor cells will tend to regress more slowly in response to a given therapy than will the faster-growing tumor cells treated at the same time.[229] In a heterogeneous cancer, therefore, the slower-growing clones are also the most kinetically resistant. These slower-growing cells should be in the minority by the time of diagnosis because, by then, they should have been overgrown by the faster-growing cells. The existence of a population of slow-growing cells may also be the consequence of the hypothetic ability of chemotherapy to differentiate cells that are not killed.[230]

The best way to treat a heterogeneous population is to treat the dominant, faster-growing populations as efficiently as possible and then to treat the numerically inferior, slower-growing populations as efficiently as possible.[163] As in the Skipper-Schabel-Wilcox model, the most efficient therapy is the most dose-dense therapy, giving as much drug as possible over as short a period as possible. This pattern of therapy is accomplished much better by sequential treatment than by strict alternation. For example, in the adjuvant breast cancer trial from Milan described above, the alternating plan, CCACCACCACCA, gave eight cycles of CMF over 30 weeks and four cycles of doxorubicin over 33 weeks.[165] The cross over, sequential plan, AAAACCCCCCCC, gave eight cycles of CMF over 24 weeks and four cycles of doxorubicin over 9 weeks. The dose density of the CMF was almost the same, but for doxorubicin the cross-over significantly improved the density. This could, by itself, account for the superiority of the AAAACCCCCCCC treatment. A similar result has also been seen in the adjuvant chemotherapy of resected osteosarcoma: doxorubicin alone was superior to doxorubicin alternating with high-dose methotrexate, presumably because the dose density of the superior agent (doxorubicin) was diluted by the alternation.[231] The results of trials in acute leukemia in adults and children[171] described above are also consistent with the concept of dose-dense sequential treatment plus dose escalation as a means of increasing dose intensity and thereby improving clinical benefit.

In the breast cancer trial from Milan,[165] the use of doxorubicin initially might have caused greater cell kill by avoiding the expression of the multi-drug resistance gene, which tends to progress over time, independent of treatment.[232,233] Conversely, the delayed use of doxorubicin might have compromised the efficacy of two other regimens described previously: ABVD following prolonged MOPP for advanced Hodgkin's disease and doxorubicin following 6 months of CMF for primary breast cancer with low degrees of nodal involvement.[150,159]

Although the invention and interpretation of clinical trials intended to test cytokinetic principles are fraught with subtleties and complexities, dose-dense sequential therapy has been successful in the laboratory. The only way to cure 10^8 L1210 cells is by induction with cytosine arabinoside plus 6-thioguanine for two or three courses, followed by one course of high doses of cyclophosphamide and carmustine (BCNU) given simultaneously.[234] In the treatment of BDF1 mice bearing the M5076 tumor, the addition of one dose of L-phenylalanine mustard (L-PAM) (a drug that by itself is only weakly active) after four doses of methyl-lomustine (CCNU) doubles the complete remission rate and the median survival.[235] The presumed mechanism for this latter effect is that the few cells left after methyl-CCNU induction are L-PAM sensitive, whereas in the untreated situation, most cells are methyl-CCNU sensitive, and L-PAM resistant. In general, alkylating agents seem particularly helpful as the crossover therapy.

Goldie and Coldman's prediction of the superiority of alternating chemotherapy assumed stringent conditions of symmetrical tumor cell numbers, growth rates, and mutation rates. Day has performed computer simulations of mutation to drug resistance under asymmetrical conditions.[236] He came to a conclusion similar to the Norton-Simon model regarding the expected superiority of a crossover, sequential plan.[237] By his worst drug rule, in a coordinated two-regimen plan, the therapy with a lower cell kill per treatment (the worst drug) should be used either first or, if it is used second, for a longer duration. However, the Norton-Simon model qualifies this to specify that the induction therapy must be sufficiently cytoreductive for the residual tumor cell burden to be low. This is another possible reason for the inferiority of ABVD following dose-reduced (and, hence, less cytotoxic) MOPP, compared with a hybrid MOPP/ABV, which could be delivered at fuller dosages.[159] Theory therefore supports an efficient induction followed in sequence by one or more aggressive chemotherapeutic crossovers. Indeed, in the treatment of acute lymphocytic leukemia in children, a classic trial demonstrated that induction by vincristine plus prednisone facilitates the anticancer activity of sequential methotrexate.[238] The Children's Cancer Study Group (CCSG) trial in childhood leukemia that gave intensive induction, consolidation, and intensification also demonstrated the importance of an efficient initial cytoreduction.[171]

CLINICAL RESULTS WITH DOSE-DENSE SEQUENTIAL THERAPY

The concept of dose-dense sequential therapy has been applied in several important clinical trials. A pilot study in breast cancer used doxorubicin following just 16 weeks of CMFVP for patients with node-positive primary disease.[239] C9344, a major adjuvant trial in node-positive breast cancer, gave doxorubicin plus cyclophosphamide with one of three dose levels of doxorubicin, followed by four cycles of paclitaxel or not.[240] The justification of crossover to paclitaxel (rather than forcing a simultaneous combination that would certainly have increased toxicity) was the concept of dose density. Although escalating the dose of doxorubicin did not improve results, the use of paclitaxel in patients with estrogen-receptor negative tumors reduced the rate of recurrence and of death to a degree comparable with the effects of CMF adjuvant chemotherapy over no therapy in the Worldwide (Oxford) Overview.[105] This trial, coordinated by the CALGB for the Intergroup, led to the US Food and Drug Administration (FDA) approval of paclitaxel for adjuvant use. The NSABP reported a confirmatory trial of similar design.[241]

Three very important adjuvant chemotherapy trials use as their backbone the positive results of the two trials described in the preceding paragraph. An Intergroup trial coordinated by the Eastern Cooperative Oncology Group (ECOG) which has recently completed accrual consists of doxorubicin plus cyclophosphamide followed either by paclitaxel or docetaxel for four cycles of 3 weeks each, or 12 weekly administrations of both taxanes. (The weekly administration is another method of increasing dose density, although the ultimate impact of this manipulation depends upon the balance between inhibition of regrowth via frequent administration and reduced cell kill because of lower doses of drug per weekly administration.)

The other two trials in this regard have recently been presented following early-reporting rules prompted by extraordinarily positive results in a joint analysis. Coordinated by the North-Central Cancer Treatment Group, one trial in HER2–over-expressing early-stage disease used doxorubicin plus cyclophosphamide followed by weekly paclitaxel with or without trastuzumab, the anti–HER2 monoclonal antibody.[242] The second was a very similar trial by the NSABP that used doxorubicin plus cyclophosphamide followed by four cycles of paclitaxel and the antibody or not each 3 weeks. These two trials were stopped early because their combined results demonstrated a significant improvement in survival with the addition of trastuzumab. Especially interesting was the observation that the arms that were most effective were the ones that combined the trastuzumab with the paclitaxel. One arm of the Intergroup trial applied trastuzumab after the completion of the paclitaxel, and this conveyed modest benefit at most. This has suggested to some investigators that the ability of the trastuzumab to inhibit re-growth between cycles of paclitaxel might have effectively increased the dose density of that drug, thereby increasing cell-kill as described in detail above. The CALGB is conducting a trial of similar design in locally advanced disease.

To build upon these results investigators at Memorial Sloan-Kettering Cancer Center are currently evaluating a dose dense regimen for HER2/neu over-expressing tumors of doxorubicin plus cyclophosphamide every 2 weeks followed by paclitaxel every 2 weeks with trastuzumab initiated at the start of paclitaxel (Dr. Chau Dang, 2004, personal communication). This may truly maximize dose density by three methods: (1) shorter inter-treatment intervals, (2) sequential therapy, and (3) inhibiting re-growth of HER2–over-expressing cells with trastuzumab.

The treatment plans that shorten inter-treatment intervals exploit the ability of hematopoietic growth factors, such as granulocyte colony–stimulating factor (G-CSF), pegfilgrastim (polyethylene glycol G-CSF) and granulocyte-macrophage (GM)-CSF[243] to minimize hematopoietic recovery times. It bears re-emphasis that this use of CSFs differs conceptually from their ability to augment other means of hematopoietic reconstitution to permit dose escalation.[244,245] In the adjuvant chemotherapy of low-risk breast cancer, the Intergroup has recently reported preliminary results of a Southwest Oncology Group (SWOG)-coordinated study of doxorubicin followed by G-CSF–supported high-dose cyclophosphamide versus a more conventional, simultaneous doxorubicin plus cyclophosphamide combination.[246] This trial showed no advantage to the dose-dense, dose-escalated sequential regimen, but interpretation is complicated by more recent observations suggesting that the efficacy of doxorubicin is capped at 60 mg/m^2 and cyclophosphamide at 600 mg/m^2. Investigators at the Memorial Sloan-Kettering Cancer Center have published data about a regimen called ATC that gives dose-dense doxorubicin followed by dose-dense paclitaxel followed by dose-dense cyclophosphamide.[247] On the basis of results that hint at considerable efficacy, this regimen was being compared with dose-escalated ABMT-supported treatment of women with stage II breast cancer and four or more involved axillary lymph nodes, but the study was terminated prematurely because of poor accrual following multiple negative reports on the efficacy of ABMT.

The cleanest proof of the usefulness of dose density has been provided by an Intergroup, CALGB-coordinated 2 by 2 factorial trial that applied several types of dose density (C9741).[248] All patients received post-operative, A (Adriamycin [doxorubicin]), C (Cytoxan [cyclophosphamide]), and T (Taxol [paclitaxel]). One axis was simultaneous AC followed by T versus sequential A followed by T followed by C. The other axis was treatment every 3 weeks (conventional scheduling) versus every 2 weeks (dose-dense scheduling) by the use of G-CSF. The dose-dense schedule resulted in a major decrease in the rates of recurrence and death with no increase in toxicity. Sequential scheduling was not inferior to simultaneous combination chemotherapy, noting that both delivered equivalent dose density because dose level and schedule were identical in both approaches. These results are entirely consistent with the modeling considerations discussed above.[249]

For diffuse large cell lymphoma, an induction regimen with doxorubicin, vincristine, and prednisone has been followed by sequential high-dose cyclophosphamide, then methotrexate (plus vincristine), then etoposide, then L-PAM (plus total body irradiation), all with GM-CSF support. In a randomized comparison against a standard aggressive combination, the induction intensification plan proved superior in complete remission rate, failure from relapse, failure from progression, and event-free survival.[250]

These cytokinetic considerations may be as applicable to radiation therapy as to chemotherapy. The Gompertzian phenomenon of rapid repopulation of clonogenic cells after cytoreductive treatment is well documented in radiobiology. Moreover, clinical data suggest an acceleration of growth of the remaining viable tumor during the second part of protracted "split-course" radiation therapy.[251,252] In the treatment of head and neck cancer, split-course treatment has been used to allow normal tissues to recuperate from radiation damage. In this treatment plan, it has been observed that an additional radiation dose is needed to overcome tumor regrowth during the rest interval between the split courses. The alternative hypothesis, that the higher radiation dose in split-course treatment could be needed because of increased radio-resistance of the tumor following the first part of the split course, is felt to be implausible.[253] In fact, the tumor is actually more completely oxygenated during the second course of treatment, which should render it more radiosensitive.[254] Hence, we are left with the likelihood of rapid regrowth between courses, more rapid than could be explained by exponential growth. The mechanism of such rapid regrowth relates to the three parameters that determine Gompertzian growth: mitotic cycle time, growth fraction, and cell loss (apoptotic) fraction. Cell cycle times of 2 to 4 days are commonly measured in head and neck cancers in the unperturbed state and after radiation therapy.[255] Nevertheless, the doubling time can decrease from 60 to 4 days because of a persistence of the clonogenic cells (ie, high growth fraction) resulting from a decrease in their tendency to differentiate or die by apoptosis (ie, low cell loss fraction). It is important to note that this increase in proliferative parameters is occurring at a time of volume regression induced by the radiotherapy, that is, the observer may see cancer shrinkage, whereas the cells may be experiencing growth acceleration as a means of compensating for the effects of therapy. The same kinetic principles applicable to chemotherapy may be needed to overcome this potential cause of treatment failure. In this regard, a review of studies of head and neck radiotherapy has calculated the dose of irradiation needed to achieve local control in half the cases.[254] This standard benchmark is consistently greater when the treatment is given over a 6-week interval than over a 4-week period,[254] which is entirely consistent with the principle of dose density.

NEW CONCEPTS

Both the Skipper–Schabel–Wilcox and Norton–Simon models are based on the observation that the rate of tumor regression is positively related to the rate of unperturbed growth. The most obvious explanation for this observation is the mitotoxicity hypothesis: tumors regress most rapidly when they are growing most rapidly because more of their cells are then synthesizing DNA and other macromolecules in preparation for mitosis. Such metabolically active cells are thereby at particular risk for cytotoxicity by drugs that interfere with such synthetic processes.[256] The intuitive notion is that poisoning the S-phase renders cells incapable of progressing successfully through the M-phase. This is a dominant idea in cytokinetic thinking, and it undoubtedly has considerable merit. Growth-stimulating substances (ie, estradiol, epidermal growth factor) increase both cell proliferation and cell kill from doxorubicin in MCF-7 cells in vitro.[257] Pharmacologic concentrations of estradiol enhance the cytotoxicity of the chemotherapeutic agent melphalan in hormone-responsive cell lines.[258] These observations have been applied clinically, and hormone recruitment schemes have indeed resulted in high local response rates in locally advanced breast cancer.[259,260] However, such treatments have proved only slightly better or no better than chemotherapy alone in metastatic breast cancer, except in data-driven subsets.[261,262] Even when benefits were seen, methodologic issues have cast doubts on the analyzability of results.[263]

We must be cautious, moreover, in interpreting laboratory data that suggest an enhancement of chemotherapeutic cytotoxicity by manipulations that increase the S-phase fraction. Tamoxifen, which can cause a G_1-S arrest in sensitive cell lines, does antagonize the cytotoxicity of melphalan and 5-fluorouracil, but it does so at dose schedules that do not affect cell proliferation.[258] Tamoxifen actually enhances the cytotoxicity of doxorubicin and the alkylating agent 4-hydroxycyclophosphamide in this system. In fact, a broad acceptance of the mitotoxicity hypothesis leaves several cytokinetic enigmas unresolved. For example, only about 5% of the cells in an average tumor in breast cancer are in the S-phase. Thus, even if we use drugs that kill G_1 and G_2 cells, only about 15 to 20% of the tumor mass could possibly be killed by a single exposure to mitotoxic therapy. To get a one-log kill (90% regression) would require more than 10 such exposures (because $[1–0.2]^{11} < 0.1$). Yet regressions greater than one log are frequently seen after just a single exposure to high-dose chemotherapy.[245] Even conventional chemotherapy, such as eight exposures to intravenous CMF, are simulated in Figure 37-2B to result in a five-log kill. It may, therefore, be implausible that such significant cytoreductions are due to mitotoxicity alone. Indeed, cytokinetic analysis of MCF-7 cells exposed to low levels of doxorubicin does not show an immediate S-phase reduction.[264] There is an accumulation of cells in late S, G_2, and M, but also a block of the G_1 to S transition starting 2 days after treatment.

Another puzzle concerns the effect of chemotherapy on normal host tissues. Chemotherapy is certainly toxic to rapidly dividing bone marrow, alimentary mucosa, and hair follicles. Yet, these tissues usually recover from the impact of chemotherapy. Some cancers, however, that are growing no more rapidly than these normal tissues may experience cytoreductions from which they never recover, that is, acute leukemias, malignant lymphomas, choriocarcinomas, and germ cell cancers may be cured by chemotherapy regimens that do not eradicate the patient's normal tissues that have comparable growth kinetics.

There is, at present, no established alternative to the mitotoxicity hypothesis that successfully relates cytokinetics to therapeutic cytotoxicity, but some intriguing concepts are under investigation. One possibility is that chemotherapy could damage G_0 cells that later exhibit their lethal injuries as they are recruited into a subsequent cycle. Another, perhaps related, possibility is suggested by the thought that the hormonal therapy of responsive cancers works by growth factor perturbation with resultant loss of viability independent of mitotoxicity.[265] Could chemotherapy share with hormone therapy this mode of action? Long-term data on the probability of breast cancer relapse after adjuvant tamoxifen and CMF[191] show similar qualitative changes.[266] Breast cancer is a particularly relevant example because it is modulated by endogenous growth factors secreted by a subset of tumor cells in an individual cancer.[267] The concept, however, may be generalizable as growth factors are now recognized to be essential for the survival of all mammalian cells. In the very genesis of cancer, malignant transformation frequently alters gene expression for growth factors, their receptors, and intracellular signal transduction proteins.[268] Leukemogenic drugs, such as alkylating agents, are known to cause cytogenetic abnormalities, frequently at loci coding for products related to growth factors.[269] It is even possible that the relation between tumor size and metastatic behavior, described in the context of the Goldie–Coldman model, is a consequence of the dependence of tumor cells on growth factors produced by the supporting stroma or the cells themselves.[270]

This discussion raises the possibility that chemotherapy, in addition to a gross mitotoxicity, might share with hormonal therapy an influence on growth factor loops.[271] When hematopoietic cells are deprived of essential growth factors, they die by apoptosis.[272,273] It has been well established that almost all chemotherapeutic drugs, as well as other lethal cytotoxins, also cause apoptosis.[274] The existence of chemotherapy-induced apoptosis by growth factor disruption could clarify several mysteries. It could explain why the histologic analysis of breast cancers regressing after chemotherapy does not always reveal a high degree of necrosis.[275] It could explain why the TLI of breast cancer appeared not to predict chemosensitivity in locally advanced disease and in the adjuvant setting.[276] By implicating host-tumor paracrine interactions, the growth factor hypothesis might explain how tumor resistance to alkylating agents could be operant in vivo but not in vitro.[277] The theory would not, moreover, be incompatible with mitotoxicity itself: rapidly growing cells that are dependent on growth factors would be expected to regress most rapidly when their growth support system is perturbed.

In the laboratory, chemotherapy can influence growth factor pathways. Doxorubicin, for example, may upregulate EGFR in HeLa and 3T3 cells.[278] Activation of protein kinase C (an intracellular signal of growth factor ligand-receptor interaction) enhances the cytotoxicity of cisplatin without increasing drug uptake.[279] In the treatment of human cancer xenografts, antibodies to EGFR, which can by themselves inhibit growth, synergize with cisplatin.[280,281] Such antibodies also synergize with doxorubicin in the treatment of A431 cells in athymic mice.[282] A major multi-institutional clinical trial has established that trastuzumab, which inactivates HER2, increases survival in early stage breast cancer in patients treated with doxorubicin plus cyclophosphamide followed by paclitaxel.[242] The ability of EGFR modulation with a small molecule to augment the cytotoxicity and hence clinical effects of chemotherapy in lung cancer is another example of the potential interplay of growth-factor modulation and chemotherapy effects.

A consideration of the impact of anticancer therapy on growth factor mechanisms must eventually encompass the diversity of cytokinetic features present in most clinical cancers. For example, clonogenic cells are those cells capable of inexhaustible proliferation, called *self renewal*.[283] These are understood to have cytokinetic parameters that are markedly different from other cancer cells with more limited proliferative capacity. Although the clonogenic stem cells are overshadowed numerically by the majority of cells in the tumor, these minority cells are the most important to eliminate in order to prevent tumor recurrence from unstable remission. Malignant clonogenic cells may cycle more quickly than nonclonogenic cells, but this is usually mitigated by a high cell loss fraction. Cell loss from the clonogenic pool is accomplished by multiple mechanisms: differentiation, apoptosis, necrosis, exfoliation, and transportation away from the tumor in blood and lymph. Clearly, these cells differ biologically and cytokinetically from other cancer cells, as determined by genotypic differences that must be exploited to affect a cancer cure.

An emerging body of work concerning the molecular biology of metastases is relevant to this discussion. One of the cardinal features of cancer cells is their abnormal mobility.[284–286] Oncogenes often deregulate both cell adhesion and mitosis.[287–291] There exist several sets of expressed genes that when combined with various weightings into signatures predict poor prognosis in breast cancer and other diseases.[292–297] Many of the indicated gene products concern the alteration of the microenvironment (such as matrix metalloproteinases, stimulators of angiogenesis, and molecules that influence cell adhesion, shape, and spatial orientation) as well as mitotic and apoptotic regulation. Indeed, a poor-prognosis signature can be created that totally excludes proliferation genes.[298,299] Furthermore, a meticulous analysis of sublines derived from a human tumor xenograft has revealed distinct gene sets that influence growth (1) in the primary site or (2) growth in the primary site and in lung metastases or (3) in bone metastases but not in the primary site.[300,301] Taken together, these observations are of considerable interest, but when interpreted in light of some of the biomathematical concepts described above they may suggest a novel and quite far-reaching hypothesis.[302] The two biomathematical concepts are (1) by Gompertzian kinetics small tumors grow relatively faster than larger tumors comprised of the same cell type, and (2) by fractal geometry small tumors are denser than larger tumors of the same cell type. The stem cell concept of the previous paragraph is also implicated.

The following hypothesis ties these disparate details together: Imagine that a cancerous mass is not one cohesive, organized collection of cells but rather a conglomerate of separate, contiguous smaller masses, each the progeny of a wandering cancer cell (perhaps a cancer stem cell) that reached its new location via direct migration or via the systemic circulation. Being a collection of small masses, one added to the other, the composite tumor would be dense (due to fractal geometry), relatively fast-growing (due to Gompertzian kinetics), disorganized histologically, invasive into surrounding tissue, sometimes multifocal, and, because each separate mass would require its own blood supply to survive, hypervascular. Furthermore, because many of the same faculties that permit the movement of a cell from its specific birth location to a different part of the body should be involved in its movement from and then back to its birth location, the same process that promotes growth in the primary site could be involved in the generation and advancement of growth in specific metastatic sites.[284,285] That is, cancerous growth could be, like the growth of a bed of weeds in a field or garden, the result of self-seeding: Each component (weed plant or new cancer locus) growing rapidly because it is low on its Gompertzian curve, but the whole tumor growing because of the continuous generation of new components.

This self-seeding hypothesis does not ignore the obvious facts that mitotic, apoptotic, and other cell-production-and-loss abnormalities are common in cancers.[303–306] But abnormalities in cell production, often seen as hyperproliferative foci, are also common in benign skin conditions and the premalignant lesions of many organs.[307–311] Malignancy may arise when a cell with proliferative deregulation acquires the ability to move and produce viable progeny in an adjacent and/or a distant site. Hence, self-seeding may relate to cytokinetics in at least two ways: By itself, the "start up" nature of new loci may produce more growth-positive cytokinetic parameters; More growth-positive cytokinetic parameters, the result of other cellular aberrations, may indicate a favorable setting for successful proliferation in new self-seeded loci.

The connection of this hypothesis with observations regarding gene sets is the following: Cancers may arise from preneoplastic changes (Gene Set P) that primarily affect cell production, increased proliferation unbalanced by increases in cell loss.[307–311] The state of malignant transformation may be associated with additional changes (Gene Set SS-T) that allow increased mobility and self-seeding in the primary tumor site.[292–297] Additional changes may promote self-seeding in the primary tumor site (Gene Set SS-T2) and distant-seeding to specific metastatic sites (Gene Sets DS-MO for bone, SS-ML for lung etc). In some cases Gene Sets SS-T and SS-M may be identical.[301] Other changes may promote self-seeding only in specific metastatic sites, where Gene Set SS-ML promotes self-seeding in the lung metastatic loci, Set SS-MB promotes self-seeding in the bone metastases and so on. It is obvious in this regard that the relationship between gene products and stroma-specific factors is critical to understanding site-specific metastatic behavior as well as growth in the primary site.[307] Ongoing work is refining this hypothesis and examining gene sets for these various functions.[300,301]

CONCLUSION

Because excess cell production is one of the most important features of all cancers, cytokinetics, the measurement and study of cell production and loss, is the fundamental physiology of cancer medicine. The field is so broad and so rapidly evolving that this chapter merely introduces its basic concepts, laboratory foundations, theoretic underpinnings, clinical relevances, and prospects for future development. Although older concepts of cancer have led to the amassing of a vast arsenal of anticancer therapies focused on the disruption of cell production, it is encouraging that the cytotoxic effects of chemotherapy might extend well beyond crude mitotoxicity. In this regard, cytokinetic analysis may play a key role in unraveling the relationships between cytotoxicity and molecular growth control, including the relationships between cancer cells and each other and their stroma. It is worthwhile to note that both intellectual aspects of cytokinetics (the study of proliferation at the cellular level and the analysis of growth curves at the macroscopic level) are relevant to this field of inquiry, and have already yielded clinical benefit.

REFERENCES

1. Howard A, Pelc, SR. Nuclear incorporation of 32p as demonstrated by autoradiographs. Exp Cell Res 1951;2:178.
2. Lajtha LG, Oliver R, Ellis F. Incorporation of 32p and adenine 14C into DNA by human bone marrow cells in vitro. Br J Cancer 1954;8:367.
3. Baak JP. A mitosis counting in tumors. Hum Pathol 1990;21:683.
4. Frei E III, Whang J, Scoggins RB, et al. The stathmokinetic effect of vincristine. Cancer Res 1964;24:1918.
5. Steel GG. Autoradiographic analysis of the cell cycle. Howard and Pelc to the present day. Int J Radiat Biol 1986;49:227.
6. Alama A, Nicolin A, Conte PF, Drewinko B. Evaluation of growth fractions with monoclonal antibodies to human alpha-DNA polymerase. Cancer Res 1987;47:1892.
7. Crocker J. Proliferation indices in malignant lymphomas. Clin Exp Immunol 1989;77:299.
8. Gerdes J, Lemke H, Brisch H, et al. Cell cycle analysis of a cell proliferation-associated human nuclear antigen defined by the monoclonal antibody Ki-67. J Immunol 1984;133:1710.
9. Simon RM, Stroot MT, Weiss GH. Numerical inversion of Laplace transforms with application to percent labeled mitoses experiments. Comput Biomed Res 1972;5:596.
10. Lala PK. Age-specific changes in the proliferation of Ehrlich ascites tumor cells grown as solid tumors. Cancer Res 1972;32:628.
11. Watson JV. The cell proliferation kinetics of the EMT6/M/AC mouse tumour at four volumes during unperturbed growth *in vivo*. Cell Tissue Kinet 1976;9:147.
12. Hastings HM, Sugihara G. Fractals. A users guide for the natural sciences. Oxford: Oxford University Press; 1993. p. 53–5.
13. Tronick SR, Aaronson SA. Growth factors and signal transduction. In: Mendelsohn J, Howley PM, Israel MA, Liotta LA, editors. The molecular basis of cancer. Philadelphia: WB Saunders; 1995. p. 117–40.
14. Pardee AB. G_1 events and regulation of cell proliferation. Science 1989;246:603.
15. Damania B, Lieberman P, Alwine JC. Simian virus 40 large T antigen stabilizes the TATA-binding protein-TFIIA complex on the TATA element. Mol Cell Biol 1998;18:3926.
16. Tevethia MJ, Lacko HA, Kierstead TD, Thompson DL. Adding an Rb-binding site to an N-terminally truncated simian virus 40 T antigen restores growth to high cell density, and the T common region in trans provides anchorage-independent growth and rapid growth in low serum concentrations. J Virol 1997;71:1888.
17. Hahn WC, Counter CM, Lunderberg AS, et al. Creation of human tumour cells with defined genetic elements. Nature 1999;400:464.
18. Ling MR, Kay JE. Lymphocyte stimulation. New York, NY: Elsevier; 1965.
19. Baserga R. Growth in size and cell DNA replication. Exp Cell Res 1984;151:1.
20. Darzynkiewicz Z, Traganos F, Melamed MR. New cell cycle compartments identified by multiparameter flow cytometry. Cytometry 1980;1:98.
21. Chaudhary PM, Roninson IB. Expression and activity of p-glycoprotein, a multidrug efflux pump, in human hematopoietic stem cells. Cell 1991;66:85.
22. Johnson LV, Walsh ML, Chen LB. Localization of mitochondria in living cells with rhodamine 123. Proc Natl Acad Sci U S A 1980;77:990.
23. Broek D, Bartlett R, Crawford K, Nurse P. Involvement of P34cdc2 in establishing the dependency of S-phase on mitosis. Nature 1991;349:388.
24. Murray AW. Remembrance of things past. Nature 1991;349:367.
25. Hartwell LH, Weinert TA. Checkpoints: controls that ensure the order of cell cycle events. Science 1989;246:629.
26. Murray AW, Kirschner MW. Dominoes and clocks. The union of two views of the cell cycle. Science 1989;246:614.
27. Laskey RA, Fairman MP, Blow JJ. S-phase of the cell cycle. Science 1989;246:609.
28. Darzynkiewicz Z. Age-specific changes in the proliferation of Ehrlich ascites tumor cells grown as solid tumors. Cancer Res 1972;32:628.
29. Gelfant S. Cycling-noncycling cell transitions in tissue aging, immunological surveillance, transformation and tumor growth. Int Rev Cytol 1981;70:1.
30. O'Farrell PH, Edgar BA, Lakich D, Lehner CF. Directing cell division during development. Science 1989;246:635.
31. Folkman J, Moscona A. Role of cell shape in growth control. Nature 1978;273:345.
32. McIntosh JR, Koonce MP. Mitosis. Science 1989;246:622.
33. LaLa PK. Age-specific changes in the proliferation of Ehrlich ascites tumor cells grown as solid tumors. Cancer Res 1972;32:628.
34. Watson JV. The cell proliferation kinetics of the EMT6/M/AC mouse tumor at four volumes during unperturbed growth in vivo. Cell Tissue Kinet 1976;9:147.
35. Baserga R. The biology of cell reproduction. Cambridge (MA): Harvard University Press; 1985.
36. Kaman EJ, Smeulders AWN, Verbeek PW, et al. Image processing for mitoses in sections of breast cancer: a feasibility study. Cytometry 1984;5:244.
37. Schipper NW, Smeulders AW, Baak JP. Automated estimation of epithelial volume in breast cancer sections. A comparison with the image processing steps applied to gynecological tumors. Pathol Res Pract 1990;186:737.
38. Dressler LG, Bartow S. A DNA flow cytometry in solid tumors: practical aspects and clinical applications. Semin Diagn Pathol 1989;6:55.
39. Kamensky LA, Melamed MR. Instrumentation for automated examination of cellular specimens. Proc IEEE 1969;57:2007.
40. VanDilla MA, Trujillo TT, Mullaney PF, Coulter JR. Cell microfluorometry. A method for rapid fluorescence measurement. Science 1969;169:1213.
41. Hedley DW, Freidlander ML, Taylor IW, et al. Method for analysis of cellular DNA content of paraffin-embedded pathological material using flow cytometry. J Histochem Cytochem 1983;31:1333.
42. Pallavicini MG. Solid tissue dispersal for cytokinetic analyses. In: Gray JW, Darzyniewicz Z, editors. Techniques for analysis of cellular proliferation. Clifton (NJ): Humana; 1986. p. 139–62.
43. Latt SA. Fluorometric detection of DNA synthesis. Possibilities for interfacing bromodeoxyuridine dye techniques with flow fluorometry. J Histochem Cytochem 1977;25:913.
44. Meyer JS, Nauert J, Koehm S, Hughes J. Cell kinetics of human tumors by in vitro bromodeoxyuridine labeling. J Histochem Cytochem 1989;37:1449.
45. Raza A, Yasin Z, Grande C. A comparison of the rate of DNA synthesis in myeloblasts from peripheral blood and bone marrows in patients with acute nonlymphocytic leukemia. Exp Cell Res 1988;176:13.
46. Hiddeman WH, Schumann J, Andreeff M, et al. A convention on nomenclature for DNA cytometry. Cytometry 1984;5:445.
47. Joensuu H, Kallioniemi OP. Different opinions on classification of DNA histograms produced from paraffin-embedded tissue. Cytometry 1989;10:711.
48. Mendelsohn ML. The growth fraction: a new concept applied to neoplasia. Science 1960;132:1496.
49. Killman SA. Acute leukemia. The kinetics of leukemic blast cells in man. Semin Hematol 1968;1:38.
50. McDivitt RW, Stone KR, Meyer JS. A method for dissociation of viable human breast cancer cells that produces flow cytometric kinetic information similar to that obtained by thymidine labeling. Cancer Res 1984;44:2628.
51. Hoffman J, Post J. In vivo studies of DNA synthesis in human normal and tumor cells. Cancer Res 1967;27:898.
52. Quastler H, Sherman FG. Cell population kinetics in the intestinal epithelium of the mouse. Exp Cell Res 1959;17:420.
53. Bruce WR, Valeriote F. Normal and malignant stem cells and chemotherapy. In: The proliferation and spread of neoplastic cells. University of Texas M. D. Anderson Hospital and Tumor Institute at Houston, 21st Annual Symposium on Fundamental Cancer Research 1967. Baltimore (MD): Williams & Wilkins; 1968. p. 409–22.
54. Till JE, McCulloch GA, Phillips RA, Siminovitch L. Aspects of the regulation of stem cell function. In: The proliferation and spread of neoplastic cells. University of Texas M. D. Anderson Hospital and Tumor Institute at Houston, 21st Annual Symposium on Fundamental Cancer Research 1967. Baltimore (MD): Williams & Wilkins; 1968. p. 235–44.
55. Hamburger A, Salmon SE. Primary bioassay of human myeloma stem cells. J Clin Invest 1977;60:846.
56. Steel GG, Lamerton LF. Cell population kinetics and chemotherapy. In: Perry S, editor. Human tumor cell kinetics. NCI; 1968. p. 29.
57. Steel GG. Cell loss as a factor in the growth rate of human tumors. Eur J Cancer 1967;3:381.
58. Guo M, Bruce AH. Cell proliferation and apoptosis. Curr Opin Cell Biol 1999;11:745.
59. Novick A, Szilard L. Experiments with the chemostat on spontaneous mutations of bacteria. Proc Natl Acad Sci U S A 1950;36:708.
60. Foulds L. The histologic analysis of mammary tumors of mice. II. The histology of responsiveness and progression. The origins of tumors. J Natl Cancer Inst 1956;17:713.
61. Iannaccone PM, Weinberg WC, Deamant FD. On the clonal origin of tumors. A review of experimental models. Int J Cancer 1987;39:778.
62. Frei E III. Models and the clinical dilemma. In: Fidler IJ, White RJ, editors. Design of models for testing therapeutic agents. New York: Van Nostrand Reinhold; 1982. p. 248–59.
63. Fidler I. Tumor heterogeneity and the biology of cancer invasion and metastases. Cancer Res 1978;38:2651.
64. Charbit A, Malaise EP, Tubiana M. Relation between the pathological nature and the growth rate of human tumors. Eur J Cancer 1971;7:307.
65. Simpson–Herren L, Sanford AH, Holmquist JP. Cell population kinetics of transplanted and metastatic Lewis lung carcinoma. Cell Tissue Kinet 1974;7:349.
66. Wegelin C. Malignant disease of the thyroid gland and its relations to goitre in man and animals. Cancer Rev 1928;3:297.
67. Neve EF. Kangri-burn cancer. BMJ 1923;2:1255.
68. Groham JH, Helvig EB. In: Graham JH, Johnson WC, Helvig EB, editors. Dermal pathology. New York: Harper & Row; 1972. p. 561–81.
69. Greenberg PL, Mara B. The preleukemic syndrome. Correlation of in vitro parameters of granulocytopoiesis with clinical features. Am J Med 1979;66:951.
70. Peterson LC, Bloomfield CD, Brunning RD. Blast crisis as an initial or terminal manifestation of chronic myeloid leukemia. Am J Med 1976;60:209.
71. Parks TG, Bussey HJR, Lockhart–Mummery HE. Familial polyposis coli associated with extracolonic abnormalities. Gut 1970;11:323.

72. De Ome KB, Medina D. A new approach to mammary tumorigenesis in rodents. Cancer 1969;24:1255.
73. Davis HH, Simons M, Davis JB. Cystic disease of the breast. Relationship to carcinoma. Cancer 1964;17:957.
74. Sandison AT. An autopsy study of the adult human breast. With special reference to the proliferative epithelial changes of importance in the pathology of the breast. Monogr Natl Cancer Inst 1962;8:1.
75. Ryser HJP. Chemical carcinogenesis. N Engl J Med 1971;285:721.
76. Glicksman AS, Pajak TF, Gottlieb AJ, et al Second malignant neoplasms in patients successfully treated for Hodgkin's disease. A Cancer and Leukemia Group B study. Cancer Treat Rep 1982;66:1035.
77. Boice JD Jr, Greene MH, Killen JY Jr, et al. Leukemia and preleukemia after adjuvant treatment of gastrointestinal cancer with semustine (methyl-CCNU). N Engl J Med 1983;309:1079.
78. Dang C, Gilewski TA, Surbone A, Norton L. Cytokinetics of chemotherapy, In Holland, Frei, editors. Cancer medicine 6th ed. Hamilton (ON): BC Decker Inc; 2003.
79. Hedley DW, Clark GM, Conrelisse CJ, et al. Consensus review of the clinical utility of DNA cytometry in carcinoma of the breast. Cytometry 1993;14:482–5.
80. 2000 Update of recommendations for the use of tumor markers in breast and colorectal cancer: clinical practice guidelines of the American Society of Clinical Oncology. J Clin Oncol 2001;6:1865–78.
81. Shawver LK, Slamon D, Ullrich A. Smart drugs. Tyrosine kinase inhibitors in cancer therapy. Cancer Cell 2002;1:117–23.
82. Steeg PS, De La Rosa A, Flatow U, et al. NM23 and breast cancer metastasis. Breast Cancer Res Treat 1993;25:175.
83. Harbeck N, Schmitt M, Kates RE, et al. Clinical utility of urokinase-type plasminogen activator and plasminogen activator inhibitor-1 determination in primary breast cancer tissue for individualized therapy concepts. Clin Breast Cancer 2002;3:196–200.
84. Anbazhagan R, Gelber RD, Bettelheim R, et al. Association of c-erbB-2 expression and S-phase fraction in the prognosis of node positive breast cancer. Ann Oncol 1991;2:47–53.
85. Fernandez Val JF, Losada J, Arregui Murua A, et al. Cell proliferation, nuclear ploidy, and EGFr and HER2/neu tyrosine kinase oncoproteins in infiltrating ductal breast carcinoma. Cancer Genet Cytogenet 2002;138:69–72.
86. French D, Pizzi C, De Marchis L, et al. Proliferative activity and genetic alterations in breast carcinoma. Proc Am Assoc Cancer Res 1993;34:3083.
87. Walker RA, Varley JM. The molecular pathology of human breast cancer. Cancer Surv 1993;16:31.
88. Paradiso A, Mangia A, Correale M, et al. Cytosol cathepsin-D content and proliferative activity of human breast cancer. Breast Cancer Res Treat 1992;23:63–70.
89. Marshman E, Streuli CH. Insulin-like growth factors and insulin-like growth factor binding proteins in mammary gland function. Breast Cancer Res 2002;4:231–9.
90. Ristimaki A, Sivula A, Lundin J, et al. Prognostic significance of elevated cyclooxygenase-2 expression in breast cancer. Cancer Res 2002;62:632–5.
91. Keyomarsi K, Tucker S, Buchholz T, et al. Cyclin E and survival in patients with breast cancer. N Engl J Med 2002;347:1566–75.
92. van't Veer LJ, Paik S, Hayes DF. Gene expression profiling of breast cancer: a new tumor marker. J Clin Oncol 2005;8:1631–5.
93. Skipper HE, Schabel FM Jr, Wilcox WS. Experimental evaluation of potential anticancer agents XIII. On the criteria and kinetics associated with "curability" of experimental leukemia. Cancer Chemother Rep 1964;35:1.
94. Giordano M, Danova M, Mazzini G, et al. Cell kinetics with in vivo bromodeoxyuridine assay, proliferating cell nuclear antigen expression and flow cytometric analysis. Prognostic significance in acute nonlymphoblastic leukemia. Cancer 1993;71:2739.
95. Skipper HE. Laboratory models. The historical perspective. Cancer Treat Rep 1986;70:3.
96. Simpson–Herren L, Lloyd HH. Kinetic parameters and growth curves for experimental tumor systems. Cancer Chemother Rep 1970;54:143.
97. Frei E III. Models and the clinical dilemma. In: Fidler IJ, White RJ, editors. Design of models for testing therapeutic agents. New York: Van Nostrand Reinhold; 1982. p. 248–59.
98. Shackney SE, McCormack GW, Guchural GJ Jr. Growth rate patterns of solid tumors and their relation to responsiveness to therapy. An analytical review. Ann Intern Med 1978;89:107.
99. Goldin A, Venditti JM, Humphreys SR, Mantel N. Influence of the concentration of leukemic innoculum on the effectiveness of treatment. Science 1956;123:840.
100. Roosa R, Weaver CF, DeLamater ED. Importance of transplant size in chemotherapeutic assay with the use of the Gardner lymphosarcoma. Proc Am Assoc Cancer Res 1957;2:243.
101. Holland JF. Clinical studies of unmaintained remissions in acute lymphocytic leukemia. In: The proliferation and spread of neoplastic cells. 21st Annual Symposium on Fundamental Cancer Research 1967. Baltimore (MD): Williams & Wilkins; 1968. p. 453–62.
102. Schabel FM. Concepts for the systemic treatment of micrometastases. Cancer 1975;35:15.
103. Shapiro DM, Fugmann RA. A role for chemotherapy as an adjunct to surgery. Cancer Res 1957;17:1098.
104. Shapiro DM, Fugmann RA. A role for chemotherapy as an adjunct to surgery. Cancer Res 1957;17:1098.
105. Early Breast Cancer Trialists' Collaborative Group. Systemic treatment of early breast cancer by hormonal cytotoxic, or immune therapy. Lancet 1992:339:1.
106. Early Breast Cancer Trialists' Collaborative Group. Treatment of early breast cancer. Worldwide evidence in 1985–1990. A systematic overview of all available randomized trials in early breast cancer of adjuvant endocrine and cytotoxic therapy. New York: Oxford University Press; 1990.
107. DeVita VT. The relationship between tumor mass and resistance to treatment of cancer. Cancer 1983;51:1209.
108. DeVita VT. Principles of chemotherapy. In: DeVita Jr T, Hellman S, Rosenberg SA, editors. Cancer: principles and practice. 3rd ed. Philadelphia: JB Lippincott; 1988. p. 279.
109. Luria SE, Delbruck M. Mutations of bacteria from virus sensitivity to virus resistance. Genetics 1943;28:491.
110. Law LW. Origin of resistance of leukaemic cells to folic acid antagonists. Nature 1952;169:628.
111. Broek D, Bartlett R, Crawford K, Nurse D. Involvement of $p34^{cdc2}$ in establishing the dependency of S-phase on mitosis. Nature 1991;349:388.
112. Hartwell LH, Weinert TA. Checkpoints. Controls that ensure the order of cell cycle events. Science 1989;246:629.
113. Murray AW, Kirschner MW. Dominoes and clocks. The union of two views of the cell cycle. Science 1989;246:614.
114. Murray AW. Remembrance of things past. Nature 1991;349:367.
115. Burchenal JH, Cremer MA, Williams BS, Armstrong RA. Sterilization of leukemic cells in vivo and in vitro. Cancer Res 1951;11:700–5.
116. Frei E III, Freireich EJ, Gehan E, et al. Studies of sequential and combination antimetabolite therapy in acute leukemia: 6-mercaptopurine and methotrexate. Blood 1961;18:431.
117. Goldie JH, Coldman AJ. A mathematic model for relating the drug sensitivity of tumors to their spontaneous mutation rate. Cancer Treat Rep 1979;63:1727.
118. Goldie JH, Coldman AJ. Application of theoretical models to chemotherapy protocol design. Cancer Treat Rep 1986;70:127
119. Goldie JH. Scientific basis for adjuvant and primary (neoadjuvant) chemotherapy. Semin Oncol 1987;14:1.
120. Kendal WS, Frost P. Metastatic potential and spontaneous mutation rates: studies with two murine cell lines and their recently induced metastatic variants. Cancer Res 1986;46:6131.
121. Poste G, Fidler IJ. The pathogenesis of cancer metastases. Nature 1980;283:139.
122. National Cancer Institute (USA). Surveillance, Epidemiology and End Results (SEER) Program, 1974–1987.
123. Rosen PP, Groshen S. Factors influencing survival and prognosis in early breast carcinoma (T1N0M0-T1N1M0). Assessment of 644 patients with median follow-up of 18 years. Surg Clin North Am 1990;70:937.
124. DeVita VT, Young RC, Cannellos GP. Combination vs. single agent chemotherapy. A review of the basis for selection of drug treatment of cancer. Cancer 1975;35:98.
125. Coldman AJ, Goldie JH. A mathematical model of drug resistance in neoplasms. In: Bruchovsky N, Goldie JH, editors. Drug and hormone resistance in neoplasia. Boca Raton (FL): CRC Press; 1982. p. 55–78.
126. Fisher RI, DeVita VT, Hubbard SM, et al. Prolonged disease-free survival in Hodgkin's disease with MOPP reinduction after first relapse. Ann Intern Med 1979;90:761.
127. Kardinal CG, Perry MC, Korzun AH, et al. Responses to chemotherapy or chemohormonal therapy in advanced breast cancer patients treated previously with adjuvant chemotherapy. A subset analysis of CALGB study 8081. Cancer 1988;61:415.
128. Valagussa P, Tancini G, Bonadonna G. Salvage treatment of patients suffering relapse after adjuvant CMF chemotherapy. Cancer 1986;58:1411.
129. Valagussa P, Brambilla C, Zambetti M, Bonadonna G. Salvage treatment after first relapse of breast cancer. A review. Proceedings, Third International Conference on Adjuvant Therapy of Primary Breast Cancer, St. Gallen, Switzerland: 1988. p. 9.
130. Iversen OH, Iversen U, Ziegler JL, Bluming AZ. Cell kinetics in Burkitt's lymphoma. Eur J Cancer 1974;10:155.
131. Bloom H, Richardson M, Harris B. Natural history of untreated breast cancer (1804–1933). Comparison of treated and untreated cases according to histological grade of malignancy. BMJ 1962;2:213.
132. Adair F, Berg J, Joubert L, Robbins GF. Long-term follow-up of breast cancer patients. The 30-year report. Cancer 1974;33:1145.
133. Ferguson DJ, Meier P, Karrison T, et al. Staging of breast cancer and survival rates. An assessment based on 50 years experience with radical mastectomy. JAMA 1982;248:1337.
134. Harris JR, Hellman S. Observations on survival curve analysis with particular reference to breast cancer. Cancer 1986;57:925.
135. Brinkley D, Haybittle JL. The curability of breast cancer. Lancet 1975;2:95.
136. Rutqvist LE, Wallgren A, Nilsson B. Is breast cancer a curable disease? A study of 14,731 women with breast cancer from the Cancer Registry of Norway. Cancer 1984;53:1793.
137. Fisher B, Redmond C, Poisson R, et al. Eight-year results of a randomized clinical trial comparing total mastectomy and lumpectomy with or without irradiation in the treatment of breast cancer. N Engl J Med 1989;320:822.
138. Ragaz J, Jackson SM, Le N, et al. Adjuvant radiotherapy and chemotherapy in node-positive premenopausal women with breast cancer. N Engl J Med 1997;337:956.
139. Overgaard M, Jensen MB, Overgaard J, et al. Postoperative radiotherapy in high-risk postmenopausal breast-cancer patients given adjuvant tamoxifen. Lancet 1999;353:1641.
140. Overgaard M, Hansen PS, Overgaard J, et al. Postoperative radiotherapy in high-risk premenopausal women with breast cancer who receive adjuvant chemotherapy. N Engl J Med 1997;337:949.
141. Hellman S. Stopping metastases at their source. N Engl J Med 1997;337:996.
142. Frei E III, Freireich EJ, Gehan E, et al. Studies of sequential and combination antimetabolite therapy in acute leukemia. 6-mercaptopurine and methotrexate. Blood 1961;18:431.
143. Ludwig Breast Cancer Study Group. Combination adjuvant chemotherapy for node positive breast cancer. N Engl J Med 1988;319:677.
144. Peters WP, Jones, RB, Vredenburgh J, et al. A large, prospective, randomized trial of high-dose combination alkylating agents with autologous cellular support as consolidation for patients with metastatic breast cancer achieving complete remission after intensive doxorubicin-based induction therapy. Proc Am Soc Clin Oncol 1996;5:149.
145. Williams S, Stablein D, Einhorn L, et al. Immediate adjuvant chemotherapy versus observation with treatment at relapse in pathological stage II testicular cancer. N Engl J Med 1987;317:1433.
146. Ragaz J, Goldie JH, Baird R, et al. Experimental basis and clinical reality of preoperative (neoadjuvant) chemotherapy in breast cancer. Recent Results Cancer Res 1989;115:28.
147. Fisher B, Bryant J, Wolmark N, et al. Effect of preoperative chemotherapy on the outcome of women with operable breast cancer. J Clin Oncol 1998;16:2672.
148. Korzun A, Norton L, Perloff M, et al. Clinical equivalence despite dosage differences of two schedules of cyclophosphamide, methotrexate, 5-fluorouracil, vincristine and prednisone (CMFVP) for adjuvant therapy of node-positive stage II breast cancer. Proc Am Soc Clin Oncol 1988;7:12.
149. Perloff M, Norton L, Korzun A, et al. Advantage of an Adriamycin combination plus Halotestin after initial CMFVP for adjuvant therapy of node-positive stage II breast cancer. Proc Am Soc Clin Oncol 1986;70:273.
150. Moliterni A, Bonadonna G, Valagussa P, et al. Cyclophosphamide, methotrexate, and fluorouracil with or without doxorubicin in the adjuvant treatment of resectable breast cancer with one to three positive axillary nodes. J Clin Oncol 1991;9:1124.
151. Wampler GL, Heim WJ, Ellison NA, et al. For the Mid-Atlantic Oncology Program. Comparison of cyclophos-

phamide, doxorubicin, and vincristine with an alternating regimen of methotrexate, etoposide, and cisplatin/cyclophosphamide, doxorubicin, and vincristine in the treatment of extensive-disease small-cell lung cancer. J Clin Oncol 1991;9:1438.

152. Longo DL, DeVita VT Jr, Duffey PL, et al. Superiority of ProMACE-CytaBOM over ProMACE-MOPP in the treatment of advanced diffuse aggressive lymphoma. Results of a prospective randomized trial. J Clin Oncol 1991;9:25.

153. Bonadonna G, Santoro A. ABVD chemotherapy in the treatment of Hodgkin's disease. Cancer Treat Rev 1982;9:21.

154. Santoro A, Bonfante V, Viviani S, et al. Salvage chemotherapy in relapsing Hodgkin's disease. Proc Am Soc Clin Oncol 1984;3:254.

155. Bonadonna G, Valagussa P, Santoro A. Alternating noncross-resistant combination chemotherapy or MOPP in stage IV Hodgkin's disease. Ann Intern Med 1986;104:739.

156. Valagussa P, Santoro A, Boracchi P, et al. Nine-year results of two randomized studies with MOPP and ABVD in Hodgkin's disease. Multiple regression analysis. Proc Am Soc Clin Oncol 1989;8:976.

157. Canellos GP, Propert K, Cooper R, et al. MOPP vs. ABVD vs. MOPP alternating with ABVD in advanced Hodgkin's disease. A prospective randomized CALGB trial. Proc Am Soc Clin Oncol 1988;7:888.

158. Longo DL, Duffey PL, DeVita VT Jr, et al. Treatment of advanced-stage Hodgkin's disease. Alternating noncross-resistant MOPP/CABS is not superior to MOPP. J Clin Oncol 191;9:1409.

159. Glick J, Tsiatis A, Schilsky R, et al. A randomized phase III trial of MOPP/ABV hybrid vs. sequential MOPP-ABVD in advanced Hodgkin's disease. Preliminary results of the Intergroup Trial. Proc Am Soc Clin Oncol 1991;10:941.

160. Hart R, Perloff M, Holland J. One-day VATH (vinblastine, Adriamycin, thiotepa, and Halotestin) therapy for advanced breast cancer refractory to chemotherapy. Cancer 1981;48:1522.

161. Aisner J, Korsun A, Perloff M, et al. A randomized comparison of CAF, VATH, and VATH alternating with CMFVP for advanced breast cancer. A CALGB study. Proc Am Soc Clin Oncol 1988;7:27.

162. Brambilla C, Rossi A, Valagussa P, Bonadonna G. Adjuvant chemotherapy in postmenopausal women. Results of sequential noncross-resistant regimens. World J Surg 1985;9:728.

163. Norton L. Implications of kinetic heterogeneity in clinical oncology. Semin Oncol 1985;12:231.

164. Buzzoni R, Bonadonna G, Valagussa P, Zambetti M. Adjuvant chemotherapy with doxorubicin plus cyclophosphamide, methotrexate, and fluorouracil in the treatment of resectable breast cancer with more than three positive axillary nodes. J Clin Oncol 1991;9:2134.

165. Bonadonna G, Zambetti M, Valagussa P. Sequential or alternating doxorubicin and CMF regimens in breast cancer with more than three positive nodes. JAMA 1995;273:542–7.

166. Cassileth PA, Lynch E, Hines JD, et al. Varying intensity of postremission therapy in acute myeloid leukemia. Blood 1992;79:1924.

167. Preisler H, Davis RB, Kirshner J, et al. Comparison of three remission induction regimens and two postinduction strategies for the treatment of acute nonlymphocytic leukemia. A Cancer and Leukemia Group B study. Blood 1987;69:1441.

168. Mayer RJ, Davis RB, Schiffer CA, et al. Intensive postremission chemotherapy in adults with acute myeloid leukemia. N Engl J Med 1994;331:896.

169. McCulloch EA, Buick RN, Curtis JE, et al. The heritable nature of clonal characteristics in acute myeloblastic leukemia. Blood 1981;58:105.

170. Bishop JF. Intensified therapy for acute myeloid leukemia [editorial]. N Engl J Med 1994;331:941.

171. Tubergen D, Gilchrist G, Coccia P, et al. The role of intensified chemotherapy in intermediate risk acute lymphoblastic leukemia (ALL) of childhood. Proc Ann Meet Am Soc Clin Oncol 1990;9:A835.

172. Frei E, Teicher BA, Holden SA, et al. Preclinical studies and clinical correlation of the effect of alkylating dose. Cancer Res 1988;48:6417.

173. Bruce WR, Meeker BE, Valeriote FA. Comparison of the sensitivity of normal hematopoietic and transplanted lymphoma colony-forming cells to chemotherapeutic agents administered in vivo. J Natl Cancer Inst 1996;37:233.

174. Griswold DP Jr, Trader MW, Frei E III, et al. Response of drug-sensitive and -resistant L1210 leukemias to high-dose chemotherapy. Cancer Res 1987;47:2323.

175. Tattersall MHN, Parker LM, Pitman SW, Frei E III. Clinical pharmacology of high-dose methotrexate. Cancer Chemother Rep (Part 3) 1975;6:25.

176. Bonadonna G, Valagussa P. Dose-response effect of adjuvant chemotherapy in breast cancer. N Engl J Med 1981;304:10.

177. Hryniuk WM. The importance of dose intensity in the outcome of chemotherapy. In: DeVita VT Jr, Hellman S, Rosenberg SA, editors. Important advances in oncology. Philadelphia: JB Lippincott; 1988. p. 121–41.

178. DeVita VT, Hubbard SM, Longo DL. The chemotherapy of lymphomas. Looking back, moving forward. Richard and Linda Rosenthal Foundation Award Lecture. Cancer Res 1987;47:5810.

179. Henderson IC, Hayes DF, Gelman R. Dose-response in the treatment of breast cancer. A critical review. J Clin Oncol 1988;6:1501.

180. Redmond C, Fisher B, Wieand HS. The methodological dilemma in retrospectively correlating the amount of chemotherapy received in adjuvant therapy protocols with disease-free survival. Cancer Treat Rep 1983;67:519.

181. Pinkel D, Hernandez K, Borella L, et al. Drug dosage and remission duration in childhood lymphocytic leukemia. Cancer 1971;27:247.

182. Samson MK, Rivlin SE, Jones SE, et al. Dose-response and dose-survival advantage for high- vs. low-dose cisplatin combined with vinblastine and bleomycin in disseminated testicular cancer. Cancer 1984;53:1029.

183. Tannock IF, Boyd NF, DeBoer G, et al. A randomized trial of two dose levels of cyclophosphamide, methotrexate, and fluorouracil chemotherapy for patients with metastatic breast cancer. J Clin Oncol 1988;6:1377.

184. Wood WC, Budman DR, Korzun AH, et al. Dose and dose intensity of adjuvant chemotherapy for stage II, node-positive breast carcinoma. N Engl J Med 1994;330:1253.

185. Fisher B, Anderson S, DeCillis A, et al. Further evaluation of intensified and increased total dose of cyclophosphamide for the treatment of primary breast cancer. Findings from National Surgical Adjuvant Breast and Bowel Project B-25. J Clin Oncol 1999;17:3374.

186. Henderson IC, Berry DA, Demetri GD, et al. Improved outcomes from adding sequential paclitaxel but not from escalating doxorubicin dose in an adjuvant chemotherapy regimen for patients with node-positive primary breast cancer . J Clin Oncol 2003;21:976–83.

187. Bruce WR, Meeker BE, Valeriote FA. Comparison of the sensitivity of normal hematopoietic and transplanted lymphoma colony-forming cells to chemotherapeutic agents administered in vivo. J Natl Cancer Inst 1966;37:233.

188. Bonadonna G, Valagussa P, Rossi A, et al. Ten-year experience with CMF-based adjuvant chemotherapy in resectable breast cancer. Breast Cancer Res Treat 1985;5:95.

189. Henderson IC, Gelman RS, Harris JR, Canellos GP. Duration of therapy in adjuvant chemotherapy trials. Monogr Natl Cancer Inst 1986;1:95.

190. Rivkin SE, Knight WA, McDivitt R, et al. Adjuvant therapy for breast cancer with positive axillary nodes designed according to estrogen receptor status. World J Surg 1985;9:723.

191. Early Breast Cancer Trialists' Collaborative Group. Systemic treatment of early breast cancer by hormonal, cytotoxic, or immune therapy. Lancet 1992;339:71.

192. Thor AD, Berry DA, Budman DR, et al. erbB-2, p53, and efficacy of adjuvant therapy in lymph node-positive breast cancer. J Natl Cancer Inst 1998;90:1346.

193. Ravdin PM. Should HER-2 status be routinely measured for all breast cancer patients? Semin Oncol 1999;26:117.

194. Paik S, Bryant J, Park C, et al. erbB-2 and response to doxorubicin in patients with axillary lymph node-positive, hormone receptor-negative breast cancer. J Natl Cancer Inst 1998;90:1361.

195. DeVita VT Jr. Dose-response is alive and well. J Clin Oncol 1986;4:1157.

196. Frei E III, Canellos GP. Dose. A critical factor in cancer chemotherapy. Am J Med 1980;69:585.

197. Collins VP, Loeffler K, Tivey H. Observations on growth rates of human tumors. Am J Radiol 1956;76:988.

198. Steel GG. Growth kinetics of tumours. Cell population kinetics in relation to the growth and treatment of cancer. Oxford (UK): Clarendon; 1977. p. 46–52.

199. Tubiana M. Tumor cell proliferation kinetics and tumor growth rate. Acta Oncol 1989;28:113.

200. Demicheli R. Growth of testicular neoplasm lung metastases. Tumor-specific relation between two Gompertzian parameters. Eur J Cancer 1980;16:1603.

201. Spratt JS, Greenberg RA, Heuser LS. Geometry, growth rates and duration of cancer and carcinoma in situ of the breast before detection by screening. Cancer Res 1986;46:970.

202. Sullivan PW, Salmon SE. Kinetics of tumor growth and regression in IgG multiple myeloma. J Clin Invest 1972;51:1697.

203. Laird AK. Dynamics of growth in tumors and normal organisms. Monogr Natl Cancer Inst 1969;30:15.

204. Norton L. Introduction to clinical aspects of preneoplasia. A mathematical relationship between stromal paracrine autonomy and population size. In: Marks PA, Turler H, Weil R, editors. Challenges of modern medicine. Vol. 1. Precancerous lesions. A multidisciplinary approach. Milan (Italy): Ares-Serono Symposia; 1993. p. 269–75.

205. Norton L. Mathematical interpretation of tumor growth kinetics. In: Greenspan EM, editor. Clinical interpretation and practice of cancer chemotherapy. New York: Raven; 1982. p. 53–70.

206. Folkman J, Shing Y. Angiogenesis. J Biol Chem 1992;267:10931–4.

207. Gilewski T, Norton L. Cytokinetics of neoplasia. In: Mendelsohn J, Howley P, Israel MA, Liotta LA, editors. The molecular basis of cancer. Philadelphia: WB Saunders; 1995.p 143–59.

208. Hastings HM, Schneider BS, Schreiber M, et al. Statistical geometry of pancreatic islets. Proc R Soc Lond B Biol Sci 1992;250:257.

209. Comroe JH. The lung. Sci Am 1966;214:56.

210. Wilson TA. Design of the bronchial tree. Nature 1967;213:668.

211. Fazzalari NL, Parkinson IH. Fractal properties of subchondral cancellous bone in severe osteoarthritis of the hip. J Bone Miner Res 1997:12:632.

212. Suwa N, Takahashi T. Morphological and morphometrical analysis of circulation in hypertension and ischemic kidney. Munich (Germany): Urban & Schwarzenberg; 1971.

213. West GB, Brown JH, Enquist BJ. A general model for the origin of the allometric scaling laws in biology. Science 1997;276:122.

214. Norton LA. Gompertzian model of human breast cancer growth. Cancer Res 1988;48:7067.

215. Heuser L, Spratt J, Polk H. Growth rates of primary breast cancer. Cancer 1979;43:1888.

216. Fisher B, Slack N, Katrych D, Wolmark N. Ten-year follow-up results in patients with carcinoma of the breast in a cooperative clinical trial evaluating surgical adjuvant chemotherapy. Surg Gynecol Obstet 1975;140:528.

217. Speer JF, Petrovsky VE, Retsky MW, Wardwell RH. A stochastic numerical model of breast cancer that simulates clinical data. Cancer Res 1984;44:4124.

218. Fisher B, Brown AM, Dimitrov NV, et al. Two months of doxorubicin-cyclophosphamide with and without interval reinduction therapy compared with 6 months of cyclophosphamide, methotrexate, and fluorouracil in positive-node breast cancer patients with tamoxifen-nonresponsive tumors. Results from the National Surgical Adjuvant Breast and Bowel Project B-15. J Clin Oncol 1990;8:1483.

219. Norton L, Simon R. Growth curve of an experimental solid tumor following radiotherapy. J Natl Cancer Inst 1977;58:1735.

220. Norton L, Simon R. Tumor size, sensitivity to therapy, and the design of treatment schedules. Cancer Treat Rep 1977;61:1307.

221. Hill RP, Stanley JA. Pulmonary metastases of the Lewis lung tumor—cell kinetics and response to cyclophosphamide at different sizes. Cancer Treat Rep 1977;61:29.

222. Paterson AHG, Lees AW, Hanson J, et al. Impact of chemotherapy on survival in metastatic breast cancer. Lancet 1980;2:312.

223. Powles TJ, Smith IE, Ford HT, et al. Failure of chemotherapy to prolong survival in a group of patients with metastatic breast cancer. Lancet 1980;1:580.

224. Tormey D, Carbone P, Band P. Breast cancer survival in single and combination chemotherapy trials since 1968. Proc Am Assoc Cancer Res 1977;18:64.

225. Bezwoda WR. Randomized, controlled trial of high dose chemotherapy versus standard dose chemotherapy for high risk, surgically treated, primary breast cancer. Proc Am Soc Clin Oncol 1999;18:4.

226. Peters WP, Rosner GL, Vredenburgh JJ, et al. Prospective, randomized comparison of high-dose chemotherapy with stem-cell support versus intermediate-dose chemotherapy after surgery and adjuvant chemotherapy in women with high-risk primary breast cancer: a report of CALGB 9082, SWOG 9114, and NCIC MA-13. J Clin Oncol 2005;10:2191.

227. The Scandinavian Breast Cancer Study Group. Results from a randomized adjuvant breast cancer study with high

dose chemotherapy with CTCb supported by autologous bone marrow stem cells versus dose escalated and tailored FEC therapy. Proc Am Soc Clin Oncol 1999;13:3.
228. Crown J, Norton L. Potential strategies for improving the results of high-dose chemotherapy in patients with metastatic breast cancer. Ann Oncol 1995;Suppl 6:21–6.
229. Norton L, Simon R. The Norton–Simon hypothesis revisited. Cancer Treat Rep 1986;70:163.
230. Ross DW, Capizzi RL. Differentiation vs. cytoreduction during remission induction in acute nonlymphoblastic leukemia treated with sequential high-dose ara-c and asparaginase. Cancer 1984;53:1651.
231. Cortes EP, Necheles TF, Holland JF, et al. Adjuvant chemotherapy for primary osteosarcoma. A Cancer and Leukemia Group B experience. In: Salmon SE, Jones SE, editors. Adjuvant chemotherapy of cancer III. New York: Grune & Stratton; 1981. p. 201–0.
232. Cordon–Cardo C, O'Brien JP. The multidrug resistance phenotype in human cancer. In: DeVita VT Jr, Hellman S, Rosenberg SA, editors. Important advances in oncology. New York: JB Lippincott; 1991. p. 19–38.
233. Goldstein LJ, Galski H, Fojo A, et al. Expression of multidrug resistance gene in human tumors. J Natl Cancer Inst 1989;81:116.
234. Skipper HE. Analyses of multiarmed trials in which animals bearing different burdens of L1210 leukemia cells were treated with two, three, and four drug combinations delivered in different ways with varying dose intensities of each drug and varying average dose intensities. South Res Inst Booklet 7 1986;42:87.
235. Griswold DP, Schabel FM Jr, Corbett TH, Dykes DJ. Concepts for controlling drug-resistant tumor cells. In: Fidler IJ, White RJ, editors. Design of models for testing cancer therapeutic agents. New York: Van Nostrand Reinhold; 1982. p. 215–24.
236. Day RS. Treatment sequencing, asymmetry, and uncertainty. Protocol strategies for combination chemotherapy. Cancer Res 1986;46:3876.
237. Norton L, Day R. Potential innovations in scheduling in cancer chemotherapy. In: DeVita VT Jr, Hellman S, Rosenberg SA, editors. Important advances in oncology. New York: JB Lippincott; 1991. p. 57–72.
238. Selawry OS, Hananian J, Wolman IJ, et al. New treatment schedule with improved survival in childhood leukemia. JAMA 1965;194:187.
239. Bhardwaj S, Holland JF, Norton L. Intensive sequenced adjuvant chemotherapy for breast cancer. Proc Am Soc Clin Oncol 1991;10:75.
240. Henderson IC, Berry DA, Demetri G, et al. Improved outcomes from adding sequential paclitaxel but not from escalating doxorubicin dose in an adjuvant chemotherapy regimen for patients with node-positive primary breast cancer. J Clin Oncol 2003;21:976–83.
241. Mamounas EP, Bryant J, Lembersky B, et al. Paclitaxel after doxorubicin plus cyclophosphamide as adjuvant chemotherapy for node-positive breast cancer: results from NSABP B-28. J Clin Oncol 2005;23:3686–96.
242. Perez E, Romond E, et al. Presented at the American Society of Clinical Oncology, May 2005.
243. Gabrilove JL. Colony-stimulating factors. Clinical status. In: DeVita VT Jr, Hellman S, Rosenberg SA, editors. Important advances in oncology. New York: JB Lippincott; 1991. p. 215–37.
244. Frei E III, Antman K, Teicher B, et al. Bone marrow autotransplantation for solid tumors. Prospects. J Clin Oncol 1989;7:515.
245. Peters WP. High dose chemotherapy and autologous bone marrow support for breast cancer. In: DeVita VT, Hellman S, Rosenberg SA, editors. Important advances in oncology. Philadelphia: JB Lippincott; 1991. p. 135–50.
246. Haskell CM, Green SJ, Sledge GW Jr, et al. Phase III comparison of adjuvant high-dose doxorubicin plus cyclophosphamide versus sequential doxorubicin followed by cyclophosphamide in breast cancer patients with 0-3 positive nodes (INT 0137). Abstract Proc Am Soc Clin Oncol 2002:142.
247. Hudis C, Lebwohl D, Crown J, et al. Dose-intensive sequential crossover adjuvant chemotherapy for women with high risk node-positive primary breast cancer. In: Salmon SE, editor. Adjuvant therapy of cancer IV. Philadelphia: JB Lippincott; 1993. p. 214–9.
248. Citron ML, Berry DA, Cirrincione C, et al. Randomized trial of dose-dense versus conventionally scheduled and sequential versus concurrent combination chemotherapy as postoperative adjuvant treatment of node-positive primary breast cancer: first report of Intergroup Trial C9741/Cancer and Leukemia Group B Trial 9741. J Clin Oncol 2003;21:1431–9.
249. Norton L. Theoretical concepts and the emerging role of taxanes in adjuvant therapy. Oncologist 2001; 3:30–5.
250. Gianni AM, Bregni M, Siena S, et al. Prospective randomized comparison of MACOP-B vs. rhGM-CSF–supported high-dose sequential myeloablative chemoradiotherapy in diffuse large cell lymphoma. Proc Am Soc Clin Oncol 1991;10:951.
251. Budihna M, Skrk J, Smid L, Furlan L. Tumor cell repopulation in the rest interval of split-course radiation treatment. Strahlentherapie 1980;156:402.
252. Withers HR, Taylor JMG, Maciejewski B. The hazard of accelerated tumor clonogen repopulation during radiotherapy. Acta Oncol 1988;27:131.
253. Andrews RJ. The radiobiology of human cancer radiotherapy. Philadelphia: WB Saunders; 1968.
254. Badib OA, Webster JH. Changes in tumour oxygen tension during radiation therapy. Acta Radiol Ther Phys Biol 1969;8:247.
255. Steel GG. Growth kinetics of tumors. Oxford (UK): Oxford University Press; 1977.
256. Valeriote F, van Putten L. Proliferation-dependent cytotoxicity of anticancer agents. A review. Cancer Res 1975;35:2619.
257. Hug V, Johnston D, Finders M, Hortobagyi G. Use of growth-stimulating hormones to improve the in vitro therapeutic index of doxorubicin for human breast cancer. Cancer Res 1986;46:147.
258. Osborne CK, Kitten L, Arteaga CL. Antagonism of chemotherapy-induced cytotoxicity for human breast cancer cells by antiestrogens. J Clin Oncol 1989;7:710.
259. Conte PF, Alama A, Bertelli G, et al. Chemotherapy with estrogenic recruitment and surgery in locally advanced breast cancer. Clinical and cytokinetic results. Int J Cancer 1987;40:490.
260. Swain SM, Sorace RA, Bagley CS, et al. Neoadjuvant chemotherapy in the combined modality approach of locally advanced nonmetastatic breast cancer. Cancer Res 1987;47:3889.
261. Conte PF, Pronzato P, Rubagotti A, et al. Conventional vs. cytokinetic polychemotherapy with estrogenic recruitment in metastatic breast cancer. Results of a randomized cooperative trial. J Clin Oncol 1987;5:339.
262. Lippman ME. Hormonal stimulation and chemotherapy for breast cancer [editorial]. J Clin Oncol 1987;5:331.
263. Lippman ME, Cassidy J, Wesley M, Young RC. A randomized attempt to increase the efficacy of cytotoxic chemotherapy in metastatic breast cancer by hormonal synchronization. J Clin Oncol 1984;2:28.
264. Bontenbal M, Sieuwerts AM, Klijn JGM, et al. Effect of hormonal manipulation and doxorubicin administration on cell cycle kinetics of human breast cancer cells. Br J Cancer 1989;60:688.
265. Lippman ME, Dickson RB. Growth control of normal and malignant breast epithelium. In: Ragaz J, Simpson–Herren J, Lippman ME, Fisher B, editors. Effects of therapy on biology and kinetics of the residual tumor. Part A. Preclinical aspects. New York: Wiley–Liss; 1990. p. 147–78.
266. Wilson AJ, Baum M, Brinkley DM, et al. Six-year result of a controlled trial of tamoxifen as single adjuvant agent in management of early breast cancer. World J Surg 1985;9:756.
267. Lippman ME, Dickson RB, Bates S, et al. Autocrine and paracrine growth regulation of human breast cancer. Breast Cancer Res Treat 1986;7:59.
268. Weinberg RA, Bishop JM, Minna JD, Sharp PA. Gene regulation and oncogenes. AACR special conference in cancer research. Cancer Res 1989;49:2188.
269. Rowley JD, Golomb AM, Vardiman JW. Nonrandom chromosomal abnormalities in acute leukemia and dysmyelopoietic syndromes in patients with previously treated malignant disease. Blood 1981;58:759.
270. Yee D, Rosen N, Favoni RE, Cullen KJ. The insulin-like growth factors, their receptors, and their binding proteins in human breast cancer. Cancer Treat Res 1991;53:93.
271. Norton L. Biology of residual breast cancer after therapy. A kinetic interpretation. In: Ragaz J, Simpson–Herren L, Lippman ME, Fisher B, editors. Effects of therapy on biology and kinetics of the residual tumor. Part A. Preclinical aspects. New York: Wiley–Liss; 1990. p. 109–32.
272. Koury MJ, Bondurant MC. Erythropoietin retards DNA breakdown and prevents programmed death in erythroid progenitor cells. Science 1990;248:378.
273. Williams GT, Smith CA, Spooncer E, et al. Haemopoietic colony stimulating factors promote cell survival by suppressing apoptosis. Nature 1990;343:76.
274. Barry MA, Behnke CA, Eastman A. Activation of programmed cell death (apoptosis) by cisplatin, other anticancer drugs, toxins and hyperthermia. Biochem Pharmacol 1990;40:2353.
275. Kennedy S, Merino MJ, Swain SM, Lippman ME. The effects of hormonal and chemotherapy on tumoral and nonneoplastic breast tissue. Hum Pathol 1990; 21:192.
276. Amadori D. Use of cell kinetics to analyze responses in combination therapy studies. New Changes in Breast Cancer Clinical Trials, November 16, 1994; Warwick Hotel, Philadelphia.
277. Teicher BA, Herman TS, Holden SA, et al. Tumor resistance to alkylating agents conferred by mechanisms operative only in vivo. Science 1990;247:1457.
278. Zuckiet G, Tritton TR. Adriamycin causes up-regulation of epidermal growth factor receptors in actively growing cells. Exp Cell Res 1983;148:155.
279. Isonishi S, Andrews PA, Howell SB. Increased sensitivity to cis-diamminedichloroplatinum (II) in human ovarian carcinoma cells in response to treatment with 12-0-tetradecanoylphorbol-13-acetate. J Biol Chem 1990;265:3623.
280. Masui H, Kawamoto T, Sato JD, et al. Growth inhibition of human tumor cells in athymic mice by antiepidermal growth factor receptor monoclonal antibodies. Cancer Res 1984;44:1002.
281. Aboud–Pirak E, Hurwitz E, Pirak ME, et al. Efficacy of antibody to epidermal growth factor receptor against KB carcinoma in vitro and in nude mice. J Natl Cancer Inst 1988;80:1605.
282. Norton L, Baselga J, Masui H, et al. Growth factor perturbation. A therapeutically exploitable mechanism for chemotherapy action. Proc Am Soc Clin Oncol 1991;10:208.
283. Al-Hajj M, Clarke MF. Self-renewal and solid tumor stem cells. Oncogene 2004;23:7274–82.
284. Hanahan D, Weinberg RA. The hallmarks of cancer. Cell 2000;100:57–70.
285. Gassmann P, Enns A, Haier J. Role of tumor cell adhesion and migration in organ-specific metastasis formation. Onkologie 2004;27:577–82.
286. Seals DF, Azucena EF Jr, Pass I, et al. The adaptor protein Tks5/Fish is required for podosome formation and function, and for the protease-driven invasion of cancer cells. Cancer Cell 2005;7:155–65.
287. Smith HS, Lu Y, Deng G, et al. Molecular aspects of early stages of breast cancer progression. J Cell Biochem Suppl 1993;17:144–52.
288. Hatsell S, Rowlands T, Hiremath M, Cowin P. Beta-catenin and Tcfs in mammary development and cancer [review]. J Mammary Gland Biol Neoplasia 2003;8:145–58.
289. Hutchinson JN, Muller WJ: Transgenic mouse models of human breast cancer. Oncogene 2000, 19:6130–7.
290. Li Y, Hively WP, Varmus HE. Use of MMTV-Wnt-1 transgenic mice for studying the genetic basis of breast cancer. Oncogene 2000;19:1002–9.
291. Hazan RB, Phillips GR, Qiao RF, Norton L, Aaronson SA. Exogenous expression of N-cadherin in breast cancer cells induces cell migration, invasion, and metastasis [published erratum appears in J Cell Biol 2000;149:236]. J Cell Biol 2000;148:779–90.
292. van de Vijver MJ, He YD, et al. A gene-expression signature as a predictor of survival in breast cancer. N Engl J Med 2002;347:1999–2009.
293. Sorlie T, Tibshirani R, Parker J, et al. Repeated observation of breast tumor subtypes in independent gene expression data sets. Proc Natl Acad Sci U S A. 2003;100:8418–23. Epub 2003 Jun 26.
294. Wadlow R, Ramaswamy S. DNA microarrays in clinical cancer research. Curr Mol Med 2005;5:111–20.
295. Van't Veer LJ, Weigelt B. Road map to metastasis. Nat Med 2003;9:999–1000.
296. Sorlie T. Molecular portraits of breast cancer: tumour subtypes as distinct disease entities. Eur J Cancer 2004;40:2667–75.
297. Hu J, Bianchi F, Ferguson M, et al. Gene expression signature for angiogenic and nonangiogenic non—small-cell lung cancer. Oncogene 2005.
298. Troester MA, Hoadley KA, Sorlie T, et al. Cell-type-specific responses to chemotherapeutics in breast cancer. Cancer Res 2004;64:4218–26.
299. Chang HY, Nuyten DS, Sneddon JB, et al. Robustness, scalability, and integration of a wound-response gene expression signature in predicting breast cancer survival. Proc Natl Acad Sci U S A 2005;102:3738–43.
300. Kang Y, Siegel PM, Shu W, et al. A multigenic program mediating breast cancer metastasis to bone. Cancer Cell 2003;3:537–49.
301. Min AJ, Gupta GP, Siegel PM, et al. Genes that mediate breast cancer metastasis to lung. Nature 2005. [In press]

302. Norton L. The Oncologist. 2005.
303. Massague J. G1 cell-cycle control and cancer. Nature 2004;432:298–306.
304. Delhalle S, Duvoix A, Schnekenburger M, Morceau F, Dicato M, Diederich M. An introduction to the molecular mechanisms of apoptosis. Ann N Y Acad Sci 2003;1010:1–8.
305. Edinger AL, Thompson CB. Death by design: apoptosis, necrosis and autophagy [review]. Curr Opin Cell Biol 2004;16:663–9.
306. Vakkila J, Lotze MT. Inflammation and necrosis promote tumour growth. Nat Rev Immunol 2004;4:641–8.
307. Rizki A, Bissell MJ. Homeostasis in the breast: it takes a village. Cancer Cell 2004;6:1–2.
308. Piet EJ, van Erp. Proliferation, differentiation, and inflammation in normal and hyperproliferative skin using multiparameter flow cytometry. In: Epidermal cells, methods and protocols. Methods in molecular biology. Vol. 289, p. 239–50.
309. Steeg PS, Zhou Q. Cyclins and breast cancer. Breast Cancer Res Treat 1998;52:17–28.
310. Wu X, Xiao Z, Chen Z, et al. Differential analysis of two-dimension gel electrophoresis profiles from the normal-metaplasia-dysplasia-carcinoma tissue of human bronchial epithelium. Pathol Int 2004;54:765–73.
311. Huang CS, O'Brien MJ, Yang S, Farraye FA. Hyperplastic polyps, serrated adenomas, and the serrated polyp neoplasia pathway. Am J Gastroenterol 2004;99:2242–55.

38

Principles of Dose, Schedule, and Combination Therapy

Emil Frei III, MD
Joseph Paul Eder, MD

The identification of novel, clinically active agents has been central to progress in cancer chemotherapy. Table 38-1 presents examples of new agents, and of areas and targets being mined for new agents. The optimal use of such agents, of which more than 40 have been identified since the 1950s, has been crucial.

Dose is a significant determinant of the antitumor activity and toxicology for the established, "classical" cytotoxic chemotherapeutic agents.[1] Higher doses (1.2 times to twice the baseline dose) made possible by growth factors (granulocyte-colony stimulating factor [G-CSF], granulocyte/macrophage-colony stimulating factor [GM-CSF]) are variably more effective. High-dose chemotherapy (4 to 10 times the baseline dose), made possible by hematopoietic stem cell transplantation, has proven that cure can be achieved for selected hematologic neoplasms. The effect of dose for biotherapeutic agents such as the interferons or interleukins and for hormones is complex and is currently under study.

Table 38-1 Molecular Targets for Cancer Treatment

The cell cycle
Cyclin-dependent kinases, cyclins, cyclin-dependent kinase inhibitors, mitotic tubule-associated proteins
Differentiation
Retinoid and vitamin D nuclear steroid receptors
Apoptosis
BCL2, NFKB1, *TP53*, *TNFSF10*, *FAS*
Angiogenesis
KDR, the endothelial integrins, *PDGFRB*
Signaling cell-surface receptors
Insulin-like growth factor receptor (IGFR1)
ERBB family of receptors
KIT
Metastasis
Matrix metalloproteinases, chemokine receptors
Intracellular signaling elements
BCR-ABL1, *ras*, *raf*, *MADD*, PI3KR5, mTOR,FRAP1, *src*, protein kinase C, focal adhesion kinase (*PTK2*: protein tyrosine kinase 2), anaplastic lymphoma kinase (*ALK*), the *STAT* family of proteins and the *MAP* family of protein kinases
Nuclear transcription factors
Eg, steroid hormone No. 4
Potential targets
Telomerase
DNA methylation (human DNA methyltransferase [MeTase])
Proteasome 20S
Farnesyltransferase
Histone deacetylase
Hsp90 (chaperone protein)
Cell surface antigens
Eg, CD20

The schedule of drug administration may be important to the therapeutic index independent of dose. For example, cytokinetic studies relating to drug schedule have led to the improved use of agents such as cytosine arabinoside (cytarabine, ara-C) in both experimental and clinical leukemia (see "Cytokinetics of Bone Marrow" later in this chapter).[2,3] Combination chemotherapy has been crucial in the development of curative regimens for hematologic malignancies, pediatric solid tumors, testicular cancer, and ovarian cancer, and for the adjuvant regimens for breast, lung, and bowel cancer, and for osteosarcomas.[4,5]

The rationale for combination chemotherapy is complex and is here discussed under the various topical headlines. The principal rationales include (1) the pragmatic: almost all therapy that has proven curative in the clinic involves the use of agents in combination (Table 38-2); and (2) the fact that genetic instability results in tumor cell heterogeneity, which manifests as drug resistance in cancer therapy.[6–8]

Although dose and combination chemotherapy are generally considered separately, they have an important and complex relationship.[9,10] Currently, an impressive increase has occurred in the number of putative molecular targets for cancer treatment development (see Table 38-1). The major clinical research challenges will be not only to maximize the effectiveness of individual agents but, particularly, to integrate drugs into optimal combination strategies.

DOSE

In controlled experimental systems, such as established tumor cells in culture, the relationship between dose and tumor cytotoxicity may be close to linear-log (ie, exponential).[11] For example, a linear increase in the dose of selected chemotherapeutic agents causes a log reduction of MCF7 human breast cancer cells in culture.[12] In Figure 38-1, dose is expressed as multiples of the IC_{90} (ie, the dose or concentration that reduces the number of tumor cells by 90%), a very good response in terms of tumor regression in a patient. The estimated total tumor burden for patients with clinically evident cancer is $5 \times 10^{11} \pm 10^{1}$ (11 ± 1 logs). Thus, a dose that produces a good partial remission (eg, 50% to 90% tumor regression) produces at most a 1-log reduction, which is less than 10% of the "exponential iceberg." Numerous factors influence the dose effect. They are presented in the subsections that follow.[13,14]

Factors Influencing the Dose Effect **Class of Chemotherapeutic Agent** The ideal therapeutic agent would maintain a linear relationship between dose and log tumor cell reduction (log-TCR) down through multiple logs of tumor cell destruction (see Figure 38-1). Ionizing radiation comes closest to this ideal.

As a group, alkylating agents are superior to the other chemotherapeutic agents in terms of maintained dose/log-TCR (see Figure 38-1). Alkylating agents exhibit major activity during the S and M periods of the cell cycle, but, unlike other chemotherapeutic agents, they maintain activity throughout the cell cycle. Although comparative studies demonstrate a dose effect in chemotherapy-sensitive tumors such as the leukemias and lymphomas, the effect of dose is less evident in solid tumors, particularly epithelial cell tumors.[15,16] Antimetabolites are active mainly in proliferating cells, and therefore pharmacokinetic resistance occurs that is overcome less by increasing dose than by increasing the duration of exposure, thus allowing more cells to enter the proliferative compartment.

Tumor Factors ***Intrinsic Tumor Cell Sensitivity*** The more sensitive the tumor is to a given agent, the steeper the dose effect. Thus, if a unit dose produces a 0.5 log-TCR, then doubling that dose may produce up to a 1.0 log tumor cell kill—which clinically represents only a partial remission. In a chemosensitive tumor, where a unit dose produces a 3 log-TCR, doubling the dose may produce up to a 6 log-TCR, depending on the degree of tumor cell heterogeneity and drug resistance (see "Drug Resistance" later in this subsection). A 6 log-TCR would produce a major clinical achievement in terms of complete response, duration of complete response, and, most important, an approach to tumor cure or eradication. Thus, for patients with a common epithelial tumor, such as breast cancer, the most that can be achieved with standard single-agent chemotherapy is a partial response (<1 log-TCR) in about 30% of patients. Combinations result in higher partial response rates and a low (10 to 20%) complete response rate. Alternatively, combination chemotherapy regimens in patients with chemosensitive tumors (eg, non-Hodgkin's lymphoma, Hodgkin's disease, and testicular cancer) may achieve multi–log-TCR as a result of combination chemotherapy.[17]

Table 38-2 Number of Agents and Curative Treatment for Childhood Acute Lymphoblastic Leukemia (ALL)

	Number of Chemotherapeutic Agents							
	1	2	3	4	5	6	7	8
Year	1948	1954	1956	1960	1965	1974	1985	1988
Agent	Methotrexate	MP	Prednisone	Vincristine	Methotrexate[a]	Adriamycin	Asparagine	ara-cytosar
CR (%)	20–40	40–92	80–95	>95	>95	>95	>95	>95
Cure (%)	0	0	0	15	5–35	55	75	80

[a]Intrathecal methotrexate.
CR = complete response; MP = 6-mercaptopurine.

Tumor Burden Tumor burden is a consistent adverse prognostic factor for response to chemotherapy. This finding was first demonstrated for transplanted tumors in mice; in these animals, macroscopic (ie, palpable) tumors often respond minimally to a given chemotherapy. The same tumor, at a microscopic tumor burden size, may be much more responsive and potentially curable.[17,18]

These observations in mice are consistent with the parallel observation that adjuvant cancer treatment is curative for patients with breast cancer, but not for those with overt metastatic breast cancer. Postulates for the delay in growth of microscopic metastases include a balanced rate of cell loss (ie, apoptosis) and of cell production. Resistant microscopic tumor may persist in most long-term survivors, an observation that has major implications for therapeutic strategy (see "Cytokinetics of the Tumor" later in this subsection).

The study of microscopic metastases in patients may become increasingly possible with modern molecular techniques for detection and characterization of minimal tumor.[17] Some of the kinetics of microscopic disease can be inferred from adjuvant chemotherapy studies (see "Adjuvant Chemotherapy" below).

Drug Resistance In the laboratory, drug resistance is usually produced by "selection pressure"—that is, by exposing target cells to progressively increasing concentrations of the selecting agent. Drug resistance usually is expressed as the concentration of drug that is required to produce 50% inhibition in a colony or growth assay (IC_{50}) for the resistant cell line, divided by the concentration required (IC_{50}) for the parent sensitive cell line. For a detailed presentation of drug resistance, see "Combination Chemotherapy" later in this chapter and Chapter 41, "Drug Resistance and its Clinical Circumvention."

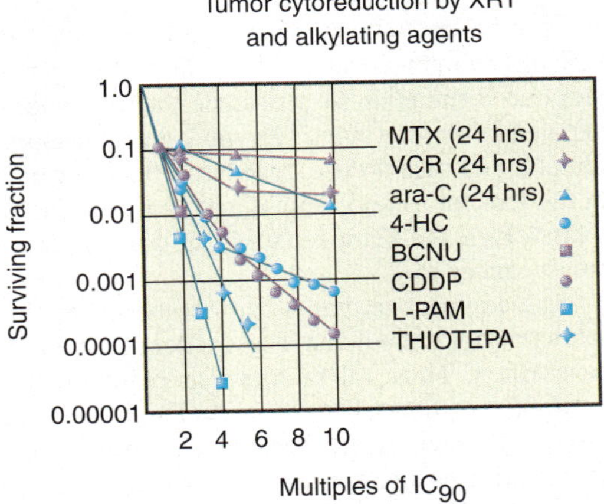

Figure 38-1 Log kill in vitro: Effect of antitumor agent concentration expressed as multiples of the IC90 (ie, the dose or concentration that reduces the number of tumor cells by 90%), on the surviving fraction of human breast cancer (MCF7) cells in culture (colony assay). 4-HC = 4-hydroxycyclophosphamide. From Frei E 3rd.[5]

Cytokinetics of the Tumor—The Growth Fraction The growth fraction (GF) of the tumor and the dose of cell cycle–specific agents has a major effect on the log-TCR of tumor cells. The generation time of cycling (ie, mitotically active) cells is much shorter than the volume doubling time.[19–23] Thus, many cells within tumors are dying or "noncycling"—that is, in G0/G1. The GF of a tumor is the ratio of the cycling cells to the total number of tumor cells.

For the common epithelial solid tumors, the GF is often less than 5%.[24,25] A solid tumor with a growth fraction of 5% would be minimally responsive to cell cycle–specific agents and variably sensitive to other chemotherapeutic agents. Repetitive treatments, however, might "recruit" cells into cycle by allowing dormant, noncycling cells access to necessary growth conditions and thus enabling them to be more effective. Prolonged exposure to cell cycle–specific agents might be effective in low–growth fraction tumors. In contrast, a high–growth fraction tumor such as Burkitt lymphoma might have a multilog response with the same treatment or even the same dose over a shorter period.[1] Specific cancer stem cells (CSCs) are responsible for the continued proliferation of a tumor. Self-renewing CSCs give rise to all progenitor and differentiated cells within a tumor, but they are a small proportion of all cells.[26] The difference between curative therapeutic regimens and those that are only palliative may be attributable to the relative sensitivities of CSCs and of the progenitor and differentiated cancer cells incapable of self-renewal. Identification of therapeutic targets within the CSC population should offer significant opportunities for more effective therapies.

Tumor Hypoxia It was in the 1950s that solid tumors were first suspected to be commonly hypoxic. Improved techniques have confirmed hypoxia in both experimental and clinical solid tumors, a condition presumably resulting from suboptimal angiogenesis and high metabolic activity (oxygen consumption). Oxygen distribution within tumors is heterogeneous and even a small fraction of hypoxic cells can profoundly affect chemotherapy responsiveness. The farther cells are from blood vessels, the lower the concentration of chemotherapeutic agents in those cells. Cellular proliferation decreases as a function of distance from blood vessels, with a significant fraction of nonproliferating cells conferring kinetic resistance to cell cycle–specific agents. Hypoxia selects for *TP53* mutants with a reduced apoptotic response to deoxyribonucleic acid (DNA) damage or cell cycle arrest. Certain cancer chemotherapy agents require oxygen as an intermediate in toxicity or in metabolism. Finally, hypoxia produces altered gene expression. There may be increased expression of adenosine triphosphate–binding cassette (ABC) proteins such as p-glycoprotein (PgP) that may confer resistance to chemotherapeutic agents. Hypoxia-inducible factor 1 stops proliferation and prevents apoptosis in the hypoxic fraction of cells. Exploiting hypoxia as a target in cancer therapy with bioreductive alkylating agents such as mitomycin C and the nitroimidazoles, which can serve as electron acceptors in lieu of oxygen, has been tried in numerous clinical circumstances since the 1960s with no or minimal benefit.[27,28]

Radiotherapy in particular requires molecular oxygen for cytotoxicity.[29] In experimental in vivo systems, oxygen-carrying perfluorocarbons and hemoglobin solutions may partially correct the hypoxia and improve the effectiveness not only of radiotherapy but also of some chemotherapeutic agents.[30,31] These laboratory observations have not been definitively tested in the clinic.

Host Factors ***Cytokinetics of Bone Marrow*** Because of the bone marrow's proliferative activity and relative lack of DNA repair capacity, myelosuppression is dose limiting for many chemotherapeutic agents. Exploiting the cytokinetic difference between marrow and tumor has been a basis for the construction of selected clinical stratigies.[3,20–23]

Normal marrow recovers within 1 to 2 weeks after cytarabine, with little cumulative myelosuppression. For many patients, recovery of acute myelogenous leukemia (AML) cells as compared with normal marrow cells between courses of cytarabine is incomplete. AML cells in vitro are less susceptible to growth factors such as G- and GM-CSF than are the cells of the normal marrow, possibly because mutations in the G-CSF receptor interfere with maturation in AML cells.[32] Thus, when marrow CSFs increase in homeostatic response to cytarabine-induced myelosuppression, the interval recovery of normal marrow may be more rapid than that demonstrated by the

AML cells, a factor that should, with successive dosing, result in a cumulative effect—hence the therapeutic advantage.

Pharmacokinetics Pharmacokinetic factors commonly affect the dose–response curve. For example, if an inactivating enzyme for the drug becomes saturated, both toxicity and antitumor effect may increase disproportionately, an effect observed with certain dose schedules of 5-fluorouracil (5-FU).[33,34]

The opposite effect may occur if a drug activation system becomes saturated. For example, ifosfamide, a pro-drug, is activated by the cytochrome P450, oxygen-dependent, drug-metabolizing enzymes in the liver to the biologically active 4-hydroxyl derivative. The 3-day conventional dose of ifosfamide is higher (1,200 to 2,400 mg/m^2 daily) than that for cyclophosphamide (600 mg/m^2) because the rate of P450 activation of ifosfamide is relatively slow. With increasing doses of cyclophosphamide, a constant fractional conversion to active 4-hydroxyl cyclophosphamide occurs. However, for ifosfamide, once the P450 enzyme system becomes saturated, a decreasing proportion of ifosfamide is converted to the active form, with a consequent loss of antitumor effect at higher doses.

CLINICAL TRIALS AND THE DOSE EFFECT Dose Selection in Patients The process for initial dose selection in phase I clinical trials is detailed in Chapter 45. In most circumstances, the dose in phase I trials and in other situations is individualized to the body surface area (BSA) of the patient. The Dubois BSA formula is useful in allometric scaling of drug dose selection between species. The expectation was that similar adjustments would reduce the variability in clearance between patients.

Clearance determines the total drug exposure (area under the curve of concentration multiplied by time [AUC]), and AUC in mice correlates with toxicity in that species. This relationship of AUC with drug exposure and toxicity also holds true in humans and can be predicted from the mouse data.[35] BSA may be helpful in selecting the dose of cytotoxic agents in childhood leukemia and was subsequently incorporated into standard usage.[36,37] Recent reviews of the literature and of individual institutional experience can find no significant correlation between BSA and clearance variability with investigational or commonly used anticancer drugs except for paclitaxel, oral busulfan, and possibly temozolomide.[38,39]

BSA is supposed to correlate with glomerular filtration rate, blood volume, and basal metabolic rate.[38] However, the variability in drug clearance introduced by these factors is small (< 25%) compared with that induced by hepatic metabolic enzymes, and there is no correlation between BSA and metabolic activity.[38] Glomerular filtration rate as estimated from serum creatinine does correlate with toxicity for topotecan, etoposide, and carboplatin. Indeed, calculated AUC from serum creatinine (Calvert formula) is now used to dose carboplatin.[37]

Enzymatic pathways are responsible for the clearance of 5-FU and 6-mercaptopurine (6-MP) and for glucuronidation via *UGT1A1* for clearance of SN-38, the active product of irinotecan (see individual chapters). Each of these enzymes has a significant incidence of polymorphisms that affect drug disposition and correlate with toxicity. Pharmacogenetic profiling offers the prospect of individualized dose selection in the future and is a frequent component in early clinical drug development. These DNA-based tests are not commercially available yet and have no clinical role at the present time.

Cytochrome P450 3A4 (family 3, subfamily A, polypeptide 4) is the most prevalent metabolic enzyme in humans and is responsible for more than 55% of drug metabolic clearance.[40] Recent studies using noncancer drugs as indicators of *CYP3A4* metabolic activity, such as the erythromycin breath test, suggest potential clinical utility with agents that are metabolized by this pathway—for example, docetaxel.[41] At present, these alternatives (except for carboplatin AUC dosing) remain under investigation, and BSA-based dosing remains the standard of clinical practice.

Real-Time Pharmacokinetics and Patient Safety Pharmacokinetic studies provide important information regarding the dose effect. In general, such studies indicate substantial variation in serum drug levels and in the AUC per given dose. For methotrexate and 6-MP in acute leukemia and for high-dose busulfan and carmustine (BCNU) in the transplant setting, the AUC level of drug or its active metabolites (or both) correlates with toxicity and therapeutic effect.[42–46]

Substantial variation in the AUC per given dose of paclitaxel was also observed in patients with solid tumor. Real-time adjustment of dose on subsequent days significantly reduced mucositis requiring morphine administration and decreased the duration of hospital stay.[47]

Dose Effect in Sensitive Tumors Few clinical studies have included dose intensity as an independent, randomized variable. In a Cancer and Leukemia Group B (CALGB) study, 596 patients with AML were randomized to receive four 5-day courses of cytarabine at one of three dose schedules: (1) 100 mg/m^2 daily ("standard arm"); (2) 400 mg/m^2 by continuous infusion; or (3) 3 g/m^2 in a 3-hour infusion every 12 hours (twice daily) on days 1, 3, and 5.[2] For patients 60 years of age or younger, the probability of remaining in continuous complete remission after 4 years was 24% in the 100 mg/m^2 group; 29% in the 400 mg/m^2 group; and 44% in the 3 g/m^2 group (p = .002), indicating a better response with increased dose. Elderly patients were less responsive. In acute lymphocytic leukemia (ALL), the dose rate of maintenance chemotherapy had a major impact on the duration of response.[48] Similarly, in studies of combination chemotherapy in small cell lung cancer, the dose effect was major.[49]

In treating individual patients, dose is a key factor if cure is possible. Thus, for leukemias, lymphomas, testicular cancer, childhood solid tumors, and conventional-dose adjuvant treatment of breast cancer, dose should not be compromised even at the risk of significant toxicity. For more resistant tumors, where palliation is the goal, dose should be adjusted primarily on the basis of toxicity.

Peripheral Blood Stem Cell and Marrow Transplantation Allogeneic bone marrow transplantation produces disease-free survival plateaus (ie, cures) in patients with acute and chronic leukemias and lymphomas, but because of the effect of graft versus leukemia, the component contributed by dose cannot be evaluated.

The most compelling evidence regarding dose–response is in high-dose, autologous stem cell rescue studies in patients with relapsed lymphoma.[50,51] Alkylating agents and total body radiotherapy-based regimens are commonly used because their dose-limiting toxicity is myelosuppression. Depending on the agent, dose can be escalated between 3 and 20 times baseline before nonmyelosuppressive toxicity becomes dose limiting. Given the considerable overlap of AUCs for serum levels of drugs at dose escalations of 2 to 4 times baseline, the escalations possible with stem cell support allow better comparisons of the effect of dose. High-dose therapy with autologous stem cell rescue produces high complete response rates and cures in non-Hodgkin's lymphoma and testicular cancer.[50,52] But because toxicity can be lethal, high-dose therapy should be limited to specialized centers.[53]

ADJUVANT CHEMOTHERAPY Randomized Studies Cytokinetics provides an experimental basis for many therapeutic designs. A brief review of the related history follows.

Skipper and colleagues established exponentiality as the fundamental relationship between drug treatment and surviving tumor fractions. It is the fractional tumor cell reduction that is constant for a given dose and drug.[11] Although this exponential relationship is modified by other factors, such as drug resistance and microenvironment, it remains the fundamental tenet of cytokinetics and chemotherapy. Norton and Simon applied Gompertzian theory and analysis to treatment during remission and demonstrated the potentially greater effectiveness of late intensification.[54] Goldie and Coldman introduced mutation to resistance theory, relating to potentiality for a cure.[55] Hryniuk and colleagues found a significant dose–response effect not only in the leukemias and lymphomas, but also in the relatively less chemosensitive tumors, such as breast cancer.[56–58]

The adjuvant setting, where the tumor burden is microscopic, should be ideal for demonstrating a dose effect. Thus, all factors that reduce tumor cytotoxicity (tumor size, decreased and abnormal vascularity, low GF, hypoxia, increased heterogeneity, and drug resistance) are less evident in the microscopic tumor (adjuvant) setting. "Standard" combination chemotherapy with cyclophosphamide, methotrexate, and 5-FU (CMF) or with cyclophosphamide, doxorubicin (Adriamycin), and 5-FU (CAF), which produce only transient partial and a few complete responses in metastatic breast cancer, reduce relapse and mortality rates by 20 to 30% in the adjuvant breast cancer setting.[59] Similar effects are seen in colon cancer.[60]

Attempts to improve disease-free survival by increasing the adjuvant chemotherapy dose in breast cancer have produced complicated results. The first statistically robust positive study was conducted by the CALGB.[15] Patients with node-positive breast cancer were randomized to one of three CAF regimens.[15] The high-dose arm involved 4 courses of CAF at doses of 600, 60, and 600 mg/m^2 respectively, every 3 to 4 weeks; in the low-dose arm, the doses were 300, 30, and 300 mg/m^2 respectively. A 10% difference in the relapse-free curve developed by 2 years and has persisted through 10 years. That result represents an approximately 20% reduction in mortality. The dose effect was seen most prominently in the 20% of patients whose tumors overexpressed *ERBB2* (formerly *HER2/neu*). For tumors without *ERBB2* overexpression, no significant dose effect was seen.[16] This subset effect would not have been identified in the absence of the molecular marker.

Two other studies conducted by the National Surgical Adjuvant Breast and Bowel Project (NSABP) failed to show that a 2 or 4 times increase in the dose of cyclophosphamide alone affected response in terms of relapse or survival in adjuvant breast cancer.[61,62] Thus, in the comparative study of CAF, the dose of Adriamycin was probably important; however, in another study of adjuvant breast cancer, patients randomized to 3 doses of Adriamycin (60, 75, and 90 mg/m^2, all given with the standard dose of cyclophosphamide) showed no difference in disease-free or overall survival. The 60 mg/m^2 is probably a threshold dose, above which no further benefit accrues.

The basis for the seemingly discordant results of dose in major clinical trials has been the subject of preclinical and mechanism-of-action studies, but it remains unexplained. We remain humble before the heterogeneity of human cancer, which permits such seemingly contradictory results. It can be speculated how often in the analysis of large comparative studies an important effect has been missed within a subset not known to exist at the time. That possibility is an important limitation in the interpretation of negative studies.

Dose-Dense Chemotherapy The concept behind dose-dense chemotherapy is to increase the intensity of drug administration by shortening the interval between treatments without increasing the total dose of drug administered. This increase is accomplished by escalating the dose or the number of cycles in a given period of time. The use of neutrophil-colony stimulating factors is an essential requirement for dose-dense therapy. Interim reports on the CALGB 9741 study, the use of dose-dense therapy with cyclophosphamide, doxorubicin, and paclitaxel in adjuvant breast cancer, either concurrently or sequentially in 2-week as opposed to the standard 3-week cycles significantly reduced the annual risk of recurrence or death. This preliminary report supports the concept of dose-dense intensification as a means to enhance chemotherapy efficacy, albeit at a cost of increased toxicity.[63]

High-Dose Therapy Requiring Stem Cell Support As mentioned earlier, the most compelling tests of dose escalation are the high-dose programs that require stem cell rescue. These programs have proven curative for a subset of hematologic neoplasms and are under investigation in epithelial solid tumors, most particularly breast cancer. The high-dose regimens generally involve combinations of alkylating agents, and include particularly CTC (cyclophosphamide, thiotepa, and carboplatin) and also CBP (cyclophosphamide, BCNU, and cisplatin), notably in breast cancer. Preliminary reports were made concerning five of the high-dose breast cancer studies; none were positive in terms of survival.[64–68] Two trials that have come to maturity have shown a reduced risk of relapse, but no improvement in overall survival—although for some patients with *ERBB2*-negative tumors, a trend toward a survival benefit was seen.[69,70] It was generally agreed that, in patients with adjuvant breast cancer, the use of high-dose chemotherapy has no established role and that such endeavors should remain investigational.[71,72]

Areas for investigation of high-dose therapy in patients with breast cancer include improved chemotherapy, improved supportive care, and the addition of biologic therapy and immunotherapy. Better identification of chemotherapy-sensitive subsets may select a more appropriate patient population.

Summary In the clinic, the effect of dose correlates generally with the basic chemosensitivity of the tumor. Thus Burkitt lymphoma, ALL, and testicular cancer are all highly sensitive and highly responsive to dose intensity, including achievement of cure. On the other hand, relatively insensitive tumors such as gastrointestinal and lung cancers and melanoma respond poorly to chemotherapy and are therefore not much affected by dose.

SCHEDULE OF DRUG ADMINISTRATION

Schedule Effects of Individual Agents

Cytarabine Skipper and colleagues performed elegant, quantitative studies of L1210 mouse leukemia of the prototype cell-cycle phase-specific agent cytarabine.[3,11] Schedule "sensitivity" was marked: that is, cytarabine given in courses of appropriate duration and with intervals that allowed for recovery of normal bone marrow produced optimal therapeutic effects. Extrapolating their work to human AML, the investigators gave patients repeated courses of a continuous infusion for 5 to 7 days separated by 2 to 3 weeks for recovery. In patients with AML, that schedule produced a 30% to 40% complete response rate as compared with 10% for other schedules, such as daily intravenous administration.[3,73,74] The addition of daunorubicin to the cytarabine further increased the complete response rate. (For details, see "Cytokinetics of Bone Marrow," earlier in this chapter.)

Gemcitabine The dose-limiting toxicity of gemcitabine, a nucleoside analogue structurally related to cytarabine, is myelosuppression.[75] Unlike cytarabine, gemcitabine has activity in solid tumors, particularly in pancreatic, breast, and nonsmall cell lung cancer. Weekly or biweekly bolus treatments are well tolerated, with toxicity largely limited to the marrow. Clinically and in experimental animal studies, gemcitabine given by continuous infusion necessitates a marked reduction in dose, particularly because of myelosuppression, but also because of gastrointestinal toxicity and, in some circumstances, hypotension.[76]

Methotrexate Intermittent methotrexate (5-day bolus courses every 3 to 4 weeks), developed by Li and colleagues for gestational choriocarcinoma, proved to be curative.[77] Goldin and colleagues demonstrated in L1210 mouse leukemia that intermittent methotrexate was superior to continuous (daily) methotrexate.[78] In a randomized, comparative study of patients with ALL in complete remission, intermittent methotrexate was significantly superior to daily therapy.[79] This empiric observation is consistent with subsequent findings by Schimke and colleagues, indicating that continuous exposure to methotrexate in vitro produces drug resistance more effectively than does intermittent methotrexate.[80] Moreover, with continuous administration, resistance results from gene amplification as compared with a transport defect following intermittent methotrexate.[80,81]

The kinetics of bone marrow recovery and mucosal cell replacement, important in cytarabine scheduling, may be important clinical determinants of scheduling with methotrexate as well.

Fluoropyrimidines In clinical studies, 5-FU is commonly administered in daily pulse doses of 350 to 450 mg/m^2 for 5 days. Using that schedule, myelosuppression is dose limiting. Twice that dose can be delivered by continuous infusion over 5 days, in which case mucositis and diarrhea become dose limiting.[82]

Fluorodeoxyuridine (FUDR) is much more toxic when delivered by continuous infusion than by intermittent bolus dosing. For example, daily doses in the range 30 to 50 mg/m^2 produce toxicity. The biochemical basis for the schedule difference is speculative. Continuous-infusion FUDR may have a greater effect on DNA synthesis; other schedules have a relatively greater effect on host tissue ribonucleic acid (RNA) and RNA synthesis.[82] Data regarding the effect of these differences in schedule on the therapeutic index are few. (Modulation with leucovorin is discussed later in this chapter.) Longer durations of systemic administration currently are under study.[83]

Thus, mechanisms of action, resistance, and cross-resistance for 5-FU appear to differ depending on the analogue chosen and the schedule of administration, among other factors.[84]

Alkylating Agents The alkylating agents are a heterogeneous group of compounds that have in common interaction with DNA. That interaction leads to transformation of mammalian cells in culture and to carcinogenesis in patients.

The alkylating agents are of equal potency in terms of antitumor effect. The difference is primarily host toxicity. This variation in toxicity is particularly true for the dichloroplatinum group of compounds, which closely resemble X-radiation in terms of antitumor effect. They are substantially different in toxicity depending on the nature of the *trans*-adducts. Most experimental data regarding alkylating agents suggest that they are schedule independent: that is, the antitumor and host effects are dose-related, independent of schedule.[85] (See "Pharmacokinetics" and "Adjuvant Chemotherapy" earlier in this chapter for discussions of specific aspects of cyclophosphamide and ifosfamides.)

There is evidence that the antiangiogenesis effect of low-dose chemotherapy may result from a cell death mechanism that differs from the mechanism in high- or standard-dose chemotherapy. This finding is consistent with evidence that resistance is much more difficult to produce experimentally in normal tissues than in tumor tissues. A popular and partial explanation is the greater DNA repair capacity of normal tissues. This difference between normal and tumor tissue has major implications for basic and clinical chemotherapy.[86,87]

Anthracyclines Cardiotoxicity is an important delayed toxicity of anthracyclines. In experimental studies, peak concentrations produced more cardiotoxicity for an equivalent dose than did lower concentrations achieved by continuous-infusion schedules. Weiss and Manthel first demonstrated that weekly doxorubicin administration produced less cardiotoxicity per total dose administered than did standard triweekly regimens.[88] Legha and colleagues demonstrated that a 4-day, continuous infusion of doxorubicin every 3 weeks is less cardiotoxic than bolus injections, an observation confirmed in randomized studies.[89–91] Infusion approaches allow a 30 to 50% increase in total cumulative dose before cardiotoxicity develops. In experimental and preliminary clinical studies, liposomal doxorubicin may be less cardiotoxic than doxorubicin.[92,93]

Etoposide An inhibitor of topoisomerase II, etoposide is selectively active against cells in cycle. Etoposide is commonly used in combination chemotherapy of solid tumors, particularly with cisplatin. Preclinical studies showed that etoposide must be present both during and immediately following cisplatin to achieve optimal effect, consistent with a possible interaction with cisplatin involving inhibition of DNA repair.

In small cell lung cancer, the optimal etoposide dose schedule of 5 daily doses every 3 to 4 weeks is consistent with the discussion earlier in this chapter of marrow and tumor cytokinetics and response to cell cycle–specific agents.[94]

Tubulin Binders Although the *Vinca* alkaloids vincristine and vinblastine are cell cycle–specific, no schedule appears superior to standard weekly dosing.[95,96] On the basis of limited data, the same is true for vinorelbine. Paclitaxel schedule considerations have been dominated by acute histamine-like toxicity, probably related to the vehicle (Cremophor EL); this toxicity is relieved by antihistamines and corticosteroids. Practical and economic considerations favoring outpatient use have resulted in 1- to 3-hour intravenous infusions, although some randomized trials suggest an advantage for infusions that are even longer.[96] Myelosuppression correlates with the duration of plasma concentrations of paclitaxel above the threshold of 0.1 mol/L.[96] Neutropenia appears to be related more to schedule than to dose, although neuropathy appears dose related.[97]

General Use of Intermittent Dosing For most chemotherapeutic agents used alone or in combination, intermittent courses (eg, four 5-day courses every 3 to 4 weeks) are generally superior to other schedules such as continuous (ie, daily) dosing. Such is the case for cyclophosphamide and methotrexate in Burkitt lymphoma, methotrexate and actinomycin D in choriocarcinoma, melphalan in myeloma, cytarabine in AML, and methotrexate in ALL.[98] It is also true for combination regimens for Hodgkin's disease, ALL, and childhood solid tumors.[95,98,99] In experimental and clinical studies alike, intermittent intensive treatment for rapidly proliferating tumors is superior. The reason may be recruitment of resting G0/G1 cells into active cycle. Continuous treatment may be superior for more indolent, low-GF tumors, but more-definitive studies are needed.[100]

Advances in supportive care now allow a novel approach to intermittent intensive chemotherapy. Leukapheresis following marrow recovery from chemotherapy and treatment with G-CSF allow the harvest of sufficient peripheral blood circulating stem cells to rescue as many as four courses of moderately intensive chemotherapy with cyclophosphamide and carboplatin.[101]

Continuous Low-Dose Administration Protracted infusions (6 weeks) of 5-FU combined with local radiotherapy in adjuvant rectal cancer demonstrated both a lower local recurrence rate in the irradiated field and a reduced incidence of metastatic relapse.[102] Capecitabine is an orally absorbable agent that undergoes biotransformation to 5-FU. Prolonged administration over 14 days of capecitabine as a single agent, repeated at 21-day intervals, shows a response rate that is superior to that of intravenous 5-FU and leucovorin, although no survival benefit accrues.[103,104] Capecitabine is also active in refractory breast cancer as monotherapy or in combination. The role of continuous fluoropyrimidine administration with capecitabine is being explored in combination chemotherapy and with radiation. The treatment interruption every 3 weeks does seem to significantly reduce toxicity with capecitabine.

For reasons related to the mechanism of action of new targeted therapies such as imatinib in chronic myelogenous leukemia and in gastrointestinal stromal tumors (which may be cytostatic rather then cytotoxic), continuous low-dose oral administration will likely become increasingly important in the future.[100,105]

COMBINATION CHEMOTHERAPY

Rationale The most compelling rationales for combination chemotherapy are (1) tumor cell heterogeneity and its implication for drug resistance, and (2) the success of combination chemotherapy in the clinic. In practical clinical terms, the selection of specific combinations in particular types of cancer depends on the individual activity of the agents in the target cancer type and the absence of overlapping toxicities. The agents with the highest single-agent activity are preferred, particularly agents that produce complete responses (if any such agents exist), with different mechanisms of action to address the theoretical heterogeneity issue.

Combination Chemotherapy in the Clinic Ample clinical precedent exists for using multiple agents. An example is the treatment of ALL in children, where eight active agents have been identified. A direct correlation is seen between the number of agents used and the cure rate (see Table 38-2). In fact, essentially all curative chemotherapy involves combinations of two and usually three or more agents (Table 38-3).

Current studies have demonstrated evidence for synergy or an additive effect between established chemotherapeutic agents and agents representing other classes. When used in combination, tamoxifen is additive and sometimes synergistic. Herceptin, a monoclonal antibody to *ERBB2,* is

Table 38-3 Cancer Chemotherapy—Number of Agents Required for Cure by Tumor Type

Tumor	Number of Agents Required for Cure	Adjuvant or Neoadjuvant	Number of Agents Required for Cure
Acute lymphoblastic leukemia (children)	4–7	Wilms' tumor	2–3
Gestational choriocarcinoma[a]			
Early	1–3	Embryonal rhabdomyosarcoma	2–3
Advanced	2–4	Osteogenic sarcoma	3
Acute myeloid leukemia	3+	Soft tissue sarcoma	3
Testicular cancer	3	Ovarian cancer	3–4
Burkitt lymphoma[b]	1–4	Breast cancer	2–4
Hodgkin's disease	4–5	Colorectal cancer	2
Diffuse histiocytic lymphoma	4–5	Nonsmall-cell lung carcinoma, stage IIIA	2
		Small-cell lung carcinoma, limited	2–4

[a]One agent is curative, but a higher cure rate results with two or more agents.
[b]One agent cures state 1 African Burkitt lymphoma, but two or more agents are better.

synergistic with doxorubicin and paclitaxel. ErbB2 is present on the cancer cell surface in 25% of patients with breast cancer. Toxicities may be substantial, however. Herceptin in combination with doxorubicin increased cardiac toxicity. A lesser risk of cardiac toxicity exists when Herceptin is included in Taxol combinations. The addition of a complement-fixing monoclonal antibody, rituximab, to cyclophosphamide, hydroxydaunomycin, vincristine sulfate (Oncovin), and prednisone chemotherapy in non-Hodgkin's lymphoma increases response without an increase in toxicity. Vincristine and prednisone represent a long-established combination that is highly potent against ALL. All-*trans*-retinoic acid and arsenic trioxide interact with acute pro-granulocytic leukemia cells with resultant differentiation and remission. Cure, however, requires the addition an anthracycline.

Tumor Cell Heterogeneity and Drug Resistance Tumors are clonal in origin, but the increasing DNA instability that accompanies the onset of neoplasia leads to increased variation in the daughter cells, called "clonal evolution to tumor cell heterogeneity." This evolution is associated with selection for progeny with greater survival capacity, which is evident as higher proliferative capacity, resistance to apoptosis, greater metastatic or invasive potential, reduced dependence on normal cellular growth factors, and angiogenesis.[106] Heterogeneity among tumor cells increases the number and diversity of potential target sites for chemotherapy and the need to combine therapeutic agents.

Initially, resistance was thought to be limited to the selecting agent (mono–drug resistance). The recognition of multi–drug resistance required a reexamination of this rationale for combination chemotherapy.[107] The ABC protein PgP, the multidrug resistance proteins, and the breast cancer–related protein confer multi–drug resistance that relates almost exclusively to natural products; however, glutathione transferase, DNA repair capacity, and topoisomerase II alterations also may be associated with multi–drug resistance.[108]

Recent studies of multicellular drug resistance indicate an altered set point for apoptosis.[109] Differences between in vitro and in vivo drug resistance are modifying the approach to combination chemotherapy.[110] Although prolonged drug exposure results in stable, resistant cell lines, acute exposure may induce short-term, reversible resistance. How the short-term resistance relates mechanistically to the long-term, presumably genetic, resistance is under study.

Cytokinetics The discovery that solid tumors contain a large number of potentially clonogenic cells in G1 or G0—presumably because of tumor hypoxia and a low GF—provided a basis for combination chemotherapy.[18,19,24] Thus, cell cycle–specific agents were employed to kill mitotically active cells, and non–cell cycle–specific agents (for example, alkylating agents) were added to damage the noncycling tumor cells. The use of repeated cycles allows normal tissues to recover, so that dose need not be compromised, and G0/G1 tumor cells can be recruited into the proliferating fraction by increased availability of nutrients, oxygen, and vascular access.

Synchronization Synchronization of tumor or normal cells in vitro and in vivo with drugs that inhibit DNA synthesis or that arrest cells in mitosis can be achieved. Experimentally, the most impressive synchronization has been achieved with hormonal agents that affect tumor, but not essential normal cells.

Some degree of tumor-cell synchrony follows this hormonal manipulation in experimental studies but the heterogeneity of human tumors with regard to the time course of recruitment and synchronization has limited this approach, and it remains investigational.[111,112]

Modulation Agents that are nontoxic may still improve the therapeutic index of an established chemotherapeutic agent, either by reducing normal-tissue toxicity—as leucovorin does for methotrexate, for example—or by preferentially enhancing antitumor efficacy—as 5-FU and leucovorin do in metastatic and adjuvant colon cancer studies.[113–124]

Biochemically, the product of 5-FU, fluorodeoxyuridine monophosphate (FdUMP), binds to the substrate site of thymidylate synthase, thus inhibiting DNA synthesis and, therefore, cellular replication. The stability and duration of this inhibition directly relate to a third agent, 5,10-methylenetetrahydrofolate, which is a metabolic product of leucovorin that also binds to thymidylate synthase (TS), producing the so-called ternary complex (FdUMP—TS—5,10-methylenetetrahydrofolate). In preclinical systems, in vitro and in vivo alike, leucovorin favorably modulated the therapeutic index of 5-FU. A number of clinical trials comparing 5-FU to 5-FU with leucovorin indicated an advantage for 5-FU/leucovorin in patients with metastatic colorectal cancer at a cost of only moderately increased mucositis and diarrhea. The combination of 5-FU with leucovorin improved survival rates in two separate studies in metastatic and adjuvant colon cancers.[123,124] In patients with head and neck cancer and with metastatic breast cancer, 5-FU modulated by leucovorin appears promising and is now under study.[125]

Bevacizumab (Avastin) is a monoclonal antibody that depletes serum vascular endothelial growth factor (VEGF). VEGF is an essential mitogenic and antiapoptotic factor for endothelial cells (see Chapter 11). Signaling through the VEGF receptor 2 (*KDR*) and platelet-derived growth factor receptor beta (*PDGFRB*) acts to increase endothelial cell permeability, which results in increased interstitial fluid pressure (IFP) within tumors. In colon, breast, lung, head and neck, cervix, and skin carcinomas, the IFP is significantly higher than in normal tissues.[126–129] Increased tumor IFP acts as a barrier for tumor transvascular transport; reduction of tumor IFP, or modulation of microvascular pressure, increases the transvascular transport of tumor-targeting antibodies or low molecular weight tracer compounds.[130,131] Growing evidence indicates that the *PDGFRB* and *KDR* tyrosine kinases play a crucial role in increased tumor IFP. That makes them candidate targets for pharmacologic intervention for tumor interstitial hypertension[132–135] and for a novel, possibly general, combination strategy that will enhance the therapeutic effects of standard chemotherapeutics. Bevacizumab reduced the IFP in patients with advanced colorectal cancer and increased the uptake of gadolinium in the tumors.[135] Combined with irinotecan, 5-FU, and leucovorin, bevacizumab produces a significant prolongation of survival in patients with metastatic colorectal cancer.[136] This modulation of IFP occurs only within tumors and provides a selective increase in drug levels to the tumor without increasing host toxicity, as was noted in both of the latter two studies. Those findings offer a general treatment strategy for solid tumors of any type.

Implications of Drug Resistance Tumor cell heterogeneity in response to the potentially cytotoxic and antiproliferative effects of cancer chemotherapeutic agents has been the stimulus for a current novel approach to combination chemotherapy. Avoiding therapeutic resistance has been from the beginning a major rationale for combination chemotherapy.

Initial observations about resistance involved reduced drug levels at the site of action because of increased efflux, alteration or amplification of the target, and cellular inactivation. Recent investigations have focused on mechanisms of drug sensitivity or resistance operative after interaction of the drug and its target receptor, including apoptosis (programmed cell death). The varying cell damage caused by various chemotherapeutic agents has the common property of triggering the apoptosis cascade in an active process that requires energy, enzymes, and cytostructure for completion.[137]

Reversal of Drug Resistance Another approach to modulation involves reversal of drug resistance, the most studied of which is multidrug resistance mediated by PgP. Verapamil and several other lipid-soluble heterocyclic drugs, including cyclosporine analogues, can inhibit PgP and thus reduce the efflux of a number of natural antitumor products (doxorubicin, vincristine, taxanes, and others) from the cell, thereby increasing cytotoxicity. PgP is increased in B-cell tumors, AML, sarcoma, and tumors previously treated with drugs that led to multidrug resistance.[138]

The modulation of alkylating agents and cisplatin also is under study. Glutathione may combine chemically with alkylating agents, thus diminishing their activity. Amifostine, a thiol that quenches DNA-damaging species, reduces the nephrotoxicity of cisplatin and the mucositis of irradiated sites.[139,140]

Molecular Biology/Targeted Therapy

Implications for Dose and Schedule The level of optimism among researchers has increased substantially as a result of recent "proof of principle" regarding the clinical effectiveness of more-targeted therapies. Evidence for unique molecu-

Table 38-4 Combination Chemotherapy versus Holotherapy

Combination	Chemotherapy	Holotherapy
Diversity of agents	Drawn from one class, antiproliferative	Drawn from all classes[a]
Number of agents	2–5	4–12+
Toxicity	Bone marrow and gastrointestinal (steep dose), cardiac, neuralgic, pulmonary	Major diversity, including that relative to dose and toxicity; toxicity commonly non-additive; limited, greater selection
Experimental design of clinical trials	Rigid, establishment	Flexible, innovative, semi-Bayesian; patient participation
Endpoints	Classical; R, dR, DFS, OS	TTP
Integration with basic science	Limited	Extensive, operational; PK, PD; targets

[a]Chemotherapy, immunotherapy, endocrinology, antiangiogenesis, antimatrix, gene therapy, control of cell cycle (anticyclins [*CDK* family], transcriptional control, antisense).
DFS = disease-free survival; dR = duration of response; OS = overall survival; PD = pharmacodynamics; PK = pharmacokinetics; R = response (partial or complete); TTP=time to tumor progression.

lar targets in cancer cells (eg, fusion genes, mutations, recombinations) and on their surfaces has led to synthesis of small molecules and monoclonal antibodies with a target specificity never before achieved in cancer therapeutics.[141–143]

Table 38-1 presents a sampling of combinations of molecules and biochemical pathways that are currently being evaluated as targets for selective antitumor agents. The magnitude of such activity and the number of active agents in preclinical systems offer remarkable opportunities for the use of agents in combination. The cumulative effect of these agents on a molecular level suggests an interaction that may result from the diversity of target interaction and a sequential or simultaneous attack on critical cell behavior.

Another important area of diversity relates to anticipated toxicity. Thus, as compared with classic chemotherapy agents, where dose-delineating toxicity usually relates to proliferating tissues and is relatively uniform, the molecular biologic agents will almost certainly express toxicity that varies from agent to agent and that largely differs from the classic antitumor agents. Molecular agents are under extensive study not only for their antitumor properties, but also most particularly for their interaction with each other and with other established antitumor agents.

Experimental Models of Combination Therapy The classic antitumor agents are limited largely to those that directly or indirectly produce DNA damage; the products of the molecular biology era markedly extend the diversity of target mechanisms. Indeed, using experimental models, a number of interesting preclinical experiments have demonstrated an additive or synergistic effect. The literature on preclinical models and computer analysis has been superbly reviewed by Rideout and Chou.[144]

The future of combination chemotherapy will be influenced substantially by the number of these compounds and their interactions. Certainly, the strategy of combining drugs whose mechanisms of action vary has been successful, even in the curative treatment of hematologic, childhood, and embryonal neoplasms.

The terms "additive" and "synergistic" are commonly used in the clinic, but are not well defined. In considering these terms, selectivity for the tumor as compared to the host—the *therapeutic index*—is key. If two agents with additive therapeutic effect have a differing dose-limiting toxicity, so that the toxicity is nonadditive, the overall antitumor effect should be described as additive. When the effects are greater than "additive," the term "synergism" may be appropriate.

Table 38-4 presents the properties and comparisons of combination chemotherapy and holotherapy. Incorporation of many more classes of agents will force more efficient experimental designs. Such designs may include, for example, a rolling phase II/phase III study design. Increasingly, quantitative molecular markers and "real time" pharmacology will be integrated operationally into clinical studies. The effectiveness of such related approaches should markedly improve the efficiency and effectiveness of clinical trials.

Oncogenes and tumor-suppressor genes may operate by modifying or exploiting abnormalities in the cell cycle such as cyclin-D, which is commonly overexpressed in some of the epithelial solid tumors, and by interfering with growth factors and angiogenesis, which are required in varying degrees for all tumors. Proteasomes, which facilitate the ubiquination of peptides and thus their removal from the cell, telomerase, and the cell cycle provide additional attractive targets for a pharmacodynamic modulatory approach. Opportunities for using such agents in combination represent major areas for preclinical and particularly clinical research.

In summary, targeted therapies provide an extension in our ability to apply and benefit from the use of cancer chemotherapeutic agents in combination.

Holotherapy—An Integrated Approach to Cancer Chemotherapy More than a half-century has elapsed since cancer chemotherapy began. The chemotherapy agents now in use originated as biologically targeted therapy. Hitchings and Elion developed specific inhibitors of purine synthesis such as 6-MP; Heidelberger targeted RNA synthesis with 5-FU; and Farber targeted the reduced folate pathway with aminopterin. These innovations not only provided the groundwork for cancer treatment, they also became tools for discovery of the basic workings of transformed cancer cells.

Natural products such as the *Vinca* alkaloids, anthracyclines, and taxanes were selected specifically for activity against cancer proliferation. These agents were combined with other classes of agents—for example, hormones, alkylating agents, and irradiation—that are active against proliferating cells. The optimal use of the new agents requires their integration into increasingly complex combinations so that a greater therapeutic index results. The same is true for the current classic chemotherapeutic agents, which largely inhibit proliferation.

Molecular biology particularly has expanded the number of classes. Thus, hormones, immunotoxins, and inhibitors of invasion and metastasis are available in addition to the classic antiproliferation compounds. Receptors of unique structure and quantity, capable of interactions with the more heterogeneous specific molecular site targets, have recently been described.[100,123]

It has become readily apparent that the vast majority of cancers will be treated successfully only with combinations of agents chosen for the highest possible individual activity against a specific type of cancer. Ideally, such drugs will have different dose-limiting toxicities. Empiricism was an essential component in the development of contemporary cancer therapy, but rational drug discovery, analogue development, preclinical modeling, precise pathologic diagnosis, careful staging of disease, and clinical trial design are the foundation for the measure of success known today.

The breakthroughs in molecular biology have presented the cancer therapist with enormous opportunities and challenges. Based on these breakthroughs, a molecular diagnosis will be able not only to determine where and how cancer originates, but also the processes that are essential to its survival. The specific processes that initiate and propagate cancer have become the targets of unprecedented rational drug development (see Table 38-1). Pharmaceutical technology provides not only small molecules, but also monoclonal antibodies, immunoconjugates, ribozymes, antisense RNA, and recombinant viruses.

The therapy of cancer now has the potential to combine agents with even more mechanisms of action to confront the heterogeneity of cancer with a wider array of therapeutics. Some of these combinations are now the standard of care, as improvements in response and survival demonstrate (see Table 38-5). The challenges to be overcome include (1) clinical development of cytostatic agents without the expectation of significant acute toxicity; (2) combining of classes of targeted agents (Table 38-5), both molecular and biologic, with regard to dose and schedule; and (3) selection of the appropriate types of cancer and individual patients for a specific therapy.

Table 38-5 Therapeutic Interaction between Agents of Different Classes

Agent	Cancer Acted On
Chemotherapy + other systemic agent	
Chemo + immunotherapy	
Cisplatin + Herceptin	Breast cancer
Taxol + Herceptin	Breast cancer
CHOP + rituximab	Lymphoma
Chemotherapy → MRT → Recovery of immunity → Vaccine	
Minitransplant chemotherapy followed by allogeneic armed lymphocyte	
Chemotherapy + hormonal therapy	
Vincristine + prednisone	Acute lymphocytic leukemia
Chemotherapy + tamoxifen	Breast cancer
Chemotherapy + differentiation agent	
Daunorubicin + ATRA	Acute progranulocytic leukemia
Chemotherapy + antiangiogenesis	
IFL + bevacizumab	Colorectal cancer

ATRA = all-*trans*-retinoic acid; IFL = irinotecan/5-fluorouracil/leucovorin.

With molecular biology playing an increasing role, the clinical and laboratory sciences that address the therapy of cancer will continue to accelerate toward cancer control.

REFERENCES

1. Frei E 3rd, Canellos GP. Dose, a critical factor in cancer chemotherapy. Am J Med 1980;69:585–94.
2. Mayer RJ, Davis RB, Schiffer CA, et al. Intensive postremission chemotherapy in adults with acute myeloid leukemia. Cancer and Leukemia Group B. N Engl J Med 1994;331:896–903.
3. Skipper HE, Schabel FM Jr, Wilcox WS. Experimental evaluation of potential anticancer agents. XXI. Scheduling of arabinosylcytosine to take advantage of its S-phase specificity against leukemia cells. Cancer Chemother Rep 1967;51:125–65.
4. Frei E 3rd. Combination cancer therapy. Cancer Res 1972;32:2593–607.
5. Frei E 3rd. Curative cancer chemotherapy. Cancer Res 1985;45:6523–37.
6. Tuberculosis Chemotherapy Trials Committee. Report to the British Medical Research Council. Various combinations of isoniazid with streptomycin or with PAS in the treatment of pulmonary tuberculosis. Br Med J 1955;435:4911.
7. Law LW. Origin of the resistance of leukemic cells to folic acid antagonists. Nature 1956;169:268–75.
8. Schnipper L. Clinical implications of tumor-cell heterogeneity. N Engl J Med 1986;314:1423–31.
9. Frei E 3rd, Elias A, Wheeler C, et al. The relationship between high-dose treatment and combination chemotherapy. The concept of summation dose intensity. Clin Cancer Res 1998;4:2027–37.
10. Hryniuk W, Frei E 3rd, Wright FA. A single scale for comparing dose-intensity of all chemotherapy regimens in breast cancer: summation dose-intensity. J Clin Oncol 1998;16:3137–47.
11. Skipper HE, Schabel FM, Jary R, Wilcox WS. Experimental evaluation of potential anticancer agents. XIII. On the criteria and kinetics associated with "curability" of experimental leukemia. Cancer Chemother Rep 1964;35:3–111.
12. Frei E 3rd, Cucchi C, Rosowsky A, et al. Alkylating agent resistance. In vitro studies of human cell lines. Proc Natl Acad Sci U S A 1985;82:2158–62.
13. Frei E 3rd, Freireich EJ. Progress and perspectives in the chemotherapy of acute leukemia. Adv Chemother 1965;2:269–89.
14. Bonadonna G. Karnofsky Memorial Lecture. Conceptual and practical advances in the management of breast cancer. J Clin Oncol 1989;7:1380–97.
15. Wood W, Budman D, Korzun A, et al. Dose and dose intensity of adjuvant chemotherapy for stage II, node-positive breast carcinoma. N Engl J Med 1994;330:1253–9.
16. Muss H, Thor A, Berry D, et al. c-*ErbB*-2 expression and response to adjuvant therapy in women with node-positive early breast cancer. N Engl J Med 1994;330:1260–6.
17. Gribben JG. Attainment of molecular remission. A worthwhile goal? J Clin Oncol 1994;12:1532–4.
18. Norton L, Simon R, Brereton HD, Bogden AE. Predicting the course of Gompertzian growth. Nature 1976;264:542–5.
19. Tannock I. Cell kinetics and chemotherapy. A critical review. Cancer Treat Rep 1978;62:1117–33.
20. Clarkson B, Ohkita T, Ota K, Fried J. Studies of cellular proliferation in human leukemia. I. Estimation of growth rates of leukemic and normal hematopoietic cells in two adults with acute leukemia given single injections of tritiated thymidine. J Clin Invest 1967;46:506–29.
21. Clarkson B, Fried J, Strife A, et al. Studies of cellular proliferation in human leukemia. 3. Behavior of leukemic cells in three adults with acute leukemia given continuous-infusions of ^{3}H-thymidine for 8 or 10 days. Cancer 1970;25:1237–60.
22. Clarkson B, Strife A, Fried J, et al. Studies of cellular proliferation in human leukemia. IV. Behavior of normal hematopoietic cells in 3 adults with acute leukemia given continuous-infusions of 3H-thymidine for 8 or 10 days. Cancer 1970;26:1–19.
23. Tannock I. Basic science of oncology. New York: McGraw–Hill; 1992. p. 139–96.
24. Steel GG. The growth kinetics of tumors in relation to their therapeutic response. Laryngoscope 1975;85:359–70.
25. Mendelsohn ML. The growth fraction. A new concept applied to tumors. Science 1960;132:1496–504.
26. Al-Hajj M, Clarke MF. Self-renewal and solid tumor stem cells. Oncogene 2004;23:7274–82.
27. Brown JM, Wilson WR. Exploiting tumor hypoxia in cancer treatment. Nat Rev Cancer 2004;4:437–47.
28. Leek RD, Stratford I, Harris AL. The role of hypoxia-inducible factor-1 in three-dimensional tumor growth, apoptosis, and regulation by the insulin-signaling pathway. Cancer Res 2005;55:4147–52.
29. Ward JF. DNA damage produced by ionizing radiation in mammalian cells: identities, mechanisms of formation, and reparability. Prog Nucleic Acid Res Mol Biol 1988;35:95–8.
30. Luk CK, Veinot-Drebot L, Tjan E, Tannock IF. Effect of transient hypoxia on sensitivity to doxorubicin in human and murine cell lines. J Natl Cancer Inst 1990;82:684–92.
31. Teicher BA, Bernal S, Holden S, Cathcart KN. Effect of fluosol-DA/carbogen on etoposide/alkylating agent antitumor activity. Cancer Chemother Pharmacol 1988;21:281–5.
32. Dong F, Brynes RK, Tidow N, et al. Mutations in the gene for the granulocyte colony-stimulating-factor receptor in patients with acute myeloid leukemia preceded by severe congenital neutropenia [see comments]. N Engl J Med 1995;333:487–93.
33. Collins JM, Dedrick RL, King FG, et al. Nonlinear pharmacokinetic models for 5-fluorouracil in man. Intravenous and intraperitoneal routes. Clin Pharmacol Ther 1980;28:235–46.
34. Schaaf LJ, Dobbs BR, Edwards IR, Perrier DG. Nonlinear pharmacokinetic characteristics of 5-fluorouracil (5-FU) in colorectal cancer patients. Eur J Clin Pharmacol 1987;32:411–8.
35. Baker SD, Verweij J, Rowinsky EK, et al. Role of body surface area in dosing of investigational anticancer agents in adults, 1991–2001. J Natl Cancer Inst 2002;94:1883–8.
36. Pinkel D. The use of body surface area as a criterion for drug dosage in cancer chemotherapy. Cancer Res 1958;18:853–6.
37. Jodrell DI, Egorin MJ, Canetta M, et al. Relationships between carboplatin exposure and tumor response and toxicity in patients with ovarian cancer. J Clin Oncol 1992;10:520–8.
38. Felici A, Verweij J, Sparreboom A. Dosing strategies for anticancer drugs: the good, the bad and the body-surface area. Eur J Cancer 2002;38:1677–84.
39. Grochow LB, Baraldi C, Noe D. Is the dose normalization to weight and body surface area useful in adults? J Natl Cancer Inst 1990;82:323–5.
40. Hasler JA, Estabrook R, Murray M, et al. Human cytochromes P450. Mol Aspects Med 1999;20:1–137.
41. Hirth J, Watkins PB, Strawderman M, et al. The effect of an individual's cytochrome CYP3A4 activity on docetaxel clearance. Clin Cancer Res 2000;6:1255–8.
42. Evans WE, Crom WR, Abromowitch M, et al. Clinical pharmacodynamics of high-dose methotrexate in acute lymphocytic leukemia. Identification of a relation between concentration and effect. N Engl J Med 1986;314:471–7.
43. Evans WE, Rodman J, Relling MV, et al. Individualized dosages of chemotherapy as a strategy to improve response for acute lymphocytic leukemia. Semin Hematol 1991;28:15–21.
44. Henner WD, Peters WP, Eder JP, et al. Pharmacokinetics and immediate effects of high dose carmustine in man. Cancer Treat Rep 1986;70:877–80.
45. Grochow LB, Jones RJ, Brundrett RB, et al. Pharmacokinetics of busulfan. Correlation with veno-occlusive disease in patients undergoing bone marrow transplantation. Cancer Chemother Pharmacol 1989;25:55–61.
46. Jones RB, Matthes S, Shpall EJ, et al. I. Acute lung injury following treatment with high-dose cyclophosphamide, cisplatin, and carmustine: pharmacodynamic evaluation of carmustine. J Natl Cancer Inst 1993;85:640–7.
47. Doroshow JH, Synold T, Somlo G, et al. Adaptive control of paclitaxel systemic exposure during high-dose chemotherapy with paclitaxel, cisplatin, cyclophosphamide, and cyclosporine A followed by stem cell rescue significantly decreases variation in hematologic recovery, mucositis, and hospital stay [abstract]. Proc Am Soc Clin Oncol 1999;18:200a.
48. Pinkel D, Hernandez K, Borella L, et al. Drug dosage and remission duration in childhood lymphocytic leukemia. Cancer 1971;27:247–56.
49. Cohen MH, Creaven PJ, Fossieck BE Jr, et al. Intensive chemotherapy of small cell bronchogenic carcinoma. Cancer Treat Rep 1977;61:349–54.
50. Philip T, Guglielmi C, Hagenbeek A, et al. Autologous bone marrow transplantation as compared with salvage chemotherapy in relapses of chemotherapy-sensitive non-Hodgkin's lymphoma [see comments]. N Engl J Med 1995;333:1540–5.
51. Gianni AM, Bregni M, Siena S, et al. High-dose chemotherapy and autologous bone marrow transplantation compared with MACOP-B in aggressive B-cell lymphoma. N Engl J Med 1997;336:1290–7.
52. Broun E, Nichols C, Kneebone P, et al. Long-term outcome of patients with relapsed and refractory germ cell tumors treated with high-dose chemotherapy and autologous bone marrow rescue. Ann Intern Med 1992;117:124–8.
53. American Society of Clinical Oncology and American Society of Hematology. Recommended criteria for the performance of bone marrow transplantation. J Clin Oncol 1990;8:563–4.
54. Norton L, Simon R. The Norton–Simon hypothesis revisited. Cancer Treat Rep 1986;70:163–9.
55. Goldie JH, Coldman AJ. A mathematic model for relating drug sensitivity of tumors to spontaneous mutation rate. Cancer Treat Rep 1979;63:1727–33.
56. Hryniuk WM, Bush H. The importance of dose intensity in chemotherapy of metastatic breast cancer. J Clin Oncol 1984;2:1281–7.
57. Hryniuk W, Levine MN. Analysis of dose intensity for adjuvant chemotherapy trials in stage II breast cancer. J Clin Oncol 1986;4:1162–70.
58. Levin L, Hryniuk WM. Dose intensity analysis of chemotherapy regimens in ovarian cancer. J Clin Oncol 1987;5:756–60.
59. Early Breast Cancer Trialists' Collaborative Group. Polychemotherapy for early breast cancer. An overview of the randomised trials. Lancet 1998;352:930–42.
60. Saltz LB, Cox JV, Blanke C, et al. Irinotecan plus 5-fluorouracil and leucovorin for metastatic colorectal cancer. N Engl J Med 2000;343:898–904.
61. Wolmark N, Fisher B, Anderson S. The effect of increasing dose intensity and cumulative dose of adjuvant cyclophosphamide in node positive breast cancer [abstract]. Breast Cancer Res Treat 1997;46:26.
62. Fisher BF, Anderson S, DeCillis A, et al. Further evaluation of intensified and increased total dose of cyclophospha-

mide for the treatment of primary breast cancer: findings from National Surgical Adjuvant Breast and Bowel Project B-25. J Clin Oncol 1999;17:3374–88.
63. Citron M, Berry D, Cirrinciione C, et al. Superiority of dose-dense (DD) over conventional scheduling (CS) and equivalence of sequential (SC) vs combination adjuvant chemotherapy (CC) for node-positive breast cancer (CALGB INT C9741) [abstract]. Breast Cancer Res Treat 2002;76(suppl 1):S15.
64. Stadtmauer EA, O'Neill A, Goldstein LJ, et al. Phase III randomized trial of high-dose chemotherapy and stem cell support shows no difference in overall survival or severe toxicity compared to maintenance chemotherapy with cyclophosphamide, methotrexate and 5-fluorouracil for women with metastatic breast cancer who are responding to conventional induction chemotherapy. The Philadelphia Intergroup study [abstract]. Proc Am Soc Clin Oncol 1999;18:1a.
65. Peters WP, Rosner G, Vredenburgh J, et al. A prospective, randomized comparison of two doses of combination alkylating agents as consolidation after CAF in high-risk primary breast cancer involving ten or more axillary lymph nodes. Preliminary results of CALGB 9082/SWOG 9114/NCIC MA-13 [abstract]. Proc Am Soc Clin Oncol 1999;18:1a.
66. Bergh J. Results from a randomized adjuvant breast cancer study with high dose chemotherapy with CTCb supported by autologous bone marrow stem cells versus dose escalated and tailored FEC therapy [abstract]. Proc Am Soc Clin Oncol 1999;18:2a.
67. Peters WP, Jones RB, Vredenburgh J, et al. A large prospective randomized trial of high-dose combination alkylating agents (CPB) with autologous cellular support as consolidation for patients with metastatic breast cancer achieving complete remission after intensive doxorubicin-based induction therapy (AFM) [abstract]. Proc Am Soc Clin Oncol 1996;15:121.
68. Lotz JP, Cure H, Janvier M, et al. High-dose chemotherapy with hematopoietic stem cells transplantation for metastatic breast cancer. Results of the French protocol Pegase 04 [abstract]. Proc Am Soc Clin Oncol 1999;18:43a.
69. Tallman MS, Gray R, Robert NJ, et al. Conventional adjuvant chemotherapy with or without high-dose chemotherapy and autologous bone marrow transplantation in high-risk breast cancer. N Engl J Med 2003;349:17–26.
70. Rodenhuis S, Bontenbal M, Beex LVAM, et al. High dose chemotherapy with hematopoietic stem-cell rescue for high-risk breast cancer. N Engl J Med 2003;349:7–16.
71. Hortobagyi GN, Buzdar AU, Champlin R, et al. Lack of efficacy of adjuvant high-dose tandem combination chemotherapy for high-risk primary breast cancer. A randomized trial [abstract]. Proc Am Soc Clin Oncol 1998;17:123.
72. Rodenhuis S, Richel KJ, van der Wall E, et al. Randomized trial of high-dose chemotherapy and hematopoietic progenitor cell support in operable breast cancer with extensive axillary lymph node involvement. Lancet 1998;352:515–21.
73. Vogler WR, Cooper LE, Groth DP. Correlation of cytosine arabinoside–induced increment in growth fraction of leukemic blast cells with clinical response. Cancer 1974;33:603–10.
74. Ho DHW, Frei E 3rd. Clinical pharmacology of 1-β-D-arabinofuranosyl cytosine. Clin Pharmacol Ther 1971;12:944–54.
75. Abbruzzese JL, Grunewald R, Weeks EA, et al. A phase I clinical, plasma, and cellular pharmacology study of gemcitabine. J Clin Oncol 1991;9:491–8.
76. Grunewald R, Kantarjian H, Du M, et al. Gemcitabine in leukemia. A phase I clinical, plasma, and cellular pharmacology study. J Clin Oncol 1992;10:406–13.
77. Li MC, Hertz R, Spencer DV. Effect of methotrexate upon choriocarcinoma and chorioadenoma. Proc Soc Exp Biol Med 1956;93:361–6.
78. Goldin A, Vendetti JM, Humphreys SB, Mantel N. Modification of treatment schedules in the management of advanced mouse leukemia with amethopterin. J Natl Cancer Inst 1956;17:203–9.
79. Selawry OS, Hananian J, Wolman IJ, et al. New treatment schedule with improved survival in childhood leukemia. JAMA 1965;194:715–24.
80. Schimke RT, Roos DS, Brown PC. Amplification of genes in somatic mammalian cells. Methods Enzymol 1987;151:85–104.
81. Rath H, Tlsty T, Schimke RT. Rapid emergence of methotrexate resistance in cultured mouse cells. Cancer Res 1984;44:3303–6.
82. Seifert P, Baker LH, Reed ML, Vaitkevicius VK. Comparison of continuously infused 5-fluorouracil with bolus injection in treatment of patients with colorectal adenocarcinoma. Cancer 1975;36:123–8.
83. Lokich J. Infusional 5-FU: historical evolution, rationale, and clinical experience. Oncology 1998;12:19–22.
84. Sobrero AF, Aschele C, Guglielmi AP, et al. Synergism and lack of cross-resistance between short-term and continuous exposure to fluorouracil in human colon adenocarcinoma cells. J Natl Cancer Inst 1993;85:1937–44.
85. Teicher BA, Holden SA, Eder JP, et al. Influence of schedule on alkylating agent cytotoxicity in vitro and in vivo. Cancer Res 1989;49:6994–8.
86. Bronner CE, Baker SM, Morrison PT, et al. Mutation in the DNA mismatch repair gene homologue h*MLH1* is associated with hereditary non-polyposis colon cancer. Nature 1994;368:258–61.
87. Fishel R, Lescoe MK, Rao MR, et al. The human mutator gene homolog *MSH2* and its association with hereditary nonpolyposis colon cancer [published erratum appears in Cell 1994;77:167]. Cell 1993;75:1027–38.
88. Weiss AJ, Manthel RW. Experience with the use of Adriamycin in combination with other anticancer agents using a weekly schedule, with particular reference to lack of cardiac toxicity. Cancer 1977;40:2046–52.
89. Legha SS, Benjamin RS, Mackay B, et al. Reduction of doxorubicin cardiotoxicity by prolonged continuous intravenous infusion. Ann Intern Med 1982;96:133–9.
90. Casper ES, Gaynor JJ, Hajdu SI, et al. A prospective randomized trial of adjuvant chemotherapy with bolus versus continuous infusion of doxorubicin in patients with high-grade extremity soft tissue sarcoma and an analysis of prognostic factors. Cancer 1991;68:1221–9.
91. Zalupski M, Metch B, Balcerzak S, et al. Phase III comparison of doxorubicin and dacarbazine given by bolus versus infusion in patients with soft-tissue sarcomas. A Southwest Oncology Group study. J Natl Cancer Inst 1991;83:926–32.
92. Rahman A, More N, Schein PS. Doxorubicin-induced chronic cardiotoxicity and its protection by liposomal administration. Cancer Res 1982;42:1817–25.
93. Alberts DS, Garcia DJ. Safety aspects of pegylated liposomal doxorubicin in patients with cancer. Drugs 1997;54:30–5.
94. Slevin ML, Clark PI, Joel SP, et al. A randomized trial to evaluate the effect of schedule on the activity of etoposide in small-cell lung cancer. J Clin Oncol 1989;7:1333–40.
95. Reiter A, Schrappe M, Ludwig WD, et al. Chemotherapy in 998 unselected childhood acute lymphoblastic leukemia patients. Results and conclusions of the multicenter trial ALL-BFM 86. Blood 1994;84:3122–33.
96. ten Bokkel Huinink WW, Eisenhauer E, Swenerton K. Preliminary evaluation of a multicenter, randomized comparative study of Taxol (paclitaxel) dose and infusion length in platinum-treated ovarian cancer. Canadian–European Taxol Cooperative Trial Group. Cancer Treat Rev 1993;19:79–86.
97. Huizing MT, Keung AC, Rosing H, et al. Pharmacokinetics of paclitaxel and metabolites in a randomized comparative study in platinum-pretreated ovarian cancer patients. J Clin Oncol 1993;11:2127–35.
98. Wolfrom C, Hartmann R, Fengler R, et al. Randomized comparison of 36-hour intermediate-dose versus 4-hour high-dose methotrexate infusions for remission induction in relapsed childhood acute lymphoblastic leukemia. J Clin Oncol 1993;11:827–33.
99. Devita VT Jr, Serpick AA, Carbone PP. Combination chemotherapy in the treatment of advanced Hodgkin's disease. Ann Intern Med 1970;73:881–95.
100. Blanke CD, von Mehrem M, Joensuu H, et al. Evaluation of the safety and efficacy of an oral molecularly-targeted therapy STI 571, in patients with metastatic or unresectable gastrointestinal stroma tumor (GIST) [abstract]. Proc Am Soc Clin Oncol 2001;20:1a.
101. Tepler I, Cannistra SA, Frei E 3rd, et al. Use of peripheral-blood progenitor cells abrogates the myelotoxicity of repetitive outpatient high-dose carboplatin and cyclophosphamide chemotherapy. J Clin Oncol 1993;11:1583–91.
102. O'Connell MJ, Martenson JA, Wieand HS, et al. Improving adjuvant therapy for rectal cancer by combining protracted-infusion fluorouracil with radiation therapy after curative surgery. N Engl J Med 1994;331:502–7.
103. Hoff PM, Ansari R, Batist G, et al. Comparison of oral capecitabine versus intravenous fluorouracil plus leucovorin as first-line treatment in 605 patients with metastatic colorectal cancer: results of randomized phase III study. J Clin Oncol 2001;19:2282–92.
104. Van Cutsem E, Twelves C, Cassidy J, et al. (Xeloda Colorectal Cancer Study Group). Oral capecitabine compared with intravenous fluorouracil plus leucovorin in patients with metastatic colorectal cancer: results of a large phase III study. J Clin Oncol 2001;19:4097–106.
105. Joensuu H, Roberts PJ, Sarlomo-Rikola M, et al. Effect of the tyrosine kinase inhibitor STI571 in a patient with metastatic gastrointestinal sarcoma tumor. N Engl J Med 2001;344:1052–6.
106. Hanahan D, Weinberg RA. The hallmarks of cancer. Cell 2000;100:57–70.
107. Ling V, Kartner N, Sudo T, et al. Multidrug-resistance phenotype in Chinese hamster ovary cells. Cancer Treat Rep 1983;67:869–74.
108. Kobayashi H, Man S, Graham CH, et al. Acquired multicellular-mediated resistance to alkylating agents in cancer. Proc Natl Acad Sci U S A 1993;90:3294–8.
109. Fisher DE. Apoptosis in cancer therapy. Crossing the threshold. Cell 1994;78:539–42.
110. Teicher BA, Herman TS, Holden SA, et al. Tumor resistance to alkylating agents conferred by mechanisms operative only in vivo. Science 1990;247:1457–61.
111. Sartorelli AC, Shansky CW, Rosman M. Biochemical approaches to the combination chemotherapy of colon cancer. Cancer 1975;36:2445–8.
112. Ruiz-Cabello J, Berghmans K, Kaplan O, et al. Hormone dependence of breast cancer cells and the effects of tamoxifen and estrogen. 31P NMR studies. Breast Cancer Res Treat 1995;33:209–17.
113. Pinkel D. Ninth annual David Karnofsky lecture. Treatment of acute lymphocytic leukemia. Cancer 1979;43:1128–37.
114. Burchenal JH. History of intrathecal prophylaxis and therapy of meningeal leukemia. Cancer Drug Deliv 1983;1:87–92.
115. Frei E 3rd, Blum RH, Pitman SW, et al. High dose methotrexate with leucovorin rescue. Rationale and spectrum of antitumor activity. Am J Med 1980;68:370–6.
116. Ackland SP, Schilsky RL. High-dose methotrexate. A critical reappraisal. J Clin Oncol 1987;5:2017–31.
117. Hande KR, Oldham RK, Fer MF, et al. Randomized study of high-dose versus low-dose methotrexate in the treatment of extensive small cell lung cancer. Am J Med 1982;73:413–9.
118. Taylor SG, McGuire WP, Hauck WW, et al. A randomized comparison of high-dose infusion methotrexate versus standard-dose weekly therapy in head and neck squamous cancer. J Clin Oncol 1984;2:1006–11.
119. Ginsberg SJ, Anderson JR, Gottlieb AJ, et al. A randomized trial of high-dose methotrexate versus standard-dose methotrexate following cyclophosphamide, doxorubicin (Adriamycin), vincristine, and prednisone with or without bleomycin in the therapy of diffuse large cell lymphoma. Preliminary report of Cancer and Leukemia Group B Study 7851. NCI Monogr 1987;5:77–80.
120. Krailo M, Ertel I, Makley J, et al. A randomized study comparing high-dose methotrexate with moderate-dose methotrexate as components of adjuvant chemotherapy in childhood nonmetastatic osteosarcoma. A report from the Children's Cancer Study Group. Med Pediatr Oncol 1987;15:69–77.
121. Gordon LI, Harrington D, Andersen J, et al. Comparison of a second-generation combination chemotherapeutic regimen (m-BACOD) with a standard regimen (CHOP) for advanced diffuse non-Hodgkin's lymphoma [see comments]. N Engl J Med 1992;327:1342–9.
122. Fisher RI, Gaynor ER, Dahlberg S, et al. Comparison of a standard regimen (CHOP) with three intensive chemotherapy regimens for advanced non-Hodgkin's lymphoma [see comments]. N Engl J Med 1993;328:1002–6.
123. Doroshow JH, Multhauf P, Leong L, et al. Prospective randomized comparison of fluorouracil versus fluorouracil and high-dose continuous-infusion leucovorin calcium for the treatment of advanced measurable colorectal cancer in patients previously unexposed to chemotherapy. J Clin Oncol 1990;8:491–501.
124. O'Connell MJ, Mailliard JA, Kahn MJ, et al. Controlled trial of fluorouracil and low-dose leucovorin given for 6 months as postoperative adjuvant therapy for colon cancer. J Clin Oncol 1997;15:246–50.
125. Dreyfuss AI, Clark JR, Wright JE, et al. Continuous-infusion high-dose leucovorin with 5-fluorouracil and cisplatin for untreated stage IV carcinoma of the head and neck. Ann Intern Med 1990;112:167–72.
126. Boucher Y, Kirkwood J, Opacic D, Jain K. Interstitial hypertension in superficial metastatic melanomas in humans. Cancer Res 1991;51:6691–4.
127. Gutmann R, Leunig M, Feyh J, et al. Interstitial hypertension in head and neck tumors in patients: correlation with tumor size. Cancer Res 1992;52:1993–5.

128. Less J, Posner M, Boucher Y, et al. Interstitial hypertension in human breast and colorectal tumors. Cancer Res 1992;52:6371–4.
129. Milosevic MF, Fyles AW, Wong R, et al. Interstitial fluid pressure in cervical carcinoma: within tumor heterogeneity, and relation to oxygen tension. Cancer 1998;82:2418–26.
130. Netti PA, Hamberg LM, Babich JW, et al. Enhancement of fluid filtration across tumor vessels: implication for delivery of macromolecules. Proc Natl Acad Sci U S A 1999;96:3137–42.
131. Tong RT, Boucher Y, Kozin SV, et al. Vascular normalization by vascular endothelial growth factor receptor 2 blockade induces a pressure gradient across the vasculature and improves drug penetration in tumors. Cancer Res 2004;64:3731–6.
132. Ferrara N, Gerber HP, LeCouter J. The biology of *VEGF* and its receptors. Nat Med 2003;9:669–76.
133. Heldin CH, Rubin K, Pietras K, Ostman A. High interstitial fluid pressure—an obstacle in cancer therapy. Nat Rev Cancer 2004;4:806–13.
134. Pietras K, Ostman A, Sjoquist M, et al. Inhibition of platelet-derived growth factor receptors reduces interstitial hypertension and increases transcapillary transport in tumors. Cancer Res 2001;61:2929–34.
135. Willett CG, Boucher Y, di Tomaso E, et al. Direct evidence that the *VEGF*-specific antibody bevacizumab has antivascular effects in human rectal cancer. Nat Med 2004;10:145–7.
136. Hurwitz H, Fehrenbacher L, Novotny W, et al. Bevacizumab plus irinotecan, fluorouracil, and leucovorin for metastatic colorectal cancer. N Engl J Med 2004;350:2335–42.
137. Kerr JF, Winterford CM, Harmon BV. Apoptosis. Its significance in cancer and cancer therapy [published erratum appears in Cancer 1994;73:3108]. Cancer 1994;73:2013–26.
138. Dalton WS, Grogan TM, Meltzer PS, et al. Drug-resistance in multiple myeloma and non-Hodgkin's lymphoma. Detection of P-glycoprotein and potential circumvention by addition of verapamil to chemotherapy [see comments]. J Clin Oncol 1989;7:415–24.
139. Kemp G, Rose P, Lurain J, et al. Amifostine pretreated for protection against cyclophosphamide-induced and cisplatin-induced toxicities. Results of a randomized control trial in patients with advanced ovarian cancer. J Clin Oncol 1996;14:2101–12.
140. Brizel D, Wasserman T, Henke M, et al. Phase III randomized trial of amifostine as a radioprotector in head and neck cancer. J Clin Oncol 2000;18: 3339–45.
141. Druker BJ, Lydon NB. Lessons learned from the development of an Abl tyrosine kinase inhibitor for chronic myelogenous leukemia. J Clin Invest 2000;105:3–7.
142. Sausville EA, Zaharevitz D, Gussio R, et al. Cyclin-dependent kinases: initial approaches to exploit a novel therapeutic target. Pharmacol Ther 1999;82:285–92.
143. Holt SE, Shay JW. Role of telomerase in cellular proliferation and cancer. J Cell Physiol 1999;180:10–8.
144. Rideout DC, Chou TC. Synergism, potentiation, and antagonism in chemotherapy. An overview. In: Chou TC, Rideout DC, editors. Synergism and antagonism in chemotherapy. San Diego (CA): Academic Press; 1991. p. 3.

Preclinical and Early Clinical Development of New Anticancer Agents

Daniel D. Von Hoff, MD, FACP
Axel-R. Hanauske, MD, PhD

Considering the rising death rates, it is obvious that there is a great need for development of new agents for treatment of patients with advanced cancer. There is also a newly perceived need for developing new agents that will be used to treat patients with "early cancer" (now referred to as intraepithelial neoplasia).[1,2] This latter approach for treating early cancer, referred to in the past as chemoprevention, represents a new concept that could have an enormous impact on the disease.[3–5]

In this chapter, we describe the fundamentals of development of new agents from discovery through the initial safety (phase I) clinical trials. Along the way, we discuss a few studies that illustrate new methodologies introduced into drug development in recent years. This chapter largely concentrates on the development of new chemical entities and not on the development of biologic agents, although many of the principles outlined here also apply to the development of those agents.

As an overview, Figure 39-1 describes the classic stages in the development of a new agent. Using this basic process, there have been over 130 agents developed for treatment of patients with a variety of malignancies as well as for treatment of early cancer. Although this is an impressive list of agents available to treat patients with a variety of cancers, it is—in the light of the biological diversity of the various types of cancer—obvious that we still need major additions to our armamentarium. Table 39-1 details all of the anticancer agents that are approved by the US Food and Drug Administration and their official approved indications. We provide that table because, as noted below, as new strategies are being developed for the proper testing of new agents, one has to be cognizant of the agents that are already approved for a specific indication. One must also be aware as to whether a new agent should be developed alone or in combination in a "frontline" setting or in a salvage or palliative setting. Table 39-1 helps allow the design of pivotal clinical trials that will lead to approval by regulatory agencies and, most importantly, become available for our patients.

EVOLUTION OF THE DISCOVERY PROCESS

Clinical Observation in the Discovery Process As this chapter is being written, the process for discovery is changing rapidly. Initial anticancer drug discovery was based on important observations by clinicians and preclinical scientists. An example of such observations, where many feel the field of chemotherapy of cancer began, was the observation by Adair and Bogg in 1931 that troops in World War I exposed to sulfur mustard developed lymphoid and bone marrow hypoplasia.[6] They then used this very toxic agent to treat a number of patients with cancer with sulfur mustard. The agent had a limited effect. Further studies of the related nitrogen mustard (of World War II) demonstrated more substantial antitumor effects, particularly in patients with lymphoma.[7,8]

Another classic example of an astute observation by clinicians was when Farber and colleagues noticed that young patients with leukemia who were treated with liver extracts or folic acid had worsening of their leukemia.[9] They then treated the patients with folic acid antagonists and described the antileukemic activity of these antagonists.

Histocytoxic Effects and Physiologic Observations Just like the observation that mustard gases cause hypoplasia of lymph nodes, spleen, and bone marrow (with subsequent clinical activity of nitrogen mustard and other alkylating agents in patients with lymphoma), there have been a number of other correlations between specific histocytotoxicity (toxicity to a particular type of tissue) and clinical activity of an agent. One of the best examples is the finding that the agent streptozocin caused destruction of the islet cells in animals (leading to diabetes).[10] Streptozocin was tried and found to have clinical activity in patients with insulinomas (a histocytotoxic effect).[11]

In early animal toxicology studies, cisplatinum caused hypoplasia of the testes and ovaries in animals and was subsequently found to have substantial activity in patients with testicular or ovarian cancer.[12–14]

As an example of a physiologic observation leading to the development of a series of new anticancer agents, the physiologic observation that rat hepatomas incorporated more uracil than the surrounding normal liver led to the Heidelberger group synthesizing the 5-fluoropyrimidines.[15,16] The observations by Elion and Hitchings, who surmised (based on the presumption that nucleic acids were in control of cell growth) that purine and pyrimidine analogs would be useful in treatment of cancers, led to the development of 6-mercaptopurine, 6-thioguanine, and many other useful anticancer agents.[17,18] Although there is still clearly room for important clinical, toxicologic, and physiologic observation, these observations will probably not dominate future drug discovery. However, readers are encouraged to keep their eyes open to clinical, histocytotoxic, and physiologic observations as described above as serendipity has historically been a pivotal step in successful drug development.

The National Cancer Institute's Drug Discovery Program as an Important Contribution in the Drug Discovery Process In the early 1960s, the US National Cancer Institute (NCI) began a major leadership role in the discovery and development of new anticancer agents. This was critical at that time because industry felt that investment in this area would not be feasible financially and that the risks were high. The NCI began its leadership by establishing the National Service Center (NSC), which served as a clearinghouse and a bank for compounds for all chemists, biologists, and other interested investigators. Compounds could be submitted to the NSC, assigned an NSC number (eg, NSC 3101139 for mitoxantrone), and tested in a series of in vitro and in vivo preclinical models. Agents that passed certain hurdles of in vitro and in vivo antitumor activity were considered by a body at the NCI called the "Decision Network" to decide whether or not to bring them into toxicology studies and eventually into clinical trials.

The very early efforts of the NCI used the KB squamous cancer cell line, originally obtained from a patient with a carcinoma of the mouth, to screen a large numbers of compounds. Compounds that were active against that cell line were further evaluated in vivo in the two murine leukemias called P388 and L1210.[19,20] These in vitro and in vivo screens did lead to compounds with clinical activity against leukemia and lymphoma (eg, vinca alkaloids, nitrosoureas). Finding agents with antitumor activity against solid tumors was much less successful.[20] In 1975, the NCI revisited their evaluation process to include in vivo evaluation of compounds against solid tumors (both autologous animal tumors and human tumors growing as xenografts in nude mice). A very important retrospective analysis of that big exper-

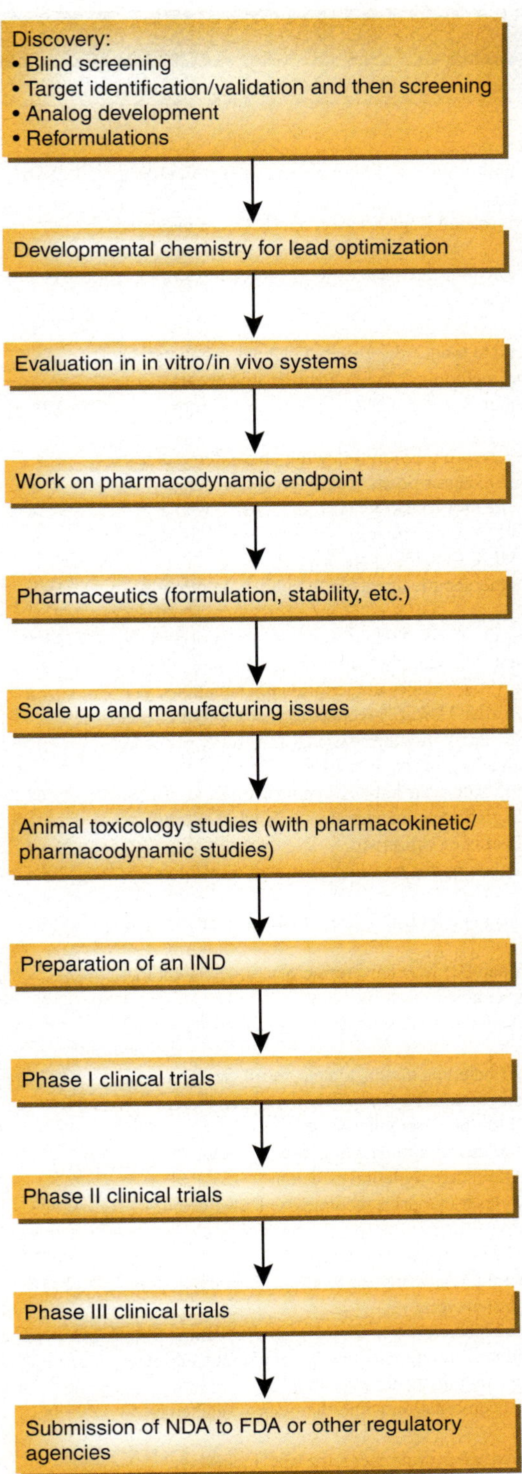

Figure 39-1 Classic stages in the development of a new anticancer agent. FDA = US Food and Drug Administration; IND = investigational new drug; NDA = new drug application.

iment was conducted by Staquet and colleagues.[21] The results of their analyses are detailed in Table 39-2.

As can be seen in the table, the P388 and L1210 mouse leukemias continued to be predictive for activity of new agents in the clinic, as did the B16 mouse melanoma solid tumor autologous model growing in immunocompetent mice. The only human tumor xenograft that appeared to be predictive for clinical antitumor activity was the MX1 mammary tumor xenograft growing in nude mice. The predictivity of these models was not tumor specific but rather in vivo activity in those systems predicted, in general, for clinical activity.[21]

Also of importance in the report by Staquet and colleagues was the finding that actual regression of established tumors in these models and the percentage of animals surviving for ≥ 45 days were even stronger predictors of eventual clinical efficacy of the agents.[21] Thus, although these in vivo evaluation systems are often maligned, when a systematic large-scale evaluation of them was examined, some models appeared to be reasonable predictors (although not tumor-specific predictors) for activity in the clinic.[22]

Of additional note in Table 39-2 is the finding that four models were judged as not predictive at all for clinical activity. Some of the models, such as the Lewis lung model, continue to be used to justify bringing many new agents into clinical trials. It is important that investigators who are contemplating bringing new agents into the clinic based on preclinical activity only in the Lewis lung, CD8, Co38, LX1, or CX1 models be mindful of the extensive prior experience demonstrating them not to be predictive for clinical activity.

To be most successful, however, it is important to remember the parameter Staquet and colleagues used for evidence of activity in the clinic (to make the correlation with the preclinical models): tumor shrinkage. Thus, their findings might not be applicable to the newer cytostatic agents being developed.

A more recent study reported on the relationship between drug activity in NCI preclinical in vitro and in vivo models and clinical activity of a new agent.[22] Of interest, for 39 agents for which there were both xenograft and phase II clinical data available, clinical activity in at least some phase II trials was observed if there was activity in at least one-third of the xenograft models tested. Of particular note was that if there was preclinical activity in one-third or more of the xenografts tested there was a 45% chance the compound would have clinical activity. In that same study, only 8 nonsmall-cell lung cancer xenografts were predictive for the clinical activity against the same histology (eg, nonsmall-cell lung cancer).

The NCI made a further revision in their evaluation strategy in 1985 when they placed a large series of 60 human tumor cell lines in place for screening purposes.[20,23–27] They have attempted to make this a more tumor type-oriented approach with inclusion of breast, lung, colon, kidney, brain, ovary, prostate, and melanoma human tumor lines.[20,24,25] At the time of introduction of this concept into the drug evaluation process, there was a great deal of discussion in the research community on how these cell lines were selected. Many investigators felt that cell lines with too rapid a doubling time were selected and did not represent the more slowly dividing solid tumors. However, this 60 cell line screening panel is the system that is currently in place. More can be learned about the 60 cell line success by visiting the Web site of the NCI at <http://dtp.nci.nih.gov/branches/btb/ivclsp.html>. Agents that are deemed active in the cell line screens (based on criteria outlined by Boyd[20] and Grever and colleagues,[25] and based on other criteria, such as disease-specific activity) are then evaluated in the traditional in vivo models to determine their therapeutic index. If they are found active, they are moved forward into preclinical toxicology studies (see below).[26,27]

The true predictivity of the NCI 60 cell line success is as yet unknown as there are no published analyses as to the true predictivity of this approach for antitumor activity in the clinic. However, many excellent analyses of the results from the NCI 60 cell lines have led to some very provocative and useful research tools.

As an initial example of a unique use of results from the 60 cell line screening, Paull and colleagues described a method (which they dubbed the COMPARE program) in which a compound evaluated in the 60 cell line screen is used as a seed and the COMPARE program is used to detect the compounds that have similar patterns (or fingerprints) of activity against the 60 cell lines.[28] A correlation coefficient is then calculated to describe the closeness of other agents to the pattern of activity of the seed compound. It appears that if two compounds have similar correlation coefficients, this will predict for comparable mechanisms of action of the compounds or even the existence of a similar intracellular target, as described by Weinstein and colleagues.[29] If the correlation coefficient of a new, active compound is low compared with the compounds evaluated in the NCI screen, it might substantially increase interest in the new compound as it is very likely to have a new (unique) mechanism of action.

Of additional importance, and of great interest to the cancer research community, the NCI 60 cell lines continue to be characterized for presence or absence of specific targets (kinases, telomerase, mismatch repair proteins, receptors).[30–32] The more precise characterization of these lines is relatively certain to help the evaluation of compounds in the lines.

Other preclinical models explored by the NCI for evaluating compounds that deserve mention were models put in place to evaluate agents against tumors taken directly from patients. There were two systems, including the in vitro human tumor cloning assay (HTCA) and the in vivo subrenal capsule system (SRC). The NCI began a program using the HTCA to screen compounds for activity against tumors taken directly from patients and growing as colonies in soft agar.[33] Although initial correlations were promising between agents detected as active in the HTCA and having subsequent antitumor activity in the clinic, the HTCA was deemed as too logistically difficult to use as an up-front screen to evaluate the vast array of compounds. However, several groups of investigators continue to use the HTCA to determine whether an agent should be taken into the clinic against a particular histologic type

Table 39-1 FDA-Approved Anticancer Agents and Their Indications[a]

Generic Name	Tradename (Company)	Indication	Year[b]
Aldesleukin	Proleukin (Chiron)	Adults with metastatic renal cell carcinoma Adults with metastatic melanoma	1992
Alemtuzumab	Campath (Berlex)	Treatment of B-cell chronic lymphocytic leukemia (B-CLL) in patients who have been treated with alkylating agents and who have failed fludarabine therapy	2001
Alitretinoin	Panretin (Ligand)	Topical treatment of cutaneous lesions in patients with AIDS-related Kaposi's sarcoma (KS), not indicated when systemic anti-KS-therapy is required	1999
Altretamine	Hexalen (MGI Pharma)	Single agent in the palliative treatment of patients with persistent or recurrent ovarian cancer following first-line therapy with a cisplatin and/or alkylating agent-based combination	1990
Aminolevulinic acid	Levulan Kerastick (Berlex)	Nonhyperkeratotic actinic keratoses of the face or scalp	1999
Anagrelide	Agrylin (Shire)	Thrombocythemia, secondary to myeloproliferative disorders, to reduce the elevated platelet count and the risk of thrombosis and to ameliorate associated symptoms including thrombohemorrhagic events	1997
Anastrozole	Arimidex (Astra Zeneca)	First-line treatment of postmenopausal women with hormone receptor-positive or hormone receptor unknown locally advanced or metastatic breast cancer. Advanced breast cancer in postmenopausal women with disease progression following tamoxifen therapy Adjuvant treatment of postmenopausal women with hormone receptor-positive early breast cancer	1995
Arsenic trioxide	Trisenox (Cell Therapeutics)	Induction of remission and consolidation in patients with acute promyelocytic leukemia (APL) who are refractory to, or have relapsed from, retinoid and anthracycline chemotherapy and whose APL is characterized by the presence of the t(15;17) translocation or PML/RAR-alpha gene expression	2000
Asparaginase	Elspar (Merck)	Acute lymphocytic leukemia, combination with other chemotherapeutic agents in the induction of remissions in pediatric patients	1978
Bacille Calmette-Guérin (BCG)	TheraCys (Aventis Pasteur) Tice BCG (Organon) PACIS (UroCor)	*TheraCys, Tice* – treatment and prophylaxis of carcinoma in situ (CIS) of the urinary bladder, prophylaxis of primary or recurrent stage Ta and/or T1 papillary tumors following transurethral resection (TUR) *PACIS* – CIS in the absence of an associated invasive cancer of the bladder in the following situations: (1) primary treatment of CIS with or without papillary tumors after TUR, (2) secondary treatment of CIS in patients failing to respond or relapsing after intravesical therapy with other agents, (3) primary or secondary treatment of CIS for patients with medical contraindications to radical surgery	1990
Betamethasone	Celestone, Celestone Soluspan (Schering)	Hypercalcemia associated with cancer, mycosis fungoides, idiopathic thrombocytopenic purpura in adults, secondary thrombocytopenia in adults, erythroblastopenia, palliative management of leukemias and lymphomas in adults, palliative management of acute leukemia of childhood	1961
Bevacizumab	Avastin	In combination with intravenous 5-fluorouracil–based chemotherapy for first-line treatment of patients with metastatic carcinoma of the colon or rectum.	2004
Bexarotene	Targetin (Ligand)	*Oral* – cutaneous manifestations of cutaneous T-cell lymphoma in patients who are refractory to at least one prior systemic therapy *Topical* – patients with cutaneous t-cell lymphoma (stage IA and IB) who have refractory or persistent disease after other therapies or who have not tolerated other therapies	1999
Bicalutamide	Casodex (Astra Zeneca)	Combination therapy with a luteinizing hormone-releasing hormone analog for the treatment of stage D2 metastatic carcinoma of the prostate	1995
Bleomycin	Blenoxane (Bristol-Myers Squibb) Bleomycin (Pharmacia)	Palliative treatment of squamous cell carcinoma: head and neck (including mouth, tongue, tonsil, nasopharynx, oropharynx, sinus, palate lip, buccal, mucosa, gingiva, epiglottis, skin, larynx), penis, cervix, and vulva Palliative treatment of lymphomas: Hodgkin's, reticulum cell sarcoma, lymphosarcoma Palliative treatment of testicular carcinoma: embryonal cell, choriocarcinoma and teratocarcinoma *Blenoxane only* – malignant pleural effusion and prevention of recurrent pleural effusions	1973
Bortezomib	Velcade (Millennium)	Treatment of multiple myeloma patients who have received at least two prior therapies and have demonstrated disease progression on the last therapy Treatment of multiple myeloma patients who have received as least one prior therapy.	2003 2005
Busulfan	Busulfex (Orphan Medical) Myleran (Glaxo SmithKline)	*Busulfex* – combination with cyclophosphamide as a conditioning regimen prior to allogeneic hematopoietic progenitor cell transplantation for chronic myelogenous leukemia *Myleran* – palliative treatment of chronic myelogenous (myeloid, myelocytic, granulocytic) leukemia	1954
Capecitabine	Xeloda (Roche)	Metastatic breast cancer resistant to both paclitaxel and an anthracycline-containing chemotherapy regimen or resistant to paclitaxel and for whom further anthracycline therapy is not indicated	1998
Carboplatin	Paraplatin (Bristol-Myers Squibb)	Initial treatment of advanced ovarian carcinoma in established combination with other approved chemotherapeutic agents Palliative treatment of patients with ovarian carcinoma recurrent after prior chemotherapy, including patients who have been previously treated with cisplatin	1989
Carmustine	BiCNU (Bristol-Myers Squibb)	Palliative therapy as a single agent or in established combination therapy with other approved chemotherapeutic agents in: glioblastoma, brainstem glioma, medulloblastoma, astrocytoma, ependymoma, and metastatic brain tumors Multiple myeloma—in combination with prednisone Hodgkin's disease—as secondary therapy in combination with other approved drugs in patients who relapse while being treated with primary therapy or who fail to respond to primary therapy Non-Hodgkin's lymphomas—as secondary therapy in combination with other approved drugs for patients who relapse while being treated with primary therapy or who fail to respond to primary therapy	1977
Cetuximab	Erbitux (Imclone)	In combination with Irinotecan for the treatment of EGFR expressing, metastatic colorectal carcinoma in patients who are refractory to Irinotecan based chemotherapy.	2004
Chlorambucil	Leukeran (Glaxo SmithKline)	Chronic lymphatic (lymphocytic) leukemia, malignant lymphomas including lymphosarcoma, giant follicular lymphoma, and Hodgkin's disease	1957
Chromic phosphate P-32	Phosphocol P-32 (Mallinckrodt)	Peritoneal or pleural effusions caused by metastatic disease, and may be injected interstitially for the treatment of cancer	1974

(Continued)

Table 39-1 FDA-Approved Anticancer Agents and Their Indications[a] *(Continued)*

Generic Name	Tradename (Company)	Indication	Year[b]
Cisplatin	Platinol-AQ (Bristol-Myers Squibb)	Metastatic testicular tumors: in established combination therapy with other approved chemotherapeutic agents in patients with metastatic testicular tumors who have already received appropriate surgical and/or radiotherapeutic procedures Metastatic ovarian tumors: in established combination therapy with other approved chemotherapeutic agents in patients with metastatic ovarian tumors who have already received appropriate surgical and/or radiotherapeutic procedures; single agent is indicated as secondary therapy in patients with metastatic ovarian tumors refractory to standard chemotherapy who have not previously received cisplatin Advanced bladder cancer: single agent for patients with transitional cell bladder cancer that is no longer amenable to local treatments such as surgery and/or radiotherapy (Nonsmall-cell lung cancer: see gemcitabine, paclitaxel, vinorelbine)	1978
Cladribine	Leustatin (Ortho Bio-Tech)	Active hairy cell leukemia as defined by clinically significant anemia, neutropenia, thrombocytopenia, or disease-related syndrome	1993
Clofarabine	Clolar (Genzyme)	Treatment of pediatric patients 1–21 years old with relapsed or refractory acute lymphoblastic leukemia after at least two prior regimens.	2004
Conjugated estrogens	Premarin (Wyeth-Ayerst)	Breast cancer (for palliation only) in appropriately selected women and men with metastatic disease Advanced androgen-dependent carcinoma of the prostate (for palliation only)	1938
Cortisone	Cortone (Merck)	Hypercalcemia associated with cancer, mycosis fungoides, idiopathic thrombocytopenic purpura in adults, secondary thrombocytopenia in adults, erythroblastopenia, palliative management of leukemias and lymphomas in adults, palliative management of acute leukemia of childhood	1950
Cyclophosphamide	Cytoxan (Bristol-Myers Squibb) Neosar (Pharmacia)	Malignant lymphomas (stages III and IV of the Ann Arbor staging system), Hodgkin's disease, lymphocytic lymphoma (nodular or diffuse), mixed-cell- type lymphoma histiocytic lymphoma, Burkitt's lymphoma Leukemias: chronic lymphocytic leukemia, chronic granulocytic leukemia (it is usually ineffective in acute blastic crisis), acute myelogenous and monocytic leukemia, acute lymphoblastic (stem cell) leukemia in children (cyclophosphamide given during remission is effective in prolonging its duration) Multiple myeloma, mycosis fungoides (advanced disease), neuroblastoma (disseminated disease), adenocarcinoma of the ovary, retinoblastoma, carcinoma of the breast	1959
Cytarabine, liposome	DepoCyt (Chiron)	Intrathecal treatment of lymphomatous meningitis	1999
Cytarabine, ara-C	Cytosar-U (Pharmacia)	Combination with other approved anticancer drugs for remission induction in acute nonlymphocytic leukemia of adults and pediatric patients; it has also been found useful in the treatment of acute lymphocytic leukemia and the blast phase of chronic myelocytic leukemia; intrathecal administration of cytarabine is indicated in the prophylaxis and treatment of meningeal leukemia	1969
Dacarbazine	DTIC-Dome (Bayer)	Metastatic malignant melanoma Hodgkin's disease as a second-line therapy when used in combination with other effective agents	1975
Dactinomycin, actinomycin D	Cosmegen (Merck)	Wilms tumor, rhabdomyosarcoma, carcinoma of testis and uterus, palliative treatment of Ewing's sarcoma and sarcoma botryoides	1964
Daunorubicin	Cerubidine (Bedford)	Combination with other approved anticancer drugs for remission induction in acute nonlymphocytic leukemia (myelogenous, monocytic, erythroid) of adults and for remission induction in acute lymphocytic leukemia of children and adults	1979
Daunorubicin citrate liposome	DaunoXome (Gilead Sciences)	First-line cytotoxic therapy for advanced HIV-associated Kaposi's sarcoma	1996
Denileukin diftitox	Ontak (Ligand)	Patients with persistent or recurrent cutaneous T-cell lymphoma whose malignant cells express the CD25 component of theIL-2-receptor	1999
Dexamethasone	Decadron (Merck)	Hypercalcemia associated with cancer, mycosis fungoides, idiopathic thrombocytopenic purpura in adults, secondary thrombocytopenia in adults, erythroblastopenia, palliative management of leukemias and lymphomas in adults, palliative management of acute leukemia of childhood	1958
Diclofenac	Solaraze (SkyePharma)	Topical treatment of actinic keratoses	2000
Docetaxel	Taxotere (Aventis)	Locally advanced or metastatic breast cancer after failure of prior chemotherapy Locally advanced or metastatic nonsmall-cell lung cancer after failure of prior platinum-based chemotherapy	1996
		In combination with prednisone as a treatment of patients with androgen independent (hormone refractory) metastatic prostate cancer.	2004
		In combination with doxorubicin and cyclophosphamide for the adjuvant treatment of patients with operable node positive breast cancer	2004
Doxorubicin	Adriamycin (Pharmacia) Rubex (Bristol-Myers Squibb)	Acute lymphoblastic leukemia, acute myeloblastic leukemia, Wilms tumor, neuroblastoma, soft tissue and bone sarcomas, breast carcinoma, ovarian carcinoma, transitional cell bladder carcinoma, thyroid carcinoma, gastric carcinoma, Hodgkin's disease, malignant lymphoma, and bronchogenic carcinoma in which the small cell histologic type is the most responsive compared to other cell types.	1974
		In combination with cyclophosphamide as a component of adjuvant therapy in patients with evidence of axillary node tumor involvement following resection of primary breast cancer.	2003
Doxorubicin liposome	Doxil (Alza)	Metastatic carcinoma of the ovary in patients with disease that is refractory to both paclitaxel- and platinum-based chemotherapy regimens AIDS-related Kaposi's sarcoma in patients with disease that has progressed on prior combination chemotherapy or in patients who are intolerant to such therapy	1995
Epirubicin	Ellence (Pharmacia)	Adjuvant therapy in patients with evidence of axillary node tumor involvement following resection of primary breast cancer	1999
Erlotinib	Tarceva (OSI)	Treatment of patients with locally advanced or metastatic nonsmall-cell lung cancer after failure of at least one prior chemotherapy regimen.	2004
Esterified estrogens	Estratab (Solvay) Menest (Monarch)	Breast cancer (for palliation only) in appropriately selected women and men with metastatic disease Advanced androgen-dependent carcinoma of the prostate (for palliation only)	1938

(Continued)

Table 39-1 FDA-Approved Anticancer Agents and Their Indications[a] *(Continued)*

Generic Name	Tradename (Company)	Indication	Year[b]
Estradiol	Estrace (Bristol-Myers Squibb)	Breast cancer (for palliation only) in appropriately selected women and men with metastatic disease Advanced androgen-dependent carcinoma of the prostate (for palliation only)	1938
Estradiol valerate	Delestrogen (Bristol-Myers Squibb)	Advanced androgen-dependent carcinoma of the prostate (for palliation only)	1938
Estramustine	Emcyt (Pharmacia)	Palliative treatment of patients with metastatic and/or progressive carcinoma of prostate	1981
Estrone	Estrone (generic)	Breast cancer (for palliation only) in appropriately selected women and men with metastatic disease Advanced androgen-dependent carcinoma of the prostate (for palliation only)	1938
Ethinyl estradiol	Estinyl (Schering)	Breast cancer (for palliation only) in appropriately selected women	1943
Etoposide	Toposar (Pharmacia) VePesid (Bristol-Myers Squibb)	*Injection* – combination therapy with other approved chemotherapeutic agents in patients with refractory testicular tumors who have already received appropriate surgical, chemotherapeutic and radiotherapeutic therapy *Injection/Oral* – combination with other approved chemotherapeutic agents as first-line treatment in patients with small-cell lung cancer	1983
Etoposide phosphate	Etopophos (Bristol-Myers Squibb)	Combination therapy with other approved chemotherapeutic agents in patients with refractory testicular tumors who have already received appropriate surgical, chemotherapeutic, and radiotherapeutic therapy Combination with other approved chemotherapeutic agents as first-line treatment in patients with small-cell lung cancer	1996
Exemestane	Aromasin (Pharmacia)	Advanced breast cancer in postmenopausal women whose disease has progressed following tamoxifen therapy	1999
Floxuridine	FUDR (Roche)	Palliative management of gastrointestinal adenocarcinoma metastatic to the liver, when given by continuous regional intra-arterial infusion in carefully selected patients who are considered incurable by surgery or other means	1970
Fludarabine phosphate	Fludara (Berlex)	Patients with B-cell chronic lymphocytic leukemia (CLL) who have not responded to or whose disease has progressed during treatment with at least one standard alkylating agent-containing regimen	1991
Fluorouracil	Adrucil (Pharmacia)	Palliative management of carcinoma of the colon, rectum, breast, stomach, and pancreas	1962
Fluorouracil	Efudex (ICN)	Topical treatment of actinic or solar keratoses; in the 5% strength, it is also useful in the treatment of superficial basal cell carcinomas when conventional methods are impractical	1962
Fluorouracil	Fluoroplex (Allergan)	Topical treatment of multiple actinic (solar) keratoses	1962
Fluoxymesterone	Halotestin (Pharmacia)	Palliation of androgen-responsive recurrent mammary cancer in women who are more than 1 year but less than 5 years postmenopausal or who have been proven to have a hormone-dependent tumor as shown by previous beneficial response to castration	1956
Flutamide	Eulexin (Schering)	Combination with LHRH agonists for the management of locally confined stage B2-C and stage D2 metastatic carcinoma of the prostate	1989
Fulvestrant	Faslodex (IPR)	Treatment of hormone receptor-positive metastatic breast cancer in postmenopausal women with disease progression following antiestrogen therapy	2002
Gefitinib	Iressa (AstraZeneca)	As monotherapy for the treatment of patients with locally advanced or metastatic nonsmall-cell lung cancer after failure of both platinum-based and docetaxel chemotherapies	2004
Gemcitabine	Gemzar (Eli Lilly)	Combination with cisplatin for the first-line treatment of patients with inoperable, locally advanced (stage IIIA or IIIB) or metastatic (stage IV) nonsmall-cell lung cancer First-line treatment of patients with locally advanced (nonresectable stage II or stage III) or metastatic (stage IV), adenocarcinoma of the pancreas; Gemzar is indicated for patients previously treated with 5-FU	1996
		In combination with paclitaxel for the first-line treatment of patients with metastatic breast cancer after failure of prior anthracycline-containing adjuvant chemotherapy, unless anthracyclines were clinically contraindicated.	2004
Gemtuzumab ozogamicin	Mylotarg (Wyeth-Ayerst)	Patients with CD33-positive acute myeloid leukemia in first relapse who are 60 years of age or older and who are not considered candidates for cytotoxic chemotherapy	2000
Goserelin acetate	Zoladex (AstraZeneca)	Palliative treatment of advanced carcinoma of the prostate in combination with flutamide for the management of locally confined stage T2b-T4 (stage B2-C) carcinoma of the prostate. Palliative treatment of advanced breast cancer in pre- and perimenopausal women	1989
Granisetron	Kytril (Roche)	Prevention of nausea and vomiting associated with initial and repeat courses of emetogenic cancer therapy, including high-dose cisplatin	1993
Hydrocortisone	Cortef, Solu-Cortef (Pharmacia) Hydrocortone (Merck)	Hypercalcemia associated with cancer, mycosis fungoides, idiopathic thrombocytopenic purpura in adults, secondary thrombocytopenia in adults, erythroblastopenia, palliative management of leukemias and lymphomas in adults, palliative management of acute leukemia of childhood	1951
Hydroxyprogesterone	Hydroxyprogesterone (Schein)	Endometrial cancer	1956
Hydroxyurea	Hydrea (Bristol-Myers Squibb)	Melanoma, resistant chronic myelocytic leukemia, and recurrent, metastatic, or inoperable carcinoma of the ovary Hydroxyurea used concomitantly with irradiation therapy is intended for use in the local control of primary squamous cell (epidermoid) carcinomas of the head and neck, excluding the lip	1967
Ibritumomab tiuxetan	Zevalin (IDEC)	Patients with relapsed or refractory low-grade, follicular, or transformed B-cell non-Hodgkin's lymphoma, including patients with rituximab refractory follicular non-Hodgkin's lymphoma	2002
Idarubicin	Idamycin (Pharmacia)	Combination with other approved antileukemic drugs for the treatment of acute myeloid leukemia in adults; this includes French-American-British classifications M1 through M7.	1990
Ifosfamide	Ifex (Bristol-Myers Squibb)	Combination with certain or other approved antineoplastic agents for third-line chemotherapy of germ cell testicular cancer; it should ordinarily be used in combination with a prophylactic agent for hemorrhagic cystitis, such as mesna	1992
Imatinib mesylate	Gleevec (Novartis)	Patients with Philadelphia chromosome positive chronic myeloid leukemia (CML) in blast crisis, accelerated phase, or in chronic phase after failure of interferon-alpha therapy; Gleevec is also indicated for the treatment of patients with Kit (CD117) positive unresectable and/or metastatic malignant gastrointestinal stromal tumors (GIST)	2001
Interferon alfa-2a	Roferon-A (Roche)	Hairy cell leukemia, AIDS-related Kaposi's sarcoma in patients 18 years of age or older, and chronic phase, Philadelphia chromosome-positive chronic myelogenous leukemia patients who are minimally pretreated (within 1 yr of diagnosis)	1986

(Continued)

Table 39-1 FDA-Approved Anticancer Agents and Their Indications[a] *(Continued)*

Generic Name	Tradename (Company)	Indication	Year[b]
Interferon alfa-2b	Intron A (Schering)	Patients 18 years of age or older with hairy cell leukemia. Adjuvant to surgical treatment in patients 18 years of age or older with malignant melanoma who are free of disease but at high risk of systemic recurrence, within 56 days of surgery Clinically aggressive follicular non-Hodgkin's lymphoma in conjunction with anthracycline-containing combination chemotherapy in patients 18 yr of age or older. Patients 18 yr of age or older with AIDS-related Kaposi's sarcoma	1986
Irinotecan	Camptosar (Pharmacia)	First-line therapy in combination with 5-fluorouracil and leucovorin for patients with metastatic carcinoma of the colon or rectum Metastatic carcinoma of the colon or rectum whose disease has recurred or progressed following initial fluorouracil-based therapy	1996
Letrozole	Femara (Novartis)	First-line treatment of postmenopausal women with hormone receptor positive or hormone receptor unknown locally advanced or metastatic breast cancer; Femara is also indicated for the treatment of advanced breast cancer in postmenopausal women with disease progression following antiestrogen therapy	1997
Leuprolide acetate	Lupron, Lupron Depot (TAP) Viadur (Bayer)	Palliative treatment of advanced prostate cancer	1985
Levothyroxine	Unithroid (Jerome Stevens)	Pituitary TSH suppression—as an adjunct to surgery and radioiodine therapy in the management of thyrotropin-dependent well-differentiated thyroid cancer	2000
Lomustine	CeeNU (Bristol-Myers Squibb)	Single agent in addition to other treatment modalities or in established combination therapy with other approved chemotherapeutic agents in: Brain tumors (both primary and metastatic) in patients who have already received appropriate surgical and/or radiotherapeutic procedures Hodgkin's disease: secondary therapy in combination with other approved drugs in patients who relapse while being treated with primary therapy or who fail to respond to primary therapy	1977
Mechlorethamine	Mustargen (Merck)	Palliative treatment of Hodgkin's disease(stages III and IV), lymphosarcoma, chronic myelocytic or chronic lymphocytic leukemia, polycythemia vera, mycosis fungoides, and bronchogenic carcinoma and metastatic carcinoma resulting in effusion	1949
Medroxyprogesterone	Depo-Provera (Pharmacia)	Adjunctive therapy and palliative treatment of inoperable, recurrent, and metastatic endometrial or renal carcinoma	1959
Medroxyprogesterone	Provera (Pharmacia)	To reduce the incidence of endometrial hyperplasia in nonhysterectomized postmenopausal women receiving 0.625 mg conjugated estrogen	1959
Megestrol acetate	Megace (Bristol-Myers Squibb)	Palliative treatment of advanced carcinoma of the breast or endometrium	1971
Melphalan	Alkeran (Glaxo SmithKline)	*Oral* – palliative treatment of multiple myeloma and nonresectable epithelial carcinoma of the ovary *Injection* – palliative treatment of patients with multiple myeloma for whom oral therapy is not appropriate	1964
Mercaptopurine	Purinethol (Glaxo SmithKline)	Remission induction and maintenance therapy of acute lymphatic leukemia Acute myelogenous (and acute myelomonocytic) leukemia	1953
Methotrexate sodium	Methotrexate (Immunex)	Treatment of gestational choriocarcinoma, chorioadenoma destruens, and hydatidiform mole In acute lymphocytic leukemia, methotrexate is indicated in the prophylaxis of meningeal leukemia and is used in maintenance therapy in combination with other chemotherapeutic agents; methotrexate is also indicated in the treatment of meningeal leukemia. Methotrexate is used alone or in combination with other anticancer agents in the treatment of breast cancer, epidermoid cancers of the head and neck, advanced mycosis fungoides, and lung cancer, particularly squamous cell and small cell types; methotrexate is also used in combination with other chemotherapeutic agents in the treatment of advanced stage non-Hodgkin's lymphomas Methotrexate in high doses followed by leucovorin rescue in combination with other chemotherapeutic agents is effective in prolonging relapse-free survival in patients with nonmetastatic osteosarcoma who have undergone surgical resection or amputation for the primary tumor	1953
Methoxsalen	8-MOP (ICN) Uvadex (Therakos)	Photopheresis in the palliative treatment of the skin manifestations of cutaneous T-cell lymphoma in persons who have not been responsive to other forms of treatment	1954
Methylprednisolone	Depo-Medrol, Medrol, Solu-Medrol (Pharmacia)	Hypercalcemia associated with cancer, mycosis fungoides, idiopathic thrombocytopenic purpura in adults, secondary thrombocytopenia in adults, erythroblastopenia, palliative management of leukemias and lymphomas in adults, palliative management of acute leukemia of childhood	1957
Methyltestosterone	Android, Testred (ICN)	Secondarily in women with advancing inoperable metastatic (skeletal) mammary cancer who are 1 to 5 yr postmenopausal	1939
Metrosyne	Demser (Merck)	Chronic treatment of patients with malignant pheochromocytoma	1979
Mitomycin, mitomycin-c	Mutamycin (Bristol-Myers Squibb)	Disseminated adenocarcinoma of the stomach or pancreas in proven combinations with other approved chemotherapeutic agents and as palliative treatment when other modalities have failed	1974
Mitotane	Lysodren (Bristol-Myers Squibb)	Inoperable adrenal cortical carcinoma of both functional and nonfunctional types	1970
Mitoxantrone	Novantrone (Immunex)	In combination with corticosteroids as initial chemotherapy for the treatment of patients with pain related to advanced hormone refractory prostate cancer. In combination with other approved drug(s) in the initial therapy of acute nonlymphocytic leukemia in adults; this category includes myelogenous , promyelocytic, monocytic, and erythroid acute leukemias	1987
Nandrolone phenpropionate	nandrolone (generic)	Secondarily in women with advanced inoperable metastatic (skeletal) mammary cancer who are 1 or 5 yr postmenopausal	1959
Nilutamide	Nilandron (Aventis)	Combination with surgical castration for the treatment of metastatic prostate cancer (stage D2)	1996
Octreotide acetate	Sandostatin, Sandostatin LAR Depot (Novartis)	Severe diarrhea and flushing episodes associated with metastatic carcinoid tumors Profuse watery diarrhea associated with vasoactive intestinal peptide (VIP)-secreting tumors	1988
Oprelvekin	Neumega (Genetics Institute)	Prevention of severe thrombocytopenia and the reduction of the need for platelet transfusions following myelosuppressive chemotherapy in patients with nonmyeloid malignancies who are at high risk of severe thrombocytopenia	2002

(Continued)

Table 39-1 FDA-Approved Anticancer Agents and Their Indications[a] *(Continued)*

Generic Name	Tradename (Company)	Indication	Year[b]
Oxaliplatin	Eloxatin (Sanofi-Synthelabo)	In combination with infusional 5-FU/LV, is indicated for the treatment of patients with metastatic carcinoma of the colon or rectum whose disease has recurred or progressed during or within 6 months of completion of first-line therapy with the combination of bolus 5-FU/LV and Irinotecan	2002
		In combination with infusional 5-Fluorouracil (5-FU) and Leucovorin (LV) for the treatment of patients previously untreated for advanced colorectal cancer.	2004
		In combination with infusional 5-FU/LV, for the adjuvant treatment of stage III colon cancer patients who have undergone complete resection of the primary tumor	2004
Oxymet holone	Anadrol-50 (Unimed)	Myelofibrosis, hypoplastic anemias owing to the administration of myelotoxic drugs	1960
Paclitaxel	Taxol (Bristol-Myers Squibb)	Treatment of patients with metastatic carcinoma of the ovary after failure of first-line or subsequent chemotherapy	1992
		Treatment of breast cancer after failure of combination chemotherapy for metastatic disease or relapse within 6 months of adjuvant chemotherapy. Prior therapy should have included an anthracycline unless clinically contraindicated	1993
		Second-line therapy for AIDS related Kaposi's sarcoma	1997
		First line treatment in advanced carcinoma of the ovary in combination with cisplatin	1998
		In combination with cisplatin indicated for the first-line treatment of nonsmall-cell lung cancer in patients who are not candidates for potentially curative surgery and/or radiation therapy	1998
		Adjuvant treatment of node-positive breast cancer administered sequentially to standard doxorubicin-containing combination chemotherapy. The benefit has been demonstrated only in patients with estrogen and progesterone receptor negative tumors	1999
Paclitaxel, protein-bound particles	Abraxane (AM Bioscience)	Treatment of breast cancer after failure of combination chemotherapy for metastatic disease or relapse within 6 months of adjuvant chemotherapy. Prior therapy should have included an anthracycline unless clinically contraindicated.	2005
Pegaspargase	Oncaspar (Enzon)	Patients with acute lymphoblastic leukemia who require L-asparaginase in their treatment regimen but have developed hypersensitivity to the native forms of L-asparaginase	1994
Pemetrexed	Alimta (Lilly)	Alimta in combination with cisplatin is indicated for the treatment of patients with malignant pleural mesothelioma whose disease is either unresectable or who are otherwise not candidates for curative surgery.	2004
		ALIMTA as a single-agent is indicated for the treatment of patients with locally advanced or metastatic nonsmall-cell lung cancer after prior chemotherapy.	
Pentostatin	Nipent (SuperGen)	Single-agent treatment of both untreated and alpha-interferon-refractory hairy cell leukemia patients with active disease as defined by clinically significant anemia, neutropenia , thrombocytopenia, or disease-related symptoms	1991
Plicamycin	Mithracin (Bayer)	Hospitalized patients with malignant tumors of the testis in whom successful treatment by surgery and/or radiation is impossible	1970
		Hypercalcemia and hypercalciuria associated with a variety of advanced neoplasms	
Polifeprosan	Gliadel (Aventis)	Adjunct to surgery to prolong survival in patients with recurrent glioblastoma multiforme for whom surgical resection is indicated	1996
Porfimer sodium	Photofrin (Axcan Scandipharm)	Palliation of patients with completely or partially obstructing esophageal cancer who, in the opinion of their physicians, cannot be satisfactorily treated with Nd:YAG laser therapy	1995
		Reduction of obstruction and palliation of symptoms in patients with completely or partially obstructing endobronchial nonsmall-cell lung cancer (NSCLC)	
		Microinvasive endobronchial NSCLC in patients for whom surgery and radiotherapy are not indicated	
Prednisolone	Prelone (Muro)	Hypercalcemia associated with cancer, mycosis fungoides, idiopathic thrombocytopenic purpura in adults, secondary thrombocytopenia in adults, erythroblastopenia, palliative management of leukemias and lymphomas in adults, palliative management of acute leukemia of childhood	1955
Prednisone	Deltasone (Pharmacia)	Hypercalcemia associated with cancer, mycosis fungoides, idiopathic thrombocytopenic purpura in adults, secondary thrombocytopenia in adults, erythroblastopenia, palliative management of leukemias and lymphomas in adults, palliative management of acute leukemia of childhood	1955
		(Multiple myeloma: see carmustine)	
Procarbazine	Matulane (Sigma-Tau)	Combination with other anticancer drugs for the treatment of stage III and IV Hodgkin's disease.	1969
		Matulane is used as part of the MOPP (nitrogen mustard, vincristine, procarbazine, prednisone) regimen	
Progesterone	Prometrium (Solvay)	Prevention of endometrial hyperplasia in nonhysterectomized postmenopausal women who are receiving conjugated estrogen tablets	1939
Rituximab	Rituxan (Genentech, IDEC)	Relapsed or refractory low grade or follicular, CD20 positive, B-cell non-Hodgkin's lymphoma	1997
Samarium-153 lexidronam pentasodium	Quadramet (Berlex)	Relief of pain in patients with confirmed osteoblastic metastatic bone lesions that enhance on radionuclide bone scan	1997
Sodium iodide I-131	Iodotope (Bracco) Sodium Iodide I-131 (CIS-US, Mallinckrodt)	Carcinoma of the thyroid	1957
Sodium phosphate P-32	Sodium Phosphate P-32 (Mallinckrodt)	Polycythemia vera, chronic myelocytic leukemia, chronic lymphocytic leukemia, and palliative treatment of selected patients with multiple areas of skeletal metastases	1952
Streptozocin	Zanosar (Pharmacia)	Metastatic islet cell carcinoma of the pancreas	1982
Strontium-89 chloride	Metastron (Nyomed Amersham)	Relief of bone pain in patients with painful skeletal metastases	1993
Talc	Sclerosol (Bryan)	Prevention of recurrence of malignant pleural effusions in symptomatic patients	1997

(Continued)

Table 39-1 FDA-Approved Anticancer Agents and Their Indications[a] *(Continued)*

Generic Name	Tradename (Company)	Indication	Year[b]
Tamoxifen citrate	Nolvadex (AstraZeneca)	Metastatic breast cancer: tamoxifen is effective in the treatment of metastatic breast cancer in women and men; in premenopausal women with metastatic breast cancer, tamoxifen is an alternative to oophorectomy or ovarian irradiation; available evidence indicates that patients whose tumors are estrogen receptor positive are more likely to benefit from tamoxifen therapy	1977
		Adjuvant treatment of breast cancer: tamoxifen is indicated for the treatment of node-positive breast cancer in postmenopausal women following total mastectomy or segmental mastectomy, axillary dissection, and breast irradiation; tamoxifen is indicated for the treatment of axillary node-negative breast cancer in women following total mastectomy or segmental mastectomy, axillary dissection, and breast irradiation	
		Ductal carcinoma in situ (DCIS): in women with DCIS, following breast surgery and radiation, tamoxifen is indicated to reduce the risk of invasive breast cancer	
		Reduction in breast cancer incidence in high-risk women: tamoxifen is indicated to reduce the incidence of breast cancer in women at high risk of breast cancer	
Temozolomide	Temodar (Schering)	Adult patients with refractory anaplastic astrocytoma, ie, patients at first relapse who have experienced disease progression on a drug regimen containing a nitrosourea and procarbazine	1999
		Adult patients with newly diagnosed glioblastoma multiforme concomitantly with radiotherapy and then as maintenance treatment	2005
Teniposide	Vumon (Bristol-Myers Squibb)	Combination with other approved anticancer agents for induction therapy in patients with refractory childhood acute lymphoblastic leukemia	1992
Testolactone	Teslac (Bristol-Myers Squibb)	Adjunctive therapy in the palliative treatment of advanced or disseminated breast cancer in postmenopausal women when hormonal therapy is indicated; it may also be used in women who were diagnosed as having had disseminated breast carcinoma when premenopausal, in whom ovarial function has been subsequently terminated	1970
Testosterone enanthate	Delatestryl (Bio-Technology General)	Secondarily in women with advancing inoperable metastatic (skeletal) mammary cancer who are 1 to 5 yr postmenopausal	1939
Thioguanine	Tabloid (Glaxo SmithKline)	Remission induction, remission consolidation, and maintenance therapy of acute nonlymphatic leukemias; although thioguanine is one of several agents with activity in the treatment of the chronic myelogenous leukemia, more objective responses are observed with busulfan, and therefore busulfan is usually regarded as the preferred drug	1966
Thiotepa	Thioplex (Immunex)	Adenocarcinoma of the breast and ovary	1959
		Intracavitary effusions secondary to diffuse or localized neoplastic diseases of various serosal cavities.	
		Superficial papillary carcinoma of the urinary bladder	
		Although now largely superseded by other treatments, thiotepa has been effective against other lymphomas, such as lymphosarcoma and Hodgkin's disease	
Topotecan	Hycamtin (Glaxo SmithKline)	Metastatic carcinoma of the ovary after failure of initial or subsequent chemotherapy	1996
		Small-cell lung cancer-sensitive disease after failure of first-line chemotherapy	
Toremifene citrate	Fareston (Schering)	Metastatic breast cancer in postmenopausal women with estrogen-receptor positive or unknown tumors	1997
Tositumomab	Bexxarf (Corixa)	Treatment of patients with CD20 positive, follicular, non-Hodgkin's lymphoma, with and without transformation, whose disease is refractory to rituximab and has relapsed following chemotherapy	2003
Trastuzumab	Herceptin (Genentech)	Single agent for the treatment of patients with metastatic breast cancer whose tumors overexpress the HER-2 protein and who have received one or more chemotherapy regimens for their metastatic disease, combination with paclitaxel for treatment of patients with metastatic breast cancer whose tumors overexpress the HER-2 protein and who have not received chemotherapy for their metastatic disease	1998
Tretinoin	Vesanoid (Roche)	Induction of remission in patients with acute promyelocytic leukemia, French-American-British classification M3 (including the M3 variant), characterized by the presence of the t(15;17) translocation and/or the presence of the *PML/RARalpha* gene who are refractory to, or who have relapsed from, anthracycline chemotherapy or for whom anthracycline-based chemotherapy is contraindicated	1971
Triamcinolone	Aristocort (Fujisawa)	Hypercalcemia associated with cancer, mycosis fungoides, idiopathic thrombocytopenic purpura in adults, secondary thrombocytopenia in adults, erythroblastopenia, palliative management of leukemias and lymphomas in adults, palliative management of acute leukemia of childhood	1957
Triptorelin pamoate	Trelstar Depot (Pharmacia)	Palliative treatment of advanced prostate cancer	2000
Valrubicin	Valstar (Medeva)	Intravesical therapy of BCG-refractory carcinoma in situ of the urinary bladder in patients for whom immediate cystectomy would be associated with unacceptable morbidity or mortality	1998
Vinblastine	Velban (Eli Lilly)	Palliative treatment of: frequently responsive malignancies: generalized Hodgkin's disease (stage III and IV, Ann Arbor modification of Rye staging system), lymphocytic lymphoma (nodular and diffuse, poorly and well differentiated), histiocytic lymphoma, mycosis fungoides (advanced stages), advanced carcinoma of the testis, Kaposi sarcoma, Letterer-Siwe disease (histiocytosis X)	1961
		Less frequently responsive malignancies: choriocarcinoma resistant to other chemotherapeutic agents, carcinoma of the breast unresponsive to appropriate endocrine surgery and hormonal therapy	
Vincristine	Oncovin (Eli Lilly) Vincasar (Pharmacia)	Acute leukemia	1963
		Combination with other oncolytic agents in Hodgkin's disease, non-Hodgkin's malignant lymphomas (lymphocytic, mixed cell, histiocytic, undifferentiated nodular, and diffuse types), rhabdomyosarcoma, neuroblastoma, and Wilms tumor	
Vinorelbine	Navelbine (Glaxo SmithKline)	Single agent or in combination with cisplatin for the first-line treatment of ambulatory patients with unresectable, advanced NSCLC; in patients with stage IV NSCLC, Navelbine is indicated as a single agent or in combination with cisplatin; in stage III NSCLC, Navelbine is indicated in combination with cisplatin	1994

[a]Please refer to approved product label for exact language regarding the approved indications.
[b]Date first FDA approval was received (any indication).

Table 39-2 The Most Predictive Animal Models: The National Cancer Institute Experience 1978–1982

Reasonably Predictive[a]	Not Predictive
P388 leukemia (mouse)	Lewis lung (mouse)
L1210 leukemia (mouse)	CD8 breast
B16 melanoma (mouse)	Co38 colon
MX-1 mammary[b]	LX1[b] lung
	CX1 colon[b]

Adapted from Staquet MJ et al.[21]
[a]Especially with regression of established tumors.
[b]Xenografts.

of malignancy (eg, gemcitabine against pancreatic cancer).[34,35] The SRC assay is a system in which tumors are taken directly from patients and are placed under the renal capsule in mice. New agents are administered to the mice to determine the effects of the agent against tumors growing under the renal capsule.[36] Once again, although initial correlations between activity in the SCR system and the clinical activity of the compound appeared promising, the logistics of evaluating a large number of compounds in this in vivo system were deemed to be too daunting. Thus, attempts using these two methods (the HTCA and the SCR systems) to evaluate large numbers of new compounds against tumors taken directly from patients (and thus not corrupted by in vitro passage in culture) were not pursued based on logistic problems (basically, the unavailability of tumors taken from patients and the technical challenges of the assays—ie, lots of manpower required). However, most investigators would agree that it would be helpful to have some way to evaluate a large number of compounds against tumors taken directly from patients.

Mechanism-Based Drug Discovery and Evaluation With the explosion of molecular techniques and knowledge of cell biology, there is now an incredible array of new methods for discovery of potential targets present in tumor cells versus normal cells.

The most recent spectacular example of a mechanistically based approach to therapy is the development of the new agent imatinib, which has substantial activity against chronic myelogenous leukemia and against gastrointestinal stromal sarcomas. To put the timeline for development of imatinib into perspective, the basic biology ground work for the discovery and development of imatinib actually began with the discovery of the Philadelphia chromosome in chronic myeloid leukemias (CMLs) in 1960.[37]

This was actually the first consistent chromosomal abnormality discovered in any type of cancer. The abnormality is a translocation involving chromosomes 9 and 22.[38] Work done from 1990 to 1993 documented that the translocation caused the *ABL* gene on the chromosome 9 (a nonreceptor tyrosine kinase) to move next to the *BCR* (breakpoint cluster region) gene on chromosome 22. This translocation codes the BCR-ABL protein p210 BCR-ABL, which is a 210-kDa transforming protein tyrosine kinase constitutively expressed and responsible for about 95% of patients with CML.[39,40] This abnormal tyrosine kinase does not exist in normal cells of the patients; therefore, it was an excellent target for development of an agent with activity against CML.

Screening was conducted to find compounds with specific activity against the BCR-ABL tyrosine kinase, and the agent (CGP57148, aka STI 571, imatinib) was found to be the most selective inhibitor by targeting the adenosine triphosphate binding site (ATP-pocket) of the enzyme.[41] The agent was further investigated in vitro and in vivo and was found to be selectively toxic to BCR-ABL–positive cells.[41–43] Phase I and II trials from 1999 to 2000 documented marked clinical activity of Gleevec against CML, particularly in the chronic phase.[44,45] As noted above, this impressive example of drug development really spanned nearly 40 years from identification of the chromosomal abnormality until documentation of clinical activity of a compound against the disease (10 years if one starts counting from the time of discovery of the target, the p120 BCR, ABL tyrosine kinase). Of note, additional work has shown that imatinib also has substantial activity against gastrointestinal stromal sarcomas, which possess abnormalities in the c-*kit* oncogene.[46] However, subsequent work showed that imatinib is not a selective inhibitor of BCR-ABL but that the compound inhibits, among others, the receptors for platelet-derived growth factor (c-sis) and macrophage colony-stimulating factor (c-fms) and that it appears to modulate diabetic nephropathy and liver fibrosis in preclinical models.[47–50]

Although not within the scope of this chapter, a variety of other mechanism-based therapeutics has also demonstrated substantial clinical antitumor activity (antiestrogens, antiandrogens, aromatase inhibitors, monoclonal antibodies to CD20, CD52, HER-2/*neu*, EGFR, and most recently the angiogenesis inhibitors particularly targeting the vascular endothelial growth factor [VEGF], etc). However, at the time of the writing of this chapter, there are also some disappointments in the area of targeting. For example, the farnesyl transferase inhibitors that have been developed to target tumors with mutations in *ras* have not shown activity against pancreatic cancer, even though they have clear clinical activity against breast cancer and acute leukemias, where *ras* mutations are not thought to be critical to the development or progression of either disease.[51–53] Another example of difficulties with targeting is the finding that despite the up-regulation of the epidermal growth factor receptor (EGFR) in a number of malignancies, the activity of small molecule inhibitors of the EGFR kinase or monoclonal antibodies to the EGFR do not appear to correlate with the increased expression of EGFR (at least by currently available methods of measuring the receptor/ kinase).[54] However, some recent brilliant work has described the fact that specific receptor mutations may help differentiate between sensitive and resistant tumors.[55–57]

Clearly, there is a great deal of work to do if targeted therapy is to succeed in major tumor types. In a recent piece of work, Druker and Lydon outlined the lessons learned from the development of imatinib.[58] These lessons provide guidelines for thinking about improved mechanism-based approaches, including the following:

1. Identification of an appropriate target molecule for drug development. The identification of the BCR-ABL tyrosine kinase as the kinase to cause CML (ie, a single molecular defect as a target) was important. The kinase was a "disease gene." For success, one probably should have a target that is critical to the disease process.
2. Availability of a validated surrogate endpoint that can be easily measured in patients to ensure that the new agent is indeed interfering with the desired target and has the desired clinical effects. For CML, this is the Philadelphia chromosome, which is monitored in blood cells (and by blood counts).
3. Improvements in techniques important for drug designs (eg, crystallography, molecular modeling) to optimize the selectivity (specificity) of compounds.

There is no question that with improvements in our understanding of the working of the cell, there will be continued efforts at developing mechanism-based agents.[58–62] However, given the terrific amount of work and substantial resources necessary to clinically develop a new agent, it is very critical that targets are selected wisely.[63]

In addition to targeting the tumor cells, it is now clear that targeting the environment of the tumor cells is taking on a whole new importance. The area of angiogenesis has given all clinicians a sense of optimism given the finding that the monoclonal antibody bevacizumab, directed against VEGF, has substantially improved (when used with chemotherapeutics) the survival of patients with colorectal cancer, nonsmall-cell lung cancer, and breast cancer. It is clear the agent also has single agent activity against renal cell and ovarian cancers.[64–68] Small molecules that target VEGF or platelet-derived growth factor (PDGF) pathways to attack the angiogenic process such as SU 11428 and BAY 43-9006 are also demonstrating important clinical antitumor activity.[69,70] Despite these unique mechanisms of action, all new agents affecting the tumor environment will still require the normal drug development process as outlined in this chapter.

It also remains of unchallenged importance that mechanism-based drug development and clinical serendipity must continue to be integrated and that only the combination of both optimize drug development strategies.

Sources of Compounds to Evaluate against Targets There is no question that the most rational way to develop a new agent against a target is to understand the crystal structure of that target and rationally design an agent to interact with that target.[58,59,63] However, for a vast majority of these targets, there is not a crystal structure identified. Fortunately, there can usually be a method developed to aid in identifying inhibitors of your targets by using molecular screening.[71]

Therefore, it is necessary for a drug development team to have access to major libraries of compounds to use against their target in a high-throughput system.

The NCI has always been a key resource for libraries of compounds, including natural products.[72] Most recently, the NCI has made the NCI Diversity Library <http://dtp.nci.nih.gov/branches/dscb/diversity_explanation.html> available to investigators. In addition, there are a number of commercial libraries available for investigator use.

One of the most interesting new methods that has become available to find initial leads against a target is a new method developed by Kauvar and colleagues called the TRAP assay.[73,74] TRAP stands for Target Recorded Affinity Profiling (or affinity fingerprinting). The theory behind the TRAP assay is that the compounds are characterized by biologic properties (their affinities to a panel of 8 to 20 reference proteins) rather than chemical structures. With the TRAP method, the number of candidate drugs can be relatively simply reduced from tens of thousands to only a few hundred that are then directly screened against the target-of-interest. If the early promise of the TRAP method is sustained, it will represent a considerable advance in rapidly finding leads against any new target. However, the overall impact on speed and quality of drug development by high-throughput assay has not yet been confirmed by structured analyses.

If one is developing a biologic agent against a cell surface receptor or against a small factor, the ability to produce a humanized monoclonal antibody appears to enable a more straightforward approach with a higher likelihood of success compared with the development of a small molecule.

PREPARATION OF AGENTS FOR CLINICAL TRIALS

Formulation Pharmaceutics or the formulation of a compound for preclinical pharmacology, toxicology, and clinical trials is an often overlooked but very important aspect of drug development. It is very desirable to have the best formulation in place that you plan to use in clinical trials before proceeding with animal pharmacology and toxicology.[75]

Difficult formulations have often led to prolonged development programs that have occasionally caused such difficulties that development of the compound was nearly discontinued. This was certainly the case with paclitaxel, which requires for solubilization a difficult Cremophor-containing combination that may result in idiosyncratic reactions in some patients.[76] A multitude of new anticancer agents (in addition to paclitaxel) have had significant formulation problems, including etoposide (solved by a formulation using 20 mg etoposide, 2 mg citric acid, 30 mg benzyl alcohol, 80 mg modified polysorbate 80/Tween 80, 650 mg polyethylene glycol 300, and 30.5% [V/V] alcohol), CPT-11 (topoisomerase I inhibitor) (solved by using a prodrug that is broken down by carboxylesterase in patients' serum and tumors), docetaxel (solved by using a formulation of polysorbate 80), geldanamycin, and several others. If one requires an exotic formulation for intravenous use, there may be a major delay in the start of clinical trials. In general, only formulations that have already been used in patients should be used to formulate a new agent.

Another major question that frequently arises in the formulation process is whether an oral route of administration would be preferable over an intravenous route. In general, for cytotoxic agents, there is a worry that there is a much greater chance for wide variability in the gastrointestinal absorption of oral agents. This variability could lead to unpredictable and potentially serious side effects in some patients and not in others. In addition, patient compliance with oral drug intake has been questioned, particularly if these drugs can cause nausea or vomiting. Therefore, in general, even if an agent can be formulated for both intravenous and oral use, it is deemed preferable to develop the intravenous formulation first. This allows one to carefully determine the pharmacology of the compound in a situation in which absorption is not an issue. An exception to this is when the compound has great schedule dependency in its preclinical activity work-up. In that situation, an oral formulation may be more desirable.[77] Also, if the drug is predicted to be taken repeatedly (eg, daily) for a prolonged period of time, development of an oral application may be advantageous. Finally, use of the oral route may now also be desirable for some of the less toxic noncytotoxic agents.

Development of an Assay for a Pharmacodynamic Endpoint (Surrogate Marker) The development of new anticancer agents has, to date, for the most part been empiric. More specifically, there has not been a prior emphasis on ensuring that the new agent actually affected the target it was designed to hit. With more mechanism-based drug design, it has been recommended to try to have some assay in place to determine whether the agent is having the desired effect on the target (ie, a pharmacodynamic endpoint). Since it is plausible to assume that any compound exerts a variety of biological effects, such an assay, of course, may not reflect the totality of a drug's biochemical or clinical properties.

This area is in its infancy, but there are some instances where assays for pharmacodynamic endpoints are being developed. For example, for the development of farnesyl transferase inhibitors, in the absence of monitoring farnesyl transferase activity in the serum or in tumor cells, there was an emphasis on analyzing inhibition of processing of farnesylated proteins such as prelamin or HDJ2 in buccal mucosa cells or in blood mononuclear cells.[78,79] Hidalgo and colleagues have also measured phosphorylation of the EGFR in skin biopsies in patients receiving EGFR antagonists.[80] It is extremely important that these surrogate markers accompany mechanism-based drug development. Without these markers, their development will be confusing, and it will not be known whether it was an inappropriate target or whether the new agent just did not affect the target (for pharmacokinetic and a variety of other possible reasons) if the compound failed.

Animal Pharmacology Animal pharmacology studies have rarely been a major part of the development of a new anticancer agent (at least in the preparation of an investigational new drug (IND) application. The exception to this is, of course, with oral anticancer agents for which bioavailability studies are required. Other important pieces of information that can be learned from pharmacology studies in animals can include (1) organ distribution of the agent, including penetration and dwell time in tumors (particularly useful for compounds that are formulated in liposomes or are new compounds formulated in nanoparticles encapsulated in albumin); and (2) penetration into the central nervous system, or other sanctuaries.[81,82]

One other very powerful piece of information that can be gleaned from animal pharmacology was described by Collins and colleagues.[83] This often (unfortunately) forgotten piece of work demonstrated that there was a direct relationship between the concentration × time (C × T) product at the LD_{10} in mice and the C × T product at the maximally tolerated dose (MTD) in patients.[83] Essentially (based on mg/m^2 basis), the C × T in mouse = C × T in humans. This important relationship appears to hold up across most animal species and can be used as a target for dose escalation in phase I trials with a new agent in patients (see below). Work by others has confirmed the relationship and has documented how that relationship can be used to determine which serum concentrations of agents will be achieved in patients (and should therefore be used in in-vitro model systems).[84,85]

Animal Toxicology Studies These studies are a critical part of any drug development program. In general, the models used for toxicology studies to date (mouse, rat, or beagle dog, used because of a biliary system closer to human) have given an excellent safety record for the development of new anticancer agents (eg, there essentially have been no catastrophes in the initial phase I clinical trials in patients). One area in which one must be a bit more careful is in the area of nucleosides and antimetabolites. As an example, the starting dose for the agent fludarabine phosphate was chosen too high, and substantial bone marrow toxicity was noted in the first dose level in patients, presumably owing to the fact that fludarabine requires activation by the enzyme deoxycytidine kinase and the levels of this enzyme are much higher in human cancer cells than they are in mouse and canine marrow cells.[86] Pemetrexed (MTA, LY231514), a multitargeted enzyme inhibitor recently approved for the treatment of patients with mesothelioma and nonsmall-cell lung cancer, had a similar problem, but with worse toxicities in animals than in patients.[87] Therefore, investigators should be alert about the possibility of discordance between animals and humans when examining results of animal toxicity studies with nucleoside analogs or other antimetabolites.

As noted above, the usual animal species required for formal toxicology studies is either a mouse or a rat plus the beagle dog.[88] For monoclonal antibodies and other biologics, a primate model is frequently required. An excellent review of toxicity requirements by the US Food and Drug Administration (FDA) has been published by DeGeorge and colleagues.[88] In Europe, there is a movement to use only two murine species (mouse and rat) as a toxicology package necessary to begin a phase I trial in patients.[89] However, if the tolerable doses in those species (based on a mg/m^2 basis) are widely divergent, additional toxicology studies in the dog are a necessity before beginning the phase I clinical trial in patients.

In general, the animal models used are reliable in predicting certain types of organ toxicities (such as myelosuppression).[90] However, the dog has been noted to be somewhat overpredictive for renal, hepatic, and gastrointestinal toxicities.[91] Neurologic, pancreatic, dermatologic, and pulmonary toxicities are generally not well predicted by the murine and canine models. The models are imperfect in predicting other organ toxicities, and occasionally, toxicities are noted in one species (eg, a murine species) but do not occur in another (eg, the dog). This is often attributable to a difference in metabolism of the agent between the species. If unacceptable toxicities are noted in mice, one should still strongly consider going into dogs or primates as they may not exhibit toxicities reported in murine models. This has been done for a few compounds that were cardiotoxic in the mouse toxicology program, but the dog correctly predicted that no serious cardiac toxicity would be noted in patients.[92] As will be outlined below, the animal toxicology package is most critical to help define the starting doses in patients beginning with the phase I trial of the agent.

Preparation of an IND (Investigational New Drug) Application Before a clinical trial can begin in the United States and most other countries, it is necessary to prepare an IND application and to submit this document to a regulatory agency (eg, the FDA). The necessary components of the IND are as outlined in Table 39-3. The clinical trial can proceed with a new agent if 30 days goes by after filing the IND package and there is no comment by the FDA. Of course, if the FDA requires additional information before the 30-day waiting period expires, that information must be supplied and approved by FDA before the first phase I clinical trial can proceed.

Table 39-3 Content and Component of an IND Application

1. Cover sheet – 1571
   a) Name, address, and telephone number of sponsor, etc
   b) Phase of clinical investigation
   c) Commitment not to begin clinical investigation until an IND is in effect
   d) Institutional Review Board commitment
   e) Commitment to follow all regulation requirements
   f) Name and title of person responsible for monitoring
   g) Name and title of person responsible for safety
   h) Any transfer obligations, ie, Clinical Research Organization
   i) Signature of sponsor
2. Table of contents
3. Introductory statement and general investigational plan
4. Reserved for FDA
5. Investigator's brochure
6. Protocols
7. CMC information
8. Pharmacology and toxicology information
9. Previous human experience with the investigational drug
10. Additional information

CMC = chemistry, manufacturing, and control; FDA = US Food and Drug Administration; IND = investigational new drug
More details can be found at the FDA Web site: <http://www.fda.gov/cder/regulatory/applications/ind_page_1.htm>

EARLY CLINICAL TRIALS

Phase I Clinical Trial This is the first trial of a new agent in patients (or in normal volunteers). Several excellent reviews have been written on phase I trial methodologies.[93–96] The objectives of the first phase I trial in humans differ as to whether the agent is first given to patients or is first given to normal volunteers.

Phase I Trial in Patients versus Normal Volunteers There is a growing interest in conducting initial phase I clinical trials of new anticancer agents in normal volunteers rather than in patients. The number one reason cited for this approach is that the normal volunteers have normal organ function not impaired by malignancy and by prior treatment of their malignancy, as in the case of patients. In addition, normal volunteers would not normally be on other concomitant medications (usually an average of 10 for patients on a phase I trial), which could complicate the pharmacokinetics and/or the side effect profile of a new agent.[97] However, clinicians caring for patients with cancer often view the conduct of the initial phase I trial in normal volunteers as a waste of precious time and a step that delays the administration of a promising agent to the very people who need it: patients with advanced cancer. However, with the development of many new cytostatics that are noncarcinogenic rather than cytotoxic agents, which are often carcinogenic, there is more and more interest in first trying the new agents in normal volunteers—just as is done in other areas of drug development such as cardiology.

For a new agent to even be considered for administration to a normal volunteer, it, of course, must be demonstrated to be noncarcinogenic and nonmutagenic in the appropriate preclinical systems. Then an initial trial in normal volunteers can begin.

The objectives of the initial clinical trial of a new anticancer agent performed in normal volunteers are more limited than if the initial clinical trial is performed in patients with advanced cancer. The objectives include the following:

1. To determine the clinical pharmacology of a single dose of the agent when given at the starting dose (and perhaps at one additional dose level, to ensure linear kinetics for the agent). This clinical pharmacology information would include peak plasma levels, half-lives of the agent, and the area under the curve (AUC) for the agent. In addition, some pharmacodynamic data could be collected, for example, whether the agent hits a target in a particular normal tissue (such as white blood cells).
2. To determine the clinical pharmacology of multiple daily doses (usually not to exceed 5 to 7 days) of the new agent at the starting dose (and perhaps at one additional dose level) to ensure that no accumulation of the agent occurs. This clinical pharmacology of the agent would include peak plasma levels, trough levels, half-lives of the agent, AUC for the agent, and steady-state plasma levels. In addition, some pharmacodynamic data could also be collected, for example, whether the agent was hitting a target in a particular normal tissue (such as white blood cells, buccal mucosal cells, saliva, hair, fingernails).
3. To determine if there are any side effects noted for these low doses of the agent in these volunteers. This is usually done by having a placebo control. This can be done by either a balanced randomization (one normal volunteer receives placebo for every one normal volunteer receiving the new agent) or by an unbalanced randomization (one normal volunteer receiving the placebo for every two or more normal volunteers receiving the new agent).

The thought for using the normal volunteer approach for the initial trials of a new antitumor agent is that the pharmacokinetic data obtained will have less variability than observed in patients with advanced cancer. It is felt that this solid information might actually shorten the phase I clinical trials for the new agent in patients and indeed allow patients with advanced cancer to actually receive more effective doses and schedules of the new agent. That information would give them a better chance of having drug activity against their tumor and subsequent clinical benefit. There can, however, be problems with taking even a new cytostatic agent—even at low doses—into a normal volunteer population. There has been a recent instance in which a cytostatic agent taken into normal volunteers and at low doses of daily administration caused a very severe cutaneous reaction (which had not been seen with the single dose). Although not life-threatening, it was cosmetically severe and actually delayed the administration of the agent to patients. In summary, the administration of new anticancer agents to normal volunteers remains somewhat controversial in oncology drug development circles.

The objectives for a phase I trial in patients with advanced malignancies include the following:

1. To determine the maximum tolerated dose (MTD) of the drug. The MTD is the dose rec-

ommended for subsequent phase II trials of the new agent.

2. To define the qualitative and quantitative toxicities of the new agent. In traditional studies, this is described by grading of toxicities according to internationally accepted tables and by observation of dose-limiting toxicities (DLTs). These tables are regularly updated and are published under <http://ctep.cancer.gov/forms/CTCAEv3.pdf>.
3. To obtain information on the clinical pharmacology of the new agent.
4. To obtain pharmacodynamic information on the new agent (eg, does a specific plasma level of the new agent interact/modulate a particular target). These studies can be done using tissue samples (normal and tumor), peripheral blood cells, skin biopsies, malignant effusions, serum proteins, buccal mucosal cells, or new imaging techniques.
5. To anecdotally document clinical antitumor activity (eg, objective responses, tumor marker decline, clinical benefit).

Selection of Schedule and Route for a Phase I Trial The schedules most commonly explored in phase I trials include (1) single dose repeated every 3 or 4 weeks, (2) daily × 5 administration repeated every 3 or 4 weeks, (3) weekly × 4 repeated every 6 weeks, (4) weekly × 3 repeated every 4 weeks, (5) 120 continuous infusion, and (6) daily × 21 repeated every 28 days. Of course, as more information (eg, pharmacokinetic/pharmacodynamic) becomes available on the new agent, it may become necessary to explore other schedules. The choice of what schedule to use (eg, the choice between a bolus versus a more frequent, eg, daily × 5 or daily × 21 schedule) is most frequently decided based on (1) the schedule—dependency for antitumor activity in the preclinical models; (2) the pharmacokinetics of the agent in the preclinical model (and eventually from data in patients); and (3) very importantly, the mechanism of action and preclinical data regarding the mechanism of action (eg, dwell time for a drug to be "on target" to have an effect). The reader is cautioned that decisions on schedule based on the most active schedule in the preclinical animal models need to take into account the fact that animal tumors have a more rapid doubling time and a much higher growth fraction than do most types of human cancers (other than leukemias or aggressive lymphomas).

As far as the route is concerned, the tried and true method for development of new agents (even if an oral route is possible with the new agent) was to proceed with the first phase I trial by the intravenous route. This intravenous trial could then be followed by the phase I oral trial. This has classically been done because (1) there is certainty of delivery of the agent with the intravenous route (patients with cancer may have abnormalities of their gastrointestinal tracts, they may have low-grade nausea from other medications [eg, pain medication], or swallowing might be difficult for them and compliance is an issue); (2) with the intravenous route, there is no question that the drug is delivered with a chance for the greatest peak plasma levels of the agent; and (3) having the correct intravenous dose first and then proceeding with the oral phase I trial of the agent allows one to assess the bioavailability of the oral form of the agent.

With the introduction of new cytostatic agents, which tend to have more schedule dependence, it is becoming more and more common to develop an agent only using the oral form of the agent (eg, tamoxifen, capecitabine, imatinib, erlotinib). With the oral form of the agent, there is more room for creativity in schedules (eg, daily × 5, 2 days off, daily × 5 and daily × 42). However, one must remember that the schedules used for the phase I trial cannot be greatly different from the schedules used in your animal toxicology package and should be manageable in a more uncontrolled clinical setting after approval of the new agent.

Calculation of the Starting Dose for the Phase I Trial The criteria for calculation of a starting dose include starting using either one-tenth the LD_{10} (or MTD) in the mouse or rat or one-sixth of the toxic dose low (TDL) in the dog. The TDL is defined as the dose in the dog that, if doubled, causes no lethality. The use of either the murine model or the dog to guide the starting dose is decided based on the dose that will give the lower or more conservative starting dose on the schedule planned to be used.[98] Because animal toxicology studies frequently give data on a mg/kg basis, it is critical to scale all doses between animals and humans using a mg/m^2 basis.[99,100] Table 39-4 details the conversion factor suggested by Freireich and colleagues for mg/kg in an animal species to a mg/m^2 scale.[99]

To demonstrate how one would calculate the starting dose for a new agent, we could use the example of the development of the topoisomerase I inhibitor CPT-11.[101] In animal toxicology studies with CPT-11, the most sensitive animal species was the mouse using a weekly schedule. For CPT-11, the MTD in the mouse given CPT-11 on the weekly schedule was 70 mg/kg. Using the conversion factor of 3 (see Table 39-4), the MTD in the mouse on a mg/m^2 level would be 70 mg/kg × 3 = 210 mg/m^2. Then, the starting dose in humans using the mouse information would be one-tenth of the MTD in mouse or one-tenth of 210 mg/m^2 or 21 mg/m^2 given weekly. If the dog had been the most sensitive animal species to CPT-11, we would have used that dog toxicology information to determine our starting dose for CPT-11.

Table 39-4 Conversion Factor for Changing mg/kg to mg/m^2 for Starting Dose in Humans

Animal Model	Appropriate Conversion Factor for Converting mg/kg to mg/m^2
Mouse	3
Rat	6
Monkey	12
Dog	20
Human	37

Adapted from Freireich EJ et al.[99]

Table 39-5 Methods for Dose Escalation in Phase I Trials

Method	Proposed by
Modified Fibonacci	Hansen et al[102]
Doubling method	Gottlieb[103] Freireich (personal communication)
Pharmacologically guided	Collins et al[83]
2 × AUC method	Evans[104]
Geometric mean + extended factor of 2	Erlichman[105]
Continual reassessment (and modified continual reassessment)	O'Quigley et al[106,107] Faries[108]
Accelerated titration design	Simon et al[109]
Selection by patient method	Freedman[111,121]

Methods for Dose Escalation The methods used for dose escalation in phase I trials had classically been the modified Fibonacci search scheme.[95,102] However, as can be seen in Table 39-5, there are now several other methods for escalation of dose in phase I trials that can be used.[103–109] Most of these other methods of dose escalation were developed to try to minimize the number of patients receiving very low, ineffective doses of a new agent to try to improve the ethics of the situation.[110–112]

The "modified Fibonacci" search scheme is the most often used method of dose escalation. However, it can result in the highest number of patients receiving ineffective doses, largely because, whereas the initial dose escalation is substantial, there is eventually a tapering off of the percent dose escalation to just 33% escalations at each subsequent dose level. Table 39-6 details a classic modified Fibonacci dose escalation scheme. The real benefit of starting a phase I clinical trial with a new agent using the modified Fibonacci scheme is that it has a superb record of safety. It is particularly the preferred method when one has an agent that has a steep dose-toxicity curve in the animal toxicology studies with the new agent. With the modified Fibonacci method, there are generally three patients entered at each dose level. This must be done carefully. In general, the first patient (patient 1) at a new dose level is entered on study and observed for 3 weeks. If no toxicities are noted in patient 1, patient 2 on the same dose level is then entered and observed for at least 2 weeks (note that, by that time, patient 1 will be well into his/her second course). If no toxicities are noted in patient 2, patient 3 can be entered after patient 2 is observed for 2 weeks. Although there is always pressure from many quarters to enter patients more quickly into a phase I trial, following this methodology provides the highest degree of safety possible and provides added protection in cases in which the new agent (or its metabolites) has a particularly long half-life or a new agent has nonlin-

Table 39-6 Modified Fibonacci Dose Escalation Scheme in Phase I Trials

n (Starting Dose)	% Increase Above Preceding Dose
n	–
2n	100
3.3n	67
5n	50
7n	40
12n	33
16n	33
etc	33

ear kinetics. One must also be careful and probably use the modified Fibonacci method when one is dealing with an agent that is a prodrug (as was CPT-11) and limited information is available on the active metabolite.

If no dose-limiting toxicity (DLT) (see definition below) is reached at a dose level, the dose is escalated for the next cohort of patients. If only one of three patients at a particular dose level is noted to have a DLT, then up to three more patients can be entered onto that dose level. If two or more patients of three to six patients are noted to have DLT's, then one has exceeded the MTD of the drug. Then additional patients are entered on the preceding dose level to ensure that one has a correct MTD—the dose to be taken into phase II trials with the new agent. It is important to note that there is no real scientific basis for the three patients per dose level used in standard phase I trials.[113] The only rationale for the three patients per dose level is that, to date, it has provided a good safety record for phase I trials.

The next dose escalation method outlined in Table 39-5 is the "doubling method." This was proposed to try to minimize the number of patients entered at ineffective dose levels. This method provides a more rapid dose escalation. Theoretically, it could lead to overshooting the dose with attendant severe toxicities (although one cannot find any examples of problems in the literature). This doubling method of dose escalation (n, 2n, 4n, 8n, 16n ...) is probably now the most commonly used method of dose escalation in phase I trials. Once grade 2 toxicity is noted in a patient at a particular dose level, the dose escalation is reduced to a 50% increase at the next dose level.

The most aggressive concept introduced to try to minimize the number of patients receiving ineffective doses of a new agent is the "continual reassessment" method (CRM) proposed by O'Quigley and colleagues in 1990, repeatedly commented on, and modified by other authors.[106–108,114–116] In this modified continual reassessment method (MCRM), a group of clinicians estimates the lower and higher limits of where clinical toxicities might be noted (based on animal toxicology data). A Bayesian approach is then used to construct a dose-toxicity curve. The phase I trial is started at one-tenth the LD_{10} or MTD in the mouse or at one-third or one-sixth of the TDL in the dog. However, the difference is that only one patient is entered at the first dose level. After the appropriate amount of follow-up (usually 2 to 3 weeks), it is judged whether the patient had toxicities (≥ grade 1). If not, then the dose toxicities curve is consulted to determine the next dose escalation. Dose escalation usually can proceed by doubling the dose as long as the dose is below the estimated MTD (on the dose-toxicity curve). The CRM/MCRM methods have now been in use for some time. There have been a few reviews of the results of trials conducted using the modified continual reassessment method.[117–119] In general, the MCRM does not save the time it takes to complete the phase I trial, nor does it actually substantially decrease the number of patients entered into the phase I trial. However, what it does do is shorten the time it takes to get to a dose that is close to the MTD for the study, and the MCRM helps decrease the number of patients who receive a potentially ineffective (< 80% of the MTD) dose in the context of a phase I study (see response rate information below).

Another method for dose escalation introduced by Simon and colleagues that also uses one patient per dose level is the "accelerated titration" design.[109] They introduced two designs (designs I and II). With design I, cohorts of one patient per dose level are treated with 40% escalations between dose levels. With the first DLT, there is an expansion of the cohort to a total of three new patients. With design II, there is only one patient per dose level, but there are dose escalations of 100% between levels, and with the first DLT, the level is also expanded to three new patients. Then escalation proceeds by 40% increments. On both designs I and II, intrapatient dose escalation is allowed if patients had grade 0 to 1 toxicity on the prior course. It is of note that very few groups advocate dose escalation within patients.[120] Dose escalation within patients can be confusing, particularly if there are cumulative toxicities with an agent (as was seen with the nitrosoureas). What is generally agreed on in this area is that if an individual patient on a phase I trial is having a beneficial effect with a new agent and is still receiving a low dose of that new agent, the patient should at least be offered the opportunity to receive a higher dose of the agent that is one level below a dose that has been deemed as safe in the phase I trial. The key is keeping the phase I patient informed of where the study is and what the safety (and efficacy) has been at higher dose levels. Unfortunately, the reality of the situation is that the average number of courses that patients receive on a phase I trial is only about two courses before they have rapid progression of their disease. This rigid progression of disease rarely permits intrapatient dose escalations.

Another phase I dose escalation methodology that is now infrequently used is the method proposed in1990 by Collins and colleagues.[83] This method is also known as the "pharmacologically guided dose escalation" method. The method is based on an important piece of work showing that the area under the C × T plasma disappearance curve (AUC) at the LD_{10} (or MTD) in the mouse is equal to the AUC at the MTD in humans. Basically, that finding provides the investigators with a target AUC. In practice, at each dose level, an AUC is determined for patients receiving that dose of the new agent. The AUC at that level is then used to determine what the next dose escalation will be (if the agent has linear kinetics). Use of this method for pharmacologically guided dose escalation requires real-time pharmacokinetics, which is sometimes problematic in a clinical situation. However, it can lead to more aggressive dose escalations. There have been some suggested improvements in the methodology that has been implemented by some phase I clinical trial groups.[118]

The other dose escalation method outlined in Table 39-5 that is of interest is the method suggested by Freedman and followed up by Daugherty and colleagues in 1998.[111,121,122] Basically, with this method, patients who are considering entry into a phase I trial are given the range of doses that are planned to be explored (usually ranging between 0.1 and 1.0 times the LD_{10} in the mouse or one-sixth to one-third of the TDL to 1.0 × TDL in the dog). Patients are then given the opportunity to select the dose that they feel they should be given. This introduces the ability of *patients* (facing the certainty that their cancer will kill them) to take control of the situation and *select their own dose*. Once the patient has received that dose, the next patient could select a dose that is higher than that. Although this may appear to be a somewhat dangerous approach, at least in one reported clinical trial it has proven to be safe enough.[122] However, in that initially reported experience (using a phase I clinical trial of a combination of agents), the authors felt that this method actually resulted in too many patients receiving lower doses of the agent (not because patients were not aggressive in selecting their doses, but because a clinical response was noted at a low-dose level, and patients hearing that opted to receive the lower dose, which, with additional experience, showed no additional activity, therefore, eventually, further dose escalations were needed).[122]

Definitions of MTD and DLTs The classic definition of an MTD is the highest dose that causes one or less of six patients to have DLT. This MTD is the dose that is generally recommended as the dose to be used in single-agent phase II trials. However, there have been different definitions of the MTD used by European research groups and it is important to carefully review the MTD definition in a protocol before working with a new agent.

The definition of a DLT is ≥ grade 3 nonhematologic or grade 4 hematologic (absolute neutrophil count < 500/µL for ≥ 7 days) toxicities according to the NCI common toxicities criteria found at the Web site <http://ctep.cancer.gov/reporting/ctc.html>.

There are frequent discussions as to whether phase I trials should always seek to define the MTD and DLTs. This question is becoming increasingly asked in clinical trials with agents that are mechanism based (eg, monoclonal antibodies, kinase inhibitors). Rather than define an MTD, there is an increasing emphasis (using pharmacodynamic measurements) on defining a biologically effective dose (BED). Of note, often the BED and the MTD are actually quite close to each other. In addition, caution is urged at stopping the phase I trial at the BED. The phase I trials with imatinib may have stopped too early if only the BED was used as a basis for stopping dose escalation. There is new evidence that one mechanism of resistance of CML cells to imatinib may be attributable to leukemia cells, which harbor less sensitive mutations.[123] It would be nice to know whether higher doses of imatinib could be used to kill these clones of tumor cells.

Selection Criteria for Patients for Phase I Trials Table 39-7 details commonly used selection criteria for inclusion in a phase I trial. These are offered as guidelines only. A few points on the exclusion criteria are worthy of discussion.

One major question is regarding whether older patients should participate in phase I trials. Of note is the study by Bowen and colleagues, which indicated that a patient's chronologic age did not impact on the toxicities experienced in phase I trials of a new agent.[124]

One of the most interesting new questions that is arising in the phase I trial arena (because of the development of more targeted agents) is whether only patients whose tumors exhibit the particular target should be entered into the phase I trial. This would seem to make sense because if the patient's tumor has the target (eg, estrogen receptor or HER2/*neu*, CD20 or CD52 positivity, or the Bcr-Abl rearrangement or mutated c-*kit*), the patient should be more likely to respond to the new agent. It is fairly clear that the presence of the target in the patient's tumor should be a criterion for entry into the study *if* the agent is *certain* to work only on tumors that possess the target, and if one is certain that the mechanism of action for the new agent is only against that particular target. In addition, one must be certain that the assay used to measure that particular target is accurate and reproducible. The selection of patients for entry on the new agent trial based on presence of the target in their tumors is certainly an entry criterion that will become a more standard criterion as we can better pinpoint the precise mechanism(s) of action of a new agent. Until then, the use of an entry criterion of the patient's tumor having the target is a bit uncertain.

Another frequent issue in selection of patients for a phase I trial is whether only patients with a certain disease should be entered into the study (eg, only patients with prostate cancer). Interestingly, this is not frequently done but will probably be done more frequently as more targeted disease-specific agents are brought into phase I trials. Until that is done, it is likely that most phase I trials will continue to allow entry of patients with a variety of malignancies.

Table 39-7 Common Selection Criteria for Entry of Patients into a Phase I Trial

1. Age ≥ 18 yrs
2. Pathologically confirmed diagnosis of any malignant solid tumor
3. Measurable disease not required
4. Life expectancy ≥ 12 wk
5. Karnofsky Performance Status of ≥ 70% (ECOG ≤ 2)
6. Adequate organ function:
   a) Neutrophils ≥ 1,500/ μL, hemoglobin ≥ 9 g/dL
   b) Platelets ≥ 100,000/μL
   c) Serum bilirubin with normal limits
   d) SGOT ≤ 2 × ULN (except if owing to disease, then ≤ 5 × ULN is acceptable)
   e) Serum creatinine within normal limits and calculated creatinine clearance ≥ 60 mL/min
   f) No atrial or ventricular arrhythmias requiring control by medication, no ischemic event experienced within the preceding 6 mo
   g) No history of seizure disorder requiring active therapy; no clinical evidence of malignancy of the central nervous system
7. Must have exhausted all therapy, which has a better chance of working for the patients (including investigational therapy) or must be in a situation for which there is no standard therapy
8. Must not have received any chemotherapy within 4 wks prior to entry (6 wks for mitomycin C or nitrosoureas) with complete recovery from toxic effects of that therapy
9. Patients must not be receiving any concomitant radiation therapy
10. Patients must have recovered from the reversible toxicities of prior therapy
11. Female patients must be of nonchildbearing potential and nonlactating and using adequate contraception with a negative pregnancy test at study entry and prior to each course of therapy
12. Male patients must also be using adequate contraception
13. No other serious concurrent medical illness or active infection should be present that would jeopardize the ability of the patient to receive (with reasonable safety) the chemotherapy outlined in this protocol
14. An effort must be made to minimize concomitant medications to those necessary for pain control, patient comfort, or life-threatening problems
15. Patients must sign an informed consent form. The patient must be aware of the neoplastic nature of his/her disease and willingly consent after being informed of the procedure to be followed, the experimental nature of the therapy, alternatives, potential benefits, side effects, risks, and discomfort

SGOT = serum glutamic-oxaloacetic transaminase; ULN = upper limits normal.

Are Phase I Clinical Trials Therapeutic? Studies have been done documenting that, indeed, conventional responses (complete and partial responses) can be seen in patients with advanced malignancies who are participating in single-agent phase I trials of a new agent.[125,126] In older reviews, the true response rate ranges from 5 to 7% (with about a 1% complete response rate).[125] However, there are also examples of considerably higher response rates, particularly in phase I combination trials.[44,127,128] Most responses are noted in a range of 80 to 120% of the MTD for the agent.

There are two recent studies that have again reviewed the benefits and risks of phase I trials.[129,130] Horstmann and colleagues reviewed all nonpediatric phase I studies sponsored by the NCI between 1991 and 2002 (460 trials with 11,935 patients). The overall response rate for the single agent phase I trials was 4.4%. The toxic death rate was 0.49%. Roberts and colleagues reviewed 213 studies (6,474 cancer patients) published in peer-reviewed journals. They noted an overall response rate of 3.8%. Of note, they found that response rates have decreased over the 12-year observation period (6.2% during the period from 1991 to 1999, 2.5% during the period from 1999 to 2002). During the time studied, the toxic death rate declined steeply from 1.1% to 0.06%. From these data the authors concluded that the ratio of risk to benefit for a patient participating in a phase I trial probably has improved.

Of increasing relevance is whether the category of stable disease will become an increasingly used measure of antitumor activity (particularly stable disease lasting ≥ 4 months). There is interest in this category of nonprogressing patients, and it is likely to be increasingly used as a criterion to determine whether a new agent is exhibiting some antitumor effect not only in a phase I setting, but also in a phase II setting.[131]

Another method that is gaining interest to determine whether a new agent is having some antitumor activity in a phase I trial is the concept of using patients as their own controls.[132] In this method, one uses the time a patient who is about to enter a new agent phase I trial has been on their prior therapeutic regimen as a control period (period A in Figure 39-2). If the patient remains on the new phase I agent for a period of time (period B) longer than he/she was on a prior therapy (period A), the agent is judged to have had some impact on the natural history of the patient's tumor. If 30% of patients on the phase I trial (who are at or near the MTD) have a period B that is longer than period A, the agent may be a promising one. Of course, this method has not been prospectively evaluated, but it is becoming a method used increasingly by many clinicians working in the phase I trial arena.

Combination of Agents in Phase I Trials Conduct of phase I trials combining a new agent along with a standard already approved agent is a phase I trial in which the ethics are more straightforward (the patient will at least be getting one agent with proven clinical activity for some patients). There is an increasing amount of clinical trial activity in this area with initial experience, with at least the monoclonal antibodies (eg, trastuzumab, rituximab) demonstrating increased clinical activity when used in combination with standard chemotherapeutic agents. This is an area of active exploration with the recent addition of cytostatic agents such as signal transduction inhibitors used in combination with standard chemotherapeutic agents.[51] Of note, in randomized trials to date, the addition of a cytostatic small molecule to a cytotoxic agent has rarely added significant clinical activity to the cytotoxic agent.[133–135]

There are many issues in the design and conduct of these combination phase I trials. However,

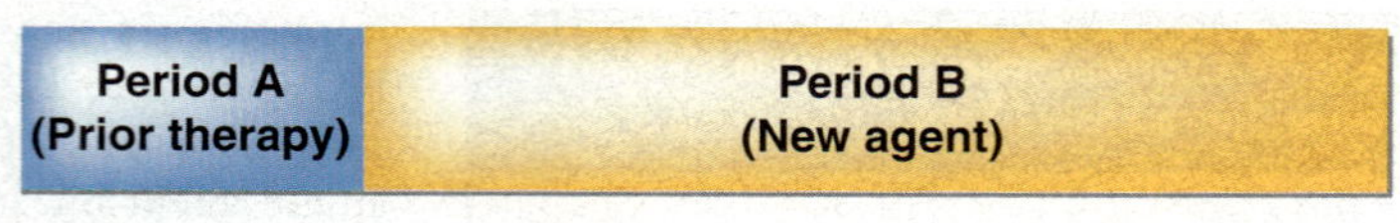

Ratio $\frac{\text{Period B}}{\text{Period A}}$ = Growth modulation index

Anything > 1.33 (33% improvement) is considered excellent (and is unexpected for second - line therapy)

Figure 39-2 The patient as his/her own control. Adapted from Von Hoff DD.[132]

general guidelines include the fact that the standard agent should generally be administered at the dose and schedule that are usually used (eg, used at their approved dose and schedule) if at all possible. This improves acceptance by investigators and patients of the study design. Sequencing of the agents should be worked out in preclinical models (if at all possible), although the predictive value of these models is not well established. By starting with the recommended/acceptable dose of the standard agent, one can then start escalation of the new agent with a fixed dose of the standard agent. In general, the starting dose for the new agent would be 25% of the MTD for the new agent alone (if there are no overlapping toxicities with the standard agent). Depending on what is seen at that initial level, the next dose levels of the new agent would be 50% of its MTD, 75% of its MTD, and then 100% of its MTD (if possible). There are also some sophisticated models that have been reported to provide additional rationales for the dose escalations used in these combination phase I studies.[136]

Issues Regarding Phase I Trials in General There are several papers written about the ethics of patient participation in phase I trials.[111,137–139] Daugherty and colleagues noted that instead of the often quoted perception by many that patients were motivated by altruism, the motivation for patients participating in phase I trials included the following:[140,141]

1. Hope for improvement in their condition (high motivation)
2. Pressure exerted by relatives and friends (high motivation)
3. They felt they had no choice (high motivation)
4. Advice or trust of physicians (low motivation)
5. Altruism (low motivation)

These findings again emphasize how important it is for the patient to have all of the facts from the clinical development team so that they can make an informed decision as to whether or not to participate in a phase I trial. One study on the impact of a phase I trial on quality of life demonstrated that participation of a patient in a phase I trial increased a patient's level of hope and appetite (measures for quality of life).[142,143]

Future Technologies Likely to Impact on Phase I Trials The rapid advances in functional imaging (eg, dynamic contrast magnetic resonance imaging, positron emission tomography, single-photon emission computed tomography) are likely to dramatically impact on the phase I clinical trial both by helping investigators assess pharmacodynamic endpoints as well as perhaps assess early evidence of an antitumor effect.

The above and other new technologies should help the phase I investigator determine more readily whether a particular new agent is helping a particular patient and improve the prospect for gain for patients who are willing to participate in phase I trials with new agents.

REFERENCES

1. O'Shaughnessy JA, Kelloff GJ, Gordon GB, et al. Treatment and prevention of intraepithelial neoplasia: an important target for accelerated new agent development. Clin Cancer Res 2002;8:314–46.
2. Alberts DS. A unifying vision of cancer therapy for the 21st century. J Clin Oncol 1999;17:13–21.
3. Bode AM, Dong Z. Targeting signal transduction pathways by chemopreventive agents. Mutat Res 2004;555:33–51.
4. Uliasz A, Spencer JM. Chemoprevention of skin cancer and photoaging. Clin Dermatol 2004;22:178–82.
5. Cohen V, Khuri FR. Chemoprevention of lung cancer. Curr Opin Pulm Med 2004;10:279–83.
6. Adair DS, Bogg HJ. Experimental and clinical studies on the treatment of cancer by dichloroethylsulfate (mustard gas). Ann Surg 1931;93:190–9.
7. Goodman LS, Wintrobe MM, Damashek W, et al. Use of methyl-bis(beta-chloroethyl)amine hydrochloride and tris(beta-chloroethyl)amine hydrochloride for Hodgkin's disease, lymphosarcoma, leukemia and certain allied and miscellaneous disorders. JAMA 1946;132:126–32.
8. Rhoads CP. Nitrogen mustards in treatment of neoplastic disease. JAMA 1946;131:656–8.
9. Farber S, Diamond LK, Mercer RD, et al. Temporary remissions in acute leukemia in children produced by folic acid antagonist 4-aminopteroyl-glutamaic acid (aminopterin). N Engl J Med 1948;238:787–93.
10. Rakatien N, Rakatien ML, Nadkarnie MR. Studies on the diabetogenic action of streptozotocin (NSC-37917). Cancer Chemother Rep 1963;29:91–8.
11. Murray-Lyon IM, Eddleston AL, Williams R, et al. Treatment of multiple-hormone-producing malignant islet-cell tumour with streptozotocin. Lancet 1968;2:895–8.
12. Schaeppi U, Heyman IA, Fleischman RW, et al. cis-Dichlorodiammineplatinum(II) (NSC-119 875): preclinical toxicologic evaluation of intravenous injection in dogs, monkeys and mice. Toxicol Appl Pharmacol 1973;25:230–41.
13. Higby DJ, Wallace HJ Jr, Albert D, Holland JF. Diamminedichloroplatinum in the chemotherapy of testicular tumors. J Urol 1974;112:100–4.
14. Wiltshaw E, Kroner T. Phase II study of cis-dichlorodiammineplatinum(II) (NSC-119875) in advanced adenocarcinoma of the ovary. Cancer Treat Rep 1976;60:55–60.
15. Rutman RJ, Cantarow A, Paschkis KE. Studies in 2-acetylaminofluorene carcinogenesis. III. The utilization of uracil-2-C14 by preneoplastic rat liver and rat hepatoma. Cancer Res 1954;14:119–23.
16. Heidelberger C. On the rational development of a new drug: the example of the fluorinated pyrimidines. Cancer Treat Rep 1981:65 Suppl 3:3–9.
17. McGinn CJ, Zalupski MM, Shureiqi I, et al. Phase I trial of radiation dose escalation with concurrent weekly full-dose gemcitabine in patients with advanced pancreatic cancer. J Clin Oncol 2001;19:4202–8.
18. Elion GB, Hitchings GH, Vanderwerff H. Antagonists of nucleic acid derivatives. VI. Purines. J Biol Chem 1951;192:505–18.
19. Driscoll JS. The preclinical new drug research program of the National Cancer Institute. Cancer Treat Rep 1984;68:63–76.
20. Boyd MR. Status of the NCI preclinical antitumor drug discovery screen. Princ Pract Oncol Updates 1989;3:1–2.
21. Staquet MJ, Byar DP, Green SB, Rozencweig M. Clinical predictivity of transplantable tumor systems in the selection of new drugs for solid tumors: rationale for a three-stage strategy. Cancer Treat Rep 1983;67:753–65.
22. Johnson JI, Decker S, Zaharevitz D, et al. Relationships between drug activity in NCI preclinical in vitro and in vivo models and early clinical trials. Br J Cancer 2001;84:1424–31.
23. Skehan P, Storeng R, Scudiero D, et al. New colorimetric cytotoxicity assay for anticancer-drug screening. J Natl Cancer Inst 1990;82:1107–12.
24. Chabner BA. In defense of cell-line screening. J Natl Cancer Inst 1990;82:1083–5.
25. Grever MR, Schepartz SA, Chabner BA. The National Cancer Institute: cancer drug discovery and development program. Semin Oncol 1992;19:622–38.
26. Hodes L. Computer-aided selection of compounds for antitumor screening: validation of a statistical-heuristic method. J Chem Inf Comput Sci 1981;21:128–32.
27. Double JA, Bibby MC. Therapeutic index: a vital component in selection of anticancer agents for clinical trial. J Natl Cancer Inst 1989:81:988–94.
28. Paull KD, Shoemaker RH, Hodes L, et al. Display and analysis of patterns of differential activity of drugs against human tumor cell lines: development of mean graph and COMPARE algorithm. J Natl Cancer Inst 1989;81:1088–92.
29. Weinstein JN, Myers TG, O'Connor PM, et al. An information-intensive approach to the molecular pharmacology of cancer. Science 1997;275:343–9.
30. Taverna P, Liu L, Hanson AJ, et al. Characterization of MLH1 and MSH2 DNA mismatch repair proteins in cell lines of the NCI anticancer drug screen. Cancer Chemother Pharmacol 2000;46:507–16.
31. O'Connor PM, Jackman J, Bae I, et al. Characterization of the p53 tumor suppressor pathway in cell lines of the National Cancer Institute anticancer drug screen and correlations with the growth-inhibitory potency of 123 anticancer agents. Cancer Res 1997;57:4285–300.
32. Scherf U, Ross DT, Waltham M, et al. A gene expression database for the molecular pharmacology of cancer. Nat Genet 2000;24:236–44.
33. Shoemaker RH, Wolpert-Defilippes MK, Kern DH, et al. Application of a human tumor colony-forming assay to new drug screening. Cancer Res 1985;45:2145–53.
34. Hanauske AR, Degen D, Marshall MH, et al. Activity of 2',2'-difluorodeoxycytidine (Gemcitabine) against human tumor colony forming units. Anticancer Drugs 1992;3:143–6.
35. Hanauske AR, Degen D, Hilsenbeck SG, et al. Effects of Taxotere and Taxol on in vitro colony formation of freshly explanted human tumor cells. Anticancer Drugs 1992;3:121–4.
36. Bogden AE, Cobb WR, Lepage DJ. The 6-day subrenal capsule assay (SRCA): its criticism, biology and review of assay/clinical correlations. Prog Clin Biol Res 1988;276:139–204.
37. Nowell PS, Hungerford DA. A minute chromocome in human granulocytic leukemia. Science 1960;132:1497.
38. Rowley JD. A new consistent chromosomal abnormality in chronic myelogenous leukaemia identified by quinacrine fluorescence and Giemsa staining [letter]. Nature 1973;243:290–3.

39. Daley GQ, Van Etten RA, Baltimore D. Induction of chronic myelogenous leukemia in mice by the P210bcr/abl gene of the Philadelphia chromosome. Science 1990;247:824–30.
40. Witte ON. Role of the BCR-ABL oncogene in human leukemia: fifteenth Richard and Hinda Rosenthal Foundation Award Lecture. Cancer Res 1993;53:485–9.
41. Druker BJ, Tamura S, Buchdunger E, et al. Effects of a selective inhibitor of the Abl tyrosine kinase on the growth of Bcr-Abl positive cells. Nat Med 1996;2:561–6.
42. Deininger MW, Goldman JM, Lydon N, Melo JV. The tyrosine kinase inhibitor CGP57148B selectively inhibits the growth of BCR-ABL-positive cells. Blood 1997;90:3691–8.
43. le Coutre P, Mologni L, Cleris L, et al. In vivo eradication of human BCR/ABL-positive leukemia cells with an ABL kinase inhibitor. J Natl Cancer Inst 1999;91:163–8.
44. Druker BJ, Talpaz M, Resta DJ, et al. Efficacy and safety of a specific inhibitor of the BCR-ABL tyrosine kinase in chronic myeloid leukemia. N Engl J Med 2001;344:1031–7.
45. Braziel RM, Launder TM, Druker BJ, et al. Hematopathologic and cytogenetic findings in imatinib mesylate-treated chronic myelogenous leukemia patients: 14 months' experience. Blood 2002;100:435–41.
46. Demetri GD, von Mehren M, Blanke CD, et al. Efficacy and safety of imatinib mesylate in advanced gastrointestinal stromal tumors. N Engl J Med 2002;347:472–80.
47. Dewar AL, Cambareri AC, Zannettino AC, et al. Macrophage colony stimulating factor receptor, c-fms, is a novel target of imatinib. Blood 2005;105:3127–32.
48. Mathew P, Thall PF, Jones D, et al. Platelet-derived growth factor receptor inhibitor imatinib mesylate and docetaxel: a modular phase I trial in androgen-independent prostate cancer. J Clin Oncol 2004;22:3323–9.
49. Lassila M, Seah KK, Allen TJ, et al. Imatinib attenuates diabetic nephropathy in apolipoprotein e-knockout mice. J Am Soc Nephrol 2004;15:2125–38.
50. Yoshiji H, Noguchi R, Kuriyama S, et al. Imatinib mesylate (STI571: Gleevec) attenuates liver fibrosis development in rats. Am J Physiol Gastrointest Liver Physiol 2004;288:G907–13.
51. Van Cutsem E, van de Velde H, Karasek P, et al. Phase III trial of gemcitabine plus tipifarnib compared with gemcitabine plus placebo in advanced pancreatic cancer. J Clin Oncol 2004;22:1430–8.
52. Johnston SR, Hickish T, Ellis P, et al. Phase II study of the efficacy and tolerability of two dosing regimens of the farnesyl transferase inhibitor, R115777, in advanced breast cancer. J Clin Oncol 2003;21:2492–9.
53. Raponi M, Belly RT, Karp JE, et al. Microarray analysis reveals genetic pathways modulated by tipifarnib in acute myeloid leukemia. BMC Cancer 2004;4:56.
54. Grunwald V, Hidalgo M. The epidermal growth factor receptor: a new target for anticancer therapy. Curr Probl Cancer 2002;26:109–64.
55. Paez JG, Janne PA, Lee JC, et al. EGFR mutations in lung cancer: correlation with clinical response to gefitinib therapy. Science 2004;304:1497–500.
56. Price DK, Figg WD. Mutations in the EGFR: the importance of genotyping. Cancer Biol Ther 2004;3:434–5.
57. Lynch TJ, Bell DW, Sordella R, et al. Activating mutations in the epidermal growth factor receptor underlying responsiveness of non-small-cell lung cancer to gefitinib. N Engl J Med 2004;350:2129–39.
58. Druker BJ, Lydon NB. Lessons learned from the development of an abl tyrosine kinase inhibitor for chronic myelogenous leukemia. J Clin Invest 2000;105:3–7.
59. Toledo LM, Lydon NB, Elbaum D. The structure-based design of ATP-site directed protein kinase inhibitors. Curr Med Chem 1999;6:775–805.
60. Gibbs JB. Anticancer drug targets: growth factors and growth factor signaling. J Clin Invest 2000;105:9–13.
61. Hanahan D, Weinberg RA. The hallmarks of cancer. Cell 2000;100:57–70.
62. Hanahan D, Folkman J. Patterns and emerging mechanisms of the angiogenic switch during tumorigenesis. Cell 1996;86:353–64.
63. Kaelin WG Jr. Choosing anticancer drug targets in the post-genomic era. J Clin Invest 1999;104:1503–6.
64. Midgley R, Kerr D. Bevacizumab—current status and future directions. Ann Oncol 2005;16:999–1004.
65. Hurwitz HI, Fehrenbacher L, Hainsworth JD, et al. Bevacizumab in combination with fluorouracil and leucovorin: an active regimen for first-line metastatic colorectal cancer. J Clin Oncol 2005;23:3502–8.
66. Ferrara N, Hillan KJ, Gerber HP, Novotny W. Discovery and development of bevacizumab, an anti-VEGF antibody for treating cancer. Nat Rev Drug Discov 2004;3:391–400.
67. Yang JC. Bevacizumab for patients with metastatic renal cancer: an update. Clin Cancer Res 2004;10:6367S–70S.
68. Yang JC, Haworth L, Sherry RM, et al. A randomized trial of bevacizumab, an anti-vascular endothelial growth factor antibody, for metastatic renal cancer. N Engl J Med 2003;349:427–34.
69. Wilhelm SM, Carter C, Tang L, et al. BAY 43-9006 exhibits broad spectrum oral antitumor activity and targets the RAF/MEK/ERK pathway and receptor tyrosine kinases involved in tumor progression and angiogenesis. Cancer Res 2004;64:7099–109.
70. Sakamoto KM. Su-11248 Sugen. Curr Opin Investig Drugs 2004;5:1329–39.
71. Johnson RK. Screening methods in antineoplastic drug discovery. J Natl Cancer Inst 1990;82:1082–3.
72. Suftness M, Newman DJ, Snyder K. Discovery and development of antineoplastic agents from natural sources. Bioorgan Marine Chem 1989;3:131.
73. Kauvar LM, Villar HO, Sportsman JR, et al. Protein affinity map of chemical space. J Chromatogr B Biomed Sci Appl 1998;715:93–102.
74. Kauvar LM, Higgins DL, Villar HO, et al. Predicting ligand binding to proteins by affinity fingerprinting. Chem Biol 1995;2:107–18.
75. Davignon JP, Craddock JS. The formulation of anticancer drugs. In: Helman K, Carter SK, editors. Fundamentals of cancer chemotherapy. New York: McGraw-Hill; 1997. p. 212–26.
76. Wiernik PH, Schwartz EL, Strauman JJ, et al. Phase I clinical and pharmacokinetic study of Taxol. Cancer Res 1987;47:2486–93.
77. Cartwright TH, Cohn A, Varkey JA, et al. Phase II study of oral capecitabine in patients with advanced or metastatic pancreatic cancer. J Clin Oncol 2002;20:160–4.
78. Adjei AA, David JN, Erlichman C. Farnesyl-transferase inhibitor: use of surrogate markers. Proc AACR-NCI-EORTC Int Conf 1999;1:145.
79. Patnaik A, Eckhardt SG, Izbicka E, et al. A phase I, pharmacokinetic, and biological study of the farnesyltransferase inhibitor tipifarnib in combination with gemcitabine in patients with advanced malignancies. Clin Cancer Res 2003;9:4761–71.
80. Hidalgo M, Siu LL, Nemunaitis J, et al. Phase I and pharmacologic study of OSI-774, an epidermal growth factor receptor tyrosine kinase inhibitor, in patients with advanced solid malignancies. J Clin Oncol 2001;19:3267–79.
81. Campbell KJ, Hesh EM, Stopeck A, et al. A phase I trial of ABI-007 administered weekly for three doses every four weeks in patients with advanced non-hematologic malignancies. Proc Am Soc Clin Oncol 2002;21:101a.
82. Von Hoff DD, Soares N, Gormley P, Poplack DG. Pharmacokinetics of ICRF-187 in the cerebrospinal fluid of subhuman primates. Cancer Treat Rep 1980;64:734–6.
83. Collins JM, Grieshaber CK, Chabner BA. Pharmacologically guided phase I clinical trials based upon preclinical drug development. J Natl Cancer Inst 1990;82:1321–6.
84. Scheithauer W, Clark GM, Salmon SE, et al. Model for estimation of clinically achievable plasma concentrations for investigational anticancer drugs in man. Cancer Treat Rep 1986;70:1379–82.
85. Davis LE, Alberts DS, Plezia PM, et al. Predictive model for plasma concentration-versus-time profiles of investigational anticancer drugs in patients. J Natl Cancer Inst 1988;80:815–9.
86. DeSouza JV, Leiby JM, Staubus AE, et al. Altered pharmacokinetics of fludarabine phosphate by 2'deoxycorformycine in the diagnosis and analysis of a rate of fludarabine activation [abstract]. Proc Am Assoc Cancer Res 1985;26:1413.
87. Rinaldi DA, Burris HA, Dorr FA, et al. Initial phase I evaluation of the novel thymidylate synthase inhibitor, LY231514, using the modified continual reassessment method for dose escalation. J Clin Oncol 1995;13:2842–50.
88. DeGeorge JJ, Ahn CH, Andrews PA, et al. Regulatory considerations for preclinical development of anticancer drugs. Cancer Chemother Pharmacol 1998;41:173–85.
89. Verweij J. Starting dose levels for phase I studies. Proc 9th NCI-EORTC Symposium on New Drugs in Cancer Therapy. 1996.
90. Grieshaber CK, Marsoni S. Relation of preclinical toxicology to findings in early clinical trials. Cancer Treat Rep 1986;70:65–72.
91. Schein P, Anderson T. The efficacy of animal studies in predicting clinical toxicity of cancer chemotherapeutic drugs. Int J Clin Pharmacol 1973;8:228–38.
92. Eckhardt SG, Baker SD, Britten CD, et al. Phase I and pharmacokinetic study of irofulven, a novel mushroom-derived cytotoxin, administered for five consecutive days every four weeks in patients with advanced solid malignancies. J Clin Oncol 2000;18:4086–97.
93. Eisenhauer EA, O'Dwyer PJ, Christian M, Humphrey JS. Phase I clinical trial design in cancer drug development. J Clin Oncol 2000;18:684–92.
94. Dent SF, Eisenhauer EA. Phase I trial design: are new methodologies being put into practice? Ann Oncol 1996;7:561–6.
95. Von Hoff DD, Kuhn J, Clark GM. Design and conduct of phase I trials. In: Staquet M, Sylvester R, Buyse M, editors. EORTC. Oxford: Oxford University Press; 1984. p. 210–20.
96. Parulekar WR, Eisenhauer EA. Phase I trial design for solid tumor studies of targeted, non-cytotoxic agents: theory and practice. J Natl Cancer Inst 2004;96:990–7.
97. Genre D, Viens P, Von Hoff DD, Clark GM. Patients who are receiving concomitant medications should not systematically be excluded from phase I studies. Anticancer Drugs 1999;10:1–7.
98. Penta JS, Rosner GL, Trump DL. Choice of starting dose and escalation for phase I studies of antitumor agents. Cancer Chemother Pharmacol 1992;31:247–50.
99. Freireich EJ, Gehan EA, Rall DP, et al. Quantitative comparison of toxicity of anticancer agents in mouse, rat, hamster, dog, monkey, and man. Cancer Chemother Rep 1966;50:219–44.
100. Schneiderman MA, Mantel N, Brown CC. From mouse to man—or how to get from the laboratory to Park Avenue and 59th Street. Ann NY Acad Sci 1975;246:237–48.
101. Rothenberg ML, Kuhn JG, Burris HA III, et al. Phase I and pharmacokinetic trial of weekly CPT-11. J Clin Oncol 1993;11:2194–204.
102. Hansen HH, Selawry OS, Muggia FM, Walker MD. Clinical studies with 1-(2-chloroethyl)-3-cyclohexyl-1-nitrosourea (NSC 79037). Cancer Res 1971;31:223–7.
103. Gottlieb JA. Phase I and phase II clinical trials: a critical reappraisal. The pharmacological basis of cancer chemotherapy. Baltimore: Williams and Wilkins; 1974.
104. Evans WE. Alternative approaches for phase I studies of anticancer drugs: a role for therapeutic drug monitoring. Ther Drug Monit 1993;15:492–7.
105. Erlichman C, Moore M, Kerr IG, et al. Phase I pharmacokinetic and pharmacodynamic study of a new anthrapyrazole, CI-937 (DUP937). Cancer Res 1991;51:6317–22.
106. O'Quigley J, Pepe M, Fisher L. Continual reassessment method: a practical design for phase I clinical trials in cancer. Biometrics 1990;46:33–48.
107. O'Quigley J, Shen LZ. Continual reassessment method: a likelihood approach. Biometrics 1996;52:673–84.
108. Faries D. Practical modifications of the continual reassessment method for phase I cancer clinical trials. J Biopharm Stat 1994;4:147–64.
109. Simon R, Freidlin B, Rubinstein L, et al. Accelerated titration designs for phase I clinical trials in oncology. J Natl Cancer Inst 1997;89:1138–47.
110. Ratain MJ, Mick R, Schilsky RL, Siegler M. Statistical and ethical issues in the design and conduct of phase I and II clinical trials of new anticancer agents [comments]. J Natl Cancer Inst 1993;85:1637–43.
111. Freedman J. The ethical analysis of clinical trials: new lessons for and from cancer research. In: Vanderpool HY, editor. The ethics of research involving human subjects. Facing the 21st century. Frederick: University Publishing Group; 1996. p. 319–38.
112. Emanuel E J. A phase I trial on the ethics of phase I trials. J Clin Oncol 1995;13:1049–51.
113. Storer BE. Small-sample confidence sets for the MTD in a phase I clinical trial. Biometrics 1993;49:1117–25.
114. Piantadosi S, Fisher JD, Grossman S. Practical implementation of a modified continual reassessment method for dose-finding trials. Cancer Chemother Pharmacol 1998;41:429–36.
115. Goodman SN, Zahurak ML, Piantadosi S. Some practical improvements in the continual reassessment method for phase I studies. Stat Med 1995;14:1149–61.
116. Mick R, Ratain MJ. Model-guided determination of maximum tolerated dose in phase I clinical trials: evidence for increased precision. J Natl Cancer Inst 1993;85:217–23.

117. Walling J, Zervos P, McCarthy S, et al. Dose escalation methodology in phase I clinical trials: a comparison of the modified continual reassessment method (mCRM) and a traditional method. Experience with the multitargeted antifolate (MTA). Proc Am Soc Clin Oncol 1997;16:209a.
118. Smith TL, Lee JJ, Kantarjian HM, et al. Design and results of phase I cancer clinical trials: three-year experience at M.D. Anderson Cancer Center. J Clin Oncol 1996;14:287–95.
119. Eckhardt SG, Siu LL, Clark G, et al. The continual reassessment method (CRM) for dose escalation in phase I trials in San Antonio does not result in more rapid study completion. Proc Am Soc Clin Oncol 1999;18:163a.
120. Korn EL, Midthune D, Chen TT, et al. A comparison of two phase I trial designs. Stat Med 1994;13:1799–806.
121. Freedman B. Cohort Specific consent: an honest approach to phase I clinical cancer studies. IRB 1990;12:5–7.
122. Daugherty CK, Ratain MJ, Minami H, et al. Study of cohort-specific consent and patient control in phase I cancer trials. J Clin Oncol 1998;16:2305–12.
123. O'Hare T, Walters DK, Stoffregen EP, et al. In vitro activity of Bcr-Abl inhibitors AMN107 and BMS-354825 against clinically relevant imatinib-resistant Abl kinase domain mutants. Cancer Res 2005;65:4500–5.
124. Bowen KJ, Eckhardt J, Clark G, et al. The impact of patient age on the outcome of phase I trials. Proc Am Soc Clin Oncol 1993;12:184.
125. Von Hoff DD, Turner J. Response rates, duration of response, and dose response effects in phase I studies of antineoplastics. Invest New Drugs 1991;9:115–22.
126. Estey E, Hoth D, Simon R, et al. Therapeutic response in phase I trials of antineoplastic agents. Cancer Treat Rep 1986;70:1105–15.
127. Druker BJ, Sawyers CL, Kantarjian H, et al. Activity of a specific inhibitor of the BCR-ABL tyrosine kinase in the blast crisis of chronic myeloid leukemia and acute lymphoblastic leukemia with the Philadelphia chromosome. N Engl J Med 2001;344:1038–42.
128. Thödtmann R, Depenbrock H, Dumez H, et al. Clinical and pharmacokinetic phase I study of multitargeted antifolate (LY231514) in combination with cisplatin. J Clin Oncol 1999;17:3009–16.
129. Horstmann E, McCabe MS, Grochow L, et al. Risks and benefits of phase 1 oncology trials, 1991 through 2002. N Engl J Med 2005;352:895–904.
130. Roberts TG Jr, Goulart BH, Squitieri L, et al. Trends in the risks and benefits to patients with cancer participating in phase 1 clinical trials. JAMA 2004;292:2130–40.
131. Dent S, Zee B, Dancey J, et al. Application of a new multinomial phase II stopping rule using response and early progression. J Clin Oncol 2001;19:785–91.
132. Von Hoff DD. There are no bad anticancer agents, only bad clinical trial designs—twenty-first Richard and Hinda Rosenthal Foundation Award Lecture. Clin Cancer Res 1998;4:1079–86.
133. Herbst RS, Giaccone G, Schiller JH, et al. Gefitinib in combination with paclitaxel and carboplatin in advanced non-small-cell lung cancer: a phase III trial—INTACT 2. J Clin Oncol 2004;22:785–94.
134. Giaccone G, Herbst RS, Manegold C, et al. Gefitinib in combination with gemcitabine and cisplatin in advanced non-small-cell lung cancer: a phase III trial—INTACT 1. J Clin Oncol 2004;22:777–84.
135. Fuster LM, Sandler AB. Select clinical trials of erlotinib (OSI-774) in non-small-cell lung cancer with emphasis on phase III outcomes. Clin Lung Cancer 2004;6 Suppl 1:S24–9.
136. Korn EL, Simon R. Using the tolerable-dose diagram in the design of phase I combination chemotherapy trials. J Clin Oncol 1993;11:794–801.
137. Sessa C, Cavalli F. Who benefits from phase I studies? Ann Oncol 1990;1:164–5.
138. Rodenhuis S, Van Den Heuvel WJA, Annyas AA, et al. Patient motivation and informed consent in a phase I study of an anticancer agent. Eur J Cancer Clin Oncol 1984;20:457–62.
139. Willems Y, Sessa C. Informing patients about phase I trials–how should it be done? Acta Oncol 1989;28:106–7.
140. Daugherty CK, Banik DM, Janish L, Ratain MJ. Quantitative analysis of ethical issues in phase I trials: a survey interview of 144 advanced cancer patients. IRB 2000;22:6–14.
141. Daugherty CK. Impact of therapeutic research on informed consent and the ethics of clinical trials: a medical oncology perspective. J Clin Oncol 1999;17:1601–17.
142. Melink TJ, Clark GM, Von Hoff DD. The impact of phase I clinical trials on the quality of life of patients with cancer. Anticancer Drugs 1992;3:571–6.
143. Berdel WE, Knopf H, Fromm M, et al. Influence of phase I early clinical trials on the quality of life of cancer patients. A pilot study. Anticancer Res 1988;8:313–21.

Pharmacology

Samir D. Undevia, MD
Mark J. Ratain, MD
William Plunkett, PhD

The clinical pharmacology of anticancer drugs was poorly understood for many years owing primarily to the lack of sensitive and specific assays for measuring the concentration of these compounds in biological fluids. The development and widespread application of high performance liquid chromatography, liquid chromatography/mass spectroscopy, and other sophisticated analytical tools allows measurements of plasma drug (and metabolite) concentrations to be performed with a high degree of precision and efficiency. Clinical pharmacokinetic studies of anticancer drugs, particularly new agents, are performed routinely in the context of phase I and II clinical trials. Although the pharmacokinetic characteristics of many drugs have been well defined, the application of this information to the clinical care of individual patients still lags behind other therapeutic areas in medicine. Plasma concentrations of digoxin, theophylline, aminoglycosides, phenytoin and many other drugs are monitored routinely to optimize efficacy and reduce toxicity; yet the measurement of doxorubicin or 5-fluorouracil (5-FU) concentrations in plasma is virtually meaningless, since there are no established relationships (of proven therapeutic utility) between pharmacokinetics and clinical effects for these or most other commonly used anticancer drugs. A notable exception is methotrexate, where delayed clearance is related to an increased risk of severe toxicity.

Pharmacokinetic-pharmacodynamic relationships are difficult to develop for many reasons. For most antineoplastic agents, there is a delay of days to weeks between measurement of drug concentrations and clinical effect. It is therefore necessary to observe patients frequently, following chemotherapy administration to accurately assess the drug effect. The maximum observed effect may be significantly less than the true maximum effect unless patients are seen daily. Although the desired effect of cancer chemotherapy is a reduction in tumor volume, usually optimized by maximizing the dose, the narrow therapeutic index of cancer chemotherapy drugs requires that most dosing strategies focus on minimizing toxicity rather than on optimizing efficacy. Despite these difficulties, significant progress has recently been made in understanding the clinical pharmacodynamics of anticancer drugs, and further studies in this area will no doubt lead to more rational administration of systemic anticancer therapy.

This chapter will focus on the principles of clinical pharmacology as they apply to systemic anticancer therapy and will attempt to illustrate how an understanding of clinical pharmacokinetics and pharmacodynamics can optimize the therapeutic index of such agents.

GENERAL MECHANISMS OF DRUG ACTION

The initial requirement for drug action is adequate drug delivery to the target site. This depends largely on blood flow in the tumor bed and the diffusion characteristics of the drug in tissue. However, delivery can also be influenced by the extent of plasma protein binding and, for orally administered drugs, by absorption, first-pass metabolism in the liver, and the requirement for activation by various mechanisms. Blood flow across a capillary bed is directly proportional to the arteriovenous pressure difference and inversely proportional to the geometric and viscous resistances. The geometric resistance to blood flow increases with increasing tumor size, a factor that may limit drug and oxygen delivery to large tumors. and thereby diminish the effectiveness of treatment with chemotherapy or radiation.[1]

The most common route of drug administration for treatment of both localized and disseminated disease is by intravenous infusion, which by definition makes 100% of the drug available in the blood. Drugs may be administered by a number of routes in addition to intravenous infusions, however, to achieve specialized pharmacologic and therapeutic goals. Regional administration may be employed to more directly target the drug to the principal tumor site and to achieve a higher drug concentration in the vicinity of the tumor. Intraperitoneal infusion of cisplatin for ovarian cancers, intrapleural administration of bleomycin in the treatment of solid tumors, and intrathecal administration of cytarabine as a means of treating leukemias are examples of intracavitary drug delivery. Alternatively, intravascular administration such as intra-arterial infusion of fluorodeoxyuridine into the hepatic artery for treatment of liver diseases has been used to achieve a pharmacologic advantage. Although oral administration is the most convenient and least expensive route of drug administration, it is associated with problems of inconsistent drug bioavailability among and within patients.[2] More consistent pharmacokinetic results are achieved with subcutaneous or intramuscular drug injections.

Delivery of the drug to the target cell is also dependent on the rate of removal from the blood. Excretion, either by the kidneys or by the biliary route, constitutes a major clearance mechanism. In addition, many drugs are cleared by metabolism to less effective or inactive metabolites as the blood passes through large body organs. Drug binding to plasma proteins can also effectively lower the concentration of free drug that is available for entry into target cells to a small fraction of the total concentration in blood.

Membrane Transport In order to produce cytotoxicity, most anticancer drugs require uptake into the cell. A number of mechanisms exist for the passage of drugs across the plasma membrane, including passive diffusion, facilitated diffusion, and active transport systems. Passive diffusion of drugs through the lipid bilayer structure of the plasma membrane is a function of the size, lipid solubility, and charge of the drug molecule. If the extracellular drug concentration is constant, then drug accumulation by the cell will continue until the rate of drug uptake from the extracellular space is equal to the rate of drug efflux from the cell. At this point, a dynamic equilibrium is reached and intracellular and extracellular drug concentrations are equal. As drug is cleared from the extracellular space, intracellular drug levels will decline if the drug is not bound or metabolized intracellularly. An important feature of the passive diffusion process is that it does not saturate. That is, as the extracellular drug concentration increases, influx into the cell increases proportionally and high intracellular drug levels can be achieved. Passive diffusion, however, is a highly inefficient and nonspecific process, although it may be a particularly important mechanism of drug uptake when carrier-mediated processes are nonfunctional, such as occurs in some cases of methotrexate resistance.

The passage of physiologically important hydrophilic compounds across the plasma membrane is usually mediated by a specific receptor, or carrier, in the plasma membrane that facilitates the translocation of the substance into or out of the cell. Carrier-mediated transport systems are distinguished from passive diffusion by having a higher degree of specificity and by being saturable at high extracellular drug concentrations owing to the presence of a finite number of receptor molecules within the membrane. Once all carrier sites become occupied, further increases in extracellular drug concentration will not produce further increments in drug influx unless a component of passive diffusion comes into play. The affinity of the carrier for the substrate can be estimated from the K_m, the drug concentration at which the influx rate is one-half maximal; the lower the K_m, the higher the carrier affinity. Although carrier-mediated systems enhance the rate of influx into the cell, not all carriers are able to translocate compounds against electrochemical forces and ultimately develop gradients such that the intracellular concentration exceeds the extracellular drug level. To do so requires the expenditure of energy and the coupling of carrier-mediated transport to an energy-requiring reaction, usually hydrolysis of adenosine triphosphate.

Many antineoplastic drugs, particularly those that are structural analogues of natural compounds, gain entry into the cell by carrier-mediated mechanisms. The functional and physiologic characteristics of several human nucleoside transporters have been characterized. However, substantial additional information is rapidly emerging as more of these molecules are cloned and their specificities are revealed.[3,4] Naturally occurring nucleosides are transported by both facilitated diffusion (equilibrative) and by concentrative mechanisms. Nucleoside analogues that are important in cancer therapy also use these transporters, but some specificity is emerging.[5] For instance, cytarabine, floxidine, and pentostatin appear to use equilibrative transporters, whereas fludarabine, gemcitabine, and cladribine are also substrates for concentrative transport systems in addition to equilibrative pathways.[6–8] Antibodies with specificity for these membrane proteins are being developed and applied to answer questions that relate the prevalence of the proteins to clinical response to nucleoside analogue therapy.[9] As many new nucleoside analogues with varied metabolic properties and mechanisms of action are currently being evaluated for antitumor activity,[10] a complete understanding of their biological activities will require an assessment of the contribution of their membrane transport. Nucleobase transporters have also been identified, but their role in the entry of useful antimetabolites such as thiopurines and 5-fluorouracil into the cell has not been established.[5] Transport of reduced folates and methotrexate is an active energy-dependent process that can be mediated by two distinct mechanisms: a membrane carrier system capable of the rapid transport of reduced folates and of 4-amino analogues of folic acid,[11,12] and a group of membrane-bound folate receptors termed the folate binding proteins that are brought into the cell by endocytosis to release ligand before recycling back to the membrane.[13] The DNA sequences for genes performing this function have now been identified, and the expressed proteins have been evaluated in cells that otherwise lack the ability to transport methotrexate.[14,15] Altered methotrexate transport features have been described in ALL blasts and in osteosarcoma as a mechanism of acquired resistance.[16] L-phenylalanine mustard uses at least two amino acid transport systems, and its influx can be inhibited by the amino acid substrates specific for these transport carriers.[17]

The importance of transmembrane movement of a drug to its pharmacologic effect depends on several factors including the rate of drug delivery to the tissue, the affinity of the transport process, and the nature of the intracellular biochemical events required for drug action. Though membrane transport can be the rate-limiting step in drug action if it governs the rate at which the drug reaches intracellular targets, this is not always the case. If drug delivery to a cell is slow relative to the influx rate, then the drug effect will be limited primarily by extracellular concentration, that is, blood flow and diffusion of the drug. Similarly, if a drug requires intracellular activation, such as phosphorylation of nucleoside analogues or polyglutamylation of methotrexate and other antifols, before they can exert a cytotoxic effect, then the rate-limiting step in drug action could be activation rather than transport—if the rate of activation is slow relative to the rate of influx into the cell.

Finally, it is important to recognize that membrane transport is frequently bidirectional with the final drug concentration in the cell representing the balance between drug influx and drug efflux. These processes may utilize different carrier systems and operate at different rates. Several efflux systems that appear to have importance in cancer chemotherapy mediate various forms of multidrug resistance. Although these have focused on efflux of complex biologically derived molecules, for example, anthracyclins and epipodophyllotoxins,[18,19] it is now clear that nucleotide analogues are also transported out of the cell by multidrug resistance-associated proteins, MRP4 and MRP5.[20,21]

Intracellular Activation Many anticancer drugs require activation before they are able to exert a cytotoxic effect. The activation process may involve chemical or enzymatic reactions in either normal or tumor tissues (Table 40-1). Cisplatin, for example, undergoes a chemical reaction with water molecules intracellularly, resulting in the generation of a positively charged aquated species that attacks nucleophilic sites on DNA.[22] In contrast, the activation of cyclophosphamide is mediated primarily by CYP2B6 (one of the P-450 enzymes), resulting in the release of active alkylating species into the systemic circulation.[23]

Intracellular activation by tumor cells is a critical determinant of effect for most antimetabolites. Nucleoside analogues such as cytarabine, fludarabine, and gemcitabine require phosphorylation to active nucleotide triphosphate forms and incorporation into DNA before they are able to exert a cytotoxic effect.[10,24–26] Nucleobase analogues such as 6-mercaptopurine and 6-thioguanine undergo phosphoribosylation to the nucleoside monophosphate forms, which are active inhibitors of de novo purine nucleotide synthesis. Amination of 6-mercaptopurine to thioguanine monophosphate followed by phosphorylation, reduction to the deoxynucleotide, and a subsequent phosphorylation results in 2'-deoxythioguanine triphosphate, which is a substrate for incorporation into DNA. Phosphoribosylation also converts 5-fluorouracil to the monophosphate, which is then phosphorylated to the diphosphate, reduced to the deoxynucleotide and dephosphorylated to the active monophosphate F-dUMP that inhibits thymidylate synthase. Additionally, the drug may be cytotoxic after incorporation of either the ribosyl or deoxyribosyl triphosphate into RNA or DNA, respectively. Although methotrexate is an effective enzyme inhibitor in its native form, intracellular conversion of the drug to polyglutamate metabolites significantly increases its potency and facilitates its binding to a number of enzymatic sites.[27] Consistent with this is the finding of a more favorable clinical outcome in acute lymphocytic leukemia patients whose blasts accumulated higher levels of methotrexate polyglutamates.[28,29] It is important to note that phosphorylation of nucleic acid analogues and polyglutamylation of methotrexate produces charged molecules that are unlikely to diffuse or to be transported out of cells.

The rate of formation of the activated drug species in the cell depends on the rate of transmembrane influx of the drug, the amount and affinity of the activating enzyme(s) in the cell, the extent of competition by the naturally occurring substrates of the activating enzymes, and the rate of degradation of the activated drug by catabolic enzymes. For many antimetabolites, membrane transport is rapid relative to enzymatic activation and is therefore not rate limiting. Once inside the cell, antimetabolites must compete with the natural substrates of metabolic enzymes for binding and activation. Finally, the activated drug then becomes a substrate for catabolic enzymes in the cell that tend to degrade it to the parent compound or to an inactive metabolite. Thus, the concentration of the active cytotoxic drug in the cell is the result of the interactions of all of these processes.

Table 40-1 Activation of Anticancer Drugs

Activation Reaction	Drug
Aquation	Cisplatin
Hydrolysis	Irinotecan
Polyglutamylation	Methotrexate
Phosphorylation	Cytarabine
	Fludarabine
	Gemcitabine
Phosphoribosylation	5-Fluorouracil
	6-Mercaptopurine
	6-Thioguanine
Microsomal oxidation	Cyclophosphamide
	Ifosphamide
	Procarbazine
Microsomal reduction	Bleomycin
Demethylation	Dacarbazine
	Hexamethylmelamine
Acetylation	Amonafide

The pyrimidine nucleoside analogue, gemcitabine, provides an excellent example of these processes. Gemcitabine is a substrate for several transport systems, but likely gains entry to the cell by a high capacity equilibrative nucleoside transport system, the velocity of which is nearly proportional to gemcitabine concentrations approaching millimolar.[30] This process is unlikely to limit gemcitabine transport into cells at the plasma concentrations (> 60 μM) achieved by standard dose rates (> 2,000 mg/m²/hr). At such plasma concentrations, however, the transport systems provide cellular concentrations of gemcitabine that saturate the rate of gemcitabine phosphorylation by deoxycytidine kinase.[31] Recognition of this lack of linearity with increasing dose rate has prompted evaluation of strategies in which gemcitabine is infused at a fixed dose rate of 10 mg/m²/min for several hours, which achieves plasma gemcitabine concentrations (~20 μM) that maximize the rate of gemcitabine phosphorylation.[32–34] Studies of circulating leukemia blasts have demonstrated that this approach increases the cellular accumulation of gemcitabine nucleotides.[35,36] Following the initial phosphorylation of gemcitabine, the monophosphate is metabolized by two successive phosphorylation reactions to the triphosphate, which, after its incorporation into replicating or repairing DNA by various DNA polymerases is inhibitory to cell growth. The initial activating enzyme, deoxycytidine kinase, is present at the lowest specific activities in human leukemic blasts[37] and is believed to be the rate-limiting step in the formation of gemcitabine triphosphate,[32] and probably for incorporation of the drug into DNA. At each phosphorylation step, gemcitabine and its metabolites compete with endogenous deoxycytidine and its nucleotides for enzyme binding. Opposing the activation of gemcitabine are cytidine deaminase and dCMP deaminase that convert the nucleoside and its monophosphate, respectively, to inactive uracil derivatives.[38] In addition, the activity of phosphatases such as 5'-nucleotidase,[26] the activities of which differ among cell types, may be important determinants of the steady-state concentrations of gemcitabine nucleotides and the rate of elimination of the triphosphate at the end of gemcitabine infusion.[39] Thus, in the case of antimetabolites, the loss or diminished affinity of an activating enzyme or enhanced activity of a catabolic enzyme may tip the balance between clinical activity and drug resistance.

Drug Targets Although cytotoxic anticancer drugs have traditionally been classified based on their mechanisms of action or their origins, they can also be grouped based on their targets. There are several major targets of drug action: nucleic acids, specific metabolic and signaling enzymes, and microtubules. When nucleic acids are the target, it is generally an action on the integrity or synthesis of DNA rather than of RNA that is presumed to cause cell death. There are several mechanisms by which drugs can bind DNA, the most well understood being alkylation of nucleophilic sites within the double helix. Most clinically effective alkylating agents have two moieties capable of developing a charged carbon that binds covalently to negatively charged sites on DNA such as the O^6 or N^7 positions of guanine. The cross-linking of the two strands of DNA produced by the bifunctional alkylating agents prevents the use of that DNA as a template for further DNA and RNA synthesis leading to inhibition of DNA replication and cell death.[40,41] Although alkylating agents are among the most widely used drugs in clinical oncology, the relationship of pharmacologic parameters to clinical effects has not been well defined for these agents. In part, this has been due to the lack of sensitive and specific techniques to detect drug-DNA binding in clinical specimens. Studies of chlorambucil-DNA binding in the tumor cells of patients with chronic lymphocytic leukemia have demonstrated considerable heterogeneity in drug-DNA binding among patient samples. However, no clear correlations have been demonstrated between the amount of drug bound and disease stage or sensitivity to treatment. In contrast, the formation of cisplatin adducts to DNA has been shown to correlate with cell kill in mammalian tumor cell lines.[43] Immunologic methods have been used to quantitate platinum-DNA adduct formation in peripheral white blood cells[44] after cisplatin. A separate study that used atomic absorption spectroscopy to quantitate total cell platinum in lymphocytes indicated a relationship between the levels of adduct after the first dose of either single-drug cisplatin or carboplatin and clinical response.[45] However, subsequent investigations have not found such a relationship between platinum-DNA adduct levels and clinical outcome.[46]

A second mechanism of drug binding to nucleic acids is intercalation, the insertion of a planar ring structure between two adjacent nucleotide bases of DNA. This mechanism is characteristic of many antitumor antibiotics. The antibiotic molecule is noncovalently, although firmly, bound to DNA and distorts the shape of the double helix, resulting in inhibition of RNA or DNA synthesis.[47,48] Many agents capable of classic intercalation, such as doxorubicin and mitoxantrone, are also inhibitors of topoisomerase II and may produce DNA strand breaks by inhibition of the religation process of this enzyme.[49,50] Indeed, a direct correlation has been noted between DNA topoisomerase II activity and cytotoxicity in doxorubicin-sensitive and resistant P388 leukemia cells.[51] A third mechanism of nucleic acid damage is illustrated by the anticancer drug bleomycin. The amino terminal tripeptide of the bleomycin molecule appears to intercalate between guanine-cytosine base pairs of DNA. The opposite end of the bleomycin peptide binds Fe (II) and serves as a ferrous oxidase, able to catalyze the reduction of molecular oxygen to superoxide or hydroxyl radicals that produce DNA strand scission.[52,53] Predictably, the levels of antioxidant enzymes such as catalase, peroxidases, and superoxide dismutase in plasma and blood are inversely correlated with chromosomal damage.[54]

Enzymes represent the second general category of targets for chemotherapeutic agents. Antimetabolites function as inhibitors of key enzymes in the purine or pyrimidine biosynthetic pathways or as inhibitors of DNA polymerases. The triphosphate of fludarabine, for instance, is known to inhibit both ribonucleotide reductase[55] and DNA ligase I.[56] After incorporation into DNA it not only inhibits the function of multiple DNA polymerases,[57] DNA primase[58] and DNA ligase I,[56] it is also resistant to removal by the proof-reading exonuclease activities associated with DNA polymerases.[57] Since these enzymes are highly active during DNA replication, antimetabolites tend to be cytotoxic only when present in sufficient concentration during the vulnerable S phase of the cell cycle; these drugs are thus frequently referred to as S phase specific. Nevertheless, because these enzymes are also required for repair of damaged DNA, it is likely that antimetabolites that inhibit these enzymes will be synergistic with agents, which elicit an incision DNA repair response that requires resynthesis of a DNA patch, regardless of cell-cycle stage.[59]

The effectiveness of enzyme inhibitors also depends on the amount of the target enzyme, its affinity for the inhibitor, and on the extent of competition by natural substrates for enzyme binding. For example, complete saturation of all dihydrofolate reductase-binding sites is required before the enzyme is effectively inhibited. As methotrexate inhibits enzymatic activity, dihydrofolate, the natural substrate, accumulates behind the metabolic block and is able to effectively compete with methotrexate for further enzyme binding.[60] Thus, large amounts of methotrexate, well in excess of the enzyme binding capacity, are required to effectively inhibit dihydrofolate reductase activity. Similarly, in the case of 5-FU, the dUMP/F-dUMP value may be an important determinant of optimal inhibition of the target enzyme thymidylate synthase, and high ratios have been associated with lack of tumor response.[61] Similarly, the amount of thymidylate synthase expression or activity is an important determinant of 5-FU activity and correlates with therapeutic response.[62] Also, polymorphisms in the thymidylate synthase gene may have prognostic value.[63,64] In addition, high basal levels of thymidine phosphorylase have been associated with lack of response to 5-FU.[65] However, screening for thymidylate phosphorylase levels is an attractive approach to selecting patients for treatment with capecitabine or doxifluridine, nucleoside analogues that require the activity of this enzyme for release of 5-FU.[66,67]

In addition to the enzymes required for purine and pyrimidine metabolism, the topoisomerases are important targets of several antineoplastic agents. Topoisomerase II relieves torsion in DNA by creating a double strand break in the molecule, facilitating the passage of adjacent DNA through the gap, followed by resealing of the break. Topoisomerase I nicks a single DNA strand, which permits the rotation on the intact strand, after which the nick is closed. Topoisomerase inhibitors bind to the respective enzymes and stabilize the reaction intermediate enzyme-DNA cleavable complex. This interference with the DNA breakage-resealing process, which is necessary for both DNA replication and RNA transcription, results in DNA strand breaks that are lethal to the cell. The epipodophyllotoxins, etoposide and teniposide, are potent inhibitors of topoisomerase II, as are a number of DNA intercalating agents, including doxorubicin, actinomycin D, and amsacrine.[49,50,68]

Two topoisomerase I inhibitors, topotecan and irinotecan, have been approved for clinical use. Whereas topotecan interacts with topoisomerase I directly, irinotecan requires activation by carboxylesterases to the active metabolite SN-38.[69] It is not yet clear whether irinotecan's antitumor effects are due primarily to intratumoral or intrahepatic activation, although there is some evidence that higher enzyme activity in tumors is associated with a greater cytotoxic effect.[70–72]

The microtubule spindle structure provides a third target for chemotherapeutic agents, classically the vinca alkaloids, vincristine and vinblastine, but more recently vinorelbine. The vinca alkaloids exert their cytotoxic effects by binding to specific sites on tubulin inhibiting of assembly of tubulin into microtubules and ultimately dissolution of the mitotic spindle structure.[73] The microtubule system in cells performs a variety of other important functions, including transport of solutes, cell movement, and chromosomal separation, and provides structural integrity, any one of which could potentially be disrupted by tubulin binding agents.[74] The taxanes are a newer class of agents, consisting of the natural plant alkaloid paclitaxel and a semisynthetic derivative docetaxel. These novel plant alkaloids inhibit cell division by stimulating tubulin polymerization, thus enhancing the formation and stability of microtubules.[75] Paclitaxel-treated cells accumulate large numbers of microtubules, free and in bundles, that disrupt microtubule function, and which ultimately cause cell death.[76,77] Although docetaxel appears to be more potent than paclitaxel, the drugs appear to have similar toxicity profiles.[78] The epothilones are nontaxane agents that also are capable of stabilizing microtubules.[79,80] Early results indicate that these compounds are active in the clinic, but have a similar spectrum of toxicity as the taxanes.

Repair of Drug-Induced Injury Cells that have been damaged by cytotoxic drugs exhibit a variety of repair mechanisms. Indeed the cytotoxic effects of a drug often represent the balance between injury and repair, and amplified repair mechanisms may account for cellular resistance to certain drugs. The cytotoxicity of alkylating agents reflects the balance between DNA adduct and cross-link formation and their removal by cellular repair processes.[81] Many cells contain specific enzymes that remove alkyl moieties from DNA, and thereby undergo direct repair of drug damage. A specific example is the protein O^6-alkylguanyltransferase that repairs DNA injury produced by chloroethylnitrosoureas. Cells containing large amounts of this protein tend to be relatively resistant to these chemotherapeutic agents. Depletion of alkyltransferase activity by exposure of cells to modified purine bases such as O^6-benzylguanine may be effective in circumventing this mechanism of resistance.[82–84] It is now clear that mammalian cells possess a family of such enzymes that are capable of repairing alkylation to specific nucleic acid bases, and that the abundance of these in a particular tissue may be responsible for conferring relative sensitivity or resistance to chemotherapeutic alkylating agents.[85–87]

The broader task of protecting the genome from a wide variety of adducts that affect replication and transcription is taken up by the nucleotide excision repair system.[88–91] The increased incidence of cancer in individuals who have genetic diseases such as xeroderma pigmentosum, which is characterized by the lack of effective nucleotide excision repair, attests to the key role this system has in suppressing carcinogenesis due to DNA damage.[92,93] This process has a broad specificity for adducts that it can remove from DNA, ranging from simple methyl groups to bulky adducts, including natural molecules such as psoralen and aminofluorene. Lesions produced by cisplatin and cyclophosphamide are also substrates; an increase in the rate of platinum adduct removal has been associated with drug resistance.[94] The mechanism of adduct removal is now clear and the various proteins involved are identified.[95,96] Basically, once a distortion in the DNA structure is detected, two incisions are made in the adduct-containing DNA strand precisely 27 or 29 nucleotides apart. This adduct-containing oligonucleotide is removed as a single piece, and new nucleotides are polymerized in the repair patch by the same DNA polymerases involved in replication. This DNA synthesis phase presents an opportunity to incorporate nucleoside analogues into DNA of cells that are not in S phase, which would otherwise not be affected. This possibility has given rise to therapeutic strategies that combine agents or modalities that elicit DNA repair with one of the newer nucleoside analogues, such as fludarabine[24] and gemcitabine,[25] which inhibit DNA synthesis by a number of different mechanisms. Blocking completion of the resynthesis step generates signaling that subsequently induces cell death.[97]

Cells also contain a variety of free radical scavenging systems that protect them from the effects of ionizing radiation and drugs that generate oxygen free radicals intracellularly. Catalase, superoxide dismutase, and glutathione peroxidase, key enzymes in the detoxification of reactive oxygen species, may be deficient in some tissues, such as cardiac muscle, leading to excessive drug toxicity. Alternatively, an increase in these protective enzymes in tumor cells may be associated with resistance to drugs that act by generating reactive oxygen species.[98] For instance, some doxorubicin-resistant cells have been shown to increase activity of superoxide dismutase and sodium-dependent glutathione peroxidase; these cells exhibit diminished susceptibility to oxygen radical injury.[99] Recent investigations have indicated the potential for therapeutic approaches that target such protective mechanisms.[100] Other studies suggest that expansion of intracellular reduced glutathione pools or increased expression of glutathione transferase may be important mechanisms of alkylating agent resistance in animal and human tumors.[101–103]

Finally, cells may be able to circumvent drug-induced injury by increased production of target enzymes. In experimental models, exposure of cells to methotrexate or 5-FU can be shown to stimulate production of dihydrofolate reductase or thymidylate synthase, respectively.[104,105] New enzyme production occurs within minutes to hours of drug exposure and is presumed to represent enhanced translation of existing mRNA rather than transcription of additional message. Amplification of DNA also occurs, however, and may be a fundamental mechanism of acquired cellular resistance to antimetabolites and natural products because of increased constitutive production of target enzymes or P-glycoprotein.[106]

As mentioned earlier, a prerequisite to drug effect at the target tissue is adequate drug delivery. Pharmacokinetics describes the concentration-time history of a drug in the body and can be used to answer fundamental questions concerning the optimal route and schedule of drug administration. The remainder of this chapter will present the principles of pharmacokinetics and pharmacodynamics and illustrate their importance in cancer chemotherapy.

PRINCIPLES OF PHARMACOKINETICS

Definitions Pharmacokinetics is the study of drug absorption, distribution, metabolism, and excretion (Figure 40-1). A fundamental concept in pharmacokinetics is drug clearance, that is, elimination of drugs from the body, analogous to the concept of creatinine clearance. In clinical practice, clearance of a drug is rarely measured directly but is calculated as either of the following:

$$\text{clearance} = \text{dose/AUC (equation 1)}$$
or
$$\text{clearance} = \text{infusion rate}/C_{ss} \text{ (equation 2).}$$

The area under the curve (AUC) represents the total drug exposure integrated over time and is an important parameter for both pharmacokinetic and pharmacodynamic analyses. As indicated in equation 1, the clearance is simply the ratio of the dose to the AUC, so that the higher the AUC for a given dose, the lower the clearance. If a drug is administered by continuous infusion and a steady state is achieved, the clearance can be estimated from a single measurement of the plasma drug concentration (C_{ss}) as in equation 2.

Clearance can conceptually be considered to be a function of both distribution and elimination. In the simplest pharmacokinetic model,

$$\text{clearance} = V\,K \text{ (equation 3),}$$

V is the volume of distribution, and K is the elimination constant. V is the volume of fluid in which

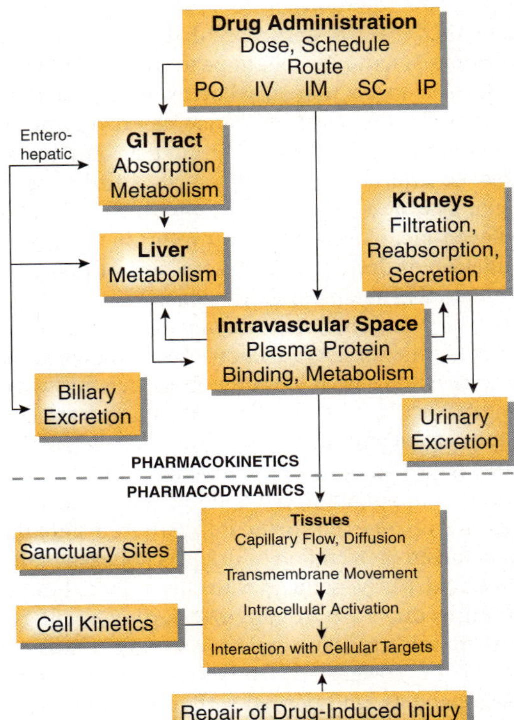

Figure 40-1 Schematic representation of pharmacokinetics and pharmacodynamics. Pharmacokinetics represents the absorption, distribution, metabolism, and excretion of drugs from the body. Pharmacodynamics describes the interaction of drugs with target tissues. GI = gastrointestinal; IM = intramuscular; IP = intraperitoneal; IV = intravenous; PO = by mouth; SC = subcutaneous.

the dose is initially diluted, and thus the higher the V, the lower the initial concentration. K is the elimination constant, which is inversely proportional to the half-life, the period of time that must elapse to reach a 50% decrease in plasma concentration. When the half-life is short, K is high and plasma concentrations decline rapidly. Thus both a high V and a high K result in relatively low plasma concentrations and a high clearance.

Linear Pharmacokinetic Models Although pharmacokinetic analysis can be conducted without specifying any mathematical models (noncompartmental methods), it is helpful to use such models as guides in therapeutic decision making. There are several important characteristics of drugs that have linear pharmacokinetics (Table 40-2). The key feature of a linear pharmacokinetic model is that

$$dC/dt = -KC \text{ (equation 4).}$$

This indicates that the instantaneous rate of change in drug concentration depends only on the current concentration. The half-life will remain constant no matter how high the concentration.

One implication of this principle is that the drug exposure (AUC) is not affected by changes in drug schedule. For example, the AUC after a 60 mg/m^2 bolus dose of doxorubicin equals the total AUC for 3 daily (or weekly) bolus doses of 20 mg/m^2, which equals the AUC for the same dose administered as a 96-hour infusion. A second implication is that the AUC is proportional to the dose. Thus, if one measures the AUC for a 60 mg/m^2 dose, one can estimate the AUC for a 90 mg/m^2 dose in the same patient as being 50% greater.

The simplest linear pharmacokinetic model, shown graphically in Figure 40-2, is

$$C(t) = \frac{\text{Dose}}{V}(e^{-kt}) \text{ (equation 5).}$$

This model assumes that the drug is administered as an instantaneous bolus and that complete distribution of the drug is also instantaneous.

These assumptions are often not valid. If the drug is administered as a slow bolus or infusion, the model must be corrected for the infusion duration. During the administration of the drug, the concentration is increasing:

$$C(t) = \frac{\text{Dose}}{VKT}(1-e^{-kt}) \text{ (equation 6).}$$

After the infusion is terminated, the drug concentration decays at the same rate as if it had been administered as an instantaneous bolus. Thus, if T represents the infusion time, then the postinfusion drug concentrations can be represented as

$$C'(t) = C(T)e^{-k(t-T)} \text{ (equation 7).}$$

Table 40-2 Characteristics of Drugs with Linear Pharmacokinetics
Area under the curve is directly proportional to dose
Half-life is independent of concentration
Clearance is independent of dose
Clearance is independent of schedule

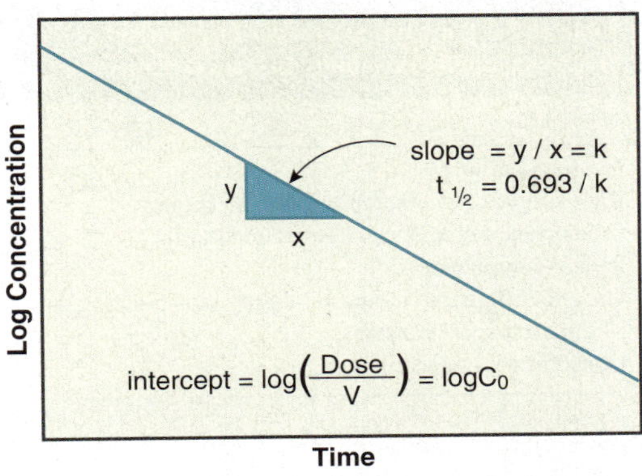

Figure 40-2 Concentration-time plot for 1-compartment linear pharmacokinetic mode. C_0 represents the initial concentration, assuming instantaneous administration and distribution. The half-life is $\log_e(2)/k$. V = volume of distribution.

Often, the pharmacokinetic data are more complex than those shown in Figure 40-2 and may be optimally fitted to a multicompartment model, usually two or three compartments (Figure 40-3). It must be emphasized that the compartments are theoretical and do not necessarily correlate with any anatomic space or physiologic process.

A large variety of computer software is available for pharmacokinetic analysis.[107–109] The interested reader is likely to benefit from hands-on experience with such programs. Several caveats need to be emphasized for the casual reader. The validity of pharmacokinetic modeling depends to a large extent on the quality of the data entered into the model. Thus, drug infusions must be precisely timed, a sufficient number of plasma samples must be drawn, the samples must be obtained on schedule, and analytic methods must be sensitive and specific. The data must be properly weighted to avoid bias due to the increased probability of analytic errors at drug concentrations near the detection limit of the assay. Results obtained using a specific model should be compared with those using noncompartmental methods. Extrapolation of models outside the known time points must be done with great caution.

Nonlinear Pharmacokinetic Models Nonlinear pharmacokinetic models imply that some aspect of the pharmacokinetic behavior of the drug is saturable. The mathematics of nonlinear models is beyond the scope of this chapter, but the

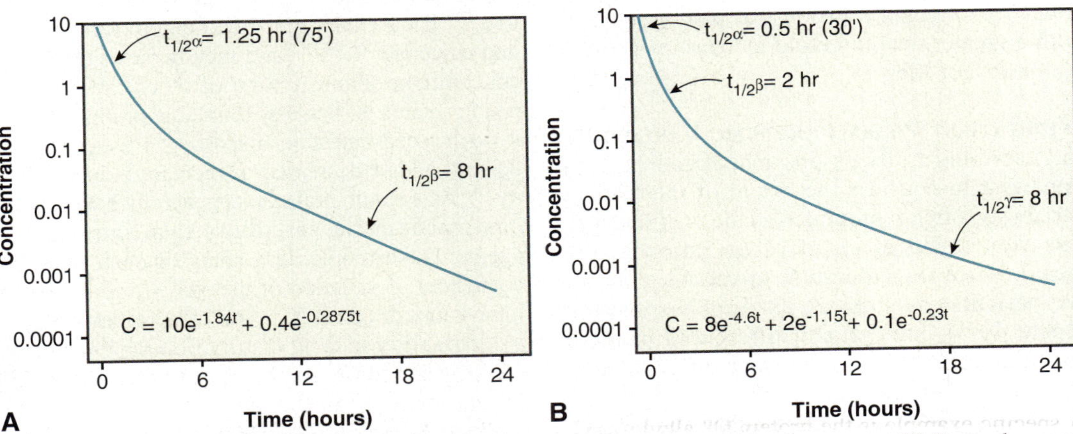

Figure 40-3 Concentration-time plots for representative 2-compartment **(A)** and 3-compartment **(B)** linear pharmacokinetic models. The two curves are very similar, with C_0 ~10 for both models. Note that for each "compartment" there is one term, and the corresponding half-life equals $t_{1/2}$ $\log_e(2)/k^n$, where k^n is the nth term.

principles are very relevant to several anticancer agents.[110–112] In contrast to the administration schedule of drugs with linear pharmacokinetics, alteration of the administration schedule of drugs that display nonlinear kinetics may markedly affect the AUC and potentially alter clinical effects.

Nonlinear pharmacokinetic behavior commonly occurs when there is saturation of a major metabolic or transport pathway. This results in decreased clearance at higher doses, with a greater-than-proportional increase in the AUC. The AUC will also increase if the infusion duration is shortened because of slower clearance at the higher peak plasma concentrations. This is clearly the case for 5-FU, probably because of saturation of its conversion to dihydrofluorouracil by the enzyme dihydropyrimidine dehydrogenase.[113–116] Schaaf and colleagues demonstrated that doubling of the 5-FU dose from approximately 7.5 mg/kg to 15 mg/kg (by IV bolus) resulted in a 135% increase in the mean AUC.[115] Since 5-FU is used on a variety of schedules, its nonlinear pharmacokinetic behavior may be one factor in its highly schedule-dependent effects. Paclitaxel has also been demonstrated to have nonlinear pharmacokinetics.[117–119] Thus, the AUC is higher, for a fixed dose, when administered by a shorter (3-hour vs 24-hour) infusion schedule, although this does not result in enhanced toxicity.[120]

The opposite situation arises when a drug's absorption from the gastrointestinal tract (or renal tubular reabsorption) is saturable. In this case, an increase in dose results in a less than proportional increase in the AUC. Gastrointestinal absorption of drugs that resemble natural compounds is frequently mediated by active transport processes that display saturable kinetics. Folate analogues such as methotrexate or leucovorin and amino acid analogues such as melphalan are examples of drugs with saturable absorption.[121–123] Cisplatin appears to have nonlinear pharmacokinetics owing to the saturation of its renal tubular reabsorption.[124,125] Forastiere and colleagues demonstrated that free plasma platinum is increased by 42% when the drug is given as a 24-hour continuous infusion, rather than as a 20-minute infusion.[124] Prolonged infusion was also associated with a greater than threefold increase in the free platinum half-life.

Interpatient Pharmacokinetic Variability

In describing a drug's pharmacokinetics, it is important to consider the extent of interpatient variability, often represented as the coefficient of variation (ratio of standard deviation to the mean). There are a multitude of variables in cancer patients that impact on drug disposition (Table 40-3). Interpatient differences in these variables can lead to significant differences in pharmacokinetic parameters.[126]

Table 40-3 Potential Sources of Interpatient Pharmacokinetic Variability in Cancer Patients

Abnormalities of Absorption
Nausea/vomiting
Prior surgery, radiotherapy, or chemotherapy
Concurrent antiemetics affecting gut motility
Patient compliance
Genetic differences in intestinal drug metabolizing and drug transport enzymes
Concomitant medications
Abnormalities of Distribution
Weight loss
Obesity
Decreased body fat (lipophilic drugs)
Pleural effusions or ascites (methotrexate)
Abnormalities of Elimination
Hepatic dysfunction because of tumor replacement or prior (or concurrent) therapy
Renal dysfunction because of malignant involvement or prior (or concurrent) therapy
Genetic differences in drug metabolizing and drug transport enzymes
Concomitant medications
Abnormalities in Protein Binding
Hypoalbuminemia
Concomitant medications

Studies of interpatient pharmacokinetic variability are potentially of great importance for optimizing antineoplastic therapy. Variability in gastrointestinal absorption is generally not considered in the use of orally administered antineoplastic agents even though drugs such as cyclophosphamide, chlorambucil, melphalan, and etoposide are commonly administered orally for a variety of malignancies.[2] The fraction of an administered dose of drug that reaches systemic circulation is referred to as its bioavailability. Alternatively, it is the ratio of the plasma AUC after oral administration to the plasma AUC after intravenous administration of the same dose. Bioavailability is influenced both by absorption barriers and the first-pass effect, which is the reduction in available drug due to metabolism in the gastrointestinal tract and liver before an orally-administered dose reaches systemic circulation. The bioavailability of the (6R) isomer of leucovorin, for example, is primarily limited by absorption. By contrast, (6S) leucovorin has limited bioavailability because of its rapid conversion to 5-methyltetrahydrofolate prior to reaching the systemic circulation.[127] Bioavailability is often highly variable and unpredictable[25,128–132] and may be accentuated by concomitant administration of other chemotherapeutic agents, particularly those that produce toxicity to the gastrointestinal mucosa.[122] Food can cause delayed and/or decreased or increased bioavaiability.[133] As a result, oral agents generally have higher pharmacokinetic variability than intravenous agents. For example, in a study of etoposide, the coefficient of variation of the AUC for oral versus intravenous drug was 58% and 28%, respectively.[134]

Variability in drug distribution may be attributed to changes in body size or to the ratio of fat to total mass.[135] In the latter case, there may be altered distribution of lipophilic drugs, which includes most of the natural product anticancer drugs and their analogues. The terminal elimination half-lives of doxorubicin, cyclophosphamide, and ifosfamide are prolonged in obese patients.[136–138] In the case of doxorubicin and cyclophosphamide, this appears to be due to a reduction in clearance, whereas in the case of ifosfamide it is related to an increased volume of distribution of the drug.[136] Drug distribution can also be altered in the setting of "third-space" fluid. The best described example of this is the delayed clearance of methotrexate due to accumulation of drug in and slow release of the drug from ascites and pleural effusions.[139]

Many patients with advanced cancer have abnormalities of liver function tests or known mass lesions within the liver, often in association with significant malnutrition. Because many antineoplastic agents are metabolized or excreted by the liver, recognizing altered elimination by the liver becomes important in the optimization of chemotherapy dosing. Unfortunately, altered hepatic metabolism or excretion of drugs is not easily predictable. Clearly, patients with severe hyperbilirubinemia due to parenchymal replacement or obstruction are likely to have altered elimination.[140,141] However, it is not often recognized that many patients with normal serum bilirubin levels may have a low drug clearance resulting in a high AUC and corresponding toxicity as a result of other liver function test abnormalities. A decrease in serum albumin (in patients with normal serum bilirubin concentrations) has been associated with a decrease in the hepatic elimination of antipyrine, a commonly used marker drug, and of vinblastine and trimetrexate.[142–145] Thus, patients with a serum albumin less than 2.5 g/dL may be at increased risk of toxicity and are potential candidates for dose reduction of agents requiring hepatic metabolism or excretion.

In contrast, alterations in renal function generally correlate with renal clearance of drugs, since renal drug clearance tends to correlate with creatinine clearance. This has been well established for carboplatin, for which a firm relationship exists between renal function and carboplatin clearance. This relationship can be used prospectively to modify the carboplatin dose and avoid excessive toxicity.[146–148]

At present, dose adjustments for hepatic and renal dysfunction are most often made empirically and manufacturer recommendations are of limited use. This is illustrated by the recommended dose reduction for capecitabine in the setting of renal impairment.[149] In an editorial regarding this recommendation,[150] Ratain noted that the recommended 25% reduction was for patients with a creatinine clearance of 31 to 50 mL/min as estimated by the Cockcroft-Gault formula, which has been criticized as inaccurate.[151–155] This formula estimates a lower creatinine clearance for women and individuals with increased serum creatinine, low weight, and increased age. Furthermore, this definition of renal impairment is not adjusted for body surface area (BSA). As a result, it is possible that a small woman would receive a dosage reduction and a large man would not, even though their BSA-normalized creatinine clearances were the same. Also, before such a dose adjustment is recommended, there must be data supporting a correlation between creatinine clearance and drug pharmacokinetics or there is the potential for subtherapeutic dosing. Because of examples such as capecitabine, there is an increasing interest in performing dose-finding and pharmacokinetic studies in patients with hepatic and renal abnormalities. This is evidenced by the formation of the National Cancer Institute Organ Dysfunction Working Group and the recent publication of several trials in these subpopulations.[140,156–160]

Abnormalities of protein binding are common, but rarely have an impact on clinical outcome. Many anticancer drugs, such as the vinca alkaloids and etoposide, are highly bound to proteins such as albumin.[141,161,162] Changes in protein binding may affect drug clearance.[163,164] More importantly, abnormal protein binding must be considered in the interpretation of measured total plasma drug concentrations, since a decrease in protein binding will result in a relative increase in the pharmacologically active "free" drug.[141,165] For a given dose, levels of unbound, active drug will be higher in the hypoalbuminemic patient as compared with the patient with normal albumin levels.

Identifying genetic differences in drug disposition (absorption, distribution, metabolism, and excretion) may be particularly important in understanding interindividual pharmacokinetic variability.[166–168] For example, SN-38 is the active metabolite of irinotecan and is primarily inactivated through biotransformation into SN-38 glucuronide (SN-38G) by UDP- glucuronosyltransferase 1A1 (UGT1A1).[169] Transcriptional efficiency of the *UGT1A1* gene is inversely correlated with the number of TA repeats in the promoter TATA box of the gene.[170] Investigators have demonstrated that the AUC for SN-38 is directly correlated with the number of TA_7 (7 TA repeats) alleles, so that individuals that are homozygous for TA_7 have higher AUC values than those who are not.[171] Clinically, these patients are at higher risk of severe neutropenia. The observed pharmacokinetic variability of other anticancer agents, such as 6-mercaptopurine,[172,173] 5-FU, and amonafide,[174–176] can also be explained, in part, by pharmacogenetic variation. The importance of this source of interpatient variability is demonstrated by the incorporation into the product labels for irinotecan[177] and 6-mercaptopurine[178] the recommendation that prescribers consider initial dosage reductions in the presence of reduced UGT1A1 and thiopurine methyltransferase (TPMT) activity, respectively.

INTRAPATIENT PHARMACOKINETIC VARIABILITY Although it is well established that interpatient pharmacokinetic variability may be significant, the importance of intrapatient variability (within a single patient) is less clear.[179] Oncologists are commonly faced with the clinical situation of increasing myelosuppression after repetitive dosing. This is generally assumed to be due to the cumulative effects of chemotherapy, making the patient more sensitive to subsequent doses. However, it is also possible that the patient's clearance of the drug(s) may have decreased, resulting in increased drug exposure.

Such a situation may arise when either hepatic or renal function changes. Renal function may change because of progressive disease (ureteral obstruction), complications of therapy (volume depletion), or as a direct toxic effect of therapy (cisplatin). Similarly, renal function may improve over time, reducing the actual drug exposure. Hepatic function may also change, producing changes in drug clearance that may result in the appearance of increased toxicity over time, as is the case for vinblastine administered by prolonged continuous infusion.[144] Thus, clinicians should carefully review the outcome of prior doses to minimize the risk of an undesirable outcome due to intrapatient pharmacokinetic variability.

Another potential source of intrapatient pharmacokinetic variability is an individual's circadian rhythm. The best studied drugs in this regard are 5-FU and 5-fluoro-2'-deoxyuridine.[180] Petit and colleagues evaluated circadian variability of 5-FU plasma concentrations during a 5-day infusion at a constant dose and demonstrated a greater than twofold difference between maximum and minimum values.[181] Similar results were obtained by Harris and colleagues who demonstrated an inverse correlation between plasma 5-FU concentration and the activity of dihydropyrimidine dehydrogenase, the major catabolic enzyme for 5-FU.[182] Investigators have explored the feasibility, toxicity, and activity of chronomodulated therapy with 5-FU, which takes advantage of the apparent circadian changes in drug clearance by increasing drug infusion during the time intervals when clearance is increased.[183–186]

DRUG-DRUG INTERACTIONS Despite the fact that anticancer drugs are almost always given as combination chemotherapy, there have been relatively few studies in this area despite the risk of pharmacokinetic interactions. For example, with the combination of paclitaxel and cisplatin, an important regimen for ovarian cancer, cisplatin reduces paclitaxel clearance if given first.[187]

Studies of modulators of drug reactions have also demonstrated that inhibition of clearance may be an unexpected outcome. In a clinical study of the effects of oral cyclosporine on irinotecan pharmacokinetics, in which subjects received irinotecan both with and without cyclosporine, investigators found a marked reduction in irinotecan clearance (from 13.4 L/h/m^2 to 5.8 L/h/m^2) with the addition of cyclosporine.[188] Moreover, the AUC of the active metabolite SN-38 was significantly increased. Similar effects of cyclosporine on clearance have been demonstrated for etoposide,[189,190] doxorubicin,[191,192] and mitoxantrone.[189]

The oncologist must be aware of the patient's prescription medication list and consider the pharmacokinetic and therapeutic consequences when prescribing a new drug. A recent drug-drug interaction with potential therapeutic implications is that of tamoxifen and selective serotonin reuptake inhibitor (SSRI) antidepressants. Both are metabolized by CYP2D6, and SSRIs are commonly prescribed for the hot flashes associated with tamoxifen therapy. Jin and colleagues recently reported the results of a prospective study of 80 breast cancer patients in which 29% were taking SSRI antidepressants after 4 months of tamoxifen therapy.[193] They found that the mean plasma concentrations of endoxifen, an active metabolite of tamoxifen, decreased by 56% ($p = .02$) with paroxetine coadministration. They also reported an interesting interaction between SSRIs and *CYP2D6* genotype in that subjects who were homozygous for the wild-type *CYP2D6* allele had a greater reduction in endoxifen concentrations as compared with those who were heterozygous (58% vs 38%). The precise clinical implications of a decrease in endoxifen concentrations is still under investigation, but these data do raise the question of whether concomitant administration of SSRI antidepressants to reduce the side effects of tamoxifen may jeopardize the efficacy of patient's anticancer therapy, and the US Food and Drug Administration is currently considering incorporating the pharmacogenetic data into the product label for tamoxifen.

In recent years, the use of herbal medicines and nutritional supplements by cancer patients has been increasing.[194] The perceived low risk of these agents and lack of knowledge about their pharmacology can result in unexpected toxic and pharmacokinetic effects when they are used concomitantly with chemotherapy. For example, St. John's Wort (*Hypericum perforatum*) is a known ligand for the pregnane X receptor (PXR).[195,196] It can therefore induce the transcription of PXR-regulated genes such as *CYP3A* and uridine diphosphate glucuronosyltransferases (UGTs).[195,197–199] Mathijssen and colleagues demonstrated that the use of St. John's Wort decreases plasma concentrations of SN-38 (active metabolite) in irinotecan-treated patients, prompting concerns that efficacy might be reduced.[200]

PRINCIPLES OF PHARMACODYNAMICS

DEFINITIONS In a general sense, pharmacodynamics is the study of dose-response relationships.[201] Thus, any laboratory or clinical study employing different doses of an agent is addressing a pharmacodynamic question. Examples include the exposure of tumor cells in vitro to varying doses of a new agent to evaluate its dose-response relationship or a phase I clinical trial to define the maximally tolerated dose and dose-limiting toxicities in patients.

In the clinical setting, the results of treatment depend on both pharmacokinetics and pharmacodynamics (see Figure 40-1). A patient may have excessive toxicity at the "standard" dose for one of two reasons. If the patient's pharmacokinetics are different from those of the typical patient (eg, decreased renal clearance of carboplatin), there may be decreased total-body clearance resulting in a higher than expected drug exposure. The second possibility is that the patient might simply be more sensitive to an average drug exposure because of prior therapy, poor nutrition, or some other less well-defined reason. It is important to distinguish between these two possibilities. In the first case, lowering the dose will result in an "average" drug exposure, whereas in the second case, lowering the dose will result in a lower-than-average drug exposure. Therefore, in the setting of dose reduction, there is a greater possibility of a response in the patient with abnormal pharmacokinetics than in the "sensitive" patient with abnormal pharmacodynamics.

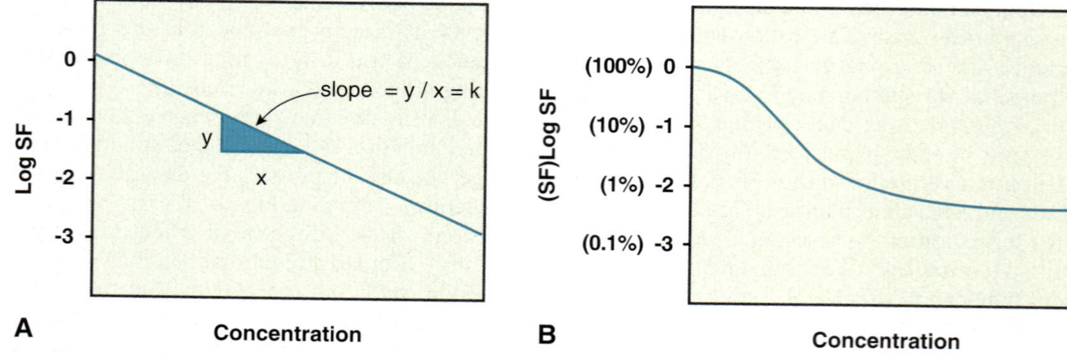

Figure 40-5 Pharmacodynamic plots for drugs with **A**, nonsaturable and **B**, saturable effects. In the simplest pharmacodynamic model (A), there is a linear relationship between dose and log kill. In B, there is a maximal effect, resulting in a plateau in the dose-response curve. SF = survival fraction.

General Pharmacodynamic Principles In the most general sense, any drug may be considered to have a maximal effect and a median dose (the dose required for 50% of the maximal effect). Wagner proposed a generalized sigmoidal model of drug effect (Figure 40-4), derived from the hypothesis that all drug effects require an initial interaction with a receptor.[202]

Most studies addressing pharmacodynamic modeling of anticancer agents have addressed phase-specific agents separately.[203,204] It may be adequate to use a simple log-linear model for nonphase-specific agents:[203,204]

Survival fraction (SF) =
No. of treated cells/No. of control cells = e^{-KC}
(equation 8).

This may be referred to as a steep dose-response curve, since the effect continues to increase proportionally as the concentration (C) increases. For any K (in equation 8), an increase in C by 2.3/K will result in a 1-log increase in antitumor effect (Figure 40-5A).

The dose-response relationships for phase-specific agents, such as the antimetabolites, are much more complicated. By definition, some cells are out of "phase" and therefore not sensitive (or relatively insensitive) to the effects of the drug during the period of drug exposure. This is not necessarily overcome by increasing the dose, but could be overcome by increasing the duration of drug exposure. The result is the appearance of a plateau in the dose-response curve (Figure 40-5B).

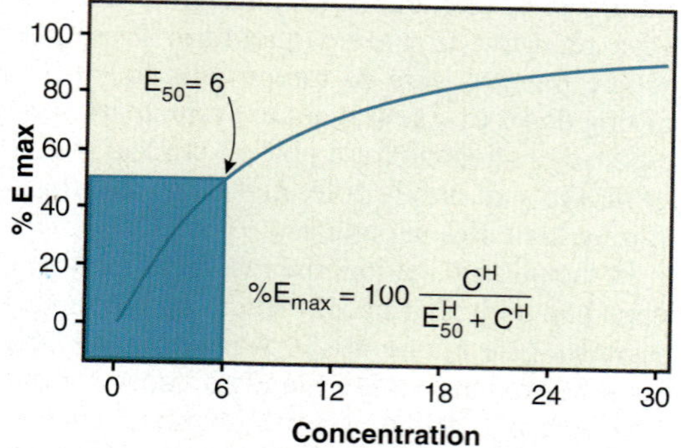

Figure 40-4 Example of E_{max} model as proposed by Wagner JG.[202] The maximum effect is 100%, and a concentration of 6 results in 50% effect. The exponent H, also known as the Hill constant, determines the shape of the curve and is usually between 1 and 2.

The effects of some antineoplastic agents depend on both the drug concentration and the duration of exposure to that concentration. For some agents, the effect is a function of the product of the concentration and exposure time, analogous to the AUC. [206] However, for antimetabolites and other phase-specific agents, the mathematical relationships are much more complex[203,204,207] and drug effect tends to be related to duration of exposure above a threshold concentration.

Plasma concentrations may be an inadequate predictor of clinical effect for those agents that undergo intracellular anabolism to active metabolites, such as is the case for cytarabine.[208] Plasma cytarabine concentrations do not appear to correlate with the rate of cellular cytarabine triphosphate (ara-CTP) accumulation or peak ara-CTP concentration in leukemia cells, although the intracellular concentration of ara-CTP is an important determinant of treatment outcome. Thus, knowledge of the plasma pharmacokinetics of cytarabine is not likely to be a useful predictor of treatment outcome for individual patients. For 6-mercaptopurine, pharmacogenetic evaluation may be potentially useful for modeling relationships between drug pharmacokinetics and clinical effects, as this drug's conversion to active intracellular 6-thioguanine metabolites by TPMT is genetically determined.[173] Studies in children with acute lymphoblastic leukemia suggest that intracellular levels of 6-thioguanine nucleotides may be an independent predictor of remission duration[172] and that heterozygosity for allelic variants of *TPMT* conferring lower enzyme activity correlates with a significantly lower rate of post-treatment minimal residual disease, an important prognostic factor.[209]

Pharmacodynamic Modeling of Cancer Chemotherapy The introduction of pharmacodynamic modeling into clinical oncology has been a slow process. The relationship between toxicity subsequent to high-dose methotrexate and that of delayed methotrexate clearance has led to the routine use of therapeutic drug monitoring of plasma methotrexate concentrations to guide leucovorin dosing.[210] Studies of other drugs have not clearly resulted in a change in clinical practice, although there has been an increase in clinical research in this area.[211]

Most early pharmacodynamic studies addressed relationships between measurements of drug exposure (AUC, C_{ss}) and toxicity. Such is the case for the leukopenia/neutropenia caused by etoposide.[165,212–218] More recently, investigators have modeled toxicity by using novel pharmacokinetic parameters, such as time above a threshold concentration for etoposide[219–221] and paclitaxel.[117,119,222,223] Other investigators have addressed the importance of active metabolites. This is of particular importance for irinotecan, a drug with both complex metabolism and toxicity patterns. Studies have suggested that irinotecan-induced diarrhea is due to direct intestinal damage by the biliary excretion of its active metabolite SN-38.[224,225] It has also been shown that neutropenia correlates strongly with SN-38 AUC.[171,226] As illustrated in Tables 40-4 and 40-5, respectively, hematologic toxicity has been easier to model than nonhematologic toxicity.

One of the best-characterized drugs is carboplatin, an analogue of cisplatin. Unlike cisplatin, the dose-limiting toxicity of carboplatin is thrombocytopenia, which is a function of drug dose, renal function, pretreatment platelet count, and prior therapy.[146] The platelet nadir produced by a dose of carboplatin is related to the carboplatin clearance, which is directly proportional to creatinine clearance. Thus, patients at high risk of severe thrombocytopenia following carboplatin therapy can be identified prospectively, and the drug doses can be modified by monitoring creatinine clearance.

There is an expanding interest in trying to optimize cancer chemotherapy by individualizing dosing on the basis of measurements of plasma or tissue drug concentrations. Investigators have attempted to optimize the dosing of etoposide,[165,227] teniposide,[228] hexamethylene bisacetamide,[229,230] etanidazole,[231] melphalan,[232] busulfan,[233,234] and 5-FU[235] by monitoring plasma drug concentrations during treatment, then using the information obtained to modify the total dose of chemotherapy administered in an attempt to avoid severe toxicity.

The targeted outcome with individualized dosing is most often toxicity. This is because of a lack of well-defined relationships between systemic exposure and efficacy for most anticancer

Table 40-4 Selected Pharmacodynamic Studies of Hematologic Toxicity

Drug	Reference	Pharmacokinetic Parameter	Toxicity
Amonafide	Ratain[175,176]	SP_m	W, P
Carboplatin	Egorin[146]	AUC	P
	Newell[148,248]	AUC	W, P
Doxorubicin	Ackland[249]	C_{ss}	W
	Piscitelli[250]	AUC	W
	Rushing[192]	AUC	W
Epirubicin	Jakobsen[251]	SP	W
Etoposide	Ratain[165]	C_{ss}	W
	Kunitoh[213]	C_{ss}	N
	Clark[221]	TAT	W, N
	Miller[214–216]	SP	W, N
	Minami[217]	C_{ss}	W, P
5-Fluorouracil	Au[252]	C_{ss}	W
	Trump[253]	C_{ss}	W
HMBA	Egorin[254]	AUC	P
	Rowinsky[255]	C_{ss}, AUC	P
Irinotecan	Innocenti[171]	AUC_m	N
	Pitot[226]	AUC_m	N
Menogaril	Egorin[256,257]	AUC	W, N
	Dodion[258]	AUC, SP	W, N
Paclitaxel	Gianni[117]	TAT	N
	Huizing[222]	TAT	W, N
	Wilson[223]	C_{ss}	N
Topotecan	Grochow[259]	AUC	N
	Stewart[260]	AUC	N, P
	Haas[129]	C_{ss}	N
Trimetrexate	Fanucchi[143]	AUC	P
	Reece[261]	AUC, C_{ss}	P
	Grochow[262,263]	AUC, SP	P, W
Vinblastine	Ratain[264]	C_{ss}	W

HMBA = hexamethylene bisacetamide; AUC = area under the curve; AUC_m = area under the curve metabolite; C_{ss} = "steady-state" concentration during continuous infusion; SP = single point; TAT = time above threshold; SP_m = single point metabolite; P =, thrombocytopenia; W = leukopenia; N = neutropenia.

agents. Such relationships, however, have been demonstrated for some drug/disease pairs. A prospective, randomized study of 182 children with acute lymphoblastic leukemia was conducted comparing standard fixed dosing versus individualized dosing of methotrexate-based therapy.[236] The latter was based on adjusting the doses to achieve plasma AUCs in the 50th to 90th percentile (based on historical controls). Researchers found that those receiving individualized therapy had an improvement in the rate of continuous complete remission (76% vs 66%) at 5 years. Pharmacodynamic relationships involving efficacy have also been found for carboplatin and ovarian cancer,[237] 5-FU and colorectal[238] and head and neck[206,239] cancer, and busulfan and allogeneic bone marrow transplantation.[240]

The Future Role of Anticancer Pharmacodynamics Should the clinical oncologist care about pharmacodynamics? Will therapeutic drug monitoring of antineoplastics be as useful as monitoring of theophylline or aminoglycoside dosing? How will these studies improve the therapeutic index? These are important issues that are currently being addressed.

Our true understanding of the dosing of most antineoplastic drugs is primitive. Body surface area (BSA) is generally the only value used to determine initial dosing; but this practice has come under increasing criticism because, for the vast majority of anticancer drugs, BSA does not correlate with pharmacokinetic or pharmacodynamic parameters.[241–246] Prior toxicity may be used to adjust dosing for subsequent cycles, although doses are more often reduced than escalated, and the magnitude of dose changes is determined empirically and often arbitrarily.

For drugs with a relatively broad therapeutic index and/or minimal interpatient pharmacokinetic or pharmacodynamic variability, individualized dosing strategies may not be necessary. However, when interpatient differences are significant, the implications on outcomes can be profound. As an example, individualized dosing of busulfan in the treatment of patients with advanced hematologic malignancies undergoing allogeneic bone marrow transplant may help to both minimize life-threatening toxicity (veno-occlusive disease) and improve survival, since there is a relationship between drug exposure and successful engraftment.[241]

A particularly exciting area of current research is pharmacogenetics. As investigators discover drug disposition polymorphisms that impact absorption, metabolism, and transport of anticancer drugs, dose individualization based on a patient's genetics will become possible. Development of this dosing strategy will require collecting DNA samples for the genotyping of candidate polymorphisms and blood samples for pharmacokinetic data in the context of large phase II and/or III clinical trials. In this way, relationships can be developed that involve not only toxicity, but also efficacy.

The next challenge will be optimizing the use of combination chemotherapy. As studies of the pharmacodynamics of single agents are completed, the next challenge will be to optimize combination chemotherapy as most cancers are treated with combinations of anticancer agents. The importance of such studies is demonstrated by the example of carboplatin and paclitaxel, where the combination results in less thrombocytopenia than carboplatin as a single agent.[247]

In conclusion, it is hoped that a better understanding of the clinical pharmacology of antineoplastic agents will improve the care of patients with cancer. At a minimum, clinicians should understand the basic principles, realizing the limitations of our current approaches.

Table 40-5 Selected Pharmacodynamic Studies of Nonhematologic Toxicity

Drug	Reference	Pharmacokinetic Parameter	Toxicity
Busulfan	Grochow[265]	AUC	H
Carmustine	Jones[266]	AUC	PU
Cisplatin	Reece[261]	SP, AUC	R
	Ayash[267]	AUC	C
Etanidazole	Coleman[231]	AUC	PN
5-Fluorouracil	Thyss[268]	AUC	NS
	van Groeningen[269]	AUC	NS
	Trump[253]	C_{ss}	MU
Irinotecan	Gupta[224]	RAUC	GI
Paclitaxel	Wilson[223]	C_{ss}	MU

AUC = area under the curve; C_{ss} = "steady-state" concentration during continuous infusion; SP = single point; RAUC = ratio of AUCs of parent drug and metabolites; R = nephrotoxicity; NS = not specified; PN = peripheral neuropathy; C = cardiac; GI = gastrointestinal; PU = pulmonary; MU = mucositis.

REFERENCES

1. Sevick EM, Jain RK. Geometric resistance to blood flow in solid tumors perfused ex vivo: effects of tumor size and perfusion pressure. Cancer Res 1989;49:3506–12.
2. DeMario MD, Ratain MJ. Oral chemotherapy: rationale and future directions. J Clin Oncol 1998;16:2557–67.
3. Damaraju VL, Damaraju S, Young JD, et al. Nucleoside anticancer drugs: the role of nucleoside transporters in resistance to cancer chemotherapy. Oncogene 2003;22:7524–36.
4. Kong W, Engel K, Wang J. Mammalian nucleoside transporters. Curr Drug Metab 2004;5:63–84.
5. Lu X, Gong S, Monks A, et al. Correlation of nucleoside and nucleobase transporter gene expression with antimetabolite drug cytotoxicity. J Exp Ther Oncol 2002;2:200–12.

6. Pastor-Anglada M, Molina-Arcas M, Casado FJ. Nucleoside transporters in chronic lymphocytic leukaemia. Leukemia. 2004;18:385–93.
7. Mangravite LM, Badagnani I, Giacomini KM. Nucleoside transporters in the disposition and targeting of nucleoside analogs in the kidney. Eur J Pharmacol 2003;479:269–81.
8. Mackey JR, Galmarini CM, Graham KA, et al. Quantitative analysis of nucleoside transporter and metabolism gene expression in chronic lymphocytic leukemia (CLL): identification of fludarabine-sensitive and -insensitive populations. Blood 2005;105:767–74.
9. Mackey JR, Jennings LL, Clarke ML, et al. Immunohistochemical variation of human equilibrative nucleoside transporter 1 protein in primary breast cancers. Clin Cancer Res 2002;8:110–6.
10. Plunkett W, Gandhi V. Purine and pyrimidine nucleoside analogs. In: Giaccone G, Schilsky R, Sondel, P, editors. Cancer chemotherapy and biological response modifiers. Annual 19. Amsterdam: Elsevier; 2001. p. 21–45.
11. McGuire JJ. Anticancer antifolates: current status and future directions. Curr Pharm Des 2003;9:2593–613.
12. Matherly LH, Goldman DI. Membrane transport of folates. Vitam Horm 2003;66:403–56.
13. Brigle KE, Seither RL, Westin EH, et al. Increased expression and genomic organization of a folate-binding protein homologous to the human placental isoform in L1210 murine leukemia cell lines with a defective reduced folate carrier. J Biol Chem 1994;269:4267–72.
14. Moscow JA, Gong M, He R, et al. Isolation of a gene encoding a human reduced folate carrier (RFC1) and analysis of its expression in transport-deficient, methotrexate-resistant human breast cancer cells. Cancer Res 1995;55:3790–4.
15. Kumar CK, Nguyen TT, Gonzales FB, Said HM. Comparison of intestinal folate carrier clone expressed in IEC-6 cells and in Xenopus oocytes. Am J Physiol 1998;274(1 Pt 1):C289–94.
16. Gorlick R, Goker E, Trippett T, et al. Defective transport is a common mechanism of acquired methotrexate resistance in acute lymphocytic leukemia and is associated with decreased reduced folate carrier expression. Blood 1997;89:1013–8.
17. Goldenberg GJ, Begleiter A. Membrane transport of alkylating agents. Pharmacol Ther 1980;8:237–74.
18. Borst P, Evers R, Kool M, Wijnholds J. A family of drug transporters: the multidrug resistance-associated proteins. J Natl Cancer Inst 2000;92:1295–302.
19. Kvackajova-Kisucka J, Barancik M, Breier A. Drug transporters and their role in multidrug resistance of neoplastic cells. Gen Physiol Biophys 2001;20:215–37.
20. Ritter CA, Jedlitschky G, Meyer zu Schwabedissen H, et al. Cellular export of drugs and signaling molecules by the ATP-binding cassette transporters MRP4 (ABCC4) and MRP5 (ABCC5). Drug Metab Rev 2005;37:253–78.
21. Borst P, Balzarini J, Ono N, et al. The potential impact of drug transporters on nucleoside-analog-based antiviral chemotherapy. Antiviral Res 2004;62:1–7.
22. Lippard SJ. New chemistry of an old molecule: cis-[Pt(NH3)2Cl2]. Science 1982;218:1075–82.
23. Roy P, Yu LJ, Crespi CL, et al. Development of a substrate-activity based approach to identify the major human liver P-450 catalysts of cyclophosphamide and ifosfamide activation based on cDNA-expressed activities and liver microsomal P-450 profiles. Drug Metab Dispos 1999;27:655–66.
24. Plunkett W, Gandhi V, Huang P, et al. Fludarabine: pharmacokinetics, mechanisms of action, and rationales for combination therapies. Semin Oncol 1993;20:2–12.
25. Plunkett W, Huang P, Searcy CE, et al. Gemcitabine: preclinical pharmacology and mechanisms of action. Semin Oncol 1996;23:3–15.
26. Galmarini CM, Jordheim L, Dumontet C. Pyrimidine nucleoside analogs in cancer treatment. Expert Rev Anticancer Ther 2003;3:717–28.
27. Allegra CJ, Chabner BA, Drake JC, et al. Enhanced inhibition of thymidylate synthase by methotrexate polyglutamates. J Biol Chem 1985;260:9720–6.
28. Whitehead VM, Rosenblatt DS, Vuchich MJ, et al. Accumulation of methotrexate and methotrexate polyglutamates in lymphoblasts at diagnosis of childhood acute lymphoblastic leukemia: a pilot prognostic factor analysis. Blood 1990;76:44–9.
29. Synold TW, Relling MV, Boyett JM, et al. Blast cell methotrexate-polyglutamate accumulation in vivo differs by lineage, ploidy, and methotrexate dose in acute lymphoblastic leukemia. J Clin Invest 1994;94:1996–2001.
30. Mackey JR, Yao SY, Smith KM, et al. Gemcitabine transport in Xenopus oocytes expressing recombinant plasma membrane mammalian nucleoside transporters. J Natl Cancer Inst 1999;91:1876–81.
31. Abbruzzese JL, Grunewald R, Weeks EA, et al. A phase I clinical, plasma, and cellular pharmacology study of 2', 2'-difluorodeoxycytidine. J Clin Oncol 1991;9:491–8.
32. Grunewald R, Abbruzzese J, Tarassoff P, Plunkett W. Saturation of 2', 2'-difluorodeoxycytidine 5'-triphosphate accumulation by mononuclear cells during a phase I trial of Gemcitabine. Cancer Chemother Pharm 1991;27:258–62.
33. Brand R, Capadano M, Tempero M. A phase I trial of weekly gemcitabine administered as a prolonged infusion in patients with pancreatic cancer and other solid tumors. Invest New Drugs 1997;15:331–41.
34. Touroutoglou N, Gravel D, Raber MN, et al. Clinical results of a pharmacodynamically-based strategy for higher dosing of gemcitabine in patients with solid tumors. Ann Oncol 1998;9:1003–8.
35. Grunewald R, Kantarjian H, Keating M, et al. Pharmacologically directed design of the dose rate and schedule of 2', 2'-difluorodeoxycytidine (Gemcitabine) administration in leukemia. Cancer Res 1990;50:6823–6.
36. Tempero M, Plunkett W, Ruiz van Haperen V, et al. Randomized phase II comparison of dose-intense gemcitabine: thirty-minute infusion and fixed dose rate infusion in patients with pancreatic adenocarcinoma. J Clin Oncol 2003;21:3402–8.
37. Shewach DS, Reynolds KK, Hertel L. Nucleotide specificity of human deoxycytidine kinase. Mol Pharmacol 1992;42:518–24.
38. Heinemann H, Xu Y-Z, Chubb S, et al. Cellular elimination of 2', 2'-difluorodeoxycytidine 5'-triphosphate: a mechanism of self-potentiation. Cancer Res 1992;52:533–9.
39. Gandhi V, Plunkett W, Du M, et al. Prolonged infusion of gemcitabine: clinical and pharmacodynamic studies during a phase I trial in relapsed acute myelogenous leukemia. J Clin Oncol 2002;20:665–73.
40. Ludeman SM. The chemistry of the metabolites of cyclophosphamide. Curr Pharm Des 1999;5:627–43.
41. Cohen SM, Lippard SJ. Cisplatin: from DNA damage to cancer chemotherapy. Prog Nucleic Acid Res Mol Biol 2001;67:93–130.
42. Bank BB, Kanganis D, Liebes LF, et al. Chlorambucil pharmacokinetics and DNA binding in chronic lymphocytic leukemia lymphocytes. Cancer Res 1989;49:554–9.
43. Terheggen PM, Emondt JY, Floot BG, et al. Correlation between cell killing by cis-diamminedichloroplatinum(II) in six mammalian cell lines and binding of a cis-diamminedichloroplatinum(II)-DNA antiserum. Cancer Res 1990;50:3556–61.
44. Reed E, Yuspa SH, Zwelling LA, et al. Quantitation of cis-diamminedichloroplatinum II (cisplatin)-DNA-intrastrand adducts in testicular and ovarian cancer patients receiving cisplatin chemotherapy. J Clin Invest 1986;77:545–50.
45. Reed E, Parker RJ, Gill I, et al. Platinum-DNA adduct in leukocyte DNA of a cohort of 49 patients with 24 different types of malignancies. Cancer Res 1993;53:3694–9.
46. Fisch MJ, Howard KL, Einhorn LH, Sledge GW. Relationship between platinum-DNA adducts in leukocytes of patients with advanced germ cell cancer and survival. Clin Cancer Res 1996;2:1063–6.
47. Binaschi M, Bigioni M, Cipollone A, et al. Anthracyclines: selected new developments. Curr Med Chem Anticancer Agents 2001 1:113–30.
48. Young RC, Ozols RF, Myers CE. The anthracycline antineoplastic drugs. N Engl J Med 1981;305:139–53.
49. Ross WE, Bradley MO. DNA double-stranded breaks in mammalian cells after exposure to intercalating agents. Biochim Biophys Acta 1981;654:129–34.
50. Moro S, Beretta GL, Dal Ben D, et al. Interaction model for anthracycline activity against DNA topoisomerase II. Biochemistry 2004;43:7503–13.
51. Deffie AM, Batra JK, Goldenberg GJ. Direct correlation between DNA topoisomerase II activity and cytotoxicity in Adriamycin-sensitive and -resistant P388 leukemia cell lines. Cancer Res 1989;49:58–62.
52. Giloni L, Takeshita M, Johnson F, et al. Bleomycin-induced strand-scission of DNA. Mechanism of deoxyribose cleavage. J Biol Chem 1981;256:8608–15.
53. Takeshita M, Grollman AP, Ohtsubo E, et al. Interaction of bleomycin with DNA. Proc Natl Acad Sci U S A 1978;75:5983–7.
54. Bolzan AD, Bianchi NO, Larramendy ML, et al. Chromosomal sensitivity of human lymphocytes to bleomycin. Influence of antioxidant enzyme activities in whole blood and different blood fractions. Cancer Genet Cytogenet 1992;64:133–8.
55. Parker WB, Bapat AR, Shen JX, et al. Interaction of 2-halogenated dATP analogs (F, Cl, and Br) with human DNA polymerases, DNA primase, and ribonucleotide reductase. Mol Pharmacol 1988;34:485–91.
56. Yang SW, Huang P, Plunkett W, et al. Dual mode of inhibition of purified DNA ligase I from human cells by 9-beta-D-arabinofuranosyl-2-fluoroadenine triphosphate. J Biol Chem 1992;267:2345–9.
57. Huang P, Chubb S, Plunkett W. Termination of DNA synthesis by 9-beta-D-arabinofuranosyl-2-fluoroadenine. A mechanism for cytotoxicity. J Biol Chem 1990;265:16617–25.
58. Catapano CV, Perrino FW, Fernandes DJ. Primer RNA chain termination induced by 9-beta-D-arabinofuranosyl-2-fluoroadenine 5'-triphosphate. A mechanism of DNA synthesis inhibition. J Biol Chem 1993;268:7179–85.
59. Yamauchi T, Nowak B, Keating MJ, Plunkett W. DNA repair initiated in chronic lymphocytic leukemia lymphocytes by 4-hydroperoxycyclophosphamide is inhibited by fludarabine and clofarabine. Clin Cancer Res 2001;7:3580–9.
60. White JC, Goldman ID. Mechanism of action of methotrexate. IV. Free intracellular methotrexate required to suppress dihydrofolate reduction to tetrahydrofolate by Ehrlich ascites tumor cells in vitro. Mol Pharmacol 1976;12:711–9.
61. Spears CP, Gustavsson BG. Methods for thymidylate synthase pharmacodynamics: serial biopsy, free and total TS, FdUMP and dUMP, and H4PteGlu and CH2-H4PteGlu assays. Adv Exp Med Biol 1988;244:97–106.
62. Johnston PG, Fisher ER, Rockette HE, et al. The role of thymidylate synthase expression in prognosis and outcome of adjuvant chemotherapy in patients with rectal cancer. J Clin Oncol 1994;12:2640–7.
63. Pullarkat ST, Stoehlmacher J, Ghaderi V, et al. Thymidylate synthase gene polymorphism determines response and toxicity of 5-FU chemotherapy. Pharmacogenomics J 2001;1:65–70.
64. Danenberg PV. Pharmacogenomics of thymidylate synthase in cancer treatment. Front Biosci 2004 1;2484–94.
65. Metzger R, Danenberg K, Leichman CG, et al. High basal level gene expression of thymidine phosphorylase (platelet-derived endothelial cell growth factor) in colorectal tumors is associated with non-response to 5-fluorouracil. Clin Cancer Res 1998;4:2371–6.
66. Tsukamoto Y, Kato Y, Ura M, et al. A physiologically based pharmacokinetic analysis of capecitabine, a triple prodrug of 5-FU, in humans: the mechanism for tumor-selective accumulation of 5-FU. Pharm Res 2001;18:1190–202.
67. Nishimura G, Terada I, Kobayashi T, et al. Thymidine phosphorylase and dihydropyrimidine dehydrogenase levels in primary colorectal cancer show a relationship to clinical effects of 5'-deoxy-5-fluorouridine as adjuvant chemotherapy. Oncol Rep 2002;9:479–82.
68. Ross W, Rowe T, Glisson B, et al. Role of topoisomerase II in mediating epipodophyllotoxin-induced DNA cleavage. Cancer Res 1984;44:5857–60.
69. Satoh T, Hosokawa M, Atsumi R, et al. Metabolic activation of CPT-11, 7-ethyl-10-[4-(1-piperidino)-1-piperidino]carbonyloxycamptothecin, a novel antitumor agent, by carboxylesterase. Biol Pharm Bull 1994;17:662–4.
70. Danks MK, Morton CL, Pawlik CA, et al. Overexpression of a rabbit liver carboxylesterase sensitizes human tumor cells to CPT-11. Cancer Res 1998;58:20–2.
71. Kojima A, Hackett NR, Ohwada A, et al. In vivo human carboxylesterase cDNA gene transfer to activate the prodrug CPT-11 for local treatment of solid tumors. J Clin Invest 1998;101:1789–96.
72. Potter PM, Pawlik CA, Morton CL, et al. Isolation and partial characterization of a cDNA encoding a rabbit liver carboxylesterase that activates the prodrug irinotecan (CPT-11). Cancer Res 1998;58:2646–51.
73. Hadfield JA, Ducki S, Hirst N, McGown AT. Tubulin and microtubules as targets for anticancer drugs. Prog Cell Cycle Res 2003;5:309–25.
74. Pellegrini F, Budman DR. Review: tubulin function, action of antitubulin drugs, and new drug development. Cancer Invest 2005;23:264–73.
75. Rowinsky EK, Cazenave LA, Donehower RC. Taxol: a novel investigational antimicrotubule agent. J Natl Cancer Inst 1990;82:1247–59.
76. Manfredi JJ, Horwitz SB. Taxol: an antimitotic agent with a new mechanism of action. Pharmacol Ther 1984;25:83–125.
77. Horwitz SB, Cohen D, Rao S, et al. Taxol: mechanisms of action and resistance. J Natl Cancer Inst Monogr 1993;15:55–61.
78. Rowinsky EK. The development and clinical utility of the taxane class of antimicrotubule chemotherapy agents. Annu Rev Med 1997;48:353–74.

79. Altmann KH. Microtubule-stabilizing agents: a growing class of important anticancer drugs. Curr Opin Chem Biol 2001;5:424–31.
80. Altaha R, Fojo T, Reed E, Abraham J. Epothilones: a novel class of non-taxane microtubule-stabilizing agents. Curr Pharm Des 2002;8:1707–12.
81. Chaney SG, Sancar A. DNA repair: enzymatic mechanisms and relevance to drug response. J Natl Cancer Inst 1996;88:1346–60.
82. Friedman HS, Dolan ME, Moschel RC, et al. Enhancement of nitrosourea activity in medulloblastoma and glioblastoma multiforme. J Natl Cancer Inst 1992;84:1926–31.
83. Friedman HS, Kokkinakis DM, Pluda J, et al. Phase I trial of O6-benzylguanine for patients undergoing surgery for malignant glioma. J Clin Oncol 1998;16:3570–5.
84. Dolan ME, Roy SK, Fasanmade AA, et al. O6-benzylguanine in humans: metabolic, pharmacokinetic, and pharmacodynamic findings. J Clin Oncol 1998;16:1803–10.
85. Sobol RW, Wilson SH. Mammalian DNA beta-polymerase in base excision repair of alkylation damage. Prog Nucleic Acid Res Mol Biol 2001;68:57–74.
86. Memisoglu A, Samson L. Base excision repair in yeast and mammals. Mutat Res 2000;451:39–51.
87. Weinfeld M, Xing JZ, Lee J, et al. Factors influencing the removal of thymine glycol from DNA in gamma-irradiated human cells. Prog Nucleic Acid Res Mol Biol 2001;68:139–49.
88. Weeda G, de Boer J, Donker I, et al. Molecular basis of DNA repair mechanisms and syndromes. Recent Results Cancer Res 1998;154:147–55.
89. Wood RD, Mitchell M, Sgouros J, Lindahl T. Human DNA repair genes. Science 2001;291:1284–9.
90. Sancar A, Lindsey-Boltz LA, Unsal-Kacmaz K, Linn S. Molecular mechanisms of mammalian DNA repair and the DNA damage checkpoints. Annu Rev Biochem 2004;73:39–85.
91. Reardon JT, Sancar A. Molecular anatomy of the human excision nuclease assembled at sites of DNA damage. Mol Cell Biol 2002;22:5938–45.
92. Cleaver, JE, Karplus, K, Sabet, M, et al. Nucleotide excision repair "a legacy of creativity." Mutat. Res 2002;485:23–36.
93. Hoeijmakers JH. Genome maintenance mechanisms for preventing cancer. Nature 2001;411:366–74.
94. Zhen W, Link CJ Jr, O'Connor PM, et al. Increased gene-specific repair of cisplatin interstrand cross-links in cisplatin-resistant human ovarian cancer cell lines. Mol Cell Biol 1992;12:3689–98.
95. Mu D, Park CH, Matsunaga T, et al. Reconstitution of human DNA repair excision nuclease in a highly defined system. J Biol Chem 1995;270:2415–8.
96. Aboussekhra A, Biggerstaff M, Shivji MK, et al. Mammalian DNA nucleotide excision repair reconstituted with purified protein components. Cell 1995;80:859–68.
97. Huang P, Plunkett W. Fludarabine- and gemcitabine-induced apoptosis: incorporation of analogs into DNA is a critical event. Cancer Chemother Pharmacol 1995;36:181–8.
98. Doroshow JH, Locker GY, Myers CE. Enzymatic defenses of the mouse heart against reactive oxygen metabolites: alterations produced by doxorubicin. J Clin Invest 1980;65:128–35.
99. Mimnaugh EG, Dusre L, Atwell J, et al. Differential oxygen radical susceptibility of Adriamycin-sensitive and -resistant MCF-7 human breast tumor cells. Cancer Res 1989;49:8–15.
100. Huang P, Feng L, Oldham EA, et al. Superoxide dismutase: a novel target for selective killing of cancer cells. Nature 2000;407:390–5.
101. Ahmad S, Okine L, Le B, et al. Elevation of glutathione in phenylalanine mustard-resistant murine L1210 leukemia cells. J Biol Chem 1987;262:15048–53.
102. Green JA, Vistica DT, Young RC, et al. Potentiation of melphalan cytotoxicity in human ovarian cancer cell lines by glutathione depletion. Cancer Res 1984;44:5427–31.
103. Moscow JA, Fairchild CR, Madden MJ, et al. Expression of anionic glutathione-S-transferase and P-glycoprotein genes in human tissues and tumors. Cancer Res 1989;49:1422–8.
104. Domin BA, Grill SP, Bastow KF, et al. Effect of methotrexate on dihydrofolate reductase activity in methotrexate-resistant human KB cells. Mol Pharmacol 1982;21:478–82.
105. Swain SM, Lippman ME, Egan EF, et al. Fluorouracil and high-dose leucovorin in previously treated patients with metastatic breast cancer. J Clin Oncol 1989;7:890–9.
106. Schimke RT. Gene amplification, drug resistance, and cancer. Cancer Res 1984;44:1735–42.
107. Laub PB, Gallo JM. NCOMP—a windows-based computer program for noncompartmental analysis of pharmacokinetic data. J Pharm Sci 1996;85:393–5.
108. Pascual B, Montoro JB. Comparative study of four different pharmacokinetic computer programs: case study of a factor VIII preparation. Eur J Clin Pharmacol 1997;52:59–64.
109. Aarons L. Software for population pharmacokinetics and pharmacodynamics. Clin Pharmacokinet 1999;36:255–64.
110. Gibaldi M, Perrier D. Pharmacokinetics. New York: Marcel Dekker; 1982.
111. Wagner JG, Szpunar GJ, Ferry JJ. A nonlinear physiologic pharmacokinetic model: I. Steady-state. J Pharmacokinet Biopharm 1985;13:73–92.
112. Yamaoka K, Takakura Y. Analysis methods and recent advances in nonlinear pharmacokinetics from in vitro through in loci to in vivo. Drug Metab Pharmacokinet 2004;19:397–406.
113. Collins JM, Dedrick RL, King FG, et al. Nonlinear pharmacokinetic models for 5-fluorouracil in man: intravenous and intraperitoneal routes. Clin Pharmacol Ther 1980;28:235–46.
114. Mukherjee K, Heidelberger C. Studies on fluorinated pyrimidines, IX. The degradation of 5-fluorouracil-6-C14. J Biol Chem 1960;235:433–7.
115. Schaaf LJ, Dobbs BR, Edwards IR, et al. Nonlinear pharmacokinetic characteristics of 5-fluorouracil (5-FU) in colorectal cancer patients. Eur J Clin Pharmacol 1987;32:411–8.
116. Wagner JG, Gyves JW, Stetson PL, et al. Steady-state nonlinear pharmacokinetics of 5-fluorouracil during hepatic arterial and intravenous infusions in cancer patients. Cancer Res 1986;46:1499–506.
117. Gianni L, Kearns CM, Giani A, et al. Nonlinear pharmacokinetics and metabolism of paclitaxel and its pharmacokinetic/pharmacodynamic relationships in humans. J Clin Oncol 1995;13:180–90.
118. Henningsson A, Karlsson MO, Viganó L, et al. Mechanism-based pharmacokinetic model for paclitaxel. J Clin Oncol 2001;19:4065–73.
119. Sonnichsen DS, Hurwitz CA, Pratt CB, et al. Saturable pharmacokinetics and paclitaxel pharmacodynamics in children with solid tumors. J Clin Oncol 1994;12:532–8.
120. Eisenhauer EA, ten Bokkel Huinink WW, Swenerton KD, et al. European-Canadian randomized trial of paclitaxel in relapsed ovarian cancer: high-dose versus low-dose and long versus short infusion. J Clin Oncol 1994;12:2654–66.
121. Alberts DS, Chang SY, Chen HS, et al. Oral melphalan kinetics. Clin Pharmacol Ther 1979;26:737–45.
122. Choi KE, Ratain MJ, Williams SF, et al. Plasma pharmacokinetics of high-dose oral melphalan in patients treated with trialkylator chemotherapy and autologous bone marrow reinfusion. Cancer Res 1989;49:1318–21.
123. Straw JA, Szapary D, Wynn WT. Pharmacokinetics of the diastereoisomers of leucovorin after intravenous and oral administration to normal subjects. Cancer Res 1984;44:3114–9.
124. Forastiere AA, Belliveau JF, Goren MP, et al. Pharmacokinetic and toxicity evaluation of five-day continuous infusion versus intermittent bolus cis-diamminedichloroplatinum(II) in head and neck cancer patients. Cancer Res 1988;48:3869–74.
125. Reece PA, Stafford I, Russell J, et al. Nonlinear renal clearance of ultrafilterable platinum in patients treated with cis-dichlorodiammineplatinum (II). Cancer Chemother Pharmacol 1985;15:295–9.
126. Undevia SD, Gomez-Abuin G, Ratain MJ. Pharmacokinetic variability of anticancer agents. Nat Rev Cancer 2005;5:447–58.
127. Schilsky RL, Ratain MJ. Clinical pharmacokinetics of high-dose leucovorin calcium after intravenous and oral administration. J Natl Cancer Inst 1990;82:1411–5.
128. Adamson PC, Pitot HC, Balis FM, et al. Variability in the oral bioavailability of all-trans-retinoic acid. J Natl Cancer Inst 1993;85:993–6.
129. Haas NB, LaCreta FP, Walczak J, et al. Phase I/pharmacokinetic study of topotecan by 24-hour continuous infusion weekly. Cancer Res 1994;54:1220–6.
130. Zimm S, Collins JM, Riccardi R, et al. Variable bioavailability of oral mercaptopurine. Is maintenance chemotherapy in acute lymphoblastic leukemia being optimally delivered? N Engl J Med 1983;308:1005–9.
131. Mani S, Iyer L, Janisch L, et al. Phase I clinical and pharmacokinetic study of oral 9-aminocamptothecin (NSC-603071). Cancer Chemother Pharmacol 1998;42:84–7.
132. de Jonge ME, Huitema ADR, Schellens JHM, et al. Population pharmacokinetics of orally administered paclitaxel formulated in Cremophor EL. Br J Clin Pharmacol 2005;59:325–34.
133. Singh BN, Malhotra, BK. Effects of food on the clinical pharmacokinetics of anticancer agents. Clin Pharmacokinet 2004;43:1127–56.
134. Hande K, Messenger M, Wagner J, et al. Inter- and intraindividual variability in etoposide kinetics with oral and intravenous drug administration. Clin Cancer Res 1999;5:2742–7.
135. Cheymol G. Drug pharmacokinetics in the obese. Fundam Clin Pharmacol 1988;2:239–56.
136. Lind MJ, Margison JM, Cerny T, et al. Prolongation of ifosfamide elimination half-life in obese patients due to altered drug distribution. Cancer Chemother Pharmacol 1989;25:139–42.
137. Rodvold KA, Rushing DA, Tewksbury DA. Doxorubicin clearance in the obese. J Clin Oncol 1988;6:1321–7.
138. Powis G, Reece P, Ahmann DL, et al. Effect of body weight on the pharmacokinetics of cyclophosphamide in breast cancer patients. Cancer Chemother Pharmacol 1987;20:219–22.
139. Chabner BA, Stoller RG, Hande K, et al. Methotrexate disposition in humans: case studies in ovarian cancer and following high-dose infusion. Drug Metab Rev 1978;8:107–17.
140. Raymond E, Boige V, Faivre S, et al. Dosage adjustment and pharmacokinetic profile of irinotecan in cancer patients with hepatic dysfunction. J Clin Oncol 2002;20:4303–12.
141. Stewart CF, Arbuck SG, Fleming RA, et al. Changes in the clearance of total and unbound etoposide in patients with liver dysfunction. J Clin Oncol 1990;8:1874–9.
142. Branch RA, Herbert CM, Read AE. Determinants of serum antipyrine half-lives in patients with liver disease. Gut 1973;14:569–73.
143. Fanucchi MP, Walsh TD, Fleisher M, et al. Phase I and clinical pharmacology study of trimetrexate administered weekly for three weeks. Cancer Res 1987;47:3303–8.
144. Ratain MJ, Vogelzang NJ, Sinkule JA. Interpatient and intrapatient variability in vinblastine pharmacokinetics. Clin Pharmacol Ther 1987;41:61–7.
145. Sotaniemi EA, Pelkonen RO, Mokka RE, et al. Impairment of drug metabolism in patients with liver cancer. Eur J Clin Invest 1977;7:269–74.
146. Egorin MJ, Van Echo DA, Tipping SJ, et al. Pharmacokinetics and dosage reduction of cis-diammine(1,1-cyclobutanedicarboxylato)platinum in patients with impaired renal function. Cancer Res 1984;44:5432–8.
147. Harland SJ, Newell DR, Siddik ZH, et al. Pharmacokinetics of cis-diammine-1,1-cyclobutane dicarboxylate platinum(II) in patients with normal and impaired renal function. Cancer Res 1984;44:1693–7.
148. Newell DR, Pearson AD, Balmanno K, et al. Carboplatin pharmacokinetics in children: the development of a pediatric dosing formula. J Clin Oncol 1993;11:2314–23.
149. Food and Drug Administration safety information on Xeloda. Available at: http://www.fda.gov/medwatch/safety/2000/xeloda.pdf (accessed August 14, 2005).
150. Ratain MJ. Dear doctor: we really are not sure what dose of capecitabine you should prescribe for your patient. J Clin Oncol 2002;20:1434–5.
151. Millward MJ, Webster LK, Toner GC, et al. Carboplatin dosing based on measurement of renal function: experience at the Peter MacCallum Cancer Institute. Aust N Z J Med 1996;26:372–9.
152. Baracskay D, Jarjoura D, Cugino A, et al. Geriatric renal function: estimating glomerular filtration in an ambulatory elderly population. Clin Nephrol 1997;47:222–8.
153. Martin L, Chatelut E, Boneu A, et al. Improvement of the Cockcroft-Gault equation for predicting glomerular filtration in cancer patients. Bull Cancer 1998;85:631–6.
154. Levey AS, Bosch JP, Lewis JB, et al. A more accurate method to estimate glomerular filtration rate from serum creatinine: a new prediction equation-modification of diet in renal disease study group. Ann Intern Med 1999;130:461–70.
155. Wright JG, Boddy AV, Highley M, et al. Estimation of glomerular filtration rate in cancer patients. Br J Cancer 2001;84:452–9.
156. Doroshow JH, Synold TW, Gandara D, et al. Pharmacology of oxaliplatin in solid tumor patients with hepatic dysfunction: a preliminary report of the National Cancer Institute Organ Dysfunction Working Group. Semin Oncol 2003;30:14–9.
157. Fleming GF, Schilsky RL, Schumm LP, et al. Phase I and pharmacokinetic study of 24-hour infusion 5-fluorouracil and leucovorin in patients with organ dysfunction. Ann Oncol 2003;14:1142–7.

158. Takimoto CH, Remick SC, Sharma S, et al. Dose-escalating and pharmacological study of oxaliplatin in adult cancer patients with impaired renal function: a National Cancer Institute Organ Dysfunction Working Group study. J Clin Oncol 2003;21:2664–72.
159. Venook AP, Egorin MJ, Rosner GL, et al. Phase I and pharmacokinetic trial of gemcitabine in patients with hepatic or renal dysfunction: Cancer and Leukemia Group B 9565. J Clin Oncol 2000;14:2780–7.
160. Venook AP, Egorin MJ, Rosner GL, et al. Phase I and pharmacokinetic trial of paclitaxel in patients with hepatic dysfunction: Cancer and Leukemia Group B 9264. J Clin Oncol 1998;16:1811–9.
161. Donigian DW, Owellen RJ. Interaction of vinblastine, vincristine and colchicine with serum proteins. Biochem Pharmacol 1973;22:2113–9.
162. Stewart CF, Pieper JA, Arbuck SG, et al. Altered protein binding of etoposide in patients with cancer. Clin Pharmacol Ther 1989;45:49–55.
163. Blair EY, Rivory LP, Clarke SJ, et al. Population pharmacokinetics of raltitrexed in patients with advanced solid tumours. Br J Clin Pharmacol 2004;57:416–26.
164. Smallwood RH, Mihaly GW, Smallwood RA, et al. Effect of a protein binding change on unbound and total plasma concentrations for drugs of intermediate hepatic extraction. J Pharmacokinet Biopharm 1988;16:529–42.
165. Ratain MJ, Schilsky RL, Choi KE, et al. Adaptive control of etoposide administration: impact of interpatient pharmacodynamic variability. Clin Pharmacol Ther 1989;45:226–33.
166. Ulrich CM, Robien K, McLeod HL. Cancer pharmacogenetics: polymorphisms, pathways and beyond. Nat Rev Cancer 2003;3:912–20.
167. Watters JW, McLeod HL. Cancer pharmacogenomics: current and future applications. Biochim Biophys Acta 2003;1603:99–111.
168. Relling MV, Dervieux T. Pharmacogenetics and cancer therapy. Nat Rev Cancer 2001;1:99–108.
169. Iyer L, King CD, Whitington PF, et al. Genetic predisposition to the metabolism of irinotecan: role of uridine diphosphate glucuronosyltransferase isoform 1A1 in the glucuronidation of its active metabolite (SN-38) in human liver microsomes. J Clin Invest 1998;101:847–54.
170. Beutler E, Gelbart T, Demina A. Racial variability in the UDP-glucuronosyltransferase 1 (*UGT1A1*) promoter: a balanced polymorphism for regulation of bilirubin metabolism? Proc Natl Acad Sci U S A 1998;95:8170–4.
171. Innocenti F, Undevia SD, Iyer L, et al. Genetic variants in the *UDP-glucuronosyltransferase 1A1* gene predict the risk of severe neutropenia of irinotecan. J Clin Oncol 2004;22:1382–8.
172. Lennard L, Lilleyman JS. Variable mercaptopurine metabolism and treatment outcome in childhood lymphoblastic leukemia. J Clin Oncol 1989;7:1816–23.
173. Lennard L, Lilleyman JS, Van Loon J, et al. Genetic variation in response to 6-mercaptopurine for childhood acute lymphoblastic leukaemia. Lancet 1990;336:225–9.
174. Ratain MJ, Mick R, Berezin F, et al. Phase I study of amonafide dosing based on acetylator phenotype. Cancer Res 1993;53:2304–8.
175. Ratain MJ, Mick R, Berezin F, et al. Paradoxical relationship between acetylator phenotype and amonafide toxicity. Clin Pharmacol Ther 1991;50:573–9.
176. Ratain MJ, Rosner G, Allen SL, et al. Population pharmacodynamic study of amonafide: a Cancer and Leukemia Group B study. J Clin Oncol 1995;13:741–7.
177. Camptosar prescribing information. Available at: http://www.pfizer.com/pfizer/download/uspi_camptosar.pdf (accessed August 14, 2005).
178. Purinethol prescribing information. Available at: http://us.gsk.com/products/assets/us_purinethol.pdf (accessed August 14, 2005).
179. Moore MJ, Erlichman C, Thiessen JJ, et al. Variability in the pharmacokinetics of cyclophosphamide, methotrexate and 5-fluorouracil in women receiving adjuvant treatment for breast cancer. Cancer Chemother Pharmacol 1994;33:472–6.
180. Hrushesky WJ, von Roemeling R, Lanning RM, et al. Circadian-shaped infusions of floxuridine for progressive metastatic renal cell carcinoma. J Clin Oncol 1990;8:1504–13.
181. Petit E, Milano G, Levi F, et al. Circadian rhythm-varying plasma concentration of 5-fluorouracil during a five-day continuous venous infusion at a constant rate in cancer patients. Cancer Res 1988;48:1676–9.
182. Harris BE, Song R, Soong SJ, et al. Relationship between dihydropyrimidine dehydrogenase activity and plasma 5-fluorouracil levels with evidence for circadian variation of enzyme activity and plasma drug levels in cancer patients receiving 5-fluorouracil by protracted continuous infusion. Cancer Res 1990;50:197–201.
183. Focan C, Levi F, Kreutz F, et al. Continuous delivery of venous 5-fluorouracil and arterial 5-fluorodeoxyuridine for hepatic metastases from colorectal cancer: feasibility and tolerance in a randomized phase II trial comparing flat versus chronomodulated infusion. Anticancer Drugs 1999;10:385–92.
184. Shimonov M, Hayat H, Chaitchik S, et al. Combined systemic chronotherapy and hepatic artery infusion for the treatment of metastatic colorectal cancer confined to the liver. Chemotherapy 2005;51:111–5.
185. Parulekar W, de Marsh RW, Wong R, et al. Phase I study of 5-fluorouracil and leucovorin by continuos infusion chemotherapy and pelvic radiotherapy in patients with locally advanced or recurrent rectal cancer. Int J Radiat Oncol Biol Phys 2004;58:1487–95.
186. Terzoli E, Garufi C, Zappala AR, et al. High-dose chronomodulated infusion of 5-fluorouracil (5-FU) and folinic acid (FA) (FF5-16) in advanced colorectal cancer patients. Cancer Res Clin Oncol 2004;130:445–52.
187. Rowinsky EK, Gilbert MR, McGuire WP, et al. Sequences of Taxol and cisplatin: a phase I and pharmacologic study. J Clin Oncol 1991;9:1692–703.
188. Chester JD, Joel SP, Cheeseman SL, et al. Phase I and pharmacokinetic study of intravenous irinotecan plus oral ciclosporin in patients with fluorouracil-refractory metastatic colon cancer. J Clin Oncol 2003;21:1125–32.
189. Lacayo NJ, Lum BL, Becton DL, et al. Pharmacokinetic interactions of cyclosporine with etoposide and mitoxantrone in children with acute myeloid leukemia. Leukemia 2002;16:920–7.
190. Lum BL, Kaubisch S, Yahanda AM, et al. Alteration of etoposide pharmacokinetics and pharmacodynamics by cyclosporine in a phase I trial to modulate multidrug resistance. J Clin Oncol 1992;10:1635–42.
191. Erlichman C, Moore M, Thiessen JJ, et al. Phase I pharmacokinetic study of cyclosporin A combined with doxorubicin. Cancer Res 1993;53:4837–42.
192. Rushing DA, Raber SR, Rodvold KA, et al. The effects of cyclosporine on the pharmacokinetics of doxorubicin in patients with small cell lung cancer. Cancer 1994;74:834–41.
193. Jin Y, Desta Z, Stearns V, et al. CYP2D6 genotype, antidepressant use, and tamoxifen metabolism during adjuvant breast cancer treatment. J Natl Cancer Inst 2005;97:30–9.
194. McCune JS, Hatfield AJ, Blackburn AA, et al. Potential of chemotherapy-herb interactions in adult cancer patients. Support Care Cancer 2004;12:454–62.
195. Moore LB, Goodwin B, Jones SA, et al. St. John's wort induces hepatic drug metabolism through activation of the pregnane X receptor. Proc Natl Acad Sci U S A 2000;97:7500–2.
196. Wentworth JM, Agostini M, Love J, et al. St. John's wort, a herbal antidepressant, activates the steroid X receptor. J Endocrinol 2000;166:R11–6.
197. Lehmann JM, McKee DD, Watson MA, et al. The human orphan nuclear receptor PXR is activated by compounds that regulate CYP3A4 gene expression and cause drug interactions. J Clin Invest 1998;102:1016–23.
198. Burk O, Koch I, Raucy J, et al. The induction of cytochrome P450 3A5 (CYP3A5) in the human liver and intestine is mediated by the xenobiotic sensors pregnane X receptor (PXR) and constitutively activated receptor (CAR). J Biol Chem 2004;279:38379–85.
199. Gardner-Stephen D, Heydel JM, Goyal A, et al. Human PXR variants and their differential effects on the regulation of human UDP-glucuronosyltransferase gene expression. Drug Metab Dispos 2004;32:340–7.
200. Mathijssen RHJ, Verweij J, de Bruijn P, et al. Effects of St. John's wort on irinotecan metabolism. J Natl Cancer Inst 2002;94:1247–9.
201. Mick R, Ratain MJ. Statistical approaches to pharmacodynamic modeling: motivations, methods, and misperceptions. Cancer Chemother Pharmacol 1993;33:1–9.
202. Wagner JG. Kinetics of pharmacologic response. I. Proposed relationships between response and drug concentration in the intact animal and man. J Theor Biol 1968;20:173–201.
203. Jusko WJ. A pharmacodynamic model for cell-cycle-specific chemotherapeutic agents. J Pharmacokinet Biopharm 1973;1:175–200.
204. Ozawa S, Sugiyama Y, Mitsuhashi J, et al. Kinetic analysis of cell killing effect induced by cytosine arabinoside and cisplatin in relation to cell cycle phase specificity in human colon cancer and Chinese hamster cells. Cancer Res 1989;49:3823–8.
205. Skipper HE, Schabel FM Jr, Mellett LB, et al. Implications of biochemical, cytokinetic, pharmacologic, and toxicologic relationships in the design of optimal therapeutic schedules. Cancer Chemother Rep 1970;54:431–50.
206. Eichholtz-Wirth H. Dependence of the cytostatic effect of Adriamycin on drug concentration and exposure time in vitro. Br J Cancer 1980;41:886–91.
207. Eichholtz H, Trott KR. Effect of methotrexate concentration and exposure time on mammalian cell survival in vitro. Br J Cancer 1980;41:277–84.
208. Liliemark JO, Plunkett W, Dixon DO. Relationship of 1-beta-D-arabinofuranosylcytosine in plasma to 1-beta-D-arabinofuranosylcytosine 5'-triphosphate levels in leukemic cells during treatment with high-dose 1-beta-D-arabinofuranosylcytosine. Cancer Res 1985;45:5952–7.
209. Stanulla M, Schaeffeler E, Flohr T, et al. Thiopurine methyltransferase (TPMT) genotype and early treatment response to mercaptopurine in childhood acute lymphoblastic leukemia. JAMA 2005;293:1485–9.
210. Ackland SP, Schilsky RL. High-dose methotrexate: a critical reappraisal. J Clin Oncol 1987;5:2017–31.
211. Kobayashi K, Jodrell DI, Ratain MJ. Pharmacodynamic-pharmacokinetic relationships and therapeutic drug monitoring. Cancer Surv 1993;17:51–78.
212. Bennett CL, Sinkule JA, Schilsky RL, et al. Phase I clinical and pharmacological study of 72-hour continuous infusion of etoposide in patients with advanced cancer. Cancer Res 1987;47:1952–6.
213. Kunitoh H, Watanabe K. Phase I/II and pharmacologic study of long-term continuous infusion etoposide combined with cisplatin in patients with advanced non-small-cell lung cancer. J Clin Oncol 1994;12:83–9.
214. Miller AA, Tolley EA. Predictive performance of a pharmacodynamic model for oral etoposide. Cancer Res 1994;54:2080–3.
215. Miller AA, Stewart CF, Tolley EA. Clinical pharmacodynamics of continuous-infusion etoposide. Cancer Chemother Pharmacol 1990;25:361–6.
216. Miller AA, Tolley EA, Niell HB, et al. Pharmacodynamics of prolonged oral etoposide in patients with advanced non-small-cell lung cancer. J Clin Oncol 1993;11:1179–88.
217. Minami H, Shimokata K, Saka H, et al. Phase I clinical and pharmacokinetic study of a 14-day infusion of etoposide in patients with lung cancer. J Clin Oncol 1993;11:1602–8.
218. Minami H, Ratain MJ, Ando Y, et al. Pharmacodynamic modeling of prolonged administration of etoposide. Cancer Chemother Pharmacol 1996;39:61–6.
219. Davidson A, Gowing R, Lowis S, et al. Phase II study of 21 day schedule oral etoposide in children. Eur J Cancer 1997;33:1816–22.
220. Sonnichsen DS, Ribeiro RC, Luo X, et al. Pharmacokinetics and pharmacodynamics of 21-day continuous oral etoposide in pediatric patients with solid tumors. Clin Pharmacol Ther 1995;58:99–107.
221. Clark PI, Slevin ML, Joel SP, et al. A randomized trial of two etoposide schedules in small-cell lung cancer: the influence of pharmacokinetics on efficacy and toxicity. J Clin Oncol 1994;12:1427–35.
222. Huizing MT, Keung AC, Rosing H, et al. Pharmacokinetics of paclitaxel and metabolites in a randomized comparative study in platinum-pretreated ovarian cancer patients. J Clin Oncol 1993;11:2127–35.
223. Wilson WH, Berg SL, Bryant G, et al. Paclitaxel in doxorubicin-refractory or mitoxantrone-refractory breast cancer: a phase I/II trial of 96-hour infusion. J Clin Oncol 1994;12:1621–9.
224. Gupta E, Lestingi TM, Mick R, et al. Metabolic fate of irinotecan in humans: correlation of glucuronidation with diarrhea. Cancer Res 1994;54:3723–5.
225. Gupta E, Mick R, Ramirez J, et al. Pharmacokinetic and pharmacodynamic evaluation of the topoisomerase inhibitor irinotecan in cancer patients. J Clin Oncol 1997;15:1502–10.
226. Pitot HC, Goldberg RM, Reid JM, et al. Phase I dose-finding and pharmacokinetic trial of irinotecan hydrochloride (CPT-11) using a once-every-three-week dosing schedule for patients with advanced solid tumor malignancy. Clin Cancer Res 2000;6:2236–44.
227. Ratain MJ, Mick R, Schilsky RL, et al. Pharmacologically based dosing of etoposide: a means of safely increasing dose intensity. J Clin Oncol 1991;9:1480–6.
228. Rodman JH, Furman WL, Sunderland M, et al. Escalating teniposide systemic exposure to increase dose intensity

for pediatric cancer patients. J Clin Oncol 1993;11:287–93.
229. Conley BA, Forrest A, Egorin MJ, et al. Phase I trial using adaptive control dosing of hexamethylene bisacetamide (NSC 95580). Cancer Res 1989;49:3436–40.
230. Conley BA, Egorin MJ, Sinibaldi V, et al. Approaches to optimal dosing of hexamethylene bisacetamide. Cancer Chemother Pharmacol 1992;31:37–45.
231. Coleman CN, Buswell L, Noll L, et al. The efficacy of pharmacokinetic monitoring and dose modification of etanidazole on the incidence of neurotoxicity: results from a phase II trial of etanidazole and radiation therapy in locally advanced prostate cancer. Int J Radiat Oncol Biol Phys 1992;22:565–8.
232. Ploin DY, Tranchand B, Guastalla JP, et al. Pharmacokinetically guided dosing for intravenous melphalan: a pilot study in patients with advanced ovarian adenocarcinoma. Eur J Cancer 1992;1311–35.
233. Grochow LB. Busulfan disposition: the role of therapeutic monitoring in bone marrow transplantation induction regimens. Semin Oncol 1993;20 Suppl 4:18–25.
234. Slattery JT, Risler LJ. Therapeutic monitoring of busulfan in hematopoietic stem cell transplantation. Ther Drug Monit 1998;20:543–9.
235. Santini J, Milano G, Thyss A, et al. 5-FU therapeutic monitoring with dose adjustment leads to an improved therapeutic index in head and neck cancer. Br J Cancer 1989;59:287–90.
236. Evans WE, Relling MV, Rodman JH, et al. Conventional compared with individualized chemotherapy for childhood acute lymphoblastic leukemia. N Engl J Med 1998;338:499–505.
237. Jodrell DI, Egorin MJ, Canetta RM, et al. Relationships between carboplatin exposure and tumor response and toxicity in patients with ovarian cancer. J Clin Oncol 1992;10:520–8.
238. Milano G, Roman P, Khater P, et al. Dose versus pharmacokinetics for predicting tolerance to 5 day continuous infusion of 5-FU. Int J Cancer 1998;41:537–41.
239. Milano G, Etienne MC, Renee N, et al. Relationship between fluorouracil systemic exposure and tumor response and patient survival. J Clin Oncol 1994;15:1291–5.
240. Bleyzac N, Souillet G, Magron P, et al. Improved clinical outcome of paediatric bone marrow recipients using a test dose and Bayesian pharmacokinetic individualization of busulfan dosage regimens. Bone Marrow Transplant 2001;28:743–51.
241. Gurney H. Dose calculation of anticancer drugs: a review of the current practice and introduction of an alternative. J Clin Oncol 1996;14:2590–611.
242. Ratain MJ. Body-surface area as a basis for dosing of anticancer agents: science, myth, or habit? [editorial]. J Clin Oncol 1998;16:2297–8.
243. Sawyer M, Ratain MJ. Body surface area as a determinant of pharmacokinetics and drug dosing. Invest New Drugs 2001;82:171–7.
244. Baker SD, Verweij J, Rowinsky EK, et al. Rose of body-surface area in dosing of investigational anticancer agents in adults, 1991–2001. J Natl Cancer Inst 2002;94:1883–8.
245. Miller AA. Body surface area in dosing anticancer agents: scratch the surface! J Natl Cancer Inst 2002;94:1822–3.
246. Egorin MJ. Horseshoes, hand grenades, and BSA-based dosing: aiming for a target. J Clin Oncol 2003;21:182–3.
247. Kearns CM, Egorin MJ. Considerations regarding the less-than-expected thrombocytopenia encountered with combination paclitaxel/carboplatin chemotherapy. Semin Oncol 1997;24(1 Suppl 2):S2–91–S2–96.
248. Newell DR, Siddik ZH, Gumbrell LA, et al. Plasma free platinum pharmacokinetics in patients treated with high dose carboplatin. Eur J Cancer Clin Oncol 1987;23:1399-405.
249. Ackland SP, Ratain MJ, Vogelzang NJ, et al. Pharmacokinetics and pharmacodynamics of long-term continuous-infusion doxorubicin. Clin Pharmacol Ther 1989;45:340-7.
250. Piscitelli SC, Rodvold KA, Rushing DA, et al. Pharmacokinetics and pharmacodynamics of doxorubicin in patients with small cell lung cancer. Clin Pharmacol Ther 1993;53:555-61.
251. Jakobsen P, Bastholt L, Dalmark M, et al. A randomized study of epirubicin at four different dose levels in advanced breast cancer. Feasibility of myelotoxicity prediction through single blood-sample measurement. Cancer Chemother Pharmacol 1991;28:465-9.
252. Au JL, Rustum YM, Ledesma EJ, et al. Clinical pharmacological studies of concurrent infusion of 5- fluorouracil and thymidine in treatment of colorectal carcinomas. Cancer Res 1982;42:2930-7.
253. Trump DL, Egorin MJ, Forrest A, et al. Pharmacokinetic and pharmacodynamic analysis of fluorouracil during 72-hour continuous infusion with and without dipyridamole. J Clin Oncol 1991;9:2027-35.
254. Egorin MJ, Sigman LM, Van Echo DA, et al. Phase I clinical and pharmacokinetic study of hexamethylene bisacetamide (NSC 95580) administered as a five-day continuous infusion. Cancer Res 1987;47:617-23.
255. Rowinsky EK, Ettinger DS, Grochow LB, et al. Phase I and pharmacologic study of hexamethylene bisacetamide in patients with advanced cancer. J Clin Oncol 1986;4:1835-44.
256. Egorin MJ, Conley BA, Forrest A, et al. Phase I study and pharmacokinetics of menogaril (NSC 269148) in patients with hepatic dysfunction. Cancer Res 1987;47:6104-10.
257. Egorin MJ, Van Echo DA, Whitacre MY, et al. Human pharmacokinetics, excretion, and metabolism of the anthracycline antibiotic menogaril (7-OMEN, NSC 269148) and their correlation with clinical toxicities. Cancer Res 1986;46:1513-20.
258. Dodion P, de Valeriola D, Crespeigne N, et al. Phase I clinical and pharmacokinetic trial of oral menogaril administered on three consecutive days. Eur J Cancer Clin Oncol 1988;24:1019-26.
259. Grochow LB, Rowinsky EK, Johnson R, et al. Pharmacokinetics and pharmacodynamics of topotecan in patients with advanced cancer. Drug Metab Dispos 1992;20:706-13.
260. Stewart CF, Baker SD, Heideman RL, et al. Clinical pharmacodynamics of continuous infusion topotecan in children: systemic exposure predicts hematologic toxicity. J Clin Oncol 1994;12:1946-54.
261. Reece PA, Stafford I, Russell J, et al. Creatinine clearance as a predictor of ultrafilterable platinum disposition in cancer patients treated with cisplatin: relationship between peak ultrafilterable platinum plasma levels and nephrotoxicity. J Clin Oncol 1987;5:304-9.
262. Grochow LB, Noe DA, Dole GB, et al. Phase I trial of trimetrexate glucuronate on a five-day bolus schedule: clinical pharmacology and pharmacodynamics. J Natl Cancer Inst 1989;81:124-30.
263. Grochow LB, Noe DA, Ettinger DS, et al. A phase I trial of trimetrexate glucuronate (NSC 352122) given every 3 weeks: clinical pharmacology and pharmacodynamics. Cancer Chemother Pharmacol 1989;24:314-20.
264. Ratain MJ, Vogelzang NJ. Phase I and pharmacological study of vinblastine by prolonged continuous infusion. Cancer Res 1986;46:4827-30.
265. Grochow LB, Jones RJ, Brundrett RB, et al. Pharmacokinetics of busulfan: correlation with veno-occlusive disease in patients undergoing bone marrow transplantation. Cancer Chemother Pharmacol 1989;25:55-61.
266. Jones RB, Matthes S, Shpall EJ, et al. Acute lung injury following treatment with high-dose cyclophosphamide, cisplatin, and carmustine: pharmacodynamic evaluation of carmustine. J Natl Cancer Inst 1993;85:640-7.
267. Ayash LJ, Wright JE, Tretyakov O, et al. Cyclophosphamide pharmacokinetics: correlation with cardiac toxicity and tumor response. J Clin Oncol 1992;10:995-1000.
268. Thyss A, Milano G, Renee N, et al. Clinical pharmacokinetic study of 5-FU in continuous 5-day infusions for head and neck cancer. Cancer Chemother Pharmacol 1986;16:64-6.
269. van Groeningen CJ, Pinedo HM, Heddes J, et al. Pharmacokinetics of 5-fluorouracil assessed with a sensitive mass spectrometric method in patients on a dose escalation schedule. Cancer Res 1988;48:6956-61.

41

Drug Resistance and its Clinical Circumvention

Jeffrey Moscow, MD
Erasmus Schneider, PhD
Branimir I. Sikic, MD
Charles S. Morrow, MD, PhD
Kenneth H. Cowan, MD, PhD

Systemic therapy with cytotoxic drugs is the basis for most effective treatments of disseminated cancers. Additionally, adjuvant chemotherapy can offer a significant survival advantage to selected patients, following the treatment of localized disease with surgery or radiotherapy, presumably by eliminating undetected minimal or microscopic residual tumor. However, the responses of tumors to chemotherapeutic regimens vary, and failures are frequent owing to the emergence of drug resistance.

The phenomenon of clinical drug resistance has prompted studies to clarify mechanisms of drug action and to identify mechanisms of antineoplastic resistance. It is expected that through such information, drug resistance may be circumvented by rational design of new noncross-resistant agents, by novel delivery or combinations of known drugs, and by the development of other treatments that might augment the activity of or reverse resistance to known antineoplastics. Multiple mechanisms of antineoplastic failure have been identified using in vitro (tissue culture) and in vivo (animal and xenograft) models of antineoplastic resistance (Table 41-1). These include anatomic and pharmacologic mechanisms that may be uniquely pertinent to individual patients as well as cellular mechanisms within tumor cells. Although mechanisms of drug resistance have been largely determined in experimental systems, many have been implicated in at least some examples of clinical studies of chemotherapeutic failure. Evidence that bears upon these mechanisms of resistance as well as strategies to circumvent them are discussed below.

GENERAL MECHANISMS OF DRUG RESISTANCE

Experimental selection of drug resistance by repeated exposure to single antineoplastic agents will generally result in cross-resistance to some related agents of the same drug class. This phenomenon is explained on the basis of shared drug transport carriers, drug metabolizing pathways, and intracellular cytotoxic targets of these structurally and biochemically similar compounds. Generally, the resistant cells retain sensitivity to drugs of different classes with alternative mechanisms of cytotoxic action.[1,2] Thus, cells selected for resistance to alkylating agents or antifolates will usually remain sensitive to unrelated drugs, such as anthracyclines. Exceptions include emergence of cross-resistance to multiple, apparently structurally and functionally unrelated drugs, to which the patient or cancer cells were never exposed during the initial drug treatment. Despite apparent differences in their presumed sites of action within cells, the drugs associated with multidrug resistance (MDR) phenotypes frequently share common metabolic pathways or efflux transport systems.

In this section, the processes related to drug resistance will be described. A more comprehensive discussion of mechanisms of resistance to specific classes of drugs will be discussed in subsequent sections.

Table 41-1 General Mechanisms of Drug Resistance

Cellular and biochemical mechanisms
Decreased drug accumulation
Decreased drug influx
Increased drug efflux
Altered intracellular trafficking of drug
Decreased drug activation
Increased inactivation of drug or toxic intermediate
Increased repair of or tolerance to drug-induced damage to:
Deoxyribonucleic acid (DNA)
Protein
Membranes
Drug targets altered (quantitatively or qualitatively)
Altered cofactor or metabolite levels
Altered downstream effectors of cytotoxicity
Altered signaling pathway and/or apoptotic responses to drug insult
Altered gene expression
DNA mutation, amplification, or deletion
Altered transcription, post-transcription processing, or translation
Altered stability of macromolecules
Mechanisms relevant in vivo
Pharmacologic and anatomic drug barriers (tumor sanctuaries)
Host-drug interactions
Increased drug inactivation by normal tissues
Decreased drug activation by normal tissues
Relative increase in normal tissue drug sensitivity (toxicity)
Host-tumor interactions

Decreased Drug Accumulation Decreased intracellular levels of cytotoxic agents is one of the most common mechanisms of drug resistance. Since polar, water-soluble drugs cannot penetrate the lipid bilayer of the cell membrane and require specific mechanisms of cell entry, resistance to these drugs is readily mediated by down-regulation of drug uptake mechanisms in tumor cells. For example, decreased influx via a high-affinity folate-transport system,[3] as well as via a reduced folate carrier,[4] are well described causes of methotrexate resistance.[5,6] For hydrophobic, nonpolar drugs that can easily diffuse across the cell membrane, decreased intracellular drug concentrations can be achieved by increasing the activities of drug efflux pumps. For example, overexpression of the P-glycoprotein (*MDR1/ABCB1*) drug efflux pump is an important example of this mechanism of resistance.[7,8]

Altered Drug Metabolism Decreased drug activation, increased drug inactivation, or alterations in necessary cofactors can also confer resistance to selected antineoplastic agents. For example, decreased conversion of nucleobase analogues to their cytotoxic nucleoside and nucleotide derivatives by alterations in specific kinases and phosphoribosyl transferase salvage enzymes can lead to resistance to these anticancer drugs.[9,10] Another example associated with resistance is decreased levels of carboxyesterase—an activity necessary to convert a topoisomerase I inhibitor, CPT-11, to its active metabolite, SN-38.[11,12] On the other hand, enhanced inactivation of pyrimidine and purine analogues by increased expression of deaminases is linked to resistance toward these agents.[13,14] Finally, alterations in cofactor levels can also modify drug toxicity. For example, optimal formation of inhibitory complexes between 5-fluorodeoxyuridine monophosphate (FdUMP) and its target enzyme, thymidylate synthase, require the cofactor 5,10-methylene tetrahydrofolate.[15] Alterations in the intracellular levels of this cofactor can lead to resistance to fluoropyrimidines.

Increased Repair or Cellular Tolerance to Drug-Induced Damage Cells contain multiple complex systems involved in the repair of damage to membranes and deoxyribonucleic acid (DNA), and changes in these repair processes can influence drug sensitivity. For example, resistance to cisplatin, a drug whose cytotoxic action involves intrastrand DNA cross-linkages (see below), is associated with increased DNA repair. Conversely, defects in mismatch repair are associated with tolerance to cisplatin-induced DNA damage.[16] In this form of platinum resistance, the repair system is apparently unable to recognize platinum-DNA adducts and fails to activate the normal, appropriate programmed cell death response.

Altered Drug Targets Qualitative changes in the enzyme targets of antineoplastic drugs can compromise drug efficacy and have been associated with resistance to inhibitors of dihydrofolate reductase,[17,18] thymidylate synthase,[19] and topoisomerases I and II.[20–25] Perhaps not surprisingly, alteration of the drug target has also been recognized as a mechanism of resistance to newer molecularly targeted chemotherapy. For example, clinical resistance to the BCR-ABL kinase inhibitor Gleevec (imatinib mesylate) results from the development of mutations in the kinase's drug-binding site.[26]

Altered Gene Expression Increased expression of target enzymes can also lead to drug resistance. These alterations may result from changes that occur at any point along the pathways of gene expression and regulation, including DNA deletion or amplification, altered transcriptional or post-transcriptional control of ribonucleic acid (RNA) levels, and altered post-translational modifications of proteins.

In addition, the same molecular mechanisms that lead to oncogenesis can also lead to drug resistance through altered expression of drug targets. For example, loss of function of the retinoblastoma (*Rb*) gene leads to accumulation of the transcription factor E2F, which, in turn, activates transcription of at least two genes involved in antifolate drug resistance, dihydrofolate reductase and thymidylate synthase (reviewed by Banerjee and colleagues[27]). Efforts to exploit these observations by using E2F as a marker of antifolate chemosensitivity have met with mixed results.[28–30]

RESISTANCE TO MULTIPLE DRUGS

De novo and acquired cross-resistance to multiple antineoplastic agents can result from several alternative factors and processes. Accordingly, we have grouped the major patterns of cross-resistance into several categories on the basis of their presumed underlying mechanisms (Table 41-2). First, MDR is frequently associated with decreased drug accumulation, usually because of increased drug efflux. MDR is generally thought to be caused by increased energy-dependent efflux of the anticancer drugs, mediated by the overexpression of ATP binding cassette (ABC) proteins. ABC proteins constitute a large family of 48 transport proteins organized into

Table 41-2 Mechanisms of Multidrug Resistance (MDR)

Resistance associated with decreased drug accumulation
- ABC transporter-mediated resistance
  - P-Glycoprotein/MDR 1/ABCB1-mediated classic MDR
  - MRP family member-mediated MDR (currently at least 3 members, MRP1, 2, and 3 in ABCC1, ABCC2, ABCC3 implicated in MDR drug efflux and detoxification)
  - BCRP (ABCG2)-mediated MDR (putative ABC half-transporter implicated in mitoxantrone and anthracycline resistance)

LRP? (lung resistance protein, a major vault protein)
Alterations in topoisomerases

seven subfamilies, *ABCA – ABCG*.[31] Of these, at least three have been directly shown to cause MDR, namely *MDR1*/P-glycoprotein (*ABCB1*), *MRP1* (*ABCC1*) and *BCRP/MXR/ABC-P* (*ABCG2*). Classic MDR associated with resistance to drugs listed in Table 41-3 is mediated by P-glycoprotein (*MDR1* or *ABCB1*). A similar but distinct MDR phenotype was attributed to the energy-dependent drug efflux activities of multidrug resistance protein (MRP) family members, including *MRP1* or *ABCC1*.[32–35] Another overlapping but discrete MDR phenotype is associated with increased expression of the recently isolated putative efflux transporter, breast cancer resistance protein (*BCRP* or *ABCG2*).[36,37] MDR has also been described in association with overexpression of the lung resistance protein (LRP). The mechanism of LRP-associated resistance is unclear, and whether LRP alone is sufficient to confer resistance is unknown. It is speculated that as a major vault protein, LRP is involved in nucleocytoplasmic transport and may be able to prevent entry of drugs into the nucleus.[38,39] Drug resistance defined by alterations in topoisomerases represents a third major category of MDR.[19–23,25,26]

Classic (*MDR1/ABCB1*-Mediated) MDR A model of MDR was described by Biedler and Riehm three decades ago.[40] Exposure of cells to any of the drugs listed in Table 41-3 can generally result in MDR phenotype.[7,8] Drug transport studies using parental and MDR cells demonstrate that the reduced cytotoxicity of these drugs is the result of decreased drug accumulation secondary to enhanced drug efflux.[41,42] The emergence of MDR

Table 41-3 Cross-Resistance Pattern of Classic (P-Glycoprotein-Mediated) MDR

Class	Drug
Anthracyclines	Doxorubicin Daunorubicin Mitoxantrone
Antibiotics	Actinomycin D Plicamycin
Antimicrotubule drugs	Vincristine Vinblastine Colchicine
Epipodophyllotoxins	Etoposide Tenoposide

was first associated with increased levels of a membrane-bound glycoprotein, P-glycoprotein. Although it is widely accepted that the *MDR1* or *ABCB1* gene encodes a protein (P-glycoprotein) that mediates an energy-dependent decrease in drug accumulation, there is considerable debate on the precise mechanism(s) involved.[8,43,44] Regardless of the mechanistic details, a great deal of evidence supports the consensus view that P-glycoprotein is an energy-dependent drug efflux pump responsible for the prevalent form of MDR. First, gene transfer experiments show that the *ABCB1* gene expression is sufficient to confer drug resistance.[45,46] Second, *ABCB1* belongs to a multigene family of transport proteins (ABC transporters), all of which share sequence homology with several bacterial transport proteins.[47,48] Third, photoaffinity labeling experiments demonstrate direct binding of drugs to P-glycoprotein.[49] Finally, the distribution of P-glycoprotein on the luminal surfaces of normal tissues, including renal tubules, colon, small intestine, and bile canaliculi is consistent with its proposed role in excretory transport.[50] Thus, P-glycoprotein appears to fulfill the requirements predicted of a membrane-bound energy-dependent drug exporter.

MDR1/ABCB1-mediated MDR displays significant phenotypic heterogeneity, and the relative degree of cross-resistance to the drugs listed in Table 41-3 varies based on the cell line and the selecting drug. Although the level of drug resistance is roughly correlated with the level of P-glycoprotein expression, *MDR1/ABCB1* mutations or polymorphisms, as well as coselections of other mechanisms of resistance may also provide phenotypic diversity.[51]

Studies have shown that high levels of *MDR1/ABCB1* expression are often associated with gene amplification and transcriptional activation.[7,8] Increased *MDR1/ABCB1* expression can also be induced transiently by heat shock,[52] heavy metals, cytotoxic drugs,[53–55] regenerating liver,[53,54] differentiating agents,[56–58] and by repeated exposure to ionizing radiation. *ABCB1* promoter activity can also be regulated by altered expression of oncogenes (*raf* and *ras*) and the tumor-suppressor gene, *TP53*.[59–63]

MDR1/ABCB1 expression has been detected in clinical samples from patients with acute and chronic leukemias,[64–68] ovarian cancer,[69] multiple myeloma,[70] breast cancer,[71–74] neuroblastoma,[75] soft tissue sarcomas,[76,77] renal cell carcinoma,[78] and others.[79] Although the numbers of patients with particular tumors in these studies were small, the results have tended to link increased *MDR/ABCB1* expression with a history of prior therapy (usually with MDR-associated drugs) and poorer treatment outcome. In general, the relationship between increased *MDR1/ABCB1* expression and adverse outcome in human cancers is strongest in hematologic malignancies. Recently, three prospective studies have shown that increased *MDR1/ABCB1* expression in patients with acute myelogenous leukemia (AML) is associated with decreased complete remission rates and reduced remission duration with use of conventional chemotherapy.[80–82] This correlation has also been demonstrated in adult multiple myeloma, lymphoma, and pediatric ALL.[83–86]

The relationship between *MDR1/ABCB1* expression and response to therapy in other cancers is less convincing.[87] In breast cancers, a meta-analysis found expression of *MDR1/ABCB1* in 30 to 40% of specimens at diagnosis, with a decreased rate of response to MDR-related cytotoxins, that is, anthracyclines and taxanes, in patients with positive tumors. Moreover, *MDR1/ABCB1* expression was more frequent in tumor specimens obtained after clinical resistance to therapy.

In patients with advanced neuroblastoma, *MDR1/ABCB1* expression has been strongly associated with aggressive biologic behavior, poor treatment response, and poor outcome.[88] However, the significance of *MDR1/ABCB1* expression in neuroblastomas is controversial as other data have suggested that increased *MDR1/ABCB1* expression is associated with more favorable clinical variables in patients with neuroblastoma.[89]

Multidrug Resistance Protein (MRP or *ABCC1*) Family Similar phenotypes of multiple resistance to antineoplastic agents have been described that are associated with the expression of other membrane proteins, including *MRP1* (multidrug resistance-associated protein 1 or *ABCC1*), which was isolated from a doxorubicin-selected MDR lung cancer cell line.[90] *ABCC1* encodes a 190-kilodalton (kDa) transmembrane protein, whose structure is strikingly homologous to P-glycoprotein (*MDR1/ABCB1*) and other members of the ATP-binding cassette (ABC) transmembrane transporter proteins.[90,91] Primary sequence analysis predicts the transmembrane structure shown in Figure 41-1. The structure, supported by immunochemical data, includes 11 plus 4 (or, alternatively, 11 plus 6) transmembrane domains with two cytosolic ATP-binding sites.[92] Increased *ABCC1* expression is associated with a MDR phenotype, while decreased *ABCC1* expression is associated with reversion to drug sensitivity. Gene transfer experiments establish that *ABCC1* can confer resistance to a variety of drugs, including anthracyclines, epipodophyllotoxins, and vinca alkaloids.[93–95] Transport studies indicate that *ABCC1* is involved in ATP-dependent efflux of some native natural product anticancer drugs. Additionally, *ABCC1* is an ATP-dependent transporter of a variety of anionic conjugates of drugs and other xenobiotics— conjugates that include glutathione conjugates, glucuronides, and sulfates.[96–101] Thus, *ABCC1* is an important xenobiotic-conjugate transport pump that is involved in efflux of a wide range of cellular poisons, including anticancer drugs and their conjugates. In contrast to *MDR1/ABCB1*, whose substrates are generally lipophilic neutral or cationic compounds, *ABCC1* preferentially recognizes amphiphilic organic anions. Although neutral, hydrophobic compounds such as vincristine are also substrates of *ABCC1*, reduced glutathione is required for their transport.[99,102] Although no covalent linkage between glutathione and vincristine is observed, it is believed that both glutathione and the neutral drug must be simultaneously present to effect efflux, and they both may be cotransported by *ABCC1*.

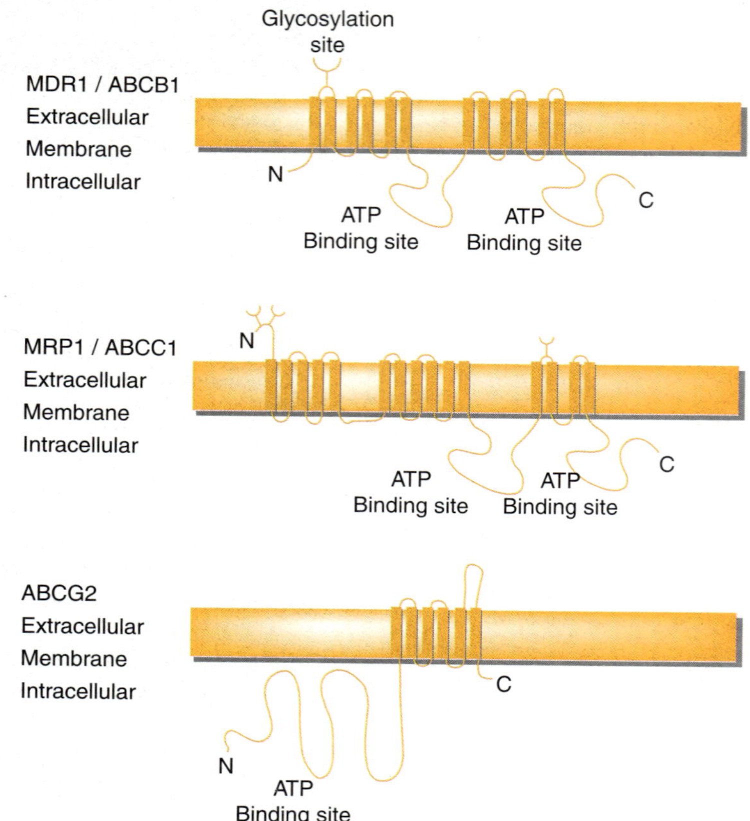

Figure 41-1 Models of multidrug resistance transporters.

Nine human MRP isoforms have been identified.[103–106] Among them, *MRP2* (*ABCC2*, *cMOAT*), and *MRP3* (*ABCC3*) are also capable of supporting efflux detoxification of cancer drugs, including epipodophyllotoxins.[33,105] Recent results indicate that *MRP1*(*ABCC1*), *MRP2* (*ABCC2*), *MRP3* (*ABCC3*), and *MRP4* (*ABCC4*) can all act as methotrexate efflux pumps and can confer resistance to methotrexate.[105,107]

***ABCG2* (Mediated MDR)** *ABCG2*-associated MDR was independently and almost simultaneously identified and described as placental ABC protein (ABC-P),[108] Breast cancer resistance protein (BCRP),[109] and mitoxantrone resistance (MXR) protein.[110] It is the second member of the ABCG subfamily of human ABC proteins and encodes a 72 kDa protein. Homologs have been found in mice,[111] rats,[112,113] pigs,[114,115] and rhesus monkeys.[116] The ABCG2 protein is a half-transporter, that is, it contains only one nucleotide-binding domain and one transmembrane domain, as opposed to the proteins encoded by *ABCB1* and *ABCC1*, which contain two each of these domains (see Figure 41-1). In cells, *ABCG2* is primarily localized to the plasma membrane,[117–119] where it forms a homodimer[120,121] or possibly a homotetramer,[122] with some evidence of even a higher order multimeric organization.[122] In the whole organism, *ABCG2* has been found at the blood brain barrier[113,115,123–126] and blood testis barrier,[127] in the placenta,[108,128–131] on the luminal or apical side of many parts of the GI tract,[128] as well as in kidney tubules,[132] liver canaliculi,[128] mammary ducts,[128] and in venous and capillary, but not arterial, endothelium.[128] Thus, it has been proposed that one of the main functions of *ABCG2* is to protect the organism from a variety of xenobiotics.[133] In addition, *ABCG2* has been suggested as a marker for the stem cell side population in a variety of tissues, including the bone marrow,[134–137] muscle,[138] liver,[112,139,140] pancreas,[141,142] lung,[143] testis,[144] heart,[145] breast,[146,147] and the limbal system of the eye.[148–151]

Like the other MDR transporters, *ABCG2* exhibits a rather promiscuous substrate specificity that shows some, though not complete, overlap with the resistance phenotype associated with *MDR1/ABCB1* and *MRP1/ABCC1*.[152] The list of substrates includes various anticancer drugs, such as irinotecan and its active metabolite SN-38, topotecan, and several of the second-generation camptothecin derivatives, and other topoisomerase I inhibitors,[153–158] mitoxantrone,[109] the anthracyclines doxorubicin, daunorubicin,[109] methotrexate,[159–162] flavopiridol,[163] tamoxifen,[164] and imatinib.[165] Furthermore, *ABCG2* has also been shown to transport a number of other substances such as rhodamine 123,[166] pheophorbide,[167] heme and porphyrins,[168,169] sulfated steroids and sterols,[164,170–172] and various HIV reverse transcriptase inhibitors.[173]

The role of *ABCG2* in clinical MDR is not clear. Initial studies examined *ABCG2* in leukemias, especially acute myelogenic leukemia (AML).[174,175] For example, among a group of 40 adult patients with AML, *ABCG2* mRNA expression varied from zero to 76 times the expression in control cells. Although there was no difference in expression between initial responders and nonresponders, among the subgroup of responders, those with the highest *ABCG2* expression had a significantly shorter overall survival (mean 38 months) compared with those with the lowest expression (mean 74 months, $p < .05$).[176] In another study of 149 adult patients with AML, *ABCG2* mRNA expression was a negative prognostic factor in patients treated with daunorubicin and mitoxantrone, but not idarubicin, which is consistent with idarubicin not being a substrate for *ABCG2*.[177,178] A similar finding was reported by Sargent and colleagues,[179] who found that in 20 either pretreated or naïve patients with AML, *ABCG2* protein expression correlated with resistance to daunorubicin, but not mitoxantrone, topotecan or doxorubicin. In another study of 20 paired clinical AML samples, *ABCG2* mRNA expression was 1.7-fold increased at relapse compared with at diagnosis, whereas neither *MDR1/ABCB1* nor *MRP1/ABCC1* expression differed in the paired samples.[180] These results suggest that high *ABCG2* expression may be a negative prognostic factor in at least a subset of patients with AML.

In contrast, several other studies failed to detect a correlation between *ABCG2* expression and clinical resistance. For example, *ABCG2* expression was undetectable in 23 of 26 AML blast cases, and there were no consistent changes over the course of the disease.[181] Similarly, van der Kolk and colleagues[182] did not detect a consistent up-regulation of *ABCG2* expression in 20 paired samples of de novo and relapsed AML. One of the inherent problems in all of these studies is the fact that *ABCG2* expression is heterogeneous among different cells with only certain subpopulations expressing high levels, such as primitive progenitor cells with the side population phenotype. Furthermore, measurements of mRNA do not necessarily correlate with associated protein levels or activity.[183,184] As a consequence, it is difficult to compare the results from the different studies, or possibly even within studies between individual patients.

Expression of *ABCG2* was also evaluated in a number of other hematologic malignancies. For example, in a small study of 30 adult patients with ALL, *ABCG2* expression was predictive of shorter disease-free survival ($p < .05$).[184] Another study of 46 patients with ALL showed that *ABCG2* expression and function was significantly higher in B-cell ALL than in T-cell ALL.[185] Two other studies specifically investigated a possible role of *ABCG2* in pediatric leukemias. In patients with T-cell ALL, there was generally a lower *ABCG2* expression then in B-cell ALL; however, there was no apparent relationship between *ABCG2* expression and clinical or in vivo resistance.[186] In contrast, *ABCG2* mRNA was more than 10 times higher in patients who failed to achieve complete remission. In this study of 59 children, higher levels of *ABCG2* expression were significantly associated with worse prognosis.[187] Furthermore, in a comparison of pediatric ALL subtypes, it was found that those with the TEL-AML1 translocation exhibited significantly higher *ABCG2* expression, which was accompanied by lower methotrexate-polyglutamate accumulation.[188]

In a study of 59 primary breast cancers, an association was observed between *ABCG2* expression and progression-free survival in a subgroup of patients with breast cancer treated with CAF, but not in those who received CMF therapy.[73] In contrast, another study reported that *ABCG2* RNA levels in 38 breast cancer patients who were treated with doxorubicin did not correlate with relapse or prognosis.[189] Similarly, there was no association of *ABCG2* expression with response to anthracycline therapy in a study of 25 primary breast carcinomas and 27 patients with preoperative therapy.[190] Interestingly, in that study, *ABCG2* protein was detected only in blood vessels and normal epithelial cells, but not in tumor cells. In another study of 72 advanced-stage nonsmall-cell lung cancers that received platinum-based therapy, response to chemotherapy, progression-free survival, and overall survival were negatively correlated with *ABCG2* positive staining by immunohistochemistry.[191]

In conclusion, it appears that *ABCG2* expression may contribute to poor chemotherapy response in AML, whereas its role in other leukemias or solid tumors is less clear.

MDR Associated with Topoisomerase Poisons Topoisomerases are nuclear enzymes that catalyze the formation of transient single- or double-stranded DNA breaks, facilitate the passage of DNA strands through these breaks, and promote rejoining of the DNA strands.[192,193] As a consequence of these activities, topoisomerases are thought to be critical for DNA replication, transcription, and recombination. The cytotoxicity of many drugs that target topoisomerases, a class of drugs here termed "topoisomerase poisons" (Table 41-4), is thought to depend on the DNA cleavage activities of topoisomerases. There are two classes of mammalian enzymes, topoisomerases I and II. Topoisomerase I catalyzes the formation of single-stranded DNA breaks, while topoisomerases II (α and β isoforms) catalyze both single- and double-stranded breaks. During the cleavage reactions, reversible DNA-topoisomerase complexes (cleavable complexes) can be stabilized by interactions with topoisomerase poisons. The formation of these stabilized DNA–topoisomerase–drug complexes is thought to initiate the production of lethal DNA strand breaks. Of the chemotherapeutic drugs that affect topoisomerase activities, the topoisomerase II poisons have been the most important clinically. A partial list of these agents, which include DNA intercalating and nonintercalating drugs, appears in Table 41-3. The topoisomerase I poisons topotecan and irinotecan are analogues of the natural plant-derived product camptothecin.

Table 41-4 Topoisomerase II Poisons

	Class	Drug
Nonintercalators	Epipodophyllotoxins	Etoposide Tenoposide
Intercalators	Anthracyclines	Doxorubicin Daunorubicin Mitoxantrone
	Acridine	m-AMSA (amsacrine)
	Anthracenedione	Mitoxantrone
	Antibiotic	Actinomycin D
	Ellipticine	9-Hydroxy ellipticine

Several laboratories have described an MDR pattern characterized by resistance of cells to several or all of the drugs listed in Table 41-3.[194,195] It is readily apparent that many topoisomerase II–targeting drugs are also members of the classic MDR phenotype (see Table 41-2). Hence, decreased drug accumulation via increased expression of *MDR1/ABCB1*, *MRP1/ABCC1*, or *ABCG2* represent common mechanisms of resistance to topoisomerase II poisons. Another important mechanism of resistance to topoisomerase II poisons is thought to involve altered topoisomerase II expression or activity. Both qualitative and quantitative changes in topoisomerase II enzyme activity have been demonstrated in resistant cell lines. Reduced levels of topoisomerase activity are associated with decreased drug-induced DNA strand breaks, as well as reduced drug cytotoxicity.[196,197] Other studies implicate intrinsic changes in drug-induced catalytic properties or associated cofactors as the basis of drug resistance in some cells.[22,198–200]

There are two mammalian isozymes of topoisomerase II, a 170 kDa form (topoisomerase IIα) and a 180 kDa form (topoisomerase IIβ), either of which may be involved in clinical drug resistance.[201–203] These isozymes differ with respect to their regulation during the cell cycle[204] and their relative sensitivities to topoisomerase II poisons.[202,203] Hence, the relative levels of the specific topoisomerase II isozymes as well as the total topoisomerase II activity may be significant determinants of the sensitivity of tumor cells to topoisomerase II drugs.

Several reports suggest the molecular basis of drug resistance associated with qualitatively altered topoisomerase II.[205] Point mutations leading to amino acid substitutions in topoisomerase IIα isolated from cells selected for resistance to topoisomerase II drugs have been described. These mutations are clustered within the conserved ATP-binding consensus sequences[206–209] or near the Tyr 804 residue involved in covalent attachment of topoisomerase IIα to DNA.[208–210] Although these topoisomerase IIα mutations are associated with drug resistance in intact cells and, in some cases, with altered enzymatic activities in vitro, the exact mechanism(s) of drug resistance and the relationship of these mutations to a specifically altered enzymatic property are incompletely understood. Moreover, the relevance for clinical drug resistance of these topoisomerase IIα mutations identified in experimentally drug-selected resistant cell lines is unknown. Indeed, one study of topoisomerase IIα derived from leukemic blasts of 15 relapsed patients failed to iden-

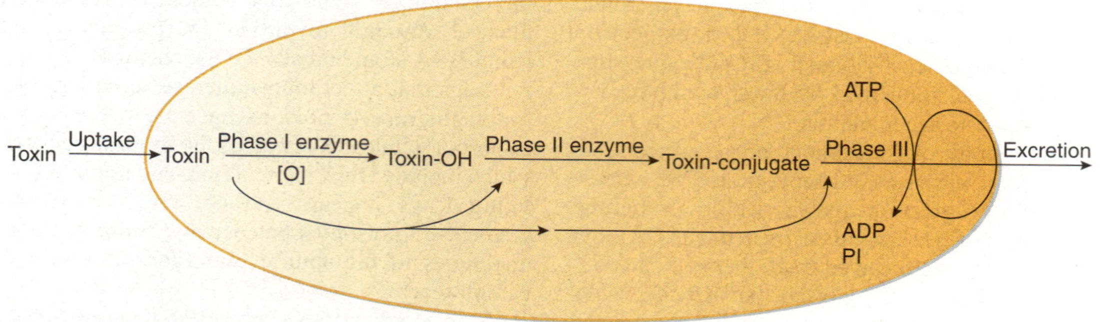

Figure 41-2 Phases I, II, and III drug detoxification.

tify mutations in either of the above two regions implicated in experimental drug resistance.[208]

The camptothecin derivatives topotecan and irinotecan enhance topoisomerase I–mediated strand breaks. These drugs have important activity in several tumor types, including colorectal, ovarian, and lung cancers.[211] Consequently, the emergence of resistance to these agents has become an increasingly important consideration. There are reports of topoisomerase I mutations derived from cell lines selected for resistance to camptothecin or its derivative, irinotecan.[24,212,213] In two of these resistant cell lines, the mutant enzyme has altered topoisomerase I activity with a reduced capacity to mediate camptothecin-induced DNA strand breaks.[212–214]

MDR Associated with Altered Expression of Drug-Metabolizing Enzymes and Drug-Conjugate Export Pumps The manner in which cells metabolize cancer drugs and other xenobiotics is often described as involving three phases of detoxification (Figure 41-2).[215] Although none of these phases are obligatory steps in the metabolism of every drug, the concept illustrated in Figure 41-2 represents a useful framework with which to view cellular detoxification mechanisms. Alterations in any of these three phases can influence the sensitivity or resistance to a particular drug or xenobiotic toxin. Phase I drug metabolism is mediated by cytochrome P-450 mixed-function oxidases. Generally, the drug or xenobiotic is rendered into a more electrophilic, reactive intermediate—a process that may enhance toxicity. These metabolites may then be converted to a less reactive, presumably less toxic, form in phase II reactions, which include the formation of drug/xenobiotic conjugations with glutathione (GSH), glucuronic acid, or sulfate—reactions that are catalyzed by multiple isozymes each of glutathione *S*-transferases (GSTs), uridine diphosphate (UDP)-glucuronosyl transferases, and sulfatases, respectively.[216–220] Phase III detoxification consists of export of the parent drug/xenobiotic or its metabolites by energy-dependent transmembrane efflux pumps, including MRP (ABCC) family members as described above.

Frequently, in cellular and animal models of drug or xenobiotic resistance, a coordinated down-regulation of phase I drug-activating enzymes and an up-regulation of specific phase II drug-conjugating enzymes is observed.[53,54,221,222] Such a programmed cellular stress response offers a versatile, generalized protective mechanism against exposure to a variety of exogenous toxins.

Of the phase II enzymes, the GSTs have been the most extensively studied. GSTs[219,220] comprise multiple soluble and membrane-associated isozymes, which catalyze the conjugation of electrophilic hydrophobic compounds (R-X) with the thiol, GSH:

$$R-X+\text{GSH} \overset{\text{GST}}{\rightarrow} R-\text{SG}+\text{H}X$$

Circumstantial evidence links the increase in specific GST isozymes or bulk GST activity in cells to resistance to alkylating agents and other drugs.[219,220,223–226] However, direct evidence that GSTs are responsible for altering drug sensitivities is limited. Another catalytic activity, selenium-independent glutathione peroxidase activity, has been attributed to some isozymes of GST:

$$R-O-OH+2\text{GSH} \overset{\text{GST}}{\rightarrow} R-OH+\text{GSSG}+H_2O$$

This and other GST-mediated reactions are of interest because of their potential to detoxify oxidative damage to membranes and DNA.

Studies using cell-free preparations of GSTs have identified a limited number of antineoplastic drug substrates of these enzymes. Table 41-5 lists these drugs and other substrates that are possibly associated with drug-mediated oxidative damage. Whether GST levels in tumor cells are sufficient to detoxify antineoplastic drugs to a clinically significant extent is a matter of considerable debate. Several cancer drugs, particularly reactive electrophilic alkylating agents, can form conjugates with glutathione—both spontaneously and in enzyme-catalyzed reactions.[227–234] However, despite these catalytic activities, the role of GSTs in drug resistance remains uncertain because of inconsistent results from different laboratories.[224,228,235–244] Indeed, some investigators have found an association between cellular resistance to some anticancer drugs and expression of a particular isozyme of GST, whereas others have found no such association.

Table 41-5 Some Important Substrates of GSTs Related to Drug Detoxification and Repair of Drug-Mediated Damage

Antineoplastic Drug	Products of Membrane and DNA Oxidation
Nitrogen mustards	Fatty acid hydroperoxides
Chlorambucil	4-Hydroxy alkenals
Melphalan	DNA hydroperoxides
Cyclophosphamide	
Thiotepa	
Nitrosoureas	
1,3-bis(2-chloroethyl)-1nitrosourea (BCNU)	
Anthracenedione	
Mitoxantrone	

The importance of drug/xenobiotic-conjugate transporters for cellular export and detoxification of certain compounds is increasingly appreciated. Conjugation frequently renders the parent drug more hydrophilic and less capable of diffusing through the plasma membrane—trapping the drug within the cell. Although conjugation with glutathionyl or glucuronosyl groups may render some drugs less toxic, these drug conjugates themselves may retain significant toxicity. For example, the glutathione conjugate formed with cisplatin is itself toxic and an inhibitor of protein synthesis.[245] Moreover, drug conjugates may inhibit their conjugating enzyme(s).[246] Thus, the relative resistance of cells expressing drug-metabolizing enzymes may depend on cellular levels of drug conjugate transporters, including the glutathione conjugate transporters,[215,247] such as the MRP (ABCC) family proteins.[35,100] Indeed, recent results using model cell lines demonstrate that combined expression of specific isozymes of GST with MRP1 is necessary to achieve full protection from the toxicities of the cancer drug chlorambucil,[248] or from the carcinogen 4-nitroquinoline 1-oxide.[249] In these studies, the expression of either GST or *MRP1* alone provided little, if any, protection from toxicity—a finding that illustrates the synergistic interaction of phase II and phase III detoxification processes in the emergence of resistance to some drugs and other xenobiotics.

Multidrug Resistance Related to Suppression of Cell Death Pathways Chemotherapeutic drugs initiate cytotoxicity through their interactions with a variety of molecular targets. For example, epipodophyllotoxins attack topoisomerases II, alkylating agents form adducts with the nucleophilic centers of DNA and proteins, and methotrexate inhibits dihydrofolate reductase, resulting in reduced pyrimidine and purine synthesis. Despite these varied primary targets, most, if not all, cancer drugs effect cell death, at least partially, via downstream events that converge upon pathways mediating type I (apoptotic) or type II (autophagic) programmed cell death or apoptosis.

Apoptosis refers to an orderly cellular death program with predictable molecular and morphologic changes, including nuclear pyknosis and fragmentation, internucleosomal endonucleolytic

DNA fragmentation, formation of cytoplasmic apoptotic bodies, and plasma membrane changes, such as transposition of phosphatidylserine to the extracellular surface.[250] Autophagy is a pathway for bulk degradation of subcellular constituents that occurs in response to stresses such as nutrient deprivation. It involves the creation of autophagosomes/autolysozymes[251] and can be inhibited by PI3 kinase inhibitors such as 3-methyladenosine and wortmannin.[251]

Apoptosis or type I programmed cell death is conveniently conceptualized in three phases. First, the initiation phase of apoptosis (eg, secondary to chemotherapy-mediated DNA damage) is characterized by its reversibility. Second, the commitment phase involves the irreversible decision to complete the death program. The commitment phase, which may involve mitochondrial changes including the permeability phase transition and the release of cytochrome c and apoptosis-inducing factor (AIF), are all hallmarks of apoptosis. Finally, the degradation or execution phase includes downstream events, including DNA fragmentation and morphologic changes. Prior to commitment, apoptosis can be modulated by regulatory elements, such as TP53 and the Bcl-2 family proteins.[250,252–254] Clearly, such regulation of the apoptotic response can have profound effects on the outcome of chemotherapy and is an area of active investigation germane to drug resistance and sensitivity.

Although apoptosis may be either TP53-dependent or -independent, frequently the cellular response to DNA damage is regulated by TP53.[252] As shown in a simplified diagram (Figure 41-3), cancer therapy–induced DNA damage is sensed by TP53 by incompletely understood mechanisms. Depending on the particular cell type and damage, TP53 expression may then initiate one of two possible pathways: apoptosis or a process of cell-cycle arrest and repair. In cells where the apoptotic pathway dominates, changes that cause dysfunction or deletion of TP53 are likely to result in reduced apoptosis in response to DNA damage, leading to relative resistance and cell survival with damage. Indeed, TP53 is required for radiation- and etoposide-induced apoptosis in thymocytes, whereas lymphoma cell lines expressing mutant TP53 were relatively resistant to DNA-damaging agents.[255–257] In cells where the TP53-dependent cell-cycle arrest and repair response dominates, deletion or mutation of *TP53* might be expected to result in decreased cell-cycle arrest and repair leading to accumulated DNA damage and hence sensitivity to the chemotherapeutic agent.[252]

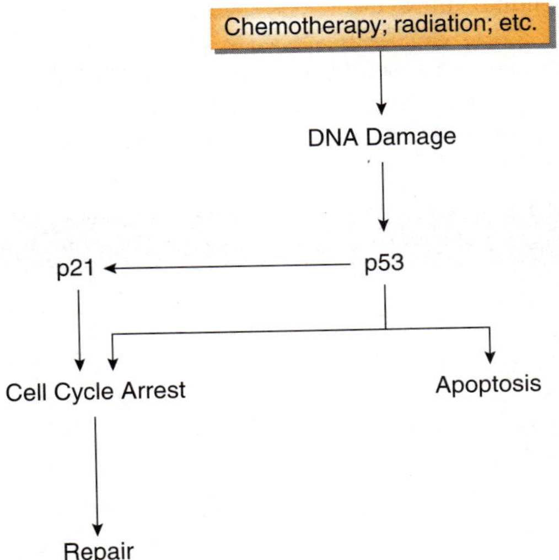

Figure 41-3 Alternative cellular responses to cancer therapeutic stress.

The mitogen-activated protein kinase (MAPK)-signaling cascades are involved in the regulation of cellular response to exogenous factors, including geno- and cytotoxic cancer treatments.[258] The extracellular stimulus-regulated kinase (ERK1/2) pathway is implicated in the proliferative response to growth factors. In cells treated with potentially cytotoxic stressors, such as radiation or anticancer drugs, the p38 and stress-activated/c-Jun *N*-terminal protein kinase (*SAPK/JNK*) pathways are implicated in mediating cell-cycle arrest or apoptosis. Modulation of these interacting pathways can have a profound effect on whether a cancer cell responds to cytotoxin challenge by activation of apoptosis or by cell-cycle arrest and repair leading to resistance to treatment.[258,259]

The Bcl-2 family proteins comprise several important regulators of apoptosis. Although their mechanism(s) of action is incompletely known, the balance of expressed antiapoptotic family members (Bcl-2, Bcl-X_L) and proapoptotic family members (Bax, Bak, Bad, and Bid) can influence the relative sensitivity of cells to toxic stressors.[253,254] Indeed, increased Bcl-2 and its antiapoptotic homologs are associated with increased resistance of lymphoid cells to the cytotoxic effects of corticosteroids, radiation, and DNA damage from chemotherapeutic drugs.[254,260–263] It has been proposed that increased levels of antiapoptotic proteins Bcl-2 or Bcl-X_L may result in reduced sensitivity to DNA-damaging cancer drugs—a resistance phenotype characterized by cell survival and increased tolerance to DNA damage and genomic instability. This genomic instability may lead to further mutations activating additional resistance mechanisms and conferring more aggressive tumor behavior.[253] Although the role of Bcl-2 family proteins and the multidomain proapoptotic members of this family in the development of type I (apoptotic) programmed cell death has been extensively characterized, recent studies indicate that these proteins also control type II (autophagy) and nonapoptotic programmed cell death.[264] Thus, the expression of mutant and wild-type TP53, Bcl-2 family members, MAPK family members, and other proteins associated with the control of apoptosis and/or autophagy may contribute significantly to the clinical sensitivity of tumor cells. These proteins are the targets of investigational agents that may become important in future strategies to overcome clinical drug resistance.

RESISTANCE FACTORS UNIQUE TO TUMOR CELLS IN VIVO: HOST-TUMOR INTERACTIONS

The failure of chemotherapy to eradicate a tumor in vivo despite exquisite sensitivity to drug in vitro might be a result of anatomic or pharmacologic sanctuaries. For example, the failure to deliver adequate amounts of many drugs across blood–brain and blood–testicular barriers probably accounts for the relatively high frequency of acute lymphoblastic leukemia relapse at these sites.[265] In large solid tumors, chemotherapeutic failures are frequently attributed to decreased drug delivery to a tumor that has overgrown its vascular supply. Additionally, development of acidosis and hypoxia in poorly perfused areas of large tumors may interfere with the cytotoxicity of some drugs. Altered prodrug activation by liver or other normal tissues may profoundly influence the efficacy of drugs such as cyclophosphamide.

Studies by Teicher and Herman[266] suggest that tumor–host interactions may influence drug pharmacokinetics and tumor resistance in unexpected ways. In this study, tumor cells selected for cyclophosphamide and cisplatin resistance in vivo were normally sensitive to drugs in vitro. When the tumor cells were reimplanted into nude mice, in vivo drug resistance was restored. These results suggest that resistant tumors may harbor cellular resistance factors that are operative only in conjunction with host factors and, therefore, mediate resistance by altered drug pharmacokinetics in vivo only. If this novel host-dependent mechanism of tumor resistance proves common, these results would provide one explanation for the failure of conventional in vitro testing to predict clinical responsiveness in all cases.

PHARMACOGENOMICS AND DRUG RESISTANCE

Integration of the knowledge of mechanisms of drug resistance with the emerging field of pharmacogenomics, the study of genetic influence on all aspects of drug therapy, has been seen as having the potential for allowing clinicians to tailor therapy on the basis of projected individual toxicity and intrinsic resistance of a tumor. Interest in the application of pharmacogenomics to the challenges of cancer drug resistance has been spurred by the success of the identification of genetic polymorphisms that can detect individuals with unusual sensitivities to drugs, such as the TPMT polymorphism that identifies patients with increased sensitivity to mercaptopurine.[267,268] The identification of genetic markers of drug resistance holds the promise of allowing clinical oncologists to practice individualized medicine, where the genetic profiles of patients and their tumors would reveal the most effective chemotherapy regimen with the fewest side effects for each patient.

However, the complexity of turning the vision of genomic medicine into a predictive tool for identifying intrinsic and acquired drug resistance creates a daunting challenge. In any predictive model, individual genetic characteristics of the host and the tumor would have to be considered. Characteristics of the host include factors that affect the classic aspects of pharmacokinetics—absorption, distribution, metabolism, and excretion of each anticancer agent. Characteristics of the tumor would include all mechanisms of pharmacodynamic interactions, including drug uptake and efflux, interaction with the site of drug action, and pathways of repair of drug damage and apoptosis.

Each aspect of pharmacokinetic and pharmacodynamic processes can involve the actions of the products of several genes, and the ultimate functional expression of these genes can be affected by hundreds of genetic factors. These genetic factors are both quantitative, usually assayed by differences in RNA or protein levels or function. Measurement of gene expression through DNA microarrays is a quantifiable surrogate for actual functional gene expression. Translational efficiency, post-translational modification, and modification of activity by other proteins all can affect ultimately quantitative function, but these parameters must be assayed separately. Using genetic analysis of SNPs to evaluate their potential or gene expression or protein function and correlating these genetic variants for drug resistance is also complex. Each gene with potential roles in drug resistance may have hundreds of SNPs, and the functional consequence of each SNP variation will require detailed analysis to determine its relevance in vitro and in vivo. Even though SNPs are often inherited in groups, in a phenomenon referred to as linkage disequilibrium, which can decrease the total number of variations present in the population, complete genetic and functional characterization of each gene is a great challenge. In addition, studies of the effect of a given SNP on drug disposition or patient outcome may not be consistent, leading to further complexity in developing predictive models based on pharmacogenomics.

For example, the *MDR1/ABCB1* gene encoding P-glycoprotein has a total of at least 216 identified SNPs.[269] Of these polymorphisms, 193 are located within introns, including 3 in the promoter region and 39 in the intron-exon border sequences, and 19 SNPs are located in the protein coding region, of which 8 result in a change of protein structure.[269] Because of linkage disequilibrium, these SNPs appear to be organized into 64 haplotypes, of which the 2 most common haplotypes account for 36% of all *MDR1/ABCB1* genes. These haplotype frequencies can vary in different ethnic populations.[269]

The most widely studied *MDR1/ABCB1* SNP occurs at nucleotide 3435, and has three variations: homozygous CC, homozygous TT, and heterozygous CT. This C3435T SNP is located in an exon, but does not result in a change in the amino acid sequence of P-glycoprotein, so any effect of inheriting an allele containing a particular polymorphism at this site would have to be due to co-inheritance of other SNPs in the allele. Several studies have shown that individuals with the TT genotype have a lower overall expression of P-glycoprotein in tissues and tumors,[270–275] although others have not.[276–283]

The potential role of *MDR1/ABCB1* SNPs in drug resistance would be suggested by the selective expression of a particular allele during drug therapy. Again, studies are conflicting on this issue, with one study showing selective expansion of cells with a particular *MDR1/ABCB1* allele in heterozygous patients,[284] although another study was unable to demonstrate this effect.[285] The clinical role of *MDR1/ABCB1* polymorphisms would also be supported by evidence that a given SNP correlated with overall clinical outcome. Again, the evidence is conflicting, with one study showing that the C3435T SNP correlated with prognosis,[286] but another study unable to demonstrate such an effect.[283]

The pharmacogenomic characterization of the cellular metabolism of the anticancer drug methotrexate further illustrates the issues involved in developing predictive models of drug resistance.[287] Methotrexate enters cells through the reduced folate carrier, undergoes polyglutamylation resulting in intracellular accumulation, and inhibits the enzyme dihydrofolate reductase (DHFR). The enzymes thymidylate synthase (TS) and methylene tetrahydrofolate reductase (MTHFR) interact in the DHFR metabolic pathway and can affect its function. Thus, there are multiple genes involved in methotrexate action, each with its own spectrum of expression levels and SNPs.

One frequently studied polymorphism is the A1298C SNP in the *MTHFR* gene. *MTHFR* regulates the relative levels of folate metabolites that are available for competing pathways for either nucleotide synthesis or DNA methylation. Two SNPs in the *MTHFR* gene, C677T and A1298C, have an impact on the relative level of 5-methyl tetrahyofolate, and therefore on the sensitivity of cells to methotrexate. This polymorphism is a potential double-edged sword, since it might be expected to increase the sensitivity of tumor cells to the drug, but also increase the potential toxicity of the drug to normal tissues. The clinical analysis of the impact of genetic polymorphism is complicated by the fact that methotrexate is given in a multitude of different regimens employing a wide range of dosages. As with the pharmacogenomic studies of *MDR1/ABCB1*, clinical studies have yielded conflicting results regarding the effect of MTHFR polymorphisms on both efficacy and toxicity.[288–291] Polymorphisms of two other genes involved in methotrexate metabolism, deletions in the untranslated region of thymidylate synthase[292,293] and the G80A SNP in the reduced folate carrier gene[291,294] also provide initial but conflicting evidence for a role of these polymorphisms in determining toxicity or outcome. In none of these genes have there been studies of allele selection in tumors, as has been attempted with *MDR1/ABCB1*, to determine a potential role of a given SNP in the development of drug resistance.

Similarly, polymorphisms in at least five genes affecting the efficacy and toxicity of irinotecan have been described.[295] Therefore, the complexity of applying pharmacogenomic information to the prediction of drug resistance and to strategies to overcome drug resistance presents an enormous challenge. New technologies may help speed the analysis of functional consequences of drug resistance–related genes.[296] However, unless truly phenotypically dominant polymorphisms are identified, such as is the case with TMPT, where activity is almost completely abrogated by an SNP, algorithms based on genetic profiles to determine optimal and nontoxic therapy are currently a potential but elusive goal.

POTENTIAL CLINICAL APPLICATION OF STRATEGIES TO AVERT OR OVERCOME DRUG RESISTANCE

Approaches to overcome chemotherapeutic failures include efforts to prevent the emergence of drug resistance (Table 41-6). An appreciation of factors that induce resistance mechanisms may lead to the choice of more efficacious treatment regimens. For example, drugs that may have only sporadic activity against a specific tumor, yet are likely to select for cross-resistance to more active agents, would be avoided. It is hoped that aggressive combination chemotherapy with noncross-reacting drugs will eliminate tumor rapidly enough to prevent the selection of tumor cell clones with multiple resistance. Another approach is to develop therapies aimed at reversing or circumventing clinical drug resistance.

Reversal of *MDR1/ABCB1*, and *MRP1/ABCC1* and *ABCG2*-Mediated Resistance Prior to the original descriptions of *MDR1/ABCB1*, Tsu-

Table 41-6 Approaches to Overcome or Circumvent Drug Resistance

Prevention	Aggressive multiple-agent therapy
	Appreciation of factors that induce resistance mechanism
Circumvention	Drug-screening programs and rational drug design
	Circumvention of drug uptake defects
	Dose escalation
	Drugs that use alternative transport mechanisms
	Agents that reverse increased efflux
	Cofactors that augment drug activation or efficacy
	Inhibition of drug inactivation
	Novel treatment modalities
	Immunotherapy
	Development of agents that target signaling and apoptotic pathways

ruo and colleagues noted that treatment with verapamil of leukemia cells made drug resistant by selection in vincristine or doxorubicin could partially restore antineoplastic drug sensitivity.[297] Furthermore, this verapamil-enhanced antineoplastic cytotoxicity, which was specific for drug-resistant but not-sensitive parental cells, was associated with increased accumulation of vincristine and doxorubicin. These results suggested that in the drug-resistant cells, vincristine and doxorubicin share a common transport system that is sensitive to modulation by verapamil. This transport system has now been identified as the P-glycoprotein drug efflux pump. Subsequently, numerous agents have been studied that can partially reverse the drug accumulation defects in classically multidrug-resistant cells, including several calcium channel blockers, calmodulin inhibitors such as phenothiazines, cyclosporin A, and cyclosporin derivatives, and other drugs.[298–304] Although the mechanism(s) by which these agents reverse MDR is incompletely understood, it is believed that direct interactions between these agents and P-glycoprotein interfere with antineoplastic drug efflux activity. Because a considerable clinical experience in the use of MDR-reversing agents has existed for the treatment of other disorders, these agents have been included in several clinical trials designed to enhance the antitumor activity of conventional cancer drugs in refractory human neoplasms.

Although there have been several encouraging studies showing the efficacy of *MDR1/ABCB1* inhibitors in murine models of MDR, most promising early clinical trials have been confined to those treating refractory or relapsed hematologic malignancies.[305–323] Studies involving the use of MDR-reversing agents in the treatment of solid human tumors have been generally disappointing.[323] Two recent phase II studies of *MDR1/ABCB1* reversal with PSC833 (valspodar),[303] a nonimmunosuppressant analogue of cyclosporine A, in combination with paclitaxel and doxorubicin in refractory ovarian cancer failed to show a convincing benefit, with complete response rates of 0% and 3%, respectively, and partial response rates of 9% and 12%, respectively. A major problem with these studies is the lack of screening of patients for *MDR1/ABCB1* expression in tumors. Since only a minority of patients entered into these trials would be expected to have tumors positive for the target, P-glycoprotein, there would be a strong dilutional effect, reducing the power of the studies to demonstrate reversal of resistance.

The largest recent phase III studies of the potential benefit *MDR1/ABCB1* reversal have focused on patients with refractory leukemia. One of these studies, in which 226 patients with AML were randomized to receive daunorubicin in a 72-hour infusion, with or without concomitant infusion of cyclosporine, showed that the addition of cyclosporine A improved relapse-free survival (34% vs 9% at 2 years; p = .031) and overall survival (22% vs 12%; p = .046).[311] It is of interest in this study that cyclosporine A did not significantly improve the remission rate and that survival improved with increasing daunorubicol concentrations in the cyclosporine-treated patients, but not in the controls, suggesting that the addition of cyclosporine enhanced the cytotoxicity of daunorubicin and eliminated resistant clones. This prospective clinical study of infusional cyclosporine and daunorubicin in AML by List and colleagues demonstrated for the first time a clear clinical benefit for the strategy of modulation of multidrug resistance.

In addition to their actions on *MDR1/ABCB1*-expressing tumor cells, MDR-reversing agents can also have profound effects on the pharmacokinetics and pharmacodynamics of cytotoxic drugs associated with MDR.[304,324] As noted above, marked increases in the area under the curve levels, decreased renal and nonrenal clearances, and increased volumes of distribution of etoposide have been observed in patients concomitantly treated with cyclosporins. These drug interactions are due in large part to inhibition of drug metabolizing enzymes and various drug transporters by cyclosporins in normal tissues, particularly the liver. Cyclosporine and its congener valspodar (PSC 833) are potent inhibitors of the mixed-function oxidase CYP 3A4, as well as the biliary drug transporter *MRP2* (*ABCC2*, *cMOAT*). Toxicities of MDR-associated drugs, such as myelosuppression, are enhanced when administered with the cyclosporine reversing agents and require appropriate reduction in the dosage of cytotoxic drugs. Because *MDR1/ABCB1* is expressed at high levels in central nervous system (CNS) endothelium and contributes to the blood–brain barrier,[325–327] concomitant administration of MDR-associated chemotherapeutic drugs and *MDR1/ABCB1* inhibitors may also enhance neurotoxicities. These pharmacologic issues must be carefully considered in future clinical trials. The extent to which *MDR1/ABCB1* inhibition alone contributes to drug interactions with cytotoxins is currently being clarified by clinical trials with zosuquidar (LY335979), a potent and specific *MDR1/ABCB1* inhibitor that has no effect of CYP 3A4 and the MRP (ABCC) family of drug transporters.[328–334]

Alternative strategies for reversing *MDR1/ABCB1*-mediated MDR include the use of monoclonal antibodies directed against extracellular epitopes of P-glycoprotein,[335] anti–P-glycoprotein antibody–toxin conjugates that target P-glycoprotein expressing MDR tumor cells,[336,337] or anti–P-glycoprotein antibodies engineered to recruit activated T-lymphocytes for the cytolysis of *MDR1/ABCB1*-expressing tumor cells.[338] Other approaches to reversing *MDR1/ABCB1*-mediated MDR include antisense and ribozyme nucleotides directed against *MDR1/ABCB1* mRNA.[323] These approaches either do not result in substantial reversal of resistance or are faced with major technical obstacles in clinical application. Even with the reduced off-target effects and drug interactions on third generation MDR modulators, such approaches will be limited by the presence of other, redundant mechanisms of resistance in human tumor cell populations.[333,339]

Similar approaches for reversing MRP (ABCC) family–mediated MDR are possible. A number of compounds inhibit *MRP1/ABCB1*-mediated efflux activity, including the organic acids probenecid and sulfinpyrazone,[93] and the cyclosporin derivative, PSC 833.[340] Finally, *MRP1/ABCC1*-mediated transport of some drugs is dependent on intracellular glutathione either as a noncovalent cofactor[99,341] or as a moiety covalently linked, nonenzymatically or by GST, to some electrophilic anticancer drugs.[248,342] Thus, depletion of tumor cell glutathione or inhibition of GST (see the section "Resistance to Free Radical–Mediated Drug Cytotoxicity" below) offer potential strategies for secondarily reversing *MRP1/ABCC1*-mediated drug resistance. Some substrates of *MRP1* are glucuronide and sulfate derivatives of the parent drug.[96,97,343,344] Thus, selective inhibition of tumor cell UDP-glucuronosyl transferases or sulfotransferases could also represent a future avenue for secondary reversal of *MRP1/ABCC1*-associated drug resistance.

Several agents have also been described that act as inhibitors of ABCG2 and may be useful as reversal agents. The most widely used of these are fumitremorgin C (FTC),[345] which is, however, too toxic for clinical use, and GF120918 (Elacridar),[156,346] which is also an inhibitor of *MDR1/ABCB1* and is currently in phase I clinical trials.[347] Other inhibitors of *ABCG2*, and thus potential reversal agents, include biricodar (VX-710),[348] novobiocin,[349,350] gefitinib,[351] and imatinib[352] (although the latter has also been found to be a substrate of *ABCG2*[165]), the Her2 neu protein inhibitor CI10333,[353] several HIV protease inhibitors,[354] and some synthetic taxanes.[355,356] Interestingly, some reports have also shown that flavonoids, especially when given as an oral cocktail, may have *ABCG2* reversing activity.[357–360]

Although fumitremorgin C and GF120918 are invaluable tools for the study of *ABCG2* in vitro and are widely used for this purpose, it is too early to judge whether the use of *ABCG2* inhibitors will also reverse MDR at the cellular level in a clinically useful way. In contrast, there is evidence that these agents can alter the oral bioavailability of drugs such as topotecan.[361,362] For example, when patients were treated with oral topotecan with coadministration of oral GF120918, the mean AUC of total topotecan more than doubled, as did the maximum plasma concentration, and the oral bioavailability increased from 40 to 97%, when compared with oral topotecan only. In contrast, coadministration of GF120918 with intravenous topotecan only had a small effect on the AUC, but no effect on the peak plasma concentration or the terminal half-life of topotecan.[361] Similar results, albeit so far only in mice, have been reported with gefitinib and irinotecan,[363] and with the fumitremorgin derivative Ko143 and topotecan.[364] These results are consistent with the apical localization of *ABCG2* in the epithelium of the small intestine and colon and a possible role of *ABCG2* in the protection of the organism from orally ingested xenobiotics.

Topoisomerase II Poisons As discussed above, resistance to topoisomerase II poisons may occur as a consequence of *MDR1/ABCB1*, *MRP1/ABCC1*, or *ABCG2* overexpression or altered topoisomerase II activities. However, none of these mechanisms will necessarily result in cross resistance to all the topoisomerase II–directed drugs listed in Table 41-3. For example, resistance to epipodophyllotoxins and anthracyclines on the basis of increased *MDR1/ABCB1* expression is not usually associated with resistance to the acridine derivative, amsacrine. Conversely, resistance to amsacrine and other intercalating drugs caused by alterations in topoisomerase II protein is not always associated with resistance to the nonintercalating, epipodophyllotoxin class of topoisomerase II poisons.[200] Therefore, these in vitro studies suggest a rationale for administering an alternative class of topoisomerase II poison in selected cases of clinical resistance to another class of topoisomerase II–directed drug. Additionally, tumor cells resistant to classic topoisomerase II poisons (see Table 41-4) frequently retain sensitivity to the cytotoxicities of the novel class of topoisomerase II–catalytic inhibitors (fostriecin, merbarone, aclarubicin, and *bis* [*2,6*-dioxopoperazines]).[205,365,366] This class of topoisomerase-directed drug offers an alternative for the treatment of topoisomerase poison–resistant tumors. Finally, structural analogues of parent topoisomerase II poisons may overcome resistance based on altered topoisomerase II.[367,368]

Resistance to Free Radical–Mediated Drug Cytotoxicity Several pathways may contribute to protection of tumor cells from anthracycline-mediated free radical damage. First, superoxide anion formation is limited in poorly vascularized, relatively hypoxemic tissues, such as may exist in the centers of large solid tumors. Second, increased intracellular levels of catalase and glutathione peroxidase (GSHPx) can deplete hydrogen peroxide, thus reducing the formation of toxic hydroxyl radicals. Indeed, in comparing parental and MDR MCF7 cells, Sinha and colleagues reported an association between increased GSHPx activity and reduced doxorubicin-stimulated hydroxyl radical formation.[369] Furthermore, lowering GSHPx activity by depleting the enzyme's cosubstrate, GSH, resulted in enhanced doxorubicin-dependent free radical formation and cytotoxicity.[370] Additionally, Kramer and colleagues found that GSH depletion with buthionine sulfoximine (BSO) could partially restore the doxorubicin sensitivity of MDR MCF7 cells, presumably by interfering with GSH-dependent reactions, including those catalyzed by GSHPx.[371] Although these results are consistent with the importance of hydrogen peroxide and hydroxyl radical formation in anthracycline cytotoxicity in MCF 7 cells, other investigators have noted that increased catalase, GSH, and GSHPx levels are not always protective of some cells from doxorubicin-mediated damage.[372]

The relative importance of free radical generation in tumor cell kill is unknown, and the protective mechanisms outlined above are speculative. Nevertheless, the GSH-dependent detoxification pathways are of particular interest because they are subject to pharmacologic manipulation. GSHPx and GST activities can be secondarily reduced by depleting tissue GSH with BSO treatment.[373,374] Furthermore, the activity of GSTs can be inhibited by the administration of competitive substrates, such as ethacrynic acid.[375] Such clinical manipulations may enhance tumoricidal activity of doxorubicin, but must be viewed cautiously as they may also potentiate drug toxicity toward normal tissues.

Alkylating Agents and Platinum Compounds Resistance to alkylating agents and platinum compounds can be described by at least three broad mechanistic categories, including decreased drug accumulation, increased drug inactivation, and enhanced repair of DNA damage.[16,376–378] Additionally, the nature of the tumor cells' response to alkylating agent damage—whether primarily apoptosis, repair, or survival with damage—will contribute significantly to the outcome of alkylating agent treatment. Preclinical studies have indicated that all these mechanisms may be circumvented, at least partially, by pharmacologic manipulations. Reactions of electrophilic alkylating agents with thiol-containing compounds represent relatively general mechanisms of antineoplastic inactivation or detoxification. For example, GSH forms conjugates with a variety of alkylating agents in both nonenzymatic and in GST-dependent reactions. Table 41-5 lists some of the compounds whose conjugation with GSH is catalyzed by GSTs in vitro.[224] Several laboratories have demonstrated an association between increased bulk GST levels or specific GST isozymes with resistance to drugs such as nitrosoureas,[379] chlorambucil, and other nitrogen mustards.[236,237,240,380,381] Additionally, increased GSH levels correlate with resistance to alkylating agents and cisplatin.[382,383] Although the electrophilic cisplatin compound can react directly with GSH, it is unknown whether GSTs can catalyze this reaction. This issue is unresolved because of conflicting results that show a correlation between elevated expression of the pi isozyme of GST and resistance to cisplatin in some cells,[384,385] but not others.[239] Perhaps more relevant to the issue of cisplatin resistance is the finding that glutathionyl-platinum complexes, which are themselves toxic, are exported by an ATP-dependent pump, probably identical to one of the glutathione conjugate pumps described previously.[245] Thus, these drug exporters should be considered in the design of treatments and formulation of strategies to enhance cisplatin efficacy.

The correlations between GSH or GST levels and drug resistance are variable. Indeed, some investigators have been unable to demonstrate a relationship between the overexpression of multiple isozymes of GST and antineoplastic resistance.[238,239,243,386] In studies that have compared paired parental and resistant cell lines, the magnitude of alkylating agent resistance associated with increased GST activity is often modest. As noted above, for some drugs such as chlorambucil, the coexpression of a glutathione conjugate efflux transporter appears to be required for the emergence of GST-mediated resistance in the MCF7 cell model system.[248] Although the clinical importance of GST and GSH in alkylating resistance is, accordingly, debated, existing preclinical data have prompted phase I trials using GST inhibitors, or the GSH synthesis inhibitor BSO, in conjunction with alkylating agents. Three phase I trials have been reported with the combination of BSO and melphalan. These trials demonstrate that it is possible to deplete glutathione levels by coadministration of BSO with alkylating agent chemotherapy. However, no phase II studies have yet been reported to demonstrate the antitumor efficacy of this approach.

Aldehyde dehydrogenase is another drug-metabolizing enzyme that is linked to cyclophosphamide-derivative resistance in murine and human models of drug resistance.[387–389] This enzyme converts aldophosphamide, a metabolite of cyclophosphamide, to the inactive compound, carboxyphosphamide, thereby preventing the decomposition of aldophosphamide to its cytotoxic derivative, phosphoramide mustard. Increased expression of aldehyde dehydrogenase is associated with resistance to cyclophosphamide in vitro. Whether inhibitors of aldehyde dehydrogenase, such as disulfiram and dimethylaminobenzaldehyde, can be used therapeutically to enhance the antitumor effect of cyclophosphamide without undue host toxicity remains to be explored.

Cisplatin toxicity is thought to be mediated primarily by the formation of lethal intrastrand DNA cross-links. Several reports suggest that either increased DNA repair or tolerance of DNA damage is associated with resistance to this compound. In a murine leukemia model, cells selected for cisplatin resistance showed enhanced ability to repair cisplatin-induced intrastrand DNA cross-links.[390,391] Aphidicolin can inhibit an enzyme implicated in DNA repair, DNA polymerase α. Treatment of ovarian carcinoma cells with aphidicolin potentiated the toxicity of cisplatin in resistant but not sensitive cells.[392] These results suggest that the coadministration of DNA polymerase α inhibitors with cisplatin may be useful in overcoming cisplatin resistance. Also implicated in platinum sensitivity and resistance are alterations in regulators of apoptosis, such as Bcl-2, Bax, or TP53.[16] Modulation of these pathways by therapeutic agents now in development represents an emerging strategy for overcoming resistance to platinum and other alkylating compounds.

Antimetabolites The antimetabolites are a clinically important group of cancer drugs used in the treatment of a variety of solid tumors and hematologic malignancies. The cytotoxicities of the antimetabolites stem from their ability to interfere with key enzymatic steps in nucleic acid metabolism. The discussion that follows concerns three particularly well-studied compounds, the antifolate methotrexate (MTX) and the pyrimidine analogues 5-fluorouracil (5-FU) and cytosine arabinoside (ara-C, 1-0-D-arabinofuranosylcytosine, cytarabine). Strategies designed to overcome the multiple described mechanisms of cellular resistance to these compounds include dose escalation, pharmacologic manipulation of drug metabolism, and rational design of new antimetabolites.[393]

MTX, the clinically important antifolate, displays significant tumoricidal activity against a variety of human neoplasms, such as acute leukemia, osteogenic sarcoma, choriocarcinoma, breast cancer, head and neck cancers, and others.[394] Consideration of MTX metabolism and sites of action (Figure 41-4) serves as the basis for understanding mechanisms of methotrexate resistance. Following uptake by the folate transport systems, MTX can bind avidly to and inhibit its primary enzyme target, dihydrofolate reductase (DHFR). In the presence of adequate thymidylate synthase activity, inhibition of DHFR results in depletion of the reduced folate pools essential for thymidylate and de novo purine synthesis. The cytotoxicity of MTX is significantly influenced by intracellular polyglutamation. MTX polyglutamates are retained preferentially by cells and bind more effectively to DHFR. Additionally, these polyglutamyl derivatives can inhibit other folate-dependent enzymes, including thymidylate synthase and 5-aminoimadazole-4-carboxamide ribonucleoside (AICAR) transformylase,[395] enzymes involved in thymidylate and de novo purine synthesis, respectively. Therefore, resistance to MTX can result from a number of alternative mechanisms, including (1) reduced MTX uptake via a defective folate transport system,[5] such as decreased expression of the reduced folate carrier[4,396] or of the folate receptors; (2) increased export via MRP family proteins[107,397] or other exporters of polyglutamatable antifolates; (3) reduced polyglutamation leading to decreased drug retention as well as reduced inhibition of thymidylate synthase and AICAR transformylase;[398] and (4) either elevated levels of DHFR or reduced affinity of DHFR for MTX.[394,399–404]

The use of high-dose MTX (HDMTX) with subsequent rescue of normal tissues by administration of the reduced folate, leucovorin (N5-formyl tetrahydrofolate) has been advocated as an approach that could theoretically circumvent most mechanisms of MTX resistance. At high systemic drug concentrations, cytocidal levels can be achieved by passive diffusion of drug into transport-defective resistant cells. Furthermore, prolonged exposure of cells to high extracellular concentrations of drug can maintain cytotoxic intracellular drug levels in the face of a drug retention defect secondary to decreased polyglutamation. Finally, increased intracellular MTX delivered by HDMTX therapy can saturate DHFR in cells whose resistance is a result of amplification of the *DHFR* gene or of lowered affinity of DHFR for MTX. Although HDMTX is of proven value in the treatment of ALL and perhaps of osteogenic sarcoma, the rationale for the use of this modality in the treatment of other cancers was recently questioned.[405,406] Indeed, some tumors, as well as normal tissues, are rescued from HDMTX toxicity by leucovorin. In these and other cases, the use of HDMTX with leucovorin rescue offers no therapeutic advantage over regimens that use conventional MTX doses. Although early studies suggested that HDMTX improved response rates to chemotherapy of osteogenic sarcoma,[407] the contribution of HDMTX therapy to the success of recent multiagent adjuvant protocols is unclear. In contrast, HDMTX is indisputably efficacious in the treatment of ALL. The success of HDMTX in this setting is probably a result of the penetration of drug across anatomic and pharmacologic barriers into tumor sanctuaries, such as testes, and, at very high MTX doses, the central nervous system.[265]

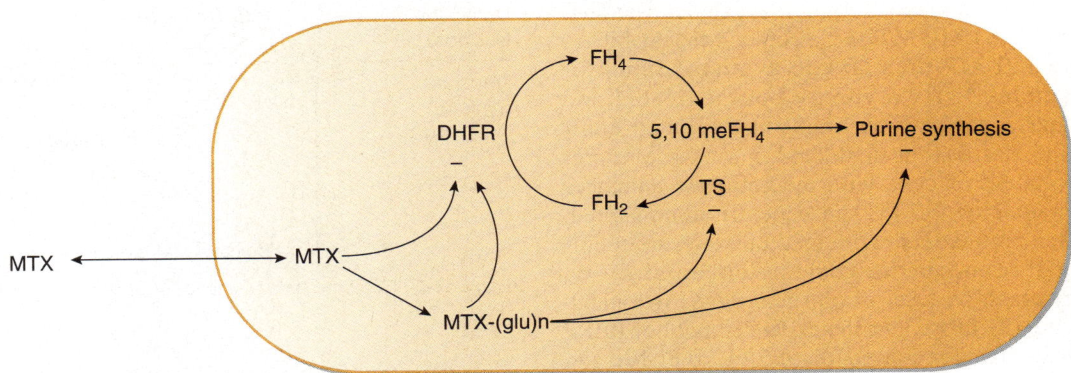

Figure 41-4 Methotrexate metabolism and toxicity. DHFR = dihydrofolate reductase; FH_2 = dihydrofolate; FH_4 = tetrahydrofolate; 5,10 $MEFH_4$ = 5,10-methylene tetrahydrofolate; MTX = methotrexate; MTX-$(glu)_n$ = plyglutamate methotrexate; TS = thymidylate synthase.

In an effort to improve drug efficacy, other inhibitors of DHFR, such as trimetrexate and piritrexim, were developed.[408–410] These lipid-soluble drugs are taken up by cells independently of the folate-carrier system; consequently, their use might obviate transport-mediated antifolate resistance. However, cells that are resistant to MTX on the basis of amplified DHFR will be cross-resistant to trimetrexate. The utility of trimetrexate is further limited by the association of classic MDR with cross-resistance to trimetrexate.[411] Cells can also overcome antifolate toxicity by increasing the salvage of nucleoside precursors. One mechanism of overcoming these mechanisms of resistance is the concomitant administration of the nucleoside transport inhibitor nitrobenzylmercaptopurine riboside (NBMPR) with antifolate drugs, which enhances antifolate cytotoxicity in rodent models.[411,412]

The pyrimidine base, 5-FU and its deoxynucleoside metabolite, 5-fluoro-2'-deoxyuridine (FdUrd) have been used in the treatment of gastrointestinal tumors, breast cancer, head and neck cancer, and some other malignancies. The metabolism of 5-FU is complex and is partially shown in Figure 41-5.[19] The best characterized mechanism of fluoropyrimidine cytotoxicity involves the inhibition of thymidylate synthase by 5-fluoro-2'-deoxyuridine monophosphate (FdUMP). Additionally, the incorporation of the metabolite, 5-fluorouridine triphosphate (FUTP) into RNA correlates with cytotoxicity in some systems. Although 5-fluoro-2'-deoxyuridine triphosphate (FdUTP) can be incorporated into DNA, the relationship between this process and the cytocidal activity of fluoropyrimidines remains undetermined. Resistance to 5-FU may be conferred by alterations in enzymes involved in fluoropyrimidine metabolism, particularly those enzymes associated with the conversion of 5-FU to the thymidylate synthase inhibitor, FdUMP.[19] Furthermore, changes in thymidylate synthase level or its affinity for FdUMP are associated with 5-FU resistance.[413–415]

Several strategies to improve fluoropyrimidine efficacy and overcome resistance have been advanced. It has been suggested that tumor cell killing may be improved by prolonged or continuous exposure to drug.[416,417] Other studies advocate the coadministration of 5-FU with the reduced folate leucovorin. The efficacy of this combination stems from leucovorin-dependent

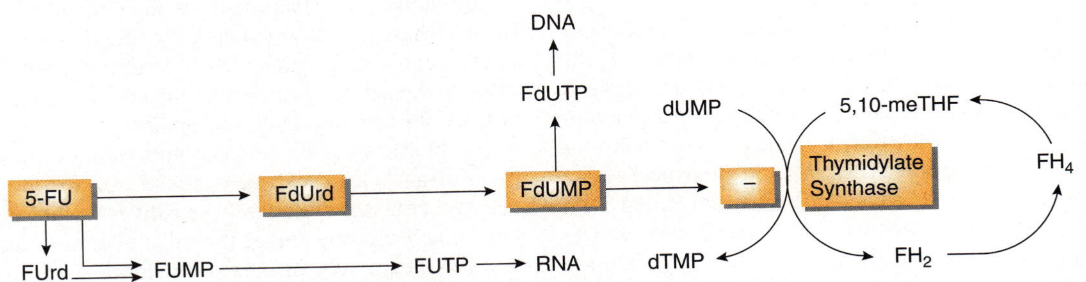

Figure 41-5 5-Fluorouracil metabolism and toxicity. 5-FU = 5-fluorouracil; FdUMP and FdUTP = 5-fluoro-2'-deoxyuridine mono- and triphosphate; FdUrd = 5-fluoro-2'-deoxyuridine.

increases in intracellular 5,10-methylene tetrahydrofolate (5,10-MTHF), a cofactor that stabilizes the FdUMP-thymidylate synthase inhibitor complex.[418,419] Synergy between 5-FU and other agents, which might be exploited clinically, has also been studied. For example, pretreatment of cells with methotrexate enhances the toxicity of 5-FU subsequently administered. Such pretreatment with methotrexate, an inhibitor of de novo purine synthesis (discussed above), increases the level of phosphoribosyl pyrophosphate (PRPP). Thus, the expanded pool of PRPP is available for conversion of 5-FU to FUMP and FUTP (see Figure 41-5). It has been suggested that the increased incorporation of FUTP into RNA that results is responsible for the improved cytotoxicity.[420,421] The inhibitor of de novo pyrimidine synthesis, *N*-phosphonacetyl-L-aspartatic acid (PALA), has been used with 5-FU in an effort to reduce pyrimidine metabolites that compete for the targets of fluoropyrimidine toxicity.[422] Finally, the synergistic interaction between interferon and halogenated pyrimidines has been investigated.[423]

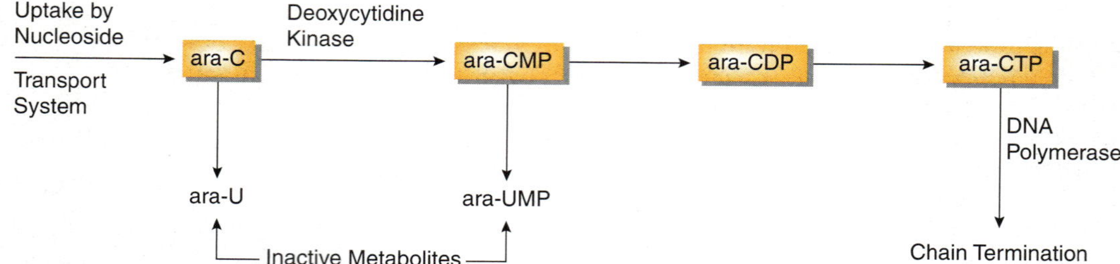

Figure 41-6 Cytosine arabinoside (ara-C) metabolism and toxicity.

Ara-C is an important nucleoside antineoplastic agent effective in the treatment of acute leukemias. Figure 41-6 presents the metabolism and mechanism of cytotoxicity of ara-C.[424] Following its uptake by the nucleoside transport system, ara-C is activated by a series of kinases to ara-CTP, a substrate of DNA polymerase that is incorporated into nascent DNA, causing premature chain termination and ultimately cell death. The rate-limiting step in ara-C activation is the S-phase specific reaction catalyzed by deoxycytidine kinase. The cytotoxic compound, ara-CTP or its precursors (ara-CMP and ara-CDP) can be catabolized by phosphatases or they (ara-C and ara-CMP) can be inactivated by deaminases. Several mechanisms of cancer cell resistance to ara-C have been demonstrated, including, but not confined to, the following. Because ara-C activation is cell-cycle dependent, quiescent cells or cells that fail to enter the S phase during the interval of treatment escape the cytotoxicity of ara-C. At suboptimal doses, otherwise drug-sensitive tumor cells located in pharmacologic or anatomic sanctuaries may survive ara-C treatment.[425] Decreased nucleoside transport has also been implicated in ara-C resistance.[426] Additionally, resistance may be conferred by altered drug metabolism, such as decreased activation by deoxycytidine kinase,[424] increased inactivation by cytidine deaminase,[14] or altered DNA polymerase affinity for ara-C.[427]

Administration of high-dose ara-C represents one approach to overcoming resistance to the drug and has been clinically useful in the treatment of some leukemias refractory to conventional doses of ara-C. Resistance based on diminished nucleoside transport and pharmacologic/anatomic sanctuaries can be circumvented with high-dose drug treatment.[425] In resistance secondary to increased drug inactivation by cytidine deaminase, coadministration of ara-C with a cytidine deaminase inhibitor such as tetrahydrouridine may reverse this mode of drug resistance.[428] Alternative pyrimidine analogues such as ara-AC (arabinofuranosyl-5-azacytosine, fazarabine) have shown activity against a broad range of tumor cells in preclinical testing and have been the subject of clinical trials.[429,430]

Resistance to Microtubule-Targeted Drugs Since the discovery of the vinca alkaloids as anticancer agents over 40 years ago, microtubule-targeted drugs (MTTD) have become one of the most important class of anticancer agents.[431,432] However, as with any other drug, their long-term efficacy is limited by resistance. Although both the vinca alkaloids and the taxanes are substrates for the ABC transporter *MDR1/ABCB1* (P-glycoprotein) and thus are affected by classic multidrug resistance, a number of microtubule specific mechanisms have also been identified.[433] These include alterations in tubulin and tubulin-binding proteins, aberrant signal transduction, and cell death pathway, which will be further described in this section.

MTTDs are broadly divided into microtubule stabilizers (the taxanes, taxol and Taxotere; the epothilones; discodermolide; eleutherobin; the sarcodictyins; and the laulimalides) and microtubule destabilizers (the vinca alkaloids vinblastine, vincristine, vindesine, vinorelbine and vinflunine; colcemid; colchicines; halichandrins; dolastatins; and hemiasterlins).[431,434] As the classification implies, the microtubule destabilizers inhibit microtubule polymer assembly by binding to the α/β-tubulin monomers, whereas the microtubule stabilizers facilitate microtubule stabilization by binding to the polymer. Accordingly, alterations in the MTTD binding sites have been found to confer resistance. For example, analysis of tubulin genes in 11 cell lines selected for resistance to vinblastine or colcemid revealed five different mutations in β-tubulin and four mutations in α-tubulin.[435] Each of these genetic changes were found to make microtubules more stable, thus conferring resistance to the action of destabilizing MTTDs. Similarly, A549 and HeLa cells selected for resistance to epothilone were found to contain mutations in β-tubulin.[436] Interestingly, these epothilone-resistant cells are collaterally sensitive to vinblastine and colchicines, suggesting that alterations in tubulins negatively affected the stability of the microtubules following exposure to microtubule destabilizers. In another set of paclitaxel-selected Chinese hamster ovary cells, a cluster of β-tubulin mutations was identified that resulted in destabilization of the microtubules, thereby conferring resistance to the stabilizer paclitaxel.[437] Thus, it appears that alterations that affect the stability of microtubules have a direct effect on a cell's sensitivity to MTTDs. Furthermore, it appears that destabilizing alterations in tubulins that can confer resistance to microtubule stabilizing drugs can also be associated with collateral sensitization to other MTTDs.

In addition to tubulin mutations that alter the stability of the microtubules, several microtubule-interacting proteins have also been identified that affect sensitivity to MTTDs, including MAP-4, stathmin, and tau.[438–441] Whereas stathmin overexpression was found to decrease microtubule polymerization and stability, overexpression of MAP-4 had the opposite effect. Thus changes in the levels of these proteins are expected to directly affect the sensitivity of cancer cells of MTTDs. Indeed, up-regulation of stathmin in breast cancer cell lines was found to decrease the polymerization of microtubules and markedly reduce taxol binding, thus decreasing the cell's sensitivity to the drug.[438] Similarly, stathmin was found to be overexpressed in two taxol-resistant ovarian cancer cells, although these also have point mutations in their β-tubulin genes.[439] Conversely to the effect of stathmin, up-regulation of MAP-4 expression was associated with increased resistance to vinca alkaloids and increased sensitivity to taxol.[441] Interestingly, both stathmin and MAP-4 activity are regulated by TP53. MAP-4 is transcriptionally repressed by wild-type TP53,[442] whereas inactivation of TP53 results in increased MAP-4 expression and a concomitant sensitization of cells to taxol and resistance to vinca alkaloids.[441] Similarly, cells expressing mutant *TP53* were found to contain high levels of stathmin and were sensitive to taxol,[438] while other studies demonstrated that exposure of cells expressing wild-type TP53 to DNA-damaging agents resulted in increased sensitivity to vinblastine and increased resistance to taxol.[443] Furthermore, ectopic expression of mutant *TP53* in J82 bladder cancer cells was associated with increased taxol cytotoxicity.[444] Similar findings were also reported with epothilone, another microtubule stabilizing agent that was more active in cells with mutant *TP53*.[445] Together, these observations indicate that the status of TP53 in cancer cells may have a profound influence on their sensitivity to MTTDs, suggesting that this can potentially be exploited when selecting antimicrotubule chemotherapy.

CONCLUSION AND FUTURE DIRECTIONS

Through the kinds of studies done largely in vitro described in this chapter, many of the mechanisms of antineoplastic drug resistance have been identified. Although several of these processes operate in vivo, their relative clinical importance must be better clarified in controlled, prospective examinations of patient tumor specimens and correlations with therapeutic responses to chemotherapy. Nevertheless, these mechanisms suggest potentially useful approaches to overcoming clinical drug resistance. These approaches include the rational choice of conventional agents or design of novel drugs that are less likely to share resistance mechanisms. Additionally, many of the pathways of antineoplastic drug inactivation or transport are targets for pharmacologic manipulations that may reverse or circumvent the resistance of tumors to some drugs. Despite these efforts, many tumors will remain refractory to conventional chemotherapeutic drugs.

REFERENCES

1. Hill BT, Price LA, Goldies JH. The value of Adriamycin in overcoming resistance to methotrexate in tissue culture. Eur J Cancer 1976;12:541–9.
2. Teicher BA, Cucchi CA, Lee JB, et al. Alkylating agents: in vitro studies of cross-resistance patterns in human cell lines. Cancer Res 1986;46:4379–83.
3. Antony AC, Kane MA, Portillo RM, et al. Studies of the role of a particulate folate-binding protein in the uptake of 5-methyltetrahydrofolate by cultured human KB cells. J Biol Chem 1985;260:14911–7.
4. Dixon KH, Lanpher BC, Chiu J, et al. A novel cDNA restores reduced folate carrier activity and methotrexate sensitivity to transport deficient cells. J Biol Chem 1994;269:17–20.
5. Sirotnak FM, Moccio DM, Kelleher LE, et al. Relative frequency and kinetic properties of transport-defective phenotypes among methotrexate-resistant L1210 clonal cell lines derived in vivo. Cancer Res 1981;41(11 Pt 1):4447–52.
6. Hill BT, Bailey BD, White JC, et al., Characteristics of transport of 4-amino antifolates and folate compounds by two lines of L5178Y lymphoblasts, one with impaired transport of methotrexate. Cancer Res 1979;39(7 Pt 1):2440–6.
7. Endicott JA, Ling V. The biochemistry of P-glycoprotein-mediated multidrug resistance. Annu Rev Biochem 1989;58:137–71.
8. Gottesman MM, Pastan I. Biochemistry of multidrug resistance mediated by the multidrug transporter. Ann Rev Biochem 1993;62:385–427.
9. Drahovsky D, Kreis W. Studies on drug resistance. II. Kinase patterns in P815 neoplasms sensitive and resistant to 1-beta-D-arabinofuranosylcytosine. Biochem Pharmacol 1970;19:940–4.
10. Brockman RW. Mechanisms of resistance to anticancer agents. Adv Cancer Res 1963;57:129–234.
11. Haaz MC, Rivory LP, Riche C, Robert J. The transformation of irinotecan (CPT-11) to its active metabolite SN-38 by human liver microsomes. Differential hydrolysis for the lactone and carboxylate forms. Naunyn Schmiedebergs Arch Pharmacol 1997;356:257–62.
12. Kanzawa F, Sugimoto Y, Minato K, et al. Establishment of a camptothecin analogue (CPT-11)-resistant cell line of human non-small cell lung cancer: characterization and mechanism of resistance. Cancer Res 1990;50:5919–24.
13. Hunt SW 3rd, Hoffee PA, Amplification of adenosine deaminase gene sequences in deoxycoformycin-resistant rat hepatoma cells. J Biol Chem 1983;258:13185–92.
14. Steuart CD, Burke PJ. Cytidine deaminase and the development of resistance to arabinosyl cytosine. Nat New Biol 1971;233:109–10.
15. Houghton JA, Maroda SJ Jr, Phillips JO, Houghton PJ. Biochemical determinants of responsiveness to 5-fluorouracil and its derivatives in xenografts of human colorectal adenocarcinomas in mice. Cancer Res 1981;41:144–9.
16. Perez RP. Cellular and molecular determinants of cisplatin resistance. Eur J Cancer 1998;34:1535–42.
17. Haber DA, Schimke RT. Unstable amplification of an altered dihydrofolate reductase gene associated with double-minute chromosomes. Cell 1981;26(3 Pt 1):355–62.
18. Haber DA, Beverley SM, Kiely ML, Schimke RT. Properties of an altered dihydrofolate reductase encoded by amplified genes in cultured mouse fibroblasts. J Biol Chem 1981;256:9501–10.
19. Armstrong RA. Fluoropyrimidine activity and resistance at the cellular level. Boca Raton (FL): CRC Press; 1989.
20. Vassetzky YS, Alghisi GC, Gasser SM. DNA topoisomerase II mutations and resistance to anti-tumor drugs. Bioessays 1995;17:767–74.
21. Rubin EH, Li TK, Duann P, Liu LF. Cellular resistance to topoisomerase poisons. Cancer Treat Res 1996;87:243–60.
22. Pommier Y, Kerrigan D, Schwartz RE, et al. Altered DNA topoisomerase II activity in Chinese hamster cells resistant to topoisomerase II inhibitors. Cancer Res 1986;46:3075–81.
23. Mirski SE, Evans CD, Almquist KC, et al. Altered topoisomerase II alpha in a drug-resistant small cell lung cancer cell line selected in VP-16. Cancer Res 1993;53:4866–73.
24. Kubota N, Kanzawa F, Nishio K, et al. Detection of topoisomerase I gene point mutation in CPT-11 resistant lung cancer cell line. Biochem Biophy Res Commun 1992;188:571–7.
25. Hinds M, Deisseroth K, Mayes J, et al. Identification of a point mutation in the topoisomerase II gene from a human leukemia cell line containing an amsacrine-resistant form of topoisomerase II. Cancer Res 1991;51:4729–31.
26. Gorre ME, Mohammed M, Ellwood K, et al. Clinical resistance to STI-571 cancer therapy caused by BCR-ABL gene mutation or amplification. Science 2001;293:876–80.
27. Banerjee D, Mayer-Kuckuk P, Capiaux G, et al. Novel aspects of resistance to drugs targeted to dihydrofolate reductase and thymidylate synthase. Biochim Biophys Acta 2002;1587:164–73.
28. Banerjee D, Gorlick R, Liefshitz A, et al. Levels of E2F-1 expression are higher in lung metastasis of colon cancer as compared with hepatic metastasis and correlate with levels of thymidylate synthase. Cancer Res 2000;60:2365–7.
29. Belvedere O, Puglisi F, Di Loreto C, et al. Lack of correlation between immunohistochemical expression of E2F-1, thymidylate synthase expression and clinical response to 5-fluorouracil in advanced colorectal cancer. Ann Oncol 2004;15:55–8.
30. Sowers R, Toguchida J, Qin J, et al. mRNA expression levels of E2F transcription factors correlate with dihydrofolate reductase, reduced folate carrier, and thymidylate synthase mRNA expression in osteosarcoma. Mol Cancer Ther 2003;2:535–41.
31. Dean M, Rzhetsky A, Allikmets R. The human ATP-binding cassette (ABC) transporter superfamily. Genome Res 2001;11:1156–66.
32. Cole SP, Deeley RG. Multidrug resistance mediated by the ATP-binding cassette transporter protein MRP. Bioessays 1998;20:931–40.
33. Cui Y, Konig J, Buchholz JK, et al. Drug resistance and ATP-dependent conjugate transport mediated by the apical multidrug resistance protein, MRP2, permanently expressed in human and canine cells. Mol Pharmacology 1999;55:929–37.
34. Kool M, de Haas M, Scheffer GL, et al. Analysis of expression of cMOAT (MRP2), MRP3, MRP4, and MRP5, homologues of the multidrug resistance-associated protein gene (MRP1), in human cancer cell lines. Cancer Res 1997;57:3537–47.
35. Loe DW, Deeley RG, Cole SP. Biology of the multidrug resistance-associated protein, MRP. Eur J Cancer 1996;32A:945–57.
36. Doyle LA, Yang W, Abruzzo LV, et al. A multidrug resistance transporter from human MCF-7 breast cancer cells. Proc Natl Acad Sci U S A 1998;95:15665–70.
37. Ross DD, Yang W, Abrusso LV, et al. Atypical multidrug resistance: breast cancer resistance protein messenger RNA expression in mitoxantrone-selected cell lines. J Natl Cancer Instit 1999;91:429–33.
38. Kickhoefer VA, Rajavel KS, Scheffer GL, et al. Vaults are up-regulated in multidrug-resistant cancer cell lines. J Biol Chem 1998;273:8971–4.
39. Izquierdo MA, Scheffer GL, Flens MJ, et al. Relationship of LRP-human major vault protein to in vitro and clinical resistance to anticancer drugs. Cytotechnology 1996;19:191–7.
40. Biedler JL, Riehm H. Cellular resistance to actinomycin D in Chinese hamster cells in vitro: cross-resistance, radioautographic, and cytogenetic studies. Cancer Res 1970;30:1174–84.
41. Juliano RL, Ling V. A surface glycoprotein modulating drug permeability in Chinese hamster ovary cell mutants. Biochim Biophys Acta 1976;455:152–62.
42. Riordan JR, Ling V. Genetic and biochemical characterization of multidrug resistance. Pharmacol Ther 1985;28:51–75.
43. Raviv Y, Pollard HV, Bruggemann EP, et al. Photosensitized labeling of a functional multidrug transporter in living drug-resistant tumor cells. J Biol Chem 1990;265:3975–80.
44. Higgins CF, Gottesman MM. Is the multidrug transporter a flippase? Trends Biochem Sci 1992;17:18–21.
45. Gros P, Ben Neriah YB, Croop JM, Housman DE. Isolation and expression of a complementary DNA that confers multidrug resistance. Nature 1986;323:728–31.
46. Ueda K, Cardarelli C, Gottesman MM, Pastan I. Expression of a full-length cDNA for the human "MDR1" gene confers resistance to colchicine, doxorubicin, and vinblastine. Proc Natl Acad Sci U S A 1987;84:3004–8.
47. Chen CJ, Chin JE, Ueda K, et al. Internal duplication and homology with bacterial transport proteins in the mdr1 (P-glycoprotein) gene from multidrug-resistant human cells. Cell 1986;47:381–9.
48. Gros P, Croop J, Housman D. Mammalian multidrug resistance gene: complete cDNA sequence indicates strong homology to bacterial transport proteins. Cell 1986;47:371–80.
49. Safa AR, Glover CJ, Meyers MB, et al. Vinblastine photoaffinity labeling of a high molecular weight surface membrane glycoprotein specific for multidrug-resistant cells. J Biol Chem 1986;261:6137–40.
50. Gottesman MM, Pastan I. Resistance to multiple chemotherapeutic agents in human cancer cells. Trends Pharmacol Sci 1988;9:54–8.
51. Choi KH, Chen CJ, Kriegler M, Roninson IB. An altered pattern of cross-resistance in multidrug-resistant human cells results from spontaneous mutations in the mdr1 (P-glycoprotein) gene. Cell 1988;53:519–29.
52. Chin KV, Tanaka S, Darlington G, et al. Heat shock and arsenite increase expression of the multidrug resistance (MDR1) gene in human renal carcinoma cells. J Biol Chem 1990;265:221–6.
53. Fairchild CR, Ivy SP, Rushmore T, et al. Carcinogen-induced mdr overexpression is associated with xenobiotic resistance in rat preneoplastic liver nodules and hepatocellular carcinomas. Proc Natl Acad Sci U S A 1987;84:7701–5.
54. Thorgeirsson SS, Huber BE, Sorrell S, et al. Expression of the multidrug-resistant gene in hepatocarcinogenesis and regenerating rat liver. Science 1987;236:1120–2.
55. Chin KV, Chauhan SS, Pastan I, Gottesman MM. Regulation of mdr RNA levels in response to cytotoxic drugs in rodent cells. Cell Growth Differ 1990;1:361–5.
56. Bates SE, Mickley LA, Chen YN, et al. Expression of a drug resistance gene in human neuroblastoma cell lines: modulation by retinoic acid-induced differentiation. Mol Cell Biol 1989;9:4337–44.
57. Mickley LA, Bates SE, Richert ND, et al. Modulation of the expression of a multidrug resistance gene (mdr-1/P-glycoprotein) by differentiating agents. J Biol Chem 1989;264:18031–40.
58. Morrow CS, Nakagawa M, Goldsmith ME, et al. Reversible transcriptional activation of mdr1 by sodium butyrate treatment of human colon cancer cells. J Biol Chem 1994;269:10739–46.
59. Goldsmith ME, Gudas JM, Schneider E, Cowan KH. Wild type p53 stimulates expression from the human multidrug resistance promoter in a p53-negative cell line. J Biol Chem 1995;270:1894–8.
60. Chen Y, Chen PL, Lee WH. Hot-spot p53 mutants interact specifically with two cellular proteins during progression of the cell cycle. Mol Cell Biol 1994;14:6764–72.
61. Chin K, Ueda K, Pastan I, Gottesman MM. Modulation of activity of the promoter of the human MDR1 gene by Ras and p53. Science 1992;255:459–62.
62. Burt RK, Garfield S, Johnson K, Thorgeirsson SS. Transformation of rat liver epithelial cells with v-H-ras or v-raf causes expression of MDR-1, glutathione-S-transferase-P and increased resistance to cytotoxic chemicals. Carcinogenesis 1988;9:2329–32.

63. Zastawny RL, Salvino R, Chen J, et al. The core promoter region of the P-glycoprotein gene is sufficient to confer differential responsiveness to wild-type and mutant p53. Oncogene 1993;8:1529–35.
64. Ma DD, Scurr RD, Davey RA, et al. Detection of a multidrug resistant phenotype in acute non-lymphoblastic leukaemia. Lancet 1987;1:135–7.
65. Sato H, Gottesman MM, Goldstein LJ, et al. Expression of the multidrug resistance gene in myeloid leukemias. Leuk Res 1990;14:11–21.
66. Rothenberg ML, Mickley LA, Cole DE, et al. Expression of the mdr-1/P-170 gene in patients with acute lymphoblastic leukemia. Blood 1989;74:1388–95.
67. Aplenc R, Lange B. Pharmacogenetic determinants of outcome in acute lymphoblastic leukaemia. Br J Haematol 2004;125:421–34.
68. Mahadevan D, List AF. Targeting the multidrug resistance-1 transporter in AML: molecular regulation and therapeutic strategies. Blood 2004;104:1940–51.
69. Bell DR, Gerlach JH, Kartner N, et al. Detection of P-glycoprotein in ovarian cancer: a molecular marker associated with multidrug resistance. J Clin Oncol 1985;3:311–15.
70. Dalton WS, Grogan TM, Meltzer PS, et al. Drug-resistance in multiple myeloma and non-Hodgkin's lymphoma: detection of P-glycoprotein and potential circumvention by addition of verapamil to chemotherapy. J Clin Oncol 1989;7:415–24.
71. Keith WN, Stallard S, Brown R. Expression of mdr1 and gst-pi in human breast tumours: comparison to in vitro chemosensitivity. Br J Cancer 1990;61:712–6.
72. Schneider J, Bak M, Efferth T, et al. P-glycoprotein expression in treated and untreated human breast cancer. Br J Cancer 1989;60:815–8.
73. Burger H, Foekens JA, Look MP, et al. RNA expression of breast cancer resistance protein, lung resistance-related protein, multidrug resistance-associated proteins 1 and 2, and multidrug resistance gene 1 in breast cancer: correlation with chemotherapeutic response. Clin Cancer Res 2003;9:827–36.
74. Leonessa F, Clarke R. ATP binding cassette transporters and drug resistance in breast cancer. Endocr Relat Cancer 2003;10:43–73.
75. Goldstein LJ, Fojo AT, Ueda K, et al. Expression of the multidrug resistance, MDR1, gene in neuroblastomas. J Clin Oncol 1990;8:128–36.
76. Chan HS, Thorner PS, Haddad G, Ling V. Immunohistochemical detection of P-glycoprotein: prognostic correlation in soft tissue sarcoma of childhood. J Clin Oncol 1990;8:689–704.
77. Oda Y, Saito T, Tateishi N, et al. ATP-binding cassette superfamily transporter gene expression in human soft tissue sarcomas. Int J Cancer 2005;114:854–62.
78. Mickisch G, Bier H, Bergler W, et al. P-170 glycoprotein, glutathione and associated enzymes in relation to chemoresistance of primary human renal cell carcinomas. Urol Int 1990;45:170–6.
79. Goldstein LJ, Galski H, Fojo A, et al. Expression of a multidrug resistance gene in human cancers. J Natl Cancer Instit 1989;81:116–24.
80. Marie JP, Zittoun R, Sikic BI. Multidrug resistance (mdr1) gene expression in adult acute leukemias: correlations with treatment outcome and in vitro drug sensitivity. Blood 1991;78:586–92.
81. Pirker R, Wallner J, Geissler K, et al. MDR1 gene expression and treatment outcome in acute myeloid leukemia. J Natl Cancer Instit 1991;83:708–12.
82. Campos L, Guyotat D, Archimbaud E, et al. Clinical significance of multidrug resistance P-glycoprotein expression on acute nonlymphoblastic leukemia cells at diagnosis. Blood 1992;79:473–6.
83. Chan HS, DeBoer G, Haddad G, et al. Multidrug resistance in pediatric malignancies. Hematol Oncol Clin North Am 1995;9:275–318.
84. Sonneveld P. Reversal of multidrug resistance in acute myeloid leukaemia and other haematological malignancies. Eur J Cancer 1996;32A:1062–9.
85. Ling V. Multidrug resistance: molecular mechanisms and clinical relevance. Cancer Chemother Pharmacol 1997;40 Suppl:S3–8.
86. Tafuri A, Gregorj C, Petrucci MT, et al. MDR1 protein expression is an independent predictor of complete remission in newly diagnosed adult acute lymphoblastic leukemia. Blood 2002;100:974–81.
87. Kaye SB. Multidrug resistance: clinical relevance in solid tumours and strategies for circumvention. Curr Opin Oncol 1998;10 Suppl 1:S15–9.
88. Chan HS, Haddad G, Thorner PS, et al. P-glycoprotein expression as a predictor of the outcome of therapy for neuroblastoma. New Engl J Med 1991;325:1608–14.
89. Ramani P, Dewchand H. Expression of mdr1/P-glycoprotein and p110 in neuroblastoma. J Pathol 1995;175:13–22.
90. Cole SP, Bhardwaj G, Gerlach JH, et al. Overexpression of a transporter gene in a multidrug-resistant human lung cancer cell line. Science 1992;258:1650–4.
91. Krishnamachary N, Center MS. The MRP gene associated with a non-P-glycoprotein multidrug resistance encodes a 190-kDa membrane bound glycoprotein. Cancer Res 1993;53:3658–61.
92. Hipfner DR, Almquist KC, Leslie FM, et al. Membrane topology of the multidrug resistance protein (MRP). A study of glycosylation-site mutants reveals an extracytosolic NH2 terminus. J Biol Chem 1997;272:23623–30.
93. Zaman GJ, Flens MJ, van Leusden MR, et al. The human multidrug resistance-associated protein MRP is a plasma membrane drug-efflux pump. Proc Natl Acad Sci U S A 1994;91:8822–6.
94. Kruh GD, Chan A, Myers K, et al. Expression complementary DNA library transfer establishes mrp as a multidrug resistance gene. Cancer Res 1994;54:1649–52.
95. Grant CE, Valdimarsson G, Hipfner DR, et al. Overexpression of multidrug resistance-associated protein (MRP) increases resistance to natural product drugs. Cancer Res 1994;54:357–61.
96. Jedlitschky G, Leier I, Buchholz U, et al. Transport of glutathione, glucuronate, and sulfate conjugates by the MRP gene-encoded conjugate export pump. Cancer Res 1996;56:988–94.
97. Zaman GJ, Cnubben NH, van Bladeren PJ, et al. Transport of the glutathione conjugate of ethacrynic acid by the human multidrug resistance protein MRP. FEBS Lett 1996;391:126–30.
98. Keppler D, Leier I, Jedlitschky G. Transport of glutathione conjugates and glucuronides by the multidrug resistance proteins MRP1 and MRP2. Biol Chem 1997;378:787–91.
99. Loe DW, Almquist KC, Deeley RG, Cole SP. Multidrug resistance protein (MRP)-mediated transport of leukotriene C4 and chemotherapeutic agents in membrane vesicles. Demonstration of glutathione-dependent vincristine transport. J Biol Chem 1996;271:9675–82.
100. Jedlitschky G, Leier I, Buchholz U, et al. ATP-dependent transport of glutathione S-conjugates by the multidrug resistance-associated protein. Cancer Res 1994;54:4833–6.
101. Muller MR, Seiler F, Thomale J, et al. Capacity of individual chronic lymphatic leukemia lymphocytes and leukemic blast cells for repair of O6-ethylguanine in DNA: relation to chemosensitivity in vitro and treatment outcome. Cancer Res 1994;54:4524–31.
102. Loe DW, Deeley RG, Cole SP. Characterization of vincristine transport by the M(r) 190,000 multidrug resistance protein (MRP): evidence for cotransport with reduced glutathione. Cancer Res 1998;58:5130–6.
103. Borst P, Elferink RO. Mammalian ABC transporters in health and disease. Annu Rev Biochem 2002;71:537–92.
104. Kool M, de Haas M, Scheffer GL, et al. Analysis of expression of cMOAT (MRP2), MRP3, MRP4, and MRP5, homologues of the multidrug resistance-associated protein gene (MRP1), in human cancer cell lines. Cancer Res 1997;57:3537–47.
105. Kool M, van der Linden M, de Haas M, et al. MRP3, an organic anion transporter able to transport anti-cancer drugs. Proc Natl Acad Sci U S A 1999;96:6914–9.
106. Ludlum DB. The chloroethylnitrosoureas: sensitivity and resistance to cancer chemotherapy at the molecular level. Cancer Invest 1997;15:588–98.
107. Hooijberg JH, Broxterman HJ, Kool M, et al. Antifolate resistance mediated by the multidrug resistance proteins MRP1 and MRP2. Cancer Res 1999;59:2532–5.
108. Allikmets R, Schriml LM, Hutchinson A, et al. A human placenta-specific ATP-Binding Cassette gene (ABCP) on chromosome 4q22 that is involved in multidrug resistance. Cancer Res 1998;58:5337–9.
109. Doyle LA, Yang W, Abruzzo LV, et al. A multidrug resistance transporter from human MCF-7 breast cancer cells. Proc Natl Acad Sci U S A 1998;95:15665–70.
110. Miyake K, Mickley L, Litman T, et al. Molecular cloning of cDNAs which are highly overexpressed in mitoxantrone-resistant cells: demonstration of homology to ABC transport genes. Cancer Res 1999;59:8–13.
111. Allen JD, Brinkhuis RF, Wijnholds J, Schinkel AH. The mouse Bcrp1/Mxr/Abcp gene: amplification and overexpression in cell lines selected for resistance to topotecan, mitoxantrone, or doxorubicin. Cancer Res 1999;59:4237–41.
112. Shimano K, Satake M, Okaya A, et al. Hepatic oval cells have the side population phenotype defined by expression of ATP-binding cassette transporter ABCG2/BCRP1. Am J Pathol 2003;163:3–9.
113. Hori S, Ohtsuki S, Tachikawa M, et al. Functional expression of rat ABCG2 on the luminal side of brain capillaries and its enhancement by astrocyte-derived soluble factor(s). J Neurochem 2004;90:526–36.
114. Eisenblatter T, Galla HJ. A new multidrug resistance protein at the blood-brain barrier. Biochem Biophys Res Commun 2002;293:1273–8.
115. Eisenblatter T, Huwel S, Galla HJ. Characterisation of the brain multidrug resistance protein (BMDP/ABCG2/BCRP) expressed at the blood-brain barrier. Brain Res 2003;971:221–31.
116. Ueda T, Brenner S, Malech HL, et al. Cloning and functional analysis of the rhesus macaque ABCG2 gene. Forced expression confers an SP phenotype among hematopoietic stem cell progeny in vivo. J Biol Chem 2005;280:991–8.
117. Rocchi E, Khodjakov A, Volk EL, et al. The product of the ABC half transporter gene ABCG2 (BCRP/MXR/ABCP) is expressed in the plasma membrane. Biochem Biophys Res Commun 2000;271:42–6.
118. Scheffer GL, Maliepaard M, Pijnenborg AC, et al. Breast cancer resistance protein is localized at the plasma membrane in mitoxantrone- and topotecan-resistant cell lines. Cancer Res 2000;60:2589–93.
119. Litman T, Jensen U, Hansen A, et al. Use of peptide antibodies to probe for the mitoxantrone resistance-associated protein MXR/BCRP/ABCP/ABCG2. Biochim Biophys Acta 2002;1565:6–16.
120. Nakanishi T, Doyle LA, Hassel B, et al. Functional characterization of human breast cancer resistance protein (BCRP, ABCG2) expressed in the oocytes of Xenopus laevis. Mol Pharmacol 2003;64:1452–62.
121. Polgar O, Robey RW, Morisaki K, et al. Mutational analysis of ABCG2: role of the GXXXG motif. Biochemistry 2004;43:9448–56.
122. Xu J, Lin Y, Yang Y, et al. Characterization of oligomeric human half-ABC transporter ATP-binding cassette G2. J Biol Chem 2004;279:19781–9.
123. Zhang W, Mojsilovic-Petrovic J, Andrade MF, et al. The expression and functional characterization of ABCG2 in brain endothelial cells and vessels. FASEB J 2003;17:2085–7.
124. Cisternino S, Mercier C, Bourasset E, et al. Expression, up-regulation, and transport activity of the multidrug-resistance protein Abcg2 at the mouse blood-brain barrier. Cancer Res 2004;64:3296–301.
125. Begley DJ. ABC transporters and the blood-brain barrier. Curr Pharm Des 2004;10:1295–312.
126. Lee YJ, Kusuhara H, Jonker JW, et al. Investigation of efflux transport of dehydroepiandrosterone sulfate and mitoxantrone at the mouse blood-brain barrier: a minor role of breast cancer resistance protein. J Pharmacol Exp Ther 2005;312:44–52.
127. Bart J, Hollema H, Groen HJ, et al. The distribution of drug-efflux pumps, P-gp, BCRP, MRP1 and MRP2, in the normal blood-testis barrier and in primary testicular tumours. Eur J Cancer 2004;40:2064–70.
128. Maliepaard M, Scheffer GL, Faneyte IF, et al. Subcellular localization and distribution of the breast cancer resistance protein transporter in normal human tissues. Cancer Res 2001;61:3458–64.
129. Kolwankar D, Glover DD, Ware H JA, Tracy TS. Expression and function of ABCB1 and ABCG2 in human placental tissue. Drug Metab Dispos 2005;33:524–9.
130. Kitano T, Iizasa H, Hwang IW, et al. Conditionally immortalized syncytiotrophoblast cell lines as new tools for study of the blood-placenta barrier. Biol Pharm Bull 2004;27:753–9.
131. Young AM, Allen CE, Audus KL. Efflux transporters of the human placenta. Adv Drug Deliv Rev 2003;55:125–32.
132. Mizuno N, et al. Impaired renal excretion of 6-hydroxy-5,7-dimethyl-2-methylamino-4-(3-pyridylmethyl) benzothiazole (E3040) sulfate in breast cancer resistance protein (BCRP1/ABCG2) knockout mice. Drug Metab Dispos 2004;32:898–901.
133. Han B, Zhang JT. Multidrug resistance in cancer chemotherapy and xenobiotic protection mediated by the half ATP-binding cassette transporter ABCG2. Curr Med Chem Anticancer Agents 2004;4:31–42.
134. Zhou S, Schuetz JD, Bunting KD, et al. The ABC transporter Bcrp1/ABCG2 is expressed in a wide variety of stem cells and is a molecular determinant of the side-population phenotype. Nat Med 2001;7:1028–34.

135. Scharenberg CW, Harkey MA, Torok-Storb B. The ABCG2 transporter is an efficient Hoechst 33342 efflux pump and is preferentially expressed by immature human hematopoietic progenitors. Blood 2002;99:507–12.
136. Kim M, Turnquist H, Jackson J, et al. The multidrug resistance transporter ABCG2 (breast cancer resistance protein 1) effluxes Hoechst 33342 and is overexpressed in hematopoietic stem cells. Clin Cancer Res 2002;8:22–8.
137. Bunting KD. ABC Transporters as phenotypic markers and functional regulators of stem cells. Stem Cells 2002;20:11–20.
138. Meeson AP, Hawke TJ, Graham S, et al. Cellular and molecular regulation of skeletal muscle side population cells. Stem Cells 2004;22:1305–20.
139. Uchida N, Leung FY, Eaves CJ. Liver and marrow of adult mdr-1a/1b(-/-) mice show normal generation, function, and multi-tissue trafficking of primitive hematopoietic cells. Exp Hematol 2002;30:862–9.
140. Nakauchi H. Isolation and clonal characterization of hematopoietic and liver stem cells. Cornea 2004;23(8 Suppl):S2–7.
141. Lechner A, Leech CA, Abraham EJ, et al. Nestin-positive progenitor cells derived from adult human pancreatic islets of Langerhans contain side population (SP) cells defined by expression of the ABCG2 (BCRP1) ATP-binding cassette transporter. Biochem Biophys Res Commun 2002;293:670–4.
142. Huang H, Tang X. Phenotypic determination and characterization of nestin-positive precursors derived from human fetal pancreas. Lab Invest 2003;83:539–47.
143. Summer R, Kotton DN, Sun X, et al. Side population cells and Bcrp1 expression in lung. Am J Physiol Lung Cell Mol Physiol 2003;285:L97–104.
144. Lassalle B, Bastos H, Louis JP, et al. 'Side Population' cells in adult mouse testis express Bcrp1 gene and are enriched in spermatogonia and germinal stem cells. Development 2004;131:479–87.
145. Martin CM, Meeson AP, Robertson SM, et al. Persistent expression of the ATP-binding cassette transporter, Abcg2, identifies cardiac SP cells in the developing and adult heart. Dev Biol 2004;265:262–75.
146. Alvi AJ, Clayton H, Joshi C, et al. Functional and molecular characterisation of mammary side population cells. Breast Cancer Res 2003;5:R1–8.
147. Clayton H. Titley I, Vivanco M. Growth and differentiation of progenitor/stem cells derived from the human mammary gland. Exp Cell Res 2004;297:444–60.
148. de Paiva CS, Chen Z, Corrales RM, et al. ABCG2 Transporter identifies a population of clonogenic human limbal epithelial cells. Stem Cells 2005;23:63–73.
149. Wolosin JM, Budak MT, Akinci MA. Ocular surface epithelial and stem cell development. Int J Dev Biol 2004;48:981–91.
150. Chen Z, de Paiva CS, Luo L, et al. Characterization of putative stem cell phenotype in human limbal epithelia. Stem Cells 2004;22:355–66.
151. Watanabe K, Nishida K, Yamato M, et al. Human limbal epithelium contains side population cells expressing the ATP-binding cassette transporter ABCG2. FEBS Lett 2004;565:6–10.
152. Litman T, Druley TE, Stein WD, Bates SE. From MDR to MXR: new understanding of multidrug resistance systems, their properties and clinical significance. Cell Mol Life Sci 2001;58:931–59.
153. Schellens JH, Maliepaard M, Scheper RJ, et al. Transport of topoisomerase I inhibitors by the breast cancer resistance protein. Potential clinical implications. Ann N Y Acad Sci 2000;922:188–94.
154. Komatani H, Kotani H, Hara Y, et al. Identification of breast cancer resistant protein/mitoxantrone resistance/placenta-specific, ATP-binding cassette transporter as a transporter of NB-506 and J-107088, topoisomerase I inhibitors with an indolocarbazole structure. Cancer Res 2001;61:2827–32.
155. Ishii M, Iwahana M, Mitsui I, et al. Growth inhibitory effect of a new camptothecin analog, DX-8951f, on various drug-resistant sublines including BCRP-mediated camptothecin derivative-resistant variants derived from the human lung cancer cell line PC-6. Anticancer Drugs 2000;11:353–62.
156. Maliepaard M, et al. Circumvention of breast cancer resistance protein (BCRP)-mediated resistance to camptothecins in vitro using non-substrate drugs or the BCRP inhibitor GF120918. Clin Cancer Res 2001;7:935–41.
157. Rajendra R, Gounder MK, Saleem A, et al. Differential effects of the breast cancer resistance protein on the cellular accumulation and cytotoxicity of 9-aminocamptothecin and 9-nitrocamptothecin. Cancer Res 2003;63:3228–33.
158. Bates SE, Medina-Perez WY, Kohlhagen G, et al. ABCG2 mediates differential resistance to SN-38 (7-ethyl-10-hydroxycamptothecin) and homocamptothecins. J Pharmacol Exp Ther 2004;310:836–42.
159. Volk EL, Farley KM, Wu Y, et al. Overexpression of wild-type breast cancer resistance protein mediates methotrexate resistance. Cancer Res 2002;62:5035–40.
160. Volk EL, Schneider E. Wild-type breast cancer resistance protein (BCRP/ABCG2) is a methotrexate polyglutamate transporter. Cancer Res 2003;63:5538–43.
161. Chen ZS, Robey RW, Belinsky MG, et al. Transport of methotrexate, methotrexate polyglutamates, and 17beta-estradiol 17-(beta-D-glucuronide) by ABCG2: effects of acquired mutations at R482 on methotrexate transport. Cancer Res 2003;63:4048–54.
162. Mitomo H, Kato R, Ito A, et al. A functional study on polymorphism of the ATP-binding cassette transporter ABCG2: critical role of arginine-482 in methotrexate transport. Biochem J 2003;373(Pt 3):767–74.
163. Robey RW, Medina-Perez WY, Nishiyama K, et al. Overexpression of the ATP-binding cassette half-transporter, ABCG2 (MXR/BCRP/ABCP1), in flavopiridol-resistant human breast cancer cells. Clin Cancer Res 2001;7:145–52.
164. Janvilisri T, Venter H, Shai S, et al. Sterol transport by the human breast cancer resistance protein (ABCG2) expressed in Lactococcus lactis. J Biol Chem 2003;278:20645–51.
165. Burger H., van Tol H, Boersma AW, et al. Imatinib mesylate (STI571) is a substrate for the breast cancer resistance protein (BCRP)/ABCG2 drug pump. Blood 2004;104:2940–2.
166. Robey RW, Honjo Y, van de Laar A, et al. A functional assay for detection of the mitoxantrone resistance protein, MXR (ABCG2). Biochim Biophys Acta 2001;1512:171–182.
167. Robey RW, Steadman K, Polgar O, et al. Pheophorbide a is a specific probe for ABCG2 function and inhibition. Cancer Res 2004;64:1242–6.
168. Krishnamurthy P, Ross DD, Nakanishi T, et al. The stem cell marker Bcrp/ABCG2 enhances hypoxic cell survival through interactions with heme. J Biol Chem 2004;279:24218–25.
169. Jonker JW, Buitelaar M, Wagenaar E, et al. The breast cancer resistance protein protects against a major chlorophyll-derived dietary phototoxin and protoporphyria. Proc Natl Acad Sci U S A 2002;99:15649–54.
170. Imai Y, Asada S, Tsukahara S, et al. Breast cancer resistance protein exports sulfated estrogens but not free estrogens. Mol Pharmacol 2003;64:610–8.
171. Suzuki M. Suzuki H, Sugimoto Y, Sugiyama Y. ABCG2 transports sulfated conjugates of steroids and xenobiotics. J Biol Chem 2003;278:22644–9.
172. Pavek P, Merino G, Wagenaar E, et al. Human breast cancer resistance protein: interactions with steroid drugs, hormones, the dietary carcinogen 2-amino-1-methyl-6-phenylimidazo(4,5-b)pyridine, and transport of cimetidine. J Pharmacol Exp Ther 2005;312:144–52.
173. Wang X, Furukawa T, Nitanda T, et al. Breast cancer resistance protein (BCRP/ABCG2) induces cellular resistance to HIV-1 nucleoside reverse transcriptase inhibitors. Mol Pharmacol 2003;63:65–72.
174. Plasschaert SL, Van Der Kolk DM, De Bont ES, et al. Breast cancer resistance protein (BCRP) in acute leukemia. Leuk Lymphoma 2004;45:649–54.
175. Abbott BL. ABCG2 (BCRP) expression in normal and malignant hematopoietic cells. Hematol Oncol 2003;21:115–30.
176. Uggla B, et al. BCRP mRNA expression v. clinical outcome in 40 adult AML patients. Leuk Res 2005;29:141–6.
177. Benderra Z, Faussat AM, Sayada L, et al. Breast cancer resistance protein and P-glycoprotein in 149 adult acute myeloid leukemias. Clin Cancer Res 2004;10:7896–902.
178. Abbott BL, et al. Low levels of ABCG2 expression in adult AML blast samples. Blood 2002;100:4594–601.
179. Sargent JM, Williamson CJ, Maliepaard M, et al. Breast cancer resistance protein expression and resistance to daunorubicin in blast cells from patients with acute myeloid leukaemia. Br J Haematol 2001;115:257–62.
180. van den Heuvel-Eibrink MM, Wiemer EA, Prins A, et al. Increased expression of the breast cancer resistance protein (BCRP) in relapsed or refractory acute myeloid leukemia (AML). Leukemia 2002;16:833–9.
181. van der Pol MA, Broxterman HJ, Pater JM, et al. Function of the ABC transporters, P-glycoprotein, multidrug resistance protein and breast cancer resistance protein, in minimal residual disease in acute myeloid leukemia. Haematologica 2003;88:134–47.
182. van der Kolk DM, Vellenga E, Scheffer GL, et al. Expression and activity of breast cancer resistance protein (BCRP) in de novo and relapsed acute myeloid leukemia. Blood 2002;99:3763–70.
183. SuvannasankhaA, Minderman H, O'Loughlin KL, et al. Breast cancer resistance protein (BCRP/MXR/ABCG2) in acute myeloid leukemia: discordance between expression and function. Leukemia 2004;18:1252–7.
184. Suvannasankha A, Minderman H, O'Loughlin KL, et al. Breast cancer resistance protein (BCRP/MXR/ABCG2) in adult acute lymphoblastic leukaemia: frequent expression and possible correlation with shorter disease-free survival. Br J Haematol 2004;127:392–8.
185. Plasschaert SLA, van der Kolk DM, de Bont ES, et al. The role of breast cancer resistance protein in acute lymphoblastic leukemia. Clin Cancer Res 2003;9:5171–7.
186. Sauerbrey A, Sell W, Steinbach D, et al. Expression of the BCRP gene (ABCG2/MXR/ABCP) in childhood acute lymphoblastic leukaemia. Br J Haematol 2002;118:147–50.
187. Steinbach D, Sell W, Voigt A, et al. BCRP gene expression is associated with a poor response to remission induction therapy in childhood acute myeloid leukemia. Leukemia 2002;16:1443–7.
188. Kager L, Cheok M, Yang W, et al. Folate pathway gene expression differs in subtypes of acute lymphoblastic leukemia and influences methotrexate pharmacodynamics. J Clin Invest 2005;115:110–7.
189. Kanzaki A, Toi M, Nakayama K, et al. Expression of multidrug resistance-related transporters in human breast carcinoma. Jpn J Cancer Res 2001;92:452–8.
190. Faneyte IF, Kristel PM, Maliepaard M, et al. Expression of the breast cancer resistance protein in breast cancer. Clin Cancer Res 2002;8:1068–74.
191. Yoh K, Ishii G, Yokose T, et al. Breast cancer resistance protein impacts clinical outcome in platinum-based chemotherapy for advanced non-small cell lung cancer. Clin Cancer Res 2004;10:1691–7.
192. Zhang H, D'Arpa P, Liu LF. A model for tumor cell killing by topoisomerase poisons. Cancer Cells 1990;2:23–7.
193. Liu LF. DNA topoisomerase poisons as antitumor drugs. Annu Rev Biochem 1989;58:351–75.
194. Gupta RS. Genetic, biochemical, and cross-resistance studies with mutants of Chinese hamster ovary cells resistant to the anticancer drugs, VM-26 and VP16-213. Cancer Res 1983;43:1568–74.
195. Glisson BS, Multidrug resistance mediated through alterations in topoisomerase II. Cancer Bull 1989;41:37–44.
196. Deffie AM, Batra JK, Goldenberg GJ. Direct correlation between DNA topoisomerase II activity and cytotoxicity in Adriamycin-sensitive and -resistant P388 leukemia cell lines. Cancer Res 1989;49:58–62.
197. Per SR, Mattern MR, Mirabelli CK, et al. Characterization of a subline of P388 leukemia resistant to amsacrine: evidence of altered topoisomerase II function. Mol Pharmacol 1987;32:17–25.
198. Danks MK, Schmidt CA, Cirtain MC, et al. Altered catalytic activity of and DNA cleavage by DNA topoisomerase II from human leukemic cells selected for resistance to VM-26. Biochemistry 1988;27:8861–9.
199. Glisson B, Gupta R, Smallwood-Kentro S, Ross W. Characterization of acquired epipodophyllotoxin resistance in a Chinese hamster ovary cell line: loss of drug-stimulated DNA cleavage activity. Cancer Res 1986;46(4 Pt 2):1934–8.
200. Zwelling LA, Hinds M, Chan D, et al. Characterization of an amsacrine-resistant line of human leukemia cells. Evidence for a drug-resistant form of topoisomerase II. J Biol Chem 1989;264:16411–20.
201. Chung TD, Drake FH, Tan KB, et al. Characterization and immunological identification of cDNA clones encoding two human DNA topoisomerase II isozymes. Proc Natl Acad Sci U S A 1989;86:9431–5.
202. Drake FH, Hofmann GA, Bartus HF, et al. Biochemical and pharmacological properties of p170 and p180 forms of topoisomerase II. Biochemistry 1989;28:8154–60.
203. Hochhauser D, Harris AL. The role of topoisomerase II alpha and beta in drug resistance. Cancer Treat Rev 1993;19:181–94.
204. Woessner RD, Mattern MR, Mirabelli CK, et al. Proliferation- and cell cycle-dependent differences in expression of the 170 kilodalton and 180 kilodalton forms of topoisomerase II in NIH-3T3 cells. Cell Growth Differ 1991;2:209–14.
205. Larsen AK, Skladanowski A. Cellular resistance to topoisomerase-targeted drugs: from drug uptake to cell death. Biochim Biophys Acta 1998;1400:257–74.

206. Bugg BY, Danks MK, Beck WT, Suttle DP. Expression of a mutant DNA topoisomerase II in CCRF-CEM human leukemic cells selected for resistance to teniposide. Proc Natl Acad Sci U S A 1991;88:7654–8.
207. Chan VT, Ng SW, Eder JP, Schnipper LE. Molecular cloning and identification of a point mutation in the topoisomerase II cDNA from an etoposide-resistant Chinese hamster ovary cell line. J Biol Chem 1993;268:2160–5.
208. Danks MK, Warmoth MR, Friche E, et al. Single-strand conformational polymorphism analysis of the M(r) 170,000 isozyme of DNA topoisomerase II in human tumor cells. Cancer Res 1993;53:1373–9.
209. Lee MS, Wang JC, Beran M. Two independent amsacrine-resistant human myeloid leukemia cell lines share an identical point mutation in the 170 kDa form of human topoisomerase II. J Mol Biol 1992;223:837–43.
210. Patel S, Fisher LM. Novel selection and genetic characterisation of an etoposide-resistant human leukaemic CCRF-CEM cell line. Br J Cancer 1993;67:456–63.
211. Giovanella BC, Stehlin JS. DNA topoisomerase I-targeted chemotherapy of human colon cancer in xenografts. Science 1989;246:1046–8.
212. Tamura H, Kohchi C, Yamada R, et al. Molecular cloning of a cDNA of a camptothecin-resistant human DNA topoisomerase I and identification of mutation sites. Nucleic Acids Res 1991;19:69–75.
213. Tanizawa A, Pommier Y. Topoisomerase I alteration in a camptothecin-resistant cell line derived from Chinese hamster DC3F cells in culture. Cancer Res 1992;52:1848–54.
214. Andoh T, Ishii K, Suzuki Y, et al. Characterization of a mammalian mutant with a camptothecin-resistant DNA topoisomerase I. Proc Natl Acad Sci U S A 1987;84:5565–9.
215. Ishikawa T. The ATP-dependent glutathione S-conjugate export pump. Trends Biochem Sci 1992;17:463–8.
216. Brierley CH, Burchell B. Human UDP-glucuronosyl transferases: chemical defense, jaundice and gene therapy. Bioessays 1993;15:749–54.
217. Brix LA, Nicoll R, Zhu X, McManus ME. Structural and functional characterisation of human sulfotransferases. Chem Biol Interact 1998;109:123–7.
218. Coughtrie MW, Sharp S, Maxwell K, Innes NP. Biology and function of the reversible sulfation pathway catalysed by human sulfotransferases and sulfatases. Chem Biol Interact 1998;109:3–27.
219. Hayes JD, Pulford DJ. The glutathione S-transferase supergene family: regulation of GST and the contribution of the isoenzymes to cancer chemoprotection and drug resistance. Crit Rev Biochem Mol Biol 1995;30:445–600.
220. Mannervik B, Danielson UH. Glutathione transferases—structure and catalytic activity. CRC Crit Rev Biochem 1988;23:283–337.
221. Cowan KH, Batist G, Tulpule A, et al. Similar biochemical changes associated with multidrug resistance in human breast cancer cells and carcinogen-induced resistance to xenobiotics in rats. Proc Natl Acad Sci U S A 1986;83:9328–32.
222. Farber E. Cellular biochemistry of the stepwise development of cancer with chemicals: G. H. A. Clowes memorial lecture. Cancer Res 1984;44(12 Pt 1):5463–74.
223. Black SM. Wolf CR. The role of glutathione-dependent enzymes in drug resistance. Pharmacol Ther 1991;51:139–54.
224. Morrow CS, Cowan KH. Glutathione S-transferases and drug resistance. Cancer Cells 1990;2:15–22.
225. Tew KD. Glutathione-associated enzymes in anticancer drug resistance. Cancer Res 1994;54:4313–20.
226. Coles B, Ketterer B. The role of glutathione and glutathione transferases in chemical carcinogenesis. Crit Rev Biochem Mol Biol 1990;25:47–70.
227. Awasthi S, Bajpai KK, Piper JT, et al. Interactions of melphalan with glutathione and the role of glutathione S-transferase. Drug Metab Dispos 1996;24:371–4.
228. Berhane K, Hao XY, Egyhazi S, et al. Contribution of glutathione transferase M3-3 to 1,3-bis(2-chloroethyl)-1-nitrosourea resistance in a human non-small cell lung cancer cell line. Cancer Res 1993;53:4257–61.
229. Bolton MG, Colvin OM, Hilton J. Specificity of isozymes of murine hepatic glutathione S-transferase for the conjugation of glutathione with L-phenylalanine mustard. Cancer Res 1991;51:2410–5.
230. Ciaccio PJ, Tew KD, LaCreta FP. Enzymatic conjugation of chlorambucil with glutathione by human glutathione S-transferases and inhibition by ethacrynic acid. Biochem Pharmacol 1991;42:1504–7.
231. Ciaccio PJ, Tew KD, LaCreta FO. The spontaneous and glutathione S-transferase-mediated reaction of chlorambucil with glutathione. Cancer Commun 1990;2:279–85.
232. Dirven HA, Dictus EL, Broeders NL, et al. The role of human glutathione S-transferase isoenzymes in the formation of glutathione conjugates of the alkylating cytostatic drug thiotepa. Cancer Res 1995;55:1701–6.
233. Dirven HA, van Ommen B, van Bladeren PJ. Involvement of human glutathione S-transferase isoenzymes in the conjugation of cyclophosphamide metabolites with glutathione. Cancer Res 1994;54:6215–20.
234. Dulik DM, Fenselau C, Hilton J. Characterization of melphalan-glutathione adducts whose formation is catalyzed by glutathione transferases. Biochem Pharmacol 1986;35:3405–9.
235. Black SM, Beggs JD, Hayes JD, et al. Expression of human glutathione S-transferases in Saccharomyces cerevisiae confers resistance to the anticancer drugs Adriamycin and chlorambucil. Biochem J 1990;268:309–15.
236. Buller AL, Clapper ML, Tew KD. Glutathione S-transferases in nitrogen mustard-resistant and -sensitive cell lines. Mol Pharmacol 1987;31:575–8.
237. Lewis AD, Hickson ID, Robson CN, et al. Amplification and increased expression of alpha class glutathione S-transferase-encoding genes associated with resistance to nitrogen mustards. Proc Natl Acad Sci U S A 1988;85:8511–5.
238. Leyland-Jones BR, Townsend AJ, Tu CP, et al. Antineoplastic drug sensitivity of human MCF-7 breast cancer cells stably transfected with a human alpha class glutathione S-transferase gene. Cancer Res 1991;51:587–94.
239. Moscow JA, Townsend AJ, Cowan KH. Elevation of pi class glutathione S-transferase activity in human breast cancer cells by transfection of the GST pi gene and its effect on sensitivity to toxins. Mol Pharmacol 1989;36:22.
240. Puchalski RB, Fahl WE. Expression of recombinant glutathione S-transferase pi, Ya, or Yb1 confers resistance to alkylating agents. Proc Natl Acad Sci U S A 1990;87:2443–7.
241. Schecter RL, et al. Expression of a rat glutathione-S-transferase complementary DNA in rat mammary carcinoma cells: impact upon alkylator-induced toxicity. Cancer Res 1993;53:4900.
242. Smith MT, Evans CG, Doane-Setzer P, et al. Denitrosation of 1,3-bis(2-chloroethyl)-1-nitrosourea by class mu glutathione transferases and its role in cellular resistance in rat brain tumor cells. Cancer Res 1989;49:2621–5.
243. Townsend AJ, Tu CP, Cowan KH. Expression of human mu or alpha class glutathione S-transferases in stably transfected human MCF-7 breast cancer cells: effect on cellular sensitivity to cytotoxic agents. Mol Pharmacol 1992;41:230–6.
244. Yang WZ, Begleiter A, Johnston JB, et al. Role of glutathione and glutathione S-transferase in chlorambucil resistance. Mol Pharmacol 1992;41:625–30.
245. Ishikawa T, Ali-Osman F. Glutathione-associated cis-diamminedichloroplatinum(II) metabolism and ATP-dependent efflux from leukemia cells. Molecular characterization of glutathione-platinum complex and its biological significance. J Biol Chem 1993;268:20116–25.
246. Meyer DJ. Significance of an unusually low Km for glutathione in glutathione transferases of the alpha, mu and pi classes. Xenobiotica 1993;23:823–34.
247. Awasthi S, Singhal SS, Srivastava SK, et al. Adenosine triphosphate-dependent transport of doxorubicin, daunomycin, and vinblastine in human tissues by a mechanism distinct from the P-glycoprotein. J Clin Invest 1994;93:958–65.
248. Morrow CS, Smitherman PK, Diah SK, et al. Coordinated action of glutathione S-transferases (GSTs) and multidrug resistance protein 1 (MRP1) in antineoplastic drug detoxification. Mechanism of GST A1-1- and MRP1-associated resistance to chlorambucil in MCF7 breast carcinoma cells. J Biol Chem 1998;273:20114–20.
249. Morrow CS, Diah S, Smitherman PK, et al. Multidrug resistance protein and glutathione S-transferase P1-1 act in synergy to confer protection from 4-nitroquinoline 1-oxide toxicity. Carcinogenesis 1998;19:109–15.
250. Hall AG. The role of glutathione in the regulation of apoptosis. Eur J Clin Invest 1999;29:238–45.
251. Bursch W. The autophagosomal-lysosomal compartment in programmed cell death. Cell Death Differ 2001;8:569–81.
252. Bellamy C.O. p53 and apoptosis. Br Med Bull 1997;53:522–38.
253. Reed JC. Bcl-2 family proteins: regulators of apoptosis and chemoresistance in hematologic malignancies. Semin Hematol 1997;34(4 Suppl 5):9–19.
254. Strasser A, Huang DC, Vaux DL. The role of the bcl-2/ced-9 gene family in cancer and general implications of defects in cell death control for tumourigenesis and resistance to chemotherapy. Biochim Biophys Acta 1997;1333:F151–78.
255. Clarke AR, et al. Thymocyte apoptosis induced by p53-dependent and independent pathways. Nature 1993;362:849.
256. Fan S, el-Deiry WS, Bae I, et al. p53 gene mutations are associated with decreased sensitivity of human lymphoma cells to DNA damaging agents. Cancer Res 1994;54:5824–30.
257. Lowe SW, Ruley HE, Jacks T, et al. p53-dependent apoptosis modulates the cytotoxicity of anticancer agents. Cell 1993;74:957–67.
258. Haq R, Zanke B. Inhibition of apoptotic signaling pathways in cancer cells as a mechanism of chemotherapy resistance. Cancer Metastasis Rev 1998;17:233–9.
259. Potapova O, Haghighi A, Bost F, et al. The Jun kinase/stress-activated protein kinase pathway functions to regulate DNA repair and inhibition of the pathway sensitizes tumor cells to cisplatin. J Biol Chem 1997;272:14041–4.
260. Miyashita T, Reed JC. bcl-2 gene transfer increases relative resistance of S49.1 and WEHI7.2 lymphoid cells to cell death and DNA fragmentation induced by glucocorticoids and multiple chemotherapeutic drugs. Cancer Res 1992;52:5407–11.
261. Miyashita T, Reed JC. Bcl-2 oncoprotein blocks chemotherapy-induced apoptosis in a human leukemia cell line. Blood 1993;81:151–7.
262. Boise LH, Gonzalez-Garcia M, Postema CA, et al. bcl-x, a bcl-2-related gene that functions as a dominant regulator of apoptotic cell death. Cell 1993;74:597–608.
263. Fisher TC, Milner AE, Gregory CD, et al. bcl-2 modulation of apoptosis induced by anticancer drugs: resistance to thymidylate stress is independent of classical resistance pathways. Cancer Res 1993;53:3321–6.
264. Shimizu S, Kanaseki T, Mizushima N, et al. Role of Bcl-2 family proteins in a non-apoptotic programmed cell death dependent on autophagy genes. Nat Cell Biol 2004;6:1221–8.
265. Poplack DG, Reaman G. Acute lymphoblastic leukemia in childhood. Pediatr Clin North Am 1988;35:903–32.
266. Teicher BA, Herman TS. Tumor resistance to alkylating agents conferred by mechanisms operative only in vivo. Science 1990;247:1457–61.
267. McLeod HL, Krynetski EY, Relling MV, Evans WE. Genetic polymorphism of thiopurine methyltransferase and its clinical relevance for childhood acute lymphoblastic leukemia. Leukemia 2000;14:567–72.
268. Relling MV, Hancock ML, Rivera GK, et al. Mercaptopurine therapy intolerance and heterozygosity at the thiopurine S-methyltransferase gene locus. J Natl Cancer Inst 1999;91:2001–8.
269. Jamroziak K, Robak T. Pharmacogenomics of MDR1/ABCB1 gene: the influence on risk and clinical outcome of haematological malignancies. Hematology 2004;9:91–105.
270. Hoffmeyer S, Burk O, von Richter O, et al. Functional polymorphisms of the human multidrug-resistance gene: multiple sequence variations and correlation of one allele with P-glycoprotein expression and activity in vivo. Proc Natl Acad Sci U S A 2000;97:3473–8.
271. Moriya Y, Nakamura T, Horinouchi N, et al. Effects of polymorphisms of MDR1, MRP1, and MRP2 genes on their mRNA expression levels in duodenal enterocytes of healthy Japanese subjects. Biol Pharm Bull 2002;25:1356–9.
272. Hitzl M, Drescher S, van der Kuip H, et al. The C3435T mutation in the human MDR1 gene is associated with altered efflux of the P-glycoprotein substrate rhodamine 123 from CD56+ natural killer cells. Pharmacogenetics 2001;11:293–8.
273. Nakamura T, Sakaeda T, Horinouchi M, et al. Effect of the mutation (C3435T) at exon 26 of the MDR1 gene on expression level of MDR1 messenger ribonucleic acid in duodenal enterocytes of healthy Japanese subjects. Clin Pharmacol Ther 2002;71:297–303.
274. Illmer T, Schuler US, Thiede C, et al. MDR1 gene polymorphisms affect therapy outcome in acute myeloid leukemia patients. Cancer Res 2002;62:4955–62.
275. Verstuyft C, Schwab M, Schaeffeler E. et al. Digoxin pharmacokinetics and MDR1 genetic polymorphisms. Eur J Clin Pharmacol 2003;58:809–12.
276. Oselin K, Gerloff T, Mrozikiewicz PM, et al. MDR1 polymorphisms G2677T in exon 21 and C3435T in exon 26 fail to affect rhodamine 123 efflux in peripheral blood lymphocytes. Fundam Clin Pharmacol 2003 17:463–9.
277. Fellay J, Marzolini C, Meaden ER, et al. Response to antiretroviral treatment in HIV-1-infected individuals with

allelic variants of the multidrug resistance transporter 1: a pharmacogenetics study. Lancet 2002;359:30–6.
278. Drescher S, Schaeffeler E, Hitzl M, et al. MDR1 gene polymorphisms and disposition of the P-glycoprotein substrate fexofenadine. Br J Clin Pharmacol 2002;53:526–34.
279. Goto M, Masuda S, Saito H, et al. C3435T polymorphism in the MDR1 gene affects the enterocyte expression level of CYP3A4 rather than Pgp in recipients of living-donor liver transplantation. Pharmacogenetics 2002;12:451–7.
280. Siegsmund M, Brinkmann U, Schaeffeler E, et al. Association of the P-glycoprotein transporter MDR1(C3435T) polymorphism with the susceptibility to renal epithelial tumors. J Am Soc Nephrol 2002;13:1847–54.
281. Sakaeda T, Nakamura T, Okumura K. MDR1 genotype-related pharmacokinetics and pharmacodynamics. Biol Pharm Bull 2002;25:1391–400.
282. Morita Y, Sakaeda T, Horinouchi M, et al. MDR1 genotype-related duodenal absorption rate of digoxin in healthy Japanese subjects. Pharm Res 2003;20:552–6.
283. Efferth T, Sauerbrey A, Steinbach D, et al. Analysis of single nucleotide polymorphism C3435T of the multidrug resistance gene MDR1 in acute lymphoblastic leukemia. Int J Oncol 2003;23:509–17.
284. Mickley LA, Lee JS, Weng Z, et al. Genetic polymorphism in MDR-1: a tool for examining allelic expression in normal cells, unselected and drug-selected cell lines, and human tumors. Blood 1998;91:1749–56.
285. van den Heuvel-Eibrink MM, Wiemer EA, de Boevere MJ, et al. MDR1 gene-related clonal selection and P-glycoprotein function and expression in relapsed or refractory acute myeloid leukemia. Blood 2001;97:3605–11.
286. Jamroziak K, Mlynarski W, Balcerczak E, et al. Functional C3435T polymorphism of MDR1 gene: an impact on genetic susceptibility and clinical outcome of childhood acute lymphoblastic leukemia. Eur J Haematol 2004;72:314–21.
287. Krajinovic M, Moghrabi A. Pharmacogenetics of methotrexate. Pharmacogenomics 2004;5:819–34.
288. Chiusolo P, Reddiconto G, Casorelli I, et al. Preponderance of methylenetetrahydrofolate reductase C677T homozygosity among leukemia patients intolerant to methotrexate. Ann Oncol 2002;13:1915–8.
289. Krajinovic M, Lemieux-Blanchard E, Chiasson S, et al. Role of polymorphisms in MTHFR and MTHFD1 genes in the outcome of childhood acute lymphoblastic leukemia. Pharmacogenomics J 2004;4:66–72.
290. Toffoli G, Russo A, Innocenti F, et al. Effect of methylenetetrahydrofolate reductase 677C—>T polymorphism on toxicity and homocysteine plasma level after chronic methotrexate treatment of ovarian cancer patients. Int J Cancer 2003;103:294–9.
291. Kishi S, Griener J, Cheng C, et al. Homocysteine, pharmacogenetics, and neurotoxicity in children with leukemia. J Clin Oncol 2003;21:3084–91.
292. Krajinovic M, Costea I, Chiasson S. Polymorphism of the thymidylate synthase gene and outcome of acute lymphoblastic leukaemia. Lancet 2002;359:1033–4.
293. Lauten M, Asgedom G, Welte K, et al. Thymidylate synthase gene polymorphism and its association with relapse in childhood B-cell precursor acute lymphoblastic leukemia. Haematologica 2003;88:353–4.
294. Laverdiere C, Chiasson S, Costea I, et al. Polymorphism G80A in the reduced folate carrier gene and its relationship to methotrexate plasma levels and outcome of childhood acute lymphoblastic leukemia. Blood 2002;100:3832–4.
295. Toffoli G, Cecchin E, Corona G, Boiocchi M. Pharmacogenetics of irinotecan. Curr Med Chem Anticancer Agents 2003;3:225–37.
296. Ishikawa T, Hirano H, Onishi Y, et al. Functional evaluation of ABCB1 (P-glycoprotein) polymorphisms: high-speed screening and structure-activity relationship analyses. Drug Metab Pharmacokinet 2004;19:1–14.
297. Tsuruo T, Iida H, Yamashiro M, et al. Enhancement of vincristine- and Adriamycin-induced cytotoxicity by verapamil in P388 leukemia and its sublines resistant to vincristine and Adriamycin. Biochem Pharmacol 1982;31:3138.
298. Boesch D, Gaveriaux C, Jachez B, et al. In vivo circumvention of P-glycoprotein-mediated multidrug resistance of tumor cells with SDZ PSC 833. Cancer Res 1991;51:4226.
299. Coley HM, Twentyman PR, Workman P. Improved cellular accumulation is characteristic of anthracyclines which retain high activity in multidrug resistant cell lines, alone or in combination with verapamil or cyclosporin A. Biochem Pharmacol 1989;38:4467–75.
300. Hu XF, Martin TJ, Bell DR, et al. Combined use of cyclosporin A and verapamil in modulating multidrug resistance in human leukemia cell lines. Cancer Res 1990;50:2953–7.
301. Nooter K, Sonneveld P, Oostrum R, et al. Overexpression of the mdr1 gene in blast cells from patients with acute myelocytic leukemia is associated with decreased anthracycline accumulation that can be restored by cyclosporin-A. Int J Cancer 1990;45:263–8.
302. Stewart DJ, Evans WK. Non-chemotherapeutic agents that potentiate chemotherapy efficacy. Cancer Treat Rev 1989;16:1–40.
303. Twentyman PR, Bleehen NM. Resistance modification by PSC-833, a novel non-immunosuppressive cyclosporin [corrected]. Eur J Cancer 1991;27:1639–42.
304. Sikic BI. Modulation of multidrug resistance: at the threshold. J Clin Oncol 1993;11:1629–35.
305. Cairo MS, Siegel S, Anas N, Sender L. Clinical trial of continuous infusion verapamil, bolus vinblastine, and continuous infusion VP-16 in drug-resistant pediatric tumors. Cancer Res 1989;49:1063–6.
306. Dalmark M, Pals H, Johnsen AH. Doxorubicin in combination with verapamil in advanced colorectal cancer. A phase II trial. Acta Oncol 1991;30:23–6.
307. Miller TP, Grogan TM, Dalton WS, et al. P-glycoprotein expression in malignant lymphoma and reversal of clinical drug resistance with chemotherapy plus high-dose verapamil. J Clin Oncol 1991;9:17–24.
308. Salmon SE, Dalton WS, Grogan TM, et al. Multidrug-resistant myeloma: laboratory and clinical effects of verapamil as a chemosensitizer. Blood 1991;78:44–50.
309. Bissett D, Kerr DJ, Cassidy J, et al. Phase I and pharmacokinetic study of D-verapamil and doxorubicin. Br J Cancer 1991;64:1168–71.
310. Ferry DR, Traunecker H, Kerr DJ. Clinical trials of P-glycoprotein reversal in solid tumours. Eur J Cancer 1996;32A:1070–81.
311. List AF, Kopecky KJ, Willman CL, et al. Benefit of cyclosporine modulation of drug resistance in patients with poor-risk acute myeloid leukemia: a Southwest Oncology Group study. Blood 2001;98:3212–20.
312. List AF, Spier C, Greer J, et al. Phase I/II trial of cyclosporine as a chemotherapy-resistance modifier in acute leukemia. J Clin Oncol 1993;11:1652–60.
313. Ozols RF, Cunnion RE, Klecker RW Jr, et al. Verapamil and Adriamycin in the treatment of drug-resistant ovarian cancer patients. J Clin Oncol 1987;5:641–7.
314. Seeber S, Osieka R, Schmidt CG, et al. In vivo resistance towards anthracyclines, etoposide, and cis-diamminedichloroplatinum(II). Cancer Res 1982;42:4719–25.
315. Skovsgaard T. Circumvention of resistance to daunorubicin by N-acetyldaunorubicin in Ehrlich ascites tumor. Cancer Res 1980;40:1077–83.
316. Slater LM, Murray SL, Wetzel MW, et al. Verapamil restoration of daunorubicin responsiveness in daunorubicin-resistant Ehrlich ascites carcinoma. J Clin Invest 1982;70:1131–4.
317. Slater LM, Sweet P, Stupecky M, et al. Cyclosporin A corrects daunorubicin resistance in Ehrlich ascites carcinoma. Br J Cancer 1986;54:235–8.
318. Solary E, Caillot D, Chauffert B, et al. Feasibility of using quinine, a potential multidrug resistance-reversing agent, in combination with mitoxantrone and cytarabine for the treatment of acute leukemia. J Clin Oncol 1992;10:1730–6.
319. Sonneveld P, Durie BG, Lokhorst HM, et al. Modulation of multidrug-resistant multiple myeloma by cyclosporin. Lancet 1992;340:255–9.
320. Tsuruo T. Reversal of acquired resistance to vinca alkaloids and anthracycline antibiotics. Cancer Treat Rep 1983;67:889–94.
321. Tsuruo T, Iida H, Kitatani Y, et al. Effects of quinidine and related compounds on cytotoxicity and cellular accumulation of vincristine and Adriamycin in drug-resistant tumor cells. Cancer Res 1984;44:4303–7.
322. Tsuruo T, Iida H, Tsukagoshi S, Sakurai Y. Overcoming of vincristine resistance in P388 leukemia in vivo and in vitro through enhanced cytotoxicity of vincristine and vinblastine by verapamil. Cancer Res 1981;41:1967–72.
323. Volm M. Multidrug resistance and its reversal. Anticancer Res 1998;18:2905–17.
324. Lum BL, Kaubisch S, Yahanda AM, et al. Alteration of etoposide pharmacokinetics and pharmacodynamics by cyclosporine in a phase I trial to modulate multidrug resistance. J Clin Oncol 1992;10:1635–42.
325. Cordon-Cardo C, O'Brien JP, Casaks D, et al. Multidrug-resistance gene (P-glycoprotein) is expressed by endothelial cells at blood-brain barrier sites. Proc Natl Acad Sci U S A 1989;86:695–8.
326. Schinkel AH, Smit JJ, van Tellingen O, et al. Disruption of the mouse mdr1a P-glycoprotein gene leads to a deficiency in the blood-brain barrier and to increased sensitivity to drugs. Cell 1994;77:491–502.
327. Thiebaut F, Tsuruo T, Hamada H, et al. Cellular localization of the multidrug-resistance gene product P-glycoprotein in normal human tissues. Proc Natl Acad Sci U S A 1987;84:7735–8.
328. Dantzig AH, Shepard RL, Law KL, et al. Selectivity of the multidrug resistance modulator, LY335979, for P-glycoprotein and effect on cytochrome P-450 activities. J Pharmacol Exp Ther 1999;290:854–62.
329. Sandler A, Gordon M, de Alwis DP, et al. A phase I trial of a potent P-glycoprotein inhibitor, zosuquidar trihydrochloride (LY335979), administered intravenously in combination with doxorubicin in patients with advanced malignancy. Clin Cancer Res 2004;10:3265–72.
330. Gerrard G, Payne E, Baker RJ, et al. Clinical effects and P-glycoprotein inhibition in patients with acute myeloid leukemia treated with zosuquidar trihydrochloride, daunorubicin and cytarabine. Haematologica 2004;89:782–90.
331. Fracasso PM, Goldstein LJ, de Alwis DP, et al. Phase I study of docetaxel in combination with the P-glycoprotein inhibitor, zosuquidar, in resistant malignancies. Clin Cancer Res 2004;10:7220–8.
332. Callies S, de Alwis DP, Mehta A, et al. Population pharmacokinetic model for daunorubicin and daunorubicinol coadministered with zosuquidar.3HCl (LY335979). Cancer Chemother Pharmacol 2004;54:39–48.
333. Thomas H, Coley HM. Overcoming multidrug resistance in cancer: an update on the clinical strategy of inhibiting p-glycoprotein. Cancer Control 2003;10:159–65.
334. Rubin EH, de Alwis DP, Pouliquen I, et al. A phase I trial of a potent P-glycoprotein inhibitor, Zosuquidar.3HCl trihydrochloride (LY335979), administered orally in combination with doxorubicin in patients with advanced malignancies. Clin Cancer Res 2002;8:3710–7.
335. Hamada H, Tsuruo T. Functional role for the 170- to 180-kDa glycoprotein specific to drug-resistant tumor cells as revealed by monoclonal antibodies. Proc Natl Acad Sci U S A 1986;83:7785–9.
336. Efferth T, Volm M. Modulation of P-glycoprotein-mediated multidrug resistance by monoclonal antibodies, immunotoxins or antisense oligodeoxynucleotides in kidney carcinoma and normal kidney cells. Oncology 1993;50:303–8.
337. FitzGerald DJ, Willingham MC, Cardarelli CO, et al. A monoclonal antibody-Pseudomonas toxin conjugate that specifically kills multidrug-resistant cells. Proc Natl Acad Sci U S A 1987;84:4288–92.
338. Van Dijk J, Tsuruo T, Segal DM, et al. Bispecific antibodies reactive with the multidrug-resistance-related glycoprotein and CD3 induce lysis of multidrug-resistant tumor cells. Int J Cancer 1989;44:738–43.
339. Sikic BI, Fisher GA, Lum BL, et al. Modulation and prevention of multidrug resistance by inhibitors of P-glycoprotein. Cancer Chemother Pharmacol 1997;40 Suppl:S13–9.
340. Leier I, Jedlitschky G, Buchholz U, et al. The MRP gene encodes an ATP-dependent export pump for leukotriene C4 and structurally related conjugates. J Biol Chem 1994;269:27807–10.
341. Loe DW, Deeley RG, Cole SP. Characterization of vincristine transport by the M(r) 190,000 multidrug resistance protein (MRP): evidence for cotransport with reduced glutathione. Cancer Res 1998;58:5130–6.
342. Barnouin K, Leier I, Jedlitschky G, et al. Multidrug resistance protein-mediated transport of chlorambucil and melphalan conjugated to glutathione. Br J Cancer 1998;**77**:201–9.
343. Hande K, Anthony L, Hamilton R, et al. Identification of etoposide glucuronide as a major metabolite of etoposide in the rat and rabbit. Cancer Res 1988;48:1829–34.
344. Jedlitschky G, Leier I, Buchholz U, et al. ATP-dependent transport of bilirubin glucuronides by the multidrug resistance protein MRP1 and its hepatocyte canalicular isoform MRP2. Biochem J 1997;327(Pt 1):305–10.
345. Rabindran SK, Ross DD, Doyle LA, et al. Fumitremorgin C reverses multidrug resistance in cells transfected with the breast cancer resistance protein. Cancer Res 2000;60:47–50.
346. de Bruin M, Miyake K, Litman T, et al. Reversal of resistance by GF120918 in cell lines expressing the ABC half-transporter, MXR. Cancer Lett 1999;146:117–126.
347. Schellens JH, Kuppens IE, Jewell RC, et al. Phase I and pharmacological study of oral topotecan and the BCRP and P-gp inhibitor elacridar [abstract]. J Clin Oncol (Meeting Abstracts), 2004;22(14 suppl):2003.

348. Minderman H, O'Loughlin KL, Pendyala L, Baer MR. VX-710 (biricodar) increases drug retention and enhances chemosensitivity in resistant cells overexpressing P-glycoprotein, multidrug resistance protein, and breast cancer resistance protein. Clin Cancer Res 2004;10:1826–34.
349. Shiozawa K, Oka M, Soda H, et al. Reversal of breast cancer resistance protein (BCRP/ABCG2)-mediated drug resistance by novobiocin, a coumermycin antibiotic. Int J Cancer 2004;108:146–51.
350. Yang CH, Chen YC, Kuo ML. Novobiocin sensitizes BCRP/MXR/ABCP overexpressing topotecan-resistant human breast carcinoma cells to topotecan and mitoxantrone. Anticancer Res 2003;23:2519–23.
351. Yanase K, Tsukahara S, Asada S, et al. Gefitinib reverses breast cancer resistance protein-mediated drug resistance. Mol Cancer Ther 2004;3:1119–25.
352. Houghton PJ, Germain GS, Harwood FC, et al. Imatinib mesylate is a potent inhibitor of the ABCG2 (BCRP) transporter and reverses resistance to topotecan and SN-38 in vitro. Cancer Res 2004;64:2333–7.
353. Erlichman C, Boerner SA, Hallgren CG, et al. The HER tyrosine kinase inhibitor CI1033 enhances cytotoxicity of 7-ethyl-10-hydroxycamptothecin and topotecan by inhibiting breast cancer resistance protein-mediated drug efflux. Cancer Res 2001;61:739–48.
354. Gupta A, Zhang Y, Unadkat JD, Mao Q. HIV protease inhibitors are inhibitors but not substrates of the human breast cancer resistance protein (BCRP/ABCG2). J Pharmacol Exp Ther 2004;310:334–41.
355. Minderman H, Brooks TA, O'Loughlin KL, et al. Broad-spectrum modulation of ATP-binding cassette transport proteins by the taxane derivatives ortataxel (IDN-5109, BAY 59-8862) and tRA96023. Cancer Chemother Pharmacol 2004;53:363–9.
356. Brooks TA, Minderman H, O'Loughlin KL, et al. Taxane-based reversal agents modulate drug resistance mediated by P-glycoprotein, multidrug resistance protein, and breast cancer resistance protein. Mol Cancer Ther 2003;2:1195–205.
357. Zhang S, Yang X, Morris ME. Combined effects of multiple flavonoids on breast cancer resistance protein (ABCG2)-mediated transport. Pharm Res 2004;21:1263–73.
358. Zhang S, Yang X, Morris ME. Flavonoids are inhibitors of breast cancer resistance protein (ABCG2)-mediated transport. Mol Pharmacol 2004;65:1208–16.
359. Yoshikawa M, Ikegami Y, Sano K, et al. Transport of SN-38 by the wild type of human ABC transporter ABCG2 and its inhibition by quercetin, a natural flavonoid. J Exp Ther Oncol 2004;4:25–35.
360. Imai Y, Tsukahara S, Asada S, Sugimoto Y. Phytoestrogens/flavonoids reverse breast cancer resistance protein/ABCG2-mediated multidrug resistance. Cancer Res 2004;64:4346–52.
361. Kruijtzer CM, Beijnen JH, Rosing H, et al. Increased oral bioavailability of topotecan in combination with the breast cancer resistance protein and P-glycoprotein inhibitor GF120918. J Clin Oncol 2002;20:2943–50.
362. Kruijtzer CM, Beijnen JH, Schellens JH. Improvement of oral drug treatment by temporary inhibition of drug transporters and/or cytochrome P450 in the gastrointestinal tract and liver: an overview. Oncologist 2002;7:516–30.
363. Stewart CF, Laggas M, Schuetz JD, et al. Gefitinib enhances the antitumor activity and oral bioavailability of irinotecan in mice. Cancer Res 2004;64:7491–9.
364. Allen JD, van Loevezijn A, Lakhai JM, et al. Potent and specific inhibition of the breast cancer resistance protein multidrug transporter in vitro and in mouse intestine by a novel analogue of fumitremorgin C. Mol Cancer Ther 2002;1:417–25.
365. Jensen PB, Sehested M. DNA topoisomerase II rescue by catalytic inhibitors: a new strategy to improve the antitumor selectivity of etoposide. Biochem Pharmacol 1997;54:755–9.
366. Withoff S, De Jong S, De Vries EG, Mulder NH. Human DNA topoisomerase II: biochemistry and role in chemotherapy resistance (review). Anticancer Res 1996;16:1867–80.
367. Baguley BC, Holdaway KM, Fray LM. Design of DNA intercalators to overcome topoisomerase II-mediated multidrug resistance. J Natl Cancer Inst 1990;82:398–402.
368. Finlay GJ, Baguley BC, Snow K, Judd W. Multiple patterns of resistance of human leukemia cell sublines to amsacrine analogues. J Natl Cancer Inst 1990;82:662–7.
369. Sinha BK, Katki AG, Batist G, et al. Differential formation of hydroxyl radicals by Adriamycin in sensitive and resistant MCF-7 human breast tumor cells: implications for the mechanism of action. Biochemistry 1987;26:3776–81.
370. Dusre L, Mimnaugh EG, Myers CE, Sinha BK. Potentiation of doxorubicin cytotoxicity by buthionine sulfoximine in multidrug-resistant human breast tumor cells. Cancer Res 1989;49:511–5.
371. Kramer RA, Zakher J, Kim G. Role of the glutathione redox cycle in acquired and de novo multidrug resistance. Science 1988;241:694–7.
372. Keizer HG, van Rijn J, Pinedo HM, Joenje H. Effect of endogenous glutathione, superoxide dismutases, catalase, and glutathione peroxidase on Adriamycin tolerance of Chinese hamster ovary cells. Cancer Res 1988;48:4493–7.
373. Alin P, Danielson UH, Mannervik B. 4-Hydroxyalk-2-enals are substrates for glutathione transferase. FEBS Lett 1985;179:267–70.
374. Ketterer B, Meyer DJ. Glutathione transferases: a possible role in the detoxification of DNA and lipid hydroperoxides. Mutat Res 1989;214:33–40.
375. Tew KD, Bomber AM, Hoffman SJ. Ethacrynic acid and piriprost as enhancers of cytotoxicity in drug resistant and sensitive cell lines. Cancer Res 1988;48:3622–5.
376. Gerson SL, Willson JK. O6-alkylguanine-DNA alkyltransferase. A target for the modulation of drug resistance. Hematol Oncol Clin North Am 1995;9:431–50.
377. Ludlum DB. The chloroethylnitrosoureas: sensitivity and resistance to cancer chemotherapy at the molecular level. Cancer Invest 1997;15:588–98.
378. Zamble DB, Lippard SJ. Cisplatin and DNA repair in cancer chemotherapy. Trends Biochem Sci 1995;20:435–9.
379. Evans CG, Bodell WJ, Tokuda K, et al. Glutathione and related enzymes in rat brain tumor cell resistance to 1,3-bis(2-chloroethyl)-1-nitrosourea and nitrogen mustard. Cancer Res 1987;47:2525–30.
380. Robson CN, Lewis AD, Wolf CR, et al. Reduced levels of drug-induced DNA cross-linking in nitrogen mustard-resistant Chinese hamster ovary cells expressing elevated glutathione S-transferase activity. Cancer Res 1987;47:6022–7.
381. Wolf CR, Hayward IP, Lawrie SS, et al. Cellular heterogeneity and drug resistance in two ovarian adenocarcinoma cell lines derived from a single patient. Int J Cancer 1987;39:695–702.
382. Hamilton TC, Ozols RF, Dabrow MB. Multidrug resistance to alkylating agents and platinum compounds: state of our knowledge. Oncology 1990;4:101–6.
383. Somfai-Relle S, Suzukaki K, Vistica BP, Vistica DT. Reduction in cellular glutathione by buthionine sulfoximine and sensitization of murine tumor cells resistant to L-phenylalanine mustard. Biochem Pharmacol 1984;33:485–90.
384. Nakagawa K, Yokota J, Wada M, et al. Levels of glutathione S transferase pi mRNA in human lung cancer cell lines correlate with the resistance to cisplatin and carboplatin. Jpn J Cancer Res 1988;79:301–4.
385. Miyazaki M, Kohno K, Saburi Y, et al. Drug resistance to cis-diamminedichloroplatinum (II) in Chinese hamster ovary cell lines transfected with glutathione S-transferase pi gene. Biochem Biophys Res Commun 1990;166:1358–64.
386. Fairchild CR, Moscow JA, O'Brien EE, Cowan KH. Multidrug resistance in cells transfected with human genes encoding a variant P-glycoprotein and glutathione S-transferase-pi. Mol Pharmacol 1990;37:801–9.
387. Bunting KD, Lindahl R, Townsend AJ. Oxazaphosphorine-specific resistance in human MCF-7 breast carcinoma cell lines expressing transfected rat class 3 aldehyde dehydrogenase. J Biol Chem 1994;269:23197–203.
388. Colvin M, Russo JE, Hilton J, et al. Enzymatic mechanisms of resistance to alkylating agents in tumor cells and normal tissues. Adv Enzyme Regul 1988;27:211–21.
389. Hilton J, Role of aldehyde dehydrogenase in cyclophosphamide-resistant L1210 leukemia. Cancer Res 1984;44:5156–60.
390. Eastman A, Schulte N. Enhanced DNA repair as a mechanism of resistance to cis-diamminedichloroplatinum(II). Biochemistry 1988;27:4730–4.
391. Sheibani N, Jennerwein MM, Eastman A. DNA repair in cells sensitive and resistant to cis-diamminedichloroplatinum(II): host cell reactivation of damaged plasmid DNA. Biochemistry 1989;28:3120–4.
392. Masuda H, Ozols RF, Lai GM, et al. Increased DNA repair as a mechanism of acquired resistance to cis-diamminedichloroplatinum (II) in human ovarian cancer cell lines. Cancer Res 1988;48:5713–6.
393. Spears CP. Clinical resistance to antimetabolites. Hematol Oncol Clin North Am 1995;9:397–413.
394. Curt GA, Carney DN, Cowan KH, et al. Unstable methotrexate resistance in human small-cell carcinoma associated with double minute chromosomes. New Engl J Med 1983;308:199–202.
395. Allegra CJ, Chabner BA, Drake JC, et al. Enhanced inhibition of thymidylate synthase by methotrexate polyglutamates. J Biol Chem 1985;260:9720–6.
396. Spinella MJ, Brigle KE, Sierra EE, Goldman ID. Distinguishing between folate receptor-alpha-mediated transport and reduced folate carrier-mediated transport in L1210 leukemia cells. J Biol Chem 1995;270:7842–9.
397. Schaub TP, Kartenbeck J, Konig J, et al. Expression of the MRP2 gene-encoded conjugate export pump in human kidney proximal tubules and in renal cell carcinoma. J Am Soc Nephrol 1999;10:1159–69.
398. Cowan KH, Jolivet J. A methotrexate-resistant human breast cancer cell line with multiple defects, including diminished formation of methotrexate polyglutamates. J Biol Chem 1984;259:10793–800.
399. Alt FW, Kellems RE, Bertino JR, Schimke RT. Selective multiplication of dihydrofolate reductase genes in methotrexate-resistant variants of cultured murine cells. J Biol Chem 1978;253:1357–70.
400. Melera PW, Lewis JA, Biedler JL, Hession C. Antifolate-resistant Chinese hamster cells. Evidence for dihydrofolate reductase gene amplification among independently derived sublines overproducing different dihydrofolate reductases. J Biol Chem 1980;255:7024–8.
401. Goldie JH, Krystal G, Hartley D, et al. A methotrexate insensitive variant of folate reductase present in two lines of methotrexate-resistant L5178Y cells. Eur J Cancer 1980;16:1539–46.
402. Flintoff WF, Essani K. Methotrexate-resistant Chinese hamster ovary cells contain a dihydrofolate reductase with an altered affinity for methotrexate. Biochemistry 1980;19:4321–7.
403. Trent JM, Buick RN, Olson S, et al. Cytologic evidence for gene amplification in methotrexate-resistant cells obtained from a patient with ovarian adenocarcinoma. J Clin Oncol 1984;2:8–15.
404. Carman MD, Schornagel JH, Rivest RS, et al. Resistance to methotrexate due to gene amplification in a patient with acute leukemia. J Clin Oncol 1984;2:16–20.
405. Ackland SP, Schilsky RL. High-dose methotrexate: a critical reappraisal. J Clin Oncol 1987;5:2017–31.
406. Kamen BA, Winick NJ. High dose methotrexate therapy: insecure rationale? Biochem Pharmacol 1988;37:2713–5.
407. Jaffe N, Link MP, Cohen D, et al. High-dose methotrexate in osteogenic sarcoma. Natl Cancer Instit Monogr 1981:201–6.
408. Bertino JR. Folate antagonists: toward improving the therapeutic index and development of new analogs. J Clin Pharmacol 1990;30:291–5.
409. Duch DS, Edelstein MP, Bowers SW, Nichol CA. Biochemical and chemotherapeutic studies on 2,4-diamino-6-(2,5-dimethoxybenzyl)-5-methylpyrido[2,3-d]pyrimidine (BW 301U), a novel lipid-soluble inhibitor of dihydrofolate reductase. Cancer Res 1982;42:3987–94.
410. Lin JT, Bertino JR. Trimetrexate: a second generation folate antagonist in clinical trial. J Clin Oncol 1987;5:2032–40.
411. Assaraf YG, Molina A, Schimke RT. Cross-resistance to the lipid-soluble antifolate trimetrexate in human carcinoma cells with the multidrug-resistant phenotype. J Natl Cancer Inst 1989;81:290–4.
412. Allay JA, Galipeau J, Blakley RL, Sorrentino BP. Retroviral vectors containing a variant dihydrofolate reductase gene for drug protection and in vivo selection of hematopoietic cells. Stem Cells 1998;16 Suppl 1:223–33.
413. Bapat AR, Zarow C, Danenberg PV. Human leukemic cells resistant to 5-fluoro-2'-deoxyuridine contain a thymidylate synthetase with lower affinity for nucleotides. J Biol Chem 1983;258:4130–6.
414. Priest DG, Ledford BE, Doig MT. Increased thymidylate synthetase in 5-fluorodeoxyuridine resistant cultured hepatoma cells. Biochem Pharmacol 1980;29:1549–53.
415. Jenh CH, Geyer PK, Baskin F, Johnson LF. Thymidylate synthase gene amplification in fluorodeoxyuridine-resistant mouse cell lines. Mol Pharmacol 1985;28:80–5.
416. Seifert P, et al. Comparison of continuously infused 5-fluorouracil with bolus injection in treatment of patients with colorectal adenocarcinoma. Cancer 1975;36:123–8.
417. Calabro-Jones PM, Byfield JA, Ward JF, Sharp TR. Time-dose relationships for 5-fluorouracil cytotoxicity against human epithelial cancer cells in vitro. Cancer Res 1982;42:4413–20.
418. Arbuck SG. 5-FU/leucovorin: biochemical modulation that works? Oncology 1987;1:61–74.
419. Grem JL, Hoth DF, Hamilton JM, et al. Overview of current status and future direction of clinical trials with 5-fluoro-

uracil in combination with folinic acid. Cancer Treat Rep 1987;71:1249–64.

420. Cadman E, Heimer R, Davis L. Enhanced 5-fluorouracil nucleotide formation after methotrexate administration: explanation for drug synergism. Science 1979;205:1135–7.
421. Cadman E, Heimer R, Benz C. The influence of methotrexate pretreatment on 5-fluorouracil metabolism in L1210 cells. J Biol Chem 1981;256:1695–704.
422. Grem JL, King SA, O'Dwyer PJ, Leyland-Jones B. Biochemistry and clinical activity of N-(phosphonacetyl)-L-aspartate: a review. Cancer Res 1988;48:4441–54.
423. Elias L, Crissman HA. Interferon effects upon the adenocarcinoma 38 and HL-60 cell lines: antiproliferative responses and synergistic interactions with halogenated pyrimidine antimetabolites. Cancer Res 1988;48:4868–73.
424. Momparler RL, Onetto-Pothier N. Drug resistance to cytosine arabinoside. In: Kessel D, editor. Resistance to antineoplastic drugs. Boca Raton (FL): CRC Press; 1989. p. 354–67.
425. Capizzi RL, Yang JL, Rathmell JP, et al. Dose-related pharmacologic effects of high-dose ara-C and its self-potentiation. Semin Oncol 1985;12(2 Suppl 3):65–74.
426. Wiley JS, Jones SP, Sawyer WH, Paterson AR. Cytosine arabinoside influx and nucleoside transport sites in acute leukemia. J Clin Invest 1982;69:479–89.
427. Tanaka M, Yoshida S. Altered sensitivity to 1-beta-D-arabinofuranosylcytosine 5'-triphosphate of DNA polymerase alpha from leukemic blasts of acute lymphoblastic leukemia. Cancer Res 1982;42:649–53.
428. Ho DH, Carter CJ, Brown NS, et al. Effects of tetrahydrouridine on the uptake and metabolism of 1-beta-D-arabinofuranosylcytosine in human normal and leukemic cells. Cancer Res 1980;40:2444–6.
429. Heideman RL, Gillespie A, Ford H, et al. Phase I trial and pharmacokinetic evaluation of fazarabine in children. Cancer Res 1989;49:5213–6.
430. Surbone A, Ford H Jr, Kelley JA, et al. Phase I and pharmacokinetic study of arabinofuranosyl-5-azacytosine (fazarabine, NSC 281272). Cancer Res 1990;50:1220–5.
431. Jordan MA, Wilson L. Microtubules as a target for anticancer drugs. Nat Rev Cancer 2004;4:253–65.
432. Zhou J, Giannakakou P. Targeting microtubules for cancer chemotherapy. Curr Med Chem Anticancer Agents 2005;5:65–71.
433. Orr GA, Verdier-Pinard P, McDaid H, Horwitz SB. Mechanisms of Taxol resistance related to microtubules. Oncogene 2003;22:7280–95.
434. He L, Orr GA, Horwitz SB. Novel molecules that interact with microtubules and have functional activity similar to Taxol. Drug Discov Today 2001;6:1153–64.
435. Hari M, Wang Y, Veeraraghavan S, Cabral F. Mutations in alpha- and beta-tubulin that stabilize microtubules and confer resistance to Colcemid and vinblastine. Mol Cancer Ther 2003;2:597–605.
436. He L, Yang CP, Horwitz SB. Mutations in beta-tubulin map to domains involved in regulation of microtubule stability in epothilone-resistant cell lines. Mol Cancer Ther 2001;1:3–10.
437. Gonzalez-Garay ML, Chang L, Blade K, et al. A beta-tubulin leucine cluster involved in microtubule assembly and paclitaxel resistance. J Biol Chem 1999;274:23875–82.
438. Alli E, Bash-Babula J, Yang JM, Hait WN. Effect of stathmin on the sensitivity to antimicrotubule drugs in human breast cancer. Cancer Res 2002;62:6864–9.
439. Balachandran R, Welsh MJ, Day BW. Altered levels and regulation of stathmin in paclitaxel-resistant ovarian cancer cells. Oncogene 2003;22:8924–30.
440. Rouzier R, et al. Microtubule-associated protein tau: a marker of paclitaxel sensitivity in breast cancer. Proc Natl Acad Sci U S A 2005;102:8315–20.
441. Zhang CC, Yang JM, White E, et al. The role of MAP4 expression in the sensitivity to paclitaxel and resistance to vinca alkaloids in p53 mutant cells. Oncogene 1998;16:1617–24.
442. Murphy M, Hinman A, Levine AJ. Wild-type p53 negatively regulates the expression of a microtubule-associated protein. Genes Dev 1996;10:2971–80.
443. Zhang CC, Yang JM, Bash-Babula J, et al. DNA damage increases sensitivity to vinca alkaloids and decreases sensitivity to taxanes through p53-dependent repression of microtubule-associated protein 4. Cancer Res 1999;59:3663–70.
444. Kielb SJ, Shah NL, Rubin MA, Sanda MG. Functional p53 mutation as a molecular determinant of paclitaxel and gemcitabine susceptibility in human bladder cancer. J Urol 2001;166:482–7.
445. Ioffe ML, White E, Nelson DA, et al. Epothilone induced cytotoxicity is dependent on p53 status in prostate cells. Prostate 2004;61:243–7.

Section 12
CHEMOTHERAPEUTIC AGENTS

42

Folate Antagonists

Peter D. Cole, MD
Barton A. Kamen, MD, PhD
Joseph R. Bertino, MD

Folic acid antagonists (antifols) are cytotoxic drugs used as antineoplastic, antimicrobial, anti-inflammatory, and immune-suppressive agents. Although several folate antagonists have been developed, methotrexate (4-amino-4-deoxy-10-N-methyl-pteroylglutamic acid; MTX; Figure 42-1) is the antifol with the most extensive history and widest spectrum of use. MTX is an essential drug in curative chemotherapy regimens used to treat patients with acute lymphoblastic leukemia, osteosarcoma, and choriocarcinoma, and is an important agent in the therapy of patients with lymphoma, breast cancer, bladder cancer, and head and neck cancer. In addition, it is used for patients with nonmalignant diseases such as rheumatoid arthritis, psoriasis, and graft-versus-host disease. This chapter will primarily review the clinical use of and metabolism of MTX and discuss several other folate antagonists that have been developed to overcome resistance or to have alternate intracellular targets.

HISTORICAL OVERVIEW

In the early 1940s, the combined observations that (1) patients with acute leukemia often have serum folate deficiency and (2) the bone marrow megaloblasts of folate-deficient patients morphologically resemble leukemic blasts prompted some investigators to postulate that acute leukemia might be a result of a deficiency of this B vitamin. The availability of crystalline pteroylglutamic acid (PGA, folic acid; see Figure 42-1), first isolated from spinach in 1941[1] and synthesized in 1945,[2] allowed the investigational administration of folate to patients with leukemia. It was rapidly recognized, however, that folic acid administration was not only ineffective, but also often accelerated the course of the disease of patients with chronic myelocytic leukemia and acute leukemia.[3]

Efforts to treat these leukemias thus turned to pharmacologically mimicking folate deficiency using folate analogues with effects antagonistic to those of the vitamin. Aminopterin (4-amino-4-deoxy PGA; AMT; see Figure 42-1) was the first of these analogues to produce temporary remissions in five of sixteen patients with acute leukemia.[4] This demonstration was a landmark in cancer chemotherapy: It provided the first demonstration that an antimetabolite could be an effective antineoplastic agent.

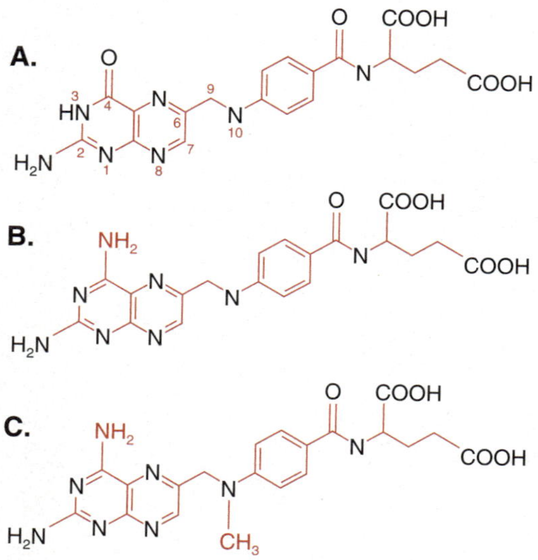

Figure 42-1 Structure of folic acid and structurally related classic antifols, AMT and MTX. **A,** Folic acid (pteroylglutamic acid; PGA). **B,** Aminopterin (4-amino-PGA). **C,** Methotrexate (4-amino-N-10-methyl PGA).

Since that initial study demonstrating the usefulness of AMT in the treatment of acute leukemia of childhood, there has been a sustained interest in, and a continued reevaluation of, this and other folate antagonists. Although known to be less potent, MTX supplanted AMT in the clinic in the early 1950s because the toxicity caused by AMT was greater and less predictable.[5–9] However, it is of interest that these two drugs have not been compared in a clinical trial. Newer antifols are rationally designed analogues of folates or MTX, synthesized either in an effort to overcome cellular resistance to MTX or to target alternative folate-dependent processes. Some of these newer antifols have been approved as antimicrobials or antineoplastic agents and others are still in clinical trial.

MECHANISM OF ACTION

Folate antagonists are cytotoxic drugs that act by interfering with one or more biosynthetic steps involving folate coenzymes. A folate analogue might function in one of several ways: by competing with folates for uptake into cells, by inhibiting the formation of folate coenzymes, or by inhibiting one or more reactions that are mediated by folate coenzymes.

Thus far, the clinically important antineoplastic folate analogues appear to work primarily by inhibiting dihydrofolate reductase (DHFR) or thymidylate synthase (TS). The prototypic antifol DHFR inhibitor is a 4-amino-substituted pterin compound (see Figure 42-1). The substitution of an amino moiety for the 4-hydroxyl results in a folate analogue with a several thousand-fold increase in affinity for DHFR. The K_i of MTX for DHFR is below 10^{-10} M, well below the K_m of the natural substrate, dihydrofolate, which is in the micromolar range.

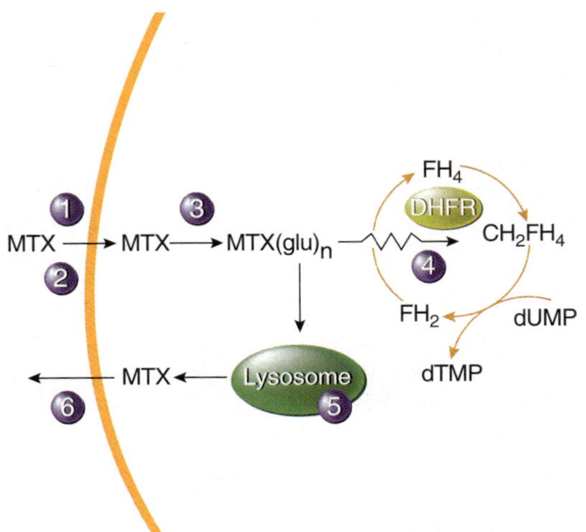

Figure 42-2 Primary site of action of MTX and MTX(glu)N. MTX enters cells by either the reduced folate carrier (1) or the membrane folate binding protein (2). MTX is then metabolized by the cytosolic enzyme folylpolyglutamate synthetase (3) to MTX(glu)N, a potent inhibitor of dihydrofolate reductase (DHFR) (4). MTX(glu)N can be hydrolyzed to MTX by the lysosomal enzyme γ-glutamyl hydrolase (GGH) (5). CH_2FH_4 = N5, N10-methylene tetrahydrofolate; dTMP = deoxythymidine monophosphate; dUMP = deoxyuridine monophosphate/deoxyuridylate; FH_2 = dihydrofolate; FH_4 = tetrahydrofolate; MTX = methotrexate; MTX(glu) N = MTX polyglutamates.

By stoichiometrically inhibiting DHFR, thereby blocking the cell's ability to replenish a supply of reduced folates necessary for de novo thymidine synthesis, MTX disrupts a critical step in the synthesis of DNA (Figure 42-2).[10] In rapidly dividing cells, the inhibition of thymidylate biosynthesis leads to a decrease in thymidine triphosphate pools, a decrease in DNA synthesis, and eventually cell death.[11,12] Inhibition of tetrahydrofolate formation leading to the inhibition of purine synthesis and rapid cell death has also been described as occurring in lymphoblasts treated with high doses of MTX.[13] The other approved antifol for the treatment of mesothelioma and non–small cell lung cancer is pemetrexed, which primarily targets TS, but also is a potent inhibitor of DHFR and glycinamide ribonucleotide transformylase (GARFT).

Intracellular metabolism of classical antifols like MTX to polyglutamate species significantly impacts their function and mechanisms of cytotoxicity.[14] The cytosolic enzyme, folylpolyglutamate synthetase (FPGS), adds glutamate residues in γ-carboxyl linkage to both folate coenzymes and classic folate antagonists (those with a glutamate moiety).[15,16] This addition of up to seven or eight additional glutamate molecules serves to add both mass and negative charge, markedly reducing efflux and increasing total intracellular accumulation at steady state.[17] Both quantitative differences in FPGS expression and qualitative differences in FPGS function[18] exist between neoplastic and nonneoplastic tissues, which may explain some of the selectivity of antifolates for neoplastic cells.[19] A relative lack of FPGS may explain the observation that a cell population with a large number of G_0 cells would be less affected by the same concentration and time of exposure to MTX than a population with more actively dividing cells.

MTX polyglutamates are more potent inhibitors of DHFR than the parent compound, because, although they bind as tightly to DHFR as MTX, they dissociate less rapidly.[20] In addition, MTX polyglutamates are also potent inhibitors of other folate-requiring enzymes, including TS[21] and two of the rate limiting steps of de novo purine synthesis: glycinamide ribonucleotide (GAR) and aminoimidazole carboxamide ribonucleotide (AICAR) transformylases.[22] Dihydrofolate polyglutamates and the formylated form of this coenzyme (10-formyl dihydrofolate), which increase after MTX blockage of DHFR, are also potent inhibitors of TS and GAR transformylase.[23] Thus, inhibition of de novo purine synthesis may be at least as necessary as DHFR inhibition for the cytotoxic effects of MTX in cancer cells[24] and for the anti-inflammatory action of MTX in patients with rheumatologic diseases.[25,26]

Two other possible mechanisms by which MTX exerts antineoplastic or anti-inflammatory action are worth mentioning. First, by inhibiting folate-dependent remethylation to methionine, MTX causes intracellular levels of homocysteine (Hcy) to rise, and a secondary elevation in S-adenosyl-homocysteine (SAH), a potent inhibitor of many folate-dependent methylation reactions. MTX exposure, therefore, can block membrane localization of ras,[27] a member of a family of critical signal transduction proteins constitutively activated in a number of human cancers.

In light of recent interest in angiogenesis as an important target for antineoplastic therapy, it is worthwhile to note that MTX has long been used as an anti-inflammatory agent at doses well below those thought to be cytotoxic.[28] It may be that this anti-inflammatory effect, and some degree of its antineoplastic activity, is due to its ability to inhibit endothelial cell proliferation at physiologically attainable concentrations, as was first documented in 1989.[29]

PHARMACOKINETICS OF MTX

MTX is one of few anticancer agents for which pharmacokinetic data are routinely used in clinical practice, especially when high doses with leucovorin rescue are employed.[30] Clinical use of pharmacokinetic data has been related to improved MTX efficacy. Retrospective analysis of children with acute lymphoblastic leukemia (ALL) shows that lower MTX clearance[31] and higher MTX concentrations[32] are associated with lower risk of relapse. Even more intriguing are data from a prospective randomized trial in patients with ALL comparing dosing by body surface area (BSA) with individualized dosing based on pharmacokinetic data, which showed significantly improved complete continuous remission rates in the individualized therapy arm.[33] It is possible, however, that these results are protocol-specific, since others have found that pharmacologically guided treatment intensification led to inferior outcomes for some subpopulations.[34]

Absorption Following oral administration, peak plasma concentrations may occur 1 to 5 hours after a dose of 15 to 30 mg/m^2. Food, nonabsorbable antibiotics, bile salts, and a shortened intestine transit time may decrease the rate and extent of MTX absorption.[35] Thus, it is suggested that the drug be taken on an empty stomach with clear liquids.

In contrast with older reports,[36] recent studies have emphasized the relatively poor and unpredictable nature of absorption of MTX after oral administration.[37,38] Nevertheless, at a dose and schedule of 25 mg/m^2, given orally every 6 hours times four doses, plasma MTX concentration greater than 0.5 μM were seen in more than 85% of pediatric patients with ALL.[39] Moreover, over an 18 month time period, there was no malabsorption as a result of therapy, which also included daily 6-mercaptopurine.

Distribution After intravenous (IV) administration of MTX, the initial volume of distribution (V_d) is approximately 0.18 L/kg of body weight. Steady-state V_d is between 0.4 and 0.8 L/kg.[40] The initial distribution phase has a $T_{1/2}$ of 30 to 45 minutes; the beta $T_{1/2}$ is 3 to 4 hours.

After high doses of MTX (> 6 g/m^2), serum concentrations in the range of 10^{-4} to 10^{-3} M are achieved.[41] At these concentrations, transmembrane transport is saturated, limiting further influx of drug to passive diffusion. These high extracellular MTX concentrations inhibit the uptake of reduced folates, including exogenous administered leucovorin (LV), explaining the need for larger doses of LV to reverse MTX action because of the competitive nature of this interaction at the transport level. Studies of MTX metabolism in lymphoblasts in vitro have also shown that too high an extracellular concentration of drug can impede metabolism of MTX to a polyglutamate.[42] The clinical significance is not known, but the observation further calls into question whether the use of high-dose MTX, other than to penetrate a sanctuary site such as the CNS or in the therapy of osteosarcoma, is worth the expense and risks.[43,44]

MTX binding to plasma proteins, especially to albumin, is approximately 50%.[45,46] The 7-hydroxymetabolite of MTX is 90% bound to plasma proteins, but apparently does not interfere with MTX binding to plasma proteins at concentrations found in patients. The highest tissue-to-plasma concentrations found in humans are in the liver and kidney, followed by the gastrointestinal tract. Prolonged plasma levels after high-dose MTX infusions in humans have been attributed to decreased transit rate secondary to gastrointestinal obstruction.

Because of the blood-brain barrier and active efflux mechanisms,[47,55] cerebrospinal fluid (CSF) MTX concentrations are approximately 1% of those in the plasma. Cytocidal concentrations are therefore not obtained in the CSF after conventional doses (15–30 mg/m^2), but can be reached with doses of 500 mg/m^2 and higher.[48,49] After high-dose systemic MTX administration, lumbar CSF and ventricular CSF concentrations were similar. High-dose MTX (HDMTX) may, therefore, be able to replace intrathecal drug for the treatment of patients with nonleukemic leptomeningeal disease.[50] However, a recent meta-analysis of CNS-directed therapy for children with acute lymphoblastic leukemia concluded that efforts to increase CSF penetration using HDMTX have not produced the desired result of lowering the rate of CNS relapse in this population.[51]

Although MTX is accumulated poorly into the CSF, even small doses of LV given orally can increase CSF folates significantly. This systemic rescue, especially if given too early after MTX, may rescue cells in the CSF compartment.[52]

When MTX is given by the lumbar route into the CSF, it distributes unreliably into the ventricles, while MTX given by an indwelling ventricular shunt provides reproducible therapeutic drug concentrations (> 10^{-6} M) for at least 48 hours.[53] An improved dose schedule utilizing the administration of multiple small doses of intrathecal MTX has been suggested.[54] Following intrathecal administration, MTX slowly exits into the systemic circulation with a $T_{1/2}$ of 8 to 10 hours.[55] Systemic toxicity can be observed if multiple doses of intrathecal MTX are administered without LV rescue. The pharmacology of intrathecal MTX and the amount of intraventricular MTX may be altered by overt meningeal leukemia and the position of the patient at the time of lumbar puncture.[56] The clinical observation that irradiation followed by MTX treatment may predispose patients to neurotoxicity may be a consequence of the effect of radiation therapy on the blood-brain barrier.[57]

Patients with pleural or peritoneal effusions may be at increased risk of developing toxicity to HDMTX as a result of "third spacing," or MTX trapping in the infusion, and slow release leading to sustained MTX concentrations in serum.[58] This phenomenon is more a problem when high doses of the drug are administered. In these circumstances, higher doses and prolonged rescue with LV may be necessary until the serum level of MTX decreases to less than 5 × 10^{-8} M.

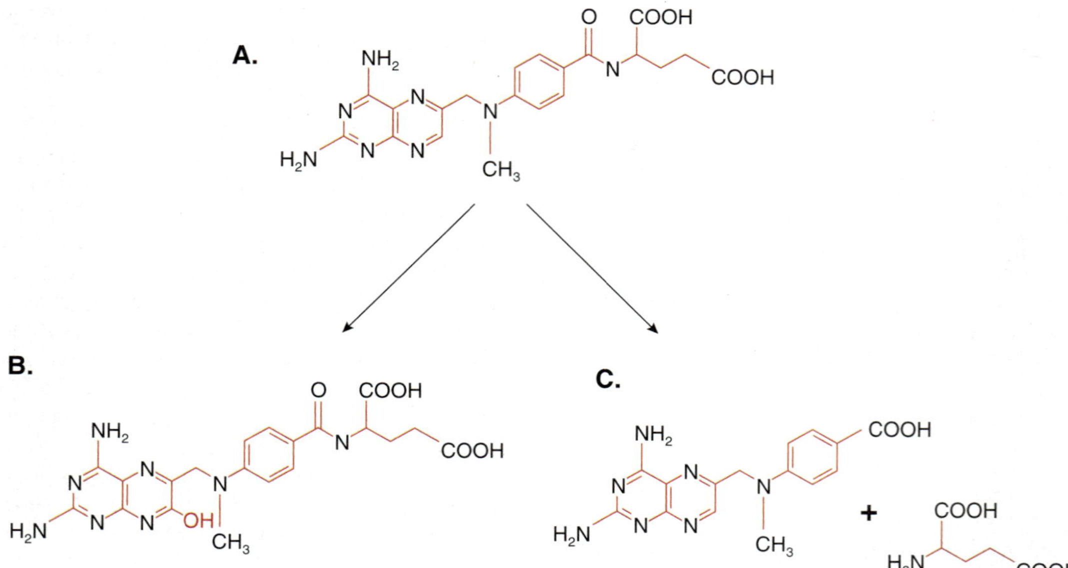

Figure 42-3 Catabolism of MTX. MTX (*A*) can be converted in the liver to 7-OH MTX (*B*). In addition, enteric bacteria will cleave the molecule to dAMPA plus glutamate (*C*).

Metabolism The major metabolite of MTX, produced by the action of hepatic aldehyde oxidase, is 7-hydroxy MTX (7-OH MTX) (Figure 42-3).[59,60] 7-OH-MTX is only 1% as potent an inhibitor of DHFR as MTX.[61,62] It is also less water soluble than MTX and may contribute to the renal toxicity frequently seen after high doses of the antifolate.[63]

A second, less important pathway of metabolism of MTX occurs in the intestine. MTX is hydrolyzed by bacteria to the pteroate (4-deoxy-4-amino-N10-methyl pteroic acid, dAMPA) and glutamic acid (see Figure 42-3).[64] dAMPA, like 7-OH MTX, is also a relatively inactive metabolite with approximately 1/200th the affinity of MTX for DHFR. dAMPA excretion in the urine accounts for only a small percentage of the dose administered (< 5%).

As mentioned, the third metabolic product of MTX that occurs via intracellular conversion is MTX polyglutamate. MTX polyglutamates are at least as potent inhibitors of DHFR as MTX and have a slower rate of disassociation from DHFR than MTX.[20] MTX polyglutamates are not found in plasma or urine because of the activity of γ-glutamyl hydrolase(s) (GGH) in plasma that convert folyl- and MTX-polyglutamates to monoglutamates. Like MTX, 7-OH MTX is also polyglutamylated intracellularly, and retention of these polyglutamate forms could contribute to MTX cytotoxicity.[65,66]

Excretion Most of administered MTX (and its metabolites 7-OH MTX and dAMPA) is excreted unchanged in the urine.[67,68] Nevertheless, there is wide interpatient variability in MTX clearance, which does not correlate perfectly with renal function.[69] Because of active secretion in the proximal tubules, renal clearance of MTX can exceed creatinine clearance.[70] MTX excretion through organic acid transporters can be inhibited by probenecid or competitively blocked by other weak organic acids, such as aspirin or penicillin G. MTX elimination is increased by drugs that block distal tubular reabsorption, such as folic acid, some cephalosporins, and sulfamethoxazole.

Following IV administration of doses of 30 to 80 mg/m^2, 0.4 to 20% of the administered dose is excreted through the canalicular multiorganic acid transporter (cMOAT; also known as ABCC2 or MRP2) into the bile. Less than 10% of MTX is recovered in the feces.[71] Abnormal MRP2 activity may affect the pharmacokinetics and pharmacodynamic profile of camptothecins, cisplatin (CDDP) and vinca alkaloids, and overexpression of MRP2 has been shown to confer resistance to MTX in vitro.[72] It may be that there are polymorphisms in MRP2 that account for the large interpatient variability in pharmacokinetics after high-dose MTX administration.

DRUG INTERACTIONS

As indicated above, several drugs used in cancer patients, including antibiotics, may alter the renal excretion of MTX, increasing toxicity or decreasing efficacy. Deleterious and even fatal reactions have been reported between MTX and nonsteroidal anti-inflammatory drugs, in particular with naproxen and ketoprofen.[73–75] This increased toxicity may be due to decreased renal elimination, possibly as a result of competition for renal secretion.[70] Other commonly used organic drugs may also potentiate MTX toxicity, such as phenylbutazone, salicylate, and probenecid.[76,77] Probenecid increased the efficacy of MTX in tumor-bearing mice, but it has not been used clinically with this goal in mind.[78]

Increased toxicity was also reported when trimethoprim, the antibacterial agent, was used together with MTX. Presumably this antifolate, with only weak binding affinity to mammalian DHFR, lowers folate stores, especially in patients with subclinical folate deficiency, making marrow cells more susceptible to MTX-induced toxicity.[79,80] Alcohol should also be avoided in patients receiving MTX because of the risk of hepatic fibrosis and cirrhosis.

PHARMACOGENOMICS

There is a growing body of data implicating inherited variation in genes for enzymes responsible for folate metabolism in interpatient variability in antifolate response or toxicity.[81,82] Functional poly-

Table 42-1 Dosage Schedules Commonly Used for Methotrexate (MTX)

Schedule and Dose	Use/Comments
Oral:	
Weekly or biweekly (15–25 mg in single or divided doses)	Mainly for nonmalignant conditions, such as psoriasis or rheumatoid arthritis
Weekly or biweekly (20–30 mg/m^2)	Maintenance therapy for ALL
Parenteral:	
Pulse weekly (30–60 mg/m^2)	Choriocarcinoma, ALL
Intermediate dose (120–500 mg/m^2 weekly)	ALL, NHL; requires LV rescue, 10–15 mg/m^2 q6h × 6–8 doses
High-dose (500–12,000 mg/m^2 weekly or every other week)	Osteosarcoma, ALL, neoplastic meningitis; requires LV rescue

ALL = acute lymphoblastic leukemia; LV = leucovorin; NHL = non-Hodgkin's lymphoma.

morphisms have been described in either the promoter or coding regions of the genes for DHFR, TS, methylenetetrahydrofolate reductase (MTHFR), methionine synthase, methionine synthase reductase, RFC, and serine hydroxymethyltransferase. Many of these polymorphisms are present at significant frequency among the population and some have been linked to higher rates of relapse or toxicity among patients with acute lymphoblastic leukemia[83,84] or rheumatoid arthritis.[85] If replicated in larger populations, these data suggest the potential for one day individualizing MTX therapy based on each patient's genotype.

CLINICAL APPLICATION

MTX has been administered on a variety of dosage schedules since its introduction into the clinic five decades ago (Table 42-1). Remarkably, there are few carefully controlled studies comparing different dose regimens. In a trial of MTX in patients with head and neck cancer treated with either 50, 500, or 5,000 mg/m^2 with LV "rescue," a trend of dose responsiveness was seen (5 of 24, 5 of 16, 9 of 18, respectively). Some responses were noted with the 5,000 mg/m^2 dose regimen in patients who failed at lower doses.[86] The importance of dosage scheduling was emphasized by an experimental study showing that resistance to high-dose pulse MTX may not extend to continuous low-dose exposure.[87]

Determining the optimum dosage schedule of MTX is complicated by the use of the drug in combination therapy. Sequencing appears to be important when MTX is used with 5-fluorouracil (5-FU) (24-hour pretreatment with MTX appears to be best), with L-asparaginase (again, 24-hour pretreatment is best), and probably with cytosine arabinoside (concurrent treatment may be optimal) and 6-mercaptopurine or 6-thioguanine (pretreatment with MTX may be optimal). Table 42-2 summarizes the use of some common drug combinations that include MTX.

CURRENT USES FOR MTX IN THE TREATMENT OF NEOPLASTIC DISEASE

Acute Leukemia MTX is used as part of nearly all therapeutic regimens for acute lymphoblastic leukemia postremission, in combination with a thiopurine[88] and/or asparaginase.[89,90] In addition, it is administered intrathecally for the prophylaxis, or treatment of, meningeal leukemia and is included in some regimens for remission induction. Early studies showed that twice-weekly therapy (20 mg/m^2) was superior to continuous daily oral administration for treatment during remission.[91] Other dosage schedules appear to be even more beneficial, including 5-day courses administered every 3 to 4 weeks, or high-dose regimens with LV rescue.[92,93] The effectiveness of an oral divided dosage (25–30 mg/m^2 given every 6 hours for 4–6 doses weekly) has also been shown.[39] It is clear that the optimum dose and schedule of MTX has not yet been defined conclusively and may vary with each disease.[43,44]

MTX has limited value in the treatment of acute nonlymphocytic leukemia, although in the 1970's, the use of MTX and L-asparaginase ("Capizzi Regimen") resulted in a significant proportion of remissions in patients with acute myelogenous leukemia (AML).[90,94] High-dose regimens with LV rescue have a transient but rapid effect on the peripheral blood count without producing marrow remissions in the large majority of these patients.[95] The lack of efficacy of MTX in this disease has been attributed to poor intracellular retention of the drug caused by a lack of polyglutamylation and an increase of the target enzyme DHFR following treatment with it.[96]

Lymphoma Based on phase II studies that indicated that moderate to high doses of MTX (200 mg/m^2 to 3 gm/m^2) with LV rescue could produce transient regressions in patients with large-cell lymphoma, MTX with LV rescue has been added to combination regimens for intermediate-grade and high-grade lymphomas.[97] In certain of these regimens (methotrexate, bleomycin, doxorubicin [Adriamycin], cyclophosphamide, vincristine [Oncovin], and dexamethasone [M-BACOD]), MTX is used with LV during the leukopenic phase of drug treatment, since the MTX/LV combination has little marrow toxicity.[98] Based on experimental studies showing that MTX and cytosine arabinoside produce additive and possibly synergistic effects,[99] this combination has also been used in regimens to treat this disease (eg, COMLA; cyclophosphamide, vincristine, MTX, cytosine arabinoside, and LV).[100]

Similarly, following documentation of responses among patients with Burkitt's lymphoma to therapy including MTX,[101,102] high-dose MTX with LV rescue has been added to cyclophosphamide, vincristine, doxorubicin (Adriamycin), and dexamethasone (CVAD), cytarabine, and intrathecal therapy,[103] as well as to other combination chemotherapy regimens[104–106] for patients with Burkitt's lymphoma.

The inclusion of high-dose MTX seems to be important in the treatment of patients with primary central nervous system (CNS) lymphomas. In a retrospective review of 226 patients with primary CNS lymphoma, those patients treated with regimens that included HDMTX followed by radiotherapy had an improved survival, with no higher risk of late neurotoxicity.[107] However, others have disputed this finding.[108]

Choriocarcinoma Choriocarcinoma is unique in that single-drug treatment with either MTX or actinomycin D produces a substantial number of cures.[109] The basis for the unusual sensitivity of this tumor to MTX is not entirely clear, but choriocarcinoma cells may accumulate and retain this drug effectively by synthesizing long-chain polyglutamates. The JAR (human choriocarcinoma) cell line was shown to have active-receptor coupled uptake (potocytosis) of folates and antifolates.[110] Current programs for the treatment of this malignancy utilize MTX in combination with other drugs, especially for "poor-risk" patients.[111]

Breast Cancer MTX as a single agent causes regressions of breast cancer in approximately 30% of patients. No single dose schedule has emerged as the optimum treatment when the drug is used as a single agent, including high-dose treatment with LV rescue. When used with fluorouracil, sequential use of MTX followed by 5-FU improved response rates to 50%; this sequential combination improved disease-free survival when used as adjuvant therapy.[112] The combination of cyclophosphamide, MTX, and 5-FU (CMF), when used as adjuvant therapy, significantly reduces the risk of relapse,[113]

Table 42-2 Combination Chemotherapy with Methotrexate (MTX)

Used With	Schedule Notes	Result	Comments
5-FU	MTX must precede 5-FU by 24 h	Synergistic	
Anthracyclines		Additive	
Bleomycin		Additive	Mucosal toxicity is increased
Corticosteroids	Used together	Synergistic	Used in ALL
Cyclophosphamide	Used together	Additive	
Cytarabine	Used together	Additive or synergistic	
L-asparaginase	If MTX precedes L-asparaginase by 24 h	Synergistic	Used in ALL, AML
	If used simultaneously	Antagonistic	
Vinca alkaloids		Additive	

ALL = acute lymphoblastic leukemia; AML = acute myelogenous leukemia; 5-FU = 5-fluorouracil.

may allow more conservative surgery among women with localized disease when used as neoadjuvant therapy,[114] and has a role in the treatment of patients with inoperable, advanced disease.[115] The combination of MTX and 5-FU with vinorelbine (VMF) instead of cyclophosphamide has also shown activity among women with advanced breast cancer.[116] An additional advantage of this combination is the diminution of long-term toxicity (infertility, carcinogenesis) compared with regimens containing alkylating agents. Finally, it is interesting to note that low-dose oral MTX (2.5 mg bid × 2d/wk) with daily oral cyclophosphamide has shown activity among heavily pretreated women with advanced metastatic breast cancer.[117]

Gastrointestinal Cancer MTX has limited effectiveness in the treatment of gastrointestinal malignancies.[118] Its role in the treatment of these diseases is mainly to modulate, and possibly improve, the effectiveness of 5-FU. By inhibiting purine synthesis, MTX pretreatment increases phosphoribosyl pyrophosphate, a precursor necessary for 5-FU nucleotide formation.[119] Data from recent trials using high-dose MTX followed by LV/5-FU in patients with colon cancer emphasize the need for a 7- to 24-hour interval between MTX and 5-FU administration.[120] Similar combinations also show activity for patients with advanced gastric cancer.[121,122]

Genitourinary Cancer MTX alone (100 mg/m^2), or in high doses (> 0.5 g/m^2) with LV rescue, is clearly active in the treatment of advanced bladder cancer. The response rate reported (approximately 30%) is similar to the response rate of the other most active single drug, cisplatin. Combinations of drugs including MTX with cisplatin, vinblastine, and doxorubicin (M-VAC) have resulted in a substantial number of long-term clinical remissions.[123] A meta-analysis of randomized trials found that neoadjuvant treatment with MTX-containing regimens conferred a clear survival advantage.[124,125]

Head and Neck Cancer MTX and cisplatin are the two most active single agents for the treatment of patients with advanced carcinoma of the head and neck region. High-dose MTX regimens with LV rescue appear to improve response rates from 30 to 50%, but remission duration and survival are not improved.[126] MTX has also been used with 5-FU in this disease, with response rates as high as 60%.[127,128] The sequence and timing of drug administration have not been shown to affect the response rate, although different patterns of toxicity were observed.[126]

Lung Cancer MTX as a single agent in conventional doses, or in high doses with LV rescue, has only marginal activity in non–small cell lung cancer.[129] This drug does have limited activity in small-cell lung cancer, and has been used in combination regimens to treat that disease.

Osteogenic Sarcoma After studies were reported indicating that high-dose MTX with LV rescue could cause regressions in patients with advanced osteogenic sarcoma, the drug was tested as adjuvant therapy in patients with disease following resection of the tumor, with encouraging results.[130] Randomized trials of pre- and post-definitive treatment have demonstrated the beneficial effect of chemotherapy that includes high-dose MTX with LV rescue,[131,132] and response may correlate with MTX dose density (defined as the amount of drug administered during a defined period of time).[133]

However, a recent report demonstrated the paradoxical finding that higher MTX exposure (higher peak concentration and higher area under the curve [AUC]) was associated with inferior outcome among patients with localized osteosarcoma.[134] Analysis of intracellular MTX in osteogenic sarcoma biopsy specimens < 24 hours after MTX administration may explain the difficulty in demonstrating clear clinical superiority of high-dose MTX. Despite 200-fold differences in dose, and 1,000-fold differences in plasma MTX concentrations, HDMTX produced only a 2.5-fold increase in intracellular MTX polyglutamates compared with repetitive oral low-dose MTX.[135] Based on the effectiveness of platinum and Adriamycin and potential renal toxicity associated with use of both MTX and platinum, some centers are eliminating the use of HDMTX unless the tumor has a poor response to initial therapy.[43]

Neoplastic Meningitis Intrathecal MTX is often a component of therapy for patients with solid-tumor neoplastic meningitis. High-dose MTX (8 g/m^2) given as the sole treatment with LV rescue may be a reasonable alternative. A recent report compared a historical control group with 16 patients with solid-tumor neoplastic meningitis given high-dose MTX alone. The study documented longer duration of cytotoxic MTX concentrations in the CSF and prolonged survival of the IV group compared with the intrathecal (IT) group.[50]

ADVERSE EFFECTS

Hematologic Toxicity Expression of many folate-dependent enzymes targeted by MTX are cell-cycle specific, consistent with their role in DNA synthesis. Tissues that are self-renewing, with a higher S-phase fraction, are therefore at highest risk of damage by the folate antagonists. Bone marrow progenitor cells of all lineages are affected by MTX, but neutropenia usually predominates. Recovery takes place 14 to 21 days following a nadir that occurs approximately 10 days after drug administration. The effects on the marrow are dose related, but there is considerable variability among patients. Subclinical folate deficiency, impaired renal function, a damaged marrow owing to previous radiation therapy, chemotherapy, or infection, and the use of trimethoprim-sulfamethoxazole for *Pneumocystis carinii* prophylaxis may predispose patients to hematologic (and gastrointestinal) toxicity. Young patients usually tolerate MTX better than do older individuals, a fact presumably related to clearance of the drug by the kidneys. The administration of LV, before 42 hours have elapsed, if in an appropriate dose, may prevent or lessen MTX toxicity and allow larger doses of the antifolate to be administered.[136]

Gastrointestinal Toxicity Mucositis is a common side effect of MTX treatment and usually becomes manifest 3 to 5 days following a dose or course of the drug. This is an early sign of MTX toxicity, and the drug should be discontinued when it occurs. More severe gastrointestinal toxicity is manifest by diarrhea, which may progress to severe bloody diarrhea. When this occurs in association with neutropenia, patients are at high risk of sepsis and death. These severe side effects generally occur in a setting of renal damage, usually a consequence of high doses of MTX, but may also occur in patients treated with conventional doses. MTX blood levels and serum creatinine levels should be followed, and appropriate doses of LV administered, along with the supportive measures instituted (see below). Nausea and vomiting, even with high doses of MTX, are usually mild to moderate.

Renal Toxicity Conventional-dose MTX regimens, not requiring LV, were occasionally reported to cause renal toxicity, presumably as a direct effect of MTX on renal tubular epithelium.[137] With the introduction of high-dose regimens requiring LV rescue, renal toxicity leading to delayed MTX clearance sometimes resulted in severe marrow and gastrointestinal toxicity, occasionally fatal, especially in adults.[43] This toxicity is believed to be due to precipitation of MTX and its less soluble metabolite, 7-OH MTX, in the tubules, as well as to a possible direct effect of this drug on the renal tubule.[63] The use of vigorous hydration, often with osmotic diuresis and alkalinization of urine to increase solubility of MTX and 7-OH MTX, has markedly ameliorated this problem. Occasional patients, even with this regimen (Table 42-3), exhibit renal impairment. Through careful monitoring of MTX and creatinine serum levels, these patients may be identified and larger doses and prolonged duration of LV employed to prevent toxicity.

Methylxanthines, such as caffeine or aminophylline, may be useful in the setting of delayed MTX clearance. MTX administration has been shown to increase adenosine content.[25] Since adenosine will decrease the glomerular filtration rate (GFR), adenosine receptor competitive antagonists, like the methylxanthines, may act as a specific diuretic to increase MTX elimination.[138]

Extremely high levels of MTX (> 10^{-3} M) are difficult to rescue, even with high doses of LV.[139] Hemodialysis and peritoneal dialysis have proved ineffective in substantially lowering MTX plasma levels. Charcoal hemoperfusion columns have been used successfully in a small number of patients.[140] Oral charcoal and cholestyramine have also been used to bind MTX in the gut, thus limiting enterohepatic recirculation and toxicity.[141] Thymidine (1–3 g/m^2/d) is also capable of rescuing patients from MTX toxicity, but this metabolite is not generally available.[142] Carboxypeptidase G1 or

Table 42-3 Supportive Care for High-Dose Methotrexate (MTX) Treatment

Pretreatment hydration and alkalinization
8 to 12 hours before treatment, patients should receive 1.5 L/m^2 of saline or 5% glucose with 100 mEq HCO_3 and 20 mEq KCl/L. Continue hydration until urine pH is 7.0 or greater before MTX administration.

Monitoring
MTX levels should be monitored at 24 hours after completion of MTX infusion. Serum creatinine should be measured pretreatment, at 24, and at 48 hours.

Additional LV rescue
Required for an MTX level greater than 10^{-6} *M* at 24 hours. Increase LV dose to 100 mg/m^2 q 6 h for levels above 10^{-6} *M* and 200 mg/m^2 q 6 h for levels above 5×10^{-6} *M*. Monitor MTX levels daily and continue LV until plasma MTX concentration is less than 10^{-8} *M*.

LV = leucovorin.

more recently, the recombinant form, G2, an enzyme capable of cleaving the peptide bond in MTX resulting in glutamate and dAMPA (see Figure 42-3), has also been used to rapidly lower MTX levels, but dAMPA is even less soluble than MTX.[143] When given in combination with thymidine and LV, carboxypeptidase G2 is highly effective in patients at high risk of developing life-threatening MTX toxicity after intravenous[144,145] or intrathecal MTX administration.[146,172]

Hepatotoxicity Chronic low-dose continuous treatment with MTX has been associated with portal fibrosis, and in some patients, with frank cirrhosis.[147] The basis for this liver damage is not known, but it may result from interference with folate homeostasis, since acute MTX hepatotoxicity in rats is reversed by choline administration.[148] Cirrhosis has been reported in patients with psoriasis, rheumatoid arthritis, and ALL treated with long-term continuous oral MTX.[149] Concurrent administration of dexamethasone may increase MTX-induced hepatotoxicity.[150] Alcohol and other hepatotoxic drugs should be avoided in these patient populations.

Intermittent schedules with pulse therapy appear to decrease the incidence of fibrosis and cirrhosis.[151] In the absence of other complicating conditions as noted above, it may be that the risk of hepatotoxicity has been somewhat exaggerated. Acute elevations of liver enzymes (serum glutamic oxaloacetic transaminase [SGOT]) commonly occur several days after treatment with high-dose MTX, but rapidly return to normal and do not appear to predict for chronic liver toxicity.[152] Based on a recent study of children with ALL, it also appears that, in the absence of hepatitis C, there are no significant permanent sequelae in patients with increased liver enzymes, even to 10 to 20 times normal.[153]

Central Nervous System Toxicity Intrathecal MTX and intravenous administration of high-dose MTX have been associated with neurotoxicity, ranging from mild to severe. In cases of inadvertent overdosing (> 100 mg intrathecally), fatalities have been reported. Greater understanding of the pathophysiology of MTX-induced neurotoxicity is now beginning to lead to therapeutic interventions to prevent or treat this complication of therapy.[154,155]

The most common immediate side effect of intrathecal MTX administration, made manifest by severe headache, fever, meningismus, vomiting, and CSF pleocytosis, is thought to be caused by a chemical arachnoiditis directly, or perhaps by the release of adenosine, which is a potent autocoid in the CNS. This effect of adenosine has been ameliorated by systemic administration of low doses of methylxanthines, such as aminophylline and theophylline, which act as competitive antagonists at adenosine receptors.[138] Acute toxicity occurring several days after high-dose systemic MTX treatment manifests with headache, paresis, aphasia, or seizures. It is usually transient, resolving within 2 to 3 days.[156,157] Dosage adjustment or switching to cytosine arabinoside may be required if these symptoms persist.

Subacute neurotoxicity (7–14 days after administration) has been observed in 5 to 18% of patients receiving intrathecal MTX and/or intravenous high-dose MTX.[158,159] At its most severe, it presents with motor paralysis of the extremities, cranial nerve palsies, seizures, and even coma. Although the pathogenesis of subacute antifolate-induced neurotoxicity is likely multifactorial, increases in Hcy may play a pivotal role. By inhibiting remethylation to methionine, MTX therapy leads to increased amounts of Hcy in the plasma and CSF of patients treated with MTX.[154] Higher CSF Hcy is observed among patients with symptoms of MTX-induced neurotoxicity than among asymptomatic patients receiving similar therapy.[160] Since Hcy is an excitotoxic amino acid (glutamate analogue) that activates the *N*-methyl-D-aspartate receptor (NMDA), it has been suggested that the subacute neurotoxicity of MTX can be ameliorated by a antagonist of the NMDA receptor, such as dextromethorphan.[160]

Delayed MTX-induced neurotoxicity may be associated with chronic demyelinating encephalopathy in as many as 80% of children with acute lymphoblastic leukemia, and the magnitude of the radiographic changes seems to correlate with number and the dose of IV MTX.[161,162] Computed tomography scans show cortical thinning, ventricular enlargement, and diffuse intracerebral calcifications.[163] Although most commonly attributed to the combination of cranial radiation with intrathecal MTX, encephalopathy has been reported in patients treated only with high-dose IV MTX. The pathogenesis of delayed neurotoxicity is not well defined, and may be a result of impairing folate-dependent methylation of components of the myelin sheath.[155,164-167] Providing an exogenous methyl donor, such as S-adenosylmethionine[168] or betaine[169] provides some benefit to patients with Alzheimer's dementia (similarly thought to be related to perturbations in methylation within the CNS[170]), but have not yet been used in patients receiving MTX.

In patients who receive an MTX overdose intrathecally (> 100 mg), immediate CSF removal with ventricolumbar perfusion is indicated.[171] Recently, intrathecal use of carboxypeptidase G2, an enzyme that cleaves MTX to glutamate plus dAMPA, was shown to decrease mortality markedly in animals given a lethal dose of MTX intrathecally, and may be the preferred therapy for this complication.[146,172] Intrathecal or systemic LV is not indicated in these cases, since it is unlikely that this toxicity is attributable to inhibition of DHFR.

Pulmonary Toxicity Although uncommon, pulmonary toxicity due to MTX has been described, and has been noted even in patients receiving low-dose oral MTX for rheumatoid arthritis.[173,174] The clinical picture usually consists of cough, dyspnea, fever, and hypoxemia. Chest radiograph findings are nonspecific, but may show patchy interstitial infiltrates. *Pneumocystis carinii* must be ruled out, especially in patients also receiving steroids. Histologic examinations show diffuse interstitial lymphocytic infiltrates, giant cells, and noncaseating granulomas. In some patients, a peripheral eosinophilia is observed, raising the possibility that this is an allergic pneumonitis. The process may progress to fibrosis, and it is important to discontinue MTX while the pulmonary toxicity is reversible. Some patients have been retreated without recurrence of the problem.

Skin Toxicity Skin toxicity to MTX occurs in 5 to 10% of patients. It manifests as an erythematous rash, characteristically noted on the neck and upper trunk. The rash may be pruritic and relatively insignificant, and usually lasts for several days. In other instances, especially when related to other signs of severe MTX toxicity, it may progress to severe bullous formation and desquamation.[175] A cutaneous vasculitis after intermediate-dose MTX has also been reported.[176]

Teratogenic and Mutagenic Effects Folate deficiency alters gene expression by causing hypomethylation of DNA, and increases DNA strand breaks by causing misincorporation of uracil instead of thymine. Consequently, folate deficiency can directly influence carcinogenesis.[177] MTX is known to be a potent abortifacient, especially if administered during the first trimester of pregnancy. Nevertheless, there is no direct evidence that MTX has any mutagenic or carcinogenic effects,[178] as there is no indication of a higher than normal incidence of fetal abnormalities in women who have been successfully treated with MTX for choriocarcinoma. Nor have these women had a higher than normal incidence of secondary malignancies.

Miscellaneous Toxicity Osteoporosis has been reported with chronic low-dose MTX administration,[179] and may result from direct inhibition of osteoblastic differentiation.[180] Fever, seizures, recall of radiation toxicity or phototoxicity, and anaphylactoid reactions have been reported with high-dose administration.[181] Pleuritic and left-upper-quadrant pain, presumably attributable to splenic capsule inflammation, has been reported with a moderately high-dose regimen. An acute hemolytic anemia owing to an IgG-3 antibody that reacts with erythrocytes only in the presence of MTX has been described.[182]

RESISTANCE TO ANTIFOLATES

Although the development of effective chemotherapeutic regimens including MTX has significantly improved the therapy of a number of different malignancies, achieving prolonged disease-free survival is still difficult even in chemotherapy-sensitive diseases. The efficacy of MTX, as with other antineoplastic agents, is ultimately limited by either inherent resistance or resistance acquired during the course of therapy. Resistance to MTX has been documented as a result of changes at each of the following steps: decreased transport into the cell, decreased metabolism to polyglutamate forms, altered interaction with the target enzyme DHFR, increased breakdown of polyglutamates, and increased efflux from the cell. Additionally, because both DHFR and FPGS activity fluctuate with cell cycle, dysregulation of cell-cycle genes may have a profound effect on antimetabolite resistance.

Intrinsic Resistance to MTX A number of lines of investigation are beginning to explain the range of intrinsic resistance to MTX seen across different tumor types both clinically and in vitro. Comparisons of leukemic blasts obtained at diagnosis from patients with AML with those obtained from patients with ALL suggest that differing ability to form long-chain MTX polyglutamates to some degree explains the relative clinical resistance of AML to MTX, compared with ALL. AML blasts have been shown to accumulate less long-chain MTX polyglutamate than ALL blasts,[183,184] with no differences in MTX transport, or in DHFR. In addition, fresh human tumor cells from patients with soft tissue sarcoma as well as certain human cancer cell lines naturally resistant to MTX, especially to short-term exposures, have been similarly found to have a low capacity to form long-chain MTX polyglutamates.[185,186]

Higher MTX-polyglutamate accumulation in B-lineage ALL blasts as compared with T-lineage blasts may be explained by the finding of higher FPGS activity in B-lineage blasts.[187,188] The possibility that different isoforms (splice variants) of FPGS are expressed in different tissues is supported by the finding of differences in FPGS affinity for MTX between AML and ALL cell lines and blast samples,[189] and between resistant and sensitive sarcoma cell lines,[190] as well as by differences between FPGS isolated from L1210 cells and murine liver in degree of inhibition by long-chain folylpolyglutamates.[18] The fact that the ratio of FPGS to GGH enzyme activity in leukemic blasts obtained at diagnosis correlates better with the ratio of long-chain to total MTX polyglutamate accumulation than the activity of either enzyme alone, suggests that the balance of the two enzymes determines the steady-state MTX polyglutamate accumulation and intrinsic MTX sensitivity.[191] However, forced overexpression of GGH in cancer cell lines does not cause MTX resistance.[192]

Impaired ability to transport MTX into cells through the reduced folate carrier also can cause intrinsic resistance. Decreased expression of *RFC* mRNA has been documented by quantitative RT-PCR in osteosarcoma samples at initial biopsy,[193] possibly explaining the clinical observation that MTX is ineffective against this disease at conventional doses, but effective in higher doses. Additionally, mutations in the *RFC* gene corresponding to altered transport function have been documented both in resistant cell lines[194] and in leukemic blasts at diagnosis.[195] Single nucleotide polymorphisms in the gene for *RFC* can result in proteins with a decreased affinity for antifolates, while maintaining sufficient affinity for folate to allow continued cell growth. Other known polymorphisms selectively increase affinity for folates and increase the intracellular folate pool. However, in one analysis of 246 pediatric leukemia patient samples, only 3 were found to have potentially functional *RFC* polymorphisms, suggesting they do not appear to play a major role in intrinsic MTX resistance in this population.[196]

Finally, lack of the retinoblastoma protein, frequently deleted or altered in many tumor types, may play a role in MTX resistance. In the absence of retinoblastoma protein, levels of the transcription factor E2F increase, resulting in an increase in transcription of several genes involved in DNA replication, including *DHFR*.[197–199]

Overexpression of p-glycoprotein does not confer resistance to MTX. However, MTX is a substrate for the related proteins, multidrug resistance proteins 1-5 (ABCC1-5)[200,201] and the breast cancer resistance protein (ABCG2).[202] ABCC5[201] and ABCG2[203] are able to transport both MTX and MTX-diglutamate. Overexpression of these proteins has been shown to be associated with MTX resistance in vitro,[201,204,205] and may affect the response to therapy among patients with leukemia.[206,207] It is not yet clear to what degree these proteins contribute to clinically relevant intrinsic resistance to MTX in other diseases.

Acquired Resistance to MTX Four predominant mechanisms of acquired resistance to MTX have been described in experimental tumors and clinical samples: an increase in DHFR activity because of amplification of this gene, altered binding of MTX to DHFR owing to DHFR mutations, and a decrease in uptake of MTX because of either a decreased influx of MTX through the RFC or a decrease of long-chain polyglutamate formation.

Unstable or reversible resistance due to gene amplification has usually been associated with the presence of "double-minute" chromosomes containing the DHFR amplicon, while high-level stable resistance has been associated with an abnormal banding region, often referred to as a homogeneously staining region (HSR).[208–210] Since the original description of DHFR gene amplification in MTX-resistant mouse tumor cells,[211] a number of mouse, hamster, and human MTX-resistant cell lines have been described, with increased DHFR and amplification of the *DHFR* gene as a mechanism of MTX resistance[212–214] Gene amplification as a mechanism of resistance occurs in some patients treated with MTX.[215–217]

Although several MTX-resistant cell lines have been found to possess an altered DHFR that has a decreased affinity for MTX, only few altered human DHFRs have been characterized in any detail.[218-222] Point mutations in DHFR in several cell lines, including human cells, have been detected that cause a change in the binding of MTX to the enzyme, and have usually involved amino acids that bind to the inhibitor by hydrophobic interaction.[223]

Although defects in polyglutamylation have been described in several MTX-resistant cell lines,[224] the resistance of these cells has usually been found to be attributable to a combination of mechanisms.[225–227] Decreased levels of MTX polyglutamates in cells may also result from increased breakdown; indeed, both intrinsic and acquired resistance to MTX in cell lines have been attributed to increased levels of GGH activity.[186,228] However, forced overexpression of GGH did not result in MTX resistance.[192] Some clinical studies have shown a strong correlation between the amount of MTX polyglutamates formed in blasts and disease-free survival in children with ALL.[229,230] This type of data is likely protocol-specific and needs to be interpreted cautiously when extrapolating to newer protocols. Indeed, more recent studies have produced contradictory data.[231,232]

At the point of entry into the cell, either mutations or deletions in the RFC could result in decreased uptake of MTX and MTX resistance. Although polymorphisms in the gene for RFC do not seem to be a common mechanism of intrinsic resistance among patients with leukemia,[196] decreased transport of MTX through the RFC has been shown to be a common mechanism of acquired resistance to MTX in leukemic blasts from patients with relapsed ALL.[233]

STRATEGIES TO OVERCOME RESISTANCE TO MTX USING NEW (OR OLDER) ANTIFOLS

Understanding the molecular basis of normal folate physiology, MTX cytotoxicity, and MTX resistance is allowing and guiding the rational design of new folate antagonists and strategies to selectively target resistant cells. Thus, to overcome resistance, the newer antifolates have been designed to have one or more of the following properties: increased transport into the cell by either increased affinity for the RFC or independence of the RFC, independence of polyglutamylation or increased polyglutamylation by virtue of increased affinity for FPGS, increased inhibition of DHFR or TS, or increased inhibition of enzymes responsible for purine synthesis. The work will undoubtedly be guided by computer graphics using crystallographic data from the target enzymes.[223] The reader is directed to recent in-depth reviews[234,235] of the rapid development of novel antifolates.

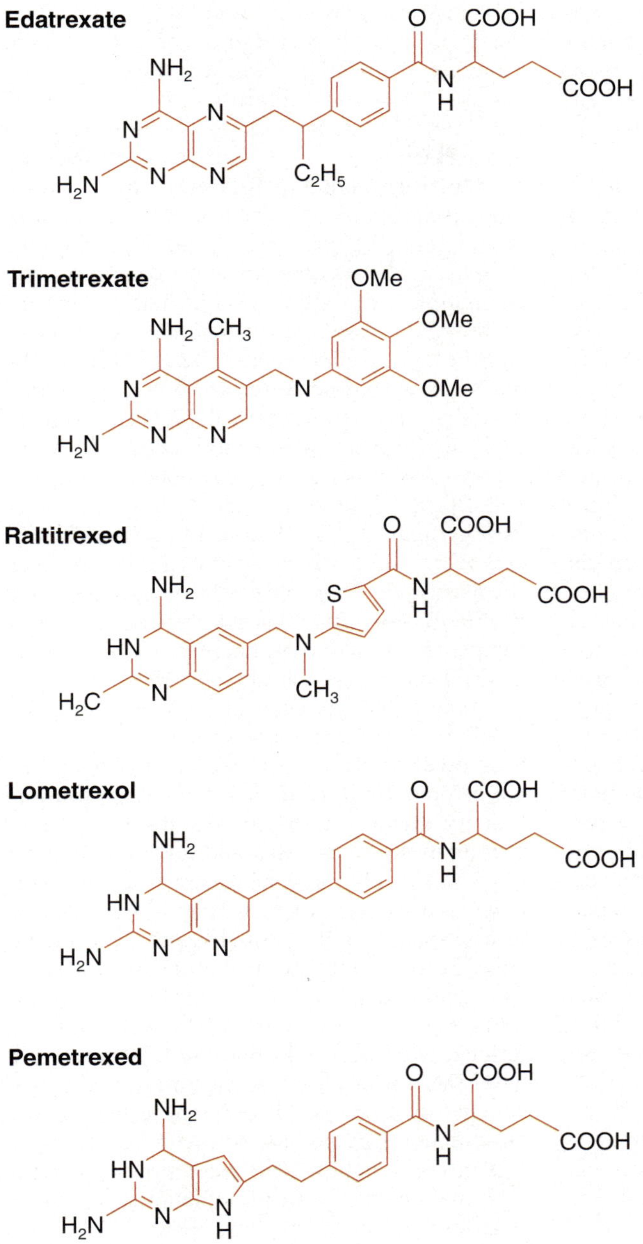

Figure 42-4 Novel folate antagonists of clinical interest.

Aminopterin (AMT) There are some recent data to support reevaluating an antifol older than MTX, 4-amino-pteroyl-glutamic acid (aminopterin; now being developed under the trade name Aminotrexate). AMT (see Figure 42-1) was the first antifolate to produce remissions among patients with leukemia.[4] AMT has several advantages over MTX, including 20 to 40 times greater clinical potency,[9,236] more efficient conversion (higher V_{max}:K_m ratio) by the enzyme folylpolyglutamate synthetase to polyglutamates,[237] leading to greater accumulation by patients' leukemic blasts in vitro,[238] and complete oral bioavailability.[239] A phase II trial of AMT in patients with refractory leukemia reaffirmed its potency, complete oral bioavailability, and potential utility, with 6 responses, including 3 complete responses (CRs), in 22 children refractory to MTX-containing regimens.[240] A phase IIb trial substituting AMT for MTX in multiagent therapy for newly diagnosed children with ALL at high risk of relapse is currently underway.[241]

Newer Inhibitors of DHFR MTX is an extremely potent inhibitor of DHFR. Although it may be possible to develop inhibitors that are more tightly bound or may irreversibly inactivate this enzyme, selectivity may not improve, unless these compounds possess other advantages (ie, more avid uptake and/or more efficient retention by malignant cells as compared with normal cells).

10-Ethyldeazaaminopterin (edatrexate; Figure 42-4), was chosen for clinical trial after detailed structure activity studies demonstrated that hydrophobic substitutions at the N10 position of AMT resulted in improved uptake and retention (polyglutamylation) by tumor cells as compared with normal cells.[242] Encouraging response rates have been noted in patients with non–small cell lung cancer, head and neck cancer, breast cancer, and malignant fibrous histiocytoma.[243–246] One limitation to its use might be that it may be relatively ineffective against MTX-resistant cells, since it uses the same carrier mechanism for transport and is polyglutamylated by the same enzyme as MTX. Further development of edatrexate was stopped when a potentially more active analogue, 10-propargyl-deazaaminopterin (PDX), was shown to be more effective than edatrexate in preclinical models,[247] likely attributable to increased uptake by the RFC folate transporter and greater intracellular polyglutamylation. PDX has shown activity in a phase II trial for patients with previously treated non–small cell lung cancer.[248]

Trimetrexate (see Figure 42-4) is a nonclassical antifolate (lacking a glutamate moiety). Like MTX, it is a potent inhibitor of DHFR, but crosses the cell membrane by passive or facilitative diffusion rather than through the RFC.[249,250] Consequently, trimetrexate (TMTX) and other nonclassical antifolates can still exert cytotoxic effects against MTX-resistant cells when the mechanism of resistance is impaired transport, decreased polyglutamylation, or even low-level amplification of DHFR.[251–253] Cells resistant to MTX owing to a mutation in DHFR leading to decreased binding of the inhibitor may or may not be cross-resistant to trimetrexate, depending on the nature of the mutation.[223] These drugs also differ from MTX in that they are not substrates for polyglutamate synthetase; therefore, retention depends on other factors. Unlike MTX, TMTX, for example, is a substrate for the p-glycoprotein efflux pump, so it may show cross-resistance to other P-glycoprotein (P-gp) substrate antineoplastic agents.[254]

One strategy for the use of trimetrexate stems from the observation that some human tumors, either intrinsically or after treatment are unable to transport reduced folates (or MTX) because of decreased expression of a functional RFC. Similar to the approach currently being taken to treat *Pneumocystis carinii* pneumonia (PCP),[255] the coadministration of trimetrexate and LV would therefore be toxic to these tumor cells, but nontoxic to the normal host tissues (capable of transporting the rescue agent LV).[256,257]

Trimetrexate is also under investigation as a modulating agent, based on preclinical data that trimetrexate followed by 5-FU and high-dose LV led to synergistic cell kill, when MTX followed by 5-FU and LV did not. Responses were noted in the phase II studies of this combination for patients with advanced gastrointestinal cancers, with manageable toxicity.[258,259] Two phase III studies have shown some evidence that this combination will delay tumor progression in patients with colorectal cancer; however, when the two studies were analyzed, there was no survival benefit when compared with 5-FU/LV treatment.[260]

Inhibitors of Other Folate-Dependent Enzymes During recent years, other targets for the development of folate antagonists have been identified, including TS, GAR, and AICAR transformylases. Potent inhibitors of TS and GAR transformylases have been synthesized and are now under active investigation (see Figure 42-4).[234,235,261]

Inhibitors of Thymidylate Synthetase The potential advantages of folate inhibitors of TS over 5-FU are that these agents are not incorporated into RNA, and that the greater deoxyuridine monophosphate (dUMP) levels that may result as a consequence of inhibition of this enzyme might increase, rather than decrease, the inhibition of TS.[262] Based on a series of structure–activity studies and toxicity studies in animals, the folate analogue, N-(5-[N-(3,4-dihydro-2-methyl-4-oxoquinazolin-6-ylmethyl)-N-methylamino]-2-thenoyl)-l-glutamic acid (D1694, raltitrexed, Tomudex; see Figure 42-4), was chosen for further clinical trials and has shown clinical activity in colorectal carcinoma.[263,264] Raltitrexed primarily targets TS, but is also a potent inhibitor of DHFR and GARFT. Of interest is that raltitrexed, even more so than MTX, is a "prodrug," in that polyglutamylation increases cytotoxicity. A phase I and pharmacokinetic trial in pediatric patients with refractory leukemia documented tolerable toxicity in this population, and 3 responses in 18 patients.[265] Among adults with colon cancer, activity comparable to 5-FU/LV has been demonstrated in phase III trials.[266–268] Raltitrexed has been licensed in Europe and Canada for use in the treatment of colon cancer. It is now being tested in combination therapy for patients with gastrointestinal malignancies.[269–271]

ZD9331 is a novel, nonpolyglutamatable antifolate inhibitor of TS.[261] Like raltitrexed, it binds with high affinity to folate receptor alpha, suggesting it will have increased activity in tumors that highly overexpress this receptor,[272] such as some ovarian cancers.

Inhibitors of Purine Synthesis 5-10-Dideazatetrahydrofolate (DDTHF; Lometrexol; see Figure 42-4) is also a prodrug. The addition of glutamates to the molecule markedly increases the inhibition of GAR transformylase. DDTHF is extremely potent, and low doses of this agent have produced delayed and prolonged marrow suppression in early clinical trials that was not predicted by rodent toxicity data.[273] This may be due to its rapid accumulation by folate receptor positive cells—and to the relatively folate-deficient state of patients in contrast to that of rodent models. DDTHF has been dropped from clinical development.

4-[2-(2-amino-4-oxo-4,6,7,8-tetrahydro-3H-pyrimidino[5,4,6][1,4]thiazin-6-yl)-(S)-ethyl]-2,5-thienoylamino-L-glutamic acid (AG2034) is a second generation GARFT inhibitor, designed using knowledge of the x-ray crystal structure of GARFT.[274] Phase I trials employing every-three-week dosing have been completed,[275,276] and its activity is being tested in phase II trials.

Multitargeted Antifolates Since much clinical resistance is related to amplification or mutation of single target enzymes, an antifol that inhibits more than one biosynthetic pathway and/or multiple steps within a single pathway has the theoretical advantage that the development of significant resistance would be less likely. The antifol analogue pemetrexed N-[4-[2-(2-amino-4,7-dihydro-4-oxo-1H-pyrrolo[2,3-d] pyrimidin-5-yl) ethyl] benzoyl]-L-glutamic acid; Alimta; see Figure 42-4) was initially developed as an inhibitor of GARFT, but was found to have inhibitory activity against AICAR transformylase, DHFR, and TS as well. It is a substrate for the reduced folate carrier (RFC), and can be polyglutamylated by FPGS. Polyglutamylation appears necessary for pemetrexed to significantly inhibit TS and GARFT but not for inhibition of DHFR.

Pemetrexed has been in clinical trials since 1995.[277] Its toxicities are similar to those seen with other antifols, with neutropenia being the major dose-limiting toxicity. Nondose-limiting toxicity includes transient elevations in serum transaminases, mucositis, and rashes. A number of phase II studies have been completed in a wide range of tumor types.[278] Among 517 patients who received pemetrexed as a single agent at 500 mg/m^2 every 21 days, with dexamethasone treatment and folic acid and vitamin B_{12} supplementation, the most common adverse events were nausea, fatigue, anorexia, and vomiting.[279] Pemetrexed has FDA approval as second-line treatment of patients with non–small cell lung cancer, based on a randomized comparison with docetaxel,[280] and in combination with cisplatin for patients with malignant pleural mesothelioma, based on superior results over cisplatin alone.[279,281]

REFERENCES

1. Mitchell HK, Snell EE, Williams RJ. The concentration of "Folic Acid". J Am Chem Soc 1941;63:2284.
2. Angier RB, Boothe JH, Hutchings BL. Synthesis of a compound identical with the L. Casei Factor. Science 1945;102:227.
3. Farber S, Cutler EC, Hawkins JW, et al. Action of pteroylglutamic conjugates on man. Science 1947;106:619–21.
4. Farber S, Diamond L, Mercer RD, et al. Temporary remissions in acute leukemia in children produced by folic acid antagonist, 4-aminopteroyl-glutamic acid (aminopterin). N Engl J Med 1948;238:787.
5. Meyer LM, Fink H, Sawitsky A, et al. Aminopterin (a folic acid antagonist) in the treatment of leukemia. Am J Clin Pathol 1949;19:119–26.
6. Sacks MS, Bradford GT, Schoenbach EB. The response of acute leukemia to the administration of the folic acid antagonists, aminopterin and amethopterin: report of 14 cases. Ann Int Med 1950;32:80–115.
7. Mills SD, Stickney JM, Hadedorn AB. Observations on acute leukemia in children treated with 4-aminopteroylglutamic acid. Pediatrics 1950;5:52–6.
8. Meyer LM, Newman A. Treatment of leukemia with aminopterin. Am J Med 1951;10:452–8.
9. Farber S, Toch R, Sears EM, et al. Advances in chemotherapy of cancer in man. In: Greenstein HA (editor): Advances in cancer research. New York: Academic Press; 1956. p. 2–73.
10. Osborne MJ, Freeman MB, Huennekens FM. Inhibition of dihydrofolic reductase by aminopterin and amethopterin. Proc Soc Exp Biol Med 1958;97:429–31.
11. Tattersall MH, Jackson RC, Jackson ST, et al. Factors determining cell sensitivity to methotrexate: studies of folate and deoxyribonucleoside triphosphate pools in five mammalian cell lines. Euro J Cancer 1974;10:819–26.
12. Fridland A. Effect of methotrexate on deoxyribonucleotide pools and DNA synthesis in human lymphocytic cells. Cancer Res 1974;34:1883–8.
13. Hryniuk WM. Purineless death as a link between growth rate and cytotoxicity by methotrexate. Cancer Res 1972;32:1506–11.
14. Chabner BA, Allegra CJ, Curt GA, et al. Polyglutamation of methotrexate. Is methotrexate a prodrug? J Clin Invest 1985;76:907–12.
15. Cichowicz DJ, Shane B. Mammalian folylpoly-gamma-glutamate synthetase. 2. Substrate specificity and kinetic properties. Biochemistry 1987;26:513–21.
16. Clarke L, Waxman DJ. Human liver folylpolyglutamate synthetase: biochemical characterization and interactions with folates and folate antagonists. Arch Biochem Biophys 1987;256:585–96.
17. Balinska M, Galivan J, Coward JK. Efflux of methotrexate and its polyglutamate derivatives from hepatic cells in vitro. Cancer Res 1981;41:2751–6.
18. Andreassi JL, 2nd, Moran RG. Mouse folylpoly-gamma-glutamate synthetase isoforms respond differently to feedback inhibition by folylpolyglutamate cofactors. Biochemistry 2002;41:226–35.
19. Koizumi S, Curt GA, Fine RL, et al. Formation of methotrexate polyglutamates in purified myeloid precursor cells from normal human bone marrow. J Clin Invest 1985;75:1008–14.
20. Jolivet J, Chabner BA. Intracellular pharmacokinetics of methotrexate polyglutamates in human breast cancer cells. Selective retention and less dissociable binding of 4-NH2-10-CH3-pteroylglutamate4 and 4-NH2-10-CH3-pteroylglutamate5 to dihydrofolate reductase. J Clin Invest 1983;72:773–8.
21. Allegra CJ, Chabner BA, Drake JC, et al. Enhanced inhibition of thymidylate synthase by methotrexate polyglutamates. J Biol Chem 1985;260:9720–6.
22. Allegra CJ, Drake JC, Jolivet J, et al. Inhibition of phosphoribosylaminoimidazolecarboxamide transformylase by methotrexate and dihydrofolic acid polyglutamates. Proc Natl Acad Sci U S A 1985;82:4881–5.
23. Baram J, Chabner BA, Drake JC, et al. Identification and biochemical properties of 10-formyldihydrofolate, a novel folate found in methotrexate-treated cells. J Biol Chem 1988;263:7105–11.
24. Allegra CJ, Hoang K, Yeh GC, et al. Evidence for direct inhibition of de novo purine synthesis in human MCF-7 breast cells as a principal mode of metabolic inhibition by methotrexate. J Biol Chem 1987;262:13520–6.
25. Cronstein BN, Naime D, Ostad E. The antiinflammatory mechanism of methotrexate. Increased adenosine release at inflamed sites diminishes leukocyte accumulation in an in vivo model of inflammation. J Clin Invest 1993;92:2675–82.
26. Johnston A, Gudjonsson JE, Sigmundsdottir H, et al. The anti-inflammatory action of methotrexate is not mediated by lymphocyte apoptosis, but by the suppression of activation and adhesion molecules. Clin Immunol 2005;114(2):154–63.
27. Winter-Vann AM, Kamen BA, Bergo MO, et al. Targeting Ras signaling through inhibition of carboxyl methylation: an unexpected property of methotrexate. Proc Natl Acad Sci U S A 2003;100:6529–34.
28. Cronstein BN. The mechanism of action of methotrexate. Rheum Dis Clin North Am 1997;23:739–55.
29. Hirata S, Matsubara T, Saura R, et al. Inhibition of in vitro vascular endothelial cell proliferation and in vivo neovascularization by low-dose methotrexate. Arthritis Rheum 1989;32:1065–73.
30. Stoller RG, Hande KR, Jacobs SA, et al. Use of plasma pharmacokinetics to predict and prevent methotrexate toxicity. N Engl J Med 1977;297:630–4.
31. Borsi JD, Moe PJ. A comparative study on the pharmacokinetics of methotrexate in a dose range of 0.5 g to 33.6 g/m^2 in children with acute lymphoblastic leukemia. Cancer 1987;60:5–13.
32. Evans WE, Crom WR, Abromowitch M, et al. Clinical pharmacodynamics of high-dose methotrexate in acute lymphocytic leukemia. Identification of a relation between concentration and effect. N Engl J Med 1986;314:471–7.
33. Evans WE, Relling MV, Rodman JH, et al. Conventional compared with individualized chemotherapy for child-

hood acute lymphoblastic leukemia. N Engl J Med 1998;338:499–505.
34. Schmiegelow K, Bjork O, Glomstein A, et al. Intensification of mercaptopurine/methotrexate maintenance chemotherapy may increase the risk of relapse for some children with acute lymphoblastic leukemia. J Clin Oncol 2003;21:1332–9.
35. Said HM, Hollander D. Inhibitory effect of bile salts on the enterohepatic circulation of methotrexate in the unanesthetized rat: inhibition of methotrexate intestinal absorption. Cancer Chemother Pharmacol 1986;16:121–4.
36. Henderson ES, Adamson RH, Oliverio VT. The metabolic fate of tritiated methotrexate. II. Absorption and excretion in man. Cancer Res 1965;25:1018–24.
37. Balis FM, Savitch JL, Bleyer WA: Pharmacokinetics of oral methotrexate in children. Cancer Res 1983;43:2342–5.
38. Kearney PJ, Light PA, Preece A, et al. Unpredictable serum levels after oral methotrexate in children with acute lymphoblastic leukaemia. Cancer Chemother Pharmacol 1979;3:117–20.
39. Winick N, Shuster JJ, Bowman WP, et al. Intensive oral methotrexate protects against lymphoid marrow relapse in childhood B-precursor acute lymphoblastic leukemia. J Clin Oncol 1996;14:2803–11.
40. Huffman DH, Wan SH, Azarnoff DL, et al. Pharmacokinetics of methotrexate. Clin Pharmacol Ther 1973;14:572–9.
41. Evans WE, Pratt CB, Taylor RH, et al. Pharmacokinetic monitoring of high-dose methotrexate. Early recognition of high-risk patients. Cancer Chemother Pharmacol 1979;3:161–6.
42. Hum MC, Smith AK, Lark RH, et al. Evidence for negative feedback of extracellular methotrexate on blasts of acute lymphoblastic leukemia in vitro. Pharmacotherapy 1997;17:1260–6.
43. Ackland SP, Schilsky RL. High-dose methotrexate: a critical reappraisal. J Clin Oncol 1987;5:2017–31.
44. Mantadakis E, Cole PD, Kamen BA. High-dose methotrexate in acute lymphoblastic leukemia: where is the evidence for its continued use? Pharmacotherapy 2005;25:748–55.
45. Steele WH, Lawrence JR, Stuart JF, et al. The protein binding of methotrexate by the serum of normal subjects. European J Clin Pharmacol 1979;15:363–6.
46. Steele WH, Lawrence JR, Stuart JF, et al. The protein binding of methotrexate in the serum of patients with neoplastic disease. Cancer Chemother Pharmacol 1981;7:61–4.
47. Rubin R, Owens E, Rall D. Transport of methotrexate by the choroid plexus. Cancer Res 1968;28:689–94.
48. Evans WE, Hutson PR, Stewart CF, et al. Methotrexate cerebrospinal fluid and serum concentrations after intermediate-dose methotrexate infusion. Clin Pharmacol Ther 1983;33:301–7.
49. Shapiro WR, Young DF, Mehta BM. Methotrexate: distribution in cerebrospinal fluid after intravenous, ventricular and lumbar injections. N Engl J Med 1975;293:161–6.
50. Glantz MJ, Cole BF, Recht L, et al. High-dose intravenous methotrexate for patients with nonleukemic leptomeningeal cancer: is intrathecal chemotherapy necessary? J Clini Oncol 1998;16:1561–7.
51. Clarke M, Gaynon P, Hann I, et al. CNS-directed therapy for childhood acute lymphoblastic leukemia: childhood ALL Collaborative Group overview of 43 randomized trials. J Clin Oncol 2003;21:1798–809.
52. Thyss A, Milano G, Etienne MC, et al. Evidence for CSF accumulation of 5-methyltetrahydrofolate during repeated courses of methotrexate plus folinic acid rescue. Br J Cancer 51989;9:627–30.
53. Mehta BM, Glass JP, Shapiro WR. Serum and cerebrospinal fluid distribution of 5-methyltetrahydrofolate after intravenous calcium leucovorin and intra-Ommaya methotrexate administration in patients with meningeal carcinomatosis. Cancer Res 1983;43:435–8.
54. Bertino JR, Sawicki WL, Lindquist CA, et al. Schedule-dependent antitumor effects of methotrexate and 5-fluorouracil. Cancer Res 1977;37:327–8.
55. Bode U, Magrath IT, Bleyer WA, et al. Active transport of methotrexate from cerebrospinal fluid in humans. Cancer Res 1980;40:2184–7.
57. Storm AJ, van der Kogel AJ, Nooter K. Effect of X-irradiation on the pharmacokinetics of methotrexate in rats: alteration of the blood-brain barrier. Euro J Cancer Clin Oncol 1985;21:759–64.
58. Wan SH, Huffman DH, Azarnoff DL, et al. Effect of route of administration and effusions on methotrexate pharmacokinetics. Cancer Res 31974;4:3487–91.
59. Fabre G, Seither R, Goldman ID. Hydroxylation of 4-aminoantifolates by partially purified aldehyde oxidase from rabbit liver. Biochem Pharmacol 1986;35:1325–30.
60. Johns DG, Loo TL. The metabolite of 4-amino-4-deoxy-N10-methylpteroylglutamic acid (methotrexate). J Pharm Sci 1967;56:356.
61. Erttmann R, Bielack S, Landbeck G. Kinetics of 7-hydroxy-methotrexate after high-dose methotrexate therapy. Cancer Chemother Pharmacol 1985;15:101–4.
62. Redetzki HM, Redetzki JE, Elias AL. Resistance of the rabbit tomethotrexate: isolation of a drug metabolite with decreased cytotoxicity. Biochem Pharmacol 1966;15:425–33.
63. Jacobs SA, Stoller RG, Chabner BA, et al. 7-Hydroxymethotrexate as a urinary metabolite in human subjects and rhesus monkeys receiving high dose methotrexate. J Clin Invest 1976;57:534–8.
64. Valerino DM, Johns DG, Zaharko DS, et al. Studies of the metabolism of methotrexate by intestinal flora. I. Identification and study of biological properties of the metabolite 4-amino-4-deoxy-N 10 -methylpteroic acid. Biochem Pharmacol 1972;21:821–31.
65. McGuire JJ, Hsieh P, Bertino JR. Enzymatic synthesis of polyglutamate derivatives of 7-hydroxymethotrexate. Biochem Pharmacol 1984;33:1355–61.
66. Rhee MS, Galivan J. Conversion of methotrexate to 7-hydroxymethotrexate and 7-hydroxymethotrexate polyglutamates in cultured rat hepatic cells. Cancer Res 1986;46:3793–7.
67. Freeman MV. The fluorometric measurement of the absorption, distribution and excretion of single doses of 4-amino-10-methyl-pteroylglutamic acid (amethopterin) in man. J Pharmacol Exp Ther 1958;122:154.
68. Calvert AH, Bondy PK, Harrap KR. Some observations on the human pharmacology of methotrexate. Cancer Treat Rep 1977;61:1647–56.
69. Joannon P, Oviedo I, Campbell M, et al. High-dose methotrexate therapy of childhood acute lymphoblastic leukemia: lack of relation between serum methotrexate concentration and creatinine clearance. Pediatr Blood Cancer 2004;43:17–22.
70. Huang KC, Wenczak BA, Liu YK. Renal tubular transport of methotrexate in the rhesus monkey and dog. Cancer Res 1979;39:4843–8.
71. Creaven PJ, Hansen HH, Alford DA, et al. Methotrexate in liver and bile after intravenous dosage in man. Br J Cancer 1973;28:589–91.
72. Koike K, Kawabe T, Tanaka T, et al. A canalicular multispecific organic anion transporter (cMOAT) antisense cDNA enhances drug sensitivity in human hepatic cancer cells. Cancer Res 1997;57:5475–9.
73. Badr MZ, Chen TS. Potentiation of methotrexate-induced gastrointestinal toxicity by non-steroidal anti-inflammatory drugs (NSAIDs) and vincristine. Toxicology 1985;34:333–40.
74. Singh RR, Malaviya AN, Pandey JN, et al. Fatal interaction between methotrexate and naproxen. Lancet 1986;1:1390.
75. Thyss A, Milano G, Kubar J, et al. Clinical and pharmacokinetic evidence of a life-threatening interaction between methotrexate and ketoprofen. Lancet 1986;1:256–8.
76. Aherne GW, Piall E, Marks V, et al. Prolongation and enhancement of serum methotrexate concentrations by probenecid. BMJ 1978;1:1097–9.
77. Liegler DG, Henderson ES, Hahn MA, et al. The effect of organic acids on renal clearance of methotrexate in man. Clin Pharmacol Ther 1969;10:849–57.
78. Sirotnak FM, Moccio DM, Young CW. Increased accumulation of methotrexate by murine tumor cells in vitro in the presence of probenecid which is mediated by a preferential inhibition of efflux. Cancer Res 1981;41:966–70.
79. Maricic M, Davis M, Gall EP. Megaloblastic pancytopenia in a patient receiving concurrent methotrexate and trimethoprim-sulfamethoxazole treatment. Arthritis Rheum 1986;29:133–5.
80. Ferrazzini G, Klein J, Sulh H, et al. Interaction between trimethoprim-sulfamethoxazole and methotrexate in children with leukemia. J Pediatr 1990;117:823–6.
81. Ulrich CM, Robien K, Sparks R. Pharmacogenetics and folate metabolism—a promising direction. Pharmacogenomics 2002;3:299–313.
82. Relling MV, Dervieux T. Pharmacogenetics and cancer therapy. Nat Rev Cancer 2001;1:99–108.
83. Aplenc R, Lange B. Pharmacogenetic determinants of outcome in acute lymphoblastic leukemia. Br J Haematol 2004;125:421–34.
84. Kager L, Cheok M, Yang W, et al. Folate pathway gene expression differs in subtypes of acute lymphoblastic leukemia and influences methotrexate pharmacodynamics. J Clin Invest 2005;115:110–7.
85. Dervieux T, Furst D, Lein DO, et al. Polyglutamation of methotrexate with common polymorphisms in reduced folate carrier, aminoimidazole carboxamide ribonucleotide transformylase, and thymidylate synthase are associated with methotrexate effects in rheumatoid arthritis. Arthritis Rheum 2004;50:2766–74.
86. Woods RL, Fox RM, Tattersall MH. Methotrexate treatment of squamous-cell head and neck cancers: dose-response evaluation. Br Med J Clin Res Ed 1981;282:600–2.
87. Pizzorno G, Mini E, Coronnello M, et al. Impaired polyglutamylation of methotrexate as a cause of resistance in CCRF-CEM cells after short-term, high-dose treatment with this drug. Cancer Res 1988;48:2149–55.
88. Bokkerink JP, Bakker MA, Hulscher TW, et al. Sequence-, time- and dose-dependent synergism of methotrexate and 6-mercaptopurine in malignant human T-lymphoblasts. Biochem Pharmacol 1986;35:3549–55.
89. Lobel JS, O'Brien RT, McIntosh S, et al. Methotrexate and asparaginase combination chemotherapy in refractory acute lymphoblastic leukemia of childhood. Cancer 1979;43:1089–94.
90. Amadori S, Tribalto M, Pacilli L, et al. Sequential combination of methotrexate and L-asparaginase in the treatment of refractory acute leukemia. Cancer Treat Rep 1980;64:939–42.
91. Anonymous. New treatment schedule with improved survival in childhood leukemia. Intermittent parenteral vs daily oral administration of methotrexate for maintenance of induced remission. Acute leukemia group B. JAMA 1965;194:75–81.
92. Favre R, Monjanel S, Alfonsi M, et al. High-dose methotrexate: a clinical and pharmacokinetic evaluation. Treatment of advanced squamous cell carcinoma of the head and neck using a prospective mathematical model and pharmacokinetic surveillance. Cancer Chemother Pharmacol 1982;9:156–60.
93. Frei E, 3rd, Blum RH, Pitman SW, et al. High dose methotrexate with leucovorin rescue. Rationale and spectrum of antitumor activity. Am J Med 1980;68:370–6.
94. Harris RE, McCallister JA, Provisor DS, et al. Methotrexate/L-asparaginase combination chemotherapy for patients with acute leukemia in relapse: a study of 36 children. Cancer 1980;46:2004–8.
95. Hryniuk WM, Bertino JR. Treatment of leukemia with large doses of methotrexate and folinic acid: clinical-biochemical correlates. J Clin Invest 1969;48:2140–55.
96. Bertino JR, Sawicki WL, Cashmore AR, et al. Natural resistance to methotrexate in human acute nonlymphocytic leukemia. Cancer Treat Rep 1977;61:667–73.
97. Rizzoli V, Mangoni L, Caramatti C, et al. High-dose methotrexate-leucovorin rescue therapy: selected application in non-Hodgkin's lymphoma. Tumori 1985;71:155–8.
98. Shipp MA, Harrington DP, Klatt MM, et al. Identification of major prognostic subgroups of patients with large-cell lymphoma treated with m-BACOD or M-BACOD. Ann Int Med 1986104:757–65.
99. Edelstein M, Vietti T, Valeriote F. The enhanced cytotoxicity of combinations of 1-beta-D-arabinofuranosylcytosine and methotrexate. Cancer Res 1975;35:1555–8.
100. Gaynor ER, Ultmann JE, Golomb HM, Sweet DL. Treatment of diffuse histiocytic lymphoma (DHL) with COMLA (cyclosphosphamide, oncovin, methotrexate, leucovorin, cytosine arabinoside): a 10-year experience in a single institution. J Clin Oncol 1985;3:1596–604.
101. Burkitt D, Hutt MS, Wright DH. The African Lymphoma: Preliminary observations on response to therapy. Cancer 1965;18:399–410.
102. Nkrumah FK, Perkins IV, Biggar RJ. Combination chemotherapy in abdominal Burkitt's lymphoma. Cancer 1977;40:1410–6.
103. Thomas DA, Cortes J, O'Brien S, et al. Hyper-CVAD program in Burkitt's-type adult acute lymphoblastic leukemia. J Clin Oncol 1999;17:2461–70.
104. Magrath IT, Janus C, Edwards BK, et al. An effective therapy for both undifferentiated (including Burkitt's) lymphomas and lymphoblastic lymphomas in children and young adults. Blood 1984;63:1102–11.
105. Sullivan MP, Ramirez I. Curability of Burkitt's lymphoma with high-dose cyclophosphamide-high-dose methotrexate therapy and intrathecal chemoprophylaxis. J Clin Oncol 1985;3:627–36.
106. Schwenn MR, Blattner SR, Lynch E, et al. HiC-COM: a 2-month intensive chemotherapy regimen for children with stage III and IV Burkitt's lymphoma and B-cell acute lymphoblastic leukemia. J Clin Oncol 1991;9:133–8.

107. Blay JY, Conroy T, Chevreau C, et al. High-dose methotrexate for the treatment of primary cerebral lymphomas: analysis of survival and late neurologic toxicity in a retrospective series. J Clin Oncol 1998;16:864–71.
108. Khan RB, Shi W, Thaler HT, et al. Is intrathecal methotrexate necessary in the treatment of primary CNS lymphoma? J Neuro-Oncol 2002;58:175–8.
109. Hammond CB, Hertz R, Ross GT, et al. Primary chemotherapy for nonmetastatic gestational trophoblastic neoplasms. Am J Obstet Gynecol 1967;98:71–8.
110. Prasad PD, Mahesh VB, Leibach FH, Ganapathy V. Functional coupling between a bafilomycin A1-sensitive proton pump and a probenecid-sensitive folate transporter in human placental choriocarcinoma cells. Biochimica et Biophysica Acta 1994;1222:309–14.
111. Newlands ES. VP-16 in combinations for first-line treatment of malignant germ-cell tumors and gestational choriocarcinoma. Sem Oncol 1985;12:37–41.
112. Marsh JC, Bertino JR, Katz KH, et al. The influence of drug interval on the effect of methotrexate and fluorouracil in the treatment of advanced colorectal cancer. J Clin Oncol 1991;9:371–80.
113. Bonadonna G, Moliterni A, Zambetti M, et al. 30 years' follow up of randomised studies of adjuvant CMF in operable breast cancer: cohort study. BMJ 2005;330:217.
114. Erol K, Baltali E, Altundag K, et al. Neoadjuvant chemotherapy with cyclophosphamide, mitoxantrone, and 5-fluorouracil in locally advanced breast cancer. Onkologie 2005;28:81–5.
115. Falo C, Moreno A, Benito E, et al. Primary chemotherapy with cyclophosphamide, methotrexate, and 5-fluorouracil in operable breast carcinoma. Cancer 2005;103:657–63.
116. Elomaa I, Joensuu H, Blomqvist C. Vinorelbine, methotrexate and fluorouracil (VMF) as first-line therapy in metastatic breast cancer: a randomized phase II trial. Ann Oncol 2003;14:699–703.
117. Colleoni M, Rocca A, Sandri MT, et al. Low-dose oral methotrexate and cyclophosphamide in metastatic breast cancer: antitumor activity and correlation with vascular endothelial growth factor levels. Ann Oncol 2002;13:73–80.
118. Anonymous. Comparison of antimetabolites in the treatment of breast and colon cancer. JAMA 1967;200:770–8.
119. Cadman E, Heimer R, Davis L. Enhanced 5-fluorouracil nucleotide formation after methotrexate administration: explanation for drug synergism. Science 1979;205:1135–7.
120. Anonymous. Superiority of sequential methotrexate, fluorouracil, and leucovorin to fluorouracil alone in advanced symptomatic colorectal carcinoma: a randomized trial. The Nordic Gastrointestinal Tumor Adjuvant Therapy Group. J Clin Oncol 1989;7:1437–46.
121. Yamao T, Shimada Y, Shirao K, et al. Phase II study of sequential methotrexate and 5-fluorouracil chemotherapy against peritoneally disseminated gastric cancer with malignant ascites: a report from the Gastrointestinal Oncology Study Group of the Japan Clinical Oncology Group, JCOG 9603 Trial. Jpn J Clin Oncol 2004;34:316–22.
122. Tahara M, Ohtsu A, Boku N, et al. Sequential methotrexate and 5-fluorouracil therapy for gastric cancer patients with peritoneal dissemination: a retrospective study. Gastric Cancer 2001;4:212–8.
123. Sternberg CN, Yagoda A, Scher HI, et al. Preliminary results of M-VAC (methotrexate, vinblastine, doxorubicin and cisplatin) for transitional cell carcinoma of the urothelium. J Urol 1985;133:403–7.
124. Anonymous. Neoadjuvant chemotherapy for invasive bladder cancer. Cochrane Database of Systematic Reviews: CD001426. 2005.
125. Sengelov L, von der Maase H, Lundbeck F, et al. Neoadjuvant chemotherapy with cisplatin and methotrexate in patients with muscle-invasive bladder tumours. Acta Oncol 2002;41:447–56.
126. Browman GP, Levine MN, Goodyear MD, et al. Methotrexate/fluorouracil scheduling influences normal tissue toxicity but not antitumor effects in patients with squamous cell head and neck cancer: results from a randomized trial. J Clin Oncol 1988;6:963–8.
127. Coates AS, Tattersall MH, Swanson C, et al. Combination therapy with methotrexate and 5-fluorouracil: a prospective randomized clinical trial of order of administration. J Clin Oncol 1984;2:756–61.
128. Browman GP, Archibald SD, Young JE, et al. Prospective randomized trial of one-hour sequential versus simultaneous methotrexate plus 5-fluorouracil in advanced and recurrent squamous cell head and neck cancer. J Clin Oncol 1983;1:787–92.
129. Sorensen JB, Hansen HH. Chemotherapy in adenocarcinoma of the lung. Cancer Surveys 1989;8:671–9.
130. Jaffe N, Frei E, 3rd, Traggis D, et al. Adjuvant methotrexate and citrovorum-factor treatment of osteogenic sarcoma. N Engl J Med 1974;291:994–7.
131. Eilber F, Giuliano A, Eckardt J, et al. Adjuvant chemotherapy for osteosarcoma: a randomized prospective trial. J Clin Oncol 1987;5:21–6.
132. Link MP, Goorin AM, Miser AW, et al. The effect of adjuvant chemotherapy on relapse-free survival in patients with osteosarcoma of the extremity. N Engl J Med 1986;314:1600–6.
133. Aquerreta I, Aldaz A, Giraldez J, et al. Methotrexate pharmacokinetics and survival in osteosarcoma. Pediatr Blood Cancer 2004;42:52–8.
134. Crews KR, Liu T, Rodriguez-Galindo C, et al. High-dose methotrexate pharmacokinetics and outcome of children and young adults with osteosarcoma. Cancer 2004;100:1724–33.
135. Winick NJ, Kamen BA, Streckfuss A, et al. Methotrexate (MTX) concentration in tumors following low-dose MTX. Cancer Chemother Pharmacol 1987;20:78–80.
136. Bertino JR. "Rescue" techniques in cancer chemotherapy: use of leucovorin and other rescue agents after methotrexate treatment. Sem Oncol 1977;4:203–16.
137. Condit PT, Chanes RE, Joel W. Renal toxicity of methotrexate. Cancer 1969;23:126–31.
138. Bernini JC, Fort DW, Griener JC, et al. Aminophylline for methotrexate-induced neurotoxicity. Lancet 1995;345:544–7.
139. Pinedo HM, Zaharko DS, Bull JM, et al. The reversal of methotrexate cytotoxicity to mouse bone marrow cells by leucovorin and nucleosides. Cancer Res 1976;36:4418–24.
140. Djerassi I, Ciesielka W, Kim JS. Removal of methotrexate by filtration-adsorption using charcoal filters or by hemodialysis. Cancer Treat Rep 1977;61:751–2.
141. Erttmann R, Landbeck G: Effect of oral cholestyramine on the elimination of high-dose methotrexate. J Cancer Res Clin Oncol 1985;110:48–50.
142. Tattersall MH, Brown B, Frei E, 3rd. The reversal of methotrexate toxicity by thymidine with maintenance of antitumour effects. Nature 21975;53:198–200.
143. McCullough JL, Chabner BA, Bertino JR. Purification and properties of carboxypeptidase G 1. J Biol Chem 1971;246:7207–13.
144. Widemann BC, Balis FM, Murphy RF, et al. Carboxypeptidase-G2, thymidine, and leucovorin rescue in cancer patients with methotrexate-induced renal dysfunction. J Clin Oncol 1997;15:2125–34.
145. Buchen S, Ngampolo D, Melton RG, et al. Carboxypeptidase G2 rescue in patients with methotrexate intoxication and renal failure. Br J Cancer 2005;92:480–7.
146. Widemann BC, Balis FM, Shalabi A, et al. Treatment of accidental intrathecal methotrexate overdose with intrathecal carboxypeptidase G2. J Natl Cancer Inst 2004;96:1557–9.
147. Zachariae H, Kragballe K, Sogaard H. Methotrexate induced liver cirrhosis. Studies including serial liver biopsies during continued treatment. Br J Dermatol 1980;102:407–12.
148. Freeman-Narrod M, Narrod SA, Custer RP. Chronic toxicity of methotrexate in rats: partial to complete projection of the liver by choline: Brief communication. J Natl Cancer Inst 1977;59:1013–7.
149. Mackenzie AH. Adverse hepatic effects of methotrexate therapy. In: Wilke WS (editor). Methotrexate therapy in rheumatic disease. New York: Dekker; 1989. p. 179.
150. Wolff JE, Hauch H, Kuhl J, et al. Dexamethasone increases hepatotoxicity of MTX in children with brain tumors. Anticancer Res 1998;18:2895–9.
151. Dahl MG, Gregory MM, Scheuer PJ. Methotrexate hepatotoxicity in psoriasis—comparison of different dose regimens. BMJ 1972;1:654–6.
152. Weber BL, Tanyer G, Poplack DG, et al. Transient acute hepatotoxicity of high-dose methotrexate therapy during childhood. NCI Monogr 1987;5:207–12.
153. Farrow AC, Buchanan GR, Zwiener RJ, et al. Serum aminotransferase elevation during and following treatment of childhood acute lymphoblastic leukemia. J Clin Oncol 1997;15:1560–6.
154. Quinn CT, Kamen BA. A biochemical perspective of methotrexate neurotoxicity with insight on nonfolate rescue modalities. J Invest Med 1996;44:522–30.
155. Vezmar S, Becker A, Bode U, et al. Biochemical and clinical aspects of methotrexate neurotoxicity. Chemotherapy 2003;49:92–104.
156. Fritsch G, Urban C. Transient encephalopathy during the late course of treatment with high-dose methotrexate. Cancer 1984;53:1849–51.
157. Jaffe N, Takaue Y, Anzai T, et al. Transient neurologic disturbances induced by high-dose methotrexate treatment. Cancer 1985;56:1356–60.
158. Mahoney DH, Jr., Shuster JJ, Nitschke R, et al. Acute neurotoxicity in children with B-precursor acute lymphoid leukemia: an association with intermediate-dose intravenous methotrexate and intrathecal triple therapy—a Pediatric Oncology Group study. J Clin Oncol 1998;16:1712–22.
159. Winick NJ, Bowman WP, Kamen BA, et al. Unexpected acute neurologic toxicity in the treatment of children with acute lymphoblastic leukemia. J Natl Cancer Inst 1992;84:252–6.
160. Drachtman RA, Cole PD, Golden CB, et al. Dextromethorphan is effective in the treatment of subacute methotrexate neurotoxicity. Pediatr Hematol Oncol 2002;19:319–27.
161. Reddick WE, Glass JO, Helton KJ, et al. Prevalence of leukoencephalopathy in children treated for acute lymphoblastic leukemia with high-dose methotrexate. Am J Neuroradiol 2005;26:1263–9.
162. Shapiro WR, Allen JC, Horten BC. Chronic methotrexate toxicity to the central nervous system. Clin Bull 1980;10:49–52.
163. Peylan-Ramu N, Poplack DG, Blei CL, et al. Computer assisted tomography in methotrexate encephalopathy. J Comput Assist Tomogr 1977;1:216–21.
164. Surtees R, Clelland J, Hann I. Demyelination and single-carbon transfer pathway metabolites during the treatment of acute lymphoblastic leukemia: CSF studies. J Clin Oncol 1998;16:1505–11.
165. Kishi T, Tanaka Y, Ueda K. Evidence for hypomethylation in two children with acute lymphoblastic leukemia and leukoencephalopathy. Cancer 2000;89:925–31.
166. Surtees R, Leonard J, Austin S. Association of demyelination with deficiency of cerebrospinal-fluid S-adenosylmethionine in inborn errors of methyl-transfer pathway. Lancet 1991;338:1550–4.
167. Hyland K, Smith I, Bottiglieri T, et al. Demyelination and decreased S-adenosylmethionine in 5,10-methylenetetrahydrofolate reductase deficiency. Neurology 1988;38:459–62.
168. Bottiglieri T, Hyland K, Reynolds EH. The clinical potential of ademetionine (S-adenosylmethionine) in neurological disorders. Drugs 1994;48:137–52.
169. Knopman D, Patterson M. An open-label, 24-week pilot study of the methyl donor betaine in Alzheimer disease patients. Alzheimer Dis Assoc Disord 2001;15:162–5.
170. Shea TB, Lyons-Weiler J, Rogers E. Homocysteine, folate deprivation and Alzheimer neuropathology. J Alzheimer's Dis 2002;4:261–7.
171. Spiegel RJ, Cooper PR, Blum RH, et al. Treatment of massive intrathecal methotrexate overdose by ventriculolumbar perfusion. N Engl J Med 1984;311:386–8.
172. Adamson PC, Balis FM, McCully CL, et al. Rescue of experimental intrathecal methotrexate overdose with carboxypeptidase-G2. J Clin Oncol 1991;9:670–4.
173. Carson CW, Cannon GW, Egger MJ, et al. Pulmonary disease during the treatment of rheumatoid arthritis with low dose pulse methotrexate. Semin Arthritis Rheum 1987;16:186–95.
174. Searles G, McKendry RJ. Methotrexate pneumonitis in rheumatoid arthritis: potential risk factors. Four case reports and a review of the literature. J Rheumatol 1987;14:1164–71.
175. Doyle LA, Berg C, Bottino G, et al. Erythema and desquamation after high-dose methotrexate. Ann Intern Med 1983;98:611–2.
176. Fondevila CG, Milone GA, Santiago P. Cutaneous vasculitis after intermediate dose of methotrexate (IDMTX). Br J Haematol 1989;72:591–2.
177. Mason JB, Levesque T. Folate: effects on carcinogenesis and the potential for cancer chemoprevention. Oncology (Huntington) 1996;10:1727–36, 1742–3; discussion 1743–4.
178. Shamberger RC, Rosenberg SA, Seipp CA, et al. Effects of high-dose methotrexate and vincristine on ovarian and testicular functions in patients undergoing postoperative adjuvant treatment of osteosarcoma. Cancer Treat Rep 1981;65:739–46.
179. Nesbit M, Krivit W, Heyn R, et al. Acute and chronic effects of methotrexate on hepatic, pulmonary, and skeletal systems. Cancer 1976;37:1048–57.
180. Uehara R, Suzuki Y, Ichikawa Y. Methotrexate (MTX) inhibits osteoblastic differentiation in vitro: possible

mechanism of MTX osteopathy. J Rheumatol 2001;28:251–6.
181. Goldberg NH, Romolo JL, Austin EH, et al. Anaphylactoid type reactions in two patients receiving high dose intravenous methotrexate. Cancer 1978;41:52–5.
182. Woolley PV, 3rd, Sacher RA, Priego VM, et al. Methotrexate-induced immune haemolytic anaemia. Br J Haematol 1983;54:543–52.
183. Lin JT, Tong WP, Trippett TM, et al. Basis for natural resistance to methotrexate in human acute non-lymphocytic leukemia. Leuk Res 1991;15:1191–6.
184. Goker E, Lin JT, Trippett T, et al. Decreased polyglutamylation of methotrexate in acute lymphoblastic leukemia blasts in adults compared to children with this disease. Leukemia 1993;7:1000–4.
185. Curt GA, Jolivet J, Carney DN, et al. Determinants of the sensitivity of human small-cell lung cancer cell lines to methotrexate. J Clin Invest 1985;76:1323–9.
186. Li WW, Waltham M, Tong W, et al. Increased activity of gamma-glutamyl hydrolase in human sarcoma cell lines: a novel mechanism of intrinsic resistance to methotrexate (MTX). Adv Exp Med Biol 1993;338:635–8.
187. Barredo JC, Synold TW, Laver J, et al. Differences in constitutive and post-methotrexate folylpolyglutamate synthetase activity in B-lineage and T-lineage leukemia. Blood 1994;84:564–9.
188. Galpin AJ, Schuetz JD, Masson E, et al. Differences in folylpolyglutamate synthetase and dihydrofolate reductase expression in human B-lineage versus T-lineage leukemic lymphoblasts: mechanisms for lineage differences in methotrexate polyglutamylation and cytotoxicity. Mol Pharmacol 1997;52:155–63.
189. Longo GS, Gorlick R, Tong WP, et al. Disparate affinities of antifolates for folylpolyglutamate synthetase from human leukemia cells. Blood 1997;90:1241–5.
190. Li WW, Lin JT, Tong WP, et al. Mechanisms of natural resistance to antifolates in human soft tissue sarcomas. Cancer Res 1992;52:1434–8.
191. Longo GS, Gorlick R, Tong WP, et al. gamma-Glutamyl hydrolase and folylpolyglutamate synthetase activities predict polyglutamylation of methotrexate in acute leukemias. Oncol Res 1997;9:259–63.
192. Cole PD, Kamen BA, Gorlick R, et al. Effects of overexpression of gamma-Glutamyl hydrolase on methotrexate metabolism and resistance. Cancer Res 2001;61:4599–604.
193. Guo W, Healey JH, Meyers PA, et al. Mechanisms of methotrexate resistance in osteosarcoma. Clin Cancer Res 1999;5:621–7.
194. Zhao R, Assaraf YG, Goldman ID. A mutated murine reduced folate carrier (RFC1) with increased affinity for folic acid, decreased affinity for methotrexate, and an obligatory anion requirement for transport function. J Biol Chem 1998;273:19065–71.
195. Jansen G, Mauritz R, Drori S, et al. A structurally altered human reduced folate carrier with increased folic acid transport mediates a novel mechanism of antifolate resistance. J Biol Chem 1998;273:30189–98.
196. Kaufman Y, Drori S, Cole PD, et al. Reduced folate carrier mutations are not the mechanism underlying methotrexate resistance in childhood acute lymphoblastic leukemia. Cancer 2004;100:773–82.
197. Fan J, Bertino JR. Functional roles of E2F in cell cycle regulation. Oncogene 1997;14:1191–200.
198. Li W, Fan J, Banerjee D, et al. Overexpression of p21(waf1) decreases G2-M arrest and apoptosis induced by paclitaxel in human sarcoma cells lacking both p53 and functional Rb protein. Mol Pharmacol 1999;55:1088–93.
199. Li W, Fan J, Hochhauser D, et al. Lack of functional retinoblastoma protein mediates increased resistance to antimetabolites in human sarcoma cell lines. Proc Natl Acad Sci U S A 1995;92:10436–40.
200. Kruh GD, Zeng H, Rea PA, et al. MRP subfamily transporters and resistance to anticancer agents. J Bioenerg Biomembr 2001;33:493–501.
201. Wielinga P, Hooijberg JH, Gunnarsdottir S, et al. The human multidrug resistance protein MRP5 transports folates and can mediate cellular resistance against antifolates. Cancer Res 2005;65:4425–30.
202. Chen ZS, Robey RW, Belinsky MG, et al. Transport of methotrexate, methotrexate polyglutamates, and 17beta-estradiol 17-(beta-D-glucuronide) by ABCG2: effects of acquired mutations at R482 on methotrexate transport. Cancer Res 2003;63:4048–54.
203. Volk EL, Schneider E. Wild-type breast cancer resistance protein (BCRP/ABCG2) is a methotrexate polyglutamate transporter. Cancer Res 2003;63:5538–43.
204. Volk EL, Farley KM, Wu Y, et al. Overexpression of wild-type breast cancer resistance protein mediates methotrexate resistance. Cancer Res 2002;62:5035–40.
205. Hooijberg JH, Broxterman HJ, Kool M, et al. Antifolate resistance mediated by the multidrug resistance proteins MRP1 and MRP2. Cancer Res 1999;59:2532–5.
206. Steinbach D, Lengemann J, Voigt A, et al. Response to chemotherapy and expression of the genes encoding the multidrug resistance-associated proteins MRP2, MRP3, MRP4, MRP5, and SMRP in childhood acute myeloid leukemia. Clin Cancer Res 2003;9:1083–86.
207. Steinbach D, Wittig S, Cario G, et al. The multidrug resistance-associated protein 3 (MRP3) is associated with a poor outcome in childhood ALL and may account for the worse prognosis in male patients and T-cell immunophenotype. Blood 2003;102:4493–98.
208. Biedler JL, Spengler BA. Metaphase chromosome anomaly: association with drug resistance and cell-specific products. Science 1976;191:185–7.
209. Kaufman RJ, Brown PC, Schimke RT. Loss and stabilization of amplified dihydrofolate reductase genes in mouse sarcoma S-180 cell lines. Mol Cell Biol 1981;1:1084–93.
210. Kaufman RJ, Schimke RT. Amplification and loss of dihydrofolate reductase genes in a Chinese hamster ovary cell line. Mol Cell Biol 1981;1:1069–76.
211. Alt FW, Kellems RE, Bertino JR, et al. Selective multiplication of dihydrofolate reductase genes in methotrexate-resistant variants of cultured murine cells. 1978. Biotechnology 1992;24:397–410.
212. Cowan KH, Goldsmith ME, Levine RM, et al. Dihydrofolate reductase gene amplification and possible rearrangement in estrogen-responsive methotrexate-resistant human breast cancer cells. J Biol Chem 1982;257:15079–86.
213. Fischer GA. Increased levels of folic acid reductase as a mechanism of resistance to amethopterin in leukemic cells. Biochem Pharmacol 1961;7:75.
214. Srimatkandada S, Medina WD, Cashmore AR, et al. Amplification and organization of dihydrofolate reductase genes in a human leukemic cell line, K-562, resistant to methotrexate. Biochemistry 1983;22:5774–81.
215. Carman MD, Schornagel JH, Rivest RS, et al. Resistance to methotrexate due to gene amplification in a patient with acute leukemia. J Clin Oncol 1984;2:16–20.
216. Curt GA, Carney DN, Cowan KH, et al. Unstable methotrexate resistance in human small-cell carcinoma associated with double minute chromosomes. N Engl J Med 1983;308:199–202.
217. Horns RC, Jr., Dower WJ, Schimke RT. Gene amplification in a leukemic patient treated with methotrexate. J Clin Oncol 1984;2:2–7.
218. Dedhar S, Hartley D, Fitz-Gibbons D, et al. Heterogeneity in the specific activity and methotrexate sensitivity of dihydrofolate reductase from blast cells of acute myelogenous leukemia patients. J Clin Oncol 1985;3:1545–52.
219. Domin BA, Cheng YC, Hakala MT. Properties of dihydrofolate reductase from a methotrexate-resistant subline of human KB cells and comparison with enzyme from KB parent cells and mouse S180 AT/3000 cells. Mol Pharmacol 1982;21:231–8.
220. Flintoff WF, Essani K. Methotrexate-resistant Chinese hamster ovary cells contain a dihydrofolate reductase with an altered affinity for methotrexate. Biochemistry 1980;19:4321–7.
221. Goldie JH, Dedhar S, Krystal G. Properties of a methotrexate-insensitive variant of dihydrofolate reductase derived from methotrexate-resistant L5178Y cells. J Biol Chem 1981;256:11629–35.
222. Melera PW, Davide JP, Oen H. Antifolate-resistant Chinese hamster cells. Molecular basis for the biochemical and structural heterogeneity among dihydrofolate reductases produced by drug-sensitive and drug-resistant cell lines. J Biol Chem 1988;263:1978–90.
223. Schweitzer BI, Dicker AP, Bertino JR. Dihydrofolate reductase as a therapeutic target. FASEB J 1990;4:2441–52.
224. Pizzorno G, Chang YM, McGuire JJ, et al. Inherent resistance of human squamous carcinoma cell lines to methotrexate as a result of decreased polyglutamylation of this drug. Cancer Res 1989;49:5275–80.
225. Cowan KH, Jolivet J. A methotrexate-resistant human breast cancer cell line with multiple defects, including diminished formation of methotrexate polyglutamates. J Biol Chem 1984;259:10793–800.
226. McCloskey DE, McGuire JJ, Russell CA, et al. Decreased folylpolyglutamate synthetase activity as a mechanism of methotrexate resistance in CCRF-CEM human leukemia sublines. J Biol Chem 1991;266:6181–7.
227. Rosowsky A, Wright JE, Cucchi CA, et al. Phenotypic heterogeneity in cultured human head and neck squamous cell carcinoma lines with low-level methotrexate resistance. Cancer Res 1985;45:6205–12.
228. Rhee MS, Wang Y, Nair MG, et al. Acquisition of resistance to antifolates caused by enhanced gamma-glutamyl hydrolase activity. Cancer Res 1993;53:2227–30.
229. Whitehead VM, Rosenblatt DS, Vuchich MJ, et al. Accumulation of methotrexate and methotrexate polyglutamates in lymphoblasts at diagnosis of childhood acute lymphoblastic leukemia: a pilot prognostic factor analysis. Blood 1990;76:44–9.
230. Whitehead VM, Vuchich MJ, Lauer SJ, et al. Accumulation of high levels of methotrexate polyglutamates in lymphoblasts from children with hyperdiploid (greater than 50 chromosomes) B-lineage acute lymphoblastic leukemia: a Pediatric Oncology Group study. Blood 1992;80:1316–23.
231. Mantadakis E, smith AK, Hynan L, et al. Methotrexate polyglutamation may lack prognostic significance in children with BCP-ALL treated with intensive oral methotrexate. J Pediatr Hematol Oncol 2002;24:636–42.
232. Mantadakis E, Smith AK, Kamen BA. Ratio of methotrexate to folate uptake by lymphoblasts in children with B-lineage acute lymphoblastic leukemia: a pilot study. J Pediatr Hematol Oncol 2000;22:221–6.
233. Gorlick R, Goker E, Trippett T, et al. Defective transport is a common mechanism of acquired methotrexate resistance in acute lymphocytic leukemia and is associated with decreased reduced folate carrier expression. Blood 1997;89:1013–8.
234. Purcell WT, Ettinger DS. Novel antifolate drugs. Curr Oncol Rep 2003;5:114–25.
235. Kamen BA, Cole P. Folate antagonists. In: Bertino JR (ed). Encyclopedia of cancer. Vol II. 2nd ed. San Diego: Academic Press; 2002. p. 235–42.
236. Dameshek W, Freedman MH, Steinberg L. Folic acid antagonists in the treatment of acute and subacute leukemia. Blood 1950;5:898–915.
237. George S, Cichowicz DJ, Shane B. Mammalian folylpoly-gamma-glutamate synthetase. 3. Specificity for folate analogues. Biochemistry 1987;26:522–9.
238. Smith A, Hum M, Winick NJ, et al. A case for the use of aminopterin in treatment of patients with leukemia based on metabolic studies of blasts in vitro. Clin Cancer Res 1996;2:69–73.
239. Ratliff AF, Wilson J, Hum M, et al. Phase I and pharmacokinetic trial of aminopterin in patients with refractory malignancies. J Clin Oncol 1998;16:1458–64.
240. Cole PD, Smith AK, Larson RA, et al. Phase II trial of oral aminopterin for adults and children with refractory acute leukemia [abstract #3715]. Proc Am Assoc Cancer Res 2002;43:749.
241. Cole PD, Drachtman RA, Masterson M, et al. Aminopterin can replace methotrexate for children with newly diagnosed acute lymphoblastic leukemia without excessive toxicity. [abstract.] Blood 2004;104:538a.
242. Sirotnak FM, Schmid FA, Samuels LL, et al. 10-Ethyl-10-deaza-aminopterin: structural design and biochemical, pharmacologic, and antitumor properties. NCI Monogr 1987;5:127–31.
243. Casper ES, Christman KL, Schwartz GK, et al. Edatrexate in patients with soft tissue sarcoma. Activity in malignant fibrous histiocytoma. Cancer 1993;72:766–70.
244. Schornagel JH, Verweij J, de Mulder PH, et al. Randomized phase III trial of edatrexate versus methotrexate in patients with metastatic and/or recurrent squamous cell carcinoma of the head and neck: a European Organization for Research and Treatment of Cancer Head and Neck Cancer Cooperative Group study. J Clin Oncol 1995;13:1649–55.
245. Shum KY, Kris MG, Gralla RJ, et al. Phase II study of 10-ethyl-10-deaza-aminopterin in patients with stage III and IV non-small-cell lung cancer. J Clin Oncol 1988;6:446–50.
246. Kuriakose P, Gandara DR, Perez EA. Phase I trial of edatrexate in advanced breast and other cancers.[see comment]. Cancer Invest 2002;20:473–9.
247. Sirotnak FM, DeGraw JI, Colwell WT, et al. A new analogue of 10-deazaaminopterin with markedly enhanced curative effects against human tumor xenografts in mice. Cancer Chemother Pharmacol 1998;42:313–8.
248. Krug LM, Azzoli CG, Kris MG, et al. 10-propargyl-10-deazaaminopterin: an antifolate with activity in patients with previously treated non-small cell lung cancer. Clin Cancer Res 2003;9:2072–8.
249. Kamen BA, Eibl B, Cashmore A, et al. Uptake and efficacy of trimetrexate (TMQ, 2,4-diamino-5-methyl-6-[(3,4,5-

trimethoxyanilino)methyl] quinazoline), a non-classical antifolate in methotrexate-resistant leukemia cells in vitro. Biochem Pharmacol 1984;33:1697–9.

250. Duch DS, Edelstein MP, Bowers SW, et al. Biochemical and chemotherapeutic studies on 2,4-diamino-6-(2,5-dimethoxybenzyl)-5-methylpyrido[2,3-d]pyrimidine (BW 301U), a novel lipid-soluble inhibitor of dihydrofolate reductase. Cancer Res 1982;42:3987–94.

251. O'Dwyer PJ, Shoemaker DD, Plowman J, et al. Trimetrexate: a new antifol entering clinical trials. Invest New Drugs 1985;3:71–5.

252. Rodenhuis S, McGuire JJ, Sawicki WL, et al. Effects of methotrexate and of the "nonclassical" folate antagonist trimetrexate on human leukemia cells. Leukemia 1987;1:116–20.

253. Taylor IW, Slowiaczek P, Friedlander ML, et al. Selective toxicity of a new lipophilic antifolate, BW301U, for methotrexate-resistant cells with reduced drug uptake. Cancer Res 1985;45:978–82.

254. Arkin H, Ohnuma T, Kamen BA, et al. Multidrug resistance in a human leukemic cell line selected for resistance to trimetrexate. Cancer Res 1989;49:6556–61.

255. Allegra CJ, Chabner BA, Tuazon CU, et al. Trimetrexate for the treatment of *Pneumocystis carinii* pneumonia in patients with the acquired immunodeficiency syndrome. N Engl J Med 1987;317:978–85.

256. Hum M, Holcenberg JS, Tkaczewski I, et al. High-dose trimetrexate and minimal-dose leucovorin: a case for selective protection? Clin Cancer Res 1998;4:2981–4.

257. Lin JT, Bertino JR. Update on trimetrexate, a folate antagonist with antineoplastic and antiprotozoal properties. Cancer Invest 1991;9:159–72.

258. Conti JA, Kemeny N, Seiter K, et al. Trial of sequential trimetrexate, fluorouracil, and high-dose leucovorin in previously treated patients with gastrointestinal carcinoma. J Clin Oncol 1994;12:695–700.

259. Blanke CD, Kasimis B, Schein P, et al. Phase II study of trimetrexate, fluorouracil, and leucovorin for advanced colorectal cancer. J Clin Oncol 1997;15:915–20.

260. Bertino JR. Modulation of 5-fluorouracil/leucovorin by trimetrexate--did it work? Ann Oncol 2002;13:10–11.

261. Newell DRA. Clinical pharmacokinetics of antitumor antifolates. Semin Oncol 1999;26:74–81.

262. Fernandes DJ, Sur P, Kute TE, et al. Proliferation-dependent cytotoxicity of methotrexate in murine L5178Y leukemia. Cancer Res 1988;48:5638–44.

263. Jackman AL, Farrugia DC, Gibson W, et al. ZD1694 (Tomudex): a new thymidylate synthase inhibitor with activity in colorectal cancer. Eur J Cancer 1995;31A:1277–82.

264. Zalcberg JR, Cunningham D, Van Cutsem E, et al. ZD1694: a novel thymidylate synthase inhibitor with substantial activity in the treatment of patients with advanced colorectal cancer. Tomudex Colorectal Study Group. J Clin Oncol 1996;14:716–21.

265. Horton TM, Blaney SM, Langevin AM, et al. Phase I trial and pharmacokinetic study of raltitrexed in children with recurrent or refractory leukemia: a pediatric oncology group study. Clin Cancer Res 2005;11:1884–9.

266. Cocconi G, Cunningham D, Van Cutsem E, et al. Open, randomized, multicenter trial of raltitrexed versus fluorouracil plus high-dose leucovorin in patients with advanced colorectal cancer. Tomudex Colorectal Cancer Study Group. J Clin Oncol 1998;16:2943–52.

267. Cunningham D, Zalcberg JR, Rath U, et al. Final results of a randomised trial comparing 'Tomudex' (raltitrexed) with 5-fluorouracil plus leucovorin in advanced colorectal cancer. "Tomudex" Colorectal Cancer Study Group. Ann Oncol 1996;7:961–5.

268. Cunningham D, Zalcberg JR, Rath U, et al. 'Tomudex' (ZD1694): results of a randomised trial in advanced colorectal cancer demonstrate efficacy and reduced mucositis and leucopenia. The 'Tomudex' Colorectal Cancer Study Group. Eur J Cancer 1995;31A:1945–54.

269. Arends JJ, Sleeboom HP, Leys MB, et al. A phase II study of raltitrexed and gemcitabine in patients with advanced pancreatic carcinoma. Br J Cancer 2005;92:445–8.

270. Ferrari VD, Amoroso V, Valcamonico F, et al. Epirubicin, cisplatin, and raltitrexed in patients with advanced gastric and hepatobiliary carcinoma: a phase II study. American J Clin Oncol 2004;27:445–8.

271. Cortinovis D, Bajetta E, Di Bartolomeo M, et al. Raltitrexed plus oxaliplatin in the treatment of metastatic colorectal cancer. Tumori 2004;90:186–91.

272. Jackman AL, Theti DS, Gibbs DD. Antifolates targeted specifically to the folate receptor. Adv Drug Deliv Rev 2004;56:1111–25.

273. Currie VE, Warrell RP, Jr., Arlin Z, et al. Phase I trial of 10-deaza-aminopterin in patients with advanced cancer. Cancer Treat Rep 1983;67:149–54.

274. Boritzki TJ, Barlett CA, Zhang C, et al. AG2034: a novel inhibitor of glycinamide ribonucleotide formyltransferase. Invest New Drugs 1996;14:295–303.

275. Bissett D, McLeod HL, Sheedy B, et al. Phase I dose-escalation and pharmacokinetic study of a novel folate analogue AG2034. Br J Cancer 2001;84:308–12.

276. Roberts JD, Shibata S, Spicer DV, et al. Phase I study of AG2034, a targeted GARFT inhibitor, administered once every 3 weeks. Cancer Chemother Pharmacol 2000;45:423–7.

277. Rinaldi DA, Burris HA, Dorr FA, et al. Initial phase I evaluation of the novel thymidylate synthase inhibitor, LY231514, using the modified continual reassessment method for dose escalation. J Clin Oncol 1995;13:2842–50.

278. O'Dwyer PJ, Nelson K, Thornton DE. Overview of phase II trials of MTA in solid tumors. Semin Oncol 1999;26:99–104.

279. Hazarika M, White RM, Jr., Booth BP, et al. Pemetrexed in malignant pleural mesothelioma. Clin Cancer Res 2005;11:982–92.

280. Hanna NH. Second-line chemotherapy for non-small-cell lung cancer: recent data with pemetrexed. Clin Lung Cancer 5 2004;Suppl 2:S75–9.

281. Vogelzang NJ, Rusthoven JJ, Symanowski J, et al. Phase III study of pemetrexed in combination with cisplatin versus cisplatin alone in patients with malignant pleural mesothelioma. J Clin Oncol 2003;21:2636–44.

Pyrimidine and Purine Antimetabolites

Giuseppe Pizzorno, PhD, PharmD
Robert B. Diasio, MD
Yung-Chi Cheng, PhD

Development of pyrimidine and purine analogs as potential antineoplastic agents evolved from an early presumption that nucleic acids are involved in growth control. Among the first analogs produced and tested for biologic activity were the 5-halogenated pyrimidines. Although in original concept these agents were targeted toward the malaria parasite, Hitchings and Elion recognized that these compounds might be valuable in the treatment of cancer, which was correctly perceived as a disease of uncontrolled growth.[1,2] These early studies focused primarily on the incorporation of analog nucleic acid bases into ribonucleic acid (RNA) or deoxyribonucleic acid (DNA) of bacteria species.[3] Concurrent studies on the metabolic activation of these heterocyclic analogs and their biochemical targets for growth inhibition, as well as the study of resistance to them, afforded many new insights into the intermediary metabolism responsible for the synthesis of DNA and RNA precursors.[4] Subsequently, it was recognized that control of these biosynthetic pathways afforded additional targets for therapeutic intervention.

Further development of these analogs was stimulated by the demonstration of quantitative, but not qualitative, differences in the activity of these pathways between normal versus neoplastic tissue. It was also realized that rapid catabolism of these agents to inactive compounds could severely limit anabolic conversion to fraudulent nucleotides. This, in itself, affords targets for the modulation of cytotoxic activity on a tissue-specific basis.

A virtually complete understanding of enzymes involved in the biosynthesis of purine and pyrimidine nucleotide precursors of RNA and DNA is now at hand.[5,6] This intricate matrix of metabolic reactions operates under a complex web of positive- and negative-feedback controls. Most purine or pyrimidine analogs are active only after metabolic activation to the nucleotide form, so these fraudulent nucleotides not only may be incorporated, but also can mimic the natural effector compounds in regulatory pathways. Alternatively, they may deplete critical intermediates, thereby generating enlarged pools of the natural precursors behind a metabolic block, producing effects that can distort the balance of ribonucleoside and deoxyribonucleoside triphosphates. A target of even greater complexity is the incorporation of triphosphates into DNA or RNA and the subsequent modification of these macromolecules. Subtle differences in the specificity and function of the polymerases generate the selectivity of certain purine and pyrimidine nucleotides as anticancer and, more importantly, antiviral agents.

PYRIMIDINE ANALOGS

Pyrimidine analogs include 5-fluorouracil, cytosine arabinoside, 5-azacytidine, and gemcitabine.

5-FLUOROURACIL **Background and Properties** A major motivation for the development of pyrimidine analogs of uracil was the early observation that preneoplastic rat liver and hepatomas incorporated uracil more actively than did the normal liver.[7] Although this may reflect a difference in the relative degradative capacity of these different tissues for uracil, it also provided a focus for the synthetic efforts of Duschinsky and colleagues that led to 5-fluorouracil (5-FU) (Figure 43-1) and related ribosides and deoxyribosides.[8] This specific site of substitution on the pyrimidine ring was selected because it might block subsequent conversion of a uracil nucleotide to thymine nucleotides with consequent inhibition of DNA synthesis and, thus, growth.

As anticipated, the pKa of 5-FU (8.1) is more acidic than that of uracil (9.6); thus, under physiologic conditions, 5-FU partially exists as an anionic species. This is undoubtedly important to the metabolic activation to the nucleotide form via the orotidylate pyrophosphorylase reaction. This uridylate analog, 5-fluorouridine monophosphate (5-FUMP), can then substitute for uridine monophosphate (UMP) in a wide spectrum of

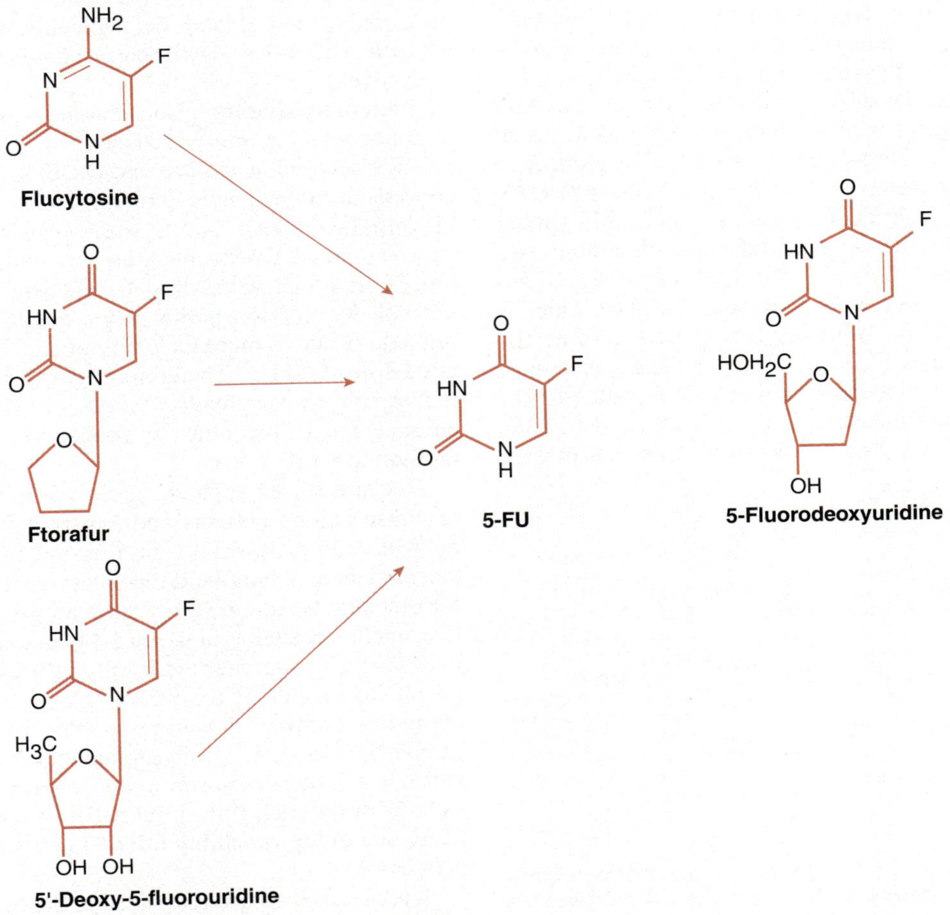

Flucytosine

Ftorafur

5'-Deoxy-5-fluorouridine

5-FU

5-Fluorodeoxyuridine

Figure 43-1 5-Fluorouracil (5-FU) and analog structures.

intermediary reactions. The product of one of these reactions, fluorodeoxyuridine monophosphate (FdUMP), plays a major role by inhibiting displacement of hydrogen from the 5-position of deoxyuridylate and replacing it with a methyl group via a tetrahydrofolate catalyzed reaction (Figure 43-2).[9] Early clinical studies showed enough promise in colon cancer and other solid tumors to sustain 50 subsequent years of further development. A primary focus of this research has been to reduce its toxicity within a variety of normal tissues, while retaining its antitumor activity. Today, 5-FU remains an important component in the therapy of several of the most common solid tumors, not only as a single agent, but also in combination with other chemotherapy agents.

Anabolism 5-FU has several possible routes of activation to the nucleotide form.[10] In normal tissues, the predominant mechanism appears to be competition with orotate for condensation with pyrophosphorylribose-5-PO_4 (PRPP) via orotidylate pyrophosphorylase to form 5-fluorouridylate.[11] In mammalian cells, this protein is a bifunctional enzyme that also catalyzes the decarboxylation of orotidylate to 5'-uridylic acid.[11]

Alternative activation routes of 5-FU follow the salvage pathways for uracil and thymine, but these are presumed to be less important in most tissues.[12–14] After formation of the nucleoside, phosphorylation by uridine kinase and adenosine triphosphate (ATP) forms 5-fluorouridine monophosphate (5-FUMP) (Figure 43-3). Further phosphorylation of 5-FUMP to 5-fluorouridine diphosphate (5-FUDP) by nucleotide kinase provides a branch point in 5-FU anabolism.[15] Additional phosphorylation of a major portion of 5-FUDP to fluorouridine triphosphate (5-FUTP) provides the substrate for RNA polymerases with consequent incorporation into several forms of RNA.[16] Alternatively, 5-FUDP can be reduced to 5-fluorodeoxyuridine diphosphate (FdUDP), which is hydrolyzed to the monophosphate FdUMP, the covalent inhibitor of thymidylate synthase.[9] Some FdUDP is phosphorylated to fluorodeoxyuridine triphosphate (FdUTP), which is an alternate substrate for deoxythymidine triphosphate (dTTP) in DNA polymerase reactions; however, high deoxyuridine triphosphate (dUTP) pyrophosphatase activity converts most of the FdUTP to FdUMP.[17] When 5-FU is incorporated into DNA, uracil *N*-glycosylase removes it, leaving an apyrimidinic sugar for the process of DNA repair. Errors in this process provide an additional basis for cytotoxicity.[18]

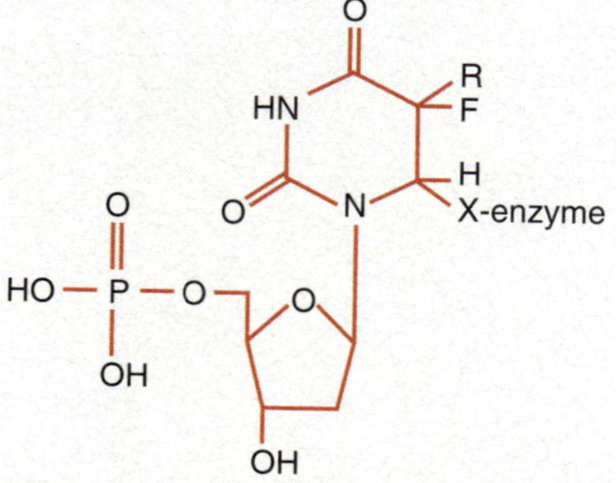

Figure 43-2 Covalent thymidylate synthase-fluorodeoxyuridylate complex; R = H or CH_2FH_4 = 5,10-methylene tetrahydrofolate.

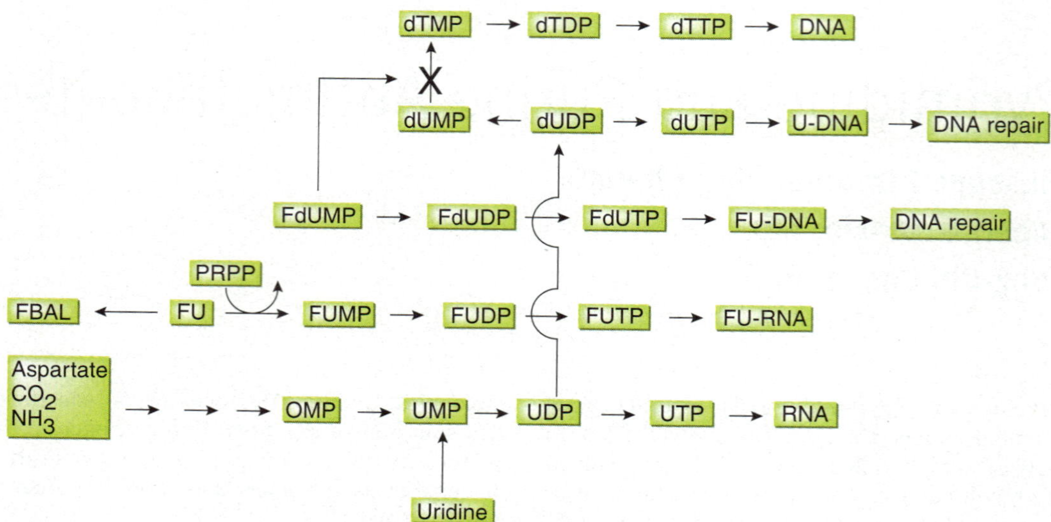

Figure 43-3 Metabolic activation and targets of fluorinated pyrimidines. CO_2 = carbon dioxide; dT = thymidine (thymine deoxyriboside); dTMP also called thymidylate; dU = deoxyuridine; dUMP = deoxyuridine monophosphate; FBAL = fluoro-β-alanine; FdU = fluorodeoxyuridine; FdUMP = fluorodeoxyuridine monophosphate; 5-FU = fluorouracil; 5-FUMP = 5-fluorouridine monophosphate (also called fluorouridylate); MP, DP, TP = mono-, di-, and triphosphate; NH_3 = ammonia; O = orotidine; OMP also called orotidylate; PRPP = phosphoribosyl pyrophosphate; U = uridine (uracil riboside); UMP also called uridylate.

Minor amounts of 5-FUDP sugar derivatives have been detected as anabolic products, but their potential to inhibit cell growth or toxicity has not been documented.[19,20] In some of the previously discussed reactions, the 5-FU nucleotide analogs are better substrates than the corresponding uracil derivatives.

Pharmacokinetics Consideration of 5-FU pharmacokinetics must focus primarily on the balance between anabolism and catabolism. The conversion to nucleotide derivatives is responsible for most, if not all, of its antineoplastic activity, even though it accounts for a very minor portion of the administered drug. Catabolism via the normal degradation pathway for uracil is the immediate fate of more than 80% of an administered dose of 5-FU.[21] Therefore, slight alterations in this pathway can greatly affect the very limited amount that is available for conversion to the nucleotide form.

Because of the apparent great variability in response among patients and apparent limited bioavailability (10–25%) via the oral route,[22] there has been a long-held recommendation that 5-FU should be administered intravenously (IV). Recent clinical studies in which 5-FU was administered orally together with ethynyluracil—a potent inactivator of the initial enzyme of the pyrimidine pathway, dihydropyrimidine dehydrogenase (DPD)—have demonstrated that 5-FU in fact has excellent absorption and bioavailability[23]; with the variability from patient to patient being due to the variability of DPD levels in the population.

Dosage used clinically in general depends on the schedule of administration.[24] The most common dosage schedules are a monthly course of one dose given on each 5 days as an IV bolus of 400 to 600 mg/m^2 or the same dosage given as a single bolus on a weekly basis.[25] The limiting toxic effect of these regimens is generally myelosuppression or mucositis. When continuous IV infusion is employed, higher doses are required (1,000–2,000 mg/m^2/d) to sustain steady-state concentrations of 5-FU (1–5 μM) in plasma, adequate to achieve therapeutic effects.[26] With this route, toxicity is most frequently mucositis, with minimal myelosuppression. Several studies have shown that this regimen is superior to the bolus regimen when 5-FU is given as a single agent.[26–28] Optimal treatment was a 48-hour infusion at weekly intervals, which improved both response and survival. Prolonged infusion of 5-FU for up to 12 weeks at 300 mg/m^2/d also produced a better response than the bolus regimen.[29,30] The most prominent toxicity in this situation was a reversible hand-and-foot syndrome.[30] It was found that during continuous IV infusions, plasma concentrations of 5-FU varied by as much as 10-fold, and subsequent studies have demonstrated that variations in dihydropyrimidine dehydrogenase may be responsible for this effect.[31] Because 5-FU is most often used in combination with other agents such as leucovorin and methotrexate, it is important to modify the dosage in each case to limit, but not eliminate, host toxicity.

Administered 5-FU has a volume of distribution of 0.20 to 0.25 L/kg, which suggests distribution into the extracellular space.[32,33] Good penetration into the cerebrospinal fluid, lymph, and neoplastic effusions have been documented.[34] Since the drug apparently freely permeates cells in culture, it is not clear why the volume of distribution approximates the extracellular space.

The rate of plasma clearance is generally first order with a half-life of 10 to 20 minutes and ranges between 500 and 1,500 mL/min.[21] Above a dosage of 800 mg/m^2, clearance may decrease rapidly. Because the primary fate of the drug is catabolism, this decreased clearance undoubtedly reflects saturation of these reactions.[35]

Intra-arterial infusion of 5-FU has been used with some success in patients with isolated hepatic metastases. As with systemic therapy, extensive single-pass clearance is achieved (19–51%), but saturation of catabolism occurs when doses are elevated.[36] Nevertheless, hepatic 5-FU concentrations considerably in excess of those tolerated systemically can be achieved. The limiting factor in high-dose regimens is cholestatic jaundice and evidence of chemical hepatitis.

The 2'-deoxyriboside of 5-FU, FdUrd, is a much more potent inhibitor of cell growth than 5-FU in cell culture.[37] This presumably reflects the ease with which this compound can be activated by thymidine kinase in a single step to FdUMP the titrating inhibitor of thymidylate synthase. In both humans and animals, IV bolus injection of FdUrd produces a dose response that is essentially that of 5-FU because it is cleaved rapidly to an equivalent amount of 5-FU that subsequently experiences the same metabolic fate as directly injected 5-FU. If, however, FdUrd is given by a 14-day continuous infusion, the maximum tolerated dose is approximately 100-fold less[36]; however, its therapeutic index is not significantly better than that of 5-FU. Even so, it can be used for isolated hepatic metastases of colon cancer by hepatic artery infusion because approximately 90% of the drug is cleared in a single pass by the liver, thus reducing systemic effects.[38] Using this route, major increases in the hepatic concentrations of intact drug are achieved relative to systemic targets of toxicity.

Catabolic Reactions The primary clearance mode of 5-FU is via catabolism along the degradative pathway for uracil.[21] The initial reaction is reduction by dihydrouracil dehydrogenase. The liver is a major site of 5-FU metabolism, and this is particularly true when the drug is given orally, intraperitoneally, or by intrahepatic arterial infusion. It is now recognized, however, that metabolism in the lung and kidneys may be of equal, or even greater, importance after IV administration.[33]

Marked circadian variations in the metabolism of 5-FU have been detected related to 24-hour cyclic variations in dihydrouracil dehydrogenase activity.[31,39] These changes are reflected in the inverse variations of plasma 5-FU concentrations during IV infusions in humans.[31,40] Means to employ these differences in the design of clinical protocols have been outlined.[41] Several clinical protocols comparing a continuous flat infusion with the circadian schedule have been conducted with 5-FU alone and in combination with leucovorin and/or platinum derivatives.[42–44] A clinical study using a 14-day continuous infusion of 5-FU and leucovorin suggests that circadian administration with a maximal infusion rate at 4 am increases the maximum tolerated dose (MTD) for both agents: 5-FU, 250 mg/m^2/d; leucovorin, 20 mg/m^2/d.[45] In patients who experienced grade 2 or higher toxicities with this schedule, the peak of their circadian infusion was moved from 9 to 10 pm. Decreased toxicity was observed (mostly diarrhea and stomatitis), and the MTD for 5-FU increased to 300 mg/m^2/d, a 50 mg increment over the MTD for a flat continuous infusion.[46]

Dihydropyrimidine dehydrogenase represents the initial rate-limiting step in the catabolism of the pyrimidines uracil, thymine, and 5-FU. More than 85% of an administered dose of 5-FU is metabolized with rapid formation of dihydrofluorouracil.[21] In a small percentage of the population, less than 3%, DPD activity is significantly below the average (below 50% of the control mean). This pharmacogenetic condition, which typically goes undetected until administration of 5-FU, can cause very serious life-threatening toxicity in patients following 5-FU-based chemotherapy; the toxicity is due to increased exposure to and activation of the anticancer agent.[47] The variability in DPD activity in normal tissues of the liver and gastrointestinal tract has been recently linked to the erratic oral bioavailability of 5-FU. DPD inhibitors, such as ethynyluracil, have been recently developed in an attempt to increase 5-FU efficacy and improve oral absorption; although, unfortunately, this has not been associated with an increase in the therapeutic index.[48–50]

The subsequent metabolic step, catalyzed by dihydropyrimidinase, yields β-fluoroureidopropionic acid. A wide variety of tumors apparently express high levels of this activity because they accumulate the subsequent degradation products β-ureidopropionic acid and β-alanine.[51]

α-Fluoro-β-alanine, the counterpart to the final product of uracil catabolism, β-alanine, is the major urinary excretion product of 5-FU.[52] In patients with cancer, this has been shown to be conjugated with bile acids and constitutes the primary biliary secretion product of 5-FU.[53] It has been suggested that the chenodeoxycholate conjugate may be responsible for the biliary toxicity seen after large-dose, intrahepatic infusion of 5-FU, and cholestasis associated with this conjugate has been demonstrated in isolated, perfused rat livers.[53] A summary of 5-FU metabolism is shown in Figure 43-3.

Mechanisms of Action Experimental evidence has suggested numerous sites for the biologic action of 5-FU (see Figure 43-3). The relative importance of each varies widely among different normal tissues and neoplasms. Commonly, the effects are divided into RNA- or DNA-directed toxicity.

RNA The predominant phosphorylated nucleoside of 5-FU, 5-FUTP, is as good a substrate as uridine triphosphate (UTP) for several RNA polymerase reactions. The degree of 5-FUTP incorporation into RNA bears a direct relationship to its concentration relative to that of the normal substrate UTP. In cell lines, greater incorporation is associated with reduced clonogenic survival.[54,55] Very substantial amounts of 5-FU replacement of uracil have been reported in each of the RNA species; the highest degree of incorporation is generally seen in the 4S-RNA.[16] Some evidence suggests that with a given cell type, the proportion of RNA incorporation in different species depends on the available form of the analog, 5-FU versus FdUrd. This result suggests compartmentalization or channeling of the analog en route to incorporation.[56]

What is less clear about incorporation into RNA is its contribution to cytotoxicity. Earlier studies indicated effects on transfer RNA acceptor activity, miscoding of protein synthesis, and inhibition of the maturation or processing of ribosomal RNA.[57] More recently, attention has focused on the inhibition of processing nuclear RNA to smaller-molecular-weight species.[58] Other post-transcriptional effects of 5-FU include inhibiting polyadenylation of messenger RNA (mRNA) and effects on DNA primase. In some model tumors and tumor lines, there is persuasive evidence that these RNA-directed events can be associated with cytotoxicity, particularly when the effects of extended exposure are monitored.[59,60]

Thymidylate Synthase The target site that can be defined most clearly is the covalent inactivation of thymidylate synthase by FdUMP.[61] Direct inhibition of the enzyme responsible for the 1-carbon transfer confirmed this site of action,[62,63] and subsequent research identified specific steps in the reaction in which a methylene group from 5,10-methylene tetrahydrofolate is transferred to the 5-position of 2'-deoxyuridylate.[9] These studies elegantly established the formation of a stable ternary covalent complex among the 5'-fluoro analog of deoxyuridylate, the reduced folate derivative, and thymidylate synthase.[64] The obvious consequence of this inhibition is an induced enzyme deficiency, depletion of dTTP, and the accumulation of deoxyuridine monophosphate (dUMP) behind the blockade.[61,65,66] More recently, it has been shown that in some tumors or normal tissues the rate-limiting factor in the formation of the abortive ternary complex with FdUMP is availability of the reduced folate derivative.[67,68] When this cofactor is limiting, it is possible to enhance inhibition by the administration of leucovorin.[69]

Recent studies have analyzed a possible correlation between TS expression and therapeutic outcome in colorectal, head and neck, and breast tumors treated with infusional 5-FU, with evidence that patients with high level of TS are less likely to respond.[70–76] A likely explanation for the lack of correlation in these studies is that factors other than TS alone may be involved. Thus, more recent clinical studies have shown that tumor response and survival are likely determined by multiple factors including TS, DPD (which controls the amount of 5-FU available for anabolism), and various enzymes in the pyrimidine anabolic pathway that control the interconversions of 5-FU anabolites.[77]

DNA Small quantities of 5-FU have been detected in internucleotide linkages within DNA.[78,79] Like dUTP, FdUTP, when it is available, is fully active as a substrate for the several DNA polymerases. But a very active glycosylase is present in most cells and excises any 5-FU or uracil that is incorporated in the place of thymine.[13,18] Mutants have been found that are relatively deficient in this editing function, and it may be that incorporation per se is not the cytotoxic event, but that the excision and repair involving a pyrimidine endonuclease generates opportunities for error-prone repair that might again reincorporate 5-FU or uracil instead of thymine nucleotides.[17,80,81] Because a considerable accumulation of dUMP occurs behind the blockade of thymidylate synthase, higher concentrations of dUTP are generated. These concentrations and any FdUTP increase the need for an editing function to remove incorporated uracil. Examination of the kinetics of this excision reaction indicates that uracil is removed as much as 30 times more rapidly than 5-FU.

It is not possible to rank the importance of these different potential mechanisms of cytotoxicity: RNA incorporation, dTTP depletion by thymidylate synthase inhibition, DNA incorporation, or damage to DNA consequent to excision of uracil or 5-FU. In fact, the relative importance of each of these sites may vary in different cell types. In some tumor lines, evidence for high sensitivity to RNA-directed effects is seen by the inability of thymidine to overcome growth inhibition, despite the presence of an active thymidine kinase.[82] In these same lines, uridine rescue is more successful than in others where thymidine effectively prevents cytotoxicity, presumably by repleting dTTP.

Resistance As with most drugs, partial or complete responses of human cancer to 5-FU are generally followed by the eventual regrowth of tumor despite sustained, or even increased, dosages. Understanding some of the factors that contribute to natural or acquired resistance has stimulated several approaches to modulating 5-FU therapy. The most prominent mechanism seen in experimental tumors is reduced anabolism of the analog to nucleotide form.[83,84] This may reflect altered condensation with PRPP or activation via the two-stage salvage pathway involving ribose-1-phosphate or deoxyribose-1-phosphate and the appropriate nucleoside phosphorylase, with subsequent phosphorylation of the resultant nucleoside by uridine or thymidine kinase. Alternatively, lack of sensitivity has been correlated with an increased disappearance rate of 5-FU nucleotides, which were documented in one case to reflect enhanced nucleotide phosphatase activity.[85] Alterations in the catabolism of 5-FU appear to affect sensitivity and predict responsiveness to the drug. DPD, the rate-limiting enzyme in the catabolism of pyrimidines, regulates the amount of 5-FU available for the activation to nucleotide forms. In hepatocellular carcinomas inherently resistant to fluoropyrimidine-based chemotherapy, DPD activity was found elevated compared with that of normal tissue.[86] DPD activity was also found to predict response to 5-FU in head and neck tumors, and DPD mRNA levels predicted resistance to the drug in colorectal cancer patients.[87,88] Other well-documented mechanisms of resistance reflect changes in the thymidylate synthase, with reduced affinity for FdUMP,[89] or increases in the rate of synthesis and activity of the enzyme, possibly associated with gene amplification or altered enzyme turnover rates.[90] The mode of exposure to the drug can result in the selection of tumor cells with different mechanisms of resistance.[91–93]

Modulation of Therapy: Leucovorin To improve the limited response rate to therapy with 5-FU, a rate of 10 to 25% in the most responsive cancers, various biochemical strategies have been investigated.[94] The degree of 5-FU activation by orotidylate pyrophosphorylase is affected by the available concentrations of PRPP. Because alterations of traffic along both the purine and pyrimidine nucleotide biosynthesis pathways affect the available concentrations of PRPP, several drug or metabolite combinations have been shown to modify the activation of 5-FU; presumably, by altering the concentration of this ribose-5'-phosphate donor.[95–97] Others have explored depletion of pyrimidine nucleotides by inhibitors of the de novo synthesis of pyrimidines. A major focus in this area has been enhancing the efficiency with which the covalent complex of FdUMP with the folate cofactor and thymidylate synthase is formed by supplementation with the reduced folate cofactor.[98]

Formation of the ternary complex of FdUMP, thymidylate synthase, and folate coenzymes may be limited by the availability of reduced folates in some cell lines and tumors.[64,99] To optimize formation of the covalent complex, large doses of leucovorin, or D,L-*N*-5-formyl tetrahydrofolate, have been employed to saturate target enzymes with L-5-10-methylene tetrahydrofolate via conversion of the l-isomer of leucovorin to 5-methyl tetrahydrofolate.[100]

5-FU cytotoxicity has been shown to be directly related to the quantity of the ternary complex formed within the cells.[59,98] Because of the enhanced inhibition of thymidylate synthase when prior supplementation with leucovorin is employed, the dose of 5-FU must be reduced by approximately 20%.[25] Under these conditions, diarrhea and mucositis remain the dose-limiting toxicities.

A wide range of clinical studies have generally confirmed the increased rate of response to 5-FU therapy in colorectal cancer when supplemented by leucovorin.[69,101,102] However, evidence for increased survival in these trials is limited.[25,101] In breast and stomach cancers, the response rate in patients who were not previously treated with 5-FU appears also to be increased by the addition of leucovorin; data for other diseases are insufficient to draw conclusions. The generally favorable results obtained in these studies have led to a rather universal addition of leucovorin to 5-FU trials in combination with other drugs. Particularly promising are three studies combining 5-FU–leucovorin with cisplatin in head and neck cancer.[69]

Oral Prodrug of 5-Fluorouracil: Capecitabine A recent meta-analysis of infusional versus bolus 5-FU has concluded that protracted low-dose infusion of 5-FU has resulted in a higher response rate, 22% versus 14%, with improvement in survival.[27] However, the long-term delivery requires a surgically implanted venous access and the use of an infusion pump. The administration of oral 5-FU could reduce the cost of treatment and be more convenient to the patient. Its oral use has been hampered by an incomplete and variable bioavailability. Over the past several years many oral fluoropyrimidines have been evaluated clinically. Although several had potentially desirable pharmacologic attributes, only capecitabine has received Food and Drug Administration (FDA) approval in the United States.

Capecitabine is an orally administered fluoropyrimidine carbamate prodrug (Figure 43-4) that is activated to 5-FU by three sequential enzymatic steps. First, hepatic carboxyesterase hydrolyses the *N*-pentyl carbamate chain to form 5'-deoxy-5-fluorocytidine, which is then deaminated to 5'-deoxy-5-fluorouridine (5'-d5-FUR) by cytidine deaminase. Then thymidine and uridine phosphorylases hydrolyze 5'-d5-FUR to produce 5-FU. The higher phosphorolytic activity expressed in human tumor tissue compared with that of the surrounding normal tissue has been suggested to result in selective activation and an improved therapeutic index. A higher concentration of 5-FU (2.9-fold) has been demonstrated in colorectal tumor specimens when compared with adjacent normal tissue of patients who received oral capecitabine 5 to 7 days prior to surgical removal of the tumor.[103] Capecitabine is typically administered bid at a total daily dosage of 2,000 to 2,500 mg/m^2/d over 14 days. This dosage generates plasma peak levels 2 hours after administration, comparable with the ones achieved with a continuous intravenous infusion of 300 mg/m^2/d of 5-FU. Toxicities were also similar to a continuous 5-FU infusion, with diarrhea, mucositis, and hand-and-foot syndrome.[104] The toxicities are for the most part tolerable, in particular at the 2,000 mg/m^2/d dosage, and reversible after a short interval off therapy.

Capecitabine was initially approved for the treatment of metastatic breast cancer resistant to chemotherapy containing both paclitaxel and anthracyclines. In this patient population, an 18.5% response rate was observed.[105]

Subsequently, capecitabine was approved for use in advanced colorectal cancer based on demonstrated equivalence in phase III studies to intravenously administered 5-FU-leucovorin (Mayo regimen).[106,107] It is of interest that coadministration of leucovorin was not required to obtain a comparable effect.

Most recently, capecitabine has been approved for combined use with docetaxel in advanced breast cancer.[108] The desirable effect of this combination may be due to up-regulation of thymidine phosphorylase by docetaxel. Several other chemotherapy agents in addition to radiation are

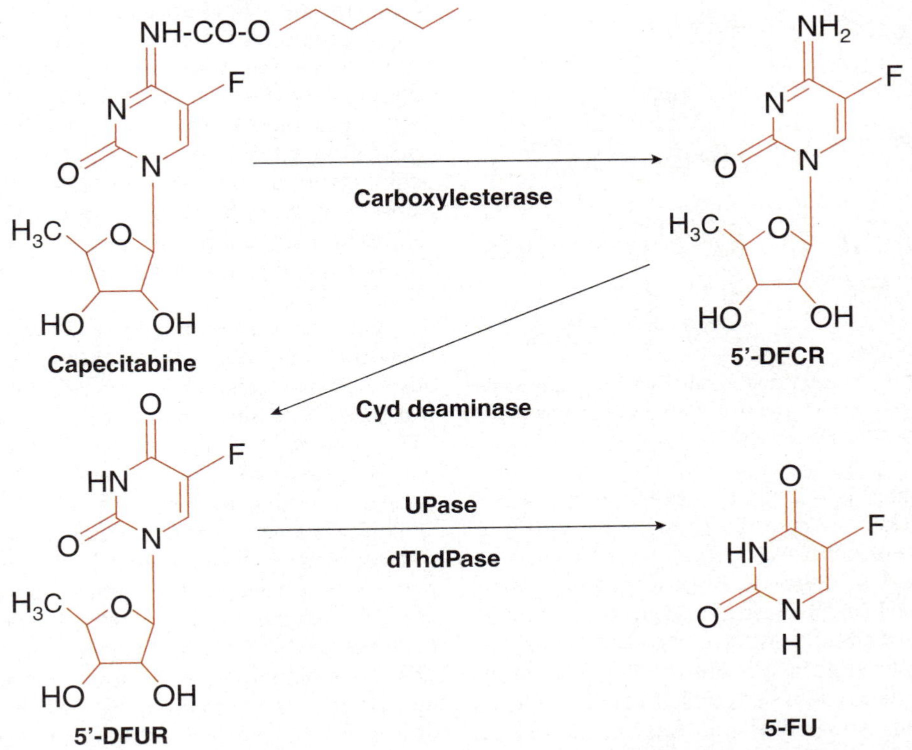

Figure 43-4 Structure and activation of capecitabine. Adapted from Xeloda product information, Roche USA. NHCO-$(CH_2)_4$ CH_3.

now recognized to up-regulate thymidine phosphorylase, thereby increasing selective intratumoral activation of capecitabine.[109]

CYTOSINE ARABINOSIDE **Background** Cytosine arabinoside (cytarabine or ara-C) is a nucleoside analog of deoxycytidine.[110] It represents one of the most important drugs in the treatment of acute myeloid leukemia. It is also active against acute lymphocytic leukemia and, to a lesser extent, is useful in chronic myelocytic leukemia and non-Hodgkin's lymphoma.[111] It has not proven to be particularly useful in the treatment of nonhematologic neoplasms. Myelosuppression and gastrointestinal epithelial injury are the primary toxic effects of ara-C. Using high-dose ara-C regimens, additional toxic effects such as intrahepatic cholestasis and central nervous system (CNS) toxicity are frequently observed.[112]

Metabolism Cytosine arabinoside is rapidly deaminated by cytidine deaminase to a much less active compound, arabinosyluracil (ara-U).[113–115] Ara-C enters cells through a carrier-mediated process or by simple diffusion.[116,117] After entering the cells, it is metabolized primarily by the enzymes that normally metabolize deoxycytidine or, in some instances, cytidine (Figure 43-5).

The enzyme that is responsible for cytosine arabinoside monophosphate (ara-CMP) synthesis is cytoplasmic deoxycytidine kinase. The amount of ara-CMP formed depends on the relative activity of cytoplasmic deoxycytidine kinase and cytidine deaminase. The enzyme responsible for conversion of ara-CMP to cytosine arabinoside diphosphate (ara-CDP) is cytidylateuridylate-deoxycytidylate (CMP-UMP-dCMP) kinase. It has been suggested that ara-CMP could be deaminated to uracil arabinoside monophosphate (ara-UMP) by dCMP deaminase.[118] Whether this pathway is functional in cells is questionable, however, because ara-CMP is a very poor substrate for dCMP deaminase compared with dCMP. Several mammalian cell lines are partially resistant to ara-C because of an increased activity of dCMP deaminase.[119,120] Enzymes responsible for the phosphorylation of ara-CDP to cytosine arabinoside triphosphate (ara-CTP) are nucleoside diphosphate (NDP) kinases. There are multiple species of NDP kinase activities in human cells, and many of them belong to the *nm23* gene family.[121]

Major attention has also been focused on the incorporation of ara-CTP into DNA in competition with deoxycytidine triphosphate (dCTP).[122–124] Elongation of DNA by polymerase α is considerably retarded by the incorporation of ara-CMP, whereas no significant impact on elongation by DNA polymerase β could be seen after incorporation of a single ara-C nucleoside residue. However, neither polymerase alone could appreciably elongate the DNA if two consecutive ara-CMP residues were incorporated. Thus, the behavior of ara-CTP on DNA polymerase is not only polymerase dependent but also sequence dependent.[125,126]

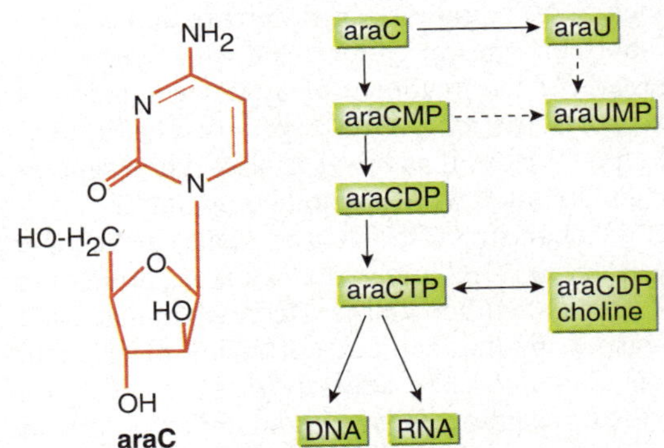

Figure 43-5 Structure and metabolism of arabinosylcytosine (ara-C). araCDP = cytosine arabinoside diphosphate; araCMP = cytosine arabinoside monophosphate; araCTP = cytosine arabinoside triphosphate; araU = arabinoxyluracil; araUMP = uracil arabinoside monophosphate; MP, DP, TP = mono-, di-, and triphosphate.

Mechanism of Action The primary action of ara-C is inhibition of nuclear DNA synthesis.[127,128] Mitochondrial DNA synthesis is not affected by ara-C, even at concentrations 10 times greater than that required to inhibit cell growth by 50%. The possibility remains, however, that the functional nature of mitochondrial DNA may be compromised through incorporation of ara-C internally.[114]

Three mechanisms have been suggested to account for the inhibition of nuclear DNA synthesis by ara-C. The relative importance of each mechanism may depend on the intracellular concentration of ara-CTP. The first mechanism is inhibition of the initiation of new replication units in chromosomes consequent to the incorporation of ara-C into the replicon–initiation primer.[129] The second mechanism is the retardation of DNA-chain elongation because of the incorporation of ara-C into DNA.[122,123] This effect is DNA polymerase and sequence dependent, as discussed earlier. Reactions catalyzed by DNA polymerase α, and perhaps DNA polymerase β, are more susceptible than other DNA polymerase activities. The third mechanism, which may become important only when a high-dose ara-C protocol is used, is the inhibition of DNA primase.[130]

In general, the inhibition of cell growth correlates well with the degree of the incorporation of ara-C into cellular DNA. The majority of incorporated ara-CMP is in internucleotide linkage in DNA. The relative ratio of ara-C in internucleotide, compared with chain-terminal positions, depends on the concentration of ara-C; the higher the concentration of ara-C to which the cells are exposed, the lower the relative amount of internucleotide ara-C residues. This could result from the higher probability of consecutive ara-CMPs being incorporated into DNA, which stops further DNA-chain elongation catalyzed by DNA polymerase α and DNA polymerase β. The amount of ara-CMP that is incorporated into DNA also depends on the relative ratio of ara-CTP to dCTP. Decreases in the intracellular pool of dCTP can increase the amount of ara-CMP that is incorporated. Exonucleases such as the recently identified TREX 1 and even TP53 could remove ara-C incorporated in terminal positions to limit the cytotoxic effects.

The mechanism of action for ara-C may be dosage dependent. At noncytotoxic concentrations, ara-C can cause human promyeloblast HL-60 cell lines to differentiate. It has been suggested that the success of low-dose ara-C therapy in patients with myelodysplastic syndrome may result from the differentiation effects of ara-C.[127] When given to patients with leukemia, high doses of ara-C cause rapid tumor-cell lysis.[131] Whether additional mechanisms of ara-C also play important roles in this protocol is unclear. In patients who receive high doses, the concentration of ara-U, the deamination product of ara-C, can exceed 100 µM in plasma.[132] The high concentrations of ara-U may act in concert with ara-C by inhibiting its metabolism, and it also may affect cell growth by mechanisms that have not yet been established.[133]

Mechanism of Resistance Cells could become resistant to ara-C because of (1) decreased activities of the carrier for ara-C transport and for cytoplasmic deoxycytidine kinase; (2) increased catabolism of ara-C through the action of cytidine deaminase; (3) increased formation of dCTP by ribonucleotide reductase and NDP kinase; or (4) decreased activity of dCMP deaminase, which could lead to increased competition between dCTP and ara-CTP for incorporation into DNA. An increased activity of 3' to 5' exonuclease, which could remove ara-CMP from the DNA-chain terminus, has also been suggested.[134]

5-AZACYTIDINE Background 5-Azacytidine (5-AC) was first synthesized in 1963, and it was later isolated as a natural product from fungal cultures.[135,136] The clinical utility of this cytidine analog is primarily in the treatment of acute myelocytic leukemia and myelodysplastic syndrome, where in low dose, it is able to cause partial or complete differentiation in hematopoiesis in the majority of patients; occasionally, clinical response has been observed in patients with solid tumors. The major toxicity of 5-AC is leukopenia and, to a lesser degree, thrombocytopenia. Hepatotoxicity has also been reported, particularly in patients with pre-existing hepatic dysfunction.[111]

Metabolism The replacement of carbon by nitrogen in position 5 of the cytidine heterocyclic ring results in a marked chemical instability. The product of the ring opening, *N*-formylamidinoribofuranosyl guanylurea, may recycle to form the parent compound, but it is also susceptible to further decomposition. This tendency to decompose not only may play a role in its mechanism of action, but also is troublesome in its clinical use.[137] Although 5-AC can be deaminated by cytidine deaminase to 5-azauridine (5-AU), a less toxic compound, the efficiency of this deamination by cytidine deaminase is less than that of cytidine. 5-AC enters mammalian cells by a facilitated nucleoside transport mechanism that is shared with other nucleosides.[138] The initial step in its activation is the conversion to 5-azacytidine monophosphate (5-ACMP) by uridine-cytidine kinase.[139] 5-ACMP is further phosphorylated to 5-AC di- and triphosphate by CMP-UMP-dCMP kinases and nucleoside diphosphate kinases, respectively. 5-AC triphosphate can be incorporated into RNA, but its pathway for incorporation into DNA is not well defined. 5-Azacytidine disphosphate (5-ACDP) likely is reduced by ribonucleotide reductase to the corresponding deoxynucleotide diphosphate. This diphosphate is phosphorylated by nucleoside diphosphate kinases to 5-azadeoxycytidine disphosphate (5-AdCTP), which can be efficiently

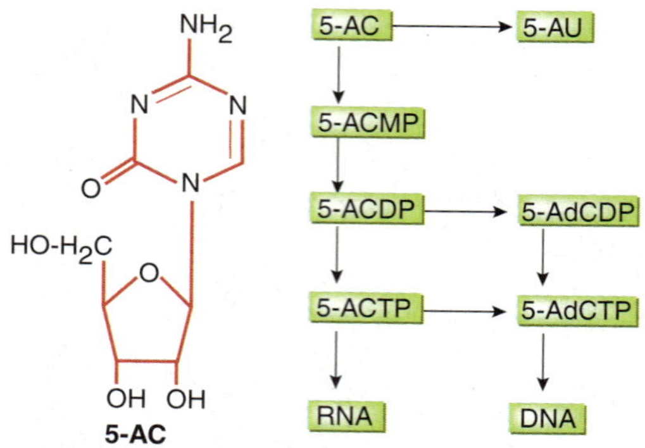

Figure 43-6 Structure and metabolism of 5-azacytidine (5-AC). 5-AdC = 5-azadeoxycytidine; 5-AU = 5-azauridine; MP, DP, TP = mono-, di-, and triphosphate.

incorporated into DNA by DNA polymerases α and β. The incorporated 5-azadeoxycytidine monophosphate (5-AdCMP) at the 3' terminus of DNA has less effect on subsequent DNA-chain elongation than the incorporated ara-CMP at the 3' terminus of DNA. 5-Azadeoxycytidine (5-AdC) is also stabilized against hydrolytic degradation by incorporation into DNA, which could result, in part, from hydrophobic shielding of the triazine ring from water and other polar nucleophiles within the DNA double helix.[126,140]

A summary of 5-AC metabolism is shown in Figure 43-6. 5-AC is most cytotoxic to cells in the DNA-synthetic phase of the cell cycle, but the exact mechanism of its cytotoxic action has not been well established. It could inhibit both DNA and RNA synthesis. Incorporation into RNA can inhibit the processing of ribosomal RNA from higher-molecular-weight species, disassembly of polyribosomes, and markedly inhibit protein synthesis. Incorporation into DNA also could inhibit DNA synthesis.[141–144] One important, well-documented effect is the inhibition of DNA methylation because of stoichiometric binding with DNA-methyltransferase after incorporation. The methylation of cytosine residues in DNA is responsible for the inactivation of specific genes; thus, treatment of cells with 5-AC leads to reduced levels of cytosine methylation and enhanced expression of selected genes that are normally suppressed. At minimally cytotoxic concentrations, 5-AC stimulates the differentiation of some tumor cell lines in culture, and it has been suggested for the treatment of hypermethylation in particular patients with myelodysplastic syndrome,[145] as well as for virus-associated cancers in combination with antiviral compounds.

Mechanism of Resistance Cells can become resistant to 5-AC by the reduction or elimination of uridine-cytidine kinase. Decreased nucleoside transport by the facilitated diffusion mechanism can also decrease sensitivity to 5-AC, and cytosine deaminase may play an important role in cell sensitivity as well. In animal models, tumor cells that are resistant to ara-C because of the deletion of cytoplasmic deoxycytidine kinase activity—a frequent mechanism of cellular resistance to ara-C—are more susceptible to 5-AC than is the parent tumor line.[146]

GEMCITABINE Background 2', 2'-difluoro-2'-deoxycytidine (dFdC) is a deoxycytidine analog with two fluorine atoms in the 2' position of the sugar moiety (Figure 43-7). First synthesized in 1986, this molecule was initially developed as an antiviral agent because of its potent inhibitory activity against both DNA and RNA viruses.[147] Subsequently, its broad spectrum of activity in murine tumors and human tumor xenografts[148] led to evaluating this antineoplastic activity in clinical trials.

dFdC was approved by the FDA in 1996 as a first-line treatment of patients with locally advanced or metastatic adenocarcinoma of the pancreas.[149,150] Subsequently, dFdC has received FDA approval for the treatment of inoperable, locally advanced or metastatic nonsmall-cell lung cancer, in combination with cisplatin.[151–154]

dFdC has been found active in the treatment of breast cancer when combined with cisplatin in patients pretreated with anthracycline and taxane.[155,156] Activity has also been shown in bladder cancer[157–160] and in ovarian cancer.[161,162] dFdC has demonstrated a promising effect in non-Hodgkin's lymphoma,[163,164] in Hodgkin's disease,[165] and in patients with relapsed or refractory cutaneous T-cell lymphoma.[166]

The dose-limiting toxicity of dFdC in both single-agent and combination studies is mild to moderate myelosuppression. The nonhematologic toxicity is mild, with nausea, vomiting, occasional skin rash, alopecia, and pneumonitis. Rare occurrences of hemolyticuremic syndrome have been reported.[167–169]

Metabolism 2', 2'-difluoro-2'-deoxycytidine requires phosphorylation by deoxycytidine kinase to exert its cytotoxic activity (see Figure 43-7). The major intracellular metabolite is 2', 2'-difluoro-2'-deoxycytidine triphosphate (dFd-CTP); lesser amounts of the monophosphate (dFdCMP) and the diphosphate (dFdCDP) are also present.[170] Cellular elimination of dFdCTP follows a biphasic course, with a short initial half-life followed by a second, slower phase of degradation.[171,172] The

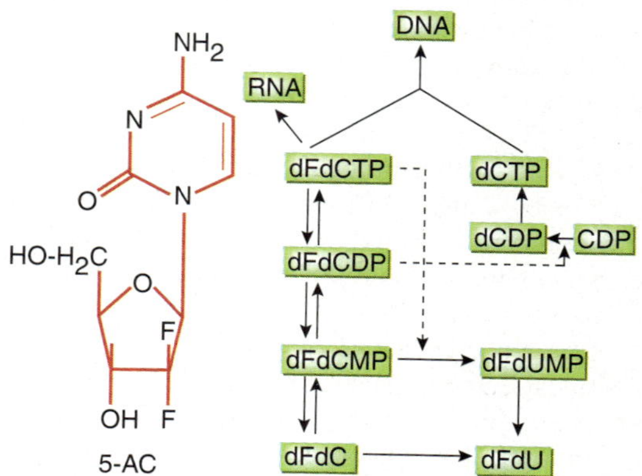

Figure 43-7 Structure, metabolism, and actions of 2', 2'-difluoro-2'-deoxycytidine (dFdC) and its nucleotides. Dashed lines indicate inhibitory actions. Modified from Heinemann et al. CDP = cytidine diphosphate; dU = deoxyuridine; MP, DP, TP = mono-, di-, and triphosphate.

biphasic elimination of dFdCTP differs from the linear monophasic kinetic that is exhibited by the triphosphate of ara-C,[173] arabinosyladenine,[174] and arabinosyl-2-fluoroadenine.[175]

Deoxycytidine deaminase inactivates dFdC to 2', 2'-difluoro-2'-deoxyuridine (dFdU), which has no antitumor activity.[170] The monophosphate of dFdC also can be deaminated to the uracil derivative 2'difluoro-deoxyridine monophosphate (dFdUMP) by deoxycytidylate deaminase.[176]

Pharmacokinetic studies during phase I clinical trials have shown a very rapid half-life (8 minutes) for dFdC because of deamination over a wide range of dosages.[177] The concentration of dFdCTP in mononuclear cells increases in proportion to the dose of dFdC infused, up to 250 mg/m^2. Above this dose, the process shows saturation in accumulation of the triphosphate derivative.

Mechanism of Action 2', 2'-difluoro-2'-deoxycytidine exerts its inhibitory activity on DNA synthesis through several distinct mechanisms. The accumulation of dFdCTP causes a reduction in the deoxyribonucleotide dCTP through direct inhibition of ribonucleotide reductase, caused mainly by dFdCDP.[178,179] Another important mechanism is the incorporation of dFdCTP into DNA. dFdCTP competes with dCTP for incorporation into the C sites of DNA as catalyzed by DNA polymerases α and ε. The primer extension pauses one deoxynucleotide after dFdCMP incorporation.[180] Moreover, the exonuclease activity of polymerase ε is unable to excise nucleotides from DNA containing dFdCMP at either the 3' end or at an internal position.[180] The cytotoxic activity of dFdC strongly correlates with the amount of monophosphate that is incorporated into cellular DNA.

Incorporation of dFdC into RNA has been detected in tumor cell lines but the extent of this incorporation was 2- to 10-fold less than that into DNA.[181]

To date, two examples of resistance to dFdC have been reported.[182,183] Human ovarian carcinoma cells exposed to increasing concentrations of dFdC became highly resistant to the drug and are cross-resistant to ara-C and 2-chlorodeoxyadenosine, and modestly resistant to doxorubicin, vincristine, and *cis*-platin. Resistant cells did not possess deoxycytidine kinase activity; therefore, they were not able to phosphorylate dFdC as well as the other two nucleoside analogs. Another mechanism of resistance has been recently reported. Human KB tumor cells could become resistant to dFdC as the result of increased expression of the M2 unit of ribonucleotide reductase. Resistance leads to elevated activity of the same enzyme, as well as an augmented intracellular dCTP pool, which could prevent the phosphorylation of dFdC by deoxycytidine kinase.[183]

PURINE ANALOGS

The original syntheses of purine antimetabolites focused on isosteric replacement of oxygen, carbon, or nitrogen in the purine ring, and they were predicated on the same logic as that used for pyrimidines.[2,3,184] The first clinically useful agent,

Mercaptopurine

Azathioprine

Thioguanine

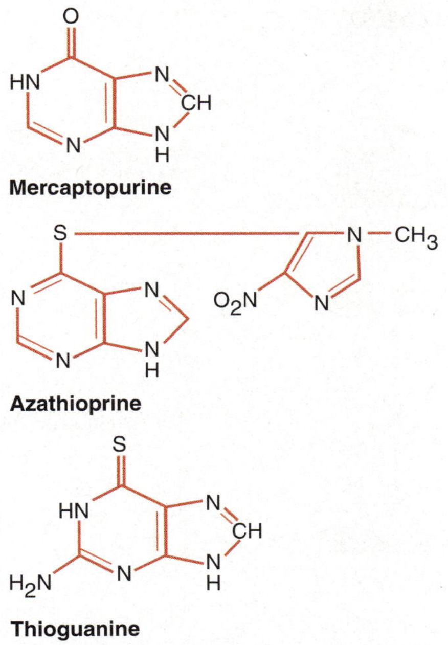

Figure 43-8 Purine antimetabolites.

however, was 6-mercaptopurine (6-MP),[185] in which the 6-OH of hypoxanthine was replaced with a thiol group (Figure 43-8). Subsequently, the equivalent analog of guanine, 6-thioguanine, was prepared.[186]

By the identification of metabolites and characterization of resistance mechanisms, early studies with 6-MP in model systems quickly demonstrated the dependence of the inhibitory activity on metabolic conversion to the corresponding nucleotide analogs.[187] Equally important to the activity of many purine analogs has been an understanding of the catabolic reactions that limit their availability. Of particular relevance are xanthine oxidase, which inactivates 6-MP and thioguanine,[188] and adenosine deaminase,[189] which is the target for deoxycoformycin and limits the action of arabinosyl adenosine.

6-Mercaptopurine (6-MP) was among the first purine analogs that demonstrated antineoplastic activity, and it remains useful in the treatment of acute leukemia.[190] Metabolic activation primarily occurs by reaction with PRPP via hypoxanthine-guanine pyrophosphorylase (HGPRT) to form 6-MP riboside 5'-phosphate, more properly called thioinosine monophosphate (TIMP).[191]

TIMP is believed to exert its major effect on purine nucleotide metabolism by inhibition of the first step in purine biosynthesis, the formation of 1-NH_2-ribose-5-PO_4, via a pseudofeedback inhibition in which TIMP mimics the regulatory action of adenine or guanine nucleoside monophosphates.[192–194] An early precursor of purine biosynthesis, 5-amino imidazol-4-carboxamide, which can be converted to the corresponding ribonucleotide, protects cells in culture against the inhibition of growth by 6-MP. This finding is consistent with the view that the primary action is limitation of an early step in de novo synthesis. TIMP also blocks the subsequent metabolism of inosinic acid, the initial purine nucleotide, to adenylic acid by inhibiting adenosylsuccinate synthase.[191] Similarly, synthesis of guanine nucleotides is reduced by inhibition of the oxidation of inosinic acid to xanthylic acid. TIMP is not incorporated into nucleic acids as such, but minor amounts are converted to thioguanylic acid, which is incorporated into both RNA and DNA. It has not been established, however, that this incorporation is significant to the toxic or antineoplastic actions of 6-MP.[1] TIMP was recently shown to be a potent inhibitor of DNA exonuclease, which could excise ara-CMP from terminal DNA. This may partly explain the synergistic interaction of 6-MP and ara-C.[195] A summary of 6-MP metabolism is presented in Figure 43-9.

6-Mercaptopurine is generally administered orally (90 mg/m^2) for several weeks. Absorption is variable, incomplete, and associated with a half-life of 20 to 45 minutes in plasma, where it is minimally bound to serum proteins.[196] The rapid turnover largely results from oxidation by xanthine oxidase, which converts it to inactive thiouric acid, the primary urinary excretion product.[197] Another metabolite, the *S*-methyl derivative of 6-MP, is found in cells as methyl mercaptopurine ribonucleotide, where it inhibits purine metabolism. It is excreted in urine as methyl mercaptopurine riboside.

The dose-limiting toxicity of 6-MP is myelosuppression. It is slow in onset, 2 to 4 weeks, and rapidly reversed after the dose is either reduced or discontinued.[198,199] All formed elements (thrombocytes, granulocytes, and erythrocytes) can be affected. Although gastrointestinal mucositis or stomatitis is minimal, approximately 25% of treated patients experience nausea, vomiting, and anorexia. A small number display hepatotoxicity.[200]

Therapeutic action depends on the formation of the nucleotide 6-MP ribonucleoside monophosphate. In experimental tumor systems, resistance commonly is associated with a decreased rate of activation to the nucleotide form, resulting from deletion or modification of HGPRT activity. Limited studies in humans, however, suggest that resistance is caused by increased activity of a 5'-phosphatase that limits the concentration and duration of intracellular 6-MP ribonucleotide.[201]

6-Mercaptopurine is effective in combination with prednisone for inducing remission in children with acute lymphoblastic leukemia. Currently, it is a regular component of consolidation and maintenance therapy for this disease. It is also of some value in adult acute lymphocytic leukemias.

Thioguanine (see Figure 43-8) is the 6-thiol derivative of guanine corresponding to 6-MP and also depends on activation via HGPRT.[190] Unlike 6-MP, however, di- and triphosphates of thioguanine ribonucleotide are formed and incorporated into RNA. After conversion to thioguanine deoxynucleotide triphosphate, it can substitute for deoxyguanosine triphosphate (dGTP) in DNA polymerase reactions.[202] This incorporation is thought to be the primary mechanism of cytotoxicity.[203] Thioguanylate monophosphate is the predominant

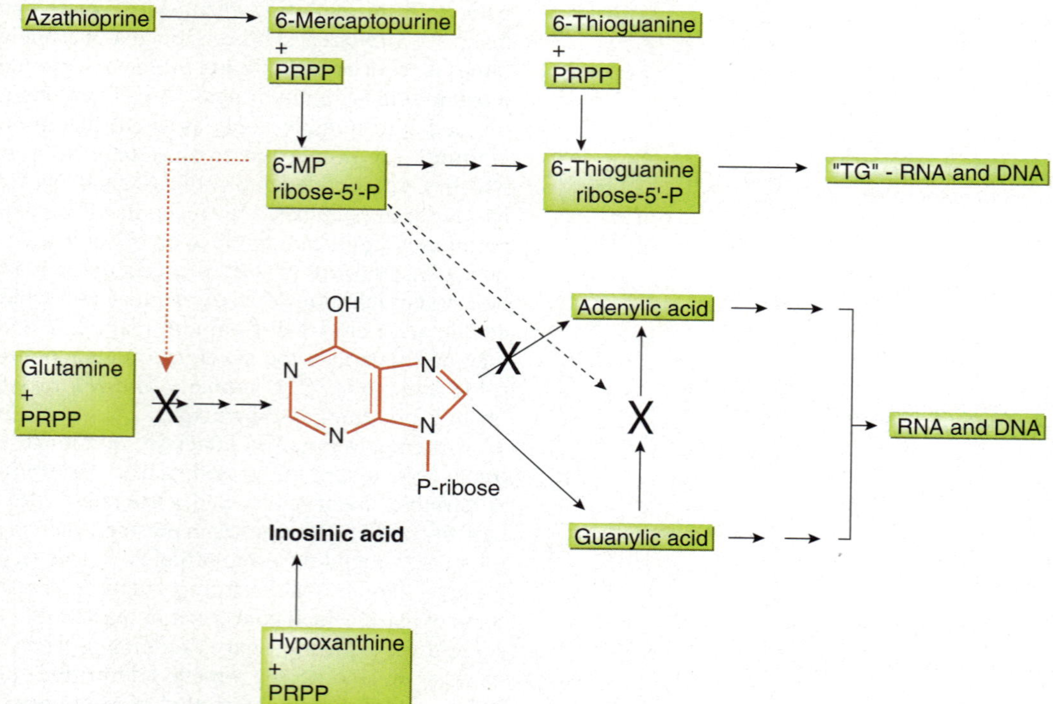

Figure 43-9 Metabolic activation and targets of thiopurines. 6-MP = 6-mercaptopurine; PRPP =pyrophosphorylribose-5-PO_4.

acid-soluble nucleotide, but it does not appear to exert the major effects on de novo purine synthesis that have been observed with 6-MP nor to deplete pools of normal purine nucleotides.

Like 6-MP, thioguanine, after deamination to thioxanthine by guanase, is readily catabolized to thiouric acid by xanthine oxidase. *S*-methylation is also observed, yielding *S*-methyl-thioguanine and thioxanthine.[204] Dethiolation contributes to metabolism as well, as evidenced by the urinary excretion of ^{35}S-SO4 after administration of ^{35}S-thioguanine. The primary use of thioguanine is in acute myeloid leukemia, where it may be combined with arabinosyl cytosine. However, recent studies question its value in this disease.[205,206] A summary of thioguanine metabolism is presented in Figure 43-9.

Allopurinol (4-hydroxypyrazolo[3,4-d]pyrimidine) is an important adjuvant to antineoplastic therapy (Figure 43-10). This agent and its primary metabolite, oxypurinol, are potent inhibitors of xanthine oxidase.[207,208] As such, they limit the formation of uric acid from the degradation of purine nucleotides and nucleic acids. In addition to this mechanism, allopurinol has been shown to inhibit purine nucleotide biosynthesis by feedback inhibition of the first reaction in the pathway and to deplete pyrophosphoryl ribose-5-PO_4, presumably by formation of the corresponding allopurinol and oxypurinol ribonucleotides.[209]

Although it was originally synthesized as an antineoplastic agent, allopurinol is widely used in the treatment of hyperuricemia that is associated with gout and other metabolic disorders.[210] Certain neoplastic states, particularly lympho- and myeloproliferative diseases, also generate hyperuricemia, and allopurinol is an effective means to avoid the associated episodes of gout or uric acid nephropathy.[211] This is particularly important in leukemias, lymphomas, and in patients with other bulky diseases when chemotherapy produces rapid tumor lysis and its attendant release of purine bases from the nucleic acids.

The elevation of hypoxanthine and xanthine concentrations in plasma by the inhibition of xanthine oxidase is less dangerous than elevated levels of uric acid. This is because these purines are more soluble and less likely to form stones or cause gout. Nevertheless, it is generally recommended that patients who are treated with allopurinol for hyperuricemia also be hydrated and alkalinized when uric acid concentrations rise significantly.

Oral dosages of 300 to 800 mg/d have been recommended and generally are well tolerated. Because allopurinol also reduces the rate of metabolic inactivation of oral 6-MP and azathioprine, doses of these purine antimetabolites must be reduced by 50 to 75% to avoid excessive toxicity.[196] Oxidation by xanthine oxidase is the primary route of allopurinol metabolism and the relevant site of action, but allopurinol can also inhibit the metabolism of drugs, such as cyclophosphamide, by the mixed function oxidases.[212]

DEOXYCOFORMYCIN Background Deoxycoformycin (pentostatin) is a natural product first isolated in 1974 from the culture of *Streptomyces antibioticus* (see Figure 43-9).[213] Its structure mimics the transitional-state form of adenosine in an adenosine deaminase–catalyzed reaction, and it is one of the most potent inhibitors of adenosine deaminase.

The initial clinical development of deoxycoformycin centered on its activity as an adenosine

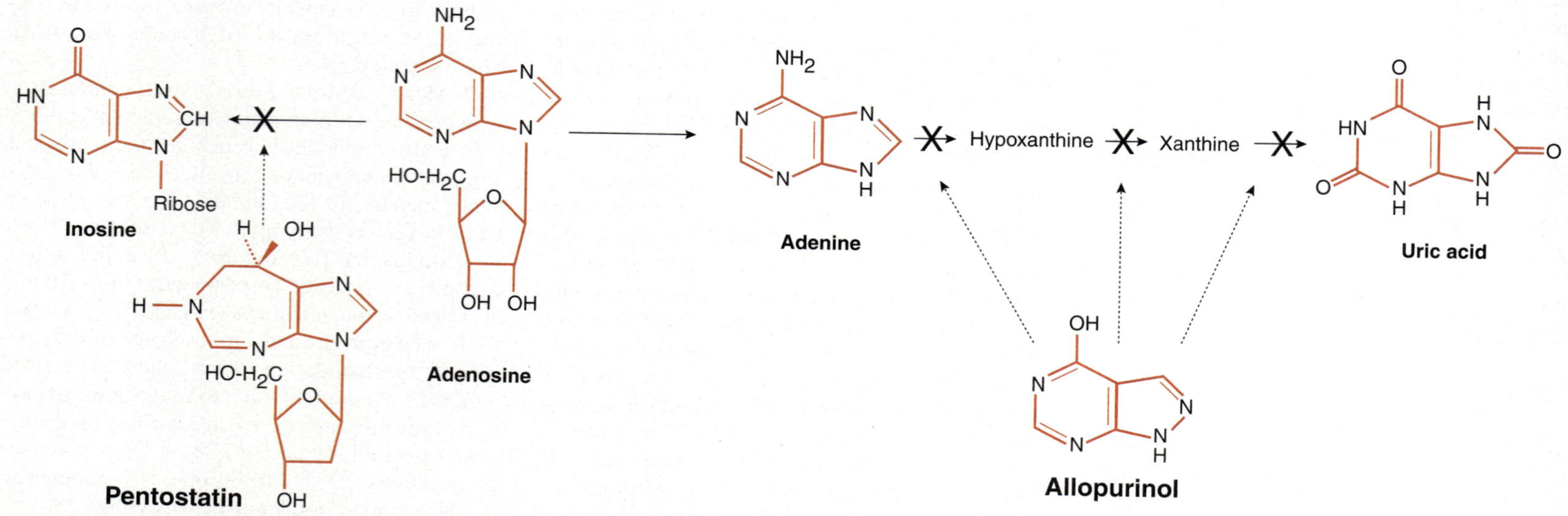

Figure 43-10 Inhibitors of purine nucleoside catabolism.

deaminase inhibitor for the potentiation of adenosine arabinoside, which was also deaminated by adenosine deaminase to yield less toxic compounds. During early phase I studies, the profound lymphotoxic effect of deoxycoformycin was noted. Other studies described a congenital syndrome of severe combined immunodeficiency associated with low or undetectable levels of adenosine deaminase in lymphocytes.[214] These results suggested the importance of adenosine deaminase in lymphocyte function, leading to intensive development of deoxycoformycin as a single agent for the treatment of lymphoproliferative diseases.

The most responsive tumor identified is hairy-cell leukemia, in which durable remissions are achieved in over 90% of patients with a relatively brief course of treatment.[215,216] Other responsive lymphoid diseases include chronic lymphocytic leukemia and prolymphocytic leukemia, mycosis fungoides, and acute T-cell leukemia/lymphoma.[217,218] Considerable variation exists in the susceptibility of patients to deoxycoformycin toxicity. This includes immunosuppression,[219,220] CNS disturbances, impaired renal function, conjunctivitis, and muscle and joint pain. Impaired renal function and poor performance status place patients at high risk of toxicity, even with low dosages of this drug.

Metabolism Deoxycoformycin enters the cell through the facilitated-diffusion nucleoside carrier. It can be phosphorylated to mono-, di-, and triphosphate nucleotides, and significant incorporation into DNA, but not RNA, has been observed.[215] Adenosine kinase and deoxycytidine kinase[213] do not appear to be responsible for the initial phosphorylation, but transphosphorylation with other purine nucleotide monophsosphates such as adenosine monophosphate (AMP) or inosine monophosphate (IMP) by 5'-nucleotidase reaction is a potential basis for nucleotide formation.

Mechanisms of Action and Resistance The primary site of action is the inhibition of adenosine deaminase. Because of the inhibition of adenosine deaminase in vivo, deoxyadenosine and adenosine cannot be catabolized efficiently. Consequently, deoxyadenosine-phosphorylated metabolites accumulate in many types of cells.[221] This imbalance in deoxynucleotide pools is known to be toxic to cells, and the antitumor activity of deoxycoformycin may result from the combination of direct effects of deoxycoformycin and its metabolites as well as the expanded pools of deoxyadenosine.

The degree of deoxyadenosine triphosphate (dATP) accumulation correlated well with cell death caused by deoxycoformycin. Thus, dATP, which is known to be an allosteric inhibitor of ribonucleotide reductase, could result in growth inhibition by the generation of an imbalance of deoxynucleotide triphosphate pools. However, additional sites of action for both deoxycoformycin and deoxyadenosine are suggested by the observation that deoxycoformycin and deoxyadenosine are cytotoxic to nondividing cells, which do not require the function of ribonucleotide reductase. One potential site is the depletion of nicotinamide adenine dinucleotide (NAD) in deoxycoformycin- and deoxyadenosine-treated cells. NAD is required for poly-ADP ribosylation, a reaction that is essential to maintain the integrity of DNA and its repair process. Depletion of NAD could reduce the capacity for DNA repair, a constant process in cells, and cause DNA breaks as well as cell death.[222,223]

The second suggested site is inhibition of *S*-adenosyl homocysteine hydrolase by deoxyadenosine.[224,225] Inhibition of this enzyme decreases the capacity of cells to perform transmethylation, a reaction that is critical for certain macromolecular functions. This mechanism does not require deoxyadenosine to be phosphorylated, and it may play an important role in the toxicity of deoxycoformycin to nonproliferating tissues, such as in the liver and CNS. The activation of mitochondrial-dependent apoptosis through the interaction of Apf and dATP could also contribute to its activity.

FLUDARABINE **Background** In the search for more effective compounds than adenine arabinoside (ara-A, vidarabine), which has limited clinical usefulness because of its rapid deamination by adenosine deaminase, 2-fluoroadenosine arabinoside (9-β-D-arabinofuranosyl-2-fluoradenine) was synthesized. It has been found to be relatively resistant to adenosine deaminase and has impressive antitumor activity.[226] Its limited solubility and consequent difficulties in formulation led to the synthesis of a prodrug, the 5'-monophosphate of 2-F-ara-A (Fludara IV).

Fludara IV entered clinical trials in 1982, and it is one of the most active agents in the treatment of chronic lymphocytic leukemia.[227,228] A high level of activity has also been observed in a variety of indolent lymphoproliferative neoplasms, including low-grade non-Hodgkin's lymphoma, cutaneous T-cell lymphoma, macroglobulinemia, and hairy-cell leukemia.[229–231] The dose-limiting toxicities during phase I trials were myelosuppression and leukopenia. Delayed onset of severe neurotoxicity was also noted with dosages of 96 mg/m^2/d for 5 to 7 days. Other toxicities noted during phase I trials included somnolence, mild to moderate nausea and vomiting, and rare but reversible interstitial pneumonitis. Fludara IV is converted by phosphatases to 2-F-ara-A within several minutes of injection; it is not further catabolized in plasma.[175]

Metabolism Transport of 2-fluoroadenosine arabinoside (F-ara-A) appears to be mediated by nonconcentrative, high- and low-affinity systems.[232] Once 2-F-ara-A is taken up by cells, it is phosphorylated to 2-fluoroadenine arabinoside monophosphate (2-F-ara-AMP), not like ara-A as a substrate of adenosine kinase, but by cytoplasmic deoxycytidine kinase.[233] Tumor cells lacking cytoplasmic deoxycytidine kinase are resistant to F-ara-A. Intracellular F-ara-AMP can be further phosphorylated to the diphosphate F-ara-ADP likely by AMP kinases. Nucleoside diphosphate kinases may be the predominant enzyme species responsible for the formation of F-ara-ATP from F-

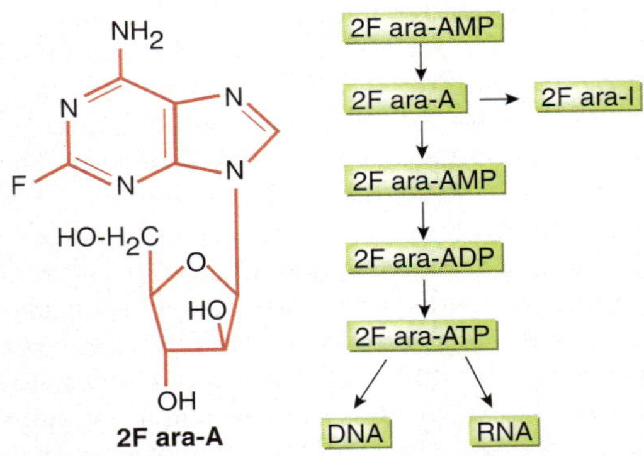

Figure 43-11 Structure and metabolism of 2-fluoroarabinosyl-adenine (2F-ara-A). 2F-ara-I represents the dominant inosine derivative. MP, DP, TP = mono-, di-, and triphosphate.

ara-ADP. F-ara-ATP can be incorporated into DNA in competition with dATP by DNA polymerases. Although DNA polymerases α, β, ε, and γ are all capable of using F-ara-ATP as a substrate, DNA polymerase α has a greater affinity for F-ara-ATP than other DNA polymerases.[234,235] Once F-ara-AMP is incorporated into the terminus of the growing DNA chain, the next step of elongation is retarded, regardless of which DNA polymerase is employed.[235,236]

In addition, F-ara-A has also been shown to be incorporated into RNA,[237,238] but which RNA polymerase is responsible has not been established. The incorporation of F-ara-A into poly (A1) RNA was 12-fold greater than that into poly (A) RNA. A summary of the metabolism of 2F-ara-A is shown in Figure 43-11.

Investigations of F-ara-A as a modulator of ara-C therapy are currently underway. When F-ara-A is given before ara-C, an increase in the accumulation of ara-CTP occurs in leukemic lymphocytes.[239] This modulation of ara-C anabolism probably results from an indirect effect of F-ara-CTP on ribonucleotide reductase, which is also responsible for dCTP synthesis de novo or deoxycytidine kinase that relates to a reduction in the deoxynucleotide pools regulating the enzyme. It may also reflect a direct effect by F-ara-CTP on the activity of deoxycytidine kinase.[239,240] The in vitro accumulation of ara-CTP has also been shown in the lymphocytes of patients with chronic lymphocytic leukemia treated with this sequential combination.[241] The results of a clinical study in individuals who are refractory to F-ara-A therapy show partial or minor responses in approximately 35% of patients.[241]

Mechanism of Action The major site of growth inhibition by F-ara-A is the inhibition of DNA synthesis. Treatment of cells with F-ara-A is associated with the accumulation of cells at the G_1–S-phase boundary and in the S phase; thus, it is a cell-cycle S-phase–specific drug.[242]

F-ara-ATP is also a potent inhibitor of ribonucleotide reductase, the key enzyme responsible for the formation of dATP. This causes a decrease of deoxynucleotides in 2F-ara-A– treated cells, which enhances the incorporation of F-ara-ATP into DNA. This may be considered to be "self-potentiation" of the inhibition of DNA synthesis by F-ara-ATP. In addition, F-ara-ATP was found to be an inhibitor of DNA primase, which is responsible for Okazaki fragment synthesis,[130] another important step in DNA synthesis. The inhibition of RNA primer formation for DNA synthesis by F-ara-ATP was recently demonstrated as well,[243] but the inhibition of Okazaki fragment formation by F-ara-ATP could conceivably play a role in the inhibition of DNA synthesis by F-ara-A. In addition, F-ara-A can inhibit mitochondrial DNA synthesis at concentrations similar to those that cause cytotoxicity; however, such inhibition does not affect cell growth for several cell generations.[243] Thus, the cytotoxicity of F-ara-A, which is usually estimated by the continuous exposure of cells to drugs for three to four generations, likely does not result from the inhibition of mitochondrial DNA.

Resistance to F-ara-A may occur because of decreased uptake, lack of deoxycytidine kinase, increased intracellular concentration of dATP, decreased susceptibility to the activity of ribonucleotide reductase, decreased affinity of DNA polymerase for F-ara-ATP, or increased efficiency of the removal of F-ara-ATP from the 3' terminus where incorporated into DNA. The potential role of the 3' to 5' exonuclease activities of DNA polymerase and other 3' and 5' exonuclease activities in removal of incorporated F-ara-AMP remains to be defined as a possible mechanism of resistance.

CLADRIBINE Background The rationale for the development of 2-chlorodeoxyadenosine (Cl-dAdo, cladribine) was that the death of lymphocytes in patients with adenosine deaminase deficiency was associated with the accumulation of deoxynucleotides. This deoxyadenosine analog was selected for its resistance to adenosine deaminase. Its specific action on lymphoid cells is attributed to the high level of deoxycytidine kinase and low 5'-nucleotidase activity in these cells.[244–246] Cladribine was shown to have potent and lasting effects in the treatment of low-grade B-cell neoplasms, such as chronic lymphocytic leukemia, non-Hodgkin's lymphoma, and hairy-cell leukemia.[247–249] In addition, Cl-dAdo has demonstrated clinical activity against acute myeloid leukemia in children, including those with leukemic blast cells in the CNS[250] and in T-cell lymphoproliferative disorders.[251] The spectrum of clinical activity is similar to that of Fludara IV; however, a few patients who do not respond to F-ara-A are sensitive to Cl-dAdo.[252] The major toxicity encountered is bone marrow suppression that is associated with severe infections. The degree of suppression relates to the rate of administration, cumulative dose, and tumor burden at the start of therapy.[247,253]

Metabolism Cladribine is transported differently in different cell types.[254] Both nitrobenzyl thioinosine (NBT)-sensitive and NBTI-insensitive nucleoside transporters are involved. Once Cl-dAdo enters cells, it can be phosphorylated by deoxycytidine (dCyd) kinase to 2-chorodeoxyadenosine mono (2Cl-dAMP),[255] which subsequently is phosphorylated to 2-chorodeoxyadenosine diphosphate (2Cl-dADP) and then to 2Cl-dATP. The enzymes involved, however, are not established. As 2Cl-dATP, it can be incorporated into DNA through the action of DNA polymerases by competing with dATP.[255] The structure and metabolism of 2-chlorodeoxyadenosine are shown in Figure 43-12.

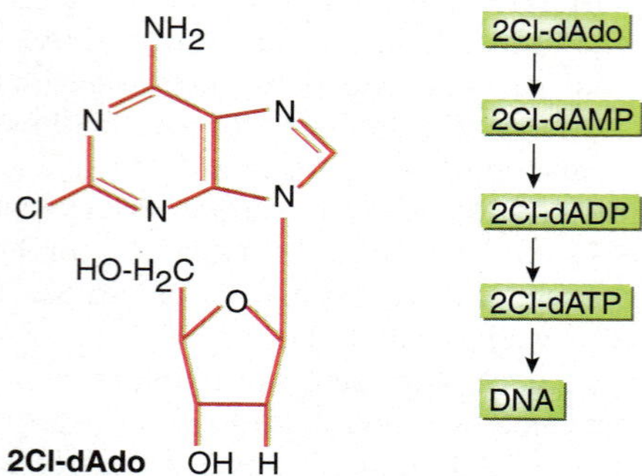

Figure 43-12 Structure and metabolism of 2-chlorodeoxyadenosine (2C1-dAdo). MP, DP, TP = mono-, di-, and triphosphate.

Mechanisms of Action 2Cl-dAdo can inhibit DNA synthesis in growing cells as well as DNA repair in resting cells.[256] When growing cells were treated with 2Cl-dAdo, an accumulation of cells in the S phase was observed, suggesting that inhibition of DNA synthesis could be responsible for the cell-killing effect of the drug. The active metabolite is 2Cl-dATP, which can compete with dATP to be incorporated into the 3'-end of the growing DNA chain. Elongation beyond the incorporated analog was significantly retarded, and this could partly contribute to its inhibitory activity against DNA synthesis. Furthermore, 2Cl-dATP is a potent inhibitor of ribonucleotide reductase.[257] Levels of intracellular deoxynucleoside triphosphates were found to decrease in cells after exposure to 2Cl-dAdo,[255] which could also contribute to its antitumor activity.

HYDROXYUREA Background Although hydroxyurea was first synthesized in 1869,[258] its biologic activity was not recognized until 60 years later, when it was discovered that hydroxyurea could produce leukopenia, anemia, and megaloblastic changes in the bone marrow of rabbits.[259] This simple molecule (Figure 43-13) has been evaluated in a number of types of cancer, but its principal uses are in myeloproliferative diseases. Currently, it is an initial therapy of choice for chronic myelogenous leukemia; it also is used as therapy for polycythemia vera and hypereosinophilic syndrome. Activity against solid tumors has been demonstrated, but in these cases, it is generally used in combination with other anticancer agents or with radiation.[260]

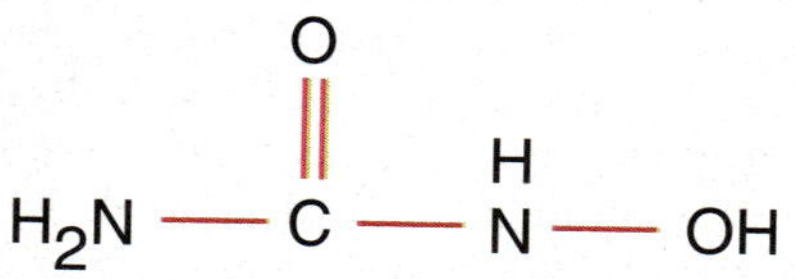

$$H_2N-\overset{\overset{\displaystyle O}{\|}}{C}-\overset{\overset{\displaystyle H}{|}}{N}-OH$$

Figure 43-13 Structure of hydroxyurea.

Hydroxyurea can be taken orally, and the half-life in plasma is approximately 4 hours.[261] It readily crosses the blood-brain barrier. It is excreted predominantly in urine, but the interpatient variability is significant. The full extent and significance of hydroxyurea metabolism in humans has not been well established. It can be degraded by intestinal bacterial urease to form hydroxylamine, which can interact with acetyl-coenzyme A to form acetohydroxamic acid; this metabolite is found in the plasma of patients receiving hydroxyurea therapy.[262]

The dose-limiting toxicity of hydroxyurea is myelosuppression. This results from inhibition of DNA synthesis in bone marrow. Toxicity begins within 2 to 5 days, and its duration is short once the drug is discontinued. Gastrointestinal side effects frequently are seen but rarely require discontinuation of therapy at the doses commonly used. Some dermatologic changes, such as hyperpigmentation, can also occur in patients after extended therapy.[260]

Mechanism of Action and Resistance Hydroxyurea is considered to enter cells by passive diffusion.[263] It inhibits cellular DNA synthesis through the inhibition of ribonucleotide reductase, which is the key enzyme responsible for the synthesis of deoxynucleotides, the building blocks of DNA.[264] The activity of ribonucleotide reductase is highly regulated by the intracellular concentration of ribonucleoside and deoxyribonucleoside triphosphates. Two models, sequential and intercalating, have been proposed for the interplay of ribonucleotide reductase and deoxynucleoside triphosphates.[265] The metabolites of deoxynucleoside analogs, such as 2F-ara-ATP and ara-ATP, are potent inhibitors of this enzyme as well. The activity of this enzyme plays a key role in controlling the intracellular concentrations of deoxynucleotide triphosphates; thus, it can influence the activation or incorporation of deoxynucleoside antimetabolites, such as ara-C, 5-FUdR, and 2F-ara-A, into DNA.

Inhibition of ribonucleotide reductase by hydroxyurea would not affect the incorporation of these antimetabolites and, therefore, could potentiate their action. Ribonucleotide reductase is composed of two types of protein subunits, M1 and M2. M1 protein does not vary with cell cycle and is responsible for the interaction with nucleotides.[266,267] M2 protein fluctuates throughout the cell cycle, with peak activity in the S phase. The alteration of ribonucleotide reductase activity through the cell cycle is primarily controlled by the amount of M2 protein that binds a stoichiometric amount of iron and a stable organic free radical localized to a tyrosine residue.[268–270] Hydroxyurea inhibits ribonucleotide reductase through the inactivation of the tyrosyl free radical on the M2 subunit.

Because of the inhibition of ribonucleotide reductase by hydroxyurea, pools of deoxynucleotide triphosphates decrease, with concomitant inhibition of DNA synthesis. The cytotoxicity of hydroxyurea is dose and time dependent. Most cells are accumulated in the S phase and at the G_1–S-phase boundary under the influence of hydroxyurea.[271,272]

Cells can become resistant to hydroxyurea because of increased ribonucleotide reductase activity, primarily resulting from increased levels of M2 protein. Levels of M1 protein increase only when high levels of resistance to hydroxyurea are generated. These increases of M1 or M2 proteins generally reflect the overexpression of the proteins because of gene amplification.[273–277]

REFERENCES

1. Clarke DA, Elion GB, Hitchings GH, Stock CC. Structure-activity relationships among purines related to 6-mercaptopurine. Cancer Res 1958;18:445–56.
2. Hitchings GH, Elion GB. The chemistry and biochemistry of purine analogs. Ann N Y Acad Sci 1954;60:195–9.
3. Elion GB, Hitchings GH, Vander-Werff H. Antagonists of nucleic acid derivatives. VI. Purines. J Biol Chem 1951;192:505–18.
4. Brockman RW. Mechanism of resistance to anticancer agents. Adv Cancer Res 1963;7:129–234.
5. Fox IH. Metabolic basis for disorders of purine nucleotide degradation. Metabolism 1981;30:616–34.
6. Jones ME. Pyrimidine nucleotide biosynthesis in animals: genes, enzymes, and regulation of UMP biosynthesis. Annu Rev Biochem 1980;49:253–79.
7. Rutman RJ, Cantarow A, Paschkis K. Studies in 2-acetylaminofluorene carcinogenesis. III. The utilization of uracil-2-C14 by preneoplastic rat liver and rat hepatoma. Cancer Res 1954;14:119–23.
8. Duschinsky R, Pleven E, Heidelberger C. The synthesis of 5-fluoropyrimidines. J Am Chem Soc 1957;79:4559–60.
9. Santi DV, McHenry CS, Sommer H. Mechanism of interaction of thymidylate synthetase with 5-fluorodeoxyuridylate. Biochemistry 1974;13:471–82.
10. Madoc-Jones H, Bruce WR. On the mechanism of the lethal action of 5-fluorouracil on mouse L cells. Cancer Res 1968;28:1976–81.
11. Reyes P, Guganig ME. Studies on a pyrimidine phosphoribosyltransferase from murine leukemia P1534J. J Biol Chem 1975;250:5097–108.
12. Cory J, Breland JB, Carter GL. Effect of 5-fluorouracil on RNA metabolism in Novikoff hepatoma cells. Cancer Res 1979;39:4905–13.
13. Houghton JA, Houghton PJ. Elucidation of pathways of 5-fluorouracil metabolism in xenografts of human colorectal adenocarcinoma. Eur J Cancer 1983;19:807–15.
14. Piper AA, Fox RM. Biochemical basis for the differential sensitivity of human T- and B-lymphocyte lines to 5-fluorouracil. Cancer Res 1982;42:3753–60.
15. Heidelberger C, Danenberg PV, Moran RG. Fluorinated pyrimidines and their nucleosides. Adv Enzymol Relat Areas Mol Biol 1983;54:58–119.
16. Glazer RI, Lloyd LS. Association of cell lethality with incorporation of 5-fluorouracil and 5-fluorouridine into nuclear RNA in human colon carcinoma cells in culture. Mol Pharmacol 1982;21:468–73.
17. Ingraham HA, Tseng BY, Goulian M. Nucleotide levels and incorporation of 5-fluorouracil and uracil into DNA of cells treated with 5-fluorodeoxyuridine. Mol Pharmacol 1982;21:211–6.
18. Ingraham HA, Tseng BY, Goulian M. Mechanism for exclusion of 5-fluorouracil from DNA. Cancer Res 1980;40:998–1001.
19. Peters GJ, Laurensse E, Lankelma J, et al. Separation of several 5-fluorouracil metabolites in various melanoma cell lines: evidence for the synthesis of 5-fluorouracilnucleotide sugars. Eur J Cancer Clin Oncol 1984;20:1425–31.
20. Peterson MS, Ingraham HA, Goulian M. 2'-Deoxyribosyl analogs of UDP-N-acetylglucosamine in cells treated with methotrexate or 5-fluorodeoxyridine. J Biol Chem 1983;258:10831–4.
21. Diasio RB, Harris BE. Clinical pharmacology of 5-fluorouracil. Clin Pharmacokinet 1989;16:215–37.
22. Christophidis N, Vajda FJE, Lucas I, et al. Fluorouracil therapy in patients with carcinoma of the large bowel: a pharmacokinetic comparison of various rates and routes of administration. Clin Pharmacokinet 1978;3:330–6.
23. Diasio RB. Clinical implications of dihydropyrimidine dehydrogenase (DPD) on 5-fluorouracil pharmacology. In: Saltz L, editor. Colorectal cancer: multimodality management. Totowa, NJ: Humana Press; 2002. p. 489–97.
24. Ansfield R, Klotz J, Nealon T, et al. A phase III study comparing the clinical utility of four regimens of 5-fluorouracil. Cancer 1977;39:34–40.
25. Erlichman C, Fine S, Wong A. A randomized trial of fluorouracil and folinic acid in patients with metastatic colorectal carcinoma. J Clin Oncol 1988;6:469–75.
26. Seifert P, Baker L, Reed ML, Vaitkevicius VK. Comparison of continuously infused 5-fluorouracil with bolus injection in treatment of patients with colorectal adenocarcinoma. Cancer 1975;36:123–8.
27. Meta-Analysis Group in Cancer. Efficacy of intravenous continuous infusion of fluorouracil compared with bolus administration in advanced colorectal cancer. J Clin Oncol 1998;16:301–8.
28. Shah A, MacDonald W, Goldie J, et al. 5-fluorouracil infusion in advanced colorectal cancer: a comparison of three dose schedules. Cancer Treat Rep 1985;69:739–42.
29. Lokich J, Ahlgren J, Gullo J, et al. A prospective randomized comparison of continuous infusion fluorouracil with a conventional bolus schedule in metastatic colorectal carcinoma: a Mid-Atlantic Oncology Program study. J Clin Oncol 1989;7:425–32.
30. Lokich J, Bothe A, Fine N, Perri J. Phase I study of protracted venous infusion of 5-fluorouracil. Cancer 1981;48:2565–8.
31. Harris BE, Ruiling S, Soong S, Diasio RB. Relationship between dihydropyrimidine dehydrogenase activity and plasma 5-fluorouracil levels with evidence for circadian variation of enzyme activity and plasma drug levels in cancer patients receiving 5-fluorouracil by protracted continuous infusion. Cancer Res 1990;50:197–201.
32. Finch RE, Bending MR, Lant AF. Plasma levels of 5-fluorouracil after oral and intravenous administration in cancer patients. Br J Clin Pharmacol 1979;7:613–7.
33. MacMillan WE, Wolberg WH, Welling PG. Pharmacokinetics of fluorouracil in humans. Cancer Res 1978;38:3479–82.
34. Clarkson B, O'Connor A, Winston L, Hutchinson D. The physiologic disposition of 5-fluorouracil and 5-fluoro-2'-deoxyuridine in man. Clin Pharmacol Ther 1964;5:581–610.
35. McDermott BJ, van der Berg HW, Murphy RF. Nonlinear pharmacokinetics for the elimination of 5-fluorouracil after intravenous administration in cancer patients. Pharmacology 1982;9:173–8.
36. Ensminger WD, Rosowsky A, Raso V, et al. A clinical pharmacological evaluation of hepatic arterial infusion of 5-fluoro-2'-deoxyuridine and 5-fluorouracil. Cancer Res 1978;38:3784–92.
37. Peters GJ, Lankelma J, Kok RM, et al. Prolonged retention of high concentrations of 5-fluorouracil in human and murine tumors as compared with plasma. Cancer Chemother Pharmacol 1993;31:269–76.
38. Sugarbaker PH, Klecker RW, Gianola FJ, Speyer JC. Prolonged treatment schedules with intraperitoneal 5-fluorouracil diminish the local-regional nature of drug distribution. Am J Clin Oncol 1986;9:1–7.
39. El Kouni MH, Naguib FNM, Cha S. Circadian rhythm of dihydrouracil dehydrogenase (DHUDase), uridine phosphorylase (UrdPase), and thymidine phosphorylase (dThdPase) in mouse liver. FASEB J 1989;3:a397.
40. Schneider M. Circadian rhythm-varying plasma concentration of 5-fluorouracil during a five-day continuous venous infusion at a constant rate in cancer patients. Cancer Res 1988;48:1676–9.
41. Hrushesky W. Circadian timing of cancer chemotherapy. Science 1985;228:73–5.
42. Bertheault-Cvitkovic F, Levi F, Soussan S, et al. Circadian rhythm-modulated chemotherapy with high dose 5-fluorouracil: a pilot study in patients with pancreatic adenocarcinoma. Eur J Cancer 1993;29:1851–4.
43. Levi F, Misset JL, Brienza S, et al. A chronopharmacologic phase II clinical trial with 5-fluorouracil, folinic acid, and oxaliplatin using an ambulatory multichannel programmable pump. Cancer 1992;69:893–900.
44. Metzger G, Massari C, Etienne MC, et al. Spontaneous or imposed circadian changes in plasma concentrations of 5-fluorouracil coadministered with folinic acid and oxaliplatin: relationship with mucosal toxicity in patients with cancer. Clin Pharmacol Ther 1994;56:190–201.
45. Bjarnason GA, Kerr IG, Doyle N, et al. Phase I study of 5-fluorouracil and leucovorin by a 14-day circadian infusion in metastatic adenocarcinoma patients. Cancer Chemother Pharmacol 1993;33:221–8.
46. Anderson N, Lokich J, Bern M, et al. A phase I clinical trial of combined fluoropyrimidines with leucovorin in a 14-day infusion. Demonstration of biochemical modulation. Cancer 1989;63:233–7.
47. Diasio RB, Beavers TI, Carpenter JT. Familial deficiency of dihydropyrimidine dehydrogenase. Biochemical basis for familial pyrimidemia and severe 5-fluorouracil-induced toxicity. J Clin Invest 1988;81:47–51.
48. Baccanari DP, Davis ST, Knick VC, Spector T. 5-Ethynyluracil (776C85): a potent modulator of the pharmacokinetics and antitumor efficacy of 5-fluorouracil. Proc Natl Acad Sci U S A 1993;90:11064–8.
49. Van Cutsem E, Sorensen J, Cassidy J, et al. International phase III study of oral eniluracil (EU) plus 5-fluorouracil (5-FU) versus intravenous (IV) 5-FU plus leucovorin (LV) in the treatment of advanced colorectal cancer (ACC) [abstract]. Proc Am Soc Clin Oncol 2001;20:522.
50. Levin J, Schilsky R, Burris H, et al. North American phase III study of oral eniluracil (EU) plus oral 5-fluorouracil (5-FU) versus intravenous (IV) 5-FU plus leucovorin (LV) in the treatment of advanced colorectal cancer (ACC) [abstract]. Proc Am Soc Clin Oncol 2001;20:523.
51. Naguib FN, el Kouni MH, Cha S. Enzymes of uracil catabolism in normal and neoplastic human tissues. Cancer Res 1985;45:5405–12.
52. Heggie GD, Sommadossi J-P, Cross DS, et al. Clinical pharmacokinetics of 5-fluorouracil and its metabolites in plasma, urine, and bile. Cancer Res 1987;7:2203–6.
53. Sweeny DJ, Barnes S, Heggie GD, Diasio RB. Metabolism fluorouracil N-choly-2-fluoro-alanine conjugate: previously unrecognized role for bile acids in drug conjugation. Proc Natl Acad Sci U S A 1987;84:5439–43.
54. Grem JL, Fischer PH. Augmentation of 5-fluorouracil cytotoxicity in human colon cancer cells by dipyridamole. Cancer Res 1985;45:2967–72.
55. Kufe DW, Major PP. 5-fluorouracil incorporation into human breast carcinoma RNA correlates with cytotoxicity. J Biol Chem 1981;256:9802–5.
56. Shani J, Danenberg PV. Evidence that intracellular synthesis of 5-fluorouridine-5'-phosphate from 5-fluorouracil and 5-fluorouridine is compartmentalized. Biochem Biophys Res Commun 1984;122:439–45.
57. Mandel HG. The incorporation of 5-fluorouracil into RNA and its molecular consequences. Prog Mol Subcell Biol 1969;1:82.
58. Parker WB, Cheng YC. Metabolism and mechanism of action of 5-fluorouracil. Pharmacol Ther 1990;48:381–95.
59. Evans RM, Laskin JD, Hakala MT. Assessment of growth-limiting events caused by 5-fluorouracil in mouse cells and in human cells. Cancer Res 1980;40:4113–22.
60. Maybaum J, Ullman B, Mandel HG, et al. Regulation of RNA- and DNA-directed actions of 5-fluoropyrimidines in mouse T-lymphoma (S-49) cells. Cancer Res 1980;40:4209–15.
61. Berger SH, Hakala MT. Relationship of dUMP and free FdUMP pools to inhibition to thymidylate synthase by 5-fluorouracil. Mol Pharmacol 1984;25:303–9.
62. Cohen SS, Flaks JG, Barner HD, et al. The mode of action of 5-fluorouracil and its derivatives. Proc Natl Acad Sci U S A 1958;44:1004–12.
63. Hartmann KU, Heidelberger C. Studies on fluorinated pyrimidines. VIII. Inhibition of thymidylate synthetase. J Biol Chem 1961;236:3006.
64. Danenberg PV, Danenberg KD. Effect of 5, 10-methylenetetrahydrofolate and the dissociation of 5-fluorodeoxyuridylate binding of human thymidylate synthetase: evidence for an ordered mechanism. Biochemistry 1978;17:4018–24.
65. Houghton JA, Weiss KD, Williams LG, et al. Relationship between 5-fluoro-2'-deoxyuridylate, 2'-deoxyuridylate, and thymidylate synthase activity subsequent to 5-fluorouracil administration in xenografts of human colon adenocarcinomas. Biochem Pharmacol 1986;35:1351–8.
66. Myers CE, Young RC, Johns DG, Chabner BA. Assay of 5-fluorodeoxyuridine 5'-monophosphate and deoxyuridine 5'-monophosphate pools following 5-fluorouracil. Cancer Res 1974;34:2682–8.
67. Evans RM, Laskin JD, Hakala MT. Effect of excess folates and deoxyinosine on the activity and site of action of 5-fluorouracil. Cancer Res 1981;41:3288–95.
68. Houghton JA, Maroda SJ Jr, Phillips JO, Houghton PJ. Biochemical determinants of responsiveness to 5-fluoroura-

cil and its derivatives in xenografts of human colorectal adenocarcinomas in mice. Cancer Res 1981;41:144–9.
69. Mini E, Trave F, Rustum YM, Bertino JR. Enhancement of the antitumor effects of 5-fluorouracil by folinic acid. Pharm Ther 1990;47:1–19.
70. Johnston PG, Fisher ER, Rockette HE, et al. The role of thymidylate synthase expression in prognosis and outcome to adjuvant chemotherapy in patients with rectal cancer. J Clin Oncol 1994;12:2640–7.
71. Leichman L, Lenz HJ, Leichman CG, et al. Quantitation of intratumoral thymidylate synthase expression predicts for resistance to protracted infusion of 5-fluorouracil and weekly leucovorin in disseminated colorectal cancers: preliminary report from an ongoing trial. Eur J Cancer 1995;31:1306–10.
72. Lenz HJ, Leichman CG, Danenberg KD, et al. Thymidylate synthase mRNA level in adenocarcinoma of the stomach: a predictor for primary tumor response and overall survival. J Clin Oncol 1996;14:176–82.
73. Peters GJ, van der Wilt CL, van Groeningen CJ, et al. Thymidylate synthase inhibition after administration of fluorouracil with or without leucovorin in colon cancer patients: implication for treatment with fluorouracil. J Clin Oncol 1994;12:2035–42.
74. Findlay MP, Cunningham D, Morgan G, et al. Lack of correlation between thymidylate synthase levels in primary colorectal tumors and subsequent response to chemotherapy. Br J Cancer 1997;75:903–9.
75. Etienne MC, Pivot X, Formento JL, et al. A multifactorial approach including tumoral epidermal growth factor receptor, p53, thymidylate synthase and dihydropyrimidine dehydrogenase to predict treatment outcome in head and neck cancer patients receiving 5-fluorouracil. Br J Cancer 1999;79:1864–9.
76. Pestalozzi BC, Peterson HF, Gelber RD, et al. Prognostic importance of thymidylate synthase expression in early breast cancer. J Clin Oncol 1997;15:1923–31.
77. Salonga D, Danenberg KD, Johnson M, et al. Gene expression levels of dihydropyrimidine dehydrogenase and thymidylate synthase together identify a high percentage of colorectal tumors responding to 5-fluorouracil. Clin Cancer Res 2000;6:1322–7.
78. Kufe DW, Major PP, Egan EM, Loh E. 5-fluoro-2'-deoxyuridine incorporation in L1210 DNA. J Biol Chem 1981;256:8885–8.
79. Morikawa K, Fan D, Denkins YM, et al. Mechanisms of combined effects of a-interferon and 5-fluorouracil on human colon cancer implanted into nude mice. Cancer Res 1989;49:799–805.
80. Caradonna SJ, Cheng Y-C. The role of deoxyuridine triphosphate nucleotide hydrolase, uracil-DNA glycosylase, and DNA polymerase in the metabolism of 5-FUdR in human tumor cells. Mol Pharmacol 1980;18:513–20.
81. Dusenbury CE, Davis MA, Lawrence TS, Maybaum J. Induction of megabase DNA fragments by 5-fluorodeoxyuridine in human colorectal tumor (HT29) cells. Mol Pharmacol 1991;39:285–9.
82. Tanaka M, Kimura K, Yoshida S. Increased incorporation of 5-fluorodeoxyuridine into DNA of human T-lymphoblastic cell lines. Gann 1984;75:986–92.
83. Mulkins MA, Heidelberger C. Biochemical characterization of fluoropyrimidine-resistant murine leukemic cell lines. Cancer Res 1982;42:965–73.
84. Mulkins MA, Heidelberger C. Isolation of fluoropyrimidine-resistant murine leukemic cell lines by one-step mutation and selection. Cancer Res 1982;42:956–64.
85. Fernandes DJ, Carroll CC. Multiple modes of resistance of human CCRF-CEM leukemic cells to 5-fluoro-2'-deoxyuridine. Cancer Res 1983;24:283.
86. Jiang W, Lu Z, He Y, Diasio RB. Dihydropyrimidine dehydrogenase activity in hepatocellular carcinoma: implication for fluorouracil-based chemotherapy. Clin Cancer Res 1997;3:395–9.
87. Diasio RB, Danenberg K, Johnson M, Danenberg P. Quantitation of dihydropyrimidine dehydrogenase expression in tumor specimens of patients treated with 5-fluorouracil using a quantitative PCR assay [abstract]. Proc Am Assoc Cancer Res 1999;39:a1286.
88. Etienne MC, Cheradame S, Fischel JL, et al. Response to fluorouracil therapy in cancer patients: the role of tumoral dihydropyrimidine dehydrogenase activity. J Clin Oncol 1995;13:1663–70.
89. Bapat AR, Zarow C, Danenberg PV. Human leukemic cells resistant to 5-fluoro-2'-deoxyuridine contain a thymidylate synthase with a lower affinity for nucleotides. J Biol Chem 1983;258:4130–6.
90. Berger SH, Jenh C-H, Johnson LF, Berger FG. Thymidylate synthase overproduction and gene amplification in fluorodeoxyuridine-resistant human cells. Mol Pharmacol 1985;28:461–7.
91. Aschele C, Sobrero A, Faderan MA, Bertino JR. Novel mechanisms of resistance to fluorouracil in human colon cancer sublines following exposure to two different clinically relevant dose schedules. Cancer Res 1992;52:1855–64.
92. Pizzorno G, Sun Z, Handschumacher RE. Effect of clinically modeled regimens on the growth response and development of resistance in human colon carcinoma cell lines. Biochem Pharmacol 1995;49:559–65.
93. Sobrero A, Aschele C, Guglielmi AP, et al. Synergism and lack of cross-resistance between short-term and continuous exposure to fluorouracil in human colon adenocarcinoma cells. J Natl Cancer Inst 1993;85:1937–44.
94. Bertino JR, Mini E. Does modulation of 5-fluorouracil by metabolites or antimetabolites work in the clinic? In: Mar-tin DS, editor. New avenues in developmental cancer chemotherapy. New York: Academic Press; 1987. p. 1–25.
95. Cadman E, Davis L, Heimer R. Enhanced 5-fluorouracil nucleotide formation following methotrexate: biochemical explanation for drug synergism. Science 1979;205:1135–7.
96. Schwartz PM, Dunigan JM, Marsh JC, Handschumacher RE. Allopurinol modification of the toxicity and antitumor activity of 5-fluorouracil. Cancer Res 1980;40:1885–9.
97. Washtien WL. Comparison of 5-fluorouracil metabolism in two human gastrointestinal tumor cell lines. Cancer Res 1984;44:909–14.
98. Ullman B, Lee M, Martin DW Jr, Santi DV. Cytotoxicity of 5-fluoro-2'-deoxyuridine: requirement for reduced folate cofactors and antagonism by methotrexate. Proc Natl Acad Sci U S A 1978;75:980–3.
99. Houghton JA, Torrance PM, Radparvar S, et al. Binding of 5-fluorodeoxyuridylate to thymidylate synthetase in human colon adenocarcinoma xenografts. Eur J Cancer Clin Oncol 1986;22:505–10.
100. Keyomarsi K, Moran R. Folinic acid augmentation of the effects of fluoropyrimidines on murine and human leukemic cells. Cancer Res 1986;46:5229–35.
101. Advanced Colorectal Cancer Meta-Analysis Project. Modulation of fluorouracil by leucovorin in patients with advanced colorectal cancer: evidence in terms of response rate. J Clin Oncol 1992;10:896–903.
102. O'Connell MJ. A phase III trial of 5-fluorouracil and leucovorin in the treatment of advanced colorectal cancer. Cancer 1989;63:1026–30.
103. Schuller J, Cassidy J, Reigner BG, et al. Tumor selectivity of Xeloda in colorectal cancer patients [abstract]. Proc Am Soc Clin Oncol 1997;16:a208.
104. Twelves C, Budman DR, Creaven PJ, et al. Pharmacokinetics and pharmacodynamics of capecitabine in two phase I studies [abstract]. Proc Am Soc Clin Oncol 1996;15:a476.
105. Blum JL. Xeloda in the treatment of metastatic breast cancer. Oncology 1999;57:16–20.
106. Hoff PM, Ansari R, Batist G, et al. Comparison of oral capecitabine versus intravenous fluorouracil plus leucovorin as first-line treatment in 605 patients with metastatic colorectal cancer: results of a randomized phase III study. J Clin Oncol 2001;19:2282–92.
107. Van Cutsem E, Twelves C, Cassidy J, et al. Oral capecitabine compared with intravenous fluorouracil plus leucovorin in patients with metastatic colorectal cancer: results of a large phase III study. J Clin Oncol 2001;19:4097–106.
108. O'Shaughnessy J. Results of a large phase III trial of Xeloda/Taxotere combination therapy versus Taxotere monotherapy in metastatic breast cancer patients [abstract]. Xeloda Breast Cancer Study Group. Breast Cancer Res Treat 2000:23a.
109. Sawada N, Ishikawa T, Sekiguchi F, et al. X-Ray irradiation induces thymidine phosphorylase and enhances the efficacy of capecitabine (Xeloda) in human cancer xenografts. Clin Cancer Res 1999;5:2948–53.
110. Talley RW, Vaitkevicius VK. Megaloblastosis produced by a cytosine antagonist, 1-D-arabinofuranosylcytosine. Blood 1963;21:252.
111. Chabner BA. Cytidine analogs. In: Chabner BA, Collins JM, editors. Cancer chemotherapy: principles and practice. Philadelphia: Lippincott; 1990. p. 154.
112. Calabresi P, Chabner BA. Antineoplastic agents. In: Gilman AG, Rall TW, Nies AS, Taylor P, editors. The pharmacological basis of therapeutics. 8th ed. New York: Pergamon Press; 1990. p. 1231–2.
113. Chabner BA, Johns DG, Coleman N, et al. Purification and properties of cytidine deaminase from normal and leukemic granulocytes. J Clin Invest 1974;53:922–31.
114. Cheng Y-C, Tan R-S, Ruth JL, Dutschman GE. Cytotoxicity of 2'-fluoro-5-iodo-1-b-d-arabinofuranosylcytosine and its relationship to deoxycytidine deaminase. Biochem Pharmacol 1983;32:726–9.
115. Chou TC, Arlin Z, Clarkson BD, Phillips FS. Metabolism of 1-d-arabinofuranosylcytosine in human leukemic cells. Cancer Res 1977;37:3561–70.
116. Paterson AR, Oliver UM. Nucleoside transport. II. Inhibition by *p*-nitrobenzylthioguanosine and related compounds. Can J Biochem 1971;49:271–4.
117. Kessel D, Hall TC, Wodinsky I. Transport and phosphorylation as factors in the antitumor action of cytosine arabinoside. Science 1967;156:1240–1.
118. Mancini WR, Cheng Y-C. Human deoxycytidylate deaminase. Substrate and regulator specificities and their chemotherapeutic implications. Mol Pharmacol 1983;23:159–64.
119. De Saint Vincent BR, Buttin G. Studies on 1-d-arabinofuranosyl-cytosine resistant mutants of Chinese fibroblasts. III. Joint resistance to arabinofuranosylcytosine and to excess thymidine—a semidominant manifestation of deoxycytidine triphosphate pool expansion. Somat Cell Genet 1979;5:67–82.
120. De Saint Vincent BR, Dechamps M, Butlin G. The modulation of the thymidine triphosphate pool of Chinese hamster cells by dCMP deaminase and UDP reductase. J Biol Chem 1980;255:162–7.
121. Cheng YC, Agarwal P, Parks RE. Erythrocytic nucleoside diphosphokinase IV. Evidence for electrophoretic heterogeneity. Biochemistry 1971;10:2139–43.
122. Furth JJ, Cohen SS. Inhibition of mammalian DNA polymerase by 1-d-arabinofuranosylcytosine and the 5'-triphosphate of 9-d-arabinofuranosyladenine. Cancer Res 1968;28:2061–7.
123. Momparler RL. Kinetic and template studies with 1-D-arabinofuranosylcytosine 5'-triphosphate and mammalian deoxyribonucleic acid polymerase. Mol Pharmacol 1972;8:362–70.
124. Valeriote F. Cellular aspects of the action of cytosine arabinoside. Med Pediatr Oncol 1982;10 Suppl 1:5–26.
125. Ohno Y, Spriggs D, Matsukage A, Kufe D. Effects of 1-darabinofuranosylcytosine incorporation on elongation of specific DNA sequences by DNA polymerase. Cancer Res 1988;48:1494–8.
126. Townsend AJ, Cheng Y-C. Sequence-specific effects of ara-5-aza-CTP and ara-CTP on DNA synthesis by purified human DNA polymerases in vitro: visualization of chain elongation on a defined template. Mol Pharmacol 1987;32:330–9.
127. Au C, Schnider W. The role of low-dosage cytosine arabinoside and aggressive chemotherapy in advanced myelodysplastic syndromes. Cancer 1989;64:1812.
128. Momparler RL. Effect of cytosine arabinoside 5'-triphosphate on mammalian DNA polymerase. Biochem Biophys Res Commun 1969;34:464–71.
129. Fridland A. Effect of cytosine arabinoside on replicon initiation in human lymphoblasts. Biochem Biophys Res Commun 1977;74:72–8.
130. Parker WB, Cheng YC. Inhibition of DNA primase by nucleoside triphosphates and their arabinofuranosyl analogs. Mol Pharmacol 1987;31:146–51.
131. Capizzi RL, Cheng YC. Sequential high-dose cytosine arabinoside and asparaginase in refractory acute leukemia. Med Pediatr Oncol 1982;10 Suppl 1:221–8.
132. Capizzi RL, Yang, J-L, Cheng E, et al. Alteration of the pharmacokinetics of high-dose ara-C by its metabolite, high ara-U in patients with acute leukemia. J Clin Oncol 1983;1:763–71.
133. Yang JL, Chang EH, Capizzi RL. Effect of uracil arabinoside on metabolism and cytotoxicity of cytosine arabinoside in 25178Y murine leukemia. J Clin Invest 1985;75:141–6.
134. Leclerc JM, Cheng Y-C. Demonstration of activities in leukemic cells capable of removing 1'-d-arabinofuranosyl cytosine (ara-C) from ara-C incorporated DNA [abstract]. Proc Am Assoc Cancer Res 1984;25:19.
135. Hanka LJ, Evans JS, Mason DJ, Dietz A. Microbiological production of 5-azacytidine: I. Production and biological activity. Antimicrob Agents Chemother 1966;6:619–24.
136. Sorm F, Piskala A, Cihak A, Vesely J. 5-azacytidine, a new highly effective cancerostatic. Experientia 1964;20:202–3.
137. Beisler J. Isolation, characterization, and properties of labile hydrolysis product of the antitumor nucleoside 5-azacytidine. J Med Chem 1978;21:204–8.
138. Plagemann PGW, Behrens M, Abraham D. Metabolism and cytotoxicity of 5-azacytidine in cultured Novikoff rat hepatoma and P388 mouse leukemia cells and their enhancement by preincubation with pyrazofurin. Cancer Res 1978;38:2458–66.

139. Drake JC, Stoller RG, Chabner BA. Characteristics of the enzyme uridine-cytidine kinase isolated from a cultured human cell line. Biochem Pharmacol 1977;26:64–6.
140. Townsend A, Leclerc J-M, Dutschman G, et al. Metabolism of 1-d-arabinofuranosyl-5-azacytosine and incorporation into DNA of human T-lymphoblastic cells (molt-4). Cancer Res 1985;45:3522–8.
141. Cihak A, Vesely J. Prolongation of the lag period preceding the enhancement of thymidine and thymidylate kinase activity in regenerating rat liver by 5-azacytidine. Biochem Pharmacol 1972;21:3257–65.
142. Li LH, Olin EJ, Buskirk HH, Reineke LM. Cytotoxicity and mode of action of 5-azacytidine on L1210 leukemia. Cancer Res 1970;30:2760–9.
143. Li LH, Olin EJ, Fraser TJ, Bhuyan BK. Phase specificity of 5-azacytidine against mammalian cells in tissue culture. Cancer Res 1970;30:2770–5.
144. Vesely J, Cihak A. 5-azacytidine: mechanism of action and biological effects in mammalian cells. Pharmacol Ther 1978;2:813.
145. Adams RL, Burdon RH. DNA methylation in eukaryotes. CRC Crit Rev Biochem 1982;13:349–84.
146. Glover AB, Leyland-Jones BR, Chun HG, et al. Azacitidine: 10 years later. Cancer Treat Rep 1987;71:737–46.
147. Delong DC, Hertel LW, Tang J, et al. Antiviral activity of 2', 2'-difluorodeoxycytidine. Washington, DC: American Society of Microbiology; March 1986.
148. Hertel LW, Boder GB, Kroin JS, et al. Evaluation of the antitumor activity of a (2'-2'-difluoro-2'-deoxycytidine). Cancer Res 1990;50:4417–22.
149. Burris HA, Moore MJ, Anderson J, et al. Improvements in survival and clinical benefit with gemcitabine as first line therapy for patients with advanced pancreas cancer: a randomized trial. J Clin Oncol 1997;15:2403–13.
150. Rothenberg ML, Moore MJ, Cripps CM, et al. A phase II trial of gemcitabine in patients with 5-FU refractory pancreas cancer. Ann Oncol 1996;7:347–53.
151. Abratt RP, Bezwoda WR, Falkson G, et al. Efficacy and safety profile of gemcitabine in nonsmall cell lung cancer: a phase II study. J Clin Oncol 1994;12:1535–40.
152. Crino L, Scagliotti G, Marangolo M, et al. Cisplatin-gemcitabine combination in advanced non-small cell lung cancer: a phase II study. J Clin Oncol 1997;15:297–303.
153. Shepherd FA. Phase I dose-escalation trial of gemcitabine and cisplatin for advanced non-small cell lung cancer: usefulness of mathematic modelling to determine maximum tolerated dose. J Clin Oncol 1996;14:1656–62.
154. Sandler AB, Nemunaitis J, Denham C, et al. Phase III trial of gemcitabine plus cisplatin versus cisplatin alone in patients with locally advanced or metastatic non-small-cell lung cancer. J Clin Oncol 2000;18:122–30.
155. Carmichael J, Possinger K, Phillip P, et al. Advanced breast cancer: a phase II trial with gemcitabine. J Clin Oncol 1995;13:2731–6.
156. Nagourney RA, Link JS, Blitzer JB, et al. Gemcitabine plus cisplatin repeating doublet therapy in previously treated, relapsed breast cancer patients. J Clin Oncol 2000;18:2245–9.
157. Pollera CF, Ceribelli A, Crecco M, et al. Weekly gemcitabine in advanced bladder cancer: a preliminary report from phase I study. Ann Oncol 1994;5:182–4.
158. Stadler WM, Kuzel T, Roth B, et al. Phase II study of single-agent gemcitabine in previously untreated patients with metastatic urothelial cancer. J Clin Oncol 1997;15:3394–8.
159. Kaufman D, Reghavan D, Carducci M, et al. Phase II trial of gemcitabine plus cisplatin in patients with metastatic urothelial cancer. J Clin Oncol 2000;18:1921–7.
160. Moore JM, Winquist EW, Murray N, et al. Gemcitabine plus cisplatin, an active regimen in advanced urothelial cancer: a phase II trial of the National Cancer Institute of Canada Clinical Trials Group. J Clin Oncol 1999;17:2876.
161. Lund B, Hansen OP, Theilade K, et al. Phase II study of gemcitabine in previously treated ovarian cancer. J Natl Cancer Inst 1994;86:1530–3.
162. Friedlander M, Millward MJ, Bell D, et al. A phase II study of gemcitabine in platinum pre-treated patients with advanced epithelial ovarian cancer. Ann Oncol 1998;9:1343–5.
163. Bernell P, Ohm L. Promising activity of gemcitabine in refractory high-grade non-Hodgkin's lymphoma. Br J Haematol 1998;101:203–4.
164. Fossa A, Santoro A, Hiddemann W, et al. Gemcitabine as a single agent in the treatment of relapsed or refractory aggressive non-Hodgkin's lymphoma. J Clin Oncol 1999;17:3788–92.
165. Santoro A, Bredenfeld H, Devizzi L, et al. Gemcitabine in the treatment of refractory Hodgkin's disease: results of a multicenter phase II study. J Clin Oncol 2000;18:2615–9.
166. Zinzani PL, Balva G, Magagnoli, et al. Gemcitabine treatment in pretreated cutaneous T-cell lymphoma experience in 44 patients. J Clin Oncol 2000;18:2603–6.
167. Brodowicz T, Breiteneder S, Wiltschke C, Zielinski CC. Gemcitabine induced hemolytic uremic syndrome: a case report. J Natl Cancer Inst 1997;89:1895–6.
168. Casper ES, Green MR, Kelaen DP, et al. Phase II trial of gemcitabine (2', 2'-difluorodeoxycytidine) in patients with adenocarcinoma of the pancreas. Invest New Drugs 1994;12:29–34.
169. Nackaerts K, Daenen M, Vansteenkiste J, et al. Hemolytic uremic syndrome caused by gemcitabine. Ann Oncol 1998;9:1355.
170. Heinemann V, Hertel LW, Grindey GB, Plunkett W. Comparison of the cellular pharmacokinetics and toxicity of 2', 2'-difluorodeoxycytidine. Cancer Res 1968;28:1976.
171. Plunkett W, Gandhi V, Chubb S, et al. 2', 2'-difluorodeoxycytidine metabolism and mechanism of action in human leukemia cells. Nucleosides Nucleotides Nucleic Acids 1989;8:775.
172. Ruiz van Haperen VWT, Veerman G, Boven E, et al. Schedule dependence of sensitivity to 2', 2'-difluorodeoxycytidine (gemcitabine) in relation to accumulation and retention of its triphosphate in solid tumour cell lines and solid tumours. Biochem Pharmacol 1994;48:1327–39.
173. Plunkett W, Iacoboni S, Estey E, et al. Pharmacologically directed ara-C therapy for refractory leukemia. Semin Oncol 1985;12 Suppl 3:20–30.
174. Shewach DS, Hahn TM, Chang E, et al. Metabolism of 2', 2'-difluoro-2-deoxycytidine and radiation sensitization of human colon carcinoma cells. Cancer Res 1994;54:3218–23.
175. Danhauser L, Plunkett W, Keating M, et al. 9-fludarabine monophosphate: a potentially useful agent in chronic lymphocytic leukemia. Nouv Rev Fr Hematol 1988;30:457.
176. Heinemann V, Xu YZ, Chubb S, et al. Cellular elimination of 2', 2'-difluorodeoxycytidine 5'-triphosphate: a mechanism of self-potentiation. Cancer Res 1992;52:533–9.
177. Abbruzzese JL, Grunewald R, Weeks EA, et al. A phase I clinical, plasma and cellular pharmacology study of gemcitabine. J Clin Oncol 1991;9:491–8.
178. Heinemann V, Xu YZ, Chubb S, et al. Inhibition of ribonucleotide reductase in CCRF-CEM cells by 2', 2'-difluorodeoxycytidine. Mol Pharmacol 1990;38:567–72.
179. Shewach DS, Plunkett W. Cellular retention of 9-d-arabinofuranosyladenine-5'-triphosphate and the pattern of recovery of DNA synthesis in Chinese hamster ovary cells. Cancer Res 1986;46:1581–4.
180. Huang P, Chubb S, Hertel LW, et al. Action of 2', 2'-difluoroxeoxycytidine on DNA synthesis. Cancer Res 1991;51:6110–7.
181. Ruiz van Haperen VW, Veerman G, Vermorken JB, Peters GJ. 2', 2'-difluorodeoxycytidine (gemcitabine) incorporation into RNA and DNA of tumour cell lines. Biochem Pharmacol 1993;46:762–6.
182. Ruiz van Haperen VW, Veerman G, Eriksson S, et al. Development and molecular characterization of a 2', 2'-difluorodeoxycytidine-resistant variant of the human ovarian carcinoma cell line A2780. Cancer Res 1994;54:4138–43.
183. Goan Y-G, Zhou B, Hu E, et al. Overexpression of ribonucleotide reductase as a mechanism of resistance to 2,2 difluorodeoxycytidine in human KB cancer cell line. Cancer Res 1999;59:4204.
184. Albert A, Brown DJ. Purine studies. Part I. Stability to acid and alkali. Solubility. Ionization. Comparison with pteridines. J Chem Soc 1954;Pt II:2060.
185. Burchenal JH, Murphy ML, Ellison RR, et al. Clinical evaluation of a new antimetabolite, 6-mercaptopurine, in the treatment of leukemia and allied diseases. Blood 1953;8:965–99.
186. Elion GB, Hitchings GH. The synthesis of 6-thioguanine. J Am Chem Soc 1955;77:1676.
187. Elion GB, Hitchings GH. Azathioprine. In: Sartorelli AC, Johns DG, editors. Handbook of experimental pharmacology. Berlin: Springer-Verlag; 1975. p. 404.
188. Paterson ARP, Tidd DM. 6-thiopurines. In: Sartorelli AD, Johns DG, editors. Handbook of experimental pharmacology. Berlin: Springer-Verlag; 1975. p. 384.
189. Agarwal RP, Spector T, Parks RE Jr. Tight-binding inhibitors: IV. Inhibition of adenosine deaminase by various inhibitors. Biochem Pharmacol 1977;26:359–67.
190. Tidd DM. Antipurines. In: Fox BW, Fox M, editors. Handbook of experimental pharmacology. Berlin: Springer-Verlag; 1984. p. 445.
191. Elion GB. Biochemistry and pharmacology of purine analogs. Fed Proc 1967;26:898–904.
192. Fernandes JF, LePage GA, Lindner A. The influence of azaserine and 6-mercaptopurine on the in vivo metabolism of ascites tumor cells. Cancer Res 1956;16:154.
193. Hill DL, Bennett LL Jr. Purification and properties of 5-phosphoribosyl pyrophosphate amidotransferase from adenocarcinoma 758 cells. Biochemistry 1969;8:122–30.
194. Skipper HE. On the mechanism of action of 6-mercaptopurine. Ann N Y Acad Sci 1954;60:315.
195. Perrino FW, Mazar DJ, Ward H, Harvey S. Exonucleases and the incorporation of aranucleotides into DNA. Cell Biochem Biophys 1999;30:331.
196. Zimm S, Collins JM, Riccardi R, et al. Variable bioavailability of oral mercaptopurine: is maintenance chemotherapy in acute lymphoblastic leukemia being optimally delivered? N Engl J Med 1983;308:1005–9.
197. Elion GB, Callahan S, Rundles RW, Hitchings GH. Relationship between metabolic fates and antitumor activities of thiopurines. Cancer Res 1963;23:1207–17.
198. Esterhay RJ Jr, Aisner J, Levi JA, Wiernik PH. High-dose 6-mercaptopurine in advanced refractory cancer. Cancer Treat Rep 1978;62:1229–31.
199. Philips FS, Sternberg SS, Hamilton L, Clarke DA. The toxic effects of 6-mercaptopurine and related compounds. Ann N Y Acad Sci 1954;60:283–96.
200. Einhorn M, Davidson I. Hepatotoxicity of 6-mercaptopurine. JAMA 1964;188:802–6.
201. Scholar EM, Calabresi P. Increased activity of alkaline phosphatases in leukemic cells from patients resistant to thiopurines. Biochem Pharmacol 1979;28:445–6.
202. LePage GA. Basic biochemical effects and mechanism of action of 6-thioguanine. Cancer Res 1963;23:1202.
203. Nelson JA, Carpenter JW, Rose LM, Adamson DJ. Mechanisms of action of 6-thioguanine, 6-mercaptopurine and 8-azaguanine. Cancer Res 1975;35:2872–8.
204. Remy CN. Metabolism of thiopyrimidines and thiopurines: s-methylation with s-adenosylmethionine transmethylase and catabolism in mammalian tissues. J Biol Chem 1963;238:1078–84.
205. Dutcher JP, Wiernik PH, Markus S, et al. Intensive maintenance therapy improves survival in adult acute nonlymphocytic leukemia: an eight-year follow up. Leukemia 1988;2:413–9.
206. Mayer RJ. Current chemotherapeutic treatment approaches to the management of previously untreated adults with de novo acute myelogenous leukemia. Semin Oncol 1987;14:384–96.
207. Elion GB. Enzymatic and metabolic studies with allopurinol. Ann Rheum Dis 1966;25:608–14.
208. Spector T, Johns DG. Stoichiometric inhibition of reduced xanthine oxidase by hydroxypyrazolo (3, 4-d) pyrimidines. J Biol Chem 1970;245:5079–85.
209. Edwards NL, Recker D, Airozo D, Fox IH. Enhanced purine salvage during allopurinol therapy: an important pharmacologic property in humans. J Lab Clin Med 1981;98:673–83.
210. Rodnan GP, Robin JA, Tolchin SF, Elion GB. Allopurinol and gouty hyperuricemia. JAMA 1975;231:1143–7.
211. Hande K, Hixon C, Chabner B. Postchemotherapy purine excretion in lymphoma patients receiving allopurinol. Cancer Res 1981;41:2273–9.
212. Vesell ES, Passananti GT, Greene F. Impairment of drug metabolism in man by allopurinol and nortriptyline. N Engl J Med 1970;283:1484–8.
213. Siaw MF, Coleman MS. In vitro metabolism of deoxycoformycin in human T lymphoblastoid cells: phosphorylation of deoxycoformycin and incorporation into cellular DNA. J Biol Chem 1984;259:9426–33.
214. Fritsch GL. Adenosine deaminase in disorders of purine metabolism and immune deficiency. Ann N Y Acad Sci 1985;451:1.
215. Kraut EH, Bouroncle BA, Grever MR. Low-dose deoxycoformycin in the treatment of hairy cell leukemia. Blood 1986;68:1119–22.
216. Spiers AS, Moore D, Cassileth PA, et al. Remissions in hairy-cell leukemia with pentostatin (2'-deoxycoformycin). N Engl J Med 1987;316:825–30.
217. Dearden CE, Hoffbrand AV, Ganeshaguru K, et al. Membrane phenotype and response to deoxycoformycin in mature T-cell malignancies. Br Med J 1987;295:873–5.
218. Grever MR, Chapman RA, Ratanatharathorn V, Slease RB. An investigation of deoxycoformycin in advanced cutaneous T-cell lymphoma. Blood 1986;66 Suppl 1:215a.
219. O'Dwyer PJ, Marsoni S. Conference on deoxycoformycin: current status and future directions. Cancer Treat Symp 1984;2:1.

220. O'Dwyer PJ, Wagner B, Leyland-Jones B, et al. 2'-deoxycoformycin (Pentostatin) for lymphoid malignancies. Ann Intern Med 1988;108:733–43.
221. Mitchell BS, Edwards NL, Koller CA. Deoxyribonucleoside triphosphate accumulation by leukemic cells. Blood 1983;62:419–24.
222. Seto S, Carrera CJ, Kubota M, et al. Mechanism of deoxyadenosine and 2-chlorodeoxyadenosine toxicity to nondividing human lymphocytes. J Clin Invest 1985;75:377–83.
223. Yu J, Matsumoto SS, Yu AL. Inhibition of transcription as a mechanism of lymphocytotoxicity induced by deoxyadenosine and 2'-deoxycoformycin. Cancer Treat Symp 1984;2:75.
224. Helland S, Ueland PM. Effect of 2'-deoxycoformycin infusion on s-adenosylhomocysteine hydrolase and the amount of s-adenosylhomocysteine and related compounds in tissues of mice. Cancer Res 1983;43:4142–7.
225. Hershfeld MS. Apparent suicide inactivation of human lymphoblast s-adenosylhomocysteine hydrolase by 2'-deoxyadenosine and adenine arabinoside: a basis for direct toxic effects of analogs of adenosine. J Biol Chem 1979;254:22.
226. Brockman RW, Schabel FM Jr, Montgomery JA. Biologic activity of 9-d-arabinofuranosyl-2-fluoradenine, a metabolically stable analog of 9-n-arabinofuranosyladenine. Biochem Pharmacol 1977;26:2193–6.
227. Grever MR, Kopecky KJ, Coltman CA, et al. Fludarabine monophosphate: a potentially useful agent in chronic lymphocytic leukemia. Nouv Rev Fr Hematol 1988;30:457–9.
228. Keating M. Fludarabine phosphate in the treatment of chronic lymphocytic leukemia. Semin Oncol 1990;17:49–62.
229. Cheson BD. Issues for the future development of fludarabine phosphate. Semin Oncol 1990;17:71–8.
230. Hochster H, Cassileth P. Fludarabine phosphate therapy of non-Hodgkin's lymphoma. Semin Oncol 1990;17:63–5.
231. Kantarjian HM, Redman JR, Keating MJ. Fludarabine phosphate therapy in other lymphoid malignancies. Semin Oncol 1990;17:66–70 .
232. Sirotnak FM, Chello PL, Dorick DM, Montgomery JA. Specificity of systems mediating transport of adenosine, 9-d-arabinofuranosyl-2-fluoradenine, and other purine nucleoside analogs in L1210 cells. Cancer Res 1983;43:104–9.
233. Brockman RW, Cheng YC, Schabel FM Jr, Montgomery JA. Metabolism and chemotherapeutic activity of 9-darabinofuranosyl-2-fluoradenine against murine leukemia L1210 and evidence for its phosphorylation by deoxycytidine kinase. Cancer Res 1980;40:3610–5.
234. Plunkett W, Huang P, Gandhi V. Metabolism and action of fludarabine phosphate. Semin Oncol 1990;17(5 Suppl 8):3–17.
235. Tseng WC, Derse D, Cheng YC, et al. In vitro activity of 9-d-arabinofuranosyl-2-fluoradenine and the biochemical actions of its triphosphate on DNA polymerases and ribonucleotide reductase from HeLa cells. Mol Pharmacol 1982;21:474–7.
236. Huang P, Chubb S, Plunkett W. Incorporation of 9-d-arabinofuranosyl-2-fluoradenine into DNA and its chain termination effect on DNA synthesis. J Biol Chem 1990;265:16617–25.
237. Huang P, Plunkett W. Preferential incorporation of arabinofuranosyl-2-fluoradenine into poly (A1) RNA and its inhibitory effects on transcription and translation [abstract]. Proc Am Assoc Cancer Res 1986;27:21.
238. Spriggs D, Robbins G, Mitchell T, Kufe D. Incorporation of 9-d-arabinofuranosyl-2-fluoradenine into HL-60 cellular RNA and DNA. Biochem Pharmacol 1986;35:247–52.
239. Gandhi V, Plunkett W. Modulation of arabinosyl nucleoside metabolism by arabinosyl nucleotides in human leukemia cells. Cancer Res 1988;48:329–34.
240. Gandhi V, Kemena A, Keating MJ, Plunkett W. Fludarabine infusion potentiates arabinosylcytosine metabolism in lymphocytes of patients with chronic lymphocytic leukemia. Cancer Res 1992;52:897–903.
241. Gandhi V, Robertson LE, Keating MJ, Plunkett W. Combination of fludarabine and arabinosylcytosine for treatment of chronic lymphocytic leukemia: clinical efficacy and modulation of arabinosylcytosine pharmacology. Cancer Chemother Pharmacol 1994;34:30–6.
242. Yang S-W, Huang P, Plunkett W, et al. Dual mode of inhibition of purified DNA ligase I from human cells by 9-d-arabinofuranosyl-2-fluoroadenosine triphosphate. J Biol Chem 1992;267:2345–9.
243. Catapano CV, Chandler KB, Fernandes DJ. Effects of anti-cancer agents on primer RNA formation in human leukemia cells [abstract]. Proc Am Assoc Cancer Res 1990;31:420.
244. Carson DA, Kaye J, Matsumoto S, et al. Biochemical basis for the enhanced toxicity of deoxyribonucleosides toward malignant human T cell lines. Proc Natl Acad Sci U S A 1979;76:2430–3.
245. Carson DA, Kaye J, Seegmiller JE. Lymphospecific toxicity in adenosine deaminase deficiency and purine nucleoside phosphorylase deficiency: possible role of nucleoside kinase(s). Proc Natl Acad Sci U S A 1977;74:5677–81.
246. Donofrio J, Coleman MS, Hutton JJ, et al. Overproduction of adenine deoxynucleosides and deoxynucleotides in adenosine deaminase deficiency with severe combined immunodeficiency disease. J Clin Invest 1978;62:884–7.
247. Carson DA, Wasson DB, Beutler E. Antileukemic and immunosuppressive activity of 2-chloro-2'-deoxyadenosine. Proc Natl Acad Sci U S A 1984;81:2232–6.
248. Piro LD, Carrera CJ, Beutler E, Carson DA. 2-chlorodeoxyadenosine: an effective new agent for the treatment of chronic lymphocytic leukemia. Blood 1988;72:1069–73.
249. Piro LD, Carrera CJ, Carson DA, Beutler E. Lasting remissions in hairy-cell leukemia induced by a single infusion of 2-chlorodeoxyadenosine. N Engl J Med 1990;322:1117–21.
250. Santana VM, Hurwitz CA, Blakley RL, et al. Complete hematologic remissions induced by 2-chlorodeoxyadenosine in children with newly diagnosed acute myeloid leukemia. Blood 1994;84:1237–42.
251. O'Brien S, Kurzrock R, Duvic M, et al. 2-chlorodeoxyadenosine therapy in patients with T-cell lymphoproliferative disorders. Blood 1994;84:733–8.
252. O'Brien S, Kantarjian H, Estey E, et al. Lack of effect of 2-chlorodeoxyadenosine therapy in patients with chronic lymphocytic leukemia refractory to fludarabine therapy. N Engl J Med 1994;330:319–22.
253. Liliemark J, Juliusson G. On the pharmacokinetics of 2-chloro-2'-deoxyadenosine in humans. Cancer Res 1991;51:5570–2.
254. Avery TL, Rehg JE, Lumm WC, et al. Biochemical pharmacology of 2 chlorodeoxyadenosine in malignant human hematopoietic cell lines and therapeutic effects of 2-bromodeoxyadenosine in drug combinations in mice. Cancer Res 1989;49:4972–8.
255. Griffig J, Koob R, Blakley RL. Mechanism of inhibition of DNA synthesis by 2-chlorodeoxyadenosine in human lymphoblastic cells. Cancer Res 1989;49:6923–8.
256. Huang M-C, Ashmun RA, Avery TL, et al. Effects of cytotoxicity of 2-chloro-2'-deoxyadenosine and 2-bromo-2'-deoxyadenosine on cell growth, clonogenicity, DNA synthesis, and cell kinetics. Cancer Res 1986;46:2362–8.
257. Parker WB, Bapat AR, Shen JX, et al. Interaction of 2-halogenated dATP analogs (F, Cl and Br) with human DNA polymerases, DNA primase, and ribonucleotide reductase. Mol Pharmacol 1988;34:485–91.
258. Dresler WFC, Stein R. Uber den Hydroxylharnstoff. Justus Liebigs Ann Chem 1869;150:242.
259. Rosenthal F, Wislicki L, Koller L. Uber die Bziehungen von schwertsen Blutgiften zu Abauprodukten des Einweisses: ein Beitrag zum Enstehungmechanismus der pernizosen Anemie. Klin Wochenschr 1928;7:972.
260. Donehower RC. Hydroxyurea. In: Chabner BA, Collins JM, editors. Cancer chemotherapy: principles and practice. Philadelphia: Lippincott; 1990. p. 154–79.
261. Belt RJ, Haas CD, Kennedy J, Taylor S. Studies of hydroxyurea administered by continuous infusion: toxicity, pharmacokinetics, and cell synchronization. Cancer 1980;46:455–62.
262. Fishbein WN, Carbone PP. Hydroxyurea: mechanisms of action. Science 1963;142:1069.
263. Tagger AY, Boux J, Wright JA. Hydroxy (14C) urea uptake by normal and transformed human cells: evidence for a mechanism of passive diffusion. Biochem Cell Biol 1987;65:925–9.
264. Cory JG. Role of ribonucleotide reductase in cell division. In: Cory JG, Cory AH, editors. Inhibitors of ribonucleoside diphosphate reductase activity. New York: Pergamon Press; 1989. p. 1.
265. Nutter LM, Cheng YC. Nature and properties of mammalian ribonucleoside diphosphate reductase. In: Cory JG, Cory AH, editors. Inhibitors of ribonucleoside diphosphate reductase activity. New York: Pergamon Press; 1989. p. 37.
266. Brissenden JE, Caras I, Thelander L, Francke U. The structural gene for the M1 subunit of ribonucleotide reductase maps to chromosome 11, band 15 in human and to chromosome 7 in mouse. Exp Cell Res 1988;174:302–8.
267. Mann GJ, Musgrove EA, Fox RM, Thelander L. Ribonucleotide reductase M1 subunit in cellular proliferation, quiescence, and differentiation. Cancer Res 1988;48:5151–6.
268. Engstrom Y, Eriksson S, Jildevik I, et al. Cell cycle-dependent expression of mammalian ribonucleotide reductase: differential regulation of the two subunits. J Biol Chem 1985;260:9114–6.
269. Eriksson S, Graslund A, Skog S, et al. Cell cycle dependent regulation of mammalian ribonucleotide reductase. J Biol Chem 1984;259:11695–700.
270. Yang-Feng TL, Barton DE, Thelander L, et al. Ribonucleotide reductase M2 subunit sequences mapped to four different chromosomal sites in humans and mice: functional locus identified by its amplification in hydroxyurea-resistant cell lines. Genomics 1987;1:77–86.
271. Kim JH, Gelbard AS, Perez AG. Action of hydroxyurea on the nucleic acid metabolism and viability of HeLa cells. Cancer Res 1967;27:1301–5.
272. Moran RE, Straus MJ. Cytokinetic analysis of L1210 leukemia after continuous infusion of hydroxyurea in vivo. Cancer Res 1979;39:1616–22.
273. Choy BK, McClarty GA, Chan AK, et al. Molecular mechanisms of drug resistance involving ribonucleotide reductase: hydroxyurea resistance in a series of clonally related mouse cell lines selected in the presence of increasing drug concentrations. Cancer Res 1988;48:2029–35.
274. Cocking JM, Tonin PN, Stokoe NM, et al. Gene for M1 subunit of ribonucleotide reductase is amplified in hydroxyurea-resistant hamster cells. Somat Cell Mol Genet 1987;13:221–33.
275. Lewis WH, Wright JA. Altered ribonucleotide reductase activity in mammalian tissue culture cells resistant to hydroxyurea. Biochem Biophys Res Commun 1974;60:926–33.
276. McClarty GA, Chan AK, Engstrom Y, et al. Elevated expression of M1 and M2 components and drug-induced post transcriptional modulation of ribonucleotide reductase in a hydroxyurea-resistant mouse cell line. Biochemistry 1987;26:8004–11.
277. Wright JA, Alam TG, McClarty GA, et al. Altered expression of M1 and M2 gene amplification in hydroxy-urea resistant hamster, mouse, rat, and human cell line. Somat Cell Mol Genet 1987;13:155–65.

44

Alkylating Agents and Platinum Antitumor Compounds

Michael Colvin, MD

The alkylating agents and the platinum antitumor compounds react with electron-rich atoms to form strong chemical bonds. In biological systems the primary cytotoxic reactions of these agents are with the atoms in proteins and DNA. The most important reactions for biological cytotoxicity are with components of DNA, and to a lesser extent with RNA and proteins. Although monofunctional reactions with DNA, RNA, and proteins occur and may have some biological effects, including generating an antigenic site on a protein or, less likely, on DNA or RNA, the therapeutic effects and most of the toxicities are produced by bifunctional reactions of these molecules to produce cross-links in DNA, which prevent separation of the DNA strands, and thus interfere with cellular replication.

The alkylating agents were the first nonhormonal compounds used successfully for the treatment of cancer. During World War I, poison gases were used as weapons, initially chlorine gas. At the battle of Ypres in Belgium, the German army released a new toxic gas, sulfur mustard, developed by a team of German scientists, whose structure is shown in Figure 44-1. Kaiser Wilhelm, the leader of Germany at the time of World War I, had built a magnificent science facility in Berlin, Germany, and many of the most brilliant scientists in the country were attracted to the facility. A team from this group of scientists developed sulfur mustard, and several members of this team later received Nobel Prizes for their subsequent scientific discoveries after the war. The principal effect of sulfur mustard is to cross-link strands of proteins and DNA, since it has two reactive arms, which react with one strand of DNA, and then in a second reaction with the other strand of DNA to prevent cellular replication, as will be discussed below.

A major effect of sulfur mustard as a weapon was to produce lymphoid aplasia and bone marrow suppression. Because of the effects of sulfur mustard in inhibiting growth, the compound was evaluated as an antitumor agent in animals and in patients[1] and was found to have an antitumor effect. However, significant work on the medical applications of these compounds did not occur until the 1940s. At that time, the less reactive and less toxic compound nitrogen mustard (Figure 44-2) was synthesized and used for the treatment of patients with lymphomas.

$$ClCH_2CH_2\text{-}S\text{-}CH_2CH_2Cl$$

Figure 44-1 Structure of sulfur mustard (bis[2-chloroethyl]sulfide).

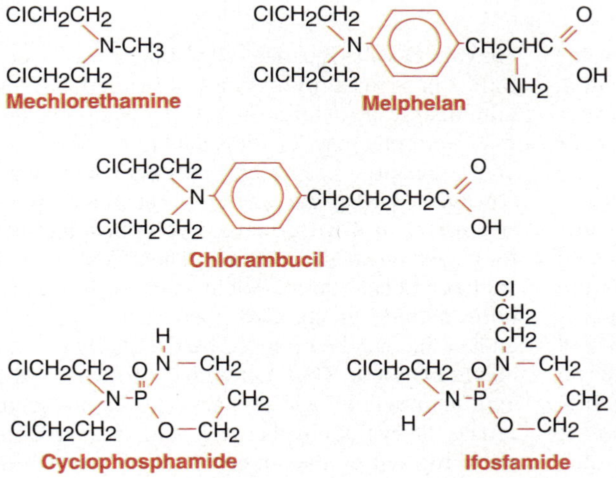

Mechlorethamine

Melphelan

Chlorambucil

Cyclophosphamide

Ifosfamide

Figure 44-2 Structures of nitrogen mustards currently used in therapy.

Most of this work was published after the end of World War II.[2–4] The clinical studies demonstrated that in patients with lymphoma, in particular, antitumor effects were seen with regression of tumors and improvement of symptoms.

CHEMISTRY OF THE ALKYLATING AGENTS

As described above, the alkylating agents react with electron-rich atoms in biological compounds, mainly nitrogen and sulfur atoms. The more reactive agents are termed SN-1 reactors, and the less reactive agents are termed SN-2 agents, as shown in Figure 44-3. The terms refer to the kinetics of the reactions; the rate of reaction of an SN-1 agent is determined only on the concentration of the reactive molecule, as illustrated in Figure 44-3, whereas the rate of reaction of an SN-2 reagent is dependent on the concentration of the alkylating agent and of the biological target. This distinction is important because the SN-1 agents are more reactive and, in general, more toxic.

A large number of chemical compounds are alkylating agents, and many such agents have been and are used clinically. This chapter will describe the compounds that are currently used clinically or represent a type of alkylating agent.

$$RX \longrightarrow R^+ + X^- \xrightarrow{Y^-} RY + X^-$$

SN 1 Reaction

$$RX + Y^- \longrightarrow [\overset{\delta^-}{Y} \cdots R \cdots \overset{\delta^-}{X}] \longrightarrow RY + X^-$$

SN 2 Reaction

Figure 44-3 SN-1 and SN-2 reactions of alkylating agents.

Types of Alkylating Agents **Nitrogen Mustards** The most frequently used alkylating agents are the nitrogen mustards, of which five are commonly used in cancer therapy currently. These compounds are Mechlorethamine (the original "nitrogen mustard"), cyclophosphamide, ifosfamide, melphelan, and chlorambucil and are illustrated in Figure 44-2. The characteristic functional component of the nitrogen mustard is the bischloroethyl group, and all of the nitrogen mustards react through an aziridine intermediate,[5] as shown in Figure 44-4.

The remainder of the molecule is important in determining the physical properties of the molecule, which affect the stability, transport, distribution, and reactivity of the agent. The importance of the entire molecule is demonstrated by cyclophosphamide. Cyclophosphamide is not a reactive compound and undergoes metabolism and activation in the body. Figure 44-5 illustrates the complex activation scheme.[6–11]

The initial activation reaction is by P-450–mediated microsomal oxidation in the liver to produce 4-hydroxycyclophosphamide, which is in spontaneous equilibrium with the open ring tautomer aldophosphamide.[6] At physiologic pH, this equilibrium is predominantly in the form of 4-hydroxycyclophosphamide.[7] This equilibrium mixture diffuses from the hepatocyte into the plasma and is distributed throughout the body. Because 4-hydroxycyclophosphamide is relatively nonpolar, it enters target cells readily by diffusion. Aldophosphamide spontaneously decomposes to produce phosphoramide mustard, which is the

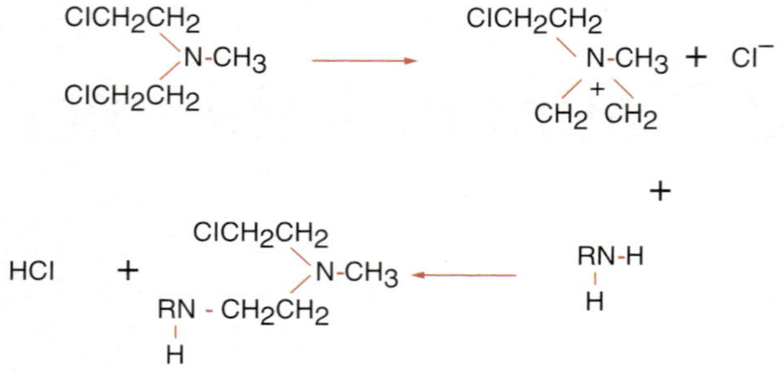

Figure 44-4 Alkylation mechanism of nitrogen mustards.

most reactive alkylating agent produced in the metabolism of cyclophosphamide. Although phosphoramide mustard is also produced extracellularly, this compound is polar and enters cells poorly, so that phosphoramide mustard in the plasma probably plays a minor role in the therapeutic and toxic effects of cyclophosphamide. Thus, 4-hydroxycyclophosphamide serves as an efficient mechanism to deliver the alkylating phosphoramide mustard into cells. Recent evidence indicates that after one of the chloroethyl groups of phosphoramide mustard cyclizes to form a chloroethylaziridinium moiety, the molecule cleaves to produce chloroethylaziridine.[8] It has been demonstrated that chloroethylaziridine is quite volatile and can diffuse between wells in in vitro studies and produce cytotoxicity in "control wells"[9] in such experiments.

The toxic compound acrolein was demonstrated to be produced by the metabolism of cyclophosphamide by Alarcon and Meienhofer,[10] but administration of didechloro-cyclophosphamide, a compound that can produce acrolein, but not cross-link, did not demonstrate antitumor activity in an animal model.[11] In 1992, Lee and colleagues[12] reported that a decrease in the enzyme O6-alkylguanine-alkyltransferase in circulating lymphocytes was produced by the administration of high doses of cyclophosphamide for bone marrow transplantation. Friedman and colleagues[13] reported that tumor cells with elevated O6-alkylguanine-alkyltransferase were sensitized to 4-hydroperoxycyclophosphamide by depletion of the enzyme. These and further studies indicate that acrolein released by cyclophosphamide metabolism forms an O6-guanyl adduct that can be removed by O6-alkylguanine-alkyltransferase. Thus, acrolein contributes to the antitumor activity and probably the carcinogenic effects of cyclophosphamide, and these effects are abrogated by the action of O6-alkylguanine-alkyltransferase.

Cyclophosphamide produces less gastrointestinal and hematopoietic toxicity than other alkylating agents. The parent compound (see Figure 44-2) is inactive and is enzymatically activated (see Figure 44-5). The basis for the decreased toxicity is the enzyme aldehyde dehydrogenase. This enzyme oxidizes aldophosphamide to carboxyphosphamide, an inactive product, which is excreted in the urine and accounts for approximately 80% of an administered dose of cyclophosphamide in any species. This enzyme is found in high concentration in the hepatic cytosol, in early hematopoietic cells, and in the stem cells and mucosal absorptive cells in the intestine.[11] Cyclophosphamide at high doses is also associated with an antidiuretic effect, which reduces urine output and produces systemic edema.[14] The dose-limiting toxicity of cyclophosphamide is a fatal cardiac lesion[15] that is now rarely seen, since the doses approaching this toxicity have been recognized and reduced.

Ifosfamide (see Figure 44-2) is a structural isomer of cyclophosphamide that is used particularly in the treatment of testicular tumors and sarcomas.[16–19] Ifosfamide undergoes the same metabolic reactions as cyclophosphamide, but the location of the chloroethyl group on the ring nitrogen produces quantitative changes in the metabolism of the drug.[19] The primary metabolite, aldoifosfamide, is also a substrate for aldehyde dehydrogenase, so that the bone marrow and gastrointestinal tract sparing properties are similar to those of cyclophosphamide. However, the oxidation of the chloroethyl side chains to produce chloroacetaldehyde is a minor pathway for cyclophosphamide (~10% of dose), but is increased to as much as 50% for ifosfamide. The increased production of chloroacetaldehyde has been implicated in the neurotoxicity of ifosfamide[19] and may contribute to the greater renal and bladder toxicity of ifosfamide. The greater side chain oxidation of ifosfamide and the lesser reactivity of ifosfamide mustard are consistent with the higher doses of ifosfamide than cyclophosphamide that are used clinically.

Melphelan (see Figure 44-2) is an alkylating agent that is used in the treatment of multiple myeloma,[20] ovarian cancer,[21,22] and breast cancer.[23] Melphelan is an amino acid analogue (see Figure 44-2) that enters cells and crosses the blood-brain barrier through active transport systems. The natural substrates for the systems are amino acids,[24] and the entry of melphelan into cells and the central nervous system[25] can be modulated by the presence of amino acids in the extracellular fluid.

Chlorambucil (see Figure 44-2) is used for the treatment of chronic lymphocytic leukemia,[26] ovarian carcinoma,[27] and lymphoma.[28] This agent is well tolerated by most patients and can be used in patients who have severe nausea and vomiting with cyclophosphamide or melphelan.

Aziridines and Epoxides Closely related to the nitrogen mustards are the aziridines, which are represented in current therapy by thiotepa and mitomycin C, and are illustrated in Figure 44-6. These agents alkylate through the same mechanism as the aziridinium intermediates produced by nitrogen mustard, but the aziridine rings formed in these compounds are uncharged and less reactive than aziridinium compounds. The two aziridine agents that are frequently used clinically are thiotepa and mitomycin C (see Figure 44-6). Like the nitrogen mustards, these compounds produce DNA interstrand cross-links. The diepoxide dianhydrogalactitol reacts with DNA in

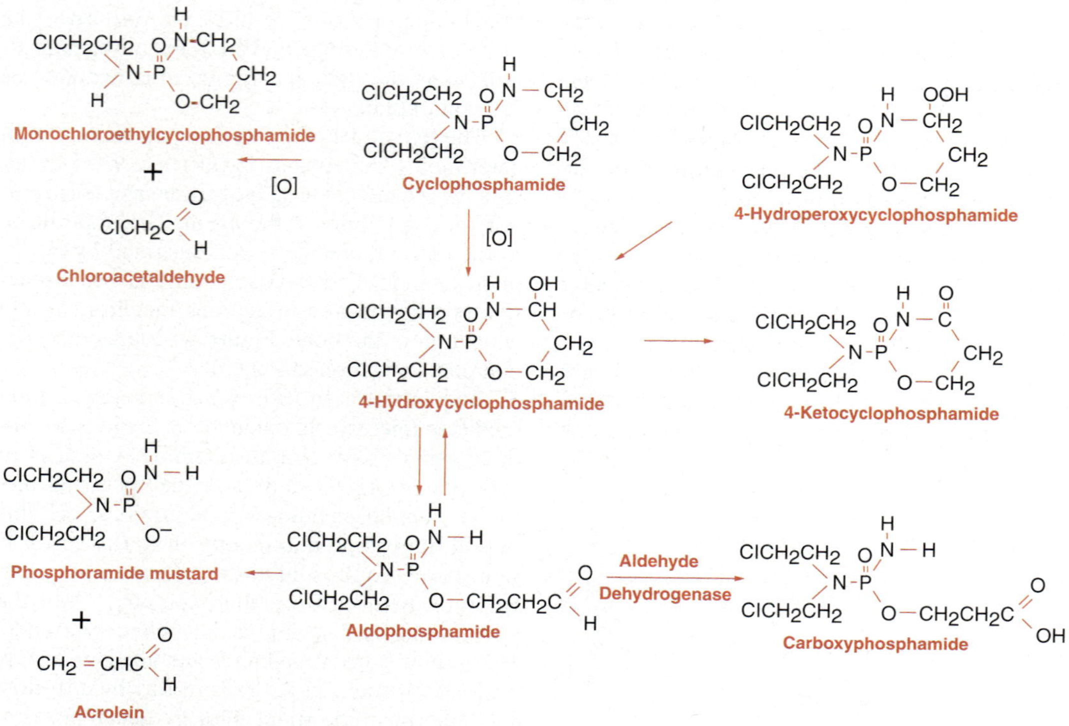

Figure 44-5 Metabolism of cyclophosphamide.

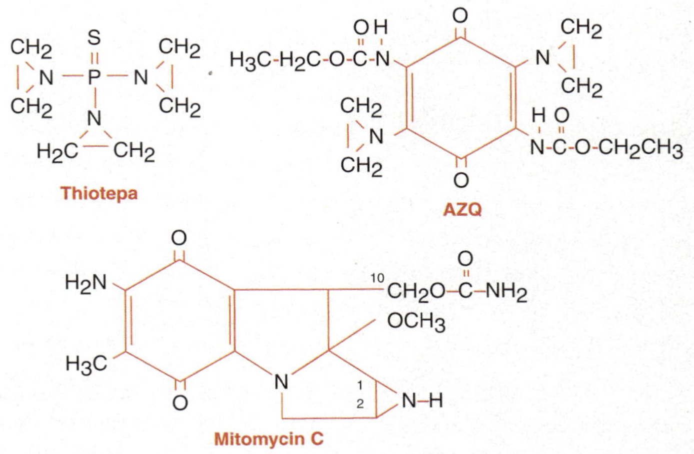

Thiotepa

AZQ

Mitomycin C

Figure 44-6 Structures of aziridine alkylating agents.

(1) -A-G-C-T / -T-C-G-A-

(2) -A-G-T-C-T / -T-C-A-G-A-

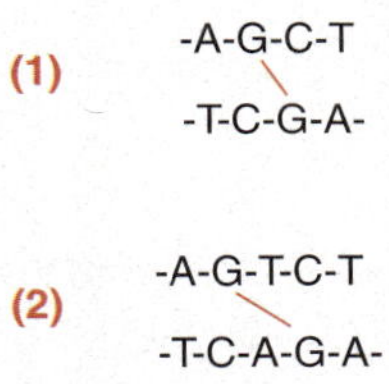

Figure 44-9 Structures of nitrosoureas.

a similar fashion to the aziridines, but has been succeeded in clinical use by dibromodulcitol, which spontaneously generates dianhydrogalactitol in vivo (Figure 44-7).

Thiotepa has been used in combination with other alkylating agents in high-dose therapy with stem cell support[29,30] for the treatment of breast cancer and for the intrathecal therapy of meningeal carcinomatosis.[31] Thiotepa is oxidatively desulfurated by hepatic microsomes to produce triethylenethiophosphoramide[32] (TEPA), which is less reactive than thiotepa.

Mitomycin C is a natural product that has been used in the treatment of breast cancer,[33] cancers of the gastrointestinal tract,[34] and head and neck cancer.[35] This compound contains an aziridine ring and appears to exert its cytotoxic effect through the cross-linking of DNA.[36] Mitomycin C undergoes reduction in cells, with enhancement of the affinity of the carbon-1 atom of the aziridine ring for nucleophiles, such as the extracyclic nitrogen atom on guanylic acid in DNA. Following this alkylation there is displacement of the activated carbamate group on the 10-carbon atom of mitomycin C by an extracyclic amino nitrogen of a guanylic acid molecule on the complementary DNA strand to produce an interstrand cross-link.[37]

The epoxides, such as dianhydrogalactitol (see Figure 44-7) are chemically related to the aziridines and alkylate through a similar mechanism of attack of a nucleophile, such an amino nitrogen, on a carbon of a strained three-membered ring in the agent. Dibromodulcitol is hydrolyzed to dianhydrogalactitol, and thus is a prodrug to an epoxide.[38] Dianhydrogalactitol and dibromodulcitol have been mainly used in Europe and have not been commonly used in the United States.

Alkyl Sulfonates The alkyl alkane sulfonate busulfan (Figure 44-8) was one of the first alkylating agents,[39] and for many years was the standard therapy for chronic myelogenous leukemia (CML), until being succeeded by the less toxic hydroxyurea and, more recently, by the molecularly targeted agent Gleevec, a specific inhibitor[40] of the *bcr-abl* oncogene expressed in CML. Busulfan has a most interesting, but not understood, selectivity and toxicity for early myeloid precursors.[41,42] Hepsulfam, an alkyl sulfonate analog of busulfan with a wider range of antitumor effects,[43] was not as active against CML. The current major use of busulfan is as a component of bone marrow ablative regimens for bone marrow and stem cell transplantation of patients with acute myeloid leukemia and other malignancies.[44] High doses of busulfan have been associated with liver damage, but this toxicity can be avoided by careful monitoring of the pharmacokinetics of the agent and appropriate dose adjustment.[45]

Nitrosoureas The nitrosoureas are a class of alkylating agents that have received considerable attention and use during the past three decades.[46] The structures of the two most frequently used nitrosoureas, carmustine (BCNU) and lomustine (CCNU), are shown in Figure 44-9. Carmustine was the first agent to demonstrate significant antitumor activity against a number of preclinical brain tumor models,[47] was active in clinical trials, is currently used for the treatment of primary brain tumors, and has shown activity against multiple myeloma. Although there are several mechanisms through which the cytotoxic activity of the nitrosoureas may occur, the putative mechanism[48–51] is that shown in Figure 44-10, a base catalyzed decomposition to an alkylating chloroethyl diazonium moiety. Lomustine (CCNU) and semustine (methyl CCNU) have demonstrated significant activity against solid tumors, including gastrointestinal tumors. Nimustine (ACNU) is more water soluble than the other nitrosoureas, and has been used for the intra-arterial and intrathecal treatment of CNS tumors. The clinical use of the nitrosoureas has been limited by the marked and prolonged hematopoietic toxicity and renal toxicity. However, because of their unique mechanism of action and activity against brain tumors, the agents have been used in drug combinations for the treatment of breast and other cancers,[52–59] and the development of nitrosoureas with a higher therapeutic index, such as fotemustine, is an important area of endeavor.

Triazenes, Hydrazines, and Related Compounds These are nitrogen-containing compounds that spontaneously decompose or can be metabolized to produce alkyl diazonium intermediates that alkylate biological molecules. Procarbazine and dacarbazine, which are illustrated in Figure 44-11, are metabolized to produce reactive methyl compounds that methylate DNA and alter its function. The metabolism of procarbazine is complex, and there are different pathways through which a reactive methyl group can be produced. The most likely pathway responsible for the DNA methylation and cytotoxicity is the generation of methylazoxyprocarbazine.[60–62] Both procarbazine and dacarbazine are used in the treatment of Hodgkin's disease[63,64] and some refractory solid tumors.[65] Temozolomide (Figure 44-12) spontaneously decomposes to generate a reactive methyl group,[66–68] which appears to produce more consistent concentrations of the reactive methyl group and has proven to be a useful agent for the treatment of brain tumors and other tumor types.[69,70] The spontaneous and the better time and spatially distributed release of the activated methyl group is probably what makes temozolomide more effective than the previous methylating agents.

Hexamethylmelamine Hexamethylmelamine is an active antitumor agent that is considered to be acting as an alkylating agent because the methyl groups are required for activity (Figure

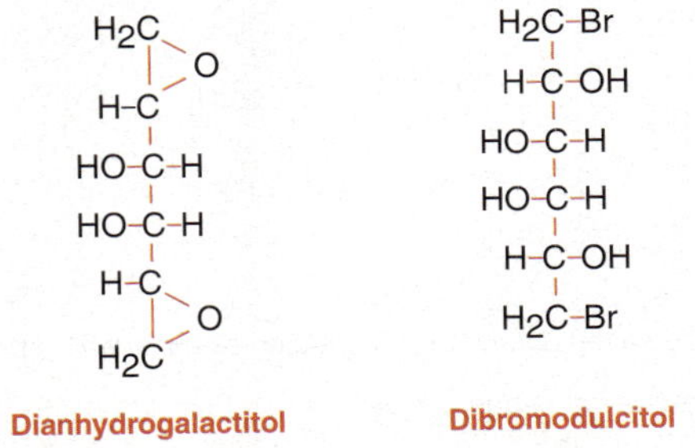

Dianhydrogalactitol

Dibromodulcitol

Figure 44-7 Structures of an epoxide alkylating agent (dianhydrogalactitol) and an epoxide prodrug (dibromodulcitol).

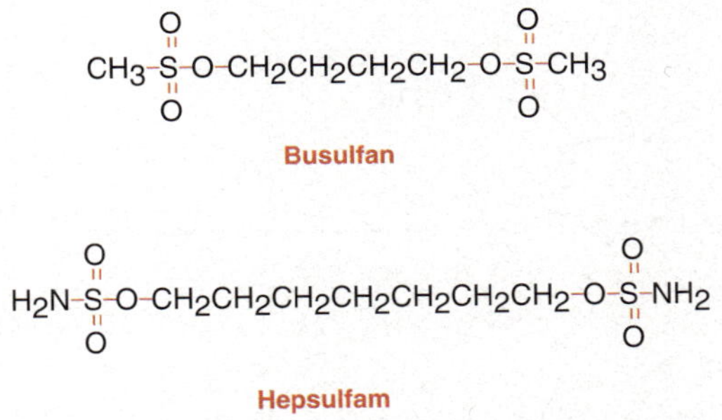

CH_3-S(O₂)-O-$CH_2CH_2CH_2CH_2$-O-S(O₂)-CH_3

Busulfan

H_2N-S(O₂)-O-$CH_2CH_2CH_2CH_2CH_2CH_2CH_2$-O-S(O₂)-$NH_2$

Hepsulfam

Figure 44-8 Structure of alkyl sulfonate (busulfan) and alkyl sulfamate (hepsulfam) agents.

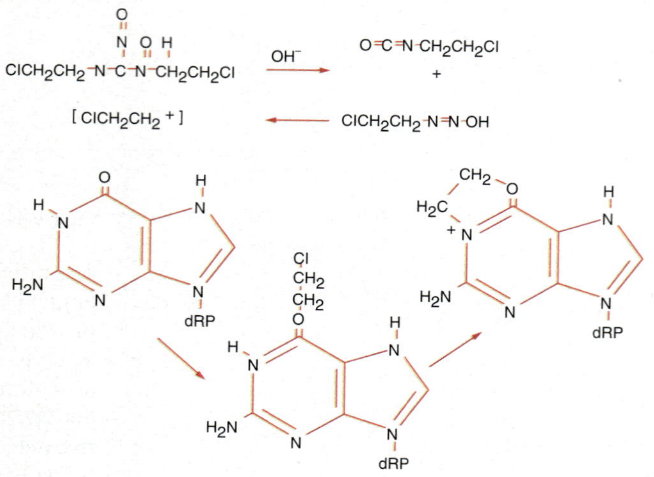

Figure 44-10 Mechanism of nitrosourea activation and alkylation of deoxyguanylic acid.

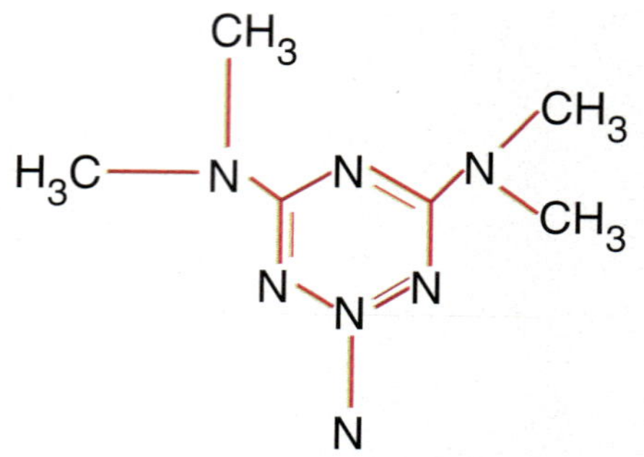

Figure 44-13 The structure of hexamethylmelamine.

44-13). The methyl groups are hydroxylated with subsequent demethylation in vivo,[71] a reaction that generates a reactive methyl group. Analogs in which the methyl groups are hydroxylated are also active. The agent does have significant antitumor activity against ovarian cancer and is used primarily in the third-line treatment of that tumor.[72]

Mechanisms of Cytotoxicity Although the alkylating agents react with a number of biologic molecules, including amino acids, thiols, and DNA, a number of lines of evidence have led to the generally accepted conclusion that the cytotoxic effects of the agents are a result of reactions with DNA. Bifunctional agents are more effective antitumor agents than monofunctional agents, but the addition of more than two alkylating groups does not further increase the cytotoxic activity. These observations[73] and the early studies of Brookes and Lawley[74,75] led to the postulation that interstrand cross-linking of DNA was responsible for the cytotoxic activity of the bifunctional alkylating agents. There is good correlation between cytotoxicity and the formation of interstrand cross-links by bifunctional alkylating agents.

Decomposition, Metabolism, and Cellular Resistance The alkylating agents react with water and are inactivated by this hydrolysis. Cellular resistance to alkylating agents is an important determinant of the effectiveness of therapy. As illustrated in Figure 44-14, there are three general types of cellular resistance. These include (1) decreased uptake[76] of agents into or increased export out of the cell, (2) increased inactivation of agents in the cell, and (3) enhanced repair of the DNA damage produced by the agents. Another mechanism of drug resistance, which only recently has been recognized, is the suppression of cellular mechanisms that produce cytotoxicity through the mechanism of apoptosis in response to cellular damage produced by antitumor agents.

The alkylating agents are inactivated by reaction with thiols such as glutathione.[77] The rate of reaction of alkylating agents with glutathione can be increased by the glutathione S-transferase enzymes,[77,78] and elevated glutathione concentrations in cells protects against the alkylating agents and may play a role in protecting normal cells from alkylating agents, but such resistance also occurs in tumor cells. Approaches to selectively increase glutathione concentrations in normal, but not tumor cells, have not been achieved.

Antitumor agents undergo microsomal and other types of xenobiotic metabolism. Such metabolism may activate agents, such as cyclophosphamide, inactivate them, or modify their physical properties without inactivating them. Nitrosoureas have been reported to be denitrosated and inactivated by microsomal metabolism.[79,80]

Chlorambucil is metabolized to bischloroethylphenylacetic acid, a less active alkylating agent, which probably continues to contribute to the therapeutic and toxic effects of chlorambucil.[81] The reactive aldophosphamide produced from cyclophosphamide is oxidized to carboxyphosphamide, an inactive metabolite (see Figure 44-5), by the enzyme aldehyde dehydrogenase, as discussed earlier.[6] This mechanism has been shown to produce cellular resistance to cyclophosphamide.[82]

The cross-linking phosphoramide mustard produced from cyclophosphamide is hydrolyzed and inactivated by the hydroxyl moiety of water and other nucleophiles. Cellular repair of monoalkylations and DNA cross-links produced by alkylating agents are carried out by cellular resistance mechanisms, and the mechanisms of such repair have been studied extensively, as described below, but are still not completely elucidated.

The best defined DNA repair resistance to alkylating agents is resistance to the nitrosoureas and other compounds that alkylate the O-6-guanine position of DNA. The protein 06-alkylguanine-DNA-alkyltransferase (O6-AT) removes alkyl groups from the O-6 position of guanine,[83–91] preventing the formation of an interstrand cross-link from a chloroethyl adduct and subsequent cross-link. The removed alkyl group is covalently and irreversibly bound to the alkyltransferase, so that the protein can catalyze the removal of only one alkyl moiety and is then rapidly catabolized. It is now obvious that elevated O6-AT is a major mechanism of resistance to nitrosoureas in human gliomas and other tumors. However, the fact that O6-alkyltranferase is irreversibly inactivated by the attachment of an alkyl group provides an

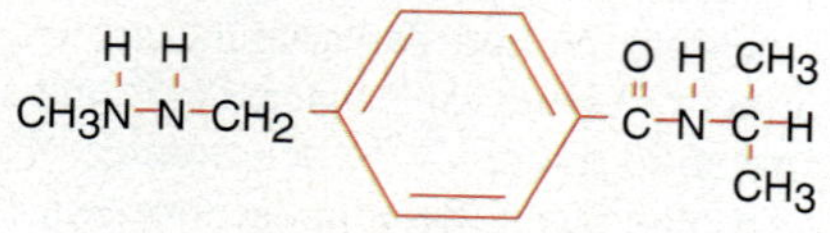

Procarbazine

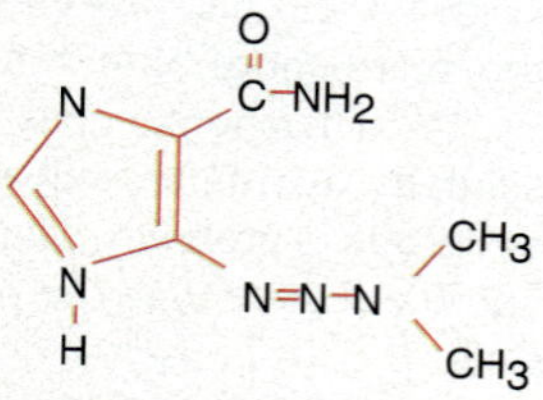

Dacarbazine

Figure 44-11 Structures of monofunctional alkylating agents.

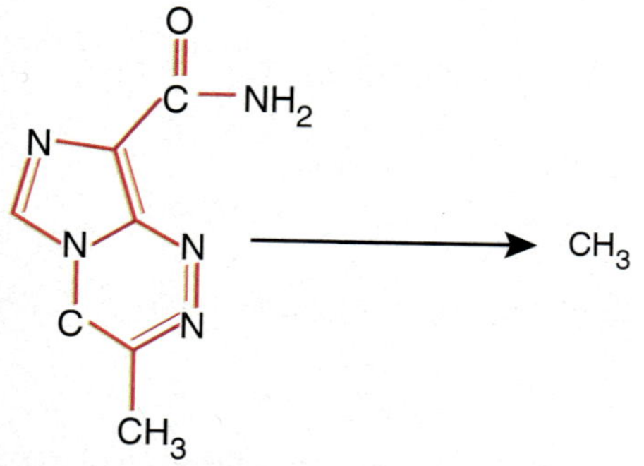

Figure 44-12 The structure of temozolomide.

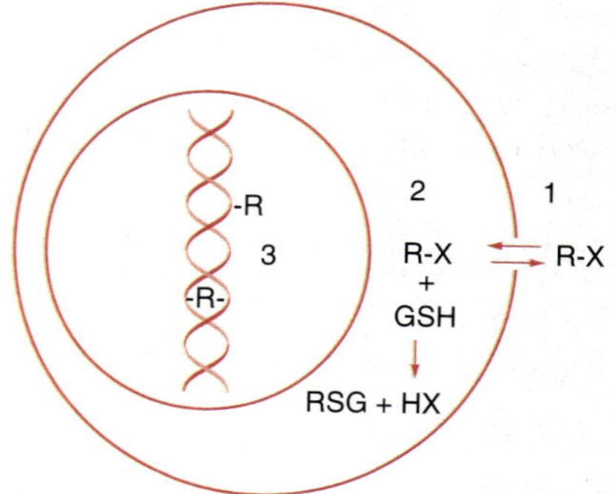

1. Decreased entry into or increased exit of agent from cell
2. Inactivation of agent in cell
3. Enhanced repair of DNA lesions produced by alkylation

Figure 44-14 Mechanisms of resistance to alkylating agents.

approach to counteracting this mechanism of resistance. If cells are treated with a monofunctional O-6 alkylating agent, such as streptozotocin, there follows a period when the O-6 alkyltransferase activity is decreased by its removal of the alkyl groups. Therefore, if therapy with alkylating agents is used during this period, the cell sensitivity has been restored. However, the bone marrow is also rendered more sensitive to alkylating agents during this period, so that lower doses of the alkylating agents should be used.

An association between increased cellular concentrations of metallothionein and resistance to platinum agents has been established,[92] which is due to binding of the agent to the multiple thiol groups of this cellular protein. Yu and colleagues have also described binding of melphelan[93] and Wei and colleagues have described phosphoramide mustard[94] to thiol groups in metallothionein, indicating that increased metallothionein in cells is another mechanism of sequestration and inactivation of alkylating agents.

The cytotoxicity of the bifunctional alkylating agents is due to a cross-link between guanylic acid nucleotides on opposite DNA strands.[95–99] The major mechanism of resistance to bifunctional alkylating agents is the excision of the cross-link.[100] Removal of interstrand cross-links from DNA in cells can be shown to occur in studies using alkaline elution and other techniques.[101] Friedman and colleagues have described a human medulloblastoma cell that is resistant to cyclophosphamide on the basis of repair of the interstrand cross-link and have defined and modeled the structure of the cross-link[97] with the rationale that accurate molecular definition of the structure will enhance the development of a less reparable cross-link. Recently, cell resistance and survival after DNA damage have been demonstrated to occur in both tumor and normal cells by endogenous inhibition of the cellular death (apoptosis) pathway. Monofunctional alkylation of a purine base in DNA can result in depurination, cleavage of the DNA,[102,103] and cell death.

There is evidence that poly(ADP ribose) polymerase is involved in the repair of nitrogen mustard lesions.[104] Also, there is convincing evidence that cells that react to alkylation damage[105] by arresting in the G_2 phase of the cell cycle can repair DNA during this period and are more resistant to alkylating agents than cells that proceed through mitosis despite alkylation damage. Such cells have increased accumulation of phosphorylated (and inactivated) cdc2 kinase associated with G_2 arrest after nitrogen mustard treatment. This alteration allows repair of DNA damage before the cell enters mitosis. Inhibitors of DNA repair have been shown to enhance the cytotoxicity of alkylating agents.[98–101] It is very likely that increased understanding of the DNA repair process will allow more effective use of alkylating agents.

In Vivo Resistance Murine tumors that are resistant to alkylating agents in vivo, but not in vitro, have been reported.[106,107] Further studies of these tumors that are resistant to cyclophosphamide, cisplatin, and thiotepa in vivo demonstrate that the tumors are also resistant to the agents in three-dimensional in vitro culture, but not in two-dimensional in vitro culture.[108] Such resistance may be acquired rapidly after drug exposure[109] and may be associated with enhanced metastatic properties. The mechanisms responsible for this type of resistance have not yet been established. There may be differences between known cellular resistance factors or between membrane properties in the three-dimensional milieu, compared with the two-dimensional configuration, and adhesion molecules may alter drug sensitivity. Other potential mechanisms for drug resistance in vivo are poor perfusion of the tumor and changes in the intracellular pH.[110]

Clinical Pharmacology **Cyclophosphamide** After the administration of a systemic dose of 50 mg/kg, plasma concentrations of the parent compound of up to 400 μmol/L can be achieved and decay with a half-life of 3 to 10 hours.[111–113] The rate of metabolism of the parent compound varies considerably between individuals and can be modulated by the administration of compounds that affect the rate of microsomal metabolism, such as phenobarbital[114] or a previous dose of cyclophosphamide.[115] After conventional doses, the clearance rate of the parent compound does not appear to significantly affect the toxicity or therapeutic effect of the agent.[116,117] This independence of effect from the rate of metabolism is probably because the parent compound is not rapidly excreted and continues to be activated, so that the AUC for systemic exposure to the active metabolite is similar after a given dose.

At the higher doses currently used in bone marrow transplantation regimens, however, the plasma concentrations of cyclophosphamide are close to the capacity of the microsomal activating enzymes. Grochow and colleagues[45] demonstrated that in patients receiving 4 g/m^2 of cyclophosphamide over 90 minutes and achieving initial plasma concentrations of greater than 500 μmol/L, saturable pharmacokinetics are seen. These investigators concluded that when the dosing rate equals or exceeds 4 g/m^2 in 90 minutes or the plasma concentration exceeds 150 μmol/L, nonlinear distribution may occur with variable exposure to the active metabolites. This study also confirmed previous reports that cyclophosphamide can induce its own metabolism.

Studies of the pharmacokinetics of the critical metabolite 4-hydroxy-cyclophosphamide were limited in the past by the difficulty of accurately measuring this labile molecule. However, more facile and specific methods are now available and the pharmacokinetics of this important metabolite are being elucidated. Anderson and colleagues measured 4-hydroxycyclophophamide in patient blood after cyclophosphamide administration by using a very specific gas chromatographic-mass spectrometric technique.[118] After a dose of cyclophosphamide of 110 mg/kg over 90 minutes, peak concentrations of 9 to 12 μmol/L and AUCs of 105 to 110 μmol/L hours were measured; a cyclophosphamide dose of 170 mg/kg given as a continuous infusion over 4 days produced plasma concentrations 1 to 5 μmol/L with a total AUC of 98 to 110 μmol/L hours.

Other studies found similar results.[119,120] All studies found a considerable patient variation in the exposure to 4-hydroxycyclophosphamide after the same dose of cyclophosphamide and differences in the exposure and ratios of cyclophosphamide/4-hydroxycyclophosphamide each day when short-duration infusions are given on subsequent days. These findings are most likely to be a result of differences in cytochrome P-450 complements in patients and the differing exposures to drugs that modulate the activities of these enzymes. These findings indicate that pharmacokinetically guided dose adjustment will be the best method to produce consistent patient exposures to the active metabolites of cyclophosphamide.

The majority of a dose of cyclophosphamide (ca 70%) is excreted in the urine as the inactive metabolite carboxyphosphamide. Renal function does not significantly affect the toxicity of cyclophosphamide[121] (most likely because spontaneous decomposition, and not renal excretion, determines the clearance of the principal active metabolites).

The clinical pharmacology of ifosfamide has been less studied than that of cyclophosphamide, but is similar to that of cyclophosphamide, except that microsomal activation is somewhat slower, and chloroethyl side chain oxidation plays a greater role in its metabolism.[122–126] Thus, for a dose of ifosfamide, lower systemic concentrations of the 4-hydroxy metabolite are achieved than for a similar dose of cyclophosphamide.[125] Both cyclophosphamide and ifosfamide are well absorbed after oral administration.[126]

Boddy and colleagues[19] demonstrated that ifosfamide, like cyclophosphamide, can induce its own metabolism. Because of the greater and more variable side chain of ifosfamide, differences in the P-450 drug metabolizing enzymes between individuals and the modulation of these enzymes by concomitantly administered agents may play a greater role in altering the clinical effects of ifosfamide than cyclophosphamide.[127,128]

Melphelan Alberts and colleagues found that peak plasma levels of 4 to 13 μmol/L of melphelan were present after intravenous administration of a 0.6 mg/kg dose of melphelan, and the half-life ($t_{1/2}$ beta) was 1.8 hours.[129,130] At this dose, the mean AUC for melphelan was 8 μmol/L hours. Similar AUC per dose and pharmacokinetics have been demonstrated by other investigators after high intravenous doses of melphelan.[131] After conventional oral doses of 0.25 mg/kg, peak plasma levels of up to 0.625 μmol/L were measured.[132,133] There is variable systemic exposure after oral dosing, and it has been shown that oral administration of food with melphelan will inhibit absorption of the agent.[134] The half-life of melphelan is prolonged in anephric dogs,[135] and it has been reported that myelosuppression from melphelan is increased in patients with decreased renal function,[136] and significant renal clearance of the parent compound in patients has been shown by Reece and colleagues.[136]

Chlorambucil After the oral administration of 0.6 mg/kg of chlorambucil, peak levels of 2 to 6 μmol/L of parent compound were found at 1 hour by Alberts and colleagues.[137] Peak plasma levels of phenylacetic acid mustard of 2 to 4 μmol/L occurred at 2 to 4 hours after chlorambucil administration. The plasma half-life of chlorambucil was 92 minutes, and that of phenylacetic acid mustard was 145 minutes. At the dose of 0.6 mg/kg of chlorambucil, the plasma AUC of chlorambucil was 3 to 9 μmol/L hours.[138]

Thiotepa The pharmacokinetics of thiotepa[139] were also studied by Henner and colleagues[140] after a continuous intravenous infusion of 12 mg/m^2. Peak plasma concentrations of about 5 μmol/L were achieved on the first day and were found to decay with a $t_{1/2}$ beta of 125 minutes. The mean AUC was 9 micromolar hours. Plasma concentrations of TEPA of up to 1 μmol/L were reached and remained in plasma longer than thiotepa. Wadler and colleagues[141] examined the plasma concentrations of thiotepa after intraperitoneal administration. Peak plasma concentrations of thiotepa of 7 μmol/L were attained on the first day, and then gradually decreased. Plasma AUC values of up to 600 μmol/L hours were achieved. When administered intraperitoneally, there was rapid loss of thiotepa from the intraperitoneal cavity and a concomitant increase in plasma concentrations to those associated with the same dose delivered intravenously. After intravenous injection, cerebrospinal fluid concentrations comparable with plasma concentrations were found.[142] Recent studies indicate that the simultaneous administration of thiotepa and cyclophosphamide will result in lower exposure to the active metabolite of cyclophosphamide, 4-hydroxycyclophosphamide, presumably because of competition for the P-450 enzymes (unpublished data, Colvin and Petros).

Nitrosoureas Levin and colleagues have studied the pharmacokinetics of BCNU.[80] After the intravenous infusion of 60 to 170 mg/m^2, peak plasma concentrations of 5 μmol/L were present and decayed with an initial half-life of 68 minutes. Henner and colleagues[143] measured the pharmacokinetics of BCNU after intravenous doses of 600 mg/m^2. The peak plasma concentration of ultrafilterable BCNU was 23% of the total plasma BCNU. The pharmacokinetics of CCNU after administration of 130 mg/m^2 to patients have also been described.[144] The parent compound could not be detected in plasma, but the monohydroxylated metabolites, *trans*-4-hydroxy CCNU and *cis*-4-hydroxy CCNU, were found in a ratio of 6:4 and at total peak concentrations of about 3 μmol/L. The plasma clearance half-lives of the hydroxy-CCNU metabolites varied from 1 to 3 hours between patients.

Busulfan Because of its insolubility in aqueous solutions, busulfan was previously available only as an oral preparation. However, an intravenous preparation is now available in a DMSO solution (Busulfex), which is increasingly used, is well tolerated, and allows more reproducible dosing and better avoidance of veno-occlusive disease without the necessity for as extensive pharmacokinetic monitoring and dose adjustment, although some variability in exposure to the agent is still seen.

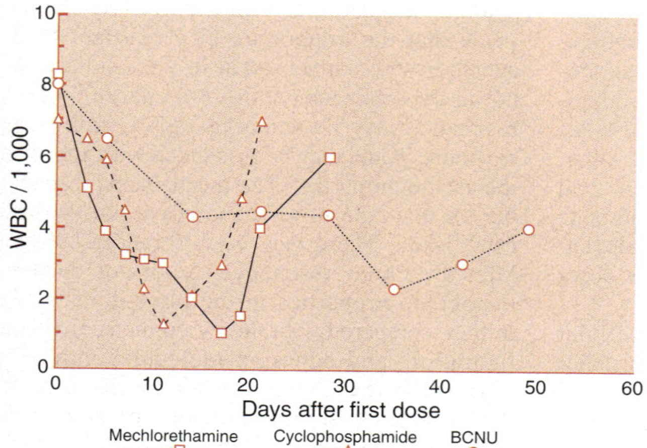

Figure 44-15 Hematopoietic toxicity of alkylating agents. WBC = white blood cells.

Toxicities The characteristic toxicities of the alkylating agents are hematopoietic, gastrointestinal, gonadal, and CNS toxicities. However, each of the agents has a characteristic set of toxicities, determined by the reactivity, metabolism, and distribution of the agent, and the clinician should be aware of the idiosyncrasies of each of the agents that he or she uses frequently.

Hematopoietic Toxicity In general, the clinical dose-limiting toxicity for an alkylating agent is hematopoietic toxicity, particularly suppression of granulocytes and platelets. The nadir of granulocyte depression after alkylating agent treatment is usually 8 to 16 days, and granulocytes usually return to normal within 20 days after a single dose of alkylating agent. Cyclophosphamide and ifosfamide are less hematopoietically toxic than are the other alkylating agents, and granulocyte numbers return to normal more rapidly, platelets are affected less, and repeated doses of cyclophosphamide and ifosfamide do not produce cumulative damage and progressive deterioration of the hematopoietic elements. The decreased hematopoietic toxicity of cyclophosphamide is due to the presence of aldehyde dehydrogenase in the hematopoietic stem cells and in early megakaryocytes, as discussed earlier. In contrast, the nitrosoureas produce severe hematopoietic toxicity and nadirs of granulocytes and platelets occur as late as 45 days.[145] Busulfan also produces severe hematopoietic depression, with a selectivity for early myeloid precursors. The variations in the cellular patterns and time courses of hematopoietic suppression after the administration of different alkylating agents indicate that the individual agents have selectivity for different hematopoietic precursor cells (Figure 44-15).

Peptide growth factors, such as granulocyte-macrophage colony-stimulating factor (GM-CSF) and granulocyte colony stimulating factor (G-CSF), which stimulate the differentiation and proliferation of hematopoietic precursors are now used effectively. The degree and duration of granulocyte depression after antitumor drug administration can be reduced by the concomitant use of these growth factors. The use of these factors with the alkylating agents is particularly attractive because of the steep dose response curve of the alkylating agents and because a considerable increase in dose may be administered before another dose-limiting toxicity is reached. For these reasons, combinations of alkylating agents have been used in association with allogeneic and autologous bone marrow transplantation.

Gastrointestinal Toxicity Damage to the gastrointestinal tract is a toxicity that frequently occurs with high-dose regimens. Mucositis, stomatitis, esophagitis, and diarrhea occur with high doses of alkylating agents, particularly after high doses of melphelan and thiotepa or combinations of alkylating agents. Significant mucositis is unusual even after high doses of cyclophosphamide or ifosfamide. This lack of gastrointestinal toxicity is caused by the presence of the enzyme aldehyde dehydrogenase in the epithelial cells of the gastrointestinal tract, which inactivates the aldophosphamide metabolite produced from the metabolism of cyclophosphamide and ifosfamide.[11] The nausea and vomiting produced by alkylating agents are, at least in part, mediated through the CNS and not caused by direct gastrointestinal toxicity.[146,147] These effects are variable between patients in that some patients tolerate high doses of alkylating agents without nausea and vomiting, while other patients are incapacitated by even low doses of alkylating agents. The frequency of nausea and vomiting does increase as the dose of an alkylating is increased. Therefore, it is important to provide the patient with adequate antiemetic medication. Such medications include phenothiazines, other antiemetics, acute doses of corticosteroids, and, more recently, antiserotonin agents.[148,149]

Veno-Occlusive Disease of the Liver This syndrome is characterized clinically by hepatomegaly, right upper quadrant pain, jaundice, ascites, and a high mortality rate from hepatic failure. Pathologically, the syndrome is characterized clinically by hepatomegaly, upper quadrant

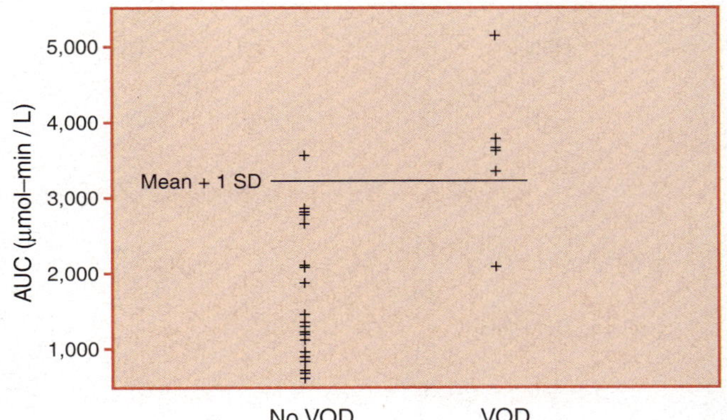

Figure 44-16 Relationship between plasma AUC of busulfan and occurrence of veno-occlusive disease of the liver.

pain, jaundice, ascites, and a high mortality rate from hepatic failure. This complication has been seen in up to 25% of patients receiving high-dose cyclophosphamide and busulfan (Figure 44-16) or cyclophosphamide and total body irradiation prior to allogeneic or autologous bone marrow transplantation for leukemia or lymphoma.[150]

Gonadal Damage A serious toxicity of the alkylating agents is gonadal damage. The characteristic lesion in men, depletion of testicular germ cells with preservation of Sertoli cells, was first described in 1948 in patients treated with mechlorethamine[151] and subsequently confirmed and better characterized[152–154] in men treated with many combinations of antitumor drugs, although the alkylating agents are probably the most potent agents in producing this effect, considering their mutagenic properties. Spermatogenesis and fertility may return after several years.[155,156] Amenorrhea, associated with disappearance of mature and primordial ovarian follicles, is seen in women treated with alkylating agents.[157,158] The frequency of this effect increases with the age of the woman and is more likely to be irreversible in older women.

Pulmonary Damage Pulmonary damage in the form of interstitial pneumonitis and fibrosis is associated with the alkylating antitumor agents. Although the exact mechanism of the pulmonary toxicity is unknown, it is presumably caused by direct toxicity of the agents to pulmonary epithelial cells. The typical presentation of this toxicity is the onset of a nonproductive cough and dyspnea, which may progress to tachypnea and cyanosis, and to pulmonary insufficiency and death. This complication was first described in association with busulfan therapy,[159] but has subsequently been described after cyclophosphamide,[160] BCNU,[161,162] and melphelan[163] and appears to be a toxicity of all the alkylating agents. A significant incidence of pulmonary toxicity has been reported in patients receiving high doses of cyclophosphamide, cisplatin, and BCNU.[164]

Hemorrhagic Cystitis The oxazaphosphorines cyclophosphamide and ifosfamide produce bladder toxicity, which is not seen with other alkylating agents. This toxicity is a hemorrhagic cystitis, which can progress to massive hemorrhage.[165] The metabolite principally responsive for this toxicity is acrolein,[166] although phosphoramide mustard and chloroacetaldehyde may contribute to the effect. Hemorrhagic cystitis is seen more commonly after ifosfamide therapy than cyclophosphamide therapy, probably because higher doses of this agent are used. Renal tubular damage has also been seen after ifosfamide, including a Fanconi-type syndrome with azotemia, elevated serum creatinine, and enzymuria.[167] The systemic administration of thiols can prevent or ameliorate the bladder damage from cyclophosphamide and ifosfamide because the thiols conjugate and inactivate the aldehyde functions of acrolein and chloroacetaldehyde. A widely used compound to prevent or ameliorate oxazaphosphorine bladder toxicity is the sodium salt of 2-mercaptoethane sulfonate (Mesna). Mesna is usually administered to all patients receiving ifosfamide and to patients receiving high-dose cyclophosphamide. Subclinical renal toxicity has been observed in patients receiving ifosfamide,[16] despite Mesna administration, so that administration of Mesna does not eliminate the need for adequate hydration and careful observation of the patient.

Antidiuresis An antidiuretic effect is commonly seen in patients receiving doses of cyclophosphamide of 50 mg/kg or greater.[168,169] This syndrome is characterized by a decrease in urine output 6 to 8 hours after drug administration, weight gain, a marked increase in urine osmolality, and a decrease in serum osmolality and sodium concentration. Pericardial and pleural effusions may be seen, and seizures caused by hyponatremia have occurred with cyclophosphamide therapy,[170] especially if low-sodium replacement fluids are administered. This antidiuretic syndrome appears to be caused by an effect of cyclophosphamide metabolites on the distal renal tubule and is self-limited, with the excess fluid excreted over a period of about 12 hours. Administration of furosemide promotes free water clearance and ameliorates the syndrome.[171]

Renal Toxicity Renal toxicity is a serious toxicity of the nitrosureas.[172,173] This effect is dose related and can produce severe renal failure and death after administration of more than 1,200 mg of BCNU. Elevation of serum creatinine and other clinical evidence of renal toxicity may not be seen until after the completion of therapy. The histology of the kidneys in patients with renal nitrosourea damage is similar to that seen in radiation nephritis. A case of acute renal failure after melphelan therapy has also been reported,[174] indicating that adequate hydration of patients undergoing treatment with any alkylating agent therapy is very important. The histology of the kidneys in patients with renal nitrosourea damage is similar to that in radiation nephritis.

Alopecia Although the association between an alkylating agent and alopecia was first described with busulfan therapy,[175] this toxicity is associated with most of the alkylating agents, and particularly with cyclophosphamide and ifosfamide therapy. The alopecia produced by these agents can be quite extensive, especially if the agent is given in combination with vincristine or doxorubicin. Regrowth of the hair occurs after cessation of therapy and may be associated with a change in the texture and color of the hair.[176] The structure-function studies of Feil and Lamoureaux[177] indicate that this toxicity is a result of entry of lipophilic metabolites into the hair follicles. This suggestion is consistent with the fact that busulfan, vincristine, and Adriamycin are lipophilic and produce severe alopecia. It is important to recognize that the growing hair develops a nick, undoubtedly from inhibition of growth of the hair at the base of the follicle at the time of drug exposure, and the hair "breaks off," rather than "falls out." The practical implication of this fact is that patients should be advised not to brush their hair during and immediately after therapy administration to avoid the breaking off of the hair.

Allergic and Hypersensitivity Reactions Because the alkylating agents react with many biologic molecules, it is not surprising that they serve as haptens and produce allergic reactions.[178–180] The most frequent reactions that have been reported have been cutaneous hypersensitivities. Anaphylactic reactions are rare, but have occurred.[181] Patterns of cross-reactivity have not been carefully defined, but cross-reactivity between agents of similar structure, such as the nitrogen mustards, have been described.[182]

Cardiotoxicity The nonhematologic dose-limiting toxicity of cyclophosphamide is a fatal cardiac toxicity characterized by specific pathologic findings[15,183] in the heart and characterized clinically by fulminant cardiac failure. The hearts of these patients are dilated, with patchy transmural hemorrhage and pericardial effusion. The microscopic findings consist of interstitial hemorrhage and edema, myocardial necrosis and vacuolar changes, and specific changes in the intramural small coronary vessels. Decreased electrocardiographic voltage and a transient increase in heart size is seen in high-dose cyclophosphamide patients without clinical symptoms, and the characteristic pathologic findings are present in patients who die of other causes following high-dose cyclophosphamide. Age greater than 50 years and previous Adriamycin exposure appear to increase the risk of cyclophosphamide cardiotoxicity.[183] To this author's knowledge, there have been no reports of pretherapy cardiac evaluation to correlate with cardiac clinical symptoms and outcome after high-dose cyclophosphamide.

Neurotoxicity In preclinical studies of alkylating agents, severe neurotoxicity was seen.[184] At the usual clinical doses, including transplant doses, frank neurotoxicity is not often seen, but drowsiness and alterations of consciousness can be seen clinically, and changes in EEG findings were detected (unpublished experience of this author) after bone marrow transplantation doses of cyclophosphamide. At BCNU doses of 1,200 mg/m^2, severe CNS toxicity has been produced,[185] and the intracarotid administration of BCNU has produced severe eye pain and blindness.[186] High-dose busulfan therapy produces seizures, and anticonvulsants are often used prophylactically.[187]

Teratogenicity Studies carried out in vivo and in embryo cultures demonstrate that all of the alkylating agents are teratogenic.[188] The teratogenic effect is the result of cytotoxic effects on the embryo by the same mechanisms through which the compounds are toxic to tumor cells.[189,190] The available clinical information indicates that there is a definite risk of a malformed infant if the mother is treated during the first trimester of pregnancy.[191] However, the administration of alkylating agents during the second and third trimesters is not associated with an increased risk of fetal malformation.[192]

Carcinogenesis Since the initial reports of acute leukemia occurring in patients treated with alkylating agents,[193,194] it has become increasingly obvious that this type of oncogenesis is a significant complication of alkylating agent therapy. Several studies indicate that the rate of acute leukemia may be 10% or higher in certain patients. Procarbazine and other methylating agents appear to be the most potent oncogenic agents.[195] Although sufficient data are not yet available to be certain, it appears that alkylating agent therapy administered over a relatively short period of time is less oncogenic than prolonged alkylating agent therapy.

Immunosuppression and Immune Enhancement The immunosuppressive effect of alkylating agents was first described by Hektoen and Corper[196] for sulfur mustard. Cyclophosphamide is particularly immunosuppressive[197] and is used for the treatment of autoimmune diseases.[198] Low doses of cyclophosphamide can enhance the immune response by selectively inhibiting immune suppressor cells,[199] and moderate doses of cyclophosphamide have been used in conjunction with immunotherapy and biological response modifiers such as interleukin-2.[200,201]

The clinical significance of the immunosuppression produced by alkylating agents in their role as antitumor agents is not certain. The two major concerns are susceptibility to infection in the immunosuppressed host and the potential interference with a host immune response to the tumor. The available evidence indicates that most intermittent antitumor regimens do not produce a profound or prolonged immunosuppression.[202]

PLATINUM ANTITUMOR COMPOUNDS

The platinum antitumor agents are complexes of platinum with ligands that can be displaced by nucleophilic (electron-rich) atoms to form strong bonds with covalent characteristics. Thus, like the alkylating agents, the platinum agents form strong chemical bonds with thiol sulfurs and animo nitrogens in nucleic acids and proteins.

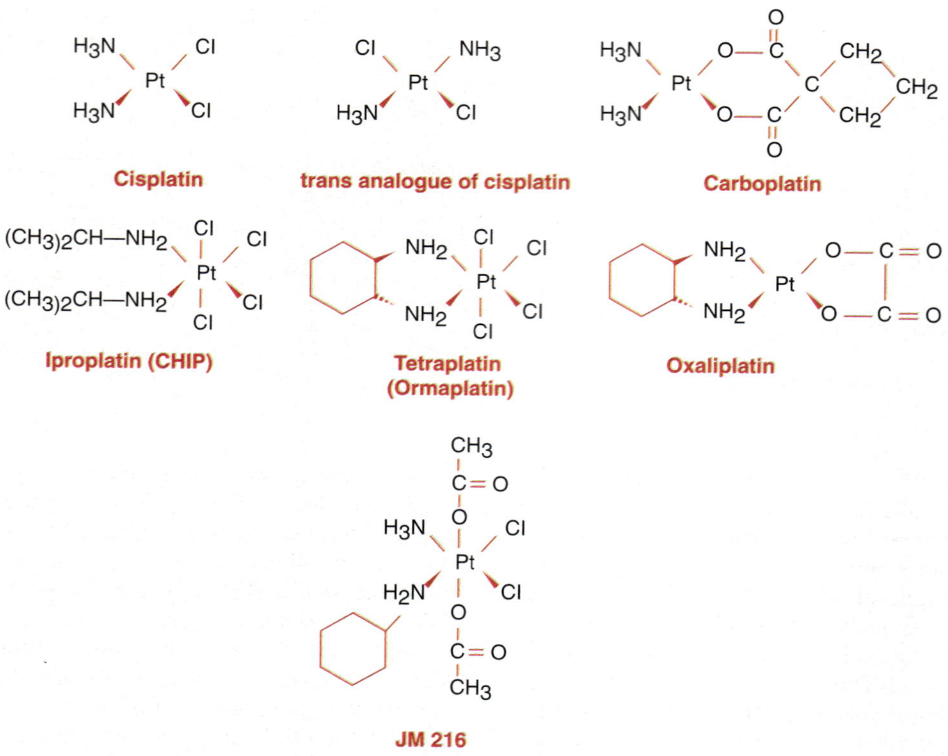

The first antitumor platinum agent was discovered by Rosenberg and colleagues[203,204] while studying the effects of electric current on bacterial growth. The growth inhibition observed was found to be caused by a platinum complex of ammonia and chloride, which was produced in the medium from the platinum electrode. These investigators found several such compounds to have antitumor activity against murine tumors in vivo.[204] The most active of these compounds was the one now known as cisplatin (Figure 44-17).

Cisplatin went into clinical trials in the early 1970s[205–207] and was found to have significant antitumor activity against testicular cancer, lymphoma, squamous cell carcinoma of the head and neck, ovarian cancer, and bladder cancer. Because of its significant therapeutic effect in these tumors and activity against a number of other solid tumors, it has become the most frequently used antitumor agent. Because of the renal and neurotoxicities of cisplatin, there were intensive efforts to devise analogs with fewer of these toxicities. This work led to the development of carboplatin, which produces primarily hematopoietic toxicity and has antitumor effects similar to those of cisplatin. Other platinum compounds have been developed and evaluated, as described later, but have not demonstrated significant advantages over cisplatinum and carboplatinum.

Cisplatin

trans analogue of cisplatin

Carboplatin

Iproplatin (CHIP)

Tetraplatin (Ormaplatin)

Oxaliplatin

JM 216

Figure 44-17 Structures of platinum antitumor agents.

Chemistry The platinum compounds that are active antitumor agents can have either four or six ligands (see Figure 44-17) with a square planar or hexahedral configuration. Those with four ligands have an oxidation state of +2, and those with six ligands, an oxidation state of +4. The chloride ligands of cisplatin and the other complexes with the +2 oxidation state can be exchanged for nucleophilic atoms in the biologic milieu, including the nitrogens of the DNA bases. The chloride ligands of the +4 compounds are much less reactive than those of the +2 compounds,[208] and it is likely that the +4 compounds are reduced in vivo to produce the reactive +2 complexes.[209] The ligand substitution reactions of the square planar complexes occur with retention of the configuration of the platinum complex. Because the *trans*-platinum compounds are essentially inactive as antitumor compounds, the ability of the *cis* compounds to form certain stereo-specific cross-links probably accounts for their antitumor activity, and specific intrastrand and interstrand cross-links have been identified.

In some *cis*-platinum compounds in clinical use, the chloride leaving ligands are replaced with carboxyl ester groups, as in carboplatin and oxaliplatin (Figure 44-18). These ligands are less readily displaced; thus, these compounds require higher concentrations for cytotoxicity. The decreased renal and neurologic toxicity of these compounds is also probably a result of their being less chemically reactive than cisplatin. Substitutions on the amino groups alter the lipophilicity and distribution of the agent.

Cellular and Molecular Pharmacology Although the chloride and carboxyester ligands can probably be directly displaced by biologic molecules, it is likely that, in the biologic milieu, the chloride or carboxy ligands are displaced by

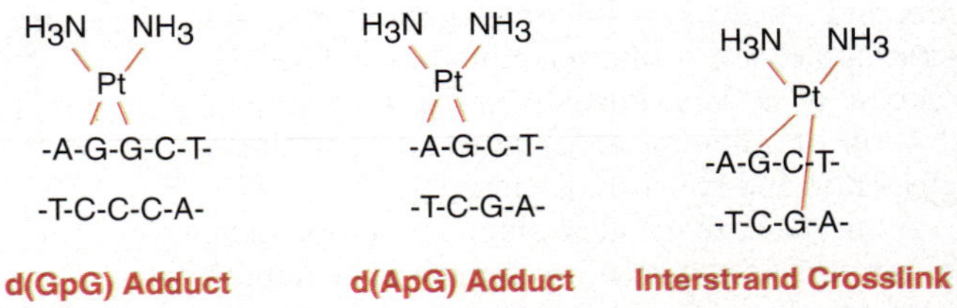

H_3N NH_3 Pt	H_3N NH_3 Pt	H_3N NH_3 Pt
-A-G-G-C-T-	-A-G-C-T-	-A-G-C-T-
-T-C-C-C-A-	-T-C-G-A-	-T-C-G-A-
d(GpG) Adduct	**d(ApG) Adduct**	**Interstrand Crosslink**

Figure 44-18 Platinum–DNA adducts.

water to form the aquo ligand, which is a better leaving group than chloride or carboxy entities. The high chloride content of the extracellular fluid should maintain the platinum compounds in the chloride and less reactive form. However, in the lower chloride content of the cell, the more reactive aquo species is formed. The loss of a proton produces the hydroxyl ligand, which is unreactive. Figure 44-19 illustrates the proposed aquation pathway for cisplatin. The platinum compounds react with many biologic molecules, but here is considerable evidence that these compounds, like the bifunctional alkylating agents, exert their cytotoxic effect by interfering with DNA replication and cell division. Roberts and Pera[210] demonstrated that the amount of platinum bound to DNA was directly related to the degree of cytotoxicity in rodent tumor cells. Zwelling and colleagues[211] demonstrated that the degree of DNA interstrand cross-linking in vitro and in vivo was directly related to the degree of cytotoxicity in rodent tumor cells.

The *cis*-platinum compounds, like the alkylating agents, react with nitrogen atoms of DNA and preferentially react with the N-7 atom of deoxyguanylic acid. Specific adducts of Pt compounds with DNA have now been characterized and studied and specific DNA intrastrand and interstrand cross-links identified.[210] The consensus of the studies is that the most frequent adducts are dGpdG and dApdG, which result from the *cis*-platinum complex linking adjacent deoxyguanylates or an adjacent deoxyadenylate and deoxyguanylate in a strand of DNA to produce an intrastrand cross-link, in both situations. A less common, but potentially more toxic lesion is one that results from binding of the platinum atom to the N-7 atom of a deoxyguanylate in the complementary strand of DNA, producing an interstrand cross-link, analogous to a nitrogen mustard interstrand cross-link. Repair of both lesions does occur, and the cytotoxicity to the cell is determined by the resultant formation and repair of the lesions[212] by the cellular DNA mismatch repair complex. Cell resistance to cross-linking agents, including cisplatin-resistant cells, often have a deficiency in the mismatch repair complex, supporting the hypothesis that an intact mismatch repair system may render cells more sensitive to cross-linking agents in that the attempt to repair results in cell death.

Mechanisms of Cellular Resistance to Platinum Agents Mechanisms of cellular resistance to platinum, which have been described, include decreased uptake of the platinum compound into cells, enhanced repair of the platinum DNA damage, and increased efflux of the agent. Elevated cellular glutathione concentrations have also been associated with cellular resistance to platinum compounds. Although decreased cellular accumulation of the platinum compounds is a mechanism of cellular resistance, the mechanism of this type of resistance appears to be variable. Several investigators have shown that tumor cells can be sensitized to the platinum agents by depletion of cellular glutathione by treatment with butathione sulfoximine, an inhibitor of glutathione synthesis.[213] Eastman[214] has demonstrated that glutathione can react with monofunctional adducts on DNA to quench the second reactive ligand and prevent cross-link formation. Resistance to platinum agents has also been associated with elevation of glutathione transferase enzyme activity. Resistance to platinum agents has also been associated with another sulfhydryl-containing protein, metallothionein.[215] Decreased cellular uptake of cisplatin into cells has also been described, which is interesting in that the uptake of cisplatin into cells does not appear to be an active process.

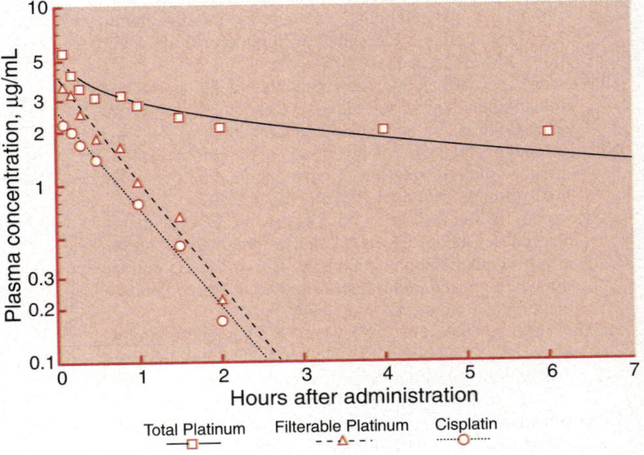

Figure 44-19 Clinical pharmacokinetics of cisplatin after single injection of 100 mg/m^2.

Clinical Pharmacology **Pharmacokinetics** The pharmacokinetics of platinum agents has been studied as total platinum, and more recently, the specific agents. In pharmacokinetic studies after cisplatin administration, total platinum in the plasma follows a triphasic pattern, with the first phase $t_{1/2}$ about 30 minutes, the second phase $t_{1/2}$ about 60 minutes, and the third phase $t_{1/2}$ greater than 24 hours.[216,217] Carboplatin exhibits similar pharmacokinetics, except that the initial half-lives are somewhat longer, less of the total platinum is protein bound, and a greater percentage of the agent is excreted by the kidneys.[218] Decreased creatinine clearance results in higher plasma levels of both cisplatin and carboplatin with potentially greater toxicity.

Toxicities **Renal** The most serious, and usually dose-limiting, toxicity of cisplatin is renal.[219,220] This toxicity presents clinically as elevated BUN and creatinine, is cumulative with continued cisplatin exposure, and is potentiated by other nephrotoxins.[221] Decreases in serum electrolytes have been associated with platinum renal toxicity, including symptomatic hypomagnesemia.[222] Although the toxicity may remain subclinical and the renal function return to normal, significant pathological damage may persist.[223] The pathology of the renal damage is characterized by focal acute tubular necrosis, dilation of convoluted tubules, thickened tubular basement membranes, formation of casts, and epithelial atypia of the collecting ducts.[223,224] High fluid intake with forced diuresis[225,226] can reduce the incidence and severity of the renal toxicity. Systemic administration of thiols can reduce renal toxicity of cisplatin in animal models, and in a clinical trial, systemic diethyldithiocarbamate appeared to reduce nephrotoxicity without affecting ototoxicity or myelosuppression.[227] The nephrotoxicity of the second generation platinum complexes, such as carboplatin iproplatin is markedly less than that of cisplatin.

Ototoxicity Ototoxicity has been a significant problem with cisplatin. This toxicity is characterized by tinnitus and hearing loss.[205,206,228] Since the higher frequencies are usually involved, the hearing loss may not be symptomatic. Vestibular toxicity does not usually occur, but can be seen.[229,230] The ototoxicity of cisplatin is dose related and is usually cumulative with subsequent courses of therapy.[231] Radiation prior to or simultaneous with the cisplatinum administration enhances the toxicity,[232] but the additive effect may be less if the cisplatin precedes the radiation.[233]

Neurotoxicity The neurotoxicity seen with the administration of cisplatin consists principally of peripheral neuropathy involving both the upper and lower extremities, with paresthesias, weakness, tremors, and loss of taste.[234] Seizures and leukoencephalopathy have been described[235] and may progress after cessation of cisplatin therapy.

Particularly severe neurotoxicity has been reported after intra-arterial infusions for head and neck cancer. Since various pharmacologic maneuvers have been able to reduce the nephrotoxicity and severe nausea and vomiting produced by cisplatin, neurotoxicity has become the dose-limiting toxicity of cisplatinum. The observation has been made that treatment of animals with an ACTH analogue will prevent neurotoxicity from cisplatin and will facilitate the recovery of established nerotoxicity,[236] but does not interfere with the antitumor effect of the agent.

Gastrointestinal Toxicity Severe nausea and vomiting have been a significant problem with cisplatin, occurring in almost all patients receiving the agent.[220,237] The cause of this toxicity is not firmly established. Work in animal models indicates that abdominal visceral innervation and 5-hydroxytryptamine. Receptors on visceral afferent nerves play a role in this toxicity, but there is also evidence that the chemoreceptor trigger zone in the medulla plays a role. The use of a dopamine antagonist, metoclopramide, prior to and during cisplatin administration has been effective in controlling this toxicity.[238,239] Dexamethasone or methylprednisolone alone or in combination with metoclopramide have been useful. More recently, antiserotonin analogues such as ondansetron and granisetron have proven highly effective in controlling nausea and vomiting. The gastrointestinal toxicities of carboplatin and iproplatin are much less than those of cisplatin.

Immune Effects In contrast to the alkylating agents, many of which are significantly immunosuppressive, cisplatin appears to have no immunosuppressive effect at the usual clinical doses and may even augment immune effect.[240]

Other Analogues in Clinical Use: Oxaliplatin Several other platinum analogues have been synthesized and evaluated clinically, including tetraplatinum and JM216. The greatest clinical impact has been observed with oxaliplatin that contains a diaminocyclohexane (DACH) carrier ligand (see Figure 44-17). Among the platinum analogues, oxaliplatin is distinctive in its activity against colorectal cancer.[241] Oxaliplatin can inhibit growth of colorectal cancer cell lines that are resistant to cisplatin and carboplatin.[242] A combination of oxaliplatin, 5-fluorouracil (5-FU) and leucovorin (FOLFOX4) produced a higher response rate, longer time to progression and better overall survival than did irinotecan, 5-FU and leucovorin (IFL) in first line therapy for metastatic colorectal cancer,[243] resulting in US FDA approval of the drug for this indication. Activity has also been observed with oxaliplatin-containing regimens in non-small cell lung, breast, gastric, bladder, renal cell, and ovarian cancers.

The dose limiting toxicity of oxaliplatin is sensory neuropathy.[244] An acute, rapidly reversible neuropathy occurs in >90% of patients that can be aggravated by exposure to cold.[245] More problematic chronic neuropathy generally relates to the cumulative dose of drug. Neuropathy has been prevented in some studies by infusion of calcium and magnesium solutions, gabapentin, carbamazepine, amifostine and glutathione. Existing neuropathy has been partially palliated by administration of calcium and magnesium solutions, gabapentin and alpha-lipoic acid.[244]

As in the case of other platinum compounds, the anti-tumor activity of oxaliplatin is thought to relate to adduct formation that produces intra- and inter-strand DNA crosslinks, as well as the binding of DNA and protein. Oxaliplatin forms fewer DNA adducts, but more DNA single strand breaks than does cisplatin.[246] Whether the greater number of single strand breaks observed with oxaliplatin results from primary interaction with DNA or the rapid induction of apoptosis is not known. Greater efficiency for inducing apoptosis, despite the formation of fewer adducts, may relate to failure of DNA repair mechanisms to recognize the DACH moieties associated with oxaliplatin adducts.[246] Mismatch repair proteins and some damage recognition proteins bind to cisplatin-GG adducts with higher affinity than to oxaliplatin-GG adducts.[247] Recently described differences in conformation for the NMR solution structures of the two types of adducts provide an explanation for the differential recognition of cisplatin- and oxaliplatin-induced DNA damage.[247]

REFERENCES

1. Adair CPJ, Bogg HJ. Experimental and clinical studies on the treatment of cancer by dichlorethylsulfide (mustard gas). Ann Surg 1931;93:190–9.
2. Goodman LS, Wintrobe MM, Dameshek W, et al. Use of methyl-bis(beta-chloroethyl)amine hydrochloride for Hodgkin's disease, lymphosarcoma, leukemia. JAMA 1946;132:263.
3. Jacobson LP, Spurr CL, Barron ESG, et al. Studies on the effects of methyl-bis(beta-chloroethyl) amine hydrochloride for Hodgkin's disease, lymphosarcoma, leukemia. JAMA 1946; 132:263.
4. Rhoads CP. Nitrogen mustards in treatment of neoplastic disease. JAMA 1946;131:656.
5. Colvin M, Chabner BA. Alkylating agents in cancer chemotherapy: principles and practice. In: Chabner BA, Collins JM, editors. Philadelphia: Lippincott; 1990. p. 276–313.
6. Fenselau C, Kan MN, Rao SS, et al. Identification of aldophosphamide as a metabolite in vitro and in vivo in humans. Cancer Res 1997;37:2538–43.
7. Zon G, Ludeman SM, Brandt JA, et al. NMR spectroscopic studies of intermediary metabolites of cyclophosphamide. A comprehensive kinetic analysis of the interconversion of cis- and trans-4-hydroxycyclophosphamide and the concomitant partitioning of aldophosphamide between irreversible conjugation pathways. J Med Chem 1984;27:466–85.
8. Shulman-Roskes EM, Noe DA, Gamcsik MP, et al. The partitioning of phosphoramide mustard and its aziridinium ions among alkylation and P-N bond hydrolysis reactions. J Med Chem 1998;41:515–29.
9. Flowers JL, Ludeman SM, Gamcsik MP, et al. Evidence for a role of chloroethylaziridine in the cytotoxicity of cyclophosphamide. Cancer Chemother Pharmacol 2000;45:335–44.
10. Alarcon RA, Meienhofer J. Formation of the cytotoxic aldehyde acrolein during the in vitro degradation of cyclophosphamide. Nat New Biol 1971;233:250–2.
11. Russo JE, Hilton J, Colvin OM. The role of aldehyde dehydrogenase isoenzymes in cellular resistance to the alkylating agent cyclophosphamide. In: Weber G, editor. Enzymology and molecular biology of carbonyl metabolism. Vol. 2. New York: Liss; 1989. p. 65.
12. Lee SM, Crowther D, Scarffe JH, et al. Cyclophosphamide decreases O6-alkylguanine-DNA transferase activity in peripheral lymphocytes of patients undergoing bone marrow transplantation. Br J Cancer 1992;66:331–6.
13. Friedman HS, Pegg AE, Johnson SP, et al. Modulation of cyclophosphamide activity by 0-6-alkylguanine-DNA alkyltransferase. Cancer Chemother Pharmacol 1999;43:80–5.
14. Bode U, Seif SM, Levine AS. Studies on the antidiuretic effect of cyclophosphamide-vasopressin release and sodium excretion. Med Pediatr Oncol 1980;8:295–303.
15. Slavin RE, Millan JC, Mullins G.M. Pathology of high dose intermittent cyclophosphamide therapy. Hum Pathol 1975;6:693–709.
16. Antman KH, Elias A, Ryan L. Ifosfamide and mesna: response and toxicity at standard and high dose schedules. Semin Oncol 1990;17:68–73.
17. Loehrer PJ Sr, Lauer R, Roth BJ, et al. Salvage therapy in recurrent germ cell cancer: ifosfamide and cisplatin plus either vinblastine or etoposide. Ann Intern Med 1988;109:540–6.
18. Pratt CB, Douglass EC, Etcubanas E, et al. Clinical studies of ifosfamide at St. Jude Children's Research Hospital, 1983–1988. Semin Oncol 1989;16 Suppl 3:51–5.
19. Boddy AV, Cole M, Pearson ADJ, Idle JR. The kinetics of the auto-induction of ifosfamide metabolism during continuous infusion. Cancer Chemother Pharmacol 1995;36:53–60.
20. Costa G, Engle RL Jr, Schilling A, et al. Melphelan and prednisone: an effective combination for the treatment of multiple myeloma. Am J Med 1973;54:589.
21. Frick JC 2nd, Tretter P, Tretter W, Hyman GA. Disseminated carcinoma of the ovary treated with L-phenylalanine mustard. Cancer 1968;21:508–13.
22. Young RC, Walton LA, Ellenberg SS, et al. Adjuvant therapy in stage I and stage II epithelial ovarian cancer. Results of two prospective randomized trials. N Engl J Med 1990;322:1021–7.
23. Fisher B, Sherman B, Rockette H, et al. L-Phenylalanine mustard (L-PAM) in the management of premenopausal patients with primary breast cancer: lack of association of disease-free survival with depression of ovarian function. Cancer 1979;44:847–57.
24. Begleiter A., Lam H-YP, Grover J, et al. Evidence for active transport of melphelan by two amino acid carriers in L5178Y lymphoblasts in vitro. Cancer Res 1979;39:353–9.
25. Greig NH, Momma S, Sweeney DJ, et al. Facilitated transport of melphelan at the rat blood-brain barrier by the large neutral amino acid carrier system. Cancer Res 1987;47:1571–6.
26. The French Cooperative Group on Chronic Lymphocytic Leukemia. A randomized clinical trial of chlorambucil versus COP in chronic lymphocytic leukemia. Blood 1990;75:1422–5.
27. Wiltshaw E. Chlorambucil in the treatment of primary adenocarcinoma of the ovary. J Obstet Bynecol Br Commonw 1964;72:586–94.
28. Portlock CS, Fischer DS, Cadman E, et al. High-dose pulse chlorambucil in advanced, low-grade non-Hodgkin's lymphoma. Cancer Treat Rep 1987;71:1029–31.
29. Goncalves A., Brand AC, Viret F, et al. High dose alkylating agents with autologous hematopoietic stem cell support and trastuzumab in ERB-B2 overexpressing metastatic breast cancer: a feasibility study. Anticancer Res 2005;25:663–7.
30. De Jonge ME, Mathot RA, Van Dam SM, et al. Extremely high exposures to thiotepa in an obese patient receiving high-dose cyclophosphamide, thiotepa and carboplatin. Cancer Chemother Pharmacol 2002;50:251–5.
31. Gutin PH, Levi JA, Wiernik PH, Walker MD. Treatment of malignant meningeal disease with intrathecal thioTEPA: a phase II study. Cancer Treat Rep 1977;61:885–7.
32. Ng SF, Waxman DJ. N,N',N''-triethylenethiophosphoramide (thio-TEPA) oxygenation by constitutive hepatic P-450 enzymes and modulation of drug metabolism and clearance in vivo by P450-inducing agents. Cancer Res 1991;51:2340–5.
33. Lyss AP, Luedke SL, Einhorn L, et al. Vindesine and mitomycin C in metastatic breast cancer. A Southeastern Cancer Study Group Trial. Oncology1989;46:357–9.
34. Wils J, Bleiberg H. Current status of chemotherapy for gastric cancer. Eur J Cancer Clin Oncol 1989;25:3–8.
35. Haffty BG, Wilson LD, Son YH, et al. Concurrent chemoradiotherapy with mitomycin C compared with porfiromycin in squamous cell cancer of the head and neck: final results of a randomized clinical trial. Int J Radiat Oncol Biol Phys 2005;61:119–28
36. Dorr RT, Bowden GT, Alberts DS, Liddil JD. Interactions of mitomycin C with mammalian DNA detected by alkaline elution. Cancer Res 1985;45:3510–6.
37. Borowy-Borowski H, Lipman R, Chowdary D, Tomasz M. Recognition between mitomycin C and specific DNA sequences for crosslink formation. Biochemistry 1990;29:2999–3006.

38. Sellei C, Ecklardt S, Horvath IP, et al. Clinical and pharmacologic experience with dibromo-dulcitol (NSC-104800), a new antitumor agent. Cancer Chemother Rep 1969;53:377–84.
39. Haddow A, Timmis GM. Myleran in chronic myeloid leukemia-chemical constitution and biological action. Lancet 1953;1:207–8.
40. Schiffer CA. STI-571: current status and future prospects. Curr Opin Investig Drugs 2001;2:1279–81.
41. Elson LA. Hematological effects of the alkylating agents. Ann N Y Acad Sci 1958;68:826–33.
42. Fried W, Kede A, Barone J. Effects of cyclophosphamide and busulfan on spleen colony-forming units and on hematopoietic stroma. Cancer Res 1977;37:1205–9.
43. Pacheco DY, Stratton NK, Gibson NW. Comparison of the mechanism of action of busulfan with hepsulfam, a new antileukemic agent, in the L1210 cell line. Cancer Res 1989;49:5108–10.
44. Santos GW, Tutschka PJ, Brookmeyer R, et al. Marrow transplantation for acute non-lymphocytic leukemia after treatment with busulfan and cyclophosphamide. N Engl J Med 1983;309:1347–78
45. Grochow LB, Jones RJ, Brundrett RB, et al. Pharmacokinetics of busulfan: correlation with veno-occlusive disease in patients undergoing bone marrow transplantation. Cancer Chemother Pharmacol 1989;25:55–61.
46. Hyde KA, Acton E, Skinner WA, et al. Potential anticancer agents-LX11. The relationship of chemical structure to antileukemia activity with analogues of 1-methyl-3-nitrosoguanidine. J Med Pharm Chem 1962;5:1
47. Schabel FM Jr, Johnston TP, McCaleb GS, et al. Experimental evaluation of potential antitumor agents: VIII. Effects of certain nitrosoureas on cerebral L1210 leukemia. Cancer Res 1963;23:226.
48. DeVita VT, Carbone PP, Owens AH Jr, et al. Clinical trials with 1,3-bis (2-chlorethyl)-1-nitrosourea, NSC-409962 (BCNU). Cancer Res 1965;25:1876.
49. Colvin M, Brundrett RB, Cowens W, et al. A chemical basis for the antitumor activity of chloroethylnitrosoureas. Biochem Pharmacol 1976;25:695–9.
50. Kohn KW. Interstrand cross-linking of DNA by 1,3-bis(2-chloroethyl)-1-nitrosourea and other 1-,3-bis(2-chloroethyl)-1-nitrosourea and other 1-(2-haloethyl)-1-nirrosoureas. Cancer Res 1977;37:1450.
51. Ludlum DB, Kramer BS, Wang J, Fenselau C. Reaction of 1,3-bis(2-chloroethyl)-1-nitrosourea with synthetic polynucleotides. Biochemistry 1975;14:5480–5.
52. Walker MD, Alexander E Jr, Hunt WE, et al. Evaluation of BCNU and/or radiotherapy in the treatment of anaplastic gliomas. A cooperative clinical trial. J Neurosurg 1978;49:333–43.
53. Presant CA, Klahr C. Adriamycin, 1,3-bis-(2-chloroethyl)-1-nitrosourea, cyclophosphamide, plus prednisone in melphelan resistant multiple myeloma. Cancer 1978;42;1222–7.
54. Peters WP, Rosner GL, Vredenburgh JJ, et al. Prospective, randomized comparison of high-dose chemotherapy with stem-cell support versus intermediate-dose chemotherapy after surgery and adjuvant chemotherapy in women with high-risk primary breast cancer: a report of CALGB 9082, SWOG 9114, and NCIC MA-13. J Clin Oncol 2005;23:2191–200.
55. Guerin C, Olivi A, Weingart JD, et al. Recent advances in brain tumor therapy: local intracerebral drug delivery by polymers. Invest New Drugs 2004;22:27–37.
56. Krouwer D, McDermott M, Prados M. Postoperative radiotherapy and radiotherapy combined with CCNU chemotherapy for treatment of brain gliomas. J Neurooncol 1990;8:189–91.
57. Clark JL, Barcewicz P, Nava HR, et al. Adjuvant 5-FU and MeCCNU improves survival following curative gastrectomy for adenocarcinoma. Am Surg 1990;56:423–7.
58. Levin VA, Chamberlain M, Silver P, et al. Phase I/II study of intraventricular and intrathecal ACNU for leptomeningeal neoplasia. Cancer Chemother Pharmacol 1989;23:301–7.
59. Roosen N, Kiwit JC, Lins E, et al. Adjuvant intraarterial chemotherapy with nimustine in the management of World Health Organization grade IV gliomas of the brain. Experience at the Department of Neurosurgery of Dusseldorf University. Cancer 1989;64:1984–94.
60. Aurback SD. Nonclassic alkylating agents. In: Chabner BA, Collins JM, editors. Cancer chemotherapy: principles and practice. Philadelphia: Lippincott; 1990. p. 314–28.
61. Erickson JM, Tweedie DJ, Ducore JM, Prough RA. Cytotoxicity and DNA damage caused by azoxy, metabolites of procarbazine in L1210 tumor cells. Cancer Res 1989;49:127–33.
62. Swaffar DS, Horstman MG, Jaw JY, et al. Methoxyprocarbazine, the active metabolite responsible for the anticancer activity of procarbazine against L1210 leukemia. Cancer Res 1989;49:2442–7.
63. Bonadonna G, Valgussa P, Santoro A, et al. Hodgkin's disease: the Milan Cancer Institute experience with MOPP and ABVD. Recent Results Cancer Res 1989;117:169–74.
64. DeVita VT Jr, Serpick AA, Carbone PP. Combination chemotherapy in the treatment of advanced Hodgkin's disease. Ann Intern Med 1970;73:881–95.
65. Flaherty LE, Redman BG, Chabot GG, et al. A phase I-II study of dacarbazine in combination with outpatient interleukin-2 in metastatic malignant melanoma. Cancer 1990;65:2471–7.
66. Auerbach SD. Nonclassic alkylating agents. In: Chabner BA, Collins JM, editors. Cancer chemotherapy: principles and practice. Philadelphia: Lippincott; 1990. p. 314–28.
67. Denny BJ, Wheelhouse RT, Stevens MF, et al. NMR and molecular modeling investigation of the mechanism of activation of the antitumor drug temozolomide and its interaction with DNA. Biochemistry 1994;33:9045–51.
68. Denny BJ, Wheelhouse RT, Stevens MF, et al. NMR and molecular modeling investigation of the mechanism of activation of the antitumor drug temozolomide and its interaction with DNA. Biochemistry 1994;33:9045–51.
69. Newlands ES, Blackledge GR, Slack JA, et al. Phase I trial of temozolomide (CCRG 81045: M&B 39831: NSC 362856). Br J Cancer 1992;65:287–91.
70. Bower M, Newlands ES, Bleehen NM, et al. Multicentre CRC phase I trial of temozolomide in recurrent or progressive high-grade glioma. Cancer Chemother Pharmacol 1997;40:484–8.
71. Rutty CJ, Abel G. In vitro cytotoxicity of the methylmelamines. Cancer Chemother Pharmacol 1980;29:235–46.
72. Greco FA, Johnson DH, Hainsworth JD. A comparison of hexamethylmelamine (altretamine), cyclophosphamide, doxorubicin and cisplatin (H-CAP) vs. cyclophosphamide, doxorubicin, and cisplatin (CAP) in advanced ovarian cancer. Cancer Res 1991;18 Suppl A:47–55.
73. Biesele JJ, Philips FS, Thiersch JB, et al. Chromosome alteration and tumor inhibition by nitrogen mustards: the hypothesis of crosslinking alkylation. Nature 1950;166:1112–4.
74. Brookes P, Lawley PD. The reaction of mono- and difunctional alkylating agents with nucleic acids. Biochem J 1961;80:486.
75. Brookes P, Lawley PD. The action of alkylating agents on deoxyribonucleic in relation to biologic effects of the alkylating agents. Exp Cell Res 1963;24 Suppl 9:512–20.
76. Goldenberg GJ, Vanstone CL, Israels LG, et al. Evidence for a transport carrier of nitrogen mustard-sensitive and -resistant L5178Y lymphoblasts. Cancer Res 1970;30:2285–91.
77. Ciaccio PJ, Tew KD, LaCreta FP. The spontaneous and glutathione S-transferase mediated reaction of chlorambucil with glutathione. Cancer Commun 1990;2:279–85.
78. Sharma M, He QY, Tomasz M. Effects of glutathione on alkylation and cross-linking of DNA by mitomycin C. Isolation of a ternary glutathione-mitomycin-DNA adduct. Chem Res Toxicol 1994;7:401–7.
79. Hill DL, Kirk MC, Struck RF. Microsomal metabolism of nitrosoureas. Cancer Res 1975;35:296–301.
80. Levin VA, Stearns J., Byrd A, et al. The effect of phenobarbital on the antitumor activity of 1,3-bis(2-chloroethyl)-1-nitrosourea (BCNU), 1-(2-chloroethyl)-3-cyclohexyl-1-nitrosourea (CCNU) and 1-(2-chloroethyl)-3-(2,6-dioxo)-3-piperidyl-1-nitrosourea (PCNU), and on the plasma pharmacokinetics and biotransformation of BCNU. J Pharmacol Exp Ther 1979;208:1–6.
81. Alberts DS, Chang SY, Chen HS, et al. Pharmacokinetics and metabolism of chlorambucil in man: a preliminary report. Cancer Treat Rev 1979;6 Suppl:9–17.
82. Hilton J. Role of aldehyde dehydrogenase in cyclophosphamide-resistant L1210 leukemia. Cancer Res 1984;44:5156–60.
83. Ewig RA, Kohn KW. DNA damage and repair in mouse leukemia 1210 cells treated with nitrogen mustard, 1,3-bis(2-chloroethyl)-1-nitrosourea, and other nitrosoureas. Cancer Res 1977;37:2114–22.
84. Erickson LC, Laurent G, Sharkey NA, Kohn KW. DNA cross-linking and monoadduct repair in nitrosourea-treated human tumor cells. Nature 1980;288:727–9.
85. Parker S, Kirk MC, Ludlum DB. Synthesis and characterization of 0-6-(chloroethyl)guanine: a putative intermediate in the cytotoxic reaction of chloroethylnitrosoureas with DNA. Biochem Biohpys Res Commun 1987;148:1124–8.
86. Pegg AE. Mammalian O6-alkylguanine-DNA alkyltransferase: regulation and importance in response to alkylating carcinogenic and therapeutic agents. Cancer Res 1990;50:6119–29.
87. Ali-Osman F, Srivenugopal K, Berger MS, Stein DE. DNA interstrand crosslinking and strand break repair in human glioma cell lines of varying [1,3-bis(2-chlorethyl)-1-nitrosourea] resistance. Anticancer Res 1990;10:677–82.
88. Felker GM, Friedman HS, Dolan ME, et al. Treatment of subcutaneous and intracranial brain tumor xenografts with O6-benzylguanine and 1,3-bis(2-chloroethyl)-1-nitrosourea. Cancer Chemother Pharmacol 1993;32:471–6.
89. Schold SC Jr, Brent TP, von Hofe E, et al. O6-alkylguanine-DNA alkyltransferase and sensitivity to procarbazine in human brain-tumor xenografts. J Neurosurg 1989;70:573–7.
90. Martin F, Solary E. Tumor cell resistance to DNA-damaging agents: from apoptosis to noesis. Curr Med Chem – Anticancer Agents 2004;4:461–3.
91. Brent TP, Houghton PJ, Houghton JA. O6-alkylguanine-DNA transferase activity correlates with the therapeutic response of human rhabdomyosarcoma xenografts to 1-(2-chloroethyl)-3-(trans-4-methylcyclohexyl)-1-nitrosourea. Proc Natl Acad Sci U S A 1985;82:2985–9.
92. Kelley SL, Basu A, Teicher BA, et al. Overexpression of metallothionein confers resistance to anticancer drugs. Science 1988;241:1813–5.
93. Yu X, Wu Z, Fenselau C. Covalent sequestration of melphelan by metallothionein alkylation of cysteines. Biochemistry 1995;34:3377–85.
94. Wei D, Fabris D, Fenselau C. Covalent sequestration of phosphoramide mustard by metallo-thionein—an in vitro study. Drug Metab Dispos 1999;27:786–91.
95. Millard JT, Raucher S, Hopkins PB. Mechlorethamine crosslinks deoxyguanosine residues at 5′-GNC sequences in duplex DNA fragments. J Am Chem Soc 1990;112:2459–60.
96. Ojwang JD, Grueneberg DA, Loechler EL. Synthesis of a duplex oligonucleotide containing a nitrogen mustard interstrand DNA-DNA cross-link. Cancer Res 1989;49:6529–37.
97. Dong Q, Barsky D, Colvin ME, et al. A structural basis for a phosphoramide mustard-induced DNA interstrand crosslink at 5′-d(GAC). Proc Natl Acad Sci U S A 1995;92:12170–4.
98. Price CC, Gaucher GM, Koneru P, et al. Relative reactivities for monofunctional nitrogen mustard alkylation of nucleic acid components. Biochim Biophys Acta 1968;166:327–59.
99. Fischhaber Pl, Gall AS, Duncan JA, Hopkins PB. Direct demonstration in synthetic oligonucleotides that N,N′-bis(2-chloroethyl)nitrosourea cross-links N-1 of deoxyguanosine to N-3 of deoxycytidine on opposite strands of duplex DNA. Cancer Res 1999;59:4363–8.
100. Kohn KW, Steigbigel NH, Spears CL. Crosslinking and repair of DNA in sensitive and resistant strains of *E. coli* treated with nitrogen mustard. Proc Natl Acad Sci U S A 1965;53:1154–61.
101. Dong Q, Bullock N, Ali-Osman F, et al. Repair analysis of 4-hydroperoxycyclophosphamide-induced DNA interstrand cross-linking in the c-myc gene in 4-hydroperoxycyclophosphamide-sensitive and -resistant medulloblastoma cell lines. Cancer Chemother Pharmacol 1996;37:242–6.
102. Verly WG. Monofunctional alkylating agents and apurinic sites in DNA. Biochem Pharmacol 1974;23:3–8.
103. Verly WG, Paquette Y. An endonuclease for depurinated DNA in *Escherichia coli* B. Can J Biochem 1972;50:217–24.
104. Stevnsner T, Ding R, Smulson M, Bohr VA. Inhibition of gene-specific repair of alkylation damage in cells depleted of poly(ADP-ribose) polymerase. Nucleic Acids Res 1994;22:4620–4.
105. O'Connor PM, Ferris DK, White GA, et al. Relationships between cdc2 kinase, DNA cross-linking, and cell cycle perturbations induced by nitrogen mustards. Cell Growth Diff 1992;3:43–52.
106. Teicher BA, Herman TA, Holden SA, et al. Tumor resistance to alkylating agents conferred by mechanisms operative only in vivo. Science 1990;247:1457–61.
107. Green SK, Frankel A, Kerbel RS. Adhesion-dependent multicellular drug resistance. Anticancer Disc 1999;14:153–68.
108. Kobayashi H, Man S, Graham CH, et al. Acquired multicellular-mediated resistance to alkylating agents in cancer. Proc Natl Acad Sci U S A 1993;90:3294–8.
109. Kerbel RS, Kobayashi H, Graham CH. Intrinsic or acquired drug resistance and metastasis: are they linked phenotypes? J Cell Biochem 1994;56:37–47.
110. Jahde E, Glussenkamp KH, Rajewsky MF. Protection of cultured malignant cells from mito-xantrone cytotoxicity

by low extracellular pH: a possible mechanism for chemoresistance in vivo. Eur J Cancer 1990;26:101–6.
111. Egorin MJ, Forrest A, Belani CP, et al. A limited sampling strategy for cyclophosphamide pharmacokinetics. Cancer Res 1989;49:3129–33.
112. Jardine I, Fenselau C, Appler M, et al. Quantitation by gas chromatography-chemical ionization mass spectrometry of cyclophosphamide, phosphoramide mustard, and nornitrogen mustard in the plasma and urine of patients receiving cyclophosphamide therapy. Cancer Res 1978;38:408–15.
113. Struck RF, Alberts DS, Horne K, et al. Plasma pharmacokinetics of cyclophosphamide and its cytotoxic metabolites after intravenous versus oral administration in a randomized, crossover trial. Cancer Res 1987;47:2723–6.
114. Jao JY, Jusko WJ, Cohen JL. Phenobarbital effects on cyclophosphamide pharmacokinetics in man. Cancer Res 1972;32:2761–4.
115. Ehrlichman C, Soldins SJ, Hardy RW, et al. Disposition of cyclophosphamide on two consecutive cycles of treatment in patients with ovarian carcinoma. Arzneimittelforschung 1988;38:839–42.
116. D'Incalci M, Bolis G, Facchinetti T, et al. Decreased half-life of cyclophosphamide in patients under continual treatment. Eur J Cancer 1979;15:7–10.
117. Chen TL, Passos-Coelho JL, Noe DA, et al. Nonlinear pharmacokinetics of cyclophosphamide in patients with metastatic breast cancer receiving high-dose chemotherapy followed by autologous bone marrow transplantation. Cancer Res 1995;55:810–6.
118. Anderson LW, Ludeman SM, Colvin OM, et al. Quantitation of 4-hydroxycyclophosphamide/aldophosphamide in whole blood. J Chromatography B Biomed Appl 1995;667:247–57.
119. Chen TL, Kennedy MJ, Anderson LW, et al. Nonlinear pharmacokinetics of cyclophosphamide and 4-hydroxycyclophosphamide/aldophosphamide in patients with metastatic breast cancer receiving high-dose chemotherapy followed by autologous bone marrow transplantation. Drug Metab Dispos 1997;25:544–51.
120. Bakke JE, Feil VJ, Fjelstul CE, Thacker EJ. Metabolism of cyclophosphamide by sheep. J Agric Food Chem 1972;20:384–8.
121. Humphrey RL, Kvols LK. The influence of renal insufficiency on cyclophosphamide-induced hematopoietic depression and recovery. Proc Am Assoc Cancer Res 1974;15:84.
122. Brade WP, Herdrich K, Varini M. Ifosfamide pharmacology, safety, and therapeutic potential. Cancer Treat Rev 1985;12:1–47.
123. Nelson RL, Allen LM, Creaven PJ. Pharmacokinetics of divided-dose ifosfamide. Clin Pharmacol Ther 1976;19:365–70.
124. Norpoth K. Studies on the metabolism of isophosphamide (NSC-109724) in man. Cancer Treat Rep 1976;60:437–43.
125. Wadler T, Heydrich D, Jork T, et al. Comparative study on human pharmacokinetics of activated ifosfamide and cyclophosphamide by a modified fluorometric test. Cancer Res Clin Oncol 1981;100:95–104.
126. Brain EG, Yu LJ, Gustafsson K, et al. Plasma pharmacokinetics of P450 dependent ifosfamide pharmacokinetics: a better understanding of drug activation in vivo. Br J Cancer 1998;77:1768–76.
127. Ducharme MP, Bernstein MI, Granvil CP, et al. Phenytoin-induced alteration in the N-dechloro-ethylation of ifosfamide stereoisomers. Cancer Chemother Pharmacol 1997;40:531–3.
128. Granville CP, Madan A, Sharkawi M, et al. Role of CYP2B6 and CYP3A4 in the in vitro N-dechlorethylation of (R)- and (S)-ifosfamide in human liver microsomes. Drug Metab Dispos 1999;27:533–41.
129. Alberts DS, Chang SY, Chen HS, et al. Kinetics of intravenous melphelan. Clin Pharmacol Ther 1979;26:73–80.
130. Alberts DS, Chang SY, Chen HS, et al. Comparative pharmacokinetics of chlorambucil and melphelan in man. Recent Results Cancer Res 1980;74:124–31.
131. Kergueris MF, Milpied N, Moreau P, et al. Pharmacokinetics of high dose melphelan in adults: influence of renal function. Anticancer Res 1994;14:2379–82.
132. Pallante SL, Fenselau C, Mennel RG, et al. Quantitation by gas chromatography-chemical ionization-mass spectrometry of phenylalanine mustard in plasma of patients. Cancer Res 1980;40:2268–72.
133. Tattersall MH, Jarman M, Newlands ES, et al. Pharmacokinetics of melphelan following oral or intravenous administration in patients with malignant disease. Eur J Cancer 1978;14:507–13.
134. Reece PA, Kotasek D, Morris RG, et al. The effect of food on oral melphelan absorption. Cancer Chemother Pharmacol 1986;16:194–7.
135. Alberts DS, Chen HS, Benz D, Mason NL. Effect of renal dysfunction in dogs on the disposition and marrow toxicity of melphelan. Br J Cancer 1981;43:330–4.
136. Reece PA, Hill HS, Green RM, et al. Renal clearance and protein binding of melphelan in patients with cancer. Cancer Chemother Pharmacol 1988;22:348–52.
137. Alberts DS, Chang SY, Chen HS, et al. Pharmacokinetics and metabolism of chlorambucil in man: a preliminary report. Cancer Treat Rev 1979;6 Suppl:9–17.
138. Hartvig P, Simonsson B, Oberg G, et al. Inter- and intraindividual differences in oral chlorambucil. Eur J Clin Pharmacol 1988;35:551–4.
139. Cohen BE, Egorin MJ, Kohlhepp EA, et al. Human plasma pharmacokinetics and urinary excretion of thiotepa and its metabolites. Cancer Treat Rep 1986;70:859–64.
140. Henner WD, Shea TC, Furlong EA, et al. Pharmacokinetics of continuous-infusion high-dose thiotepa. Cancer Treat Rep 1987;71:1043–7.
141. Wadler S, Egorin MJ, Zuhowski EG, et al. Phase 1 clinical and pharmacokinetic study of thiotepa administered intraperitoneally in patients with advanced malignancies. J Clin Oncol 1989,7:132–9.
142. Strong JM, Collins JM, Lester C, Poplack DG. Pharmacokinetics of intraventricular and intravenous N,N',N" triethylenethiophosphoramide (thiotepa) in rhesus monkeys and humans. Cancer Res 1986;46(12 Pt 1):6101–4.
143. Henner WD, Peters WP, Eder JP, et al. Pharmacokinetics and immediate effects of high-dose carmustine in man. Cancer Treat Rep 1986;70:877–80.
144. Lee FY, Workman P, Roberts JT, Bleehen NM. Clinical pharmacokinetics of oral CCNU (lomustine). Cancer Chemother Pharmacol 1985;14:125–31.
145. Reyes ES, Talley RW, O'Bryan RM, Gastesi RA. Clinical evaluation of 1,3-bis-(2-chloroethyl)-1-nitrosourea (BCNU; NSC-409962) with fluoxymesterone (NSC-12165) in the treatment of solid tumors. Cancer Chemother Rep 1973;57:225–30.
146. Borison HL, Brand ED, Orland RK. Emetic action of nitrogen mustard (mechlorethamine hydrochloride) in dogs and cats. Am J Physiol 1958;192:410–6.
147. Fetting JH, McCarthy LE, Borison HL, Colvin M. Vomiting induced by cyclophosphamide and phosphoramide mustard in cats. Cancer Treat Rep 1982;66:1625–9.
148. Carden PA, Mitchell SL, Waters KD, et al. Prevention of cyclophosphamide/cytarabine-induced emesis with ondansetron in children with leukemia. J Clin Oncol 1990;8:1531–5.
149. Getz E, Sulkes A, Ochayon L, et al. Methylprednisolone versus metoclopramide as antiemetic treatment in patients receiving adjuvant cyclophosphamide, methotrexate, 5-fluorouracil (CMF) chemotherapy: a randomized crossover blind study. J Chemother 1989;1:365–8.
150. Jones RJ, Lee KS, Beschorner WE, et al. Venoocclusive disease of the liver following bone marrow transplantation. Transplantation 1987;44:778–83.
151. Spitz S. The histological effects of nitrogen mustards on human tumors and tissues. Cancer 1948;1:383.
152. Miller DG. Alkylating agents and human spermatogenesis. JAMA 1971;217:1662–5.
153. Sherins RJ, DeVita VT Jr. Effect of drug treatment for lymphoma on male reproductive capacity. Ann Intern Med 1973;79:216–20.
154. Blake DB, Heller RH, Hsu SH, Shacter BZ. Return of fertility in a patient with cyclophosphamide-induced azoospermia. Johns Hopkins Med J 1976;139:20–2.
155. Hinkes E, Plotkin D. Reversible drug-induced sterility in a patient with acute leukemia. JAMA 1973;223:1490–1.
156. Miller JJ 3rd, Williams GF, Leissring JC. Multiple late complications of therapy with cyclophosphamide, including ovarian destruction. Am J Med 1971;50:530–5.
157. Rose DP, Davis TE. Ovarian function in patients receiving adjuvant chemotherapy for breast cancer. Lancet 1977;1:1174–6.
158. Kyoma H, Wada T, Nishizawa T, et al. Cyclophosphamide-induced ovarian failure and its therapeutic significance in patients with breast cancer. Cancer 1977;39:1403–9.
159. Oliner H, Schwartz R, Rubio F Jr, Dameshek W. Interstitial pulmonary fibrosis following busulfan therapy. Am J Med 1961;31:134–9.
160. Patel AR, Shah PC, Rhee HL, et al. Cyclophosphamide therapy and interstitial pulmonary fibrosis. Cancer 1976;38:1542–9.
161. Bailey CC, Marsden HB, Jones PH. Fatal pulmonary fibrosis following 1,3-bis(2-chloroethyl)-1-nitrosourea (BCNU) therapy. Cancer 1978;42:74–6.
162. Holoye PY, Jenkins DE, Greenberg SD. Pulmonary toxicity in long-term administration of BCNU. Cancer Treat Rep 1976;60:1691–4.
163. Codling BW, Chakera TM. Pulmonary fibrosis following therapy with melphelan for multiple myeloma. J Clin Pathol 1972;25:668–73.
164. Todd NW, Peters WP, Ost AH, et al. Pulmonary drug toxicity in patients with primary breast cancer treated with high-dose combination chemotherapy and autologous bone marrow transplantation. Am Rev Resp Dis 1993;147:1264–70.
165. Forni AM, Koss LG, Geller W. Cytological study of the effect of cyclophosphamide on the epithelium of the urinary bladder in man. Cancer 1964;17:1348–55.
166. Cox PJ. Cyclophosphamide cystitis-identification of acrolein as the causative agent. Biochem Pharm Pharmacol 1979;28:2045–9.
167. Van Dyk JJ, Falkson HC, Van der Merwe AM, Falkson G. Unexpected toxicity in patients treated with iphosphamide. Cancer Res 1972;32:921–4.
168. DeFronzo RA, Braine HG, Colvin M, Davis PJ. Water intoxication in man after cyclophosphamide therapy. Time course and relation to drug activation. Ann Intern Med 1973;78:861–9.
169. Bode U, Seif SM, Levine AS. Studies on the antidiuretic effect of cyclophosphamide: vasopressin release and sodium excretion. Med Pediatr Oncol 1980;8:295–303.
170. Harlow PJ, DeClerck YA, Shore NA, et al. A fatal case of inappropriate ADH excretion induced by cyclophosphamide therapy. Cancer 1979;44:896–8.
171. Green TP, Mirkin BL. Prevention of cyclophosphamide-induced antidiuresis by furosemide infusion. Clin Pharmacol Ther 1981;29:634–42.
172. Harmon WE, Cohen HJ, Schneeberger EE, Grupe WE. Chronic renal failure in children treated with methyl CCNU. N Engl J Med 1979;300:1200–3.
173. Schacht RG, Baldwin DS. Chronic interstitial nephritis and renal failure due to nitrosourea (NU) therapy. Kidney Intl 1978;14:661.
174. Kashimura M, Kondo M, Abe T, et al. A case report of acute renal failure induced by melphelan in a patient with cancer. Gan To Kagaku Ryoho 1986;34:2010.
175. Bierman HR, Kelly KH, Knudson AG Jr, et al. The influence of 1,4-dimethylsulfonoxy-1,4-dimethylbutane in neoplastic disease. Ann NY Acad Sci 1958;68:1211–22.
176. Ganci L, Serrou B. Changes in hair pigmentation associated with cancer chemotherapy. Cancer Treat Rep 1980;64:193.
177. Feil VS, Lamoureaux CH. Alopecia activity of cyclophosphamide metabolites and related compounds in sheep. Cancer Res 1974;34:2596–8.
178. Cornwell GG 3rd, Pajak TF, McIntyre OR. Hypersensitivity reactions to IV melphelan during treatment of multiple myeloma: cancer and leukemia Group B experience. Cancer Treat Rep 1979;63:399–403.
179. Lakin JD, Cahill RA. Generalized urticaria to cyclophosphamide: type 1 hypersensitivity to an immunosuppressive agent. J Allergy Clin Immunol 1976;58(1 Pt 2):160–71.
180. Ross WE, Chabner BA. Allergic reaction to cyclophosphamide in a mechlorethamine-sensitive patient. Cancer Treat Rep 1977;61:495–6.
181. Karchmer RK, Hansen BL. Possible anaphylactic reaction to intravenous cyclophosphamide. JAMA 1977;237:475.
182. Kim HC, Kesarwala HH, Colvin M, Saidi P. Hypersensitivity reaction to a metabolite of cyclophosphamide. J Allergy Clin Immunol 1985;76:591–4.
183. Steinherz LJ, Steinherz PG. Cyclophosphamide cardiotoxicity. Cancer Bull 1985;37:231–4.
184. Steinberg SS, Philips FS, Scholler J. Pharmacological and pathological effects of alkylating agents. Ann N Y Acad Sci 1958;68:811–25.
185. Takvorian T, Parker LM, Hochberg FH, et al. Single high dose of BCNU with autologous bone marrow (ABM). Proc AACR Am Soc Clin Oncol 1980;21:341.
186. Yamada K, Bremer AM, West CR, et al. Intra-arterial BCNU therapy in the treatment of metastatic brain tumor from lung carcinoma. Cancer 1979;44:2000–7.
187. Vassal G, Deroussent A, Hartmann O, et al. Dose-dependent neurotoxicity of high-dose-busulfan in children: a clinical and pharmacological study. Cancer Res 1990;50:6203–7.
188. Murphy ML, Del Moro A, Lacon C. The comparative effects of five poly-functional alkylating agents on the rat fetus, with additional notes. Ann N Y Acad Sci 1958;68:762–81.
189. Hales BF. Effects of phosphoramide mustard and acrolein, cytotoxic metabolites of cyclophosphamide, on mouse limb development in vitro. Teratology 1989;40:11–20.
190. Little SA, Mirkes PE. DNA cross-linking and single-strand breaks induced by teratogenic concentrations of 4-hydro-

peroxycyclophosphamide and phosphoramide mustard in postimplantation rat embryos. Cancer Res 1987;47:5421–6.
191. Nicholson HO. Cytotoxic drugs in pregnancy. Review of reported cases. J Obstet Gynaecol Br Commonw 1968;75:307–12.
192. Ortega J. Multiple agent chemotherapy including bleomycin of non-Hodgkin's lymphoma during pregnancy. Cancer 1977;40:2829–35.
193. Hochberg MC, Shulman LE. Acute leukemia following cyclophosphamide therapy for Sjögren's syndrome. Johns Hopkins Med J 1978;142:211–4.
194. Kyle RA, Pierce RV, Bayrd ED. Multiple myeloma and acute myelomonocytic leukemia. N Engl J Med 1970;283:1121–5.
195. Dorr FA, Coltman CA Jr. Second cancers following antineoplastic therapy. Curr Probl Cancer 1985;9:1–43.
196. Hektoen L, Corper HJ. The effect of mustard gas (dichloroethyl-sulphide) on antibody formation. J Infect Dis 1920;28:279–85.
197. Makinodan T, Santos GW, Quinn RP. Immunosuppressive drugs. Pharmacol Rev 1970;22:189–247.
198. Barratt TM, Soothill JF. Controlled trial of cyclophosphamide in steroid-sensitive relapsing nephrotic syndrome of childhood. Lancet 1970;2:279–82.
199. Berd D, Mastrangelo MJ. Active immunotherapy of human melanoma exploiting the immunopotentiating effects of cyclophosphamide. Cancer Invest 1988;6:337–49.
200. Berd D, Mastrangelo MJ. Effect of low-dose cyclophosphamide on the immune system of cancer patients: depletion of CD4+, 2H4+ suppressor-inducer T-cells. Cancer Res 1988;48:1671–5.
201. Mitchell MS, Kempf RA, Harel W, et al. Effectiveness and tolerability of low-dose cyclophosphamide and low-dose intravenous interleukin-2 in disseminated melanoma. J Clin Oncol 1988;6:409–24.
202. Mullins GM, Anderson PN, Santos GW. High dose cyclophosphamide therapy in solid tumors. Cancer 1975;36:1950–8.
203. Rosenberg B, Van Camp L, Krigas T. Inhibition of cell division in *Escherichia coli* by electrolysis products from a platinum electrode. Nature 1965;698–9.
204. Rosenberg B, VanCamp L, Trosko JE, Mansour VH. Platinum compounds: a new class of potent antitumor agents. Nature 1969;222:385–6.
205. Higby DJ, Wallace HJ Jr, Albert DJ, Holland JF. Diamminedichloroplatinum: a phase I study showing responses in testicular and other tumors. Cancer 1974;33:1219–5.
206. Higby DJ, Wallace HJ Jr, Holland JF. *Cis*-diamminedichloroplatinum (NSC-119875): a phase I study. Cancer Chemother Rep 1973;57:459–63.
207. Lippman AJ, Helson C, Helson L, Krakoff IH. Clinical trials of *cis*-diamminedichloroplatinum (NSC-119875). Cancer Chemother Rep 1973;57:191–200.
208. Blatter EE, Vollano JE, Krishnan BS, Dabrowiak JC. Interaction of the antitumor agents *cis,cis,trans*-Pt(NH3)C12(OH)2 and *cis,cis,trans*-Pt IV[(CH3)2-CHNH2]2Cl2(OH)2 and their reduction products with PM2 DNA. Biochemistry 1984;23:4817–20.
209. Pendyala L, Cowens JW, Chheda GB, et al. Identification of *cis*-dichloro-bis-isopropylamine platinum (II) as a major metabolite of iproplatin in humans. Cancer Res 1988;48:3533–6.
210. Roberts JJ, Pera MF. DNA as a target for anticancer coordination compounds. In: Lippard SJ, editor. Platinum, gold, and other metal chemotherapeutic agents. Washington, DC: American Chemical Society; 1983. p. 3.
211. Zwelling LA, Anderson T, Kohn KW. DNA-protein and DNA interstrand cross-linking by *cis*- and *trans*-platinum (II) diamminedichloride in L1210 mouse leukemia cells and relation to cytotoxicity. Cancer Res 1979;39:365–9.
212. Plooy AC, van Dijk M, Berends F, Lohman PH. Formation and repair of DNA interstrand cross-links in relation to cytotoxicity and unscheduled DNA synthesis induced in control and mutant human cells treated with *cis*-diamminedichloroplatinum (II). Cancer Res 1985;45:4178–84.
213. Hromas RA, Andrews PA, Murphy MP, Burns CP. Glutathione depletion reverses cisplatin resistance in murine L1210 leukemia cells. Cancer Lett 1987;34:9–13.
214. Eastman A. Cross-linking of glutathione to DNA by cancer chemotherapeutic platinum coordination complexes. Chem Biol Interact 1987;61:241–8.
215. Andrews PA, Murphy MP, Howell SB. Metallothionein mediated cisplatin resistance in human ovarian carcinoma cells. Cancer Chemother Pharmacol 1987;19:149–54.
216. Himmelstein KJ, Patton TF, Belt RJ, et al. Clinical kinetics on intact cisplatin and some related species. Clin Pharmacol Ther 1981;29:658–64.
217. Belt RJ, Himmelstein KJ, Patton TF, et al. Pharmacokinetics of non–protein-bound platinum species following administration of *cis*-dichlorodiammineplatinum (II). Cancer Treat Rep 1979;63:1515–21.
218. Oguri S, Sakakibara T, Mase H, et al. Clinical pharmacokinetics of carboplatin. J Clin Pharmacol 1988;28:208–15.
219. Gottlieb JA, Drewinko B. Review of the current clinical status of platinum coordination complexes in cancer chemotherapy. Cancer Chemother Rep 1975;59:621–8.
220. Piel IJ, Perlia CP. Phase II study of *cis*-dichlorodiammineplatinum (II) (NSC-119875) in combination with cyclophosphamide (NSC-26271) in the treatment of human malignancies. Cancer Chemother Rep 1975;59:995–9.
221. Dentino M, Luft FC, Yum MN, et al. Long term effect of *cis*-diamminedichloride platinum (CDDP) on renal function and structure in man. Cancer 1978;41:1274–81.
222. Schilsky RL, Anderson T. Hypomagnesemia and renal magnesium wasting in patients receiving cisplatin. Ann Intern Med 1979;90:929–31.
223. Gonzales-Vitale JC, Hayes DM, Cvitkovic E, Sternberg SS. The renal pathology in clinical trials of *cis*-platinum (II) diamminedichloride. Cancer 1977;39:1362–71.
224. Madias NE, Harrington JT. Platinum nephrotoxicity. Am J Med 1978;65:307–14.
225. Chary KK, Higby DJ, Henderson ES, Swinerton KD. Phase I study of high-dose *cis*-dichlorodiammineplatinum (II) with forced diuresis. Cancer Treat Rep 1977;61:367–70.
226. Hayes DM, Cvitkovic E, Golbey RB, et al. High dose cis-platinum diammine dichloride: amelioration of renal toxicity by mannitol diuresis. Cancer 1977;39:1372–81.
227. Berry JM, Jacobs C, Sikic B, et al. Modification of cisplatin toxicity with diethyldithiocarbamate. J Clin Oncol 1990;8:1585–90.
228. Skinner R, Pearson AD, Amineddine HA, et al. Ototoxicity of cisplatinum in children and adolescents. Br J Cancer 1990;61:927–31.
229. Black FO, Myers EN, Schramm VL, et al. Cisplatin vestibular ototoxicity: preliminary report. Laryngoscope 1982;92:1363–8.
230. Wright CG, Schaefer SD. Inner ear histopathology in patients treated with *cis*-platinum. Laryngoscope 1982;92:1408–13.
231. Hadjilaskari P, Fengler R, Hartmann R, Henze G. [Ototoxicity of cisplatin in children with malignant diseases.] Klin Padiatr 1989;201:316–21.
232. Granowetter L, Rosenstock JG, Packer RJ. Enhanced *cis*-platinum neurotoxicity in pediatric patients with brain tumors. J Neurooncol 1983;1:293–7.
233. Kretschmar CS, Warren MP, Lavally BL, et al. Ototoxicity of preradiation cisplatin for children with central nervous system tumors. J Clin Oncol 1990;8:1:1191–8.
234. Von Hoff DD, Schilsky R, Reichert CM, et al. Toxic effects of *cis*-dichlorodiammineplatinum (II) in man. Cancer Treat Rep 1979;63:1527–31.
235. Bruck W, Heise E, Friede RL. Leukoencephalopathy after cisplatin therapy. Clin Neuropathol 1989;8:263–5.
236. Gerritsen van der Hoop R, Hamers FP, Neijt JP, et al. Protection against cisplatin-induced neurotoxicity by ORG 2766: histological and electrophysiological evidence. J Neurol Sci 1994;126:109–15.
237. Prestayko AW. Cisplatin and analogues: a new class of anticancer drugs. In: Crooke ST, Prestayko AW, editors. Cancer and chemotherapy. Vol. III, antineoplastic agents. New York: Academic Press; 1981. p. 133.
238. Gralla RJ, Itri LM, Pisko SE, et al. Antiemetic efficacy of high-dose metoclopramide: randomized trials with placebo and prochlorperazine in patients with chemotherapy-induced nausea and vomiting. N Engl J Med 1981;305:905–9.
239. Kahn T, Elias EG, Mason GR. A single dose of metoclopramide in the control of vomiting from *cis*-dichlorodiammineplatinum (II) in man. Cancer Treat Rep 1978;62:1106–7.
240. Reed E, Kohn KW. Platinum analogues. In: Chabner BA, Collins JM, editors. Cancer chemotherapy: principles and practice. Philadelphia: Lippincott; 1990. p. 475.
241. Venook A. Critical evaluation of current treatments in metastatic colorectal cancer. The Oncologist 2005; 250–61.
242. Rixe O, Ortuzar W, Alvarez M et al. Oxaliplatin, tetraplatin, cisplatin and carboplatin: spectrum of activity in drug-resistant cell lines of the National Cancer Institute's Anticancer Drug Screen panel. Biochem Pharmacol 1996; 52:1855–65.
243. Goldberg RM, Sargent DJ, Norton RF et al. A randomized controlled trial of fluorouracil plus leucovorin, irinotecan and oxaliplatin combinations in patients with previously untreated metastatic colorectal carcinoma. J Clin Oncol 2004; 22:23–30.
244. Cersosimo RJ. Oxaliplatin-associated neuropathy. Ann Pharmacotherapy 2005; 39:128–35.
245. Grothey A. Oxaliplatin safety profile: neurotoxicity. Semin Oncol 2003; 30(supplement 15): 5–13.
246. Raymond E, Faivre S, Chaney E et al. Cellular and molecular pharmacology of oxaliplatin. Mol Cancer Ther 2002; 1:227–35.
247. Chaney SG, Campbell SL, Bassett E, Wu Y. Recognition and processing of cisplatin- and oxaliplatin-DNA adducts. Crit Rev Oncol Hematol 2005; 53:3–11.

45

Drugs That Target DNA Topoisomerases

Eric H. Rubin, MD
William N. Hait, MD, PhD

The epipodophyllotoxins, deoxyribonucleic acid (DNA) intercalators, and camptothecins are considered together in this chapter because they share a common cellular target: DNA topoisomerases. Accordingly, mutations in topoisomerases can cause resistance to several drugs of unrelated structure. These drugs represent some of the most active agents in the treatment of a wide variety a cancers, and they share a similar spectrum of untoward side effects that limit their therapeutic index.

TOPOISOMERASE BIOLOGY

Double-stranded DNA can be too loosely wound (negatively supercoiled) or too tightly wound (positively supercoiled) relative to its lowest energy state. Protein complexes that track along DNA, such as transcription or replication complexes, produce alterations in DNA supercoiling that are regulated by ubiquitous topoisomerase enzymes.[1] The genomes of prokaryotes typically encode four topoisomerases. One of these enzymes, DNA gyrase, is the target of several antimicrobial agents, including the quinolone antibiotics.[2] The genomes of eukaryotes typically encode four or more topoisomerases, with the human genome currently known to contain five family members: topoisomerase I, topoisomerase IIα and IIβ, and topoisomerase IIIα and IIIβ.

Although the relative roles of these enzymes in mammalian DNA metabolism are not yet clear, loss of topoisomerase I, IIβ (and probably IIα), or IIIα is lethal, indicating that each enzyme serves an irreplaceable function.[3] Mice lacking topoisomerase IIIβ are viable, but have histologic lesions in multiple organs and a shortened lifespan.[4] Studies in both yeast and mammalian cells show that topoisomerase I is found in transcription and replication complexes, suggesting that topoisomerase I commonly provides the "DNA swivel" required for DNA tracking by ribonucleic acid (RNA) and DNA polymerases.[5,6]

By contrast, topoisomerase II enzymes seem to function predominantly after replication, during separation of daughter DNA strands or remodeling of chromatin structure.[7–10] Distinct roles for the IIα and IIβ isoforms of topoisomerase II are not yet known, although these enzymes differ in nuclear localization[11] and cell-cycle regulation.[12]

Less is known regarding the role of topoisomerase III isozymes in mammalian cells. However, in yeast, topoisomerase III associates with Sgs1,[13] a protein homologous to the Bloom and Werner's syndrome proteins, which are helicases involved in genomic stability and aging, respectively.[14,15] In addition, loss of the murine topoisomerase IIIβ enzyme results in aneuploidy in sperm and loss of fertility.[16]

Topoisomerases are also distinguishable biochemically. For example, topoisomerase I and III are classified as type I enzymes because they alter DNA supercoiling by cleaving a single strand of the DNA duplex. The topoisomerase II enzymes are classified as type II enzymes and cleave both strands. Detailed structural and biochemical data have clarified the mechanisms by which these enzymes accomplish the seemingly treacherous task of breaking and then resealing DNA. In type I and II enzymes alike, a hydroxyl group in a tyrosine residue is used in a transesterification reaction involving the DNA phosphate backbone. The result is the formation of a transient reaction intermediate involving the covalent linkage of the protein to the DNA backbone. The topoisomerase–DNA link can be at the 3' end of the DNA break (topoisomerase I), or at the 5' end of the break (topoisomerase II). Based on data obtained from structural analyses of topoisomerase I–DNA complexes, a model of the cleavage of DNA by the enzyme has been proposed (Figure 45-1).[17] In the covalent topoisomerase I–DNA complex, the 5' end of the nick is not bound tightly by the enzyme, with rotation of the nicked strand around the noncleaved strand resulting in alterations in DNA supercoiling.[17]

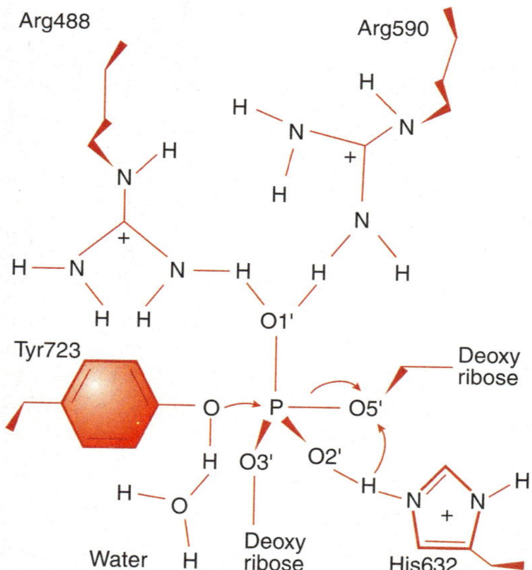

Figure 45-1 Model of DNA strand cleavage by topoisomerase I. Formation of the covalent bond involving tyrosine 723 is shown, as are other active site amino acids believed to function in the cleavage process. Reproduced with permission from Stewart L et al.[17]

In contrast to type I enzymes, type II enzymes function as homo- or heterodimers (eg, IIα:IIβ) and require adenosine triphosphate (ATP) for catalysis. Type II enzyme catalysis involves binding of one DNA duplex by the dimer, followed by formation of an ATP-dependent clamp around another DNA duplex (Figure 45-2).[18] Cleavage of the first duplex occurs in conjunction with, or after formation of, the clamp. Passage of the second duplex through the gap in the first duplex alters DNA topology. The clamp mechanism minimizes the risk of improper resealing of the transient double-strand break made by the enzyme.[18]

HOW DRUGS "POISON" TOPOISOMERASES

Many organisms synthesize compounds that convert topoisomerases into DNA-damaging agents, thereby exploiting the toxic effects inherent in a reaction that requires breaking and resealing DNA. Currently, topoisomerase I and topoisomerase IIα and IIβ are known to be targets of naturally occurring plant alkaloids and yeast fermentation products. Similar targeting of topoisomerase III is likely but not yet proven.[19]

Elegant studies performed in the genetically tractable organism *Saccharomyces cerevisiae* indicate that topoisomerase-targeting compounds kill cells not simply by inhibiting topoisomerase catalysis, but by stabilizing the normally transient reaction intermediate in which the enzyme is covalently linked to DNA.[20] Thus, these compounds are often called topoisomerase "poisons"[21] and either increase the rate of DNA cleavage or decrease the rate of DNA religation by the topoisomerase. Topoisomerase poisons are believed to bind to DNA, the topoisomerase, or both molecules concurrently at or near the region of the enzyme involved in the formation of the DNA–protein covalent linkage.

Many topoisomerase poisons, such as the anthracyclines and actinomycin D, are relatively planar hydrophobic compounds that bind to DNA with high affinity by intercalation, which involves stacking of the compound between adjacent base pairs. Nonintercalating DNA binders can also poison topoisomerases, exemplified by the effects of the DNA minor-groove

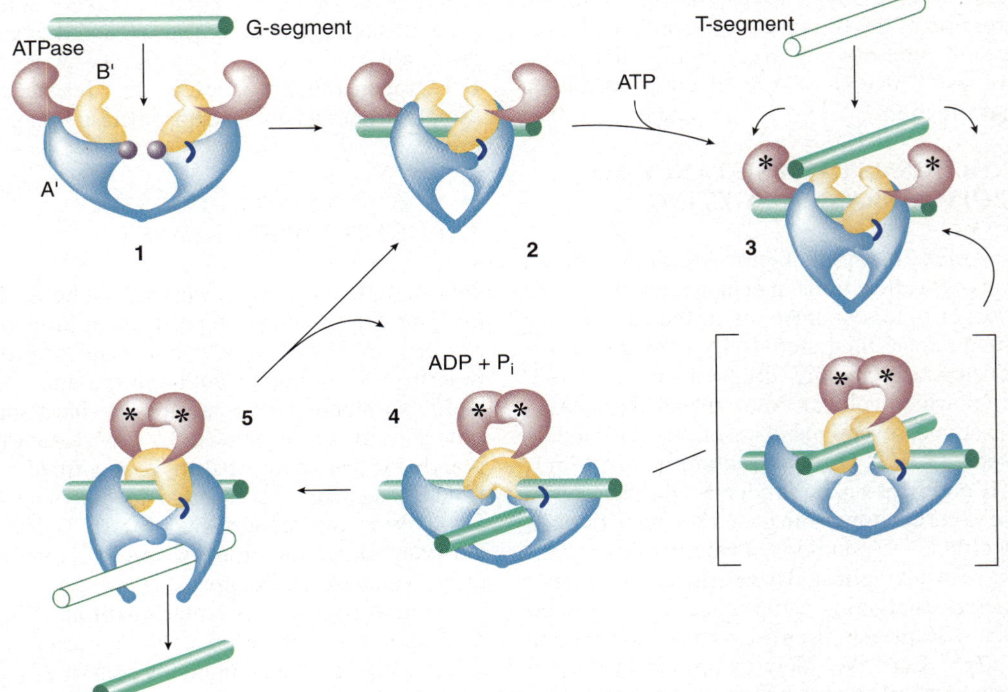

Figure 45-2 Model of topoisomerase II catalysis. The DNA duplex that undergoes cleavage is called the G-segment (for "gate") and the other DNA duplex is called the T-segment (for "transported"). Binding of the G-segment (step 1) results in a conformational change (step 2) in which the active-site tyrosines (shown as purple circles) are brought into position for cleavage of the G-segment. After binding of the T-segment and adenosine triphosphate (ATP), a "clamp" is formed around the T-segment (step 3), which is then transported though the gap in the G-segment (step 4). Subsequently, the G-strand is religated and the T-segment is released (step 5). After ATP hydrolysis, the "clamp" is opened, and the cycle can repeat. Modified from Berger JM et al.[18]

ligand Hoechst 33358 on topoisomerase I.[22] However, DNA binding is neither necessary nor sufficient for topoisomerase poisoning. For example, neither camptothecin nor etoposide bind DNA stably, yet both are potent topoisomerase I and II poisons, respectively.

A crystal structure of a drug–topoisomerase I–DNA complex is now available[23] and provides great insight into the mechanism of topoisomerase poisoning by anticancer drugs. In this complex, the drug mimics a DNA base pair and stacks into the DNA duplex at the topoisomerase I cleavage site (Figure 45-3). The stacking prevents religation of the DNA by the enzyme.

Molecular models of topoisomerase II–DNA–drug ternary complexes are not yet available. Nevertheless, the structures of fragments of DNA gyrase and of the *Saccharomyces cerevisiae* topoisomerase II are known, permitting structural mapping of residues implicated in catalysis or drug interactions.[18,24]

Despite the structural differences of topoisomerase II poisons such as doxorubicin and etoposide (see below), several mutations that confer resistance to both drugs map to the adenosine triphosphatase (ATPase) domain of topoisomerase II. Because the ATPase domain is important in the formation of a topoisomerase II–DNA covalent complex, these data suggest that impairment of DNA cleavage activity by the enzyme may confer resistance to drugs that, although structurally distinct, act by a common mechanism of trapping the covalent topoisomerase II–DNA complex.[25]

A novel mechanism of poisoning topoisomerase II was recently identified for bisdioxopiperazines, such as ICRF-187.[26] Rather than stabilizing the enzyme–DNA covalent bond, these compounds bind to a region of the enzyme that, in the presence of ATP, forms a circular clamp around DNA. By inhibiting the ATPase activity of the enzyme, these compounds prevent the topoisomerase II clamp from opening, resulting in a unique cytotoxic lesion in DNA.[27]

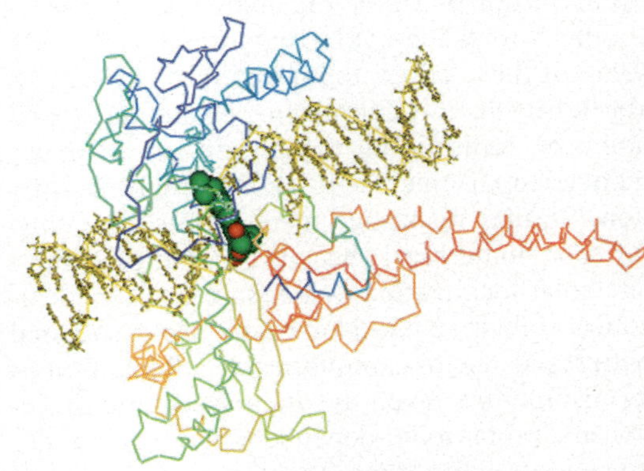

Figure 45-3 Structure of a topotecan–DNA–topoisomerase I covalent complex. The image was generated using iMol software (<http://www.pirx.com/iMol/>) and coordinates from Staker et al,[24] obtained from the Protein Data Bank (<http://www.rcsb.org/pdb/>). The DNA duplex is shown in yellow, with topoisomerase I shown in wire format. The drug molecule (topotecan) is in the center of the figure and is shown as green and red spheres.

Although this chapter focuses on drugs that target topoisomerases, several types of natural or induced DNA damage can also poison topoisomerase I or II. For example, abasic sites, which occur frequently in cells, lead to stabilization of both topoisomerase I and II covalent complexes.[28,29] Base mismatches or other DNA structural alterations, such as pyrimidine dimers or platinum adducts, can also poison topoisomerases.[30–32] Incorporation of nucleoside analogues such as cytosine arabinoside[33] and 2'-deoxy-2',2'-difluorocytidine (gemcitabine)[34] induces topoisomerase I-mediated DNA cleavage, suggesting that topoisomerase I may be involved in the anticancer activity of these drugs. Oxidative stress may also poison topoisomerase II, either through oxidative DNA damage or perhaps by directly modifying the enzyme.[35]

CELLULAR RESPONSE TO TOPOISOMERASE-MEDIATED DNA DAMAGE

The creation of drug-stabilized topoisomerase–DNA covalent complexes (ternary complexes) is not sufficient to kill cells. For example, treatment of cells with the DNA polymerase inhibitor aphidicolin protects cells from the cytotoxicity induced by brief exposure to either topoisomerase I or II poisons.[36] The effect is more pronounced for topoisomerase I poisons. Because topoisomerase I cleavage complexes involve single-strand breaks, whereas topoisomerase II cleavage complexes involve double-strand breaks, Hsiang and colleagues were led to propose a replication fork collision model for topoisomerase I poisons (Figure 45-4).[37] In that model, replication forks generate lethal double-strand breaks upon encountering drug–topoisomerase I–DNA ternary complexes. A similar phenomenon likely occurs upon collision of RNA polymerase II transcription complexes with topoisomerase I–DNA–drug ternary complexes.[38] This transcription-based effect may explain the finding that camptothecins may also kill non–S-phase cells.[39,40]

Certain DNA repair processes also determine the cytotoxic effects of topoisomerase poisons. Hypersensitivity to both topoisomerase I and II drugs occurs in cells in which repair of DNA double-strand breaks is defective.[41] Furthermore, cells lacking proteins involved in transcription-coupled DNA repair, such as in Cockayne's syndrome, are specifically hypersensitive to topoisomerase I poisons.[42] Loss of proteins involved in DNA damage checkpoints, such as the ataxia telangiectasia or Chk1 proteins, also confers hypersensitivity to topoisomerase I poisons.[43,44] In addition, Nash and colleagues identified a tyrosyl–DNA phosphodiesterase that can hydrolyze the tyrosine–DNA phosphodiester bonds that link topoisomerase I

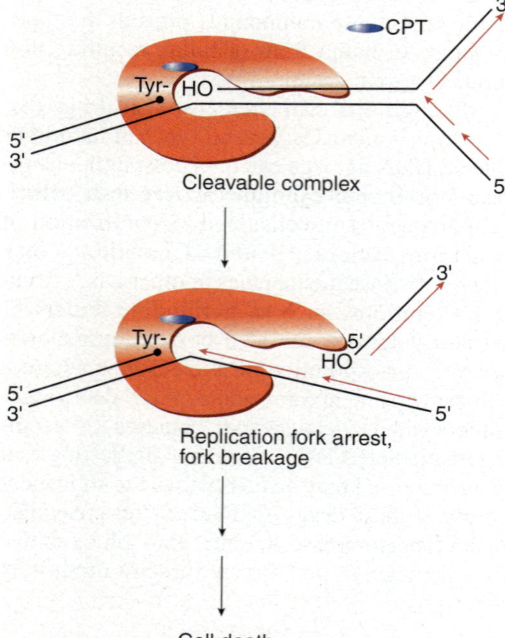

Figure 45-4 Generation of DNA double-strand breaks from collision of a replication fork with a camptothecin–DNA–topoisomerase I ternary complex. The covalent linkage of the active site tyrosine (Tyr) with the cleaved DNA strand is shown, as is the presence of a 5'-hydroxyl (HO) on the cleaved strand. Courtesy of Li TK and Liu LF.

molecules to DNA, suggesting that this phosphodiesterase is involved in the repair of topoisomerase-mediated DNA damage.[45] Indeed, overexpression of this protein was shown to reduce the DNA damage produced by treating cells with topoisomerase-targeting agents such as camptothecin or etoposide.[46] Topoisomerases are also modified in response to DNA damage. Those modifications include ubiquitination and conjugation to the small ubiquitin-like protein SUMO.[47–50] Ubiquitination of topoisomerases may lead to proteasome-mediated degradation, which by removing the target may limit the DNA damage produced by topoisomerase-targeting drugs.

In addition to causing cell death, topoisomerase-mediated DNA damage may, under certain circumstances, lead to neoplastic transformation. Epidemiologic studies link etoposide therapy to secondary leukemias,[51] and in vitro studies demonstrate that both topoisomerase I and II can mediate illegitimate recombination as a result of incorrect ligation of a DNA strand to an enzyme-linked DNA break.[52,53] Furthermore, the 11q23 chromosomal translocation involving the *mll* oncogene that occurs commonly in leukemias occurring secondary to chemotherapy and childhood leukemias contains a breakpoint sequence that is a preferred topoisomerase II cleavage site.[54] Thus, it is possible that topoisomerase II is involved in leukemogenesis. Topoisomerase I was also found to be involved in a chimeric fusion protein that includes the nucleoporin gene *NUP98,* created by a t(11;20)(p15;q11) translocation.[55] This translocation is associated with secondary myelodysplastic syndromes; forced expression of the fusion protein confers a leukemogenic phenotype,[56] suggesting that topoisomerase I may also be involved in neoplastic transformation.

MECHANISMS OF RESISTANCE TO TOPOISOMERASE TARGETING

Resistance to topoisomerase-targeting drugs can involve alterations in drug accumulation, in the target topoisomerase, or in the response to topoisomerase-mediated DNA damage. Many topoisomerase-targeting drugs are natural products for which cellular efflux mechanisms exist. For example, several members of the ATP-binding cassette (ABC) family—including the Mdr1, Mrp1, and Mrp2 gene products—produce resistance to certain topoisomerase II poisons through drug efflux.[57–59] Similarly, a variety of transporters have been implicated in resistance to the topoisomerase I-targeting camptothecins, most notably the ABC protein Bcrp (also known as Mxr and Abcg2).[60] Bcrp is widely expressed in normal human tissues, including the placenta, brain, small intestine, testis, ovary, colon, and liver.[61] Increased expression of Bcrp was recently implicated in resistance to induction therapy in children with acute myeloid leukemia.[62] Overexpression of Bcrp confers resistance to some, but not all, camptothecin analogs.[63]

Altered topoisomerases have been described in many drug-resistant cell lines. Those alterations include point mutations in a topoisomerase[64] and defects in topoisomerase phosphorylation—the latter having been implicated in the regulation of catalytic activity.[65,66] For both topoisomerase I and topoisomerase II, a single-point mutation can confer resistance to structurally distinct drugs. This phenomenon underscores the mechanistic similarity of topoisomerase-targeting drugs and is often called "atypical" multidrug resistance.[67]

Alteration of topoisomerase II localization by mutation or other mechanisms represents another resistance-conferring alteration.[68–72] In some of these cases, topoisomerase II localizes aberrantly in the cytoplasm, producing resistance by minimizing the possibility of drug-induced topoisomerase II–DNA complex formation. Similar resistance mechanisms may exist for topoisomerase I, because a change from a nucleolar localization to a diffuse nuclear localization of yeast topoisomerase I is associated with resistance to camptothecin.[73] Reduction of topoisomerase levels by increased ubiquitination and proteasome-dependent protein degradation has also been implicated as a drug-resistance mechanism.[48]

Resistance mechanisms that exist "downstream" from the formation of topoisomerase–DNA cleavage complexes also need to be considered. As discussed earlier, certain DNA repair enzymes may process topoisomerase-mediated DNA damage. Loss of proteins involved in the repair of DNA double-strand breaks results in hypersensitivity to topoisomerase I- and II-targeting drugs alike.[74] By contrast, overexpression of the DNA repair protein Xrcc1 confers resistance to camptothecins but not to topoisomerase II-targeting drugs.[75]

INTERCALATING DRUGS THAT TARGET TOPOISOMERASES

The Anthracyclines **History** The anthracyclines are fermentation products of *Streptomyces peucetius* var. *caesius* and were originally described as antitumor antibiotics. Daunomycin and doxorubicin were first shown to have antitumor activity in the 1960s.[76,77] Subsequently, a search for less-toxic derivatives identified additional drugs that have added to the repertoire available to the modern oncologist. Today, the anthracyclines constitute several of our most effective anticancer regimens.

Structure–Activity Relationships Figure 45-5 shows the structures of the clinically used anthracyclines. The compounds consist of a planar, hydrophobic tetracycline ring linked to a daunosamine sugar through a glycosidic linkage. All drugs are positively charged at physiologic pH, favoring intercalation into DNA. In addition, the anthracyclines possess quinone moieties on adjacent rings that allow them to participate in electron-transfer reactions and to generate oxygen free radicals.

Daunomycin and doxorubicin differ by only a single hydroxyl at position C14, yet have distinct spectra of antitumor activity. Idarubicin is a semisynthetic derivative of daunomycin (4-demethoxydaunorubicin) lacking the 4-methoxy group present on the parent compound. Epirubicin is an epimer of doxorubicin, having the C4' hydroxyl group on the amino sugar in the equatorial rather than the axial position, which increases lipophilicity as compared with doxorubicin. A liposome-encapsulated formulation of doxorubicin (Doxil) was approved for use in acquired immunodeficiency syndrome (AIDS)–related Kaposi's sarcoma. Despite differences in the pharmacokinetics of Doxil and doxorubicin (eg, Doxil has a lower volume of distribution and greater area under the curve [AUC]), major differences in activity have not been seen between Doxil and conventional formulations of doxorubicin.

Mechanism of Action The anthracyclines are highly reactive in solution and create a panoply of effects on biologic systems. Much of their cytotoxicity results from topoisomerase II poisoning (see above). Anthracyclines also intercalate into double-stranded DNA and produce structural changes that interfere with DNA and RNA synthesis. Before the effects of the anthracyclines on topoisomerase II were fully appreciated, it was their ability to participate in oxidation and reduction reactions that was believed to produce cytotoxicity. Anthracyclines generate reactive oxygen species—including oxygen free radicals, hydroxyl radicals, and hydrogen peroxide—

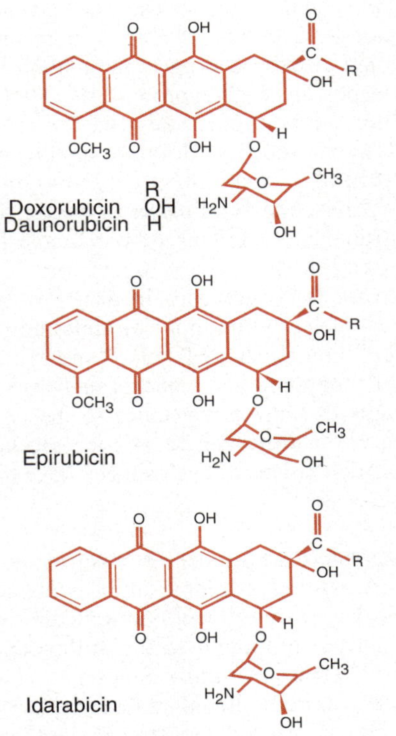

Figure 45-5 Structures of anthracyclines.

that damage DNA, messenger RNA (mRNA), proteins, and lipids. The peroxidation of lipids may account for much of the cardiac toxicity characteristic of these drugs.[78,79]

Clinical Pharmacology ***Dose and Administration*** Anthracyclines can be given at varying doses and schedules. Lower weekly doses or low-dose continuous infusions over 96 hours result in decreased toxicity without adverse effects on efficacy.[80] Lower doses produce lower peak plasma concentrations that are believed to correlate with decreased cardiac toxicity. In contrast, efficacy correlates best with AUC. Changing the dose and schedule from a higher-dose bolus to a lower-dose continuous infusion increases the incidence and severity of mucositis but decreases myelosuppression, nausea, and vomiting. Most clinicians reduce the dose of anthracyclines by 50% and 75% in patients having plasma bilirubin concentrations of 1.2 to 3.0 mg/dL and 3.1 to 5.0 mg/dL respectively.

As a single agent, doxorubicin (Adriamycin, Rubex) is given intravenously at a recommended dose of 40 to 75 mg/m^2. Care should be taken to avoid extravasation. Doxorubicin is indicated in the treatment of many solid tumors (eg, breast, sarcoma, bladder, thyroid, gastric, ovary, and small cell lung cancers) and in the treatment of Hodgkin's and non-Hodgkin's lymphoma, as well as in the treatment of acute lymphoblastic and myeloblastic leukemias. A liposomal formulation of doxorubicin (Doxil) is also available and was shown to be effective in the treatment of refractory ovarian cancer.[81] In this formulation, the liposomes are coated with polyethylene glycol to reduce clearance by the mononuclear phagocyte system. The liposomal formulation of doxorubicin may enhance accumulation of the drug at metastatic cancer sites as a result of alterations in tumor vasculature.[82]

Daunorubicin (Cerubidine) is given intravenously at a recommended dose of 30 to 60 mg/m^2 daily for 3 days. Care should be taken to avoid extravasation. Daunorubicin is indicated for the treatment of acute lymphocytic and myelogenous leukemias. It has limited activity against solid tumors and non-Hodgkin's lymphoma.

Idarubicin (Idamycin) is given intravenously at a recommended dose of 12 mg/m^2 daily for 3 days in combination with cytosine arabinoside for the treatment of acute myelogenous leukemia.

Epirubicin (Ellence) is given intravenously at a recommended dose of 100 to 120 mg/m^2 by bolus injection every 3 weeks. It is a vesicant and must be given with caution. A variety of other schedules have been evaluated, including an intravenous injection of 40 to 50 mg/m^2 on 2 consecutive days.[83]

Following intravenous administration, anthracyclines are rapidly cleared from the plasma, where they reach all tissues except the brain and testes. Approximately 75% of the drug remaining in the plasma is bound to plasma proteins.[84] Within tissues, the drugs are tightly bound to DNA. Tissue concentrations of anthracycline correlate with content of DNA and are 10- to 500-fold greater than concentrations in plasma.[85] Tumor concentrations of drug have rarely been measured. In one study, patients receiving a 96-hour infusion showed concentrations of up to 10 μmol/L in myeloma cells.[86]

Anthracyclines are metabolized in the liver and excreted in the bile. Less than 10% of an administered dose can be found in the urine, except in the case of epirubicin (see below). Reduction of the 13-keto group to the enol by aldoketoreductase produces active metabolites. Idarubicin is metabolized more rapidly than other anthracyclines. The resulting idarubicinol has activity similar to the parent compound. Because of the dependence on hepatic metabolism and clearance into the bile, dose reductions are recommended for patients with impaired hepatic function.

Epirubicin is conjugated with glucuronide on the 4' equatorial hydroxyl and excreted in the bile. Ten percent of an administered dose of epirubicin is found in the urine as epirubicinol and as conjugates of the glucuronide aglycone.[87] Its metabolism is decreased in the presence of liver metastases, with or without hepatic dysfunction.[88]

Anthracyclines are eliminated primarily by biliary excretion and to a lesser extent through the kidneys. Disappearance of anthracyclines from the plasma is multiphasic. A rapid initial phase of redistribution is followed by prolonged 0- and *y*-phase terminal elimination. The prolonged terminal phase accounts for most of the AUC and results in sustained therapeutic concentrations in the plasma following a bolus injection.[84]

Anthracyclines produce myelosuppression, mucositis, alopecia, nausea, vomiting, and increased skin pigmentation. Myelosuppression is the acute dose-limiting toxicity. After administration of a bolus dose, the white blood cell count begins to fall in 7 days. The count reaches a nadir at 10 to 14 days and recovers 1 to 2 weeks later. Thrombocytopenia and anemia are less severe. Dose- and schedule-related toxicities include mucositis, nausea and vomiting, diarrhea, and alopecia. Erythema at the injection site ("flare reaction") is benign, in contrast to extravasation, which can lead to serious local complications such as severe necrosis of surrounding tissues. Inflammation at sites of previous radiation ("radiation recall") can lead to unanticipated complications, including pericarditis, pleural effusion, and skin rash. The incidence of nausea and vomiting, alopecia, and cardiac toxicity is less with epirubicin than with doxorubicin. Cardiac effects occur at higher doses, and congestive heart failure has been reported less frequently. Cardiac toxicity, manifested by arrhythmias, tachycardia, and congestive heart failure, is described in detail below.

Activity The anthracyclines are indicated for use against both solid and hematologic malignancies. Doxorubicin has the broadest spectrum of activity. Its introduction in the 1960s and its incorporation into combination regimens led to curative treatments for non-Hodgkin's lymphoma (cyclophosphamide, hydroxydaunomycin [doxorubicin], Oncovin [vincristine], and prednisone: CHOP) and less-toxic treatments for Hodgkin's disease (Adriamycin, bleomycin, vinblastine, dacarbazine: ABVD). Doxorubicin is also active against Ewing's, osteogenic, and other soft-tissue sarcomas.

Doxorubicin is one of the most active agents in the treatment of breast cancer. Single-agent activity is similar to that of paclitaxel[70] and is comparable with combination chemotherapy in patients with metastatic disease. Also, in the adjuvant setting, doxorubicin-containing regimens are more active than are non–anthracycline-containing regimens.[89–91] Doxorubicin has limited but demonstrable activity against thyroid cancer, ovarian cancer, and small cell lung cancer. Finally, it has also demonstrated activity against endometrial carcinoma; cancer of the testis, prostate, cervix, and head and neck; and multiple myeloma.

Daunomycin is used mostly for the treatment of acute lymphocytic and myelocytic leukemias. Although it has some activity against pediatric solid tumors, it has little activity against adult solid malignancies. Idarubicin is used predominantly in the treatment of adult acute myelogenous leukemia.

Epirubicin has broad-spectrum antitumor activity in preclinical models. In the clinic, it has activity against melanoma; breast, colorectal, renal, gastric, pancreatic, hepatocellular, ovarian, and lung cancers; and soft-tissue sarcomas. In addition, it is part of active regimens against

Hodgkin's disease and non-Hodgkin's lymphoma.[92] Epirubicin is indicated in the adjuvant treatment of breast cancer, where it has activity similar to that of doxorubicin.[93]

Cardiac Toxicity All anthracyclines produce cardiac damage that can result in serious and even life-threatening complications.[94] Cardiac toxicity is more common with doxorubicin and daunorubicin than with epirubicin or idarubicin. Acutely, anthracyclines can produce arrhythmias and ST-T wave changes that are usually not serious and that resolve spontaneously. In rare cases, a syndrome resembling acute pericarditis myocarditis can occur. The syndrome is characterized by a fall in cardiac ejection fraction, conduction abnormalities, pericardial effusion, and congestive heart failure.

Congestive heart failure from congestive cardiomyopathy is more common and of greater clinical significance than are the acute cardiac effects. Mortality rates of more than 30% have been reported.[95,96] The anthracyclines produce myocardial damage by several mechanisms. Perhaps the most important is generation of reactive oxygen species during electron transfer from the semiquinone to quinone moieties of the molecule. The generation of hydrogen peroxide and the peroxidation of myocardial lipids contribute to myocardial damage. The heart may be uniquely susceptible to cardiac damage from oxidation reactions. For example, the low activity of catalase in cardiac tissue renders the myocardium dependent on glutathione peroxidase for detoxification of hydrogen peroxide. Anthracyclines deplete glutathione, thereby leaving the heart vulnerable to oxidative attack.

The incidence of cardiomyopathy is related to both cumulative dose and schedule of administration. Cardiac toxicity is best correlated with peak plasma concentration of the parent drug rather than with the AUC. Greater cumulative doses of doxorubicin can be given to patients receiving low-dose continuous infusions than to those receiving higher-dose bolus injections every 3 to 4 weeks. Predisposition to cardiac damage includes a previous history of heart disease, hypertension, radiation to the mediastinum, age younger than 4 years, and prior use of anthracyclines or other cardiac toxins.[96] Recently, the addition of trastuzumab (Herceptin) to either epirubicin or doxorubicin produced an unexpected increase in congestive heart failure at cumulative anthracycline doses below those anticipated to produce cardiac damage.[97]

Table 45-1 lists the incidence of clinically detectable congestive heart failure when doxorubicin is given at doses of 40 to 75 mg/m^2 as a bolus injection every 3 to 4 weeks. When doxorubicin is given by a low-dose weekly regimen (10 to 20 mg/m^2/wk) or by slow continuous infusion over 96 hours, cumulative doses of more than 500 mg/m^2 can be given. However, careful monitoring of cardiac function is still required and should increase in frequency at higher cumulative doses.[77,80] Doses of daunorubicin below 1,000 mg/m^2 (equivalent to 550 mg/m^2 doxorubicin) are considered safe. Doses of idarubicin below 290 mg/m^2 do not produce clinical congestive heart failure despite changes in cardiac ejection.[98] Epirubicin appears to be as active as doxorubicin and has less cardiac toxicity.[99]

Table 45-1 Incidence of Clinically Detectable Congestive Heart Failure as a Function of Cumulative Doxorubicin Dose

Cumulative Dose (mg/m^2)	Incidence of Congestive Heart Failure (%)
< 350	< 1
550	7
600	15
700	30

Cardiac function can be monitored during treatment with anthracyclines by electrocardiography, echocardiography, or radionuclide scans.[100] Numerous studies demonstrate the danger of embarking on anthracycline therapy in patients with underlying cardiac disease (eg, a baseline left ventricular ejection fraction of less than 50%) and of continuing therapy after a documented decrease in ejection fraction by more than 10% (if this decrease falls below the lower limit of normal) or by 20% regardless of the absolute value.

Certain drugs may abrogate the damaging effects of anthracyclines on the heart. For example, dexrazoxane (ADR-529) is a metal chelator that decreases the myocardial toxicity of doxorubicin in breast cancer patients and has recently been approved for that use by the US Food and Drug Administration (FDA).[101] Dexrazoxane chelates iron and copper, thereby interfering with the redox reactions that generate free radicals and damage myocardial lipids. Similar protective effects have been suggested for amifostine, an organic thiophosphate that is dephosphorylated to form a reactive thiol (*N*-2-mercaptoethyl-1,3,-diaminopropane), a free-radical scavenger. However, insufficient clinical data are available to recommend amifostine for cardioprotection.[101]

The cardiac toxicity of liposomal doxorubicin appears to be less than that of the free compound. For example, in a phase III trial, cardiac toxicity from doxorubicin appeared at a cumulative dose of about 500 mg/m^2, whereas doses of up to 600 mg/m^2 of the liposomal compound were not associated with a significant change in left ventricular ejection fraction.[102] This finding is consistent with retrospective analyses in which median cumulative doses of liposomal doxorubicin ranging from 465 mg/m^2 to 1,700 mg/m^2 were not found to produce significant cardiac toxicity and confirms an earlier phase II trial.[103]

Mechanisms of Resistance The general mechanisms of resistance to topoisomerase poisoning are covered above. The resistance of cancer cells to anthracyclines has received enormous attention.[104] Several plausible mechanisms exist, including decreased drug accumulation because of transport by P-glycoprotein, the *MDR1* gene product, and Mrp-1, the *ABCC1* (formerly *MRP1*) gene product. Both are members of the ATP-binding cassette family that includes *CFTR*, the gene implicated in cystic fibrosis. Additional mechanisms of resistance include down-regulation of or mutations in topoisomerase II,[64] increases in drug-neutralizing species, such as glutathione or glutathione transferase,[105] mutations in *TP53*,[106] and overexpression of antiapoptotic molecules such as Bcl-2.[107] Attempts to reverse resistance to the anthracyclines with multidrug resistance modulators, such as derivatives of cyclosporin, have had limited success.[108]

The Anthracenediones **Mitoxantrone** ***History*** A search for anthracycline analogues with less cardiac toxicity identified mitoxantrone, the most active compound in the anthracenedione series.[109] The antitumor spectrum of mitoxantrone is more limited than that of doxorubicin. Early clinical trials demonstrated significant differences from the anthracyclines in terms of spectrum of activity and cardiac toxicity. Diminished cardiac toxicity is believed to be caused by the decreased ability of mitoxantrone to participate in the generation of oxygen free radicals. In addition, the potential for extravasation injury and nausea and vomiting is less.

Structure Anthracenediones differ from anthracyclines by the lack of the glycoside substituents present in the latter. Figure 45-6 shows the structure of mitoxantrone, an amino anthracenedione.

Mechanism of Action Mitoxantrone produces double-stranded DNA breaks by poisoning topoisomerase II.[110] Unlike the anthracyclines, mitoxantrone is less likely to participate in one-electron reduction reactions and is therefore less effective in forming free radicals.

Clinical Pharmacology Mitoxantrone is given by intravenous injection at a dose of 12 mg/m^2 for 3 days with cytosine arabinoside to patients with acute myelogenous leukemia and at a dose of 12 to 14 mg/m^2 once every 3 weeks to patients with solid tumors. The drug is given over a period of 30 minutes and is rarely associated with extravasation injury.

Following intravenous administration, mitoxantrone is rapidly cleared from the plasma. Its

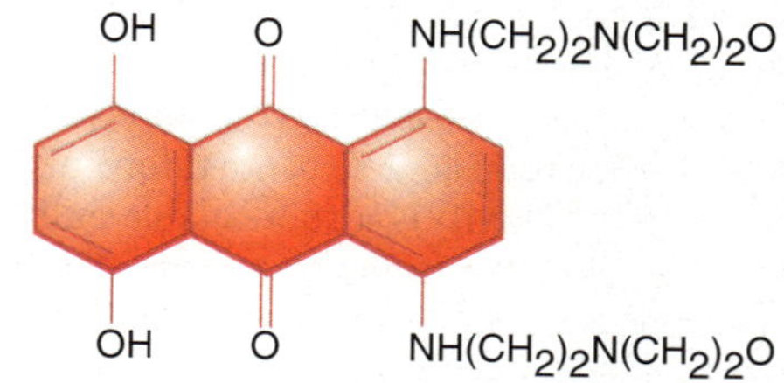

Figure 45-6 Structure of mitoxantrone.

clearance is best described by a three-compartment model, with an initial α-phase t½ of 2 to 15 minutes attributable to rapid uptake by formed elements of the blood; a 0 phase of between 17 minutes and 3 hours that is the consequence of redistribution back into the blood and into most tissues of the body; and a terminal y t½ of 5 to 6 days.[111–113] As is the case with the anthracyclines, a high proportion of mitoxantrone is found in tissues tightly bound to DNA and in plasma bound to plasma proteins. Mitoxantrone is metabolized to the monocarboxylic and dicarboxylic acids formed by oxidation of the terminal hydroxyl groups on the alkyl side chain. Mitoxantrone may also be conjugated to glutathione.[114] Most of the drug is excreted in the feces, with less than 10% recovered in the urine. Dose reduction is recommended for patients with severe hepatic dysfunction (bilirubin > 3 mg/dL).

Myelosuppression is the dose-limiting side effect. Mucositis, nausea and vomiting, and alopecia are less common than with doxorubicin. Cardiac toxicity is seen at cumulative doses exceeding 160 mg/m^2 in patients not receiving prior therapy with an anthracycline or other cardiotoxic drug.[115]

Activity Mitoxantrone is indicated for the treatment of acute leukemias. It is also used to treat breast and prostate cancer. When used in combination with cytosine arabinoside, response rates in acute myelogenous leukemia range from 50 to 70%.[116–118]

Mitoxantrone produces an overall response rate of 17 to 35% in metastatic breast cancer.[119] When used in combination with 5-fluorouracil and leucovorin, the response rate was 45 to 65%.[120] Mitoxantrone has activity similar to that of doxorubicin in patients with previously treated breast cancer but produces significantly less cardiac toxicity.[117] In combination with prednisone, mitoxantrone had been considered the "gold standard" for the treatment of hormone-refractory prostate cancer, but newer docetaxel-containing regimens may be somewhat better).[121–123]

Mechanism of Resistance Unlike the anthracyclines, mitoxantrone is not avidly transported by P-glycoprotein or Mrp1.[124] Resistance occurs through alterations in topoisomerase II, and the action of the breast cancer resistance protein (Bcrp/Abcg2).[125]

Actinomycin D (Dactinomycin, Cosmegen) ***History*** Actinomycins were the first antibiotics isolated from the culture broth of *Streptomyces* by Waksman and Woodruff in 1940, and they have activity against gram-positive and gram-negative bacteria and some fungi.[126] Toxicity precluded their use as anti-infection agents. Dactinomycin and other related antibiotics were subsequently found to have both antineoplastic and antibacterial activities.

Structure The actinomycins are "chromopeptides," consisting of a planar phenoxazone actinocin ring (which produces the yellow-red color of the drug), attached to two peptide side chains (Figure 45-7).

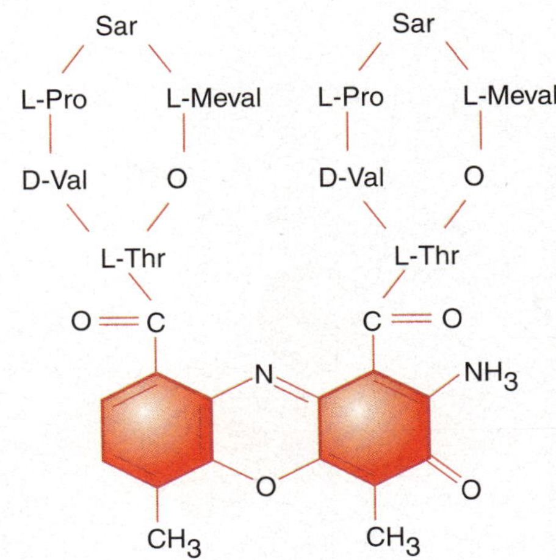

Figure 45-7 Structure of actinomycin D.

Mechanism of Action Dactinomycin intercalates into DNA. Crystallographic radiography and nuclear magnetic resonance studies revealed that the interaction between actinomycin D and DNA occurs between the drug and deoxyguanosine.[127–129] The phenoxazone ring intercalates between adjacent guanine–cytosine bases, and the polypeptide chains extend along the minor groove of the helix, thereby stabilizing the drug–DNA complex.

Although inhibition of DNA-mediated RNA polymerase is believed to be the primary mechanism of action, poisoning of topoisomerase II and the production of double-strand DNA breaks may also be important.[130] DNA breaks can also occur through the generation of free radicals.

Clinical Pharmacology Dactinomycin is administered by intravenous injection or by isolation and perfusion of involved limbs or body areas. The usual adult daily dose is 10 to 15 μg/kg daily for 5 days, repeated at intervals of 4 to 6 weeks, or 400 to 600 μg/m^2 once weekly (maximum 2 mg/wk) for 3 weeks. The usual pediatric dose is 10 to 15 μg/kg or 450 μg/m^2 daily (up to 500 μg/d) for a maximum of 5 days, or a total dose of 2.5 mg/m^2 in divided daily doses over a 7-day period. The dose can usually be repeated every 3 to 6 weeks. Dactinomycin can also be administered by isolation perfusion at 50 μg/kg for lower extremities or pelvis or 35 μg/kg for upper extremities.

Following intravenous administration, dactinomycin is rapidly bound to tissues. It undergoes minimal biotransformation and is found excreted unchanged in the bile and urine. The terminal t½ is 36 hours.[131] Dactinomycin does not cross the blood–brain barrier. Because of limited pharmacologic data, no firm guidelines have been established for using the drug in the presence of hepatic or renal dysfunction.

Myelosuppression occurs approximately 7 to 10 days following administration. Other important toxicities are mucositis (including esophagitis, ulceration, and proctitis), nausea, vomiting, alopecia, erythema, desquamation, and increased inflammation and pigmentation of skin in irradiated areas ("radiation recall"). Dactinomycin is a severe vesicant and must be administered with caution.

Activity The most important indication for dactinomycin is in the treatment of Wilms tumor, where it is curative in combination with surgery, radiation, and vincristine.[132] It is also effective in the treatment of rhabdomyosarcoma in combination with cyclophosphamide and vincristine (VAC). Other uses include Kaposi's sarcoma, sarcoma botryoides, gestational trophoblastic tumors, and testicular cancer.

Mechanism of Resistance Dactinomycin was one of the first drugs shown to be transported by P-glycoprotein.[133] Other mechanisms of resistance remain poorly understood.

NONINTERCALATING TOPOISOMERASE-TARGETING DRUGS

The Epipodophyllotoxins **History** The epipodophyllotoxins were synthesized in an effort to improve the activity of podophyllotoxin, an antimicrotubule agent that is present in mandrake plant extracts. A subtle structural change (the removal of a methyl group from the pendant aromatic ring of podophyllotoxin) abrogates tubulin binding, but confers the ability to poison topoisomerase II (Figure 45-8).[134] The epipodophyllotoxins etoposide (VP-16) and teniposide (VM-26) were in clinical use long before their mechanisms of action were understood. Although early studies indicated that cells treated with these drugs exhibited DNA strand breaks,[135] topoisomerase II was not identified as the target until the early 1980s.[136,137]

Structure–Activity Relationships A model for epipodophyllotoxin binding to the topoisomerase II–DNA complex does not yet exist, despite the availability of crystal structures for eukaryotic topoisomerase II[16] and the related prokaryotic DNA gyrase.[24] Nevertheless, the structure of the pendant aromatic ring is critical for activity; alterations in either the substituents of that ring or the stereochemical relationship between it and the tetracyclic ring system can greatly affect the topoisomerase poisoning activity of the drugs.[138,139] Subtle alterations in the tetracyclic ring may also significantly alter activity, but the glycosidic substituent can be replaced by a variety of other groups without affecting activity.[140] These data led to a model whereby the planar polycyclic component of epipodophyllotoxins stacks into the cleavage site of topoisomerase II–DNA complexes, with the pendant ring binding to either the enzyme or a DNA groove.[141]

Mechanism of Action Epipodophyllotoxins are nonintercalating topoisomerase II poisons.

Etoposide and Etoposide Phosphate ***Clinical Pharmacology*** Etoposide is approved in the United States for the treatment of testicular and small cell lung carcinomas. Etoposide phosphate is more water soluble than etoposide and is a prodrug that is rapidly converted to etoposide in vivo.[142] Intravenous and oral formulations of etoposide and etoposide phosphate are both avail-

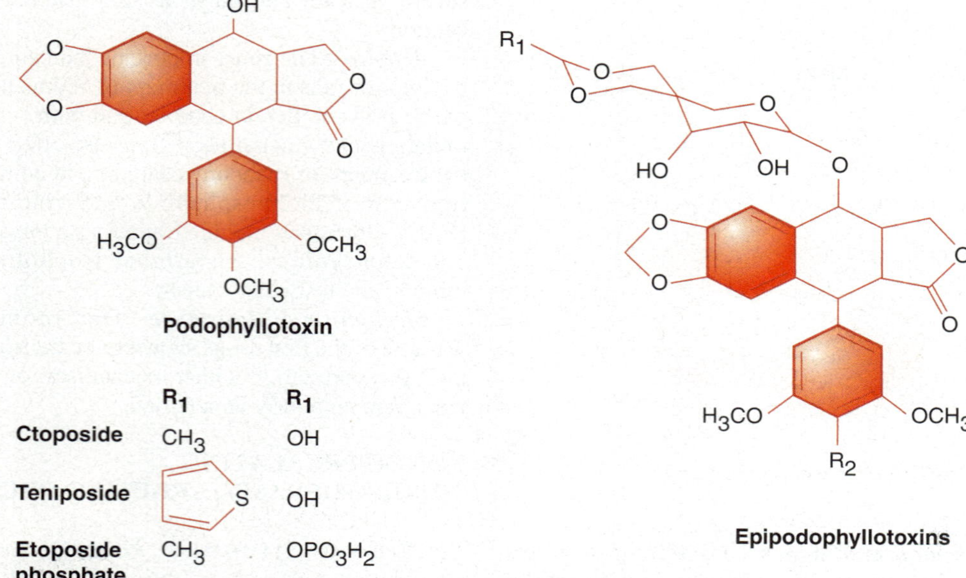

Figure 45-8 Structures of podophyllotoxin and epipodophyllotoxins.

able. Schedules using prolonged or frequent intermittent dosing appear to be more effective than single-dose regimens.[143] Etoposide is commonly administered as a 1-hour intravenous infusion using multiple daily doses of 100 mg/m^2. That dose is associated with a t½ of about 9 hours.[144] Approximately 96% of etoposide is bound to plasma proteins,[145] with a significant proportion of the drug excreted unchanged by the kidney.[146] A 30% dose reduction is recommended in patients with impaired renal function.[147] Although a small percentage of etoposide and etoposide metabolites are excreted in the bile, dose adjustment may not be required in patients with hepatic dysfunction.[148] When administered intravenously, etoposide should be infused slowly, because rapid infusion may result in hypotension. Etoposide phosphate can be administered more rapidly. When given orally, etoposide is often administered daily for 14 to 21 days. Bioavailability of oral etoposide is approximately 50%. Intestinal P-glycoprotein may efflux etoposide and is thus important in the intestinal absorption of the drug.[149]

Myelosuppression is the major toxicity associated with the administration of etoposide, either intravenously or orally. Infrequent toxicities include allergic or other infusional reactions manifested as fever, bronchospasm, and hypotension. Toxicities associated with oral etoposide include nausea, vomiting, and mucositis.

Activity Etoposide is commonly used in combination with other drugs in the treatment of testicular cancer, small cell and non–small cell lung cancer, Hodgkin's and non-Hodgkin's lymphomas, acute myeloid leukemia, gastric cancer, and soft-tissue sarcomas.

Teniposide ***Clinical Pharmacology*** Teniposide is less commonly used than etoposide. It is approved for the treatment of refractory childhood acute lymphocytic leukemia. Teniposide is also used in the treatment of gliomas.[150] In teniposide, a thiophene group replaces the methyl group present on the glucose moiety of etoposide (see Figure 45-8). The alteration affects both the interaction with topoisomerase II and clinical pharmacology.

Teniposide is a more potent in vitro poison of topoisomerase II than etoposide is.[137] In addition, a greater fraction of teniposide is protein bound relative to etoposide,[151] and renal function is less relevant to teniposide clearance.[152] As is the case with etoposide, myelosuppression is the dose-limiting toxicity for teniposide. Cremophor is used in teniposide formulations, which may explain the greater frequency of hypersensitivity reactions observed with teniposide than with etoposide.[153]

Camptothecins ***History*** Camptothecin is an alkaloid (molecular weight: 348 kDa) produced by the Chinese tree *Camptotheca acuminata*. It was identified as an antineoplastic agent in the 1960s by Wall and Wani.[154] Early studies with camptothecin indicated that cellular exposure to the drug resulted in DNA breaks; the interaction with topoisomerase I was identified by Hsiang and colleagues in the 1980s.[155] Because the camptothecin alkaloid is relatively insoluble in aqueous solutions, initial clinical trials with camptothecin used a sodium salt derivative.[156,157]

Although responses occurred during those trials, severe myelosuppression or cystitis was frequently observed, and the drug was deemed too toxic for clinical use. Subsequently, it was discovered that, in the salt derivatives, the lactone at position 20 in camptothecin is hydrolyzed to a carboxylic acid. The resultant opening of the lactone ring significantly decreased the activity of the compound.[158] Further development of camptothecins led to two water-soluble derivatives, topotecan and irinotecan, that can be delivered as lactones and that are currently approved for the treatment of cancer. Several other camptothecin analogues are in clinical development.

Structure–Activity Relationships Camptothecin is a five-ringed heterocyclic alkaloid (Figure 45-9). Certain substitutions in the A ring may augment topoisomerase poisoning, presumably by increasing drug binding to the topoisomerase I–DNA cleavage complex.[159] By contrast, substitutions in the E ring often abrogate activity. Indeed, the stereochemistry of C20 in the E ring is critical, with the *R*-isomer inactive.[160] Irinotecan is a prodrug; the piperidino group present at C10 is hydrolyzed by plasma or tissue carboxylesterases to SN-38, which is much more active than irinotecan in inducing topoisomerase I-mediated DNA damage.

Other notable derivation strategies have produced drugs currently in clinical testing: (1) 7 silyl congeners, designed to enhance lipophilicity and to stabilize the E ring lactone;[161] (2) 20 esters, designed as prodrugs to prevent hydrolysis of the E ring;[162] and (3) homocamptothecins, which contain a seven-membered E ring that is less susceptible to hydrolysis in plasma.[163]

Mechanism of Action Camptothecins are topoisomerase I poisons that do not bind DNA in the absence of the enzyme.

Topotecan ***Clinical Pharmacology*** Topotecan is approved for the treatment of ovarian cancer[164] and small cell lung cancer.[165] Typically, it is administered intravenously at a dose of 1.5 mg/m^2 as a 30-minute infusion daily for 5 days, followed by a 2-week period of rest. Several alternative dosing schedules have been explored, including a 1-month continuous intravenous infusion.[166] Those schedules do not seem to be associated with activity that is significantly better than the activity observed with the 5-day schedule.

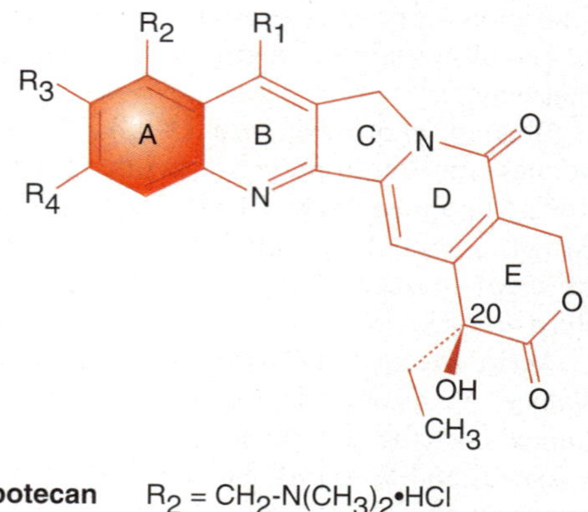

Figure 45-9 Structures of camptothecins.

The topotecan E ring[167] lactone is rapidly hydrolyzed in plasma, with approximately 50% of the drug present as the inactive open-ring carboxylate 15 minutes after infusion.[168] Renal function is important in topotecan clearance; approximately 30% of the drug is excreted unchanged in the urine.[169] Dose reduction is recommended for patients with renal impairment, but does not appear necessary for patients with hepatic dysfunction.[170,171]

Myelosuppression is the most common toxicity observed with daily administration of topotecan. Although severe nonhematologic toxicities are uncommon after administration of topotecan, mucositis was dose limiting in trials that used a 5-day continuous infusion in patients with leukemia.[172]

Activity Topotecan is active as a single agent in the treatment of ovarian cancer, small cell and non–small cell lung cancer, acute myelocytic leukemia, and myelodysplastic syndromes. The combination of topoisomerase I-targeting drugs with other cytotoxic agents was often additive or synergistic in preclinical models, and a variety of drug combination strategies are being investigated in the clinic.[173–175] Combinations of topotecan with topoisomerase II inhibitors or cisplatin appear particularly promising.[176–178] Recent evidence suggests that topotecan effectively crosses the blood–brain barrier and may be effective in treating brain metastases from a variety of sources.[179]

Irinotecan ***Clinical Pharmacology*** Irinotecan is usually administered intravenously as a weekly infusion of 125 mg/m^2 for 4 weeks, with a 2-week rest period.[180] An alternative dosing schedule, commonly used in Europe, uses 90-minute infusions of 240 to 350 mg/m^2 every 3 weeks.[181] Notably, xenograft studies suggest that the schedule of administration may be a critical determinant of efficacy for this drug, and it is not clear that either of these schedules is optimal for antitumor efficacy in patients.[182]

Irinotecan is rapidly metabolized by carboxylesterases to SN-38. Studies suggest that this metabolism may vary among body tissues (including malignant tissues).[183] With irinotecan, as compared with other camptothecins, a relatively greater proportion of SN-38 is maintained in plasma as the active lactone. This phenomenon may be related to stabilization of the SN-38 lactone by human albumin.[184]

In addition to being converted to SN-38, irinotecan is excreted in urine and bile. Biliary excretion of SN-38, following glucuronide conjugation in the liver (at least in part by the *UGT1A1* enzyme isotype), is a major clearance mechanism for this metabolite.[185] Reduction in the glucuronidation of SN-38 is associated with an increased risk of severe diarrhea following treatment with irinotecan.[186] Similarly, inherited defects in hepatic glucuronide transferases, which occur in patients with the Gilbert or Crigler-Najjar syndromes, may predispose to severe toxicity with conventional doses of irinotecan.[185,187] Patients with certain *UGT1A1* genetic polymorphisms are also at higher risk for developing diarrhea after irinotecan treatment.[188–190] Additional studies of irinotecan and SN-38 suggest that biliary excretion of both the conjugated and unconjugated forms of these drugs may depend upon the Mrp-2 (*ABCC3*) ATP-dependent transporter, which is defective in patients with Dubin-Johnson syndrome.[191]

The most common toxicities associated with weekly infusion schedules of irinotecan are diarrhea and myelosuppression. Two mechanisms are involved in irinotecan-induced diarrhea: (1) acute cholinergic effects produced by inhibition of acetylcholinesterase by the drug,[192] and (2) delayed mucosal cytotoxicity. The former toxicity may be treated by administration of atropine; the latter responds to early and aggressive administration of loperamide.[193]

Activity Irinotecan is active in the treatment of several malignancies, including colorectal cancer,[194,195] small cell and nonsmall cell lung cancer,[196–199] gastric cancer,[200] and cervical cancer.[201]

REFERENCES

1. Wang JC. DNA topoisomerases. Ann Rev Biochem 1996;65:635–92.
2. Froelich-Ammon SJ, Osheroff N. Topoisomerase poisons: harnessing the dark side of enzyme mechanism. J Biol Chem 1995;270:21429–32.
3. Nitiss JL. Investigating the biological functions of DNA topoisomerases in eukaryotic cells. Biochem Biophys Acta 1998;1400:63–81.
4. Kwan KY, Moens PB, Wang JC. Infertility and aneuploidy in mice lacking a type IA DNA topoisomerase III beta. Proc Natl Acad Sci U S A 2003;100(5):2526–31.
5. Brill SJ, DiNardo S, Voelkel-Meiman K, Sternglanz R. Need for DNA topoisomerase activity as a swivel for DNA replication or transcription of ribosomal RNA. Nature 1987;326:414–6.
6. Kim RA, Wang JC. Function of DNA topoisomerases as replication swivels in *Saccharomyces cerevisiae*. J Mol Biol 1989;208:257–67.
7. DiNardo S, Voelkel K, Sternglanz R. DNA topoisomerase II mutant of *Saccharomyces cerevisiae*: topoisomerase II is required for segregation of daughter molecules at the termination of DNA replication. Proc Natl Acad Sci U S A 1984;81:2616–20.
8. Holm C, Goto T, Wang JC, Botstein D. DNA topoisomerase II is required at the time of mitosis in yeast. Cell 1985;41:553–63.
9. Uemura T, Ohkura H, Adachi Y, et al. DNA topoisomerase II is required for condensation and separation of mitotic chromosomes in *S. pombe*. Cell 1987;50:917–25.
10. Varga-Weisz PD, Wilm M, Bonte E, et al. Chromatin-remodelling factor CHRAC contains the ATPases ISWI and topoisomerase II. Nature 1997;388:598–602.
11. Negri C, Scovassi AI, Braghetti A, et al. DNA topoisomerase IIbeta: stability and distribution in different animal cells in comparison to DNA topoisomerase I and IIa. Exp Cell Res 1993;206:128–33.
12. Woessner RD, Mattern MR, Mirabelli CK, et al. Proliferation- and cell cycle–dependent differences in expression of the 170 kilodalton and 180 kilodalton forms of topoisomerase II in NIH-3T3 cells. Cell Growth Differ 1991;2:209–14.
13. Gangloff S, McDonald JP, Bendixen C, et al. The yeast type I topoisomerase Top3 interacts with Sgs1, a DNA helicase homolog: a potential eukaryotic reverse gyrase. Mol Cell Biol 1994;14:8391–8.
14. Ellis NA, Groden J, Ye TZ, et al. The Bloom's syndrome gene product is homologous to RecQ helicases. Cell 1995;83:655–66.
15. Yu CE, Oshima J, Fu YH, et al. Positional cloning of the Werner's syndrome gene. Science 1996;272:258–62.
16. Kwan KY, Moens PB, Wang JC. Infertility and aneuploidy in mice lacking a type IA DNA topoisomerase III beta. Proc Natl Acad Sci U S A 2003;100:2526–31.
17. Stewart L, Redinbo MR, Qiu X, et al. A model for the mechanism of human topoisomerase I. Science 1998;279:1534–41.
18. Berger JM, Gamblin SJ, Harrison SC, Wang JC. Structure and mechanism of DNA topoisomerase II [published erratum appears in Nature 1996;380:179]. Nature 1996;379:225–32.
19. Li W, Wang JC. Mammalian DNA topoisomerase IIIα is essential in early embryogenesis. Proc Natl Acad Sci U S A 1998;95:1010–3.
20. Reid RJ, Benedetti P, Bjornsti MA. Yeast as a model organism for studying the actions of DNA topoisomerase-targeted drugs. Biochem Biophys Acta 1998;1400:289–300.
21. Liu LF. DNA topoisomerase poisons as antitumor drugs. Ann Rev Biochem 1989;58:351–75.
22. Chen AY, Yu C, Gatto B, Liu LF. DNA minor groove-binding ligands: a different class of mammalian DNA topoisomerase I inhibitors. Proc Natl Acad Sci U S A 1993;90:8131–5.
23. Staker BL, Hjerrild K, Feese MD, Behnke CA, Burgin AB Jr, Stewart L. The mechanism of topoisomerase I poisoning by a camptothecin analog. Proc Natl Acad Sci U S A 2002;99(24):15387–92.
24. Morais Cabral JH, Jackson AP, Smith CV, et al. Crystal structure of the breakage-reunion domain of DNA gyrase. Nature 1997;388:903–6.
25. Wasserman RA, Wang JC. Mechanistic studies of amsacrine-resistant derivatives of DNA topoisomerase II. J Biol Chem 1994;269:20943–51.
26. Roca J, Ishida R, Berger JM, et al. Antitumor bisdioxopiperazines inhibit yeast DNA topoisomerase II by trapping the enzyme in the form of a closed protein clamp. Proc Natl Acad Sci U S A 1994;91:1781–5.
27. Wessel I, Jensen LH, Jensen PB, et al. Human small cell lung cancer NYH cells selected for resistance to the bisdioxopiperazine topoisomerase II catalytic inhibitor ICRF-187 demonstrate a functional R162Q mutation in the Walker A consensus ATP binding domain of the alpha isoform. Cancer Res 1999;59:3442–50.
28. Kingma PS, Osheroff N. Apurinic sites are position-specific topoisomerase II poisons. J Biol Chem 1997;272:1148–55.
29. Pourquier P, Pilon AA, Kohlhagen G, et al. Trapping of mammalian topoisomerase I and recombinations induced by damaged DNA containing nicks or gaps. Importance of DNA end phosphorylation and camptothecin effects. J Biol Chem 1997;272:26441–7.
30. Lanza A, Tornaletti S, Rodolfo C, et al. Human DNA topoisomerase I-mediated cleavages stimulated by ultraviolet light-induced DNA damage. J Biol Chem 1996;271:6978–86.
31. Pourquier P, Ueng LM, Kohlhagen G, et al. Effects of uracil incorporation, DNA mismatches, and abasic sites on cleavage and religation activities of mammalian topoisomerase I. J Biol Chem 1997;272:7792–6.
32. van Waardenburg RC, de Jong LA, van Eijndhoven MA, et al. Platinated DNA adducts enhance poisoning of DNA topoisomerase I by camptothecin. J Biol Chem 2004;279:54502–9.
33. Pourquier P, Takebayashi Y, Urasaki Y, et al. Induction of topoisomerase I cleavage complexes by 1-beta-D-arabinofuranosylcytosine (Ara-C) in vitro and in Ara-C-treated cells. Proc Natl Acad Sci U S A 2000;97:1885–90.
34. Pourquier P, Gioffre C, Kohinagen G, et al. Gemcitabine (2,2'-difluoro-2'-deoxyeytidine); an antimetabolite that poisons topoisomerase I. Clin Cancer Res 2002;8:2499–504.
35. Li TK, Chen AY, Yu C, et al. Activation of topoisomerase II-mediated excision of chromosomal DNA loops during oxidative stress. Genes Dev 1999;13:1553–60.
36. D'Arpa P, Beardmore C, Liu LF. Involvement of nucleic acid synthesis in cell killing mechanisms of topoisomerase poisons. Cancer Res 1990;50:6919–24.
37. Hsiang Y, Lihou M, Liu L. Arrest of replication forks by drug-stabilized topoisomerase I–DNA cleavable complexes as a mechanism of cell killing by camptothecin. Cancer Res 1989;49:5077–82.
38. Wu J, Liu LF. Processing of topoisomerase I cleavable complexes into DNA damage by transcription. Nucleic Acids Res 1997;25:4181–6.
39. O'Connor PM, Nieves-Neira W, Kerrigan D, et al. S-phase population analysis does not correlate with the cytotoxicity of camptothecin and 10,11-methylenedioxycamptothecin in human colon carcinoma HT-29 cells. Cancer Commun 1991;3:233–40.
40. Morris EJ, Geller HM. Induction of neuronal apoptosis by camptothecin, an inhibitor of DNA topoisomerase I: evidence for cell cycle-independent toxicity. J Cell Biol 1996;134:757–70.

41. Nitiss J, Wang JC. DNA topoisomerase-targeting antitumor drugs can be studied in yeast. Proc Natl Acad Sci U S A 1988;85:7501–5.
42. Squires S, Ryan AJ, Strutt HL, Johnson RT. Hypersensitivity of Cockayne's syndrome cells to camptothecin is associated with the generation of abnormally high levels of double strand breaks in nascent DNA. Cancer Res 1993;53:2012–9.
43. Smith PJ, Makinson TA, Watson JV. Enhanced sensitivity to camptothecin in ataxia-telangiectasia cells and its relationship with the expression of DNA topoisomerase I. Int J Radiat Biol 1989;55:217–31.
44. Wan S, Capasso H, Walworth NC. The topoisomerase I poison camptothecin generates a Chk1-dependent DNA damage checkpoint signal in fission yeast. Yeast 1999;15:821–8.
45. Pouliot JJ, Yao KC, Robertson CA, Nash HA. Yeast gene for a Tyr–DNA phosphodiesterase that repairs topoisomerase I complexes. Science 1999;286:552–5.
46. Barthelmes HU, Habermeyer M, Christensen MO, et al. *TDP1* overexpression in human cells counteracts DNA damage mediated by topoisomerases I and II. J Biol Chem 2004;279:55618–25.
47. Desai SD, Liu LF, Vazquez-Abad D, D'Arpa P. Ubiquitin-dependent destruction of topoisomerase I is stimulated by the antitumor drug camptothecin. J Biol Chem 1997;272:24159–64.
48. Desai SO, Li TK, Rodrigues-Bowman A, et al. Ubiquitin/265 proteasome-mediated degradation of topoisomerase 1 as a resistance mechanism to camptothecin in tumor cells. Cancer Res 2001;61:5926–32.
49. Mao Y, Sun M, Desai SD, Liu LF. SUMO-1 conjugation to topoisomerase I: a possible repair response to topoisomerase-mediated DNA damage. Proc Natl Acad Sci U S A 2000;97:4046–51.
50. Desai SD, Zhang H, Rodriguez-Bauman A, et al. Transcription-dependent degradation of topoisomerase I-DNA covalent complexes. Mol Cell Biol 2003;23:2341–50.
51. Ratain MJ, Rowley JD. Therapy-related acute myeloid leukemia secondary to inhibitors of topoisomerase II: from the bedside to the target genes [see comments]. Ann Oncol 1992;3:107–11.
52. Halligan BD, Davis JL, Edwards KA, Liu LF. Intra- and intermolecular strand transfer by HeLa DNA topoisomerase I. J Biol Chem 1982;257:3995–4000.
53. Bae YS, Kawasaki I, Ikeda H, Liu LF. Illegitimate recombination mediated by calf thymus DNA topoisomerase II in vitro. Proc Natl Acad Sci U S A 1988;85:2076–80.
54. Felix CA, Lange BJ, Hosler MR, et al. Chromosome band 11q23 translocation breakpoints are DNA topoisomerase II cleavage sites. Cancer Res 1995;55:4287–92.
55. Ahuja HG, Felix CA, Aplan PD. The t(11;20)(p15;q11) chromosomal translocation associated with therapy-related myelodysplastic syndrome results in an NUP98-TOP1 fusion. Blood 1999;94:3258–61.
56. Gurevich RM, Aplan PD, Humphries RK. NUP98-topoisomerase I acute myeloid leukemia-associated fusion gene has potent leukemogenic activities independent of an engineered catalytic site mutation. Blood 2004;104:1127–36.
57. Gros P, Ben Neriah YB, Croop JM, Housman DE. Isolation and expression of a complementary DNA that confers multidrug resistance. Nature 1986;323:728–31.
58. Cole SPC, Chanda ER, Dicke FP, et al. Non-P-glycoprotein-mediated multidrug resistance in a small cell lung cancer cell line: evidence for decreased susceptibility to drug-induced DNA damage and reduced levels of topoisomerase II. Cancer Res 1991;51:3345–52.
59. Koike K, Kawabe T, Tanaka T, et al. A canalicular multispecific organic anion transporter (cMOAT) antisense cDNA enhances drug sensitivity in human hepatic cancer cells. Cancer Res 1997;57:5475–9.
60. Allen JD, Brinkhuis RF, Wijnholds J, Schinkel AH. The mouse *BCRP1/MXR/ABCP* gene: amplification and over-expression in cell lines selected for resistance to topotecan, mitoxantrone, or doxorubicin. Cancer Res 1999;59:4237–41.
61. Doyle LA, Yang W, Abruzzo LV, et al. A multidrug resistance transporter from human MCF-7 breast cancer cells. Proc Natl Acad Sci U S A 1998;95:15665–70.
62. Steinbach D, Sell W, Voigt A, et al. *BCRP* gene expression is associated with a poor response to remission induction therapy in childhood acute myeloid leukemia. Leukemia 2002;16:1443–7.
63. Rajendra R, Gounder MK, Saleem A, et al. Differential effects of the breast cancer resistance protein on the cellular accumulation and cytotoxicity of 9-aminocamptothecin and 9-nitrocamptothecin. Cancer Res 2003;63:3228–33.
64. Rubin EH, Li T, Duan P, Liu LF. Cellular resistance to topoisomerase poisons. In: Hait WN, editor. Drug resistance. Norwell (MA): Kluwer Academic; 1996. p. 243–60.
65. Takano H, Kohno K, Ono M, et al. Increased phosphorylation of DNA topoisomerase II in etoposide-resistant mutants of human cancer KB cells. Cancer Res 1991;51:3951–7.
66. DeVore RF, Corbett AH, Osheroff N. Phosphorylation of topoisomerase II by casein kinase II and protein kinase C: effects on enzyme-mediated DNA cleavage/religation and sensitivity to the antineoplastic drugs etoposide and 4'-(9-acridinylamino)methane-sulfon-m-anisidide. Cancer Res 1992;52:2156–61.
67. Beck WT, Cirtain MC, Danks MK, et al. Pharmacological, molecular, and cytogenetic analysis of "atypical" multidrug-resistant human leukemic cells. Cancer Res 1987;47:5455–60.
68. Feldhoff PW, Mirski SE, Cole SP, Sullivan DM. Altered subcellular distribution of topoisomerase II alpha in a drug-resistant human small cell lung cancer cell line. Cancer Res 1994;54:756–62.
69. Mirski SEL, Cole SPC. Cytoplasmic localization of a mutant Mr 160,000 topoisomerase IIa is associated with the loss of putative bipartite nuclear localization signals in a drug-resistant human lung cancer cell line. Cancer Res 1995;55:2129–34.
70. Harker WG, Slade DL, Parr RL, Holguin MH. Selective use of an alternative stop codon and polyadenylation signal within intron sequences leads to a truncated topoisomerase II alpha messenger RNA and protein in human HL-60 leukemia cells selected for resistance to mitoxantrone. Cancer Res 1995;55:4962–71.
71. Wessel I, Jensen PB, Falck J, et al. Loss of amino acids 1490Lys-Ser-Lys1492 in the COOH-terminal region of topoisomerase II alpha in human small cell lung cancer cells selected for resistance to etoposide results in an extranuclear enzyme localization. Cancer Res 1997;57:4451–4.
72. Engel R, Valkov NI, Gump JL, et al. The cytoplasmic trafficking of DNA topoisomerase II alpha correlates with etoposide resistance in human myeloma cells. Exp Cell Res 2004;295:421–31.
73. Edwards TK, Shaman JA, Dennis T, et al. Role for nucleolin/Nsr1 in the cellular localization of topoisomerase I. 1999. J Biol Chem 2000;275:36181–8.
74. Nitiss JL, Rose A, Sykes KC, et al. Using yeast to understand drugs that target topoisomerase. Ann NY Acad Sci 1996;803:32–43.
75. Park SY, Lam W, Cheng YC. X-ray repair cross-complementing gene I protein plays an important role in camptothecin resistance. Cancer Res 2001;62:459–65.
76. Zunino F, Gambetta R, DiMarco A, et al. Effects of the stereochemical configuration on the interaction of some daunomycin derivatives with DNA. Biochem Biophys Res Commun 1976;69:744–50.
77. Arcamone F, Cassinelli G, Fantini G, et al. Adriamycin, 14-hydroxy-daunomycin, a new antitumor antibiotic from *S. peucetius* var. *caesius*. Biotechnol Bioeng 1969;11:1101–10.
78. Doroshow JH. Role of hydrogen peroxide and hydroxyl radical formation in the killing of Ehrlich tumor cells by anticancer quinones. Proc Natl Acad Sci U S A 1986;83:4514–8.
79. Sinha BK, Katki AG, Batist G, et al. Differential formation of hydroxyl radical by Adriamycin in sensitive and resistant MCF-7 human breast tumor cells: implication for the mechanism of action. Biochemistry 1987;26:3776–81.
80. Legha SS, Benjamin RS, Mackay B, et al. Reduction of doxorubicin cardiotoxicity by prolonged continuous intravenous infusion. Ann Intern Med 1982;96:133–9.
81. Gordon AN, Tonda M, Sun S, Rackoff W. Long-term survival advantage for women treated with pegylated liposomal doxorubicin compared with topotecan in a phase 3 randomized study of recurrent and refractory epithelial ovarian cancer. Gynecol Oncol 2004;95:1–8.
82. Harrington KJ, Mohammadtaghi S, Uster PS, et al. Effective targeting of solid tumors in patients with locally advanced cancers by radiolabeled pegylated liposomes. Clin Cancer Res 2001;7:243–54.
83. Kolaric K, Potrebica V, Cervek J. Phase II clinical trial of 4'-epidoxorubicin in metastatic solid tumors. J Cancer Res Clin Oncol 1983;106:148–52.
84. Greene R, Collins J, Jenkins J, et al. Plasma pharmacokinetics of Adriamycin and Adriamycinol: implications for the design of in vitro experiments and treatment protocols. Cancer Res 1983;43:3417–21.
85. Terasaki T, Iga T, Sugiyama Y, et al. Experimental evidence of characteristic tissue distribution of Adriamycin: tissue DNA concentration as a determinant. J Pharm Pharmacol 1982;34:597–600.
86. Speth PAJ, Linssen PCM, Holdrinet RSG, et al. Plasma and cellular Adriamycin concentrations in patients with myeloma treated with 96-hour continuous infusion. Clin Pharmacol Ther 1987;41:661–5.
87. Weenen H, Lankelma J, Penders PGM, et al. Pharmacokinetics of 4'-epidoxorubicin in man. Invest New Drugs 1983;1:59–64.
88. Ganzina F. 4'-Epidoxorubicin, a new analogue of doxorubicin: a preliminary overview of preclinical and clinical data. Cancer Treat Rev 1983;10:1–22.
89. Jones RB, Holland JF, Bhardwaj S, et al. A phase I–II study of intensive-dose Adriamycin for advanced breast cancer. J Clin Oncol 1987;5:172–7.
90. Ahmann DL, Schaid DJ, Bisel HF, et al. The effect on survival of initial chemotherapy in advanced breast cancer: polychemotherapy versus single drug. J Clin Oncol 1987;5:1928–32.
91. Polychemotherapy for early breast cancer: an overview of randomised trials. Early Breast Cancer Trialists Collaborative Group. Lancet 1998;352:930–42.
92. Sledge GW, Neuberg D, Ingle J, et al. Phase III trial of doxorubicin (A) vs paclitaxel (T) vs doxorubicin + paclitaxel (A + T) as first-line therapy for metastatic breast cancer (MBC): an intergroup trial [abstract]. Proc Am Soc Clin Oncol 1997;16:1a.
93. Bontenbal M, Andersson M, Wildiers J, et al. Doxorubicin vs epirubicin, report of a second-line randomized phase II/III study in advanced breast cancer. EORTC Breast Cancer Cooperative Group. Br J Cancer 1998;77:2257–63.
94. VonHoff DD, Layard MW, Basa P, et al. Risk factors for doxorubicin-induced congestive heart failure. Ann Intern Med 1979;91:710–7.
95. Bristow MR, Billingham ME, Mason JW, Daniels JR. Clinical spectrum of anthracycline antibiotic cardiotoxicity. Cancer Treat Rep 1978;62:873–9.
96. Lefrak EA, Pitha J, Rosenheim S, et al. Clinicopathologic analysis of Adriamycin cardiotoxicity. Cancer 1973;32:302–14.
97. Slamon D, Leyland-Jones B, Shak S, et al. Addition of Herceptin to first-line chemotherapy for *HER2* overexpressing metastatic breast cancer markedly increases anti-cancer activity: a randomized, multinational controlled phase III trial [abstract]. Proc Am Soc Clin Oncol 1998;17:377a.
98. Anderlini P, Benjamin RS, Wong FC, et al. Idarubicin cardiotoxicity: a retrospective study in acute myeloid leukemia and myelodysplasia. J Clin Oncol 1995;13:2827–34.
99. Launchbury AP, Habboubi N. Epirubicin and doxorubicin: a comparison of their characteristics, therapeutic activity and toxicity. Cancer Treat Rev 1993;19:197–228.
100. Alexander J, Dainiak N, Berger HJ, et al. Serial assessment of doxorubicin cardiotoxicity with quantitative radionuclide angiocardiography. N Engl J Med 1979;300:278–83.
101. Hensley ML, Schuchter LM, Lindley C, et al. American Society of Clinical Oncology clinical practice guidelines for the use of chemotherapy and radiotherapy protectants. J Clin Oncol 1999;17:3333–55.
102. O'Brien ME, Wigler N, Inbar M, et al. Reduced cardiotoxicity and comparable efficacy in a phase III trial of pegylated liposomal doxorubicin HCl (CAELYX/Doxil) versus conventional doxorubicin for first-line treatment of metastatic breast cancer. Ann Oncol 2004;15:440–9.
103. Muggia FM, Hainsworth JD, Jeffers S, et al. Phase II study of liposomal doxorubicin in refractory ovarian cancer: antitumor activity and toxicity modification by liposomal encapsulation. J Clin Oncol 1997;15:987–93.
104. Hait W. Drug resistance. In: Freireich E, editor. Cancer treatment and research. Vol. 87. Boston: Kluwer Academic Publishers; 1996. p. 243–60.
105. Raha A, Tew KD. Glutathione-*S*-transferase. In: Hait W, editor. Drug resistance. Vol. 87. Boston: Kluwer Academic Publishers; 1996. p. 83–122.
106. Lowe SW, Bodis S, McClatchey A, et al. P53 status and the efficacy of cancer therapy in vivo. Science 1994;266:807–10.
107. Tu Y, Xu FH, Liu J, et al. Upregulated expression of *BCL-2* in multiple myeloma cells induced by exposure to doxorubicin, etoposide, and hydrogen peroxide. Blood 1996;88:1805–12.
108. Advani R, Visani G, Milligan D, et al. Treatment of poor prognosis AML patients using PSC833 (valspodar) plus mitoxantrone, etoposide, and cytarabine (PSC-MEC). Adv Exp Med Biol 1999;457:47–56.
109. Murdock KC, Wallace RE, Durr FE, et al. Antitumor agents: I. 1,4-Bis[(aminoalkyl)amino]-9,10-anthracenediones. J Med Chem 1979;22:1024–30.

110. Crepsi MO, Ivanier SE, Genovese J, et al. Mitoxantrone affects topoisomerase activities in human breast cancer cells. Biochem Biophys Res Comm 1986;136:521–8.
111. Savaraj N, Lu K, Manuel V, Loo TL. Pharmacology of mitoxantrone in cancer patients. Cancer Chemother Pharmacol 1982;8:113–7.
112. Alberts DS, Peng YM, Bowden GT, et al. Pharmacology of mitoxantrone: mode of action and pharmacokinetics. Invest New Drugs 1985;3:101–7.
113. Alberts DS, Peng YM, Leigh S, et al. Disposition of mitoxantrone in cancer patients. Cancer Res 1985;45:1879–84.
114. Wolf CR, MacPherson JS, Smyth JF. Evidence for the metabolism of mitoxantrone by microsomal glutathione transferases and 3-methylcholanthrene-inducible glucuronosyl transferases. Biochem Pharmacol 1986;35:1577–81.
115. Shenkenberg TD, Von Hoff DD. Mitoxantrone: a new anticancer drug with significant clinical activity. Ann Intern Med 1986;105:67–81.
116. Arlin ZA, Silver R, Cassileth P, et al. Phase I–II trial of mitoxantrone in acute leukemia. Cancer Treat Rep 1985;69:61–4.
117. Paciucci PA, Ohnuma T, Cuttner J, et al. Mitoxantrone in patients with acute leukemia in relapse. Cancer Res 1983;43:3919–22.
118. Dutcher JP, Wiernik PH, Strauman JJ, et al. Mitoxantrone (MITOX) and cytosine arabinoside (ARA-C) in acute non-lymphocytic leukemia (ANLL) and blast crisis of chronic myelogenous leukemia (CML-B) [abstract]. Proc Am Soc Clin Oncol 1985;4:170.
119. Neidhart JA, Gochnour D, Roach R, et al. A comparison of mitoxantrone and doxorubicin in breast cancer. J Clin Oncol 1986;4:672–7.
120. Hainsworth JD, Andrews MB, Johnson DH, Greco FA. Mitoxantrone, fluorouracil, and high-dose leucovorin: an effective, well-tolerated regimen for metastatic breast cancer [see comments]. J Clin Oncol 1991;9:1731–5.
121. Petrylak DP, Tangen CM, Hussain MH, et al. Docetaxel and estramustine compared with mitoxantrone and prednisone for advanced refractory prostate cancer. N Engl J Med 2004;351:1513–20.
122. Dagher R, Li N, Abraham S, et al. Approval summary: docetaxel in combination with prednisone for the treatment of androgen-independent hormone-refractory prostate cancer. Clin Cancer Res 2004;10:8147–51.
123. Tannock IF, de Wit R, Berry WR, et al. Docetaxel plus prednisone or mitoxantrone plus prednisone for advanced prostate cancer. N Engl J Med 2004;351:1502–12.
124. Nakagawa M, Schneider E, Dixon KH, et al. Reduced intracellular drug accumulation in the absence of P-glycoprotein (Mdr1) overexpression in mitoxantrone-resistant human MCF-7 breast cancer cells. Cancer Res 1992;52:6175–81.
125. Ee PL, He X, Ross DD, Beck WT. Modulation of breast cancer resistance protein (*BCRP/ABCG2*) gene expression using RNA interference. Mol Cancer Ther 2004;3:1577–83.
126. Waksman SA, Woodruff HB. Bacteriostatic and bactericidal substances produced by a soil *Actinomyces*. Proc Soc Exp Biol Med 1940;45:609.
127. Sobell HM, Jain SC. Stereochemistry of actinomycin D binding to DNA: II. Detailed molecular model of actinomycin–DNA complex and its implications. J Mol Biol 1972;68:21–34.
128. Liu X, Chen H, Patel DJ. Solution structure of actinomycin–DNA complexes: drug interaction at isolated G-C sites. J Biomol NMR 1991;1:323–47.
129. Yu C, Tseng YY. NMR study of the solution confirmation of actinomycin D. Eur J Biochem 1992;209:181–7.
130. Ross WE, Bradley MO. DNA double-strand breaks in mammalian cells after exposure to intercalating agents. Biochem Biophys Acta 1981;654:129–34.
131. Tattersall NHM, Sodergren JE, Dengupta SK. Pharmacokinetics of actinomycin D in patients with malignant melanoma. Clin Pharmacol Ther 1975;17:701–8.
132. Farber S. Chemotherapy in the treatment of leukemia and Wilm's tumor. JAMA 1966;198:826–36.
133. Biedler J, Riehm H. Cellular resistance to actinomycin D in Chinese hamster cells in vitro: cross resistance, radioautographic and cytogenetic studies. Cancer Res 1970;30:1174–84.
134. Chen GL, Yang L, Rowe TC, et al. Nonintercalative antitumor drugs interfere with the breakage-reunion reaction of mammalian DNA topoisomerase II. J Biol Chem 1984;259:13560–6.
135. Wozniak AJ, Ross WE. DNA damage as a basis for 4'-demethyl epipodophyllotoxin-9-(4,6-*O*-ethylidene-p-D-glucopyranoside) (etoposide) toxicity. Cancer Res 1983;43:120–4.
136. Ross WE, Rowe T, Glisson B, et al. Role of topoisomerase II in mediating epipodophyllotoxin-mediated DNA cleavage. Cancer Res 1984;44:5857–60.
137. Long BH, Musial ST, Brattain MG. Single- and double-strand DNA breakage and repair in human lung adenocarcinoma cells exposed to etoposide and teniposide. Cancer Res 1985;45:3106–12.
138. Long BH, Musial ST, Brattain MG. Comparison of cytotoxicity and DNA breakage activity of congeners of podophyllotoxin including VP16–213 and VM26: a quantitative structure–activity relationship. Biochemistry 1984;23:1183–8.
139. Leteurtre F, Madalengoitia J, Orr A, et al. Rational design and molecular effects of a new topoisomerase II inhibitor, azatoxin [published erratum appears in Cancer Res 1992;52:6136]. Cancer Res 1992;52:4478–83.
140. Anyanwutaku IO, Guo X, Chen HX, et al. Activities of novel nonglycosidic epipodophyllotoxins in etoposide-sensitive and -resistant variants of human KB cells, P-388 cells, and in vivo multidrug-resistant murine leukemia cells. Mol Pharmacol 1996;49:721–6.
141. Macdonald TL, Lehnert EK, Loper JT, et al. On the mechanism of interaction of topoisomerase II with chemotherapeutic agents. In: Potmesil M, Kohn KW, editors. DNA topoisomerases in cancer. New York: Oxford University Press; 1991. p. 199–214.
142. Schacter LP, Igwemezie LN, Seyedsadr M, et al. Clinical and pharmacokinetic overview of parenteral etoposide phosphate. Cancer Chemother Pharmacol 1994;34:S58–63.
143. Slevin ML, Clark PI, Joel SP, et al. A randomized trial to evaluate the effect of schedule on the activity of etoposide in small-cell lung cancer. J Clin Oncol 1989;7:1333–40.
144. Arbuck SG, Douglass HO, Crom WR, et al. Etoposide pharmacokinetics in patients with normal and abnormal organ function. J Clin Oncol 1986;4:1690–5.
145. Stewart CF, Pieper JA, Arbuck SG, Evans WE. Altered protein binding of etoposide in patients with cancer. Clin Pharmacol Ther 1989;45:49–55.
146. Sinkule JA, Hutson P, Hayes FA, et al. Pharmacokinetics of etoposide (VP16) in children and adolescents with refractory solid tumors. Cancer Res 1984;44:3109–13.
147. Joel SP, Shah R, Slevin ML. Etoposide dosage and pharmacodynamics. Cancer Chemother Pharmacol 1994;34:S69–75.
148. Hande KR, Wolff SN, Greco FA, et al. Etoposide kinetics in patients with obstructive jaundice [see comments]. J Clin Oncol 1990;8:1101–7.
149. Leu BL, Huang JD. Inhibition of intestinal P-glycoprotein and effects on etoposide absorption. Cancer Chemother Pharmacol 1995;35:432–6.
150. Brandes AA, Rigon A, Zampieri P, et al. Carboplatin and teniposide concurrent with radiotherapy in patients with glioblastoma multiforme: a phase II study. Cancer 1998;82:355–61.
151. Petros WP, Rodman JH, Relling MV, et al. Variability in teniposide plasma protein binding is correlated with serum albumin concentrations. Pharmacotherapy 1992;12:273–7.
152. Clark PI, Slevin ML. The clinical pharmacology of etoposide and teniposide. Clin Pharmacokinet 1987;12:223–52.
153. O'Dwyer PJ, King SA, Fortner CL, Leyland-Jones B. Hypersensitivity reactions to teniposide (VM-26): an analysis. J Clin Oncol 1986;4:1262–9.
154. Wall ME, Wani MC. Camptothecin and Taxol: discovery to clinic. Thirteenth Bruce F. Cain memorial award lecture. Cancer Res 1995;55:753–60.
155. Hsiang Y, Hertzberg R, Hecht S, Liu LF. Camptothecin induces protein-linked DNA breaks via mammalian DNA topoisomerase I. J Biol Chem 1985;260:14873–8.
156. Muggia FM, Creaven PJ, Hansen JJ, et al. Phase I clinical trial of weekly and daily treatment with camptothecin (NSC-100880): correlation with preclinical studies. Cancer Chemother Rep 1972;56:515–21.
157. Moertel CG, Schutt AJ, Reitemeier RJ, Hahn RG. Phase II study of camptothecin (NSC-100880) in the treatment of advanced gastrointestinal cancer. Cancer Chemother Rep 1972;56:95–101.
158. Hertzberg RP, Carafana MJ, Holden KG, et al. Modification of the hydroxy lactone ring of camptothecin: inhibition of mammalian topoisomerase I and biological activity. J Med Chem 1989;32:715–20.
159. Jaxel C, Kohn KW, Wani MC, et al. Structure–activity study of the actions of camptothecin derivatives on mammalian topoisomerase I: evidence for a specific receptor site and a relation to antitumor activity. Cancer Res 1989;49:1465–9.
160. Wall ME, Wani MC, Natschke SM, Nicholas AW. Plant antitumor agents. 22. Isolation of 11-hydroxycamptothecin from *Camptotheca acuminata* Decne: total synthesis and biological activity. J Med Chem 1986;29:1553–5.
161. Pollack IF, Erff M, Bom D, et al. Potent topoisomerase I inhibition by novel silatecans eliminates glioma proliferation in vitro and in vivo. Cancer Res 1999;59:4898–905.
162. Wadkins RM, Potter PM, Vladu B, et al. Water soluble 20(*S*)-glycinate esters of 10,11-methylenedioxycamptothecins are highly active against human breast cancer xenografts. Cancer Res 1999;59:3424–8.
163. Bailly C. Homocamptothecins: potent topoisomerase I inhibitors and promising anticancer drugs. Crit Rev Oncol Hematol 2003;45:91–108.
164. ten Bokkel Huinink W, Gore M, Carmichael J, et al. Topotecan versus paclitaxel for the treatment of recurrent epithelial ovarian cancer [see comments]. J Clin Oncol 1997;15:2183–93.
165. Ardizzoni A, Hansen H, Dombernowsky P, et al. Topotecan, a new active drug in the second-line treatment of small-cell lung cancer: a phase II study in patients with refractory and sensitive disease. The European Organization for Research and Treatment of Cancer Early Clinical Studies Group and New Drug Development Office, and the Lung Cancer Cooperative Group. J Clin Oncol 1997;15:2090–6.
166. Hochster H, Liebes L, Speyer J, et al. Phase I trial of low-dose continuous topotecan infusion in patients with cancer: an active and well-tolerated regimen. J Clin Oncol 1994;12:553–9.
167. Markman M, Blessing JA, Alvarez Rd, et al. Phase II evaluation of 24 h continuous infusion topotecan in recurrent potentially platinum-sensitive ovarian cancer. A Gynecologic Oncology Group study. Gynecol Oncol 2000;77:122–5.
168. Rowinsky E, Grochow L, Hendricks C, et al. Phase I and pharmacologic study of topotecan: a novel topoisomerase I inhibitor. J Clin Oncol 1992;10:647–56.
169. Grochow LB, Rowinsky EK, Johnson R, et al. Pharmacokinetics and pharmacodynamics of topotecan in patients with advanced cancer. Drug Metab Dispos 1992;20:706–13.
170. O'Reilly S, Rowinsky EK, Slichenmyer W, et al. Phase I and pharmacologic study of topotecan in patients with impaired renal function [see comments]. J Clin Oncol 1996;14:3062–73.
171. O'Reilly S, Rowinsky E, Slichenmyer W, et al. Phase I and pharmacologic studies of topotecan in patients with impaired hepatic function. J Natl Cancer Inst 1996;88:817–24.
172. Kantarjian HM, Beran M, Ellis A, et al. Phase I study of topotecan, a new topoisomerase I inhibitor, in patients with refractory or relapsed acute leukemia. Blood 1993;81:1146–51.
173. Kano Y, Suzuki K, Akutsu M, et al. Effects of CPT-11 in combination with other anti-cancer agents in culture. Int J Cancer 1992;50:604–10.
174. Whitacre CM, Zborowska E, Gordon NH, et al. Topotecan increases topoisomerase IIa levels and sensitivity to treatment with etoposide in a schedule-dependent process. Cancer Res 1997;57:1425–8.
175. Gupta E, Toppmeyer D, Zamck R, et al. Clinical evaluation of sequential topoisomerase targeting in the treatment of advanced malignancy. Cancer Ther 1998;1:292–301.
176. Rowinsky EK, Kaufmann SH, Baker SD, et al. Sequences of topotecan and cisplatin: phase I, pharmacologic, and in vitro studies to examine sequence dependence. J Clin Oncol 1996;14:3074–84.
177. Tolcher AW, O'Shaughnessy JA, Weiss RB, et al. A phase I study of topotecan followed sequentially by doxorubicin in patients with advanced malignancy. Clin Cancer Res 1997;3:755–60.
178. Crump M, Lipton J, Hedley D, et al. Phase I trial of sequential topotecan followed by etoposide in adults with myeloid leukemia: a National Cancer Institute of Canada Clinical Trials Group Study. Leukemia 1999;13:343–7.
179. Wong ET, Berkenblit A. The role of topotecan in the treatment of brain metastases. Oncologist 2004;9:68–79.
180. Rothenberg ML, Eckardt JR, Kuhn JG, et al. Phase II trial of irinotecan in patients with progressive or rapidly recurrent colorectal cancer. J Clin Oncol 1996; 14:1128–35.
181. Rougier P, Bugat R, Douillard JY, et al. Phase II study of irinotecan in the treatment of advanced colorectal cancer in chemotherapy-naive patients and patients pre-treated with fluorouracil-based chemotherapy. J Clin Oncol 1997;15:251–60.

182. Thompson J, Stewart CF, Houghton PJ. Animal models for studying the action of topoisomerase I targeted drugs. Biochem Biophys Acta 1998;1400:301–19.
183. Ahmed F, Vyas V, Cornfield A, et al. In vitro activation of irinotecan to SN-38 by human liver and intestine. Anticancer Res 1999;19:2067–71.
184. Burke TG, Munshi CB, Mi Z, Jiang Y. The important role of albumin in determining the relative human blood stabilities of the camptothecin anticancer drugs. J Pharm Sci 1995;84:518–9.
185. Iyer L, King CD, Whitington PF, et al. Genetic predisposition to the metabolism of irinotecan (CPT-11). Role of uridine diphosphate glucuronosyltransferase isoform 1A1 in the glucuronidation of its active metabolite (SN-38) in human liver microsomes. J Clin Invest 1998;101:847–54.
186. Gupta E, Mick R, Ramirez J, et al. Pharmacokinetic and pharmacodynamic evaluation of the topoisomerase inhibitor irinotecan in cancer patients. J Clin Oncol 1997;15:1502–10.
187. Wasserman E, Myara A, Lokiec F, et al. Severe CPT-11 toxicity in patients with Gilbert's syndrome: two case reports. Ann Oncol 1997;8:1049–51.
188. Iyer L, Das S, Janisch L, et al. UGT1A1*28 polymorphism as a determinant of irinotecan disposition and toxicity. Pharmacogenomics J 2002;2:43–7.
189. Mathijssen RH, Marsh S, Karlsson MO, et al. Irinotecan pathway genotype analysis to predict pharmacokinetics. Clin Cancer Res 2003;9:3246–53.
190. Marcuello E, Altes A, Menoyo A, et al. UGT1A1 gene variations and irinotecan treatment in patients with metastatic colorectal cancer. Br J Cancer 2004;91:678–82.
191. Chu XY, Kato Y, Ueda K, et al. Biliary excretion mechanism of CPT-11 and its metabolites in humans: involvement of primary active transporters. Cancer Res 1998;58:5137–43.
192. Morton CL, Wadkins RM, Danks MK, Potter PM. The anticancer prodrug CPT-11 is a potent inhibitor of acetylcholinesterase but is rapidly catalyzed to SN-38 by butyrylcholinesterase. Cancer Res 1999;59:1458–63.
193. Pitot HC, Wender DB, O'Connell MJ, et al. Phase II trial of irinotecan in patients with metastatic colorectal carcinoma. J Clin Oncol 1997;15:2910–9.
194. Douillard JY, Cunningham D, Roth AD, et al. Trinotecan combined with fluorouracil compared with fluorouracil alone as first-line treatment for metastatic colorectal cancer: a muticenter randomised trial. Lancet 2000;355:1041–7.
195. Saltz LB, Cox JV, Blanke C, et al. Irinotecan plus fluorouracil and leucovorin for metastatic colorectal cancer. Irinotecan Study Group. N Engl J Med 2000;343:905–14.
196. Noda K, Nishiwaki Y, Kawahara M, et al. Irinotecan plus cisplatin compared with etoposide plus cisplatin for extensive small-cell lung cancer. N Engl J Med 2002;346:85–91.
197. Fukuoka M, Niitani H, Suzuki A, et al. A phase II study of CPT-11, a new derivative of camptothecin, for previously untreated non–small-cell lung cancer. J Clin Oncol 1992;10:16–20.
198. Masuda N, Matsui K, Negoro S, et al. Combination of irinotecan and etoposide for treatment of refractory or relapsed small-cell lung cancer. J Clin Oncol 1998;16:3329–34.
199. Kudoh S, Fujiwara Y, Takada Y, et al. Phase II study of irinotecan combined with cisplatin in patients with previously untreated small-cell lung cancer. West Japan Lung Cancer Group. J Clin Oncol 1998;16:1068–74.
200. Shirao K, Shimada Y, Kondo H, et al. Phase I–II study of irinotecan hydrochloride combined with cisplatin in patients with advanced gastric cancer. J Clin Oncol 1997;15:921–7.
201. Verschraegen CF, Levy T, Kudelka AP, et al. Phase II study of irinotecan in prior chemotherapy-treated squamous cell carcinoma of the cervix. J Clin Oncol 1997;15:625–31.

Microtubule-Targeting Natural Products

Eric K. Rowinsky, MD

The treatment of many diseases owes much to the importance of medicines that have been derived from natural sources, and the treatment of malignant disease is no exception. After several plant-derived compounds demonstrated prominent anticancer activity in patients with advanced malignancies in the 1950s and 1960s, the microtubule was recognized as a subcellular target of major strategic importance. The first widely used class of antimicrotubule agents, the vinca alkaloids, has been the mainstay of both palliative and curative regimens for treating both hematopoietic and lymphoid malignancies for several decades. The addition of the plant-derived taxanes, which possess a unique mechanism of antimicrotubule action and antitumor spectra, to our therapeutic arsenal several decades later has resulted in renewed interest in the microtubule as a target, as well as in the identification of other natural products, to treat cancers. More recently, a large number of plant- and marine-derived compounds with yet even more distinctive antimicrotubule and anticancer activities have been identified and are undergoing clinical evaluation. This chapter focuses on the microtubule as a target for therapeutic development, relevant antimicrotubule agents that play a major role in cancer therapeutics, particularly the vinca alkaloids and taxanes, and several new classes of antimicrotubule agents, such as the epothilones and other agents targeting kinesins, mitotic kinases, and other critical microtubule elements.

MICROTUBULES AS STRATEGIC TARGETS AGAINST CANCER

Microtubules are highly regulated and integral components of the cellular cytoskeleton that can be disrupted by the vinca alkaloids, taxanes, and an increasingly known number of natural products and synthetic compounds.[1–5] Although the most important functions of microtubules in proliferative cells are through their actions as components of the mitotic spindle, they are also involved in many other essential functions throughout the cell cycle of both malignant and nonmalignant cells, including intracellular transport, locomotion, adhesion, anchorage of subcellular organelles and receptors, and signal transduction and antimicrotubule agents may disrupt many of these essential functions.[1–6]

Microtubules are composed of dimeric subunits made up of α- and β-tubulin monomers, each of which consists of approximately 450 amino acids. Tubulin dimers assemble into microtubules by forming linear protofilaments.[1–6] Each microtubule is composed of 9 to 13 protofilaments that form a cylindrical wall around a hollow core, with the α-tubulin subunit of one dimer in contact with the β-tubulin subunit of the next, as shown in Figure 46-1. The microtubule has a distinct polarity, which is conferred by the alignment of protofilaments in parallel, with one end, termed the plus end at which assembly is rapid and net elongation occurs, and one end, termed the negative end, at which assembly is slow and net shortening occurs.

The unique functions of microtubules are related to their polymerization dynamics, involving a complex and dynamic equilibrium between an intracellular pool of α-β-tubulin dimers and the microtubule polymer, and a simultaneous release of the α-β-tubulin dimers into the soluble tubulin pool.[1–7] Tubulin polymerization occurs by a nucleation-elongation mechanism, in which the slow formation of a short microtubule "nucleus" is followed by rapid elongation of the microtubule at its ends by the reversible, noncovalent addition of α-β-tubulin dimers. The dynamic equilibrium between free α-β-tubulin dimers and the microtubule occurs simultaneously at both ends of the microtubule.[1,5–7] The assembly process utilizes energy provided by the hydrolysis of guanosine triphosphate (GTP).[8] Tubulin binds GTP with high affinity, and as tubulin-GTP is added to the ends of growing microtubules, GTP is gradually hydrolyzed to guanosine diphosphate (GDP) and P_i.[9] The P_i ultimately dissociates from the microtubule, leaving a microtubule core that consists of tubulin bound to GDP. The GDP nucleotide remains nonexchangeable until the tubulin subunit dissociates from the microtubule. Although tubulin polymerization and dissociation, and consequently microtubule elongation and shortening, occur simultaneously at each end, the net changes in length at the more kinetically dynamic plus end are much larger over time than those at the minus end. If the polymerization reaction is followed in vitro, an initial lag phase is noted, after which microtubules form rapidly until a plateau phase is reached. In the intact cell, microtubules usually grow from a specific nucleating site or the microtubule organizing complex (MTOC), which is located centrally near the nucleus and consists of a centrosome, a lattice of microtubule-associated proteins (MAPs), γ-tubulin, and a pair of centrioles.[10]

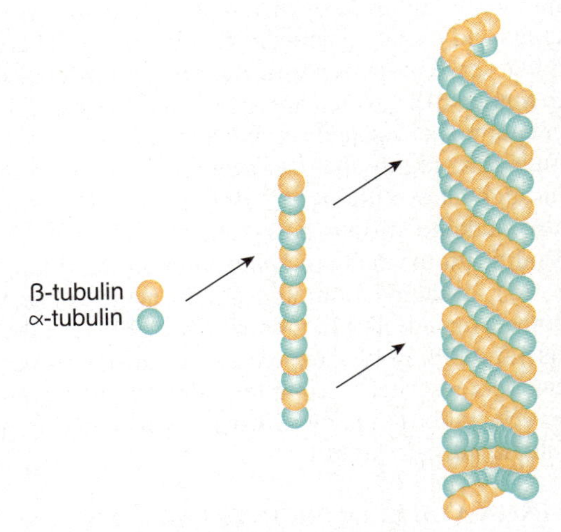

Figure 46-1 Schematic model of the α-β tubulin dimer with the monomers represented by shades of gray and white. The dimers associate linearly to form protofilaments that then in turn associate laterally to form the hollow cylindrical wall of the microtubule. Protofilaments can twist slowly around the microtubule axis, although these shown here are in parallel as in microtubules containing 13 protofilaments. Throughout most of the microtubule, lateral contacts involve α-α and β-β monomer interactions. Monomers of each type thus are in contact along a shallow spiral path around the microtubule.

Two principal processes govern microtubule dynamics in vivo.[1–7] The first, known as treadmilling, is the net growth at one end of the microtubule and the net shortening at the opposite end.[11] Treadmilling plays a role in many microtubule functions, especially the polar movement of the chromosomes during the anaphase stage of mitosis. The second dynamic process, termed dynamic instability, is a process in which the plus ends of microtubules switch spontaneously between states of slow sustained growth and rapid shortening.[11–14]

At the onset of mitosis, the interphase array of microtubules, which are attached to the MTOC by their minus ends with their plus ends radiating out toward the cell periphery, disassemble and are replaced by a new population of spindle microtubules that are much more dynamic.[2,12,15,16] As the spindle-shaped array of newly assembled microtubules is organized, the nuclear envelope breaks down and releases the now condensed chromosomes, and the centrosomes, which were duplicated before mitosis, separate into the poles of the forming mitotic spindle. The rate of dynamic instability is accelerated during mitosis, resulting in the formation and attachment of the mitotic spindles to the chromosomes. In most cells, mitosis progresses rapidly and the highly dynamic microtubules that comprise the mitotic spindle render them sensitive to the vinca alkaloids, taxanes, and other antimicrotubule agents.[3,12]

Dynamic instability and treadmilling are vital to the assembly and function of the mitotic spindle, and the high dynamaticity of mitotic spindle microtubules is required for the precise alignment of the chromosomes and their attachment to the spindle during metaphase, as well as chromosome separation during anaphase. These processes enable the microtubules of the mitotic spindle to make vast growing and shortening excursions, essentially probing the cytoplasm, until they become attached to a chromosome at its kinetochore. If even a single chromosome is unable to achieve a bipolar attachment to the spindle, perhaps because of drug-induced suppression of microtubule dynamics, the cell will not traverse beyond a prometaphase/metaphase-like state, which eventually triggers apoptosis. Although mitotic spindles can form in the presence of low concentrations of antimicrotubule agents, mitosis cannot progress beyond the mitotic checkpoint at the metaphase/anaphase transition or is delayed in this stage.[12,15] Such perturbations in mitotic spindle dynamics may delay cell-cycle progression at critical mitotic checkpoints, ultimately triggering apoptosis.[7,12,15] In the unperturbed normal state, oscillations of the duplicated chromosomes, dynamic instability, and microtubule treadmilling, in which there is addition of tubulin to the spindle at the kinetochore and loss of tubulin at the spindle poles, exert considerable tension on the chromosomes in metaphase and facilitate progression to anaphase.[17] In anaphase, microtubules that are attached to the chromosomes undergo shortening, while another subpopulation of microtubules called interpolar microtubules lengthen, resulting in polar movement of the chromosomes. Suppression of spindle-microtubule treadmilling and dynamic instability by antimicrotubule agents reduce spindle tension and impede progression from metaphase to anaphase, triggering cell death.[2–4,18,19]

The net direction of the dynamic equilibrium between the intracellular pool of tubulin and the microtubule polymer is influenced by several factors, including GTP, the ionic environment, cell-cycle modulators, and a family of proteins that regulate tubulin polymerization and microtubule function called microtubule-associated proteins (MAPs).[1,8,18,20] MAPs are partly responsible for the functional diversity of microtubules in different tissues. The major classes of MAPs include tau proteins (molecular weights, 40,000–60,000 daltons) and high-molecular-weight (200,000–300,000 daltons) proteins whose members include MAP1, MAPc (an adenosine triphosphatase [ATPase]), MAP2, MAP4, and the motor proteins dynein (a GTPase) and kinesin (an ATPase). Both classes of MAPs possess two binding domains, one of which binds to microtubules. Since this domain also binds to free tubulin molecules simultaneously, MAPs facilitate the initial nucleation step of tubulin polymerization. The other domain may be involved in linking the microtubule to other cellular constituents. Some MAPs, such as the dyneins and kinesins, function as microtubule motors, transmitting chemical energy to mechanical force and moving various solutes and subcellular organelles along the microtubule.[1,18] Motor proteins play critical roles in mitosis, premeiotic events, and organelle transport, and are being evaluated as strategic targets for anticancer therapeutic development.[20,21]

Catharanthine nucleus

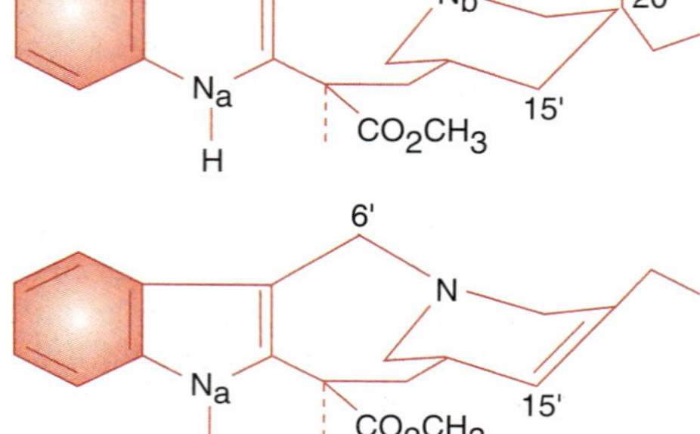

	R_1	R_2	R_3
Vindesine	$-CH_3$	$-CONH_2$	$-OH$
Vincristine	$-CHO$	$-CO_2CH_3$	$-OCOCH_3$
Vinblastine	$-CH_3$	$-CO_2CH_3$	$-OCOCH_3$
Vinorelbine	$-CH_3$	$-CO_2CH_3$	$-OCOCH_3$

Vindoline nucleus

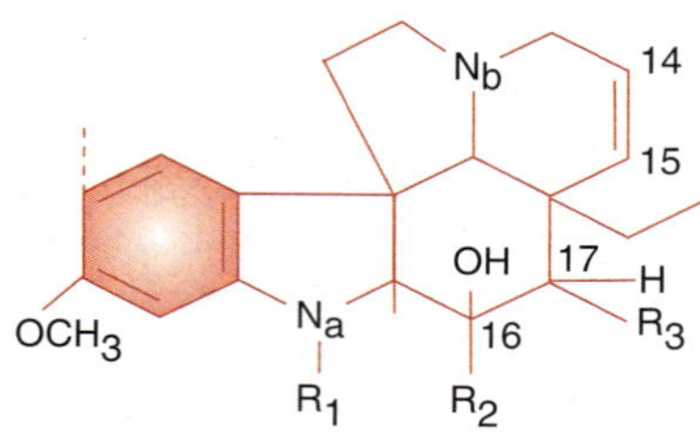

Figure 46-2 Chemical structures of the vinca alkaloids.

In addition to MAPs, the functional diversity of microtubules among various tissues and tumors is conferred by differences in tubulin isotypes and post-translational modifications. There are at least six isotypes of both α- and β-tubulin in human cells, which are distinguished by different amino acid sequences and encoded by a large, multigene family that has been highly conserved throughout evolution.[22–25] Both forms of tubulin also undergo various post-translational chemical modifications, including phosphorylation, tyrosination, glutamylation, and others, which confer both structural and functional diversity.[26] Analysis of tubulin isotype expression in various tissues has demonstrated a complex, albeit highly conserved, pattern of isotype distribution, suggesting functional specificity.

VINCA ALKALOIDS: INTRODUCTION AND INDICATIONS

The vinca alkaloids are naturally occurring or semisynthetic nitrogenous bases extracted from the pink periwinkle plant *Catharanthus roseus* G. Don.[27–29] The early medicinal uses of this plant led to the screening of these compounds for their hypoglycemic activity, which was of little importance compared with their cytotoxic effects. Many vinca alkaloids have been extensively evaluated, but only vincristine (VCR), vinblastine (VBL), and vinorelbine (VRL) are approved for use in the United States. The vinca alkaloids have dimeric structures composed of two basic multiringed units (Figure 46-2), an indole nucleus (catharanthine), and a dihydroindole nucleus (vindoline), joined together with other complex systems. Structurally, VCR and VBL are identical except for a single substitution on the vindoline nucleus, where VCR and VBL possess formyl and methyl groups, respectively. Although this minor difference does not fundamentally alter the mechanisms and tubulin-binding properties of these agents, the antitumor and toxicologic profiles of VCR and VBL differ significantly.[27,28,30–32]

VCR is used more commonly to treat pediatric malignancies, which likely reflects a higher level of sensitivity of pediatric malignancies to VCR and better tolerance of therapeutic VCR doses in children. In both children and adults, however, VCR is an essential component of the chemotherapy regimens used to treat acute lymphocytic leukemia, lymphoid blast crisis of chronic myeloid leukemia, and both Hodgkin's and non-Hodgkin's lymphomas. VCR also plays a role in some multimodality therapies of Wilms' tumor, Ewing's sarcoma, neuroblastoma, and rhabdomyosarcoma, as well as in the treatment of multiple myeloma, particularly as a component of the VAD regimen (VCR, doxorubicin, and doxorubicin), small-cell lung cancer, and soft-tissue and bone sarcomas.[29] In addition, VCR has been reported to be effective in treating nonmalignant immunologically-mediated hematologic disorders such as refractory autoimmune thrombocytopenia, hemolytic uremic syndrome, and thrombotic thrombocytopenia purpura.[27–29]

VBL has been a mainstay component of chemotherapy regimens for germ cell malignancies and some types of advanced lymphomas.[29] Until recently, a regimen termed PVB, consisting of cisplatin, VBL, and bleomycin, was the standard therapy for advanced germ cell carcinomas.[23] However, VBL has largely been replaced by etoposide in this combination, particularly in patients with favorable disease characteristics, because of the more favorable toxicity profile of the cisplatin-etoposide regimen. For Hodgkin's lymphoma, VBL is often used in combination with doxorubicin, bleomycin, and dacarbazine (ABVD). This regimen is either administered alone or alternated with MOPP (nitrogen mustard, VCR, procarbazine, and prednisone), which is non–cross-resistant to ABVD.[29] A MOPP/ABV hybrid regimen that includes both VCR and VBL has also been extensively studied. Antineoplastic activity is also observed with VBL as a single agent or in combination with other antineoplastic drugs in carcinomas of the breast, bladder, and lung, Kaposi's sarcoma, choriocarcinoma, terminal phase of chronic myelogenous leukemia, mycosis fungoides, Letterer-Siwe disease (histiocytosis X), and choriocarcinomas that are resistant to other chemotherapy agents.[29] Infusions of VBL or VBL-loaded platelets have been effective in some cases of refractory autoimmune thrombocytopenia because of its avidity to platelets.[29] VBL has also been used alone or in combination with other agents to treat Kaposi's sarcoma and bladder, breast, and some types of central nervous system malignancies.

The semisynthetic VBL derivative vinorelbine (5'-norhydro VBL; VRL), which is structurally modified on its catharanthine nucleus, resulting in substantially greater lipophilicity as compared with the other vinca alkaloids, is approved in the United States for treating non–small cell lung cancer as either a single agent or in combination with cisplatin, and has been registered to treat patients with advanced breast cancer elsewhere.[29,33–37] The agent has also demonstrated relevant clinical activity in advanced ovarian carcinoma and lymphoma, but a unique role in the treatment of these cancers has not been defined. VRL has also been demonstrated to confer high therapeutic indices to patients with advanced breast and lung cancers who are elderly or have diminished performance abilities.[29,33–37]

Another widely studied vinca alkaloid, vindesine (VDS, desacetyl VBL caroxyamide), a semisynthetic derivative and human metabolite of VBL, was introduced in the 1970s.[29,31,32] In some reports, response rates in non–small-cell lung cancer with combinations of VDS and cisplatin or mitomycin appear to be superior to those achieved with standard combinations or with either agent alone.[29,31,32] In addition, antineoplastic activity has been seen in acute lymphocytic leukemia, blast crisis of chronic myeloid leukemia, malignant melanoma, pediatric solid tumors, and metastatic renal, breast, esophageal, and colorectal carcinomas; however, a unique role for VDS in oncology remains to be defined. Recently, vinflunine, which is a novel bifluorinated vinca alkaloid that appears to have unique antitumor and toxicity properties, has demonstrated notable clinical activity in bladder and other cancers.[38,39]

Mechanism of Action The vinca alkaloids principally induce cytotoxicity by disrupting microtubule function, particularly affecting microtubules comprising the mitotic spindle apparatus, leading to metaphase arrest.[2–4,6,12,27–29,40–46] However, they are also capable of many other biochemical activities that may or may not be related to their effects on microtubules, including inhibiting synthesis of proteins and nucleic acids, elevating oxidized glutathione, altering lipid metabolism and membrane lipids, elevating cyclic adenosine monophosphate (cAMP), and inhibiting calcium–calmodulin-regulated cAMP phosphodiesterase.[46] Many of the effects that do not involve microtubule disruption occur only after treatment with superpharmacological concentrations, whereas nanomolar concentrations, which are readily achievable in clinical practice, induce typical antimicrotubule effects. The vinca alkaloids also disrupt the structural integrity of platelets and other nonmalignant cells, which are rich in tubulin and depend on microtubules for structure. In addition to mitotic disruption, the vinca alkaloids and other antimicrotubule agents affect cells in nonmitotic cell-cycle phases, which is not surprising because microtubules are involved in many nonmitotic functions.[29,45,46]

The vinca alkaloids bind rapidly and reversibly to sites on tubulin (called the vinca domain), which are distinct from those of the taxanes, colchicine, podophyllotoxin, and GTP, but similar to those of maytansine and other plant alkaloids.[2,5–7,28,29,38,39,41,43,44,47,48] The vinca alkaloids appear to bind to two microtubule binding sites with different affinities.[1,2,4,5,12,38,39,43,44,48–53] High-affinity sites (K_d, 1–2 μmol) are at the ends of microtubule, whereas low-affinity sites (K_d, 0.25–3.0 mmol) are along the sides. Binding of the vinca alkaloids to the high-affinity sites is responsible for the potent suppression of tubulin exchange at low concentrations (< 1 μmol). At low concentrations, microtubule dynamics (treadmilling and dynamic instability) are disrupted, but microtubule mass is not affected. The overall result is a potent mitotic block at the metaphase/anaphase boundary. Binding of the vinca alkaloids to low-affinity sites appears to be responsible for reduced microtubule mass due to tubulin depolymerization and the splaying of microtubules into spiral aggregates or spiral protofilaments that form paracrystals, ultimately leading to microtubule disintegration. These effects occur at high drug concentrations (> 1 to 2 μmol) by a self-propagated mechanism, initially involving drug binding to a limited number of sites, which progressively weakens the lateral interactions between the protofilaments, thereby exposing new sites.

The vinca alkaloids induce a potent block in mitosis at the metaphase/anaphase transition.[2,45,54] Following nuclear envelop breakdown, the vinca alkaloids block mitotic spindle formation and reduce the tension at the kinetochores of the chromosomes. Although chromosomes may condense, they remain scattered in the cells. The chromosomes separate along their lengths, but still remain attached at their centromeres.[2,12,16,19,45,46,55] Mitotic progress is delayed in a metaphase-like state with chromosomes "stuck" at the spindle poles, unable to move to the spindle equator. The cell-cycle signal to the anaphase-promoting complex, which is required for the cell to transition from metaphase to anaphase, is blocked and the cells eventually undergo apoptosis. Cell-cycle progression in the absence of anaphase or cytokinesis may occur, resulting in chromatin decondensation and formation of multilobed nuclei.[2,12,19] Disruption of spindle microtubule dynamics without microtubule depolymerization ultimately leads to apoptosis, which involves the inactivation of anti-apoptotic proteins and activation of proapoptotic genes (see, in the section "Taxanes" below, "Mechanism of Action" and "Mechanisms of Resistance").[2,12,16,17,19,38,39,55–58] The induction of apoptosis, however, does not depend on the presence of an intact TP53 checkpoint.[17,56,57,59] The loss of p21, a protein that controls entry into mitosis at the G_2/M checkpoint, enhances sensitivity of tumor cells to both vinca alkaloids and taxanes, possibly by hastening entry of drug-damaged cells into mitosis.[17,56–58]

The relationships between the effects of vinca alkaloids on cell proliferation, mitotic arrest, mitotic spindle disruption, and depolymerization of microtubules have been characterized in a series of studies that indicate that the drug concentration that inhibits cell proliferation is directly related to the concentration that induces metaphase arrest.[45] The inhibition of proliferation and blockage of cells in metaphase at the lowest effective drug concentrations occur with little or no microtubule depolymerization or disorganization of the mitotic spindle apparatus. With increasing drug concentrations, the organization of microtubules and chromosomes in arrested mitotic spindles deteriorates in a manner that is similar for most antimicrotubule agents.[2,3,12,13]

In addition to their direct cytotoxic effects on tumor cells, the vinca alkaloids, taxanes, and other antimicrotubule agents inhibit angiogenesis with surprising potency.[60] However, the relative contribution of these antiangiogenic effects to the clinical antitumor activity of the vinca alkaloids is unclear.

The disparate sensitivity of various tissues and tumors to the vinca alkaloids is multifactorial. One possible explanation is the differential sensitivity of tissues with varying tubulin isotype composition, which may affect intracellular drug accumulation and binding to tubulin binding.[24,61] In addition, differences in the type and concentration of MAPs and post-translational tubulin modifications, which may influence drug interactions with tubulin, as well as variability in cellular permeability and retention, may affect the formation and stability of complexes formed between the vinca alkaloids and tubulin. Other putative factors include differences in the tissue GTP content, rates of GTP hydrolysis, and cellular permeability.[61–76]

Mechanisms of Resistance In most preclinical models, resistance to the vinca alkaloids develops rapidly and is associated with decreased drug accumulation and retention. At least two major mechanisms of resistance to the vinca alkaloids have been characterized in tissue-culture experiments. The first mechanism typifies the "classic" pleiotropic or multidrug-resistant (MDR) phenotype that can be either innate (primary) or acquired. Although many proteins that mediate MDR have been characterized, the most well known are the ATP-binding cassette (ABC) transporters that belong to the largest known transporter gene family and translocate a wide range of substrates across cellular compartments.[77] These intracellular and extracellular membrane-spanning proteins, which transport both endobiotics and xenobiotics, confer resistance to the vinca alkaloids and other structurally bulky natural products in vitro. The best characterized ABC transporters responsible for drug resistance are the permeability glycoproteins (Pgp) or the *MDR1* encoded gene product MDR1 (ABC Subfamily B1) and the multidrug resistance protein (MRP; ABC Subfamily C2).[77]

MDR1 is a 170-kDa Pgp energy-dependent transmembrane pump that regulates the efflux of a wide range of bulky hydrophobic substances.[77] The protein is constitutively overexpressed in various normal tissues, which include renal tubule epithelium, colonic mucosa, and adrenal medulla, as well as tumors derived from these tissues. Pgp, an ATPase, functions to bind and extrude the vinca alkaloids from the tumor cell in a process that requires energy in the form of adenosine triphosphate (ATP). The MDR phenotype also confers varying degrees of cross-resistance to other structurally bulky natural products such as the taxanes, anthracyclines, epipodophyllotoxins, and colchicine; however, resistance is most prominent against the principal agent in which selection pressure was established in vitro. The specific Pgp associated with vinca alkaloid resistance shows slight antigenic and amino acid sequence differences and a different amino acid map after digestion than does Pgp from cells selected for resistance to colchicines or taxanes.[78–81] In fact, two forms of the protein have been demonstrated to be produced by a single clone of VCR-resistant cells, and these forms undergo post-translational *N*-glycosylation and phosphorylation, which leads to further structural diversity and may explain the greater degree of resistance for the specific agent used compared with the resistance of other drugs conferred by MDR, and may also account for the variable patterns of resistance among MDR cells. The clinical ramifications of this resistance mechanism are not known; however, VCR resistance measured in vitro did not correlate with Pgp overexpression in one study in childhood acute lymphoblastic leukemia.[82]

MRP1, a 190 kD membrane-spanning protein that shares 15% amino acid homology with MDR1, also confers resistance to the vinca alkaloids in vitro.[30,77,83-86] MRP1 expression has been found in many types of tumors and has been implicated as a component of the MDR phenotype in cancers of the lung, colon, breast, bladder, and prostate, as well as leukemia. MRP1 transports glutathione conjugates of alkylating agents and several types of xenobiotics such as etoposide and doxorubicin, but only confers resistance to the latter agents. The MRP1 resistance profile also includes the vinca alkaloids and methotrexate.[30,77,83–86] Although many other ABC transporters have been identified and several confer cellular resistance to the vinca alkaloids in vitro, their roles in conferring inherent or acquired drug resistance in the clinic are even less clear than those of MDR1 and MRP1.

Drug resistance conferred by MDR1 and MRP in vitro is reversible after treatment with various agents that have distinctly different structural and functional characteristics, such as the calcium-channel blockers, calmodulin inhibitors, detergents, progestational and antiestrogenic agents, antibiotics, antihypertensives, antiarrhythmics, antimalarials, and immunosuppressives, which has become a source of clinical interest.[30,77,87,88] These reversal agents bind directly to Pgp, thereby blocking the efflux of the cytotoxic drugs and increasing intracellular drug concentrations. However, clinical studies of resistance modulation have been confounded by the fact that MDR modulators, particularly MDR1 reversal agents, also enhance drug uptake in normal cells, decrease biliary elimination and drug clearance, and lead to enhanced toxicity.[30,77,87,88] Overall, strategies aimed at reversing resistance to the vinca alkaloids in the clinic with pharmacologic modulators of both MDR1 and MRP have been disappointing, most likely owing to the fact that the *MDR1* expression is capable of producing a large number of alternate resistance proteins.[77]

Structural and functional alterations in α- and β-tubulins, resulting from either genetic mutations, post-translational modifications, or differential expression of tubulin isotypes, particularly the β-III isotype of β-tubulin, have also been identified in tumor cells with resistance to the vinca alkaloids.[89–95] Vinca alkaloid resistance, which results in increased microtubule stability, is also associated with increased expression of MAPs, particularly MAP4.[96] Alterations in α- and β-tubulin promote resistance to agents that inhibit microtubule assembly by enhancing microtubule stability, possibly by promoting longitudinal interdimer and intradimer interactions and/or lateral interactions between protofilaments. Furthermore, these "hyperstable" microtubules are collaterally sensitive to the taxanes (see in the section "Taxanes" below, "Mechanisms of Resistance"). Although such tubulin modifications have been demonstrated repeatedly in tumor cells that are continuously exposed to the vinca alkaloids in vitro, the relevance of "hyperstable tubulin" caused by alterations in tubulins or MAPs is not known.

Variability in cellular permeation and retention may also influence the formation and stability of vinca alkaloid-tubulin complexes.[38,39,65–67,69–74] The vinca alkaloids are rapidly taken up into cells and then accumulate intracellularly, with intracellular to extracellular concentrations ratios as high as 5- to 500-fold, depending on the cell type.[65,66] In murine leukemia cells, the intracellular concentrations of VCR are 5- to 20-fold higher than the extracellular concentrations, and ratios ranging from 150- to 500-fold have been reported with other vinca alkaloids.[66,67,97] There are also marked differences in cellular uptake and retention between the vinca alkaloids, the latter of which may relate to potency and the duration of drug action. For example, VRL is more rapidly taken up and metabolized than other vinca alkaloids in isolated human hepatocytes,[74] and the greater potency of VCR during exposures of short duration compared with VBL was related to the greater cellular retention of VCR in another model system. An important determinant of drug accumulation and retention is lipophilicity. The differences in the catharanthine ring of VRL render it a more lipophilic agent and increase its retention in tissues, which may explain why it is more effective at disrupting the microtubules of the mitotic spindles compared with axonal microtubules.[73] The differential effects of the vinca alkaloids on axonal microtubules due to variable cellular retention and lipophilicity may explain why VRL treatment results in less neurotoxicity than other vinca alkaloids. The mechanisms responsible for the intracellular accumulation of the vinca alkaloids and other agents that bind to tubulin are not fully known, but may relate to their tubulin-binding properties and several other factors. Differential drug uptake among different tumor types may also relate to tubulin isotype expression, differential uptake, efflux pump mechanisms, and intracellular reservoirs for drug accumulation.

Pharmacology **Cellular Pharmacology** Temperature-independent, nonsaturable mechanisms, analogous to simple diffusion, most likely account for most transport of the vinca alkaloids, and temperature-dependent saturable processes are less important.[74] Although the drug concentration and duration of treatment are important determinants of both drug accumulation and cytotoxicity, the duration of drug exposure above a critical threshold concentration is perhaps the most important determinant of cytotoxicity.[65,76] Cytotoxicity is directly related to the extracellular concentration of drug when the duration of treatment is kept constant; for prolonged exposure to VCR, the concentration yielding 50% inhibition lies in the range of 1 to 5 nmol/L.[76]

Clinical Pharmacology ***General*** Information about the clinical pharmacology of the vinca alkaloids, which were largely studied

Table 46-1 Vinca Alkaloids: Comparative Pharmacokinetic and Toxicologic Characteristics

	Vincristine	Vinblastine	Vindesine	Vinorelbine
Standard adult dose range (mg/m^2/wk)	1–2	6–8	3–4	15–30
Pharmacokinetic behavior	Triphasic	Triphasic	Triphasic	Triphasic
Plasma half-lives				
α (minutes)	< 5	< 5	< 5	< 5
β (minutes)	50–155	53–99	55–99	49–168
γ (hours)	23–85	20–64	20–24	18–49
Clearance (L/h/kg)	0.16	0.74	0.25	0.4–1.29
Primary route	Hepatic metabolism and biliary elimination	Hepatic metabolism and biliary elimination	Hepatic metabolism and biliary elimination	Hepatic metabolism and biliary elimination
Principal toxicity	Neurotoxicity	Neutropenia	Neutropenia	Neutropenia
Other toxicities	Constipation, SIADH	Alopecia neurotoxicity, mucositis	Alopecia, neurotoxicity	Neurotoxicity vomiting, constipation, mucositis

SIADH = syndrome of inappropriate secretion of antidiuretic hormone.

decades ago, must take into account the fact that sensitive, specific, and reliable analytic assays capable of measuring the minute plasma concentrations resulting from the administration of milligram quantity doses were not available. Pharmacologic studies were performed initially with radiolabeled drugs; however, interpretation of the results has been confounded by the chemical instability of these agents. Several vinca alkaloids, particularly VCR and VBL, may undergo spontaneous degradation under mild conditions, forming degradative products that can be separated using high-pressure liquid chromatography (HPLC).[96] Radiolabeled compounds coupled to HPLC were later used for improved separation of the various chemical moieties. More recently, radioimmunoassay (RIA) and enzyme-linked immunosorbent assay (ELISA) methods using antisera capable of detecting picomolar drug concentrations have been developed; however, polyclonal antisera raised against the vinca alkaloids cannot distinguish between the parent compounds and related derivatives, and, therefore, may not provide sufficient quantitative information about degradation products and metabolites. To meet the challenge, more refined RIA and ELISA methods using monoclonal antibodies with considerably greater sensitivity and specificity have been developed. Furthermore, recent technical advances in extraction and detection methodologies have increased the sensitivity and specificity of chromatographic methods. For example, tandem mass spectroscopy in conjunction with HPLC has greatly enhanced the sensitivity and specificity of chromographic methods.

Table 46-1 summarizes the pharmacokinetic characteristics of the vinca alkaloids. The vinca alkaloids generally exhibit triphasic clearance from plasma following intravenous administration as a bolus infusion or brief injection. The pharmacokinetic behavior of these agents is typified by large volumes of distribution, high early clearance rates, long terminal half-lives, extensive hepatic metabolism, and biliary/fecal elimination. The relatively short α and β distribution phases, which are likely a result of rapid distribution and uptake into peripheral tissues and formed blood elements, are similar for all vinca alkaloids. However, the terminal (γ) phase, which is relatively long because of the avid tissue sequestration and slow release of drug, has been reported to differ by approximately four-fold.

Vincristine VCR is rapidly distributed to the peripheral compartment following administration. There is extensive binding to both plasma proteins and formed blood elements, particularly platelets, which contain large quantities of tubulin. This served as the rationale for using VCR-loaded platelets for treating disorders of platelet consumption such as idiopathic thrombocytopenia purpura.[29] In contrast, penetration of VCR across the blood-brain barrier is poor, probably because of the molecule's large size and is an avid substrate for ABC transporter pumps that maintain the integrity of the blood brain barrier. Following administration of conventional doses (1.4 mg/m^2), given as a brief intravenous infusion, peak plasma levels approach 0.4 μmol.[29,67,75,98–102] Total VCR clearance is slow, which reflects avid tissue binding and slow release, and terminal half-lives in the range of 23 to 85 hours have been reported.[29,67,75,98–102] VCR is metabolized and excreted primarily by the hepatobiliary system. Seventy-two hours after the administration of radiolabeled VCR, approximately 12% of the radioactivity is recovered in the urine (50% of which consists of metabolites), and approximately 70% is recovered from feces (40% of which consists of metabolites).[29,67,75,76,98–104] As many as 6 to 11 metabolites have been detected in studies performed in both humans and animals.[105] The structures of most, however, have not been identified. The metabolites, 4-deacetylVCR, and both 4'-deoxy-3'-hydroxyVCR and 3',4'- epoxyVCR *N*-oxide have been identified after incubation of VCR with bile.[29,67,75,76,96,98–105] The nature of the VCR metabolites identified to date, such as 4-deacetylVCR and *N*-deformylVCR, which have been isolated from human bile, and 4'-deoxy-3'-hydroxyVCR and 3',4'- epoxyVCR *N*-oxide following incubation of VCR with bile, indicate that the agent is principally metabolized by hepatic cytochrome P-450 CYP3A. There has been conflicting, albeit sparse, evidence that peak plasma concentration and systemic exposure are major pharmacologic determinants of VCR-induced neurotoxicity.[106]

Vinblastine The pharmacologic behavior of VBL is similar to that of VCR.[29,67,75,107] Following rapid intravenous injection of VBL at standard doses, peak plasma drug concentrations are approximately 0.4 μmol/L. Tissue distribution is also extensive. Like VCR, binding of VBL to plasma proteins and formed elements of blood is considerable. Furthermore, distribution is rapid, with half-life values of approximately 4 minutes and 1.6 hours for α and β phases, respectively. Terminal half-life values ranging from 20 to 24 hours have been reported. Like VCR, VBL disposition is principally through the hepatobiliary system. The principal mode of VBL disposition is hepatic metabolism and biliary excretion. Fecal excretion of the parent compound is low, indicating that metabolism is substantial. The cytochrome P-450 CYP3A isoform appears to be principally responsible for its biotransformation.[74] At least one metabolite, 4-deacetylVBL, or VDS, which appears to be as active as the parent compound, has been identified in humans, and small quantities have been detected in both urine and feces.

Vinorelbine The pharmacologic behavior of VRL is similar to those of the other vinca alkaloids, and plasma concentrations decline in a biexponential or triexponential manner. Immediately following intravenous administration, plasma concentrations decline rapidly followed by much slower elimination phases ($t_{1/2\gamma}$, 18–49 h).[29,35,36,108,109] Plasma protein binding has been reported to range from 80% to 91%, with binding primarily to α_1-acid glycoprotein, albumin, and lipoproteins.

VRL is widely distributed with extensive sequestration in virtually all tissues, except brain. The drug is also extensively bound to platelets. The wide distribution of VRL may reflect the agent's lipophilicity, which is among the highest of the vinca alkaloids. Tissue to plasma ratios range from 20 to 80, although VRL concentrations in human lung have been reported to be 300-fold greater than plasma concentrations and 3.4- to 13.8-fold higher than lung concentrations achieved with VDS and VCR, respectively. Hepatic metabolism and biliary excretion of metabolites and VRL are the predominant modes of drug disposition.[29,35,36,108,109] Approximately 33 to 80% of the administered dose of VRL is excreted into the feces, whereas urinary excretion represents only 16 to 30% of total drug disposition, the majority of which is metabolized VRL. Cytochrome P-450 isoform CYP3A is principally involved in biotransformation in humans.[35,37,110–115] The principal metabolites appear to be 4-*O*-deacetyl-VRL, 3,6-epoxy-VRL, and several hydroxy-VRL isomers. Most metabolites are inactive. Although 4-*O*-deacetyl-VRL may be as active as VRL, this finding is of minor importance since concentrations are minute.

The total body clearance of VRL (1.2 L/hour/kg) and $t_{1/2}\gamma$ values of approximately 26 hours were found to be the same in elderly and younger patients with normal hepatic function in one study.[114] Clearance has been found to be adversely affected in patients who have liver metastases that involve more than 75% of the organ; clearance can be predicted in such patients by the monoethylglycinexylidide clearance test, which assesses CYP3A4 function.[115] Although VRL clearance is not accurately predicted by bilirubin concentrations in serum, markedly elevated levels have been associated with significant reductions in clearance in the few patients studied.

VRL is active when given orally. In animal studies, 100% of total radioactivity is absorbed after the ingestion of tritium-labeled VRL, whereas human studies using powder-filled, liquid-filled, and gelatin-filled capsules have shown that the bioavailability of the parent compound is 43% for the powder-filled and 27% for the liquid-filled capsules; the bioavailability of the gel-filled capsule was negligibly affected by food.[108,116,117] C_{peak} values are achieved within 1 to 2 hours after oral treatment, and interindividual variability is moderate.

Drug Interactions The vinca alkaloids, particularly VCR and VBL, have been demonstrated to enhance methotrexate accumulation in tumor cells in vitro, an effect mediated by a vinca alkaloid-induced blockade of drug efflux; however, the minimal drug concentrations of VCR required to achieve this effect (0.1 µmol/L) are achieved transiently in vivo.[118–120] The vinca alkaloids also inhibit the cellular influx and cytotoxicity of the epipodyllotoxins in vitro, but the clinical ramifications of this effect are unknown.[121] L-asparaginase may reduce the hepatic clearance of the vinca alkaloids, particularly VCR, which may result in increased toxicity. To minimize the possibility of this interaction, it is recommended that VCR be given 12 to 24 hours before L-asparaginase.

Treatment with the vinca alkaloids has precipitated seizures associated with subtherapeutic plasma phenytoin concentrations, most likely due to the induction of CYP3A-mediated clearance of phenytoin.[122–125] Reduced plasma phenytoin levels have been noted from 24 hours to 10 days after treatment with both VCR and VBL. Administration of the vinca alkaloids with erythromycin, itraconazole, and other pharmacologic inhibitors of CYP3A may lead to severe toxicity.[122,126] Concomitantly administered drugs, such as pentobarbital and H_2-receptor antagonists, may also influence VCR clearance by modulating hepatic cytochrome P-450 metabolic processes.[122,127] Another potential drug interaction may occur in patients who have Kaposi's sarcoma related to acquired immunodeficiency syndrome and are receiving concurrent treatment with 3' azido-3'-deoxythymidine (AZT) and the vinca alkaloids, as the vinca alkaloids may inhibit glucuronidation of AZT to its 5'-O-glucuronide metabolite.[128] Based on a report of a constellation of severe toxicities, including syndrome of inappropriate secretion of antidiuretic hormone (SIADH), bilateral cranial nerve palsies, peripheral neuropathy, cranial nerve palsies, heart failure, and cardiovascular effects following VCR treatment in pediatric patients with acute lymphocytic leukemia who had been receiving treatment with nifedipine and itraconazole, it is possible that these medications may enhance the neurologic and cardiovascular effects of the vinca alkaloids.[127] Lastly, the significant interindividual and intraindividual variability of VCR pharmacokinetics in children has been attributed to the variable induction of P-450 metabolism due to concurrent use of P-450-inducing corticosteroids.[124,125]

The use of mitomycin C in combination with the vinca alkaloids has been associated with pulmonary toxicity as described in the section "Toxicity" below, "Miscellaneous."

Toxicity The principal toxicities of the vinca alkaloids differ despite their structural and pharmacologic similarities. Peripheral neurotoxicity is the predominant toxicity of VCR, whereas myelosuppression predominates with VBL, VDS, and VRL. Nevertheless, peripheral neurotoxicity is often noted following cumulative treatment with VBL, VDS, and VRL, inadvertent high-dose treatment, and in patients who are inherently susceptible (see section on Neurotoxicity). Nevertheless, VCR can cause myelosuppression under the similar conditions.

Neurotoxicity Although the vinca alkaloids are similar from a structural standpoint, their toxicologic profiles differ significantly. All of the vinca alkaloids induce a characteristic peripheral neurotoxicity, but VCR is most potent in this regard. The neurotoxicity is principally characterized by a peripheral, symmetric mixed sensory-motor, and autonomic polyneuropathy.[28,32,37,129–132] The primary pathologic effect is axonal degeneration and decreased axonal transport, most likely caused by a drug-induced perturbation of microtubule function. At onset, only symmetric sensory impairment and paresthesia in a length-dependent manner (distal extremities first) is often encountered. Neuritic pain and loss of deep tendon reflexes may develop with continued treatment, which may be followed by foot drop, wrist drop, motor dysfunction, ataxia, and paralysis. Back, bone, and limb pains may occur. Electrophysiologic studies typically reveal normal nerve conduction velocities; however, diminished amplitude of sensory and motor nerve action potentials and prolonged distal latencies, resembling axonal degeneration, may be noted.[28,32,37,129–132] Rarely, cranial nerves are affected, resulting in hoarseness, diplopia, jaw pain, facial palsies, and laryngeal paralysis.[133] The uptake of VCR into the brain is low, and central nervous system effects, such as confusion, mental status changes, depression, hallucinations, agitation, insomnia, seizures, coma, SIADH, and visual disturbances, may occur in rare situations.[37,134,135] Acute, severe autonomic neurotoxicity is uncommon, but may arise as a consequence of high-dose therapy (greater than 2 mg/m^2) or in patients with diminished drug clearance because of altered hepatic function.[131,132,134–139] Toxic manifestations of autonomic neurotoxicity include constipation, abdominal cramps, paralytic ileus, urinary retention, orthostatic hypotension, and hypertension.[131,132,134–139]

In adults treated with VCR, the neurotoxic effects may begin with cumulative doses as little as 5 to 6 mg, and manifestations may be profound after cumulative doses of 15 to 20 mg. Although it has been remarked that children are less susceptible to neurotoxicity than adults, and that the elderly are particularly prone, these apparent age-related differences may, in fact, be caused by previously inaccurate dose calculation using body weight in children and adults and using body surface area in infants.[133,140] In infants, VCR doses are calculated now according to body weight, which may be more accurate from a pharmacologic standpoint because of ubiquitous tissue distribution. Patients with antecedent neurologic disorders, such as Charcot-Marie-Tooth disease, hereditary and sensory neuropathy type I, Guillain-Barré syndrome, and childhood poliomyelitis, are highly predisposed to neurotoxicity.[141–143] VCR treatment in patients with hepatic dysfunction or obstructive liver disease is associated with an increased risk of developing neuropathy because of impaired drug metabolism and delayed biliary excretion.[144]

The only known effective intervention for vinca alkaloid neurotoxicity is discontinuing treatment or reduction of the dose or frequency of drug administration.[136,144,145] Although a number of antidotes, including thiamine, vitamin B_{12}, folinic acid, pyridoxine, and neuroactive agents (eg, sedatives, tranquilizers, anticonvulsants), have been used, these treatments have not been clearly shown to be effective.[106,146–149] Folinic acid protects mice against otherwise lethal doses of the vinca alkaloids, and there are anecdotal reports of its successful use following VCR overdosage in man; however, prospective studies have never been performed.[147,148] Suggested dosages for folinic acid for the treatment of overdosage are 15 mg every 3 hours for 24 hours and then every 6 hours for at least 48 hours. Recent results with other protective agents appear more promising. In one randomized, double-blind trial, coadministration of glutamic acid and VCR was associated with less neurotoxicity.[149] The adrenocorticotropin analogue ORG 2766 also demonstrated protection against VCR-induced neuropathy in an animal model, and in a double-blind, placebo-controlled pilot study in cancer patients.[29] Several other agents, including nerve growth factor, insulin-like growth factor I, and amifostine, appear to alter the natural course of neurotoxicity in experimental models, but there has been no definitive evidence that these agents may be effective in the clinic.

The manifestations of neurotoxicity are similar for all vinca alkaloids; however, severe neurotoxicity is observed less frequently with VBL, VDS, and VRL, as compared with VCR.[52,150] VRL has a lower affinity for axonal microtubules than either VCR or VBL, which seems to be confirmed by clinical observations.[29,35,37,73,150]

Myelosuppression Neutropenia is the principal dose-limiting toxicity of VBL, VDS, and VRL. Thrombocytopenia and anemia are usually less common and less severe. The onset of neutropenia is usually 7 to 11 days after treatment, and recovery is generally by days 14 to 21. Myelosuppression is not typically cumulative. Although VCR is rarely associated with hematologic toxicity, severe myelosuppression has been observed in situations resulting in increased drug exposure, such as following inadvertent overdose, and hepatic insufficiency.

Gastrointestinal Gastrointestinal toxicities, aside from those caused by autonomic dysfunction, may also occur.[28,29,32,37,106,151,152] Gastrointestinal autonomic dysfunction, as manifested by bloating, constipation, and abdominal pain, occurs most commonly with VCR, high doses of the other vinca alkaloids, or settings associated with high drug exposure (eg, hepatic dysfunction, overdosages). An initial manifestation of autonomic dysfunction due to poor intestinal transit may be impaction of stool in the upper colon. An empty rectum may be noted on digital examination or an abdominal radiograph may be useful in diagnosing this condition, which may be responsive to high enemas and laxatives. A routine prophylactic regimen to prevent constipation is therefore recommended for all patients receiving VCR. Severe autonomic toxicity may lead to paralytic ileus, particularly in children, intestinal necrosis, and even intestinal perforation. The ileus, which may mimic a "surgical abdomen," usually resolves with conservative measures after termination of treatment. Patients who receive high dosages of VCR or have hepatic dysfunction may be especially prone to develop severe gastrointestinal complications due to autonomic neurotoxicity. Although success with drugs used prophylactically to minimize toxicity, including lactulose, caerulein, metoclopramide, and the cholecystokinin analogue sincalide, has been reported anecdotally, these agents also may alter the pharmacokinetic behavior of the vinca alkaloids by affecting biliary excretion and/or enterohepatic recirculation, which may ultimately result in increased drug clearance.[29]

Mucositis, stomatitis, and pharyngitis occur more frequently with VBL than VRL or VDS, and are least common with VCR. Nausea, vomiting, and diarrhea may also occur to a lesser extent. Asymptomatic and brief elevations in serum levels of hepatic transaminases and alkaline phosphatase have been noted. Pancreatitis has also been reported rarely with VRL.[151]

Miscellaneous The vinca alkaloids are potent vesicants and may cause profound tissue damage if extravasation occurs. If extravasation is suspected, treatment should be discontinued immediately and aspiration of any residual drug remaining in the tissues should be attempted.[153–156] In experimental studies, cold packs have been shown to increase toxicity, while heat appears to limit damage. The application of local heat immediately for 1 hour four times daily for 3 to 5 days and the injection of hyaluronidase, 150 to 1,500 units (15 units/mL in 6 mL of 0.9% sodium chloride solution) subcutaneously, through 6 clockwise injections in a circumferential manner using a 25-gauge needle (changing the needle with each injection) into surrounding tissues is the treatment of choice in minimizing both discomfort and latent cellulitis.[156] The use of calcium leucovorin, diphenhydramine, hydrocortisone, isoproterenol, sodium bicarbonate, and vitamin A cream have been ineffective in animal models.[154] An immediate surgical consultation to consider early debridement is recommended. Discomfort and signs of phlebitis may also occur along the course of an injected vein, with resultant sclerosis, but phlebitis may be minimized if the vein is adequately flushed after treatment.

Mild and reversible alopecia occurs in approximately 10% and 20% of patients treated with VRL and VCR, respectively. Acute cardiac ischemia, chest pains without evidence of ischemia, fever without an obvious source, Raynaud's phenomenon, and palmar-plantar erythrodysthesia (hand-foot syndrome) have also been reported with the vinca alkaloids.[157–159]

Respiratory reactions, characterized by dyspnea, have been reported in approximately 5% of patients, particularly when vinca alkaloids are combined with mitomycin C.[160,161] The onset of pulmonary toxicity may be acute, with bronchospasm and dyspnea as the predominant manifestations, resembling an allergic reaction. The second type of toxicity is a subacute reversible reaction associated with cough and dyspnea and occasionally with interstitial infiltrates. This reaction typically occurs within 1 hour after treatment. The use of steroids has been felt to be beneficial in severe cases, and several patients have been retreated without sequelae. There is no clear evidence that implicates VRL as a cause of chronic pulmonary toxicity.

All of the vinca alkaloids have been implicated as a cause of SIADH, and patients who are receiving an intensive hydration regimen are particularly prone to severe hyponatremia secondary to SIADH.[27–29,37,106] This entity has been associated with elevated plasma levels of antidiuretic hormone and usually remits in 2 to 3 days. Hyponatremia generally responds to fluid restriction, as with hyponatremia associated with SIADH from other causes. VBL may cause photosensitivity reactions, possibly due to corneal irritation, and muscular effects.[162]

The inadvertent intrathecal administration of the vinca alkaloids causes an ascending myeloencephalopathy that is usually fatal. Reports of immediate cerebrospinal fluid withdrawal and lavage with Ringer's lactate solution supplemented with fresh frozen plasma (15 mL/L) at a rate of 55 mL/hour for 24 hours has provided encouraging results, with 2 affected patients surviving with significant paraplegia, but intact cerebral function.[163] To prevent this mistake, intrathecal methotrexate and intravenous VCR in the same setting should not be administered in the same setting, and the drugs should not be delivered together to staff.

Administration, Dose, and Schedule It is recommended that the vinca alkaloids be administered by rapid intravenous injection, possibly through a running parenteral infusion. Inadequate flushing following treatment may increase the risk of phlebitis and injection site reactions, and, therefore, the catheter should not be removed before the vein is flushed.

VCR is commonly administered to children weighing more than 10 kg as a bolus intravenous injection at a dosage of 1.5 to 2.0 mg/m^2 weekly, although 0.05 to 0.65 mg/kg weekly is commonly used in smaller children. For adults, the conventional weekly dose is 1.4 to 2.0 mg/m^2. A restriction of the absolute dose of VCR to 2.0 to 2.5 mg in children and 2.0 mg in adults, which is often referred to as "capping," has been generally adopted based on early reports of substantial gastrointestinal toxicity in small numbers of patients treated at higher doses. However, there is very little pharmacologic or toxicologic evidence to support this practice, and available evidence suggests that it should be reconsidered, particularly in light of the wide interpatient variability in pharmacokinetic behavior and tolerance.[144,164,165] There is significant interpatient variability in the clearance of VCR (as much as 11-fold), and some patients are able to tolerate much higher doses with little or no toxicity. Moreover, the safety and efficacy of treatment regimens that do not employ capping at 2.0 mg have been documented in adults.[164] In any case, doses should not be reduced for mild peripheral neurotoxicity, particularly if the agent is being used in a potentially curative setting. Instead, doses should be modified for manifestations indicative of more serious neurotoxicity, including severe symptomatic sensory changes, motor and cranial nerve deficits, and ileus, until toxicity resolves. In clearly palliative situations, dose reductions, lengthening dosing intervals, or selecting an alternative agent may be justified in the event of moderate neurotoxicity. A routine prophylactic regimen to prevent the serious consequences of severe autonomic toxicity, particularly severe constipation, is also recommended.

The most commonly used schedule for VBL in combination chemotherapy regimens uses a rapid intravenous injection at a dosage of 6 mg/m^2 weekly. Approved dosing recommendations for weekly dosing are 2.5 and 3.7 mg/m^2 for children and adults, respectively, followed by gradual escalation in increments of 1.8 and 1.25 mg/m^2 weekly based on hematologic tolerance. It is recommended that weekly VBL doses of 18.5 mg/m^2

in adults and 12.5 mg/m^2 in children not be exceeded as a single agent; however, these doses are substantially higher than most patients can tolerate because of myelosuppression, even on less frequent schedules of administration. Because the severity of leukopenia that may occur with identical VBL doses varies widely, VBL should probably not be given more frequently than once each week. Five-day continuous infusions of VBL have been used at dosages ranging from 1.5 to 2.0 mg/m^2 per day, which achieves biologically relevant plasma concentrations of approximately 2.0 nmol/L, but the overall advantages of using protracted infusions for a drug that is widely distributed and avidly bound to peripheral tissues may be minimal.

VRL is usually administered at a dosage of 30 mg/m^2 on a weekly or biweekly schedule as a 6- to 10-minute intravenous injection through a side-arm port into a running infusion (alternatively, a slow bolus injection followed by flushing the vein with 5% dextrose or 0.9% sodium chloride solutions) or as a short infusion over 20 minutes. It appears that the more rapid infusions are associated with less local venous toxicity. Oral dosages of 80 to 100 mg/m^2 given weekly are generally well tolerated, but an acceptable oral formulation has not yet been approved. Other dosing schedules that have been evaluated include chronic oral administration of low doses, intermittent high doses, and prolonged intravenous infusion schedules.

Because of their remarkable vesicant properties, the vinca alkaloids should not be administered intramuscularly, subcutaneously, intravesically, or intraperitoneally. Direct intrathecal injection of VCR and other vinca alkaloids, which has occurred as inadvertent clinical mishaps, induces a severe myeloencephalopathy characterized by ascending motor and sensory neuropathies, encephalopathy, and death (see the section "Toxicity" above, "Neurotoxicity").

Although specific dosing guidelines for patients with hepatic dysfunction have not been thoroughly evaluated, the major role of the liver in the disposition of the vinca alkaloids implies that dose modifications should be considered for patients with hepatic dysfunction, particularly hepatic excretory dysfunction.[165] A 50% dose reduction is often recommended for patients with total bilirubin levels between 1.5 and 3.0 mg/dL (50% dose reduction for bilirubin levels between 2.0 and 3.0 mg/dL is recommended for VRL), and at least a 75% dose reduction for plasma total bilirubin levels above 3.0 mg/dL. Dose reduction for renal insufficiency is not indicated.

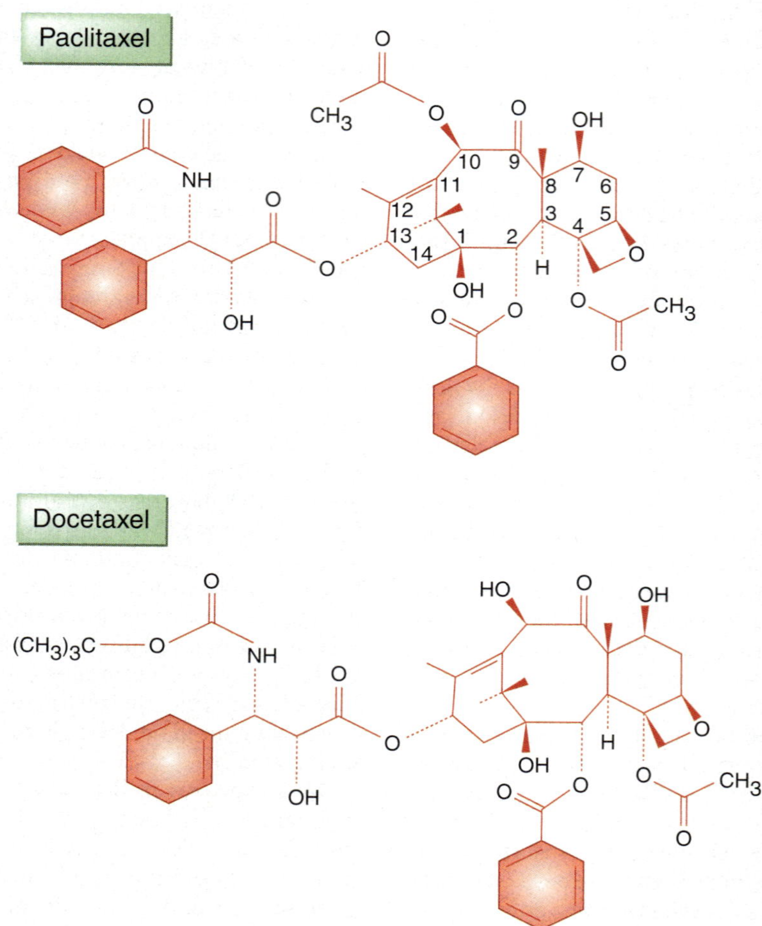

Figure 46-3 Chemical structures of the taxanes, paclitaxel and docetaxel.

TAXANES

Although the taxanes affect microtubules, they are substantially different from the vinca alkaloids in terms of their principal mechanisms of action, pharmacology, clinical indications, and toxicity profiles. Interest in the taxanes began in 1963, when a crude extract of the bark of the Pacific yew tree, *Taxus brevifolia,* demonstrated broad activity in preclinical tumor models.[166] In 1971, Monroe Wall and colleagues identified paclitaxel as the active constituent of the bark extract.[166] Paclitaxel's early development was delayed by the limited supply of its primary source that was exclusively derived from the Pacific yew tree; the difficulties inherent in large-scale isolation, extraction, and preparation of bulk compound for a natural product; and its poor aqueous solubility. Interest was maintained during this time by the characterization of its novel mechanism of action and the availability of an adequate drug supply for requisite preclinical and limited clinical evaluations. The early search for taxanes derived from more abundant and renewable resources led to the semisynthesis of docetaxel by the addition of a side chain to 10-deacetylbaccatin III, an inactive taxane precursor found in the needles and other components of more abundant yew species.[167] The supply of paclitaxel is no longer preclusive of the development of a feasible semisynthetic process. A wide variety of taxane analogues, as well as paclitaxel formulations, have been evaluated. Recently, a paclitaxel-protein-bound particle formulation (ABI-007) has received regulatory approval in the United States.

Figure 46-3 shows the structures of paclitaxel and docetaxel, which are complex esters consisting of a 15-member taxane ring system linked to an unusual 4-member oxetan ring. The taxane rings of both paclitaxel and docetaxel, but not 10-deacetylbaccatin III, are linked to an ester side chain attached to the C-13 position of the ring, which is essential for antimicrotubule and antitumor activity.[168] The structures of paclitaxel and docetaxel differ in substitutions at the C-10 taxane ring position and on the ester side chain attached at C-13, which render docetaxel slightly more water soluble and potent than paclitaxel. However, the clinical ramifications of these differences are not clear.

Clinical Indications Paclitaxel initially received regulatory approval in the United States and many other countries for the treatment of patients with ovarian cancer after failure of first-line or subsequent chemotherapy.[166] Its use in combination with a platinum compound as primary induction therapy in suboptimally debulked stage III or IV ovarian cancer has demonstrated a survival advantage in randomized phase 3 studies.[169] In the United States, paclitaxel is also indicated for treatment of patients with metastatic breast cancer after failure of combination chemotherapy for metastatic disease or at relapse within 6 months of adjuvant chemotherapy, with prior therapy that includes an anthracycline unless clinically contraindicated.[170] Recently, the combination of gemcitabine and paclitaxel demonstrated superior survival to paclitaxel alone in the first-line treatment of metastatic breast cancer, and gemcitabine as a component of this doublet received regulatory approval.[171] Additionally, regulatory approval for treating patients with stage II breast cancer following standard doxorubicin-based adjuvant chemotherapy after the early results of a phase 3 study suggested that the addition of the taxane conferred superior progression-free and overall survival; however, a survival advantage was not apparent with longer follow-up.[172–174] Compelling early results have been noted following treatment of patients with stage II breast cancer with alternative taxane-containing regimens, particularly "dose-dense" regimens, but randomized studies to determine the effects of these approaches on survival are being carried out.[172,173,175] Paclitaxel has also received regulatory approval in the United States for second-line treatment of Kaposi's sarcoma associated with the acquired immunodeficiency syndrome, and in combination with cisplatin as primary treatment of patients with non–small cell lung cancer who are not candidates for radiation therapy or potentially curative surgery.[176,177]

Docetaxel initially received regulatory approval in the United States for patients with metastatic or locally advanced breast cancer after failure of anthracycline-based chemotherapy, which was later broadened to a general second-line indication.[167,173] Subsequently, the combination of capecitabine and docetaxel demonstrated superior survival over docetaxel alone after failure of an anthracycline in patients with locally advanced or metastatic breast cancer.[167,173] More recently, regulatory approval was granted for docetaxel's use in combination with cyclophosphamide and doxorubicin in the adjuvant treatment of patients with local breast cancer following definitive local treatment.[173] In non–small cell lung cancer, docetaxel initially received regulatory approval for treatment of unresectable locally advanced or metastatic disease after demonstrating increased survival after failure of cisplatin-based therapy, and the combination of docetaxel and cisplatin was later granted regulatory approval as first-line treatment of such patients.[178] Both paclitaxel and docetaxel have demonstrated notable activity in patients with hormone-refractory prostate cancer (HRPC) and regulatory approval was recently granted for docetaxel in combination with prednisone for this indication as the regimen demonstrated superior survival over mitoxantrone and prednisone.[179,180]

ABI-007, the newest taxane to be added to the clinician's armamentarium after receiving regulatory approval for the treatment of breast cancer after failure of anthracycline-based chemotherapy for metastatic disease or relapse within 6 months of adjuvant therapy, is a formulation of paclitaxel in 3 to 4% human serum albumin, similar to the concentration of albumin in the blood in contrast to earlier formulations of paclitaxel in polyoxyethylated castor oil.[181,182]

It is important to note that the antitumor spectra for paclitaxel and docetaxel are identical, with activity noted in many other diverse cancers including head and neck, esophageal, gastric, endometrial, bladder, small cell lung, and germ cell carcinomas, and lymphoma and melanoma. The extent to which apparent differences in response rates, other endpoints, and regulatory indications granted, in part reflect differences in regulatory strategies, study design, dose, and schedule, but not necessarily the inherent superiority of any specific taxane.

Mechanism of Action The binding site for paclitaxel on microtubules is different from the binding sites for exchangeable GTP, colchicine, podophyllotoxin, and vinblastine. Paclitaxel binds to the N-terminal 31 amino acids of the β-tubulin subunit of the tubulin polymers, although additional sites may be involved.[166,183–188] Paclitaxel sits in a pocket that is lined by several hydrophobic residues and is situated on the luminal side of the microtubule wall, roughly in the middle of the monomer along the protofilament direction.[7,189,190] Docetaxel, which most likely shares the same binding site as paclitaxel, appears to have a 1.9-fold higher affinity for the site, and the tubulin assembly process induced by docetaxel proceeds with a critical protein concentration that is 2.1-fold lower than that of paclitaxel.[188,191–194] However, it is not clear whether these differences translate into greater therapeutic indices for docetaxel in relevant clinical settings because greater potency may result in more severe toxicity at identical drug concentrations in vivo. Nevertheless, the results of both preclinical and clinical studies indicate that the taxanes may not be completely cross-resistant, but these results may reflect differences in delivered dose and schedule.

Although both the vinca alkaloids and taxanes produce similar disruptive effects on the mitotic spindle apparatus, their principal mechanisms of action differ. The taxanes alter the tubulin rate dissociation constants at both ends of the microtubules by reducing the critical tubulin concentration required for microtubule assembly and promoting both nucleation and elongation phases of the polymerization reaction, thereby stabilizing microtubules against depolymerization and enhancing polymerization.[2–6,15,40–42,183–185,194,195] Binding of the taxanes to polymerized tubulin strengthens the microtubule. At substoichiometric concentrations, the taxanes suppress microtubule dynamics without appreciably increasing the rate of formation of polymerized tubulin.[2,3,12,19,40,42,183,184] At much higher concentrations, which are readily achieved in the clinic, the taxanes induce tubulin polymerization and increase microtubule mass. The microtubules of taxane-treated cells are extraordinarily stable, resisting depolymerization by cold, calcium ions, GTP, and depolymerizing antimicrotubule agents. These actions result in the suppression of treadmilling and dynamic instability, which are essential for normal microtubule dynamics during both mitotic and nonmitotic phases of the cell cycle.[2,3,12,15,19,190,195,196] Both stoichiometric and substoichiometric binding of the taxanes inhibit the proliferation of cells, principally by inducing a sustained mitotic block at the metaphase/anaphase boundary; however, morphologic findings, such as the formation of microtubule bundles during the nonmitotic phases of the cell cycle, suggest that the interphase microtubules in nonproliferating cells may also be affected. Nevertheless, microtubule dynamics are highest in mitosis in the course of mitotic spindle formation, and therefore the cell is most sensitive to the taxanes during this phase.

Perturbations of mitotic processes and the induction of mitotic arrest by the taxanes trigger apoptosis; however, the precise mechanisms by which these perturbations result in cell death have not been determined. Nevertheless, the taxanes do interact with numerous regulatory proteins and oncogenes that relate to the integrity of mitosis and several different mechanisms that potentially link the mitotic arrest induced by the taxanes and other antimicrotubule agents to the initiating event in the intrinsic pathway of apoptosis have been characterized.[17,19,59,197–210] For example, microtubule disruption induces the tumor suppressor gene *TP53* and inhibitors of cyclin-dependent kinases (eg, p21/Waf-1), and modulates several protein kinases.[19,17,197,208,210] As a consequence, cells are arrested in G_2/M, after which time they may either undergo apoptosis or traverse through G_2/M and divide.[207] The apoptotic initiating events also include activation of the proapoptotic molecules Bax and Bad and inactivation of the antiapoptotic regulators Bcl-2 and Bcl_{XL}.[208,209] Various kinases have been implicated in the phosphorylation of Bcl-2 induced by the taxanes and other antimicrotubule agents, including Jun N-terminal kinase (JNK) and its proapoptotic effector Bim, c-Raf, extracellular signal regulated kinase (ERK) -1 and -2, cyclin-dependent kinase (CDK)-1, cAMP-dependent protein kinase A, and protein kinase Cα.[57,198,208,209] Phosphorylation (inactivation) of Bcl-2 family members and phosphorylation of pro-apoptotic molecules (activation) stimulate the intrinsic pathway of apoptosis and downstream effector caspases.[207,211] The antimitotic effects of the taxanes and other antimicrotubule agents may be linked to apoptosis through other modulatory events such as the phosphorylation of the proapoptotic protein Bad by activating CDK1.[210]

The taxanes also perturb interphase microtubules in nonproliferating cells. Taxanes induce the formation of microtubule bundles.[195,212] Paclitaxel has also been reported to induce transcription factors and enzymes that mediate proliferation, apoptosis, and inflammation.[200,210,213,214] In addition, these agents enhance the effects of ionizing radiation in vitro and in vivo, which may be related to the inhibition of cell-cycle progression in G_2 and the mitotic phases, which are the most radiosensitive phases of the cell cycle.[215–219] In angiogenesis inhibition assays, they also inhibit parameters indicative of angiogenesis at concentrations below those that induce cytotoxicity, but the contribution of these effects to the overall antitumor actions of the taxanes is not clear.[206,220,221]

The taxanes have been demonstrated to induce many other cellular effects that may or may not relate to their disruptive effects on microtubule dynamics. Although the taxanes primarily block cell-cycle traverse in the mitotic phases, the agents prevent G_0 to S-phase transition in both normal and malignant cells.[212,222] Explanations that have been proposed to account for the nonmitotic actions of the taxanes include disruptive effects on tubulin in the cell membrane, the interphase cytoskeleton, and microtubules that are involved in growth factor signaling.[29,223]

The taxanes inhibit specific functions in nonmalignant tissues, which may be mediated through their disruptive effects on microtubule dynamics.[29] For example, paclitaxel inhibits relevant morphologic and biochemical processes in human neutrophils, including chemotaxis, migration, spreading, polarization, hydrogen peroxide generation, and killing of phagocytized microorganisms.[29] Paclitaxel also antagonizes the effects of microtubule-disrupting drugs on lymphocyte function, cAMP metabolism, and inhibits the proliferation of stimulated human lymphocytes.[29] Paclitaxel mimics the effects of endotoxic bacterial lipopolysaccharide on macrophages, which results in a rapid decrement in tumor necrosis factor-α (TNF-α) receptors and TNF-α release.[209,213,214] The agent also induces expression of the gene for TNF-α, but these activities are not related to paclitaxel's disruptive effects on microtubule assembly, which raises the issue of the role of cytokines in the antitumor activities of the taxanes.[213] Additionally, paclitaxel has been demonstrated to inhibit chorioretinal fibroblast proliferation and contractility in an in vitro model of proliferative vitreoretinopathy, as well as neointimal smooth muscle cell proliferation after angioplasty.[224,225] Cardiac arterial stents coated with paclitaxel received regulatory approval in the United States and elsewhere because of a significantly decreased incidence of restenosis from fibroblast proliferation and intimal hyperplasia.[226] Finally, paclitaxel inhibits secretory functions in many specialized cells, such as insulin secretion in isolated rat islets of Langerhans, protein secretion in rat hepatocytes, and the nicotinic receptor-stimulated release of catecholamines from chromaffin cells of the adrenal medulla.[29]

Mechanisms of Resistance Two general mechanisms of acquired taxane resistance have been described in cells made resistant by prolonged drug treatment at low concentrations. The best-characterized mechanism is the MDR phenotype, which can be mediated by several ABC multidrug transporter family members. The most important ABC transporter with respect to conferring taxane resistance is the 170-kDa Pgp efflux pump or the *MDR1* encoded gene product MDR1 (ABC subfamily B1; ABCB1) and MDR2 (ABC subfamily ABCB4) (see the section "Vinca Alkaloids: Introduction and Indications" above, "Mechanisms of Resistance").[77,185,227,228] In addition, low-level taxane resistance appears to be conferred by the bile salt export protein (BSEP, also known as ABCC11).[77] Unlike the vinca alkaloids, ABCC1 (MRP1) and ABCC2 (MRP2) do not appear to be involved in transporting the taxanes.[229,230] In murine systems, the particular species of Pgp found in paclitaxel-resistant cells is similar, but not identical, to that found in VBL- and colchicine-resistant cells derived from the same parental line.[77,200] These cells are cross-resistant with many other natural products, and resistance to both paclitaxel and docetaxel conferred by MDRl can be reversed by many classes of membrane-active drugs, including the calcium channel blockers, tamoxifen, cyclosporine A, and antiarrhythmic agents.[77,200] Even the principal component of the vehicles used to formulate paclitaxel and docetaxel—polyoxyethylated castor oil and polysorbate-80, respectively, can reverse taxane resistance in vitro.[231,232] In fact, plasma concentrations of polyoxyethylated castor oil achieved with paclitaxel on clinically relevant dose schedules are sufficient to reverse MDR, whereas sufficient modulatory concentrations of polysorbate-80 are not achieved with docetaxel in the clinic. However, strategies aimed at reversing resistance to taxanes and other MDR substrates in the clinic have resulted in low impact at best, but most studies have been performed with MDR modulators that reduce taxane clearance and increase toxicity (eg, verapamil, cyclosporine A), thereby confounding interpretation of the inherent effects of these agents on MDR modulation. However, MDR modulators that do not affect taxane clearance and toxicity, such as the cyclosporine analogue PSC 833 and the MDR/MRP modulator VX-710, have not been demonstrated to enhance antitumor activity to a relevant degree.[77,233,234]

Similar to the vinca alkaloids, several human cell lines rendered taxane resistant by treatment with high drug concentrations for protracted periods have structurally altered α- and β-tubulins and an impaired ability to polymerize tubulin dimers into microtubules (see the section "Vinca Alkaloids: Introduction and Indications" above, "Mechanisms of Resistance").[90–92,235–238] These cells lack normal microtubules in their interpolar mitotic spindles and have an inherently slow rate of microtubule assembly when grown in the absence of drug. The continuous presence of the taxanes is required for microtubule assembly to proceed. Furthermore, these mutants are also collaterally sensitive to the vinca alkaloids. In some experimental systems, paclitaxel-resistant cells had mutated β-tubulin alleles, with mutations involving the putative taxane binding sites; specifically, leucines at positions 215, 217, and 228 were mutated to histidine, arginine, or phenylalanine.[239,240] Low-level expression resulted in drug resistance, whereas, high-level expression of these mutations caused impairment of microtubule assembly, cell-cycle arrest, and failure to proliferate, all of which were reversed by incubation with paclitaxel.

There is evidence indicating that alterations in tubulin content, tubulin isotype profiles, and tubulin polymerization dynamics may confer taxane resistance in preclinical systems and in the clinic. For example, paclitaxel-resistant tumors have been demonstrated to have significantly higher levels of class I, III, and IVa isotypes of β-tubulin.[17,93,239–243] High intratumoral levels of the β_{III} isotype, which is a minor component of cellular β-tubulin and increases the dynamic instability of microtubules, impedes microtubule assembly, and confers resistance to the taxanes, has been demonstrated in tumor biopsies sampled from patients with taxane-resistant tumors and cell lines with acquired taxane resistance.[244–247] Higher levels of class β_{III} tubulin RNA levels have also been reported in non–small cell lung cancers of patients who did not respond to taxane-based treatment, which is in line with in vitro findings.

Mutations of tubulin isotype genes, gene amplifications, and isotype switching have also been reported in taxane-resistant cell lines.[59,90,200,201,238,240,244–246,248] Although clinical data from patients with non–small cell lung cancer indicate that mutations in β-tubulin are associated with taxane resistance, these observations have not been confirmed and these findings may have been caused by amplification of pseudogenes.

Growth factor signaling may contribute to taxane resistance by raising the cell's threshold for taxane-induced apoptosis. Insulin-like growth factor-I, for example, appears to protect responsive breast cancer cell lines from the cytotoxic effects of the anthracyclines and taxanes, possibly by activating the phosphatidylinositol 3-kinase (PI3K) pathway and inducing phosphorylation (inactivation) of antiapoptotic factors.[249] Other mediators that may influence the cell's threshold for drug-induced apoptosis include TP53, erbB-2, auora 2-kinase, survivin, and BRAC1. The centromere-associated serine/threonine kinase, aurora 2-kinase, which is involved in centrosome separation, biopolar spindle formation, and chromosomal kinetochore attachment to the mitotic spindle, appears to override the mitotic assembly checkpoint and induce taxane resistance.[2] In addition, the overexpresssion of survivin, a member of the inhibitor of apoptosis family of proteins, inhibits caspase activity and apoptosis induced by antimicrotubule agents. The disruption of the tumor-suppressor gene, *BRAC1*, which is implicated in maintaining genomic stability through DNA repair and appears to be involved in hereditary breast and ovarian cancers, appears to play a role in conferring resistance to paclitaxel and the inducible expression of BRAC1 may enhance paclitaxel-induced apoptosis.[2] The mutational loss of the TP53 tumor suppressor does not confer resistance to microtubule polymerizing agents in contrast to DNA-disruptive agents. Also, there was no relationship evident between paclitaxel sensitivity and TP53 status in the National Cancer Institute's 60-tumor type-specific drug screening panel.[19] Additionally, cells lacking wild-type TP53 display increased sensitivity to paclitaxel.

MAPs have been implicated in mechanisms of resistance to apoptosis induced by the taxanes and other antimicrotubule agents, as illustrated by the observation that MAP4, which is negatively regulated by wild-type *TP53*, increases sensitivity to paclitaxel.[250,251] The suppression of dynamic instability by low concentrations of microtubule polymerizing agents may also enhance the nuclear accumulation of TP53 and the induction of proapoptotic TP53–up-regulated modulator of apoptosis.[2] This may represent a TP53-dependent mechanism of apoptosis induced by antimicrotubule agents in cells that harbor functional TP53.[19] Finally, overexpression of p21, a downstream effector of TP53, appears to impede cell-cycle traverse in G_2, thereby blocking progression into the more drug-vulnerable mitotic phase and decreasing taxane sensitivity.[252,253]

Transfection of cells with erbB-2, a member of the epidermal growth factor receptor family that is amplified and overexpressed in approximately 30% of breast cancers, has been demonstrated to increase taxane resistance, and high expression of erbB-2 in vitro relates to taxane resistance.[252,253] Overexpression of erbB-2 can also inhibit CDK1 either by inducing p21, which participates in the G_2/M checkpoint and contributes to resistance to apoptosis induced by antimicrotubule agents, or directly phosphorylating (inactivating) CDK1, which may block taxane-mediated entry into mitosis and apoptosis.[2] Consistent with this relationship, down-regulation of erbB-2 by the anti–erbB-2 antibody trastuzumab sensitizes breast cancer cells to the taxanes, and the combination of trastuzumab and either paclitaxel or docetaxel is associated with increased survival compared with the taxanes alone.[253,254] Nevertheless, the presence of *erbB-2* amplification does not adversely influence response to first-line chemotherapy with either epirubicin-paclitaxel or epirubicin-cyclophosphamide.[255] Furthermore, the taxane-containing regimen may preferentially benefit women with erbB-2-expressing breast cancer.

Table 46-2 Taxanes: Comparative Pharmacokinetic and Toxicologic Characteristics

Parameter	Paclitaxel	Docetaxel	ABI-007
Standard adult dose	135 (24-h infusion)	75–100 (1-h infusion)	260 (30-min infusion)
Range (mg/m²/3 week)	175–225 (3-h infusion)		
(mg/m²/week)	80	30–36	
Pharmacokinetic behavior (clinically-relevant doses)	Triphasic	Triphasic Dose-proportional to 115 mg/m²	Biphasic Dose-proportional
(> 175 mg/m²)	Saturable taxane elimination and distribution; pseudo nonlinearity due to vehicle		
Plasma half-lives (terminal)	10–20 h	10–20 h	27 h
Clearance	20–25 L/h*	36 L/h	15 L/h/m²
Primary route	Hepatic metabolism and biliary elimination	Hepatic metabolism and biliary elimination	Hepatic metabolism and biliary elimination
Principal toxicity	Neutropenia	Neutropenia	Neutropenia
Other toxicities	Alopecia, neurotoxicity, myalgia, hypersensitivity reactions, asthenia	Alopecia, skin and nail toxicity, asthenia, myalgia, fluid retention neurotoxicity, hypersensitivity reactions	Alopecia, asthenia, myalgia, injection-site reactions, hypersensitivity reactions

*175 mg/m² over 3 hours (dose-schedule).

Clinical Pharmacology **General** The taxanes are most commonly administered intravenously at dosages ranging from 175 to 225 mg/m² over 3 hours (paclitaxel), 75 to 100 mg/m² over 1 hour (docetaxel), or 260 mg/m² over 30 minutes (ABI-007) every 3 weeks, but other schedules, particularly weekly schedules, are commonly used (see the section "Administration, Dose, and Schedule" below). The oral bioavailability of both paclitaxel and docetaxel is poor, which is due, in part, to the constitutive overexpression of Pgp and P-450 metabolizing capability of enterocytes and/or first-pass metabolism in the liver and/or intestines; however, oral bioavailability can be enhanced if the taxanes are administered orally following treatment with oral cyclosporine or other modulators of Pgp and cytochrome P-450 mixed-function oxidases.[256] As shown in Table 46-2, paclitaxel and docetaxel share the following pharmacologic characteristics: large volumes of distribution, rapid and avid binding to all tissues except for the unperturbed central nervous system, long terminal half-lives and substantial hepatic metabolism, biliary excretion, and fecal elimination.

Paclitaxel More recent pharmacologic evaluations of paclitaxel, which involved shorter administration schedules and highly sensitive analytical assays, indicate that its pharmacokinetic behavior is nonlinear or pseudononlinear.[232,257–261] Nonlinear behavior is more apparent with shorter infusions that result in higher plasma paclitaxel concentrations and more effective saturation of both drug elimination and tissue distribution processes. Both saturable distribution and elimination processes may be, in part, responsible for paclitaxel's nonlinear behavior, with tissue distribution becoming effectively saturated at lower drug concentrations (achieved with paclitaxel dosages of less than 175 mg/m² over 3 h) as compared with elimination processes that are saturated at higher concentrations (achieved with paclitaxel dosages > 175 mg/m² over 3 h). A potential ramification of true nonlinearity is that dose escalation may result in a disproportionate increase in drug exposure and toxicity, whereas dose reduction may result in a disproportionate decrease in drug exposure. However, the use of shorter infusion schedules also results in higher plasma concentrations of paclitaxel's polyoxyethylated castor oil vehicle, which may simulate nonlinearity (pseudononlinearity) by binding paclitaxel and inhibiting drug disposition.[261,262]

The pharmacologic behavior of paclitaxel in plasma appears to be triphasic and its volume of distribution is much larger than the volume of total body water, indicating extensive drug binding to plasma proteins or other tissue elements, possibly tubulin.[232] Plasma protein binding is high (> 95%) and readily reversible. Albumin and α_1-acid glycoprotein contribute equally to drug binding with a minor contribution from lipoproteins.[263-265] None of the drugs that are commonly administered with paclitaxel, including ranitidine, dexamethasone, diphenhydramine, doxorubicin, 5-fluorouracil, and cisplatin, appear to significantly alter protein binding.[264] Drug binding to platelets is extensive and saturable, and animal distribution studies with radiolabeled paclitaxel indicate extensive drug uptake and retention by virtually all tissues, except for normal sanctuary sites such as the normal brain and testes.[266,267]

Clearance is closely related to body surface area, providing a rationale for dosing based on this parameter. In humans, peak plasma concentrations achieved with 3- to 96-hour schedules (more than 0.05–10 μmol/L) and drug concentrations in third-space fluid collections such as ascites (more than 0.1 μmol/L), are capable of inducing relevant biologic effects in vitro, but drug penetration into the unperturbed central nervous system is negligible.[232,267,268] The principal mode of paclitaxel disposition is hepatic metabolism and biliary excretion. The liver metabolizes and excretes both paclitaxel and paclitaxel metabolites into the bile.[232,266,269–275] In rats treated with radiolabeled paclitaxel, 98% of radioactivity is recovered from feces collected for 6 days, and approximately 71% of an administered dose of paclitaxel is excreted in the feces over 5 days as either parent compound or metabolites in humans, with 6α-hydroxypaclitaxel being the largest component, accounting for 26% of the dose; unmetabolized paclitaxel accounts for only 5% of the dose. Renal clearance of paclitaxel and metabolites may account for up to 14% of the administered dose.[232] In humans, cytochrome P-450 mixed-function oxidases are responsible for the bulk of drug disposition, specifically the isoenzymes CYP2C8 and CYP3A4, which metabolize paclitaxel to 6α-hydroxypaclitaxel (major) and another hydroxylated metabolite, both of which are much less active than paclitaxel in vivo, possibly due to their greater polarity which precludes intracellular uptake.[232,269–273] There is considerable interindividual variability in paclitaxel metabolism that can be attributed to pharmacogenetic differences in P-450 metabolism and concurrent medications that alter metabolism.[232,272–275]

Pharmacodynamic analyses demonstrate that several pharmacokinetic parameters indicative of drug exposure relate to the principal toxicities of paclitaxel, the most important and consistent of which is the relationship between the severity of neutropenia and the duration of drug exposure above biologically relevant plasma concentrations ranging from 0.05 to 0.1 μmol/L.[232,257,259,272] A prospective analysis of pharmacokinetic determinants of outcome in several hundred patients with advanced non–small cell lung cancer treated with the combination of cisplatin and paclitaxel at either 135 or 250 mg/m^2 over 24 hours demonstrated that the magnitude of the steady-state plasma paclitaxel concentration correlates poorly with antitumor activity, disease-free survival, and overall survival.[276]

Docetaxel The pharmacokinetics of docetaxel (1-h schedule) in plasma are triphasic and linear at doses of 115 mg/m^2 or less.[167,277–282] Terminal half-lives ranging from 11.1 to 18.5 hours have been reported. In one population study, plasma concentration data revealed triphasic pharmacokinetics, and the following pharmacokinetic parameters: $t_{1/2\gamma}$ of 12.4 hours, clearance of 1 L/h/m^2, and steady-state volume of distribution of 74 L/m^2.[167,277–282] The most important determinants of docetaxel clearance were body surface area, hepatic function, and plasma α_1-acid glycoprotein concentration, whereas age and plasma albumin level had significant, albeit minor, influences on clearance. Like paclitaxel, plasma protein binding is high (> 80–90%), and binding is primarily to α_1-acid glycoprotein, albumin, and lipoproteins.[167,277–282] Like paclitaxel, docetaxel is widely distributed, but does not enter the unperturbed central nervous system.[283,284] In both dogs and mice treated with radiolabeled drug, fecal excretion accounts for 70 to 80% of total radioactivity, whereas urinary excretion accounts for 10% or less.[283] The hepatic cytochrome P-450 mixed-function oxidases, particularly CYP3A, the activity of which, in adults, is represented by the combined activities of CYP3A4, CYP3A5, CYP3A7, and CYP3A43, is responsible for most of docetaxel's metabolism.[285–287] In contrast to paclitaxel, the C13 side chain, instead of the taxane ring, is metabolized.[285,286,288] These metabolites seem to be much less active than docetaxel.

The principal pharmacokinetic determinants of toxicity, particularly neutropenia, are drug exposure and the time that plasma concentrations exceed biologically relevant concentrations.[282] A population pharmacodynamic analysis of determinants of outcome in phase II trials of docetaxel revealed that the most important determinants of the time to progression in patients with metastatic breast cancer are the pretreatment plasma concentration of α_1-acid glycoprotein, number of prior chemotherapy regimens, and number of disease sites, whereas both drug exposure and the pretreatment plasma concentration of α_1-acid glycoprotein were positive determinants of time to progression in patients with advanced lung cancer treated with docetaxel.[278,280] Conversely, the pretreatment plasma level of α_1-acid glycoprotein was negatively, albeit significantly, related to the probability of experiencing both severe neutropenia and febrile neutropenia. The rate of docetaxel clearance has also been related to CYP3A4 activity, as assessed by the [^{14}C-N-methyl] erythromycin breath test.[286]

ABI-007 In clinical studies following the administration of ABI-007 doses ranging from 80 to 360 mg/m^2, paclitaxel pharmacokinetics were dose-proportional. At the recommended dose of 260 mg/m^2, total clearance averaged 15 liters/hour/m^2 and the mean volume of distribution was 632 L/m^2. Approximately 89 to 98% of paclitaxel is protein-bound in vitro. Metabolic studies demonstrate a similar metabolic profile as paclitaxel in polyoxyethylated castor oil formulations. Fecal and urinary excretion accounts for approximately 20% and 4% of the total dose of ABI-007 administered.

In a study that examined plasma pharmacokinetics and partitioning of radiolabeled paclitaxel from ABI-007 and a polyoxyethylated paclitaxel formulation into red blood cells and tumor tissue for 24 hours following tail vein injection of 20 mg/kg paclitaxel in an MX-1 human breast cancer xenograft model, the distribution of ABI-007 was rapid and extensive, as shown by a 5-fold larger volume of distribution and much lower peak plasma concentrations (C_{max}) and area under the concentration time curve (AUC) values compared with a polyoxyethylated castor oil formulation.[289,290] Furthermore, ABI-007 demonstrated a significantly lower plasma/blood ratio of paclitaxel across all time points and distributed more effectively into MX-1 tumors. Tumor AUC values of paclitaxel were 1.6-fold higher, on average, with ABI-007 and terminal half-life values for ABI-007 were significantly longer than from the polyoxyethylated castor oil formulation (17.1 vs 4.0 h). The prolonged half-life for ABI-007 could be attributed to red blood cell penetration and temporary storage of paclitaxel for ABI-007, releasing paclitaxel as plasma levels decrease.

Drug Interactions Both sequence-dependent pharmacokinetic and toxicologic interactions between taxanes and several other chemotherapy agents have been noted.[291] The most prominent sequence-dependent effects relate to the platinum compound and the taxanes, particularly with protracted taxane administration schedules. Sequence dependence has been primarily reported with paclitaxel, which most likely relates to the fact that docetaxel has been evaluated on a shorter (1-h) schedule. The sequence of cisplatin followed by paclitaxel (24-h schedule) induces more profound neutropenia than the reverse sequence, which is explained by a 33% reduction in the clearance of paclitaxel following cisplatin.[292,293] The least toxic sequence, paclitaxel before cisplatin, was demonstrated to induce more cytotoxicity in vitro, and therefore it was selected for clinical development.[292] Sequence-dependence does not appear to be a clinically relevant phenomenon with the taxanes on shorter schedules. The modulation of cytochrome P-450–dependent paclitaxel-metabolizing enzymes by cisplatin may, in part, explain these findings. Treatment with paclitaxel on either a 3- or 24-hour schedule followed by carboplatin was demonstrated to produce equivalent neutropenia and less thrombocytopenia as compared with carboplatin as a single agent, which is not explained by pharmacokinetic interactions.[272,294,295] Both neutropenia and mucositis are more severe when paclitaxel on a 24-hour schedule is administered before doxorubicin, as compared with the reverse sequence, which is most likely caused by an approximately 32% reduction in the clearance of doxorubicin and doxorubicinol when the agent is administered after paclitaxel.[296–298] Neither sequence-dependent pharmacologic nor toxicologic interactions between doxorubicin and paclitaxel on a shorter (3-h) schedule have been noted; however, the doxorubicin clearance is reduced with both sequences, and the combination of paclitaxel (3-h schedule) and doxorubicin (bolus infusion) produces a much higher rate of congestive cardiotoxicity than would have been expected from an equivalent cumulative doxorubicin dose given without paclitaxel (see the section "Toxicity," below, for a discussion of cardiotoxicity).[296,297] Although similar decrements in the clearance of epirubicin and its metabolites have been reported in studies of paclitaxel combined with epirubicin, an increased incidence of cardiotoxicity has not been observed.[299] The precise etiology for these interactions is unclear. The pharmacokinetic interactions may not be of sufficient magnitude to account for the enhanced cardiotoxicity of the combination, and there are experimental data indicating that paclitaxel enhances the metabolism of doxorubicin to cardiotoxic metabolites, such as doxorubicinol, in cardiomyocytes. Docetaxel does not appear to influence doxorubicin pharmacokinetics but, like paclitaxel, docetaxel can enhance the metabolism of doxorubicin to toxic species in the human heart.[300] Competition for the hepatic or biliary Pgp transport of the anthracyclines with paclitaxel or its polyoxyethylated castor oil vehicle (or both) is an alternate explanation.[231,291,296] Similar effects have not been noted with docetaxel, which is not formulated in polyoxyethylated castor oil.

Hematologic toxicity has been more profound with the sequence of cyclophosphamide before paclitaxel (24-h schedule) than with the reverse sequence.[301] Sequence-dependent cytotoxic effects have been reported when the taxanes are combined with 5-fluorouracil, etoposide, cytosine arabinoside, fludarabine, flavopiridol, and other antineoplastic agents in vitro.[291] In human tumor xenografts, both paclitaxel and docetaxel have been demonstrated to induce thymidine phosphorylase activity, which may increase the metabolic activation of the oral fluoropyrimidine prodrug capecitabine.[301,302]

Interactions between the taxanes and other classes of drugs, particularly those dependent on cytochrome P-450–dependent metabolism, have been documented.[302] Several inducers of cytochrome P-450 mixed-function oxidases, such as the anticonvulsants phenytoin and phenobarbital, accelerate the metabolism of both paclitaxel and docetaxel in human microsomes in vitro and in both children and adults who are concurrently receiving treatment with these anticonvulsants, as manifested by rapid drug clearance and tolerance of high drug doses.[232,269,271,273,291,303–307] There is preclinical evidence to suggest that docetaxel has a markedly reduced propensity to cause drug interactions that may entail hepatic CYP3A4 induction.[275] Conversely, many types of agents that inhibit cytochrome P-450 mixed-function oxidases, such as orphenadrine, erythromycin, cimetidine, testosterone, ketoconazole, fluconazole, midazolam, polyoxyethylated castor oil, and corticosteroids, interfere with the metabolism of paclitaxel and docetaxel in human microsomes in vitro; however, the inhibitory concentrations of these agents exceed those achieved in clinical practice, and the clinical relevance of these findings is not known. Besides the potent inhibitors of CYP3A listed above, other well-established inhibitors and inducers of CYP3A, including grapefruit juice and herbal products (eg, St. John's wort and Echinacea), may potentially induce pharmacokinetic interactions with the taxanes. Although there has been concern that the use of different H_2-receptor antagonists with variable cytochrome P-450 inhibitory activities as components of premedication regimens may differentially affect drug clearance and hence toxicity, neither toxicologic nor pharmacologic differences between the agents were noted in a randomized clinical trial.[308] A review of early clinical trial results with docetaxel has not demonstrated significant alterations in docetaxel clearance by corticosteroids. In addition, interactions between warfarin and the taxanes, possibly due to protein-binding displacement effects, have been reported.[309]

The incidence of congestive heart failure has also been higher in breast cancer patients treated with the combination of trastuzumab and paclitaxel than with paclitaxel alone, but the explanation for this observation has not been determined.[310,311]

Toxicity Myelosuppression is the principal toxicity of the taxanes. However, despite similar structures, these agents possess modest differences in their toxicity spectra.

Paclitaxel Neutropenia is the principal toxicity of paclitaxel.[312] The onset is usually on days 8 to 10, and recovery typically occurs by days 15 to 21. The main clinical determinant for the severity of neutropenia is the extent of prior myelosuppressive therapy; however, the neutropenia is typically noncumulative and the duration of severe neutropenia, even in heavily pretreated patients, is generally brief. Pharmacokinetic parameters of paclitaxel in plasma that reflect drug exposure, particularly the duration that plasma concentrations are maintained above biologically relevant levels (0.05–0.10 µmol/L; see the section "Clinical Pharmacology" above) relate to the severity of neutropenia, which may explain why neutropenia is more severe with longer infusion schedules.[313,314] But because paclitaxel distributes widely and avidly even following treatment on short schedules, protracted schedules may not portend superior antitumor activity. At paclitaxel dosages exceeding 175 mg/m^2 on a 24-hour schedule and 225 mg/m^2 on a 3-hour schedule, neutrophil counts typically decrease to below 500/µL for fewer than 5 days in most courses, even in untreated patients. Even patients who have received extensive prior therapy can usually tolerate paclitaxel dosages in the range of 175 to 200 mg/m^2 administered over 3 or 24 hours. More frequent schedules, particularly weekly treatment with 80 to 100 mg/m^2, have resulted in less severe neutropenia than single-dosing schedules (see the section "Administration, Dose, and Schedule" below). Severe thrombocytopenia and anemia are unusual, except in heavily pretreated patients.

The incidence of major hypersensitivity reactions (HSRs) in early phase I trials approached 30%, but the incidence is approximately 1 to 3% following the advent and broad adoption of effective prophylaxis.[312,315–321] Most major reactions are characterized by dyspnea with bronchospasm, urticaria, and hypotension, which typically occur within the first 10 minutes after the first, and less frequently after the second, treatment. Major HSRs generally resolve completely after stopping treatment and occasionally after treatment with antihistamines, fluids, and vasopressors. Patients who have major reactions have been rechallenged successfully after receiving high doses of corticosteroids, but this approach is not always successful.[315,316,318,322] Patients who have experienced paclitaxel-related HSRs have also received docetaxel uneventfully.[323] Less severe manifestations of hypersensitivity phenomena, such as flushing and rashes, have been noted in as many as 40% of patients, and it is particularly important to note that minor HSRs do not portend the development of major reactions. The HSRs are most likely caused by a nonimmunologically mediated release of histamine or histamine-like substances in the polyoxyethylated castor oil vehicle, but the taxane moiety may also be contributory. In some cases, complement activation has been demonstrated.[320] Although the incidence of major HSRs is reduced with lower administration rates and longer infusion durations, the rates of major reactions are low on both 3- and 24-hour schedules when patients are premedicated with corticosteroids and both H_1-histamine and H_2-histamine antagonists (see the section "Administration, Dose, and Schedule" below). In an assessment of the relative safety of two different paclitaxel schedules (24 vs 3 h), the rates of major reactions were low and similar (2.1% vs 1.0%) in patients receiving paclitaxel for 3 or 24 hours, respectively, with premedication.[312,324]

A peripheral neuropathy dominated by sensory manifestations, such as numbness and paresthesia, in a glove-and-stocking distribution is the principal neurotoxic effect of paclitaxel.[312,325] There is often symmetric distal loss of sensation carried by both large (proprioception, vibration) and small (temperature, pinprick) fibers. Symptoms may begin as soon as 24 to 72 hours after treatment with higher doses (≥ 250 mg/m^2), but usually occur only after multiple courses at 135 to 250 mg/m^2 every 3 weeks or 80 to 100 mg/m^2 weekly, and are cumulative thereafter. Severe neurotoxicity precludes chronic treatment with paclitaxel at dosages above 250 mg/m^2 over 3 or 24 hours, but severe neurotoxicity is uncommon at conventional doses (< 200 mg/m^2) of paclitaxel alone even in patients who previously received other neurotoxic agents such as cisplatin. It appears that patients treated with paclitaxel over shorter (eg, 3-h) schedules are more prone to the neurotoxic effect of paclitaxel as compared with those treated with longer (eg, 24- or 96-h) schedules, which argues that peak concentrations may be a principal pharmacologic determinant of neurotoxicity. The incidence of neurotoxicity has been particularly high in patients receiving paclitaxel as a 3-hour infusion combined with cisplatin.

The distal, symmetric, length-dependent neurologic deficits suggest that paclitaxel causes a sensory and motor axonal loss similar to the dying-back neuropathies that may have their origin in the cell body or in axonal transport, but a few patients have the simultaneous onset of symptoms in the arms and legs, involvement of the face (perioral numbness), the predominance of large fiber loss, and diffuse areflexia suggestive of a neuronopathy. Both types of neuropathy depend on the dose of paclitaxel or its combination with cisplatin.[293,326] Motor and autonomic dysfunction may also occur, especially at high doses and in patients with preexisting neuropathies caused by diabetes mellitus and alcoholism. Although several measures, such as the administration of amifostine, glutamate, pyridoxine, sulfhydryl group scavenger drugs, and anticonvulsants, appear to reduce the neurotoxic effects of paclitaxel in some experimental models, anecdotal reports, or insufficiently powered randomized trials, there is no convincing evidence that any specific measure is effective at ameliorating existing manifestations or preventing the development or worsening of neurotoxicity.[327,328]

Optic nerve disturbances, characterized by scintillating scotomata, may also occur.[259] Acute encephalopathy, which can progress to coma and death, has been reported following treatment with high doses (> 600 mg/m^2).[329,330] A transient acute encephalopathy following paclitaxel treatment in patients who receive prior cranial irradiation occurs rarely.[331,332]

Paclitaxel may produce transient myalgia without physical or biochemical evidence of myositis. Myalgia is typically experienced 2 to 5 days after treatment with doses above 170 mg/m^2.[333] A constellation of muscular and neuropathic effects also often precludes continuous treatment with paclitaxel administered on a weekly schedule, requiring the institution of rest periods. In general, nonsteroidal anti-inflammatory agents are minimally effective in palliating and preventing symptoms, and narcotics are usually administered prophylactically post-treatment on days 2 to 5 in patients who have been symptomatic. Antihistamines have also been anecdotally reported to prevent acute myalgia. Several investigators have reported that treatment with corticosteroids, specifically prednisone 10 mg twice daily for 5 days beginning 24 hours after treatment, is effective at reducing myalgia and arthralgia, and gabapentin, glutamate, and antihistamines could be used for management or prevention.

In early studies in which routine cardiac monitoring was performed because of the high rate of major HSRs, paclitaxel was noted to cause cardiac rhythm disturbances, the overwhelming majority of which were not associated with symptoms or sequelae; therefore, the clinical relevance of these effects is not known.[312,334] The most common rhythm disturbance appears to be transient bradycardia. The cumulative experience to date suggests that isolated asymptomatic bradycardia without hemodynamic effects is not an indication for discontinuing paclitaxel. More important bradyarrhythmias, including Mobitz type I (Wenckebach syndrome), Mobitz type II, and third-degree heart block, have been noted, but the incidence in a large National Cancer Institute database was only 0.1%.[335] Most documented episodes have been asymptomatic. Because such events were noted in patients enrolled in early trials that required continuous cardiac monitoring, second- and third-degree heart block are likely under-reported because cardiac monitoring is not usually performed. Interestingly, reports of similar disturbances in both animals and humans who ingested various species of yew plants and related taxanes affecting cardiac automaticity and conduction suggest that the bradyarrhythmias are caused by paclitaxel. Myocardial infarction, cardiac ischemia, atrial arrhythmias, and ventricular tachycardia have been noted, but whether there is a causal relationship between paclitaxel and these events is uncertain. There is no evidence that chronic, long-term treatment with paclitaxel causes progressive cardiac dysfunction. Routine cardiac monitoring during paclitaxel therapy is not necessary, but is recommended for those patients who may not be able to tolerate bradyarrhythmias, such as those with atrioventricular conduction disturbances or ventricular dysfunction. Although patients with a wide range of cardiac abnormalities and cardiac histories were broadly and empirically restricted from participating in early clinical trials, paclitaxel treatment has been reported to be well tolerated in a small series of gynecologic cancer patients with major cardiac risk factors.[336] On the other hand, repetitive treatment of patients with the combined regimen of paclitaxel on a 3-hour schedule and doxorubicin as a brief infusion is associated with a higher frequency of congestive cardiotoxicity than would be expected to occur with the same cumulative doxorubicin dose given without paclitaxel (see the section "Taxanes" above, "Drug Interactions").[296] In one study in previously untreated women with advanced breast cancer treated with escalating doses of paclitaxel as a 3-hour infusion and doxorubicin 60 mg/m^2 to a cumulative dose of 480 mg/m^2, which would be predicted to result in a less than 5% incidence of congestive cardiotoxicity in patients treated with doxorubicin alone, the incidence of congestive cardiotoxicity was approximately 25%.[296] However, the incidence of cardiotoxicity was less than 5% when similar patients received identical schedules of paclitaxel and doxorubicin, but the cumulative doxorubicin dose did not exceed 360 mg/m^2.[337,338] Both experimental and early clinical results suggest that deferoxamine may reduce the cardiotoxicity of the doxorubicin paclitaxel combination.[265] The incidence of congestive heart failure was also significantly higher in breast cancer patients treated with the combination of trastuzumab and paclitaxel than in those treated with paclitaxel alone in a randomized phase III trial; consequently, careful monitoring of patients receiving this combination is warranted.[254,310,311]

Gastrointestinal toxicities, including nausea, vomiting, and diarrhea, are uncommon. Higher paclitaxel doses may cause mucositis, especially in patients with leukemia who may be more prone to mucosal barrier breakdown or in patients receiving protracted infusions. Rare cases of neutropenic enterocolitis and gastrointestinal necrosis have been noted, particularly in patients given high doses of paclitaxel in combination with doxorubicin or cyclophosphamide.[339,340] Severe hepatotoxicity and pancreatitis have also been noted, but these events are rare Acute bilateral pneumonitis has been reported in less than 1% of patients treated on a 3-hour schedule in one series, and both interstitial and parenchymal pulmonary toxicity have been reported, but clinically significant pulmonary effects are uncommon.[319,341]

Paclitaxel also induces reversible alopecia of the scalp, but all body hair is usually lost with cumulative therapy. Alopecia appears to be dose related and occurs only following repetitive treatment with weekly administration schedules. Although the agent is often not considered a vesicant, extravasation of large volumes can cause moderate soft-tissue injury. Inflammation at the injection site and along the course of an injected vein may occur. Nail disorders have been reported, particularly in patients treated on weekly schedules.[342] Recall reactions in previously irradiated sites have also been noted.

Docetaxel Similar to paclitaxel, neutropenia is the principal toxicity of docetaxel.[167,343,344] At dosages ranging from 75 to 100 mg/m^2 administered as a 1-hour infusion, neutrophil counts usually decrease to below 500/µL. The onset of neutropenia is usually noted on day 8 and complete resolution typically occurs by days 15 to 21. Neutropenia is significantly less when low doses are administered frequently, such as on a weekly schedule (see the section 'Administration, Dose, and Schedule" below). The most important determinant of neutropenia is the extent of prior therapy, but α_1-acid glycoprotein and the duration of drug exposure above biologically relevant concentrations appear to be important determinants (see the section "Clinical Pharmacology" above). Significant effects on platelets and red blood cells are uncommon.

Even though docetaxel is not formulated in polyoxyethylated castor oil, HSRs have been reported in approximately 31% of patients receiving docetaxel without premedications.[167,343,344] However, most of these reactions are not major. Nevertheless, major reactions, characterized by dyspnea, bronchospasm, and hypotension, particularly during the first two courses and within minutes after the start of treatment, have been reported. Manifestations generally resolve within 15 minutes after cessation of treatment, and docetaxel is usually able to be reinstituted without consequences, occasionally after treatment with an H_1-histamine antagonist. Both the incidence and severity of HSRs appear to be reduced significantly by premedication with corticosteroids and both H_1- and H_2-histamine antagonists (see the section "Administration, Dose, and Schedule" below). Like paclitaxel, patients who experience major HSRs have been re-treated successfully after resolution of symptoms and following treatment with corticosteroids and H_1-histamine antagonists. Although patients who have experienced HSRs following paclitaxel treatment have been re-treated successfully with docetaxel, this strategy has not been studied in a rigorous fashion.

In early studies, a unique fluid retention syndrome, characterized by edema, weight gain, and third-space fluid collection, was noted in patients treated with multiple courses of docetaxel and was related to the absolute cumulative dose.[167,343–346] Fluid retention did not appear to be related to hypoalbuminemia or cardiac, renal, or hepatic dysfunction, but to increased capillary permeability. Capillary filtration studies revealed a two-stage process with progressive congestion of the interstitial space by proteins and water, starting between the second and fourth course that progressed to insufficient lymphatic drainage. In early studies in which prophylactic medication was not used, fluid retention was not usually significant at cumulative docetaxel doses below 400 mg/m^2; however, the incidence and severity of fluid retention increased sharply at cumulative doses of 400 mg/m^2 or greater, and often resulted in the delay or termination of treatment. Prophylactic treatment with corticosteroids with or without H_1- and H_2-histamine antagonists reduces the overall incidence of fluid retention and increases the number of courses and cumulative docetaxel dose before the onset of this toxicity (see the section "Administration, Dose, and Schedule" below).[345] In fact, drug-induced fluid retention has been uncommon following the broad adoption of corticosteroid premedication. Fluid retention resolves slowly after docetaxel is stopped, with complete resolution occurring several months after treatment in patients with severe toxicity. Aggressive and early treatment with progressively more potent diuretics, starting with potassium sparing diuretics, has been successfully used to manage fluid retention. The incidence of fluid retention appears to be lower in studies that used lower doses (60–75 mg/m^2) of docetaxel during each course, but this may be a result of the administration of lower overall cumulative doses, and the effects of lower doses on antitumor activity are unknown.

Although both neurosensory and neuromuscular effects due to docetaxel are similar to paclitaxel, they are less common and appear to be less severe compared with paclitaxel.[167,343,344,347] In a phase III trial, patients with advanced ovarian carcinoma receiving first-line treatment with docetaxel and carboplatin experienced significantly less severe and less total neurotoxicity than did those receiving treatment with paclitaxel and carboplatin.[348] Mild to moderate peripheral neurotoxicity is observed in approximately 40% of previously untreated patients. Previous treatment with cisplatin appears to increase the likelihood of developing neurotoxicity. The neurotoxicity is qualitatively similar to that of paclitaxel, with sensory effects predominating. Patients typically complain of paresthesia and numbness, but peripheral motor disturbances may also occur. Severe toxicity is unusual following repetitive treatment with docetaxel doses less than 100 mg/m^2, except in patients with antecedent disorders such as alcohol abuse.

Although cardiovascular effects, including angina, arrhythmia, conduction disturbances, congestive heart failure, hypertension, and hypotension, have been noted rarely in the pretreatment period, there is no convincing evidence that directly links docetaxel to these events. Stomatitis appears to occur more frequently with docetaxel than paclitaxel, particularly with prolonged infusions that are used rarely. Nausea, vomiting, and diarrhea have also been observed infrequently, but severe manifestations are rare. Empiric use of antiemetic premedication does not appear to be warranted. Phlebitis along the course of the infused veins and local inflammation at the injection site are occasionally noted; however, severe tissue damage following drug extravasation is not generally observed. Transient arthralgia and myalgia without inflammatory manifestations are occasionally noted within days following treatment. Malaise, often referred to as asthenia, has been a prominent complaint in patients who have been treated with large cumulative doses, particularly when docetaxel is administered on a continuous weekly schedule.[349,350]

Skin toxicity may occur in as many as 50 to 75% of patients[138,139,273,278,279]; however, premedication may reduce the overall incidence of this toxicity. An erythematous pruritic maculopapular rash that affects the forearms, hands, and/or feet is typical. Desquamation of the hands and feet, which is a component of a more general palmar-plantar syndrome that may respond to pyridoxine or cooling, and onychodystrophy characterized by brown discoloration, ridging, onycholysis, soreness, and brittleness and loss of the nail plate have been reported.[342,351,352] Skin and nail changes appear to be most prominent in patients treated frequently with low doses (ie, weekly schedules). Excessive lacrimation, occasionally due to cannicular stenosis, may also occur.[353] Other rare events that may or may not be related to docetaxel itself include confusion, erythema multiforme, neutropenic enterocolitis, hepatitis, ileus, interstitial pneumonia, seizures, pulmonary fibrosis, hepatitis, radiation recall, and visual disturbances.

ABI-007 The toxicity profile of ABI-007 is similar to that of paclitaxel, with neutropenia as the principal dose-limiting toxicity.[181,289,290] The majority of other paclitaxel-related toxicities have been observed; however, relationships between the rate of individual toxicities and dose differ. The rate of HSRs, particularly major reactions, appears much less than that of paclitaxel, most likely because of the absence of polyoxyethylated castor oil in the formulation. No premedication regimen to prevent HSRs is recommended.

ADMINISTRATION, DOSE, AND SCHEDULE **Paclitaxel** Discerning the optimal dose and schedule for the taxanes, principally paclitaxel, has been a major focus of many evaluations over the last decade.[313] The collective results of these efforts indicate that paclitaxel has prominent antitumor activity on multiple schedules and that no particular schedule is superior from an efficacy standpoint across all tumor types; however, toxicity profiles may be vastly different. The earliest clinical studies of paclitaxel were limited to the 24-hour schedule, largely as a consequence of an apparent increased rate of severe HSRs on shorter schedules, but the development of effective premedication regimens led to evaluation of a broad range of dosing schedules. Although paclitaxel 135 mg/m^2 on a 24-hour schedule was initially approved for patients with refractory and recurrent ovarian cancer, regulatory approval was later obtained for paclitaxel 175 mg/m^2 on a 3-hour schedule in these and other indications. In patients with advanced breast and ovarian cancers, the collective results of randomized studies in patients treated with paclitaxel on 3-, 24-, and 96-hour-every-3-weeks administration schedules indicate that they are largely equivalent, particularly with regard to event-free and overall survival, although response rates have occasionally been higher with more protracted schedules.[313,354] The extensive distribution of the taxanes to peripheral tissues, as well as the avid and protracted tissue binding of these agents, may explain the lack of substantial differences in antitumor activity between short and more protracted administration schedules despite substantial differences in vitro.

There has also been considerable interest in intermittent schedules, particularly those in which paclitaxel is administered as a 1-hour infusion weekly, which results in substantially less myelosuppression than every-3-week schedules.[349,355,356] Furthermore, there have been reports of impressive and superior activity of weekly compared with every-3-week schedules in several disease settings, particularly in treatment of advanced and metastatic breast cancer patients.[355–357] However, there is no convincing evidence that weekly treatment results in robust activity in tumors unresponsive to the taxanes on every-3-week schedules. Nevertheless, the weekly schedule may be advantageous for patients who are at high risk of developing severe myelosuppression, but there appears to be a higher incidence of neuromuscular effects.

Paclitaxel is indicated and generally administered at a dosage of 175 mg/m^2 over 3 hours or, less frequently, 135 to 175 mg/m^2 over 24 hours every 3 weeks. Several randomized trials in patients with advanced lung, head and neck, and ovarian cancers have consistently failed to show that paclitaxel dosages above 135 to 175 mg/m^2 on a 24-hour schedule are superior to conventional doses.[313,354] Nearly identical results have been obtained in a phase III study in patients with metastatic breast cancer, in which greater efficacy was not observed in patients treated with paclitaxel dosages above 175 mg/m^2 on a 3-hour schedule.[358] The following dosages have been recommended on less conventional schedules: 200 mg/m^2 over 1 hour as either a single dose or 3 divided doses every 3 weeks; 140 mg/m^2 over 96 hours every 3 weeks; and 80 to 100 mg/m^2 weekly. The most common schedules evaluated in patients with Kaposi's sarcoma caused by the acquired immunodeficiency syndrome are paclitaxel 135 mg/m^2 over 3 or 24 hours every 3 weeks and 100 mg/m^2 every 2 weeks.[191] Paclitaxel has also been administered into the pleural and peritoneal cavities. Biologically relevant plasma concentrations have been achieved with intraperitoneal administration, and concentrations in the peritoneal cavity are several orders of magnitude higher than plasma concentrations.

The following premedication is recommended to prevent major HSRs: dexamethasone 20 mg orally or intravenously, 12 and 6 hours before treatment; an H_1-histamine antagonist (such as diphenhydramine, 50 mg intravenously) 30 minutes before treatment; and an H_2-histamine antagonist (such as cimetidine, 300 mg; famotidine, 20 mg; or ranitidine, 150 mg intravenously) 30 minutes before treatment. A single dose of a corticosteroid (dexamethasone 20 mg intravenously) administered 30 minutes before treatment also appears to confer effective prophylaxis of major HSRs.

Hepatic metabolism and biliary excretion are the principal modes of drug disposition, paclitaxel and dose modifications are required in patients with hepatic dysfunction. However, official recommendations have not been formulated, and study results are somewhat conflicting because of differences in the definitions of dose-limiting toxicity between various studies. Prospective studies indicate that patients with moderate to severe elevations in serum concentrations of hepatocellular enzymes and/or bilirubin are more likely to develop severe toxicity than patients without hepatic dysfunction.[359,360] Therefore, it is recommended that paclitaxel doses be reduced by at least 50% in patients with moderate or severe hepatic excretory dysfunction (hyperbilirubinemia) and/or substantial elevations in hepatic transaminases. Renal clearance contributes minimally to overall clearance (5–10%), and patients with severe renal dysfunction do not appear to require dose modification.[232,361] Based on the pharmacologic behavior, particularly the wide distributive properties of the taxanes, dose modifications are not required solely for peripheral edema and third-space fluid collections.

Contact of the paclitaxel-polyoxyethylated castor oil formulation with plasticized polyvinyl chloride (PVC) equipment or devices must be avoided because of the risk of patient exposures to plasticizers that may be leached from PVC infusion bags or sets. Paclitaxel solutions should be diluted and stored in glass or polypropylene bottles or suitable plastic bags (polypropylene or polyolefin) and administered through polyethylene-lined administration sets that include an in-line filter with a microporous membrane not greater than 0.22 microns.

Docetaxel In the United States, docetaxel is indicated at a dosage range of 60 to 100 mg/m^2 and 75 mg/m^2 over 1 hour in patients with breast and non–small cell lung cancers, respectively, but most early clinical trials in advanced breast, ovarian, and non–small cell lung cancers evaluated doses at the higher end of this range (75–100 mg/m^2), with scant data available for patients treated with docetaxel 60 mg/m^2.[167] Although some untreated or minimally pretreated patients generally tolerate docetaxel at a dose of 100 mg/m^2 without severe toxicity, emerging data indicate poorer tolerance in more heavily pretreated patients, in whom 75 mg/m^2 appears to be more reasonable from a toxicologic perspective.[362] Docetaxel 75 mg/m^2 is associated with a survival benefit in patients with non–small cell lung cancer following first-line treatment. Like paclitaxel, docetaxel has also been administered as a 1-hour infusion weekly.[350] Although a clear benefit of chronic weekly drug administration over the conventional schedule in terms of antitumor activity is not evident at this time, prospective randomized trials are in progress to address this issue. However, hematologic toxicity is much less with weekly dose schedules than with conventional dose schedules. Both cumulative asthenia and neurotoxicity are the principal toxicities of docetaxel administered weekly, precluding administration of dosages exceeding 36 mg/m^2/wk. Despite the use of a polysorbate-80 formulation instead of polyoxyethylated castor oil, which is used to formulate paclitaxel, a relatively high rate of HSRs and profound fluid retention in patients who did not receive premedication has led to the use of several effective premedication regimens, the most popular of which is dexamethasone 8 mg orally twice daily for 3 or 5 days starting 1 or 2 days, respectively, before docetaxel, with or without both H_1- and H_2-histamine antagonists given 30 minutes before docetaxel.[344,345] Administration of docetaxel without corticosteroids is not recommended, even in patients who do not develop HSRs, because drug-related fluid retention, which is a chronic toxicity, requires drug discontinuation.

A retrospective review of docetaxel pharmacokinetics in patients without hyperbilirubinemia demonstrated that docetaxel clearance is reduced by approximately 25% in patients with elevations in serum concentrations of both hepatic transaminases (1.5-fold or greater) and alkaline phosphatase (2.5-fold or greater), regardless of whether the elevations are a result of hepatic metastases.[278–280] Therefore, dose reductions by at least 25% are recommended for such individuals. More substantial reductions (50% or greater) may be required in patients who have moderate or severe hepatic excretory dysfunction (hyperbilirubinemia). Similar to paclitaxel (see the section "Taxanes" above, "Administration, Dose, and Schedule"), there is no rationale for dose modification solely for renal deficiency and/or third-space fluid accumulation. Also similar to the case with paclitaxel (see the section "Taxanes" above, "Administration, Dose, and Schedule"), glass bottles or polypropylene or polyolefin plastic products should be used for preparation and storage, and docetaxel should be administered through polyethylene-lined administration sets.

ABI-007 The agent, ABI-007, received regulatory approval in the United States for the treatment of patients with metastatic breast cancer after failure of combination chemotherapy for metastatic disease or relapse within 6 months of adjuvant chemotherapy. The recommended dosage schedule for this indication is 260 mg/m^2 as a 30-minute IV infusion. No premedication to prevent HSRs is required prior to administration. The use of PVC-free containers and administration sets is not necessary, and the use of an in-line filter is not recommended.

NOVEL ANTIMICROTUBULE AGENTS IN EARLY CLINICAL DEVELOPMENT

The clinical success of the taxanes has led to a search for other drugs that enhance tubulin polymerization, yielding several promising compounds that may confer a therapeutic advantage over the taxanes, including the epothilones (isolated from myxobacterium *Sorangium cellulosum*), discodermolide (isolated from the Caribbean sponge *Discodermia dissoluta*), the sarcodictyins, eleutherobin (isolated from the soft coral *Eleutherobia sp*) and laulimalide (isolated from the marine sponge *Cacospongia mycofijiensis*), and sarcodictyins (isolated from the Mediterranean stoloniferan coral *Sarcodictyon roseum*), (Figure 46-4). Some of these compounds compete with paclitaxel for binding to microtubules and appear to bind at or near the taxane site (epothilones, discodermolide, eleutherobins, and sarcodictyins), but others, such as laulimalide, seem to bind to unique sites on microtubules.[2,4,5,188,192] All of these compounds possess either low-level or no substrate affinity for ABC transporters, and retain various degrees of activity against taxane-resistant cells in vitro, but the clinical implications of these characteristics are not clear.

Of the aforementioned, the epothilones are the furthest along in development. Not only do they promote tubulin polymerization and induce mitotic arrest, but several epothilones possess much greater cytotoxic potency than either paclitaxel or docetaxel.[2,4,5,188,190,192,363–366] In contrast to the taxanes and vinca alkaloids, overexpression of Pgp minimally affects the cytotoxicity of epothilones A and B. Furthermore, various point mutations in β-tubulin, which confer resistance to the taxanes in vitro, do not necessarily confer resistance to the epothilones.[364,366,367] Several epothilone B analogs, including ixabepilone (BMS-247550) and patupiline (EPO906), are currently undergoing clinical evaluation. The principal mode of disposition for ixabepilone is via cytochrome P-450 metabolism and biliary excretion, whereas patupiline is metabolized via carboxyesterases.[366,368–371] The pharmacological characteristics are typified by marked tissue uptake, avid and protracted tissue binding, and long terminal half-lives of elimination. Furthermore, their principal toxicities differ, namely diarrhea for patupiline and both myelosuppression and neurotoxicity for ixabepilone.[366] In early clinical trials, responses have been noted in patients with advanced carcinomas of the breast, lung, prostate, and ovary, some of whom experienced recurrent disease following or during treatment with the taxanes. However, the magnitude of their activity in taxane-refractory malignancies needs to be addressed. Of note, patupiline has demonstrated antitumor activity in advanced colorectal and renal carcinomas, which are almost always inherently resistant to antimicrotubule agents, but the magnitude of appreciable activity in cancers with primary or acquired resistance to the taxanes is negligible.[366,372] An epothilone D, desoxyepotholone B (KOS862) that has demonstrated at least equivalent potency and less toxicity than the taxanes and epothilone B analogues in preclinical studies, is in early clinical development.[47,364,373] Additional modifications of naturally occurring epothilones have been made in an effort to improve solubility, such as those leading to the development of BMS-310705, which is a C-21 derivative of epothilone B.[370,374]

Similar to the epothilones A and B, discodermolide-induced tubulin polymers are quite stable to treatment with calcium and are composed of short microtubules instead of tubulin spirals.[365,375] In addition to low-level cross-resistance to Pgp overexpressing cancer cells, paclitaxel and epothilone-resistant human tumor cells that express mutant β-tubulin, retain sensitivity to discodermolide. Furthermore, discodermolide and paclitaxel have demonstrated synergistic cytotoxicity in vitro, suggesting that their tubulin binding sites and microtubule effects are not identical.[375,376] However, unforeseen pulmonary toxicity has been seen in early clinical studies of a completely synthetic discodermolide (XAA296).[377] Because eleutherobin, epothilones A and B, and discodermolide, competitively inhibit [^{3}H]paclitaxel binding to microtubules, a common pharmacophore was sought and identified, which may enable the development of hybrid constructs with more desirable biological characteristics.[188,192]

Other natural and semisynthetic agents under evaluation bind to the vinca or colchicine-binding domains. Among the most potent are the dolastatins, which constitute a series of oligopeptides isolated from the sea hare, *Dolabela auricularia*.[378,379] Two of the most potent dolastatins, dolastatin-10 and -15, noncompetitively inhibit binding of vinca alkaloids to tubulin, inhibit tubulin polymerization, and tubulin-dependent GTP hydrolysis, stabilize the colchicine-binding activity of tubulin, and possess

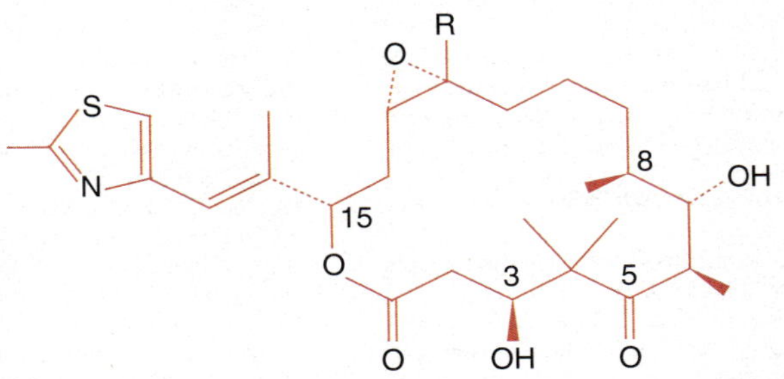

Epothilone A (R=H)
Epothilone B (R=Me)

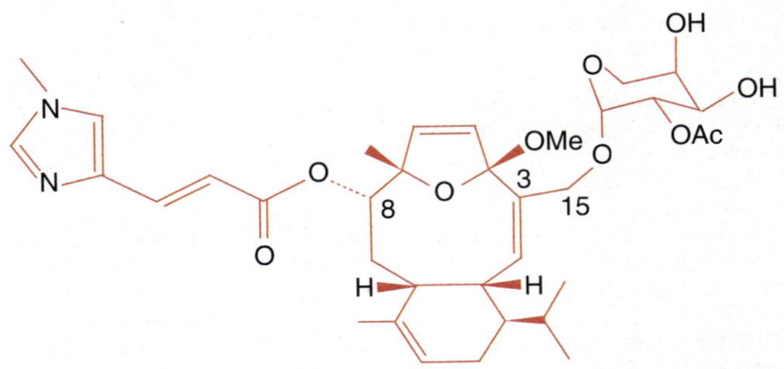

Eleutherobin

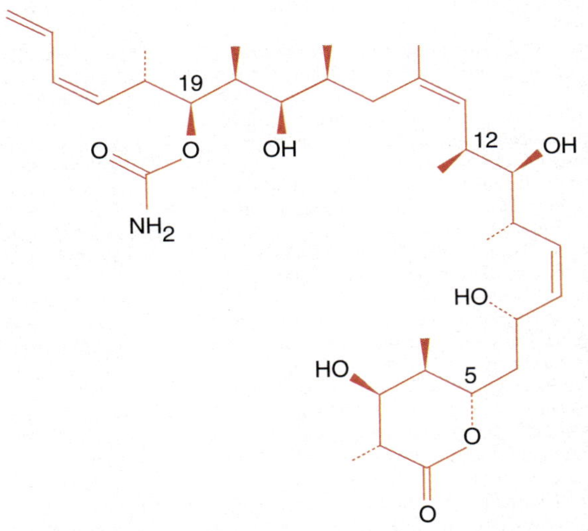

(+)-Discodermolide

Figure 46-4 Chemical structures of several natural products that induce tubulin polymerization and share mechanistic features with the taxanes: epothilone A and B, eleutherobin (*middle*), and discodermolide.

cytotoxic activity in the picomolar to low nanomolar range. Dolastatin-10 and semisynthetic dolastatin analogues (synthadotin [ILX-651] and TZT-1027), which binds in the vinca domain, are undergoing clinical evaluation.[2,4,380,381]

Phomopsin A, halichondrin B, homohalichondrin B, and spongistatin 1, which competitively inhibit vinca alkaloid binding to tubulin, are being evaluated in preclinical or early clinical evaluations. E7389, a macrocyclic ketone analogue of the marine natural product halichondrin B originally isolated from the marine sponge *Halicondrin okadai*, and two less complex synthetic macrocyclic ketone analogues, ER-076349 and ER-086526 are in early clinical evaluations. These compounds bind to tubulin, inhibit tubulin polymerization, disrupt mitotic spindle formation, induce mitotic arrest, and possess growth inhibitory properties in the subnanomolar range and marked activity in preclinical studies. Several biochemical correlates of apoptosis are also observed following E7389 treatment, including phosphorylation of the antiapoptotic protein Bcl-2, cytochrome c release from mitochondria, proteolytic activation of caspase-3 and -9, and cleavage of the caspase-3 substrate poly(ADP-ribose) polymerase. The agent is currently in phase I-II evaluations in patients with advanced solid malignancies.

Also in clinical development is HTI-286, a synthetic form of hemiasterlin, which is a natural product derived from marine sponges.[382] Hemiasterlin and its analogues bind to the vinca-peptide site in tubulin, disrupt normal microtubule dynamics, and, at stoichiometric amounts, depolymerize microtubules. HTI-286 is a much weaker substrate for Pgp than the vinca alkaloids and taxanes. It has excellent in vivo antitumor activity in human xenograft models, including tumors that express Pgp. The agent is cross-resistant with other vinca peptide-binding agents, including hemiasterlin A, dolastatin-10, and vinblastine (7- to 28-fold), and DNA-damaging drugs, including doxorubicin and mitoxantrone (16- to 57-fold), but is minimally cross-resistant with the taxanes, epothilones, or colchicine (1- to 4-fold). However, resistance appears to be at least partially mediated by mutation of α-tubulin and by an ATP-binding cassette drug pump distinct from P-glycoprotein, ABCG2, MRP1, or MRP3.

Most efforts targeting the tumor vasculature are aimed at the development of agents that inhibit the process of angiogenesis, but recently, several antimicrotubule agents have been demonstrated to rapidly shut down existing tumor vasculature.[383–385] Since the late 1990s, the combretastatins and *N*-acetylcolchicinol-*O*-phosphate, compounds that resemble colchicine and bind to the colchicine domain on tubulin, have undergone extensive development as antivascular agents. Several of them (combretastatin-A-4 3-*O*-phosphate, combrestatin A-1-phosphate (CA-1-P), ZD6126 and AVE8062A are in clinical trials.[386–388] Although objective antitumor activity in preliminary evaluations has been noted, cardiovascular toxicity has been problematic.

Targeting Mitotic Kinesins and Kinases

Although tubulin is the most abundant protein component of the mitotic spindle apparatus, many additional proteins, such as mitotic kinesins, play critical roles in the mechanics of mitosis and in progression through the premitotic cell-cycle checkpoint. Kinesins are motor proteins that translate chemical energy released by the hydrolysis of ATP into mechanical force for movement along microtubules, transport of a wide variety of cargoes, and the intracellular organization of the mitotic spindle and other microtubule-containing structures.[20,389–391]

The mitotic kinesins are a subgroup of kinesin motor proteins that function exclusively in mitosis in proliferating cells.[389–391] During mitosis, different, highly specialized mitotic kinesins play critical roles in various aspects of mitotic spindle assembly, including the establishment of spindle bipolarity, spindle pole organization, chromosome alignment and segregation, and regulation of microtubule dynamics. The establishment of mitotic spindle bipolarity is among the earliest events in spindle assembly, and it requires the function of a specific kinesin motor protein KSP (also known as Eg5), which has no known role outside of mitosis. The expression profiles of KSP mRNA in normal tissues are consistent with preferential expression of KSP in proliferating cells relative to normal adjacent tissue and postmitotic neurons. As essential elements in mitotic spindle assembly and function, KSP and mitotic kinesins provide attractive targets for intervention into the cell cycle.[20,389–391] CK0106023 (SB-715992) a polycyclic, nitrogen-containing heterocycle and allosteric inhibitor of KSP motor domain ATPase with a Ki of 12 nM and a potent KSP inhibitor that causes mitotic arrest, is entering clinical trials.[391–393] The compound, which is 10,000-fold more selective for KSP relative to other members of the kinesin superfamily, has been shown to block assembly of a functional mitotic spindle, thereby causing cell-cycle arrest in mitosis and subsequent cell death.[391] In tumor-bearing mice, the agent exhibited antitumor activity comparable to or exceeding that of paclitaxel and caused the formation of monopolar mitotic figures identical to those produced in cultured cells.[391] In addition, a more potent KSP inhibitor with apparently higher therapeutic indices than SB715992, SB743921, is in phase I clinical investigations.

A host of mitotic kinases are also being assessed as strategic targets for anticancer therapeutic development. For example, the aurora kinases (A, B, C) are essential for the regulation of chromosome segregation and cytokinesis during mitosis, and aberrant expression and activity of these kinases occur in a wide range of human tumors and lead to aneuploidy and tumorigenesis.[394,395] Recently, a highly potent and selective small-molecule inhibitor of the aurora kinases, VX-680, has been demonstrated to block cell-cycle progression and induce apoptosis in a diverse range of human tumor types.[396] This compound causes profound inhibition of tumor growth in a variety of in vivo xenograft models, leading to regression of leukemia, and colon and pancreatic tumors at well-tolerated doses, and is entering clinical trials.

REFERENCES

1. Gelfand VI, Bershadsky AD. Microtubule dynamics: mechanism, regulation, and function. Annu Rev Cell Biol 1991;7:93.
2. Jordan MA, Wilson L. Microtubules as a target for anticancer drugs. Nat Rev Cancer 2004;4:253.
3. Jordan MA. Mechanism of action of antitumor drugs that interact with microtubules and tubulin. Curr Med Chem Anticancer Agents 2002;2:1.
4. Kavallaris M, Verrillis NM, Hill BT. Anticancer therapy with novel tubulin-interacting drugs. Drug Resist Updat 2001;4:392.
5. Pinz H. Recent advances in the field of tubulin polymerization inhibitors. Expert Rev Anticancer Ther 2002;2:695.
6. Correia JJ, Lobert S. Physiochemical aspects of tubulin-interacting antimitotic drugs. Curr Pharm Des 2001;7:1213.
7. Nogales E, Whittaker M, Milligan RA, Downing KH. High-resolution model of the microtubule. Cell 1999;96:79.
8. Carlier M-F. Role of nucleotide hydrolysis in the polymerization of actin and tubulin. Cell Biophys 1998;12:105.
9. Mitchison TJ. Localization of exchangeable GTP binding site at the plus end of microtubules. Science 1993;261:1044.
10. Zheng Y, Jung MK, Oakley BR. Gamma-tubulin is present in Drosophila melanogaster and Homo sapiens and is associated with the centrosome. Cell 1991;65:817.
11. Margolis RL, Wilson L. Microtubule treadmilling: what goes around comes around. Bioessays 1998;20:830.
12. Wilson L, Panda D, Jordan MA. Modulation of microtubule dynamics by drugs: a paradigm for the actions of cellular regulators. Cell Struc Funct 1999;24:329.
13. Mitchison T, Kirschner M. Dynamic instability of microtubule growth. Nature 1984;312:232.
14. Erickson HP, O'Brien ET. Microtubule dynamic instability and GTP hydrolysis. Annu Rev Biophys Biomol Struct 1992;21:145.
15. Wilson L, Jordan MA. Pharmacological probes of microtubule function. Biochemistry. 1993;59:185.
16. Zhai Y, Kronebusch PJ, Simon PM, Borisy GG. Microtubule dynamics at the G2/M transition: abrupt breakdown of cytoplasmic microtubules at nuclear envelope breakdown and implications for spindle morphogenesis. J Cell Biol 1996;135:201.
17. Olmsted JB. Microtubule-associated proteins. Annu Rev Cell Biol 1986;2:421.
18. Bhalla KN. Microtubule-targeted anticancer agents and apoptosis. Oncogene 2003;22:9075.
19. Jordan MA, Wendell KL, Gardiner S, et al. Mitotic block induced in HeLa cells by low concentrations of paclitaxel (Taxol) results in abnormal mitotic exit and apoptotic cell death. Cancer Res 1996;56:816.
20. Vallee RB, Bloom GS, Theurkauf WE. Microtubule associated proteins: subunits of the cytomatrix. J Cell Biol 1984;99:38s.
21. Vale RD, Milligan RA. The way things move: looking under the hood of molecular motor proteins. Science 2000;288:88.
22. Khan A, Luduena F. Different effects of vinblastine on the polymerization of isotypically purified tubulins from bovine brain. Invest New Drugs 2003;21:3.
23. Raff EC. The role of multiple tubulin isoforms in cellular microtubule function. In: Hyams JF, Lloyd CD, editors. Microtubules. New York: Wiley-Liss; 1993. p. 89.
24. Luduena RF. Multiple forms of tubulin: different gene products and covalent modifications. Int Rev Cytol 1998;178:207.
25. Luduena RF. Are tubulin isotypes functionally significant? Mol Biol Cell 1983;4:445.
26. Schulze E, Asai DJ, Bulinski JC, et al. Post-translational modification and microtubule stability. J Cell Biol 1987;105:2167.
27. Johnson IS. Historical background of vinca alkaloid research and areas of future interest. Cancer Chemother Rep 1968;52:455.
28. Johnson IS, Armstrong JG, Gorman M et al. The vinca alkaloids: a new class of oncolytic agents. Cancer Res 1963;23:1390.
29. Rowinsky EK, Donehower RC. The clinical pharmacology and use of antimicrotubule agents in cancer chemotherapeutics. Pharmacol Ther 1992;52:35.
30. Betrand Y, Capdeville R, Balduck N, et al. Cyclosporin A used to reverse drug resistance increases vincristine neurotoxicity. Am J Hematol 1992;40:158.
31. Dancey J, Steward WP. The role of vindesine in oncology—recommendations after 10 years' experience. Anticancer Drugs 1995;6:625.
32. Joel S. The comparative clinical pharmacology of vincristine and vindesine: Does vindesine offer any advantage in clinical use? Cancer Treat Rev 1996;21:513.
33. Gridelli C, De Vivo R. Vinorelbine in the treatment of non-small cell lung cancer. Curr Med Chem 2002;9:879.
34. Domenech GH, Vogel CL. Single agent vinorelbine as first-line chemotherapy in elderly patients with advanced breast cancer. Anticancer Res 2003;23:1657.
35. Budman DR. Vinorelbine (Navelbine): a third-generation vinca alkaloid. Cancer Invest 1997;15:475.
36. Curran MP, Plosker GL. Vinorelbine: a review of its use in elderly patients with advanced non-small cell lung cancer. Drugs Aging 2002;19:695.
37. Johnson SA, Harper P, Hortobagyi GN, Pouillart P. Vinorelbine: an overview. Cancer Treat Rev 1996;22:127.
38. Kruczynski A, Hill BT. Vinflunine, the latest Vinca alkaloid in clinical development. A review of its preclinical anticancer properties. Crit Rev Oncol Hematol 2001;40:159.
39. Ngan V, Bellman K, Hill B, et al. Novel actions of the antitumor drugs vinflunine and vinorelbine on microtubules. Mol Pharmacol 2001;60:225.
40. Derry WB, Wilson L, Jordan MA. Substoichiometric binding of Taxol suppresses microtubule dynamics. Biochem 1995;34:2203.
41. Wilson L, Jordan MA. Microtubule dynamics: taking aim at a moving target. Chem Biol 1995;2:569.
42. Jordan MA, Toso RJ, Thrower D, Wilson L. Mechanism of mitotic block and inhibition of cell proliferation by Taxol at low concentrations. Proc Natl Acad Sci U S A 1993;90:9552.
43. Donoso RJ, Jordan MA, Farrell KW, et al. Kinetic stabilization of the microtubule dynamic instability in vitro by vinblastine. Biochem 1993;32:185.
44. Himes RH, Kersey RN, Heller-Bettinger I, Sampson FE. Action of the vinca alkaloids, vincristine and vinblastine, and desacetyl vinblastine amide on microtubules in vitro. Cancer Res 1976;36:3798.
45. Tucker RW, Owellen RJ, Harris SB. Correlation of cytotoxicity and mitotic spindle dissolution by vinblastine in mammalian cells. Cancer Res 1977;37:4346.
46. Bruchovsky N, Owen AA, Becker AJ, et al. Effects of vinblastine on the proliferative capacity of L cells and their progress through the division cycle. Cancer Res 1965;25:1232.
47. Chou TC, Zhang XG, Harris CR, et al. Desoxyepothilone B is curative against human tumor xenografts that are refractory to paclitaxel. Proc Natl Acad Sci U S A 1998;95:15798.
48. Jordan MA, Thrower D, Wilson L. Mechanism of inhibition of cell proliferation by the vinca alkaloids. Cancer Res 1991;51:2212.
49. Himes RH. Interactions of the Catharanthus (vinca) alkaloids with tubulin and microtubules. Pharmacol Ther 1991;51:256.
50. Jordan MA, Margolis RL, Himes RH, Wilson LJ. Identification of a distinct class of vinblastine binding sites on microtubules. J Mol Biol 1986;187:61.
51. Jordan MA, Wilson L. Kinetic analysis of tubulin exchange at microtubule ends at low vinblastine concentrations. Biochem 1990;29:2730.
52. Singer WD, Jordan MA, Wilson L, Himes RH. Binding of vinblastine to stabilized microtubules. Mol Pharmacol 1989;36:366.
53. Donoso JA. Effect of microtubule proteins on the interaction of vincristine and microtubules and tubulin. Cancer Res 1979;39:1604.
54. Beck WT. Alkaloids. In: Fox BW, Fox M, editors. Antitumor drug resistance. Berlin: Springer-Verlag; 1984. p. 589.
55. Palmer CG, Livengood D, Warren AK, et al. The action of the vincaleukoblastine on mitosis in vitro. Exp Cell Res 1960;20:198.
56. Fan S, Cherney B, Reinhold W, et al. Disruption of p53 function in immortalized human cells does not affect survival or apoptosis after Taxol or vincristine treatment. Clin Cancer Res 1998;4:1047.
57. Blagosklonny MV, Robey R, Bates S, et al. Pretreatment with DNA-damaging agents permits selective killing of checkpoint-deficient cells by microtubule-active drugs. J Clin Invest 2000;105:533.
58. Jordan MA, Thrower D, Wilson L. Effects of vinblastine, podophyllotoxin and nocodazole on mitotic spindles. Implications for the role of microtubule dynamics in mitosis. J Cell Sci 1992;102:401.
59. Zhang CC, Yang JM, Bash-Babula J, et al. DNA damage increases sensitivity to vinca alkaloids and decreases sensitivity to taxanes through p53-dependent repression of microtubule-associated protein 4. Cancer Res 1999;59:3663.
60. Vacca A, Iurlaro M, Ribatti D, et al. Antiangiogenesis is produced by nontoxic doses of vinblastine. Blood 1999;94:4143.
61. Sullivan KF. Structure and utilization of tubulin isotypes. Annu Rev Cell Biol 1988;4:687.
62. Lobert S, Correia JJ. Energetics of vinca alkaloid interactions with tubulin. Methods Enzmol 2000;323:77.
63. Lobert S, Vulevic B, Correria JJ. Interaction of vinca alkaloids with tubulin: a comparison of vinblastine, vincristine, and vinorelbine. Biochem 1996;35:6806.
64. Bowman LC, Houghton JA, Houghton PJ. Formation and stability of vincristine-tubulin complex in kidney cytosols. Role of GTP and GTP hydrolysis. Biochem Pharmacol 1988;37:1251.
65. Ferguson PJ, Cass CE. Differential cellular retention of vincristine and vinblastine by cultured human promyelocytic leukemia HL-60/C-1 cells: the basis of differential toxicity. Cancer Res 1985;45:5480.
66. Bleyer WA, Frisby SA, Oliverio VT. Uptake and binding of vincristine by murine leukemia cells. Biochem Pharmacol 1975;24:633.
67. Rahmani R, Zhou XJ, Placidi M, et al. In vivo and in vitro pharmacokinetics and metabolism of vinca alkaloids in rat. I. Vindesine (4-deacetyl-vinblastine 3-carboxyamide). Eur J Drug Metab Pharmacokinet 1990;15:49.
68. Zhou XJ, Martin M, Placidi M, et al. In vivo and in vitro pharmacokinetics and metabolism of vinca alkaloids: II. Vinblastine and vincristine. Eur J Drug Metab Pharmacokinet 1990;15:323.
69. Ferguson PJ, Phillips JR, Steiner M, et al. Differential activity of vincristine and vinblastine against cultured cells. Cancer Res 1984;45:5480.
70. Houghton JA, Williams LG, Houghton PJ. Stability of vincristine complexes in cytosols derived from xenografts of human rhabdomyosarcoma and normal tissues of the mouse. Cancer Res 1985;45:3761.

71. Bowman LC, Houghton JA, Houghton PJ. GTP influences the binding of vincristine in human tumor cytosols. Biochem Biophys Res Commun 1986;135:695.
72. Gout PW, Noble RL, Bruchovsky N, Beer CT. Vinblastine and vincristine growth-inhibitory effects correlate with their retention by cultured Nb2 node lymphoma cells. Int J Cancer 1984;34:245.
73. Ferguson PJ, Philips JR, Seiner M, Cass CE. Biochemical effects of Navelbine on tubulin and associated proteins. Cancer Res 1984;44:3307.
74. Zhou XJ, Placidi M, Rahmani R. Uptake. Uptake and metabolism of vinca alkaloids by freshly isolated human hepatocytes in suspension. Anticancer Res 1994;14:1017.
75. Rahmani R, Zhou XJ. Pharmacokinetics and metabolism of vinca alkaloids . Cancer surveys 1993;17:269.
76. Jackson DV, Bender RA. Cytotoxic thresholds of vincristine in a murine and human leukemia cell line in vitro. Cancer Res 1979;39:4346.
77. Lockhart A, Tirona G Kim B. Pharmacogenetics of ATP-binding cassette transporters in cancer and chemotherapy. Mol Ther 2003;2:685.
78. Safa AR, Glover CJ, Meyers MB, et al. Vinblastine photoaffinity labeling of a high molecular weight surface membrane glycoprotein specific for multidrug-resistant cells. Biochem 1987;262:13685.
79. Grant CE, Validmarsson G, Hipfner R, et al. Overexpression of multidrug resistance associated protein (MRP) increases resistance to natural product drugs. Cancer Res 1994;54:356.
80. Greenberger LM, Williams SS, Horwitz SB. Biosynthesis of heterogeneous forms of multidrug resistance associated glycoproteins. J Biol Chem 1987;262:13685.
81. Choi K, Chen C, Kriegler M, Roninson IB. An altered pattern of cross-resistance in multidrug-resistant human cells results from spontaneous mutations in the mdr1 (P-glycoprotein) gene. Cell 1988;53:519.
82. Pieters R, Hongo T, Loonen AH, et al. Different types of non-P-glycoprotein mediated multiple drug resistance in children with relapsed acute lymphoblastic leukaemia. Br J Cancer 1992;65:691.
83. Nooter K, Westerman AM, Flens MJ, et al. Expression of the multidrug resistance-associated protein (MRP) in human tissues and adult solid cancers. Clin Cancer Res 1995;1:1301.
84. Kruh GD, Gaughan KT, Godwin A, Chan A. Expression pattern of MRP in human tissues and adult solid tumor cell lines. J Natl Cancer Inst 1995;87:1256.
85. Hipner DR, Deeley RG, Cole SP. Structural, mechanistic, and clinical aspects of MRP1. Biochim Biopsy Acta 1999;1461:359.
86. Zaman GJ, Floens JM, van Leusden MR, et al. The human multidrug resistance-protein MRP is a plasma membrane drug-efflux pump. Proc Natl Acad Sci U S A 1994;91:8822.
87. Pinkerton CR. Multidrug resistance reversal in childhood malignancies: potential for a real step forward? Eur J Cancer 1996;32A:641.
88. List AF, Kopecky KJ, Willman CL, et al. Benefit of cyclosporine modulation of drug resistance in patients with poor-risk acute myeloid leukemia: a Southwest Oncology Group Study. Blood 2004;98:3212.
89. Minotti AM, Barlow SB, Cabral F. Resistance to antimitotic drugs in Chinese hamster ovary cells correlates with changes in the level of polymerized tubulin. J Biol Chem 1991;266:3987.
90. Cabral FR, Barlow SB. Resistance to the antimitotic agents as genetic probes of microtubule structure and function. Pharmacol Ther 1991;52:159.
91. Cabral FR, Barlow SB. Mechanisms by which mammalian cells acquire resistance to drugs that affect microtubule assembly. FASEB J 1989;3:1593.
92. Cabral FR, Brady RC, Schiber MJ. A mechanism of cellular resistance to drugs that interfere with microtubule assembly. Ann N Y Acad Sci 1986;466:748.
93. Hari M, Wang Y, Veeraraghavan S. Mutations in alpha- and beta-tubulin that stabilize microtubules and confer resistance to Colcemid and vinblastine. Mol Cancer Ther 2003;2:597.
94. Ranganathan S, Dexter DW, Benetatos CA et al. Cloning and sequencing of human βIII-tubulin cDNA: induction of betaIII isotype in human prostate carcinoma cells by acute exposure to antimicrotubule agents. Biochim Biophys Acta 1998;1395:237.
95. Kavallaris M, Tait AS, Walsh BJ, et al. Multiple microtubule alterations are associated with vinca alkaloid resistance in human leukemia cells. Cancer Res 2001;61:5803.
96. Sethi VS, Thimmaiah KN. Structural studies of the degradation products of vincristine dihydrogen sulfate. Cancer Res 1985;45:4386.
97. Jordan MA, Himes RH, Wilson L. Comparison of the effects of vinblastine, vincristine, vindesine, and vinepidine on microtubule dynamics and cell proliferation in vitro. Cancer Res 1985;45:2741.
98. Bender RA, Castle MC, Margileth DA, Oliverio VT. The pharmacokinetics of [3H]-vincristine in man. Clin Pharmacol Ther 1977;22:430.
99. Nelson RL, Dyke RW, Root MA. Comparative pharmacokinetics of vindesine, vincristine, and vinblastine in patients with cancer. Cancer Treat Rev 1980;7(Suppl):17.
100. Sethi VS, Jackson DV, White CT, et al. Pharmacokinetics of vincristine sulfate in adult cancer patients. Cancer Res 1981;41:3551.
101. Owellen RJ, Root MA, Hains FO. Pharmacokinetic of vindesine and vincristine in humans. Cancer Res 1977;37:2603.
102. Owellen RJ, Donigian DW. ^{3}H-Vincristine: preparation. and preliminary pharmacology. J Med Chem 1972;15:894.
103. Castle MC, Margileth DA, Oliverio VT. Distribution and excretion of [3H]vincristine in the rat and the dog. Cancer Res 1976;36:3684.
104. Jackson DV, Castle MC, Bender RA. Biliary excretion of vincristine. Clin Pharmacol Ther 1978;24:101.
105. Sethi VS, Castle MC, Surratt P, et al. Isolation and partial characterization of human urinary metabolites of vincristine sulfate. Proc Am Assoc Cancer Res 1981;22:173.
106. Gidding CE, Kellie SJ, Kamps WA, de Graaf SS. Vincristine revisited. Crit Rev Oncol Hematol 1999;29:267.
107. Owellen RJ, Hartke CA, Hains FO. Pharmacokinetics and metabolism of vinblastine in humans. Cancer Res 1977;37:2597.
108. Rowinsky EK, Noe DA, Lucas VS, et al. A phase I, pharmacokinetic and absolute bioavailability study of oral vinorelbine (Navelbine) in solid tumor patients. J Clin Oncol 1994;12:1754.
109. Jehl F, Quoix E, Leveque D, et al. Pharmacokinetic and preliminary metabolic fate of Navelbine in humans as determined by high performance liquid chromatography. Cancer Res 1991;51:2073.
110. Levêque D, Jehl F. Clinical pharmacokinetics of vinorelbine. Clin Pharmacokinet 1996;31:184.
111. Rahmani R, Gueritte F, Martin M, et al. Comparative pharmacokinetics of antitumor *vinca* alkaloids: intravenous bolus injections of Navelbine and related alkaloids to cancer patients and rats. Cancer Chemother Pharmacol 1986;16:223.
112. Levêque D, Merle-Melet M, Bresler L, et al. Biliary elimination and pharmacokinetics of vinorelbine in micropigs. Cancer Chemother Pharmacol 1993;32:487.
113. Krikorian A, Rahmani R, Bromet M, et al. Pharmacokinetics and metabolism of Navelbine. Semin Oncol 1989;16(Suppl 4):21.
114. Sorio R, Robieux I, Galligioni E, et al. Pharmacokinetics and tolerance of vinorelbine in elderly patients with metastatic breast cancer. Eur J Cancer 1997;33:301.
115. Robieux I, Sorio R, Borsatti E, et al. Pharmacokinetics of vinorelbine in patients with liver metastases. Clin Pharmacol Ther 1996;59:32.
116. Bugat R, Variol P, Roche H, et al. The effects of food on the pharmacokinetic profile of oral vinorelbine. Cancer Chemother Pharmacol 2002;50:285.
117. Zhou XJ, Zhou-Pan XR, Favre R, Rahmani R. Relative bioavailability of two oral formulations of Navelbine in cancer patients. Biopharm Drug Dispos 1994;15:577.
118. Bender RA, Bleyer WA, Frisby SA. Alteration of methotrexate uptake in human leukemia cells by other agents. Cancer Res 1975;35:1305.
119. Zager RF, Frisby SA, Oliverio VT. The effects of antibiotics and cancer chemotherapeutic agents on the cellular transport and antitumor activity of methotrexate in L1210 murine leukemia. Cancer Res 1973;33:1670.
120. Bender RA, Nichols AP, Norton L, et al. Lack of therapeutic synergism of vincristine and methotrexate in L1210 murine leukemia in vivo. Cancer Treat Rep 1978;62:997.
121. Yalowich JC. Effect of microtubule inhibition on etoposide accumulation and DNA damage in human K562 cells in vitro. Cancer Res 1987;47:1010.
122. Chan JD. Pharmacokinetic drug interactions of vinca alkaloids. Summary of case reports. Pharmacother 1998;18:1304.
123. Bollini R, Riva R, Albani R, et al. Decreased phenytoin levels during antineoplastic therapy: a case report. Epilepsia 1983;24:75.
124. Jarosinski PF, Moscow JA, Alexander MS, et al. Altered phenytoin clearance during intensive chemotherapy for acute lymphoblastic leukemia. J Pediatr 1988;112:996.
125. Villikka K, Kivistö KT, Mäenpää H, et al. Cytochrome P-450-inducing antiepileptics increase the clearance of vincristine in patients with brain tumors. Clin Pharmacol Ther 1999;66:589.
126. Tobe SW, Siu LL, Jamal SA, et al. Vinblastine and erythromycin: an unrecognized serious drug interaction. Cancer Chemother Pharmacol 1995;35:188.
127. Sathiapalan RK, El-Soth H. Enhanced vincristine neurotoxicity from drug interactions: case report and review of literature. Pediatr Hematol Oncol 2001;18:543.
128. Rajaonarison JF, Lacarelle B, Catalin J, et al. Effect of anticancer drugs on the glucuronidation of 3'azido-3'-deoxythymidine in human liver microsomes. Drug Metab Dispos 1993;21:823.
129. Legha SS. Vincristine neurotoxicity. Pathophysiology and management. Med Toxicol 1986;1:421.
130. Bradley WG, Lassman LP, Pearce GW. The neuromyopathy of vincristine in man: clinical electrophysiological and pathological studies. J Neurol Sci 1970;10:107.
131. Quasthoff S, Hartung HP. Chemotherapy-induced peripheral neuropathy. J Neurol 2002;249:9.
132. Casey EB, Jellife AM, Le Quesne PM, Millett YL. Vincristine neuropathy, clinical and electrophysiological observations. Brain 1973;96:69.
133. Burns BV, Shotton JC. Vocal fold palsy following vinca alkaloid treatment. J Laryngol Otol 1998;112:485.
134. Greig NH, Soncrant TT, Shetty HU, et al. Brain uptake and anticancer activities of vincristine and vinblastine are restricted by their low cerebrovascular permeability and binding to plasma constituents in rat. Cancer Chemother Pharmacol 1990;26:263.
135. Carpentieri R, Lockhart LH. Ataxia and athetosis as side effects of chemotherapy with vincristine in non-Hodgkin's lymphomas. Cancer Treat Rep 1978;62:561.
136. Peltier AC, Russell JW. Recent advances in drug-induced neuropathies. Curr Opin Neurol 2002;15:633.
137. Hironen HE, Saknu TT, Heinonen E, et al. Vincristine treatment of acute lymphoblastic leukemia induces transient autonomic cardioneuropathy. Cancer 1988;64:801.
138. Gottlieb RJ, Cuttner J. Vincristine-induced bladder atony. Cancer 1971;28:674.
139. Carmichael SM, Eagleton L, Ayers CR, Mohler D. Orthostatic hypotension during vincristine therapy. Arch Intern Med 1970;126:290.
140. Woods WG, O'Leary M, Nesbit ME. Life-threatening neuropathy and hepatotoxicity in infants during induction therapy for acute lymphoblastic leukemia. J Pediatr 1981;98:642.
141. Chauvenet AR, Shashi V, Selsky C, et al. Vincristine-induced neuropathy as the initial presentation of Charcot-Marie-Tooth disease in acute lymphoblastic leukemia: a Pediatric Oncology Group study. J Pediatr Hematol Oncol 2003;25:316.
142. Orejana-Garcia AM, Pascual-Huerta J, Perez-Melero A. Charcot-Marie-Tooth disease and vincristine. J Am Podiatr Med Assoc 2003;93:229.
143. Trobaugh-Lotrario AD, Smith AA, Odom LF. Vincristine neurotoxicity in the presence of hereditary neuropathy. Med Pediatr Oncol 2003;40:39.
144. Desai ZR, Van den Berg HW, Bridges JM, et al. Can severe vincristine neurotoxicity be prevented? Cancer Chemother Pharmacol 1982;8:211.
145. Boyle FM, Wheeler HR, Shenfield GM. Glutamate ameliorates experimental vincristine neuropathy. JPharmacol Exp Ther 1996;279:410.
146. Jackson DV Jr, McMahan RA, Pope EK, et al. Clinical trial of folinic acid to reduce vincristine neurotoxicity. Cancer Chemother Pharmacol 1986;17:281.
147. Grush OC, Morgan SK. Folinic acid rescue for vincristine toxicity. Clin Toxicol 1979;14:71.
148. Helmann K, Hutchinson GE, Henry K. Reduction of vincristine toxicity by Cronassial. Cancer Chemother Pharmacol 1987;20:21.
149. Jackson DV, Wells HB, Atkins JN, et al. Amelioration of vincristine neurotoxicity by glutamic acid. Am J Med 1988;84:1016.
150. Binet S, Fellous A, Lataste H, et al. In situ analysis of the action of Navelbine on various types of microtubules using immunofluorescence. Semin Oncol 1989;16(Suppl 4):5.
151. Tester W, Forbes W, Leighton J. Vinorelbine-induced pancreatitis: a case report. J Natl Cancer Inst 1997;89:1631.
152. Sharma RK. Vincristine and gastrointestinal transit. Gastroenterol 1988;95:1435.
153. Dorr RT, Alberts DS. Vinca alkaloid skin toxicity: antidote and drug disposition studies in the mouse. J Natl Cancer Inst 1985;74:113.

154. Dorr T. Antidotes to vesicant chemotherapy extravasation. Blood Rev 1990;4:41.
155. Bellone JD. Treatment of vincristine extravasation. JAMA 1981;245:343.
156. Pattison J. Managing cytotoxic extravasation. Nurs Times 2002;98:32.
157. Subar M, Muggia FM. Apparent myocardial ischemia associated with vinblastine administration. Cancer Treat Rep 1986;70:690.
158. Hansen SW, Helweg-Larsen S, Trajoborg W. Long-term neurotoxicity in patients treated with cisplatin, vinblastine, and bleomycin for metastatic germ cell cancer. J Clin Oncol 1989;7:1457.
159. Hantel A, Rowinsky EK, Donehower RC. Nifedipine and oncologic Raynaud's phenomenon. Ann Intern Med 1988;108:767.
160. Ballen KK, Weiss ST. Fatal acute respiratory failure following vinblastine and mitomycin administration for breast cancer. Am J Med Sci 1988;295:558.
161. Hohneker JA. A summary of vinorelbine (Navelbine) safety data from North American clinical trials. Semin Oncol 1994;21(Suppl 10):42.
162. Blain PG. Adverse effects of drugs on skeletal muscle. Adverse Drug React Bull 1984;104:384.
163. Stenfanou A, Dooley M. Simple method to eliminate the risk of inadvertent intrathecal vincristine administration. J Clin Oncol 2003;21:2044.
164. Sulkes A, Collins JM. Reappraisal of some dosage adjustment guidelines. Cancer Treat Rep 1987;71:229.
165. Van den Berg HW, Desai ZR, Wilson R, et al. The pharmacokinetics of vincristine in man: reduced drug clearance associated with raised serum alkaline phosphatase and dose-limiting elimination. Cancer Chemother Pharmacol 1982;8:215.
166. Rowinsky EK, Donehower RC. Drug therapy: paclitaxel (Taxol). N Engl J Med 1995;332:1004.
167. Cortes JE, Pazdur R. Docetaxel. J Clin Oncol 1995;13:2643.
168. Gueritte-Voegelein F, Guenard D, Lavelle F, et al. Relationships between the structures of Taxol analogues and their antimitotic activity. J Med Chem 1991;34:992.
169. McGuire WP, Hoskins WJ, Brady MF, et al. Cyclophosphamide and cisplatin compared with paclitaxel and cisplatin in patients with stage III and IV ovarian cancer. N Engl J Med 1996;334:1.
170. Siedman AD. Monotherapy options in the management of metastatic breast cancer. Semin Oncol 2003;2(Suppl 3):6.
171. Moinpour C, Wu J, Donaldson G, et al. Gemcitabine plus paclitaxel (GT) versus paclitaxel (T) as first-line treatment of anthracycline pre-treated metastatic breast cancer (MBC): quality of life (QoL) and pain palliation results from the global phase III study. Proc Am Soc Clin Oncol 2004;22:14S.
172. Citron ML, Berry DA, Cirrincione C, et al. Randomized trial of dose-dense versus conventionally scheduled and sequential versus concurrent combination chemotherapy as postoperative adjuvant treatment of node-positive primary breast cancer: first report of Intergroup Trial C9741/Cancer and Leukemia Group B Trial 9741. J Clin Oncol 2003;21:1432.
173. Nowak AK, Wilcken NR, Stockler MR, et al. Systematic review of taxane-containing versus non-taxane-containing regimens for adjuvant and neoadjuvant treatment of early breast cancer. Lancet Oncol 204;5:372.
174. Henderson IC, Berry D, Demetri G, et al. Improved outcomes from adding sequential paclitaxel but not from escalating doxorubicin dose in an adjuvant chemotherapy regimen for patients with node-positive primary breast cancer. J Clin Oncol 2003;21:976–83.
175. Hudis CA, Schmitz N. Dose-dense chemotherapy in breast cancer and lymphoma. Semin Oncol 2004;31(Suppl 8):19.
176. Bonomi P, Kim K, Fariclough D, et al. Comparison of survival and quality of life in advanced non-small cell lung cancer patients treated with two dose levels of paclitaxel combined with cisplatin versus etoposide with cisplatin: results from an Eastern Cooperative Oncology Group trial. J Clin Oncol 2000;18 :623.
177. Jie C, Tulpule A, Zheng T, et al. Treatment of epidemic AIDS-related Kaposi's sarcoma. Curr Opin Oncol 1997;9:433.
178. Simon GR, Bunn PA Jr. Taxanes in the treatment of advanced (stages III and IV) non-small cell lung cancer (NSCLC): recent developments. Cancer Invest 2003;21:87.
179. Eisenberger MA, De Wit R, Berry W, et al. A multicenter phase III comparison of docetaxel (D) + prednisone (P) and mitoxantrone (MTZ) + P in patients with hormone-refractory prostate cancer (HRPC). Proc Am Soc Clin Oncol 2004;22:14S.
180. Petrylak DP, Tangen C, Hussain M, et al. SWOG 99-16: Randomized phase III trial of docetaxel (D)/estramustine (E) versus mitoxantrone(M)/prednisone(p) in men with androgen-independent prostate cancer (AIPCA). Proc Am Soc Clin Oncol 2004;22:14S.
181. O'Shaughnessy J, Tjuldanin S, Davidson N, et al. ABI-007 (ABRAXANE^{TM}), a nanoparticle albumin-bound (nab) paclitaxel demonstrates superior efficacy vs Taxol in metastatic breast cancer: a phase III trial. Proc Annual San Antonio Breast Cancer Conference 2003;26:44.
182. Rowinsky EK, Calvo E. Novel agents that target tubulin and related elements. Semin Oncol 2005;in press.
183. Manfredi JJ, Parness J, Horwitz SB. Taxol binds to cellular microtubules. J Cell Biol 1982;94:688.
184. Schiff PB, Fant J, Horwitz SB. Promotion of microtubule assembly in vitro by Taxol. Nature 1979;22:665.
185. Horwitz SB, Cohen D, Rao S, et al. Taxol: mechanisms of action and resistance. J Natl Cancer Inst Monogr 1993;15:55.
186. Rao S, Krauss NE, Heerding JM, et al. 3'-(p-Azidobenzamido)Taxol photolabels the N-terminal 31 amino acids of b-tubulin. J Biol Chem 1994;269:3132.
187. Rao S, Orr GA, Chaudhary AG, et al. Characterization of the Taxol binding site on the microtubule: 2-(m-azidobenzoyl)Taxol photolabels a peptide (amino acids 217-231) of beta tubulin. J Biol Chem 1995;270:20235.
188. Ojima I, Chakravarty S, Inoue T, et al. A common pharmacophore for cytotoxic natural products that stabilize microtubules. Proc Nat Acad Sci U S A 1999;96:4256.
189. Nogales E, Wolf SG, Khan IA, et al. Structure of tubulin at 6.5Å and location of the Taxol-binding site. Nature 2004;375:424.
190. Jordan A, Hadfield JA, Lawrence NJ, McGowan AT. Tubulin as a target for anticancer drugs which interact with the mitotic spindle. Med Res Rev 1998;18:259.
191. Diaz JF, Andreu JM. Assembly of purified GDP-tubulin into microtubules induced by Taxol and Taxotere: reversibility, ligand stoichiometry, and competition. Biochem 1993;32:2747.
192. Giannakakou P, Gussio R, Nogales E, et al. A common pharmacophore for epothilone and taxanes: molecular basis for drug resistance conferred by tubulin mutations in human cancer cells. Proc Natl Acad Sci U S A 2000;97:2904.
193. Caplow M, Shanks J, Ruhlen R. How Taxol modulates microtubule disassembly. J Biol Chem 1994;269:23399.
194. Ringel I, Horwitz SB. Studies with RP56976 (Taxotere): a semisynthetic analogue of Taxol. J Natl Cancer Inst 1991;83:288.
195. Schiff PB, Horwitz SB. Taxol stabilizes microtubules in mouse fibroblast cells. Proc Natl Acad Sci U S A 1980;77:1561.
196. Yvon A-M, Wadsworth P, Jordan MA. Taxol suppresses dynamics of individual microtubules in living human tumor cells. Mol Biol Cell 1999;10:947.
197. Bhalla K, Ibrado AM, Tourkina E, et al. Taxol induces internucleosomal DNA fragmentation associated with programmed cell death in human myeloid leukemia cells. Leukemia 1993;7:563.
198. Poruchynsky MS, Wang EE, Rudin CM, et al. Bcl-xL is phosphorylated in malignant cells following microtubule disruption. Cancer Res 1998;58:3331.
199. Wang LG, Liu XM, Kreis W, Budman DR. The effect of antimicrotubule agents on signal transduction pathways of apoptosis: a review. Cancer Chemother Pharmacol 1999;44:355.
200. Dumontet C, Sikic B. Mechanism of action and resistance to antitubulin agents: microtubule dynamics, drug transport, and cell death. J Clin Oncol 1999;17:1061.
201. Strobel T, Swanson L, Korsmeyer S, Cannistra SA. BAX enhances paclitaxel-induced apoptosis through a p53-independent pathway. Proc Natl Acad Sci U S A 1996;93:14094.
202. Scatena CD, Stewart ZA, Mays D, et al. Mitotic phosphorylation of Bcl-2 during normal cell cycle progression and Taxol-induced cell growth arrest. J Biol Chem 1998;273:30777.
203. Torres K, Horwitz SB. Mechanisms of Taxol-induced cell death are concentration dependent. Cancer Res 1998;58:3620.
204. Fernlini C, Raspaglio G, Mozzetti S. Bcl-2 down-regulation is a novel mechanism of paclitaxel resistance. Mol Pharmacol 2003;64:51.
205. Moss PJ, Fitzpatrick FA. Taxane-mediated gene induction is independent of microtubule stabilization: induction of transcription regulators and enzymes that modulate inflammation and apoptosis. Proc Natl Acad Sci U S A 1998;95:3896.
206. Griffon-Etienne G, Boucher Y, Brekken C, et al. Taxane-induced apoptosis decompresses blood vessels and lowers interstitial fluid pressure in solid tumors: clinical implications. Cancer Res 1999;59:776.
207. Ganansia-Leymarie V, Bischoff P, Bergerat JP. Signal transduction pathways of taxanes-induced apoptosis. Curr Med Chem Anticancer Agents 2003;3:291.
208. Blagosklonny MV, Schulte TW, Nguyen P, et al. Taxol-induction of p21 WAF1 and p53 requires c-raf-1. Cancer Res 1995;55:4623.
209. Blagosklonny MV. Unwinding the loop of Bcl-2 phosphorylation. Leukemia 2001;15:869.
210. Konishi Y, Lehtinen M, Donovan N, Bonni A. Cdc2 phosphorylation of BAD links the cell cycle to the cell death machinery. Mol Cell 2002;9:1005.
211. Moos PJ, Fitzpatrick FA. Taxane-mediated gene induction is independent of microtubule stabilization: induction of transcription regulators and enzymes that modulate inflammation and apoptosis. Proc Natl Acad Sci U S A 1998;95:3896.
212. Rowinsky EK, Donehower RC, Jones RJ, Tucker RW. Microtubule changes and cytotoxicity in leukemic cell lines treated with Taxol. Cancer Res 1988;48:4093.
213. Burkhart CA, Berman JW, Cwindell CS, et al. Relationship between Taxol and other taxanes on induction of tumor necrosis factor-a gene expression and cytotoxicity. Cancer Res 1994;54:5779.
214. Ding AH, Porteu F, Sanchez E, et al. Shared actions of endotoxin and Taxol on TNF receptors and TNF release. Science 1990;248:370.
215. Creane M, Seymour CB, Colucci S. Radiobiological effects of docetaxel (Taxotere): a potential radiation sensitizer. Int J Radiat Biol 1999;75:731.
216. Niero A, Emiliani E, Monti G, et al. Paclitaxel and radiotherapy: sequence-dependent efficacy preclinical model. Clin Cancer Res 1999;5:2213.
217. Mason KA, Hunter NR, Milas M, et al. Docetaxel enhances tumor radioresponse in vivo. Clin Cancer Res 1997;3:2431.
218. Tishler RB, Geard CR, Hall EJ, Schiff PB. Taxol sensitizes human astrocytoma cells to radiation. Cancer Res 1992;52:3595.
219. Fettel MR, Grossman SA, Fisher J, et al. Pre-irradiation paclitaxel in glioblastoma multiforme (GBM): efficacy, pharmacology, and drug interactions. J Clin Oncol 1997;15:3121.
220. Belotti D, Vergani V, Drudis T, et al. The microtubule-affecting drug paclitaxel has antiangiogenic activity. Clin Cancer Res 1996;2:1843.
221. Klauber N, Paragni S, Flynn E, et al. Inhibitor of angiogenesis and breast cancer in mice by the microtubule inhibitors 2-methoxyestradiol and Taxol. Cancer Res 1997;57:81.
222. Roberts JR, Allison DC, Dooley WC, et al. Effects of Taxol on cell cycle traverse: Taxol-induced polyploidization as a marker for drug resistance. Cancer Res 2990;50:710.
223. Quillen M, Castello C, Krishan A, et al. Cell surface tubulin in leukemic cells: molecular structure surface binding, turnover, cell cycle expression, and origin. J Cell Biol 1985;101:2345.
224. Sollott SJ, Cheng L, Pauly RR, et al. Taxol inhibits neointimal smooth muscle cell accumulation after angioplasty in the rat. J Clin Invest 1995;95:1869.
225. Van Bockxmeer FM, Martin CE, Thompson DE, et al. Taxol for the treatment of proliferative vitreoretinopathy. Invest Ophthalmol Vis Sci 1985;26:1140.
226. Laroia ST, Laroia AT. Drug-eluting stents. A review of the current literature. Cardiol Rev 2004;12:37.
227. Orr, GA Verdier-Pinard P, McDaid H, Horwitz SB. Mechanisms of Taxol resistance related to microtubules. Oncogene 2003;22:7280.
228. Roy SN, Horwitz SB. A phosphoglycoprotein with Taxol resistance in J774.2 cells. Cancer Res 1985;45:3856.
229. Cole SPC, Sparks KE, Fraser K, et al. Pharmacological characterization of multidrug resistant MRP-transfected human tumor cells. Cancer Res 1994;54:5902.
230. Lorico A, Rappa G, Flavell RA, et al. Double knockout of the MRP gene leads to increased drug sensitivity in vitro. Cancer Res 1996;56:5351.
231. Webster LK, Cosson EJ, Stokes KH, Millward MJ. Effect of the paclitaxel vehicle, Cremophor EL, on the pharmacokinetics of doxorubicin and doxorubicinol in mice. Br J Cancer 1996;73:522.
232. Rowinsky EK. Pharmacology and metabolism. In: McGuire W, Rowinsky E, editors. Paclitaxel in cancer treatment. New York: Marcel-Dekker; 1995. p. 91.

233. Rowinsky EK, Smith L, Chaturvedi P, et al. Pharmacokinetic and toxicologic interactions between the multidrug resistance reversal agent VX-710 and paclitaxel in cancer patients. J Clin Oncol 1998;16:2964.
234. Patnaik A, Oza AM, Warner E, et al. A phase I dose-finding and pharmacokinetic study of paclitaxel and carboplatin with oral valspodar in patients with advanced solid tumors. J Clin Oncol 2000;18:3677.
235. Cabral F, Wible L, Brenner S, Brinkley BR. Taxol-requiring mutants of Chinese hamster ovary cells with impaired mitotic spindle activity. J Cell Biol 1983;97:30.
236. Druckman S, Kavallaris M. Microtubule alterations and resistance to tubulin-binding agents. Int J Oncol 2002;21:621.
237. Haber M, Burkhart CA, Regl DL, et al. Altered expression of Mb2, the class II b-tubulin isotype, in a murine J774.2 cell line with a high level of Taxol resistance. J Biol Chem 1995;270:31269.
238. Kavallaris M, Kuo DYS, Burkhart CA, et al. Taxol-resistant epithelial ovarian tumors are associated with altered expression of specific beta-tubulin isotypes. J Clin Invest 1997;100:1282.
239. Giannakakou P, Sackett DL, Kang YK, et al. Paclitaxel-resistant human ovarian cancer cells have mutant beta-tubulins that exhibit impaired paclitaxel-driven polymerization. J Biol Chem 1997;272:17118.
240. Gonzalez-Garay ML, Chang L, Blade K, et al. A β-tubulin leucine cluster involved in microtubule assembly and paclitaxel resistance. J Biol Chem 1999;274:23875.
241. Hari M, Yang H, Zeng C, et al. Expression of class III beta-tubulin reduces microtubule assembly and confers resistance to paclitaxel. Cell Motil Cytoskeleton 2003;56:45.
242. Kavallaris M, Burkhart CA, Horwitz SB. Antisense oligonucleotides to class III beta-tubulin sensitize drug resistant cells to Taxol. Br J Cancer 1999;80:1020.
243. Ranganathan S, Dexter DW, Hudes GR. Modulation of endogenous β-tubulin isotype expression as a result of human β III cDNA transfection into prostate carcinoma cells. Br J Cancer 2001;85:735.
244. Monzo M, Rosell R, Sánchez JJ, et al. Paclitaxel resistance in nonsmall cell lung cancer associated with beta tubulin gene mutations. J Clin Oncol 1999;17:1786.
245. Kelley MJ, Li S, Harpole DH. Genetic analysis of the β-tubulin gene, TUBB, in non-small cell lung cancer. J Natl Cancer Inst 2001;93:1886.
246. Blade K, Menick DR, Cabral F. Overexpression of class I, II, or IVb beta-tubulin isotypes in CHO cells is insufficient to confer resistance to paclitaxel. J Cell Sci 1999;112:2213.
247. Rosell R, Fossella F, Milas L. Molecular markers and targeted therapy with novel agents: prospects in the treatment of non-small cell lung cancer. Lung Cancer 2002;38(Suppl 4):43.
248. Verrills NM, Flemming CL, Liu M, et al. Microtubule alterations and mutations induced by desoxyepothilone B: implications for drug-target interactions. Chem Biol 2003;10:597.
249. Gooch JL, Van Den Berg CL, Yee D. Insulin-like growth factor (IGF)-I rescues breast cancer cells from chemotherapy-induced cell death-proliferative and anti-apoptotic effects. Breast Cancer Res Treat 1999;56:1.
250. Murphy M, Hinmann A, Levine AJ. Wild-type p53 negatively regulates the expression of a microtubule-associated protein. Genes Dev 1996;10:2971.
251. Zhang CC, Yang JM, White E, et al. The role of MAP4 expression in the sensitivity to paclitaxel and resistance to vinca alkaloids in p53 mutant cells. Oncogene 1998;16:1617.
252. Yu D, Liu B, Jing T, et al. Overexpression of both p185$^{c\text{-}erB2}$ and p170$^{mdr\text{-}1}$ renders breast cancer cells highly resistant to Taxol. Oncogene 1998;16:2087.
253. Yu D, Liu B, Tan M, et al. Overexpression of c-erbB-2/neu in breast cancer cells confers increased resistance to Taxol via mdr-1-independent mechanisms. Oncogene 1996;13:1359.
254. Slamon DJ, Leyland-Jones B, Shak S, et al. Use of chemotherapy plus a monoclonal antibody against HER2 for metastatic breast cancer that overexpresses HER2. N Engl J Med 2001;344:783.
255. Konecny GE, Thomssen C, Luck HJ, et al. Her-2/neu gene amplification and response to paclitaxel in patients with metastatic breast cancer. J Natl Cancer Inst 2004;96:1141.
256. Malingre MM, Beijnen JH, Schellens JHM. Oral delivery of the taxanes. Invest New Drugs 2001;19:155.
257. Huizing MT, Keung ACF, Rosing H, et al. Pharmacokinetics of paclitaxel and metabolites in a randomized comparative study in platinum-pretreated ovarian cancer patients. J Clin Oncol 1993;11:2127.
258. Gianni L, Kearns C, Gianni A, et al. Nonlinear pharmacokinetics and metabolism of paclitaxel and its pharmacokinetic/pharmacodynamic relationships in humans. J Clin Oncol 1995;13:180.
259. Sonnichsen D, Hurwitz C, Pratt C, Relling MV. Saturable pharmacokinetics and paclitaxel pharmacodynamics in children with solid tumors. J Clin Oncol 1994;12:532.
260. Ohtsu T, Sasaki Y, Tamura T, et al. Clinical pharmacokinetics and pharmacodynamics of paclitaxel: a 3-hour infusion versus a 24-hour infusion. Clin Cancer Res 1995;1:599.
261. Van Tellingen O, Huizing MT, Panday VR, et al. Cremophor EL causes (pseudo) nonlinear pharmacokinetics of paclitaxel in patients. Br J Cancer 1999;81:330.
262. Sparreboom A, van Zuylen L, Brouwer E, et al. Cremophor EL-mediated alterations of paclitaxel distribution in human blood: clinical pharmacokinetic implications. Cancer Res 1999;59:1454.
263. Gelderblom H, Mross K, ten Tije AJ, et al. Comparative pharmacokinetics of unbound paclitaxel during 1- and 3-hour infusions. J Clin Oncol 2002;20:574.
264. Kumar GN, Walle UK, Bhalla KN, et al. Binding of Taxol to human plasma, albumin, and alpha 1-acid glycoprotein. Res Commun Chem Pathol Pharmacol 1993;80:337.
265. Henningsson A, Sparreboom A, Sandstrom, et al. Population pharmacokinetic modelling of unbound and total plasma concentrations of paclitaxel in cancer patients. Eur J Cancer 2003;39:1105.
266. Walle T, Walle UK, Kumar GN, Bhalla KN. Taxol metabolism and disposition in cancer patients. Drug Metab Dispos 1995;23:506.
267. Lesser G, Grossman SA, Eller S, Rowinsky EK. The neural and extra-neural distribution of systemically administered [3H]paclitaxel in rats: a quantitative autoradiographic study. Cancer Chemother Pharmacol 1995;34:173.
268. Glantz MJ, Choy H, Kearns CM, et al. Paclitaxel disposition in plasma and central nervous systems of humans and rats with brain tumors. J Natl Cancer Inst 1995;87:1077.
269. Cresteil T, Monsarrat B, Alvinerie P, et al. Taxol metabolism by human liver microsomes: identification of cytochrome P450 isoenzymes involved in its biotransformation. Cancer Res 1994;54:386.
270. Monsarrat B, Alvinerie P, Dubois J, et al. Hepatic metabolism and biliary clearance of Taxol in rats and humans. J Natl Cancer Inst Monogr 1993;15:39.
271. Monsarrat B, Chatelut E, Royer I, et al. Modification of paclitaxel metabolism in a cancer patient by induction of cytochrome P450 3A4. Drug Metab Dispos 1998;26:229.
272. Kearns CM, Egorin MJ. Considerations regarding the less-than-expected thrombocytopenia encountered with combination paclitaxel/carboplatin chemotherapy. Semin Oncol 1997;24(Suppl 2):S2.
273. Harris JW, Rahman A, Kim B-R, et al. Metabolism of Taxol by human hepatic microsomes and liver slices: participation of cytochrome P450 3A4 and an unknown P450 enzyme. Cancer Res 1994;15:4026.
274. Nallani SC, Goodwin B, Maglich JM. Introduction of cytochrome P450 3A by paclitaxel in mice: pivotal role of the nuclear xenobiotic receptor, pregnane X receptor. Drug Metab Dispos 2003;31:681.
275. Nallani SC, Goodwin B, Buckley AR, et al. Differences in the induction of cytochrome P450 3A4 by taxane anticancer drugs, docetaxel and paclitaxel, assessed employing primary human hepatocytes. Cancer Chemother Pharmacol 2004;54:219.
276. Rowinsky EK, Bonomi P, Jiroutek M, et al. Paclitaxel steady-state plasma concentration as a determinant of disease outcome and toxicity in lung cancer patients treated with paclitaxel and cisplatin. Clin Cancer Res 1999;5:767.
277. Clarke SJ, Rivory LP. Clinical pharmacokinetics of docetaxel. Clin Pharmacokinet 1999;36:99.
278. Bruno R, Hille D, Riva A, et al. Population pharmacokinetic/pharmacodynamics of docetaxel in phase II studies in patients with cancer. J Clin Oncol 1998;16:186.
279. Bruno R, Sanderink GJ. Pharmacokinetics and metabolism of Taxotere (docetaxel). In: Workman P, Graham MA, editors. Cancer Surveys. New York: Cold Spring Harbor Laboratory Press; 1993. p. 535.
280. Bruno R, Vivier N, Veyrat-Follet C, et al. Population pharmacokinetics and pharmacokinetic-pharmadynamic relationships for docetaxel. Invest New Drugs 2001;19:163.
281. McLeod HL, Kearns CM, Kuhn JG, Bruno R. Evaluation of the linearity of docetaxel pharmacokinetics. Cancer Chemother Pharmacol 1998;42:155.
282. Baker SD, Zhao M, Lee CK, et al. Comparative pharmacokinetics of weekly and every-three-weeks docetaxel. Clin Cancer Res 2004;10:1976.
283. Marland M, Gaillard C, Sanderink G, et al. Kinetics, distribution, metabolism and excretion of radiolabeled Taxotere (14C-RPR 56976) in mice and dogs. Proc Am Assoc Cancer Res 1993;34:393.
284. Ten Tije AJ, Loos WJ, Zhao M, et al. Limited cerebrospinal fluid penetration of docetaxel. Anticancer Drugs 2004;15:715.
285. Royer I, Bonsarrat B, Sonnier M, et al. Metabolism of docetaxel by human cytochromes P450: interactions with paclitaxel and other antineoplastic agents. Cancer Res 1996;56:58.
286. Hirth J, Watkins PB, Strawderman M, et al. The effect of an individual's cytochrome CYP3A4 activities on docetaxel clearance. Clin Cancer Res 2000;6:1255.
287. Sparreboom A, Van Tellingen O, Scherrenburg EJ, et al. Isolation, purification and biological activity of major docetaxel metabolites from human feces. Drug Metab Dispos 1996;24:655.
288. Shou M, Martinet M, Korzekwa KR, et al. Role of cytochrome P450 3A4 and 3A5 in the metabolism of Taxotere and its derivatives: enzyme specificity, interindividual distribution and metabolic contribution in human liver. Pharmacogenetics 1998;8:8391.
289. Ibrahim NK, Desai N, Legha S, et al. Phase I and pharmacokinetic study of ABI-007, a Cremophor-free, protein-stabilized, nanoparticle formulation of paclitaxel. Clin Cancer Res 2002;8:1038.
290. Nyman DS, Campbell KJ, Hersh E, et al. A phase I trial of ABI-007, nanoparticle paclitaxel, administered to patients with advanced non-hematologic malignancies. Proc Am Soc Clin Oncol 2004;22:2027.
291. Vigano L, Locatelli A, Grasselli G, Gianni L. Drug interactions of paclitaxel and docetaxel and their relevance for the design of combination therapy. Invest New Drugs 2001;19:197.
292. Rowinsky EK, Citardi M, Noe DA, Donehower RC. Sequence-dependent cytotoxicity between cisplatin and the antimicrotubule agents Taxol and vincristine. J Cancer Res Clin Oncol 1993;119:737.
293. Rowinsky EK, Gilbert M, McGuire WP, et al. Sequences of Taxol and cisplatin: a phase I and pharmacologic study. J Clin Oncol 1991;9:1692.
294. Belani CP, Kearns CM, Zuhowski EG, et al. Phase I trial, including pharmacokinetic and pharmacodynamic correlations, of combination paclitaxel and carboplatin in patients with metastatic non-small-cell lung cancer. J Clin Oncol 1999;17:676.
295. Daga H, Isobe T, Miyazaki M, et al. Investigating the relationship between serum thrombopoietin kinetics and the platelet-sparing effect: a clinical pharmacological evaluation of combined paclitaxel and carboplatin in patients with non small cell lung cancer. Oncol Rep 2004;11:2225.
296. Gianni L, Munzone E, Capri G, et al. Paclitaxel by 3-hour infusion in combination with bolus doxorubicin in women with untreated metastatic breast cancer: high antitumor efficacy and cardiac effects in a dose-finding and sequence-finding study. J Clin Oncol 1995;13:2688.
297. Gianni L, Vigano L, Locatelli A, et al. Human pharmacokinetic characterization and in vitro study of the interactions between doxorubicin and paclitaxel in patients with breast cancer. J Clin Oncol 1997;15:1906.
298. Holmes FA, Madden T, Newman RA, et al. Sequence-dependent alteration of doxorubicin pharmacokinetics by paclitaxel in a phase I study of paclitaxel and doxorubicin in patients with metastatic breast cancer. J Clin Oncol 1996;14:2713.
299. Gennari A, Salvadori B, Donati S, et al. Cardiotoxicity of epirubicin/paclitaxel-containing regimens: role of cardiac risk factors. J Clin Oncol 1999;11:3596.
300. Perotti A, Cresta S, Grasselli G. Cardiotoxic effects of anthracycline-taxane combinations. Expert Opin Drug Saf 2003;2:59.
301. Kennedy MJ, Zahurak ML, Donehower RC, et al. Phase I and pharmacologic study of sequences of paclitaxel and cyclophosphamide supported by granulocyte colony-stimulating factor in women with previously treated metastatic breast cancer. J Clin Oncol 1995;14:783.
302. Sarvada N, Ishikawa T, Fukase Y, et al. Induction of thymidine phosphorylase activity and enhancement of capecitabine efficacy by Taxol/Taxotere in human cancer xenografts. Clin Cancer Res 1998;4:1013.
303. James-Dow CA, Klecker RW, Katki AG, et al. Metabolism of Taxol by human and rat liver in vitro. A screen for drug

interactions and interspecies differences. Cancer Chemother Pharmacol 1995;36:107.
304. Klecker RW, Jamis-Dow CA, Egorin MJ, et al. Effect of cimetidine, probenecid, and ketoconazole on the distribution, biliary secretion, and metabolism of ^{3}H-Taxol in the Sprague-Dawley rat. Drug Metab Dispos Biol Fate 1994;22:254.
305. Desai PB, Duan JZ, Zhu YW, Kouzi S. Human liver microsomal metabolism of paclitaxel and drug interactions. Eur J Drug Metab Pharmacokinet 1998;23:417.
306. Prados MD, Schold SC, Spence AM, et al. Phase II study of paclitaxel in patients with recurrent malignant glioma. J Clin Oncol 1996;14:2316.
307. Bun SS, Ciccolini J, Bun H. Drug interactions of paclitaxel metabolism in human liver microsomes. J Chemother 2003 Jun;15(3):266–74.
308. Slichenmyer W, McGuire W, Donehower R, et al. Pretreatment H2 receptor antagonists that differ in P450 modulation activity: comparative effects on paclitaxel clearance rates. Cancer Chemother Pharmacol 1995;36:227.
309. Thompson ME, Highley MS. Interaction between paclitaxel and warfarin. Ann Oncol 2003;14:500.
310. Jeriah S, Keegan P. Cardiotoxicity associated with paclitaxel/trastuzumab combination chemotherapy. J Clin Oncol 1999;17:1647.
311. Pegram MD, Konecny GE, O'Callaghan C, et al. Rational combinations of trastuzumab with chemotherapeutic drugs used in the treatment of breast cancer. J Natl Cancer Inst 2004;96:759.
312. Rowinsky EK, Eisenhauer EA, Chaudhry V, et al. Clinical toxicities encountered with Taxol. Semin Oncol 1993;20(Suppl 3):1.
313. Rowinsky EK. The taxanes: dosing and scheduling considerations. Oncology 1997;11(Suppl 2):7.
314. Kerns CM, Gianni L, Egorin M. Paclitaxel pharmacokinetics and pharmacodynamics. Semin Oncol 1995;22:16.
315. Bookman MA, Kloth DD, Kover PE, et al. Short-course intravenous prophylaxis for paclitaxel-related hypersensitivity reactions. Ann Oncol 1997;8:611.
316. Kloover JS, den Bakker MA, Gelderblom H, van Meerbeeck JP. Fatal outcome of a hypersensitivity reaction to paclitaxel: a critical review of premedication regimens. Br J Cancer 2004;90:305.
317. Olson JK, Sood AK, Sorosky JI, et al. Taxol hypersensitivity: rapid retreatment is safe and cost effective. Gynecol Oncol 1996;68:25.
318. Peereboom D, Donehower RC, Eisenhauer EA, et al. Successful retreatment with Taxol after major hypersensitivity reactions. J Clin Oncol 1993;11:885.
319. Ramanathan RK, Belani CP. Transient pulmonary infiltrates: a hypersensitivity reaction to paclitaxel. Ann Intern Med 1996;124:278.
320. Szebeni J, Muggia FM, Alving CR. Complement activation by Cremophor EL as a possible contributor to hypersensitivity to paclitaxel: an in vitro study. J Natl Cancer Inst 1998;90:300.
321. Weiss R, Donehower RC, Wiernik PH, et al. Hypersensitivity reactions from Taxol. J Clin Oncol 1990;8:1263.
322. Price KS, Castells MC. Taxol reactions. Allergy Asthma Proc 2002;23:205.
323. Bernstein BJ. Docetaxel as an alternative to paclitaxel after acute hypersensitivity reactions. Ann Pharmacother 2000;34:1332.
324. Eisenhower E, ten Bokkel Huinink W, Swenerton KD, et al. European-Canadian randomized trial of Taxol in relapsed ovarian cancer: high vs low dose and long vs short infusion. J Clin Oncol 1994;12:2654.
325. Rowinsky EK, Chaudhry V, Cornblath DR, Donehower RC. The neurotoxicity of Taxol. Monogr Natl Cancer Inst 1993;15:107.
326. Chaudhry V, Rowinsky EK, Sartorious SE, et al. Peripheral neuropathy from Taxol and cisplatin combination chemotherapy: clinical and electrophysiological studies. Ann Neurol 1994;35:490.
327. Vahdat L, Papadopoulos K, Lange D, et al. Reduction of paclitaxel-induced per neuropathy with glutamine. Clin Cancer Res 2004;7:1192.
328. Gelmon K, Eisenhauer E, Bryce C, et al. Randomized phase II study of high-dose paclitaxel with or without amifostine in patients with metastatic breast cancer. J Clin Oncol 1999;17:3038.
329. Capri G, Munzone E, Tarenzi E, et al. Optic nerve disturbances: a new form of paclitaxel neurotoxicity. J Natl Cancer Inst 1994;86:1099.
330. Hofstra LS, de Vries EG, Willemse PH. Ophthalmic toxicity following paclitaxel infusion. Ann Oncol 1997;8:1053.
331. Nieto Y, Cagnoni PJ, Bearman SI, Shpall EJ. Acute encephalopathy: a new toxicity associated with high-dose paclitaxel. Clin Cancer Res 1999;5:501.
332. Ziske CG, Schottker B, Gorschluter M, et al. Acute transient encephalopathy after paclitaxel infusion: report of three cases. Ann Oncol 2002;13:629.
333. Garrison JA, McCune JS, Livingston RB, et al. Myalgias and arthralgias associated with paclitaxel. Oncology 2003;17:271.
334. Rowinsky EK, McGuire WP, Guarnieri T, et al. Cardiac disturbances during the administration of Taxol. J Clin Oncol 1991;9:1704.
335. Arbuck SG, Strauss H, Rowinsky EK, et al. A reassessment of the cardiac toxicity associated with Taxol. Monogr Natl Cancer Inst 1993;15:117.
336. Markman M, Kennedy A, Webser K, et al. Paclitaxel administration to gynecologic cancer patients with major cardiac risk factors. J Clin Oncol 1998;16:3483.
337. Della Torre P, Imondi AR, Bernardi C, et al. Cardioprotection by dexrazoxane in rats treated with doxorubicin and paclitaxel. Cancer Chemother Pharmacol 1999;44:138.
338. Sparano JA, Speyer J, Gradishar WJ, et al. Phase I trial of escalating doses of paclitaxel plus doxorubicin and dexrazoxane in patients with advanced breast cancer. J Clin Oncol 1999;17:880.
339. Pestalozzi BC, Sotos GA, Choyke PL, et al. Typhlitis resulting from treatment with Taxol and doxorubicin in patients with metastatic breast cancer. Cancer 1993;71:1797.
340. Seewaldt VL, Cain JM, Goff BA, et al. A retrospective review of paclitaxel-associated gastrointestinal necrosis in patients with epithelial ovarian cancer. Gynecol Oncol 1997;67:137.
341. Ayoub JP, North L, Greer J, et al. Pulmonary changes in patients with lymphoma who receive paclitaxel. J Clin Oncol 1997;15:2476.
342. Minisini AM, Tosti A, Sobrero AF, et al. Taxane-induced nail changes: incidence, clinical presentation and outcome. Ann Oncol 2003;14:333.
343. Schrijvers D, Wanders, J Dirix L, et al. Coping with toxicities of docetaxel (Taxotere). Ann Oncol 1993;4:610.
344. Markman M. Managing taxane toxicities. Support Care Cancer 2003;11:144.
345. Piccart MJ, Klijn J, Paridaens R, et al. Corticosteroids significantly delay the onset of docetaxel-induced fluid retention: final results of a randomized study of the European Organization for Research and Treatment of Cancer, Investigational Drug Branch for Breast Cancer. J Clin Oncol 1997;15:149.
346. Semb KA, Aamdal S, Oian P. Capillary protein leak syndrome appears to explain fluid retention in cancer patients who receive docetaxel treatment. J Clin Oncol 1998;16:3426.
347. Hilkens PH, Verweij J, Stoter G, et al. Peripheral neurotoxicity induced by docetaxel. Neurology 1996;46:104
348. Vasey PA. Survival and long-term toxicity results of the SCOTROC study: docetaxel-carboplatin (DC) vs. paclitaxel-carboplatin (PC) in epithelial ovarian cancer. Proc Am Soc Clin Oncol 1992;21:202A.
349. Greco FA, Thomas M, Hainsworth JD. One-hour paclitaxel infusions: review of the safety and efficacy. Cancer Sci Am 1999;5:179.
350. Hainsworth JD, Burris HA, Greco FA. Weekly administration of docetaxel (Taxotere): summary of clinical data. Semin Oncol 1999;26(Suppl 10):19.
351. Luftner D, Flath B, Akrivakis C, et al. Dose-intensified weekly paclitaxel induces multiple nail disorders. Ann Oncol 1996;9:1139.
352. Wasner G, Hilpert F, Schattschneider J. Docetaxel-induced nail changes—a neurogenic mechanism: a case report. J Neurooncol 2002;58:167.
353. Esamaeli B, Hortobagyi G, Esteva F. Canalicular stenosis secondary to weekly docetaxel: a potentially preventable side effect. Ann Oncol 2002;13:218.
354. Takimoto CH, Rowinsky EK. Dose-intense paclitaxel: deja vu all over again? J Clin Oncol 2003;21:2810.
355. Seidman AD, Berry D, Cirrincione C, et al. CALGB 9840: phase III study of weekly (W) paclitaxel (P) via 1-hour(h) infusion versus standard (S) 3h infusion every third week in the treatment of metastatic breast cancer (MBC), with trastuzumab (T) for HER2 positive MBC and randomized for T in HER2 normal MBC [abstract 512]. Proc Am Soc Clin Oncol 2004;22:6s.
356. Seidman AD, Hudis CA, Albanel J, et al. Dose-dense therapy with weekly 1-hour paclitaxel infusions in the treatment of metastatic breast cancer. J Clin Oncol 1998;16:3353.
357. Green MC, Buzdar AU, Smith T, et al. Weekly paclitaxel followed by FAC as primary systemic chemotherapy of operable breast cancer improves pathologic complete remission rates when compared to every 3-week paclitaxel therapy followed by FAC-final results of a prospective randomized phase III study. Proc Am Soc Clin Oncol 2002;21:35a.
358. Winer EP, Berry DA, Woolf S, et al. Failure of higher-dose paclitaxel to improve outcome in patients with metastatic breast cancer: cancer and leukemia group B trial 9342. J Clin Oncol 2004;22:2061.
359. Venock AP, Egorin MJ, Rosner GL, et al. Phase I and pharmacokinetic trial of paclitaxel in patients with hepatic dysfunction. Cancer and leukemia group B 9264. J Clin Oncol 1998;16:1811.
360. Baker SD, Ravdin P, Aylesworth C, et al. A phase I and pharmacokinetic study of docetaxel in cancer patients with liver dysfunction due to malignancies. Proc Am Soc Clin Oncol 1998;17:192.
361. Kinzel PE, Dorr RT. Anticancer drug renal toxicity and elimination: dosing guidelines for altered renal function. Cancer Treat Rev 1995;21:33.
362. Salminen E, Bergman M, Huhtala S, et al. Docetaxel: standard recommended dose of 100 mg/m2 is effective but not feasible for some metastatic breast cancer patients heavily pretreated with chemotherapy—a phase II single-center study. J Clin Oncol 1999;17:1127.
363. Kowalski RJ, Giannakakou P, Hamel E. Activities of the microtubule-stabilizing agents epothilones A and B with purified tubulin and in cells resistant to paclitaxel (Taxol). J Biol Chem 1997;272:2534.
364. Bollag DM, McQueney PA, Zhu, J. et al. Epothilones, a new class of microtubule-stabilizing agents with a Taxol-like mechanism of action. Cancer Res 1995;55:2325.
365. Dabydeen DA, Florence GJ, Paterson I, Hamel E. A quantitative evaluation of the effects of inhibitors of tubulin assembly on polymerization induced by discodermolide, epothilone B, and paclitaxel. Cancer Chemother Pharmacol 2004;53:397.
366. Goodin S, Kane MP, Rubin EH. Epothilones: mechanism of action and biologic activity. J Clin Oncol 2004;22:2015.
367. Stachel SJ, Biswas K, Danishefsky SJ. The epothilones, eleutherobins, and related types of molecules. Curr Pharm Des 2001;7:1277.
368. Lee FY, Borzilleri R, Fairchild CR, et al. BMS-247550: a novel epothilone analog with a mode of action similar to paclitaxel but possessing superior antitumor efficacy. Clin Cancer Res 2001;7:1429.
369. Abraham J, Agrawal M, Bakke S, et al. Phase I trial and pharmacokinetic study of BMS-247550, an epothilone B analog, administered intravenously on a daily schedule for five days. J Clin Oncol 2003;21:1866.
370. Lee FY, Vite G, Hofle G, et al. The discovery of BMS-310705: a water-soluble and chemically stable semisynthetic epothilone possessing potent parenteral and oral antitumor activity against models of taxane-sensitive and -resistant human tumors in vivo [abstract 3928]. Proc Am Assoc Cancer Res 2002;43:792.
371. Mani S, McDaid H, Hamilton A, et al. Phase I clinical and pharmacokinetic study of BMS-247550, a novel derivative of epothilone B, in solid tumors. Clin Cancer Res 2004;10:1289.
372. Rothermel J, Wartmann M, Chen T, Hohneker J. EPO906 (epothilone B): a promising novel microtubule stabilizer. Semin Oncol 2003;30:51.
373. Chou TC, Zhang XG, Balog A, et al. Desoxyepothilone B: an efficacious microtubule-targeted antitumor agent with a promising in vivo profile relative to epothilone B. Proc Natl Acad Sci U S A 1998;95:9642.
374. Mekhail T, Chung C, Holden S, et al. Phase I trial of novel epothilone B analog BMS-310705 IV q21 days [abstract 515]. Proc Am Soc Clin Oncol 2003;22:129.
375. Martello LA, McDaid HM, Regl DL, et al. Taxol and discodermolide represent a synergistic drug combination in human carcinoma cell lines. Clin Cancer Res 2000;6:1978.
376. Honore S, Kamath K, Braguer D, et al. Synergistic suppression of microtubule dynamics by discodermolide and paclitaxel in non-small cell lung carcinoma cells. Cancer Res 2004;64:4957.
377. Mita AA, Lockhart C, Chen T-L, et al. A phase I pharmacokinetic (PK) trial of XAA296A (Discodermolide) administered every 3 wks to adult patients with advanced solid malignancies [abstract 205]. Proc Am Soc Clin Oncol 2004;23:133.
378. Poncet J. The dolastatins, a family of promising antineoplastic agents. Curr Pharm Des 1999;5:139.

379. Bai R, Pettit GR, Hamel E. Dolastatin 10, a powerful cytostatic peptide derived from a marine animal. Inhibition of tubulin polymerization mediated through the *Vinca* alkaloid binding domain. J Biol Chem 1990;265:17141.
380. Hammond LA, Ruvuna F, Cunningham CC. Phase (Ph) I evaluation of the dolastatin analogue synthadotin (SYN-D; ILX651): pooled data analysis of three alternate schedules in patients (pts) with advanced solid tumors [abstract 3068]. Proc Am Soc Clin Oncol 2004;23:212.
381. Schoffski P, Thate B, Beutel G, et al. Phase I and pharmacokinetic study of TZT-1027, a novel synthetic dolastatin 10 derivative, administered as a 1-hour intravenous infusion every 3 weeks in patients with advanced refractory cancer. Ann Oncol 2004;15:671.
382. Loganzo F, Discafani CM, Annable T, et al. HTI-286, a synthetic analogue of the tripeptide hemiasterlin, is a potent antimicrotubule agent that circumvents P-glycoprotein-mediated resistance in vitro and in vivo. Cancer Res 2003;63:1838.
383. Kanthou C, Tozer GM. The tumor vascular targeting agent combretastatin A-4-phosphate induces reorganization of the actin cytoskeleton and early membrane blebbing in human endothelial cells. Blood 2002;99:2060.
384. Tozer GM, Kanthou C, Parkins CS, Hill SA. The biology of the combretastatins as tumour vascular targeting agents. Int J Exp Pathol 2002;83:21.
385. Thorpe PE. Vascular targeting agents as cancer therapeutics. Clin Cancer Res. 2004;10;415.
386. Cooney MM, Radivoyevitch T, Dowlati A, et al. Cardiovascular safety profile of combretastatin a4 phosphate in a single-dose phase I study in patients with advanced cancer. Clin Cancer Res 2004;10:96.
387. Davis PD, Dougherty GJ, Blakey DC. ZD6126: a novel vascular-targeting agent that causes selective destruction of tumor vasculature. Cancer Res 2004;62:7247.
388. Stevenson JP, Rosen M, Sun W, et al. Phase I trial of the antivascular agent combretastatin A4 phosphate on a 5-day schedule to patients with cancer: magnetic resonance imaging evidence for altered tumor blood flow. J Clin Oncol 2003;21:4428.
389. Wood KW, Cornwell WD, Jackson JR. Past and future of the mitotic spindle as an oncology target. Curr Opin Pharmacol 2001;4:370.
390. Goldstein LS, Philip AV. The road less traveled: emerging principles of kinesin motor utilization. Annu Rev Cell Dev Biol 1999;15:141.
391. Sakowicz R, Finer JT, Beraud C, et al. Antitumor activity of a kinesin inhibitor. Cancer Res 2004;64:3276.
392. Chu QS, Holen KD, Rowinsky EK, et al. Phase I trial of novel kinesin spindle protein (KSP) inhibitor SB-715992 IV Q 21 days [abstract 2078]. Proc Am Soc Clin Oncol 2004;22:146.
393. Burris HA, Lorusso P, Jones S, et al. Phase I trial of novel kinesin spindle protein (KSP) inhibitor SB-715992 IV days 1, 8, 15 q 28 days [abstract 2004]. Proc Am Soc Clin Oncol 2004;22:128.
394. Carmena M, Earnshaw WC. The cellular geography of aurora kinases. Nat Rev Mol Cell Biol 2003;11:842.
395. Warner SL, Bearss DJ, Han H, Von Hoff DD. Targeting aurora-2 kinase in cancer. Mol Cancer Ther 2003;2: 589.
396. Harrington EA, Bebbington D, Moore J, et al. VX-680, a potent and selective small-molecule inhibitor of the Aurora kinases, suppresses tumor growth in vivo. Nat Med 2004;10:262.

47

Small-Molecule Inhibitors of Protein Kinases in the Treatment of Human Cancer

Michael C. Heinrich, MD
Charles D. Blanke, MD
Christopher L. Corless, MD, PhD
Brian J. Druker, MD

Over the last several decades it has become clear that the phenotypic hallmarks of cancer are a consequence of perturbations in normal cellular homeostatic mechanisms.[1] These cellular processes frequently depend on signaling mechanisms that transmit information concerning extracellular or cytoplasmic conditions to the nucleus, thereby influencing gene transcription and/or deoxyribonucleic acid (DNA) synthesis. A ubiquitous and critical component of these signal transduction pathways is the large family of protein kinases.[2] Based on the data from the Human Genome Project it is estimated that the human genome contains approximately 550 protein kinases and an additional 130 protein phosphatases that regulate the activity of the various protein kinases.[3] The protein kinases are classified as tyrosine kinases, with specific activity for tyrosine residues only, serine/threonine kinases with activity for serine and threonine residues only, and kinases with activity for all three residues. Tyrosine kinases can be further subdivided into proteins that have an extracellular ligand binding domain (receptor tyrosine kinases, [RTKs]) and enzymes that are confined to the cytoplasm and/or nuclear cellular compartment (nonreceptor tyrosine kinases, [NRTKs]).[4]

Abnormal activation of specific protein kinases can be demonstrated in most human neoplasms and many nonmalignant inflammatory states.[2,5,6] There are multiple mechanisms that can result in this aberrant activation: (1) over-expression because of gene amplification or enhanced gene transcription; (2) chromosomal translocation resulting in expression of a protein that contains the catalytic domain of a tyrosine kinase fused to protein motifs encoded by a different gene; (3) autocrine or paracrine stimulation of growth factor RTKs by cognate ligand; (4) loss of tumor-suppressor genes that negatively regulate signal-transduction pathways involving protein kinases; (5) loss of regulatory phosphatases; and (6) activating mutations, including point mutations, insertions, and deletions in the kinase itself.

STRATEGIES TO INHIBIT TYROSINE KINASES

Based on the association of certain human cancers with dysregulation of specific pathways involving protein tyrosine kinases (Table 47-1), it has long been hypothesized that specific inhibitors of these protein kinases might be effective anticancer agents.[7,8] There are two broad strategies for inhibiting tyrosine kinase activity: (1) inhibition of protein expression; and (2) inhibition of enzymatic activity (Table 47-2). Whereas methods to inhibit

Table 47-1 Tyrosine Kinases Associated with Human Cancers

Tyrosine Kinase	Mechanisms of Activation	Associated Human Cancers
ABL	Chromosomal translocation	CML; ALL
ALK	Chromosomal translocation	ALCL; IMT
ARG	Chromosomal translocation	AML
EGFR (HER1, ErbB1)	Over-expression; extracellular domain deletions	Glioblastoma multiforme; NSCLC; HNSCC
	Gain-of-function mutations	NSCLC
FGFR1	Chromosomal translocation	AML; MPD; lymphoma
FGFR2	Gain-of-function point mutations	Gastric cancer
FGFR3	Over-expression; gain-of-function point mutations	Multiple myeloma; papillary bladder cancer
FLT3	Gain-of-function mutations of juxtamembrane or activation loop domains	AML; MLL-rearranged ALL
HER2 (Neu, ErbB2)	Over-expression (genomic amplification)	Breast cancer; ovarian cancer
	Gain-of-function mutations of TK2	NSCLC
HER3 (ErbB3)	Over-expression	Breast cancer
HER4 (ErbB4)	Over-expression	Breast cancer
JAK2	Chromosomal translocation	ALL; AML; atypical CML
	Gain-of-function mutation	PRV; MF; ET; MPD NOS
KIT	Gain-of-function mutations of extracellular, juxtamembrane, TK1 or TK2 domains	GIST; AML; seminoma; mastocytosis; sinonasal NK/T-cell lymphoma
LCK	Chromosomal translocation; gain-of-function point mutations	T-cell ALL
PDGFRA	Over-expression; chromosomal translocation	Gliomas; glioblastoma multiforme; variant CML (BCR-PDGFRA); Hypereosinophilic syndrome/variant mastocytosis (FIP1L1-PDGFRA)
PDGFRB	Chromosomal translocation; autocrine loop	CMML; DFSP
RET	Chromosomal translocation; gain-of-function point mutations	Papillary thyroid cancers; medullary thyroid carcinoma; parathyroid hyperplasia
TRKA	Chromosomal translocations	Papillary thyroid cancers; neuroblastoma
TRKC	Chromosomal translocations	Congenital fibrosarcoma; AML; secretory breast cancer; mesoblastic nephroma

Abbreviations: ALCL = anaplastic large cell lymphoma; ALL = acute lymphoblastic leukemia/lymphoma; AML = acute myelogenous leukemia; CML = chronic myelogenous leukemia; DFSP = dermatofibrosarcoma protuberans; GIST = gastrointestinal stromal tumor; HNSCC = head and neck squamous cell carcinoma; IMT = inflammatory myofibroblastic tumor; MPD = myeloproliferative disorder; NOS = not otherwise specified; NSCLC = non–small-cell lung carcinoma.

Table 47-2 Approaches to Targeting Tyrosine Kinases

Strategies to inhibit the expression of tyrosine kinases
Nucleic acids
Antisense oligonucleotides
Interfering ribonucleic acids
Monoclonal antibodies
Inhibitors of molecular chaperones (eg, heat shock protein 90)
Strategies to inhibit the activity of tyrosine kinases
Monoclonal antibodies
Soluble receptor (to bind ligand)
Monomeric ligand (to block dimerization of receptor tyrosine kinases)
Small-molecule adenosine triphosphate antagonists
Small molecule inhibitors of protein substrate binding

kinase expression have been demonstrated in the laboratory, this strategy has yet to be translated successfully to the clinic (with the exception of monoclonal antibodies, which, in some cases may induce degradation of the targeted kinase).[9] The two methods for inhibiting tyrosine kinases that have achieved clinical success are RTK-specific monoclonal antibodies and small molecule inhibitors that block the binding of adenosine triphosphate (ATP) to tyrosine kinases. Two monoclonal antibodies targeting RTKs have been Food and Drug Administration (FDA) approved: trastuzumab (Herceptin), a monoclonal antibody to HER2, for the treatment of breast carcinomas that overexpress HER2,[10,11] and cetuximab (Erbitux), a monoclonal antibody against the epidermal growth factor receptor (EGFR) for advanced colorectal cancer in combination with chemotherapy.[12] A third monoclonal antibody, bevacizumab (Avastin), targets vascular endothelial growth factor (VEGF), the ligand for the VEGF receptor (VEGFR). It has been FDA approved for patients with advanced colorectal cancer in combination with fluorouracil-containing regimens and has activity in combination with chemotherapy against a broad range of tumor types.[13] Presumably, bevacizumab functions by preventing the binding of VEGF to its receptor, thereby preventing the activation of the receptor. Because monoclonal antibodies are most effective against extracellular epitopes, they are better suited for targeting RTKs than NRTKs. These monoclonal antibodies are discussed in other chapters of this textbook.

Small-molecule antagonists of ATP binding to tyrosine kinases have proven to be effective drugs for inhibiting tyrosine kinase activity. All tyrosine kinases share a similar enzymatic activity—transfer of a phosphate group from ATP to a tyrosine residue—and are therefore highly homologous in their kinase domains. Despite the high degree of conservation of the ATP binding domain in all protein kinases, there are variations in the protein conformations around the ATP binding pocket that have allowed the development of inhibitors with surprising specificity and affinity. The specificity is achieved in part through interaction of the inhibitors with amino acids that are different than those directly involved in binding ATP.[14] This chapter focuses on general issues regarding the development of kinase inhibitors and provides several examples of agents currently in the clinic.

TYROSINE KINASE INHIBITORS

Targeting Considerations Whether a cancer can be treated effectively with a tyrosine kinase inhibitor (TKI) may depend largely on the extent to which the growth of the tumor cells is dependent on the targeted tyrosine kinase(s). This principle can be illustrated by hypothetical tumor cells whose growth is dependent on tyrosine kinase A, kinase B, or both kinases A + B (Figure 47-1). This model is based on experimental observations with factor-dependent human acute myeloid leukemia (AML) cells.[15] The growth of tumor cells that are dependent on a single kinase would be inhibited by treatment with the appropriate TKI. In contrast, there would be no effect on proliferation when cells dependent on kinase A are treated with an inhibitor against kinase B, or vice versa. In the case of tumor cells that are dependent on both kinases A + B, therapy with an inhibitor against one of the kinases would reduce proliferation by only 50%. Complete inhibition of such cells could be achieved only when both kinases are inhibited. In some cancers, the situation may be even more complex, with tumor cell survival dependent on three or more kinases. In such cases, it could be necessary to target all of the kinases, or to inhibit downstream effectors that were shared between all or most of the kinases.

The implications of this model are that monotherapy with a TKI will be most effective when the growth of a tumor is dependent on only one tyrosine kinase. As described in this chapter, chronic myelogenous leukemia (CML) and gastrointestinal stromal tumor (GIST) both fit this description. It is likely that early in the development of a tumor, single genetic defects are more common, while in advanced malignancies, multiple, redundant pathways support the growth and survival of the tumor. For this reason, monotherapy with a TKI may be most useful in the earlier stages of disease, if activation of a specific tyrosine kinase is critical to the development of the tumor.[16,17] In this regard, the most attractive cancers for monotherapy with a TKI are those diseases in which there is a genomic mechanism of target activation (see Table 47-1).

In the above model it should be noted that a biologic effect does not necessarily equate with a clinical benefit. For example, in the case of a tumor that is codependent on kinase A and B, treatment with an inhibitor specific to kinase A would decrease proliferation by 50% (a biologic effect). However, because slowing the growth rate would not decrease the tumor size, this result would be regarded as "progressive disease." If the end point of the clinical trial is tumor shrinkage, the inhibitor would be dismissed as an ineffective therapy. However, end points such as delay in time to progression or prolongation of survival might reveal a therapeutic benefit. Additional studies that combined the kinase A inhibitor with other treatments (kinase B inhibitors, cytotoxics, immune treatments, etc) that could impact the other 50% of proliferation might result in improved clinical efficacy. An example of improved results combining a kinase inhibitor with chemotherapy has been observed in the clinical trials of sorafenib (BAY 43-9006), a RAF, VEGFR inhibitor in patients with metastatic melanoma.[18,19]

These issues demonstrate some of the difficulties faced in the development of targeted agents such as TKIs. Specifically, single-agent TKIs may have minimal activity using standard end points in patients with advanced malignancies and there may be a need to combine TKIs with other agents to see significant clinical activity. Besides the need to consider alternative end points, it is also crucial to include measurement of kinase activation before and during therapy. For example, if the targeted kinase is not inhibited in the tumor, this raises the possibility of poor tumor penetration or lack of potency of the agent. If, however, the kinase is inhibited and no measurable response is observed, this suggests that either the kinase is

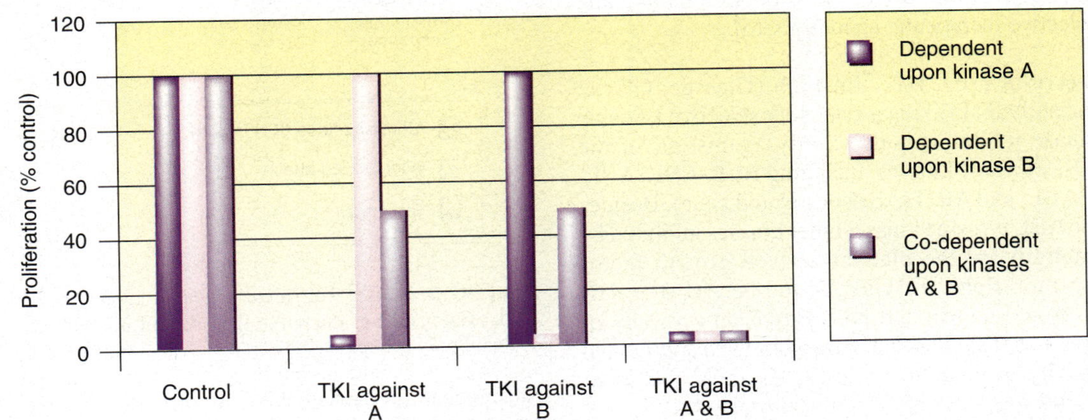

Figure 47-1 Effect of tyrosine kinase inhibitors (TKIs) against kinase A or kinase B in tumors dependent on A and/or B for proliferation. The clinical effect of monotherapy with a given TKI is determined by the dependence of the tumor cells on the targets inhibited by that agent. In tumors dependent on more than one kinase for survival, therapies must inhibit all of the critical kinases for maximal therapeutic effect.

not required for the growth and survival of the cancer and that an agent targeting this kinase will not be clinically useful, or that an incorrect end point was selected to determine response. It is also possible that only a subset of patients whose cancer expresses a target will respond to therapy. Thus, clinical studies of kinase inhibitors need to integrate sophisticated correlative studies with various clinical end points to draw meaningful conclusions about monotherapy and to guide development of combination therapy studies.

BCR-ABL as a Therapeutic Target Of all the diseases associated with activated tyrosine kinases, the best-validated target is the BCR-ABL tyrosine kinase in CML. The pathogenetic role of this kinase in CML was firmly established by a series of discoveries over the last 40 years.[20,21] Virtually all patients with CML exhibit a reciprocal translocation between the long arms of chromosomes 9 and 22, t(9;22)(q34;q11).[22] This translocation results in fusion of the *ABL* oncogene from chromosome 9 with sequences from chromosome 22, the breakpoint cluster region (*BCR*), giving rise to a chimeric *BCR-ABL* gene.[23,24] This fusion gene is transcribed and translated into a protein that functions as a constitutively activated tyrosine kinase.[25,26] Depending on the site of the breakpoint in *BCR*, one of two different fusion proteins are produced, p185 (185 kilodaltons [kDa]) and p210 (210 kDa). The p210 protein is present in approximately 95% of patients with CML and in up to 20% of adult patients with de novo acute lymphoblastic leukemia (ALL), whereas the p185 form is seen in approximately 10% of adult patients with ALL and in the majority of pediatric patients with *BCR-ABL*-positive ALL (5% of pediatric ALL cases).[27–29] Expression of BCR-ABL in primary hematopoietic cells and a variety of myeloid and lymphoid cell lines renders these cells growth factor independent for proliferation.[30–32] However, even more convincing evidence for the leukemogenic potential of BCR-ABL is its ability to induce myeloproliferative disorders in animal models.[33–36] Because all of the transforming activities of BCR-ABL are dependent on its tyrosine kinase activity,[37] an inhibitor of the BCR-ABL kinase would be predicted to be an effective and selective therapeutic agent for CML.

Imatinib and CML Imatinib (Gleevec, Glivec, formerly STI571) is a relatively selective tyrosine kinase inhibitor, with activity against all of the ABL tyrosine kinases, including BCR-ABL, ABL, v-ABL, and ARG (Abelson-related gene). Besides the ABL tyrosine kinase, other kinases inhibited by imatinib are the platelet-derived growth factor receptor alpha (PDGFRA) and beta (PDGFRB) tyrosine kinases, and KIT. Based on a variety of preclinical studies that showed in vitro and in vivo activity of imatinib against CML cells, this compound was advanced to clinical trials.[38,39]

In a standard dose-escalation, phase I study, conducted in patients with CML, imatinib was well tolerated.[16,17] Despite dose escalation from 25 mg to 1,000 mg in 14 cohorts of patients, a maximally tolerated dose (MTD) could not be defined. Imatinib was administered once daily and pharmacokinetics showed a half-life of 13 to 16 hours.[40] Significant clinical benefits were observed at doses of 300 mg per day and above. In patients with chronic-phase disease who were interferon resistant or intolerant, 53 of 54 (98%) achieved a complete hematologic response and 96% of these responses lasted beyond 1 year.[17] In patients with myeloid blast crisis, 21 of 38 (55%) patients responded, with 18% having responses lasting beyond 1 year.[16]

The success of the phase I studies prompted phase II studies in which single-agent imatinib was tested further in patients with chronic-phase disease who were interferon-refractory or intolerant, as well as accelerated-phase patients and patients with CML in myeloid blast crisis and *BCR-ABL*-positive ALL. These studies accrued more than 1,000 patients at 30 centers in 6 countries over a period of 6 to 9 months. Figure 47-2 summarizes the published results from these studies with 18 months of follow-up.[41–44] These studies served as the basis for accelerated FDA approval of imatinib in May 2001 for the above indications.

A phase III randomized study comparing 400 mg per day of imatinib to interferon plus cytarabine in newly diagnosed patients with chronic-phase disease accrued over 1,000 patients in a 7-month period. With a median follow-up of 18 months, patients randomized to imatinib had statistically significant better results than patients treated with interferon plus cytarabine in all parameters measured, including rates of complete hematologic response, major and complete cytogenetic response, tolerance of therapy, and freedom from disease progression (Table 47-3).[45] With 42 months of follow-up, disease progression has occurred in only 16% of patients treated initially with imatinib, with an overall survival of 91%.[46] Disease progression was defined as death, progression to accelerated or blastic phases, loss of a complete hematologic response, or loss of a major (Philadelphia [Ph] chromosome-positive metaphases less than 35%) or complete cytogenetic response (no Ph chromosome-positive metaphases). For patients who have achieved a complete cytogenetic response, the relapse rate is 2% per year and for patients with a 3-log or greater decrease in quantitative reverse transcriptase-polymerase chain reaction (RT-PCR) for *BCR-ABL* transcripts, the relapse rate is only 0.5% per year.[46,47]

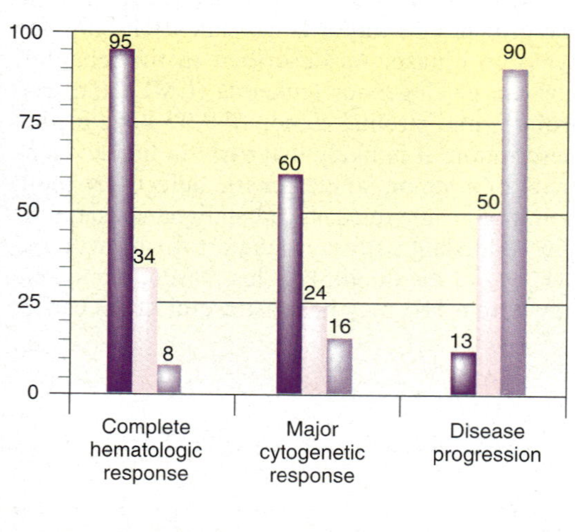

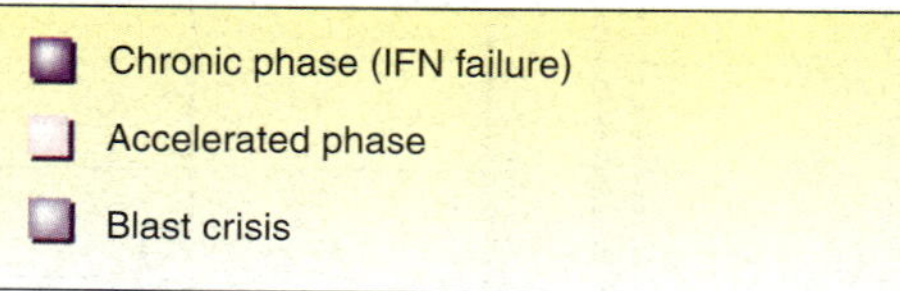

Figure 47-2 Phase II clinical trials of imatinib for CML. The results of the phase II studies of imatinib are shown. Study groups included patients in chronic-phase, who were resistant or intolerant of interferon, and patients with accelerated-phase or blast crisis. Results shown are with a median follow up of up to 30 months and the rate of disease progression is at 24 months.[41,43,44] Major cytogenetic response includes patients with Ph chromosome positive metaphases of less then or equal to 35%.

Table 47-3 Phase III Results of Imatinib versus IFN-α Plus Cytarabine for Newly Diagnosed Chronic Phase Patients with CML[45]

	Imatinib 400 mg/d, $n = 553$	IFN-α + Ara-C, $n = 553$
CHR	97%	69%
MCR	87%	35%
CCR	76%	14%
Intolerance	3%	31%
Progressive disease	3%	8.5%

Results are with a median follow-up of 18 months. Abbreviations: CHR, complete hematologic response; MCR, major cytogenetic response; CCR, complete cytogenetic response. Intolerance leading to discontinuation of first-line therapy. Progressive disease to accelerated phase or blast crisis. (All of these differences are highly statistically significant with $p < .001$).

MECHANISMS OF RELAPSE/ RESISTANCE TO IMATINIB

Response rates to imatinib in CML patients with chronic-phase disease are quite high and thus far, have been durable. Response rates are also quite high in patients with advanced-phase disease, but relapses, despite continued therapy with imatinib, are common. A coordinated approach to analyzing potential mechanisms of relapse or resistance to imatinib began with an analysis of the expression of the target (Figure 47-3). In all patients with CML who relapsed on imatinib therapy, the BCR-ABL kinase remains present. Next, it was determined whether there was persistent inhibition of the BCR-ABL kinase (see Figure 47-3). Patients with persistent inhibition of the BCR-ABL kinase would be predicted to have additional molecular abnormalities besides BCR-ABL driving the growth and survival of the malignant clone. In contrast, patients with reactivation of the kinase would be postulated to have resistance mechanisms that either prevent imatinib from reaching the target or render the target insensitive to BCR-ABL. In the former category

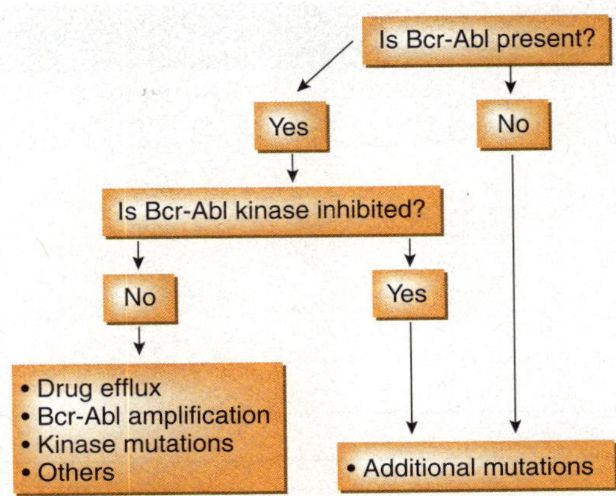

Figure 47-3 Distinguishing between potential mechanisms of relapse.

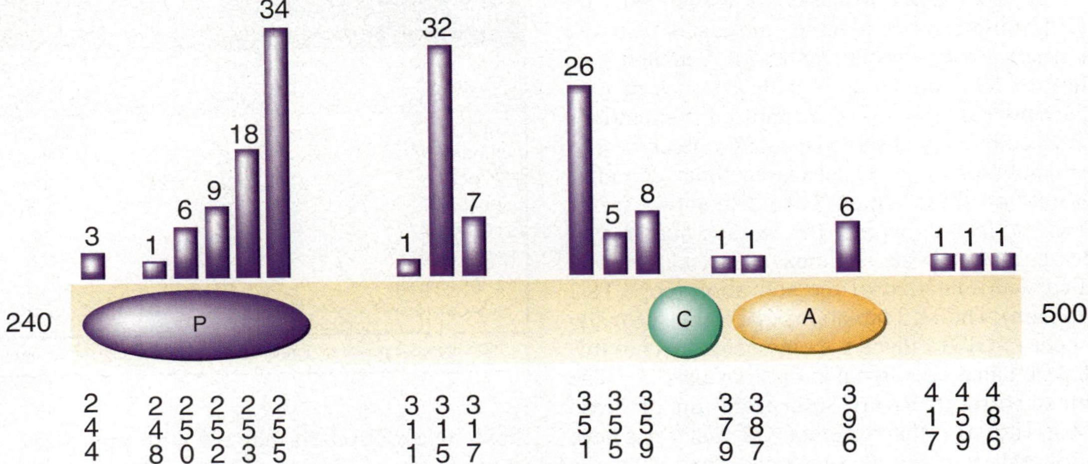

Figure 47-4 Schematic of point mutations in the ABL kinase domain. The ABL kinase domain, from amino acid 240 to 500, is shown with the ATP binding domain (*P*), the catalytic domain (*C*), and the activation loop (*A*). The numbers below the kinase domain are amino acids that are mutated in patients who relapsed on therapy with imatinib. The vertical lines above the kinase domain indicate the number of times each amino acid has been found to be mutated as compiled from the literature.[49,51,57,172,173] Adapted from Shah NP et al.[56]

are mechanisms such as drug efflux or protein binding of imatinib. In the latter category would be mutations of the BCR-ABL kinase that render BCR-ABL insensitive to imatinib and amplification of the BCR-ABL protein.

In the largest studies of resistance or relapse, several consistent themes have emerged. In the majority of patients who respond to imatinib but subsequently relapse while remaining on therapy, the BCR-ABL kinase has been reactivated.[48] BCR-ABL kinase activity was analyzed by assessing tyrosine phosphorylation of CRKL, a direct substrate of the BCR-ABL kinase, and the major tyrosine phosphorylated protein in samples from patients with CML.[49,50] In these studies, between 50 and 90% of relapsed patients have BCR-ABL point mutations in over 25 different amino acids scattered throughout the ABL kinase domain (Figure 47-4).[51–57] Some other patients have amplification of *BCR-ABL* at the genomic or transcript level. In contrast, in patients with primary resistance, that is, patients who do not respond to imatinib therapy, BCR-ABL-independent mechanisms are most common.[53]

In patients who relapse as a consequence of reactivation of the BCR-ABL kinase, the BCR-ABL kinase remains a good target. Alternate ABL kinase inhibitors have already been synthesized and two have advanced to clinical trials. One of these compounds, AMN107 was synthesized based on the knowledge of the crystal structure of the ABL kinase in complex with imatinib. This information was used to synthesize an ABL inhibitor that is approximately 30-fold more potent than imatinib.[58,59] An alternate approach was to profile existing compounds for activity against the ABL kinase. This led to the recognition that many SRC inhibitors are also inhibitors of the ABL kinase.[60,61] One of these dual SRC/ABL inhibitors, dasatanib (BMS-354825), is over 100-fold more potent against ABL than imatinib.[58,62] Both AMN107 and dasatanib inhibit most of the common imatinib-resistant BCR-ABL kinase domain mutations except T315I.[58,59,62] AMN107 has variable activity against the mutants, but generally retains its 30-fold greater potency against the various mutants.[58,59] Dasatinib, by virtue of its smaller size and ability to bind ABL in both its active and inactive conformations, inhibits most of the mutants with an IC50 of 10 nmol/L or less.[58,63] Both compounds have shown significant activity in phase I trials in imatinib-resistant patients and have advanced to phase II studies.[63,64]

KIT AS A THERAPEUTIC TARGET

KIT (also known as c-KIT) is a type III receptor tyrosine kinase that has strong sequence homology to the other members of this RTK family—specifically, PDGFRA, PDGFRB, FLT3 (STK1, FLK2), and c-FMS (CSF-1R). All members of this family have a shared protein structure consisting of five extracellular, immunoglobulin-like domains, a hydrophobic transmembrane domain, and a tyrosine kinase domain that is split into two halves by a hydrophilic insert (Figure 47-5).[65] Interestingly, this family of kinases shares some homology with the ABL kinase, and three of its members (KIT, PDGFRA and PDGFRB) are sensitive to inhibition by imatinib, while the remainder of the kinases of this family (FLT3, FMS) are not.[66,67] The ligand for KIT is Steel factor (SLF) also known as KIT ligand, stem cell factor and mast cell growth factor. The importance of KIT in normal developmental processes is highlighted by the phenotypes of mice deficient in either KIT or SLF. These mice have deficiencies in erythropoiesis, pigmentation, mast cells, germ cells, and interstitial cells of Cajal. Complete absence of KIT or SLF expression results in embryonic lethality caused by severe anemia.[68,69]

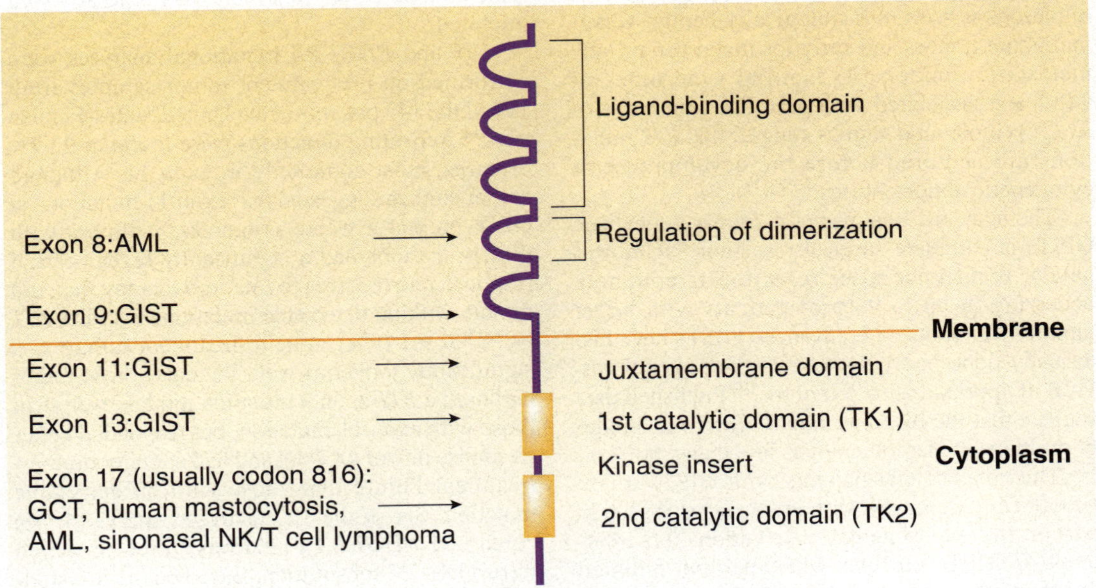

Figure 47-5 Schematic of activating mutations in the KIT receptor tyrosine kinase. The sites of activating mutations of KIT that are associated with human cancers are indicated by arrows. As shown, extracellular or intracellular (kinase and nonkinase domains) mutations can result in ligand-independent activation of KIT kinase activity.

Several human diseases are associated with KIT mutations that have increased tyrosine kinase activity (see Figure 47-5). A notable feature of KIT mutations is their association with particular diseases. For example, the mutations most commonly observed in GISTs affect the juxtamembrane or proximal extracellular domains. Rarely do these tumors have a mutation in the TK1 or TK2 domain.[70] In contrast, human systemic mastocytosis is almost universally associated with mutation of the activation loop (TK2 domain). The TK2 mutations that do occasionally occur in GISTs involve amino acids that are different than those altered in mastocytosis.[70,71] The most straightforward interpretation of these observations is that different KIT mutations have different signaling consequences, the oncogenic effects of which are heavily influenced by the cellular context. Of note, KIT mutations vary in their sensitivity to imatinib.

GISTs as a Model Disease for a KIT TKI GISTs are mesenchymal neoplasms that can arise from any organ in the gastrointestinal tract or from the mesentery or omentum. Although GISTs morphologically resemble leiomyosarcomas and nerve sheath tumors, they are a distinct entity.[72] Compared to these other mesenchymal neoplasms, GISTs have relatively simple karyotypes (partial or complete loss of chromosomes 1, 9, 14, 15, and 22, but no consistent additions or translocations).[73] In addition, approximately 95% of GISTs express KIT, and biochemical evidence of its activation can be found in almost all GISTs.[70] In approximately 80% of cases, this activation is linked to somatic mutations of *KIT*, most commonly in exons 9 or 11.[70] Interestingly, a subset of GISTs (approximately 7%) harbor mutations in the PDGFRA, which can function as an oncogenic substitute for KIT.[74]

Several lines of evidence indicate that *KIT* mutations are an early pathogenetic event in GISTs: (1) a similar frequency and spectrum of mutations is seen in histologically benign versus malignant tumors and early/localized versus late/metastatic tumors; (2) familial syndromes of GIST are associated with germline mutations of *KIT*; (3) molecular studies suggest that *KIT* mutations are acquired before the development of cytogenetic abnormalities.[70,73,75]

The standard treatment for primary, localized GISTs is complete surgical resection.[76] Unfortunately, recurrence after resection is common, occurring in up to 90% of patients with larger tumors.[77] Patients with advanced GISTs have historically done poorly, with a median overall survival of approximately 9 months.[78] Published data suggest that the response rate of GISTs to single- or multiagent chemotherapy is less than 5%.[79]

The concept that patients with GISTs might benefit from treatment with imatinib was based in part on two experimental observations: (1) treatment of GIST cell lines with imatinib inhibited proliferation and induced apoptosis; and (2) several GIST-associated mutant KIT isoforms were potently inhibited by imatinib in vitro at concentrations similar to wild-type KIT.[80,81] Based on these observations, a patient with metastatic, chemotherapy-resistant GIST was treated with 400 mg per day of imatinib in a proof-of-concept study. The tumor in this patient expressed an exon 11 mutant KIT isoform and the patient responded dramatically, with a symptomatic, pathologic, and objective response by standard CT and PET scan criteria.[82]

Table 47-4 Therapeutic Trials of Imatinib in Gastrointestinal Stromal Tumor

Trial	Phase	Dose (mg/d)	Objective Response (PR+CR, %)	Tumor Control (PR+CR+SD, %)
EORTC[170]	I	400–1,000	63	90
EORTC[106]	II	800	71	89
EORTC[87]	III	400	50	82
EORTC[87]	III	800	54	86
US-Finnish[171]	II	400	66	83
US-Finnish[171]	II	600	66	83
US-Canadian[83]	III	400	48	75
US-Canadian[83]	III	800	48	74

PR = objective partial response; CR = objective complete response; SD = stable disease.

The strong preclinical rationale, coupled with the clinical success in this solitary patient, led to several phase I and/or II studies in which imatinib doses ranged from 400 to 1,000 mg per day. Response rates in these trials ranged from 54 to 71% (Table 47-4). An additional 16 to 37% of treated patients demonstrated prolonged stable disease and importantly, the survival of these patients was equivalent to that of patients with partial responses by standard RECIST criteria.[83] Primary resistance was rare, occurring in only 5 to 12% of patients. Although secondary resistance did eventually occur in a substantial fraction of patients, overall clinical benefit, in general, was durable. With a median follow-up of 34 months, 46% of patients on the United States-Finnish study were alive and still on therapy.[84] Nearly all patients on the early phase trials experienced toxicity, but treatment was generally well tolerated.

KIT and *PDGFRA* mutational analyses were performed on pretreatment tumor samples from 121 of the 147 patients in the United States-Finnish trial.[84] Activating mutations were found in 92.9% of cases, most commonly in exon 11. Although earlier studies suggested that exon 11 mutations in GIST predict a worse prognosis,[85] tumors with these mutations had a significantly higher partial response rate (83.5%) to imatinib therapy than did tumors with no detectable mutations in either *KIT* or *PDGFRA* (0%); time-to-treatment failure was significantly longer as well. Patients whose tumor harbored a *KIT* exon 9 mutation did less well than those with exon 11 mutation, but responded better (response rate of 48.7%), and had a longer time-to-treatment failure than those with no detectable mutation. Six of the 127 analyzed GISTs (4.7%) contained *PDGFRA* mutations, three of which were a D842V substitution. Based on in vitro studies, this isoform of PDGFRA is highly resistant to imatinib.[84,86] Correspondingly, none of the three patients with this specific mutation responded to imatinib.

Several additional studies have addressed important issues regarding the use of imatinib in GIST. The North American Sarcoma Intergroup and a consortium made up of the European Organization for Research and Treatment of Cancer (EORTC), Italian Sarcoma Group, and Australiasian Gastrointestinal Cancer Trials Group conducted nearly identical randomized phase III trials comparing 400 mg or 800 mg per day of imatinib (see Table 47-3).[83,87] Both studies allowed crossover from the lower to higher dose at the time of progression. The primary objective of the EORTC trial (946 patients) was progression-free survival (PFS), whereas the North American study (746 patients) looked at both PFS and overall survival. Both included toxicity assessment as a secondary objective. In the North American Intergroup trial, response rates, PFS, and overall survival were statistically indistinguishable between the lower- and higher-dose arms (see Table 47-3).[83] In the EORTC trial, no differences were seen in response rates (50% and 54% respectively, for 400 versus 800 mg per day), or primary resistance rates (13 and 9%). Two-year survival was similar at 69 and 74%. In contrast to the North American study, however, the EORTC study showed a statistically significant PFS advantage of the higher dose. At two years, 56% on lower-dose and only 48% on higher-dose imatinib had failed (progression or death).[87] The reason for the difference in efficacy outcomes is unclear. It may represent greater power to detect a real change on the European study (larger number of patients), a biologic difference between populations, or other factors. At this time, most experts still recommend a starting dose of 400 mg of imatinib daily in newly diagnosed patients with metastatic GIST.

Duration of imatinib therapy, both in responding and progressing patients with GIST, remains of interest. Blay and associates treated patients with incurable GIST for one year. At that time, patients achieving at least stable disease were randomized to either continuing imatinib or stopping drug until progression and then restarting. With a median follow-up of 21 months after randomization, 21 of 32 pts (66%) who discontinued therapy versus 4 of 26 pts (15%) who remained on continuous therapy experienced progressive disease. Imatinib interruption was associated with a significantly reduced PFS ($p < 10^{-4}$), but overall survival was similar as imatinib reintroduction allowed tumor control in 11 of 14 patients

(79%).[88] The authors concluded that continuous imatinib is associated with improved PFS, even in patients achieving a complete response.

Another significant issue is whether patients progressing on imatinib should remain on the drug. Theoretically, some malignant clones might be controlled by drug whereas others have become resistant. Supporting this theory, Van den Abbeele and associates studied metabolic activity in imatinib-resistant GIST using FDG-PET.[89] As part of a clinical trial of SU11248, a multi-targeted kinase inhibitor with potent activity against KIT, PDGFRA, PDGFRB, and VEGFR2, 11 patients with imatinib-refractory GIST underwent FDG-PET scanning before and after cessation of imatinib, prior to initiation of SU11248. There was highly significant difference between the log standardized uptake value (SUV) means of tumors before and after termination of imatinib therapy ($p = .0005$). Nine of the eleven patients had at least one lesion with an SUV increase of greater than 25% after stopping drug. The authors concluded that terminating imatinib, even in patients with drug-refractory GIST, results in a tumor "flare" phenomenon.[89] They suggested there are tumor cell populations for which imatinib remains effective, even in patients demonstrating progression on the drug. Based on similar evidence, the National Comprehensive Cancer Network has formally recommended continuing imatinib therapy in patients with documented progression, assuming they are not rapidly deteriorating or they have no options for participation in a clinical trial <http://www.nccn.org/professionals/physician_gls/PDF/sarcoma.pdf>. Adjuvant and neoadjuvant use of imatinib is another area of great interest. Several cooperative group trials to assess these uses are accruing patients or have recently been completed in the United States and Europe.[90]

The median time to disease progression in imatinib-treated patients with advanced GIST is approximately two years.[87] A number of studies have examined mechanisms of imatinib-resistance using biopsy specimens obtained from progressing lesions.[87,91–94] Similar to the situation in CML, many imatinib-resistant tumors have acquired kinase mutations in the ATP binding pocket of KIT (exons 13 and 14), or the activation loop (exon 17). However, resistance mechanisms in GISTs are more heterogeneous than those seen in chronic-phase CML as some tumors actually lose KIT expression, presumably due to a "switch" to a different oncogenic mechanism. Other tumors become imatinib-resistant without acquisition of secondary kinase mutations—most notably in the case of primary resistance of GISTs with *KIT* exon 9 mutations or wild-type *KIT/PDGFRA* genotypes.

A number of kinase inhibitors have been tested for activity against imatinib-resistant GIST tumors. The most developed of these agents is sunitinib (formerly SU11248), a multi-targeted inhibitor of the KIT, PDGFRA, PDGFRB, FLT3, CSF-1R, VEGFR1, and VEGFR2 RTKs.[95,96] This agent has the potential to inhibit the growth of imatinib-resistant tumors either by direct inhibition of tumor-associated oncogenic kinases and by disruption of the tumor-associated vascular supply. In a phase I/II study involving 97 patients, objective responses were observed in 8% of patients with an additional 37% having stable disease for greater than 6 months. In this study, the median time-to-treatment failure and overall survival were 8 and 20 months, respectively. There was a striking correlation between pre-imatinib tumor genotype and response to sunitinib, with a median time-to-treatment failure for patients with *KIT* exon 9 or no *KIT/PDGFRA* mutations of 14 months compared with only 5 months for patients whose GIST had a *KIT* exon 11 mutation. Notably, the relationship between kinase mutations and clinical outcome was the converse of that seen with imatinib, where patients with *KIT* exon 11 mutations have the best clinical outcomes.[97] These results further highlight the underlying biologic heterogeneity among GISTs and the complex interaction between tumor biology and different kinase inhibitors in determining clinical responses to these agents. Based on these promising results, sunitinib was tested in a randomized, placebo-controlled phase III study of patients with imatinib-resistant GIST. Patients treated with sunitinib had superior time-to-treatment failure and overall survival as compared with patients receiving placebo.[98]

OTHER DISEASES TARGETED BY IMATINIB

In addition to CML and GIST, imatinib has been tested as a monotherapy in a large number of other human malignancies, based in part on evidence of KIT or PDGFR expression. These include carcinoma of the prostate, breast, and lung (small cell), adenoid cystic carcinoma, melanoma, and a variety of non-GIST sarcomas. These cancers, which do not harbor *KIT* or *PDGFR* mutations, are unresponsive to imatinib.[99–106]

In contrast, imatinib does have activity in neoplasms that are caused by oncogenic activation of PDGFRs. This includes the subset of patients with chronic myelomonocytic leukemia that results from fusion of the *EVT6* (*TEL*) and *PDGFRB* genes.[107,108] Similarly, dermatofibrosarcoma protuberans, a low-grade sarcoma of the dermis, is characterized by a (17;22) translocation involving the *COL1A1* and *PDGF-B* genes, which results in over-production of fusion COL1A1-PDGF-BB ligand and consequent hyperactivation of PDGFRB.[109] Patients with this tumor also respond to imatinib.[110,112] Hypereosinophilic syndrome is another example of an imatinib-sensitive disease. In this case a *PDGFRA* fusion gene product (FIP1L1-PDGFRA) is the activated target.[113–115] Interestingly, patients with disease respond to as little as 100 mg of imatinib,[116] one fourth the effective dose in CML and GIST, providing yet another example of the critical relationship between kinase mutation type and drug sensitivity.

Besides GIST, there are a number of other human cancers associated with *KIT* mutations, including mastocytosis, seminoma, and AML, that might be effectively treated with a KIT TKI. However, *KIT* mutations are detectable in only 25% of cases of seminoma and less than 5% of adult patients with AML[15]. Design of clinical trials for these diseases will likely require determination of *KIT* mutational status as a condition of trial eligibility. Equally important, the mutations in these tumors—most commonly detected in the TK2 domain (exon 17)—result in KIT isoforms that are biochemically resistant to imatinib.[117] *KIT* mutations are present in 95% of mast cell disease, but again, the most common mutation (D816V) is fully resistant to imatinib.[117] Thus, it will be necessary to develop other TKIs with activity against these particular mutations. This point demonstrates the importance of assessing the activity of TKIs against the full spectrum of mutant alleles that are observed clinically to best guide clinical trials.

EGFR AS A THERAPEUTIC TARGET

The EGFR is expressed in a wide variety of human malignancies, including carcinomas of the lung, breast, colon, ovary, bladder, prostate, head and neck, as well as gliomas and a subset of sarcomas.[118,119] The EGFR can be activated through gene amplification, overexpression of its ligands (EGF, transforming growth factor-α), and somatic mutation. The concept that blocking EGFR signaling might be effective in the treatment of cancers was introduced in the early 1980s with the development of EGFR-specific antibodies.[120] Enthusiasm for the therapeutic potential of this target grew with the observation that EGFR expression correlates with resistance to chemotherapy and worse outcome in a number of different cancers, particularly carcinomas of the head and neck, esophagus, bladder, cervix, and ovary.[121] Amplification of the *EGFR* gene is common in gliomas, but less so in other tumors. Approximately half of glioblastomas express mutant isoforms of the EGFR that have extracellular domain deletions.[122] These types of mutation appear to be rare in other cancers, but mutations in the EGFR kinase domain have recently been discovered in adenocarcinomas of the lung and colon.[123–125]

A chimeric antibody that recognizes the EGFR (cetuximab) was approved by the FDA in 2004 for use in combination with chemotherapy for the treatment of advanced colorectal adenocarcinomas. Several additional monoclonal human or humanized EGFR antibodies are in clinical development (ABX-EGF, EMD-72000, h-R3). These agents are discussed in detail in another chapter of this volume. Small molecule ATP-binding inhibitors with activity against the EGFR include relatively specific agents (gefitinib, erlotinib, EKB-569), and compounds that inhibit other members of the EGFR family (lapatinib, CI-1033), including HER2/ERBB2. Additional EGFR-targeted drugs are in preclinical or early clinical development. Two EGFR inhibitors (gefitinib and erlotinib) have recently been approved by the FDA for the treatment of non-small-cell lung cancer (NSCLC) and will be further discussed.

Table 47-5 Therapeutic Trials of Gefitinib and Erlotinib in Non-Small-Cell Lung Cancer

Study	Phase	Study Arms (*n*)	Response Rate	Stable Disease	Overall Survival
Monotherapy trials					
IDEAL1[174]	II	Gefitinib 250 mg/d (103) *vs* 500 mg/d (106)	18% *vs* 19%	39%	7.6 *vs* 8 mo
IDEAL2[127]	II	Gefitinib 250 mg/d (102) *vs* 500 mg/d (114)	12% *vs* 9%	31% *vs* 27%	6.5 *vs* 5.9 mo
Perez-Soler[175]	II	Erlotinib 150 mg/d (57)	12%	39%	8.4 mo
ISEL	III	Gefitinib 250 mg/d *vs* placebo (total 1692)	8.2%	—	5.6 *vs* 5.1 mo
Shepherd et al.[126]	III	Erlotinib 150 mg/d (488) *vs* placebo (243)	8.9%	—	6.7 *vs* 4.7 mo*
Combination trials					
INTACT 1[176]	III	Gemcitabine & cisplatin +/– gefitinib 250 or 500 mg/d (total 1093)	47%, 51%, 50%	—	10.9, 9.9, 9.9 mo
INTACT 2[177]	III	Paclitaxel & carboplatin +/– gefitinib 250 or 500 mg/d (total 1037)	29%, 30%, 30%	—	9.9, 9.8, 8.7 mo
TALENT[178]	III	Gemcitabine & cisplatin +/– erlotinib 150 mg/d (total 1172)	30%, 31%	—	10.9, 9.9 mo
TRIBUTE[179]	III	Paclitaxel & carboplatin +/– erlotinib 150 mg/d (total 1059)	19% vs 21%	—	10.6 *vs* 10.8 mo

*Statistically significant.

Initial excitement over gefitinib and erlotinib was generated during phase II trials in patients with chemotherapy-refractory NSCLC, the results of which are summarized in Table 47-5. Although the overall response rates were low, some patients showed dramatic improvement and more than one third enjoyed symptomatic relief. Interestingly, the response rate to gefitinib was substantially higher among Japanese patients than in the United States cohort.

Despite provocative findings in the phase II trials, a survival advantage over placebo was not observed in a phase III trial of gefitinib for NSCLC post chemotherapy (see Table 47-5). Although a similar phase III trial of erlotinib did yield a statistically significant increase in overall survival, the benefit was relatively small (31% versus 22% at 1 year).[126] Further disappointment emerged from combination trials, in which it was found that the addition of either gefitinib or erlotinib to standard chemotherapy did not provide a measurable benefit to NSCLC patients undergoing treatment for stage III or IV disease (see Table 47-5). Thus, the overall clinical trial results with gefitinib and erlotinib did not match initial hopes. Nevertheless, a small percentage of patients clearly benefited from treatment with these inhibitors. Subset analyses revealed that the best responses were observed in East Asian patients, women, never-smokers, and patients with adenocarcinoma showing bronchioloalveolar features.[127,128] Interestingly, EGFR expression, as assessed by immunohistochemistry, was not strongly correlated with responses.[129]

EGFR MUTATIONS AND RESPONSE TO EGFR TKIS

In April 2004, two landmark studies uncovered a relationship between gain-of-function mutations in the EGFR and response to gefitinib.[123,125] Combining the data from these two reports, mutations were found in 13 of 14 gefitinib-responsive tumors and in 0 of 11 non-responsive tumors. In vitro experiments confirmed that the mutant isoforms of EGFR were constitutively activated and could be fully inhibited by the drug.[123,125] Furthermore, the sensitivity of NSCLC cell lines to gefitinib also correlated with the presence of EGFR mutations.[125] The relationship between EGFR mutations and gefitinib response was quickly confirmed in a third, independent report, which also extended the observation to erlotinib-responsive tumors.[130] Thus, it appears that both inhibitors are most effective against NSCLC tumors that are EGFR 'addicted,' as evidenced by the presence of oncogenic mutations.

Follow-up studies from a number of institutions worldwide have established that the most common mutations in *EGFR* are in-frame deletions (or deletion-substitutions) in exon 19 and a point mutation (L858R) in exon 21.[131–135] Additional mutations have been described in exons 18 and 20; occasional tumors have two mutations. Based on these studies, *EGFR* mutations are most common in East Asians patients (up to 40%), women and never-smokers, and they are limited to adenocarcinomas (particularly tumors with bronchioloalveolar features). As noted above, these clinicopathologic features are independent predictors of gefitinib response. More importantly, a small study from Japan ($n = 21$) showed a trend toward an overall survival advantage for gefitinib-treated patients whose tumors harbored an EGFR mutation, and this was statistically validated in a second Japanese series ($n = 56$).[135,136] In a Korean study of 90 patients treated with gefitinib, both the time to progression (21.7 versus 1.8 months) and overall survival (30.5 versus 6.6 months) were significantly longer in patients with mutation-positive tumors.[137] It is likely that the prolonged survival of these patients was a direct benefit of gefitinib, because there is no difference in the overall survival of untreated patients with EGFR-mutant versus non-mutant NSCLC.[134]

The relationship between *EGFR* mutations and response to EGFR TKIs closely parallels the experience with imatinib and its oncogenically activated targets in CML and GISTs. Perhaps not surprisingly, secondary drug resistance in NSCLC patients who initially respond well to either gefitinib or erlotinib has been linked to the acquisition of a new point mutation (T790M) that directly interferes with drug binding in the ATP pocket.[138,139] This observation substantiates the importance of EGFR signaling in NSCLCs that contain *EGFR* mutations, but it also suggests that the effectiveness of monotherapy with TKIs in NSCLC patients may be limited by the selection of drug-resistant isoforms of EGFR.

The role of TKIs in the treatment of NSCLC without *EGFR* mutations is another important issue. In approximately 15 to 20% of NSCLC patients who have a partial response to gefitinib or erlotinib, no *EGFR* mutations are detected.[123,125,135,137] This may be due in part to technical issues, but it is also possible that other TKI targets are activated in this subset of cases. Thus, assays for *EGFR* mutations are not absolutely predictive of drug response. It is also important to note that *EGFR* mutations are not found in approximately 30% of patients who experience disease stabilization and symptomatic relief on gefitinib or erlotinib. In the case of erlotinib, the benefit of this effect translated to a small but statistically significant survival advantage for chemotherapy-refractory NSCLC patients treated in a phase III trial (see Table 47-5). Although mutation data are not available from that study, it has been argued that the results could not have been influenced by the low frequency of *EGFR* mutations expected in the North American population that was treated. Given its favorable side effect profile, erlotinib can be considered as a second-line therapy in cases without *EGFR* mutation.

Identification of *EGFR* mutations will clearly be important in the design and interpretation of future clinical trials with EGFR TKIs. In this regard, another gene of interest is *KRAS*. *EGFR* and *KRAS* mutations appear to be mutually exclusive in NSCLC,[132,140] and one report suggests that tumors with *KRAS* mutations do not respond to gefitinib and erlotinib.[140] As KRAS is a downstream signaling protein of the EGFR, this makes biologic sense. In future years, screening for *KRAS* and *EGFR* mutations may become routine in the diagnosis and management of NSCLC.

OTHER TARGETS AND OTHER INHIBITORS

As delineated in Table 47-1, there are numerous tyrosine kinases implicated in a variety of human tumors. Inhibitors of many of these kinases are in preclinical and early clinical trials.[141] For example, FLT3 inhibitors are being tested in AML[142–144] and a variety of VEGFR inhibitors are also in clinical trials.[145] Besides tyrosine kinases, there are numerous serine/theonine kinases that have critical roles in malignancies. This includes B-RAF mutations in the majority of melanomas, some colon cancers, and others.[146–148] AKT, which is activated in tumors with PTEN deficiency and by a variety of growth-stimulatory pathways, is also an attractive target.[149] Similarly, a variety of cell cycle kinase inhibitors are in preclinical and clinical development.[150,151] Lastly, lipid kinases, notably phosphoinositol 3-kinase, is mutated in colon and breast cancers,[152–154] and inhibitors of these kinases are being developed.[155] For all of these targets, the lessons learned from the clinical development of the specific agents described in this chapter apply.

TOXICITY OF TKIs

Given the ubiquitous expression of tyrosine kinases such as KIT, PDGFR, and EGFR, one might predict that inhibition of any one of them with a TKI would result in significant, perhaps even fatal, complications. Mice that are KIT or PDGFR null have an embryonic lethal phenotype,[69,156–158] and EGFR null animals manifest a variety of severe defects.[159] Surprisingly, TKIs are well tolerated in humans. This may reflect differences in kinase dependence between adult and embryonic tissues.[160] Alternatively, humans may have redundant gene function that minimizes the effect of suppressing common kinases. It is also possible that residual kinase activity may persist during TKI therapy and this may be sufficient to protect dependent tissues. If this latter explanation is correct, then side effects might become more apparent as more potent kinase inhibitors are generated. Regardless, the paucity of serious side effects has important implications for clinical trial design as discussed below.

In a clinical trial of imatinib for patients with chronic-phase CML, only 2% of patients discontinued therapy with imatinib due to adverse events.[41] In both CML and GIST patients, the most common imatinib side effects have been mild and include nausea, periorbital edema, muscle cramps, fatigue, and diarrhea.[17,161] Serious adverse events, which are rare, include skin rash, fluid retention, and elevated liver function tests, but these are readily managed by dose reduction or interruption in most patients. Among patients with GIST treated in the EORTC phase III trial, grade 3 to 5 adverse effects were significantly more common in the 800 mg group than in the 400 mg group.[87] However, such effects were less likely to occur if the dose was escalated to 800 mg after patients were on 400 mg for a period of time. Interestingly, the incidence of myelosuppression is much greater in patients with CML than in patients with solid tumors.[161] This suggests that myelosuppression is a therapeutic effect in patients with CML where hematopoiesis is predominantly contributed by the BCR-ABL-positive clone. In contrast, severe gastrointestinal/intraabdominal bleeding is a complication seen primarily in patients with GIST, most likely due to tumor necrosis in the setting of mucosal ulceration.

Gefitinib and erlotinib have very similar side effect profiles, consisting predominantly of grade 1 or 2 rash (43–75%) and diarrhea (49–54%). However, rare cases of interstitial lung disease (0.3–0.6% in the United States; 2% in Japan) have been documented for both drugs, and up to a third of these cases are fatal.[162,163] Interestingly, even kinase inhibitors with relatively broad specificity, such as dasatinib, which inhibits PDGFR, KIT, ABL, and SRC, have been relatively well-tolerated in early clinical trials.[64] Whether this favorable toxicity profile will be maintained with long-term therapy and whether this will be true of all kinase inhibitors remains to be determined. However, the good tolerability of kinase inhibitors has allowed speculation about the utility of inhibitors with less specificity, as they may be capable of targeting more tumors.[150]

CONSIDERATIONS IN CLINICAL TRIAL DESIGN FOR TKIs

The development of imatinib, gefitinib, and erlotinib offers several lessons for the design of clinical trials of TKIs. The traditional end point of a phase I trial for a new chemotherapy agent has been the determination of the MTD. This end point is justified on the assumption that "more is better" in terms of the clinical efficacy of traditional chemotherapy agents in treating cancer. In contrast, "less may be more" when using small-molecule kinase inhibitors. This is because the specificity of TKIs tends to decrease at higher doses. For example, imatinib is highly selective for the ABL, KIT and PDGFR kinases at doses of less than 5 μmol/L but has broader, nonselective effects at doses of 20 to 50 μmol/L.[38] Because almost complete inhibition of BCR-ABL activity (and presumably maximal clinical activity in CML) is achieved at plasma levels of 2 to 5 μmol/L, there is little justification for further escalation of the dose. Thus, in phase I trials of TKIs the stopping dose should not necessarily be determined by toxicity, but rather by other end points: (1) the dose that consistently achieves the target plasma level for maximal kinase inhibition (as predicted from preclinical studies); (2) direct confirmation of target kinase inhibition at test doses; and (3) failure to improve response rate with continued dose escalation. Of course, safety and tolerability continue to be critical components of any phase I trial of a new agent, including a TKI.

There are a number of methods for determining the pharmacodynamic effects of a kinase inhibitor. The most direct is biochemical measurement of target activation in a tumor specimen. This may be straightforward in cases in which tumor cells can be obtained by skin biopsy or phlebotomy, but this approach creates difficulties in cases where tumor specimens can be obtained only by more invasive procedure such as percutaneous biopsy of liver metastases. Even in cases where tumor specimens can be readily obtained, measurement of the activation status of the target may be technically difficult due to limitations in assay sensitivity. For example, in the case of CML, it is difficult to directly measure BCR-ABL phosphorylation or kinase activity in neutrophils obtained from peripheral blood.[49,164]

An alternative approach to assessing the pharmacodynamic effect of a TKI is measurement of a surrogate marker. In the case of CML, the measurement of phospho-CRKL has proven to be useful in assessing the effectiveness of imatinib in inhibiting BCR-ABL activity in CML cells.[17,49] Likewise, some studies of EGFR inhibitors have measured EGFR phosphorylation and/or ERK activation in biopsies of normal skin as a surrogate for effects on the EGFR in tumor cells.[165,166] Functional imaging is proving increasingly valuable in assessing TKI activity. For example, PET scans during early treatment with imatinib are predictive of long-term response to imatinib.[167] In the case of VEGFR inhibitors, it may prove feasible to assess drug effect by measurement of vascular permeability using dynamic MRI or other novel imaging techniques.[168,169]

Another important issue in designing trials for TKIs is the selection of patients for enrollment in a clinical trial of a TKI. Figure 47-6A shows a hypothetical set of clinical trials in which monotherapy with a TKI results in an 80% clinical response rate *if and only if* the target is present in the tumor. In the four examples shown in this figure, the target frequency varies from 90 to 10%, and the corresponding overall response rates vary from 72 to 8%. Without knowledge of the target frequency in a treated population, one might conclude that the trial with a 72% response rate was successful but the trial with an 8% response rate was a failure. However, in both cases, the therapy was equally effective in patients who expressed the target (80% in both cases). Thus, determination of target status in clinical specimens obtained from enrolled patients is crucial to the meaningful interpretation of clinical trial results. Indeed, the best results may be obtained when patient eligibility for a trial is made contingent on target status.

The above example is the simplest possibility for clinical trial design, with target expression sufficient to predict responses. However, a more complicated situation is portrayed in Figure 47-6B. In this example, target expression is not sufficient to predict responses; rather, some evidence for target activation is required and only a subset of patients with target expression would respond. In this example, the target expression is 100%, but target activation varies from 90 to 10%. In patients with target expression and activation, the response rate is again 80%. Thus, the overall response varies from 72 to 8%. If the target expression and activation is high, it might be concluded erroneously that expression is sufficient for response; whereas, if expression is high and activation is low, one might conclude correctly that expression does not correlate with response, but conclude erroneously that the agent lacks activity.

The examples in Figure 47-6B are directly applicable to the clinical trials of imatinib in GIST and gefitinib and erlotinib in NSCLC. In the former, the majority of patients expressed an activating *KIT* mutation that is imatinib-sensitive. Accordingly, the overall response rate was quite

A

	Target frequency	Target response rate	Observed response rate
100 patients	90% →	80% →	72%
100 patients	50% →	80% →	40%
100 patients	25% →	80% →	20%
100 patients	10% →	80% →	8%

B

	Target Expression	Target Activation	Target response rate	Observed response rate
100 patients	100% →	90% →	80% →	72%
100 patients	100% →	50% →	80% →	40%
100 patients	100% →	25% →	80% →	20%
100 patients	100% →	10% →	80% →	8%

Figure 47-6 Responses in a clinical trial of a molecularly targeted agent. **A,** Response is determined by target expression. In this set of clinical trials, the response rate is 80% in patients whose tumors express the appropriate target. As the target frequency varies from 10 to 90%, the overall clinical response ranges from 8 to 72%. **B,** Response depends on expression and activation. In this example, the target is expressed in all patients, but is activated in 10 to 90% of patients. The response rate to the agent is again 80%, but only in patients with target expression and activation, thus, the overall clinical response ranges from 8 to 72%. In the absence of information concerning target frequency and/or activation, the results of the clinical trials cannot be meaningfully compared and interpreted.

high.[84] However, closer inspection of the data clearly showed that it was *KIT* mutational status that best correlated with response to imatinib. In contrast, the response rate to the EFGR kinase inhibitors was low, despite the fact that the majority of patients enrolled in the clinical trials of these agents expressed the EGFR. It is now known that patients with EGFR mutations have the best responses to gefitinib and erlotinib.[123,125] Thus, this represents an example where the target expression is high, but frequency of activation is low. However, this subgroup of patients has an extremely high response rate and demonstrates that in this subgroup of patients that their tumors are dependent on the activity of the mutated EGFR.

Although TKIs have been used successfully in the treatment of several cancers, the development of TKIs for many malignancies may be quite complex. Adequately designed clinical trials of TKIs need to assess for the presence and activation of a target before and during therapy. These trials may need to use end points other than objective response, particularly in advanced disease, where multiple redundant pathways mediate tumor growth and survival. However, by combining assessments of kinase inhibition with appropriately designed end points, it should be possible to determine whether a specific kinase contributes to the growth and survival of a particular cancer.

REFERENCES

1. Hanahan D, Weinberg RA. The hallmarks of cancer. Cell 2000;100:57–70.
2. Blume-Jensen P, Hunter T. Oncogenic kinase signalling. Nature 2001;411:355–65.
3. Lander ES, Linton LM, Birren B, et al. Initial sequencing and analysis of the human genome. Nature 2001;409:860–921.
4. Hubbard SR, Till JH. Protein tyrosine kinase structure and function. Annu Rev Biochem 2000;69:373–98.
5. Cohen P. Protein kinases—the major drug targets of the twenty-first century? Nat Rev Drug Discov 2002;1:309–15.
6. Sridhar R, Hanson-Painton O, Cooper DR. Protein kinases as therapeutic targets. Pharm Res 2000;17:1345–53.
7. Levitzki A, Gazit A. Tyrosine kinase inhibition: an approach to drug development. Science 1995;267:1782–8.
8. Yaish P, Gazit A, Gilon C, Levitzki A. Blocking of EGF-dependent cell proliferation by EGF receptor kinase inhibitors. Science 1988;242:933–5.
9. Baselga J, Albanell J. Mechanism of action of anti-HER2 monoclonal antibodies. Ann Oncol 2001;12 Suppl 1:35–41.
10. Baselga J. Phase I and II clinical trials of trastuzumab. Ann Oncol 2001;12(Suppl 1):49–55.
11. Smith IE. Efficacy and safety of Herceptin in women with metastatic breast cancer: results from pivotal clinical studies. Anticancer Drugs 2001;12(Suppl 4):3–10.
12. Goldberg RM. Cetuximab. Nat Rev Drug Discov 2005; Suppl:10–1.
13. Ferrara N, Hillan KJ, Gerber HP, Novotny W. Discovery and development of bevacizumab, an anti-VEGF antibody for treating cancer. Nat Rev Drug Discov 2004;3:391–400.
14. Fabbro D, Ruetz S, Buchdunger E, et al. Protein kinases as targets for anticancer agents: from inhibitors to useful drugs. Pharmacol Ther 2002;93:79–98.
15. Heinrich MC, Blanke CD, Druker BJ, Corless CL. Inhibition of KIT tyrosine kinase activity: A novel molecular approach to the treatment of KIT positive malignancies. J Clin Oncol 2002;20:1692–703.
16. Druker BJ, Sawyers CL, Kantarjian H, et al. Activity of a specific inhibitor of the Bcr-Abl tyrosine kinase in the blast crisis of chronic myeloid leukemia and acute lymphoblastic leukemia with the Philadelphia chromosome. N Engl J Med 2001;344:1038–42.
17. Druker BJ, Talpaz M, Resta D, et al. Efficacy and safety of a specific inhibitor of the Bcr-Abl tyrosine kinase in chronic myeloid leukemia. N Engl J Med 2001;344:1031–7.
18. Eisen T, Ahmad T, Gore ME, et al. Phase I trial of BAY 43-9006 (sorafenib) combined with dacarbazine (DTIC) in metastatic melanoma patients. J Clin Oncol, 2005 ASCO Annual Meeting Proceedings 2005;23(Suppl):712.
19. Flaherty KT, Brose M, Schuchter L, et al. Phase I/II trial of BAY 43-9006, carboplatin (C) and paclitaxel (P) demonstrates preliminary antitumor activity in the expansion cohort of patients with metastatic melanoma. J Clin Oncol, 2004 ASCO Annual Meeting Proceedings 2004;22(Suppl):711.
20. Druker BJ. Imatinib as a paradigm of targeted therapies. Adv Cancer Res 2004;91:1–30.
21. Nowell PC. Progress with chronic myelogenous leukemia: a personal perspective over four decades. Annu Rev Med 2002;53:1–13.
22. Rowley JD. A new consistent chromosomal abnormality in chronic myelogenous leukaemia identified by quinacrine fluorescence and Giemsa staining. Nature 1973;243:290–3.
23. de Klein A, van Kessel AG, Grosveld G, et al. A cellular oncogene is translocated to the Philadelphia chromosome in chronic myelocytic leukemia. Nature 1982;300:765–7.
24. Heisterkamp N, Stam K, Groffen J, et al. Structural organization of the bcr gene and its role in the Ph' translocation. Nature 1985;315:758–61.
25. Ben-Neriah Y, Daley GQ, Mes-Masson A-M, et al. The chronic myelogenous leukemia-specific P210 protein is the product of the bcr/abl hybrid gene. Science 1986;233:212–4.
26. Konopka JB, Watanabe SM, Witte ON. An alteration of the human c-abl protein in K562 leukemia cells unmasks associated tyrosine kinase activity. Cell 1984;37:1035–42.
27. Clark SS, McLaughlin J, Timmons M, et al. Expression of a distinctive BCR-ABL oncogene in Ph1-positive acute lymphocytic leukemia (ALL). Science 1988;239:775–7.
28. Deininger MW, Goldman JM, Melo JV. The molecular biology of chronic myeloid leukemia. Blood 2000;96:3343–56.
29. Shtivelman E, Lifshitz B, Gale RP, Canaani E. Fused transcript of abl and bcr genes in chronic myelogenous leukaemia. Nature 1985;315:550–4.
30. Daley GQ, Baltimore D. Transformation of an interleukin 3-dependent hematopoietic cell line by the chronic myelogenous leukemia-specific P210bcr/abl protein. Proc Natl Acad Sci U S A 1988;85:9312–6.
31. Gishizky ML, Witte ON. Initiation of deregulated growth of multipotent progenitor cells by bcr-abl in vitro. Science 1992;256:836–9.
32. Young JC, Witte ON. Selective transformation of primitive lymphoid cells by the BCR/ABL oncogene expressed in long-term lymphoid or myeloid cultures. Mol Cell Biol 1988;8:4079–87.
33. Daley GQ, Van Etten RA, Baltimore D. Induction of chronic myelogenous leukemia in mice by the P210bcr/abl gene of the Philadelphia chromosome. Science 1990;247:824–30.
34. Heisterkamp N, Jenster G, ten Hoeve J, et al. Acute leukaemia in bcr/abl transgenic mice. Nature 1990;344:251–3.
35. Huettner CS, Zhang P, Van Etten RA, Tenen DG. Reversibility of acute B-cell leukaemia induced by BCR-ABL1. Nat Genet 2000;24:57–60.
36. Kelliher MA, McLaughlin J, Witte ON, Rosenberg N. Induction of a chronic myelogenous leukemia-like syndrome in mice with v-abl and BCR/ABL. Proc Natl Acad Sci U S A 1990;87:6649–53.
37. Lugo TG, Pendergast AM, Muller AJ, Witte ON. Tyrosine kinase activity and transformation potency of bcr-abl oncogene products. Science 1990;247:1079–82.
38. Druker BJ, Tamura S, Buchdunger E, et al. Effects of a selective inhibitor of the ABL tyrosine kinase on the growth of BCR-ABL positive cells. Nature Med 1996;2:561–6.
39. Deininger M, Buchdunger E, Druker BJ. The development of imatinib as a therapeutic agent for chronic myeloid leukemia. Blood 2005;105:2640–53.
40. Peng B, Hayes M, Resta D, et al. Pharmacokinetics and pharmacodynamics of imatinib in a phase I trial with chronic myeloid leukemia patients. J Clin Oncol 2004;22:935–42.
41. Kantarjian H, Sawyers C, Hochhaus A, et al. Hematologic and cytogenetic responses to imatinib mesylate in chronic myelogenous leukemia. N Engl J Med 2002;346:645–52.
42. Ottmann OG, Druker BJ, Sawyers CL, et al. A phase 2 study of imatinib in patients with relapsed or refractory Philadelphia chromosome-positive acute lymphoid leukemias. Blood 2002;100:1965–71.
43. Sawyers CL, Hochhaus A, Feldman E, et al. Imatinib induces hematologic and cytogenetic responses in patients with chronic myeloid leukemia in myeloid blast crisis: results of a phase II study. Blood 2002;99:3530–9.
44. Talpaz M, Silver RT, Druker BJ, et al. Imatinib induces durable hematologic and cytogenetic responses in patients with accelerated phase chronic myeloid leukemia: results of a phase 2 study. Blood 2002;99:1928–37.
45. O'Brien SG, Guilhot F, Larson RA, et al. Imatinib compared with interferon and low-dose cytarabine for newly diagnosed chronic-phase chronic myeloid leukemia. N Engl J Med 2003;348:994–1004.
46. Guilhot F, on behalf of the IRIS (International Randomized IFN vs STI571 Study Group). Sustained durability of responses plus high rates of cytogenetic responses result in long-term benefit for newly diagnosed chronic-phase

chronic myeloid leukemia (CML-CP) treated with imatinib (IM) therapy: update from the IRIS study [abstract]. Blood 2004;104:10.

47. Hughes TP, Kaeda J, Branford S, et al. Frequency of major molecular responses to imatinib or interferon alfa plus cytarabine in newly diagnosed chronic myeloid leukemia. N Engl J Med 2003;349:1423–32.
48. Shah NP, Sawyers CL. Mechanisms of resistance to STI571 in Philadelphia chromosome-associated leukemias. Oncogene 2003;22:7389–95.
49. Gorre ME, Mohammed M, Ellwood K, et al. Clinical resistance to STI-571 cancer therapy caused by BCR-ABL gene mutation or amplification. Science 2001;293:876–80.
50. Oda T, Heaney C, Hagopian J, et al. CRKL is the major tyrosine phosphorylated protein in neutrophils from patients with chronic myelogenous leukemia. J Biol Chem 1994;269:22925–8.
51. Al-Ali HK, Heinrich MC, Lange T, et al. High incidence of BCR-ABL kinase domain mutations and absence of mutations of the PDGFR and KIT activation loops in CML patients with secondary resistance to imatinib. Hematol J 2004;5:55–60.
52. Branford S, Rudzki Z, Walsh S, et al. High frequency of point mutations clustered within the adenosine triphosphate-binding region of BCR/ABL in patients with chronic myeloid leukemia or Ph-positive acute lymphoblastic leukemia who develop imatinib (STI571) resistance. Blood 2002;99:3472–5.
53. Hochhaus A, Kreil S, Corbin AS, et al. Molecular and chromosomal mechanisms of resistance to imatinib (STI571) therapy. Leukemia 2002;16:2190–6.
54. Hofmann WK, Jones LC, Lemp NA, et al. Ph(+) acute lymphoblastic leukemia resistant to the tyrosine kinase inhibitor STI571 has a unique BCR-ABL gene mutation. Blood 2001;99:1860–2.
55. Roche-Lestienne C, Soenen-Cornu V, Grardel-Duflos N, et al. Several types of mutations of the Abl gene can be found in chronic myeloid leukemia patients resistant to STI571, and they can pre-exist to the onset of treatment. Blood 2002;100:1014–8.
56. Shah NP, Nicoll JM, Nagar B, et al. Multiple BCR-ABL kinase domain mutations confer polyclonal resistance to the tyrosine kinase inhibitor imatinib (STI571) in chronic phase and blast crisis chronic myeloid leukemia. Cancer Cell 2002;2:117–25.
57. von Bubnoff N, Schneller F, Peschel C, Duyster J. BCR-ABL gene mutations in relation to clinical resistance of Philadelphia-chromosome-positive leukaemia to STI571: a prospective study. Lancet 2002;359:487–91.
58. O'Hare T, Walters DK, Stoffregen EP, et al. In vitro activity of Bcr-Abl inhibitors AMN107 and BMS-354825 against clinically relevant imatinib-resistant Abl kinase domain mutants. Cancer Res 2005;65:4500–5.
59. Weisberg E, Manley PW, Breitenstein W, et al. Characterization of AMN107, a selective inhibitor of native and mutant Bcr-Abl. Cancer Cell 2005;7:129–41.
60. Dorsey JF, Jove R, Kraker AJ, Wu J. The pyrido[2,3-d]pyrimidine derivative PD180970 inhibits p210Bcr-Abl tyrosine kinase and induces apoptosis of K562 leukemic cells. Cancer Res 2000;60:3127–31.
61. La Rosee P, Corbin AS, Stoffregen EP, et al. Activity of the Bcr-Abl kinase inhibitor PD180970 against clinically relevant Bcr-Abl isoforms that cause resistance to imatinib mesylate (Gleevec, STI571). Cancer Res 2002;62:7149–53.
62. Shah NP, Tran C, Lee FY, et al. Overriding imatinib resistance with a novel ABL kinase inhibitor. Science 2004;305:399–401.
63. Giles F, Kantarjian H, Wassmann B, et al. A phase I/II study of AMN107, a novel aminopyrimidine inhibitor of Bcr-Abl, on a continuous daily dosing schedule in adult patients with imatinib-resistant advanced phase chronic myeloid leukemia (CML) or relapsed/refractory Philadelphia chromosome (Ph+) acute lymphocytic leukemia (ALL) [abstract]. Blood 2004;104:10.
64. Sawyers CL, Shah NP, Kan arjian HM, et al. Hematologic and cytogenetic respons in imatinib-resistant chronic phase chronic myeloid le kemia patients treated with the dual SRC/ABL kinase hibitor BMS-354825: results from a phase I dose esc ation study [abstract]. Blood 2004;104:4.
65. Andre C, Martin E, Cornu et al. Genomic organization of the human c-kit gene: e lution of the receptor tyrosine kinase subclass III. Onc ene 1992;7:685–91.
66. Buchdunger E, Cioffi Cl Law N, et al. Abl protein-tyrosine kinase inhibit STI571 inhibits in vitro signal transduction mediat by c-kit and platelet-derived growth factor receptors. J Pharmacol Exp Ther 2000;295:139–45.
67. Hanks SK, Quinn AM, Hunter T. The protein kinase family: conserved features and deduced phylogeny of the catalytic domains. Science 1988;241:42–52.
68. Russell ES. Hereditary anemias of the mouse: a review for geneticists. Adv Genet 1979;20:357–459.
69. Zsebo KM, Williams DA, Geissler EN, et al. Stem cell factor is encoded at the Sl locus of the mouse and is the ligand for the c-kit tyrosine kinase receptor. Cell 1990;63:213–24.
70. Rubin BP, Singer S, Tsao C, et al. KIT activation is a ubiquitous feature of gastrointestinal stromal tumors. Cancer Res 2001;61:8118–21.
71. Longley BJ, Reguera MJ, Ma Y. Classes of c-KIT activating mutations: proposed mechanisms of action and implications for disease classification and therapy. Leuk Res 2001;25:571–6.
72. Fletcher CD, Berman JJ, Corless C, et al. Diagnosis of gastrointestinal stromal tumors: A consensus approach. Hum Pathol 2002;33:459–65.
73. Heinrich MC, Rubin BP, Longley BJ, Fletcher JA. Biology and genetic aspects of gastrointestinal stromal tumors: KIT activation and cytogenetic alterations. Hum Pathol 2002;33:484–95.
74. Heinrich MC, Corless CL, Duensing A, et al. PDGFRA activating mutations in gastrointestinal stromal tumors. Science 2003;299:708–10.
75. Corless CL, McGreevey L, Haley A, et al. KIT mutations are common in incidental gastrointestinal stromal tumors one centimeter or less in size. Am J Pathol 2002;160:1567–72.
76. Blanke CD, Eisenberg BL, Heinrich MC. Gastrointestinal stromal tumors. Curr Treat Options Oncol 2001;2:485–91.
77. Ng EH, Pollock RE, Romsdahl MM. Prognostic implications of patterns of failure for gastrointestinal leiomyosarcomas. Cancer 1992;69:1334–41.
78. van Glabbeke M, Hogendoorn PC, Mouridsen H, et al. Progression free rate as the principal end-point for phase II trial on soft tissue sarcoma: What should be the target? A retrospective study of the EORTC Soft Tissue and Bone Sarcoma (STBSG) database [abstract]. Proc Am Soc Clin Oncol 2001;20:354.
79. DeMatteo RP, Heinrich MC, El-Rifai WM, Demetri G. Clinical management of gastrointestinal stromal tumors: before and after STI-571. Hum Pathol 2002;33:466–77.
80. Heinrich MC, Griffith DJ, Druker BJ, et al. Inhibition of c-kit receptor tyrosine kinase activity by STI 571, a selective tyrosine kinase inhibitor. Blood 2000;96:925–32.
81. Tuveson DA, Willis NA, Jacks T, et al. STI571 inactivation of the gastrointestinal stromal tumor c-KIT oncoprotein: biological and clinical implications. Oncogene 2001;20:5054–8.
82. Joensuu H, Roberts PJ, Sarlomo-Rikala M, et al. Effect of the tyrosine kinase inhibitor STI571 in a patient with a metastatic gastrointestinal stromal tumor. N Engl J Med 2001;344:1052–6.
83. Rankin C, von Mehren M, Blanke C, et al. Dose effect of imatinib (IM) in patients (pts) with metastatic GIST - Phase III Sarcoma Group Study S0033. J Clin Oncol, 2004 ASCO Annual Meeting Proceedings 2004;22(Suppl):819.
84. Heinrich MC, Corless CL, Demetri GD, et al. Kinase mutations and imatinib response in patients with metastatic gastrointestinal stromal tumor. J Clin Oncol 2003;21:4342–9.
85. Hirota S, Isozaki K, Moriyama Y, et al. Gain-of-function mutations of c-kit in human gastrointestinal stromal tumors. Science 1998;279:577–80.
86. Corless CL, Schroeder A, Griffith D, et al. PDGFRA mutations in gastrointestinal stromal tumors: frequency, spectrum and in vitro sensitivity to imatinib. J Clin Oncol 2005.
87. Verweij J, Casali PG, Zalcberg J, et al. Progression-free survival in gastrointestinal stromal tumours with high-dose imatinib: randomised trial. Lancet 2004;364:1127–34.
88. Le Cesne A, Perol D, Ray-Coquard I, et al. Interruption of imatinib (IM) in GIST patients with advanced disease: Updated results of the prospective French Sarcoma Group randomized phase III trial on survival and quality of life. J Clin Oncol, 2005 ASCO Annual Meeting Proceedings 2005;23(Suppl):823.
89. Van Den Abbeele AD, Badawi RD, Manola J, et al. Effects of cessation of imatinib mesylate (IM) therapy in patients (pts) with IM-refractory gastrointestinal stromal tumors (GIST) as visualized by FDG-PET scanning. J Clin Oncol, 2004 ASCO Annual Meeting Proceedings 2004;22(Suppl):198.
90. Blay JY, Bonvalot S, Casali P, et al. Consensus meeting for the management of gastrointestinal stromal tumors. Report of the GIST Consensus Conference of 20–21 March 2004, under the auspices of ESMO. Ann Oncol 2005;16:566–78.
91. Antonescu CR, Besmer P, Guo T, et al. Acquired resistance to imatinib in gastrointestinal stromal tumor occurs through secondary gene mutation. Clin Cancer Res 2005;11:4182–90.
92. Debiec-Rychter M, Cools J, Dumez H, et al. Mechanisms of resistance to imatinib mesylate in gastrointestinal stromal tumors and activity of the PKC412 inhibitor against imatinib-resistant mutants. Gastroenterology 2005;128:270–9.
93. Chen LL, Trent JC, Wu EF, et al. A missense mutation in KIT kinase domain 1 correlates with imatinib resistance in gastrointestinal stromal tumors. Cancer Res 2004;64:5913–9.
94. Fletcher JA, Corless CL, Dimitrijevic S, et al. Mechanisms of resistance to imatinib mesylate (IM) in advanced gastrointestinal stromal tumor (GIST) [abstract]. Proc Am Soc Clin Oncol 2003;22:815.
95. Sun L, Liang C, Shirazian S, et al. Discovery of 5-[5-fluoro-2-oxo-1,2- dihydroindol-(3Z)-ylidenemethyl]-2,4- dimethyl-1H-pyrrole-3-carboxylic acid (2-diethylaminoethyl)amide, a novel tyrosine kinase inhibitor targeting vascular endothelial and platelet-derived growth factor receptor tyrosine kinase. J Med Chem 2003;46:1116–9.
96. Mendel DB, Laird AD, Xin X, et al. In vivo antitumor activity of SU11248, a novel tyrosine kinase inhibitor targeting vascular endothelial growth factor and platelet-derived growth factor receptors: determination of a pharmacokinetic/pharmacodynamic relationship. Clin Cancer Res 2003;9:327–37.
97. Maki RG, Fletcher JA, Heinrich MC, et al. Results from a continuation trial of SU11248 in patients with imatinib (IM)-resistant gastrointestinal stromal tumor (GIST). J Clin Oncol, 2005 ASCO Annual Meeting Proceedings 2005;23(Suppl):818.
98. Demetri GD, Van Oosterom AT, Blackstein M, et al. Phase 3, multicenter, randomized, double-blind, placebo-controlled trial of SU11248 in patients (pts) following failure of imatinib for metastatic GIST. J Clin Oncol, 2005 ASCO Annual Meeting Proceedings 2005;23(Suppl):308.
99. Hotte SJ, Winquist EW, Lamont E, et al. Imatinib mesylate in patients with adenoid cystic cancers of the salivary glands expressing c-kit: a Princess Margaret Hospital phase II consortium study. J Clin Oncol 2005;23:585–90.
100. Johnson BE, Fischer T, Fischer B, et al. Phase II study of imatinib in patients with small cell lung cancer. Clin Cancer Res 2003;9:5880–7.
101. Krug LM, Crapanzano JP, Azzoli CG, et al. Imatinib mesylate lacks activity in small cell lung carcinoma expressing c-kit protein: a phase II clinical trial. Cancer 2005;103:2128–31.
102. Modi S, Seidman AD, Dickler M, et al. A phase II trial of imatinib mesylate monotherapy in patients with metastatic breast cancer. Breast Cancer Res Treat 2005;90:157–63.
103. Rao K, Goodin S, Levitt MJ, et al. A phase II trial of imatinib mesylate in patients with prostate specific antigen progression after local therapy for prostate cancer. Prostate 2005;62:115–22.
104. Tiffany NM, Wersinger EM, Garzotto M, Beer TM. Imatinib mesylate and zoledronic acid in androgen-independent prostate cancer. Urology 2004;63:934–9.
105. van Oosterom AT, Judson IR, Verweij J, et al. Update of phase I study of imatinib (STI571) in advanced soft tissue sarcomas and gastrointestinal stromal tumors: a report of the EORTC Soft Tissue and Bone Sarcoma Group. Eur J Cancer 2002;38(Suppl 5):83–7.
106. Verweij J, van Oosterom A, Blay JY, et al. Imatinib mesylate (STI-571 Glivec, Gleevec) is an active agent for gastrointestinal stromal tumours, but does not yield responses in other soft-tissue sarcomas that are unselected for a molecular target. Results from an EORTC Soft Tissue and Bone Sarcoma Group phase II study. Eur J Cancer 2003;39:2006–11.
107. Apperley JF, Gardembas M, Melo JV, et al. Response to imatinib mesylate in patients with chronic myeloproliferative diseases with rearrangements of the platelet-derived growth factor receptor beta. N Engl J Med 2002;347:481–7.
108. Magnusson MK, Meade KE, Nakamura R, et al. Activity of STI571 in chronic myelomonocytic leukemia with a platelet-derived growth factor beta receptor fusion oncogene. Blood 2002;100:1088–91.
109. Simon MP, Pedeutour F, Sirvent N, et al. Deregulation of the platelet-derived growth factor B-chain gene via fusion with collagen gene COL1A1 in dermatofibrosarcoma protuberans and giant-cell fibroblastoma. Nat Genet 1997;15:95–8.
110. McArthur GA, Demetri GD, van Oosterom A, et al. Molecular and clinical analysis of locally advanced dermatofibrosarcoma protuberans treated with imatinib: Imatinib Target Exploration Consortium Study B2225. J Clin Oncol 2005;23:866–73.

111. Maki RG, Awan RA, Dixon RH, et al. Differential sensitivity to imatinib of 2 patients with metastatic sarcoma arising from dermatofibrosarcoma protuberans. Int J Cancer 2002;100:623–6.
112. Rubin BP, Schuetze SM, Eary JF, et al. Molecular targeting of platelet-derived growth factor B by imatinib mesylate in a patient with metastatic dermatofibrosarcoma protuberans. J Clin Oncol 2002;20:3586–91.
113. Gotlib J, Cools J, Malone JM, 3rd, et al. The FIP1L1-PDGFRalpha fusion tyrosine kinase in hypereosinophilic syndrome and chronic eosinophilic leukemia: implications for diagnosis, classification, and management. Blood 2004;103:2879–91.
114. Griffin JH, Leung J, Bruner RJ, et al. Discovery of a fusion kinase in EOL-1 cells and idiopathic hypereosinophilic syndrome. Proc Natl Acad Sci U S A 2003;100:7830–5.
115. Cools J, Stover EH, Boulton CL, et al. PKC412 overcomes resistance to imatinib in a murine model of FIP1L1-PDGFRalpha-induced myeloproliferative disease. Cancer Cell 2003;3:459–69.
116. Gleich GJ, Leiferman KM, Pardanani A, et al. Treatment of hypereosinophilic syndrome with imatinib mesilate. Lancet 2002;359:1577–8.
117. Ma Y, Zeng S, Metcalfe DD, et al. The c-KIT mutation causing human mastocytosis is resistant to STI571 and other KIT kinase inhibitors; kinases with enzymatic site mutations show different inhibitor sensitivity profiles than wild-type kinases and those with regulatory-type mutations. Blood 2002;99:1741–4.
118. Mendelsohn J, Baselga J. Status of epidermal growth factor receptor antagonists in the biology and treatment of cancer. J Clin Oncol 2003;21:2787–99.
119. Salomon DS, Brandt R, Ciardiello F, Normanno N. Epidermal growth factor-related peptides and their receptors in human malignancies. Crit Rev Oncol Hematol 1995;19:183–232.
120. Sato JD, Kawamoto T, Le AD, et al. Biological effects in vitro of monoclonal antibodies to human epidermal growth factor receptors. Mol Biol Med 1983;1:511–29.
121. Nicholson RI, Gee JM, Harper ME. EGFR and cancer prognosis. Eur J Cancer 2001;37(Suppl 4):9–15.
122. Nishikawa R, Ji XD, Harmon RC, et al. A mutant epidermal growth factor receptor common in human glioma confers enhanced tumorigenicity. Proc Natl Acad Sci U S A 1994;91:7727–31.
123. Lynch TJ, Bell DW, Sordella R, et al. Activating mutations in the epidermal growth factor receptor underlying responsiveness of non-small-cell lung cancer to gefitinib. N Engl J Med 2004;350:2129–39.
124. Nagahara H, Mimori K, Ohta M, et al. Somatic mutations of epidermal growth factor receptor in colorectal carcinoma. Clin Cancer Res 2005;11:1368–71.
125. Paez JG, Janne PA, Lee JC, et al. EGFR mutations in lung cancer: correlation with clinical response to gefitinib therapy. Science 2004;304:1497–500.
126. Shepherd FA, Pereira J, Ciuleanu TE, et al. A randomized placebo-controlled trial of erlotinib in patients with advanced non-small cell lung cancer (NSCLC) following failure of 1st line or 2nd line chemotherapy. A National Cancer Institute of Canada Clinical Trials Group (NCIC CTG) trial. J Clin Oncol, 2004 ASCO Annual Meeting Proceedings 2004;22(Suppl):622.
127. Kris MG, Natale RB, Herbst RS, et al. Efficacy of gefitinib, an inhibitor of the epidermal growth factor receptor tyrosine kinase, in symptomatic patients with non-small cell lung cancer: a randomized trial. JAMA 2003;290:2149–58.
128. Miller VA, Kris MG, Shah N, et al. Bronchioloalveolar pathologic subtype and smoking history predict sensitivity to gefitinib in advanced non-small-cell lung cancer. J Clin Oncol 2004;22:1103–9.
129. Parra HS, Cavina R, Latteri F, et al. Analysis of epidermal growth factor receptor expression as a predictive factor for response to gefitinib ('Iressa', ZD1839) in non-small-cell lung cancer. Br J Cancer 2004;91:208–12.
130. Pao W, Miller V, Zakowski M, et al. EGF receptor gene mutations are common in lung cancers from "never smokers" and are associated with sensitivity of tumors to gefitinib and erlotinib. Proc Natl Acad Sci U S A 2004;101:13306–11.
131. Huang SF, Liu HP, Li LH, et al. High frequency of epidermal growth factor receptor mutations with complex patterns in non-small cell lung cancers related to gefitinib responsiveness in Taiwan. Clin Cancer Res 2004;10:8195–203.
132. Kosaka T, Yatabe Y, Endoh H, et al. Mutations of the epidermal growth factor receptor gene in lung cancer: biological and clinical implications. Cancer Res 2004;64:8919–23.
133. Marchetti A, Martella C, Felicioni L, et al. EGFR mutations in non-small-cell lung cancer: analysis of a large series of cases and development of a rapid and sensitive method for diagnostic screening with potential implications on pharmacologic treatment. J Clin Oncol 2005;23:857–65.
134. Shigematsu H, Lin L, Takahashi T, et al. Clinical and biological features associated with epidermal growth factor receptor gene mutations in lung cancers. J Natl Cancer Inst 2005;97:339–46.
135. Tokumo M, Toyooka S, Kiura K, et al. The relationship between epidermal growth factor receptor mutations and clinicopathologic features in non-small cell lung cancers. Clin Cancer Res 2005;11:1167–73.
136. Mitsudomi T, Kosaka T, Endoh H, et al. Mutations of the epidermal growth factor receptor gene predict prolonged survival after gefitinib treatment in patients with non-small-cell lung cancer with postoperative recurrence. J Clin Oncol 2005;23:2513–20.
137. Han SW, Kim TY, Hwang PG, et al. Predictive and prognostic impact of epidermal growth factor receptor mutation in non-small-cell lung cancer patients treated with gefitinib. J Clin Oncol 2005;23:2493–501.
138. Kobayashi S, Boggon TJ, Dayaram T, et al. EGFR mutation and resistance of non-small-cell lung cancer to gefitinib. N Engl J Med 2005;352:786–92.
139. Pao W, Miller VA, Politi KA, et al. Acquired resistance of lung adenocarcinomas to gefitinib or erlotinib is associated with a second mutation in the EGFR kinase domain. PLoS Med 2005;2:e73.
140. Pao W, Wang TY, Riely GJ, et al. KRAS mutations and primary resistance of lung adenocarcinomas to gefitinib or erlotinib. PLoS Med 2005;2:e17.
141. Arora A, Scholar EM. Role of tyrosine kinase inhibitors in cancer therapy. J Pharmacol Exp Ther 2005.
142. Fiedler W, Serve H, Dohner H, et al. A phase 1 study of SU11248 in the treatment of patients with refractory or resistant acute myeloid leukemia (AML) or not amenable to conventional therapy for the disease. Blood 2005;105:986–93.
143. Stone RM, DeAngelo DJ, Klimek V, et al. Patients with acute myeloid leukemia and an activating mutation in FLT3 respond to a small-molecule FLT3 tyrosine kinase inhibitor, PKC412. Blood 2005;105:54–60.
144. Sattler M, Scheijen B, Weisberg E, Griffin JD. Mutated tyrosine kinases as therapeutic targets in myeloid leukemias. Adv Exp Med Biol 2003;532:121–40.
145. Ahmed SI, Thomas AL, Steward WP. Vascular endothelial growth factor (VEGF) inhibition by small molecules. J Chemother 2004;16(Suppl 4):59–63.
146. Davies H, Bignell GR, Cox C, et al. Mutations of the BRAF gene in human cancer. Nature 2002;417:949–54.
147. Garnett MJ, Marais R. Guilty as charged: B-RAF is a human oncogene. Cancer Cell 2004;6:313–9.
148. Sebolt-Leopold JS, Herrera R. Targeting the mitogen-activated protein kinase cascade to treat cancer. Nat Rev Cancer 2004;4:937–47.
149. Sansal I, Sellers WR. The biology and clinical relevance of the PTEN tumor suppressor pathway. J Clin Oncol 2004;22:2954–63.
150. Klein S, McCormick F, Levitzki A. Opinion: Killing time for cancer cells. Nat Rev Cancer 2005.
151. Senderowicz AM. Targeting cell cycle and apoptosis for the treatment of human malignancies. Curr Opin Cell Biol 2004;16:670–8.
152. Philp AJ, Campbell IG, Leet C, et al. The phosphatidylinositol 3'-kinase p85alpha gene is an oncogene in human ovarian and colon tumors. Cancer Res 2001;61:7426–9.
153. Samuels Y, Wang Z, Bardelli A, et al. High frequency of mutations of the PIK3CA gene in human cancers. Science 2004;304:554.
154. Campbell IG, Russell SE, Choong DY, et al. Mutation of the PIK3CA gene in ovarian and breast cancer. Cancer Res 2004;64:7678–81.
155. Luo J, Manning BD, Cantley LC. Targeting the PI3K-Akt pathway in human cancer: rationale and promise. Cancer Cell 2003;4:257–62.
156. Fruttiger M, Karlsson L, Hall AC, et al. Defective oligodendrocyte development and severe hypomyelination in PDGF-A knockout mice. Development 1999;126:457–67.
157. Betsholtz C, Karlsson L, Lindahl P. Developmental roles of platelet-derived growth factors. Bioessays 2001;23:494–507.
158. Hellstrom M, Kalen M, Lindahl P, et al. Role of PDGF-B and PDGFR-beta in recruitment of vascular smooth muscle cells and pericytes during embryonic blood vessel formation in the mouse. Development 1999;126:3047–55.
159. Threadgill DW, Dlugosz AA, Hansen LA, et al. Targeted disruption of mouse EGF receptor: effect of genetic background on mutant phenotype. Science 1995;269:230–4.
160. Mendelsohn J, Baselga J. The EGF receptor family as targets for cancer therapy. Oncogene 2000;19:6550–65.
161. Demetri GD, von Mehren M, Blanke CD, et al. Efficacy and safety of imatinib mesylate in advanced gastrointestinal stromal tumors. N Engl J Med 2002;347:472–80.
162. Giaccone G. Epidermal growth factor receptor inhibitors in the treatment of non-small-cell lung cancer. J Clin Oncol 2005;23:3235–42.
163. Shah NT, Kris MG, Pao W, et al. Practical management of patients with non-small-cell lung cancer treated with gefitinib. J Clin Oncol 2005;23:165–74.
164. Druker BJ, Lydon NB. Lessons learned from the development of an abl tyrosine kinase inhibitor for chronic myelogenous leukemia. J Clin Invest 2000;105:3–7.
165. Albanell J, Rojo F, Averbuch S, et al. Pharmacodynamic studies of the epidermal growth factor receptor inhibitor ZD1839 in skin from cancer patients: histopathologic and molecular consequences of receptor inhibition. J Clin Oncol 2002;20:110–24.
166. Albanell J, Codony-Servat J, Rojo F, et al. Activated extracellular signal-regulated kinases: association with epidermal growth factor receptor/transforming growth factor alpha expression in head and neck squamous carcinoma and inhibition by anti-epidermal growth factor receptor treatments. Cancer Res 2001;61:6500–10.
167. Van den Abbeele AD, Badawi RD. Use of positron emission tomography in oncology and its potential role to assess response to imatinib mesylate therapy in gastrointestinal stromal tumors (GISTs). Eur J Cancer 2002;38(Suppl 5):60–5.
168. Mross K, Drevs J, Muller M, et al. Phase I clinical and pharmacokinetic study of PTK/ZK, a multiple VEGF receptor inhibitor, in patients with liver metastases from solid tumours. Eur J Cancer 2005;41:1291–9.
169. Morgan B, Thomas AL, Drevs J, et al. Dynamic contrast-enhanced magnetic resonance imaging as a biomarker for the pharmacological response of PTK787/ZK 222584, an inhibitor of the vascular endothelial growth factor receptor tyrosine kinases, in patients with advanced colorectal cancer and liver metastases: results from two phase I studies. J Clin Oncol 2003;21:3955–64.
170. van Oosterom AT, Judson I, Verweij J, et al. Safety and efficacy of imatinib (STI571) in metastatic gastrointestinal stromal tumours: a phase I study. Lancet 2001;358:1421–3.
171. von Mehren M, Blanke CD, Joensuu H, et al. High incidence of durable responses induced by imatinib mesylate (Gleevec) in patients with unresectable and metastatic gastrointestinal stromal tumors (GISTs) [abstract]. Proc Am Soc Clin Oncol 2002;21:403.
172. Barthe C, Gharbi MJ, Lagarde V, et al. Mutation in the ATP-binding site of BCR-ABL in a patient with chronic myeloid leukaemia with increasing resistance to STI571. Br J Haematol 2002;119:109–11.
173. Branford S, Rudzki Z, Walsh S, et al. Detection of BCR-ABL mutations in patients with CML treated with imatinib is virtually always accompanied by clinical resistance, and mutations in the ATP phosphate-binding loop (P-loop) are associated with a poor prognosis. Blood 2003;102:276–83.
174. Fukuoka M, Yano S, Giaccone G, et al. Multi-institutional randomized phase II trial of gefitinib for previously treated patients with advanced non-small-cell lung cancer (The IDEAL 1 Trial). J Clin Oncol 2003;21:2237–46.
175. Perez-Soler R, Chachoua A, Hammond LA, et al. Determinants of tumor response and survival with erlotinib in patients with non--small-cell lung cancer. J Clin Oncol 2004;22:3238–47.
176. Giaccone G, Herbst RS, Manegold C, et al. Gefitinib in combination with gemcitabine and cisplatin in advanced non-small-cell lung cancer: a phase III trial--INTACT 1. J Clin Oncol 2004;22:777–84.
177. Herbst RS, Giaccone G, Schiller JH, et al. Gefitinib in combination with paclitaxel and carboplatin in advanced non-small-cell lung cancer: a phase III trial--INTACT 2. J Clin Oncol 2004;22:785–94.
178. Gatzemeier U, Pluzanska A, Szczesna, et al. Results of a phase III trial of erlotinib (OSI-774) combined with cisplatin and gemcitabine (GC) chemotherapy in advanced non-small cell lung cancer (NSCLC). J Clin Oncol 2004;22:619s.
179. Herbst RS, Prager D, Hermann R, et al. TRIBUTE - A phase III trial of erlotinib HCl (OSI-774) combined with carboplatin and paclitaxel (CP) chemotherapy in advanced non-small cell lung cancer (NSCLC). J Clin Oncol 2004;22:619s.

Section 13

BIOTHERAPEUTICS

48

Interferons

Ernest C. Borden, MD

Interferons (IFNs) were the first biologic and protein therapeutic agent to achieve regulatory approval for prolongation of survival of cancer patients. IFNs are now licensed worldwide not only as therapeutic agents for cancer but also as antiviral agents and for multiple sclerosis. IFNs have been a prototype for dissecting the biologic and clinical effects of cytokines. IFNs are a family of molecules that include more than 15 expressed genes and a number of pseudogenes coded on human chromosome 9 (except IFN-γ on chromosome 12). Cellular action follows binding to a relatively small (< 2,000/cell) number of high-affinity receptors. Signal-transducing nuclear regulatory proteins then modulate gene expression, resulting in production of induced proteins. These proteins, induced by IFNs, underlie the pleiotropic biologic effects: virus inhibition, immunomodulation, slowing of cell proliferation, apoptosis, angiogenesis inhibition, and alterations in differentiation. However, which induced cellular proteins result in the various biologic and therapeutic effects remain undefined, as do the specific cellular mechanism(s) of antitumor action. In more than a dozen cancers, IFNs result in regression or control of the disease process (Table 48-1). The spectrum of single-agent activity of IFNs compares favorably with other systemic antitumor modalities. As a human protein that regulates gene transcription, IFNs are a unique form of cancer therapy.

MOLECULES: THEIR INDUCTION, RECEPTORS, AND GENE REGULATION

IFNs are a family of proteins, each encoded at a specific genetic locus. Three major classes of IFNs (α, β, and γ) were defined initially on the basis of chemical, antigenic, and biologic differences. These families have now been confirmed to result from significant differences in primary amino acid sequence. With advances in molecular biology, sequencing technology, and genome mapping, complete sequences for 20 expressed human IFN proteins have been defined.[1,2] Both IFN-α and IFN-β are 166 amino acids in length, with an additional 20–amino acid secretory peptide present on the aminoterminal end. Comparison of the sequences of IFN-α and IFN-β has defined approximately 45% homology of nucleotides and 29% homology of amino acids. Each of the nonallelic human IFN-α genes differs by approximately 10% in nucleotide sequence and 15 to 25% in amino acid sequence (Table 48-2). IFN-γ, 143 amino acids in length, is located on chromosome 12 and also contains a 20–amino acid secretory peptide. IFN-γ has only minimal sequence homology with IFN-α or IFN-β (see Table 48-2). Three other human IFN classes, ω, ε, and κ, have subsequently been defined,[2–4] the latter as a result of a genome search. Although IFN-β and IFN-γ, produced by eukaryotic cells, are glycosylated, biologic differences from the unglycosylated IFN-α2 produced in *Escherichia coli* have not yet been identified. All IFNs have the defining biologic effect of induction of intracellular resistance to replication of both ribonucleic acid (RNA) and deoxyribonucleic acid (DNA) viruses.

INTERFERON INDUCTION

Conceptually, it is important to distinguish IFN production and action (Figure 48-1). Viruses remain the prototypical inducers of expression of IFNs. Although all body cells probably have the capacity to produce IFN-α and IFN-β, the primary cells of origin are dendritic cells. IFN-γ was identified after exposure of lymphocytes to mitogens or sensitized lymphocytes to specific antigens. Interleukin (IL)-2, tumor necrosis factors (TNFs), IL-12, IL-15, and a 15 kDa protein induced by IFN-α and IFN-β are also potent inducers of IFN-γ, under some circumstances resulting in substantial titers.[5–7] Production of IFNs is part of host defense mechanisms for resistance to neoplasia; experimental suppression of IFN in mice results in increased lethality from tumors.[8]

The first chemically defined inducers of IFNs were double-stranded polyribonucleotides, which are potent IFN inducers and immunomodulators in mice but not in humans. Low-molecularweight inducers of IFNs have been identified in different animal species, and several low-molecular-weight inducers have been introduced into clinical trials.[9–12] Orally active inducers, such as the acridines, halopyrimidinones, or substituted quinolones, would be convenient and useful not only for therapeutic purposes but also as chemopreventive agents.[13] Halopyrimidinones are clinically effective for low-grade transitional carcinomas of the bladder.[12] Almost all inducers activate Toll-like receptor (TLR) signaling pathways; TLRs on plasmacytoid dendritic cells are probably the primary regulator for most systemic IFN production.

Table 48-1 Interferons: Current Status
Regulation of gene transcription
Biologic response modulatory effects defined in humans
Phase II antitumor activity confirmed in more than 12 human cancers
Phase III trials demonstrate improved quality and quantity of life, cancer, virus diseases, multiple sclerosis

RECEPTORS

The cellular response to IFNs requires the interaction of only a small number of molecules with high-affinity, species-specific dimeric cell surface receptors. The gene for the receptor for human IFN-α and IFN-β is on chromosome 21, whereas a gene on chromosome 6 codes for the human

Table 48-2 Family of Interferon Molecules

Family	Chr (Hu)	Types, *n*	*n*	Amino Acid Homology, %*
Alpha†	9	13	165–166	75–85
Beta	9	1	166	30
Gamma	12	1	143	1
Omega	9	> 1	173	50
Kappa	9	1	207	30
Lambda	19	3	175	15–20
Epsilon	9	1	187	< 10

Chr (Hu) = human chromosome on which the gene is found.

*Compared with interferon (IFN)-α.

†The IFN licensed for clinical use is IFN-α2a (Hoffmann-LaRoche, Nutley NJ), and it differs from IFN-α2b (Schering-Plough, Kenilworth, NJ) by a single amino acid 23 (lysine in IFN-α2a; arginine in IFN-α2b). IFN-α2 is 165 amino acids with a deletion at amino acid 44 of an aspartate residue.

IFN-γ receptor. IFN receptors confer almost absolute species restrictions. IFN-α and IFN-β share and compete for the same receptor, although IFN-β binds with higher affinity and forms a more stable complex.[14,15] Although down-regulation of receptors occurs with IFN-α2 administration, neither this event nor receptor number has clearly correlated with therapeutic effects in hematologic malignancies.[16,17]

Studies on binding and cross-linking of radiolabeled IFNs to the cell surface have identified the existence of a dimeric structure for the receptor for IFN-α and IFN-β. To elicit a cellular response, IFN-α and IFN-β require two subunits, IFNAR (IFN-alpha receptor)-1 and IFNAR-2. Human IFNAR-1 is a glycoprotein of 557 amino acids.[18] A 515–amino acid form of human IFNAR-2 has been identified as the universal ligand binding subunit of the IFN-α and IFN-β receptors. The known structure of other members of the human cytokine receptor II family has enabled the three-dimensional structure of the extracellular domains of IFNAR-1 and IFNAR-2 to be modeled. IFN-β shares only 30% identity with the IFN-α subtypes and appears to engage the receptor heterodimer differently. This can result in the greater activation by IFN-β of subsets of genes,[19–23] possibly through serine phosphorylation of signal transducer and activator of transcription (STAT)-1 and/or activation of other transcription factors.[21]

SIGNAL TRANSDUCTION

After receptor binding, specific tyrosine kinases, tyk2 (not part of the receptor), together with one or more additional tyrosine kinases, Janus-activated kinase (JAK)-1 and JAK-2, are phosphorylated. These activated tyrosine kinases activate the signal-transducing peptides[24] (Figure 48-2) and induce the formation of a complex of protein subunits (interferon-stimulated gene factor [ISGF]-3α) consisting of STAT-1α or STAT-1β and STAT-2. The proteins STAT-1α and STAT-1β are alternatively spliced products of the same gene. The

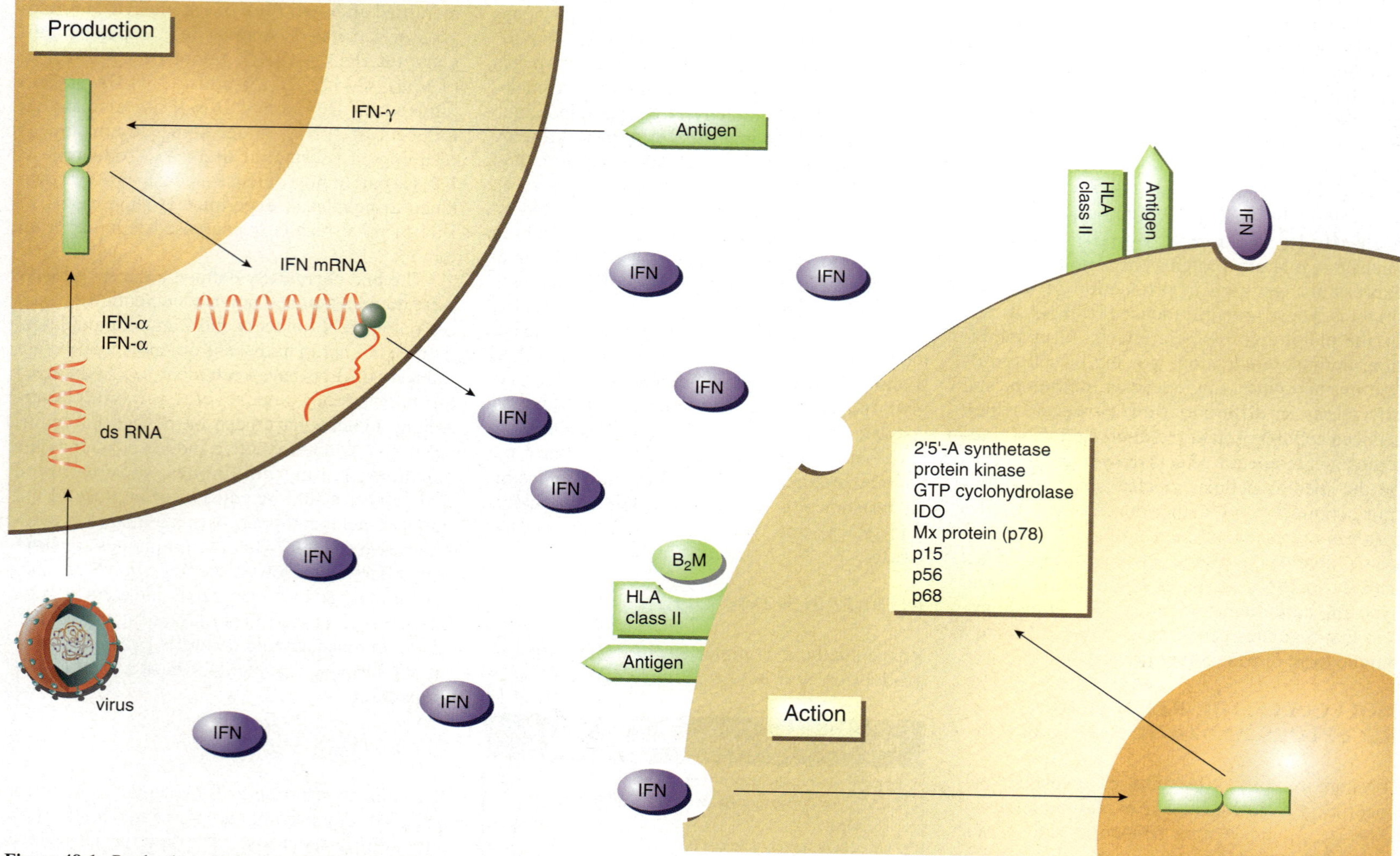

Figure 48-1 Production of interferon (IFN)-α or IFN-β is stimulated by viruses through a final common pathway of double-stranded ribonucleic acid or, in the case of IFN-γ, exposure to specific antigens. The action of IFNs is mediated via binding to a specific receptor on the cell surface with induction of cell surface proteins (human leukocyte antigen [HLA] classes I and II, β2-microglobulin, tumor-associated antigens) and intracellular proteins (2'5'-synthetase, protein kinase R, guanosine triphosphate [GTP] cyclohydrolase, indoleamine dioxygenase, interferon-stimulate gene 15 [ISG15], promyelocytic leukemia [PML], and others).

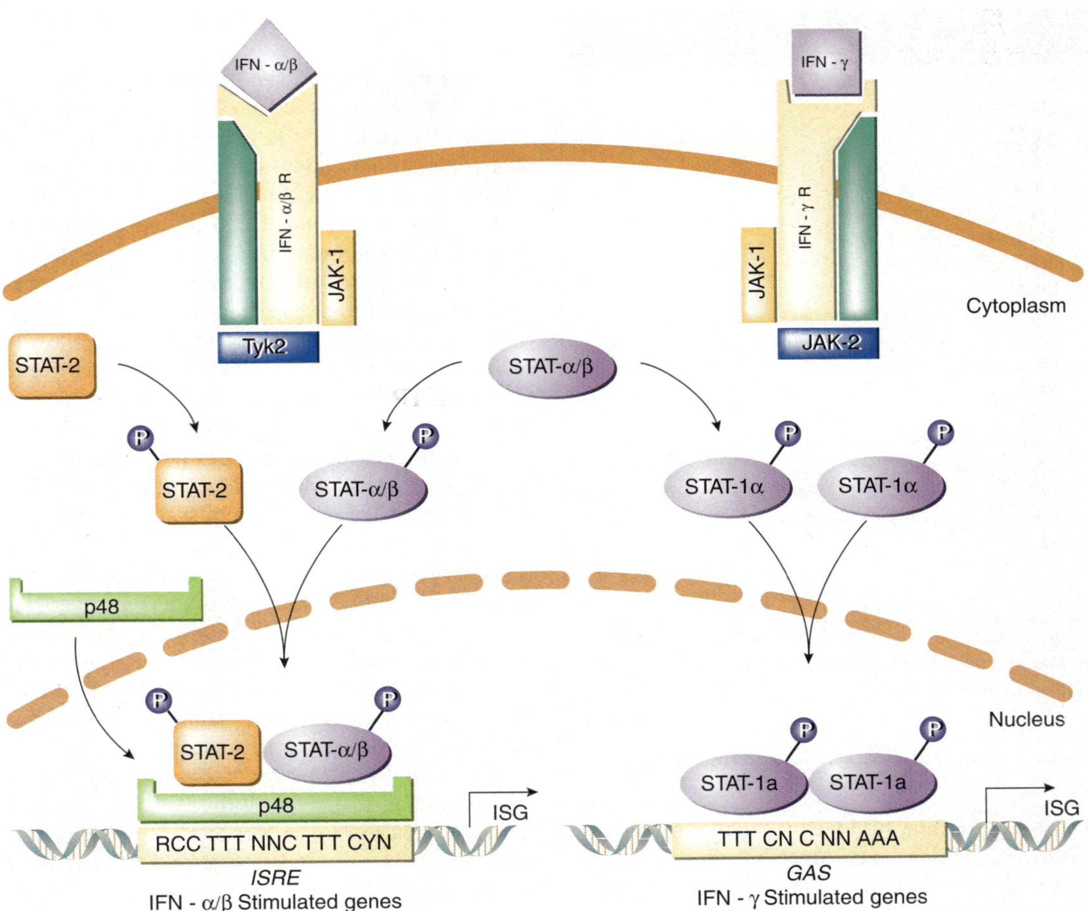

Figure 48-2 Pathway of signal transduction by interferons (IFNs). After binding to specific receptors, tyrosine kinases (JAK-1, JAK-2, Tyk2) are activated. These tyrosine kinases phosphorylate inactive transcription factors (STAT-1a, STAT-1p, STAT-2), which form a transcriptional factor, interferon-stimulated gene factor (ISGF)-3 or STAT-1α dimer. The interferon-stimulated response element (ISRE) or gamma activation site (GAS) has shared nucleotides for all IFN-stimulated genes. N = nucleotide; Y = pyrimidine.

STAT-1α protein contains 39 additional amino acids at its carboxyl end. The phosphorylated ISGF-3α complex is translocated to the nucleus and forms (with the addition of a fourth subunit, p48 or interferon-regulatory factor [IRF]-9) a DNA-binding complex specific for the IFN-stimulated response element. IFN-γ receptor activation results in a similar sequence of events, although the transcriptional regulatory complex consists of a homodimer of STAT-1 that binds to DNA elements termed gamma activation sites. Other signaling cascades are also activated by IFNs, including activation of phosphatidylinositol 3-kinase and the mitogen-activated protein (MAP) kinase cascades.[21,25,26]

Inhibitory for action of IFNs at the receptor level is a family of suppressor of cytokine signaling (SOCS) proteins.[27,28] SOCS proteins may be effectors of a negative feedback mechanism that shuts down response following IFN stimulation. Also inhibitory are two phosphatases, SHP-1 and SHP-2, that influence receptor-activated tyrosine kinase signaling. Because both of these phosphatases are negative regulators of signaling by IFNs and other cytokines, inhibitors have been evaluated and proven effective in augmenting antitumor activities.[29,30]

INDUCED GENES AND ANTITUMOR ACTIONS

IFNs are pleiotropic cellular modulators (Table 48-3). Antitumor effects result from either a direct effect on viability and proliferation or antigenic composition of tumor cells and/or from an indirect effect on modulation of immune effector cell populations with tumor cell specificities. IFNs regulate gene expression, modulate expression of proteins on the cell surface, and induce synthesis of new enzymes. Alterations in gene expression result in modulation of levels of receptors for other cytokines, concentration of regulatory proteins on the surface of immune effector cells, and activities of enzymes that modulate cellular growth and function. On a cellular basis, these effects translate into alterations of the state of differentiation, rate of proliferation and cell death, and functional activity of many cell types.

A problem in attributing the effects of IFNs to specific gene products has been the evidence that they induce hundreds of genes. This has resulted in identification by gene profiling of marked increases in specific messenger RNA from treatment of human primary and malignant cell lines with IFN-α, IFN-β, or IFN-γ.[19,20,31] Over a hundred of these genes induced by type I IFNs are involved in apoptosis, including protein kinase R (PKR), promyelocytic leukemia (PML), RAP46/Bag-1, phospholipid scramblase, and tumor necrosis factor–related apoptosis-inducing ligand (TRAIL).[19,20] Not only may these genes induce biologic effects themselves, they may also interact to augment biologic effects with other cytokines. Apoptosis can be augmented by combinations of IFNs with apoptosis-inducing agents such as TRAIL.[21,32]

The enzymes 2',5'-oligoadenylate synthetase (2',5'-A synthetase), a PKR, and indoleamine 2,3-dioxygenase are among the enzymes induced by IFNs (Table 48-4). 2'5'-A synthetases are multiple isoform products of a three-gene family[33] that provide relatively specific markers of IFN system activation. A latent ribonuclease, RnaseL, is activated by the oligonucleotides synthesized by 2',5'-A synthetase. One result of induction of these enzymes is inhibition of protein synthesis. The level of the RNaseL increases in growth-arrested cells and during cellular differentiation.[34] Apoptosis is suppressed in RNaseL null mice treated with different apoptotic agents.[35] Germline mutations in RNaseL are associated with familial prostate carcinoma, further validating the postulate that an influence on RNA levels by RNaseL may be important in oncogenesis.[36]

A constitutive serine-threonine kinase, PKR, with a unique requirement for double-stranded RNA undergoes induction and activation by IFNs.[37] The major function of this kinase is growth control; it can also induce apoptosis.[38] Cells expressing PKR mutants formed colonies in soft agar and produced large tumors after injection into nude mice.[39] PKR and STAT-1 were both required for IFN-mediated down-regulation of c-*myc*.[40] PKR expression may be partially controlled by an IFN-induced transcription factor, IRF-1.[41] Because IRF-1 increases rapidly in growth-arrested cells, it may influence expression of genes involved in negative control of cell growth and may mediate the antiproliferative effects of IFNs. A second transcription factor, IRF-2, identified in murine cells, has sequence

Table 48-3 Pleiotropic Biologic Effects of Interferons

Microbial inhibition	Immunomodulatory
RNA viruses	Cytotoxicity
DNA viruses	T cell
Intracellular pathogens	Natural killer/lymphokine-activated killer cells
Protein induction	Monocytes
Adhesion proteins	Antibody dependent
Enzyme induction	Antigen processing
Chemokines	Vascular
Cell modulation	Angiogenesis inhibition
Oncogene depression	Lipoprotein reduction
Slow mitotic cycle	Antitumor
Differentiation	Mouse
Apoptosis	Human

DNA = deoxyribonucleic acid; RNA = ribonucleic acid.

Table 48-4 Modulation of Gene Expression by Interferons*

Antigen processing	Enzymes and other proteins
LMP-2	2'5'-A synthetase[†]
HLA complex	TRAIL[†]
Class I (A, B, C)[†]	XAF-1
Class II (DR, DP, DQ)[†]	Protein kinase R
β2-Microglobulin[†]	Indoleamine dioxygenase[†]
Invariant chain	Guanylate-binding proteins[†]
Tumor-associated antigens	GTP cyclohydrolase[†]
TAG72	Metallothionein II
CEA[†]	Mn^{2+} superoxide dismutase
TRAIL	ISG-15
Myeloblastin	Phospholipid scramblase
Adhesion proteins	PML
Intercellular adhesion module 1	p56
Leu-13	Transcription factors
Depressed functional activities	IRF-1 (ISGF-2)
Ornithine decarboxylase	IRF-2
Oncogenes	IFN consensus sequence-binding protein
c-*myc*, c-Ha-*ras*, c-*fos*	Stat-1
P-450 microsomal enzymes	
Fibroblast growth factor	

CEA = carcinoembryonic antigen; GTP = guanosine triphosphate; HLA = human leukocyte antigen; IFN = interferon; IRF = interferon-regulatory factor; ISG = interferon-stimulated gene; ISGF = interferon-stimulated gene factor; LMP =proteosome subunits; TAG = tumor associated glycoprotein; TRAIL = tumor necrosis factor–related apoptosis-inducing ligand.

*Representative of over 300 genes augmented at a transcriptional level.

[†]Modulation demonstrated in patients after interferons.

homology to IRF-1 and is a functional antagonist of IRF-1. On constitutive expression, IRF-2 can result in cell transformation, which is inhibited by IRF-1.[41]

At least three families of guanosine triphosphatases (GTPases) are induced by IFNs. The best characterized is the Mx family. The Mx proteins belong to the dynamin superfamily of large GTPases, proteins involved in endocytosis, vesicle transport, cell cycle progression, and metastasis suppression [42,43] Other families of GTPases are some of the most abundant proteins in IFN-treated human cells.[44]

Several additional IFN-induced genes may influence apoptosis. Among these is the gene PML. PML knockout mice were used to demonstrate that PML is necessary for programmed cell death induced by IFN-α and IFN-β.[45] Phospholipid scramblase flips phosphatidylserine from the inner layer of the plasma membrane to the outer layer.[46] The appearance of phosphatidylserine on the outer layer of the cell membrane has been observed in apoptotic cells. In IFN-sensitive, but not IFN-resistant, melanoma cells, TRAIL/Apo2L was induced, as were other proteins implicated in apoptosis.[31,47] These IFN-stimulated proteins initiated the apoptotic cascade with alterations in mitochondrial membrane potential and changes in bcl-2 levels.[32,47,48] Molecular interactions between TRAIL and IFNs suggest that these two molecules may synergize in induction of apoptosis.[32,47,49] IFNs down-regulate expression of the multidrug resistance gene (*MDR1*) in human colon carcinoma cells, suggesting that IFNs might increase apoptosis after cellular stresses.[50]

Measurement of IFN-induced genes or the quantitation of immune effector cell function can be used to define biologically active molecules, doses, schedules, and routes of administration. Most biologic response modulatory effects peak at 24 to 48 hours, after intravenous or subcutaneous administration, which contrasts with maximal serum levels that peak in minutes to hours.[51,52] After intravenous bolus administration, the $t_{1/2}\alpha$ of IFN-α2 is short (< 60 minutes). Induced proteins and their products can be identified on cells and in the serum of treated patients (see Table 48-4). The mean terminal half-life is 4 to 5 hours, with no serum levels measurable at 12 hours. After intramuscular or subcutaneous administration, peak levels are 3 to 8 hours.[53] The pharmacologic hallmark of IFN-β is virtual absence of serum levels with subcutaneous or intramuscular administration, yet biologic response modulatory and therapeutic effects occur.[51]

Pegylated IFNs have markedly different kinetics than do unmodified IFNs.[54–56] Once-weekly administration has resulted in measurable serum levels of IFN-α2 at 7 days at doses in excess of those required for gene induction and cellular effects in vitro and has resulted in tumor responses in metastatic renal carcinoma and chronic myelogenous leukemia (CML). Although pegylated IFNs may be modestly better tolerated, their greater therapeutic effectiveness has resulted in regulatory approvals in chronic active hepatitis.[57,58] Clinical effectiveness against a hepatitis C virus serotype previously unresponsive to unmodified IFN-α2[57,58] suggests that the altered pharmacokinetics and pharmacodynamics result in a drug with different cellular and clinical actions. This greater effectiveness may be important in decreasing the frequency of development of hepatocellular carcinoma after hepatitis virus infection.[59,60]

MECHANISMS OF ANTITUMOR ACTION

Antiproliferative, Apoptotic, and Differentiative Effects IFN-α and IFN-β can affect all phases of the cell cycle. When fibroblasts are stimulated by serum, epidermal growth factor, or insulin, IFNs cause a prolongation of the G_1 phase, a reduced rate of entry into the S phase, and a lengthening of the S and the G_2 phases.[61,62] The cumulative effects of prolongation of the cell cycle of both normal and tumor cells by IFNs result in cytostasis, an increase in cell size, and apoptosis.[47,48,62,63] Proto-oncogenes regulated by IFNs include c-*myc*, *bcl-2*, c-Ha-*ras*, and c-*src*.[40,64–66] An important checkpoint protein mutated in many cancers is the retinoblastoma protein (Rb). Underphosphorylated Rb (the active form) specifically binds and inhibits the transcription factor E2F, thus inhibiting cell cycle progression. The primary influence of IFN-α on Rb is inhibition of its hyperphosphorylation.[67,68] Inhibition of Rb hyperphosphorylation by IFN-α resulted from rapid reduction of the expression of cyclin D3, which decreased formation of cyclin D–cdk4 and cyclin D–cdk6 kinase complexes.[69] E2F controls a number of cell cycle–related genes, such as c-*myc* and *cdc2*. In addition, IFN-α converted the E2F-Rb complex into a transcription repressor by inducing the dephosphorylation of Rb.[70] IFN-α reduction of transcription of c-*myc* is at least in part a consequence of IFN reduction in DNA binding of the transcription factor E2F, which binds to the c-*myc* promoter.[71] Downstream of Rb and E2F, IFN-α reduced the amount of the cdc25 tyrosine phosphatase, resulting in the loss of activation of cyclin E–cdk2 and cyclin A–cdk2 kinase complexes.[69] Also, the cdk inhibitor $p21^{WAF1}$ was induced,[72] which negatively regulated the cyclin E–cdk2 complex. Mouse 3T3 cells transformed with the human Ha-*ras-1* gene and cultured continuously in the presence of murine IFN-α or IFN-β produced revertant colonies in which transcription of the *ras* gene was inhibited. Most cells retained the revertant phenotype during many cell generations despite renewed high levels of transcription of the *ras* gene and of p21 ras protein.[73]

Clinical effectiveness in CML has spurred investigations of potential mechanisms in that disorder. IFN-α may restore defective adhesion of CML progenitors to bone marrow stroma, thereby allowing normal growth inhibitory signals to regulate stem cell and early precursor proliferation.[74] An IFN-induced transmembrane protein associated with cell adhesion and antiproliferative effects has been correlated with improved survival in CML.[75] Proliferation of CML stem cells and myeloid series elements may be inhibited by IFN-α.[76,77] Fas can be up-regulated by IFN-α, an event that resulted in Fas-mediated apoptosis.[78] Both Fas expression and stem cell proliferation in vitro correlated with clinical response.[76,77] Loss in mice of expression of a transcription factor gene interferon consensus sequence-binding protein (ICSBP) resulted in a myeloproliferative syndrome phenotypically similar to CML.[79] ICSBP expression was found to be low in patients with both acute and chronic myeloid leukemias.[79] Treatment with IFN-α2 over several months resulted in normalization of ICSBP expression. Resistance in CML has also been correlated with constitutive expression of SOCS3.[80] An IFN-stimulated protein, myeloblastin, has been associated with a specific T-cell response in IFN-α responsive patients, suggesting an immune component to the effects of IFN-α.[81] This latter protein was not induced by imatinib.[80] Prolonged treatment with imatinib in vitro, however, resulted in greater sensitivity to IFN-α as a result of loss of a regulatory phosphatase.[82]

IMMUNE EFFECTOR CELLS

IFNs augment the effectiveness of all immune effector cell types that have the potential to kill tumor target cells. These include cytotoxic T cells, natural killer (NK)/lymphokine-activated killer cells, and monocytes (see Table 48-3). IFNs can also boost antibody-dependent cell-mediated cytotoxicity, mediated by subpopulations of these effectors. In addition to augmenting expression of human leukocyte antigen (HLA) molecules (see below in this section), IFNs directly augment T-cell functions relevant to tumor cell cytotoxicity.[83–85] The ability of IFNs to augment NK cell activity and monocyte function has been demonstrated both in vitro and in vivo.[86–89] Addition of IFNs to NK cells, even those of depressed lytic activity, can result in augmented tumor cell cytotoxicity.[86,87] Patients given IFNs have augmented NK cell and monocyte activity 24 to 72 hours after IFN administration.[86,87]

Unique augmenting effects on dendritic cell maturation and function, differing from those of granulocyte-macrophage colony-stimulating factor, have been identified.[90–93] These have included strong promotion of a T helper cell 1 response and IL-15, CD83, and CD25 induction.[91–93] An increase in response to chemokines with up-regulation of CCR7 and an enhanced chemotactic response has also been observed.[91] Dendritic cell function may be partially mediated by interferon-stimulated gene 15 (*ISG15*), which is secreted by tumor cells.[94] When IFN-α2 was used in combination with ex vivo pulsing of human immunodeficiency virus (HIV), an enhanced response to HIV antigens resulted in severe combined immunodeficiency disease mice.[95] IFN-β may be effective in conjunction with other cytokines to stimulate an immune response.[96]

Equivalent antitumor effectiveness of IFNs in mice has been identified for tumor cells sensitive or resistant to antiproliferative effects of IFNs in vitro.[97] Additional evidence supporting a role for host immune effector cell response to IFNs comes from studies in which mice with Friend leukemia, syngeneic tumor, or human prostate and HeLa tumor xenografts received an antibody to murine IFN.[8,98] These mice, in the absence of exogenous IFN, experienced enhanced tumor growth and transplantability, suggesting that neutralization of endogenous IFN removes aspects of host defense to tumor. When treated with exogenous IFN-α, $stat1^{-/-}$ mice could not reject $stat1^{+/+}$ melanomas; conversely, equivalent survival resulted in wild-type mice implanted with $stat1^{+}$ or $stat1^{-}$ tumors.[99] However, studies in nude mice with human tumor xenografts also demonstrated the antitumor effects of exogenous human IFNs.[100,101] This demonstrates, in view of the strict species specificity of IFNs, that the direct effects can also limit tumor growth in vivo.

Host modulatory effects of IFNs are part of the network of cytokine and cellular interactions. Induced gene modulation with subsequent production of specific proteins must underlie the immune regulatory effects of IFNs (see Table 48-4). IFNs enhance cell surface expression of major histocompatibility complex (MHC) antigens, tumor-associated antigens (TAAs), and Fc receptors. All IFNs augment MHC class I expression, and IFN-γ enhances MHC class II expression on tumor cells as well.[101–103] An increase in MHC expression may enhance monocyte or macrophage antigen-presenting functions. Following IFN-γ, respiratory activity in macrophages has increased with production of toxic oxygen intermediates, such as hydrogen peroxide and superoxide anion.[90,100] Monocytes stimulated by IFNs secrete monokines, including colony-stimulating factor, TNF, and IL-1, as well as plasminogen activator, complement, and a variety of enzymes and other cytotoxic mediators.[100,104,105]

Enhancement of expression of TAAs, such as tumor-associated glycoprotein 72 and carcinoembryonic antigens, has both diagnostic and therapeutic implications.[106,107] No increase in TAA occurs on normal cells. Enhanced expression of TAA and HLA classes I and II may lead to improved tumor cell recognition by host immune cells, with resultant enhancement of killing. In addition, accurate localization of primary and metastatic tumor by monoclonal antibodies directed against appropriate TAAs could allow more directed therapy by using monoclonal antibodies as a carrier for radionuclides or cytotoxic agents.

ANGIOGENESIS INHIBITION

Another component of IFN-mediated antitumor effects is inhibition of angiogenesis.[108] Following IFN treatment, tumor endothelial cells exhibit microvascular injury and a pattern of coagulation necrosis.[109] Systemic administration of IFN-α reduced tumor cell growth in IFN-sensitive cells by directly inhibiting the expression of the angiogenic protein basic fibroblast growth factor (bFGF).[110] IFN-α and IFN-β also down-regulate bFGF in other human carcinomas.[111,112] Interruption of the angiogenic signal by IFNs precedes the antiproliferative effect and is detectable between 24 and 48 hours after tumor inoculation.[101] IFN down-regulation of bFGF correlates with reduced vascularization and reduced growth of tumors in nude mice.[110] IL-8 has also proven to be a potent mediator of angiogenesis and, consequently, of tumorigenesis.[113] IFN inhibits IL-8 production.[114] In addition to inhibiting angiogenic proteins, IFN-γ up-regulates the expression of an angiostatic protein, IP-10.[115] IP-10 is an IFN-γ–induced C-X-C chemokine with the ability to repress the angiogenic activities of both bFGF and IL-8.[115]

Clinically, IFN-α2 treatment has successfully induced regression of bulky hemangiomas, tumors consisting of abnormal endothelial cells, and Kaposi's sarcoma.[116,117] IFN-α2 was beneficial in life-threatening hemangiomas of infancy, leading to angioma regression in more than 80% of children treated.[116] Not only did hemangiomas regress, but their life-threatening complications, including consumptive coagulopathy and high-output cardiac failure, were controlled.[116] These observations provide the rationale for assessment of IFN-α2 in other neoplastic disorders with endothelial cell proliferation, angiosarcoma, and giant cell tumor of bone.[118]

ANTITUMOR EFFECTS IN HUMANS

IFNs have achieved a role in clinical medicine well beyond that of the selective antiviral agent envisioned at discovery. Clinically, beneficial therapeutic activity of IFN-α2 as a single agent has been demonstrated in more than a dozen malignancies (Table 48-5). These findings have led to regulatory approvals around the world. Augmenting therapeutic effectiveness could lead to wider adoption for other malignancies, such as ovarian, breast, bronchogenic, bladder, and gastrointestinal carcinomas and acute leukemias, in which phase I or phase II clinical trials have suggested potential benefit.

The unique molecular and cellular effects of IFNs complement the mechanisms of actions of other therapies. When combined with other therapies in cell and animal models, IFNs have augmented effectiveness for malignancies of diverse histologies. A reduction in cell number or tumor size and prolongation of survival have, in most cases, been additive and often synergistic. Building on these observations, the single-agent clinical activity in hematopoietic malignancies and solid tumors and second-generation IFNs or inducers, IFN therapeutic applications could substantially increase.

Table 48-5 Antitumor Effectiveness of Interferon-α in Phase II Trials

Chronic leukemias	Malignant melanoma†
Myeloid*†	Midgut carcinoids
Hairy cell*†	Renal carcinomas†
Myeloproliferative syndromes*	Kaposi's sarcomas
Lymphomas	Ovarian carcinomas‡
Follicular*†	Basal cell carcinomas‡
T cell*	Bladder carcinomas‡
Large cell	Breast carcinomas
Multiple myeloma	

*Response rates > 40%.
†Improved survival in phase III trials.
‡Also intralesional or regional administration.

HEMATOLOGIC MALIGNANCIES

The degree of activity and improvement in quality of life of patients with hairy cell leukemia resulted in the first licensed approval for an IFN in the United States. More than 85% of patients have objective evidence of a partial or complete hematologic response to IFN-α2.[119] Following IFNs, there was a gradual decrease in bone marrow infiltration with hairy cells and a normalization of peripheral hematologic parameters. This resulted in reduced morbidity from the disease process, a reduction in red cell and platelet transfusion requirements, and a decreased frequency of infection,[120] effects that increased with continuous treatment.[121] Although now supplanted in clinical use by other, even more effective drugs, US Food and Drug Administration approval in hairy cell leukemia opened the way for expanded clinical trials of IFN-α2 in other disease states.

In CML, IFN-α2 resulted in a sustained therapeutic response in a majority (> 75%) of newly diagnosed patients.[122,123] Untreated patients or patients with disease of less than 1 year duration have been more likely to respond.[123] In addition to a reduction in leukemic cell mass, a reduction has occurred in the frequency of cells bearing the underlying 9 to 22 chromosomal translocation.[123] With continued treatment, approximately 25% of patients will develop a cytogenetic complete response with loss of expression of the Philadelphia chromosome–expressing cells. Equivalence and/or superiority of IFN-α2 to busulfan and hydroxyurea for CML were demonstrated.[124–126] Continued treatment resulted in 30% of all patients treated for 8 or more years being alive.[127] Median and 10-year survival data demonstrate a significant and cost-effective advantage for IFN-α2 when compared with chemotherapy,[127,128] although with increased toxicity, an increase in cytogenetic response frequency occurred with the addition of cytosine arabinoside alone or in combination with IFN-α2.[129–131] The activity of the second-generation pegylated IFN-α2 with convenience of weekly administration has been confirmed with suggestion of greater activity. Whether IFN-α2 will be used to clinical advantage with the therapeutic advance in CML, which has resulted from imatinib mesylate, is just beginning to be assessed.[132,133] However, in vitro, the two modalities have synergistic effectiveness in inhibiting CML precursor proliferation.[134,135] Thrombocytosis associated with myeloproliferative disorders, whether Philadelphia chromosome positive or negative, can also be effectively controlled by IFN-α2.[136–138] Similarly, polycythemia vera can be clinically palliated with a reduction in the need for periodic phlebotomies.[139] The clonal, life-threatening hypereosinophilic syndrome and chronic eosinophilic leukemia with chromosomal translocation, sometimes even in patients refractory to other therapies, can also be effectively controlled.[140,141]

Response rates of 10 to 20% occur in patients with advanced multiple myeloma treated with various schedules.[142] When patients who had received 12×10^6 U/m^2 of IFN-α2 intramuscularly daily were analyzed according to previous therapy, 50% of previously untreated patients had responded.[143] Similarly, patients who had received only phenylalanine mustard and prednisone had a 40% response rate.[142] In patients who had a tumor response, levels of serum immunoglobulins were restored, an effect infrequently seen with chemotherapy.[143] Alternate cycles of IFN-α2 and chemotherapy for induction, when evaluated in the randomized setting, produced a significant increase in complete response frequency and response duration compared with chemotherapy alone; however, no impact on overall survival emerged.[144] Studies have identified prolonged survival in some but not all trials when IFN-α2 has been used as maintenance therapy for patients stable or responding to induction chemotherapy, but this has not been confirmed in all trials[145–152] Because mechanisms of response and resistance are better defined on a molecular level, IFNs could be part of an effective combination therapy for this disease.

In lymphomas of various histologies and of both B- and T-cell phenotypes, IFN-α may have a therapeutic role.[153] IFNα2, 50×10^6 units three times a week, was effective in 45% of patients with advanced cutaneous T-cell lymphoma.[154] In nodular, poorly differentiated B-cell lymphomas, a greater than 45% response frequency occurred with IFN-α2, even in patients previously treated with combination chemotherapy.[153,155] Responses can persist for more than 6 months after cessation of therapy. For B-cell lymphomas, the significant single-agent activity of IFN-α2 has been integrated into effective combined-modality treatments for both low- and intermediate-grade non-Hodgkin's lymphoma.[156–162] Prolonged disease-free survival in low-grade lymphomas has resulted from IFN-α2 used either as induction or maintenance in combination with cyclophosphamide, vincristine, and prednisone in randomized multicenter trials.[159,160] Combination with doxorubicin-based regimens has prolonged both disease-free survival and overall survival in two prospectively randomized trials.[157,158,161,162] In one trial for intermediate- and high-grade lymphomas, patients received IFN-α2 for no more than 30 days during the first 6 months of treatment as a sensitizing effect for chemotherapy; therapeutic benefit has been maintained with 10 years of observations.[161] Despite a careful design to ensure that effective chemotherapy doses would not be compromised, total cytotoxic chemotherapy doses were reduced by participating investigators in the IFN-containing arm; despite this, a positive therapeutic impact of IFN-α2 was evident.[161] Somewhat surprisingly, an impact was seen only on progression-free but not overall survival if IFNs were used as maintenance for low-grade lymphoma.[163,164] Because IFNs can increase both HLA class I and antibody-dependent cellular cytotoxicity, a relatively low dose of IFN-α2 was combined with rituximab in a phase II trial with an increase in progression-free survival.[165] A high frequency of deletion of IFN-α genes has been identified in posttransplant lymphoproliferative disease.[166] Thus, in addition to the effects of IFN on B-cell proliferation, rationale exists for clinical trials. Indeed when used primarily for individual patients in this setting, a high frequency of response has been observed.[167]

SOLID TUMORS

For metastatic melanoma and renal carcinomas, IFN-α2 has resulted in therapeutic effects exceeding or equivalent to available treatments. Response rates of melanoma to IFN-α2 have ranged from 2 to 29%; the cumulative response totaled from three series of 124 patients involving patients who used recombinant IFN-α2 was 15% (10% partial and 5% complete), a level comparable to results with cytotoxic agents,[168,169] although combinations of IFNs with other active modalities, such as chemotherapy and/or IL-2, might increase response rates.[170–176] Although higher response rates were identified, the critical parameters of progression-free survival and overall survival have not been markedly prolonged.[177–179] Thus, IFN-α2 in combination with chemotherapy may increase tumor regression frequency but with a significant increase in toxicity and without an impact on eventual outcome. In contrast to the results in metastatic melanoma, prolongation of disease-free survival, and often of overall survival, has emerged from the use of IFN-α2 as an adjuvant to surgery for melanoma for patients at high risk of disease recurrence (stage IIB or stage III).[180–185] Benefit appears to be greatest for those patients treated at the high doses used in US cooperative group studies. In the most recent of these trials, a comparison with a ganglioside vaccine resulted in a 48% decrease in the risk of death for those patients receiving IFN-α2 ($p < .01$).[185] Pegylation has resulted in responses in metastatic melanoma, leading to innovative, long-duration trial designs with doses adjusted for maintenance of activity.[56,186]

Response rates from 4 to 26% have been reported in trials of IFN-α2 for metastatic renal carcinoma, with a mean response of 15% in a cumulative summary of several trials.[187] In one of the initial trials, either 2 or 20×10^6 U/m^2 was administered daily.[188] No objective responses occurred at the lower dose, but at the higher dose, 4 of 15 patients responded. Subsequently, additional patients were treated at 20×10^6 U/m^2 with 8 of 26 responses. The median duration of response was 3 months, but a dose reduction was required in 50% of the patients.[188] When compared with other modalities in randomized phase III trials, a significant benefit was observed when IFN-α2 was used for metastatic renal carcinoma. In a randomized trial of 226 patients that compared IFN-α2 with medroxyprogesterone, a significant 2½-month increase in survival was identified.[189] A second trial randomized patients to either vinblastine or vinblastine and IFN-α2a. A 7½-month prolongation of survival resulted in the patients receiving vinblastine and IFN-α2a when compared with vinblastine alone.[190] These findings are supported by an earlier meta-analysis that suggested that patients receiving IFN-α had a beneficial effect on survival compared with control regimens.[191] Two randomized trials support the conclusion that survival prolongation may be greatest for those patients who have nephrectomies despite the presence of metastases and who then receive IFN-α2.[192,193] Although these results suggest that, as with melanoma, a beneficial effect might occur with IFN-α2 used as an adjunct to surgery for those patients at the highest risk of recurrence, a trial using a low dose of IFN-α2 for 3 months did not show a benefit.[194] Possibly, the higher serum levels that occur with pegylated IFN-α2 might result in the types of effects seen in adjuvant use in melanoma.

Clinical trials of IFN-α in endocrine pancreatic tumors have identified a high objective rate (75%) of a reduction in tumor-produced peptides.[195,196] Midgut carcinoid tumors, although often behaving in an indolent fashion, produce symptoms such as flushing and diarrhea, which may interfere with daily activities. In trials of IFN-α in midgut carcinoid tumors, a mean response rate of approximately 50% (improvement in symptoms or a decrease in 5-hydroxyindoleacetic acid) has been reported.[195] Objective tumor regression occurs less frequently, being observed in approximately 15% of patients, but can include both primary tumors and hepatic metastases.[196] Other solid tumors, such as ovarian, bladder, and basal cell carcinomas, have responded to IFN-α administered regionally, particularly in patients with less tumor bulk.[197–199]

SIDE EFFECTS

Like other potent physiologic mediators, such as glucocorticoids, IFNs have toxicities when administered with pharmacologic intent (Table 48-6). The side effects with the initial dose are predominantly constitutional.[200,201] These are dominated by malaise, fever, and chills, which begin a few hours after the commonly used subcutaneous route and last for 2 to 8 hours. These influenza-like symptoms occur uniformly following the initial injection, with subsequent development of tachyphylaxis with additional daily injections. Flu-like symptoms can be partially controlled with acetaminophen. Chronic fatigue may necessitate dose reduction; tolerance can be improved with lower doses and intermittent scheduling. Fatigue and anorexia are the dose-limiting toxicities with chronic administration;

Table 48-6 Clinical Side Effects of Interferons

Acute	Chronic
Fever	Fatigue
Chills	Anorexia
Malaise	Weight loss
Myalgias	Mild neutropenia
Headaches	Transaminase elevations
Nausea	Depression, mental slowing

Less common: confusion, hair shedding, thrombocytopenia, diarrhea, and nausea and vomiting.

weight loss occurs and may be significant (> 10%). In general, older patients have greater difficulty with these side effects than do younger patients. Nausea and vomiting have usually been mild and of short duration. The most frequent neurologic side effects (other than the possible relationship of the fatigue) are somnolence, confusion, and depression. A small randomized trial has suggested that paroxetine may partially ameliorate the depression.[202]

Hematologic effects include mild granulocytopenia with a reduction by 40 to 60%,[204–217] followed by rapid rebound to normal after discontinuation of therapy. No increase in infectious sequelae has occurred during IFN-induced leukopenia, and granulocytopenia is rarely dose limiting. Anemia occurs with chronic therapy but is rarely severe. This may reflect an influence on the erythropoiesis because recovery of normal hematocrit has often required weeks or months. Mild thrombocytopenia has occurred in 5 to 50% of patients and is influenced by marrow infiltration with tumor. Elevation of transaminases, which is usually mild, has occurred more commonly in the presence of pretreatment hepatic abnormalities and is dose related. Although little or no IFN can be identified in urine, renal failure reduces, but does not eliminate, clearance, suggesting that catabolism by renal tubular cells is one degradation pathway.[203] With improved understanding of the mechanism of action and clinical introduction of other members of the IFN-α family and second-generation IFNs,[218,219] it can be anticipated that the therapeutic index of IFNs will improve.

With chronic administration, a minority of patients develop neutralizing antibody to the administered IFN-α2 and IFN-β.[204,205] Antibody development is a function of dose, schedule, route, and, possibly, underlying disease. Antibodies have rarely been identified with < 4 months of IFN administration. Particularly when present in high titer, neutralizing antibodies may be correlated with disease progression.

PERSPECTIVE

IFNs have improved therapeutic approaches for malignancies and viral diseases. They are the first human proteins to be effective as a cancer treatment modality. The full spectrum of actions and interactions, mechanism of antitumor effects, and optimal dose, schedule, and type of IFN for specific clinical indications have still only been partially delineated (Table 48-7). As the first clinical product of recombinant DNA technology for oncology, IFNs, both themselves and as a prototype for other therapeutic proteins, opened an era of biologic therapies for malignancies. Innovative approaches to potentiate the effects of IFNs suggest that the therapeutic potential has just begun to be fully realized (see Table 48-7).

Reaching the full potential of IFNs as therapeutics for cancer will result from additional understanding of the mechanisms of antitumor action, the molecular and cellular pathways influencing tumor cell resistance, use of second-generation IFNs, and identifying potentiating interactions with other modalities of cancer treatment. Furthermore, suppression of the IFN system of the host in and by malignant cells is emerging as an important contributor to the development of the clinical disease. Mutation of a gene in the IFN response pathway RNaseL increases the risk of prostate cancer.[36,206] Gene expression profiling and cytogenetic analyses have identified decreases in IFN-stimulated genes in melanoma, colon, breast, and hematologic malignancies.[75,207–216] Epigenetic and genetic silencing of IFN-stimulated gene expression also likely influences tumor development.[217–219] In addition to being a primary source for production of IFNs, dendritic cell maturation is also influenced.[91–93] Activation of the IFN system, as has been used in chronic hepatitis to decrease the risk of hepatocellular carcinoma, suggests that IFNs or inducers may play a role in clinical chemoprevention.[12,13,220,221]

Second-generation IFNs and inducers have already begun to demonstrate clinical advantage. Randomized, double-blind, placebo-controlled, and dose-escalating phase I trials have identified better toleration and tumor responses for the only other recombinant IFN-α evaluated.[222,223] Pegylation of IFN-α2 has resulted in advantageous pharmacokinetics, improved clinical outcomes for patients with chronic active hepatitis, and tumor response in renal carcinoma, melanoma, and CML.[56,224] With further definition of the role of each of the pleiotropic molecular and cellular effects, substantial opportunities exist to improve therapeutic outcomes for a number of malignancies by use of IFNs or IFN inducers.

Table 48-7 Research to Result in More Effective Use of Interferons in Cancer

- Molecules
  - Inducers
  - Structure-function relationships
  - Effects of new types
- Mechanism of action
  - Genes induced
  - Protein modulation
  - Immunomodulatory effects
  - Antiproliferative/apoptotic
  - Differentiation effects
  - Angiogenesis inhibition
- Cellular activation mechanisms
  - Receptors
  - Transcription regulation
  - Function of induced proteins
- Clinical strategies
  - Biologic modulation
  - Dose/schedule optimization
  - Combination therapies
  - Second generation
  - New disease targets
  - Minimizing side effects

REFERENCES

1. Pestka S. The human interferon-alpha species and hybrid proteins. Semin Oncol 1997; (3 Suppl 9):S9-18-S9-40
2. Kontsek P, Karayainni-Vasconcelos G, Kontsekova E. The human interferon system: characterization and classifica-

tion after discovery of novel members. Acta Virol 2003;47:201–15.

3. LaFleur DW, Nardelli B, Tsareva T, et al. Interferon-kappa, a novel type I interferon expressed in human keratinocytes. J Biol Chem 2001;276:39765–71.
4. Adolf GR. Human interferon omega—a review. Mult Scler 1995;8 Suppl 1:S44–7.
5. Chan SH, Perussia B, Gupta JW, et al. Induction of interferon production by natural killer cell stimulatory factor: characterization of the responder cells and synergy with other inducers. J Exp Med 1991;173:869–79.
6. Lotze MT, Matory YL, Ettinghausen SE, et al. In vivo administration of purified human interleukin-2: half-life, immunologic effects, and expansion of peripheral lymphoid cells in vivo with recombinant IL-2. J Immunol 1985;135:2865–74.
7. Recht M, Borden EC, Knight E Jr. A human 15-kDa IFN-induced protein induces the secretion of IFN-γ. J Immunol 1991;147:2617–23.
8. Gresser I, Belardelli F, Maury C, et al. Injection of mice with antibody to interferon enhances the growth of transplantable murine tumors. J Exp Med 1983;158:2095–107.
9. Litton G, Hong R, Grossberg SE, et al. Biological and clinical effects of the oral immunomodulator 3,6-bis(2-piperidinoethoxy)acridine trihydrochloride in patients with advanced malignancy. J Biol Response Mod 1990;9:61–70.
10. Urba WJ, Longo DL, Weiss RB. Enhancement of natural killer activity in human peripheral blood by flavone acetic acid. J Natl Cancer Inst 1988;80:521–5.
11. Witt PL, Ritch PS, Reding D, et al. Phase I trial of an oral immunomodulator and interferon inducer in cancer patients. Cancer Res 1993;53:5176–80.
12. Borden E, Sidky Y, Erturk E, et al. Protection from carcinogen-induced murine bladder carcinoma by interferons and an oral interferon-inducing pyrimidinone, bropirimine. Cancer Res 1990;50:1071–4.
13. Sarosdy MF, Lowe BA, Schelhammer PF, et al. Oral bropirimine immunotherapy of carcinoma in situ of the bladder: results of a phase II trial. Urology 1996;48:21–7.
14. Ruzicka FJ, Jach ME, Borden EC. Binding of recombinant-produced interferon beta ser to human lymphoblastoid cells: evidence for two binding domains. J Biol Chem 1987;262:16142–9.
15. Russell-Harde D, Wagner TC, Perez HD, Croze E. Formation of a uniquely stable type I interferon receptor complex by interferon beta is dependent upon particular interactions between interferon beta and its receptor and independent of tyrosine phosphorylation. Biochem Biophys Res Commun 1999;255:539–44.
16. Billard C, Ferbus D, Diez RA, et al. Correlation between the biological and therapeutic effects of interferon-alpha in low-grade nodular non-Hodgkin's lymphoma: lack of in vivo down-regulation and reduced affinity of IFN-alpha receptors in unresponsive patients. Leuk Res 1991;15:121–8.
17. Faltynek CR, Princler GL, Rossio JL, et al. Relationship of the clinical response and binding of recombinant interferon alpha in patients with lymphoproliferative diseases. Blood 1986;67:1077–82.
18. Uze G, Lutfalla G, Gresser I. Genetic transfer of a functional human interferon alpha receptor into mouse cells: cloning and expression of its cDNA. Cell 1990;60:225–34.
19. Der SD, Zhou A, Williams BR, Silverman RH. Identification of genes differentially regulated by interferon alpha, beta or gamma using oligonucleotide arrays. Proc Natl Acad Sci U S A 1998;95(26):15623–8.
20. Leaman DW, Chawla-Sarkar M, Jacobs B, et al. Novel growth and death related interferon- stimulated genes (ISGs) in melanoma: greater potency of IFN-beta compared with IFN-alpha2. J Interferon Cytokine Res 2003;23:745–56.
21. Sanceau J, Hiscott J, Delattre O, Wietzerbin J. IFN-beta induces serine phosphorylation of Stat-1 in Ewing's sarcoma cells and mediates apoptosis via induction of IRF-1 and activation of caspase-7. Oncogene 2000;19:3372–83.
22. Rani MR, Asthagiri AR, Singh A, et al. A role for NF-kappa B in the induction of beta-R1 by interferon-beta. J Biol Chem 2001;276:44365–8.
23. Lewerenz M, Mogensen KE, Uze G. Shared receptor components but distinct complexes for alpha and beta interferons. J Mol Biol 1998;282:585–99.
24. Stark G, Kerr I, Williams B, et al. How cells respond to interferons. Annu Rev Biochem 1998;67:227–64.
25. David M, Petricoin E III, Benjamin C, et al. Requirement for MAP kinase (ERK2) activity in interferon alpha-and interferon beta-stimulated gene expression through STAT proteins. Science 1995;269:1721–3.
26. Uddin S, Yenush L, Sun XJ, et al. Interferon-alpha engages the insulin receptor substrate-1 to associate with the phosphatidylinositol 3'-kinase. J. Biol Chem 1995;270:15938–41.
27. Nicholson SE, Hilton DJ. The SOCS proteins: a new family of negative regulators of signal transduction. J Leukoc Biol 1998;63:665–8.
28. Yoshimura A. The CIS/JAB family: novel negative regulators of JAK signaling pathways. Leukemia 1998;12:1851–7.
29. David M, Chen HE, Goelz S, et al. Differential regulation of the alpha/beta interferon-stimulated Jak/Stat pathway by the SH2 domain-containing tyrosine phosphatase SHPTP1. Mol Cell Biol 1995;15:7050–8.
30. Yi T, Pathak MK, Lindner JD, et al. Anti-cancer activity of sodium stibogluconate in synergy with IFNs. J Immunol 2002;169:5978–85.
31. Silva AJ, Brickelmaier M, Majeau GR, et al. Comparison of gene expression patterns induced by treatment of human umbilical vein endothelial cells with IFN-alpha 2b vs. IFN-beta 1a: understanding the functional relationship between distinct type I interferons that act through a common receptor. J Interferon Cytokine Res 2002;2:173–88.
32. Chawla-Sarkar M, Leaman DW, Jacobs BS, Borden EC. IFN-beta pretreatment sensitizes human melanoma cells to TRAIL/Ap02 ligand-induced apoptosis. J Immunol 2002;169:847–55.
33. Rebouillat D, Hovanessin A. The human 2',5' oligoadenylate synthetase family: activation by 2-5A. J Interferon Cytokine Res 1999;19:295–308.
34. Zhou A, Paranjape J, Brown TL, et al. Interferon action and apoptosis are defective in mice devoid of 2',5'-oligoadenylate–dependent RNase L. EMBO J 1997;16:6355–63.
35. Wang LZA, Vasavada S, Dong B, et al. Elevated levels of 2',5'-linked oligoadenylate-dependent ribonuclease L occur as an early event in colorectal tumorigenesis. Clin Cancer Res 1995;1:1421–8.
36. Carpten J, Nupponen N, Isaacs S, et al. Germline mutations in the ribonuclease L gene in families showing linkage with HPCI. Nat Genet 2002;30:181–4.
37. Hovanessian AG. Interferon-induced dsRNA-activated protein kinase (PKR): antiproliferative, antiviral and antitumoral functions. Semin Virol 1993;4:237–45.
38. Balachandran S, Kim CN, Yeh WC, et al. Activation of the dsRNA-dependent protein kinase PKR induces apoptosis through FADD-mediated death signaling. EMBO J 1998;17:6888–902.
39. Koromilas AE, Roy S, Barber GN, et al. Malignant transformation by a mutant of the IFN-inducible dsRNA-dependent protein kinase. Science 1992;257:1685–9.
40. Ramana CV, Grammatikakis N, Chernov M, et al. Regulation of c-*myc* expression by IFN-gamma through Stat1-dependent and -independent pathways. EMBO J 2000;19:263–72.
41. Harada H, Fujita T, Miyamoto M, et al. Structurally similar but functionally distinct factors, IRF-1 and IRF-2, bind to the same regulatory elements of IFN and IFN-inducible genes. Cell 1989;58:729–39.
42. Kochs G, Haener M, Aebi U, Haller O. Self-assembly of human MxA GTPase into highly ordered dynamin-like oligomers. J Biol Chem 2002;177:14172–6.
43. Mushinski JF, Nguyen P, Khanna C, et al. The interferon-inducible GTPase MxA is a metastasis suppressor. Eur J Cancer 2004;Suppl 2:46.
44. Cheng Y;Supp 2:S, Colonno RJ, Yin FH. Interferon induction of fibroblast proteins with guanylate binding activity. J Biol Chem 1983;258:7746–50.
45. Wang ZG, Ruggero D, Ronchetti S, et al. PML is essential for multiple apoptotic pathways. Nat Genet 1998;20:266–72.
46. Zhou Q, Zhao J, Al-Zoghaibi F, et al. Transcriptional control of the human plasma membrane phospholipid scramblase 1 gene is mediated by interferon-alpha. Blood 2000;95:2593–9.
47. Chawla-Sarkar M, Leaman DW, Borden EC. Preferential induction of apoptosis by interferon (IFN)-beta compared with IFN-alpha2: correlation with TRAIL/Ap02L induction in melanoma cell lines. Clin Cancer Res 2001;7:1821–31.
48. Chen Q, Gong B, Mahmoud-Ahmed AS, et al. Ap02L/TRAIL and Bcl-2-related proteins regulate type I interferon-induced apoptosis in multiple myeloma. Blood 2001;98:2183–92.
49. Kumar-Sinha C, Varambally S, Sreekumar A, Chinnaiyan AM. Molecular cross-talk between the TRAIL and interferon signaling pathways. J Biol Chem 2002;277:575–85.
50. Stein U, Walther W, Shoemaker RH. Modulation of mdr1 expression by cytokines in human colon carcinoma cells: an approach for reversal of multidrug resistance. Br J Cancer 1996;74:1384–91.
51. Goldstein D, Sielaff KM, Storer BE, et al. Human biologic response modification by interferon in the absence of measurable serum concentrations: a comparative trial of subcutaneous and intravenous interferon beta serine. J Natl Cancer Inst 1989;81:1061–8.
52. Merritt JA, Ball LA, Sielaff KM, et al. Modulation of 2',5'-oligoadenylate synthetase in patients treated with alpha-interferon: effects of dose, schedule, and route of administration. J Interferon Res 1986;6:189–98.
53. Gutterman JU, Fine S, Quesada J, et al. Recombinant leukocyte A interferon: pharmacokinetics, single-dose tolerance, and biologic effects in cancer patients. Ann Intern Med 1982;96:549–55.
54. Motzer RJ, Rakhit A, Ginsberg M, et al. Phase I trial of 40-kd branched pegylated interferon alfa-2a for patients with advanced renal cell carcinoma. J Clin Oncol 2001;19:1312–9.
55. Talpaz M, O'Brien S, Rose E, et al. Phase I study of polyethylene glycol formulation of interferon a-2b (Schering 54031) in Philadelphia chromosome positive chronic myelogenous leukemia. Blood 2001;98:1708–13.
56. Bukowski RM, Tendler C, Cutler D, et al. Treating cancer with PEG intron: pharmacokinetic profile and dosing guidelines for an improved interferon-alpha-2b formulation. Cancer 2002;95:389–96.
57. Lindsay KL, Trepo C, Heintges T, et al. A randomized, double-blind trial comparing pegylated interferon alfa-2b to interferon alfa-2b as initial treatment for chronic hepatitis C. Hepatology 2001;34:395–403.
58. Zeuzem S, Feinman SV, Rasenack J, et al. Peginterferon alfa-2a in patients with chronic hepatitis C. N Engl J Med 2000;343:1666–72.
59. Hayashi N, Kasahara A. Interferon for decreasing the incidence of hepatocellular carcinoma in patients with chronic hepatitis C. Oncology 2002;62 Suppl 1:87–93.
60. Nishiguchi S, Shiomi S, Nakatani S, et al. Prevention of hepatocellular carcinoma in patients with chronic active hepatitis C and cirrhosis. Lancet 2001;357:196–7.
61. Balkwill F, Taylor-Papadimitriou J. Interferon affects both G1 and S+G2 in cells stimulated from quiescence to growth. Nature 1978;274:798–800.
62. Gewert DR, Moore G, Tilleray VJ, Clemens MJ. Inhibition of cell proliferation by interferons: 1. Effects on cell division and DNA synthesis in human lymphoblasts (Daudi) cells. Eur J Biochem 1984;139:619–25.
63. Otsuki T, Yamada O, Sakaguchi H, et al. Human myeloma cell apoptosis induced by interferon-a. Br J Haematol 1998;103:518–29.
64. Raveh T, Hovanessian AG, Meurs EF, et al. Double-stranded RNA-dependent protein kinase mediates c-myc suppression induced by type I interferons. J Biol Chem 1996;271:25479–84.
65. Koshiji M, Adachi Y, Sogo S, et al. Apoptosis of colorectal adenocarcinoma (COLO 201) by tumour necrosis factor-alpha (TNF-α) and/or interferon-gamma (IFN-γ), resulting from down-regulation of Bcl-2 expression. Clin Exp Immunol 1998;111:211–8.
66. Samid D, Chang EH, Friedman RM. Biochemical correlates of phenotypic reversion in interferon-treated mouse cells transformed by a human oncogene. Biochem Biophys Res Commun 1984;119:21–8.
67. Kumar R, Atlas I. Interferon a induces the expression of retinoblastoma gene product in human Burkitt lymphoma Daudi cells: role in growth regulation. Proc Natl Acad Sci U S A 1992;89:6599–603.
68. Resnitzky D, Tiefenbrun N, Berissi H, Kimchi A. Interferons and interleukin 6 suppress phosphorylation of the retinoblastoma protein in growth-sensitive hematopoietic cells. Proc Natl Acad Sci U S A 1992;89:402–6.
69. Tiefenbrun N, Melamed D, Levy N, et al. Alpha interferon suppresses the cyclin D3 and cdc25A genes, leading to a reversible G0-like arrest. Mol Cell Biol 1996;16:3934–44.
70. Iwase S, Furukawa Y, Kikuchi J, et al. Modulation of E2F activity is linked to interferon-induced growth suppression of hematopoietic cells. J Biol Chem 1997;272:12406–14.
71. Melamed D, Tiefenbrun N, Yarden A, Kimchi A. Interferons and interleukin-6 suppress the DNA-binding activity of E2F in growth-sensitive hematopoietic cells. Mol Cell Biol 1993;13:5255–65.
72. Subramaniam PS, Cruz PE, Hobeika AC, Johnson HM. Type I interferon induction of the Cdk-inhibitor p21WAF1 is accompanied by order G1 arrest, differentiation and apop-

tosis of the Daudi B-cell line. Oncogene 1998;16:1885–90.
73. Samid D, Flessate DM, Greene JJ, et al. Persisting revertant after interferon treatment of oncogene-transformed cells. In: Stewart WI, Schellekens H, editors. The biology of the interferon system. Amsterdam: Elsevier; 1986. p. 327.
74. Bhatia R, McCarthy JB, Verfaillie CM. Interferon-α restores normal R-1 integrin-mediated inhibition of hematopoietic progenitor proliferation by the marrow microenvironment in chronic myelogenous leukemia. Blood 1996;87:3883–91.
75. Akyerli CB, Beksec M, Holko M, et al. Expression of IFITM1 in chronic myeloid leukemia patients. Leuk Res 2005;29:283–6.
76. Cornelissen JJ, Ploemacher RE, Wognum BW, et al. An in vitro model for cytogenetic conversion in CML. Interferon-alpha preferentially inhibits the outgrowth of malignant stem cells preserved in long-term culture. J Clin Invest 1998;102:976–83.
77. Gordon M, Marley SB, Lewis JL, et al. Treatment with interferon-alpha preferentially reduces the capacity for amplification of granulocyte-macrophage progenitors (CFU-GM) from patients with chronic myeloid leukemia but spares normal CFU-GM. J Clin Invest 1998;102:710–5.
78. Selleri C, Maciejewski J, Pane F, et al. Fas-mediated modulation of bcr/abl in chronic myelogenous leukemia results in differential effects on apoptosis. Blood 1998;92:981–9.
79. Holtschke T, Lohler J, Kanno Y, et al. Immunodeficiency and chronic myelogenous leukemia-like syndrome in mice with a targeted mutation of the ICSBP gene. Cell 1996;87:307–17.
80. Sakai I, Takeuchi K, Yamauci H, et al. Constitutive expression of SOCS3 confers resistance to IFN-alpha in chronic myelogenous leukemia cells. Blood 2002;100:2926–31.
81. Buchert A, Wolfl S, Schmidt M, et al. Interferon-alpha, but not the ABL-kinase inhibitor imatinib (STI-571), induces expression of myeloblastin and a specific T cell response in chronic myeloid leukemia. Blood 2003;101:259–64.
82. Shimuzu T, Miyakawa Y, Oda A, et al. STI-571-resistant KT-1 cells are sensitive to interferon-alpha accompanied by the loss of T-cell protein tyrosine phosphatase and prolonged phosphorylation of Stat1. Exp Hematol 2003;31:601–8.
83. Kayagaki N, Yamaguchi N, Nakayama M, et al. Type I interferons regulate tumor necrosis factor-related apoptosis-inducing ligand (TRAIL) expression on human T cells: a novel mechanism for the antitumor effects of type I IFNs. J Exp Med 1999;189:1451–60.
84. Belardelli F, Gresser I. The neglected role of type I interferon in the T-cell response. Immunol Today 1996;17:369–72.
85. Astsaturov I, Petrella T, Bagriacik EU, et al. Amplification of virus-induced antimelanoma T-cell reactivity by high-dose interferon-alpha 2b: implications for cancer vaccines. Clin Cancer Res 2003;9:4347–55.
86. Herberman R, Djeu JY, Ortaldo JR, et al. Role of interferon in augmentation of natural and antibody-dependent cytotoxicity. Cancer Treat Rep 1978;62:1893–6.
87. Edwards BS, Hawkins MJ, Borden EC. Comparative in vivo and in vitro activation of human natural killer cells by two recombinant alpha interferons differing in antiviral activity. Cancer Res 1984;44:3135–9.
88. Kleinerman ES, Kurzrock R, Wyatt D, et al. Activation or suppression of the tumoricidal properties of monocytes from cancer patients following treatment with human recombinant γ-interferon. Cancer Res 1986;46:5401–5.
89. Nathan C, Prendergast TJ, Wiebe ME. Activation of human macrophages: comparison of other cytokines to interferon-alpha. J Exp Med 1984;160:600–5.
90. Chen X, Regn S, Raffegerst S, et al. Interferon alpha in combination with GM-CSF induces the differentiation of leukemic antigen-presenting cells that have the capacity to stimulate a specific anti-leukemic cytotoxic T-cell response from patients with chronic myeloid leukemia. Br J Haematol 2000;111:596–607.
91. Parlato S, Santini SM, Lapenta C, et al. Expression of CCR-7, MIP-3beta, and Th-1 chemokines in type I IFN-induced monocyte-derived dendritic cells: importance for the rapid acquisition of potent migratory and functional activities. Blood 2001;98:3022–9.
92. Radvanyi LG, Banerjee A, Weir M, Messner H. Low levels of interferon-alpha induce CD86 (B7.2) expression and accelerate dendritic cell maturation from human peripheral blood mononuclear cells. Scand J Immunol 1999;50:499–509.
93. Moschella F, Bisikirska B, Maffei A, et al. Gene expression profiling and functional activity of human dendritic cells induced with IFN-alpha2b: implications for cancer immunotherapy. Clin Cancer Res 2003;9:2022–31.
94. Padovan E, Terracciano L, Certa U, et al. Interferon-stimulated gene 15 constitutively produced by melanoma cells induces E-cadherin expression on human dendritic cells. Cancer Res 2002;62:3453–8.
95. Santini S, Lapenta C, Logozzi M, et al. Type I interferon as a powerful adjuvant for monocyte-derived dendritic cell development and activity in vitro and in Hu-PBL-SCID mice. J Exp Med 2000;191:1777–88.
96. Buelens C, Bartholome EJ, Amraoui Z, et al. Interleukin-3 and interferon beta cooperate to induce differentiation of monocytes into dendritic cells with potent helper T-cell stimulatory properties. Blood 2002;99:993–8.
97. Reid TR, Race ER, Wolff BH, et al. Enhanced in vivo therapeutic response to IFN in mice with an in vitro interferon-resistant B-cell lymphoma. Cancer Res 1989;49:4163–9.
98. Reid LM, Minato N, Gresser I, et al. Influence of anti-mouse interferon serum on the growth and metastasis of tumor cells persistently infected with virus and of human prostatic tumors in athymic nude mice. Proc Natl Acad Sci U S A 1981;78:1171–5.
99. Lesinski GB, Anghelina M, Zimmerer J, et al. The antitumor effects of IFN-alpha are abrogated in a STAT1-deficient mouse. J Clin Invest 2003;112:170–80.
100. Balkwill FR, Moodie EM, Freedman V, Fantes KH. Human interferon inhibits the growth of established human breast tumours in the nude mouse. Int J Cancer 1982;30:231–5.
101. Sidky Y, Borden EC. Inhibition of angiogenesis by interferons: effects on tumor- and lymphocyte-induced vascular responses. Cancer Res 1987;47:5155–61.
102. Basham TY, Bourgeade MF, Creasey AA, Merigan TC. Interferon increases HLA synthesis in melanoma cells: interferon-resistant and -sensitive cell lines. Proc Natl Acad Sci U S A 1982;79:3265–9.
103. Fellous M, Nir U, Wallach D, et al. Interferon-dependent induction of mRNA for the major histocompatibility antigens in human fibroblasts and lymphoblastoid cells. Proc Natl Acad Sci U S A 1982;76:3082–6.
104. Nathan C. Secretory products of macrophages. J Clin Invest 1987;79:319–26.
105. Arenzana-Seisdedos F, Virelizier JL, Fiers W. Interferons as macrophage-activating factors. III. Preferential effects of interferon-gamma on the interleukin 1 secretory potential of fresh or aged human monocytes. J Immunol 1985;134:2444–8.
106. Greiner JW, Fisher PB, Pestka S, Schlom J. Differential effects of recombinant human leukocyte interferons on cell surface antigen expression. Cancer Res 1986;46:4984–90.
107. Borden EC. Augmented tumor-associated antigen expression by interferons. J Natl Cancer Inst 1988;80:148–9.
108. Lindner DJ. Interferons as anti-angiogenic agents. Curr Oncol Rep 2002;4:510–4.
109. Dvorak HF, Gresser I. Microvascular injury in pathogenesis of interferon-induced necrosis of subcutaneous tumors in mice. J Natl Cancer Inst 1989;81:497–502.
110. Dinney CP, Bielenberg DR, Perrotte P, et al. Inhibition of basic fibroblast growth factor expression, angiogenesis, and growth of human bladder carcinoma in mice by systemic interferon-alpha administration. Cancer Res 1998;58:808–14.
111. Singh RK, Gutman M, Bucana CD, et al. Interferons alpha and beta down-regulate the expression of basic fibroblast growth factor in human carcinomas. Proc Natl Acad Sci U S A 1995;92:4562–6.
112. Slaton J, Perrote P, Inoue K, et al. Interferon-α-mediated down-regulation of angiogenesis-related genes and therapy of bladder cancer are dependent on optimization of biological dose and schedule. Clin Cancer Res 1999;5:2726–34.
113. Koch AE, Polverini PJ, Kunkel SL, et al. Interleukin-8 as a macrophage-derived mediator of angiogenesis. Science 1992;258:1798–801.
114. Reznikov LL, Puren AJ, Fantuzzi G, et al. Spontaneous and inducible cytokine responses in healthy humans receiving a single dose of IFN-α2b: increased production of interleukin-1 receptor antagonist and suppression of IL-1-induced IL-8. J Interferon Cytokine Res 1998;18:897–903.
115. Strieter RM, Kunkel SL, Arenberg DA, et al. Interferon gamma-inducible protein 10 (IP-10), a member of the C-X-C chemokine family, is an inhibitor of angiogenesis. Biochem Biophys Res Commun 1995;210:51–7.
116. Ezekowitz A, Mulliken JB, Folkman J. Interferon alfa-2a therapy for life-threatening hemangiomas of infancy. N Engl J Med 1992;326:1456–63.
117. Krown SE. Interferon-α: evolving therapy for AIDS-associated Kaposi's sarcoma. J Interferon Cytokine Res 1998;18:209–14.
118. Budd GT. Management of angiosarcoma. Curr Oncol Rep 2002;4:515–9.
119. Quesada J, Hersh EM, Manning J, et al. Treatment of hairy-cell leukemia with recombinant alpha interferon. Blood 1985;1986:493–7.
120. Golomb HM, Jacobs A, Fefer A, et al. Alpha-2 interferon therapy of hairy-cell leukemia: a multicenter study of 64 patients. J Clin Oncol 1986;4:900–5.
121. Ratain MJ, Golomb HM, Bardawil RG, et al. Durability of responses to interferon alpha-2b in advanced hairy cell leukemia. Blood 1987;69:872–7.
122. Kantarjian HM, Deisseroth A, Kurzrock R, et al. Chronic myelogenous leukemia: a concise update. Blood 1993;82:691–703.
123. Talpaz M. Use of interferon in the treatment of chronic myelogenous leukemia. Semin Oncol 1994;21:3–7.
124. Hehlmann R, Heimpel H, Hasford J. Randomized comparison of interferon-α with busulfan and hydroxyurea in chronic myelogenous leukemia. The German CML Study Group. Blood 1994;84:4064–77.
125. Italian Cooperative Study Group on Chronic Myeloid Leukemia. Interferon-alpha 2a as compared with conventional chemotherapy for the treatment of chronic myeloid leukemia. N Engl J Med 1994;330:820–5.
126. Silver R, Woolf SH, Hehlmann R, et al. An evidence-based analysis of the effect of busulfan, hydroxyurea, interferon, and allogeneic bone marrow transplantation in treating the chronic phase of chronic myeloid leukemia: developed for the American Society of Hematology. Blood 1999;94:1517–36.
127. Italian Cooperative Study Group on Chronic Myeloid Leukemia. Long-term follow-up of the Italian trial of interferon-alpha versus conventional chemotherapy in chronic myeloid leukemia. Blood 1998;92:1541–8.
128. Liberato NL, Quaglini S, Barosi G. Cost-effectiveness of interferon alfa in chronic myelogenous leukemia. J Clin Oncol 1997;15:2673–82.
129. Guilhot F, Chastang C, Michallet M, et al. Interferon alfa-2b combined with cytarabine versus interferon alone in chronic myelogenous leukemia. French Chronic Myeloid Leukemia Study Group. N Engl J Med 1997;337:223–9.
130. Giles FJ, Kantarjian H, O'Brien S, et al. Results of therapy with interferon alpha and cyclic combination chemotherapy in patients with Philadelphia chromosome positive chronic myelogenous leukemia in early chronic phase. Leuk Lymphoma 2001;41:309–19.
131. Sacchi SKH, Smith TL, O'Brien S, et al. Early treatment decisions with interferon-alfa therapy in early chronic-phase chronic myelogenous leukemia. J Clin Oncol 1998;16:882–9.
132. Wassmann B, Scheuring U, Pfeifer H, et al. Efficacy and safety of imatinib mesylate (Gleevec) in combination with interferon-alpha (IFN-alpha) in Philadelphia chromosome-positive acute lymphoblastic leukemia (Ph+ ALL). Leukemia 2003;17:1919–24.
133. Baccarani M, Martinelli G, Rosti G, et al, GIMEMA Working Party on Chronic Myeloid Leukemia. Imatinib and pegylated human recombinant interferon-alpha2b in early chronic phase chronic myeloid leukemia. Blood 2004;104(13);4245–51.
134. Thiesing JT, Ohno-Jones S, Kolibaba KS, Druker BJ. Efficacy of STI571, an Abl tyrosine kinase inhibitor, in conjunction with other antileukemic agents against Bcr-Abl-positive cells. Blood 2000;96:3195–9.
135. Kano Y, Akutsu M, Tsunoda S, et al. In vitro cytotoxic effects of a tyrosine kinase inhibitor STI571 in combination with commonly used antileukemic agents. Blood 2001;97:1999–2007.
136. Ludwig H, Cortelezzi A, Van Camp BG. Treatment with recombinant IFN-α-2c: multiple myeloma and thrombocythaemia in myeloproliferative diseases. Oncology 1985;42 Suppl 1:19–25.
137. Talpaz M, Kurzrock R, Kantarjian H, et al. Recombinant IFN-a therapy of chromosome-negative myeloproliferative disorders with thrombocytosis. Am J Med 1989;86:554–8.
138. Gilbert H. Long-term treatment of myeloproliferative disease with interferon-α-2b: feasibility and efficacy. Cancer 1998;83:1205–13.
139. Silver R. Interferon-alpha2b: a new treatment for polycythemia vera. Ann Intern Med 1993;119:1091–2.
140. Butterfield J, Gleich GJ. Interferon-α treatment of six patients with the idiopathic hypereosinophilic syndrome. Ann Intern Med 1994;121:648–53.

141. Yamada O, Kitahara K, Imamura K, et al. Clinical and cytogenetic remission by interferon-alpha in a patient with chronic eosinophilic leukemia associated with a unique t(3;9;5) translocation. Am J Hematol 1998;58:137–41.
142. Costanzi JJ, Cooper MR, Scarffe JH, et al. Phase II study of recombinant alpha-2 interferon in resistant multiple myeloma. J Clin Oncol 1985;3654–9.
143. Quesada JR, Hawkins M, Horning S, et al. Collaborative phase I-II study of recombinant DNA-produced leukocyte interferon (clone A) in metastatic breast cancer, malignant lymphoma, and multiple myeloma. Am J Med 1984;77:427–32.
144. Oken MM, Kyle RA, Greipp PR, et al. Complete remission induction with combined VBMCP chemotherapy and interferon (rIFN alpha 2b) in patients with multiple myeloma. Leuk Lymphoma 1996;20:447–52.
145. Borden EC. Innovative treatment strategies for non-Hodgkin's lymphoma and multiple myeloma. Semin Oncol 1994;21:14–22.
146. Mandelli F, Avvisati G, Amadori S, et al. Maintenance treatment with recombinant interferon alpha-2b in patients with multiple myeloma responding to conventional induction chemotherapy. N Engl J Med 1990;322:1430–4.
147. Group NMS. Interferon-alpha 2b added to melphalan prednisone for initial and maintenance therapy in multiple myeloma. Ann Intern Med 1996;124:212–22.
148. Cunningham D, Powles R, Malpas J, et al. A randomized trial of maintenance interferon following high-dose chemotherapy in multiple myeloma: long-term follow-up results. Br J Haematol 1998;1998:495–502.
149. Browman GP, Bergsagel D, Sicheri D, et al. Randomized trial of interferon maintenance in multiple myeloma: a study of the National Cancer Institute of Canada Clinical Trials Group. J Clin Oncol 1995;13:2354–60.
150. Alexanian R, Weber D, Dimopoulos M, et al. Randomized trial of γ-interferon or dexamethasone as maintenance treatment for multiple myeloma. Am J Hematol 2000;65:204–9.
151. Salmon SE, Crowley JJ, Balcerzak SP, et al. Interferon versus interferon plus prednisone remission maintenance therapy for multiple myeloma: a Southwest Oncology Group Study. J Clin Oncol 1998;16:890–6.
152. Drayson MT, Chapman CE, Dunn JA, et al. MRC trial of alpha 2b-interferon maintenance therapy in first plateau phase of multiple myeloma. Br J Haematol 1998;101:195–202.
153. Armitage JO, Coiffier B. Activity of interferon-alpha in relapsed patients with diffuse large B-cell and peripheral T-cell non-Hodgkin's lymphoma. Ann Oncol 2000;11:359–61.
154. Bunn P, Foon KA, Ihde DC, et al. Recombinant leukocyte A interferon: an active agent in advanced cutaneous T-cell lymphomas. Ann Intern Med 1984;101:484–7.
155. Foon KA, Sherwin SA, Abrams PG, et al. Treatment of advanced non-Hodgkin's lymphoma with recombinant leukocyte A interferon. N Engl J Med 1984;311:1148–52.
156. O'Connell M, Colgan JP, Oken MM, et al. Clinical trial of recombinant leukocyte A interferon as initial therapy for favorable histology non-Hodgkin's lymphomas and chronic lymphocytic leukemia. An Eastern Cooperative Oncology Group pilot study. J Clin Oncol 1986;4:128–36.
157. Solal-Celigny P, Lepage E, Brousse N, et al. Doxorubicin containing regimen with or without interferon alfa-2b for advanced follicular lymphomas: final analysis of survival and toxicity in the Groupe d'etude des lymphomes folliculaires 86 trial. J Clin Oncol 1998;16:2332–8.
158. Smalley RV, Andersen JW, Hawkins MJ, et al. Interferon alfa combined with cytotoxic chemotherapy for patients with non-Hodgkin's lymphoma. N Engl J Med 1992;327:1336–41.
159. Hagenbeek A, Carde P, Meerwaldt JH, et al. Maintenance of remission with human recombinant interferon alfa-2a in patients with stages III and IV low-grade malignant non-Hodgkin's lymphoma. J Clin Oncol 1998;16:41–7.
160. Arranz R, Garcia-Alfonso P, Sobrino P, et al. Role of interferon alfa-2b in the induction and maintenance treatment of low-grade non-Hodgkin's lymphoma: results from a prospective, multicenter trial with double randomization. J Clin Oncol 1998;16:1538–46.
161. Smalley RV, Weller E, Hawkins MJ, et al. Final analysis of the ECOG I-COPA trial (E6484) in patients with non-Hodgkin's lymphoma treated with interferon alfa (IFN-(x2a) plus an anthracycline-based induction regimen. Leukemia 2001;15:1118–22.
162. Rohatiner AZS, Gregory WM, Peterson B, et al. A meta-analysis to evaluate the role of interferon (IFN-α2) in follicular lymphoma. J Clin Oncol 2005. [In press]
163. Fisher RI, Dana BW, LeBlanc M, et al. Interferon alfa consolidation after intensive chemotherapy does not prolong the progression-free survival of patients with low-grade non-Hodgkin's lymphoma: results of the Southwest Oncology Group Randomized Phase III Study 8809. J Clin Oncol 2000;18:2010–6.
164. Rohatiner A, Radford J, Deakin D, et al. A randomized controlled trial to evaluate the role of interferon as initial and maintenance therapy in patients with follicular lymphoma. Br J Cancer. 2001;85(1):29–35.
165. Davis TA, Maloney DG, Grillo-Lopez AJ, et al. Combination immunotherapy of relapsed or refractory low-grade or follicular non-Hodgkin's lymphoma with rituximab and interferon-γ-2a1. Clin Cancer Res 2000;6:2644–52.
166. Wood A, Angus B, Kestevan P, et al. Alpha interferon gene deletions in post-transplant lymphoma. Br J Haematol 1997;98:1002–3.
167. Faro A. Interferon-alpha and its effects on post-transplant lymphoproliferative disorders. Springer Semin Immunopathol 1998;20:425–36.
168. Creagan E, Ahmann DL, Green SJ. Phase II study of recombinant leukocyte interferon (rIFN-alpha-A) in disseminated malignant melanoma. Cancer 1984;54:2844–9.
169. Robinson W, Mughal TI, Thomas MR, et al. Treatment of metastatic melanoma with recombinant interferon alpha 2. Immunobiology 1986;172:275–82.
170. Rosenberg SA, Lotze MT, Yang JC, et al. Combination therapy with interleukin-2 and alpha-interferon for the treatment of patients with advanced cancer. J Clin Oncol 1989;7:1863–74.
171. Legha SS, Ring S, Eton O, et al. Development and results of biochemotherapy in metastatic melanoma: the University of Texas M.D. Anderson Cancer Center experience. Cancer J Sci Am 1997;3 Suppl 1:S9–15.
172. Antoine E, Benhammouda A, Bernard A, et al. Salpetriere Hospital experience with biochemotherapy in metastatic melanoma. Cancer J Sci Am 1997;3 Suppl 1:S16–21.
173. Thompson JA, Gold PJ, Markowitz DR, et al. Updated analysis of an outpatient chemoimmunotherapy regimen for treating metastatic melanoma. Cancer J Sci Am 1997;3 Suppl 1:S29–34.
174. Legha SS, Ring S, Eton O, et al. Development of a biochemotherapy regimen with concurrent administration of cisplatin, vinblastine, dacarbazine, interferon alfa, and interleukin-2 for patients with metastatic melanoma. J Clin Oncol 1998;16:1752–9.
175. Richards J, Gale D, Mehta N, Lestingi T. Combination of chemotherapy with interleukin-2 and interferon alfa for the treatment of metastatic melanoma. J Clin Oncol 1999;17:651–7.
176. Flaherty LE, Atkins M, Sosman J, et al. Outpatient biochemotherapy with interleukin-2 and interferon alfa-2b in patients with metastatic malignant melanoma: results of two phase II cytokine working group trials. J Clin Oncol 2001;19:3194–202.
177. Eton O, Legha SS, Bedikian AY, et al. Sequential biochemotherapy versus chemotherapy for metastatic melanoma: results from a phase III randomized trial. J Clin Oncol 2002;20:2045–52.
178. Ridolfi R, Chiarion-Sileni V, Guida M, et al. Cisplatin, dacarbazine with or without subcutaneous interleukin-2, and interferon alpha-2b in advanced melanoma outpatients: results from an Italian multicenter phase III randomized clinical trial. J Clin Oncol 2002;20:1600–7.
179. Atzpodien J, Neuber K, Kamanabrou D, et al. Combination chemotherapy with or without s.c. IL-2 and IFN-alpha: results of a prospectively randomized trial of the Cooperative Advanced Malignant Melanoma Chemoimmunotherapy Group (ACIMM). Br J Cancer 2002;86:179–84.
180. Kirkwood JM, Strawderman MH, Ernstoff MS, et al. Interferon alfa-2b adjuvant therapy of high-risk resected cutaneous melanoma: the Eastern Cooperative Oncology Group Trial EST 1684. J Clin Oncol 1996;14:7–17.
181. Cole BF, Gelber RD, Kirkwood JM, et al. Quality-of-life adjusted survival analysis of interferon alfa-2b adjuvant treatment of high-risk resected cutaneous melanoma: an Eastern Cooperative Oncology Group study. J Clin Oncol 1996;14:2666–73.
182. Pehamberger H, Soyer HP, Steiner A, et al. Adjuvant interferon alfa-2a treatment in resected primary stage II cutaneous melanoma. Austrian Malignant Melanoma Cooperative Group. J Clin Oncol 1998;16:1425–9.
183. Grob JJ, Dreno B, de la Salmoniere P, et al. Randomised trial of interferon alpha-2a as adjuvant therapy in resected primary melanoma thicker than 1.5 mm without clinically detectable node metastases. French Cooperative Group on Melanoma. Lancet 1998;351:1905–10.
184. Kirkwood JM, Ibrahim JG, Sondak VK, et al. High- and low-dose interferon alfa-2b in high-risk melanoma: first analysis of Intergroup trial E1690/S9111/C9190. J Clin Oncol 2000;18:2444–58.
185. Kirkwood JM, Ibrahim JG, Sosman JA, et al. High-dose interferon alfa-2b significantly prolongs relapse-free and overall survival compared with the GM2-KLH/QS-21 vaccine in patients with resected stage IIB-III melanoma: results of Intergroup trial E1694/S9512/C509801. J Clin Oncol 2001;19:2370–80.
186. Eggermont AM, Punt CJ. Does adjuvant systemic therapy with interferon alpha for stage II-III melanoma prolong survival? Am J Clin Dermatol 2003;4:531–36.
187. Bukowski RM. Cytokine therapy for metastatic renal cell carcinoma. Semin Urol Oncol 2001;19:148–54.
188. Quesada J, Rios A, Swanson D, et al. Antitumor activity of recombinant-derived interferon alpha in metastatic renal cell carcinoma. J Clin Oncol 1985;3:1522–8.
189. Members of the MRC Renal Cancer Collaborators. Interferon-α and survival in metastatic renal carcinoma: early results of a randomized controlled trial. Lancet 1999;353(9146):14–7.
190. Pyrhonen S, Salminen E, Ruutu M, et al. Prospective randomized trial of interferon alfa-2a plus vinblastine versus vinblastine alone in patients with advanced renal cell carcinoma. J Clin Oncol 1999;17:2859–67.
191. Hernberg M, Pyrhonen S, Muhonen T. Regimens with or without interferon-alpha as treatment for metastatic melanoma and renal cell carcinoma: an overview of randomized trials. J Immunother 1999;22:145–54.
192. Mickisch GH, Garin A, van Poppel H, et al. Radical nephrectomy plus interferon-alfa-based immunotherapy compared with interferon alfa alone in metastatic renal-cell carcinoma: a randomized trial. Lancet 2001;358:966–70.
193. Flanigan RC, Salmon SE, Blumenstein BA, et al. Nephrectomy followed by interferon alfa-2b compared with interferon alfa-2b alone for metastatic renal-cell cancer. N Engl J Med 2001;345:1655–9.
194. Pizzocaro G, Piva L, Colavita M, et al. Interferon adjuvant to radical nephrectomy in Robson stages II and III renal cell carcinoma: a multicentric randomized study. J Clin Oncol 2001;19:425–31.
195. Moertel C, Rubin J, Kvols LK. Therapy of metastatic carcinoid tumor and the malignant carcinoid syndrome with recombinant leukocyte A IFN. J Clin Oncol 1989;7:865–8.
196. Oberg K. Chemotherapy and biotherapy in the treatment of neuroendocrine tumours. Ann Oncol 2001;12 Suppl 2:S111–4.
197. Greenway H, Cornell RC, Tanner DJ, et al. Treatment of basal cell carcinoma with intralesional interferon. J Acad Dermatol 1986;15:437–43.
198. Belldegrun A, Franklin JR, O'Donnell MA, et al. Superficial bladder carcinoma: the role of interferon alpha. J Urol 1998;159:1793–801.
199. Berek J, Markman M, Stonebraker B, et al. Intraperitoneal interferon-alpha in residual ovarian carcinoma: a phase II Gynecologic Oncology Group study. Gynecol Oncol 1999;75:10–4.
200. Weiss K. Safety profile of interferon-alpha therapy. Semin Oncol 1998;25 (1 Suppl 1):9–13.
201. Kirkwood JM, Bender C, Agarwala S, et al. Mechanisms and management of toxicities associated with high-dose interferon alfa-2b therapy. J Clin Oncol 2002;20:3703–18.
202. Musselman DL, Lawson DH, Gumnick JF, et al. Paroxetine for the prevention of depression induced by high-dose interferon alfa. N Engl J Med 2001;344:961–6.
203. Gotoh A, Hara I, Fujiwawa M, et al. Pharmacokinetics of natural human IFN-a in hemodialysis patients. J Interferon Cytokine Res 1999;19:1117–23.
204. Freund M, von Wussow P, Diedrich H, et al. Recombinant human interferon (IFN) alpha-2b in chronic myelogenous leukemia: dose dependence of response and frequency of neutralizing anti- interferon antibodies. Br J Haematol 1989;72:350–6.
205. Itri LM, Sherman MI, Palleroni AV, et al. Incidence and clinical significance of neutralizing antibodies inpatients receiving recombinant IFN-alpha-2a. J Interferon Res 1989;9(Suppl):S9–15.
206. Casey G, Neville PJ, Plummer SJ, et al. RNASEL Arg462Gln variant is implicated in up to 13% of prostate cancer cases. Nat Genet 2002;32:581–3.
207. Fountain JW, Karayiorgou M, Ernstoff MS, et al. Homozygous deletions within human chromosome band 9p21 in melanoma. Proc Natl Acad Sci U S A 1992;89:10557–61.

208. Olopade OI, Buchhagen DL, Malik K, et al. Homozygous loss of the interferon genes defines the critical region on 9p that is deleted in lung cancers. Cancer Res 1993;53:2410–5.

209. Cairns P, Tokino K, Eby Y, Sidransky D. Homozygous deletions of 9p21 in primary human bladder tumors detected by comparative multiplex polymerase chain reaction. Cancer Res 1994;54:1422–4.

210. Johnsen A, France J, Sy MS, Harding CV. Down-regulation of the transporter for antigen presentation, proteasome subunits, and class I major histocompatibility complex in tumor cell lines. Cancer Res 1998;58:3660–7.

211. Green WB, Slovak ML, Chen IM, et al. Lack of IRF-1 expression in acute promyelocytic leukemia and in a subset of acute myeloid leukemias with del(5)(q31). Leukemia 1999;13:1960–71.

212. Ross DT, Scherf U, Eisen MB, et al. Systematic variation in gene expression patterns in human cancer cell lines. Nat Genet 2000;24:227–35.

213. Shou J, Soriano R, Hayward SW, et al. Expression profiling of a human cell line model of prostatic cancer reveals a direct involvement of interferon signaling in prostate tumor progression. Proc Natl Acad Sci U S A 2002;99:2830–5.

214. Seliger B, Atkins D, Bock M, et al. Characterization of human lymphocyte antigen class I antigen-processing machinery defects in renal cell carcinoma lesions with special emphasis on transporter-associated with antigen-processing down-regulation. Clin Cancer Res 2003;9:1721–7.

215. Hoek K, Rimm DL, Williams KR, et al. Expression profiling reveals novel pathways in the transformation of melanocytes to melanomas. Cancer Res 2004;64:5270–82.

216. Pitha-Rowe I, Petty WJ, Feng Q, et al. Microarray analyses uncover UBE1L as a candidate target gene for lung cancer chemoprevention. Cancer Res 2004;64:8109–15.

217. Karpf AR, Peterson PW, Rawlins JT, et al. Inhibition of DNA methyltransferase stimulates the expression of signal transducer and activator of transcription 1, 2, and 3 genes in colon tumor cells. Proc Natl Acad Sci U S A 1999;96:14007–12.

218. Lu R, Au WC, Yeow WS, et al. Regulation of the promoter activity of interferon regulatory factor-7 gene. Activation by interferon and silencing by hypermethylation. J Biol Chem 2000;275:31805–12.

219. Kulaeva OI, Draghici S, Tang L, et al. Epigenetic silencing of multiple interferon pathway genes after cellular immortalization. Oncogene 2003;22:4118–27.

220. Nakaii M, Yano Y, Ninomiya T, et al. IFN-alpha prevents the growth of pre-neoplastic lesions and inhibits the development of hepatocellular carcinoma in the rat. Carcinogenesis 2004;25:389–97

221. Honda K, Yanai H, Negishi H, et al. IRF-7 is the master regulator of type-I interferon-dependent immune responses. Nature 2005;434:772–7.

222. Hawkins MJ, Borden EC, Merritt JA, et al. Comparison of the biologic effects of two recombinant human interferons alpha (rA and rD) in humans. J Clin Oncol 1984;2:221–6.

223. Masci P, Bukowski R, Patten P, et al. New and modified interferons alpha: preclinical and clinical data. Current Oncol Reports 2003;5:108–13.

224. Michallet M, Mal;oisel F, Delain M, et al, PEG-Intron CML Study Group. Pegylated recombinant interferon alpha-2b vs recombinant interferon alpha-2b for the initial treatment of chronic-phase chronic myelogenous leukemia: a phase III study. Leukemia 2004;18:309–15.

49

Cytokines and Hematopoietic Growth Factors

Suhendan Ekmekcioglu, PhD
Elizabeth A. Grimm, PhD
Razelle Kurzrock, MD

Cytokines are a large family of more than 160 soluble intercellular signaling peptides produced by almost every cell in the body, including various cancer cells. Some cytokines are growth stimulatory, and others are inhibitory. Cytokines with clinical relevance to cancer include those subclassified further as interleukins, monokines, chemokines, and hematopoietic growth factors. Attempts to elicit immune activation in cancer patients using immunostimulatory interleukins, and most notably interleukin (IL)-2, have provided some success in cancer therapy. Teleologically, the fact that metastatic human cancers exist in patients with otherwise generally adequate immune systems indicates that such tumors are functionally nonimmunogenic. Presuming antigens exist on tumor cells, various immunostimulatory cytokines, and particularly interleukins, are now administered to patients in an attempt to initiate, augment, or otherwise stimulate a weak or previously nonexistent antitumor immune response. In addition to immune response stimulation, some interleukins have been used to stimulate the growth and differentiation of various subpopulations of blood cells after chemotherapy or bone marrow transplantation in a restorative role.

Interleukin designates any soluble protein or glycoprotein product of leukocytes that regulates the responses of other leukocytes. Often called the "hormones of the immune response," interleukins produce their effects primarily through paracrine interactions. The cascades of interleukins that are generated by both pathogen exposure and antigen-specific interactions are primarily local, with the functions of individual interleukins mediated by paracrine interaction with specific receptors expressed differentially on different cell types, including hematopoietic and immunologic cells, but also including endothelial and other cells. The paracrine immune effects of these interleukins include the initiation, amplification, maintenance, and termination of various phases of the immune response. Interleukins are designated by "IL" followed by their designated number in order of discovery.

It is now clear that the pleiotropic nature of many cytokines allows them to influence virtually all organ systems (Figure 49-1). In addition to their vital role in promoting hematopoietic cell growth, differentiation, and activity, these molecules are vital to the proper functioning of the central nervous system, cardiorespiratory system, alimentary tract, and liver, as well as to bone remodeling, lipid metabolism, and embryogenesis and maintenance of pregnancy. Interestingly, many of these molecules have pleiotropic effects on numerous organ systems, for example, stem cell factor influences neurogenesis and prolactin promotes erythropoiesis. Cytokines may have their own private receptor but may also share a "public" receptor with other cytokines (Tables 49-1 and 49-2).[1]

The biologic characterization of the known clinically relevant interleukins and selected cytokines, the rationale for their use in therapy for patients with cancer, and the accumulated clinical experience represent the subjects of this chapter.

HEMATOPOIESIS AND THE ROLE OF GROWTH FACTORS

Through a series of well-orchestrated divisions, hematopoietic stem cells give rise to all the blood elements: mature lymphocytes, granulocytes, monocytes, erythrocytes, and megakaryocytes/platelets. Functionally, these early progenitors are capable of self-renewal as well as proliferation and differentiation. Self-renewal occurs when a cell enters the cell cycle and undergoes one round of mitosis, giving rise to daughter cells at the same stage of development. Differentiation defines the sequence of events by which cells mature. There is a loss of self-renewal capacity as lineage commitment progresses, though some regenerative capacity may be maintained.

The development, homeostasis, trafficking, and response capacity of the hematopoietic system are tightly regulated by a complex communications network that is mediated by intercellular signals. These signals are triggered by direct cell-to-cell or cell-to-matrix contact or by the release of soluble cytokine mediators. Cytokines act on cells by interacting with specific receptors on the cell surface. This interaction promotes signal transmission across the cell membrane and activates intercellular signaling cascades that are integrated at the gene expression level. The vast majority of the soluble cytokine ligands can elicit a wide array of biologic responses. At the same time, there is considerable overlap in function between many of these cytokines.

The identification and cloning of hematopoietic growth factors have revolutionized hematology practice. Raising white blood cell counts in neutropenic patients was unimaginable until the advent of granulocyte (G)-CSF and granulocyte macrophage (GM)-CSF. Today, growth factors are routinely used to alleviate neutropenia and, to a lesser extent, thrombocytopenia and anemia after chemotherapy. They can also help mobilize stem cells for transplantation, reverse cytopenias in a variety of nonmalignant illnesses, and may have the potential to mobilize the immune system against infection or cancer.

ERYTHROPOIETIN

Erythropoietin (EPO) is the major hormone regulator of erythropoiesis. It has an established role in the treatment of anemia associated with a variety of illnesses (Table 49-3[2–7]).

Biologic Activities of EPO EPO provides a proliferative signal to early erythroid progenitors (burst forming unit-erythroid [BFU-E]) and a differentiation signal to a later erythroid precursor (colony forming unit-erythroid [CFU-E]). EPO can also promote megakaryocyte differentiation, B-cell proliferation, and endothelial cell chemotaxis.

EPO and Human Disease On the one hand, high levels of endogenous EPO are often found in patients with anemia due to cancer, especially hematologic malignancies. On the other hand, in many patients with anemia, even anemia due to cancer, there is a relative deficiency in endogenous EPO. In other words, though the levels of this molecule are elevated, they are not as high as they should be for the degree of anemia.

Certain cases of familial erythrocytosis have been attributed to the presence of EPO-hypersensitive cells. This heightened EPO response results from the formation of a truncated EPO receptor, which is missing a negative regulatory domain.[5]

EPO in the Clinic EPO is most useful in those anemias where there is an absolute or a relative deficiency in endogenous EPO levels. First used successfully as replacement therapy to correct the anemia associated with chronic renal failure, EPO is also effective at increasing hemoglobin in some patients with both solid tumors and hematologic malignancies as well as in those with a variety of other conditions (see Table 49-3).[6]

The quality of life for patients with anemic renal failure or cancer who respond to EPO is clearly improved. Although EPO has generally

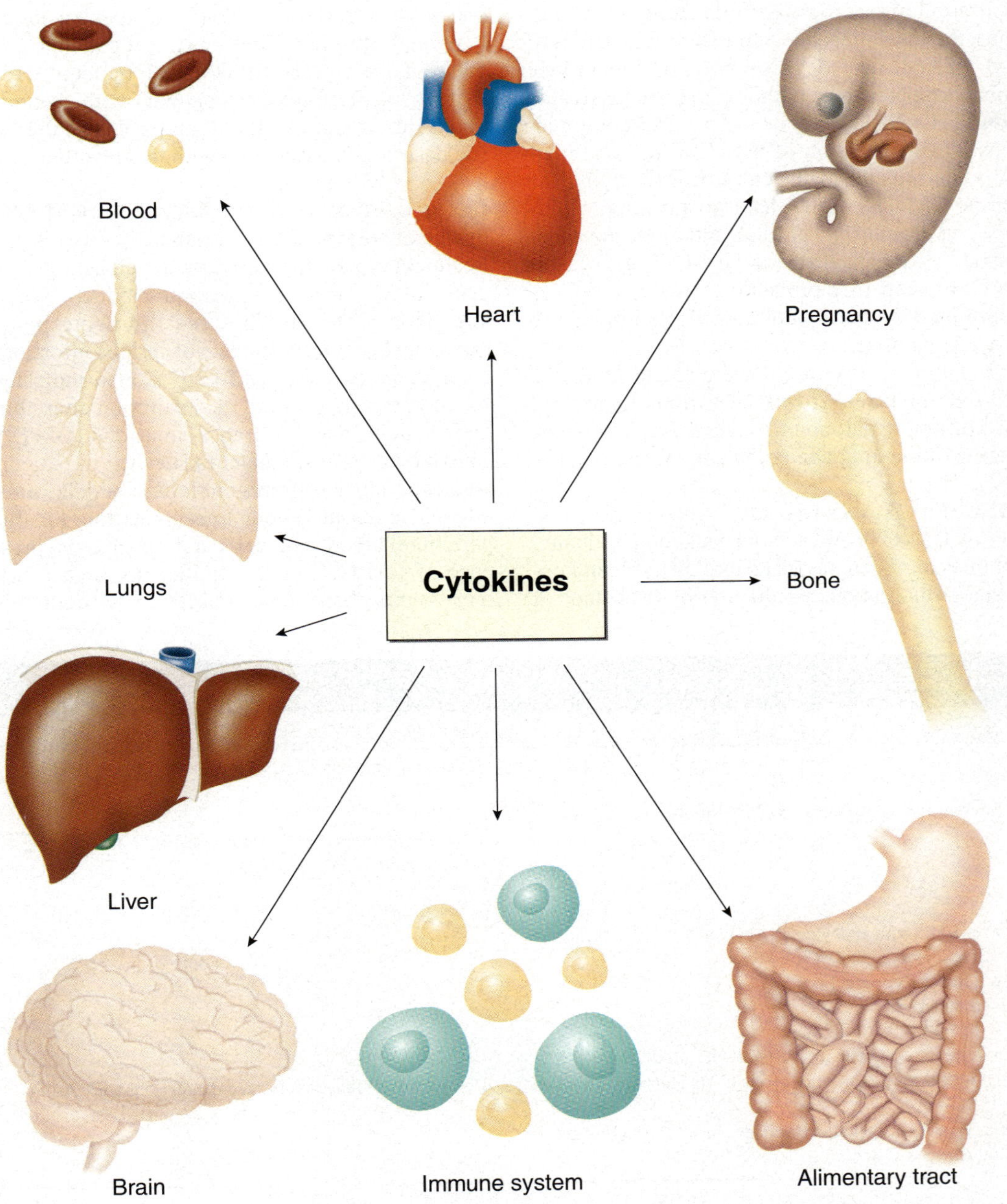

Figure 49-1 In addition to their effects on hematopoiesis and immunocompetence, "hematopoietic" growth factors influence multiple organ systems, including (but not limited to) bone remodeling, cardiorespiratory function, hepatic function, and the gastrointestinal tract.

been used for patients with hemoglobin < 10 gm/dL, the maximum improvement of quality of life actually occurs at higher levels—11 to 13 gm/dL.[7] In the case of cancer, however, not all patients respond, and those with the highest levels of endogenous EPO are probably less likely to benefit. Also, experience in patients with renal failure has revealed a state of "functional iron deficiency." Relative (or functional) iron deficiency occurs when erythropoiesis is stimulated to the point that iron cannot be mobilized rapidly enough from stores to adequately supply the erythron. Under these circumstances, percent transferrin saturation may decrease to less than 20% (though ferritin levels may be high), and hypochromic red blood cells/reticulocytes appear in the circulation despite the presence of normal or even increased iron stores. Once transferrin saturation drops, supplemental iron administration is necessary. Oral iron dosing may be inadequate for this purpose and parenteral iron administration is often necessary. For many patients on hemodialysis, aggressive parenteral iron supplementation results in substantial reductions in EPO dosage. Whether or not, and to what extent "functional iron deficiency" complicates EPO therapy of the anemia of cancer is unclear.

GRANULOCYTE-MACROPHAGE COLONY-STIMULATING FACTOR

Granulocyte-macrophage colony-stimulating factor (GM-CSF) was the first CSF to enter clinical trials. It has now been approved in many countries for treatment of neutropenia after chemotherapy or transplantation, for treatment of graft failure, and for peripheral blood stem cell mobilization (Table 49-4[8–11]).

Major Biologic Activities of GM-CSF

GM-CSF stimulates proliferation of multilineage progenitors and the growth of BFU-E, granulocyte, macrophage, and eosinophil colonies. GM-CSF also enhances the functional activity of most phagocytes, including neutrophils, macrophages, and eosinophils. In GM-CSF–deficient mice, the major morbidity results from the absence of normal phagocytic function rather than from a failure to produce phagocytes. Indeed, there is no compelling evidence that GM-CSF alone induces neutrophilic differentiation in the absence of G-CSF. It is, therefore, likely that the neutrophilic leukocytosis seen after GM-CSF treatment reflects the ability of GM-CSF to induce other growth factors, such as IL-1, which then stimulates production of G-CSF.

Experimental overexpression of GM-CSF protein has been achieved using transgenic mice

Table 49-1 Types of Hematopoietic Growth Factor Receptors[1]

Type	Characteristics	Receptor Examples
Type 1 cytokine receptor	Does not possess intrinsic kinase activity. Receptor acts as docking site for adaptor molecules, which leads to phosphorylation of cellular substrates	IL-1, IL-2, IL-3, IL-4, IL-5, IL-6, IL-7, IL-9, IL-13, IL-18, IL-21, GM-CSF, G-CSF, EPO, TPO, leukemia inhibitory factor
Type II cytokine receptor	Contains extracellular fibronectin III type domain	Interferon and IL-10
Receptors with tyrosine Kinase domains (Type III)	Large extracellular immunoglobulin-like domain, single Transmembrane spinning region, and a cytoplasmic tyrosine kinase domain(s)	fms (M-CSF receptor), FLT-3, c-kit (SCF receptor), PDGFR
Chemokine receptor	Seven transmembrane spanning G protein-linked regions	IL-8
Tumor necrosis factor family	Cysteine-rich repeats in the extracellular domain, and cytoplasmic 80 amino acid "death domain"	Tumor necrosis factor and Fas

EPO = erythropoietin; G-CSF = granulocyte colony-stimulating factor; GM-CSF = granulocyte macrophage colony-stimulating factor; IL = interleukin; M-CSF = macrophage colony-stimulating factor; SCF = stem cell factor; TPO = thrombopoietin.

Table 49-2 Receptor Subunits Shared among Cytokines[1]

Some Cytokines Using Subunit	Receptor Subunit Shared
IL-3, IL-5, and GM-CSF	β subunit
IL-2, IL-4, IL-7, IL-9, IL-15, and IL-21	IL-2 receptor γc chain
IL-2 and IL-15	β chain of IL-2 receptor
IL-4 and IL-13	IL-4Rα and IL-13Rα1
IL-6, oncostatin M, leukemia inhibitory factor, IL-11, IL-27, IL-31	gp130
IL10, IL-22, IL-28, IL-29	IL-10Rβ
IL-17, IL-25	IL-17BR
IL-19, IL-20, IL-24	IL-20Rα, IL-20Rβ
IL-20, IL-22, IL-24	IL-22Rα
IL-12, IL-23	IL-12Rβ1

GM-CSF = granulocyte macrophage colony-stimulating factor; IL = interleukin.

or by insertion of retroviral vectors expressing GM-CSF into the bone marrow of mice. The transgenic mice exhibit blindness (caused by accumulation of macrophages in the eye) and infiltration of macrophages into striated muscles. Thus, the local presence of high concentrations of GM-CSF during development of the mouse embryo appears to be pathologic. Humans treated with GM-CSF do not develop these complications. Overexpression of GM-CSF in bone marrow cells infected with retroviruses carrying the murine GM-CSF cDNA leads to a myeloproliferative syndrome that is fatal, although non-neoplastic.[8] Expression of the GM-CSF gene itself does not lead to neoplastic transformation as determined by subsequent transplantation of cells into normal mice.

A number of reports have also substantiated GM-CSF–induced growth of various tumor cell lines of nonhematopoietic origin: small-cell carcinoma of the lung and colon adenocarcinoma.

GM-CSF in Human Disease Autocrine expression of GM-CSF in myeloid leukemia cells and cell lines has been proposed to play a role in neoplasia.[9] Autonomous production by the tumor of GM-CSF (or G-CSF) has also been implicated as one possible pathophysiologic mechanism underlying leukemoid reactions in cancer patients.[10] In addition, the presence of GM-CSF biologic activity in synovial fluid from patients with rheumatoid arthritis suggests that it may enhance the tissue destruction associated with this disorder.

Clinical Indications for GM-CSF GM-CSF has been shown to be safe and effective in the treatment of patients with acute myelogenous leukemia (AML) who are undergoing induction therapy. This molecule shortens the neutropenic period and decreases the rate of serious infections in older individuals. GM-CSF is also indicated for accelerating myeloid reconstitution after allogeneic bone marrow transplantations (BMTs). This molecule also enhances survival in patients who experience engraftment failure or delay after allogeneic or autologous transplantation. Finally, peripheral blood stem cells mobilized in the presence of GM-CSF yield significantly higher colony counts than those mobilized without this

Table 49-3 Erythropoietin*

	Characteristic[2–7]	Comment
Chromosomal localization[3]	7q21	
Major production sites	Kidney, liver	Induced by hypoxia
Selected biologic activities	Promotes the proliferation, differentiation, and survival of erythroid precursors	
Receptor	EPO receptor	Class I cytokine receptor encoded at 19p13 and utilizing JAK2 and STAT5 signaling
Natural antagonists	Soluble EPO receptor	
Major clinical indications	Anemia of renal failure	
	Anemia of zidovudine therapy of HIV (with endogenous EPO level < 500 mU/mL)	
	Anemia of cancer, especially after chemotherapy of solid tumors	
	Reduction of blood transfusions in elective surgery	
	Potentiation of autologous blood donation	
	Anemia of prematurity	
	Maximum quality-of-life improvement is at hemoglobin of 11–13 gm/dL	
	Hyperglycosylated EPO (darbopoietin alfa) has prolonged half-life and can be administered less frequently	Correction of "functional iron deficiency" is important
	Postulated to offer neuroprotection after neurological damage since EPO/EOP receptors are present in the central nervous system	

EPO = erythropoietin; HIV = human immunodeficiency virus.
*Reviewed in Cazzola M.[2]

Table 49-4 Granulocyte Macrophage Colony-Stimulating Factor

	Characteristic[8–11]	Comment
Chromosomal localization[3]	5q31.1	Located 9 kb downstream of IL-3
Forms	14–35 kDa	May be variably glycosylated. Removal of the carbohydrate increases the specific activity
Production sites	T and B cells, macrophages, mast cells, thymic epithelial cells, fibroblasts, endothelial cells, mesothelial cells, osteoblasts	
Selected biologic activities	Stimulates growth of multilineage progenitors, BFU-E, granulocyte, macrophage, and eosinophil colonies	
	Induces migration and proliferation of vascular endothelial cells	
	Activates mature phagocytes (neutrophils, macrophages, eosinophils)	
Receptor	Type I receptor with alpha and beta subunits	α subunit = CD116 on Xp22.32 and Yp11.3 in the pseudoautosomal region β subunit = CDw131 at 22q12.2-13.1 β subunit shared by IL-3 and IL-5
Major clinical indications	Neutropenia due to myelosuppressive chemotherapy or BMT	
	Peripheral blood stem cell mobilization	
	Graft failure	
	After induction therapy for AML	

BFU-E = burst-forming unit erythroid; BMT = bone marrow transplantation.

Table 49-5 Granulocyte Colony-Stimulating Factor

	Characteristic[12–21]	Comment
Chromosomal localization[3]	17q11.2-q12	
Major production sites	Stromal cells, endothelial cells, fibroblasts, monocytes	Induced by TNF-α and IL-1
Forms	Differential splicing produces two forms of biologically active G-CSF	
	Two forms of G-CSF differ by three amino acids	
Selected biologic activities	Regulates production and function of neutrophils	
Receptor	G-CSF receptor	G-CSF receptor = CD114 on chromosome 1p35-34. Cytoplasmic region transduces proliferative and survival signals; C-terminal transduces differentiation signals
Major clinical indications	Neutropenia due to chemotherapy or BMT	Pegylated G-CSF is long-acting and requires only one dose per chemotherapy cycle
	Chronic and cyclic neutropenia	
	AIDS-related neutropenia	
	Autoimmune neutropenia	
	Peripheral blood stem cell mobilization	
	G-CSF reduces morbidity from high-risk febrile neutropenia treated with antibiotics	

AIDS = acquired immune deficiency syndrome; BMT = bone marrow transplantation; G-CSF = granulocyte colony-stimulating factor; TNF = tumor necrosis factor.

molecule and, after transplantation, recipients of GM-CSF–mobilized progenitors have quicker neutrophil, platelet, and red blood cell recovery and shorter hospital stays.

Although the use of GM-CSF to alleviate mucositis has been proposed, a double-blind study in which GM-CSF was administered topically failed to demonstrate salutary activity in this condition.[11]

GRANULOCYTE COLONY-STIMULATING FACTOR

Granulocyte colony-stimulating factor (G-CSF) has revolutionized the treatment of neutropenia and its sequelae (infection). It has been used by over two million patients worldwide and has been found to be remarkably effective and virtually devoid of side effects (Table 49-5[12–21]).[12,13]

Biologic Activities of G-CSF G-CSF is a relatively specific stimulator of the growth and differentiation of hematopoietic progenitor cells committed to the neutrophil lineage. It also protects neutrophils from apoptosis and enhances their function (chemotaxis, phagocytosis, oxidative responses, and microbicidal activity). Finally, G-CSF moves mature neutrophils from the marrow into the circulation.

G-CSF in Human Disease In healthy persons, mean ± SD G-CSF levels are 25 ± 19.7 pg/mL. G-CSF levels increase by 30-fold in infection and by 10,000-fold in septic shock.[18] Some patients with solid tumors present with significantly increased leukocyte counts (leukemoid reaction). In several of these individuals, elevated serum levels of G-CSF (or GM-CSF) have been demonstrated and probably account for the rise in white blood cell count.[10] Presumably, G-CSF (or GM-CSF) is produced by the tumor itself.

Point mutations in the gene for the G-CSF receptor have been described in patients with AML, which evolved from severe congenital neutropenia. These mutations truncate the C-terminal cytoplasmic region of the G-CSF receptor and hence are presumed to disrupt the maturation signal of the receptor.[14]

Clinical Indications for G-CSF G-CSF promotes a rapid increase in neutrophilic leukocytes, which lasts about 24 hours. Despite the multitude of patients who have received G-CSF, few toxicities have been reported. Even very long-term G-CSF administration appears fairly innocuous; the most common side effect is bone pain.

Studies of G-CSF as an adjunct to standard-dose cytotoxic chemotherapy for solid tumors and lymphomas demonstrate that the duration of neutropenia, the number of days of hospitalization, and the number of days of antibiotic treatment are reduced significantly during G-CSF cycles. Placebo-controlled studies in patients with small-cell lung cancer showed a clinically significant protective effect of G-CSF against febrile neutropenia.[15] Significantly more patients recovered from chemotherapy-induced neutropenia in time to receive their next chemotherapy dose while on G-CSF cycles, compared with non–G-CSF cycles. After high-dose chemotherapy (both myeloablative and nonmyeloablative), recovery from neutropenia and its associated complications is more rapid when patients receive G-CSF. These studies suggest that the dose intensity of nonmyeloablative chemotherapy (in terms of total dose per unit time) can be increased with G-CSF support, by allowing higher doses of cytotoxic agents to be administered, by compressing the duration of chemotherapy cycles, or both. The efficacy of adding G-CSF to broad-spectrum antibiotics in patients with high-risk neutropenia has recently also been demonstrated.[18]

In the transplantation setting, the administration of G-CSF results in reductions in neutropenia and infection.[16] G-CSF also mobilizes autologous peripheral blood progenitor cells; these cells are used to accelerate hematopoietic recovery in patients who have received myeloablative or myelosuppressive chemotherapy.[17]

In patients with de novo AML, G-CSF administration is associated with reductions in the time to neutrophil recovery and the duration of fever.[19] However, there are no statistically significant differences between the G-CSF–treated and the placebo-treated groups, in terms of treatment outcome parameters—complete remission or relapse-free survival.

More than 90% of patients with severe chronic neutropenias (congenital, cyclic, or idiopathic) show increases in absolute neutrophil count and reductions in the incidence of fevers, mouth ulcers, and other infection-related events after G-CSF treatment.[12,20] Finally, in patients with acquired immune deficiency syndrome (AIDS), G-CSF reverses and prevents zidovudine-induced neutropenia.[21] Of interest, G-CSF may also be useful in enhancing the defenses of non-neutropenic patients with AIDS who have bacterial infections. Studies have, however, shown only modest benefit for G-CSF in the setting of non-neutropenic infection in normal individuals.[13]

A new form of G-CSF has recently been developed—a conjugate of G-CSF and monomethoxy-polyethylene glycol. Pegylated G-CSF has a prolonged half-life because of its reduced renal clearance. Serum clearance is directly related to neutrophil number. As a result, only a single SC dose of pegylated G-CSF (Neulasta) is required after chemotherapy. Based on the results of randomized, blinded trials, this molecule is indicated to decrease the incidence of infection in patients with nonmyeloid malignancies receiving myelosuppressive chemotherapy with a significant incidence of febrile neutropenia.[21]

MACROPHAGE COLONY-STIMULATING FACTOR

The existence of a macrophage colony-stimulating factor (M-CSF) was first recognized by Robinson and colleagues in 1969.[22] Although M-CSF is now known to affect a variety of organ systems, its cardinal effect remains its ability to influence most aspects of monocyte/macrophage development and function (Table 49-6[22–26]).

Biologic Activities of M-CSF M-CSF stimulates differentiation of progenitor cells to mature monocytes, and prolongs the survival of mono-

Table 49-6 Macrophage Colony-Stimulating Factor

	Characteristic[22–26]	Comment
Chromosomal localization[3]	1p21-p13	
Forms	Three forms produced: soluble M-CSF, proteoglycan form, and membrane-bound form	Proteoglycan form binds to low density lipoprotein
Major production sites	Monocytes/macrophages Fibroblasts Epithelial cells Vascular endothelium Osteoblasts	
Selected biologic activities	Influences most aspects of monocyte/macrophage development and function Stimulates hematopoiesis Induces osteoclast production Helps maintain pregnancies Lowers cholesterol levels Affects microglial function	
Receptor	Fms	Fms is a proto-oncogene product located at 5q33-34
Major clinical trials	Enhances hematopoietic recovery after chemotherapy or transplantation Attenuates neutropenia in chronic neutropenia Lowers serum cholesterol May be useful in therapy of fungal infections	

cytes. It enhances cytotoxicity, superoxide production, phagocytosis, chemotaxis, and secondary cytokine production (G-CSF, IL-6, and IL-8) in monocytes and macrophages. In addition to stimulation of hematopoiesis, M-CSF also promotes differentiation and proliferation of osteoclast progenitor cells and has profound effects on lipid metabolism.

M-CSF is important in pregnancy. Physiologically, a large amount of this molecule is produced in the placenta, and it is believed to play an essential role in trophoblast differentiation (see Table 49-6).[24] The elevated serum M-CSF levels of early pregnancy may participate in the immunologic mechanisms responsible for the maintenance of the pregnancy.[25]

Many of the biologic effects of M-CSF are underscored by experiments with genetically engineered mice. Indeed, mice lacking M-CSF suffer from a deficiency of macrophages and osteoclasts, hematopoietic failure, and osteopetrosis.

M-CSF in Human Disease M-CSF is intricately involved in atherosclerosis, but information about its role remains contradictory. For instance, M-CSF administration lowers cholesterol levels. Paradoxically, it appears that an absence of M-CSF protects against atherosclerosis even in the presence of hyperlipidemia.[25]

M-CSF and Fms are expressed in the brain. This cytokine induces microglial proliferation, activation, and survival. Furthermore, M-CSF has been implicated in the pathogenesis of Alzheimer's disease.

M-CSF contributes to the viability of pregnancies. Levels of this cytokine are high in normal pregnancy and reduced in nonpregnant women who suffer from recurrent spontaneous abortions.

In malignancy, mutations in Fms (the M-CSF receptor) have been reported at codon 969 in about 10% of cases of human myeloid malignancies (including myelodysplasia and AML).

M-CSF in the Clinic In a large-scale double-blind controlled study, it has been shown that the administration of M-CSF to AML patients after consolidation chemotherapies shortens the periods of neutropenia and thrombocytopenia after chemotherapy and reduces the incidence and shortens the duration of febrile neutropenia.[24] Similar benefits have been reported after chemotherapy or bone marrow transplantation. M-CSF can elevate neutrophil counts in children with chronic neutropenia. Finally, preliminary results in uncontrolled trials suggest that this molecule may improve outcome after fungal infections.[26]

STEM CELL FACTOR

Stem cell factor (SCF) is also known as kit ligand, mast cell growth factor, or steel factor. It functions as a hematopoietic cytokine that triggers its biologic effect by binding to c-kit (the SCF receptor) (Table 49-7[27–38]).[27]

Biologic Activities of SCF Elizabeth Russell first suggested that the murine W and Sl loci may encode a receptor-ligand pair critical for murine hematopoiesis in vivo.[32] As mentioned above, SCF is constitutively produced by marrow stromal elements. It is now well established that SCF acts on hematopoietic stem cells and, in some lineages, mature cells.

SCF synergizes with other cytokines (including EPO, IL-3, GM-CSF, and G-CSF) to support

Table 49-7 Stem Cell Factor

	Characteristic[27–38]	Comment
Chromosomal localization[3]	12q22-12q24	
Natural forms of SCF	Transmembrane and soluble	Both forms are biologically active
Major sites of production	Marrow stroma Hematopoietic cells Gut epithelial cells Central nervous system Thymus Skin keratinocytes	IL-1 and TNF increase stromal SCF production
Selected biologic activities	Promotes hematopoiesis at multiple levels Influences primordial germ cell and melanocyte migration during embryonic life Affects immunoregulatory cells (B and T cells, mast cells, NK cells, dendritic cells) Influences hematopoietic cell adhesive properties	
Receptor	c-kit	Also known as CD117: Encoded on 4q11-q13 (piebald locus)
Natural antagonists	Soluble c-kit receptor	Kit is mutated in gastrointestinal stromal tumors
Major clinical trials	Peripheral blood progenitor mobilization (SCF + G-CSF better than SCF alone) Aplastic anemia (trilineage responses seen after SCF)	STI571 (Gleevec) targets the activated Kit Kinase activity and produces striking responses in gastrointestinal stromal tumors with Kit mutations

G-CSF = granulocyte colony stimulating factor; IL-1 = interleukin-1; NK = natural killer; SCF = stem cell factor; TNF = tumor necrosis factor.

the direct colony growth of BFU-E, CFU-GM, and CFU-granulocyte/erythroid/macrophage/megakaryocyte (GEMM) in semisolid media, and current data suggest that SCF can act on a more primitive cell (pre–CFU-C) capable of generating the direct colony-forming cells. SCF can also promote progenitor cell survival, accelerate stem cell entry into cell cycle, and function as a chemotactic and chemokinetic factor for these cells. Synergistic proliferative effects on megakaryocytic progenitor cells are observed when SCF is combined with thrombopoietin (TPO) or IL-3.[29]

In regard to lymphopoiesis, SCF enhances the proliferative response of pre-B cells to IL-7 and plays a role in the early stages of T-lymphocyte development as well as in mature T-cell function. In addition, CD34+ human hematopoietic cells can differentiate into natural killer (NK) cells in vitro in the presence of SCF plus IL-2. (NK cells are a subset of large granular lymphocytes, which are important for the immune response to viral infection and to tumor.) SCF can also amplify dendritic cell progenitor numbers in vitro; these cells are efficient at antigen presentation and play a role in T-cell immunity. The presence of SCF is probably a prerequisite for mast cell proliferation, differentiation, activation, secretory function, and chemotaxis.

SCF is also involved in processes of cell adhesion and trafficking. SCF induces progenitor cell adhesion to fibronectin, a process that may involve alteration of integrin avidity through an inside-out signal initiated in response to c-kit receptor kinase activation after ligand binding. Alternatively, it is possible that the transmembrane form of SCF displayed on fibroblasts binds directly to the c-kit receptor on the surface of hematopoietic cells and, thus, helps to anchor the hematopoietic cells in the microenvironment.[29]

Supporting the role of SCF in cellular trafficking are experiments demonstrating that primates treated with SCF show a 10- to 100-fold increase in the number of circulating progenitor cells. The effects of SCF when combined with G-CSF are even more pronounced.[34] Phase I clinical studies show that treatment with SCF increases the numbers of progenitor cells of many types (including BFU-E, CFU-GM, CFUMeg, and CFU-GEMM) in the marrow.[35]

SCF and c-kit in Human Disease The concentration of SCF in normal human serum is, on average, 3.3 ng/mL. Serum SCF levels are not elevated in patients with aplastic anemia, myelodysplasia, chronic anemia, or after marrow ablative therapy.[29] Thus, the level of SCF in the circulation, unlike the level of EPO, is not inversely related to the hematocrit.

Alterations in the local distribution of SCF within the skin have been implicated in the pathogenesis of cutaneous mastocytosis.[29] Point mutations in the c-kit receptor cytoplasmic domain have been identified in murine and human mast cell lines and in hematopoietic cells from patients with mast cell disorders.[29] Mutations in the c-kit receptor have also been found in patients with the autosomal dominant disorder piebaldism. (Human piebaldism is characterized by a white hair forelock and hypopigmented patches on the trunk and extremities, possibly because of failure of melanocyte migration during embryogenesis). Finally, activating mutations in kit characterize a type of leiomyosarcoma known as gastrointestinal stromal tumors.

Neoplastic human hematopoietic cells (in AML, anaplastic large cell lymphoma, and Hodgkin's disease) can also display the c-kit receptor. Receptor density is highest in erythroleukemia cell lines, which may express up to 50,000 to 100,000 c-kit receptors per cell. Solid tumor cell lines (including small-cell lung cancer, breast cancer, and neuroblastoma) as well as a variety of fresh human tumor tissues (particularly small-cell lung cancer, testicular seminoma, glioblastoma, and some breast cancers) also express c-kit receptor protein.[29]

SCF in the Clinic Clinical trials of SCF in a number of situations have been undertaken. SCF factor seems to be reasonably well tolerated, with the predominant side effects being transient local erythema and long-lasting hyperpigmentation (because of increased melanization) at injection sites. The most worrisome toxicity is a mast cell effect resulting in allergic-like reactions characterized by urticaria, with or without respiratory symptoms.[29] The side effects of SCF, including the allergic phenomenon, appear to be dose-dependent.

Clinical trials of SCF plus G-CSF are also underway. The incidence of allergic-like reactions was approximately 2% in 400 SCF-treated patients.[36] A randomized study in breast cancer patients demonstrated that SCF plus G-CSF is a more effective peripheral blood progenitor cell mobilization regimen than G-CSF alone.[37] Use of SCF alone and together with G-CSF has also resulted in trilineage responses in aplastic anemia patients.[38] Few side effects were seen in either study, possibly because of premedication of patients with antihistamines.

Of special interest is the role of mutations in the SCF-receptor (kit) in gastrointestinal stromal tumors. These mutations activate the kinase enzymatic activity of kit. A kinase inhibitor targeted against kit (STI571 or Gleevec) has been found to be dramatically effective in these notoriously chemotherapy-resistant tumors.[33]

THROMBOPOIETIN

The humoral basis of megakaryocyte and platelet production has been more enigmatic than that of other lineages. Factors that have now been implicated in at least some aspects of thrombocyte development include IL-3, IL-6, IL-9, IL-11, G-CSF, GM-CSF, SCF, leukemia inhibiting factor, and TPO. The latter molecule is believed to be of paramount importance in the physiologic regulation of platelet production. Unfortunately, however, compared with the striking effects of the granulopoietic factors in neutropenic patients, use of the thrombopoietic molecules in the clinic setting has met with less success. Of interest, a random-peptide-screening approach has recently permitted the identification of a 29-amino acid peptide that promotes megakaryocyte growth and platelet formation by stimulating the TPO receptor (Table 49-8[39–50]).[39]

Biologic Properties of TPO That TPO participates in hematopoiesis in general, in addition to thrombopoiesis, is supported by experiments demonstrating that genetic elimination of TPO or its receptor causes a 65 to 95% reduction in the numbers of transplantable stem cells. The survival of TPO in the circulation is longer than that of other hematopoietic growth factors (half-life = 30 hours). Consequently, when TPO is administered to animals or humans, the platelet count begins to increase after 3 to 5 days, depending on the dose and the species. In animals treated with nonablative doses of chemotherapeutic agents, radiation, or both, TPO results in higher nadir platelet counts and accelerates platelet recovery by 7 to 14 days. It also has favorable effects on the recovery of erythrocytes and granulocytes.[41]

TPO and Human Disease High serum levels of TPO have been found in patients with autosomal dominant hereditary thrombocythemia.[43] Overproduction has been attributed to a splice donor mutation in the gene for TPO, which leads to a shortened 5'-untranslated region that is more efficiently translated than its normal counterpart.[43] Because platelets themselves regulate the level of circulating TPO, high levels of TPO are also found in patients with bone marrow failure states. Homozygous elimination of c-mpl (TPO receptor) results in congenital amegakaryocytic thrombocytopenia.

TPO in the Clinic Two forms of TPO have entered clinical trials.[41,42] These forms are termed (1) TPO (the full-length polypeptide) and (2) polyethylene glycol- (PEG-) conjugated recombinant human megakaryocyte growth and development factor (PEG-rHuMGDF) (a truncated protein containing only the receptor-binding region chemically modified by the addition of PEG).

Because its biologic action is prolonged (as a result of its action on both primitive and mature hematopoietic cells and its slow clearance from plasma), parenteral administration of TPO for 7 to 10 days results in increased platelet production 6 to 16 days later.[44] Results of clinical trials of PEG-rHuMGDF or recombinant human TPO in patients with cancer who were receiving chemotherapy, albeit with regimens that produce only moderate thrombocytopenia, suggest that platelet counts return to baseline significantly faster and the nadir platelet counts are higher.[45,46] However, the effectiveness of these molecules in accelerating platelet recovery after myeloablative therapy has not been impressive.[47] Furthermore, in patients with delayed platelet recovery after peripheral-blood stem-cell or bone marrow transplantation, recombinant human TPO did not significantly raise platelet counts in most patients.[48] This study was, however, compromised by the limited number of doses given to each patient (one to five injections per month). Because

Table 49-8 Thrombopoietin

	Characteristic[39–50]	Comment
Chromosomal localization[3]	3q27-q28	
Major sites of production	Liver Kidney Smooth muscle Marrow stroma Brain	
Selected biologic properties	Major regulator of platelet production Acts in synergy with EPO to stimulate growth of erythroid progenitors Acts in synergy with IL-3 and SCF to stimulate proliferation and prolong	Homologous to murine myeloproliferative leukemia virus
Receptor	Mpl	Located on chromosome 1p34
Recombinant forms for clinical trials	TPO (the full-length polypeptide	
Major clinical trials	Accelerates platelet recovery after chemotherapy Increases platelet yield from normal donors for platelet transfusions Enhances mobilization of peripheral blood progenitor cells by G-CSF Nonimpressive effects on platelet recovery after myeloablative therapy	Trials of PEG-conjugated recombinant human megakaryocyte growth and development factor have been suspended because of antibody formation

EPO = erythropoietin; G-CSF = granulocyte colony-stimulating factor; IL-3 = interleukin-3; PEG = polyethylene glycol; PEG-rHuMGDF = PEG-conjugated recombinant human megakaryocyte growth and development factor; SCF = stem cell factor; TPO = thrombopoietin.

of the finding that platelets can remove TPO from the circulation, an issue that should be considered in future trials is the possibility that platelet transfusions may dampen the recovery of megakaryocytes after myelosuppressive therapy and may blunt response to exogenously administered TPO. Therefore, early treatment with this molecule may be more beneficial than treatment later during hematopoietic recovery.[41] Finally, TPO can result in multilineage mobilization of peripheral blood progenitor cells. The kinetics of progenitor release differs from that after G-CSF. Following G-CSF peripheral blood progenitors increase almost immediately, peak at day 5 to 6, and decrease with G-CSF cessation. In contrast, Peg-MGDF resulted in a late and sustained increase in progenitors, with levels first detected on day 8, and climbing on day 12, despite cytokine discontinuation.[50]

PEG-rHuMGDF has also been given to normal subjects in a single dose of 3 mg per kilogram of body weight. Administration of this molecule increased the yield of platelets by a factor of nearly 4 and was associated with a quadrupling of platelet counts in the recipients of the apheresed platelets.[49] Even so, because of the development of neutralizing antibodies and subsequent thrombocytopenia in some patients, clinical studies with the PEGylated molecule have been terminated.

In conclusion, the issue of whether clinically relevant thrombocytopenia can be ameliorated after chemotherapy of solid tumors may be moot, since severe thrombocytopenia is not commonly encountered in this setting. In leukemias and after transplantation, future studies will need to address dose-timing issues. Finally, since thrombocytopenia is a major cause of morbidity and mortality in bone marrow failure states (myelodysplasia, aplastic anemia, graft failure), investigations of TPO in these illnesses are urgently needed.

INTERLEUKIN-1

Interleukin-1 (IL-1α and IL-1β) is the prototypic pleiotropic cytokine (Table 49-9[51–63]).[51,52] This molecule influences nearly every cell type. Because

Table 49-9 Interleukin-1

	Characteristic[51–63]	Comment
Chromosomal localization[3]	2q13	
Natural forms	IL-1α and IL-1β (Extended family of 10 members)	
Selected biologic activities	Promotes acute phase response Induces production of multiple cytokines Up-regulates cell-surface cytokine expression Synergizes with other cytokines to stimulate hematopoietic progenitor proliferation Influences immune regulation (T- and B-cell responses) Modulates endocrine function Affects bone formation IL-1R acts as a cofactor in neural transmission IL-1 is probably not critical for normal hematopoiesis; it is, however, central in disease states	IL-1 acts on nearly every organ system[50,51] Both pro-IL-1α and IL-1α are biologically active; function intracellularly; bind to the nucleus Pro-IL-1β is not fully biologically active; after cleavage by ICE, it is excreted extracellularly where it exerts its effects
Receptors	IL-1RI and IL-1RII (Extended family of 10 members including IL-18R)	IL-1RI = CD121a at 2q12; IL-1RII = CDw121b at 2q12-q22 IL-1RI transduces a signal; IL-1RII does not
Natural antagonists	Soluble IL-1RI and IL-1RII and IL-1RA	IL-1RA binds to IL-1 receptor but has not agonist activity (acts as antagonist). Intracellular pool of IL-1RA may compete for nuclear IL-1 binding sites. Soluble receptors can bind to IL-1α, IL-1β and IL-1RA (thus antagonizing both IL-1 and its antagonist [IL-1RA]).
Major clinical trials	IL-1α and IL-1β Modest reduction in postchemotherapy neutropenia or thrombocytopenia; numerous side effects No significant antitumor activity in melanoma or renal cell carcinoma IL-1RA No clear-cut reduction in mortality in sepsis patients Amelioration of rheumatoid arthritis and graft-versus-host disease	IL-1α and IL-1β Significant toxicities encountered IL-1RA well tolerated

ICE = interleukin-1 converting enzyme; IL-1 = interleukin-1; IL-1R = interleukin-1 receptor; IL-1RA = interleukin-1 receptor antagonist of rheumatoid arthritis and graft-versus-host disease.

IL-1 is a highly inflammatory cytokine, the margin between salutary effects and serious toxicity in humans is exceedingly narrow. Compounds that attenuate the production and/or activity of IL-1 are therefore also being explored in clinical trials.

Biologic Effects of IL-1 The basis for the protean effects of IL-1 is the ability of this cytokine to modulate the expression of a wide variety of genes and surface receptors. Indeed, IL-1 can increase the expression of itself as well as many other cytokines (including IL-1RA), cytokine receptors (including IL-2, IL-3, IL-5, GM-CSF, c-kit), inflammatory mediators (such as cyclo-oxygenase and inducible nitric oxide synthase), hepatic acute phase reactants, growth factors (including, but not limited to, fibroblast growth factor, keratinocyte growth factor, hepatocyte growth factor, nerve growth factor, insulin-like growth factor, activan), clotting factors, neuropeptides, lipid-related genes, extracellular matrix molecules, and oncogenes (eg, c-*jun*, c-*abl*, c-*fms*, c-*myc*, c-*fos*).[51] IL-1 can decrease the expression of certain genes including albumin, TNF receptor p55, IL-1 receptor type 1, PDGF-α receptor, TGF-β-1, and CD34 on endothelium.[51]

IL-1 and Hematopoiesis IL-1 is able to increase the production of various CSFs and stem cell factors, either by increasing their transcription or by stabilizing their mRNA. IL-1 may have protective effects after irradiation or cytotoxic drugs. In addition, IL-1 synergizes with CSFs for expansion of bone marrow. However, evidence in mice with specifically targeted gene deletions indicates that normal hematopoiesis can take place in the absence of IL-1–converting enzyme (ICE), IL-1β, or IL-1RI. Therefore, it appears that IL-1 is not necessary for normal hematopoiesis but plays a role in hematopoietic responses to disease states. In support of this contention is the observation that spontaneous expression (sans exogenous stimulation) of IL-1 in circulating blood cells from normal volunteers cannot be detected even using sensitive polymerase chain reaction methods.[55]

IL-1 and Human Disease The IL-1 family has been implicated in the function and the dysfunction of virtually every human organ system. Indeed, increased IL-1 production has been reported in patients with infections (viral, bacterial, fungal, and parasitic), intravascular coagulation, cancer (both solid tumors and hematologic malignancies), Alzheimer's disease, autoimmune disorders, trauma (surgery), ischemic diseases (myocardial infarction), pancreatitis, graft-versus-host disease, transplant rejection, and in healthy subjects after strenuous exercise.[51] IL-1 may also participate in the development of atherosclerotic lesions.

Recently, it has been suggested that it is really the balance between IL-1 and its naturally occurring antagonists that is most relevant to illness.[53] This balance may be altered in different ways, depending on the disease. For instance, after myocardial infarction or surgery, and in asymptomatic persons infected with human immunodeficiency virus (HIV)-1, markedly elevated levels of IL-1RA are present in the circulation without elevated IL-1β. On the one hand, in body fluids from patients with infectious, inflammatory, or autoimmune disease, the molar "ratio" of endogenous IL-1RA to IL-1β is often 10 to 100, and levels of IL-1RA may be a better indicator of disease severity than are levels of IL-1β. On the other hand, in AML, IL-10 is spontaneously expressed, but IL-1RA gene expression is suppressed even when stimulated with GMCSF.[56,57] In chronic myelogenous leukemia (CML), patients with advanced disease and poor survival have suppressed IL-1RA accompanied by high IL-1β.[58] Similarly, in patients with acute Lyme arthritis, the duration of joint inflammation is longer in persons with lowest joint fluid levels of IL-1RA.

In AML and CML patients, IL-1β acts as an autocrine growth factor; exposure to molecules that decrease the activity of IL-1 suppresses leukemic proliferation.[59,60] Constitutive production of IL-lα, IL-1β, and/or IL-1RA in solid tumors (melanomas, hepatoblastoma, sarcomas, squamous cell carcinomas, transitional cell cancers, and ovarian carcinomas) has been described as well and may, in some cases, contribute to metastatic potential. However, the relationship between IL-1 and tumor growth is complex. Indeed, for some cell types, IL-1 can have growth inhibiting properties.

Finally, several presumptive autoimmune disorders (psoriasis, inflammatory bowel disease, diabetes mellitus) are associated with a polymorphism in the IL-1RA gene. Likewise, polymorphism has also been found in the promoter region of IL-1RI in patients with autoimmune diabetes.

IL-1 in the Clinic IL-lα and IL-1β have both been administered in clinical cancer trials.[51] In general, the acute toxicities of either isoform of IL-1 were greater after intravenous injection compared with subcutaneous injection. Subcutaneous injection was associated with significant local pain, erythema, and swelling. Dose-related chills and fever were observed in nearly all patients, and even a 1 ng/kg dose was pyrogenic. Nearly all patients receiving intravenous IL-1 at doses of 100 ng/kg or greater experienced significant hypotension, probably because of induction of nitric oxide.

IL-1 infusion into humans significantly increased circulating IL-6 levels and resulted in a rise in leukocyte counts, even at doses as low as 1 or 2 ng/kg. Increases in platelets were also observed in patients with normal marrow reserves. In addition, peripheral monocyte count and phorbol-induced superoxide production increased significantly.

In contrast to the results in patients with good marrow function, patients with aplastic anemia treated with 5 daily doses of IL-lα (30–100 ng/kg) had no increases in peripheral blood counts or bone marrow cellularity.[61] However, after chemotherapy, two doses of IL-10 significantly shortened the duration of neutropenia,[62] and IL-lα (5 days) significantly reduced thrombocytopenia.[63] Overall, the benefits of IL-1 therapy were compromised by its toxicity.

IL-1RA has also been administered to humans. When given intravenously to healthy volunteers, it is without side effects or changes in biochemical, hematologic, or endocrinologic parameters. These studies support the concept that there is no role for IL-1 in the regulation of body temperature, blood pressure, or hematopoiesis in health. IL-1RA has been administered to patients with sepsis in several studies, but without clear-cut reduction in mortality (though certain subgroups may benefit). Improvement after IL-1RA administration has been seen in patients with rheumatoid arthritis and with graft-versus-host disease.

INTERLEUKIN-2

Originally described as a T-cell growth factor, the function of IL-2 extends beyond lymphocyte activation and population expansion, though T cells still appear to be its major target (Table 49-10[64–68]).[64]

Table 49-10 Interleukin-2

	Characteristic[64–68]	Comment
Chromosomal localization[3]	4q26-q27	
Production sites	T cells	
Selected biologic activities	Induces proliferation and activation of T cells, B cells, and NK cells	
Receptor	αβγ heterotrimeric complex	α chain (p55) = CD25 at 10p14-p15 β chain (p75) = CD122 at 22q11.2-q13 Ψ chain (p64) = CD132 at Xq13 β chain shared by IL-2 and IL-15 γ chain shared by IL-2, IL-4, IL-7, IL-9, and IL-15
Major clinical indications	Antitumor activity in melanoma and renal cell carcinoma IL-2 diphtheria fusion toxin (DAB-IL-2) approved for use in cutaneous T-cell lymphomas	IL-2 use associated with significant toxicity

IL = interleukin; NK = natural killer.

Table 49-11 Interleukin-3

	Characteristic[77–84]	Comment
Chromosomal localization[3]	5q31	
Major product sites	Activated T cells NK cells Stimulated mast cells	
Selected biologic activities	Stimulation of multilineage hematopoietic progenitors, especially when used in combination with other cytokines (SCF, IL-1, IL-6, G-CSF, GM-CSF, EPO, TPO	
Receptor	IL-3 receptor (heterodimer of IL-3 specific α subunit and β subunit)	IL-3Rα = CDw123 at Xp22.3, Yp13.3 β subunit = CDw131 at 22q12-q13 β subunit used by receptors for GM-CSF and IL-5
Major clinical trials	Increases stem cell mobilization when used with G-CSF or GM-CSF In combination with GM-CSF, hastens bone marrow recovery after transplant Sequential IL-3 and GM-CSF produce multilineage responses in some marrow failure patients[72] Induces occasional sustained remissions in Diamond-Blackfan anemia	

EPO = erythropoietin; G-CSF = granulocyte colony-stimulating factor; GM-CSF = granulocyte macrophage colony-stimulating factor; IL = interleukin; NK = natural killer; SCF = stem cell factor; TPO = thrombopoietin.

Biologic Activities of IL-2 IL-2 primarily acts as a T-cell growth factor, but B cells, NK cells, and lymphokine-activated killer cells are also responsive to this cytokine. Following binding of IL-2 with the trimeric receptor complex, internalization occurs and cell-cycle progression is induced in association with the expression of a defined series of genes.[69] A second functional response occurs through the IL-2βγ dimeric receptor, also known as the intermediate affinity dimeric complex (kDa, 10^{-9}) and involves the differentiation of several subclasses of lymphocytes into lymphokine-activated killer (LAK) cells.[70] This response occurs in patients with cancer who receive IL-2[71,72] and was originally considered to be a critical part of the anticancer effect of IL-2. LAK cells recognize and kill tumor cells, irrespective of the histocompatibility expression status on fresh human tumor cells tested.[73] The multiple biologic effects of IL-2 on immune cells include the induced proliferation of antigen-stimulated T cells and induction of cytotoxicity in major histocompatibility complex (MHC)-restricted, antigen-specific T lymphocytes, NK cells leading to non–MHC-restricted LAK cell activity, and activation of tumoricidal monocytes; it is not clear what role any of these effector systems have in vivo.[74,75]

However, IL-2 knockout mice do not suffer from lymphopenia or immune deficiency, suggesting that IL-2 is not required for lymphopoiesis per se. (Even so, the results of knockout mice experiments should be interpreted cautiously, since it is plausible that a cytokine deficiency present in the embryonic stage could be compensated for by up-regulation of one or more other cytokines/receptors with overlapping functions. In contrast, in a normal adult animal the cytokine might play a critical role in certain biologic processes and the ability to compensate for its loss may be diminished or absent.)

IL-2 knockout mice develop a syndrome of generalized inflammatory disease involving multiple organs often with severe fatal colitis.[66] Animals made deficient in the IL-2RA gene manifest a similar phenotype. Mice lacking the IL-2Rβ chain (shared by IL-2 and IL-15) display spontaneously activated T cells, increased differentiation of B cells into plasma cells with high serum concentrations of immunoglobulins IgG and IgE, as well as autoantibodies that cause hemolytic anemia. Therefore, the essential role of IL-2 in vivo, which is not compensated for by other cytokines may be the maintenance of self-tolerance and activation-induced cell death.

IL-2 in the Clinic IL-2 has been used to treat several different cancers. There is evidence of antitumor activity in diseases such as melanoma and kidney cancer, albeit with relatively low response rates and at the cost of considerable toxicity. For instance, overall response rates of renal cell cancer to IL-2 are in the range of 15 to 25% with a complete remission rate of 5 to 10%. Complete response rates and response duration appear to favor high- rather than low-dose regimens. In melanoma biochemotherapy, regimens combing interleukin-2 and interferon-α with, for instance, cisplatin, vinblastine, and dacarbazine, produce response rates of up to 60%, but this has yet to be translated into a confirmed survival impact.[67] IL-2 has also been given to leukemic patients in a variety of doses and schedules, with hints that it might be useful in remission maintenance.[67]

Development of second-generation IL-2 analogs that do not induce the same high levels of secondary cytokines provides promise for further reduction of the toxicities, providing that the efficacy is not dependent on these secondary effects.[76] Preclinical development of IL-2 analogs is proceeding rapidly, and such molecules could be in the clinic within a few years.

Another approach to therapy has been to use IL-2 attached to a toxin to target and kill cancer cells bearing the IL-2 receptor. DAB389IL-2 is an IL-2 receptor (IL-2R) specific fusion protein. It contains the enzymatic and translocation domains of the diphtheria toxin fused to human IL-2. This chimera is able to direct the cytocidal action of the diphtheria toxin enzymatic region only to cells that bear the IL-2R. DAB389IL-2 has recently been approved for therapy of cutaneous T-cell lymphomas. Antitumor effects may also be seen in patients with other lymphoid diseases bearing the IL-2 receptor.[68]

INTERLEUKIN-3

IL-3 was first described by Lee and Ihle as a T-cell product involved in the pathogenesis of Moloney leukemia-virus-induced T-cell lymphomas.[77] This molecule is of interest because of its in vitro ability to stimulate multilineage hematopoietic progenitors (Table 49-11[77–84]).[78,79]

Biologic Properties of IL-3 The multilineage response of normal hematopoietic progenitor cells to IL-3 has been demonstrated both in vitro and in vivo. In vitro, IL-3, in combination with other cytokines, such as SCF, IL-6, IL-1, G-CSF, GM-CSF, EPO, or TPO, induces the proliferation of CFU-GM, CFU-Eo, CFU-Baso, BFU-E, and CFU-GEMM in semisolid medium, and stimulates the proliferation of purified CD34+ cells in suspension culture.[78] Indeed, in combination with other cytokines, in particular SCF, IL-6, IL-1, FL, G-CSF, and/or EPO, IL-3 is included in almost all protocols to expand hematopoietic stem and progenitor cell in vitro.

IL-3 in Human Disease In vitro data from supernatants of long-term bone marrow cultures suggest that marrow stromal cells produce reduced levels of IL-3 in patients with aplastic anemia.[81]

IL-3 mRNA has been detected in allergen-induced type I responses in the nasal mucosa as well as in late-phase cutaneous reactions of atopic subjects, being coordinately expressed with GM-CSF, IL-5, and IL-4. The eosinophilia in tissues from chronic hyperplastic sinusitis was found to correlate with IL-3 and GM-CSF mRNA detected by in situ hybridization.[79]

Finally, IL-3 has also been implicated in acute lymphocytic leukemia (ALL) with a t(5:14)(q31;q32) translocation.[82] In two such patients, the translocation resulted in juxtaposition of the IL-3 gene and the Ig heavy chain gene, and excess IL-3 transcripts were produced by the leukemic cells, perhaps explaining the eosinophilia seen in these patients.

IL-3 in the Clinic IL-3 has been used in a variety of clinical trials: peripheral blood stem cell mobilization, postchemotherapy and transplantation, and

Table 49-12 Interleukin-4 and Interleukin-13

	Characteristic[86–95]	Comment
Chromosomal localization[3]	5q31	The IL-13 gene is located 12 kb 5' upstream to IL-4 and is linked to it in a "tail-to-head" fashion
Major production sites	IL-4 T cells (Th0 and Th2), basophils, mast cells, eosinophils IL-13 T cells (Th0, Th1, and Th2), basophils, mast cells, B cells	
Selected biologic activities	Both IL-4 and IL-13 are involved in allergic reaction(induce switch to IgE)	IL-4, but not IL-13, promotes T-cell growth and differentiation (perhaps because T cells lack IL-13 receptors)
Receptor	IL-4 and IL-13 receptors share subunits Type I IL-4 receptor (IL-4Rα and IL-2 receptor γc chain subunits) transduce IL-4; type II IL-4 receptor (IL-4Rα and the IL-13Rα1 subunits) transduce IL-4 and IL-13; IL-4Rα and IL-13Rα2 complex or two IL-13Rα transduce IL-13	IL-4Rα = CD124 at 16p11-p12; γc chain = CD132 at Xq13 IL-2 receptor γc chain is common to receptors for IL-2, IL-4, IL-7, IL-9, and IL-15
Natural antagonists	Soluble IL-4 and IL-13 exist	
Major clinical trials	Only minor antitumor activity has been seen in a variety of human cancers of IL-4	IL-4 is well tolerated

IL = interleukin.

bone marrow failure states. The majority of studies show only modest effects of IL-3 by itself; however, in conjunction with other growth factors, significant salutary effects are demonstrated. For instance, in the mobilization studies, treatment with IL-3 did not mobilize by itself but significantly potentiated G-CSF–induced yield of all progenitor cell types used to restore hematopoiesis after high-dose chemotherapy. After transplantation, the combination of IL-3 and GM-CSF proved more efficient to support bone marrow engraftment than IL-3 or GM-CSF alone. The combination of IL-3 and GM-CSF was more efficient than G-CSF for supporting platelet recovery, but was of similar benefit for the reconstitution of myelopoiesis. Following chemotherapy, IL-3 was found to attenuate neutropenia and/or thrombocytopenia in some but not all clinical studies. A significant benefit of IL-3 as compared with G-CSF or GM-CSF after chemotherapy has not yet been established.

In a recent European multicenter study, 3 of 40 patients with Diamond-Blackfan anemia achieved sustained remission off all therapy, for 3 years in one case.[83] Modest increases in platelets, hemoglobin, and neutrophil counts have also occasionally been seen in patients with myelodysplasia or aplastic anemia treated with IL-3.[84] Significantly better results have been observed in patients with bone marrow failure treated with IL-3 followed by GM-CSF. At IL-3 dosages > 1.2 μg/kg/d, 7 of 16 patients (44%) with severe pancytopenia had multilineage responses with normalization or near-normalization of blood counts. Although prolonged therapy was necessary to achieve maximal hematopoietic recovery, responses were durable for up to 4 years after discontinuation of treatment.[80,85]

Side effects of IL-3 include dose-dependent fever, rash, fatigue, diarrhea, rigor, musculoskeletal pain, chills, headache, conjunctivitis, edema, chest pain, dyspnea, decreases in platelet counts, increases in basophilic counts, marrow fibrosis, and pulmonary edema. The tolerance to IL-3 appears to be several-fold better in patients with bone marrow failure states, as compared with those treated after chemotherapy.[80]

INTERLEUKIN-4 AND INTERLEUKIN-13

IL-4, identified in 1982, and IL-13, discovered several years later, are closely related.[86–88] They share biologic and immunoregulatory functions on B cells, monocytes, dendritic cells, and fibroblasts. Both IL-4 and IL-13 genes are located in the same vicinity on chromosome 5. The major regulatory sequences in the IL-4 and IL-13 promoters are identical, thus explaining their restricted expression pattern in activated T cells and mast cells. Furthermore, the IL-4 and IL-13 receptors are multimeric and share at least one common chain—IL-4RA. This, together with similarities in IL-4 and IL-13 signal transduction, explains the striking overlap of biologic properties between these two cytokines (Table 49-12[86–95]). The inability of IL-13 to regulate T-cell differentiation due to a lack of IL-13 receptors on T lymphocytes, however, represents a major difference between these cytokines. Therefore, despite the impact redundancy of these two molecules, regulatory mechanisms are in place to guarantee their distinct functions.

Biologic Activities of IL-4 and IL-13 IL-13 elicits many, but not all, of the biologic actions of IL-4. IL-4 is, however, distinguished from IL-13 by its T-cell growth factor activity and its ability to drive differentiation of Th0 precursors toward the Th2 lineage. (Th2 cells secrete IL-4 and IL-5 and lead to a preferential stimulation of humoral immunity. In contrast, Th1 cells, which produce IL-2 and interferon [IFN]-γ, lead to a preferential stimulation of cellular immunity.)

IL-4 and IL-13 in Human Disease IL-4 and IL-13 play a key role in the development of the allergic reaction at the effector level by inducing the switch toward IgE. Atopic blood mononuclear cells display an increased capacity to produce IL-4 and allergen immunotherapy greatly reduces IL-4 production. Furthermore, spontaneous IgE synthesis in vitro by lymphocytes from patients with atopic dermatitis is partially inhibited by anti–IL-4 and anti–IL-13 antibodies.

In vitro and animal models show that IL-4 and IL-13 also have anti-inflammatory effects, which have been demonstrated on synovium from rheumatoid arthritis. IL-4 can also inhibit the production of IL-6 and leukemia inhibitory factor. Finally, IL-4 can suppress stromal cell proliferation in vitro in long-term bone marrow cultures, suggesting its possible utility in myelofibrosis.[90]

IL-4 and IL-13 possess potent antitumor activity in vivo in mice. Tumorigenic IL-4-transfected plasmacytoma cell lines fail to grow in nude mice, and these IL-4 producing tumor cells inhibit the growth of other tumors.[91] Finally, IL-4 can inhibit the proliferation of some human cancer cell lines (including various hematologic malignancies as well as nonsmall-cell lung cancer, colon cancer, head and neck carcinomas, glioblastomas) in vitro as well as in vivo in nude mice. A similar antiproliferative effect of IL-13 on human breast cancer cells has been described. Moreover, a chimeric protein composed of IL-13 and a truncated form of *Pseudomonas* exotoxin A exhibits specific cytotoxic activity toward human renal cell carcinoma, but not against normal hemopoietic cells.[92] Similarly, a recombinant IL-4 *Pseudomonas* exotoxin effectively targets IL-4 receptors on glioblastomas in animal models.

Clinical Trials of IL-4 Despite the preclinical promise of IL-4, to date, clinical trials of this molecule in humans demonstrated that although the molecule is safe and nontoxic, only sporadic antitumor activity in a variety of cancers, including melanoma, lung cancer, and AIDS-related Kaposi's sarcoma, is observed.[93–95]

INTERLEUKIN-5

IL-5 is a T-cell–derived cytokine involved in the pathogenesis of atopic diseases. It specifically controls the production, activation, and localization of eosinophils. Eosinophils mediate allergic and asthmatic symptoms. T cells purified from the bronchoalveolar lavage (BAL) and peripheral blood of asthmatics secrete an elevated amount of IL-5. Therefore, agents that suppress either the production or the activity of IL-5 would be expected to ameliorate the pathologic effects of the allergic response (Table 49-13[96–103]).[96]

Biologic Activities of IL-5 IL-5 plays a central role in the control of eosinophilia. This cytokine affects the production and function of eosinophils and their tissue migration and localization. In addition, IL-5 promotes eosinophil survival by inhibiting their apoptosis.[98] Although eosinophils are involved in a wide range of dis-

Table 49-13 Interleukin-5

	Characteristic[96–103]	Comment
Chromosomal localization[3]	5q31	Part of gene cluster encoding IL-3, IL-4, and GM-CSF
Structure	Structurally related to IL-3, IL-4, M-CSF, and GM-CSF	
Major production sites	Activated CD4+ T cells, mast cells, CD8+ T cells	Mostly produced by Th2 cells
Selected biologic activities	Regulates production, function, survival, and migration of eosinophils Enhances basophil number and function	
Receptor	Consists of IL-5Rα (IL-5-specific) and a β subunit β subunit is common to IL-3 and GM-CSF complexes	IL-5Rα = CDw125 located at 3p26-24 β subunit = CD2131 at 22q12-q13
Potential clinical application	IL-5 antagonists may be useful in treatment of allergy and asthma; however, trial of monoclonal antibody against IL-5 was not effective in asthma	

GM-CSF = granulocyte macrophage colony-stimulating factor; IL = interleukin.

eases, their numbers are significantly increased in both helminthic infections and allergy.

IL-5 also enhances basophil numbers and can prime human basophils for histamine release; and leukotriene production and specific receptors have been shown on the cell surface.

Another target for IL-5 is the T cell itself. Interestingly, IL-5 enhances IL-2–dependent differentiation and proliferation of T cells, although no receptors for IL-5 have been demonstrated on these cells.

IL-5 and Human Disease T cells in the bronchial alveolar lavage of atopic asthmatics show elevated expression of IL-4 and IL-5. In contrast, T cells purified from peripheral blood of non-atopic asthmatics secrete elevated amounts of IL-5, but not IL-4, as compared with normal controls. Monoclonal antibodies against IL-5 have been shown to reduce eosinophil influx and decrease bronchial hyperreactivity in animal models.[99] However, such an antibody failed to show responses in a clinical trial of allergen-induced airway diseases. The implications of these trials on the role of IL-5 and eosinophils in asthma are still being debated.[99]

Interestingly, IL-5 is secreted from Reed-Sternberg cells and may, therefore, be the cause of eosinophilia in patients with Hodgkin's disease.[100]

IL-5 also promotes eosinophil infiltration and parasite killing in helminthic infections.[101] Finally, in bullous pemphigoid, IL-5 production may lead to eosinophil infiltration and activation resulting in basement membrane damage.[103]

INTERLEUKIN 6

IL-6 was first cloned in 1986.[104] It is a typical cytokine, exhibiting functional pleiotropy and redundancy (Table 49-14[104–120]). IL-6 is involved in the immune response, inflammation, and hematopoiesis. Indeed, prior to its complete characterization, this molecule was variously referred to as interferon-β2, B-cell stimulatory factor 2, human plasmacytoma growth factor, or hepatocyte stimulatory factor. IL-6 is a 21- to 30-kDa glycoprotein of 212 amino acids that binds to a specific receptor that requires the same 130-kDa membrane glycoprotein for mediation of signal transduction, as has been described for several cytokines, including IL-2.[121,122] The biologic effects of IL-6 include synthesis of acute phase reactants in the liver, as well as effects on the hypothalamic-pituitary axis, bone resorption, and on both the humoral and cellular arms of the immune system.[123–127] As a major inducer of the acute-phase response, this cytokine may play a role in the pathogenesis of sepsis.

Biologic Activities of IL-6 IL-6 is a potent and essential factor for the normal development and function of both B and T lymphocytes.[107] This molecule is also involved in a panoply of other biologic activities: (1) differentiation of myeloid leukemic cell lines into macrophages, (2) megakaryocyte maturation, (3) neural differentiation, (4) osteoclast development, and (5) acute-phase protein synthesis in hepatocytes (see Table 49-14).[108]

IL-6 and Human Disease IL-6 acts as a growth factor for myeloma/plasmacytoma, keratinocytes, mesangial cells, renal cell carcinoma, and Kaposi's sarcoma and promotes the growth of hematopoietic stem cells. On the other hand, IL-6 also inhibits the growth of myeloid leukemic cell lines and certain carcinoma cell lines. IL-6 transgenic mice

Table 49-14 Interleukin-6

	Characteristic[104–120]	Comment
Chromosomal localization[3]	7p21	
Major production sites	Activated B and T cells Monocytes Fibroblasts Endothelial cells Keratinocytes Synovial cells Stromal cells	Inducers: IL-1, lipopolysaccharide, IFN-gamma, platelet-derived growth factor, GM-CSF, and TNF Inhibitors: Glucocorticoids
Selected biologic activates	B- and T-cell development and function Thrombopoiesis Acute phase protein synthesis Inhibition of hepatic albumin excretion Osteoclastic bone resorption Neural differentiation	
Receptor	IL-6Rα together with gp130	IL-6Rα = CD126 at 1q21 gp130 = CD130 at 5q11 gp130 is also used by leukemia inhibitory factor and IL-11 Soluble IL-6 receptors exist but have agonist action. Can interact with cells that have gp130 but not IL-1Rα.
Major clinical trials	Response rates = 8–14% in melanoma and renal cell carcinoma Modest platelet-enhancing ability post-chemotherapy or autologous transplant with significant toxicity Antibody to block IL-6 is entering clinical trial	

GM-CSF = granulocyte macrophage colony-stimulating factor; IFN = interferon; IL = interleukin; TNF = tumor necrosis factor.

Table 49-15 Interleukin-7

	Characteristic[129–137]	Comment
Chromosomal localization[3]	8q12-q13	
Major production sites	Stroma of thymus and bone marrow, keratinocytes, intestinal epithelium, liver, dendritic cells (not produced by lymphocytes)	
Selected biologic activities	Critical for T- and B-cell development	
Receptor	Composed of IL-7Rα (CD127) and the common γc chain subunits	IL-7Rα = CD127 at 5p13 γc chain = CD132 at Xq13 γc chain is common to receptors for IL-2, IL-4, IL-7, IL-9, and IL-15

IL = interleukin; IL-7R = interleukin-7 receptor.

or mice bearing a retrovirus vector expressing IL-6 show massive plasmacytosis, hypergammaglobulinemia, an increase in acute-phase proteins, and eventually develop plasmacytoma.[109]

Significant correlations between serum IL-6 activity and serum levels of acute-phase proteins have been demonstrated in a variety of inflammatory conditions. IL-6 may be involved in the abnormalities seen in patients with cardiac myxoma who show hypergammaglobulinemia. Abnormal IL-6 production may participate in the pathophysiology of rheumatoid arthritis and aberrant expression of the IL-6 receptor is seen in several autoimmune diseases.[110]

IL-6 has been implicated as a mediator of B symptoms in lymphoma.[111] Elevated serum IL-6 levels have also been associated with an adverse prognosis in both Hodgkin's and non-Hodgkin's lymphoma.[105,112–115] In diffuse large-cell lymphoma, IL-6 levels were found to be the single most important independent prognostic factor selected in multivariate analysis for predicting complete remission rate and relapse-free survival.[115] IL-6 levels may also be exploitable as a prognostic factor in renal cell carcinoma and multiple myeloma, and high levels are observed in prostate and ovarian cancer as well. IL-6 probably also plays an etiologic role in the systemic manifestations of the lymphoproliferative disorder Castleman disease.[116] High IL-6 levels are also an adverse prognostic factor in pancreatic cancer.[128]

Finally, it should be mentioned that IL-6 levels are high in a variety of infections as well as in other inflammatory conditions, such as burns. Soluble IL-6 receptors have also been demonstrated to be high in many of these conditions.

IL-6 in the Clinic In patients undergoing chemotherapy or autologous transplantation, IL-6 has minimal to no platelet-enhancing activity at tolerable doses. Toxicity includes fever and anemia.[117–119]

IL-6 has also been tested as an antitumor agent in melanoma and renal cell carcinoma. Response rates have been low (< 15%).[108] Because high levels of IL-6 correlate with an adverse outcome in many cancers and functions as an autocrine/paracrine growth factor in some tumors, clinical studies of an IL-6 inhibitor may be worthwhile.

INTERLEUKIN-7

IL-7 was identified and cloned on the basis of its ability to induce proliferation of B-cell progenitors in the absence of stromal cells (Table 49-15[129–137]).[129] It is now known that this cytokine is secreted by stromal cells in the bone marrow and thymus and is irreplaceable in the development of both B and T cells.[130–132] Indeed, the nonredundant nature of IL-7 is underscored by the observation that ablation of IL-7 or parts of the IL-7 receptor in gene knockout mice ineluctably leads to a profound defect in lymphocyte development.

Biologic Activities of IL-7/IL-7 Receptor The major sites for the production of T and B cells are the thymus and the bone marrow, respectively. The T cells of the thymus are the progeny of progenitors initially generated in the bone marrow. Numerous cytokines play a role in B- and T-cell development. However, most single cytokine knockout mice show relatively normal B- and T-cell compartments (though immune function may be compromised), indicating that many cytokine functions are redundant. In contrast, IL-7–deficient mice present with striking lymphocyte depletion in both the thymus and bone marrow. Collectively, these genetic experiments identify clearly distinct in vivo roles for various lymphoid factors. IL-2 and IL-4 function by influencing mature lymphocyte populations during immune responses, whereas IL-7 plays a singularly dominant role for the production and expansion of lymphocytes.

All lymphocytes are derived from hematopoietic stem cells. The up-regulation of the IL-7R occurs at the stage of the clonogenic common lymphoid progenitor, a recently identified population that can give rise to all lymphoid lineages at a single cell level.[135] There are at least three principal means by which IL-7R–mediated signals act in lymphocyte development: enhancement of proliferation, triggering of lineage-specific developmental programs, and maintenance of viability of appropriately selected cells. After the common lymphoid progenitor commits to either the T- or the B-cell lineage, the IL-7R apparently begins to mediate different nonredundant signals for each lineage. The most important intracellular event for lymphoid commitment is the variable, diversity, joining recombination of immunoglobulin and T-cell receptor genes. These rearrangements allow lymphocytes to acquire the diversity of variable domains necessary for antigen recognition. The IL-7R plays a critical role in the rearrangement process.[131] IL-7 signaling also promotes the survival of developing thymocytes and mature T cells, presumably by up-regulating Bcl-2.[135]

IL-7 and Human Disease High IL-7 levels are found in states of T-cell depletion and may, therefore, play a role in promoting T-cell expansion.[136] High levels of IL-7 are also found in chronic lymphocytic leukemia and in Burkitt's lymphoma, and transgenic mice overexpressing the IL-7 gene show dramatic changes in lymphocyte development, which, in some instances, can result in the formation of lymphoid tumors.[137]

INTERLEUKIN-8

IL-8 was first identified in 1987 as a potent, proinflammatory chemokine that induces trafficking of neutrophils across the vascular wall (chemotaxis) (Table 49-16[138–146]).[138] This molecule belongs to a chemokine superfamily whose members include neutrophil-activating peptide-2, platelet factor-4, growth-related cytokine (GRO) (also known as melanoma growth-stimulating activity), and interferon inducible protein-10, all of which are responsible for the directional migration of various cells.[139] Interestingly, IL-8 receptor demonstrates strong homology to a gene encoded by human herpesvirus-8 (HHV-8) (implicated in the etiology of Kaposi's sarcoma).[140,141]

Biologic Activity of IL-8 The chemotactic agents generated by inflammatory stimuli recruit the circulating leukocytes, in particular neutrophils, for defensive purposes and direct them to injury sites. The migration of circulating leukocytes is viewed as a multistep process, which consists of (1) leukocyte rolling along the endothelial lining, (2) accelerated activation of leukocyte integrins, (3) adhesion of the cells to endothelial ligands, and (4) diapedesis (migration across the vascular wall). The leukocytes follow the IL-8 concentration gradient and accumulate at the location of elevated concentration. These processes play a fundamental role in the host defense since activated leukocytes act to kill and engulf invading bacteria at the site of injury.

Among the neutrophil-affecting chemokines, IL-8 is one of the most potent.[143] On exposure to a chemokine, neutrophils are activated, and within seconds, their shapes are changed. The process of shape change is crucial. It is modulated by perturbations of cellular integrins and the actin cytoskeleton. The activation and up-regulation of integrins also permits the adherence of the neutrophils to the endothelial cells of the vessel wall so as to allow for subsequent migration into the tissues. The actin molecules polymerize and break down to form the lamellipodia, which assists in the migration of cells by acting like arms and legs.

Table 49-16 Interleukin-8

	Characteristic[138–146]	Comment
Chromosomal localization[3]	4q12-q13	
Forms	8 kDa molecule. Four forms (79, 77, 72, and 69 amino acids) exist	Forms are tissue specific
Major production sites	Monocytes, neutrophils, T cells, fibroblasts, endothelial cells, epithelial cells	Up-regulators IL-1α, IL-1β, TNF-α, IL-3, microorganisms, hypoxia, acidosis, nitric oxide Suppressors IL-4, TGF-β, glucocorticoids
Selected biologic activities	Potent chemoattractant agent for a variety of leukocytes, especially neutrophils Suppresses colony formation of immature myeloid progenitors Increases keratinocyte and endothelial cell proliferation Increases adhesiveness of melanoma cells	
Receptor	IL-8Rα and IL-8Rβ exist	IL-8Rα and IL-8Rβ reside at 2q35 IL-8 receptor is homologous to a gene encoded by HHV-8
Potential clinical application	Antibodies to block IL-8 are entering clinical trial	

HHV-8 = human herpesvirus-8; IL = interleukin; TGF = transforming growth factor; TNF = tumor necrosis factor.

Although neutrophil activation appears to be the major task of IL-8, the production of this cytokine by a large variety of cells is indicative of functional pleiotropy. Indeed, basophils, T lymphocytes, and endothelial cells have also been found to show chemotactic responses to IL-8. Moreover, IL-8 can activate integrins in monocytes and eosinophils, hence contributing to their adhesion to endothelial cells.

IL-8 in Human Disease In the synovium of patients suffering from rheumatoid arthritis, IL-8 is part of the cytokine cascade. The production of IL-8 in large quantities has also been associated with other inflammatory diseases: asthma, leprosy, psoriasis, inflammatory bowel disease, atherosclerosis, cystic fibrosis, and in various respiratory syndromes.[139] Consonant with these observations is the demonstration, in animal models, that compounds interfering with the chemokine system can be exploited for anti-inflammatory therapy.[144]

IL-8 can induce tumor growth, an effect attributed to its angiogenic activity, a property that promotes vascularization. On the one hand, the administration of anti–IL-8 to SCID mice bearing xenografts of IL-8–expressing human lung cancer has been shown to have beneficial effects.[145] On the other hand, antitumor effects of IL-8 have also been reported. Of interest in this regard is the fact that increased levels of IL-8 have been discerned in lung carcinomas and in melanomas. IL-8 may be a growth factor for pancreatic cancer and for melanoma.[139] In melanomas, IL-8 levels correlate with the growth and metastatic potential of the tumor cells, and exposure of the cells to interferon (an agent with known antitumor activity in melanoma) decreases IL-8 levels and cancer cell proliferation.[146] Blocking IL-8 or IL-8R has been suggested as a therapeutic strategy.[139]

INTERLEUKIN-9

Human IL-9 was initially identified and cloned by Yang and colleagues as a mitogenic factor for a human megakaryoblastic leukemia.[147] More recently, IL-9 targets were found to encompass a wide range of cells (Table 49-17[147–150]).[148,149]

Biologic Activities of IL-9 Cellular elements responsive to IL-9 include erythroid progenitors, human T cells, B cells, fetal thymocytes, thymic lymphomas, and immature neuronal cell lines.[148]

IL-9 can support the clonogenic maturation of erythroid progenitors in the presence of EPO. By contrast, granulocyte or macrophage colony formation (CFU-GM, CFU-G, or CFU-M) is usually not influenced by IL-9. Experiments comparing the effects of IL-9 on fetal and adult progenitors have shown that IL-9 is more effective on fetal cells. Cells, which are activated, are also more likely to be responsive to this cytokine. In addition to its proliferative activity, IL-9 also seems to be a potent regulator of mast cell effector molecules. It should also be mentioned that there is frequent synergy between IL-9 and other cytokines, such as IL-2 (for fetal thymocytes and lymphomas), IL-4 (for immunoglobulin production), EPO (for erythroid differentiation), and IL-3 (for mast cell proliferation).

A role for hematopoietic cytokines in the differentiation of neuronal cells has been suggested by studies on immortalized murine embryonic hippocampal progenitor cell lines. In combination with basic fibroblast growth factor and transforming growth factor-a, IL-9 enhanced neurite outgrowth as well as other morphologic modifications and conferred electrical excitability to these cells.[150]

IL-9 in Human Disease There is an interesting paradox between the unresponsiveness of normal T cells to IL-9 and the potent activity of this molecule on lymphoma cells. This contrast is illustrated by the observation that murine T cells acquire the ability to respond to IL-9 after a long period of in vitro culture, while they simultaneously acquire characteristics of tumor cell lines. Observations made with transgenic mice also demonstrate the oncogenic potential of dysregulated IL-9 production since 5 to 10% of mice that overexpress this cytokine develop lymphoblastic lymphomas.[149] In line with these data, constitutive IL-9 production by human Hodgkin's lymphomas and large-cell anaplastic lymphomas has now been clearly documented.[148] Even so, the pathophysiologic role of IL-9 remains elusive.

The activity of IL-9 as a mast cell differentiation factor and its potential role in IgE production also raise the hypothesis that IL-9 could be involved in some allergic processes, such as asthma.

INTERLEUKIN-10

IL-10 is a pleiotropic cytokine discovered in 1989 as an activity produced by murine type 2 helper T cells (Th2) (Table 49-18[151–163]).[151,152] It was initially designated as cytokine synthesis inhibitory factor because of its ability to inhibit the production of certain cytokines by (Th1).[153] Of interest, IL-10 exhib-

Table 49-17 Interleukin-9

	Characteristic[147–150]	Comment
Chromosomal localization[3]	5q31.1	
Major production sites	Activated Th2 cells	
Selected biologic activities	Supports clonogenic maturation of erythroid progenitors Acts as a mast cell differentiation factor Protects lymphomas from apoptosis Cooperates with IL-4 in B-cell responses Enhances neuronal differentiation	Has more pronounced effect on fetal vs adult cells Transformed or activated T cells much more responsive to IL-9 than normal, resting T cells
Receptor	IL-9 receptor	Located on subtelomeric (pseudoautosomal) region of chromosomes X (Xq28) and Y (Yq12)

IL = interleukin.

Table 49-18 Interleukin-10

	Characteristic[151–163]	Comment
Chromosomal localization[3]	1q31-q32	
Structure	Strongly homologous to BCRF1 of the Epstein-Barr virus genome	BCRF1 protein is viral IL-10; IL-19, IL-20, IL-22, IL-24, and IL-26 are homologous to IL-10
Major production sites	CD4+ cells (Th0, Th1, and Th2), CD8+ cells, monocytes, macrophages, B cells	Th2 cells are main source
Selected biologic activities	Inhibits cytokine synthesis by Th1 cells and monocytes/macrophages	Inhibits IL-1, IL-2, IL-6, IL-8, IL-10, IL-12, TNF, GM-CSF, G-CSF, IFN-γ, and lymphotoxin
	Stimulates B cell proliferation	Up-regulates IL-1RA and soluble IL-1
	Involved in transformation of B cells by EBV and TNF receptors	
Receptor	IL-10 receptor interferon receptors	Localized to 11q23
Clinical studies	Trend toward efficacy in rheumatoid arthritis, inflammatory bowel disease, and autoimmune diseases	Well tolerated

EBV = Epstein-Barr virus; G-CSF = granulocyte colony-stimulating factor; GM-CSF = granulocyte macrophage colony-stimulating factor; IFN = interferon; IL = interleukin; TNF = tumor necrosis factor.

its strong DNA and amino acid sequence homology to an open reading frame—BCRF1—in the Epstein-Barr virus (EBV) genome.[153] Indeed, the BCRF1 protein product displays many of the biologic properties of cellular IL-10 and has, therefore, been termed viral IL-10.

Biologic Activities of IL-10 IL-10 inhibits the synthesis of Th1-derived cytokines, including IL-2, IFN-γ, GM-CSF, and lymphotoxin, and of monocyte-derived IL-1α and -β, IL-6, IL-8, TNF-α, GM-CSF, and G-CSF. Exogenous IL-10 can also suppress expression of IL-10.[152] At the same time, IL-10 induces the synthesis of the IL-1 receptor antagonist by macrophages. IL-10 also suppresses the CD28 co-stimulatory pathway, and hence, acts as a decisive mechanism in determining if a T cell will contribute to an immune response or become anergic.

From the molecular standpoint, IL-10 suppresses cytokine expression at a transcriptional level and also at a post-transcriptional level (by enhancing mRNA degradation).[154] Both these mechanisms appear to require new protein synthesis. At a cellular level, Th1 cytokines synthesis inhibition is mediated indirectly through the effect of IL-10 on antigen-presenting cells (APC), since suppression occurs when macrophages, but not B cells, are used as antigen-presenting cells.[155]

In the presence of monocytes/macrophages, IL-10 inhibits proliferation of resting T cells, including Th0, Th1, and Th2 CD4+ T-cell clones. This inhibition can only be partially reversed by high concentrations of IL-2, suggesting that the reduced proliferation is only partially a reflection of reduced IL-2 production. IL-10 can also enhance the cytotoxic activity of CD8+ T cells. All these effects support an important role of IL-10 in regulating inflammatory responses.

In contrast to the inhibitory effects on other lineages, IL-10 has a stimulatory effect on B cells and mast cells.[156] For instance; IL-10 strongly stimulates proliferation and differentiation of activated B cells.

IL-10 and Human Disease The protein product of BCRF1 (viral IL-10) exhibits properties similar to those of human IL-10. The ability of EBV to transform human B cells may be, at least in part, a ramification of the ability of viral IL-10 to stimulate B-cell proliferation. The *bcrf1* gene is transcribed late in the process of viral infection, when newly formed viral particles are produced.[157] Since IFN-γ is an important mediator of the antiviral activity of T cells and NK cells, the cytokine synthesis inhibitory activity of IL-10 may also contribute to tumorigenesis by allowing viral infection to proceed. Thus, IL-10 may have a role in the development of lymphoma through two mechanisms: its proliferation-stimulating properties on B cells, and its immunosuppressive properties that impair viral control and tumor immunosurveillance. This role has been demonstrated in a severe combined immunodeficiency (SCID) mouse model for lymphomagenesis.[158] Eighty percent of such mice injected intraperitoneally with human peripheral blood lymphocytes from healthy EBV-seropositive individuals developed EBV-lymphoproliferative disease.

Of interest, primary B lymphoma cells from both HIV-positive and HIV-negative lymphoma (NHL) patients secrete substantial amounts of IL-10. Indeed, several groups of investigators have evaluated the role and prognostic significance of IL-10 in patients with NHL.[159–163] A series of studies has demonstrated that (1) IL-10 levels are elevated in lymphoma patients; and (2) high IL-10 levels correlate with prognosis, if an assay that detects both human and viral IL-10 is used. Assays, which detect only human IL-10, yield no correlation with prognosis. These studies raise additional questions about the participation of EBV in lymphomagenesis.

INTERLEUKIN-11

Originally characterized as a thrombopoietic factor, IL-11 is now known to be expressed and have activity in a multitude of other systems, including the gut, testes, and the central nervous system (Table 49-19[164–172]).[164,165] Clinically, this cytokine has been approved by the US Food and Drug Administration for amelioration of chemotherapy-induced thrombocytopenia.

Biologic Activities of IL-11 IL-11 was originally isolated from cells derived from the hematopoietic microenvironment and may act as a paracrine or autocrine growth factor in this environment. IL-11 acts synergistically with other early- and late-acting

Table 49-19 Interleukin-11

	Characteristic[164–172]	Comment
Chromosomal localization[3]	19q13.3-q13.4	
Major production sites	Gut, testis, central nervous system, stromal elements, osteoblasts, leukemic cell lines, melanoma cell lines	Can be induced by IL-1α and other cytokines
Selected biologic activities	Best known as a thrombopoietic factor	
	Stimulates multilineage progenitors, erythropoiesis, myelopoiesis, and lymphopoiesis	
	Decreases mucositis in animal models	
	Stimulates osteoclast development	
	Inhibits adipogenesis	
	Stimulates proliferation of neuronal cells	
Receptor	IL-11Rα and gp130 subunits gp130 = CD130 on 5q11	IL-11Rα on 9p13
	IL-6, oncostatin M, and leukemia inhibitory factor also use gp130 subunit	
Major clinical trials	Approved for use to prevent chemotherapy-induced thrombocytopenia	Most common side effect is fluid accumulation

IL = interleukin; IL-11R = interleukin-11 receptor.

Table 49-20 Interleukin-12

	Characteristic[173–179]	Comment
Chromosomal localization[3]	IL-12A: 3p12-q13.2 IL-12B: 5q31.1-q33.1	
Structure	Composed of IL-12A (p40) and IL-12B (p35)	IL-12A and IL-12B are encoded by two distinct genes
Major production sites	Macrophages Stimulated monocytes, neutrophils, and dendritic cells EBV-infected B cells	
Selected biologic activities	Proinflammatory cytokine important in resistance to infections Th1 development Stimulatory and inhibitory effects on hematopoiesis	
Receptor	IL-12Rβ1 and IL-12Rβ2 chains are related to gp130	IL-12Rβ1 at 19p13.1 IL-12Rβ2 at 1p31.2
Natural antagonists	IL-12 p40 homodimers	
Major clinical trials	Potential use in vaccine development No benefit in hepatitis C trial Modest antitumor activity with significant toxicity in melanoma and renal cell carcinoma	Significant toxicities may limit use

EBV = Epstein-Barr virus; IL-12 = interleukin-12; IL-12R = interleukin-12 receptor.

growth factors to stimulate various stages and lineages of hematopoiesis.[164] In synergy with IL-3, IL-4, IL-7, IL-12, IL-13, SCF, FLT-3 ligand, and GM-CSF, IL-11 stimulates the proliferation of primitive stem cells and their commitment in to multilineage progenitors as well as their differentiation. The synergistic effects of IL-11 and TPO on multilineage cells may be mediated in part by SCF/c-kit interactions.

IL-11 acts synergistically with IL-3, TPO, or SCF to stimulate various stages of megakaryocytopoiesis and thrombopoiesis.[167,168] IL-11, alone or in combination with other cytokines (IL-3, SCF, or EPO), can stimulate multiple stages of erythropoiesis. IL-11 also modulates the differentiation and maturation of myeloid progenitor cells. IL-11 in combination with SCF stimulates myeloid colony formation. The combination of IL-11 with IL-13 or IL-14 can reduce the proportion of granulocytes and blasts in myeloid colonies, with a concomitant increase in macrophages. Although in vivo IL-11 increases the cycling rates and absolute number of myeloid progenitors of normal mice, it has no effects on peripheral leukocyte counts when administered to normal rodents and nonhuman primates.

IL-11 in combination with SCF or IL-4 effectively supports the generation of B cells in primary cultures. IL-11 and IL-4 can also reverse the inhibitory effect of IL-3 on early B-lymphocyte development. The promotion of B-cell differentiation may be mediated by T cells.

In vitro studies show that IL-11 can directly interact with gastrointestinal epithelial cells and reversibly inhibit proliferation of the intestinal crypt stem cell lines.[169] Subcutaneous administration of IL-11 effectively attenuated mucositis induced by 5-fluorouracil in animals. Survival in IL-11–treated animals was significantly better than controls.[165]

IL-11 in combination with lα,25-dihydroxyvitamin D 3 (lα,25[OH]2D3) and parathyroid hormone has been shown to stimulate osteoclast development. Exogenous IL-11 also stimulates the proliferation of hippocampal neuronal progenitor cells (H19-7) in a dose-dependent fashion.

IL-11 in Human Disease As mentioned above, alveolar and bronchial epithelial cells produce large amounts of IL-11. The up-regulation of IL-11 production by inflammatory cytokines, respiratory syncytial virus, and retinoic acid suggests that IL-11 may play an important role in pulmonary inflammation.

IL-11 acts as a synergistic factor with IL-3, GM-CSF, and SCF to stimulate proliferation of human primary leukemia cells, myeloid leukemia cell lines, megakaryoblastic cell lines, and erythroleukemic cell lines and to stimulate leukemic blast colony formation. IL-11 mRNA expression in leukemic cells and inhibition of leukemic cell growth by IL-11 antisense oligonucleotides suggest that IL-11 may function as an autocrine growth factor in leukemic cell lines.[171] Although IL-11 stimulates the proliferation of murine plasmacytoma cells and murine hybridoma cells, the effect of IL-11 on the growth of human myeloma/plasmacytoma cells is controversial.[164]

Clinical Use of IL-11 A multicenter, randomized, placebo-controlled clinical trial of IL-11 has been conducted in 93 cancer patients who had received at least one platelet transfusion during a prior chemotherapy cycle (secondary prophylaxis design).[155] These patients were given an additional cycle of the same chemotherapy without dose reduction and were randomized to receive either IL-11 (at a dose of 25 or 50 μg/kg) or placebo. The patients treated with IL-11 in this study were less likely to require platelet transfusions than the patients receiving placebo ($p < .05$). Edema was the most common clinical problem associated with IL-11. Some patients developed pleural effusions, shortness of breath, and/or atrial arrhythmias.[165] Lower dosages of IL-11 (10 μg/day SC) have been reported to be safe and to effectively raise platelet counts in patients suffering from a variety of bone marrow failure states.[170]

INTERLEUKIN-12

IL-12 was first identified as an NK-cell stimulatory factor.[173] Subsequently, it was demonstrated that IL-12 is crucial to the development of Th1 cells.[174] Indeed, there appears to be a common pathway leading from the innate immune response to adaptive immunity—intracellular pathogens stimulate macrophages to produce IL-12, which then promotes the development of Th1 cells from a naïve cell population. This pathway may be exploitable in the design of novel immunotherapies and vaccines (Table 49-20[173–179]).

Biologic Activities of IL-12 and Role in Disease IL-12 is a potent proinflammatory molecule, which is essential for resistance to bacterial, fungal, and parasitic infections. It is produced within a few hours of infection, activates NK cells, and, through its ability to induce IFN-γ production, enhances the phagocytic and bacteriocidal activity of phagocytic cells and their ability to release proinflammatory cytokines, including IL-12 itself.

IL-12 is also a key immunoregulatory molecule, especially of Th1 responses. It is produced during the early phases of infection and inflammation and sets the stage for the ensuing antigen-specific immune response, favoring differentiation and function of the Th1 T cells, while inhibiting the differentiation of the Th2 T cells. Indeed, the type of Th-cell differentiation after pathogen exposure is most likely determined by the balance between IL-12 and IL-4, which favor Th1 and Th2 development, respectively.

IL-12 does not induce proliferation of resting peripheral blood T cells or NK cells; it does potentiate the proliferation of T cells induced by various mitogens and has a direct proliferative effect on preactivated T and NK cells. IL-12 is effective at lower concentrations than IL-2 but is not as potent a proliferative agent as the latter molecule. IL-12 also enhances the generation of cytotoxic T cells and lymphokine-activated killer cells.

IL-12 synergizes with other hematopoietic factors to promote survival and proliferation of early multipotent hematopoietic progenitor cells and lineage-committed precursor cells.[177] Although in vitro IL-12 has mostly stimulatory effects on hematopoiesis, in vivo IL-12 treatment results in decreased bone marrow hematopoiesis and both transient anemia and neutropenia, an effect mediated by IFN-γ.

Table 49-21 Interleukin-15

	Characteristic[180–185]	Comment
Chromosomal localization[3]	4q31	
Major production sites	Monocytes/macrophages, fibroblasts, keratinocytes, epithelial cells, placenta, skeletal muscle, heart, lung, liver, kidney	Not expressed by resting or activated T cells
Selected biologic activities	Triggers proliferation and immunoglobulin production in preactivated B cells Number of CD8+ memory T cells may be controlled by balance of IL-15 (stimulatory) and IL-12 (inhibitory) Stimulates proliferation of NK cells and activated CD4+ or CD8+ T cells Facilitates the induction of LAK cells and CTLs Stimulates mast cell proliferation Promotes proliferation of hairy-cell leukemia and chronic lymphocytic leukemia cells	Shares biologic effects with IL-2
Receptor	High affinity receptor requires IL-2Rβ and γ chains and IL-15Rα chain	IL-2Rβ = CD122 at 22q11.2-q13 IL-2Rγ = CD132 at Xq13 IL-15Rα at 10p14-p15

CTL = cytolytic T lymphocyte; IL-2R = interleukin-2 receptor; LAK = lymphokine activated killer; NK = natural killer.

IL-12 in the Clinic IL-12 has potential for exploitation in allergy and as an adjuvant for infectious disease therapy.[178] Additionally, the ability of IL-12 to revert existing states of tolerance or anergy makes it a candidate for use in the composition of vaccines for infectious agents or tumors. Phase I clinical trials have been started in the last few years in oncology (with an emphasis on melanomas, renal cell carcinomas, and cutaneous T-cell lymphomas) as well as in the setting of HIV infection and chronic hepatitis B and C. To date, administration of IL-12 to patients with chronic hepatitis C does not appear advantageous.[179] What is more worrisome is, in cancer patients treated with high doses of IL-12, acute hematopoietic, hepatic, and gastrointestinal toxicities were observed and several deaths were reported. In long-term treatments, toxicity was mostly pulmonary. It has been suggested that some of the severe toxicity of IL-12 can be attenuated if a single injection is administered 1 to 2 weeks before initiating daily dosing.[175]

INTERLEUKIN-15

IL-15 shares biologic activities with IL-2 (Table 49-21[180–185]).[180]

Biologic Activities of IL-15 Similar to IL-2, IL-15 is able to trigger both proliferation of and immunoglobulin production by normal B lymphocytes. These biologic functions may be acquired, however, only when B cells have been preactivated in vitro with polyclonal mitogens or when they are cultured in association with other stimuli. IL-15 also stimulates the proliferation of NK cells and activated CD4+ and CD8+ T cells, and facilitates the induction of cytolytic effector cells (such as lymphokine-activated killer cells). Finally, the numbers of CD8+ memory T cells is maintained in animals by a balance between the stimulatory effect of IL-15 and the suppressive effects of IL-12.[184]

IL-15 and Human Disease High levels of IL-15 have been observed in rheumatoid arthritis, and IL-15 triggers T-cell growth in sarcoidosis. In addition, IL-15 responsiveness distinguishes malignant B cells from normal B lymphocytes. In contrast to normal B lymphocytes, which require preactivation in order to proliferate in response to IL-15, leukemic cells from patients with chronic B-cell malignancies (chronic lymphocytic leukemia and hairy-cell leukemia) proliferate in response to IL-15 regardless of in vitro preactivation. The proliferation elicited by IL-15 in chronic lymphocytic leukemia and hairy-cell leukemia is mainly related to the presence of the β and γ chains of the IL-2R system on the malignant B lymphocytes.[180] Even so, IL-15 cannot be considered an autocrine factor in these leukemias, since it is not produced by the leukemic cells themselves. Rather, the major reservoir of IL-15 in these patients is from cells belonging to the monocyte/macrophage lineage.[180]

INTERLEUKIN-16

Cruikshank and Center first described IL-16 in 1982 (Table 49-22[186,187]).[185] They found that this molecule was a lymphocyte chemo attractant factor expressed by mitogen-stimulated human peripheral blood mononuclear cells.[185]

Biologic Activities of IL-16 IL-16 is a proinflammatory and immunomodulatory cytokine. It is a potent chemo attractant for all CD4+ cells including T cells, monocytes, and eosinophils and, as such, has been identified at inflammatory sites characterized by infiltrating CD4+ cells.[186] In addition to cell motility, IL-16 induces cell-cycle progression and cytokine synthesis in CD4+ T cells.

Although responsive to IL-2, IL-16–treated cells cannot be stimulated through the T-cell receptor. These findings are consistent with the concept that CD4 functions as a regulator molecule for lymphocyte activation, capable of facilitating either antigen-induced activation or cytokine-directed cellular activation.[187] It has been postulated that IL-16 contributes to a general antigen-independent, nonclonal recruitment and priming of CD4+ cells in an inflammatory process. Although the recruited cells are responsive to cytokine stimulation, they are refractory to antigen-specific stimulation. This process would allow higher numbers of cells to be recruited to an inflammatory focus by decreasing the susceptibility of these cells to antigen-specific induced cell death (known as activation-induced cell death).[186]

IL-16 in Human Disease IL-16 may be involved in asthma because the airway epithelium from asthmatics produces IL-16 after histamine stimulation, although similar epithelium from normals does not.[185] Also, IL-16 may play a role

Table 49-22 Interleukin-16

	Characteristic[186,187]	Comment
Chromosomal localization[3]	15q26.1	
Forms	17 kDa peptide	Biologic activity requires cleavage of pro–IL-16 by caspase 3 and autoaggregation into tetrameric form Main source is CD8+ cells
Major production sites	CD4+ and CD8+ T cells, airway epithelium (from asthmatics), eosinophils, mast cells	
Selected biologic activities	Chemoattractant for CD4+ cells (T cells, monocytes, eosinophils) May be involved in asthma and in granulomatous inflammation Has antiviral effects on HIV-1	
Receptor	Requires CD4 for biologic activities	
Potential clinical trials	May have potential use in HIV infection	

HIV = human immunodeficiency virus.

Table 49-23 Interleukin-17

	Characteristic[188–196]	Comment
Chromosomal localization[3]	2q31	
Major production sites	CD4+ activated memory T cells (CD45+, Ro+)	
Selected biologic activities	May mediate, in part, T-cell contribution to inflammation	Homologous to open reading frame 13 of *Herpesvirus saimiri*[172]
	Stimulates epithelial, endothelial, fibroblastic and macrophage cells to express a variety of inflammatory cytokines	
	Promotes the capacity of fibroblasts to sustain hematopoietic progenitor growth	
	Promotes differentiation of dendritic cell progenitors	
	May be involved in the pathogenesis of rheumatoid arthritis and graft rejection	
Receptor	IL-17 receptor	Ubiquitously expressed on hematopoietic and epithelial cells Located at 22q111.22-23

IL-17 = interleukin-17.

in granulomatous inflammation; high IL-16 levels are found in the lymph nodes and lungs of sarcoidosis patients and in the BAL material from patients with *Mycobacterium tuberculosis.* Since IL-16 is a T-cell chemoattractant, IL-16 inhibitors may have therapeutic implications in suppressing T-cell–mediated inflammation.

In addition, IL-16 has antiviral effects on HIV-1 replication and, at the same time, can promote growth of CD4+ T cells. Both these activities are required for immune reconstitution in individuals infected with HIV-1 and suggest another possible clinical application for this molecule.[186]

INTERLEUKIN-17

Human IL-17 was originally identified by Rouvier and colleagues (Table 49-23[188–196]).[188] Of interest, this molecule has 72% overall sequence identity at the amino acid level with open reading frame 13 of *Herpesvirus saimiri.*[189]

Biologic Activities of IL-17 Although limited in number, studies suggest that IL-17 may be a soluble factor by which T cells induce or contribute to inflammation (see Table 49-23).[193] IL-17 can also stimulate epithelial, endothelial, and fibroblastic cells, and macrophages to express a variety of cytokines.[177] The cytokines released after exposure to IL-17 appear to be cell specific. For instance, fibroblast cells produce IL-1, G-CSF, IFN-γ, IL-6, and IL-8 in response to IL-17, and macrophages produce TNF-α, IL-1β, IL-1Rα, IL-6, IL-10, and IL-12.[195]

IL-17 also exhibits indirect hematopoietic activity by enhancing the capacity of fibroblasts (through stimulation of growth factor release) to sustain the proliferation of CD34+ hematopoietic progenitors and their differentiation into neutrophils.[190,193] IL-17 can also promote the maturation of dendritic cell progenitors.[196]

IL-17 in Human Disease In rheumatoid arthritis synovial tissue, high levels of IL-17 contribute to IL-6 production by synoviocytes and to local inflammatory reactions.[192] Because IL-17 acts to differentiate early dendritic cells, it has been implicated in host T-cell allostimulation and graft rejection.[196]

INTERLEUKIN-18

IL-18 (IFN-inducing factor) was first described as a serum activity that induced IFN-γ production in mouse spleen cells.[197] It is related to the IL-1 family of genes (Table 49-24[54,197–204]).

Structure of IL-18 IL-18 has a molecular weight of 18 to 19 kDa and has homology to IL-1.[198,199] Like IL-1β, IL-18 is initially synthesized as an inactive precursor molecule (pro–IL-18) lacking a signal peptide and is cleaved by ICE to yield an active molecule.[200,201]

Biologic Activities of IL-18 T lymphocytes, NK cells, and macrophages are primary targets for IL-18 (see Table 49-24). For example, IL-18 directly stimulates production of TNF in human blood CD4+ T lymphocytes and NK cells and plays an important role in promoting a long-lasting T-helper type-1 (Th1) lymphocyte response to viral antigens. (A vigorous Th1 response against viruses results in the generation of viral antigen-targeted cytotoxic T lymphocytes.)

IL-18 does not appear to be an endogenous pyrogen, but may nevertheless contribute to inflammation and fever because it is a potent inducer of TNF, chemokines, and IFN.[202] In the case of IFN-γ induction, IL-18 acts as a costimulant with mitogens or IL-2. Indeed, mice deficient in ICE, the molecule, which cleaves pro–IL-18 to its mature form, fail to produce IFN-γ in response to endotoxin.

INTERLEUKIN-19

IL-19 is one of the members of the human IL-10 family of cytokines (Table 49-25[205]). IL-19 shares 21% amino acid identity with IL-10, and the exon/intron structure of IL-19 is similar to that of the human IL-10 gene, comprising five exons and four introns within the coding region of the IL-19 cDNA.[205] The expression of IL-19 messenger ribonucleic acid (mRNA) can be induced in monocytes by lipopolysaccharides or GM-CSF.

INTERLEUKIN-20

IL-20 was discovered as another IL-10–related cytokine. It induces keratinocyte proliferation and causes aberrant epidermal differentiation in the skin.[206] IL-20 receptor complex is described as a heterodimer of two orphan class II cytokine receptor subunits named IL-20Rα and IL-20Rβ (Table 49-26[206–208]). Recombinant IL-20 binds to its receptor on keratinocytes and stimulates a STAT3-containing signal transduction pathway.[208] Experimental evidence suggests a role for IL-20 and its receptor in psoriasis, a multigenic skin disease characterized by increased keratinocyte proliferation and differentiation. Clinical applications are currently under consideration.

Table 49-24 Interleukin-18

	Characteristic[54,197–204]	Comment
Chromosomal localization[3]	11q22.2-q22.3	
Structure	Shows homology to IL-1	ICE cleaves inactive pro–IL-18 to mature IL-18
Selected biologic activity	Promotes production of IFN-γ, TNF	
	Targets are T cells, NK cells, and macrophages	
	Promotes Th1 responses to virus	
Receptor	IL-18R	
Natural antagonists	IL-18–binding protein exists	Poxvirus carries a version of IL-18–binding protein, which blunts host response to infection

ICE = IL-1–converting enzyme; IFN = interferon; IL-1Rrp = IL-1 receptor-related protein; TNF = tumor necrosis factor.

Table 49-25 Interleukin-19

	Characteristic[205]	Comment
Chromosomal localization[3]	1q32	
Structure	Shows homology to IL-10	Belongs to IL-10 cytokine family
	Molecular weight ~ 21 kDa	
Selected biologic activities	Induces IL-6 and TNF-α	
Receptor	IL-20R1 and IL-20R2	
Major production sites	Monocytes and B cells at very low levels	No T-cell production has been found

IL = interleukin; TNF = tumor necrosis factor.

INTERLEUKIN-21

IL-21, a cytokine most closely related to IL-2 and IL-15 (Table 49-27[207,209,210]), is involved in the proliferation and maturation of NK-cell populations from bone marrow, as well as in the proliferation of mature B-cell and T-cell populations.[209] IL-21 has been implicated in the activation of innate immune responses and in the Th1 response. IL-21 also plays a critical role in regulating immunoglobulin production of B cells.[210]

INTERLEUKIN-22

IL-22 was originally described as an IL-9–inducible gene and called IL-TIF.[211] IL-22 activities include induction of the acute phase response in hepatocytes. These activities are mediated through a heterodimeric receptor composed of the IL-22R subunit and the β chain of IL-10R.[212] In addition to its cellular receptor, IL-22 binds to a secreted class II cytokine receptor family member that acts as a natural IL-22 antagonist (Table 49-28[211,212]). To date, IL-22 has not been applied clinically.

INTERLEUKIN-23

IL-23 is a member of the IL-6 family of cytokines and is closely related in structure to IL-12. These cytokines are heterodimeric cytokines, which share the p40 subunit, and both have unique second subunits, IL-23p19 and IL-12p35 (Table 49-29[213,214]). In addition to the close structural relationship between IL-23 and IL-12, their heterodimeric receptors share the IL-12Rb1 chain and these cytokines have been shown to have similar properties.[213,214]

INTERLEUKIN-24

IL-24 was originally named melanoma differentiation-associated gene-7 (mda-7) when it was discovered in 1995. It was identified by subtractive hybridization after the treatment of melanoma cells with IFN-β and mezerein, which caused their terminal differentiation and growth arrest.[215] In 2001, it was realized that mda-7 encodes a secreted protein that exhibits significant homology to IL-10 as another member of the IL-10 family (Table 49-30[207,216–220]). This molecule was officially designated as IL-24.[216] Human IL-24 is secreted by activated peripheral blood mononuclear cells and is the ligand for two heterodimeric receptors, IL-22R1/IL-20R2 and IL-20R1/IL-20R2.[217] IL-24 also acts as a tumor-suppressor gene and the protein product was found to be constitutively expressed by melanocytes, nevus cells, and some primary melanomas, but not metastatic lesions of melanoma.[218,219] This is possibly the first example of a tumor-suppressor gene exhibiting immune stimulatory properties.[220]

IL-24 in the Clinic Because of the tumor suppressor characteristics of IL-24, it may poten-

Table 49-26 Interleukin-20

	Characteristic[206–208]	Comment
Chromosomal localization[3]	1q32	Belongs to IL-10 cytokine family
Signal transduction pathway	Activation of the JAK-STAT3 pathway	
Selected biologic activates	Induction of genes involved in inflammation such as TNF-α, MRP14 and MCP-1	
Potential clinical trials	May have potential for chronic inflammatory skin disease	Low levels of production have been seen in skin, trachea
Receptor	IL20R1 and IL20R2	

IL = interleukin; JAK = janus activated kinases; MCP = monocyte chemoattractant protein; MRP = myeloid related proteins; STAT = signal transducer and activator of transcription.

Table 49-27 Interleukin-21

	Characteristic[207,209,210]	Comment
Chromosomal localization[3]	4q26-27	Belongs to IL-2 cytokine family
Structure	Shows homology to IL-15	They share about 25% amino acid identity
Selected biologic activities	Mainly, regulates T-cell proliferation and differentiation	In general, it modulates the proliferation and differentiation of not only T cells, but also B cells, NK cells, and dendritic cells
	Regulates cell-mediated immunity and the clearance of tumors	
Signal transduction pathway	IL-21 binding stimulates activation of JAK1/JAK3 and the subsequent phosphorylation of STAT1, as well as STAT3 and STAT5	
Major production sites	Expressed preferentially in CD4+ T cells	
Receptor	IL-21R	
Potential clinical application	Since it controls adaptive immune responses, its use in a clinical setting may prove efficacious for the treatment of cancer and infectious disease	

IL = interleukin; JAK = janus activated kinases; NK = natural killer; STAT = signal transducer and activator of transcription.

Table 49-28 Interleukin-22

	Characteristic[211,212]	Comment
Chromosomal localization[3]	12q14	Belongs to IL-10 cytokine family
Structure	Shows homology to IL-10	
	Molecular weight ~ 25–40 kDa	
Selected biologic activities	Up-regulates the production of acute phase reactans	Involvement in inflammatory and perhaps immune responses
	Induces the production of ROS in resting B cells	
Major production sites	Constitutive expression in thymus and brain	Cytokine can be induced by IL-9 in thymic lymphoma cells, T helper cells and mast cells
Receptor	IL-22R1 and IL-10R2	

IL = interleukin; ROS = reactive oxygen species.

Table 49-29 Interleukin-23

	Characteristic[213,214]	Comment
Chromosomal localization[3]	12q13	
Structure	Molecular weight ~ 40 kDa	Belongs to IL-12 cytokine family
Selected biologic activities	A unique function of IL-23 is the preferential induction of proliferation of the memory subset of T cells	Its biological activities share many functions with IL-12. All induce T-cell IFN-g production
Signal transduction pathway	JAK2 constitutively associates with IL-23 receptor, and ligand binding results in the activation of JAK2, TYK2, STAT1, STAT3, STAT4, and STAT5	
Receptor	IL-12Rb1 and IL-23R	The IL-23R is expressed at low levels on T cells, NK cells, monocytes, and DCs

DC = dendritic cells; IFN = interferon; IL = interleukin; JAK = janus activated kinases; NK = natural killer; STAT = signal transducer and activator of transcription; TYK = tyrosine kinases.

Table 49-30 Interleukin-24

	Characteristic[207,216–220]	Comment
Chromosomal localization[3]	1q32	
Structure	Shows homology to IL-10	Belongs to IL-10 cytokine family
Selected biologic activities	Induces IL-6, TNF-α, IL-1b, IL-12 and GM-CSF Functionally it has opposite effects with IL-10 Infection with Ad-IL-24 results in down-regulation of Bcl-2 and Bcl-XL (antiapoptotic proteins) and up-regulation of Bax and Bak (proapoptotic proteins) in cancer cells	At low concentration, functions as a cytokine; however, over-expression induces apoptosis selectively in cancer cells
Major production sites	Human monocytes Its expression can be up-regulated in monocytes by LPS or in T cells by anti-CD3 MoAb	Expression could be induced in human PBMC Upon treatment with PHA or LPS
Receptor	IL-20R1 and IL-20R2 IL-22R1 and IL-20R2	

IL = interleukin; GM-CFS = granulocyte-macrophage colony stimulating factors; LPS = lipopolysaccharide; PBMC = peripheral blood mononuclear cells; PHA = phytohemagglutinin; TNF = tumor necrosis factor.

Table 49-31 Interleukin-25

	Characteristic[223]	Comment
Chromosomal localization[3]	14q11	
Structure	Shows significant homology to IL-17	Belongs to IL-17 cytokine family
Selected biologic activities	IL-25 induces IL-4, IL-5, and IL-13 gene expression and protein production	
Clinical functions	Potent inflammatory activity and its association with various human disease states suggest this cytokine family as an important contributor to the pathophysiology of pulmonary diseases	
Receptor	IL-17BR	

IL = interleukin.

Table 49-32 Interleukin-26

	Characteristic[207,224]	Comment
Chromosomal localization[3]	12q14	
Structure	Shows homology with IL-10 Molecular weight ~ 19 kDa	Some cluster with IFN-g and IL-22
Selected biologic activities	Immune-protective role against viral infection	
Major production sites	IL-26 mRNA is specifically overexpressed by T cells after HSV transformation	Expression could be induced in NK and T cells upon stimulation
Receptor	Unknown	

HSV = *Herpesvirus saimiri*; IFN = interferon; IL = interleukin; NK = natural killer.

tially be used for cancer treatments in the clinic. Gene transfer of IL-24 has been studied in the phase I setting using intratumoral injections of Ad-mda7/IL-24 (INGN 241) in 28 patients with resectable solid tumors.[221] It has been reported that intratumoral administration of INGN 241 is well tolerated and induced apoptosis in a large percentage of tumor cells.[221,222]

INTERLEUKIN-25

IL-25 was recently identified as a cytokine that is structurally related to IL-17 and induces IL-4, IL-5, and IL-13 gene expression (Table 49-31[223]). The induction of these cytokines results in Th2-like responses marked by increased serum IgE, IgG1, and IgA levels, blood eosinophilia, and epithelial-cell hyperplasia. As a newly discovered cytokine, little is known about IL-25 besides the fact that it is derived from Th2 T cells, and it is capable of amplifying allergic-type inflammatory responses by its actions on other cells.

INTERLEUKIN-26

Subtraction hybridization coupled with representational differential analysis identified IL-26/AK155 as a gene up-regulated in human T cells following infection with *Herpesvirus saimiri* (HVS). It has the capacity to transform these cells in culture (Table 49-32[207,224]). The IL-26 protein has 24.7% amino acid identity and 47% amino acid similarity with human IL-10. Structural analysis revealed that IL-26 contains six helices with four highly conserved cysteine residues, which are assumed to be relevant for dimer formation as is the case with IL-10. It was determined that IL-26 mRNA is specifically overexpressed by T cells after HVS transformation.

INTERLEUKIN-27

In 2002, Pflanz and colleagues[225] described a new heterodimeric cytokine, related to IL-12. This cytokine was designated IL-27. It acts together with IL-12 to trigger IFN-γ production by naïve $CD4^+$ T cells (Table 49-33[225–227]). They also identified IL-27 as the ligand for TCCR/WSX-1, a novel member

Table 49-33 Interleukin-27

	Characteristic[225–227]	Comment
Chromosomal localization[3]	12q13	Belongs to IL-12 cytokine family
Structure	Shows homology to IL-12	
Selected biologic activities	Early Th1 initiation Synergizes with IL-12 in inducing IFN-g production by T cells and NK cells	All IL-12, 23, and 27 induce T-cell IFN-g production
Major production sites	IL-27 production is restricted to myeloid cells with the highest levels found in LPS-activated monocytes and monocyte-derived dendritic cells	
Receptor	TCCR/WSX-1 and GP130	WSX-1 is expressed mainly on T cells

IFN = interferon; IL = interleukin; NK = natural killer.

Table 49-34 Interleukin-28A, 28B, and 29

	Characteristic[228]	Comment
Chromosomal localization[3]	19q13	Distantly related to Type 1 IFNs and IL-10 cytokine family
Signal transduction pathway	Can signal through ISRE regulatory sites	
Selected biologic activities	Antiviral activities	
Receptor	IL-28R1 and IL-10R2	
Potential clinical applications	Alternative therapeutic choice to Type IFNs	

IFN = interferon; IL = interleukin; ISRE = interferon stimulated response element.

of the class I cytokine receptor family shown to be important for Th1 development.[226] Recent studies revealed that IL-27 has the ability to induce tumor-specific antitumor activity and protective immunity and that the antitumor activity is mediated mainly through CD8+ T cells, and IFN-γ.[227]

INTERLEUKIN-28 AND INTERLEUKIN-29

The IL-28 family has been identified from the human genomic sequence, designated interleukin 28A (IL-28A), IL-28B, and IL-29. These molecules are distantly related to type I IFNs and the IL-10 family. IL-28 and IL-29 are induced by viral infection and show antiviral activity. Moreover, IL-28 and IL-29 interact with a heterodimeric class II cytokine receptor that consists of IL-10Rβ and an orphan class II receptor chain, designated IL-28Rα. This newly described cytokine family may serve as an alternative to type I IFNs in providing immunity to viral infection (Table 49-34[228]).

INTERLEUKIN-31

As the latest addition to the list, IL-31 has been identified as a four-helix bundle cytokine that is preferentially produced by T helper type 2 cells. IL-31 signals through a receptor composed of IL-31 receptor A and oncostatin M receptor. Expression of IL-31 receptor A and oncostatin M receptor mRNA is induced in activated monocytes, whereas epithelial cells expressed both mRNAs constitutively (Table 49-35[229]). More specifically, the data indicate that IL-31 may be involved in promoting the dermatitis and epithelial responses that characterize allergic and nonallergic diseases.

OTHER HEMATOPOIETIC GROWTH FACTORS

Some of the growth factors discussed have already found their place in clinical medicine.[230–237] However, many other cytokines also have the ability to affect hematopoietic growth and development and are now being explored. These include early-acting, multipotential factors such as FLT-3 ligand, factors that may act indirectly such as TNF-α, and molecules such as insulin-like growth factors that were initially discovered by virtue of their effects on unrelated tissues (Table 49-36[230–237]). In addition, because of its increasing importance, FLT-3 ligand will be discussed in depth below.

FLT-3 Ligand FLT-3 (Fms-like tyrosine kinase 3) is also known as FLK-2 (fetal liver kinase-2) and STK-1 (human stem cell kinase-1) (Table 49-37[238,239]).[238] The ligand for FLT-3 was cloned in 1993.

Biologic Activity of FLT-3 Ligand Both the membrane-bound and soluble forms can activate the tyrosine kinase enzymatic activity of the receptor and stimulate growth of progenitor cells in the marrow and blood. However, like stem cell factor, FLT-3 ligand does not efficiently induce proliferation of normal myeloid and lymphoid progenitors by itself, but rather strongly synergizes with other hematopoietic growth factors and interleukins. FLT-3 ligand is a growth factor for immature myeloid cells and stem cells and can expand CD34+ cell populations. The FLT-3 ligand also plays an important role in immune response.

FLT-3 Ligand in Human Disease FLT-3 is expressed at high levels in a spectrum of hematologic malignancies, including subsets of patients with acute myelogenous leukemia, B precursor cell, acute lymphoblastic leukemia, and a fraction of T-cell ALL and chronic myelogenous leukemia in lymphoid blast crisis. Interestingly, FLT-3 mutations have been described in about 30% of patients with AML, making these mutations the most common anomaly in AML. These have also been reported, albeit with lower frequency, in myelodysplastic syndrome but are rarely detected in ALL. The mutations result in activation of FLT-3 kinase enzymatic activity.

FLT-3 Ligand in the Clinic Since FLT-3 can stimulate proliferation of early progenitors, its administration to leukemia patients will need to be undertaken with circumspection. However, FLT-3 ligand may also enhance antitumor immunity, and may be exploitable in this venue. Perhaps the most promising focus for development of the FLT-3 system relates to the advent of FLT-3 inhibitors, which suppress the enzymatic activity of the mutated receptor (FLT-3). This is especially pertinent to AML because, as mentioned

Table 49-35 Interleukin-31

	Characteristic[229]	Comment
Chromosomal localization[3]	12q24	
Signal transduction pathway	Signals through STAT 1, 3 and 5	
Selected biologic activities	Responsible for promoting the dermatitis and epithelial responses that characterize allergic and nonallergic diseases	
Tissue distribution	Low expression of mRNA in testis, bone marrow, skeletal muscle, kidney, colon, thymus, small intestine, and trachea	
Major production sites	Activated CD4+ T cells and lower expression in activated CD8+ cells	
Receptor	IL-31RA and oncostatin M receptor	Homology of IL-31RA to gp130 places this cytokine in the gp130-IL-6 cytokine family

IL = interleukin; STAT = signal transducer and activator of transcription.

Table 49-36 Other Hematopoietic Growth Factors

Molecule	Characteristics
TNF-α	Predominant effects may be indirect through induction of expression of other cytokines
	In vivo, stimulates granulopoiesis and inhibits erythropoiesis
IGF-1	Induces erythroid colony formation even in the absence of EPO
LIF	Induces differentiation of murine myeloid leukemia line
	Constitutively expressed by bone marrow stroma
	May enhance colony formation, especially if combined with other cytokines

EPO = erythropoietin; IGF-1 = insulin like growth factor-1; IL = interleukin; LIF = leukemia inhibitory factor; NK = natural killer; TNF-α = tumor necrosis factor-α.

above, activating mutations of FLT-3 are seen in about one-third of patients with this leukemia.

USE OF HEMATOPOIETIC GROWTH FACTORS AFTER CHEMOTHERAPY

The use of hematopoietic growth factors as supportive care after chemotherapy revolves around several issues. These include the degree to which they are actually needed with standard-dose chemotherapy, whether or not high-dose chemotherapy with cytokine support is advantageous as compared with standard-dose chemotherapy, and the cost of the growth factors.[230]

Hematopoietic Growth Factors and Standard-Dose Chemotherapy of Solid Tumors The risks of myelosuppression were initially reported in relation to the sequelae of chemotherapeutic induction regimens used to treat acute leukemias. Life-threatening infections and bleeding accompanied severe and prolonged myelosuppression and compromised the overall favorable impact of cytotoxic therapy for leukemia. The model of leukemia treatment was subsequently extrapolated to the care of patients with solid tumors, although in these cancers, oncologists rarely induce hematologic toxicities comparable with those observed in the induction therapy of acute leukemia.

It is generally felt that the routine use of hematopoietic growth factors as primary prophylaxis in all patients with nonmyeloid malignancies treated with any myelosuppressive chemotherapy is wasteful. Furthermore, prospective randomized data have shown that, on the one hand, there is no indication for the "therapeutic" use of G-CSF in patients with uncomplicated (afebrile) neutropenia. On the other hand, although further study is needed, administration of these molecules to support high-risk populations (eg, the very elderly and those with severe comorbid disease) has been judged appropriate by the American Society of Clinical Oncology (ASCO) Guidelines Committee.[231] Several randomized trials have also shown that when control groups have an incidence of febrile neutropenia of at least 40%, primary prophylactic administration of CSFs reduces the incidence of this complication by half. Routine use of growth factors has therefore been deemed of value after regimens that are expected to produce this degree of myelosuppression.

Secondary prophylaxis appears to be a reasonable application for hematopoietic growth factors. In patients with a history of poor tolerance to chemotherapy, and specifically in those individuals who have previously experienced an episode of febrile neutropenia, administration of growth factor support may prevent the need to reduce chemotherapy doses. However, this strategy is considered most effective for curable tumors. In the setting of other tumors, dose reduction should be considered because published data do not show survival benefit with dose maintenance and secondary prophylaxis.

Hematopoietic Growth Factors and High-Dose Chemotherapy in Solid Tumors At one time, it was taken as axiomatic that higher doses of chemotherapy would result in better responses, if toxicity could be avoided. This view was based on observations in animal models as well as published studies, which supported a dose threshold below which optimal responses are not seen.

Nearly all clinical trials have demonstrated an increased ability of patients to tolerate higher "dose intensities" of chemotherapy with equivalent toxicities, if adjunctive growth factor (usually G-CSF or GM-CSF) support is utilized. To date, reasonably good data have been generated to support the use of very high dose therapy with stem cell support in leukemia, relapsed intermediate to high-grade lymphomas, and multiple myeloma. Even so, for the vast majority of the more common human solid tumors, dose escalation of chemotherapy to the degree requiring the routine support of hematopoietic cytokines has not yet been prospectively proven to be of worth. Therefore, the ASCO Guidelines Committee concluded that dose- or schedule-based intensification of chemotherapy should be undertaken only in the context of clinical research trials.[231]

Use of Hematopoietic Growth Factors in Febrile and Afebrile Neutropenic Patients On the one hand, there is no indication for the use of CSFs in patients with uncomplicated neutropenia. On the other hand, G-CSF (or GM-CSF) is often used as an adjunct to empiric antibiotics in patients with febrile neutropenia, even though in the modern era of broad-spectrum parenteral antibiotics, mortality from febrile neutropenia is quite rare in patients with solid tumors. Most studies have shown that in the setting of uncomplicated febrile neutropenia, routine use of CSFs as adjuvants is not justified. However, the use of CSFs has been deemed reasonable in certain high-risk febrile neutropenic patients, for example, those with pneumonia, hypotension, multiorgan dysfunction, or fungal infection.[231]

Hematopoietic Growth Factors in Leukemic Patients Concern has been raised about the potential of growth factors to stimulate the proliferation of myeloid leukemia cells. Randomized trials have not, however, shown this to be clinically relevant. Indeed, the use of CSFs to support the intensive myelotoxic chemotherapy of leukemia has been one of the first "label expansions" for these agents on the basis of the strength of more recent clinical trial data.[204] Overall, there is evidence from several studies that administration of CSFs shortly after completion of AML induction therapy can achieve modest decreases in the duration of neutropenia and perhaps amelioration of infectious complications in older patients (although response rates and long-term outcome are not changed). Primary administration of CSFs in patients over 55 years old is therefore considered reasonable.[231] It also appears likely that these results are applicable to younger individuals. In ALL induction therapy, use of G-CSF is also justified by the evidence.[231] Use of CSFs for priming leukemic cells before chemotherapy has not, to date, been found worthwhile.

Colony-Stimulating Factor Regimes (Timing and Duration) Existing data suggest that for optimal neutrophil recovery, G-CSF or GM-CSF should be started between 24 and 72 hours

Table 49-37 FLT-3 Ligand

	Characteristics[238,239]	Comment
Forms	Soluble and membrane-bound	
Major production sites	Hematopoietic bone marrow microenvironment	
Selected biologic activities	Synergizes with other hematopoietins to promote progenitor growth	
	Can expand CD34+ cells	
	Increases dendritic and natural killer cells	
Receptor	FLT-3	
Potential clinical trials	FLT-3 inhibitors are being tested in AML	Activating FLT-3 mutations are found in ≈ 30% of AML

AML = acute myelogenous leukemia.

after chemotherapy. The recommended dosage of G-CSF is 5 μg/kg (SC) daily; GM-CSF, 250 μg/m^2/d. Doses of G-CSF may be increased in increments of 5 μg/kg for each chemotherapy cycle, if the duration and severity of neutropenia warrant it. CSFs are generally continued until an absolute neutrophil count of 10,000/μL is achieved, though earlier discontinuation may be reasonable and cost effective. Issues regarding the pros and cons of using G-CSF versus GM-CSF cannot, in general, be addressed by currently available studies. Recently, a pegylated G-CSF (Neulasta) with a prolonged half-life has been approved for clinical use. Clearance of this molecule is via neutrophil receptor binding and, hence, is directly related to neutrophil counts. Therefore, a single dose of pegylated G-CSF can be used after chemotherapy. In general, a dose of pegylated G-CSF (6 mg SC) should be given at least 24 hours after chemotherapy. It is indicated in patients with nonmyeloid malignancies receiving myelosuppressive drugs with a significant incident of febrile neutropenia.

Non-Myeloid Growth Factors Currently, the only nonmyeloid growth factors approved for clinical use by the United States Federal Drug Administration (FDA) are EPO and IL-11. Given the difficulty in identifying patients who should receive G-CSF/GM-CSF, it is clear that the task is magnified significantly when other hematologic cell lineages are taken into account. Furthermore, the availability of blood components (red blood cells and platelets) for transfusion further complicates the issue.

The use of EPO and IL-11 has not been addressed in the ASCO Clinical Practice Guidelines. Since efficacy of IL-11 was demonstrated in patients who experienced marked lowering of platelet counts following the previous chemotherapy cycle, however, this molecule is approved in the United States for the prevention of severe thrombocytopenia following myelosuppressive chemotherapy in patients with nonmyeloid malignancies who are at high risk for this problem. Dosing with IL-11 should generally commence 6 to 24 hours following the completion of chemotherapy. The recommended dosage is 50 μg/kg/d subcutaneously. Dosing is continued until the postplatelet nadir reaches ≥ 50,000 cells/μL (generally 10–21 days). Fluid retention is the most common side effect.

In regard to EPO, the potential to reduce red cell transfusion requirements and to increase quality of life are therapeutic goals. EPO has been shown to increase hematocrit and decrease transfusion requirements after the first month of chemotherapy (months 2 and 3) in anemic cancer patients. On this basis, EPO has been FDA-approved in the United States for the treatment of anemia in patients with nonmyeloid malignancies where the anemia is due to the effect of chemotherapy. Baseline endogenous serum EPO levels vary among such patients, and in general, individuals with lower baseline levels respond more vigorously. Although no specific serum EPO levels can be stipulated above which patients will not respond to EPO, those with levels above 200 mU/L are considered much less responsive. The recommended starting dosage of EPO is 150 μg/kg given subcutaneously three times per week. Because of the length of time required for erythropoiesis, a clinically significant increase in hematocrit may not be seen for several weeks. The dose of EPO can be doubled after 8 weeks if response is not satisfactory. If the hematocrit exceeds 40%, EPO should be withheld. Recently, a hyperglycosylated EPO (darbopoeitin α) has been approved. It can be given every 1 to 2 weeks for chemotherapy-related anemia. Functional iron deficiency (transferrin saturation ≤ 20%) has been found to occur in renal failure patients, despite normal to elevated total body iron stores. Parenteral iron administration in such patients significantly improves response to EPO. The extent to which a similar phenomenon complicates EPO therapy of cancer is not yet established.

HEMATOPOIETIC GROWTH FACTORS IN THE TRANSPLANTATION SETTING

Worldwide, three recombinant CSFs have been accepted for use in the transplant recipient: G-CSF and GM-CSF (worldwide) and M-CSF (in Japan).[232] In brief, CSFs can be routinely recommended as adjuncts to allogeneic and autologous progenitor cell transplants, both for mobilization of peripheral blood progenitor cells and as a means to speed hematopoietic reconstitution after transplantation with bone marrow or peripheral blood progenitors. Administration of CSFs to patients who experience delayed or inadequate neutrophil engraftment also appears warranted.[231]

G-CSF Several trials have been performed confirming that patients who receive G-CSF achieve an absolute neutrophil count (ANC) of ≥ 500 cells/μL earlier than controls following autologous or allogeneic BMT. Neutrophil recovery to 500 cells/μL is generally 7 days earlier, platelet recovery is not affected, infection is either not affected or is less frequent, and hospital stay is not affected or is of shorter duration in G-CSF–treated patients. No adverse effects of G-CSF on graft-versus-host disease, rate of relapse, survival, or the occurrence of graft failure or infection has been observed. The dosage of G-CSF used is usually 10 μg/kg/d administered subcutaneously. G-CSF is often started one or more days after infusion of bone marrow progenitors and continued until neutrophils attain a level ≥ 1,000 to 1,500 cells/μL for 3 consecutive days, and then tapered (though this cutoff point is fairly arbitrary). A transient fall in neutrophils may occur after G-CSF is discontinued.

In regard to peripheral blood stem cell transplantation, both neutrophil and platelet recovery are enhanced and hospital stay is shortened with the infusion of peripheral blood progenitors harvested after a short course of G-CSF (10 μg/kg/d). No effect on incidence of documented infection was observed in most trials. G-CSF is generally given for at least 4 days before the first leukapheresis procedure and continued until the last leukapheresis for peripheral blood stem cell collection. Dose modifications should be made in those individuals who develop a white blood cell count > 100,000/μL.

GM-CSF GM-CSF has similar activity to G-CSF, but toxicity (low-grade fevers, myalgias, bone pains, abdominal pains) is greater. Enhanced macrophage function is observed in patients receiving GM-CSF and is theoretically of benefit to patients with infection.

Efficacy of GM-CSF has been demonstrated following myeloablative chemotherapy in patients undergoing autologous or allogeneic transplantation and for mobilization of progenitors. Patients who develop graft delay or graft failure after autologous or allogeneic transplantation also appear to derive benefit from the use of GM-CSF. The primary advantages are reductions in the rates of infection and in the duration of hospitalization. In general, no effect was observed on the incidence or duration of acute graft-versus-host disease (GVHD), rate of relapse, or survival in patients receiving GM-CSF, as compared with placebo after allogeneic or autologous transplantation, but the rate of chronic graft-versus-host-disease may be increased.

M-CSF M-CSF has been sparsely explored in the United States. It has received approval in Japan to enhance neutrophil recovery following allogeneic transplantation, dose-intensive therapy for ovarian cancer, and after consolidation chemotherapy for AML. It appears that the purified product used in Japan has a similar effect as recombinant G-CSF or GM-CSF after autologous transplantation. It may also have a similar or, possibly, greater effect than GM-CSF on enhancing macrophage function.

THROMBOPOIETIC AGENTS IN THE CLINIC: AN OVERVIEW

Reliably raising platelet counts in thrombocytopenic humans has proven much more difficult than ameliorating neutropenia. Cytokines that stimulate platelet production may act on early progenitors promoting their commitment along the megakaryocytic lineage or may enhance survival of already committed megakaryocytes. During the 1990s, a series of molecules with thrombopoietic potential have been tested in clinical trials: IL-3, IL-6, SCF, IL-11, and TPO. Overall, the results have been disappointing.

Currently, the only thrombopoietic molecule approved for clinical use in the United States is IL-11. A phase III study of IL-11 in conjunction with a diuretic (to prevent fluid accumulation) demonstrated a reduction in thrombocytopenia after chemotherapy.[172] The favorable results of this trial prompted the FDA to approve the use of IL-11 for this indication (as discussed above). Even so, the effect of IL-11 on platelets appears to be much less dramatic than that of G-CSF on leukocytes and with considerably more side effects. However, the other thrombopoietic molecules have fared even worse in clinical trials.

Phase I/II studies of IL-3 given to cancer patients after chemotherapy or autologous bone marrow transplantation showed only modest augmentation of platelet recovery. Furthermore, these changes occurred at doses that were difficult to tolerate.[233–235] Interestingly, much higher doses of IL-3 were well tolerated in patients with thrombocytopenia due to aplastic anemia, graft failure, or myelodysplasia.[84] Furthermore, though these patients rarely responded to IL-3 alone, over one-third had major trilineage recovery when IL-3 and GM-CSF were given sequentially for prolonged periods of time.[79] In some individuals, responses were durable even after discontinuation of therapy.[85]

SCF has also been administered after chemotherapy, again with modest salutary effects on neutrophils and platelet counts and a high incidence of transient allergic reactions.[233] Furthermore, though SCF, especially when combined with G-CSF, has shown efficacy at mobilizing stem cells (which were later reinfused), this regimen did not improve platelet recovery.[37] In aplastic anemia patients, however, use of SCF alone and together with G-CSF has resulted in trilineage responses.[38] As with the sequential IL-3/GM-CSF studies mentioned above, prolonged therapy was necessary to see responses, and recovery was durable in some individuals even after treatment was stopped.

PIXY321 is a fusion protein that consists of the active domains of GM-CSF and IL-3. Although attenuation of thrombocytopenia in PIXY321-treated sarcoma patients was reported in a phase II trial, several subsequent randomized studies have failed to confirm any benefit.

Clinical trials of IL-6 have also shown minimal to no platelet-enhancing activity when this molecule was administered to patients undergoing chemotherapy or autologous transplantation.[117–119] Combining this molecule with G-CSF also did not yield statistically significant improvements. It has been suggested that increased platelet counts require doses above the maximum tolerated level.

At the time of discovery of TPO, this molecule was trumpeted as the true platelet growth factor. However, it too has proven problematic. The PEGylated version of TPO (produced by Amgen Corp) resulted in significantly increased platelet yields in normal subjects[49] but was, nevertheless, abandoned because of the development of antibodies in some of the recipients.

HEMATOPOIETIC GROWTH FACTORS IN BONE MARROW FAILURE STATES

Hematopoietic Growth Factors in Myelodysplastic Syndrome According to the ASCO guidelines, intermittent use of colony stimulating factors in severely neutropenic myelodysplastic syndrome patients with recurrent infection may be considered.[231] Data supporting their long-term continuous use are, however, lacking. Randomized studies have not shown an increased risk of progression to leukemia; nevertheless, in one such study, overall survival was shorter in the G-CSF arm than in the supportive-care arm in patients with refractory anemia with excess blasts.[231]

In regard to EPO, meta-analyses suggest that about 15% of patients with myelodysplasia will respond to this molecule. Patients with endogenous serum EPO levels of greater than 200 mU/mL are unlikely to respond.

Aplastic Anemia G-CSF is often utilized as an adjunct to immunosuppressive therapy in the frontline management of aplastic anemia. This molecule, as well as GM-CSF, is sometimes used to raise neutrophil counts in patients with this disorder, though individuals with very severe disease may not respond. Of interest, investigational studies have demonstrated that the dose of CSF needed to raise neutrophil counts may be minuscule compared with that used following chemotherapy.[236]

A variety of growth factors have been administered to patients with aplastic anemia in an attempt to achieve multilineage recovery.[84] Most of these trials have demonstrated only modest, if any, responses. More recently, trials with combinations of growth factors have also been performed. Use of GM-CSF or G-CSF together with EPO may stimulate bilineage recovery, with most hemoglobin responses occurring in patients with serum EPO levels < 2,000 mU/mL.[236,237] Of more interest, durable multilineage recovery has been reported with the use of sequential IL-3 followed by GM-CSF, as well as with SCF combined with G-CSF.[38,80] Prolonged therapy (several months) is often necessary to achieve response, and in the case of these early-acting factors, high doses appear more effective. However, molecules such as IL-3 and SCF remain investigational.

Severe Chronic Neutropenia G-CSF is indicated in patients with a diagnosis of congenital, cyclic, or idiopathic neutropenia. In congenital neutropenia, the recommended daily starting dosage is 6 μg/kg twice daily administered by subcutaneous injection. In idiopathic or cyclic neutropenia, the starting dosage is 5 μg/kg/d. Chronic daily administration is needed, with the target absolute neutrophil counts being 1,500 to 10,000/μL.

FUTURE PERSPECTIVES

From the inchoate understanding of cytokines of a decade ago has now emerged a complex picture of interacting stimulatory and inhibitory factors. Many of the molecules that govern this process have been cloned and have entered clinical trials. It is now clear that regulatory cytokines are characteristically pleiotropic and, at the same time, exhibit significant functional redundancy.

The history of medicine is replete with examples that show how innovative technologies improve clinical outcomes. The genetic engineering techniques that permitted the rapid cloning of newly identified cytokines and their translation into clinical therapies in hematology and oncology are an exciting example of this phenomenon.[230] However, it should be remembered that many, if not most, cytokines and their respective natural inhibitors are ubiquitously expressed and have myriad biologic properties that influence virtually every organ system (see Figure 49-1). It is already apparent that these molecules may also be effective in allergic and inflammatory conditions. Furthermore, the emerging understanding of their role and the availability of recombinant molecules for clinical therapeutics suggest that their exploitation is still in the nascent stages and will ultimately impact most fields of medicine.

REFERENCES

1. Ozaki K, Leonard WJ. Cytokine and cytokine receptor pleiotropy and redundancy. J Biol Chem 2002;277:29355–8.
2. Cazzola M. How and when to use erythropoietin. Curr Opin Hematol 1998;5:103–8.
3. National Center for Biotechnology Information. Online Mendelian inheritance in man: gene map. Available at: http://www.ncbi.nlm.nih.gov/Omim/getmap.cgi (accessed June 17, 2005).
4. Zhu Y, D'Andrea AD. The molecular physiology of erythropoietin and the erythropoietin receptor. Curr Opin Hematol 1994:1:113–8.
5. De La Chapelle A, Sistonen P, Lehvaslaiho H, et al. Familial erythrocytosis genetically linked to erythropoietin receptor gene. Lancet 1993:341:82–4.
6. Adamson JW. Epoietin alfa: into the new millennium. Semin Oncol 1998;25:76–9.
7. Crawford J, Cella D, Cleeland CS, et al. Relationship between changes in hemoglobin level and quality of life during chemotherapy in anemic cancer patients receiving epoetina therapy. Cancer 2002;95:888–95.
8. Johnson GR, Gonda TJ, Metcalf D. A lethal myeloproliferative syndrome in mice transplanted with bone marrow cells infected with a retrovirus expressing granulocyte-macrophage colony stimulating factor. EMBO J 1986;8:441–5.
9. Gasson JC. Molecular physiology of granulocyte-macrophage colony-stimulating factor. Blood 1991;77: 1131–45.
10. Wetzler M, Estrov Z, Talpaz M, et al. Granulocyte-macrophage colony-stimulating factor as a cause of paraneoplastic leukaemoid reaction in advanced transitional cell carcinoma. J Intern Med 1993;234:417–20.
11. Carter L, Petros WP, Rosner GL, et al. Evaluation of GMCSF mouthwash for the prevention of chemotherapy-induced mucositis: a randomized, double-blind, dose-finding study. Cytokine 1995;7:471–7.
12. Bonilla MA, Dale D, Zeidler C, et al. Long-term safety of treatment with recombinant human granulocyte colony-stimulating factor (r-metHuG-CSF) in patients with severe congenital neutropenia. Br J Haematol 1994;88:723–30.
13. Root RK, Dale DC. Granulocyte colony-stimulating factor and granulocyte-macrophage colony stimulating factor: comparisons and potential for use in the treatment of infections in nonneutropenic patients. J Infect Dis 1999;179 Suppl 2:S342–52.
14. Dong F, Brynes RK, Tidow N, et al. Mutations in the gene for the granulocyte colony-stimulating-factor receptor in patients with acute myeloid leukemia preceded by severe congenital neutropenia. N Engl J Med 1995;333:487–93.
15. Crawford J, Ozer H, Stoller R, et al. Reduction by granulocyte colony-stimulating factor of fever and neutropenia induced by chemotherapy in patients with small-cell lung cancer. N Engl J Med 1991;325:164–70.
16. Stahel RA, Jost LM, Cerny T, et al. Randomized study of recombinant human granulocyte colony-stimulating factor after high-dose chemotherapy and autologous bone marrow transplantation for high-risk lymphoid malignancies. J Clin Oncol 1994;12:1931–8.
17. Schmitz N, Linch DC, Dreger P, et al. Randomised trial of filgrastim-mobilised peripheral blood progenitor cell trans-plantation versus autologous bone-marrow transplantation in lymphoma patients. Lancet 1996;347:353–7.
18. Hubel K, Dale DC, Liles WC. Therapeutic use of cytokines to modulate phagocyte function for the treatment of infectious diseases: current status of granulocyte-macrophage colony-stimulating factor, granulocyte-macrophage colony-stimulating factor, macrophage colony-stimulating factor, and interferon-gamma. J Infect Dis 2002;185:1490–501.
19. Heil G, Hoelzer D, Sanz MA, et al. A randomized, double-blind, placebo-controlled, phase III study of filgrastim in remission induction and consolidation therapy for adults with de novo acute myeloid leukemia. Blood 1997;90:4710–8.
20. Kuritzkes DR, Parenti D, Ward DJ, et al. Filgrastim prevents severe neutropenia and reduces infective morbidity in patients with advanced HIV infection: results of a randomized, multicenter, controlled trials. AIDS 1998;12:65–74.

21. Crawford J. Clinical uses of pegylated pharmaceuticals in oncology. Cancer Treat Rev 2002;28Suppl A:7–11.
22. Robinson WA, Stanley ER, Metcalf D. Stimulation of bone marrow colony growth in vitro. Blood 1969;33:396–9.
23. Sherr CJ, Rettenmier CW, Sacca R, et al. The c-fms protooncogene product is related to the receptor for the mononuclear phagocyte growth factor, CSF-1. Cell 1985;41:665–76.
24. Motoyoshi K. Biological activities and clinical application of M-CSF. Int J Hematol 1998;67:109–22.
25. Flanagan AM, Lader CS. Update on the biologic effects of macrophage colony-stimulating factor. Curr Opin Hematol 1998;5:181–2.
26. Nemunaitis J. Use of macrophage colony-stimulating factor in the treatment of fungal infections. Clin Infect Dis 1998;26:1279–81.
27. Williams DE, Eisenman J, Baird A, et al. Identification of a ligand for the c-kit proto-oncogene. Cell 1990;63:167–74.
28. Anderson DM, Williams DE, Tushinski R, et al. Alternate splicing of mRNAs encoding human mast cell growth factor and localization of the gene to chromosome 12q22q24. Cell Growth Differ 1991;2:373–8.
29. Broudy VC. Stem cell factor and hematopoiesis. Blood 1997;90:1345–58.
30. Ullrich A, Schlessinger J. Signal transduction by receptors with tyrosine kinase activity. Cell 1990;61:203–5.
31. Matsui Y, Zsebo KM, Hogan BLM. Embryonic expression of a haematopoietic growth factor encoded by the Sl locus and the ligand for c-kit. Nature 1990;347;667–9.
32. Russell ES. Hereditary anemias of the mouse: a review for geneticists. Adv Genet 1979;20:357–459.
33. Demetri GD, von Mehran M, Blanke CD, et al. Efficacy and safety of imatinib mesylate in advanced gastrointestinal stromal tumors. N Engl J Med 2002;347:472–80.
34. Andrews RG, Briddell RA, Knitter GH, et al. Rapid engraftment by peripheral blood progenitor cells mobilized by recombinant human stem cell factor and recombinant human granulocyte colony-stimulating factor in nonhuman primates. Blood 1995;85:15–20.
35. Tong J, Gordon MS, Srour EF, et al. In vivo administration of recombinant methionyl human stem cell factor expands the number of human marrow hematopoietic stem cells. Blood 1993;82:784–91.
36. Tricot G, Jagannath S, Desikan KR, et al. Superior mobilization of peripheral blood progenitor cells (PBPC) with r-metHuSCF (SCF) and r-metHuG-SCF (Filgrastim) in heavily pretreated multiple myeloma (MM) patients. Blood 1996;88:388a–93a.
37. Shpall EJ, Wheeler CA,Turner SA, et al. A randomized phase 3 study of peripheral blood progenitor cell mobilization of stem cell factor and filgrastim in high risk breast cancer patients. Blood 1999;93:2491–501.
38. Kurzrock R, Gratwohl A, Paquette R, et al. Trilineage responses seen with stem cell factor (STEMGEN, SCF) and filgrastim (G-CSF) treatment in aplastic anemia (AA) patients (Pts) [abstract]. Br J Haematol 1998;102:1.
39. Cwirla SE, Balasubramanian P, Duffin DJ, et al. Peptide agonist of the thrombopoietin receptor as potent as the natural cytokine. Science 1997;276:1696–9.
40. Metcalf D. Thrombopoietin—at last. Nature 1994;369:519–20.
41. Kaushansky K, Drachman JG. The molecular and cellular biology of thrombopoietin: the primary regulator of platelet production. Oncogene 2002;21:3359–67.
42. Hofmann WK, Ottmann OG, Hoelzer D. Megakaryocytic growth factors: is there a new approach for management of thrombocytopenia in patients with malignancies? Leukemia 1999;13:S14–18.
43. Wiestner A, Schlemper RF, van der Maas AP, Skoda RC. An activating splice donor mutation in the thrombopoietin gene causes hereditary thrombocythaemia. Nat Genet 1998;18:49–52.
44. Vadhan-Raj S, Murray LJ, Bueso-Ramos C, et al. Stimulation of megakaryocyte and platelet production by a single dose of recombinant human thrombopoietin in patients with cancer. Ann Intern Med 1997;126:673–81.
45. Fanucchi M, Glaspy J, Crawford J, et al. Effects of polyethylene glycol-conjugated recombinant human megakaryocyte growth and development factor on platelet counts after chemotherapy for lung cancer. N Engl J Med 1997;336:404–9.
46. Basser RL, Rasko JE, Clarke K, et al. Randomized, blinded, placebo-controlled phase I trial of PEGylated recombinant human megakaryocyte growth and development factor with filgrastim after dose-intensive chemotherapy in patients with advanced cancer. Blood 1997;90:2513–8.
47. Glaspy J, Vredenburgh J, Demetri GD, et al. Effects of PEGylated recombinant human megakaryocyte growth and development factor (PEG-rHuMGDF) before high dose chemotherapy (HDC) with peripheral blood progenitor cell (PBPC) support [abstract]. Blood 1997;90 Supp 1:580a.
48. Nash R, Kurzrock R, DiPersio J, et al. Safety and activity of recombinant human thrombopoietin (rhTPO) in patients (pts) with delayed platelet recovery (DPR) [abstract]. Blood 1997;90 Suppl 1:262a.
49. Kuter D, McCullough J, Romo J, et al. Treatment of platelet (PLT) donors with PEGylated recombinant human megakaryocyte growth and development factor (PEG-rHuMGDF) increases circulating PLT counts (CTS) and PLT apheresis yields and increases platelet increments in recipients of PLT transfusions [abstract]. Blood 1997;90 Suppl 1:579a.
50. Kuter DJ, Begley CG. Recombinant human thrombopoietin: basic biology and evaluation of clinical studies. Blood 2002;100(10):3457–69.
51. Dinarello CA. Interleukin-1, interleukin-1 receptors and interleukin-1 receptor antagonist. Intern Rev Immunol 1998;16:457–99.
52. Veltri S, Smith JW. Interleukin-1 trials in cancer patients: a review of the toxicity, antitumor, and hematopoietic effects. Stem Cells 1996;13:164–76.
53. Arend WP. Cytokine imbalance in the pathogenesis of rheumatoid arthritis: the role of interluekin-1 receptor antagonist. Semin Arthritis Rhem 2001;30(5 Suppl 2):1–6.
54. Sims JE. IL-1 and IL-18 receptors, and their extended family. Curr Opin Immunol 2002;14:117–22.
55. Mileno MD, Margolis NH, Clark BD, et al. Coagulation of whole blood stimulates interleukin-1 beta gene expression: absence of gene transcripts in anticoagulated blood. J Infect Dis 1995;172:308–11.
56. Granowitz EV, Santos A, Poutsiaka DD, et al. Circulating interleukin-1 receptor antagonist levels during experimental endotoxemia in humans. Lancet 1991;338:1423–8.
57. Rambaldi A, Torcia M, Bettoni S, et al. Modulation of cell proliferation and cytokine production in acute myeloblastic leukemia by interleukin-1 receptor antagonist and lack of its expression by leukemic cells. Blood 1991;78:3248–53.
58. Wetzler M, Kurzrock, Estrov Z, et al. Altered levels of interleukin-l beta and interleukin-1 receptor antagonist in chronic myelogenous leukemia: clinical and prognostic correlates. Blood 1994;84:3142–7.
59. Estrov Z, Kurzrock R, Estey E, et al. Inhibition of acute myelogenous leukemia blast proliferation by interleukin-1 (IL-1) receptor antagonist and soluble IL-1 receptors. Blood 1992;79:1938–45.
60. Estrov Z, Kurzrock R, Wetzler M, et al. Suppression of chronic myelogenous leukemia colony growth by interleukin-1 (IL-1) receptor antagonist and soluble IL-1 receptors: a novel application for inhibitors of IL-1 activity. Blood 1991;78:1476–84.
61. Walsh CE, Liu JM, Anderson SM, Rossio JL. A trial of recombinant human interleukin-1 in patients with severe refractory aplastic anaemia. Br J Haematol 1992;80:106–11.
62. Iizumi T, Sato S, Iiyama T, et al. Recombinant human interleukin-1 beta analogue as a regulator of hematopoiesis in patients receiving chemotherapy for urogenital cancers. Cancer 1991;68:1520–3.
63. Smith JW, Longo D, Alford WG, et al. The effects of treatment with interleukin-1α on platelet recovery after high-dose carboplatin. N Engl J Med 1993;328:756–61.
64. Smith KA. Interleukin-2: inception, impact, and implications. Science 1988;240:1169–76.
65. Gomez J, Gonzales A, Martinez-A C, Rebollo A. IL-2-induced cellular events. Crit Rev Immunol 1998;18:185–220.
66. Sadlack, B, Merz H, Schorle H, et al. Ulcerative colitis-like disease in mice with disrupted interleukin-2 gene. Cell 1993;75:253–61.
67. Atkins MB. Interleukin-2: clinical applications. Semin Oncol 2002;3(Suppl 7):12–7.
68. Nichols J, Foss F, Kuzel TM, et al. Interleukin-2 fusion protein: an investigational therapy for interleukin-2 receptor expressing malignancies. Eur J Cancer 1997;33:S34–36.
69. Stern JB, Smith KA. Interleukin-2 induction of T-cell G1 progression and c-*myb* expression. Science 1986;233:203–6.
70. Grimm EA, Owen-Schaub LB, Londaon WG, Yagita M. Lymphokine-Activated Killer Cells. Induction and function. Ann N Y Acad Sci 1988;532:380–6.
71. Yang SC, Grimm EA, Parkinson DR, et al. Clinical and immunomodulatory effects of combination immunotherapy with low-dose interleukin 2 and tumor necrosis factor alpha in patients with advanced non–small-cell lung cancer: a phase I trial. Cancer Res 1991;51:3669–76.
72. Yang SC, Owen-Schaub LB, Grimm EA, Roth JA. Induction of lymphokine activated killer cytotoxicity with interleukin-2 and tumor necrosis factor alpha against primary lung cancer target. Cancer Immunol Immunother 1989;29:193–6.
73. Grimm EA, Mazumder A, Zhang HZ, Rosenberg SA. The lymphokine-activated killer cell phenomenon: lysis of NK-resistant fresh solid tumor cells by IL-2 activated autologous human peripheral blood lymphocytes. J Exp Med 1982;155:1823–41.
74. Mier JW, Vachino G, Van Der Meer JWM, et al. Induction of circulating tumor necrosis factor (TNF alpha) as the mechanism for the febrile response to interleukin-2 (IL-2) in cancer patients. J Clin Immunol 1988;8:426–36.
75. Owen-Schaub LB, de Mars M, Murphy EO Jr, Grimm EA. IL-2 dose regulates TNF-α mRNA transcription and protein secretion in human peripheral blood lymphocytes. Cell Immunol 1991;132:193–200.
76. Heaton K, Ju G, Grimm EA. Human interleukin-2 analogs that preferentially bind the intermediate-affinity IL-2 receptor lead to reduced secondary cytokine secretion. Cancer Res 1993;53:2597–602.
77. Lee JC, Ihle JN. Chronic immune stimulation is required for Moloney leukemia virus-induced lymphomas. Nature 1981;289:407–9.
78. Eder M, Geissler G, Ganser A. IL-3 in the clinic. Stem Cells 1997;15:327–33.
79. Lindemann A, Mertelsmann R. Interleukin-3 and its receptor. Cancer Treat Res 1995;80:107–42.
80. Talpaz M, Patterson M, Kurzrock R. Sequential administration of IL-3 and GM-CSF in bone marrow failure patients: a phase I study [abstract 100]. Blood 1994;84 Suppl 1:28a.
81. Gibson FM, Scopes, J, Daly S, et al. Haemopoietic growth factor production by normal and aplastic anaemia stroma in long-term bone marrow culture. Br J Haematol 1995;91:551–61.
82. Mecker TC, Hardy D, Willman C, et al. Activation of the interleukin-3 gene by chromosome translocation in acute lymphocytic leukemia with eosinophilia. Blood 1990;76:285–9.
83. Ball SE, Tchernia G, Wranne L, et al. Is there a role for interleukin-3 in Diamond-Blackfan anaemia? Results of a European multicentre study. Br J Haematol 1995;91:313–8.
84. Kurzrock R, Talpaz M, Estrov Z, et al. Phase I study of recombinant human interleukin-3 in patients with bone marrow failure. J Clin Oncol 1991;9:1241–50.
85. Wu HH, Talpaz M, Champlin RE, et al. Sequential interleukin 3 and granulocyte-macrophage-colony stimulating factor therapy in patients with bone marrow failure with long-term follow-up of responses. Cancer 2004;98:2410–9.
86. Howard M, Farrar J, Hilfiker M, et al. Identification of a T-cell derived B cell growth factor distinct from interleukin-2. J Exp Med 1982;155:914–21.
87. Brown KD, Zurawski SM, Mosmann TR, et al. A family of small inducible proteins secreted by leukocytes are members of a new superfamily that includes leukocyte and fibroblast-derived inflammatory agents, growth factors, and indicators of various activation process. J Immunol 1989;142:679–87.
88. McKenzie ANJ, Culpepper JA, de Waal Malefyt R, et al. Interleukin-13, a novel T cell-derived cytokine that regulates human monocyte and B cell function. Proc Natl Acad Sci U S A 1993;90:3735–9.
89. Chomarat P, Banchereau J. Interleukin-4 and interleukin-13: their similarities and discrepancies. Intern Rev Immunol 1998;17:1–52.
90. Wetzler M, Kurzrock R, Estrov A, et al. Suppressed formation of bone marrow adherent layers derived from acute myeloid leukemia patients after in vitro exposure to interleukin-4. Leuk Res 1997;21:519–27.
91. Tepper RI, Pattengale PK, Leder P. Murine interleukin-4 displays potent anti-tumor activity in vivo. Cell 1989;57:503–12.
92. Puri RK, Leland P, Obiri NI, et al. Targeting of interleukin-13 receptor on human renal cell carcinoma cells by a recombinant chimeric protein composed of interleukin-13 and a truncated form of Pseudomonas exotoxin A (PE38QQR). Blood 1996;87:4333–9.
93. Leach MW, Rybak ME, Rosenblum IY. Safety evaluation of recombinant human interleukin-4 in clinical studies. Clin Immunol Immunopathol 1997;893:12–4.
94. Whitehead RP, Unger JM, Goodwin, et al. Phase II trial of recombinant human interleukin-4 in patients with dis-

seminated malignant melanoma: a Southwest Oncology Group study. J Immunol 1998;21:440–6.

95. Tulpule A, Joshi B, DeGuzman N, et al. Interleukin-4 in the treatment of AIDS-related Kaposi's sarcoma. Ann Oncol 1997;8:79–83.

96. Karlen S, De Boer ML, Lipscombe RJ, et al. Biological and molecular characteristics of interleukin-5 and its receptor. Intern Rev Immunol 1998;16:227–47.

97. Sakamaki K, Miyajima I, Kitamura T, Miyajima A. Critical cytoplasmic domains of the common beta subunit of the human GM-CSF, IL-3 and IL-5 receptors for growth, signal transduction and tyrosine phosphorylation. EMBO J 1992;11:3541–9.

98. Yamaguchi Y, Hayashi Y, Sumaga Y, et al. Highly purified murine interleukin-5 (IL-5) stimulates eosinophil function and prolongs in vitro survival. Il-5 as an eosinophil chemotactic factor. J Exp Med 1988;167:1737–42.

99. O'Byrne PM, Inman MD, Parameswaran K. The trials and tribulations of IL-5, eosinophils, and allergic asthma. J Allergy Clin Immunol 2001;108:503–8.

100. Pinto A, Aldinucci D, Gloghini A, et al. The role of eosinophils in the pathobiology of Hodgkin's disease. Ann Oncol 1997;8 Suppl 2:89–96.

101. Lange AM, Yutanawiboonchai W, Scott P, Abraham D. IL-4 and IL-5 dependent protective immunity to Onchocerca volvulus infective larvae in BALB/cBYJ mice. J Immunol 1994;153:205–11.

102. Baba T, Sonozaki H, Seki K, et al. An eosinophil chemotactic factor present in blister fluids of bullous pemphigoid patients. J Immunol 1976;116:112–6.

103. Lalani T, Simmons RK, Ahmed AR. Biology of IL-5 in health and disease. Ann Allergy Asthma Immunol 1999;82:317–33.

104. Hirano T, Yasukawa K, Harada H, et al. Complementary DNA for a novel human interleukin (BSF-2) that induces B lymphocytes to produce immunoglobulin. Nature 1986;324;73–6.

105. Seymour JF, Kurzrock R. Interleukin-6: biologic properties and role in lymphoproliferative disorders. In: Kurzrock R, Talpaz M, editors. Cytokines: interleukins and their receptors. Norwell (MA): Kluwer Academic Publishers; 1995. p.123–32.

106. Hirano T. Interleukin 6 and its receptor: ten years later. Int Rev Immunol 1998;16:249–84.

107. Muraguchi A, Hirano T, Tang B, et al. The essential role of B cell stimulatory factor 2 (BSF-2/IL-6) for the terminal differentiation of B cells. J Exp Med 1988;167:332–44.

108. Veldhuis GJ, Willemse PHB, Mulder NJ, et al. Potential use of recombinant human interleukin-6 in clinical oncology. Leuk Lymph 1996;20:373–9.

109. Suematsu S, Matsusaka T, Matsuda T, et al. Generation of transplantable plasmacytomas with t(12;15) in IL-6 transgenic mice. Proc Natl Acad Sci U S A 1992;89:232–5.

110. Hirano T, Matsuda T, Turner M, et al. Excessive production of interleukin 6/B cell stimulatory factor-2 in rheumatoid arthritis. Eur J Immunol 1988;18:1797–801.

111. Kurzrock R, Redman J, Cabanillas F, et al. Serum interleukin 6 levels are elevated in lymphoma patients and correlate with survival in advanced Hodgkin's disease and with B symptoms. 1993;53:2118–22.

112. Seymour JF, Talpaz M, Cabanillas F, et al. Serum interleukin-6 levels correlate with prognosis in diffuse large cell lymphoma. J Clin Oncol 1995;13:575–82.

113. Fayad L, Cabanillas F, Talpaz M, et al. High serum interleukin-6 levels correlate with a shorter failure-free survival in indolent lymphoma. Leuk Lymph 1998;30:563–71.

114. Seymour JF, Talpaz M, Hagemeister FB, et al. Clinical correlates of elevated serum levels of interleukin-6 in patients with untreated Hodgkin's disease. Am J Med 1997;102:21–8.

115. Seymour JF, Talpaz M, Cabanillas F, et al. Serum interleukin-6 levels correlate with prognosis in diffuse large-cell lymphoma. J Clin Oncol 1995;13:575–82.

116. Hsu S-M, Waldron JA, Xie S-S, Barlogie B. Expression of interleukin-6 in Castleman's disease. Hum Pathol 1993;24:833–9.

117. D'Hondt V, Humblet Y, Guillaume T, et al. Thrombopoietic effects and toxicity of interleukin-6 in patients with ovarian cancer before and after chemotherapy: a multi-centric placebo-controlled, randomized phase Ib study. Blood 1995;85:2347–53.

118. Budd GT, Pelley R, Samuels T, et al. Phase II randomized trial of simultaneous rhIL-6 and G-CSF following MAID chemotherapy in patients with sarcomas: preliminary results [abstract]. Proc Am Soc Clin Oncol 1995;14:256.

119. Lazarus HM, Winton EF, Williams SF, et al. Phase I multicenter trial of interleukin-6 therapy after autologous bone marrow transplantation in advanced breast cancer. Bone Marrow Transplant 1995;19:935–42.

120. Jones SA, Horiuchi S, Topley N, et al. The soluble interleukin 6 receptor: mechanisms of production and implications in disease. FASEB J 2001;15:43–58.

121. Tagga T, Hibi M, Hirata Y, et al. Interleukin-6 triggers the association of its receptor with a possible signal transducer gp 130. Cell 1989;58:573–81.

122. Yanasaki K, Taga T, Hirata Y, et al. Cloning and expression of the human interleukin-6 (BSF-2/IFNB2) receptor. Science 1988;241:825–8.

123. Tosato G, Pike S. Interferon B2/interleukin-6 is a costimulant for human T lymphocytes. J Immunol 1988;141:1556–62.

124. Geiger T, Andus T, Klapproth J, et al. Induction of rat acute phase proteins by interleukin-6 in vivo. Eur J Immunol 1988;18:717–21.

125. Hirano T, Kishimoto T. Purification to homogeneity and characterization of human B-cell differentiation factor (BCDF or BSF p-2). Proc Natl Acad Sci U S A 1985;82:5490–4.

126. Jilka RL, Hangoc G, Grasole G, et al. Increase osteoclast development after estrogen loss: mediation by interleukin-6. Science 1992;257:88–91.

127. Spangelo BL, Judd AM, Isakson PC, et al. Interleukin-6 stimulates anterior pituitary hormone release in vivo. Endocrinology 1989;125:575–7.

128. Ebrahimi B, Tucker SL, Li D, et al. Cytokines in pancreatic carcinoma: correlation with phenotypic characteristics and prognosis. Cancer 2004;101(12):2727–36.

129. Namen AE, Lupton S, Hjerrild K, et al. Stimulation of B-cell progenitors by cloned murine interleukin-7. Nature 1988;333:571–3.

130. Pillai M, Torok-Storb B, Iwata M. Expression and function of IL-7 receptors in marrow stromal cells. Leuk Lymphoma 2004;45:2403–8.

131. Peschon JJ, Morrissey PJ, Grabstein KH, et al Early lymphocyte expansion is severely impaired in interleukin 7 receptor-deficient mice. J Exp Med 1994;180:1955–60.

132. Torigoe K, Ushio S, Okura T, et al. Purification and characterization of the human interleukin-18 receptor. J Biol Chem 1997;272:25737–42.

133. Goodwin RG, Friend D, Ziegler SF, et al. Cloning of the human and murine interleukin-7 receptors: demonstration of a soluble form and homology to a new receptor superfamily. Cell 1990;60:941–6.

134. Murray R. Physiologic roles of interleukin-2, interleukin-4, and interleukin-7. Curr Opin Hematol 1996;3:230–4.

135. Akashi K, Kondo M, Weissman IL. Role of interleukin-7 in T-cell development from hematopoietic stem cells. Immunol Rev 1998;165:13–28.

136. Fry TJ, Mackall CL. Interleukin-7: from bench to clinic. Blood 2002;99:3892–904.

137. Mertsching E, Meyer V, Linares J, et al. Interleukin-7, a nonredundant potent cytokine whose over-expression massively perturbs B-lymphopoiesis. Int Rev Immunol 1998;16:285–308.

138. Walz A, Peveri P, Aschauer H, Baggiolini M. Purification and amino acid sequencing of NAF, a novel neutrophilactivating factor produced by monocytes. Biochem Biophys Res Comm 1987;149:755–61.

139. Xie K. Interleukin-8 and human cancer biology. Cytokine Growth Factor Rev 2001;12:375–91.

140. Guo HB, Browing P, Nicholas J, et al. Characterization of a chemokine receptor-related gene in human herpesvirus 8 and its expression in Kaposi's sarcoma. Virology 1997;228:371–8.

141. Arvanitakis L, Geras-Raaka E, Varma A, et al. Human herpesvirus KSHV encodes a constitutively active G-protein-coupled receptor linked to cell proliferation. Nature 1997;385:296–7.

142. Rahman, A, Harvey K, Siddiqui RA. Interleukin-8: an autocrine inflammatory mediator. Curr Pharm Design 1999;5:241–53.

143. Baggiolini M, Clark-Lewis I. Interleukin-8, a chemotactic and inflammatory cytokine. FEBS Lett 1992;307:97–101.

144. Heath H, Qin S, Rao P, et al. Chemokine receptor usage by human eosinophils. The importance of CCR3 demonstrated using an antagonistic monoclonal antibody. J Clin Invest 1997;99:178–84.

145. Strieter RM, Polverini PJ, Arenberg DA, et al. Role of X-X-C chemokines as regulators of angiogenesis in lung cancer. J Leuk Biol 1995;57:752–62.

146. Bar EM. Role of interleukin-8 in tumor growth and metastasis of human melanoma. Pathobiology 1999;67:12–8.

147. Yang Y, Ricciardi S, Ciarletta A, et al. Expression cloning of a cDNA encoding a novel human hematopoietic growth factor: human homologue of murine T-cell growth factor P40. Blood 1989;74:1880–4.

148. Renauld JC. Interleukin-9: structural characteristics and biologic properties. In: Kurzrock R, Talpaz M, editors. Cytokines: interleukins and their receptors. Norwell (MA): Kluwer Academic Publishers; 1995. p.47–62.

149. Demoulin JB, Renauld JC. Interleukin 9 and its receptor: an overview of structure and function. Int Rev Immunol 1998:16:345–58.

150. Mehler MF, Rozental R, Dougherty M, et al. Cytokine regulation of neuronal differentiation of hippocampal progenitor cells. Nature 1993;362:62–5.

151. Fiorentino DF, Bond MW, Mosmann TR. Two types of mouse T helper cell, IV. Th2 clones secrete a factor that inhibits cytokine production by the Th1 clones. J Exp Med 1989;170:2081–95.

152. Cortes J, Kurzrock R. Interleukin-10 in non-Hodgkin's lymphoma. Leuk Lymph 1997;26:251–9.

153. Moore KW, Vieira P, Fiorentino DF, et al. Homology of cytokine synthesis inhibitory factor (IL-10) to the Epstein-Barr virus gene BCRF1. Science 1990;248:1230–4.

154. Williams LM, Ricchetti G, Sarma U, et al. Interleukin-10 suppression of myeloid cell activation: a continuing puzzle. Immunology 2004;113:281–92.

155. Akdis CA, Blaser K. Mechanisms of interleukin-10 mediated immune suppression. Immunol 2001;103(2):131–6.

156. Rousset F, Garcia E, Defrance T, et al. IL-10 is a potent growth and differentiation factor for activated human B lymphocytes. Natl Acad Sci U S A 1992;89:1890–3.

157. Dumoutier L, Renauld JC. Viral and cellular interleukin-10 (IL-10)-related cytokines: from structures to functions. Eur Cytokine Netw 2002;13(1):5–15.

158. Barocchi RA, Ross ME, Tan JC, et al. Lymphomagenesis in the SCID-hu mouse involves production of human interleukin-10. Blood 1995;85:1063–74.

159. Blay JY, Burdin N, Rousset F, et al. Serum interleukin-10 in non-Hodgkin's lymphoma: a prognostic factor. Blood 1993;82:2169–74.

160. Stasi R, Zinzani PL, Galieni P, et al. Detection of soluble interleukin-2 receptor and interleukin-10 in the serum of patients with aggressive non-Hodgkin's lymphoma. Cancer 1994;74:1792–800.

161. Stasi R, Zinzani PL, Galieni, et al. Prognostic value of serum IL-10 and soluble IL-2 receptor levels in aggressive non-Hodgkin's lymphoma. Br J Haematol 1994;88:770–7.

162. Cortes JE, Talpaz M, Cabanillas F, et al. Serum levels of interleukin-10 in patients with diffuse large cell lymphoma: lack of correlation with prognosis. Blood 1995;85:2516–20.

163. Blay JY, Voorzanger N, Favrot M, et al. Presence of Epstein-Barr virus viral interleukin-10 in the serum of patients with non-human immunodeficiency virus related diffuse large-cell non-Hodgkins' lymphomas [letter]. Blood 1995;86:4702–7.

164. Du X, Willaims DA. Interleukin-11: review of molecular, cell biology, and clinical use. Blood 1997;89:3897–908.

165. Sonis S, Edwards I, Lucey C. The biological basis for the attenuation of mucositis: the example of interleukin-11. Leukemia 1999;13:831–4.

166. Hilton DJ, Hilton AA, Raicevic A, et al. Cloning of a murine IL-11receptor alpha-chain; requirement for gp130 for high affinity binding and signal transduction. EMBO J 1994;13:4765–75.

167. Brougy VC, Lin NL, Kaushansky K. Thrombopoietin (cmpl ligand) acts synergistically with erythropoietin, stem cell factor, and interleukin-11 to enhance murine megakaryocyte colony growth and increased megakaryocyte ploidy in vitro. Blood 1995;85:1719–24.

168. Kaushansky K, Broudy VD, Lin N, et al. Thrombopoietin, the Mpl ligand is essential for full megakaryocyte development. Proc Natl Acad Sci U S A 1995;92:3234–7.

169. Booth C, Potten CS. Effects of IL-11 on the growth of intestinal epithelial cells in vitro. Cell Prolif 1995;28:581–6.

170. Kurzrock R, Cortes J, Thomas DA, et al. Pilot study of low-dose interleukin-11 in patients with bone marrow failure. J Clin Oncol 2001;19(21):4165–72.

171. Kobyashi S, Teramura M, Sugawara I, et al. Interleukin-11 acts as an autocrine growth factor for human megakaryoblastic cell lines. Blood 1993;81:889–93.

172. Isaacs C, Robert NJ, Bailey FA, et al. Randomized placebo-controlled study of recombinant human interleukin-11 to prevent chemotherapy-induced thrombocytopenia in patients with breast cancer receiving dose-intensive cyclophosphamide and doxorubicin. J Clin Oncol 1997;15:3368–77.

173. Kobayashi M, Fitz L, Ryan M, et al. Identification and purification of natural killer cell stimulatory factor (NKSF), a cytokine with multiple biologic effects on human lymphocytes. J Exp Med 1989;170:827–46.

174. Hisieh C, Macatonia SE, Tripp CS, et al. Listeria-induced Th1 development in ab-TCR transgenic CD4' T cells

occurs through macrophage production of IL-12. Science 1993;260:547–9.
175. Trinchieri G, Scott P. Interleukin-1 basic principles and clinical applications. Curr Top Microbiol Immunol 1999;238:57–78.
176. Golab J, Zagodozdzon R. Antitumor effects of interleukin-12 in preclinical and early clinical studies. Int J Mol Med 1999;3:537–44.
177. Jacobsen SEW. IL-12, a direct stimulator and indirect inhibitor of hematopoiesis. Res Immunol 1995;146:506–14.
178. Trinchieri G. Interleukin-12: a cytokine at the interface of inflammation and immunity. Adv Immunol 1998;70:83–243.
179. Zeuzem S, Hopf U, Carreno V, et al. A phase I/II study of recombinant human interleukin-12 in patients with chronic hepatitis C. Hepatology 1999;29:1280–7.
180. Trentin L, Zambello R, Facco M, et al. Interleukin-15: a novel cytokine with regulatory properties on normal and neoplastic B lymphocytes. Leuk Lymph 1997;27:35–42.
181. Grabstein KH, Eisenman J, Shanebeck K, et al. Cloning of a T-cell growth factor that interacts with the b chain of the interleukin-2 receptor. Science 1994;264:965–8.
182. Burton JD, Bamford RN, Peters C, et al. A lymphokine, provisionally designated interleukin T and produced by a human adult T-cell leukemia line, stimulates T-cell proliferation and the induction of lymphokine-activated killer cells. Proc Natl Acad Sci U S A 1994;91:4935–9.
183. Waldmann T, Tagaya Y, Bamford R. Interleukin-2, interleukin-15, and their receptors. Int Rev Immunol 1998;16:205–26.
184. Ku CC, Murakami M, Sakamoto A, et al. Control of homeostasis of CD8+ memory T-cells by opposing cytokines. Science 2000;288:675–8.
185. Cruikshank W, Center DM. Modulation of lymphocyte migration by human lymphokines. II. Purification of a lymphotactic factor (LCF). J Immun 1982;128:2569–74.
186. Cruikshank WW, Kornfeld H, Center DM. Signaling and functional properties of interleukin-16. Int Rev Immunol 1998;16:523–40.
187. Bowers K, Pitcher C, Marsh M. CD4: a co-receptor in the immune response and HIV infection. Int J Biochem Cell Biol 1997;29:871–5.
188. Rouvier EM, Lucianai MF, Mattei MG, et al. CTLA-8, cloned from an activated T cell, bearing AU-rich messenger RNA instability sequences, and homologous to a Herpesvirus saimiri gene. J Immunol 1993;150:5445–9.
189. Yao Z, Fanslow WC, Seldin MF, et al. Herpesvirus saimiri encodes a new cytokine. Immunity 1995;3:811–6.
190. Fossiez F, Djossou O, Chomarat P, et al. T cell interleukin-17 induces stromal cells to produce proinflammatory and hematopoietic cytokines. J Exp Med 1996;183:2593–603.
191. Yao Z, Fanslow WC, Seldin MF, et al. Herpesvirus saimiri encodes a new cytokine, IL-17, which binds to a novel cytokine receptor. Immunity 1995;3:811–21.
192. Chabaud M, Durand JM, Buchs N, et al. Human interleukin-17: a T cell-derived proinflammatory cytokine produced by the rheumatoid synovium. Am Coll Rheumatol 1999;42:963–70.
193. Yao Z, Painter SL, Fanslow WC, et al. Human IL-17: a novel cytokine derived from T cells. J Immunol 1995;155:5483–6.
194. Aarvak T, Chabaud M, Miossec P, Natvig JB. IL-17 is produced by some proinflammatory Th1/Th0 cells but not by Th2 cells. J Immunol 1999;162:1246–51.
195. Schwarzenberger P, La Russa, Miller A, et al. IL-17 stimulates granulopoiesis in mice: use of an alternate, novel gene therapy-derived method for in vivo evaluation of cytokines. J Immunol 1998;161:6383–9.
196. Antonysamy MA, Fanslow WC, Fu F, et al. Evidence for a role of IL-17 in alloimmunity: a novel IL-17 antagonist promotes heart graft survival. Transplant Proc 1999;31:93.
197. Nakamura K, Okamura H, Wada M, et al. Endotoxin-induced serum factor that stimulates gamma interferon production. Infect Immun 1989;57:590–5.
198. Okamura H, Nagata K, Komatsu T, et al. A novel costimulatory factor for gamma interferon induction found in the livers of mice causes endotoxic shock. Infect Immun 1995;63:3966–72.
199. Bazan JF, Timans JC, Kaselein RA. A newly defined interleukin-1? Nature 1996;379:591–6.
200. Sekut L, Talanian R, Paskind M, et al. Caspase-1 processes IFN-inducing factor and regulates LPS-induced IFN-gamma production. Nature 1997;386:619–23.
201. Gu Y, Kuida K, Tsutsui H, et al. Activation of interferon-g inducing factor mediated by interleukin-1g converting enzyme. Science 1997;275:206–9.
202. Dinarello CA. Interleukin-1 beta, interleukin-18, and the interleukin-1 beta converting enzyme Ann NY Acad Sci 1998;856:1–11.
203. Parnet P, Garka KE, Bonnert TP, et al. IL-1Rrp is a novel receptor-like molecule similar to the type I interleukin-1 receptor and its homologues TI/ST2 and IL-1R AcP. J Biol Chem 1996;271:183–6.
204. Novick D, Dinarello CA, Rubinstein M. Soluble IL-18 receptor in human urine: characterization and purification [abstract]. Cytokine 1997;9:963.
205. Gallagher G, Dickensheets H, Eskdale J, et al. Cloning, expression and initial characterization of interleukin-19 (IL-19), a novel homologue of human interleukin-10 (IL-10). Genes Immunol 2000;1:442–50.
206. Blumberg H, Conklin D, Xu WF, et al. Interleukin 20: discovery, receptor identification, and role in epidermal function. Cell 2001;104:9–19.
207. Pestka S, Krause CD, Sarkar D, et al. Interleukin-10 and related cytokines and receptors. Annu Rev Immunol 2004;22:929–79.
208. Dumoutier L, Leemans C, Lejeune D, et al. Cutting edge: STAT activation by IL-19, IL-20 and mda-7 through IL-20 receptor complexes of two types. J Immunol 2001;167:3545–9.
209. Parrish-Novak J, Dillon SR, Nelson A, et al. Interleukin 21 and its receptor are involved in NK cell expansion and regulation of lymphocyte function. Nature 2000;408:57–63.
210. Ozaki K, Spolski R, Feng CG, et al. A critical role for IL-21 in regulating immunoglobulin production. Science 2002;298:1630-4.
211. Dumoutier L, Louahed J, Renauld JC. Cloning and characterization of IL-10-related T cell-derived inducible factor (IL-TIF), a novel cytokine structurally related to IL-10 and inducible by IL-9. J Immunol 2000;164:1814–9.
212. Kotenko SV, Izotova LS, Mirochnitchenko OV, et al. Identification of the functional interleukin-22 (IL-22) receptor complex: the IL-10R2 chain (IL-10Rbeta) is a common chain of both the IL-10 and IL-22 (IL-10-related T cell-derived inducible factor, IL-TIF) receptor complexes. J Biol Chem 2001;276:2725–32.
213. Oppmann, B, Lesley R, Blom B, et al. Novel p19 protein engages IL-12p40 to form a cytokine, IL-23, with biological activities similar as well as distinct from IL-12. Immunity 2000;13:715–25.
214. Parham C, Chirica M, Timans J, et al. A receptor for the heterodimeric cytokine IL-23 is composed of IL-12Rb1 and a novel cytokine receptor subunit, IL-23R. J Immunol 2002;168:5699–708.
215. Jiang H, Lin JJ, Su ZZ, et al. Subtraction hybridization identifies a novel melanoma differentiation associated gene, mda-7, modulated during human melanoma differentiation, growth and progression. Oncogene 1995;11:2477–86.
216. Caudell EC, Mumm JB, Poindexter N, et al. The protein product of the tumor suppressor gene, melanoma differentiation-associated gene 7, exhibits immunostimulatory activity and is designated IL-24. J Immunol 2002;168:6041–6.
217. Wang M, Tan Z, Zhang R, et al. Interleukin 24 (MDA-7/MOB-5) signals through two heterodimeric receptors, IL-22R1/IL-20R2 and IL-20R1/IL-20R2. J Biol Chem 2002;277:7341–7.
218. Ekmekcioglu S, Ellerhorst J, Mhashilkar AM, et al. Down-regulated melanoma differentiation associated gene (mda-7) expression in human melanomas. Int J Cancer 2001;94:54–9.
219. Ellerhorst JA, Prieto VG, Ekmekcioglu S, et al. Loss of MDA-7 expression with progression of melanoma. J Clin Oncol 2002;20:1069–74.
220. Chada S, Mhashilkar AM, Ramesh R, et al. Bystander activity of Ad-mda7: human MDA-7 protein kills melanoma cells via an IL-20 receptor-dependent but STAT3-independent mechanism. Mol Ther 2004;10:1085–95.
221. Cunningham CC, Chada S, Merritt JA, et al. Clinical and local biological effects of an intratumoral injection of *mda-7* (IL24; INGN 241) in patients with advanced carcinoma: a phase I study. Mol Ther 2005;11:149–59.
222. Tong AW, Nemunaitis J, Su D, et al. Intratumoral injection of INGN 241, a nonreplicating adenovector expressing the melanoma-differentiation associated gene-7 (*mda-7*/IL24): biologic outcome in advanced cancer patients. Mol Ther 2005;11:160–72.
223. Fort MM, Cheung J, Yen D, et al. IL-25 induces IL-4, IL-5, and IL-13 and Th2-associated pathologies in vivo. Immunity 2001;15:985–95.
224. Knappe A, Hor S, Wittmann S, Fickenscher H. Induction of a novel cellular homolog of interleukin-10, AK155, by transformation of T lymphocytes with herpes virus saimiri. J Virol 2000;74:3881–7.
225. Pflanz S, Timans JC, Cheung J, et al. IL-27, a heterodimeric cytokine composed of EBI3 and p28 protein, induces proliferation of naive CD4$^+$ T cells. Immunity 2002;16:779–90.
226. Chen Q, Ghilardi N, Wang H, et al. Development of Th1-type immune responses requires the type I cytokine receptor TCCR. Nature 2000;407:916–20.
227. Hisada M, Kamiya S, Fujita K, et al. Potent antitumor activity of interleukin-27. Cancer Res 2004;64:1152–6.
228. Sheppard P, Kindsvogel W, Xu W, et al. IL-28, IL-29 and their class II cytokine receptor IL-28R. Nature Imm 2003;4:63–8.
229. Dillon SR, Sprecher C, Hammond A, et al. Interleukin 31, a cytokine produced by activated T cells, induces dermatitis in mice. Nature Imm 2004;5:752–60.
230. Demetri GD. Evidence-based use of hematopoietic cytokines in clinical oncology. In: Wingard JR, Demetri GD, editors. Clinical applications of cytokines and growth factors. Norwell (MA): Kluwer Academic Publishers; 1999. p. 1–407.
231. Update of recommendations for the use of hematopoietic colony-stimulating factors: evidence-based clinical practice guidelines. 2000. Available at: http://www.ASCO.org (accessed June 17, 2005).
232. Nemunaitis J. The use of cytokines during blood and marrow transplantation. In: Wingard JR, Demetri GD, editors. Clinical applications of cytokines and growth factors. Norwell (MA): Kluwer Academic Publishers; 1999. p. 382–402.
233. Maslak P, Nimer SD. The efficacy of IL-3, SCF, IL-6, and IL-11 in treating thrombocytopenia. Semin Hematol 1998;35:253–60.
234. D'Hondt V, Weynants P, Humblet YP, et al. Dose-dependent interleukin-3 stimulation of thrombopoiesis and neutropoiesis in patients with small-cell lung carcinoma before and following chemotherapy: a placebo-controlled randomized phase Ib study. J Clin Oncol 1993:11:2063–71.
235. Fibbe WE, Raemaekers J, Verdonck LF, et al. Recombinant human interleukin-3 after autologous bone mar-row transplantation for malignant lymphoma: a phase I/II multicenter study [abstract]. Blood 1991;78 Suppl 1:163a.
236. Kurzrock R, Talpaz M, Gutterman JU. Very low doses of GM-CSF administered alone or with erythropoietin in aplastic anemia. Am J Med 1992;93:41–8.
237. Bessho M, Hirashima K, Asano S, et al. Treatment of the anemia of aplastic anemia patients with recombinant human erythropoietin in combination with granulocyte colony-stimulating factor: a multicenter randomized controlled study. Eur J Haematol 1996;58:265–72.
238. Gilliland G, Griffin JD. The roles of FLT3 in hematopoiesis and leukemia. Blood 2002;100(5):1532–42.
239. Sawyers C. Finding the next Gleevec: FLT3 targeted kinase inhibitor therapy for acute myeloid leukemia. Cancer Cell 2002;1:413–5.

50

Monoclonal Serotherapy

Robert C. Bast Jr, MD
Michael R. Zalutsky, PhD
Robert J. Kreitman, MD
Arthur E. Frankel, MD

Following the initial report of Kohler and Milstein,[1] the monoclonal antibody technology has exerted a prompt and substantial impact on laboratory investigation. Over the last 25 years, the availability of monoclonal reagents has permitted the development of novel markers for in vitro applications, including monitoring response to treatment, detecting malignant cells histochemically, identifying subsets of patients with particularly favorable or unfavorable prognoses, and distinguishing some tumors of unknown origin. Application of monoclonal antibodies for the in vivo treatment of human cancer has been more gradual, but serotherapy with monoclonal antibodies and their conjugates now has an established role in the management of certain leukemias, lymphomas, breast cancers, and colon cancers.[2–4]

The United States Food and Drug Administration (FDA) has approved 18 monoclonal antibodies, radionuclide conjugates or targeted toxins, for therapeutic indications, including transplant rejection, coronary thrombosis, respiratory syncytial virus infection, rheumatoid arthritis, Crohn's disease, psoriasis, asthma, and cancer.[5] Nine of the sixteen have been approved for the treatment of cancer (Table 50-1). Among the unmodified monoclonal antibodies, rituximab (Rituxan) is now marketed for relapsed or refractory low-grade non-Hodgkin's lymphoma (NHL), trastuzumab (Herceptin) for breast cancers that overexpress HER-2 receptors, alemtuzumab (Campath) for B-cell chronic lymphocytic leukemia (B-CLL) and cetuximab (Erbitux) and bevacizumab (Avastin) for colon cancer. With the general availability of these agents, it appears that monoclonal serotherapy now has an established role in clinical oncology.

In an attempt to exert greater antitumor activity in vivo, monoclonal antibodies have been linked to cytotoxic drugs, radionuclides, and immunotoxins. Extensive preclinical and clinical studies have now been performed with each type of immunoconjugate. Gemtuzumab ozogamicin (Mylotarg), a conjugate of the cytotoxic antibiotic calicheamicin with a humanized anti-CD33 antibody, has received regulatory approval for the treatment of relapsed acute myelogenous leukemia (AML) in patients over 60 years of age. Ibritumomab tiuxetan (Zevalin), a conjugate of ^{90}Y with the murine monoclonal antibody from which rituximab was humanized, was the first radioimmunotherapeutic agent to be approved by the FDA based on its activity in relapsed or refractory follicular lymphoma, including lymphomas resistant to rituximab.[6] ^{131}I-tostuzumab (Bexxar) is a radioimmunoconjugate containing ^{131}I linked to another anti-CD20 antibody that has proven superior to anti-CD20 antibody alone and has also been approved for use in the United States. Several toxin-antibody conjugates appear promising. Although technically not a monoclonal antibody, denileukin diftitox (Ontak), a fusion protein that contains interleukin (IL)-2 and diphtheria toxin, is a targeted toxin that binds to the IL-2 receptor and has FDA approval for the treatment of cutaneous T-cell leukemia. This chapter considers some of the possibilities for, and limitations of, monoclonal reagents, radionuclide conjugates, and targeted toxins for the treatment of cancer patients.

THERAPY WITH UNMODIFIED MONOCLONAL ANTIBODIES

Treatment In Vivo

Lymphoma and Leukemia With rare exceptions, murine monoclonal antibodies raised against human neoplasms recognize tumor-associated antigens, which are also expressed by normal adult or fetal tissues. Some antigens, however, are expressed by only a small number of normal cells that may not be essential to a patient's well being.

Anti-idiotypic Antibodies One of the most promising reports remains that of Levy and colleagues, who prepared tumor-specific murine monoclonal antibodies against the unique idiotopes associated with the cell surface membrane immunoglobulin present on human B-cell lymphomas but expressed by, at most, a very small subset of normal B cells.[7,8] The original patient treated with a specific anti-idiotypic antibody remained in complete remission for 72 months and survived for more than 17 years.[5] Treatment of 18 lymphoma patients with anti-idiotypic antibodies alone produced an objective response rate of 67% with little toxicity.[5] In subsequent trials, anti-idiotypic antibodies were combined with interferon (IFN)-α, chlorambucil, or IL-2. Overall, a response rate of 63% was observed in 52 patients, with several complete responses extending beyond 10 years.[5] Most of the antibodies that produced responses in vivo were of the murine immunoglobulin G1 (IgG1) isotype, which is generally least efficient in fixing complement or participating in antibody-dependent cell-mediated cytotoxicity (ADCC). Anti-idiotypic antibodies that bind to the B-cell receptor complex appear to induce apoptosis (programmed cell death) by delivering a death signal. In a fraction of patients treated with anti-idiotypic antibodies, recurrence is associated with loss of the relevant antigen. Genes encoding the cell surface membrane immunoglobulin continue to undergo point mutations, resulting in the loss of idiotypic determinants.[9] Use of anti-idiotypic antibodies has provided a critical proof of concept, but widespread application has been hindered by the logistic challenge of developing reagents for each patient.

Rituximab Monoclonal antibodies against differentiation antigens that are shared by cancer cells from different patients have also been used to treat NHL, as well as acute and chronic leukemias. One target that has proven useful is CD20, a 35-kDa phosphoprotein calcium channel that is expressed on the surface of all normal B cells and in 80% of NHLs but not on other normal tissues. Repeated weekly administration of a chimeric mouse/human IgG1 anti-CD20 antibody, rituximab, produced a 48 to 50% response rate in patients with relapsed low-grade follicular NHL, with a median time to progression of 10.2 to 13.2 months.[10,11] In 37 newly diagnosed patients, treatment with rituximab (375 mg/m^2 weekly for 4 infusions) produced an overall response rate of 72%, with 36% complete responses and median time to disease progression of 2.2 years.[12] Consequently, rituximab can be used to treat patients at relapse after chemotherapy, the indication for which it is currently approved, or it might be used as an alternative to observation in patients with a low tumor burden of indolent non-Hodgkin's lymphoma.[13]

Treatment with rituximab has generally been well tolerated. Most side effects were infusion-related and occurred within the first few hours, particularly during the first infusion. Adverse events generally lasted for minutes to hours and included chills, fever, nausea, fatigue, headache, pruritus, and the sensation of throat swelling.[14] Normal B-lymphocyte counts can decrease to zero after the initial infusion; recovery begins by 6 months and is complete by 9 to 12 months.

Table 50-1 Monoclonal Antibodies, Radionuclide Conjugates, and Targeted Toxins Approved in the United States for Treatment of Cancer

Antibody	Product Name	FDA Approved	Type	Antigenic Target	Indication
Rituximab	Rituxan	1997	Chimeric	CD20	Relapsed or refractory follicular and low grade non-Hodgkin's lymphoma
Trastuzumab	Herceptin	1998	Humanized	HER-2	Metastatic breast cancers that overexpress HER-2
Denileukindefitox	Ontak	1999	Humanized	CD25	Cutaneous T-cell leukemia
Gemtuzumab	Mylotarg	2000	Humanized	CD33	Relapsed acute myelogenous leukemia in elderly patients
Alemtuzumab	Campath	2001	Humanized	CD52	B-cell chronic lymphocytic leukemia
^{90}Y-ibritumomab tiuxetan	Zevalin	2002	Murine	CD20	Relapsed or refractory follicular and low grade non-Hodgkin's lymphomas in elderly patients and rituximab resistant disease
^{131}I-tostuzumab	Bexxar	2003	Murine	CD20	Relapsed or refractory follicular and low grade non-Hodgkin's lymphomas in elderly patients and rituximab resistant disease
Cetuximab	Erbitux	2004	Chimeric	EGFR	Colorectal cancer
Bevacizumab	Avastin	2004	Humanized	VEGF	Colorectal cancer

Immunoglobulin levels, however, are maintained, and intercurrent infections requiring hospitalization occurred in only 2% of patients during 1 year of follow-up. Following approval by the FDA in 1997, more than 125,000 patients have been treated with rituximab in the United States.[10] Among these individuals, only eight deaths have been associated with treatment related to the development of paraneoplastic pemphigus, Stevens-Johnson syndrome, and toxic epidermal necrolysis.[15]

Since regulatory approval for the treatment of patients with recurrent or refractory follicular or indolent NHL, indications have been extended to provide 8 rather than 4 weekly courses and to retreat patients who had previously responded.[16] After relapse, re-treatment with a similar course of rituximab produced an overall response rate of 38% in 60 patients, with 10% complete remissions. Median time to progression exceeded 15 months.[17] Combination of rituximab with cyclophosphamide, doxorubicin, vincristine, and prednisone (CHOP) chemotherapy in 40 patients with low-grade follicular lymphoma, some of whom had been previously treated, resulted in an overall response of 100%, with 58% complete remissions and 42% partial remissions. Median time to progression exceeded 40.5 months.[18] Preliminary reports suggest that the addition of rituximab to cyclophosphamide, vincristine, and prednisone (CVP) chemotherapy prolonged time to progression in patients with follicular NHL[19] and that maintenance rituximab improves outcome after treatment with CVP alone.[20] Ongoing studies are attempting to define the optimal schedule of administration,[21] the importance of maintenance therapy,[22] and how to best integrate rituximab treatment before, during, or after chemotherapy for treatment of follicular lymphoma.

More aggressive diffuse large-cell NHL has been less responsive to rituximab alone. Among 54 patients with disease in relapse, the overall response rate to 8 cycles of rituximab was 31%, including 9% complete remissions with a median time to progression in responders of 8 or more months.[23] A trial has been conducted by the Groupe d'Etude des Lymphomes de l'Adulte (GELA) in 400 elderly patients with more aggressive diffuse large-cell NHL who were randomized to receive CHOP plus rituximab or CHOP alone.[23] A complete response rate of 76% was observed with the combination, compared with 60% with CHOP alone. Event-free survival ($p < .005$) and overall survival ($p < .01$) were significantly prolonged by the addition of rituximab. If these promising observations can be confirmed, the addition of rituximab to CHOP may provide the first improvement in the systemic treatment of diffuse large-cell lymphoma in the last 20 years. When subset analysis was performed on the GELA trial, the greatest benefit was observed against lymphomas that overexpressed the antiapoptotic protein BCL2.[24]

Treatment with rituximab, alone or in combination with fludarabine, has been extended to chronic lymphocytic leukemia (CLL).[25] In early studies, only a very modest response rate (15%) was observed with now standard doses of rituximab, possibly related to the lower concentration of CD20 on the CLL cell surface and to the shedding of soluble CD20, creating an "antigenic sink."[26] Treatment with higher doses of rituximab or thrice weekly administration has, however, achieved an overall response rate of 46% in CLL, with an even higher response rate in previously untreated patients.[26] A Cancer and Leukemia Group B (CALGB) trial of fludarabine and rituximab in 42 patients with CLL yielded a 100% response rate, with 48% of patients achieving a complete remission.[27]

The mechanism(s) by which rituximab kills leukemia and lymphoma cells is not completely understood but probably involves antibody-dependent cell mediated cytotoxicity (ADCC), complement-mediated cytotoxicity, and the direct effect of CD20 ligation.[28] In cancer cells, cross-linking CD20 can induce cell cycle arrest, inhibit DNA synthesis, activate caspases, and induce apoptosis.[27] Both natural killer (NK) cells and polymorphonuclear leukocytes can be important effectors for ADCC,[27] and a correlation has been observed between clinical response to rituximab and a specific allelic polymorphism in the FcγRI IIa receptor for IgG required for ADCC.[29] With regard to complement-mediated cytotoxicity, the response to rituximab is impaired in mice genetically deficient in C1q that lack the first component of the complement pathway, but that have intact ADCC.[30] Clinical resistance to rituximab treatment rarely involves loss of CD20 expression but can be associated with upregulation of complement resistance proteins CD55 and CD59.[31] Interestingly, different patterns of gene expression have been observed in lymphoma cells obtained prior to treatment from responders and non-responders to rituximab.[32] Gene expression in tumors that failed to respond resembled that in normal lymphoid tissues and exhibited higher expression of genes encoding certain complement components and genes involved in cytokine, T-cell and tumor necrosis factor signaling.

Anti-CD10 and Anti-CD5 In early studies of CD10-positive acute lymphoblastic leukemia (ALL), anti-CD10 antibody induced prompt modulation of the common ALL antigen, preventing effective therapy.[33] Intravenous infusion of anti-CD5 also produced antigenic modulation and only transient, partial regression in a fraction of patients with T-cell leukemia/lymphoma and CLL.[34] In one of the first studies of serotherapy with monoclonal reagents, a serum-blocking factor was demonstrated that prevented binding of the monoclonal antibody to circulating lymphosarcoma cells, consistent with the presence of shed tumor antigen.[35]

Alemtuzumab Other antigens have proven to be better targets for leukemic cells. CD52 is a 21- to 28-kDa nonmodulating cell surface glycophosphatidylinositol-linked glycoprotein that is abundantly expressed on most normal and malignant lymphocytes and monocytes. The CAMPATH-1 family includes three monoclonal antibodies that bind to CD52 and that can mediate cell lysis with human complement and effectors for ADCC.[36] Campath-1M is a rat IgM, Campath-1G is a rat IgG2b, and Campath-1H (alemtuzumab) is a humanized IgG1. Campath-1M has been used to purge normal T cells from human bone marrow prior to allogeneic transplantation, and CAMPATH-1G has been administered to marrow recipients prior to transplantation to reduce subsequent graft-versus-host disease (GVHD).[37,38]

In 15 patients with T-cell prolymphocytic leukemia (T-PLL), alemtuzumab treatment produced 60% complete remissions and 13% partial remissions for an overall response rate of 73%.[39] By contrast, deoxycoformycin, the best available chemotherapeutic agent, achieved an overall response rate of 40%, with only 12% complete remissions among 25 historical controls. Sensitivity of T-PLL to alemtuzumab may relate to high levels of CD52 expression or the susceptibility of cells to damage by complement or ADCC.

Responses to alemtuzumab were, however, relatively short lived, with a median of 9 months. Consequently, alemtuzumab may be only one component of a successful plan for treatment of this disease. In 14 heavily pretreated peripheral T-cell lymphoma patients, alemtuzumab produced an overall response rate of 36% with three complete and two partial remissions.[40] The median duration of complete response was 6 months.

In B-CLL, alemtuzumab produced responses in 30 to 42% of heavily pretreated patients and in 89% of 9 previously untreated patients.[41,42] Responses in previously untreated patients were durable, extending for some individuals beyond 2 years. Disease in the blood and bone marrow responded more frequently than did nodal disease.[43] As CLL cells can co-express CD52 and CD20, investigators are currently exploring the combined use of anti-CD52 alemtuzumab and anti-CD20 rituximab.[44]

Treatment with alemtuzumab is associated with a "first dose" reaction, consisting of fever, rigors, rash, nausea, vomiting, and dyspnea related to release of tumor necrosis factor (TNF)-α and IL-6.[43] Prolonged depression of normal T- and B-lymphocyte levels predisposes to opportunistic infection including cytomegalovirus (CMV) and fungal infections. Infections can be partly prevented by prophylaxis with acyclovir, cotrimoxazole, and itraconazole, but the infections are a significant risk.[43] Cardiac toxicity has also been reported with congestive heart failure and arrhythmias that improved when the drug was discontinued in patients with mycosis fungoides/Sézary syndrome.[45]

Solid Tumors The HER family of transmembrane tyrosine kinase growth factor receptors has provided targets for serotherapy in solid tumors. As outlined in Chapter 5, "Signal Transduction," interaction of peptide growth factor ligands with HER family receptors triggers signaling through the Ras–mitogen activated protein (MAP) kinase pathway and the phosphatidylinositol 3 (PI3)-kinase pathways, enhancing cell-cycle progression, proliferation, and survival in normal cells and cancer cells. Of the four HER family receptors, most attention has been given to HER-1 (epidermal growth factor receptor) and to HER-2.

Cetuximab Several monoclonal antibodies have been prepared against the extracellular domain of the 170-kDa epidermal growth factor receptor (EGFR) that is overexpressed in a number of carcinomas, including non–small-cell lung cancer, head and neck cancer, pancreatic cancer, and 70% of colorectal cancers. Cetuximab is a humanized monoclonal antibody that blocks the ligand-binding site of EGFR, preventing receptor activation and signaling. In experimental systems, treatment of human cancer cells with cetuximab produces cell cycle arrest in G_0-G_1, induces p21, directs hypophosphorylation of Rb, inhibits proliferation, and blocks the production of angiogenic factors such as vascular endothelial growth factor (VEGF).[46] In addition, treatment with cetuximab potentiates the activity of doxorubicin, paclitaxel, topotecan, and irinotecan as well as radiation therapy in nude mouse heterografts of human cancer. Potentiation of cytotoxic chemotherapy and radiation therapy may relate to inhibition of MAP kinase and PI3 kinase with induction of BAX, activation of caspase 8, and downregulation of BCL-2 and NFκB, rendering cancer cells more sensitive to apoptotic stimuli.[47] Weekly treatment with cetuximab alone produced partial remissions in 9% of 57 patients with chemotherapy-refractory colorectal cancer.[48] Side effects in a majority of patients included an acneiform rash, predominantly on the face and upper torso, and a composite syndrome of asthenia, fatigue, and malaise or lethargy.

In two trials, a combination of irinotecan and cetuximab was used to treat a total of 450 patients with documented metastases from EGFR-positive colorectal cancer that had previously received irinotecan.[49,50] A combination of cetuximab and irinotecan produced a partial response in 17 to 23% compared with 11% in patients re-treated with irinotecan alone. In one study progression-free, but not overall, survival was significantly prolonged with the combination (4.1 vs 1.1 months). Interestingly, the level of EGFR expression did not correlate with response to the cetuximab-based therapy. Consistent with this observation, 4 of 16 previously treated patients (25%) with EGFR immunohistologically negative cancers responded to a combination of cetuximab and irinotecan.[51] Consequently, patients should not be excluded from treatment based on immunohistochemical evaluation of EGFR.

Promising phase II trials have also been conducted in head and neck cancer and in pancreatic cancer.[52,53] A combination of gemcitabine and cetuximab was administered to 58 patients with metastatic pancreatic cancer.[54] Five patients (12%) achieved a partial response and 26 (63%) had stable disease. Median time to progression was 3.8 months and median overall survival was 7.1 months. One year progression-free and overall survival rates were 12% and 32%, comparing favorably with previous studies with gemcitabine alone.

Trastuzumab Approximately 20 to 30% of breast cancers overexpress the 185-kDa tyrosine kinase growth factor receptor *c-erbB2* (HER-2).[55] While HER-2 lacks a functioning ligand-binding domain, it is the preferred dimerization partner for the other HER family members including EGFR, HER-3 and HER-4.[56] Overexpression of HER-2 by breast cancer cells is associated with a poor prognosis, particularly in node-positive disease, as well as with resistance to paclitaxel, CMF, and tamoxifen, but with an improved response to doxorubicin.[56,57] Resistance to systemic therapy, increased risk of recurrence and shortened survival reflect the biological consequences of HER-2 overexpression, including increased proliferation, increased cell survival, increased invasion and metastasis, and increased angiogenesis. Monoclonal antibodies directed against the extracellular domain of this receptor can inhibit growth of cancer cells that overexpress HER-2.[58,59] In addition, treatment with anti–HER-2 antibodies can increase the susceptibility of cancer cells to platinum compounds, taxanes, doxorubicin, and 4-hydroperoxy-cyclophosphamide.[60,61] Interestingly, binding of anti–HER-2 antibodies to the HER-2 receptors in the juxtamembrane region[62] can activate the tyrosine kinase[59] but may prevent ligand-driven interaction of HER-2 with HER-3 to activate the PI3 kinase pathway, decreasing the antiapoptotic activity of phospho-AKT.[59,63,64] Binding of trastuzumab to the extracellular domain of HER-2 can also downregulate the HER-2 receptor. In vivo, inhibition of proangiogenic factors and mediation of ADCC may also play a role.

In clinical studies, the humanized murine anti–HER-2 IgG1 monoclonal antibody trastuzumab (Herceptin) produced objective regression of recurrent breast carcinoma in 12 to 15% of 269 heavily pretreated women.[65,66] Although cisplatin has demonstrated marginal activity against breast cancer in previous studies, a combination of cisplatin and trastuzumab produced an objective clinical response in 24% of 37 patients, with a median duration of 8.4 months.[67] A critical international multi-institutional study was performed in 469 women with recurrent breast cancer.[68] Patients who had not previously received adjuvant therapy with doxorubicin were randomized to doxorubicin (or epirubicin) and cyclophosphamide, with or without trastuzumab. Women who had received adjuvant doxorubicin were randomized to paclitaxel with or without trastuzumab. The addition of trastuzumab to chemotherapy was associated with a longer time to disease progression (median 7.4 vs 4.6 months; $p < .001$), a higher objective response rate (50% vs 32%; $p < .001$), a longer duration of response (median 9.1 vs 6.1 months; $p < .001$), and longer survival (median 25.1 vs 20.3 months; $p = .01$). This study resulted in the approval of trastuzumab by the FDA in 1998 for the treatment of recurrent HER-2-overexpressing breast cancers. Adjuvant trials are currently underway. Recent studies have documented that trastuzumab enhances the response rate to Navelbine and gemcitabine in metastatic breast cancer.[69–72] Based on laboratory studies, two phase II trials were undertaken that documented a 58 to 72% overall response in two groups of 62 patients with times to progression of 9.9 to 12.7 months following treatment with platinum salts, docetaxel, and trastuzumab.[73] Large randomized phase III trials are in progress to evaluate this regimen for recurrent disease and in an adjuvant setting.

In most studies, only those breast cancers with strong expression of HER-2 driven by amplification of the gene responded to the antibody alone or to a combination of antibody with chemotherapy. Immunohistochemistry can provide an initial screen for HER-2 overexpression, but 2+-3+ reactions should be confirmed with the more reliable fluorescence in situ hybridization assay.[74] One recent report suggests that HER-2 gene amplification can be acquired as breast cancers progress, arguing for repeated testing for HER-2 overexpression.[75] Because only a fraction of patients respond, overexpression of HER-2 is necessary, but not sufficient reason to assure response to trastuzumab. Lack of response to trastuzumab correlated with lack of expression of the PTEN phosphatase, the enzyme that removes phosphate groups from PI3 and interrupts signaling through AKT.[76] Treatment with trastuzumab increased PTEN membrane localization and phosphatase activity by reducing PTEN tyrosine phosphorylation through inhibition of Src that could no longer dock on the HER-2 receptor.

Treatment with trastuzumab is well tolerated and is associated with low-grade fever, chills, and fatigue that are most frequently observed with the first administration. In most studies, trastuzumab has been administered weekly, but it has been administered every 3 weeks at higher dosage with acceptable toxicity and trough levels.[77] When trastuzumab has been combined with doxorubicin or paclitaxel, increased cardiotoxicity has been observed. In the pivotal trial that demonstrated the efficacy of trastuzumab, American Heart Association class III and IV cardiac dysfunction occurred in 27% of the group given trastuzumab with anthracycline and cyclophosphamide compared with 8% of the group given anthracycline and cyclophosphamide alone.[78] A similar degree of cardiac dysfunction was observed in 13% of patients who received paclitaxel and trastuzumab compared with 1% who received paclitaxel alone. Cardiac dysfunction generally responded to medical management,[78] but the mechanism remains obscure. Only low levels of HER-2 are found on cardiac myocytes, but trastuzumab can localize to the myocardium, and the ligand heregulin that binds to HER-2-HER-3 and HER2-HER-4 dimers appears critical to the fetal development and survival of cardiac tissue under apoptotic stress.[79] Use of less cardiotoxic anthracyclines in combination with trastuzumab offers one alternative. Recently, a neoadjuvant trial has been reported where epirubicin, paclitaxel, and trastuzumab produced a significantly higher pathological complete response rate than did chemotherapy alone (67% vs 25%) without development of clinically evident congestive heart failure.[80]

Targeting HER-2 with a different antibody, pertuzumab (Omnitarg, 2C4), prevents ligand-induced dimerization of HER-2 with other HER-family members.[81,82] Use of pentuzumab in combination with trastuzumab synergistically inhibited survival of a breast cancer cell line that overexpressed HER-2 associated with increased apoptosis and blockade of signaling through AKT, but not through MAP kinase.[83]

Edrocolomab Several clinical trials have used the 17-1A murine IgG2a antibody (edrecolomab), which reacts with human gastrointestinal carcinomas.[84–87] Responses have been reported in colorectal and pancreatic carcinoma, although evidence of tumor regression has often been equivocal and the role of the antibody difficult to define. In one study, 6 of 22 patients (27%) did experience an objective response to prolonged treatment.[84] Injection of 17-1A has evoked a human antimurine immunoglobulin response, and some of the patients' antibodies have had anti-idiotypic specificity. Development of antimurine immunoglobulin antibodies has generally been regarded as an undesirable consequence of injecting a foreign protein because they shorten the circulating half-life of the monoclonal antibody. Anti-idiotypic antibodies can, however, bear the internal image of the antigen and stimulate endogenous immunity in recipients.[88–91] Development of specific immunity may be one of the factors contributing to the outcome of a prospective concurrently controlled trial in 189 patients with resected Duke's C (stage III) colon cancer randomized to adjuvant therapy with edrecolomab or to observation.[92] With 7 years of follow-up, treatment with unconjugated edrecolomab decreased recurrence by 23% ($p < .04$) and improved overall survival ($p < .01$).[93] In a larger multinational study of 2,761 patients, the addition of edrecolomab to 5-flurouracil and folinic acid did not improve overall or disease-free survival, and edrecolomab monotherapy was associated with significantly shorter overall and disease-free survival than treatment with fluorouracil and folinic acid.[94] However, in another large concurrently controlled trial of 1,839 patients treated with 5-flurouracil leucovorin or 5-fluorouracil-levamisole, with or without edrecolomab, the addition of the antibody produced a 27% relative improvement in overall survival that was statistically significant.[95] At present, the role of edrecolomab in the management of colorectal cancer remains uncertain.

Anti-Ganglioside Antibodies Unmodified murine monoclonal antibodies have produced regression of metastases from malignant melanoma. Intravenous administration of antibodies against GD3, a prominent ganglioside on the surface of melanoma cells, produced objective responses in 14% of 51 patients.[96] Inflammatory reactions were noted around tumor sites. Biopsies demonstrated infiltration with lymphocytes and mast cells, degranulation of the mast cells, and deposition of complement components. Studies ex vivo suggest that a threshold level of GD3 expression may be required for susceptibility to host effector mechanisms.[97] Antibodies capable of mediating ADCC and complement cytotoxicity were most effective. Clinical trials have attempted to combine anti-GD3 antibodies with different cytokines that might enhance effector function for ADCC.[98] Administration of R24 anti-GD3 antibody prior to IL-2 produced only 1 response in 20, whereas administration of R24 2 weeks after the initiation of IL-2 treatment produced 10 responses in 32 patients.[99] Combination of R24 with IFN-α, granulocyte-macrophage colony-stimulating factor (GM-CSF), or M-CSF was ineffective, but a tumor lysis syndrome was observed in one melanoma patient treated with TNF-α and R24.[100] Intravenous administration of different antibodies against GD2 ganglioside produced responses in only 2 of 42 patients with melanoma. Contact of antibodies with tumor cells can be enhanced by direct intratumoral injection. Intratumoral injection of a human IgM monoclonal antibody reactive with the GD2 ganglioside produced partial and complete regression of injected cutaneous melanoma nodules in 4 of 8 patients[75] (Figures 50-1 and 50-2). Tumor nodules that failed to respond to repeated injection had relatively lower levels of antigen than did nodules that regressed. A mononuclear infiltrate was observed at the sites of antibody injection.

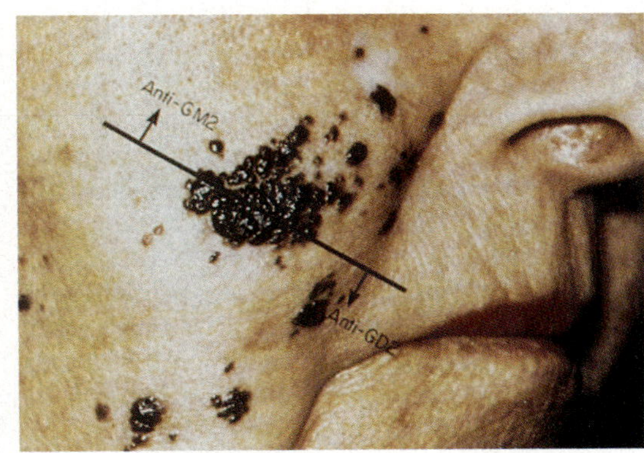

Figure 50-1 Recurrent melanoma, unresponsive to radiotherapy, prior to immunotherapy with intralesional injections of human monoclonal antibody to GM2 or GD2.

Bevacizumab Angiogenesis is critical for normal fetal growth and wound healing, but it is also required for tumor growth and metastasis.[101] Novel approaches to inhibiting angiogenesis have exploited the presence of antigens displayed on tumor-associated endothelium or on proangiogenic factors produced by tumor cells. Bevacizumab (Avastin) binds to the proangiogenic vascular endothelial growth factor (VEGF) that has also been characterized as vascular permeability factor (VPF). Blockade of VEGF/VPF can inhibit tumor-driven angiogenesis in heterografts.[102] Expression of VEGF/VPF has correlated with formation of ascites in mice with ovarian cancer heterograft models.[103] Treatment with bevacizumab can completely inhibit ascites formation.[104]

The majority of sporadic renal cell cancers exhibit inactivation of the von Hippel Lindau (VHL) gene and consequent overexpression of VEGF.[105] In a randomized phase II trial that compared 2 doses of bevacizumab (3 or 10 mg/kg every 2 weeks) with placebo in patients with renal cell carcinoma, a significant prolongation of disease-free survival was observed when high-dose bevacizumab was compared with placebo ($p < .01$).[106] The probability of being progression-

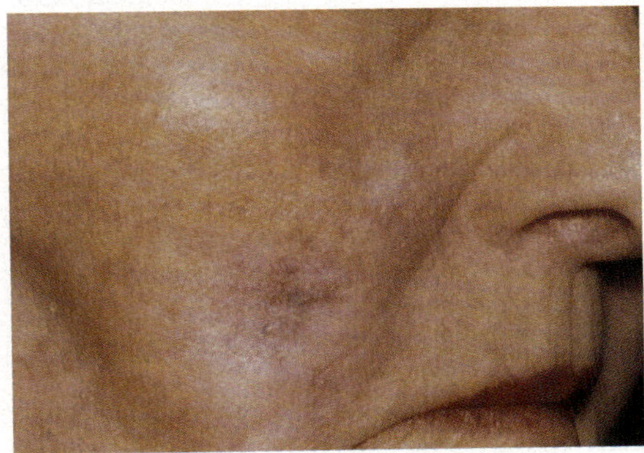

Figure 50-2 The same patient as in Figure 50-1, 2 years later, after complete regression of all disease.

free for patients with high-dose antibody, low-dose antibody and placebo was 64%, 39%, and 20% at 4 months and 30%, 14%, and 5% at 8 months. Interferon-alpha is a standard initial therapy for renal cell cancer with a modest response rate and a survival advantage demonstrated in randomized trials. A phase III trial is underway to compare treatment with interferon-alpha and bevacizumab to interferon-alpha alone in previously untreated patients with renal cell cancer.[107] The antivascular effect of bevacizumab has been demonstrated after preoperative treatment of 6 patients with primary and locally advanced carcinoma of the rectum. A single infusion of bevacizumab decreased tumor perfusion, vascular volume, microvascular density, interstitial fluid pressure, and the number of viable, circulating endothelial and progenitor cells.[108] In patients with previously untreated metastatic colorectal carcinoma, the addition of bevacizumab to irinotecan, fluorouracil, and leukovorin increased the overall response rate (44.8% vs 34.8%) and significantly prolonged median progression-free survival (10.4 vs 7.4 months) and median overall survival (20.3 vs 15.6 months).[109] In a randomized phase II trial, the addition of bevacizumab to carboplatin and paclitaxel was associated with an increased response rate (32% vs 19%), prolonged median time to progression (7.4 vs 4.2 months), and overall survival (17.7 vs 14.9 months) in patients with non–small-cell lung cancer.[110] In patients with breast cancer previously treated with anthracyclines and taxanes, the addition of bevacizumab to capecitabine significantly increased the response rate (20% vs. 9%), but not progression free survival (4.9 vs 4.2 months) and overall survival (15.1 vs 14.5 months).[111]

In patients with renal cell, colorectal and breast cancer, bevacizumab administration has been well tolerated. Grade 3 hypertension has been observed more frequently in patients who receive the anti-VEGF antibody, but has been easily managed.[109] In patients with non–small-cell lung cancer, minor mucocutaneous hemorrhage and major hemoptysis was observed, associated with four deaths among 35 patients.[110] Major hemoptysis was associated with squamous cell histology, tumor necrosis and cavitation, as well as disease close to major vessels.

Barriers to Successful Serotherapy **Antigen Specificity** Few, if any, monoclonal antibodies react only with tumor cells and fail to react with normal tissues. The remarkable efficacy and modest toxicity of anti-idiotypic antibodies reflect, at least in part, their limited reactivity with the vast majority of human B cells. The toxicity of CAMPATH-1 reflects reactivity with normal lymphocytes and monocytes. To treat cancers in some organs, such as ovary or thyroid, tissue-specific antbodies rather than tumor-specific antibodies may suffice because all normal tissue is removed during primary therapy.

Antigenic Modulation Antigens that modulate and are shed into the circulation, such as CD10 in ALL, have generally proven to be poor targets for serotherapy. An exception to this generalization has been observed with trastuzumab treatment of breast cancers that overexpress HER-2. The extracellular domain of HER-2 is cleaved and has been used as a marker for receptor overexpression.

Heterogeneity of Antigen Expression Heterogeneity has been observed in antigen expression within and between cancers from different individuals. Cells that lack antigen expression cannot be effectively targeted. With unconjugated antibodies that lack "bystander" activity, a combination of several reagents may be required to target all cells. In the case of different breast cancers, a combination of five monoclonal reagents can target more than 90% of cells in more than 90% of cancers from different individuals.[112]

Effective Delivery of Antibody to Tumor Cells Most attempts to develop effective serotherapy have utilized IgG antibodies with an Mr of 150 kDa. By contrast, most conventional cytotoxic drugs have a mass of less than 1 kDa. Consequently, monoclonal antibodies have slower kinetics of distribution and less tissue penetration than do conventional drugs.[113] For example, intravenous injection of an IgG2a murine monoclonal antibody against a 250-kDa melanoma-associated chondroitin sulfate proteoglycan core protein resulted in selective localization of antibody in metastatic nodules of malignant melanoma.[114] The greater the amount of antibody administered, the greater was the accumulation of murine immunoglobulin that could be demonstrated immunohistochemically in biopsied material. Even after the infusion of 500 mg of antibody, complete saturation of antigenic sites was not achieved in all patients, consistent with limited access of antibody to tumor cells outside the vascular compartment. The success of an antibody to localize to tumors depends on several factors. The ability of monoclonal antibodies to reach tumor cells can be limited by abnormal vascularity, elevated interstitial pressure, and relatively large distances for transport of immunoglobulins through the interstitium.[115,116] Disordered tumor vessels permit greater leakage of albumin and other plasma proteins into the interstitial space around cancer cells. Blockage of lymphatic outflow by tumor cells prevents clearance of interstitial protein, increasing oncotic pressure and fluid accumulation. Increased interstitial pressure impedes effective translocation of antibody. Biodistribution studies indicate that distance from blood vessels is an important factor affecting antigen recognition and binding. The central areas of bulky disease not only have increased fluid pressure, but are also poorly perfused, making these regions less accessible to antibodies.[117] In addition, large tumor masses can act as antigenic sinks, decreasing drug delivery to other tumor sites.[118] Modeling studies led Juweid and colleagues to formulate the hypothesis of the binding-site barrier, which postulated that antibody molecules could be prevented from penetrating tumors by the very fact of their successful binding to peritumoral antigen.[119] Subsequent experimental studies have supported this hypothesis. Intracavitary therapy has been used in an attempt to improve access of antibody to tumor cells, but antibody generally penetrates only a few millimeters beneath the serosal surface.

Immune Response to Foreign Immunoglobulin Substantial effort has been expended on the development of human monoclonal antibodies that should be less immunogenic, but their titer, specificity, isotype, and affinity continue to limit the clinical utility of these reagents.[120–122] Because a large number of antibodies used clinically are derived from mice, they can induce the development of human antimouse antibodies (HAMAs). The presence of HAMAs can prevent effective delivery of murine monoclonal antibodies to tumor cells, particularly when multiple doses must be administered to obtain optimal antitumor activity. Genetic manipulation of murine monoclonal antibodies has been used to generate less immunogenic reagents. Chimeric (60% human) and humanized (95% human) antibodies have been engineered to retain the murine antigen-binding complementarity regions in association with human framework regions.[120] Although the immunogenicity of such antibodies can be substantially reduced and HAMA responses can be limited, their injection can still evoke an anti-idiotypic response. The availability of antibodies derived entirely from humans, isolated from combinatorial libraries using the process of phage display, has revolutionized therapeutic strategies.[122] Unlike murine antibodies, human or humanized antibodies that contain the human Fc antibody portion trigger ADCC and complement-dependent cytotoxicity. An array of novel affinity maturation techniques such as bacterial cell-surface scFv display and cell-free ribosome display are emerging to isolate rare high-affinity clones.[123] Genetic engineering has also been used to produce single-chain antigen-binding proteins that may have more favorable pharmacokinetic properties than intact immunoglobulin or Fab fragments.[124]

Potency of Effector Mechanisms To the extent that unmodified monoclonal antibodies inhibit tumor growth, several mechanisms may be important for antitumor activity, including direct growth inhibition, induction of apoptosis, inhibition of angiogenesis, complement-dependent lysis, and ADCC, in addition to possible intervention in the specific immunoregulatory network of the host. Antibodies that react with the EGFR or with HER-2 can inhibit the growth of tumor cells ex vivo in the absence of complement components or host effector cells.[125,126] Antibodies that block EGF binding to the EGFR such as cetuximab affect growth more readily than do antibodies that bind to other sites on the receptor. Inhibition of ligand binding appears important for the inhibition of anchorage-dependent, but not anchorage-independent, growth. Antibodies have been described that produce apoptosis in some lymphoid cell lines, activated T cells, and certain carcinoma cell lines.[127] Murine antibodies of the IgM, IgG2a, and IgG3 isotypes can fix human complement, but often rather poorly. The rat monoclonal antibody CAMPTH-1G is an important exception to this generalization in that the antibody can mediate lysis of human cells that bear the appropriate antigen in the presence of human complement components.[128] Murine antibodies of IgG3, IgG2a, and IgG2b have been reported to mediate ADCC in which large granular lymphocytes (LGLs), monocytes, macrophages, or polymorphonuclear leukocytes are bound to tumor cells through Fc receptors after antibody has bound to specific antigenic determinants on the tumor cell surface. IgG3 appears to be particularly important for ADCC with LGLs, whereas IgG2a may interact more effectively with human monocytes.[129] In some instances, it has been possible to arm mononuclear leukocytes with antibody prior to interaction with tumor targets. In vivo, ADCC may be compromised in cancer patients due to a paucity of appropriate effector cells or to the presence of circulating immune complexes that occupy or downregulate Fc receptors. Antibodies that react against GD3 on melanoma cells can also bind to GD3 on the surface of T cells, enhancing their cytotoxic and proliferative responses.[130] Hybrid antibodies have been generated with one binding site for T-cell-associated antigens and one binding site for tumor-associated antigens.[131] Such hybrid antibodies enhance tumor cell killing by IL-2–activated T cells, possibly by encouraging contact between effector cells and tumor targets.[132]

Therapy with Drug–Monoclonal Antibody Conjugates Murine monoclonal antibodies have been coupled to a variety of conventional cytotoxic agents, including antifolates, anthracyclines, vinca alkyloids, and alkylating agents. Prepolymerization of some drugs such as doxorubicin prior to conjugation can achieve higher ratios of drug to antibody. Drugs can be bound to the amino side chains of lysine residues, provided that the most reactive residues are not found in the antigen-binding site. Linkage of drugs to antibody through the carbohydrate moieties of the murine immunoglobulin has provided site-specific conjugation that generally does not impair antibody binding.[133,134]

One concern raised by some investigators is based on the observation that many cell surface antigens have fewer than 10^5 copies per cell. Release of 1 to 3×10^6 drug molecules at the cell surface might or might not be sufficient to eliminate tumor. Another concern relates to the ability of large immunoglobulin carrier complexes to translocate across tumor capillaries. In preclinical studies, however, drug–monoclonal antibody conjugates proved substantially more effective than did the free drug. Only some of these conjugates are more potent, but many are less toxic, providing an improved therapeutic index. Therapeutic advantage may relate to different rates or patterns of drug uptake when linked with monoclonal reagents. In some instances, novel linkages have been devised that would release drug at low pH or only in the presence of lysosomal proteases. Not all drug–antibody conjugates must enter cells to provide effective antitumor therapy in nude mouse heterograft models. BR96-DOX, used an anti-LewisY (Ley) antibody linked to multiple doxorubicin molecules with an acid-labile bond.[135] In phase I studies, upper gastrointestinal toxicity was noted consistent with the known distribution of LeY determinants and the ability of the Fc domain to activate immunologic effector mechanisms.

Gemtuzumab Ozogamicin Calicheamicin has been conjugated with an anti-CD33 antibody.[136] CD33 is a 67-kDa glycoprotein expressed on the surface of more than 90% of AMLs and on early myeloid progenitor cells but not on normal pluripotent stem cells. Gemtuzumab ozogamicin, a conjugate of humanized anti-CD33 antibody and the cytotoxic antibiotic calicheamycin, is rapidly internalized by myeloblasts and induces apoptosis.[137] Three multicenter trials evaluated gemtuzumab ozogamicin in 142 patients with CD33 + AML in first relapse, administering two doses of 9 mg/m^2 on days 1 and 15 by 2-hour intravenous infusion.[138] Complete remission, with or without full platelet recovery, was observed in 30% of the patients. Because CD33 is expressed on hematopoietic precursors, grade 3 or 4 neutropenia and thrombocytopenia were observed in 99% of 101 patients age 60 years or above. Infections (27%) and mucositis (4%) were less frequently observed.[139] Veno-occlusive disease occurred, however, in 14 of 119 patients (12%) who received gemtuzumab ozogamicin-based regimens, including 5 patients who had not previously undergone stem cell transplantation.[140] Current studies are incorporating gemtuzumab ozogamicin into front-line therapy.[141]

Other investigators have explored the use of drug-containing liposomes coated with monoclonal antibodies to deliver larger aliquots of drug.[142,143] Stealth liposomes avoid deposition in normal liver, spleen, and lung after intravenous injection. In the future, antibody-coated nanoparticles might permit intravenous administration of targeted therapy.

Radioimmunotherapy of Cancer Radioimmunotherapy (RIT) involves the targeted delivery of an antibody labeled with a radionuclide emitting cytotoxic radiation to tumor cells. The development of monoclonal reagents has permitted more specific targeting, as well as large-scale production of conjugates for clinical trials. The limited efficacy of unmodified monoclonal antibodies has prompted their use as carriers of radionuclides, drugs, or toxins. Drug conjugates and immunotoxins kill only the targeted cell, whereas radionuclide conjugates can exert a bystander effect, destroying adjacent cells that lack antigen expression. There are two types of bystander effects. The first relates to the fact that the physical range of alpha and beta particles is multicellular, so cells not taking up the labeled molecule can still be hit. Recently, a second mechanism, the radiation-induced biological bystander effect, has been identified, in which cells not directly hit by radiation can also be killed.[144]

Choice of Radioisotope With external beam therapy, only a limited area of the body is irradiated. RIT, like cytotoxic chemotherapy, is a systemic treatment that, in principle, can eliminate metastatic disease throughout the body. In RIT, the biological effect is mediated by energy absorbed from the emissions of the radionuclide. To take advantage of tumor targeting, relatively short path lengths are desirable. Consequently, radionuclides have been chosen that emit alpha particles or beta particles, rather that gamma rays. The maximum path of beta emissions in tissue can range from 1 to 10 millimeters, while alpha particles have a much shorter path length, equivalent to only a few cell diameters. In addition to path length, other factors that must be considered in the selection of radionuclides for RIT include radiation quality, physical half-life, radiochemistry, and commercial availability.[145]

Beta Emitters Most clinical RIT have utilized radionuclides that decay by the emission of beta particles. Given the length of their path, beta emissions are most appropriate for treating tumors larger than 0.5 cm. In addition, not every cell needs to be targeted with a radionuclide conjugate. Bombardment of adjacent tumor cells by multiple beta particles results in enhanced killing through cross fire, partially compensating for a lack of homogeneity of antigen expression from cell to cell. In theory, one might choose among beta emitters based on the size of the tumor, or consider using a radionuclide cocktail consisting of radionuclides emitting radiation of a different range. Shorter-range beta emitters such as ^{131}I and ^{67}Cu might be used to treat micrometastatic disease, where a greater fraction of their decay energy would be deposited within small tumor cell clusters. Conversely, more energetic, longer-range beta emitters such as ^{90}Y and ^{188}Re could destroy larger tumor deposits and eliminate tumor cells that had escaped direct targeting due to lack of antigen expression or poor vascularity.[146]

The extent of heterogeneity of dose deposition in tumor is highly dependent on both the antibody characteristics and radionuclide properties and can enhance therapeutic efficacy through the selective dose delivery to the radiosensitive areas of tumor. Radionuclide characteristics can affect the heterogeneity of dose deposition within viable and necrotic areas of a tumor. When ^{131}I- and ^{90}Y-labeled radioconjugates were compared directly, ^{131}I generally delivered a higher dose throughout the tumor, even though the instantaneous dose-rate distribution for ^{90}Y was more uniform.[147] Although the long range of beta emitters can compensate for heterogeneous delivery of antibodies to malignant cell populations, this characteristic also increases the irradiation of normal tissues. Particularly problematic is the fact that beta decay from circulating radionuclide conjugates can irradiate bone marrow cells producing dose-limiting myelosuppression.[148]

Alpha-Emitters Alpha particles generally have higher energies than beta particles and exhibit very short path lengths (< 100 μm) in tissue. They are considered to be radiations of high linear energy transfer (LET), which have a high probability of producing cytotoxic DNA double-strand breaks.[149] Alpha particle-emitting radionuclides that have been most widely investigated for use in RIT include 61-min ^{212}Bi, 46-min ^{213}Bi, 7.2-h ^{211}At, and 10-day ^{225}Ac.[150] Because of their short range, alpha emitters may be most effective in RIT directed against blood-borne tumor cells, micrometastatic disease, and cancer cells near the surface of cavities, such as ovarian carcinoma.[151] Clinical trials with alpha emitters have begun and will be described in a later section of this chapter.

RIT in Hematologic Malignancies Currently, the only radiolabeled monoclonal antibodies approved for cancer treatment are ^{90}Y-iritumomab tiuxetan and ^{131}I-tositumomab, both registered for the therapy of follicular low-grade NHL. Lymphomas are particularly attractive targets for RIT because of their inherent radiosensitivity as well as the presence of differentiation antigens at the lymphoma cell surface that can be used for targeting. In most studies, however, radionuclide conjugates have been used to treat patients who have failed conventional treatment with cytotoxic chemotherapy and, in some cases, external beam radiotherapy. Consequently, the outcome of these trials may underestimate the potential of RIT if radioimmunoconjugates were used to treat minimal residual disease earlier in a patient's course.

^{90}Y-iritumomab Tiuxetan ^{90}Y-iritumomab (Zevalin) consists of an anti-CD20 murine monoclonal antibody covalently linked to the pure beta-emitting radionuclide ^{90}Y. The CD20 molecule is highly expressed by a high percentage of malignant B-cells as well as normal B-cells. For this reason, important aspects of the administration protocol are predosing with cold antibody in an attempt to saturate normal cell populations and a dose of ^{111}In-labeled antibody to determine dosimetry.[152, 153] Although the antibody alone has some therapeutic effect, addition of the radionuclide significantly increases the therapeutic response. In a randomized trial that compared treatment with ^{90}Y-iritumomab tiuxetan to treatment with rituximab in 143 patients with relapsed lymphoma, ^{90}Y-iritumomab tiuxetan produced an 80% response rate compared with 56% with rituximab (p = .002).[154] Treatment of 54 patients with rituximab-refractory disease with ^{90}Y-iritumomab tiuxetan resulted in an overall response rate of 74%, with 15% achieving a complete remission. Treatment of patients with ^{90}Y-iritumomab tiuxetan did result in frequent grade 3 and 4 hematological toxicities, and 22% of patients required platelet transfusions.[155]

^{131}I-tositumomab The second CD20-targeted radiotherapeutic that has recently become available for the treatment of follicular NHL is ^{131}I-tositumomab (Bexxar). Clinical experience with ^{131}I-tositumomab has been summarized in a recent review.[156] In a pivotal study of 60 patients with chemotherapy-refractory low-grade or transformed low-grade NHL, treatment with ^{131}I-tositumomab was compared with the patients' last qualifying chemotherapy (LQC).[157] The overall response rate to a single course of ^{131}I-tositumomab was 65% compared with 28% with the patients' LQC ($p < .001$). Complete responses were observed in 20% after RIT and in 3% after the LQC ($p < .001$), with median durations of response of 6.5 and 3.4 months ($p < .001$), respectively. For complete responders, however, the median duration of response after the LQC was 6.1 months, whereas after RIT the median duration of response was more than 47 months. These results are comparable with those from an earlier study at the University of Michigan in which 7 of 53 patients remained in a complete response after ^{131}I-tositumomab for 3 to 5.7 years.[158] Extension of this treatment strategy to newly diagnosed lymphoma patients is also being evaluated, and the results have been very encouraging with about 75% of patients achieving generally durable complete responses.[159]

In the current design of the ^{131}I-tositumomab regimen,[156] a dose of 450 mg of unlabeled tositumomab combined with 35 mg of tositumomab labeled with 5 mCi of ^{131}I are first administered and then whole-body images are obtained over the next week in order to calculate patient specific dosimetry. Then, about a week later, a second dose of 450 mg of unlabeled tositumomab combined with 35 mg of tositumomab labeled with sufficient mCi of ^{131}I to yield the desired total body radiation absorbed dose is administered. In this protocol, the administered mCi varies, while the targeted radiation dose is held constant, similar to external beam therapy. Toxicities associated with this therapy have primarily been hematopoietic[160] and dependent in part on the extent of previous treatments.

Other Antibodies for Lymphoma RIT Other lymphoma-associated antigens have been investigated in clinical RIT studies. Lym-1 targets the β-chain of HLA-DR expressed on malignant and a fraction of normal lymphocytes. Lym-1 labeled with ^{131}I has induced responses in 52% of 21 heavily pretreated patients with NHL who entered a trial, with complete remissions in 33% for a mean duration of 14 months.[161] Lym-1 has also been radiolabeled with ^{67}Cu or with ^{90}Y and the effect of the three different isotopes compared in clinical trials.[162,163] The ^{67}Cu-labeled construct, and less consistently the ^{90}Y-labeled construct, exhibited greater uptake and longer retention in tumor, resulted in a higher radiation dose, and improved the therapeutic index relative to ^{131}I-labeled constructs.[163–165] Unfortunately, the ^{67}Cu radionuclide is rarely produced, making the preferred approach impractical.

Based on the fact that tenascin-C is overexpressed by NHL, Rizzieri and colleagues[166] have evaluated the antitenascin antibody chimeric 81C6 in 9 NHL patients. Sites of tumor retained the ^{131}I radiolabel longer than normal organs and the mean absorbed dose to tumor was 963 cGy compared with 67 cGy for whole-body absorbed dose. Even at doses of 30 to 40 mCi, one patient attained a complete remission and one a partial remission. Unlike CD20, the tenascin-C molecular target is generally overexpressed on more aggressive diffuse lymphomas, making antitenascin targeted RIT a potentially complementary treatment to the anti-CD20 reagents that are currently commercially available.

RIT In Solid Tumors The successful treatment of solid tumors with RIT has been much more difficult to achieve and this is due to a number of factors. Compared with hematological malignancies, most solid tumors are considerably less radiation sensitive, so considerably higher and sustained levels of labeled antibody are needed to achieve a similar effect. Because many patients have bulky disease at the time of presentation, the delivery of curative levels of radiation to all regions of the tumor is a difficult task. Trials involving patients with solid tumors, including breast, gastrointestinal, and prostate cancers, produced variable antitumor responses, but these were not as impressive as the responses observed in hematological malignancies.[147,167] Some of the most encouraging results have been obtained with locoregional RIT in brain tumors.

Colorectal Cancer A variety of different oncofetal and differentiation antigens have been targeted with RIT in human colorectal cancer. Behr and colleagues focused on targeting carcinoembryonic antigen (CEA) with ^{131}I-labeled humanized antibodies producing some objective responses.[168] Using ^{90}Y as the radiolabel, the anti-CEA antibody T84.66 has been evaluated in both nonmyeloablative and myeloablative trials, but results to date have not been encouraging.[169,170] Radioiodinated antibodies reactive with the A33 antigen, a transmembrane glycoprotein that is rapidly internalized, also have been evaluated, but no significant tumor responses were observed.[171,172] CC49 is a murine antibody that reacts with an adenocarcinoma antigen, TAG-72. Iodine-131-labeled CC49 or a conjugate with the human/mouse chimeric version of the antibody did not produce any significant clinical responses in patients with colorectal carcinoma.[173] Because conventionally radioiodinated antibodies can be rapidly dehalogenated in vivo, the same antibody was labeled with ^{90}Y and used in a phase I trial. Tissue biopsies of tumor targets and organs at risk were obtained to validate estimates of dosimetry. The study detected only low tumor-to-normal tissue ratios and raised doubts about the potential of ^{90}Y-conjugated CC49 antibody for RIT of solid tumors.[174]

Ovarian Cancer Given the distinctive pattern of spread of ovarian cancer within the abdominal cavity, RIT can be administered via the intraperitoneal route, maximizing exposure of tumor cells on serosal surfaces while minimizing irradiation of normal organs outside the cavity. The anti-human milk fat globule protein (anti-MUC 1) antibody HMFG1 (pemtumomab R1549; Antisoma) has been labeled with ^{90}Y and used in a clinical study to treat patients with advanced ovarian cancer following conventional surgery and chemotherapy.[175,176] In a pilot study of women with minimal residual disease, half of the patients were free from disease and in complete remission several years after treatment, consistent with the possible activity of RIT against minimal residual on the surface of the peritoneal cavity. Among 21 patients who achieved complete remission following surgery, chemotherapy, and intraperitoneal RIT, 78% survived for longer than 10 years, and the median survival had not been reached with a maximum follow-up of 12 years.[177,178] An international multi-institution randomized concurrently controlled phase III clinical trial of ^{90}Y-R1549 was then performed in patients who had no gross residual disease after conventional therapy. Unfortunately, the results were no better than the control arm, so product development was halted in the middle of 2004. Interestingly, a significantly greater number of extraperitoneal recurrences was observed in the radioimmunotherapy arm.

Several other radiolabeled antibodies have been evaluated for RIT in ovarian cancer, and the results obtained appear to be critically dependent on the volume of disease at the time of treatment. For example, with ^{177}Lu-labeled CC49 antibody, only 1 of 13 patients with gross disease responded to treatment, whereas 4 of 5 patients with occult disease did respond.[179] The response of patients with ovarian cancer following RIT with intravenously administered ^{131}I-labeled chimeric monoclonal antibody MOv18 directed against a tumor-associated folate receptor is also currently being evaluated.[180] To date, results have shown that ^{131}I-labeled chimeric MOv18 can be given safely to patients with normal bone marrow reserves and may have therapeutic potential, particularly in patients with minimal residual disease.

Prostate Cancer Prostate cancer is an attractive target for RIT. As summarized by Smith-Jones,[181] the prostate is not an essential organ, permitting targeting of tissue-specific antigens, metastases generally are small in volume and isolated in the bone marrow and lymph nodes, facilitating access of labeled antibodies from the blood pool. TAG-72 was one of the first antigens to be targeted with radiolabeled antibodies, but no major responses were observed in prostate cancer patients.[182,183] Prostate-specific membrane antigen (PSMA) is an attractive molecular target for prostate cancer RIT because it is expressed on nearly all primary and metastatic prostate cancers and is not shed into the circulation.[181] Earlier studies of anti-PSMA RIT utilized the 7E11/CY356 antibody were not successful, consistent with the fact that the epitope being targeted on the PSMA molecules was inside the cells, and thus, not available for antibody targeting.[184] A more promising tactic is to utilize an antibody such as J591 that reacts with an extracellular epitope of PSMA.[185] Phase I clinical trials evaluating the therapeutic potential of J591 antibody radiolabeled with the beta emitting radionuclides ^{177}Lu and ^{90}Y are currently underway, and preliminary results show excellent targeting of radionuclide to bone and soft tissue lesions.[181]

Renal Cancer A promising molecular target for the treatment of renal cell carcinomas is carbonic anhydrase IX because this enzyme is overexpressed in more than 80% of tumors of this type.[186] Thirty-three patients with measurable metastatic renal cell carcinoma have been treated with ^{131}I-labeled G250, a murine monoclonal antibody (G250).[187] There were no major responses. On the basis of external imaging, ^{131}I-labeled mouse monoclonal antibody G250 showed excellent localization to all tumors that were 2 cm or more. Of the patients studied, 17 of 33 had stable disease, with tumor shrinkage observed in 2. Antibody immunogenicity restricted therapy to a single infusion. For this reason, a human/mouse chimeric G250 was developed. This antibody has been labeled with ^{131}I and is currently being evaluated in a fractionated dose protocol in patients with renal cell carcinoma.[188]

Brain Tumors Glioblastoma multiforme (GBM) is a malignancy with an extremely poor prognosis that generally kills through local invasion. Because brain tumors in adults rarely metastasize outside the cranium, locoregional approaches for RIT can be utilized, where the labeled antibody is injected directly into a surgically created tumor resection cavity or into nonresected tumor. More than 500 brain tumor patients have been treated to date with radiolabeled antibodies that bind to tenascin-C, an extracellular matrix glycoprotein that is overexpressed in more than 90% of GBM biopsies, with the level of expression increasing with advancing tumor grade.[189] The efficacy and toxicity of a single dose of ^{131}I-labeled murine antitenascin antibody 81C6 (120 mCi) infused directly into the resection cavity has been assessed in 33 patients with previously untreated malignant glioma.[190] Median survival for all malignant brain tumor patients was 86.7 weeks, and for GBM patients, was 79.4 weeks, exceeding that for historic controls treated with conventional postoperative radiotherapy and chemotherapy. Reversible hematological toxicity was observed in 27% of patients, and symptomatic neurological toxicity occurred in 15%, but only a single patient required reoperation for radionecrosis. These observations suggest that a randomized phase III study would be of value. Because tenascin-C is also expressed on normal tissues such as liver, it is not an ideal molecular target for RIT. In contrast, the epidermal growth factor receptor variant III (EGFRvIII) is characterized by a deletion in its extracellular domain, and is found in GBM but not normal tissues, including those that express high levels of the wild type receptor. Antibodies have been developed that are specific for EGFRvIII, as well as labeling methodologies that minimize the release of radionuclide from the tumor cell due to intracellular processing of the internalized receptor.[191]

Strategies for Improved RIT The success of RIT in NHL has demonstrated the feasibility of this approach to cancer therapy. However, the more modest results to date in patients with solid tumors suggest that more sophisticated strategies may be needed to improve therapeutic outcomes for patients with these malignancies. Approaches under investigation include multiple dose RIT protocols,[192] vasoactive agents[193,194] and hyperthermia[195,196] for increasing antibody tumor accumulation, targeting tumor vasculature,[197] and use of gene therapy techniques for increasing expression levels of the target antigen.[198] Two strategies that show particular promise for increasing the efficacy of RIT are pretargeting and the use of alpha-particle emitting radionuclides.

Pretargeting An advantage of using intact antibodies for RIT is that their binding to tumor is both higher and more prolonged than that of antibody fragments, thereby resulting in higher tumor radiation dose. On the other hand, the larger molecular size of whole immunoglobulin decreases the rate of tumor accumulation and impedes diffusion within the tumor. Pretargeting approaches are attractive because they offer the possibility of obtaining the benefits of intact antibodies while minimizing the disadvantages.[199] In pretargeting procedures, the antibody is administered first, and after a sufficient delay period to achieve sufficient uptake in the tumor, a radiolabeled lower molecular weight compound is injected. By shifting the label from the antibody to a smaller molecule, more rapid normal tissue clearance and tumor penetration can be achieved.

The most widely explored pretargeting strategy exploits the high affinity (~10^{13} to 10^{15} M^{-1}) binding of the ~60-kDa proteins avidin and streptavidin to the 244-Da water-soluble vitamin, biotin. A number of different regimens have been investigated including injection of a radiolabeled biotin derivative after pretargeting of a streptavidin-antibody conjugate, and pretargeting of a biotinylated antibody, followed by streptavidin, followed by radiolabeled biotin. In some cases, a clearing agent is used before injection of the labeled biotin conjugate. Clinical investigations with streptavidin-biotin pretargeting have been performed in patients with lung, ovarian, and colorectal carcinomas, as well as other types of cancer.[199]

Encouraging results have been obtained with a three-step protocol—biotinylated antitenascin antibody, avidin and streptavidin, and finally, ^{90}Y-labeled biotin—all administered via a catheter placed in the surgical resection cavity of recurrent patients with anaplastic astrocytoma (AA) ($n = 8$) and GBM ($n = 16$).[200] Patients received two cycles of treatment and the median survival for AA and GBM patients was 19 and 11.5 months, respectively. The efficacy of this pretargeting RIT protocol has also been evaluated in an adjuvant setting in newly diagnosed patients, 17 with AA and 20 with GBM.[201] All patients received surgery and external beam radiation; then, 19 patients received the three reagents in the sequence described above, with the remaining 18 patients serving as controls. In this trial, all reagents were administered via the intravenous route instead of directly into the surgical resection cavity. The median survival estimated for GBM patients was 8 months in the control group ($n = 12$) and 33.5 months in the treated group ($n = 8$). Phase III trial of this promising pretargeting RIT protocol is being planned.

A second pretargeting approach that has also been investigated involves the use of bispecific antibodies. In this method, one arm of the construct binds to a tumor-associated molecular target while the other is directed at a small molecule such as a radiometal-chelate complex.[202] An intriguing variation is to utilize a radiolabeled, stabilized peptide that contains two copies of the antigenic template.[203,204] In this way, it should be possible to promote binding to tumor cells, where antigen concentration is high, cross-linking two bispecific antibodies through a peptide bridge. Results in animal models have been very positive; however, it remains to be ascertained if this method provides any practical therapeutic advantage in the clinical setting.

Alpha-Particle RIT The most attractive feature of alpha particle emitting radionuclides for RIT is their markedly increased potency compared with other types of radiation. Studies in cell culture have demonstrated that human tumor cells can be killed after only a few alpha particles traverse a cell.[205] Furthermore, the cytotoxicity of alpha particles is nearly independent of dose rate, oxygen concentration, and cell-cycle stage.[149] While the conceptual advantages of alpha particles for RIT were known for a long time, practical investigation in patients required developments in radionuclide production, protein-labeling chemistry, and radiation dosimetry.[206–209]

The first RIT agent labeled with an alpha-particle emitting radionuclide to be evaluated in patients was ^{213}Bi-labeled HuM195, a humanized antibody reactive with the CD33 antigen that is overexpressed on human leukemia cells.[210] A phase I trial was conducted in 18 patients with relapsed and refractory acute myelogenous leukemia or chronic myelomonocytic leukemia. Because of the 46-min half-life of ^{213}Bi, the labeled antibody was administered in multiple doses (3–7) in order to achieve total administered activities ranging from 602 to 3,515 MBq. Absorbed dose ratios between potential tumor sites (bone marrow, liver, and spleen) and whole body were about 1,000 times higher than seen previously when this antibody was labeled with β-emitters. Large leukemia volume reductions were achieved in many patients; however, no complete remissions were observed. A phase I/II is currently underway to evaluate the therapeutic potential of ^{213}Bi-labeled HuM195 in patients treated with cytarabine before receiving the labeled antibody at doses of 18.5 to 46.25 MBq/kg.[211] Complete and partial responses were seen in some patients treated at the two highest dose levels and prolonged myelosuppression was found to be dose limiting at the highest dose level.

A phase I trial is currently being performed to determine the maximum tolerated dose, pharmacokinetics and objective responses to ^{211}At-labeled chimeric 81C6 antitenascin monoclonal antibody administered into surgically created glioma resection cavities in recurrent glioma patients.[212] The 7.2-h half-life alpha-particle emitting radiohalogen ^{211}At was produced at the Duke University Medical Center cyclotron, and the antibody was labeled using the *N*-succinimidyl 3-[^{211}At]astatobenzoate method.[209] To date, 17 patients (3 anaplastic oligodendroglioma, 14 GBM) have received escalating activities (74 MBq, $n = 5$; 148 MBq, $n = 6$; 248 MBq, $n = 5$; 370 MBq, $n = 1$) of ^{211}At-labeled chimeric antibody 81C6. Serial blood counts and imaging indicated very low levels of leakage of ^{211}At from the surgical resection cavity, confirming the stability of the labeled antibody in vivo. The average estimated radiation dose to the tumor cavity margin was 2,986 Gy, compared with less than 10 cGy received by normal brain, liver, spleen, and bone marrow. The median survival for these recurrent brain tumor patients was 54 weeks, a significant increase compared with conventional treatments (~25–30 weeks). A particularly encouraging result was that 2 patients with recurrent GBM survived for 151 and 153 weeks after ^{211}At-labeled 81C6 monoclonal antibody therapy.

Targeted Toxins Targeted toxins are hybrid protein drugs consisting of ligands that bind to the surface of cancer cells and deliver toxin inhibitors of protein synthesis that induce cell death. The ligand (haptophore) may be a hormone, cytokine, monoclonal antibody, or antibody fragment. Toxins (toxophores) that have been used clinically include diphtheria toxin, *Pseudomonas* exotoxin, ricin, gelonin, saporin, and pokeweed antiviral protein. A major challenge in the construction of targeted toxin conjugates is to identify adequately specific ligands and to reduce the nonspecific binding of the toxin moiety to normal tissues. The two components (haptophore and toxophore) are covalently linked, either with a heterobifunctional linker or by genetic fusion.

A number of haptophores have been found that bind with high affinity to antigens or receptors on neoplastic tissues and have been developed for systemic administration to patients with malignancies that have become resistant to standard cytotoxic agents (Table 50-2).[213–252] None of the targets is truly tumor specific; most are differentiation antigens or growth factor receptors. Nevertheless, initial clinical data suggest that, in certain cases, either cancer cells exhibit a higher concentration of targets or the loss of the normal cells that bear the target does not produce serious side effects. After binding the target, the ligand must internalize by receptor-mediated endocytosis to permit the toxin to gain entry from endosomes into the cytosol.[253] Many targets have had to be abandoned prior to in vivo or clinical testing because they lack this crucial property. Nevertheless, a number of targeted toxins have been made that both bind to tumor cells and are internalized in a selective fashion. Once produced in sufficient quantities, many of these have been tested clinically. Encouraging results with systemic targeting of the IL-2 receptor and CD22 in hematopoietic neoplasms, along with local targeting of IL-4 receptors, IL-13 receptors, and transferrin receptors in brain tumors suggest that sufficient drug delivery can be achieved to attain clinical benefit.

Toxins that inhibit protein synthesis must be modified to remove normal tissue binding sites and to add a tumor-selective ligand. Diphtheria toxin is a 58-kDa Mr protein with three domains. An N-terminal domain catalyzes ADP-ribosylation of elongation factor-2 (EF-2), inactivating cellular protein synthesis. A hydrophobic middle domain is responsible for translocating the ADP-ribosylation domain from endosomes to the cytosol. A C-terminal domain binds the toxin to receptors on normal cells triggering internalization into endosomes.[254] Diphtheria toxin has been genetically modified for use in targeted toxin synthesis by either (1) a point mutation in the binding domain, altering a critical Ser525 to a phenylalanine (CRM107) or (2) deletion of the 147-amino acid residue cell-binding domain (DT388 or DAB389).[255,256] *Pseudomonas* exotoxin is a 68-kDa Mr polypeptide with an N-terminal cell-binding domain followed by an amphipathic helix-containing translocation domain and a C-terminal ADP-ribosylation domain.[257] *Pseudomonas* exotoxin has been altered to eliminate normal tissue binding by deleting amino acid residues 1 to 252 and 365 to 380, yielding PE38.[258] Ricin toxin is a 64-kDa Mr heterodimer consisting of two subunits linked by a disulfide bond. The A subunit has rRNA N-glycosidase enzyme activity that inactivates ribosomes and blocks cell protein synthesis. The B subunit is a lectin that binds to normal oligosaccharides at the mammalian cell surface.[259] Ricin is prepared for targeted toxin synthesis by reduction and removal of the cell-binding B subunit so that only the A subunit (RTA) is used[260] or by chemically blocking the lectin-binding sites of the B subunit with reactive glycopeptides to create a blocked ricin molecule (bR).[261] Gelonin, saporin, and pokeweed antiviral protein are also ribosomal RNA N-glycosidases capable of inactivating protein synthesis.[262] Because they lack cell-binding moieties, each can be used directly to construct targeted toxins without modification. Currently, there is insufficient information to choose one toxin over another for treatment of particular cancers. The ligand and modified toxins are linked together chemically or genetically, and the conjugates or fusion proteins are purified, usually by chromatographic separation. Once purified, selective cytotoxicity for malignant cells is tested in tissue culture and in animal models. Studies of the molecular mechanisms for intoxication by these targeted toxins suggest that they use the same intracellular pathways as their parent toxins (Figure 50-3).

Subsequently, many targeted toxins have been scaled up for clinical studies. A number of clinical trials have been conducted with immunotoxins and fusion toxins over the last 20 years. These studies defined a number of pharmacologic and toxicologic barriers that needed to be overcome. Table 50-3 lists these clinical studies, as well as current clinical trials of targeted toxins, with a description of the compound, the diseases for which it is being tested, the response rate, and the toxicities where known. Some of these drugs have exhibited significant anticancer activity in phase I and II clinical studies, primarily in patients with chemotherapy-refractory cancers. The original rationale for the production and testing of these reagents was that they had a different mecha-

Table 50-2 Haptophores Used in Clinically Tested Targeted Toxins

Ligands	Receptor/Antigen	Toxin	Linker	Name
B3 Mab	Lewis a	PE	C	LMB-1[213]
B3 sFv	Lewis a	PE	G	LMB-7[214]
BR96 sFv	Lewis a	PE	G	B96(sFv)PE40[215]
B3 dsFv	Lewis a	PE	G	LMB-9[216]
RFB4 Mab	CD22[b]	Ricin	C	IgG-RFB4-dgA[217]
RFB4 Fab'	CD22[b]	Ricin	C	Fab'-RFB4-dgA[218]
RFB4 dsFv	CD22[b]	PE	G	BL22[219]
HD37 Mab	CD19[b]	Ricin	C	IgG-HD37-dgA[220]
B43 Mab	CD19[b]	PAP	C	B43-PAP2[21]
Anti-B4 Mab	CD19[b]	Ricin	C	Anti-B4-bR[222]
IL2	IL2R[b]	DT	G	ONTAK[223]
Anti-Tac Mab	CD25[b]	PE	C	Anti-Tac-PE[224]
RFT5 Mab	CD25[b]	Ricin	C	RFT5-dgA2[25]
IL3	IL3R	DT	G	DT_{388}IL3[226]
Anti-Tac sFv	CD25[b]	PE	G	LMB-2[227]
Tf	TfR	DT	C	HN6600[228]
454A12 Mab	TfR	Ricin	C	454A12-rA[229]
IL4	IL4R	PE	G	IL4(38-37)PE38KDEL[230]
HuM195 Mab	CD33[b]	Gel	C	HuM195-rGel[231]
GM-CSF	GM-CSFR	DT	C	DT_{388}GMCSF[232]
N901 Mab	CD56[b]	Ricin	C	N901-bR2[33]
TGFα	EGFR	PE	G	TP40[234]
TGFα	EGFR	PE	G	TP38[335]
EGF	EGFR	DT	G	DAB389EGF[236]
791T/36 Mab	72 kD Mr antigen	Ricin	C	Xomazyme-791[237]
260F9 Mab	55 kD Mr antigen	Ricin	C	260F9-rA[238]
Ber-H2 Mab	CD30[b]	SAP	C	Ber-H2-SO6[239]
Ki-4 Mab	CD30	Ricin	C	Ki-4-dgA[340]
T101 Mab	CD5[b]	Ricin	C	T101-RTA[241]
H65 Mab	CD5[b]	Ricin	C	H65-RTA[242]
XMMME-001	Proteoglycan	Ricin	C	XMMME-001-Mab-RTA[243]
OVB3 Mab	Ovarian antigen	PE	C	OVB3-PE[244]
3A1 Mab	CD7[b]	Ricin	C	3A1-dgRTA[245]
TXU Mab	CD7[b]	PAP	C	TXU-PAP[246]
e23 dsFv	erbB-2[c]	PE	G	Erb-38[247]
FRP sFv	ErbB-2	PE	G	scFv(FRP5)-ETA[248]
SPV-T3a Mab	CD3[b]	Ricin	C	SPV-53a-dgA+WT1-dgA[249]
SS1 dsFv	Mesothelin	PE	G	SS1(dsFv)-PE38[250]
IL13	IL13R	PE	G	IL13PE38QQR[251]
OKT10 Mab	CD38[b]	SAP	C	OKT10-saporin[252]

C=chemical conjugate; CD3, CD5,CD7, CD19, CD22, CD25, CD30, CD 33, CD 38, and CD56 are "cluster-designation" cell surface antigens; dsFv=disulfide stabilized sFv; EGF=epidermal growth factor; erbB-2 is the Her-2/neu gene product; Fab'=Fab antibody fragment, G=genetic fusion; GM-CSF=granulocyte-macrophage colony-stimulating factor; GMCSFR=GM-CSF receptor; Gel=gelonin; kD=kilodaltons; Lewis a is a carbohydrate antigen; Mab=monoclonal antibody; PAP=pokeweed antiviral protein; PE=*Pseudomonas* exotoxin; sFv=single chain Fv antibody; SO6=saporin; Tf=transferrin; TfR=transferrin receptor; TGFα=transforming growth factor alpha.

nism of action than DNA or cell division-damaging therapeutics, and thus might be effective either alone or in combination in patients with chemotherapy-resistant cancers. This rationale appears to be at least partly validated. Examples of targeted toxins with 30% or more complete remission and partial remission rates include Ontak (denileukin diftitox) DAB389IL2 for refractory cutaneous T-cell lymphomas, LMB2 and BL22 for refractory hairy cell leukemia, as well as HN6600, IL4(38-37)PE38KDEL, and IL13PE38QQR for interstitial therapy of high-grade gliomas.

Efficacy in Leukemia and Lymphoma With different targeted toxins, a significant fraction of responses has been observed in patients with cutaneous T-cell leukemia, hairy cell leukemia, and other lymphoid neoplasms that express CD25 or CD22.

Denileukin Diftitox The fusion protein of diphtheria toxin and IL-2 targets cancer cells and normal cells that bear IL-2 receptors (CD25). When 9 or 18 μg/kg/d of denileukin diftitox (Ontak) was administered daily for 5 consecutive days every 3 weeks for up to eight cycles, a 30% objective response rate was observed in 71 patients with refractory stage IB to IV chronic T-cell lymphoma.[223] The median response lasted 6.9 months, with a range of 2.7 to 23.7 months. Among patients with advanced disease (stage > IIB), responses were more common at the higher dose (38% vs 10%; $p = .07$). Decreased tumor burden correlated with amelioration of symptoms measured by a quality-of-life questionnaire. In addition, 52% of patients classified as having stable disease showed a 50% decrease in tumor burden at some point during the study, although these responses lasted for less than 6 weeks. Denileukin diftitox was administered at 18 μg/kg daily for 5 days every 3 weeks up to 8 cycles to 45 B-cell NHL patients.[263] There were 3 complete responses (CRs) (6.7%) and 8 partial responses (PRs) (17.8%) for a total response rate of 24.5%. Median response duration was 7 months. Toxicities were low grade and transient. Thirty patients with steroid refractory acute graft versus host disease (GVHD)

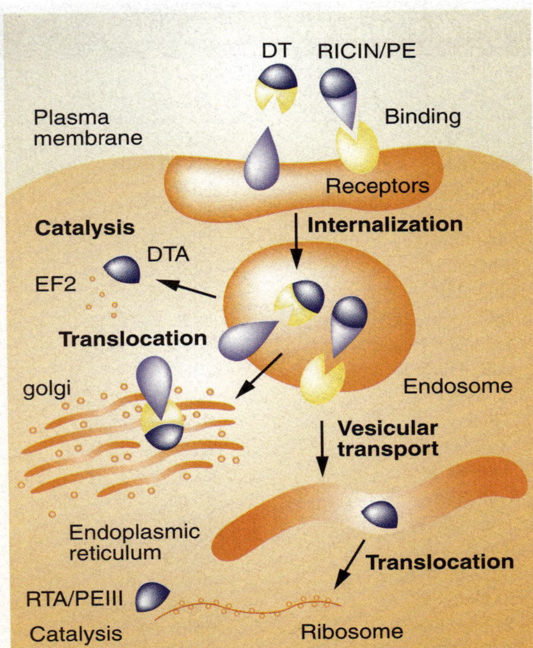

Figure 50-3 Model of cell intoxication by toxins and targeted toxins. Receptors for targeted toxins differ from parent toxin, but post-binding steps appear to match between the targeted toxin and the parent toxin. Toxins bind cell surface receptors; the complex internalizes to endosomes; the toxin reaches a translocation-competent compartment (endosomes for Diphtheria toxin and endoplasmic reticulum for PE and ricin); the catalytic domain of the toxin crosses the membrane to the cytosol; cytosolic toxin inactivates protein synthesis.

received 9 μg/kg denileukin diftitox on days 1,5 or 1,3,5,15,17,19 or 1 to 5 and 15 to 19.[264] There were 12 CRs and 5 PRs for a total 71% response rate. Dose limiting toxicity (DLT) was transient transaminasemia. A total of 27 CLL patients received denileukin diftitox at 18 μg/kg daily for 5 days every 3 weeks for up to 8 cycles in three different pilot phase II studies.[265–267] One CR and 6 PRs were observed for an overall response rate of 26%. A vascular leak syndrome (VLS) was the major toxicity.

LMB-2 (Anti-Tac(Fv)-PE38) LMB-2 is a fusion construct that incorporates *Pseudomonas* exotoxin (PR38) and an antibody fragment reactive with CD25. LMB-2 has been administered to 35 patients with different lymphomas at doses of 2 to 63 μg/kg intravenously over 30 minutes every other day × 3.[227] A complete remission was observed in one patient that was ongoing at 20 months. There were seven partial remissions in patients with several different neoplasms, including hairy cell leukemia (3 patients), chronic T cell lymphoma (1 patient), CLL (1 patient), Hirschsprung disease (1 patient), and adult T-cell leukemia (1 patient). Responders received at least 60 μg/kg total dose of LMB-2 per cycle. The median duration of remission has not been determined, but responses exceed 6 and 20 months in two patients. Responding patients had clearance of circulating malignant cells, improvement in skin lesions, and regression of adenopathy and splenomegaly.

BL22 BL22, consisting of a disulfide-stabilized anti-CD22 Fv fused to PE38, was given at doses of 3 to 50 μg/kg intravenously over 30 minutes every other day for a total of 3 doses to 16

Table 50-3 Targeted Toxin Clinical Trials*

Name	Disease	Response Rate (CR+PR/Total)	Toxicities
ONTAK	CTCL	22/71	VLS[223]
ONTAK	GVHD	17/24	VLS[264]
ONTAK	NHL	11/45	VLS[263]
ONTAK	CLL	7/27	VLS[265-267]
HN6600	Gliomas	12/44	CNS[228]
LMB-2	HCL	8/35	Liver[227]
B43-PAP	ALL	5/17	VLS[221]
IgG-RFB4-dgA	NHL	11/54	VLS[217,259,260]
Fab'-RFB4-dgA	NHL	5/14	VLS[239]
BER-H2-SO6	HD	5/12	VLS[239]
Ki-4-dgA	HD	1/15	VLS[240]
TP40	Bladder cancer	8/43	None[234]
Anti-B4-bR	NHL	8/59	Liver[222,261]
Anti-B4-bR	CLL	0/11	Liver[282]
H65-RTA	CTCL	4/14	VLS[242]
3A1-dgRTA	T-LGL, T-ALL	2/11	VLS[245]
$DAB_{486}IL2$	CTCL	4/19	Liver[262]
IgG-HD37-dgA	NHL	3/32	VLS, Acrocyanosis[220]
LMB-1	Carcinomas	2/38	VLS[213]
Xomazyme-791	Colon cancer	2/16	VLS[237]
T101-RTA	CLL	2/18	VLS[241]
Anti-CD25-dgA	HD	2/15	VLS[225]
N901-bR	SCLC	1/21	VLS251[233]
260F9-rA	Breast cancer	1/9	Schwann, VLS[238]
XMMME-001-RTA	Melanoma	1/22	VLS[243]
Erb-38	Carcinomas	0/8	Liver[247]
OVB3-PE	Ovarian cancer	0/23	CNS[244]
LMB-7	Carcinomas	0/54	Liver, kidney[214]
Anti-Tac-PE	ATL	0/4	Liver[224]
454A12-rA	Adenocarcinoma	0/20	CNS[229]
454A12-rA	Leptomeningeal cancer	0/8	Arachnoid[229]
$DAB_{389}EGF$	Breast cancer	0/43	Liver[236]
BL22	HCL	13/16	HUS[219]
$DT_{388}GMCSF$	AML	4/35	Liver[232]
IL4(38-37)PE38KDEL	Gliomas	6/9	CNS[230]
SPV-T3a-dgA+WT1-dgA	GVHD	2/4	None[276]
IL13PE38QQR	Gliomas	13/39	CNS[286]
SS1(dsFv)PE38	Mesothelioma, ovarian cancer	2/23	VLS[250]
BR96(sFv)PE40	Breast cancer	0/46	GI[215]
LMB-9	Carcinomas	0/10	Renal[216]
TXU-PAP	HIV infection	0/6	None[246]
ScFv(FRP5)-ETA	Carcinoma, melanoma	6/11	None[248]
TP38	Glioma	3/15	CNS[235]
HuM195-rGel	AML	TE	—

*AML=acute myeloid leukemia; ATL=adult T-cell leukemia; CLL=chronic lymphocytic leukemia; CNS=central nervous system; CR = complete response; CTCL=cutaneous T-cell lymphoma; GVHD=graft-versus-host disease; HCL=hairy cell leukemia; HUS=hemolytic uremic syndrome; HD=Hodgkin's disease; NHL=non-Hodgkin's lymphoma; PR = partial response; TALL=T-cell acute lymphoblastic leukemia; TE=too early; T-LGL=T-cell large granular lymphocyte leukemia; SCLC=small-cell lung carcinoma; VLS=vascular leak syndrome.

patients with purine analog resistant hairy cell leukemia.[219] There were 13 responses (81%), including 11 complete remissions (69%). The 3 non-responders either received low doses or had pre-existing toxin-neutralizing antibodies. Remissions were durable, with only 3 of 11 responders relapsing after 10 to 23 months. Retreatment could produce second complete remissions. Thus, BL22 immunotoxin appears to be the current best salvage treatment for relapsed HCL patients.

Other Targeted Toxins With other targeted toxins, responses have been observed in chemotherapy-refractory patients in phase I trials for leukemia and lymphoma, but at rates of less than 30%. Haptophores have targeted CD19, CD22, and the GM-CSF receptor. Toxophores have included PAP, deglycosylated ricin A chain and DT. There are ongoing studies with HuM195-rGel, DT388IL3, IL4(38-37)-PE38KDEL, IL13PE38QQR, TXU-PAP, BR96(sFv)-PE40, and B43-PAP, but it is too early to assess response rates.

Efficacy in Solid Tumors Although targeted toxins have been used to treat a variety of solid tumors, the most promising results have been observed with brain tumors in which locoregional therapy has been possible.

HN6600 (Tf-CRM107) HN6600 (Tf-CRM107), a transferrin-binding site mutant diphtheria toxin, was infused interstitially via one and/or two catheters implanted into the tumor beds of 44 patients with high-grade gliomas.[228] HN6600 was delivered by convection over 5 days. There were 12 responders as determined by MRI (27%), with median survival of more than 71 weeks.

IL4(38–37) PE38KDEL IL4 (38–37) PE38KDEL was administered by 1 to 3 stereotactic catheters over 4 to 8 days to 9 patients with recurrent high-grade gliomas.[230] Six of 9 patients showed tumor necrosis by MRI and histopathology. There was one unmaintained complete remission lasting over 18 months.

IL13-PE38QQR IL13-PE38QQR was administered intra-tumorally by convection-enhanced delivery to malignant gliomas and 13 of 39 patients had remissions lasting 7 to 117+ weeks.[251] Toxicity was observed with tumor necrosis and cerebral edema. The targeted toxin has been infused intratumorally in glioma patients by convection-enhanced delivery at 0.4 mL/hr over 50 hours through 2 catheters with systemic corticosteroids. There were 3 out of 15 remissions, including 1 CR of > 83 weeks.

Other Targeted Toxins Minimal antitumor activity has been observed with several other targeted toxins when administered to patients with a variety of solid tumors. N901-bR (anti-CD56-blocked ricin) was given for 7 days by continuous infusion and produced 1 partial remission in 21 patients with refractory small-cell lung cancer.[233] LMB-1 (anti-Ley-PE38) was administered by single intravenous bolus infusion to 38 patients with advanced solid tumors.[213] There was 1 complete remission and 1 partial remission lasting 2 and over 7 months, respectively. Phase I/II studies have been conducted with SGN-10 (BR96sFv-PE40),[215] LMB-7 (B3Fv-PE38), and LMB-9 (B3[dsFv]PE38) without response.[214,216] After GI prophylaxis, liver and renal toxicity was dose limiting. SS1(dsFv)PE38 was administered to 23 patients with mesothelioma, ovarian cancer, or pancreas cancer. The drug was infused every other day up to 6 doses at doses up to 18 µg/kg and yielded resolution of ascites in 2 patients for 6 and 30+ months. VLS was observed.[250]

Toxicities In some instances, the receptor/ antigen recognized by the targeted toxin is present on normal tissues and, in retrospect, predictable side effects have occurred. LMB-7 binds the Ley antigen that is expressed on normal stomach mucosa. Initial dose-limiting toxicity consisted of nausea, vomiting, and diarrhea. Endoscopy confirmed gastritis with apoptotic cells in the body and fundus. Prophylaxis with omeprazole, antiemetics, and loperamide greatly reduced the side effects and permitted dose escalation. DT388GMCSF binds the GM-CSF receptor present on liver macrophages (Kupffer cells), and dose-limiting toxicity to the liver was observed. Erb-38-bound receptors were present on normal hepatocytes and caused hepatotoxicity at low dose. OVB3-PE and 260F9-rA reacted with antigen present in the central nervous system and Schwann cells, respectively, and produced dose-limiting neurotoxicities. Preliminary work suggests that HN66000 (Tf-CRM107) binds transferrin receptors present on normal brain capillaries. Peritumoral focal brain injury occurred in some infused patients 2 to 4 weeks after treatment. Stereotypic changes were observed consisting of serpentine strips of increased signal in the peritumoral cortex evident on unenhanced T_1-weighted MRI scans. Biopsy results confirmed thrombosed cortical venules and/or capillaries. By lowering the concentration of HN6600 in the infusate and lowering the volume infused, toxicity to normal adjacent cortex was ameliorated.

Toxicities that are independent of ligand binding have been observed with most targeted toxins. These include either hepatocyte injury causing abnormal liver function tests or vascular endothelial damage with resultant VLS. Both the hepatic lesion and the vascular lesion may relate to nonspecific uptake of targeted toxins by normal human tissues. The normal tissue mediating these injuries may be the tissue showing the observed toxicity (liver or vascular endothelium) or may be macrophages that secondarily release cytokines, producing liver and blood vessel damage. Data support both hypotheses.

Hepatocytes have been exposed to targeted toxins in cell culture. Targeted toxins can bind to the hepatocyte cell surface dependent on the pI of the ligand in the conjugate.[268] Animals have been treated with toxins, and release of cytokines by macrophages has been demonstrated.[269] Cytokines, including TNF-α , can also directly injure hepatocytes. Which mechanism is more responsible for the transaminasemia in patients treated with fusion toxins cannot be determined from currently available data, but several mechanisms may operate simultaneously. Use of targeted toxins with lower nonspecific binding appears warranted as do efforts to block macrophage cytokine release.

VLS is characterized by weight gain, increased vascular permeability, hypoalbuminemia, myalgias, mild renal and pulmonary insufficiency, hypotension, and, in some cases, aphasias and pulmonary edema. The syndrome occurs transiently, but at times severely, after targeted toxin treatment. VLS usually occurs 4 to 6 days after initiating therapy and lasts 4 to 10 days. The cause of the endothelial lesion is unknown. Again, both uptake by vascular endothelium and macrophages have been postulated as triggering events. Several studies have shown apoptosis of endothelial cells in culture after toxin conjugate exposure.[270]A slight increase in loss of endothelial surface relative to replacement could lead to a significant leak. Endothelial cells may be uniquely sensitive due to exposure to high concentrations of the targeted toxin in the bloodstream. A correlation between AUC (blood concentration of conjugate × time) and VLS has been reported.[271] Smaller fusion toxins or recombinant immunotoxins with shorter circulating half-lives in vivo may yield less VLS at comparable doses. Vitetta and colleagues have identified a tripeptide disintegrin motif (xDy, where x = L, I, G, or V and y = V, L, or S) present on the surface of peptide toxins and interleukin-2 which can bind endothelial cell receptors and trigger increased vascular permeability.[272] Immunotoxins prepared with blocked disintegrin sites produce less VLS in vivo.[272] Clinical trials with such modified immunotoxins are eagerly anticipated. Alternatively, inflammatory cytokines released by toxin-ingested macrophages could also produce profound systemic alterations in vascular integrity. Although no animal model reproduces human VLS, a syndrome of hydrothorax, hypoalbuminemia, hemoconcentration, and neutrophilia developed in rats after intravenous injections of anti-Ley Fv-PE40.[273] Rats treated with PE40 alone or IL6-PE4E also developed a VLS-like syndrome.[274] The syndrome in rats was prevented by prophylaxis with steroids or nonsteroidal anti-inflammatory drugs (NSAIDs). This may result from the blocking of macrophage cytokine release by these agents. To date, however, no clinical data have documented an elevation in circulating inflammatory cytokines. However, it still appears prudent to select smaller targeted toxins. The role of steroid prophylaxis is less certain, as anecdotal reports suggest either protection or lack of protection in humans.

Other side effects have been reported with targeted toxins. Mild constitutional symptoms can occur when drug is infused rapidly (< 30–60 min), including fever, chills, myalgias, headaches, chest discomfort, and transient hypotension. The infusion may be stopped and the patient treated symptomatically. The drug infusion can then be restarted at a slower rate, generally without complications. Corticosteroid prophylaxis appears to prevent these constitutional symptoms. Rarely, patients may have an anaphylactoid response to targeted toxin. As these are proteins, rare hypersensitivity reactions are not unexpected. However, the occurrence of this complication mandates administration of targeted toxins in a setting where diagnosis and treatment of anaphylaxis are routine. Therapy may include 0.3 mL of epinephrine, 100 mg of solumedrol, and 25 mg of diphenhydramine, all given intravenously along with supplemental boluses of intravenous normal saline, nasal prong or face mask oxygen, and continuous cardiac monitoring until resolution of signs and symptoms. Patients should not be retreated with the same targeted toxin, if anaphylaxis is due to the drug, because the reaction is likely to recur with further exposure.

Pharmacology Recent advances in disease selection and targeted toxin design have led to an improvement in tumor localization and reduced immunogenicity. However, there remain important pharmacologic barriers. The circulating half-life varies with the size of the molecule. Larger molecules have longer half-lives, with 24 hours for Combotox and N901-bR and 9 hours for LMB-1. Each of these molecules consists of whole IgGs coupled to peptide toxins. Smaller molecules, including the single-chain immunotoxins LMB-2 and LMB-7 and the cytokine fusion toxin Ontak (DAB389IL2), have shorter half-lives of 5 hours, 2 hours, and 1 hour respectively. Some of the clearance of the smaller molecules (near 60 kDa) may be through the renal glomerulus. However, most of the clearance of these foreign proteins is likely by the liver or reticuloendothelial system. No clinical protocols have been reported that comprehensively correlate the percentage of extravascular tumor cell saturation with the dose of targeted toxin. The assumption has been made that toxicities, including VLS, hepatotoxicity, or neurotoxicities, reflect the administration of sufficient doses to saturate extravascular tumor sites. In vitro studies with multicellular tumor spheroids and mathematical models using data from other proteins suggest that smaller-sized fusion toxins and permeability enhancers such as cisplatin or hyaluronidase may improve tumor uptake.[275,276] Clinical responses with targeted toxins in lymphomas and leukemias may be due in part to a significant fraction of circulating malignant stem cells in these diseases.

Targeted toxins have generated humoral immune responses in all recipients, with the exception of patients with CLL. Clearly, the development of neutralizing antibodies is detrimental to targeted toxin antitumor efficacy. In many trials, retreatment has been limited to a few cycles because of the development of neutralizing antibodies. Even when the antibodies generated are nonneutralizing, they may form immune complexes that accelerate clearance of the targeted toxin from the circulation, reducing clinical benefit. Rituximab is being administered in combination with LMB-1 in an attempt to reduce the immune response to the immunotoxin.[213] Other methods include co-administration of 15-deoxyspergualin or CTLA4 Iq and have, to date, only been tried in animal models.[277] Immunodominant epitopes may be modified.[278] Finally, the use of human ribonuclease as a toxophore may be an additional method for reducing conjugate immunogenicity.[279]

Conclusions The potential for targeted toxins, as postulated by Paul Ehrlich one century ago, has not been fully realized to date.[280] However, over the last 20 years, with the advent of genetic engineering and advances in receptor physiology, we have progressed to the point where several targeted toxins have demonstrated clinical activity. Over the next decade, further ligand-receptor systems can be defined that extend the applications of targeted toxins to additional disease states. Control of the nonspecific toxicities and immune responses with various prophylactic maneuvers should further improve the therapeutic index of these molecules. Finally, combination therapy trials with cytotoxic chemotherapeutic agents are likely to yield even higher response rates with more durable responses. Combinations of radionuclide conjugates and targeted toxins have demonstrated synergy in heterograft models and deserve further evaluation in the clinic.[281] The next decade should see exciting advances in the development of these reagents and in their application to more effective treatment of patients with cancer.

REFERENCES

1. Kohler G, Milstein C. Continuous cultures of fused cells secreting antibody of predefined specificity. Nature 1975;256:495–7.
2. Dillman RO. Monoclonal antibodies in the treatment of malignancy: basic concepts and recent developments. Cancer Invest 2001;19:833–41.
3. Jurcic JG. Antibody based treatments for leukemia and lymphoma. ASCO annual meeting summaries. 2002. p. 180–6.

4. Harris M. Monoclonal antibodies as therapeutic agents for cancer. Lancet 2004; 5:292–302.
5. Levy R. Karnofsky lecture: immunotherapy of lymphoma. J Clin Oncol 1999;17:7–12.
6. Press OW. Radiolabeled antibody therapy of B-cell lymphomas. Semin Oncol 1999;26 (5 Suppl 14):58–65.
7. Miller RA, Maloney DG, Warnke R, Levy R. Treatment of B-cell lymphoma with monoclonal anti-idiotype antibody. N Engl J Med 1982;306:517–22.
8. Levy R, Miller RA. Therapy of lymphoma directed at idiotypes. Natl Cancer Inst Monogr 1990;10:61–8.
9. Raffeld M, Neckers L, Longo DL, Cossman J. Spontaneous alteration of idiotype in a monoclonal B-cell lymphoma. Escape from detection by anti-idiotype. N Engl J Med 1985;312:1653–8.
10. Maloney D, Grillo-Lopez A, White C, et al. IDEC-C2B8 (rituximab) anti-CD20 monoclonal antibody therapy in patients with relapsed low-grade non-Hodgkin's lymphoma. Blood 1997;90:2188–95.
11. McLaughlin P, Grillo-Lopez A, Link B, et al. Rituximab chimeric anti-CD20 monoclonal antibody therapy for relapsed indolent lymphoma: half of patients respond to a four-dose treatment program. J Clin Oncol 1998;16:2825–33.
12. Witzig TE, Vukov AM, Habermann TM, et al. Rituximab therapy for patients with newly diagnosed, advanced-stage, follicular grade I non-Hodgkin's lymphoma: a phase II trial in the North Central Cancer Treatment Group. J Clin Oncol 2005;23:1103–8.
13. Horning SJ. Optimizing rituximab in B-cell lymphoma. J Clin Oncol 2005;23:1056–8.
14. Grillo-Lopez A, White C, Varns, C, et al. Overview of the clinical development of rituximab: first monoclonal antibody approved for the treatment of lymphoma. Semin Oncol 1999;26(5 Suppl 14):66–73.
15. Grillo-Lopez AJ, Hedrick E, Rashford M, Benyunes M. Rituximab: ongoing and future clinical development. Semin Oncol 2002;29:105–12.
16. Piro LD, White CA, Grillo Lopez AJ, et al. Extended rituximab (anti-CD20 monoclonal antibody) therapy for relapsed or refractory low-grade or follicular non-Hodgkin's lymphoma. Ann Oncol 1999;10:655–61.
17. Davis T, Levy R, White C, et al. Rituximab: phase II (PII) retreatment (Rerx) study in patients (pts) with low-grade or follicular (LG/F) NHL [abstract]. Blood 1998;92(Suppl):414a.
18. Czuczman MS, Grillo-Lopez AJ, White C, et al. Treatment of patients with low-grade B-cell lymphoma with the combination of chimeric anti-CD20 monoclonal antibody and CHOP chemotherapy. J Clin Oncol 1999;17:268–78.
19. Marcus R, Imrie K, Belch A, et al. CVP chemotherapy plus rituximab compared with CVP firstline treatment for advanced follicular lymphoma. Blood 2005;105:1417–23.
20. Hochster HS, Weller E, Ryan T. Results of E1496: a phase III trial of CVP with or without maintenance rituximab in advanced indolent lymphoma. Proc Clin Oncol 2003;22:6502.
21. Gordan LN, Grow WB, Pusateri A, et al. Phase II trial of individualized rituximab dosing for patients with CD-20 positive lymphoproliferative disorders. J Clin Oncol 2005;23:1096–102.
22. Hainsworth JD, Litchy S, Shaffer DW, et al. Maximizing therapeutic benefit of rituximab: maintenance therapy versus re-treatment at progression in patients with indolent non-Hodgkin's lymphoma. J Clin Oncol 2005;23:1088–95.
23. Coiffier B. Rituximab in the treatment of diffuse large B-cell lymphomas. Semin Oncol 2002;29:30–5.
24. Mounier N, Briere J, Gisselbrecht C, et al. Rituximab plus CHOP (R-CHOP) overcomes bcl-2 associated resistance to chemotherapy in elderly patients with diffuse large B-cell lymphoma (DLBCL). Blood 2003;101:4279–84.
25. Mavromatis B, Cheson BD. Monoclonal antibody therapy of chronic lymphocytic leukemia. J Clin Oncol 2003;21:1874–81.
26. Keating MJ, O'Brien S, Albitar M. Emerging information on the use of rituximab in chronic lymphocytic leukemia. Semin Oncol 2002;29:70–4.
27. Byrd JC, Peterson B, Park K, et al. Rituximab added to fludarabine improves response in previously untreated chronic lymphocytic leukemia: preliminary results from CALGB 9712 [abstract]. Proc Am Soc Clin Oncol 2001;20:280a.
28. Eisenbeis CF, Caligiuri MA, Byrd JC. Rituximab: converging mechanisms of action in non-Hodgkin's lymphoma? Clin Can Res 2003;9:5810–12.
29. Cartron G, Dacheux L, Salles G, et al. Therapeutic activity of humanized anti-CD20 monoclonal antibody and polymorphism in IgG Fc receptor FcgammaRIIIa gene. Blood 2002;99:754–8
30. DiGaetano N, Cittera E, Nota R, et al. Complement activation determines the therapeutic action of rituximab in vivo. J Immunol 2003;171:1581–7.
31. Maloney DG, Smith B, Rose A. Rituximab: mechanism of action and resistance. Semin Oncol 2002;29:2–9.
32. Bohen SP, Troyanskaya OG, Alter O, et al. Variation in gene expression pattern in follicular lymphoma and the response to rituximab. Proc Natl Acad Sci 2003;100:1926–30.
33. Ritz J, Pesando JM, Notis-McConarty J, et al. Use of monoclonal antibodies as diagnostic and therapeutic reagents in acute lymphoblastic leukemia. Cancer Res 1981;41:4771–5.
34. Dillman RO, Shawler DL, Dillman JB, Royston I. Therapy of chronic lymphocytic leukemia and cutaneous T-cell lymphoma with T101 monoclonal antibody. J Clin Oncol 1984;2:881–91.
35. Nadler LM, Stashenko P, Hardy R, et al. Serotherapy of a patient with a monoclonal antibody directed against a human lymphoma associated antigen. Cancer Res 1980;40:3147–54.
36. Dyer MJS. The role of CAMPATH-1 antibodies in the treatment of lymphoid malignancies. Semin Oncol 1999;26(5 Suppl 14):52–7.
37. Naparstek E, Delukina M, Or R, et al. Engraftment of marrow allografts treated with Campath-1 monoclonal antibodies. Exp Hematol 1999;7:1210–8.
38. Hale G, Zhang MJ, Bunjes D, et al. Improving the outcome of bone marrow transplantation by using CD52 monoclonal antibodies to prevent graft-versus-host disease and graft rejection. Blood 1998;92:4581.
39. Pawson R, Dyer MJ, Barge R, et al. Treatment of T-cell prolymphocytic leukemia with human CD52 antibody. J Clin Oncol 1997;15:2667–72.
40. Enblad G, Hagberg H, Erlanson M, et al. A pilot study of alemtuzumab (anti-CD52 monoclonal antibody) therapy for patients with relapsed or chemotherapy-refractory peripheral T-cell lymphomas. Blood 2004;103:2920–4.
41. Keating M, Flinn I, Jain V, et al. Therapeutic role of alemtuzumab (Campath-1H) in patients who have failed fludarabine: results of a large international study. Blood 1999;99:3554–61.
42. Osterborg A, Fassas AS, Anagnostopoulos A, et al. Humanized CD52 monoclonal antibody Campath-1H as first-line treatment in chronic lymphocytic leukaemia. Br J Haematol 1996;93:151–3.
43. Flynn JM, Byrd JC. Campath-1H monoclonal antibody therapy. Curr Opin in Oncol 2000;12:574–81.
44. Nabhan C, Rosen ST. Conceptual aspects of combining rituximab and Campath-IH in the treatment of chronic lymphocytic leukemia. Semin Oncol 2002;29:75–80.
45. Lenihan DJ, Alencar AJ, Yang D, et al. Cardiac toxicity of alemtuzumab in patients with mycosis fungoides/Sézary syndrome. Blood 2004;104:655–8.
46. Mendelsohn J. Targeting the epidermal growth factor receptor for cancer therapy. J Clin Oncol 2002;20:1–13.
47. Ellis LM, Hoff PM. Targeting the epidermal growth factor receptor: an important incremental step in the battle against colorectal cancer. J Clin Oncol 2004;22:1177–9.
48. Saltz LB, Meropol NJ, Loehrer PJ Sr, et al. Phase II trial of cetuximab in patients with refractory colorectal cancer that expresses the epidermal growth factor receptor. J Clin Oncol 2004;22:1201–8.
49. Saltz L, Rubin M, Hochster H, et al. Cetuximab (IMCC225) plus irinotecan (CPT-11) is active in CPT-11-refractory colorectal cancer (CRC) that expresses epidermal growth factor receptor (EGFR). Proc of ASCO 2001;30:3a.
50. Cunningham D, Humblet Y, Siena S, et al. Cetuximab monoclonal and cetuximab plus irinotecan in irinotecan-refractory metastatic colorectal cancer. N Engl J Med 2004;351:337–45.
51. Chung KY, Shia J, Kemeny NE, et al. Cetuximab shows activity in colorectal cancer patients tumors that do not express the epidermal growth factor receptor by immunohistochemistry. J Clin Oncol 2005;23:1803–10.
52. Herbst RS, Hong WK. IMC-225, an antiepidermal growth factor receptor monoclonal antibody for treatment of head and neck cancer. Semin Oncol 2002;29:18–30.
53. Abbruzzese JL, Xiong HQ. Epidermal growth factor receptor-targeted therapy for pancreatic cancer. Semin Oncol 2002;29:31–7.
54. Xiong HQ, Rosenberg A, LoBuglio A, et al. Cetuximab, a monoclonal antibody targeting the epidermal growth factor receptor, in combination with Gemcitabine for advanced pancreatic cancer: a multicenter phase II trial. J Clin Oncol 2004;22:2610–6.
55. Slamon DJ, Godolphin W, Jones LA, et al. Studies of the HER-2/neu protooncogene in human breast and ovarian cancer. Science 1989;244:707–12.
56. Sledge GW. HERe-2 stay: the continuing importance of translational research in breast cancer. J Nat Can Instit 2004;96:725–7.
57. Bast RC Jr, Ravdin P, Hayes DF. 2000 update of recommendations for the use of tumor markers in breast and ovarian cancer. J Clin Oncol 2001;19:1865–78.
58. Drebin JA, Link VC, Greene MI. Monoclonal antibodies specific for the neu oncogene product directly mediate anti-tumor effects in vivo. Oncogene 1988;2:387–94.
59. Xu FJ, Rodriguez GC, Whitaker R, et al. Antibodies against immunochemically distinct epitopes on the extracellular domain of HER-2/neu (*c-erbB-2*) inhibit growth of breast and ovarian cancer cell lines. Int J Cancer 1993;53:401–8.
60. Baselga J, Norton L, Albanell J, et al. Recombinant humanized anti-HER2 antibody (Herceptin) enhances the antitumor activity of paclitaxel and doxorubicin against HER2/neu overexpressing human breast cancer. Cancer Res 1999;59:2020.
61. Pegram MD, Konecny GE, O'Callaghan C, et al. Rational combinations of trastuzumab with chemotherapeutic drugs used in the treatment of breast cancer. J Natl Cancer Inst 2004;96:739–49.
62. Cho HS, Mason K, Ramyar KX, et al. Structure of the extracellular region of HER2 alone and in complex with the Herceptin fab. Nature 2003;421:756–60.
63. Kumar R, Mandal M, Vadlamudi R. New insights into anti-HER-2 receptor monoclonal antibody research. Semin Oncol 2000;27:84–91.
64. Yakes FM, Chinratanalab W, Ritter CA, et al. Herceptin-induced inhibition of phosphatidylinositol-3 kinase and Akt is required for antibody-mediated effects on p27, cyclin D1, and antitumor action. Cancer Res 2002;62:4132–41.
65. Baselga J, Tripathy D, Mendelsohn J, et al. Phase II study of weekly intravenous trastuzumab (Herceptin) in patients with HER2/neu overexpressing metastatic breast cancer. Semin Oncol 1999;26(4 Suppl 12):78–83.
66. Cobleigh MA, Vogel CL, Tripathy NJ, et al. Multinational study of the efficacy and safety of humanized anti-HER2 monoclonal antibody in women who have HER2-overexpressing metastatic breast cancer that has progressed after chemotherapy for metastatic disease. J Clin Oncol 1999;17:2639–48.
67. Pegram MD, Slamon DJ. Combination therapy with trastuzumab (Herceptin) and cisplatin for chemoresistant metastatic breast cancer: evidence for receptor-enhanced chemosensitivity. Semin Oncol 1999;26 Suppl 12:89–95.
68. Slamon DJ, Leyland-Jones B, Shak S, et al. Use of chemotherapy plus a monoclonal antibody against HER2 for metastatic breast cancer that overexpresses HER2. N Engl J Med 2001;344:783–92.
69. Ligibel JA, Winer EP. Trastuzumab/chemotherapy combinations in metastatic breast cancer. Semin Oncol 2002;29:38–43.
70. Qu G, Perez EA. Gemcitabine and targeted therapy in metastatic breast cancer. Semin Oncol 2002;29 Suppl 11:44–52.
71. Burstein HJ, Harris LN, Marcom PK, et al. Trastuzumab and vinorelbine as first-line therapy for HER2-overexpressing metastatic breast cancer: multicenter phase II trial with clinical outcomes, analysis of serum tumor markers as predictive factors, and cardiac surveillance algorithm. J Clin Oncol 2003;21:2889–95.
72. Stein S, DeMichele A, Domchek S, Fox K. Gemcitabine and trastuzumab combinations for patients with metastatic breast cancer overexpressing HER2/neu. Clin Breast Cancer 2004;3:S117–20.
73. Pegram MD, Pienkowski T, Northfelt DW, et al. Results of two open-label, multicenter phase II studies of docetaxel, platinum slats, and trastuzumab in HER2-positive advanced breast cancer. J Natl Cancer Inst 2004;96:725–7.
74. Pauletti G, Dandekar SF, Rong H, et al. Testing for HER-2/neu in breast cancer: is fluorescence in situ hybridization superior in predicting outcome? An assessment of methods for tissue-based detection of their HER-2/neu alterations in human breast cancer: a direct comparison of fluorescence in situ hybridization and immunohistochemistry. J Clin Oncol 2000;18:3651–64.
75. Meng S, Tripathy D, Shete S, et al. HER-2 gene amplification can be acquired as breast cancer progresses. PNAS 2004;25:9393–98.
76. Nagata Y, Lan KS, Zhou X, et al. PTEN activation contributions to tumor inhibition by trastuzumab, and loss of PTEN predicts trastuzumab resistance in patients. Cancer Cell 2004;6:117–27.

77. Leyland-Jones B, Glemon K, Ayoub JP, et al. Pharmacokinetics, safety, and efficacy of trastuzumab administered every three weeks in combination with paclitaxel. J Clin Oncol 2003;21:3965–71.
78. Perez EA, Rodeheffer R. Clinical cardiac tolerability of trastuzumab. J Clin Oncol 2004;22:322–9.
79. Schneider JW, Chang AY, Garratt A. Trastuzumab cardiotoxicity: speculations regarding pathophysiology and targets for further study. Semin Oncol 2002;29:22–8.
80. Buzdar AU, Ibrahim NK, Francis D, et al. Significantly higher pathologic complete remission rate after neoadjuvant therapy with trastuzumab, paclitaxel and epirubicin chemotherapy: results of a randomized trial in human epidermal growth factor receptor 2 positive operable breast cancer. J Clin Oncol 2005;23:3676-85.
81. Badache A, Hynes NE. A new therapeutic antibody masks ErbB2 to its partners. Cancer Cell 2004;5:299–301.
82. Franklin MC, Carey KD, Vajdos FF, et al. Insights into ErbB signaling from the structure of the ErbB2-pertuzumab complex. Cancer Cell 2004;5:317–28.
83. Nahta R, Hung MC, Esteva FJ. The HER-2 targeting antibodies trastuzumab and pertuzumab synergistically inhibit the survival of breast cancer cells. Cancer Res 2004;64:2343–6.
84. Blottiere HM, Maurel C, Douillard JY. Immune function of patients with gastrointestinal carcinoma after treatment with multiple infusions of monoclonal antibody 17-1A. Cancer Res 1987;47:5238–41.
85. LoBuglio AF, Saleh M, Peterson L, et al. Phase I clinical trial of CO17-1A monoclonal antibody. Hybridoma [Suppl]. 1986;5:117–23.
86. Mellstedt H, Frauodin JE, Ragnhammar P, et al. The clinical use of monoclonal antibodies MAb 17-1A in the treatment of patients with metastatic colorectal carcinoma. Med Oncol Tumor Pharmacol 1989;6:99–107.
87. Sears HF, Herlyn D, Steplewski Z, Koprowski H. Effects of monoclonal antibody immunotherapy on patients with gastrointestinal adenocarcinoma. J Biol Response Mod 1984;3:138–50.
88. Herlyn D, Ross AH, Koprowski H. Anti-idiotypic antibodies bear the internal image of a human tumor antigen. Science 1986;232:100–2.
89. Herlyn D, Wettendorff M, Schmoll E, et al. Anti-idiotype immunization of cancer patients: modulation of the immune response. Proc Natl Acad Sci U S A 1987;84:8055–9.
90. Mittelman A, Chen ZJ, Kageshita T, et al. Active specific immunotherapy in patients with melanoma: a clinical trial with mouse antiidiotypic monoclonal antibodies elicited with syngeneic anti-high-molecular-weight melanoma-associated antigen monoclonal antibodies. J Clin Invest 1990;86:2136–44.
91. Wettendorff M, Iliopoulos D, Tempero M, et al. Idiotypic cascades in cancer patients treated with monoclonal antibody CO17-1A. Proc Natl Acad Sci U S A 1989;86:3787–91.
92. Riethmuller G, Schlimok G, Schneider-Gadicke E, et al. University of Munich, Department of Immunology and German 17-1A Study Group. Monoclonal antibody (MAB) treatment of resected Dukes C colorectal carcinoma (CRC): a prospective randomized trial. Proc Am Soc Clin Oncol 1994;13:199.
93. Riethmulller G, Holz E, Schlimok G, et al. Monoclonal antibody therapy for resected Dukes' C colorectal cancer: seven-year outcome of a multicenter randomised trial. J Clin Oncol 1998;16:1788–94.
94. Punt CJ, Nagy A, Douillard JY, et al. Edrecolomab alone or in combination with fluorouracil and folinic acid in the adjuvant treatment of stage III colon cancer: a randomized study. Lancet, 2002;360:671–7.
95. Fields AL, Keller AM, Schwartzberg L, et al. Edrecolomab (17-1A antibody) (EDR) in combination with 5-fluorouracil (FU) based chemotherapy in the adjuvant treatment of stage III colon cancer: results of a randomised North American phase III study. ASCO 2002;31:508a.
96. Houghton AN, Chapman PB. Melanoma. In: DeVita VT, Hellman S, Rosenberg SA, editors. Biologic therapy of cancer. Philadelphia (PA): Lippincott; 1995. p. 576.
97. Cheresh DA, Honsik CJ, Staffileno LK, et al. Disialoganglioside GD3 on human melanoma serves as a relevant target antigen for monoclonal antibody-mediated tumor cytolysis. Proc Natl Acad Sci U S A 1985;82:5155–9.
98. Bajorin DF, Chapman PB, Dimaggio J, et al. Phase I evaluation of a combination of monoclonal antibody R24 and interleukin 2 in patients with metastatic melanoma. Cancer Res 1990;50:7490–5.
99. Creekmore S, Urba W, Koop W, et al. Phase IB/II trial of R24 antibody and interleukin-2 (IL2) in melanoma. Proc Am Soc Clin Oncol 1992;186:345.1.
100. Minasian LM, Szatrowski TP, Rosenblum M, et al. Hemorrhagic tumor necrosis during a pilot trial of tumor necrosis factor-α and anti-GD3 ganglioside monoclonal antibody in patients with metastatic melanoma. Blood 1993;83:56–74.
101. Folkman J. Angiogenesis in cancer, vascular, rheumatoid and other disease. Nature Medicine 1995;1:27–31.
102. Skobe M, Rockwell P, Goldstein N, et al. Halting angiogenesis suppresses carcinoma cell invasion. Nat Med 1997;3:1222–7.
103. Yoneda J, Kuniyasu H, Crispens MA, et al. Expression of angiogenesis-related genes and progression of human ovarian carcinomas in nude mice. J Natl Cancer Inst 1988;90:447–54.
104. Mesiano S, Ferrara N, Jaffe RB. Role of vascular endothelial growth factor in ovarian cancer. Am J Pathol 1998;153:1249–56.
105. Rini BI, Small EJ. Biology and clinical development of vascular endothelial growth factor-targeted therapy in renal cell carcinoma. J Clin Oncol 2005;23:1028–43.
106. Yang JC, Haworth L, Sherry RM, et al. A randomized trial of bevacizumab, and anti-vascular endothelial growth factor antibody, for metastatic renal cancer. N Engl J Med 2003;349:427–34.
107. Rini BI, Halabi S, Taylor J, et al. Cancer and leukemia group B 90206: a randomized phase III trial of interferon-alpha or interferon-alpha plus anti-vascular endothelial growth factor antibody in metastatic renal cell carcinoma. Clin Cancer Res 2004;10:2584–6.
108. Willett CG, Boucher Y, Tomaso E, et al. Direct evidence that the VEGF-specific antibody bevacizumab has antivascular effects in human rectal cancer. Nature Medicine 2004;10:145–7.
109. Hurwitz H, Fehrenbacher L, Novotny W, et al. Bevacizumab plus irinotecan, fluorouracil, and leucovorin for metastatic colorectal cancer. N Engl J Med 2004;350:2335–42.
110. Johnson DH, Fehrenbacher L, Novotny WF, et al. Randomized phase II trial comparing bevacizumab plus Carboplatin and paclitaxel with Carboplatin and paclitaxel alone in previously untreated locally advanced or metastatic non-small cell lung cancer. J Clin Oncol 2004;22:2184–91.
111. Miller KD, Chap LI, Holmes FA, et al. Randomized phase III trial of capecitabine compared with bevacizumab plus capecitabine in patients with previously treated metastatic breast cancer. J Clin Oncol 2005;23:792–9.
112. Boyer CM, Borowitz MJ, McCarty KS Jr, et al. Heterogeneity of antigen expression in benign and malignant breast and ovarian epithelial cells. Int J Cancer 1989;43:55–60.
113. Dillman RO. Human antimouse and antiglobulin responses to monoclonal antibodies. Antibody Immunocon Radiopharm 1990;3:1.
114. Schroff RW, Woodhouse CS, Foon KA, et al. Intratumor localization of monoclonal antibody in patients with melanoma treated with antibody to a 250,000-dalton melanoma-associated antigen. J Natl Cancer Inst 1985;74:299–306.
115. Jain RK. Transport of molecules in the tumor interstitium: a review. Cancer Res 1987;47:3039–51.
116. Jian RK. Physiological barriers to delivery of monoclonal antibodies and other macromolecules in tumors. Cancer Res 1990;50:814s–9s.
117. Boxer GM, Begent RHJ, Kelly AMB, et al. Factors influencing variability of localisation of antibodies to carcinoembryonic antigen (CEA) in patients with colorectal carcinoma—implication for radioimmunotherapy. Br J Cancer 1992;65:825–31.
118. Van Osdol W, Fujimori K, Weinstein JN. An analysis of monoclonal antibody distribution in microscopic tumor nodules: consequences of a "binding site barrier." Cancer Res 1991;51:4776–84.
119. Juweid M, Swayne LC, Sharkey RM, et al. Prospects of radioimmunotherapy in epithelial ovarian cancer: results with iodine-131-labeled murine and humanized MN-14 anti-carcinoembryonic antigen monoclonal antibodies. Gynecol Oncol 1997;67:259–71.
120. Weiner L. Monoclonal antibody therapy of cancer. Semin Oncol 1999;26 Suppl 4:43–51.
121. Goldenberg DM. Challenges to the therapy of cancer with monoclonal antibodies. J Natl Cancer Inst 1991;83:78–9.
122. Reichmann L, Clark M, Waldmann H, Winter G. Reshaping antibodies for therapy. Nature 1988;332:323–7.
123. Hanes J, Pluckthun A. In vitro selection and evolution of functional proteins by using ribosome display. Proc Natl Acad Sci U S A 1997;94:4937–42.
124. Colcher D, Bird R, Roselli, et al. In vivo imaging of a recombinant single-chain antigen-binding protein. J Natl Cancer Inst 1990;82:1191–7.
125. Mendelsohn J. Growth factor receptors as targets for antitumor therapy with monoclonal antibodies. Prog Allergy 1988;45:147–60.
126. Xu FJ, Rodriguez GC, Whitaker R, et al. Antibodies against immunochemically distinct epitopes on the extracellular domain of HER-2/neu (c-erbB-2) inhibit growth of breast and ovarian cancer cell lines. Int J Cancer 1993;53:401–8.
127. Debatin KM, Goldmann CK, Bamford R, et al. Monoclonal-antibody-mediated apoptosis in adult T-cell leukaemia. Lancet 1990;335:497–500.
128. Waldmann H, Cobbold S, Wilson A, et al. Rat monoclonal antibodies for bone marrow transplantation—the CAMPATH series. Adv Exp Med Biol 1985;186:869–75.
129. Steplewski Z, Lubeck MD, Koprowski H. Human macrophages armed with murine immunoglobulin G2a antibodies to tumors destroy human cancer cells. Science 1983;221:865–7.
130. Hersey P, MacDonald M, Burns C, Cheresh DA. Enhancement of cytotoxic and proliferative responses of lymphocytes from melanoma patients by incubation with monoclonal antibodies against ganglioside GD3. Cancer Immunol Immunother 1987;24:144–50.
131. Clark M, Gilliland L, Waldmann H. Hybrid antibodies for therapy. Prog Allergy 1988;45:31–49.
132. Mezzanzanica D, Canevari S, Menard S, et al. Human ovarian carcinoma lysis by cytotoxic T cells targeted by bispecific monoclonal antibodies: analysis of the antibody components. Int J Cancer 1988;41:609–15.
133. McKearn TJ, Lopes AD, Radcliffe RD. In vivo efficacy of site-specific anti-folate monoclonal antibody conjugates. Presented at Third International Conference on Monoclonal Antibody Immunoconjugates. San Diego (CA): Cancer UCSD Cancer Center; 1988. p. 17.
134. Rodwell JD, Alvarez VL, Lee C, et al. Site-specific covalent modification of monoclonal antibodies: in vitro and in vivo evaluations. Proc Natl Acad Sci U S A 1986;83:2632–6.
135. Trail PA, Willner D, Lasch SJ, et al. Cure of xenografted human carcinomas by BR96-doxorubicin immunoconjugates. Science 1993;261:212–5.
136. Hinman LM, Hamann PR, Wallace R, et al. Preparation and characterization of monoclonal antibody conjugates of the calicheamicins: a novel and potent family of antitumor antibiotics. Cancer Res 1993;53:3336–42.
137. Linenberger ML. CD33-directed therapy with gemtuzumab ozogamicin in acute myeloid leukemia: progress in understanding cytotoxicity and potential mechanisms of drug resistance. Leukemia 2005,19:176–82.
138. Sievers EL, Larson RA, Stadtmauer EA, et al. Efficacy and safety of gemtuzumab ozogamicin in patients with CD33-positive acute myeloid leukemia in first relapse. J Clin Oncol 2001;19:3244–54.
139. Larson RA, Boogaerts M, Estey E, et al. Antibody-targeted chemotherapy of older patients with acute myeloid leukemia in first relapse using Mylotarg. Leukemia 2000;16:1627–36.
140. Giles FJ, Kantarjian HM, Kornblau SM, et al. Mylotarg (gemtuzumab ozogamicin) therapy is associated with hepatic venoocclusive disease in patients who have not received stem cell transplantation. Cancer 2001;92:406–13.
141. Giles F, Estey E, O'Brien S. Gemtuzumab ozogamicin in the treatment of acute myeloid leukemia. Cancer 2003;98:2095–104.
142. Connor J, Sullivan S, Huang L. Monoclonal antibody and liposomes. Pharmacol Ther 1985;28:341–65.
143. Matthay KK, Heath TD, Badger CC, et al. Antibody-directed liposomes: comparison of various ligands for association, endocytosis, and drug delivery. Cancer Res 1986;46:4904–10.
144. Mothersill C, Seymour C. Radiation-induced bystander effects: past history and future directions. Radiat Res 2001;155:759–67.
145. Zalutsky MR, Lewis J. Radiolabeled antibodies for tumor imaging and therapy. In: Welch MJ, Redvanly C., editors. Handbook of Radiopharmaceuticals: radiochemistry and Applications. Chichester, UK: Wiley; 2003. p. 685–714.
146. Flynn AA, Pedley RB, Green AJ et al. Antibody and radionuclide characteristics and the enhancement of the effectiveness of radioimmunotherapy by selective dose delivery to radiosensitive areas of tumour. Int J Radiat Biol 2002;78:407–15.
147. Jhanwar YS, Divgi C. Current status of therapy of solid tumors. J Nucl Med 2005;46:141S–50S.
148. Kampf G. Steps towards cancer therapy with radionuclides--a review including radiation biophysical aspects. Radiobiol Radiother (Berl) 1990;31:215–29.

149. Jurcic JG, Larson SM, Sgouros G, et al. Targeted alpha particle immunotherapy for myeloid leukemia. Blood 2002;100:1233–9.
150. Mulford DA, Scheinberg DA, Jurcic JG. The promise of targeted α-particle therapy. J Nucl Med 2005; 46:199S-204S.
151. Zalutsky MR, Pozzi OR. Radioimmunotherapy with α-particle emitting radionuclides. Q J Nucl Med Mol Imaging 2004;48:289–95.
152. Wagner HN Jr, Wiseman GA, Marcus CS, et al. Administration guidelines for radioimmunotherapy of non-Hodgkin's lymphoma with ^{90}Y-labeled anti-CD20 monoclonal antibody. J Nucl Med 2002;43:267–72.
153. Fink-Bennett DM, Thomas K. ^{90}Y-Ibritumomab tiuxetan in the treatment of relapsed or refractory B-cell non-Hodgkin's lymphoma. J Nucl Med Technol 2003;31:61–68.
154. Witzig TE, White CA, Gordon LI, et al. Final results of a randomized controlled study of the Zevalin radioimmunotherapy regimen versus a standard course of rituximab immunotherapy for B cell NHL [abstract]. Blood 2000;96:831a.
155. Zevalin (ibritumomab tiuxetan) [package insert]. San Diego (CA): IDEC pharmaceuticals Corporation; 2002.
156. Wahl RH. Tositumomab and ^{131}I therapy in Non-Hodgkin's lymphoma. J Nucl Med 2005;46:128S–40S.
157. Kaminski M, Zelentz AD, Press OW, et al. Pivotal study of iodine 131-tositumomab for chemotherapy refractory low-grade or transformed low-grade B cell non-Hodgkin's lymphomas. J Clin Oncol 2001;19:3908–11.
158. Kaminski MS, Estes J, Zasadny KR, et al. Radioimmunotherapy with iodine (131)I tositumomab for relapsed or refractory B-cell non Hodgkin's lymphoma: updated results and long term follow-up of the University of Michigan experience. Blood 2000;96:1259–66.
159. Press OW, Unger JM, Braziel RM, et al. A phase 2 trial of CHOP chemotherapy followed by tositumomab/iodine I131 tositumomab for previously untreated follicular non-Hodgkin's lymphoma: Southwest Oncology Group Protocol S9911. Blood 2003;102:1606 –12.
160. Bexxar (tositumomab and ^{131}I-tositumomab) [package insert]. Seattle (WA): Corixa Corporation and Philadelphia (PA): GlaxoSmithKline; 2003.
161. DeNardo GL, DeNardo SJ, Goldstein DS, et al. Maximum-tolerated dose, toxicity, and efficacy of ^{131}I-Lym-1 antibody for fractionated radioimmunotherapy of non-Hodgkin's lymphoma. J Clin Oncol 1998;16:3246–56.
162. O'Donnell RT, DeNardo GL, Kukis DL, et al. A clinical trial of radioimmunotherapy with ^{67}Cu-2IT-BAT-Lym-1 for non-Hodgkin's lymphoma. J Nucl Med 1999;40:2014–20.
163. DeNardo GL, Kukis DL, O'Donnell RT, et al. Are radiometal-labeled antibodies better than ^{131}I-labeled antibodies: comparative pharmacokinetics and dosimetry of copper-67-, iodine-131 and yttrium-90-labeled Lym-1 antibody in patients with non-Hodgkin's lymphoma. Clin Lymphoma 2000;1:118–26.
164. DeNardo SJ, DeNardo GL, Kukis DL, et al. ^{67}Cu-2IT-BAT-Lym-1 pharmacokinetics, radiation dosimetry, toxicity and tumor regression in patients with lymphoma. J Nucl Med 1999;40:302–10.
165. DeNardo SJ, Kukis DL, Shen S, et al. ^{67}Cu versus ^{131}I-labeled Lym-1 antibody: comparative pharmacokinetics and dosimetry in patients with non-Hodgkin's lymphoma. Clin Cancer Res 1999;5:533–41.
166. Rizzieri DA, Akabani G, Zalutsky MR, et al. Phase 1 trial study of ^{131}I-labeled chimeric 81C6 monoclonal antibody for the treatment of patients with non-Hodgkin's lymphoma. Blood 2004;104:642–8.
167. Sharkey RM, Goldenberg DM. Perspectives on cancer therapy with radiolabeled monoclonal antibodies. J Nucl Med 2005;46:115S–27S.
168. Behr TM, Salib AL, Liersch T, et al. Radioimmunotherapy of small volume disease of colorectal cancer metastatic to the liver: preclinical evaluation in comparison to standard chemotherapy and initial results of a phase I clinical study Clin Cancer Res 1999;5:3232s–42s.
169. Wong JYC, Chu DZ, Yamauchi DM, et al. A phase I radioimmunotherapy trial evaluating ^{90}yttrium-labeled anti-carcinoembryonic antigen (CEA) chimeric T84.66 in patients with metastatic CEA-producing malignancies. Clin Cancer Res 2000;6:3855–63.
170. Wong JY, Shibata S, Williams LE, et al. A phase I trial of ^{90}Y-anti-carcinoembryonic antigen chimeric T84.66 radioimmunotherapy with 5-fluorouracil in patients with metastatic colorectal cancer. Clin Cancer Res 2003;9:5842–52.
171. Welt S, Divgi CR, Kemeny N et al., Phase I/II study of iodine 131-labeled monoclonal antibody A33 in patients with advanced colon cancer. J Clin Oncol 1994;12:1561–71.
172. Welt S, Scott AM, Divgi CR, et al. Phase I/II study of iodine 125-labeled monoclonal antibody A33 in patients with advanced colon cancer. J Clin Oncol 1996;14:1787–97.
173. Meredith RF, Khazaeli MB, Plott WE, et al. Comparison of two mouse/human chimeric antibodies in patients with metastatic colon cancer. Antibody Immunocon Radiopharmacol 1992;5:75–80.
174. Tempero M, Leichner P, Baranoeska J, et al. High-dose therapy with ^{90}Yttrium-labeled monoclonal antibody CC49: a phase I trial. Clin Cancer Res 2000;6:3095–102.
175. Hird V, Steward JS, Snook D, et al. Intraperitoneally administered ^{90}Y-labeled monoclonal antibodies as a third line of treatment in ovarian cancer. A phase 1-2 trial: problems encountered and possible solutions. Br J Cancer 1990;62:48–51.
176. Hird V, Maraveyas A, Snook D, et al. Adjuvant therapy of ovarian cancer with radioactive monoclonal antibody. Br J Cancer 1993;68:403–6.
177. Nicholson S, Gooden CS, Hird V, et al. Radioimmunotherapy after chemotherapy compared to chemotherapy alone in the treatment of advanced ovarian cancer: a matched analysis. Oncol Rep 1998;5:223–6.
178. Epenetos AA, Hird V, Lambert H, et al. The long-term survival of patients with ovarian cancer treated with radioimmunotherapy. Int. J Gynecol Cancer 2000;10:44–6.
179. Alvarez RD, Partridge EE, Khazaeli MB, et al. Intraperitoneal radioimmunotherapy of ovarian cancer with 177Lu-CC49: a phase I/II study. Gynecol Oncol 1997;65:94–101.
180. van Zanten-Przybysz I, Molthoff CF, Roos JC, et al. Radioimmunotherapy with intravenously administered ^{131}I-labeled chimeric monoclonal antibody MOv18 in patients with ovarian cancer. J Nucl Med 2000;41:1168–76.
181. Smith-Jones PM. Radioimmunotherapy of prostate cancer. Q J Nucl Med Mol Imaging 2004;48:297–304.
182. Myers RB, Meredith RF, Schlom J, et al. Tumor associated glycoprotein-72 is highly expressed in prostatic adenocarcinomas. J Urol 1994;152:243–6.
183. Meredith RF, Bueschen AJ, Khazaeli MB, et al. Treatment of metastatic prostate carcinoma with radiolabeled antibody CC49. J Nucl Med 1994;35:1017–22.
184. Kahn D, Austin JC, Maguire RT, et al. A phase II study of [^{90}Y] yttrium-capromab pendetide in the treatment of men with prostate cancer recurrence following radical prostatectomy. Cancer Biother Radiopharm 1999;14:99-111.
185. Bander NH, Nanus DM, Milowsky MI, et al. Targeted systemic therapy of prostate cancer with a monoclonal antibody to prostate-specific membrane antigen. Semin Oncol 2003;30:667–76.
186. Oosterwijk E, Bander NH, Divgi CR, et al. Antibody localization in human renal cell carcinoma: a phase I study of monoclonal antibody G250. J Clin Oncol 1993;11:738 – 50.
187. Divgi CR, Bander NH, Scott AM, et al. Phase I/II radioimmunotherapy trial with iodine-131-labeled monoclonal antibody G250 in metastatic renal cell carcinoma. Clin Cancer Res 1998;4:2729–39.
188. Divgi CR, O'Donoghue JA, Welt S, et al. Phase I clinical trial with fractionated radioimmunotherapy using ^{131}I-labeled chimeric G250 in metastatic renal cancer. J Nucl Med 2004;45:1412–21.
189. Zalutsky MR. Targeted radiotherapy of brain tumours. Br J Cancer 2004;90:1469–73.
190. Reardon DA, Akabani G, Coleman RE, et al. Phase II trial of murine ^{131}I-labeled antitenascin monoclonal antibody 81C6 administered into surgically created resection cavities of patients with newly diagnosed malignant gliomas. J Clin Oncol 2002;20:1389–97.
191. Vaidyanathan G, Affleck DJ, Bigner DD, Zalutsky MR. Improved xenograft targeting of tumor-specific anti-epidermal growth factor receptor variant III antibody labeled using *N*-succinimidyl 4-guanidinomethyl-3-iodobenzoate. Nucl Med Biol 2002;29:1–11.
192. DeNardo GL, Schlom J, Buchsbaum DJ, et al. Rationales, evidence, and design considerations for fractionated radioimmunotherapy. Cancer 2002;94:1332–48.
193. Pedley RB, Hill SA, Boxer GM, et al. Eradication of colorectal xenografts by combined radioimmunotherapy and combretastatin a-4 3-O-phosphate. Cancer Res 2001;61:4716–22.
194. Pedley RB, El-Emir E, Flynn AA, et al. Synergy between vascular targeting agents and antibody-directed therapy. Int J Radiat Oncol Biol Phys 2002;54:1524–31.
195. Hauck ML, Zalutsky MR. Enhanced tumour uptake of radiolabelled antibodies by hyperthermia: part I: time of injection relative to hyperthermia. Int J Hyperthermia 2005;21:1–11.
196. Hauck ML, Zalutsky MR. Enhanced tumour uptake of radiolabelled antibodies by hyperthermia: part II: application of the thermal equivalency equation. Int J Hyperthermia 2005;21:13–27.
197. Akabani G, McLendon RE, et al. Vascular targeted endoradiotherapy using alpha-particle emitting compounds: theoretical analysis. Int J Radiat Oncol Biol Phys 2002;1259–75.
198. Buchsbaum DJ. Imaging and therapy of tumors induced to express somatostatin receptor by gene transfer using radiolabeled peptides and single chain antibody constructs. Semin Nucl Med 2004;34:32– 46.
199. Boerman OC, van Schaijk FG, Oyen WJ, et al. Pretargeted radioimmunotherapy of cancer: progress step by step. J Nucl Med 2003;44:400–11.
200. Paganelli G, Bartolomei M, Ferrari M, et al. Pre-targeted locoregional radioimmunotherapy with ^{90}Y-biotin in glioma patients: phase I study and preliminary therapeutic results. Cancer Biother Radiopharm 2001;16:227–35.
201. Grana C, Chinol M, Robertson C, et al. Pretargeted adjuvant radioimmunotherapy with yttrium-90-biotin in malignant glioma patients: a pilot study. Br J Cancer 2002;21; 86:207–12.
202. Goodwin DA, Meares CF. Advances in pretargeting biotechnology. Biotechnol Adv. 2001;19:435–50.
203. Rossi EA, Sharkey RM, McBride W, et al. Development of new multivalent bispecific agents for pretargeting tumor localization and therapy. Clin Cancer Res 2003;9:3886S–96S.
204. Sharkey RM, McBride WJ, Karacay H, et al. A universal pretargeting system for cancer detection and therapy using bispecific antibody. Cancer Res 2003;63:354–63.
205. Zalutsky MR, Vaidyanathan G. Astatine-211-labeled radiotherapeutics: an emerging approach to targeted alpha particle therapy. Current Pharm Design 2000;6:1433–55.
206. McDivitt MR, Finn RD, Ma D, et al. Preparation of α-emitting ^{213}Bi-labeled antibody constructs for clinical use. J Nucl Med 1999;40:1722–7.
207. Akabani G, Kennel SJ, Zalutsky MR. Microdosimetric analysis of alpha particle emitting targeted radiotherapeutics using histological images. J Nucl Med 2003;44:792–805.
208. McLendon RE, Archer GE, Larsen RH, et al. Radiotoxicity of systemically administered ^{211}At labeled human/mouse chimeric monoclonal antibody: a long term survival study with histologic analysis. Int J Radiat Oncol Biol Phys 1999;45:491–9.
209. Zalutsky MR, Zhao XG, Alston KL, et al. High-level production of alpha-particle-emitting ^{211}At and preparation of ^{211}At-labeled antibodies for clinical use. J Nucl Med 2001;42:1508–15.
210. Jurcic JG, Larson SM, Sgouros G, et al. Targeted alpha particle immunotherapy for myeloid leukemia. Blood 2002;100:1233–9.
211. Burke JM, Jurcic JG, Divgi CR, et al. Sequential cytarabine and alpha-particle immunotherapy with bismuth-213-labeled anti-CD33 monoclonal antibody HuM195 in acute myeloid leukemia (AML) [abstract]. Blood 2002;100:339.
212. Zalutsky M, Reardon D, Akabani G, et al. Astatine-211 labeled human/mouse chimeric antitenascin monoclonal antibody via surgically created resection cavities for patients with recurrent glioma: phase I study [abstract]. NeuroOncol 2002;4:S10.
213. Hassan R, Williams-Gould J, Watson T, et al. Pretreatment with rituximab does not inhibit the human immune response against the immunogenic protein LMB-1. Clinical Cancer Res 2004;10:16–18.
214. Pai LH, Wittes R, Setser A, et al. Phase I trial of recombinant immunotoxin LMB-7[B3(Fv)PE38] for adult solid tumors. Proc AACR 1997;38:85.
215. Posey JA, Khazaeli MB, Bookman MA, et al. A phase I trial of the single-chain immunotoxin SGN-10 (BR96sFv-PE40) in patients with advanced solid tumors. Clinical Cancer Res 2002;8:3092–9.
216. Hausner PF, Karp JE, Edelman MJ, et al. Phase I study of LMB-9 (B3(dsFv)PE38), a recombinant disulfide stabilized anti-Lewis Y immunotoxin administered by continuous infusion. Proc ASCO 2003;22:184.
217. Amlot PL, Stone MJ, Cunningham D, et al. A phase I study of an anti-CD22-deglycosylated ricin A chain immunotoxin in the treatment of B-cell lymphomas resistant to conventional therapy. Blood 1993;82:2624–33.

218. Vitetta ES, Stone M, Amlot P, et al. Phase I immunotoxin trial in patients with B-cell lymphoma. Cancer Res 1991;51:4052–8.
219. Kreitman RJ, Wilson WH, Bergeron K, et al. Efficacy of the anti-CD22 recombinant immunotoxin BL22 in chemotherapy-resistant hairy cell leukemia. N Engl J Med 2001;345:241–7.
220. Stone MJ, Sausville EA, Fay JW, et al. A phase I study of bolus versus continuous infusion of the anti-CD19 immunotoxin, IgGHD37-dgA, in patients with B-cell lymphoma. Blood 1996;88:1188–97.
221. Uckun F. Immunotoxin for the treatment of leukaemia. Br J Haematol 1993;85:435.
222. Grossbard ML, Lambert JM, Goldmacher VS, et al. Anti-B4-blocked ricin: a phase I trial of 7-day continuous infusion in patients with B-cell neoplasms. J Clin Oncol 1993;11:726–37.
223. Olsen E, Duvic M, Frankel A, et al. Pivotal phase III trial of two dose levels of DAB389IL2 (ONTAK) for the treatment of cutaneous T-cell lymphoma. J Clin Oncol 2001;19:376–88.
224. Waldmann T, Pastan I, Gansow O, et al. The multi-chain interleukin-2 receptor: a target for immunotherapy. Ann Intern Med 1992;116:148–60.
225. Schnell R, Vitetta ES, Schindler J, et al. Clinical trials with an anti-CD25 ricin A-chain experimental and immunotoxin (RFT5-SMPT-dgA) in Hodgkin's lymphoma. Leuk Lymph 1998;30:525–37.
226. Misra, D, Frankel, AE, Hall, P, et al. The use of DT388-IL3 fusion protein in patients with refractory acute myeloid leukemia (AML). Blood 2004;104:212b.
227. Kreitman RJ, Wilson WH, White, JD, et al. Phase I trial of recombinant immunotoxin anti-Tac(Fv)-PE38 (LMB-2) in patients with hematologic malignancies. J Clin Oncol 2000;18:1622–36.
228. Oldfield, EH, Broaddus WC, Bruce J, et al. Phase II trial of convection-enhanced distribution of recombinant immunotoxin in patients with recurrent malignant gliomas. Proc Am Assoc Neurol Surg 2000;18:94–5.
229. Laske DW, Muraszko KM, Oldfield EH, et al. Intraventricular immunotoxin therapy for leptomeningeal neoplasia. Neurosurgery 1997;41:1039–49.
230. Rand RW, Kreitman RJ, Patronas N, et al. Intaventricular administration of recombinant circularly permuted interleukin-4-Pseudomonas exotoxin in patients with high grade gliomas. Clin Cancer Res 2000;6:2157–65.
231. Pagliaro LC, Liu B, Munker R, et al. Humanized M195 monoclonal antibody conjugated to recombinant gelonin: an anti-CD33 immunotoxin with antileukemic activity. Clin Cancer Res 1998;4:1971–6.
232. Frankel AE, Powell BL, Hall PD, et al. Phase I trial of a novel diphtheria toxin/GM-CSF fusion protein (DT388GMCSF) for refractory or relapsed acute myeloid leukemia (AML). Clin Cancer Res 2002;8:1004–13.
233. Lynch TJ, Lambert JM, Coral F, et al. Immunotoxin therapy of small-cell lung cancer: a phase I study of N901-blocked ricin. J Clin Oncol 1997;15:723–34.
234. Goldberg MR, Heimbrook DC, Russo P, et al. Phase I clinical study of the recombinant oncotoxin TP40 in superficial bladder cancer. Clin Cancer Res 1995;1:57–61.
235. Sampson JH, Akabani G, Archer GE, et al. Progress report of a phase I study of the intracerebral microinfusion of a recombinant chimeric protein composed of transforming growth factor (TGF)-alpha and a mutated form of the Pseudomonas exotoxin termed PE-38 (TP-38) for the treatment of malignant brain tumors. J Neurooncol 2003;65:27–35.
236. Bacha P, Shaw J, Baselga J, et al. Phase I dose-escalation studies of the safety and tolerability of DAB389EGF in patients with epidermal growth factor receptor (EGF-R) expressing solid tumors. Proc Fourth Intl Symp Immunotoxins 1995;138.
237. Byers VS, Rodvien R, Grant K, et al. Phase I study of monoclonal antibody-ricin A chain immunotoxin XomaZyme-791 in patients with metastatic colon cancer. Cancer Res 1989;49:6153–60.
238. Gould BJ, Borowitz MJ, Groves ES, et al. Phase I study of an anti-breast cancer immunotoxin by continuous infusion: report of a targeted toxic effect not predicted by animal studies. J Natl Cancer Inst 1989;81:775–81.
239. Falini B, Bolognesi A, Flenghi L, et al. Response of refractory Hodgkin's disease to monoclonal anti-CD30 immunotoxin. Lancet 1992;339:1195–6.
240. Schnell R, Borchmann P, Staak JO, et al. Clinical evaluation of ricin A-chain immunotoxins in patients with Hodgkin's lymphoma. Ann Oncol 2003;14:729–36.
241. Hertler A, Schlossman D, Borowitz M, et al. An Anti-CD5 immunotoxin for chronic lymphocytic leukemia: enhancement of cytotoxicity with human serum albumin-monensin. Int J Cancer 1989;43:215–9.
242. LeMaistre CF, Rosen S, Frankel A, et al. Phase I trial of H65-RTA immunoconjugate in patients with cutaneous T-cell lymphoma. Blood 1991;78:1173–82.
243. Spitler LE, del Rio M, Khentigan A, et al. Therapy of patients with malignant melanoma using a monoclonal antimelanoma antibody-ricin A chain immunotoxin. Cancer Res 1987;47:1717–23.
244. Pai L, Bookman M, Ozols R, et al. Clinical evaluation of intraperitoneal Pseudomonas exotoxin immunoconjugate OVB3-PE in patients with ovarian cancer. J Clin Oncol 1991;9:2095–103.
245. Frankel AE, Laver JH, Willingham MC, et al. Therapy of patients with T-cell lymphomas and leukemias using an anti-CD7 monoclonal antibody-ricin A chain immunotoxin. Leuk Lymph 1997;26:287–98.
246. Uckun FM, Bellomy K, O'Neill K, et al. Toxicity, biological activity, and pharmacokinetics of TXU (anti-CD7)-pokeweed antiviral protein in chimpanzees and adult patients infected with human immunodeficiency virus. J Pharmacol Exp Therapeutics 1999;291:1301–7.
247. Pai-Scherf LH, Villa J, Pearson D, et al. Hepatotoxicity in cancer patients receiving Erb-38, a recombinant immunotoxin that targets the erbB2 receptor. Clin Cancer Res 1999;5:2311–5.
248. Azemar M, Djahansouzi S, Jager E, et al. Regression of cutaneous tumor lesions in patients intratumorally injected with a recombinant single-chain antibody toxin targeted to ErbB2/HER2. Breast Cancer Res Treatment 2003;82:155–64.
249. van Oosterhout YVJM, van Ernst L, Schattenberg AVMB, et al. A combination of anti-CD3 and anti-CD7 ricin A-immunotoxins for the in vivo treatment of acute graft versus host disease. Blood 2000;95:3693–701.
250. Hassan R, Bullock S, Kreitman RJ, et al. Targeted therapy of mesothelin expressing mesotheliomas (MM), ovarian cancer (OC), and pancreatic cancer (PC): results of phase I study of SS1(dsFv)PE38 (SS1P). Proc ASCO 2004;22 Suppl 15:3035.
251. Kunwar S. Convection enhanced delivery of IL13-PE38QQR for treatment of recurrent malignant glioma: presentation of interim findings from ongoing phase I studies. Acta Neurochir Suppl 2003;88:105–11.
252. Flavell DJ, Boehm DA, Noss A, et al. Therapy of human T-cell acute lymphoblastic leukaemia with a combination of anti-CD7 and anti-CD38-SAPORIN immunotoxins is significantly better than therapy with each individual immunotoxin. Br J Cancer 2001;84:571–8.
253. Bjorn MJ, Ring D, Frankel A. Evaluation of monoclonal antibodies for the development of breast cancer immunotoxins. Cancer Res 1985;45:1214–21.
254. Choe, S, Bennett, M, Fujii, G, et al. The crystal structure of diphtheria toxin. Nature 1992;357:216–22.
255. Greenfield L, Johnson VG, Youle RJ. Mutations in diphtheria toxin separate binding from entry and amplify immunotoxin selectivity. Science 1987;238:536–9.
256. Williams D, Snider CE, Strom TB, Murphy JR. Structure/function analysis of interleukin-2-toxin (DAB486IL-2). Fragment B sequences required for the delivery of fragment A to the cytosol of target cells. J Biol Chem 1990;265:11885–9.
257. Hwang J, FitzGerald D, Adhya S, Pastan I. Functional domains of *Pseudomonas* exotoxin identified by deletion analysis of the gene expressed in *E. coli.* Cell 1987;48:129–36.
258. Pastan I, Pai LH, Brinkmann U, FitzGerald DJ. Recombinant toxins: new therapeutic agents for cancer. Ann NY Acad Sci 1995;758:345–54.
259. Montfort W, Villafranca J, Monzingo A, et al. The three-dimensional structure of ricin at 2.8 angstroms. J Biol Chem 1987;262:5398–403.
260. Jansen FK, Blythman HE, Carriere D, et al. Immunotoxins: hybrid molecules combining high specificity and potent cytotoxicity. Immunol Rev 1982;62:185–216.
261. Lambert JM, Goldmacher VS, Collinson AR, et al. An immunotoxin prepared with blocked ricin: a natural plant toxin adapted for therapeutic use. Cancer Res 1991;78:3306.
262. Irvin JD. Pokeweed antiviral protein. Pharmacol Ther 1983;21:371–87.
263. Dang NH, Hagemeister FB, Pro B, et al. Phase II study of denileukin diftitox for relapsed/refractory B-cell non-Hodgkin's lymphoma. J Clin Oncol 2004;22:4095–102.
264. Ho VT, Zahrieh D, Hochberg E, et al. Safety and efficacy of denileukin diftitox in patients with steroid refractory acute graft-versus-host disease after allogeneic hematopoietic stem cell transplantation. Blood 2004;104:1224–6.
265. Frankel AE, Fleming DR, Hall PD, et al. A phase II study of DT fusion protein denileukin diftitox in patients with fludarabine-refractory chronic lymphocytic leukemia. Clin Cancer Res 2003;9:3555–61.
266. Seymour JF, Morgan SJ, Wolf MM, et al. Denileukin diftitox (Ontak), an interleukin-2 (IL-2) fusion toxin, has significant activity in fludarabine-refractory chronic lymphocytic leukemia (CLL). Blood 2003;102:673a.
267. Kuriakose P, Turturro F, Berdeja JG, et al. A phase II study of denileukin diftitox (ONTAK) in patients with fludarabine refractory B-cell chronic lymphocytic leukemia. Blood 2004;104:289b.
268. Heestand G, Robbin DH, Onda M, et al. Recombinant toxins containing Pseudomonas exotoxin directly injure hepatocytes in the absence of Kupffer cells. Blood 2005. [In press]
269. Schumann J, Angermuller S, Bang R, et al. Acute hepatotoxicity of *Pseudomonas aeruginosa* exotoxin A in mice depends on T cells and TNF. J Immunol 1998;161:5745–54.
270. Soler-Rodriguez A, Ghetie M, Oppenheimer-Marks N, et al. Ricin A-chain and ricin A-chain immunotoxins rapidly damage human endothelial cells: implications for vascular leak syndrome. Exp Cell Res 1993;206:227–34.
271. Baluna, R, Rizo, J, Gordon, BE, et al. Evidence for a structural motif in toxins and interleukin-2 that may be responsible for binding to endothelial cells and initiating vascular leak syndrome. Proc Natl Acad Sci U S A 1999;96:3957–62.
272. Smallshaw JE, Ghetie V, Rizo J, et al. Genetic engineering of an immunotoxin to eliminate pulmonary vascular leak in mice. Nature Biotech 2003;21:387–91.
273. Siegall C, Liggitt D, Chace D, et al. Prevention of immunotoxin-mediated vascular leak syndrome in rats with retention of antitumor activity. Proc Natl Acad Sci U S A 1994;91:9514–8.
274. Rozemuller H, Rombouts WJ, Touw IP, et al. Treatment of acute myelocytic leukemia with interleukin-6 Pseudomonas exotoxin fusion protein in a rat leukemia model. Leukemia 1996;10:1796–803.
275. Wenning, LA, Murphy, RM. Coupled cellular trafficking and diffusional limitations in delivery of immunotoxins to multicellular tumor spheroids. Biotechnol Bioeng 1999;62:562–75.
276. Sung C, van Osdol W. Effects of molecular weight and intracellular processing on tumor penetration of immunotoxins. Proc Fourth Intl Symp Immunotoxins 1995;107.
277. Pai L, FitzGerald D, Tepper M, et al. Inhibition of antibody response to Pseudomonas exotoxin and an immunotoxin containing Pseudomonas exotoxin by 15-deoxyspergualin in mice. Cancer Res 1990;50:7750–3.
278. Castelletti D, Fracasso G, Righetti S, et al. A dominant linear B-cell epitope of ricin Achain is the target of a neutralizing antibody response in Hodgkin's lymphoma patients treated with an anti-CD25 immunotoxin. Clin Exp Immunol 2004;136:365–72.
279. Rybak S, Hoogenboom H, Meade H, Youle R. Humanization of immunotoxins. Proc Natl Acad Sci U S A 1992;89:3165–9.
280. Ehrlich P. The relationship existing between chemical constitution, distribution and pharmacological action. In: Himmelweite IF, Dale H, editors. The collected papers of Paul Ehrlich. Vol. I. London, UK: Pergammon Press; 1956. p. 596.
281. Xu F, Leadon SA, Yu Y, et al. Synergistic interaction between anti-p185HER-2 ricin A chain immunotoxins and radionuclide conjugates for inhibiting growth of ovarian and breast cancer cells that overexpress HER-2. Clin Cancer Res 2000;6:3334–41.
282. lTsimberidou AM, Giles FJ, Kantarjian HM, et al. Anti-B4 blocked ricin post chemotherapy in patients with chronic lymphocytic leukemia—long term followup of a monoclonal antibody based approach to residual disease. Leuk Lymphoma 2003;44:1719–25.

51

Vaccines and Immunostimulants

James W. Hodge, PhD
Jeffrey Schlom, PhD
Scott I. Abrams, PhD

The discipline of tumor immunology, once limited to a basic understanding of the immune system under normal and pathologic conditions, has evolved to include potential clinical applications toward the immunotherapy of malignancy. In turn, tumor immunotherapy has evolved to the point that the immune system may now be appropriately manipulated or modulated against neoplastic disease or the neoplastic process. For immunotherapy to be effective, however, it must satisfy the following major premises: (1) the host immune system is competent and contains the relevant precursor cells and functional antigen-presenting cell (APC) populations; (2) tumor cells express antigens that selectively or specifically distinguish them from normal host tissues for effective immune recognition and attack after vaccination; and (3) under conditions of peripheral T-cell anergy, such immunotherapeutic strategies must be able to overcome or "break" potential tolerance mechanisms, without inducing unacceptable autoimmune toxicities.

The use of cancer vaccines for the potential treatment of human malignancies has reached several new milestones in scientific discovery. Areas of intense investigations include the development and characterization of (1) tumor-associated antigens (TAAs) or tumor-specific antigens (TSAs) selectively expressed or overexpressed by malignant cells as compared with normal adult tissues; (2) novel vaccine delivery systems for the induction of endogenous host antitumor immune responses; (3) cytokines and other immunostimulants to further augment immunogenic properties of vaccine preparations; and (4) adoptive immunotherapy approaches employing dendritic cells (DCs) expressing relevant tumor-rejection antigens or effector cells, which activate or mediate antitumor responses, respectively. The combination of gene discovery with each of those areas has accelerated the rate of both basic mechanistic findings and potential clinical applications. For example, (1) gene discovery has led to the identification of new tumor antigens and will undoubtedly also spur the detection of new cytokines, chemokines and T-cell costimulatory molecules; and (2) knowledge of T-cell activation and tumor–host interactions will improve our understanding of how to better use immunotherapies. At the preclinical stage, the construction and analysis of transgenic mouse models, which better mirror the human cancer situation, may not only strengthen our understanding of the neoplastic process, but also help guide the application of both active and passive immunotherapy strategies in the clinic.

TARGETS FOR VACCINE THERAPY

Many potential targets for cancer immunotherapy were identified recently (Table 51-1). It is important to note that when an antigen is a target for vaccine therapy, the activated T cells, induced by vaccination, recognize peptide–MHC (major histocompatibility complex) complexes of the tumor antigen on the cell surface. T cells do not recognize the surface protein—only the peptide–MHC complex. Thus, targets of vaccine therapy need not be cell-surface proteins. These targets can be grouped into two major categories: TSAs and TAAs.

Tumor-Specific Antigens TSAs comprise gene products that are uniquely expressed in tumors, such as point-mutated *ras* oncogenes, mutated *p53* suppressor genes, anti-idiotype antibodies (Abs), and products of ribonucleic acid (RNA) splice variants and gene translocations.

Three mutations at codon 12 represent the vast majority of *ras* mutations, which are found in approximately 20 to 30% of human tumors. In other words, in the United States alone, approximately 140,000 new cases of cancer each year involve *ras* mutations, and upwards of 800,000 current patients with cancer have tumors that contain *ras* mutations.[1] Because the ras protein is not found on the cell surface, one can envision vaccine therapy directed against peptide–MHC complexes on the cell surface. One good reason to consider *ras* gene products as targets for immunotherapy is that *ras* mutations occur early in the transformation process.

Although mutations in the *p53*-suppressor gene are attractive targets for immunotherapy, their use is not without several disadvantages. One drawback in particular is the vast number of mutations that span across four exons, which leads to a situation in which almost every patient would require a specific immunotherapy regimen. It is now known that the normal *p53* gene is overexpressed in tumors containing *p53* gene mutations. Therefore, overexpression of the normal or wild-type p53 protein may be a more promising target for immunotherapy.[2]

B-cell lymphomas overexpress a single immunoglobulin variant on their cell surface; therefore, each B-cell lymphoma displays a

Table 51-1 Examples of Targets for Cancer Vaccine Therapy*

Carcinoma-associated antigens	
HER-2/*neu*	PSMA (prostate-specific membrane antigen)
CEA (carcinoembryonic antigen)	p53 (point mutated and overexpressed)
PSA (prostate-specific antigen)	ras (point mutated)
MUC-1	EGF-R (epidermal growth factor receptor)
PAP	VEGF (vascular endothelial growth factor)
PSMA	mesothelin
CA125 (cancer antigen 125)	PAGE-4
sTn	TARP
KSA (17-1A)	
Melanoma antigens	
MAGE	GD2
MART	GM2
gp100	GD3
Tyrosinase	
Leukemia/lymphoma	
Anti-idiotype antibodies	CD36
CD20	Aberrant class II
CD19	B1
CD22	CD25 (interleukin [IL]-2R) (anti-TAC)
Viral antigens	
Human papillomavirus (HPV)	
Endogenous retroviral gene products	
HERV-K	

* This represents only a partial list of current and potential targets for vaccine therapy.
HERV-K = human endogenous retrovirus type k; PAP = prostatic acid phosphatase; PSMA = prostate-specific membrane antigen.

unique target for immunotherapy[3–5] The gene products of RNA splice variants and deoxyribonucleic acid (DNA) translocations also represent unique fusion proteins that can be specific targets for immunotherapy, including c-erb-B2 RNA splice variants and the bcr/abl product of DNA translocation of chronic myelogenous leukemia. Although these somatic mutations are exquisitely specific targets for therapy, their use gives rise to several issues that need to be addressed. For example, in each case, only a certain percentage of tumors may express the mutation.

Therefore, tailored immunotherapies for individual patients or groups of patients would be required. Other potential issues are (1) the functional expression level of these mutant gene products may not be sufficient on the cell surface of the tumor as a peptide–MHC complex to serve as a target of T–cell-mediated immunotherapy; (2) the products of these mutations may not contain immunogenic epitopes; and (3) some of these products may not be required to maintain the transformed state and, therefore, may be lost in metastatic variants.

Tumor-Associated Antigens TAAs can be categorized into five major groups: oncofetal antigens, oncogene products, tissue-lineage antigens, viral antigens, and "new targets." Oncofetal antigens, which include carcinoembryonic antigen (CEA), the breast cancer mucin MUC-1, and prostate-specific membrane antigen (PSMA), can be overexpressed in tumors and may be expressed in some normal tissues. These antigens are also found in fetal tissues. Thus, two opposing arguments can be made against using oncofetal antigens as targets: because these antigens are expressed in fetal tissue, a state of thymic and/or peripheral tolerance to them in the host may exist; on the other hand, too much immunity to these antigens, as a consequence of vaccination, may lead to autoimmune states.

Oncogene and suppressor gene products, such as nonmutated HER-2/*neu* and p53, are analogous to oncofetal antigens in that they can be overexpressed in tumors and may be expressed in some fetal tissues. Similarly, telomerase, an enzyme important in cellular replication and chromosomal stability, is much more active in malignant cells as compared with most normal cells. Epitopes derived from human telomerase have been reported, and presumably may be overexpressed by neoplastic cells.

Tissue-lineage antigens such as prostate-specific antigen (PSA) and melanocyte antigens, MART-1/Melan A, tyrosinase, gp100, and TRP-1 (gp75) are expressed in a tumor of a given type and the normal tissue from which it is derived. Tissue-lineage antigens are potentially useful targets for immunotherapy if the normal organ/tissue in which they are expressed is not essential, such as the prostate, breast, or melanocyte. Several viruses are associated with the etiology of some cancers. An excellent example of this connection is the human papilloma virus (HPV) and cervical cancer.

The Human Genome Project and advances in proteomics have led to the discovery of literally dozens of new TSA and TAA candidates. A major challenge of the future will be to sort out which of these products is worth pursuing on the long and costly path to the development of new cancer immunotherapeutics.

Table 51-2 Vaccine Modalities

Vaccine Modalities
Tumor cells
Whole tumor cells (x-irradiated)
Gene modified tumor cells (GM-CSF, costimulatory molecules, lymphotactin)
Cell extracts and oncolysates
Direct injection of tumor with cytokine or costimulatory gene
Protein/molecule-based
Protein
Peptide
Glycopeptide
Glycolipid
Anti-idiotype MAb
MAb fusion proteins
Antigen-presenting cells
Dendritic cells
Unmodified
Gene modified
Peptide pulsed
RNA transfected
Loaded with tumor lysates
Fused with tumor cells
B cells
Vector-based
Viral vectors
Replication-competent:
Vaccinia
Adenovirus
RNA viruses (replicons)
Replication-defective:
Avipox: fowlpox, canarypox
MVA
Adenovirus
Bacterial vectors
Listeria
Salmonella
BCG
Yeast vectors
Plasmid DNA

BCG = bacillus Calmette-Guerin; DNA = deoxyribonucleic acid; GM-CSF = granulocyte-macrophage colony stimulating factor; MAb = monoclonal antibody; MVA = modified vaccinia Ankara; RNA = ribonucleic acid.

Types of Vaccines Numerous vaccine-delivery systems have been analyzed in experimental models and many of these are now being evaluated in the clinic (Table 51-2). Each of these systems has its advantages and disadvantages; moreover, one may eventually find that some of these modalities are most beneficial when used in combination or in tandem.

Whole Tumor Cell Vaccines There are two major categories of whole tumor cell vaccines: (1) autologous (ie, manipulating the tumor from a patient into a vaccine for that patient) and (2) allogeneic (ie, in which tumor cells from other patients, usually from established tumor cell lines, are used). The major advantage of using whole tumor cell vaccines is that several TSAs or TAAs, yet undefined, may be present in the vaccine preparation. However, this approach has major disadvantages as well, including (1) the actual amount of any TAA or TSA would be diluted by normal cellular components; (2) the vast majority of human tumors, with the exception of hematopoietic malignancies, do not express costimulatory molecules and thus would not activate naïve T cells to levels capable of inducing therapeutic responses; and (3) one does not know, when using this approach, what the immunogenic proteins or epitopes are. Therefore, it is difficult to measure immune responses and to amplify those specific responses. Nonetheless, as detailed below, preclinical and clinical use of whole tumor cell vaccines, albeit modified, have already met with some success.

Autologous Whole Tumor Cell Vaccines As stated earlier, the advantage of this approach is that the putative TSAs or TAAs of that tumor would also be present in the vaccine preparation. For example, if a patient's tumor is found to have a unique p53 mutation or splice variant, an autologous whole tumor cell vaccine may be the only vaccine therapy that is efficacious. However, preparing this vaccine requires an enormous amount of effort. Fresh tumor specimens need to be obtained at surgery and prepared in a similar manner for each patient. In addition, tumor masses will differ in terms of percentage of tumor cells, degree of necrosis, and other factors. Indeed, a great deal of effort has been expended in preparing a vaccine consisting of whole tumor cells obtained at surgery, x-irradiated, and administered to patients admixed with bacille Calmette-Guérin (BCG; see below). Although the vaccines are efficacious for antitumor activity, a lesson learned from these studies is that a central laboratory is required to prepare these vaccines from tumors that are obtained at surgery from several institutions.

Allogeneic Whole Tumor Cell Vaccines These vaccines, which usually employ one or more tumor cell lines, are relatively easy to prepare when compared with autologous vaccines. These preparations may also contain several TSAs and/or TAAs. Moreover, the cell lines used in the preparations can be infected with vectors that express cytokine genes (such as granulocyte-macrophage colony-stimulating factor [GM-CSF])[6] or costimulatory molecule genes, such as B7-1,[7] to enhance the immunogenicity of the tumor cell. A disadvantage in the use of allogeneic vaccines prepared from whole tumor cells is that they do not constitutively express costimulatory molecules, as described above. Moreover, one can always make the case that because allogeneic cells are used, alloimmunity to non-self components may develop. However, this was not the case in early clinical trials, which include studies using oncolysates (ie, tumor cell preparations that had been infected with vaccinia virus and then lysed in an effort to enhance their immunogenicity).[8] More recent studies used cell lines infected with GM-CSF with some success,[8] as well as allogeneic neuroblastoma cells transduced with the genes for IL-2 and lymphotactin.[9]

Direct Injection of Cytokine Genes or Costimulatory Molecule Genes into Tumor Two signals are known to be required for the efficient activation of T cells. The first signal is mediated through a peptide–MHC complex on the cell surface of the APC, which binds to the

T-cell receptor (TCR) on the surface of the T cell. In most cases, in the absence of interleukin (IL)-2 production, this interaction alone will lead to a state of T-cell anergy or nonresponsiveness. The second signal involves the interaction of a T-cell costimulatory molecule on the surface of the APC with its ligand on the surface of the T cell. To date, the most studied of the T-cell costimulatory molecules is B7-1, which interacts with two ligands on the T-cell surface (CD28 for upregulation of T-cell function, and CTLA-4 for downregulation of T-cell function). Numerous preclinical studies show that the addition of B7-1 to a weakly immunogenic tumor will make it more immunogenic.[7] This phenomenon has also occurred when other costimulatory molecules, such as intercellular adhesion molecule (ICAM)-1 and lymphocyte function-associated antigen (LFA)-3, have been added to tumors. Thus, one can envision the direct injection of a vector containing a costimulatory molecule into a tumor mass to induce an antitumor immune response. It should be pointed out that a costimulatory molecule must be on the surface of the tumor to induce an immune response, but it does not necessarily have to be present on the tumor for the T cell to kill the tumor cell. The advantage of this direct-injection approach is that the "vaccine" is the patient's own tumor, which may express a unique TSA or TAA profile. In ongoing studies, vaccinia- and avipox-based recombinants expressing the B7-1 costimulatory molecule are being directly injected into melanoma or carcinoma lesions. Clinical studies are ongoing in which recombinant vaccinia- and recombinant avipox-TRICOM vectors containing a triad of costimulatory molecules (B7-1, ICAM-1, and LFA-3; designated TRICOM) are being directly injected into tumor lesions. Cytokines can also be introduced into the tumor mass using vectors as delivery vehicles, as in the case of a recombinant vaccinia virus expressing GM-CSF that was directly injected into melanoma lesions.[10]

Proteins Proteins, fusion proteins, glycoproteins, and even glycolipids have been used as vaccines for human cancers. These protein-based vaccines have the advantage of not containing normal cellular components, as do whole tumor cell vaccines. However, one of the disadvantages of this approach is the cost associated with producing and purifying these proteins. Proteins and glycoproteins are usually given with some type of immunostimulant or adjuvant formulation to enhance immune responses or help their incorporation into professional APCs. In some cases, combinations of proteins are used as immunogens.[11] Studies along these lines include the use of PSA in liposomes,[12] CEA protein in combination with GM-CSF,[13] sTn glycoprotein,[14] and GD2, GM2, and GD3.[15,16] These latter preparations, given to melanoma patients, have shown efficient induction of Ab responses that may be extremely important, in some cases, in the induction of antitumor immunity.[15]

Peptides Two major types of peptides induce an immune response by interacting with the appropriate class of the MHC molecule on the APC surface. Peptides of approximately 8 to 11 amino acids in length, if they possess the appropriate binding motifs, will bind to MHC class I molecules. These peptide–MHC complexes will interact with the TCR to activate CD8$^+$ T cells. In experimental models, CD8$^+$ T cells, termed cytotoxic T lymphocytes (CTLs), are usually responsible for lytic destruction of tumors. Peptides of approximately 11 to 15 amino acids in length, if they contain the appropriate binding motifs, will bind to MHC class II molecules on the surface of T cells. This will lead to the activation of CD4$^+$, or "helper," T cells.[17,18] The principal function of CD4$^+$ T cells is to produce cytokines and to help promote activation of CD8$^+$ T cells. These "MHC-restricted" responses are thus effective only if the appropriate MHC allele is present in a patient. The most studied MHC restriction element in the human population is the MHC class I allele, HLA-A2, which is found in approximately 50% of the Caucasian population. Peptide-binding motifs to HLA-A2 molecules have been identified. Many clinical trials are being carried out in which a given cohort of individuals possess the HLA-A2 allele; thus, T-cell responses to a particular defined peptide can be quantified. Numerous preclinical studies have shown that both CD8$^+$ and CD4$^+$ T cells are usually activated for a vigorous antitumor effect. However, studies do exist in which either a CD8$^+$ T-cell response alone or a CD4$^+$ T-cell response alone can provide an antitumor effect. Oligopeptides that contain both class I and class II epitopes can also be used. In a unique set of circumstances, an oligopeptide of the repeat sequences of the MUC-1 mucin has been shown to crosslink TCRs in an MHC unrestricted manner to activate T cells.[19]

Using peptides as immunogens has many advantages, including: (1) whole proteins may contain parts of the molecule that are shared with normal cellular proteins, and the use of peptides minimizes the potential for induction of autoimmunity; (2) preparation is relatively easy and affordable; (3) because the immunogen is extremely well defined, the immune response can be analyzed in several ways and quantitated; (4) tetramers, which are molecules that contain specific peptides bound to MHC components, can be used to bind to, and isolate, antigen-specific T cells induced and amplified in the host; (5) tumors can be stripped of peptide–MHC complexes, and those peptides displayed on the surface of tumors can be identified; and (6) peptides can be modified to be more immunogenic in the generation of peptide agonists.

Agonist Peptides Peptide agonists fall into two general categories. In the first category, amino acids of the peptide that bind to the MHC on the APC are modified. More vigorous MHC binding (ie, higher affinity for the MHC molecule) often leads to the generation of a more vigorous T-cell response. An example of this is the alteration in the CEA peptide.[20] The second category of agonist has been termed a TCR agonist. In this case, an amino acid of the peptide that interacts with the TCR on the T cell is modified; this can also result in a more vigorous induction of the T-cell response. An example of this is the generation of the TCR agonist for CEA.[21]

The same property that makes a peptide vaccine attractive (ie, its specificity) can also be a disadvantage. For example, a CTL epitope peptide may induce a CTL response that is short-lived because of the lack of "help" provided by helper peptides. Moreover, peptides are useful only in the vaccination of patients who have that specific allele (eg, for only ≤ 50% of the population that has the HLA-A2 allele for an HLA-A2–reactive peptide). Combinations of antigenic peptides with reactivities for multiple HLA alleles would circumvent this limitation. A large clinical experience in the use of peptides as cancer vaccines is now emerging. Some peptides under study include HPV,[22] ras,[23,24] HER-2/*neu*,[25] MAGE,[26] MART-1, tyrosinase,[27] gp100,[20,28] CEA,[29] MUC-1,[30] and PSMA,[31,32] among others.

Anti-idiotypes The idiotypic network is involved in the control of immune regulation. B-cell lymphomas present unique immunoglobulins on their cell surface, which make exquisite targets for immunotherapy. Anti-idiotype MAb vaccines have been quite successful clinically for this malignancy.[3,4,33–36] But the specificity inherent in these vaccine strategies is both an advantage and disadvantage; different B-cell lymphomas will display unique idiotypes on their cell surface, making their preparation for each patient labor-intensive.

The concept of exploiting the idiotypic network has also carried over to the treatment of carcinomas. In the clinic, treatment with an anti-idiotype MAb that was prepared against an anti-CEA MAb has been used as a vaccine approach.[37,38] In preclinical studies,[39] this vaccine approach has demonstrated antitumor activity.

In clinical studies,[37,38] the use of the anti-CEA anti-idiotype MAb has led to the generation of anti-CEA Ab responses and anti-CEA proliferative T-cell responses in patients with colon carcinoma. Stable disease has also been noted in these patients. The injection of an anti-CA125 MAb in patients with ovarian cancer has led to the induction of Ab2 and Ab3 anti-idiotype Abs. The Ab3 antibodies were shown to kill ovarian tumor cells via an Fc-mediated mechanism.[40]

Vectors Vectors are one of the more flexible means of vaccine delivery. Several major categories of both viral and bacterial vectors are now in use in the clinic (see Table 51-2). Each vector category and each vector type has its own advantages and disadvantages. Review articles have been written on the potential merits of these vectors.[41–46] In general, the advantages of a vector-based vaccine are that (1) the entire tumor antigen gene, or parts of that gene can be inserted; (2) multiple genes (including genes for costimulatory molecules and cytokines) can be inserted into some types of vectors; (3) the relative cost of this type of production is low, when compared with the preparation and purification of proteins or whole tumor cell vaccines; and (4) many vectors have the ability to infect professional APCs so that the antigens they express can be processed.

Replication-Competent Vectors One of the most studied groups of all vaccine vectors is the poxvirus group. Vaccinia virus, which was derived from a benign pox disease in cows, has been administered to more than 1 billion people and is responsible for the worldwide eradication of smallpox.[47] As a result, smallpox vaccinations in the United States and most Western countries were halted approximately 30 years ago. However, most cancer patients are older than age 30 and, therefore, have some level of a preexisting immunity to vaccinia virus. For this reason, recombinant vaccinia viruses most likely cannot be given multiple times in vaccine protocols. Early studies of recombinant vaccinia viruses containing human immunodeficiency virus (HIV) transgenes showed that vaccinia virus-immune patients could not make as potent an immune response as vaccinia virus-naïve patients.[48] Subsequent studies show that when higher doses of recombinant vaccinia viruses are used, vaccinia virus-immune patients can mount a vigorous response to the transgene after vaccination. However, this response is greatly diminished at the second and third vaccination.[49] Thus, preclinical and recent clinical[50] studies show that optimal use of recombinant vaccinia viruses may be to prime the immune response, followed by boost vaccinations with other vectors (such as replication-defective avipox vectors), peptides, or proteins. A major advantage to using vaccinia virus or the replication incompetent poxviruses is that large amounts of foreign DNA can be inserted into the vector. To date, as many as seven transgenes have been expressed in one vaccinia virus vector. Another major advantage is that proteins expressed in vaccinia virus tend to be more immunogenic than the native protein, which is most likely a result of the inflammatory responses triggered against highly immunogenic vaccinia virus proteins. Other advantages of poxviruses, such as vaccinia virus, modified vaccinia Ankara (MVA), and avipox viruses (see below) include wide host range, stable recombinants, accurate replication, and efficient posttranslational processing of the inserted gene. Several clinical trials with recombinant vaccinia containing TAAs, such as CEA,[50] PSA,[51] and HPV,[22,52] have been completed; others are ongoing.

Adenovirus has also been proposed as an attractive vector for application in recombinant vaccine design because its viral genome can be altered to accept foreign genes that are stably integrated. Furthermore, to produce recombinant adenovectors, endogenous viral DNA sequences are typically deleted from replication-competent regions, which results in an attenuated form of the virus with potentially improved safety. Recombinant adenoviruses have been widely used in gene therapy protocols, and a number of vaccine protocols for the induction of immune responses have already been carried out.[53–56] In preclinical studies, immunization of mice with a recombinant adenovirus expressing a model TAA led to the induction of an antigen-specific CTL response and regression of established pulmonary metastases. In clinical trials, recombinant adenoviruses encoding MART-1 or gp100 genes were administered to patients with malignant melanoma. The vaccine, given at multiple routes, doses and frequencies, did not produce significant adverse effects. However, immunologic findings did not reveal a consistent pattern of induction of TAA-specific T-cell responses, as determined by IFN-γ production in response to MART-1 or gp100-associated peptides, presumably because of the high levels of preexisting and/or inducible neutralizing Abs found in this patient population. Thus, recombinant adenoviruses may eventually best be used in diversified prime and boost protocols.

Replication-Defective Viral Vectors The poxvirus family contains the replication-competent vaccinia virus and a derivative of vaccinia virus termed MVA.[41] A major attribute of this vector is its potential lack of toxicity, because it can infect mammalian cells but cannot replicate. Other replication-defective members of the poxvirus family are the avipox vectors (fowlpox and canarypox/ALVAC).[42] These avipox vectors infect human cells and express their transgenes for 2 to 3 weeks followed by cell death; they are incapable of re-infecting cells. Recent clinical studies have shown that avipox-based CEA vectors can be given numerous times to patients with a resulting increase in CEA-specific T-cell responses.[57]

Bacterial and Yeast Vectors Bacterial vectors, such as *Salmonella*[58,59] and *Listeria*,[46] offer an advantage in that they have tropism for professional APCs, such as macrophages. Whereas these vectors are potentially virulent in humans, several attenuated strains are now being developed for possible human use. *Listeria* monocytogenes, for example, is of particular interest for both clinical and immunologic reasons. From a clinical perspective, recombinant *Listeria* monocytogenes-based vectors may be administered orally. From an immunologic perspective, these recombinant bacterial vectors might activate both MHC class II-restricted $CD4^+$ and MHC class I-restricted $CD8^+$ T-cell responses, due in large part to the microorganism's unique two-phase life cycle. After infection or phagocytosis of *Listeria* monocytogenes by monocytes/macrophages, the bacterium occupies a phagolysosome, which also coincides with a major site of MHC class II antigen processing and presentation. Subsequently, *Listeria* monocytogenes produces listeriolysin O, an enzyme that disrupts the integrity of the phagolysosomal membrane and, thus, permits access of the bacterium into the cytosol, which also turns out to be a major site of MHC class I antigen processing and presentation. Moreover, infected macrophages produce IL-12, which is an important cytokine that favors cell-mediated immunity. Recently, preclinical studies using a yeast vector-based vaccine have also been reported.[60]

Plasmid DNA These vectors represent a potentially powerful vaccine delivery system.[61] Polynucleotide vaccines are easy to prepare, but the mode of action of these vectors in inducing an immune response is not fully understood because most studies have involved intramuscular inoculations, and it is not known how antigens get to professional APCs. Many preclinical studies using infectious disease agents and cancer antigens have been carried out with DNA vectors. To date, however, few clinical trials using polynucleotide vaccines in cancer have been reported.[62–64]

RNA Virus Vectors One new and promising experimental approach for improving the immunogenicity of polynucleotide or genetic vaccines is to endow them with "self-replicating" ability. To achieve this effect, a gene encoding an RNA replicase, an enzyme produced from alphaviruses such as Sindbis virus or Semliki forest virus, is introduced into the RNA vector.[65,66] In preclinical studies using model TAAs, such RNA viral vectors have been shown to be strongly immunogenic for the induction of antigen-specific Ab and CTL responses, and effective in tumor prevention and tumor-therapy settings in vivo.[67] Additional studies revealed that cells infected with self-replicating RNA vectors transiently synthesize large amounts of antigenic materials before undergoing apoptotic cell death. Apoptosis is thought to result from the formation of double-stranded RNA intermediates which, interestingly, may also have a secondary consequence and promote activation of resident DCs.[67] Thus, the proinflammatory effects of such RNA intermediates may play a role in further potentiating immunogenicity, over and above what is observed with conventional plasmids.

Dendritic Cell Vaccines The DC is considered the most potent APC and, therefore, one of the most attractive means of immunization.[68,69] One can employ DCs by (1) loading with a peptide, protein, or anti-idiotype Ab, (2) infecting with a viral vector, (3) loading with apoptotic bodies from tumor cells, or (4) fusing with a tumor cell.[70–73] The major disadvantages of this approach are the great cost and effort involved. One must obtain large amounts of peripheral blood mononuclear cells (PBMCs) from patients via leukapheresis. The PBMCs must then be cultured for several days in the presence of cytokines such as GM-CSF, IL-4, and/or TNF-α, and then reinfused into the patient. This must be done for each patient. However, DC biology is a rapidly growing field with much promise. In clinical trials, DCs loaded with anti-idiotype Abs for B-cell lymphoma cancer patients have proved quite successful, resulting in clinical remissions.[3,35] Other clinical studies that use peptide-loaded DCs in a range of human malignancies are under way.[29,32,68,74–76] Generally, DC-based vaccinations are safe and induce antigen-specific T-cell responses and remissions, at least in subsets of patients with advanced disease. A particularly intriguing strategy involves immunization with DCs that had been "fused" with the host's own tumor cells, resulting in a DC-tumor cell hybrid vaccine.[77,78] Significant antitumor responses were observed in both preclinical animal studies,[72,79] as well as in patients with metastatic renal cell carcinoma.[73] The use of exosomes, that is, substructures of DCs, also may prove to be a valuable vaccine delivery vehicle.[80]

Fusion Proteins and Immunoglobulins The use of these MAb-based reagents represents an intermediate modality between passive Ab therapy and active vaccine therapy. Activation of T cells via CD28 leads to increased T-cell function, and binding to CTLA-4 leads to diminished T-cell function. MAbs to CTLA-4 have been used in preclinical studies to show antitumor effects in some murine models.[81,82] Anti–CTLA-4 MAb was recently used with a peptide vaccine in a melanoma trial. Ab–cytokine fusion proteins offer the ability to pair an antitumor Ab with a cytokine such as IL-2. Preclinical studies have shown that antitumor MAb IL-2 fusion proteins can activate T cells at the tumor site.[83] Clinical trials using this approach have begun. Ab–IL-12 fusion proteins have also demonstrated efficacy in preclinical studies.[84,85]

Immunostimulants/Cytokines An expanding principle in the field of immunology and immunotherapy is that the DC is central to the initiation of the adaptive immune response. However, to make the DC functionally useful for this essential role, the DC requires prior activation by elements of the innate immune response. Thus, the DC is thought to be the cellular bridge linking innate and adaptive immunity. If therapeutic strategies can be developed to augment activation and maturation of the DC, it would then be conceivable to improve immunogenicity of a weak TAA. One way to achieve this outcome is through the use of immunostimulants, which will likely play an important role in virtually all aspects of immunotherapy, especially cancer vaccine development.

TAA and TSA are by definition weak immunogens because tumors develop, persist and grow in the presence of an intact immune system, as described earlier. This was originally thought to be due to "tolerance" mechanisms. However, there is considerable support for the idea that a "danger" signal is most important for initiating an immune response.[86] Evidence exists that a poor immunogen, such as a TAA, can be rendered more immunogenic by either its mode of presentation to the immune system or its use in combination with an immunostimulant. A list of such immunostimulants is shown in Table 51-3. The term immunostimulant encompasses several groups of agents that can work in a variety of ways. Proteins and peptides rapidly dissipate from the injection site if administered alone. Conventional adjuvants such as incomplete Freund's adjuvant (IFA) will allow the immunogen to be maintained at the injection site (the so-called "depot effect") so that infiltrating APCs and effector cells can initiate a more vigorous immune response. Immunostimulants also work by crossing membrane barriers. In this case, proteins must be taken up by professional APCs and presented in the context of MHC molecules for effective presentation to the immune system. Adjuvants with lipophilic components and liposomes[87] facilitate this process.

Microbial products, such as those present in certain adjuvants (eg, IFA, BCG and even poxviruses), also are potent activators of DCs partly because they contain agonists of toll-like receptors (TLRs). TLR are expressed by DCs (and other innate immune cell types), and comprise a family of approximately 10 to 15 receptors that bind to a number of different microbial components,

Table 51-3 Immunostimulants for Cancer Immunotherapy

Type	Example(s)
Adjuvants	Incomplete Freund adjuvant, Detox, QS-21, alum
Cytokine (local)	GM-CSF
Cytokines (systemic)	IL-2
Fusion proteins	Antitumor MAb–IL-2
Chemokine	M1P-1α
"Danger signal"	TLR-agonists–CpGs, Aldara
	Viral or bacterial vectors
T-cell costimulatory molecules	
Vector-expressed	B7-1, ICAM-1, LFA-3
Blockade (MAb)	Anti–CTLA-4 MAb
Cyclophosphamide	
BCG	
Liposomes	
Flt-3L	

BCG = bacillus Calmette-Guerin; CTLA-4 = cytotoxic T lymphocyte antigen-4; GM-CSF = granulocyte-macrophage colony stimulating factor; ICAM-1 = intercellular adhesion molecule-1; IL-2 = interleukin-2; LFA-3 = leukocyte function-associated antigen-3; MAb = monoclonal antibody; TLR = toll-like receptor.

namely lipopolysaccharide (LPS), RNA species and CpG motifs.[88,89] Activation of DCs via their TLRs augments expression of adhesion, chemokine and chemokine receptor molecules, which, in turn, regulate cellular trafficking to sites of inflammation and pathogenic encounters. Thus, the biological consequences of TLR engagement lead to inflammation, characterized by the recruitment of key immune and non-immune effector cells to mediate pathogen destruction. In regard to TLR agonists, CpG motifs constitute the most studied of these sequences.[90–93] Purified CpG sequences have been admixed with peptide immunogens to enhance immune responses in preclinical studies. Clinical studies are now in progress to explore their utility in cancer immunotherapy.[92] It is thought that some of the immunogenic properties of vectors, such as BCG, poxviruses and plasmid DNA constructs, can be credited to the fact that they also contain numerous CpG motifs.

In addition, certain cytokines and chemokines have been shown to enhance the level of APC function either locally or systemically. For example, GM-CSF has been reported to enhance antigen-specific T-cell responses, such as proliferative, CTL, delayed-type hypersensitivity reactions or antitumor responses.[94–101] It should be noted, however, that GM-CSF most likely acts indirectly via recruitment and activation of host APC populations, such as macrophages and DCs.[102,103] Increased APC capacity correlates with heightened levels of MHC, adhesion, and costimulatory molecules, which seem to improve immune system interactions overall. Local GM-CSF at the vaccination site has been shown to increase the infiltration of DC in regional nodes.[96] Clinical studies using GM-CSF along with protein immunogens have shown an enhancement of the antigen-specific immune response.[33,104] Flt-3L administration has been shown to enhance the number of DCs systemically, both in animal models and clinically.[105,106] Finally, several cytokines and chemokines have been shown to play a critical role in enhancing T-cell function.[107–111] The most studied of these is IL-2.[112,113] When used as a single agent, IL-2 has been shown to have antitumor effects in melanoma patients[112,114] and, as recently reported, to enhance the effectiveness of melanoma-based peptide vaccines.[20] Other cytokines, such as IL-7, IL-12 and IL-15, have been shown to enhance T-cell responses in experimental models and may have more potential clinical utility than IL-2.[108,115–117]

VACCINE CLINICAL TRIALS

It has been demonstrated that patients with advanced cancers can be administered vaccines directed against "self" antigens, which are overexpressed on tumors as compared with normal tissues, and mount an immune response to those self-antigens. Overall, the actual method of presentation of the self-antigen to the immune system via the vaccine has proven to be an important factor in breaking "tolerance." As described above, the strategies of employing modified whole tumor cells, peptide-pulsed DCs, recombinant vectors, altered peptides, and vaccines given in combination with cytokines and/or T-cell costimulatory molecules are now playing an important role in clinical trial design and development. Below is a partial description of previous and ongoing vaccine clinical trials.

Melanoma The vast majority of vaccine clinical trials to date have been conducted in patients with melanoma. This is attributable to several reasons, among them (1) interferon (IFN) and IL-2 have both shown clinical responses in melanoma, indicating that the immune response to melanoma-associated antigens may be involved in therapeutic responses; (2) melanoma lesions are readily accessible, and thus can be studied for immune infiltrate; (3) melanoma lesions can be grown in culture to obtain both tumor cells and TILs for adoptive transfer; (4) numerous melanoma-associated antigens have been identified; and (5) of all solid tumor types, perhaps the most potent in vitro immune responses are directed against melanoma-associated antigens. Previous adoptive transfer clinical studies with TILs demonstrated that immune T cells directed against melanoma-associated antigens, in the presence of IL-2, can kill melanoma cells in situ.[118]

Table 51-4 Cancer Vaccine Trials with Reported Survival Benefit

Vaccine Type	Comment	Tumor	Trial Phase	Survival Benefit	Ref.
Autologous whole-tumor cell	Unmodified	Renal	III	5 year survival: 78% in vaccine arm vs. 67% for no treatment arm ($p = .02$)	(283)
Autologous whole-tumor cell	GM-CSF modified	NSCLC	I/II	Median survival of 17 months (95% CI) vs. historical controls	(284)
Autologous whole-tumor cell	BCG modified	Colon	III	5.8-year overall survival in Dukes Stage II: Significantly improved overall survival adjuvant to surgery vs. surgery alone ($p < .05$)	(140)
Autologous whole-tumor cell	Unmodified	HCC	II	2 year recurrence of 29% in vaccine arm vs. 54% in the control group ($p < .05$)	(285)
Autologous whole-tumor cell	IFN-gamma treated	Sarcomas	I/II	Progression-free survival at 14 months: 95% in vaccine arm	(286)
Autologous whole-tumor cell	Lysate	Renal	II	5-year overall survival: 86% in vaccine arm vs. 71% for no treatment arm ($p = .0059$)	(287)
Autologous whole-tumor cell	Unmodified	Melanoma	II	5-year overall survival: 39% in vaccine arm vs. 19% for no vaccine arm ($p = .0009$)	(138)
Autologous whole-tumor cell	Unmodified	Melanoma	II	5-year overall survival Stage III: 49% in vaccine arm vs. 20% for non vaccine arm ($p = .0001$)	(288)
Allogeneic whole-tumor cell	BCG modified	Melanoma	II	Median Survival Time: 37 months for vaccine arm vs. 17 months for no treatment arm ($p = .0277$)	(136)
Allogeneic whole-tumor cell	B7-1 modified	NSC lung carcinoma	II	Media survival for all vaccine patients is 18 months (90% CI vs control)	(289)
Protein	STn (KLH modified)	Breast	I/II	Median survival of 19.7 months (vaccine with cyclophosphamide) vs 12.6 months (without cyclophosphamide); $p = .017$)	(151)
Peptide	Unmodified	Melanoma	I/II	22% of patients relapse free for > 42 months	(290)
Vectors (viral)	Vaccinia CEA ALVAC-CEA	CEA expressing tumors	I/II	Overall survival for patients in vaccine arm was 56% for patients in the vaccinia prime/Alvac boost arm (VAAA) vs. 11% for patients in the Alvac arm (AAAV), ($p = .05$)	(291)
Vectors (viral)	Fowlpox/ Vaccinia-CEA/MUC-1/ TRICOM	Pancreatic	I	Overall survival ongoing, at analysis >7.3 months vs. 3 months for historical controls	(292)
Vectors (viral)	Fowlpox/ Vaccinia-CEA(6D)/ TRICOM	CEA expressing tumors	I/II	Total: 58 patients 60% of patients with stable disease for > 6 months. Increased 2 year survival with patients in vaccine + GM-CSF arm	(143)
Vectors (viral)	Vaccinia cell lysates	Melanoma	III	10 year survival: 53.4% in vaccine arm vs. 41% for no treatment arm ($p = .68$)	(293)
Vectors (viral)	Fowlpox-PSA	Prostate	II	78.1 % clinical progression free survival	(165)
Dendritic cell	DC loaded with PAP-GM-CSF	Prostate	III	Median overall survival of 25.9 months in vaccine arm vs. 22 months in placebo arm ($p = .02$). At 36 months 33% of patients in the vaccine arm were alive vs. 11% of placebo patients ($p = .003$)	(294)
Dendritic cell	DC loaded with autologous tumor	Melanoma	II	48% progression-free survival (Interim analysis)	(295)
Dendritic cell	DC loaded with autologous tumor	Melanoma	II	Survival was significantly increased over that noted with control patients ($p < .001$)	(296)
Anti-idiotypic antibody	CA-125 antigen	Ovarian	I/II	Median survival: 19.4 months for vaccine arm vs 4.9 months for control arm ($p = .0001$)	(183)

A = ALVAC-CEA; ALVAC = recombinant canarypox virus; BCG = bacillus Calmette-Guerin; CA-125 = cancer antigen 125; CEA = carcinoembryonic antigen; CI = confidence interval; DC = dendritic cell; GM-CSF = granulocyte-macrophage colony stimulating factor; HCC = hepatocellular carcinoma; IFN = interferon; NSCLC = non-small cell lung carcinoma; PAP = prostatic acid phosphatase; PSA = prostate-specific antigen; STn (KLH) = Sialyl-Tn (keyhole limpet hemocyanin); TRICOM = triad of costimulatory molecules; V = vaccinia-CEA.

Clinical trials have been conducted using various peptides derived from melanoma-associated antigens, including tyrosinase, MART-1, gp100, Melan-A (a modified gp100 epitope[20], and members of the MAGE family.[20,119–123] Vaccination induced immune responses as well as clinical benefits were reported. Another peptide approach is vaccination with autologous tumor-derived heat shock protein/peptide complexes[124] or peptides contained within autologous tumor cell lysates.[125] Immune responses and clinical responses have also been observed using melanoma peptide vaccination in conjunction with anti-CTLA-4,[126] melanoma peptide-pulsed dendritic cells,[120,127] tumor RNA-transfected dendritic cells,[128] as well as intratumoral administration of autologous dendritic cells.[129] Recent research indicates that immunization with hybrids of tumor- and antigen-presenting cells can induce protective immunity and rejection of established tumors in various rodent models. Kugler and colleagues[73] reported that heterokaryon vaccination (autologous melanoma tumor cells and allogeneic dendritic cells) induced clinical responses in 40% of patients, with 23% of patients completely resolving all metastatic tumor lesions.

Recombinant viral vectors encoding melanoma transgenes have been utilized clinically, including an adenovirus encoding MART-1 and gp100[56] and an ultraviolet (UV)-inactivated nonreplicating recombinant vaccinia virus encoding epitopes from Melan-A, MART-1, gp100, and tyrosinase. Immunization with plasmid DNAs encoding either gp100[130] or tyrosinase[131] have not demonstrated significant clinical responses.

Several clinical studies have employed autologous melanoma cells as vaccine. Clinical responses were observed when these melanoma cell vaccines were preceded by cyclophosphamide.[132,133] Clinical responses were also observed when autologous melanoma cells were transduced with GM-CSF and given as vaccine.[134,135] In addition, intratumoral administration of recombinant vaccinia encoding GM-CSF in patients with cutaneous melanoma has been reported to induce antitumor immune responses.[10]

Several randomized phase II trials have been carried out using either autologous[136,137] or allogeneic[138] melanoma vaccine in patients with resected melanoma (Table 51-4). In these trials, there is evidence of improved disease-free survival in the vaccine arm vs. control or no treatment groups.

Gastrointestinal Carcinoma A prospective randomized clinical trial has been carried out in 254 patients with stage II and stage III colon cancer using autologous tumor cell vaccine with BCG. A 5.3-year median follow-up showed 40 recurrences in the control group and 25 in the vaccine group. The vaccine showed a statistically significant clinical benefit in patients with surgically resected stage II colon cancer, but not stage III colon cancer.[139] In another study, vaccination with an autologous tumor cell-BCG vaccine post-surgery demonstrated a significant survival benefit over surgery alone (see Table 51-4).[140]

Several clinical trials have been conducted employing CEA-based vaccines. Results of vaccination of patients with recombinant vaccinia virus,[49] recombinant avipox virus[57,141,142] or a prime with recombinant vaccinia (rV)-CEA and multiple boosts with avipox-CEA[143] have demonstrated the generation of CEA-specific immune responses in patients with advanced gastrointestinal (GI) carcinomas and other CEA-expressing carcinomas. A randomized trial using both vaccinia and avipox CEA vaccines containing a triad of T-cell costimulatory molecules has indicated improved survival in patients receiving the prime boost regimen plus GM-CSF (see Table 51-4); 40% had stable disease for at least 4 months, with 61% of these patients having prolonged stable disease (> 6 months).[143] CEA peptide-pulsed DCs have also been employed in clinical studies using a modified CEA agonist peptide.[144] Two of 12 patients with advanced cancers experienced tumor regression, 1 patient had a mixed response, and 2 had stable disease. Clinical responses correlated with the expansion of CEA-specific T cells. Clinical studies have also been carried out using anti-idiotype antibodies directed against anti-CEA monoclonal antibodies. These studies have demonstrated the induction of immune responses,[145] slowed disease progression and prolonged survival.[146]

Allogeneic whole tumor cell vaccines modified to secrete GM-CSF have also been employed in a phase I trial in patients with pancreatic cancer. Evidence of vaccine-induced immune responses were observed as measured by delayed-type hypersensitivity.[147,148] Clinical studies are ongoing in patients with GI carcinomas using a viral vector vaccine employing p53 as the target antigen.[149]

Breast Cancer Several different breast cancer and carcinoma-associated antigens have been employed as targets for vaccine clinical trials in patients with advanced breast cancer. STn is a glycopeptide contained in carcinoma-associated mucin. Patients were randomized to receive vaccine (sTn coupled to keyhole limpet hemocyanin [KLH]) with or without cyclophosphamide. Patients treated with vaccine and cyclophosphamide were reported to have lived significantly longer (projected median survival of 19.7 months versus actual median survival of 12.6 months; $p = .017$)[150] than those treated with the same vaccine without cyclophosphamide (see Table 51-4). Additionally, sTn KLH vaccine has also been administered to breast and ovarian cancer patients after an autologous stem-cell transplant (following high-dose chemotherapy). Vaccinated patients appeared more likely to survive and less likely to relapse, but further studies are required.[151] Several clinical trails have been carried out using the MUC-1 mucin as a target, including the use of MUC-1 peptides,[19,152,153] recombinant vaccinia virus encoding MUC-1 and IL-2,[154] modified vaccinia virus (MVA) expressing human MUC-1,[155] and mannan–MUC-1 fusion protein.[156] In other trials, this MUC-1 fusion protein induced greater immune responses when administered with cyclophosphamide.[157] Studies carried out with the *HER-2/neu* peptides with or without GM-CSF have demonstrated the ability of patients with breast cancer to generate HER-2–specific immune responses.[158–160]

Avigan has shown that fusion cell vaccination of patients with metastatic breast and renal cancer induces both immunological and clinical responses.[77] An anti-idiotype antibody that mimics the human milk fat globule antigen has also been utilized as a breast cancer vaccine in conjunction with autologous stem cell transplantation. In that study, the 3-year overall survival rate was 48% (95% confidence interval (CI), 32–64%), whereas the progression-free survival rate was 32% (95% CI, 19–45%).[161]

Prostate Cancer Clinical trials in patients with advanced prostate cancer and rising PSA have been carried out using a recombinant vaccinia virus expressing PSA (rV-PSA). PSA levels in 14 of 33 men treated were stable for at least 6 months after primary vaccination. Nine patients remained stable for 11 to 25 months.[51] PSA-specific immune responses have been observed[51,162] as well as "epitope spreading" to other prostate-associated antigens.[163,164] A randomized phase II study combining rV-PSA with a vaccine containing a single T-cell costimulatory molecule (rV-B7-1) with standard definitive radiotherapy in patients with localized prostate cancer has been completed. In that study, 13 of 17 patients had increases in PSA-specific T cells of at least threefold versus no detectable increases in the radiotherapy-only arm ($p < .0005$). A randomized phase II clinical trial examined the use of a prime/boost vaccine strategy using rV-PSA as a prime vaccination and a fowlpox virus expressing PSA (rF-PSA) in patients with biochemical progression after local therapy for prostate cancer. Of those patients who were evaluated, 45.3% remained free of PSA progression at 19.1 months and 78.1% demonstrated clinical progression-free survival.[165] A randomized phase II study has compared vaccine therapy with second line hormone therapy (nilutamide). The vaccine employed there is rV-PSA admixed with rV-B7-1 for the prime, followed by boosting with rF-PSA.[166] The trial was randomized for second-line hormone therapy (nilutamide) versus vaccine with a crossover at disease progression so that each arm would receive combination vaccine plus hormone therapy. Time to treatment failure was prolonged in patients initially receiving vaccine alone and then receiving vaccine plus nilutamide.[167] Cellular immune responses to PSA in patients with advanced prostate cancer have also been observed using recombinant PSA protein formulated in liposomes.[168]

Several other prostate-associated antigens are also currently being targeted in vaccine trials. Dendritic cells pulsed with a prostatic acid phosphatase peptide have been used. Eleven of 21 patients developed T-cell responses to the homologous prostatic acid phosphatase (PAP) antigen, and 6 of 21 patients had clinical stabilization of their previously progressing prostate cancer.[144] Clinical trials have also been carried out using peptide-pulsed DCs loaded with peptides of human PAP[169] and PSMA, with and without GM-CSF,[169–172] as well as DCs transfected with PSA tumor RNA.[173] In these studies, antigen-specific immune responses have been observed and some decreases in serum PSA have also been noted.

In addition to the numerous studies that have demonstrated the ability of patients to mount immune responses to "self" prostate-associated antigens, it should also be pointed out that androgen withdrawal in patients with prostate cancer has led to the induction of T-cell infiltration in prostate tissue.[174] Thus, vaccine with androgen ablation may have implications for future immunotherapeutic treatment of prostate cancer.

Leukemia/Lymphoma The variable regions of B-cell receptor immunoglobulins on lymphomas are excellent targets for vaccines. These idiotypes have now been used successfully in the treatment of B-cell lymphomas.[33,175,176] An idiotype protein vaccine was used in 20 patients after a chemotherapy-induced first clinical complete remission. After vaccination, tumor-specific T-cell responses were found in 19 of 20 patients. Vaccination was associated with clearance of residual tumor cells from blood and long-term disease-free survival. The addition of GM-CSF to the vaccine was of extreme importance.[33] Clinical responses have also been observed using idiotype vaccine in patients with multiple myeloma.[35] For patients with chronic myelogenous leukemia, vaccination with bcr-abl oncogene breakpoint fusion peptides has generated specific immune responses.[177]

Other Tumor Types Intravesical BCG has been used successfully in the treatment of bladder cancer, implicating immune mechanisms.[178] Intravesical administration of wild-type vaccinia virus has now been shown to be safe, and 3 of 4 patients treated were free of disease at 4-year follow-up.[179] The response of renal carcinoma to high-dose IL-2 and IFN-α also implicates immune mechanisms in therapeutic responses.[180] An autologous renal cell carcinoma (RCC) tumor-cell vaccine that was genetically modified to overexpress B7-1 to provide costimulation to tumor-reactive T cells was employed.[181] In that trial, 26% (4 of 15) of patients had either a partial response or stable disease, whereas 9 patients continued to have progressive disease.

Vaccination of pediatric solid tumor patients with tumor–lysate-pulsed DCs expanded specific T cells and mediated some tumor regression.[182] In addition, clinical trials have examined vaccination of glioma patients with DC/glioma fusions and fusion cell vaccination of patients with metastatic breast and renal cancer.[77,78] Clinical findings have also been reported in patients with advanced ovarian cancer using a vaccine consisting of an MAb directed against the tumor antigen CA125.[40] A phase II study examining an anti-idiotypic antibody vaccine that functionally imitated the CA125 antigen reported survival benefit; median survival of the vaccine group was 19.4 months versus 4.9 months for the control arm (see Table 51-4).[183]

Considerations in the Analyses of Clinical Trial Results It has now been demonstrated that appropriate vaccine delivery systems and vaccine strategies can elicit immune responses in patients with advanced cancer to TAAs and, in some cases, can mediate prolonged survival, prolonged disease-free interval, drops in serum tumor markers, and/or regression of metastatic disease. The trials outlined in Table 51-4 provide only initial indications of prolonged survival benefit. It should be pointed out, however, that only large-scale randomized phase III trials can prove the efficacy of such vaccines. As mentioned above, patients with advanced cancers are perhaps the least appropriate population to demonstrate the efficacy of a potential cancer vaccine; thus, future clinical trials should be carried out in patients with less advanced cancers. To do so will require the use of vaccines immediately prior to, during, or immediately following adjuvant therapy. Several such studies are ongoing.

Thus, the overall goal is the use of vaccine regimens in combination with front-line cancer therapies, thereby reducing the interval between disease diagnosis and the initiation of vaccine; this hopefully will bring the use of cancer vaccines closer to its original intention, for use in patients in the minimal disease setting.

COMBINATION THERAPIES

Anti-tumor effects induced by cancer vaccines may be difficult to obtain with large tumor masses for three different reasons: (1) tumor cells produce immunoregulatory molecules that have the ability to anergize T cells, (2) large tumor masses are difficult to penetrate by T cells, and (3) the quantity of T cells generated by the host immune system would be far outnumbered by the cells in a large tumor mass. Vaccines would most probably show the greatest efficacy in the adjuvant or neo-adjuvant setting, where tumor burden is minimal. A great deal of effort is now being put into the use of vaccines with conventional therapies such as local radiation of tumor, chemotherapeutic agents, hormones, and monoclonal antibodies.

Vaccine Plus Radiation Radiation is the standard of care for many cancer types and has conventionally been exploited for its direct cytotoxic effect on tumors or palliative effects in patients. Local radiation of tumor has also been shown to alter tumor architecture, resulting in more effective drug delivery. Recently, however, it has been reported that local radiation of tumor cells given at doses insufficient to kill tumor will modulate numerous classes of genes and consequently alter the phenotype of the tumor cell.[184–186] Several genes that have been shown to be upregulated in both murine and human tumors post-irradiation are Fas, MHC Class I, ICAM-1, and the tumor-associated antigens CEA, MUC-1, HER-2/*neu*, p53, and CA 125. The upregulation of any one of these genes has the ability to render a tumor cell more susceptible to T-cell mediated immune attack. For example, Fas, a member of the tumor necrosis factor (TNF) receptor family, is a death receptor that induces apoptosis on binding to its natural ligand (FasL). Fas-mediated apoptosis has been shown to play an important role in tumor cell destruction along with granzyme-mediated killing. Recent preclinical studies have shown for the first time that the regulation of Fas expression in tumor cells via sublethal local tumor irradiation significantly improved the therapeutic efficacy of a recombinant anti-cancer vaccine in a preclinical model.[186] Subsequent studies also showed that the use of sublethal doses of irradiation of human colorectal, lung, and prostate cancer cells altered numerous genes and led to the upregulation of Fas and other molecules, rendering these tumor cells more susceptible to killing by human CTL.[184] Although the mechanism of enhanced immunogenicity of x-irradiated tumor cells is not fully understood, it is also known that low doses of gamma rays can induce stress genes and increase reactive oxygen species. A recent clinical study has reported on the combined use of a recombinant cancer vaccine with standard definitive radiotherapy in patients with localized prostate cancer.[164] There is an excellent review on immune modulation by ionizing radiation and its implication for cancer therapy.[187]

Vaccine Plus Chemotherapy If cancer vaccines are to be used early in the disease process, they would most likely need to be used in combination with certain chemotherapeutic agents. While counterintuitive, it has recently been shown that vaccine therapy may not only be compatible with certain chemotherapies, but also may actually be synergistic. It has been previously established that drugs such as interferon can upregulate both MHC Class I and numerous tumor-associated antigens on the surface of tumor cells. It has also been shown, however, that drugs commonly used in cancer chemotherapy can also upregulate tumor antigens and/or histocompatibility antigens. For example, 5-fluorouracil treatment of tumor cells has been shown to upregulate CEA and MHC Class I. Thalidomide and a potent thalidomide analog were both shown to enhance virus-specific CD8 cytokine production and cytolytic activity. Systemic cyclophosphamide combined with local intratumoral injection of DCs led to complete tumor regression in an experimental melanoma model.[188] Adriamycin has also been shown to increase effector T-cell activity. In preclinical models, the chemotherapy agents cyclophosphamide, doxorubicin, and paclitaxel have been shown to enhance the antitumor immune response of a whole tumor cell vaccine.[189]

Several things are important to point out in considering the use of chemotherapy with vaccine: (1) the combined use of vaccine and chemotherapy early on in the disease process should not be confused with the use of vaccines following multiple regimens of different chemotherapeutic agents in the advanced disease setting, where the immune system would most likely be impaired; (2) not all chemotherapeutic agents will be compatible with vaccine; (3) dose scheduling of vaccine when used with chemotherapy may be extremely important. Obviously, future studies will be required to optimize the combined use of vaccine and chemotherapy. An excellent review on combining anti-neoplastic drugs with tumor vaccines has recently appeared.[190]

Vaccine Plus Hormone Therapy The use of vaccines with anti-androgen therapy represents an intriguing possibility for the treatment of prostate cancer. It has previously been shown that androgen ablative therapy induces profuse T-cell infiltration of benign glands and tumors in the human prostate. T-cell infiltration was readily apparent after 1 to 3 weeks of therapy. Also, T cells within the treated prostate exhibited restricted TCR usage consistent with a local oligoclonal response.[191] These studies thus have important implications for the potential use of vaccine in combination with androgen ablative therapy in prostate cancer, as well as implications for other hormone-sensitive malignancies including breast cancer.[191] A recent clinical trial in prostate cancer patients who had received prior hormonal therapy but had an increasing serum PSA without radiographic evidence of metastases was carried out. The trial was randomized for second-line hormone therapy (nilutamide) versus vaccine with a crossover at disease progression so that each arm would receive combination vaccine plus hormone therapy. Time to treatment failure was prolonged in patients initially receiving vaccine alone and then receiving vaccine plus nilutamide. Further studies are obviously needed to validate such observations, but these studies clearly demonstrate the potential for the combined use of vaccine and hormone therapy.[167]

Vaccine Plus Monoclonal Antibodies There are several different ways in which vaccine and monoclonal antibodies can be used in combination. These include (1) the use of therapeutic antibodies such as herceptin or rituxan in combination with vaccine, in which each acts independently, (2) the use of anti-tumor antibody cytokine fusion proteins such as anti-tumor antibody/IL-2 to enhance T-cell activity at the site of tumor, (3) the use of monoclonal antibodies such as anti-CTLA-4, which will block negative regulatory immune signals and thus enhance immune responses, and (4) the use of monoclonal antibodies or fusion proteins directed against regulatory T cells.

RECENT INNOVATIONS IN VACCINE DESIGN AND DELIVERY

There have been numerous recent advances in our basic understanding of immune mechanisms, tumor immunology and vaccinology. Table 51-5 outlines some of these as they relate to cancer vaccine design and development.

Mechanism of T-cell Activation Recent studies have shown that a range of effector cells can be involved in anti-tumor effects. In most preclinical studies the $CD8^+$ CTL is involved in anti-tumor effects and the $CD4^+$ helper T cell is important for supplying "help" via cytokines to further activate the CTL. Other effector cells, however, can be involved, including macrophages and NK cells, and studies have also shown that in certain cases the generation of anti-tumor antibodies can mediate anti-tumor effects via antibody-dependent cell-mediated cytotoxicity.[192] T-cell activation has been shown to be a complex phenomenon involving the interaction of the peptide–MHC complex on the antigen-presenting cell with the T-cell receptor on the T cell; for weak antigens such as tumor-associated antigens,

Table 51-5 Areas of Active Investigation in Vaccine Design and Development

Gene discovery: tumor-associated antigen (TAA) and tumor-specific antigen (TSA)
Identification of mode of action of T-cell subsets
New assays to analyze vaccines' ability to enhance specific T-cell responses
ELISPOT (enzyme-linked immunosorbent spot assay) for IFN, granzyme
Intracellular cytokine (flow cytometry)
FastImmune
RNase protection
Avidity assays for T cells (cytolytic assay, CD107a)
RT-PCR of T-cell subsets
Proliferation of T-cell subsets
Dendritic-cell biology and dendritic-cell subsets
Costimulatory molecules
Two or more signals required
Important for weak antigens like TAA
Agonist epitopes to enhance immunogenicity
Cytokine and chemokine biology
Diversified prime and boost immunization protocols
Awareness that vaccines may be most efficacious in a limited disease setting
Inhibition of suppressor cell subsets

IFN = interferon; RT-PCR = reverse transcriptase polymerase chain reaction.

however, accessory molecules are necessary for efficient T-cell activation. These have been termed "T-cell costimulatory molecules." At this time over a dozen of such costimulatory molecules have been identified. Costimulatory molecules are found on professional antigen presenting cells, such as dendritic cells, but are not found on the vast majority of solid tumors. It has also recently been shown that combinations of these costimulatory molecules act synergistically to further enhance T-cell activation.[193] The most studied of costimulatory molecules are B7-1 and B7-2; several other costimulatory molecules that have also been extensively studied are ICAM-1, LFA-3, and CD40, each with its own ligand on T cells.[194–198] Costimulatory molecules have been introduced into tumors in experimental models by retroviral, adenovirus, vaccinia, and avipox vectors.[7,95,199–204] Most preclinical studies have demonstrated that when costimulatory molecules are placed into a tumor cell that is weakly immunogenic or nonimmunogenic in a host, the transduced tumor cell may become immunogenic to the point that it elicits antitumor immunity.[205] Genes for costimulatory molecules can also be placed into vectors along with tumor-antigen genes for use in more conventional vaccines. Preclinical studies have shown that simply admixing a recombinant vaccinia virus expressing a TAA with a recombinant vaccinia virus expressing a costimulatory molecule can enhance antigen-specific T-cell responses and antitumor immunity.[206,207] Preclinical studies have shown that either recombinant vaccinia virus or recombinant avipox vectors, each containing three different costimulatory molecules (B7-1, ICAM-1, and LFA-3), can enhance T-cell responses and antitumor immunity to far greater levels than those recombinants containing only one costimulatory molecule.[193]

Recent studies have also shown that it is not necessarily the quantity of T cells that are generated, but their quality, that is, their avidity.[208–210] This is measured by the ability of different populations of T cells to actually kill targets. It has recently been shown that the use of vaccines with T-cell costimulation and certain cytokines can actually enhance T-cell avidity.[209] Mechanistically, it has also been shown that when T cells are activated, they actually acquire, through an immunologic synapse, costimulatory molecules and peptide–MHC complex from the APCs[211]; this acquisition has been shown to actually sustain the activation of T cells. T-cell activation has also been shown to be enhanced by the inhibition of regulatory signals through the use of reagents such as anti-CTLA-4 antibody.[198,212,213]

Regulatory T Cells Several different types of regulatory T cells have now been identified.[214–217] The evolutionary reason for their existence is most likely to reduce autoimmune phenomena. Since TAAs for the most part are self-antigens, regulatory T cells appear to have a major role in reducing immune responses to TAAs. Three main types of regulatory T cells that have now been identified are: $CD4^+$ $CD25^+$, immature macrophages, and $CD4^+$ NKT^+ cells.[216,217] Studies are ongoing employing reagents that can potentially reduce the activity of these regulatory T cells including the fusion protein Ontak,[218] cyclophosphamide,[150,157,219] and anti-CD25 antibodies.[220,221] The inhibition of these cells will most likely be a part of cancer vaccine therapy in the future.

Antigen Cascade The phenomenon of antigen cascade is now evolving as an important facet in the evaluation of cancer vaccines. This has been studied through a phenomenon termed "cross presentation of antigens." This was first defined using the term "epitope spreading," in which a given peptide was used as a vaccine and the host immune response post-vaccination was not only directed to that epitope, but also to other epitopes of the same tumor antigen.[186,221,222] This phenomenon has now been expanded using the term "antigen cascade," in which a given antigen is used as a vaccine, and the host immune response post-vaccination is not only directed against the antigen in the vaccine, but also to other antigens in the tumor. These phenomena can be explained by the fact that as a consequence of some tumor cell destruction induced by the vaccine, APCs will engulf tumor fragments and then "cross-present" those tumor fragments to T cells, thus initiating the antigen cascade phenomenon. This has now been observed in several preclinical models and in clinical trials, and may eventually be correlated with anti-tumor activity.

Diversified Prime and Boost Immunization Strategies Although each of the various methods of immunization described above (see Table 51-2) has advantages and disadvantages, the most effective immunization protocol may involve priming with one type of immunogen and boosting with another. This method may be advantageous because (1) two different arms of the immune system may be enhanced by using two different modalities (ie, $CD4^+$ and then $CD8^+$ T cells); (2) one methodology may be more effective in priming naïve cells, while another modality may be more effective in enhancing memory cell function; and (3) some of the most effective methods of immunization, like the use of recombinant vaccinia virus or adenoviruses, can be used only a limited number of times because of host anti-vector responses. These vectors may be most effective when used as priming agents, followed by boosts with other agents. Numerous preclinical studies demonstrate the advantages of diversified prime and boost protocols.[62,223–226] Recent clinical studies show that priming with a recombinant vaccinia virus and boosting with recombinant avipox viruses is more effective than using either recombinant vector alone.[50,57,143]

Route of Vaccination Conventional vaccinations involve subcutaneous or intradermal inoculations. It has recently been shown in several preclinical models and some clinical studies that intratumoral and/or intranodal vaccination may be more efficacious in some cases. Indeed, in a recent study, it has been shown that the sequential use of primary vaccination s.c. followed by booster vaccination intratumorally is more efficacious in terms of anti-tumor effects than the sustained use of either route.[227]

ISSUES IN CANCER VACCINE DEVELOPMENT

Several issues inevitably slow the development of new immunotherapies. One such issue is the relevance of preclinical models. Many models to date have consisted of the use of transplanted murine tumors that grow rapidly. However, most human tumors do not grow as quickly and do not represent the percent of body mass that murine tumors do. Little is known about how the degree of vasculature in a transplanted tumor compares with the degree in many metastatic human tumors. Moreover, the rapid growth of murine tumors leads to two problem areas: (1) immunosuppression of the host, which has been associated with the downregulation or alteration of components of the TCR (eg, zeta-chain) of T cells in mice with progressive transplanted tumors, and (2) the short time span does not permit multiple booster vaccinations. For example, only a few weeks separate the time of tumor transplant and the time of a moribund animal. As a result, very few cycles of vaccine immunotherapy can be given. This situation is in stark contrast with the potential optimal use of vaccine therapy in a patient with minimal residual disease, whose tumor burden represents a relatively small fraction of body mass and who can receive many cycles of immunotherapy over 1, 2, or several years.

Transgenic animal models that form spontaneous cancers were recently developed. Several types of transgenic models have been constructed and analyzed in immunotherapy paradigms: eg, HER-2/*neu*,[228] CEA,[229] MUC-1,[230] and TRAMP (in prostate cancer).[231] Even in these models, tumor growth occurs within a few months after birth; in many cases, animals are dead of their tumors in 4 to 9 months. The additional time window between tumor development, progression, and death in transgenic mice with spontaneously arising neoplasms as compared with nontransgenic mice in transplanted tumor settings, however, provides a somewhat greater opportunity to evaluate novel and diversified immunotherapies. In many cases, transgenic mice receiving active or passive immunotherapies indeed undergo therapeutic responses without overt autoimmunity.

Another issue involves the appropriate disease state at which to administer immunotherapeutics. Standard practice and medical ethics dictate that all new phase I immunotherapies and many phase II trials be administered to patients with advanced metastatic disease who have failed conventional therapy. A mindset prevails in some that one must see the elimination of large tumor masses by traditional staging technologies (ie, radiography or computed tomography) before an immunotherapy can proceed to the adjuvant setting. However, a patient population with "measurable" disease may be the worst group in which to define the efficacy of a new immunotherapy, because of (1) potential immunosuppressive factors caused by the tumor, which have been elegantly demonstrated by the fact that advanced cancer patients possess a T helper cell 2 (Th2) phenotype in advanced disease as compared with a Th1 phenotype in early disease[232–234]; (2) potential regulatory or "suppressor" T cells that bear a unique $CD4^+CD25^+$ phenotype and may exist in the circulation, lymphoid compartments and at sites of tumor growth that might downregulate productive antitumor immune responses[235–237]; (3) immunosuppression caused by previous therapy (ie, radiation, chemotherapy); and (4) tumor penetrance of the immunotherapeutic, which may be distinct from tumor penetrance of small molecules. It is hoped that the field will eventually mature to the point where, for example, vaccines that are shown to be safe and to elicit specific immune responses in advanced cancer patients will be analyzed in patients in the adjuvant setting. Two studies lend credence to this argument. In one study, monoclonal antibody (MAb) 17-1A was shown to have little biologic effect in patients with advanced disease. When administered to colorectal cancer patients with minimal residual disease, it was shown to be clinically effective, and just as effective as chemotherapy.[238,239] Larger confirmatory studies are in progress. In the second study, which was a vaccine trial using an irradiated whole tumor-cell vaccine with BCG in colorectal cancer, the vaccine was shown to be ineffective in patients with Dukes C cancer and effective in patients with Dukes B.[139] The downside of using immunotherapies in a minimal residual disease setting is the long period required to determine efficacy as measured in disease-free interval or survival, which is often 3 to 8 years. In this case, one must rely heavily on surrogate markers to determine the potential efficacy of a given therapy. These markers include a drop in serum antigens such as CEA and PSA; polymerase chain reaction (PCR) analysis of tumor cells in the blood and, in vaccine therapy, the generation of immunogen-specific Ab or T-cell immune responses.

As with all aspects of cancer therapy, immunotherapy has its share of obstacles and challenges, some of which have already been addressed above. A fundamental consideration for the use of immunotherapy reflects the nature of the patient population. The original intention of immunotherapy was to use it in patients with metastatic cancer or disease refractory to conventional treatments. From an ethical standpoint, it was both reasonable and appropriate to enlist such patients in newer experimental therapies because such patient populations have already failed "standard-of-care" treatment. From a scientific or practical standpoint, however, such patient populations may be the worst to test experimental immunotherapies because disease progression or prior therapies may have already compromised immune function. By its very nature, immunotherapy requires a functional immune system and, therefore, it is vitally important to assess immune and/or performance status of selected patient populations.

A second fundamental consideration rests with appreciating the sophistication of the host-tumor relationship. By the time cancer is clinically detectable, it likely had already evolved to the point where it can efficiently evade host immune recognition and attack. Potential chronic, persistent and long-term interactions with the host immune system may enforce selective pressures that, in turn, influence the outgrowth of the clinically detectable tumor mass. In fact, studies in mouse models of spontaneous and chemically induced tumor formation support this notion, which has been termed "cancer immunoediting"[240,241] and reflects a refinement of the original concept of "cancer immunosurveillance."[242] Thus, although cancer is considered a genetic disease,[243,244] interactions with the immune system or other host factors during tumor development and progression may serve to select and reshape the immunogenic repertoire of neoplastic clones that eventually emerge and constitute the clinically detectable malignant lesion.

Given these factors, the third challenge is how best to employ or construct cancer vaccines to activate a meaningful anti-neoplastic T-cell response. This is further complicated, however, by the discovery that many defined tumor antigens are self-proteins (see Table 51-1) and therefore generally fail to initiate strong anti-neoplastic T-cell responses altogether. Thus, a key issue with cancer vaccines is how to overcome potential mechanisms of immune suppression, or central or peripheral tolerance against antigenic, but weakly immunogenic neoplasms. Central tolerance refers to the complete absence or depletion of relevant T-cell clones, whereas peripheral tolerance refers to the functional suppression of preexisting antitumor T-cell clones via host- or tumor-induced mechanisms.[245,246] However, based on preclinical studies in transgenic mice expressing self-TAA[100,231,247–249] and in human clinical studies,[250,251] it appears more likely that tumor-specific lymphoid precursors do exist in the periphery, but remain in a peripherally unresponsive (tolerant) state.

The failure to activate immunity, therefore, does not necessarily mean that cancerous cells are not antigenic, as just pointed out. On the contrary, neoplastic cells are antigenic (ie, they express TAA or TSA), but generally are not immunogenic; that is, they tend to lack expression of costimulatory molecules and/or lack the capacity to create a pro-inflammatory environment necessary to sustain efficient T-cell activation and clonal expansion following TCR engagement of the MHC/antigen complex.[86,103,246,252] Briefly, costimulatory signals are provided by professional APC, such as DCs. These signals include cell surface expression of a family of B7 molecules, as well as the production of inflammatory cytokines, namely IL-12, that ultimately promote T-cell activation. Such DCs have the capacity to process and present tumor antigens to both $CD4^+$ and $CD8^+$ T cells, and simultaneously supply the appropriate costimulatory signals necessary for full T-cell activation. However, because the host-tumor microenvironment is also highly immunosuppressive,[236,253–255] and may not be readily infiltrated with relevant APC populations expressing the necessary costimulatory properties, it is unlikely that efficient T-cell activation can be achieved. Cancer vaccines, therefore, are constructed to enhance tumor immunogenicity and to promote such pro-inflammatory reactions, namely via (1) the recruitment and modulation of APCs to express both the TAA and appropriate costimulatory molecules for activation of antigen-specific T cells or (2) the genetic modification of tumor cells *ex vivo* to express pertinent costimulatory or inflammatory properties for use as whole tumor cell vaccines.[103,246,248,252,256–259]

Adoptive cellular immunotherapy may circumvent these types of early immune interactions, since the selection and expansion of desirable in vivo–generated T-cell populations, such as TIL, are conducted under defined in vitro conditions, in the absence of any negative regulatory influences of the in vivo tumor microenvironment.[251] However, upon adoptive transfer, such effector/memory T cells must still be able to traffic to and accumulate at sites of tumor deposits and execute anti-neoplastic activity in the face of other possible types of tumor-induced barriers, which are outlined below. Adoptive transfer studies, however, are extremely costly, labor intensive, and have been carried out in only a few centers in the last 20 years since first reported. A vaccine-induced T-cell response also confronts some roadblocks at the effector phase of the immune reaction, as does adoptive transfer. For example, during the effector phase of the host-tumor interaction, neoplastic cells may evade the immune system as a consequence of (1) reduced expression of MHC determinants, β-2-microglobulin protein or adhesion (eg, ICAM-1) molecules, thereby diminishing T cell–target conjugate formation and triggering of critical effector functions[260–262]; (2) production of tumor-derived inhibitory factors, such as interleukin-10 (IL-10), vascular endothelial growth factor (VEGF), transforming growth factor-β (TGF-β) and prostaglandins,[236,254,255] which abrogate cell-mediated immune reactions; (3) failure to elicit Ag-specific T-cell responses because of tumor-induced alterations in TCR signaling[253,263,264]; (4) resistance to immune attack, owing to the inability of effector T cells to efficiently mediate Fas-dependent death[265–267]; (5) Fas ligand (FasL) expression, which has been suggested to eliminate infiltrating Fas^+, $CD4^+$ or $CD8^+$ T lymphocytes, although this latter possibility remains controversial[268–270]; (6) tumor-induced alterations in T-cell subtype cytokine profiles that are unfavorable for productive cellular immune reactions[234,271]; (7) negative regulatory influences or suppressor cell types, such as $CD4^+CD25^+$ Treg cells[272] that may exist in the circulation or at sites of tumor growth[237,273,274] and/or $CD4^+$ NKT cells that produce IL-13, which, in turn stimulates immature macrophages (termed $Gr\text{-}1^+CD11b^+$ cells) to secrete TGF-β[275]; and (8) inefficient tumor penetrance of the Ag-specific T cells, particularly in the treatment of large tumor masses. This latter issue, however, will most likely not be a significant factor in the treatment of small tumor masses and micrometastases in minimal residual disease.

Finally, in the event a therapeutic T-cell response is initiated and executed, the possibility also exists in some cases for the development of undesirable immune reactions as well. For example, if vaccines are directed against a given TAA, the induction of immunity toward the tumor may also eventually lead to the induction of immunity to normal tissues also expressing that TAA. This has been the case in immune responses to some melanoma-associated antigens, where vitiligo has been induced, in both experimental and clinical studies.[251,276] It is of interest to note that, in preclinical vaccine studies, the induction of antitumor immunity in transgenic mice expressing TAAs has not led to the induction of autoimmunity in normal tissues expressing those same TAAs.[71,228,247,248,277,278] Moreover, in the vast majority of clinical trials using vaccines directed against carcinomas, no autoimmunity has been observed (except in the case of melanoma), including those cases in which clinical antitumor effects have been demonstrated.[139]

In summary, in human cancer numerous TAAs have now been defined, which has enabled the development and application of both active and passive immunotherapies in the clinic. The fundamental basis of effective immunotherapy, however, will undoubtedly require a fuller understanding of the host-tumor interaction, including strategies to optimize both quantitative and qualitative elements of the T-cell mediated immune response in the face of constant genetic and epigenetic influences governing tumor development, survival and progression. This becomes particularly important in settings where weak T-cell responses may be induced that lack adequate potency to achieve therapeutic efficacy and/or induced T-cell responses may influence the emergence of more aggressive tumorigenic phenotypes. Perhaps combination therapies, which are described in further detail here, involving vaccination with other oncological treatments, such as radiation,[186,279] chemotherapy,[189,251] cytokines (eg, IFN, IL-2, IL-12, IL-15),[108,251,280] passive administration of tumor-specific monoclonal antibodies,[100] or non-steroidal anti-inflammatory drugs (eg, cyclooxygenase-2 inhibitors),[281,282] may prove even more beneficial to facilitate long-term clinical regressions concomitant with a lower risk toward the generation of aggressive tumor escape variants.

PARADIGM SHIFTS

The field of cancer vaccines is currently in a state of active preclinical and clinical investigation. Traditional vaccines are employed to prevent infectious diseases. Cancer vaccines are currently being evaluated to treat patients already diagnosed with cancer. Thus, a new paradigm needs to be established, which bridges the evaluation of conventional vaccines for infectious diseases and the evaluation of cytotoxic agents for the treatment of cancer.

Preclinical and clinical studies have now demonstrated several important points in the evaluation of cancer vaccines: (1) The majority of cancer vaccines are directed against antigens that are overexpressed in tumors, but are also found to some extent on either embryonic tissues or to a lower level on some normal adult tissues. It was previously thought that patients could not mount an immune response to such antigens. Numerous studies, however, have shown this is indeed not the case, and that patients with cancer can indeed mount an immune response to their tumor when given an appropriate vaccine. (2) Lack of toxicity. It was previously thought that since some tumor antigens are also expressed on some normal adult tissues, there would be an immune response resulting in toxicity. With the exception of some vaccines directed against some melanoma antigens, toxicities associated with cancer vaccines have been relatively mild, especially when compared to cytotoxic anti-cancer agents.

The evaluation of cancer vaccines in clinical trials may well necessitate a new paradigm, as follows: (1) Cancer vaccines and cytotoxic drugs act completely differently in terms of mode of action. Cytotoxic drugs either kill or do not kill tumor cells. Lack of efficacy is due to either drug resistance by tumor cells, inadequate amounts of drug delivered to the tumor, and/or drug-induced toxicity in the host. Thus, if a patient's disease is progressing on a cytotoxic drug, that drug is immediately withdrawn. The use of a cancer vaccine involves a dynamic process in which the patient's own immune system is activated. It is clear from decades of preclinical studies and now clinical trials that to maximize the host immune response, one must not only give a primary vaccination but also multiple booster vaccinations. Multiple vaccinations are especially important because factors may be given off by the tumor that will blunt the immune response. Thus it is quite conceivable that a patient's disease will continue to progress following early vaccinations only to see disease stabilization or a reduction in tumor burden following multiple vaccinations. Thus, the paradigm of "drug withdrawal upon progression" should be revisited with the use of cancer vaccines. (2) The phase I, II, III paradigm. Clinical trials with a new drug are traditionally evaluated in patients with advanced tumors (many times with a large tumor burden) who have failed prior cytotoxic therapies. Objective clinical responses are evaluated by RECIST criteria looking for a greater than 50% reduction in tumor volume. Since the generation of an immune response to a vaccine is a dynamic process, in which T cells can be continually generated upon booster vaccines, a more appropriate endpoint for evaluation should be time to progression and, more importantly, survival. Also, since only a finite amount of T cells can be generated, it may be inappropriate to evaluate a cancer vaccine by its ability to drastically reduce a large tumor burden; this is especially true in patients whose immune system has been compromised due to numerous rounds of prior chemotherapy. A more appropriate setting would be the evaluation of cancer vaccines earlier in the disease setting in patients with either a small tumor burden or a high probability of disease progression. This should particularly be considered in light of the relatively low level of toxicity seen in the use of cancer vaccines. Thus, survival should be the principal endpoint for the analysis of cancer vaccines. One is all too familiar with claims of activity of cytotoxic drugs, in which there is a reduction of tumor burden by RECIST criteria in a minority of cases, only to see no statistical difference in survival. Unfortunately, there is still a "paradigm paralysis" by some holding on to the old paradigm used for the evaluation of cytotoxic drugs. (3) Combination therapies. One of the major advantages in the use of cancer vaccines is their reduced toxicity. One of the "conventional wisdom" paradigms that is now being reevaluated is that one cannot use cancer vaccines in combination with chemotherapy or radiation therapy. Preclinical studies, and now several clinical studies, have shown that patients can mount an immune response to cancer vaccine when given in combination with certain cytotoxic drugs, hormones or local radiation of tumor. Indeed, recent preclinical studies have shown that when tumor cells are exposed to radiation or certain chemotherapeutic agents at levels insufficient to kill tumor, the phenotype of tumor cells is actually modulated to make them more susceptible to T-cell mediated killing.

In conclusion, (1) not all cancer vaccines are created equal, (2) a new paradigm should be employed in the clinical evaluation of cancer vaccines, (3) strategies should be employed in which cancer vaccines are employed with other conventional cancer therapies earlier in the disease process, and (4) the development of cancer vaccines should be considered as an immunologic platform building on preclinical and clinical knowledge of gene discovery, vectorology, cytokines, and the mechanism of activation of the immune response.

CONCLUSION

Finally, rapid achievements in the areas of molecular biology and immunology have led to the development of recombinant vaccines encoding TSAs, TAAs, and also T-cell costimulatory molecules or cytokines in monovalent and polyvalent constructs for use in active immunotherapy. Unraveling basic mechanisms of antigen recognition, antigen processing, antigen presentation, and tumor escape processes has led to the identification and exploitation of DCs, costimulatory molecules, and antigen-specific T cells for use in diverse aspects of immunotherapy. Although considerable knowledge has been acquired to this point, the steady influx of new information as a result of basic studies, translational studies, and clinical trials will most likely further translate the science of tumor immunology into clinical modalities for a range of human cancers and, perhaps, strategies for the prevention of certain neoplasms.

ACKNOWLEDGMENTS

The authors gratefully acknowledge the assistance of Debra Weingarten in the preparation of this chapter.

REFERENCES

1. Abrams SI, Hand PH, Tsang KY, Schlom J. Mutant *ras* epitopes as targets for cancer vaccines. Semin Oncol 1996;23:118–34.
2. Nikitina EY, Chada S, Muro-Cacho C, et al. An effective immunization and cancer treatment with activated dendritic cells transduced with full-length wild-type p53. Gene Ther 2002;9:345–52.
3. Hsu FJ, Benike C, Fagnoni F, et al. Vaccination of patients with B-cell lymphoma using autologous antigen-pulsed dendritic cells. Nat Med 1996;2:52–8.
4. Kwak LW, Thielemans K, Massaia M. Idiotypic vaccination as therapy for multiple myeloma. Semin Hematol 1999;36:34–7.
5. Ruffini PA, Kwak LW. Immunotherapy of multiple myeloma. Semin Hematol 2001;38:260–7.
6. Hobeika AC, Clay TM, Mosca PJ, et al. Quantitating therapeutically relevant T-cell responses to cancer vaccines. Crit Rev Immunol 2001;21:287–97.
7. Hodge JW, Abrams S, Schlom J, Kantor JA. Induction of antitumor immunity by recombinant vaccinia viruses expressing B7-1 or B7-2 costimulatory molecules. Cancer Res 1994;54:5552–5.
8. Wallack MK, Sivanandham M, Balch CM, et al. Surgical adjuvant active specific immunotherapy for patients with stage III melanoma: the final analysis of data from a phase III, randomized, double-blind, multicenter vaccinia melanoma oncolysate trial. J Am Coll Surg 1998;187:69–77;discussion 9.
9. Rousseau RF, Haight AE, Hirschmann-Jax C, et al. Local and systemic effects of an allogeneic tumor cell vaccine combining transgenic human lymphotactin with interleukin-2 in patients with advanced or refractory neuroblastoma. Blood 2003;101:1718–26.
10. Mastrangelo MJ, Maguire HC, Jr, Eisenlohr LC, et al. Intratumoral recombinant GM-CSF-encoding virus as gene therapy in patients with cutaneous melanoma. Cancer Gene Ther 1999;6:409–22.
11. Bystryn JC. Vaccines for melanoma. Design strategies and clinical results. Dermatol Clin 1998;16:269–75.
12. Harris DT, Matyas GR, Gomella LG, et al. Immunologic approaches to the treatment of prostate cancer. Semin Oncol 1999;26:439–47.
13. Samanci A, Yi Q, Fagerberg J, et al. Pharmacological administration of granulocyte/macrophage-colony- stimulating factor is of significant importance for the induction of a strong humoral and cellular response in patients immunized with recombinant carcinoembryonic antigen. Cancer Immunol Immunother 1998;47:131–42.
14. Sandmaier BM, Oparin DV, Holmberg LA, et al. Evidence of a cellular immune response against sialyl-Tn in breast and ovarian cancer patients after high-dose chemotherapy, stem cell rescue, and immunization with Theratope STn-KLH cancer vaccine. J Immunother 1999;22:54–66.
15. Livingston PO, Wong GY, Adluri S, et al. Improved survival in stage III melanoma patients with GM2 antibodies: a randomized trial of adjuvant vaccination with GM2 ganglioside. J Clin Oncol 1994;12:1036–44.
16. Chapman PB, Wu D, Ragupathi G, et al. Sequential immunization of melanoma patients with GD3 ganglioside vaccine and anti-idiotypic monoclonal antibody that mimics GD3 ganglioside. Clin Cancer Res 2004;10:4717–23.
17. Ruiz M, Kobayashi H, Lasarte JJ, et al. Identification and characterization of a T-helper peptide from carcinoembryonic antigen. Clin Cancer Res 2004;10:2860–7.
18. Kobayashi H, Omiya R, Ruiz M, et al. Identification of an antigenic epitope for helper T lymphocytes from carcinoembryonic antigen. Clin Cancer Res 2002;8:3219–25.
19. Finn OJ, Jerome KR, Henderson RA, et al. MUC-1 epithelial tumor mucin-based immunity and cancer vaccines. Immunol Rev 1995;145:61–89.
20. Huarte E, Sarobe P, Lu J, et al. Enhancing immunogenicity of a CTL epitope from carcinoembryonic antigen by selective amino acid replacements. Clin Cancer Res 2002;8:2336–44
21. Zaremba S, Barzaga E, Zhu M, et al. Identification of an enhancer agonist cytotoxic T lymphocyte peptide from human carcinoembryonic antigen. J. Natl. Cancer Inst 1997;57:4570–7.
22. van Driel WJ, Kenter GG, Fleuren GJ, et al. Immunotherapeutic strategies for cervical squamous carcinoma. Hematol Oncol Clin North Am 1999;13:259–73.
23. Abrams SI, Hodge JW, McLaughlin JP, et al. Adoptive immunotherapy as an *in vivo* model to explore antitumor mechanisms induced by a recombinant anticancer vaccine. J. Immunother 1997;20:48–59.
24. Gjertsen MK, Bakka A, Breivik J, et al. *Ex vivo ras* peptide vaccination in patients with advanced pancreatic cancer: results of a phase I/II study. Int J Cancer 1996;65:450–3.
25. Disis ML, Grabstein KH, Sleath PR Cheever MA. Generation of immunity to the HER-2/neu oncogenic protein in patients with breast and ovarian cancer using a peptide-based vaccine. Clin Cancer Res 1999;5:1289–97.
26. Marchand M, van Baren N, Weynants P, et al. Tumor regressions observed in patients with metastatic melanoma treated with an antigenic peptide encoded by gene MAGE-3 and presented by HLA- A1. Int J Cancer 1999;80:219–30.
27. Jager E, Ringhoffer M, Dienes HP, et al. Granulocyte-macrophage-colony-stimulating factor enhances immune responses to melanoma-associated peptides in vivo. Int J Cancer 1996;67:54–62.
28. Salgaller ML, Marincola FM, Cormier JN, Rosenberg SA. Immunization against epitopes in the human melanoma antigen gp100 following patient immunization with synthetic peptides. Cancer Res 1996;56:4749–57.
29. Morse MA, Deng Y, Coleman D, et al. A Phase I study of active immunotherapy with carcinoembryonic antigen peptide (CAP-1)-pulsed, autologous human cultured dendritic cells in patients with metastatic malignancies expressing carcinoembryonic antigen. Clin Cancer Res 1999;5:1331–8.
30. Goydos JS, Elder E, Whiteside TL, et al. A phase I trial of a synthetic mucin peptide vaccine. Induction of specific immune reactivity in patients with adenocarcinoma. J Surg Res 1996;63:298–304.
31. Murphy GP, Elgamal AA, Su SL, et al. Current evaluation of the tissue localization and diagnostic utility of prostate specific membrane antigen. Cancer 1998;83:2259–69.
32. Murphy GP, Tjoa BA, Simmons SJ, et al. Infusion of dendritic cells pulsed with HLA-A2-specific prostate- specific membrane antigen peptides: a phase II prostate cancer vaccine trial involving patients with hormone-refractory metastatic disease. Prostate 1999;38:73–8.
33. Bendandi M, Gocke CD, Kobrin CB, et al. Complete molecular remissions induced by patient-specific vaccination plus granulocyte-monocyte colony-stimulating factor against lymphoma. Nat Med 1999;5:1171–7.
34. Kwak LW, Campbell MJ, Czerwinski DK, et al. Induction of immune responses in patients with B-cell lymphoma against the surface-immunoglobulin idiotype expressed by their tumors. N Engl J Med 1992;327:1209–15.
35. Reichardt VL, Okada CY, Liso A, et al. Idiotype vaccination using dendritic cells after autologous peripheral blood stem cell transplantation for multiple myeloma--a feasibility study. Blood 1999;93:2411–9.
36. Liso A, Stockerl-Goldstein KE, Auffermann-Gretzinger S, et al. Idiotype vaccination using dendritic cells after autologous peripheral blood progenitor cell transplantation for multiple myeloma. Biol Blood Marrow Transplant 2000;6:621–7.
37. Foon KA, Chakraborty M, John WJ, et al. Immune response to the carcinoembryonic antigen in patients treated with an anti-idiotype antibody vaccine. J Clin Invest 1995;96:334–42.
38. Foon KA, John WJ, Chakraborty M, et al. Clinical and immune responses in advanced colorectal cancer patients treated with anti-idiotype monoclonal antibody vaccine that mimics the carcinoembryonic antigen. Clin Cancer Res 1997;3:1267–76.
39. Pervin S, Chakraborty M, Bhattacharya-Chatterjee M, et al. Induction of antitumor immunity by an anti-idiotype antibody mimicking carcinoembryonic antigen. Cancer Res 1997;57:728–34.
40. Schultes BC, Baum RP, Niesen A, et al. Anti-idiotype induction therapy: anti-CA125 antibodies (Ab3) mediated tumor killing in patients treated with Ovarex mAb B43.13 (Ab1). Cancer Immunol Immunother 1998;46:201–12.
41. Moss B. Genetically engineered poxviruses for recombinant gene expression, vaccination, and safety. Proc Natl Acad Sci U S A 1996;93:11341–8.
42. Paoletti E. Applications of pox virus vectors to vaccination: an update. Proc Natl Acad Sci U S A 1996;93:11349–53.
43. Carroll MW, Moss B. Poxviruses as expression vectors. Curr Opin Biotechnol 1997;8:573–7.
44. Rolph MS, Ramshaw IA. Recombinant viruses as vaccines and immunological tools. Curr Opin Immunol 1997;9:517–24.
45. Weiskirch LM, Paterson Y. Listeria monocytogenes: a potent vaccine vector for neoplastic and infectious disease. Immunol Rev 1997; 158159–69.
46. Kaufmann SH, Hess J. Impact of intracellular location of and antigen display by intracellular bacteria: implications for vaccine development. Immunol Lett 1999;65:81–4.
47. Fenner F, Henderson DA, Arita I, et al. Smallpox and its eradication. Geneva: World Health Organization; 1988.
48. Cooney EL, Collier AC, Greenberg PD, et al. Safety of and immunological response to a recombinant vaccinia virus vaccine expressing HIV envelope glycoprotein [see comments]. Lancet 1991;337:567–72.
49. Tsang KY, Zaremba S, Nieroda CA, et al. Generation of human cytotoxic T cells specific for human carcinoembryonic antigen epitopes from patients immunized with recombinant vaccinia-CEA vaccine. J Natl Cancer Inst 1995;87:982–90.
50. Marshall JL, Hoyer RJ, Toomey MA, et al. Phase I study in advanced cancer patients of a diversified prime-and-boost vaccination protocol using recombinant vaccinia virus and recombinant nonreplicating avipox virus to elicit anti-carcinoembryonic antigen immune responses. J Clin Oncol 2000;18:3964–73.
51. Eder JP, Kantoff PW, Roper K, et al. A phase I trial of a recombinant vaccinia virus expressing prostate-specific antigen in advanced prostate cancer. Clin Cancer Res 2000;6:1632–8.
52. Borysiewicz LK, Fiander A, Nimako M, et al. A recombinant vaccinia virus encoding human papillomavirus types 16 and 18, E6 and E7 proteins as immunotherapy for cervical cancer. Lancet 1996;347:1523–7.
53. Juillard V, Villefroy P, Godfrin D, et al. Long-term humoral and cellular immunity induced by a single immunization with replication-defective adenovirus recombinant vector. Eur J Immunol 1995;25:3467–73.
54. Chen PW, Wang M, Bronte V, et al. Therapeutic antitumor response after immunization with a recombinant adenovirus encoding a model tumor-associated antigen. J Immunol 1996;156:224–31.
55. Xiang ZQ, Yang Y, Wilson JM, Ertl HC. A replication-defective human adenovirus recombinant serves as a highly efficacious vaccine carrier. Virology 1996;219:220–7.
56. Rosenberg SA, Zhai Y, Yang JC, et al. Immunizing patients with metastatic melanoma using recombinant adenovi-

ruses encoding MART-1 or gp100 melanoma antigens. J Natl Cancer Inst 1998;90:1894–900.
57. Marshall JL, Hawkins MJ, Tsang KY, et al. Phase I study in cancer patients of a replication-defective avipox recombinant vaccine that expresses human carcinoembryonic antigen. J Clin Oncol 1999;17:332–7.
58. Curtiss R 3rd, Kelly SM, Tinge SA, et al. Recombinant Salmonella vectors in vaccine development. Dev Biol Stand 1994;82:23–33.
59. Schodel F, Curtiss R 3rd. Salmonellae as oral vaccine carriers. Dev Biol Stand 1995;84:245–53.
60. Lu Y, Bellgrau D, Dwyer-Nield LD, et al. Mutation-selective tumor remission with Ras-targeted, whole yeast-based immunotherapy. Cancer Res 2004;64:5084–8.
61. Pardoll DM, Beckerleg AM. Exposing the immunology of naked DNA vaccines. Immunity 1995;3:165–9.
62. Restifo NP, Rosenberg SA. Developing recombinant and synthetic vaccines for the treatment of melanoma. Curr Opin Oncol 1999;11:50–7.
63. Conry RM, LoBuglio AF, Kantor J, et al. Immune response to a carcinoembryonic antigen polynucleotide vaccine. Cancer Res 1994;54:1164–8.
64. Conry RM, LoBuglio AF, Curiel DT. Polynucleotide-mediated immunization therapy of cancer. Semin Oncol 1996;23:135–47.
65. Leitner WW, Ying H, Restifo NP. DNA and RNA-based vaccines: principles, progress and prospects. Vaccine 1999;18:765–77.
66. Schlesinger S, Dubensky TW. Alphavirus vectors for gene expression and vaccines. Curr Opin Biotechnol 1999;10:434–9.
67. Ying H, Zaks TZ, Wang RF, et al. Cancer therapy using a self-replicating RNA vaccine. Nat Med 1999;5:823–7.
68. Steinman RM, Dhodapkar M. Active immunization against cancer with dendritic cells: the near future. Int J Cancer 2001;94:459–73.
69. Banchereau J, Schuler-Thurner B, Palucka, et al. Dendritic cells as vectors for therapy. Cell 2001;106:271–4.
70. Chen D, Xia J, Tanaka Y, et al. Immunotherapy of spontaneous mammary carcinoma with fusions of dendritic cells and mucin 1-positive carcinoma cells. Immunology 2003;109:300–7.
71. Gong J, Chen D, Kashiwaba M, et al. Reversal of tolerance to human MUC1 antigen in MUC1 transgenic mice immunized with fusions of dendritic and carcinoma cells. Proc Natl Acad Sci U S A 1998;95:6279–83.
72. Tanaka Y, Koido S, Chen D, et al. Vaccination with allogeneic dendritic cells fused to carcinoma cells induces antitumor immunity in MUC1 transgenic mice. Clin Immunol 2001;101:192–200.
73. Kugler A, Stuhler G, Walden P, et al. Regression of human metastatic renal cell carcinoma after vaccination with tumor cell-dendritic cell hybrids. Nat Med 2000;6:332–6.
74. Nestle FO, Alijagic S, Gilliet M, et al. Vaccination of melanoma patients with peptide- or tumor lysate-pulsed dendritic cells. Nat Med 1998;4:328–32.
75. Palucka K, Banchereau J. Dendritic cells: a link between innate and adaptive immunity. J Clin Immunol 1999;19:12–25.
76. Timmerman JM, Levy R. Dendritic cell vaccines for cancer immunotherapy. Annu Rev Med 1999;50:507–29.
77. Avigan D, Vasir B, Gong J, et al. Fusion cell vaccination of patients with metastatic breast and renal cancer induces immunological and clinical responses. Clin Cancer Res 2004;10:4699–708.
78. Kikuchi T, Akasaki Y, Abe T, et al. Vaccination of glioma patients with fusions of dendritic and glioma cells and recombinant human interleukin 12. J Immunother 2004;27:452–9.
79. Koido S, Tanaka Y, Chen D, et al. The kinetics of in vivo priming of CD4 and CD8 T cells by dendritic/tumor fusion cells in MUC1-transgenic mice. J Immunol 2002;168:2111–7.
80. Vincent-Schneider H, Stumptner-Cuvelette P, Lankar D, et al. Exosomes bearing HLA-DR1 molecules need dendritic cells to efficiently stimulate specific T cells. Int Immunol 2002;14:713–22.
81. Leach DR, Krummel MF, Allison JP. Enhancement of antitumor immunity by CTLA-4 blockade. Science 1996;271:1734–6.
82. Yang YF, Zou JP, Mu J, et al. Enhanced induction of antitumor T-cell responses by cytotoxic T lymphocyte-associated molecule-4 blockade: the effect is manifested only at the restricted tumor-bearing stages. Cancer Res 1997;57:4036–41.
83. Xiang R, Lode HN, Dreier T, et al. Induction of persistent tumor-protective immunity in mice cured of established colon carcinoma metastases. Cancer Res 1998;58:3918–25.
84. Gillies SD, Lan Y, Wesolowski JS, et al. Antibody-IL-12 fusion proteins are effective in SCID mouse models of prostate and colon carcinoma metastases. J Immunol 1998;160:6195–203.
85. Lode HN, Xiang R, Duncan SR, et al. Tumor-targeted IL-2 amplifies T cell-mediated immune response induced by gene therapy with single-chain IL-12. Proc Natl Acad Sci U S A 1999;96:8591–6.
86. Matzinger P. The danger model: a renewed sense of self. Science 2002; 296:301–5.
87. Alving CR, Koulchin V, Glenn GM, Rao M. Liposomes as carriers of peptide antigens: induction of antibodies and cytotoxic T lymphocytes to conjugated and unconjugated peptides. Immunol Rev 1995;145:5–31.
88. Okamoto M, Sato M. Toll-like receptor signaling in anticancer immunity. J Med Invest 2003;50:9–24.
89. Iwasaki A, Medzhitov R. Toll-like receptor control of the adaptive immune responses. Nat Immunol 2004;5:987–95.
90. Krieg AM. Immune effects and mechanisms of action of CpG motifs. Vaccine 2000;19:618–22.
91. Jahrsdorfer B, Weiner GJ. CpG oligodeoxynucleotides for immune stimulation in cancer immunotherapy. Curr Opin Investig Drugs 2003;4:686–90.
92. Wooldridge JE, Weiner GJ. CpG DNA and cancer immunotherapy: orchestrating the antitumor immune response. Curr Opin Oncol 2003;15:440–5.
93. Prud'homme GJ. DNA vaccination against tumors. J Gene Med 2005;7:3–17.
94. Disis ML, Bernhard H, Shiota FM, et al. Granulocyte-macrophage colony-stimulating factor: an effective adjuvant for protein and peptide-based vaccines. Blood 1996;88:202–10.
95. Hurwitz AA, Townsend SE, Yu TF, et al. Enhancement of the anti-tumor immune response using a combination of interferon-gamma and B7 expression in an experimental mammary carcinoma. Int J Cancer 1998;77:107–13.
96. Kass E, Panicali DL, Mazzara G, et al. Granulocyte/macrophage-colony stimulating factor produced by recombinant avian poxviruses enriches the regional lymph nodes with antigen-presenting cells and acts as an immunoadjuvant. Cancer Res 2001;61:206–14.
97. Borrello I, Pardoll D. GM-CSF-based cellular vaccines: a review of the clinical experience. Cytokine Growth Factor Rev 2002;13:185–93.
98. Dranoff G. GM-CSF-based cancer vaccines. Immunol Rev 2002;188:147–54.
99. Schneeberger A, Luhrs P, Kutil R, et al. Granulocyte-macrophage colony-stimulating factor-based melanoma cell vaccines immunize syngeneic and allogeneic recipients via host dendritic cells. J Immunol 2003;171:5180–7.
100. Wolpoe ME, Lutz ER, Ercolini AM, et al. HER-2/neu-specific monoclonal antibodies collaborate with HER-2/neu-targeted granulocyte macrophage colony-stimulating factor secreting whole cell vaccination to augment $CD8^+$ T cell effector function and tumor-free survival in Her-2/neu-transgenic mice. J Immunol 2003;171:2161–9.
101. Yang AS, Monken CE, Lattime EC. Intratumoral vaccination with vaccinia-expressed tumor antigen and granulocyte macrophage colony-stimulating factor overcomes immunological ignorance to tumor antigen. Cancer Res 2003;63:6956–61.
102. Pardoll DM. Cancer vaccines. Nat Med 1998;4:525–31.
103. Emens LA, Jaffee EM. Cancer vaccines: an old idea comes of age. Cancer Biol Ther 2003;2:S161–8.
104. Ullenhag GJ, Frodin JE, Jeddi-Tehrani M, et al. Durable carcinoembryonic antigen (CEA)-specific humoral and cellular immune responses in colorectal carcinoma patients vaccinated with recombinant CEA and granulocyte/macrophage colony-stimulating factor. Clin Cancer Res 2004;10:3273–81.
105. Maraskovsky E, Brasel K, Teepe M, et al. Dramatic increase in the numbers of functionally mature dendritic cells in Flt3 ligand-treated mice: multiple dendritic cell subpopulations identified. J Exp Med 1996;184:1953–62.
106. Lynch DH, Andreasen A, Maraskovsky E, et al. Flt3 ligand induces tumor regression and antitumor immune responses in vivo. Nat Med 1997;3:625–31.
107. Pertl U, Luster AD, Varki NM, et al. IFN-gamma-inducible protein-10 is essential for the generation of a protective tumor-specific CD8 T cell response induced by single-chain IL-12 gene therapy. J Immunol 2001;166:6944–51.
108. Wigginton JM, Park JW, Gruys ME, et al. Complete regression of established spontaneous mammary carcinoma and the therapeutic prevention of genetically programmed neoplastic transition by IL-12/pulse IL-2: induction of local T cell infiltration, Fas/Fas ligand gene expression, and mammary epithelial apoptosis. J Immunol 2001;166:1156–68.
109. Crittenden M, Gough M, Harrington K, et al. Expression of inflammatory chemokines combined with local tumor destruction enhances tumor regression and long-term immunity. Cancer Res 2003;63:5505–12.
110. Flanagan K, Glover RT, Horig H, et al. Local delivery of recombinant vaccinia virus expressing secondary lymphoid chemokine (SLC) results in a CD4 T-cell dependent antitumor response. Vaccine 2004;22:2894–903.
111. Klebanoff CA, Finkelstein SE, Surman DR, et al. IL-15 enhances the in vivo antitumor activity of tumor-reactive CD8+ T cells. Proc Natl Acad Sci U S A 2004;101:1969–74.
112. Rosenberg SA. Progress in the development of immunotherapy for the treatment of patients with cancer. J Intern Med 2001;250:462–75.
113. Dudley ME, Rosenberg SA. Adoptive-cell-transfer therapy for the treatment of patients with cancer. Nat Rev Cancer 2003;3:666–75.
114. Royal RE, Steinberg SM, Krouse RS, et al. Correlates of Response to IL-2 Therapy in Patients Treated for Metastatic Renal Cancer and Melanoma. Cancer J Sci Am 1996;2:91.
115. Waldmann TA, Dubois S, Tagaya Y. Contrasting roles of IL-2 and IL-15 in the life and death of lymphocytes: implications for immunotherapy. Immunity 2001;14:105–10.
116. Fry TJ, Moniuszko M, Creekmore S, et al. IL-7 therapy dramatically alters peripheral T-cell homeostasis in normal and SIV-infected nonhuman primates. Blood 2003;101:2294–9.
117. Dranoff G. Cytokines in cancer pathogenesis and cancer therapy. Nat Rev Cancer 2004;4:11–22.
118. Rosenberg SA. Adoptive cellular therapy: clinical applications. In: DeVita VT Jr, Hellman S, Rosenberg SA, editors, Biologic therapy of cancer. Philadelphia: JB Lippincott; 1991 p. 214–36.
119. Slingluff CL Jr, Petroni GR, Yamshchikov GV, et al. Clinical and immunologic results of a randomized phase II trial of vaccination using four melanoma peptides either administered in granulocyte-macrophage colony-stimulating factor in adjuvant or pulsed on dendritic cells. J Clin Oncol 2003;21:4016–26.
120. Mackensen A, Herbst B, Chen JL, et al. Phase I study in melanoma patients of a vaccine with peptide-pulsed dendritic cells generated in vitro from CD34(+) hematopoietic progenitor cells. Int J Cancer 2000;86:385–92.
121. Slingluff CL Jr., Yamshchikov G, Neese P, et al. Phase I trial of a melanoma vaccine with gp100(280-288) peptide and tetanus helper peptide in adjuvant: immunologic and clinical outcomes. Clin Cancer Res 2001;7:3012–24.
122. Wang F, Bade E, Kuniyoshi C, et al. Phase I trial of a MART-1 peptide vaccine with incomplete Freund's adjuvant for resected high-risk melanoma. Clin Cancer Res 1999;5:2756–65.
123. Schaed SG, Klimek VM, Panageas KS, et al. T-cell responses against tyrosinase 368–376(370D) peptide in HLA*A0201+ melanoma patients: randomized trial comparing incomplete Freund's adjuvant, granulocyte macrophage colony-stimulating factor, and QS-21 as immunological adjuvants. Clin Cancer Res 2002;8:967–72.
124. Belli F, Testori A, Rivoltini L, et al. Vaccination of metastatic melanoma patients with autologous tumor-derived heat shock protein gp96-peptide complexes: clinical and immunologic findings. J Clin Oncol 2002;20:4169–80.
125. Chakraborty NG, Sporn JR, Tortora AF, et al. Immunization with a tumor-cell-lysate-loaded autologous-antigen-presenting-cell-based vaccine in melanoma. Cancer Immunol Immunother 1998;47:58–64.
126. Phan GQ, Yang JC, Sherry RM, et al. Cancer regression and autoimmunity induced by cytotoxic T lymphocyte-associated antigen 4 blockade in patients with metastatic melanoma. Proc Natl Acad Sci U S A 2003;100:8372–7.
127. Banchereau J, Palucka AK, Dhodapkar M, et al. Immune and clinical responses in patients with metastatic melanoma to CD34(+) progenitor-derived dendritic cell vaccine. Cancer Res 2001;61:6451–8.
128. Su Z, Dannull J, Heiser A, et al. Immunological and clinical responses in metastatic renal cancer patients vaccinated with tumor RNA-transfected dendritic cells. Cancer Res 2003;63:2127–33.
129. Triozzi PL, Khurram R, Aldrich WA, et al. Intratumoral injection of dendritic cells derived in vitro in patients with metastatic cancer. Cancer 2000;89:2646–54.
130. Rosenberg SA, Yang JC, Sherry RM, et al. Inability to immunize patients with metastatic melanoma using plas-

mid DNA encoding the gp100 melanoma-melanocyte antigen. Hum Gene Ther 2003;14:709–14.

131. Tagawa ST, Lee P, Snively J, et al. Phase I study of intranodal delivery of a plasmid DNA vaccine for patients with Stage IV melanoma. Cancer 2003;98:144–54.

132. Berd D, Maguire HC Jr, McCue P, Mastrangelo MJ. Treatment of metastatic melanoma with an autologous tumor-cell vaccine: clinical and immunologic results in 64 patients. J Clin Oncol 1990;8:1858–67.

133. Elias EG, Suter CM, Fabian DS. Adjuvant immunotherapy in melanoma with irradiated autologous tumor cells and low dose cyclophosphamide. J Surg Oncol 1997;64:17–22.

134. Kusumoto M, Umeda S, Ikubo A, et al. Phase 1 clinical trial of irradiated autologous melanoma cells adenovirally transduced with human GM-CSF gene. Cancer Immunol Immunother 2001;50:373–81.

135. Soiffer R, Lynch T, Mihm M, et al. Vaccination with irradiated autologous melanoma cells engineered to secrete human granulocyte-macrophage colony-stimulating factor generates potent antitumor immunity in patients with metastatic melanoma. Proc Natl Acad Sci U S A 1998;95:13141–6.

136. Hsueh EC, Essner R, Foshag LJ, et al. Active immunotherapy by reinduction with a polyvalent allogeneic cell vaccine correlates with improved survival in recurrent metastatic melanoma. Ann Surg Oncol 2002;9:486–92.

137. Morton DL, Hsueh EC, Essner R, et al. Prolonged survival of patients receiving active immunotherapy with Canvaxin therapeutic polyvalent vaccine after complete resection of melanoma metastatic to regional lymph nodes. Ann Surg 2002;236:438–48; discussion 48–9.

138. Hsueh EC, Essner R, Foshag LJ, et al. Prolonged survival after complete resection of disseminated melanoma and active immunotherapy with a therapeutic cancer vaccine. J Clin Oncol 2002;20:4549–54.

139. Vermorken JB, Claessen AM, van Tinteren H, et al. Active specific immunotherapy for stage II and stage III human colon cancer: a randomised trial. Lancet 1999;353:345–50.

140. Uyl-de Groot CA, Vermorken JB, Hanna MG Jr, et al. Immunotherapy with autologous tumor cell-BCG vaccine in patients with colon cancer: a prospective study of medical and economic benefits. Vaccine 2005;23:2379–87.

141. Horig H, Lee DS, Conkright W, et al. Phase I clinical trial of a recombinant canarypoxvirus (ALVAC) vaccine expressing human carcinoembryonic antigen and the B7.1 co-stimulatory molecule. Cancer Immunol Immunother 2000;49:504–14.

142. von Mehren M, Arlen P, Gulley J, et al. The influence of granulocyte macrophage colony-stimulating factor and prior chemotherapy on the immunological response to a vaccine (ALVAC-CEA B7.1) in patients with metastatic carcinoma. Clin Cancer Res 2001;7:1181–91.

143. Marshall JL, Gulley JL, Arlen PM, et al. Phase I study of sequential vaccinations with fowlpox-CEA(6D)-TRICOM alone and sequentially with vaccinia-CEA(6D)-TRICOM, with and without granulocyte-macrophage colony-stimulating factor, in patients with carcinoembryonic antigen-expressing carcinomas. J Clin Oncol 2005;23:720–31.

144. Fong L, Brockstedt D, Benike C, et al. Dendritic cell-based xenoantigen vaccination for prostate cancer immunotherapy. J Immunol 2001;167:7150–6.

145. Foon KA, John WJ, Chakraborty M, et al. Clinical and immune responses in resected colon cancer patients treated with anti-idiotype monoclonal antibody vaccine that mimics the carcinoembryonic antigen. J Clin Oncol 1999;17:2889–5.

146. Samonigg H, Wilders-Truschnig M, Kuss I, et al. A double-blind randomized-phase II trial comparing immunization with antiidiotype goat antibody vaccine SCV 106 versus unspecific goat antibodies in patients with metastatic colorectal cancer. J Immunother 1999;22:481–8.

147. Jaffee EM, Hruban RH, Biedrzycki B, et al. Novel allogeneic granulocyte-macrophage colony-stimulating factor-secreting tumor vaccine for pancreatic cancer: a phase I trial of safety and immune activation. J Clin Oncol 2001;19:145–56.

148. Thomas AM, Santarsiero LM, Lutz ER, et al. Mesothelin-specific CD8(+) T cell responses provide evidence of in vivo cross-priming by antigen-presenting cells in vaccinated pancreatic cancer patients. J Exp Med 2004;200:297–306.

149. van der Burg SH, Menon AG, Redeker A, et al. Induction of p53-specific immune responses in colorectal cancer patients receiving a recombinant ALVAC-p53 candidate vaccine. Clin Cancer Res 2002;8:1019–27.

150. MacLean GD, Miles DW, Rubens RD, et al. Enhancing the effect of THERATOPE STn-KLH cancer vaccine in patients with metastatic breast cancer by pretreatment with low-dose intravenous cyclophosphamide. J Immunother Emphasis Tumor Immunol 1996;19:309–16.

151. Holmberg LA, Oparin DV, Gooley T, et al. Clinical outcome of breast and ovarian cancer patients treated with high-dose chemotherapy, autologous stem cell rescue and THERATOPE STn-KLH cancer vaccine. Bone Marrow Transplant 2000;25:1233–41.

152. Musselli C, Ragupathi G, Gilewski T, et al. Reevaluation of the cellular immune response in breast cancer patients vaccinated with MUC1. Int J Cancer 2002;97:660–7.

153. Brossart P, Wirths S, Stuhler G, et al. Induction of cytotoxic T-lymphocyte responses in vivo after vaccinations with peptide-pulsed dendritic cells. Blood 2000;96:3102–8.

154. Scholl SM, Balloul JM, Le Goc G, et al. Recombinant vaccinia virus encoding human MUC1 and IL2 as immunotherapy in patients with breast cancer. J Immunother 2000;23:570–80.

155. Rochlitz C, Figlin R, Squiban P, et al. Phase I immunotherapy with a modified vaccinia virus (MVA) expressing human MUC1 as antigen-specific immunotherapy in patients with MUC1-positive advanced cancer. J Gene Med 2003;5:690–9.

156. Karanikas V, Hwang LA, Pearson J, et al. Antibody and T cell responses of patients with adenocarcinoma immunized with mannan–MUC1 fusion protein. J Clin Invest 1997;100:2783–92.

157. Karanikas V, Thynne G, Mitchell P, et al. Mannan Mucin-1 Peptide Immunization: Influence of Cyclophosphamide and the Route of Injection. J Immunother 2001;24:172–83.

158. Disis ML, Gooley TA, Rinn K, et al. Generation of T-cell immunity to the HER-2/neu protein after active immunization with HER-2/neu peptide-based vaccines. J Clin Oncol 2002;20:2624–32.

159. Knutson KL, Schiffman K Disis ML. Immunization with a HER-2/neu helper peptide vaccine generates HER-2/neu CD8 T-cell immunity in cancer patients. J Clin Invest 2001;107:477–84.

160. Knutson KL, Schiffman K, Cheever MA, Disis ML. Immunization of cancer patients with a HER-2/neu, HLA-A2 peptide, p. 369–377, results in short-lived peptide-specific immunity. Clin Cancer Res 2002;8:1014–8.

161. Reece DE, Foon KA, Chatterjee MB, et al. Use of the Anti-idiotype Breast Cancer Vaccine 11D10 in Conjunction with Autologous Stem Cell Transplantation in Patients with Metastatic Breast Cancer. Clin Breast Cancer 2003;3 Suppl 4:152–7.

162. Sanda MG, Smith DC, Charles LG, et al. Recombinant vaccinia-PSA (PROSTVAC) can induce a prostate-specific immune response in androgen-modulated human prostate cancer. Urology 1999;53:260–6.

163. Cavacini LA, Duval M, Eder JP, Posner MR. Evidence of determinant spreading in the antibody responses to prostate cell surface antigens in patients immunized with prostate-specific antigen. Clin Cancer Res 2002;8:368–73.

164. Gulley JL, Arlen PM, Bastian A, et al. Combining a recombinant cancer vaccine with standard definitive radiotherapy in patients with localized prostate cancer. Clin Cancer Res 2005;11:3353–62.

165. Kaufman HL, Wang W, Manola J, et al. Phase II randomized study of vaccine treatment of advanced prostate cancer (E7897): a trial of the Eastern Cooperative Oncology Group. J Clin Oncol 2004;22:2122–32.

166. Arlen PM, Gulley JL, Tsang KY, Schlom J. Strategies for the development of PSA-based vaccines for the treatment of advanced prostate cancer. Expert Rev Vaccines 2003;2:483–93.

167. Arlen P, Gulley J, Todd N, et al. Antiandrogen, vaccine and combination therapy in patients with nonmetastatic hormone refractory prostate cancer. J Urol 2005;174:539–46.

168. Meidenbauer N, Harris DT, Spitler LE, Whiteside TL. Generation of PSA-reactive effector cells after vaccination with a PSA-based vaccine in patients with prostate cancer. Prostate 2000;43:88–100.

169. Small EJ, Fratesi P, Reese DM, et al. Immunotherapy of hormone-refractory prostate cancer with antigen-loaded dendritic cells. J Clin Oncol 2000;18:3894–903.

170. Lodge PA, Jones LA, Bader RA, et al. Dendritic cell-based immunotherapy of prostate cancer: immune monitoring of a phase II clinical trial. Cancer Res 2000;60:829–33.

171. Simmons SJ, Tjoa BA, Rogers M, et al. GM-CSF as a systemic adjuvant in a phase II prostate cancer vaccine trial. Prostate 1999;39:291–7.

172. Tjoa BA, Simmons SJ, Elgamal A, et al. Follow-up evaluation of a phase II prostate cancer vaccine trial. Prostate 1999;40:125–9.

173. Heiser A, Maurice MA, Yancey DR, et al. Induction of polyclonal prostate cancer-specific CTL using dendritic cells transfected with amplified tumor RNA. J Immunol 2001;166:2953–60.

174. Mercader M, Bodner BK, Moser MT, et al. T cell infiltration of the prostate induced by androgen withdrawal in patients with prostate cancer. Proc Natl Acad Sci U S A 2001;98:14565–70.

175. Kwak LW, Young HA, Pennington RW, Weeks SD. Vaccination with syngeneic, lymphoma-derived immunoglobulin idiotype combined with granulocyte/macrophage colony-stimulating factor primes mice for a protective T-cell response. Proc Natl Acad Sci U S A 1996;93:10972–7.

176. Timmerman JM, Czerwinski DK, Davis TA, et al. Idiotype-pulsed dendritic cell vaccination for B-cell lymphoma: clinical and immune responses in 35 patients. Blood 2002;99:1517–26.

177. Pinilla-Ibarz J, Cathcart K, Korontsvit T, et al. Vaccination of patients with chronic myelogenous leukemia with bcr-abl oncogene breakpoint fusion peptides generates specific immune responses. Blood 2000;95:1781–7.

178. Hurle R, Losa A, Manzetti A, Lembo A. Intravesical bacille Calmette-Guérin in Stage T1 grade 3 bladder cancer therapy: a 7-year follow-up. Urology 1999;54:258–63.

179. Gomella LG, Mastrangelo MJ, McCue PA, et al. Phase I study of intravesical vaccinia virus as a vector for gene therapy of bladder cancer. J Urol 2001;166:1291–5.

180. Lopez Hanninen E, Kirchner H, Atzpodien J. Interleukin-2 based home therapy of metastatic renal cell carcinoma: risks and benefits in 215 consecutive single institution patients. J Urol 1996;155:19–25.

181. Antonia SJ, Seigne J, Diaz J, et al. Phase I trial of a B7-1 (CD80) gene modified autologous tumor cell vaccine in combination with systemic interleukin-2 in patients with metastatic renal cell carcinoma. J Urol 2002;167:1995–2000.

182. Geiger JD, Hutchinson RJ, Hohenkirk LF, et al. Vaccination of pediatric solid tumor patients with tumor lysate-pulsed dendritic cells can expand specific T cells and mediate tumor regression. Cancer Res 2001;61:8513–9.

183. Reinartz S, Kohler S, Schlebusch H, et al. Vaccination of patients with advanced ovarian carcinoma with the anti-idiotype ACA125: immunological response and survival (phase Ib/II). Clin Cancer Res 2004;10:1580–7.

184. Garnett CT, Palena C, Chakarborty M, et al. Sublethal irradiation of human tumor cells modulates phenotype resulting in enhanced killing by cytotoxic T lymphocytes. Cancer Res 2004;64:7985–94.

185. Chakraborty M, Abrams SI, Camphausen K, et al. Irradiation of tumor cells up-regulates Fas and enhances CTL lytic activity and CTL adoptive immunotherapy. J Immunol 2003;170:6338–47.

186. Chakraborty M, Abrams SI, Coleman CN, et al. External beam radiation of tumors alters phenotype of tumor cells to render them susceptible to vaccine-mediated T-cell killing. Cancer Res 2004;64:4328–37.

187. Friedman EJ. Immune modulation by ionizing radiation and its implications for cancer immunotherapy. Curr Pharm Des 2002;8:1765–80.

188. Tong Y, Song W, Crystal RG. Combined intratumoral injection of bone marrow-derived dendritic cells and systemic chemotherapy to treat pre-existing murine tumors. Cancer Res 2001;61:7530–5.

189. Machiels JP, Reilly RT, Emens LA, et al. Cyclophosphamide, doxorubicin, and paclitaxel enhance the antitumor immune response of granulocyte/macrophage-colony stimulating factor- secreting whole-cell vaccines in HER-2/neu tolerized mice. Cancer Res 2001;61:3689–97.

190. Terando A, Mule JJ. On combining antineoplastic drugs with tumor vaccines. Cancer Immunol Immunother 2003;52:680–5.

191. Kwon ED, Hurwitz AA, Foster BA, et al. Manipulation of T cell costimulatory and inhibitory signals for immunotherapy of prostate cancer. Proc Natl Acad Sci U S A 1997;94:8099–103.

192. Sondel PM, Hank JA. Antibody-directed, effector cell-mediated tumor destruction. Hematol Oncol Clin North Am 2001;15:703–21.

193. Hodge JW, Sabzevari H, Yafal AG, et al. A triad of costimulatory molecules synergize to amplify T-cell activation. Cancer Res 1999;59:5800–7.

194. Wingren AG, Parra E, Varga M, et al. T cell activation pathways: B7, LFA-3, and ICAM-1 shape unique T cell profiles. Crit Rev Immunol 1995;15:235–53.

195. Schultze J, Nadler LM, Gribben JG. B7-mediated costimulation and the immune response. Blood Rev 1996;10:111–27.

196. Schwartz RH. Models of T cell anergy: is there a common molecular mechanism? J Exp Med 1996;184:19–29.
197. Swain SL, Croft M, Dubey C, et al. From naive to memory T cells. Immunol Rev 1996; 150: 143–67.
198. Allison JP, Hurwitz AA, Leach DR. Manipulation of costimulatory signals to enhance antitumor T–cell responses. Curr Opin Immunol 1995;7:682–6.
199. Melero I, Bach N, Chen L. Costimulation, tolerance and ignorance of cytolytic T lymphocytes in immune responses to tumor antigens. Life Sci 1997;60:2035–41.
200. Gilboa E. Immunotherapy of cancer with genetically modified tumor vaccines. Semin Oncol 1996;23:101–7.
201. Li Y, Hellstrom KE, Newby SA, Chen L. Costimulation by CD48 and B7-1 induces immunity against poorly immunogenic tumors. J Exp Med 1996;183:639–44.
202. Gilligan MG, Knox P, Weedon S, et al. Adenoviral delivery of B7-1 (CD80) increases the immunogenicity of human ovarian and cervical carcinoma cells. Gene Ther 1998;5:965–74.
203. Townsend SE Allison JP. Tumor rejection after direct costimulation of CD8+ T cells by B7- transfected melanoma cells [see comments]. Science 1993; 259: 368–70.
204. Baskar S, Azarenko V, Garcia Marshall E, et al. MHC class II-transfected tumor cells induce long-term tumor-specific immunity in autologous mice. Cell Immunol 1994;155:123–33.
205. Hodge JW, Schlom J. Comparative studies of a retrovirus versus a poxvirus vector in whole tumor-cell vaccines. Cancer Res 1999;59:5106–11.
206. Hodge JW, McLaughlin JP, Abrams SI, et al. Admixture of a recombinant vaccinia virus containing the gene for the costimulatory molecule B7 and a recombinant vaccinia virus containing a tumor-associated antigen gene results in enhanced specific T-cell responses and antitumor immunity. Cancer Res 1995;55:3598–603.
207. Akagi J, Hodge JW, McLaughlin JP, et al. Therapeutic antitumor response after immunization with an admixture of recombinant vaccinia viruses expressing a modified MUC1 gene and the murine T-cell costimulatory molecule B7. J Immunother 1997;20:38–47.
208. Rubio V, Stuge TB, Singh N, et al. Ex vivo identification, isolation and analysis of tumor-cytolytic T cells. Nat Med 2003;9:1377–82.
209. Hodge JW, Chakraborty M, Kudo-Saito C, et al. Multiple costimulatory modalities enhance CTL avidity. J Immunol 2005;174:5994–6004.
210. Oh S, Hodge JW, Ahlers JD, et al. Selective induction of high avidity CTL by altering the balance of signals from APC. J Immunol 2003;170:2523–30.
211. Tatari-Calderone Z, Semnani RT, Nutman TB, et al. Acquisition of CD80 by human T cells at early stages of activation: functional involvement of CD80 acquisition in T cell to T cell interaction. J Immunol 2002;169:6162–9.
212. Santin AD, Bellone S, Gokden M, et al. Vaccination with HPV-18 E7-pulsed dendritic cells in a patient with metastatic cervical cancer. N Engl J Med 2002;346:1752–3.
213. Goldstone SE, Palefsky JM, Winnett MT, Neefe JR. Activity of HspE7, a novel immunotherapy, in patients with anogenital warts. Dis Colon Rectum 2002;45:502–7.
214. Boehncke W–H, Takeshita T, Pendleton CD, et al. The importance of dominant negative effects of amino acid side chain substitution in peptide–MHC molecule interactions and T cell recognition. J Immunol 1993;150:331–41.
215. Ahlers JD, Takeshita T, Pendleton CD, Berzofsky JA. Enhanced immunogenicity of HIV-1 vaccine construct by modification of the native peptide sequence. Proc Natl Acad Sci U S A 1997;94:10856–61.
216. Serafini P, De Santo C, Marigo I, et al. Derangement of immune responses by myeloid suppressor cells. Cancer Immunol Immunother 2004;53:64–72.
217. Kusmartsev S, Gabrilovich DI. Immature myeloid cells and cancer-associated immune suppression. Cancer Immunol Immunother 2002;51:293–8.
218. Foss FM. Interleukin-2 fusion toxin: targeted therapy for cutaneous T cell lymphoma. Ann N Y Acad Sci 2001;941:166–76.
219. Lutsiak ME, Semnani RT, De Pascalis R, et al. Inhibition of CD4(+)25+ T regulatory cell function implicated in enhanced immune response by low-dose cyclophosphamide. Blood 2005;105:2862–8.
220. Shimizu J, Yamazaki S, Sakaguchi S. Induction of tumor immunity by removing CD25+CD4+ T cells: a common basis between tumor immunity and autoimmunity. J Immunol 1999;163:5211–8.
221. Kudo-Saito C, Schlom J, Hodge JW. The requirement of multimodal therapy (vaccine, local tumor radiation, and reduction of suppressor cells) to eliminate established tumors. Clin Cancer Res 2005;11:4533–44.
222. Ribas A, Timmerman JM, Butterfield LH Economou JS. Determinant spreading and tumor responses after peptide-based cancer immunotherapy. Trends Immunol 2003;24:58–61.
223. Bei R, Kantor J, Kashmiri SV, et al. Enhanced immune responses and anti-tumor activity by baculovirus recombinant carcinoembryonic antigen (CEA) in mice primed with the recombinant vaccinia CEA. J Immunother Emphasis Tumor Immunol 1994;16:275–82.
224. Hodge JW, McLaughlin JP, Kantor JA, Schlom J. Diversified prime and boost protocols using recombinant vaccinia virus and recombinant non-replicating avian pox virus to enhance T-cell immunity and antitumor responses. Vaccine 1997;15:759–68.
225. Irvine KR, Chamberlain RS, Shulman EP, et al. Enhancing efficacy of recombinant anticancer vaccines with prime/boost regimens that use two different vectors. J Natl Cancer Inst 1997;89:1595–601.
226. Murata K, Garcia-Sastre A, Tsuji M, et al. Characterization of in vivo primary and secondary CD8+ T cell responses induced by recombinant influenza and vaccinia viruses. Cell Immunol 1996;173:96–107.
227. Kudo-Saito C, Schlom J, Hodge JW. Intratumoral vaccination and diversified subcutaneous/ intratumoral vaccination with recombinant poxviruses encoding a tumor antigen and multiple costimulatory molecules. Clin Cancer Res 2004;10:1090–9.
228. Esserman LJ, Lopez T, Montes R, et al. Vaccination with the extracellular domain of p185neu prevents mammary tumor development in neu transgenic mice. Cancer Immunol Immunother 1999;47:337–42.
229. Kass E, Schlom J, Thompson J, et al. Induction of protective host immunity to carcinoembryonic antigen (CEA), a self-antigen in CEA transgenic mice, by immunizing with a recombinant vaccinia-CEA virus. Cancer Res 1999;59:676–83.
230. Soares MM, Mehta V, Finn OJ. Three different vaccines based on the 140-amino acid MUC1 peptide with seven tandemly repeated tumor-specific epitopes elicit distinct immune effector mechanisms in wild-type versus MUC1-transgenic mice with different potential for tumor rejection. J Immunol 2001;166:6555–63.
231. Hurwitz AA, Foster BA, Kwon ED, et al. Combination immunotherapy of primary prostate cancer in a transgenic mouse model using CTLA-4 blockade. Cancer Res 2000;60:2444–8.
232. Romagnani S. Lymphokine production by human T cells in disease states. Annu Rev Immunol 1994;12:227–57.
233. Pellegrini P, Berghella AM, Del Beato T, et al. Disregulation in TH1 and TH2 subsets of CD4+ T cells in peripheral blood of colorectal cancer patients and involvement in cancer establishment and progression. Cancer Immunol Immunother 1996;42:1–8.
234. Clerici M, Shearer GM, Clerici E. Cytokine dysregulation in invasive cervical carcinoma and other human neoplasias: time to consider the TH1/TH2 paradigm. J Natl Cancer Inst 1998;90:261–3.
235. Onizuka S, Tawara I, Shimizu J, et al. Tumor rejection by in vivo administration of anti-CD25 (interleukin-2 receptor alpha) monoclonal antibody. Cancer Res 1999;59:3128–33.
236. Woo EY, Chu CS, Goletz TJ, et al. Regulatory CD4(+)CD25(+) T cells in tumors from patients with early- stage non-small cell lung cancer and late-stage ovarian cancer. Cancer Res 2001;61:4766–72.
237. Woo EY, Yeh H, Chu CS, et al. Cutting edge: Regulatory T cells from lung cancer patients directly inhibit autologous T cell proliferation. J Immunol 2002;168:4272–6.
238. Riethmuller G, Schneider-Gadicke E, Schlimok G, et al. Randomised trial of monoclonal antibody for adjuvant therapy of resected Dukes' C colorectal carcinoma. German Cancer Aid 17-1A Study Group. Lancet 1994;343:1177–83.
239. Riethmuller G, Holz E, Schlimok G, et al. Monoclonal antibody therapy for resected Dukes' C colorectal cancer: seven-year outcome of a multicenter randomized trial. J Clin Oncol 1998; 16: 1788–94.
240. Shankaran V, Ikeda H, Bruce AT, et al. IFNgamma and lymphocytes prevent primary tumour development and shape tumour immunogenicity. Nature 2001;410:1107–11.
241. Dunn GP, Old LJ Schreiber RD. The three Es of cancer immunoediting. Annu Rev Immunol 2004;22:329–60.
242. Burnet FM. The concept of immunological surveillance. Prog Exp Tumor Res 1970;13:1–27.
243. Hanahan D, Weinberg RA. The hallmarks of cancer. Cell 2000;100:57–70.
244. Vogelstein B, Kinzler KW. Cancer genes and the pathways they control. Nat Med 2004;10:789–99.
245. Van Parijs L, Abbas AK. Homeostasis and self-tolerance in the immune system: turning lymphocytes off. Science 1998;280:243–8.
246. Pardoll D. Does the immune system see tumors as foreign or self? Annu Rev Immunol 2003;21:807–39.
247. Greiner JW, Zeytin H, Anver MR, Schlom J. Vaccine-based therapy directed against carcinoembryonic antigen demonstrates antitumor activity on spontaneous intestinal tumors in the absence of autoimmunity. Cancer Res 2002;62:6944–51.
248. Hodge JW, Grosenbach DW, Aarts WM, et al. Vaccine therapy of established tumors in the absence of autoimmunity. Clin Cancer Res 2003;9:1837–49.
249. Sakai Y, Morrison BJ, Burke JD, et al. Vaccination by genetically modified dendritic cells expressing a truncated neu oncogene prevents development of breast cancer in transgenic mice. Cancer Res 2004;64:8022–8.
250. Arlen P, Tsang KY, Marshall JL, et al. The use of a rapid ELISPOT assay to analyze peptide-specific immune responses in carcinoma patients to peptide vs. recombinant poxvirus vaccines. Cancer Immunol Immunother 2000;49:517–29.
251. Dudley ME, Wunderlich JR, Robbins PF, et al. Cancer regression and autoimmunity in patients after clonal repopulation with antitumor lymphocytes. Science 2002;298:850–4.
252. Finn OJ. Cancer vaccines: between the idea and the reality. Nat Rev Immunol 2003;3:630–41.
253. Horiguchi S, Petersson M, Nakazawa T, et al. Primary chemically induced tumors induce profound immunosuppression concomitant with apoptosis and alterations in signal transduction in T cells and NK cells. Cancer Res 1999;59:2950–6.
254. Levitsky HI. Augmentation of host immune responses to cancer: overcoming the barrier of tumor antigen-specific T-cell tolerance. Cancer J Sci Am 2000;6 Suppl 3:281–90.
255. Siegel PM, Massague J. Cytostatic and apoptotic actions of TGF-beta in homeostasis and cancer. Nat Rev Cancer 2003;3:807–20.
256. Hodge JW, Rad AN, Grosenbach DW, et al. Enhanced activation of T cells by dendritic cells engineered to hyperexpress a triad of costimulatory molecules. J Natl Cancer Inst 2000;92:1228–39.
257. Tsang KY, Zhu M, Even J, et al. The infection of human dendritic cells with recombinant avipox vectors expressing a costimulatory molecule transgene (CD80) to enhance the activation of antigen-specific cytolytic T cells. Cancer Res 2001;61:7568–76.
258. Merad M, Sugie T, Engleman EG, Fong L. In vivo manipulation of dendritic cells to induce therapeutic immunity. Blood 2002;99:1676–82.
259. Nair SK, Morse M, Boczkowski D, et al. Induction of tumor-specific cytotoxic T lymphocytes in cancer patients by autologous tumor RNA-transfected dendritic cells. Ann Surg 2002; 235: 540–9.
260. Rivoltini L, Carrabba M, Huber V, et al. Immunity to cancer: attack and escape in T lymphocyte-tumor cell interaction. Immunol Rev 2002;188:97–113.
261. Khong HT, Wang QJ, Rosenberg SA. Identification of multiple antigens recognized by tumor-infiltrating lymphocytes from a single patient: tumor escape by antigen loss and loss of MHC expression. J Immunother 2004;27:184–90.
262. Spiotto MT, Rowley DA, Schreiber H. Bystander elimination of antigen loss variants in established tumors. Nat Med 2004;10:294–8.
263. Finke J, Ferrone S, Frey A, et al. Where have all the T cells gone? Mechanisms of immune evasion by tumors. Immunol Today 1999;20:158–60.
264. Taylor DD, Gercel-Taylor C, Lyons KS, et al. T-cell apoptosis and suppression of T-cell receptor/CD3-zeta by Fas ligand-containing membrane vesicles shed from ovarian tumors. Clin Cancer Res 2003;9:5113–9.
265. Djerbi M, Screpanti V, Catrina AI, et al. The inhibitor of death receptor signaling, FLICE-inhibitory protein defines a new class of tumor progression factors. J Exp Med 1999;190:1025–32.
266. Medema JP, de Jong J, van Hall T, et al. Immune escape of tumors in vivo by expression of cellular FLICE- inhibitory protein. J Exp Med 1999;190:1033–8.
267. Bergmann-Leitner ES, Abrams SI. Differential role of Fas/Fas ligand interactions in cytolysis of primary and metastatic colon carcinoma cell lines by human antigen-specific CD8+ CTL. J Immunol 2000;164:4941–54.
268. Favre-Felix N, Fromentin A, Hammann A, et al. Cutting edge: the tumor counterattack hypothesis revisited: colon

cancer cells do not induce T cell apoptosis via the Fas (CD95, APO-1) pathway. J Immunol 2000;164:5023–7.
269. Restifo NP. Not so Fas: Re-evaluating the mechanisms of immune privilege and tumor escape. Nat Med 2000;6:493–5.
270. Khong HT, Restifo NP. Natural selection of tumor variants in the generation of "tumor escape" phenotypes. Nat Immunol 2002;3:999–1005.
271. Ito N, Nakamura H, Tanaka Y, Ohgi S. Lung carcinoma: analysis of T helper type 1 and 2 cells and T cytotoxic type 1 and 2 cells by intracellular cytokine detection with flow cytometry. Cancer 1999;85:2359–67.
272. Shevach EM. $CD4^+$ $CD25^+$ suppressor T cells: more questions than answers. Nat Rev Immunol 2002;2:389–400.
273. Sutmuller RP, van Duivenvoorde LM, van Elsas A, et al. Synergism of cytotoxic T lymphocyte-associated antigen 4 blockade and depletion of CD25(+) regulatory T cells in antitumor therapy reveals alternative pathways for suppression of autoreactive cytotoxic T lymphocyte responses. J Exp Med 2001;194:823–32.
274. Curiel TJ, Coukos G, Zou L, et al. Specific recruitment of regulatory T cells in ovarian carcinoma fosters immune privilege and predicts reduced survival. Nat Med 2004;10:942–9.
275. Terabe M, Matsui S, Park JM, et al. Transforming growth factor-beta production and myeloid cells are an effector mechanism through which CD1d-restricted T cells block cytotoxic T lymphocyte-mediated tumor immunosurveillance: abrogation prevents tumor recurrence. J Exp Med 2003;198:1741–52.
276. Overwijk WW, Theoret MR, Finkelstein SE, et al. Tumor regression and autoimmunity after reversal of a functionally tolerant state of self-reactive CD8+ T cells. J Exp Med 2003;198:569–80.
277. Shibata MA, Jorcyk CL, Liu ML, et al. The C3(1)/SV40 T antigen transgenic mouse model of prostate and mammary cancer. Toxicol Pathol 1998;26:177–82.
278. Gendler SJ Mukherjee P. Spontaneous adenocarcinoma mouse models for immunotherapy. Trends Mol Med 2001;7:471–5.
279. Cao ZA, Daniel D, Hanahan D. Sub-lethal radiation enhances anti-tumor immunotherapy in a transgenic mouse model of pancreatic cancer. BMC Cancer 2002;2:11.
280. Waldmann TA. IL-15 in the life and death of lymphocytes: immunotherapeutic implications. Trends Mol Med 2003;9:517–21.
281. Haller DG. COX-2 inhibitors in oncology. Semin Oncol 2003;30:2–8.
282. Zeytin HE, Patel AC, Rogers CJ, et al. Combination of a poxvirus-based vaccine with a cyclooxygenase-2 inhibitor (celecoxib) elicits antitumor immunity and long-term survival in CEA.Tg/MIN mice. Cancer Res 2004;64:3668–78.
283. Jocham D, Richter A, Hoffmann L, et al. Adjuvant autologous renal tumour cell vaccine and risk of tumour progression in patients with renal-cell carcinoma after radical nephrectomy: phase III, randomised controlled trial. Lancet 2004;363:594–9.
284. Nemunaitis J, Sterman D, Jablons D, et al. Granulocyte-macrophage colony-stimulating factor gene-modified autologous tumor vaccines in non-small-cell lung cancer. J Natl Cancer Inst 2004;96:326–31.
285. Peng BG, Liang LJ, He Q, et al. Tumor vaccine against recurrence of hepatocellular carcinoma. World J Gastroenterol 2005;11:700–4.
286. Dillman R, Barth N, Selvan S, et al. Phase I/II trial of autologous tumor cell line-derived vaccines for recurrent or metastatic sarcomas. Cancer Biother Radiopharm 2004;19:581–8.
287. Repmann R, Goldschmidt AJ, Richter A. Adjuvant therapy of renal cell carcinoma patients with an autologous tumor cell lysate vaccine: a 5-year follow-up analysis. Anticancer Res 2003;23:969–74.
288. Morton DL. Immune response to postsurgical adjuvant active immunotherapy with Canvaxin polyvalent cancer vaccine: correlations with clinical course of patients with metastatic melanoma. Dev Biol (Basel) 2004;116:209–17; discussion 29–36.
289. Raez LE, Cassileth PA, Schlesselman JJ, et al. Allogeneic vaccination with a B7.1 HLA-A gene-modified adenocarcinoma cell line in patients with advanced non-small-cell lung cancer. J Clin Oncol 2004;22:2800–7.
290. Letsch A, Keilholz U, Fluck M, et al. Peptide vaccination after repeated resection of metastases can induce a prolonged relapse-free interval in melanoma patients. Int J Cancer 2005;114:936–41.
291. Slack R, Ley L, Chang P, et al. Association between CEA-specific T cell responses (TCR) following treatment with vaccinia-CEA (V) and Alvac-CEA (A) and survival in patients (Pts) with CEA-bearing tumors. [abstract 1086] American Society of Clinical Oncology, Proceedings 2001.
292. Schuetz T, Marshall JL, Kaufmann HL, et al. Two phase I studies of prime-boost vaccinations with vaccinia-fowlpox vaccines expressing CEA, MUC-1, and TRICOM costimulatory molecules (B7.1/ICAM-1/LFA-3) in patients with advanced pancreatic cancer. [abstract 2564] American Society of Clinical Oncology, Proceedings 2004.
293. Hersey P, Coates AS, McCarthy WH, et al. Adjuvant immunotherapy of patients with high-risk melanoma using vaccinia viral lysates of melanoma: results of a randomized trial. J Clin Oncol 2002;20:4181–90.
294. Small EJ, Schellhammer PF, Higano CS, et al. Results of a placebo-controlled phase III trial of immunotherapy with APC8015 for patients with hormone refractory prostate cancer (HRPC). [abstract 4500] American Society of Clinical Oncology, Proceedings 2005.
295. Dillman R, Selvan S, Schiltz P, et al. Phase I/II trial of melanoma patient-specific vaccine of proliferating autologous tumor cells, dendritic cells, and GM-CSF: planned interim analysis. Cancer Biother Radiopharm 2004;19:658–65.
296. O'Rourke MG, Johnson M, Lanagan C, et al. Durable complete clinical responses in a phase I/II trial using an autologous melanoma cell/dendritic cell vaccine. Cancer Immunol Immunother 2003;52:387–95.

Section 14

ENDOCRINE THERAPY

52

Hypothalamic and Other Peptide Hormones

Andrew V. Schally, PhD, DSc, MD (hc)
Ana Maria Comaru-Schally, MD, MS*

ANALOGUES OF PEPTIDE HORMONES

Hypothalamo-Hypophysial Relationship, Hypothalamic Hormones, and Other Peptides It has been known since the 1930s that the anterior pituitary gland secretes several hormones that stimulate the thyroid, the gonads, and the adrenal cortex and that regulate various bodily processes. However, the mechanisms of the control of pituitary function were still not completely understood even in the 1950s, and several theories existed concerning this control. Harris[1] assembled anatomic and physiologic evidence that the hypothalamic portion of the brain secreted neurohormones that traversed the portal vessels to regulate the secretion of pituitary hormones. In the mid-1950s, one of the authors (A.V.S.) became interested in the hypothalamus and set about to prove Harris's neurohormonal theory. This work extended over 23 years.

It is well known now that the hypothalamic hormones stimulate or inhibit the release of various anterior pituitary hormones.[2–4] The discovery of several of these hypothalamic hormones, their isolation, structural identification, and synthesis, and the physiologic and clinical studies with synthetic hormones firmly established the concept of hypothalamic control of the pituitary gland.[2–5] Hypothalamic hormones are known to influence growth, reproduction, lactation, metabolism, gastrointestinal function, and the response to stress. Basal release of some hypothalamic hormones, including luteinizing hormone-releasing hormone (LHRH), into hypophysial portal blood is pulsatile, and surges occur before such events as ovulation.[3,5] Some hypothalamic peptide hormones are also produced in the extrahypothalamic brain areas (where they may serve as neurotransmitters) and in endocrine-like cells of non-neural tissues. Thus, somatostatin is present in discrete cells of the pancreas, gastric mucosa, duodenum, and other tissues and may, through paracrine control, play an important role in the regulation of the endocrine pancreas and gastrointestinal tract. LHRH, growth hormone-releasing hormone (GHRH), and their messenger ribonucleic acids (mRNAs) are also found in some tumors.[5,7,8] Mammalian bombesin-like peptides, such as gastrin-releasing peptide (GRP) and neuromedin B, are present in the gastrointestinal tract, the brain (including the hypothalamus), and various tumors and appear to produce mitogenic effects.[3,9,10] Understanding the functions of these peptide hormones and the effects of synthetic analogues should enable the clinician to better diagnose and treat a variety of cancers.

AGONISTS OF LHRH

Early Studies and the Basis of Oncologic Applications Thirty-four years have passed since our laboratory accomplished the isolation, determination of structure, and synthesis of the hypothalamic hormone controlling the secretion of both LH and follicle-stimulating hormone (FSH) from the anterior pituitary gland.[4] The discovery of LHRH, also called gonadotropin-releasing hormone (GnRH), had a major impact on medicine and has led to many practical clinical uses.[2–6] A strong interest in medical applications of LHRH derivatives stimulated the synthesis of agonistic, antagonistic, and recently, cytotoxic analogues of LHRH.[5,8,11] In the past 34 years, more than 3,000 analogues of LHRH have been synthesized.[5,6,8] The investigation of the effects of LHRH analogues on various cancers began in the late 1970s. LHRH analogues proved to have a variety of applications, including major uses in oncology.[5,8]

A number of LHRH analogues substituted in positions 6, 10, or both are much more active than LHRH.[3,5,6] Among the agonists being used clinically are [D-Trp^6]LHRH (triptorelin), [D-Leu^6, Pro^9-NHEt]LHRH (leuprolide), [D-Ser(Bu^t)^6, Pro^9-NHEt]LHRH (buserelin), [D-Ser(Bu^t)^6, Aza-Gly^{10}]LHRH (goserelin), and [D-Nal(2)^6]LHRH (nafarelin) (Table 52-1). These agonists are 50 to 100 times more potent than LHRH and also possess prolonged activity.[3,5,6]

Although an acute injection of superactive agonists of LHRH induces a marked and sustained release of LH and FSH, chronic administration produces inhibitory effects through a process of "down-regulation" of pituitary receptors for LHRH leading to a suppression of circulating levels of FSH and LH (bioactive but not always radioimmunoactive) and of sex steroid levels[3,5,6,8] (see the section "Mode of Action of LHRH Analogues" below). Thus, the inhibition of pituitary and gonadal function that occurs after chronic administration of agonists of LHRH and that creates a state of sex steroid deprivation by eliminating the stimulatory effects of estrogen or testosterone is the main basis for the oncologic application of LHRH agonists.[3,5,6,8]

Development of Sustained Delivery Systems Initially, superagonists of LHRH were given daily by the subcutaneous (SC) or intranasal route.[3–5] Subsequently, long-acting delivery systems for [D-Trp^6]LHRH and other agonists in microcapsules of poly(DL-lactide-co-glycolide) (PLG) or a different biodegradable, biocompatible polymer, designed to release a controlled dosage of the peptide (usually 100 μg) over a 30-day period were developed.[3,5,6,12–14] For administration, the microcapsules or microgranules are suspended in an injection vehicle containing 2% carboxymethylcellulose or D-mannitol and 1% Tween 20 or 80 in water and injected intramuscularly (IM).[5] In addition to 1- to 3-month release formulations of Triptorelin[5], 1- to 4-month prep-

*Deceased.

Table 52-1 Luteinizing Hormone-Releasing Hormone Agonists in Clinical Use

	Structure[a]									
	1	2	3	4	5	6	7	8	9	10
	pyro-Glu	His	Trp	Ser	Tyr	Gly	Leu	Arg	Pro	Gly-NH_2
Buserelin (Hoechst, Marion-Roussel)						D-Ser(But)				Ethylamide
Nafarelin (Syntex)						D-(2-Nal)				
Leuprolide (Abbott-Takeda, TAP Pharm)						D-Leu				Ethylamide
Goserelin (Astra-Zeneca						D-Ser(But)				Az-Gly-NH_2
Triporelin (Ipsen-Beaufour; Ferring, Aché)						D-Trp				

Az-Gly = AZA-glycine; But = o-tert butyl; Ethylamide = NH-Ch_2-Ch_3 (NHEt in text); LHRH = luteinizing hormone-releasing hormone; NAL(2) = 3-(2-naphthyl)alanine.
[a]The abbreviations of the amino acids are in accord with the recommendations of the IUPAC-IUB JCBN.

arations of Lupron Depot (containing 3.75–30 mg of leuprolide[13]) injectable IM and of Zoladex (goserelin, 3.6–10.8 mg) in subcutaneous implants of the polymer PLG[14] are also available.[5] Sustained delivery formulations are capable of maintaining therapeutic levels of peptides for 4 to 16 weeks. Delayed delivery systems developed for periodic administration are efficacious, reliable, and convenient and also increase the patient's compliance.

Current Uses of LHRH Agonists Chronic administration of LHRH agonists is being used to induce the regression of endocrine-dependent malignant neoplasms, especially prostate and breast cancer.[3–5,8,13,14,16–20] Suppression of pituitary-gonadal axis by LHRH agonists can also be used for the treatment of central precocious puberty.[6] The inhibition of LH and ovarian steroidogenesis provides the basis for the therapeutic use of LHRH agonists in diseases and conditions that result from inappropriate hormone levels or that can be treated by the suppression of estrogens. These applications include endometriosis, uterine fibroids (leiomyomas), polycystic ovarian disease (PCOD), dysfunctional uterine bleeding, and hirsutism.[6,21] LHRH agonists are also extensively used in assisted reproductive technology for in vitro fertilization and embryo transfer (IVF-ET).[6,22]

Pharmacokinetics and Metabolism LHRH agonists are degraded and eliminated from plasma several times more slowly than natural LHRH, the half-life of which is 2 to 4 minutes in humans.[5] The binding affinity of [D-Trp^6]LHRH to LHRH receptors is about 10 times higher than that of LHRH,[5,23] and its plasma half-life is 7.6 hours. A single IM injection of the 3.75 mg of depot preparation of microcapsules liberating 100 µg/d results, after an initial peak, in [D-Trp^6]LHRH concentrations of 200 to 500 pg/mL lasting for about 4 to 5 weeks.[5] Labeled LHRH analogues accumulate primarily in the liver and kidneys (the main degrading organs) and the pituitary, the biologic target.[5]

Side Effects and Toxicology The main side effects caused by chronic administration of LHRH agonists are those that can be attributed to sex-hormone deficiency.[5] These consist of impotence and loss of libido in men and "hot flashes" or climacteric-like vasomotor phenomena and osteopenia in both sexes.

LHRH ANTAGONISTS

LHRH antagonists represent another class of peptide analogues with important oncologic and gynecologic applications.[3,5,6,8] These antagonists act on the same receptor sites as LHRH and cause an immediate inhibition of the release of gonadotropins and sex steroids.[5,8,21] Although a repeated administration of LHRH agonists is necessary for the inhibition of LH and sex steroids, this effect can be induced with a single injection of a potent LHRH antagonist.[5] Because the antagonists induce an immediate suppression, their use prevents "flare-up" phenomena, which can occur in some cancer patients.[3,5,8] Antagonistic analogues of LHRH were made at first for contraception.[5,23] Since 1972, hundreds of LHRH antagonists have been synthesized and assayed in animals. Some of the more potent early antagonists were also found to be active in humans.[5] Insertion of D-arginine into position 6 of LHRH antagonists increased the inhibitory activity, but induced histamine liberation, resulting in transient edema and other anaphylactoid reactions.[5,23,24] To eliminate the undesirable edematogenic effects, new analogues with D-ureidoalkyl amino acids such as D-Cit and D-Hci at position 6 were synthesized in our laboratory and tested.[5,24] Among these antagonists, SB-75 Cetrorelix (Table 52-2) was the most active in vivo in rats and did not exert any edematogenic effects, even at a dose of 1.5 mg/kg.[22,24]

Other groups introduced different structural modifications that also diminish anaphylactoid reactions. Antagonists such as Antide[25] and Nal-Glu antagonist[26] were potent although the latter caused some side effects in clinical trials. Among other antagonists are Azaline B,[27] Ganirelix,[28] and Abarelix[29] (see Table 52-2 for structures).

Current Clinical Status of LHRH Antagonists In phase I clinical studies, single and multiple SC injections as well as IV infusions of Cetrorelix were given to more than 200 healthy subjects of both sexes.[5,22] The dose range for single doses was 0.25 to 20 mg SC.[22] Gonzales-Barcena and colleagues[30] reported a decrease lasting 12 to 24 hours in serum LH, FSH, and testosterone levels in normal men after SC administration of 300 µg Cetrorelix. Behre and colleagues[31] and Klingmuller and colleagues[32] studied the effects of Cetrorelix in normal men and found 73 to 91% testosterone suppression after SC injection of 1 to 5 mg Cetrorelix.[22] Cetrorelix seemed to have a higher suppressive rate than other antagonists, such as Nal-Glu or Detirelix, and even in large doses of up to 10 mg only occasionally caused minimal erythema, in contrast to Nal-Glu antagonist, which produced local side effects.[22,30–32] In healthy premenopausal women, Cetrorelix administered between days 6 and 10 of the menstrual cycle in doses of 3 to 5 mg caused an immediate decrease in

Table 52-2 Luteinizing Hormone-Releasing Hormone Antagonists[a]

Trivial Name	Sequence
Cetrorelix (SB-75)	[Ac-D-Nal)^1, D-Phe(4Cl)^2, D-Pal(3)^3, DCit^6, D-Ala^{10}]-LHRH
Antide	[N-Ac-D-Nal(2)^1, D-Phe(4Cl)^2, D-Pal(3)^3, Lys (nic)^5, D-Lys(Nic)^6, Lys (iPr)8, D-Ala^{10}]-LHRH antagonist
Nal-Glu	[Ac-D-Nal(2)^1, D-Phe(4Cl)^2, D-Pal(3)^3, Arg^5, D-Glu^6(AA), D-Ala^{10}]-LHRH
Azaline B	[Ac-D-Nal^1, D-Phe(4Cl)^2, D-Pal^3, Aph^5(Atz), Aph^6(Atz), Ilys^8, D-Ala^{10}]-GnRH
Ganirelix	[N-Ac-D-Nal(2)^1, D-Phe(4Cl)^2, D-Pal(3)^3, D-hArg(Et_2)^6, L-hArg(Et_2)^8, D-Ala^{10}]-GnRH
Abarelix	[N-Ac-D-Nal(2)-D-(p-Cl-Phe-D-Pal(3)-Ser-NM-Tyr-Asn-Leu-Ilys-Pro-Gly-NH_2]

Ac = acetyl; Cit = citrulline (2-amino-5-ureidopentanoic acid); D-Glu6(AA) = 4-(p-methoxy-benzoyl-D-2-aminobutyric acid; hArg = homoarginine; Ilys = Ne-isopropyllsine; LHRH = luteinizing hormone-releasing hormone; Lys-(iPr) = Ne-isopropyllysine; Lys(Nic) = Ne-nicotinoyllysine; Nal(2) = 3-(2-naphthyl)alanine; NM = N-methyl; Pal(3) = 3-(3-pyridyl)alanine; Phe(4Cl) = 4-chlorophenylalanine.
[a]The abbreviations of the amino acids are in accord with the recommendations of the IUPAC-IUB JCBN.
For comparison with the amino acids sequence of LHRH see Table 52-1.

serum LH, FSH, and estradiol.[33] Cetrorelix given IV, SC, or IM in doses of 300 to 1,200 μg also inhibited LH and FSH release in postmenopausal women and caused no side effects.[30]

In patients with benign prostatic hyperplasia (BPH) or advanced prostate carcinoma, treatment with Cetrorelix produced an inhibition of serum LH and FSH levels and a fall in serum testosterone levels[34,35] (for prostate cancer, see the respective section below). In the first study in men with benign prostatic hyperplasia, Cetrorelix was given SC for 4 weeks at dosages of 500 μg bid to 11 patients presenting with prostatism and urinary outflow obstruction.[34] There was a clear clinical improvement after the first week of therapy, and the prostatic volume showed a significant decrease that was maintained in some patients after discontinuation of therapy.[34]

In the second study, 13 patients with symptomatic BPH were treated with a loading dosage of Cetrorelix, 5 mg bid SC for 2 days, followed by 1 mg/day SC for 2 months.[35] Treatment with Cetrorelix produced a 53% decline in the International Prostate Symptom Score, a 46% improvement in the quality-of-life score, a rapid 27% reduction in prostatic volume, and an increase in peak urinary flow rates. Serum testosterone fell to castration levels on day 2 but was inhibited only by 64 to 74% during maintenance therapy; after cessation of treatment, levels returned to normal. During long-term follow-up, most patients continued to show progressive improvement in urinary symptoms and enhancement of sexual function, and prostatic volume remained normal. These studies demonstrate that in patients with symptomatic BPH, treatment with Cetrorelix is safe and produces long-term improvement.[35] These findings were extended in large phase IIb trials using two different depot formulations. Cetrorelix offers a therapeutic alternative to patients with BPH who are considered poor surgical risks.[35]

Cetrorelix has also been used successfully in women undergoing IVF-ET procedures to prevent premature LH surge.[6,22] Following phase II/III trials in several hundred patients, Cetrorelix was approved in Europe and the United States for use in controlled ovarian stimulation programs.[22] Sustained-release formulations of Cetrorelix (depot) have been developed by Zentaris (Frankfurt on Main, Germany). LHRH antagonists are likewise used for other clinical indications, such as leiomyomas and endometriosis, in which inhibition of sex steroids is desirable.[6,22] Depot formulations of Cetrorelix and Abarelix are now available. In ongoing clinical trials with Cetrorelix, low dosage regimens are used to induce transient suppression of sex steroids for the treatment of BPH, endometriosis, and myomas.

LHRH Analogues Carrying Cytotoxic Radicals An additional new class of antitumor drugs has been developed based on LHRH analogues bearing cytotoxic radicals, such as doxorubicin and its derivative 2-pyrrolino-doxorubicin.[3,4,36,37] LHRH analogues carrying these cytotoxic radicals are designed as targeted chemotherapeutic agents intended for the treatment of cancers that contain receptors for LHRH. Thus, we linked [D-Lys[6]]LHRH through the ε-amino group of its D-Lys moiety to the 14-OH group of doxorubicin to form cytotoxic LHRH analogue AN-152.[11,36,37] A still more potent cytotoxic analogue (AN-207) was synthesized by conjugating 2-pyrrolino-doxorubicin (AN-201), a daunosamine-modified derivative of doxorubicin that is at least 100 times more active in vivo than its parent compound, to the same [D-Lys[6]]LHRH carrier.[11,36,37] The antiproliferative activity of the cytotoxic radicals and the high binding affinity of the carrier to LHRH receptors are both fully preserved in the cytotoxic LHRH analogues AN-152 and AN-207.[37] AN-152 and AN-207 are less toxic and much more effective in vivo than their respective radicals in inhibiting tumor growth in LHRH-receptor-positive models of human ovarian, mammary, endometrial, and prostatic cancers, as well as melanomas and renal cell carcinomas xenografted into nude mice.[36] Thus, cytotoxic LHRH analogues could be considered for treatment of these cancers. Such analogues act as chemotherapeutic agents targeted to the tumor cells by their peptide portions for which binding sites are present on the tumor cell membranes. Because the antitumor action may be exerted to a greater degree locally or at least at more selective sites that have the cell membrane receptors, the peripheral toxicity on normal cells that do not bind cytotoxic analogues would be reduced. A peptide containing a cytotoxic radical is bound to the membrane receptors and internalized.[36] An internalization was shown in human breast, endometrial, and ovarian cancers,[11,36] which contain receptors for LHRH. After endocytosis, such a compound could interfere with intracellular events in cancer cells.

The damage inflicted by cytotoxic analogues to pituitary LH- and FSH-secreting cells would not be deleterious to the cancer patient, since hypophysectomy has been used for treatment of some cancers. Our work in the pituitary cell superfusion system indicates that cytotoxic LHRH analogues selectively affect LH cells but not growth hormone (GH) and thyrotropin cells.[36] A possible damage to other cells (eg, corticotrophs) could also be alleviated by replacement therapy.[36] Cytotoxic compounds linked to hormonal peptides such as LHRH that can be targeted to certain cancers possessing receptors for those peptides and that are more selective for killing cancer cells could be of major therapeutic importance. This approach could extend the utility of analogues of LHRH from the current palliation toward an eventual cure. Phase-I/II clinical trials with cytotoxic LHRH analog AN-152 in patients with breast and ovarian cancer are in progress.

MODE OF ACTION OF LHRH ANALOGUES

Pituitary-Gonadal Axis LHRH agonists are widely used in oncology and gynecology. The mechanism of action of these analogues is mainly based on the inhibition of pituitary and gonadal function, but direct effects on various tumors may also play a role.[5,6,21] Continuous treatment with LHRH agonists causes a down-regulation (a decrease in the number) of LHRH receptors and an uncoupling of the LHRH signal transduction mechanism.[5,21,38] This results in a desensitization of gonadotrophs and a marked reduction in the secretion of bioactive LH and FSH.[5,6,11] This state is reversible and is called "selective medical hypophysectomy."[5,21] The decrease in circulating LH and FSH, together with down-regulation of gonadal receptors for LH and FSH, produces a complete inhibition of testicular or ovarian function and a fall in sex steroid levels. This state is called "chemical or medical castration."[5,21,39] The key advantage of the medical castration achieved by LHRH agonists is its reversibility.[5,21] In addition, various extrapituitary tissues, including the prostate, breast, uterus, and ovaries, as well as many tumors, contain specific receptors for LHRH, which might permit direct inhibitory actions of LHRH analogues.[5,8,21,36,40–42]

The principal mechanism of action of LHRH antagonists is the competitive occupancy of LHRH receptors, but recent experimental evidence documents that treatment with the LHRH antagonist Cetrorelix also down-regulates pituitary LHRH receptors in rats and decreases the levels of mRNA for LHRH receptors.[5,8,21,43] These phenomena may also occur clinically.[5,8,22] The down-regulation of pituitary LHRH receptors is also reversible, and a complete recovery occurs 1 to 2 months after cessation of treatment with antagonists.[5,21]

The mechanism of pituitary LH release in response to LHRH is not completely understood. The first step in the action of LHRH involves its binding to a plasma membrane receptor, which causes a microaggregation of receptors and complex formation.[38,44] The complex formed is then internalized and degraded although this internalization is not necessary for the liberation of the gonadotropins. Calcium and the products of phosphoinositide metabolism have been implicated as second messengers[38,44] The LHRH receptor is coupled to a guanosine triphosphate (GTP)-binding protein (G protein) that can activate phospholipase C, which leads to the production of diacylglycerol and the activation of protein kinase C.[38,44] Recent studies show that multiple G proteins are involved in the action of LHRH on the gonadotrope. Activation of G protein stimulates LH release and inositol phosphate production.[38,44] The complete mechanisms still remain to be elucidated.

Direct Effects Clinical evidence indicates that in patients with advanced breast or prostate cancer, medical castration produced by the chronic administration of LHRH analogues accounts for most benefits derived from the treatment.[5,21,44] However, there is also evidence that LHRH agonists and antagonists can exert direct effects on tumor cells.[5,21] This view is based on clinical results, the detection of high-affinity binding sites for LHRH in various cancers, and the effects on tumor cell lines in cultures.

Medical castration should not benefit postmenopausal women with breast cancer. However, various investigators[5,21,44–46] have reported responses in postmenopausal women with breast cancer treated with LHRH agonists. Saphner and colleagues obtained an 11% response rate in postmenopausal women treated with Zoladex.[47] Similarly, medical castration should not benefit breast cancer patients with estrogen receptor (ER)-negative tumors, but responses in ER-negative premenopausal patients treated with leuprolide or Zoladex have been recorded.[16,18]

Receptors for LHRH in Various Tumors Direct effects of LHRH analogues are mediated by receptors found on tumor cells. Specific membrane receptors for LHRH have been found in various animal and human cancers.[8,40–42] Binding sites for LHRH were detected in LNCaP and DU 145 human prostate cancer lines.[48,49] More than 80% of human prostate cancer specimens exhibit high-affinity receptors for [D-Trp^6]LHRH.[5,8,41] Various investigators found LHRH receptors in several human mammary carcinoma cell lines.[5,8,44,49,50] LHRH membrane receptor sites were also detected in 260 of 500 samples of human breast cancer (52%).[40] LHRH receptors were found in 78% of human ovarian epithelial cancer specimens and in EFO-21, EFO-27, and OV-1063 human ovarian cancer lines.[21,42] Similarly, in nearly 80% of human endometrial carcinomas and in HEC-1A and Ishikawa endometrial cancer lines, the presence of receptors for [D-Trp^6]LHRH was established.[21] LHRH receptors are also found in human pancreatic cancers.[3,5,51] The expression of LHRH receptor gene in human breast, ovarian, and prostate cancer cell lines and melanomas and renal cell carcinomas was also demonstrated.[5,21,52–54] These findings provide a rationale for therapeutic approaches based on LHRH analogues in malignancies in which specific receptors for LHRH are found.

Inhibition of Growth of Tumor Cell Lines Observations on growth inhibition of cultured tumor cells by LHRH analogues support the concept of their direct effects. Significant inhibition of human breast and prostatic cancer cells by LHRH agonists in vitro is now well documented.[5,8,48–50,52,55] The LHRH antagonist Cetrorelix also causes a marked inhibition of proliferation of mammary, ovarian, and endometrial cancer cell lines.[5,8,21,44,55,56] These results suggest a regulatory role of LHRH-like peptides in tumor growth. LHRH is not present in the general circulation in significant concentrations, but the presence of LHRH immunoreactivity and mRNA for LHRH in human mammary cancer cells suggests that local LHRH may play a role in the growth of mammary tumors.[52] Subsequently, the evidence for production of an LHRH-like peptide and/or expression of mRNA for LHRH was obtained in human prostatic, endometrial, and ovarian cancer lines.[5,44,53,54] These LHRH-like peptides could function as local regulators of tumor growth. LHRH agonists and antagonists might inhibit the growth of tumor cells in part by nullifying the action of endogenous LHRH-like peptides.

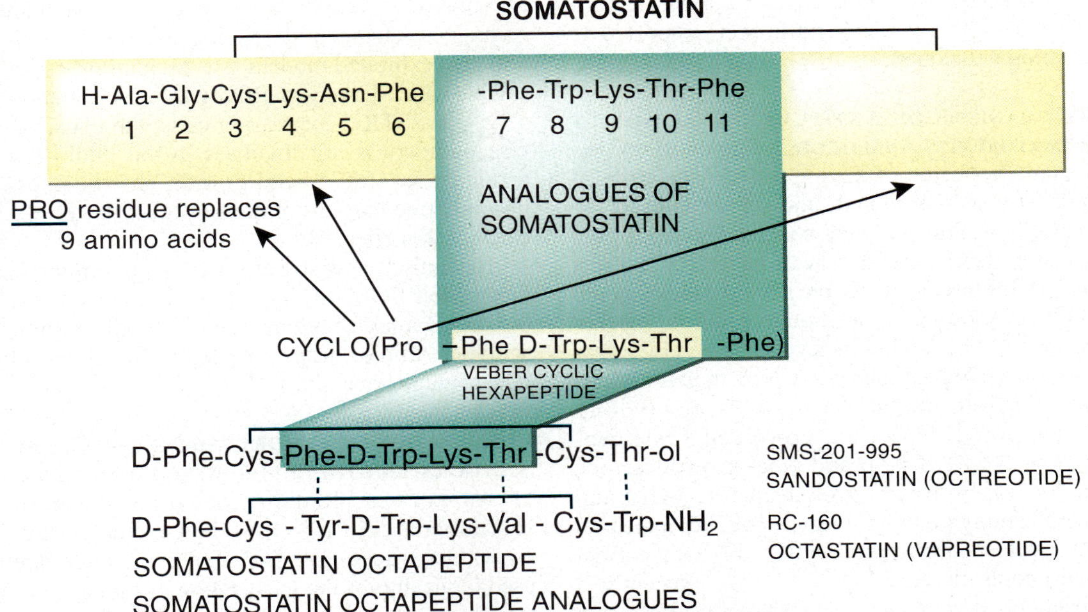

Figure 52-1 Structural relationship of somatostatin, Veber hexapeptide, and octapeptide analogs Sandostatin and Octastatin.

SOMATOSTATIN ANALOGUES

Tetradecapeptide somatostatin (Figure 52-1) has many biologic actions, inhibits a large variety of cells, and appears to be an endogenous antiproliferative agent.[3,8,57,58] The clinical potential of somatostatin has been appreciated for some 30 years. Various studies demonstrated the inhibitory effects of somatostatin in patients with acromegaly; endocrine pancreatic tumors, such as insulinomas and glucagonomas; ectopic tumors, such as gastrinomas; and vasoactive intestinal peptide (VIP)-producing tumors.[8,58] However, the half-life of somatostatin is very short; thus, its therapeutic use is impractical.[8,58]

Several groups synthesized somatostatin analogues with more selective and prolonged activities.[59–61] On the basis of conformational analysis, Veber and colleagues replaced 9 of the 14 amino acids of somatostatin with a single proline residue (see Figure 52-1).[61] The hexapeptide analog cyclo(-Pro-Phe-D-Trp-Lys-Thr-Phe) was much more potent than somatostatin in inhibiting GH, insulin, and glucagon release.[58,61] Bauer and colleagues synthesized highly potent octapeptide analogues of somatostatin.[59] They incorporated the sequence 7 to 10 of somatostatin, Phe-D-Trp-Lys-Thr, proposed as essential,[61] into a series of analogues of which D-Phe-Cys-Phe-D-Trp-Lys-Thr-Cys-Thr-OL, containing a C-terminal amino alcohol, was the most active (see Figure 52-1).[59] This analogue, designated SMS-201-995 (Sandostatin, octreotide), was about 50 times more potent than somatostatin in tests on inhibition of GH secretion and more selective.

Many analogues of somatostatin, designed specifically for antitumor activity, were synthesized by our group,[3,58,60] incorporating Tyr and Val in positions corresponding to residues 7 and 10, respectively, of somatostatin-14 (SS-14). Thus, the analogues RC-121 RC-160 (see Figure 52-1) were about 100 times more potent than SS-14 in tests for inhibition of GH release in vivo in rats and possessed a prolonged duration of action. RC-160 has been shown to be a powerful tumor growth suppressor in various experimental models of pancreatic, prostatic, renal, colorectal, gastric, and mammary cancers[3,8,58,62–66] as well as glioblastomas and small-cell and nonsmall-cell lung carcinomas.[3,8,63] Sandostatin is known to selectively inhibit the growth of various endocrine tumors and is the analogue of somatostatin most extensively investigated in clinical trials.[57] Sandostatin and other somatostatin analogues, such as RC-160 and BIM-23014 (Lanreotide; 3(2-naphthyl)-D-Ala-Cys-Tyr-D-Trp-Lys-Val-Cys-Thr-NH_2), have been used for the treatment of acromegaly, endocrine tumors of the gastroenteropancreatic system (including carcinoid tumors), insulinomas, glucagonomas, gastrinomas, and VIPomas.[8,57,58,67] Long-acting preparations of Sandostatin LAR Depot and lanreotide for once-monthly administration are now available. Attempts have been made to use modern somatostatin analogues for the therapy of various human cancers such as prostatic, breast, pancreatic, and lung cancers,[3,8,33,51,57,58,62,64,68–70] but relevant palliative benefits have been obtained so far only in hepatocellular carcinoma.[71] (See the sections on specific neoplasms below.)

Side Effects The side effects of somatostatin analogues consist mainly of steatorrhea, which can be controlled; diarrhea and loose stools; malabsorption; gastrointestinal cramps; and occasional nausea. Somatostatin inhibits gallbladder contractions, and about 27% of patients treated chronically with Sandostatin were reported to develop gallstones.

Mechanisms of Antitumoral Action of Somatostatin Analogues Somatostatin analogues, by virtue of having a wide spectrum of activities (which include the suppression of the secretions of the pituitary, pancreas, stomach, and gut; interference with growth factors; and direct antiproliferative effects on some tissues), could inhibit various tumors through multiple mechanisms.[8,58] The fall in GH levels induced by somatostatin analogues causes a reduction in the secretion of hepatic insulin-like growth factor I (IGF-I), which could inhibit the growth of some cancers.[3,7] IGF-I, IGF-II, and other growth factors, including epidermal growth factor (EGF) and transforming growth factor-α (TGF-α), appear to be involved in the proliferation of both normal and neoplastic cells.[3,7,8,51,58,68,72–75] Recently, a strong positive association was reported between plasma IGF-I levels and risk of prostatic, breast, colorectal, and lung cancers.[76–80] Various observations indicate that some somatostatin analogues act as growth inhibitors in cancer cells through the activation of tyrosine phosphatase (see the section "Receptors for Somatostatin" below).[3,8,58,81–83] Thus, somatostatin analogues exert their effects by several mechanisms involving interference with the transmission of intracellular signals that regulate cell growth.[8,58,81–83]

Receptors for Somatostatin Somatostatin induces its biologic effects by interacting with specific receptors that are coupled to a variety of signal transduction pathways involving adenylate cyclase, Ca^{2+} channels, and protein dephosphorylation.[3,81,82] High- or low-affinity SS-14 receptors were identified in various normal human tissues and in human neoplasms, including such brain tumors as meningiomas and differentiated glia-derived tumors (astrocytomas and oligodendrogliomas); pituitary tumors; hormone-producing gastrointestinal tumors; small-cell and nonsmall-cell lung carcinomas; and lymphomas and breast, pancreatic, colorectal, prostatic, renal, and ovarian cancers.[8,40,41,57,68,72,75,84–89]

So far, five subtypes of somatostatin receptor, SSTR-1 to SSTR-5, have been cloned and functionally characterized.[8,36,81,82] They belong to the guanine nucleotide-binding regulatory protein (G-protein)-linked receptor family. They all bind somatostatin-14 and somatostatin-28 with similar affinity but show major differences in their affinities for various somatostatin analogues.[8,81,82] Sandostatin (octreotide) and RC-160 have a high binding affinity for somatostatin receptor subtype SSTR-2 and can induce a stimulation of tyrosine phosphatase activity and an inhibition of the proliferation of the cells expressing *SSTR-2* gene.[81] This implicates tyrosine phosphatase as a transducer of the growth inhibition signal. Since mRNAs of receptor subtypes are variably expressed in different cancers,[8,11] this indicates the necessity for a precise determination of receptor subtypes in tumor tissue before therapy with analogues. Octapeptide analogues such as RC-160 also exhibited moderate-to-high affinities for SSTR-3 and -5 and low affinity for SSTR-1 and -4.[36,82] In SSTR-5-expressing cells, the phosphatase pathway is not involved in the inhibitory action of RC-160 on cell growth, and the phosphoinositide/calcium pathway could be implicated in this effect.[82]

Recently, a new somatostatin peptidomimetic designated SOM230 has been synthesized that possessed a high binding activity to all receptor subtypes. Clinical trials revealed its high GH and IGF-I inhibitory activity.[90]

Localization of Tumors and Metastases by Scintigraphy with Radiolabeled Somatostatin Analogues Radioiodinated analogues of somatostatin, such as [^{111}In-DTPA-D-Phe^1]-octreotide (Octreoscan) and [^{123}I-Tyr^3]-octreotide, are used clinically for the localization of tumors containing receptors for somatostatin.[8,84,85,89,91] Thus, the presence of somatostatin receptors permits the localization of some tumors and metastases using scanning techniques.[8,84,85,91] Information about membrane receptor levels makes feasible the planning of therapy with analogues. Lamberts and colleagues used [^{123}I-Tyr^3]-octreotide for the scanning of five patients with endocrine pancreatic tumors and found this procedure valuable in the localization of primary tumors as well as their often clinically unrecognized metastases.[91] Krenning and colleagues[85] carried out somatostatin receptor scintigraphy in more than 1,000 patients and reported that various primary tumors, both neuroendocrine or non-neuroendocrine, containing high numbers of somatostatin receptors can be localized in vivo.

Metastases can be also visualized by scintigraphy with Octreoscan.[85] Neuroendocrine tumors readily localized with Octreoscan included GH- and TSH-producing pituitary tumors, gastrinomas, insulinomas, glucagonomas, unclassified apudomas, medullary thyroid carcinomas, neuroblastomas, pheochromocytomas, carcinoids, and small-cell lung cancer.[8,85] Non-neuroendocrine tumors that contained somatostatin receptors and that could be localized by in vivo scintigraphy included nonsmall-cell lung cancer, meningiomas, breast cancer, and astrocytomas, but not exocrine pancreatic tumors.[85] The value of scintigraphy as a conventional diagnostic technique for tumors such as breast cancer still has to be established.[85] Scintigraphy in therapeutic trials with somatostatin analogues should help to determine which patients are likely to benefit from the treatment. In many cases, a positive scintigram predicted a good response to treatment with octreotide.[85]

Use of Radiolabeled Somatostatin Analogues for Local Tumor Therapy Work is also in progress on applying somatostatin analogues labeled with appropriate radionuclides such as ^{111}indium, ^{123}iodine, ^{188}rhenium, ^{177}lutetium, or ^{90}yttrium in cancer therapy. Radiolabeled somatostatin analogues could allow treatment of somatostatin receptor-positive tumors by delivering a radioactive isotope to the cancer cell. ^{111}In-radiolabeled [DTPA^0, Tyr^3]octreotide, [DTPA^0,Tyr^3]octreotate, pentetreotide (Octreoscan) and ^{90}Y-labeled-DOTA-D-Phe^1, Tyr^3 octreotide, [^{177}Lu-DOTA^0, Tyr^3]octreotate were reported as promising for in situ radionuclide therapy of SS receptor-positive tumors [92–94] (see under specific tumors).

Cytotoxic Analogues of Somatostatin The presence of binding sites for somatostatin in certain cancers can also be used for targeting chemotherapeutic agents linked to somatostatin analogues. We synthesized a series of modern targeted cytotoxic analogues of SST.[11,36,95] These conjugates consist of doxorubicin or 2-pyrrolino-doxorubicin (AN-201) linked covalently to carrier SST octapeptide analogues[11,36,95] and possess both the receptor affinity and the cytotoxic activity. In a highly active targeted cytotoxic somatostatin analogue AN-238, AN-201 is linked to octapeptide carrier RC-121. AN-238 inhibits growth of experimental prostatic, renal, pancreatic, breast, ovarian, and lung cancers, as well as lymphomas and brain tumors and their metastases expressing SSTR-2 or -5, and it can be used for targeted chemotherapy.[8,11,36]

ANTAGONISTS OF BOMBESIN AND GASTRIN-RELEASING PEPTIDE

The bombesin-like peptides make up a large family of peptides found in amphibians and mammals, including humans. The tetradecapeptide bombesin (Table 52-3) was isolated from the skin of the frog *Bombina* in 1970.[3,8,9,10] Subsequently, two mammalian bombesin-like peptides were characterized: gastrin-releasing peptide (GRP), which is related to bombesin, and neuromedin B, which is related to amphibian ranatensin.[9] Much evidence suggests that bombesin-like peptides function as growth factors and, through autocrine or paracrine mechanisms, modulate the growth of some benign and neoplastic tissues. Bombesin can release gastrin and exert other pharmacologic effects on the gastrointestinal tract in mammals.[3,10] Bombesin-like immunoreactivity is widely distributed in mammalian brain (including the hypothalamus), lung, and gastrointestinal (GI) tract.[8,10] GRP is a 27-amino acid peptide isolated from porcine stomach.[9,10] The carboxyl-terminal decapeptide of GRP is identical to that of bombesin, except that residue number 20 in GRP is histidine instead of glutamine, found in position 7 of bombesin (see Table 52-3). GRP and GRP (14-27) possess all the biologic and immunologic activities of bombesin.[8,10] GRP is widely distributed in human fetal lung and GI tract and in rat brain, especially the hypothalamus.[8,10] Neuromedin B, isolated from the porcine spinal cord, exists both in short form (10 amino acids) and long form (32 amino acids) and has phenylalanine in the penultimate position from the C-terminus, instead of the leucine found in bombesin and GRP (see Table 52-3).

Table 52-3 Structures of Bombesin, Gastrin-Releasing Peptide, and Neuromedin B[a]

Bombesin														
pGlu -	Gln -	Arg -	Leu -	Gly -	Asn -	Gln -	Trp -	Ala -	Val -	Gly -	His -	Leu -	Met -	NH^2
1	2	3	4	5	6	7	8	9	10	11	12	13	14	
Gastrin-releasing peptide (human)														
Val -	Pro -	Leu -	Pro -	Ala -	Gly -	Gly -	Gly -	Thr -	Val -	Leu -	Thr -	Lys		
Met -	Tyr -	Pro -	Arg -	Gly -	Asn -	His -	Trp -	Ala -	Val -	Gly -	His -	Leu -	Met -	NH_2
14	15	16	17	18	19	20	21	22	23	24	25	26	27	
Neuromedin B														
Gly -	Asn -	Leu -	Trp -	Ala -	Thr -	Gly -	His -	Phe -	Met -	NH_2				
1	2	3	4	5	6	7	8	9	10					

[a]Sequence homologies relative to bombesin are underlined.

In analogs, (psi) indicates a reduced (pseudo) peptide bond ($-CH_2-NH-$).

From an oncologic point of view, the most important action of bombesin/GRP and neuromedin B is their ability to act as growth factors in tumoral tissues. The link between bombesin/GRP and small-cell lung cancer (SCLC) was discovered by Cuttitta and colleagues, who found that SCLC cells both secrete and respond to bombesin-like peptides.[96,97] Many SCLC lines express neuromedin B and its receptors.[9] Since bombesin-like peptides are produced also in other cancers, such as breast, prostatic, and pancreatic cancer, and could act as growth factors involved in tumor progression,[98,99] the development of hormonal therapy based on bombesin antagonists should be considered.[3,8,9,51,62,63,65,100]

Receptors for Bombesin/Gastrin Releasing Peptide Four receptor subtypes associated with the bombesin-like peptides have been described and cloned.[9,101] They are classified as the GRP-preferring subtype; the neuromedin B-preferring subtype; the bombesin receptor subtype 3, present in lung cancer cell lines, the natural ligand of which is not yet known; and amphibian bombesin receptor subtype 4 (BRS-4 or BB-4), which has a higher affinity for bombesin than for GRP.[101] GRP receptor subtypes bind GRP and bombesin with high affinity and neuromedin B with lower affinity. Subtypes 1 through 3 are coupled through G proteins to effectors, including phospholipase C.[9] Specific receptors for bombesin/GRP have also been demonstrated in human breast and prostate cancer biopsies[102] and in various breast and pancreatic cancer cell lines.[39,98,103] The expression of bombesin/GRP receptors may be related to malignant transformation.[104]

The activation of protein kinase C is involved in the transduction of the mitogenic signal of bombesin/GRP. Binding of bombesin/GRP to the receptors causes a rapid mobilization of Ca^{2+} from intracellular stores and an increase in the concentration of cytosolic Ca^{2+}.[9,10]

Antagonists of Bombesin/Gastrin-Related Peptide The discovery that bombesin/GRP function as autocrine growth factors for SCLC and other tumors stimulated the development of antagonists for the hormonal treatment of these malignancies. Several laboratories synthesized antagonists based on the sequence of bombesin or GRP.[65,100,106–107] In addition to SCLC, bombesin/GRP antagonists might also find application in the treatment of colorectal, gastric, pancreatic, mammary, prostatic, and other cancers.[3,51,62,63,65] Early bombesin antagonists were analogues of substance P, such as [D-Arg^1, D-Phe^5, D-Trp^{7,9}, Leu^{11}] substance P, which had relatively low potency.[3,106] More specific bombesin/GRP receptor antagonists were based on the replacement of Met-14 residue by Leu and the introduction of a reduced peptide bond between positions 13 and 14.[107] Shorter-chain nonapeptide analogues of bombesin (6-14) with reduced 13-14 peptide bond, such as D-Phe^6, Leu$^{13}\Psi(CH_2NH)$Leu^{14}-bombesin (6-14), were even more potent.[107]

Various bombesin antagonists with different modifications at positions 6, 7, and 14 were synthesized in our laboratory. D-tetrahydrocarbolinecarboxylic (D-Tpi) acid residue, a constrained structural analogue of Trp, was introduced in position 6, producing such analogues as D-Tpi^6, Leu^{13}, $\Psi(CH_2NH)$-Leu^{14}-bombesin (6-14) (RC-3095).[3,100] Bombesin/GRP antagonist RC-3095 and related analogues blocked the binding of bombesin to the receptors and suppressed the growth of various human cancer lines, such as HT-29 colon cancer; PC-82, PC-3, and DU 145 prostate cancer; MKN-45 gastric carcinoma; CFPAC-1 pancreatic cancer; H69 SCLC; and MCF-7-MIII breast cancer xenografted into nude mice.[3,8,62,63,65,100,103] The antitumor effects of RC-3095 could be linked to a significant decrease in the binding capacity of EGF receptors in these tumors.[3,62,63,65,101,103,108] Several bombesin pseudononapeptides with modified C- and N-termini such as, Hca^6, Leu^{13}, $\Psi(CH_2N)$Tac^{14}-BN(6–14) (RC-3940-II) were also synthesized,[105] which showed a greater antitumor activity than RC-3095.[108] Ongoing phase I/II clinical trials will determine the possible application of bombesin/GRP antagonists such as RC-3095 and RC-3940-II in the treatment of various cancers.

Cytotoxic Analogues of Bombesin Since receptors for bombesin-like peptides are present on a wide variety of tumors, cytotoxic bombesin octapeptide analogues, such as AN-215 containing 2-pyrrolino-doxorubicin, were developed.[36,109] AN-215 powerfully inhibited growth of H-69 SCLC, PC-3 androgen-independent prostate cancers and U-87 human glioblastomas and had a lower toxicity than the anthracycline itself.[8,36] Cytotoxic bombesin analogues might also find application in the treatment of colorectal, gastric, and pancreatic cancers. Bombesin/GRP analogs labeled with radionuclides are also being developed for cancer imaging and treatment.

ANTAGONISTS OF GROWTH HORMONE-RELEASING HORMONE

Growth hormone-releasing hormone was first isolated from human pancreatic tumors that caused acromegaly and only later from animal and human hypothalami.[7,8] Two major forms were characterized: GHRH (1-44)NH_2 and GHRH (1-40).[7,8] Virtually full intrinsic biologic activity is present in the 29 N-terminal amino acid residues (GHRH [1–29]NH_2) (Table 52-4).[7] The presence of biologically and immunologically active GHRH and mRNA for GHRH in human breast, endometrial, and ovarian cancers, SCLC, and gliomas suggests that locally produced GHRH may play a functional role in the proliferation of these tumors.[7,8] That replacement of Ala in position 2 of GHRH by D-Arg leads to antagonists was discovered by Robberecht and colleagues.[110] The GHRH antagonist [N-Ac-Tyr^1, D-Arg^2]hGHRH (1-29)NH_2 (see Table 52-4) was able to suppress GH release in rats.[7,8] We initially synthesized and tested various antagonists of hGHRH (1-29), which contained D-Arg^2, Phe(4Cl)^6, Abu^{15}, Nle^{27}, and Agm^{29} substituents, such as MZ-4-71 and MZ-5-156 (see Table 52-4), which had higher antagonistic activity in vivo.[7,111] Subsequently, we incorporated other changes and a new sequence at the C-terminus, namely, D-Arg^{28} -Har^{29} -NH_2, producing highly potent and long-acting GHRH antagonists JV-1-36 and JV-1-38 (see Table 52-4).[7,8,112] Specific antagonists of human GHRH are needed clinically for the treatment of disorders caused by the excessive secretion of growth hormone, for example, acromegaly.[7,8] However, the main applications of GHRH antagonists might be in the field of cancer.[7,8] Thus, GHRH antagonists were designed to block the binding and action of GHRH, which stimulates the secretion of GH. In turn, GH activates the production of IGF-I by the liver and other tissues.[7,8] By suppressing GH secretion, antagonists of GHRH decrease the synthesis of hepatic IGF-I[7,8] and reduce the level of IGF-I in serum. Thus, the inhibitory effects of GHRH antagonists on growth of some tumors are

Table 52-4 Growth Hormone-Releasing Hormone[a] and Its Antagonistic Analogues

GHRH (1-29)NH_2	Tyr-Ala-Asp-Ala-Ile-Phe-Thr-Asn-Ser-Tyr-Arg-Lys-Val-Leu-Gly-Gln-Leu-Ser-Ala-Arg-Lys-Leu-Leu-Gln-Asp-Ile-Met-Ser-Arg-NH_2
Standard antagonist	[Ac-Tyr^1, D-Arg^2]hGHRH(1-29)NH_2
MZ-4-71	[Ibu-Tyr^1, D-Arg^2, Phe(4CI)^6, Abu^{15}, Nle^{27}]hGHRH(1-28)Agm
MZ-5-156	[PhAc-Tyr^1, D-Arg^2, Phe(4-CI)^6, Abu^{15}, Nle^{27}]hGHRH(1-28)Agm
JV-1-36	[PhAc-Tyr^1, D-Arg^2, Phe(4-CI)^6, Arg^9, Aub^{15}, Nle^{27}, D-Arg^{28}, Har^{29}]hGHRH(1-29)NH_2
JV-1-38	[PhAc-Tyr^1, D-Arg^2, Phe(4-CI)^6, Har^9, Tyr(Me)^{10}, Abu^{15}, Nle^{27}, D-Arg^{28}, Har^{29}]hGHRH(1-29)NH_2

[a]GHRH(1-29)NH_2.

Reproduced with permission from Schally AV, Barga J.[7]

produced in part by indirect pathways through suppression of hepatic (endocrine) IGF-I secretion. IGF-I can act as an endocrine, paracrine, or autocrine growth factor for various human cancers.[8,58] The involvement of IGF-I in breast, prostate, colon, renal, and lung cancers, bone tumors, and other malignancies is well established.[7,8,58,68,73,74,76–80] The presence of receptors for IGF-I in various human tumors, including breast, lung (both SCLC and non-SCLC), colon, pancreatic, and prostate cancers, osteogenic sarcomas, and brain tumors[7,8,58,68,72–74] may be related to the malignant transformation and proliferation of these cancers.[7,8,68,72,73] GHRH antagonists appear to inhibit growth of various tumors influenced by endocrine secretion of IGF-I as well as by autocrine and/or paracrine production of IGF-I and -II. After therapy with GHRH antagonists studies showing a major reduction in tumor IGF-II concentration and IGF-II mRNA expression, parallel to tumor inhibition of renal carcinomas, prostatic, pancreatic, and colorectal cancers xenografted into nude mice, indicate direct effects.[7,8]

GHRH antagonists also exert a direct inhibitory action on tumor growth, mediated through specific GHRH receptors on tumors, by blocking the mitogenic effect of GHRH, which is produced locally by various human cancers such as endometrial, ovarian, breast, and pancreatic.[8] Hence, a wide range of cancers can be inhibited by GHRH antagonists.[8] The relative importance of these mechanisms could be different in various tumors.[8] Because GHRH antagonists inhibit IGF-II–dependent tumors, they should be superior to the GH antagonist pegvisomant, since the synthesis of IGF-II is not controlled by GH. GHRH antagonists could be useful also for suppression of tumors that do not express somatostatin receptors. Further development of GHRH antagonists should lead to new therapeutic antitumor agents.

GHRELIN

GH secretion has been assumed to be mainly regulated by GHRH, which stimulates the release, and by somatostatin, which inhibits it. Recently, however, a peptide named ghrelin was isolated from stomach of rat and human and shown to possess very high GH-releasing activity both in animals and man.[113] Ghrelin has 28-amino acids and an-octanoyl modification at Ser in position 3. This peptide appears to be the natural ligand of the GH secretagogue receptor (GHS-R), which was an "orphan" receptor. GH secretagogues, also called growth hormone-releasing peptides, are synthetic hexapeptides related to Met-enkephalin that can stimulate the release of GH from the pituitary by acting both in the hypothalamus and directly on the anterior pituitary. Ghrelin is present in human plasma at considerable levels. It is likely that this molecule, produced in and secreted from the stomach, can circulate in the bloodstream and act on the pituitary. Thus the release of GH from the pituitary might be regulated not only by hypothalamic GH-releasing hormone, but also by ghrelin derived from the stomach and hypothalamus.[113] Ghrelin appears to influence metabolism and obesity and may be involved in the growth of some neoplasms. Recently, receptors for ghrelin different from GSR-1A receptors were identified in some tumors, including human breast cancers and in breast cancer lines such as MCF-7.[115] In these cell lines, ghrelin caused a significant inhibition of cell proliferation. These findings warrant further investigations of the possible role of ghrelin in the regulation of tumor growth.

TREATMENT OF VARIOUS TUMORS WITH PEPTIDE ANALOGUES

PROSTATE CANCER Clinically Localized Prostate Cancer For the past 20 years, LHRH agonists have been used mostly for the palliative treatment of patients with advanced prostate cancer[5,8,12,13,15,17,115–122] More recently, LHRH agonists with or without antiandrogens have been used prior to or following various local treatments in patients with clinically localized prostate cancer and at high risk of disease recurrence.[123–125] The treatment options for patients with clinically localized prostate cancer (stage T1-T2N0M0) include watchful waiting, radical prostatectomy, radiation therapy, and hormonal therapy.[116,123,126] Watchful waiting (observation alone) with subsequent delayed hormonal therapy at disease progression is a reasonable choice for patients with a life expectancy of less than 10 years who present with small and well-differentiated cancers.[116,126] Potentially curative treatments such as radical prostatectomy or radiation therapy are recommended for those men who have a life expectancy of more than 10 years.[116,126] Nevertheless, the optimal primary therapy for patients with clinically localized prostate cancer still remains to be determined.[116,123–126] In some patients, especially in those at high risk of recurrence (eg, large prostate gland, high-grade tumors, positive surgical margins at prostatectomy), complete cancer control cannot be achieved with present therapies.[116,123–126] A rise in serum prostate-specific antigen (PSA) levels has been documented in a significant number of patients following various local treatments.[116,123–126] It has also been estimated that about 20% of patients receive second cancer treatment within 3 years following different primary treatments for localized prostate cancer.[125] The likelihood of receiving second treatment may be lowest in patients initially treated with radical prostatectomy.[125] In order to improve the clinical outcome of patients at greater risk of local recurrence and tumor progression, LHRH agonists alone and in combination with an antiandrogen have been used prior to or after prostatectomy.[116,123–125,127] Androgen deprivation prior to radical prostatectomy can lower the incidence of positive surgical margins, but it does not appear to increase the survival.[123] Radiation therapy for positive margins similarly does not alter survival.[123] Treatment with LHRH agonists is now recommended in men with a rising PSA level after surgery or radiotherapy. However, long-term follow-up is needed to determine the benefits of adjuvant hormonal treatment in terms of local control, disease progression, and improvement in patient survival.[116,123–126]

Locally Advanced Prostate Cancer The optimum treatment of patients with locally advanced (T3) nonmetastatic prostate cancer also remains to be established.[116,123,125–129] Cancers that have spread beyond the capsule of the prostate have a much lower chance of cure with radical prostatectomy or radiation therapy.[116,123,125,128,129] A complete tumor removal in patients with locally advanced prostate cancer is frequently not possible, and other evidence suggests that radiotherapy alone does not provide long-term control of prostate cancer.[116,123,127–129] Patients with stage T3 disease, especially those with poorly differentiated tumors, should be treated with adjuvant hormonal therapy combined with surgery or nonsurgical modalities.[116,125,127–129] A promising effect of treatment with LHRH agonist in combination with an antiandrogen flutamide prior to radical prostatectomy has been demonstrated in patients with T3 prostate cancer.[127] In addition, adjuvant therapy with LHRH agonists started at the beginning of external irradiation treatment and continued for 3 years can improve the 5-year overall survival of patients with locally advanced prostate cancer.[128]

Advanced Prostate Cancer Carcinoma of the prostate is androgen dependent in about 70% of cases.[5,8,13,116–121] Twenty to 30 percent of patients with prostate cancer already have metastatic disease when first diagnosed.[118] The management of advanced prostate cancer is palliative and is based on therapies that produce androgen deprivation.[5,8,116–122] The aim of endocrine therapy is to improve the quality of life and prolong survival.[116,118] Chronic administration of LHRH agonists, with and without an antiandrogen, or surgical removal of the testes (orchiectomy) is the standard therapy for advanced prostate cancer.[8,116,117,120–122] Approximately 70 to 80% of patients with prostate cancer achieve symptomatic and objective responses with androgen ablation.[116–121] However, all hormonal therapies aimed at androgen deprivation provide remission of only limited duration.[116–122] Androgen deprivation is associated with a decrease in libido, impotence, "hot flashes," and osteopenia.[116–121] Surgical castration has a psychologic impact, and most patients prefer the treatment with LHRH analogues.[115,116,118,119] Therapy with LHRH agonists is as effective as orchiectomy and offers the advantage of avoiding castration.[115–117] Diethylstilbestrol (DES) was used extensively in the past but caused serious cardiovascular, hepatic, and mammotropic side effects.

Use of LHRH Agonists Alone and in Combination with Antiandrogens Based on the finding of Redding and Schally in 1981 that [D-Trp[6]]LHRH inhibited the growth of transplantable rat prostatic tumors,[130] the first successful palliation with LHRH analogues in patients with advanced prostate cancer was achieved in our collaborative trial at the Royal Victoria Hospital in Montreal.[131] This demonstration that LHRH analogues were safe and effective alternatives to orchiectomy was followed by many confirmations, which have been reviewed.[5,13] However, early daily injections were inconvenient and occasionally produced compliance problems. The development of long-acting sustained-release formulations permitted injections on a monthly basis.[5,12,13,115,117,120,121]

It is now well established that chronic administration of the potent long-acting agonistic analogue of LHRH, such as leuprolide, Decapeptyl, or Zoladex, provides effective palliative therapy in patients with advanced prostate cancer.[5,13,115–118,120,121] Acceptance of LHRH analogues is excellent, and in a survey of patients with prostatic cancer who were offered a choice between orchidectomy and LHRH agonists, the analogues were selected by more than 70% of the patients as primary treatment.[115] Nevertheless, since superactive agonists of LHRH initially induce a marked release of LH, FSH, and sex steroids, some episodes of occasional temporary flare-up of the disease during the first week of administration have been reported.[15,116,132,133] The initial increase in plasma testosterone has been associated with an elevation in prostatic acid phosphatase and an increase in bone pain (flare) in 5 to 10% of patients treated for T4M/b disease.[15,116,132] The worsening of clinical symptoms during the few weeks of treatment is a concern in patients with vertebral metastases and/or urinary obstruction, which if aggravated, may lead to neurologic problems or to an increase in urinary obstruction.[116,132] Administration of antiandrogen such as flutamide, cyproterone acetate, nilutamide, or bicalutamide prior to and during early therapy with agonists can prevent disease flare-up in prostate cancer patients treated with LHRH agonists.[132,133]

The combination of orchiectomy with surgical adrenalectomy to eliminate adrenal androgens was proposed by Huggins and Scott more than 50 years ago.[117,120] The concept was that adrenal androgen may stimulate the growth of prostate tumors. Antiandrogens, which neutralize the effect of endogenous androgens, have been used for many years in the management of prostate cancer.[120] Labrie and colleagues[133] reintroduced the concept of maximal androgen blockade (MAB) and proposed combining an LHRH agonist with an antiandrogen for treating advanced prostate cancer. However, the benefits of MAB are of questionable clinical importance.[122] Although two large trials reported a significant improvement in survival with MAB,[15,120] many other trials have not shown significant benefit on meta-analysis.[117,122] In addition, complete androgen blockade may be associated with a higher toxicity rate and decreased quality of life. Thus, the data available do not support routine use of antiandrogens in combination with medical or surgical castration as first-line hormonal therapy in patients with metastatic prostate cancer.[122]

Recently, intermittent androgen suppression (IAS) with LHRH agonist and flutamide or cyproterone acetate has been introduced for treatment of advanced prostate cancer.[119] Although results of these trials confirm that IAS cycles can improve quality of life during off-treatment, the efficacy of this modality of treatment needs to be determined in randomized controlled trials.[119]

Use of LHRH Antagonists in Men with Prostate Cancer In nude mice bearing xenografts of PC-82 human prostate adenocarcinoma LHRH antagonist Cetrorelix caused a greater decrease in tumor growth, serum testosterone, and PSA levels than the agonist [D-Trp[6]]LHRH.[8,5,22]

Since 1988, we have been carrying out various clinical studies with the antagonist Cetrorelix in patients with advanced prostate cancer.[3,5,8,34,35,132] The first study indicated that a persistent inhibition of testosterone levels can be maintained in patients with advanced prostatic cancer treated with 500 μg Cetrorelix bid for several months.[5,34] After the first week of therapy, a significant decrease in bone pain, relief in urinary outflow obstruction, and reversal of the signs of prostatism were observed.[34] Subjective improvement continued during the following weeks of treatment so that the patients no longer required analgesics. The serum levels of PSA, acid, and alkaline phosphatase gradually fell, achieving nearly normal values at 6 weeks. In patients with stage C disease, there was a large decrease in prostate size as measured by ultrasonography.[34] Another study involved 36 patients with advanced prostate cancer, elevated levels of PSA, and bone pain. Group I consisted of 16 patients who received 500 μg Cetrorelix bid SC for up to 37 months.[5,22] Thirteen patients showed a clinical remission, but 5 patients relapsed later. Group II included 20 patients who received a loading dosage of Cetrorelix 5 mg bid SC for the first 2 days and thereafter 800 μg bid SC for up to 20 months. The loading dose can immediately suppress testosterone to castration levels.[22] Nineteen patients showed a clinical remission, but 3 relapsed later. We also evaluated the response to Cetrorelix in 5 patients with advanced carcinoma of the prostate and paraplegia due to metastatic compression of spinal cord or cauda equina.[132] Cetrorelix was given at dosages of 500 μg bid or 5 mg bid for 2 days and then 800 μg bid. In all patients, the neurologic symptoms regressed. The neurologic improvement continued during the treatment, and at 3 months, all the patients were able to walk with the aid of a cane. In 1 patient, myelography showed that the spinal cord compression had disappeared. Bladder function greatly improved in all 5 patients during treatment with Cetrorelix. The inhibition of gonadotropins and testosterone was maintained during the 3 months of therapy,[132] and the high levels of PSA gradually decreased by 42 to 96%. Abarelix depot was also evaluated in phase III trials because initial hormonal therapy in men with prostate cancer and a restricted new drug application was filed.[34] Overall results show that LHRH antagonists might be particularly useful for patients with prostate cancer and metastases in the brain, spine, liver, and bone marrow, in whom the LHRH agonists cannot be used as single drugs because of the possibility of flare-up.[5,132]

Relapse from Androgen Control It has been documented in thousands of patients with advanced prostate carcinomas that LHRH agonists provide effective palliative therapy resulting in objective stable disease or partial remission.[5,115–117] However, all hormonal therapies aimed at androgen deprivation, including orchiectomy, antiandrogens, LHRH analogues, and their combination, provide remissions of only limited duration. Most patients with advanced prostatic carcinoma relapse in 18 to 36 months.[5,13,115–117] The relapse is manifested clinically, radiologically, and biochemically by serially increasing serum PSA values.[135] These patients finally die, apparently of androgen-independent prostatic cancer. The molecular mechanisms implicated in the development and progression of this malignancy are incompletely understood. The relapse of prostate cancer may involve selective proliferation of clones of androgen-independent cancer cells that were present within a predominantly androgen-sensitive but heterogeneous tumor.[136] Although hormone-dependent tumor cells stop growing after androgen elimination, the testosterone-insensitive cells are capable of proliferation and eventually become predominant.[136] This topic was recently reviewed.[135]

Growth factors, including EGF, TGF-α, TGF-β, IGF-I, IGF-II, and bombesin, may play a role in the growth and progression of prostate cancer.[3,5,7,8,36,58,76,77,99,104] Several human prostate cancer cell lines were shown to secrete and respond to EGF and TGF-α.[3,8] Several studies indicate a strong and statistically positive association between serum IGF-I levels and risk of prostate cancer.[7,76,77] Receptors for EGF, IGF-I, and bombesin/GRP have been demonstrated on prostate cancer cells[7,58,104] and may be involved in neoplastic transformation. Interference with the action, secretion, signal transmission, and receptors of endogenous growth factors by somatostatin analogues, bombesin/GRP antagonists, and GHRH antagonists or by the use of cytotoxic analogues could inhibit the growth of androgen-independent prostate cancers and delay the relapse.[3,7,8] These new approaches were evaluated in experimental studies.

In nude mice bearing xenografts of the androgen-independent human prostate cancer cell lines PC-3 or DU 145, tumor growth was significantly reduced by bombesin antagonists RC-3095 and RC-3940-II, with a concomitant down-regulation of EGF receptors.[3,8] GHRH antagonists MZ-4-71, MZ-5-156, and JV-1-38 likewise suppressed growth of PC-3 and DU 145 prostate cancers, reduced serum IGF-I, and diminished the levels of IGF-II and expression of IGF-II mRNA in tumor tissue.[7,8] GHRH antagonists may inhibit the growth of androgen-independent prostate cancers by reducing hepatic secretion of IGF-I, the production of IGF-I and IGF-II by the tumor tissue and the effects of locally produced GHRH.[7,8] GHRH antagonists also enhance tumor growth inhibition induced by androgen deprivation in androgen-dependent models of prostatic cancer. Targeted cytotoxic LHRH analogue AN-152 and AN-207 inhibited the growth of LHRH receptor-positive MDA-PCa-2b, LNCaP, C4-2 and PC-82 human prostate cancer in nude mice.[11,137] In addition, we demonstrated in nude mice bearing PC-3 prostatic cancer that cytotoxic somatostatin analogue AN-238 could be targeted to human primary and metastatic prostate carcinomas that express SSTR-2 and SSTR-5.[8,138] AN-238 decreased growth of xenografted tumors, and in a metastatic model implanted orthotopically with PC-3 cells, reduced the weight of primary tumors and prevented the lymphatic spread of cancer.[138] AN-238 likewise inhibited growth of human androgen-sensitive prostate cancers and androgen-independent intraosseous tumors.[11] Targeted chemotherapy with cytotoxic bombesin analog AN-215 also suppresses proliferation of human prostate cancers in nude mice and AN-215 could benefit patients with relapsed prostate cancers.

Phase I and II trials with bombesin/GRP antagonists and cytotoxic LHRH analogs are in progress. We similarly evaluated the effects of administration of the octapeptide analog of somatostatin RC-160 Vapreotide at the time of relapse in patients with androgen-independent prostate cancer.[139] Our results indicate that therapy with the somatostatin analog Vapreotide at the time of relapse can induce a remission with a fall in serum PSA in some patients with prostate cancer who no longer respond to androgen deprivation.[139] Recently, objective clinical responses and symptomatic improvement with the combination therapy of the somatostatin analog Lanreotide, LHRH analog triptorelin (Decapeptyl) and dexamethasone in patients with relapsed metastatic prostatic cancer stage D3 have also been reported by Koutsilieris and colleagues.[140] However, experimental results suggest that cytotoxic analogs of somatostatin are likely to result in greater improvements in the clinical management of relapsed prostate cancer than those that can be produced by the octapeptide somatostatin analogs. Evaluation of various approaches aimed at delaying relapse time and prolonging survival in patients with prostate cancer who no longer respond to androgen-deprivation therapy must be continued.

Perspectives for Improvement of Therapy with Peptide Analogues LHRH agonists and antagonists that safely produce medical castration are now available.[3,5,8,22,34,132] Future clinical studies using combinations of LHRH analogues with bombesin/GRP antagonists or GHRH antagonists might reveal effective combinations of peptides that could delay the relapse. Cytotoxic peptides could be an important addition to the oncologic armamentarium since more than 80% of human prostate cancer samples express receptors for LHRH, somatostatin, and bombesin.[5,8,11,36,41,139] Experimental studies demonstrate that cytotoxic analogues can inhibit growth of tumors and their metastates and even cause tumor regression.[5,8,11,36,41,139] Targeted chemotherapy may permit an escalation of doses and improve the tumor treatment outcome.

Breast Cancer Breast cancer is the most common malignancy among American women and is responsible for about 44,000 deaths annually in the United States. Approximately 30% of unselected premenopausal patients with breast cancers have estrogen-dependent tumors and can be treated by hormonal manipulations, which include surgical oophorectomy.[5,21] The antiestrogen tamoxifen has provided a useful therapy in premenopausal women with advanced breast cancer, specifically those with ER-positive tumors.[20] Tamoxifen has shown clear benefits in postmenopausal women with breast cancer,[20] probably because of direct inhibition of the action of extraovarian estrogens on tumors,[20] and when used for chemoprevention, it was also reported to reduce the risk of breast cancer. However, tamoxifen does not completely antagonize the effect of estrogens[20] and contributes to an increase in endometrial carcinomas. Surgical oophorectomy is invasive and irreversible;[21] consequently, new approaches to produce rapid estrogen deprivation are being explored. Several antiestrogens, such as raloxifene and toremifene, are being evaluated clinically.[141] An array of aromatase inhibitors is clinically active (see Chapter 108, "Malignant Melanoma").

Experimental studies in rat and mouse models of mammary tumors showed that agonists of LHRH, by creating a state of sex steroid deficiency, would be useful for the treatment of estrogen-dependent breast cancer.[3,5,8,19] Clinical trials conducted since 1982 with Decapeptyl, Buserelin, Zoladex, or leuprolide in women with metastatic breast cancer revealed frequent objective responses in premenopausal patients with ER-positive tumors.[5,8,14,18,19,21] Responses to LHRH analogues in a small percentage (8–11%) of postmenopausal women[5,18,21,45–47] can be tentatively explained by a direct effect of LHRH agonists on tumors.[21]

At present, LHRH agonists are mainly targeted at premenopausal women with breast cancer in whom a clear suppression of ovarian estrogen can be obtained.[19] This indication is supported by recent studies. Tumor remissions after Zoladex therapy occurred primarily in about 50% of women with well-differentiated, slow-growing, ER-positive disease.[14,19] A large trial by Kaufmann and colleagues in premenopausal women with breast cancer, using depot implants of Zoladex, demonstrated 53% objective tumor responses.[16] Santen and colleagues summarized these various studies and calculated a 41% objective response rate in unselected premenopausal patients and 51% in women with ER-positive tumors.[20] Overall results suggest that "medical oophorectomy" with LHRH agonists is effective in women with estrogen-dependent breast cancers.[20,141,142]

Combination Therapy The combination of an LHRH analogue with an antiestrogen in the treatment of breast cancer might provide complete "estrogen blockade."[141,142] Recently Klijn and colleagues[142] demonstrated that the combination of LHRH agonist buserelin with tamoxifen was more effective and resulted in longer overall survival in premenopausal patients with advanced breast cancer than treatment with either drug alone. The use of aromatase inhibitors in combination with LHRH agonists has also been suggested in patients who relapse on treatment with LHRH agonists alone.[21,141] The combination of hormonal ablation based on LHRH analogues with chemotherapy is also being investigated in ER-positive disease.[141]

Future Directions: LHRH Antagonists, Somatostatin Analogues, Bombesin/GRP Antagonists, GHRH Antagonists, and Cytotoxic Peptide Analogues Growth factors such as EGF, IGF-I and -II, bombesin-like peptides, GH and GHRH may be involved in breast cancer growth.[3,7,8,58,72] IGF-I and -II, acting through IGF-I receptor, might influence growth of human breast cancers by endocrine, autocrine, or paracrine mechanisms.[7] There is a positive correlation between circulating IGF-I levels and risk of breast cancer in premenopausal women.[78] Various strategies for lowering IGF-I levels, such as tamoxifen, somatostatin analogues, and GHRH antagonists are being considered.[7,78,143] Receptors for somatostatin were found in about 30% of human breast cancer specimens.[40] Somatostatin receptor subtypes SST-2 and -5 are expressed in normal and malignant breast tissue.[87,88] The presence of receptors for somatostatin (SS-R) in human breast cancer is associated with a good prognosis.[72,75] The relapse-free survival for patients with tumors containing SS-R was significantly longer than for patients with SS-R–negative tumors; after 5 years, 82% versus 46% were disease-free.[72] Manni and colleagues showed that combined somatostatin analogue octreotide and bromocriptine therapy suppressed GH, IGF-I, and PRL secretion in postmenopausal women with advanced breast cancer,[69] but only 1 patient experienced disease stabilization. In 135 postmenopausal women with metastatic breast cancer, combination of tamoxifen and octreotide produced a greater reduction in serum IGF-I levels than tamoxifen alone but was not more efficacious therapeutically.[143]

The gene for human EGF-receptor 2 (*HER-2*), also known as *ErbB-2*, is amplified in 25 to 30% of breast cancers and in other cancers and in those cases where the encoded receptor protein is overexpressed in malignant cells.[144] A recombinant monoclonal antibody against *HER-2*, trastuzumab (Herceptin) has been developed.[144] Clinical evaluations showed that this antibody can produce responses in women with metastatic breast cancer that overexpress *HER-2*. Phase III clinical trials demonstrated that the efficacy of targeted therapy with Herceptin is increased when it is combined with chemotherapy.[144]

Another approach to *HER-2*–positive disease could be based on bombesin/GRP antagonists. Various studies demonstrate that bombesin/GRP may be involved in the function and growth of human breast cancer.[3,8,103,104] Bombesin stimulates proliferation of MCF-7-MIII and MDA-MB-231 human breast cancer lines[104] and this effect can be inhibited by bombesin/GRP antagonists. Specific receptors for bombesin/GRP have been demonstrated in 33 of 100 human breast specimens and in various human breast cancer cell lines.[103,104] Bombesin/GRP antagonists RC-3095 and RC-3940-II inhibit the growth of estrogen-dependent and independent MXT mammary cancer in mice and various human breast cancers in nude mice.[3,145] The inhibitory effect of bombesin antagonists on the growth of these breast cancers is linked with a major decrease in EGF receptor levels in tumors.[8] Inhibition of growth of estrogen-independent MDA-MB-231 breast cancers in nude mice, induced by treatment with bombesin antagonists RC-3095 and RC3940-II was also associated with a substantial reduction in the expression of mRNA for HER-2 and 3 and in the levels of HER-2- and 3 receptor proteins.[145] Bombesin receptor antagonists might be useful for therapy of ER-negative, HER-2–positive breast cancers and phase I/II clinical trials are in progress.

Antagonists of GHRH also offer a new approach to the treatment of breast cancer. Various GHRH antagonists reduced serum IGF-I levels and inhibited growth of MXT estrogen-independent mouse mammary cancers and estrogen-independent MDA-MB-468 human breast cancers xenografted into nude mice.[7] In vitro, GHRH antagonists reduced the proliferation of MDA-MB-468 cell line and IGF-II secretion. These results suggest that GHRH antagonists inhibit breast cancer growth through interference with hepatic and tumoral production of IGFs.[7]

Antagonistic analogues of LHRH, such as Cetrorelix, also await therapeutic trials in women with breast cancer to establish their clinical efficacy[5,22] Cytotoxic analogues of LHRH, such as AN-152 and AN-207, bind with high affinity to human breast cancers.[5,8,36] AN-152 and AN-207 caused a regression of MX-1 hormone-independent doxorubicin-resistant human breast cancers in nude mice.[11,36,146] We have also shown that cytotoxic LHRH analog AN-207 inhibited tumor growth and prevented metastatic disease in estrogen independent MDA-MB-231 and MDA-MB-435 human breast cancers xenografted into nude mice.[8] This suggests that targeted cytotoxic LHRH analogues such as AN-207 could be considered for treatment of LHRH receptor-positive advanced or metastatic breast cancers in women.[5,8,36,146] The effects of targeted cytotoxic somatostatin analogue (AN-238) on tumor growth were studied in nude mice with xenografts of MDA-MB-231, MX-1, and MCF-7-MIII human breast cancers.[147] Treatment with AN-238 reduced the volume of MCF-7-MIII and MDA-MB-231 tumors and caused a complete regression of MX-1 tumors in 50% of animals.[147] These results demonstrate that cytotoxic somatostatin analogue AN-238 effectively inhibits growth of human breast cancers expressing SSTR-2 and -5 and could be used in patients for receptor-targeted chemotherapy.[8,36,147]

Epithelial Ovarian Cancer Epithelial ovarian cancer is the most common cause of death from gynecologic cancer in the United States.[5,8] Treatment based on surgery, chemotherapy, and steroids is suboptimally effective, and new approaches must be explored.[5,21,148] Ovarian cancer may be dependent on LH and FSH.[3,5,21,56] Inhibition of the growth of experimental ovarian epithelial cancers, produced by LHRH analogs, may be due in part to suppression of gonadotropins.[3,5,21,148] However, some of the inhibitory effects of LHRH analogs could be direct since specific binding sites for LHRH have been found in 80% of surgically removed human ovarian carcinoma specimens as well as in OV-1063, EFO-21, and EFO-27 human ovarian cancer cell lines.[21,42,44] The expression of mRNA for LHRH and for LHRH receptors in these cell lines[53] supports the view that local LHRH-like substances may be involved in the proliferation of ovarian cancer.[44] Bombesin receptors are also widely distributed in human ovarian carcinomas, and bombesin/GRP-receptor antagonists inhibit growth of experimental ovarian cancers. IGF-I and -II, EGF, and endothelin can also influence ovarian cancers.[3,5,21,56]

Although it was initially reported that chronic treatment with [D-Trp^6]LHRH could induce the regression of advanced ovarian cancer,[21,148] no beneficial effects of therapy with microcapsules of [D-Trp^6]LHRH could be found in a large controlled trial including 200 patients with advanced ovarian cancer who received surgical cytoreduction and chemotherapy.[149] In animal studies the LHRH antagonist Cetrorelix inhibited growth of human ovarian cancers better than agonist [D-Trp^6]LHRH,[3,5,56] and therefore it was tried clinically. In phase I/II clinical trials in patients with advanced ovarian cancer after first-line chemotherapy, 3 of 17 evaluable patients showed a partial remission and 4 showed a stabilization of disease following therapy with Cetrorelix.[22] The effects of targeted cytotoxic LHRH analogues on growth of experimental ovarian cancers were also evaluated. Cytotoxic analogues AN-152 and AN-207 inhibited significantly the growth of LHRH receptor-positive OV-1063 ovarian tumors in nude mice while equivalent doses of doxorubicin and radical AN-201 were ineffective and toxic.[8,36,150] The growth of LHRH receptor-negative UCI-107 human ovarian carcinoma was not inhibited, indicating that the presence of receptors is essential for the targeted cytotoxic therapy. Cytotoxic bombesin analog AN-215 also inhibited the growth of experimental ovarian cancer. Targeted chemotherapy based on cytotoxic analogues such as AN-152 and AN-207 may improve the management of ovarian cancer. Phase I clinical trials with AN-152 are in progress.

Endometrial Carcinoma Endometrial carcinoma is the fourth most common cancer in American women.[3,21,141] Surgery or radiotherapy is successful in 75% of patients, but new methods are needed for advanced (International Federation of Gynecology and Obstetrics [FIGO] stage III or IV) or relapsed cases.[21] The involvement of estrogens in the pathogenesis of endometrial adenocarcinoma is well recognized.[3,5,21] LHRH analogues inhibit endometrial cancer by producing estrogen deprivation and through direct effect on tumors. Approximately 80% of human endometrial carcinomas show specific high-affinity membrane receptors for LHRH.[5,21] Bioactive and immunoreactive LHRH, binding sites for LHRH and the expression of mRNA for LHRH were also found in HEC-1A and Ishikawa human endometrial cancer cell lines,[5,21,44] and [D-Trp^6]LHRH and antagonist Cetrorelix significantly inhibited their proliferation.[21,44] In a phase II trial in patients with recurrent endometrial cancer, administration of depot leuprolide or goserelin led to a partial or complete remission in 6 patients (35%).[151] Phase II trials with Cetrorelix are planned. Cytotoxic LHRH analogs AN-152 and AN-207 powerfully inhibit the growth of experimental human endometrial cancers, which express LHRH receptors and might provide a new treatment modality for women with advanced endometrial carcinoma.[11] Clinical trials are in progress. GHRH antagonists can also inhibit the growth of HEC-1A human endometrial cancers xenografted into nude mice, probably through a direct effect on the tumoral GHRH receptors.

Exocrine Pancreatic Cancer Carcinoma of the pancreas has a poor prognosis, and the 5-year survival rate is about 2%.[3,8,51,58,64,70] Only 15 to 20% of tumors are resectable, and radiation and chemotherapy are of limited effectiveness.[39,51,58,70] Consequently, it is essential to develop more effective therapy. Various experimental and clinical findings indicate that the growth of exocrine pancreatic cancer may be influenced by GI hormones, growth factors such as EGF, IGF-I, IGF-II, and sex steroids.[39,51,64,66] That the growth of experimental pancreatic tumors can be inhibited by hormonal manipulations, such as the administration of analogues of LHRH and somatostatin, was first reported by Redding and Schally in 1984.[152] Attempts are being made to develop a hormonal therapy for exocrine cancer of the pancreas based on somatostatin analogues, bombesin/GRP antagonists, LHRH analogues, and GHRH antagonists.[3,7,8,36,51,58,64,66,70,98] Somatostatin analogues suppress the secretion and/or action of GI hormones (gastrin, secretin, and cholecystokinin) that might influence the growth of the malignant cells of the pancreas.[58,64] Somatostatin analogues inhibit EGF, TGF-α, and IGF-I, which appear to be involved in neoplastic processes.[3,8,66]

A marked inhibition of tumor growth was demonstrated in hamsters with BOP-induced pancreatic cancer and in nude mice bearing xenografted MIA PaCa-2, CFPAC-1, and SW-1990 human pancreatic cancer lines after treatment with somatostatin analogue RC-160, [D-Trp^6]LHRH, or antagonist Cetrorelix.[3,51,66,98] Treatment with RC-160 plus 5-fluorouracil (5-FU) also produced greater tumor inhibition than 5-FU or the analogue alone.[3,51,66]

Bombesin and GRP can influence the release of GI hormones, promote pancreatic secretion and growth, and stimulate pancreatic carcinogenesis.[39,51,98] Thus, bombesin stimulates the growth of CFPAC-1 and other human pancreatic cancer cells in vitro through high-affinity binding sites for bombesin found on these cells; this effect was inhibited by RC-3095.[98] The inhibitory effect of bombesin/GRP antagonist RC-3095 and RC-3940-II on hamster ductal pancreatic cancers was invariably linked to a major down-regulation of EGF receptors.[3,8,66] Antagonist RC-3095 and RC-3940-II also inhibited the growth of CFPAC-1, SW-1990, and other human pancreatic cancer cells transplanted into nude mice.[51,153] Our recent findings indicate that GHRH antagonists inhibit growth of experimental pancreatic cancers, likely by decreasing the production and levels of IGF-II in tumors.[7]

On the basis of experimental observations that administration of [D-Trp^6]LHRH inhibits the growth of pancreatic cancers, this analogue and Buserelin were tried clinically in patients with inoperable pancreatic cancer. The increase in survival time produced by [D-Trp^6]LHRH was small[51] and Buserelin caused no remissions. In phase I/II clinical trials, somatostatin analogue RC-160 was used as a single drug at doses of 1.5 to 6 mg/day in patients with inoperable pancreatic cancer.[51] Nearly 30% of patients showed radiologic evidence of tumor stabilization for up to 6 months, but RC-160 could not induce an effective palliation in most patients.[51] Sandostatin and other somatostatins also produced disappointing results, although Rosenberg and colleagues[70] reported that a combination of Sandostatin with tamoxifen prolonged the survival of patients with pancreatic cancer. The overall poor therapeutic results with octapeptide somatostatin analogues are likely due to the fact that in human exocrine pancreatic cancers, there is a loss of gene expression for somatostatin receptor subtype 2 (SSTR-2), which is the preferred subtype for these analogues.[8,11,81,82,154] Other studies indicate that in human pancreatic cancers, the somatostatin receptors on the cell surface may not be functional.[154] Visualization of exocrine pancreatic tumors by SST-receptor scintigraphy with ^{111}indium-DTPA-Phe^1-octreotide is difficult.[85] However, the expression of subtypes 5 (SST-5) and 3 (SST-3)[90] in pancreatic cancer should make possible therapy with cytotoxic somatostatin analogues[36,95] or somatostatin analogues labeled with various radioisotopes.[92,93]

Cytotoxic somatostatin analogues and cytotoxic bombesin analogues containing doxorubicin and/or AN-201 that can be targeted to pancreatic cancers have been shown to be effective in inhibiting growth of human pancreatic cancer lines xenografted into nude mice.[8,11,36,95,109] Such cytotoxic analogues could be considered for the study in patients with advanced pancreatic cancer who do not respond to other therapies.

Colorectal Cancer Advanced disseminated colon cancer is difficult to treat, and new treatment modalities are needed.[3,65] GI hormones, especially gastrin and bombesin/GRP; growth factors, such as EGF, IGF-I and -II, and TGF-α; and sex steroids may be involved in tumorigenesis of the colon.[3,7,58,65] IGF-I receptors were found in human colon carcinomas.[7,58,79] The incidence of colon cancer is increased in acromegalics, suggesting that excessive secretion of GH or IGF-I may be a factor.[3,7] There is an association between elevated plasma levels of IGF-I and risk of colorectal cancer.[79] Approaches based on the use of analogues of somatostatin, antagonists of GHRH or antagonists of bombesin/GRP and aimed at inhibiting GI hormones, and growth factors are being tried in colorectal cancer.[3,7,8,65] Binding sites for bombesin/GRP are found in human colon cancer cell lines, and bombesin antagonists RC-3095 and RC-3440 strongly inhibit the growth of HT-29 human colon cancers in nude mice.[65] GHRH antagonists also strongly suppress in vitro and in vivo proliferation of HT-29 colon cancers and block IGF-II production.[7,8] Somatostatin analogue RC-160 inhibits the growth of experimental human colon cancers in vivo,[3,65] and although the expression of SST-2 receptor subtype in human colorectal cancer is low, SST-5 can be used for targeting of cytotoxic somatostatin analogs.[90] The resistance of colorectal cancers to chemotherapy is related to mutations in the *TP53* tumor suppressor gene, but cytotoxic somatostatin analog AN-238 was able to suppress the growth of SST-5–containing HCT-15 and HT-29 colorectal cancers that express mutant *TP53*. GHRH antagonists, and cytotoxic somatostatin analogues could be considered for the development of new hormonal therapies of colon cancer. Recently Avastin (bevacizumab), a recombinant monoclonal antibody targeting vascular endothelial growth factor (VEGF), was reported to improve overall survival of patients with colorectal cancers when combined with standard chemotherapy.[155]

Gastric Cancer Patients with unresectable stomach cancer have a poor prognosis, and new therapeutic approaches are needed.[3] GI hormones, especially gastrin and bombesin/GRP, and growth factors such as EGF, TGF-α, and IGF-I are implicated in the growth of human gastric adenocarcinoma.[8,58,62] Somatostatin analogues such as RC-160 and Sandostatin inhibit the growth of MKN-45 human gastric cancer xenografts in nude mice.[3,62] Bombesin receptors are present in human gastric cancer as well as in MKN-45 and Hs746T gastric cancer cell lines, and bombesin stimulates the growth of Hs746T cells in vitro.[3,8,62] Bombesin/GRP antagonists inhibit the growth of MKN-45 and Hs746T human gastric cancer cells implanted in nude mice or cultured in vitro.[3,62] Cytotoxic analog AN-238 can suppress the growth of human gastric cancers that have SST-2 and SST-5 receptor subtypes.

Brain Tumors Brain tumors are responsible for about 13,000 deaths annually in the United States.[3,63,141] Therapeutic modalities glioblastomas and astrocytomas need improvement. That brain tumors are hormone sensitive is supported by much evidence.[3,8,58,63]

The presence of receptors for EGF and IGF-I and -II in human brain tumors[3,7,58,63] suggests that they may be involved in the proliferation of these tumors. Various brain tumors also contain significant levels of high-affinity receptors for somatostatin, especially SST-2 subtype[57,84–86] and receptors for bombesin/GRP.[63] Radioiodinated somatostatin analogues can label somatostatin receptors in diverse tumors in vivo, including meningiomas and astrocytomas, and can be used for tumor localization.[84,85] Investigations on the effects of peptide analogues on the growth of brain tumors demonstrated that somatostatin analogue RC-160, bombesin/GRP antagonists RC-3095 and RC-3940-II, and antagonists of GHRH inhibit the proliferation of various human glioblastomas transplanted into nude mice or cultured in vitro.[3,7,63] Recent studies show that cytotoxic somatostatin analogue AN-238 can be targeted to SST-2 receptors on experimental U-87MG human glioblastomas to produce a powerful inhibition of growth.[156] Cytotoxic bombesin analog AN-215 also suppresses growth of human glioblastomas in nude mice.[7,8,11] Merlo and colleagues[94] used intratumoral injection of ^{90}Y-labeled DOTA^0-D-Phe^1-Tyr^3-octreotide for receptor targeting in 11 glioma patients and obtained six disease stabilizations and shrinkage of a cystic low-grade astrocytoma component. Cytotoxic bombesin analogs and radiolabeled or cytotoxic somatostatin analogues could be considered for the development of new approaches to the treatment of some brain tumors.

Lung Cancer Lung cancer is the leading cause of cancer-related deaths in the United States and in the Western world.[3,8,11,108] SCLC accounts for 20 to 25% of all cases of lung cancer.[97,109] Most cases of SCLC are already metastatic at the time of diagnosis, and although chemotherapy can be used, long-term survival is infrequent.[97] The outlook for patients with advanced non-SCLC is likewise poor.[97] Therefore, new therapeutic modalities are needed for both SCLC and non-SCLC.

The development of hormonal therapy based on bombesin/GRP antagonists, GHRH antagonists, or cytotoxic analogues could be considered for SCLC.[3,7,8] SCLC can secrete bombesin-like peptides, including GRP and neuromedin B, that function like autocrine growth factors and stimulate the growth of this tumor.[96,97] GHRH could also be a growth factor in SCLC.[7,8] High-affinity receptors for bombesin-like peptides and mRNA for receptor subtypes 2 and 3 have been identified in several SCLC lines.[3,9,157] Potent bombesin/GRP antagonists that can inhibit the growth of SCLC in vivo and in vitro have been synthesized.[3,8,100,105–108] We reported that bombesin/GRP antagonists RC-3095 and RC-3940-II suppressed the growth of H-69 SCLC by decreasing the concentration of receptors for bombesin and EGF.[108]

Growth factors, such as EGF, TGF-α, and IGF-I, also appear to play a role in the proliferation and progression of lung cancer.[3,7,8,58,68,73] It has been demonstrated that several human SCLC and non-SCLC cell lines secrete and respond to IGF-I, EGF, and TGF-α through specific receptors.[3,7,8,73] High plasma levels of IGF-I are associated with an increased risk of lung cancer.[80] Somatostatin receptors are also expressed in SCLC.[89] It has been demonstrated that octreotide reduces IGF-I levels in patients with SCLC.[68] Scintigraphy with ^{111}In-pentetreotide can localize primary tumors in patients with SCLC and non-SCLC.[85,89] Treatment with cytotoxic somatostatin analog AN-238 induces a powerful inhibition of human SCLC and non-SCLC tumors in nude mice.[8,11] GHRH antagonists can inhibit the growth of both SCLC and non-SCLC xenografts in nude mice by reducing serum IGF-I levels, the concentration of IGF-I and -II in tumors,[7,8,158] and the actions of autocrine GHRH. They might find application in the treatment of a wider range of lung cancers. When cytotoxic bombesin analogue AN-215 was targeted to experimental H-69 SCLC xenografts, it also significantly suppressed tumor growth.[157] It is likely that approaches based on peptide analogues can be developed for treatment of lung cancer with markedly reduced side effects as compared with systemic chemotherapeutic agents.[3,7,89] Phase II clinical trials with bombesin antagonists are in progress.

Bone Cancers The most common primary tumors of bone and cartilage are typified by osteogenic sarcomas and chondrosarcomas.[7,8] The treatment of these sarcomas includes chemotherapy, radiotherapy, and radical surgery, but there is much room for therapeutic improvement. The growth of osteosarcomas and chondrosarcomas appears to be dependent on IGF-I or GH.[8,74] Receptors for IGF-I are present on osteosarcomas.[8,74] The proliferation of osteosarcomas in cell cultures is enhanced by IGF-I. An approach to lower IGF-I secretion based on somatostatin analogues[3,58] or antagonists of GHRH[7] might be beneficial for the treatment of osteosarcomas. However, somatostatin analogues do not adequately suppress IGF-I levels,[74] and somatostatin receptors are absent in some osteosarcomas.[74] Recent results show that GHRH antagonists inhibit the growth of human MNNG/HOS osteosarcomas and SK-ES-I Ewing's sarcomas transplanted into nude mice or cultured in vitro, possibly by interfering with the secretion of IGF-I.[7,8] The findings suggest that GHRH antagonists should be considered for study in osteosarcomas and other bone tumors.

Renal Cancer Renal cell carcinoma (RCC) is the most common malignancy of the kidney, accounting for about 85% of all renal neoplasms.[7,159] Current available therapeutic regimens have a modest impact on survival,[7,159] and new therapeutic approaches are needed. The etiology of RCC is poorly understood. Expression of the receptors for EGF, IGF-I, and somatostatin has been reported in RCC.[88] Recently, we demonstrated the inhibition of the growth of CAKI-I human renal adenocarcinoma in nude mice following therapy with LHRH antagonist Cetrorelix, somatostatin analogue RC-160, or bombesin antagonists, accompanied by a marked decrease in the number of EGF receptors.[160] Another study showed that GHRH antagonist MZ-4-71 also effectively inhibits growth of CAKI-I RCC.[7,8] This effect was linked to a reduction in serum GH and IGF-I and -II levels in tumors. The most powerful inhibition of the growth of human RCC lines and inhibition of metastases in nude mice was obtained with cytotoxic somatostatin analog AN-238.[8,11,161] Human RCC specimens and RCC cell lines also express LHRH receptors and RCC tumors are inhibited by cytotoxic LHRH analogs. These findings support further evaluation of these cytotoxic peptides for the therapy of advanced RCC.

Hepatocellular Carcinoma Hepatocellular carcinoma (HCC) is the most common type of primary hepatic carcinoma.[162] HCC is rare in the United States and Western Europe but common in Asia and Africa. The prognosis of HCC is poor, and treatment options for HCC apart from surgical resection are limited.[162] Recently, two studies reported the use of analogues of somatostatin for the treatment of HCC.[71,163] In a randomized study comprising 58 patients with advanced HCC, therapy with octreotide at a dosage of 250 μg bid increased the median survival to 13 months, compared with 4 months for the untreated patients.[71] A successful treatment of an advanced HCC with the analogue lanreotide was also described.[163] The presence of receptors for somatostatin in HCC was not clearly demonstrated, and the mechanism of action of the somatostatin analogues in HCC is not known. Additional clinical trials with octreotide and vapreotide (Octastatin) are in progress.

TUMORS PRODUCING HYPOTHALMIC HORMONES

Most somatostatinomas are malignant and the mortality rate for patients with metastatic disease is high (reviewed by Schally and colleagues[8]). It is possible that an analysis of the SST receptor subtypes in tumor samples of patients with somatostatinomas may help identify those patients who could respond to novel therapies based on somatostatin analogues linked to cytotoxic compounds or radionuclides.

Ectopic secretion of corticotropin releasing hormone (CRH) is a very rare disorder and is seen mostly in patients with well-differentiated bronchial carcinoid tumors.[8] The tumor is usually not resectable at the time of diagnosis. It is conceivable that the cytotoxic analogues of somatostatin might be useful for treating those patients with unresectable CRH or ACTH-secreting tumors whose lesions can be localized by somatostatin receptor scintigraphy.[8] The possible involvement of TRH in the pathogenesis of TSH producing tumors is not known.[8]

The prognosis for patients with GHRH-producing tumors is generally poor and the use of standard chemotherapy is generally unsuccessful. Administration of somatostatin analogues to patients with nonresectable GHRH-secreting tumors improves some of the clinical manifestations of acromegaly and reduces GH levels (reviewed by Schally and colleagues[8]). The administration of an early GHRH antagonist was also reported to reduce GH-hypersecretion in a patient with metastatic GHRH-secreting carcinoid tumor, but the effect lasted only 3 to 4 hours.[164] New generations of GHRH antagonists or cytotoxic somatostatin analogues might prove to be of benefit in patients with acromegaly due to metastatic GHRH-secreting tumors.

Gonadotroph adenomas are usually clinically nonfunctioning pituitary tumors that often cause significant morbidity (reviewed by Schally and colleagues[8]), including visual impairment, hypopituitarism, and headache. The expression of LHRH mRNA and mRNA for LHRH receptors was also detected in gonadotroph tumors. Treatment with octreotide can produce a reduction in tumor size in some patients. LHRH antagonists such as Cetrorelix might be more effective in reducing gonadotroph adenoma size before transsphenoidal surgery as well as after operation in those patients who continue to have significant residual tumor. Some hypothalamic hamartomas contain LHRH neurosecretory neurons and cause true precocious puberty. Medical therapy with the LHRH agonists and not surgery is considered the preferred approach. LHRH antagonist Cetrorelix may also prove to be useful for the management of patients with precocious puberty due to pituitary hamartomas.

REFERENCES

1. Harris GW. Neural control of the pituitary gland. London: Arnold; 1955.
2. Schally AV. Aspects of hypothalamic regulation of the pituitary gland. Science 1978;202:18–28.
3. Schally AV. Hypothalamic hormones: from neuroendocrinology to cancer therapy. Anticancer Drugs 1994;5:115–30.
4. Schally AV, Kastin AJ, Arimura A. Hypothalamic FSH and LH-regulating hormone. Structure, physiology and clinical studies. Fertil Steril 1971;22:703–21.

5. Schally AV. LHRH analogues: their impact on the control of tumorigenesis. Peptides 1999;20:1247–62.
6. Schally AV. LHRH analogues: I. their impact on reproductive medicine. Gynecol Endocrinol 1999;13:401–9.
7. Schally AV, Varga J. Antagonistic analogues of growth hormone-releasing hormone (GHRH): new potential antitumor agents. Trends Endocrinol Metab 1999;10:383–91.
8. Schally AV, Comaru-Schally AM, Nagy A, et al. Hypothalamic hormones and cancer. Front Neuroendocrinol 2001, 22:248–91.
9. Spindel ER, Giladi E, Segerson TP, Nagalla S. Bombesin-like peptides: of ligands and receptors. Recent Prog Horm Res 1993;48:365–91.
10. Sunday ME, Kaplan LM, Motoyama E, et al. Biology of disease, gastrin-releasing peptide (mammalian bombesin) gene expression in health and disease. Lab Invest 1988;59:5–24.
11. Schally AV, Nagy A. Chemotherapy targeted to cancers through tumoral hormone receptors. Trend Endocrinol Metab 2004;15:300–10.
12. Parmar H, Lightman SL, Allen L, et al. Randomised controlled study of orchidectomy vs. long-acting D-Trp-6-LHRH microcapsules in advanced prostatic carcinoma. Lancet 1985;2:1202–5.
13. Sharifi R, Soloway M. Leuprolide Study Group: clinical study of leuprolide depot formulation in the treatment of advanced prostate cancer. J Urol 1990;143:68–72.
14. Walker KJ, Walker RF, Turkes A, et al. Endocrine effects of combination anti-oestrogen and LHRH agonist therapy in premenopausal patients with advanced breast cancer. Eur J Cancer Clin Oncol 1989;25:651–4.
15. Crawford ED, Eisenberger MA, McLeod DG, et al. A controlled trial of leuprolide with and without flutamide in prostatic carcinoma. N Engl J Med 1989;321:419–24.
16. Kaufmann M, Jonat W, Kleeburg U, et al. The German Zoladex trial group: goserelin, a depot gonadotropin releasing hormone agonist in the treatment of premenopausal patients with metastatic breast cancer. J Clin Oncol 1989;7:1113–9.
17. Keuppens F, Denis L, Smith P, et al. Zoladex and flutamide versus bilateral orchiectomy. Cancer 1990;66:1045–57.
18. Manni A, Santen R, Harvey H, et al. Treatment of breast cancer with gonadotropin-releasing hormone. Endocr Rev 1986;7:89–94.
19. Nicholson RI, Walker KJ, Walker RF, et al. Review of the endocrine actions of LHRH analogues in premenopausal women in breast cancer. Horm Res 1989;32:198–224.
20. Santen RJ, Manni A, Harvey H, Redmond C. Endocrine treatment of breast cancer in women. Endocr Rev 1990;11:221–65.
21. Emons G, Schally AV. The use of luteinizing hormone releasing hormone agonists and antagonists in gynecological cancers. Hum Reprod 1994;9:1364–79.
22. Reissmann T, Schally AV, Bouchard P, et al. The LHRH-antagonist Cetrotide® (Cetrorelix). A review. Hum Reprod 2000, 6:322–31.
23. Karten MJ, Rivier JE. Gonadotropin-releasing hormone analogue design. Structure-function studies toward the development of agonists and antagonists: rationale and perspective. Endocr Rev 1986;7:44–66.
24. Bajusz S, Csernus VJ, Janaky T, et al. New antagonists of LHRH: II. Inhibition and potentiation of LHRH by closely related analogues. Int J Pept Protein Res 1988;32:425–35.
25. Ljungqvist A, Feng DM, Hook W, et al. Antide and related antagonists of luteinizing hormone release with long action and oral activity. Proc Natl Acad Sci U S A 1988;85:8236–40.
26. Rivier JE, Porter J, Rivier CL, et al. New effective gonadotropin releasing hormone antagonists with minimal potency for histamine release in vitro. J Med Chem 1986;29:1846–51.
27. Jiang G, Miller C, Koerber SC, et al. Betidamino acid scan of the GnRH antagonist Acyline. J Med Chem 1997;40:3739–48.
28. Nelson LR, Fujimoto VY, Jaffe RB, Monroe SE. Suppression of follicular phase pituitary-gonadal function by a potent new gonadotropin-releasing hormone antagonist with reduced histamine-releasing properties (Ganirelix). Fertil Steril 1995;63:963–9.
29. Molineaux CJ, Sluss PM, Bree MP, et al. Suppression of plasma gonadotropins by Abarelix: a potent new LHRH antagonist. Mol Urol 1998;2:265–8.
30. Gonzalez-Barcena D, Vadillo-Buenfil M, Garcia Procel E, et al. Inhibition of luteinizing hormone, follicle-stimulating hormone and sex steroid levels in men and women with a potent antagonist analogue of luteinizing hormone-releasing hormone, Cetrorelix (SB-75). Eur J Endocrinol 1994;131:286–92.
31. Behre HM, Klein B, Steinmeyer E, et al. Effective suppression of luteinizing hormone and testosterone by single doses of the new gonadotropin-releasing hormone antagonist Cetrorelix (SB-75) in normal men. J Clin Endocrinol Metab 1992;75:393–398.
32. Klingmuller D, Schepke M, Enzweiler C, Bidlingmaier F. Hormonal responses to the new potent GnRH antagonist Cetrorelix. Acta Endocrinol 1993;128:15–8.
33. Leroy I, d'Acremont MF, Brailly-Tabard S, et al. A single injection of a gonadotropin-releasing hormone (GnRH) antagonist (Cetrorelix) postpones the luteinizing hormone (LH) surge: further evidence for the role of GnRH during the LH surge. Fertil Steril 1994;62:461–7.
34. Gonzalez-Barcena D, Vadillo-Buenfil M, Gomez Orta F, et al. Responses to the antagonistic analogue of LHRH (SB-75) (Cetrorelix) in patients with benign prostatic hyperplasia and prostatic cancer. Prostate 1994;24:84–92.
35. Comaru-Schally AM, Brannan W, Schally AV, et al. Efficacy and safety of luteinizing hormone-releasing hormone antagonist Cetrorelix in the treatment of symptomatic benign prostatic hyperplasia. J Clin Endocrinol Metab 1998;83:3826–31.
36. Schally AV, Nagy A. Cancer chemotherapy based on targeting of cytotoxic peptide conjugates to their receptors on tumors. Eur J Endocrinol 1999;140:1–14.
37. Nagy A, Schally AV, Armatis P, et al. Cytotoxic analogs of luteinizing hormone-releasing hormone containing doxorubicin or 2-pyrrolinodoxorubicin, a derivative 500–1000 times more potent. Proc Natl Acad Sci U S A 1996;93:7269–73.
38. Hawes BE, Conn PM. Assessment of the role of G proteins and inositol phosphate production in the action of gonadotropin-releasing hormone. Clin Chem 1993;39:325–32.
39. Redding TW, Schally AV. Inhibition of prostate tumor growth in two rat models by chronic administration of D-Trp-6-LHRH. Proc Natl Acad Sci U S A 1981;78:6509–12.
40. Fekete M, Wittliff JL, Schally AV. Characteristics and distribution of receptors for [D-Trp6]-luteinizing hormone-releasing hormone, somatostatin, epidermal growth factor, and sex steroids in 500 biopsy samples of human breast cancer. J Clin Lab Anal 1989;3:137–47.
41. Halmos G, Arencibia JM, Schally AV, et al. High incidence of receptors for luteinizing hormone-releasing hormone (LHRH) and LHRH receptor gene expression in human prostate cancers. J Urol 2000;103:623–9.
42. Srkalovic G, Schally AV, Wittliff JL, et al. Presence and characteristics of receptors for [D-Trp^6]-luteinizing hormone-releasing hormone and epidermal growth factor in human ovarian cancer. Int J Oncol 1998;12:489–98.
43. Pinski J, Lamharzi N, Halmos G, et al. Chronic administration of luteinizing hormone-releasing hormone (LHRH) antagonist Cetrorelix decreases gonadotrope responsiveness and pituitary LHRH receptor messenger ribonucleic acid levels in rats. Endocrinology 1996;137:3430–6.
44. Emons G, Ortmann O, Schulz K-D, Schally AV. Growth-inhibitory actions of analogues of luteinizing hormone releasing hormone on tumor cells. Trends Endocrinol Metab 1997;8:355–62.
45. Harris AL, Carmichael J, Cantwell BMJ, Dowsett M. Zoladex endocrine and therapeutic effects in post-menopausal breast cancer. Br J Cancer 1989;59:97–9.
46. Plowman PN, Nicholson RI, Walker KJ. Remission of postmenopausal breast cancer during treatment with the luteinizing hormone releasing hormone agonist ICI 118630. Br J Cancer 1986;54:903–9.
47. Saphner T, Troxel AB, Tormey DC, et al. Phase II study of goserelin for patients with postmenopausal metastatic breast cancer. J Clin Oncol 1993;11:1529–35.
48. Limonta P, Dondi D, Moretti RM, et al. Antiproliferative effects of luteinizing hormone-releasing hormone agonists on the human prostatic cancer cell line LNCaP. J Clin Endocrinol Metab 1992;75:207–12.
49. Eidne KA, Fanagan CA, Harris NS, Millar RP. Gonadotropin-releasing hormone (GnRH)-binding sites in human breast cancer cell lines and inhibitory effects of GnRH antagonists. J Clin Endocrinol Metab 1987;64:425–32.
50. Miller WR, Scott WN, Morris R, et al. Growth of human breast cancer cells inhibited by a luteinizing hormone-releasing hormone agonist. Nature 1985;313:231–3.
51. Schally AV, Szepeshazi K, Qin Y, et al. Antitumor effects of analogues of somatostatin and antagonists of bombesin/GRP in experimental models of pancreatic cancer. Int J Pancreatol 1994;16:246–9.
52. Harris NS, Dutlow C, Eidne K, et al. Gonadotropin-releasing hormone gene expression in MDA-MB-231 and ZR-75-1 breast carcinoma cell lines. Cancer Res 1991;51:2577–81.
53. Irmer G, Bürger C, Müller R, et al. Expression of the messenger ribonucleic acids for luteinizing hormone-releasing hormone and its receptor in human ovarian epithelial carcinoma. Cancer Res 1995;55:817–22.
54. Limonta P, Dondi D, Moretti RM, et al. Expression of luteinizing hormone-releasing hormone mRNA in the human prostatic cancer cell line LNCaP. J Clin Endocrinol Metab 1993;76:797–800.
55. Sharoni Y, Bosin E, Miinster A, et al. Inhibition of growth of human mammary tumor cells by potent antagonists of luteinizing hormone-releasing hormone. Proc Natl Acad Sci U S A 1989;86:1648–51.
56. Yano T, Pinski J, Halmos G, et al. Inhibition of growth of OV-1063 human epithelial ovarian cancer xenografts in nude mice by treatment with luteinizing hormone-releasing hormone antagonist SB-75. Proc Natl Acad Sci U S A 1994;91:7090–4.
57. Lamberts SWJ. The role of somatostatin and its analogues in the diagnosis and treatment of tumors. Endocr Rev 1991;12:450–82.
58. Schally AV. Oncological application of somatostatin analogues. Cancer Res 1988;48:6977–85.
59. Bauer W, Briner U, Doepfner W, et al. SMS-201-995. A very potent and selective octapeptide analogue of somatostatin with prolonged action. Life Sci 1982;31:1133–40.
60. Cai R-Z, Szoke B, Lu R, et al. Synthesis and biological activity of highly potent octapeptide analogues of somatostatin. Proc Natl Acad Sci U S A 1986;83:1896–900.
61. Veber DF, Freidinger RM, Schwenk-Perlow D, et al. A potent cyclic hexapeptide analogue of somatostatin. Nature 1981;292:55–8.
62. Pinski J, Halmos G, Yano T, et al. Inhibition of growth of MKN45 human gastric-carcinoma xenografts in nude mice by treatment with bombesin/gastrin-releasing-peptide antagonist (RC-3095) and somatostatin analogue RC-160. Int J Cancer 1994;57:574–80.
63. Pinski J, Schally AV, Halmos G, et al. Somatostatin analogues and bombesin/gastrin-releasing peptide antagonist RC-3095 inhibit the growth of human glioblastomas in vitro and in vivo. Cancer Res 1994;54:5895–901.
64. Radulovic S, Comaru-Schally AM, Milovanovic S, Schally AV. Somatostatin analogue RC-160 and LHRH antagonist SB-75 inhibit growth of MIA PaCa-2 human pancreatic cancer xenografts in nude mice. Pancreas 1993;8:88–97.
65. Radulovic S, Schally AV, Reile H, et al. Inhibitory effects of antagonists of bombesin/gastrin-releasing peptide (GRP) and somatostatin analogue (RC-160) on growth of HT-29 human colon cancers in nude mice. Acta Oncol 1994;33:693–701.
66. Szepeshazi K, Halmos G, Schally AV, et al. Growth inhibition of experimental pancreatic cancers and sustained reduction in epidermal growth factor receptors during therapy with hormonal peptide analogues. J Cancer Res Clin Oncol 1999;125:444–52.
67. Kvols LD, Moertel CG, O'Connell MJ, et al. Treatment of the malignant carcinoid syndrome. N Engl J Med 1986;315:663–6.
68. Macaulay VM, Smith LE, Everard MJ, et al. Experimental and clinical studies with somatostatin analogue octreotide in small cell lung cancer. Br J Cancer 1991;64:451–6.
69. Manni A, Boucher AE, Demers LM, et al. Endocrine effects of combined somatostatin analogue and bromocriptine therapy in women with advanced breast cancer. Breast Cancer Res Treat 1989;14:289–98.
70. Rosenberg L, Barkun AN, Denis MH, Pollak M. Low dose octreotide and tamoxifen in the treatment of adenocarcinoma of the pancreas. Cancer 1995;75:23–8.
71. Kouroumalis E, Skordilis P, Thermos K, et al. Treatment of hepatocellular carcinoma with octreotide: a randomised controlled study. Gut 1998;42:442–7.
72. Foekens JA, Portengen H, van Putten WLJ, et al. Prognostic value of receptors for insulin-like growth factor 1, somatostatin, and epidermal growth factor in human breast cancer. Cancer Res 1989;49:7002–9.
73. Macaulay VM, Everard MJ, Teale D, et al. Autocrine function of insulin-like growth factor I in human small cell lung cancer cell lines and fresh tumor cells. Cancer Res 1990;50:2511–7.
74. Pollak M, Polychronakos C, Richard M. IGF-I is a potent mitogen for human osteogenic sarcoma. J Natl Cancer Inst 1990;82:301–5.
75. Reubi JC, Torhorst J. The relationship between somatostatin, epidermal growth factor, and steroid hormone receptors in breast cancer. Cancer 1989;64:1254–60.

76. Chan JM, Stampfer MJ, Giovannucci E, et al. Plasma insulin-like growth factor-I and prostate cancer risk: a prospective study. Science 1998;279:563–6.
77. Wolk A, Mantzoros CS, Andersson SO, et al. Insulin-like growth factor-I and prostate cancer risk: a population-based, case-control study. J Natl Cancer Inst 1998;90:911–5.
78. Hankinson SE, Willett WC, Colditz GA, et al. Circulating concentrations of insulin-like growth factor-I and risk of breast cancer. Lancet 1998;351;1393–6.
79. Ma J, Pollak MN, Giovannucci E, et al. Prospective study of colorectal cancer risk in men and plasma levels of insulin-like growth factor (IGF)-I and IGF-binding protein-3. J Natl Cancer Inst 1999;91:620–5.
80. Yu H, Spitz MR, Mistry J, et al. Plasma levels of insulin-like growth factor-I and lung cancer risk: a case-control analysis. J Natl Cancer Inst 1999;91:151–6.
81. Buscail L, Delesque N, Estève JP, et al. Stimulation of tyrosine phosphatase and inhibition of cell proliferation by somatostatin analogues: mediation by human somatostatin receptor subtypes SSTR1 and SSTR2. Proc Natl Acad Sci U S A 1994;91:2315–9.
82. Buscail L, Estève JP, Saint-Laurent N, et al. Inhibition of cell proliferation by the somatostatin analogue RC-160 is mediated by SSTR2 and SSTR5 somatostatin receptor subtypes through different mechanisms. Proc Natl Acad Sci U S A 1995;92:1580–4.
83. Liebow C, Reilly C, Serrano M, Schally AV. Somatostatin analogues inhibit growth of pancreatic cancer by stimulating tyrosine phosphatase. Proc Natl Acad Sci U S A 1989;86:2003–7.
84. Krenning EP, Breeman WAP, Kooij PPM, et al. Localisation of endocrine-related tumors with radioiodinated analogue of somatostatin. Lancet 1989;1:242–4.
85. Krenning EP, Kwekkeboom DJ, Bakker WH, et al. Somatostatin receptor scintigraphy with [^{111}In-DTPA-D-Phe^{1}]- and [^{123}I-Tyr^{3}]-octreotide: the Rotterdam experience with more than 1000 patients. Eur J Nucl Med 1993;20:716–31.
86. Reubi JC, Maurer R, Klijn JGM, et al. High incidence of somatostatin receptors in human meningiomas: biochemical characterization. J Clin Endocrinol Metab 1986;63:433–8.
87. Evans AA, Crook T, Laws SAM, et al. Analysis of somatostatin receptor subtype mRNA expression in human breast cancer. Br J Cancer 1997;75:798–803.
88. Vikic-Topic S, Raisch KP, Kvols LK, Vuk-Pavlovic S. Expression of somatostatin receptor subtypes in breast carcinoma, carcinoid tumor, and renal cell carcinoma. J Clin Endocrinol Metab 1995;80:2974–9.
89. O'Byrne KJ, Halmos G, Pinski J, et al. Somatostatin receptor expression in lung cancer. Eur J Cancer 1994;30A:1682–7.
90. Lewis I, Bauer W, Albert R, et al. A novel somatostatin mimic with broad somatotropin release inhibitory factor receptor binding and superior therapeutic potential. J Med Chem 2003;46:2334–44.
91. Lamberts SWJ, Hofland LJ, van Koetsveld PM, et al. Parallel in vivo and in vitro detection of functional somatostatin receptors in human endocrine pancreatic tumors: consequences with regard to diagnosis, localization and therapy. J Clin Endocrinol Metab 1990;71:566–74.
92. Otte A, Mueller-Brand J, Dellas S, et al. Yttrium-90-labelled somatostatin-analogue for cancer treatment. Lancet 1998;351:417–8.
93. McCarthy KE, Woltering EA, Espenan GD, et al. In situ radiotherapy with ^{111}In-pentetreotide: initial observations and future directions. Cancer J Sci Am 1998;4:94–102.
94. Merlo A, Hausmann O, Wasner M, et al. Locoregional regulatory peptide receptor targeting with the diffusible somatostatin analogue ^{90}Y-labeled DOTA^{0}-D-Phe^{1}-Tyr^{3}-octreotide (DOTATOC): a pilot study in human gliomas. Clin Cancer Res 1999;5:1025–33.
95. Nagy A, Schally AV, Halmos G, et al. Synthesis and biological evaluation of cytotoxic analogs of somatostatin containing doxorubicin or its intensely potent derivative, 2-pyrrolinodoxorubicin. Proc Natl Acad Sci U S A 1998;95:1794–9.
96. Cuttitta F, Carney DN, Mulshine JW, et al. Bombesin-like peptides can function as autocrine growth factors in human small cell lung cancer. Nature 1985;316:823–6.
97. Minna JD. Neoplasms of the lung. In: Braunwald E, Isselbacher KJ, Petersdorf RG, editors. Harrison's principles of internal medicine. 11th ed. New York: McGraw-Hill; 1987. p. 1115–23.
98. Wang QJ, Knezetic JA, Schally AV, et al. Bombesin may stimulate proliferation of human pancreatic cancer cells through an autocrine pathway. Int J Cancer 1996;68:1–7.
99. Aprikian AG, Han K, Guy L, et al. Neuroendocrine differentiation and the bombesin/gastrin-releasing peptide family of neuropeptides in the progression of human prostate cancer. Prostate 1998;8:52–61.
100. Radulovic S, Cai R-Z, Serfozo P, et al. Biological effects and receptor binding affinities of new pseudononapeptide bombesin/GRP receptor antagonists with N-terminal D-Trp or D-Tpi. Int J Pept Protein Res 1991;38:593–600.
101. Nagalla SR, Barry BJ, Creswick KC, et al. Cloning of a receptor for amphibian [Phe^{13}] bombesin distinct from the receptor for gastrin-releasing peptide: identification of a fourth bombesin receptor subtype (BB4). Proc Natl Acad Sci U S A 1995;92:6205–9.
102. Halmos G, Wittliff JL, Schally AV. Characterization of bombesin/GRP receptors in human breast cancer and their relationship to steroid receptor expression. Cancer Res 1995;53:280–7.
103. Yano T, Pinski T, Groot K, Schally AV. Stimulation by bombesin and inhibition by bombesin/gastrin-releasing peptide antagonist RC-3095 of growth of human breast cancer cell lines. Cancer Res 1992;52:4545–7.
104. Markwalder R, Reubi JC. Gastrin-releasing peptide receptors in the human prostate: relation to neoplastic transformation. Cancer Res 1999;59:1152–9.
105. Cai R-Z, Reile H, Armatis P, Schally AV. Potent bombesin antagonists with C-terminal Leu $c(CH_2N)$-Tac-NH_2 or its derivatives. Proc Natl Acad Sci U S A 1994;91:12664–8.
106. Langdon S, Seithi T, Ritchie A, et al. Broad spectrum neuropeptide antagonists inhibit the growth of small cell lung cancer in vivo. Cancer Res 1992;52:4554–7.
107. Coy DH, Taylor JE, Jiang N-Y, et al. Short-chain pseudopeptide bombesin receptor antagonists with enhanced binding affinities for pancreatic acinar and Swiss 3T3 cells display strong antimitotic activity. J Biol Chem 1989;264:14691–7.
108. Koppan M, Halmos G, Arencibia JM, et al. Bombesin/gastrin-releasing peptide antagonists RC-3095 and RC-3940-II inhibit tumor growth and decrease the levels and mRNA expression of epidermal growth factor receptors in H-69 small cell lung carcinoma. Cancer 1998;83:1335–43.
109. Nagy A, Armatis P, Cai R-Z, et al. Design, synthesis, and in vitro evaluation of cytotoxic analogs of bombesin-like peptides containing doxorubicin or its intensely potent derivative, 2-pyrrolinodoxorubicin. Proc Natl Acad Sci U S A 1997;94:652–6.
110. Robberecht P, Coy DH, Waelbroeck M, et al. Structural requirements for the activation of rat anterior pituitary adenylate cyclase by growth hormone-releasing factor (GRF): discovery of (N-Ac-Tyr^{1}, D-Arg^{2})-GRF (1-29)-NH_2 as a GRF antagonist on membranes. Endocrinology 1985;117:1759–64.
111. Zarandi M, Horvath JE, Halmos G, et al. Synthesis and biological activities of highly potent antagonist of growth hormone-releasing hormone. Proc Natl Acad Sci U S A 1994;91:12298–303.
112. Varga JL, Schally AV, Horvath JE, et al. Increased activity of antagonists of growth hormone-releasing hormone substituted at positions 8, 9 and 10. Proc Natl Acad Sci 2004;101:1708–13.
113. Kojima M, Hosod H, Date Y, et al. Ghrelin is a growth hormone releasing acylated peptide from stomach. Nature 1999;402:656–60.
114. Cassoni P, Papotti M, Ghe C, et al. Identification, characterization and biological activity of specific receptors for natural (ghrelin) and synthetic growth hormone secretagogues and analogs in human breast carcinomas and cell lines. J Clin Endocrinol Metab 2001;86:1738–45.
115. Crawford DE. Hormonal therapy of prostatic carcinoma. Defining the challenge. Oncology 1990;66:1035–8.
116. Oh WK, Hurwitz M, D'Amico AV, et al. Neoplasms of the prostate. In: Holland JF, Frei E III, Bast RC, et al, editors. Cancer Medicine 5. Hamilton (ON): BC Decker; 2000. p. 1559–88.
117. Prostate Cancer Trialists' Collaborative Group. Maximum androgen blockade in advanced prostate cancer: an overview of 22 randomized trials with 3283 deaths in 5710 patients. Lancet 1995;346:265–9.
118. Rosendahl I, Kiebert GM, Curran D, et al. Quality-adjusted survival (Q-TWiST) analysis of EORTC trial 30853: comparing goserelin acetate and flutamide with bilateral orchiectomy in patients with metastatic prostate cancer. Prostate 1999;38:100–9.
119. Theyer G, Hamilton G. Current status of intermittent androgen suppression in the treatment of prostate cancer. Urology 1998;52:353–9.
120. Denis LJ, Carneiro de Moura JL, Bono A, et al. Goserelin acetate and flutamide versus bilateral orchiectomy: a phase III EORTC trial (30853). Urology 1993;42:119–30.
121. Eisenberger MA, Crawford ED, Wolf M, et al. Prognostic factors in stage D2 prostate cancer: important implications for future trials: results of a Cooperative Intergroup study (INT .0036). Semin Oncol 1994;21:613–9.
122. Laufer M, Denmeade SR, Sinibaldi VJ, et al. Complete androgen blockade for prostate cancer: what went wrong? J Urol 2000;164:3–9.
123. Soloway MS, Sharifi R, Wajsman Z, et al. Randomized prospective study comparing radical prostatectomy alone versus radical prostatectomy preceded by androgen blockade in clinical stage B2 (T2bNxM0) prostate cancer. J Urol 1995;154:424–8.
124. Bourdin S, Karam G, Clemain P, et al. Clinical experience with leuprorelin acetate before radiotherapy for prostatic cancer. J Int Med Res 1990;18 Suppl 1:74–8.
125. Grossfeld GD, Stier DM, Flanders SC, et al. Use of second treatment following definitive local therapy for prostate cancer: data from the caPSURE database. J Urol 1998;160:1398–404.
126. Steinberg GD, Bales GT, Brendler CB. An analysis of watchful waiting for clinically localized prostate cancer. J Urol 1998;159:1431–6.
127. Schulman CC. Neoadjuvant androgen blockade prior to prostatectomy: a retrospective study and critical review. Prostate Suppl 1994;5:9–14.
128. Bolla M, Gonzalez D, Warde P, et al. Improved survival in patients with locally advanced prostate cancer treated with radiotherapy and goserelin. N Engl J Med 1997;337:295–300.
129. van den Ouden D, Hop WCJ, Schroder FH. Progression in and survival of patients with locally advanced prostate cancer (T3) treated with radical prostatectomy as monotherapy. J Urol 1998;160:1392–7.
130. Redding TW, Schally AV. Inhibition of prostate tumor growth in two rat models by chronic administration of D-Trp-6-LH-RH. Proc Natl Acad Sci U S A 1981;78:6509–12.
131. Tolis G, Ackman D, Stellos A, et al. Tumor growth inhibition in patients with prostatic carcinoma treated with luteinizing hormone-releasing agonists. Proc Natl Acad Sci U S A 1982;79:1658–62.
132. Gonzalez-Barcena B, Vadillo-Buenfil M, Cortez-Morales A, et al. LH-RH antagonist SB-75 (cetrorelix) as primary single therapy in patients with advanced prostatic cancer and paraplegia due to metastatic invasion of spinal cord. Urology 1995;45:275–81.
133. Labrie F, Dupont A, Belanger A, Lachance R. Flutamide eliminates the risk of disease flare in prostatic cancer patients treated with a luteinizing hormone-releasing hormone agonist. J Urol 1987;138:804–6.
134. Trachtenberg J, Gittleman M, Steidle C, et al. A phase 3, multicenter, open label, randomized study of abarelix versus leuprolide plus daily antiandrogen in men with prostate cancer. J Urol. 2002;167:1670–4.
135. Oh WK, Kantoff PW. Management of hormone refractory prostate cancer: current standards and future prospects. J Urol 1998;160:1220–9.
136. Isaacs JT. The timing of androgen ablation therapy and/or chemotherapy in the treatment of prostatic cancer. Prostate 1984;5:1–17.
137. Plonowski A, Schally AV, Nagy A, et al. Inhibition of in vivo proliferation of MDA-PCa-2b human prostate cancer by a targeted cytotoxic analog of luteinizing hormone-releasing hormone AN-207. Cancer Lett 2002;176:57–63.
138. Plonowski A, Schally AV, Nagy A, et al. Inhibition of PC-3 human androgen-independent prostate cancer and its metastases by cytotoxic somatostatin analog AN-238. Cancer Res 1999;59:1947–53.
139. Gonzales-Barcena D, Schally AV, Vadillo-Buenfil M, et al. Response of patients with advanced prostatic cancer to administration of somatostatin analog RC-160 (vapreotide) at the time of relapse. The Prostate 2003;56:183–91.
140. Koutsilieris M, Mitsiades C, Dimopoulos T, et al. A combination therapy of dexamethasone and somatostatin analog reintroduces objective clinical responses to LH-RH analog in androgen ablation-refractory prostate cancer patients. J Clin Endocrinol Metab 2001;86:5729–36.
141. Vogel CL. Hormonal approaches to breast cancer treatment and prevention: an overview. Semin Oncol 1996;23 Suppl 9:2–9.
142. Klijn JG, Beex LV, Mauriac L, et al. Combined treatment with buserelin and tamoxifen in premenopausal meta-

static breast cancer: a randomized study. J Natl Cancer Inst 2000;92:903–11.

143. Ingle JN, Suman VJ, Kardinal CG, et al. A randomized trial of tamoxifen alone or combined with octreotide in the treatment of women with metastatic breast carcinoma. Cancer 1999;85:1284–92.

144. Slamon DJ, Leyland-Jones B, Shak S, et al. Use of chemotherapy plus a monoclonal antibody against *HER2* for metastatic breast cancer that overexpresses *HER2.* N Engl J Med 2001;344:783–92.

145. Bajo AM, Schally AV, Krupa M, et al. Bombesin antagonists inhibit growth of MDA-MB-435 estrogen independent breast cancers and decrease the expression of ErbB-2/HER-2 oncoprotein and c-*jun* and c-*fos* oncogenes Proc Nat Acad Sci U S A 2002;99:3836–41.

146. Kahan Z, Nagy A, Schally AV, et al. Complete regression of MX-1 human breast cancer xenografts after targeted chemotherapy with a cytotoxic analog of luteinizing hormone-releasing hormone AN-207. Cancer 1999;85:2608–15.

147. Kahan Z, Nagy A, Schally AV, et al. Inhibition of growth of MX-1, MCF-7-MIII and MDA-MB-231 human breast cancer xenografts after administration of a targeted cytotoxic analog of somatostatin, AN-238. Int J Cancer 1999;82:592–8.

148. Parmar H, Phillips RH, Rustin G, et al. Therapy of advanced ovarian cancer with D-Trp^{6}-LH-RH (Decapeptyl) microcapsules. Biomed Pharmacother 1988;42:531–8.

149. Emons G, Ortmann O, Tiechert HM, et al. Luteinizing hormone-releasing hormone agonist triptorelin in combination with cytotoxic chemotherapy in patients with advanced ovarian carcinoma: a prospective double blind randomized trial. Cancer 1996;78:1452–60.

150. Miyazaki M, Schally AV, Nagy A, et al. Targeted cytotoxic analog of luteinizing hormone-releasing hormone AN-207 inhibits growth of OV-1063 human epithelial ovarian cancers in nude mice. Am J Obstet Gynecol 1999;180:1095–103.

151. Gallagher CJ, Oliver RTD, Oram DH, et al. A new treatment for endometrial cancer with gonadotrophin-releasing hormone analogue. Br J Obstet Gynaecol 1991;98:1037–41.

152. Redding TW, Schally AV. Inhibition of growth of pancreatic carcinomas in animal models by analogs of hypothalamic hormones. Proc Natl Acad Sci U S A 1984;81:248–52.

153. Qin Y, Ertl T, Cai R-Z, et al. Antagonists of bombesin/gastrin releasing peptide inhibit growth of SW-1990 human pancreatic adenocarcinoma and production of cyclic AMP. Int J Cancer 1995;63:257–62.

154. Fisher WE, Doran TA, Muscarella P II, et al. Expression of somatostatin receptor subtype 1-5 genes in human pancreatic cancer. J Natl Cancer Inst 1998;90:332–4.

155. McCarthy M. Antiangiogenesis drug promising for metastatic colorectal cancer. Lancet 2003;361:1959.

156. Kiaris H, Schally AV, Nagy A, et al. Regression of U-87MG human glioblastomas in nude mice after treatment with a cytotoxic somatostatin analog AN-238. Clin Cancer Res 2000;6:709–17.

157. Kiaris H, Schally AV, Nagy A, et al. Targeted cytotoxic analog of bombesin/gastrin-releasing peptide inhibits the growth of H-69 human small cell lung carcinoma in nude mice. Br J Cancer 1999;81:966–71.

158. Pinski J, Schally AV, Jungwirth A, et al. Inhibition of growth of human small-cell and non–small-cell lung carcinomas by antagonists of growth hormone-releasing hormone (GH-RH). Int J Oncol 1996;9:1099–105.

159. Motzer RJ, Bander NH, Nanus DM. Renal cell carcinoma. N Engl J Med 1996;335:865–75.

160. Jungwirth A, Schally AV, Halmos G, et al. Inhibition of the growth of Caki-I human renal adenocarcinoma in vivo by luteinizing hormone-releasing hormone antagonist Cetrorelix, somatostatin analog RC-160, and bombesin antagonist RCC-3940-II. Cancer 1998;82:909–17.

161. Plonowski A, Schally AV, Nagy A, et al. Inhibition of metastatic renal cell carcinomas expressing somatostatin receptors by a targeted cytotoxic analog of somatostatin AN-238. Cancer Res 2000;60:2996–3001.

162. Fried MW. Treatment of hepatocellular carcinoma: medical options. Liver Transplant Surg 1998;4:592–7.

163. Raderer M, Hejna MHL, Kurtaran A, et al. Successful treatment of an advanced hepatocellular carcinoma with the long acting somatostatin analog lanreotide. Am J Gastroenterol 1999;94:278–9.

164. Jaffe CA, DeMott-Friberg R, Frohman LA, Barkan AL. Suppression of growth hormone (GH) hypersecretion due to ectopic GH-releasing hormone (GH-RH) by a selective GH-RH antagonist. J Clin Endocrinol Metab 1997;82:634–7.

53

Corticosteroids

Lorraine I. McKay, PhD
John A. Cidlowski, PhD

HORMONES OF THE ADRENAL CORTEX

The history of corticosteroid biology began over 150 years ago and is well documented in a number of reviews (for example, see Munck[1] for a complete description). This chapter will briefly summarize the history of corticosteroid biology, chemistry, and clinical use. It will also review the pharmacology and physiology of these hormones and their analogs and discuss their use in the treatment of neoplasms. Finally, it will present the currently understood mechanism of action of corticosteroids in the context of their therapeutic efficacy, and it will touch on current efforts to dissociate efficacy from the deleterious side effects of corticosteroids.

In 1849, Addison observed that a lack of functional adrenal glands is fatal. Subsequent research categorized the effects of adrenal insufficiency into those due to electrolyte imbalance and those due to altered carbohydrate metabolism. From that time through the first half of the twentieth century, understanding of adrenal function expanded, with Cushing's identification of hypercorticalism in 1932, followed by the identification of adrenocorticotropic hormone (ACTH) from the anterior pituitary and its description as a regulator of the adrenal cortex. Several bioactive steroids, including cortisol and aldosterone, were isolated from the adrenal cortex and characterized. In 1949, Hench first reported the efficacy of cortisol and ACTH in the treatment of rheumatoid arthritis, an observation that set in motion a burgeoning application of these "miracle drugs" for a wide variety of inflammatory diseases. Intense investigation of these compounds was spurred by this widespread clinical interest, and in the subsequent decade, most of the biochemistry of the synthesis and metabolism of adrenocortical steroids was elucidated.[1] The field of corticosteroid therapy rapidly advanced at this time, with the development of the majority of currently available synthetic corticosteroid analogs as well as identification of practical methods for plasma cortisol determination.[2]

Since the 1950s, corticosteroid analogs that separate anti-inflammatory and electrolyte balance effects have been developed. However, despite continual effort, clinically meaningful separation of efficacy from side effects has proven elusive. Consequently, use of these powerful drugs is limited by their slow, cumulative side-effect profile. Damage associated with chronic corticosteroid therapy may not become apparent until the consequences are catastrophic.[2]

Adrenal Anatomy and Secreted Steroids

There are three zones of the adrenal cortex: the zonae glomerulosa, fasciculata, and reticularis. Aldosterone is synthesized in the outermost zona glomerulosa, a region of the adrenal cortex regulated primarily by circulating sodium, potassium, and angiotensin. Cortisol and corticosterone are produced by the inner zonae fasciculata and reticularis, regions of the adrenal regulated by ACTH released from the anterior pituitary.

Although five classes of steroid hormones are produced in the adrenal cortex (glucocorticoids, mineralocorticoids, progestins, androgens, and estrogens), the amount of progestin, androgen, and estrogen produced by the adrenal is a minor fraction of the total amount of these steroids produced in the body. By contrast, glucocorticoids and mineralocorticoids are produced almost exclusively in the adrenal cortex. Glucocorticoids (in humans the primary glucocorticoid is cortisol, in rodents, corticosterone) have a broad physiologic role that includes both regulation of glucose metabolic pathways and modulation of the immune system. Mineralocorticoids (aldosterone is the major bioactive mineralocorticoid in humans) are key regulators of mineral and water balance.

Biosynthetic Pathways Corticosteroid biosynthesis has been well characterized, and is presented in simplified form in Figure 53-1. Cholesterol, the precursor to all steroid biosynthetic pathways, is converted to a variety of steroid molecules in a series of reactions catalyzed by several cytochrome P-450 (cyp 450) enzymes. Although some cholesterol can be synthesized within the adrenal cortex, the vast majority of cholesterol used in steroid biosynthesis is taken up from a pool of circulating cholesterol bound to low-density lipoproteins in the plasma. After synthesis, corticosteroids are rapidly secreted. Because corticosteroids are not stored in the adrenal cortex, the rate of secretion from the adrenal gland reflects the rate of steroid synthesis.

CONTROL OF CORTICOSTEROID SECRETION

Glucocorticoids ACTH, a peptide hormone synthesized and secreted by the corticotrophs (basophilic cells) of the anterior pituitary gland, maintains the adrenal glands and controls the rate of corticosteroid synthesis. The three zones of the adrenal cortex are regulated by ACTH to varying extents. Elevated ACTH can result in adrenocortical hypertrophy and sustained high output of cortisol and corticosterone, whereas ACTH deficiency results in adrenocortical atrophy and reduced secretion of glucocorticoids. Aldosterone levels are not significantly affected by ACTH, because the zona glomerulosa is relatively unresponsive to ACTH.

ACTH, like other peptide hormones, functions through G-protein–coupled receptors (GPCR). ACTH binding and activation of cognate GPCRs in the adrenal cell membrane increases intracellular levels of cyclic adenosine monophosphate (cAMP) and other second messengers, which increases the rate of conversion of cholesterol to pregnenolone (the first step in the steroid biosynthetic pathway) and consequently increases the synthesis and secretion of steroid hormones.[3] ACTH regulates the conversion of cholesterol to pregnenolone in two ways: by increasing the synthesis of the cyp 450 side chain cleavage enzyme,[4,5] and by increasing the number of low-density lipoprotein (LDL) receptors that provide the cholesterol substrate of the enzyme.[6]

ACTH secretion from the pituitary is regulated by corticotropin-releasing factor (CRF), secreted by the median eminence of the hypothalamus in response to neural signals. CRF, which reaches the pituitary via a vascular connection with the hypothalamus, induces synthesis and release of the ACTH precursor molecule pro-opiomelanocortin (POMC). POMC is cleaved into ACTH and other bioactive peptides including β-endorphin and β-lipotropin before secretion by the corticotrophs. Glucocorticoids negatively feed back on ACTH levels both at the level of the hypothalamus and the pituitary.[7] They suppress the synthesis of POMC, decrease stores of ACTH in secretory granules, and at high levels can cause degeneration of the corticotrophs. In adrenalectomized or Addison's disease patients, glucocorticoid levels are low and ACTH remains high. However, ACTH levels can still be increased by CRF, demonstrating that ACTH remains under control of the nervous system in the absence of negative feedback. In addition to endocrine feedback loops, the hypothalamic-pituitary-adrenal (HPA) axis is subject to immune regulation via the action of cytokines (eg, interleukins 1β and 6, tumor necrosis factor-α, and interferons α and γ), which regulate POMC expression, CRF secretion and function, and function of the adrenal cortex.

Plasma cortisol levels fluctuate, with 7 to 13 spontaneous increases in the rate of cortisol secretion per day.[8] Although irregular, these

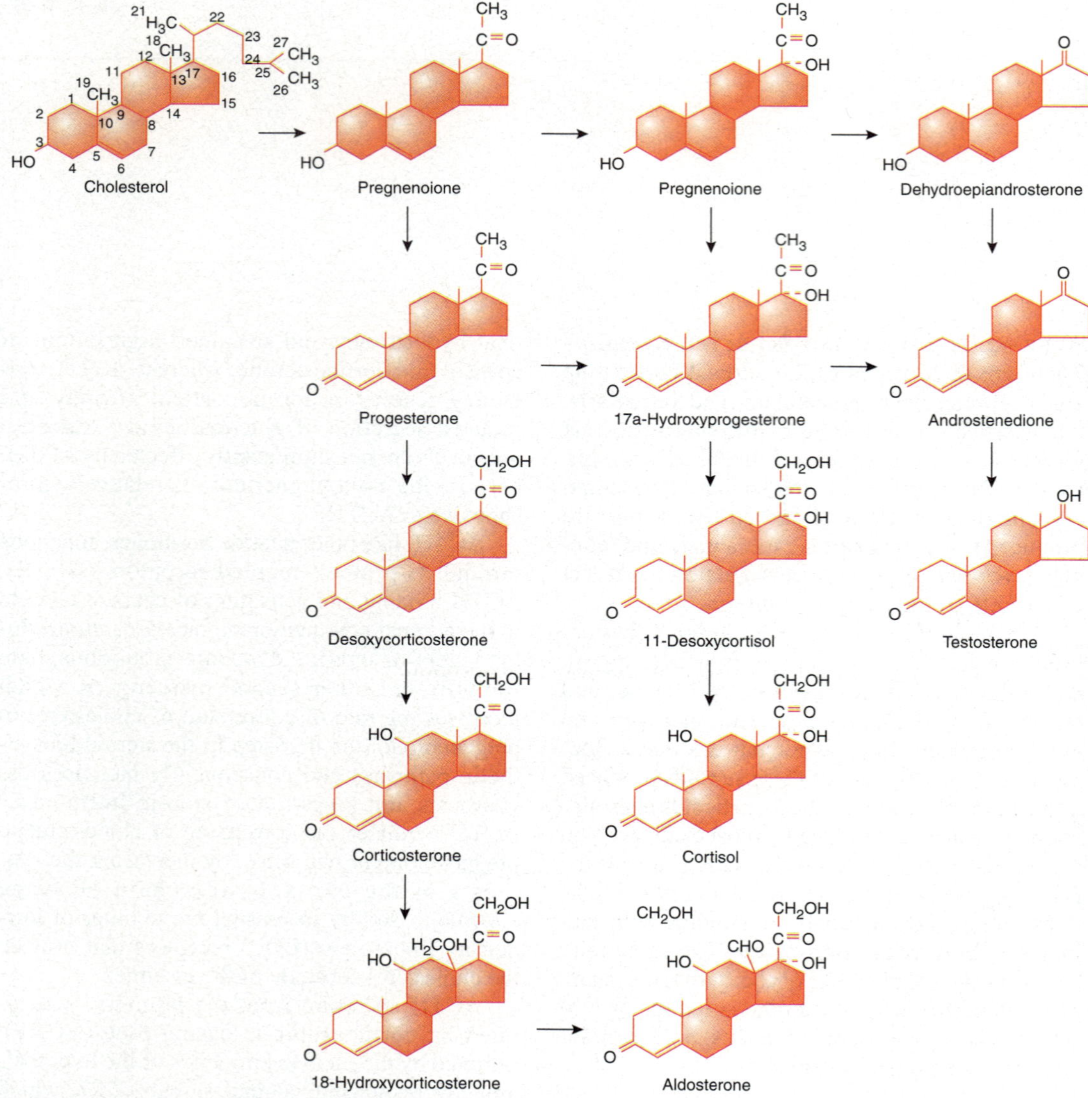

Figure 53-1 Principal pathways of adrenocorticosteroid biosynthesis. (Reproduced with permission from Haynes RC Jr and Murad F.[110])

changes occur in reproducible pattern, with a consistent slope of rise in secretion rate for any given person. The average slope of rise in secretion is 50 mg/min, with a semi-log decay in cortisol peaks that indicates an on/off mechanism of spontaneous secretion. The total amount of cortisol secreted each day is largely determined by the number of episodes of high secretion that occur, and not by the rate of secretion. The spontaneous rhythm of secretion results in a nadir of plasma cortisol 1 to 2 hours after the onset of sleep, followed by a rise to maximal levels upon awakening and a drop in plasma cortisol over the course of the day. This secretion pattern is due to intrinsic hypothalamic function and is not subject to negative feedback by glucocorticoids. Although the mechanism of the rhythm is unclear, the major factors that influence the pattern are the timing of sleep, feeding, and light exposure.

Stress (physical or psychological) is a key regulator of the production of ACTH and the secretion of adrenal steroids, with the magnitude of the adrenal response in direct proportion to the intensity of the stress.[9] If the sensory connections that mediate stressful stimuli are blocked, the adrenal response does not occur.[10] Glucocorticoid exposure before stress can dampen the stress response due to negative feedback on the HPA axis.[11]

Mineralocorticoids The major physiologic regulator of aldosterone levels is the renin-angiotensin system.[12] Renin, synthesized in the kidney, converts angiotensinogen to angiotensin I (AT I). The AT I peptide is subsequently converted to the active peptide angiotensin II (AT II) and its bioactive degradation products AT III and AT IV, by the action of angiotensin-converting enzymes (ACE). AT II (and probably AT III and AT IV) stimulates aldosterone biosynthesis through interaction with GPCRs in the zona glomerulosa, a process regulated by a variety of factors including plasma potassium level, intracellular calcium, and release of nitric oxide (NO) and atrial natriuretic peptide.[13] AT II also increases peripheral arterial resistance, which results in increased blood pressure.[14] Changes in blood pressure then feed back on the secretion of renin, a process regulated by the interaction of kidney baroreceptors, renal nerves, NO synthesis, and the balance of calcium, potassium, and sodium in the serum.[15]

Sodium and potassium levels are an additional modulator of mineralocorticoid synthesis. Increased serum potassium acts directly on the adrenal gland, up-regulating early steps in adrenal steroid biosynthesis and resulting in increased aldosterone secretion. Low serum sodium can also increase aldosterone secretion, but this mechanism does not appear to be a major contributor to mineralocorticoid secretion, because serum sodium concentration changes little with changes in total blood volume.

PHARMACOKINETICS OF CORTICOSTEROIDS

Rate of Secretion Cortisol is secreted at a rate of 15 to 20 mg/day in men (in women, the rate is about 10% lower),[16] while corticosterone is secreted at a rate of 4 mg/day. ACTH stimulation can increase corticosterone secretion to 40 mg/d. The two main mineralocorticoids, aldosterone and deoxycorticosterone, are secreted at the rates of 50 to 200 and 16 to 40 mg/d, respectively.

Metabolism Corticosteroids are metabolized through enzymatic transformations that diminish their physiologic activity and increase water solubility to enhance their urinary excretion.[17] Most of the serum cortisol is reduced to dihydrocortisol, followed by conversion to tetrahydrocortisol, which is then conjugated to glucuronic acid. Approximately 10% of cortisol is converted to the 17-ketosteroid, which is then conjugated to sulfate. Circulating aldosterone is converted to the tetrahydroglucuronide derivative. Corticosteroid metabolism occurs primarily in the liver, and certain diseases of the liver result in elevated free hormone due to decreased corticosteroid metabolism and a reduction in serum steroid-binding proteins.

Plasma Clearance The plasma clearance of cortisol is rapid, with a half-life of 66 minutes at normal hormone levels.[8] With large steroid loads, the half-life increases to 120 minutes. The volume of distribution (VD) changes in a similar fashion, with a VD of 10 L under normal conditions and a VD that can be greater than total body water with large steroid loads. Corticosterone turns over even more rapidly than cortisol, and the clearance rates of both steroids are unaffected by acute stress or adrenal insufficiency. The plasma half-life of aldosterone is less than 20 minutes.

Excretion Cortisol excretion in urine is relatively low (100 μg/d), because 80 to 90% of filtered cortisol is reabsorbed from the distal tubule of the kidney.[18] In contrast, conjugated metabolites are filtered and excreted with no reabsorption. More than 90% of secreted glucocorticoid is ultimately excreted in urine. Less than 10% of secreted aldosterone appears in the urine in the free form. The majority is excreted as glucuronide derivatives.

Transport in Blood Most of the circulating cortisol is bound to liver-derived corticosteroid binding globulin (CBG) or albumin, with only a small amount in free form. At normal plasma levels, (a relatively constant 40 mg/L or 0.8 μmol) CBG binds about 70% of plasma cortisol (14 μg/dL). However, plasma CBG levels are dynamically regulated. For example, during pregnancy, plasma levels of CBG rise dramatically, while acute stresses, such as burn injury or sepsis, can lead to dramatic decreases in plasma CBG. Cortisol binds to CBG with high affinity (kDa 2.4×10^{-7} M; half-life of steroid binding = 5 days). Other steroids, including progesterone, prednisolone, and aldosterone, can compete for binding sites on CBG, and high levels of one steroid will displace the others. For example, therapeutic levels of prednisone displace 35% of CBG-bound cortisol. Many synthetic glucocorticoids, including dexamethasone, do not bind CBG. Albumin circulates in plasma at a concentration of 40 g/L (0.5 to 0.6 mmol) and has low affinity for cortisol (kDa 5×10^{-5} M). Only 20% of plasma cortisol is bound to albumin. At low serum cortisol levels, most of the cortisol is bound to CBG. However, the binding capacity of CBG is saturated at a cortisol concentration of 28 μg/dL, a level that is frequently exceeded in stressed patients. With elevations in plasma cortisol, there is an increased proportion of albumin-bound and free cortisol, whereas the amount of CBG-bound cortisol remains constant. The concentration of free cortisol is 1 μg/dL at a normal total plasma cortisol of 20 μg/dL, although this value can rise to as high as 15 to 50 μg/dL after ACTH stimulation. Free cortisol is considered to be the active form and because there is a rapid equilibration between the bound and free fractions of cortisol, the bound fraction acts as a reservoir. Thus, increases in plasma CBG, such as occur during pregnancy, can greatly increase the amount of cortisol reserves available at a constant rate of synthesis, whereas short-term decreases in plasma CBG during acute stress can significantly increase the pool of free cortisol. That total plasma cortisol falls below 5 μg/dL at night exemplifies how rapidly cortisol can leave the plasma. Aldosterone does not have a specific binding protein, but binds weakly to albumin. A normal plasma aldosterone level is 0.006 μg/dL (0.17 nmol). Other steroids with mineralocorticoid activity, such as corticosterone and 11-deoxycorticosterone, do bind CBG. CBG-bound corticosteroids are resistant to metabolism.

Table 53-1 Relative Potencies and Equivalent Doses of Corticosteroids

Anti-Inflammatory Compound	Relative Potency	Relative Sodium-Retaining Potency	Duration of Action*	Approximate Equivalent Dose† (mg)
Cortisol	1	1	S	20
Cortisone	0.8	0.8	S	25
Corticosterone	0.4	15	S	—
Fludrocortisone	10	125	S	—
Prednisone	4	0.8	I	5
Prednisolone	4	0.8	I	5
6a-methylprednisolone	5	0.5	I	4
Triamcinolone	5	0	I	4
Paramethasone	10	0	L	2
Betamethasone	25	0	L	0.75
Dexamethasone	25	0	L	0.75
Deoxycorticosterone	0.2	100	—	—
Aldosterone	0.3	3000	—	—

*I = intermediate or 12- to 36-h biologic half-life; L = long or 36- to 72-h biologic half-life; S = short or 8- to 12-h biologic half-life.

†These dose relationships apply only to oral or intravenous administration; relative potencies may differ greatly when injected intramuscularly or into joint spaces. From Haynes RC Jr and Murad F.[110]

STEROID SYNTHESIS INHIBITORS

Several inhibitors of steroid biosynthesis are used clinically to treat hypercorticism. One category of inhibitors block the 11β-hydroxylation of steroids, terminating synthesis after the formation of the cortisol precursor 11-deoxycortisol and therefore resulting in decreased cortisol, aldosterone, and androgen with accumulation of upstream pathway components such as pregnenolone and 11β-deoxycortisol. Under such conditions, sodium balance is maintained by the mineralocorticoid activity of 11-deoxycortisone. Ketoconazole is effective as monotherapy and considered to be the most effective and best tolerated of the 11β-hydroxylase inhibitors. It also directly antagonizes the glucocorticoid receptor and may directly inhibit ACTH release. Although metyrapone also inhibits 11-β hydroxylase, there is often a compensatory ACTH secretion that can necessitate increasing doses of the drug. Mitotane selectively destroys adrenocortical cells by accumulating in the cell membrane and damaging membrane ion transporters, and it causes a rapid decrease in plasma corticosteroid levels. Aminoglutethimide inhibits the conversion of cholesterol to 20α-hydroxycholesterol, blocking synthesis of cortisol, aldosterone, and other classes of steroid hormones such as estrogens. Aminoglutethimide is sometimes used as monotherapy for hypercorticism, but its use as an inhibitor of estrogen synthesis has been largely displaced by aromatase inhibitors, which are more potent and specific for blocking estrogen production and do not create the need for corticosteroid replacement.[19]

PHARMACEUTICAL DERIVATIVES

The molecular structure of steroid hormones is a critical determinant of their activities. Structure–activity relationships of steroids have driven the synthesis of a myriad of cortisol analogs with varying potencies that effectively separate the glucocorticoid and mineralocorticoid activities of the natural corticosteroids. This has made synthetic glucocorticoids clinically useful, even though it has not yet been possible to separate glucocorticoid activity from the toxic side effects of these molecules to a clinically meaningful extent. Table 53-1 lists some of the available natural and synthetic corticosteroids with their relative ratio of specificity and equivalent doses. Corticosteroids are absorbed readily from the gastrointestinal tract. Water-soluble esters are given intravenously (IV) to achieve absorption rapidly, while intramuscular injection provides more prolonged effects. Corticosteroids are also well absorbed from several sites of topical application, and large doses can lead to systemic absorption.

Patient-to-patient variations in corticosteroid absorption, plasma protein binding, and clearance rates exist. There is wide interpatient variability in the free fraction of synthetic steroids at comparable total plasma concentrations. There is also variability in patient sensitivity to generation of Cushing's-like symptoms. These differing sensitivities are reflected in different plasma corticosteroid concentrations, suggestive of pituitary resistance to corticosteroid feedback. Differences in the pharmacokinetics of glucocorticoids between men, women, and children should also be considered when designing therapeutic regimens.[20]

PHYSIOLOGIC AND PHARMACOLOGIC EFFECTS OF CORTICOSTEROIDS

Corticosteroids are key regulators of whole-body homeostasis that provide an organism with the capacity to resist environmental changes and invasion of foreign substances. The effects of corticosteroids are broad, including profound alterations in carbohydrate, protein, and lipid metabolism, and the modulation of electrolyte and water balance. Corticosteroids affect all of the major systems of the body, including the cardiovascular, musculoskeletal, nervous, and immune systems, and play critical roles in fetal development, including the maturation of the fetal lung. Because so many systems are corticosteroid responsive, tight regulatory control is exerted on the system. Direct corticosteroid effects are sometimes difficult to separate from their complex relationship with other hormones, in part due to the permissive action of low levels of corticosteroid on the effectiveness of other hormones, including catecholamines and glucagon. Nevertheless, the effects of corticosteroids can be classified into two general categories: glucocorticoid (intermediary metabolism, inflammation, immunity, wound healing, myocardial, and muscle integrity) and mineralocorticoid (salt, water, and mineral metabolism). Although the following section discusses the separate effects of glucocorticoids and mineralocorticoids, it must be emphasized that natural steroids possess both glucocorticoid and mineralocorticoid activity. The ratio between the two activities ranges from all glucocorticoid and almost no mineralocorticoid activity (cortisol) to all mineralocorticoid and almost no glucocorticoid activity (aldosterone).

Intermediary Metabolism Glucocorticoids stimulate the conversion of protein to carbohydrate through gluconeogenesis and promote the storage of carbohydrate as glycogen. The increase in urinary nitrogen after an increase in glucocorticoids is the result of amino acid mobilization from protein and its subsequent breakdown as a source of carbon during gluconeogenesis. Adrenalectomized animals are able to function normally as long as food (ie, free amino acids) is available. Upon starvation, however, these animals cannot mobilize amino acids from muscle or serum protein, elucidating a role for cortisol mobilization.[21] Glucocorticoids stimulate the process of hepatic gluconeogenesis, resulting in elevated plasma glucose, which leads to deposition of liver glycogen. Increased hepatic gluconeogenesis/glycogenesis is due to direct effects of glucocorticoids on the hepatic expression of genes that code for enzymes required for glucose and glycogen biosynthesis. Prolonged exposure to glucocorticoids leads to a diabetic-like state due to the increase in plasma glucose and a decreased insulin sensitivity, while low glucocorticoid concentrations lead to hypoglycemia, decreased glycogen stores, and hypersensitivity to insulin. Glucocorticoids also decrease facilitated uptake of glucose in peripheral tissues to provide more glucose for glycogen formation in the liver. This effect is particularly prevalent in leukocytes and may be a major contributing factor to the rapid elevation in blood glucose after steroid administration. The complex mechanisms for the peripheral effects of glucocorticoids are still unclear, but chronic administration can result in the atrophy of lymphatic tissue and muscle, osteoporosis, and thinning of the skin.

Glucocorticoids are closely involved with lipid metabolism and our understanding of the nature and mechanisms of these lipid effects is still growing. One well established lipid effect is glucocorticoid facilitation of lipolytic agents: mobilization of fat from peripheral depots by epinephrine and other lipolytics is severely blunted in the absence of glucocorticoids, because they facilitate the response of adipocytes to the rise in cAMP induced by these lipolytics.[22] Sustained glucocorticoid excess results in a redistribution of body fat from the periphery to a more central pattern of deposition, resulting in the characteristic "cushingoid" fat distribution: excess fat in the upper trunk and face, with very little fat in the extremities. The mechanism for this paradoxical effect on body fat is not well understood, but there may be differences in the number of glucocorticoid receptors in different types of fat cells, so that cells with fewer receptors are less responsive to glucocorticoid regulation of glucose transport. Glucose and triglyceride accumulation would occur in low-GR cells in response to a rise in insulin levels, while adipocytes with higher levels of receptor (perhaps in the periphery) would respond to the high glucocorticoid level by decreasing glucose uptake and would not accumulate triglycerides. Recent investigation into the metabolic syndrome has suggested another mechanism for glucocorticoid effects on fat distribution. Metabolic syndrome is characterized by insulin resistance, hyperlipidemia, diabetes, and a fat distribution comparable to that of Cushing's disease, but without elevated plasma cortisol or an HPA axis disruption. Recent studies suggest that the enzyme 11-β hydroxysteroid dehydrogenase type 1 (11β HSD1) amplifies the concentration of active glucocorticoid by 11-ketoreduction of inactive steroids in tissues where it is expressed, thus creating local hypercorticism in the context of normal plasma cortisol regulation. Such a mechanism could also explain different glucocorticoid sensitivities in different adipocyte populations.[23]

Electrolyte and Water Balance The major function of mineralocorticoids is the regulation of electrolyte balance and blood pressure. Aldosterone increases sodium reabsorption and excretion of potassium and hydrogen in the renal tubule. Mineralocorticoid excess causes positive sodium balance, increased extracellular fluid volume, normal or slightly high plasma sodium, hypokalemia, and alkalosis. Hypocorticism results in renal loss of sodium, hyponatremia, hyperkalemia, and a decrease in extracellular fluid volume and cellular hydration. The 1% decrease in sodium reabsorption that occurs in hypocorticism is enough to cause profound cardiovascular changes, resulting in circulatory collapse, renal failure, and ultimately, death. Aldosterone modulates sodium levels by activating mineralocorticoid receptors (MR) in the kidney distal tubules, increasing aprical membrane permeability of the cells lining the cortical collecting tube. There is also evidence for a rapid, non-genomic up-regulation of sodium-hydrogen exchange by aldosterone that may be modulated by a membrane-bound MR. Aldosterone also increases sodium/potassium ATPase activity in the serosal membrane. These changes increase sodium reabsorption and generate a higher negative potential in the lumen, which is the driving force for increased potassium and hydrogen excretion. Mineralocorticoids also increase calcium and magnesium excretion, probably due to volume expansion. Prolonged aldosterone treatment results in sodium "escaping," a cessation of sodium changes, with a continued potassium and hydrogen loss. The mechanism for this effect is unknown but may involve MR down-regulation and consequent mineralocorticoid insensitivity.

Glucocorticoid effects on the kidney differ from mineralocorticoid effects. Glucocorticoids increase water diuresis, glomerular filtration rate, and renal plasma flow. Cortisol increases sodium retention and potassium excretion, without an increase in hydrogen excretion. The major renal complications of glucocorticoid therapy are nephrocalcinosis, nephrolithiasis, and increased stone formation as a result of increased urinary calcium and uric acid.

Electrolyte changes in response to mineralocorticoid treatment also occur in the gastrointestinal mucosa, salivary and sweat glands, and exocrine pancreas. In these tissues, a longer onset period is required to detect significant responses to aldosterone, and no sodium "escape" occurs after prolonged hormone administration. In the intestine, aldosterone does not cause changes in intestinal electrolyte absorption, but glucocorticoids increase sodium and water absorption and potassium secretion. Both glucocorticoid and mineralocorticoid receptors are present in the mucosa, and dexamethasone can bind to both receptor types whereas aldosterone can only bind to its own receptor. Cortisol also increases gastric acid secretion and blood flow to the gastric mucosa, while decreasing the rate of gastric cell proliferation. High doses of glucocorticoids may cause peptic ulceration or aggravate preexisting ulcers (for a complete review of mineralocorticoid biology, see Argawal and Mirshashi[24]).

Endocrine System Corticosteroids have multiple effects on endocrine homeostasis in addition to modulation of ACTH secretion. Cortisol increases growth hormone secretion in patients with acromegaly, while spontaneous secretion of growth hormone is inhibited in hypercorticism. Growth failure in children with prolonged glucocorticoid treatment is apparently a result of decreased epiphyseal plate maturation and long-bone growth.[25] Corticosteroids depress the secretion of thyroid-stimulating hormone in patients with myxedema[26] and reduce the physiologic effectiveness of thyroxine. High doses of steroid decrease luteinizing hormone release in response to luteinizing hormone-releasing hormone,[25] potentiate the adrenergic effects of catecholamines, and stimulate the synthesis of epinephrine. Other systemic effects of high doses of glucocorticoids include adrenocortical insufficiency upon glucocorticoid removal, steroid-induced diabetes, hyperlipidemia, elevated glucagon, and hypocalcemia.[27]

Cardiovascular System The major cardiovascular effects of corticosteroids are related to their regulation of epinephrine, angiotensin, plasma volume, and electrolyte retention, which act in concert to maintain normal blood pressure and cardiac output. However, hypotension induced by hypocorticism is not solely due to these factors. Corticosteroids also impact on myocardial responsiveness, arteriolar tone, and capillary permeability; hypocorticism increases capillary permeability, diminishes vasomotor response, and decreases cardiac output and cardiac size. Hypercorticism results in chronic arterial hypertension caused by sustained excessive sodium retention, a mineralocorticoid-specific effect.[28] Aldosterone affects ion transport in the vascular smooth muscle and the central nervous system,[29] possibly altering sympathetic output by influencing the periventricular area of the hypothalamus, where information about cardiovascular status, and electrolyte and fluid balance are integrated. Hypertension can also be induced by glucocorticoids, although the mechanism for this response is not well defined. Glucocorticoids influence many factors that modulate blood pressure: they influence kidney function by increasing filtration fraction and glomerular hypertension, as well as the synthesis of angiotensinogen and atrial natriuretic peptide. They decrease prostaglandin synthesis, thereby decreasing vasodilation, and simultaneously increase responsiveness to vasopressors. They modulate vascular tone by decreasing expression of calcium-activated potassium channels, and there is evidence that glucocorticoids potentiate atherosclerosis and thromboembolic complications.[30]

Musculoskeletal System Normal corticosteroid levels are required for muscle maintenance, but corticosteroid imbalance can lead to myopathies. Elevated aldosterone causes muscle weakness because of hypokalemia, while high glucocorticoid levels cause muscle wasting due to increased protein catabolism. Hypocorticism results in decreased work capacity of striated muscle, weakness, and fatigue. This response reflects an inadequacy of the circulatory system rather than electrolyte and carbohydrate imbalances.

Chronic glucocorticoid administration results in osteoporosis, a serious limiting factor in the clinical use of steroids. Glucocorticoid-induced bone loss is a multifaceted process. Glucocorticoids reduce bone remodeling by directly modulating osteoclast, osteoblast, and osteocyte function and lifespan. They increase renal calcium excretion and decrease gastrointestinal calcium absorption, resulting in reduced serum calcium. Parathyroid hormone (PTH), a stimulator of osteoclasts, is elevated in response to reduced serum calcium. Glucocorticoids also increase PTH sensitivity. Other effects of high doses of glucocorticoids on the musculoskeletal system include aseptic or avascular necrosis of bone and spontaneous tendon rupture, due to increased collagen metabolism.[31]

Central Nervous System Corticosteroids affect the nervous system indirectly by maintaining plasma glucose levels, adequate circulation, and normal electrolyte levels. Direct effects of corticosteroids on the central nervous system occur, but are not well defined. Corticosteroid levels influence mood, behavior, electroencephalograph patterns, memory consolidation, and brain excitability. Chronic glucocorticoid treatment causes cell death in hippocampal neurons, and elevated glucocorticoid is thought to play a role in altered cognition, dementia, and depression in aging humans.[32] Patients with Addison's disease are subject to apathy, depression, irritability, and psychosis, symptoms that are alleviated by glucocorticoid, but not mineralocorticoid, therapy. Cushing's disease patients sometimes develop neuroses and psychoses that are reversible with the removal of excess hormone. Increases in brain excitability in hypercorticism and after mineralocorticoid treatment are a result of electrolyte imbalances. However, increased brain excitability induced by cortisol is not due to changes in sodium concentration. Chronic glucocorticoid treatment can also result in pseudotumor cerebri, primarily in children.[33]

Hematologic Effects Corticosteroids increase hemoglobin and red cell content of blood, possibly by retarding erythrophagocytosis. This effect is demonstrated by the occurrence of polycythemia in Cushing's disease and mild normochromic anemia in Addison's disease. Corticosteroids also affect circulating white cells. Glucocorticoid treatment results in increased polymorphonuclear leukocytes in blood as a result of increased rate of entrance from marrow and a decreased rate of removal from the vascular compartment. In contrast, the lymphocytes, eosinophils, monocytes, and basophils decrease in number after administration of glucocorticoids. A single dose of cortisol results in a 70% decrease in lymphocytes and a 90% decrease in monocytes, occurring 4 to 6 hours after treatment and persisting for about 24 hours. Cell numbers then rise 24 to 72 hours after treatment.[34] The decrease in lymphocytes, monocytes, and eosinophils is generally thought to be a consequence of redistribution of these cells, as well as glucocorticoid-induced apoptosis in some cell types. T lymphocytes are more sensitive to glucocorticoid-induced apoptosis than are B lymphocytes, and T-cell subpopulations differ in their glucocorticoid sensitivity. A decrease in basophils occurs by an unknown mechanism.[35]

Anti-Inflammatory Effects Glucocorticoids prevent or suppress the full inflammatory reaction to infectious, physical, or immunologic agents, inhibiting early inflammatory events such as edema, cellular exudation, fibrin deposition, capillary dilatation, migration of leukocytes into the area, and phagocytic activity. Later events, such as capillary and fibroblast proliferation, deposition of collagen, and cicatrization, are also inhibited. The anti-inflammatory mechanism of glucocorticoids, while not completely understood, is of great therapeutic relevance and is the subject of intense scientific investigation. A major effect of glucocorticoids on the inflammatory process is inhibition of recruitment of neutrophils and monocytes. Glucocorticoids dampen the ability of neutrophils to adhere to capillary endothelial cells by a dual mechanism. They block the normal increase in expression of endothelial adhesion molecules (ELAM-1) and intercellular adhesion molecules (ICAM-1), and they induce lipocortin, a protein inhibitor of phospholipase A2 (PLA2). Because PLA2 is an enzyme involved in prostaglandin synthesis, glucocorticoids ultimately decrease the synthesis and release of prostaglandin mediators of cell adhesion. Glucocorticoids also inhibit synthesis of plasminogen activator and migration inhibitory factor, stabilize lysosomes (thereby decreasing the release of hydrolytic enzymes and histamine), and decrease binding of chemokines that attract white blood cells. Glucocorticoids slow wound healing by blocking the normal inflammatory reaction of breaking down and disorganizing collagen (reviewed in Paliogianni and Boumpas[35] and Pitzalis and colleagues[36]).

Adaptive Immune System It is well known that hypocorticism results in hypertrophy of lymphoid tissue (ie, thymus, spleen, lymph nodes) and hypercorticism leads to diminution or total loss of these tissues. Glucocorticoids induce rapid apoptosis in lymphatic tissue in rats and mice, but these effects seem to occur only at pharmacologic doses in man. The effects seen in humans, therefore, may be due to changes in the rate of formation or destruction of lymphoid cells that become evident over a longer period of time. More acute effects of glucocorticoid on lymphoid cells in man are probably caused by sequestration of the cells rather than by cell lysis, although certain types of activated T lymphocytes are likely to be susceptible to glucocorticoid-induced apoptosis. In contrast to normal human lymphocytes, acute lymphocytic leukemias and other malignancies respond to glucocorticoid treatment by apoptosis, as is seen in rodents. Glucocorticoids decrease the secretion of interleukin 1 and other mediators of immune response, inhibit lymphocyte participation in delayed hypersensitivity reactions, and interfere with the rejection of immunologically incompatible graft tissue. This is probably a consequence of decreases in leukocyte recruitment. High doses of glucocorticoids inhibit immunoglobulin synthesis, kill B cells, and decrease production of components of the complement system.[37]

Other Effects Other effects of prolonged glucocorticoid therapy include ophthalmologic (posterior subcapsular cataracts, increased intraocular pressure) and dermatologic (redistribution of subcutaneous fat, hirsutism, alopecia, impaired wound healing, purpura, purple striae, and acneiform eruptions) problems. Long-term glucocorticoid treatment, with the concomitant immunosuppression, also leaves patients susceptible to invasive diseases such as Kaposi's sarcoma and fungal infections.[38] Recent data suggest that glucocorticoids may also be important positive regulators of innate immunity.[39]

CORTICOSTEROIDS IN THE TREATMENT OF NEOPLASMS

The first experimental observation of glucocorticoid efficacy in cancer was that cortisone caused tumor regression in a transplantable mouse lymphosarcoma.[40] Soon, this observation extended to a wide variety of murine lymphatic tumors, and corticosteroid effects were also evaluated on many nonendocrine and nonlymphoid transplantable rodent tumors. Pharmacologic doses of steroid inhibited growth of various tumor systems.[41] Tissue culture studies confirmed that lymphoid cells were the most sensitive to glucocorticoids and responded to treatment with decreases in DNA, ribonucleic acid (RNA), and protein synthesis.[42] Studies of proliferating human leukemic lymphoblasts supported the hypothesis that glucocorticoids have preferential lymphocytolytic effects. The mechanism of action was initially thought to be caused by impaired energy use via decreased glucose transport and/or phosphorylation; it was later discovered that glucocorticoids induce apoptosis, or programmed cell death, in certain lymphoid cell populations.[43,44] Despite a still incomplete understanding of glucocorticoid mechanism of action, they are of great clinical value in the treatment of lymphoid neoplasms. They are also sometimes used in therapeutic regimens for other endocrine-responsive cancers, are efficacious in the treatment of several frequently occurring side effects of malignancies, and are widely used for general palliative therapy.

Neoplasms Treated with Corticosteroids

Acute Lymphoblastic Leukemia Glucocorticoids are a mainstay of acute lymphoblastic leukemia (ALL) treatment protocols because they are powerful inducers of blast cell apoptosis. The important role of glucocorticoids in ALL therapy is underscored by the observation that polymorphisms in genes related to corticosteroid function that decrease corticosteroid sensitivity are correlated with poor prognosis and risk of early relapse, and "poor pred response" has recently been identified as the most predictive marker of relapse in ALL.[45,46]

Treatment of ALL with prednisone alone was found to yield significant clinical improvement and 50% remission rates,[47] but remission was short (1 year) and relapse, most often of a steroid-resistant phenotype, inevitable. Therefore, multiple drug therapy combining prednisone with other cytotoxic agents is now used. Under regimens containing vincristine and prednisone or prednisolone, more than 90% of children[48,49] and up to 80% of adults[50] achieve remission. The inclusion of agents such as daunorubicin, L-asparaginase, cytosine arabinoside, doxorubicin, and cyclophosphamide appears to prolong remission, but whether it increases the rate of remission is unclear. Dexamethasone is thought to be a more potent antileukemic agent than prednisone at conventional equivalent doses, but it also induces more toxicity.[51] In one study, prednisone pretreatment before initiation of combination therapy improved the rate of complete remission in adult patients.[52]

After remission is achieved, a 2- to 3-year program of maintenance therapy follows that involves regular intensive chemotherapy sessions that include glucocorticoids.[53] Prophylactic treatment to prevent relapse in the central nervous system is often administered; the treatment consists of cranial radiotherapy and intrathecal treatment with prednisone, methotrexate, and cytosine arabinoside.[54,55] With this approach, more than 80% of children appear to be cured (5-year event-free survival). The success rate is considerably lower in adults; only 15 to 30% of adults appear to be cured.

In refractory cases, or in cases of relapse, which occurs in approximately 20% of children with acute lymphoblastic leukemia, re-induction involves more aggressive combination chemotherapy, again including a glucocorticoid.[56] Treatment with high doses of methylprednisolone (1 g/m^2 for 5 to 8 days) is also used and may be more effective than conventional-dose prednisolone, with little toxicity.[57,58] However, overall survival rates after relapse remain fairly low, averaging 35 to 65% in children and less in adults.

Acute Myeloid Leukemia Glucocorticoids appear to have little value in the treatment of acute myeloid leukemia. Although they have been included in some combination chemotherapies, their importance in such regimens is unclear.[58]

Chronic Lymphocytic Leukemia Current frontline therapy for chronic lymphocytic leukemia (CLL) consists of either combination chemotherapy including cyclophosphamide, doxorubicin, vincristine, and prednisolone (CHOP), or the purine analog fludarabine, sometimes in combination with steroids and alkylating agents. Fludarabine appears to be effective in both untreated and refractory cases of chronic lymphocytic leukemia. Rituximab, a monoclonal antibody against the cell surface antigen CD20, is a newer therapeutic alternative active as monotherapy or in addition to conventional chemotherapeutic regimens. Recent studies indicate that a combination of rituximab with fludarabine may prove to be the most effective available therapy to attain improved complete response rates.[59] Corticosteroids are particularly useful in a treatment regimen if the neoplasm is associated with autoimmune hemolytic anemia, neutropenia, and thrombocytopenia with hemorrhagic complications.[60] Glucocorticoids alleviate the lymphadenopathy and hepatosplenomegaly that are often associated with this condition.

Chronic Myeloid Leukemia Imatinib, a specific BCR-ABL tyrosine kinase inhibitor, has rapidly become the gold standard in the treatment of chronic myeloid leukemia (CML).[61] Although patients who are resistant to imatinib and not candidates for stem cell transplantation may receive interferon alpha or conventional chemotherapy, CML presents no indication for corticosteroids today.

Hodgkin's Lymphoma Hodgkin's lymphoma is a solid tumor that is now considered curable by chemotherapy. Consequently, considerations in the choice of current treatment options revolve around selecting therapy that preserves fertility and minimizes toxicity and therapy-induced secondary malignancies. Corticosteroids alone can achieve worthwhile objective results in 66% of Hodgkin's lymphoma patients resistant to alkylating agents. Combination therapy with mechlorethamine, Oncovin (vincristine), procarbazine, prednisone (MOPP), developed in 1964, was the first treatment to effectively cause complete remission, and probably cures, in a majority of patients. Subsequent regimens, most of which employ a glucocorticoid, are as effective as MOPP. Adriamycin (doxorubicin), bleomycin, vinblastine, and dacarbazine (ABVD), a nonglucocorticoid regimen, has a favorable toxicity profile similar to that of MOPP and is now considered a superior first-line therapy.[62]

Treatment of early-stage Hodgkin's lymphoma with a combination of radiotherapy and chemotherapy may be most effective. The NOVP (Novantrone [mitoxantrone], Oncovin [vincristine], vinblastine, prednisone) treatment regimen in combination with radiotherapy shows promise as an effective yet minimally toxic treatment of early Hodgkin's disease, with all patients in a preliminary study achieving complete remission and 5-year overall survival rates of 95%.[63] Advanced-stage disease treated with MOPP, ABVD, or other similar combinations exhibits a complete response rate of 55 to 75%.[64–66] Aggressive salvage therapies for relapsed or refractory Hodgkin's disease that contain a glucocorticoid have a complete response rate around 30 to 50%.[67–69] It should be noted that targeted immunotherapy (rituximab) also shows preliminary promise as a therapy because of its apparent combination of efficacy with minimal toxicity.

Non-Hodgkin's Lymphoma Corticosteroids used as single-agent therapy produce temporary responses in patients with non-Hodgkin's lymphoma (NHL); they are therefore included in virtually every complex regimen used for the treatment of NHL. Many new NHL regimens also include rituximab, either first-line, or in subsequent maintenance therapy. Although there is evidence for improved response rates with the inclusion of this monoclonal antibody, the evidence of better long-term survival rates is not yet available.[70] Regimens differ according to lymphoma histologic subtype and stage. Patients with disseminated lymphomas treated with recent generations of drug combinations have 3- to 4-year survival rates of 30 to 70%. One study indicates that the use of interferon-α2b in combination with a typical glucocorticoid-containing drug regimen produces good results (85% overall response rate and 86% 3-year survival rate).[71] For tumors within the central nervous system, dexamethasone is preferred instead of prednisone to decrease tumor swelling.

Multiple Myeloma Therapeutic approach to multiple myeloma (MM) depends on the patient's eligibility for stem-cell transplant (usually limited to patients younger than 70). When transplant is indicated, one of the following therapies is commonly employed as an induction phase prior to the transplant.[72] Combination therapy with melphalan and prednisolone, the standard therapy for MM for decades and still the standard therapy for older patients, results in a 50% response rate, but without complete remission and with a median survival of only 24 to 30 months. A combination of vincristine, Adriamycin, and dexamethasone (VAD) is also used, especially in refractory disease, but affords no survival advantage, while treatment with intermittent dexamethasone administration leads to an overall response rate of 43%, a lower response than with VAD therapy, but with a much lower incidence of serious complications. Very high doses of glucocorticoids alone are temporarily useful, albeit toxic, in cases of progressive or resistant disease, when rapid cytoreduction is necessary, or if bone marrow reserve is limited. These doses can be as high as 1 g/m^2/d for prednisone and 40 mg/m^2/d for dexamethasone.[73] Interferons have been used as single agent or combination therapy with steroids with limited success.[72]

Breast Cancer The highly malignant nature of breast cancers dictates aggressive systemic therapeutic regimens. Although estrogen receptor positive cancers are most often treated with newer, endocrine-based therapies, chemotherapy remains the only option for endocrine-resistant metastatic breast cancer. Although never used as the sole treatment of breast cancer, glucocorticoids have been included in various combination chemotherapies. Cyclophosphamide, methotrexate, and 5-fluorouracil (CMF)-type regimens, with and without prednisone, result in tumor regression in 50 to 80% of patients and complete response in 15 to 20%.[74,75] Although palliation of symptoms occurs in a majority of patients, only a small percentage benefit by prolonged survival. The role of prednisone in the effectiveness of the CMF and prednisone (CMFP) regimen is unclear, with some trials indicating no difference in response rates to CMFP or CMF, and another indicating that inclusion of prednisone resulted in a longer time to treatment failure and a longer survival time. A trial of radiation treatment plus or minus prednisone indicated that inclusion of prednisone improved disease-free and overall survival in premenopausal women older than age 45 years.[76] A trial of high-dose 11-drug combination chemotherapy including prednisone resulted in a very high response rate (overall response, 92%; complete response, 73%), but median survival time was not markedly increased from other studies.[77] An 8-drug combination with autologous bone marrow transplantation and locoregional radiotherapy tested on patients with at least 5 involved lymph nodes resulted in a 5-year disease-free survival rate of 84%.[78] The efficacy of the glucocorticoids in such regimens may be due, at least in part, to the improved tolerance of cytotoxic drugs. There is evidence that dexamethasone has hematopoietic protective effects in chemotherapeutic regimens and in animals bearing human breast cancer xenografts dexamethasone increases efficacy of chemotherapeutic agents.[79] For patients who do not consent to aggressive cytotoxic chemotherapy, the alternative combination of mitoxantrone, leucovorin, 5-fluorouracil, and prednisone induced tumor regression in 67% of patients with a complete response in 25%.[81] Standard therapy, however, includes anthracyclines, taxanes and cyclophosphamide with or without fluorouracil, without the use of steroids except for their use in the prevention of allergic reaction and emesis.

Other Uses Hydrocortisone replacement (approximately 40 mg/d) is indicated after surgical or chemical adrenalectomy as performed to eliminate circulating steroids in cases ectopic ACTH excess. Hemangiomas in infants are often treated with injections of glucocorticoids.[82] Thymomas are often treated with glucocorticoids either alone or in combination with cytotoxic drugs.[82] Other tumors that have been treated with combination chemotherapy involving a glucocorticoid include medulloblastoma, primitive neuroectodermal tumors, and ependymomas.[83,84]

Symptomatic Uses of Corticosteroids **Palliative Care** Glucocorticoid treatment produces rapid symptomatic improvements in critically ill patients, including relief of fever, sweats, lethargy, weakness, and other nonspecific effects of cancer. Glucocorticoids also cause mild euphoria, a general feeling of well being, and a stimulation of appetite.[85,86] These effects are transient, and only short-term treatment is possible due to side effects of the high doses. In addition, glucocorticoid withdrawal can result in adrenocortical insufficiency. For these reasons, corticosteroid treatment is appropriate only for patients whose life expectancy is brief (a few weeks or less). Although doses of 25 mg/d prednisolone can be used, with a decrease to 7.5 to 15 mg/d for maintenance of effects, other options for pain management in terminally ill patients makes the use of glucocorticoids in this context relatively rare.

Hypercalcemia Hypercalcemia, a common complication of many malignancies,[87] is often caused by increased bone resorption and renal calcium reabsorption. This effect is thought to be a consequence of factors secreted by tumors, particularly tumors of lymphoid origin. Although glucocorticoids do not lower normal calcium levels, high-dose glucocorticoid has efficacy in the treatment of hypercalcemia (100 mg/d prednisolone, 400 mg/d hydrocortisone). The mechanisms of glucocorticoid action in reduction of serum calcium are thought to be cytolytic effects on lymphoid cells, decreased lymphokine secretion, and inhibition of vitamin D action on calcium metabolism. Glucocorticoids are most effective on hypercalcemia that is secondary to high vitamin D levels, and least effective in patients with solid tumors. Results in treatment of multiple myeloma patients are inconsistent. Therefore, glucocorticoids are a poor treatment modality except in cases of vitamin D-mediated hypercalcemia, and other medications are utilized, particularly the bisphosphonates.

Central Nervous System Tumors Neurologic symptoms from primary and metastatic brain and spinal cord tumors are partially caused by peritumoral edema.[88] Glucocorticoids can ameliorate these symptoms in approximately 70 to 80% of cases after several days of treatment,[89] likely by inducing both decreased edema production and increased edema reabsorption. Dexamethasone is the recommended steroid for this treatment because it contains no mineralocorticoid activity and is highly potent. A dose of 16 mg/d is used with an increase to 100 mg/d if no response occurs. This dose is continued until the maximum response is obtained, then decreased gradually and maintained at the lowest effective dose. Recent findings suggest that currently used doses may be excessive, however, because 2 to 4 mg of dexamethasone per day is sufficient for controlling edema during radiotherapy for brain metastases.[90–92] Glucocorticoid effects on the brain and spinal cord are short-lived and only increase survival time slightly unless other measures, such as radiotherapy and surgery, are taken. Glucocorticoids are often administered during these therapies to alleviate the edema that is normally induced by these treatments. It has been observed that glucocorticoids can decrease the amount of a cytotoxic drug that gets to a tumor, possibly by decreasing capillary permeability. For this reason, a recent pilot study eliminated dexamethasone from the standard high-dose methotrexate protocol for children with brain tumors. The results indicated that dexamethasone could be eliminated from such treatment protocols without serious brain edema or increased toxicity, and with a reduction in the incidence of liver toxicity.[93]

Antiemetic Action Glucocorticoids decrease the severity and frequency of both chemotherapy-induced and post-surgical emesis. Dexamethasone (8 to 20 mg) and methylprednisolone (125 to 250 mg) are widely employed for this indication, with vomiting episodes reduced by as much as 74%.

Glucocorticoids are most effective when used at low doses to enhance the antiemetic efficacy of other drugs. The combination of dexamethasone with a serotonin receptor antagonist (eg, ondansetron, granisetron, tropisetron) is so effective that it is now the standard antiemetic prophylaxis for many chemotherapeutic agents.[94] The mechanism of glucocorticoid-mediated antiemesis is unknown. The effect may be associated with decreases in prostaglandin synthesis, or glucocorticoids may act directly on the chemoreceptor trigger zone by modifying capillary permeability or stabilizing lysosomal membranes.

Other Uses of Glucocorticoids Acute upper airway obstruction, from direct tumor growth or by compression from thyroid, lung, and esophageal cancers, can be reduced by glucocorticoid treatment either alone or with radiotherapy.[95] Glucocorticoids can partially relieve other cancer-related obstructions (including superior vena cava syndrome; lymphedema; liver metastases; masses in the pelvis, mediastinum, or retroperitoneum; and blockages of the large bowel or ureter) by reducing peritumoral inflammation and edema. Pain from bone metastases or metastatic arthralgia from solid tumors often responds to glucocorticoid treatment. Several chemotherapeutic agents (mitomycin, bleomycin, busulfan, carmustine), as well as radiotherapy, are associated with pulmonary toxicity. Preventive glucocorticoid administration during chemotherapy, for example, dexamethasone administration during mitomycin chemotherapy for non–small-cell lung cancer,[96]can prevent lung injury. However, decreased antineoplastic effects of mitomycin in such a context suggests that further study of this application is warranted. Loss of vision associated with pseudotumor cerebri can be treated with glucocorticoids.[97]Glucocorticoids are also used prophylactically for pre-and postadministration of taxane-containing chemotherapy to reduce the incidence of acute hypersensitivity reactions and anaphylactic responses. Such premedication greatly reduces, but does not completely eliminate, these acute reactions. There is evidence, however, that the small subpopulation in which hypersensitivity is not prevented are presenting with a hypersensitivity response of a nonallergic nature, in contrast to those who respond positively to steroid treatment.[98]

Mechanism of Glucocorticoid Action The majority of the biologic effects of steroid hormones are mediated by intracellular receptors specific for each class of steroid. The human glucocorticoid receptor is actually a group of variant receptors expressed from a single *GR* gene via alternative splicing or initiation events.[99] GRα, the classical, most well understood of the human GR forms, is a 98-kilodalton cytoplasmic protein present in all tissues that are targets of glucocorticoid action. Mice with a disrupted *GR* gene lack a functional receptor and die shortly after birth, indicating that a functional glucocorticoid signaling pathway is essential for life. Glucocorticoid receptors are required for most glucocorticoid-induced changes to occur, but hormonal sensitivity is not guaranteed by the presence of receptors. Although a good correlation between cellular concentration of glucocorticoid receptors and sensitivity to glucocorticoids exists, other factors (including nonfunctional or modified receptors and other cellular factors that modify receptor function) modulate glucocorticoid sensitivity.

A model for our current understanding of glucocorticoid action is described in Figure 53-2. Free glucocorticoid is thought to diffuse into the cell, and then bind noncovalently and with high affinity to the cytoplasmic GR. GR, held in a ligand-binding competent conformation by its association with regulatory proteins, including heat shock protein 90, becomes activated upon ligand binding. Activation is not completely understood, but is known to involve a conformational change in GR, increased phosphorylation of the receptor, and release of associated regulatory proteins. Activated steroid-receptor complex translocates to the nucleus, binds as a homodimer to specific DNA sequences called glucocorticoid-responsive elements (GREs), and alters the transcription rate of specific genes associated with the GRE. Figure 53-3 depicts a classical glucocorticoid-responsive gene. The GRE, shown with the consensus DNA sequence, is located in the 5'-regulatory region of the gene. GR dimer bound to this GRE can interact with transcriptional cofactors, as well as with DNA-binding transcription factors that bind to other regulatory elements located in the 5' region, such as the TATA and CAAT boxes. By this mechanism, glucocorticoids acting via the GR can increase the transcription rate of a positive GRE-containing gene, or decrease the transcription rate of a negative GRE-containing gene. Alterations in the transcription rate lead to changes in the amount of messenger RNA and, ultimately, the level of protein that is synthesized from these genes, and thus alter cellular functions. GRs also negatively regulate the transcription of genes indirectly by interfering with the activity of other transcriptional activators, such as AP-1 and NFκB. These repressive actions are thought to be the result of protein-protein, rather than protein-DNA, interactions. GR interacts, either directly or via associated factors, with AP-1 heterodimers of fos and jun, thereby inhibiting the transcriptional activity of AP-1. Via this mechanism, GR modulates transcription of genes that lack a GRE but are AP-1 responsive. GR exhibits similar negative interactions with the transcription factor NFκB. In this case, the p65 subunit of NFκB interacts with GR. This interaction changes multiple interactions between the transcriptional machinery, the transcriptional cofactors that are recruited to the NFκB responsive gene promoter, and GR and/or NFκB. An important aspect of receptor regulation that is especially relevant to glucocorticoid therapy is glucocorticoid-induced down-regulation of the GR. The ability of glucocorticoid to down-regulate its own receptor is mediated by the receptor itself.[100] A maximal 50 to 75% decrease

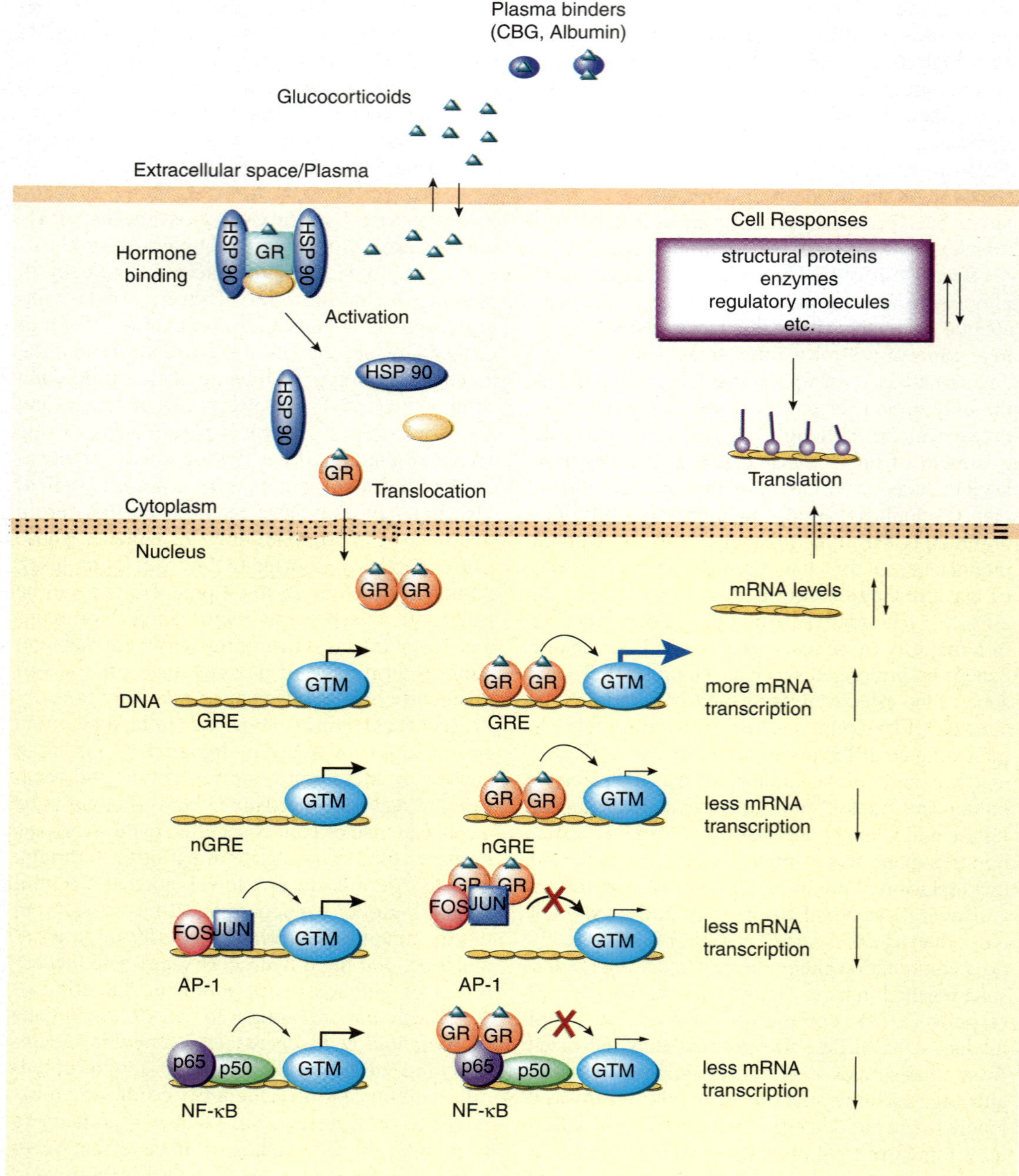

Figure 53-2 Mechanism of action for the glucocorticoid signaling pathway. AP-1 = AP-1 responsive element; GR = glucocorticoid receptor; GRE = glucocorticoid responsive element; GTM = general transcriptional machinery; HSP = heat shock protein; NFκB = NFκB responsive element; nGRE = negative GRE.

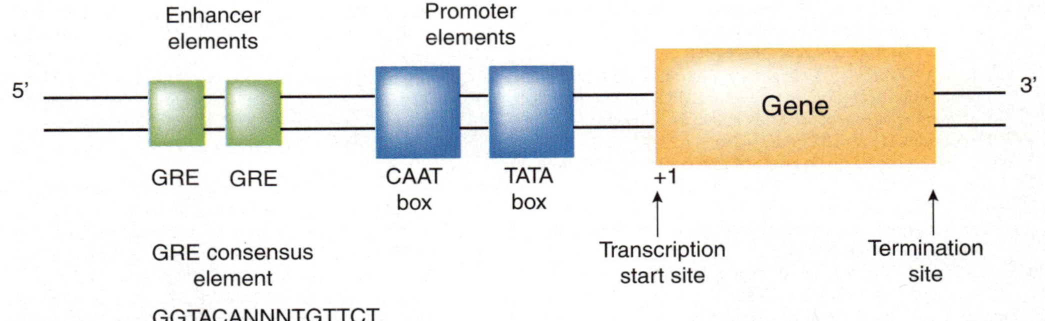

Figure 53-3 Structural characteristics of a classical glucocorticoid-responsive gene. GRE = glucocorticoid-responsive element; N = unspecified nucleoside.

in receptor protein, mediated by a decrease in receptor messenger RNA, occurs within 24 hours of treatment. Long-term administration of glucocorticoids, associated with down-regulation of the glucocorticoid receptor, decreases function of many glucocorticoid-sensitive genes, suggesting that continuous glucocorticoid treatment can have widespread deleterious effects on cell function. This may explain why alternate day glucocorticoid therapy presents less risk of unwanted side effects[101] and suggests that it may be important to administer therapeutic doses of glucocorticoids in a manner that simulates the natural diurnal rhythm of glucocorticoid secretion to maximize efficacy and safety.

Although the majority of known glucocorticoid effects are via receptor-mediated transcriptional modulation, there is also evidence for other glucocorticoid actions, including post-transcriptional regulation of the expression of some inflammatory cytokines and so-called "non genomic" glucocorticoid effects (on ion fluxes, for example) that occur too rapidly to be attributed to transcriptional regulation. These are areas of glucocorticoid function that are less clearly understood.[102]

Anticorticosteroids Steroid receptor antagonists have been synthesized that inhibit the action of receptor ligands. Most of these antagonists are modified steroids that are competitive inhibitors of the receptor. The antagonist forms a complex with the receptor and then interferes with one or more of the normal functions of a ligand-bound receptor (nuclear translocation, association with GREs, interaction with transcriptional cofactors, transcriptional modulation).

Selective GR antagonists are a currently active area of investigation, but one of the best-characterized antiglucocorticoids is the antiprogestin mifepristone (RU-486). The antiprogestin effects of RU-486 are used clinically for the induction of abortions, but the antiglucocorticoid effects afford its occasional use as a treatment of hypercorticism. RU-486 has been evaluated as an antineoplastic agent for meningioma, breast cancer, prostate cancer, and hepatoma, but the relative importance of the antiprogestin to antiglucocorticoid effects in these contexts is unclear.

Antimineralocorticoids like spironolactone and the more selective aldosterone receptor antagonist eplerenone, have demonstrated great success in reducing mortality in severe heart failure and opened a new area in the management of hypertension.[103]

Corticosteroid Resistance In addition to the multiple GR variants already described, several mutations of the glucocorticoid receptor have been identified in vivo that result in either general or tissue-localized cortisol resistant phenotypes. Many other GR mutations that cause impaired function have been induced in vitro in leukemic cell lines by chemotherapeutic agents (reviewed in Hala and colleagues[104]). It is well known that a subpopulation of leukemia patients is resistant to glucocorticoid therapy, and other patients develop such resistance over the course of treatment. Therefore investigators have long tried to understand the relationship between GR function, receptor concentration, and clinical responsiveness. No consistent relationship has been found between glucocorticoid receptor number and sensitivity to apoptosis: the strongest correlation exists for acute lymphocytic leukemia and non-Hodgkin's lymphoma,[105] acute myeloid leukemia shows no correlation, and inconsistent results have been found with other leukemias. This lack of relationship between receptor number and responsiveness to glucocorticoid therapy suggests that factors other than the presence of glucocorticoid receptors mediate the susceptibility of lymphoid cells to glucocorticoid-induced apoptosis.

In terms of GR function, resistant human leukemia cell lines were not initially found to contain major defects in their glucocorticoid receptor. Molecular analysis of the glucocorticoid receptor gene from resistant variants of the human T-cell–derived CEM cell line, however, identified GR mutations.[106] These mutations are often subtle, in some cases involving a single nucleotide base pair change.

A better understanding of the mechanisms of corticosteroid resistance may result from current research to develop a more complete understanding of the variant forms of the human glucocorticoid receptor. Perhaps of most interest is the beta form of hGR (hGRβ). This isoform is identical to the classical hGRα through the first 727 amino acids, but diverges at the carboxy terminus. This variant of GR, like hGRα, is widely expressed. Unlike hGRα, hGRβ does not bind hormone, is localized to the cell nucleus independent of hormone status, and does not activate glucocorticoid responsive genes. In vitro studies suggest that hGRβ functions as a dominant negative repressor of hGRα-mediated transactivation. Cell type specific expression patterns for hGRα and hGRβ may be a key modulator of glucocorticoid sensitivity: the ratio of hGRα: hGRβ may be a more important determinant of hormone responsiveness than the absolute number of glucocorticoid receptors.[107]

Glucocorticoid-Induced Apoptosis Glucocorticoid-induced lymphocytolysis in rats and mice, resulting in significant reductions in the size of the thymus, spleen, and lymph nodes, is a widely studied phenomenon. The specific process by which large populations of immature thymocytes in the rodent thymus die rapidly after glucocorticoid treatment is known as apoptosis, or programmed cell death. Apoptosis is associated with many physiologic processes, including embryogenesis, morphogenesis, normal tissue turnover, and cell-mediated immunity, and is induced by many different signals in these various systems. Morphologic characteristics of apoptosis include cellular condensation and internucleosomal chromatin degradation, followed by fragmentation into apoptotic bodies that are phagocytosed by neighboring cells or circulating macrophages.

Glucocorticoid-induced apoptosis occurs primarily in lymphocytes and is mediated by the GR. However, not all lymphocytes are sensitive. Immature T cells and some B cells are very sensitive to apoptosis, whereas mature T cells are not. In rodents, responsive cell populations start to die within 8 hours of glucocorticoid treatment in vivo. Nearly all immature thymocytes are dead within 48 hours of treatment.

The sensitivity of human lymphocytes to glucocorticoid-induced apoptosis appears to differ. Although human lymphocytes respond to glucocorticoids, they do not die with the same kinetics as rodent cells. The marked lymphocytopenia observed after glucocorticoid treatment is mostly due to redistribution of lymphocytes into other tissues and is returned to normal within 24 hours. Although human lymphocytes are generally more resistant to apoptosis, certain subpopulations (including cortical and medullary thymocytes, mature T-helper cells, natural killer cells, cytotoxic T lymphocytes, and immature B cells) do die in response to glucocorticoids. More importantly, several malignant hematopoietic cells are sensitive to glucocorticoid-induced apoptosis. These include multiple myeloma, acute lymphoblastic leukemia, and chronic lymphocytic leukemia.[104] Some human leukemic cells, notably acute and chronic lymphocytic leukemia, show morphologic and biochemical signs of apoptosis upon death.[109] The difference between normal and malignant human lymphocytes that causes the increased susceptibility of malignant cells to apoptosis is unknown. Targeted apoptosis is developing into an important tool in the repertoire of cancer therapy techniques. Active study on the phenomenon of apoptosis and cell type specific inducers of apoptosis as potential anticancer therapies continues.

REFERENCES

1. Munck A. Glucocorticoid biology—a historical perspective. In: Goulding NJ, Flower RJ, editors. Glucocorticoids. Basel: Birkhauser Verlag; 2001. p. 17–33.
2. Parente L. The development of synthetic glucocorticoids. In: Goulding NJ, Flower RJ, editors. Glucocorticoids. Basel: Birkhauser Verlag; 2001. p. 35–51.
3. Haynes RC Jr. The activation of adrenal phosphorylase by the adrenocorticotropic hormone. J Biol Chem 1958;233:1220–2.
4. Gwynne JT, Mahaffee D, Brewer HB, Ney RL. Adrenal cholesterol uptake from plasma lipoproteins; regulation by corticotropin. Proc Natl Acad Sci U S A 1976;73:4329–33.
5. Simpson ER, Mason JI, John ME, et al. Regulation of the biosynthesis of steroidogenic enzymes. J Steroid Biochem 1987;27:801–5.
6. Brown MS, Kovanen PT, Goldstein JL. Receptor-mediated uptake of lipoprotein-cholesterol and its utilization for steroid synthesis in the adrenal cortex. Recent Prog Horm Res 1979;35:215–57.
7. Gann DS, Dallman MF, Engleland WC. Reflex control and modulation of ACTH and corticosteroids. Int Rev Physiol 1981;24:157–99.
8. Weitzman ED, Fukushima D, Nogeire C, et al. Twenty-four hour pattern of the episodic secretion of cortisol in normal subjects. J Clin Endocrinol Metab 1971;33:14–22.
9. Vaughan GM, Becker RA, Allen JP, et al. Cortisol and corticotrophin in burned patients. J Trauma 1982;22:263–73.
10. George JM, Reier CE, Lanese RR, Rower JM. Morphine anesthesia blocks cortisol and growth hormone response to surgical stress in humans. J Clin Endocrinol Metab 1974;38:736–41.
11. Copinschi G, L'Hermite M, LeClerq R, et al. Effects of glucocorticoids on pituitary hormone responses to hypoglycemia. Inhibition of prolactin release. J Clin Endocrinol Metab 1975;40:442–9.
12. Davis JD. Regulation of aldosterone secretion. In: Eisenstein AB, editor. The adrenal cortex. Boston: Little, Brown; 1967.
13. Lumbers ER. Angiotensin and aldosterone. Regul Pept 1999;80(3):91–100.
14. Blair-West JR, Coghlan JP, Denton DA, et al. A dose-response comparison of the actions of angiotensin II and angiotensin III in sheep. J Endocrinol 1980;87:409–17.
15. Wagner C, Kurtz A. Regulation of renal renin release. Curr Opin Nephrol Hypertens 1998;7(4):437–41.
16. New MI, Seaman MP, Peterson RE. A method for the simultaneous determination of the secretion rates of cortisol, 11-desoxycortisol, corticosterone, 11-desoxy-corticosterone and aldosterone. J Clin Endocrinol Metab 1969;29:514–22.
17. Bondy PK. The adrenal cortex. In: Bondy PK, Rosenberg LE, editors. Metabolic control and disease, 8th ed. Philadelphia: Saunders; 1980. p. 1427.
18. Scurry MT, Sheart L. Stop-flow analysis of the reabsorption of cortisol. Endocrinology 1969;84:681–2.
19. Wolkowitz OM, Reus VI. Treatment of depression with antiglucocorticoid drugs. Psychosom Med 1999;61:698–711.
20. Ito S, Kusunoki Y, Oka T, et al. Pharmacokinetics of high-dose methylprednisolone in children. Dev Pharmacol Ther 1992;19:99–105.
21. Kaplan SA, Nagareda Shimizu CS. Effects of cortisol on amino acids in skeletal muscle and plasma. Endocrinology 1963;72:267–72.
22. Shafrir E, Steinberg D. The essential role of the adrenal cortex in the response of plasma free fatty acids, cholesterol and phospholipids to epinephrine injection. J Clin Invest 1960;39:310–9.
23. Seckl JR. 11-β hydroxysteroid dehydrogenase: changing glucocorticoid action. Curr Opin Pharmacol 2004;4:597–602.
24. Argawal MK, Mirshashi M. General overview of mineralocorticoid hormone action. Pharmacol Ther 1999;84:273–326.
25. Sakakura M, Takebe K, Nakagawa S. Inhibition of luteinizing hormone secretion by synthetic LHRH by long-term treatment with glucocorticoids in human subjects. J Clin Endocrinol Metab 1975;40:774–9.
26. Wilber JF, Utiger RD. The effect of glucocorticoids on thyrotropin secretion. J Clin Invest 1969;48:2096–103.
27. Eberlein WR, Bongiovanni AM, Rodriguez CS. Diagnosis and treatment: the complications of steroid treatment. Pediatrics 1967;40:279–82.
28. Krakoff LR. Glucocorticoid excess syndromes causing hypertension. Cardiol Clin 1988;6:537–45.
29. Gomez Sanchez EP. Central hypertensive effects of aldosterone. Front Neuroendocrinol 1997;18(4):440–62.
30. David DS, Grieco MH, Cushman P Jr. Adrenal glucocorticoids after twenty years–a review of their clinically relevant consequences. J Chron Dis 1970;22:637–711.
31. Cohen D, Adachi JD. The treatment of glucocorticoid-induced osteoporosis. J Steroid Biochem and Molecular Biol 2004;88:337–49.
32. Pomara N, Greenberg WM, Branford MD, Doraiswamy PM. Therapeutic implications of HPA axis abnormalities in Alzheimer's disease: review and update. Psychopharmacol Bulletin 2003 Spring;37(2):120–34.
33. Weisberg LA, Chatorian AM. Pseudotumor cerebri of childhood. Am J Dis Child 1977;131:1243–8.
34. Pountain GD, Keogan MT, Hazleman BL, Brown DL. Effect of single dose compared with three days' prednisolone treatment of healthy volunteers: contrasting effects on circulating lymphocyte subsets. J Clin Pathol 1993;46:1089–92.
35. Paliogianni F, Boumpas DT. Molecular and cellular aspects of cytokine regulation by glucocorticoids. In: Goulding NJ, Flower RJ, editors. Glucocorticoids. Basel: Birkhauser Verlag; 2001. p. 81–101.
36. Pitzalis C, Pipitone N, Perretti M. Glucocorticoids and leukocyte adhesion. In: Goulding NJ, Flower RJ, editors. Glucocorticoids. Basel: Birkhauser Verlag; 2001. p. 105–18.
37. Caren LD, Rosenberg LT. Steroids and serum complement in mice: influence of hydrocortisone, diethylstilbestrol, and testosterone. Science 1966;152:782–3.
38. Kirwan JR. Systemic glucocorticoids in chronic arthritis. In: Goulding NJ, Flower RJ, editors. Glucocorticoids. Basel: Birkhauser Verlag; 2001. p. 175–90.
39. Hermoso MA, Matsuguchi T, Smoak K, Cidlowski JA. Glucocorticoids and tumor necrosis factor alpha cooperatively regulate toll-like receptor-2 gene expression. Mol Cell Biol 2004:24(11):4743–56.
40. Heilman FR, Kendall EC. The influence of 11-dehydro-17-hydroxycorticosterone (compound E) on the growth of malignant tumor in the mouse. Endocrinology 1944;34:416–26.
41. Vollmer EP. A viewpoint on animal tumors as test systems for steroids. In: Hormonal steroids, biochemistry, pharmacology, and therapeutics. Proc First Int Cong Horm Steroids 1965;2:351.
42. Baxter GD, Collins RJ, Harmon BV, et al. Cell death by apoptosis in acute leukemia. J Pathol 1989;158:123–9.
43. Rosen JM, Fina JJ, Millholland RJ, Rosen F. Inhibition of glucose uptake in lymphosarcoma 1798 by cortisol and its relationship to the biosynthesis of deoxyribonucleic acid. J Biol Chem 1970;245:2074–80.
44. Cohen JJ. Lymphocyte death induced by glucocorticoids. In: Schleimer RP, Claman HN, Oronsky AL, editors. Anti-inflammatory steroid action: basic and clinical aspects. San Diego: Academic; 1989. p. 110.
45. Fleury I, Primeau M, Doreau A, et al. Polymorphisms in genes involved in the corticosteroid response and the outcome of childhood acute lymphoblastic leukemia. Am J Pharmacogenomics 2004:4(5):331–41.
46. Schrappe M. Evolution of BFM Trials for childhood ALL. Ann Hematol 2004;83 Suppl 1:S121–3.
47. Vietti TJ, Sullivan MP, Berry DH, et al. The response of acute childhood leukemia to an initial and a second course of prednisone. J Pediatr 1965;66:18–26.
48. Koizumi S, Fujimoto T. Improvement in treatment of childhood acute lymphoblastic leukemia: a 10-year study by the Children's Cancer and Leukemia Study Group. Int J Hematol 1994;59:99–112.
49. Yang CP, Lin ST, Liang DC, et al. Treatment of childhood acute lymphoblastic leukemia with protocol TCL-842 in Taiwan: the Taiwan Children's Cancer Study Group. J Formos Med Assoc 1993;92:431–9.
50. Weiss M. Induction therapy of adult acute lymphocytic leukemia without the use of vincristine or prednisone. Hematol Oncol North Am 2001 Feb. 15(1):1–7.
51. Belgaumi AF, Al-Bakrah M, Al-Mahr M, et al. Dexamethasone-associated toxicity during induction chemotherapy for childhood acute lymphoblastic leukemia is augmented by concurrent use of daunomycin. Cancer 2003;97:2898–903.
52. Annino L, Vegna M, Camera A, et al. Treatment of adult acute lymphoblastic leukemia: long-term follow up of the GIMEME ALL0288 randomized study. Blood 2002;99(3):863–71.
53. Sabbath KD, Weitberg AB, Calabresi P. Potentially curable neoplasms. Dis Mon 1986;32:593–652.
54. Winick NJ, Smith SD, Shuster J, et al. Treatment of CNS relapse in children with acute lymphoblastic leukemia: a Pediatric Oncology Group study. J Clin Oncol 1993;11:271–8.
55. Buhrer C, Hartmann R, Fengler R, et al. Importance of effective central nervous system therapy in isolated bone marrow relapse of childhood acute lymphoblastic leukemia. BFM (Berlin-Frankfurt-Munster) Relapse Study Group. Blood 1994;83:3468–72.
56. Ryalls MR, Pinkerton CR, Meller ST, et al. High-dose methylprednisolone sodium succinate as a single agent in relapsed childhood acute lymphoblastic leukaemia. Med Pediatr Oncol 1992;20:119–23.
57. Yetgin S, Gurgey A, Tuncer AM, et al. A comparison of the effect of high-dose methylprednisolone with conventional-dose prednisolone in acute lymphoblastic leukemia patients with randomization. Leuk Res 1998;22(6):485–93.
58. Nagura E, Kimura K, Yamada K, et al. Nationwide randomized comparative study of daunorubicin and aclarubicin in combination with behenoyl cytosine arabinoside, 6-mercaptopurine, and prednisolone for previously untreated acute myeloid leukemia. Cancer Chemother Pharmacol 1994;34:23–9.
59. Byrd JC, Rai K, Peterson BL, et al. Addition of rituximab to fludarabine may prolong progression-free survival and overall survival in patients with previously untreated chronic lymphocytic leukemia: an updated retrospective comparative analysis of CALGB 9712 and CALGB 9011. Blood 2005;105(1):49–53.
60. Johnson LE. Chronic lymphocytic leukemia. Am Fam Physician 1988;38:167–76.
61. Stone RM. Optimizing treatment of chronic myeloid leukemia: a rational approach. The Oncologist 2004;9:259–70.
62. Connors J, Noordijk E, Horning S. Hodgkin's lymphoma: basing the treatment on the evidence. Hematology 2001;178–93.
63. Tormo M, Terol L, Marugan I, et al. Treatment of stage I and II Hodgkin's disease with NOVP and radiotherapy. Leuk Lymphoma 1999;34(1 and 2):137–42.
64. Canellos GP, Anderson JR, Propert KJ, et al. Chemotherapy of advanced Hodgkin's disease with MOPP, ABVD, or MOPP alternating with ABVD. N Engl J Med 1992;327:1478–84.
65. Cullen MH, Stuart NS, Woodroffe C, et al. ChlVPP/ PABlOE and radiotherapy in advanced Hodgkin's disease. The Central Lymphoma Group. J Clin Oncol 1994;12:779–87.
66. Somers R, Carde P, Henry-Amar M, et al. A randomized study in stage IIIB and IV Hodgkin's disease comparing eight courses of MOPP versus an alteration of MOPP with ABVD: a European Organization for Research and Treatment of Cancer Lymphoma Cooperative Group and Groupe Pierre-et-Marie-Curie controlled clinical trial. J Clin Oncol 1994;12:279–87.
67. Pfreundschuh MG, Rueffer U, Lathan B, et al. Dexa-BEAM in patients with Hodgkin's disease refractory to multidrug chemotherapy regimens: a trial of the German Hodgkin's Disease Study Group. J Clin Oncol 1994;12:580–6.
68. Fairey AF, Mead GM, Jones HW, et al. CAPE/PALE salvage chemotherapy for Hodgkin's disease patients relapsing within 1 year of ChlVPP chemotherapy. Ann Oncol 1993;4:857–60.
69. Smith MR, Khanuja PS, al-Katib A, et al. Continuous infusion ABDIC therapy for relapsed or refractory Hodgkin's disease. Cancer 1994;73:1264–9.
70. Seymour JF. New Treatment approaches to indolent non-Hodgkin's lymphoma. Semin Oncol 2004;1 Suppl 2:27–32.
71. Solal-Celigny P, Lepage E, Brousse N, et al. Recombinant interferon alfa-2b combined with a regimen containing doxorubicin in patients with advanced follicular lymphoma. Groupe d'Etude des Lymphomes de l'Adulte. N Engl J Med 1993;329:1608–14.
72. Sirohi B. Powles R. Multiple myeloma. Lancet 2004;363:875–87.
73. Palumbo A, Boccadoro M, Garino LA et al. Interferon plus glucocorticoids as intensified maintenance therapy prolongs tumor control in relapsed myeloma. Acta Haematol 1993; 90:71–6.

74. Ludwig Breast Cancer Study Group. A randomized trial of adjuvant combination chemotherapy with or without prednisone in premenopausal breast cancer patients with metastases in one to three axillary lymph nodes. Cancer Res 1985;45:4454–9.
75. Tormey DC, Kline JC, Palta M. Short-term high-density systemic therapy for metastatic breast cancer. Breast Cancer Res Treat 1985;5:177–88.
76. Meakin JW, Allt WEC, Beale FA. Ovarian irradiation and prednisone following surgery and radiotherapy for carcinoma of the breast. Breast Cancer Res Treat 1983;3:S45–8.
77. Tormey DC, Kline JC, Palta M. Short-term high-density systemic therapy for metastatic breast cancer. Breast Cancer Res Treat 1985;5:177–88.
78. De Graaf H, Willemse PH, de Vries EG, et al. Intensive chemotherapy with autologous bone marrow transfusion as primary treatment in women with breast cancer and more than five involved axillary lymph nodes. Eur J Cancer 1994;30A:150–3.
79. Wang H, Li M, Rinehart JJ, Zhang R. Pretreatment with dexamethasone increases antitumor activity of carboplatin and gemcitabine in mice bearing human cancer xenografts: in vivo activity pharmacokinetics, and clinical implications for cancer chemotherapy. Clinical Cancer Res 2004;10(5):1633–44.
80. Carmo-Pereira J, Costa FO, Henriques E. Mitoxantrone, folinic acid, 5-fluorouracil and prednisone as first-line chemotherapy for advanced breast carcinoma. A phase II study. Eur J Cancer 1993;29A:1814–6.
81. Iwanaka T, Tsuchida Y, Hashizume K, et al. Intralesional corticosteroid injection with short-term oral prednisolone for infantile hemangiomas of the eyelid and orbit. J Pediatric Surg 1994;29:482–6.
82. Park HS, Shin DM, Lee JS, et al. Thymoma. A retrospective study of 87 cases. Cancer 1994;73:2491–8.
83. Wang KC, Lee JI, Cho BK, et al. Treatment outcome and prognostic factors of medulloblastoma. J Korean Med Sci 1994;9:64–73.
84. Geyer JR, Zeltzer PM, Boyett JM, et al. Survival of infants with primitive neuroectodermal tumors or malignant ependymomas of the CNS treated with eight drugs in one day: a report from the Children's Cancer Group. J Clin Oncol 1994;12:1607–15.
85. Tchekmedyian NS. Clinical approaches to nutritional support in cancer. Curr Opin Oncol 1993;5:633–8.
86. Lai YL, Fang FM, Yeh CY. Management of anorexic patients in radiotherapy: a prospective randomized comparison of megestrol and prednisolone. J Pain Symptom Management 1994;9:265–8.
87. Attie MF. Treatment of hypercalcemia. Endocrinol Metab Clin North Am 1987;18:807–28.
88. Edwards MSB, Prados M. Current management of brain stem gliomas. Pediatr Neurosci 1987;13:309–15.
89. Weissman DE. Glucocorticoid treatment for brain metastases and epidural spinal cord compression: a review. J Clin Oncol 1988;6:543–51.
90. Sorensen S, Helweg-Larsen S, Mouridsen H, Hansen HH. Effect of high-dose dexamethasone in carcinomatous metastatic spinal cord compression treated with radiotherapy: a randomised trial. Eur J Cancer 1994;30A:22–7.
91. Hildebrand J, Gangji D. Supportive care of neurologic complications. Curr Opin Oncol 1992;4:632–41.
92. Vech CJ, Hovestadt A, Verbiest HB, et al. Dose-effect relationship of dexamethasone on Karnofsky performance in metastatic brain tumors: a randomized study of doses of 4, 8, and 16 mg per day. Neurology 1994;44:675–80.
93. Wolff JEA, Hauch H, Kuhl J, et al. Dexamethasone increases hepatotoxicity of MTX in children with brain tumors. Anticancer Res 1998;18(4B):2895–9.
94. Italian Group for Antiemetic Research. Randomized, double-blind, dose-finding study of dexamethasone in preventing acute emesis induced by anthracyclines, carboplatin, or cyclophosphamide. J. Clin Oncol 2004;22:725–9.
95. Walsh TD, West TS. Controlling symptoms in advanced cancer. BMJ 1988;296:477–81.
96. Spain RC. The case for mitomycin in non-small cell lung cancer. Oncology 1993;50(Suppl 1):35–50.
97. Liu GT, Glaser JS, Schatz NJ. High-dose methylprednisolone and acetazolamide for visual loss in pseudo-tumor cerebri. Am J Ophthalmol 1994;118:88–96.
98. Ardavanis A, Tryfonopoulos I, Yiotis G, et al. Non-allergic nature of docetaxel-induced acute hypersensitivity reactions. Anti-Cancer Drugs 2004;15:581–5.
99. Lu NZ, Cidlowski JA. The origin and functions of multiple human glucocorticoid receptor isoforms. Ann NY Acad Sci 2004;1024:102–23.
100. Burnstein KL, Cidlowski JA. Regulation of gene expression by glucocorticoids. Annu Rev Physiol 1989;51:683–99.
101. Walton J, Watson BS, Ney RL. Alternate-day versus shorter-interval steroid administration. Arch Intern Med 1970;126:601–7.
102. Goulding NJ. The molecular complexity of glucocorticoid actions in inflammation—a four ring circus. Curr Opin Pharmacol 2004;4:629–36.
103. Weinberger MH. Eplerenone: a new selective aldosterone receptor antagonist. Drugs of Today 2004;40(6):481–5.
104. Hala M, Hartmann BL, Bock G, et al. Glucocorticoid receptor gene defects and resistance to glucocorticoid-induced apoptosis in human leukemic cell lines. Int J Cancer 1996;68(5):663–8.
105. Quddus FF, Levanthal BG, Boyet JM, et al. Glucocorticoid receptors in immunological subtypes of child-hood acute lymphocytic leukemia cells: a Pediatric Oncology Group study. Cancer Res 1985;45:6482–6.
106. Bray PJ, Cotton RGH. Variations of the human glucocorticoid receptor gene (*NR3C1*): pathological in vitro mutations and polymorphisms. Human Mutation 2003;21:557–68.
107. McKay LI, Cidlowski JA. Molecular control of immune/inflammatory responses: interactions between nuclear factor-icB and steroid receptor signaling pathways. Endocr Rev 1999;20:435–59.
108. Alnemri ES, Fernandes TF, Haldar S, et al. Involvement of Bcl-2 in glucocorticoid-induced apoptosis of human pre-B-leukemias. Cancer Res 1992;52:491–5.
109. Galili U, Leizerowitz R, Moreb J, et al. Metabolic and ultrastructural aspects of the in vitro lysis of chronic lymphocytic leukemia cells by glucocorticoids. Cancer Res 1982;42:1433–40.
110. Haynes RC Jr, Murad F. Adrenocorticotropic hormone; adrenocortical steroids and their synthetic analogs; inhibitors of adrenocortical steroid biosynthesis. In: Gilman AG, Goodman LS, Rall TW, Murad F, editors. The pharmacological basis of therapeutics, 7th ed. New York: Macmillan; 1985. p. 1459–89.

54

Estrogen, Antiestrogens, and Aromatase Inhibitors

Aman U. Buzdar, MD
Harold A. Harvey, MD
V. Craig Jordan, OBE, PhD, DSc

INTRODUCTION

The importance of the reproductive endocrine system in breast cancer treatment began to be appreciated at the turn of nineteenth century. It was around this time that it was realized that approximately one-third of premenopausal women with advanced breast cancer would respond to oophorectomy.[1] However, it was only when the estrogen receptor (ER) was discovered that it was possible to fully appreciate the mechanisms underlying the activity of ovarian ablation and other associated treatments for breast cancer such as ovarian irradiation, adrenalectomy, and hypophysectomy.[2] Establishing the role of the ER pathway in breast cancer growth, and the dissection of the cellular components associated with its activity, led to the realization that the ER pathway represented a promising target for therapeutic intervention.[2] As a result, a number of endocrine agents have been identified that are directed toward either markedly reducing the level of circulating and intratumoral estrogen (the aromatase inhibitors) or to directly inhibiting the activity of the ER (the antiestrogens).

This chapter discusses recent advances in our knowledge of the molecular biology and physiology underlying the different approaches that target the ER pathway, and examines preclinical studies and results of clinical trials that support the use of each approach in the treatment of hormone-dependent breast cancer.

BIOLOGY OF ESTROGEN PRODUCTION AND MODE OF ACTION IN NORMAL AND NEOPLASTIC BREAST TISSUE

Role of Estrogen Estrogens are believed to modulate cell growth by causing an increase in stimulatory growth factors (eg, transforming growth factor-alpha [TGF-α]) and a decrease in inhibitory growth factors (eg, the TGF-β family).[3] These growth factors are thought to initiate, or prevent, progress through the cell cycle by interaction with their respective membrane receptors, with the regulatory mechanism functioning as an autocrine loop. There are also paracrine (cell-cell) influences of growth factors (eg, insulin-like growth factor-1 [IGF-1]) that can play a role in modulating the replication of epithelial cells.

Biosynthesis of Estrogen **Aromatase Structure and Regulation** Aromatase catalyzes three separate steroid hydroxylations involved in the conversion of androstenedione to estrone. The first two give rise to 19-hydroxy and 19-aldehyde structures, and the third, although still controversial, probably also involves the C-19 methyl group with release of formic acid.[4]

Aromatase consists of a complex containing a cytochrome P-450 heme-containing protein (P-450 AROM), as well as the flavoprotein nicotinamide adenine dinucleotide phosphate (NADPH) cytochrome P-450 reductase.[5] The aromatase gene encodes a polypeptide of 503 amino acids with a molecular weight of 55 kilodaltons (kDa), which exhibits approximately 30% homology with other cytochrome P-450 proteins. As aromatase has low overall homology with other members of the P-450 superfamily, it belongs to a separate gene family designated *CYP19*.

Aromatase expression occurs in many organs, including the ovary, placenta, hypothalamus, liver, muscle, adipose tissue, and the cancerous breast tissue itself.[6] Aromatase expression is controlled by multiple agents, including cytokines, cyclic adenosine monophosphate (cAMP), gonadotropins, phorbol esters, glucocorticoids, and growth factors.[7] Such regulation is associated with comparable changes in the levels of P-450 AROM messenger ribonucleic acid.[5,6] In contrast, the NADPH cytochrome P-450 reductase component is much less markedly affected. At least four major promoter sites have been identified, which account for the tissue-specific regulation of the human *P-450 AROM* gene.[7]

Sites of Estrogen Biosynthesis **Ovary** In premenopausal women, the ovary is the most important site of aromatase and estrogen production. Luteinizing hormone (LH) controls the production of androstenedione by the theca cell compartment, while follicle-stimulating hormone (FSH) up-regulates aromatase expression in granulosa cells. Acting in concert, LH stimulates production of the substrate for aromatase, whereas FSH increases the amount of aromatase so that estradiol production can increase by 8- to 10-fold at the time of ovulation. Attempts to interrupt ovarian estrogen biosynthesis with first-generation aromatase inhibitors have failed because of the reflex increases in FSH and LH secretion, which counteract the inhibitory action of the drug[8] (Figure 54-1). It is conceivable that with the introduction of more potent aromatase inhibitors, it may be possible to block ovarian steroidogenesis.

Extraglandular Aromatase In postmenopausal women, estrogen synthesis takes place nearly exclusively in extraglandular tissues. Androstenedione, produced primarily by the adrenal and, to a negligible extent, by the ovary, is converted to estrone by aromatase in the periphery, such as in adipose tissue.[9] The enzyme 17-hydroxysteroid dehydrogenase then converts estrone to estradiol. Estrone can also be conjugated into estrone sulfate to form a slowly turning-over storage pool, with a potential for back-conversion to estrone. Through the androstenedione to estrone pathway, postmenopausal women produce approximately 100 mg of estrone per day, and more if they are obese.[10] A substantial fraction of estrone is converted to estradiol to produce circulating concentrations of 10 to 20 pg/mL (Figure 54-2).

Local Estrogen Synthesis in Breast Tumors The levels of estradiol in human breast tumor tissues are an order of magnitude higher (4- to 6-fold) than those in plasma.[11] The mechanisms responsible for maintenance of high tissue estradiol concentrations are not completely defined, but are likely to involve local production of estradiol by the tumor itself.[12] Several investigators have identified aromatase activity in human breast tumors,[13,14] and aromatase expression has been shown to be a potential marker of endocrine responsiveness. Approximately two-thirds of human breast cancers contain appreciable levels of aromatase activity. However, as discussed below, aromatase expression is heterogeneous, such that high activity is present in focal clusters of specific cell types.

An additional pathway of local estrogen production by the tumor could involve steroid sulfatase, which hydrolyzes estrone sulfate to estrone. The levels of steroid sulfatase are actually higher in human breast tumors than those of aromatase, although the affinity of sulfatase for the substrate is much lower than that of aromatase.[12] Although the relative importance of steroid sulfatase versus aromatase in human breast cancer tissue remains to be defined, it is interesting to note that steroid sulfatase expression has been shown to be associated with an increased risk of recurrence and worsened outcome.[15]

Heterogenous Cellular Expression of Aromatase by Normal and Malignant Breast Tissue The quantification of P-450 AROM transcripts in breast adipose tissue from mastectomy specimens has indicated that the highest trans-

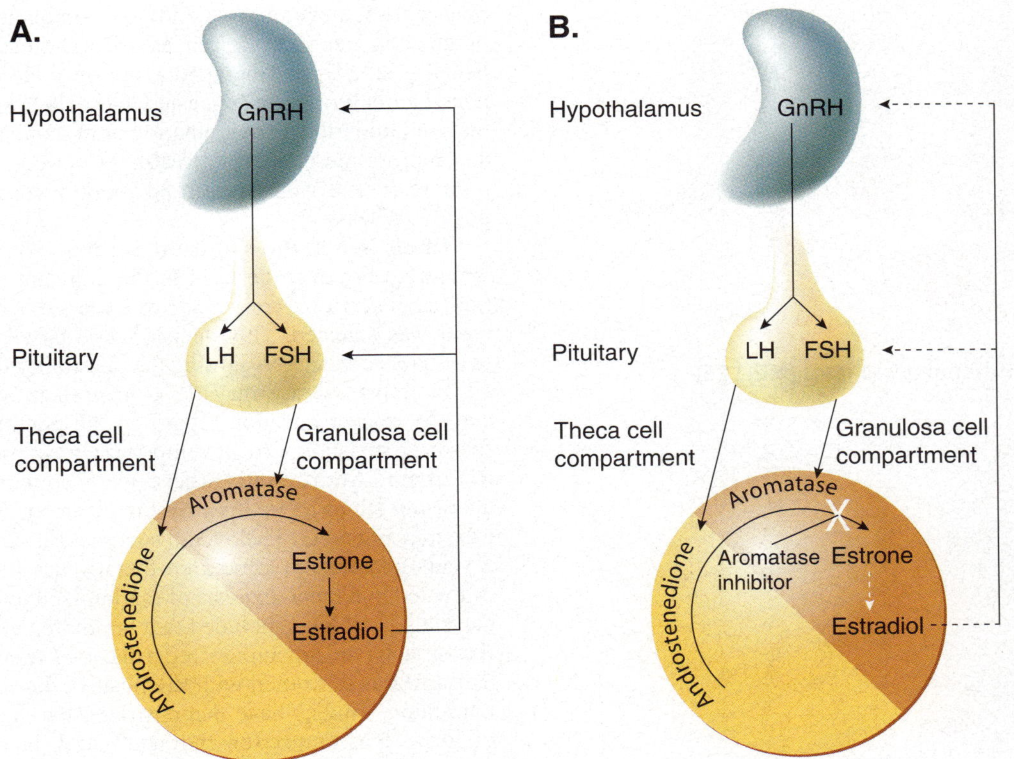

Figure 54-1 **A,** The hypothalamic-pituitary-ovarian axis. The triangle represents the hypothalamus; the ovoid, the pituitary; and the circle, the ovary. As indicated, the ovary is divided into the theca-cell compartment, where androstenedione is synthesized, and the granulosa-cell compartment, which contains the majority of the aromatase enzyme. **B,** Blockade of aromatase interrupts the negative feedback inhibition by estradiol of GnRH, LH, and FSH. Consequently, LH increases and stimulates greater production of androstenedione. FSH stimulates increased production of the aromatase enzyme. These two actions are generally sufficient to overcome the inhibitory effects of most aromatase inhibitors.

cript levels were localized to tumor-bearing quadrants, which also contained the highest proportion of adipose cells.[7] These data suggest that regional differences in the relative proportions of different histologic components of the breast tissue (ie, adipocytes vs stromal cells) may be the primary cause of estrogenic concentration gradients, because regions containing a higher number of stromal cells are the sites of elevated P-450 AROM transcript levels. The authors postulate that once neoplastic transformation has occurred, locally increased estrogen levels promote tumor growth. A positive feedback loop may be created, whereby locally produced estrogens and tumor-derived factors act in a paracrine-autocrine fashion to sustain tumor growth and development. A similar physiologic construct is also suggested by Santen and colleagues, who observed that the highest degree of aromatase expression occurred in stromal spindle cells, whereas tumor epithelial, stromal inflammatory, and normal breast elements contained lesser amounts. Furthermore, a statistically significant correlation was found between biochemical measurements of aromatase and the stromal spindle cell histologic score.[16] Heterogeneity in aromatase expression by human breast cancers has also been reported by other investigators, at both the message and protein levels.[17,18] Taken together, these observations provide further support for the possibility that human breast tumors contain biologically relevant amounts of aromatase, exerting autocrine or paracrine effects.

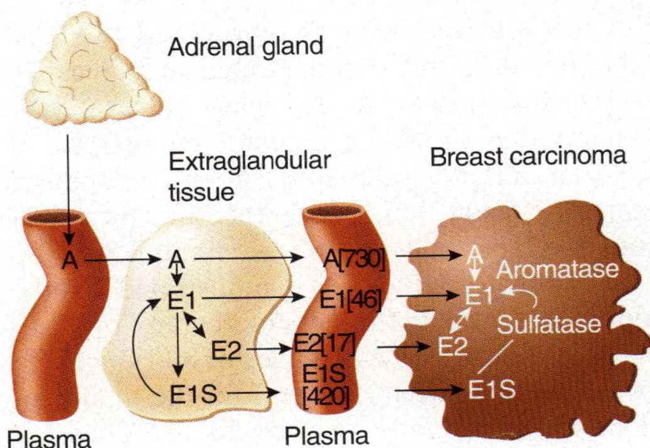

Figure 54-2 Sources of estrogen in postmenopausal women. The adrenal gland secretes androstenedione (A), which enters plasma and then tissue. Extraglandular and breast tumor tissues contain the enzymes necessary to convert A to estrone (E1), and to estradiol (E2), or to estrone sulfate (E1S). These steroids circulate in the plasma at levels indicated within the brackets and are expressed as pg/mL.

ANTIESTROGENS

Background As our knowledge of the role of estrogen in breast cancer developed, a number of antiestrogens were identified and synthesized[19] (Figure 54-3). This process has sometimes been problematical, with the development of some antiestrogens, such as MER25, being halted because of tolerability problems, while clomiphene (Clomid), although acting as an antifertility agent in rodents, was found to actually induce ovulation in women.[20] However, the antiestrogen tamoxifen demonstrated efficacy combined with a low incidence of side effects and so was developed further.[21]

Tamoxifen **Mode of Action** Tamoxifen is the trans-geometric isomer of a substituted triphenylethylene with well-characterized antifertility[22] and antitumor[23] activity in the rat. As a group, the triphenylethylene-type antiestrogens have an interesting species-specific pharmacology.[24] In short-term tests in the mouse, tamoxifen can cause increases in uterine wet weight and vaginal cornification. In contrast, tamoxifen is classified as a pure antiestrogen in the chick. Tamoxifen exhibits the properties of a partial estrogen agonist/antagonist in rats and women. It is this balance of biologic properties that is key to the current strategies for the use of tamoxifen.

Tamoxifen is a competitive inhibitor of estradiol binding to the ER.[19] Estradiol causes the proliferation of ER-positive breast cancer cells in culture, and tamoxifen can reversibly prevent estrogen-stimulated growth.[25] Similarly, tamoxifen will prevent estrogen-stimulated growth of ER-positive breast cancer cells transplanted into immune deficient (athymic) mice.[26] Antiestrogens, such as tamoxifen, negate the stimulatory effects of estrogen by blocking the ER, causing the cell to be held at the G_1 phase of the replicative cycle.[27] Tamoxifen also causes a decrease in the circulating levels of IGF-1.[28]

Clinical Pharmacology Tamoxifen treatment schedules vary depending on the country and its initial clinical trials evaluating the drug. Schedules of 10 mg twice daily or 20 mg once daily are recommended in the United States, although 10 mg three times daily and 20 mg twice daily have been used in other countries. There is a low incidence of side effects, the most frequent of which are hot flashes[24] and, in general, the high therapeutic index has permitted wide variations in dosage.

Tamoxifen is rapidly absorbed and attains steady-state serum levels within 4 to 6 weeks.[29] The drug is extensively metabolized to *N*-desmethyltamoxifen (major metabolite) and 4-hydroxytamoxifen (minor metabolite). Both metabolites have the potential[30] to be converted to 4-hydroxy-*N*-desmethyltamoxifen, which is also a minor metabolite[31,32] that has a high affinity for the ER[33] and may contribute to the antitumor actions of tamoxifen.[34] Tamoxifen has a long serum half-life of 7 days, and the metabolite *N*-desmethyltamoxifen has an even longer serum half-life of 14 days.[35] These long serum half-lives are probably why a withdrawal response has not been routinely documented when tamoxifen therapy is discontinued.

Tamoxifen exhibits weak estrogen-like properties in postmenopausal women.[24,36] There is a partial decrease in LH and FSH levels, increases in sex hormone-binding globulin (SHBG) levels, decreases in antithrombin III, some changes in vaginal cytology, and hyperplasia of the endometrium. Tamoxifen causes ovarian stimulation

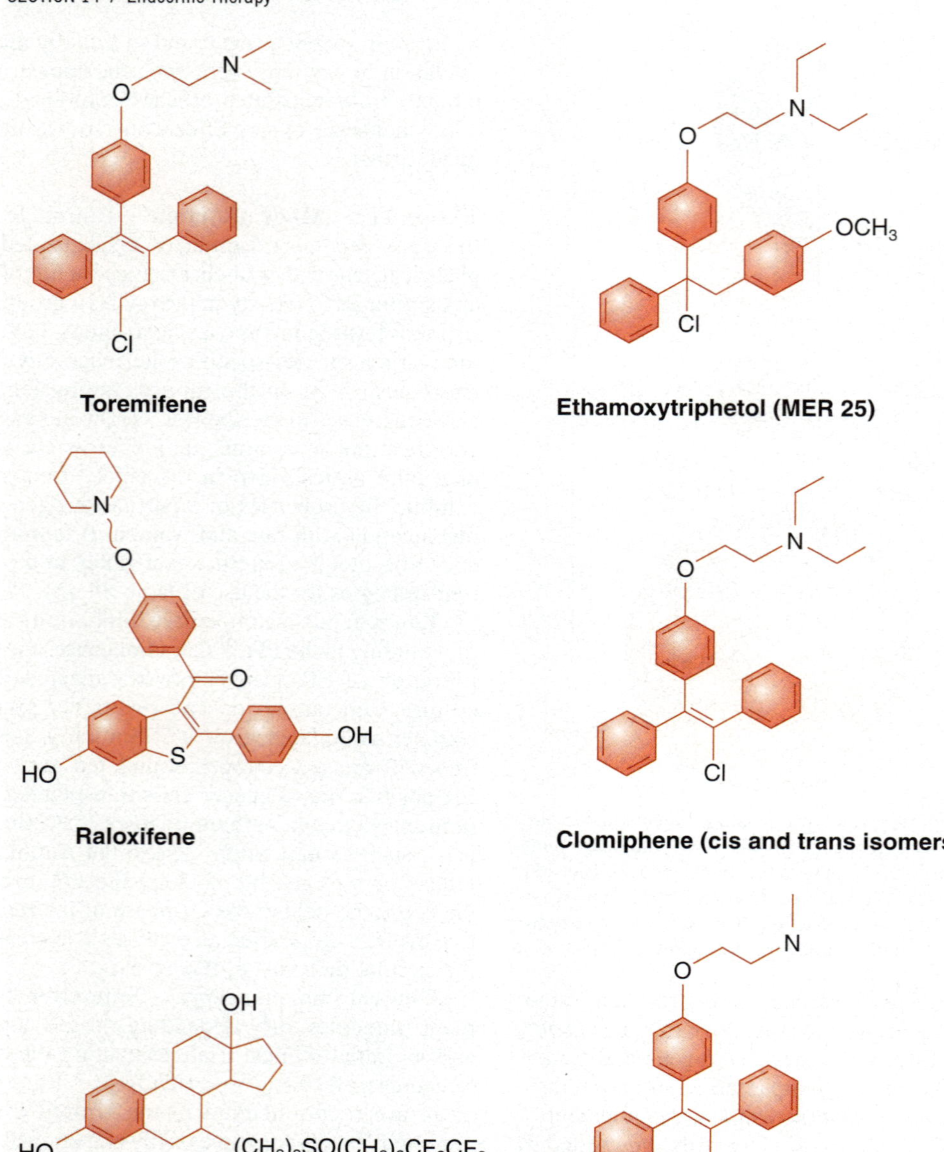

Figure 54-3 Structure of antiestrogens.

in premenopausal women with ovulatory cycles and increases in steroidogenesis.[37-41] Women are at risk of pregnancy during tamoxifen therapy, and patients should be informed about the need for barrier contraception. Tamoxifen is not recommended if a woman is pregnant, although clinical cases of teratogenesis have not been reported with tamoxifen.

Tamoxifen in Advanced Breast Cancer Tamoxifen is an endocrine option for metastatic disease in postmenopausal patients.[24] Approximately one-third of patients respond to tamoxifen therapy and the response rate is similar to that seen with diethylstilbestrol (DES) therapy.[42] However, tamoxifen exhibits fewer side effects compared with DES, with hot flashes being the side effect most commonly reported during tamoxifen therapy (less common, but more serious, side effects are discussed further in the section "Tolerability of Antiestrogens" below). Patients with ER-positive disease are more likely to benefit from tamoxifen therapy.[24] Correlation of clinical response and ER status indicates that 48% (159 of 333) of patients with ER-positive disease had partial or complete responses, whereas only 13% (17 of 129) of ER-negative patients had responses. A variety of combinations of other hormonal agents and combination chemotherapy have been examined, but tamoxifen is usually administered as monotherapy.

Tamoxifen is effective in the treatment of advanced disease in premenopausal women.[37,39] Small randomized trials have demonstrated that tamoxifen produces a response rate and overall survival similar to what is seen after oophorectomy.[43,44] However, with the development of effective luteinizing hormone-releasing hormone (LHRH) agonists such as goserelin (Zoladex) (to reduce ovarian steroidogenesis by preventing LH release from the pituitary gland), the combination of goserelin and tamoxifen has become established as an effective therapeutic option.[45] Hence, recent guidelines have suggested that LHRH agonists or tamoxifen, in combination or in sequence, are appropriate endocrine treatment options for premenopausal women with hormone receptor-positive disease.[46]

Tamoxifen in the Adjuvant Setting When tamoxifen began to be used in the adjuvant setting, a conservative course of 1 or 2 years of treatment was selected. This decision was based on reasonable concerns regarding the possibility that ER-negative disease may develop prematurely, and the related question regarding the potential for drug resistance to develop with prolonged treatment. Additionally, there were concerns about the ethics of treating people in whom disease may not recur. The overall success of 1, 2, or 5 years of adjuvant tamoxifen therapy has been evaluated in a meta-analysis of randomized clinical trials,[47] which concluded that tamoxifen confers a survival advantage regardless of menopausal status in women with ER-positive disease. Laboratory studies have demonstrated the value of long-term tamoxifen therapy[48] and, in the meta-analysis, 5 years of tamoxifen was superior to 2 years of tamoxifen for ER-positive pre- or postmenopausal women.[47] One year of tamoxifen has little or no benefit, and the drug is virtually ineffective as an adjuvant in patients with ER-negative disease. The benefit of more than 5 years of treatment with tamoxifen has been discussed,[47] with the conclusion that the long-term follow-up of a large number of patients is required before a definitive conclusion can be reached. These data are currently unavailable and, as a result, the value of more than 5 years of tamoxifen continues to be uncertain.

Chemotherapy Plus Tamoxifen Data relating to the combination of chemotherapy with tamoxifen are somewhat inconclusive. The Eastern Cooperative Oncology Group (ECOG) has evaluated the duration of tamoxifen therapy in postmenopausal patients, all of whom received combination chemotherapy (cyclophosphamide plus methotrexate plus 5-fluorouracil [CMF]). An initial analysis[49] demonstrated an increase in disease-free survival with 5 years versus 1 year of tamoxifen. However, a combined analysis of this trial, and a similar study in premenopausal women, did not find a difference in survival or time to relapse between the two treatments.[50]

A report from Italy has demonstrated that the addition of combination chemotherapy of CMF (6 cycles followed by 4 courses of epirubicin) to long-term tamoxifen (5 years) for the treatment of ER-positive, node-positive disease does not seem to significantly improve the clear-cut effectiveness of tamoxifen alone in preventing recurrence.[51] In contrast, the National Surgical Adjuvant Breast and Bowel Project (NSABP) protocol B-16 shows a benefit for tamoxifen-treated postmenopausal patients with the addition of an Adriamycin-containing chemotherapy regimen.[52]

A recent examination of long-term findings from NSABP trials B-14 and B-20 shows that over 12 years the benefit from the combination of CMF and tamoxifen was greater than that for tamoxifen alone (hazard ratio [HR] for recurrence-free survival [RFS] 0.52, $p < .0001$; HR for overall survival 0.78, $p = .063$).[53] These trials were performed in 6,490 women with primary breast cancer, negative axillary lymph nodes, and ER-positive disease.

Recent evidence suggests that tamoxifen given sequentially following cyclophosphamide, doxorubicin, and 5-fluorouracil (CAF) combination chemotherapy is more beneficial than concurrent CAF with tamoxifen.[54] Sequential administration of CAF and tamoxifen was found to produce significant improvements in disease-free survival and overall survival compared with concurrent administration or tamoxifen alone.

OTHER ANTIESTROGENS **Toremifene** Toremifene (Fareston; see Figure 54-3) is a structural derivative of tamoxifen with similar antiestrogenic and estrogenic properties demonstrated in laboratory animals. In general, toremifene is highly protein bound, which could explain its long serum half-life. Toremifene is less potent than tamoxifen and, consequently, clinical studies have evaluated doses of toremifene up to 240 mg/day. Toremifene is cross-resistant with tamoxifen, but clinical trials have shown that it exhibits a similar efficacy and side-effect profile to tamoxifen, and so may be used as an alternative to treat advanced breast cancer, and it could represent a useful option in the adjuvant setting.[55,56]

Raloxifene Raloxifene (Evista) is an antitumor agent in animals[57] but is not available for the treatment of breast cancer. The drug has not been tested successfully for any stage of the disease. Raloxifene maintains bone density in rats[58,59] and postmenopausal women[60] and is available for the treatment and prevention of osteoporosis. Raloxifene reduces serum cholesterol[61] and is being tested for the reduction of risk of coronary heart disease in high-risk women. An exploratory study in postmenopausal women with primary breast cancer has indicated that raloxifene is associated with significant antiproliferative effects in ER-positive disease.[62] The Multiple Outcomes of Raloxifene Evaluation (MORE) trial included 7,705 postmenopausal women with osteoporosis, and has shown that the risk of invasive breast cancer was decreased by 76% ($p < .001$) during 3 years of treatment.[63] The MORE trial has been extended, with data now indicating that the reduction in invasive breast cancer risk continues beyond 4 years.[64] Raloxifene is currently being tested against tamoxifen for the reduction of breast cancer in 22,000 high-risk postmenopausal women (the Study of Tamoxifen and Raloxifene [STAR] trial). Raloxifene should not be used in premenopausal women until more complete data are available to support its use in this patient group.

The side effects of raloxifene are consistent with other antiestrogens; hot flashes, leg cramps, and an increase in vascular events have been reported. Raloxifene appears to demonstrate uterine safety in early evaluations,[65] but because endometrial cancer is rare, uterine safety can only be assured through the results of ongoing long-term prevention trials.[64]

Trilostane Trilostane (Modrenal) is an antiadrenal drug that is usually used for short-term adrenal suppression in the treatment of Cushing's syndrome. However, trilostane's ability to modify the binding of estrogen to the ER has prompted interest in its potential to block breast tumor cell proliferation. A meta-analysis of several small studies investigating the use of trilostane in postmenopausal women with advanced breast cancer reported clinical benefit with this agent, and further trials are needed to evaluate its worth as an endocrine therapy for advanced breast cancer.[66]

Fulvestrant Fulvestrant (Faslodex) is an ER antagonist that, unlike tamoxifen, has no agonist effects. Fulvestrant binds to the ER, inhibiting deoxyribonucleic acid (DNA) binding and so promoting the rapid degradation of the ER. This results in a dramatic loss of cellular ER levels,[67,68] which is also associated with a significant reduction in progesterone receptor (PgR) expression.[69,70]

Fulvestrant (250 mg intramuscular [IM] injection once monthly) has been compared with anastrozole (Arimidex) (1 mg orally once daily) in two phase III trials in postmenopausal women with advanced breast cancer who had progressed on prior tamoxifen therapy.[71,72] The trials demonstrated that fulvestrant was well tolerated and was at least as effective as anastrozole. A prospective, combined analysis of the two trials indicated that, after a median follow-up of 15.1 months, the median times to progression [TTP] were 5.5 months versus 4.1 months, and overall response rates were 19.2% versus 16.5% for fulvestrant versus anastrozole, respectively. The median durations of response were 16.7 months for fulvestrant and 13.7 months for anastrozole.[73] An extended follow-up has demonstrated that the mean duration of response for all randomized patients (from onset or response to progression) was significantly greater for fulvestrant compared with anastrozole, with a ratio of average response durations of 1.30 (95% confidence intervals [CI] 1.13, 1.50; $p < .01$). Based on these and other data, fulvestrant has been approved for the treatment of hormone receptor-positive, metastatic breast cancer in postmenopausal women progressing on prior antiestrogen therapy.[74]

Fulvestrant is well tolerated, with generally mild side effects, the most frequent of which are hot flashes, and very few patients withdraw from the clinical trials because of drug-related events. Although fulvestrant 250 mg/month is clearly effective, the good tolerability of fulvestrant means that a loading doses regimen may be a clinical option to allow steady state levels to be achieved more rapidly. This may allow treatment responses to be achieved and recognized earlier. Such regimens are currently being evaluated in phase III clinical trials.

The different mechanism of action of fulvestrant, compared with other antiestrogens, may mean that resistance to prior endocrine therapies is not reflected in cross-resistance to fulvestrant. This question has been examined in retrospective analyses, with data indicating that patients who respond to fulvestrant but later progress may retain sensitivity to other endocrine agents.[75] A similarly retrospective study has indicated that fulvestrant may be a useful option in the treatment of postmenopausal women with visceral metastases.[76] The appropriate positioning of fulvestrant within sequential endocrine therapies will need careful consideration.

TOLERABILITY OF ANTIESTROGENS **Osteoporosis** Estrogen is important in maintaining bone health in premenopausal women. After menopause, hormone replacement therapy is often recommended to prevent the development of osteoporosis. Clearly, the long-term administration of an antiestrogen has the potential to precipitate premature osteoporosis.

Animal studies show that tamoxifen has estrogenic effects in bone.[59,77] Clinical studies show that 2 years of adjuvant tamoxifen therapy does not decrease bone density[78–80] and there is evidence to suggest that tamoxifen is beneficial and maintains bone in the lumbar spine and the neck of the femur.[81–83] Tamoxifen showed a nonsignificant decrease in fractures in the NSABP prevention study; however, it must be stressed that this was not a primary endpoint and that the study population was not at risk of osteoporosis.[84]

Atherosclerosis Estrogen lowers low-density lipoprotein (LDL) cholesterol levels and raises high-density lipoprotein (HDL) cholesterol levels. It is possible that this change in blood lipids is responsible for the decrease in myocardial infarction observed in premenopausal women compared with men. Following menopause, women are at the same risk of coronary heart disease as men. It can be argued that the long-term administration of an antiestrogen could produce a population at risk of premature coronary heart disease. However, the estrogen-like effects of tamoxifen [24] lower the circulating levels of cholesterol in female patients.[85–91]

A meta-analysis of 52,929 women showed a significant decrease in fatal myocardial infarction,[92] as did an analysis of a Scottish clinical trial of 5 years of adjuvant tamoxifen.[93] However, an NSABP study in a small series of women not at risk of coronary heart disease showed only a nonsignificant decrease in coronary heart disease.[94]

Ophthalmic Effects Certain antiestrogens, including tamoxifen, have been shown to produce cataracts in preclinical models.[24] An evaluation[95] of patients receiving tamoxifen, 10 to 20 mg 2 or 3 times daily for up to 2 years, noted no ocular changes. Nevertheless, high-dose tamoxifen therapy is associated with retinal changes (keratopathy and multiple paramacular refractile lesions in the nerve fiber and inner plexiform layers).[96] It is, therefore, possible that accumulated toxicity will occur with decades of tamoxifen therapy. Although there is no evidence that severe ocular changes occur, there is evidence that tamoxifen is associated with a modest increase in the incidence of cataracts and cataract operations.[84,97,98] Patients with pre-existing macular degeneration should be carefully evaluated when starting tamoxifen therapy.[99]

Thromboembolic Disorders A number of recent reports have demonstrated an association between the use of tamoxifen and subsequent thromboembolic episodes. In the preventative setting, tamoxifen has been shown to be associated with a significantly increased risk of developing a major venous thromboembolism.[100] Similarly, a systematic review of studies published between 1966 and 2003 indicated that both chemopreventative tamoxifen, and tamoxifen used in the treatment of early-stage disease, were associated with an increased risk of venous thromboembolism.[101] An analysis of NSABP clinical trials[84] showed a significant increase in thromboembolic disorders in postmenopausal women. This is comparable with increases noted with hormone replacement therapy or raloxifene.[61] Patients with a known history of thromboembolic disorders should be carefully evaluated before a decision is made to use long-term tamoxifen therapy.

Uterine Stimulation Tamoxifen is known to produce some estrogen-like effects in postmenopausal women.[24] Research has demonstrated that increases in endometrial thickness, hyperplasia, and fibroids may follow several years of tamoxifen therapy.[61,102] Endometrial thickening is associated with the stromal component of the uterus rather than the epithelial component.[103] Transvaginal ultrasonography is, however, an unreliable tool for the evaluation of patients taking tamoxifen.[104]

Endometrial carcinoma has been reported to occur in patients receiving tamoxifen therapy, with long-term tamoxifen use being associated with a poorer prognosis, seemingly because of less favorable histology and higher stage.[105] Indeed, the Stockholm[106] and NSABP[107] adjuvant trials of tamoxifen noted an increase in endometrial carcinoma, compared with rates in a control arm. Similarly, the Early Breast Cancer Trialists' Group overview of women with early breast cancer demonstrated that tamoxifen was associated with a significant increase in the incidence of endometrial cancer.[47] The NSABP P-1 Breast Cancer Prevention trial noted that the increased risk of endometrial cancer was predominantly in women of 50 years or older, and was evident early in the follow-up period.[84] Premenopausal women are not at risk of an increase in endometrial cancer. All cases of persistent vaginal bleeding should be followed up with a gynecologic examination and an endometrial biopsy. It is important to bear in mind that the benefits associated with tamoxifen outweigh the increased risk of endometrial cancer. However, some consideration will need to be given to the risk of endometrial cancer when tamoxifen is used as a preventative agent in healthy women.

Liver Carcinogenesis Tamoxifen produces DNA adducts in the livers of both rats[108] and monkeys,[109] and lifetime treatment with > 3 g/kg causes carcinogenesis in the liver.[110,111] The relevance of these laboratory findings for the treatment of human disease has been discussed[112]; however, an increase in human hepatocellular carcinoma has not been noted since tamoxifen was introduced into the market in 1978,[113] and no increase in liver tumors is noted in the overview analysis.[47]

AROMATASE INHIBITORS

In postmenopausal or castrated women, the major source of estrogen derives not from the ovaries, but from the conversion of the adrenal hormones androstenedione and, to a lesser extent, testosterone to estrone (see Figure 54-2). This enzymatic conversion occurs at extra-adrenal or peripheral sites, such as fat, liver, and muscle, and is catalyzed by the aromatase enzyme complex. Some breast cancer tissues also contain aromatase. Potent aromatase inhibitors that further lower the levels of both circulating and intratumoral estrogens are now recognized as effective agents in the treatment of postmenopausal women with hormone-sensitive breast cancer.

Increasing use of aromatase inhibitors has essentially eliminated the need for major endocrine ablative procedures, such as adrenalectomy or hypophysectomy, as palliative therapy for metastatic breast cancer. Importantly, they now challenge tamoxifen as the preferred first-line choice in the treatment of postmenopausal women with advanced disease, and are becoming part of the adjuvant therapy of early-stage disease.

Development of Early Aromatase Inhibitors Because aminoglutethimide is the prototype of later aromatase inhibitors, it is useful to briefly consider the information gleaned from the early experimental and clinical experience with this agent.

Aminoglutethimide, a derivative of the sedative agent glutethimide, was initially introduced into clinical medicine as an anticonvulsant and was later recognized to be an inhibitor of cytochrome P-450 N-mediated steroid hydroxylations.[114] Aminoglutethimide was initially thought to produce a "medical adrenalectomy," but it was later recognized that the estrogen-lowering effect induced by the aminoglutethimide and glucocorticoid regimen was primarily a result of inhibition of the aromatase enzyme.[115,116] The effects of this compound, however, are rather nonspecific, because the drug affects a number of hydroxylation steps in the metabolic conversion of cholesterol to active steroid products and, overall, the use of aminoglutethimide plus glucocorticoid in women with breast cancer produces results similar to those expected from other forms of endocrine therapy.

Patients receiving the standard dose of aminoglutethimide (1,000 mg/day) experience a wide range of side effects during the induction of therapy; the major problems include drug rash, fever, and lethargy. Many patients also require mineralocorticoid replacement with 9α-fluorohydrocortisone (Florinef) because of the inhibition of aldosterone production[117] or thyroxine supplementation because of the inhibitory effects of aminoglutethimide on thyroid hormone synthesis, a cytochrome P-450 N-dependent process.[118] The frequency and severity of side effects from aminoglutethimide, particularly when compared with tamoxifen, provided impetus to the development of less-toxic aromatase inhibitors that could be easily utilized for prolonged periods of time.

Development of Improved Aromatase Inhibitors and Their Classification The problems associated with aminoglutethimide (multiple actions, side effects, the need for exogenous glucocorticoids) emphasized the need to develop second- and third-generation aromatase inhibitors. These newer compounds demonstrate increased potency, greater specificity, and reduced toxicity, compared with aminoglutethimide. Several new compounds have been studied, and the recent data for the clinically important ones (anastrozole, letrozole, and exemestane) are reviewed below. These data derive from studies in the advanced (first- and second-line), adjuvant, and neoadjuvant (preoperative) settings.

A convenient classification divides the aromatase inhibitors into the mechanism-based inhibitors (type I) and those that are competitive inhibitors (type II) (Figure 54-4).

Mechanism-Based Aromatase Inhibitors Mechanism-based aromatase inhibitors (also known as suicide inhibitors) initially compete with the natural substrate (ie, androstenedione and testosterone) for binding to the active site of the enzyme. The enzyme then specifically acts on the inhibitor to yield reactive alkylating species, which form covalent bonds at or near the active site of the enzyme. Through this mechanism, the enzyme is irreversibly inactivated.

Second-Generation Mechanism-Based Aromatase Inhibitors ***Formestane*** Formestane (4-hydroxyandrostenedione, Lentaron) is a second-generation steroidal aromatase inhibitor that is given by deep intramuscular injection. Preliminary in vivo studies showed superiority over tamoxifen,[119] and formestane is active in postmenopausal women with advanced breast cancer who have progressed on tamoxifen,[120] with efficacy similar to that of megestrol acetate.[121] Formestane has also demonstrated clinical benefit in patients who have progressed on nonsteroidal aromatase inhibitors,[122] although larger trials are required to clarify the position of this drug in the treatment of advanced breast cancer.

Third-Generation Mechanism-Based Aromatase Inhibitors ***Exemestane*** Exemestane (6-methylene-androsta-1,4-diene-3,17-dione, Aromasin) is an irreversible (type I or mechanism-based) aromatase inhibitor.[123,124] Exemestane's inhibitory constant (K_i) for competitive

First generation
non-steroidal competitive inhibitors

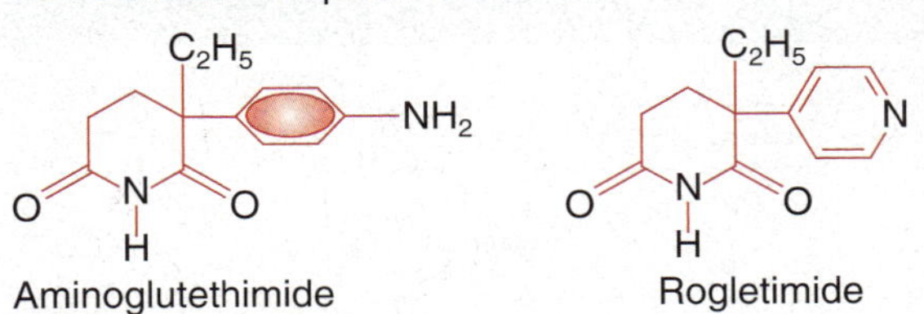

Second generation
A. Steroidal, mechanism based inhibitors

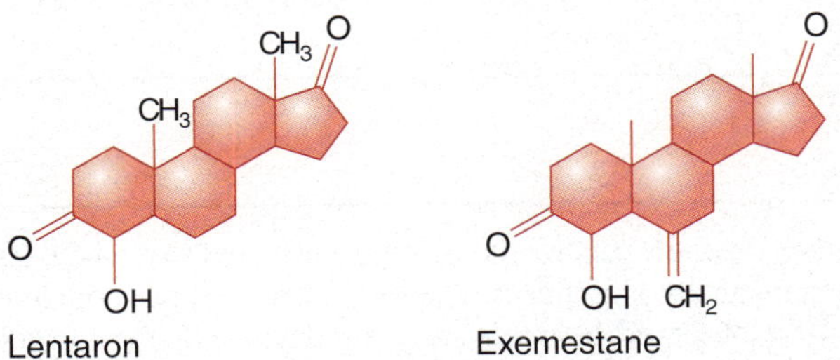

B. Non-steroidal competitive inhibitors

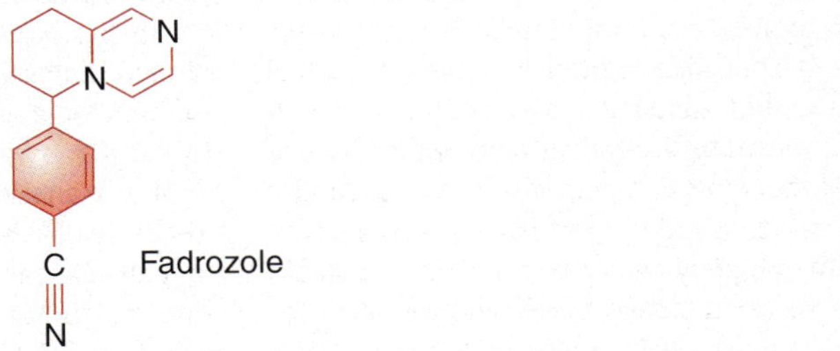

Third generation
Non-steroidal, mechanism based inhibitors

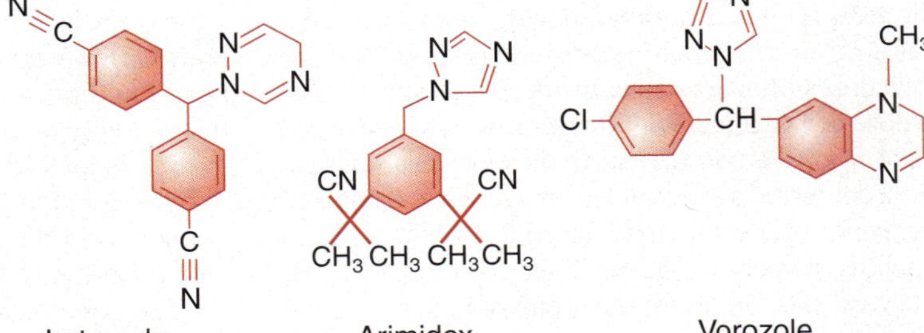

Figure 54-4 Structure and classification of representative aromatase inhibitors. Compounds are shown in approximate order of increasing specificity and potency of aromatase inhibition.

inhibition is 10.2 nmol/L, and for irreversible inactivation is 26 nmol/L. Single-dose administration reveals a major reduction of plasma estrogens with this compound,[124] with a dose of 25 mg/day inhibiting aromatase activity by 97.9%, as documented by the isotope kinetic technique.

Second-Line Exemestane Phase II clinical trials of exemestane in postmenopausal patients with metastatic breast cancer showed very promising results with response rates ranging from 11 to 28%, depending on the extent of prior endocrine therapy.[125,126] In a large, randomized phase III trial conducted in 769 postmenopausal patients with metastatic breast cancer no longer responding to tamoxifen, exemestane 25 mg/day PO was compared with megestrol acetate 40 mg 4 times daily. Patient and disease characteristics were similar between the two arms of the trial. Kaufman and colleagues reported a 15% objective response rate (ORR) among the 366 women receiving exemestane, which was similar to the 12.4% ORR for the women treated with megestrol acetate. An additional 22% of women in each treatment group experienced stabilization of their disease. Exemestane produced a statistically significant increase in the median duration of overall clinical benefit (60.1 vs 49 weeks, $p = .025$), as well as in the median time to tumor progression. Furthermore, in this trial, the authors reported that the median survival was also significantly longer in patients receiving exemestane. Table 54-1 summarizes these results. Side effects associated with exemestane treatment were mild and included hot flashes, nausea, and fatigue in relatively few patients. Undesirable weight gain was also less frequent among women receiving exemestane, compared with that observed in women treated with megestrol acetate.[127]

First-Line Exemestane A phase II study has compared exemestane (25 mg/day) with tamoxifen (20 mg/day) as first-line treatment of metastatic breast cancer in postmenopausal women (n = 93) (Table 54-2).[128] Mature data from the trial indicate that the median duration of response for exemestane (n = 61) was 16 months compared with 22 months for tamoxifen (n = 59). The ORR (complete response plus partial response) was 41% for exemestane versus 17% for tamoxifen. It was concluded that exemestane was well tolerated and active in the first-line treatment of metastatic disease and, as a result, the study was extended into phase III.[129] Exemestane was well tolerated and was associated with a significantly longer progression-free survival compared with tamoxifen (10.9 vs 6.7 months, respectively).

COMPETITIVE AROMATASE INHIBITORS Competitive inhibitors bind reversibly to the active site of the aromatase enzyme and prevent product formation only as long as the inhibitor occupies the catalytic site. The available mechanism-based inhibitors are exclusively steroidal in structure, whereas the competitive inhibitors are nonsteroidal compounds (see Figure 54-4).

Second-Generation Nonsteroidal, Competitive Aromatase Inhibitors ***Fadrozole*** Fadrozole (CGS 16949A; 4-[5,6,7,8-tetrahydroimidazo-(1,5-a)-pyridin-5yl] benzonitrile) is a highly potent inhibitor of aromatase with a K_i of 0.19 nmol, which compares with 600 nM for aminoglutethimide.[130,131]

Clinical data from several phase II trials of fadrozole demonstrated an overall ORR in postmenopausal patients with advanced breast cancer that ranged from 3 to 23%. In one trial, objective regressions were recorded in 20% of 54 patients[132] and 28% of 18 patients treated by Possinger and colleagues experienced an objective response.[133] Falkson's group reported an ORR of 23% among 78 patients.[134] All studies reported a higher rate of disease stabilization, and the median time to treatment failure ranged from 4 to 16 months. It should be noted that most patients enrolled in these early trials had received several prior endocrine and other therapies.

Toxicity attributed to fadrozole is mild and consists mainly of nausea, anorexia, fatigue, and hot flashes. Two large multicenter phase III trials have compared fadrozole with megestrol acetate in patients who had received only tamoxifen as prior hormone therapy. No significant differences were observed between the two treatment arms of the trials with respect to TTP, ORRs, response duration, or overall survival. Nausea was more frequent for fadrozole than megestrol acetate in both trials (22% vs 13%, and 36% vs 11%, respectively). In contrast, edema was more common with megestrol acetate than with fadrozole (21% vs 12%, and 19% vs 12%, respectively) as was weight gain.[135] Fadrozole represents a major improvement over aminoglutethimide and the drug is approved in Japan for the treatment of patients with breast cancer.

Third-Generation Nonsteroidal Competitive Aromatase Inhibitors Third-generation aromatase inhibitors are the most potent and highly

Table 54-1 Combined Data from Phase III Trials Comparing Anastrozole, Letrozole, and Exemestane with Megestrol Acetate in Postmenopausal Women Previously Treated with Tamoxifen

	Combined Data		Initial Trial		Second Trial		Initial Trial	
	Anastrozole	Megestrol Acetate	Letrozole	Megestrol Acetate	Letrozole	Megestrol Acetate	Exemestane	Megestrol Acetate
No. patients	263	253	174	189	199	201	366	403
Objective response[a], %	12.6	12.2	23.6	16.4	16.1	14.9	15	12
Clinical benefit[b], %	42.2	40.3	34.5	31.7	26.7	23.4	37	35
Progression, %	57.4	59.3	53.4	56.1	51.3	50.7	48	53
Median TTP, months	5	5	5-6	5.5	3	3	5	5
Median duration of benefit, months	18.3	15.7	33	18	17.5	15.4	15	12
Median survival, months	28.7	21.5	25.3	21.5	28.6	26.2	NA	28

TTP = time to progression; NA = not available.
[a]Objective response = complete response plus partial response.
[b]Clinical benefit = complete response plus partial response plus stable disease for ≥ 6 months.

selective members of this class of drugs. Anastrozole, letrozole, and vorozole have undergone extensive clinical study and are discussed below.

Anastrozole Anastrozole (Arimidex) is a potent and selective benzyltriazole derivative. At a concentration of 15 nmol/L anastrozole inhibits aromatase activity by 50%. In rodents, maximal hormonal suppression is achieved with an oral dose of 0.1 mg/kg. Studies conducted in monkeys demonstrate similar inhibitory potency when expressed on a mg/m^2 basis and assessed by measurement of plasma estradiol. Studies in women demonstrated suppression of plasma estrogen to levels approaching the limits of assay sensitivity. Anastrozole produced no effects on aldosterone, cortisol, or thyroxine synthesis. The estimated elimination half-life in humans is 32.2 hours.[136]

Second-Line Anastrozole Anastrozole was the first aromatase inhibitor to be approved in the United States for the management of advanced breast carcinoma in postmenopausal women. This approval was based on results from two pivotal trials that together accrued a total of 764 patients randomized to receive either anastrozole (1 mg/day PO) or anastrozole (10 mg/day PO) or megestrol acetate 40 mg 4 times daily.[137] These patients had metastatic disease that was progressing following therapy with tamoxifen, given either in the adjuvant setting or as first-line endocrine therapy for metastatic disease. Patients in the three arms of the trial had similar prognostic characteristics including age, ER status, disease-free interval, and sites of metastases. Results from these important trials showed similar ORRs in either dose of anastrozole or megestrol acetate. No statistically significant dose-response differences were observed between the 1 mg/day and 10 mg/day dosage. ORRs, including complete and partial response rates and stabilization of disease of > 6 months (ie, total clinical benefit), averaged 35%. It should be noted that recent studies demonstrate that disease stabilization for > 6 months is a meaningful clinical parameter because patients experiencing this response survive equally as long as patients undergoing partial response.[138] Patients with complete or partial responses or stable disease survive longer than those with disease progression. In initial reports, anastrozole was considered superior to megestrol acetate because it was better tolerated. It was associated with less undesirable weight gain, dyspnea, fever, and thromboembolic events, when compared with megestrol acetate.[137] As there were no differences between the two doses of anastrozole, the drug was approved at a dose of 1 mg/day. With further maturity, combined data from the two pivotal trials show that anastrozole conferred a survival advantage when compared with the progestin (median 26.7 months vs 22.5 months, respectively) (see Table 54-1). The 2-year survival was 56.1% for the group of patients receiving anastrozole (1 mg/day), compared with 46.3% for patients treated with megestrol acetate.[139]

First-Line Anastrozole As first-line therapy in postmenopausal women with advanced breast cancer, anastrozole (1 mg/day) was compared with tamoxifen (20 mg/day) in two international, multicenter trials involving 1,145 patients[140,141] (see Table 54-2). Patients were randomized in a double-blind, double-dummy trial designed to determine whether or not the two treatments had equivalent efficacy in this patient population. The primary endpoints of the trials were TTP, ORR, and tolerability.

In the North American trial carried out in the United States and Canada,[141] median TTP was 11.1 months for anastrozole and 17 months for tamoxifen (p = .005; two-sided). Clinical benefit rates were 59% for anastrozole and 46% for tamoxifen (p = .0098; two-sided retrospective analysis), suggesting that anastrozole is superior to tamoxifen in the first-line treatment of advanced breast cancer. In the European trial,[140] median TTP was 8.2 and 8.3 months, and ORR was 32.9% and 32.6% in the anastrozole and tamoxifen arms, respectively, confirming that anastrozole was at least as effective as tamoxifen in terms of the primary efficacy endpoints. However, it should be noted that the European trial enrolled fewer women with ER-positive disease compared with the North American trial (~45% vs 89% of patients, respectively). Hence the difference in the TTP results between the two trials is mainly attributed to the percentage of patients with confirmed ER-positive tumors.

The combined analysis of both trials was performed after a median follow-up of 18.5 months and included 551 patients who received anastrozole and 510 who received tamoxifen.[142] Median TTP was 8.5 months for anastrozole versus 7.0 months for tamoxifen (p = .103; two-sided). The ORR was 29.0% for anastrozole and 27.1% for tamoxifen. Clinical benefit rates were 57.1% for anastrozole

Table 54-2 Efficacy Data from Trials Comparing Anastrozole, Letrozole, and Exemestane with Tamoxifen in the First-Line Treatment of Postmenopausal Women with Metastatic Breast Cancer

	Phase II Study				Phase III Studies			
	Letrozole	Tamoxifen	Exemestane	Tamoxifen	Anastrozole[a]	Tamoxifen[a]	Anastrozole[b]	Tamoxifen[b]
No. patients	453	454	61	59	170	182	340	453
Objective response, %	30	20[c]	41	14	21	17	33	30
Clinical benefit, %	49	38[c]	56	42	59	46[c]	56	56
TTP, months	9	6[c]	9	5	11	6[c,d]	8	8
TTF, months	9	6[c]	NR	NR	8	5	6	6

TTF = time to failure; TTP = time to progression.
[a]North American Study.
[b]European study.
[c]Difference is statistically significant.
[d]Nonprotocol analysis; NR, not recorded.

and 52% for tamoxifen ($p = .1129$; two-sided retrospective analysis). For patients with hormone receptor-positive tumors (59.8% of patients), median TTP was 10.7 months for anastrozole versus 6.4 months for tamoxifen ($p = .022$; two-sided). Anastrozole was associated with significantly fewer venous thromboembolic events than tamoxifen.

Letrozole The second aromatase inhibitor to gain approval in the United States with the indication for management of postmenopausal women with metastatic breast cancer was letrozole (Femara). Letrozole is also a potent nonsteroidal competitive aromatase inhibitor and possesses considerable selectivity for aromatase. When administered orally to adult female rats at a dose of 1 mg/L/day for 14 days, letrozole decreased uterine weight to that observed after a surgical ovariectomy.[143] Letrozole also causes significant regression of dimethylbenzanthracene-induced rat mammary tumors.

Clinical studies in normal healthy volunteers, as well as dose-seeking phase I trials in postmenopausal women with advanced breast cancer, showed that letrozole in a dose as little as 0.25 mg/day PO caused maximal suppression of plasma and urinary estrogens. Using a highly sensitive recombinant DNA-based estradiol bioassay, levels of estradiol were shown to decrease by 95% to levels of 0.05–0.07 pmol/L. This observation underscores the limitation of standard radioimmunoassays for detection of estradiol levels in patients given highly potent aromatase inhibitors.[144] Early trials of letrozole in heavily pretreated postmenopausal women with metastatic breast cancer demonstrated both clinical efficacy and lack of significant toxicity.[145] Approval of this agent was based on the results of two large, multicenter, randomized trials similar in design to the studies involving anastrozole, which are described below.

Second-Line Letrozole In a pivotal trial, 555 postmenopausal women with metastatic breast carcinoma progressing after treatment with tamoxifen were randomized to receive letrozole 0.5 mg/day or 2.5 mg/day, or standard doses of megestrol acetate. The women in the three treatment groups were comparable in all respects. The 2 doses of letrozole caused similar prompt and profound suppression of plasma and urinary estrogens. Letrozole (2.5 mg/day) yielded ORRs of 36% and 35%, respectively, compared with 27% and 33%, respectively, for letrozole (0.5 mg/day) and 32% for megestrol acetate. The median duration of response for letrozole (2.5 mg/day) was 33 months, compared with 18 months for both megestrol acetate and letrozole 0.5 mg/day. Similarly, there was a trend in time to tumor progression and survival that favored letrozole 2.5 mg/day (see Table 54-1).[146] The second multinational study enrolled 602 patients; all patients had advanced or metastatic breast cancer, with evidence of disease progression while receiving continuous adjuvant antiestrogen therapy, had experienced relapse within 12 months of stopping adjuvant antiestrogen therapy given for at least 6 months, or had experienced disease progression while receiving antiestrogen therapy for advanced disease. There were no statistically significant differences among the three treatment groups for overall objective tumor response. Patients treated with letrozole 0.5 mg/day had improvements in disease progression ($p = .044$) and a decreased risk of treatment failure ($p = .018$) compared with patients treated with megestrol acetate. Letrozole 0.5 mg/day showed a trend for survival benefit compared with megestrol acetate ($p = .053$).

In a second, similar study involving 555 postmenopausal patients with advanced breast cancer progressing after tamoxifen therapy, letrozole was compared with aminoglutethimide (250 mg twice daily) and hydrocortisone. Letrozole 2.5 mg once daily produced an ORR of 19.5% versus 12.4% for aminoglutethimide.[147] The median response duration was 21 months for letrozole compared with 14 months for aminoglutethimide, and there was a statistically significant improvement in overall survival for the patients receiving letrozole. Moreover, letrozole produced less somnolence and skin rash.

First-Line Letrozole A large, multicenter, double-blind, first-line phase III clinical trial in postmenopausal women ($n = 907$) with locally advanced or metastatic breast cancer compared letrozole (2.5 mg/day) with tamoxifen (20 mg/day).[148] The primary endpoint was TTP and secondary endpoints included ORR, time to treatment failure (TTF), time to response, and survival. Sixty-five percent of patients had ER-positive/PgR-positive status. TTP was significantly longer for letrozole than for tamoxifen (median 41 vs 26 weeks). Letrozole was superior to tamoxifen in TTF ($p = .0001$), with a median of 40 weeks for letrozole and 25 weeks for tamoxifen. ORR was significantly higher for letrozole patients at 30%, compared with 20% for tamoxifen-treated patients ($p = .0006$) (see Table 54-2). Prior adjuvant tamoxifen in this trial was seen to have an adverse impact on subsequent response to treatment with tamoxifen therapy. These data were confirmed in a follow-up study that updated the efficacy results.[149] The updated study also examined survival, finding that median overall survival was 34 months for letrozole and 30 months for tamoxifen. If appropriate, patients were permitted to cross over to the alternative treatment upon disease progression or discontinuation, and it was reported that patients who initially received letrozole exhibited a longer duration on endocrine therapy compared with those who initially received tamoxifen (median of 16 months vs 9 months, respectively).

Vorozole Vorozole (R83842; R76713; 6-[(S)4-Chlorophenyl)-1H-1,2,4-triazol-1-ylmethyl]-1-methyl-1H-benzotriazole) represents another specific aromatase inhibitor that has shown little toxicity in animal studies. Phase I clinical studies revealed an acute reduction of plasma estradiol to undetectable levels in normal men receiving one 10 mg dose and a 64% reduction in premenopausal women.[150] A phase II study in postmenopausal women with metastatic breast cancer indicated that vorozole-related side effects were mild, with a profound suppression of serum estradiol and estrone from pretreatment levels. Of 27 evaluable patients, 3 (11%) had partial remission of their disease and 14 achieved disease stabilization for a median duration of 12 months.[151] In addition, vorozole was well tolerated and produced a higher response rate (20% vs 15%,) and longer TTP (18 months vs 12 months) than megestrol acetate in a phase III randomized clinical trial in postmenopausal patients with metastatic breast cancer progressing on tamoxifen.[152] However, despite these clinical results, vorozole has now been withdrawn from further clinical development.

Neoadjuvant Studies with Aromatase Inhibitors Neoadjuvant treatment is intended to downstage a tumor before primary locoregional therapy with surgery, thus allowing breast-conserving therapy in a greater number of patients, or making surgery possible in cases that were considered inoperable. As the third-generation aromatase inhibitors have demonstrated efficacy in the treatment of advanced and early disease, it is important to examine the benefits these agents may bring to the preoperative setting.

Anastrozole A small, randomized, double-blind, single-center study was performed in which anastrozole (1 mg/day and 10 mg/day, for 3 months) was used as neoadjuvant therapy in 23 postmenopausal women with newly diagnosed, ER-rich, locally advanced, or large (> 3 cm) operable breast tumors.[153] Of 17 patients who would have required mastectomy at the initiation of treatment, 15 were suitable for breast conservation after 3 months of treatment with anastrozole. These results suggest that anastrozole is effective as neoadjuvant therapy in postmenopausal women with ER-rich breast tumors.

Two recent studies have compared neoadjuvant treatment with anastrozole and tamoxifen for 12 weeks in postmenopausal women with large operable or inoperable (including locally advanced) hormone receptor-positive breast cancers. The Immediate Preoperative Arimidex, Tamoxifen, or Combined with Tamoxifen (IMPACT) trial enrolled 330 women and, of the 124 women considered to require a mastectomy at baseline, significantly more became eligible for breast-conserving surgery after 3 months of treatment with anastrozole compared with tamoxifen (46% vs 22%, respectively; $p = .03$).[154] The PReOperative Arimidex Compared with Tamoxifen (PROACT) trial involved 451 women and reported that 43% versus 31% of women receiving anastrozole or tamoxifen, respectively, became eligible for surgery or for less invasive surgery ($p = .04$).[155] Anastrozole was well tolerated in both trials. A prospectively planned, combined analysis of these two trials has been performed. The analysis demonstrated that a significantly greater proportion of patients with inoperable disease or who required a mastectomy at trial entry who received anastrozole, had an improvement in feasible surgery from baseline to actual surgery at 3 months, compared with those receiving tamoxifen. These data indicate that anastrozole is an effective and well-tolerated neoadjuvant therapy for postmenopausal women with hormone receptor-positive breast cancer.

Letrozole Letrozole (2.5 mg/day, n = 12; 10 mg/day, n = 12) was administered to 24 patients with ER-positive breast tumors as primary systemic therapy.[156] The resulting median reduction in tumor volume was 81%. Fifteen patients who would have been considered for mastectomy before letrozole therapy were found to be suitable for breast conservation after 3 months of letrozole treatment. In a double-blind, randomized, multicenter study, letrozole (2.5 mg/day) was compared with tamoxifen (20 mg/day) as neoadjuvant treatment of 337 postmenopausal women with ER-positive primary breast cancer, over a 4-month period.[157] All patients at baseline were considered ineligible for breast-conserving surgery. The primary endpoint was tumor response. ORRs were 55% for letrozole (n = 154) versus 36% for tamoxifen (n = 170), a difference that was statistically significantly different ($p < .001$; Mantel-Haenszel log-rank test). After 4 months of therapy, 45% of letrozole-treated patients underwent a lumpectomy/quadrantectomy versus 35% of tamoxifen-treated patients ($p = .022$). It was concluded that letrozole was significantly superior to tamoxifen in terms of tumor reduction, which resulted in a superior rate of breast-conserving surgery in the letrozole-treated group. These data have been supported by additional biologically based trials. In one study, letrozole has been shown to be more effective than tamoxifen in the neoadjuvant treatment of patients with ER-positive, epidermal growth factor receptor-1 (ErbB-1)-positive and or ErbB-2 (HER2/neu)-positive primary breast cancer.[158] Following on from this, a more recent trial in postmenopausal women with ER-positive locally advanced disease has indicated that, unlike tamoxifen, the inhibition of proliferation induced by letrozole in the neoadjuvant setting was independent of ErbB status.[159]

Exemestane A small study has examined the efficacy of exemestane in the neoadjuvant setting. Thirteen postmenopausal women with untreated large or locally advanced ER-rich tumors were treated with exemestane (25 mg/day for 3 months). One patient died during the study because of an unrelated cause. Before treatment, 10 of the remaining 12 patients were considered to require a mastectomy; after treatment, only 2 patients underwent a mastectomy and 10 patients received breast-conserving surgery.[160] More recently, exemestane (25 mg/day for 6 months) has been shown to be an effective and well-tolerated neoadjuvant therapy for elderly patients, allowing conservative surgery to be used in patients who were considered ineligible for surgery at trial entry.[161,162]

Adjuvant Studies with Aromatase Inhibitors Tamoxifen remains the most widely used endocrine agent for the adjuvant therapy of early breast cancer in postmenopausal women. Nevertheless, tamoxifen does have limitations in use, most notably its recognized pharmacologic properties and side effects. As discussed earlier, tamoxifen is associated with an increased risk of both thromboembolic events and endometrial changes, including endometrial cancer.[47,105] It is reasonable to conclude that other endocrine agents can provide at least equivalent, if not superior, efficacy together with improved tolerability in patients with early disease. In this context, it is important to consider data from adjuvant trials of the newer generation aromatase inhibitors.

Initial Treatment of Early Disease Anastrozole is currently the only aromatase inhibitor that has mature data as initial adjuvant therapy in postmenopausal women with early breast cancer. The 'Arimidex,' Tamoxifen, Alone or in Combination (ATAC) trial is a randomized, double-blind trial designed to compare the efficacy and tolerability of 5 years of treatment with tamoxifen with that of anastrozole versus the combination of anastrozole and tamoxifen.[163–165] The primary endpoints are time to recurrence and safety; other criteria for evaluation include time to distant metastases, survival, and occurrence of contralateral breast cancer.

The ATAC trial enrolled 9,366 postmenopausal women with invasive breast cancer who had completed primary therapy (surgery). The mean age of the patients was similar in each of the three treatment arms: 64.1 years in both single-agent arms and 64.3 years in the combination arm. The treatment arms were well balanced in terms of hormone receptor status of the tumors. After an initial median follow-up of 33.3 months and treatment duration of 30.7 months, 317 of the 3,125 women in the anastrozole group suffered a relapse in their breast cancer or died, compared with 379 of 3,116 women in the tamoxifen group. This 17% improvement in disease-free survival was statistically significant ($p = .0129$). In the combination arm, 383 of 3,125 women had a relapse of their breast cancer or died as a first event.[163]

The first efficacy update was performed after a median follow-up period of 47 months and confirmed the findings of the initial analysis.[164] Of the first events, 84 patients in the anastrozole arm had locoregional disease, compared with 101 in the tamoxifen arm and 1,071 in the combination therapy arm. Twenty patients who received anastrozole had invasive contralateral disease, compared with 35 in the tamoxifen arm and 30 in the combination therapy arm. Disease-free survival in the ER-positive population produced an HR of 0.86 for anastrozole versus tamoxifen, representing a 14% reduction with anastrozole compared with treatment with tamoxifen ($p = .03$). In the combination therapy arm, the HR was 1.04, or nearly equivalent to tamoxifen alone ($p = .7$).

In a safety analysis performed after a median duration of treatment of 36.9 months, predefined adverse events favoring tamoxifen included a reduction in musculoskeletal disorders and there was a specific side effect of arthralgia associated with aromatase inhibitors. There was also an excess of fractures in absolute terms in the anastrozole arm compared with tamoxifen (fracture rates were 7.1% vs 4.4% in anastrozole and tamoxifen arms, respectively). However, in favor of anastrozole was the reduction in the incidence of hot flashes (–5.3%), and a significant difference in the incidence of vaginal bleeding (–3.9%) and vaginal discharge (–9.2%). There was also a significant reduction in the risk of endometrial cancer (–0.6%), with the rates of the anastrozole group very similar to the rates that might be expected in a similar untreated population. Endometrial cancer was detected in 15 women receiving tamoxifen and in 3 women receiving anastrozole. There was a significant reduction in ischemic cerebrovascular accidents (–1.2%), venous thromboembolic events (–1.6%), and deep-vein thrombosis (–0.7%). Anastrozole was associated with a reduction in the risk of contralateral breast cancer. The odds ratio of anastrozole versus tamoxifen is 0.62, which represents a 38% reduction in the incidence of contralateral breast cancers over tamoxifen.

A recent analysis from the ATAC trial has been conducted after a median follow-up of 68 months, at which point only 8% of patients remained on treatment.[165] The data confirm that patients treated with anastrozole continue to exhibit prolonged disease-free survival and time to recurrence, and reduced distant metastases compared with tamoxifen (Table 54-3). As tamoxifen is associated with higher rates of recurrence and increased numbers of adverse events and treatment withdrawals, it is important that patients receive treatment with the most effective and well-tolerated therapy at the earliest opportunity. Five years of anastrozole should, therefore, be considered the preferred initial treatment of choice in the adjuvant setting.

Newly Diagnosed Postmenopausal Women with Hormone Receptor-Positive Disease: the BIG 1-98 Trial The Breast International Group 1-98 (BIG 1-98) trial randomized 8,028 postmenopausal women with newly diagnosed hormone receptor-positive breast cancer. BIG 1-98 includes two primary adjuvant arms comparing 5 years of letrozole with 5 years of tamoxifen, and two sequential treatment arms comparing 2 years of letrozole followed by 3 years of tamoxifen and 2 years of tamoxifen followed by 3 years of letrozole. Patients from all four arms were included in the primary core analysis, but events in the sequential arms were only counted up to the time of the treatment switch plus 30 days. At a median follow-up of 25.8 months, a significant benefit was seen in favor of letrozole over tamoxifen in terms of disease-free survival (HR 0.81, 95% CI 0.70, 0.93; $p = .003$). There was a significantly greater incidence of bone fractures in patients receiving letrozole compared with those receiving tamoxifen (odds ratio 1.44; $p = .0006$). Patients in the tamoxifen group had significantly more grade 3-5 thromboembolic events (odds ratio 0.38; $p < .0001$) than patients in the letrozole group. The overall incidence of adverse events was similar in the two treatment groups. Fifty-five patients on letrozole and 38 patients on tamoxifen died without recurrence ($p = .08$); there were more cerebrovascular and cardiac deaths in patients receiving letrozole compared with those receiving tamoxifen (7 vs 1 and 26 vs 13, respectively).

Table 54-3 Efficacy Data from Studies of Aromatase Inhibitors in the Adjuvant Treatment of Postmenopausal Women with Early Breast Cancer

	Initial Therapy	Post-Tamoxifen Therapy		
	ATAC Trial Anastrozole vs Tamoxifen	MA 17 Trial Letrozole vs Placebo	IES Trial Exemestane vs Tamoxifen	ITA Trial Anastrozole vs Tamoxifen
Median follow-up	68 months	2.4 years	30.6 months	24 months
No. patients	9366	5187	4742	426
	DFS	Death, recurrence or CLBC	Risk of recurrence	Death
	HR 0.87	HR 0.61	HR 0.68	HR 0.18
	(95% CI 0.78, 0.97; p = .01)	(95% CI 0.47, 0.79; p ≤.001)	(95% CI 0.56, 0.82; p = .00005)	(95% CI 0.02, 1.57; p = .07)
	TTP	Recurrence or CLBC	Survival free of distant metastases	Relapse
	HR 0.79	HR 0.57	HR 0.66	HR 0.36
	(95% CI 0.70, 0.90; p = .0005)	(95% CI 0.43, 0.75; p = .00008)	(95% CI 0.52, 0.83; p = .0004)	(95% CI 0.17, 0.75; p = .006)
	CLBC		CLBC	
	OR 0.58		HR 0.44	
	(95% CI 0.38, 0.88; p = .01)		(95% CI 0.20, 0.98; p = .04)	

CI = confidence intervals; CLBC = contralateral breast cancer; DFS = disease-free survival; HR = hazard ratio; OR = odds ratio; TTP = time to progression.

Post-Tamoxifen Treatment Although anastrozole has the most mature data compared with tamoxifen as primary adjuvant therapy, letrozole has been examined as an adjuvant therapy for women who have already received initial adjuvant therapy with tamoxifen.[166] The MA 17 trial was a randomized, double-blind, extended adjuvant, placebo-controlled trial in 5,187 postmenopausal women who had received 5 years of adjuvant treatment with tamoxifen (see Table 54-3). Although the trial was controversially unblinded earlier than intended, it did demonstrate that, after a median follow-up of 2.4 years, women receiving letrozole exhibited a significantly longer disease-free survival rate compared with those receiving placebo (93% vs 87%, respectively; p ≤ .001). The HR for local or metastatic recurrence, or new contralateral breast cancer in the letrozole versus the placebo group was 0.57 (95% CI 0.52, –0.75; p = .00008).

Letrozole was found to be well tolerated and was associated with a lower incidence of vaginal bleeding and an increase in low-grade hot flashes, arthritis, arthralgia, and myalgia, compared with placebo. However, the premature termination of the study means that longer follow-up is required to fully establish the adverse-event profile of letrozole in the adjuvant setting. In particular, it will be important to determine letrozole's cardiovascular effects and to assess the long-term impact of treatment on bone metabolism. The latter is particularly relevant, since a diagnosis of new-onset osteoporosis and fractures occurred in a significantly higher number of women in the letrozole group, compared with placebo (8% vs 6%, respectively; p = .003).[167]

Switching from Tamoxifen The Intergroup Exemestane Study (IES) has examined the question of what is the optimal endocrine therapy after a woman has received 2 to 3 years of tamoxifen therapy.[168] The trial enrolled 4,742 patients who were randomly assigned to continue with tamoxifen, or to switch to exemestane for the remainder of the 5-year treatment period. Three years after randomization, the data indicate that switching to exemestane was associated with a significant improvement in disease-free survival compared with continuing with tamoxifen (91.5% vs 86.8%, respectively) (see Table 54-3). Overall survival was not significantly different between the two groups, and contralateral breast cancer occurred in 20 patients receiving tamoxifen, compared with 9 patients receiving exemestane (p = .04).

Anastrozole has also been examined as an adjuvant option in postmenopausal women who had received treatment with tamoxifen for ≥ 2 years in the Italian Tamoxifen Anastrozole (ITA) trial.[169] Women (n = 426) were randomized to either continue to receive tamoxifen for 5 years, or to switch to anastrozole 1 mg/day for a similar length of time. After a median follow-up of 24 months, the data indicated that switching patients to anastrozole appeared to decrease their risk of relapse and death (see Table 54-3). For women switching to anastrozole, the HR for relapse was 0.36 (95% CI 0.17, 0.75; p = .006) and the HR for death was 0.18 (95% CI 0.02, 1.57; p = .07). In addition, serious adverse events were found to be more common for women who continued to receive tamoxifen, compared with those treated with anastrozole (29 vs 14 events, respectively).

The Austrian Breast and Colorectal Cancer Study Group (ABCSG) 95 and Arimidex-Nolvadex (ARNO) 95 trials have examined the efficacy of switching adjuvant therapy from tamoxifen to anastrozole. These studies included a combined total of 3,123 postmenopausal women with hormone receptor-positive early breast cancer, and a prospectively planned combined analysis indicated that the HR for recurrence-free survival was 0.59 (95% CI 0.42, 0.82; p < .0018) for anastrozole versus tamoxifen.[170] These data, therefore, support the results of the ITA trial and suggest that postmenopausal women who have received 2 years of treatment with adjuvant tamoxifen should switch to anastrozole.

Tolerability of Aromatase Inhibitors **Bone Effects** Both anastrozole and letrozole have been shown to be associated with an increase in fractures and joint disorders.[164–166] However, only the ATAC trial has long-term data and these indicate that the fracture rate in women receiving anastrozole stabilizes after the initial 2 years of treatment.[171] Indeed, the most recent analysis of data from the ATAC trial, performed after a median follow-up of 68 months, confirms that the safety profile of anastrozole remains unchanged during the 5-year treatment period.[165] These data indicate that fracture rates per 1,000 women-years were 22.6 for anastrozole versus 15.6 for tamoxifen (HR 1.44; 95% CI 1.21, 1.68; p < .0001), although incidence of hip fractures was low and similar between the two treatments.

More specifically, the effects of anastrozole on markers of bone turnover have been studied in two clinical trials, one in women with advanced disease[172] and one in patients with early disease.[173] The study in postmenopausal patients with advanced breast cancer indicated that treatment with anastrozole (1 mg/day for 12 weeks) produced significant increases in markers of bone formation and bone resorption.[172] However, it was noted that the presence of bone metastases was correlated with increases in the markers of bone turnover (bone-specific alkaline phosphatase [bone-ALP] and urinary type-I collagen N-telopeptides [NTX]). A sub-protocol of the ATAC study has examined changes in the markers of bone turnover after 1 year of treatment, and reported that anastrozole 1 mg/day was associated with an increase in NTX and bone-ALP, while tamoxifen (20 mg/day) was associated with decreases in these markers.[173,174]

Treatment with letrozole (2.5 mg/day) for 6 months in healthy postmenopausal women resulted in a significant increase in bone resorption, as measured by urinary pyridinoline and deoxypyridinoline, compared with baseline (p < .005 for both markers).[175] A study published by Harper-Wynne and colleagues has shown that 3-month treatment with letrozole resulted in increases in bone resorption (measured by C-terminal).[176] However, there are currently no published data available on the effects of letrozole on markers of bone turnover in women with advanced or early breast cancer.

Treatment with exemestane for 8 weeks has also been shown to produce significant increases in a marker of bone formation (bone-ALP) and resorption (serum type-I collagen C-telopeptide).[177] In addition, two other studies have indicated that exemestane produces increases in markers of bone resorption and formation, one in 13 postmenopausal patients with advanced disease and disease progression on one nonsteroidal aromatase inhibitor,[178] and another in postmenopausal women with low-risk early breast cancer.[179]

Overall, in the absence of head-to-head studies between aromatase inhibitors, it is not possible to determine whether they have any different effects on bone resorption, because the duration of treatment was different, as were the bone markers and sex of the volunteers. In addition, although mature follow-up data are available for anastrozole, comparable data are not yet available for the other aromatase inhibitors, letrozole or exemestane. The ability of bisphosphonates to prevent or reverse bone loss associated with aromatase inhibitors is starting to be examined in trials such as the Zometa/Femara Adjuvant Synergy Trials (Z-FAST/ZO-FAST). In these trials, postmenopausal women with hormone receptor-positive early-stage disease will receive letrozole 2.5 mg daily and be randomized to one of two zoledronic acid treatment arms: zoledronic acid 4 mg every 6 months starting when letrozole treatment commences, or zoledronic acid 4 mg every 6 months beginning only if the patient's bone mineral density decreases below −2.0 standard deviations. Studies such as this will provide insight into the effectiveness of bisphosphonates in postmenopausal women receiving aromatase inhibitors for the treatment of early breast cancer.

Effects on Lipid Anastrozole does not markedly alter lipid profiles (when compared with baseline measures); data derived from patients (n = 952 at study entry) recruited into two large advanced breast cancer trials comparing anastrozole and tamoxifen showed that anastrozole (1 mg/day) did not affect nonfasting lipids in women with advanced breast cancer (measurements taken every 12 weeks for > 2 years).[180] In a smaller, more recent study of postmenopausal patients (n = 27) who were compared with baseline measures, treatment with anastrozole did not significantly alter mean serum levels of apolipoprotein A-1 and B after 6 months of treatment.[181] This confirmed a previous report that indicated that treatment with anastrozole (median duration of 76 weeks) did not significantly alter any lipid profile.[182]

Letrozole (2.5 mg/day) had an unfavorable effect on fasting lipids in 20 women with advanced breast cancer, after 8 and 16 weeks of treatment,[183] with letrozole treatment resulting in significant increases in total (p = .05) and LDL-cholesterol (p < .01), and apolipoprotein B (p = .05) levels. In addition, 9 weeks of treatment with exemestane in postmenopausal women with advanced breast cancer resulted in a significant decrease in total cholesterol (p < .01), HDL-cholesterol (p < .01), and total triglyceride (p = .023),[184] which are in a favorable direction with respect to total cholesterol and triglycerides, but in an unfavorable direction with respect to HDL-cholesterol. However, the results of the European Organization of Research and Treatment of Cancer (EORTC) trial (n = 122) showed that 24 weeks of exemestane had no impact on serum lipids.[185]

Of course, lipid profiles are surrogate endpoints, with the most appropriate being the incidence of cardiovascular events over the longer term. The ATAC trial demonstrates that long-term adjuvant treatment with anastrozole resulted in significantly fewer thromboembolic and cerebrovascular events compared with tamoxifen.[165] However, equivalent data are not currently available for letrozole or exemestane, and so it is important that the results for anastrozole are not extrapolated to the other aromatase inhibitors, since the agents appear to exhibit varying effects on lipid profiles.

SELECTION OF PATIENTS FOR THERAPY WITH AROMATASE INHIBITORS

Postmenopausal Women Endocrine therapy is usually offered to patients with metastatic disease who have ER- or PgR-positive or receptor-unknown disease. In addition to the level of receptors, clinical features that might suggest a favorable response include a long disease-free interval after initial surgery or the presence of nodal, soft tissue, bone, pleural, or nodular lung metastases. Patients with central nervous system involvement, extensive liver disease, lymphangitic spread of tumor in the lungs, or rapidly progressing and life-threatening disease are not ordinarily considered candidates for hormone therapy. Earlier clinical experience and data from the literature suggested that most endocrine therapies, with the possible exceptions of androgens and glucocorticoids, are equally efficacious. The decision to choose one endocrine therapy over another depended on the menopausal status of the patient, considerations of efficacy, ease of administration, cost, and side effects. Historically, of all the earlier endocrine therapies, tamoxifen was associated with the fewest side effects. The aromatase inhibitors, however, lack the partial estrogen agonist effect of tamoxifen. The available data confirm the superiority of aromatase inhibitors as the drug of first choice in metastatic breast cancer.

In the adjuvant setting, the availability of more mature data now suggests that anastrozole, and not tamoxifen, should be the preferred choice for the initial treatment of early disease. This conclusion has been confirmed in the recent American Society of Clinical Oncology (ASCO) Technology Assessment.[186]

Premenopausal Women Considerations of efficacy, cost, toxicity, and ease of administration also dictate the choice of endocrine therapy in premenopausal patients. On the basis of these considerations, first-line therapy includes either tamoxifen or oophorectomy. Effective castration can be accomplished either by surgery, pelvic irradiation, or the use of LHRH agonists. Because the ovaries are resistant to aromatase inhibition (see Figure 54-1), aromatase inhibitors have traditionally been tested in postmenopausal patients. However, the activity of the very potent third-generation aromatase inhibitors makes it likely that these compounds can be used in combination with an LHRH agonist. In a small study, 16 patients with metastatic (n = 13) or locally advanced primary breast cancer (n = 3) received goserelin and anastrozole for up to 32 months. Clinical benefit was observed in 89% of the women, with 7 of the 13 women displaying clinical benefit for a year or longer.[187] A second trial has recently examined the efficacy and tolerability of goserelin plus anastrozole in 22 premenopausal women with measurable recurrent or metastatic, hormone receptor-positive disease. Preliminary data from 18 patients indicate that clinical benefit was observed in 13 patients (72%).[188] These early data suggest that the combination of an LHRH agonist with an aromatase inhibitor may be an active therapeutic option in the treatment of premenopausal women, but additional studies are needed to further define the role of anastrozole in this subgroup of patients.

Male Breast Cancer Male breast cancer, although a rare condition, is frequently an estrogen-dependent tumor. Although tamoxifen is often used in the management of this disease, only anecdotal reports are available concerning the activity of aromatase inhibitors in this setting. In a small series of five patients, clinical benefit with anastrozole was observed in men with breast cancer following antiestrogen therapy.[189] However, limited data have indicated that exemestane appears to stimulate tumor growth in men with prostate cancer,[190] and so caution should be exercised before using exemestane for the treatment of male breast cancer. Further additional studies are needed to define the role of aromatase inhibitors in male patients with breast cancer because of the very limited data regarding their safety and efficacy.

FUTURE PERSPECTIVES IN THE CLINICAL DEVELOPMENT OF ANTIESTROGEN AND AROMATASE INHIBITOR THERAPIES FOR BREAST CANCER

Chemoprevention Tamoxifen has been shown to prevent carcinogenesis in rodent models of mammary cancer.[191,192] These laboratory data, in conjunction with the efficacy of tamoxifen in preventing the appearance of second primary breast cancers,[106,193] has lead to increased enthusiasm for the use of tamoxifen as a preventive agent in women at risk of breast cancer. The carcinogenic insult that initiates breast cancer probably occurs during the reproductive years. An overview of the main outcomes from the five main breast cancer prevention trials, covering more than 28,000 patients, has shown that tamoxifen produced a 38% reduction in breast cancer incidence (p < .0001).[194] There was no effect on ER-negative disease (p = .21), but ER-positive cancers were reduced by 48% (p < .0001). However, endometrial cancer rates were increased (consensus relative risk 2.4; p = .0005) in patients receiving preventive tamoxifen,

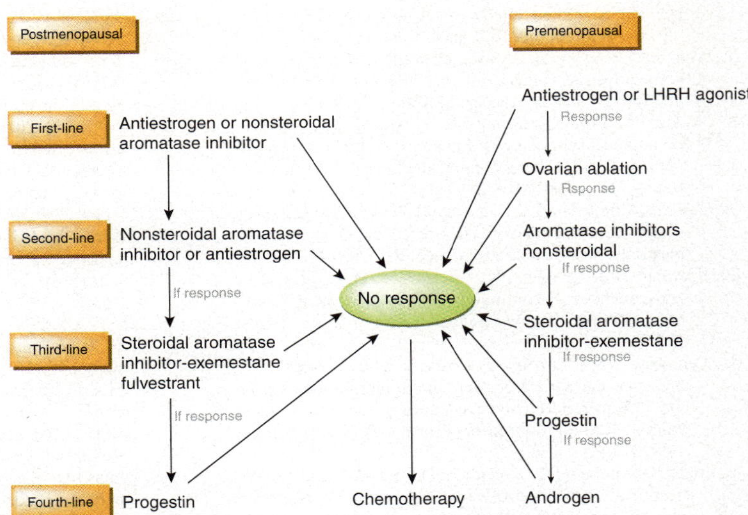

Figure 54-5 Potential sequential endocrine options for patients with metastatic breast cancer.

as were venous thromboembolic events (relative risk 1.9; $p < .0001$). As a result, tamoxifen cannot be used as a true preventive because the timing of the event is unknown and the unrestricted use of tamoxifen in young women of reproductive age (15–30 years) would be unwise. An exception to this is when tamoxifen is used for the reduction of breast cancer risk in high-risk women, for which it is the first medicine to be approved by the US Food and Drug Administration.

The side effects associated with tamoxifen mean that it will be important to evaluate the action of the aromatase inhibitors in the preventive setting. Estrogens are clearly carcinogenic, possibly because of their proliferative effects on normal breast epithelium as well as the genotoxic effects of certain estrogen metabolites. By lowering tissue levels of estrogen, aromatase inhibitors might block both initiation and promotion of breast cancer. Aromatase inhibitors might be ideal agents to investigate in the chemoprevention of breast cancer. Coombes and colleagues reported that 4-hydroxyandrostenedione prevents N-methyl-N-nitrosourea-induced rat mammary carcinoma.[195] Similar observations with other aromatase inhibitors and animal models suggest that inhibitors of estrogen biosynthesis can prevent breast cancer. Results from the ATAC trial after a median follow-up of 68 months showed that anastrozole adjuvant therapy was associated with 53% further reduction in the risk of development of contralateral disease in women with hormone-receptor positive disease ($p = .001$), compared with adjuvant tamoxifen therapy.[165] These results highlight the need to evaluate aromatase inhibitors as chemopreventive agents, since their safety profile is more favorable than tamoxifen for most endpoints. Moreover, aromatase inhibitors are not associated with endometrial carcinoma in women and, therefore, may become preferred to antiestrogens in the chemoprevention of breast cancer. This question is being examined in the second International Breast cancer Intervention Study (IBIS). The trial aims to recruit 4,000 women with locally excised ductal carcinoma in situ, who will be randomized to receive either anastrozole or placebo.[196]

Combination versus Sequential Therapy A few clinical studies have attempted to combine different classes of endocrine agents, but generally there are no large bodies of data to support the combination approach as superior to the sequential use of hormone therapies to treat metastatic breast cancer. Furthermore, combinations of agents might lead to unfavorable pharmacologic interactions. Sequential use of endocrine therapies takes advantage of the availability of a number of agents that do not exhibit cross-resistance. For example, patients exhibit responses to aromatase inhibitors, tamoxifen, and progestins after progression on fulvestrant, and the steroidal aromatase inhibitor exemestane has exhibited activity in patients who have progressed on prior treatment with a nonsteroidal aromatase inhibitor, such as anastrozole.[197] This extends the period of time during which endocrine therapy can be used, thus postponing the need for cytotoxic chemotherapy.[198] For women with metastatic hormone-dependent breast cancer, a potential sequence of endocrine therapy is presented in Figure 54-5.

Hormonal Resistance and Breast Cancer In clinical practice, the sequential use of hormonal agents can produce long-term palliation of hormone-dependent breast cancer. Eventually, however, the problem of hormone resistance is encountered. The mechanisms by which tumors become resistant to hormones, in general, are only partially understood.[199] Refractoriness to therapy with aromatase inhibitors is related not to the failure of these agents to suppress estradiol levels, but rather because of alterations in other cellular components, such as the growth factor receptor pathways.[200] Our increasing understanding of these processes, and the development of target-orientated therapies, such as gefitinib (Iressa) or trastuzumab (Herceptin), are interesting areas of future research that should make novel therapeutic approaches available for the treatment of endocrine resistance.

SUMMARY

A number of therapeutic options are now available that target the stimulatory effects of estrogen, either by disrupting estrogen-receptor binding or by inhibiting the production of estrogen. Tamoxifen has been ubiquitous as the front-line antiestrogen therapy for the treatment of all stages of breast cancer, and remains the central choice for the treatment of premenopausal women. However, the identification of newer antiestrogens, and the development of noncross-resistant aromatase inhibitors, means that tamoxifen should no longer be considered the "gold standard" therapy for postmenopausal women with hormone-sensitive breast cancer. For these women, the results of the first-line comparative trials of anastrozole and letrozole now support the use of these aromatase inhibitors in the first-line treatment of advanced disease in postmenopausal women. Similarly, substantial data support the use of aromatase inhibitors in the adjuvant setting, either as the initial treatment of choice (anastrozole), or after treatment with tamoxifen (anastrozole, exemestane, and letrozole).

There appear to be differences between the three main aromatase inhibitors in terms of pharmacokinetics and their effects on plasma lipids, bone, and adrenosteroidogenesis. Although extensive data are available for anastrozole, until equivalent results are available for all the agents, it cannot be assumed that each of the aromatase inhibitors will display the same tolerability and safety profiles when given for extended periods of time in the adjuvant setting. Thus, at present it is difficult to fully establish the comparative risk:benefit ratio for each of the drugs.

Lastly, as more antihormonal therapies become available, and our understanding of the molecular pathways underpinning resistance increases, it is essential that the optimal sequence of endocrine agents be established in the treatment of breast cancer. This may prolong the time during which endocrine therapies can be used, so postponing the time when cytotoxic chemotherapy becomes a necessary option.

REFERENCES

1. Beatson GT. On the treatment of inoperable cases of carcinoma of the mamma: suggestions for a new method of treatment, with illustrative cases. Lancet 1896;2:105–7.
2. Jensen EV, Jordan VC. The estrogen receptor: a model for molecular medicine. Clin Cancer Res 2005;9:1980–9.
3. Dickson RB, Lippman ME. Estrogenic regulation of growth and polypeptide growth factor secretion in human breast carcinoma. Endocr Rev 1987;8:29–43.
4. Fishman J, Hahn EF. The nature of the final oxidative step in the aromatization sequence. Steroids 1987;50:339–45.
5. Simpson ER, Merrill JC, Hollub AJ, et al. Regulation of estrogen biosynthesis by human adipose cells. Endocr Rev 1989;10:136–48.
6. Abul-Hajj YJ, Iverson R, Kiang DT. Aromatization of androgens by human breast cancer. Steroids 1979;33:205–22.
7. Bulun SE, Simpson ER. Regulation of aromatase expression in human tissues. Breast Cancer Res Treat 1994;30:19–29.
8. Santen RJ, Samojlik E, Wells SA. Resistance of the ovary to blockade of aromatization with aminoglutethimide. J Clin Endocrinol Metab 1980;51:473–7.

9. Judd HL, Judd GE, Lucas WE, et al. Endocrine function of the postmenopausal ovary: concentration of androgens and estrogens in ovarian and peripheral vein blood. J Clin Endocrinol Metab 1974;39:1020–4.
10. Kirschner MA, Schneider G, Ertel NH, et al. Obesity, androgens, estrogens, and cancer risk. Cancer Res 1982;42:3281s–5s.
11. Fishman J, Nisselbaum JS, Menendez-Botet CJ, et al. Estrone and estradiol content in human breast tumors: relationship to estradiol receptors. J Steroid Biochem 1977;8:893–6.
12. Santen RJ, Leszczynski D, Tilson-Mallet N, et al. Enzymatic control of estrogen production in human breast cancer: relative significance of aromatase versus sulfatase pathways. Ann NY Acad Sci 1986;464:126–37.
13. Lipton A, Santner SJ, Santen RJ, et al. Aromatase activity in primary and metastatic human breast cancer. Cancer 1987;59:779–82.
14. O'Neill JS, Miller WR. Aromatase activity in breast adipose tissue from women with benign and malignant breast diseases. Br J Cancer 1987;56:601–4.
15. Suzuki T, Nakata T, Miki Y, et al. Estrogen sulfotransferase and steroid sulfatase in human breast carcinoma. Cancer Res 2003;63:2762–70.
16. Santen RJ, Martel J, Hoagland M, et al. Stromal spindle cells contain aromatase in human breast tumors. J Clin Endocrinol Metab 1994;79:627–32.
17. Esteban JM, Warsi Z, Haniu M, et al. Detection of intratumoral aromatase in breast carcinomas. An immunohistochemical study with clinicopathologic correlation. Am J Pathol 1992;140:337–43.
18. Koos RD, Banks PK, Inkster SE, et al. Detection of aromatase and keratinocyte growth factor expression in breast tumors using reverse transcription-polymerase chain reaction. J Steroid Biochem Mol Biol 1993;45:217–25.
19. Jordan VC. Biochemical pharmacology of antiestrogen action. Pharmacol Rev 1984;36:245–76.
20. Greenblatt RB, Barfield WE, Jungck EC, et al. Induction of ovulation with MRL/41. Preliminary report. JAMA 1961;178:101–4.
21. Jordan VC. Tamoxifen: a most unlikely pioneering medicine. Nat Rev Drug Discov 2003;2:205–13.
22. Harper MJ, Walpole AL. A new derivative of triphenylethylene: effect on implantation and mode of action in rats. J Reprod Fertil 1967;13:101–19.
23. Jordan VC, Dowse LJ. Tamoxifen as an anti-tumour agent: effect on oestrogen binding. J Endocrinol 1976;68:297–303.
24. Furr BJ, Jordan VC. The pharmacology and clinical uses of tamoxifen. Pharmacol Ther 1984;25:127–205.
25. Lippman ME, Bolan G. Oestrogen-responsive human breast cancer in long term tissue culture. Nature 1975;256:592–93.
26. Osborne CK, Hobbs K, Clark GM. Effect of estrogens and antiestrogens on growth of human breast cancer cells in athymic nude mice. Cancer Res 1985;45:584–90.
27. Osborne CK, Boldt DH, Clark GM, et al. Effects of tamoxifen on human breast cancer cell cycle kinetics: accumulation of cells in early G1 phase. Cancer Res 1983;43:3583–5.
28. Colletti RB, Roberts JD, Devlin JT, et al. Effect of tamoxifen on plasma insulin-like growth factor I in patients with breast cancer. Cancer Res 1989;49:1882–4.
29. Jordan VC. Metabolites of tamoxifen in animals and man: identification, pharmacology, and significance. Breast Cancer Res Treat 1982;2:123–38.
30. Robinson SP, Langan-Fahey SM, Jordan VC. Implications of tamoxifen metabolism in the athymic mouse for the study of antitumor effects upon human breast cancer xenografts. Eur J Cancer Clin Oncol 1989;25:1769–76.
31. Lien EA, Solheim E, Kvinnsland S, et al. Identification of 4-hydroxy-N-desmethyltamoxifen as a metabolite of tamoxifen in human bile. Cancer Res 1988;48:2304–8.
32. Lien EA, Solheim E, Lea OA, et al. Distribution of 4-hydroxy-N-desmethyltamoxifen and other tamoxifen metabolites in human biological fluids during tamoxifen treatment. Cancer Res 1989;49:2175–83.
33. Jordan VC, Collins MM, Rowsby L, et al. A monohydroxylated metabolite of tamoxifen with potent antioestrogenic activity. J Endocrinol 1977;75:305–16.
34. Etienne MC, Milano G, Fischel JL, et al. Tamoxifen metabolism: pharmacokinetic and in vitro study. Br J Cancer 1989;60:30–5.
35. Patterson JS, Settatree RS, Adam HK, et al. Serum concentrations of tamoxifen and major metabolite during long-term Nolvadex therapy, correlated with clinical response. Eur J Cancer 1980;Suppl 1:89–92.
36. Jordan VC, Fritz NF, Tormey DC. Long-term adjuvant therapy with tamoxifen: effects on sex hormone binding globulin and antithrombin III. Cancer Res 1987;47:4517–9.
37. Manni A, Pearson OH. Antiestrogen-induced remissions in premenopausal women with stage IV breast cancer: effects on ovarian function. Cancer Treat Rep 1980;64:779–85.
38. Ravdin PM, Fritz NF, Tormey DC, et al. Endocrine status of premenopausal node-positive breast cancer patients following adjuvant chemotherapy and long-term tamoxifen. Cancer Res 1988;48:1026–9.
39. Sawka CA, Pritchard KI, Paterson AH, et al. Role and mechanism of action of tamoxifen in premenopausal women with metastatic breast carcinoma. Cancer Res 1986;46:3152–6.
40. Sherman BM, Chapler FK, Crickard K, et al. Endocrine consequences of continuous antiestrogen therapy with tamoxifen in premenopausal women. J Clin Invest 1979;64:398–404.
41. Veronesi A, Maisonneuve P, Costa A, et al. Prevention of breast cancer with tamoxifen: preliminary findings from the Italian randomised trial among hysterectomised women. Italian Tamoxifen Prevention Study. Lancet 1998;352:93–7.
42. Ingle JN, Ahmann DL, Green SJ, et al. Randomized clinical trial of diethylstilbestrol versus tamoxifen in postmenopausal women with advanced breast cancer. N Engl J Med 1981;304:16–21.
43. Buchanan RB, Blamey RW, Durrant KR, et al. A randomized comparison of tamoxifen with surgical oophorectomy in premenopausal patients with advanced breast cancer. J Clin Oncol 1986;4:1326–30.
44. Ingle JN, Krook JE, Green SJ, et al. Randomized trial of bilateral oophorectomy versus tamoxifen in premenopausal women with metastatic breast cancer. J Clin Oncol 1986;4:178–85.
45. Klijn JG, Blamey RW, Boccardo F, et al. Combined tamoxifen and luteinizing hormone-releasing hormone (LHRH) agonist versus LHRH agonist alone in premenopausal advanced breast cancer: a meta-analysis of four randomized trials. J Clin Oncol 2001;19:343–53.
46. National Comprehensive Cancer Network. Breast Cancer. Clinical Practice Guidelines in Oncology v.1.2004. Available at: http://www.nccn.org/physician_gls/f_guidelines.html (accessed May 19, 2004).
47. Early Breast Cancer Trialists' Collaborative Group. Tamoxifen for early breast cancer: an overview of the randomised trials. Lancet 1998;351:1451–67.
48. Jordan VC. Laboratory studies to develop general principles for the adjuvant treatment of breast cancer with antiestrogens: problems and potential for future clinical applications. Breast Cancer Res Treat 1983;3(Suppl):S73–86.
49. Falkson HC, Gray R, Wolberg WH, et al. Adjuvant trial of 12 cycles of CMFPT followed by observation or continuous tamoxifen versus four cycles of CMFPT in postmenopausal women with breast cancer: an Eastern Cooperative Oncology Group phase III study. J Clin Oncol 1990;8:599–607.
50. Tormey DC, Gray R, Falkson HC. Postchemotherapy adjuvant tamoxifen therapy beyond five years in patients with lymph node-positive breast cancer. Eastern Cooperative Oncology Group. J Natl Cancer Inst 1996;88:1828–33.
51. Boccardo F, Rubagotti A, Amoroso D, et al. Chemotherapy versus tamoxifen versus chemotherapy plus tamoxifen in node-positive, oestrogen-receptor positive breast cancer patients. An update at 7 years of the 1st GROCTA (Breast Cancer Adjuvant Chemo-Hormone Therapy Cooperative Group) trial. Eur J Cancer 1992;28:673–80.
52. Fisher B, Redmond C, Legault-Poisson S, et al. Postoperative chemotherapy and tamoxifen compared with tamoxifen alone in the treatment of positive-node breast cancer patients aged 50 years and older with tumors responsive to tamoxifen: results from the National Surgical Adjuvant Breast and Bowel Project B-16. J Clin Oncol 1990;8:1005–18.
53. Fisher B, Jeong JH, Bryant J, et al. Treatment of lymph-node-negative, oestrogen-receptor-positive breast cancer: long-term findings from National Surgical Adjuvant Breast and Bowel Project randomised clinical trials. Lancet 2004;364:858–68.
54. Albain K, Barlow W, O'Malley F, et al. Concurrent (CAFT) versus sequential (CAF-T) chemohormonal therapy (cyclophosphamide, doxorubicin, 5-fluorouracil, tamoxifen) versus T alone for postmenopausal, node-positive, estrogen (ER) and/or progesterone (PgR) receptor-positive breast cancer: mature outcomes and new biologic correlates on phase III intergroup trial 0100 (SWOG-8814). Abstract 37 LB presented at the 27th Annual San Antonio Breast Cancer Symposium; 2004 Dec 8–11; San Antonio (TX).
55. Holli K, Valavaara R, Blanco G, et al. Safety and efficacy results of a randomized trial comparing adjuvant toremifene and tamoxifen in postmenopausal patients with node-positive breast cancer. Finnish Breast Cancer Group. J Clin Oncol 2000;18:3487–94.
56. Pyrhonen S, Ellmen J, Vuorinen J, et al. Meta-analysis of trials comparing toremifene with tamoxifen and factors predicting outcome of antiestrogen therapy in postmenopausal women with breast cancer. Breast Cancer Res Treat 1999;56:133–43.
57. Gottardis MM, Jordan VC. Antitumor actions of keoxifene and tamoxifen in the N-nitrosomethylurea-induced rat mammary carcinoma model. Cancer Res 1987;47:4020–4.
58. Black LJ, Sato M, Rowley ER, et al. Raloxifene (LY139481 HCI) prevents bone loss and reduces serum cholesterol without causing uterine hypertrophy in ovariectomized rats. J Clin Invest 1994;93:63–9.
59. Jordan VC, Phelps E, Lindgren JU. Effects of anti-estrogens on bone in castrated and intact female rats. Breast Cancer Res Treat 1987;10:31–5.
60. Delmas PD, Bjarnason NH, Mitlak BH, et al. Effects of raloxifene on bone mineral density, serum cholesterol concentrations, and uterine endometrium in postmenopausal women. N Engl J Med 1997;337:1641–7.
61. Walsh BW, Kuller LH, Wild RA, et al. Effects of raloxifene on serum lipids and coagulation factors in healthy postmenopausal women. JAMA 1998;279:1445–51.
62. Dowsett M, Bundred NJ, Decensi A, et al. Effect of raloxifene on breast cancer cell Ki67 and apoptosis: a double-blind, placebo-controlled, randomized clinical trial in postmenopausal patients. Cancer Epidemiol Biomarkers Prev 2001;10:961–6.
63. Cummings SR, Eckert S, Krueger KA, et al. The effect of raloxifene on risk of breast cancer in postmenopausal women: results from the MORE randomized trial. Multiple Outcomes of Raloxifene Evaluation. JAMA 1999;281:2189–97.
64. Martino S, Cauley JA, Barrett-Connor E, et al. Continuing outcomes relevant to Evista: breast cancer incidence in postmenopausal osteoporotic women in a randomized trial of raloxifene. J Natl Cancer Inst 2004;96:1751–61.
65. Cohen FJ, Watts S, Shah A, et al. Uterine effects of 3-year raloxifene therapy in postmenopausal women younger than age 60. Obstet Gynecol 2000;95:104–10.
66. Leonard RCF, Bundred N, Buzdar A, et al. Multi-center clinical trials of trilostane (Modrenal) for advanced breast cancer in post-menopausal women [abstract 431]. Breast Cancer Res Treat 2003;87(Suppl 1).
67. Fawell SE, White R, Hoare S, et al. Inhibition of estrogen receptor-DNA binding by the "pure" antiestrogen ICI 164,384 appears to be mediated by impaired receptor dimerization. Proc Natl Acad Sci U S A 1990;87:6883–7.
68. McClelland RA, Gee JM, Francis AB, et al. Short-term effects of pure anti-oestrogen ICI 182780 treatment on oestrogen receptor, epidermal growth factor receptor and transforming growth factor-alpha protein expression in human breast cancer. Eur J Cancer 1996;32A:413–6.
69. DeFriend DJ, Howell A, Nicholson RI, et al. Investigation of a new pure antiestrogen (ICI 182780) in women with primary breast cancer. Cancer Res 1994;54:408–14.
70. Robertson JFR, Nicholson RI, Bundred NJ. Comparison of the short-term biological effects of fulvestrant (ICI 182, 780) with tamoxifen in postmenopausal women with primary breast cancer. Breast Cancer Res Treat 2000;59:99.
71. Howell A, Robertson JFR, Quaresma Albano J, et al. Fulvestrant, formerly ICI 182,780, is as effective as anastrozole in postmenopausal women with advanced breast cancer progressing after prior endocrine treatment. J Clin Oncol 2002;20:3396–403.
72. Osborne CK, Pippen J, Jones SE, et al. Double-blind, randomized trial comparing the efficacy and tolerability of fulvestrant versus anastrozole in postmenopausal women with advanced breast cancer progressing on prior endocrine therapy: results of a North American trial. J Clin Oncol 2002;20:3386–95.
73. Robertson JF, Osborne CK, Howell A, et al. Fulvestrant versus anastrozole for the treatment of advanced breast carcinoma in postmenopausal women—a prospective combined analysis of two multicenter trials. Cancer 2003;98:229–38.
74. Bross PF, Cohen MH, Williams GA, et al. FDA drug approval summaries: fulvestrant. Oncologist 2002;7:477–80.
75. Vergote I, Robertson JFR, Kleeberg U, et al. Postmenopausal women who progress on fulvestrant ('Faslodex') remain sensitive to further endocrine therapy. Breast Cancer Res Treat 2003;79:207–11.

76. Mauriac L, Pippen JE, Quaresma Albano J, et al. Fulvestrant (Faslodex) versus anastrozole for the second-line treatment of subgroups of postmenopausal women with visceral and non-visceral metastases: combined results from two multicentre trials. Eur J Cancer 2003;39:1228–33.
77. Turner RT, Wakley GK, Hannon KS, et al. Tamoxifen inhibits osteoclast-mediated resorption of trabecular bone in ovarian hormone-deficient rats. Endocrinology 1988;122:1146–50.
78. Love RR, Mazess RB, Tormey DC, et al. Bone mineral density in women with breast cancer treated with adjuvant tamoxifen for at least two years. Breast Cancer Res Treat 1988;12:297–302.
79. Powles TJ, Hardy JR, Ashley SE, et al. A pilot trial to evaluate the acute toxicity and feasibility of tamoxifen for prevention of breast cancer. Br J Cancer 1989;60:126–31.
80. Turken S, Siris E, Seldin D, et al. Effects of tamoxifen on spinal bone density in women with breast cancer. J Natl Cancer Inst 1989;81:1086–8.
81. Kristensen B, Ejlertsen B, Dalgaard P, et al. Tamoxifen and bone metabolism in postmenopausal low-risk breast cancer patients: a randomized study. J Clin Oncol 1994;12:992–7.
82. Love RR, Mazess RB, Barden HS, et al. Effects of tamoxifen on bone mineral density in postmenopausal women with breast cancer. N Engl J Med 1992;326:852–6.
83. Ward RL, Morgan G, Dalley D, et al. Tamoxifen reduces bone turnover and prevents lumbar spine and proximal femoral bone loss in early postmenopausal women. Bone Miner 1993;22:87–94.
84. Fisher B, Costantino JP, Wickerham DL, et al. Tamoxifen for prevention of breast cancer: report of the National Surgical Adjuvant Breast and Bowel Project P-1 Study. J Natl Cancer Inst 1998;90:1371–88.
85. Bertelli G, Pronzato P, Amoroso D, et al. Adjuvant tamoxifen in primary breast cancer: influence on plasma lipids and antithrombin III levels. Breast Cancer Res Treat 1988;12:307–10.
86. Bruning PF, Bonfrer JM, Hart AA, et al. Tamoxifen, serum lipoproteins and cardiovascular risk. Br J Cancer 1988;58:497–9.
87. Caleffi M, Fentiman IS, Clark GM, et al. Effect of tamoxifen on oestrogen binding, lipid and lipoprotein concentrations and blood clotting parameters in premenopausal women with breast pain. J Endocrinol 1988;119:335–9.
88. Bagdade JD, Wolter J, Subbaiah PV, et al. Effects of tamoxifen treatment on plasma lipids and lipoprotein lipid composition. J Clin Endocrinol Metab 1990;70:1132–5.
89. Love RR, Newcomb PA, Wiebe DA, et al. Effects of tamoxifen therapy on lipid and lipoprotein levels in postmenopausal patients with node-negative breast cancer. J Natl Cancer Inst 1990;82:1327–32.
90. Love RR, Wiebe DA, Feyzi JM, et al. Effects of tamoxifen on cardiovascular risk factors in postmenopausal women after 5 years of treatment. J Natl Cancer Inst 1994;86:1534–9.
91. Love RR, Wiebe DA, Feyzi JM, et al. Effects of tamoxifen on cardiovascular risk factors in postmenopausal women after 5 years of treatment. J Natl Cancer Inst 1994;86:1534–9.
92. Braithwaite RS, Chlebowski RT, Lau J, et al. Meta-analysis of vascular and neoplastic events associated with tamoxifen. J Gen Intern Med 2003;18:937–47.
93. McDonald CC, Stewart HJ. Fatal myocardial infarction in the Scottish adjuvant tamoxifen trial. The Scottish Breast Cancer Committee. BMJ 1991;303:435–7.
94. Costantino JP, Kuller LH, Ives DG, et al. Coronary heart disease mortality and adjuvant tamoxifen therapy. J Natl Cancer Inst 1997;89:776–82.
95. Longstaff S, Sigurdsson H, O'Keeffe M, et al. A controlled study of the ocular effects of tamoxifen in conventional dosage in the treatment of breast carcinoma. Eur J Cancer Clin Oncol 1989;25:1805–8.
96. Kaiser-Kupfer MI, Lippman ME. Tamoxifen retinopathy. Cancer Treat Rep 1978;62:315–20.
97. Gorin MB, Day R, Costantino JP, et al. Long-term tamoxifen citrate use and potential ocular toxicity. Am J Ophthalmol 1998;125:493–501.
98. Paganini-Hill A, Clark LJ. Eye problems in breast cancer patients treated with tamoxifen. Breast Cancer Res Treat 2000;60:167–72.
99. Pavlidis NA, Petris C, Briassoulis E, et al. Clear evidence that long-term, low-dose tamoxifen treatment can induce ocular toxicity. A prospective study of 63 patients. Cancer 1992;69:2961–4.
100. Duggan C, Marriott K, Edwards R, et al. Inherited and acquired risk factors for venous thromboembolic disease among women taking tamoxifen to prevent breast cancer. J Clin Oncol 2003;21:3588–93.
101. Deitcher SR, Gomes MP. The risk of venous thromboembolic disease associated with adjuvant hormone therapy for breast carcinoma: a systematic review. Cancer 2004;101:439–49.
102. Kedar RP, Bourne TH, Powles TJ, et al. Effects of tamoxifen on uterus and ovaries of postmenopausal women in a randomised breast cancer prevention trial. Lancet 1994;343:1318–21.
103. Decensi A, Fontana V, Bruno S, et al. Effect of tamoxifen on endometrial proliferation. J Clin Oncol 1996;14:434–40.
104. Fung MF, Reid A, Faught W, et al. Prospective longitudinal study of ultrasound screening for endometrial abnormalities in women with breast cancer receiving tamoxifen. Gynecol Oncol 2003;91:154–9.
105. Bergman L, Beelen ML, Gallee MP, et al. Risk and prognosis of endometrial cancer after tamoxifen for breast cancer. Comprehensive Cancer Centres' ALERT Group. Assessment of Liver and Endometrial cancer Risk following Tamoxifen. Lancet 2000;356:881–7.
106. Fornander T, Rutqvist LE, Cedermark B, et al. Adjuvant tamoxifen in early breast cancer: occurrence of new primary cancers. Lancet 1989;1:117–20.
107. Fisher B, Costantino JP, Redmond CK, et al. Endometrial cancer in tamoxifen-treated breast cancer patients: findings from the National Surgical Adjuvant Breast and Bowel Project (NSABP) B-14. J Natl Cancer Inst 1994;86:527–37.
108. Han XL, Liehr JG. Induction of covalent DNA adducts in rodents by tamoxifen. Cancer Res 1992;52:1360–3.
109. Shibutani S, Suzuki N, Laxmi YR, et al. Identification of tamoxifen-DNA adducts in monkeys treated with tamoxifen. Cancer Res 2003;63:4402–6.
110. Greaves P, Goonetilleke R, Nunn G, et al. Two-year carcinogenicity study of tamoxifen in Alderley Park Wistar-derived rats. Cancer Res 1993;53:3919–24.
111. Williams GM, Iatropoulos MJ, Djordjevic MV, et al. The triphenylethylene drug tamoxifen is a strong liver carcinogen in the rat. Carcinogenesis 1993;14:315–7.
112. Jordan VC, Morrow M. Should clinicians be concerned about the carcinogenic potential of tamoxifen? Eur J Cancer 1994;30A:1714–21.
113. Muhlemann K, Cook LS, Weiss NS. The incidence of hepatocellular carcinoma in US white women with breast cancer after the introduction of tamoxifen in 1977. Breast Cancer Res Treat 1994;30:201–4.
114. Cash R, Brough AJ, Cohen MN, et al. Aminoglutethimide (Elipten-Ciba) as an inhibitor of adrenal steroidogenesis: mechanism of action and therapeutic trial. J Clin Endocrinol Metab 1967;27:1239–48.
115. Chakraborty J, Hopkins R, Parke DV. Inhibition studies on the aromatization of androst-4-ene-3,17-dione by human placental microsomal preparations. Biochem J 1972;130:19P–20P.
116. Thompson EA, Jr., Siiteri PK. The involvement of human placental microsomal cytochrome P-450 in aromatization. J Biol Chem 1974;249:5373–8.
117. Cocconi G. First generation aromatase inhibitors—aminoglutethimide and testololactone. Breast Cancer Res Treat 1994;30:57–80.
118. Santen RJ, Wells SA, Cohn N, et al. Compensatory increase in TSH secretion without effect on prolactin secretion in patients treated with aminoglutethimide. J Clin Endocrinol Metab 1977;45:739–46.
119. Brodie AM, Marsh D, Brodie HJ. Aromatase inhibitors--IV. Regression of hormone-dependent, mammary tumors in the rat with 4-acetoxy-4-androstene-3,17-dione. J Steroid Biochem 1979;10:423–9.
120. Coombes RC, Goss P, Dowsett M, et al. 4-Hydroxyandrostenedione in treatment of postmenopausal patients with advanced breast cancer. Lancet 1984;2:1237–9.
121. Freue M, Kjaer M, Boni C, et al. Open comparative trial of formestane versus egestrol acetate in postmenopausal patients with advanced breast cancer previously treated with tamoxifen. Breast 2000;9:9–16.
122. Carlini P, Frassoldati A, De Marco S, et al. Formestane, a steroidal aromatase inhibitor after failure of non-steroidal aromatase inhibitors (anastrozole and letrozole): is a clinical benefit still achievable? Ann Oncol 2001;12:1539–43.
123. Evans TR, di Salle E, Ornati G, et al. Phase I and endocrine study of exemestane (FCE 24304), a new aromatase inhibitor, in postmenopausal women. Cancer Res 1992;52:5933–9.
124. Lønning PE. Pharmacological profiles of exemestane and formestane, steroidal aromatase inhibitors used for treatment of postmenopausal breast cancer. Breast Cancer Res Treat 1998;49 (Suppl 1):S45–52.
125. Jones S, Belt R, Coppin CM. A phase study of antitumor efficacy and safety of exemestane as second-line hormonal treatment of postmenopausal patients with metastatic breast cancer refractory to tamoxifen. Breast Cancer Res Treat 1998;50:304.
126. Jones S, Vogel C, Fehrenbacher L. Proc Am Soc Clin Oncol 1998;17:150a.
127. Kaufmann M, Bajetta E, Dirix LY, et al. Exemestane is superior to megestrol acetate after tamoxifen failure in postmenopausal women with advanced breast cancer: results of a phase III randomized double-blind trial. The Exemestane Study Group. J Clin Oncol 2000;18:1399–411.
128. Paridaens R, Dirix L, Lohrisch C, et al. Mature results of a randomized phase II multicenter study of exemestane versus tamoxifen as first-line hormone therapy for postmenopausal women with metastatic breast cancer. Ann Oncol 2003;14:1391–8.
129. Paridaens R, Therasse P, Dirix L, et al. First-line hormonal treatment (HT) for metastatic breast cancer (MBC) with exemestane (E) or tamoxifen (T) in postmenopausal patients (pts)—A randomized phase III trial of the EORTC Breast Group [abstract 515]. Proc Am Soc Clin Oncol 2004;23:6.
130. Schieweck K, Bhatnagar AS, Matter A. CGS 16949A, a new nonsteroidal aromatase inhibitor: effects on hormone-dependent and -independent tumors in vivo. Cancer Res 1988;48:834–8.
131. Schieweck K, Bhatnagar AS, Batzl C, et al. Anti-tumor and endocrine effects of non-steroidal aromatase inhibitors on estrogen-dependent rat mammary tumors. J Steroid Biochem Mol Biol 1993;44:633–6.
132. Harvey HA, Lipton A, Santen RJ. Clinical trials with the aromatase inhibitor CGS16949A in advanced breast cancer: the US experience. In: Jonat W, Santen RJ, eds. Aromatase inhibition present and future. New York: Parthenon; 1991. p. 89–96.
133. Possinger K, Lanzalone S. The role of aromatase inhibition in the treatment of metastatic breast cancer. In: Aromatase inhibition present and future. New York: Parthenon; 1991. p. 29–34.
134. Falkson CI, Falkson HC. A randomised study of CGS 16949A (fadrozole) versus tamoxifen in previously untreated postmenopausal patients with metastatic breast cancer. Ann Oncol 1996;7:465–9.
135. Buzdar AU, Smith R, Vogel C, et al. Fadrozole HCL (CGS-16949A) versus megestrol acetate treatment of postmenopausal patients with metastatic breast carcinoma: results of two randomized double blind controlled multi-institutional trials. Cancer 1996;77:2503–13.
136. Dowsett M, Yates RA, Lindsay A, et al. Endocrine effects of Arimidex, a potent aromatase inhibitor, in men and postmenopausal women. Breast Cancer Res Treat 1993;27:152.
137. Buzdar A, Jonat W, Howell A, et al. Anastrozole, a potent and selective aromatase inhibitor, versus megestrol acetate in postmenopausal women with advanced breast cancer: results of overview analysis of two phase III trials. Arimidex Study Group. J Clin Oncol 1996;14:2000–11.
138. Howell A, Mackintosh J, Jones M, et al. The definition of the 'no change' category in patients treated with endocrine therapy and chemotherapy for advanced carcinoma of the breast. Eur J Cancer Clin Oncol 1988;24:1567–72.
139. Buzdar AU, Jonat W, Howell A, et al. Anastrozole versus megestrol acetate in the treatment of postmenopausal women with advanced breast carcinoma: results of a survival update based on a combined analysis of data from two mature phase III trials. Arimidex Study Group. Cancer 1998;83:1142–52.
140. Bonneterre J, Thürlimann B, Robertson JF, et al. Anastrozole versus tamoxifen as first-line therapy for advanced breast cancer in 668 postmenopausal women: results of the Tamoxifen or Arimidex Randomized Group Efficacy and Tolerability study. J Clin Oncol 2000;18:3748–57.
141. Nabholtz JM, Buzdar A, Pollak M, et al. Anastrozole is superior to tamoxifen as first-line therapy for advanced breast cancer in postmenopausal women: results of a North American multicenter randomized trial. Arimidex Study Group. J Clin Oncol 2000;18:3758–67.
142. Bonneterre J, Buzdar A, Nabholtz JM, et al. Anastrozole is superior to tamoxifen as first-line therapy in hormone receptor positive advanced breast carcinoma. Cancer 2001;92:2247–58.
143. Bhatnagar AS, Hausler A, Schieweck K, et al. Highly selective inhibition of estrogen biosynthesis by CGS 20267, a new non-steroidal aromatase inhibitor. J Steroid Biochem Mol Biol 1990;37:1021–7.
144. Klein KO, Demers LM, Santner SJ, et al. Use of ultrasensitive recombinant cell bioassay to measure estrogen levels in women with breast cancer receiving the aromatase inhibitor, letrozole. J Clin Endocrinol Metab 1995;80:2658–60.

145. Iveson TJ, Smith IE, Ahern J, et al. Phase I study of the oral nonsteroidal aromatase inhibitor CGS 20267 in postmenopausal patients with advanced breast cancer. Cancer Res 1993;53:266–70.
146. Dombernowsky P, Smith I, Falkson G, et al. Letrozole, a new oral aromatase inhibitor for advanced breast cancer: double-blind randomized trial showing a dose effect and improved efficacy and tolerability compared with megestrol acetate. J Clin Oncol 1998;16:453–61.
147. Gershanovich M, Chaudri HA, Campos D, et al. Letrozole, a new oral aromatase inhibitor: randomised trial comparing 2.5 mg daily, 0.5 mg daily and aminoglutethimide in postmenopausal women with advanced breast cancer. Letrozole International Trial Group (AR/BC3). Ann Oncol 1998;9:639–45.
148. Mouridsen H, Gershanovich M, Sun Y, et al. Superior efficacy of letrozole versus tamoxifen as first-line therapy for postmenopausal women with advanced breast cancer: results of a phase III study of the International Letrozole Breast Cancer Group. J Clin Oncol 2001;19:2596–606.
149. Mouridsen H, Gershanovich M, Sun Y, et al. Phase III study of letrozole versus tamoxifen as first-line therapy of advanced breast cancer in postmenopausal women: analysis of survival and update of efficacy from the International Letrozole Breast Cancer Group. J Clin Oncol 2003;21:2101–9.
150. De Coster R, Wouters W, Bowden CR, et al. New non-steroidal aromatase inhibitors: focus on R76713. J Steroid Biochem Mol Biol 1990;37:335–41.
151. Goss PE. Pre-clinical and clinical review of vorozole, a new third generation aromatase inhibitor. Breast Cancer Res Treat 1998;49(Suppl 1):S59–65.
152. Goss PE, Winer EP, Tannock IF, et al. Randomized phase III trial comparing the new potent and selective third-generation aromatase inhibitor vorozole with megestrol acetate in postmenopausal advanced breast cancer patients. North American Vorozole Study Group. J Clin Oncol 1999;17:52–63.
153. Dixon JM, Renshaw L, Bellamy C, et al. The effects of neoadjuvant anastrozole (Arimidex) on tumor volume in postmenopausal women with breast cancer: a randomized, double-blind, single-center study. Clin Cancer Res 2000;6:2229–35.
154. Smith I, Dowsett M, on behalf of the IMPACT Trialists. Comparison of anastrozole vs tamoxifen alone and in combination as neoadjuvant treatment of estrogen receptor-positive (ER+) operable breast cancer in postmenopausal women: the IMPACT trial [abstract 1]. Breast Cancer Res Treat 2003;82(Suppl 1):S6.
155. Cataliotti L, Buzdar A, Noguchi S, et al. Efficacy of PReOperative Arimidex (anastrozole) Compared with Tamoxifen (PROACT) as neoadjuvant therapy in postmenopausal women with hormone receptor-positive breast cancer [abstract 46]. Eur J Cancer Suppl 2004;2:69.
156. Dixon JM, Love CD, Bellamy CO, et al. Letrozole as primary medical therapy for locally advanced and large operable breast cancer. Breast Cancer Res Treat 2001;66:191–9.
157. Eiermann W, Paepke S, Appfelstaedt J, et al. Preoperative treatment of postmenopausal breast cancer patients with letrozole: A randomized double-blind multicenter study. Ann Oncol 2001;12:1527–32.
158. Ellis MJ, Coop A, Singh B, et al. Letrozole is more effective neoadjuvant endocrine therapy than tamoxifen for ErbB-1- and/or ErbB-2-positive, estrogen receptor-positive primary breast cancer: evidence from a phase III randomized trial. J Clin Oncol 2001;19:3808–16.
159. Ellis MJ, Coop A, Singh B, et al. Letrozole inhibits tumor proliferation more effectively than tamoxifen independent of HER1/2 expression status. Cancer Res 2003;63:6523–31.
160. Dixon JM, Anderson T, Miller WR. Phase IIb study of neoadjuvant exemestane (EXE) in locally advanced breast cancer [abstract 1908]. Proc Am Soc Clin Oncol 2001;20:40b.
161. Gil M, Barnadas A, Cirera L, et al. Exemestane as neoadjuvant treatment in patients > 65 years with T > 3cm; preliminary results of a multicenter Spanish phase II trial [abstract 272]. Breast Cancer Res Treat 2002;76(Suppl 1):S77.
162. Gil M, Barnadas A, Cirera L, et al. Primary hormonal therapy with exemestane in patients with breast tumors > 3 cm in diameter: Results of a Spanish multicenter phase II trial [abstract 603]. Proc Am Soc Clin Oncol 2004;22.
163. The ATAC Trialists' Group. Anastrozole alone or in combination with tamoxifen versus tamoxifen alone for adjuvant treatment of postmenopausal women with early breast cancer: first results of the ATAC randomised trial. Lancet 2002;359:2131–9.
164. The ATAC Trialists' Group. Anastrozole alone or in combination with tamoxifen versus tamoxifen alone for adjuvant treatment of postmenopausal women with early-stage breast cancer. Results of the ATAC (Arimidex, Tamoxifen, Alone or in Combination) trial efficacy and safety update analyses. Cancer 2003;98:1802–10.
165. The ATAC Trialists' Group. Results of the ATAC (Arimidex, Tamoxifen, Alone or in Combination) trial after completion of 5 years' adjuvant treatment for breast cancer. Lancet 2005;365:60–2.
166. Goss PE, Ingle JN, Martino S, et al. A randomized trial of letrozole in postmenopausal women after five years of tamoxifen therapy for early-stage breast cancer. N Engl J Med 2003;349:1793–802.
167. Goss PE. NCIC CTG MA.17 Final analysis of updated data: A placebo-controlled trial of letrozole following tamoxifen as adjuvant therapy in postmenopausal women with early breast cancer. Available at: http://www.asco.org/ac/1,1003,_12-002511-00_18-0026-00_19-0011301,00.asp (accessed November 10, 2004).
168. Coombes RC, Hall E, Gibson LJ, et al. A randomized trial of exemestane after two to three years of tamoxifen therapy in postmenopausal women with primary breast cancer. N Engl J Med 2004;350:1081–92.
169. Boccardo F, Rubagotti A, Amoroso D, et al. Anastrozole appears to be superior to tamoxifen in women already receiving adjuvant tamoxifen treatment [abstract 3]. Breast Cancer Res Treatment 2003;82(Suppl 1):S6.
170. Jakesz R, Kaufmann M, Gnant M, et al. Benefits of switching postmenopausal women with hormone-sensitive early breast cancer to anastrozole after 2 years adjuvant tamoxifen: combined results from 3,123 women enrolled in the ABCSG Trial 8 and the ARNO 95 Trial [abstract 2]. Breast Cancer Res Treat 2004;88(Suppl 1):S7.
171. Locker GY, Eastell R. The time course of bone fractures observed in the ATAC ('Arimidex,' Tamoxifen, Alone or in Combination) trial [abstract 98]. Proc Am Soc Clin Oncol 2003;22:25.
172. Bajetta E, Martinetti A, Zilembo N, et al. Biological activity of anastrozole in postmenopausal patients with advanced breast cancer: effects on estrogens and bone metabolism. Ann Oncol 2002;13:1059–66.
173. Coleman RE. Association between prior chemotherapy and the adverse event profile of adjuvant anastrozole and tamoxifen: a retrospective analysis of data from the ATAC ('Arimidex,' Tamoxifen, Alone or in Combination) trial on behalf of the ATAC trialists' group. Poster 243 presented at the 29th European Society of Medical Oncology Congress; 2004 Oct 2–Nov, Vienna, Austria.
174. Eastell R, Adams J. Results of the 'Arimidex' (anastrozole, A), Tamoxifen (T), Alone or in Combination (C) (ATAC) trial: effects on bone mineral density (BMD) and bone turnover (ATAC Trialists' Group) [abstract 113]. Ann Oncol 2002;13(Suppl 5):32.
175. Heshmati HM, Khosla S, Robins SP, et al. Endogenous residual estrogen levels determine bone resorption even in late menopausal women. J Bone Mineral Res 1997;12:S121.
176. Harper-Wynne C, Ross G, Sacks N, et al. Effects of the aromatase inhibitor letrozole in healthy postmenopausal women rationale for prevention. Proc Am Soc Clin Oncol 2001;20:335b.
177. Martinetti A, Zilembo N, Ferrari L, et al. Bone turnover markers and insulin-like growth factor components in metastatic breast cancer: results from a randomised trial of exemestane vs megestrol acetate. Anticancer Res 2003;23:3485–91.
178. Ferrari L, Bajetta E, Martinetti A, et al. Could exemestane affect insulin-like growth factors, interleukin 6 and bone metabolism in postmenopausal advanced breast cancer patients after failure on aminoglutethimide, anastrozole or letrozole? Int J Oncol 2003;22:1081–9.
179. Geisler J, Lonning P, Krag LE, et al. Estrogens and bone metabolism in postmenopausal women with early breast cancer at low risk treated with exemestane: a randomized placebo-controlled study [abstract 531]. Proc Am Soc Clin Oncol 2004;23:9.
180. Dewar J, Nabholtz J, Bonneterre J, et al. The effect of anastrozole ('Arimidex') on serum lipids: a randomized comparison of anastrozole (AN) vs. Tamoxifen (TAM) in postmenopausal women with advanced breast cancer [abstract 164]. Breast Cancer Res Treat 2000;64(Suppl):S51.
181. Wojtacki J, Lesniewski-Kmak K, Piotrowska M, et al. Effect of anastrozole on serum levels of apolipoprotein A-I and B in patients with early breast cancer: additional data on lack of atherogenic properties [abstract 6053]. Breast Cancer Res Treat 2004;88:S238.
182. Wojtacki J, Lesniewski-Kmak K, Pawlak W, et al. Anastrozole therapy and lipid profile: an update [abstract 297]. Eur J Cancer Suppl 2004;2:142.
183. Elisaf MS, Bairaktari ET, Nicolaides C, et al. Effect of letrozole on the lipid profile in postmenopausal women with breast cancer. Eur J Cancer 2001;37:1510–3.
184. Engan T, Krane J, Johannessen DC, et al. Plasma changes in breast cancer patients during endocrine therapy—lipid measurements and nuclear magnetic resonance (NMR) spectroscopy. Breast Cancer Res Treat 1995;36:287–97.
185. Lohrisch C, Paridaens R, Dirix LY, et al. No adverse impact on serum lipids of the irreversible aromatase inactivator, Aromasin [exemestane (E)] in 1st-line treatment of metastatic breast cancer (MBC): companion study to a European Organization of Research and Treatment of Cancer (Breast Group) Trial with Pharmacia Upjohn [abstract 167]. Proc Am Soc Clin Oncol 2001;20:43a.
186. Winer EP, Hudis C, Burstein HJ, et al. American Society of Clinical Oncology Technology Assessment on the use of aromatase inhibitors as adjuvant therapy for postmenopausal women with hormone receptor–positive breast cancer: status report 2004. J Clin Oncol 2005;23:619–29.
187. Forward D, Cheung KL, Jackson L, et al. Combined use of goserelin (Zoladex) and anastrozole (Arimidex) in premenopausal women with metastatic breast cancer (MBC). Proc Am Soc Clin Oncol 2000;19:147a.
188. Carlson N, Schurman CM, Rivera E, et al. Goserelin plus anastrozole for the treatment of premenopausal women with hormone receptor-positive recurrent/metastatic breast cancer. Breast Cancer Res Treat 2004;88(Suppl 1):S237–8.
189. Giordano SH, Valero V, Buzdar AU, et al. Efficacy of anastrozole in male breast cancer. Am J Clin Oncol 2002;25:235–7.
190. Bonomo M, Mingrone W, Brauchli P, et al. Exemestane seems to stimulate tumour growth in men with prostate carcinoma. Eur J Cancer 2003;39:2111–2.
191. Jordan VC. Effect of tamoxifen (ICI 46,474) on initiation and growth of DMBA-induced rat mammary carcinomata. Eur J Cancer 1976;12:419–24.
192. Jordan VC, Lababidi MK, Mirecki DM. Anti-oestrogenic and anti-tumour properties of prolonged tamoxifen therapy in C3H/OUJ mice. Eur J Cancer 1990;26:718–21.
193. Fisher B, Costantino J, Redmond C, et al. A randomized clinical trial evaluating tamoxifen in the treatment of patients with node-negative breast cancer who have estrogen-receptor-positive tumors. N Engl J Med 1989;320:479–84.
194. Cuzick J, Powles T, Veronesi U, et al. Overview of the main outcomes in breast-cancer prevention trials. Lancet 2003;361:296–300.
195. Coombes RC, Wilkinson JR, Bliss JM, et al. 4-Hydroxyandrostenedione in the prophylaxis of N-methyl-N-nitrosourea induced mammary tumourigenesis. Br J Cancer 1991;64:247–50.
196. Cuzick J. Aromatase inhibitors in prevention—data from the ATAC (Arimidex, Tamoxifen Alone or in Combination) trial and the design of IBIS-II (the second International Breast Cancer Intervention Study). Recent Results Cancer Res 2003;163:96–103.
197. Lønning PE, Bajetta E, Murray R, et al. Activity of exemestane in metastatic breast cancer after failure of nonsteroidal aromatase inhibitors: a phase II trial. J Clin Oncol 2000;18:2234–44.
198. Carlson RW, Henderson IC. Sequential hormonal therapy for metastatic breast cancer after adjuvant tamoxifen or anastrozole. Breast Cancer Res Treat 2003;80(Suppl 1):S19–26.
199. Jordan VC. Selective estrogen receptor modulation: concept and consequences in cancer. Cancer Cell 2004;5:207–13.
200. Nicholson RI, Gee JMW, Knowlden J, et al. The biology of antihormone failure in breast cancer. Breast Cancer Res Treat 2003;80(Suppl 1):S29–34.

55

Progestins

Kenneth S. McCarty Jr, MD, PhD
Mark D. Nichols, PhD
Pamela A. Hershberger, PhD
Justin C. McCarty
Kenneth S. McCarty Sr, PhD*

Progestins are involved in the regulation of development and differentiation, proliferation, apoptosis, and metabolism in many target tissues. Progestins have broad implications in neoplasia. Some of the progestin effects on target tissues are mediated by transcription, whereas other effects are more rapid and do not involve direct transcriptional effects. Target tissue effects include secretory changes in the uterine epithelium, maintenance of the reproductive tract in females, proliferation and differentiation in the breast, quantitative changes in sex steroid receptor proteins, and effects on both mesenchymal and epithelial elements, involving, in addition, effects on inflammation and fluid balance. It is now clear that progestins exert their effect through several mechanisms, including classic gene regulation by nuclear steroid receptors that are ligand-dependent transcription factors, as well as by rapid effects on a variety of signal transduction molecules and pathways, including some involving the plasma membrane. It is now thought that a subpopulation of the conventional nuclear steroid receptor, localized at the cell membrane, may mediate some of the rapid signaling effects of progestins; in addition, novel membrane receptors for these steroid hormones have been implicated in some rapid signaling effects. Most tissue responses to progestins, but far from all, are the result of the molecular interaction of the steroid with the nuclear progesterone receptor (PR). These receptors can be demonstrated to concentrate in the nuclei of target cells. Progesterone interaction with its receptor is only the first phase of a complex series of events involved in the regulatory mechanisms that determine the response to this hormone. In addition to the sequence of events in the assembly of a preinitiation complex of ribonucleic acid (RNA) polymerase II and general transcription factors, a series of proteins serve to modulate the response to progestins in target tissues. These proteins that modulate transcriptional activity are referred to as coregulators (coactivators, corepressors, and cointegrators), and they produce a series of protein–deoxyribonucleic acid (DNA), protein–RNA, and protein–protein interactions to either enhance or repress gene transcription. This complex interaction of PR with bound progestin and coregulator proteins provides potential selectivity to the interaction with promoter and response elements in different tissues.[1,2]

Steroid receptor interactions with multiple coregulator proteins provide a partial explanation of how target tissues function differently under specific physiologic conditions and disease states. Progestin function should no longer be regarded as limited to that of a differentiation sex steroid. It is critical to provide molecular mechanisms to explain how some tissues respond to progestins with cell proliferation, whereas in other tissues, the same progestins inhibit proliferation and are associated with cell differentiation. We have yet to account for the dramatic differences in progesterone-induced changes observed in tissues such as the breast and uterus. These differences are seen in both epithelial and stromal elements and seemed paradoxical prior to the recognition of the complexity of the role of coregulatory proteins in steroid hormone signaling.[1,2] Proliferation of breast epithelium is associated with progesterone,[3] whereas in the uterus, estrogen is dominant in proliferation and progesterone inhibits proliferation.[4] Despite this diametric effect on proliferation in these organs, progestins affect secretory differentiation and activity in both tissues after estrogen priming. Progestins also alter glandular epithelium and smooth muscle in other organs and tissues, including effects on vascular repair and fibrosis, as well as reticuloendothelial elements and inflammation.

Progestins also demonstrate rapid effects on signal transduction pathways, as do all classes of steroid hormones. Rapid actions occur in a time frame of seconds, which is far too rapid to have involved gene transcription. Further, inhibitors of gene transcription do not affect these rapid actions. These rapid effects include changes in second-messenger production or activity, protein kinase activity, and ion channels.[5,6] As a result of these observations, four types of nuclear hormone receptors are described to include (1) subpopulations of the conventional steroid receptor that associates with signaling complexes in the cytoplasm or plasma membrane; (2) modified forms of the receptor that preferentially localize to the plasma membrane; (3) transmembrane receptors for peptide hormones or neurotransmitters that are allosterically modulated by steroid hormones; and (4) novel transmembrane receptors unrelated to the classic nuclear steroid receptor.[6]

PHYSIOLOGY

The dominant naturally occurring progestin is progesterone (Figure 55-1). Progesterone is produced early in the scheme of the synthetic pathway involving the conversion of cholesterol to androgens, progestins, and estrogens. After menopause, in the absence of hormone replacement, the adrenal gland becomes the principal source of progestins as well as other sex steroids. In the premenopausal woman, progesterone is principally derived from the corpus luteum of the ovary, but in pregnancy after the eighth week of gestation, the placental progesterone production greatly exceeds ovarian-derived progesterone. The placental trophoblast is the dominant cell responsible for progesterone production by the placenta. The development of a secretory endometrium in which the blastocyst can implant requires progesterone. Progesterone is synthesized by the adrenal glands through conversion of pregnenolone. Progesterone levels of 25 ng/mL are usual in the luteal phase of the menstrual cycle, whereas levels to 150 ng/mL are seen in late pregnancy. High levels of progesterone (in

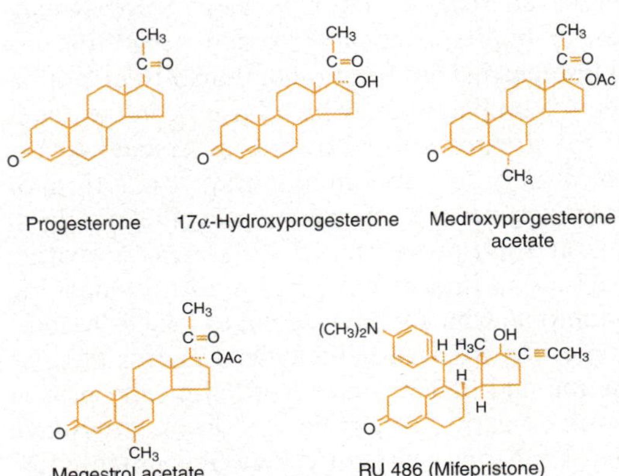

Figure 55-1 Structures of progesterone and related compounds. RU-486 is the most commonly used antiprogestin, and it also has antiglucocorticoid activity.

*Deceased.

the range of 100 to 150 ng/mL) are associated with tissue responses that have implications for treatment of other conditions. Progesterone clearly also has actions in the central nervous system, including sexual behavior, luteinizing hormone–releasing hormone response in the hypothalamus in the menstrual cycle regulation of ovulation, and neuroprotective effects, including amelioration of seizure activity. Progesterone metabolites, such as allopregnanolone and other reduced progesterone metabolites, may act locally in the central nervous system in a paracrine function, and these reduced progesterone metabolites have potent analgesic, sedative, and anticonvulsive effects mediated by allosteric enhancement of γ-aminobutyric acid (GABA) with its receptor.[7] Thus, although the conventional PR is present in specific sites in the brain, including the amygdala and limbic system, many of the effects, including antiseizure activity, do not appear to involve the classic PR.[6]

Progesterone has significant effects on immune function and has been shown to inhibit T-lymphocyte cell-mediated immune response, prostaglandin formation, and smooth muscle contractility.[8] There exists ample evidence of progesterone's effects on the cardiovascular system. PR is expressed in endothelial cells and in vascular smooth muscle cells and mediates both rapid effects and endothelial cell proliferation.[6,9,10] Progesterone also appears to act synergistically with estrogen to induce vasodilation.[6,10,11]

PHARMACOLOGY

Progestins are often prescribed in contraception and in conjunction with estrogen in postmenopausal hormone replacement therapy (HRT). In postmenopausal HRT, progestins are added to estrogen replacement principally to minimize the risk of uterine cancer associated with estrogen-only therapy, although the effects of adding progestins to estrogen on the risk of breast cancer have become of increasing concern.[12] The recommendation for adding progestin to estrogen replacement therapy in the climacteric places new emphasis on understanding the mechanism of progesterone action in settings other than contraception, particularly in populations with an increased risk of endometrial and breast cancer.[4,13] In premenopausal women, progestins and antiprogestins are used predominantly in contraceptive preparations, which have been the focus of the greatest effort toward understanding the pharmacology and mechanism of action of progesterone, as well as various synthetic progestins and antiprogestins.[14] Progestins are often used alone in selected women with climacteric symptoms who are advised not to take estrogens. Progestins are used in the endocrine treatment of uterine and breast cancer with clinically proven antineoplastic properties.[15,16] Progestins have also been of therapeutic benefit in meningiomas,[17] pulmonary lymphangiomyomatosis,[18] uterine leiomyomas,[19] and endometriosis,[20] producing tumor stabilization or reduction, disease remission, or disease inhibition. Some degree of antineoplastic effects has also been suggested in other neoplasms, such as ovarian carcinoma,[21] esophageal carcinoma,[22] cervical carcinoma,[23] and endometrial stromal sarcoma,[24] but controlled clinical trials have yet to prove the efficacy of progesterone in these tumors.

Progesterone is poorly absorbed when given orally, although transdermal administration has shown some efficacy.[25] When injected, progesterone must be administered with an oil carrier. A number of synthetic progestins are available that are well absorbed in the gastrointestinal tract. Synthetic progestins are derivatives of the steroid structure of either progesterone or testosterone. This derivative relationship provides the basis for the classification of the synthetic progestins. The synthetic progestins most often encountered include 17-hydroxyprogesterone, medroxyprogesterone (Provera), medroxyprogesterone acetate, megestrol acetate (Megace) (see Figure 55-1), norethindrone, norethindrone enanthate, norethindrone acetate, norethynodrel, norgestrel, desogestrel, and gestodene. In view of their importance in contraception and their therapeutic use in the climacteric and in neoplastic disease, new synthetic progestational compounds are under continued development and evaluation.

The poor absorption of progesterone has been overcome with some of the synthetic derivative progestins but at the cost of adverse effects on plasma lipid levels,[26] and alternate derivatives or alternate administration routes continue to be sought. Medroxyprogesterone given as a single intramuscular injection of 25 to 50 mg shows alteration of the estrogen-stimulated endometrium, with secretory morphology and a reduction in proliferative change, for just over 2 weeks, although increases in basal body temperature from such treatment may last 6 weeks or more. Depo-medroxyprogesterone has a period of action that is considerably longer. Oral medroxyprogesterone and oral megestrol acetate are well absorbed. Medroxyprogesterone produces a luteal effect in anovulatory patients, with an oral dose of 5 to 10 mg daily for 5 days. A dose of 5 to 10 mg/d for 10 days is typically recommended for anovulatory patients and in programs of cyclic estrogen-progesterone therapy for the climacteric. If daily progesterone is used in conjunction with estrogen replacement, a dose of 2.5 mg daily is recommended.

A 19-norsteroid, RU-486, is an antiprogesterone that has been used clinically in the last several years for its effects on pregnancy (see Figure 55-1). This compound is effectively absorbed orally and appears to bind to the PR with high affinity and to effect altered coregulator protein interaction after binding. RU-486 also has significant antiglucocorticoid activity and weak antiandrogen activity, being an effective contragestational agent.[27]

Quantitative increases in PR concentration in target cells are induced by preovulatory estrogen surges. This has the effect of priming target cells to respond to the progesterone rise produced by the corpus luteum after ovulation. Loss of the function of the corpus luteum (luteolysis) is associated with a rapid decrease in progesterone and estradiol. Associated with this rapid decrease in progesterone and estrogen is the disintegration of the endometrium. Since progesterone activity is often dependent on an intact functional PR, the molecular mechanism likely involved in RU-486 action is an inhibition of normal PR function and protein interactions (see below). However, in addition to conventional steroid receptors, membrane G protein–coupled–like receptor activity has been identified, specifically in progesterone-induced oocyte maturation,[28] as well as in other systems.[6] In ovarian granulosa cells, a novel membrane protein related to the ligand binding domain of the conventional PR has been observed to mediate both the antimitotic and the antiapoptotic effects of progesterone.[6]

In addition to the epithelial effects of progesterone, the effects on mesenchymal tissue, bone metabolism, water retention, lipid metabolism, and the central nervous system must all be considered in developing treatment strategies using progestins.[6,29,30]

BASIC MECHANISM OF PR LIGAND-DEPENDENT TRANSCRIPTION

Activation Function, Heat Shock Proteins, and Postsynthetic Modifications

Progesterone functions in RNA transcription regulation through a complex series of interactions that is initiated by binding of the hormone to its cognate receptor (Figure 55-2).[1,2] In the absence of hormone, PR monomers are associated with a complex of heat shock proteins (HSPs) 90, 70, 60, and 40, among others, and are transcriptionally inactive.[31–33] This complex of proteins appears to continuously associate and dissociate partner components as they move from nucleus to cytoplasm and back. When the ligand is bound, these HSPs are released or, more likely, fail to reassociate with PR.[31–33]

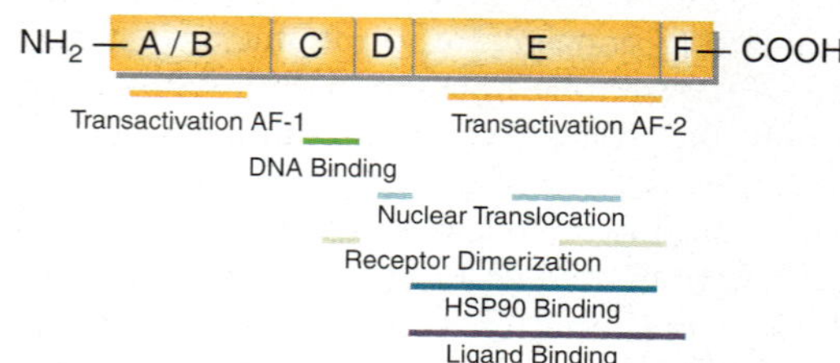

Figure 55-2 Schematic diagram of the functional protein domains of nuclear steroid receptors, such as the progesterone receptor (PR). Transactivation domain activation function (AF)-2 activity is hormone dependent, whereas AF-1 activity is hormone independent. The position of helix 12 at the C-terminus of AF-2 is noted in *black*. The central deoxyribonucleic acid (DNA) binding domain has the two zinc-finger structures that are characteristic of the nuclear receptor superfamily. The hormone binding domain has numerous overlapping functions as shown.

After ligand binding, the receptors are then able to form homodimers and remain localized in the nucleus. Although the chaperone function of the HSP90 complex is intimately associated with the inactive or "repressed state" of the steroid receptor, it is probably maintaining the receptor in a prestate that can recognize and bind progesterone. Steroid receptors are not able to effectively bind their cognate ligands in the absence of HSPs, presumably owing to unfolding. The binding of progesterone to PR reconfigures the hormone binding domain into a conformation that also activates the conserved transcriptional activation function (AF)-2 at its carboxy terminus. AF-2 function amplifies the transcription signal from PR at progesterone-responsive genes. This occurs by release of the chaperone protein(s) and corepressor proteins from PR followed by binding of coactivator proteins that enhance RNA polymerase II activity at the gene. In the absence of progesterone or HSPs, the PR is functionally inactive. Results suggest that in human breast cancers, an HSP designated HSP27 may be involved in cell growth, arrest, and enhanced differentiation.[34] HSP70 also appears to be involved in cell proliferation.

The function of the HSP has also been associated with cell death or apoptosis and differentiation.[1,2] The synthesis of HSP27 is modulated in the endometrium during different phases of the menstrual cycle. The synthesis of HSP90 that stabilizes the inactive form of the receptor is modulated by environmental or other stress, resulting in increased cellular concentrations. Higher concentrations of HSP90 appear to suppress sex steroid receptor–dependent transcription in general.[35]

Post-translational modification, such as phosphorylation, has also been implicated in PR function. One phosphorylation signal from mitogen-activated protein kinase (MAPK) at serine 294 of the PR is shown to lead to increased degradation of the PR at the proteosome.[36] A number of phosphorylation modifications have been mapped on the PR and others of the steroid receptors,[37,38] as well as recent evidence of meaningful signal sites on the coregulator proteins, yet the biologic consequences are still not fully understood. The rapid activation of the Src/ras/raf/MAPK pathway, in conjunction with the study of the interaction of estrogen receptor (ER) and PR, suggests that Src is a central component in the coupling of extracellular membrane–initiated signals.[6] The Src/MAPK signaling is affected by progesterone (and estrogen) in various cell types, with an effect on proliferation and survival. This insight begins to shed light on how the transcriptional regulators estrogen and progesterone have such profound effects on proliferation in certain target tissues. Human PR interaction with Src appears to be through a mechanism different from ER. The polyproline sequence of the PR from amino acids 421 to 428 creates a direct interaction with the SH3 domain of Src and sister signaling molecules.[6,39]

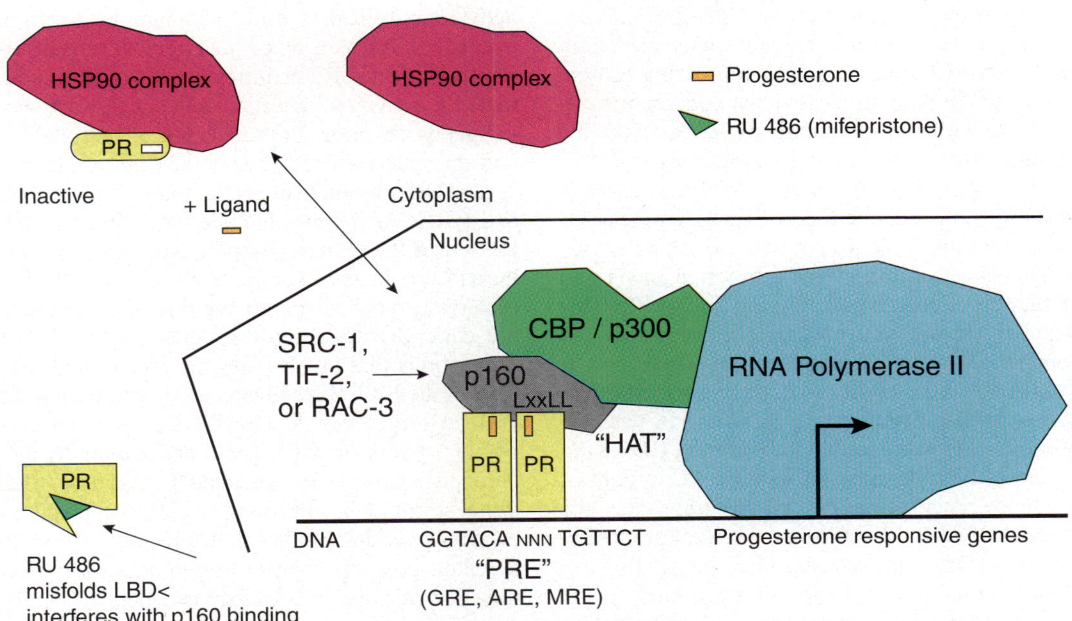

Figure 55-3 Progesterone receptors (PRs) are ligand-activated transcription factors. In the absence of hormone, PR monomers are associated with a complex of heat shock proteins and are transcriptionally inactive. This complex of proteins appears to associate and dissociate partner components as they move from nucleus to cytoplasm and back. Binding of progesterone to PR reconfigures the hormone binding domain (HBD) into a conformation that allows PR to homodimerize, bind progesterone response elements (PREs) in the nucleus, and activate activation function 2 (AF-2) to bind p160 coactivator proteins. Coactivators contain conserved leucine-rich amino acid motifs (LxxLL) that are key in binding to nuclear receptors. These coactivators also show histone acetyltransferase (HAT) activity, which modifies histones and opens chromatin near regulated genes, increasing ribonucleic acid (RNA) transcription by RNA polymerase II. If RU-486 is bound to PR, the HBD has an alternative conformation that does not bind p160 coactivators but instead binds corepressors that block transcription. The consensus binding sites for the glucocorticoid, androgen, and mineralocorticoid receptors are the same as PREs.

Structure of the DNA Binding Domain

The DNA binding domain (DBD) (see Figure 55-2) of the nuclear hormone receptors that respond to lipophilic signals is the most highly conserved feature of the superfamily.[1,2,40,41] The consensus sequence of the DBD cores is composed of 66 amino acids that include nine perfectly conserved cysteines. All but one is part of two highly conserved zinc fingers, each of which has one zinc coordinated by four cysteines. One of these fingers appears to be involved in required dimer formation, whereas the other specifies nucleotide sequence recognition in the major groove of the DNA of progesterone response elements (PREs) in front of progesterone-responsive genes.[40–42] Activation of PR by progesterone binding allows dimerization and unmasks the DBD for binding.[40–42] The sequence surrounding the PRE also influences how active the enhancer will be and which other proteins may help or inhibit PR transcription from that given site at that gene.

Function of PR Coregulators (Coactivators and Corepressors) on Transcription

On binding of progesterone, the PR changes its conformation in the ligand binding domain (LBD) in such a way that it decreases affinity for corepressors and increases the recruitment of coactivators (Figure 55-3). The increase in transcription activity results from the interaction with coactivators that include steroid receptor coactivator 1 (SRC-1), transcription intermediary factor 2, and retinoic acid coactivator 3, among others.[1,2,5,6] The SRC-1 interacts with the N-terminal AF-1 and the C-terminal AF-2 of the PR. This serves to emphasize that SRC-1 functions to synergize the ligand-independent amino terminal AF-1 with the ligand-responsive carboxyl terminal AF-2 of the PR. This resulting enhanced transcription is referred to as transactivation.[1,2]

PR has been shown to contain a repressor domain that binds to a corepressor, such as N-CoR, when the PR is bound by hormone antagonists.[43] For example, the antagonist RU-486 results in an inactive receptor-ligand complex. Thus, it is proposed that coactivators function by interacting positively with general transcription factors (GTFs) to activate target gene transcription, whereas corepressors interact with the same GTFs to repress the receptor-ligand complex.[2] In both situations, the HSP90, HSP70, and others have already dissociated from the PR complex when it binds either coactivators or corepressors. This suggests that the function of the coregulators is to modulate the interaction of the GTFs and the hormone response elements (HREs) at the TATA promoter in the transcription of specific genes.[2]

Corepressor binding is associated with a conformation of the receptor that prevents the complex from binding to its DNA binding element through the DBD. Even though the receptor can be shown to dimerize after ligand binding, unless the corepressor is displaced, transcription is not stimulated. Antagonist ligands such as RU-486 misfold the LBD to inhibit coactivator binding and enhance corepressor binding.[43,44] Recent x-ray crystal structure work has confirmed two distinct forms of the receptor when bound by hormones versus antihormones.[45,46] The surface generated for protein interaction is different, leading to either activating or repressing protein binding.[45,46] Numerous reviews and reports are available with regard to many of the details of the function of receptor–ligand interactions.[1,2,6,44–47]

An interesting observation for PR was made on a form in which the C-terminal 42 amino acids were deleted.[47] This removes all of helix 12, which is key for normal AF-2 function and is part of the direct coactivator binding site to PR. This form of PR was activated by antiprogestins and was not activated by progesterone. These activities reflected the ability to bind PR; RU-486 was able to bind and abnormally activate PR, whereas progesterone was not able to bind the LBD owing to loss of binding contacts in helix 12. In light of the more recent x-ray crystal structure data, the absence of helix 12 explains the lack of progesterone activation, and its absence apparently precludes interaction of repressing proteins on PR that would normally inactivate it when bound by RU-486. These "reversed ligand" phenotypic features of steroid receptors seem to be general for other family members also.

Potential Function of the Coactivator SRC-1 on Chromatin Remodeling Steroid hormones have long been known to affect chromatin structure. As the chromatin complex, eukaryotic DNA is efficiently packaged into arrays of nucleosomes that contain about 145 base pairs of DNA tightly wrapped as 1.7 turns around a histone octamer. This complex is likely to remain inaccessible to the steroid receptor–transcription complex. The nucleosome histone octamer is held together through the positively charged lysines on histone N-termini interacting with the negatively charged DNA residues. Recent evidence has shown that p160 coactivators such as SRC-1 have enzymatic activity as histone acetyltransferases (HATs) (see Figure 55-3), as does cyclic adenosine monophosphate response element binding protein.[48–50] HAT activity results in less tightly bound nucleosomes and more active transcription. Thus, SRC-1 enhances the ligand-dependent, receptor-dependent, and cell-free transcription of chromatin.[50] Conversely, corepressors are known to recruit histone deacetylases, which have the opposite effect and increase nucleosome affinity and repression of gene activity.[2]

Specific Target Selection of Progesterone Function Target cells not only must distinguish progesterone in the presence of other steroids, present in small amounts, they also must distinguish progesterone from other hydrophobic molecules that are frequently found in 100-fold or greater excess. Thus, although progesterone may affect a number of physiologic processes, such a high degree of discrimination is limited to differentiated cells that possess PR proteins and activatable PREs in their genome.[1,2,6]

PR is a prototypic member of a superfamily of transcriptional regulatory proteins. The target gene regulation is primarily dependent on progesterone activation of PR that results in a complex series of events.[1,2,6] As with other members of this superfamily, activated PR acquires the capacity to modulate the activity of specific target genes. Some target genes are under the regulation of both the PR and the glucocorticoid receptor because the consensus DNA binding site is the same for both PRE and GRE. Such genes include ER, human metallothionein IIA,[51] uteroglobulin, vitellogenin,[52] and human pregnancy–specific β-glycoprotein.[53] The molecular mechanisms to provide discrimination are dependent on highly specific protein–DNA interactions that involve specific amino acid residues of the PR DBD and nucleotide residues of the PRE at target genes. The PRE sequences of a whole network of target genes are potentially recognized by the *trans*-activated PR.[2] These PRE gene sequences are further characterized as enhancers in that neither their precise orientation nor their position appears to be critical for function. The response mechanism is dependent on the steps, beginning with hormone recognition, followed by activation of the DBD and then interaction of the DBD with chromosomal DNA target-gene PRE sequences. The surrounding nucleotides will affect net activity and affinity, as well as neighboring bound proteins and spacing.

Analyses of the DNA sequences also demonstrate that most progesterone-responsive target genes not only have multiple PRE copies but also are able to bind other steroid receptors, especially glucocorticoid receptor. Many of these HREs result in competition that modifies the function of PR. This knowledge of the existence of multiple and overlapping PREs and HREs provides for a plausible mechanism to account for the clinical observation that both the dose and hormone history have a profound effect on the clinical response of patients' tumors to hormone manipulation. As a specific example, it is frequently observed that the administration of different levels of progesterone enhances the cooperative binding to HREs and that a number of hormone combinations both down- and up-regulate progesterone-responsive genes.

PR Function and PR Mutations Progesterone response is dependent on the presence of functionally intact PR. Progestin-induced activity is only initiated when the steroid is bound to the carboxy terminal or progesterone-binding domain to induce *trans*-activation of transcription.[1,2,6] An absence of hormone response will result from either the absence of the PR protein altogether or its inability to bind hormone. The physical presence of PR by immunohistochemistry with a monoclonal antibody does not ensure that it will respond to ligand. Point mutations or deletions in the PBD of the PR can occur that result in constitutively active or inactive PR. There is also evidence of inactivated receptors as a consequence of mutations in what are now recognized as coregulator binding sites.[6,54]

Functional Significance of the Presence of Multiple PR Isoforms In humans, PR is composed of two PR isoforms, PRA and PRB, encoded by a single gene.[55] The expression of the human PR is reported to be controlled by two different transcription start sites that direct the synthesis of two transcripts and result in the two receptor protein isoforms. The PRA is N-terminally truncated by 164–amino acid residues and therefore is slightly smaller than PRB.[55] The PRA and PRB coexpress in many of the same cells and appear to be synthesized in equal proportions. There are reports of what appears to be functional differences between PRA and PRB in the transcriptional activation of target genes.[56] In breast cancers, PRA is expressed at high levels in some tumors, with the suggestion that PRA may act as a *trans*-dominant inhibitor of PRB.[56]

Further work on the two PR isoforms has made use of knockout mouse experiments in which only the PRA or the PRB form is missing.[57] The mice that had no PRA had major defects in the ovaries and uterus and were sterile. The mammary glands and thymus were normal. On the other hand, the PRB defective mice were fertile, with normal ovaries, uterus, and thymus, but they exhibited reduced mammary ductal morphology. The conclusions from this work are that PRA is primarily involved in fertility, whereas PRB has more function in mammary development. Interestingly, the two forms seem to activate different subsets of genes as opposed to simply being expressed in one cell type versus another.[57]

Function of Estrogen-Induced PR Synthesis In breast epithelial tissue, differentiation is dependent on the synthesis and activation of both PR and ER. The synthesis of either PR or ER requires both a specific signal response and a permissive chromosomal configuration in the region of the steroid receptor gene. This permissive state requires that a number of nuclear events have occurred, including the synthesis of *trans*-activating nuclear proteins, demethylation of the DNA, estrogen up-regulation of PR, and postsynthetic modification of a number of specific nuclear proteins.[2,5,6] PR and ER activation, then, are dependent not only on receptor synthesis and ligand binding affinity but equally on associations with at least a spectrum of additional proteins, including several classes of transcription-specific protein stimulators.

Tissue-Specific Modulation of Receptor Activity The progesterone response mediated by *trans*-activated PR represents critical interactions with chromatin and its complement of associated proteins. Most abundant among these are the histones[49] and the HMG1 and HMG2 chromosomal proteins,[58] which have been shown to interact directly with steroid receptors.[58] HMGB1 aids PR binding to PREs by some sevenfold and further selectively enhances its transcriptional stimulation.[58,59] These HMG proteins are postsynthetically modified by both histone kinases and acetylases.[60]

PR not only functions in its binding to *cis*-activating PREs at upstream DNA sequences of a number of progesterone-responsive genes, it also has the capacity to function as a down-regulator of the synthesis of other hormone receptors, for example, ER.[61,62] PR should be considered a target gene for estrogen response in that a functional ER is required to up-regulate the synthesis of PR.[63] This mechanism may also account for the modulation of PR synthesis in response to glucocorticoid competition for DNA response elements.

Postsynthetic modifications involve both subtle alterations in the PR structure and *cis*- and *trans*-activating factors. Modifications include (1) phosphorylation and acetylation of chromosomal proteins, such as histones HMG1 and HMG2; (2) postsynthetic modification of the binding of HSPs to PR; (3) phosphorylation of both of these proteins; and (4) coregulator-associated enzymatic activities. In addition to the multiple *cis*-activating components described for HRE, *trans*-activating elements are also required for RNA transcription critical for the hormone response.[1,2,6,7]

PR as a Member of the Superfamily of Receptor Proteins The superfamily of receptor proteins that interact with many lipophilic ligands have a number of features in common with PR (see Figure 55-2).[6] Early studies using proteolytic digestion of PR proteins demonstrated a loss of DNA binding in spite of retention of the specific ligand binding. These proteolytic receptor digests were referred to as meroreceptor fragments. A number of highly conserved regions for the receptor protein genes have been observed through cloning of receptor proteins. The structures of the receptor proteins for progesterone, estrogen, and glucocorticoid show a striking homology with other hydrophobic signal proteins, including thyroid receptor, retinoic acid receptors, and vitamin D_3 receptor.[5,6]

Intracellular Localization Progesterone is a hydrophobic signaling molecule and is thus unrestricted by plasma or nuclear membranes, being free to diffuse through membranes to interact with specific proteins. Whereas it is clear that the specificity attained by a hydrophilic signal is dependent on its interaction with cell surface receptors, the precise intracellular localization of all hydrophobic steroid molecules is unresolved. The use of antireceptor antibodies to PR and ER demonstrates these proteins in the nucleus, whereas immunoreactive glucocorticoid receptor in the absence of ligand is found in the cytoplasm. After complexing with their specific ligands, all steroid receptors are detected only in the nucleus. The presence of the specific ligand is a primary signal for nuclear translocation and retention. The interaction of progesterone with the plasma membrane is even more complex.[6]

CLINICAL OBSERVATIONS ON PROGESTIN RECEPTOR AND TARGET TISSUE RESPONSES TO PROGESTINS

Progestins are involved in benign physiologic changes ranging from differentiated secretory activity to edematous changes in stromal tissues of the breast. Progestins are also significant considerations in neoplastic disease, being associated with both a decreased risk of endometrial neoplasms and a slightly increased risk of breast neoplasms when used in conjunction with estrogen replacement for menopause. Progesterone is also associated with a number of clinically important responses in target tissues. Progestins have a critical role in the support of the products of conception: the differentiation of the endometrium and the promotion of the secretory phase of the endometrium; the maturation and cornification of the vaginal mucosal epithelium; the suppression of ovulation; the inhibition of gonadotropin release; the proliferation of breast epithelium and the induction of secretory activity in breast epithelium; and a natriuretic effect on the kidneys. A number of these biologic effects of progesterone are seen only in concert with priming of the target tissues with estrogen, whereas other effects appear to be interrelated with the actions of other steroid hormones, peptide hormones, and/or growth factors. Both progesterone and estrogen influence the response when superpharmacologic doses are used. Possible interactions between progesterone, estrogen, and growth factors must be taken into account when constructing treatment strategies.

THE UTERUS

Normal Uterus The cyclic response of the uterus to estrogen and progesterone is among the best studied examples of hormonal modulation of tissue response. There is clear evidence of cyclic regulation of ER and PR proteins in the endometrial epithelium, myometrium, and endometrial stroma. The induction of PR by estrogen has been shown both in vitro and in vivo. An increase in PR at the end of the proliferative phase of the menstrual cycle occurs in the stromal or myometrial tissue 24 to 48 hours before the observed peak of PR levels in endometrial epithelial tissue.[13] This cyclic change can be aborted by the administration of 10 mg of medroxyprogesterone for 5 to 10 days, associated with regression of the epithelium. Epithelial hyperplasia of the uterus exposed to progestins first shows acanthomatous or squamous metaplastic changes (changes wherein the cells resemble squamous cells), followed by secretory differentiation and, finally, regression of the hyperplastic change, with eventual atrophy after 10 to 14 days.

Uterine Carcinoma Uterine carcinoma is a localized disease in the majority of cases. There is a several-fold increased incidence of adenocarcinoma of the uterus when a woman is given unopposed estrogen in physiologic doses, and this increased frequency is reduced to that of the population not receiving estrogen if progestins are also given. Progestins can be effectively given in several ways. Among these options is that progestins be given for the last 10 days of the estrogen replacement cycle or at a lower dose throughout the cycle.

When diagnosed, adenocarcinoma of the uterus is cured by local therapy in 80% of cases. In the event of recurrence, exogenous progestin is an effective treatment in a significant fraction of cases: more than 30% of patients with recurrent disease demonstrate an objective response to exogenous progestins. ER and PR can be measured in these tumors, and the presence of these receptors correlates with differentiation of the tumor, prognosis for the patient, and response to progestins. The duration of response is not predicted by the presence of a receptor and varies from months to years. Tumors that lack ER and PR respond objectively to progestins in fewer than 10% of cases. Tumors that have been treated with radiotherapy have a greater tendency to be PR negative than tumors that have not been treated with radiation. Because of the low toxicity of progestins, trials of progestin therapy are often warranted even if receptors have not been measured in the tumor or appear to be absent in recurrent or inoperable endometrial carcinoma.

The effective use of progestins in treating endometrial hyperplasia associated with unopposed estrogen and in patients with receptor-rich well-differentiated adenocarcinomas further supports the role of progestins in suppressing proliferation of the endometrium. The use of hormone therapy has readily demonstrable effects on endometrial histology.[4]

Other Neoplasms of the Uterus Pharmacologic progestin has a clearly beneficial effect on uterine leiomyomas, and significant levels of PR have been demonstrated in these proliferations of mesenchymal origin.[19] Uterine sarcomas, including stromal sarcomas and leiomyosarcomas, have a variable response to progesterone.[24] PR is not consistently observed in these tumors.

PR has been reported in some studies of squamous carcinoma of the uterine cervix (up to 41% of tumors).[23] Cervical epithelial maturation was correlated with progesterone secretion (ovulation). PR was not found in the majority of tumors in other studies, and no firm evidence of clinical or histologic correlation of the presence of PR has been shown.

THE BREAST

Normal Breast Progestin response in the human breast is complex and influences both proliferation and differentiated function. The luteal phase of the menstrual cycle (progesterone dominant) is characterized by both active secretion and the peak of proliferative activity in the normal breast.[14] Epidemiologic data appear to implicate progestins in proliferative disorders and cancers of the breast in a more direct fashion than had been previously thought. The observations of increased risk of breast cancer with the addition of progestins to estrogen replacement therapy resulted in the cessation of the Women's Health Initiative trial of estrogen plus progestin.[12,64] It has been recognized from the earliest studies of ER and PR in breast epithelial systems that progesterone action, mediated through PR, resulted in down-regulation of the ER in breast epithelium. This observation suggested that the influence of estrogen would be to stimulate proliferation of the breast epithelium and that the effect of progesterone might be to inhibit proliferation, similar to the effect seen in the uterus. Whereas the effect on regulation of ER appears to be similar, the effect of progestins and specifically progesterone in physiologic amounts is not similar. This must be considered in recommending sex steroid replacement therapy in the climacteric because this risk is statistically significant.[6] Thought should be given to the fact that adding progestin to estrogen replacement therapy does not reduce the risk of breast cancer and in several studies appears to increase the risk to some extent.[6,64]

Breast Cancer PRs have been studied extensively in cancerous human breast tissue. Patients whose tumors are PR positive have a higher probability of responding to endocrine therapy (not necessarily progestins) and in most series show a somewhat better prognosis with respect to both survival and disease-free interval.[57] Considerable controversy exists with respect to the effect of menstrual cycle phase at surgery on the evaluation of tissue for receptor and to whether there is an effect of this timing on prognosis.[63,65–68] PR, in contrast to ER, does not show increasing levels with increasing age of the population studied.[63]

Progestin therapy for metastatic breast cancer has been used principally as a second- or third-line therapy following selective ER modifiers such as tamoxifen and, more recently, aromatase inhibitors in postmenopausal patients. The principal progestin used for metastatic breast cancer has been megestrol acetate. The response of metastatic breast cancer to megestrol is predicted by the presence of ER and/or PR but is best predicted by the observation of an objective response to previous hormonal therapy. One of the more interesting aspects of progestin therapy for metastatic breast cancer is the observation of a dose-response increase in efficacy. Patients who have relapsed or progressed on conventional therapeutic doses of medroxyprogesterone (100–200 mg/d) or megestrol (160 mg/d) may show an additional response with increased dose (to 2,000 mg/d for medroxyprogesterone or to 1,600 mg/d for megestrol). A beneficial side effect of the progestin is increased appetite and weight gain, although some of the weight gain can be associated with fluid retention. The mechanism of the increased appetite and actual weight gain is poorly understood, although this property of appetite enhancement has been used clinically to treat cancer-associated anorexia and cachexia. A number of other central nervous system effects of progestins have been characterized, including beneficial effects on climacteric symptoms.[6,12,30]

Other Tumors of the Breast PRs have been reported in fibroadenomas, phyllodes tumors, and breast sarcomas. There is no convincing evidence for a biologic response to progestin manipulation of either cystosarcoma phyllodes or stromal sarcoma of the breast.

THE OVARY

Epidemiologic data have shown an effect on the incidence of ovarian epithelial carcinoma in patients who have used estrogen-progesterone preparations to inhibit ovulation. PR is observed in 30 to 40% of ovarian carcinomas.[21] Although some studies have observed a trend toward better survival in patients with PR-positive carcinomas, no convincing data to indicate objective response to progestin therapy have been reported.

OTHER TISSUES

PR and response to progestins have been repeatedly reported in meningiomas and pulmonary lymphangioleiomyomatosis, renal cell carcinomas, and squamous cell carcinoma of the head and neck. The presence of PRs in meningiomas is consistently observed, and clinical trials have shown a response to progestins. In squamous cell carcinoma of the head and neck, the presence of progestin receptors has been detected, but in these tumors, as in renal cell carcinoma, an objective response to progestin treatment has not been convincingly shown. In contrast, progestin therapy has become an important option in the treatment of pulmonary lymphangioleiomyomatosis, which was a uniformly fatal condition before progestin-hormone therapy was shown to be effective.[18] In cases in which pulmonary lymphangiomyomatosis is treated early in the course of the disease, before extensive chylous effusion is present, an objective response to continued progesterone therapy is noted in the majority of patients. This response appears to require that the progestin be continued. Responses at greater than 5 years have been observed; in some patients, however, the disease progresses after a period of remission despite continued progesterone.

CONCLUSION

It is now abundantly clear that progestins have broad implications for tissue development and differentiation, as well as proliferation and apoptosis control in target tissues. The mechanism of action of progestins is not limited to nuclear receptor–mediated transcriptional regulation. Many of the paradoxes of the nuclear receptor model become clarified through the recognition of the interaction of progestins (and estrogens) with other signaling pathways, including evidence of membrane-mediated effects. The different responses that progestins induce in specific target tissues and how such differences can exist in the face of what appears to involve the same PR isoforms, the same ligand, and the same or similar PREs have emerged as a critical area for understanding the role of progestins in both the development and differentiation of breast and endometrium and the development and control of neoplastic processes in these tissues. The broad spectrum of tissue response to progesterone has been shown to involve subtle differences in the competition of the liganded PR for an array of coregulators in the signaling pathway.[1,2,5,6,61] The PR–chromatin interaction is only part of what determines the differentiated function induced by progesterone. Many of the molecular details of progesterone induction of specific gene activation of RNA transcription have now been identified, whereas others remain elusive. Binding of progesterone to PR causes a refolding of the LBD to an active conformation that dissociates repressive HSP complexes and associates coactivators.[1,2,5,6] They interact with AF-1 and AF-2 to amplify transcription at PR-responsive genes. Antagonists such as RU-486 simply misfold the LBD, inhibit coactivator binding, and increase corepressor binding. Coactivators, corepressors, isoforms, and postsynthetic modifications all contribute to the complex regulation of response to these steroids. Progestins also influence cell proliferation and can be seen to play a role in the treatment of a number of neoplasms, primarily those of the endometrium and breast. The molecular mechanisms involved in the progestin treatment response are complex and involve complex signaling systems, which offer a number of targets that may be considered in treatment design.[69]

REFERENCES

1. Nettles KW, Green GL. Ligand control of coregulator recruitment to nuclear receptors. Annu Rev Physiol 2005;67:309–33.
2. McKenna NJ, O'Malley BW. Combinatorial control of gene expression by nuclear receptors and coregulators. Cell 2002;108:465–74.
3. Anderson T, Howell A, Williams G. Oral contraceptive use increases proliferation and decreases oestrogen receptor content of epithelial cells in the normal human breast. Int J Cancer 1991;48:206–10.
4. Writing Group for the PEPI Trial. Effects of hormone replacement therapy on endometrial histology in postmenopausal women: the Postmenopausal Estrogen/Progestin Interventions (PEPI) Trial. JAMA 1996;275:370–5.
5. Cheskis BJ. Regulation of cell signaling cascades by steroid hormones. J Cell Biochem 2004;93:20–7.
6. Edwards DP. Regulation of signal transduction pathways by estrogen and progesterone. Annu Rev Physiol 2005;67:335–76.
7. Reddy DS, Castaneda DC, O'Malley BW, Rogawski MA. Anticonvulsant activity of progesterone and neurosteroids in progesterone receptor knockout mice. J Pharmacol Exp Ther 2004;310:230–9.
8. Szekeres-Bartho J, Barakonyi A, Polgar B, et al. The role of gamma delta T cells in progesterone mediated immunomodulation during pregnancy: a review. Am J Reprod Immunol 1999;42:44–8.
9. Vazquez F, Rodriquez-Manzaneque JD, Lydon JP, et al. Progesterone regulates proliferation of endothelial cells. J Biol Chem 1999;274:2185–92.
10. Karas RH, van Eickels M, Lydon JP, et al. A complex role for the progesterone receptor in the response to vascular injury. J Clin Invest 2001;108:611–8.
11. Minshall RD, Pavcnik D, Browne DL, Hermsmeyer K. Nongenomic vasodilator action of progesterone on primate coronary arteries. J Appl Physiol 2002;92:701–8.
12. Women's Health Initiative Investigators. Risks and benefits of estrogen plus progestin in healthy postmenopausal women. JAMA 2002;288:321–3.
13. McCarty KS Jr. Proliferative stimuli in the normal breast: estrogens or progestins. Hum Pathol 1989;20:1137.
14. Baulieu EE. A novel approach to human fertility control: contragestion by the anti-progesterone RU 486. Eur J Obstet Gynecol Reprod Biol 1988;28:125.
15. Robertson JFR, William MR, Todd J, et al. Factors predicting the response of patients with advanced breast cancer to endocrine (Megace) therapy. Eur J Clin Oncol 1989;25:469.
16. Nyholm HC. Estrogen and progesterone receptors in endometrial cancer. Clinicopathological correlations and

prognostic significance [review]. APMIS Suppl 1996;65:5–33.
17. Halper J, Colvard DS, Scheithauer BW, et al. Estrogen and progesterone receptors in meningiomas: comparison of nuclear binding, dextran-coated charcoal and immunoperoxidase staining assays. Neurosurgery 1989;25:546.
18. Berger U, Khaghani A, Pomerance A, et al. Pulmonary lymphangioleiomyomatosis and steroid receptors. An immunocytochemical study. Am J Clin Pathol 1990;93:609.
19. Maheux R. Treatment of uterine leiomyomata: past, present and future. Horm Res 1989;32:125.
20. Lessey BA, Metzger DA, Haney AF, McCarty KS Jr. Immunohistochemical analysis of estrogen and progesterone receptor in endometriosis; comparison with normal endometrium during the menstrual cycle and the effect of medical therapy. Fertil Steril 1989;27:515.
21. Harding M, Cowan S, Hole D, et al. Estrogen and progesterone receptors in ovarian cancer. Cancer 1990;65:486.
22. Berg NJ, Colvard DS, Neel HB III, et al. Progesterone receptors in carcinomas of the upper aerodigestive tract. Otolaryngol Head Neck Surg 1989;101:527.
23. Hunter RE, Longcope C, Keough P. Steroid hormone receptors in carcinoma of the cervix. Cancer 1987;60:392.
24. Keen CE, Phillip G. Progestin-induced regression in low-grade endometrial stromal sarcoma. Case report and literature review. Br J Obstet Gynaecol 1989;96:1435.
25. Crook D, Crust MP, Gangar KF, et al. Comparison of transdermal and oral estrogen-progestin replacement therapy: effects on serum lipids and lipoproteins. Am J Obstet Gynecol 1992;166:950–5.
26. Ottosson UB, Johansson BG, Shultz B. Subfraction of high density lipoprotein cholesterol during estrogen replacement therapy: a comparison between progestin and natural progesterone. Am J Obstet Gynecol 1985;6:746.
27. Baulieu EE. Contragestation and other clinical applications of RU 486, an antiprogesterone at the receptor. Science 1989;245:1351.
28. Thomas P, Zhu Y, Pace M. Progestin membrane receptors involved in the meiotic maturation of teleost oocytes: a review with some new findings. Steroids 2002;67:511–7.
29. Tremollieres F, Pouilles JM, Ribot C. Effect of long-term administration of progestogen on post menopausal bone loss: result of a two-year, controlled randomized study. Clin Endocrinol (Oxf) 1993;38:627–31.
30. Lobo RA, Gibbons WE. The role of progestin therapy in breast disease and central nervous system function. J Reprod Med 1982;27:515.
31. Smith DF. Chaperones in progesterone receptor complexes. Semin Cell Dev Biol 2000;11:45–52.
32. Kosano H, Stensgard B, Charlesworth MC, et al. The assembly of progesterone receptor-hsp90 complexes using purified proteins. J Biol Chem 1998;273:32973–9.
33. Hernandez MP, Chadli A, Toft DO. HSP40 binding is the first step in the HSP90 chaperoning pathway for the progesterone receptor. J Biol Chem. 2002;277:11873–81.
34. Vargas-Roig LM, Fanelli MA, Lopez LA, et al. Heat shock proteins and cell proliferation in human breast cancer biopsy samples. Cancer Detect Prev 1997;21:441–51.
35. Sabbah M, Radanyi C, Rredeuilh G, Baulieu EE. The 90 kDa heat-shock protein (hsp90) modulates the binding of the oestrogen receptor to its cognate DNA. Biochem J 1996;314:205–13.
36. Lange CA, Shen T, Horwitz KB. Phosphorylation of human progesterone receptors by mitogen-activated protein kinase at Ser-294 signals their degradation by the 26S proteosome. Proc Natl Acad Sci U S A 2000;97:1032–7.
37. Knotts TA, Orkiszewski RS, Cook RG, et al. Identification of a phosphorylation site in the hinge region of the human progesterone receptor and additional amino-terminal phosphorylation sites. J Biol Chem 2001;276:8475–83.
38. Weigel NL. Steroid hormone receptors and their regulation by phosphorylation. Biochem J 1996;319:657–67.
39. Boonyaratanakornkit V, Scott MP, Ribon V, et al. Progesterone receptor contains a proline-rich motif that directly interacts with SH3 domains and activates c-Src family tyrosine kinases. Mol Cell 2001;8:269–80.
40. Evans RM, Hollenberg SM. Zinc fingers: gilt by association. Cell 1988;52:1.
41. Miesfeld RL. The structure and function of steroid receptor proteins. Crit Rev Biochem Mol Biol 1989;24:101.
42. Green S, Chambon P. Nuclear receptors enhance our understanding of transcription regulation. Trends Genet 1988;4:309.
43. Graham JD, Bain DL, Richer JK, et al. Thoughts on tamoxifen resistant breast cancer. Are coregulators the answer or just a red herring? J Steroid Biochem Mol Biol 2000;74:255–9.
44. Edwards DP, Leonhardt SA, Gass-Handel E. Novel mechanisms of progesterone antagonists and progesterone receptor. J Soc Gynecol Investig 2000;7:S22–4.
45. Williams SP, Sigler PB. Atomic structure of progesterone complexed with its receptor. Nature 1998;393:392–6.
46. Tanenbaum DM, Wang Y, Williams SP, Sigler PB. Crystallographic comparison of the estrogen and progesterone receptor's ligand binding domains. Proc Natl Acad Sci U S A 1998;95:5998–6003.
47. Vegeto E, Allan GF, Schrader WT, et al. The mechanism of RU486 antagonism is dependent on the conformation of the carboxy-terminal tail of the human progesterone receptor. Cell 1992;69:703–13.
48. Kelner DN, McCarty KS Sr. Porcine liver nuclear histone acetyltransferase: partial purification and basic properties. J Biol Chem 1984;259:3413.
49. Spencer TE, Jenster G, Burcin MM, et al. Steroid receptor coactivator-1 is a histone acetyltransferase. Nature 1997;389:194–8.
50. Liu Z, Wong J, Tsai SY, et al. Steroid receptor coactivator-1 (SRC-1) enhances ligand-dependent and receptor-dependent cell-free transcription of chromatin. Proc Natl Acad Sci U S A 1999;96:9485–90.
51. Slater EP, Cato AC, Karin M, et al. Progesterone induction of metallothionein-IIA gene expression. Mol Endocrinol 1988;2:485.
52. Wahli W. Evolution and expression of vitellogenin genes. Trends Genet 1988;4:227.
53. Chilton BS, Mani SK, Bullock DW. Servomechanism of prolactin and progesterone in regulating uterine gene expression. Mol Endocrinol 1988;2:1169.
54. Dobson AD, Conneely OM, Beattie W, et al. Mutational analysis of the chicken progesterone receptor. J Biol Chem 1989;264:4207.
55. Kastner P, Krust A, Turcotte B, et al. Two distinct estrogen-regulated promoters generate transcripts encoding the two functionally different human progesterone receptor forms A and B. EMBO J 1990;9:1603.
56. McGowan E, Clarke C. Effect of overexpression of progesterone receptor A on endogenous progestin-sensitive endpoints in breast cancer cells. Mol Endocrinol 1999;13:1657–71.
57. Conneely OM, Mulac-Jericevic B, DeMayo F, et al. Reproductive functions of progesterone receptors. Recent Prog Horm Res 2002;57:339–55.
58. Bernues J, Querol E. Non-random reconstitution of HMG1 and HMG2 in chromatin. Determination of the histone contacts. Biochem Biophys Acta 1989;1008:52–61.
59. Verrijdt G, Haelens A, Schoenmakers E, et al. Comparative analysis of the influence of the high-mobility group box 1 protein on DNA binding and transcriptional activation by the androgen, glucocorticoid, progesterone and mineralocorticoid receptors. Biochem J 2002;361:97–103.
60. Mold DE, McCarty KS Sr. A Chinese hamster ovary cell histone deacetylase that is associated with a unique class of mononucleosomes. Biochemistry 1987;26:8257.
61. Nardulli AM, Greene GL, O'Malley BW, Katzenellenbogen BS. Regulation of progesterone receptor messenger ribonucleic acid and protein levels in MCF-7 cells by estradiol: analysis of estrogen's effect on progesterone receptor synthesis and degradation. Endocrinology 1988;122:935.
62. Ree AH, Landmark BF, Eskild W, et al. Autologous down-regulation of messenger ribonucleic acid protein levels for estrogen receptors in MCF-7 cells: an inverse correlation to progesterone receptor levels. Endocrinology 1989;124:2577.
63. McCarty KS Jr, Silva JS, Cox EB, et al. Relationship of age and menopausal status to estrogen receptor content in primary carcinoma of the breast. Ann Surg 1983;197:123–30.
64. Fletcher, SW, Colditz, GA. Failure of estrogen plus therapy for prevention. JAMA 2002;288:366–8.
65. Osborne CK. Steroid hormone receptors in breast cancer management. Breast Cancer Res Treat 1998;51:227–38.
66. Bawde RA, Gregory WM, Chaudary MA, et al. Timing of surgery during the menstrual cycle and survival of premenopausal women with operable breast cancer. Lancet 1991;337:1261–4.
67. McGuire WL, Hilsenbeck S, Clark GM. Optimal mastectomy timing. J Natl Cancer Inst 1992;84:346–8.
68. Nathan B, Bates T, Anbazhagan R, et al. Timing of surgery for breast cancer in relation to the menstrual cycle and survival of premenopausal women. Br J Surg 1993;80:43–8.
69. Lange CA, Richer J, Horwitz KB. Hypothesis: progesterone primes breast cancer cells for cross-talk with proliferative or antiproliferative signals [review]. Mol Endocrinol 1999;13:829–36.

Androgen Deprivation Strategies in the Treatment of Advanced Prostate Cancer

Samuel R. Denmeade, MD

Since the pioneering studies of Charles Brenton Huggins nearly 60 years ago, it has been known that prostate cancer cells, like certain normal prostate epithelial cells, can be chronically dependent on a critical level of androgenic stimulation for their net continuous growth and survival.[1] It is on this basis that androgen ablation has been used as standard systemic therapy for metastatic prostate cancer. It has been estimated that in 2005, 31,000 males in the United States will die from prostate cancer.[2] Essentially, all of these patients will have received treatment with a variety of androgen ablation techniques. Presently, there are a multitude of excellent means of ablating serum androgens, and these include surgical orchiectomy and chronic treatment with luteinizing hormone–releasing hormone (LH-RH) analogues, alone and in combination with antiandrogens. In this chapter, a review of the present state of knowledge regarding the biology of androgen activity in prostate tissue and the use of new methods of androgen deprivation therapy to treat prostate cancer is presented. Although androgen ablation therapy has been used to treat advanced prostate cancer for almost 60 years, debate continues to this day as to the optimal methods and timing of androgen deprivation therapy. These controversial questions include the following: (1) Is combined androgen blockade (CAB) superior to monotherapy? (2) Will the use of intermittent androgen suppression (IAS) replace continuous therapy? (3) Should androgen deprivation be initiated early in the course of disease or delayed to minimize toxicities? (4) How should toxicities of androgen blockade be properly managed? (5) What is the proper use of second-line hormonal therapies? (6) How do we increase accrual to clinical trials prior to or during initiation of hormonal therapy? These topics will be explored in an attempt to provide information that will allow physicians to counsel patients to select the best available hormonal treatments.

DEFINITION OF ANDROGEN RESPONSIVENESS ON A CELLULAR BASIS

Androgens are the major regulators of proliferation and death for the normal prostate. This is because androgens regulate the total prostatic epithelial cell number by chronically stimulating the rate of cell proliferation (ie, agonistic ability of androgen) while simultaneously inhibiting the rate of cell death (ie, antagonistic ability of androgen) of specific subsets of androgen-sensitive and -dependent epithelial cells and endothelial cells within the prostate.[3–5] If a sufficient systemic androgen level is not chronically maintained (eg, following androgen ablation), then the subset of androgen-dependent prostatic epithelial and endothelial cells dies rapidly via the activation of an energy-dependent cascade of biochemical and morphologic changes, collectively referred to as programmed cell death or apoptosis.

Within the normal prostate, the glandular epithelial and a subset of endothelial cells are androgen dependent because without sufficient levels of circulated androgen, their rate of cells proliferating is lower than their rate of cell death.[3–5] These dependent cells are thus eliminated by androgen ablation. In contrast, the prostatic basal cells are not androgen dependent because they are not eliminated following castration.[6] Indeed, the stem cells within this basal cell compartment are androgen independent in that their rates of proliferation and death are unaffected by androgen ablation.[3,7,8] Also, in this basal cell compartment are amplifying cells, and although they are not androgen dependent (ie, not eliminated by androgen ablation), their rate of cell proliferation is enhanced by androgen over their rate of cell death (ie, these cells are androgen sensitive but not androgen dependent). Indeed, the androgen sensitivity of these amplifying cells allows exogenous androgen replacement to induce the proliferative restoration of the androgen-dependent glandular cell compartment in the involuted prostate of previously castrated hosts.[7,8]

Thus, the prostate is heterogeneously composed of a limited number of androgen-independent stem cells, which, besides maintaining their own limited numbers, give rise to a larger subset of progeny that differentiate into the androgen-independent, but -sensitive, amplifying cells. When sufficient androgen is not present (ie, following androgen ablation), the amplifying cells are maintained (ie, rate of proliferation = rate of cell death) but do not expand into transit cells. In contrast, when physiologically normal levels of androgen are exogenously replaced in a previously castrated host, the majority of these androgen-sensitive amplifying cells differentiate into androgen-dependent transit (ie, glandular) epithelial cells. Once the normal number of these androgen-dependent transit (glandular) cells is reached, their rate of cell proliferation balances their rate of cell death such that neither prostatic regression nor continuous glandular overgrowth occurs. Thus, in the presence of physiologic androgen, the normal prostate is in a steady-state, self-renewing, maintenance condition, heterogeneously composed of androgen-independent, -sensitive, and -dependent epithelial cells. Owing to the clonally expansive nature of this hierarchical stem cell organization, the vast majority of the epithelial compartment is composed of androgen-dependent glandular cells, with lower numbers of androgen-sensitive basal cells and a limited number of androgen-independent basal stem cells.[7,8]

MECHANISM OF ANDROGEN ACTION

Studies at the molecular level have demonstrated that androgens function via binding to their cognate nuclear receptors, inducing conformational changes in the occupied androgen receptor (AR). ARs exhibit a prototypic multidomain structure containing an N-terminal activation domain, a C-terminal ligand binding domain, and a centrally located DNA binding region with two zinc finger motifs.[9–14] Specific interaction with androgenic ligands results in the conformational activation of AR. This allows the binding of the occupied AR with additional nuclear proteins (ie, coactivator proteins and general transcription factors) to produce transcriptional complexes, which can activate or repress specific gene expression by binding to the androgen-responsive elements present in the promoter regions in a series of androgen-regulated genes.[15] It does this by forming an active transcriptional complex, resulting in site-directed chromatin remodeling and enhancement of target gene expression.[15] *SRC1* is a coactivator for AR; it functions in transcriptional activation through its histone acetyltransferase activity (HAT) and multiple interactions with agonist-bound receptors; other coactivators, such as CBP or P300; other HAT, such as p/CAF; and some GTFs, such as TBP and TIFIIB.[15] *SRC1* is a member of a gene family that includes *SRC1*, *TIF2* (also termed *GRIP1* and *SRC2*), and P/*CIP* (also termed *RAC*3, *ACTR*, *AIBI*, and *SRC3*).[15] Cell-free in vitro transcription and in vivo experiments have indicated that the *SRC1* family members enhance AR-dependent transactivation of nuclear genes.[15] The regulation of the expression of these genes both stimulates prostate cell proliferation and inhibits prostate cell death.[3]

OVERVIEW OF REGULATION OF SYSTEMIC ANDROGEN LEVELS

The organs involved in the regulation of androgen production are the hypothalamus, pituitary gland,

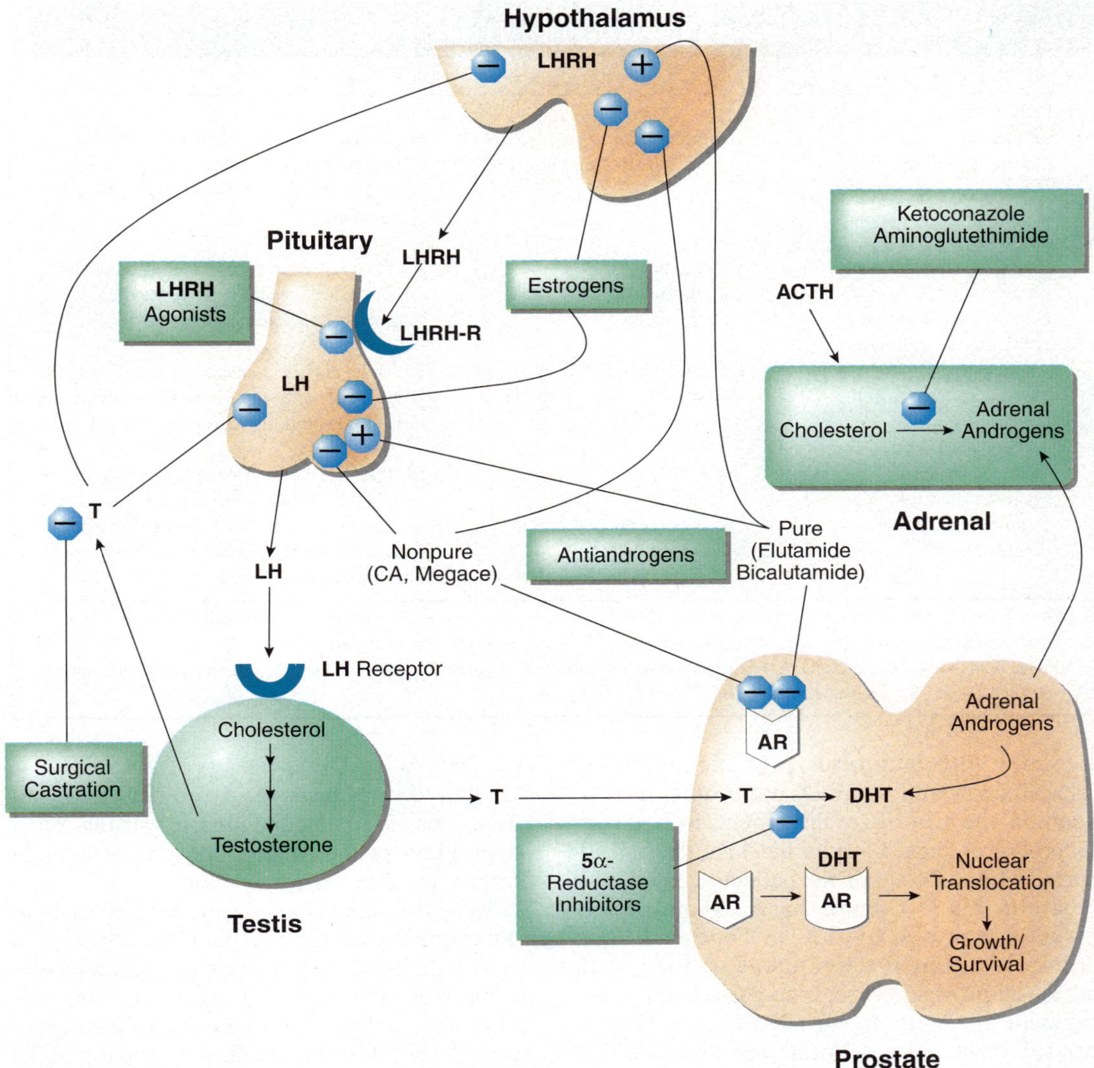

Figure 56-1 Regulation of androgen production and sites of blockade of androgen action. AR = androgen receptor; CA = cyproterone acetate; DHT = dihydrotestosterone; LH = luteinizing hormone; LH-RH = luteinizing hormone–releasing hormone; T = testosterone.

testes, and adrenal glands (Figure 56-1). The peptide hormones, LH-RH, and corticotropin-releasing factor are produced by the hypothalamus. These releasing hormones reach the anterior pituitary gland via the hypothalamic-pituitary vascular network, where they stimulate, respectively, the release of luteinizing hormone (LH) and adrenocorticotropic hormone (ACTH) into the blood (see Figure 56-1). LH and ACTH, via the blood, stimulate the testes and adrenal glands, respectively. The Leydig cells of the testes, under the influence of LH, produce 95% of the circulating testosterone (T), whereas the adrenal gland, under the influence of ACTH, produces androstenedione and dehydroepiandrosterone, which can be converted within prostatic tissues to more active androgens.[16] More than 95% of the circulating T is bound to T-estradiol binding globulin and plasma albumin.[17] Feedback loops serve to modify the secretion of the anterior pituitary gland and the hypothalamus. Thus, serum T exerts a negative feedback in both the hypothalamus and the pituitary gland on the release of LH-RH and LH, respectively. Serum cortisol feeds back on the hypothalamus and pituitary gland and inhibits further production of corticotropin-releasing factor and ACTH. Adrenal androgens appear to be quite weak and do not appear to exert any negative feedback on the hypothalamic-pituitary axis.[17]

The goal of androgen ablation therapy in prostate cancer is to deprive the androgen-dependent cancer cells of androgenic stimulation. This can be achieved by one or more combinations of four mechanisms:

1. Surgical removal of the testes (ie, bilateral orchiectomy) to eliminate testicular androgens and by hypophysectomy or adrenalectomy to eliminate adrenal androgens
2. Suppression of pituitary LH release, thereby inhibiting T production by the testes
3. Inhibition of androgenic synthesis in the testes and adrenal glands
4. Inhibition of androgen action at the level of androgen-dependent prostate cancer cells

At present, the "gold standard" for androgen ablation therapy is bilateral orchiectomy.[1] Surgical removal of the testes results in a 95% reduction of circulating T.[16] The advantages of this surgical approach include efficacy, assurance of patient compliance, cost-effectiveness, minimal morbidity from the procedure, and rapidity of symptomatic response. The disadvantages include the side effects of loss of libido, erectile impotence, hot flashes, occasional breast tenderness, and possible psychological trauma of "disfiguring" surgery. On the basis of these disadvantages, most men with metastatic prostate cancer in the United States choose alternative pharmacologic approaches that produce androgen ablation. Presently, there are a large variety of pharmacologic agents to achieve androgen ablation. These agents can be divided into two basic groups. The first group of agents produces androgen ablation indirectly by lowering the extracellular supply of androgen to the prostate cancer cells by means of lowering the level of androgen in the blood. These agents include LH-RH agonists, estrogenic compounds, progestational agents, and androgen synthesis inhibitors of various types. The second group of agents produces androgen ablation by inhibiting the intracellular response to androgen within androgen-dependent prostate cancer cells. Quantitatively, the major circulating androgen in the blood is T. Within prostate cancer cells, however, T is converted to a series of metabolites, the major one being 5α-dihydrotestosterone (DHT).[18,19] The enzyme responsible for the irreversible conversion of T to DHT is the membrane-bound nicotinamide adenine dinucleotide phosphate–dependent 5α-oxidoreductase (5α-reductase).[20] Once formed by the 5α-reductase enzymes, DHT binds to the intracellular AR.[21] This DHT–AR binding results in the trophic stimulation of proliferation and blockage of death of the hormone-dependent prostate cancer cells.[22] Thus, androgen ablation can be achieved at the prostate cancer cell level either by inhibiting the production of DHT via 5α-reductase inhibitors or by preventing the binding of DHT to its receptor owing to competitive inhibition by antiandrogen antagonists.

PHARMACOLOGIC APPROACHES TO LOWER CIRCULATING ANDROGEN

LH-RH Analogues LH-RH is a decapeptide (ie, ^{5}-oxo-L-prolyl^1-L-histidyl^2-L-tryptophyl^3-L-seryl^4-L-tyrosyl^5-glysyl^6-L-leucyl^7-L-arginyl^8-L-prolyl^9-L-glysyl^{10}) that stimulates the release of LH protein by the anterior pituitary gland. LH stimulates the testes to release T (see Figure 56-1). Substitutions at the sixth, ninth, or tenth position of the decapeptide LH-RH result in synthetic agonist analogues with prolonged half-life and potency. For example, the LH-RH agonist analogue leuprolide has a D-leucine at position 6 and an *N*-ethyl-L-prolinamide at position 9, whereas the agonist analogue buserelin has a D-(t-butyl) serine at position 6 and an *N*-ethyl-L-prolinamide at position 9. Initial administration of these agonist analogues results in stimulation on LH and follicle-stimulating hormone production, such that T levels rise 140 to 170% within several days.[23,24] This rise in serum T can result in patients with metastatic prostate cancer undergoing a "flare" response.[24,25] This flare response can result in increased bone pain, urinary obstruction, lymphedema, or spinal cord compression. The flare response can be blocked by administering an antiandrogen for 1 week before the start of LH-RH agonist treatment.[26,27]

With chronic LH-RH agonist administration (ie, after approximately 4 weeks of treatment), castratation levels of T are produced. This paradoxical T suppression by LH-RH agonist analogues results from (1) alterations in the central feedback control of LH release, (2) desensitization of the testes to LH owing to a decrease in LH receptor content; and (3) direct testicular steroid enzyme inhibition. LH-RH agonists are not active orally but can be administered as nasal sprays, subcutaneous injections daily, or deep intramuscular depot injections monthly. In the United States, the most commonly used LH-RH agonists are leuprolide acetate (Lupron) and goserelin acetate (Zoladex). These agents are available in depot forms that can be administered monthly or at longer intervals (leuprolide also is available in a 4-month depot) (Table 56-1). Leuprolide acetate is formulated in microspheres for intramuscular injection, and goserelin acetate is formulated as a cylindrical plug for subcutaneous injection. Recently, a 12-month leuprolide acetate implant (Viadur) has become available.[28,29] Surgically inserted subcutaneously, the 4 × 45 mm implant uses osmotic pressure to deliver leuprolide continuously at a controlled rate and can effectively achieve castration levels of T for 1 year.[28,29]

The advantage of the LH-RH agonists over surgical castration is that the androgen ablation is reversible if the agonist is discontinued. The side effects are tolerable, although they include hot flashes, muscle wasting, erectile impotence, and decreased libido.[30] The long-term side effects of LH-RH agonists include osteoporosis and anemia (see Table 56-1).[31] The major disadvantages of the agonists are that (1) chronic administration of LH-RH agonists is required to inhibit LH release and to reduce the serum androgens to castration levels; (2) such chronic agonist treatment can induce an initial flare response[32,33]; (3) chronic administration leads to osteoporosis and osteopenia[31]; (4) the treatment is very costly (ie, over US $5,000/year/patient compared with diethylstilbestrol's [DES] cost of $36/year).[32] Despite these disadvantages, owing to its low cardiovascular toxicity, time-release depot preparations of LH-RH agonists have become the most commonly used method to achieve castration-level T, even with the cost disadvantage.

In contrast to LH-RH agonists, LH-RH antagonists do not induce a flare response. A 1-month depot formulation of an LH-RH antagonist, Abarelix, has been most extensively tested in patients with prostate cancer. In two recent phase III studies comparing Abarelix depot with leuprolide and with leuprolide plus bicalutamide, Abarelix lowered serum T more quickly.[33] In addition, the majority of the patients treated with leuprolide or leuprolide plus bicalutamide had a T surge, whereas none of the patients treated with Abarelix did.[33] On this basis, Abarelix was recently approved by the US Food and Drug Administration for treatment of men with advanced prostate cancer who cannot take other types of hormone therapy. Further studies are needed, however, to delineate the clinical utility and long-term safety of these LH-RH antagonists as both initial therapy and therapy for patients with androgen-independent prostate cancer that may still express LH-RH receptors.

Table 56-1 Hormonal Agents Commonly Used in Treatment of Prostate Cancer

Agent	Dosage*	Toxicities
LH-RH agonists		
Leuprolide (Lupron)	7.5 mg/mo–22.5 mg/3 mo (IM)	For the class: hot flashes, decreased libido, impotence, gynecomastia, fatigue, edema, muscle waning, osteoporosis, anemia, disease flare
Goserelin (Zoladex)	3.6 mg/mo–10.8 mg/3 mo (SC)	
Antiandrogens		
Flutamide (Eulexin)	250 mg tid	For the class: decreased libido, gynecomastia, hot flashes, hepatotoxicity, diarrhea
Bicalutamide (Casodex)	50 mg daily	
Nilutamide (Nilandron)	150 mg daily	Nilandron-impaired night vision
Adrenal enzyme inhibitors		
Aminoglutethimide (Cytadren)	250 mg qid + HC 20–30 mg qd	Lethargy, dizziness, nausea, rash, weight gain, hypoaldosteronism, hypothyroidism, nausea, vomiting; requires acidic pH
Ketoconazole (Nizoral)	400 mg tid + HC 20–30 mg qd	
Miscellaneous agents		
Diethylstilbesterol	1 mg daily	DVT, stroke, cardiac ischemia (more common at higher doses), gynecomastia, fluid retention, weight gain, DVT, impotence, gynecomastia, loss of libido, decreased HDL, side effects associated with hypercortisolism
Megesterol acetate (Megace)	40 mg qid	
Cyproterone acetate	Dose varies 50–100 mg tid	
Prednisone	7.5–10 mg daily	

DVT = deep venous thrombosis; HC = hydrocortisone; HDL = high-density lipoprotein; IM = intramuscular; LH-RH = luteinizing hormone–releasing hormone; qd = daily; qid = four times daily; SC = subcutaneous; tid = three times daily.

*Dosage from Swain SM, Lippman ME. Endocrine therapies of cancer. In: Chabner BA, Collins JM, editors. Cancer chemotherapy: principles and practice. Philadelphia (PA): Lippincott; 1990. p. 59–109.

ANTIANDROGENS Antiandrogens compete with androgens for binding sites on the AR. Two classes of antiandrogens are used clinically: the "pure" and the "nonpure" type.[34] A pure antiandrogen functions as an androgen antagonist by competitively inhibiting the binding of DHT or T with the ARs within target cells, without decreasing serum T systemically (see Figure 56-1). The pure antiandrogens used most commonly in the United States are the nonsteroidal antiandrogens flutamide (Eulexin) and bicalutamide (Casodex) (see Table 56-1). Nilutamide (Nilandron) is a newer nonsteroidal antiandrogen that is also approved for use (see Table 56-1).[34] Flutamide was initially approved because it blocked the flare from LH-RH agonists, and bicalutamide was approved on the basis of a comparative trial showing antitumor equivalence and an improved safety profile relative to flutamide.[35] Flutamide must be administered in multiple daily doses because of its short half-life, whereas bicalutamide has a longer half-life that permits once-a-day dosing. Toxicities of this class include diarrhea, elevations in serum transaminases, and gynecomastia (see Table 56-1). The advantage of these agents is that they do not have the same degree of hot flashes, loss of libido, and muscle wasting. Most importantly for the patient, they can potentially preserve potency when used alone.

Since the pure antiandrogens bind not only to ARs in prostate cancer cells but also to the ARs in the hypothalamus and pituitary gland, these compounds block the negative feedback of androgens at the hypothalamic-pituitary level (see Figure 56-1).[34] Thus, treatment with pure antiandrogens eventually increases the level of LH released into circulation.[36] This eventually leads to an increase in the serum T level, which results in increased tissue levels of T and DHT, which diminishes the ability of the pure antiandrogen antagonist to compete for AR binding. In general, serum T concentrations increase by a mean of 50 to 100%, with peak concentrations occurring after 1 to 9 months.[37] T concentrations, although elevated, remain within the normal range, possibly because the increased concentration of estradiol limits increases in LH secretion.[38] Therefore, pure antiandrogens have rarely been used as monotherapy. They are usually combined either with surgical castration or with LH-RH analogues.[39–42] Recently, however, a number of large randomized studies have reported similar efficacy of high-dose antiandrogens as monotherapy compared with castration, and these studies are reviewed below.

The nonpure agents are classified as steroidal antiandrogens and include cyproterone acetate and megesterol acetate (Megace).[34] These nonpure agents have progestational and glucocorticoid activity in addition to their effects as antiandrogens.[34] Cyproterone acetate is a potent progestational agent and, therefore, through feedback mechanisms, inhibits the release of LH-RH and LH from the pituitary gland (see Figure 56-1).[42] Cyproterone acetate still retains its androgen antagonist ability to directly compete with DHT for binding to the AR (see Figure 56-1).[43] Thus, cyproterone acetate functions to both decrease serum T systemically and act as an AR inhibitor within androgen-dependent prostate cancer cells.

Estrogens When the blood level of estrogen rises to a pharmacologically sufficient concentration, inhibition of the release of LH from the pituitary gland results, thus decreasing T synthesis and release from the testes (see Figure 56-1). Therefore, chronic maintenance of pharmacologic blood levels of estrogen can depress serum T to the same minimal level as that observed following surgical orchiectomy.[44] When given orally, naturally occurring estrogens (ie, 17β-estradiol and estrone) are rapidly metabolized by the liver and are not able to sufficiently elevate the blood estrogen levels to depress serum T. DES is a synthetic compound that has potent estrogenic abilities and is capable of reaching sufficient blood levels following oral delivery to suppress LH release.

Androgen Synthesis Inhibiting Agents Ketoconazole, commonly used as a broad-spectrum antifungal agent, inhibits the conversion of lanenterol to ergosterol in fungi and to cholesterol in man via its ability to inhibit the testicular and adrenal cytochrome P-450 enzymes (see Figure 56-1). It produces very rapid and sustained decreases in testicular and adrenal androgen production. At the usual dose of 400 mg every 8 hours, ketoconazole reduces serum T to castratation levels in less than 24 hours in 75% of men.[45–48] High-dose ketoconazole (ie, 400 mg three times daily orally), although effective in lowering serum T, is not commonly used as first-line androgen ablation therapy. This is because of the necessity of a strict every-8-hour regimen to compensate for the short duration of its action, coupled with poor compliance owing to gastric intolerance. Aminoglutethimide can also be used as second-line therapy to block adrenal androgen production, once progression after testicular androgen ablation has occurred, but is not often used owing to significant side effects, which include hypotension, nausea and vomiting, fatigue, anorexia, depression, edema, and skin rashes (see Table 56-1).

5α-Reductase Inhibitors DHT is believed to be the active intracellular androgen in stimulating growth and inhibiting cell death of androgen-dependent normal prostatic cells and presumably prostate cancer cells.[49] Inhibiting DHT production without decreasing systemic T levels could be advantageous. T itself, without conversion to DHT, is capable of maintaining the anabolic effects of androgen on muscle mass, male libido, and sperm maturation.[50] Theoretically, 5α-reductase inhibitors could inhibit the DHT-induced stimulation of androgen-dependent prostate cancer growth without negating the effects of T on muscle mass, libido, or erectile potency. Owing to these quality of life issues, there is a great deal of clinical interest in developing effective and specific 5α-reductase inhibitors. In experimental and human studies, the substrate inhibitor finasteride has been demonstrated to inhibit the 5α-reductase activity and to decrease the serum and tissue DHT content.[51,52] In vivo treatment with finasteride eventually leads not only to a decrease in tissue DHT but also an increase in tissue T concentration.[52] Presently, clinical trials are under way to test the efficiency of finasteride as single-agent therapy for metastatic prostate cancer.

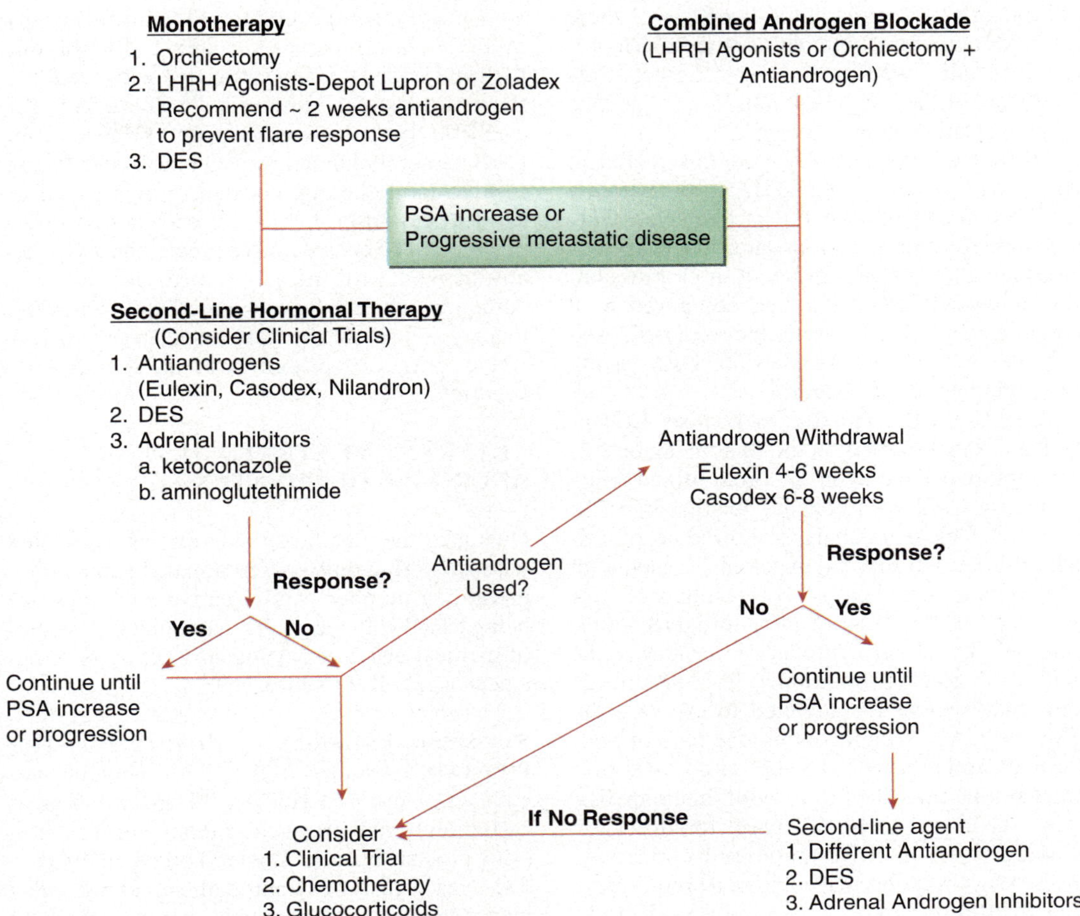

Figure 56-2 Algorithm for use of hormonal therapies in treatment of recurrent or metastatic prostate cancer. (See text for a discussion of monotherapy versus combined androgen blockade and optimal timing of therapy initiation.)

ANDROGEN DEPRIVATION STRATEGIES FOR THE TREATMENT OF RECURRENT AND METASTATIC PROSTATE CANCER

LH-RH Agonists as Monotherapy Since the development of depot LH-RH agonists, oral estrogens are rarely used as primary hormonal therapy owing to the increased number of side effects. The LH-RH agonists leuprolide and goserelin are available in the United States. Both agents have been investigated in phase II and randomized phase III trials. These agents were found to be equivalent to DES and orchiectomy. Another LH-RH agonist used outside the United States, buserelin, is also comparable with orchiectomy in response and survival. Overall, the monotherapy studies with LH-RH agonists, DES, or orchiectomy have been associated with objective and subjective improvement in 60 to 85% of patients, a median progression-free survival of 12 to 18 months, and a median survival of 24 to 30 months. Although chronic use of these agents is considerably more expensive than orchiectomy, most patients now prefer the depot LH-RH agonists because of the psychological implications of loss of the testicles.[53] In addition, the recent increased popularity of intermittent hormonal therapy, even though yet unproven, has made orchiectomy an even less likely choice for most patients (Figure 56-2). Long-term use of LH-RH agonists is associated with loss of bone density, and this can be prevented by addition of bisphosphonates.[54,55]

Combined Androgen Blockade Labrie and colleagues originally suggested that following androgen ablation, prostate cancer cells could adapt to decreased concentrations of androgens.[56,57] They proposed that the levels of androgens of adrenal origin were sufficient to maintain the hormone-dependent growth of these adapted prostate cancer cells. To inhibit the effect of these adrenal gland–derived androgens, these investigators combined surgical or medical castration with a nonsteroidal antiandrogen. In a preliminary pilot study, this CAB approach produced remarkable improvements in outcome compared with historical controls.[56] On the basis of these initial results, a large number of randomized prospective studies were performed to further study the effects of the combined approach in patients with metastatic prostate cancer.[58]

Overall, 27 prospectively randomized clinical trials involving approximately 8,000 patients have been conducted over the past 15 years. Only three of these studies demonstrated that CAB produced a significant improvement in progression-free or overall survival when compared with monotherapy. The majority of the studies showed no benefit to CAB, with some studies suggesting that monotherapy was better.[58]

In 1995, the Prostate Cancer Trialists' Collaborative Group reported on the first meta-analysis that included data from 22 randomized trials comparing CAB with gonadal ablation in 5,710 patients.[59] This meta-analysis showed no significant difference in survival in patients treated with CAB versus monotherapy. The results were not influenced by the type of antiandrogens (flutamide, nilutamide, or cyproterone acetate) or the method of gonadal ablation.[59] Two additional meta-analyses were conducted to evaluate the effects of CAB trials involving one type of nonsteroidal antiandrogen. Caubet and colleagues selected nine published trials with flutamide that were considered to be adequate for overview analysis,[60] whereas Bertagna and colleagues selected seven studies that compared orchiectomy plus nilutamide with orchiectomy alone.[61] Although both reports suggest a significant survival advantage with CAB, there are major concerns about these analyses because they included only selected studies.[58] The criteria for study selection, limited patient number, and short-term follow-up are among the potential limitations of these two meta-analyses that serve to reduce the significance of these reports.[58]

Finally, the Agency for Health Care Policy and Research (AHCPR) published on the Internet (<http://www.ahcpr.gov/clinic/index.html evidence>; AHCPR report No.99-E012) the results of a comprehensive meta-analysis based on all published CAB studies. This meta-analysis found no difference in 2-year survival. Only 10 of the 27 trials reported 5-year survival figures, and preliminary results suggest a minimal difference in favor of CAB.[58]

Despite the fact that the three reported positive studies represented only a small fraction of the trials, these positive findings were sufficient to cause a major shift over the last decade toward the use of CAB as the preferred treatment of metastatic prostate cancer by some practitioners. However, on the basis of the findings in 24 of 27 randomized trials and 2 large meta-analyses, it can be concluded that CAB is not associated with a clinically meaningful improvement in survival over surgical or medical castration alone in patients with metastatic prostate cancer.[58] In addition, in INT-0015, quality of life was prospectively evaluated, and this study demonstrated that although improvement in quality of life over baseline was seen in both arms, the improvement was more pronounced in the monotherapy group.[62] This difference in quality of life was due to the increased toxicity associated with the use of the antiandrogen flutamide.[62] Therefore, the available data suggest minimal to no benefit for CAB versus monotherapy.[58] On the basis of these results, monotherapy consisting of medical or surgical castration to achieve castratation levels of T should be considered adequate first-line therapy in men with metastatic prostate cancer.[58] Antiandrogens can be used initially as short-term therapy to prevent the flare associated with LH-RH agonists or added later as second-line agents.[58]

ALTERNATIVE STRATEGIES FOR ANDROGEN DEPRIVATION

Owing to the significant side effects associated with LH-RH agonist–based gonadal suppression therapy, a number of alternative strategies are being tested with the goal of lessening the toxicity of medical castration while still depriving prostate cancer cells of androgen.[63]

Revisiting Estrogen as Monotherapy for Prostate Cancer In the 1940s, Huggins and colleagues first reported on the use of surgical castration or oral estrogen as treatment for metastatic prostate cancer.[1] Bilateral orchiectomy produces rapid onset of symptomatic relief with minimal side effects and, therefore, has been the gold standard in prostate cancer therapy. As an alternative to surgery, DES was demonstrated to be as effective as orchiectomy in lowering T to castratation levels.[1] In 1967, the Veterans Administration Cooperative Urological Research Group (VACURG) reported on the use of DES with or without orchiectomy in the treatment of prostate cancer.[64] Byar and Corle reported on the long-term results of estrogen therapy for prostate cancer on the basis of the studies of the VACURG.[65] They concluded that (1) estrogen therapy provides significant palliation in most patients with advanced prostate cancer; (2) orchiectomy plus DES is no better than orchiectomy or DES alone; (3) 1 mg/d of DES was equivalent in its effect on prostate cancer survival as DES 5 mg/d; however, DES 1 mg/d is not sufficient to depress serum T to castratation levels; and (4) DES 1 mg/d was associated with a decreased cardiovascular risk compared with DES 5 mg/d but still produced significant risk, especially for elderly men with increased nonestrogen risk factors. The VACURG results were later confirmed by the European Organisation for Research and Treatment of Cancer (EORTC) trial 30805 demonstrating that DES 1 mg therapy was equivalent to orchiectomy.[66]

Unfortunately, the side effects of pharmacologic amounts of estrogen are numerous: nausea, vomiting, headaches, fluid retention, gynecomastia, impotence, pedal edema, thrombophlebitis, myocardial infarction, and stroke.[67–69] Because of the significantly increased risk of cardiovascular complications associated with oral estrogens, many physicians no longer prescribe them to their patients with prostate cancer. The toxicity of oral estrogens appears to be due to "first-pass" effects through the liver when absorption is via the portal route. These toxic effects can be ameliorated if estrogens are given parenterally, not orally. This has been clearly established by a large Finnish study of 477 men with prostate cancer, which demonstrated that increased cardiovascular risks can be eliminated with parenteral depot estrogens.[70] This study demonstrated that when 160 mg/mo of polyestradiol phosphate (PEP) (eg, Estradurin) is given as a slow-release intramuscular depot, the treatment is effective for prostate cancer control and patients had significantly fewer cardiovascular deaths than those treated with orchiectomy or combination intramuscular and oral estrogen therapy. In addition, in this study, parenteral PEP had a protective effect on cardiovascular deaths. This may be due to the fact that when given as a once-monthly intramuscular injection, parenteral PEP caused an increase in serum triglycerides and low-density lipoprotein triglycerides.[70–72] In a large randomized study of 915 men, the Scandinavian Prostatic Cancer Group compared the effect on overall survival of CAB (ie, orchiectomy or LH-RH agonist and flutamide) with that of parenteral estrogen (PEP).[73] At a median follow-up of 18.5 months, ~58% of men in both groups had died and no signs of a difference in overall survival were observed between the two groups. No differences in cardiovascular mortality were observed in the two groups. The incidence of hot flashes was 30.1% in the PEP-treated group and 74.3% in the CAB-treated group, and the frequency and distress owing to hot flashes were also significantly lower than in the CAB group.[74] In addition, the use of estrogen and selective estrogen receptor modulators does not lead to development of osteoporosis that is associated with long-term use of LH-RH agonist.[75,76] Thus, the use of a parenteral depot of estrogens given monthly as an intramuscular injection is an inexpensive and effective pharmacologic approach to androgen ablation that should be reconsidered as an effective alternative to LH-RH agonists.

Nonsteroidal Antiandrogens as Monotherapy Because of the potential for preserving potency, antiandrogens have been tested as monotherapy. Several randomized studies have compared antiandrogens with gonadal suppression. In one small study, flutamide was compared with DES and was found to have an equivalent response rate but an inferior survival (28 vs 43 months).[77] A second study compared bicalutamide (50 mg daily) with surgical castration and found prostate-specific antigen (PSA) normalization in 17% of the bicalutamide group and 47% of the castrated group. Even though survival was not significantly different between the two groups, the authors of this study concluded that standard-dose bicalutamide was not as effective as castration for treatment of patients with metastatic disease.[78]

Other studies have evaluated a higher dose of bicalutamide (150 mg) as monotherapy.[79] High-dose bicalutamide has been compared with gonadal suppression in two large, open-label, randomized studies. Combined data from these studies demonstrated that bicalutamide was inferior to castration in patients with metastatic disease with respect to time to progression and overall survival, although the median survival between the two groups was only 6 weeks.[80,81] For patients with rising PSA levels only, the two treatments were equivalent with respect to time to progression and overall survival.[80,81] Bicalutamide monotherapy was well tolerated, and patients had increased sexual interest and physical capacity when compared with the castrated group. In a small subgroup of one of these studies (n = 29), there was no decrease in bone mineral density compared with age-matched controls, whereas clinically significant reductions in bone mineral density were seen in castrated patients.[82] This result needs to be confirmed in larger randomized studies. The incidence of gynecomastia in the bicalutamide treated group was approximately 50%.[79] These data suggest that high-dose antiandrogen blockade may be a viable alternative in patients with nonmetastatic disease.

High-dose bicalutamide has also been evaluated as adjuvant therapy by the Early Prostate Cancer Program, which consisted of three randomized, double-blind, placebo-controlled trials prospectively designed for combined analysis.[83,84] In these combined trials, 8,113 men with T1b–T4, M0, any N (N0 in one trial) prostate cancer were randomized to bicalutamide 150 mg/d (n = 4,052) or placebo (n = 4,061) in addition to standard care (radical prostatectomy, radiotherapy, or watchful waiting). At a median 5.4 years of follow-up (21.6% progression events), bicalutamide significantly improved progression-free survival in the overall population, with positive results in two of the three trials.[84] Patients with locally advanced disease gained the most benefit from bicalutamide in terms of progression-free survival, irrespective of underlying therapy. Overall survival in these trials was similar in the bicalutamide and placebo groups across the program and in each trial. Among watchful waiting patients, survival appeared to be improved with bicalutamide in those with locally advanced disease, whereas survival appeared to be reduced with bicalutamide in those with localized disease. The most common adverse events with bicalutamide were gynecomastia and breast pain. The authors of these studies concluded from their analysis that bicalutamide may provide benefit in patients with locally advanced disease.[84] However, the current data from these trials suggest that early or adjuvant hormonal therapy for patients at low risk of disease progression, such as those with localized disease, is not appropriate.[84]

INTERMITTENT ANDROGEN SUPPRESSION

IAS is being used with increasing frequency in an attempt to minimize the adverse effects associated with long-term androgen deprivation.[85] The rationale for this approach was initially based on the results of experiments in animal tumor models, which suggested that IAS could delay, but not prevent, progression to androgen independence.[86,87] These studies also demonstrated that in both animal models and men with prostate cancer, apoptosis could be induced multiple times with successive cycles of androgen withdrawal and replacement.

To date, 15 studies using IAS have been reported in the literature.[85] These studies had small patient populations distributed in different stages (ie, local, locoregional, and metastatic).[85] In many of these studies, androgen ablation is achieved using CAB with an LH-RH agonist and an antiandrogen.[88–90] Although the treatment design has varied somewhat, in general, the approach has been to start patients on androgen deprivation and continue until the PSA level reaches a nadir or becomes undetectable. At this point, the androgen withdrawal is stopped, and patients are followed up with serial PSA measurements. When the PSA reaches a prescribed level (eg, 10 ng/mL) or returns to the patient's baseline level, the androgen suppression is re-initiated. In most patients treated in this manner, serum T returned to the normal range within 5 to 20 weeks of discontinuing treatment.[91] The off-treatment periods in these studies have been associated with an improvement in the patient's sense of well-being and the recovery of libido and potency in those who reported normal sexual function before the start of therapy.[85] These preliminary studies, in aggregate, have demonstrated that repeated cycles of androgen suppression could induce repeated PSA responses. Daliani and colleagues observed significant interpatient variability in the duration of the PSA response after each cycle of IAS in a small number of patients and concluded that owing to this interpatient variability, randomized studies will be needed to adequately explore the efficacy of individualized IAS.[92]

These preliminary studies have led to several ongoing, large, multi-institutional, randomized studies comparing IAS with continuous androgen suppression. A National Cancer Institute–sponsored study led by the Southwest Oncology Group (SWOG 9346) randomized approximately 1,500 men with stage IV prostate cancer to either intermittent or continuous androgen deprivation with goserelin and bicalutamide. A second study sponsored by the National Cancer Institute of Canada randomized approximately 1,300 men with PSA progression following radiotherapy to either intermittent or continuous androgen deprivation with an LH-RH agonist (buserelin, goserelin, or leuprolide) and an antiandrogen (flutamide, bicalutamide, or nilutamide). Because of the potential improvement in quality of life, patient enthusiasm for IAS is understandable. These large randomized trials will provide the data needed to determine the role of IAS in the treatment of prostate cancer. Until this information is available, however, patients must be informed that the long-term safety and efficacy of this approach are unknown and should be considered experimental.[81]

Second-Line Hormonal Therapy Eventually, all patients responding to initial androgen deprivation therapy will develop progressive disease, as manifested by rising PSA levels, the appearance of new lesions on imaging studies, or worsening symptoms. The treatment of hormone-refractory prostate cancer remains a challenge for the clinician owing to the lack of a clearly defined standard therapy. One important approach involves secondary hormonal manipulation following failure of primary androgen deprivation (see Figure 56-2).[93,94]

Prostate cancer cells can be classified on the basis of responsiveness to androgen deprivation. Androgen-dependent cells are those that respond to androgen withdrawal by cessation of proliferation and activation of apoptosis. Within hormone-refractory metastatic sites, there is a heterogeneous collection of cells with relative degrees of androgen independence. One subset of cells is those that are androgen sensitive in that they have an increased proliferative rate in the presence of androgen. These cells are able to continue to proliferate, albeit more slowly, in the absence of androgen. These androgen-sensitive cells are also less likely to undergo apoptosis on androgen withdrawal. True androgen-independent cells do not alter their proliferative rates in the presence or absence of androgen.

Several studies have demonstrated that androgen-independent tumors can derive a further growth advantage on exposure to androgens.[95,96] This continued sensitivity is due to the continued presence of the subset of androgen-sensitive prostate cancer cells in hormone-refractory patients. Therefore, continued androgen suppression should be considered the standard of care for hormone-refractory patients.[97]

AR is a key mediator of androgen function within normal and malignant prostate cells. AR is nearly universally expressed in primary and metastatic sites in untreated and androgen ablation recurrent patients, suggesting that AR is required for the progression of prostate cancer to the androgen-unresponsive metastatic stage.[98–100] Molecular analysis demonstrated that amplification of the Xq11-q13 region in which the AR gene is located is common in prostate cancer recurring during androgen ablation therapy.[100,101] AR amplification has been detected in ~30% of recurrent prostate cancers but none in the specimens taken from the same patients prior to therapy.[100,101] Combining these results suggests that in approximately one-third of patients, failure of androgen ablation therapy may be caused by clonal outgrowth of prostate cancer cells with increased AR expression.

In addition to amplification, mutations in the gene can cause AR dysfunction, including alterations of AR specificity, binding affinity, and expression.[102–104] AR mutations occur in low frequency in primary prostate cancer.[105] In contrast, cells in the distant metastases and androgen ablation recurrent prostate cancer often contain AR mutations.[103–105] Functional studies indicate that, in many cases, these mutated receptors are not inhibited but rather can be stimulated by some antiandrogens.[103–105] These studies demonstrating AR amplification or mutation in patients failing primary androgen deprivation therapy may, in part, explain the clinical benefit observed in a subset of patients treated with some form of second-line hormonal therapy. Second-line hormone therapy can be divided into several categories (see Figure 56-2)[94]:

1. Antiandrogen withdrawal
2. Addition of an antiandrogen in patients failing gonadal suppression
3. Inhibition of adrenal steroidogenesis
4. Use of glucocorticoids or other alternative steroids

Antiandrogen Withdrawal The majority of patients with advanced prostate cancer are treated initially with an antiandrogen in combination with gonadal suppression or are given an antiandrogen after progression while gonadally suppressed. This approach was initially proposed by Labrie and colleagues and was based on the hypothesis that adrenal androgens may provide additional stimulation to hypersensitive prostate cancer cells.[56,57] Recent data also suggest that amplification of the AR can occur in a subset of prostate cancer cells following androgen deprivation.[100,101] This subset, therefore, may respond to additional androgen blockade. The use of antiandrogens in patients as second-line therapy is associated with a significant response rate and is discussed in the following section.[93,94]

Kelley and Scher, in 1993, were the first to observe that withdrawal of the antiandrogen flutamide from patients with hormone-refractory prostate cancer could result in symptomatic and objective improvement.[106] These investigators termed this phenomenon "antiandrogen withdrawal syndrome." Although initially observed in patients on flutamide,[106–108] PSA declines and symptomatic benefits have also been described after withdrawal of both bicalutamide[109,110] and nilutamide.[111,112] Discontinuation responses have also been seen after removal of the steroidal antiandrogens megesterol acetate[113] and DES.[114] In the studies reported to date, withdrawal responses have been observed in 15 to 30% of patients.[106–116] No particular clinical variable predicts the likelihood of a withdrawal response.[115,117] With flutamide, the length of treatment seems to be associated with the likelihood of a response, although this finding has not been seen in every study.[115,117] Patients treated with an antiandrogen for as short a period as 2 months can have a withdrawal response.[117]

Most patients responding to flutamide withdrawal will experience a decrease in PSA within 4 weeks.[115,117] Responses may occur later (ie, 6–8 weeks) with bicalutamide and nilutamide owing to their longer half-life.[116] The median duration of response to antiandrogen withdrawal is approximately 4 months, although prolonged responses have been observed.[115–117]

The recognition of the antiandrogen withdrawal response has significantly altered the treatment of hormone-refractory patients. A trial of antiandrogen withdrawal has become standard practice in patients on combined androgen therapy because it is nontoxic and can benefit a significant number of patients (see Figure 56-2). In addition, all clinical trials assessing the response to new agents now require an adequate period of antiandrogen withdrawal prior to enrollment to avoid confusion in evaluating response rates.

Use of Antiandrogens Most patients in the United States with advanced prostate cancer receive either medical or surgical castration, with or without an antiandrogen as primary hormonal therapy. On the basis of recent results demonstrating that CAB is not superior to monotherapy, patients increasingly are treated with an LH-RH agonist until the PSA levels begin to rise, and then they are given an antiandrogen as initial second-line hormonal therapy. Data from only a few studies are available, but existing evidence suggests that patients treated initially with gonadal suppression can benefit from the later addition of an antiandrogen, with response rates ranging from 15 to 50%.[118–121]

In patients demonstrating progression after primary therapy with combined androgen suppression, the recommended first maneuver is to withdraw the antiandrogen and assess for a response. Two clinical studies have investigated the effect of adding a bicalutamide following flutamide withdrawal. Scher and colleagues reported on 10 of 26 patients (38%) who had previous flutamide therapy and had a greater than 50% decrease in PSA after high-dose bicalutamide.[120] Responses were observed in patients with and without a previous withdrawal response to flutamide. Similarly, Joyce and colleagues reported a 23% response rate to bicalutamide (150 mg/d), with the majority of responders having received prior flutamide.[121] It appears, therefore, that bicalutamide may induce further responses in patients previously treated with flutamide.

Adrenal Androgen Inhibitors The adrenal gland is the source of 5 to 10% of peripheral T.[19] Labrie and colleagues proposed that, following androgen ablation, a subset of prostate cancer cells can become hypersensitive to androgens.[56,57] Therefore, the low level of androgens produced by the adrenal glands may be sufficient to provide continued stimulation. The most commonly used agent to inhibit adrenal androgen production is ketoconazole. Because it can inhibit mineralocorticoid production, hydrocortisone is often given in combination with ketoconazole. Small and colleagues reported that 62.5% of men treated with high-dose ketoconazole (1,200 mg daily) and hydrocortisone after flutamide withdrawal had a > 50% decrease in PSA.[122] In both of these studies, the median duration of response has been 3 to 4 months.[123,124] These studies and others have defined a role for ketoconazole as a potentially effective second-line hormonal agent; however, like the antiandrogens, response durations have been short.[94]

Other Second-Line Agents Several other agents have been tested and may be useful as secondary therapy in hormone-refractory patients. Glucocorticoids have been used for some time as a palliative treatment in end-stage prostate cancer. Recently, Tannock and colleagues treated patients with 7.5 to 10 mg prednisone and observed that nearly 40% patients reported an improved quality of life at 1 month and that 20% maintained this improvement for 4 months.[125] In a larger randomized study comparing mitoxantrone and prednisone with prednisone alone, 21% of patients randomized to prednisone alone had improved quality of life and 22% had a greater than 50% decrease in PSA levels.[126] Smith and colleagues treated 21 hormone-refractory patients with low-dose DES (1 mg/d) and reported a 43% PSA response rate.[127] They concluded that oral DES should be considered an active second-line agent. Megace has also been tested as a second-line agent, but response rates in several studies have been lower than comparable studies using other second-line agents.[94] Interestingly, withdrawal of Megace may result in a decline in PSA level, even in those receiving low-dose (20–40 mg daily) therapy for hot flashes.[123]

TIMING OF ANDROGEN DEPRIVATION THERAPY

Immediate versus Delayed Androgen Ablation The question of when to initiate androgen deprivation therapy has been debated almost since the introduction of this therapy by Huggins and colleagues. Until the results of the VACURG study were published in 1967, early endocrine therapy was the treatment of choice for patients who were not amenable to surgical cure.[85] The VACURG study randomized patients into four treatment groups: (1) placebo, (2) bilateral orchiectomy, (3) DES 5 mg/d, and (4) orchiectomy plus DES.[67] In this study, the placebo group was given hormonal therapy at the time of progression. Therefore, this study evolved into a comparison of early versus delayed therapy. On initial analysis of the data, the investigators concluded that delaying hormonal therapy does not appear to compromise survival.[67] A second VACURG study randomized patients to placebo versus increasing amounts of DES and also demonstrated no difference between early versus delayed therapy.[65] These data continue to serve as the rationale for delaying hormonal therapy until there are signs of skeletal metastases.

From a later reanalysis of the VACURG survival data, Byar and Corle concluded that younger patients with high-grade tumors (Gleason score 7–10) and stage D disease appeared to derive a survival benefit from the initiation of hormonal therapy at the time of diagnosis.[65] Little benefit was seen in older patients and for patients with low-grade and lower-stage disease.

In 1997, the Medical Research Council (MRC) of the United Kingdom published the results of a randomized study comparing early versus delayed androgen deprivation in patients who were not surgical candidates or who had failed radiation therapy.[128] This study included 938 patients with M0, Mx, or M1 prostate cancer.[128] This study demonstrated a decreased rate of local progression, pathologic fracture, cord compression, and ureteral obstruction.[128] Most importantly, cancer-specific survival was superior (p = .02) in the immediate-therapy arm for all patients and an even more pronounced benefit was seen in the patients with M0 disease (54% vs 70%).[129] A more recent abstract with longer-term data from the MRC trial reported that although immediate therapy continued to improve overall disease-specific survival, overall survival differences were becoming much smaller.[129] This study has been criticized owing to a lack of uniform staging data. In addition, this study relied on bone scan and symptom assessment to define progression. It is, therefore, difficult to extrapolate these results obtained in patients with more advanced disease to patients in the United States who are seen more frequently and may have PSA levels obtained as often as every 3 months.

In a nonrandomized study of patients with stage D1 prostate cancer who had undergone bilateral pelvic lymphadenectomy and radical prostatectomy, Zincke demonstrated a disease progression rate of only 10% in patients who had immediate orchiectomy versus 50% for those who received delayed orchiectomy.[130] The rates of nonprogression at 5 and 10 years for patients who had immediate orchiectomy were 84% and 80%, respectively, compared with 48% and 38%, respectively, for patients who had delayed therapy.

Messing and colleagues reported on the results of a phase III randomized study comparing early versus delayed hormonal therapy in men who had undergone a radical prostatectomy and pelvic lymphadenectomy and were found to be node positive (Table 56-2).[131] Ninety-eight men were randomized with a mean follow-up of 7.2 years.[131] This study demonstrated that early initiation of androgen deprivation significantly delays progression and prolongs survival compared with observation and delayed hormonal therapy (summarized in Table 56-2).[131] Although this result was significant, this study was performed on a small number of patients and was criticized for the high mortality rate in the untreated controls over the study period and for a lack of central review of pathology specimens.[132]

Although this study provides compelling evidence in favor of early androgen deprivation in node-positive patients, little information is available on the optimal timing of hormonal therapy in the rapidly increasing subset of patients who are PSA-only failures. Currently, an increasing number of patients are treated early with hormone therapy on the basis of a rising PSA, without evidence of radiographic metastases. Many of these patients often develop a rising PSA while on hormone therapy and still have negative radiographic evidence for metastases.[85] No data yet exist to help decide whether patients with PSA-only recurrence will derive any benefit from immediate hormonal therapy. Because of the hot flashes, muscle wasting, and impotence associated with androgen deprivation, many patients understandably wish to delay therapy.

Walsh and colleagues characterized, in a retrospective analysis, the time course of disease progression in 1,997 men with biochemical recurrence after radical prostatectomy.[133] Of the 1,997 men, 315 (15%) developed biochemical PSA elevation, and 34% of these developed metastatic disease within the study period.[133] The median actuarial time to metastases was 8 years from the time of PSA level elevation, and, once the patients developed metastatic disease, the median time to death was 5 years.[133] The prognostic factors associated with a high probability of remaining metastases free were a Gleason score of 5 to 7, PSA recurrence more than 2 years after prostatectomy, and a PSA doubling time of > 10 months (Table 56-3). In patients with all three good prognostic factors, the probability of remaining metastases free at 7 years was 82% (see Table 56-3). In contrast, for patients with poor prognostic factors (ie, Gleason score 8–10 and PSA recurrence < 2 years), the probability at 7 years was only 21% (see Table 56-3). These authors provided an algorithm to help physicians counsel their patients on the risks of recurrence based on these three factors.[133] These data suggest that for patients with good prognostic factors, early hormonal therapy would unlikely be of benefit. In contrast, patients with a poor prognosis would more likely benefit from early initiation of hormonal therapy.

These conclusions were further supported by recent reports from D'Amico and colleagues.[134] This group evaluated outcomes in 8,669 patients with prostate cancer treated with surgery (5,918) or radiation (2,751) and demonstrated that a short post-treatment PSA doubling time of less than 3 months following radical prostatectomy or radiation therapy was significantly associated with time to prostate cancer–specific mortality.[132] On this basis, this group concluded that patients with a PSA doubling time of less than 3 months should be considered for early initiation of androgen suppression therapy (or clinical trial) to delay the imminent sequelae of metastatic bone disease.[134]

These data will be useful in the design of future studies comparing early versus delayed hormonal therapy. Additional data are also needed to determine the course of action in the new class of patients with "PSA-only hormone-refractory prostate cancer."[104] These questions need to be addressed in well-designed randomized studies, some of which are currently ongoing. Until such data are available, the optimal timing for initiation of hormone therapy in PSA-only recurrences is unknown.

CONCLUSION

As reviewed, there are now a number of alternative pharmacologic approaches that can be used to produce androgen ablation. Recent shifts in treatment philosophy have caused a move from maximum therapy with CAB toward strategies, such as IAS, that try to minimize toxicities while still providing adequate treatment. Large randomized studies should answer several important treatment questions regarding the optimal timing of therapy, the role of IAS, and the use of potential potency-preserving therapies, such as high-dose antiandrogens as first-line treatment. The discovery of the antiandrogen withdrawal response has also stimulated renewed interest in the use of second-line hormonal approaches and forced us to rethink the term "hormone-refractory prostate cancer."

Although these new androgen deprivation approaches offer expanded treatment options for

Table 56-2 Results of a Phase III Study Comparing Immediate versus Delayed Hormonal Therapy*

	n	Total Deaths	PC Deaths	Overall	Progression Objective	PSA Only
Immediate	46	6 (13.0)	2 (4.3)	9 (19.6)	4 (8.7)	5 (10.9)
Delayed	52	18 (34.6)	16 (30.8)	39 (75.0)	29 (55.8)	10 (19.2)

PC = prostate cancer; PSA = prostate-specific antigen.
*In patients with node-positive disease following radical prostatectomy.[152]

Table 56-3 Probability of Being Free of Metastatic Prostate Cancer on the Basis of Gleason Score, Time to PSA Recurrence, and PSA Doubling Time

	% Probability Metastatic Disease Free					
	Gleason 5–7 PSA Recurrence				Gleason 8–10	
	> 2 Years			< 2 Years	> 2 Years	< 2 Years
Metastatic Disease-Free Period, yr	PSA Doubling Time, mo > 10 (*n* = 106)	< 10 (*n* = 18)	> 10 (*n* = 55)	< 10 (*n* = 28)	(*n* = 44)	(*n* = 53)
3	95	82	79	81	77	53
5	86	69	76	35	60	31
7	82	60	59	15	47	21

Adapted from Pound CR et al.[133]
PSA = prostate-specific antigen.

patients with potentially less toxicity, it must be kept in mind that the annual death rate from metastatic prostate cancer has not changed significantly since androgen ablation was introduced as standard therapy over 50 years ago. Androgen deprivation provides excellent palliation for metastatic bone disease and may, in many cases, prolong survival. However, androgen-independent cells eventually develop that are resistant to androgen deprivation therapy, regardless of the pharmacologic approach used.[135] Unfortunately, no therapy has yet proven effective in prolonging survival in patients whose disease progresses while they are on hormonal therapy. Significant progress is still needed in the development of nonandrogen ablative approaches for treating androgen-independent prostate cancer.[135] Agents that can directly activate apoptosis, growth factor antagonists, antiangiogenesis agents, and immunomodulatory therapies are several promising areas currently being evaluated in the laboratory and in the clinic. Combinations of these new agents with androgen deprivation therapy need to be tested in well-designed clinical trials. Combination therapies may represent the next step toward the development of curative therapy for prostate cancer.

REFERENCES

1. Huggins C, Stevens RE, Hodges CV. Studies of prostatic cancer: II. The effects of castration on advanced carcinoma of the prostate gland. Arch Surg 1941;42:209–23.
2. Jemal A, Murray T, Ward E, et al. Cancer statistics, 2005. CA Cancer J Clin 2005;55:10–30.
3. Denmeade SR, Lin XD, Isaacs JT. Role of programmed (apoptotic) cell death during the progression and therapy for prostate cancer. Prostate 1996;28:251.
4. Joseph IBJK, Isaacs JT. Potentiation of the antiangiogenic ability of linomide by androgen ablation involves down-regulation of vascular endothelial growth factor in human androgen responsive prostatic cancers. Cancer Res 1997;57:1054.
5. Joseph IBJK, Nelson JB, Denmeade SR, et al. Androgens regulate vascular endothelial growth factor content in normal and malignant prostatic tissue. Clin Cancer Res 1997;3:2507.
6. Verhagen APM, Aadlers TW, Ramaeker FCS, et al. Differential expression of keratins in the basal and luminal compartments of rat prostatic epithelium during degeneration and regeneration. Prostate 1988;13:25.
7. Isaacs JT. Control of cell proliferation and cell death in the normal and neoplastic prostate: a stem cell model. In: Rogers CH, Coffey DS, Cunha G, et al, editors. Benign prostatic hyperplasia. Bethesda (MD): National Institutes of Health, Department of Health and Human Services; 1987. p. 85. Report No.: INH 87-2881.
8. Isaacs JT, Coffey DS. Etiology of BPH. Prostate Suppl 1989;2:33.
9. Chen S, Song CS, Lavrovsky Y, et al. Catalytic cleavage of the androgen receptor messenger RNA and functional inhibition of androgen receptor activity by a hammerhead ribozyme. Mol Endocrinol 1998;12:1558.
10. Choong CS, Sturm MJ, Strophair JA, et al. Partial androgen insensitivity caused by an androgen receptor mutation at amino acid 907 (Gly–Arg) that results in decreased ligand binding affinity and reduced androgen receptor messenger ribonucleic acid levels. J Clin Endocrinol Metab 1996;81:236.
11. Culig Z, Hobisch A, Cronauer MV, et al. Mutant androgen receptor detected in an advanced-stage prostatic carcinoma is activated by adrenal androgens and progesterone. Mol Endocrinol 1993;7:1541.
12. Lee WH, Morton RA, Epstein JI, et al. Cytidine methylation of regulatory sequences near the p-class glutathione-S-transferase gene accompanies human prostate cancer carcinogenesis. Proc Acad Natl Sci U S A 1994;91:11733.
13. Nazareth LV, Weigel NL. Activation of the human androgen receptor through a protein kinase A signaling pathway. J Biol Chem 1996;271:19900.
14. Tilley WD, Buchana G, Hickey TT, et al. Mutations in the androgen receptor gene are associated with progression of human prostate cancer to androgen independent. Clin Cancer Res 1996;2:277.
15. Xu J, Qin Y, DeMayo FJ, et al. Partial hormone resistance in mice with disruption of the steroid receptor coactivator-1 (SRC-1) gene. Science 1998;279:1922.
16. Coffey DS. The biochemistry and physiology of the prostate and seminal vesicles. In: Walsh PC, Gittes RF, Perlmutter AD, Stamey TA, editors. Campbell's urology. 5th ed. Philadelphia (PA): W.B. Saunders; 1986. p. 233–74.
17. Swerdloff RS. Physiology of male reproduction: hypothalamic-pituitary function. In: Walsh PC, Gittes RF, Perlmutter AD, Stamey TA, editors. Campbell's urology. 5th ed. Philadelphia (PA): W.B. Saunders; 1986. p. 186–200.
18. Brendler CB, Isaacs JT, Follansbee AL, Walsh PC. The use of multiple variables to predict response to endocrine therapy in carcinoma of the prostate: a preliminary report. J Urol 1984;131:694–700.
19. Klein H, Bressel M, Kastendieck H, Voigt KD. Quantitative assessment of endrogenous testicular and adrenal sex steroids of steroid metabolizing enzymes in untreated human prostatic cancerous tissue. J Steroid Biochem 1988;30:119–30.
20. Bruchovsky N, Wilson JD. The conversion of testosterone to 5α-androstan-17β-ol-3-one by rat prostate in vivo and in vitro. J Biol Chem 1968;243:2012–21.
21. Anderson KM, Liao S. Selective retention of dihydrotestosterone by prostatic nuclei. Nature 1968;219:27–9.
22. Kyprianou N, English HF, Isaacs JT. Programmed cell death during regression of PC-82 human prostate cancer following androgen ablation. Cancer Res 1990;50:3748–53.
23. Tolis G, Menta A, Kinch R, et al. Suppression of sex steroids by an LH-RH analogue in man. Clin Res 1980;28:676–80.
24. Leuprolide Study Group. Leuprolide versus diethylstilbestrol for metastatic prostatic cancer. N Engl J Med 1984;311:1281–6.
25. Waxman J, Man A, Hendry WF, et al. Importance of early tumor exacerbation in patients treated with long acting analogues of gonadotropin releasing hormone for advanced prostatic cancer. BMJ 1985;291:1387–8.
26. Svensson M, Varenhorst E, Kagedal B. Initial administration of cyproterone acetate to prevent the rise of testosterone concentration during treatment with an LH-RH agonist in prostatic cancer. Anticancer Res 1986;6:379–84.
27. Kuhn J-M, Billebaud T, Navratil H, et al. Prevention of the transient adverse effects of a gonadotropin-releasing hormone analog (buserelin) in metastatic prostate carcinoma by administration of an antiandrogen (nilutamide). N Engl J Med 1989;321:413–8.
28. Fowler JE Jr, Gottesman JE, Reid CF, et al. Safety and efficacy of an implantable leuprolide delivery system in patients with advanced prostate cancer. J Urol 2000;164(3 Pt 1):730–4.
29. Fowler JE, Flanagan M, Gleason DM, et al. Evaluation of an implant that delivers leuprolide for 1 year for the palliative treatment of prostate cancer. Urology 2000;55:639–42.
30. Eisenberger MA, O'Dwyer PJ, Friedman MA. Gonadotropin hormone-releasing hormone analogues: a new therapeutic approach for prostatic cancer. J Clin Oncol 1986;5:414–24.
31. Stege R. Potential side-effects of endocrine treatment of long duration in prostate cancer. Prostate 2000;10:38–42.
32. Bayoumi AM, Brown AD, Garber AM. Cost-effectiveness of androgen suppression therapies in advanced prostate cancer. J Natl Cancer Inst 2000;92:1731–9.
33. Stricker HJ. Luteinizing hormone-releasing hormone antagonists in prostate cancer. Urology 2001;58(2 Suppl 1):24–7.
34. Steinberg GD, Isaacs JT. Pharmacological approaches to the management of metastatic prostate cancer. In: Hickman JA, Tritton TR, editors. Cancer chemotherapy. Oxford (UK): Blackwell Scientific Publications; 1993. p. 322–43.
35. Oesterling J, Fuks Z, Lee CT, Scher HI. Cancer of the prostate. In: DeVita VT, Hellman S, Rosenberg SA, editors. Cancer: principles and practice of oncology. Philadelphia (PA): Lippincott-Raven; 1997. p. 1363–8.
36. Knuth UA, Hano R, Nieschllag E. Effect of flutamide or cyproterone acetate on pituitary and testicular hormones in normal men. J Clin Endocrinol Metab 1984;59:963–9.
37. Tyrrell CJ, Denis L, Newling D, et al. Casodex 10-200mg daily, used as monotherapy for the treatment of patients with advanced prostate cancer. Eur Urol 1998;33:39–53.
38. Verhelst J, Denis L, Van-Vliet P, et al. Endocrine profiles during administration of the new non-steroidal anti-androgen Casodex in prostate cancer. Clin Endocrinol 1994;41:525–30.
39. Schroeder FH, Lock TM, Chadha DR, et al. Metastatic cancer of the prostate managed with buserelin versus buserelin plus cytoterone acetate. J Urol 1987;137:912–8.
40. Beland G, Elhilali M, Fradet Y, et al. A controlled trial of castration with and without nilutamide in metastatic prostatic carcinoma. Cancer 1990;66:1074–9.
41. Iverson P, Suciu S, Sylvester R, et al. Zoladex and flutamide versus orchiectomy in the treatment of advanced prostatic cancer. Cancer 1990;66:1067–73.
42. Tyrell CJ, Altwein JE, Klippel F, et al. A multicenter randomized trial comparing the luteinizing hormone-releasing hormone analogue goserelin acetate alone and with flutamide in the treatment of advanced prostate cancer. J Urol 1991;146:1321–6.
43. Sufrin G, Coffey DA. Flutamide: mechanisms of action of a new nonsteroidal antiandrogen. Invest Urol 1976;13:429–34.
44. Mackler MA, Liberti JP, Smith MJV, et al. The effect of orchiectomy and various doses of stilbestrol on plasma testosterone levels in patient with carcinoma of the prostate. Invest Urol 1972;9:423–5.
45. Trachtenberg J, Halpern N, Pont A. Ketoconazole: a novel and rapid treatment of advanced prostatic cancer. J Urol 1983;130:152–3.
46. Trachtenberg J. Ketoconazole therapy in advanced prostatic carcinoma. J Urol 1984;132:61–3.
47. Pont A. Long-term experience with high-dose ketoconazole therapy in patients with stage D2 prostatic carcinoma. J Urol 1987;137:902–4.
48. Johnson DE, Babaion RJ, Eschenbach A, et al. Ketoconazole therapy for hormonally refractive metastatic prostate cancer. Urology 1988;31:132–4.
49. Gao J, Isaacs JT. Development of an androgen receptor null model for identifying the site of initiation for androgen stimulation of proliferation and suppression of programmed (apoptotic) death of PC-82 human prostate cancer cells. Cancer Res 1998;58:3299.
50. George FW, Johnson L, Wilson JD. The effect of a 5α-reductase inhibitor on androgen physiology in the immature rat. Endocrinology 1989;125:2434–8.
51. Vermeulen A, Schelfhout W, Desy W. Plasma androgen levels after subcapsular orchiectomy or estrogen treatment for prostatic carcinoma. Prostate 1982;3:115–21.
52. Brooks JR, Berman C, Primka RL, et al. 5α-Reductase inhibitory and anti-androgenic activities of some 4-azasteroids in the rat. Steroids 1986;47:1–19.
53. Cassileth BR, Soloway MS, Vogelzang NJ, et al. Patients' choice of treatment in stage D prostate cancer. Urology 1989;33 Suppl:57–62.
54. Smith MR, McGovern FJ, Zietman AL, et al. Pamidronate to prevent bone loss during androgen-deprivation therapy for prostate cancer. N Engl J Med 2001;345:948–55.
55. Lipton A, Small E, Saad F, et al. The new bisphosphonate, Zometa (zoledronic acid), decreases skeletal complications in both osteolytic and osteoblastic lesions: a comparison to pamidronate. Cancer Invest 2002;20 Suppl 2:45–54.
56. Labrie F, Dupont A, Belanger A, et al. Combination therapy with flutamide and castration (LHRH agonists or orchiectomy) in advanced prostate cancer: a marked improvement in response and survival. J Steroid Biochem 1985;23:833–41.
57. Labrie F, Veillux R, Fournier A. Low androgen levels induce the development of androgen-hypersensitive cell clones in shionogi mammary carcinoma cells in culture. J Natl Cancer Inst 1988;80:1138–47.
58. Laufer M, Carducci M, Blumenstein B, Eisenberger MA. Combined androgen blockade (CAB) for the treatment of patients with metastatic prostate cancer: summary of 15 years of clinical research. Update Series Vol XVIII Lesson 29. AUA; 1999.
59. Prostate Cancer Trialists' Collaborative Group. Maximum androgen blockade in advanced prostate cancer: an overview of 22 randomized trials with 3238 deaths in 5710 patients. Lancet 1995;346:265–9.
60. Caubet JF, Tosteson TD, Dong EW, et al. Maximum androgen blockade in advanced prostate cancer: a meta-analysis of published randomized controlled trials using nonsteroidal antiandrogens. Urology 1997;49:71–8.
61. Bertagna C, DeGery A, Hucher M, et al. Efficacy of the combination of nilutamide plus orchiectomy in patients with metastatic prostate cancer. A meta-analysis of 7 randomized double-blind trials (1056 patients). Br J Urol 1994;73:396–402.
62. Moinpour CM, Savage MJ, Troxel A, et al. Quality of life in advanced prostate cancer: results of a randomized therapeutic trial. J Natl Cancer Inst 1998;90:1537–44.

63. Hellerstedt BA, Pienta KJ. The current state of hormonal therapy for prostate cancer. CA Cancer J Clin 2002;52:154–79.
64. Veterans Administration Cooperative Urological Research Group. Treatment and survival of patients with cancer of the prostate. Surg Gynecol Obstet 1967;124:1011.
65. Byar DP, Corle DK. Hormone therapy for prostate cancer: results of the Veterans Administration Cooperative Urological Research Group Studies. NCI Monogr 1988;7:165–70.
66. Robinson MRG. A further analysis of European Organization for Research and Treatment of Cancer Protocol 3085: orchidectomy versus orchidectomy plus cyproterone acetate versus low-dose diethylstilbestrol. Cancer 1993;72 Suppl 12:3855.
67. Balckard CE. The Veterans Administration Cooperative Urological Research Group studies of carcinoma of the prostate: a review. Cancer Chemother Rep 1975;59:225–7.
68. Hedlund PO, Gustafsson H, Sogren S. Cardiovascular complications to treatment of prostatic cancer. Scand J Urol Nephrol 1980;55 Suppl:103–5.
69. Glashan RW, Robinson MRG. Cardiovascular complications in the treatment of prostatic cancer. Br J Urol 1981;53:624–31.
70. Aro J. Cardiovascular and all-cause mortality in prostatic cancer patients treated with estrogens or orchiectomy as compared to the standard population. Prostate 1991;18:131–7.
71. Agardh CD, Nilsson-Ehle P, Lundgren R, Gustafson A. The influence of treatment with estrogens and estramustine phosphate on platelet aggregation and plasma lipoproteins in non-disseminated prostatic carcinoma. J Urol 1984;132:1021–4.
72. Rossner S, Hedlund PO, Jogerstrand T, Sawe U. Treatment of prostatic cancer: effects on serum lipoproteins and the cardiovascular system. J Urol 1985;133:53–7.
73. Hedlund PO, Henriksson P. Parenteral estrogen versus total androgen ablation in the treatment of advanced prostate carcinoma: effects on overall survival and cardiovascular mortality. The Scandinavian Prostatic Cancer Group (SPCG)-5 Trial Study. Urology 2000;55:328–33.
74. Spetz AC, Hammar M, Lindberg B, et al, Scandinavian Prostatic Cancer Group-5 Trial Study. Prospective evaluation of hot flashes during treatment with parenteral estrogen or complete androgen ablation for metastatic carcinoma of the prostate. J Urol 2001;166:517–20.
75. Scherr D, Pitts WR Jr, Vaughn ED Jr. Diethylstilbesterol revisited: androgen deprivation, osteoporosis and prostate cancer. J Urol 2002;167(2 Pt 1):535–8.
76. Ke HZ, Qi H, Crawford DT, et al. Lasofoxifene (CP-336,156), a selective estrogen receptor modulator, prevents bone loss induced by aging and orchidectomy in the adult rat. Endocrinology 2000;141:1338–44.
77. Chang A, Yeap B, Blum R, et al. A double blind randomized study of primary treatment for stage D2 prostate cancer: diethylstilbesterol (DES) versus flutamide (F). Proc Am Soc Clin Oncol 1992;11:202.
78. Sharifi R. Casodex versus castration in treatment of stage D2 prostate cancer: prostate specific antigen (PSA) as a measure of outcome. Proc Am Soc Clin Oncol 1993;12:241.
79. Iversen P. Antiandrogen monotherapy: indications and results. Urology 2002;60 Suppl 3A:64–71.
80. Chodak G, Sharifi R, Kasimis B, et al. Single agent therapy with bicalutamide: a comparison with medical or surgical castration in the treatment of prostate cancer. Urology 1995;46:849.
81. Blackledge GRP. High-dose bicalutamide monotherapy for the treatment of prostate cancer. Urology 1996;47:44.
82. Tyrell CJ, Blake GM, Iversen P, et al. "Casodex" may preserve bone mineral density of patients with advanced prostate cancer [abstract]. BJU Int 1986;Suppl 3:220–1.
83. See WA, Wirth MP, McLeod DG, et al. Bicalutamide as immediate therapy either alone or as adjuvant to standard care of patients with localized or locally advanced prostate cancer: first analysis of the Early Prostate Cancer Program. J Urol 2002;168:429–35.
84. Wirth MP, See WA, McLeod DG, et al, Casodex Early Prostate Cancer Trialists' Group. Bicalutamide 150 mg in addition to standard care in patients with localized or locally advanced prostate cancer: results from the second analysis of the Early Prostate Cancer Program at median followup of 5.4 years. J Urol 2004;172:1865–70.
85. Moul JW. Contemporary hormonal management of advanced prostate cancer. Oncology (Huntingt) 1998;12:499–505.
86. Gleave M, Bruchovsky N, Bowden M, et al. Intermittent androgen suppression prolongs time to androgen-independent progression in the LNCaP prostate tumor model. J Urol 1994;151:457A.
87. Akakura K, Bruchovsky N, Goldenberg SL, et al. Effects of intermittent androgen suppression on androgen-dependent tumors: apoptosis and serum prostate specific antigen. Cancer 1993;71:2782.
88. Horwich A, Huddart RA, Gadd J, et al. A pilot study of intermittent androgen deprivation in advanced prostate cancer. Br J Urol 1998;81:96–9.
89. Goldenberg SL, Bruchovsky N, Gleave ME, et al. Intermittent androgen suppression in the treatment of prostate cancer: a preliminary report. Urology 1995;45:839.
90. Higano CS, Ellis W, Russell K, Lange PH. Intermittent androgen suppression with leuprolide and flutamide for prostate cancer: a pilot study. Urology 1996;48:800–4.
91. Oefelein MG. Serum testosterone-based luteinizing hormone-releasing hormone agonist redosing schedule for chronic androgen ablation: a phase I assessment. Urology 1999;54:694–9.
92. Daliani D, Bui C, Logothetis C. The significance of variability in PSA responses on individualized intermittent androgen suppression (IAS) for prostate cancer: results of a pilot study [abstract]. Proc Am Soc Clin Oncol 1998;17:323a.
93. Small EJ, Vogelzang NJ. Second-line hormonal therapy for advanced prostate cancer: a shifting paradigm. J Clin Oncol 1997;15:382–8.
94. Reese DM, Small EJ. Secondary hormonal manipulations in hormone refractory prostate cancer. Urol Clin North Am 1999;26:311–21.
95. Fowler JE, Whitmore WF. The response of metastatic adenocarcinoma of the prostate to exogenous testosterone. J Urol 1981;126:372–5.
96. Manni A, Bartholomew M, Caplan R, et al. Androgen priming and chemotherapy in advanced prostate cancer: evaluation of determinants of clinical outcome. J Clin Oncol 1988;6:1456–66.
97. Taylor CD, Elson P, Trump DL. Importance of continued testicular suppression in hormone refractory prostate cancer. J Clin Oncol 1996;14:1756–64.
98. Hobisch A, Culig Z, Radmayr C, et al. Distant metastases from prostate carcinoma express androgen receptor protein. Cancer Res 1995;55:3068.
99. Hobisch A, Culig Z, Radmayr C, et al. Androgen receptor status of lymph node metastases from prostate cancer. Prostate 1996;28:129.
100. Koivisto P, Kononen J, Palmberg C, et al. Androgen receptor gene amplification: a possible molecular mechanism for androgen deprivation therapy failure in prostate cancer. Cancer Res 1997;57:314.
101. Viskorpi T, Hyytinen E, Koivisto P, et al. In vivo amplification of the androgen receptor gene and progression of human prostate cancer. Nat Genet 1995;9:401.
102. Choong CS, Sturm MJ, Strophair JA, et al. Partial androgen insensitivity caused by an androgen receptor mutation at amino acid 907 (Gly–Arg) that results in decreased ligand binding affinity and reduced androgen receptor messenger ribonucleic acid levels. J Clin Endocrinol Metab 1996;81:236.
103. Culig Z, Hobisch A, Cronauer MV, et al. Mutant androgen receptor detected in an advanced-stage prostatic carcinoma is activated by adrenal androgens and progesterone. Mol Endocrinol 1993;7:1541.
104. Taplin ME, Bubley GJ, Shuster TD, et al. Mutation of the androgen-receptor gene in metastatic androgen-independent prostate cancer. N Engl J Med 1995;332:1393–8.
105. Tilley WD, Buchanan G, Hickey TE, et al. Mutations in the androgen receptor gene are associated with progression of human prostate cancer to androgen independence. Clin Cancer Res 1996;2:277–85.
106. Kelly WK, Scher HI. Prostate specific antigen decline after antiandrogen withdrawal. J Urol 1993;149:607–9.
107. Scher HI, Kelly WK. Flutamide withdrawal syndrome: its impact on clinical trials in hormone-refractory prostate cancer. J Clin Oncol 1993;11:1566–72.
108. Herrada J, Dieringer P, Logothetis CJ. Characterization of patients with androgen-independent prostatic carcinoma whose serum prostate specific antigen decreased following flutamide withdrawal. J Urol 1996;155:620–3.
109. Nieh PT. Withdrawal phenomenon with the antiandrogen Casodex. J Urol 1995;153:1070–3.
110. Small EJ, Carroll PR. Prostate-specific antigen decline after Casodex withdrawal: evidence for an antiandrogen withdrawal syndrome. Urology 1994;43:408–10.
111. Gomella LG, Ismail M, Nathan FE. Antiandrogen withdrawal syndrome with nilutamide. J Urol 1997;157:1366.
112. Huan SD, Gerridzen RG, Yau JC, et al. Antiandrogen withdrawal syndrome with nilutamide. Urology 1997;49:620–3.
113. Dawson NA, McLeod DG. Dramatic prostate specific antigen decrease in response to discontinuation of megesterol acetate in advanced prostate cancer: expansion of the antiandrogen withdrawal syndrome. J Urol 1995;153:1946–7.
114. Bissada NK, Kaczmarek AT. Complete remission of hormone refractory adenocarcinoma of the prostate in response to withdrawal of diethylstilbesterol. J Urol 1995;153:1944–5.
115. Scher HI, Zhang Z-F, Cohen L, et al. Hormonally relapsed prostatic cancer: lessons from the flutamide withdrawal syndrome. Adv Urol 1995;8:61–95
116. Schellhammer P, Venner P, Haas G, et al. Prostate specific antigen decreases after withdrawal of antiandrogen therapy with bicalutamide or flutamide in patients receiving combined androgen blockade. J Urol 1997;157:1731–5.
117. Small EJ, Srinvas S. The antiandrogen withdrawal syndrome: experience in a large cohort of unselected patients with advanced prostate cancer. Cancer 1995;76:1428–34.
118. Sogani PC, Vagaiwala MR, Whitmore WF Jr. Experience with flutamide in patients with advanced prostatic cancer without prior endocrine therapy. Cancer 1984;54:744.
119. Jacobi GH, Altwein JE, Kurth KH, et al. Treatment of advanced prostatic cancer with parenteral cyproterone acetate: a phase II randomized trial. Br J Urol 1980;52:208–15.
120. Scher HI, Liebertz C, Kelly WK, et al. Bicalutamide for advanced prostate cancer: the natural versus treated history of disease. J Clin Oncol 1997;15:2928–38.
121. Joyce R, Fenton MA, Rode P, et al. High dose bicalutamide for androgen independent prostate cancer: effect of prior hormonal therapy. J Urol 1997;159:149–53.
122. Dowsett M, Shearer RJ, Ponder BAJ, et al. The effects of aminoglutethimide and hydrocortisone, alone and combined, on androgen levels in post-orchiectomy prostatic cancer patients. Br J Cancer 1988;57:190–2.
123. Sartor O, Cooper M, Weinberger M, et al. Surprising activity of flutamide withdrawal, when combined with aminoglutethimide, in treatment of "hormone-refractory" prostate cancer. J Natl Cancer Inst 1994;86:222–7.
124. Small EJ, Baron AD, Fippin L, et al. Ketoconazole retains activity in advanced prostate cancer patients with progression despite flutamide withdrawal. J Urol 1997;4:1204–7.
125. Tannock I, Gospodarowicz M, Meakin W, et al. Treatment of metastatic prostate cancer with low-dose prednisone: evaluation of pain and quality of life as pragmatic indices of response. J Clin Oncol 1989;7:590–7.
126. Tannock I, Osoba D, Stockler M, et al. Chemotherapy with mitoxantrone plus prednisone or prednisone alone for symptomatic hormone-resistant prostate cancer: a Canadian randomized study with palliative endpoints. J Clin Oncol 1996;14:1756–64.
127. Smith DC, Redman BG, Flaherty LE, et al. A phase II trial of oral diethylstilbesterol as a second-line hormonal agent in advanced prostate cancer. Urology 1998;52:257–60.
128. Medical Research Council Prostate Cancer Working Party Investigators Group. Immediate versus deferred treatment for advanced prostate cancer: initial results of the Medical Research Council trial. Br J Urol 1997;79:235–46.
129. Medical Research Council Prostate Cancer Working Party Investigators Group. Immediate versus deferred hormone therapy for prostate cancer: how safe is androgen deprivation? BJU Int 2000;86:2000.
130. Zincke H. Extended experience with surgical treatment of stage D1 adenocarcinoma of prostate: significant influences of immediate adjuvant hormonal treatment (orchiectomy) on outcome. Urology 1989;33 Suppl:27–35.
131. Messing EM, Manola J, Sarosdy M, et al. Immediate hormonal therapy compared with observation after radical prostatectomy and pelvic lymphadenectomy in men with node-positive prostate cancer. N Engl J Med 1999;341:1781-8.
132. Eisenberger MA, Walsh PC. Early androgen deprivation for prostate cancer? N Engl J Med 1999;341:1837–8.
133. Pound CR, Partin AW, Eisenberger MA, et al. Natural history of progression after PSA elevation following radical prostatectomy. JAMA 1999;281:1591–7.
134. D'Amico AV, Moul J, Carroll PR, et al. Prostate specific antigen doubling time as a surrogate end point for prostate cancer specific mortality following radical prostatectomy or radiation therapy. J Urol 2004;172:S42–6.
135. Isaacs JT. The biology of hormone refractory prostate cancer: why does it develop? Urol Clin North Am 1999;26:263–73.

Section 15

GENE THERAPY

57

Cancer Gene Therapy

Sunil J. Advani, MD
Ralph R. Weichselbaum, MD
Donald W. Kufe, MD

Advances in our understanding of the genetic alterations that accumulate in the progression to a malignant cell have provided unforeseen opportunities for the development of new therapeutic strategies. Cancer gene therapy is an emerging field that was initially received with unbridled enthusiasm as one such opportunity to take advantage of the genetic differences between normal and transformed cells. Limitations in our ability to deliver genes to every cancer cell, however, have dampened interest in developing approaches to inactivate oncogenes or replace nonfunctioning tumor-suppressor genes. Nonetheless, other therapeutic strategies have emerged that exploit the presently available delivery systems and our understanding of alterations that distinguish the cancer cell. This chapter defines the principles of gene therapy and their application to the treatment of cancer.

Gene therapy can be broadly defined as the transfer of genetic material into a cell to transiently or permanently alter the cellular phenotype. Introduction of a nucleic acid or target gene (transgene) directly into cells is referred to as transfection. Alternatively, transduction refers to the introduction of a transgene into a cell through a viral vector system. Gene transfer can be performed by transfection or transduction of target cells in vitro and then administration of the modified cells to an animal or patient. In vivo gene transfer is accomplished by direct transfection or transduction of target cells in the patient. The introduction of genes that encode proteins with potential antitumor effects has been described as therapeutic gene transfer. The mechanistic effects of the therapeutic gene product and the stability of transgene expression are factors of importance to the different approaches that now constitute cancer gene therapy. Of equal importance is delivery of the therapeutic gene to the target cell. The delivery system, or vector, generally consists of a nucleic acid sequence or promoter that drives expression of the transgene and a polyadenylation signal that stabilizes the transcribed messenger ribonucleic acid (mRNA). The vector is usually inserted into a bacteriophage for propagation in vitro or integrated into a virus.

The delivery of therapeutic genes to cancer cells poses the greatest challenge to the successful application of cancer gene therapy in humans. As such, considerable effort is being devoted to the development of more selective and efficient vectors. In particular, vectors that target specific tumor cell populations, or that contain promoters that are selectively activated in tumor cells, are at the forefront of progress in the cancer gene therapy field. An extension of the cancer gene therapy paradigm is the use of replication-competent viruses (viral oncolysis). Replication-competent viruses are beginning to overcome some of the hurdles of inefficient delivery that plague other gene transfer methods. This chapter begins with a description of the available vector systems and then discusses the therapeutic genes that are presently under study. Although not involving the transfer of genes to cancer cells, certain other strategies, such as the administration of recombinant vaccines, indirectly target the tumor cell, and although considered in the context of cancer gene therapy, are described here and in the chapters on tumor immunology and active specific immunotherapy with vaccines.

GENE DELIVERY SYSTEMS

Viral and nonviral vector systems are being employed in gene therapy approaches to cancer. The following sections describe the RNA and deoxyribonucleic acid (DNA) viruses and the nonviral vectors that are being used to deliver transgenes to tumor cells.

Retroviruses Retroviruses are single-stranded RNA viruses that consist of the 5' and 3' long-terminal repeats (LTRs) and the *gag*, *pol*, and *env* structural genes. *Gag* encodes three proteins that form the shell of the virion. *Pol* encodes reverse transcriptase, integrase, and ribonuclease H (RNaseH), which are necessary for viral integration into host chromosomal DNA. The *env* gene encodes the envelope glycoprotein that extends from the lipid membrane of the virion and functions as a ligand for the cellular viral receptor. Viruses deleted of one or more of their structural genes (eg, *env)* are fully infectious when propagated in a viral producer cell that expresses the missing gene.[1] When a transgene is inserted into the deleted virus and that virus infects a target cell, viral sequences containing the transgene integrate into the host genome and confer expression of both viral genes and the transgene. The deleted viral vector, however, is incapable of undergoing viral replication because the deleted structural gene that is necessary for this process is not expressed by the target cell. As such, the deleted viral vector transfers and expresses the transgene but is incapable of establishing an active infection in the host. Other studies show that the 5' and 3' LTRs and a short sequence just 5' to the *gag* initiation codon (the packaging sequence) are sufficient to confer packaging when all of the structural genes are expressed by the producer cell. Transfection of these producer cell lines with a minimal vector containing the desired transgene results in the production of a defective recombinant retrovirus. The transduction of target cells with recombinant retroviruses that are defective in viral gene expression also minimizes the development of an antiviral immune response.

Retroviruses integrate into target cell DNA and thus achieve stable integration of the transgene. Theoretically, stable integration should provide long-term expression, although methylation of the LTR often results in down-regulation of transgene transcription.[2] The receptor for the Moloney murine leukemia retrovirus (MoMuLV) is found on most human cells. Thus, although cell type is not limiting for vector transduction, a potential disadvantage is the ubiquitous distribution of the receptor, and thereby little target cell selectivity. To address this issue of selective target cell transduction, hybrid envelope proteins have been generated by fusing a portion of the *env* gene to a sequence encoding a ligand for a specific cell surface receptor. For example, fusions to the erythropoietin domain that binds to the erythropoietin receptor have generated recombinant retroviral vectors that selectively target those cells expressing the receptor. Identification of the crystal structure of the murine retroviral envelope protein should facilitate the development of vectors with modifications of this structure and restricted target cell tropisms.[3]

An important limitation of the MoMuLV-based retroviral vectors is that they integrate only into actively dividing cells. As most solid tumors have low growth fractions, it is unlikely that these retroviral vectors would transduce a significant proportion of the tumor. By contrast, the human immunodeficiency virus type-1 replicates in nondividing cells,[4,5] and thus may represent a more effective vector for the transduction of tumors. In addition, retroviralvector-mediated insertional mutagenesis could result in transformation of the transduced target cell. Although no murine retrovirus has been pathogenic in humans, a study in nonhuman primates demonstrated the development of hematologic malignancies following treatment with high doses of retroviral vectors containing replication-competent helper viruses.[6] On the basis of these limitations, MoMuLV-based retroviruses are considered best suited for in vitro transduction of specific target cells that can be isolated and stimulated to undergo proliferation. The eventual utility of retroviral vectors for in vivo transduction is uncertain.

ADENOVIRUSES Adenoviruses are nonenveloped, linear, double-stranded DNA viruses. Approximately 50 serotypes of adenovirus have been identified and grouped from A to F on the basis of genome size, composition, homology, and organization. The most studied adenoviruses are the group C serotypes 1, 2, 5, and 6. The prototype adenoviral vector for gene therapy is based on adenovirus type 5 (Ad5).

Adenoviral attachment to cells is mediated by fibers that extend from the 12 vertices of the outer capsid. The adenoviral genome is approximately 36 kilobases (kb) and is conventionally represented as 100 map units (1 map unit = 360 base pairs [bp]). Each end of the viral genome is flanked by 100 to 150 bp of repeated DNA sequence (inverted terminal repeat). Viral gene expression occurs in a sequential cascade. Adenoviral genes are grouped as early (E) genes whose expression precedes viral DNA replication and the transcription of late (L) genes at 6 to 8 hours after infection. The E genes encode regulatory proteins for viral replication and the L genes encode structural proteins necessary for assembly of progeny virions. Among the E genes, the E1A and E1B products of the E1 gene are the first viral proteins produced after infection and are critical for viral replication.

Adenoviral vectors have been based on the observation that deletion of the E1A and part of the E1B gene results in replication-deficient viruses. Such viruses can be propagated in helper cell lines that express the E1 gene products. For example, the 293 helper cell line was prepared from human embryonic cells stably transformed with Ad5 DNA fragments that constitutively express the E1 proteins.[7] The amount of DNA that can be effectively packaged into adenovirus virions is ~105% of the wild-type genome and thus allows for the insertion of ~2 kb of foreign DNA. With the E1A-deleted viruses, it has been possible to insert 5 to 6 kb of DNA. An additional 2 kb of DNA can be inserted by deletion of the E3 gene. The E3 gene product functions in abrogating the host immune response to the virus by preventing cytolysis mediated through cytotoxic T cells and tumor necrosis factor. E3 is not required for viral growth in tissue culture, and E3-deleted viruses appear to be fully infectious.

Adenoviral vectors have a number of potential advantages over retroviral vectors. Most human cell types are susceptible to adenoviral infection and are subject to efficient transduction. Additionally, adenoviruses can deliver transgenes to both dividing and nondividing cells. This property is of particular significance in the setting of tumors that contain a heterogenous cell population of both cycling and noncycling cells. Because adenoviruses are relatively stable and resistant to physical manipulations, vectors can be concentrated to high titers (10^{11} to 10^{12} PFU/mL) and frozen for use at later times (a property that is generally not possible with retroviruses because of their fragility under physical stresses such as freezing). Another advantage of adenoviral vectors is that the adenoviral life cycle does not require integration into the host cell genome. Because adenoviral DNA is episomal, insertional mutagenesis is much less a concern than it is for retroviral vectors. Also, a promoter of choice can be used to drive the inserted transgene, affording the opportunity for tissue selective expression or inducibility. By contrast, the use of heterologous promoters in retroviral vectors is often problematic because the promoter can be overridden by strong constitutive activity of the retroviral LTR.

A major disadvantage of current adenoviral vectors is the induction of a significant host immune response. A T-cell–mediated response against adenoviral proteins causes a local inflammatory reaction that can result in lysis of the transduced cells and a shorter duration of adenoviral-mediated transgene expression. The immune response is partly a result of E1-deleted adenoviruses expressing other E and L genes and initiating viral DNA replication. As such, vectors are needed that exhibit silencing of viral gene expression and DNA replication and thereby prolong transgene expression. Another concern with adenoviral vectors is the development of virus-neutralizing antibodies. In this setting, attempts to rechallenge immunocompetent animals with adenoviral constructs have resulted in diminished transgene expression. As most humans have been exposed to wild-type adenovirus and harbor neutralizing antibodies, these vectors may be quickly cleared when administered in clinical trials. As noted above, adenoviral vectors are limited by the size of the transgene. With current vectors, 8.5 kb appears to be the limit of foreign DNA that can be inserted. Also of concern in the propagation of E1-deleted viruses in helper cell lines is the generation of replication-competent adenoviruses. In this regard, recombination can occur between the E1-deleted adenovirus and the E1 region present in the 293 helper cell line.

HERPES SIMPLEX VIRUSES Herpes simplex viruses (HSVs) are large enveloped double-stranded DNA viruses classified as either α, β, or γ, based on viral characteristics. HSV-1 is a herpes virus that is naturally neurotropic and also infects epithelial cells. A characteristic of HSV-1 infection is the establishment of a latent ("dormant") state in sensory neurons that, in the presence of certain stimuli, results in reactivation of the virus and entry into the lytic cycle.

HSV attachment to cells is mediated by binding of glycoproteins expressed at the viral envelope to cellular membrane receptors.[8] The HSV-1 genome is approximately 150 kb and encodes about 90 proteins. The sequence is represented by two stretches of DNA, unique long and unique short, flanked by inverted repeat segments. Genes in the unique region are present as single copies, whereas those in the repeat segments are present as two copies. HSV-1 viral genes have been classified as either essential or nonessential depending on whether deletion of the gene allows for growth of the mutated virus in cell culture. Nonetheless, genes considered nonessential in cell culture may be functional in optimizing viral replication in vivo. Viral gene expression is coordinately regulated with the α genes (involved in regulatory functions) expressed first, followed by β genes (involved in nucleic acid metabolism and viral DNA replication) and then γ genes (encoding structural proteins). Viral DNA replication proceeds in a concatameric fashion in which individual viral DNA genomes are cleaved by signals in the terminal α sequence and packaged into preformed viral capsids.

Replication-deficient HSV-1–based vectors are categorized as helper virus dependent and independent. Helper virus-dependent vectors have also been termed amplicons. Amplicons are defective HSV genomes that arise spontaneously by recombination and are amplified by serial passage at high multiplicities of infection.[9] At a minimum, the defective genome (amplicon) consists of a terminal a sequence and an origin of viral DNA synthesis. A viral origin of DNA synthesis allows for propagation of the amplicon, and the a sequence is needed to cleave concatameric DNA and package the amplicon. As amplicons are largely devoid of coding sequences, viral structural proteins and those involved in viral DNA replication and exocytosis must be provided by a "helper" virus. One such helper virus was generated by deletion of an essential HSV-1 gene, α4. In this system, an α4-expressing complementary cell line is transfected with the amplicon and then superinfected with the α4-deleted HSV-1. In theory, amplicons could accommodate as much as 150 kb (the size of the HSV-1 genome) because the backbone of the amplicon is usually < 15 kb. Moreover, amplicons efficiently express integrated transgenes[10] for relatively long periods as there is no associated latency shutdown of viral gene expression. Despite these advantages, there are certain problems that exist with the amplicon approach. First, because helper viruses are needed to encode the missing viral proteins, amplicons become contaminated with helper viral DNA. This problem has been solved in part by the generation of helper viruses that fail to package.[11] Second, the yields of amplicons are several orders of magnitude less than that achieved with wild-type viruses, and the ratio of amplicon to helper virus is low. Last, amplicons tend to be unstable with serial passage because there is a selective advantage for smaller amplicons.[12]

Helper virus-independent HSV-1 viral vectors have deletions in essential viral genes. Because of deletion of one or more essential genes, such viruses need to be grown in appropriate cell lines that complement the defects. These HSV-1 vectors replicate to high titers. In addition, although dependent on the viral genes that are deleted, up to 40 kb of foreign DNA can be inserted (at least fourfold greater than can be achieved with adenoviral vectors). HSV-1 vectors can also deliver genes to a wide range of cell types. With regard to disadvantages, many of the essential viral genes encode multifunctional proteins. For example, α4 is both a transcriptional activator and repressor. Thus, deletion of α4 may influence viral gene expression in a manner detrimental to a gene therapy vector. Also, as with E1-deleted adenoviruses, expression of the remaining viral genes in the infected cell may lead to the induction of an antiviral immune response. As found with defective viruses that are grown in complementing cell lines, there is the possibility of recombination and reversion to a wild-type phenotype. Given that wild-type HSV-1 infection is associated with neurologic sequelae, recombination is of concern in using the helper virus-independent HSV-1–based vectors. However, as the molecular basis for HSV-1 neurovirulence is better defined, such vectors may gain more widespread use. Moreover, as discussed below, genetically engineered replication-competent HSV-1 viruses are currently being studied in a phase I trial for glioma patients with no apparent adverse effects.

Adeno-Associated Virus Adeno-associated viruses (AAVs) are small, nonenveloped, linear single-stranded DNA parvoviruses that are naturally replication deficient. Four of the six known AAV serotypes are human isolates (AAV-2, AAV-3, AAV-5, and AAV-6), whereas AAV-1 and AAV-4 are of simian origin. AAV-2 is the predominant serotype used in gene therapy approaches. Infection with AAV results in either a latent or productive infection phase. Productive infection is dependent on the presence of a helper virus (adenovirus, herpes virus, or vaccinia) or on exposure to genotoxic stress. In the absence of a helper virus or genotoxic stress, AAV integrates into the long arm of chromosome 19 (q19.3-qter), known as the AAVS1 site, and enters a latent phase.

The genome of AAV is approximately 4.7 kb. The DNA is flanked by inverted terminal repeats (ITRs) of 145 bases. The ITRs serve as origins of DNA replication and are required for packaging recombinant AAV into infectious virus. Also, the ITRs are the only *cis* elements essential to the AAV replicative life cycle. Between the ITRs are two sets of open reading frames (ORFs), Rep and Cap. The Rep ORF encodes four nonstructural proteins that regulate AAV replication and site-specific integration. The Cap ORF encodes three structural proteins (VP1 to 3).

Recombinant AAVs (rAAVs) for gene therapy are constructed by deleting the Rep and Cap ORFs and replacing the deleted DNA with a transgene between the ITRs. To propagate rAAV in cell culture, rAAV vectors containing the ITRs and transgene are cotransfected with a plasmid expressing the Rep and Cap genes. The transfected cells are then infected with adenovirus to provide the helper function and thereby efficient rAAV replication. As such, the rAAV must subsequently be purified from the adenovirus in a setting in which the rAAV titers are often low relative to the adenovirus contamination. As the helper function of the adenovirus resides in the E1a, E1b, E2a, E4, and VA1 proteins, expression of these genes by 293 cells provides the requisite helper effect in the absence of adenoviral infection. This approach has also been reported to increase rAAV titers.[13,14]

rAAVs have certain advantages as gene therapy vectors. rAAVs are naturally replication defective and are considered nonpathogenic. Also, deletion of the Rep and Cap ORFs, and thereby expression of viral proteins, decreases immunogenicity. rAAVs have a broad tissue tropism (ie, lung, muscle, central nervous system, liver, and retina) as a consequence of attachment of AAV-2 to the ubiquitously expressed cell surface heparan sulfate proteoglycan (HSPG). The αVβ5 integrin and the fibroblast growth factor 1 receptor have also been shown to act as cofactors for the binding and entry of AAV-2 into cells.[15,16] Unlike retroviruses, rAAVs transduce both replicating and nonreplicating cells. Deletion of the Rep ORF, however, abolishes the site-specific integration of AAV into chromosome 19.[17,18] In addition, despite deletion of the Rep ORF, rAAV can accommodate only 4 kb of DNA insert.

Nonviral Gene Delivery Viral vectors, having evolved to enter cells by receptor-mediated processes and to escape from endosomes with delivery of their DNA to nuclei, are highly efficient in gene transduction. Disadvantages of viral vectors include immune recognition of viral proteins with destruction of the infected cells and with an inability for repeated viral administration. Other limitations of viral vectors include the potential for insertional mutagenesis, restrictions in the size of the transgene, and difficulties encountered in large-scale production for clinical trials. Nonviral delivery systems have thus been explored to overcome some of these obstacles.

Two commonly used laboratory techniques for transfecting plasmid DNA into cells involve calcium phosphate precipitation and electroporation. In calcium phosphate precipitation, plasmid DNA complexed to calcium phosphate crystals enters the cell by endocytosis and is then transported to the nucleus. In electroporation, brief high-voltage electrical pulses are applied to cells to induce the formation of transient pores in the cell membrane. DNA enters the cell through these pores. Both methods of transfection are restricted to cells in culture.

Direct microinjection of genes into nuclei of cells is another method of transfection that abrogates the exposure of DNA to the acidic conditions of endosomes. Although tedious, microinjection is particularly useful for delivering DNA to embryonic cells or oocytes. Direct injection of DNA into skeletal or cardiac muscle is associated with uptake by cells and expression of the transgene. Similar findings have been obtained following injection of DNA into solid tumors growing in nude mice. In this setting, reporter gene expression has been stable for 5 days and can persist for up to 10 days after injection.[19] Significantly, intratumoral injection of the interferon (IFN)-γ gene is associated with inhibition of tumor growth.[20]

Direct DNA injection by the "gene gun" refers to particle-mediated gene transfer in which DNA is delivered by physical force. In this approach, DNA is commonly coated onto gold particles. Acceleration of the DNA-coated particles into tissues or target cells is followed by release of the DNA in the nucleus.[21] The gene gun has been used to deliver immunomodulatory genes to tumor cells in vitro and in animal models.[21,22] Gene gun delivery, like direct DNA injection, is limited by low transfection efficiencies and transfection of both tumor and normal cells.

Cationic liposomes form artificial membranes that complex with DNA and confer the transfection of DNA into cells by endocytosis.[23] Complexes of cationic liposomes and DNA have been used to deliver DNA into tumor cells in culture, into tumor xenografts in mice, and into tumors in patients.[24–27] Liposome-mediated gene transfer is limited by aggregation of the DNA in endosomes and thereby destruction in the acidic environment or by nuclease digestion during transfer of the DNA from the cytoplasm to the nucleus.[23]

"Synthetic viruses" were developed to exploit the efficiency of viral vectors and the advantages of liposomes.[28] DNA is condensed and packaged by poly-L-lysine and targeted to specific cells by conjugating a ligand for a cell surface receptor to the polylysine-DNA complex. Ligands include transferrin, basic fibroblast growth factor, and integrin-binding domains.[29,30] The polylysine-DNA complex is internalized by receptor-mediated endocytosis into endosomes. Fusogenic peptides have been incorporated into the complex to release the DNA from the endosomal compartment.[28,31] The N-terminal sequence of the influenza virus hemagglutinin subunit HA-2 induces destabilization of the endosomal membrane at acidic pH and releases internalized DNA from the endosomes. GALA, another fusogenic peptide, forms a random coil at pH 7.5 and an amphipathic helix at acidic pH. As such, in the acidic environment of the endosome, GALA destabilizes the endosomal membrane.[31] Thus, conjugation of the polylysine-DNA complex to both a ligand and a fusogenic peptide confers cell receptor-specific transfection and efficient transfer of DNA to the nucleus.

Virus-like coats have also been used to package and deliver DNA to cells. For example, an adenoviral-based dodecahedron has been constructed from the structural proteins, penton base, and fiber.[32] In this system, which is devoid of the viral genome, the penton base and fiber mediate efficient cell attachment, internalization, and release from the endosome.

In summary, although providing an alternative approach for cancer gene therapy, nonviral gene delivery is not as efficient as that achieved with viral vectors. Nonviral delivery systems, nonetheless, provide certain advantages in settings, such as immunomodulation strategies, in which transfection of only a fraction of the target cell population can be sufficient to achieve the requisite response. By contrast, more efficient transduction as achieved with viral vectors is necessary in the setting of treatment with therapeutic genes.

THERAPEUTIC GENES

In cancer gene therapy, the replacement of mutated tumor-suppressor genes or other strategies to correct the transformed phenotype requires the transduction of every tumor cell. Given the limitations of the available gene transfer systems to achieve that goal, therapeutic approaches have been developed to exploit the potential for transduction or transfection of only limited populations of tumor cells. In this context, gene therapy for cancer has been focused on the delivery of genes that encode proteins that activate prodrugs and thereby induce cytotoxicity of both transduced and neighboring tumor cells. The delivery of genes that encode proteins that disrupt cell-cycle progression and induce apoptosis represents another area of focus. In addition, genes that modulate the immune response can be delivered to tumor or normal cell populations to induce antitumor immunity.

Virus-Directed Enzyme/Prodrug Therapy

Several cancer gene therapy strategies employ the delivery to tumor cells of genes encoding drug-converting enzymes and then treatment with systemic administration of the respective nontoxic prodrug. This approach of expressing drug-susceptibility genes in tumor cells has been termed "suicide gene therapy." Cells transduced to express the prodrug enzyme confer conversion of the prodrug to active metabolites and thereby selective cytotoxicity. In the setting of treatment with conventional chemotherapeutic agents, the achievement of high local tumor drug concentrations is limited by systemic toxicity. By contrast, virus-directed enzyme/prodrug therapy improves the therapeutic ratio by administration of high systemic concentrations of the prodrug and conversion to the cytotoxic metabolite only within the transduced tumor microenvironment.

Table 57-1 Enzyme/Prodrug Combinations

Converting Enzyme	Prodrug	Action of Drug
HSV-thymidine kinase	Ganciclovir, acyclovir, bromovinyl-deoxyuridine	Antimetabolite
E. coli cytosine deaminase	5-Fluorocytosine	Antimetabolite
Human cytochrome P-450 2B1	Cyclophosphamide, ifosfamide	Alkylator
E. coli XGPRT	6-thioxanthine	Antimetabolite
E. coli DeoD	6-methylpurine-2'-deoxyribonucleoside	Antimetabolite
E. coli nitroreductase	CB1954 (5-aziridin-1-yl)-2,4-dinitrobenzamide	Alkylator

Essential to virus-directed enzyme/prodrug therapy is the identification of therapeutically effective converting enzyme/prodrug combinations. Transduction of tumor cells to express nonmammalian enzymes or to overexpress mammalian enzymes has been employed to selectively increase conversion of prodrugs to their toxic metabolites. Most of the strategies have employed transduction of genes encoding nonmammalian enzymes. Enzyme/prodrug combinations have been in large part based on the experience of treating tumors with conventional chemotherapeutic agents. For example, certain prodrugs have been converted to active antimetabolites that target replicating cells or to cell-cycle–active, phase-nonspecific, alkylating agents (Table 57-1).

HSV-Thymidine Kinase In contrast to mammalian thymidine kinase, HSV-thymidine kinase (HSV-tk) preferentially phosphorylates the antiherpetic nucleoside analogs ganciclovir, acyclovir, and bromovinyl-deoxyuridine to monophosphates. In turn, cellular kinases phosphorylate the monophosphorylated nucleotides to triphosphates, which are then incorporated into replicating DNA by DNA polymerase α. Incorporation of the nucleotide analogs into DNA is associated with chain termination and the induction of DNA single-strand breaks. Compared with cells transduced to express HSV-tk, mammalian cells are relatively resistant to the toxic effects of these agents in vitro and in vivo.

Retroviral and adenoviral vectors have been used to directly transduce tumor cells with HSV-tk. Systemic administration of ganciclovir in the setting of HSV-tk–transduced tumor models is associated with substantial regressions.[33] Significantly, complete eradication of certain tumors is achieved despite transduction of only 10 to 70% of the tumor cell population. These observations contributed to identification of the "bystander effect."[34] Multiple mechanisms may be responsible for this effect. For example, studies have implicated the transfer of phosphorylated ganciclovir nucleotides from HSV-tk–transduced cells to surrounding cells via intracellular gap junctions.[35] Such a mechanism of eliciting a bystander effect is in concert with the finding in tissue culture of a requirement for cell-to-cell contact. In addition, interleukin (IL)-6 and IL-1 secreted by HSV-tk–transduced tumor cells treated with ganciclovir may function as paracrine factors in the induction of nontransduced cell death. The bystander effect has also been attributed to the transfer of signals from dying HSV-tk–transduced cells that induce apoptosis of adjacent cells. In this regard, the association of HSV-tk/ganciclovir treatment with aggregation of death receptors (CD95) and activation of caspases could transduce proapoptotic signals to neighboring cells.[36]

Cytosine Deaminase Cytosine deaminase (CD) is expressed in bacteria and fungi but not in mammalian cells. CD deaminates cytosine to uracil and thereby converts the nontoxic prodrug 5-fluorocytosine (5-FC) to 5-fluorouracil (5-FU). 5-FU is metabolized to the deoxynucleotide monophosphate (FdUMP) in cells, inhibits thymidylate synthase, and blocks methylation of uridylate to thymidylate. DNA synthesis is, in turn, inhibited by the decrease in thymidylate pools. Conversion of 5-FU to fluorouridine triphosphate (FUTP) and incorporation into RNA also disrupts ribosomal RNA and mRNA function. As 5-FU is an effective, but potentially toxic, anticancer agent, transduction of tumor cells to express CD and then administration of 5-FC can obviate normal tissue toxicity by increasing concentrations of 5-FU selectively in the tumor.

An advantage of the CD/5-FC combination is a potentially substantial bystander effect that can compensate for the low transduction efficiencies of the available delivery systems. 5-FU readily diffuses in and out of cells by a nonfacilitated diffusion mechanism. Thus, cells near those transduced to express CD are exposed to a concentration gradient of 5-FU that decreases with increasing distance. Significantly, with as few as 2% of the tumor cells transduced to express CD, significant tumor regressions are induced by administration of 5-FC.[37] Also, CD/5-FC therapy has been reported to be effective in tumor models (ie, gliomas) not sensitive to 5-FU.[38] A potential disadvantage of the CD/5-FC combination derives from diffusion of 5-FU into normal surrounding tissues. Nonetheless, 5-FU is predominantly toxic to dividing, as compared with quiescent, cells; thus, the CD/5-FC combination could be more effective against tumors, such as gliomas, hepatomas, and sarcomas, that reside in mitotically quiescent tissues. In addition, as 5-FU is a known radiosensitizer, the higher local tumor concentrations of this agent that are achieved with CD/5-FC therapy could provide a selective increase in sensitivity to irradiation. In this context, CD/5-FC therapy has been associated with radiosensitization in the treatment of human tumor xenografts.[39,40]

Cytochrome P-450 2B1 Cyclophosphamide and ifosfamide are nontoxic to cells in the absence of conversion by cytochrome P-450 2B1 to their active metabolites. For example, cyclophosphamide is activated by hepatic cytochrome P-450 2B1 to 4-hydroxycyclophosphamide and thereby production of phosphoramide mustard (a DNA alkylator) and acrolein (a protein alkylator).[41] These metabolites circulate systemically to both tumor and normal tissue and result in toxicity to normal cell populations, such as hematopoietic cells and the gastrointestinal mucosa, with a high proliferative index. Cytochrome P-450 2B1 is expressed by hepatocytes and generally not by tumor cells. Thus, transduction of tumor cells to express cytochrome P-450 2B1 results in the direct intratumoral metabolism of cyclophosphamide or ifosphamide. This approach has been used to sensitize gliomas expressing cytochrome P-450 2B1 to cyclophosphamide.[42] In addition, this approach is associated with a bystander effect induced by diffusion of cyclophosphamide metabolites and is not dependent on cell-to-cell contact.[43]

Additional Suicide Genes The *Escherichia coli gpt* gene encodes the xanthine-guanine phosphoribosyl transferase (XGPRT), which converts the xanthine analog 6-thioxanthine to 6-thioxanthine monophosphate by the addition of a ribose phosphate. Within the cell, 6-thioxanthine monophosphate is demethylated to 6-thioguanine monophosphate, a potent inhibitor of nucleic acid synthesis.[44]

The *E. coli DeoD* gene encodes a purine nucleoside phosphorylase (PNP) that, in contrast to mammalian PNP, can hydrolyze the nontoxic 6-methylpurine-2'-deoxyribonucleoside to the toxic purine analog 6-methylpurine.[45]

The *E. coli* nitroreductase (NTR) activates the prodrug CB1954, which is a weak mono-functional alkylating agent. CB1954 is bioreduced by NTR to the 4-hydroxylamino derivative, which is then converted by thioesters (ie, coenzyme A) into a potent bifunctional alkylating agent.[46] As bioreduction of CB1954 is more efficient with NTR than with the cellular DT diaphorase, transduction of tumor cells to express NTR confers sensitivity to the active CB1954 metabolite.

Gene Therapy Directed at Cell-Cycle Control and Apoptosis The discovery of cellular proteins that regulate cell-cycle progression and the induction of apoptosis has provided opportunities to exploit their expression in cancer gene therapy strategies. The following are three such approaches that have been explored by transduction of tumor cells with cellular genes that, when constitutively expressed, disrupt proliferation and induce apoptosis.

p53 The p53 tumor suppressor is induced in the cellular response to genotoxic agents, oxidative stress, hypoxia, and oncogene expression.[47] In the response to DNA damage, p53 activates genes involved in (1) cell-cycle arrest (p21), (2) DNA repair (PCNA, GADD45), and (3) induction of apoptosis (Bax, IGF-bp3). p53 may also induce apoptosis by a mechanism independent of transcriptional activation. Whether p53 induces cell-cycle arrest and DNA repair or apoptosis is thought to be cell-type specific and dependent on the apoptotic threshold of the cell. Importantly, the induction of tumor cell apoptosis by cancer chemotherapeutic agents and radiation is dependent on normal p53 function.[48,49] In addition, the findings that p53 is mutated in approximately 50% of human tumors provide support for developing gene therapy strategies that confer expression of the normal p53 protein.

Several studies demonstrate that transduction of p53 into tumor cells induces cell-cycle arrest or apoptosis in culture and inhibits growth of tumor xenografts in mice.[50–52] Given the limitations of the available gene delivery systems, combining p53 gene therapy with conventional anticancer treatment may be important to achieving complete tumor cell kill. In this context, the combination of p53 gene therapy and cisplatin or radiation increases the apoptotic response of tumor cells and control of tumor xenografts.[13,53,54] Translation of these findings to clinical trials has demonstrated the feasibility of delivering p53 by replication-incompetent retroviral and adenoviral vectors into tumors of patients with non–small-cell lung cancer (NSCLC). In a phase I study, adenovirus-mediated p53 gene transfer was accomplished by computed tomography-guided percutaneous fine-needle injection or by bronchoscopy in 28 NSCLC patients.[55] Evaluation of post-treatment tumor biopsy specimens demonstrated the adenoviral vector in 86% by polymerase chain reaction (PCR) and vector-specific expression of p53 in 46% by reverse transcriptase (RT)-PCR. These studies show that adenoviral-mediated p53 gene therapy is feasible and that, given the safety of this approach, subsequent trials will be performed to assess efficacy.

E2F-1 E2F-1 is a member of the E2F family of transcription factors that regulate the expression of gene products that are primarily involved in S-phase progression.[56] Although E2F-1 is oncogenic,[57] other evidence supports a role as a tumor suppressor. For example, overexpression of E2F-1 can result in apoptosis.[58] Also, E2F-1–deficient mice develop spontaneous tumors.[59,60] Based on these observations, an adenoviral vector was developed to deliver E2F-1 to glioma cells.[61] The results of these studies demonstrate that transduction of E2F-1 induces glioma cell apoptosis and inhibits glioma xenograft growth in nude mice. Thus, E2F-1 gene therapy, like that with p53, provides an approach to inhibit tumor cell growth and induce apoptosis.

p21 *p21* is a cyclin-dependent kinase (cdk) inhibitor. By binding to and inhibiting the activity of cyclin/cdk complexes, *p21* blocks cell-cycle progression. Of importance to cancer gene therapy, transfer of the *p21* gene into tumor cells suppresses tumorigenicity[19,62] and induces apoptosis.[63]

Down-Regulation of Genes Involved in Tumor Progression Another approach to suppress the malignant phenotype involves down-regulation of oncogenes and other genes that contribute to tumor progression. Triple-helix formation, antisense oligonucleotides, ribozymes, and RNA-mediated interference (RNAi) have been developed to target the expression of specific genes. Although down-regulation of genes to treat cancer is theoretically attractive, the available approaches are limited by the need to achieve sufficient suppression of the targeted gene to reverse the transformed phenotype or to induce cell death.

Triple-Helix Formation Triple-helix–forming oligonucleotides (TFOs) bind to duplex DNA in a sequence-specific manner and, as a third strand, block gene transcription (Figure 57-1). The polypurine or polypyrimidine TFO binds to the purine-rich strand in the major DNA groove through Hoogsteen hydrogen bonds.[64] A, C, or G in the TFO binds to G in the purine stretch of duplex DNA. Conversely, T or A in the TFO binds to A in the purine stretch of duplex DNA. To use TFOs as anticancer agents, a target sequence rich in purines must be identified that is involved in regulating the transcription of an oncogene. A complementary TFO is constructed that binds to the target sequence and thereby results in down-regulation of oncogene transcription. TFO binding results in both conformational changes in the major groove and steric effects that block DNA-protein interactions. As a consequence of TFO binding, transcription factors, such as Sp 1 and NFκB, are unable to interact with the altered pro-

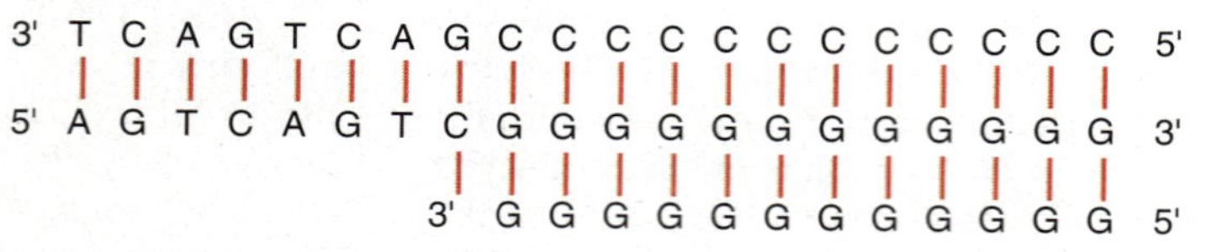

Figure 57-1 Triple-helix formation to block gene transcription.

moter elements. TFOs can also disrupt gene transcription by blocking transcriptional elongation. Another role for TFOs is in directing targeted mutagenesis.[65] For example, linking the TFO to a mutagenic agent, such as psoralen, targets the mutagen to the sequence-specific binding site and induces site-specific mutations.

The first use of a TFO to inhibit oncogene expression was directed at a 27-base–long purine-rich sequence in the P1 region of the c-*myc* promoter.[66] The H-*ras, Her2/neu, IGF1-R, TNF,* and *GM-CSF* genes also have purine-rich sequences that serve as targets for TFOs.[67–72] Importantly, TFO-induced decreases in mRNAs of certain target genes are associated with suppression of growth factor-dependent cell growth (ie, *IGF1-R, TNF, GM-CSF*). Thus, although TFOs target specific gene sequences and, as such, require fewer molecules than when targeting RNA or protein, a requirement for purine-rich regulatory sequences limits this approach. Also, binding affinity needs to be improved to increase the stability of decreasing oncogene expression. In this context, free amino groups have been added to the 3' end of the TFO to decrease susceptibility to nuclease digestion. Intercalating agents (ie, acridine) have been conjugated to TFOs to stabilize binding to duplex DNA. In addition, to ensure adequate intracellular levels of the TFO, these sequences have been incorporated into plasmids or vectors for transfection or transduction of the target cell.

Antisense Antisense (AS) oligonucleotides and complementary DNAs (cDNAs) block translation of target mRNAs in a sequence-specific manner by the formation of complementary base-pairing between the AS molecule and the mRNA (Figure 57-2). AS molecules have been generated as single-stranded RNAs or DNAs with lengths as short as 15 to 20 bases (oligos) or as long as a sequence complementary to the entire mRNA. For AS oligonucleotides, the region of the mRNA to be targeted is crucial and is based on accessibility of that site to the AS molecule. RNA molecules are sensitive to nucleases and have half-lives of 15 to 30 minutes in serum. Therefore, most AS molecules are the more nuclease-resistant deoxynucleotides. To afford further protection against nuclease digestion, AS deoxyoligonucleotides are synthesized as phosphorothioates in which one of the nonbridging oxygens surrounding the phosphate group of the deoxynucleotide is replaced with a sulfur atom.[73] AS molecules designed to bind to the entire mRNA are made by inserting the cDNA into the expression plasmid in the opposite or antisense orientation. AS molecules can function by blocking translation initiation factors from binding near the 5' cap site of the mRNA or by interfering with interaction of the mRNA and ribosomes. In addition, binding of the AS deoxyoligonucleotide to the mRNA creates a hybrid that is sensitive to digestion by RNaseH and thereby degradation of the mRNA.[74]

A 13-base AS deoxyoligonucleotide complementary to Rous sarcoma virus sequences was used more than 20 years ago to inhibit viral translation and replication.[75,76] Since then, the *myb* protooncogene has been targeted by an 18-base AS deoxyoligonucleotide to inhibit the growth of hematopoietic and melanoma cells.[77,78] To target the c-*fos* protooncogene, a retrovirus encoding AS c-*fos* was used to transduce breast carcinoma cells and thereby decrease c-*fos* mRNA levels and inhibit growth.[79] This strategy with the AS c-*fos* retrovirus has been studied in clinical trials.[80] Other AS targets have included cyclin G1 and insulin-like growth factor-1 receptor.[81,82]

Inhibition of tumor angiogenesis represents a promising target for AS therapy because the genetically stable endothelial cells rely on growth factors produced by the tumor cell. In this context, vascular endothelial growth factor (VEGF), an angiogenic factor that is produced by tumor cells, has been targeted for AS-mediated down-regulation.[83-85] Transduction of tumor cells with a vector encoding an AS complementary to VEGF decreased VEGF mRNA and protein levels, decreased microvessel density, decreased tumor growth, and increased tumor necrosis.

Ribozymes Ribozymes (RNA enzymes) are RNA molecules that catalyze site-specific cleavage of RNA (Figure 57-3).[86,87] The activity of ribozymes is dependent on divalent cations, usually Mg2+, which contribute to folding and structural stability.[88] Most naturally occurring ribozymes function in a *cis* manner by cleaving intramolecular RNA. However, RNA in RNAseP, which is involved in transfer ribonucleic acid (tRNA) processing, acts intramolecularly by a *trans* mechanism.[89] The catalytic domains of the ribozymes are named after their secondary structure and include hammerhead, hairpin, axehead, and pseudoknot motifs. Hammerhead ribozyme, which is the most extensively studied ribozyme, consists of three helical stems with the core catalytic domain being adjacent to helix II and flanked by two targeting sequences (helix I and III) that bind to the complementary RNA. The hammerhead cleaves RNA at the 3' end of a NUN triplet (N = any nucleotide) and prefers a G in the first position of the triplet (see Figure 57-3).

The therapeutic potential of ribozymes resides in their ability to cleave mRNA in a sequence-specific manner. For example, to target a certain oncogene, a GUN triplet and flanking sequences are identified in the corresponding mRNA. A hammerhead ribozyme is constructed to target the GUN site by linking the catalytic core and helix II to flanking sequences that are complementary to those in the oncogenic mRNA. Thus, the flanking sequences of the recombinant ribozyme form base pairs with the target RNA and thereby contact the ribozyme catalytic core with the mRNA GUN site.

Expression of the c-*fos* protooncogene is suppressed by a c-fos mRNA-specific ribozyme.[90] Another target for ribozymes is the multidrug resistance gene-1 (*MDR-1*) mRNA,[91] which has a GUC triplet at the –6 to –4 position (upstream to the translation start site). Ribozyme-mediated down-regulation of MDR-1 expression increases the chemosensitivity of otherwise resistant tumor cells. Additional genes targeted by ribozymes include the pleiotrophin growth factor for melanomas and the hepatocyte growth factor for gliomas.[92,93] These ribozyme-mediated approaches target both malignant and normal cells.

Tumor-specific mRNA targets include *bcr-abl,* H-*ras,* and the aberrantly spliced epidermal growth factor receptor. The *bcr-abl* fusion gene has a GUU triplet at the 3' end of exon 3 of the *bcr* gene, which is adjacent to the fusion site in the c-*abl* exon 2.[94] As the flanking sequences of the GUU site reside in both the *bcr* and c-*abl* genes, the ribozyme specifically cleaves the *bcr-abl* fusion mRNA. Activating mutations of the H-*ras* gene have been identified in codons 12, 13, and 61. In codon 12, the normal GGU triplet is mutated to GUU, which serves as a cleavage site for the hammerhead ribozyme.[95] In gliomas, the epidermal growth factor receptor (EGFR) mRNA is aberrantly spliced such that the transcript lacks exons II to VI. Adjacent to the fusion site of exon I to exon VII is a GUA site that is cleaved by a hammerhead ribozyme containing flanking sequences that recognize exon I and exon VII.[96] Thus, this ribozyme can be used to specifically target the aberrantly spliced, but not the intact, EGFR transcript.

RNAi RNAi is a post-transcriptional gene silencing mechanism conserved in nature from plants to mammals. The hints of such a process came from studies of transgenic plants in which overexpression of genes resulted in a paradoxical reduction in expression of the transgene. Such a mechanism was eventually elucidated in mammalian cells and has been developed as a powerful new approach to achieve gene-specific suppression. RNAi is a process in which small interfering RNAs (siRNAs) form double-stranded structures with complementary RNA molecules and mediate their degradation.[97] Cells produce siRNAs by degrading double-stranded RNA molecules (dsRNA) into 21–23 nucleotide base pairs with

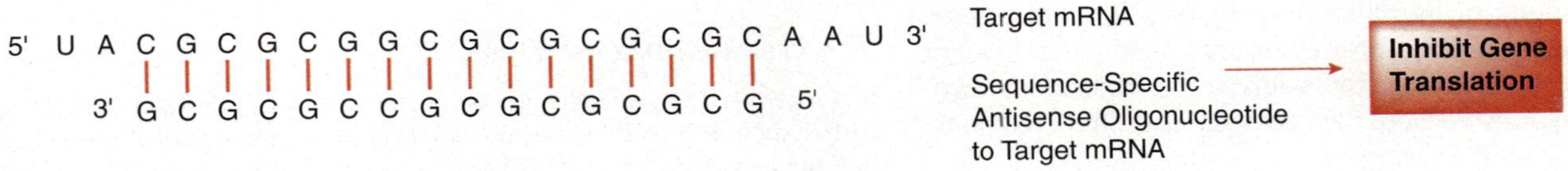

Figure 57-2 Antisense oligonucleotide to block mRNA translation.

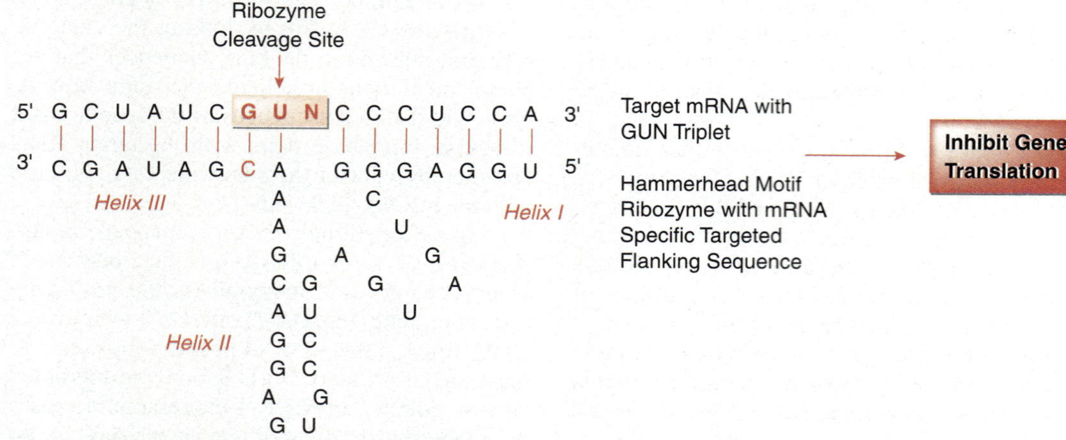

Figure 57-3 Ribozyme-mediated cleavage of mRNA.

2–3 nucleotide overhangs on the 3' end through the action of a ribonuclease termed Dicer (Figure 57-4). One strand of the siRNA then associates with an RNA-induced silencing complex (RISC). The siRNA serves as a template for complementary mRNA resulting in sequence-specific degradation of mRNA (transcriptional inhibition) by RISC. The target RNA is cleaved 10 nucleotides from the 5' end of the anti-sense siRNA sequence. The nuclease activity of RISC is due to eIF2C, a member of the argonaute family of proteins.[98] It has also been reported that the RISC complex can block translation from mRNA. Viruses often produce dsRNA during the course of replication, and RNAi serves as a cellular antiviral mechanism. In principle, RNAi is reminiscent of antisense technology, however, RNAi results in more complete gene suppression than can be achieved with antisense approaches.

The ability to exploit RNAi for gene therapy was initially hampered by activation of interferon pathways after delivery of dsRNA molecules. RNA molecules greater than 30 nucleotides in length activate interferon-mediated signaling cascades resulting in global suppression of protein translation. However, transferring chemically synthesized 21-nucleotide base pair siRNAs into mammalian cells induced gene-specific suppression.[99] Delivering siRNAs for cancer gene therapy strategies may be limited by their degradation in blood and extracellular fluids as well as inefficient delivery methods to tumor cells of siRNA molecules. To overcome such obstacles, DNA vector-based approaches of RNAi have been developed.[100] Plasmids are constructed to express the target RNAi sequence as a palindromic sequence separated by a hairpin loop. These short hairpin RNAs (shRNA) are then processed by Dicer into siRNAs (see Figure 57-4). Additionally, DNA-based RNAi vectors can be incorporated into more efficient viral-based delivery vectors. RNAi has proven to be a powerful technique in the laboratory to identify novel genes involved in the development of cancer, since gene-specific expression can be knocked "down" rapidly without the necessity of producing knockout cell lines.

Strategies have also been devised to employ RNAi as an anticancer therapy. As for antisense, TFO and ribozymes, gain of function mutations (ie, oncogenes) need to be identified that can be targeted and blocked by RNAi. The last few years have seen a rapid expansion in the application of RNAi as a therapeutic agent in experimental tumor models. Here we will provide a few recent examples that demonstrate the different potential uses of RNAi in cancer gene therapy. Liposomal delivery of chemically synthesized siRNAs targeting fatty acid synthase was shown to induce apoptosis in prostate cancer cells, whereas no effect was noted on normal fibroblasts.[101] This study also validates fatty acid synthase as a therapeutic target for certain tumors. Transfection of multidrug-resistant (MDR) leukemic cells with plasmids encoding shRNA for the MDR P-glycoprotein resulted in reduced cell surface expression of P-glycoprotein as well as restored sensitivity to certain chemotherapy agents compared with parental therapy-resistant tumor cells.[102] Although these studies show siRNA can be potentially beneficial in cancer therapy, clinical situations require the ability to efficiently deliver and activate RNAi in pre-existing tumors.

Plasmids encoding shRNAs have been delivered to tumor by different strategies, including viral and nonviral systems. Pegylated liposomes containing shRNA plasmids have been targeted to specific cell membranes and have demonstrated efficacy against intracranial gliomas in murine models.[103] In this study, the pegylated liposome was complexed with antibodies to the mouse transferrin receptor (binding tumor vasculature) and the human insulin receptor (targeted to human glioma cells). This "immunoliposome" was used to deliver a plasmid encoding a shRNA to the oncogenic EGFR receptor found on glioma cells. Interestingly, intravenous delivery of such vector to mice bearing intracranial gliomas significantly increased survival. Nonreplicating viral vectors have also been used to activate RNAi. The HIV lentiviral based vector has been used to target the activating MAPK pathway mutant BRAF (V599E) in melanomas through RNAi.[104] Melanoma cells with mutant BRAF (V599E) were specifically targeted compared with melanoma cells that did not harbor such a mutation by the shRNA. However, replication-deficient viral vectors have been plagued by low transduction efficiency of tumors. To overcome this barrier, replication-competent viral vectors have been

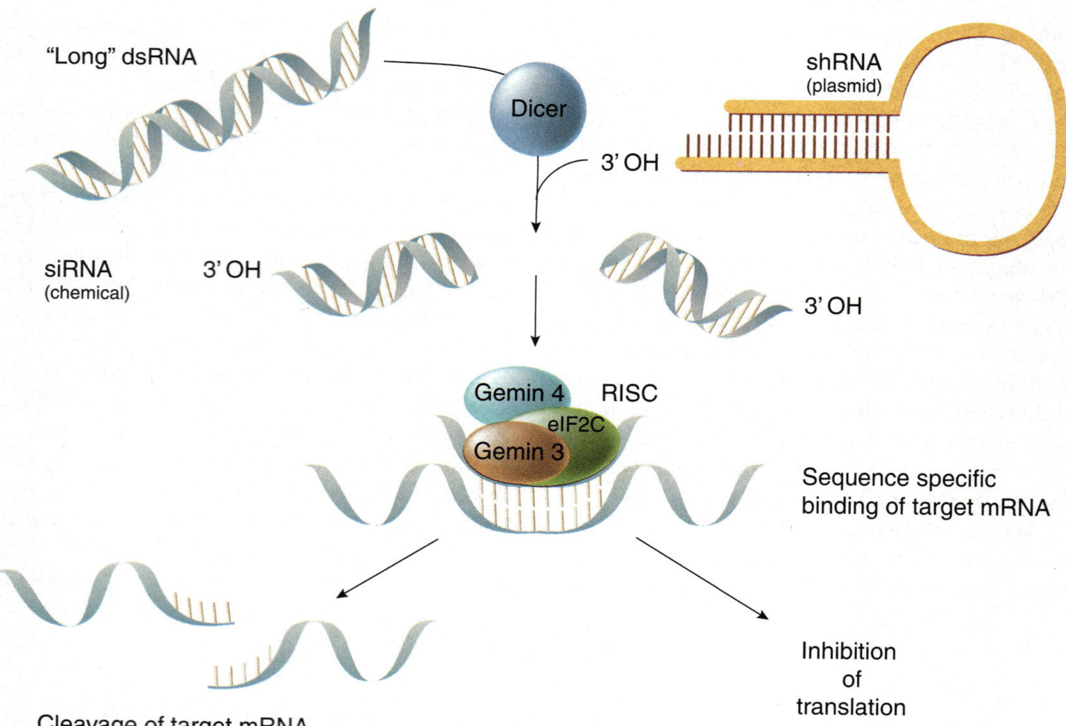

Figure 57-4 RNA interference. dsRNA or a short hairpin RNA (shRNA) is processed by the ribonuclease Dicer into siRNA molecules. siRNAs can also be chemically synthesized and bypass Dicer. siRNA binds to the RNA-induced silencing complex (RISC) to mediated sequence-specific degradation of target mRNA.

investigated for cancer gene therapy (see "Viral Oncolysis" later in this chapter). Replication-competent viruses, however, may encode defense mechanisms to overcome RNAi, since RNAi has been implicated as a cellular antiviral strategy. Studies with replication-competent adenoviruses have shown that such viruses can be employed to deliver plasmid based shRNAs and activate gene-specific RNAi-mediated silencing.[105] This opens the possibility of combining viral oncolysis with RNAi to enhance tumor cell killing.

Immunomodulatory Genes The premise of cancer immunotherapy is based on the assumption that tumor-associated antigens (TAAs) exist and that the host immune system can recognize expression of these antigens by tumor cells. A significant advantage of immunotherapy is thus the ability to recruit the immune system to attack disseminated tumor cells and thereby eliminate both local and metastatic disease. In recent years, the identification of human TAAs and elucidation of the mechanisms responsible for the induction of antitumor immunity have provided the requisite background for bringing to bear the potential of immunotherapy in the treatment of cancer. Importantly, the marriage of immunotherapy and gene therapy has provided an opportunity to induce immunity against specific TAAs and to selectively activate the immune response in the tumor microenvironment. Immunomodulatory genes include those encoding cytokines, costimulatory molecules, and TAAs.

Genetic immunotherapy has been developed to induce the immune recognition of TAAs as "foreign" antigens. In ex vivo approaches, autologous tumor cells transfected in culture to express an immunomodulatory gene encoding a cytokine or costimulatory molecule are reimplanted into the patient. In in vivo therapy, the gene is delivered directly into the tumor or, with certain vaccines, into normal tissues. The identification of specific TAAs is not required when tumor cells are used as the source of antigen; however, in this setting, immunity can be induced to epitopes from both TAAs and normal antigens. Alternatively, vaccination with a gene encoding a TAA, while requiring TAAs that are known, induces antitumor immunity that is antigen specific. Although initial studies focused on the delivery of single immunomodulatory genes, experience supports the combination of genes encoding cytokine, costimulatory molecules, and TAAs to maximally reverse immunologic unresponsiveness or tolerance to tumors.

Cytokine Genes The identification and cloning of cytokine genes has enabled the characterization of the pleiotropic effects of cytokines on the immune system and inflammatory cells. The systemic administration of IL-2 is associated with tumor regressions in subsets of patients with renal cell carcinomas and melanomas; however, systemic delivery of cytokines, such as IL-2, that nonspecifically activate the immune system, is limited by substantial toxicity. As with the delivery of genes encoding prodrug-converting enzymes, cytokine-based gene therapy can restrict expression of the cytokine to the tumor microenvironment. The continuous production of the cytokine by transduced tumor cells also overcomes the disadvantages of circulating peak and trough cytokine levels associated with systemic administration. Of note, cytokine gene immunotherapy functions in the activation of antitumor immunity and is dependent on the expression of TAAs.

Cytokine genes studied in the induction of antitumor immunity include IL-1, IL-2, IL-4, IL-6, IL-12, granulocyte-macrophage colony-stimulating factor (GM-CSF), tumor necrosis factor (TNF), IFN-α, and IFN-γ. The adoptive transfer approach involves transduction of cytokine genes into tumor explants and then lethal irradiation of the tumor cells. For example, prostate cancer tissue is excised, transduced in culture with a retrovirus expressing GM-CSF, irradiated, and then used to vaccinate the patient.[106] Production of GM-CSF recruits dendritic cells to the immunization site for presentation of tumor antigens to CD4+ and CD8+ T cells. Malignant melanomas have also been targeted by this approach using IL-2 as the cytokine.[107]

Direct in vivo delivery of genes into tumors represents an alternative approach. An IFN-γ encoding plasmid directly injected into tumors as naked DNA or in a cationic liposome has resulted in the production of IFN-γ for 7 days.[20] IFN-γ activates T cells, natural killer (NK) cells, and macrophages and induces major histocompatibility complex (MHC) class I and II expression. Gene gun-mediated intratumoral delivery has been used for plasmids expressing IFN-γ, IL-6, TNF, and IL-2.[21] In addition, intramuscular injection of plasmid DNA encoding IFN-α is associated with reductions in tumor growth and in the development of metastases by a CD8+ T-cell–dependent mechanism.[108] IFN-α activates the immune system, decreases tumor cell proliferation, decreases angiogenesis, induces a T-helper pathway, and up-regulates MHC class I expression. A variation on this approach is to add autologous irradiated tumor cells (as a source of antigen) to fibroblasts transfected to express cytokine encoding plasmids. This strategy is advantageous when tumor explants are difficult to culture and transfect ex vivo and has been employed in murine tumor models and phase I clinical trials.[22,109]

Costimulatory Genes The effective activation of T cells is dependent on at least two signals. The first, mediated by MHC molecules, involves antigen-specific interactions with the T-cell receptor (TCR). The second involves costimulation provided by the interaction of B7 molecules (B7-1, B7-2) with CD28 or CTLA4 on the T cell surface. The antigen-TCR interaction can select antigen-specific cytolytic T cells (CTL); however, costimulation is needed for appropriate signaling and clonal expansion of a CTL population. Although most cells express MHC class I molecules for antigen presentation, costimulatory molecules are predominantly found on professional antigen-presenting cells (APCs), such as dendritic cells, Langerhan cells, B cells, monocytes, and macrophages. The lack of costimulatory molecules on tumor cells results in MHC class I presentation of tumor antigens in the absence of costimulation and thereby T cell anergy. Thus, one mechanism for generating antitumor CTL is through the delivery of costimulatory genes to tumor cells such that antigens are presented in the context for CTL activation.

Recombinant vaccinia virus has been used to transduce weakly immunogenic syngeneic murine tumor cells in vitro with genes encoding B7-1 or B7-2.[110] The finding that tumor growth is inhibited following implantation of the transduced tumor cells into immunocompetent mice indicated that costimulation by B7 molecules is sufficient to induce antitumor CTL activity. By contrast, mice immunosuppressed by irradiation failed to reject the B7-transduced tumor cells. Importantly, mice that rejected the transduced tumor also rejected a subsequent challenge with parental nontransduced tumor cells. Other studies demonstrate that B7 costimulation is needed to induce tumor-specific CTL in naive mice, but is not required for tumor rejection upon rechallenge.[111] These findings suggest that transduction of B7 genes into one tumor site could confer rejection of B7-negative tumors at other sites. Transduction of multiple myeloma cells with a recombinant AAV expressing B7-1 or B7-2 also induces specific antitumor CTL activity as measured by T-cell proliferation, production of IL-2 and IFN-γ, and lysis of target cells.[112]

CD40 ligand (CD40L) is selectively expressed on CD4+ T helper cells and stimulates APCs through binding to the CD40 receptor. As the interaction of CD40L with CD40 stimulates antigen-specific T-cell responses, transduction of tumor cells with the CD40L gene can confer more efficient presentation of TAA and enhanced antitumor immunity. For example, intratumoral delivery of an adenovirus expressing CD40L is associated with CD8+ T-cell–mediated antitumor immunity and inhibition of tumor growth in murine models.[113]

Activation of T cells is dependent on multiple factors. Thus, delivery of a single immunomodulatory gene will probably be insufficient to activate effective antitumor immunity. As certain cytokines are involved in expansion of T-cell clones, gene therapy strategies delivering both a cytokine and costimulatory gene could prove synergistic in inducing antitumor immunity. In this context, adenoviral-mediated transduction of both *IL-2* and *B7-1* genes has resulted in a greater than additive antitumor effect in a breast cancer model.[114]

Tumor-Associated Antigen Genes Gene therapy with recombinant vectors that express a TAA has been developed as vaccines for the induction of active specific immunotherapy. Genes that express TAA can be distinguished as (1) endogenous, nonmutated genes that are often overexpressed in tumors; (2) endogenous genes that are mutated and thereby express an altered protein; and (3) exogenous genes. Examples of nonmutated genes associated with tumors include melanoma/melanocyte differentiation antigens (MART-1/MelanA, gp100, tyrosinase, TRP-1, and TRP-2), testicular cancer/testes antigens (MAGE, BAGE, GAGE, and NY-ESO-1), carcinoembryonic antigen (CEA), PSA, and DF3/MUC1.[26,115] TAAs expressed by endogenous mutated genes include p53, cdk4, caspase 8, and β-catenin.[116-118] TAAs from exogenous sources are often derived from viral transformation as exemplified in human papillomaviruspositive cervical cancer.

Gene therapy-based tumor vaccination induces immunity against specific TAAs and is distinguished from the nonspecific immune stimulation associated with transfer of cytokine or costimulatory genes. One method of vaccination involves delivery of the TAA-encoding gene directly into the patient by viral or nonviral systems. Another approach is accomplished through in vitro transfection or transduction of cells, generally APCs, with the TAA gene and reintroduction of these cells to the patient. Direct delivery of the TAA gene at subcutaneous or intradermal sites is used more widely than the ex vivo approach. Expression of the TAA in the epidermis is associated with processing of the TAA by Langerhans cells and thereby with presentation of TAA peptides to T cells.

Vaccination with genes encoding TAAs has been accomplished by transfection and viral transduction. For example, immunization of mice with naked DNA encoding a TAA was achieved by direct intramuscular injection.[119] The immunized mice are protected against challenge with tumor cells expressing the TAA. In clinical trials, recombinant vaccinia virus expressing CEA has been administered intradermally.[120] Peripheral blood lymphocytes from certain vaccinated patients responded to stimulation with CEA in vitro.[120,121] Genes encoding the melanoma/melanocyte differentiation antigens MART-1 and gp100 have been used to vaccinate patients with metastatic melanoma.[122] A long-term complete response was achieved in one patient vaccinated with an adenovirus expressing MART-1. Another phase I trial of a recombinant PSA expressing vaccinia virus vaccine (PROSTVAC) in men with advanced prostate cancer has demonstrated induction of anti-PSA immunity and stabilization of the disease course in certain patients.[123]

Multiple genes encoding TAAs can be constructed in a single plasmid or the genes can be coadministered in separate plasmids. In this context, a potential disadvantage of immunization against a single TAA is that expression of the antigen can be down-regulated in tumors. Thus, immunization against multiple TAAs could decrease the potential for the development of immunologic resistance by the tumor cell. In this strategy, multiple TAAs for a tumor must be known; however, at present, there are few well-characterized TAAs for most tumors. Another approach has been to codeliver the B7-1 gene with the TAA gene to maximize the antitumor immune response. Recombinant vaccinia viruses encoding B7-1 or CEA have been administered as a mixture at a ratio of 1:3 to further stimulate the anti-CEA response.[124] Similar findings have been obtained following vaccination with mixtures of vaccinia viruses expressing B7-1 and MUC1.[125] More advanced vaccinia and fowlpox vector systems have been developed to express B7-1, intercellular adhesion molecule (ICAM), and lymphocyte function-associated antigen (LFA)-3 in a single virus for coadministration with vectors expressing TAAs.[126]

SELECTIVE GENE EXPRESSION

A substantial limitation of conventional cancer chemotherapy and radiotherapy is the toxicity of these agents to normal tissue. The nonselectivity of the available gene delivery systems also renders cancer gene therapy strategies potentially toxic to normal cell populations. Selectivity of gene therapy for tumors has been achieved to date largely by direct intratumoral administration of recombinant vectors. Indeed, the ongoing cancer gene therapy clinical trials are, for the most part, limited to treatment of localized disease. Given that many localized cancers are amenable to surgical resection, and gene therapy of metastatic disease is presently unapproachable, the clinical presentations in which cancer gene therapy could be efficacious are presently few. As such, strategies are under development to increase selectivity of the available vectors by restricting transduction to tumor cells and by employing promoters that are activated in transformed, but not normal cell populations.

Tumor-Selective Retroviruses Retroviruses are classified as either amphotropic or ecotropic on the basis of their species specificity. Amphotropic retroviruses infect most mammalian cells, whereas ecotropic viruses are restricted to murine cells because of specific interaction of a viral glycoprotein and a murine cell surface cationic amino acid transporter. Ecotropic retroviruses have been genetically altered to express a modified glycoprotein and thereby target retroviral gene delivery (Figure 57-5).[127] In one approach to target human breast carcinoma cells with an envelope-modified ecotropic MoMuLV, heregulin, a ligand for the human epidermal growth factor receptor (HER) family, was inserted into the viral glycoprotein.[128] As HER-2 is overexpressed in 20 to 30% of human breast cancers,[129] virus expressing the heregulin chimeric glycoprotein is being developed to selectively target those cells.

Tumor-Selective Adenoviruses Adenoviruses express trimeric fibers that extend from the vertices of the capsid. The fibers terminate into globular knob domains that interact with the cellular coxsackie-adenovirus receptor (CAR).[130] CAR is an integral membrane protein that is widely expressed on diverse cell types. After the fiber knob binds to CAR, internalization of the virus is mediated by arginine-glycine-aspartic acid (RGD) domains in the penton base of the virus that interact with integrins on the cell surface.

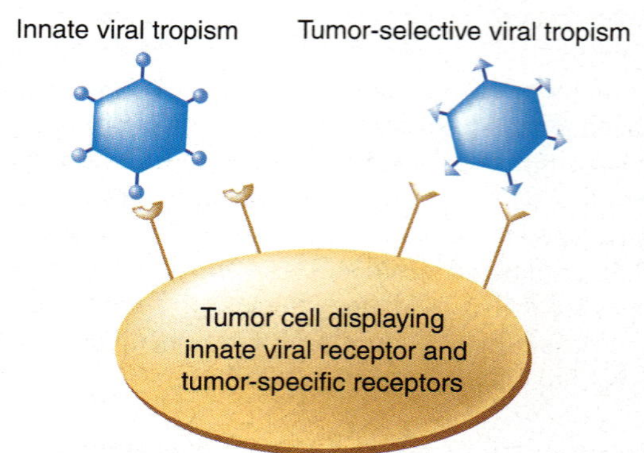

Figure 57-5 Genetic modification of viral receptor proteins to target tumor-specific receptors.

In the "adenobody" approach, an adenoviral neutralizing antibody is fused to a ligand of a specific cell receptor. The antibody–ligand fusion protein binds to the adenoviral fiber and blocks interaction with CAR. The ligand fused to the antibody then redirects the virus to cells expressing that ligand binding receptor (Figure 57-6). For example, epidermal growth factor (EGF) has been linked to an adenoviral antibody to target viral infection of cells that express the EGF receptor.[131] In addition, a bispecific antibody has been used that binds to both the adenovirus and the precarcinoma epithelial cell adhesion molecule (EpCAM).[132] EpCAM is expressed on breast, ovarian, lung, and colon carcinomas. Ovarian carcinoma cells have also been targeted by the adenobody approach by using an antibody fused to the ligand of the basic fibroblast growth factor receptor[2,133,134] As the adenobody approach is dependent on in vitro incubation of the fusion antibody and virus before tumor inoculation, a more appealing strategy is to genetically alter the adenoviral fibers to directly recognize receptors overexpressed on tumor cells. To this end, adenoviral chimeric fibers have been generated that alter adenoviral tropism,[135] and peptide epitopes have been inserted into the H1 loop of the adenoviral fiber domain.[136]

Importantly, certain tumors express low levels of CAR and are thereby resistant to adenoviral gene transfer.[137] To bypass CAR-dependent attachment, adenoviral vectors have been constructed that incorporate an RGD peptide within

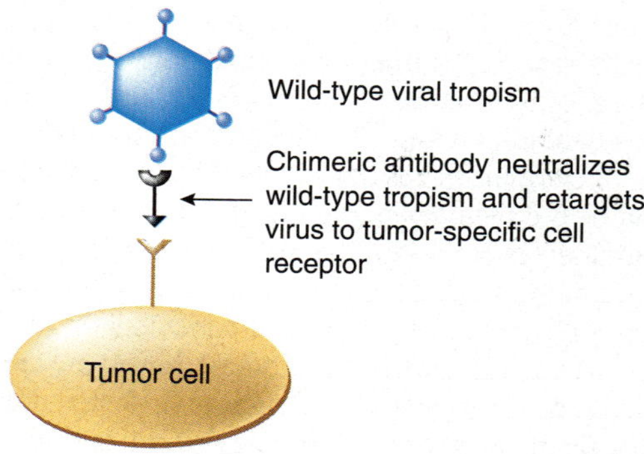

Figure 57-6 Chimeric antibodies to alter viral tropism for tumor cells.

the H1 loop of the adenoviral fiber knob domain.[138] Certain tumors overexpress classes of RGD-binding integrins. For example, the α2β1 and α3β1 integrins are commonly overexpressed by squamous cell carcinomas of the head and neck. The RGD-containing adenoviral vectors have been reported to selectively target both head and neck cancer and ovarian cancer cells.[139,140]

Tumor-Selective Adeno-Associated Virus AAV has been genetically altered to express modified capsid proteins.[141] A 14-aminoacid–peptide sequence containing the RGD motif has been inserted into AAV2 capsid proteins. The capsid-modified AAV2 infects cells resistant to AAV2 infection by integrin-mediated binding. Although this approach does not directly translate to tumor targeting, the results support the concept that AAV capsid modifications will provide another strategy to selectively target gene transfer to tumor cells.

Tumor-Selective Promoters/Enhancers Viral vectors have been generated that infect a broad spectrum of cell types but only express the transgene in selected cells. Such selectivity of gene expression has been achieved by constructing these vectors with promoters/enhancers that confer tumor- or tissue-selective transcription (Figure 57-7). Tissue-restricted transcriptional control elements include the α1-antitrypsin and albumin promoters (hepatocyte-selective), tyrosine hydrolase promoter (melanocytes), villin promoter (intestinal epithelium), glial fibrillary acidic protein promoter (astrocytes), myelin basic protein (glial cells), and the immunoglobulin gene enhancer (B lymphocytes). If a tissue, such as the prostate, is nonessential, then tissue-selective promoters that target both tumor and normal cells can be used for cancer gene therapy. Alternatively, if only the tumor can be targeted and the surrounding normal tissue of an essential organ must be spared, then the approach necessitates use of tumor-selective promoters. Tumor-selective promoter elements have been identified in the following genes: α-fetoprotein (hepatoma), DF3/MUC1 (breast and other carcinomas), thyroglobulin (thyroid carcinoma), prostate-specific antigen (prostate carcinoma), and carcinoembryonic antigen (breast, lung, and colorectal carcinomas). In this context, the DF3/MUC1 promoter has been incorporated into retroviral and adenoviral vectors to selectively drive the expression of transgenes in human carcinomas that overexpress the MUC1 gene.[142–145] Also, as the Myc/Max family of transcription factors are overexpressed in certain tumor cells, the promoter elements of these genes have been used to selectively drive transgene expression in Myc/Max-overexpressing tumors. The identification of new genes that are transcriptionally activated in tumor, as compared with normal, cells should be rapidly advanced by the recent developments in DNA chip technologies and thereby the definition of new classes of tissue- and tumor-selective promoters for cancer gene therapy.

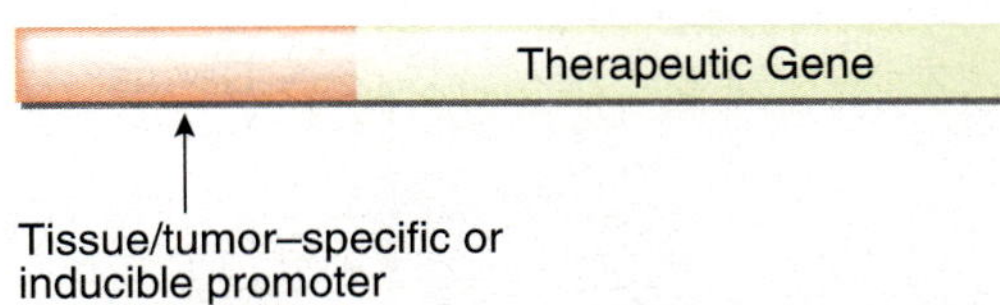

Figure 57-7 Transcriptional regulation of the delivered therapeutic gene through selective promoters and enhancers.

Inducible Promoters Another strategy for regulating transgene expression is through the use of inducible promoters (see Figure 57-7). In the tetracycline repressor system, the bacterial tet operon mediates transcriptional repression of a heterologous promoter in the presence of the tet repressor (tetR) protein. The tetR gene is expressed by another vector or by another coding sequence in the same vector. Transcriptional repression is relieved by exposure to tetracycline, which binds to tetR and thereby prevents its interaction with the tet operon. Release from transcriptional repression in mammals is achieved at doses of tetracycline significantly lower than those used for antimicrobial purposes. This approach, although potentially amenable to regulating the level of transgene expression, activates transcription in both transduced tumor and normal cells and, thus, has no impact on selectivity.

Another targeted gene therapy strategy has been developed with cancer therapy inducible promoters. One of the cellular responses to cancer therapeutic agents is transcriptional up-regulation of genes.[146] Such genes products dictate the cellular response to the perceived insult. Upon delivery of ionizing radiation (IR) to cells, the early growth response-1 (Egr-1) gene is induced.[147] One implication of this result is that the promoter of Egr-1 can act as a "molecular switch" to activate a ligated transgene following IR (Figure 57-8). TNFα is known to be tumoricidal, however, systemic toxicity of TNFα is a limiting factor. By placing the cDNA for TNFα upstream of the Egr-1 promoter, expression of TNFα can be placed under the control of IR.[148] This treatment paradigm has been incorporated with a replication-defective adenovirus (designated TNFerade).[149] TNFα gene expression is restricted by 2 mechanisms. First, the replication-defective virus is delivered directly to the tumor bed via intratumoral inoculation and taken up by the surrounding tumor cells. Second, TNFα expression is activated in the targeted irradiated field (Figure 57-9). An advantage of the radiation-inducible promoters is that transgene expression can be regulated in both a spatial and temporal manner. Both the location expression and the timing of transgene expression are restricted to the targeted irradiated field. Any plasmids delivered to cells located outside of the irradiated field, in principle, have low, if any, expression of the transgene. The replication-defective adenovirus containing the EGR-TNFα construct has entered phase I/II clinical trials in combination with radiation in a variety of tumors.[150]

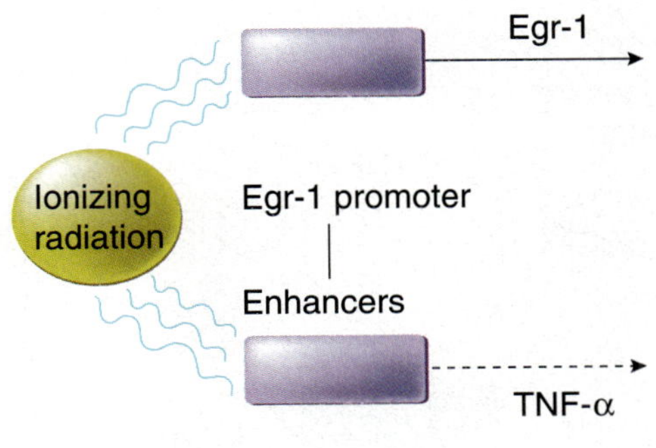

Figure 57-8 Creating ionizing radiation-activated therapeutic genes. Ionizing radiation (IR)-induced gene promoters are identified and then ligated to cDNA sequences whose gene products have antitumor activity.

Although IR-mediated gene therapy is designed for improving local tumor control, the paradigm has been expanded to incorporate chemotherapy for systemic cancer therapy. IR activates the Egr-1 promoter through the production of free radical oxygen species.[147] Therefore, any agent capable of producing intracellular free radical oxygen species can activate the Egr-1 promoter (Figure 57-10). More recent studies demonstrated activation of the EGR-TNF construct by cisplatin and other genotoxic chemotherapeutic agents.[151,152] Another gene product activated by chemotherapeutic agents is mdr1.[153] In a similar vein to TNFerade, the chemotherapeutic response elements within the mdr promoter were ligated to TNFα.[154] In the above examples, not only is TNFα transcription regulated by IR/chemotherapy, but also the newly produced TNFα interacts synergistically with the inducing cancer agents for enhanced tumor cell kill (see Figure 57-10). Importantly, the above combinations have been shown to target not only tumor cells, but in addition the surrounding tumor vasculature.[155] The advantages of this are at least twofold. First, the relative genetic stability of endothelial cells suggests that resistance to this therapeutic approach will not develop. Second, diverse histologic tumors may be amenable to such therapy by targeting the common vasculature instead of varied tumor types.

The Cre recombinase/loxP system is a more recently developed approach to target gene transcription in tumor cells (Figure 57-11). In this system, DNA sequences are targeted ("floxed") with 34 bp palindromes or loxP sites. The Cre recombinase binds to the loxP sites and, through homologous recombination, deletes the sequences between those sites. This system has been exploited for suicide gene therapy of thyroid cancer.[156] The Cre gene is placed under control of the thyroglobulin promoter and is transcribed in thyroglobulin-expressing cells. The therapeutic gene is placed in a second plasmid under the control of a constitutive promoter; however, the promoter and therapeutic gene are separated by a loxP-marked DNA sequence that prevents transcription. Thus, under these conditions, there is no

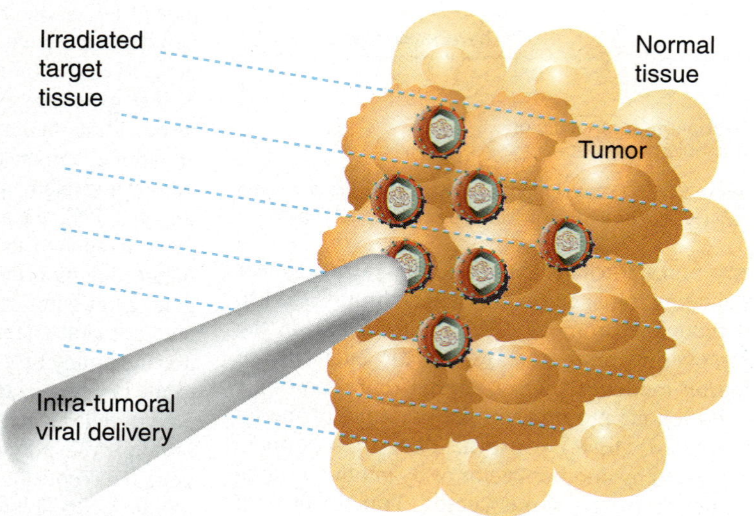

Figure 57-9 Spatial and temporal control of gene therapy by ionizing radiation (IR) is physically targeted to the tumor target volume. Intratumoral delivery of genetic constructs further restricts the spatial effects of combined therapy. In addition, temporal control of gene therapy is achieved by controlling the activity of gene therapy upon timing delivery of IR.

expression of the therapeutic gene. When a thyroid cancer cell is transduced to express both the Cre recombinase plasmid and the therapeutic gene plasmid, the following occur: (1) the Cre recombinase is expressed by activation of the thyroglobulin promoter, (2) the Cre recombinase deletes the loxP-targeted sequence that prevents transcription of the therapeutic gene, and (3) the therapeutic gene is then transcribed under control of the constitutive promoter. This strategy has also been reported for CEA-expressing tumor cells by placing the Cre recombinase under control of the CEA promoter.[157]

VIRAL ONCOLYSIS

The use of a replicating virus as an antitumor agent is based on the premise that as a consequence of successful viral replication, multiple viral progeny are released from the destroyed cell to infect surrounding cells. Inoculation of a tumor with a competent virus thus results in death of infected tumor cells as the virus replicates throughout the tumor (viral oncolysis). Replication-competent viruses overcome one of the major limitations of replication-deficient viruses, that is, the ability to infect an entire tumor cell population. In principle, initial infection of only a few tumor cells would initiate a chain reaction, such that surrounding tumor cells become infected by viral progeny released from the initially infected cells. Once the virus reaches and infects the surrounding normal tissue, replication of a virus that is selective for tumor cells would be aborted, sparing normal tissue from the pathogenic effects of the wild-type parental virus.

The concept of viral oncolysis was introduced at the beginning of the twentieth century. In 1904, Dock reported a dramatic remission of leukemia in a woman following a presumed infection by influenza virus.[158] The first experimental demonstration of viral oncolysis is attributed to Levaditi and Nicolau, who showed that vaccinia virus was able to inhibit tumors in both mice and rats.[159] In the 1950s and 1960s, trials were conducted with multiple viruses that had been selected in tissue culture for their ability to replicate in tumor cells. However, no such clinically active viruses were identified and enthusiasm waned.

More recently, the replicative life cycle of many viruses has been elucidated at the molecular level, including the sequence of viral genomes and the functions of viral proteins. In a similar vein, mutations occurring in the transformation from wild-type to cancer cell have also begun to be unraveled. With such knowledge, the concept of viral oncolysis has reemerged with a more "rational" approach. A common theme emerging from studying the interaction of viruses with cells is the presence of viral proteins whose function is to overcome host-cell antiviral defenses (Figure 57-12A). Two examples of cellular antiviral defenses include double-strand RNA-dependent protein kinase (PKR) and the tumor-suppressor protein p53. Upon viral infection, double-stranded RNA production results in the autophosphorylation and activation of PKR, which mediates antiviral defenses, including the phosphorylation and inactivation of the translation initiation factor, eIF-2α. Viral proteins, such as the herpes simplex virus-1 encoded $\gamma_1$34.5, reverse the inhibition of translation initiation and thereby allow viral protein synthesis to proceed. Viruses also encode proteins to inactivate p53 including the adenoviral protein E1B. Curiously, the malignant cell phenotype evolves with mutations that inactivate cellular antiviral proteins. Activating mutations in Ras are implicated in inhibiting PKR. Inactivation of p53 in tumor cells occurs by mutations in p53 itself or in the proteins regulating p53. In principle, attenuated replication-competent viruses could be constructed to target tumor cells that harbor such mutations by deleting the viral protein that corresponds to the mutated cellular protein (Figure 57-12B). Such a mutant virus could replicate in tumor cells with disarmed cellular defenses and produce attenuated viral progeny to infect surrounding tumor cells. However, the mutant virus would be unable to grow in wild-type cells because it lacks the viral protein necessary to counteract a particular cellular antiviral defense. In general, this is the current paradigm for constructing replication-competent tumor-selective viruses.

With the use of live, attenuated viruses for cancer therapy, certain safety considerations are warranted. The attenuated virus should be genetically stable such that mutants do not revert to wild-type phenotypes. Engineering multiple mutations into the therapeutic virus can minimize reversion of attenuated viruses to wild-type viruses. Employing nonintegrating viruses prevents untoward consequences of genetic mutations in the host cell. Finally, the pathology induced by the virus should be well characterized and minimal. Effective anti-

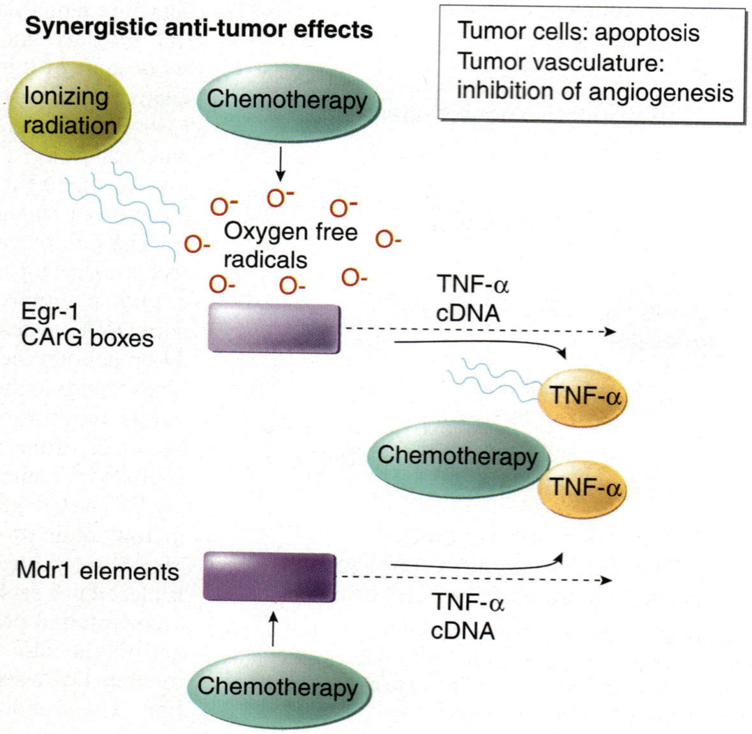

Figure 57-10 Local/systemic therapy to activate and synergize gene therapy. IR and chemotherapy activate gene expression through responsive promoter elements. Moreover, the transcribed therapeutic gene products interact synergistically with chemotherapy/IR to enhance tumor kill by targeting both tumor cells and the tumor vasculature.

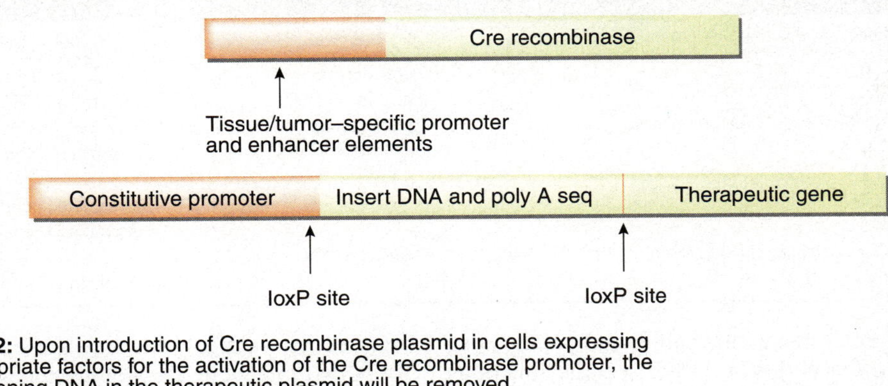

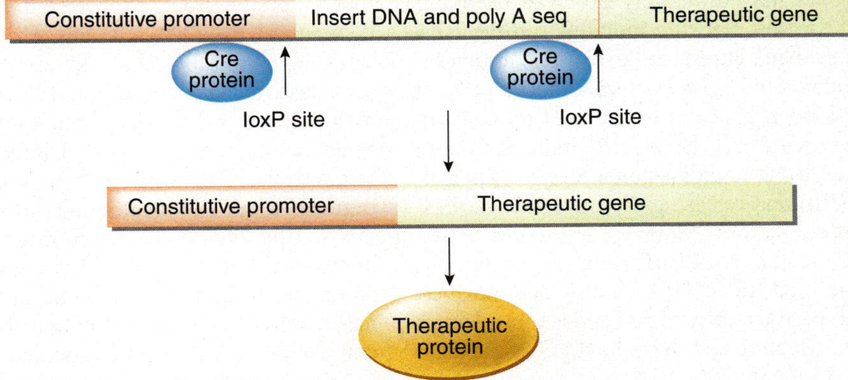

Figure 57-11 Cre recombinase/loxP system for cancer gene therapy.

viral drugs should be available in the event of toxicity from the viral therapy. The following are examples of oncolytic viruses currently being pursued in the laboratory and the clinic (Table 57-2).

Oncolytic Adenovirus The basic biology of adenoviruses was briefly introduced above. Important in the development of replication-competent adenoviruses are two early adenoviral gene products, E1A and E1B. Although both viral proteins are multifunctional, two well-characterized functions have played a pivotal role in the development of oncolytic adenoviruses. E1A binds to Rb pocket proteins and releases E2F proteins to induce S-phase gene synthesis, facilitating viral replication.[160] In response to adenoviral infection and the effects of E1A, p53 is activated and induces cell-cycle arrest or apoptosis, presumably as mechanisms to prevent viral replication. E1B is involved in transcriptionally silencing and degrading p53 and thereby blocks p53 antiviral effects. Because p53 is mutated or deleted in approximately 50% of human tumors, p53-mediated antiviral defense mechanisms are not available to those cells. To exploit this tumor cell phenotype, an adenovirus (*dl*1520; ONYX-015) with a deletion in the 55-kilodalton (kDa), E1B gene was created.[161] *dl*1520 was predicted to replicate preferentially in cells with nonfunctional p53, but not in cells expressing functional p53. As such, the virus would continuously replicate in and lyse tumor cells harboring nonfunctional p53. When the virus encounters normal tissue, replication is abrogated by p53-dependent defense mechanisms. Conflicting results, however, have been reported in the relationship between replication of the E1B-deleted virus and tumor cell p53 status.[162–164] A partial resolution to these apparently conflicting results lies in understanding the regulation of p53 stability and function by the p53-Mdm2 autoregulatory loop (Figure 57-13).

In cells with wild-type p53 gene, p53 protein has a relatively short half-life in unstressed cells and is also functionally silent. A major regulator of p53 function and stability is the protooncogene Mdm2.[165] Mdm2 inhibits p53 function by blocking

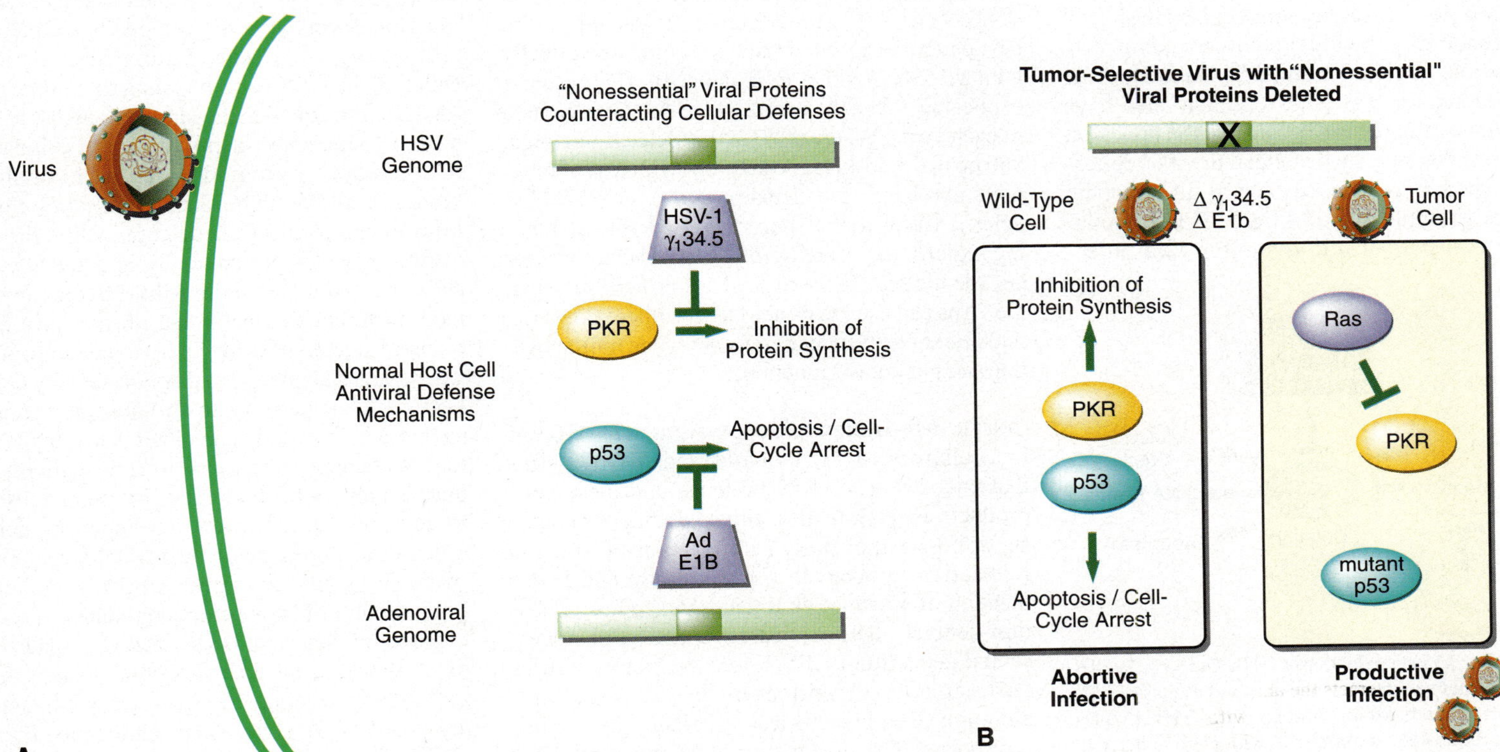

Figure 57-12 Creating replication-conditional oncolytic viruses. **A,** Specific viral gene products are involved in counteracting host cell antiviral defense mechanisms. **B,** Deletion of these viral gene products creates a virus that can only replicate in tumor cells with specific mutations.

Table 57-2 Representative Replication-Competent Tumor-Selective Viruses

Parental Virus	Selective Virus	Viral Gene(s) Deleted/Mutated	Cellular Protein Target	Tumor Cell Selectivity
Adenovirus	*dl*1520 (Onyx-015)	E1B	Inactivates p53	Nonfunctional p53
	eg, *dl*922-947	E1A	Inactivates pRb	Disrupted G1S checkpoint
Herpes simplex virus-1	hrR3	UL39 (ribonucleotide reductase)	Creates deoxynucleotides	Cycling cells
	G207	γ134.5	Dephosphorylates eIF-2	? Activating Ras mutation
		UL39		
	R7020 (NV1020)	UL24	?	Attenuated neurovirulence
		UL56	?	Attenuated virulence
		Internal invert region (one copy of 134.5 0 and 4)	Dephosphorylates eIF-2	
Reovirus	Wild-type	None		Activating Ras mutation

p53 transcriptional activity, exporting p53 to the cytoplasm, and acting as an E3 ubiquitin ligase to promote proteasome-dependent p53 degradation. Mdm2 could be thought of as a functional homolog of the 55-kDa E1B in terms of inactivating p53 (see Figure 57-13). Also included in the regulatory pathway of p53 is p14ARF, a member of the INK4 tumor-suppressor proteins. p14ARF promotes the stability of p53 by binding to and blocking the E3 ubiquitin ligase activity of Mdm2. Mdm2 is amplified in 7% of human tumors and can further suppress the activity of p53. Deletion or inactivating mutations of p14ARF in tumor cells results in the unopposed action of Mdm2, again resulting in functionally inactive p53. Therefore, *dl*1520 may be able to preferentially replicate in tumor cells with inactivating mutations in p53 or p14ARF, as well as in cells with activating mutations in Mdm2. Mutations in any three of these proteins could result in the same phenotype, that is, nonfunctional p53. In support of this hypothesis, *dl*1520 was shown to replicate preferentially in colon carcinoma and mesothelioma cell lines that have loss of p14ARF.[166]

In creating *dl*1520, 827 base pairs were deleted from the E1B gene region. Because of their limited coding capacity, viruses have maximized the utility of their genome, with viral proteins encoding multiple functions. Deletion of the 55-kDa E1B, while done to target the p53 path-way, may also have unexpected consequences because of the knockout of functions that may be beneficial to viral replication and thereby reduce efficacy as an oncolytic agent. For example, the 55-kDa E1B also modulates the transport of mRNA during viral infection.[167] Point mutations within viral proteins may result in the ability to target specific functions, while sparing other functions of the viral protein. Such viruses may ultimately prove to be better oncolytic viruses. Specific mutations in the E1A protein have been introduced to test this principle.

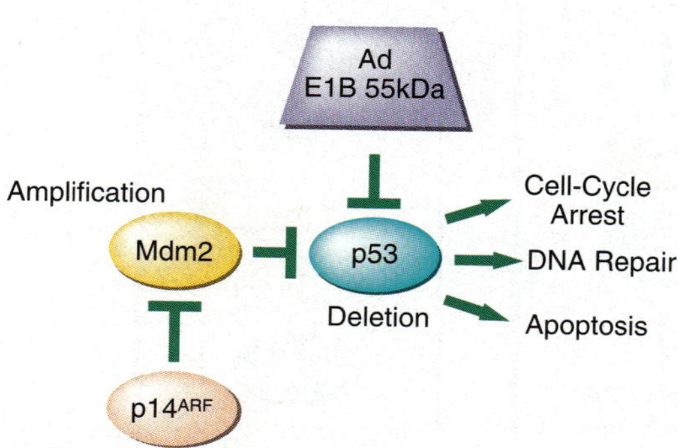

Figure 57-13 p53 and adenovirus E1B. The 55-kDa E1B adenoviral protein counteracts the antiviral effects of p53. In principle, an adenoviral mutant with E1B 55 kDa deleted can replicate in a tumor cell with (1) p53 deleted/nonfunctional, (2) Mdm2 amplified, or (3) p14ARF deleted/nonfunctional.

The adenoviral E1A protein encodes at least two functions, S-phase induction and transactivation of adenoviral early genes. E1A induces S phase by binding to the retinoblastoma family of pocket proteins (Rb) and releasing the inhibition on E2F transcription factors. Mapping studies revealed amino acids 121 to 127 of the E1A protein are required to bind Rb.[168] E1A binding and inactivation of Rb permits adenovirus replication in either quiescent or cycling cells by inducing S-phase gene synthesis. Deletion of the E1A amino acids responsible for Rb binding blocks E2F transactivation and inhibits adenoviral replication in quiescent cells. Such a mutant virus preferentially replicates in cycling cells and it may replicate more efficiently in tumor cells, which routinely contain inactivating mutations of G1/S checkpoint proteins. Two groups recently created such an E1A mutant virus with $<$ 30 bp deleted from the E1A region, delta24 and *dl*922-947.[169,170] The *dl*922-947 virus appears to be a better oncolytic virus when compared directly with *dl*1520 (55-kDa E1B deleted). This result is explicable, given the nature of the deletions created in each virus. Whereas *dl*1520 is deleted of almost 900 bp in the 55-kDa E1B region (with loss of functions unrelated to p53 inactivation), *dl*922-947 is deleted in only a small portion of E1A (the Rb binding region). Importantly, *dl*922-947 mutant viruses encode the remainder of the E1A protein such that the virus can use the protein for its other known (ie, p300 binding and adenoviral early gene transactivation) and unknown functions.

Oncolytic Herpes Simplex Virus-1 HSV-1 is a relatively large double-stranded DNA virus that encodes at least 89 proteins, and these gene products are classified as either essential or nonessential. Essential proteins are required for viral replication to occur in tissue culture, and hence deletion of essential viral genes generates replication-deficient herpes viruses. Deletion of nonessential genes from HSV-1 genome creates viruses still capable of replicating in tissue culture, although usually with less efficiency than wild-type virus. The designation of nonessential for these gene products is something of a misnomer. Invariably, deletion of nonessential genes results in viruses that are highly attenuated in animal models of HSV-1 infection. Many of the nonessential viral gene products are homologous to cellular proteins that are preferentially expressed in cycling cells as compared with quiescent cells. Examples of such viral genes are thymidine kinase, ribonucleotide reductase, dUTPase, and uracil DNA glycosylase. Wild-type HSV-1 encodes such homologs because in the natural course of HSV-1 infection, the virus infects quiescent, postmitotic sensory neurons and requires a pool of nucleotides to replicate viral DNA. Elucidating the function of essential and nonessential genes of HSV-1 along with the virus' ability to infect both quiescent and cycling cells has resulted in the development of replication-competent, tumor-selective attenuated HSV-1.

The first example of the creation of a genetically engineered, replication-competent HSV-1 exploited the differences of the intracellular environment of quiescent and cycling cells (ie, tumor cells) as an oncolytic agent for glioblastoma multiforme (GBM). Because GBM grow in an environment surrounded by quiescent terminally differentiated neurons, an attenuated replication-competent HSV-1 was designed to infect replicating glioma cells, but not terminally differentiated noncycling cells (surrounding neural tissue). Deleting the HSV gene encoding thymidine kinase (tk, UL23) resulted in the viral mutant dlsptk.[171] To replicate efficiently, dlsptk requires a cellular pool of nucleotides created by cellular thymidine kinase. Cellular thymidine kinase functions in *trans* to complement the deletion within the virus. dlsptk replicates preferentially in actively cycling cells expressing thymidine kinase but not in terminally differentiated cells that do not have excess pools of nucleotides for DNA replication. A considerable disadvantage of dlsptk is that, by deleting HSV-1-tk, sensitivity to the common antiviral agents acyclovir and ganciclovir is lost in the event that it becomes necessary to treat patients with unacceptable viral toxicities. To retain sensitivity to acyclovir, viruses were developed by deleting other viral genes involved in DNA replication. Inactivating the viral gene UL39, encoding the large subunit of ribonucleotide reductase, resulted in the tumor-selective HSV-1 hrR3.[172] Inactivation of UL39 was achieved by inserting the gene for lac Z. Similarly, deleting the HSV-1 gene UL2, encoding uracil DNA glycosylase, also created a virus (3616UB) that selectively replicates in cycling cells, which can complement for the function of the deleted viral protein.[173]

A major concern in the use of replication-competent HSV-1 in gene therapy is its neurovirulence with ensuing encephalitis. An ideal oncolytic virus would be non-neurovirulent. One HSV-1 gene involved in neurovirulence is γ134.5. Deleting both copies of the γ134.5 gene (virus R3616), present in the repeat regions, reduced HSV-1 neurovirulence by greater than five orders of magnitude in murine models.[174] The γ134.5 gene product (ICP 34.5) is involved in counteracting cellular antiviral machinery. A common innate host cell viral defense mechanism is activation of double-stranded RNA-dependent protein kinase, which phosphorylates the alpha subunit of translation initiation factor 2 (eIF-2α) and blocks translation of viral mRNA (see Figure 57-14). ICP 34.5 effectively reverses the effects of PKR on eIF-2α by binding to cellular protein phosphatase-1 (PP1), dephosphorylating eIF-2α, and preventing protein synthesis shutoff.[175,176] R3616 is both safe and effective in the treatment of experimental gliomas in murine models.[177,178] How is R3616 capable of replicating in tumor cells when protein synthesis is shutoff by PKR in infected cells? Part of the answer may involve the Ras signaling pathway in tumor cells compared with normal cells.[179] Tumor cells routinely contain activating mutations in the Ras signaling pathway.[180] Thus, activated Ras in tumor cells may complement the deletion of γ134.5 in HSV-1 to allow tumor-selective viral replication (see Figure 57-14).

Although viruses deleted for γ134.5 are safe, they replicate sluggishly in tumor cells. To create a more robust virus, second-site mutant viruses of R3616 have been isolated that circumvent the protein synthesis shutoff phenotype of γ134.5 deletion viruses.[181] One compensatory second-site mutation in R3616 involves the US11 gene and the US12 promoter. The US11 gene product binds to RNA and is expressed with late (γ) kinetics, whereas the US12 gene is regulated as an immediate-early (α) gene. Second-site R3616 mutants that overcome PKR-mediated protein synthesis shutoff link the US11 gene with the US12 promoter. US11 expressed with immediate-early kinetics compensates for deletions in γ134.5, in that eIF-2α is not phosphorylated and protein translation is not inhibited.[182] Viruses deleted in γ134.5, but expressing US11 with α kinetics, replicate to higher titers compared with γ134.5 null virus, R3616, and have greater efficacy as oncolytic agents.[183,184]

G207 was generated by deleting the ribonucleotide reductase and γ134.5 genes of HSV-1.[185] With deletions in two genes, this virus has a lower probability of reversion to a wild-type phenotype, thereby increasing its safety profile. Also, there are two mechanisms of targeting tumor cells. The deletion of ribonucleotide reductase targets the virus to cycling cells, and deletion of the γ134.5 gene may target cells with an activated Ras pathway.

The attenuated herpes virus R7020 was designed as a potential vaccine for HSV-1 and HSV-2.[186] R7020 was constructed by deleting the internal inverted repeat sequence of HSV-1 and replacing this region with glycoproteins from HSV-2. Theoretically, cells infected with R7020 would express both HSV-1 and HSV-2 glycoproteins, and antibodies would be generated to both viruses. Because R7020 was designed as a vaccine for healthy individuals, it underwent stringent safety studies followed by limited clinical trials. However, R7020 did not prove efficacious as a vaccine. Nonetheless, with the extensive safety profile, R7020 was studied as a potential antitumor agent. Studies demonstrate that R7020 (also known as NV1020) replicates efficiently in a variety of tumor xenografts, and there is no evidence for tumor resistance to repeated inoculation.[187,188]

Oncolytic Reovirus Reovirus (respiratory enteric orphan virus) is a double-stranded RNA virus that is associated with mild upper respiratory infections or enteritis. No specific disease is associated with reovirus infection, and hence the designation of "orphan." Reovirus infection of permissive cells results in activation of transcription factors (NF1cB), MAP kinase pathways, and cell-cycle arrest, as well as apoptosis.[189] Being a double-stranded RNA virus, replication of the viral genome activates double-stranded RNA-activated protein kinase (PKR). As mentioned above, activated PKR phosphorylates the translation initiation factor, eIF-2α, resulting in the cessation of protein synthesis (Figure 57-14). For reovirus replication to occur, the actions of PKR need to be inhibited. Important to the application of reovirus as an oncolytic agent was the observation that certain permissive cell lines (in which protein synthesis was not shut off) had activating mutations in the Ras signaling pathway. Cell lines resistant to reovirus infection in culture could be made sensitive to infection by transfecting genes encoding proteins that activate the Ras pathway, that is, EGFR, v-erbB oncogene, or SOS.[190–192] These data suggest the Ras pathway counteracted PKR and enabled reovirus replication. How Ras activation allows reovirus replication to proceed remains unclear; however, evidence suggests that Ras activation induces an inhibitor of PKR.[177]

The translation of these observations in employing reovirus as an oncolytic virus is coupled with the fact that 30% of human tumors have Ras-activating mutations.[181] Such mutations include activating mutations within Ras itself, or activating mutations in receptor tyrosine kinases (EGFR or platelet-derived growth factor receptor [PDGFR]). Tumors harboring such mutations would be predicted to permit reovirus replication. Initial results in tumor models appear to support such a hypothesis. Tumors with activated Ras (ie, gliomas, colorectal, and ovarian cancers) are sensitive to reovirus infection.[193–195] The interest in reovirus oncolytic therapy rests in its natural safety profile, with a lack of associated disease pathology upon wild-type reovirus infection.

Transcriptionally Targeted Oncolytic Viruses Another technique to achieve tumor-specific cytotoxicity with replication-competent viruses is to place expression of viral essential genes under the transcriptional control of tumor-specific promoter/enhancer sequences. Essential viral genes are absolutely required to be expressed for viral replication to proceed. Normally these genes are placed under the control of ubiquitous cellular transcription factors and/or viral transactivators (Figure 57-15A). However, as mentioned previously, therapeutic gene constructs for cancer have been placed under the transcriptional control of tumor/tissue-specific or -inducible promoter sequences. Such a strategy restricts expression of the therapeutic gene to cell types that express requisite transcription factors for the promoter. In an analogous strategy, the replicating virus can be thought of as one large therapeutic gene construct. Placing the expression of a viral essential gene under the control of tumor/tissue-specific promoter/enhancer elements restricts viral replication to the targeted tumor/tissue type (Figure 57-15B). Viral infection of other cells that do not express the necessary transcription factor(s) results in nonexpression of the essential gene and an abortive infection without progeny virus. Transcriptionally targeted replicating viruses have been created using either adenovirus or HSV-1.

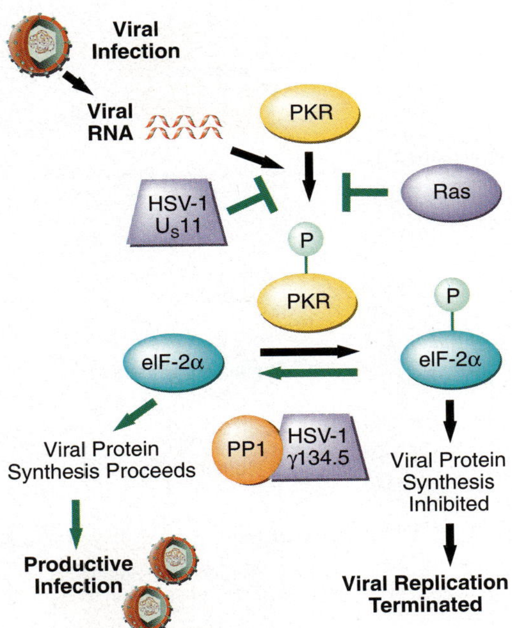

Figure 57-14 PKR and HSV-1. Activation of PKR by double-stranded RNA results in cessation of viral protein synthesis *(gray arrows)*. The HSV-1 viral genes US11 or γ134.5 inhibit the action of PKR *(black arrows)*. Activating mutations in Ras can also inhibit activation of the PKR pathway upon viral infection and thereby allow tumor-selective HSV-1 to replicate.

The E1 region (E1A and E1B) of adenovirus encodes proteins required for viral gene expression. By controlling expression of the E1 region with a tumor-selective promoter, viral replication can be restricted to tumor cells. For example, to target hepatocellular carcinoma cells, the promoter/enhancer of the α-fetoprotein gene has been placed upstream to the E1 sequences.[196] This virus replicates selectively in hepatocellular carcinoma cells that overexpress α-fetoprotein, but not in α-fetoprotein–negative tumor cells. Similarly, an adenovirus was generated to specifically target prostate cancer cells. The engineered adenovirus, CN706, was constructed by placing the promoter/enhancer region of the PSA gene upstream of the E1A gene.[197] This virus repli-

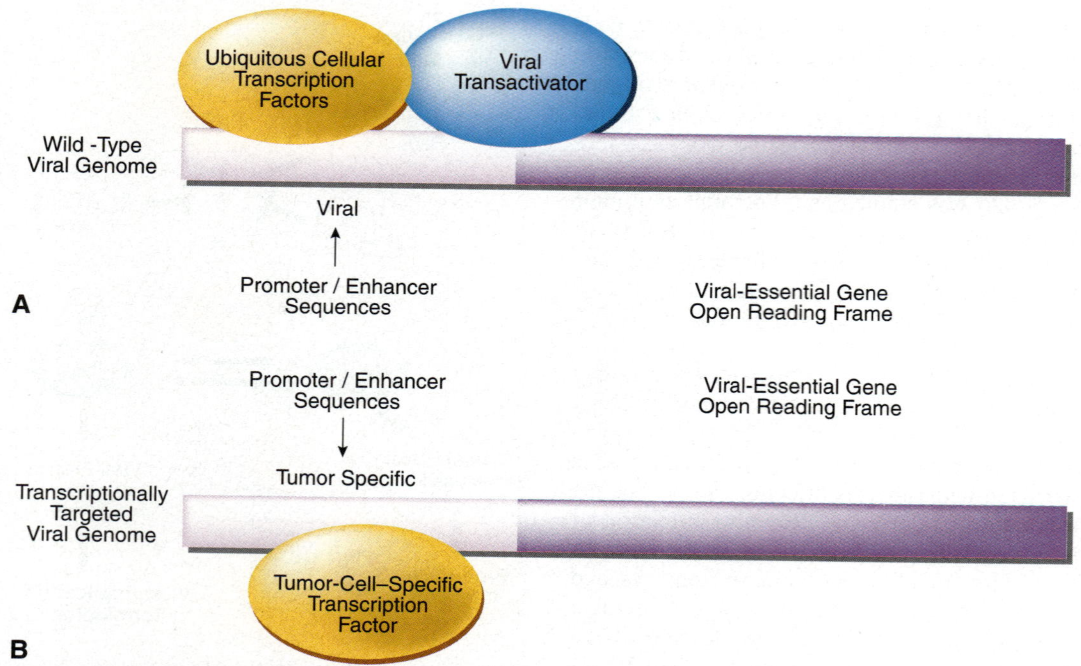

Figure 57-15 Transcription-targeted oncolytic viruses. **A**, In wild-type viral genomes, viral-essential genes are under the control of ubiquitous cellular transcription factors that allow replication to proceed in multiple cell histologies. **B**, In transcription-targeted tumor viruses, viral-essential genes are placed under the control of tumor-specific transcription factors that allow replication to occur only in specific tumor histologies.

cates to high titers in prostate cancer cells overexpressing PSA and not in cancer cells that do not express PSA. To target MUC1-positive tumor cells (ie, breast tumor), the E1A gene has been placed under the control of the DF3/MUC1 promoter/enhancer sequences described above.[198]

The HSV-1 viral mutant d120 is deleted of the viral essential gene α4 and does not replicate upon infecting cells.[199] The transcriptionally targeted HSV-1 G92A was created by placing the α4 gene under the transcriptional control of the albumin enhancer/promoter elements and restricted viral replication to albumin expressing cells.[200] Wild-type HSV-1 replicated efficiently in cells irrespective of albumin expression, while virus G92A replicated more efficiently in albumin-expressing cell lines compared to nonalbumin-expressing cell lines. In a similar vein, the calponin promoter has also been used to control expression of HSV-1 α4.[201] Calponin mRNA is overexpressed in soft-tissue/bone tumors, thereby providing a means to target such tumors with replication-conditional viruses.

The drawback of the above-mentioned transcription-targeted approaches is that individualized viruses have to be created for each tumor type. Also, tumors within a given tissue type also can vary in their expression of specific transcription factors, limiting the utility of such viruses for broad tissue types. To circumvent these problems, an adenovirus was constructed that targets tumor endothelial cells.[202] The benefits of targeting the tumor vasculature are twofold: genetic stability and a common process among multiple solid tumors. The process of angiogenesis by endothelial cells involves the up-regulation of multiple endothelial cell receptor complexes such as VEGF and transforming growth factor (TGF)-β. By placing the adenoviral E1A and E1B genes under the transcriptional control of the Flk-1 (VEGFR-2) and endoglin (CD105/TGF-β receptor component) promoter/enhancer sequences, the adenovirus preferentially replicates in dividing endothelial cells compared with tumor cells.

Therapeutic Gene Delivery with Replication-Competent Viruses Previously the delivery of therapeutic gene products with replication-defective viral vectors was discussed. Strategies described earlier in "Therapeutic Genes" have also been employed with replication-selective tumor viruses as well. These strategies have included the delivery of immunomodulatory genes, prodrug-converting enzymes (suicide gene therapy), and cytotoxic genes. Replication-competent HSV-1 has been created to express the immunostimulatory IL-12 gene and the prodrug-converting enzyme cytosine deaminase gene.[203,204] Conditionally replicating adenoviruses have been created that express the cytotoxic TNF-α gene and the genes encoding the prodrug-converting enzymes cytosine deaminase and thymidine kinase.[198,205] Delivery of a cytotoxic gene in combination with a replication-competent virus seems counterintuitive. However, these gene-delivery approaches appear to enhance the therapeutic effect of antitumor therapy schedules in murine experimental tumor model systems. The therapeutic gene delivered may enhance tumor cell kill by eliciting a bystander effect and result in the cell death of neighboring tumor cells that are not infected by the virus.

Combination Chemotherapy/Radiotherapy with Replication-Competent Finally, studies have also begun to assess the utility of combining standard anticancer agents with replication-competent viruses. Combining different therapeutic modalities has been a mainstay of cancer therapy. Viral lysis of tumor cells presents an alternative means to destroy cells in addition to chemo/radiotherapy. Adding gene therapy to standard tumor therapies has many potential benefits. Since chemo/radiotherapy and oncolytic viruses target cellular destruction differently, resistant tumor cells are less likely to emerge. Also, lower doses of each therapy may be utilized to achieve a comparable degree of tumor cell kill to monotherapy, resulting in decreased normal tissue toxicity of the individual agents.

Of greater interest is the combination of oncolytic viruses with ionizing radiation (IR)/chemotherapy resulting in synergistic tumor cell kill. IR enhances the therapeutic potential of mutant oncolytic adenoviruses and HSV-1 in part by increasing the replication potential of the viruses.[205–208] A variety of chemotherapeutic agents have also been reported to augment the efficacy of replication-conditional adenovirus and HSV-1.[209–212] Especially intriguing in this treatment paradigm are results of a phase II clinical trial for recurrent head and neck cancer treated with E1B-deleted adenovirus (ONYX-015) in combination with 5-FU and cisplatin.[213] Preliminary results suggest that the chemotherapy augments the therapeutic effect of replicating-conditional adenovirus in patients' tumors.

Studies have begun to address how chemotherapy/IR enhance the ability of viruses to replicate. In creating oncolytic viruses, viral genes are deleted, resulting in relative tumor specificity of the mutant virus (see Figure 57-12). One way to enhance viral replication is to provide the deleted viral function in *trans* by a cellular protein homologue. For the HSV-1 mutant G207 (see Table 57-2), both deleted viral genes (ie, large subunit of ribonucleotide reductase [RR] and γ134.5) have cellular counterparts that are up-regulated by IR/chemotherapy.[214,215] IR induces cellular RR activity that complements the viral RR deletion.[216] Also, IR induces the growth arrest and DNA damage inducible genes, Gadd.[217] One of these genes, Gadd34, shares significant homology to the carboxy terminus of γ134.5.[218,219] As the name implies, Gadd34 is induced by genotoxic agents, including IR and chemotherapy. Therefore, IR and chemotherapy may be able to increase transcomplementation of virally deleted gene functions (Figure 57-16). One other implication of these observations is that viral oncolysis may also be regulated in a spatial and temporal manner by IR (see Figure 57-9). Cellular homologues can be induced within the targeted irradiated tumor field enhancing viral replication and tumor kill. However, when the mutant virus reaches nonirradiated, normal cells, there is a lack of transcomplementation and viral replication ceases.

These examples demonstrate how knowledge of cell and viral molecular biology has provided the basis for the construction of genetically engineered viruses that selectively replicate in tumor

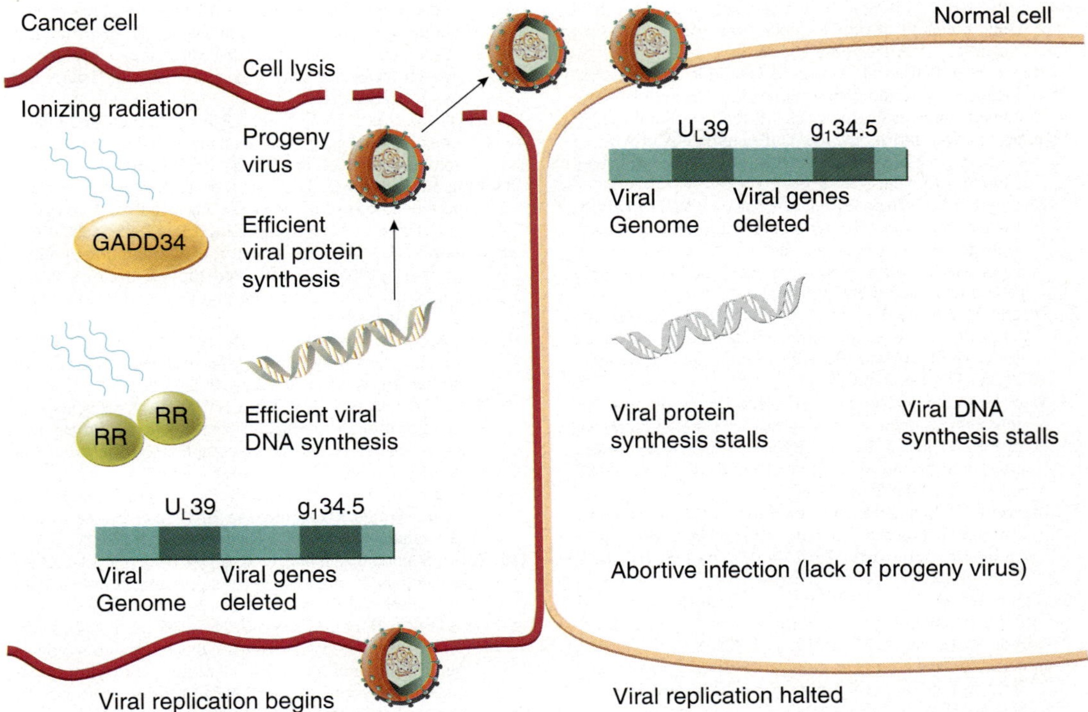

Figure 57-16 IR enhancing the oncolytic capacity of attenuated, replication-competent viruses. IR activates cellular genes/proteins that provide transcomplementation to virally deleted genes. Spatial restriction of IR to cancer cells provides a mechanism by which attenuated viruses can replicate more robustly in tumor cells compared with normal cells outside of the targeted irradiated volume.

cells. Other replication-competent viruses under study include Newcastle disease virus and parvoviruses. Multiple clinical trials are underway to determine the therapeutic efficacy of the current generation of replication-conditional viruses. At the same time, further basic science research in both tumor and viral biology is providing means to create more potent oncolytic viruses with increased safeguards to specifically target the tumor. The majority of current studies have focused on the use of replication-conditional viruses for regional therapy (ie, direct tumor inoculation); however, studies are also evolving that use the virus as a systemic therapeutic agent that could target metastases. This would involve the virus surviving the systemic circulation and then homing in on malignant cells. Such viruses could bind selectively to tumor-cell–specific receptors to gain entry and have their gene expression driven by tumor cell–specific transcription factors.

REFERENCES

1. Miller A. Retroviral vectors. Curr Top Microbiol Immunol 1993;158.
2. Challita P, Kohn D. Lack of expression from a retroviral vector after transduction of murine hematopoietic stem cells is associated with methylation in vivo. Proc Natl Acad Sci U S A 1994;91:2567–71.
3. Fass D, Davey R, Hamson C, et al. Structure of a murine leukemia virus receptor-binding glycoprotein at 2.0 angstrom resolution. Science 1997;277:1662–6.
4. Lewis P, Hensel M, Emerman M. Human immunodeficiency virus infection of cells arrested in the cell cycle. EMBO J 1992;11:3053–8.
5. Weinberg J, Matthews T, Cullen B, Malim M. Productive human immunodeficiency virus type 1 (HIV-1) infection of nonproliferating human monocytes. J Exp Med 1991;174:1477–82.
6. Donahue R, Kessler S, Bodine D, et al. Helper virus induced T cell lymphoma in nonhuman primates after retroviral mediated gene transfer. J Exp Med 1992;176:1125–35.
7. Graham FL, Smiley J, Russel WC, Nairn R. Characteristics of a human cell line transformed by DNA from human adenovirus type 5. J Gen Virol 1977;36:59–72.
8. Geraghty R, Krummenacher C, Cohen G, et al. Entry of alpha herpes viruses mediated by poliovirus receptor-related protein 1 and poliovirus receptor. Science 1998;280:1618–20.
9. Frenkel N, Jacob R, Honess R, et al. Anatomy of herpes simplex virus DNA III. Characterization of defective DNA molecules and biological properties of virus populations containing them. J Virol 1975;16:153–67.
10. Kwong A, Frenkel N. The herpes simplex virus amplicon IV. Efficient expression of a chimeric chicken ovalbumin gene amplified within defective virus genomes. Virology 1985;142:421–5.
11. Fraefel C, Song S, Lim F, et al. Helper virus-free transfer of herpes simplex virus type 1 plasmid vectors into neural cells. J Virol 1996;70:7190–7.
12. Kwong A, Frenkel N. Herpes simplex virus amplicon: effect of size on replication of constructed defective genomes containing eucaryotic DNA sequences. J Virol 1984;51:595–603.
13. Fujiwara T, Grimm E, Mukhopadhyay T, et al. Induction of chemosensitivity in human lung cancer cells in vivo by adenovirus-mediated transfer of the wild-type p53 gene. Cancer Res 1994;54:2287–91.
14. Collaco R, Cao X, Trempe J. A helper virus-free packaging system for recombinant adeno-associated virus vectors. 1999;238:397–405.
15. Summerford C, Bartlett J, Samulski R. AlphaVbeta5 integrin: a co-receptor for adeno-associated virus type 2 infection. Nat Med 1999;5:78–82.
16. Qing K, Mah C, Hansen J, Zhou S, et al. Human fibroblast growth factor receptor 1 is a co-receptor for infection by adeno-associated virus 2. Nat Med 1999;5:71–7.
17. Kearns W, Afione S, Fulmer S, et al. Recombinant adeno-associated virus (AAV-CFTR) vectors do not integrate in a site-specific fashion in an immortalized epithelial cell line. Gene Ther 1996;3:748–55.
18. Flotte T, Carter B. Adeno-associated virus vectors for gene therapy. Gene Ther 1995;2:357–62.
19. Yang Z, Perkins N, Ohno T, et al. The p21 cyclin-dependent kinase inhibitor suppresses tumorigenicity in vivo. Nat Med 1995;1:1052–6.
20. Nomura T, Yasuda K, Yamada T, et al. Gene expression and antitumor effects following direct interferon (IFN)-gamma gene transfer with naked plasmid DNA and DC-chol liposome complexes in mice. Gene Ther 1999;6:121–9.
21. Sun W, Burkholder J, Sun J, et al. In vivo cytokine gene transfer by gene gun reduces tumor growth in mice. Proc Natl Acad Sci U S A 1995;92:2889–93.
22. Turner J, Tan J, Crucian B, et al. Broadened clinical utility of gene gun-mediated, granulocyte-macrophage colony-stimulating factor cDNA-based tumor cell vaccines as demonstrated with a mouse myeloma model. Hum Gene Ther 1998;9:1121–30.
23. Zabner J, Fasbender A, Moninger T, et al. Cellular and molecular barriers to gene transfer by a cationic lipid. J Biol Chem 1995;270:18997–9007.
24. Nabel GJ, Nabel EG, Yang ZY, et al. Direct gene transfer with DNA-liposome complexes in melanoma: expression, biologic activity, and lack of toxicity in humans. Proc Natl Acad Sci U S A 1993;90:11307–11.
25. Blezinger P, Freimark B, Matar M, et al. Intratracheal administration of interleukin 12 plasmid-cationic lipid complexes inhibits murine lung metastases. Hum Gene Ther 1999;10:723–31.
26. Chen Q, Kumar D, Stass S, Mixson AJ. Liposomes complexed to plasmids encoding angiostatin and endostatin inhibit breast cancer in nude mice. Cancer Res 1999;59:3308–12.
27. Zou Y, Zong G, Ling Y, et al. Effective treatment of early endobronchial cancer with regional administration of liposome-p53 complexes. J Natl Cancer Inst 1998;90:1130–7.
28. Wagner E, Plank C, Zatloukal K, et al. Influenza virus hemagglutinin HA-2 N-terminal fusogenic peptides augment gene transfer by transferrin-polylysine-DNA complexes: toward a synthetic virus-like gene-transfer vehicle. Proc Natl Acad Sci U S A 1992;89:7934–8.
29. Hoganson D, Chandler L, Fleurbaaij G, et al. Targeted delivery of DNA encoding cytotoxic proteins through high-affinity fibroblast growth factor receptors. Hum Gene Ther 1998;9:2565–75.
30. Hart S, Arancibia-Carcamo C, Wolfert M, et al. Lipid-mediated enhancement of transfection by a nonviral integrin-targeting vector. Hum Gene Ther 1998;9:575–85.
31. Simoes S, Slepushkin V, Gasper R, et al. Gene delivery by negatively charged ternary complexes of DNA, cationic liposomes and transferrin or fusigenic peptides. Gene Ther 1998;5:955–64.
32. Fender P, Ruigrok R, Gout E, et al. Adenovirus dodecahedron, a new vector for human gene transfer. Nat Biot 1997;15:52–6.
33. Smythe C, Newport JW. Coupling of mitosis to the completion of S phase in Xenopus occurs via modulation of the tyrosine kinase that phosphorylates p34cdc2. Cell 1992;68:787.
34. Freeman S, Abboud C, Whartenby K, et al. The "bystander effect": tumor regression when a fraction of the tumor mass is genetically modified. Cancer Res 1993;53:5274–83.
35. Elshami A, Saavedra A, Zhang H, et al. Gap junctions play a role in the bystander effect of the herpes simplex virus thymidine kinase/ganciclovir system in vitro. Gene Ther 1996;3:85–92.
36. Beltinger C, Fulda S, Kammertoens T, et al. Herpes simplex virus thymidine kinase/ganciclovir-induced apoptosis involves ligand-independent death receptor aggregation and activation of caspase. Proc Natl Acad Sci U S A 1999;96:8699–704.
37. Huber B, Austin E, Good S, et al. In vivo antitumor activity of 5-fluorocytosine on human colorectal carcinoma cells genetically modified to express cytosine deaminase. Cancer Res 1993;53:4619–26.
38. Dong Y, Wen P, Manome Y, et al. In vivo replication-deficient adenovirus vector-mediated transduction of the cytosine gene sensitizes glioma cells to 5-fluorocytosine. Hum Gene Ther 1996;7:713–20.
39. Hanna N, Mauceri H, Wayne J, et al. Virally directed cytosine deaminase/5-fluorocytosine gene therapy enhances radiation response in human cancer xenografts. Cancer Res 1997;57:4205–9.
40. Pederson L, Buchsbaum D, Vickers S, et al. Molecular chemotherapy combined with radiation therapy enhances killing of cholangiocarcinoma cells in vitro and in vivo. Cancer Res 1997;57:4325–32.
41. Chang JD, Xu Y, Raychowdhury MK, Ware JA. Molecular cloning and expression of a cDNA encoding a novel isoenzyme of protein kinase C (nPKC). J Biol Chem 1993;268:14208–14.
42. Wei M, Tamiya T, Chase M, et al. Experimental tumor therapy in mice using the cyclophosphamide-activating cytochrome P450 2B1 gene. Hum Gene Ther 1994;5:969–78.

43. Wei M, Tamiya T, Rhee R, et al. Diffusible cytotoxic metabolites contribute to the in vivo bystander effect associated with the cyclophosphamide/cytochrome P450 2B1 cancer gene therapy paradigm. Clin Cancer Res 1995;1:1171–7.
44. Mroz P, Moolten F. Retrovirally transduced Escherichia coli gpt genes combine selectability with chemosensitivity capable of mediating tumor eradication. Hum Gene Ther 1993;4:589–95.
45. Sorscher E, Peng S, Bchok Z, et al. Tumor cell bystander killing in colonic carcinoma utilizing the Escherichia coli DeoD gene to generate toxic purines. Gene Ther 1993;1:233–8.
46. McNeish I, Green N, Gilligan M, et al. Virus directed enzyme produg therapy for ovarian and pancreatic cancer using retrovirally delivered E. coli nitroreductase and CB1954. Gene Ther 1998;5:1061–9.
47. Levine AJ. p53, the cellular gatekeeper for growth and division. Cell 1997;88:323–31.
48. Lowe SW, Ruley HE, Jacks T, Housman DE. p53-dependent apoptosis modulates the cytotoxicity of anticancer agents. Cell 1993;74:957–67.
49. Lowe SW, Schmitt EM, Smith SW, et al. p53 is required for radiation-induced apoptosis in mouse thymocytes. Nature 1993;362:847–9.
50. Badie B, Drazan K, Kramar M, et al. Adenovirus-mediated p53 gene delivery inhibits 9L glioma growth in rats. Neurol Res 1995;17:209–16.
51. Gomez-Manano C, Fueyo J, Kyritsis A, et al. Adenovirus-mediated transfer of the p53 gene produces rapid and generalized death of human glioma cells via apoptosis. Cancer Res 1996;56:694–9.
52. Li Z, Rakkar A, Katayose Y, et al. Efficacy of multiple administrations of a recombinant adenovirus expressing wild-type p53 in an immune-competent mouse tumor model. Gene Ther 1998;5:605–13.
53. Spitz F, Nguyen D, Skibber J, et al. Adenoviral-mediated wild-type p53 gene expression sensitizes colorectal cancer cells to ionizing radiation. Clin Cancer Res 1996;2:1665–71.
54. Gallardo D, Drazan K, Mcbride W. Adenovirus-based transfer of wild-type p53 gene increases ovarian tumor radiosensitivity. Cancer Res 1996;56:4891–3.
55. Swisher S, Roth J, Nemunaitis J, et al. Adenovirus-mediated p53 gene transfer in advanced non-small-cell lung cancer. J Natl Cancer Inst 1999;91:763–71.
56. Johnson DG, Schwarz JK, Cress WD, Nevins JR. Expression of transcription factor E2F-1 induced quiescent cells to enter S phase. Nature 1993;365:349–52.
57. Singh P, Wong S, Hong W. Overexpression of E2F-1 in rat embryo fibroblasts leads to neoplastic transformation. EMBO J 1994;13:3329–38.
58. Qin X-Q, Livingston DM, Kaelin WG Jr, Adams PD. Deregulated transcription factor E2F-1 expression leads to S-phase entry and p53-mediated apoptosis. Proc Natl Acad Sci U S A 1994;91:10918–22.
59. Field S, Tsai F, Kuo F, et al. E2F-1 functions in mice to promote apoptosis and suppress proliferation. Cell 1996;85:549–61.
60. Yamasaki L, Jacks T, Bronson R, et al. Tumor induction and tissue atrophy in mice lacking E2F-1. Cell 1996;85:537–48.
61. Fueyo J, Gomez-Manzano C, Yung W, et al. Overexpression of E2F-1 in glioma triggers apoptosis and suppresses tumor growth in vitro and in vivo. Nat Med 1998;4:685–90.
62. Ohno T, Yang Z, Ling X, et al. Combination gene transfer to potentiate tumor regression. Gene Ther 1997;4:361–6.
63. Tsao Y, Huang S, Chang J, et al. Adenovirus-mediated p21 (WAF1/SDII/CIP1) gene transfer induces apoptosis of human cervical cancer cell lines. J Biol Cell 999;73:4983–90.
64. Chan P, Glazer P. Triplex DNA: fundamentals, advances, and potential applications for gene therapy. J Mol Med 1997;75:267–82.
65. Havre P, Gunther E, Gasparro F, Glazer P. Targeted mutagenesis of DNA using triple helix-forming oligonucleotides linked to psoralen. Proc Natl Acad Sci U S A 1993;90:7879–83.
66. Cooney M, Czernuszewicz G, Postel E, et al. Site-specific oligonucleotide binding represses transcription of the human c-myc gene in vitro. Science 1988;241:456–9.
67. Mayfield C, Ebbinghaus S, Gee J, et al. Triplex formation by the human Ha-ras promoter inhibits Spl binding and in vitro transcription. J Biol Chem 1994;269:18232–9238.
68. Noonberg S, Scott G, Hunt C, et al. Inhibition of transcription factor binding to the HER2 promoter by triplex-forming oligodeoxyribonucleotides. Gene 1994;149:123–6.
69. Rininsland F, Johnson T, Chericky C, et al. Suppression of insulin-like growth factor type I receptor by a triplex-helix strategy inhibits IGF-I transcription and tumorgenic potential of rat C6 glioblastoma cells. Proc Natl Acad Sci U S A 1997;94:5854–9.
70. Aggarwal B, Schwarz L, Hogan M, Rando R. Triplex helix-forming oligodeoxyribonucleotides targeted to the human tumor necrosis factor (TNF) gene inhibit TNF production and block the TNF-dependent growth of human glioblastoma tumor cells. Cancer Res 1996;56:5156–64.
71. Kochetkova M, Iverson P, Lopez A, Shannon M. Deoxyribonucleic acid triplex formation inhibits granulocyte macrophage colony-stimulating factor gene expression and suppresses growth in juvenile myelomonocytic leukemic cells. J Clin Invest 1997;99:3000–8.
72. Porumb H, Gousset H, Letellier R, et al. Temporary ex vivo inhibition of the expression of the human oncogene HER2 (NEU) by a triple helix-forming oligonucleotide. Cancer Res 1996;56:515–22.
73. Stein C, Cohen J. Oligodeoxynucleotides as inhibitors of gene expression: a review. Cancer Res 1988;48:2659–68.
74. Walder R, Walder J. Role of RNase H in hybrid-arrested translation by antisense oligonucleotide. Proc Natl Acad Sci U S A 1988;85:5011–15.
75. Zamecnik P, Stephenson M. Inhibition of Rous sarcoma virus replication and cell transformation by a specific oligodeoxynucleotide. Proc Natl Acad Sci U S A 1978;75:280–4.
76. Stephenson M, Zamecnik P. Inhibition of rous sarcoma viral RNA translation by a specific oligodeoxynucleotide. Proc Natl Acad Sci U S A 1978;75:285–8.
77. Gewirtz A, Calabretta B. A c-myb antisense oligodeoxynucleotide inhibits normal human hematopoiesis in vitro. Science 1988;242:1303–6.
78. Hijiya N, Zhang J, Ratajczak M, et al. Biologic and therapeutic significance of MYB expression in human melanoma. Proc Natl Acad Sci U S A 1994;91:4499–503.
79. Arteaga C, Holt J. Tissue-targeted antisense c-fos retroviral vector inhibits established breast cancer xenografts in nude mice. Cancer Res 1996;56:1098–103.
80. Holt J, Arteaga C, Robertson D, Moses H. Gene therapy for the treatment of metastatic breast cancer by in vivo transduction with breast-targeted retroviral vector expressing antisense c-fos RNA. Hum Gene Ther 1996;7:1367–80.
81. Skotzko M, Wu L, Anderson W, et al. Retroviral vector-mediated gene transfer of antisense cyclin G1 (CYCG1) inhibits proliferation of human osteogenic sarcoma cells. Cancer Res 1995;55:5493–8.
82. Liu X, Turbyville T, Fritz A, Whitesell L. Inhibition of insulin-like growth factor I receptor expression in neuroblastoma cells induces the regression of established tumors in mice. Cancer Res 1998;58:5432–8.
83. Saleh M, Stacker S, Wilks A. Inhibition of growth of C6 glioma cells in vivo by expression of antisense vascular endothelial growth factor sequence. Cancer Res 1996;56:393–401.
84. Cheng S, Huang H, Nagane M, et al. Suppression of glioblastoma angiogenicity and tumorgenicity by inhibition of endogenous expression of vascular endothelial growth factor. Proc Natl Acad Sci U S A 1996;93:8502–7.
85. Oku T, Tjuvajev J, Miyagawa T, et al. Tumor growth modulation by sense and antisense vascular endothelial growth factor gene expression: effects on angiogenesis, vascular permeability, blood volume, blood flow, fluorodeoxyglucose uptake, and proliferation of human melanoma intracerebral xenografts. Cancer Res 1998;58:4185–92.
86. Piche A, Rancour C. A role for intracellular immunization in chemosensitization of tumor cells? Gene Ther 1999;6:1202–9.
87. Scanlon K, Ohta Y, Ishida H, et al. Oligonucleotide-mediated modulation of mammalian gene expression. FASEB 1995;9:1288–96.
88. Pyle A. Ribozyme: a distinct class of metalloenzymes. Science 1993;261:709–14.
89. James H, Gibson I. The therapeutic potential of ribozymes. Blood 1998;91:371–82.
90. Scanlon K, Jiao L, Funato T, et al. Ribozyme-mediated cleavage of c-fos mRNA reduces gene expression of DNA synthesis enzymes and metallothionein. Proc Natl Acad Sci U S A 1991;88:10591–5.
91. Kiehntopf M, Brach M, Licht T, et al. Ribozyme-mediated cleavage of the MDR-1 transcript restores chemosensitivity in previously resistant cancer cells. EMBO J 1997;13:4645–52.
92. Czubayko F, Schulte A, Berchem G, Wellstein A. Melanoma angiogenesis and metastasis modulated by ribozyme targeting of the secreted growth factor pleiotrophin. Proc Natl Acad Sci U S A 1996;87:14753–8.
93. Abounader R, Ranganathan S, Lal B, et al. Reversion of human glioblastoma malignancy by U1 small nuclear RNA/ribozyme targeting of scatter factor/hepatocyte growth factor and c-met expression. J Natl Cancer Inst 1999;91:1548–56.
94. Snyder D, Wu Y, Wang J, et al. Ribozyme-mediated inhibition of bcr-abl gene expression in a Philadelphia chromosome-positive cell line. Blood 1993;82:600–5.
95. Feng M, Cabrera G, Deshane J, et al. Neoplastic reversion accomplished by high efficiency adenoviral-mediated delivery of an anti-ras ribozyme. Cancer Res 1995;55:2024–8.
96. Yamazaki H, Kijima H, Ohnishi Y, et al. Inhibition of tumor growth by ribozyme-mediated suppression of aberrant epidermal growth factor receptor gene expression. J Natl Cancer Inst 1998;90:581–7.
97. Fire A, Xu S, Montgomery MK, et al. Potent and specific genetic interference by double-stranded RNA in Caenorhabditis elegans. Nature 1998;391:806–11.
98. Rand TA, Ginalski K, Grishin NV, Wang X. Biochemical identification of Argonaute 2 as the sole protein required for RNA-induced silencing complex activity. Proc Natl Acad Sci U S A 2004;101:14385–9.
99. Elbashir SM, Harborth J, Lendeckel W, et al. Duplexes of 21-nucleotide RNAs mediate RNA interference in cultured mammalian cells. Nature 2001;411:494–8.
100. Sui G, Soohoo C, Affar E, et al. A DNA vector-based RNAi technology to suppress gene expression in mammalian cells. Proc Natl Acad Sci U S A 2002;99:5515–20.
101. De Schrijver E, Brusselmans K, Heyns W, et al. RNA interference-mediated silencing of the fatty acid synthase gene attenuates growth and induces morphological changes and apoptosis of LNCaP prostate cancer cells. Cancer Res 2003;63:3799–804.
102. Yague E, Higgins CF, Raguz S. Complete reversal of multidrug resistance by stable expression of small interfering RNAs targeting MDR1. Gene Ther 2004;11:1170–4.
103. Zhang Y, Zhang YF, Bryant J, et al. Intravenous RNA interference gene therapy targeting the human epidermal growth factor receptor prolongs survival in intracranial brain cancer. Clin Cancer Res 2004;10:3667–77.
104. Sumimoto H, Miyagishi M, Miyoshi H, et al. Inhibition of growth and invasive ability of melanoma by inactivation of mutated BRAF with lentivirus-mediated RNA interference. Oncogene 2004;23:6031–9.
105. Carette JE, Overmeer RM, Schagen FH, et al. Conditionally replicating adenoviruses expressing short hairpin RNAs silence the expression of a target gene in cancer cells. Cancer Res 2004;64:2663–7.
106. Simons J, Mikhak B, Chang J, et al. Induction of immunity to prostate cancer antigens: results of a clinical trial of vaccination with irradiated autologous prostate tumor cells engineered to secrete granulocyte-macrophage colony-stimulating factor using ex vivo gene transfer. Cancer Res 1999;59:5160–8.
107. Palmer K, Moore J, Everard M, et al. Gene therapy with autologous, interleukin 2-secreting tumor cells in patients with malignant melanoma. Hum Gene Ther 1999;10:1261–8.
108. Horton H, Anderson D, Hernandez P, et al. A gene therapy for cancer using intramuscular injection of plasmid DNA encoding interferon alpha. Proc Natl Acad Sci U S A 1999;96:1553–8.
109. Sobol R, Shawler D, Carson C, et al. Interleukin 2 gene therapy of colorectal carcinoma with autologous irradiated tumor cells and genetically engineered fibroblasts: a phase I study. Clin Cancer Res 1999;5:2359–65.
110. Hodge JW, Abrams S, Schlom J, Kantor JA. Induction of antitumor immunity by recombinant vaccinia viruses expressing B7-1 or B7-2 costimulatory molecules. Cancer Res 1994;54:5552–5.
111. Baskar S, Clements V, Glimcher L, et al. Rejection of MHC class II-transfected tumor cells requires induction of tumor-encoded B7-1 and/or B7-2 costimulatory molecules. J Immunol 1996;156:3821–7.
112. Wendtner C, Nolte A, Mangold E, et al. Gene transfer of the costimulatory molecules B7-1 and B7-2 into human multiple myeloma cells by recombinant adeno-associated virus enhances the cytolytic T cell response. Gene Ther 1997;4:726–35.
113. Kikuchi T, Crystal R. Anti-tumor immunity induced by in vivo adenovirus vector-mediated expression of CD40 ligand in tumor cells. Hum Gene Ther 1999;10:1375–87.
114. Emtage P, Wan Y, Bramson J, et al. A double recombinant adenovirus expressing the costimulatory molecule B7-1 (murine) and human IL-2 induces complete tumor regression in a murine breast adenocarcinoma model. J Immunol 1998;160:2531–8.

115. Rosenberg S. A new era for cancer immunotherapy based on the genes that encode cancer antigens. Immunity 1999;10:281–7.
116. Wolfel T, Hauer M, Schneider J, et al. A p16INK4a-insensitive CDK4 mutant targeted by cytolytic T lymphocytes in a human melanoma. Science 1995;269:1281–4.
117. Mandruzzato S, Brasseur F, Andry G, et al. A CASP-8 mutation recognized by cytolytic T lymphocytes on a human head and neck carcinoma. J Exp Med 1997;186:785–93.
118. Robbins P, El-Gamil M, Li Y, et al. A mutated beta-catenin gene encodes a melanoma-specific antigen recognized by tumor infiltrating lymphocytes. J Exp Med 1996;183:1185–92.
119. Wang B, Merva M, Dang K, et al. Immunization by direct DNA inoculation induces rejection of tumor cell challenge. Hum Gene Ther 1995;6:407–18.
120. Tsang KY, Zaremba S, Nieroda CA, et al. Generation of human cytotoxic T cells specific for human carcinoembryonic antigen epitopes from patients immunized with recombinant vaccinia-CEA vaccine. J Natl Cancer Inst 1995;87:982–90.
121. Conry RM, LoBuglio AF, Loechel F, et al. A carcinoembryonic antigen polynucleotide vaccine has in vivo antitumor activity. Gene Ther 1995;2:59–65.
122. Rosenberg S, Zhai Y, Yang J, et al. Immunizing patients with metastic melanoma using recombinant adenovirus encoding MART-1 or gp100 melanoma antigens. J Natl Cancer Inst 1998;90:1894–900.
123. Eder JP, Kantoff PW, Roper K, et al. A phase I trial of a recombinant vaccinia virus expressing prostate-specific antigen in advanced prostate cancer. Clin Cancer Res 2000;6:1632–8.
124. Hodge J, Mclaughlin J, Abrams S, et al. Admixture of a recombinant vaccinia virus containing the gene for the costimulatory molecule B7 and a recombinant vaccinia virus containing a tumor-associated antigen and antitumor immunity. Cancer Res 1995;55:3598–603.
125. Akagi J, Hodge JV, McLaughlin JP, et al. Therapeutic antitumor response after immunization with an admixture of recombinant vaccinia viruses expressing a modified MUC1 gene and the murine T-cell costimulatory molecule B7. J. Immunotherapy 1997;20:38–47.
126. Hodge J, Sabzevari H, Yafal A, et al. A triad of costimulatory molecules synergize to amplify T-cell activation. Cancer Res 1999;59:5800–7.
127. Kasahara N, Dozy A, Kan Y. Tissue-specific targeting of retroviral vectors through ligand-receptor interactions. Science 1994;266:1373–6.
128. Han X, Kasahara N, Kan Y. Ligand-directed retroviral targeting of human breast cancer cells. Proc Natl Acad Sci U S A 1995;92:9747–51.
129. Slamon D, Clark G, Wong S, et al. Human breast cancer: correlation of relapse and survival with amplification of the HER-2/neu oncogene. Science 1987;235:177–82.
130. Bewley M, Springer K, Zhang Y, et al. Structural analysis of the mechanism of adenovirus binding to its human cellular receptor, CAR. Science 1999;286:1579–83.
131. Watkins S, Mesyanzhinov V, Kurochkina L, Hawkins R. The 'adenobody' approach to viral targeting: specific and enhanced adenoviral gene delivery. Gene Ther 1997;4:1004–12.
132. Haisma H, Pinedo H, Rijswijk A, et al. Tumor-specific gene transfer via an adenoviral vector targeted to the pan-carcinoma antigen EpCAM. Gene Ther 1999;6:1469–74.
133. Rancourt C, Rogers B, Sosnowski B, et al. Basic fibroblast growth factor enhancement of adenovirus-mediated delivery of the herpes simplex virus thymidine kinase gene results in augmented therapeutic benefit in a murine model of ovarian cancer. Clin Cancer Res 1998;4:2455–61.
134. Doukas J, Hoganson D, Ong M, et al. Retargeted delivery of adenoviral vectors through fibroblast growth factor receptors involves unique cellular pathways. FASEB J 1999;13:1459–66.
135. Krasnykh V, Mikheeva G, Douglas J, Curiel D. Generation of recombinant adenovirus vectors with modified fibers for altering viral tropism. J Virol 1996;70:6839–46.
136. Krasnykh V, Dmitriev I, Mikheeva G, et al. Characterization of an adenovirus vector containing a heterologous peptide epitope in the HI loop of the fiber knob. J Virol 1998;72:1844–52.
137. Li Y, Pong R, Bergelson J, et al. Loss of adenoviral receptor expression in human bladder cancer cells: a potential impact on the efficacy of gene therapy. Cancer Res 1999;59:325–30.
138. Dmitriev I, Krasnykh V, Miller C, et al. An adenovirus vector with genetically modified fibers demonstrates expanded tropism via utilization of a coxsackievirus and adenovirus receptor-independent cell entry mechanism. J Virol 1998;72:9706–13.
139. Kasono K, Blackwell J, Douglas J, et al. Selective gene delivery to head and neck cancer cells via an integrin targeted adenoviral vector. Clin Cancer Res 1999;5:2571–9.
140. Vanderkwaak T, Wang M, Gomez-Navarro J, et al. An advanced generation of adenoviral vectors selectively enhances gene transfer for ovarian cancer gene therapy approaches. Gynecol Oncol 1999;74:227–34.
141. Girod A, Ried M, Wobus C, et al. Genetic capsid modifications allow efficient re-targeting of adeno-associated virus type 2. Nat Med 1999;5:1052–6.
142. Abe M, Kufe D. Characterization of cis-acting elements regulating transcription of the human DF3 breast carcinoma-associated antigen (MUC1) gene. Proc Natl Acad Sci U S A 1993;90:282–6.
143. Manome Y, Abe M, Hagen MF, et al. Enhancer sequences of the DF3 gene regulate expression of the herpes simplex virus thymidine kinase gene and confer sensitivity of human breast cancer cells to ganciclovir. Cancer Res 1994;54:5408–13.
144. Chen L, Chen D, Manome Y, et al. Breast cancer selective gene expression and therapy mediated by recombinant adenoviruses containing the DF3/MUC1 promoter. J Clin Invest 1995;96:2775–82.
145. Chen L, Pulsipher M, Chen D, et al. Selective transgene expression for detection and elimination of contaminating carcinoma cells in hematopoietic stem cell sources. J Clin Invest 1996;98:2539–48.
146. Weichselbaum RR, Kufe DW, Hellman S, et al. Radiation-induced tumour necrosis factor-alpha expression: clinical application of transcriptional and physical targeting of gene therapy. Lancet Oncol 2002;3:665–71.
147. Datta R, Taneja N, Sukhatme V, et al. Reactive oxygen intermediates target CArG sequences to mediate activation of the immediate early transcription factor EGR-1 by ionizing radiation. Proc Natl Acad Sci U S A 1993;90:2419–22.
148. Hallanhan D, Mauceri H, Seung L, et al. Spatial and temporal control of gene therapy using ionizing radiation. Nat Med 1995;1:786–91.
149. Rasmussen H, Rasmussen C, Lempicki M, et al. TNFerade Biologic: preclinical toxicology of a novel adenovector with a radiation-inducible promoter, carrying the human tumor necrosis factor alpha gene. Cancer Gene Ther 2002;9:951–7.
150. Senzer N, Mani S, Rosemurgy A, et al. TNFerade biologic, an adenovector with a radiation-inducible promoter, carrying the human tumor necrosis factor alpha gene: a phase I study in patients with solid tumors. J Clin Oncol 2004;22:592–601.
151. Yamini B, Yu X, Gillespie GY, et al. Transcriptional targeting of adenovirally delivered tumor necrosis factor alpha by temozolomide in experimental glioblastoma. Cancer Res 2004;64:6381–4.
152. Park JO, Lopez CA, Gupta VK, et al. Transcriptional control of viral gene therapy by cisplatin. J Clin Invest 2002;110:403–10.
153. Chaudhary PM, Roninson IB. Induction of multidrug resistance in human cells by transient exposure to different chemotherapeutic drugs. J Natl Cancer Inst 1993;85:632–9.
154. Walther W, Wendt J, Stein U. Employment of the mdr1 promoter for the chemotherapy-inducible expression of therapeutic genes in cancer gene therapy. Gene Ther 1997;4:544–52.
155. Mauceri HJ, Hanna NN, Wayne JD, et al. Tumor necrosis factor alpha (TNF-alpha) gene therapy targeted by ionizing radiation selectively damages tumor vasculature. Cancer Res 1996;56:4311–4.
156. Nagayama T, Nishihara E, Iitaka M, et al. Enhanced efficacy of transcriptionally targeted suicide gene/prodrug therapy for thyroid carcinoma with the Cre-LoxP system. Cancer Res 1999;59:3049–52.
157. Kijima T, Osaki T, Nishino K, et al. Application of the Cre recombinase/loxP system further enhances antitumor effects in cell type-specific gene therapy against carcinoembryonic antigen-producing cancer. Cancer Res 1999;59:4906–11.
158. Dock G. Influence of complicating diseases upon leukaemia. J Med Sci 1904;127:563–92.
159. Levaditi C, Nicolau S. Affinite du virus herpetique pour les neoplasmes epitheliaux. Comptes Rendus Societe Biologie 1922;87:498–500.
160. Whyte P, Buchkovich KJ, Horowitz JM, et al. Association between an oncogene and an anti-oncogene: the adenovirus E1A proteins bind to the retinoblastoma gene product. Nature 1988;334:124–9.
161. Bischoff J, Kirn D, Williams A, et al. An adenovirus mutant that replicates selectively in p53-deficient human tumor cells. Science 1996;274:373–6.
162. Hall A, Dix B, O'Carroll S, Braithwaite A. p53-dependent cell death/apoptosis is required for a productive adenovirus infection. Nature Med 1998;4:1068–72.
163. Rothmann T, Hengstermann A, Whitaker N, et al. Replication of ONYX-015, a potential anticancer adenovirus is independent of p53 status in tumor cells. J Virol 1998;72:9470–8.
164. Goodrum F, Ornelles D. p53 status does not determine outcome of E1B 55-kilodalton mutant adenovirus lytic infection. J Virol 1998;72:9479–90.
165. Alarcon-Vargas D, Ronai Z. p53-Mdm2--the affair that never ends. Carcinogenesis 2002;23:541–7.
166. Ries SJ, Brandts CH, Chung AS, et al. Loss of p14ARF in tumor cells facilitates replication of the adenovirus mutant dl1520 (ONYX-015). Nat Med 2000;6:1128–33.
167. Pilder S, Moore M, Logan J, Shenk T. The adenovirus E1B-55K transforming polypeptide modulates transport or cytoplasmic stabilization of viral and host cell mRNAs. Mol Cell Biol 1986;6:470–6.
168. Whyte P, Williamson NM, Harlow E. Cellular targets for transformation by the adenovirus E1A proteins. Cell 1989;56:67–75.
169. Fueyo J, Gomez-Manzano C, Alemany R, et al. A mutant oncolytic adenovirus targeting the Rb pathway produces anti-glioma effect in vivo. Oncogene 2000;19:2–12.
170. Heise C, Kirn DH. Replication-selective adenoviruses as oncolytic agents. J Clin Invest 2000;105:847–51.
171. Martuza R, Malick A, Markert J, et al. Experimental therapy of human glioma by means of a genetically engineered virus mutant. Science 1991;252:854–6.
172. Mineta T, Rabkin S, Yazaki T, et al. Attenuated multi-mutated herpes simplex virus-1 for treatment of malignant gliomas. Nat Med 1995;1:938–43.
173. Pyles RB, Warnick RE, Chalk CL, et al. A novel multiply-mutated HSV-1 strain for the treatment of human brain tumors. Hum Gene Ther 1997;8:533–44.
174. Chou J, Kern E, Whitley R, Roizman B. Mapping of herpes simplex virus neurovirulence to gamma 134.5, a gene nonessential for growth in culture. Science 1990;250:1262–6.
175. Chou J, Chen JJ, Gross M, Roizman B. Association of a M(r) 90,000 phosphoprotein with protein kinase PKR in cells exhibiting enhanced phosphorylation of translation initiation factor eIF-2 alpha and premature shutoff of protein synthesis after infection with gamma 134.5- mutants of herpes simplex virus 1. Proc Natl Acad Sci U S A 1995;92:10516–20.
176. He B, Gross M, Roizman B. The gamma(1)34.5 protein of herpes simplex virus 1 complexes with protein phosphatase 1alpha to dephosphorylate the alpha subunit of the eukaryotic translation initiation factor 2 and preclude the shutoff of protein synthesis by double-stranded RNA-activated protein kinase. Proc Natl Acad Sci U S A 1997;94:843–8.
177. Chambers R, Gillespie G, Soroceanu L, et al. Comparison of genetically engineered herpes simplex viruses for the treatment of brain tumors in a scid mouse model of human malignant glioma. Proc Natl Acad Sci U S A 1995;92:1411–5.
178. Andreansky S, Soroceanu L, Flotte ER, et al. Evaluation of genetically engineered herpes simplex viruses as oncolytic agents for human malignant brain tumors. Cancer Res 1997;57:1502–9.
179. Farassati F, Yang AD, Lee PW. Oncogenes in Ras signalling pathway dictate host-cell permissiveness to herpes simplex virus 1. Nat Cell Biol 2001;3:745–50.
180. Mundschau LJ, Faller DV. Oncogenic ras induces an inhibitor of double-stranded RNA-dependent eukaryotic initiation factor 2 alpha-kinase activation. J Biol Chem 1992;267:23092–8.
181. Mohr I, Gluzman Y. A herpesvirus genetic element which affects translation in the absence of the viral GADD34 function. EMBO J 1996;15:4759–66.
182. Cassady KA, Gross M, Roizman B. The second-site mutation in the herpes simplex virus recombinants lacking the gamma134.5 genes precludes shutoff of protein synthesis by blocking the phosphorylation of eIF-2alpha. J Virol 1998;72:7005–11.
183. Mohr I, Sternberg D, Ward S, et al. A herpes simplex virus type 1 gamma34.5 second-site suppressor mutant that exhibits enhanced growth in cultured glioblastoma cells is severely attenuated in animals. J Virol 2001;75:5189–96.
184. Todo T, Martuza RL, Rabkin SD, Johnson PA. Oncolytic herpes simplex virus vector with enhanced MHC class I

presentation and tumor cell killing. Proc Natl Acad Sci U S A 2001;98:6396–401.
185. Mineta T, Rabkin SD, Yazaki T, et al. Attenuated multi-mutated herpes simplex virus-1 for the treatment of malignant gliomas. Nat Med 1995;1:938–43.
186. Meignier B, Martin B, Whitley RJ, Roizman B. In vivo behavior of genetically engineered herpes simplex viruses R7017 and R7020. II. Studies in immunocompetent and immunosuppressed owl monkeys (Aotus trivirgatus). J Infect Dis 1990;162:313–21.
187. Advani SJ, Chung SM, Yan SY, et al. Replication-competent, nonneuroinvasive genetically engineered herpes virus is highly effective in the treatment of therapy-resistant experimental human tumors. Cancer Res 1999;59:2055–8.
188. Delman KA, Bennett JJ, Zager JS, et al. Effects of preexisting immunity on the response to herpes simplex-based oncolytic viral therapy. Hum Gene Ther 2000;11:2465–72.
189. Tyler KL, Clarke P, DeBiasi RL, et al. Reoviruses and the host cell. Trends Microbiol 2001;9:560–4.
190. Strong J, Tang D, Lee P. Evidence that the epidermal growth factor receptor on host cells confers reovirus infection efficiency. Virology 1993;197:405–11.
191. Strong J, Coffey M, Tang D, et al. The molecular basis of viral oncolysis: usurpation of the Ras signaling pathway by reovirus. EMBO J 1998;17:3351–62.
192. Strong J, Lee P. The v-erbB oncogene confers enhanced cellular susceptibility to reovirus infection. J Virol 1996;70:612–6.
193. Coffey M, Strong J, Forsyth P, Lee P. Reovirus therapy of tumors with activated Ras pathway. Science 1998;282:1332–4.
194. Wilcox ME, Yang W, Senger D, et al. Reovirus as an oncolytic agent against experimental human malignant gliomas. J Natl Cancer Inst 2001;93:903–12.
195. Hirasawa K, Nishikawa SG, Norman KL, et al. Oncolytic reovirus against ovarian and colon cancer. Cancer Res 2002;62:1696–701.
196. Hallenbeck P, Chang Y, Hay C, et al. A novel tumor-specific replication-restricted adenoviral vector for gene therapy of hepatocellular carcinoma. Hum Gene Ther 1999;10:1721–33.
197. Rodriguez R, Schuur E, Lim H, et al. Prostate attenuated replication competent adenovirus (ARCA) CN706: a selective cytotoxic for prostate-specific antigen-positive prostate cancer cells. Cancer Res 1997;57:2559–63.
198. Kurihara T, Brough DE, Kovesdi I, Kufe DW. Selectivity of a replication-competent adenovirus for human breast carcinoma cells expressing the MUC1 antigen. J Clin Invest 2000;106:763–71.
199. DeLuca NA, McCarthy AM, Schaffer PA. Isolation and characterization of deletion mutants of herpes simplex virus type 1 in the gene encoding immediate-early regulatory protein ICP4. J Virol 1985;56:558–70.
200. Miyatake S-I, Tani S, Feigenbaum F, et al. Hepatoma-specific antitumor activity of an albumin enhancer/promoter regulated herpes simplex virus in vivo. Gene Ther 1999;6:564–72.
201. Yamamura H, Hashio M, Noguchi M, et al. Identification of the transcriptional regulatory sequences of human calponin promoter and their use in targeting a conditionally replicating herpes vector to malignant human soft tissue and bone tumors. Cancer Res 2001;61:3969–77.
202. Savontaus MJ, Sauter BV, Huang TG, Woo SL. Transcriptional targeting of conditionally replicating adenovirus to dividing endothelial cells. Gene Ther 2002;9:972–9.
203. Parker JN, Gillespie GY, Love CE, et al. Engineered herpes simplex virus expressing IL-12 in the treatment of experimental murine brain tumors. Proc Natl Acad Sci U S A 2000;97:2208–13.
204. Nakamura H, Mullen JT, Chandrasekhar S, et al. Multimodality therapy with a replication-conditional herpes simplex virus 1 mutant that expresses yeast cytosine deaminase for intratumoral conversion of 5-fluorocytosine to 5-fluorouracil. Cancer Res 2001;61:5447–52.
205. Rogulski KR, Wing MS, Paielli DL, et al. Double suicide gene therapy augments the antitumor activity of a replication-competent lytic adenovirus through enhanced cytotoxicity and radiosensitization. Hum Gene Ther 2000;11:67–76.
206. Blank SV, Rubin SC, Coukos G, et al. Replication-selective herpes simplex virus type 1 mutant therapy of cervical cancer is enhanced by low-dose radiation. Hum Gene Ther 2002;13:627–39.
207. Chen Y, DeWeese T, Dilley J, et al. CV706, a prostate cancer-specific adenovirus variant, in combination with radiotherapy produces synergistic antitumor efficacy without increasing toxicity. Cancer Res 2001;61:5453–60.
208. Advani SJ, Sibley GS, Song PY, et al. Enhancement of replication of genetically engineered herpes simplex viruses by ionizing radiation: a new paradigm for destruction of therapeutically intractable tumors. Gene Ther 1998;5:160–5.
209. Chahlavi A, Todo T, Martuza RL, Rabkin SD. Replication-competent herpes simplex virus vector G207 and cisplatin combination therapy for head and neck squamous cell carcinoma. Neoplasia 1999;1:162–9.
210. Heise C, Sampson-Johannes A, Williams A, et al. ONYX-015, an E1B gene-attenuated adenovirus, causes tumor-specific cytolysis and antitumoral efficacy that can be augmented by standard chemotherapeutic agents. Nature Med 1997;3:639–45.
211. You L, Yang CT, Jablons DM. ONYX-015 works synergistically with chemotherapy in lung cancer cell lines and primary cultures freshly made from lung cancer patients. Cancer Res 2000;60:1009–13.
212. Toyoizumi T, Mick R, Abbas AE, et al. Combined therapy with chemotherapeutic agents and herpes simplex virus type 1 ICP34.5 mutant (HSV-1716) in human non-small cell lung cancer. Hum Gene Ther 1999;10:3013–29.
213. Khuri FR, Nemunaitis J, Ganly I, et al. A controlled trial of intratumoral ONYX-015, a selectively-replicating adenovirus, in combination with cisplatin and 5-fluorouracil in patients with recurrent head and neck cancer. Nat Med 2000;6:879–85.
214. Stanziale SF, Petrowsky H, Joe JK, et al. Ionizing radiation potentiates the antitumor efficacy of oncolytic herpes simplex virus G207 by upregulating ribonucleotide reductase. Surgery 2002;132:353–9.
215. Bennett JJ, Delman KA, Burt BM, et al. Comparison of safety, delivery, and efficacy of two oncolytic herpes viruses (G207 and NV1020) for peritoneal cancer. Cancer Gene Ther 2002;9:935–45.
216. Kuo ML, Kinsella TJ. Expression of ribonucleotide reductase after ionizing radiation in human cervical carcinoma cells. Cancer Res 1998;58:2245–52.
217. Fornace AJ Jr, Nebert DW, Hollander MC, et al. Mammalian genes coordinately regulated by growth arrest signals and DNA-damaging agents. Mol Cell Biol 1989;9:4196–203.
218. Hollander MC, Zhan Q, Bae I, Fornace AJ Jr. Mammalian GADD34, an apoptosis- and DNA damage-inducible gene. J Biol Chem 1997;272:13731–7.
219. Chou J, Roizman B. Herpes simplex virus 1 gamma(1)34.5 gene function, which blocks the host response to infection, maps in the homologous domain of the genes expressed during growth arrest and DNA damage. Proc Natl Acad Sci U S A 1994;91:5247–51.

Section 16

BONE MARROW TRANSPLANTATION

58

Hematopoietic Cell Transplantation

Roy Jones, PhD, MD
Elizabeth Shpall, MD
Richard Champlin, MD

Hematopoietic cell transplantation involves engraftment of stem cells, which can be collected from the bone marrow, peripheral blood, or umbilical cord blood. Allogeneic transplants are obtained from another individual. Autologous transplants involve use of a patient's own hematopoietic cells, usually after cryopreservation. Syngeneic transplants are between genetically identical twins.

Hematopoietic transplantation is an effective treatment for many life-threatening hematologic, immune, metabolic, and neoplastic diseases (Table 58-1).[1,2] Hematopoietic transplantation has been studied in animal models since the late 1940s as a means to rescue recipients exposed to lethal irradiation or myeloablative drugs. Allogeneic transplantation was first successfully used in humans for treatment of children with severe combined immune deficiency.[2] Allogeneic transplants are used for treatment of bone marrow failure states, hemoglobinopathies, immune deficiencies, and inborn errors of metabolism by establishing a new, normally functioning hematopoietic and immune system. The most common use of allogeneic and autologous hematopoietic transplantation is for treatment of malignancies.

Donnall Thomas was awarded the Nobel Prize for his pioneering work in the development of hematopoietic cell transplantation, particularly for acute myelogenous leukemia.[3] Over time the use of transplantation has expanded to include at least the variety of indications included in Table 58-1 and its scientific basis has been more clearly refined to emphasize intensive chemoradiotherapy treatment of malignancy, immune replacement or augmentation for a variety of conditions, or genetic replacement.[4–7]

The basis for autologous hematopoietic cell transplantation is to use patient-derived hematopoietic stem cells to prevent otherwise lethal myelosuppression from intensive treatment. The primary use of this technique is to eradicate malignant cells or tumors resistant to less intense treatment. Recently, this technique is being explored as a method to deplete autoimmune cells associated with diverse diseases such as multiple sclerosis[8] or scleroderma.[9]

The basis of allogeneic hematopoietic transplantation is the engraftment of donor-derived stem cells; in the recipient these cells reconstitute hematopoiesis and immunity. Following successful transplantation, recipients are considered chimeras with hematopoietic and immune cells derived from the donor. Mesenchymal and epithelial tissues remain predominantly host derived. Recently, it has become established that bone marrow stem cells are capable of limited differentiation into nonhematopoietic tissues[10] including mesenchymal cells,[11,12] liver,[13,14] cardiovascular tissues,[15] and, possibly, neural tissue.[16] There is considerable interest in stem cell transplantation for restoration of damaged or diseased organs and tissues.[17,18]

Table 58-1 Diseases Treated with Hematopoietic Transplantation
Malignant
Acute myelogenous leukemia
Myelodysplastic syndromes
Acute lymphoblastic leukemia
Chronic myelogenous leukemia and myeloproliferative disorders
Chronic lymphocytic leukemia
Non-Hodgkin's lymphoma
Hodgkin's disease
Multiple myeloma and amyloidosis
Solid tumors: breast, testicular, ovarian, and small cell lung cancer
Pediatric solid tumors: neuroblastoma, Ewing sarcoma, medulloblastoma, renal cell cancer, melanoma
Nonmalignant
Aplastic anemia and related bone marrow failure states
Hemoglobinopathies: thalassemia, sickle cell anemia
Congenital disorders of hematopoiesis: Fanconi anemia and related syndromes
Congenital immune deficiencies: severe combined immune deficiency, Wiskott-Aldrich syndrome, chronic granulomatous disease, and related syndromes
Inborn errors of metabolism
Autoimmune disorders

METHODS OF TRANSPLANTATION

In most cases, transplanted hematopoietic cells are infused following intensive chemotherapy, irradiation, or other therapies such as antibodies. With chemotherapy, it is critical to delay the cell infusion until substantial disappearance of cytotoxic agent so as not to damage the infused cells. In the case of autologous transplantation, intensive treatment is the critical therapeutic principle and always precedes the cell infusion. Allogeneic transplantation can be designed to utilize a wider variety of therapeutic principles and thus the content of the pre-cell infusion treatments is more variable. As initially designed by Thomas and[19–21] Santos,[22] intensive chemotherapy with or without irradiation was used in a manner similar to autotransplants. This treatment was conceived with three goals in mind: (1) eradication of malignancy, (2) host immune ablation to allow acceptance of foreign cells, and (3) creation of "space" to allow engraftment. Over time a variety of chemotherapeutic agents has been explored for use in transplantation, emphasizing the alkylating agents cyclophosphamide, busulfan, melphalan, thiotepa, and carmustine (BCNU). The goal was to administer the highest doses of treatment that produced tolerable extrahematopoietic toxicity and, hopefully, maximal antitumor effect. It was established that total body irradiation could be delivered in a maximal dose of 1200–1400 cGy.[20,23]

More recently, the existence of graft-versus-malignancy (GVM) effect has been shown and established a therapeutic activity for allotransplantation independent of the pre-cell infusion treatment.[24] As with any treatment, GVM activity produces its own toxicity, immunosuppression, because of its close association with graft-versus-host disease (GVHD). With this new treatment, reduced-intensity pre-cell infusion treatment (nonmyeloablative allotransplantation) has been explored as a means of reducing the risk of allotransplantation. Additionally, infusions of donor lymphocytes (DLI) following transplantation can be used to augment the GVM effect.[25]

HEMATOPOIETIC TRANSPLANTATION AS TREATMENT FOR MALIGNANCIES

Most hematopoietic transplants have been performed for treatment of hematologic malignancies.[26] Many chemotherapy drugs (predominantly alkylating agents[27]) and irradiation produce a dose-dependent antitumor response. Higher doses produce greater cytoreduction and may overcome low-level drug resistance. Myelosuppression is the dose limiting toxicity of many chemotherapeutic agents and whole body irradiation. Doses of some agents can be markedly escalated three- to five-fold above conventional maximally tolerated dose if followed by autologous or allogeneic transplantation to restore hematopoiesis (Figure 58-1). Dose-intensive therapy with hematopoietic transplantation is an effective treatment for a wide range of hematologic malignancies and selected solid tumors.

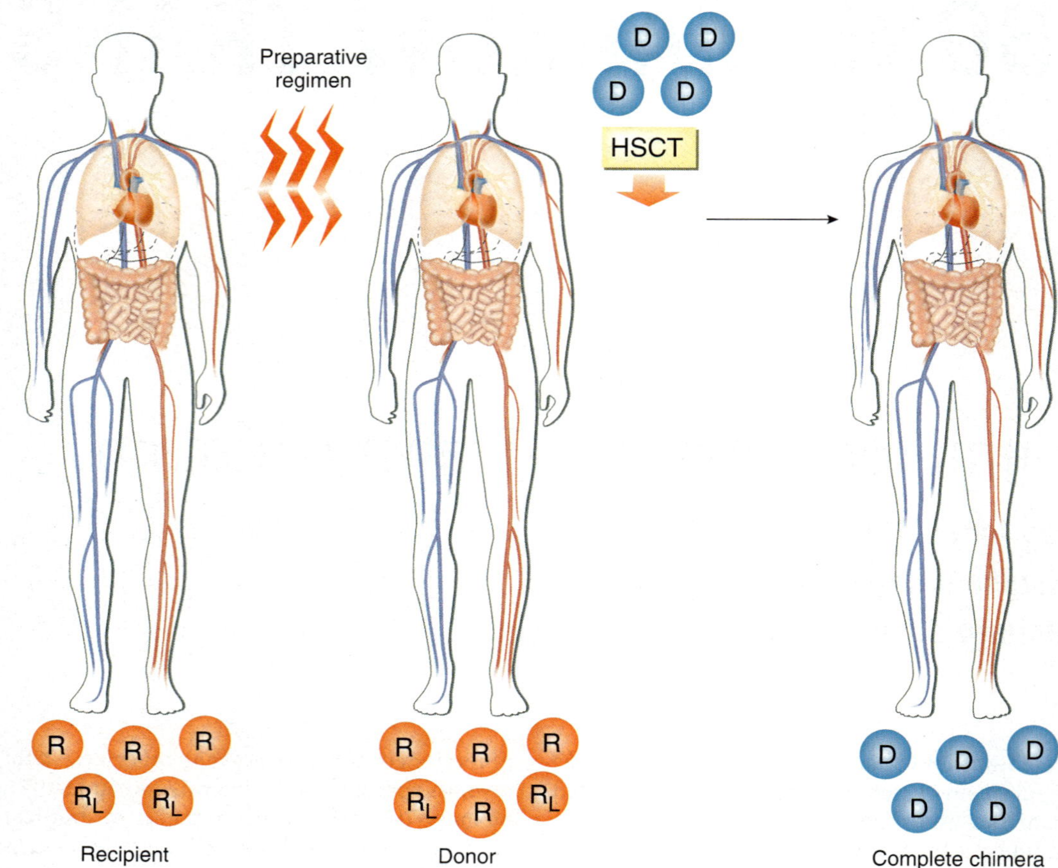

Figure 58-1 Scheme of allogeneic hematopoietic transplantation. The recipient receives a myeloablative preparative regimen designed to eradicate malignant and normal cells. The recipient then receives donor hematopoietic cells that restore hematopoiesis. D = donor hematopoietic cells; HSCT = hematopoietic stem cell transplant; R = recipient's normal bone marrow cells; RL = recipient's leukemia cells in bone marrow.

AUTOLOGOUS TRANSPLANTATION Autologous transplantation is generally designed to exploit the concept of dose intensity as described, and has been used to produce killing of tumor following relapse from conventional treatment or in a setting where conventional treatments are known to have little or no probability of tumor eradication. As a general rule, autologous hematopoietic transplantation is most effective in patients with malignancies shown to be responsive to conventional treatment immediately prior to the transplant regimen.[28] Other factors known to predispose to relapse include higher-volume residual tumor[29,30] tumor types not known to exhibit a steep dose-killing relationship,[30] or treatment of patients at high risk for toxicities from the proposed treatment regimen

During and for months following the transplant process significant immune suppression occurs as a result of depletion of immune cells from the patient and slow regrowth of the transplant.[31,32] The extent to which antitumor immunity aids in control of minimal tumor is controversial. Immune augmentation strategies used in the post-transplant setting are being actively explored to avoid this potential weakness.[33] An additional factor which might predispose to relapse using this technique is contamination of the harvested cells with tumor. Although limited investigation using gene-marked tumor cells has shown that cryopreserved tumor cells can engraft and contribute to relapse, the clinical importance of this phenomenon is unclear.[34] Numerous studies have failed to demonstrate benefit from depletion of tumor cells from grafts, but only partial depletion was usually achieved in those studies.[35] Further research awaits development of high-level tumor depletion technologies.

Malignancies shown to be cured by autologous hematopoietic cell transplantation include intermediate grade lymphoma,[36] Hodgkin's disease,[37] acute lymphoblastic leukemia,[21,38] and acute myelogenous leukemia.[39,40] Although not proven to be curative, major improvement in survival in myeloma patients receiving autologous transplantation have made the technique a standard treatment for appropriate patients with this condition.[41,42] Benefit for patients with breast,[43] and ovarian[44] cancers, germ cell cancers,[45] low grade lymphomas,[46] and a variety of pediatric solid tumors[47] are more controversial but are being actively studied.

ALLOGENEIC TRANSPLANTATION Allogeneic hematopoietic transplants also confer an immune-mediated graft-versus-malignancy (GVM) effect. Donor-derived lymphoid cells may react against and eradicate malignant cells that survive high-dose cytotoxic therapy.[48,49] The risk of relapse of the malignancy after high-dose therapy and hematopoietic transplantation is increased in syngeneic transplants compared to allogeneic transplants.[50,51] Relapse risk is also increased if the putative effector cells, T lymphocytes, are depleted from an allogeneic transplant for prevention of GVHD.[52] Patients with acute or chronic GVHD have reduced risk of relapse, suggesting a relationship between GVM and GVHD.[53,54] High doses of immunosuppressive therapy have been associated with an increased risk of relapse, and withdrawal of immunosuppressive treatment can occasionally produce remission in patients relapsing after transplantation.[55] The most direct evidence for GVM comes from the observation that donor lymphocyte infusion (DLI) can reinduce remission in patients who relapse post-transplant.[56,57]

There are major differences among malignancies in their susceptibility to GVM effects. Indolent myeloid and lymphoid malignancies are highly sensitive to this process, as evidenced by durable remissions after modulation of immunosuppression or donor lymphocyte infusions in patients who have relapsed after an allogeneic transplant. GVM effects have been best documented in patients with chronic myelogenous leukemia. The majority of patients who relapse into chronic phase following an allogeneic transplant achieve durable complete remission with donor lymphocyte infusions.[55] Follicular lymphomas, mantle cell lymphoma, and chronic lymphocytic leukemia (CLL) also appear very sensitive to graft-versus-malignancy effects.[58,59] Allogeneic transplants are associated with a substantially lower relapse rate than purged autologous transplants. Selected patients with CLL or low-grade lymphoma have responded to donor lymphocyte infusions or modification of immunosuppressive therapy.

Graft-versus-malignancy effects also occur but with lesser intensity against other hematologic malignancies including acute myelogenous leukemia (AML), multiple myeloma, Hodgkin's disease and intermediate-grade lymphoma. In these diagnoses, allogeneic transplants produce a greater frequency of durable remissions than syngeneic or autologous transplants, but these disorders respond less frequently to DLI and responses are usually transient. Acute lymphoblastic leukemia and high-grade lymphoma appear relatively insensitive to graft-versus-leukemia (GVL) effects,[60] although patients with GVHD do have a reduced risk of relapse.[53]

Graft-versus-malignancy effects may also affect some solid tumors, particularly renal cell carcinoma; approximately one-third of patients have achieved complete and partial remissions.[61] Selected patients with breast cancer and other solid tumors have also responded.[62]

GVM effects may be directed against a number of potential target antigens. This may involve immune reactivity against broadly expressed major or minor histocompatibility antigens; targets which overlap with GVHD. GVM could also result from reactivity against minor histocompatibility antigens restricted to hematopoietic cells, a graft-versus-hematopoietic effect. This may explain the occurrence of GVM effects without GVHD in hematologic diseases. Malignancy-specific antigens, such as the products of mutated genes or over-expressed cellular antigens may also be involved. Development of methods to separate GVM effects and GVHD, and generate antigen-specific antitumor responses is a major goal of ongoing research.

DONOR SELECTION

Autologous Transplantation Autologous transplants use the patient as their own donor. In the closely related special case, syngeneic transplants are donations from a genetically identical twin. Autologous transplants require no histocompatibility matching but often come from patients who have received extensive prior chemotherapy. This treatment often produces compromise of marrow stem cell function. As a general rule, the more extensive the pre-harvest chemotherapy, the greater the probability that the harvest will be unsatisfactory. Because the harvested patient has already been screened for suitability as a transplant patient, comorbid factors preventing the patient from being harvested are unlikely. Thus, adequacy of the harvested cells is the single critical factor in this process. Two factors limit suitability of harvested cells: (1) engraftment potential, and (2) extent of tumor contamination. Both of these factors are discussed later in the chapter. Patients undergo collection of bone marrow or peripheral blood progenitor cells that are then cryopreserved in a viable state. Patients subsequently receive high-dose myelosuppressive therapy to eradicate the malignancy, followed by reinfusion of the stored autologous cells to reconstitute hematopoiesis. Autologous transplants have the advantage that the hematopoietic cells will not be rejected or produce GVHD. However, autologous transplants may be contaminated by malignant cells and do not confer a GVM effect. Unmodified autologous transplants cannot be used for genetic or acquired diseases in which the hematopoietic cells are injured or defective, although autologous hematopoietic cells can potentially be used as vehicles for gene therapy designed to correct deficiency states.

Allogeneic Transplantation Allogeneic transplants are collected from a related or unrelated donor. The human leukocyte antigen (HLA) system is the major histocompatibility complex (MHC) in man, and the results of allogeneic transplantation depend on the histocompatibility between donor and recipient. The HLA system is encoded by several closely linked loci on the short arm of chromosome 6.[63] Class I loci include HLA-A, -B, and -C alleles. The class II region includes DR, DQ, and DP loci. Compatibility was initially defined by serologic assays. The serologic groups have recently been further divided into specific alleles by molecular oligonucleotide typing.

Most transplants have been from HLA-identical sibling donors. The HLA genes are inherited as a haplotype with one haplotype derived from each parent. There is approximately a one in four chance that any given sibling will be HLA matched with a potential recipient. Unfortunately, most patients lack an HLA-identical sibling. Related donor-recipient pairs that are mismatched for only one A, B, or DR HLA locus have a higher incidence of GVHD and graft failure, but survival is similar to transplants between HLA-identical siblings. Registries of potential unrelated donors have been established to provide hematopoietic transplants for patients lacking a histocompatible relative. HLA gene frequencies vary considerably among racial and ethnic groups, and patients are likely to find transplants among potential donors of their own genetic background. Linkage disequilibrium occurs such that some common haplotypes occur, but approximately half of the populations have rare haplotypes. There are now over 5 million potential unrelated bone marrow donors accessible in registries worldwide, and approximately half of patients can access an HLA-A, -B, and -DR–identical donor. Unrelated donor transplants are often successful, although the incidence and severity of graft-versus-host disease is increased, compared to transplants from HLA-identical siblings.[64,65] This is related in part to greater genetic disparity for non-HLA antigens among unrelated individuals; these pairs are also more likely to be mismatched for HLA molecular variants. Recent studies in which unrelated donors were selected using molecular allele typing methods have had a reduced risk of GVHD, and results are approaching those seen with transplants from HLA-identical siblings.[66–68]

Transplant recipients who are mismatched for two or more loci have relatively poor results, with a high risk of graft rejection, GVHD, and associated complications.[69] Haploidentical donors are readily available for most patients. Aggressive T-cell depletion (4 to 5 log reduction) of the donor hematopoietic cells can prevent GVHD, but results in a higher rate of graft failure.[70,71] Results have been improved with the use of "megadoses" of T-cell–depleted peripheral blood progenitor cells and an intensive myeloablative preparative regimen.[72] Delayed immune reconstitution and a high frequency of opportunistic infections remain major complications. Because these difficulties have resisted substantial improvement, umbilical cord blood (UCB) is now frequently used.[73] Constraints for HL-A matching of UCB are much less than that for other cell sources, with mismatches at 2 of 6 HL-A A, B, and DR loci acceptable.[74] Owing to the size of the units, cord blood transplants have been most successful in children, but are also under investigation in adults.[75] Recent data suggest that outcomes may be improving rapidly, and could be equivalent to survival for patients receiving serologically matched unrelated cell donations.

ENGRAFTMENT OF HEMATOPOIETIC TRANSPLANTS

Autologous Transplants Autologous hematopoietic cells can be obtained from either bone marrow or after "mobilization" from peripheral blood. Peripheral blood-derived cells are now routinely used for autologous transplantation because they engraft more rapidly. Mobilization is accomplished by administration of granulocyte-stimulating hematopoietic growth factors alone or in combination with chemotherapy. The combination clearly produces higher yields of precursor cells but is more time consuming and requires doses of chemotherapy that produce transient pancytopenia and risk of infection. Selection of mobilization technique requires estimation of the likely quality of the patient's progenitor cells as has been reviewed.[76] Hematopoietic transplantation requires collection of sufficient numbers of hematopoietic stem cells for reconstitution of hematopoiesis and immunity.[77,78] A major area of ongoing research is to characterize the phenotype and function of hematopoietic stem cells. Human repopulating stem and progenitor cells express the CD34 cell surface antigen that comprises $< 1\%$ of the bone marrow.[79] Highly enriched CD34 positively selected cells have been used for autologous or allogeneic hematopoietic transplantation, resulting in rapid hematologic recovery.[79] Stem cells also express *c-Kit*,[80] thy-1,[81] and AC133.[82] More primitive CD34-negative stem cells have been described which can differentiate into CD34+ progenitors.[83,84] Recent data indicate that CD34 expression is reversibly expressed by activated stem cells.[60] Common lymphoid and myeloid progenitors have recently been described that contribute to initial engraftment and early reconstitution of lymphoid and myeloid cells, respectively.

Hematopoietic stem cells reside primarily in the bone marrow, and initially, hematopoietic transplantation used unfractionated bone marrow cells. Donors undergo general or regional anesthesia. One to 1.5 liters of marrow is harvested by multiple aspirations; usually from the posterior superior iliac crests.[85] Adequate collections include 2 to 5×10^8 nucleated cells/kg and 0.5 to 3×10^6 CD34+ cells/kg. The procedure is generally safe for the donor. Hematopoietic cells are rapidly regenerated and there are no long-term adverse consequences for the donors. Rare complications may occur, primarily relating to general anesthesia and to infection or injury at the site of marrow aspirations.

Hematopoietic stem cells circulate in low frequency in the peripheral blood and peripheral blood progenitor cells (PBPC) have been used as an alternative source of hematopoietic cells for transplantation.[86,87] Hematopoietic stem cells are "mobilized" from the marrow during recovery from myelosuppressive chemotherapy and by treatment with various cytokines.[88,89] Treatment with G-CSF increases the frequency of CD34+ cells 25-fold, allowing collection of an adequate dose for transplantation by apheresis.[90]

The rate of hematopoietic recovery post transplant correlates with the number of CD34+ cells/kg infused. The minimum number of cells necessary for transplantation is not well defined, but optimal hematopoietic recovery with PBPC requires $> 5 \times 10^6$ CD34+ cells/kg.[91] After the therapy is completed, the hematopoietic cells are infused intravenously. The cells circulate transiently and sufficient numbers of stem cells home to the bone marrow to restore hematopoiesis. Peripheral blood counts are profoundly suppressed following high-dose chemotherapy, but generally recover within 2.5 to 4 weeks following bone marrow transplantation. The date of engraftment is generally defined as the first of three consecutive days with an absolute neutrophil count $> 0.5 \times 10^9$/L. Hematopoietic growth factors granulocyte colony-stimulating factor (G-CSF) or granulocyte-macrophage colony-stimulating factor (GM-CSF) accelerate recovery of granulocyte counts, but have no effect on erythrocytes or platelets. Transplantation of PBPC generally produces more rapid hematopoietic recovery than bone marrow, and they accelerate recovery of platelets as well as granulocytes. Granulocyte recovery following PBPC infusion generally occurs within 10 to 14 days.[76]

Tumor Cell Contamination and Purging For autologous transplantation, the patient must first undergo collection of hematopoietic stem cells and cryopreservation.[92,93] Cryopreservation can be reliably performed, and the stored cells remain viable for more than 5 years. Hematopoietic cell collection should ideally occur at a time when the bone marrow is normally cellular and the blood and marrow do not contain malignant cells. Malignant cells may contaminate autologous stem cell products; the likelihood varies with the diagnosis and disease stage. Mobilized peripheral blood stem cells tend to have a lower frequency of tumor cell contamination than bone marrow harvests.[94] Peripheral blood stem cell transplants can be performed in patients in whom marrow harvesting is not feasible, such as those with prior pelvic radiotherapy.

Tumor cells can be identified in histologically normal product by a variety of techniques, including cell culture, flow cytometry, immunohistochemistry, and polymerase chain reaction for amplification of clone-specific markers, such as a typical translocation or immunoglobulin gene rearrangement. Gene marking studies using retroviral gene vectors have shown that tumor cells contained in the graft can contribute to relapse in patients with leukemia, neuroblastoma, and presumably other diagnoses.[95–97] Numerous clinical studies have shown that tumor cell contamination of the autograft is associated with shortened disease-free survival.[98–100] Purging methods have been developed to deplete the autograft of tumor cells in an attempt to improve outcomes.[91] Purging methods most often use monoclonal antibodies combined with complement, immunomagnetic beads, or conjugated toxins. Positive selection of CD34+ cells is another widely used approach,[101,102] and combined methods are investigated as a potentially better purging strategy. Pharmacological purging include ex vivo treatment of the autograft with chemotherapeutic agents such as 4-hydroxycyclophosphamide.[103,104]

The clinical benefit of purging is not well documented. Successful purging of marrow harvests of patients with follicular lymphoma or with breast cancer was associated with superior outcome.[98] However, the presence of tumor cells in the autograft may correlate with the extent of systemic residual disease, and this is not direct evidence that reinfused tumor cells caused relapse. Most patient's relapse in sites of prior disease, and inadequate systemic cytoreduction is believed to be the major cause of relapse post-autologous transplantation. An alternative explanation is that tumor cells in the graft home preferentially to sites of prior disease where the microenvironment supports their growth. There are no randomized studies documenting reduced relapse rates using purged versus unpurged autologous transplants, and the role of purging remains controversial.

Allogeneic Transplantation A pretransplant immunosuppressive treatment, often termed the "preparative regimen," or "conditioning," is necessary to prevent rejection of an allogeneic hematopoietic transplant. More intensive pretransplant immunosuppression is required for hematopoietic transplantation than is necessary to prevent rejection of solid organ allografts such as kidney, liver, or heart. The immunosuppressive preparative treatment administered prior to transplantation must markedly suppress the recipient's T lymphocyte and natural killer (NK) cell function. The intensity of immunosuppressive therapy required for engraftment varies depending on the immunocompetence of the recipient and the composition of the transplanted cells. High doses of donor stem cells and T cells present in the allograft also enhance engraftment by an alloreactive graft-versus-host hematopoietic effect.[72,105]

Allogeneic engraftment of donor cells can be documented by acquisition of donor-type cell surface antigens, isoenzymes, chromosome markers, or DNA–restriction fragment length polymorphisms. Following successful transplantation, cells of the hematologic and immunologic systems are primarily derived from the donor, although in some cases mixed chimerism occurs in which both donor and recipient derived cells are present. Mixed chimerism is more frequent after T-cell depletion of the donor graft and after nonmyeloablative conditioning.

Granulocyte recovery after PBPC or bone marrow allotransplantation occurs with timing similar to autologous transplantation. PBPC contains approximately one log more T cells than a bone marrow harvest that affects the immunologic effects after allogeneic transplantation.[106] In most studies, the incidence and severity of acute GVHD is unchanged with PBPC compared to bone marrow,[107,108] but the rate of chronic GVHD has been increased.[40,108] Recent studies have reported improved early survival after allogeneic transplantation of PBPC compared to bone marrow in high risk recipients.[109,110]

Umbilical cord blood has recently been proposed as an alternative source of hematopoietic stem cells for transplantation from related or unrelated donors. The umbilical cord contains 50 to 100 mL of fetal blood, which can be collected after delivery of the placenta and separation from the fetus. Cord blood is a rich source of hematopoietic stem and progenitor cells.[111,112] The major limitation is the small number of hematopoietic cells that can be collected from a single umbilical cord, less than 10% of the cell dose administered in a typical bone marrow transplant. The advantage with cord blood transplantation is that the rate of GVHD is reduced compared to bone marrow transplantation;[113] this reduction allows transplantation into partially HLA-mismatched, related and unrelated recipients. Many unrelated cord blood registries and collection centers have been established.[114] Transplant results have been related to the cell dose transplanted per kg recipient body weight, with the best results if $> 3 \times 10^7$ nucleated cells/kg are infused.[115,116] The time to engraftment and hematologic recovery after cord blood transplantation depends on the cell dose administered and may be very prolonged, > 6 weeks in some patients.

Nonablative Hematopoietic Transplant The recipient (R), a patient with normal and malignant leukemia cells (RL) in the bone marrow, receives a nonmyeloablative preparative regimen designed to prevent rejection of the transplant. The patient receives hematopoietic cells from the donor, which, after engraftment, produces a state of mixed chimerism in which both donor and recipient derived cells coexist. A subsequent graft-versus-hematopoietic effect may then occur which eradicates residual normal and malignant cells of host origin, resulting in complete chimerism (presence of only donor derived hematopoietic and immune cells). A donor lymphocyte infusion (DLI) may be administered to augment the graft-versus-malignancy effect.

SELECTION OF AUTOLOGOUS OR ALLOGENEIC TRANSPLANTATION

Selection of the type of transplantation for a patient, autologous or allogeneic, depends on the type of malignancy, age of the recipient, availability of a suitable donor, the ability to collect a tumor-free autograft, the stage and status of disease (bone marrow involvement, bulk of disease, chemosensitivity to conventional chemotherapy), and the malignancy's susceptibility to GVM effects.

Autologous transplantation is readily available, and there is no need to identify an HLA-matched donor. Autologous transplants have a lower risk of life-threatening complications; there is no risk of GVHD and no need for immunosuppressive therapy to prevent GVHD and graft rejection. Immune reconstitution is more rapid than after an allogeneic transplant and there is a lower risk of opportunistic infections. Graft failure occurs rarely. Treatment-related mortality is lower than 5% in most studies, and elderly patients can tolerate treatment relatively well.[117,118]

However, autologous transplants have several drawbacks. Since malignant cells may involve the blood and bone marrow, the autograft may be contaminated with clonogenic tumor cells that can contribute to relapse. Autologous transplantation relies solely on the effect of high-dose cytoreductive treatment and lacks the immune-mediated GVM effect resulting after allogeneic transplantation. In most malignancies, relapse rates are higher after autologous transplants than after allogeneic transplantation, although this is often offset by a lower rate of treatment-related mortality. Prior therapy, especially with multiple courses of alkylating agents or purine analogs, produce cumulative myelosuppression and may result in poor stem cell collection and persistent pancytopenia after transplant.[119] Patients with extensive prior therapy are at high risk for developing myelodysplasia and secondary acute leukemia after autologous hematopoietic transplantation.[120,121]

Allogeneic transplantation has the advantage that the graft is free of contaminating tumor cells. The graft also includes donor-derived immunocompetent cells, which may produce an immune GVM effect. There is generally a lower risk for disease recurrence after allogeneic transplants compared to autologous transplantation. However, allogeneic transplants may be associated with a number of potentially fatal complications such as regimen-related organ toxicity, graft failure, and GVHD. Immune reconstitution is slower after allogeneic transplantation and opportunistic infections are more frequent. Treatment-related mortality is significantly higher than with autologous transplantation and is increased with mismatched or unrelated allogeneic transplants compared to transplantation from an HLA-identical sibling donor.

Allogeneic hematopoietic transplantation has usually been restricted to younger patients in good general condition because of the increased risk of regimen-related toxicity and GVHD with advanced age. Most malignancies that are effectively treated by allogeneic transplantation are more common in elderly patients. The development of non-ablative preparative regimens, as well as improvement in supportive care, infection control, and immunosuppressive therapy now enable many centers to treat older patients, > 65 years of age.[122–124]

In general, allogeneic transplants have been used in the treatment of leukemias and myelodysplastic syndromes. Autologous transplants have been used more often in solid tumors, lymphoma, and myeloma, although non-ablative allogeneic transplants are under evaluation in these disorders as a means to induce GVM effects.

The outcome of transplantation relates to the selection of patients and timing of transplant during the natural history of the malignancy. The best results occur when the transplant is performed early in the disease course, when the malignancy is still sensitive to chemoradiotherapy treatment, and when the tumor burden is low. Conversely, transplants done as a last resort are associated with high rates of both relapse and treatment-related toxicity. The malignancy may also be complicated by development of infections, organ toxicity, or poor performance status over time, which markedly increases the risk of transplant-related complications. Many malignancies can be initially controlled with relatively nontoxic standard forms of chemotherapy, and transplants are best employed after failure of initial treatment. In general, transplantation should be offered early in the course to patients with diseases that are at high risk for relapse or transformation to aggressive form, or to patients with early disease recurrence. The possibility of future transplant should be considered early in the course of appropriate malignancies, and early identification of a potential donor is advisable so that a transplant can be promptly performed should the disease recur.

Responsiveness to conventional-dose chemotherapy is a major predictive factor for the outcome of hematopoietic transplant. The best results have been achieved in patients with chemosensitive relapse or when transplant is performed in high-risk patients as consolidation of response, particularly in patients with minimal disease at the time of transplant. Patients with partial response to initial chemotherapy are also good candidates. Primary resistance can sometimes be overcome by dose-intense treatment, such as in patients with acute leukemia, Hodgkin's disease, or multiple myeloma who have failed to achieve an initial remission. However, patients with bulky disease, refractory relapse, or multiple relapses of their malignancy have a poor prognosis.

PRETRANSPLANT THERAPY

Autologous Transplantation Early autologous treatment regimens were copied from the allogeneic experience and utilized cyclophosphamide plus either total body irradiation (TBI) or busulfan. TBI has the advantage of being able to be delivered in precise dose and with protection of vulnerable organs such as lungs and kidneys. TBI is suboptimal for the treatment of bulk tumor masses where hypoxia and resistance may characterize deep-seated tumor cells. In contrast, chemotherapy agents such as busulfan penetrate tumor vascularity and reaches deep-seated tumors more effectively. Thus, although TBI is still used in autotransplantation and can be very effective in patients with leukemia or non-bulky tumor, regional radiotherapy is used increasingly as an adjunct to chemotherapy treatments to areas of bulk tumor.

Alkylating agents are the most commonly used drugs in transplant regimens because they usually kill tumor cells in direct proportion to increasing dose.[1] Ironically cyclophosphamide, the first agent used in transplantation, only does so if the rate of drug dosing is less than the activating capacity of the liver, as cyclophosphamide is a prodrug incapable of killing tumor without activation.[6] The other most commonly used alkylating agents include melphalan, busulfan, BCNU, and thiotepa. The platinum derivatives carboplatin[125] and cisplatin[126] are also used extensively. Other commonly used non-alkylator are etoposide (VP-16), cytosine arabinoside, and fludarabine. As a general rule, drugs explored for use with transplantation must be able to have their doses escalated several fold above conventional dose range.

The most frequently used chemotherapy regimen is BEAM (BCNU, etoposide, Ara-C, and melphalan), commonly used for Hodgkin's disease and lymphomas.[127] The ICE regimen (ifosfamide, carboplatin, etoposide) is also used for these diseases.

In recent years, monoclonal antibodies have proven to be useful when added to standard treatments for leukemia and lymphoma. Gemtuzumab (Mylotarg) is being studied as part of transplant regimens.[128] Rituximab, shown to improve the survival of patients with intermediate grade lymphoma when combined with cyclophosphamide, doxorubicin, vincristine, and prednisone (CHOP) chemotherapy, is being studied as a component of transplant regimens.[129] Radiolabeled monoclonal antibodies are also being explored in this setting as are radioisotopes chelated by bone-seeking small molecules capable of targeted treatment to tumor involving bone and bone marrow.[130]

Allogeneic Transplantation For the treatment of malignancies, the preparative regimen may be directed to eradicating the malignancy or the defective hematopoietic tissue. The preparative regimen generally involves chemotherapy drugs alone, perhaps using newer agents as previously described for autotransplants, or combined with TBI. The classical "myeloablative" regimens used in the treatment of leukemia are designed to ablate both hematopoiesis and immunity in the recipient and typically involves the combination of high-dose cyclophosphamide with either TBI[131,132] or high-dose busulfan.[133,134] These regimens are sufficient to produce engraftment of > 98% of allogeneic transplants from HLA-identical siblings. More intensive immunosuppression is necessary for transplants from HLA-nonidentical siblings or if T cells are depleted from the allograft in order to prevent GVHD; addition of other myelosuppressive or immunosuppressive drugs such as anti-thymocyte globulin (ATG) have been employed to enhance engraftment in these settings.

The toxicity of high-dose myeloablative therapy limits the use of this modality to relatively young patients in good medical condition. The discovery of the curative potential of the immune mediated GVM effect has led to a novel approach using lower-dose, non-ablative preparative regimens as a means to reduce the toxicity of allogeneic hematopoietic transplantation. These nonmyeloablative conditioning regimens have been designed not to eradicate the malignancy, but rather to provide sufficient immunosuppression to achieve engraftment and to allow induction of GVM (Figure 58-2).[124,135,136] These regimens can be tolerated by older patients and those with co-morbidities who were not eligible to receive an ablative preparative regimen. Nonablative regimens are now being investigated as an alternative strategy to reduce transplant-related morbidity in a variety of settings. Most non-ablative regimens include a purine analog, such as fludarabine, combined with an alkylating agent (cyclophosphamide, melphalan, or busulfan) or low-dose total body irradiation. Engraftment has been achieved in most patients, and this approach is effective against a range of hematologic malignancies and possibly selected solid tumors such as renal carcinoma.

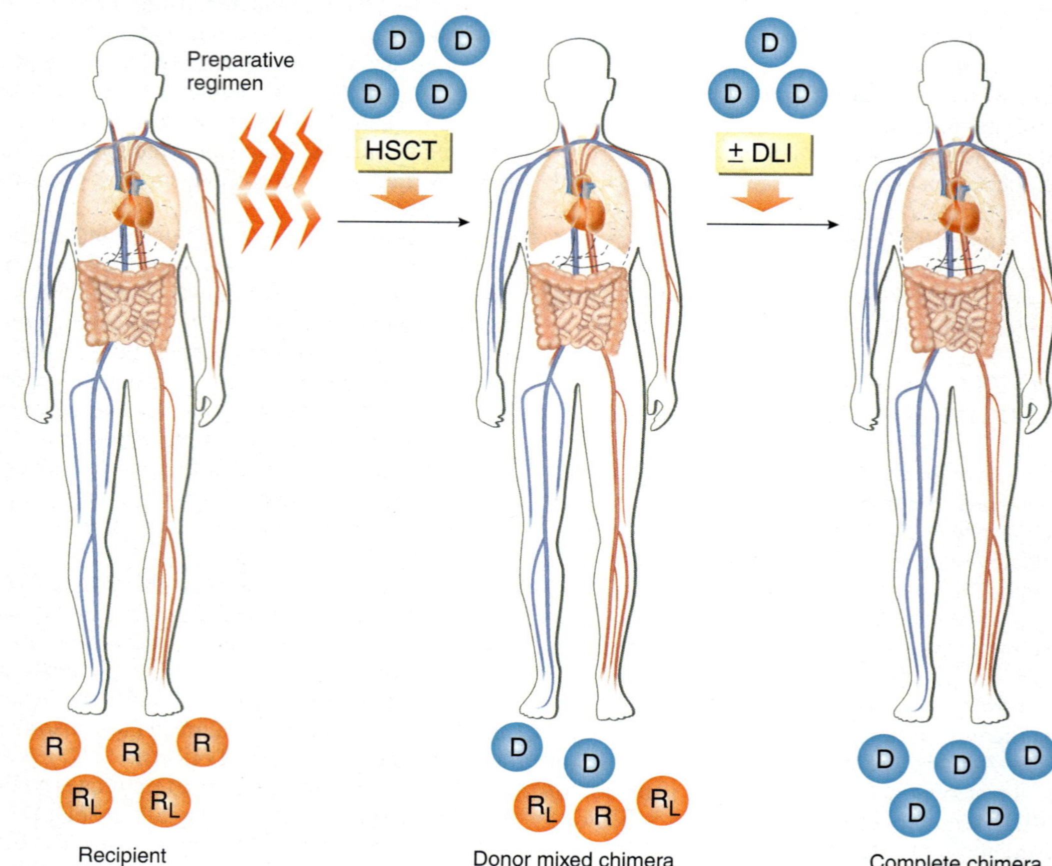

Figure 58-2 Scheme of non-ablative allogeneic hematopoietic transplantation. D = donor hematopoietic cells; DLI = donor lymphocyte infusion; HSCT = hematopoietic stem cell transplant; R = recipient's normal bone marrow cells; RL = recipient's leukemia cells in bone marrow.

COMPLICATIONS OF HEMATOPOIETIC TRANSPLANTATION

Intensive chemoradiotherapy and hematopoietic transplantations may be associated with a number of serious complications as listed in Table 58-2. These include immune-mediated processes such as graft rejection and GVHD, toxicities resulting from the pretransplant conditioning regimen, infections due to neutropenia, and post-transplant immune deficiency.

GRAFT REJECTION AND GRAFT FAILURE

Graft failure is defined as the failure to establish hematopoietic engraftment (primary graft failure) or loss of an established graft (secondary graft failure). This is defined as granulocytes failing to recover to > 0.5×10^9/L or falling below this level for > 3 days after initial recovery. Graft failure after autologous transplant occurs rarely and is most often related to infusion of an inadequate number of viable stem cells. Purging techniques, which may injure or reduce the numbers of hematopoietic stem cells, increase the risk of graft failure. It is recommended that an untreated, autologous backup marrow or peripheral blood stem cell collection be stored for patients receiving purged grafts; this backup collection can be infused to rescue patients if poor hematologic recovery or graft failure occurs.

Graft failure after allogeneic transplantation is most commonly due to immunologic rejection. Graft rejection is caused by host-derived cytotoxic T lymphocytes, NK cells, or antibodies directed against donor hematopoietic cells.[137,138] With current regimens, rejection occurs in fewer than 2% of transplants from an HLA-identical sibling. The risk is increased in recipients of HLA-mismatched or matched unrelated donor transplants.[72,139,140] Donor CD8+ T lymphocytes provide a graft-facilitating effect, and T lymphocyte depletion from the allogeneic graft increases the risk of graft failure.[141,142] Other accessory cells with graft-facilitating activity also exist.[142] Infusion of a larger number of stem cells[72] and increasing the myeloablative and immunosuppressive intensity of the preparative regimen[73] enhances engraftment.

Graft failure or poor graft function may be caused by administration of myelosuppressive

Table 58-2 Complications after Hematopoietic Transplantation

Immune complications
Graft rejection
Acute and chronic graft-versus-host disease
Regimen-related toxicity of the preparative regimen
Mucositis and gastroenteritis
Veno-occlusive disease of the liver
Diffuse alveolar hemorrhage and interstitial pneumonitis
Hemorrhagic cystitis
Hematologic complications
Hemolytic anemia
Thrombotic thrombocytopenic purpura hemolytic disorders
Infections and immunodeficiency
EBV associated lymphoproliferative disease
Late complications
Growth disturbances
Hypothyroidism
Sterility and hypogonadism
Cataracts
Avascular necrosis
Secondary malignancies

EBV = Epstein-Barr virus.

drugs, GVHD, and infections in the early post transplant period. Ganciclovir, given for prevention or treatment of cytomegalovirus infections, is the most common drug producing graft failure; this is generally reversible when the drug is discontinued. Trimethoprim-sulfamethoxazole given to prevent *Pneumocystis carinii* infections is modestly myelosuppressive and only rarely produces graft failure. Cytomegalovirus,[143] parvovirus,[144] human herpesvirus 6,[145] and mycobacterial and fungal infections may also compromise the graft. Poor engraftment may also result from microenvironment or marrow stroma dysfunction related to the patient's underlying disease or prior therapy.

Graft failure that is not due to rejection can often be successfully treated with growth factors G-CSF or GM-CSF[146] or second hematopoietic stem cell infusion from the same donor or an alternative donor.

Table 58-3 Clinical Staging and Grading of GVHD

Acute GVHD

Stage	Skin[a]	Liver[b]	Gut[b]
1	maculopapular rash < 25%	bilirubin 2–3 mg/dL	diarrhea 500–1,000 mL or persistent nausea[c]
2	maculopapular rash 25–50%	bilirubin 3–6 mg/dL	diarrhea 1,000–1,500 mL
3	generalized erythroderma	bilirubin 6–15 mg/dL	diarrhea > 1,500 mL
4	desquamation and bulla	bilirubin > 15 mg/dL	Severe abdominal pain or ileus

[a] extents determined by rule of nines or burn chart
[b] downgrade one stage for additional causes of elevated bilirubin or diarrhea
[c] requires histologic evidence of GVHD in the stomach or duodenum
GVHD = graft-versus-host disease.

Overall Grade[a]	Severity	Skin		Liver		Gut
0	None	0		0		0
I	Mild	1-2		0		0
II	Moderate	3	or	1 or	or	1
III	Severe			2–3 or		2–3
IV[b]	Life threatening	4 or	or	4 or	or	4

Sources: Glucksberg H, et al,[150] Przepiorka D, et al.[107]
[a]Minimal organ stage required to determine grade.
[b]Grade IV may also be determined with lower organ involvement with extreme decrease in performance status.

Grading of Chronic GVHD

Limited	Localized skin involvement and/or hepatic dysfunction
Extensive	1. Generalized skin involvement or 2. Localized skin involvement and/or hepatic dysfunction, plus any of the following: a. Liver histology showing chronic aggressive hepatitis, bridging necrosis or cirrhosis b. eye involvement (Schirmer's test < 5 mm wetting) c. involvement of mucosalivary glands or oral mucosa d. involvement of any other target organ

Source: Sullivan KM, et al.[161]

GRAFT-VERSUS-HOST DISEASE

Graft-versus-host disease (GVHD) is a major, potentially life threatening complication of allogeneic hematopoietic transplantation. Acute and chronic GVHD are distinct, but interrelated syndromes. Acute GVHD typically occurs within the first 100 days post transplant and results from reactivity of mature donor T lymphocytes present in the graft directed against disparate major or minor histocompatibility antigens of the recipient (the host). Chronic GVHD is a syndrome of disordered immune regulation that resembles a number of autoimmune diseases. The classical manifestations of chronic GVHD generally develop between day 80 and 2 years post-transplant.

The pathophysiology of acute GVHD involves three phases.[147] The first involves conditioning-regimen–related tissue injury resulting in cytokine release, up-regulation of HLA molecules, activation of macrophages, and generation of a pro-inflammatory state. In the second phase, alloreactive T cells recognize allogeneic antigens presented on host dendritic cells, become activated, and expand. The third phase involves generation of effector cells and cytokines that produce tissue injury. Acute GVHD requires donor T lymphocytes and recipient antigen-presenting cells to occur.[148] A corollary of these activation mechanisms is that conditioning regimens producing greater tissue injury may produce more intense GVHD.

Acute GVHD involves the skin, gastrointestinal (GI) tract, and liver as the primary target tissues. The hematopoietic and immune systems are also involved. It is unclear why other tissues are not directly affected by GVHD. A maculopapular rash is usually the first presentation and is typically pruritic and confluent. When severe, generalized erythroderma, bullae, and desquamation may occur. Acute GVHD of the liver targets the biliary epithelium and produces cholestatic hepatitis with marked elevation of bilirubin and alkaline phosphatase. Synthetic function is usually preserved early in the course. GVHD can affect the entire GI tract, targeting epithelial cells. GI GVHD characteristically produces secretory diarrhea, abdominal pain, and on rare occasions, ileus. Upper GI GVHD produces nausea, vomiting, and anorexia, all which may occur without lower GI tract or other tissue involvement.[149] Conjunctivitis and other ocular manifestations, anemia, and thrombocytopenia may also occur.

The diagnosis of acute GVHD is based on clinical assessment, supported by biopsies of involved tissues.[150,151] The staging and grading of acute GVHD is based on the severity of involvement of the various tissues and is outlined in Table 58-3. In general, grade I is mild and does not require treatment. Grade II is moderate and requires systemic treatment, and grades III and IV are severe and life threatening, respectively. Severe GVHD is associated with a poor prognosis because of direct tissue damage, debilitation, and severe immunodeficiency caused by the GVHD process itself and by its treatment with immunosuppressive drugs.

The most important factor predicting the risk of GVHD is HLA disparity between the donor and recipient.[69,152] With current immunosuppressive prophylaxis, acute GVHD occurs in 25 to 50% of patients after transplants from an HLA-identical sibling; this may be related to disparity between minor histocompatibility antigens. A higher incidence, up to 60 to 90% has been reported following transplants from mismatched and unrelated donors. Results are improving for unrelated donor transplantation with the use of more precise molecular histocompatibility typing to identify donors. Older age is associated with an increased incidence of acute and chronic GVHD. Male-related minor histocompatibility antigens, H-Y, are potential targets of GVHD[153] and sex-mismatched grafts from female donors into male recipients have a higher rate of acute GVHD, particularly if the female donor is sensitized to male antigens by prior pregnancy or blood transfusions.[154] Some studies show a history of herpesviruses infection is associated with an increased risk of GVHD.[155] Less intensive, nonmyeloablative conditioning regimens may also limit the severity of GVHD, presumably due to the limitation of the pro-inflammatory phase that facilitates development of GVHD.

Pharmacologic immunosuppression is generally administered for the first six months post transplant to reduce the incidence and severity of GVHD. The current standard of care combines either cyclosporine or tacrolimus with a short course of methotrexate.[156–158] Cyclosporine and tacrolimus prevent activation of T cells, whereas methotrexate targets proliferating T cells that were activated at the early post transplant phase by host antigens. Addition of corticosteroids is the first line of therapy in patients who develop acute GVHD. Approximately half of patients have a sustained response[159] and the steroid dose can be gradually tapered off. Steroid-resistant GVHD has an unfavorable prognosis although 30 to 40% of the patients will respond to a second line therapy such as ATG.[160] The prognosis is best for GVHD limited to the skin. Acute GVHD involving the liver or multiple organs has a poorer prognosis than other sites. Newer investigational agents for treatment of acute GVHD include monoclonal anti–T-cell antibodies, sirolimus, and a number of investigational cytokine inhibitors. Photopheresis, employing extracorporeal ultraviolet (UV) irradiation of blood after administration of a UV absorbing agent systemically can also be effective in selected patients.

The most effective method for prevention of GVHD is depletion of T lymphocytes from the graft.[52] This approach has not been shown to improve survival in HLA-matched sibling or matched unrelated donor transplants due to increased risk of graft failure, relapse, and opportunistic infections. Transplantation from haploidentical donors has a very high risk of acute GVHD, and the best results have been achieved using T-cell depleted transplants. Post transplant immunosuppressive therapy is not required to prevent GVHD if $< 10^5$ T cells/kg are infused for HLA-matched sibling transplants, and $< 10^4$ T cells/kg for HLA-mismatched cases.

Chronic GVHD is a related syndrome affecting 25 to 60% of recipients of allogeneic transplantation who survive more than 6 months after transplant.[161] It most often occurs between 80 and 200 days after transplant, but the onset may be delayed to the second year. Chronic GVHD is more common in older patients and in patients with prior acute GVHD although approximately one third of affected patients have a de novo presentation without prior acute GVHD.[162] Chronic GVHD may be more prevalent after transplants with peripheral blood stem cells than with marrow transplantation.[163]

Chronic GVHD has protean clinical manifestation similar to those seen in several autoimmune disorders such as progressive systemic sclerosis, Sjögren syndrome, and primary biliary cirrhosis.[130] It is a syndrome of immune dysregulation with generation of auto-reactive T cells directed against shared MHC determinant and production of autoantibodies. Chronic GVHD is associated with thymic dysfunction and failure of the thymus to delete auto-reactive cells and induce tolerance. Chronic GVHD is associated with profound immunosuppression and the major risk to the patients relates to high incidence of opportunistic infections.

Chronic GVHD most frequently involves the skin, liver, oral cavity, and eyes. Skin involvement consists of erythema, hyperkeratosis, and desquamation. Its onset is often insidious with gradual thickening and tightness of the subcutaneous tissues and limitation of joint flexibility. Additional symptoms include sicca syndrome with dry eyes, dry mouth, and lichenoid changes in the mouth. Liver involvement is characterized by cholestatic changes. Bronchiolitis obliterans may occur without other major manifestations of chronic GVHD. Intestinal involvement with anorexia, dysphagia, malabsorption, and wasting may occur. Polymyositis, serositis, and autoimmune manifestation occur rarely. Secondary infections are common causes of morbidity and mortality, and antimicrobial prophylaxis is warranted. Chronic GVHD may become a chronic debilitating disease affecting quality of life and remains the major determinant of late transplant-related morbidity. Chronic GVHD is classified as "limited" if only minor skin or liver involvement occurs, or "extensive" if there is diffuse involvement of the skin or multiple organs or when the liver histology indicates advanced changes. Progressive onset of extensive chronic GVHD from acute GVHD and the presence of thrombocytopenia are poor prognostic factors.[164]

Corticosteroids are the first line of therapy for chronic GVHD.[165] The chronic nature of this syndrome requires long-term therapy for at least 6 to 9 months, using the lowest steroid doses, which control symptoms. Alternate day dosage may be preferable to minimize the complications resulting from chronic steroid therapy. Cyclosporine or tacrolimus may be used in combination with corticosteroids in high-risk patients.[166–168] Combinations of immunosuppressive agents may improve control of the direct manifestations of chronic GVHD, but they increase the risk of infectious morbidity and mortality. Mycophenolate mofetil has some efficacy and can be employed as a steroid-sparing agent.[169,170]

REGIMEN-RELATED TOXICITY

Myeloablative preparative regimens used to cytoreduce the malignancy approach the limit of tolerance for several tissues. The gastrointestinal tract, kidneys, lungs, and liver are the most susceptible to toxic damage, but severe toxicity may also involve the heart, bladder, nervous system, and other tissues. The actual risk for toxicity varies among regimens and their relative dose intensity, is related to the toxicity profiles of the involved agents and their interactions and is affected by coexisting organ dysfunction, the effects of the diseases and prior therapy, and infections. Most toxicities are experienced during the first 30 days post-transplant, but regimen-related hepatic injury (hepatic veno-occlusive disease), pulmonary toxicity, and neurologic effects may be delayed for several months.

Veno-occlusive disease (VOD) of the liver frequently occurs after TBI, busulfan, BCNU, thiotepa, carboplatin, and etoposide-containing regimens.[171] The relative incidence varies widely but may approach 40 to 50% with very intensive treatments. VOD involves an injury to hepatic venules and hepatocytes, which is characteristic and can be diagnosed by transvenous liver biopsy even in the presence of thrombocytopenia. The clinical syndrome is characterized by painful hepatic enlargement, ascites, generalized fluid retention, and striking elevation of serum bilirubin. There is no proven treatment other than supportive care, and factors predicting the probability of a fatal outcome from VOD have been described.[172] Pulmonary toxicity directly related to drug injury is most commonly caused by BCNU, the frequency varying from 5 to 60% with increasing dose.[173] Virtually every alkylating agent used in transplantation has been associated with pulmonary toxicity, though much less commonly than with BCNU. This injury typically occurs between 3 to 12 weeks following transplant and usually produces progressive shortness of breath, cough, and diffuse interstitial abnormalities on chest radiograph or CT scan. If infection is excluded, steroid treatment can produce total reversal of this side effect.[173] Central neurotoxicity, most commonly manifest by subtle cognitive dysfunction, has been frequently reported. Severe nonfocal toxicity, including stupor and coma, has been associated with regimens containing high doses of BCNU and thiotepa, both of which penetrate the central nervous system (CNS) well. In addition, the immunosuppressives cyclosporine and tacrolimus can cause both focal and nonfocal CNS dysfunction that often responds to temporary discontinuation of the drug.[174] These agents also produce sporadic peripheral neuropathy, which is slow to resolve after drug discontinuation. Cardiac toxicity, usually manifests temporary myocardial injury and decline in cardiac ejection fraction, is also produced by a variety of alkylating agent regimens. Although most commonly asymptomatic and lasting only 1 to 3 months, it can occur in 20 to 40% of patients in selected regimens.[175] Irreversible cardiac failure can be seen but is much less common.

HEMATOLOGIC COMPLICATIONS

Hemolytic reactions may result from ABO blood group incompatibility between the donor and recipient.[176] The incompatibility may be major when the recipient plasma contains isohemagglutinins against donor red blood cells (RBC) or minor when the donor plasma contains isohemagglutinins against recipient RBC. ABO incompatibility is not a contraindication for allogeneic transplant. Red blood cells should be removed from the donor graft to prevent acute hemolytic reaction in cases with major ABO incompatibility and plasma should be removed in pairs with minor ABO incompatibility.

Thrombotic thrombocytopenic purpura (TTP) may occur after hematopoietic transplantation and is more common after allogeneic than autologous transplants.[177] Factors implicated in initiating endothelial injury include chemotherapeutic agents, irradiation, cyclosporine and tacrolimus, cytomegalovirus (CMV) and fungal infections, and cytokine-release syndromes. TTP occurring post-autologous or -allogeneic hematopoietic transplantation has a poor prognosis. Treatment with plasma exchange results in response in some patients.[178,179]

IMMUNODEFICIENCY AND INFECTIONS

Recipients of hematopoietic transplants have a severe immunodeficiency involving both T and B-cells.[180–182] Intensive preparative regimens ablate the host immune system. Myeloid cells, macrophage/monocytes, and lymphocytes are subsequently produced from precursor cells present in the graft. The most profound abnormalities occur within the first 6 months followed by slow recovery over the first year.[183] HLA-mismatched or unrelated donor transplants have a more severe immunodeficiency and risk for opportunistic infections, particularly if T-cell depletion is used to prevent GVHD.[184] Patients receiving umbilical cord blood transplants are at particular risk for profound and prolonged immunodeficiency because of the immature nature of the infused cells and the small size of the graft. Recipients of autologous and syngeneic transplants also have a period of immunodeficiency, but their recovery is usually more rapid and post-transplant infections are less frequent and severe than after allogeneic transplantation. Patients with acute and chronic GVHD have a profound immunodeficiency state for prolonged periods and are highly susceptible to unusual infections.[185] Recipients of hematopoietic transplants may be susceptible to unusual opportunistic infections and also to acute overwhelming infections. Prophylactic strategies against an array of potential infections and rapid recognition and treatment of infections are an essential part of successful management of transplant recipients.[186] Immunoglobulin replacement therapy should be considered in patients with documented immunoglobulin deficiency. Re-vaccinations should be performed upon immune recovery and are typically carried out 1 year post-transplant.[187] Isolation measures and especially meticulous hand washing are important in prevention of nosocomial acquisition of infections.

Post-transplant lymphoproliferative disease (PTLD) is a life-threatening complication of allogeneic transplantation.[188] It is more prevalent in recipients of T-cell depleted marrow grafts, transplants from unrelated donors, in patients with GVHD, and especially in those treated with aggressive immunosuppressive treatment including ATG. PTLD in hematopoietic transplant recipients arises from the transformation of donor-derived B-lymphocytes by Epstein-Barr virus (EBV) infection. Patients who are seronegative against EBV prior to transplant may develop PTLD early in the course due to primary EBV infection, and the disease may be rapidly progressive. Seropositive patients may develop a more indolent form as a late complication of prolonged immunosuppression. PTLD presents with systemic symptoms, adenopathy, and frequently with extranodal lesions in the GI tract, liver, and CNS. Treatment includes withdrawal of immunosuppression and administration of the antiCD20 monoclonal antibody, rituximab. Cellular therapy with donor lymphocyte infusion, at relatively low cell numbers, has dramatic results in controlling PTLD.[189] More recently methods have been developed to generate EBV-specific cytotoxic lymphocytes for the treatment of this complication.[190] Patients with increasing levels of EBV deoxyribonucleic acid are at highest risk for lymphoproliferative disease and are candidates for preemptive immunotherapy.

Late Effects Late complications of hematopoietic transplantation include delayed effects of high-dose therapy, indolent infections, transfusion-related complications, and chronic GVHD. Late toxicity of high-dose therapy can produce cataracts, pulmonary fibrosis, dental abnormalities, hypothyroidism, and hypogonadism, growth retardation, osteoporosis, and avascular necrosis of the hip or other bones.[161] Permanent sterility occurs in most patients.

There is an increased risk of solid and hematologic secondary tumors after hematopoietic transplantation.[30,31] Solid tumors, mostly head and neck cancers, squamous cell carcinomas, melanomas, and brain and thyroid cancers may be more common in recipients of TBI-containing regimens and the cumulative incidence is up to 7% at 15 years. Myelodysplasia and secondary leukemia occur more commonly after autologous transplant, occurring in 4 to 18% of patients within 2.5 to 8.5 years of transplant.[191,192] There are data to suggest that myelodysplasia is associated more with extensive prior therapy than with the high-dose chemotherapy given prior to the transplant.

INDICATIONS FOR HEMATOPOIETIC TRANSPLANTATION

Acute Myeloid Leukemia Hematopoietic cellular transplantation has been extensively evaluated for the treatment of patients with AML.[193,194] Myeloablative transplants have been used in younger patients. AML is more common with advanced age, but about 30% of the patients are younger than 55 years. Most patients have received preparative regimens involving high-dose cyclophosphamide and total body irradiation or the combination of busulfan and cyclophosphamide. Most studies showed no difference in outcome between the two regimens, but one randomized study showed an advantage for TBI.[195,196] Most patients achieve complete remission after high-dose therapy and hematopoietic transplantation. The major causes of treatment failure are GVHD, regimen-related toxicity, infections, and recurrent leukemia. More intensive regimens designed to have greater antileukemic activity by increasing the TBI dose or adding additional chemotherapeutic agents have produced additional toxicity, and overall survival has not improved.[197] The outcome after allogeneic transplantation is primarily dependent on the disease status (remission versus relapse), cytogenetic abnormality of the leukemia, patient age, and histocompatibility between donor and recipient.[198]

Nonmyeloablative regimens have also been investigated as a means to decrease regimen-related toxicity. This has been effective in patients transplanted while in remission, but there is a high relapse rate in patients with overt leukemia.[135] Novel approaches include the inclusion of anti-myeloid monoclonal antibodies, which are radiolabeled or conjugated to toxins that can target the malignant cells with little systemic toxicity.[199]

Autologous bone marrow transplantation has also been evaluated as treatment for AML.[200,201] Patients undergo procurement and cryopreservation of bone marrow cells while in remission. They may then receive similar marrow ablative chemoradiotherapy followed by reinfusion of the cryopreserved hematopoietic cells to restore hematopoiesis. A major limitation is the high likelihood that the "remission" bone marrow may be contaminated by small numbers of leukemic cells, which would be cryopreserved and reinfused with the autologous marrow. Additionally, no GVL effect accompanies this treatment. Nonetheless, 30 to 50% of patients have achieved prolonged remissions after autologous transplants performed in first or second remission. A number of techniques have been explored to deplete occult leukemic cells from the harvested bone marrow in vitro prior to cryopreservation. Immunologic approaches using anti-AML monoclonal antibodies[202] or pharmacologic agents, such as *cis-4*-hydroperoxycyclophosphamide[104] or mafosfamide[103] have been studied. Although some of the best results are reported in series using purged marrow, no controlled studies have been done, and the efficacy of purging remains to be determined.

The best results are achieved when allogeneic or autologous transplantation is given to patients in first remission where long-term disease-free survival is 40 to 60%.[203,204] It remains an unresolved question whether patients with a sibling donor should receive allogeneic transplant while in first remission or at the time of relapse. There are numerous studies comparing allogeneic hematopoietic transplantation with autologous transplantation and consolidation chemotherapy in patients with AML in first remission.[194,205,206] Results have been conflicting, in part because of various regimens used, different type, intensity, and number of consolidation cycles prior to transplant, and because only a portion of patients received the assigned treatment in each study. In general, most studies have shown a significantly lower relapse rate in patients receiving allogeneic transplantation. Relapse rates after autologous transplantation is higher, but still superior to chemotherapy in most studies. Survival has not been significantly improved in most studies in adults, because some patients may be salvaged with allogeneic transplantation after relapse. Most centers recommend allogeneic transplants in first remission for patients with intermediate or high-risk cytogenetic abnormalities and clinical features, but not for patients with a favorable prognosis, such as those with the $t^{8;21}$, inv 16, or $t^{15;17}$ abnormalities.

Elderly patients have a higher rate of regimen-related toxicity and GVHD. Most centers have limited transplantation to patients less than 55 to 60 years of age who have an HLA-identical sibling donor. However, AML is more common with advanced age. Elderly patients are more likely to have adverse cytogenetics and antecedent hematologic disorders and thus an unfavorable outcome. The use of nonmyeloablative regimens for induction of GVL as the main goal of treatment has opened the option of allogeneic transplantation to patients up to 75 years of age with chemotherapy-sensitive disease.[124,136]

The risks of allogeneic transplantation are increased in patients without an HLA-identical sibling donor. Transplants from a matched unrelated donor or related mismatched donor should be considered in patients after relapse, those with poor-risk cytogenetic abnormalities, or patients with an antecedent hematologic disorder.[207,208] Haploidentical transplants using high doses of CD34+ selected stem cells, which are depleted of T lymphocytes or umbilical cord blood, have a high risk of treatment related mortality, but have been successful in patients with advanced AML. A marked antileukemic effect has been related to donor-derived alloreactive NK cells. Sensitive molecular assays have recently been established to detect minimal numbers of leukemia cells; these may allow selection of patients at high risk to relapse and possibly guide selection of therapy.

MYELODYSPLASTIC SYNDROMES

Myelodysplastic syndromes (MDS) are a group of clonal hematologic disorders, manifested by peripheral cytopenias and a high risk of transformation to AML. They may occur de novo or secondary to prior chemotherapy for another malignancy. MDS most often occur in elderly patients, but about 10% of patients are young.

Outcome is determined by the French-American-British morphological classification. Patients with refractory anemia or refractory anemia with ringed sideroblasts have longer survival than patients with refractory anemia with excess myeloblasts or chronic myelomonocytic leukemia (advanced MDS). The International Prognostic Score (IPPS) score defines low-, intermediate-, and high-risk groups based on marrow blast percentage, cytopenias, and karyotype.[209] The median survival of patients with low-risk IPPS scores is 5.7 years, but it is only 0.4 years for high-risk patients.

Allogeneic transplantation is a potentially curative treatment for MDS[210–214]; however, the timing of transplantation is controversial. Patients with high-risk disease, excess blasts, severe neutropenia, transfusion dependency, and high-risk cytogenetic abnormalities are considered candidates. Stable patients with low-risk disease may have extended survival with conservative therapy and should generally not be offered transplant until disease progression. The conditioning regimens used are similar to those used for AML. Nonmyeloablative transplants have been successful in some patients, and DLI can restore remission in some patients with post-transplantation relapse.

The outcome is related to the MDS morphology or IPPS score.[215] The relapse rate after transplant for early MDS is less than 10%, and long-term disease-free survival is 50 to 60%. The risk of relapse for patients with RAEB/RAEB-T is approximately 30% with 30 to 40% long-term survival. Survival is better for young patients and when transplant is given early after diagnosis, but is worse after transplants from an unrelated donor. The relapse rate after transplant for therapy-related MDS is similar to de novo MDS, but treatment-related complications occur more often, probably because these patients are usually heavily pretreated for their primary malignancy.[213,215] There are anecdotal reports of use of autologous transplants for MDS.[216] Some patients have normal stem cells that coexist with the abnormal clone, like patients with de novo AML. These patients can achieve non-clonal remission with intensive chemotherapy, and theoretically, normal stem cells can be collected at recovery from chemotherapy. Detection of residual disease in the autograft may be difficult. Too few autologous transplants have been performed to allow conclusions.

ACUTE LYMPHOBLASTIC LEUKEMIA

Hematopoietic transplantation is an effective treatment for acute lymphoblastic leukemia (ALL).[217–221] Intensive chemotherapy regimens have resulted in cure of approximately 70% of children with ALL. There has also been a substantial improvement in the treatment of adult ALL with similar regimens; 80 to 90% achieve complete response (CR) with induction regimens and 30 to 35% can be cured.[222] Consequently, hematopoietic transplantation has generally been reserved for patients after relapse, patients who fail to achieve remission with initial chemotherapy, and for a subset of patients in first remission with a high risk for recurrence of the disease.

Transplantation in first remission is controversial.[223,224] Most studies have shown no survival advantage for such patients having hematopoietic transplantation because a reduced relapse rate is offset by treatment-related mortality. Patients with Philadelphia chromosome positive ALL have an extremely poor prognosis, with < 10% achieving long-term disease-free survival. Allogeneic transplantation in first remission can cure 30 to 40%, and should be considered the standard of care for these patients.[225,226] The use of other adverse prognostic factors to select patients for transplantation in first remission is controversial.

Hematopoietic transplantation is indicated for most patients with relapsed disease.[227,228] Children with relapse occurring more than 36 months after first remission, or more than 12 months after completion of maintenance chemotherapy may still be cured with chemotherapy.[229] The outcome of most adults with relapsing disease is dismal, and they should be considered for hematopoietic transplantation.[218,230] About 20 to 30% of patients with primary refractory ALL can be salvaged with allogeneic transplant. The prognosis of patients with chemotherapy resistant relapse is poor.

The most common preparative regimen used for transplants in ALL includes high-dose cyclophosphamide and total body irradiation with or without other chemotherapeutic agents. TBI-containing regimens may be associated with improved disease-free survival, in comparison to non–TBI-containing regimens.[231] Intensification of irradiation or addition of other agents to TBI has generally not improved overall outcome, and development of more effective regimens would be desirable.

Autologous hematopoietic transplantation has also been evaluated in patients with ALL, mostly in children.[232–234] A number of monoclonal antibodies to leukemia-associated antigens are available in ALL; these antigens are nonreactive with normal hematopoietic progenitors. These include antibodies to the common ALL antigen (CD10) or a number of T-cell antigens. A number of patients have received autologous transplants using bone marrow that was treated ex vivo with one or more of these antibodies and complement. Limitations to this technique include probable antigenic heterogeneity among neoplastic cells, and it is unclear if leukemic stem cells express these cell surface antigens. Although selected patients with ALL in second remission have achieved prolonged remissions after receiving intensive chemotherapy, total body irradiation, and autologous transplantation using antiCD10 antibody and complement-treated marrow, long-term disease-free survival is < 20% in most series. These data are difficult to interpret because many of the successful cases involved patients having a relatively good prognosis with conventional treatment.

CHRONIC MYELOID LEUKEMIA

Chronic myeloid leukemia (CML) is a hematologic malignancy characterized by excessive clonal proliferation of myeloid cells and their progenitors. In greater than 90% of cases, the Philadelphia chromosome, $t^{9;22}$ is a marker of the malignant clone and results from rearrangement of the *BCR* and *ABL* genes, producing a fusion protein with abnormal tyrosine kinase activity. CML is more common with advanced age, and the median age of onset is 60 years.

The disease can be divided into two phases: an initial chronic phase in which cell maturation is normal followed by transformation to accelerated or acute phase (blast crisis). Blast crisis is characterized by maturation arrest at the level of the myeloblast or lymphoblast and resembles acute leukemia.

CML has been treated with chemotherapy, interferon-based therapies, and hematopoietic transplantation. The recent development of imatinib mesylate, a selective inhibitor of the BCRABL tyrosine kinase, has changed the standard of care for this disease.[235] Imatinib mesylate has produced a high rate of cytogenetic complete remissions in initial trials.[236] Responding patients typically still have minimal residual disease detectable by polymerase chain reaction assays, and the impact of this agent on the natural history of CML and survival is still uncertain. The role of hematopoietic transplantation is being re-evaluated as long-term data with tyrosine kinase inhibitors become available.

Allogeneic hematopoietic transplantation is a highly effective treatment for CML, capable of producing cure of the disease.[237,238] Most patients have received busulfan and cyclophosphamide or cyclophosphamide and total body irradiation as the preparative regimen. Both regimens appear equally effective.[239,240] The oral busulfan formulation is erratically absorbed; toxicity and antileukemic effects are dependent on the levels of busulfan achieved.[241,242] The new intravenous busulfan has more reliable pharmacokinetics and appears to have less toxicity. It has not been possible to improve the antileukemic effect of the preparative regimen with additional chemotherapy or higher doses of irradiation without a concomitant increase in toxicity.[242]

The major determinants of transplant outcome are the stage of the disease at the time of transplant, age of recipient, type of donor, and interval from diagnosis to transplantation. The best results have been reported for patients receiving transplant while in chronic phase, with a disease-free survival of approximately 60 to 80% beyond 5 years. If the transplant is performed within the first 1 to 2 years of diagnosis, and from an HLA-identical sibling, survival may be 80 to 90%.[237,238] Hematopoietic transplantation is the only treatment that potentially allows long-term survival in accelerated or blastic CML. Patients who are in an accelerated phase have a 35% chance of prolonged survival. For patients undergoing transplantation during blast crisis, only approximately 10 to 20% become long-term survivors. The major cause of treatment failure in advanced CML is leukemia relapse.

Younger patients have better tolerance of myeloablative treatment and lower rates of GVHD than the elderly. Recently, nonmyeloablative regimens have allowed successful treatment of elderly patients. With improved donor selection using molecular histocompatibility testing, the results of unrelated donor transplants are approaching those achieved with a matched sibling donor.[65]

The high dose preparative regimen may not completely eliminate all malignant cells and a graft-versus-leukemia effect is necessary to prevent relapse. Most patients may still have small numbers of Philadelphia chromosome positive cells identified by cytogenetics or polymerase chain reaction analysis up to 6 to 12 months posttransplant[243]; typically, these cells are gradually eliminated due to the GVL effect. Relapse after transplant can be clinically overt or diagnosed only by cytogenetic or molecular analysis. CML is the most sensitive malignancy to graft-versus-leukemia effects; infusion of additional donor T lymphocytes can reinduce durable remission in 80 to 90% of patients with early relapse.[60,244,245] Relapse in advanced phase is less likely to respond to DLI. Patients receiving DLI may become pancytopenic at the time of response. This is more common in patients with a high percentage of host-derived hematopoiesis at the time of DLI.[245] Recovery of donor-derived hematopoiesis usually follows, but some patients require infusion of additional donor stem cells to support hematopoietic recovery. GVHD is a major risk after DLI; its risk can be minimized by starting with a low T-cell dose of 5 to 10×10^6/kg and subsequently escalating the dose until response occurs.

Hematopoietic transplantation has been used for the treatment of other myeloproliferative disorders.[246–248] The appropriate timing of transplantation is not well defined. Most researchers require the patient to be transfusion-dependent to justify the risks inherent with hematopoietic transplantation.[249]

CHRONIC LYMPHOCTIC LEUKEMIA

CLL is an indolent lymphoid malignancy; median survival exceeds 10 years.[250,251] Chronic lymphocytic leukemia is a clonal disorder of B cells, characterized by the accumulation of small mature-appearing lymphocytes, although rare T-cell variants also occur. The Rai and the Binet systems separate CLL patients into prognostic groups.[252] The National Cancer Institute-sponsored Working Group recommends use of the "3-risk group" modification of the original five-stage Rai staging system.[253] The median survival is > 14 years for the low-risk group, 8 years for the intermediate group, and 4 years for the high-risk group. Adverse prognostic factors are recent absence of immunoglobulin gene rearrangement, expression of CD38, and higher levels of beta2-microglobulin.[254]

Chemotherapy is generally recommended if the disease causes symptoms or impaired performance status.[253] Chemotherapy involving fludarabine combined with alkylating agents such as cyclophosphamide is effective to control symptoms, reduce bulk of disease, and has palliative benefit.[255,256] More recent trials have employed rituximab as well, and complete clinical response of high-risk CLL are becoming more frequent.[256] Responses are transient, however, and overall survival has not been substantially improved; this disease is considered incurable. The prognosis is poorer once disease progression occurs after initial chemotherapy. Results depend on the response to salvage chemotherapy. The overall survival is 2.5 to 4 years.

Several studies of high-dose chemoradiotherapy with autologous hematopoietic transplantation have been reported using marrow collected after a fludarabine induced remission.[257,258] The autograft can be purged by monoclonal antibodies directed against B lymphocytes, and elimination of detectable systemic malignant cells is associated with improved survival.[259] The role and optimal timing of autologous transplantation is controversial. The results of autologous transplants have been best when performed early in the disease, but the impact on survival in this selected group of lower-risk patients is unknown. Only transient remissions have been achieved in heavily pretreated patients with advanced disease.

Allogeneic transplantation has been studied predominantly in younger patients with advanced disease and poor prognosis.[260–262] Patients with chemosensitive disease have better outcome following transplant. An International Bone Marrow Transplant Registry (IBMTR) analysis showed a 3-year survival of 46%, but also a high risk for transplant-related mortality.[263] A graft-versus-leukemia effect has been shown in this disease,[264] and this has led to studies using nonmyeloablative conditioning to reduce toxicity and to extend the use of allogeneic transplantation options to the treatment of patients up to age 75.[50] Encouraging preliminary results have been reported by many groups using this strategy.

The optimal timing of allogeneic transplantation is controversial. Given the risks of allogeneic transplantation and the indolent course of newly diagnosed patients, it is generally recommended that the procedure be considered only after failure of initial therapy. The prognosis is relatively poor if the procedure is delayed until after multiple relapses or after development of refractoriness to chemotherapy.[48]

NON-HODGKIN'S LYMPHOMA

The non-Hodgkin's lymphomas are a heterogeneous group of malignancies with indolent to highly aggressive natural histories. Treatment with both standard and transplant-based therapies depends on the histologic subtype and prognostic factors operative in each patient. A number of classification systems have been proposed. A Revised European-American Lymphoma classification is widely used and incorporates immunophenotype as well as morphologic criteria,[265] and a World Health Organization classification has recently been proposed.[241] These disorders result from malignant transformation and clonal proliferation of lymphoid cells and their progenitors. Each histologic type is associated with characteristic cytogenetic and molecular abnormalities.[266–268]

Lymphoid malignancies can be grouped into major categories: low-, intermediate-, and high-grade. The low-grade lymphomas—small lymphocytic lymphoma, follicular small cleaved cell lymphoma, and follicular mixed cell lymphoma—are indolent diseases but incurable with standard forms of chemotherapy. Follicular small-cleaved cell lymphoma and follicular mixed cell lymphoma are the most common categories included among low-grade lymphomas. These diseases are associated with the $t^{14;18}$, resulting in rearrangement of the *BCL2* gene. Low-grade lymphoma patients have a median survival of 7 to 9 years.[269] The major factors influencing prognosis include stage, lactic dehydrogenase, and beta2- microglobin level.

High-dose chemotherapy with autologous hematopoietic transplantation has been extensively evaluated for low-grade lymphoma, producing rates of complete remission over 80%. Since these disorders characteristically involve the bone marrow, many studies have used marrow or blood stem-cell autografts depleted of malignant cells by using anti–B-cell monoclonal antibodies, a process which may achieve prolonged remissions.[100,270,271] Achievement of molecular complete remissions in which *BCL2* rearrangement is undetectable by polymerase chain reaction analysis has been associated with prolonged disease-free survival. There is controversy, however, regarding the role of autologous transplantation in this disease. Long-term survival is similar after autologous hematopoietic transplantation and with conservative forms of standard-dose chemotherapy.[272] There is a risk of secondary myelodysplasia and acute leukemia after autotransplants in this disease, particularly in heavily pretreated patients.[121,273,274]

Allogeneic bone marrow transplantation has also been evaluated in patients with low-grade lymphoma. High-dose cyclophosphamide and TBI, with or without other agents, or the combination of carmustine, etoposide, ara-C, and melphalan (BEAM) are the most commonly used preparative regimens. Several groups have reported extended disease-free survival in patients with far advanced disease. Relapse rates after allogeneic transplants have been substantially lower than with transplantation of purged autologous transplants, most likely due to the graft-versus-lymphoma effect.[275,276] The recent encouraging results using nonmyeloablative preparative regimens for allogeneic transplantation may reduce the risk of treatment-related mortality; approximately 85% were alive and disease free.[136] This option should be considered for patients after failure of initial chemotherapy.

Mantle cell lymphoma is associated with a poor prognosis. Autologous hematopoietic transplants may be effective in chemoresponsive patients in first remission, but patients with resistant or recurrent disease have a high rate of treatment failure.[277,278] Allogeneic hematopoietic transplants have been promising in this disease.[279,280] Khouri and colleagues reported a series of 16 patients treated with allogeneic blood or marrow transplantation achieving 55% disease-free survival at three years.[278] These preliminary data indicate that allogeneic hematopoietic transplantation using an ablative or nonmyeloablative regimen can induce durable remission in patients with mantle cell lymphoma. Allogeneic transplantation appears promising in patients who fail to respond to initial chemotherapy or relapse; its role in newly diagnosed patients needs to be determined. Further clinical trials are needed.

Intermediate- and high-grade lymphomas are aggressive malignancies with a short natural history in the absence of effective therapy. These disorders are responsive to combination chemotherapy, and a fraction of patients achieve durable remissions. Standard chemotherapy for large cell lymphoma results in cure in approximately 40% for newly diagnosed patients with diffuse large cell lymphoma. High-, intermediate- and low-risk groups have been defined.

High-dose chemotherapy and autologous transplantation improve cure rates for patients with recurrent large cell lymphoma who respond to salvage chemotherapy.[281,282] The Parma study randomized patients younger than 60 years, with chemosensitive relapse and no marrow or CNS involvement, either to continued salvage chemotherapy or to high-dose chemotherapy and autologous bone marrow transplantation.[283] The 5-year event-free survival was 46% in the transplant group, and 12% in the standard chemotherapy group; overall survival was also improved. Autologous hematopoietic transplantation can therefore be considered the preferred treatment for that group of patients. Patients with chemotherapy resistant disease and those with multiple relapses have poor results, with less than 20% durable remissions.

Patients achieving only a partial response to initial chemotherapy are rarely cured with chemotherapy and are appropriate candidates for autologous HCT; however, patients who continue to progress through initial treatment only rarely achieve prolonged remission if autologous hematopoietic transplantation is attempted at that time.[284] One study showed that patients with a slow antitumor response might do as well with continuing induction chemotherapy as those with early hematopoietic transplant.[285]

High-dose chemotherapy with autologous hematopoietic transplantation has also been studied in high-risk patients with intermediate-grade lymphoma in first remission. Two studies reported that high-dose chemotherapy with autologous hematopoietic transplantation improved event-free survival of patients with intermediate- or high-risk prognostic features,[286,287] but other studies failed to confirm this benefit.[288] Ongoing clinical trials are addressing this issue.

High-dose therapy with allogeneic transplantation has been examined in a number of phase I and II studies in patients with intermediate- or high-grade lymphoma. Several studies reported a decreased recurrence rate compared to autologous transplants, but the benefit is off-set by higher rates of treatment-related mortality.[289] Many physicians have reserved allotransplantation for patients having a poor prognosis with alternative modalities, such as a relatively poor response to chemotherapy, or patients in which autologous transplants were not feasible.

Hodgkin's Disease Hodgkin's disease is a chemotherapy responsive malignancy, but 20 to 30% of patients with advanced disease may fail to achieve complete remission and approximately one-third of responders will subsequently relapse. For patients with recurrent Hodgkin's disease, high-dose chemotherapy and autologous hematopoietic transplantation results in a complete remission rate > 50 to 80% and a 40 to 60% disease-free survival at 3 to 5 years post-transplant.[290–292] The BEAM and cyclophosphamide carmustine etoposide preparative regimens have been most frequently used. Numerous phase II studies have suggested that high-dose chemotherapy improves disease-free survival and possibly overall survival compared to standard chemotherapy in this setting. Patients recurring after an initial remission that is shorter than 1 year have superior disease-free survival with high-dose chemotherapy compared to standard dose-salvage treatment, and most researchers recommend high-dose therapy for those patients. Controversy remains regarding patients with a long first remission. For patients in second or subsequent relapse and considered incurable with standard dose chemotherapy, autologous transplantation is recommended.

Patients who fail to achieve complete remission with initial chemotherapy have a poor outcome, however, 20 to 40% can be salvaged by HCT.[292] Patients with partial response fare better than patients with bulky progressive disease. Ongoing studies are evaluating the role for high-dose therapy with autologous hematopoietic transplantation as part of the initial therapy for patients with high-risk features.

Late relapses and a high incidence of secondary myelodysplasia (approximately 15%) continue to be major problems among long-term survivors. Late infections and cardiac and pulmonary toxicity may also occur.

Relatively few allogeneic transplants have been performed in patients with Hodgkin's disease.[293] High-dose therapy with allogeneic transplantation is associated with a high treatment-related mortality in patients with Hodgkin's disease, exceeding 50% in some studies. Studies of patients with advanced disease not suitable for autologous transplant have shown a 15 to 20% salvage rate with HLA-matched sibling trans-plantation. Use of nonmyeloablative regimens to reduce treatment-related mortality is currently being investigated, and the preliminary results are encouraging.[294,295]

Multiple Myeloma Multiple myeloma is a common hematologic malignancy that occurs in increasing frequently with advancing age. Standard chemotherapy can control the disease for variable periods, but only 5% achieve complete remission, and the median survival is approximately 3 years.[296] In a randomized study of newly diagnosed multiple-myeloma patients, high-dose chemoradiotherapy with autologous hematopoietic transplantation was superior to standard chemotherapy[297]; 52% of the patients randomized to the transplant were alive and 28% were progression free at 5 years, compared to 12% and 10%, respectively, for the standard chemotherapy group. High-dose chemotherapy with autologous hematopoietic transplantation is now considered standard treatment for patients with intermediate- or high-tumor-mass multiple myeloma. High-dose therapy and autologous transplantation delays relapse, but is not curative, and almost all patients ultimately develop recurrent disease.

Chemosensitivity of the tumor is a major determinant of transplant outcome. Patients with chemosensitive disease who received transplants within the first year had a more favorable outcome, and 40 to 50% may achieve CR. Encouraging results have also been achieved in patients with primary refractory disease if transplanted early in the course of disease,[298,299] but treatment is of only limited value in advanced resistant disease, and especially in patients with refractory relapse.[300] Advanced age, high beta2-microglobulin level, and cytogenetic abnormalities involving chromosome 13 are the most prominent adverse prognostic factors.[301,302]

With the introduction of peripheral blood progenitor cell transplants and better supportive care, autologous hematopoietic transplants have become considerably safer. Treatment-related mortality is typically less than 5%, even for elderly patients up to 70 years of age. The most common regimen used includes high-dose melphalan. A recent randomized trial failed to demonstrate any advantage with the addition of TBI to high-dose melphalan.

The timing of autologous transplant remains controversial. Most studies have suggested a better outcome when autologous hematopoietic transplantation is performed early, within 1 year of diagnosis. Others advocate early collection of stem cells, but delaying high-dose chemotherapy itself to subsequent progression. A randomized French study of early versus late transplant did not show any survival difference, but patients randomized to early transplant enjoyed longer periods of time without a need for chemotherapy.[303] A major problem is that myeloma characteristically involves the bone marrow and minimal residual disease is present in most patients at the time of autologous cell collection. One approach is to try to deplete the autograft of contaminating myeloma cells. One technique is to positively select CD34+ stem/progenitor cells, a procedure capable of depleting tumor cells by more than 3 logs (99.9%). Although this can eliminate detectable cells in the autologous transplant in most patients, this approach has not been shown to improve remission duration or survival rates.[102] Most patients presumably relapse due to residual resistant systemic disease. Improved treatment for cytoreduction is needed. Novel approaches include investigation of tumor vaccines[304] and post-transplant maintenance treatment.

Allogeneic hematopoietic transplants have been studied, primarily in young patients with myeloma who have relapsed or progressed during standard chemotherapy.[305] Allogeneic transplantation provides a tumor-free graft and also an immune graft-versus-myeloma effect. Relapse occurs almost invariably after autologous HCT, but may be less common after allogeneic transplant. Donor lymphocyte infusions have reinduced remission in a few patients relapsing after allogeneic transplant, consistent with the presence of a graft-versus-myeloma effect.[306,307] However the reduced relapse rate is offset by a high treatment-related mortality rate approaching 50% in heavily pretreated myeloma patients. Three-year progression-free survival is approximately 30 to 40%. Most comparative studies have shown that autologous transplants have a better overall survival than allografts, at least during the first few years after transplant.[308,309] Encouraging results have recently been reported using an autologous transplant for tumor cytoreduction followed by an non-ablative allogeneic transplant several months later to induce an immune graft-versus-myeloma effect.[310]

Other plasma cell dyscrasias have also been effectively treated with high-dose melphalan and autologous hematopoietic transplantation. This has become the treatment of choice for primary amyloidosis, a related, invariably fatal disease.[311]

Solid Tumors High-dose chemotherapy with autologous hematopoietic transplantation has been studied in a number of chemotherapy responsive solid tumors to exploit the dose-response effects of many chemotherapeutic agents. Breast cancer has been the most common disease treated by high-dose chemotherapy and autologous transplantation. There remains, however, considerable controversy regarding the efficacy of high-dose therapy in this disease and the role of hematopoietic transplant based therapies. The most effective high-dose chemotherapy regimens used include combinations of alkylating agents and related drugs, including cyclophosphamide, melphalan, thiotepa, carmustine, cisplatin, or carboplatin.[312,313] Taxanes are also being studied in preparative regimens.[313] Studies in patients with chemotherapy responsive metastatic breast cancer have documented that this approach significantly increases the CR rate to > 50 percent with long-term disease-free survival in approximately 20%.[314] Although these results appear superior to those achieved with standard-dose chemotherapy, much of the apparent benefit can be explained by patient selection bias.[315] A recent randomized trial showed no benefit for high-dose chemotherapy in patients with metastatic breast cancer,[316] but this study did not adequately evaluate patients with low-bulk disease who appear most likely to benefit in phase II studies. Autologous transplantation has also been used as adjuvant therapy in patients with local regional breast cancer at high risk of relapse. This has generally been defined as stage II and III disease. In phase II studies approximately 50 to 85% of these high-risk patients survive free of relapse at 5 years. Recent studies comparing high-dose chemotherapy with autologous transplantation to standard treatment in this setting have had conflicting results, and longer follow up of these controlled studies is necessary for definitive analysis.[317,318]

Relapse remains a major problem and use of biologic or immunologic therapies for minimal residual breast cancer after autologous transplantation needs to be evaluated.[34] Clinical studies using allogeneic transplantation are exploring the potential of graft-versus-malignancy effect in this disease.[62]

Dose-intensive chemotherapy is being increasingly used for treating ovarian cancer.[319–321] Like breast cancer, this tumor is sensitive to alkylating agents, platinum-based chemotherapy agents, taxanes, and topoisomerase I inhibitors. Transplants have not been used commonly in the adjuvant setting, but have a role for patients with low-bulk disease after a second-look laparotomy and for patients with chemotherapy-sensitive low-bulk relapsed disease.

A similar approach with autologous transplantation has been used for the treatment of other chemotherapy-responsive solid tumors in adults, including testicular or germ cell carcinomas, and small cell carcinoma of the lung. Testicular carcinoma is a chemotherapy-responsive malignancy that is frequently cured using standard chemotherapy. Patients failing first- and second-line chemotherapy regimens have received high-dose chemotherapy and autologous transplants. Response rates are high, and a fraction have achieved long-term remissions.[322]

Autologous transplants have been extensively studied in small cell lung cancer.[323] Patients with extensive disease or relapsed carcinoma have generally had only brief responses and modest clinical benefit. Better results have been obtained as consolidation therapy for patients with limited small cell lung cancer with prolongation of remission duration in some studies. Few patients are long-term survivors, and the efficacy of this approach remains to be established.

Autologous transplants have been studied in a range of pediatric solid tumors such as neuroblastoma and Ewing sarcoma, tumors which are highly sensitive to chemotherapy and irradiation, yet have a poor prognosis in patients with advanced disease.[324,325]

Allogeneic hematopoietic transplants have recently been studied in renal cell carcinoma. This is considered a chemotherapy resistant malignancy. Nonablative allogeneic transplantation has been studied as a means to induce the immunotherapeutic graft-versus-tumor effect and approximately 40% of patients with metastatic disease have achieved complete and partial responses.[326] Most responses have occurred in patients with graft-versus-host disease and after withdrawal of immunosuppressive therapy. Ongoing research is directed at identifying the target antigens for this graft-versus-tumor effect.

Nonmalignant Indications **Aplastic Anemia** Aplastic anemia (AA) is an uncommon disease producing primary bone marrow failure with pancytopenia and hypocellular bone marrow. Severe aplastic anemia is defined as marrow cellularity of less than 25%, with either neutrophil count $< 0.5 \times 10^9$/L, platelet count $< 20 \times 10^9$/L, or total reticulocyte count $< 40 \times 10^9$/L. Without effective therapy, more than 50% of patients with severe AA may die within 6 months of diagnosis. Effective treatments for AA include immunosuppressive therapy (such as cyclosporine and ATG)[327] and hematopoietic transplantation.

Historically, graft rejection was a major complication of allogeneic transplantation for AA, occurring in up to 30% of recipients.[328] Multiple blood transfusions may sensitize the recipient against the donor and increase the risk of rejection. Cyclophosphamide alone or in combination with ATG is the most commonly used preparative regimen for bone marrow transplantation from a matched sibling donor.[329] Late graft rejection may occur after the post-transplant immunosuppression is withdrawn. With current regimens, early transplant, a judicious transfusion policy, and improved supportive care systems, less than 10% reject the grafts and long-term survival can be achieved in 80 to 90% of recipients of marrow from an HLA-matched sibling donor.

Hematopoietic transplantation from a partially matched related donor or a phenotypically matched unrelated donor requires additional immunosuppression for prevention of rejection, but the mode and dose have not been established.[330,331] Fewer than 50% are long-term survivors.[332,333]

Several studies have compared the effectiveness of allogeneic transplantation and immunosuppressive therapy. Most studies have shown a survival advantage for patients younger than 40 who have allogeneic transplantation from an HLA-matched sibling. Immunosuppressive therapy has a higher risk for late complications, such as relapse or development of myelodysplasia or AML. However, for patients above age 40 to 50, there is a higher risk of complications with allogeneic transplantation, and it should be reserved for those who fail immunosuppressive therapy. Patients lacking an HLA-identical related donor should receive a trial of immunosuppressive therapy; alternative donor transplants should be considered only in those who fail to respond.

Allogeneic bone marrow transplantation is also an effective treatment for paroxysmal nocturnal hemoglobinuria and other nonmalignant bone marrow failure states.[334]

Congenital Metabolic and Immune Disorders Allogeneic transplantation is a potentially curative treatment in a number of congenital disorders of the hematopoietic and immune systems. Thalassemia[335] and sickle cell anemia[333] are among the most common nonmalignant hematological disorders curable with transplant. Results in patients with thalassemia have been more favorable when performed early, and in patients who are not heavily transfused and with no sign of severe hepatic iron overload or portal fibrosis. Most patients received busulfan and cyclophosphamide to avoid the many toxic effects of TBI in young children. Fanconi anemia has been treated similarly to aplastic anemia, but with very low-dose conditioning regimen due to the known sensitivity of these patients to the effects of irradiation and alkylating agents.[336,337] Patients are not cured of the non-hematologic manifestations of the disease, and many develop secondary solid tumors.

Allogeneic transplantation has been the treatment of choice for infants with severe combined immunodeficiency.[338] Engraftment can be achieved in many patients even without conditioning in this disorder. Allogeneic transplantation has been able to reverse the bone sclerosis in osteopetrosis.[339] The results in storage diseases have been inconsistent.[340] T-cell depletion may be useful in preventing GVHD. For patients without a matched sibling, both unrelated donor transplants, or mismatched related transplants, have been successful.[341] In most disorders outcome was better when transplants were given early, and promising results have been reported for transplants in utero.[342] In the future, gene modification of autologous cells may be a curative approach for some of these disorders.[343]

There has been increasing interest over the last few years in autologous transplantation with or without T-cell depletion of the graft for the treatment of autoimmune disorders.[344] The goal is to ablate the abnormal immune response and reconstitute immunity from hematopoietic stem cells and progenitors. Encouraging results have been reported in a limited number of patients with rheumatoid arthritis, systemic lupus erythematosus, multiple sclerosis, myasthenia gravis, and other disorders.[5,345]

FUTURE DIRECTIONS

Over the last decade hematopoietic transplantation has become a much safer procedure, applicable to a larger patient population in a variety of disease processes. The use of hematopoietic transplantation is likely to evolve with the development of molecularly directed anticancer therapies and with improved methods to selectively target and modulate immunity. Targeted radiation therapies, such as monoclonal antibody–radionuclide immunoconjugates and bone-seeking isotopes, are under active evaluation as a means to target radiotherapy to the tumor; this approach has little systemic toxicity other than myelosuppression. It may be possible to further improve results by using strategies to overcome drug resistance mechanisms, strategies such as administration of inhibitors to P-glycoprotein or other mechanisms of drug resistance.

The immune graft-versus-malignancy effect associated with allogeneic transplants illustrates the capability of the immune system in eradicating cancer. Strategies to enhance immune antitumor mechanisms with both allogeneic and autologous transplants are under active investigation. The major goal is to separate the beneficial graft-versus malignancy effect from the graft-versus-host disease. Tumor vaccines have been generated by ex vivo transfection of tumors with genes (to improve presentation of antigens), co-stimulatory molecules, and various cytokines to enhance the immune response directed against the tumor. Autologous antigen-presenting cells either pulsed with tumor antigens or used by themselves when they originate from the malignant clone, have also been used in vitro or in vivo to stimulate and expand cytotoxic T lymphocytes and other effectors for cellular immunotherapy. Ongoing research efforts seek to generate antigen-specific immune cells directed against tumors and major pathogens, but sparing normal donor tissues.

The collection of bone marrow or peripheral blood hematopoietic cells offers the potential for ex vivo genetic therapy to improve treatment results. Transfection of genes for drug resistance, such as from the multidrug-resistance gene *MDR1,* into normal marrow cells or transfer of genes into lymphocytes to modify the immune response may improve patient outcomes.

In the allogeneic transplant setting, efforts are directed at expanding the donor pool, reducing the toxicity of the procedure, and improving the methods to deliver immunotherapy. The majority of patients who are candidates for allogeneic transplant do not have an HLA-matched sibling donor. Further development of international unrelated donor registries for bone marrow, blood stem cells, and cord blood will increase the likelihood of finding a donor. Special attention is given to representation of ethnic minorities in these registries. New molecular methods to improve the precision of histocompatibility matching may decrease the risk of rejection and GVHD. Another approach is to use related partially matched donors. The risk of graft failure and GVHD can been minimized by infusions of large numbers of stem cells and aggressive T-cell depletion, but this type of transplant is still limited by delayed immune reconstitution after transplant and high risk of infections. Strategies are being investigated to find ways to delete alloreactive T-cell subsets, but retain subsets that contribute to graft facilitation, GVL, and infection control.

Considerable progress has been achieved in supportive care to make allogeneic transplants increasingly safe over time by preventing infections and transplant-related complications. The finding that GVL is responsible for much of the therapeutic potential of allogeneic transplants has opened the way for the use of nonmyeloablative regimens as a means to allow engraftment of donor cells with reduced toxicity. Providing GVL as the primary treatment requires carefully planned prospective clinical trials to define the role of this strategy, the diseases, and the patient population for which it will be useful.

REFERENCES

1. Thomas ED, Storb R, Clift RA, et al. Bone-marrow transplantation (second of two parts). N Engl J Med 1975;292:895–902.
2. Gatti RA, Meuwissen HJ, Allen HD, et al. Immunological reconstitution of sex-linked lymphopenic immunological deficiency. Lancet 1968;2:1366–9.
3. Thomas ED, Buckner CD, Banaji M, et al. One hundred patients with acute leukemia treated by chemotherapy, total body irradiation, and allogeneic marrow transplantation. Blood 1977;49:511–33.
4. Gratwohl A, Tyndall A. From autoimmunity to stem cell transplantation. Crit Rev Oncol Hematol 1999;30:159–72.
5. Burt RK, Traynor AE, Pope R, et al. Treatment of autoimmune disease by intense immunosuppressive conditioning and autologous hematopoietic stem cell transplantation. Blood 1998;92:3505–14.
6. Brenner MK. Gene transfer to hematopoietic cells. N Engl J Med 1996;335:337–9.
7. Bonini C, Ferrari G, Verzeletti S, et al. HSV-TK gene transfer into donor lymphocytes for control of allogeneic graft-versus-leukemia. Science 1997;276:1719–24.
8. Fassas A. Autologous stem cell transplants in treatment of multiple sclerosis: where we stand and future prospects [review]. International Journal of Hematology 2002;76 Suppl 1:223–5.
9. Espigado I, Marin-Niebla A, Rovira M, et al. Phase I/II trials of autologous peripheral blood stem cell transplantation in autoimmune diseases resistant to conventional therapy: preliminary results from the Spanish experience. Transplantation Proceedings 2003;35:742–3.
10. Anderson DJ, Gage FH, Weissman IL. Can stem cells cross lineage boundaries? Nat Med 2001;7:393–5.
11. Deans RJ, Moseley AB. Mesenchymal stem cells: biology and potential clinical uses. Exp Hematol 2000;28:875–84.
12. Fibbe WE. Mesenchymal stem cells. A potential source for skeletal repair [review]. Annals of the Rheumatic Diseases 2002;61 Suppl 2:29–31ii.
13. Alison MR, Poulsom R, Jeffery R, et al. Hepatocytes from non-hepatic adult stem cells. Nature 2000;406:257.
14. Krause DS, Theise ND, Collector MI, et al. Multi-organ, multi-lineage engraftment by a single bone marrow-derived stem cell. Cell 2001;105:369–77.
15. Abbott JD, Giordano FJ. Stem cells and cardiovascular disease review]. Journal of Nuclear Cardiology 2003;10:403–12.
16. Antel JP, Nalbantoglu J, Olivier A. Neuronal progenitors-learning from the hippocampus. Nat Med 2000;6:249–50.
17. Korbling M, Katz RL, Khanna A, et al. Hepatocytes and epithelial cells of donor origin in recipients of peripheral-blood stem cells. N Engl J Med 2002;346:738–46.

18. Prockop DJ. Further proof of the plasticity of adult stem cells and their role in tissue repair [review]. Journal of Cell Biology 2003;160:807–9.
19. Thomas ED, Storb R, Clift RA, et al. Bone-marrow transplantation. N Engl J Med 1975;292:832–43.
20. Thomas ED. Total body irradiation regimens for marrow grafting. Int J Radiat Oncol Biol Phys 1990;19:1285–8.
21. Thomas ED, Buckner CD, Banaji M, et al. One hundred patients with acute leukemia treated by chemotherapy, total body irradiation and allogeneic marrow transplantation. Blood 1977;49:511–33.
22. Santos GW, Yeager AM, Jones RJ. Autologous bone marrow transplantation. Ann Rev Med 1989;40:99–112.
23. Clift RA, Buckner CD, Applebaum FR, et al. Long-term follow-up of a randomized trial of two irradiation regimens for patients receiving allogeneic marrow transplants during first remission of acute myeloid leukemia. Blood 1998;92:1455–6.
24. Slavin S, Morecki S, Weiss L, Or R. Donor lymphocyte infusion: the use of alloreactive and tumor-reactive lymphocytes for immunotherapy of malignant and nonmalignant diseases in conjunction with allogeneic stem cell transplantation. J Hematother Stem Cell Res 2002;11:265–76.
25. Thomas ED. Karnofsky Memorial Lecture. Marrow transplantation for malignant diseases. J Clin Oncol 1983;1:517–31.
26. Frei E 3rd, Holden SA, Gonin R, et al. Antitumor alkylating agents: in vitro cross-resistance and collateral sensitivity studies. Cancer Chemother Pharmacol 1993;33:113–22.
27. Rahman ZU, Frye DK, Buzdar AU, et al. Impact of selection process on response rate and long-term survival of potential high-dose chemotherapy candidates treated with standard-dose doxorubicin-containing chemotherapy in patients with metastatic breast cancer. J Clin Oncol 1997;15:3171–7.
28. Peters WP, Jones RB, Vredenburgh J, et al. A large, prospective, randomized trial of high-dose combination alkylating agents (CPB) with autologous cellular support (ABMS) as consolidation for patients with metastatic breast cancer achieving complete remission after intensive doxorubicin-based induction therapy (AFM) (Meeting abstract). Breast Cancer Res Treat 201996; 37 (Suppl):35 1996; 37(Suppl):35.
29. Appelbaum FR, Deisseroth AB, Graw RG Jr, et al. Prolonged complete remission following high dose chemotherapy of Burkitt's lymphoma in relapse. Cancer 1978;41:1059–63.
30. Nieto Y, Shpall EJ. Autologous stem-cell transplantation for solid tumors in adults. Hematol Oncol Clin North Am 13:939–68.
31. Olsen GA, Gockerman JP, Base RC Jr, et al. Altered immunologic reconstitution after standard-dose chemotherapy or high-dose chemotherapy with autologous bone marrow support. Transplantation 1988;46:57.
32. Vellenga E, Sizoo W, Hagenbeck A, Lowenberg B. Different repopulation kinetics of erythroid (BFU-E), myeloid (CFU-GM) and T lymphocyte (TC-CFU) progenitor cells after autologous and allogeneic bone marrow transplantation. Br J Haematol 1987;65:137.
33. Borrello I, Sotomayor EM, Rattis FM, et al. Sustaining the graft-versus-tumor effect through posttransplant immunization with granulocyte-macrophage colony-stimulating factor (GM-CSF)-producing tumor vaccines. Blood 2000;95:3011–19.
34. Brenner MK, Rill DR, Moen RC, et al. Gene-marking to trace origin of relapse after autologous bone-marrow transplantation. Lancet 1993;34185–6.
35. Shpall EJ, Lemaistre CF, Holland K, et al. A prospective randomized trial of buffy coat versus CD34- selected autologous bone marrow support in high-risk breast cancer patients receiving high-dose chemotherapy. Blood 1997;90:4313–20.
36. Vose JM, Rowlings PA, Lazarus HM, et al. Autotransplants for intermediate grade and immunoblastic non-Hodgkin's lymphoma (NHL) at first relapse (REL1) or in second remission (CR2): a report from the Autologous Blood and Marrow Transplant Registry North America (ABMTR)). Proc Annu Meet Am Soc Clin Oncol 1996;15:1273a.
37. Chopra R, McMillian AK, Linch DC, et al. The place of high-dose BEAM therapy and autologous bone marrow transplantation in poor-risk Hodgkin's disease. A single center eight-year study of 155 patients. Blood 1993;81:1137–45.
38. Ramsay NK, Kersey JH. Indications for marrow transplantation in acute lymphoblastic leukemia. Blood 1990;75:815–18.
39. Candoni A, Sperotto A, Tomadini V, et al. Autologous stem cell transplantation as post-remission therapy for acute myeloid leukemia. Risk factors at diagnosis can predict the outcome. Leuk Lymphoma 2003;44:1083–5.
40. Novitzky N, Thomas V, Stubbings H. Intensified myeloablative therapy and autologous stem-cell transplantation for patients with AML: single center experience. Cytotherapy 2003;5:139–46.
41. Attal M, Harousseau J-L, Stoppa A-M, et al. A prospective, randomized trial of autologous bone marrow transplantation and chemotherapy in multiple myeloma. N Engl J Med 1996;335:91–7.
42. Lahuerta JJ, Grande C, Martinez-Lopez J, et al. Tandem transplants with different high-dose regimens improve the complete remission rates in multiple myeloma. Results of a Grupo Espanol de Sindromes Linfoproliferativos/Trasplante Autologo de Medula Osea phase II trial. Br J Haematol 2003;120:296–303.
43. Peters WP, Rosner GL, Vredenburgh JJ, et al. Prospective, randomized comparison of high-dose chemotherapy with stem-cell support versus intermediate-dose chemotherapy after surgery and adjuvant chemotherapy in women with high-risk primary breast cancer a report of CALGB 9082, SWOG 9114, and NCIC MA-13. J Clin Oncol 2005;23:2191–200.
44. Donato ML, Gershenson DM, Wharton JT, et al. High-dose topotecan, melphalan, and cyclophosphamide (TMC) with stem cell support: a new regimen for the treatment of advanced ovarian cancer. Gynecol Oncol 2001;82:420–6.
45. Rick O, Kollmannsberger C, Beyer J, et al. Current aspects of high-dose chemotherapy in germ-cell tumors. Crit Rev Oncol Hematol 2003;47:237–48.
46. Lenz G, Dreyling M, Schiegnitz E, et al. Myeloablative radiochemotherapy followed by autologous stem cell transplantation in first remission prolongs progression-free survival in follicular lymphoma: a results of a prospective, randomized trial of the German low-grade lymphoma study group. Blood 2004;104:2667–74.
47. Meyers PA. High-dose therapy with autologous stem cell rescue for pediatric sarcomas. [Review] [38 refs]. Curr Opin Oncol 2004;16(2):120–5.
48. Champlin R, Khouri I, Shimoni A, et al. Harnessing graft-versus-malignancy: non-myeloablative preparative regimens for allogeneic hematopoietic transplantation, an evolving strategy for adoptive immunotherapy. Br J Hematol 2000;111:18–29.
49. Horowitz MM, Gale RP, Sondel PM, et al. Graft-versus-leukemia reactions after bone marrow transplantation. Blood 1990;75:555–62.
50. Gale RP, Champlin RE. How does bone-marrow transplantation cure leukemia? Lancet 1984;2:28–30.
51. Gale RP, Horowitz MM, Ash RC, et al. Identical-twin bone marrow transplants for leukemia. Ann Intern Med 1994;120:646–52.
52. Marmont AM, Horowitz MM, Gale RP, et al. T-cell depletion of HLA-identical transplants in leukemia. Blood 1991;78:2120–30.
53. Sullivan KM, Weiden PL, Storb R, et al. Influence of acute and chronic graft-versus-host disease on relapse and survival after bone marrow transplantation from HLA-identical siblings as treatment of acute and chronic leukemia. Blood 1989;73:1720–8.
54. Weiden PL, Sullivan KM, Flournoy N, et al. Antileukemic effect of chronic graft-versus-host disease: contribution to improved survival after allogeneic marrow transplantation. N Engl J Med 1981;304:1529–33.
55. Collins RH Jr, Rogers ZR, Bennett M, et al. Hematologic relapse of chronic myelogenous leukemia following allogeneic bone marrow transplantation: apparent graft-versus leukemia effect following abrupt discontinuation of immunosuppression. Bone Marrow Transplant 1992;10:391–5.
56. Kolb HJ, Schattenberg A, Goldman JM, et al. Graft-versus leukemia effect of donor lymphocyte transfusions in marrow grafted patients. European Group for Blood and Marrow Transplantation Working Party Chronic Leukemia. Blood 1995;86:2041–50.
57. Collins RH Jr, Shpilberg O, Drobyski WR, et al. Donor leukocyte infusions in 140 patients with relapsed malignancy after allogeneic bone marrow transplantation. J Clin Oncol 1997;15:433–44.
58. van Besien KW, de Lima M, Giralt SA, et al. Management of lymphoma recurrence after allogeneic transplantation: the relevance of graft-versus-lymphoma effect. Bone Marrow Transplant 1997;19:977–82.
59. Khouri IF, Saliba RM, Giralt SA, et al. Nonablative allogeneic hematopoietic transplantation as adoptive immunotherapy for indolent lymphoma: low incidence of toxicity, acute graft-versus-host disease, and treatment-related mortality. Blood 2001;98:3595–9.
60. Collins RH Jr, Goldstein S, Giralt S, et al. Donor leukocyte infusions in acute lymphocytic leukemia. Bone Marrow Transplant 2000;26:511–16.
61. Childs R, Chernoff A, Contentin N, et al. Regression of metastatic renal-cell carcinoma after nonmyeloablative allogeneic peripheral-blood stem-cell transplantation. N Engl J Med 2000;343:750–8.
62. Ueno NT, Rondon G, Mirza NQ, et al. Allogeneic peripheral- blood progenitor-cell transplantation for poor-risk patients with metastatic breast cancer. J Clin Oncol 1998;16:986–93.
63. Hansen JA, Choo SY, Geraghty DE, Mickelson E. The HLA system in clinical marrow transplantation. Hematol Oncol Clin North Am 1990;4:507–15.
64. Kernan NA, Bartsch G, Ash RC, et al. Analysis of 462 transplantations from unrelated donors facilitated by the National Marrow Donor Program. N Engl J Med 1993;328:593–602.
65. McGlave PB, Shu XO, Wen W, et al. Unrelated donor marrow transplantation for chronic myelogenous leukemia: 9 years' experience of the national marrow donor program. Blood 2000;95:2219–25.
66. Hansen JA, Gooley TA, Martin PJ, et al. Bone marrow transplants from unrelated donors for patients with chronic myeloid leukemia. N Engl J Med 1998;338:962–8.
67. Petersdorf EW, Mickelson EM, Anasetti C, et al. Effect of HLA mismatches on the outcome of hematopoietic transplants. Curr Opin Immunol 1999;11:521–6.
68. Beatty PG, Clift RA, Mickelson EM, et al. Marrow transplantation from related donors other than HLA-identical siblings. N Engl J Med 1985;313:765–71.
69. Anasetti C, Amos D, Beatty PG, et al. Effect of HLA compatibility on engraftment of bone marrow transplants in patients with leukemia or lymphoma. N Engl J Med 1989; 320:197–204.
70. Champlin RE, Passweg JR, Zhang MJ, et al. T-cell depletion of bone marrow transplants for leukemia from donors other than HLA-identical siblings: advantage of T-cell antibodies with narrow specificities. Blood 2000;95:3996–4003.
71. Aversa F, Tabilio A, Terenzi A, et al. Successful engraftment of T-cell-depleted haploidentical "three-loci" incompatible transplants in leukemia patients by addition of recombinant human granulocyte colony-stimulating factor mobilized peripheral blood progenitor cells to bone marrow inoculum. Blood 1994;84:3948–55.
72. Bachar-Lustig E, Rachamim N, Li HW, et al. Mega dose of T cell-depleted bone marrow overcomes MHC barriers in sublethally irradiated mice. Nat Med 1995;1:1268–73.
73. Kurtzberg J, Graham M, Casey J, et al. The use of umbilical cord blood in mismatched related and unrelated hematopoietic stem cell transplantation. Blood Cells 1994;20:275–83.
74. Laughlin MJ, Eapen M, Rubinstein P, et al. Outcomes after transplantation of cord blood or bone marrow from unrelated donors in adults with leukemia. N Engl J Med 2004;351:2265–75.
75. Rocha V, Labopin M, Sanz G, et al. Transplants of umbilical cord blood or bone marrow from unrelated donors in adults with acute leukemia. N Engl J Med 2004;351:2276–85.
76. Shpall EJ, Champlin R, Glaspy JA. Effect of CD34+ peripheral blood progenitor cell dose on hematopoietic recovery. Biol Blood Marrow Transplant 1998;4:84–92.
77. Weissman IL. Stem cells: units of development, units of regeneration, and units in evolution. Cell 2000;100:157–68.
78. Weissman IL. Stem cells—scientific, medical, and political issues. N Engl J Med 2002;346:1576–9.
79. Berenson RJ, Bensinger WI, Hill RS, et al. Engraftment after infusion of CD34+ marrow cells in patients with breast cancer or neuroblastoma. Blood 1991;77:1717–22.
80. Kawashima I, Zanjani ED, Almaida-Porada G, et al. CD34+human marrow cells that express low levels of Kit protein are enriched for long-term marrow-engrafting cells. Blood 1996;87:4136–42.
81. Baum CM, Weissman IL, Tsukamoto AS, et al. Isolation of a candidate human hematopoietic stem-cell population. Proc Natl Acad Sci U S A 1992;89:2804–8.
82. Yin AH, Miraglia S, Zanjani ED, et al. AC133, a novel marker for human hematopoietic stem and progenitor cells. Blood 1997;90:5002–12.
83. Osawa M, Hanada K, Hamada H, Nakauchi H. Long-term lymphohematopoietic reconstitution by a single CD34-low/negative hematopoietic stem cell. Science 1996;273:242–5.
84. Zanjani ED, Almeida-Porada G, Livingston AG, et al. Human bone marrow CD34– cells engraft in vivo and undergo multilineage expression that includes giving rise to CD34+ cells. Exp Hematol 1998;26:353–60.

85. Thomas ED, Storb R. Technique for human marrow grafting. Blood 1970;36:507–15.
86. Champlin RE. Peripheral blood progenitor cells: a replacement for marrow transplantation? Semin Oncol 1996;23(2 Suppl 4):15–21.
87. Hartmann O, Le Corroller AG, Blaise D, et al. Peripheral blood stem cell and bone marrow transplantation for solid tumors and lymphomas: hematologic recovery and costs. A randomized, controlled trial. Ann Intern Med 1997;126:600–7.
88. Socinski MA, Cannistra SA, Sullivan R, et al. Granulocyte macrophage colony-stimulating factor induces the expression of the CD11b surface adhesion molecule on human granulocytes in vivo. Blood 1988;72:691–7.
89. Sheridan WP, Begley CG, Juttner CA, et al. Effect of peripheral- blood progenitor cells mobilized by filgrastim (GCSF) on platelet recovery after high-dose chemotherapy. Lancet 1992;339:640–4.
90. Anderlini P, Korbling M, Dale D, et al. Allogeneic blood stem cell transplantation: considerations for donors. Blood 1997;90:903–8.
91. Shpall EJ, Champlin R, Glaspy JA. Effect of CD34+ peripheral blood progenitor cell dose on hematopoietic recovery. Biol Blood Marrow Transplant 1998;4:84–92.
92. Attarian H, Feng Z, Buckner CD, et al. Long-term cryopreservation of bone marrow for autologous transplantation. Bone Marrow Transplant 1996;17:425–30.
93. Rowley SD, Bensinger WI, Gooley TA, Buckner CD. Effect of cell concentration on bone marrow and peripheral blood stem cell cryopreservation. Blood 1994;83:2731–6.
94. Ross AA, Cooper BW, Lazarus HM, et al. Detection and viability of tumor cells in peripheral blood stem cell collections from breast cancer patients using immunocytochemical and clonogenic assay techniques. Blood 1993;82:2605–10.
95. Brenner MK, Rill DR, Moen RC, et al. Gene-marking to trace origin of relapse after autologous bone-marrow transplantation. Lancet 1993;341:85–86.
96. Deisseroth AB, Zu Z, Claxton D, et al. Genetic marking shows that Ph+ cells present in autologous transplants of chronic myelogenous leukemia (CML) contribute to relapse after autologous bone marrow in CML. Blood 1994; 83:3068–76.
97. Rill DR, Santana VM, Roberts WM, et al. Direct demonstration that autologous bone marrow transplantation for solid tumors can return a multiplicity of tumorigenic cells. Blood 1994;84:380–3.
98. Gribben JG, Freedman AS, Neuberg D, et al. Immunologic purging of marrow assessed by PCR before autologous bone marrow transplantation for B-cell lymphoma. N Engl J Med 1991;325:1525–33.
99. Vredenburgh JJ, Peters WP, Rosner G, A et al. Detection of tumor cells in the bone marrow of stage IV breast cancer patients receiving high-dose chemotherapy: the role of induction chemotherapy. Bone Marrow Transplant 1995;16:815–21.
100. Sharp JG, Kessinger A, Mann S, et al. Outcome of high dose therapy and autologous transplantation in non-Hodgkin's lymphoma based on the presence of tumor in the marrow or infused hematopoietic harvest. J Clin Oncol 1996;14:214–19.
101. Shpall EJ, Lemaistre CF, Holland K, et al. A prospective randomized trial of buffy coat versus CD34-selected autologous bone marrow support in high-risk breast cancer patients receiving high-dose chemotherapy. Blood 1997;90:4313–20.
102. Vescio R, Schiller G, Stewart AK, et al. Multi-center phase III trial to evaluate CD34 (+) selected versus unselected autologous peripheral blood progenitor cell transplantation in multiple myeloma. Blood 1999;93:1858–68.
103. Gorin NC, Aegerter P, Auvert B, et al. Autologous bone marrow transplantation for acute myelocytic leukemia in first remission: a European survey of the role of marrow purging. Blood 1990;75:1606–14.
104. Yeager AM, Kaizer H, Santos GW, et al. Autologous bone marrow transplantation in patients with acute non-lymphocytic leukemia, using ex vivo marrow treatment with 4-hydroperoxycyclophosphamide. N Engl J Med 1986;315:141–7.
105. Lapidot T, Faktorowich Y, Lubin I, Reisner Y. Enhancement of T-cell-depleted bone marrow allografts in the absence of graft-versus-host disease is mediated by CD8+ CD4-and not by CD8– CD4+ thymocytes. Blood 1992;80:2406–11.
106. Korbling M, Huh YO, Durett A, et al. Allogeneic blood stem cell transplantation: peripheralization and yield of donor derived primitive hematopoietic progenitor cells (CD34+ Thy-1dim) and lymphoid subsets, and possible predictors of engraftment and graft-versus-host disease. Blood 1995;86:2842–8.
107. Przepiorka D, Smith TL, Folloder J, et al. Risk factors for acute graft-versus-host disease after allogeneic blood stem cell transplantation. Blood 1999;94:1465–70.
108. Bensinger WI, Clift R, Martin P, et al. Allogeneic peripheral blood stem cell transplantation in patients with advanced hematologic malignancies: a retrospective comparison with marrow transplantation. Blood 1996;88:2794–2800.
109. Champlin RE, Schmitz N, Horowitz MM, et al. Blood stem cells compared with bone marrow as a source of hematopoietic cells for allogeneic transplantation. IBMTR Histocompatibility and Stem Cell Sources Working Committee and the European Group for Blood and Marrow Transplantation (EBMT). Blood 2000;95:3702–9.
110. Bensinger WI, Martin PJ, Storer B, et al. Transplantation of bone marrow as compared with peripheral-blood cells from HLA-identical relatives in patients with hematologic cancers. N Engl J Med 2001;344:175–81.
111. Broxmeyer HE. Questions to be answered regarding umbilical cord blood hematopoietic stem and progenitor cells and their use in-transplantation. Transfusion 1995;35:694–702.
112. Cairo MS, Wagner JE. Placental and/or umbilical cord blood: an alternative source of hematopoietic stem cells for transplantation. Blood 1997;90:4665–78.
113. Rocha V, Wagner JE Jr, Sobocinski KA, et al. Graft-versus host disease in children who have received a cord-blood or bone marrow transplant from an HLA-identical sibling. Eurocord and International Bone Marrow Transplant Registry Working Committee on Alternative Donor and Stem Cell Sources. N Engl J Med 2000;342:1846–54.
114. Rubinstein P, Carrier C, Scaradavou A, et al. Outcomes among 562 recipients of placental-blood transplants from unrelated donors. N Engl J Med 1998;339:1565–77.
115. Gluckman E, Rocha V, Boyer-Chammard A, et al. Outcome of cord-blood transplantation from related and unrelated donors. Eurocord Transplant Group and the European Blood and Marrow Transplantation Group. N Engl J Med 1997;337:373–81.
116. Kurtzberg J, Laughlin M, Graham ML, et al. Placental blood as a source of hematopoietic stem cells for transplantation into unrelated recipients. N Engl J Med 1996;335:157–66.
117. Kusnierz-Glaz CR, Schlegel PG, Wong RM, et al. Influence of age on the outcome of 500 autologous bone marrow transplant procedures for hematologic malignancies. J Clin Oncol 1997;15:18–25.
118. Miller CB, Piantadosi S, Vogelsang GB, et al. Impact of age on outcome of patients with cancer undergoing autologous bone marrow transplant. J Clin Oncol 1996;14:1327–32.
119. Bensinger W, Appelbaum F, Rowley S, et al. Factors that influence collection and engraftment of autologous peripheral-blood stem cells. J Clin Oncol 1995;13:2547–55.
120. Friedberg JW, Neuberg D, Stone RM, et al. Outcome in patients with myelodysplastic syndrome after autologous bone marrow transplantation for non-Hodgkin's lymphoma. J Clin Oncol 1999;17:3128–35.
121. Marolleau JP, Brice P, Morel P, Gisselbrecht C. Secondary acute myeloid leukemia after autologous bone marrow transplantation for malignant lymphomas. J Clin Oncol 1993;11:590–1.
122. McSweeney PA, Storb R. Mixed chimerism: preclinical studies and clinical applications. Biol Blood Marrow Transplant 1999;5:192–203.
123. Slavin S, Nagler A, Naparstek E, et al. Nonmyeloablative stem cell transplantation and cell therapy as an alternative to conventional bone marrow transplantation with lethal cytoreduction for the treatment of malignant and nonmalignant hematologic diseases. Blood 1998;91:756–63.
124. Champlin R, Khouri I, Komblau S, et al. Reinventing bone marrow transplantation. Nonmyeloablative preparative regimens and induction of graft-vs-malignancy effect. Oncology (Huntingt) 1999;13:621–8.
125. Antman K, Ayash L, Elias A, et al. A phase II study of high-dose cyclophosphamide, thiotepa, and carboplatin with autologous marrow support in women with measurable advanced breast cancer responding to standard dose therapy. J Clin Oncol 1992;10:102–10.
126. Peters WP, Shpall EJ, Jones RB et al. High-dose alkylating agents with bone marrow support as initial treatment for metastatic breast cancer. J Clin Oncol 1988;1368–76.
127. Chopra R, McMillan AK, Linch DC, et al. The place of high-dose BEAM therapy and autologous bone marrow transplantation in poor-risk Hodgkin's disease. A single-center eight-year study of 155 patients. Blood 1993;81:1137–45.
128. Giles FJ, Kantarjian HM, Kornblau SM, et al. Mylotarg (gemtuzumab ozogamicin) therapy is associated with hepatic venoocclusive disease in patients who have not received stem cell transplantation. Cancer 2001;92:406–13.
129. Rapoport AP, Meisenberg B, Sarkodee-Adoo C, et al. Autotransplantation for advanced lymphoma and Hodgkin's disease followed by post-transplant Rituxan/GM-CSF or radiotherapy and consolidation chemotherapy. Bone Marrow Transplantation 2002;29:303–12.
130. Appelbaum FR, Brown P, Sandmeier B, et al. Use of holmium-166-EDTMP (Ho-166-EDTMP) for marrow ablation prior to marrow transplantation. Exp Hematol 1988;16:494.
131. Thomas ED. Total body irradiation regimens for marrow grafting. Int J Radiat Oncol Biol Phys 1990;19:1285–8.
132. Shank B. Total body irradiation for marrow or stem-cell transplantation. Cancer Invest 1998;16:397–404.
133. Santos GW, Tutschka PJ, Brookmeyer R, et al. Marrow transplantation for acute non-lymphocytic leukemia after treatment with busulfan and cyclophosphamide. N Engl J Med 1983;309:1347–53.
134. Tutschka PJ, Copelan EA, Klein JP. Bone marrow transplantation for leukemia following a new busulfan and cyclophosphamide regimen. Blood 1987;70:1382–8.
135. Giralt S, Estey E, Albitar M, et al. Engraftment of allogeneic hematopoietic progenitor cells with purine analog-containing chemotherapy: harnessing graft-versus-leukemia without myeloablative therapy. Blood 1997;89:4531–6.
136. Khouri IF, Keating M, Korbling M, et al. Transplant-lite: induction of graft-versus-malignancy using fludarabine based nonablative chemotherapy and allogeneic blood progenitor-cell transplantation as treatment for lymphoid malignancies. J Clin Oncol 1998;16:2817–24.
137. Kernan NA, Bordignon C, Heller G, et al. Graft failure after T-cell-depleted human leukocyte antigen identical marrow transplants for leukemia: I. Analysis of risk factors and results of secondary transplants. Blood 1989;74:2227–36.
138. Fleischhauer K, Kernan NA, O'Reilly RJ, et al. Bone marrow- allograft rejection by T lymphocytes recognizing a single amino acid difference in HLA-B44. N Engl J Med 1990;323:1818–22.
139. Petersdorf EW, Longton GM, Anasetti C, et al. Association of HLA-C disparity with graft failure after marrow transplantation from unrelated donors. Blood 1997;89:1818–23.
140. Davies SM, Ramsay NK, Haake RJ, et al. Comparison of engraftment in recipients of matched sibling of unrelated donor marrow allografts. Bone Marrow Transplant 1994;13:51–7.
141. Martin PJ. Donor CD8 cells prevent allogeneic marrow graft rejection in mice: potential implications for marrow transplantation in humans. J Exp Med 1993;178:703–12.
142. Kaufman CL, Colson YL, Wren SM, et al. Phenotypic characterization of a novel bone marrow-derived cell that facilitates engraftment of allogeneic bone marrow stem cells. Blood 1994;84:2436–46.
143. Simmons P, Kaushansky K, Torok-Storb B. Mechanisms of cytomegalovirus-mediated myelosuppression: perturbation of stromal cell function versus direct infection of myeloid cells. Proc Natl Acad Sci U S A 1990;87:1386–90.
144. Schleuning M, Jager G, Holler E, et al. Human parvovirus B19-associated disease in bone marrow transplantation. Infection 1999;27:114–7.
145. Carrigan DR, Knox KK. Human herpes virus 6 (HHV-6) isolation from bone marrow: HHV-6-associated bone marrow suppression in bone marrow transplant patients. Blood 1994;84:3307–10.
146. Nemunaitis J, Singer JW, Buckner CD, et al. Use of recombinant human granulocyte-macrophage colony-stimulating factor in graft failure after bone marrow transplantation. Blood 1990;76:245–53.
147. Ferrara JL, Deeg HJ. Graft-versus-host disease. N Engl J Med 1991;324:667–74.
148. Shlomchik WD, Couzens MS, Tang CB, et al. Prevention of graft versus host disease by inactivation of host antigen presenting cells. Science 1999;285:412–5.
149. Weisdorf DJ, Snover DC, Haake R, et al. Acute upper gastrointestinal graft-versus-host disease: clinical significance and response to immunosuppressive therapy. Blood 1990;76:624–9.
150. Glucksberg H, Storb R, Fefer A, et al. Clinical manifestations of graft-versus-host disease in human recipients of marrow from HL-A-matched sibling donors. Transplantation 1974;18:295–304.

151. Przepiorka D, Weisdorf D, Martin P, et al. 1994 Consensus Conference on Acute GVHD Grading. Bone Marrow Transplant 1995;15:825–8.
152. Gajewski J, Gjertson D, Cecka M, et al. The impact of T-cell depletion on the effects of HLA DR beta 1 and DQ beta allele matching in HLA serologically identical unrelated donor bone marrow transplantation. Biol Blood Marrow Transplant 1997;3:76–82.
153. Rufer N, Wolpert E, Helg C, et al. HA-1 and the SMCY derived peptide FIDSYICQV (H-Y) are immunodominant minor histocompatibility antigens after bone marrow transplantation. Transplantation 1998;66:910–6.
154. Flowers ME, Pepe MS, Longton G, et al. Previous donor pregnancy as a risk factor for acute graft-versus-host disease in patients with aplastic anemia treated by allogeneic marrow transplantation. Br J Haematol 1990;74:492–6.
155. Bostrom L, Ringden O, Jacobsen N, et al. A European multicenter study of chronic graft-versus-host disease. The role of cytomegalovirus serology in recipients and donors–acute graft-versus-host disease, and splenectomy. Transplantation 1990;49:1100–5.
156. Nash RA, Pineiro LA, Storb R, al. FK506 in combination with methotrexate for the prevention of graft-versus-host disease after marrow transplantation from matched unrelated donors. Blood 1996;88:3634–41.
157. Przepiorka D, Ippoliti C, Khouri I, et al. Tacrolimus and Mini-dose methotrexate for prevention of acute graft-versus-host disease after matched unrelated donor marrow transplantation. Blood 1996;88:4383–9.
158. Storb R, Pepe M, Deeg HJ, et al. Long-term follow-up of a controlled trial comparing a combination of methotrexate plus cyclosporine with cyclosporine alone for prophylaxis of graft-versus-host disease in patients administered HLA-identical marrow grafts for leukemia. Blood 1992;80:560–1.
159. Martin PJ, Schoch G, Fisher L, et al. A retrospective analysis of therapy for acute graft-versus-host disease: initial treatment. Blood 1990;76:1464–72.
160. Martin PJ, Schoch G, Fisher L, et al. A retrospective analysis of therapy for acute graft-versus-host disease: secondary treatment. Blood 1991;77:1821–8.
161. Sullivan KM, Agura E, Anasetti C, et al. Chronic graft-versus- host disease and other late complications of bone marrow transplantation. Semin Hematol 1991;28:250–9.
162. Atkinson K, Horowitz MM, Gale RP, et al. Risk factors for chronic graft-versus-host disease after HLA-identical sibling bone marrow transplantation. Blood 1990;75:2459–64.
163. Champlin RE, Schmitz N, Horowitz MM, et al. Blood stem cells compared with bone marrow as a source of hematopoietic cells for allogeneic transplantation. IBMTR Histocompatibility and Stem Cell Sources Working Committee and the European Group for Blood and Marrow Transplantation (EBMT). Blood 2000;95:3702–9
164. Pepe MS, Longton G, Pettinger M, et al. Summarizing data on survival, relapse, and chronic graft-versus-host disease after bone marrow transplantation: motivation for and description of new methods. Br J Haematol 1993;83:602–7.
165. Siadak M, Sullivan KM. The management of chronic graft versus-host disease. Blood Rev 1994;8:154–60.
166. Sullivan KM, Witherspoon RP, Storb R, et al. Alternating day cyclosporine and prednisone for treatment of high risk chronic graft-v-host disease. Blood 1988;72:555–61.
167. Tzakis AG, Abu-Elmagd K, Fung JJ, et al. FK 506 rescue in chronic graft-versus-host-disease after bone marrow transplantation. Transplant Proc 1991;23:3225–7.
168. Vogelsang GB. How I treat chronic graft-versus-host disease. Blood 2001;97:1196–1201.
169. Vogelsang GB, Arai S. Mycophenolate mofetil for the prevention and treatment of graft-versus host disease following stem cell transplantation: preliminary findings. Bone Marrow Transplantation 2001;27:1255–62.
170. Busca A, Saroglia EM, Lanino E, et al. Mycophenolate mofetil (MMF) as therapy for refractory chronic GVHD (cGVHD) in children receiving bone marrow transplantation. Bone Marrow Transplantation 2000;25:1067–71.
171. Schulman HM, Hinterberger W. Hepatic veno-occlusive disease- liver toxicity syndrome after bone marrow transplantation. Bone Marrow Transplant 1992;10:197–214.
172. Bearman SI, Anderson GI, Mori M, et al. Venoocclusive disease of the liver: development of a model for predicting fatal outcome after marrow transplantation. J Clin Oncol 1993;11:1729–36.
173. Jones RB, Matthes S, Shpall EJ, et al. Acute lung injury following high-dose cyclophosphamide, cisplatin and BCNU. Pharmacodynamic evaluation of BCNU. J Natl Cancer Institute 1993;85:640–7.
174. Openshaw H, Slatkin NE. Neurological complications. In: Thomas ED, Blume KG, Forman SJ, editors. Hematopoietic cell transplantation. Malden, MA: Blackwell Science, Inc, 1999: 659–73.
175. Gottdiener JS, Applebaum FR, Ferrand VJ, et al. Cardiotoxicity associated with high-dose cyclophosphamide therapy. Arch Int Med 1981;141:758–63.
176. Gajewski JL, Petz LD, Calhoun L, et al. Hemolysis of transfused group O red blood cells in minor ABO-incompatible unrelated donor bone marrow transplants in patients receiving cyclosporine without posttransplant methotrexate. Blood 1992;79:3076–85.
177. Moake JL, Byrnes JJ. Thrombotic microangiopathies associated with drugs and bone marrow transplantation. Hematol Oncol Clin North Am 1996;10:485–97.
178. Fuge R, Bird JM, Fraser A, et al. The clinical features, risk factors and outcome of thrombotic thrombocytopenic purpura occurring after bone marrow transplantation. Br J Haematol 2001;113:58–64.
179. Roy V, Rizvi MA, Vesely SK, George JN. Thrombotic thrombocytopenic purpura-like syndromes following bone marrow transplantation: an analysis of associated conditions and clinical outcomes. Bone Marrow Transplant 2001;27:641–6.
180. Aotsuka N, Asai T, Oh H, et al. Lymphocyte subset reconstitution following human allogeneic bone marrow transplantation: differences between engrafted patients and graft failure patients. Bone Marrow Transplant 1991;8:345–9.
181. Keever CA, Small TN, Flomenberg N, et al. Immune reconstitution following bone marrow transplantation: comparison of recipients of T-cell depleted marrow with recipients of conventional marrow grafts. Blood 1989;73:1340–50.
182. Guinan EC, Molrine DC, Antin JH, et al. Polysaccharide conjugate vaccine responses in bone marrow transplant patients. Transplantation 1994;57:677–84.
183. Douek DC, Vescio RA, Betts MR, et al. Assessment of thymic output in adults after hematopoietic stem-cell transplantation and prediction of T-cell reconstitution. Lancet 2000;355:1875–81.
184. Bacigalupo A, Mordini N, Pitto A, et al. Transplantation of HLA-mismatched CD34+ selected cells in patients with advanced malignancies: severe immunodeficiency and related complications. Br J Haematol 1997;98:760–6.
185. Brochu S, Rioux-Masse B, Roy J, et al. Massive activation induced cell death of alloreactive T cells with apoptosis of bystander post-thymic T cells prevents immune reconstitution in mice with graft-versus-host disease. Blood 1999;94:390–400.
186. Powles R, Singhal S, Treleaven J, et al. Identification of patients who may benefit from prophylactic immunotherapy after bone marrow transplantation for acute myeloid leukemia on the basis of lymphocyte recovery early after transplantation. Blood 1998;91:3481–6.
187. Dykewicz CA. Summary of the Guidelines for Preventing Opportunistic Infections among Hematopoietic Stem Cell Transplant Recipients. Clin Infect Dis 2001;33:139–4.
188. Curtis RE, Travis LB, Rowlings PA, et al. Risk of lymphoproliferative disorders after bone marrow transplantation: a multi-institutional study. Blood 1999;94:2208–16.
189. Papadopoulos EB, Ladanyi M, Emanuel D, et al. Infusions of donor leukocytes to treat Epstein-Barr virus–associated lymphoproliferative disorders after allogeneic bone marrow transplantation. N Engl J Med 1994;330:1185–91.
190. Gottschalk S, Heslop HE, Rooney CM. Treatment of Epstein–Barr virus–associated malignancies with specific T cells. Ad Cancer Res 2002;84:175–201.
191. Abruzzese E, Radford JE, Miller JS, et al. Detection of abnormal pretransplant clones in progenitor cells of patients who developed myelodysplasia after autologous transplantation. Blood 1999;94:1814–9.
192. Armitage JO. Myelodysplasia and acute leukemia after autologous bone marrow transplantation. J Clin Oncol 2000;18:945–6.
193. Clift RA, Buckner CD. Marrow transplantation for acute myeloid leukemia. Cancer Invest 1998; 16:53–61.
194. Zittoun RA, Mandelli F, Willemze R, et al. Autologous or allogeneic bone marrow transplantation compared with intensive chemotherapy in acute myelogenous leukemia. European Organization for Research and Treatment of Cancer (EORTC) and the Gruppo Italiano Malattie Ematologiche Maligne dell'Adulto (GIMEMA) Leukemia Cooperative Groups. N Engl J Med 1995;332:217–23.
195. Appelbaum FR. Is there a best transplant conditioning regimen for acute myeloid leukemia? Leukemia 2000;14:497–501.
196. Blaise D, Maraninchi D, Archimbaud E, et al. Allogeneic bone marrow transplantation for acute myeloid leukemia in first remission: a randomized trial of a busulfan-Cytoxan versus Cytoxan-total body irradiation as preparative regimen: a report from the Group d'Etudes de la Greffe de Moelle Osseuse. Blood 1992;79:2578–82.
197. Clift RA, Buckner CD, Appelbaum FR, et al. Long-term follow- Up of a randomized trial of two irradiation regimens for patients receiving allogeneic marrow transplants during first remission of acute myeloid leukemia. Blood 1998;92:1455–6.
198. Champlin R, Gale RP. Acute myelogenous leukemia: recent advances in therapy. Blood 1987;69:1551–62.
199. Matthews DC, Appelbaum FR, Eary JF, et al. Phase I study of (131)I-anti-CD45 antibody plus cyclophosphamide and total body irradiation for advanced acute leukemia and myelodysplastic syndrome. Blood 1999;94:1237–47.
200. Burnett AK, Goldstone AH, Stevens RM, et al. Randomized comparison of addition of autologous bone-marrow transplantation to intensive chemotherapy for acute myeloid leukemia in first remission: results of MRC AML 10 trial. UK Medical Research Council Adult and Children's Leukemia Working Parties. Lancet 1998;351:700–8.
201. Cassileth PA, Andersen J, Lazarus HM, et al. Autologous bone marrow transplant in acute myeloid leukemia in first remission. J Clin Oncol 1993;11:314–9.
202. Ball ED, Rybka WB. Autologous bone marrow transplantation for adult acute leukemia. Hematol Oncol Clin North Am 1993;7:201–31.
203. Appelbaum FR, Fisher LD, Thomas ED. Chemotherapy v marrow transplantation for adults with acute non-lymphocytic leukemia: a five-year follow-up. Blood 1988;72:179–84.
204. Champlin RE, Ho WG, Gale RP, et al. Treatment of acute myelogenous leukemia. A prospective controlled trial of bone marrow transplantation versus consolidation chemotherapy. Ann Intern Med 1985;102:285–91.
205. Burnett AK. Transplantation in first remission of acute myeloid leukemia. N Engl J Med 1998;339:1698–1700.
206. Reiffers J, Stoppa AM, Attal M, et al. Allogeneic vs autologous stem cell transplantation vs chemotherapy in patients with acute myeloid leukemia in first remission: the BGMT 87 study. Leukemia 1996;10:1874–82.
207. Anasetti C. Transplantation of hematopoietic stem cells from alternate donors in acute myelogenous leukemia. Leukemia 2000;14:502–4.
208. Champlin R. Bone marrow transplantation for leukemia utilizing HLA-matched unrelated donors. Bone Marrow Transplant 1993;11 Suppl 1:74–7.
209. Greenberg PL. Risk factors and their relationship to prognosis in myelodysplastic syndromes. Leuk Res 1998;22 Suppl 1:3–6s.
210. de Witte T, Gratwohl A. Bone marrow transplantation for myelodysplastic syndrome and secondary leukemias. Br J Haematol 1993;84:361–4.
211. de Witte T, Hermans J, Vossen J, et al. Hematopoietic stem cell transplantation for patients with myelodysplastic syndromes and secondary acute myeloid leukemias: a report on behalf of the Chronic Leukemia Working Party of the European Group for Blood and Marrow Transplantation (EBMT). Br J Haematol 2000;110:620–30.
212. Deeg HJ, Shulman HM, Anderson JE, et al. Allogeneic and syngeneic marrow transplantation for myelodysplastic syndrome in patients 55 to 66 years of age. Blood 2000;95:1188–94.
213. Witherspoon RP, Deeg HJ, Storer B, et al. Hematopoietic stem-cell transplantation for treatment-related leukemia or myelodysplasia. J Clin Oncol 2001;19:2134–41.
214. Appelbaum FR, Anderson J. Allogeneic bone marrow transplantation for myelodysplastic syndrome: outcomes analysis according to IPSS score. Leukemia 1998;12 Suppl 1:S25–9.
215. Yakoub-Agha I, de La SP, Ribaud P, et al. Allogeneic bone marrow transplantation for therapy-related myelodysplastic syndrome and acute myeloid leukemia: a long-term study of 70 patients-report of the French society of bone marrow transplantation. J Clin Oncol 2000;18:963–71.
216. de Witte T, van Biezen A, Hermans J, et al. Autologous bone marrow transplantation for patients with myelodysplastic syndrome (MDS) or acute myeloid leukemia following MDS. Chronic and Acute Leukemia Working Parties of

the European Group for Blood and Marrow Transplantation. Blood 1997;90:3853–7.
217. Borgmann A, Schmid H, Hartmann R, et al. Autologous bone-marrow transplants compared with chemotherapy for children with acute lymphoblastic leukemia in a second remission: a matched-pair analysis. The Berlin-Frankfurt- Munster Study Group. Lancet 1995;346:873–6.
218. Barrett AJ, Horowitz MM, Gale RP, et al. Marrow transplantation for acute lymphoblastic leukemia: factors affecting relapse and survival. Blood 1989;74:862–71.
219. Horowitz MM, Messerer D, Hoelzer D, et al. Chemotherapy compared with bone marrow transplantation for adults with acute lymphoblastic leukemia in first remission. Ann Intern Med 1991;115:13–18.
220. Martin TG, Gajewski JL. Allogeneic stem cell transplantation for acute lymphocytic leukemia in adults. Hematol Oncol Clin North Am 2001;15:97–120.
221. Martin TG, Linker CA. Autologous stem cell transplantation for acute lymphocytic leukemia in adults. Hematol Oncol Clin North Am 2001;15:121–43.
222. Kantarjian HM, O'Brien S, Smith TL, et al. Results of treatment with hyper-CVAD, a dose-intensive regimen, in adult acute lymphocytic leukemia. J Clin Oncol 2000;18:547–61.
223. Zhang MJ, Hoelzer D, Horowitz MM, et al. Long-term follow- up of adults with acute lymphoblastic leukemia in first remission treated with chemotherapy or bone marrow transplantation. The Acute Lymphoblastic Leukemia Working Committee. Ann Intern Med 1995;123:428–31.
224. Forman SJ, Blume KG. Allogeneic bone marrow transplantation for acute leukemia. Hematol Oncol Clin North Am 1990;4:517–33.
225. Barrett AJ, Horowitz MM, Ash RC, et al. Bone marrow transplantation for Philadelphia chromosome-positive acute lymphoblastic leukemia. Blood 1992;79:3067–70.
226. Forman SJ, O'Donnell MR, Nademanee AP, et al. Bone marrow transplantation for patients with Philadelphia chromosome-positive acute lymphoblastic leukemia. Blood 1987;70:587–8.
227. Forman SJ, Schmidt GM, Nademanee AP, et al. Allogeneic bone marrow transplantation as therapy for primary induction failure for patients with acute leukemia. J Clin Oncol 1991;9:1570–4.
228. Kersey JH, Weisdorf D, Nesbit ME, et al. Comparison of autologous and allogeneic bone marrow transplantation for treatment of high-risk refractory acute lymphoblastic leukemia. N Engl J Med 1987;317:461–7.
229. Herzig RH, Bortin MM, Barrett AJ, et al. Bone-marrow transplantation in high-risk acute lymphoblastic leukemia in first and second remission. Lancet 1987;1:786–9.
230. Champlin R, Gale RP. Acute lymphoblastic leukemia: recent advances in biology and therapy. Blood 1989;73:2051–66.
231. Davies SM, Ramsay NK, Klein JP, et al. Comparison of preparative regimens in transplants for children with acute lymphoblastic leukemia. J Clin Oncol 2000;18:340–7.
232. Brenner MK. Autologous bone-marrow transplantation in childhood acute lymphoblastic leukemia. Lancet 1995;346:856–7238.
233. Doney K, Buckner CD, Fisher L, et al. Autologous bone marrow transplantation for acute lymphoblastic leukemia. Bone Marrow Transplant 1993;12:315–21.
234. Sallan SE, Niemeyer CM, Billett AL, et al. Autologous bone marrow transplantation for acute lymphoblastic leukemia. J Clin Oncol 1989;7:1594–1601.
235. Druker BJ, Tamura S, Buchdunger E, et al. Effects of a selective inhibitor of the Abl tyrosine kinase on the growth of Bcr-Abl positive cells. Nat Med 1996;2:561–6.
236. Druker BJ, Talpaz M, Resta DJ, et al. Efficacy and safety of a specific inhibitor of the BCR-ABL tyrosine kinase in chronic myeloid leukemia. N Engl J Med 2001;344:1031–7.
237. Goldman JM, Szydlo R, Horowitz MM, et al. Choice of pretransplant treatment and timing of transplants for chronic myelogenous leukemia in chronic phase. Blood 1993;82:2235–8.
238. Thomas ED, Clift RA. Indications for marrow transplantation in chronic myelogenous leukemia. Blood 1989;73:861–4.
239. Clift RA, Radich J, Appelbaum FR, et al. Long-term follow-up of a randomized study comparing cyclophosphamide and total body irradiation with busulfan and cyclophosphamide for patients receiving allogeneic marrow transplants during chronic phase of chronic myeloid leukemia. Blood 1999;94:3960–2.
240. Clift RA, Buckner CD, Appelbaum FR, et al. Allogeneic marrow transplantation in patients with chronic myeloid leukemia in the chronic phase: a randomized trial of two irradiation regimens. Blood 1991;77:1660–5.
241. Slattery JT, Clift RA, Buckner CD, et al. Marrow transplantation for chronic myeloid leukemia: the influence of plasma busulfan levels on the outcome of transplantation. Blood 1997;89:3055–60.
242. Andersson BS, Thall PF, Madden T, et al. Busulfan systemic exposure related toxicity and acute graft-versus host disease: defining a therapeutic window for i.v. BuCy2 in chronic myelogenous leukemia. Biol Blood Marrow Transplant 2002;8:477–85.
243. Radich JP, Gehly G, Gooley T, et al. Polymerase chain reaction detection of the BCR-ABL fusion transcript after allogeneic marrow transplantation for chronic myeloid leukemia: results and implications in 346 patients. Blood 1995;85:2632–8.
244. Dazzi F, Szydlo RM, Craddock C, et al. Comparison of single-dose and escalating-dose regimens of donor lymphocyte infusion for relapse after allografting for chronic myeloid leukemia. Blood 2000;95:67–71.
245. Van Rhee F, Lin F, Cullis JO, et al. Relapse of chronic myeloid leukemia after allogeneic bone marrow transplant: the case for giving donor leukocyte transfusions before the onset of hematologic relapse. Blood 1994;83:3377–83.
246. Anderson JE, Sale G, Appelbaum FR, et al. Allogeneic marrow transplantation for primary myelofibrosis and myelofibrosis secondary to polycythaemia vera or essential thrombocytosis. Br J Haematol 1997;98:1010–6.
247. Przepiorka D, Giralt S, Khouri I, et al. Allogeneic marrow transplantation for myeloproliferative disorders other than chronic myelogenous leukemia: review of forty cases. Am J Hematol 1998;57:24–8.
248. Guardiola P, Esperou H, Cazals-Hatem D, et al. Allogeneic bone marrow transplantation for agnogenic myeloid metaplasia. French Society of Bone Marrow Transplantation. Br J Haematol 1997;98:1004–9.
249. Barosi G. Myelofibrosis with myeloid metaplasia: diagnostic definition and prognostic classification for clinical studies and treatment guidelines. J Clin Oncol 1999;17:2954–70.
250. O'Brien S, Del Giglio A, Keating M. Advances in the biology and treatment of B-cell chronic lymphocytic leukemia. Blood 1995;85:307–18.
251. Foon KA, Rai KR, Gale RP. Chronic lymphocytic leukemia: new insights into biology and therapy. Ann Intern Med 1990;113:525–39.
252. Rai KR, Sawitsky A, Cronkite EP, et al. Clinical staging of chronic lymphocytic leukemia. Blood 1975;46:219–34.
253. Rai KR, Han T. Prognostic factors and clinical staging in chronic lymphocytic leukemia. Hematol Oncol Clin North Am 1990;4:447–56.
254. Damle RN, Wasil T, Fais F, et al. Ig V gene mutation status and CD38 expression as novel prognostic indicators in chronic lymphocytic leukemia. Blood 1999;94:1840–7.
255. Flinn IW, Byrd JC, Morrison C, et al. Fludarabine and cyclophosphamide with filgrastim support in patients with previously untreated indolent lymphoid malignancies. Blood 2000;96:71–75.
256. Keating MJ, O'Brien S, Albitar M. Emerging information on the use of rituximab in chronic lymphocytic leukemia. Seminars in Oncology 2002;29(1 Suppl 2):70–4.
257. Dreger P, von Neuhoff N, Kuse R, et al. Early stem cell transplantation for chronic lymphocytic leukemia: a chance for cure? Br J Cancer 1998;77:2291–7.
258. Khouri IF, Keating MJ, Vriesendorp HM, et al. Autologous and allogeneic bone marrow transplantation for chronic lymphocytic leukemia: preliminary results. J Clin Oncol 1994;12:748–58.
259. Provan D, Bartlett-Pandite L, Zwicky C, et al. Eradication of polymerase chain reaction-detectable chronic lymphocytic leukemia cells is associated with improved outcome after bone marrow transplantation. Blood 1996;88:2228–35.
260. Khouri I, Champlin R. Allogenic bone marrow transplantation in chronic lymphocytic leukemia. Ann Intern Med 1996;125:780.
261. Khouri IF, Przepiorka D, van Besien K, et al. Allogeneic blood or marrow transplantation for chronic lymphocytic leukemia: timing of transplantation and potential effect of fludarabine on acute graft-versus-host disease. Br J Haematol 1997;97:466–73.
262. Rabinowe SN, Soiffer RJ, Gribben JG, et al. Autologous and allogeneic bone marrow transplantation for poor prognosis patients with B-cell chronic lymphocytic leukemia. Blood 1993;82:1366–76.
263. Michallet M, Archimbaud E, Bandini G, et al. HLA-identical sibling bone marrow transplantation in younger patients with chronic lymphocytic leukemia. European Group for Blood and Marrow Transplantation and the International Bone Marrow Transplant Registry. Ann Intern Med 1996;124:311–5.
264. Rondon G, Giralt S, Huh Y, et al. Graft-versus-leukemia effect after allogeneic bone marrow transplantation for chronic lymphocytic leukemia. Bone Marrow Transplant 1996;18:669–72.
265. Harris NL, Jaffe ES, Stein H, et al. A revised European-American classification of lymphoid neoplasms: a proposal from the International Lymphoma Study Group. Blood 1994;84:1361–92.
266. Dierlamm J, Michaux L, Criel A, et al. Genetic abnormalities in chronic lymphocytic leukemia and their clinical and prognostic implications. Cancer Genet Cytogenet 1997;94:27–35.
267. Matutes E, Oscier D, Garcia-Marco J, et al. Trisomy 12 defines a group of CLL with atypical morphology: correlation between cytogenetic, clinical and laboratory features in 544 patients. Br J Haematol 1996;92:382–8.
268. Juliusson G, Oscier DG, Fitchett M, et al. Prognostic subgroups in B-cell chronic lymphocytic leukemia defined by specific chromosomal abnormalities. N Engl J Med 1990;323:720–4.
269. Horning SJ. Natural history of and therapy for the indolent non-Hodgkin's lymphomas. Semin Oncol 1993;20(5 Suppl 5):75–88.
270. Rohatiner AZ, Johnson PW, Price CG, et al. Myeloablative therapy with autologous bone marrow transplantation as consolidation therapy for recurrent follicular lymphoma. J Clin Oncol 1994;12:1177–84.
271. Negrin RS, Kusnierz-Glaz CR, Still BJ, et al. Transplantation of enriched and purged peripheral blood progenitor cells from a single aphaeresis product in patients with non-Hodgkin's lymphoma. Blood 1995;85:3334–41.
272. Johnson PW, Rohatiner AZ, Whelan JS, et al. Patterns of survival in patients with recurrent follicular lymphoma: a 20-year study from a single center. J Clin Oncol 1995;13:140–7.
273. Milligan DW, Ruiz de Elvira MC, et al. Secondary leukemia and myelodysplasia after autografting for lymphoma: results from the EBMT. EBMT Lymphoma and Late Effects Working Parties. European Group for Blood and Marrow Transplantation. Br J Haematol 1999;106:1020–6.
274. Krishnan A, Bhatia S, Slovak ML, et al. Predictors of therapy- related leukemia and myelodysplasia following autologous transplantation for lymphoma: an assessment of risk factors. Blood 2000;95:1588–93.
275. van Besien K, Thall P, Korbling M, et al. Allogeneic transplantation for recurrent or refractory non-Hodgkin's lymphoma with poor prognostic features after conditioning with thiotepa, busulfan, and cyclophosphamide: experience in 44 consecutive patients. Biol Blood Marrow Transplant 1997;3:150–6.
276. Freedman AS, Neuberg D, Gribben JG, et al. High-dose chemoradiotherapy and anti-B-cell monoclonal antibody purged autologous bone marrow transplantation in mantle- cell lymphoma: no evidence for long-term remission. J Clin Oncol 1998;16:13–18.
277. Khouri IF, Romaguera J, Kantarjian H, et al. Hyper-CVAD and high-dose methotrexate/cytarabine followed by stem-cell transplantation: an active regimen for aggressive mantle-cell lymphoma. J Clin Oncol 1998;16:3803–9.
278. Khouri IF, Lee MS, Romaguera J, et al. Allogeneic hematopoietic transplantation for mantle-cell lymphoma: molecular remissions and evidence of graft-versus-malignancy. Ann Oncol 1999;10:1293–9.
279. Adkins D, Brown R, Goodnough LT, et al. Treatment of resistant mantle cell lymphoma with allogeneic bone marrow transplantation. Bone Marrow Transplant 1998;21:97–9.
280. Corradini P, Ladetto M, Astolfi M, et al. Clinical and molecular remission after allogeneic blood cell transplantation in a patient with mantle-cell lymphoma. Br J Haematol 1996;94:376–8.
281. van Besien K, Tabocoff J, Rodriguez M, et al. High-dose chemotherapy with BEAC regimen and autologous bone marrow transplantation for intermediate grade and immunoblastic lymphoma: durable complete remissions, but a high rate of regimen-related toxicity. Bone Marrow Transplant 1995;15:549–55.
282. Bosly A, Coiffier B, Gisselbrecht C, et al. Bone marrow transplantation prolongs survival after relapse in aggressive-lymphoma patients treated with the LNH-84 regimen. J Clin Oncol 1992;10:1615–23.
283. Philip T, Guglielmi C, Hagenbeek A, et al. Autologous bone marrow transplantation as compared with salvage chemotherapy in relapses of chemotherapy-sensitive non-Hodgkin's lymphoma. N Engl J Med 1995;333:1540–5.
284. Philip T, Hartmann O, Biron P, et al. High-dose therapy and autologous bone marrow transplantation in partial remission after first-line induction therapy for diffuse non-Hodgkin's lymphoma. J Clin Oncol 1988;6:1118–24.

285. Martelli M, Vignetti M, Zinzani PL, et al. High-dose chemotherapy followed by autologous bone marrow transplantation versus dexamethasone, cisplatin, and cytarabine in aggressive non-Hodgkin's lymphoma with partial response to front-line chemotherapy: a prospective randomized Italian multi-center study. J Clin Oncol 1996;14:534–42.
286. Gianni AM, Bregni M, Siena S, F et al. High-dose chemotherapy and autologous bone marrow transplantation compared with MACOP-B in aggressive B-cell lymphoma. N Engl J Med 1997;336:1290–7.
287. Haioun C, Lepage E, Gisselbrecht C, et al. Benefit of autologous bone marrow transplantation over sequential chemotherapy in poor-risk aggressive non-Hodgkin's lymphoma: updated results of the prospective study LNH87-2. Groupe d'Etude des Lymphomes de l'Adulte. J Clin Oncol 1997;15:1131–7.
288. Verdonck LF, van Putten WL, Hagenbeek A, et al. Comparison of CHOP chemotherapy with autologous bone marrow transplantation for slowly responding patients with aggressive non-Hodgkin's lymphoma. N Engl J Med 1995;332:1045–51.
289. Chopra R, Goldstone AH, Pearce R, et al. Autologous versus allogeneic bone marrow transplantation for non-Hodgkin's lymphoma: a case-controlled analysis of the European Bone Marrow Transplant Group Registry data. J Clin Oncol 1992;10:1690–5.
290. Bierman PJ, Vose JM, Armitage JO. Autologous transplantation for Hodgkin's disease: coming of age? Blood 1994;83:1161–4.
291. Jagannath S, Armitage JO, Dicke KA, et al. Prognostic factors for response and survival after high-dose cyclophosphamide, carmustine, and etoposide with autologous bone marrow transplantation for relapsed Hodgkin's disease. J Clin Oncol 1989;7:179–85.
292. Lazarus HM, Rowlings PA, Zhang MJ, et al. Autotransplants for Hodgkin's disease in patients never achieving remission: a report from the Autologous Blood and Marrow Transplant Registry. J Clin Oncol 1999;17:534–45.
293. Gajewski JL, Phillips GL, Sobocinski KA, et al. Bone marrow transplants from HLA-identical siblings in advanced Hodgkin's disease. J Clin Oncol 1996;14:572–8.
294. Carella AM, Cavaliere M, Lerma E, et al. Autografting followed by nonmyeloablative immunosuppressive chemotherapy and allogeneic peripheral-blood hematopoietic stem-cell transplantation as treatment of resistant Hodgkin's disease and non-Hodgkin's lymphoma. J Clin Oncol 2000;18:3918–24.
295. Anderlini P, Giralt S, Andersson B, et al. Allogeneic stem cell transplantation with fludarabine-based, less intensive conditioning regimens as adoptive immunotherapy in advanced Hodgkin's disease. Bone Marrow Transplant 2000;26:615–20.
296. Gore ME, Selby PJ, Viner C, et al. Intensive treatment of multiple myeloma and criteria for complete remission. Lancet 1989;2:879–82.
297. Attal M, Harousseau JL, Stoppa AM, et al. A prospective, randomized trial of autologous bone marrow transplantation and chemotherapy in multiple myeloma. Intergroupe Francais du Myelome. N Engl J Med 1996;335:91–7.
298. Alexanian R, Dimopoulos MA, Delasalle KB, et al. Myeloablative therapy for primary resistant multiple myeloma. Stem Cells 1995;13 Suppl 2:118–21.
299. Alexanian R, Dimopoulos MA, Hester J, et al. Early myeloablative therapy for multiple myeloma. Blood 1994;84:4278–82.
300. Alexanian R, Dimopoulos M, Smith T, et al. Limited value of myeloablative therapy for late multiple myeloma. Blood 1994;83:512–6.
301. Tricot G, Sawyer JR, Jagannath S, et al. Unique role of cytogenetics in the prognosis of patients with myeloma receiving high-dose therapy and autotransplants. J Clin Oncol 1997;15:2659–66.
302. Jagannath S, Barlogie B, Dicke K, et al. Autologous bone marrow transplantation in multiple myeloma: identification of prognostic factors. Blood 1990;76:1860–6.
303. Fermand JP, Ravaud P, Chevret S, et al. High-dose therapy and autologous peripheral blood stem cell transplantation in multiple myeloma: up-front or rescue treatment? Results of a multi-center sequential randomized clinical trial. Blood 1998;92:3131–6.
304. Kwak LW, Thielemans K, Massaia M. Idiotypic vaccination as therapy for multiple myeloma. Semin Hematol 1999;36(1 Suppl 3):34–7.
305. Gahrton G, Bjorkstrand B. Progress in hematopoietic stem cell transplantation for multiple myeloma. J Intern Med 2000;248:185–201.
306. Tricot G, Vesole DH, Jagannath S, et al. Graft-versus-myeloma effect: proof of principle. Blood 1996;87:1196–8.
307. Verdonck LF, Lokhorst HM, Dekker AW, et al. Graft-versus myeloma effect in two cases. Lancet 1996;347:800–1.
308. Bjorkstrand BB, Ljungman P, Svensson H, et al. Allogeneic bone marrow transplantation versus autologous stem cell transplantation in multiple myeloma: a retrospective case-matched study from the European Group for Blood and Marrow Transplantation. Blood 1996;88:4711–8.
309. Gahrton G, Svensson H, Bjorkstrand B, et al. Syngeneic transplantation in multiple myeloma—a case-matched comparison with autologous and allogeneic transplantation. European Group for Blood and Marrow Transplantation. Bone Marrow Transplant 1999;24:741–5.
310. Gertz MA, Lacy MQ, Dispenzieri A. Myeloablative chemotherapy with stem cell rescue for the treatment of primary systemic amyloidosis: a status report. Bone Marrow Transplant 2000;25:465–70.
311. Khouri I, Giralt S, Champlin R. Non-myeloablative allogeneic hematopoietic transplantation and induction of graft-versus-malignancy. Cancer Treat Res 2002;110:137–47.
312. Antman K, Ayash L, Elias A, et al. A phase II study of high-dose cyclophosphamide, thiotepa, and carboplatin with autologous marrow support in women with measurable advanced breast cancer responding to standard-dose therapy. J Clin Oncol 1992;10:102–10.
313. Stemmer SM, Cagnoni PJ, Shpall EJ, et al. High-dose paclitaxel, cyclophosphamide, and cisplatin with autologous hematopoietic progenitor-cell support: a phase I trial. J Clin Oncol 1996;14:1463–72.
314. Antman KH, Rowlings PA, Vaughan WP, et al. High-dose chemotherapy with autologous hematopoietic stem-cell support for breast cancer in North America. J Clin Oncol 1997;15:1870–9.
315. Rahman ZU, Frye DK, Buzdar AU, et al. Impact of selection process on response rate and long-term survival of potential high-dose chemotherapy candidates treated with standard-dose doxorubicin-containing chemotherapy in patients with metastatic breast cancer. J Clin Oncol 1997;15:3171–7.
316. Stadtmauer EA, O'Neill A, Goldstein LJ, et al. Conventional-dose chemotherapy compared with high-dose chemotherapy plus autologous hematopoietic stem-cell transplantation for metastatic breast cancer. Philadelphia Bone Marrow Transplant Group. N Engl J Med 2000;342:1069–76.
317. Antman KH, Heitjan DF, Hortobagyi GN. High-dose chemotherapy for breast cancer. JAMA 1999;282:1701–3.
318. Baynes RD, Dansey RD, Klein JL, et al. High-dose chemotherapy and hematopoietic stem cell transplantation for breast cancer: past or future? Semin Oncol 2001;28:377–88.
319. Legros M, Dauplat J, Fleury J, et al. High-dose chemotherapy with hematopoietic rescue in patients with stage III to IV ovarian cancer: long-term results. J Clin Oncol 1997;15:1302–8.
320. Stiff PJ, Bayer R, Kerger C, et al. High-dose chemotherapy with autologous transplantation for persistent/relapsed ovarian cancer: a multivariate analysis of survival for 100 consecutively treated patients. J Clin Oncol 1997;15:1309–17.
321. Donato ML, Gershenson DM, Wharton JT, et al. High-dose topotecan, melphalan, and cyclophosphamide (TMC) with stem cell support: a new regimen for the treatment of advanced ovarian cancer. Gynecol Oncol 2001;82:420–6.
322. Nichols CR, Rosti G. Dose-intensive therapy for germ cell neoplasms. Semin Oncol 1992;19(1 Suppl 2):145–9.
323. Elias A. Hematopoietic stem cell transplantation for small cell lung cancer. Chest 1999;116(6 Suppl):531–8s.
324. Matthay KK, O'Leary MC, Ramsay NK, Villablanca J, Reynolds CP, Atkinson JB et al. Role of myeloablative therapy in improved outcome for high risk neuroblastoma: review of recent Children's Cancer Group results. Eur J Cancer 1995;31A:572–5.
325. Shuster JJ, Cantor AB, McWilliams N, et al. The prognostic significance of autologous bone marrow transplant in advanced neuroblastoma. J Clin Oncol 1991;9:1045–9.
326. Childs RW, Clave E, Tisdale J, et al. Successful treatment of metastatic renal cell carcinoma with a nonmyeloablative allogeneic peripheral-blood progenitor-cell transplant: evidence for a graft-versus-tumor effect. J Clin Oncol 1999;17:2044–9.
327. Bacigalupo A, Bruno B, Saracco P, et al. Antilymphocyte globulin, cyclosporine, prednisolone, and granulocyte colony-stimulating factor for severe aplastic anemia: an update of the GITMO/EBMT study on 100 patients. European Group for Blood and Marrow Transplantation (EBMT) Working Party on Severe Aplastic Anemia and the Gruppo Italiano Trapianti di Midolio Osseo (GITMO). Blood 2000;95:1931–4.
328. Champlin RE, Horowitz MM, van Bekkum DW, et al. Graft failure following bone marrow transplantation for severe aplastic anemia: risk factors and treatment results. Blood 1989;73:606–13.
329. Storb R, Etzioni R, Anasetti C, et al. Cyclophosphamide combined with antithymocyte globulin in preparation for allogeneic marrow transplants in patients with aplastic anemia. Blood 1994;84:941–9.
330. Anasetti C, Storb R, Longton G, et al. Donor buffy coat cell infusion after marrow transplantation for aplastic anemia. Blood 1988;72:1099–1100.
331. Deeg HJ, Anasetti C, Petersdorf E, et al. Cyclophosphamide plus ATG conditioning is insufficient for sustained hematopoietic reconstitution in patients with severe aplastic anemia transplanted with marrow from HLA-A, B, DRB matched unrelated donors. Blood 1994;83:3417–8.
332. Hows J, Szydlo R, Anasetti C, et al. Unrelated donor marrow transplants for severe acquired aplastic anemia. Bone Marrow Transplant 1992;10 Suppl 1:102–6.
333. Davies SM, Wagner JE, DeFor T, et al. Unrelated donor bone marrow transplantation for children and adolescents with aplastic anemia or myelodysplasia. Br J Haematol 1997;96:749–56.
334. Saso R, Marsh J, Cevreska L, et al. Bone marrow transplants for paroxysmal nocturnal haemoglobinuria. Br J Haematol 1999;104:392–6.
335. Lucarelli G, Galimberti M, Polchi P, et al. Bone marrow transplantation in patients with thalassemia. N Engl J Med 1990;322:417–21.
336. Walters MC, Storb R, Patience M, et al. Impact of bone marrow transplantation for symptomatic sickle cell disease: an interim report. Multi-center investigation of bone marrow transplantation for sickle cell disease. Blood 2000;95:1918–24.
337. Flowers ME, Zanis J, Pasquini R, et al. Marrow transplantation for Fanconi anemia: conditioning with reduced doses of cyclophosphamide without radiation. Br J Haematol 1996;92:699–706.
338. Socie G, Gluckman E, Raynal B, et al. Bone marrow transplantation for Fanconi anemia using low-dose cyclophosphamide/ thoraco abdominal irradiation as conditioning regimen: chimerism study by the polymerase chain reaction. Blood 1993;82:2249–56.
339. Fischer A, Haddad E, Jabado N, et al. Stem cell transplantation for immunodeficiency. Springer Semin Immunopathol 1998;19:479–92.
340. Gerritsen EJ, Vossen JM, Fasth A, et al. Bone marrow transplantation for autosomal recessive osteoporosis. A report from the Working Party on Inborn Errors of the European Bone Marrow Transplantation Group. J Pediatr 1994;125:896–902.
341. Krivit W, Lockman LA, Watkins PA, et al. The future for treatment by bone marrow transplantation for adrenoleukodystrophy, met achromatic leukodystrophy, globoid cell leukodystrophy and Hurler syndrome. J Inherit Metab Dis 1995;18:398–412.
342. Filipovich AH, Shapiro RS, Ramsay NK, et al. Unrelated donor bone marrow transplantation for correction of lethal congenital immunodeficiencies. Blood 1992;80:270–6.
343. Flake AW, Roncarolo MG, Puck JM, et al. Treatment of X-linked severe combined immunodeficiency by in utero transplantation of paternal bone marrow. N Engl J Med 1996;335:1806–10.
344. Kohn DB, Hershfield MS, Carbonaro D, et al. T lymphocytes with a normal ADA gene accumulate after transplantation of transduced autologous umbilical cord blood CD34+ cells in ADA-deficient SCID neonates. Nat Med 1998;4:775–80.
345. van Bekkum DW. Autologous stem cell therapy for treatment of severe inflammatory autoimmune diseases. Neth J Med 1998;53:130–3.

Part V

Principles of Multidisciplinary Management

Section 17
PSYCHO-ONCOLOGY

59

Principles of Psycho-Oncology

Jimmie C. Holland, MD
Alexandra Sacks, BA

"We are not ourselves when nature, being oppressed, commands the mind to suffer with the body."
—King Lear, Act II, Sc.IV

Quality of life (QOL), or patient reported outcomes (PROs), has received increasing attention in recent years. More concern has also been directed toward recognizing and treating the distressed patient or family member. Stresses on oncologists have also been identified, particularly the effect of dealing daily with serious illness and death. Research is more actively exploring social, behavioral, and psychological contributions to cancer prevention, early detection, and survival. Psycho-oncology, which has emerged slowly since 1975 as a subspecialty of oncology, focuses on these psychosocial issues along the continuum from prevention to cure, at all stages of disease. A body of information is now available, training programs exist, a research agenda has been formulated, and clinical practice guidelines based on evidence from research have been developed.[1,2]

Psycho-oncology addresses the two psychological dimensions of cancer: first, the psychological response to cancer of patients, at all stages of disease, their families, and the medical team. This aspect, so vitally dependent on communication, affects the care of all patients, at all visits, with all sites and stages of cancer and all treatments. The second dimension addresses psychological, behavioral, and social factors that influence cancer risk, detection, and survival. Clinicians and clinical investigators, from psychology, psychiatry, social work, nursing, and clergy, make up members of the psychosocial teams that exist in many cancer centers and hospitals. These teams provide consultation, teach psychosocial issues to oncology staff, raise awareness of this dimension of care, and collaborate in studies in which quality of life is important. Active research in brain, immune, and endocrine links is occurring, particularly around the role of cytokines in producing "sickness behavior" that may provide a biologic basis for common symptoms of fatigue, depression, anxiety, weakness, and cognitive changes.[3,4]

Most cancer centers and oncology divisions now have a psycho-oncology or psychosocial unit whose role is to treat distressed patients and family members, and to serve as a psychosocial teaching resource for oncology staff. Only a few centers have programs that include research and training. Trained volunteers, particularly those who have experienced cancer personally or in their families, play an increasingly important role as well. Links between advocacy organizations, such as the National Coalition for Cancer Survivors (NCCS), are collaborating with the American Psychosocial Oncology Society (APOS), the only multidisciplinary national organization representing this subspecialty of oncology, to address health policy barriers to care (Web site: www.apos.org).

This chapter describes the development of psycho-oncology, psychiatric disorders, the common psychosocial problems, the range of interventions available, and the research directions to improve the science and practice of psycho-oncology.[5]

HISTORICAL PERSPECTIVE

The stigma that cancer equals death, which has been attached to the disease for centuries, led to the long respected dictum that doctors should not tell patients that they had cancer. To do so was considered cruel, and would take away patients' hope (Table 59-1). For centuries there was indeed no treatment, and both doctors and patients had a fatalistic attitude as they awaited the inevitable outcome. The advent of anesthesia and antisepsis led

Table 59-1 Historical Attitudes About Cancer and Development of Psycho-Oncology

1800s	Prevailing attitude was cancer equals death Fatalistic acceptance of diagnosis Diagnosis never revealed to patient
1900–20	American Cancer Society formed to fight fatalism and educate public that early treatment by surgery could be curative
1937	National Cancer Institute formed to seek a cure for cancer
1950s	First studies of psychological response to cancer reported
1960s	Combined modalities lead to increased survival in Hodgkin's disease, ALL and childhood tumors
1960-70	Debate about telling or not telling diagnosis and change to revealing the diagnosis; federally mandated guidelines for informed consent
1980	Prevalence studies of psychiatric and psychological sequelae in cancer Psycho-oncology units develop in larger cancer centers Education of public about lifestyle and cancer prevention; behavioral research in changing habits (eg, smoking), diet and lifestyle
1990	Health-related Quality of Life assessment was accepted as an outcome measure in clinical trials Intervention studies undertaken to impact quality of life and reduce distress
2000	Standards for psychosocial care developed and clinical practice treatment guidelines for management of common types of psychiatric disorders and psychosocial forms of distress. Exploration of genetic factors in vulnerability to development of fatigue; cognitive dysfunction with chemotherapy; biologic contribution of proinflammatory cytokines to symptoms of fatigue, depression, and cognitive problems.

to possible surgical removal of some tumors. Near the end of the nineteenth century, and early in the twentieth century, it became important to counter the public's fatalistic attitudes because surgical cure was possible, but only if the cancer was detected in an early stage. The American Cancer Society was formed in 1913 to teach the warning symptoms of cancer to the public and to reduce their immobilizing fears. As radiation and surgery were combined to treat cancer, more cures were affected. The establishment of the National Cancer Institute in 1937 reflected new enthusiasm for seeking a cause and cure of cancer. The addition of chemotherapy to the combined modalities resulted in the cure of several childhood tumors. This led to an increase in interest in medical outcomes of long-term survivors of cancer and provided the first opportunity for exploring patients' psychological responses to cancer.

By the early 1970s, as survival improved and patients became more willing to reveal they had been treated for cancer, the diagnosis of cancer began to be more frequently revealed to patients. At about the same time, concern for more humane care of patients at the end of life was seen, with the development of the hospice movement and greater interest in pain management and palliative care. Greater openness in revealing the diagnosis, increased concern for the dying, and enhanced concern about QOL and the rights of patients led to more attention for the supportive and psychological aspects of care. Evidence for the link of environmental exposures to cancer, particularly cigarette smoking, gave new impetus to examine the role of psychological and behavioral factors in cancer prevention.

Around this same period, psychosomatic medicine developed within the field of psychiatry, leading to a powerful movement that sought to identify psychological factors as the major cause of several chronic diseases, particularly asthma, peptic ulcer, rheumatoid arthritis, and cancer. None of these suppositions has proved true. Patients with cancer often feared that they had "caused their own cancer." Beliefs such as this have led to societal attitudes of "blaming the victim" that have made coping with cancer even harder. Patients are often reluctant to ask for counseling because they fear the stigma of mental illness.

By 1980, the stage was set to increase the study of psychological problems of patients with cancer. However, valid tools to assess these variables were few. Early investigators were forced to develop new instruments or modify those originally developed to assess patients with major psychiatric disorders. Investigators with knowledge of research methods in both cancer and social science were few. Nevertheless, a small group of investigators largely associated with cancer centers around the world, primarily in the United States, the United Kingdom, and Sweden, began to identify themselves as psycho-oncologists and they began to study prevalence of psychiatric comorbidity in cancer, and to address key psychosocial questions. The field continued to grow as some groups developed training programs that began to train young clinicians and investigators. This brief history underscores the relative youth of psycho-oncology that began in the mid 1970s. It also points out the degree to which historical attitudes toward cancer have contributed to the reluctance of patients to identify their emotional problems to their oncologists, even today.

COMMON PSYCHOLOGICAL RESPONSES

Reactions to Diagnosis of Cancer

Patients often respond with anxiety and dread when they recognize that tests are being done to rule out cancer. If the doctor delivers the news that the diagnosis *is* cancer, an existential crisis occurs which requires an individual to call upon all inner psychological resources to cope. The common concerns can be remembered as 4 Ds: Death (with pain), Disability, Dependence on others, and Disfigurement (physical changes in body). How the doctor delivers the bad news is a factor in the patient's response. Insensitivity in giving bad news is often recalled years later. The importance of good communication skills is a critical aspect of quality cancer care.[6] Research has given rise to practice guidelines in how to present the information, how to be sensitive to the patient's response, and the importance of presenting a treatment plan in conjunction with the bad news.[7–11]

Most people in our society do not think very often about death, but the first thought on learning a cancer diagnosis frequently is "I could die of this." This creates both a psychological and an existential crisis. The person seeks to cope with the challenge and maintain emotional control. This is often done by trying to put the information in a context that yields a tolerable meaning.[12–14] Park and Folkman (1997) described how stressful information is processed cognitively by individuals, first by confronting the situation and changing it if possible; however, finding it can't be changed, individuals search for a tolerable understanding that reconciles their life values and goals with their new situation.[12] For many, searching for meaning may result in exploring prior religious and spiritual beliefs that give a context in which the threat to life and the possibility of death can be understood.[15]

The diagnosis creates a period of expected crisis and normal emotional upheaval (Table 59-2).[1] The initial phase is often characterized by disbelief and denial that the news is true. For example, the assumption may be: "They must have mixed up the slides." High anxiety levels make it hard to process information, at the very time that critical treatment decisions must be made. Feeling "numb" and being unable to concentrate may require that information must be repeated several times.

Phase II of response to the diagnosis is usually characterized by emotional turmoil and dysphoria during which the reality is slowly acknowledged. The person is anxious and depressed, has a short attention span, anorexia and insomnia, and inability to maintain daily activities. Thoughts of illness and death intrude repeatedly and cannot be dispelled. This period may last 1 to 2 weeks, ordinarily diminishing as the person begins treatment that leads to a sense of regaining control. A therapeutic alliance with the doctor and a treatment plan makes the future seem more hopeful.

Phase III represents the longer-term adaptation to illness, lasting from weeks to months, in which the patient adjusts to the diagnosis and treatment, finds reason for optimism, and returns to normal routines and ways of coping that were characteristic and successful in the past. The quality of adaptation depends on the patient's prior level of adjustment and emotional maturity. It is important that family, friends, and staff be aware that there is no single best way to cope. Individuals have developed their own coping styles that, for better or worse, have gotten them through prior life crises. There is a strong tendency in parts of today's society to demand that individuals with cancer have a positive attitude to beat it. Such patients are made to feel guilty if they do not cope in this way, and they often are told that the absence of a positive attitude leads to worse outcomes. Although a "positive thinking" strategy works well for some individuals, it does not for others. The doctor's understanding of and respect for each individual's way of coping is critically important.[16,17] This sequence of disbelief, turmoil, and adaptation reappears with each new crisis in the course of illness. Depression becomes more prominent at time of progression or treatment failure.

FACTORS IN ADAPTATION TO CANCER

It is important to recognize psychological and social factors that predict good or poor adjustment, enabling early identification of vulnerable individuals. Factors that contribute to adaptation derive from three areas: (1) society-derived,

Table 59-2 Normal Responses to Crises Encountered with Cancer

Phase	Symptoms	Time Interval
Phase I: Initial Response	Disbelief or denial or despair ("I knew it all along")	Usually less than 1 week
Phase II: Dysphoria	Anxiety, depressed mood, anorexia, insomnia, poor concentration, inability to function	Usually 1 to 2 weeks, but varies
Phase III: Adaptation	Accepts validity of information and begins dealing with options available Finds reasons for optimism and resumes usual activities	Usually by 2 weeks, but adaptation continues over months; may or may not be successful

Table 59-3 Factors That Determine Psychological Adjustment to Cancer

Society-derived
- Open discussion of diagnosis vs. unrevealed secret
- Knowledge of treatment options, prognosis, and participation as partner in treatment
- Popular beliefs (stress causes cancer)

Patient-derived
- Intrapersonal
  - Developmental stage at time of cancer and meaning of curtailed goals (eg, marriage, children)
  - Coping ability; emotional maturity at time of cancer; philosophic, spiritual, or religious beliefs that influence coping
- Interpersonal
  - Spouse, family, friends (social support)
  - Socioeconomic/social class

Cancer-derived
- Site, stage, symptoms (especially pain) and prognosis
- Treatment required (surgery, radiation, chemotherapy) and sequelae (immediate and delayed)
- Altered body structure or function, rehabilitation/restoration available
- Psychological management by the treating staff

Table 59-4 Developmental Stages and Cancer

Stage	Tasks	Disruption	Intervention
Children			
Childhood (early)	Motor	Developmental slowing	Physical/social stimulation
	Speech	Regression	Structured play
	Cognition	Separation anxiety	Increasing family contact
	Family bonding	Withdrawal	Continuity of staff
	Socialization	Increasing fears (pain)	Trust of staff
	Confidence	Being "different"	Maintain appearance
Childhood (late)	Prepubertal	School phobia	Minimize absences
	Peer relations	Death fears	Discuss illness and monitor responses
	Intellectual and physical prowess		
Adolescents and Adults			
Adolescence	Menarche/puberty	Alopecia/amputation	Maintain appearance
	Peer acceptance	"Differentness"	Maintain peer contact
		Decreasing school/physical performance	
	Increasing independence	Increasing dependence	Support independence
	Sexual experimentation	Conflicts about self and sexuality	Counseling
	Formation of identity	Impact of illness	Counseling
	Intimacy	Decreasing attractiveness	Maintain appearance
	Marriage	Sterility/impotence	Sex counseling
	Parental role	Decreasing family role	Homemaker
			Support children
	Work role	Disruption of job performance	Decreasing job interruptions
Adult (middle)	Changing hormonal status/menopause	Altered appearance	Maintain appearance
	Older children	Disrupted marital/family role	Counseling (patient and family)
	"Empty nest"		
	Peak of career	Disrupted achievements	Financial planning
Adult (old)	Aging changes	Increasing physical/emotional losses	Health-related
	Physical limitations	Services to maintain	Care of self
	Adjustment to increasing losses	Increasing dependence on others	Social support system
	Increasing social support needed	Increasing isolation	Promote social/familial network
	Retirement	Decreasing financial security	Financial planning

which are the social attitudes and beliefs about cancer that affect the patient; (2) patient-derived, which are the individual attributes the person brings to illness; and, (3) cancer-derived, which represent the clinical reality of the illness to which the patient must adapt (Table 59-3).

Society-Derived Factors The society-derived factors are constantly changing since they reflect society's attitudes toward cancer and its treatment, as well as perceptions and knowledge of cancer at a given time. Long feared and stigmatized, cancer is somewhat less frightening today. The diagnosis is routinely given in the United States, and the public is better informed about the treatments; they are justifiably more optimistic about outcome. Coupled with current standards of informed consent and legal mandates for patients' knowledge of treatment options, better communication between doctor and patient has been a positive spin-off. This has resulted, however, in an added burden for the patient because of the fuller knowledge of the realistic expectation associated with each treatment option. In addition, patients who have finished cancer treatment are followed far more carefully today with frequent scans and markers to detect recurrent cancer. Follow-up visits and scans are preceded by a period of increased anxiety and fears. Thus, uncertainty about the future is far greater today then in the past when reassurance was firmly given.

An additional burden is the widely popularized belief that stress causes cancer. Some patients mistakenly feel that grief, depression, a stressful event, or their personalities caused their cancer. Repeated reassurance that this is not true is necessary. Johansen's group in Denmark, using the Danish national cancer registry, has unambiguously shown that depression, personality, and grief do not increase risk of cancer.[18,19]

Patient-Derived Factors The patient-derived factors that affect adaptation come from three sources: the intrapersonal (developmental stage and coping ability); interpersonal (the social support from others); and socioeconomic and social class (the material resources available).

The developmental stage of the person at the time that cancer is diagnosed determines in part the meaning of an illness or treatment-related loss. Jeopardy to fertility or altered appearance, such as hair loss for example, may affect patients differently, depending upon the time of life when the event occurs. An awareness of the individual's developmental stage and the biologic, psychological, and social tasks that usually pertain to it help to understand the impact of cancer and to derive interventions for each age. Table 59-4 outlines the developmental stages, the normal tasks that must be achieved at each age, the disruption in achieving expected life goals, and the interventions to minimize the deleterious effects of illness.[20] It is particularly important in treating childhood and adolescent cancer to assure that, as nearly as possible, normal developmental milestones are reached and maintained.[21]

The strategies that patients use to cope with cancer must accomplish several goals: (1) to keep distress within manageable levels; (2) to maintain a sense of personal worth; (3) to restore or maintain relations with significant others; (4) to enhance recovery and physical function; and (5) to work out a socially acceptable post-illness status with maximal physical function.[13] Taken overall, good coping strategies are important in maintaining a sense of control, optimism, humor, and acceptance of the facts, whereas seeking constructive positive approaches to illness and treatment. Spiritual beliefs and religion provide a view of life, death, and illness for some; a community of like-minded individuals who share their views may also help in coping.[15]

In terms of prior experience, individuals at greater risk of distress are those who have had a prior psychiatric problem; those who have experienced death of a family member to cancer, particularly if it is from the same type of cancer; and, those who have had an extreme trauma earlier in life (eg, Holocaust survivors or survivors of physical abuse).[22] A recurrence of post-traumatic stress disorder (PTSD) symptoms may develop which complicate coping with cancer. Table 59-5 outlines the major predictors of poor coping.[21] The use of rapid short or single item screens to identify these vulnerable individuals are increasingly being validated and used in clinical settings.[23,24]

The patient's social environment provides the important interpersonal resources of a spouse or

Table 59-5 Predictors of Poor Coping with Cancer

Social isolation
Low socioeconomic status
Alcohol or drug abuse
Prior psychiatric history
Prior experience with cancer (eg, death of a relative)
Recent losses/bereavement
Inflexibility and rigidity of coping
Pessimistic philosophy of life
Absence of a belief/value system, from which to view life and death
Multiple obligations

Adapted from Holland and Rowland.[21]

partner, family, and friends. Increasing evidence suggests the central role that social support plays in both coping and survival. Isolated individuals have more trouble coping with illness, and have a higher age-matched mortality.[25–27]

A third patient-derived factor is that of socioeconomic resources and social class. Increasing evidence points to the effect on both morbidity and mortality; not only by limited access to appropriate care but also because of poorer education and fewer resources that affect cancer treatment availability and outcome.[28,29] Research points to a social class gradient across the five social classes, based on education and income, in which higher mortality correlates with lower social class.[30]

Cancer-Derived Factors The cancer-derived factors that contribute to adaptation are the clinical facts themselves of stage of disease at diagnosis; site; presence of symptoms (especially pain); prognosis; the type(s) of treatment required and their immediate and long-term impact on function; and, the extent of rehabilitation that is possible. These are the "givens," along with the psychological management by the oncology team. The sensitive oncologist and nurse are key sources of psychological support for the patient and family. Concern, compassion, and "caring" in the context of professional ministrations are invaluable aids to the patient's ability to cope with illness.[31]

PSYCHOLOGICAL ISSUES BY STAGE OF DISEASE

Psychological issues change in relation to stage of disease. They can be considered in four broad categories: (1) patients receiving active treatment with cure as a goal; (2) patients receiving palliative care, with the treatment of cancer aimed at long-term control or short-term comfort; (3) problems of patients who have completed active treatment and who are survivors; and (4) asymptomatic, healthy individuals who have a known enhanced genetic risk of cancer by family history, genetic testing, or by positive tumor markers.

Adaptation to Active Treatment In patients undergoing treatment aimed at cure, the goal of psychosocial intervention is to support the ability to cope with the demands of treatment and side effects, to reduce distress, and to assist in symptom management (eg, anxiety, pain, nausea and vomiting).[32–37] Some sites of cancer, particularly pancreatic, are associated with greater physical symptoms and depression, bringing into question whether proinflammatory cytokines may be a factor.[3,4,38]

Oncologists often underestimate levels of anxiety and depression.[31] Hospitalized patients have higher frequency of both psychosocial problems and psychiatric disorders due to level of illness.[39,40] Ambulatory patients who have been screened in the waiting room for level of distress show that from a quarter to almost half (depending on tumor type and prognosis) have significant distress (mixed anxiety and depressive symptoms) and should be referred to a mental health professional.[23,24,41,42]

The goal of cure encourages most individuals to tolerate the temporary discomfort and side effects of surgery, chemotherapy, and radiation, and to adapt to the permanent physical changes that are necessary to achieve a cure.[43] Control of anxiety, depression, delirium, pain, nausea, and vomiting helps patients to adhere to treatment. McQuellon and colleagues have used an orientation program for new patients that gave them added information about what to expect. Anxiety and depression symptoms were reduced as compared to the usual care group.[44] Counseling, support groups, cognitive-behavioral interventions, and psychopharmacologic agents all are useful to control distress. The status of psychosocial interventions has been reviewed in an Institute of Medicine monograph.[45]

Adaptation to Palliative Care The transition from a curative approach to a palliative one is extremely difficult for the patient, family, and the oncologist who has often worked with the patient through months of arduous treatment. The combination of physical symptoms, psychological distress, and the existential crisis constitutes the "suffering" associated with advanced cancer.[46] Patients have a period of high distress on learning that the goal has shifted from cure to control of their cancer; however, they adapt remarkably well to the altered goal. Today, the perception that recurrent cancer can be a chronic disease, particularly in those living with advanced prostate and breast cancer, helps to maintain hope for control if not a cure. This phase may last for years. It is only when treatments and investigational therapies begin to fail that end of life issues more clearly emerge.

Assurance of the physician's commitment to continued care and symptom control becomes more important. Appointing a health proxy and discussion of wishes about resuscitation and life-sustaining measures are best discussed early rather than late. Decisions about where continuing care will be given must be discussed, as well as assessing whether end-of-life care can be managed at home. When it is possible, both patient and family benefit psychologically from these conversations.[47–49] Considerable information exists today about symptom control in advanced stages of illness, with better control of pain, anorexia, nausea, constipation, dyspnea, weakness, cachexia, and suffering (distress).[50–53] Portenoy and colleagues studied prevalence of symptoms in patients with advanced cancer and found fatigue, weakness, pain, and emotional distress present in over two-thirds of patients.[43] Palliative care in children is also better defined.[54]

There are growing numbers of controlled trials of medication, behavioral, and psychological interventions, including clinical practice guidelines in their use at end of life, to treat the psychosocial and psychiatric disorders which are common in advanced stages of illness: anxiety, depression, and confusion (delirium).[48,50,55,56] Psychotherapeutic approaches have been devised for patients facing the existential crisis of the end of life. Chochinov has described "dignity-conserving" psychotherapy to help the person feel valued and esteemed: "It targets maintenance of dignity as a therapeutic objective and as a principle of bedside care for patients nearing death."[57] Breitbart and colleagues have developed a "meaning-centered" therapy, based on the principles of logotherapy developed by Viktor Frankl.[58] Other studies have identified the role of the psychiatrist in managing psychiatric disorders associated with terminal cancer, particularly depression.[46,59,60] Requests for physician-assisted suicide require careful consideration in the context of control of the physical, psychological, and spiritual aspects.[60–63] Concern for family, especially the caregiver and children must be a part of palliative care. Rauch and Muriel have described a clinical consultation for parents during treatment to guide them in talking with their children. Table 59-6 shows what children can understand at different ages and Table 59-7 provides ways the oncologist can advise and facilitate children's coping when a parent has cancer.[64,65]

Adaptation to Being a Survivor Common concerns of survivors are fears of recurrence, worry about delayed physical effects, risk of second cancers, and sterility (Table 59-8 outlines the psychosocial sequelae).[66] Cancer survivors are important advocates for improving cancer care, representing the nine million United States survivors. Patient advocates are now members of committees in the National Cancer Institute's policy bodies and cooperative groups. An Institute of Medicine monograph on childhood survivors presents the current status of our knowledge; a similar report on adult survivors is in preparation.[67]

Cognitive deficits occur with radiation to the brain and with several types of chemotherapy in adults and in children. Recent reviews by Ahles and others suggest that even adjuvant chemotherapy for breast cancer produces subtle cognitive deficits that are apparent months and even years after treatment.[68,69] These cognitive changes, long identified by patients as "chemo-brain," are the subject of greater investigation currently. Ahles has proposed, from preliminary data, that the presence of the APOE4 allele, known to be associated with Alzheimer's, may predispose

Table 59-6 Child Development and Experience of a Parent's Illness

Infancy (0–2 years)
- Does not understand the meaning of illness
- Experiences parental absence, distracted mood of caretakers, and changes in environment and schedule

Preschool age (3–6 years)
- Combination of egocentric perspective and associative, idiosyncratic logic leads the child to believe s/he caused the cancer or can get the cancer
- Misplaced feelings of blame/guilt can lead to behavioral outbursts or increased anxiety
- Fantasy/imaginative play helps children work through worries
- Children may be reactive to inconsistent rules about bedtime, food choices, attending preschool

Latency (7–12 years)
- Simple cause and effect logic may lead the child to assume a specific cause of the cancer (eg, cigarette smoking or cancer is contagious)
- Normal school-age emphasis on rules and fairness may lead to the expectation that if a parent follows all the treatment recommendations, they will automatically be cured.
- Importance of "fitting in" may cause discomfort with the parent's appearance in front of peers (eg, a mother without hair)

Adolescence (13–21 years)
- Abstract thinking enables the child to reflect on the possible outcomes of a serious illness and its impact on different family members, yet a child may continue to be largely self-centered
- Normal teenage wishes for greater independence are complicated by parental needs and expectations in the context of the illness
- Mood symptoms, risk-taking behavior, and substance abuse may be veiled responses to the parental illness

Adapted from Rauch P and Muriel A.[64,65]

Table 59-7 Maximizing Childhood Coping When a Parent Has Cancer

Support the child
- Maintain usual daily routines
- Utilize a small number of familiar caretakers as much as possible
- Ask about the details of a child's day
- Allow children who want to visit a sick parent in the hospital to do so, but prepare the child for what he or she will see
- For hospital visits, bring a familiar adult who is willing to leave the hospital room with the child when the child is ready to leave

Protect family time
- Continue family rituals and activities
- Designate a close friend or relative to organize community and neighborhood support
- Encourage adult friends and family not to call to ask about the parent's illness during family time

Facilitate parent and child communication
- Use simple, developmentally appropriate language to describe the cancer, but be honest. Euphemisms lead to confusion and more anxiety
- Give news bulletins about any new information that might be overheard
- Welcome all questions warmly
- Take the time to understand what underlies a child's question
- Questions need not be answered immediately
- Remind children not to worry alone
- Note the settings that most often facilitate questions and discussion
- Respect a child's wish not to talk

Adapted from Rauch P and Muriel A.[64,65]

Table 59-8 Psychosocial Sequelae in Cancer Survivors

- Positive effect of appreciating life more
- Major psychiatric disorders are uncommon (15–20% score in significantly distressed range)
- Subtle psychological distress is common
- Anxiety about recurrence/illness/death (Damocles syndrome)
- Greater sense of vulnerability (less control, lower self-esteem)
- Reminders (smells, sights) of chemotherapy produce anxiety and nausea
- Post-traumatic stress disorder (PTSD) (around 15%), (including PTSD symptoms, around 25%)
- Sexual problems related to treatment: less sense of attractiveness, lower sexual desire, poorer sexual performance
- Career goals altered negatively (fewer risks; less ability to change jobs)
- Job and health insurance problems

patients after chemotherapy to greater cognitive problems in the spatial and visual memory and executive function.[70]

Another area for potential psychological translational research is the finding of a genetic pattern that predicted greater fatigue and poorer QOL in patients who were tested before beginning treatment for stage IV colon cancer. The over-expression of *DP4D* gene, the only endogenous source of neurotransmitter B-alanine, was significantly associated with greater patient-reported fatigue (p = .008).[71] This area demands attention from clinical investigators in children and adults since fatigue is a troubling and common symptom that warrants study.

Studies of young adult survivors of Hodgkin's disease,[72] of acute leukemia, and of testicular cancer reveal several psychosocial issues that apply to survivors across tumor sites (see Table 59-8).[72,73] Most psychologically healthy individuals emerge from cancer treatment without serious psychological sequelae or significant psychiatric disorders. There is a subset of survivors, however, around 15 to 20%, who do show significant problems including PTSD symptoms. Usually, these are patients who report greater physical sequelae of treatment and who have fewer social supports.

Survivors report persistent fears of recurrence and death (Damocles syndrome), a greater sense of uncertainty and vulnerability about the future, and lower self-esteem. A minor physical symptom is feared as a sign of recurrent cancer; anxiety and even panic is common before follow-up visits. Anxiety diminishes over time, but it continues to exacerbate at times of medical visits. Gonadal toxicity results in infertility in both sexes, and in women, symptoms of premature menopause and sexual dysfunction occur. Even when no treatment-related gonadal toxicity is present, there often is lower sexual desire and poorer sexual satisfaction and performance for both men and women.[74,75] A study from Canada found, however, that the population-based rate of sexual dysfunction (50%) of women survivors of breast cancer was not different from matched postmenopausal women who had not had cancer.[76,77]

Career goals suffer from difficulty in changing jobs and pursuing a chosen career, based in part on realistic concerns about health insurance and prejudice about having had cancer. Many survivors report subtle forms of discrimination.[72] A study by Maunsell and colleagues in Quebec found that 646 women, 3 years after breast cancer, were only slightly more often unemployed than an equally large (890) comparison group.[76] The data suggest that working-women complete primary treatment and return to an unchanged job situation, which provides a more optimistic perspective.[77]

Chemotherapy results in long-lasting, conditioned, Pavlovian responses to reminders of the treatment situation where nausea and vomiting occurred with cyclic chemotherapy.[32,78] Cella and colleagues found that smells, tastes, and sights that were reminders of treatment, even as long as 11 years later, resulted in a sudden sense of unexplained anxiety and nausea (but rarely vomiting).[79]

An increasing interest is occurring in the salutary effects of exercise on both physical and mental function of cancer patients, particularly for survivors.[80] Better-controlled randomized trials are needed to provide a stronger evidence base.

Anxiety is seen after aggressive cancer treatment, particularly stem cell transplant, in the form of PTSD. Symptoms of hypervigilance, flashbacks, anxiety, depressive symptoms, poor self-esteem, and poor concentration are reported.[22,81,82] Studies suggest that about 10 to 15% of survivors of transplant have PTSD, but another 10 to 15% have some of the symptoms of PTSD without reaching full criteria for the diagnosis. Kornblith and colleagues in CALGB have found that women who are 20 year breast cancer survivors have low levels of anxiety about cancer, but a significant subgroup of about 20% still had

PTSD symptoms related to memories of treatment.[83] Cognitive-behavioral therapy with or without medication, is the current treatment.

Adaptation to Increased Genetic Risk of Cancer Healthy individuals increasingly recognize that they are at risk of a particular type of cancer by virtue of the cancer history in their families.[84,85] They are informed today about the increased risk of breast, colon, ovarian, and prostate cancer among first-degree relatives as well as of melanoma and endocrine tumors (MENS I and II).[86] The psychological impact of this knowledge results in an increasing number of individuals who are physically healthy but constitute the "worried well": they must deal with knowledge of enhanced risk despite good health. Some perceive themselves as "walking time-bombs." In a study by Kash and colleagues of women with two or more first-degree relatives with breast cancer, those most anxious were least able to carry out regular breast self-examination or have mammograms, despite the importance of surveillance.[87] Studies have been conducted to explore how to counsel those at risk.[88,89] People usually overestimate their actual risk, and genetic counseling is helpful to give them accurate information about actual risk.

Most studies have explored psychological responses to breast, ovarian, and colon cancer genetic risk.[84–96] The potential for discrimination in the workplace, health and life insurance, and breach of privacy regarding this information are concerns for the patient and for family members. In addition, there are many yet unidentified gene mutations so that results are often far from definitive. The potential harm to minors is particularly worrisome, except when an intervention could be life saving, as in MENS I and II, when it is appropriate to involve minors in the information. Pre-testing counseling must identify the psychologically vulnerable individuals for additional attention. Severe psychological sequelae have not been reported and most individuals who learn their genetic results, whether positive or negative, tolerate the information well, even when the clinical significance of results are ambiguous. More studies are needed of the impact on family members who indirectly learn of their own risk and in handling family conflicts that sometimes follow disclosures. The Institute of Medicine and the Human Genome Project have led in examining the social policy issues.

SCREENING FOR DISTRESS AND CLINICAL PRACTICE GUIDELINES

As oncology care has shifted to ambulatory settings, and as managed care has mandated shorter visits, under-recognition and under-treatment of psychiatric and psychosocial problems has increased.[97] The Panel for Management of Psychosocial Distress, appointed by the National Cancer Centers Network (NCCN), has addressed this issue by developing standards and guidelines[2] These are the first in the United States, following Australia's national guidelines for psychosocial care.[98] The NCCN Panel identified the barriers causing under-recognition as coming from patients' and physicians' attitudes about psychological issues. Patients with cancer are reluctant to ask for help for fear of the "psychiatric" or "psychological" label. The Panel, comprised of psychiatrists, psychologists, oncologists, nurses, social workers, clergy, and patient advocates, proposed that the word "distress" be used as a more acceptable and non-stigmatizing "umbrella" word. The assumption is that a level of distress is normal if one has cancer, but severity can increase until it reaches a level of disabling symptoms of anxiety or depression.[2,24] The Panel defined distress as: "An unpleasant emotional experience of a psychological (cognitive, behavioral, emotional), social, and/or spiritual nature that may interfere with the ability to cope effectively with cancer and its treatment. Distress extends along a continuum, ranging from common normal feelings of vulnerability, sadness, and fears to problems that can become disabling, such as depression, anxiety, panic, social isolation, and spiritual crisis."[2]

Table 59-9 Standards of Care for Management of Distress

Distress should be recognized, monitored, documented and treated promptly at all stages of disease
All patients should be screened for distress at their initial visit and as clinically indicated
Screening should identify the level and nature of the distress
Distress should be assessed and managed by clinical practice guidelines

NCCN Practice Guidelines.[2]

The panel then developed standards for psychosocial care, similar to those developed to improve pain management (Table 59-9). The goal is to rapidly screen and identify patients with distress using a single item or short screening tool in the waiting room, using pencil and paper or a touch screen. At Johns Hopkins Cancer Center, all patients fill out a short questionnaire that is scanned and patients with scores indicative of high distress are called at home and given an appointment to see the social worker.[99] The NCCN Panel proposed use of a simple item Distress Thermometer, a 0 to 10 scale, asking, "How distressed have you been this week?"; the patient marks the level (Figure 59-1). This is based on the successful use of the 0 to 10 scale used widely to ask patients to rate their pain. Studies by several investigators have validated the Distress Thermometer and a score of 4 to 5 is recommended as the cut-off for the level of distress that should be evaluated further.[23,41] Thus, 4 to 5 provides the "trigger" for further questioning by the nurse or social workers, as the first stage of a two-stage screening with a fuller evaluation done at a second stage.[2] The Thermometer is accompanied by a Problem List on which the patient indicates the major sources of distress: physical, psychological, social or practical problems (eg, finances) or spiritual (see Figure 59-1). The type of problem identified indicates the psychosocial resource needed. If the problem is physical, then it is addressed by the oncologist, as well as mild psychosocial problems. Figures 59-1 and 59-2 show the guidelines for triage and the Thermometer and Problem List recommended. (For additional studies, see references 42,100–102). This provides a model in which counseling is integrated into total care.

However, oncologists often note the difficulty in identifying mental health professionals in their communities who are skilled in working with patients who have cancer. The American Psychosocial Oncology Society (APOS) has addressed this need by developing a directory of counselors who are trained in psycho-oncology. The directory can be accessed by a call to the help line: 1-866-APOS-4-HELP or through the APOS Web site at <www.apos-society.org>.

PSYCHIATRIC DISORDERS

The key clinical question for the oncologist is how to identify the point at which the normal distress associated with cancer (eg, fear, worry, and sadness) has become a treatable psychiatric disorder. Most psychiatric disturbances in patients with cancer relate to illness or treatment side effects.[103] Taken overall, about a third of patients

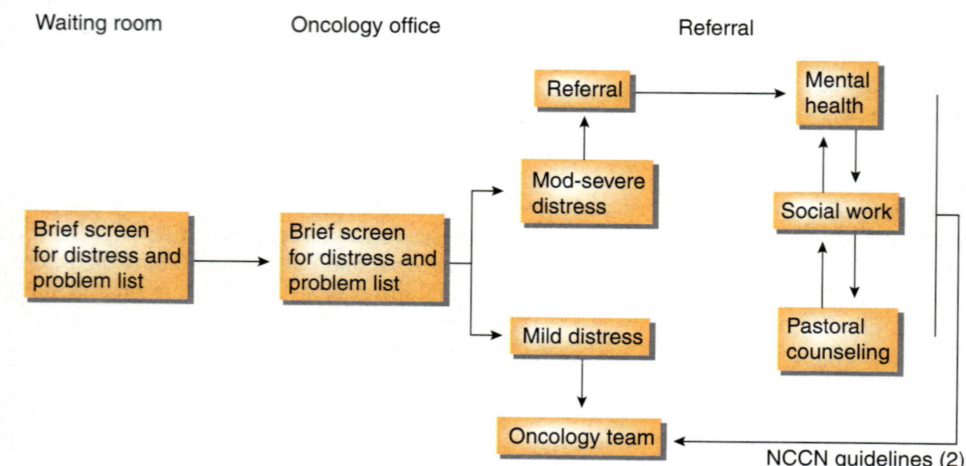

Figure 59-1 Evaluation/treatment guidelines in oncology clinic.

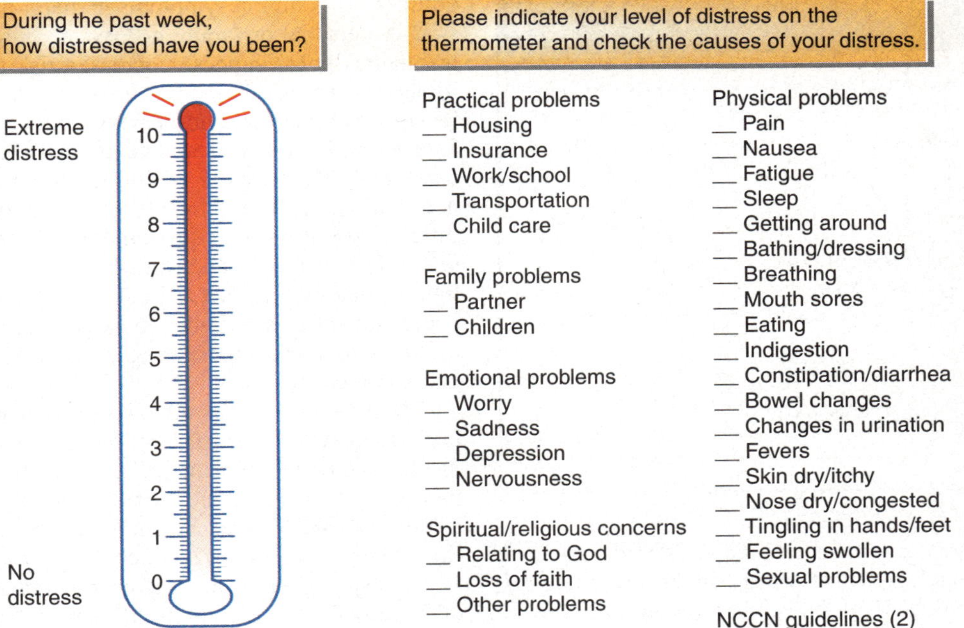

Figure 59-2 Thermometer and Problem List.

have distress at a level that should be evaluated and treated [45,103–105] The percentage is even greater among younger patients; those with sites of cancer with poorer prognosis, for example, brain, pancreas, lung; and those who are hospitalized with greater level of illness causing confusional states and greater anxiety and depression.[99,106]

Anxiety Disorders Anxiety is the most common form of distress related to anxiety provoking situations, medical causes and medications (Tables 59-10 and 59-11). It occurs with abnormal metabolic states: hypoxia, pulmonary embolus, sepsis, delirium, bleeding, cardiac arrhythmia, and hypoglycemia. Hormone-secreting tumors that produce anxiety are: pheochromocytoma, thyroid tumors, carcinoid, parathyroid adenoma, ACTH-producing tumors, insulinoma, and paraneoplastic disorders (remote CNS effect).

Several drugs produce symptoms of anxiety: corticosteroids, neuroleptics, bronchodilators, thyroxine, and psychostimulants. Metoclopramide or other neuroleptics given for the control of chemotherapy-related nausea and vomiting produce restlessness, akathisias, and dystonias. A benzodiazepine promptly reduces the restless movements, anxiety, and agitation. Withdrawal states from alcohol, narcotic analgesics, and sedative-hypnotics produce anxiety as a prominent symptom.

Some patients undergoing cyclic chemotherapy using an emetogenic regimen begin to develop anticipatory anxiety, nausea, and vomiting by about the third cycle, a few days to hours in advance of receiving the next cycle of treatment.[32,107,108] This is a learned, conditioned, Pavlovian autonomic response to the repeated chemotherapy-related experience of nausea and vomiting (described earlier in survivors). More effective antiemesis regimens have reduced the frequency and severity of this problem. However, behavioral interventions and anti-anxiety medication are sometimes needed.

Patients who have pre-existing phobias, panic attacks, generalized anxiety, post-traumatic stress disorder (PTSD), or obsessive-compulsive disorder are at risk of their symptoms exacerbating during cancer treatment (see Table 59-10).[109] Phobias of needles, blood, hospitals, claustrophobia, or agoraphobia complicate the ability to tolerate hospital procedures. Panic attacks often occur in patients who already have shortness of breath or tachycardia for medical reasons, complicating these physical symptoms.[103,110] Patients who have had prior traumatic events may have flashbacks of painful memories that have been quiescent for many years.[20,22]

Obsessive compulsive disorder (OCD) is a complicating psychiatric disorder during cancer treatment, which leads to indecisiveness about treatment decisions and difficulty with the inability to control the situation. Fears of the future, phobias, and rigidity, make it difficult for patients with OCD to cope with illness and they often reject psychotropic drugs.

The treatment of anticipatory anxiety is usually handled by good communication and adequate information, allowing the person to "rehearse" the feared event (Table 59-12). Enlisting the oncology nurse or social worker is often helpful in giving additional information and offering reassurance.

For persistent or distressing anxiety, three types of treatment are available, often used in combination: (1) psychotherapy and counseling, (2) cognitive-behavioral interventions, and (3) psychopharmacologic medications. Counseling or formal psychotherapy using a psychoeducational, cognitive-behavioral, or supportive intervention model is helpful[111–114] (see Table 59-12). Fawzy and colleagues outlined the range of psychosocial interventions that have been proven efficacious in controlled trials.[45] A meta-analysis of randomized controlled trials showed that a range of interventions are efficacious in improving QOL and decreasing distress, but data do not show an effect upon survival.[115]

There are several forms of psychotherapy that have been tested and more are in development: psychoeducational, interpersonal psychotherapy (IPT), supportive, cognitive-behavioral, and existential or meaning-centered therapies. Several behavioral interventions are effective. Relaxation

Table 59-10 Causes of Anxiety in Patients with Cancer

- Situational
  - Diagnosis of cancer, prognosis discussion
  - Crisis, illness/treatment
  - Conflicts with family or staff
  - Anticipating a frightening procedure
  - Awaiting results of tests
  - Fears of recurrence *after* completing treatment
- Disease-related
  - Poorly controlled pain
  - Abnormal metabolic states
  - Hormone secreting tumors
  - Paraneoplastic syndromes (remote CNS effects)
- Treatment-related
  - Frightening or painful procedures (MRI, scans, wound debridement)
  - Anxiety-producing drugs (antiemetic neuroleptics, bronchodilators)
  - Withdrawal states (opioids, benzodiazepines, alcohol)
  - Conditioned (anticipatory) anxiety, nausea, and vomiting with cyclic chemotherapy
- Exacerbation of preexisting anxiety disorder
  - Phobias (needles, claustrophobia)
  - Panic or generalized anxiety disorder
  - Post-traumatic stress disorder (Holocaust survivors, Vietnam veterans, recall of the death of a relative with cancer)
  - Obsessive compulsive disorder

Table 59-11 Anxiety Related to Common Medical Problems in Cancer

Medical Problems	Examples
Poorly controlled pain	Unresponsive or under-treated pain
Abnormal metabolic states	Hypoxia, pulmonary embolus, sepsis, fever, delirium, hypoglycemia, hypercalcemia, bleeding, coronary occlusion and heart failure, cardiac arrhythmia
Hormone-secreting tumors	Pheochromocytoma, thyroid tumors, carcinoid, parathyroid adenoma, ACTH-producing tumors, insulinoma
Anxiety-producing drugs	Corticosteroids, neuroleptics used as antiemetics, thyroxine, bronchodilators, β-adrenergic stimulants, antihistamines, (paradoxic reactions), withdrawal states (alcohol, narcotic analgesics, sedative-hypnotics)
Side effects of treatment	Allergic skin rash to antibiotics, unexpected toxicity (eg, diarrhea)

Table 59-12 Treatment of Anxiety Disorders

Treatment Modality	Components
Supportive psychotherapy	Providing information, rehearsal of feared events, reassurance
	Individual therapy
	Support group
Behavioral	Relaxation, hypnosis
	Systematic desensitization
Psychopharmacologic	Benzodiazepines
	Short acting (alprazolam, lorazepam, oxazepam)
	Long acting (diazepam, clorazepate, clonazepam)
	Selective Serotonin Reuptake Inhibitors (SSRIs) (paroxetine, sertraline, citalopram, escitalopram, fluoxetine)
	β-Blockers (propranolol)
	Antihistamines
	Neuroleptics (thioridazine, trifluoperazine, haloperidol)
	Buspirone
Combinations of the above	

exercises with guided imagery and hypnosis are most frequently employed. These methods are particularly helpful to patients who wish to maintain and enhance their beleaguered sense of control. Relaxation and meditation are useful adjunctive treatments for anxiety related to pain and for control of conditioned chemotherapy-related nausea and vomiting.[108,116,117]

Significant anxiety symptoms are most often treated pharmacologically by sedative-hypnotics from the benzodiazepine class of drugs, by the serotonin reuptake inhibitors (SSRIs), by antidepressants that affect depression and anxiety (often present together), as well as by antihistamines, beta-blockers, and neuroleptics in low dose. Table 59-13 outlines the benzodiazepines commonly used and their starting and therapeutic doses. A shorter half-life provides better control and less likelihood of poor elimination and oversedation. Insomnia responds to a bedtime dose of temazepam 15 mg; clonazepam, 1 mg; or zolpidem, 5 mg. The antidepressants trazodone 50 mg, and mirtazapine 15 mg are also useful for bedtime sedation. Daytime anxiety responds to lorazepam, 0.5 mg; alprazolam, 0.25 to 0.50 mg tid or qid. Clonazepam, 0.5 mg bid, or diazepam 5 mg bid are longer acting. It is important to taper these medications to prevent a mild rebound in anxiety or withdrawal symptoms. Buspirone is useful, because it has no sedating effects and no addictive qualities. Low dose neuroleptics are useful in older patients, using risperidone, olanzapine, or quetiapine during the day or bedtime.

Mood Disorders It is important to keep in mind that depression does respond to treatment and should not be left untreated because it is "based on reality" in patients with cancer. Depressive symptoms occur as reactive depression (often with anxiety); dysthymia (chronic or minor depression); major depression and bipolar disorder. Bipolar disorder and dysthymia usually pre-exist the cancer diagnosis.

Depression is difficult to diagnose in patients with cancer because the neoplastic disease itself may produce the vegetative symptoms of cancer: fatigue, weakness, loss of libido, insomnia, loss of interest, poor concentration, and motivation.[118] The oncologist must depend on the psychological symptoms of dysphoric mood, helplessness, hopelessness, worthlessness, loss of pleasure (anhedonia), and suicidal thoughts.[119] Table 59-14 outlines the common symptoms in major depression. A personal or family history of depression or bipolar illness suggests increased risk during illness as well as having poor social support, being socially isolated and having experienced a recent loss. Evaluation should explore mental status, mood, hopelessness, feeling of being a burden, and suicidal ideation. Insomnia, anorexia, fatigue, agitation, or psychomotor retardation may relate to illness and must be interpreted in light of that fact. In fact, all these symptoms are being studied as a possible consequence of proinflammatory cytokines, suggesting a possible biologic contribution.[3,4]

Table 59-15 outlines the medical-related risk factors: greater level of debilitation, advanced disease and presence of another chronic illness or disability. Several medications frequently contribute: steroids, some chemotherapeutic agents (interferon, interleukin 2, vincristine, procarbazine, L-asparaginase), and medications given for other reasons.[119] Depression is seen with organ failure and with some nutritional, endocrine, and neurologic complications of cancer. Depression is

Table 59-13 Common Anti-Anxiety Agents

Drug	Brand Name	Starting Dose/Day	Therapeutic Dose/Day
Selective serotonin reuptake inhibitors			
Sertraline	Zoloft	25–50 mg AM	50–150 mg
Fluoxetine	Prozac	10–20 mg AM	20–60 mg
Paroxetine	Paxil	10–20 mg	20–60 mg
Citalopram	Celexa	10–20 mg	20–60 mg
Escitalopram	Lexapro	5–10 mg	10–30 mg
Benzodiazepines			
Alprazolam, XR	Xanax	0.25–0.5 mg	0.5–2.0 mg
Clonazepam, wafers	Klonopin	0.25–0.5 mg	0.5–2.0 mg
*Lorazepam	Ativan	0.25–0.5 mg	0.5–2.0 mg
*Diazepam	Valium	2 mg	5–20 mg
Hypnotics			
Temazepam	Restoril	15 mg	15–45 mg
Zolpidem	Ambien	5 mg	5–20 mg

* Also IV, IM.

Table 59-14 Evaluation of Depression and Predisposing Factors

Evaluative Category	Findings
Family history	Depression; suicide
Personal history	Previous depression, bipolar disorder, suicide attempt, alcoholism, substance abuse
Signs and symptoms	Recent bereavement
	Psychologic
	Dysphoric mood (eg, sad, depressed, anxious, crying, diurnal mood change)
	Feelings of hopelessness; helplessness
	Loss of interest and pleasure; anhedonia
	Guilt, burden on others, worthlessness
	Poor concentration
	Mood incongruent to disease outlook
	Suicidal thoughts or plans
	Delusional thoughts (psychotic symptoms rare, except in organic affective syndrome)
	Somatic (less interpretable in more physically impaired patients)
	Insomnia
	Anorexia and weight loss
	Fatigue
	Psychomotor retardation or agitation
	Constipation
	Decreased libido

Table 59-15 Medical-Related Risk Factors for Depression in Patients with Cancer

- Poorly controlled pain
- Other chronic disease/disability; advanced stage
- Medications
  - Corticosteroids
  - Prednisone, dexamethasone
  - Interferon and Interleukin-2
  - Chemotherapeutic agents
    - Vincristine, vinblastine, procarbazine, L-asparaginase
- Other medications
  - Cimetidine
  - Indomethacin
  - Levodopa
  - Methyldopa
  - Pentazocine
  - Phenmetrazine
  - Phenobarbital
  - Propranolol
  - Rauwolfia alkaloids
  - Tamoxifen
  - Antibiotics (amphotericin B)
- Other medical conditions
  - Metabolic (anemia; hypercalcemia)
  - Nutritional (B_{12} or folate)
  - Endocrine (hyper-hypothyroidism; adrenal insufficiency)
  - Neurologic (paraneoplastic syndrome)
- Sites of cancer
  - Pancreatic, small cell lung, breast cancer, lymphoma (producing remote central nervous system effects)

Table 59-16 Commonly Used Antidepressants in Cancer

Drug	Brand Name	Starting Daily Dosage PO (mg)	Therapeutic Daily Dosage PO (mg)
Selective serotonin-reuptake inhibitors			
Sertraline	Zoloft	25–50 mg AM	50–150 mg
Fluoxetine	Prozac	10–20 mg AM	20–60 mg
Paroxetine	Paxil	10–20 mg AM	20–60 mg
Citalopram	Celexa	10–20 mg AM	20–60 mg
Escitalopram	Lexapro	5–10 mg	10–20 mg
Tricyclics (neuropathic pain management primarily)			
Nortriptyline	Pamelor	25–50 mg	50–200 mg
Amitriptyline	Elavil	25–50 mg	50–200 mg
Desipramine	Norpramin	25–50 mg	50–200 mg
Other agents			
Venlafaxine	Effexor	18.75–37.5 mg	75–225 mg
Trazodone	Desyrel	50–100 mg	100–200 mg
Bupropion (XL, SR)	Wellbutrin, Zyban	50–75 mg	150–400 mg
Mirtazapine	Remeron	15 mg HS	15–45 mg
Psychostimulants			
Methylphenidate	Ritalin	5–10 mg (8 AM & Noon)	10–30 mg
Modafinil	Provigil	50–100 mg (8 AM & Noon)	100–400 mg
Dextroamphetamine	Dexedrine	5–10 mg (8 AM & Noon)	10–20 mg

Lithium and mood stabilizers only for bipolar disorder; MAOIs not recommended.

a common symptom of pancreatic cancer, which has led to speculation about a tumor-induced mood change, possibly though alteration of brain serotonergic function through the effect of proinflammatory cytokines.[38,120,121] These disease-related major depressions are called Mood Disorder Related to Medical Condition.

Depression is managed first by establishing good rapport with the patient and assuring support from available family or friends. Supportive psychotherapeutic, behavioral interventions, and psychotropic agents are often combined in treatment.[122,123] Cognitive behavioral interventions encourage the patient to reframe problems more constructively and often reduce uncontrolled, distressing emotions.

Psychotropic drugs are effective in controlling depressive symptoms with cancer.[123] Table 59-16 lists the most frequently used antidepressant medications in patients with cancer and their starting and maintenance doses. The antidepressants commonly used today are selective serotonin-reuptake inhibitors (SSRIs). Today, tricyclics are used primarily for adjuvant pain management and peripheral neuropathy. Psychostimulants are widely used to promote well-being and counteract the fatigue from advanced illness and opioids. Dextroamphetamine, methylphenidate, and modafinil are useful. All antidepressants should be started in low dose in elderly and debilitated patients and titrated upward as tolerated.

Suicide and Cancer The incidence of suicide is increased in patients with cancer compared to the general population, but it is not as high as often is assumed. Suicide by overdose at home during the terminal stages of cancer is doubtless under-diagnosed and under-reported due to stigma.[124–126] Suicide is more likely to occur in advanced disease, when depression, hopelessness, and the presence of poorly controlled symptoms (especially pain) are greatest. Table 59-17 outlines risk factors and Table 59-18 outlines assessment of suicidal risk. Key questions are the nature of suicidal thoughts (passive or active); past history of psychiatric problems, particularly depression or suicide attempts; recent bereavement; and family history of depression or suicide, and presence of poorly controlled pain. Availability of family and social support are integral to assume adequate surveillance at home.

Evaluation of suicidal thoughts takes into account disease stage and prognosis (Table 59-19). Almost all patients who receive a diagnosis of cancer, even when the prognosis is good, carry a "secret" thought that "I won't die in pain with advanced cancer—I'll kill myself first." With some patients, they maintain a hidden supply of a drug, which is kept for this purpose. It usually serves as a "steam valve" with which the person is able to maintain a sense of ultimate control over the disease and feared intolerable pain. The thought actually serves as a protective coping device.

Serious ruminating about suicide in a patient for whom the disease is in remission or in whom a good prognosis exists requires careful evaluation.[126] A study of all suicides in Finland in 1 year found that 4.3% had cancer.[127] Surprisingly, half of the patients with cancer were in remission at the time of the suicide. They had greater prior psychiatric problems, particularly substance abuse. It is important that these patients be recognized and aggressively treated for depression and suicidal risk, including psychiatric hospitalization if necessary.

Patients with a poor prognosis, advanced disease, and poorly controlled symptoms often have thoughts of suicide that are more likely to be viewed as rational.[128] They may request help from a physician to write a prescription for a drug to use to commit suicide. A treatable major depression may be fueling their suicidal ideation. Chochinov and colleagues[61,63] found that the persistent desire for death in the terminally ill is closely associated with the diagnosis of depression. It is particularly important to evaluate the presence of hopelessness that is a greater predictor of suicidal risk than depression itself.[126]

Attention to any uncontrolled physical symptom, especially pain, is important. Adequate pain

Table 59-17 Risk Factors for Suicide in Cancer

- Personal
  - Prior history of depression or suicide attempt (personal or family)
  - Prior psychiatric disorder
  - Prior alcohol or drug abuse
  - Depression and hopelessness
  - Recent loss/bereavement
  - Socially isolated
- Medical
  - Pain
  - Delirium with poor impulse control
  - Advanced illness
  - Debilitation, exhaustion, fatigue

Table 59-18 Evaluation of Suicidal Risk

- Establish rapport
- Ask about symptoms (pain, discomfort, and adequacy of their control)
- Ask about depression and suicidal thoughts at present or in the past
- Ask about suicidal thoughts (Are they passive ["I wish I could die"] or active ["I am thinking of ways to do it"])
- Ask about family or friends and sense of support from others
- Ask about any recent loss of close person, especially if by cancer
- Ask about understanding of illness, presence of confusion, fatigue
- Asking does not cause suicidal thoughts; the patient is usually relieved to express them

Table 59-19 Suicide in Relation to Stage of Disease

Patients at all stages of cancer
- Suicidal thoughts are common and serve as a means to maintain a sense of control over the disease
- Carrying out the act is viewed as for "the future when I need to do it"
- Some maintain a means of suicide (eg, drugs) to assure ultimate control over feared intolerable symptoms

Patients in remission, with good prognosis
- Serious suicidal thoughts represent underlying psychiatric disorder (depression, substance abuse)
- Unlikely to appear "rational"; treat aggressively, including hospitalization

Patients with poor prognosis and poorly controlled symptoms
- Thoughts of suicide often appear "rational"
- May request advice about physician-assisted suicide
- Need evaluation for presence of treatable depression
- Need attention to quality-of-life issues and comfort
- Suicidal wishes usually diminish with control of distressing symptoms
- Adequate symptom control by physician may hasten death (dual effect) but is not actual physician-assisted suicide

Patients in terminal stage
- May request euthanasia by lethal injection from physician
- Request often reflects poor quality of life, hopelessness, and depression
- Need for control of symptoms, even when hastens death

control may have the dual effect of hastening death, but few physicians have difficulty in carrying out such a treatment aimed at comfort. Most physicians do not regard this as assisted suicide but as best medical care geared to maximal comfort.[57]

Patients who are in the terminal stages and are too weak to carry out a suicidal act are those most likely to request euthanasia. Although the societal debate has been intense, support for legalized euthanasia has not occurred. In Oregon, where physician-assisted suicide by giving the patient a prescription has been legalized, the numbers who request help remain small and the controversy continues over the state's right to continue over federal action that prohibits the use of FDA controlled substances for this purpose. This controversy will come before the Supreme Court for resolution.

Poorly controlled pain in patients with beginning organ failure and a mild metabolic encephalopathy results in poor judgment and poor impulse control and may lead to an impulsive suicidal attempt.[129] Such patients in the hospital should be given a 24-hour companion, a nurse or a family member who understands the patient's compromised state.

Delirium Delirium, or encephalopathy, is a non-focal global cerebral dysfunction characterized by waxing and waning levels of consciousness, disordered thinking, mood change, disorientation and confusion, psychomotor slowing or agitation, altered behavior, judgment, and altered sleep-wake cycles. It is often worse at night, hence the term "sundowning." It is usually contrasted with dementia by being reversible; however, in advanced stages of cancer, due to organ failure and metabolic derangements, it is often not reversible. The goal is first to control behaviors that may be harmful to the patient or others (eg, pulling out lines, combative behavior). Family members should be told that the cause of the behavior is brain dysfunction, not a mental aberration, and given guidance in understanding the patient's states.

In patients with cancer, especially those in advanced stages, a sudden change in mood or behavior is most often related to a change in neurologic, vascular, or metabolic status; a psychological basis is far less likely. In fact, up to three-quarters of terminally ill patients may develop a delirium before death. Common causes of delirium in cancer are outlined in Table 59-20. A change in behavior in which the person becomes irritable, uncooperative, agitated, or somnolent, and misinterprets sounds or objects is apt to represent early signs of delirium. This picture may be followed by delusions, usually paranoid ("there are people here trying to hurt me"), frank hallucinations, and difficulty in being maintained in bed or hospital rooms (Table 59-21). Mood can change markedly with irritability or depression with suicidal ideation.

Management begins with attention to the patient's safety. It is important to have one-to-one observation, preferably by a person present who can correct misinterpretations of what is happening. Limiting the number of new faces and experiences is useful while enhancing awareness of time and place. Older patients are most prone to become confused, and delirium may be superimposed on early mild dementia. Physical restraints must sometimes be used to prevent removal of vital IV lines and bandages, and to prevent falls. Chemical restraint may be necessary. The management regimen is low-dose haloperidol, a potent dopamine blocker, 0.5 to 1.0 mg bid to qid. Lorazepam given with a neuroleptic reduces agitation in doses of 0.5 to 1.0 mg tid to qid; however, given alone, it may increase confusion. Haloperidol and lorazepam often are given together to reduce confusion and diminish agitation.[131] Olanzapine is a highly effective anti-delirium drug given by mouth and by intramuscular route. Table 59-22 outlines the drugs that are useful and their route of administration. Correcting the underlying metabolic or neurologic problem is not always possible, however, and comfort for the patient and family may depend materially on being able to control the symptoms of confusion and agitation. Patients with psychomotor slowing may safely be observed without treatment, but significant degrees of confusion with agitation must be treated.[59,129] This is often seen in terminal stages and achieving sedation may be the goal to provide comfort and safety for the patient and family.

PSYCHIATRIC AND PSYCHOSOCIAL INTERVENTIONS

There has been a great increase in controlled trials of well defined psychotherapies which show efficacy in terms of decreased distress and

Table 59-20 Common Causes of Delirium in Cancer

Causes	Examples
Metabolic encephalopathy because of vital organ failure	Liver, kidney, lung (hypoxia), thyroid, adrenal
Electrolyte imbalance	Sodium, potassium, calcium, glucose
Treatment side effects	Narcotic/analgesics
	Anticholinergics
	Phenothiazines
	Antihistamines
	Chemotherapeutic agents
	Steroids
	Radiation therapy to brain
Infection	Septicemia
Hematologic abnormalities	Microcytic and macrocytic anemias, coagulopathies
Nutritional	General malnutrition, thiamine, folic acid, vitamin B_{12}
Paraneoplastic syndromes	Remote effects of tumors
Metastatic or primary brain tumor	Hormone-producing tumors

Table 59-21 Behavioral Symptoms of Delirium in Patients with Cancer

State	Symptom
Early, mild	Change in sleep pattern with restlessness, attempts to get out of bed, transient periods of disorientation
	Unexplained anxiety and sense of dread
	Increased irritability, anger, temper outbursts
	Withdrawal, refusal to talk to staff or relatives
Late, severe with behavioral changes	Forgetfulness, not previously present
	Refusal to cooperate with reasonable requests; pulling out tubes and lines
	Angry, swearing, shouting, abusive
	Demanding to go home, pacing corridor
	Illusions (misidentifies staff, visual and sensory clues)
	Delusions (misinterprets events, usually paranoid, fears of being harmed)
	Hallucinations (visual and auditory)

Table 59-22 Medications for Managing Delirium in Cancer Patients

Drug	Brand Name	Approximate Daily Dosage
Neuroleptics		
Haloperidol	Haldol	0.5–5 mg every 2–12 h, PO, IV, SC, IM
Chlorpromazine	Thorazine	12.5–50 mg every 4–12 h, PO, IV, IM
Risperidone	Risperdal	1–3 mg every 12 h, PO
Olanzapine	Zyprexa	2.5–5 mg every 6–8 h, PO
Quetiapine	Seroquel	12.5–50 mg every 12 h, PO
Benzodiazepines		
Lorazepam	Ativan	0.5–2.0 mg every 1–4 h, PO, IV, IM
Midazolam*		30–100 mg every 24 h, IV, SC
Anesthetics		
Propofol*		10–50 mg every hour, IV

* Usually IV continuous infusion in intensive care setting.

improved QOL, an effect that persists for months.[113,114,132,134] Brief crisis counseling[134] and combined psychosocial and educational interventions have proven of value in coping.[135] Problem-solving counseling is a cognitive approach that is helpful for patients and family members.[116] Twillman and Manetto[37] have shown efficacy of concurrent psychotherapy and pharmacotherapy in management of depression and anxiety. Other studies have compared antidepressants.[136–138] Kissane and colleagues have taken a cognitive-existential approach for women with breast cancer that acknowledges the awareness of the crisis of meaning.[139] Chochinov has described "dignity-conserving" psychotherapy to assist patients in feeling valued and esteemed as they approach end of life.[57] Group counseling models have been developed from trials directed at both early and advanced disease with evidence of efficacy.[35,139–142] They are effective in reducing distress and in helping to control pain.

The widespread use of groups has led to questions of whether psychosocial interventions can extend life. A meta-analysis conducted by Petticrew and colleagues[142] found little support for any association between psychological coping styles and recurrence and survival from cancer. There is little doubt that effective coping assures adherence to treatment and indirectly affects survival. Studies done over a decade ago by Spiegel and colleagues[143] and by Fawzy[144] reported a positive impact on survival, but this has not been demonstrated in subsequent studies. Goodwin and colleagues have reported a carefully designed replication of Spiegal's study in a multicenter trial in Canada.[145] They confirmed the reduction of distress and enhanced QOL, but they did not show a survival advantage. Although other studies of group intervention have also shown no survival advantage,[140,146] the Goodwin study is the most definitive in terms of being a large, randomized trial.[145] Kissane has conducted a similar large trial and found better treatment compliance and a trend towards increased survival, suggesting that group therapy may enhance compliance.[147]

Behavioral interventions have been well tested and accepted in cancer patients. Relaxation, meditation, and systematic desensitization are all effective in reducing anxiety, conditioned responses from chemotherapy-induced nausea and vomiting, and pain.[80] These behavioral interventions are often coupled with cognitive therapy approaches.[116] The value of art therapy in helping patients cope has also been shown in both hospitalized and ambulatory patients.[148]

With the explosion of complementary and alternative medicine (CAM), there has been a tendency for behavioral and CAM therapies to overlap.[149] A study by Burstein and colleagues,[150] and a commentary on it,[151] explored use of CAM by women in the year following initial breast cancer treatment. Women who had used CAM were more depressed, more worried about the future, and had poorer QOL, suggesting that many were not recognized as distressed by their oncologist and hence were not referred; or, that complementary therapies were more positively viewed than psychological interventions.

QUALITY-OF-LIFE ASSESSMENT

The definition of health-related QOL is the level of performance in the major domains of life function as reported by patient-self-report.[47,152] In the 1990s, clinical trials have increasingly included the assessment of QOL. Interest in QOL grew after 1984, when the US Food and Drug Administration demanded that the efficacy of new anticancer agents be demonstrated by improved survival or evidence of enhanced QOL, which led to development of more valid measurement tools. Karnofsky and Burchenal actually described in 1949 that, in addition to survival, subjective improvement was equally important in the evaluation of patients' responses to treatment.[154] Despite that early observation, however, only selected trials assess QOL, usually when there is a small likely treatment advantage (eg, trials of chemotherapy agents in pancreatic cancer) or when a highly effective new treatment has significant side effects (eg, stem cell transplant). The term QOL has been proposed to be replaced by the term Patient Reported Outcomes that is a much better term.[155]

Six domains are included in multidimensional quality-of-life measures: physical, functional, psychologic, social, sexual, and work (Table 59-23). No "gold standard" of measurement currently exists, but the EORTC instruments in Europe and those developed by Cella in the United States are widely used in many languages. Historically, the Functional Living Index-Cancer (FLIC) was the first.[156] The Cancer Rehabilitation Evaluation System (CARES) consists of 139 items that queries the six quality-of-life domains.[157] A series of quality of life measures related to cancer site were developed and tested by the European Organization for Research and Treatment of Cancer (EORTC).[158] The scales have a core of questions that are applicable to the QOL for all patients and modules which query the specific issues related to a disease site or stage (eg, prostate, breast, lung cancer).

A similar approach has been used by Cella and colleagues[159] in development of the Functional Assessment of Cancer Therapy (FACT), which adds an aspect of patient assessment regarding the discrepancy between prior and present function. In addition to the FACT-General, the core questions, Cella has developed modules for the major cancer sites and for common problems such as nausea, vomiting, pain, spiritual beliefs, and fatigue. Aside from the Karnofsky Performance Rating Scale, Spitzer and colleagues' Quality of Life Index (QL-index) is the major observer-rated measure of QOL that is used with any frequency.[160]

Additional scales, not developed specifically for cancer but widely used, are the Psychosocial Adjustment to Illness Scale (PAIS) and the Sickness Impact Profile (SIP).[161,162] The PAIS in particular has been used extensively with several chronic illnesses, including cancer. The SIP scale is similar in format to CARES in that it lists 136 problems that can result from illness that affect QOL. Symptom Inventory is a measure of symptom distress.[163] The MOS General Health Survey instruments have the advantage of being used with other diseases and short and longer valid forms are available.[164]

Recent efforts in quality of life research have concentrated on development of a unitary measure that combines length of survival and QOL, referred to as "quality-adjusted life years" or QALY. "TWIST" (Time Without Symptoms or Toxicity), is another QALY method. These methods, coupled with economic analysis, are providing increasing information to assist patients and doctors in making decisions about cancer treatments.

FAMILY ISSUES AND BEREAVEMENT

Families have emerged as a significant overburdened and under-recognized component of health care today. Families of patients seen in focus

Table 59-23 Quality-of-Life Measurement: Functional Areas of Living Assessed

Physical	Symptoms of disease and treatment of side effects
Functional	Ability to perform usual activities
Psychologic	Mood, sense of well-being
Sexual	Desire, performance
Social	Family, friends, leisure
Work	Usual level of activity

groups reported that hospital staff saw them as "difficult."[165] Yet, families must care for patients at home today with high levels of illness. The demand that they give physical care and carry out medical procedures is far greater than previously. An estimated 25 million households are caring for a chronically ill family member—many in homes of the economically deprived.[166]

Attention is slowly being given to the greater needs of families today by health policy planners. However, in addition to economic issues, there are profoundly stressful psychological and social consequences. These issues are compounded when the care at home is being given for advanced and terminal stages of cancer.[49] Oncologists' responsibility to the patient extends to evaluation of the caregiver as well, and the ability of that key person to cope with the demands. Children in the household also require attention, and guidance for the adult caregiver about answering children's questions is important (see Tables 59-6, 59-7).[64,65]

GRIEF IN SURVIVING FAMILY MEMBERS

Oncologists who treat patients with cancer often come to know family members well, especially during terminal stages of illness. They are in a unique position to support the family when the patient dies and to assure care for grief in the surviving caregiver and family members, especially children.[167] They need to recognize abnormal reactions and refer the grieving relative for bereavement counseling. Hospice programs include this as part of their services. It is important to be aware in one's community of both support groups for the bereaved and of mental health professionals who offer bereavement counseling. Severe, protracted, or complicated grief reactions require treatment since they often lead to major depression. Data overall suggest that 80% of people experience normal grieving but around 20% will have complicated or abnormal grief.

There has been much interest in the question of whether psychosocial factors like grief, stress, depression, or personality result in increased risk of cancer or progression. Studies have found no higher mortality from cancer among parents in Israel who had lost a child by accident or war 10 years earlier[168] or in parents in Denmark who had experienced death of their child by cancer.[19] Similar negative results were found for depression[169] and for personality.[18,19]

These findings suggest that, based on epidemiological data, grief does not increase risk of cancer nor lead to its recurrence or progression in survivors. This information is reassuring for individuals who fear that experiencing a loss makes them more vulnerable to cancer or its progression.

STRESS AND BURNOUT IN ONCOLOGY STAFF

A topic of increasing concern is the impact of repeated losses and stresses upon oncologists and nurses that produces burnout. Nurses experience more burnout and job dissatisfaction when their work load is excessive.[171] The impact of the daily giving of bad news to patients and families takes its own toll.[172] In 1991, Whippen and Canellos did a survey of ASCO oncologists. About 60% expressed feelings of burnout due to the stress of too much paper work, administrative matters, too little time for family, too heavy a workload, and dealing with patients receiving palliative care.[173] Unpublished, a second survey 10 years later confirms the continuing concern.

A study at Memorial Sloan Kettering reported house staff with the highest burnout scores had greater emotional exhaustion, felt "distanced" from patients, and had a sense of diminished professional accomplishment. Having some religious beliefs, good communication skills, and good patient relationships appeared to counter burnout development, as did having a "hardy" personality.[174] Continuing examination of the impact of clinical practice on oncologists and their primary team is necessary.

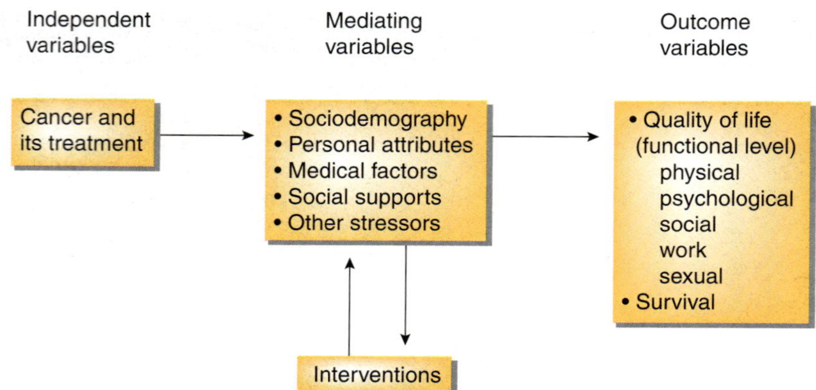

Figure 59-3 Research model for psychiatric and quality of life research in oncology.

SUMMARY

The subspecialty of psycho-oncology began in the last quarter of the twentieth century, reflecting the increased interest in psychiatric, psychological, and social factors in cancer prevention, the "human" side of the care of patients with cancer at all stages, and the impact of cancer on family members and on medical and nursing staff. Early identification of vulnerable patients is important through a rapid screen which can lead to a second stage evaluation to recognize and diagnose the common psychiatric disorders of anxiety, depression, and delirium, the latter often caused by medications and metabolic complications of cancer. The modalities available to treat these symptoms are psychotherapeutic, behavioral, pharmacologic, and complementary therapies. Having a mental-health professional familiar with the psychological aspects of cancer who is available for evaluation and treatment of patients is an important resource, and best when part of the primary team (see Figure 59-1).

The measurement of health-related QOL (now referred to as PROs) that assesses patients' functioning in the major domains of living has been a valuable addition to clinical trial research, permitting assessment not only of survival, but the quality of the time lived. This merger of data from the two diverse areas of survival time and quality of life augurs well for future research in oncology that addresses the "total" patient. The model for research in psycho-oncology incorporates the independent variables of cancer and treatment; the outcome variables of survival and QOL; and, the mediating variables which constitute the areas in which psycho-oncology seeks to intervene by psychological, social, and pharmacological means (Figure 59-3).[5]

REFERENCES

1. Holland JC. Psycho-oncology. New York: Oxford University Press, 1998.
2. Holland JC, Andersen B, et al. NCCN distress management clinical practice guidelines in oncology. Journal of the National Comprehensive Cancer Network 2003;1:344–74.
3. Cleeland CS, Bennett GJ, Dantzen, R. Are the symptoms of cancer and cancer treatment due to a shared biologic mechanism? Cancer 2003;97:2919–25.
4. Musselman DL, Miller AH, et al. Higher than normal interleukin-6 concentrations in cancer patients with depression: preliminary findings. Am J Psychiatry 2001;158:1252–7.
5. Holland, JC. History of psycho-oncology: overcoming attitudinal and conceptual barriers. Psychosom Med 2002;64:206–21.
6. Hagerty RG, Butour PN, et al. Communicating with realism and hope: incurable cancer patients' views on the disclosure of prognosis. J Clin Oncol 2005;23:1278–88.
7. Ptacek JT, Fries EA, Eberhardt JL, Ptacek JJ. Breaking bad news to patients: physicians' perceptions of the process. Support Care Cancer 1999;7:13–20.
8. National Health + Medical Research Council Psychosocial Clinical Practice Guidelines: Information, Support, and Counseling for Women with Breast Cancer. National Medical & Research Council Australia, 2000.
9. Girgis A, Sanson-Fisher RW. Breaking bad news: consensus for medical practitioners. J Clin Oncol 1995;9:2445–56.
10. Back AL, Arnold RM, et al. Approaching difficult communication tasks in oncology. CA: A Cancer Journal for Clinicians 2005;55:164–77.
11. Baile WF, Kudelka AP, Beale EA, et al. Communication skills training in oncology: description and preliminary outcomes of workshops on breaking bad news and managing patient reactions to illness. Cancer 1999;86:887–97.
12. Park C, Folkman S. Meaning in the context of stress and coping. Rev Gen Psych 1997;1:115–44.
13. Spencer S, Carver C, Price A. Psychological and social factors in adaptation. In: Holland JC, editor. Psycho-oncology. New York: Oxford University Press, 1998. p. 211–22.
14. Watson M, Greer S. Personality and coping. In: Holland JC, editor. Psycho-oncology. New York: Oxford University Press, 1998. p. 91–8.
15. Holland JC, Passik S, Kash KM, et al. The role of religious and spiritual beliefs in coping with malignant melanoma. Psycho-Oncology 1999;8:14–26.

16. Akizuki N, Yamawaki S, et al. Development of an impact thermometer to use in combination with the distress thermometer as a brief screening goal for adjustment disorders and/or major depression in cancer patients. J Pain Symptom Manage 2005;29:91–9.
17. Holland J, Lewis S. The human side of cancer. New York: Harper Collins; 2000.
18. Li J, Hanson D. Cancer incidence in parents after loss of a child: a nationwide study. Cancer 2002;95:2237–42.
19. Dalton SO, Boeson EH, et al. Mind and cancer: do psychological factors cause cancer? Euro J Cancer 2002;38:1313–23.
20. Rowland JH. Intrapersonal resources: developmental stage of adaptation: adult model. In: Holland JC, Rowland JH, editors. Handbook of psycho-oncology: psychological care of the patient with cancer. New York: Oxford University Press; 1989. p. 25–43.
21. Owen JE, Kawashima T, et al. Pain prevalence and retrospective incidence in childhood cancer survivors: childhood cancer survivor study. Psycho-Oncology 2005;14(Suppl):517.
22. Peretz T, Baider L, Ever-Hadani P, De-Nows AK. Psychological distress in female cancer patients with holocaust experience. Gen Hosp Psychiatry 1994;16:413–8.
23. Zabora J, BrintzenhofeSzoc K, Jacobsen, P, et al. A new psychosocial screening tool. Psychosomatics 2001;42:241–6.
24. Jacobsen P, Donovan K, Trask M, et al. Screening for psychological distress in ambulatory cancer patients: a multicenter evaluation of the distress thermometer. Cancer 2005;103:1494–02.
25. Baider L, Walach N, Perry S, Kaplan De-Nour A. Cancer in married couples: higher or lower distress? J Psychosom Res 1998;45:239–48.
26. Berkman L. The role of social relations in health promotion. Psychosom Med 1995; 57:245–54.
27. Helgeson V. Social support and quality of life. Qual Life Res Rev 2003;12(Suppl 1):25–31.
28. Marmot M. Status syndrome: how your social standing directly affects your health and life expectancy. London: Bloomburt & Henry Holt; 2004.
29. Steptoe A, Wardle J, Marmot M. Positive affect and health-related neuroendocrine, cardiovascular, and inflammatory processes. Proc Natl Acad Sci U S A 2005;102:6508–12.
30. Marmot M. Social determinants of health inequalities. Lancet 2005;365:1099–104.
31. Newell S, Sanson-Fisher R, Girgis A, Bonaventura A. How well do medical oncologist's perceptions reflect their patients' reported physical and psychosocial problems? Cancer 1998;83:1640–51.
32. Jacobsen PB, Bovbjerg DH, Schwartz M, et al. Conditioned emotional distress in women receiving chemotherapy for breast cancer. J Consult Clin Psychol 1995;63:108–114.
33. Van't-Spijker A, Trijsburg RW, Duivenvoorden HJ. Psychological sequelae of cancer diagnosis: a meta-analysis review of 58 studies after 1980. Psychosom Med 1997;59:280–93.
34. Musselman D, Lawson D, Gumnick J et al. Paroxetine for prevention of depression induced by high dose interferon alfa. N Engl J Med 2001;344:961–966.
35. Kissane D, Bloch S, Swath G, et al. Cognitive existential group psychotherapy for women with primary breast cancer: a randomized controlled trial. Psycho-Oncology 2003;12:532–546.
36. Nordin K, Glimelius B. Psychological reactions in newly diagnosed gastrointestinal cancer patients. Acta Oncologica 1997;36:803–10.
37. Twillman RK, Manetto C. Concurrent psychotherapy and pharmacotherapy in the treatment of depression and anxiety in cancer patients. Psycho-Oncology 1998;7:285–90.
38. Ebrahimi B, Tucker SL, et al . Cytokines in pancreatic carcinoma. Cancer 2004;101:2727–36.
39. Cassem E, Chochinov H, Breitbart W, editors. Care and management of the patient at the end of life. In: Handbook of psychiatry in palliative care. New York: Oxford University Press; 2000.
40. Aass SD, Fossa AA, Dahl, Moe TJ. Prevalence of anxiety and depression in cancer patients seen at the Norwegian Radium Hospital. Eur J Cancer 1997;33:1597–1604.
41. Roth AJ, Kornblith AB, Batel-Copel L, et al. Rapid screening for psychologic distress in men with prostate carcinoma: a pilot study. Cancer 1998;82:1904–8.
42. Payne DK, Hoffman RG, Theodoulou M, et al. Screening for anxiety and depression in women with breast cancer. Psychiatry and medical oncology gear up for managed care. Psychosomatics 1999;40:64–9.
43. Portenoy RK, Thaler HT, Kornblith AB, et al. Symptom prevalence, characteristics and distress in a cancer population. Qual Life Res 1994;3:189–94.
44. McQuellon RP, Wells M, Hoffman S, et al. Reducing distress in cancer patients with an orientation program. Psycho-Oncology 1998;7:207–17.
45. Hewitt M, Herdman R, Holland J, editors. Meeting psychosocial needs of women with breast cancer. Washington (DC): Institute of Medicine, National Academies Press; 2004.
46. Lee V, Cohen R, Edgar L. Clarifying "meaning" in the context of cancer research: a systematic literature review. Palliative Supportive Care 2004;2:291–303.
47. Grassi L, Indelli M, Marzola M, et al. Depressive symptoms and quality of life in home care-assisted cancer patients. J Pain Symptom Manage 1996;12:300–7.
48. Goldenberg D, Holland J, Schacter S. Palliative care in the chronically mentally ill. In: Breibart W, Chochinov H, editors. Psychiatric issues in palliative care. New York: Oxford University Press; 1999.
49. Schacter S, Coyle N. Palliative home care—impact on families. In: Holland JC, editor. Psycho-oncology. New York: Oxford University Press; 1998. p. 1004–15.
50. Chochinov H, Breitbart W, editors. Handbook of psychiatry in palliative medicine. New York: Oxford University Press; 2000.
51. Breitbart W, Payne D. Pain. In: Holland JC, editor. Psycho-oncology. New York: Oxford University Press; 1998. p. 450–67.
52. Fleishman S. Cancer cachexia. In: Holland JC, editor. Psycho-oncology. New York: Oxford University Press; 1998. p. 468–75.
53. Eccleston MS, Williams A. systematic review and meta-analysis of randomized controlled trials of cognitive behavior therapy, and behavior therapy for chronic pain in adults, excluding headache. Pain 1999;80:1–13.
54. Field N, Behrman R, editors. When children die: improving palliative and end-of-life care of children and their families. Washington DC: Institute of Medicine, The National Academies Press; 2003.
55. Assessing Treatment Impact Using Patient Reported Outcomes (PROs): Challenges in Study Design, Conduct, and Analysis. Meeting Report, Paris, May 10–11, 2004. Special Issue 3, Patient-Reported Outcomes Spring, 2005.
56. Holland J, Chertkov L. Clinical practice guidelines for the management of psychosocial and physical symptoms of cancer. In: Foley KM, Gelband H, editors. Improving palliative care for cancer. Washington (DC): National Academy Press; 2001. p. 199–232.
57. Chochinov HM. Dignity-conserving care—a new model for palliative care: helping the patient feel valued. J Am Med Assoc 2002;287:2253–60.
58. Greenstein M, Breitbart W. Cancer and the experience of meaning: a group psychotherapy program for people with cancer. Am J Psychotherapy 2000;54:486–500.
59. Breitbart, W. Spirituality and meaning-centered group psychotherapy interventions in advanced cancer. Supportive Care Cancer 2002;10:272–80.
60. Block SD, Billings JA. Patient request for euthanasia and assisted suicide in terminal illness. the role of the psychiatrist. Psychosomatics 1995;36:445–57.
61. Chochinov HM, Wilson KG, Ennis M, et al. Desire for death in the terminally ill. Am J Psychiatry 1995; 152:1185–91.
62. Chochinov HM, Wilson KG, Ennis M, Lander S. Are you depressed? Screening for depression in the terminally ill. Am J Psychiatry 1997;154:155.
63. Chochinov HM, Wilson KG, Ennis M, Lander S. Depression, hopelessness, and suicidal ideation in the terminally ill. Psychosomatics 1998;39:366–70.
64. Rauch P, Muriel A, Cassem N. Parents with cancer: who's looking after the children? J Clin Oncol 2002;20:4399–402.
65. Rauch P, Muriel A. The importance of parenting concerns among patients with cancer. Crit Rev Oncol Hematol 2004;49:37–42.
66. Kornblith A. Psychosocial adaptation of cancer survivors. In: Holland JC, editor. Psycho-oncology. New York: Oxford University Press; 1998. p. 223–56.
67. Hewitt M, Weiner SL, Simone JV, editors. Institute of Medicine. Childhood cancer survivorship: improving care and quality of life. Washington (DC): National Academies Press; 2003.
68. Ahles T, Saykin A, Furstenberg C, et al. Neuropsychologic impact of standard dose systemic chemotherapy in long term survivors of breast cancer and lymphoma. J Clin Oncol 2002;20:485–93.
69. Shagen SB, van Dam FS, Muller MJ, et al. Cognitive deficits after postoperative adjuvant chemotherapy for breast carcinoma cancer. Cancer 1999;85:640–50.
70. Ahles T, Saykin A. Mechanisms and vulnerabilities for chemotherapy-induced cognitive decline. Psycho-Oncology 2003;12(Suppl).
71. Sloan J, McLeod H, Sargeat J, et al. Preliminary evidence of relationship between genetic markers and oncology: patient quality of life (QOL) prior to treatment. Psycho-Oncology 2005;14(Suppl 519).
72. Kornblith AB, Anderson J, Cella DF, et al. Quality of life assessment of Hodgkin's disease survivors: a model for cooperative clinical trials. Oncology 1990;4:93–8.
73. Greenberg D, Kornblith A, Hendon J, et al. Quality of life for adult leukemia survivors treated on clinical trials of cancer and leukemia group B during the period 1971–1988: predictors for later psychological distress. Cancer 1997;80:1936–44.
74. Andersen BL, Woods XA, Copeland LJ. Sexual self-schema and sexual morbidity among gynecologic cancer survivors. J Consult Clin Psychol 1997;65:221–9.
75. Syrjala KL, Roth-Roemer SL, Abrams JR, et al. Prevalence and predictors of sexual dysfunction in long-term survivors of marrow transplantation. J Clin Oncol 1998;16:3148–57.
76. Maunsell E, Drolet M, Brisson C. Work situation after breast cancer: results from a population-based study. J Natl Cancer Inst 2004;96:1813–22.
77. Schover L. Myth busters: telling the true story of breast cancer survivorship. J Natl Cancer Inst 2004;96:1800–1.
78. Morrow G, Roscoe J, Hickok J. Nausea and vomiting. In: Holland JC, editor. Psycho-oncology. New York: Oxford University Press; 1998. p. 476–84.
79. Cella DF, Pratt A, Holland JC. Persistent anticipatory nausea, vomiting, and anxiety in cured Hodgkin's disease patients after completion of chemotherapy. Am J Psychiatry 1986;143:641.
80. Knowls R, Aaronson N, Uebelhart D. Physical exercise in cancer patients during and after medical treatment: a systematic review of randomized and controlled trials. J Clin Oncol 2005;23:3830–42.
81. Andrykowski MA, Cordova MJ. Factors associated with PTSD symptoms following treatment for breast cancer: test of the Andersen model. J Trauma 1998;11:189–203.
82. Reynolds M, Brewin CR. Intrusive memories in depression and posttraumatic stress disorder. Behav Res Ther 1999;37:201–15.
83. Kornblith A, Herudon J, Weiss R. Longterm adjustment of early stage breast cancer 20 years after adjuvant chemotherapy. Cancer 2003;98:679–689.
84. Robinson GE, Rosen BP, Bradley LN, et al. Psychological impact of screening for familial ovarian cancer: reactions to initial assessment. Gynecol Oncol 1997;65:197–205.
85. Croyle RT, Smith KR, Botkin JR, et al. Psychological responses to BRCA1 mutation testing: preliminary findings. Health Psychology 1997;16:63–72.
86. Meiser B. Psychological impact of genetic testing for cancer susceptibility: an update of the literature. Psycho-Oncology 2005;14:1–15.
87. Kash KM, Holland JC, Halper S, Miller DG. Psychological distress and surveillance behaviors of women with a family history of breast cancer. J Natl Cancer Inst 1992;84:24–30.
88. Lerman C, Kash K, Stefanek M. Younger women and increased risk for breast cancer: perceived risk, psychological well-being and surveillance behaviors. Monogr Natl Cancer Inst 1994;16:171–7.
89. Mandelblatt J, Schecter C, Yabriff K, et al. Benefits and costs of interventions to improve breast cancer outcomes in African American women. J Clin Oncol 2004;22:2554–66.
90. Watson M, Foster C, Eccles, R et al. Psychosocial impact of breast/ovarian (BRCA 1/2) cancer-predictive genetic testing in a UK multicentre cohort. J Breast Cancer 2004;91:1787–94.
91. Audrain J, Schwartz MD, Lerman C, et al. Psychological distress in women seeking genetic counseling for breast-ovarian cancer risk: the contributions of personality and appraisal. Ann Behav Med 1998;19:370–7.
92. Wainberg S, Husted J. Utilization of screening and preventative surgery among unaffected carriers of BRCA1 and BRCA2 gene mutation. Cancer Epidemial Biomarkers Prevention 2004;13:1989–95.
93. Jacobsen PB, Valdimarsdottier HB, et al. Decision-making about genetic testing among women at familial risk for breast cancer. Psychosom Med 1997;59:459–66.
94. Kash K, Holland J, et al. Psychological counseling strategies for women at risk of breast cancer. J Natl Cancer Inst Monogr 1995;17:73–8.
95. Lerman C, Hughes C, Lemon SJ, et al. What you don't know can hurt you: adverse psychological effects in members

of BRCA1-linked and BRCA2-linked families who decline genetic testing. J Clin Oncol 1998;16:1650–4.
96. Andrews LB, Fullerton JE, Holtzman NA, Motulsky AG. Assessing genetic risk: implications for health and social policy. Washington, DC: National Academy Press, 1994.
97. Hoffman B, Zevon M, et al. Screening for distress in cancer patients: The NCCN rapid screening measure. Psycho-Oncology 2004;13:1–8.
98. Turner J, Zapart S, Pedersen, K. Clinical Practice guidelines for psychosocial care of adults with cancer. Psycho-Oncology 2005;14:159–74.
99. Zabora J. The prevalence of psychological distress by cancer site. Psycho-Oncology 2001;10:19–28.
100. Passik SD, Dugan W, McDonald MV, et al. Oncologists' recognition of depression in their patients with cancer. J Clin Oncol 1998;16:1594–600.
101. Dugan W, McDonald MV, Passik SD, et al. Use of the Zung Self-Rating Depression Scale in cancer patients: feasibility as a screening tool. Psycho-Oncology 1999;7:483–93.
102. Derogatis LR, Morrow GR, Fetting D, et al. The prevalence of psychiatric disorders among cancer patients. JAMA 1983;249:751.
103. Strain J. Adjustment disorders. In: Holland JC, editor. New York: Oxford University Press; 1998. p. 509–17.
104. Barg FK, Cooley M, Pasacreta J, et al. Development of a self-administered psychosocial cancer screening tool. Cancer Practice 1994;2:288–96.
105. Farber DM, Wienerman BH, Kuypers JA. Psychosocial distress in oncology outpatients. J Psychosoc Oncol 1984;2:109.
106. Bukberg J, Penman D, Holland JC. Depression in hospitalized cancer patients. Psychosom Med 1984;46:199.
107. Andrykowski MA, Redd WH. Longitudinal analysis of the development of anticipatory nausea. J Consult Clin Psychol 1987;55:36.
108. Redd WH, Jacobsen PB, Die-Trill M, et al. Cognitive/attentional distraction in the control of conditioned nausea in pediatric oncology patients receiving chemotherapy. J Consult Clin Psychol 1987;55:391.
109. Payne D, Massie M. Anxiety in palliative care. In: Chochinov H, Breitbart W, editors. Handbook of psychiatry in palliative medicine. New York: Oxford University Press; 2000.
110. Noyes R, Jr., Holt C, Massie M. Anxiety disorders. In: Holland JC, editor. Psycho-oncology. New York: Oxford University Press, 1998. p. 548–63.
111. Burton MV, Parker RW, Farrell A, et al. A randomized controlled trial of preoperative psychological preparation for mastectomy. Psycho-Oncology 1995;4:1–19.
112. Fawzy FI, Fawzy NW. A structured psychoeducational intervention for cancer patients. Gen Hosp Psychiatry 1994;16:149–92.
113. Moorey S, Greer S, Watson M, et al. Adjuvant psychological therapy for patients with cancer: outcome at one year. Psycho-Oncology 1994;3:1–10.
114. Moorey S, Greer S, Bliss J, Law M. A comparison of adjuvant psychological therapy and supportive counseling in patients with cancer. Psycho-Oncology 1998;7:218–28.
115. Meyer T, Mark M. Effects of psychosocial interventions with adult cancer patients: a meta-analysis of randomized experiments. Health Psychology 1995;14:101–8.
116. Jacobsen PB, Hann D. Cognitive-behavioral interventions. In: Holland JC, editor. Psycho-oncology. New York: Oxford University Press; 1998. p. 717–29.
117. Kabat-Zinn J, Massion AO, Hebert J, Rosenbaum E. Meditation. In: Holland JC, editor. Psycho-oncology. New York: Oxford University Press; 1998. p. 767–79.
118. Roth AJ, Holland JC. Treatment of depression in cancer patients. Primary Care and Cancer 1994;14,23–9.
119. Coups E, Winell J, Holland J. Depression in the context of cancer. In: Lucinio J, Ma-LeWong W, editors. Volume 1. Biology of depression: from novel insights to therapeutic strategies. Weinheim (Germany): Wiley; 2005. p. 365–85.
120. McDaniel JS, Musselman DL, Porter MR. Depression in cancer: diagnosis, biology, and treatment. Gen Psych 1995;52:89–99.
121. Lerner DM, Stoudemire A, Rosenstein DL. Cytokine-induced neuropsychiatric toxicity. In: Holland SM, editor. Cytokine therapeutics in infectious diseases. Philadelphia: Lippincott/Williams and Wilkins; 2001. p. 323–32.
122. Breitbart W, Payne D. Psychiatric aspects of pain management in patients with adrenal cancer and AIDS. In: Chochinov H, W Breitbart, editors. Handbook of psychiatry in palliative medicine. New York: Oxford University Press; 2000. p. 131–61.
123. Wilson K, Chochinov H, de Faye B, et al. Diagnosis and management of depression in palliative care. In: Chochinov H, Breitbart W, editors. Handbook of psychiatry in palliative medicine. New York: Oxford University Press; 2000. p. 25–51.
124. Bolund C. Suicide and cancer. I: Demographical and suicidological description of suicides among cancer patients in Sweden. J Psychosoc Oncol 1985;3:17.
125. Bolund C. Suicide and cancer. II: Medical and care factors in suicide by cancer patients in Sweden, 1973–1976. J Psychosoc Oncol 1986;3:31.
126. Rosenfeld B, Krevo S, Breitbart W, et al. Suicide, assisted suicide, and euthanasia in the terminally ill. In: Chochinov H, Breitbart W, editors. Handbook of psychiatry in palliative medicine. New York: Oxford University Press; 2000. p. 51–63.
127. Hietanen P, Lonnqvist J. Cancer and suicide. Ann Oncol 1991;2:19.
128. Conwell Y, Caine ED. Rational suicide and the right to die: reality and myth. N Engl J Med 1991;325:1100.
129. Breitbart W, Cohen K. Delirium. In: Holland JC, editor. Psycho-oncology. New York: Oxford University Press; 1998. p. 564–75.
130. Musselman DL, Lawson DH, Gumnick JF, et al. Paroxetine for the prevention of depression induced by high-dose interferon alpha. N Engl J Med 2001;344:961–6.
131. Breitbart W, Marotta R, Platt M, et al. A double-blind trial of haloperidol, chlorpromazine and lorazepam in treatment of delirium in hospitalized AIDS patients. Am J Psychiatry 1996;153:231–7.
132. Moynihan C, Bliss JM, Davidson J, et al. Evaluation of adjuvant psychological therapy in patients with testicular cancer: randomized controlled trial. BMJ 1998;316:429–35.
133. Burton M, Watson M. Counseling People with cancer. New York: John Wiley & Sons; 1998.
134. Loscalzo M, BrintzenhofeSzoc K. Brief crisis counseling. In: Holland JC, editor. Psycho-oncology. New York: Oxford University Press; 1998. p. 662–75.
135. Fawzy F, Fawzy N. Psychoeducational interventions. In: Holland JC, editor. Psycho-oncology. New York, NY: Oxford University Press; 1998, p. 676–93.
136. Holland JC, Romano SJ, Heiligenstein JH, et al. A controlled trial of fluoxetine and desipramine in depressed women with advanced cancer. Psycho-Oncology 1998;7:291–300.
137. Bruera E, Neumann, CM. The uses of psychotropics in symptom management in advanced cancer. Psycho-Oncology 1998;7:346–58.
138. Breitbart W. Psychotropic adjuvant analgesics for pain in cancer and AIDS. Psycho-Oncology 1998;7:333–45.
139. Kissane DW, Bloch S, Miach P, et al. Cognitive-existential group therapy for patients with primary breast cancer—techniques and themes. Psycho-Oncology 1997;6:25–33.
140. Edmonds CVI, Lockwood GA, Cunningham AJ. Psychological response to long term group therapy: a randomized trial with metastatic breast cancer patients. Psycho-Oncology 1999;8:74–91.
141. Boesen E, Ross L, Frederiksen K, Thomsen B. Psychoeducational intervention for patients with cutaneous malignant melanoma: a replication study. J Clin Oncol 2005;23:1270–7.
142. Petticrew M, Bell R, Hunter D. Influence of psychological coping on survival and recurrence in people with cancer: systematic review. BMJ 2002;325:1066.
143. Spiegel D, Kraemer H, Bloom JR, Gottheil D. Effect of psychosocial treatment on survival of patients with metastatic breast cancer. Lancet 1989;2:8.
144. Fawzy FI, Fawzy NW, Hyun CS, et al. Malignant melanoma: effects of early unstructured psychiatric intervention coping and affective state of recurrence and survival 6 years later. Arch Gen Psychiatry 1993;50:681.
145. Goodwin PJ, Leszcz M, Ennis M, Koopmans J, et al. The effect of group psychosocial support on survival in metastatic breast cancer. N Engl J Med. 2001;345:1719–26
146. Gellert GA, Maxwell RM, Siegel BS. Survival of breast cancer patients receiving adjunctive psychosocial support therapy: a 10-year follow-up study. J Clin Oncol 1993;11:66.
147. Kissane D, Grabsch B. Supportive-expressive group therapy: the transformation of existential ambivalence into creating living while enhancing adherence to anti-cancer therapies. Psycho-Oncology 2004;13:155–69.
148. Luzzatto P, Gabriel B. Art psychotherapy. In: Holland JC, editor. Psycho-oncology. New York: Oxford University Press; 1998. p. 743–57.
149. Eisenberg DM, Davis RB, Ettner ST, et al. Trends in alternative medicine use in the united states, 1990–1970: results of a follow-up national survey. JAMA 1998;280:1569–75.
150. Burstein HJ, Gelber S, Guadagnoli E, Weeks JC. Use of alternative medicine by women with early stage breast cancer. N Engl J Med 1999;340:1733–9.
151. Holland JC. Use of alternative medicine–a marker for distress? N Engl J Med 1999;340:1758–9.
152. Jacobsen PB, Hann DM. Cognitive-behavioral interventions. In: Holland JC, editor. Psycho-oncology. New York, NY: Oxford University Press; 1998. p. 717–29.
153. Outcome Measurement Working Group. (COMCUG). NCL, outcomes assessment in cancer: measures, methods, and applications. J Lipscomb C. Gotacy C Snyder, editors. Cambridge University Press, 2005. When Do They Add Value? Meeting Report, Assessing Treatment Impact Using Patient Reported Outcomes (PROs): Challenges in Study Design, Conduct; an Analysis. Paris, May 10–11, 2004.
154. Karnofsky DA, Burchenal JH. The clinical evaluation of chemotherapeutic agents in cancer. In: McLeod CM, editor. Evaluation of chemotherapeutic agents. New York: Columbia University Press; 1949. p. 191.
155. Lipscomb J, Gotay CG, Snyder C, editors. Outcomes assessment in cancer: measures, methods, and applications. Cambridge: Cambridge University Press; 2005.
156. Schipper H, Clinch J, McMurray A, Levitt M. Measuring the quality of life of cancer patients: the functional living index-cancer development and validation. J Clin Oncol 1984;2:472.
157. Schag CC, Heinrich RL. CARES. Cancer Rehabilitation Evaluation System: Development of a comprehensive quality of life measurement tool. Oncology 1990;4:135–8.
158. Aaronson NK, Bakker W, Stewart AL, et al. Multidimensional approach to the measurement of quality of life in lung cancer clinical trials. In: Aaronsen NK, Beckmann J, editors. The quality of life of cancer patients. New York: Raven Press; 1987. p. 63–82.
159. Cella D, Tulsky D, Gray G, et al. The functional assessment of cancer therapy scale: development and validation of the general measurement. J Clin Oncol 1993;11:570.
160. Spitzer WO, Dobson AJ, Hall J, et al. Measuring the quality of life of cancer patients: a concise QL-index for use by physicians. J Chron Dis 1981;34:585.
161. Bergner M, Bobbitt RA, Carter WB, Gilson BS. The Sickness Impact Profile: development and final revision of a health status measure. Med Care 1981;19:787.
162. Derogatis LR, Lopez M. PAIS and PAIS-SR: administration, scoring, and procedures manual. I. Baltimore: In Clinical Psychometric Research, 1983.
163. Cleeland CS, Mendoza TR, Wang, XS, et al. Assessing symptom distress in cancer patients: The MD Anderson symptom inventory. Cancer 2000;89:1634–46.
164. Stewart AL, Hays RD, Ware JE. The MOS Shortform General Health Survey: reliability and validity in a patient population. Med Care 1988;26:724.
165. Speice J, Harkness J, Laneri H, et al.. Involving Family members in cancer care: focus group considerations of patients and oncological providers. Psycho-Oncology: Journal of the Psychological, Social and Behavioral Dimensions of Cancer 2000;9,101–12.
166. Levine C. Rough crossings: family caregivers—odysseys through the health care system. New York: United Hospital Fund; 1998. p. 66.
167. Shear K, Frank E. Treatment of complicated grief: a randomized controlled trial. JAMA 2005; 293:2601–8.
168. Levav I, Kohn R, Iscovich J, et al. Cancer incidence and survival following bereavement. Am J Public Health 2000;90:1601–7.
169. Oksbjerg, S, Dalton, L, Mellenkjaer, J et al. Depression and cancer risk: a register-based study of patients hospitalized with affective disorders. Am J Epidemiol 2002;155:1088–95.
170. Schapiro, I, Folgaard, N, Jergensen, T et al. Personality and risk for cancer. Am J Epidemiol 2001;153:757–63.
171. Aiken LH, Clarke SP, Sloane DM, et al. Hospital nurse staffing and patient mortality, nurse burnout and job dissatisfaction. JAMA 2002;288:1987–93.
172. Mount BM. Dealing with our losses. J Clin Oncol 1986;4:1127–34.
173. Whippen DA, Canellos GP. Burnout syndrome in the practice of oncology: results of a random survey of 1,000 oncologists. J Clin Oncol 1991;9:1916–20.
174. Kash KM, Holland JC, et al. Stress and burnout in oncology. Oncology 2000;14:1621–33.

Section 18

ONCOLOGY NURSING

60

Principles of Oncology Nursing

Paula Trahan Rieger, RN, MSN, AOCN, FAAN

Cancer management is an interdisciplinary endeavor; thus, an understanding of the principles of oncology nursing is fundamental to the effective practice of all other oncology subspecialties. Oncology nurses are engaged in collaborative practice with all members of the health care team to provide optimal management of patients with cancer. Their professional practice requires detailed knowledge of the biologic and psychosocial dimensions of cancer as a disease and its impact on the lives of patients and their loved ones. Oncology nurses have key roles as caregivers, as well as providers of patient and family education, in clinical cancer research, in health care administration, and as advanced oncology nurse practitioners. Cancer nurses also are continuously involved in the enhancement of nursing practice through research, continuing education, and advanced education.

ONCOLOGY NURSING AS A SPECIALTY

Historically, nurses have had a special role in the care of patients with cancer, a role that was especially significant in those few institutions devoted exclusively to cancer care before the National Cancer Act of 1971. However, the expanded research and treatment program against cancer that has occurred during the past quarter-century has been a catalyst for the development of oncology nursing as a separate specialty.[1–5] The recognition of cancer as a major national health problem was key to formally establishing the specialty of oncology nursing. This increased attention to cancer coincided with and complemented a major new emphasis in the nursing profession toward expanded roles in comprehensive patient care. Many oncology nurses first worked as both nurses and data managers for cancer research studies. As oncology called for increasingly more complex therapy, the collaborative relationship between nurse and physician became, and continues to be, the best way to provide uniquely comprehensive patient care.[6,7]

The Oncology Nursing Society (ONS) was established by a small group of nurses working primarily in research settings with medical oncologists involved in clinical research.[4,8] Its initial goals were to provide a forum for discussing practice issues in cancer nursing and to develop mechanisms for nurses to contribute to this new and evolving specialty area. There was a need to promote the practice of oncology nurses in different care settings, to promote advanced practice, to develop national and local networking, and to develop continuing education programs. Research in cancer nursing subsequently became a high priority of the ONS. The success of this national organization has contributed to the recognition of oncology nursing as a valued specialty.[4]

Today, the ONS has a membership of more than 31,000 registered nurses (RNs) and other health care professionals and 220 chapters across the United States. The majority of members (65%) provide direct patient care.[9] Educational conferences, publications, activities related to health policy, and research initiatives are just a few of the concentrated areas of effort. The ONS Foundation, which was established in 1981, has awarded more than $14 million (US) in research grants, scholarships, and awards since its inception. The ONS Foundation is the largest funder of oncology nursing research outside the US government.[10]

The development of nursing standards has been a primary purpose of the American Nurses Association (ANA) since the late 1960s, and the ANA published the first nursing standards of practice in 1973.[11] These first nursing standards were generic in nature and focused on the nursing process. The standards were the catalyst toward defining quality nursing care. Shortly thereafter, many nursing organizations developed standards of practice specific to the various specialty practices that exist within the nursing profession. In 1979, ONS, in collaboration with ANA, published *Outcome Standards for Cancer Nursing Practice*.[12] A second collaborative effort in 1987 led to the development of *Standards of Oncology Nursing Practice*,[11] and this document was revised in 1996 to form the *Statement on the Scope and Standards of Oncology Nursing Practice*.[13] In 2004, to reflect the dynamic changes present in oncology nursing practice, ONS published the 2004 *Statement on the Scope and Standards of Oncology Nursing Practice* (Table 60-1).[14] ONS has also developed advanced practice standards (Table 60-2).[15,16] These standards serve as a definition of the highest quality of oncology nursing practice.

CERTIFICATION

In 1985, ONS established the Oncology Nursing Certification Corporation (ONCC) to provide an examination for the formal certification of oncology nurses. Certification in oncology nursing promotes continuing education and communicates to the public and other professionals that an oncology nurse has specialized knowledge and expertise. Nurses who pass the generalist certification examination may use the oncology certified nurse (OCN) credential with their signature. After OCNs earn the credential by testing, they have the option of using ONC-PRO for all subsequent renewals, provided that they do not let their certification lapse. The ONC-PRO program allows the renewal candidate to accrue points through continuing education, academic education, publications, and presentations or by participation in test item writing for the certification examination. Renewal by retesting is an option if that is the nurse's preference. As of May 2005, more than 21,000 oncology nurses have been certified.[17] In the fall of 1999, the ONCC began to offer pediatric oncology nursing certification and the certified pediatric oncology nurse (CPON) credential.

Table 60-1 Standards of Oncology Nursing Practice

Standards of Care

I. Assessment: The oncology nurse systematically and continually collects data regarding the health status of the client.

II. Diagnosis: The oncology nurse analyzes assessment data in determining nursing diagnoses.

III. Outcome identification: The oncology nurse identifies expected outcomes individualized to the patient.

IV. Planning: The oncology nurse develops an individualized and holistic plan of care that prescribes interventions to attain expected outcomes.

V. Implementation: The oncology nurse implements the plan of care to achieve the identified expected outcomes for the patient.

VI. Evaluation: The oncology nurse systematically and regularly evaluates the patient's responses to interventions to determine progress toward achievement of expected outcomes.

Standards of Professional Performance

I. Quality of care: The oncology nurse systematically evaluates the quality of care and effectiveness of oncology nursing practice within all practice settings.

II. Practice evaluation: The oncology nurse consistently evaluates his or her own nursing practice in relation to job-specific performance expectations, statewide regulatory requirements, and national oncology nursing professional standards.

III. Education: The oncology nurse acquires and improves his or her current knowledge base related to cancer care and oncology nursing that fosters enhanced competence and critical thinking skills.

IV. Collegiality: The oncology nurse contributes to the professional development of unlicensed and licensed peers and interdisciplinary colleagues.

V. Ethics: The oncology nurse uses ethical principles as a basis for decision making and patient advocacy.

VI. Collaboration: The oncology nurse partners with patients, families, the interdisciplinary team, and community resources to provide optimal care.

VII. Research: The oncology nurse contributes to the scientific base of nursing practice, education, and management via multiple venues: identifying clinical dilemmas and problems appropriate for rigorous study, collecting data, critiquing existing research, and making use of research.

VIII. Resource utilization: The oncology nurse considers factors related to safety, effectiveness, and cost in planning and delivering client care.

IX. Leadership: The oncology nurse anticipates the dynamic nature of cancer care and readies herself or himself and colleagues for an evolving future.

Adapted from Brant JM and Wickham RS.[14]

Table 60-2 Standards of Advanced Oncology Nursing Practice

Standard I. Assessment

The oncology APN collects comprehensive clinical and research data from patients and their families.

Standard II. Diagnosis

The oncology APN synthesizes and critically analyzes assessment data to determine diagnoses/problems.

Standard III. Outcomes

The oncology APN identifies expected outcomes derived from evidence-based clinical outcome data.

Standard IV. Plan

The oncology APN develops an individualized, holistic, and comprehensive plan of care for patients based on the diagnoses/problems that includes ongoing assessment and management of identified problems in collaboration with other members of the health care team.

Standard V. Implementation

The oncology APN prescribes and implements interventions and treatments consistent with the plan of care to achieve expected outcomes.

Standard Va. Case Management/Coordination of Care

The oncology APN coordinates and provides both evidence-based care and overall case management.

Standard Vb. Consultation

The oncology APN provides consultation to professional colleagues, patients, and families regarding clinical, research, and administrative nursing issues.

Standard Vc. Health Promotion, Health Maintenance, and Health Education

The oncology APN promotes, maintains, and improves the health of patients with cancer and their families as related to the potential or actual cancer diagnosis, treatment, and subsequent late effects. The oncology APN prevents and minimizes illness and injury with regard to a potential or actual cancer diagnosis and treatment.

Standard Vd. Prescriptive Authority and Treatments

The oncology APN uses prescriptive authority and treatments in accordance with institutional, state, and federal laws and regulations to manage the potential or actual cancer diagnosis, treatment, and late effects of treatment.

Standard Ve. Referral

The oncology APN facilitates appropriate referrals when the need for further evaluation and additional resources is identified.

Standard VI. Evaluation

The oncology APN evaluates responses to the comprehensive treatment plan and determines whether the outcomes were achieved.

Standards of Professional Performance

Standard I: Quality of Care

The oncology APN uses quality of care criteria for clinical outcomes and for determining the effectiveness of clinical care.

Standard II. Self-Evaluation

The oncology APN continuously evaluates his or her advanced nursing practice in an effort to provide competent, evidence-based clinical care.

Standard III. Education

The oncology APN in practice demonstrates a well-rounded, theoretic, research-based, state-of-the science, clinically strong knowledge base in oncology nursing and related disciplines.

Standard IV. Leadership

The oncology APN serves as a leader, role model, and mentor for the professional development of peers and colleagues.

Standard V. Ethics

The oncology APN demonstrates ethical behavior during all interactions with patients, families, organizations, and communities.

Standard VI. Multidisciplinary Process

The oncology APN promotes a multidisciplinary approach to providing advanced oncology nursing care to patients and families related to potential or actual cancer diagnoses and treatments.

Standard VII. Research

The oncology APN utilizes evidence to identify, examine, validate, and evaluate knowledge, theories, and creative approaches to health care.

Adapted from Jacobs LA.[16]
APN = advanced practice nurse.

Today more than 978 nurses are certified as CPONs.

ONS was the first nursing specialty organization to provide certification for advanced practice nurses (APNs). In 1994, 1998, and 2003, the ONCC conducted role delineation studies to distinguish advanced practice nursing from basic nursing practice in oncology and to describe the professional roles and practice behaviors of advanced oncology nurses.[18,19] The first advanced certification, the advanced oncology certified nurse (AOCN) test, was based on the results of these studies. Unique to the advanced examination is the requirement that an oncology nurse must have at least a master's degree. Nurses who passed the advanced examination were allowed to use the AOCN credential with their signature. As of 2005, there are more than 1,495 AOCNs.

In April 2004, the ONCC Board of Directors approved significant changes to advanced certification in oncology nursing. Beginning in January 2005, ONCC will offer role-specific advanced practice certification examinations: the advanced oncology certified nurse practitioner (AOCNP) and the advanced oncology certified clinical nurse specialist (AOCNS). The most important factors weighed in the decision were the results of the role delineation study of advanced practice nursing, which was completed in 2003. The study revealed that although oncology NPs and oncology clinical nurse specialists (CNSs) share a common knowledge base, discernible differences exist in their work responsibilities. Nurses who currently are AOCN certified may renew their credential through the ONC-PRO program for as long as they desire to keep the AOCN credential.[20] Table 60-3 describes the eligibility criteria

Table 60-3 Eligibility Criteria for Oncology Nursing Certification

Oncology Certified Nurse (OCN) Certified Pediatric Oncology Nurse (CPON)	Advanced (AOCN) Certificate (Renewal Only)	Advanced Oncology Certified Nurse Practitioner (AOCNP)	Advanced Oncology Certified Clinical Nurse Specialist (AOCNS)
Current RN license	Current RN license	Current RN license	Current RN license
Minimum of 1 yr experience as an RN within 3 yr prior to application	A master's or higher degree in nursing, preferably with a focus in oncology	A master's or higher degree in nursing	A master's or higher degree in nursing
Minimum of 1,000 h of oncology nursing (pediatric for CPON) practice within 2½ yr before application	Minimum of 2½ yr experience as an RN within the 5 yr prior to application	Successful completion of a nurse practitioner program	Minimum of 500 h of supervised practice in an advanced practice role in oncology nursing
Completion of a minimum of 10 contact h of continuing education in the specialty of oncology nursing or an academic elective in oncology nursing (for initial certification only)	Minimum of 2,000 h of oncology nursing practice within the 5 yr before application	Minimum 500 h of supervised clinical practice as an oncology nurse practitioner	

Adapted from Oncology Nursing Certification Corporation.[21]
RN = registered nurse.

for oncology nursing certification at both the generalist and advanced levels.[21]

ONCOLOGY NURSING EDUCATION

Educational curricula have been developed and implemented to provide oncology nurses with an appropriate understanding of genetics, cancer biology, epidemiology, prevention, detection and diagnosis, treatment and symptom management, nursing practice issues, and trends in cancer care. Cancer nursing texts[22–27] and journals, such as *Oncology Nursing Forum*, *Clinical Journal of Oncology Nursing*, *Cancer Nursing*, and *Seminars in Oncology Nursing*, focus on these topics. Cancer nursing is part of the general undergraduate curricula, and more than 25 graduate nursing educational curricula offer a master's degree with a specialty in oncology. In addition, doctoral programs and oncology nursing professorships have been established.

Approximately 36% of ONS members have a bachelor's degree in nursing, 24% have an associate degree, and 13% have a diploma. Over 17% of ONS members have a master's degree or higher. Membership in the ONS offers opportunities for the study and education necessary to qualify for the OCN, AOCNP, and AOCNS credentials by passing the certification examinations. Increasingly, educational preparation at the master's level is specified in many oncology job descriptions. For example, a master's degree is required for oncology CNSs and NPs. Typically, over 12% of ONS members are pursuing additional education at the baccalaureate or graduate level.[9]

ONCOLOGY NURSING RESEARCH

The evolution of oncology nursing research as a foundation for oncology nursing practice has been extraordinary since the inception of the specialty. From a modest beginning in the 1970s, nursing research evolved in the 1980s to the identification of research priorities, companion studies in cooperative group clinical trials, and initial programs of research and funding. In the 1990s, continued advances have included increased funding sources, research through state-of-the-knowledge conferences, and major areas of studies (eg, fatigue, quality of life, pain), which are having a noteworthy impact on cancer care.[28] ONS has conducted five research priority surveys since 1981. The top 20 research priorities, in rank order, from the most recent survey were, quality of life, participation in decision making about treatment in advanced disease, patient/family education, participation in decision making about treatment, pain, tobacco use and exposure, screening/early detection of cancer, prevention of cancer/cancer risk reduction, palliative care, evidence-based practice, nurses as advocates, fatigue/lack of energy, cancer recurrence, curative treatment/care, patient outcomes of cancer care, cognitive impairment/mental status changes, late effects of treatment, hospice/end of life, initial cancer diagnosis, and ethical issues.[29]

As a result of today's health care environment, the nursing profession is challenged by insurers, health policy makers, and managed care organizations to demonstrate the effectiveness of nursing care through research that examines the link between specific nursing interventions and patient outcomes. In 2003, ONS developed a definition of "oncology nursing sensitive patient outcomes" and a strategic plan for ONS in relation to outcomes of care for individuals with cancer that are sensitive to nursing. Outcomes, which focus on how patients and their health care problems are affected by nursing interventions, have been identified and are described as nursing-sensitive patient outcomes and result in changes in patients' symptom experience, functional status, safety, psychological distress, and/or costs. Since the inception of ONS, more than 300 nursing research studies have been funded. ONS and the National Cancer Institute sponsor two cancer nursing research short courses each year to help nurses with their study designs and to address use of research findings. Additionally, ONS has a research agenda to identify the types of research needed, areas that need additional research, and resources necessary to achieve research goals.[30]

HEALTH POLICY

Historically, professional nurses have been extensively involved in political advocacy. Professional nursing organizations provide opportunities for nurses to collectively address health care issues and to influence the development of sound public policy. ONS's involvement with health policy began with its incorporation as a specialty nursing professional organization in 1975. Today ONS is recognized, alongside other professional organizations, as an important voice on issues related to cancer care. For each Congressional session, the ONS Board develops a health policy agenda and actively advocates on Capitol Hill for those issues on behalf of patients and the profession. Increasingly, ONS members are participating in equal parity with professionals of other health care disciplines to promote development of health policy and associated regulations and serve as consultants, providing their unique perspective on proposed legislation. ONS members have been appointed to the National Cancer Advisory Board, the National Cancer Institute Board of Scientific Advisors, and the Institute of Medicine's National Cancer Policy Board. ONS has sponsored educational sessions at its annual congress on health policy and advocacy skills for members and regional workshops on health policy skills.[31]

ROLE OF THE ONCOLOGY NURSE

Oncology nurses practice in a variety of settings, including acute care hospitals, ambulatory care clinics, private oncologists' offices, radiation therapy facilities, home health care agencies, and community agencies. They practice in association with a number of oncologic disciplines, including surgical oncology, radiation oncology, gynecologic oncology, pediatric oncology, and medical oncology. The majority of ONS members are involved in direct patient care and practice at the generalist level, with approximately 40% working in an inpatient setting, 9% in a hospital-based outpatient clinic, 16% in physician offices, and 9% in hospice or home care.[9] Positions in the outpatient and home care setting continue to increase as the preference for patient treatment remains outside the hospital setting.[32,33] The roles of the oncology nurse vary from the intensive care focus of bone marrow transplantation to the community focus of cancer screening, detection, and prevention.

As the health care delivery system changes and new scientific discoveries are integrated into cancer care, the role of the oncology nurse will continue to evolve. Oncology nurses currently work in a variety of roles and settings that were unheard of 10 years ago but are now increasingly commonplace. In the ambulatory setting, oncology nurses function in nurse-run clinics that provide services such as long-term follow-up care to patients with cancer, prescreening prior to chemotherapy administration, the management of fatigue, or general symptom management. As the field of cancer genetics has developed, so have roles for APNs in the provision of cancer genetic counseling and risk assessment.[34] Oncology nurses serve in numerous leadership positions, such as chief executive officers, directors of cancer service lines, and directors of admission services, at hospitals and clinics.

The following discussion on the role of the oncology nurse focuses on patient assessment, patient education, coordination of care, direct patient care, symptom management, and supportive care. To illustrate how varied the role may be and its importance across the continuum of cancer care, examples related to the role of the oncology nurse in direct patient care, symptom management, and supportive care are provided.

PATIENT ASSESSMENT

Nurses are expected to be expert in assessing a patient's physical and emotional status, health history, health practices, and both the patient's and the family's knowledge of the disease and its treatment. The oncology nurse reviews the treatment plan with the oncologist, is aware of expected outcomes and possible complications, and independently assesses the patient's general physical and emotional status. It is essential that a detailed nursing history and physical examination be completed. An oncology nurse is expected to be aware of the results and general implications of all relevant laboratory, pathology, and imaging studies. Assessment of the patient's understanding of the disease and proposed treatment is fundamental in allaying anxiety and formulating a care plan. Obtaining this information will help avoid misunderstanding and confused expectations. Thorough patient preparation improves compliance with treatment programs and may impact treatment outcomes as well. A nursing care plan is developed in response to the particular needs identified from the assessment.[14] At a minimum, this plan promotes (1) the patient's understanding of therapy goals, treatment schedules, and possible side effects of therapy; (2) physical and psychological preparation for therapy; (3) physical and psychological comfort; and (4) compliance.

PATIENT EDUCATION

The nurse often has a better opportunity than any other member of the health care team to develop the required rapport for effective educational efforts with patients and their families. Patient and family education starts before therapy and continues during and after therapy. Continual reinforcement throughout the treatment course helps ensure success. Appropriate written and visual teaching aids may be used, as well as referrals to other professionals or community programs, such as cancer support groups. Such education includes structured and unstructured experiences to assist patients with coping with their diagnosis, long-term adjustments, and symptoms; to gain information about prevention, diagnosis, and care; and to develop skills, knowledge, and attitudes to maintain or regain health status. This planned education uses a combination of methods that best meet the needs, capabilities, and learning style of the patient.[35] The ONS has enhanced this definition by recommending the following patient education outcome criteria[36]: the patient and/or family should be able to (1) describe the state of the disease and therapy at a level consistent with the patient's educational and emotional status; (2) participate in the decision-making process pertaining to the plan of care and life activities; (3) identify appropriate community resources that provide information and services; (4) describe appropriate actions for highly predictable problems, oncologic emergencies, and major side effects of the disease and/or therapy; and (5) describe the schedule when ongoing therapy is predicted.

The change to outpatient administration of chemotherapy has increased the necessity for accurate and thorough patient and family education. This requires nurses to understand the possible side effects of each antineoplastic agent and the self-care activities for reducing their severity. Describing the side effects or problems that patients might experience from the regimen as a whole is more effective than focusing on each separate drug. Patients often express more concern about the occurrence and management of side effects than the mechanism of action of particular agents. Reiteration of important points will assist in achieving the desired outcome. Identifying a time sequence in which side effects generally occur may allay patient anxiety and will assist nurses in selecting the appropriate interventions. This may help distinguish the side effects of chemotherapy from other possible causes of similar symptoms. Patient education is facilitated when the side effects are classified as immediate, early, delayed, and late.

A variety of teaching tools and methods are available, the choice of which is based on individual patient needs and abilities. Printed, visual, and audiovisual educational materials are used in conjunction with discussion and continued reinforcement. With the increased development of the Internet, more and more cancer patients and family members are accessing the World Wide Web to gain information about cancer. Chat groups are serving as a source of information and support. This method of communication will continue to be an increasing source of knowledge for consumers.

Patients should be encouraged to keep personal, written, daily diaries that record treatment dates, symptoms, test dates, and questions. A personal diary provides additional written documentation of the onset of specific phenomena and accurate dates of therapy, in case the patient's medical record is not available.

COORDINATION OF CARE

The oncology nurse plays a vital role in coordinating the multiple and complex technologies now commonly employed in cancer diagnosis and treatment. This coordination encompasses direct patient care; documentation in the medical record; participation in therapy across care settings; symptom management; organization of referrals to other health care providers; and both patient and family education, as well as counseling throughout diagnosis, therapy, and follow-up. The nurse often serves as the patient's first line of communication. Many patients travel long distances, so the importance of communication by telephone must be emphasized. It allows continuous patient communication, early recognition of emergencies, and regular emotional support. Many institutions have developed guidelines for triaging telephone calls and problems. These guidelines provide basic steps that are helpful in identifying patient problems over the telephone before consulting with the physician and relaying specific instructions for follow-up care.[37]

Modern cancer care is performed at multiple sites by a variety of personnel at a pace that is accelerated by a cost-conscious staff. Communication between personnel at different facilities may be suboptimal, and the communication and coordination that the oncology nurse can provide represent an invaluable service to patients and families.

DIRECT PATIENT CARE

The majority of ONS members provide direct patient care, which often involves the administration of chemotherapy. National certification for chemotherapy currently does not exist. Each institution or practice should have written policies for chemotherapy certification, administration of antineoplastic drugs (all routes), safe drug handling and disposal, management of untoward reactions, such as allergic reactions, and methods for documentation. ONS currently offers a chemotherapy trainers course. These trainers may then offer chemotherapy training courses in the community to oncology nurses based on ONS guidelines and curriculum.

An important responsibility of nurses involved in the delivery of chemotherapy is to ensure that the correct dose and the correct drug are administered by the correct route to the right patient. Because of the complexity of chemotherapy regimens, requirements for supportive care drugs, and the physiologic vulnerability of patients owing to their malignancies and intensive therapies, patients with cancer should be the focus of interdisciplinary medication error prevention programs. Nurses play a critical role in patient safety and the implementation of preventive and risk-reducing interventions to improve the drug delivery process.[38] A report from the Institute of Medicine noted that more people die annually from medication errors than from workplace injuries. A national agenda with state and local implications for reducing medical errors and improving patient safety has been set forth. Recommendations are devoted to a safer health care system.[39] In 2001, ONS published its position statement on the prevention and reporting of medication errors, which provides recommendations for practice, policy, systems, education, and research for the delivery of safe care.[40] It is recommended that individual institutional guidelines include a reporting system for errors and a systematic way to review current practice to provide changes to prevent repetition of errors.

SYMPTOM MANAGEMENT

Oncology nurses are challenged on a daily basis to deal with the numerous symptoms that patients with cancer and their families encounter as a result of the cancer or its treatment. Nurses triage patient problems and assist in the evaluation of symptoms and initiation of interventions. For example, subjective and objective data, including information about the last chemotherapy treatment and knowledge of the patient's history, guide the nurse in determining the patient's disposition and treatment. Much progress has been made in managing the side effects of chemotherapy, and nurses and nursing research have contributed significantly to this success. For example, nausea and vomiting are two of the most common symptoms associated with chemotherapy. Control of these symptoms has been a nursing research priority. Multiple studies have helped define nausea and vomiting and develop tools to measure occurrence, distress, and individual experiences associated with these symptoms.[40,41] This information assists in the treatment of nausea and vomiting and evaluation of the effectiveness of prescribed treatments.[42]

Fatigue is the most distressing side effect reported by patients and is a cancer-related symptom that nurses have played a major role in managing. Nurse researchers have contributed significantly to the definition, measurement, and management of fatigue.[43–49] ONS has played a major role in cancer fatigue management through several activities. In 1994, the organization sponsored a state-of-the knowledge conference on cancer-related fatigue. The published report of this conference provides a list of practice and research guidelines.[50] In conjunction with the pharmaceutical corporation OrthoBiotech, ONS coordinated the FIRE (Fatigue Initiative on Research and Education) project to increase the awareness of this problem. The FIRE project included funds for nursing research, professional education, and public education. The FIRE project has served as a model for subsequent programs within the ONS. The first National Cancer Fatigue Awareness Day was held in 1998. Nurses continue to address this underreported, underdiagnosed, and undertreated cancer-related symptom.

SUPPORTIVE CARE

Oncology nurses are closely involved with numerous supportive care issues encountered by cancer patients and their families. This chapter does not provide a detailed discussion of the numerous areas of supportive and palliative care, but two areas deserve special mention: the involvement of nurses in pain management and in survivorship. Because nurses spend more time with patients experiencing pain than does any other health professional, it is of the utmost importance that the nurse be knowledgeable about pain assessment and both pharmacologic and nonpharmacologic management of pain to provide good pain control as well as patient and family education.[51–53] However, as with other health care professions, barriers to providing effective pain control exist within nursing as well. The major problems are misconceptions and fears about addiction, drug tolerance, sedation, and respiratory depression; lack of knowledge about pain assessment and analgesics; and undertreatment with analgesics.[54] This is understandable when one considers the minimal time that is devoted to pain control in traditional undergraduate nursing curricula. Fortunately, these problems are now being addressed, and the education programs and resources available have improved considerably. State cancer pain initiatives, guidelines, and organizational position statements have been excellent efforts toward improving pain management. ONS developed a position paper on cancer pain that delineated the scope of practice for nurses with different levels of expertise.[55] Even the Joint Commission for Accreditation for Healthcare Organizations has recognized the problem of inadequate pain management and incorporates pain management in standards.[56]

More than 50% of individuals who are diagnosed with invasive cancer will live beyond 5 years, and the majority will be considered cured. Thus, issues of survivorship and living with the effects of cancer and its treatment are a significant concern. This is evidenced by an increasing emphasis on rehabilitation for cancer survivors. ONS was the first professional group to provide a practical definition of cancer rehabilitation as a "process by which individuals within their environments are assisted to achieve optimal functioning within the limits imposed by cancer" and published a position statement with the association of rehabilitation nurses in 1999, which was updated in 2003.[57] ONS has a special interest group focused on this area as well. Cancer rehabilitation espouses the goal of maximizing independence and dignity and reducing the extent to which cancer interferes with an individual's physical, psychosocial, and economic functioning. The rehabilitation process should begin at the time of diagnosis or definitive medical intervention and should continue until the individual is able to maintain the desirable level of independence.

ADVANCED PRACTICE IN ONCOLOGY NURSING

Advanced practice oncology nurses play a critical role in leading efforts to improve health care access, promote clinical excellence and quality of life, document outcomes, and increase cost-effectiveness. APNs are RNs who have acquired specialized knowledge and skills by completing a master's or doctorate degree in their specialty. The ONS, American Nurses Association, American Association of Colleges of Nursing, and National Council of State Boards of Nursing officially adopted the title "advanced practice nurse" as the single designation for CNSs and nurse practitioners NPs. Congress recognized the role of APNs in meeting the nation's health care needs when it enacted Section 4511 of the Balanced Budget Act of 1997. The act extended Medicare coverage for professional services provided by CNSs and NPs.[58] The APN has acquired advanced, in-depth knowledge and preceptored clinical experiences in oncology that enable her or him to exhibit a high degree of independent and collaborative judgment and clinical skill in providing nursing care to patients with cancer and their families.[16] The advanced practice of oncology nursing is used throughout the cancer care continuum, with APNs functioning in the acute care setting, private physician practices, ambulatory clinics, long-term follow-up clinics, prevention centers, the provision of cancer genetic counseling, and the provision of supportive and palliative care.

Of the four traditional advanced practice nursing roles (ie, clinical nurse midwife, nurse anesthetist, CNS, and NP), those of the CNS and NP are most commonly seen in cancer care. In all of these roles, there is emphasis on providing nursing care at an advanced level to patients and families through comprehensive health assessments; the identification of normal and abnormal health characteristics; treatment of a variety of human responses throughout the cancer care continuum according to practice guidelines, protocols, or standing orders; initiation of appropriate care; and the continuous evaluation of outcomes. The range of competencies includes direct care, coaching, consultation, collaboration, ethical decision making, research use, and leadership.[59] Table 60-4 reviews the roles of the CNS and the NP.[60–62]

Oncology NPs will generally spend a greater percentage of time as a direct caregiver than will CNSs. Depending on the state in which an APN is licensed, the scope of practice includes varying degrees of prescriptive authority and physician supervision required and title recognition. In only a few states do APNs have Drug Enforcement Agency licensure. The APN must be licensed in her or his state as an RN and is subject to that state's legal constraints and regulations for recognition and licensure of advanced practice. Oncology NPs can effectively meet both the medical and nursing needs of patients by functioning in a collaborative practice model supported by a

Table 60-4 Role Functions of Clinical Nurse Specialist and Nurse Practitioners

Role	Definition	Education	Role Functions
Nurse practitioners[60,61]	Nurse practitioners are primary care providers who practice in ambulatory, acute, and long-term care. They are registered nurses with specialized advanced education and clinical competency to provide health and medical care for diverse populations in a variety of primary, acute, and long-term care settings. A master's degree is required for entry-level practice. The nurse practitioner participates as a team member in the provision of health and medical care, interacting with professional colleagues to provide comprehensive care.	Graduate degree (master's or doctoral) or a post–master's degree certificate Meets all other board of nursing requirements to practice as a nurse practitioner (may include the need for certification as a nurse practitioner).	Nurse practitioners assess and manage both medical and nursing problems. Their practice emphasizes health promotion and maintenance, disease prevention, and the diagnosis and management of acute and chronic diseases. This includes taking histories; conducting physical examinations; ordering, performing, and interpreting appropriate diagnostic and laboratory tests; prescription of pharmacologic agents; and treatments and nonpharmacologic therapies for the management of the conditions that they diagnose. The nurse practitioner serves as a primary care provider and consultant for individuals, families, and communities in a variety of ambulatory and inpatient settings.
Clinical nurse specialists (CNS)[62]	A CNS independently provides theory and research-based care to clients in facilitating attainment of health goals, works with nurses to advance nursing practice to improve outcomes cost-effectively, and/or provides clinical expertise to affect system-wide changes in organizations to improve programs of care.	Graduate degree (master's or doctoral) or post–master's degree certificate. Training includes a minimum of 500 clinical practice hours in the CNS specialty that is accredited by a board-accepted national nursing accrediting body and meets all other (state board of nursing) requirements to practice as a clinical nurse specialist as identified by the state board of nursing in which the nurse practices.	Direct care services: (1) integrates advanced knowledge of disease and medical treatments in a holistic assessment of the person while focusing on the diagnosis of symptoms, functional problems, and risk behaviors that have etiologies requiring nursing interventions; (2) uses assessment data, research, and theoretic knowledge to design, implement, and evaluate nursing interventions that integrate delegated medical treatments as needed; (3) is authorized to prescribe or order durable medical equipment when such equipment is a self-care assistive device or assists nurses in the delivery of quality nursing care. Additionally, the CNS who has fulfilled the requirements for prescriptive authority in a specialty area is authorized to prescribe, administer, and distribute medications or pharmaceutical agents in the area of specialty practice. Indirect patient care: (1) serves as a consultant to other nurses and health care professionals in managing highly complex patient care problems or in achieving quality, cost-effective outcomes across settings; (2) serves as a leader in the appropriate use of research in practice innovations that improve patient care; (3) develops, plans, guides, and directs programs of care for populations of patients and provides direction to nursing personnel and others in these programs of care; (4) evaluates patient outcomes and cost-effectiveness of care to identify needs for practice improvements within the clinical specialty or program; (5) serves as a leader of multidisciplinary groups in designing and implementing alternative solutions to patient care issues across the continuum of care.

shared philosophy of practice, written agreements delineating shared responsibilities and accountability, incorporation of the role into day-to-day practice, and regular evaluation and readjustment of goals.

Changes in the health care system have challenged professionals to improve the delivery of cancer care services. As a result of these demands, the role of the oncology APN has continued to expand. ONS believes that APNs are a vital component of the health care team that provides care to patients with cancer and that barriers to full use of APNs must be addressed. Two consistent barriers that remain are reimbursement and prescriptive authority. To promote quality cancer care and to adequately manage the symptoms, such as pain, that can affect a patient's quality of life, the oncology APN must be granted prescriptive authority for medications, blood products, and nutritional supplements. The inclusion of controlled substances within the scope of prescriptive authority for APNs is a vital component to ensure optimal symptom management in patients with cancer.[58]

To advance quality cancer care, it is critical that the fields of medicine and nursing form collaborative partnerships that recognize and mutually respect the contributions of each discipline to quality cancer care. As nursing roles have expanded, the traditional boundaries between the two disciplines have blurred. To fully collaborate, professional partners must be secure in their individual professional identities to fully support and promote each partner's professional integrity and contribution to quality patient care. Barriers that must be overcome to achieve full collaboration are a lack of education regarding role effectiveness, stereotyping of nursing roles, a lack of clinical and interpersonal competence, physician resistance to acceptance of the role, and conflicting values between the professionals involved.

NURSING SHORTAGE

According to a July 2002 report by the Health Resources and Services Administration, 30 states were estimated to have shortages of RNs in 2000. The shortage is projected to intensify over the next two decades, with 44 states plus the District of Columbia expected to have RN shortages by 2020. The report *Projected Supply, Demand, and Shortages of Registered Nurses: 2000-2020* is available on-line.[63] According to projections from the US Bureau of Labor Statistics published in the February 2004 *Monthly Labor Review*, more than 1 million new and replacement nurses will be needed by 2012. For the first time, the US Department of Labor has identified registered nursing as the top occupation in terms of job growth through 2012.[64] Currently, hospitals are coping with a significant shortage, which is predicted only to increase in the coming years. By 2020, the RN workforce is forecast to be roughly the same size as it is today, declining nearly 20% below projected RN workforce requirements. The primary factor that has led to the aging of the RN workforce appears to be the decline in younger women choosing nursing as a career during the last two decades. Unless this trend is reversed, the RN workforce will continue to age and eventually shrink, and will not meet projected long-term workforce requirements. The current shortage is garnering much needed attention from hospital administrators, nursing and other professional organizations, legislatures, and the public.[65]

As the pool of nurses continues to shrink, the number of nurses available for oncology care dwindles as well. Therefore, it is imperative to attract individuals to the nursing field. Many efforts are under way to address the shortage, including those that address recruitment strategies to attract individuals to enter the nursing profession and retention strategies. The nursing shortage is high on the list of priorities for ONS as a professional organization, especially how the shortage might affect patient outcomes. To maintain quality care, the nation needs not just oncology nurses but nurses who are highly trained, skilled professionals. The shortage is no single entity's responsibility. This is everyone's issue, both public and private. ONS has supported legislation targeting the nursing shortage, has collaborated with other nursing professional organizations in addressing the shortage, and has conducted a study on the oncology nursing workforce.[66,67] Oncologists can play a key role in fostering a workplace environment that is respectful of the contributions of oncology nurses and promotes a collaborative working relationship. This will promote both retention of nurses and recruitment of men and women into the field of nursing.

SUMMARY

The progress of professional oncology nursing parallels the progress made in the surgical, radiologic, and medical approaches to the treatment of cancer. The oncology nurse has become an integral component of the cancer care team. Oncology nurses have earned the respect of physicians, other health care professionals, and, most importantly, patients and their families. As the health care delivery system continues to change, both the settings in which care is provided and the integration of new discoveries into cancer care, oncology nurses and advanced practice oncology nurses will continue to move into an ever-expanding variety of new roles as levels of knowledge, experience, and expertise advance.

REFERENCES

1. Hilkemeyer R. A historical perspective in cancer nursing. Oncol Nurs Forum 1985;12 Suppl:6–15.
2. Yarbro CH. The history of cancer nursing. In: McCorkle R, Grant M, Frank-Stromborg M, Baird SB, editors. Cancer nursing. 2nd ed. Philadelphia: WB Saunders; 1996. p. 12–24.
3. Johnson J, Baird S, Hilderley L, editors. It took courage, compassion, and curiosity. Pittsburgh (PA): Oncology Nursing Press; 2001.
4. Mayer DK, editor. Celebrating our past, creating our future. Oncol Nurs Forum 2000;28 Suppl: 1–32.
5. O'Mara A, Bakos A. Preparing oncology nurse scientists: opportunities at the National Cancer Institute. Oncol Nurs Forum 2003;30:745–6.
6. Houldin AD, Naylor MD, Haller DG. Physician-nurse collaboration in research in the 21st century. J Clin Oncol 2004;22:774–6.
7. Moore P. Achieving quality cancer care requires collaboration among all oncology professionals: we each contribute in a unique way. ONS News 1998;13:18.
8. Yarbro CH. ONS the early days: four smiles and a post office box. Oncol Nurs Forum 1984;11:79–85.
9. Oncology Nursing Society. Demographics report, as of October 1, 2004. Pittsburgh (PA): Oncology Nursing Society; 2004.
10. Oncology Nursing Society Foundation. Available at: http://www.onsfoundation.org/ (accessed May 31, 2005).
11. American Nurses Association and the Oncology Nursing Society. Standards of oncology nursing practice. Washington (DC): American Nurses Association; 1987.
12. American Nurses Association and the Oncology Nursing Society (ONS). Outcomes Standards for cancer nursing practice. . Washington DC: American Nurses Association; 1979
13. American Nurses Association and the Oncology Nursing Society. Statement on the scope and standards of oncology nursing practice. Washington (DC): American Nurses Publishing; 1996.
14. Brant JM, Wickham RS, editors. Oncology Nursing Society. Statement on the scope and standards of oncology nursing practice. Pittsburgh (PA): Oncology Nursing Society Publishing Division; 2004.
15. Oncology Nursing Society. Statement on the scope and standards of advanced practice in oncology nursing. Pittsburgh (PA): Oncology Nursing Press; 1997.
16. Jacobs LA, editor. Oncology Nursing Society: statement on the scope and standards of advanced practice in oncology nursing. 3rd ed. Pittsburgh (PA): Oncology Nursing Society Publishing Division; 2003.
17. Oncology Nursing Certification Corporation. Demographics report as of May 2005. Pittsburgh (PA): Oncology Nursing Certification Corporation; 2005.
18. McMillan SC, Heusinkveld KB, Spray JA, Murphy CM. Revising the blueprint for the AOCN examination using a role delineation study for advanced practice oncology nursing. Oncol Nurs Forum 1999;26:529–37.
19. Oncology Nursing Certification Corporation. 2005 Options in advanced oncology nursing certification: AOCNS - AOCNP - AOCN®. Available at: www.oncc.org (accessed May 31, 2005).
20. Ponto J, Murphy CM. Advanced nursing certification to become role specific. Clin J Oncol Nurs 2004;8:447-8.
21. Oncology Nursing Certification Corporation. 2005 Certification bulletin. Pittsburgh (PA): Oncology Nursing Certification Corporation; 2005. Available at: www.oncc.org (accessed May 31, 2005).
22. Yarbro CH, Frogge MH, Goodman M, Groenwald SL, editors. Cancer nursing: principles and practice. 6th ed. Sudbury (MA): Jones and Bartlett; 2005.
23. Otto S, editor. Oncology nursing clinical reference. St. Louis (MO): Mosby; 2004.
24. Varricchio CG, editor. A cancer source book for nurses. 8th ed. Sudbury (MA): Jones and Bartlett; 2004.
25. Yarbro CH, Frogge MH, Goodman M, editors. Cancer symptom management. 3rd ed. Sudbury (MA): Jones and Bartlett; 2004.
26. Rieger PT, editor. Biotherapy: a comprehensive overview. 2nd ed. Sudbury (MA): Jones and Bartlett; 2001.
27. Itano J, Taoka JN, editors. Core curriculum for oncology nursing. 3rd ed. Philadelphia: Saunders; 1998.
28. McGuire DB, Ropka ME. Research and oncology nursing practice. Semin Oncol Nurs 2000;16:35-46.
29. Berger AM, Berry DL, Christopher KA, et al. Oncology Nursing Society Year 2004 Research Priorities Survey. Oncol Nurs Forum 2005;32: 281–90.
30. Oncology Nursing Society–Research. Available at: http://www.ons.org/research/ (accessed May 31, 2005).
31. Rieger PT, Moore P. Professional organizations and role in advocacy. Semin Oncol Nurs 2002;18:276–89.
32. Bruce SD. Ambulatory/office setting offers nurses new rewards…and new challenges. ONS News 2003;18:1, 4–5.
33. Buchsel PC, editor. Oncology nursing in the ambulatory setting. 2nd ed. Sudbury (MA): Jones & Bartlett; 2005.
34. Calzone KA, Masny A. Genetics and oncology nursing. Semin Oncol Nurs 2004;20:178–85.
35. Padberg RM, Padberg LF. Patient education and support. In: Yarbro Ch, Frogge MH, Goodman M, editors. Cancer nursing principles and practice. 5th ed. Sudbury (MA): Jones and Bartlett; 2000. p. 1609–31.
36. Blecher CS, editor. Oncology Nursing Society standards of oncology education: patient/significant other and public. 3rd ed. Pittsburgh (PA): Oncology Nursing Publishing Division; 2002.
37. Preston FA. Telephone triage. Clin J Oncol Nurs 2000;4:294–6.
38. Boyle DA, Schulmeister L, Lajeunesse JD, Anderson RW. Medication misadventures in cancer care. Semin Oncol Nurs 2002;18:109–20.
39. Kohn L, Corrigan J, Donaldson M, editors, for Committee on Quality of Health Care in America, Institute of Medicine. To err is human: building a safer health system. Washington (DC): Academy Press; 2000.
40. Smith MC, Holcombe JK, Stullenbarger E. A meta-analysis of intervention effectiveness for symptom management in oncology nursing research. Oncol Nurs Forum 1994;21:1201–9; discussion 1209–10.
41. Rhodes VA, McDaniel RW, Homan SS, et al. An instrument to measure symptom experience. Symptom occurrence and symptom distress. Cancer Nurs 2000;23:49–54.
42. Marek C. Antiemetic therapy in patients receiving cancer chemotherapy. Oncol Nurs Forum 2003;30:259–71.
43. Stricker CT, Drake D, Hoyer KA, Mock V. Evidence-based practice for fatigue management in adults with cancer; exercise as an intervention. Oncol Nurs Forum 2004;31:963–76.
44. Patrick DL, Ferketich SL, Frame PS, et al. National Institutes of Health State-of-the-Science Panel. National Institutes of Health state-of-the-science conference statement: symptom management in cancer: pain, depression, and fatigue, July 15–17, 2002. J Natl Cancer Inst Monogr 2004;32:9–16.
45. Mock V, Olsen M. Current management of fatigue and anemia in patients with cancer. Semin Oncol Nurs 2003;19(4 Suppl 2):36–41.
46. Gomez E. Nursing leads the way in cancer-related fatigue on the Web. ONS News 2003;18:7.
47. Wu HS, McSweeney M. Measurement of fatigue in people with cancer. Oncol Nurs Forum 2001;28:1371–84; quiz 1385–6.
48. Hockenberry-Eaton M, Hinds PS. Fatigue in children and adolescents with cancer: evolution of a program of study. Semin Oncol Nurs 2000;16:261–72; discussion 272–8.
49. Winningham ML, Barton Burke M, editors. Fatigue in cancer: a multidimensional approach. Sudbury (MA): Jones and Bartlett; 1999.
50. Winningham ML, Nail LM, Burke MB, et al. Fatigue and the cancer experience: the state of the knowledge. Oncol Nurs Forum 1994;21:23–36.
51. Fine PG, Miaskowski C, Paice JA. Meeting the challenges in cancer pain management. J Support Oncol 2004;2(6 Suppl 4):5–22.
52. Kim JE, Dodd M, West C, et al. The PRO-SELF pain control program improves patients' knowledge of cancer pain management. Oncol Nurs Forum 2004;31:1137–43.
53. McGuire DB, Yarbro CH, Ferrell B, editors. Cancer pain management. 2nd ed. Sudbury (MA): Jones and Barlett; 1995.
54. Yeager K, McGuire DB, Scheidler VR. Assessment of cancer pain. In: Yarbro CH, Frogge MH, Goodman M, editors. Cancer nursing principles and practice. 5th ed. Sudbury (MA): Jones and Bartlett; 2000. p. 633–56.
55. Oncology Nursing Society. Cancer pain management. Oncol Nurs Forum 2001;28:439–40.
56. Joint Commission on Accreditation of Healthcare Organizations. 2005 Comprehensive accreditation manual for hospitals: the official handbook (CAMH). Oak Brook Terrace (IL): Joint Commissions Resources Publications; 2005.
57. Oncology Nursing Society. Position on rehabilitation of people with cancer. Available at: http://www.ons.org/publications/positions/Rehabilitation.shtml (accessed Jan 8, 2005).
58. Oncology Nursing Society. The role of the advanced practice nurse in oncology care. Available at: http://www.ons.org/publications/positions/AdvancePractice.shtml (accessed Jan 8, 2005).
59. Spross JA, Hearney CA. Shaping advanced nursing practice in the new millennium. Semin Oncol Nurs 2000;16:12–24.
60. American Academy of Nurse Practitioners. Nurse practitioners as an advanced practice nurse role position statement. Austin (TX): American Academy of Nurse Practitioners; 2002. Available at: www.aanp.org (accessed Jan 8, 2005).
61. American Academy of Nurse Practitioners. Scope of practice. Available at: www.aanp.org (accessed Jan 8, 2005).
62. National Association of Clinical Nurse Specialists. Model rules and regulations for CNS title protection and scope of practice 2004. Available at: www.nacns.org (accessed Jan 8, 2005).
63. Health Resources and Services Administration. Projected supply, demand, and shortages of registered nurses: 2000-2020. Available at: http://bhpr.hrsa.gov/healthworkforce/reports/rnproject/default.html (accessed Jan 8, 2005).
64. Bureau of Labor and Statistics. Monthly labor review. 2004. Available at: www.bls.gov/news.release/ecopro.toc.htm (accessed May 31, 2005).
65. Ponte PR. The American health care system at a crossroads: an overview of the American Organization of Nurse Executives monograph. Online J Issues Nurs 2004 31;9:3. Available at: http://nursingworld.org/ojin/topic24/tpc24_2.htm (accessed Jan 8, 2005).
66. Lamkin L, Rosiak J, Buerhaus P, et al. Oncology nursing society workforce survey. Part I.: perceptions of the nursing workforce environment and adequacy of nurse staffing in outpatient and inpatient oncology settings. Oncol Nurs Forum 2001;28:1545–52.
67. Lamkin L, Rosiak J, Buerhaus P, et al. Oncology Society Workforce Survey. Part II: perceptions of the nursing workforce environment and adequacy of nurse staffing in outpatient and inpatient oncology settings. Oncol Nurs Forum 2002;29:93–100.

Section 19

CANCER REHABILITATION MEDICINE

61

Principles of Cancer Rehabilitation Medicine

David C. Thomas, MD
Kristjan T. Ragnarsson, MD

Medical advances in the diagnosis and management of cancer have markedly increased survival rates. Although the treatment for some patients may now result in complete cure and no perceived physical deficits, for others, an aggressive definitive treatment may result in significant physical impairment or disability. To ensure quick restoration of optimal function, early and continued aggressive rehabilitation interventions should be provided, including physical and occupational therapy, prosthetic and orthotic devices, and assistive equipment. Application of rehabilitation techniques frequently results in a swift functional improvement and a reduction in subjective complaints, even when the prognosis for life is considered poor. It has always been difficult to predict with a degree of certainty the life expectancy of an individual with cancer. Modern diagnostic techniques and effective treatment of malignant neoplastic diseases have invalidated old statistics and dogmas regarding life expectancy and thus made accurate prognostication even more difficult for the clinician. No cancer patient, even one with widespread metastases, should be denied the benefits of aggressive treatment, including appropriate surgical intervention, chemotherapy, radiation, and comprehensive rehabilitation. These interventions, when offered in an integrated and timely fashion, prolong life, protect organs and residual healthy tissue, reduce pain, and maximize self-care and mobility skills, helping reduce the stigma of cancer and physical impairment while providing dignity and a better quality of life for the cancer patient.

Early referral for rehabilitation services and good communication among the oncologist, the surgeon, the rehabilitation specialist (physiatrist), and the other members of the cancer rehabilitation team are essential to the patient's successful return to optimal function. A comprehensive and well-coordinated rehabilitation approach that concurrently deals with the physical, psychological, and social problems caused by the malignancy and the consequent disability usually yields the best results. Most important for success, however, is the patient's personal interest and ability to participate in the rehabilitation program and to pursue the established functional goals, supported by family, friends, and caregivers.

APPLICATION OF REHABILITATION CONCEPTS

Many persons afflicted by cancer develop some form of functional impairment or disability that will interfere with self-care, mobility, and a smooth transition to their former lifestyle. Cancer rehabilitation can be broadly defined as the maximum restoration of physical, psychological, social, vocational, recreational, and economic functions within the limits imposed by the malignancy and its treatment. To make a significant and timely impact on such a wide variety of functions and needs, the efforts of a well-coordinated and goal-oriented multidisciplinary cancer rehabilitation team are required (Table 61-1). Because of the patient's often uncertain prognosis, most cancer rehabilitation programs focus on quick gains in mobility and self-care skills and the provision of psychosocial support to the patient and family.

Table 61-1 Interdisciplinary Cancer Rehabilitation Team

Physician (physiatrist)	Speech-language pathologist
Rehabilitation nurse	Social worker
Physical therapist	Psychologist
Occupational therapist	Chaplain
Prosthetist-orthotist	Vocational counselor
Nutritionist	Recreational therapist

Flexibility in goal setting is unavoidable because of the patient's changing needs, stamina, and medical status.

Several studies show that cancer rehabilitation programs result in measurable benefits when individualized, specific, and realistic goals are set.[1,2] Comprehensive inpatient rehabilitation services may be economically provided for disabled cancer patients who are considered "cured or controlled," but precise short-term rehabilitation interventions may enable even those with a poor prognosis to gain the mobility and self-care skills that facilitate early hospital discharge.[3]

The physical impairment experienced by cancer patients may result from tissue destruction caused by the cancer itself, prolonged bed rest, or inactivity or from definitive treatment, such as surgery, radiation, or chemotherapy. The exact nature of the impairment may vary, but, in essence, it is no different from impairment caused by trauma or noncancerous disease and is customarily managed by the rehabilitation team. A specific rehabilitation goal must be established for each patient and an individualized program prescribed that is designed to obtain measurable early results. The main rehabilitation goals for all people with physical disabilities are, first, to develop maximum skills in the activities of daily living (ADL) (Table 61-2) allowed by the disability and, second, to obtain independent mobility with or without assistive devices, such as wheelchairs, prostheses, orthoses, walkers, crutches, or canes. To reach these goals, the therapist uses physical exercise to improve muscle strength, endurance, joint flexibility, and self-care skills, as well as to apply physical modalities to decrease pain and swelling. Prescription, fabrication, and fitting of prosthetic and orthotic devices and other assistive equipment, followed by training in their use, are essential for amputees and individuals

Table 61-2 Activities of Daily Living*

Eating and drinking	Moving in bed
Dressing and undressing	Changing position
Bathing and grooming	Walking
Toileting	Climbing stairs
Managing bladder and bowel functions	General wheelchair skills
Manipulating small objects	Using a manual wheelchair
Caring for health and fitness	Using a powered wheelchair

*Rehabilitation indicators: skill indicators.

with significant muscle weakness, paralysis, or unstable skeletal structures.

It is essential to provide rehabilitation interventions that also aim at the often profound psychological, sexual, social, and vocational consequences of the cancer and the physical impairment. Preferably, the anticipated psychosocial difficulties should be addressed when the initial diagnosis is made and when treatment is begun. The goal of cancer care is not just to eradicate or control the malignancy and extend the patient's life but to maintain or reestablish a life of quality.

The rehabilitation goals of cancer patients may be broadly classified according to the different stages of the disease. Preventive rehabilitation therapy is started early after the diagnosis of cancer is made, that is, before or immediately after surgery, radiotherapy, and/or chemotherapy. At this stage, no significant physical impairment exists, but therapy is started to prevent functional loss. Restorative rehabilitation therapy is directed at the comprehensive restoration of maximum function for patients considered "cured or controlled" but who have a residual physical impairment and disability. Supportive rehabilitation therapy attempts to increase the self-care skills and mobility of the cancer patient with growing cancer and progressive impairment and disability by the application of quick, effective methods, for example, providing appropriate assistive devices and the teaching of simple techniques for self-care.[4] Supportive rehabilitation therapy also includes physical exercises to prevent the effects of immobilization, such as joint contractures, muscle atrophy, weakness, and pressure sores. Palliative rehabilitation therapy aims to increase or maintain the comfort and function of patients with terminal cancer by using physical modalities, simple orthotic devices, and assistive equipment to manage pain, joint contractures, and pressure sores and to provide at least partial self-sufficiency.[4]

CANCER REHABILITATION AND ADAPTATION TEAM

Organized cancer rehabilitation programs can significantly improve a patient's physical function and community reintegration.[3,5] An integral part of such programs is an interdisciplinary cancer rehabilitation and adaptation team (see Table 61-1). The exact composition of the team may vary considerably, depending on the program's philosophy and size, the type of institution, and the range of disabilities encountered. The team is led by a physician who is either an oncologist or, more commonly, a physiatrist.[5] An oncology nurse, social worker, psychologist, physical therapist, occupational therapist, vocational counselor, chaplain, and nutritionist are present on most teams. Other rehabilitation professionals may contribute to the rehabilitation of cancer patients, depending on each patient's specific physical impairment, including a prosthetist, an orthotist, a speech-language pathologist, a driver's trainer, and a recreational therapist. The roles of the various team members are described below.

The *physiatrist,* the medical specialist who usually directs the cancer rehabilitation team, needs to be knowledgeable in oncology in addition to having expertise in the field of physical medicine and rehabilitation. To establish realistic goals and prescribe an appropriate rehabilitation program, the physiatrist needs to know (1) details of the cancer diagnosis with respect to organ site, histology, and grade of anaplasia; (2) the cancer's anatomic staging (primary site only, involvement of regional nodes, or metastases); (3) the patient's life expectancy, that is, whether the patient is "cured or controlled" and, if not, the anticipated rapidity of the cancer's progression; and (4) the definitive treatment plan for the cancer, that is, the timing of surgery, chemotherapy, or radiation and its anticipated efficacy and potential side effects. The physiatrist discusses this information with the rehabilitation team as the basis for developing a specific and realistic plan of preventive, restorative, supportive, and palliative therapies. The physiatrist introduces the patient and caregivers to the goals of the cancer rehabilitation team and meets regularly with the team, as well as with the patient and caregivers, to direct and coordinate their efforts while taking into account the patient's progress and changing needs.

The *rehabilitation oncology nurse* serves primarily as an easily accessible resource to the nursing staff, giving care to the cancer patient, as well as to the patient and the caregivers. The nurse evaluates the patient's specific nursing needs, plans the patient's care, helps obtain nursing supplies, and educates other nurses, the patient, and their caregivers about nursing techniques and the principles of cancer treatment while monitoring and assisting in the discharge process.

The *physical therapist* teaches the patient to perform specific exercises to strengthen muscles, increase stamina, and maintain or improve joint range of motion and trunk flexibility. When indicated, training is provided to improve balance and coordination, as well as functional skills: transfers into and out of bed, wheelchair locomotion, and ambulation with or without assistive devices. Task-oriented exercises, such as ambulation or training in self-care, may improve function and safety by repetition and prolonged therapy.

The *occupational therapist* focuses on upper extremity exercises and training in self-care activities(see Table 61-2). Different adaptive equipment may be provided to make the patient more proficient in self-care and activities related to work and recreation.

The *nutritionist* evaluates the patient's nutritional condition, assesses the additional metabolic demands that the cancer places on the body, and recommends the optimal diet with respect to specific clinical condition, caloric intake, food ingredients of choice, optimal consistency for easy swallowing, and the individual's tastes.

The *prosthetist* or *orthotist* makes artificial limbs (prostheses) or special braces (orthoses) for patients in need of such devices.

The *speech-language pathologist* evaluates and provides therapy for impaired oral communication and works closely with the occupational therapist and nutritionist in the assessment and care of swallowing disorders.

The *social worker* has many important roles in the rehabilitation of the cancer patient, but especially with respect to discharge planning, facilitating a smooth transition from the hospital to the community, ensuring continuity of care, and securing appropriate follow-up services after discharge. The *psychologist* assesses the patient's cognition and behavior, including intelligence, personality (ie, ideational, emotional, behavioral, and character patterns), personal history, motivation, and reaction to the illness, and assists the patient and the caregivers in coping.[6–8]

A chaplain or religious counselor is often included in the cancer rehabilitation team.

A vocational counselor should participate in the care of physically impaired cancer patients who have any potential of returning to work.

The *recreational therapist* offers activities to meet the different needs and interests of disabled individuals both in and out of the hospital, such as art therapy, music therapy, attending art shows and sports events, going to theaters, eating at restaurants, and shopping.

FUNCTIONAL ASSESSMENT

Unlike other fields of medicine, the outcome of rehabilitation interventions cannot be measured by survival or by the disappearance of symptoms. The effectiveness of rehabilitation interventions is judged by the patient's degree of functional independence. The revised International Classification of Functioning, Disability and Health (ICIDH-2) offers a framework for understanding the complex interaction between disease and disability.[9]

To assess and monitor function accurately, the performance in different activities of self-care, mobility, and communication must be numerically rated according to the patient's level of independence: completely independent, independent with devices, requires assistance (supervision, "spotting," reminding, physical help), or completely dependent. This requires the collection of numerous diverse data by various means, including physical examination, observation, and a review of records and reports from the various rehabilitation team members, as well as the gathering of information directly from the patient and caregivers. The functional evaluation scale that currently is gaining the widest acceptance by rehabilitation professionals is the Functional Independence Measure (FIM) (Table 61-3),[10–12] but for cancer patients, the Karnofsky Performance Status Scale is the most widely used evaluation scale (Table 61-4).[13]

The Cancer Rehabilitation Evaluation System (CARES) is another scale developed specifically to measure quality of life and functional outcome for patients with cancer. It is valid, reliable, and sensitive to changes in status.[14,15]

REHABILITATION PROCESS

Rehabilitation services are frequently requested too late in the care of the cancer patient. The physiatrist should be consulted as soon as it may be anticipated that the cancer will result in a physical disability. The rehabilitation interventions may thus be planned and explained to the patient before, during, or immediately following definitive treatment. Physical and occupational therapy is initially provided at the bedside, but the patient should be mobilized out of bed as soon as possible and escorted to the rehabilitation area, where facilities and equipment are conducive to better performance. Other members of the rehabilitation team become involved in the care of the disabled cancer patient as deemed appropriate by the physiatrist. If these interventions allow the patient to become self-sufficient and ambulatory, then the patient should be discharged home directly from the acute service, when medically indicated, having received proper instructions, equipment, and referrals for specific nursing interventions.

A more comprehensive and intensive rehabilitation program on an inpatient rehabilitation service is provided for physically disabled cancer patients who do not swiftly gain independence in ADL and mobility with daily therapy on the acute service, who are medically capable of actively participating in the program for at least 3 hours daily, and who are motivated and mentally capable of following instructions and learning the different tasks.

The inpatient rehabilitation unit should be in a hospital with an in-house physician on call and the various medical and surgical consultation services available at all times. Here the disabled cancer patient is reevaluated by the physiatrist, who obtains a detailed medical and social history and performs a careful physical examination to assess the general medical and precise musculoskeletal and neurologic condition, as well as the current functional ability. The physiatrist writes the routine medical orders for nursing care, medications, and disability-specific diagnostic tests, including radiologic studies, urologic evaluation, pulmonary function tests, and electrodiagnostic studies. The physiatrist prescribes the specific exercises and training methods to be given by the physical and occupational therapists, as well as interventions by the other members of the interdisciplinary team.

The rehabilitation program begins promptly after transfer to the inpatient rehabilitation ser-

Table 61-3 Functional Independence Measure (FIM)

LEVELS		
	7 Complete Independence (Timely, Safely) 6 Modified Independence (Device)	NO HELPER
	Modified Dependence 5 Supervision 4 Minimal Assist (Subject = 75+) 3 Moderate Assist (Subject = 50%+) Complete Dependence 2 Maximal Assist (Subject = 25%+) 1 Total Assist (Subject = 0%)	HELPER

	ADMIT	DISCHG	FOL-UP
Self Care			
A. Eating			
B. Grooming			
C. Bathing			
D. Dressing-Upper Body			
E. Dressing-Lower Body			
F. Toileting			
Sphincter Control			
G. Bladder Management			
H. Bowel Management			
Mobility			
Transfer:			
I. Bed, Chair, Wheelchair			
J. Toilet			
K. Tub, Shower			
Locomotion			
L. Walk/wheel Chair	w c	w c	w c
M. Stairs			
Communication			
N. Comprehension	a v	a v	a v
O. Expression	v n	v n	v n
Social Cognition			
P. Social Interaction			
Q. Problem Solving			
R. Memory			
Total F/M			

NOTE: Leave no blanks; enter 1 if patient not testable due to risk

Table 61-4 Karnofsky Performance Status Scale

General	Index	Specific Criteria
Able to carry on normal activity; no special care needed	100	Normal; no complaints; no evidence of disease
	90	Able to carry on normal activity; minor signs or symptoms of disease
	80	Normal activity with effort; signs or symptoms of disease
Unable to work; able to live at home and care for most personal needs; varying amount of assistance needed	70	Cares for self; unable to carry on normal activity or to do work
	60	Requires occasional assistance from others, but able to care for most needs
	50	Requires considerable assistance from others; needs frequent medical care
Unable to care for self; requires institutional or hospital care or equivalent; disease may be rapidly progressing	40	Disabled; requires special care and assistance
	30	Severely disabled; hospitalization indicated; death not imminent
	20	Very sick, hospitalization necessary; active supportive treatment necessary
	10	Moribund
	0	Dead

vice. Several hours each day are spent in an active therapy program in addition to different ward activities, such as self-care training, management of bowel and bladder dysfunction, and educational and recreational activities. When serious medical complications arise during the course of rehabilitation that interfere with the patient's ability to attend the rehabilitation program for at least 3 hours a day for more than 3 consecutive days, the patient should be transferred to the appropriate medical or surgical service for definitive care.

Within 1 week of admission, an initial team conference is held at which the patient's medical, functional, psychologic, social, vocational, and recreational status, as well as the rehabilitation potential and prognosis, are presented and discussed. More specific rehabilitation goals are set, the needs for equipment and personal assistance are assessed, and a discharge date is predicted. Soon after this conference, the physiatrist meets with the patient and the caregivers to discuss these issues and answer questions regarding the patient's medical condition and rehabilitation program. Team rehabilitation conferences are held biweekly to discuss the patient's progress and plans for discharge. Although the patient is making continuous and measurable progress toward the set functional goals of independence in ADL and mobility, continued inpatient stay may be justified.[16] When a patient is discharged home, it is most important to ensure that needed equipment and supplies have been obtained, caregivers or home health aides have been instructed and trained in the patient's care, follow-up by the visiting nurse service has been arranged, and referrals have been made for continued therapy and visits with various physicians, including the oncologist, surgeon, physiatrist, and family doctor.

CANCER OF THE BRAIN

Brain damage may result from primary tumors of the brain, metastatic disease, or treatment of the cancer—surgery, radiation, or, more rarely, chemotherapy. The symptoms and disability that may result vary extensively but, in essence, are similar to those that are seen in patients who have sustained traumatic brain injury or a stroke involving different parts of the brain (Table 61-5). The main difference, however, is the potentially progressive or recurrent nature of the brain cancer and its uncertain prognosis. The greatest deficits are frequently seen immediately after surgery or during radiation and chemotherapy, after which remarkable improvement may occur. Late brain injury from radiation with infarction or necrosis also may occur, but the resulting disability has a less favorable prognosis for recovery. All patients with brain cancer and impaired function in mobility or ADL should be referred for rehabilitation services. Many, regardless of tumor type, can be helped with simple rehabilitation measures, whereas others may require comprehensive inpatient rehabilitation, which should be provided when longer life expectancy allows.[17] Following definitive treatment of primary brain tumors in children, rehabilitation significantly improves outcome in self-care activities, transfers into and out of bed, and locomotion by a wheelchair or walking.[18]

Table 61-5 Rehabilitation Problems Associated with Cancer of the Brain

Paralysis	Dysarthria
Spasticity	Aprosodia
Joint contractures	Dysphagia
Pain	Ataxia
Sensory deficits	Visual-perceptual deficits
Visual field deficits	Cognitive and behavioral deficits
Diplopia	Psychosocial-vocational problems
Aphasia	

Most commonly, the rehabilitation intervention starts after surgical resection or removal of the brain tumor. When medically stable, the patient should be helped to sit up, get out of bed, and start on an active restoration program that is designed according to the patient's general condition. The location and size of the cerebral lesion clearly determine the clinical symptoms encountered. The variability of the symptoms precludes a standard rehabilitation approach but demands an individual evaluation and treatment plan. Broadly, the problems of patients with cancer of the brain are physical, psychological, social, and vocational. Table 61-5 lists the most common problems, which are briefly discussed below.

Paralysis, often in the form of hemiplegia, can be a conspicuous consequence of brain cancer. Although the paralysis is most profound just after the brain surgery, a certain return of motor power is common and may continue for several weeks or months.

Mobilization training starts when the patient is ready to be transferred out of bed. Depending on the extent of the paralysis, the patient may be taught to ambulate with assistive devices or to maneuver a wheelchair. As the body balance improves and the patient has learned to lean consistently to his or her good side, ambulation outside the parallel bars can begin, with the patient using an appropriate ambulation aid carried in the unaffected upper extremity. Usually, some knee extensor strength returns, providing the patient with adequate knee support, but the ankle dorsiflexors and invertors still may be weak. Here a plastic ankle-foot orthosis (AFO) may be prescribed to prevent the foot dragging during the swing phase of gait. This orthosis is easily inserted into most shoes. It is cosmetically superior to the old metal orthoses and usually provides equal or better function. If knee extensor strength does not return, fabrication of a knee-ankle-foot orthosis may be considered, but the prognosis for functional ambulation with such a device is poor.

The major goal in the rehabilitation of the patient with cancer of the brain is independence in ADL, which may be obtained through training, prescription of proper assistive devices, and possibly modification of the patient's clothing and the architecture of the patient's home.

Spasticity frequently interferes with mobility and performance of ADL. Factors that may aggravate the spasticity (eg, skin lesions, infections, and anxiety) need to be identified and treated. Thorough stretching of all joints should be performed daily. Medications (ie, dantrolene sodium, baclofen, or diazepam) may be of some benefit but should be used sparingly in view of their potential side effects. Selected nerve blocks with dilute solutions of phenol or motor point blocks with botulinum toxin are usually effective in reducing local spasticity, but surgical procedures for reduction of spasticity in patients with cancer of the brain are rarely indicated.

Joint contractures, whether owing to muscle imbalance, spasticity, improper bed positioning, or an inadequate exercise program, may change the rehabilitation prognosis significantly. A 10° flexion contracture of the knee, for example, will greatly increase oxygen consumption during ambulation and thus markedly reduce endurance. Knee contractures that exceed 15° will usually make functional ambulation impossible for the patient with brain cancer and hemiplegia. Development of a frozen shoulder may make independent dressing impossible. Prevention of contractures by proper joint range of motion exercises is imperative from the onset of the disability because treatment of contracture is relatively ineffective.

Pain in different parts of the body may be experienced in patients with neurologic deficits caused by cancer of the brain. Dysesthetic thalamic pain is notably refractory to treatment, although various centrally acting agents may be helpful. Pain with motion of the hemiplegic shoulder is common, perhaps owing to muscle imbalance at the shoulder girdle and recurrent minor trauma to the periarticular structures. Shoulder support by an arm sling or a lapboard, administration of analgesics, application of heat or cold modalities, and gentle range of motion and strengthening exercises may all help reduce the pain and improve shoulder function. Complex regional pain syndrome, formerly known as *reflex sympathetic dystrophy,* may occur and requires similar treatment, but more effective relief may be obtained by simply administering oral steroids, for example, prednisone 5 mg four times a day for 2 to 3 weeks.[19] Sympathetic nerve blocks may be performed when symptoms are more persistent.

Sensory deficits of varying degrees are commonly seen in patients with brain cancer, either in the distribution of the cranial nerves or on one or both sides of the body. Cancer affecting the parietal lobes of the brain may cause severe sensory loss with little muscle weakness. This may interfere with balance and mobility because the patient who cannot feel motion is unable to control it. Although physical exercise cannot decrease the sensory loss, training with adaptive gait aids (ie, canes, crutches, or a walker and wearing of proper shoes) may help the patient ambulate functionally again.

Visual deficits, such as double vision or visual field deficits, are commonly seen as a result of cancer in the lower brain or above the tentorium, respectively. Although double vision may improve spontaneously, the use of unilateral or alternating eye patches or special prism glasses may be helpful. The value of exercises for retraining the eye muscles is uncertain. Homonymous hemianopsia—blindness to the affected side of the body caused by a contralateral brain tumor—rarely resolves spontaneously. Whereas a patient with a left brain lesion usually learns easily to compensate for hemianopsia through scanning of the environment, the patient with a right brain lesion may experience severe difficulties owing to accompanying anosognosia, that is, lack of awareness of the affected left side of the body and of the surroundings. Specialized programs of cognitive remediation have been found to be effective with these patients.[20]

Aphasia may be seen in patients with cancer in the left dominant hemisphere of the brain. This is an impairment of the central language process, with reduced capacity for interpretation and formulation of the symbols for communication. Although all components of language—listening, speaking, reading, and writing—are usually affected, they are not affected to an equal extent; thus, several types of aphasia are recognized.[21,22] Expressive or nonfluent aphasia is caused by lesions in the Broca area of the brain and is characterized by reduced language production, vocabulary, and use of grammar. The patient is well aware of these difficulties and becomes very frustrated. Less well known is receptive or fluent aphasia, which is caused by lesions in the Wernicke area of the brain. Here the patient primarily has difficulty in understanding language, both his or her own and that of others. The patient thus may be able to speak continuously at normal speed and with normal intonation without giving any pertinent information or being aware of the errors. The efficiency of speech therapy is debated because most patients will have a degree of spontaneous improvement. Nonetheless, speech therapy is indicated, whenever available, not only for psychological support but also to provide the necessary stimulation for the patient to use his or her maximum speech ability, to adjust to new circumstances, and to instruct the caregiver in proper communication with the patient by using short, simple sentences at a normal voice volume, gestures, and facial expressions, always with respect, optimism, patience, and encouragement.

Dysarthria is a motor disturbance of speech, which implies weakness, slowness, or incoordination of the muscles that produce speech. Understanding written or spoken language is, therefore, never a problem. Articulation is usually the main problem, but speed, rhythm, sound, and intonation may also be disturbed. Mild dysarthria accompanies many brain cancers that involve cranial nerves and the cerebrum and affect the facial musculature, but dysarthria is particularly prominent in brainstem tumors. If speech remains completely unintelligible, other communication methods are introduced, such as writing, typing, sign language, or pictures.

Dysphagia, or impaired swallowing, is frequently seen in patients with brain cancer, especially when the brainstem is involved. In its most severe form, the patient may be totally unable to swallow, but in milder cases, there may only be difficulty with the swallowing of liquids. Serial radiographic swallowing studies should be done for proper monitoring of the condition until it is resolved or until other safer means of nutrition are established. A swallowing training program may be instituted by the speech or occupational therapist in which the patient attempts to swallow food of different consistency using different techniques and positions. A nasogastric tube can be used for several weeks while waiting for spontaneous recovery, but a more persistent dysphagia warrants insertion of a gastrostomy tube for prolonged feeding.

Neuropsychological changes may be prominent when cancer affects the cerebral hemispheres. Reduced memory and judgment frequently make successful rehabilitation impossible because the patient may be unable to remember instructions. Visual perceptual deficits, caused by a central disturbance in organizing visual stimuli from the environment, frequently accompany right brain damage even when visual field and acuity are normal. These patients may experience difficulty in recognizing the three dimensions: depth and distances, the relationship of lines and objects, and vertical and horizontal lines. Patients with lesions in the left hemisphere, on the other hand, usually act and learn slowly, make few mistakes, and are aware of their deficits, which frustrate them severely. In recent years, neuropsychological training programs designed to help patients overcome the visual, perceptual, and cognitive deficits have been reported as being successful.[23,24] In addition, repeated neuropsychological evaluations have been found to be sensitive indicators of recurrence.[25]

CANCER OF THE SPINE

The spine is the most common site for skeletal metastases.[26] At autopsy, 70% of patients who die from cancer demonstrate vertebral metastases[27] and more than 5% have evidence of metastatic compression of the spinal cord.[28] This is usually an extradural anterior mass that involves bone. Intradural extramedullary tumors are usually histologically benign meningiomas or neurofibromas. Gliomas (ie, ependymomas, astrocytomas, and medulloblastomas) are usually intramedullary, although occasionally they are also found in an extramedullary site. Although the response to treatment is quite different for all of these histologically distinct tumors, the neurologic symptoms, signs, and rehabilitation interventions are quite similar.

Injury to the spinal cord and peripheral nerves is a recognized risk of therapeutic radiation that may not become manifest for many months or even years.[29] A transient radiation myelopathy primarily involving sensory neurons may occur in 10 to 15% of patients receiving mantle radiation for Hodgkin's disease.[30] This condition is usually associated only with sensory symptoms, such as paresthesias and Lhermitte's sign, and resolves in 1 to 9 months.[30] Delayed radiation myelopathy is an irreversible and progressive neurologic condition that may affect motor, sensory, and sphincter functions and has a reported incidence of 1 to 12%.[31]

Clinical Presentation By far the most frequent presenting symptom of a tumor of the spine is pain. The pain may be localized, diffuse, or radicular in nature. It is characteristically made worse by activity and by straining. Different from more benign back pain, the pain caused by tumors tends to be persistent, tends to be present or even worse at night, and is not relieved by rest. Additional symptoms at presentation may be weakness of the legs, difficulty in walking, and urinary sphincteric problems leading to incontinence.

Neurologic deficits may develop insidiously or occur suddenly, depending on the tumor's rate of growth and location or on the occurrence of a sudden pathologic fracture. Slowly progressive neurologic dysfunction is often seen with tumors of the lower spine that encroach on the cauda equina, whereas tumors of the thoracic spine may cause the sudden collapse of a vertebral body with direct compression of the spinal cord or of its blood supply. Although only half of all tumors of the spine are located in the thoracic region, these cause 70% of all spinal cord compressions that result in paraplegia. Frequently, the neurologic lesion is incomplete, with sensation and motor function preserved to varying degrees, as may be rated by the ASIA Impairment Scale.[32] Impaired bladder and bowel control at first may present clinically as urinary urgency or hesitancy, but with progressive cord compression, urinary retention or bowel and bladder incontinence may occur.

Treatment Proper rehabilitation management planning and intervention depend on an accurate diagnosis and staging of the tumor, just as does medical and surgical management. Most patients with spinal metastases can and should be managed nonsurgically with radiation, chemotherapy, and orthotic stabilization of the spine because it has been demonstrated that radiation alone provides results that are similar to those of surgery followed by radiation.[33] In general, laminectomy with decompression is of limited use compared with radiation because the compressive lesion is usually located anteriorly to the cord and the surgical procedure itself contributes to spinal instability. However, profound neurologic deficits, especially when occurring rapidly, may warrant surgical decompression, which preferably should be done by an anterior approach followed by surgical stabilization of the spine. Surgical decompression of the spinal cord is not very effective once the patient has become completely paraplegic. Surgical stabilization may often be indicated when gross spinal instability is present because two of the three "columns" (anterior, middle, and posterior) of the spine have been destroyed by the tumor.[34]

Spinal metastases and myelomatous lesions, even when accompanied by compression fractures and minor or modest spinal instability, can be successfully managed by spinal orthotic support and radiation. Both modalities may significantly

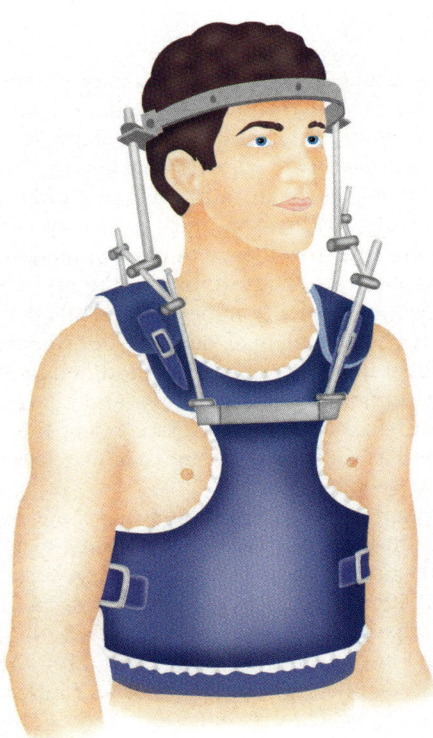

Figure 61-1 Halo-orthosis. Reproduced with permission from Ragnarsson KT. Orthotics and shoes. In: DeLisa JA, editor. Rehabilitation medicine: principles and practice. Philadelphia: Lippincott; 1988. p. 326.

decrease pain. Lesions in the cervical spine are most rigidly immobilized by a halo brace (Figure 61-1) but also may be adequately supported by a sternal-occipital-mandibular immobilizer (SOMI brace) (Figure 61-2). When such lesions are present in the upper thoracic spine, spinal orthoses may not be necessary because this part of the spine is stabilized inherently by the rib cage. Lesions in the more mobile lower thoracic and lumbar spine are often associated with severe pain. An adjustable thoracolumbosacral (TLS) orthosis (Figure 61-3) with posterior stays may provide sufficient support for less severe lesions, decrease pain, and allow greater mobility. Larger lesions and postoperative conditions may require fabrication of a custom-molded plastic TLS brace, a two-piece removable orthosis (Figure 61-4) that firmly grabs the pelvis below and the chest above.

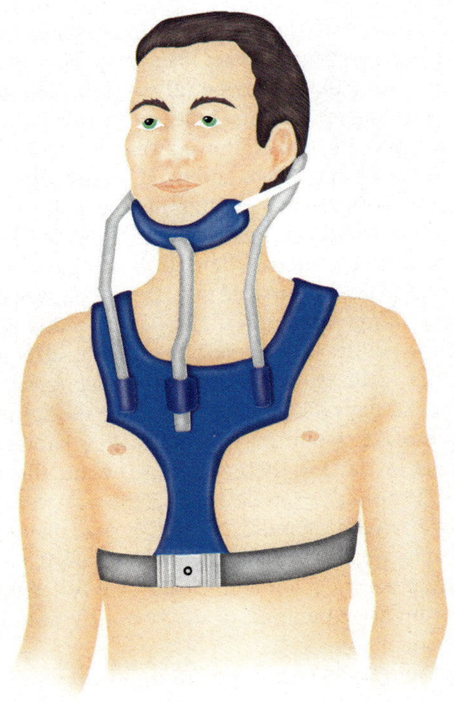

Figure 61-2 Sternal-occipital-mandibular immobilizer (SOMI orthosis). Reproduced with permission from Ragnarsson KT. Orthotics and shoes. In: DeLisa JA, editor. Rehabilitation medicine: principles and practice. Philadelphia: Lippincott; 1988. p. 326.

When neurologic loss has occurred, the rehabilitation therapy must be carefully individualized, on the basis of the extent of the neurologic dysfunction, the medical or surgical condition, and the patient's life expectancy. Spinal cord dysfunction with severe or complete paralysis and sensory loss, and perhaps bladder and bowel dysfunction, warrants a comprehensive but relatively short-term rehabilitation program involving as many members of the rehabilitation team as judged appropriate by the physiatrist. The rehabilitation programs should be designed to address each of the many clinical complications and conditions that may be seen in individuals with spinal cord dysfunction of traumatic origin (Table 61-6). Early intervention should include bedside physical and occupational therapy, establishment of bowel and bladder training programs, and the application of nursing principles to prevent complications, such as pressure sores and joint contractures, that increase morbidity, worsen the functional prognosis, and prolong the rehabilitation phase. Proper positioning of the patient in bed and turning at least every 2 hours is of paramount importance in this regard. The patient and caregivers are given emotional support and are educated in the medical aspects of spinal cord dysfunction and management. If the prognosis is poor, the patient is instructed early in the ADL skills, which the patient can quickly learn to perform, and is provided with the necessary assistive devices, such as a wheelchair, nursing supplies, and personal assistance. As soon as medically appropriate, discharge from the hospital to the home or a nursing facility can be accomplished. When life expectancy is greater than 3 months and the general criteria for admission to the inpatient rehabilitation service are met, the patient should be transferred there for a more comprehensive and intensive rehabilitation program to improve mobility and self-care skills.[35,36]

CANCER OF THE HEAD AND NECK

Definitive treatment of cancer that arises from the skin of the face and neck or tissues of the nose, mouth, throat, and larynx may result in impairments in cosmesis, oral communication, feeding, and respiration, as well as affect the senses of sight, hearing, taste, and smell. These

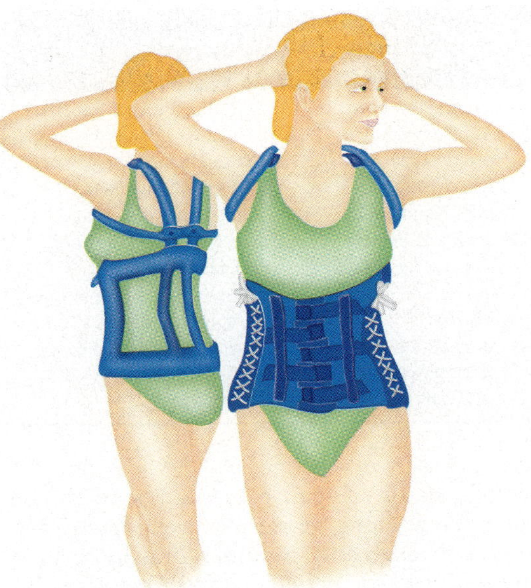

Figure 61-3 Thoracolumbosacral orthosis (Knight-Taylor brace). Reproduced with permission from Ragnarsson KT. Rehabilitation of patients with physical disabilities caused by tumors of the musculoskeletal system. In: Lewis MM, editor. Musculoskeletal oncology: a multidisciplinary approach. Philadelphia: WB Saunders; 1992. p. 463.

functional deficits may have major psychological, social, and vocational consequences if not adequately addressed early and managed properly. Sensory deficits and radiation-induced skin changes require careful grooming and hygiene to prevent further skin damage by using nonirritating soaps and cosmetic products, an

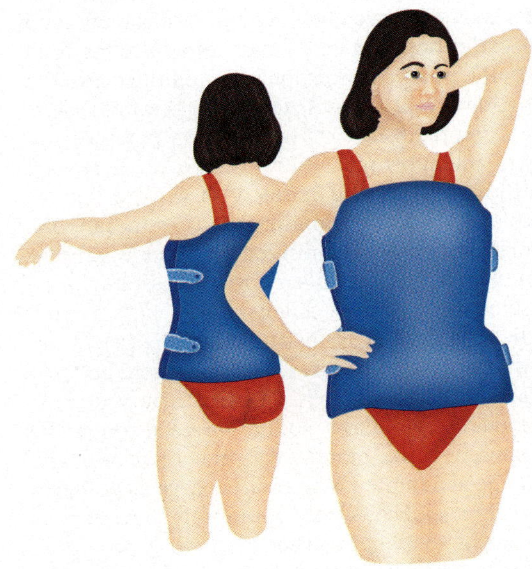

Figure 61-4 Custom-molded thoracolumbosacral orthosis (TLSO), a two-piece removable plastic orthosis ("body jacket"). Reproduced with permission from Ragnarsson KT. Rehabilitation of patients with physical disabilities caused by tumors of the musculoskeletal system. In: Lewis MM, editor. Musculoskeletal oncology: a multidisciplinary approach. Philadelphia: WB Saunders; 1992. p. 463.

Table 61-6 Conditions and Complications Associated with Spinal Cord Dysfunctions

Loss of motor power	Metabolic disturbances
Loss of sensation	Negative calcium balance
Pressure sores	Negative nitrogen balance
Urinary dysfunction	Hormonal imbalance
Bowel dysfunction	Circulatory disturbances
Sexual dysfunction	Orthostatic hypotension
Autonomic hyperreflexia	Edema
Pain	Deep vein thrombophlebitis
Spasticity	Respiratory disturbances
Joint contractures	Psychological problems
Heterotopic ossifications	Social problems
Vocational problems	

electric razor instead of a blade, lukewarm water for washing, loose-fitting garments, and similar measures. Meticulous oral hygiene is essential, and the patient should frequently use diluted mouthwash with 3% hydrogen peroxide but avoid all irritating agents (ie, alcohol, tobacco, and astringent toothpaste) and should limit denture wear. A noxious taste and dry mouth may be reduced by the use of artificial saliva and by increasing fluid intake. Mobilizing exercises for the mouth, jaw, neck, and shoulders should be emphasized to prevent adhesions and contractures.

Cosmetic defects of the face are primarily treated by surgical reconstruction, but different types of maxillofacial prostheses may be custom-made from plastic materials to closely match the facial contours and complexion. Surgical resection of cancer involving the mouth, pharynx, and larynx may result in impaired functions of chewing, swallowing, and speaking in different proportions. Following resection of the tongue and mandible, physical exercise of the residual muscles may improve chewing and swallowing, and special tubes or utensils may help place the food into the pharynx or esophagus and thus ease the swallowing process. Total laryngectomy results in a complete loss of voice and a permanently open tracheostomy.[37] Preoperatively, a speech pathologist should meet with the patient to explain ways to communicate postoperatively. Communication is initiated postoperatively by using writing materials, communication boards, or electronic typing gadgets, but as early as possible, the patient is instructed in the use of an artificial electrolarynx. Here a handheld battery-powered "diaphragm" is placed firmly against the neck to transmit sound waves through the tissues into the mouth, where it resonates and may be articulated with relative ease as comprehensible speech. Greater training, however, is required to become proficient in esophageal speech, which is generated by trapping air in the upper esophagus by the tongue and releasing it suddenly into the pharynx, thus producing a "burp-like" low-pitched sound that may be articulated into words. In some cases, a tracheopharyngeal shunt may be surgically reconstructed to restore a more normal voice.[38] Because of the open tracheostomy, the laryngectomized patient is unable to strain during lifting, pushing, or defecation, except by manually closing the stoma. The permanent tracheostomy requires not only good local care but also inhalation of humidified air through a stoma cover made of a piece of gauze that acts as a sieve for dust and other foreign materials.

Radical neck dissection may involve the removal of several neck muscles and temporary or permanent damage of the spinal accessory nerve that supplies the sternocleidomastoid and the trapezius muscles. This is likely to result in gross asymmetry of the neck and shoulders, restriction of motion, overstretching of remaining muscles, and persistent pain if not treated early. During the rehabilitation of these patients, it is of primary importance to unload the shoulder immediately postoperatively, reduce shoulder and neck pain, and prevent stretch fibrosis of the trapezius and contracture of the unopposed pectoralis muscles, as well as provide strengthening exercises for the residual muscles in the neck and shoulder girdle to compensate for lost muscles.[39] Sleeping on the back is preferable, with proper support provided by pillows placed between the scapulae and under the posterior neck. Lying on the affected side is to be avoided, and when lying on the unaffected side, the affected arm should be slightly raised and supported on a pillow. Occasionally, it may be helpful to wear a sling, or even a shoulder orthosis, to compensate for trapezius paralysis. Therapeutic exercises are initially passive but gradually progress to active-assistive and eventually resistive exercises, as tolerated by the patient. Strenuous physical activities, such as lifting, carrying, pulling, and pushing, should be avoided initially but may be resumed in the course of time as the physical condition improves.

CANCER OF THE LUNG

The physical disabilities associated with lung cancer and its treatment include respiratory insufficiency, shoulder pain and stiffness, scoliosis, and the remote effects of certain lung cancers that cause a neuromuscular disorder that becomes manifest as weakness and incoordination. However, the functional limitations associated with lung cancer frequently do not receive adequate attention and intervention because of the high mortality and short life expectancy associated with the disease.

Reduced respiratory capacity after lung resection or pneumonectomy, especially when combined with preexisting chronic obstructive pulmonary disease, may result in respiratory complications and insufficiency during both the postoperative period and the long-term follow-up. As the patient recuperates and becomes ambulatory, shoulder range of motion, general strengthening, and endurance exercises, as well as postural training, are added to the therapy program to increase strength and stamina and prevent post-thoracotomy scoliosis and scapulohumeral displacement.[40]

CANCER OF THE BREAST

Breast cancer that is treated with mastectomy or with lumpectomy followed by radiation, and/or with chemotherapy may result in considerable physical disability. Radical mastectomy with removal of the pectoralis muscles, although now rarely performed, may cause shoulder weakness and, together with axillary node dissection, may produce swelling of the ipsilateral arm. Stiffness of the shoulder and hand may limit reach and manual dexterity. Fortunately, the recent trend of performing modified radical mastectomies or lumpectomies and routinely providing proper postoperative rehabilitation therapy has reduced the frequency and severity of these problems.

Postoperative rehabilitation has three main goals: prevention of physical disability, restoration of cosmetic appearance, and psychosocial and vocational readjustment. Physical rehabilitation aims at improving muscle strength and mobility at the shoulder, minimizing arm swelling, and facilitating resumption of all functional activities—ADL, recreation, and work. Following radical mastectomy, the arm should be kept slightly elevated, with the shoulder abducted to 80 to 90° and externally rotated, keeping the elbow free.[41] The entire arm is compressed by a well-wrapped elastic Ace bandage, which is reapplied every 8 hours to reduce the swelling. Substantially less physical rehabilitation is necessary following modified radical mastectomy and axillary dissection, an operation that spares the pectoralis major and usually the pectoralis minor. Lumpectomy with axillary dissection requires even less physical rehabilitation, which may proceed at a more rapid pace. Depending on the extent of the mastectomy, physical exercises may be started within 2 to 5 days postoperatively. Gentle exercises are started at this time, with the patient actively moving all of the unaffected limbs, as well as the elbow, wrist, and hand on the affected side, and isometrically contracting the distal muscles (hand squeezing) while supine and with the affected arm elevated. When the drains have been removed from the surgical site, the exercises may become more demanding. The patient starts performing gentle active exercises of the affected shoulder while still in a supine position. Approximately 10 days postoperatively, when the sutures are removed, active or active-assistive shoulder exercises in the upright position are begun, that is, "wall climbing" exercises using the uninvolved arm or an overhead pulley system to ease the task. On discharge, the patient receives a series of exercises to perform at home to ensure that full shoulder mobility and maximum strength will be regained.

Lymphedema of the arm after radical mastectomy is seen in approximately 10 to 15% of patients, although relatively mild or moderate arm swelling is much more common, especially in the early postoperative days. Lymphedema is less common after modified radical mastectomy and rare after lumpectomy, even though both procedures do have axillary dissection. When lymphedema is severe, it may result in both a significant disability and a disfigurement. Although surgical removal of lymph nodes and lymph vessels or their destruction by radiation undoubtedly is the major etiologic factor, a number of other contributing factors may play a role, including infection, inflammation, scar formation, obesity, thrombophlebitis, arm dominance, and habitual dependent position of the arm. The greatest incidence of lymphedema has been noted among those who received high-dose radiation or had a history of one or more infections.[42,43] Prevention of lymphedema with proper postoperative care and initiation of an exercise program, referred to as complex decongestive physiotherapy, is most important because treatment of persisting lymphedema is relatively ineffective. Such treatment usually involves different physical interventions: performing, several times a day, sets of isometric exercises of all of the arm muscles while the arm is maintained in an elevated position, compression bandaging, manual lymphatic drainage, and skin care with patient education. These modalities help pump the fluid from the hand and distal arm toward the body. Compression therapy by manual massage of both the edematous[44,45] and the contralateral arm[46] has also been advocated but is considered by some to be time-consuming and inefficient.[47] Between periods of use, the arm should be carefully wrapped with elastic bandages, and when maximum reduction of the edema has been obtained, a custom-fitted elastic support sleeve should be fabricated and worn continuously. The entire limb should be guarded against even trivial trauma, which may be caused by constricting garments and excessive heat or exercise, to minimize swelling. Treatment with these physical modalities and exercise benefits the majority of patients with postoperative lymphedema and is more effective than diuretics, salt restriction diets, benzopyrones, or surgical procedures.[46–49] Benzopyrone reportedly causes a slow but safe reduction of high-protein lymphedema of the extremities by stimulating proteolysis by macrophages.[50]

CANCER OF THE GASTROINTESTINAL TRACT

The cancer rehabilitation team is involved in the care of the patient who has cancer limited to the gastrointestinal tract when the definitive surgical treatment has resulted in an ostomy. The enterostomal therapist (ET nurse) plays a major role in helping the cancer patient with an ostomy (ie, colostomy, ileostomy, or urostomy) understand the principles of ostomy care, learn the different aspects of ostomy management, and adjust to the altered self-image.

Colostomy The surgical treatment of cancer of the rectum usually mandates the creation of a colostomy by using the sigmoid colon. A cancer higher in the colon can frequently be resected and the bowel reconnected by anastomosis. Before undergoing a surgical procedure for cancer that will result in a colostomy, the surgeon needs to discuss the plans carefully with the patient. Subsequently, the ET nurse should meet with the patient and family members to explain in simple but clear terms the nature of the colostomy, for example, where the stoma will be located on the abdominal wall, how it will look, what coverings and collection appliances will be needed, how evacuation will occur, and so on. A positive attitude on the part of the medical and nursing staff is important at this time, although the patient's fears and concerns regarding function, appearance, and sexual activity need to be acknowledged and discussed. A visit by a person who is successfully managing his or her colostomy may be very helpful. Good preoperative preparation reduces the patient's fears and builds confidence, both of which will facilitate postoperative rehabilitation.

Postoperatively, protecting the skin and collecting the drainage should be the primary goals. This is accomplished by a properly fitted appliance. Modern appliances with protective skin barriers cut to fit the exact size of the stoma will avoid postoperative peristomal skin excoriation and keep the patient dry and odor free. A person with a colostomy has a choice of allowing the bowels to function normally or to irrigate as a method of attempting to control bowel movements. Often the bowel habits return to normal patterns, and a well-fitting appliance may be emptied or changed as needed.

Numerous clinical problems may arise at any time after the creation of a colostomy. These may include constipation, diarrhea, odor, skin excoriation and maceration, skin infections (fungi or bacteria), and stomal bleeding. Sexual dysfunction after abdominoperineal resection is common, not owing to the colostomy per se but to damage to the autonomic nerves in the pelvis sustained during extensive surgery. The altered self-image often associated with the colostomy can cause temporary sexual dysfunction, although sexual desire is not lessened.[51] Sexual counseling for both partners, good communication, and the teaching of new techniques for mutual gratification can do much to restore successful sexual activity. The colostomy patient may experience a reactive depression or grief and subsequently go through the different stages of adaptation that are associated with any kind of major personal loss. The colostomy's negative influence on the patient's self-image is best counteracted by the physician and the ET nurse when they are able to make an accurate assessment of the patient's complaints and condition, plan actions and interventions accordingly, and provide supportive counseling on an individual basis.[52]

Ileostomy The principles and techniques of ileostomy care are similar to those of colostomy. The stools are of a loose consistency and drain continuously from the ileostomy. It is, therefore, necessary that the collecting pouch be worn at all times and that it be properly fitted by an ET nurse. Small bowel contents contain active digestive enzymes, which can cause severe peristomal skin excoriation if leakage occurs. Because the fluid loss through ileostomy is greater than with colostomy, fluid intake must be increased to prevent dehydration. In general, the psychosocial adjustment and rehabilitation outcome for an individual with ileostomy are similar to those after any surgery that requires alteration of elimination habits and results in living with a stoma.

CANCER OF THE GENITOURINARY SYSTEM

Invasive cancer of the bladder frequently requires radical cystectomy and the creation of a new outlet for urine. More than 40 years ago, Bricker developed the ileal conduit procedure by connecting the ureters to an isolated segment of ileum, which is surgically closed at one end but opens at the other as a stoma on the abdominal wall, allowing free elimination of the urine. This procedure has become the traditional form of long-term urinary diversion. The management principles of ileal conduit stoma care are similar to those of colostomy and ileostomy. Because urine flows continuously from the stoma, the collecting system must be well fitted and watertight to prevent leakage. Skin or stoma problems from the urine are not uncommon and may be caused by alkaline urine. Many physicians prescribe vitamin C, 1,000 mg daily, to keep the urine slightly acidic. The intake of 8 to 10 glasses of fluid daily is important. In recent years, the continent urostomy has gained considerable popularity when used with compliant patients. The Kock pouch and the Indiana pouch, with several modifications of both procedures, result in an internal reservoir.[53–58] The patient inserts a catheter into the stoma every 4 to 6 hours to empty the internal pouch contents. This procedure eliminates the need for external devices.

Genital Cancer The cancer rehabilitation team may occasionally be asked to provide care for a patient with cancer involving the genital organs or when the cancer and its treatment have caused sexual dysfunction. Rehabilitation interventions usually involve carefully planned reconstructive surgery and psychological and sexual counseling. The form of surgical reconstruction varies, depending on the type of the cancer and the extent of the surgical resection but also on the specific needs of the patient. The woman who has undergone radical gynecologic surgery with resection of the vagina may benefit from vaginal reconstruction that allows resumption of sexual intercourse.[59] The man who is unable to achieve penile erection can be prescribed medications (ie, sildenafil), taught intrapenile injection of vasodilating drugs to cause erection when desired, or, rarely nowadays, have a penile prosthesis implanted.[60] The choice of prosthesis is between semirigid silicone rod implants and a system of inflatable cylinders implanted into the shaft of the penis, with the scrotal pump and fluid reservoir placed in the abdominal wall.[61–63] The implantation of the semirigid rod is a relatively simple surgical procedure with few mechanical problems, but the penis stays semierect permanently. The inflatable prosthesis provides a more normal appearance of the penis both when flaccid and erect, but mechanical problems with the system often arise.

Cancer of the testes is usually treated with prompt surgical excision of one or both of the testicles, followed by radiation and/or chemotherapy. Surgical implantation of a prosthetic testicle at a later date may be gratifying for patients concerned about their appearance and self-image.

Sexual Rehabilitation Sexual rehabilitation is not limited to those who have cancer affecting the genital organs but should be available for anyone who experiences sexual dysfunction for physical or psychological reasons as a result of cancer and its treatment. Different members of the rehabilitation team collaborate in providing sexual counseling for patients with different forms of cancer, both on an individual basis and by organizing courses and seminars on the physiology and anatomy of sexual function, on human sexuality, and on ways of adjusting to sexual dysfunction. Male sexual impotence compounds the reactive depression associated with the diagnosis of cancer and adds to the stigma of any physical disability. This condition is frequently met with prejudice and poor understanding on the part of both the patient and the patient's sexual partner. Sexual rehabilitation emphasizes that sexuality is considered part of the whole person and cannot be lost because of an illness or injury. Physical disability, in contrast to a physical illness, does not decrease sexual drive, although it may affect sexual function both physically and psychologically. The anatomy and physiology of sexual function should be carefully explained to the disabled patient and his or her partner and general guidelines for success given. Good communication and strengthening of relationships between sexual partners are emphasized. The different physical aspects of sexual performance are explained to make expectations compatible with performance capability. For most cancer patients with a physical disability, impairment of mobility, sensation, continence, and erection should not interfere with building a solid personal relationship, with having sensitivity to the partner's desires, or with being able to please and enjoy. Sexual rehabilitation is built on the concept that if sexual comfort is taught, sexual competence may result.[64] Manual and oral sexual acts may be appropriate for both sexes. No treatment or rehabilitation of the patient with cancer can be considered complete until the clinician has adequately addressed the impact of the condition on sexual function. Sexual health cannot be separated from total health. The extra time spent considering sexual adequacy and providing guidelines for help can benefit the patient for years.

CANCER OF THE LIMBS

Primary malignant tumors of the limbs require surgical treatment. The main surgical goal is to remove the tumor, either by an excision with wide margins through a site well clear of any malignant growth or by radical removal of the entire bone or the compartment afflicted by the tumor. A subsequent surgical goal is to reconstruct the resulting defect for optimal function and cosmesis. Although limb amputation has been practiced for centuries, in recent years, limb salvage by extended local or regional excision and reconstruction has been the principal goal. The survival and disease-free survival after both types of surgical approaches are similar and have been vastly improved in recent years by the use of chemotherapy, radiation, or both. The return to optimal function can best be ensured by a multidisciplinary rehabilitation team approach that includes the surgeon, the medical and radiation oncologists, the physiatrist, and all of the members of the rehabilitation team.[65]

Skeletal metastases are more common than primary bone tumors.[66] Metastases to the limb bones are less common than those to the spine. Although some patients may complain of localized pain, others are essentially asymptomatic until a pathologic fracture occurs. Such fractures occur in approximately 10 to 15% of patients who have radiographic evidence of skeletal metastasis. Pathologic fractures are most debilitating and often result in diminished survival for otherwise stable patients.[26] At particular risk of pathologic fractures are women with metastatic breast cancer, patients with advanced metastatic disease, and those with a large single lytic lesion eroding the bony cortex.[67] Active rehabilitation and physical mobilization do not seem to increase the fracture risk significantly. When prognosis suggests many months of anticipated function, prophylactic surgery for impending fracture of the femoral neck or shaft often diminishes the total disability consequent to pathologic fracture and more difficult surgical repair. Prophylactic surgery is otherwise generally not warranted, but radiation may have some effect in reducing pain and limiting tumor growth.[68] If pathologic fracture occurs, open surgical treatment with adequate internal fixation and conjunctive use of methylmethacrylate may be employed successfully to relieve pain, restore mobility, ease nursing care, and provide psychological reassurance.[69] Postoperative immobilization should be brief, and aggressive physical therapy should be started early to return the patient swiftly to previous function and to minimize hospitalization.

Preoperative Rehabilitation Rehabilitation care should start immediately after the diagnosis of primary cancer of a limb is established, regardless of whether amputation or limb-sparing surgery is planned for cancer removal or whether chemotherapy and radiation are to be instituted pre- or postoperatively. The implications of surgery and the postoperative course should be discussed at this time with the patient and caregivers. Simultaneously, an appropriate physical exercise program should begin. Although it is important that the positive aspects of the surgical treatment be explained (ie, that it is a swift, lifesaving technique and that modern technology and training allow significant restoration of function), it is best for the physician to resist overly optimistic predictions and to discourage unrealistic hopes until postoperative rehabilitation success has been ensured. On the other hand, pessimistic statements as to what the patient will never be able to do are needless and are usually inaccurate. Peer counseling by a successfully rehabilitated amputee may further help the patient anticipate postoperative events and function.

When amputation or limb-sparing surgery is planned, the exact level of amputation and the surgical approach should be thoughtfully chosen, taking into account not only the location and type of cancer but also the probability of good wound healing and the successful fitting of a prosthesis when required. It may be helpful for the surgeon to consult with the physiatrist and prosthetist for this purpose. Preoperatively, strengthening exercises should be started for muscles in the uninvolved extremities and the trunk, as well as for muscles to be spared in the affected limb. Specifically, the patient should learn to perform isometric exercises for the quadriceps and gluteal muscles. Strengthening exercises for the unaffected limbs should focus specifically on shoulder depressors and elbow extensors, which are critical for ambulation with crutches or walkers. Trunk-strengthening and balancing exercises may further ensure postoperative ambulation success. Ambulation with a walker or a pair of crutches, non–weight bearing on the affected limb, should be practiced preoperatively while the patient has no fear of falling because of a lack of limb support and is not impaired by incisional pain, medications, or postoperative complications. Such preoperative therapy not only will help the patient succeed swiftly in postoperative ambulation and self-care activities, but a quick restoration of function will ease the emotional adjustment to the disability, whether it be amputation or limb sparing with an internal prosthesis.

Limb Amputation Limb amputation for cancer at one time was discouraged because the prevailing opinion was that poor life expectancy did not justify the expense of surgery and prosthetic fitting. However, the 5-year survival rate for patients who have undergone amputations for limb cancer (49%) compares favorably with the survival rate of patients with amputations for limb ischemia,[70] and the functional skills of cancer amputees are reportedly better than the skills of those patients who have had amputations for other reasons.[71]

Until recently, amputations for cancer were done in a radical fashion and left little, if any, residual limb, except when amputating for very distal limb tumors, because the basic clinical rule was to amputate proximally to the joint immediately above the tumor site. Lower limb amputations for cancer involving the knee joint or thigh thus were frequently performed by a hip disarticulation or hemipelvectomy and upper limb amputations by shoulder disarticulation or interscapulothoracic (forequarter) amputations. Modern diagnostic techniques now can demonstrate the presence or absence of metastases with a high degree of accuracy. According to a recent survey, because of the use of adjuvant chemotherapy, sarcomatous metastases are not as common as was previously thought.[72] Thus, less extensive amputation techniques can now be employed, such as cross-bone amputations with 3 to 4 inches of normal bone left as the margin. Greater residual limb length thus results, and functional outcome is better for most patients. Accordingly, primary cancer in the distal femur now permits an amputation through the proximal femur, a cancer in the proximal tibia permits amputation in the mid- or distal femur, and cancer in the distal tibia allows a below-knee (B-K) amputation. Analogous amputation levels may be appropriately considered for cancer of the upper limbs.

Although maximum preservation of limb length compatible with eradication of the cancer is desirable, certain amputation levels may result in residual limbs that are difficult to fit and, therefore, best avoided, such as the hind foot, the distal third of the leg, and the femoral supracondylar region. It is critical to preserve the knee joint, if possible, to ensure smoothness of gait, lower energy cost, and better function. Whenever possible, 12 to 18 cm of tibia should be retained for optimal prosthetic fitting, but even a very short B-K amputation that retains the tibial tubercle will preserve knee extension by the quadriceps muscle, and preservation of the knee joint will provide the needed position sense. This amputation level is, therefore, better than amputating above the knee. When the fibula is retained, it should be cut slightly shorter than the tibia. Disarticulation at the knee is also preferable to above-knee (A-K) amputation because it provides a wide weight-bearing surface, a long lever arm, and proprioception. Unfortunately, this level often cannot be chosen owing to intra-articular spread of cancer located in the mid- or proximal tibia. It is preferable to have the A-K amputated residual limb as long as possible to preserve maximal adduction power. Prosthetic knee joints can accommodate any length of femur. A residual femoral length that is less than 8 cm from the greater trochanter to the tip functions poorly. As a rule, hip disarticulation is preferred to an amputation level above the lesser trochanter. Hip disarticulation and hemipelvectomy need reconstruction with a long posterior flap to create a proper sitting area on the prosthesis.[73] When provided with a well-fitting plastic laminated socket and an endoskeletal modular-design prosthesis, persons with hip disarticulation are able to stand, walk, and sit quite comfortably. Hemicorporectomy (translumbar amputation) has been performed on rare occasions on patients with widespread cancer of the pelvis but without metastases elsewhere. This procedure is a challenging alternative to the nonsurgical approach and has been shown to have a good rehabilitation outcome.[74] Cancers in the upper limbs unfortunately are primarily found in the proximal humerus and require shoulder disarticulation or interscapulothoracic amputation. Here it is important to retain quality skin and maximum muscle mass for padding the shoulder, but retention of the humeral head, if possible, will result in better prosthetic fitting.

Successful prosthetic use depends to a large extent on proper surgical techniques of amputation.[75] It is not adequate to provide only a long residual limb, although this is important for both leverage and large total contact area for weight bearing. Optimally, the residual limb should be firm and tapered or cylindrical in shape, with all bone ends well padded. The skin must have good innervation and vascular supply and not be adherent to bone or have sensitive scars.

Postoperative care should ensure optimal wound healing, minimize limb swelling, prevent joint contractures, and improve muscle strength and function. Application of appropriate dressing and external pressure on the residual limb is very important.[76] Wrapping with the customary elastic bandages must be done skillfully with frequent reapplications to maintain maximum sustained pressure and to avoid a tourniquet effect. Different forms of semirigid dressings have been used, such as Unna paste dressings, custom-made elastic "socks," plastic films, and inflatable air splints, each of which has advantages and disadvantages. Inflatable and removable air splints, recently popularized, are made of clear plastic and have a zipper, which allows easy inspection, attachments, and removal.

An elastic plaster bandage may be applied to the residual limb immediately after the amputation. This immediate postsurgical fitting is a rigid form of dressing that can effectively reduce edema and postoperative pain. A prosthetic pylon and foot can be attached directly to the plaster to allow standing within 2 days postoperatively. Initially, only minimal weight bearing is allowed, but progressive ambulation is continued, and full weight bearing may be possible in 3 to 4 weeks.[77] Several disadvantages of this technique have made it difficult to implement. The removable rigid dressing provides for easier inspection of the residual limb, dressing change, and adjustment for progressive shrinkage and may even allow attachment of a temporary adjustable prosthesis.[78,79]

Postoperative Exercise Program Physical and occupational therapy should be initiated within 2 days after the amputation. The preoperative exercise program is resumed for muscle strengthening and joint mobilization. Knee flexion contractures may easily develop after B-K amputation, whereas hip flexion and abduction contractures are frequently seen with short A-K amputation. Mobilization is started at the bedside, but within a few days, the patient is taken to the therapy area, and ambulation in parallel bars or with a walker is started. The skillful amputee is subsequently provided with a pair of crutches; however, when prosthetic fitting has been completed, a single cane will usually suffice. Different types of ready-made or prefabricated temporary prosthetic devices exist for the earliest ambulation efforts, but a custom-fitted provisional prosthesis should be provided as soon as the surgical incision has healed. The amputee, however, may be discharged from the hospital even without a prosthesis if the patient is ambulating safely with assistive gait devices and is independent in ADL. Transfer to the inpatient rehabilitation unit for more intensive therapy may be advisable at any time before these two goals are reached if the amputee is otherwise medically stable.

Prescription of an Artificial Limb The physician needs to consider multiple factors when prescribing a limb prosthesis. The amputation level and limb condition clearly are of primary importance, but prosthetic candidacy may be affected by numerous other factors, including associated medical conditions, other physical disabilities, life expectancy, muscle strength and coordination, stamina, various psychological factors (ie, motivation, emotional adjustment, and cognition), and individual lifestyle factors (ie, age, weight, family support, recreational interest, environment, and type of work). The extent of prosthetic use is, to some degree, predictable because each symptomatic medical problem adversely affects functional prognosis. The ability of the patient to ambulate with a walker or a pair of crutches but without a prosthesis strongly suggests prosthetic candidacy. After carefully considering these different factors, the physiatrist may have to choose between a prosthesis that provides relatively greater safety with stability and one with greater function and mobility and between durability and low prosthetic weight, besides considering differences in cost and cosmesis.

Most prostheses are currently fabricated from metals and plastics. The customary B-K prosthesis consists of a socket, shank, and ankle-foot components, as well as a suspension system. The socket usually has a patellar tendon–bearing design and total contact with the residual limb for maximum pressure distribution.[80] Modern liners that add comfort and protect sensitive skin are usually made of silicone gel and may be designed to provide a suction suspension system with an attached distal pin that locks into a receptacle in the bottom of the socket or shank.[81] The shank is either of an endoskeletal design with an internal metal pylon or an exoskeletal structure made from laminated plastic. The solid-ankle cushioned-heel foot is simple, durable, lightweight, and cosmetic and is still most commonly prescribed, despite the arrival of a variety of new energy-storing prosthetic feet, such as the Seattle and FLEX feet designs. The B-K prosthesis is usually attached to the residual limb by a supracondylar cuff, although several other alternatives exist. The A-K amputee traditionally obtains a prosthesis with a rigid quadrilateral socket and a posterior ischial seat for additional weight bearing. More modern socket designs promise greater comfort in sitting and better control during ambulation.[82] The popular single-axis knee joint with constant friction is simple and durable, whereas the more costly and complex polycentric or hydraulic knee units can provide better function for young, physically active amputees. Stability of the knee joint during stance may be increased by posterior placement of the knee axis, but for maximum safety, manual or automatic knee locks may be added. The A-K prosthesis optimally is suspended by total suction or by partial suction and a Silesian bandage or a pelvic band. An endoskeletal pylon connects the knee unit above to the prosthetic foot below. After a hip disarticulation, the amputee receives the Canadian-type prosthesis, which has a plastic laminated socket encircling the pelvis. This provides a resting surface for the ischial tuberosity for weight bearing. With proper molding, it is suspended from the iliac crest. A similar prosthesis is worn after hemipelvectomy, with the rib cage providing the weight-bearing surface.

Cancer in the upper limb frequently requires shoulder disarticulation or interscapular thoracic amputation, both of which make fitting the patient with a functional body-powered prosthesis difficult or impossible. Myoelectrically controlled and externally powered prostheses may provide some gross function, but such prostheses are relatively expensive, are heavy, and require repair more often than body-powered prostheses.

In recent years, prosthetic techniques for all types of amputations have advanced significantly, especially with respect to evaluation methods, socket design, ankle-foot components, and cosmesis.[83,84]

Prosthetic Fitting and Training Before completion of the prosthesis, the amputee needs to visit the prosthetist several times to ensure optimal fit, function, and comfort. When fabrication has been completed, the prescribing physician checks the prosthesis for fit and comfort, socket stability, joint motions, appearance, and function. The lower limb amputee receives gait training, with or without gait aids, depending on motor skills, instructions in attachment and removal techniques, and exercises to increase muscle strength, joint range of motion, balance, and posture. The upper limb amputee learns to open and close the terminal device, position the arm, manipulate objects, and perform self-care tasks. Initially, a prosthesis may not be worn comfortably for more than 15 to 30 minutes at a time. The amputee thus requires frequent rest periods and short therapy sessions. After each wear, the skin of the residual limb must be examined for signs of excessive pressure or poor socket fit. At the beginning of prosthetic wear, confrontational situations may develop between the amputee and the health professional, especially when the patient's expectations do not match the actual situation.

Lower limb amputees ambulate at greater energy costs than do persons with no disability.[85,86] The B-K amputee expends 23 to 68% more energy per unit distance than does a person without amputation, and the A-K amputee expends 52 to 124% more.[87] However, to save energy, most amputees decrease their speed of ambulation, which is approximately 2.0 to 2.5 mph for B-K and 1.0 to 1.5 mph for A-K amputees compared with a normal speed of 3 to 4 mph for persons without amputation. The lower energy cost and greater speed of ambulation for the B-K amputee clearly show the importance of sparing the knee joint whenever possible. Patients with hip disarticulation or hemipelvectomy ambulate with lower energy expenditure if they use axillary crutches without a prosthesis compared with prosthetic use.[87]

Various clinical problems may occur as the result of the amputation and consequent prosthetic wear, including pain, skin lesions, swelling, joint contractures, and depression. Most amputees experience phantom sensation, which is a painless awareness of the amputated part. In contrast, phantom pain may be described as burning, crushing, cramping, or shooting sensations in the amputated phantom limb. The reported incidence of phantom pain has varied between 10 and 85%.[88] This variation may be due to differences in classification of the types of pain,[89] the fear of presumed mental illness if a phantom pain is reported,[88] and the time delay since surgery.[90] The pain may be aggravated by limb contact and different physical activities, but the exact cause remains unknown because no detectable pathology is usually discovered. Phantom pain[91] may be preventable or effectively managed by careful preoperative explanations of the nature of the phantom phenomenon, good surgical techniques, regular examinations postoperatively, and frequent manual handling and good care of the residual limb, as well as by effective treatment of infections and early provision of a functional prosthesis. Definitive treatment, however, is difficult, but symptoms usually improve when a relatively normal situation has been restored. Other beneficial interventions include desensitization by frequent self-inspection and manipulation of the residual limb, application of superficial heat or cold, deep heating with diathermy, massage, vibration, transcutaneous electrical nerve stimulation, imaginary exercises of the phantom limb, active exercises of the entire body, local anesthesia, and psychological interventions. Analgesic medications are relatively ineffective, but agents acting on the central nervous system may be helpful.

LIMB-SPARING SURGICAL RECONSTRUCTION

Local resection of cancer with limb-sparing reconstruction may result in survival, disease-free survival equal to that for amputation, and function that is superior to that for amputation.[92,93] Amputation, however, is still a primary treatment for many limb tumors because it may, at times, be impossible to perform a proper resection while preserving key nerves and vessels and to reconstruct a functional limb.

Limb-sparing reconstructive surgery obviously is an attractive alternative to amputation for both cosmetic and emotional reasons, but it should be undertaken only if it will restore better and longer-lasting function than amputation with subsequent prosthetic fitting.[94] Depending on the location and size of the tumor, it may be a difficult procedure in which muscles, bone, and even joints are removed with the tumor. The cancerous bone may be replaced by transplanting a fresh-frozen cadaveric bone allograft or an autologous graft but more commonly by installing a synthetic metallic prosthetic implant.[95–97] An expandable and adjustable prosthesis may now be installed in growing children, who formerly were felt to fare better with amputation.[98] Rehabilitation interventions preferably should begin preoperatively when physical and/or occupational therapists should first teach the patient the muscle-strengthening, range of motion, and ambulation exercises that will be resumed postoperatively. Following lower limb–sparing surgery, the patient may begin exercising the uninvolved limbs on the first postoperative day, but the initiation, pace, and intensity of exercises and the amount of weight bearing for the affected limb depend on the exact mode of reconstruction and the postoperative course. During rehabilitation and a 2.5-year follow-up of 17 children who underwent resection of malignant bone tumors in the lower limbs with insertion of expandable prostheses, 7 of these children walked without any assistive devices, but 10 required knee orthoses, crutches, or both for ambulation.[99] Following upper limb–saving surgery, active hand and isometric shoulder muscle exercises are started on the first postoperative day, but if humeral resection is performed, active elbow and shoulder exercises should not begin for 2 or 8 weeks postoperatively, depending on whether a metallic implant or allografts or autografts, respectively, are used. It is thus of primary importance that the rehabilitation staff know exactly which muscles, nerves, and bones were resected and what the reconstruction entailed to plan a safe and effective rehabilitation program. Training in ADL is initiated approximately 1 week postoperatively.

CONCLUSION

Management of cancer appropriately focuses on prevention, early diagnosis, and cure, but following effective treatment, many cancer patients experience some physical impairment that results in a physical disability or a handicap. As the prognosis for cancer improves, it becomes more important to ensure that all cancer patients regain maximum function in the broadest sense to ensure return to all former roles. Multidisciplinary rehabilitation, therefore, is an integral part of the total management of the cancer patient. The exact functional deficits need to be identified for each patient and proper rehabilitation interventions started promptly or at the same time as other treatments.

REFERENCES

1. Marciniak CM, Sliwa JA, Spill G, et al. Functional outcome following rehabilitation of the cancer patient. Arch Phys Med Rehabil 1996;77:892–5.
2. Dietz JH. Rehabilitation oncology. New York: Wiley; 1981. p. 69–75.

3. Cole RP, Scialla SJ, Bednarz L. Functional recovery in cancer rehabilitation. Arch Phys Med Rehabil 2000;81:623–7.
4. Hinterbuchner C. Rehabilitation of a physical disability in cancer. N Y State J Med 1978;78:1066–9.
5. Harvey RF, Jellinek HM, Habeck RV. Cancer rehabilitation: an analysis of 36 program approaches. JAMA 1982;247:2127–31.
6. Thistle HG, Hislop HJ, Moffroid M, Lowman EW. Isokinetic contraction. A new concept of resistive exercises. Arch Phys Med Rehabil 1967;48:279–82.
7. Gordon WA, Freidenbergs I, Diller L, et al. The efficacy of psychosocial intervention with cancer patients. J Consult Clin Psychol 1980;48:743–59.
8. Holland JC, Rowland JH. Handbook of psychooncology. Psychological care of the patient with cancer. New York: Oxford University Press; 1989.
9. World Health Organization. International classification of impairment, disabilities and handicaps. A manual or classification relating to consequences of disease. Geneva: World Health Organization; 1980.
10. Dodds TA, Martin DP, Stolow WC, Deyo RA. A validation of the functional independence measurement and its performance among rehabilitation inpatients. Arch Phys Med Rehabil 1993;74:531–6.
11. Grenger CV, Hamilton BB, Shriver SF. Guide for the use of the uniform data system for medical rehabilitation. Buffalo (NY): State University of New York; 1986.
12. Heinemann AW, Linacre JM, Wright BD, et al. Relationship between impairment and physical disability as measured by the functional independence measure. Arch Phys Med Rehabil 1993;74:566–73.
13. Mor V, Laliberte L, Morris JN, Wiemann M. The Karnofsky Performance Status Scale: an examination of its reliability and validity in a research setting. Cancer 1984;53:2002–7.
14. Schag CA, Ganz BA, Heinrich RL. Cancer Rehabilitation Evaluation System—Short Form (CARES-SF). A cancer specific rehabilitation and quality of life instrument. Cancer 1991;68:1406–13.
15. Schag CA, Heinrich RL. Development of a comprehensive quality of life measurement tool: CARES. Oncology 1990;4:135–8.
16. Thomas DC, Kreizman IJ, Melchiorre P, Ragnarsson KT. Rehabilitation of the patient with chronic critical illness. In: Nierman D, Nelson J, editors. Critical care clinics. Philadelphia: WB Saunders; 2002. p. 18:695–715.
17. Marciniak CM, Sliwa JA, Heinemann AW, Semik PE. Functional outcomes of persons with brain tumors after inpatient rehabilitation. Arch Phys Med Rehabil 2001; 82:457–63.
18. Philip PA, Ayyangar R, Vanderbilt J, Gaebler-Spira DJ. Rehabilitation outcome in children after treatment of primary brain tumor. Arch Phys Med Rehabil 1994;75:36–9.
19. Davis SW, Petrillo CR, Eichberg RD, Chu DS. Shoulder-hand syndrome in a hemiplegic population: a five-year retrospective study. Arch Phys Med Rehabil 1977;58:353–6.
20. Gordon WA, Hibbard M, Egelko S, et al. Perceptual remediation in patients with right brain damage: a comprehensive program. Arch Phys Med Rehabil 1985;66:353–9.
21. Albert ML, Helm-Estabrooks N. Diagnosis and treatment of aphasia. Part I and part II. JAMA 1988;259:1043–7,1205–10.
22. Geschwind N. Current concepts, aphasia. N Engl J Med 1971;284:654–6.
23. Ross ED, Mesulam MM. Dominant language functions of the right hemisphere. Prosody and emotional gesturing. Arch Neurol 1979;36:144–8.
24. Gordon WA, Hibbard MR, Kreutzer J. Cognitive remediation issues in research and practice. J Head Trauma Rehabil 1989;4:76–85.
25. Lieberman AN, Foo SH, Ransohoff J, et al. Long-term survival among patients with malignant brain tumors. Neurosurgery 1982;10:450–3.
26. Aaron AD. The management of cancer metastatic to bone. JAMA 1994;272:1206–9.
27. Harrington KD. Metastatic disease of the spine. J Bone Joint Surg Am 1986;68:1110–5.
28. Barron KD, Hirano A, Araki S, Ferry RD. Experiences with metastatic neoplasms involving the spinal cord. Neurology 1959;9:91–106.
29. Garden FH. Radiation injuries to the spinal cord and peripheral nerves. Phys Med Rehabil State Art Rev 1994;8:405–11.
30. Word JA, Kalokhe UP, Aron BS, et al. Transient radiation myelopathy (Lhermitte's sign) in patients with Hodgkin's disease treated by mantle irradiation. Int J Radiat Oncol Biol Phys 1980;6:1731–40.
31. Dropcho EJ. Central nervous system injury by therapeutic irradiation. Neurol Clin 1991;9:969–88.
32. Ditunno JF, Young W, Donovan WH, Creasey G. The International Neurological Standards booklet for neurological and functional classification of spinal cord injury. Paraplegia 1994;32:70–80.
33. Gilbert RW, Kim JH, Posner JB. Epidural spinal cord compression from metastatic tumor: diagnosis and treatment. Ann Neurol 1978;3:40–51.
34. Errico TJ, Kostuik JP. Diagnosis and treatment of metastatic disease of the spinal column: a review. Contemp Orthop 1986;13:15–26.
35. McKinley WO, Conti-Wyneken AR, Vokac CW, Cifu DX. Rehabilitative functional outcome of patients with neoplastic spinal cord compression. Arch Phys Med Rehabil 1996;77:892–5.
36. McKinley WO, Huang ME, Tewksbury MA. Neoplastic vs. traumatic spinal cord injury: an inpatient rehabilitation comparison. Am J Phys Med Rehabil 2000;79:138-44.
37. Keith RL, Darley FL. Laryngectomy rehabilitation. Boston: College Hill Press; 1986.
38. Juarbe C, Shemen L, Eberle R, et al. Primary tracheoesophageal puncture for voice restoration. Am J Surg 1986;152:464–6.
39. Villanueva R, Ajmani C. The role of rehabilitation medicine in physical restoration of patients with head and neck cancer. Cancer Bull 1977;29:46–54.
40. Sinclair JD. Exercise in pulmonary disease. In: Basmajian JW, editor. Therapeutic exercise. 3rd ed. Baltimore: Williams and Wilkins; 1978. p. 565–90.
41. Degenshein GA. Mobility of the arm following radical mastectomy. Surg Gynecol Obstet 1977;145:77.
42. Levinson SF. Rehabilitation of the patient with cancer or human immunodeficiency virus. In: DeLisa J, editor. Rehabilitation medicine: principles and practice. 2nd ed. Philadelphia: Lippincott; 1993. p. 916–33.
43. Segerstrom K, Bjerle P, Graffman S, Nystrom A. Factors that influence the incidence of brachial edema after treatment of breast cancer. Scand J Plast Reconstr Surg Hand Surg 1992;26:223–7.
44. Cheville AL, McGarvey CL, Petrek JA, et al. Lymphedema management. Semin Radiat Oncol 2003;13:290–301.
45. Elkins E. Effect of various procedures on the flow of lymph. Arch Phys Med Rehabil 1953;34:31–9.
46. Foldi E, Foldi M, Clodius L. The lymphedema chaos: a lancet. Ann Plast Surg 1989;22:505–15.
47. Grabois M. Breast cancer: post-mastectomy lymphedema. Phys Med Rehabil State Art Rev 1994;8:267–77.
48. Zeissler RH, Rose GB, Nelson PA. Post mastectomy lymphedema: late results of treatment in 385 patients. Arch Phys Med Rehabil 1972;53:159–66.
49. Casley-Smith JR, Boris M, Weindorf S, Lasinski B. Treatment for lymphedema of the arm, the Casley-Smith method: a noninvasive method produces continued reduction. Cancer 1998;83(12 Suppl Am):2843–60.
50. Casley-Smith JR, Morgan RG, Piller NB. Treatment of lymphedema of the arms and legs with 5,6-benzo-(a)-pyrone. N Engl J Med 1993;329:1158–63.
51. Gottesman JE. Male sexual dysfunction. Ostomy Q 1981;19:18–9.
52. Brogna L. Self-concept and rehabilitation of the person with an ostomy. J Enterostomal Ther 1985;12:205–9.
53. Brogna L, Lakaszawski M. Nursing management. The continent urostomy. J Enterostomal Ther 1986;13:139–47.
54. Carroll PR, Presti JC Jr, McAninch JW, Tanagho EA. Functional characteristics of the continent ileocecal urinary reservoir: mechanisms of urinary continence. J Urol 1989;142:1032–6.
55. Kock NG, Nilson AE, Nilsson LO, et al. Urinary diversion via continent ileal reservoir: clinical results in twelve patients. Urology 1982;128:469–75.
56. Rowland RG, Mitchell ME, Bihrle R. The cecoileal continent urinary reservoir. World J Urol 1985;3:185–90.
57. Rowland RG, Mitchell ME, Bihrle R, et al. Indiana continent reservoir. J Urol 1987;137:1136–9.
58. Skinner D, Boyd SD, Lieskovsky G. Clinical experience with a Kock continent ileal reservoir for urinary diversion. J Urol 1984;132:1101–7.
59. Edwards CL, Loeffler M, Rutledge FN. Vaginal reconstruction. In: Von Eschenbach AC, Rodriguez DB, editors. Sexual rehabilitation of the urologic cancer patient. Boston: Hall; 1981. p. 250–65.
60. Sparwasser C, Drescher P, Pust RA, Madsen PO. Long-term results of therapy with intracavernous injections and penile venous surgery in chronic erectile dysfunction. Scand J Urol Nephrol 1994;157 Suppl:107–12.
61. Finney RP. The treatment of erectile impotence with semi-rigid penile prosthesis. In: Von Eschenbach AC, Rodriguez DB, editors. Sexual rehabilitation of the urologic cancer patient. Boston: Hall; 1981. p. 228–9.
62. Pearman RO. Treatment of organic impotence by implantation of a penile prosthesis. J Urol 1976;97:716–9.
63. Scott FB, Bradley WE, Timm GW. Management of erectile impotence: use of implantable inflatable prosthesis. Urology 1973;2:80–2.
64. Comfort A. Sexual consequences of disability. Philadelphia: Stickley; 1978.
65. Ragnarsson KT. Rehabilitation of patients with physical disabilities caused by tumors of the musculoskeletal system. In: Lewis MM, editor. Musculoskeletal oncology—a multidisciplinary approach. Philadelphia: Saunders; 1992. p. 429–48.
66. Neff JR. Metastatic disease to bone. In: Lewis MM, editor. Musculoskeletal oncology: a multidisciplinary approach. Philadelphia: Saunders; 1992. p. 377–99.
67. Bunting R, Lamont-Havers W, Schweon D, Kliman A. Pathologic fracture risk in rehabilitation of patients with bony metastases. Clin Orthop 1985;192:222–7.
68. Schocker JD, Brady LW. Radiation therapy for metastasis. Clin Orthop 1982;169:38–43.
69. Sherry HS, Levy RN, Siffert RS. Metastatic disease of bone in orthopaedic surgery. Clin Orthop 1982;8:44–52.
70. Subbarao JV, McPhee MC. Prosthetic rehabilitation. Comparison of the outcome in patients with cancer and vascular amputations of the extremities. Orthop Rev 1982;11:43–51.
71. Kegel B, Carpenter ML, Burgess EM. Functional capabilities of lower extremity amputees. Arch Phys Med Rehabil 1978;59:109–20.
72. Gebhardt MC, Mankin HJ. Osteosarcomas: the treatment controversy, part II. Surg Rounds Orthop 1988; :25–42.
73. Enneking WF, Dunham WK. Resection and reconstruction of a primary neoplasm involving the innominate bone. Am J Bone Joint Surg 1978;60:731–46.
74. Frieden FH, Gertler M, Tosberg W, Rusk HA. Rehabilitation after hemicorporectomy. Arch Phys Med Rehabil 1969;50:259–63.
75. Burgess EM, Zettl JH. Amputations below the knee. Artif Limbs 1969;13:1–12.
76. Katz RT, Wu Y. Postoperative and pre-prosthetic management of the below knee amputee. Contemp Orthop 1985;10:53–63.
77. Burgess EM, Romano RL. Management of lower extremity amputees using immediate post surgical prostheses. Clin Orthop 1968;57:137–56.
78. Gottschalk F, Mooney V, McClellan B, Carlton A. Early fitting of the amputee with plastic temporary adjustable below knee prosthesis. Contemp Orthop 1986;13:15–8.
79. Wu Y, Keagy RD, Krick HJ, et al. An innovative removable rigid dressing technique for below the knee amputation. Am J Bone Joint Surg 1979;61A:724–9.
80. Edwards ML. Below knee prosthetic socket designs and suspension systems. Phys Med Rehabil Clin N Am 2000;11:585–93, vi.
81. Leonard JA, Meier RH. Upper and lower extremity prosthetics. In: DeLisa JA, Gans BM, editors. Rehabilitation medicine: principles and practice. Philadelphia: Lippincott-Raven; 1998. p. 669–96.
82. Schuch CM. Transfemoral amputation: prosthetic management. In: Bowker JH, Michael JW, editors. Atlas of limb prosthetics: surgical, prosthetic and rehabilitation principles. St. Louis (MO): Mosby; 1992. p. 509–33.
83. Staats TB. Advanced prosthetic techniques for below knee amputations. Orthopaedics 1985;8:249–58.
84. Huang ME, Levy CE, Webster JB. Acquired limb deficiencies. 3. Prosthetic components, prescriptions and indications. Arch Phys Med Rehabil 2001;82(3 Suppl 1):S17–24.
85. Gonzalez EG, Corcoran PJ, Reyes RL. Energy expenditure in below knee amputees: correlation with stump length. Arch Phys Med Rehabil 1974;55:111–9.
86. Traugh GH, Corcoran PJ, Reyes RL. Energy expenditure of ambulation in patients with above knee amputations. Arch Phys Med Rehabil 1975;56:67–71.
87. Gonzalez EG, Edelstein JE. Energy expenditure during ambulation. In: Gonzalez EG, Myers SJ, Edelstein JE, et al, editors. The physical basis of rehabilitation medicine. Boston: Butterworth-Heinemann; 2001. p. 417–47.
88. Davis RW. Phantom sensation, phantom pain, and stump pain. Arch Phys Med Rehabil 1993;74:79–91.
89. Weinstein SM. Phantom pain. Oncology (Huntingt) 1994;8:65–70.
90. Houghton AD, Nicholls G, Houghton AL, et al. Phantom

pain: natural history and association with rehabilitation. Ann R Coll Surg Engl 1994;76:22–45.
91. Harwood DD, Hanumanthu S, Stoudemire A. Pathophysiology and management of phantom limb pain. Gen Hosp Psychiatry 1992;14:107–18.
92. Simon MA, Aschliman MA, Thomas N, Mankin HJ. Limb salvage treatment versus amputation for osteosarcoma of the distal end of the femur. J Bone Joint Surg Am 1986;68:1331–7.
93. Davis AM, Devlin M, Griffin AM, et al. Functional outcome in amputation versus limb sparing of patients with lower extremity sarcoma: a matched case-control study. Arch Phys Med Rehabil 1999;80:615–8.
94. Lewis MM. Bone tumor surgery. Limb-sparing techniques. Philadelphia: Lippincott; 1988.
95. Barbera C, Lewis MM. Surgical considerations in tumors about the knee. In: Lewis MM, editor. Musculoskeletal oncology: a multidisciplinary approach. Philadelphia: Saunders; 1992. p. 327–42.
96. Kenan S, Kleinbart FA, Lewis M. Tumors and tumor like conditions of the shoulder girdle. In: Lewis MM, editor. Musculoskeletal oncology: a multidisciplinary approach. Philadelphia: Saunders; 1992. p. 283–306.
97. Mankin HJ, Gebhardt MC. Allografts in the management of bone tumors: part II. Surg Rounds Orthop 1988;24–40.
98. Frieden RA, Ryniker D, Kenan S, Lewis MM. Assessment of patient function after limb sparing surgery. Arch Phys Med Rehabil 1993;74:38–43.
99. Ditunno JF, Young WS, Donovan WH, et al. Standards for neurological classification of spinal injury patients. Chicago: American Spinal Injury Association; 1992.

Section 20

MULTIDISCIPLINARY MANAGEMENT

62

Principles of Multidisciplinary Management

James F. Holland, MD, ScD (hc)
Emil Frei III, MD
Donald W. Kufe, MD
Robert C. Bast Jr, MD
Raphael E. Pollock, MD, PhD, FACS
Ralph R. Weichselbaum, MD
Waun Ki Hong, MD
William N. Hait, MD, PhD

Most cancer patients, and society in general, would like to think that the entire team of doctors, nurses, and specialists is cooperatively involved in solving their medical problems. Patients have little awareness of turf battles, professional egos, personal animosities, or medical fads, but if they knew of their existence, they would have little tolerance for them. Oncologists of all disciplines and health professionals who interact with them are human beings, not unemotional automatons. Happily, the energies they squander in picayune or counterproductive activities are small compared to their constructive, positive efforts to seek improved (not just new) approaches to cancer.

The keystone for a successful interdisciplinary management team is attitude: humility, tolerance, adaptability, and appreciation of alternative approaches. None of us is so skilled that he or she can be as expert in every discipline as a highly competent exponent of that particular specialty. No one is omniscient. We are, and must be, interdependent, so it is important to work with individuals who are trustworthy and friendly. More failures of interdisciplinary management teams seem to occur because of personality conflicts than because of intellectual disagreements. In the heat of confrontational oratory, emotional preferences may win out over reasoned accord. Resorting to the literature should shed more light on a problem, not more heat. A selective literature survey can often be construed to support either side of an acrimonious dispute. Facts trump opinions.

In actual clinical practice, decisions are often implemented by the oncologic specialist who first encounters the patient. A much better way is to work with trusted colleagues and consultants whose opinions, where appropriate, are solicited before the first irreversible step is taken. Actions already taken can seldom be undone. A formal tumor conference (never really possible or necessary for every patient) serves the purpose of institutionalizing a forum for discussion, thereby diminishing the impact of bias and previous anecdotal experience. A conference serves the additional function of allowing oncologists of several disciplines to recognize individuals of other disciplines whose opinions and consultations appear to be the most learned and whose personalities are compatible. A tumor conference occasionally alters the primary oncologist's opinions and plans and, thus, the therapeutic approach for a specific patient. A conference may surface unfamiliar data, with references, that can change the course. An important contribution of a conference is the establishment of dialogue, which impacts on the future disposition of similar clinical problems. Managed care programs undeniably intrude on this concept, however, with limitation of referrals to plan members and the pressure of economic constraints to spend less time with and on each patient.

A second oncologic specialist of a different discipline, whose encounter with the patient occurs after the first oncologist has already changed the tumor and the patient, may rightly point out a better approach for the future. A medical oncologist or radiation oncologist can better know and eventually better treat a patient who has been seen before definitive surgical treatment rather than after. A surgical oncologist (and the patient) would be ill-treated if a patient were prepared for surgery by staff in chemotherapy or radiation therapy without the surgeon's examining the tumor and the patient beforehand. In diseases in which radiotherapy and chemotherapy both play a role, joint planning is mandatory.

In the absence of absolute oncologic truths, there is much room for diverse opinions. Interdisciplinary oncology implies that each discipline performs a complementary function. The best analogy is to a symphony: each instrument is played harmoniously on the same score, rather than all on the same note, or each to a different tune. And as in a symphony's output of music, interdisciplinary oncology requires belief in the probability that better outcomes will result, thus validating the extra commitment in time.

THE PRIMARY PHYSICIAN

No universal blood or urine tests exist that can diagnose asymptomatic cancer. Occasional patients may present abnormal protein patterns or marker alterations, but except for the prostate-specific antigen (PSA) test, such tests are not yet sufficiently sensitive or specific to justify their use for screening. Many cancers can be found in asymptomatic status by periodic, careful physical examinations. These are cancers of the skin, subcutaneous tissues, oral cavity, thyroid, lymph nodes, breast, gynecologic tract, penis, testes, anus, prostate, and rectum. Some asymptomatic cancers are announced by conditions revealed through simple laboratory tests often done for other purposes: leukocytosis, anemia, microscopic hematuria, hyperglobulinemia, and chest radiography or computed tomography (CT). Specific examinations proved to be of value in screening for cancer, such as cervical cytology, fecal occult blood testing, regular mammography, systematic colonoscopy, and PSA, are discussed in detail in Chapter 28, "Cancer Screening and Early Detection." Furthermore, some diagnoses can be made before cancer cells invade. Asymptomatic cancers tend to be smaller than symptomatic ones and often imply a better prognosis. Regrettably, for most sites, diagnoses when cancers are asymptomatic are still uncommon.

Until reliable diagnostic blood tests for visceral cancers are invented, probably tumor by tumor, history taking remains the most important diagnostic tool. Most cancers are discovered when the patient no longer has other simple explanations and remedies for a new significant symptom and finally seeks medical attention. Most such symptoms of cancer are readily confused with symptoms of common benign diseases. By attentive consideration of every minor symptom, a good primary doctor must sift out the symptom that could be due to cancer from that which is not likely to be. The constellation of symptoms, their duration, and associated findings lead the alert physician to consider cancer. Cough, dyspepsia, anorexia, hoarseness, constipation, diarrhea, menorrhagia, weight loss, fever, fatigue, a lump, or pain, any one of which persists for 2 weeks and cannot be readily explained, requires consideration of cancer in the differential diagnosis. Other possible causes may exist and lead to other diagnoses, but cancer that is not thought of early is always diagnosed too late. It is the physician's job to be suspicious and to exclude the diagnosis of cancer, rather than to be complacent, and finally arrive at the diagnosis of cancer when the patient's complaints are severe and unambiguous. Suspicion is a virtue when looking for cancer. Early cancer symptoms are usually intermittent. Any pain at the outset is ordinarily not constant and may be poorly localized or even migratory. Subcutaneous masses and nodes can even seem to regress temporarily. Systemic dysfunction may be so mild as to be easily rationalized or overlooked by the patient.

Histories that are taken are more valuable than histories that are given. On suspecting cancer, the primary physician is often able to order the appropriate tests for histologic or cytologic confirmation of that suspicion. At this point, the interdisciplinary process should start. Studies that do not establish a diagnosis of cancer could be the wrong studies. Oncologic consultation might suggest other procedures of value. The primary physician often sends a patient to a surgeon for biopsy, which, when positive, may be followed by resection without further consultation. The proper time for discussion with representatives from the many disciplines who might eventually become involved is after a diagnosis is suspected or after it is proved but before the inauguration of definitive therapy. Psycho-oncologic consultation and formal rehabilitation may not be necessary for every patient but, when needed, should be arranged before the therapeutic program is initiated. Pathology consultation is always needed and is best obtained in person, at the pathologist's double-headed microscope with the slide in view.

The surgeon, medical oncologist, and radiation oncologist should, in many cases, have protocols for therapy of common cancers. Where possible, these protocols should be part of designed studies that will accumulate sufficient numbers from which conclusions can be drawn. Sometimes this involves a single institution (or even a single practice); whenever possible, it should be part of institutional or national protocols designed to answer fundamental questions concerning the management of cancer. When multiple protocols exist, a consensus must be reached to prioritize the sequence in which they will be offered to patients. Where no protocol exists, agreement that defines the procedures and the sequence for a particular patient should be sought ahead of time. The family physician should be a full partner in all of these decisions.

The family physician may also be a principal member of the follow-up team for a cancer patient and can identify any change from well-being that signals possible tumor activity. At this point, the participation of an oncologist is called for. Alternatively, oncologic surveillance can fall to the medical oncologist. The primary physician must also assess the possible familial risk and supervise the appropriate survey of family members in conjunction with the medical oncologist.

THE RADIOLOGIST

Imaging specialties are essential in the diagnosis and staging of cancer. An oncologist should review all relevant imaging studies with the appropriate radiologist, sonographer, or nuclear medicine physician. A written report is mandatory, but it is much increased in value by the oncologist's personal viewing of the images with the radiologist. Although it is commonplace to order standard menus (CT or magnetic resonance imaging [MRI]), a radiologist can suggest the best techniques for particular problems. Special CT scans with thinner slices can provide better definition of small lesions, or special MRI views with or without fat suppression or gadolinium may provide optimal visualization. Follow-up examinations using dynamic flow scanning, single photon emission CT, positron emission tomography, sonographic or CT-guided needle biopsy, and similar procedures always require the professional input of an imaging specialist.

Oncologists can request that the imaging specialist not give an interpretation directly to the patient. Thoughtless reporting of radiologic findings to patients before they are known by the responsible oncologist can cause significant difficulty in management, for both the oncologist and the patient. The radiologist is a consultant to the oncologist, not to the patient. The responsibility for the interpretation of findings to the patient, and for the support that often must go with it, rests with the oncologist.

THE PATHOLOGIST

The pathologist is an indispensable member of every interdisciplinary team. The function of the entire team is dependent on a proper diagnosis; therefore, pathology is a defining control. When the team pathologist is uncertain of a diagnosis, other local pathologists can be consulted for their opinions. Furthermore, the Armed Forces Institute of Pathology and several prominent universities and cancer centers are justly famed for their consultations.

The ready access of most of the gastrointestinal tract to endoscopic inspection and biopsy, easy access to the genitalia in both sexes, the accessibility of the tracheobronchial tree to fiberoptic bronchoscopy, and safe intraoperative biopsies mean that preoperative or intraoperative pathologic confirmation of diagnosis should be available for nearly every tumor. Based on clinical studies and the presence of tumor-associated markers, renal and testicular masses are typically removed without first establishing histologic proof. This is justified by the desire to avoid tumor spillage that can occur during a biopsy. For other diseases, radical surgery without a preceding pathologic diagnosis is unnecessary and dangerous. Similarly, an inadequate surgical procedure performed because the nature of the pathologic process was not appreciated suggests insufficient or mistaken intraoperative consultation. Amputation of a breast or an extremity without pre- or intraoperative pathologic diagnosis constitutes malpractice. However, on the basis of surgical judgment, a surgeon may conscientiously and competently sacrifice adjacent, dispensable, normal tissue—organs such as the spleen, kidney, and adrenal gland or a segment of gut, diaphragm, bladder, or vaginal wall—that appears to be involved by cancer without histologically establishing invasion. In other circumstances, the pathologist's imprimatur is necessary to justify cancer therapies. The same restrictions apply to primary radiation therapy or chemotherapy.

The pathologist is responsible for giving as definitive a description of the tumor as determined effort can provide: its extent, its relationship to surgical margins and normal structures, and the involvement of lymph nodes, lymphatics, and blood vessels. Wherever possible, a specimen of fresh tissue should be maintained frozen because, increasingly, new immunodiagnostic, molecular biologic, and biochemical techniques allow classification of tumors for receptors, oncogenes, tumor suppressor genes, and antigens that may some day provide prognostic information of great value. In selected circumstances, fresh tissue can be used for assays that predict chemotherapeutic or immunotherapeutic sensitivity.

In addition to tissue preservation for more sophisticated studies, pathology now allows better classification of tumors. Immunopathology and cytochemistry should be able to distinguish among most anaplastic neoplasms by studies of markers such as common leukocyte antigen, cytokeratins, vimentin, mucin, neuron-specific enolase, and S-100 protein, which are often used as panels of reagents to decide whether the tumor is a lymphoma, squamous cell carcinoma, sarcoma, adenocarcinoma, neuroectodermal tumor, or melanoma. Communication ahead of time with the pathologist can refine the choice of reagents and can provide extant or ancillary pathologic materials and information to aid in reaching the correct diagnosis. In their anaplastic state, all of the tumors mentioned may resemble one another in hematoxylin-eosin staining. If any suggestion exists that pathologic classification might be elusive, in addition to a specimen for freezing (which could later be subjected to molecular biologic study and possible genetic classification), a small fresh sample of representative neoplasm should be placed in glutaraldehyde fixative in the operating room for eventual electron microscopy. Today's research classifications may well become tomorrow's standard rubric and nomenclature. Oncologists should encourage the most discriminating description and classification of tumors because new therapeutic considerations may prove to be applicable as discoveries are made.

When doubt exists concerning the nature of a neoplasm, additional opinions are always appropriate. Pathologic uncertainty is a shaky foundation on which to build therapeutic strategy.

THE SURGICAL ONCOLOGIST

The surgical oncologist is most often the first among oncologic specialists to see the patient. The primary physician most commonly pursues a diagnosis, and in circumstances in which this requires biopsy, the surgeon is called. For decades, any surgeon was considered competent to exercise all surgical skills, including cancer surgery. Indeed, although most surgeons may be acceptably competent, the specialty of surgical oncology is increasingly becoming recognized. Surgical oncologists are clinical scientists with knowledge of and experience in cancer surgery that come from additional training, limitation of the scope of general surgical practice, familiarity with the biology and natural history of cancers, and familiarity with the role of the other oncologic specialties in their diagnosis and management. Until surgical oncology becomes recognized by the proper accrediting agencies, other oncologists must exercise their judgment about the oncologic qualifications of their surgical confreres. Some of the appropriate criteria are membership in the Society of Surgical Oncology, postgraduate training in a cancer institute or university program under a mentor known for cancer surgical expertise, concentration of surgical practice on cancer and related diseases, and published work.

Since a general surgeon may perform the biopsy, a surgical oncologist is sometimes called on to supersede the first surgeon on the case. Herein lie some of the problems because the primary cancer operation is of the utmost importance for proper staging and for achieving surgical cure. In this regard, biopsy of any mass should be considered only in the context of whether the operating surgeon will be the best choice for eventual definitive surgical therapy. Since a considerable portion of their activity deals with neoplasia, thoracic surgeons, urologic surgeons, and neurosurgeons must be chosen for their specific interest and general expertise because there is not likely to be an oncologic subspecialty in the near future for those specific organ systems. On the other hand, gynecologic oncology, orthopedic oncology, otorhinolaryngologic oncology, and surgical oncology are well defined, and the general gynecologist, orthopedist, otorhinolaryngologist, or surgeon is unlikely to be as well qualified as the oncologist within the specialty.

Because the implications for a proven, potentially resectable neoplasm entail many other considerations to optimize curability, the prudent surgical oncologist surveys the potential contributions of medical oncology, radiation oncology, and other specialties before proceeding with the operation.

Where appropriate and possible, patients should be entered into clinical investigative trials. There is so much that is unknown about cancer that investigative activities should still be of prime concern to all oncologists. In institutions where investigative programs are not employed, sober consideration of joining in this effort through a community oncology program or in alliance with some other active institution should be exercised.

In the absence of a structured protocol, joint assessment is appropriate to determine whether chemotherapy or radiotherapy prior to surgery may improve outcome. Most often, this entails direct consultation with medical and radiation oncologists. An opportunity for the three specialties to see the patient in the native, unaltered state is of great value for subsequent planning. The treatment of breast cancer, rectal cancer, head and neck cancer, lung cancer, bone and soft tissue sarcoma, and brain tumors is most often best approached by multidisciplinary components from all three specialties. Whereas specific diseases may be treated well by single-modality approaches, bidisciplinary or tridisciplinary opinion is usually advantageous. Sentinal node biopsy in breast cancer and melanoma is a surgical innovation requiring nuclear medicine and pathologic collaboration. Surgical oncologists must work collaboratively with plastic surgeons to undertake breast reconstruction and sometimes in the course of facial reconstruction.

Surgical oncologists must also be available for surgical aspects of management later in the course of disease. Venous access devices may be required, depending on the drugs to be used and the status of peripheral veins. End-staging laparoscopy or laparotomy may, in many instances, make more sense than earlier operation so that the medical oncologist may be certain that a complete clinical remission is pathologically confirmed rather than wait for a lymphoma or ovarian cancer to relapse. Intestinal obstruction in the course of cancer may require operative surgical management. A medical or radiation oncologist may discover a suspicious mass or infiltration that needs biopsy and pathologic assessment.

Palliative surgery is an area in which medical and radiation oncologists often present problems to the surgeon in the hope of potential operative remedy. Debulking, diverting, and pain-relieving operations may all be appropriate procedures in the proper circumstance.

Surgical oncologists also have legitimate interests in adjuvant chemotherapy and immunotherapy. For those willing to devote the time required for this undertaking, use of established drugs in adjuvant programs can be an improvement over surgical procedures alone. Indeed, the National Surgical Adjuvant Breast and Bowel Project has contributed significantly to our knowledge of adjuvant therapy for these diseases. Surgical oncologic investigators have also been among the pioneers of immunologic cancer research. The rarity of surgical oncologists in practice, however, ordinarily precludes these activities for surgeons because so much of their time is ordinarily invested in pre- and postoperative care and in actual surgery. Medical oncologists must stand ready to assume primary responsibility for subsequent oncologic management. Orthopedic oncologists, otorhinolaryngologic oncologists, and neurosurgical oncologists ordinarily ally themselves with a medical oncologist who has specialized interests and expertise in the treatment of neoplasms of their particular discipline.

THE ANESTHESIOLOGIST

Intraoperative management of a cancer patient is similar to that for any major surgery. Since anesthesiologists often manage recovery rooms and even intensive care units, their role has expanded. Assurance of effective pain control in the immediate postoperative period is fundamental. Alcohol nerve block and rhizotomy have been superseded by this reversible method. Patient-controlled epidural analgesia postoperatively is the province of anesthesiology. Epidural block by continuous administration of narcotic and anesthetic solutions may also be indispensable for refractory pain in the course of metastatic cancer. Patient-controlled analgesia by intravenous or subcutaneous narcotics at other times for efficient pain control is a technique of importance to all branches of oncology, however, and should not be considered a proprietary anesthesiologic exclusive. Most patients can achieve pain control on oral medications. Anesthesiologists are important members of pain teams.

THE MEDICAL ONCOLOGIST

The medical oncologist usually serves the traditional role of internist in the interdisciplinary management of cancer. Whereas the surgical procedure or the radiotherapeutic treatment course is of short duration, the medical oncologist has continuing responsibility that may stretch over months or years of therapy and decades of follow-up, depending on the neoplasm.

There is an understandable but regrettable tendency for every specialist who has interacted with a patient to schedule follow-up appointments, which may entail many more visits and much greater expense than is necessary or prudent. A combined-modality follow-up clinic avoids this problem but may not be adaptable to most office practices. Each therapist is entitled to see the results of the particular treatment regimen that has been applied. The region of previous disease is only a portion of the patient's overall health concerns, however. The search for remediable disease in regional and distant areas and a continuing assessment of the impact of the disease and its treatment on the patient as a whole are ordinarily considered medical tasks. A useful approach for medical oncologists is to send the findings at a follow-up visit, including laboratory and radiologic results, to the primary physician, surgeon, and radiation oncologist (or other appropriate specialist) so that what is going on is communicated to all. The medical oncologist is also most often the conduit to the patient for announcing program change, such as the appearance of metastases, the necessity for more therapy of whatever kind, and sometimes the shift to a palliative approach. The medical oncologist may also superintend both the medical activities of the patient that are not addressed by the primary physician and the general oncologic assessments that are of importance to the surgeon, radiation oncologist, and medical oncologist alike. When regional concerns arise that are in the purview of the other specialties, the medical oncologist should facilitate early real-time consultation.

The medical oncologist should participate in decisions concerning choice of therapy and in the clinical staging, which may determine operability. The medical oncologist should be responsible for evaluating the potential for induction (primary, neoadjuvant) chemotherapy and for the choice of regimen for postoperative chemotherapeutic or immunotherapeutic management.

Since our knowledge base is still incomplete, wherever possible, patients should enter research protocols. Data are emerging that emphasize the value of neoadjuvant (primary or induction) chemotherapy in the care of tumors classically considered first for regional surgical or radiotherapeutic approaches. Osteosarcoma and several pediatric tumors, stage III breast cancer, stage III non–small cell lung cancer, advanced head and neck carcinoma, rectal cancer, and, arguably, some other cancers have benefited from chemotherapeutic impact on the presumptive micrometastases and on the primary tumor. The chemotherapeutic effect on the primary tumor serves as an in vivo bioassay of drug effect, allowing shift to a different regimen if ineffectual. Complete pathologic regression of primary tumors from chemotherapy has been associated with improved results for osteosarcoma, breast cancer, and head and neck cancer. Treatment of the primary neoplasm may be simplified, and lesions once considered inoperable are now potentially curable. This changing paradigm may increase the applicability of radiotherapy and surgery with intent to cure.

The medical oncologist is most often the physician to reassure the patient when there is no evident cancer. Although the absence of a tumor may, in fact, be a tumor in eclipse, the medical oncologist must keep the patient from dwelling incessantly and anxiously on imminent relapse. Reassurance should never involve a lie, just a reasoned basis for hope that relapse will not occur. Osler's admonition to live life in day-tight packages is helpful.

The medical oncologist is the responsible physician when therapeutic options for disease control become progressively restricted as a cancer patient approaches death. Although selective interventions by surgical or radiation oncologists or other specialists may be required, the overall responsibility for the patient's palliative care, pain control, nutrition, psychosocial adaptation, and coping with the actual dying process falls on the medical oncologist. A competent medical oncologist is an expert in palliative care.

THE RADIATION ONCOLOGIST

Radiation oncology is entirely devoted to the study of cancer because radiation is no longer used in the treatment of benign diseases. The radiation oncologist must, therefore, be in a position to make an overall oncologic evaluation, as well as specific recommendations for radiotherapy.

In the case of diseases that radiotherapy can sometimes cure, such as localized lymphomas, cancer of the tongue and oral cavity, cancer of the cervix, and cancer of the prostate, the radiation oncologist must have equal early access to the patient to set forth the possible indications for and accomplishments of radiation therapy for such tumors. Cordial interactive liaison with surgical and medical oncologists is crucial to allow this delineation of options before the patient is committed to and is changed by another treatment approach.

Controversy exists over the relative debilities and late toxicities of surgery and radiotherapy. Where equal curative potential exists, there is additional reason to assess the disruption of anatomy and the dysfunction that might occur from surgery or radiotherapy. There is no consensus because each discipline often champions its own approach. The major improvement in immediate reconstructive techniques has made surgery around the face much less disfiguring. Surgeons point out dry mouth and dysgeusia as late undesirable toxicities of radiation, whereas radiotherapists decry the organ loss, physiologic distortions, and cosmetic problems of surgery. Similar controversy attends vaginal dysfunction after radiation treatment for early carcinoma of the cervix compared with total hysterectomy. In carcinomas of the bladder, the discordance is even greater because total cystectomy diminishes the quality of life, but American urologists often question whether radiation therapy is equally effective, stage for stage. Although radiotherapy for T2 and T3 bladder cancers is reportedly highly effective in Europe, there has been little clinical investigation of this approach in the United States. Radical surgery for carcinoma of the prostate, with problems of capsular invasion, impotence, and incontinence, has not been directly compared with interstitial radiotherapy and teletherapy, which have complications of their own. A definitive comparison in early-stage prostate cancer is overdue once there is consensus about which patients do not need immediate treatment at all.

For operable oral, pharyngeal, cervical, bladder, and prostate cancer, closer cooperation of the radiation oncologist and surgeon before decisions are finalized might provide for greater organ preservation and less dysfunction when therapy is equivalent stage for stage. The great problem, however, is to overcome the prejudice that the results will not be the same, with each specialty nearly equally persuaded and equally unpersuasive. Randomized clinical trials are sorely needed but may never be done because of the evolution of the combined-modality approaches.

In combined-modality approaches, chemotherapy is a major component, together with radiotherapy and surgery. Many reports indicate that chemotherapy induces major regressions when used as primary therapy for head and neck cancer, bladder cancer, breast cancer, pediatric sarcomas, and lymphomas. So, too, does hormonal therapy for prostate cancer. Primary chemotherapy, with its major theoretic advantage of decreasing the number of cells to be killed by radiation or to be removed by surgery, is under active study. Until proven otherwise, radiation field sizes and surgical boundaries cannot be safely reduced below the original extent of the tumor, where residual cells may remain after chemotherapy. A major advantage of primary chemotherapy, in addition to a decrease in primary tumor burden, is an early attack against undetected micrometastatic disease. Furthermore, when the tumor vasculature is intact, unimpaired by radiation angiopathy or surgical disruption, there is a greater chance of delivering a chemotherapeutically effective dose. Last, the regression of tumor seen in the primary neoplasm reinforces confidence in using the same chemotherapeutic regimen for presumed micrometastases during the adjuvant period. Indeed, when complete regression of tumor occurs, as demonstrated pathologically, outcomes are much improved in osteosarcoma and breast cancer.

For tumors that are regionally invasive beyond resectability in the pharynx, esophagus, pancreas, cervix, and prostate, radiation is usually employed as primary therapy and sometimes after chemotherapy or hormone therapy. The dismal results often seen in these advanced tumors unfairly taint the potential contributions of radiation oncology in the treatment of less advanced tumors. Pilot efforts are needed to construct combined-modality approaches for tumors that are regionally inoperable at first encounter but that might become resectable after chemotherapy and/or radiation therapy. On the basis of negative functional and anatomic imaging studies and multiple biopsies showing no residual tumor, some might not require surgery at all. Creation of such regimens, with some success, would allow their transfer to less advanced problems in comparison with surgery.

Primary brain tumors are usually best treated by primary surgery followed by radiotherapy, often with chemotherapy. When surgery is unfeasible, new techniques of stereostatic radiotherapy—delivering precisely localized radiation from several angles so as to spare normal brain—offer promise. Stereostatic radiation has been used in other sites. Intensity-modulated radiation therapy is a computer-dependent technique of minimizing exposure of normal tissues during treatment.

Radiotherapy can cure localized and regionalized lymphomas of certain types. The advantages and disadvantages of combined-modality therapy or of the use of chemotherapy alone are presented in detail for the specific diseases. There continues to be a clear indication for combined chemotherapy and radiotherapy in patients whose lymphomas are large and where the certainty of tumor eradication by either modality alone is not ensured. Radiotherapy may be a critical component in salvage regimens for relapsed leukemias and lymphomas, for which maximal chemotherapy, together with autologous or allogeneic stem cell transplantation, is undertaken.

For palliation and pain relief, radiation therapy is indispensable to the practice of oncology. Radiotherapy can usually offer relief from the pain of tumor infiltration in bone, regardless of tumor type. Although the extent of tumor regression (as a measure of radiosensitivity) varies, this may determine the length of remission rather than initial pain relief.

THE GYNECOLOGIC ONCOLOGIST

Gynecologic oncologists as a class may belong to the most integrated oncologic specialty. They are fully qualified to diagnose and treat neoplasia of the female genital organs by surgery and chemotherapy and to share in radiotherapeutic planning and execution to a considerable degree, particularly for brachytherapy. Highly skilled gynecologic oncologists are divided on whether gastrointestinal complications of ovarian or other cancers should be handled by surgical oncologists, general surgeons, or gynecologic oncologists. Much of this depends on local custom rather than expertise at performing lysis of adhesions or enteroenterostomies. The preoperative preparation for and execution of procedures that involve urinary tract manipulation are almost invariably conducted cooperatively with urologists.

Many medical oncologists treat gynecologic neoplasms with chemotherapy in investigational and clinical settings. This is true for adjuvant therapy as well as treatment of manifest clinical metastasis. In many academic institutions, medical and gynecologic oncologists have collaborated in the study of the biology and treatment of gynecologic cancers. Local custom, the surgical obligations of gynecologic oncologists, and collaborative undertakings involving both specialties determine the allocation of work. Medical oncologists should be actively involved when a gynecologist without specific oncologic expertise or interest has undertaken to perform the surgery.

THE NEUROSURGEON

The longer survival of patients with many types of cancer has led to a higher frequency of patients presenting with one or two brain metastases that can be resected. Metastases to one or two adjacent vertebral bodies with pain, vertebral collapse, or impending cord compression also appear to be more common. In such instances, surgical correction must be considered, as well as radiation therapy, because neurosurgery often may provide better palliation. In addition, neurosurgical procedures for pain control are crucial as last-resort measures.

THE PEDIATRIC ONCOLOGIST

Pediatric oncologists generally maintain independence from adult oncologic specialties. Radiotherapists and surgeons in major centers subspecialize in pediatric neoplasms. Some gynecologists and urologists have particular interests in pediatric diseases. Orthopedic oncologists devote much of their time to pediatric sarcomas; thus, there is no specialized subset for pediatric neoplasms. In major centers, pediatric counterparts to all of the medical oncologic resources, such as pediatric neurologists, radiologists, and even pathologists, illustrate the specificity of pediatric oncologic information. Nearly every child in the United States can have access to programs of the newly consolidated Children's Oncology Group. The dramatic progress in cancer therapeutics in children derives, in part, from the universal recognition that childhood cancer is a terrible tragedy and that every effort must be made to derive all possible information from every case. This allows the child with cancer to benefit from all of the information that has gone before and creates a new database for those who will come after. The unique features of pediatric oncology are presented in Section 37.

THE PSYCHO-ONCOLOGIST

The mind is the only organ system that is affected in every patient with cancer. Nonetheless, all patients do not need formal psychiatric help. Because general psychiatrists often lack full understanding of the organic aspects of cancers and the therapeutic procedures that are commonly employed, their effectiveness in dealing with these real-life problems is lessened. Psycho-oncologists have, by dint of special education and experience, a better foundation from which to undertake supervision of those patients whose psychiatric problems are too pervasive for oncologists of other disciplines to manage. Psycho-oncologists implement much of their influence by interaction with staff in addition to patients.

Helping train oncologists to deal sensitively and empathetically with patients is a continuing task for psycho-oncologists. It is important for oncologists to recognize the fact that a patient's cancer is usually the greatest challenge that he or she has ever faced. Staring into the abyss, often for the first time, requires more equanimity and fortitude than many patients can muster. There are sensitive and insensitive ways to communicate bad news to a patient. Training can make a difference. Psycho-oncology's best offerings teach doctors how to handle their own inadequacies, how to tolerate their own frustrations and failures, and how to convey a humanitarian dimension to the grim reality of many cancer treatments. Not all medicine comes in a bottle.

Psycho-oncologists have stressed objective methods of quantifying emotions and subjective judgment that determine the quality of life. The pain thermometer has been paralleled by the distress thermometer, which may serve as a triggering indicator for medication to allay anxiety or depression. Major elevation of the stress thermometer indicates the need for psychiatric or psychological intervention.

THE REHABILITATION SPECIALIST

Rehabilitation specialists provide patients with the opportunity for self-reliance. Cutting the bonds of dependency can be the best of all remedies. Whether in speech, ambulation, ostomy care, physical appearance, occupational rehabilitation, or sexual expression, oncologists must maintain as a goal that patients should lead pain-free lives with minimal, if any, deficits in normal function. Early and vigorous rehabilitation efforts can make life more worth living. Oncologists could and should consult rehabilitation medicine specialists earlier and more often.

THE ONCOLOGY NURSE

An oncology nurse has become one of the team's indispensable specialists. An oncologist's nightmare is to have a complex cancer patient admitted to a general service floor. The unique medications, procedures, and tests for oncology patients are themselves adequate justification for the specialty of oncology nursing. Oncology nurses have a greater than ordinary understanding of cancer pain and a perception of the psychological stresses that cancer patients suffer. These two precious insights allow a much more aggressive advocacy for pain control and a humanistic and realistic support of patients and families during their crises. Oncology nurses in ambulatory settings become telephone specialists in patient management and triage, to the great advantage and comfort of cancer patients—and to the great advantage and efficiency of oncologists.

Oncology nurses have become the prime movers in home care, rendering active therapy or supervision of palliative measures. Because of it, home hospice care has become more common, more economical, and more desirable.

THE ONCOLOGY PHARMACIST

The very nature of oncologic drugs imparts a special responsibility for their appropriate and safe use. The special postgraduate training of an oncology pharmacist and the conscientious practice of his or her profession significantly benefits every cancer patient. Knowledge of appropriate doses, pharmacokinetics, incompatibilities, special administration procedures, acute and cumulative toxic manifestations, unique databases, alternative drugs and routes of administration, and avoidance of personal exposure is an attribute brought to the interdisciplinary team by an oncology pharmacist. Meticulous record keeping in computerized files is an indispensable backup for the clinical chart. Any installation treating several patients each day can ill afford not to have a specialized oncology pharmacist. For the smaller practice, premixed drugs prepared by a central oncology pharmacist add a layer of convenience and security.

NONMEDICAL PROFESSIONALS

A few additional people are crucial in the oncologic approach to advanced cancer at home. A social worker familiar with the great stresses of cancer on every member of the family is a treasured asset. The complexities in social, insurance, economic, and service spheres can be greatly simplified by the compassionate and professional interest of an oncology social worker. Additional, often critical, community resources, such as the American Cancer Society, Cancer Care, veteran patient support groups, Meals on Wheels, companion visits, and home health care aides, may seem to be effortlessly mobilized by a social worker.

For those who have been guided by religious tenets and who have practiced their religion, the clergy can be extremely helpful. Religious practices can be strengthening; however, death-bed conversions are uncommon. For those who have not made religion a significant portion of their lives, visits of the clergy or allusions to an afterlife provide little comfort.

Competent business associates who manage the complexities of third-party payers, precertifications, collections, write-offs, and purchases can be worth their weight in gold. Indeed, the success or failure of an oncology practice depends in large part on an undiscounted revenue stream and prudent cost control.

FAMILY MEMBERS

The principal support throughout the cancer experience comes from a loving family. All else may pale in comparison with the radiant affection of a spouse or other family member. The loving one who recognizes that all of the good that can be done must be done creates the palpable substance of being loved for the patient. In addition to benefit for the patient, such behavior creates comforting memories for the doer and future self-satisfaction that in the ultimate crisis he or she was steadfast.

Cancer and Pregnancy

Phuong Khanh H. Morrow, MD
Richard L. Theriault, DO, MBA, FACP
Gabriel N. Hortobagyi, MD, FACP

The diagnosis of cancer during pregnancy presents a complex set of challenges for the patient, family members, and physicians. Often the welfare of the mother is perceived to be threatened by the pregnancy owing to concerns regarding the disease, the diagnostic and therapeutic procedures required for treatment, and a desire to avoid harm to the fetus during treatment for the mother's malignancy. Indeed, a frequent recommendation in the past has been to terminate the pregnancy. For those patients wishing to maintain the pregnancy, concern for the welfare of the fetus and neonate dominates the process of diagnosis and treatment. Many have perceived that treatment may require compromise of the well-being of the mother or fetus. In some circumstances, fetal death may be an unavoidable consequence of cancer treatment. Frequently, however, judicious decision making not only can provide cancer care for the pregnant woman but also will preserve the pregnancy through successful labor and delivery.

Many issues arise in the realm of concurrent cancer and pregnancy (Table 63-1). The data for specific tumor types, diagnostic procedures, therapeutic interventions, and long-term cancer outcomes have been derived primarily from case reports, small case series, and retrospective reviews. Controlled studies are rare, and prospective data are rarer still. Data on labor and delivery outcomes for patients completing pregnancy remain scarce, as are long-term data on the growth and development of children exposed to cancer treatment in utero. Decision making for patients and physicians is complex and must take into consideration not only medical issues but also moral, religious, ethical, and legal concerns.[1,2] Informed decisions are difficult when little information is available. The historical record, as imperfect as it may be, serves as the basis for patient care in the unusual circumstance of the concurrent diagnosis of cancer and pregnancy.

Table 63-1 Issues Related to Cancer and Pregnancy (A Few)

Issues
Impact of cancer on pregnancy
Impact of pregnancy on cancer
Termination of pregnancy/fetal death with cancer treatment
Diagnostic procedures and staging during pregnancy
Cancer treatment, maternal effects
Cancer treatment, fetal effects
Placental metastasis
Transplacental malignancy
Long-term outcome for children
Ethical, moral, legal concerns
The unknown

CANCER AND PREGNANCY EPIDEMIOLOGY

The diagnosis of cancer during pregnancy is rare. For example, the published data for breast cancer estimates that 1 in 3,000 to 3 in 10,000 deliveries occur in women with a diagnosis of breast cancer.[3–6] The most frequent cancer diagnoses in association with pregnancy were reported by Smith and colleagues in a retrospective review of 3,168,911 deliveries in California from 1992 to 1997.[7] In this review, 2,247 cases of primary malignancy were reported. They found 7.1 cases per 10,000 live singleton births; among these cases, the cancer diagnosis occurred in the prenatal period, at the time of delivery, or up to 12 months postpartum. There were 1.8 cases per 10,000 live singleton births for the prenatal period. Per 10,000 live singleton births, the most common tumor types were breast (1.3), thyroid (1.2), cervical (0.8), Hodgkin's disease (0.5), ovarian (0.5), acute and chronic leukemia (0.37), and lymphoma (0.28). As the trend toward delayed childbearing continues, it has been surmised that cancers whose incidence increases with age may be more frequently seen concurrent with pregnancy.[7–9]

In a retrospective review spanning 24 years, Sayedur and colleagues reported an ovarian cancer incidence of 0.08 in 1,000 deliveries.[10] Komurcu and colleagues reported a slightly greater incidence of colorectal carcinoma in association with pregnancy, with an estimated 1 case per 13,000 live-born deliveries.[11] Cervical cancer during pregnancy is rare—1 per 1,200 to 10,000 pregnancies—and presents difficult management choices with regard to surgical and radiation treatment. Similar to the California study, Kaiser and colleagues estimated the incidence of cancer in pregnancy as 1 in 1,000, with cervical cancer being the most frequent.[12] This finding is consistent with the observations of Allen and colleagues, who reported an incidence of 0.26 per 1,000 pregnancies for cervical cancer, noting that cervical cancer was the most common malignancy to complicate pregnancy.[13] However, cancer from nearly any anatomic location can occur with pregnancy (Table 63-2).

DIAGNOSIS AND STAGING

A biopsy, with review of cytologic and histologic material, is required for the diagnosis of any malignancy during pregnancy. The type of biopsy is determined by the accessibility of the disease site and the quantity of material required.

If a surgical biopsy if required, the anatomic location of the biopsy and the gestational age of the fetus are factors to be considered prior to proceeding. A surgical biopsy can be performed safely.[14,15] It is imperative that adequate material for pathologic diagnosis and required studies be obtained; for example, hormone receptors and *HER2/neu* status are necessary for the proper evaluation of breast cancer, and morphologic and immunophenotyping of lymphomas and leukemias is essential to their optimal assessment and treatment.

Staging provides guidance for discussions regarding cancer prognosis, recommended locoregional and/or systemic therapies, and potential risks of treatment in relation to benefit and outcome for the patient. Frequently, staging assessment in the nonpregnant patient involves exposure to ionizing radiation, which is to be avoided whenever possible during pregnancy. The impact of radiation on the fetus varies with respect to fetal gestational age. Preimplantation and organogenesis are most sensitive to the negative effects of radiation exposure.[16] Fetal exposures of < 5 cGy are not thought to be harmful.[17] With a number of procedures, exposure to radiation is negligible; examples are the chest radiograph (2.6 millirads) and intravenous pyelogram (500–800 millirads).[18] With chest computed tomography (CT), radiation exposure increases up to 3,000 millirads; for abdominal CT, exposure may be as high as 9,000 millirads.[18] As a consequence of known fetal toxicity associated with exposure to ionizing radiation during pregnancy, abdominal shielding and nonionizing techniques should be used whenever possible during these imaging procedures.[19,20] Ultrasonography for breast, liver, and other abdominal organs can also contribute to the staging evaluation.[18] Magnetic resonance imaging (MRI) can be used to assess for bone and liver disease, as well as fetal abnormalities, if required.[21–27] Accurate determination of disease stage is essential in ensuring accurate cancer treatment decisions, and findings during the staging process also may influence the woman's decision regarding the maintenance of her pregnancy.

Table 63-2 Tumor Types Reported During Pregnancy (Partial List)

Acoustic neuroma[138]	Hepatocellular[139]
Acute leukemia, lymphoid and myeloid[105,140]	Hodgkin's disease[29,80,81]
Adenocarcinoma of cervix[141]	Melanoma[142]
Adenocarcinoma of the papilla of Vater[143]	Multiple myeloma[144]
Bladder[145]	Mycosis fungoides[146]
Breast[54,55]	Neuroectodermal[147]
Burkitt's lymphoma[92,93]	Non-Hodgkin's lymphoma[78,84,85]
Cervix[13,68,72]	Non–small cell lung[148]
Chronic lymphocytic leukemia[110,111]	Ovary[10]
Chronic myelogenous leukemia[114–117]	Pancreas[143]
Colon[11]	Pheochromocytoma[149]
Craniopharyngioma[150]	Rectal[151]
Endometrial[152]	Renal[153]
Fallopian tube carcinoma[154]	Sarcoma[155]
Gastric[156]	T-cell leukemia[157]
Hairy cell leukemia[158]	Thyroid[62,64,159,160]
Head/neck[161]	Vulvar[162]

CANCER TREATMENT DURING PREGNANCY

The optimal treatment of cancer during pregnancy requires a meticulously coordinated multidisciplinary approach. Careful and repeated consultation with the obstetrician and/or maternal fetal medicine specialist is essential during the course of the pregnancy. Accurate assessment of fetal age, maturation, and the expected delivery date must be performed prior to treatment planning. The therapeutic options for the pregnant patient do not differ from those of the nonpregnant patient with cancer, but the application of treatment may be more complex.

SURGERY

Surgery remains the mainstay for treatment of solid tumors, and pregnancy is not a contraindication for cancer surgery. Mazze and Kallen reported on a registry series of 5,405 pregnant patients on whom surgery was performed.[14] They did not observe an increased incidence of congenital malformations or stillbirths in women who had surgical procedures while pregnant.[14] An increased frequency of low and very low birth weight infants was noted and attributed to prematurity and intrauterine growth retardation. No specific type of surgical procedure or anesthesia was associated with an increase in adverse reproductive outcomes. In a case-control study, Duncan and colleagues did not observe an increase in congenital anomalies in 2,565 pregnant women who had surgery while pregnant when compared with control patients who did not have surgery.[15] If warranted by tumor type and disease stage, surgery should proceed and should be coordinated with the obstetrician, anesthesiologist, and neonatal specialist.

RADIATION

Pregnancy has been considered an absolute contraindication to radiation therapy for cancer. Radiation therapy for cervical cancer during pregnancy usually leads to fetal death and spontaneous abortion.[28] The fetus is most sensitive to malformation from radiation exposure 2 to 8 weeks after conception, whereas exposure from 8 to 25 weeks of gestation has the greatest risk of mental retardation.[16] Nevertheless, successful radiation therapy of pregnant women with Hodgkin's disease has been reported.[29] If radiation is warranted, appropriate fetal shielding, careful dosimetry calculations, and estimates of fetal dose exposure are necessary.[30–34] Radiation therapy for breast cancer, following mastectomy or breast conservation surgery, can usually be delayed until the postpartum period. The National Commission on Radiation Protection has established recommended guidelines for total radiation exposure during pregnancy.[17] Less than 5 cGy is considered safe. If fetal exposure exceeds > 15 cGy, termination of pregnancy has been recommended.[17]

SYSTEMIC THERAPY

For many malignancies, systemic therapy is used as primary or adjuvant treatment. Many different agents have been reported to have been used in pregnancy. Representative chemotherapeutic, hormonal, and biologic agents are listed in Table 63-3.

Systemic therapy is of concern because of the potential deleterious effects on the fetus. Physiologic changes associated with pregnancy (elevated blood volume, increased cardiac output, amplified glomerular filtration rate, and changes in circulating protein levels) make predictions about drug pharmacokinetics uncertain at best.[35] In addition, systemic agents are designed to be antiproliferative compounds, and their administration during pregnancy poses a genuine risk to the developing fetus. Potential concerns include stillbirth, spontaneous abortion, fetal malformations or teratogenesis, organ-specific toxicities, intrauterine growth retardation with low birth weight, and premature delivery.[36]

The fetal risks related to chemotherapy appear to be greatest during the first trimester of pregnancy. Doll and colleagues reviewed antineoplastic agents and fetal malformations in relation to the trimester of pregnancy.[36] They reported that in utero exposure to systemic agents was associated with fetal malformation risks of 14% and 19% for alkylating agents and antimetabolites, respectively. A similar review of second- and third-trimester exposure demonstrated a 1.3% incidence of fetal malformation. Thus, they concluded that single-agent or combination chemotherapy could be given during the second and third trimesters with low risk of fetal malformation, but these agents should be avoided during the first trimester of pregnancy. Similarly, in a review of cytotoxic agents used during pregnancy, Ebert and colleagues collected 217 cases from the literature published between 1983 and 1995.[35] They classified the use of the agents by disease category and analyzed the outcome of pregnancy in relation to agent, dose, and gestational age at exposure. There were 94 cases of leukemia, 57 cases of lymphoma, 26 cases of breast or ovarian cancer, 16 cases of cytotoxic therapy used for rheumatic diseases, and 22 cases of cytotoxic therapy used for various severe illnesses, including Ewing's sarcoma, liver carcinoma, and melanoma. Eighteen newborns were reported to have congenital developmental abnormalities. Of these 18 newborns, 15 neonates had been exposed to cytotoxic drugs during the first trimester. Chromosomal abnormalities were noted in two neonates who had experienced exposure to cytotoxic agents during the first trimester. Antimetabolite use was found in 50% of the neonates with congenital abnormalities following first-trimester exposure to chemotherapy. Of the reviewed cases, 82.3% of leukemia patients, 75.4% of lymphoma patients, and 75% of breast or ovary cancer patients with associated pregnancies were reported to have live births with normally developed neonates. Germann and colleagues collected data involving 160 patients who received anthracyclines during pregnancy.[37] In this group, five cases of fetal malformations (3%) were found, with three cases occurring with the use of chemotherapy in the first trimester. The remaining two cases of fetal malformation occurred after chemotherapy administration in the second trimester; one involved Down syndrome unrelated to chemotherapy, and the other involved a congenital adherence of the iris to the cornea that demonstrated no clinical consequence. The combination chemotherapy regimens associated with fetal malformations included cytosine arabinoside or cyclophosphamide. Systemic treatment, especially with antimetabolites, should be avoided during the first trimester of pregnancy except in circumstances in which a delay in cancer treatment would jeopardize the life of the patient (acute leukemia).

Erythropoietin use during pregnancy was reported by Scott and colleagues.[38] No maternal or fetal toxicities have been noted. Dale and colleagues found that the use of filgrastim during pregnancy was not associated with a change in neonatal outcome when compared with untreated patients.[39]

SPECIFIC CANCERS

Breast Cancer The diagnosis of breast cancer during pregnancy is often delayed, presum-

Table 63-3 Drugs Reported to Have Been Used During Pregnancy

MACOP-B	Hydroxyurea	α Interferon	Prednisone
MOPP-ABVD	All-*trans* retinoic acid	Rituximab	Tamoxifen
FAC	Methotrexate	Erythropoietin	
CMF	Doxorubicin/epirubicin	Filgrastim	
AC	Cyclophosphamide, nitrogen mustard	Trastuzumab	
VACOP-B	Vincristine, triethylene melamine		
	Bleomycin		
	Cisplatin		
	Vinorelbine, vinblastine, vincristine		
	Paclitaxel		
	Docetaxel		
	Etoposide		
	Idarubicin, daunorubicin		
	Cytosine arabinoside		
	5-Fluorouracil, busulfan		
	Teniposide		
	6-Mercaptopurine		
	Dacarbazine		
	Aminopterin		
	Actinomycin D		
	Procarbazine		
	Amsacrine		
	L-Asparaginase		

ABVD = Adriamycin (doxorubicin), bleomycin, vinblastine, and dacarbazine; AC = Adriamycin (doxorubin) and cyclophosphamide; CMF = cyclophosphamide, methotrexate, and 5-fluorouracil; FAC = 5-fluorouracil, Adriamycin (doxorubicin), and cyclophosphamide; MACOP-B = methotrexate, Adriamycin (doxorubicin), cyclophosphamide, Oncovin (vincristine), prednisone, and bleomycin; MOPP = mechlorethamine, Oncovin (vincristine), procarbazine, and prednisone; VACOP-B = VePesid (etoposide), Adriamycin (doxorubicin), Cytoxan (cyclophosphamide), Oncovin (vincristine), prednisone, and bleomycin.

ably owing to the anatomic and physiologic changes in the pregnant breast.[40,41] However, women with breast cancer during pregnancy have demonstrated the same survival rates, stage for stage, as nonpregnant patients with breast cancer.[42,43] Imaging of the breast in women with a palpable mass or thickening is warranted. Mammography and ultrasonography may confirm the presence of a malignant mass. Although Max and Klamer reported normal mammograms in six of eight women with breast cancer during pregnancy, others reported abnormal mammograms in the majority of women with pregnancy and breast cancer (18 of 23 and 5 of 8).[44–46]

There are limited data on ultrasonography; Liberman and colleagues reported positive findings in six of six patients, and Samuels and colleagues found positive findings in two of four patients.[45,46] Ultrasonography may be useful for guiding either fine-needle aspiration (FNA) or core biopsy to confirm a diagnosis of malignancy.[47–49]

Staging evaluation can be tailored to clinical findings. If clinically suspicious regional nodes are identified on physical examination or by imaging techniques, FNA that is guided by palpation or ultrasonography can be used to confirm metastases. Chest radiography, liver ultrasonography, and MRI of the thoracic or lumbar spine can be used to assess for extant organ metastasis.[18,21,22] The theoretic dosage of radiation that would be absorbed by the fetus following sentinel lymph node biopsy has been calculated to be less than 5 cGy.[50,51]

Local regional treatment with mastectomy and axillary lymph node dissection has been considered standard.[52] Breast-conserving surgery is possible with postpartum breast irradiation.[53] Pre- or postoperative chemotherapy is used with the same criteria for selection of therapy as in the nonpregnant patient. Berry and colleagues reported on a prospective study using 5-fluorouracil, doxorubicin, and cyclophosphamide in pregnant women with breast cancer.[54] No spontaneous abortions, stillbirths, or congenital malformations were noted. Complications for the neonate included (1) prematurity (delivered at 29 weeks owing to maternal preeclampsia), (2) neutropenia, (3) tachypnea of the newborn, (4) and respiratory distress syndrome. An update of this series (39 patients) again noted no spontaneous abortions, stillbirths, or congenital malformations. One case of spontaneous cryptogenic intracranial hemorrhage occurred. All complications had resolved.[55]

A retrospective survey of breast cancer treated during pregnancy has been reported by Giacalone and colleagues.[56] They reported 17 live births, 2 spontaneous abortions, and 1 stillbirth in 20 patients. A variety of chemotherapy agents were used, including alkylating agents and anthracyclines. Complications of labor and delivery were not reported.

The treatment of advanced breast cancer with tamoxifen is common. Of the six case reports of tamoxifen use during pregnancy, four women delivered healthy infants.[57] In one case, however, a female child was born with ambiguous genitalia. In another of the six cases, an infant who had been exposed to numerous potentially toxic agents (cocaine, marijuana, and radioactive technetium diphosphonate) in utero, in addition to tamoxifen, was born with a congenital craniofacial defect. A single report of docetaxel to treat metastatic breast cancer during pregnancy noted no fetal malformations.[58] Two case reports have documented the use of paclitaxel for breast cancer during pregnancy, with delivery of healthy infants.[59,60] Recently, a single case of the use of trastuzumab, in combination with vinorelbine, in the treatment of metastatic breast cancer in a pregnant female was reported. The patient delivered a healthy male infant at 34 weeks gestation.[61]

Thyroid Cancer Thyroid cancer is more common in women than in men. In pregnant women, it presents most often as an asymptomatic nodule in the neck. Ultrasound evaluation can confirm the size and solid character of the nodule. FNA biopsy is the most reliable diagnostic test and is safe and accurate during pregnancy.[62–64] Most often, pregnancy-associated thyroid cancers are well-differentiated tumors. Radioiodine scans and therapeutic radioiodine should not be given during pregnancy and can be safely delayed until after parturition.[65] Thyroid surgery can be delayed until after delivery for many patients, especially if the diagnosis is made during the third trimester of pregnancy.[65] If warranted, thyroid resection can be done under local anesthesia with "light sedative and narcotics."[66] In a case-control study, Moosa and Mazzaferi reported on 61 pregnant patients with thyroid cancer and 528 age-matched nonpregnant controls.[67] They reviewed the diagnosis, treatment, and outcome for the two cohorts. Seventy-four percent of the pregnant patients had been discovered to possess an asymptomatic thyroid nodule during routine examinations. Twenty percent of the pregnant patients underwent thyroid surgery during the second trimester, whereas 77% of patients underwent surgery following delivery. Thirty percent of the patients received postoperative iodine 131 therapy; all of these treatments were administered postpartum. The presence of pregnancy or delayed surgery conferred no differences in cancer recurrence, distant recurrence, or death. Based on these findings, Moosa and Mazzaferi concluded that treatment for thyroid cancer during pregnancy may be delayed until after delivery in most patients.

Cervical Cancer In the California series, cervical cancer was the third most common cancer diagnosed during pregnancy and the postpartum period.[7] Nguyen and colleagues stated that all pregnant women should have cytologic screening of the cervix and, as appropriate, colposcopy, biopsy, and selective conization.[68]

Evaluation of the extent of disease for diagnosed cervix cancer includes physical examination and assessment of pelvic anatomic structures by MRI. A report of laparoscopic lymph node staging at 16 weeks of pregnancy demonstrates the feasibility of this technique.[69] Treatment options vary with disease stage, gestational age at diagnosis, and the desires of the patient. For stage I disease, Sorosky and colleagues reported a favorable outcome with only planned follow-up observation until the third trimester.[70] They followed eight women with stage I disease, < 2.5 cm in dimension, for a mean interval of 109 days. All patients underwent delivery via cesarean delivery, followed by radical hysterectomy. Serial MRI was used to follow the disease for two patients, and no clinical disease progression was noted. After treatment, all patients were alive and free of disease at a mean follow-up of 37 months.

In a review of 22 patients with cervical cancer diagnosed during pregnancy or within 12 months postpartum, Allen and colleagues noted 20 live deliveries and only 1 disease recurrence.[13] Nine of 11 patients with microinvasive disease were treated with core biopsy only. Ten patients with stage IB or IIA disease were treated with radical hysterectomy, and one patient with stage IIIB disease received chemotherapy, radiation therapy, and simple hysterectomy as treatment. Allen and colleagues recommended that all pregnant women undergo cervical cytologic evaluation. Cone biopsy is safe in pregnancy and may be adequate treatment for microinvasive disease.

Outcome and recurrence risk have been assessed in relation to the method of delivery for women diagnosed with cervical cancer during pregnancy or within 6 months postpartum. Sood and colleagues followed 83 pregnant women with cervical cancer; 56 of these patients were diagnosed with cervical cancer during pregnancy, and 27 patients were diagnosed with cervical malignancy postpartum.[71] Since the risk of recurrence was increased in those diagnosed postpartum who delivered vaginally, Sood and colleagues concluded that women with cervical cancer should be delivered by cesarean. However, van der Vange and colleagues, in a case-control study, reported that the mode of delivery had no effect on survival.[72] Overall, they noted no difference in the survival of pregnant patients with cervical cancer compared with the nonpregnant group. For cervical malignancies diagnosed at delivery and during the immediate postpartum period, episiotomy site recurrence of cancer has been reported.[73] Systemic chemotherapy for cervical cancer can be effective when given during pregnancy. For example, Marana and colleagues reported on a 26-year-old patient with stage IIB cervix cancer diagnosed at 14 weeks of gestation.[74] She was treated with cisplatin and bleomycin and delivered a normal infant at 38 weeks gestation. Indeed, cisplatin has been the most frequently used agent in case reports of cervical cancer chemotherapy. In addition, a case report noted the delivery of a normal infant following systemic treatment of a pregnant patient with a combined regimen of cisplatin and paclitaxel.[75]

Treatment of the pregnant patient with cervical cancer requires careful consideration of disease stage and gestational age. Early in pregnancy with early-stage disease, pregnancy termination followed by cancer treatment may be appropriate. Alternatively, a planned delay in cancer treatment with careful monitoring of the disease may allow for successful completion of the pregnancy.[70] Radiation therapy will cause fetal death and usually results in spontaneous abortion.[28]

Since a significant population of patients are diagnosed with cervical cancer while in childbearing age, the concern for preservation of fertility has led to the use of radical vaginal trachelectomy with pelvic lymphadenectomy, instead of radical hysterectomy, in selected patients with stage I cervical cancer. Burnett and colleagues made this procedure available to 21 patients over a period of 6 years.[76] Following the procedure, eight patients demonstrated no residual cervical disease. Eight patients had minimal residual cancer without lymph vascular space invasion. Two patients demonstrated lymph vascular space invasion but negative margins and lymph nodes. Two patients required completion of radical vaginal hysterectomy to successfully obtain negative margins. The last patient had lymph vascular space invasion and a positive margin present within the surgical specimen. The latter three patients underwent postoperative pelvic radiation therapy. Therefore, 18 of 21 patients received radical trachelectomy to preserve fertility. Within this group, one patient gave birth to healthy twins, delivered at 24 weeks, following superovulation treatment. One patient delivered a singleton term infant via cesarean hysterectomy; no residual disease was found in the cervix. The last patient most likely became pregnant in the week prior to the radical vaginal trachelectomy. She had spontaneous rupture of membranes at 20 weeks gestation, requiring hysterotomy for evacuation of the uterus with subsequent neonatal demise.

No prospective studies have assessed the impact of pregnancy on cervical cancer prognosis or of cervical cancer on pregnancy outcome. Nguyen and colleagues concluded that tumor characteristics and maternal survival were not adversely affected by pregnancy, nor was pregnancy adversely affected by cervical cancer.[68] Similar conclusions were reached by van der Vange and colleagues in a case-control study.[72] They reported on 23 patients diagnosed during pregnancy and 24 patients diagnosed within 6 months postpartum. Thirty-nine patients had early-stage disease. No difference in survival was noted for cases compared with controls. They noted that the delivery method had no effect on survival, thus concluding that the prognosis for early-stage cervix cancer is similar in pregnant and nonpregnant women. Zemlickis and colleagues reported on a long-term follow-up of cervical cancer outcome in a case-control study of pregnant women.[77] No survival differences were observed. When compared with matched controls, invasive cervical cancer patients were more likely to give birth to children who had lower birth weights. No adverse impact of pregnancy on cervical cancer outcome could be demonstrated.

Hodgkin's Disease and Non-Hodgkin's Lymphoma The presentation of Hodgkin's disease during pregnancy does not differ from that of the nonpregnant patient, with lymphadenopathy being the most common method of presentation.[78] The diagnosis is established by lymph node biopsy, with obtainment of sufficient material to confirm the specific type of disease.[79] Staging assessment, in addition to medical history and physical examination, can include abdominal shielded chest radiography, abdominal ultrasonography, and MRI to document disease location and extent and to assist treatment planning. For supradiaphragmatic disease, radiation therapy can be completed successfully while maintaining the pregnancy with uterine and fetal shielding.[29,31,79–81] Radiation therapy during pregnancy for stage IA and IIA Hodgkin's disease was reported by Woo and colleagues.[29] Sixteen patients received radiation to the neck (2), neck and mediastinum (3), or mantle (11). Fetal radiation dose estimates were determined for nine patients. Reported doses ranged from 1.4 to 5.5 cGy for photon therapy and 10 to 13.6 cGy for cobalt therapy. There were 16 normal full-term infants, and the 10-year patient survival rate was 71%. This outcome is similar to that in an earlier report by Jacobs and colleagues, who reported on the use of radiation therapy involving the neck and mediastinum during the second and third trimesters of pregnancy.[81] Supradiaphragmatic radiation therapy can be accomplished while maintaining a viable pregnancy. There are limited data regarding the impact of Hodgkin's disease on pregnancy or on the effects of pregnancy on prognosis. Anselmo and colleagues concluded that the prognosis of Hodgkin's disease was not affected by pregnancy.[82] Tawil and colleagues, reporting on their experience with 12 patients with Hodgkin's disease and pregnancy, concluded that pregnancy did not significantly affect the course of the malignancy, and the presence of this malignancy did not affect pregnancy outcome.[80] Examining pregnancy outcome, Zuazu and colleagues found no increase in the complication rate of pregnancy in 56 patients with leukemia or lymphoma.[83] In those patients treated with systemic chemotherapy, there was no increase in the incidence of fetal malformations. In the Gelb and colleagues series, patients were treated with a variety of systemic chemotherapy agent combinations, including MOPP (mechlorethamine, Oncovin [vincristine], procarbazine, prednisone), ABV (Adriamycin [doxorubicin], bleomycin, vinblastine), COP (cyclophosphamide, Oncovin [vincristine], prednisone), and CHOP (cyclophosphamide, doxorubicin, Oncovin [vincristine], prednisone).[78] No fetal malformations were reported. Fifteen patients were alive and disease free. Gelb and colleagues concluded that otherwise indicated systemic therapy should not be delayed because of pregnancy.

Non-Hodgkin's lymphoma (NHL) during pregnancy presents at a more advanced stage and has more aggressive biologic behavior than Hodgkin's disease during pregnancy.[78,84,85] The clinical behavior of NHL appears to be the same with or without pregnancy.[78] Because the majority of patients present with advanced-stage disease, systemic chemotherapy is warranted. Combination chemotherapy has been reported to be used with some success. Agents used have included epirubicin, vincristine, prednisone, etoposide, cyclophosphamide, doxorubicin, and bleomycin in various combinations VACOP-B (VePesid [etoposide], Adriamycin [doxorubicin], Cytoxan [cyclophosphamide], Oncovin [vincristine], prednisone, and bleomycin), and MACOP-B Cytoxan (methotrexate, Adriamycin [doxorubicin], [cyclophosphamide], Oncovin [vincristine], prednisone, and bleomycin).[86–88] Two separate publications have reported the use of rituximab in the treatment of NHL during pregnancy. Herold and colleagues used a combination of rituximab, doxorubicin, vincristine, and prednisolone to treat a female with bulky stage IIA NHL.[89] At the time of initiation of therapy, the patient was in her twenty-first week of pregnancy. She demonstrated an excellent response to the regimen, with good tolerance. The patient then delivered a healthy infant at 35 weeks via cesarean section; the child demonstrated a normal B-cell population. Kimby and colleagues treated a patient with stage IIB NHL with weekly rituximab for four cycles.[90] The patient reported conception occurrence between the first and second infusions of rituximab. She delivered a healthy baby girl at 40 weeks. The infant demonstrated a low granulocyte count at birth, but her hematologic parameters had recovered by 18 months of age.

Aviles and colleagues reported the outcome of 16 patients treated for NHL during pregnancy, including 8 during the first trimester.[91] No congenital malformations were noted, and normal deliveries were reported. They concluded that pregnancy was not a contraindication to treating NHL and that long-term remission was possible. Burkitt's lymphoma, anaplastic large cell lymphoma, and T-cell lymphoma have all been reported in association with pregnancy.[92–97]

Ovarian Cancer Ovarian cancer during pregnancy is rare. In a review of adnexal masses during pregnancy, one ovarian cancer was found in 125 patients.[98] There were 40 dermoids, 15 endometriomas, 14 cysts, 13 cystoadenomas, 9 tubal cysts, and 4 fibroids—a 0.8% malignancy rate.[98]

In a retrospective review, Sayedur and colleagues identified 9 cases of ovarian cancer and pregnancy over 24 years, an incidence of 0.08 in 1,000 pregnant women.[10] For pregnant women, adnexal masses are more frequent and likely to be benign, and management decisions are becoming more complex. Ultrasonography, percutaneous aspiration, and surgical intervention are possible.

In a study by Platek and colleagues, 31 patients of 43,372 deliveries were found to have adnexal masses > 6 cm persistent beyond 16 weeks of gestation.[99] No ovarian cancers were diagnosed. When malignancies have been found, germ cell tumors and epithelial cancers of low malignant potential were most common.[100] The pathology of ovarian cancer during pregnancy was reviewed by Dgani and colleagues.[101] They recorded data on 23 patients over a 24-year period. Borderline carcinomas were most frequent (35%), followed by invasive epithelial tumors (30%), dysgerminomas (17%), and granulosa cell tumors (13%). Early-stage disease was common; 74% of patients were stage I.

In the series of Sayedur and colleagues, seven of the nine patients had stage I epithelial tumors.[10] Five patients were treated with salpingo-oophorectomy, three with total abdominal hysterectomy and bilateral salpingo-oophorectomy with omentectomy. They reported 100% survival for stage I disease and 78% 5-year survival overall. Conservative surgery for early-stage disease and low malignant potential tumors may preserve fertility. In the Dgani and colleagues series, 14 of the 23 patients delivered live neonates.[101] These authors concluded that the overall prognosis for ovarian cancer during pregnancy is better than ovarian tumors in general because of early stage at diagnosis and tumors of low malignant potential.

Chemotherapy for more advanced-stage disease has been reported primarily as case reports. Cisplatin, carboplatin, doxorubicin, bleomycin, cyclophosphamide, and, most recently, paclitaxel have all been given for treatment of ovarian cancer during pregnancy.[75,102–104]

Acute and Chronic Leukemia **Acute Leukemia** Acute leukemia occurring during pregnancy presents unique circumstances because of bone marrow failure and the attendant cytopenias that may occur. Myeloid leukemias are more common than lymphoid. The presenting signs and symptoms are not different from those of the nonpregnant patient. The diagnosis is made by bone marrow aspiration, and standard classification is used for subtyping. In a series from the Mayo Clinic, 17 patients with acute leukemia were seen in a 37-year period. Fifteen of the 17 patients were diagnosed with acute myeloid disease. The majority of these individuals presented during the first or second trimester of pregnancy. Five of nine patients treated with chemotherapy during pregnancy had long-term complete remissions, whereas three of four patients who delayed treatment until after delivery died of disease. No fetal malformations were noted in those treated with chemotherapy during pregnancy.[105]

Cardonick and Iacobucci performed an analysis of 152 patients who were treated for acute lymphoblastic leukemia (63 cases) or acute myelogenous leukemia (89 cases).[106] They found that 6 neonates developed congenital abnormalities and 12 neonates demonstrated intrauterine growth retardation. There were 11 cases of intrauterine fetal death and 2 neonatal deaths. All cases of abnormalities occurred in association with first-trimester use of cytarabine or thioguanine, as monotherapy or in combination with an anthracycline. However, combinations of vincristine, mercaptopurine, doxorubicin or daunorubicin, cyclophosphamide, prednisone, and methotrexate were used in all trimesters without anomalies.

Acute promyelocytic leukemia is of special interest because of the use of all-*trans* retinoic acid in the treatment program. Retinoids have known teratogenic effects.[107] However, a number of case reports have documented fetal safety and favorable patient outcome with the use of all-*trans* retinoic acid for acute promyelocytic leukemia.[108,109]

Chronic Leukemia Pregnancy with chronic lymphocytic leukemia (CLL) is extraordinarily rare.[110,111] Welsh and colleagues reported a case of CLL with pregnancy and noted a substantial decrease in white blood cells after delivery.[111] They noted that this apparent hematologic remission was not accompanied by clonal remission. Gurman described a case of a patient who became pregnant shortly after her diagnosis of CLL.[112] She received no cytotoxic therapy and delivered a healthy infant at 39 weeks gestation. Her third trimester was complicated by gestational diabetes and preeclampsia. Unlike the Welsh and colleagues report, which demonstrated elevated numbers of lymphocytes in the intervillous space, the latter case demonstrated no lymphocytic infiltration of the placenta. Ali and colleagues treated a patient who was diagnosed with CLL during her seventeenth week of gestation.[113] She received three courses of leukapheresis at the twenty-fifth, thirtieth, and thirty-eighth week of gestation to maintain her white blood cell count below 100×10^9/L. She delivered a normal infant at 39 weeks of gestation.

Chronic myeloid leukemia has been treated during pregnancy with interferon-α, hydroxyurea and leukapheresis, and leukapheresis alone.[114–117] No untoward effects on fetal growth and development or complications of labor and delivery have been reported.

Sustaining the pregnancy until delivery is feasible. No fetal malformations with the use of interferon or hydroxyurea have been reported. Limited data suggest that pregnancy has no effect on the long-term outcome of chronic myeloid leukemia; however, there are no case-control studies. No clinical data on the use of imatinib during pregnancy have been reported. However, data from animal studies indicate that imatinib can cause fetal abnormalities.

TRANSPLACENTAL MALIGNANCY AND PLACENTAL METASTASIS

A number of case reports have noted transplacental passage of malignancy from mother to neonate (Table 63-4).[118–125] Catlin and colleagues reported a neonatal death related to the transplacental passage of maternal natural killer cell lymphoma.[118] Successful treatment of maternal transplacental small cell lung cancer has been noted.[125] Teksam and colleagues presented a striking case of a 33-week neonate who was emergently delivered after her mother was diagnosed with lung cancer.[126] Owing to the presence of placental metastases, the infant underwent initial screening with brain MRI and chest and abdomen CT, both of which were apparently normal.

Table 63-4 Transplacental Malignancy (Partial List)
Choriocarcinoma[124]
Leukemia[121,123]
Melanoma[120]
Natural killer cell lymphoma[118]
Small cell lung cancer[125]

Unfortunately, serial examinations demonstrated development of a cerebellar tumor that significantly improved after chemotherapy, but the mass progressed a few months afterward. Biopsy and resection confirmed that the neoplasm was metastatic lung cancer. Additional metastatic lesions were identified in the frontal and temporal lobes on follow-up MRI.

Leukemia cell identification in circulation in a neonate born to a mother with acute lymphocytic leukemia has also been reported. However, leukemic cell engraftment and neonatal disease were not observed.[123] Acute monocytic leukemia transmission from mother to fetus has been documented.[121]

Alexander and colleagues reviewed 87 cases of fetal or placental metastases; they found that malignant melanoma affected 31% of these patients, making melanoma the most common malignancy to involve both the fetus and the placenta.[122]

Dildy and colleagues reviewed placental metastases and reported 52 cases in 1989.[127] Solid tumors and hematologic malignancies have been noted to involve the placenta (Table 63-5).[94,128–135] Systematic evaluation of the placenta at the time of delivery of the pregnant woman with cancer has not been routine.[135]

Table 63-6 Multidisciplinary Approach to the Pregnant Patient with Cancer

Confirm Diagnosis	Cytology, Histology
Assess extent of disease	Staging, physical examination, organ function, metastatic disease
Disease-related prognosis independent of pregnancy	
Assess pregnancy	Comorbidities: age, diabetes
	Gestational age
	Expected delivery data
Review treatment options	Patient
	Anticipated benefits for the patient
	"Cure," prolongation of life, improve or delay symptoms
Anticipated risks for the patient	
Review treatment options	Fetus
	Anticipated outcome
	Maintaining pregnancy
	Anticipated risks for the fetus
Plan and implement treatment plan	
Reevaluate patient and fetus at frequent intervals	
Multidisciplinary treatment team members	Patient
	Obstetrician
	Surgical oncologists, radiation oncologists, medical oncologists, gynecologic oncologists, and radiation oncologists
	Nurses
	Ethicists
	Social service
	Pastoral care

OUTCOME OF CHILDREN EXPOSED TO CANCER THERAPY IN UTERO

Neurodevelopment of children exposed to chemotherapy in utero has not been systematically assessed. Few long-term data have been reported other than anecdotal reports noting "normal" development. Delayed effects on cognitive function and on neurologic and behavioral development are lacking.[136] A long-term report on children exposed to chemotherapy in utero during treatment of mothers for a variety of hematologic malignancies was presented by Aviles and Neri.[137] They described 84 children followed a median of 18.7 years. Thirty-eight had been exposed to chemotherapy in utero during the first trimester of pregnancy. Fertility was reported to be preserved, with some of the chemotherapy-exposed children having become parents. No learning, neurologic, or psychological problems were reported for any of the in utero chemotherapy-exposed subjects.

CONCLUSION

Cancer during pregnancy presents a unique opportunity for multispecialty oncologic and prenatal care. The gathering and discussion of data to be used in treatment planning require careful coordination with obstetric, surgical, and anesthesiologist colleagues. Given the concern for the well-being of both mother and fetus, support for and reassurance of the patient during the decision process become a paramount duty for physicians. It is possible to have a favorable outcome for mother and child. An outline of a sequential approach to multispecialty management for cancer and pregnancy is presented in Table 63-6.

Table 63-5 Placental Metastases

Small cell lung cancer[125]
Melanoma[127]
Pancreas[129]
Breast[131]
Medulloblastoma[128]
Large cell lung cancer[130]
B-cell lymphoma[133]
T-cell lymphoma[134]
Non-Hodgkin's lymphoma[135]
Large cell lymphoma[94]

REFERENCES

1. Theriault RL, Stallings CB, Buzdar AU. Pregnancy and breast cancer: clinical and legal issues. Am J Clin Oncol 1992;15:535–9.
2. Iseminger KA, Lewis MA. Ethical challenges in treating mother and fetus when cancer complicates pregnancy. Obstet Gynecol Clin North Am 1998;25:273–85.
3. Reis LAG, Hankey BF, Miller BA, et al. Cancer statistics review 1973-1988. III.39, 91-2789. Bethesda (MD): National Cancer Institute; 1991. NIH Publication.
4. White TT. Prognosis of breast cancer for pregnant and nursing women: analysis of 1,413 cases. Surg Gynecol Obstet 1955;700:661–6.
5. Saunders CM, Baum M. Breast cancer and pregnancy: a review. J R Soc Med 1993;86:162–5.
6. Anderson JM. Mammary cancers and pregnancy. BMJ 1979;1:1124–7.
7. Smith LH, Dalrymple JL, Leiserowitz GS, et al. Obstetrical deliveries associated with maternal malignancy in California, 1992 through 1997. Am J Obstet Gynecol 2001;184:1504–12.
8. Ventura S. First births to older mothers. Am J Public Health 1989;79:1675–84.
9. Kelsey J, Berkowitz G. Breast cancer epidemiology. Cancer Res 1988;48:5615–23.
10. Sayedur RM, Al Sibai MH, Rahman J, et al. Ovarian carcinoma associated with pregnancy. A review of 9 cases. Acta Obstet Gynecol Scand 2002;81:260–4.
11. Komurcu S, Ozet A, Ozturk B, et al. Colon cancer during pregnancy. A case report. J Reprod Med 2001;46:75–8.
12. Kaiser HE, Nawab E, Nasir A, et al. Neoplasms during the progression of pregnancy. In Vivo 2000;14:277–85.
13. Allen DG, Planner RS, Tang PT, et al. Invasive cervical cancer in pregnancy. Aust N Z J Obstet Gynaecol 1995;35:408–12.
14. Mazze RI, Kallen B. Reproductive outcome after anesthesia and operation during pregnancy: a registry study of 5405 cases. Am J Obstet Gynecol 1989;161:1178–85.
15. Duncan PG, Pope WD, Cohen MM, Greer N. Fetal risk of anesthesia and surgery during pregnancy. Anesthesiology 1986;64:790–4.
16. Nakagawa K, Aoki Y, Kusama T, et al. Radiotherapy during pregnancy: effects on fetuses and neonates. Clin Ther 1997;19:770–7.
17. Pregnancy and medical radiation. Ann ICRP 2000;30(1):iii–43.
18. Rosene-Montella K, Larson L. Obstetric monitoring: maternal and fetal testing: diagnostic testing. In: Lee RV, Rosene-Montella K, Barbour LA, et al, editors. Medical care of the pregnant patient. Philadelphia: American College of Physicians; 2000. p. 103–16.
19. Fenig E, Mishaeli M, Kalish Y, Lishner M. Pregnancy and radiation. Cancer Treat Rev 2001;27:1–7.
20. Kusama T, Ota K. Radiological protection for diagnostic examination of pregnant women. Congenit Anom Kyoto 2002;42:10–4.
21. Larson RE, Semelka RC. Magnetic resonance imaging of the liver. Top Magn Reson Imaging 1995;7:71–81.
22. Sanal SM, Flickinger FW, Caudell MJ, Sherry RM. Detection of bone marrow involvement in breast cancer with magnetic resonance imaging. J Clin Oncol 1994;12:1415–21.
23. Jones AL, Williams MP, Powles TJ, et al. Magnetic resonance imaging in the detection of skeletal metastases in patients with breast cancer. Br J Cancer 1990;62:296–8.
24. Gosfield E, Alavi A, Kneeland B. Comparison of radionuclide bone scans and magnetic resonance imaging in detecting spinal metastases. J Nucl Med 1993;34:2191.
25. Duncan KR. The development of magnetic resonance imaging in obstetrics. Br J Hosp Med 1996;55:178–81.
26. Mattison DR, Angtuaco T. Magnetic resonance imaging in prenatal diagnosis. Clin Obstet Gynecol 1988;31:353–89.
27. Kirkinen P, Partanen K, Vainio P, Ryynanen M. MRI in obstetrics: a supplementary method for ultrasonography. Ann Med 1996;28:131–6.
28. Sood AK, Sorosky JI, Mayr N, et al. Radiotherapeutic management of cervical carcinoma that complicates pregnancy. Cancer 1997;80:1073–8.
29. Woo SY, Fuller LM, Cundiff JH, et al. Radiotherapy during pregnancy for clinical stages IA-IIA Hodgkin's disease. Int J Radiat Oncol Biol Phys 1992;23:407–12.
30. Kouvaris JR, Antypas CE, Sandilos PH, et al. Postoperative tailored radiotherapy for locally advanced breast carcinoma during pregnancy: a therapeutic dilemma. Am J Obstet Gynecol 2000;183:498–9.

31. Cygler J, Ding GX, Kendal W, Cross P. Fetal dose for a patient undergoing mantle field irradiation for Hodgkin's disease. Med Dosim 1997;22:135–7.
32. Islam MK, Saeedi F, Al-Rajhi N. A simplified shielding approach for limiting fetal dose during radiation therapy of pregnant patients. Int J Radiat Oncol Biol Phys 2001;49:1469–73.
33. Antypas C, Sandilos P, Kouvaris J, et al. Fetal dose evaluation during breast cancer radiotherapy. Int J Radiat Oncol Biol Phys 1998;40:995–9.
34. Greskovich JF Jr, Macklis RM. Radiation therapy in pregnancy: risk calculation and risk minimization. Semin Oncol 2000;27:633–45.
35. Ebert U, Loffler H, Kirch W. Cytotoxic therapy and pregnancy. Pharmacol Ther 1997;74:207–20.
36. Doll DC, Ringenberg QS, Yarbro JW. Antineoplastic agents and pregnancy. Semin Oncol 1989;16:337–46.
37. Germann N, Goffinet F, Goldwasser F. Anthracyclines during pregnancy: embryo-fetal outcome in 160 patients. Ann Oncol 2004;15:146–50.
38. Scott LL, Ramin SM, Richey M, et al. Erythropoietin use in pregnancy: two cases and a review of the literature. Am J Perinatol 1995;12:22–4.
39. Dale DC, Cottle TE, Fier CJ, et al. Severe chronic neutropenia: treatment and follow-up of patients in the Severe Chronic Neutropenia International Registry. Am J Hematol 2003;72:82–93.
40. Byrd BF, Bayer DS, Robertson JC, et al. Treatment of breast tumors associated with pregnancy and lactation. Ann Surg 1962;155:940–7.
41. Bunker ML, Peters MV. Breast cancer associated with pregnancy and lactation. Am J Obstet Gynecol 1963;85:312–9.
42. Lethaby A, O'Neill M, Mason B. Overall survival from breast cancer in women pregnant or lactating at or after diagnosis. Auckland Breast Cancer Study Group. Int J Cancer 1996;67:751–5.
43. Ezzat A, Raja MA, Berry J, et al. Impact of pregnancy on non-metastatic breast cancer: a case control study. Clin Oncol (R Coll Radiol) 1996;8:367–70.
44. Max MH, Klamer TW. Pregnancy and breast cancer. South Med J 1983;76:1088–90.
45. Liberman L, Giess C, Dershaw D, et al. Imaging of pregnancy-associated breast cancer. Radiology 1994;191:245–8.
46. Samuels TH, Liu FF, Yaffe M, Haider M. Gestational breast cancer. Can Assoc Radiol J 1998;49:172–80.
47. Gupta RK, McHutchinson AGR, Dowle CS, Simpson JS. Fine-needle aspiration cytodiagnosis of breast masses in pregnant and lactating women and its impact on management. Diagn Cytopathol 1993;19:156–9.
48. Bottles K, Taylor RN. Diagnosis of breast masses in pregnant and lactating women by aspiration cytology. Obstet Gynecol 1985;66(3 Suppl):76S–8S.
49. Gupta RK. The diagnostic impact of aspiration cytodiagnosis of breast masses in association with pregnancy and lactation with an emphasis on clinical decision making. Breast J 1997;3:131–4.
50. Keleher A, Wendt R III, Delpassand E, et al. The safety of lymphatic mapping in pregnant breast cancer patients using Tc-99m sulfur colloid. Breast J 2004;10:492–5.
51. Gentilini O, Cremonesi M, Trifiro G, et al. Safety of sentinel node biopsy in pregnant patients with breast cancer. Ann Oncol 2004;15:1348–51.
52. Collins JC, Liao S, Wile AG. Surgical management of breast masses in pregnant women. J Reprod Med 1995;40:785–8.
53. Kuerer HM, Gwyn K, Ames FC, Theriault RL. Conservative surgery and chemotherapy for breast carcinoma during pregnancy. Surgery 2002;131:108–10.
54. Berry DL, Theriault RL, Holmes FA, et al. Management of breast cancer during pregnancy using a standardized protocol. J Clin Oncol 1999;17:855–61.
55. Gwyn K, Theriault RL, Sahin A, et al. Treatment of breast cancer during pregnancy using a standard protocol: update of the M.D. Anderson experience. Proc Am Soc Clin Oncol 2001;20:18b.
56. Giacalone P-L, Laffargue F, Benos P. Chemotherapy for breast carcinoma during pregnancy. Cancer 1999;86:2266–72.
57. Barthelmes L, Gateley CA. Tamoxifen and pregnancy. Breast 2004;13:446–51.
58. De Santis M, Lucchese A, De Carolis S, et al. Metastatic breast cancer in pregnancy: first case of chemotherapy with docetaxel. Eur J Cancer Care (Engl) 2000;9:235–7.
59. Gonzalez-Angulo AM, Walters RS, Carpenter RJ Jr, et al. Paclitaxel chemotherapy in a pregnant patient with bilateral breast cancer. Clin Breast Cancer 2004;5:317–9.
60. Gadducci A, Cosio S, Fanucchi A, et al. Chemotherapy with epirubicin and paclitaxel for breast cancer during pregnancy: case report and review of the literature. Anticancer Res 2003;23:5225–9.
61. Fanale M, Uyei A, Theriault RL, et al. Treatment of metastatic breast cancer with trastuzumab and vinorelbine during pregnancy. Clin Br Cancer 2005. [In press]
62. Choe W, McDougall IR. Thyroid cancer in pregnant women: diagnostic and therapeutic management. Thyroid 1994;4:433–5.
63. Morris PC. Thyroid cancer complicating pregnancy. Obstet Gynecol Clin North Am 1998;25:401–5.
64. Hamburger JI. Thyroid nodules in pregnancy. Thyroid 1992;2:165–8.
65. Driggers RW, Kopelman JN, Satin AJ. Delaying surgery for thyroid cancer in pregnancy. A case report. J Reprod Med 1998;43:909–12.
66. Hisham AN, Aina EN. A reappraisal of thyroid surgery under local anaesthesia: back to the future? Aust N Z J Surg 2002;72:287–9.
67. Moosa M, Mazzaferri EL. Outcome of differentiated thyroid cancer diagnosed in pregnant women. J Clin Endocrinol Metab 1997;82:2862–6.
68. Nguyen C, Montz FJ, Bristow RE. Management of stage I cervical cancer in pregnancy. Obstet Gynecol Surv 2001;55:633–43.
69. Hertel H, Possover M, Kuhne-Heid R, Schneider A. Laparoscopic lymph node staging of cervical cancer in the 19th week of pregnancy. A case report. Surg Endosc 2001;15:324.
70. Sorosky JI, Squatrito R, Ndubisi BU, et al. Stage I squamous cell cervical carcinoma in pregnancy: planned delay in therapy awaiting fetal maturity. Gynecol Oncol 1995;59:207–10.
71. Sood AK, Sorosky JI, Mayr N, et al. Cervical cancer diagnosed shortly after pregnancy: prognostic variables and delivery routes. Obstet Gynecol 2000;95(6 Pt 1):832–8.
72. van Der Vange N, Weverling GJ, Ketting BW, et al. The prognosis of cervical cancer associated with pregnancy: a matched cohort study. Obstet Gynecol 1995;85:1022–6.
73. Cliby WA, Dodson MK, Podratz KC. Cervical cancer complicated by pregnancy: episiotomy site recurrences following vaginal delivery. Obstet Gynecol 1994;84:179–82.
74. Marana HRC, deAndrade JM, Mathes A, et al. Chemotherapy in the treatment of locally advanced cervical cancer and pregnancy. Gynecol Oncol 2001;80:272–4.
75. Sood AK, Shahin MS, Sorosky JI. Paclitaxel and platinum chemotherapy for ovarian carcinoma during pregnancy. Gynecol Oncol 2001;83:599–600.
76. Burnett AF, Roman LD, O'Meara AT, Morrow CP. Radical vaginal trachelectomy and pelvic lymphadenectomy for preservation of fertility in early cervical carcinoma. Gynecol Oncol 2003;88:419–23.
77. Zemlickis D, Lishner M, Degendorfer P, et al. Maternal and fetal outcome after invasive cervical cancer in pregnancy. J Clin Oncol 1991;9:1956–61.
78. Gelb AB, van de Rijn M, Warnke RA, Kamel OW. Pregnancy-associated lymphomas: a clinicopathologic study. Cancer 1996;78:304–10.
79. Nisce LZ, Tome MA, He S, et al. Management of coexisting Hodgkin's disease and pregnancy. Am J Clin Oncol 1986;9:146–51.
80. Tawil E, Mercier JP, Dandavino A. Hodgkin's disease complicating pregnancy. J Can Assoc Radiol 1985;36:133–7.
81. Jacobs C, Donaldson SS, Rosenberg SA, Kaplan HS. Management of the pregnant patient with Hodgkin's disease. Ann Intern Med 1981;95:669–75.
82. Anselmo AP, Cavalieri E, Enrici RM, et al. Hodgkin's disease during pregnancy: diagnostic and therapeutic management. Fetal Diagn Ther 1999;14:102–5.
83. Zuazu J, Julia A, Sierra J, et al. Pregnancy outcome in hematologic malignancies. Cancer 1991;67:703–9.
84. Lishner M, Zemlickis D, Sutcliffe SB, Koren G. Non-Hodgkin's lymphoma and pregnancy. Leuk Lymphoma 1994;14:411–3.
85. Ioachim HL. Non-Hodgkin's lymphoma in pregnancy. Three cases and review of the literature. Arch Pathol Lab Med 1985;109:803–9.
86. Goldwasser F, Pico JL, Cerrina J, et al. Successful chemotherapy including epirubicin in a pregnant non-Hodgkin's lymphoma patient. Leuk Lymphoma 1995;20:173–6.
87. Rodriguez JM, Haggag M. VACOP-B chemotherapy for high grade non-Hodgkin's lymphoma in pregnancy. Clin Oncol 1995;7:319–20.
88. Nantel S, Parboosingh J, Poon M-C. Treatment of an aggressive non-Hodgkin's lymphoma during pregnancy with MACOP-B chemotherapy. Med Pediatr Oncol 1990;18:143–5.
89. Herold M, Schnohr S, Bittrich H. Efficacy and safety of a combined rituximab chemotherapy during pregnancy. J Clin Oncol 2001;19:3439.
90. Kimby E, Sverrisdottir A, Elinder G. Safety of rituximab therapy during the first trimester of pregnancy: a case history. Eur J Haematol 2005;72:292–5.
91. Aviles A, Diaz-Maqueo JC, Torras V, et al. Non-Hodgkin's lymphomas and pregnancy: presentation of 16 cases. Gynecol Oncol 1990;37:335–7.
92. Antic N, Colovic M, Cemerikic V, et al. Disseminated Burkitt's-like lymphoma during pregnancy. Med Oncol 2000;17:233–6.
93. Barnes MN, Barrett JC, Kimberlin DF, Kilgore LC. Burkitt lymphoma in pregnancy. Obstet Gynecol 1998;92(4 Pt 2):675–8.
94. Meguerian-Bedoyan Z, Lamant L, Hopfner C, et al. Anaplastic large cell lymphoma of maternal origin involving the placenta: case report and literature survey. Am J Surg Pathol 1997;21:1236–41.
95. Aviles A. Peripheral T-cell lymphoma involving the placenta. Cancer 1993;72:300–1.
96. Lesesve J-F, Buisine J, Gregoire M-J, et al. Leukaemic small cell variant anaplastic large cell lymphoma during pregnancy. Clin Lab Haematol 2000;22:297–301.
97. Lees CC, Tsirigotis M, Carr JVL, Richards MA. T-cell non-Hodgkin's lymphoma presenting in the first trimester of pregnancy. Postgrad Med J 1994;70:371–2.
98. Bromley B, Benacerraf B. Adnexal masses during pregnancy: accuracy of sonographic diagnosis and outcome. J Ultrasound Med 1997;16:447–52.
99. Platek DN, Henderson CE, Goldberg GL. The management of a persistent adnexal mass in pregnancy. Am J Obstet Gynecol 1995;173:1236–40.
100. Zanotti KM, Belinson JL, Kennedy AW. Treatment of gynecologic cancers in pregnancy. Semin Oncol 2000;27:686–98.
101. Dgani R, Shoham Z, Atar E, et al. Ovarian carcinoma during pregnancy: a study of 23 cases in Israel between the years 1960 and 1984. Gynecol Oncol 1989;33:326–31.
102. Bayhan G, Aban M, Yayla M, et al. Cisplatinum combination chemotherapy during pregnancy for mucinous cystadenocarcinoma of the ovary. Eur J Cancer 1999;20:231–2.
103. King LA, Nevin PC, Williams PP, et al. Treatment of advanced epithelial ovarian carcinoma in pregnancy with cisplatin-based chemotherapy. Gynecol Oncol 1991;41:78–80.
104. Malfetano JH, Goldkrand JW. Cisplatinum combination chemotherapy during pregnancy for advanced epithelial ovarian carcinoma. Obstet Gynecol 1990;75:545–7.
105. Greenlund LJ, Letendre L, Tefferi A. Acute leukemia during pregnancy: a single institutional experience with 17 cases. Leuk Lymphoma 2001;41:571–7.
106. Cardonick E, Iacobucci A. Use of chemotherapy during human pregnancy. Lancet Oncol 2004;5:283–91.
107. Lammer EJ, Chen DT, Hoar RM, et al. Retinoic acid embryopathy. N Engl J Med 1985;313:837–41.
108. Stentoft J, Nielsen JL, Hvidman LE. All-trans retinoic acid in acute promyelocytic leukemia in late pregnancy. Leukemia 1994;8:1585–8.
109. Hansen WF, Fretz P, Hunter SK, Yankowitz J. Leukemia in pregnancy and fetal response to multiagent chemotherapy. Obstet Gynecol 2001;97(5 Pt 2):809–12.
110. Chrisomalis L, Baxi LV, Heller D. Chronic lymphocytic leukemia in pregnancy. Am J Obstet Gynecol 1996;175:1381–2.
111. Welsh TM, Thompson J, Lim S. Chronic lymphocytic leukemia in pregnancy. Leukemia 2000;14:1155.
112. Gurman G. Pregnancy and successful labor in the course of chronic lymphocytic leukemia. Am J Hematol 2002;71:208–10.
113. Ali R, Ozkalemkas F, Ozkocaman V, et al. Successful labor in the course of chronic lymphocytic leukemia (CLL) and management of CLL during pregnancy with leukapheresis. Ann Hematol 2004;83:61–3.
114. Celiloglu M, Altunyurt S, Undar B. Hydroxyurea treatment for chronic myeloid leukemia during pregnancy. Acta Obstet Gynecol Scand 2000;79:803–4.
115. Baykal C, Zengin N, Coskun F, et al. Use of hydroxyurea and alpha-interferon in chronic myeloid leukemia during pregnancy: a case report. Eur J Gynaecol Oncol 2000;21:89–90.
116. Haggstrom J, Adriansson M, Hybbinette T, et al. Two cases of CML treated with alpha-interferon during second and third trimester of pregnancy with analysis of the drug in the new-born immediately postpartum. Eur J Haematol 1996;57:101–2.
117. Strobl FJ, Voelkerding KV, Smith EP. Management of chronic myeloid leukemia during pregnancy with leukapheresis. J Clin Apheresis 1999;14:42–4.

118. Catlin EA, Roberts JD Jr, Erana R, et al. Transplacental transmission of natural-killer-cell lymphoma. N Engl J Med 1999;341:85–91.
119. Carosell ED, Dausset J, Rouas-Freiss N. Transplacental transmission of natural-killer-cell lymphoma. N Engl J Med 1999;341:1937.
120. Moller D, Ipsen L, Asschenfeldt P. Fatal course of malignant melanoma during pregnancy with dissemination to the products of conception. Acta Obstet Gynecol Scand 1986;65:501–2.
121. Osada S, Horibe K, Oiwa K, et al. A case of infantile acute monocytic leukemia caused by vertical transmission of the mother's leukemic cells. Cancer 1990;65:1146–9.
122. Alexander A, Samlowski WE, Grossman D, et al. Metastatic melanoma in pregnancy: risk of transplacental metastases in the infant. J Clin Oncol 2003;21:2179–86.
123. vanderVelden V, Willemse MJ, Mulder MF, et al. Clearance of maternal leukaemic cells in a neonate. Br J Haematol 2001;114:104–6.
124. McNally OM, Tran M, Fortune D, Quinn MA. Successful treatment of mother and baby with metastatic choriocarcinoma. Int J Gynecol Cancer 2002;12:394–8.
125. Tolar J, Coad JE, Neglia JP. Transplacental transfer of small-cell carcinoma of the lung. N Engl J Med 2002;346:1501–2.
126. Teksam M, McKinney A, Short J, et al. Intracranial metastasis via transplacental (vertical) transmission of maternal small cell lung cancer to fetus: CT and MRI findings. Acta Radiol 2004;45:577–9.
127. Dildy GA III, Moise KJ Jr, Carpenter RJ Jr, Klima T. Maternal malignancy metastatic to the products of conception: a review. Obstet Gynecol Surv 1989;44:535–40.
128. Baergen RN, Johnson D, Moore T, Benirschke K. Maternal melanoma metastatic to the placenta: a case report and review of the literature. Arch Pathol Lab Med 1997;121:508–11.
129. Brossard J, Abish S, Bernstein ML, et al. Maternal malignancy involving the products of conception: a report of malignant melanoma and medulloblastoma. Am J Pediatr Hematol Oncol 1994;16:380–3.
130. Eltorby M, Khane V, Osborne P, Shanklin D. Placenta metastasis from maternal carcinoma: a report of three cases. J Reprod Med 1995;40:399–403.
131. Salamon MA, Sherer DM, Saller DN, et al. Placental metastases in a patient with recurrent breast carcinoma. Am J Obstet Gynecol 1994;171:573–4.
132. Dunn JS Jr, Anderson CD, Brost BC. Breast carcinoma metastatic to the placenta. Obstet Gynecol 1999;94(5 Pt 2):846.
133. Nishi Y, Suzuki S, Otsubo Y, et al. B-cell-type malignant lymphoma with placental involvement. J Obstet Gynaecol Res 2000;26:39–43.
134. Kurtin PJ, Gaffey TA, Habermann TM. Peripheral T-cell lymphoma involving the placenta. Cancer 1992;70:2963–8.
135. Tsujimura T, Matsumoto K, Aozasa K. Placental involvement by maternal non-Hodgkin's lymphoma. Arch Pathol Lab Med 1993;117:325–7.
136. Nulman I, Laslo D, Fried S, et al. Neurodevelopment of children exposed in utero to treatment of maternal malignancy. Br J Cancer 2001;85:1611–8.
137. Aviles A, Neri N. Hematological malignancies and pregnancy: a final report of 84 children who received chemotherapy in utero. Clin Lymphoma 2001;2:173–7.
138. Kachhara R, Devi CG, Nair S, et al. Acoustic neurinomas during pregnancy: report of two cases and review of literature. Acta Neurochir (Wien) 2001;143:587–91.
139. Lau WY, Leung WT, Ho S, et al. Hepatocellular carcinoma during pregnancy and its comparison with other pregnancy-associated malignancies. Cancer 1995;75:2669–76.
140. Morishita S, Imai A, Kawabata I, Tamaya T. Acute myelogenous leukemia in pregnancy: fetal blood sampling and early effects of chemotherapy. Int J Gynaecol Obstet 1994;44:273–7.
141. Hoffman JS, Bazzurini L, Laird L, et al. Term delivery following conservative treatment for villoglandular papillary adenocarcinoma of the uterine cervix: report of a case and analysis of the literature. Gynecol Oncol 2001;81:310–3.
142. Slingluff CL Jr, Reintgen DS, Vollmer RT, Seigler HF. Malignant melanoma arising during pregnancy. A study of 100 patients. Ann Surg 1990;211:552–7.
143. Ruano R, Hase EA, Bernini C, et al. Pancreaticoduodenectomy as treatment of adenocarcinoma of the papilla of Vater diagnosed during pregnancy. A case report. J Reprod Med 2001;46:1021–4.
144. Sakata H, Karamitsos J, Kundaria B, DiSaia PJ. Case report of interferon alfa therapy for multiple myeloma during pregnancy. Am J Obstet Gynecol 1995;172:217–9.
145. Loughlin KR, Ng B. Bladder cancer during pregnancy. Br J Urol 1995;75:421–2.
146. Echols KT, Gilles JM, Diro M. Mycosis fungoides in pregnancy: remission after treatment with alpha-interferon in a case refractory to conventional therapy: a case report. J Matern Fetal Med 2001;10:68–70.
147. Varveris H, Mazonakis M, Damilakis J, et al. Peripheral primitive neuroectodermal tumour during pregnancy. Br J Radiol 2002;75:543–7.
148. Mujaibel K, Benjamin A, Delisle MF, Williams K. Lung cancer in pregnancy: case reports and review of the literature. J Matern Fetal Med 2001;10:426–32.
149. Wijeyaratne CN, Sheriffdeen AH, Seneviratne HR. Bilateral phaeochromocytoma during pregnancy. Ceylon Med J 2001;46:24–6.
150. Magge SN, Brunt M, Scott RM. Craniopharyngioma presenting during pregnancy 4 years after a normal magnetic resonance imaging scan. Neurosurgery 2001;49:1014–7.
151. Parry BR, Tan BK, Chan WB, Goh HS. Rectal carcinoma during pregnancy. Aust N Z J Surg 1994;64:618–20.
152. Ichikawa Y, Takano K, Higa S, et al. Endometrial carcinoma coexisting with pregnancy, presumed to derive from adenomyosis: a case report. Int J Gynecol Cancer 2001;11:488–90.
153. Sainsbury DC, Dorkin TJ, Macphail S, Soomro NA. Laparoscopic radical nephrectomy in first-trimester pregnancy. Urology 2004;64:1231.
154. Adolph A, Le T, Khan K, Biem S. Recurrent metastatic fallopian tube carcinoma in pregnancy. Gynecol Oncol 2001;81:110–2.
155. Shufaro Y, Uzieli B, Pappo O, Abramov Y. Pregnancy and delivery in a patient with metastatic embryonal sarcoma of the liver. Obstet Gynecol 2002;99(5 Pt 2):951–3.
156. Maeta M, Yamashiro H, Oka A, et al. Gastric cancer in the young, with special reference to 14 pregnancy-associated cases: analysis based on 2,325 consecutive cases of gastric cancer. J Surg Oncol 1995;58:191–5.
157. Utsumi T, Tsuda A, Hirano H, et al. A case of pregnancy with adult T-cell leukemia. J Obstet Gynaecol Res 1996;22:599–601.
158. Alothman A, Sparling TG. Managing hairy cell leukemia in pregnancy. Ann Intern Med 1994;120:1048–9.
159. Herzon FS, Morris DM, Segal MN, et al. Coexistent thyroid cancer and pregnancy. Arch Otolaryngol Head Neck Surg 1994;120:1191–3.
160. Vini L, Hyer S, Pratt B, Harmer C. Management of differentiated thyroid cancer diagnosed during pregnancy. Eur J Endocrinol 1999;140:404–6.
161. Ferlito A, Devaney SL, Carbone A, et al. Pregnancy and malignant neoplasms of the head and neck. Ann Otol Rhinol Laryngol 1998;107(11 Pt 1):991–8.
162. Gitsch G, van Eijkeren M, Hacker NF. Surgical therapy of vulvar cancer in pregnancy. Gynecol Oncol 1995;56:312–5.

Cancer and Aging

Arti Hurria, MD
Hyman B. Muss, MD
Harvey J. Cohen, MD

Cancer is a disease that disproportionately affects older patients. People age 65 and older have an 11-fold increase in the incidence of cancer and a 15-fold increase in cancer mortality in comparison to people younger than age 65 (Tables 64-1 and 64-2).[1,2] Sixty percent of all cancers occur in people ≥ age 65. The number of older people with cancer is continuously growing as the population is aging. In the United States, in 1900, 3.1 million people were age 65 and older. Over the century, this number increased approximately 10-fold, so that in the year 2000 there were 35 million people age 65 and older. This number is expected to double yet again, thus in 2030, it is projected that there will be 70.2 million people over the age of 65, accounting for 20% of the population (Table 64-3).[1,3]

Among those over age 65, there has been an age shift over time, leading to an increase in the older segment of the population. For example, during the 1990s the number age 85 and older increased by 38%, the number age 75 to 84 increased by 23%, and the number age 65 to 74 increased by less than 2%.[3] By 2030, the number ≥ age 85 is expected to double.[1] Those who live to age 100 and beyond, the "centenarians," are the fastest growing segment of the older population. Data from the US Census bureau demonstrate that were 72,000 centenarians in the United States in 2000. This number is projected to increase 10-fold by 2050, so that there will be 834,000 centenarians in the United States.[4] The four countries that share the highest percentage of the older population are China, the United States, India, and Japan, accounting for > 43% of the world population aged 75 and older.[1] Based on these statistics, oncologists inevitably care for a large number of older patients. There is no standard chronological age at which a person is considered "older." Historically, aged ≥ 65 was used for two reasons: (1) this was the traditional age for retirement, and (2) people in the United States become eligible for entitlement programs (Social Security, Medicare). As our population ages, we see much heterogeneity in the aged ≥ 65 population, with many individuals continuing to work and function similarly to younger counterparts. Therefore, this chapter will focus on defining characteristics to understand "functional age," rather than "chronological age" to distinguish the "older" patient. This chapter will also be dedicated to discussing the unique issues and considerations in caring for an older patient with cancer.

Table 64-1 11-Fold Increase in Cancer Incidence and 15-Fold Increase in Cancer Mortality with Age ≥ 65

Age	Incidence (per 100,000)	Mortality (per 100,000)
< age 65	204.1	73.3
≥ age 65	2255.1	1080.3

LIFE EXPECTANCY AND AGING

Statistics regarding average life expectancy are useful to consider when caring for an older patient. The average life expectancy at birth is 76.5 years. As an individual ages, the average projected life expectancy increases. For example, a person who lives to 65 years of age has an average life expectancy of 17.7 years, placing their projected age of death at 82.7 years. A person who lives to 80 years of age, has an average projected life expectancy of 8.5 years, placing the projected age of death at 88.5 years. Even the 100-year old person has an average life expectancy of 2.5 years, placing their average projected age of death at 102.5 years. One may think of this as a "survival of the fittest" phenomenon, in which the absolute life expectancy increases as one ages (Table 64-4).[5] In addition, this projected life expectancy will be impacted by other comorbid (co-existing) medical problems (Table 64-5).

THE BIOLOGY OF CANCER AND AGING

Aging can be defined as "the process that converts healthy adults into frail ones with diminished reserves in most physiologic systems and an exponentially increasing vulnerability to disease and death."[6] Despite the universality of this definition, aging is clearly a heterogeneous process. Each individual ages at a unique pace and demonstrates varying manifestations of vulnerability. The mechanisms of both aging and neoplasia are incompletely understood and therefore theories about the association of these two processes are an area of active research.

Several theories of the association with aging and neoplasia have been described. One theory is based on the multi-step model of carcinogenesis. With time there is increased exposure to possible carcinogens and an accumulation of cellular events, leading to a development of a malignant cell. With this model of neoplasia, the older patient is more vulnerable, as a function of time, to progress through the different stages of neoplasia. In addition, older patients have had a longer duration of exposure to carcinogens.[7]

Another theory of the association of aging and neoplasia is an association between alterations in growth regulatory gene function with aging. Thus, aging is a process in which certain genes are activated and others are suppressed, leading to an increase in oncogene activation or a decrease in tumor suppressor gene activity. Once a mutation occurs, an aged cell may have decreased ability for DNA repair.[7]

Although each of these theories is plausible, they don't explain why an individual is more or less susceptible to the development of neoplasia, especially in the absence of carcinogen exposure. In addition, these theories do not explain why

Table 64-2 Incidence of Ten Major Tumors in Patients Under and Over 65 Years of Age

Tumor Site	Patients Aged Under 65 Years (%)	Patients Aged Over 65 Years (%)	Number of Cases
Prostate	23.1	76.9	179,300
Colon	26.1	73.9	94,700
Pancreas	27.0	73.0	28,600
Urinary Bladder	28.6	71.4	54,200
Stomach	30.4	69.6	21,900
Lung	34.2	65.8	171,600
Rectum	34.6	65.4	34,700
Non-Hodgkin Lymphoma	49.0	51.0	56,800
Breast (women)	52.5	47.5	175,000
Ovary	54.1	45.9	25,200

Reprinted with permission from Yancik and Ries.[2]

Table 64-3 The Growing US Population Age 65 and Older[1,2]

Year	Million	% of Population
1900	3.1	4.1
2000	35	12.4
2030	70.2	20.1

among the oldest old patients, there may be a drop-off in cancer incidence in the oldest segment of the population. Autopsy studies have suggested that among older patients, there is a difference in the incidence of cancer in the centenarians in comparison to younger patients. In a study of 507 patients over 75 years of age, the prevalence of cancer at the time of autopsy decreased with increasing age (35% age 75 to 79, 20% age 95 to 99, and 16% in centenarians). Cancer was the cause of death in fewer older patients (67% of patients aged 75 to 90 and in 41% of patient aged 95 and older), and there was a decreased incidence of metastatic disease, with increasing age.[8]

PHYSIOLOGIC CHANGES WITH AGING

Physiologic changes occur in each organ system with aging, independent of disease. Most organ systems show a linear physiological decline beginning at 30 years of age. This decline occurs at variable rates between individuals and across organ systems. The consequence of these changes during normal activity is minimal; however, during times of stress the decreased reserve becomes more apparent.[9]

As the cardiovascular system ages, there is a decrease in cardiac output, decrease in maximal heart rate, and prolonged recovery following exertion. During times of stress, there is a decreased response to catecholamines. As the pulmonary system ages, there is a decreased response to hypoxemia or hypercapnia, decreased elasticity in the lung tissue, increased ventilation-perfusion mismatch, and decreased forced expiratory volume. Endocrine changes with aging include a decrease in certain hormone levels and an increase in others. For example, there is a decrease in insulin-like growth factor, growth hormone, renin, aldosterone, dehydroepiandrosterone, and sex steroids, and increase in insulin, norepinephrine, parathyroid hormone, vasopressin, and atrial natriuretic peptide. Changes to the neurological system with aging include neuronal loss, decrease in brain weight, decreased vision, loss in high frequency and low frequency hearing, and alterations in both taste and smell. Changes in the immune system manifest as decrease in thymic mass, decreased production of thymic hormones, decrease in naive lymphocytes, and a decrease in antibody response.[9]

Table 64-4 Average Life Expectancy

Age Now	Life Expectancy	Age of Death
65	17.7	82.7
70	14.3	84.3
75	11.2	86.2
80	8.5	88.5
85	6.3	91.3
90	4.5	94.5
95	3.3	98.3
100	2.5	102.5

*Data derived from the National Vital Statistics Report.[5]

There is a decrease in hepatic and renal mass with aging. Autopsy studies demonstrate a decrease in liver volume with aging by approximately 25 to 50%. In addition, there is decreased hepatic blood flow, estimated at a 10 to 15% decrease in liver perfusion, even after taking into account the decrease in liver volume.[10–12] Renal mass decreases by 25 to 30% over the lifespan, leading to a decreased number of functional nephrons. Renal blood flow decreases by 1% per year after 50 years of age and glomerular filtration decreases by 1 mL/minute/year after the age of 40.[10,12]

Hematopoietic changes with aging include a decrease in bone marrow mass and increase in bone marrow fat. Despite this, peripheral blood cell concentrations in healthy older patients are similar to those of younger patients.[13]

THE FRAIL OLDER PATIENT

The term "frail" is used to describe a subset of older patients with a critically reduced functional reserve that places them at risk for dependency, institutionalization, illness, hospitalization, and mortality. It is estimated that approximately 10 to 25% of people aged 65 and older are "frail." Despite the large number of patients who are described as "frail," no standard definition identifies these patients prior to the development of an adverse outcome.[14] A proposed definition of frailty is "a state of age-related physiologic vulnerability resulting from impaired homeostatic reserve and reduced capacity of the organism to withstand stress." Therefore, the clinical syndrome of frailty is proposed to be a dynamic consequence of a negative energy balance; for example, starting with undernutrition that leads to loss of muscle and bone mass and contributes to further decline in activity level and strength. This, in combination with decreased reserve, contributes to the increased vulnerability of the frail patient. The end result is failure to thrive, which is a syndrome of unexplained weight loss, decreased muscle mass, and metabolic abnormalities including a decrease in albumin, creatinine, cholesterol, and hemoglobin. Immune dysfunction and chronic inflammation may play a role in frailty. Research by Cohen and colleagues demonstrates that markers of inflammation are associated with aging and frailty including the cytokine interleukin 6 (IL 6) and the acute phase reactant, C-reactive protein (CRP). In addition, elevations in plasma D dimer have been associated with age. Both IL 6 and D dimer have been predictive of mortality and functional decline.[14,15]

The following clinical characteristics are often used to describe a frail older person: aged > 85 years, dependence in activities of daily living, comorbid (co-existing) medical conditions (including serious cardiovascular, respiratory, or cerebrovascular conditions), and one or more geriatric syndromes (dementia, delirium, urinary or fecal incontinence, history of osteoporotic fractures, failure to thrive, neglect, and abuse).[16] Frail older patients with cancer represent a unique subset of patients that pose challenging therapeutic decisions. An important initial step in evaluation of the frail patient is to determine whether the cancer is likely to decrease the patient's life expectancy. In a model proposed by Balducci and colleagues, one would consider treatment of the cancer if it was impacting the patient's life expectancy or if it was causing a compromise in quality of life. The goal of treatment must be determined: life prolonging verses palliation. Treatment decisions involve weighing the risks and benefits with the patient and caregiver. As the nation is aging, there will be a rise in the number of frail older patients with cancer. Clinical trials focusing on efficacy and tolerability of treatment within this patient population are needed.[16]

Table 64-5 Baseline Life Expectancy for Patients with Various Ages and Comorbidity Levels

Age	Healthy	Average	Sick
65	20.0	18.5	9.7
70	15.8	14.8	8.6
75	12.1	11.5	7.3
80	8.8	8.4	5.9
85	6.1	5.9	4.5

From Extermann, Balducci, and Lyman,[59] with permission.

EVALUATION OF THE OLDER PATIENT: GERIATRIC ASSESSMENT

The term "geriatric assessment" was defined at a consensus conference in 1989, as "a multi-dimensional inter-disciplinary patient evaluation that leads to the identification of patient's problems."[17] The assessment includes an evaluation of the older person's functional status (ability to live independently at home and in the community), comorbid medical conditions, cognition, psychological status, social functioning and support, medication review, and nutritional status (Table 64-6). This comprehensive assessment allows for identification of areas of vulnerability and a multi-disciplinary plan to address these areas. In addition, geriatric assessment provides valuable information regarding prognostic factors for morbidity and mortality in the older patient. Each

Table 64-6 Key Components of a Comprehensive Geriatric Assessment

Functional status
Comorbid (co-existing) medical conditions
Cognition
Psychological status
Social functioning and support
Socioeconomic issues
Medication review
Nutritional status

Table 64-7 Functional Status Assessment

Activities of Daily Living	Instrumental Activities of Daily Living
Bathing	Telephone
Dressing	Traveling
Toileting	Shopping
Transfer	Preparing meals
Continence	Housework
Eating	Medication management
	Money management

domain of a geriatric assessment will be reviewed below.

FUNCTIONAL STATUS

Assessment of functional status includes an evaluation of an individual's ability to live independently at home and in the community. Traditional assessment measures are "Activities of Daily Living" (ADL) and "Instrumental Activities of Daily Living" (IADL) (Table 64-7). Activities of daily living are basic self-care skills, such as ability to bathe, dress, toilet, transfer, maintain continence, and feed oneself. These activities are essential in order for one to maintain independence in the home. Dependence in activities of daily living has been predictive of survival, nursing home placement, prolonged hospital stay, worsening of function in the hospital, and greater home care use.[18,19] An individual who is dependent in one or more activities of daily living has an average life expectancy of less than three years.[20]

Instrumental activities of daily living include those self-care skills that allow one to live independently in the community. These include ability to telephone, shop, travel, prepare meals, do housework, take medications, and manage one's finances. In a study by Reuben and colleagues of 282 patients aged 64 and older, dependence in instrumental activities of daily living (such as housework, shopping, and driving, scored as a continuous variables), was an independent predictor of mortality ($p < .0001$).[21] Dependence in instrumental activities of daily living is predictive of risk of cognitive impairment.[22] Individuals who are dependent in instrumental activities of daily living often need assistance to maintain independence in the community.

Cancer in an older patient is associated with increased dependence in functional status. In a large study of older patients, individuals with cancer had more limitations in activities of daily living and instrumental activities of daily living than individuals without cancer and required more healthcare use.[23] In a study of women with breast cancer, normal levels of functioning were re-established over the year following diagnosis; however, the rate of recuperation was slower among older women in comparison to younger women.

COMORBID MEDICAL CONDITIONS

Comorbidity is defined as a concurrent medical problem that is a competing source of morbidity or mortality. In a study by Yancik and colleagues, summary data on comorbidity were collected on 7,600 patients aged ≥ 55 years. The most common concurrent medical problems included hypertension (42.9%), heart-related conditions (39.1%), and arthritis (34.9%). The number of comorbid conditions increased with age. Patients aged 55 to 64 had an average of 2.9 comorbid conditions, patients aged 65 to 74 had 3.6 comorbid conditions, and those 75 and older had 4.2 medical conditions (Table 64-8).[1] In a study by Extermann and colleagues of 203 patients with cancer (median age 75; range 63–91), comorbidity and functional status were found to be independent.[24] Therefore, each is an important domain to assess.

The level of comorbidity has been shown to affect functional recovery following surgical treatment for breast cancer. In a study of older women with breast cancer, women with > 2 comorbid conditions were less likely to become independent in completing instrumental activities of daily living and more likely to experience difficulty completing tasks requiring upper body strength.[25]

The impact of comorbidity on overall survival has been demonstrated. In a study by Satariano and colleagues, patients with breast cancer who had ≥ three of seven selected comorbid conditions had a 20-fold higher rate of mortality from a comorbid medical condition than from breast cancer. These findings were independent of a number of other factors including age, race, treatment, tumor stage, tumor histology, tumor size, social, or behavioral factors. Patients with three or more comorbid conditions had a four-fold increase in mortality in comparison to those with no comorbid medial conditions.[26] The impact of age on the relative risk of mortality from a concurrent, comorbid illness in comparison to a newly diagnosed illness is illustrated in Figure 64-1.[66]

The potential impact of a new disease as a competing cause of mortality decreases with increasing age secondary to the decrease in absolute projected life expectancy. For example, consider the impact of a disease with a projected 50% mortality over 5 years in a 65-year old person in comparison to an 85-year old person. This disease will decrease the 65-year old person's average life expectancy by approximately 10 years, whereas it will decrease an 85-year old person's average life expectancy by about 2 years, because the absolute projected life expectancy of an 85-year old person is less than that of a 65-year old person and therefore the potential impact of a new disease on affecting life expectancy is smaller.[66]

Table 64-8 Rank Order of Major Condition, >10% of Study Sample

Condition	Percent
Hypertension	42.9
Heart-related conditions	39.1
Arthritis	34.9
Gastrointestinal problems	31.0
Anemia	22.6
Eye problems	19.0
Urinary tract	18.0
Previous cancers	15.4
Gallbladder problems	14.9
Chronic obstructive pulmonary disease	14.5
Diabetes	12.8
Fracture	10.8
Gland disorders	10.6

From Yancik R,[1] with permission.

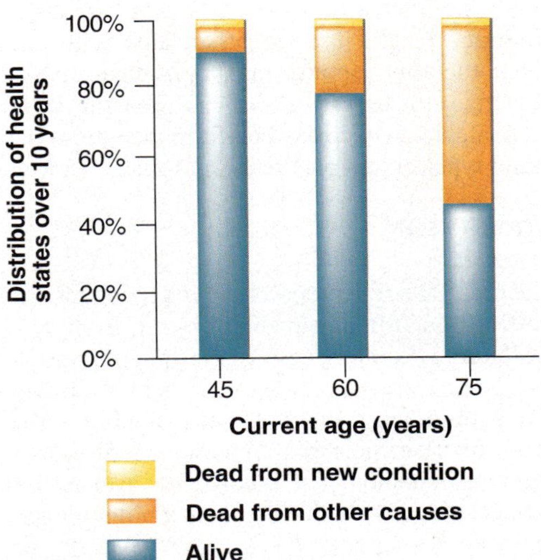

Figure 64-1 This example considers the distribution of health states over 10 years for women newly diagnosed with a disease for which the 10-year disease-related mortality is 10%.[66]

NUTRITION

Poor nutritional status is an independent predictor of functional dependency and survival. In a prospective cohort study of 214 older community-dwelling adults, a low body mass index, defined as a body mass index < 22 kg/m^2 was associated with dependency in activities of daily living [odds ratio 1.21; 95% confidence interval (CI) 1.01–1.45]. After adjusting for potential confounding factors including age, gender, mental status, comorbidity and functional dependency, body mass index < 22 kg/m^2 was associated with decreased one year survival [relative risk (RR) 0.85, 95% CI 0.74–0.97].[28]

Weight change over a three-year period was recorded in a study of 4,714 community-dwelling adults, aged 65 and older. Weight change, defined as a 5% or greater loss or gain in weight over a three-year period, occurred in 34.6% of women and 27.3% of men. A higher proportion of participants lost weight, than gained weight. Weight loss, and not weight gain, was associated with an increased risk of mortality (Hazard ratio = 1.67, 95% CI = 1.29–2.15). This study suggests that even a small amount of weight loss is a significant prognostic indicator of mortality.[29]

The prognostic effect of unintentional weight loss in patients with cancer was evaluated in a study of 3,047 patients enrolled in Eastern Cooperative Oncology Group chemotherapy trials.[24] Weight loss during the 6 months prior to chemotherapy was associated with poorer survival (statistically significant in 9 out of 12 tumor types). In addition, weight loss was associated with lower chemotherapy response rates (significant only in patients with breast cancer). Decreasing weight correlated with decreased performance status in all tumor types except pancreatic and gastric cancer.[30]

COGNITION

The presence of dementia is an independent prognostic indicator of survival.[31,32] In a study by Wolfson and colleagues, 10,263 people aged 65 and older were screened for dementia. Of these 821 people had a diagnosis of probable Alzheimer's disease, possible Alzheimer's disease, or vascular dementia. The median survival of these patients was 3.3 years (3.1 years if a diagnosis of probable Alzheimer's disease, 3.5 years if possible Alzheimer's disease, and 3.3 years if vascular dementia).[32] This study demonstrated that the median survival of a person with dementia was shorter than previously estimated.

A baseline assessment of cognition in an older patient with cancer is important for several reasons. First, if a person has a rapid change in memory or new cognitive deficits, metastatic disease to the brain should be excluded. Secondly, the degree of cognitive impairment will need to be considered when devising a treatment plan. For example, all oral medications and especially chemotherapy drugs should be used with caution in patients with cognitive impairment. Correct dosing for oral chemotherapy is as important as with intravenous chemotherapy, so that if the patient takes an incorrect dose, the side effects could be serious or even fatal. The role of the patient's family or caregiver is critical in maintaining safety. A patient with cognitive impairment will need assistance in remembering instructions regarding use of supportive medications such as anti-emetics. A caregiver will need to be aware of potential side effects of treatment that would necessitate medical attention.

PSYCHOLOGICAL STATE AND SOCIAL SUPPORT

Older patients with cancer often demonstrate better psychological functioning in comparison to younger patients. Following a diagnosis of breast cancer, older women demonstrate better mental health and well being in comparison to younger patients.[33] In women $<$ aged 65, a recent diagnosis of breast cancer produced a marked increase in anxiety and depression and decreased morale in comparison to people of the same age who had a diagnosis over 5 years prior. In comparison, for women $\geq$ 65 years of age, a more recent diagnosis did not affect their level of anxiety, depression, or morale in comparison to age counterparts with a diagnosis greater than 5 years ago.[34]

The presence of social support plays an important role in the psychological functioning of the older patient. Significant predictors of severe psychological distress in women of breast cancer of any age include being divorced or separated and having less social support.[36] Therefore, social support can serve as a buffer against the psychological impact of a stressful life event.

In addition, social isolation is an independent predictor of mortality. This was demonstrated in a study by Seeman and colleagues in which they examined the importance of four measures of social support: (1) marital status, (2) close contact with two or more close friends/relatives, (3) regular church attendance, and (4) membership in other types of groups. The presence of social ties was related to survival, independent of age, so that during the 5-year follow-up, the relative hazard for five-year mortality among men and women in three community-based cohorts ranged from 1.97 to 3.06 for participants with no social ties in comparison to those with all four social ties.[36] In another study of 282 patients aged 65 and older, living alone was independently predictive of risk of death.[21]

MEDICATION REVIEW: EVALUATION FOR POLYPHARMACY

A review of the patient's medication list is an important part of the geriatric assessment. In addition, one must consider whether newly prescribed medications may cause an adverse effect or drug interaction. Older patients are more vulnerable to adverse drug events than younger patients. Approximately one-fifth of hospital admissions in older patients are secondary to adverse drug events.[10] This is partly because older patients use three-fold more medications than younger patients. The average number of medications taken by an older patient is 4 drugs. Ninety percent of older patients take at least one drug.

Contributing to the risk of adverse drug events are the changes in pharmacokinetics and pharmacodynamics that occur with aging. These changes should be considered with the dosing of any medication, including chemotherapy. There are age-related changes in the gastrointestinal tract such as decreased acid secretion and fewer villi in mucosal surfaces. Despite these changes, there is no significant change in drug absorption with aging. There are significant changes in volume of distribution. These include, increased body fat (leading to slower metabolism of lipid soluble drugs), decrease in total body water (leading to an increase in the plasma level of water-soluble drugs), decrease in lean body mass, decrease in serum albumin, and decrease in hemoglobin.[11]

Hepatic metabolism changes with aging, secondary to decreased liver volume and decreased hepatic blood flow. Phase I hepatic reactions (oxidation, deamination, hydroxylation) decrease with aging. These include reactions mediated via cytochrome P-450, decreasing by approximately 30% in older patients. There is no significant change in phase II hepatic reactions (conjugation: acetylation, glucuronidation, sulfation) with aging.[10–12]

Renal mass decreases by 25 to 30% over the lifespan, leading to a decreased number of functional nephrons. Consequently there is a decrease in glomerular filtration, tubular secretion, and reabsorption with aging. Renal blood flow decreases by 1% per year after the age of 50 and glomerular filtration decreases by 1 mL/minute/year after the age of 40.[10–12] Therefore, drugs dependent on renal clearance have a longer half-life in older patients and drug dosing may need to be adjusted based on creatinine clearance. A study of older patients with breast cancer receiving CMF (cyclophosphamide, methotrexate, and 5-fluorouracil) demonstrated that age related trends in toxicity could be eliminated by dosing the drugs based on creatinine clearance.[37]

COMPREHENSIVE GERIATRIC ASSESSMENT

Geriatric assessment is a comprehensive approach to the evaluation of the older patient, with an evaluation of the domains described above: functional status, comorbidity, cognition, nutritional status, psychological state and social support, and medication review. Studies regarding the value of this assessment have been conflicting; however, a meta-analysis of the controlled trials by Stuck and colleagues suggests a benefit to geriatric assessment. This meta-analysis of 28 controlled trials comprising 4,959 participants and 4,912 controls, randomized to one of five comprehensive geriatric assessment programs demonstrated that a geriatric evaluation and management unit (inpatient unit for geriatric assessment and rehabilitation) reduced mortality by 35% at 6 months and a home assessment service (in-home geriatric assessment) reduced mortality by 14% at 36 months via early identification and treatment of problems.[38] A more recently published multi-site randomized, controlled trial of inpatient and outpatient geriatric evaluation and management demonstrated that geriatric evaluation and management-reduced functional decline and improved mental health but had no effect on survival.[39]

The role of geriatric assessment in care of the older cancer patient is an area under active research. Balducci and colleagues studied geriatric assessment in the evaluation of the older patient with cancer and found that this assessment helped to characterize patients of the same chronological age by identifying impairment in the following areas: dependency in functional status (18% ADL, 72% IADL), serious comorbidity (36% by Charlson scale, 94% by Cumulative Illness Rating Scale - Geriatrics), memory impairment (22%), poor nutrition (19%), and polypharmacy (41%).[40] Therefore, this assessment could be useful in understanding a patient's "biological age," in contrast to their "chronological age." Garman and colleagues performed a retrospective chart review of older patients with cancer admitted to an inpatient Geriatric Evaluation and Management Unit, in which a comprehensive geriatric assessment was used to identify goals of care. These goals were accomplished in over 75% of cases: 73% in symptom management, 79% in functional improvement, and 100% in disposition and caregiver support.[67]

The impact of geriatric assessment in predicting a patient's risk of toxicity to chemotherapy has not been determined; however, this informa-

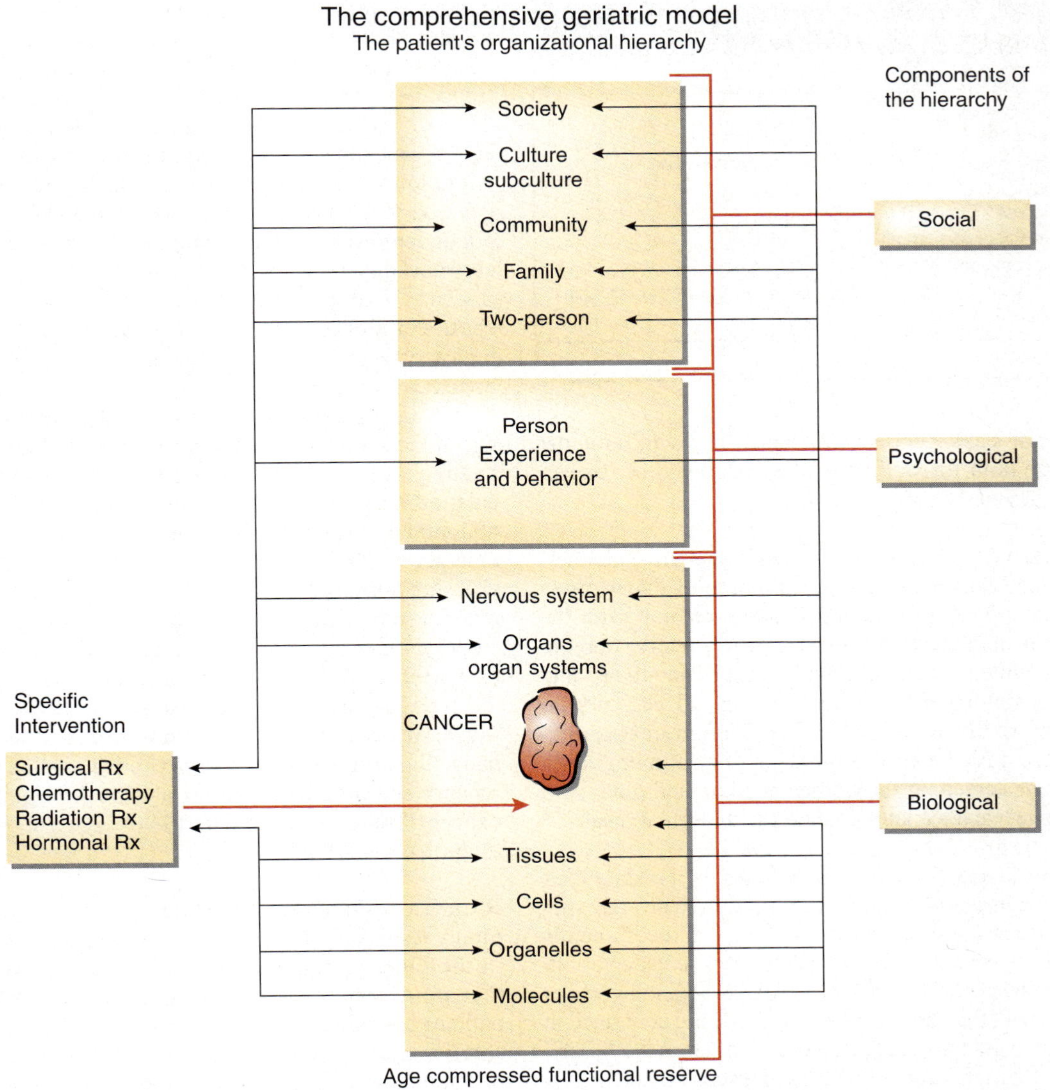

Figure 64-2 The Comprehensive Geriatric Model. From Cohen and DeMaria,[42] with permission.

tion would be potentially valuable to oncologists for several reasons. First, it would help the clinician get a sense of the "functional age" of the patient. Second, it would identify patients at high risk for functional decline or toxicity to treatment, for whom targeted intervention may be beneficial. Third, it would provide valuable information regarding older patients in clinical trials, allowing us to standardize patient characteristics across studies and to control for possible confounding factors contributing to mortality.

A traditional comprehensive geriatric assessment is a multi-disciplinary assessment that takes 2 hours to perform. Because of the time-intensive nature, it is often not feasible in a busy oncology practice. Therefore, other means of performing geriatric assessment are under study. The Cancer and Leukemia Group B is developing a short geriatric assessment tool. Pilot data demonstrated that this brief but comprehensive, mainly self-administered geriatric assessment questionnaire is feasible in the setting of an outpatient oncology clinic. The mean time to complete the assessment was 27 minutes; 78% completed the self-administered portion without assistance. There was no association of age ($p = .56$) or educational level ($p = .99$) with ability to complete the assessment without assistance. Eighty-three percent of patients stated that the assessment was easy to understand, and 100% stated that no items were upsetting. Ninety percent were satisfied with the length of the questionnaire.[68] This information will be collected as baseline information in subsequent clinical trials. Ingram and colleagues reported on the feasibility of a self-reported assessment tool, including an evaluation of the following 10 domains: demographics, comorbid conditions, activities of daily living, functional status, pain, financial well-being, social support, emotional state, spiritual well-being, and quality of life. Seventy-seven percent of patients who received the survey and kept their appointment returned the survey. Therefore, self-report may be a feasible way of collecting this information.[41]

A proposed framework depicting the factors to consider in decision-making for an older patient with cancer is described in the Comprehensive Geriatric Model, developed by Cohen and DeMaria (Figure 64-2).[42] This model summarizes the key aspects critical to the care of the older patient including social, psychological, and biological factors which may impact on the host, the disease, and the outcomes from treatment. In this model, chronological age plays a role by defining the decreased functional reserve that can occur with aging, but subsequent factors including biological, social, and psychological factors unique to the individual patient are factored into decision-making. This is a dynamic process in which alterations in one domain can subsequently impact upon the other domains within the model.

KNOWLEDGE ABOUT OLDER CANCER PATIENTS: UNDER-REPRESENTATION ON CLINICAL TRIAL

Despite the aging population and the association of cancer with aging, data regarding the benefits and risks of treatment of the older cancer patient are limited. This is secondary to limited involvement of older patients on clinical trials. The Southwest Oncology Group analyzed 164 clinical trials from 1993 to 1996, comprised of 16,396 patients. They found that only 25% of the patients on clinical trial were aged 65 and older. This under-representation was across 15 cancer types, except lymphoma. Older patients with breast cancer were the least represented, with only 9% of patients over the age of 65.[43]

Similar data regarding the under-representation of the older patient are seen in Canadian trials. Enrollment on clinical trials by age was analyzed from 1993 to 1996. Fifty-eight percent of the Canadian population with cancer is ≥ age of 65, whereas only 22% of patients enrolled on trial were ≥ age of 65.[44]

The representation on clinical trials worsens with increasing age. The National Cancer Institute analyzed enrollment of patients ≥ age of 65 and patients ≥ age of 75. Data from 23,000 patients across 500 therapeutic trials were analyzed. They found an under-representation of patients over the age of 65 on clinical trial; however, this was even more pronounced for patients ≥ age of 75. Only 11% of men on clinical trial were over the age of 75 and only 5% of women were over the age of 75. There was a striking under-representation of older patients with breast cancer, with only 2.7% being over the age of 75. This study demonstrated that with increasing age, there is even less representation on clinical trial.[45]

The National Institute of Aging responded to the limited involvement of older patients in cancer clinical trials by supporting a series of program announcements and initiatives focusing on the older patient (Table 64-9). Through this support, the body of knowledge regarding care of the older cancer patient will grow.

UNDERSTANDING BARRIERS TO CLINICAL TRIAL ENROLLMENT

The Cancer and Leukemia Group B (CALGB) Committee on Cancer in the Elderly developed a study to understand barriers to participation of older patients on cancer treatment trials. Women

Table 64-9 National Institutes of Aging Program Announcements and Initiatives

Focus	Number	Title
Breast	PA-96-034	Aging, women, and breast cancer
Prostate	PA-97-019	Aging, race, and ethnicity
	PA-99-081	Biology, development, and progression of malignant prostate disease
Pharmacology	PA-98-089	Cancer pharmacology
Multiple tumors	PA-99-030	Aging and old age as risk factors for multiple tumors
	PA-02-169	Integrating aging and cancer research
Cooperative groups	October, 1998	Studies of older cancer patients in the NCI Clinical Trials Cooperative Group
Cancer centers	CA-03-504	Planning and development (p20) grant integrating aging and cancer research in NCI-designated cancer centers

From Muss, Cohen, and Lichtman,[56] with permission.

with breast cancer, < age of 65 and ≥ age of 65, were paired by physician and stage. The trial sought to determine the frequency with which each group was offered enrollment on clinical trial and likelihood of accepting treatment on trial. The results demonstrated that older women were less likely to be offered enrollment onto clinical trial than younger women (51% < age 65 vs 35% ≥ age 65; $p = .06$): however, if offered, older women would be as likely to accept enrollment on trial as younger women (56% < age 65 vs 50% ≥ age 65; $p = .67$). The study also sought to determine the reason why patients refused entry onto clinical trial and the reasons why physicians did not offer clinical trials to patients. The reasons why physicians did not offer a clinical trial to older patients in comparison to younger patients differed because of two reasons: (1) physicians were concerned about the toxicity of treatment in older patients; and (2) physicians were concerned regarding the impact of comorbid diseases.[46] The most common physician recommendations of ways to improve accrual of older patients to clinical trials, include providing clinic personnel to explain trials to older patients and their families, providing educational materials about clinical trials for patients and families, and providing transportation to make it easier for older patients to participate in clinical trials.[60]

CANCER SCREENING IN THE ELDERLY

National organizations publish screening recommendations for the public as a whole; however, few provide guidelines for cancer screening in the elderly. The American Geriatrics Society (AGS) recommends that cancer screening be individualized, rather than setting guidelines strictly by age, taking into account the patient's preferences, life expectancy, and the risks and benefits of the screening test.[61] General guidelines to help steer these discussions with patients at average risk for developing these cancers are summarized below.

Breast Cancer Breast cancer screening traditionally consists of mammography, clinical breast exam, and breast self-exam. The American Cancer Society (ACS) recommends continuing breast cancer screening as long as a woman is in good health and is a candidate for treatment.[62] The AGS recommends annual mammography or at least biennial mammography until the age of 75, and biennially or at least every 3 years thereafter, with no upper age limit for women with an estimated life expectancy of 4 or more years.[63]

Cervical Cancer The ACS guidelines for cervical cancer screening recommend that women aged 70 and older may cease screening with the Papanicolaou (Pap) smear if there are three or more documented, consecutive, normal Pap smears and no abnormal smears within the 10 year period before the age of 70.[62] The US Preventative Service Task Force recommends discontinuing cytologic screening for women aged 65 and older who have had adequate screening with normal results.[62]

Prostate Cancer Screening for prostate cancer consists of a digital rectal exam and prostate specific antigen (PSA) test. The ACS recommends offering annual screening for prostate cancer, with digital rectal exam and PSA test, beginning at the age of 50 in patients at average risk and continued in men who have a life expectancy of at least 10 years. The benefits and limitations of testing should be discussed with the patient so that an informed decision regarding screening is made.[62] The US Preventative Service Task Force clinical guidelines state that men with a life expectancy of less than 10 years are unlikely to benefit from prostate cancer screening.[64]

Colon Cancer The ACS recommends that adults at average risk begin screening for colorectal cancer at 50 years of age. There are many options for colon cancer screening including annual fecal occult blood testing, flexible sigmoidoscopy every 5 years, annual fecal occult blood testing plus flexible sigmoidoscopy every 5 years, colonoscopy every 10 years, or double-contrast barium enema every 5 years.[62] The US Preventative Services Task Force acknowledges the appropriate age at which to discontinue colorectal cancer screening is unknown, because screening studies have generally been restricted to patients younger than the age of 80. They recommend discontinuing screening in patients whose age or comorbid conditions limit life expectancy.[65]

TREATMENT TOLERANCE OF THE OLDER PATIENT

Surgery Surgery is the primary treatment for the majority of solid tumors. Failure to obtain definitive surgical treatment is associated with an increased mortality from disease regardless of age. For example, in a study performed by the Cancer Research UK Breast Cancer Trials Group, 455 women older than 70 years of age, with operable breast cancer, were randomized to treatment with tamoxifen alone versus tamoxifen plus surgery. At 12.7 years of follow-up, women who did not undergo surgery had an increase in breast cancer mortality (Hazard ratio 1.68; 95% CI 1.15–2.47).[47] Therefore if possible, older women should undergo primary surgical removal of breast cancer in order to decrease their risk of breast cancer mortality.

Several studies have demonstrated that advanced age alone should not be a reason to deny surgical treatment for colorectal cancer.[48–51] Risk of surgical morbidity and mortality is increased with intra-abdominal surgery or those performed under an emergency situation; however, even in these high-risk situations, older patients benefit from surgical management. In a study of emergency colorectal surgery, older and younger patients had a similar primary resection rate (95% > age 70, 89% ≤ age 70; $p = .70$) and primary anastomosis rate (84% > age 70, 78% ≥ age 70; $p = .64$). Older patients had a higher incidence of postoperative cardiopulmonary complications, but no statistically significant difference in mortality (9% > age 70, 5% ≥ age 70; $p = .48$).[48]

Radiation Therapy Radiation therapy is commonly used for both curative and palliative intent in the older patient. Studies have demonstrated that treatment tolerance in younger and older patients is similar.[52,53] In a study of 1,208 patients receiving thoracic irradiation, age had no impact on the acute or late radiation toxicities. Patients were divided into 6 age groups, ranging from < 50 to > 70. There was no significant difference in acute toxicities such as nausea, dyspnea, esophagitis, or weakness and there was no significant difference in survival between age groups ($p = .82$). Older patients were more likely to experience weight loss than younger patients ($p = .002$).[53] Therefore, close attention should be paid to nutritional status in older patients receiving radiation.

Treatment tolerance to radiation and efficacy of radiation therapy in the "oldest old" patient has also been demonstrated. In a retrospective review of 191 patients ≥ age of 80, 94% were able to complete treatment without complications. A response to treatment was seen in 77% of patients treated for curative intent and 81% of patients treated for palliative intent. Six percent of patients required treatment interruption, secondary to weight loss from diarrhea, dysphagia, or progressive disease. This occurred more commonly in patients who were treated with large treatment fields. Of patients receiving treatment for aero-digestive tract cancer, 20% of patients had grade 3 mucositis and 2% of patients had grade 4 mucositis, reinforcing the need for careful attention to nutritional status and weight loss in older patients.[54]

Other studies have sought to determine whether there is a subgroup of older patients with low risk disease in which radiation therapy can be eliminated. A study performed by the Cancer and Leukemia Group B randomized 636 women aged 70 and older with clinical stage I, estrogen-receptor-positive breast cancer who underwent a lumpectomy to: treatment with radiation to the affected breast and tamoxifen, or tamoxifen alone. The women treated with tamoxifen alone had more locoregional recurrences at 5 years of follow-up: 4% in the tamoxifen alone arm verses 1% in the tamoxifen and radiation arm ($p < .001$). All locoregional recurrences were managed with additional surgery and there was no difference in breast-cancer-specific mortality or 5-year rates of overall survival: 86% in the tamoxifen-alone arm verses 87% in the tamoxifen and radiation arm ($p = .94$). The results suggest that radiation therapy is beneficial in decreasing the risk of locoregional recurrence in older women who have low-risk tumors; however, no impact on survival has been demonstrated to date. This study has been reported with 5 years of follow-up. Therefore, if a patient has an estimated life expectancy of greater than 5 years, radiation therapy should be strongly considered.[55]

Chemotherapy Several studies have sought to determine whether treatment on chemotherapy trials is more toxic for older patients.[56] A study by the Piedmont Oncology Association was a case control study of women with metastatic breast cancer enrolled on clinical trials. The women were divided into three groups, by age: <50, 50 to 69, and >70. The study demonstrated that older women receiving treatment on clinical trial had no significant difference in the incidence of toxic effects, dose delivery, or dose delays in comparison to younger women. In addition, there was no difference in response, time to disease progression, or survival. Therefore, older women who received treatment on clinical trial not only tolerated the treatment as well, but also equally benefited from this treatment.[57] An analysis of phase II trials at Illinois Cancer Center found similar results. Older and younger patients had no difference in toxic effects, need for dose reduction, or need for treatment interruption or delay. In addition, there was no difference in response to treatment.[58]

These studies suggest that selected older patients tolerate treatment similarly to younger patients. One caveat is that it is not clear is whether the older patients who were represented on these clinical trials were healthier than the general older population. Since so few older patients are offered entry on clinical trial, the older patients represented on clinical trials may have a younger "functional age." Therefore, incorporating geriatric assessment into clinical trials would be a valuable way of standardizing possible confounding factors across patients of the same chronological age, helping to determine the "functional age" of the patients represented. Clinical trials focusing on the older patient are needed in order to optimize care of this patient population. Developing a registry of older patients with selected diseases (breast cancer, colon cancer, intermediate grade lymphoma, etc) and treated with chemotherapy with curative intent would provide a database with which to evaluate patterns of care and outcomes.

CONCLUSIONS

Cancer is a disease that disproportionately affects older patients. Data regarding the care of these patients are limited secondary to the under-representation of older patients on clinical trials. In moving forward, an effort should be made to include older patients on clinical trial, in order to increase our understanding about the optimal way to care for this growing population. Incorporation of geriatric assessment in the care of the older patient will provide information regarding prognostic factors that distinguish two individuals of the same chronological age, thereby helping us understand "functional age." Brief, comprehensive geriatric assessment screening tools for older oncology patients are currently under development.

REFERENCES

1. Yancik, R. Cancer burden in the aged. Cancer 1997;80:1273–83.
2. Yancik R, Ries, LA. Aging and Cancer in America: Demographics and Epidemiologic Perspectives. Hematology/Oncology Clinics of North America 2000;14:17–23.
3. US Census Bureau, Census 2000 Summary File 1; 1990 Census of Population, General Population Characteristics, United States (1990 CP-1-1). Available at: http://www.census.gov/prod/2001pubs/c2kbr01-10.pdf (accessed 28 June 2005).
4. Day JC, 1996, Population Projections of the United States by Age, Sex, Race, and Hispanic Origin: 1995 to 2050, U.S. Bureau of the Census, Current Population Reports, P25-1130, U.S. Government Printing Office, Washington, DC.
5. Anderson RN, United States Life Table, 1997. National Vital Statistics Report from the Center for Disease Control and Prevention. 1999;47. Available at: http://www.cdc.gov/nchs/ (accessed 28 June 2005).
6. Miller RA. The Biology of Aging and Longevity. In: Principles of Geriatric Medicine and Gerontology. Hazzard WR, Blass JP, Ettinger WH, Halter JB, Ouslander JG, editors. New York: McGraw-Hill, 1999. p. 3–19.
7. Cohen HJ. Oncology and Aging: General Principles of Cancer in the Elderly. In: Principles of Geriatric Medicine and Gerontology. Hazzard WR, Blass JP, Ettinger WH, Halter JB, Ouslander JG editors. New York: McGraw-Hill,1999. p. 117–30.
8. Stanta G, Campagner L, Cavallieri F, Giarelli L. Cancer of the oldest old. What we have learned from autopsy studies. Clin Geriatr Med 1997;13:55–68.
9. Cohen, HJ. Cancer Care in the Older Population: Physiology of Aging. American Society of Clinical Oncology Curriculum 2002.
10. Vestal RE. Aging and pharmacology. Cancer 1997;80:1302–10.
11. Avorn J, Gurwitz, JH. Principles of Pharmacology. In: Geriatric Medicine, 3rd edition. Cassel C, Cohen HJ, Larson EB, Meier DE, Resnick NM, Rubenstein L, editors. New York: Springer-Verlag; 1997. p. 55–70.
12. Lichtman SM, Villani G. Chemotherapy in the elderly: pharmacologic considerations. Cancer Control 2000;7:548–56.
13. Baraldi-Junkins CA, Beck AC, Rothstein G. Hematopoiesis and Cytokines: Relevance to Cancer and Aging. Hematology/Oncology Clinics of North America 2000;14:45–61.
14. Fried LP, Walston J. Frailty and Failure to Thrive. In: Principles of Geriatric Medicine and Gerontology. Hazzard WR, Blass JP, Ettinger WH, Halter JB, Ouslander JG, editors. New York: McGraw-Hill, 1999.p. 1387–1402.
15. Cohen HJ. In search of the underlying mechanisms of frailty. J Gerontol A Biol Sci Med Sci 2000;55:706–8m.
16. Balducci L, Stanta G. Cancer in the frail patient. A coming epidemic. Hematol Oncol Clin North Am 2000;14:235–50.
17. Repetto L, Comandini D. Cancer in the elderly: assessing patients for fitness. Crit Rev Oncol Hematol 2000;35:155–60.
18. Naglie G. Frailty. In: Oxford Textbook of Geriatric Medicine. Evans, JG, Williams, TF, Beattie, BL, Michel JP, Wilcok GK, editors. New York: Oxford University Press, Inc., 2000. p. 1181–92.
19. Narain P, Rubenstein LZ, Wieland GD, et al. Predictors of immediate and 6 month outcomes in hospitalized elderly patients. The importance of functional status. J Am Geriatr Society 1988; 36:775–83.
20. Balducci L, Extermann M. Management of cancer in the older person: A practical approach. Oncologist 2000;5:224–37.
21. Reuben DB, Rubenstein LV, Hirsch SH, Hays RD. Value of functional status as a predictor of mortality: results of a prospective study. Am J Med 1992;93:663–9.
22. Barberger-Gateau P, Fabrigoule C, Helmer C, et al.. Functional impairment in instrumental activities of daily living: an early clinical sign of dementia? J Am Geriatr Soc 1999;47:456–62.
23. Stafford RS, Cyr PL. The impact of cancer on the physical function of the elderly and their utilization of health care. Cancer 1997;80:1973–80.
24. Extermann M, Overcash J, Lyman GH, et al. Comorbidity and functional status are independent in older cancer patients. JCO 1998;16:1582–7.
25. Satariano WA. Comorbidity and functional status in Older Women with Breast Cancer: Implications for Screening, Treatment, and Prognosis. The Journals of Gerontology 1992;47:24–31.
26. Satariano WA, Ragland DR. The effect of comorbidity on 3-year survival of women with primary breast cancer. Annals of Internal Medicine 1994;120:104–10.
27. Welch HG, Albertsen PC, Nease RF, et al. Estimating treatment benefits for the elderly: the effect of competing risks. Ann Intern Med 1996;124:577–84.
28. Landi F, Giuseppe G, Gambassi G, et al. Body Mass Index and Mortality among Older People Living in the Community. Journal of the American Geriatric Society 1999;47:1072–6.
29. Newman AB, Yanez D, Harris T, et al. Weight change in old age and its association with mortality. Journal of the American Geriatrics Society 2001;49:1309–18.
30. Dewys WD, Begg C, Lavin PT, et al. Prognostic effect of weight loss prior to chemotherapy in cancer patients. The American Journal of Medicine 1980;68:491–7.
31. Eagles JM, Beattie JAG, Restall DB, et al. Relationship between cognitive impairment and early death in the elderly. Br Med Journal 1990;300:239–40.
32. Wolfson C, Wolfson DB, Asgharian M, et al. A reevaluation of the duration of survival after the onset of dementia. N Engl J Med 2001;344:1111–16.
33. Vinokur AD, Threatt BA, Vinokur-Kaplan D, Satariano WA. The process of recovery from breast cancer for younger and older patients. Changes during the first year. Cancer 1990;65:1242–54.
34. Vinokur AD, Threatt BA, Caplan RD, Zimmerman BL. Physical and psychosocial functioning and adjustment to breast cancer. Long-term follow-up of a screening population. Cancer 1989;63:394–405.
35. Kornblith AB, Herndon JE, Zuckerman E, et al. Social support as a buffer to the psychological impact of stressful life events in women with breast cancer. Cancer 2001;91:443–54.
36. Seeman TE, Berkman LF, Kohout F, et al. Intercommunity Variations in the Association between Social Ties and Mortality in the Elderly. A Comparative Analysis of Three Communities. Ann Epidemiol 1993;3:325–35.
37. Gelman RS, Taylor SG. Cyclophosphamide, methotrexate, and 5-fluorouracil chemotherapy in women more than 65 years old with advanced breast cancer: the elimination of age trends in toxicity by using doses based on creatinine clearance. J Clin Oncol 1984;2:1404–13.
38. Stuck AE, Siu AL, Wieland GD, et al. Comprehensive geriatric assessment: a meta-analysis of controlled trials. Lancet 1993;342:1032–6.
39. Cohen HJ, Feussner JR, Weinberger M, et al. A controlled trial of inpatient and outpatient geriatric evaluation and management. N Engl J Med 2002;346:905–12.
40. Balducci, L. The geriatric cancer patient: equal benefit from equal treatment. Cancer Control. 2001;8(2 Suppl):1–25.
41. Ingram SS, Seo PH, Martell RE, et al. Comprehensive Assessment of the Elderly Cancer Patient: The Feasibility of Self-Report Methodology. JCO 2002;20:770–5.
42. Cohen HJ, DeMaria L. Comprehensive cancer care: special problems of the elderly. In: Physician's Guide to Cancer

Care Complications. Edited by Laszlo J. New York: Marcel Dekker, 1986: pp 237-75.

43. Hutchins LF, Unger JM, Crowley JJ, et al. Underrepresentation of patients 65 years of age or older in cancer- treatment trials. N Engl J Med 1999;341:2061–7.
44. Yee K, Pater JL, Pho L, et al. Enrollment of older patients in cancer treatment trials in Canada: Why is age a barrier? J Clin Oncol 2003:21:1618–23.
45. Trimble EL, Carter CL, Cain D, et al. Representation of older patients in cancer treatment trials. Cancer 1994;74:2208–14.
46. Kemeny MM, Peterson BL, Kornblith AB, et al. Barriers to Clinical Trial Participation by Older Women with Breast Cancer. J Clin Oncol 2003;21:2268–75.
47. Fennessy M, Bates T, MacRae K, et al. Late follow-up of a randomized trial of surgery plus tamoxifen versus tamoxifen alone in women aged over 70 with operable breast cancer. British Journal of Surgery 2004; 91(6): 699-704.
48. Kemeny MM, Busch-Devereaux E, Merriam LT, O'Hea BJ. Cancer Surgery in the Elderly. Hematology/Oncology Clinics of North America 2000;14:169–92.
49. Poon RT, Law WL, Chu KW, Wong J. Emergency resection and primary anastomosis for left-sided obstructing colorectal carcinoma in the elderly. Br J Surg 1998;85:1539–42 .
50. Makela JT, Kiviniemi H, Laitinen S. Survival after operations for colorectal cancer in patients aged 75 years or over. Eur J Surg 2000;166:473–9.
51. Hessman O, Bergkvist L, Strom S. Colorectal cancer in patients over 75 years of age--determinants of outcome. Eur J Surg Oncol 1997;23:13–9.
52. Zachariah B, Balducci L. Radiation therapy of the older patient. Hematol Oncol Clin North Am 2000;14:131–67.
53. Pignon T, Gregor A, Schaake Koning C, et al. Age has no impact on acute and late toxicity of curative thoracic radiotherapy. Radiother Oncol 1998;46:239–48.
54. Zachariah B, Balducci L, Venkattaramanabalaji GV, et al. Radiotherapy for cancer patients aged 80 and older: a study of effectiveness and side effects. Int J Radiat Oncol Biol Phys 1997;39:1125–9.
55. Hughes KS, Schnaper LA, Berry D, et al. Lumpectomy Plus Tamoxifen with or Without Irradiation in Women 70 Years of Age or Older with Early Breast Cancer. New Engl J Med 2004;351:971–7.
56. Muss HB, Cohen HJ, Lichtman SM. Clinical research in the older cancer patient. Hematology/Oncology Clinics of North America 2000;14:283–91.
57. Giovanazzi-Bannon S, Rademaker A, Lai G, Benson AB. Treatment Tolerance of Elderly Patients Entered onto Phase II Clinical Trials: An Illinois Cancer Center Study. JCO 1994;12:2447–52.
58. Christman K, Muss HB, Case LD, Stanley V. Chemotherapy of metastatic breast cancer in the elderly. The Piedmont Oncology Association Experience. JAMA 1992;268:57–62.
59. Extermann M, Balducci L, Lyman GH. What threshold for adjuvant therapy in older breast cancer patients? J Clin Oncol 2000;18:1709–17.
60. Kornblith AB, Kemeny M, Peterson BL, et al. Survey of Oncologists' Perceptions of Barriers to Accrual of Older Patients with Breast Carcinoma to Clinical Trials. Cancer 2002;95:989–96.
61. AGS Ethics Committee. AGS Position Paper: Health Screening Decisions for Older Adults. Available at: ahttp://www.americangeriatrics.org/products/poitionpapers/stopscreeningPF.shtml (accessed December 24, 2004).
62. Smith, RA, Cokkinides V, Eyre, HJ. American Cancer Society Guidelines for the Early Detection of Cancer, 2004. CA Cancer J Clin 2004;54:41–52.
63. AGS Clinical Practice Committee. American Geriatrics Society (AGS) Position Statement: Breast Cancer Screening in Older Women. Available at: www.americangeriatrics.org/staging/products/poitionpapers/brstcncrPF.shtml (accessed December 24, 2004).
64. Harris R, Lohr K. Screening for Prostate Cancer: An Update of the Evidence for the US Preventative Services Task Force. Ann Intern Med. 2002; 137:917–29.
65. US Preventative Services Task Force. Screening for colorectal cancer: recommendations and rationale. Ann Inter Med. 2002;137:129–31.
66. Welch HG, Albertsen PC, Nease RF, et al. Estimating Treatment Benefits for the Elderly. Ann Intern Med. 1996;124:577–84.
67. Garman KS, McConnell ES, Cohen HJ. Inpatient care for elderly cancer patients: the role for Geriatric Evaluation and Management Units in fulfilling goals of care. Crit Rev Oncol Hematol 2004;51:241–7.
68. Hurria A, Gupta S, Zauderer M, et al. Developing a cancer-specific geriatric assessment: a feasibility study. Cancer 2005;104(9):1998–2005 [Epub ahead of print].

Integrative Oncology: Complementary Therapies in Cancer Care

Barrie R. Cassileth, PhD, MS
Gary Deng, MD, PhD
K. Simon Yeung, RPh, MBA, LAc

EVOLUTION OF COMPLEMENTARY AND ALTERNATIVE MEDICINE

The long history of nonmainstream therapies in cancer medicine helps place today's activities in perspective and illustrates differences and some surprising similarities over the years.[1] Major ideologies that ran contrary to contemporaneous mainstream medical science developed along with modern medicine itself. Thompsonianism, popular in the early nineteenth century, espoused the belief that all disease results from a single cause (cold) and can be cured with a single remedy (heat) and decried the "tyranny" of doctors.[1,2] Homeopathy, which remains of substantial public interest today, 150 years after its formal development, still holds to the "law of Similia" (like cures like) but rarely refers back to its companion founding belief that disease results from "psora," or suppressed itch.[1,3]

In the late nineteenth century, naturopathy achieved a level of popularity that is equalled today. It held that disease results from violation of the "natural" laws of living and that worthwhile remedies included natural activities, such as diets and colonic irrigation, rather than drugs, which were denounced as harmful.[1,4] The nineteenth century was known then as the "golden age" of quackery.[5]

Quasimedicinals dominated questionable or alternative cancer medicine in the early twentieth century. A wide variety of pills, potions, and ointments were touted as cancer cures at that time. Promoted in newspaper advertisements and elsewhere, these products included the likes of Chamlee's Cancer-Specific Purifies-the-Blood Cure, Radol, Cancerol, BF Bye cancer cure, and many others.[6] In succeeding decades, Koch's glyoxylide, the Hoxsey cancer treatment, Krebiozen, and then laetrile led the list of questionable methods.[7]

Striking similarities between today's popular questionable remedies and some that previously dominated include an emphasis on natural, self-care alternatives to what critics then, as now, termed an impersonal medical system.[2] Today, however, there is a substantive difference in the reaction of mainstream medicine. Increasing amounts of scientific research, as well as political activity and public pressure, have created a new environment: mainstream openness and interest. Although outrageous claims for "alternative therapies" remain, many complementary cancer therapies are now studied in the most respectable institutions.

This chapter reviews the current status of unconventional medicine and specific alternative and complementary practices, as well as their use, value, and toxicities; delineates mainstream acceptance, concerns, and regulatory issues; and discusses the implications of the deepening trend in health care represented by this growth industry. Resources for additional information are also provided.

TERMINOLOGY AND DEFINITIONS

The vast collection of disparate treatments and questionable cancer therapies includes a broad spectrum of treatments, from unproven cancer cures to soothing adjunctive regimens (Table 65-1). Complicating the situation, this array of dissimilar therapies, some harmful, many helpful, is known by the same terms: *complementary medicine*, *alternative medicine*, and *complementary and alternative medicine* (CAM).

Terminology applied to questionable cancer therapies has changed dramatically over the decades. Reflecting varying degrees of disapproval over time, these have included "unorthodox," "unconventional," "questionable," "unproven," and even "quackery," the American Cancer Society's 1914 reproach. Recently, however, the term *integrative oncology* has been applied to research-based complementary therapies in cancer care.

All but 2% of people who use unconventional remedies did so to complement, rather than replace, mainstream care according to a large survey.[8] In cancer medicine, alternative therapies typically are promoted as independent treatments—literal alternatives—for use instead of surgery, chemotherapy, and radiation. They are often invasive and biologically active, unproven or disproved, expensive, and potentially harmful. They may harm directly through biologic activity or indirectly when patients postpone receipt of mainstream care. Examples include the metabolic therapies available in Tijuana, Mexico, high-dose vitamins, and other products sold over the counter or delivered intravenously in alternative clinics, electromagnetic cures, and many other products and regimens.[9]

Although research evidence is scanty,[10] it appears that a small proportion, probably less than 10% of tissue biopsy–diagnosed cancer patients, seek alternative rather than mainstream care initially. Specific complementary and alternative therapies are discussed below.

IMPACT ON THE HEALTH CARE SYSTEM

The acceptance of unconventional therapies, along with the advent of managed care, advances in biotechnology, and other significant medical and societal events, marked health care in the 1990s and was among the significant changes that occurred during that time. The popularity of CAM has affected every component of the health care system and all specialties of medicine, including oncology. It has left its mark on the thinking and practice of physicians and other health professionals and contributed to patients' broadened involvement and influence in their own care.

No longer a collection of covert practices, unconventional cancer medicine today is highly visible, and information about it is widely available to the general public. It is a multibillion-dollar business in the United States and of equivalent impact and importance throughout the developed world.

CAM USE AND USERS

Prevalence and Preferred CAM Therapies Internationally, including in North America, the use of CAM for cancer is widespread. A systematic review of relevant published data located 26 surveys of cancer patients from 13 countries, including 5 from the United States.[11] The average prevalence across all studies was 31%. Therapies most commonly used included dietary treatments, herbs, homeopathy, hypnotherapy, imagery or visualization, meditation, megavitamins, relaxation, and spiritual healing. New investigations substantiate these results.[12–14] All but one of the US surveys obtained information about specific therapies employed. Patients used Laetrile, metabolic therapies, diets, spiritual healing, megavitamins, imagery, and "immune

Table 65-1 For Patients: Complementary Therapies to Smooth the Way during Cancer Treatment and Recovery

Anxiety and Stress

Acupressure: Use the fingers of one hand to press inside the wrist of the other hand. Press for a minute or two approximately 1 inch above the hand crease. Pressing this acupoint relieves nausea as well as anxiety and stress.

Aroma therapy: Put a few drops of "essential oil" of rosemary, lavender, or chamomile (available in health food stores and pharmacies) in the bath or light a scented candle while relaxing. The fragrance is luxurious and calming.

Meditation and other relaxation techniques: These are opportunities for minivacations in the mind. Close your eyes and see yourself in a pleasant, peaceful place. Breathe deeply and slowly. Or lie down, eyes closed. Start at the tip of your toes and gradually move up your body as you consciously relax each body part. Your body and mind will relax accordingly.

Music therapy: Music has important physiologic and emotional benefits. It calms, distracts, and soothes at a very fundamental level of being.

Therapeutic massage: Visit a licensed, certified massage therapist experienced with people undergoing cancer therapy or arrange for that person to visit you. Or have a friend or family member gently massage your neck and shoulders, hands, and feet. Weekly therapeutic massages will keep you feeling good.

Valerian: Make a tea from 1 to 2 teaspoons of the dried root from this herb. You may prefer capsules because the tea does not have a pleasant odor (health food stores and pharmacies have both). It is nonaddictive, effectively reduces anxiety, and brings about sleep.

Yoga: Take a class, rent a videotape, borrow a book, and practice postures along with deep breathing techniques. Anyone can do it—even while bedridden. It is said to bring mind, body, and spirit together in a peaceful union. However it works, yoga relaxes.

Backache or Muscle Ache

Capsicum cream: Hot red peppers contain a powerful pain-relieving chemical called capsaicin. It is the active ingredient in many rub-on pharmaceutic pain relievers. Blend or mash a red pepper. Add some of the mashed red pepper to white body lotion or cold cream until the lotion turns pink. Rub it on the sore spots.

Hydrotherapy: A warm bath or Jacuzzi should help.

Massage: Try a professional massage by a licensed, certified massage therapist or a careful muscle massage by a friend or relative. Patients with lymphatic cancers should avoid touch massage.

Willow tea: The bark of the willow tree contains salicin, an active ingredient similar to aspirin. (Avoid this herb if aspirin causes upset stomach, if you take an anticoagulant such as warfarin, or if your doctor told you to use an aspirin substitute.)

Colds and Flu

Garlic: Eat raw or cooked garlic or try deodorized garlic capsules.

Echinacea: This herb has been used to reduce the duration and symptoms of colds, but recent research failed to support its benefit for these indications.

Eucalyptus or camphor: Place it in a steam vaporizer; inhaling may help reduce symptoms of congestion.

Zinc lozenges: Studies show that they may reduce the duration of a cold or flu.

Constipation

Fluid extracts or capsules of senna work well. Plantago seed, also called psyllium seed, is an effective herbal bulk laxative. Take it with plenty of water.

Prune juice, alone or flavored with apple juice, lemon, and honey, is a delicious way to solve the problem.

Water (6 to 8 glasses a day) and fiber (fruit, bran cereal, prunes) consumed regularly should keep this problem away, and regular exercise is also helpful.

Depression

Light therapy consists of bright-light boxes placed at eye level on a desk or table. Light boxes are made specifically to reduce depression and are especially effective in northern parts of the world, where sunlight is rare, or during winter months in the northern hemisphere. Light boxes are used in mainstream medicine and recommended by psychiatrists to treat seasonal affective disorder.

Meditation and yoga are very helpful for depression and anxiety (see "Anxiety" above).

Tai chi is a gentle exercise program practiced daily by millions of older Chinese and popular in the United States as well. Follow the slow motions, which typically mimic animal movements, as displayed in books, videotapes, and classes. Research shows that tai chi not only lifts depressed mood, it also improves bodily balance, reduces falls, and increases physical strength.

Diarrhea

Peppermint tea and yogurt.

Headache

Acupressure: Press the acupoint between your eyebrows or in the hollows at the base of the skull on both sides of the spine.

Heartburn

Herb teas, especially ginger and peppermint. Salad items, including artichoke, lettuce, onion, garlic, and olives, as well as fennel and caraway seeds.

Nausea

Acupressure: Press inside of the wrist with the fingers of the other hand (see "Anxiety" above).

Peppermint tea.

Ginger tea, capsules, or candy. Shave fresh ginger and add it to boiled water to make tea or add sugar and gelatin to the boiled ginger water and let it cool. Cut into cubes and eat as candy. Ginger ale or cookies, if made with real ginger and not flavoring, work too.

Chronic Pain

Acupuncture: See your Yellow Pages for a licensed, accredited acupuncture doctor. Properly trained acupuncturists use disposable stainless steel needles and do a virtually painless job.

Biofeedback: This requires equipment and a trained biofeedback therapist. Check the telephone book. Many pain clinics and pain management experts in hospitals use biofeedback or can make referrals.

Useful herbs: External capsicum (see "Backache" above) and willow bark tea (avoid if you should not take aspirin or if on anticoagulants).

Hypnotherapy: Some people can get rid of chronic pain or reduce it substantially with hypnosis. Pain clinics, the telephone book, and your nurse or doctor are good referral sources for certified hypnotherapists.

Massage (see "Anxiety" above).

Sleep Problems

Relax in a warm bath scented with lavender oil.

Massage.

Meditation.

Make tea of fresh or dried lemon balm or valerian root.

system stimulants."[11] Across samples, the prevalence of CAM use in the United States ranges from 7 to 90%. A survey focusing on alternative cancer therapies included responses from 33 countries, including the United States, China, Australia, Zimbabwe, Brazil, Latvia, Malaysia, Thailand, and Japan. An extraordinary number and variety of different alternative treatments were reported; specific therapies varied geographically (eg, Di Bella therapy in Italy and other Mediterranean countries, Essiac in Canada). Many therapies are associated with a single unconventional practitioner in a single country. The treatments reported most often included dietary therapies, shark products, vitamin therapies, and botanicals.[15]

Prevalence rates from all CAM studies conducted in the United States and internationally vary from less than 10% to more than 90%. This broad range, with its apparent discrepancies, may be attributed primarily to variable understandings and definitions of CAM. Often surveys do not define CAM or, more typically, define it extremely broadly, resulting in the inclusion of lifestyle activities, such as weight loss efforts, exercise, and church attendance, and support activities, such as group counseling, which creates bloated figures for CAM use.

The profound influence of 1994 legislation allowing herbal medicines and other "food supplements" to be sold over the counter without US Food and Drug Administration (FDA) review is evident in the increased use of herbal remedies from 3% in 1991, to 17% in 1997, to more than 20% in 1999.[16] It is estimated that sales of dietary supplements have more than doubled since passage of the 1994 law.

Virtually all studies conducted to date of cancer patients and of the general public internationally show that those who seek CAM therapies tend to be better educated, of higher socioeconomic status, female, and younger than those who do not. They tend to be more health conscious and to use more mainstream medical services than people who do not use CAM.

CAM Use among Pediatric Cancer Patients The use of CAM methods among pediatric oncology patients represents a special and understudied issue. CAM therapies are used by 31 to 84% of children with cancer, including many children enrolled in clinical trials.[17] Of particular interest is the type of CAM received: prayer, exercise, and spiritual healing accounted for more than 96% of CAM used. A recent study of pediatric cancer patients in Washington state reported that 73% of a sample of 75 patients had used CAM. Although use of dietary supplements and botanical medicines was common, 60% of users had seen a practitioner since diagnosis, and this was predominantly for the treatment of cancer or cancer therapy–related symptoms.[18] In neither study was CAM used as a substitute for conventional medicine. However, excluded from this sample by definition are the pediatric patients removed from conventional hospitals and brought for alternative treatment to clinics in the United States, Mexico, or elsewhere. Patients who receive only alternative cancer therapies do not appear in CAM surveys because all but one of these surveys[10] were conducted in mainstream clinics or hospitals.

Public Access to Information In contrast to the situation 20 years ago, when even determining the whereabouts of CAM practitioners required underground investigation, today CAM is very much an open and public issue, widely discussed and readily found on the Internet. Magazines provide the general public with details about new CAM therapies. The Yellow Pages of telephone books in most cities and towns typically list various types of practitioners. Information available to the public varies widely in accuracy. Many Web sites and publications that appear to be objective actually are sponsored by commercial enterprises that promote and sell the products they report. (Reputable Web sites are listed at the end of this chapter.)

Misinformation about health issues is widespread. In 1999, the US Federal Trade Commission (FTC) announced that it had identified hundreds of Web sites promoting and selling phony cures for cancer and other serious ailments.[19] At the same time, the FTC established "Operation Cureall," an effort to stop bogus Internet health claims.[20] The US Department of Health and Human Services released a report in 1999 on communication and health expressing concern about the lack of assistance to enable consumers to properly evaluate the credibility of Internet health information.

Today, the key words "alternative" and "cancer" elicit more than 8 million hits on Google (January 2005). It is difficult, if not impossible, for most patients to distinguish between reputable sources of information and those backed by vested interests.

National Institutes of Health Activity In addition to its acceptance by public sources of information, CAM has entered mainstream medicine in an unprecedented fashion. The Office of Alternative Medicine (OAM) was established at the National Institutes of Health (NIH) by Congressional mandate in 1992, its stated purpose to investigate unconventional medical practices.[21] In 1998, Congress elevated the OAM to the National Center for Complementary and Alternative Medicine, allocating $50 million for its support. Its current budget approaches $118 million. In 1998, an Office of Cancer Complementary and Alternative Medicine was established to coordinate and enhance the CAM-related activities of the National Cancer Institute (NCI).

Medical Schools and Medical Centers Another marker of mainstream interest is the emergence of medical school courses in CAM. Elective courses in CAM and portions of required courses were taught in 75 medical schools in the United States in 1997,[22] and the number has increased since then.[23]

In addition, numerous hospitals, medical centers, and major cancer centers have developed research and clinical service programs in complementary therapies. Services range from mind-body or massage therapy sessions only to acupuncture, exercise, the study or provision of herbs and food supplements, and more. Some clinical programs are repackaged support services, previously available to patients as spiritual care, group and individual counseling, art therapy, nutritional guidance, and so on.

Recognition by Mainstream Journals and Physicians A survey of 295 family physicians in the Maryland-Virginia region revealed that up to 90% of family physicians view complementary therapies such as diet and exercise, behavioral medicine, and hypnotherapy as legitimate medical practices.[24] A majority of them refer patients to nonphysicians for these therapies or provide the services themselves. Homeopathy, Native American medicine, and traditional Oriental medicine, however, were not seen as legitimate practices.

Two hundred Canadian general practitioners held similar views.[25] A survey of physicians in Massachusetts, Washington state, New Mexico, and Israel showed that primary care physicians are more likely than other specialists to use and refer patients to alternative therapies.[26] An early survey revealed that mainstream physicians practicing alternative medicine tended to consist almost exclusively of family practitioners and psychiatrists.[10]

In addition to increasing coverage of CAM services by health insurers, a final marker of mainstream interest noted here is the publication of CAM research articles in major mainstream medical journals. Articles about CAM in major journals shifted from commentaries through the 1970s expressing realistic concern about quackery,[27–29] to surveys of patients' knowledge and use of unproven methods in the 1980s,[30–32] to reports of actual research results starting primarily in the mid-1990s.

Mainstream Disapproval Despite broad public acceptance of alternative and complementary therapies in North America, the professional oncology community is hardly unanimous in its approval. Not all mainstream physicians are pleased with current efforts to integrate CAM and mainstream medicine or with a separate NIH research entity for CAM.[33–35] It is unfortunate that the value of rational, useful therapies sometimes is diminished by the deviation from basic scientific principles of some approaches, such as homeopathy and therapeutic touch.

CAM THERAPIES AND PRACTITIONERS

CAM therapies may be categorized in a variety of ways. The seven categories applied here are based on those developed by the OAM[36]: (1) diet and nutrition; (2) mind-body techniques; (3) bioelectromagnetics; (4) alternative medical systems; (5) pharmacologic and biologic treatments; (6) manual healing methods; and (7) herbal medicine. Currently popular therapies within each of these categories are discussed in the following sections. Many of these approaches are unproved methods promoted as alternatives to mainstream cancer treatment. Helpful complementary or adjunctive therapies are given in Table 65-1.

Diet and Nutrition Advocates of dietary cancer treatments typically extend mainstream assumptions about the protective effects of fruits, vegetables, fiber, and avoidance of excessive dietary fat in reducing cancer risk to the idea that foods or vitamins can cure cancer. Proponents of this belief make their claims in books with titles such as *The Food Pharmacy: Dramatic New Evi-*

dence that Food Is Your Best Medicine, *Prescription for Nutritional Healing*, and *New Choices in Natural Healing*. The chapter on cancer in a popular tome, *Alternative Medicine*, after criticizing chemotherapy, radiation, and surgery as "highly invasive…[that] may shorten the patient's life," recommends that therapy instead address the entire body and employ a "nontoxic approach…incorporating treatments that rely on biopharmaceutical, immune enhancement, metabolic, nutritional, and herbal, nontoxic methods."[37]

Metabolic Therapies and Detoxification Metabolic therapies continue to draw patients from North America to the many clinics in Tijuana, Mexico. These therapies involve practitioner-specific combinations of diet plus vitamins, minerals, enzymes, and "detoxification." One of the best known sites for metabolic therapy is the Gerson Clinic, where treatment is based on the belief that the toxic products of cancer cells accumulate in the liver, leading to liver failure and death. The Gerson treatment aims to counteract liver damage with a low-salt, high-potassium diet, coffee enemas, and a gallon of fruit and vegetable juice daily.[38] The clinic's use of liquefied raw calf liver injections was suspended in 1997 following sepsis in a number of patients.

Other Tijuana clinics and practitioners provide their own versions of metabolic therapy, applying individualized dietary and "detoxification" regimens. Metabolic regimens are based on a belief in the importance of detoxification, which is thought necessary for the body to heal itself. Practitioners view cancer and other illnesses as symptoms of the accumulation of toxins. This is a nonphysiologic but venerable concept that originated in ancient Egyptian, ayurvedic, and other early efforts to understand illness and death, both of which were believed to be caused by the putrefaction of food in the colon. Decay and purging were major themes in the therapeutic regimens of early cultures. Neither the presence of toxins nor the benefit of eliminating them has been documented.

Megavitamin and Orthomolecular Therapy The popular use of nutritional supplements as treatments contrasts ironically with alternative medicine's simultaneous emphasis on "natural" foods and therapies. Some patients and alternative practitioners believe that large doses of vitamins—typically hundreds of pills a day—or intravenous infusions of high-dose vitamin C can cure disease.

In 1968, Nobel laureate Linus Pauling coined the term *orthomolecular* to describe the treatment of disease with large quantities of nutrients. His claims that massive doses of vitamin C could cure cancer were disproved in clinical trials,[39,40] but megavitamin and orthomolecular therapies—the latter adds minerals and other nutrients—remain popular among cancer patients. Perhaps the simplicity of this approach and the fact that patients can prescribe and obtain their own over-the-counter therapy contribute to its appeal. There is no evidence that megavitamin or orthomolecular therapy is effective in treating any disease.

Some patients with treatable cancers turn to megavitamin therapy instead of mainstream care. A major US television news program aired a segment about one of its own producers, a young woman just diagnosed with early-stage breast cancer, who opted for hundreds of vitamin and mineral pills daily instead of surgery. This program did not present a follow-up report of her death, thus leaving the public with the impression that alternatives to mainstream care—in this case, megavitamin therapy—are viable options for cancer patients.

Macrobiotic Diet The macrobiotic diet was developed in the 1930s by George Ohsawa, a Japanese philosopher who sought to integrate traditional Oriental medicine, Christian teachings, and aspects of Western medicine.[41] The diet is embedded in a fanciful concept of human physiology and disease that holds, for example, that blood cells are produced not in the bone marrow but in the stomach, where they are birthed by a "mother red blood cell." Macrobiotic diagnostic techniques, including iridology and pulse diagnoses, are similarly misguided. Macrobiotics Web sites are extremely persuasive and attractive, which probably contributes to an apparent resurgence of interest in this dietary fad. There is no evidence that the macrobiotic diet is beneficial for patients diagnosed with cancer.

Mind-Body Techniques The potential to influence our health with our minds is an appealing concept in the United States. It affirms the power of the individual, a belief intrinsic to American culture. Some mind-body interventions, such as hypnosis, meditation, and relaxation techniques, have moved into mainstream medicine as their merits were studied and published.[42–44] Randomized trials have demonstrated the positive effects of relaxation therapy on anxiety, depression, or mood in newly diagnosed cancer patients.[45–47] Relaxation training and hypnosis decrease anxiety during treatment procedures, such as chemotherapy or bone marrow aspiration, in most[48,49] but not all[50] randomized trials. In addition, hypnosis has been found effective for the treatment of anticipatory nausea in children.[51] Trials have also generally found hypnosis and relaxation training to be beneficial against chemotherapy-induced nausea in adults,[52,53] although some studies found no differences between groups.[54]

Music therapy is provided by professional musicians who are also trained music therapists. Typically, they hold graduate degrees in music therapy and are trained to deal with the psychosocial and clinical issues faced by patients and family members. Music therapy is particularly effective in palliative care, with randomized trials indicating benefit for reducing anxiety,[55–57] depression,[58,59] and pain.[60]

Some proponents argue that patients can use mental attributes and mind-body work to prevent or cure cancer. This belief is attractive because it ascribes to patients almost complete control over the course of their illness.[61,62] A 1989 *Lancet* article reported that women with breast cancer who attended weekly support group sessions had improved survival compared with women who did not attend,[62] but prospective replications of this randomized study have failed to find survival differences.[63–65]

Attending to the psychological health of cancer patients is a fundamental component of good cancer care. Support groups, a good doctor-patient relationship, and the emotional and instrumental help of family and friends are vital. However, the idea that patients can influence the course of their disease through mental or emotional work is not substantiated and can evoke feelings of guilt and inadequacy when disease continues to advance despite patients' best spiritual or mental efforts.[61]

Bioelectromagnetics Bioelectromagnetics is the study of interactions between living organisms and their electromagnetic fields. According to proponents, magnetic fields penetrate the body and heal damaged tissues, including cancers and pain originating from localized musculoskeletal injuries.[66] These are bogus claims with no merit.

Alternative Medical Systems This category includes ancient systems of healing typically based on concepts of human physiology that differ from those accepted by modern science. Two of the most popular healing systems are traditional Chinese medicine and India's ayurvedic medicine, popularized by best-selling author Deepak Chopra.[67]

The term *ayurveda* comes from the Sanskrit words *ayur* (life) and *veda* (knowledge). Ayurveda's ancient healing techniques are based on the classification of people into one of three predominant body types, with specific remedies for disease and regimens to promote health for each. This system has a strong mind-body component and uses techniques such as yoga and meditation to keep the body in balance. Ayurveda also emphasizes regular detoxification and cleansing through all bodily orifices.

Traditional Chinese medicine explains the body in terms of its relationship to the environment and the cosmos. Concepts of human physiology and disease are interwoven with geographic features of ancient China and with the forces of nature. Qi (pronounced chee), the life force said to run through all of nature, flows in the human body through vertical energy channels known as meridians. Qi must flow in the correct strength and quality through each of the meridians and organs for health to be maintained. The best known method of altering the flow of qi is acupuncture, the insertion of needles at special points on the meridians (Figure 65-1). Given modern understanding, acupuncture points appear to correspond to physiologic and anatomic features such as peripheral nerve junctions or trigger points, which are areas of increased sensitivity within muscles that cause the characteristic patterns of referred pain. Although the very existence of qi or a "vital energy force" remains unproved, a substantial quantity of scientific research supports the value of acupuncture for the relief of pain and other symptoms.

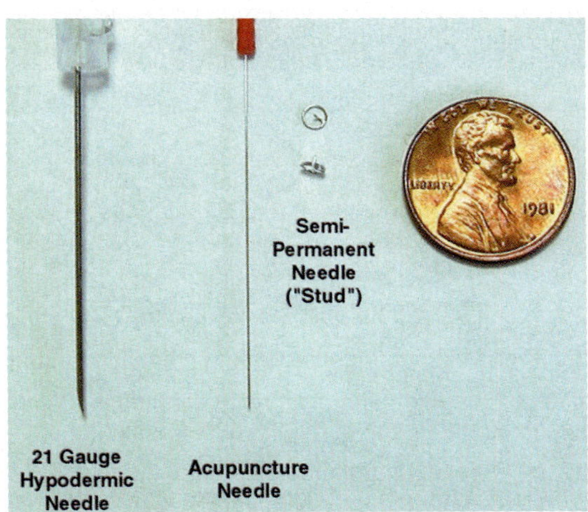

Figure 65-1 An example of needles used during acupuncture.

One of the most intensively researched areas is nausea and vomiting, where randomized, blinded, placebo-controlled trials consistently support the effectiveness of acupuncture as an antiemetic in pregnancy,[68] after anesthesia,[68,69] during chemotherapy,[67,68,70] and to prevent postoperative vomiting in pediatric patients.[71]

Evidence from systematic reviews of randomized trials indicates that acupuncture is effective for both acute[72] and chronic pain.[73] Acupuncture for chronic cancer pain has been studied. Several single-arm studies report that approximately half of patients in significant pain, despite receiving optimal pharmacologic management, obtain clinically relevant, persisting pain relief from acupuncture.[74–77]

A randomized placebo-controlled trial tested auricular acupuncture for patients whose pain remained despite stable pain medication treatment.[78] Ninety patients were randomized to have needles placed at correct acupuncture points (treatment group) or at nonacupuncture points or pressure applied at nonacupuncture points. Pain intensity decreased by 36% at 2 months from baseline in the treatment group, a statistically significant difference compared with the two control groups, for whom little pain reduction was seen. Skin penetration per se showed no significant analgesic effect.

One explanation for the analgesic effects of acupuncture is that it stimulates release of endogenous opioids and other neurotransmitters. Seminal research conducted in the 1970s demonstrated that acupuncture induced analgesia in mice that could be blocked by naloxone.[79] Moreover, mice deficient in opiate receptors show poor electroacupuncture analgesia.[80] Levels of endogenous opioids in the cerebrospinal fluid increase following acupuncture in humans.[81]

Preliminary evidence suggests that acupuncture may lead to changes in the expression of opioids, an observation that may provide a basis for understanding its persisting effects.[82] Functional magnetic resonance imaging technology is now applied to examine the specific nervous pathways involved in acupuncture. True acupuncture can induce brain activation in the hypothalamus and nucleus accumbens and deactivation in the anterior cingulate cortex, amygdala, and hippocampus. Such changes are not observed in control stimulations, which affect only sensory cortex change. Deactivation of the amygdala and hippocampus has also been observed with electroacupuncture. These data suggest modulation of the affective-cognitive aspect of pain perception.[83] A correlation between signal intensities and analgesic effects has been reported.[84]

In addition to acupuncture, basic therapeutic approaches developed initially as part of traditional Chinese medicine include acupressure, qi gong, and tai chi. Tai chi is a well-documented, effective, gentle exercise technique, particularly useful in preventing falls among the frail or elderly.[85] Traditional Chinese medicine also includes a full herbal pharmacopoeia with remedies for most ailments, including cancer.[86] The potential anticancer benefits of herbal remedies are under investigation,[87–89] but herb-drug interactions remain a serious concern.[9,90]

Pharmacologic and Biologic Treatments This group of alternative treatments is invasive and biologically active. Among the popular pharmacologic therapies today is antineoplastons, developed by Stanislaw Burzynski and available in his clinic in Houston, Texas.[91] Laboratory analysis conducted by a respected scientist concluded that antineoplastons did not normalize tumor cells. Early promising anecdotal reports encouraged a limited clinical trial for pediatric patients with brain tumors, but a joint research effort by the NIH Office of Alternative Medicine (now the National Center for Complementary and Alternative Medicine) and the NCI failed to accrue sufficient numbers of patients, and none of the six patients assessable for response showed tumor regression.[92] Further research at the Burzynski Institute was permitted under an investigational new drug permit, but preliminary data were criticized by respected mainstream scientists as uninterpretable and the therapy as useless and toxic.[93]

For the public, the effectiveness of this treatment remains unclear. Although the therapy is unproved and outside the realm of mainstream medicine, patients report anecdotal success, and case reports have been published. In the last decade, however, Burzynski and colleagues published case reports and case series but no controlled trials.[94–96]

Immunoaugmentative therapy (IAT), developed by the late Lawrence Burton, remains available in his clinic in the Bahamas. Injected IAT is said to balance four protein components in the blood and to strengthen the patient's immune system. According to proponent literature, Burton claimed that IAT was particularly effective in treating mesothelioma.[97] Documentation of IAT's efficacy remains anecdotal.

Interest in shark cartilage as a cancer therapy was activated by a 1992 book by I. William Lane, *Sharks Don't Get Cancer*. Advocates base their therapy on its putative antiangiogenic properties, but research has failed to document clinical benefit. The dwindling commercial success of shark cartilage as a treatment for cancer led to its promotion for "aging bone conditions." A phase I-II trial found no clinical benefit.[98]

Cancell, also called Entelev, Cantron, and Protocel, is another well-known biologic remedy that appears to be especially popular in Florida and the midwestern United States. Proponents claim that it reverts cancer cells to a "primitive state" from which they can be digested and rendered inert. FDA laboratory studies showed this product to be composed of common chemicals, including nitric acid, sodium sulfite, potassium hydroxide, sulfuric acid, and catechol, and found no basis for any proponent claims.[99]

Manual Healing Methods Osteopathic and chiropractic doctors were among the earliest groups to use manual methods. The value of chiropractic treatment for low back pain was supported by an NIH consensus conference,[100] but its value is widely disputed by mainstream physicians, and oncologists tend to recommend against its use for cancer patients.[101]

Important among today's manipulation techniques is hands-on massage, its benefits, documented in randomized trials,[102,103] suggesting that therapeutic massage reduces anxiety in a variety of groups, including cancer patients.[104] Data also indicate that massage improves psychological end points in cancer patients. In a large study, 87 hospitalized cancer patients were randomized to foot massage or control. Pain and anxiety scores fell with massage, with differences between groups achieving both statistical and clinical significance.[105]

Therapeutic touch is another popular manual healing method that, despite its name, involves no direct contact. Instead, healers move their hands a few inches above a patient's body and sweep away "blockages" to the patient's energy field. Although a study published in *JAMA* showed that experienced therapeutic touch practitioners were unable to detect the investigator's "energy field,"[106] and despite mainstream scientists' unwillingness to accept its fundamental premises, therapeutic touch is taught in North American nursing schools and is widely practiced by nurses in the United States and other countries.[107]

Herbal Remedies for Cancer Herbal remedies are an essential part of traditional and folk healing methods with long histories of use. Herbal medicine is found in virtually all areas of the world and across all cultures historically. Although many herbal remedies are claimed to have anticancer effects, only a few have gained substantial popularity. Following a summary review of herbal remedies with limited or no utility, more promising herbal treatments are discussed.

Essiac has remained popular for decades, especially in North America. Developed initially by a Native healer from southwestern Canada, it was popularized by a Canadian nurse, Rene Caisse (Essiac is Caisse spelled backward). Essiac comprises four herbs: burdock, Turkey rhubarb, sorrel, and slippery elm. Researchers at the NCI and elsewhere found that it has no anticancer effect.

Iscador, a derivative of mistletoe, is a popular cancer remedy in Europe, where it is said to have been in continuous use as folk treatment since the time of the Druids. Iscador is available in many mainstream European cancer clinics. No survival benefit has been found in studies of patients with malignant melanoma[108] or head and neck cancer.[109] A small trial in glioma reported statistically significant differences between groups for one outcome in one subgroup but is flawed by multiple testing.[110]

Pau d'arco tea is said to be an Incan remedy for many illnesses, including cancer. Made from the bark of an indigenous South American evergreen tree, its active ingredient, lapachol, has been isolated. Although lapachol showed antitumor activity in animal studies conducted in the 1970s, it does not appear to affect human malignancies. The tea does induce nausea and vomiting. Despite the absence of efficacy, pau d'arco tea is sold as a cancer remedy in health food stores, by mail, and on the Internet.

Asian herbal remedies show greater promise in oncology. Several mushroom-derived compounds are approved for use as cancer treatments in Japan, and there is evidence of effectiveness in randomized phase III trials. Polysaccharide kureha (PSK), an extract of the mushroom *Coriolus versicolor*, or schizophyllan has been subjected to a number of studies. Trials typically compared chemotherapy or radiotherapy plus mushroom extract or conventional treatment alone and found superior survival with PSK compared with controls in both gastrectomy[111,112] and esophagectomy patients.[113]

Two randomized trials of PSK extract given after curative resection for colorectal cancer have been conducted. In the first (N = 120), median survival in the PSK group was approximately 5 years compared with slightly over 4 years in controls.[114] A subsequent trial randomized 462 colorectal cancer patients scheduled for curative resection to chemotherapy with or without PSK.[115] Disease-free and overall survival rates were significantly higher in the PSK group. In recent randomized trials, oral PSK with tegafururacil reduced recurrence and increased survival in stage III patients with colorectal cancer.[116,117] The results are less encouraging in breast cancer[118,119] and leukemia.[120]

PC-SPES (PC for prostate cancer; SPES is the Latin word for hope), a combination of eight herbs, all but one from traditional Chinese medicine, reduces prostate-specific antigen levels in men with advanced prostate cancer regardless of whether the disease is androgen dependent.[121–123] Improvements in quality of life also have been reported.[122] PC-SPES was suspended from the market in early 2002 when undisclosed contamination with anxiolytic and antithrombotic agents was uncovered.

Table 65-2 Herbal Products with Toxic Effects

Herbs	Purported Uses	Adverse Effects
Chaparral tea	Pain	Liver failure
Comfrey	Bruises, ulcers	Hepatotoxicity and possibly lead to death
Kava kava	Anxiety, insomnia	Hepatotoxicity and liver failure
Ma huang (ephedra) (banned by the FDA)	Asthma, weight loss	Hypertension, cardiac failure, and stroke
St. John's wort	Depression	Increased drowsiness
Yohimbe	Sexual dysfunction	Seizures, kidney failure, and death
Aristolochia	Weight loss	Nephrotoxicity

FDA = US Food and Drug Administration.

Sho-saiko-to is a traditional Asian medicine for liver disease composed of seven botanicals. It has marked antiproliferative effects on various cancer lines, particularly hepatoma.[124] In a phase III randomized trial, 260 patients with cirrhosis were randomized to treatment with sho-saiko-to or a control.[125] At 5 years, sho-saiko-to led to a one-third reduction in the incidence of hepatocellular carcinoma (23% vs 34%) and a 40% reduction in deaths (24% vs 40%).

In a separate study, Sun Soup, a formula of 19 selected vegetables from traditional Chinese medicine believed to have antitumor activity, was added to the diets of 12 patients with stages III and IV non–small cell lung cancer.[126] Thirteen clinically similar patients were selected as controls. All patients received conventional therapies. The median survival of control patients was 4 months (mean 4.8 months). The median survival of patients who received the vegetable remedy was 15.5 months (mean 15 months). This nontoxic vegetable brew was reported to improve quality of life.

These investigations suggest that historical herbal cancer remedies, pretested to ensure the purity and consistency of the product and studied carefully, may produce potentially useful, nontoxic cancer treatments. The difficulty with time-honored herbal remedies is that they are rarely tested for purity, examined for consistency, or studied carefully. They are, nonetheless, in common use.

Cancer patients commonly use over-the-counter herbal products in addition to or instead of those promoted specifically as cancer treatments. It is therefore important to recognize herbal remedies that may help cancer patients (see Table 65-1) and those that are toxic (Table 65-2) or interact with other medications (Table 65-3). Because neither the FDA nor any other government agency examines herbal remedies for safety and effectiveness prior to their marketing, few products have been formally tested for side effects or quality control, but information is beginning to emerge on the basis of public experience with over-the-counter supplements.

Recent reports in the literature describe severe liver and kidney damage from some herbal remedies (see Table 65-2). These reports underscore the fact that "natural" products, contrary to apparent consumer belief, are not necessarily safe or harmless.[127] Most members of the public apparently are not aware that herbs are dilute pharmaceuticals, natural drugs that contain scores of different chemicals, most of which have not been documented. The effects are not always predictable.

Moreover, the potential for herb-drug interaction is sufficiently problematic that patients on chemotherapy should be told to stop using herbal remedies prior to and during treatment. Similar cautions are necessary for patients receiving radiation because some herbs photosensitize the skin and cause severe reactions. Patients scheduled for surgery should be alerted to the fact that some herbs produce dangerous blood pressure swings and other unwanted interactions with anesthetics.[9,90] Herbs such as feverfew, garlic, ginger, and ginkgo have anticoagulant effects and should be avoided by patients on warfarin, heparin, aspirin, and related agents. The risk of herb-drug interactions appears to be greatest for patients with kidney or liver problems.[9,90,128]

REGULATORY AND SAFETY ISSUES: HERBAL REMEDIES AND OTHER FOOD SUPPLEMENTS

Dietary supplements, which include vitamins and minerals, homeopathic remedies, herbal treatments, antioxidants, and other over-the-counter products, are commonly used today by cancer patients and by the public in general. Sales in 2003 of dietary supplements were approximately $10 billion.[129]

No legal standards exist for the processing or packaging of herbs. Quality control standards and reviews are needed. Because they are not mandatory, however, few food supplement companies voluntarily self-impose quality evaluation and control. Consumer protection and enforcement agencies cannot provide protection against contaminated or falsely advertised products. Current federal regulations do not permit such oversight, and regulatory capability would prohibit full analysis and ongoing oversight of the estimated 20,000 food supplement items now sold over the counter.

Nonetheless, Canada is establishing a federal office to evaluate and regulate herbal remedies,

Table 65-3 Commonly Used Botanicals and Their Potential Interactions with Cancer Therapies

Botanicals	Cancer Drugs/Therapies	Potential Problems
Astragalus	Immunosuppressants	Antagonistic effects
Dong quai	Anticoagulants	Additive effects; prolongs PT/INR
Garlic	Anticoagulants, antiplatelet agents	Prolongs PT/INR
	Cytochrome P-450 substrates	Increases cytochrome P-450 activities
Ginkgo	Anticoagulants, antiplatelet agents	Prolongs PT/INR
	Cytochrome P-450 substrates	Affects cytochrome P-450 activities
Ginseng	Anticoagulants	Additive effects, prolongs PT/INR
Grape seed extract	Certain chemotherapeutic agents	Antioxidant effects may interfere with chemotherapeutic agents
Kava kava	Sedatives	Additive effects
	Cytochrome P-450 substrates	Inhibits cytochrome P-450 activities
	Drugs that are hepatotoxic	Hepatotoxicity
Soy	Hormonal therapy	May have mild estrogenic effects
	Tamoxifen	May antagonize the effects of tamoxifen
St. John's wort	Sedatives	Additive effects
	Cytochrome P-450 substrates	Induces cytochrome P-450 activities
	P-glycoprotein substrates	Induces P-glycoprotein activities
Valerian	Sedatives	Additive effects

Adapted from Memorial Sloan-Kettering Cancer Center Integrative Medicine Information Program. Available at: www.mskcc.org/abouth-erbs (accessed Jan 4, 2005).

INR = international normalized ratio; PT = prothrombin time.

which it will treat as a new category distinct from drugs and foods. In the United States, organizations such as the American Medical Association and the American Cancer Society have produced position papers, and FDA hearings have been held on food supplement issues. The magnitude and seriousness of the problem probably will result in the establishment of government oversight programs of some kind, despite anticipated efforts on the part of the food supplement industry to block efforts that could lead to regulation.

CAM PRACTITIONERS AND PRACTICES

Training and Licensure of CAM Practitioners Major categories of CAM practitioners outside mainstream medicine include chiropractors, naturopaths, and acupuncturists, who often practice a broader range of traditional Chinese medicine involving herbal therapeutics.[130]

Chiropractic requires 4 years of training and prepares students to provide primary clinical services, including wellness maintenance, diagnosis of illness, and primary care, in addition to musculoskeletal care. Fifteen percent of clinical training is devoted to organ systems other than the musculoskeletal system. All 50 states plus the District of Columbia have licensure programs for chiropractors. The accrediting agency for chiropractic medicine was established in 1971, and a standardized national examination was created in 1982.[130,131]

Naturopathic doctoral degrees are awarded after 4 years of training. Naturopathic education is designed to prepare primary care providers. Training emphasizes health promotion, disease prevention, and the use of natural remedies, such as botanicals. As of January 2005, all 13 states that license naturopaths permit the designation ND—doctor of naturopathic medicine.[132] The accrediting agency for naturopathy was established in 1978, and standardized tests were first offered in 1986.

Practitioners of acupuncture and herbal medicine are trained for 3 to 4 years. They learn to diagnose disease, using pulse diagnosis and other traditional Chinese medicine techniques, and to treat common problems with acupuncture and herbal remedies. Acupuncturists are recognized and licensed in 39 states.[133] Acupuncturists were accredited, and their standardized national test was created in 1982.[134]

CAM Research Issues More than 40 CAM journals have been established in recent years. Most represent a second tier of publication, in which peer review often means evaluation by CAM proponents who have little training or experience in research. Although they are included in *MEDLINE*, the validity and reliability of articles in these publications do not necessarily meet standards of mainstream peer-reviewed journals and should be read with caution and attention to methodology and the reliability of conclusions. Few articles in these journals stand the test of scientific scrutiny.

SUMMARY

Fraudulent products and regimens abound; there are no viable "alternatives" to mainstream cancer care. Complementary therapies, conversely, are rational, evidence-based therapies used adjunctively to relieve symptoms and enhance quality of life. Massage therapy, acupuncture, music therapy, meditation, self-hypnosis, and other mind-body therapies are examples of complementary interventions that effectively reduce the physical and emotional symptoms experienced by cancer patients. These should be made available by certified practitioners trained to treat patients with cancer. Herbs and other botanicals, many of which hold great promise and are currently under study, should be avoided by patients under active treatment or on prescription medications.

REFERENCES

1. Cassileth B, Brown H. Unorthodox cancer medicine. CA Cancer J Clin 1988;38:176–92.
2. Starr P. The social transformation of American medicine. New York: Basic Books; 1982.
3. Kaufman M. Homeopathy in America: the rise and fall of a medical heresy. Baltimore: Johns Hopkins Press; 1971.
4. Kellogg J. The natural diet of man. Battle Creek (MI): Modern Medicine Publishing; 1923.
5. Janssen WF. Cancer quackery—the past in the present. 1979;6:526–36.
6. Cramp A. Nostrums and quackery and pseudo-medicine. Chicago: American Medical Association; 1912.
7. Cassileth BR. Sounding boards. After laetrile, what? N Engl J Med 1982;306:1482–4.
8. Society for Integrative Oncology. Available at: http://www.IntegrativeOnc.org (accessed Dec 29, 2004).
9. Memorial Sloan-Kettering Cancer Center. Available at: http://www.mskcc.org/mskcc/html/11570.cfm (accessed May 25, 2005).
10. Cassileth BR, Lusk EJ, Strouse TB, Bodenheimer BJ. Contemporary unorthodox treatments in cancer medicine: a study of patients, treatments and practitioners. Ann Intern Med 1984;101:105–12.
11. Ernst E, Cassileth BR. The prevalence of complementary/alternative medicine in cancer: a systematic review. Cancer 1998;83:777–82.
12. Miller M, Boyer MJ, Butow PN, et al. The use of unproven methods of treatment by cancer patients. Frequency, expectations and cost. Support Care Cancer 1998;6:337–47.
13. Crocetti E, Crotti N, Feltrin A, et al. The use of complementary therapies by breast cancer patients attending conventional treatment. Eur J Cancer 1998;34:324–8.
14. Fernandez CV, Stutzer CA, MacWilliam L, Fryer C. Alternative and complementary therapy use in pediatric oncology patients in British Columbia: prevalence and reasons for use and nonuse. J Clin Oncol 1998;16:1279–86.
15. Cassileth BR, Schraub S, Robinson E, Vickers A. Alternative medicine use worldwide: the International Union Against Cancer survey. Cancer 2001;91:1390–3.
16. Druss BG, Rosenheck RA. Association between use of unconventional therapies and conventional medical services. JAMA 1999;282:651–6.
17. Kelly KM. Complementary and alternative medical therapies for children with cancer. Eur J Cancer 2004;40:2041–6.
18. Neuhouser ML, Patterson RE, Schwartz SM, et al. Use of alternative medicine by children with cancer in Washington state. Prev Med 2001;33:347–54.
19. Stolberg S. Trade agency finds Web slippery with snake oil. New York Times, Section A, Page 16, June 25, 1999.
20. Federal Trade Commission. Available at: http://www.ftc.gov/cureall/ (accessed May 26, 2005).
21. Unconventional Medical Practices. Senate Appropriations Committee Report. Washington, D.C.: Government Printing Office (GPO); 1992. p.141.
22. Wetzel MS, Eisenberg DM, Kaptchuk TJ. Courses involving complementary and alternative medicine at US medical schools. JAMA 1998;280:784–7.
23. Brokaw JJ, Tunnicliff G, Raess BU, Saxon DW. The teaching of complementary and alternative medicine in U.S. medical schools: a survey of course directors. Acad Med 2002;77:876–81.
24. Berman BM, Singh BK, Lao L, et al. Physicians' attitudes toward complementary or alternative medicine: a regional survey. J Am Board Fam Pract 1995;8:361–6.
25. Verhoef MJ, Sutherland LR. General practitioners' assessment of and interest in alternative medicine in Canada. Soc Sci Med 1995;41:511–5.
26. Borkan J, Neher JO, Anson O, Smoker B. Referrals for alternative therapies. J Fam Pract 1994;39:545–50.
27. Soffer A. Chihuahuas and laetrile, chelation therapy, and honey from Boulder, Colo [editorial]. Arch Intern Med 1976;136:865–6.
28. Jukes TH. Laetrile for cancer. JAMA 1976;236:1284–6.
29. Ingelfinger FJ. Quenchless quest for questionable cure [editorial]. N Engl J Med 1976;295:838–9.
30. Pendergrass TW, Davis S. Knowledge and use of "alternative" cancer therapies in children. Am J Pediatr Hematol Oncol 1981;3:339–45.

31. Eidinger RN, Schapira DV. Cancer patients' insight into their treatment, prognosis, and unconventional therapies. Cancer 1984;53:2736–40.
32. Fulder SJ, Munro RE. Complementary medicine in the United Kingdom: patients, practitioners, and consultations. Lancet 1985;2:542–5.
33. Park R, Goodenough U. Buying snake oil with tax dollars. New York Times, Section A, Page 15, Column 2, January 3, 1996.
34. Quackwatch. Available at: http://www.quackwatch.org/ (accessed May 20, 2005).
35. Angell M, Kassirer JP. Alternative medicine—the risks of untested and unregulated remedies. N Engl J Med 1998;339:839–41.
36. Workshop on Alternative Medicine. Alternative medicine: expanding medical horizons. A report to the National Institutes of Health on alternative medical systems and practices in the United States. Washington (DC): US Government Printing Office; 1992.
37. Group. BG. Alternative medicine: the definitive guide. Puyallup (WA): Future Publishing; 1993.
38. Green S. A critique of the rationale for cancer treatment with coffee enemas and diet. JAMA 1992;268:3224–7.
39. Creagan ET, Moertel CG, O'Fallon JR, et al. Failure of high-dose vitamin C (ascorbic acid) therapy to benefit patients with advanced cancer. A controlled trial. N Engl J Med 1979;301:687–90.
40. Moertel CG, Fleming TR, Creagan ET, et al. High-dose vitamin C versus placebo in the treatment of patients with advanced cancer who have had no prior chemotherapy. A randomized double-blind comparison. N Engl J Med 1985;312:137–41.
41. Kushi M. The macrobiotic approach to cancer. New York: Avery, Penguin Putnam; 1991.
42. Sellick SM, Zaza C. Critical review of 5 nonpharmacologic strategies for managing cancer pain. Cancer Prev Control 1998;2:7–14.
43. Integration of behavioral and relaxation approaches into the treatment of chronic pain and insomnia. NIH Technology Assessment Panel on Integration of Behavioral and Relaxation Approaches into the Treatment of Chronic Pain and Insomnia. JAMA 1996;276:313–8.
44. Syrjala KL, Donaldson GW, Davis MW, et al. Relaxation and imagery and cognitive-behavioral training reduce pain during cancer treatment: a controlled clinical trial. 1995;63:189–98.
45. Bridge LR, Benson P, Pietroni PC, Priest RG. Relaxation and imagery in the treatment of breast cancer. BMJ 1988;297:1169–72.
46. Bindemann S, Soukop M, Kaye SB. Randomised controlled study of relaxation training. Eur J Cancer 1991;27:170–4.
47. Walker LG, Walker MB, Ogston K, et al. Psychological, clinical and pathological effects of relaxation training and guided imagery during primary chemotherapy. Br J Cancer 1999;80:262–8.
48. Kazak AE, Penati B, Boyer BA, et al. A randomized controlled prospective outcome study of a psychological and pharmacological intervention protocol for procedural distress in pediatric leukemia. J Pediatr Psychol 1996;21:615–31.
49. Zeltzer L, LeBaron S. Hypnosis and nonhypnotic techniques for reduction of pain and anxiety during painful procedures in children and adolescents with cancer. J Pediatr 1982;101:1032–5.
50. Wall VJ, Womack W. Hypnotic versus active cognitive strategies for alleviation of procedural distress in pediatric oncology patients. Am J Clin Hypnosis 1989;31:181–91.
51. Zeltzer LK, Dolgin MJ, LeBaron S, LeBaron C. A randomized, controlled study of behavioral intervention for chemotherapy distress in children with cancer. Pediatrics 1991;88:34–42.
52. Morrow GR, Morrell C. Behavioral treatment for the anticipatory nausea and vomiting induced by cancer chemotherapy. N Engl J Med 1982;307:1476–80.
53. Vasterling J, Jenkins RA, Tope DM, Burish TG. Cognitive distraction and relaxation training for the control of side effects due to cancer chemotherapy. J Behav Med 1993;16:65–80.
54. Arakawa S. Use of relaxation to reduce side effects of chemotherapy in Japanese patients. Cancer Nurs 1995;18:60–6.
55. Augustin P, Hains AA. Effect of music on ambulatory surgery patients' preoperative anxiety. AORN J 1996;63:750–8.
56. Kaempf G, Amodei ME. The effect of music on anxiety. A research study. AORN J 1989;50:112–8.
57. White JM. Effects of relaxing music on cardiac autonomic balance and anxiety after acute myocardial infarction. Am J Crit Care 1999;8:220–30.
58. Hanser SB, Thompson LW. Effects of a music therapy strategy on depressed older adults. J Gerontol 1994;49:P265–9.
59. Lai YM. Effects of music listening on depressed women in Taiwan. Issues Ment Health Nurs 1999;20:229–46.
60. Zimmerman L, Pozehl B, Duncan K, Schmitz R. Effects of music in patients who had chronic cancer pain. West J Nurs Res 1989;11:298–309.
61. Cassileth BR. The social implications of mind-body cancer research. Cancer Invest 1989;7:361–4.
62. Spiegel D, Bloom JR, Kraemer HC, Gottheil E. Effect of psychosocial treatment on survival of patients with metastatic breast cancer. Lancet 1989;2:888–91.
63. Cunningham AJ, Edmonds CV, Jenkins GP, et al. A randomized controlled trial of the effects of group psychological therapy on survival in women with metastatic breast cancer. Psychooncology 1998;7:508–17.
64. Gellert GA, Maxwell RM, Siegel BS. Survival of breast cancer patients receiving adjunctive psychosocial support therapy: a 10-year follow-up study. J Clin Oncol 1993;11:66–9.
65. Goodwin PJ, Leszcz M, Ennis M, et al. The effect of group psychosocial support on survival in metastatic breast cancer. N Engl J Med 2001;345:1719–26.
66. Pujol J, Pascual-Leone A, Dolz C, et al. The effect of repetitive magnetic stimulation on localized musculoskeletal pain. Neuroreport 1998;9:1745–8.
67. Chopra D. Ageless body, timeless mind. New York: Harmony Books; 1993.
68. Vickers AJ. Can acupuncture have specific effects on health? A systematic review of acupuncture antiemesis trials. J R Soc Med 1996;89:303–11.
69. Lee A, Done ML. The use of nonpharmacologic techniques to prevent postoperative nausea and vomiting: a meta-analysis. Anesth Analg 1999;88:1362–9.
70. Shen J, Wenger N, Glaspy J, et al. Electroacupuncture for control of myeloablative chemotherapy-induced emesis: a randomized controlled trial. JAMA 2000;284:2755–61.
71. Somri M, Vaida SJ, Sabo E, et al. Acupuncture versus ondansetron in the prevention of postoperative vomiting. A study of children undergoing dental surgery. Anaesthesia 2001;56:927–32.
72. Ernst E, Pittler MH. The effectiveness of acupuncture in treating acute dental pain: a systematic review. Br Dent J 1998;184:443–7.
73. Melchart D, Linde K, Fischer P, et al. Acupuncture for recurrent headaches: a systematic review of randomized controlled trials. Cephalalgia 1999;19:779–86.
74. Filshie J, Redman D. Acupuncture and malignant pain problems. Eur J Surg Oncol 1985;11:389–94.
75. Leng G. A year of acupuncture in palliative care. Palliat Med 1999;13:163–4.
76. Alimi D, Rubino C, Leandri EP, Brule SF. Analgesic effects of auricular acupuncture for cancer pain. J Pain Symptom Manage 2000;19:81–2.
77. Deng G, Cassileth BR, Yeung KS. Complementary therapies for cancer-related symptoms. J Support Oncol 2004;2:419–26; discussion 427–9.
78. Alimi D, Rubino C, Pichard-Leandri E, et al. Analgesic effect of auricular acupuncture for cancer pain: a randomized, blinded, controlled trial. J Clin Oncol 2003;21:4120–6.
79. Pomeranz B, Chiu D. Naloxone blockade of acupuncture analgesia: endorphin implicated. Life Sci 1976;19:1757–62.
80. Peets JM, Pomeranz B. CXBK mice deficient in opiate receptors show poor electroacupuncture analgesia. Nature 1978;273:675–6.
81. Clement-Jones V, McLoughlin L, Tomlin S, et al. Increased beta-endorphin but not met-enkephalin levels in human cerebrospinal fluid after acupuncture for recurrent pain. Lancet 1980;2:946–9.
82. Guo HF, Tian J, Wang X, et al. Brain substrates activated by electroacupuncture of different frequencies (I): comparative study on the expression of oncogene c-fos and genes coding for three opioid peptides. Brain Res Mol Brain Res 1996;43:157–66.
83. Wu MT, Hsieh JC, Xiong J, et al. Central nervous pathway for acupuncture stimulation: localization of processing with functional MR imaging of the brain—preliminary experience. Radiology 1999;212:133–41.
84. Zhang WT, Jin Z, Cui GH, et al. Relations between brain network activation and analgesic effect induced by low vs. high frequency electrical acupoint stimulation in different subjects: a functional magnetic resonance imaging study. Brain Res 2003;982:168–78.
85. Ross MC, Presswalla JL. The therapeutic effects of tai chi for the elderly. J Gerontol Nurs 1998;24:45–7.
86. Hsu HY. Treating cancer with Chinese herbs. Los Angeles: Oriental Healing Arts Institute; 1982.
87. Bushman JL. Green tea and cancer in humans: a review of the literature. Nutr Cancer 1998;31:151–9.
88. Kurashige S, Jin R, Akuzawa Y, Endo F. Anticarcinogenic effects of shikaron, a preparation of eight Chinese herbs in mice treated with a carcinogen, N-butyl-N'-butanolnitrosoamine. Cancer Invest 1998;16:166–9.
89. Oh WK, Kantoff PW, Weinberg V, et al. Prospective, multicenter, randomized phase II trial of the herbal supplement, PC-SPES, and diethylstilbestrol in patients with androgen-independent prostate cancer. J Clin Oncol 2004;22:3705–12.
90. Cassileth B, Lucarelli C. Herb-drug interactions in oncology. Hamilton (ON): BC Decker; 2003.
91. Burzynski SR, Kubove E. Initial clinical study with antineoplaston A2 injections in cancer patients with five years' follow-up. Drugs Exp Clin Res 1987;13 Suppl 1:1–11.
92. Buckner JC, Malkin MG, Reed E, et al. Phase II study of antineoplastons A10 (NSC 648539) and AS2-1 (NSC 620261) in patients with recurrent glioma. Mayo Clin Proc 1999;74:137–45.
93. Experts say interpretable results unlikely in Burzynski's antineoplastons studies. Cancer Lett 1998;24:1–16.
94. Burzynski SR, Lewy RI, Weaver RA, et al. Phase II study of antineoplaston A10 and AS2-1 in patients with recurrent diffuse intrinsic brain stem glioma: a preliminary report. Drugs R D 2003;4:91–101.
95. Burzynski SR, Kubove E, Burzynski B. Treatment of hormonally refractory cancer of the prostate with antineoplaston AS2-1. Drugs Exp Clin Res 1990;16:361–9.
96. Burzynski SR, Weaver RA, Lewy RI, et al. Phase II study of antineoplaston A10 and AS2-1 in children with recurrent and progressive multicentric glioma: a preliminary report. Drugs R D 2004;5:315–26.
97. Moss RW. Cancer therapy: the independent consumer's guide. New York: Equinox Press; 1992.
98. Miller DR, Anderson GT, Stark JJ, et al. Phase I/II trial of the safety and efficacy of shark cartilage in the treatment of advanced cancer. J Clin Oncol 1998;16:3649–55.
99. Butler K. A consumer's guide to alternative medicine. Buffalo (NY): Prometheus Books; 1992.
100. Lawrence DJ. Report from the Consensus Conference on the Validation of Chiropractic Methods. J Manipulative Physiol Ther 1990;13:295–6.
101. Shekelle PG. What role for chiropractic in health care? N Engl J Med 1998;339:1074–5.
102. Field TM. Massage therapy effects. Am Psychol 1998;53:1270–81.
103. Ahles TA, Tope DM, Pinkson B, et al. Massage therapy for patients undergoing autologous bone marrow transplantation. J Pain Symptom Manage 1999;18:157–63.
104. Cassileth BR, Vickers AJ. Massage therapy for symptom control: outcome study at a major cancer center. J Pain Symptom Manage 2004;28:244–9.
105. Grealish L, Lomasney A, Whiteman B. Foot massage. A nursing intervention to modify the distressing symptoms of pain and nausea in patients hospitalized with cancer. Cancer Nurs 2000;23:237–43.
106. Rosa L, Rosa E, Sarner L, Barrett S. A close look at therapeutic touch. JAMA 1998;279:1005–10.
107. O'Mathuna DP. Evidence-based practice and reviews of therapeutic touch. J Nurs Scholar 2000;32:279–85.
108. Kleeberg UR, Suciu S, Brocker EB, et al. Final results of the EORTC 18871/DKG 80-1 randomised phase III trial. rIFN-alpha2b versus rIFN-gamma versus ISCADOR M versus observation after surgery in melanoma patients with either high-risk primary (thickness >3 mm) or regional lymph node metastasis. Eur J Cancer 2004;40:390–402.
109. McNamee D. Mistletoe extract ineffective in melanoma (news). Lancet 1999;354:1101.
110. Lenartz D, Dott U, Menzel J, et al. Survival of glioma patients after complementary treatment with galactoside-specific lectin from mistletoe. Anticancer Res 2000;20:2073–6.
111. Niimoto M, Hattori T, Tamada R, et al. Postoperative adjuvant immunochemotherapy with mitomycin C, futraful and PSK for gastric cancer. An analysis of data on 579 patients followed for five years. Jpn J Surg 1988;18:681–6.
112. Nakazato H, Koike A, Saji S, et al. Efficacy of immunochemotherapy as adjuvant treatment after curative resection of gastric cancer. Study Group of Immunochemotherapy with PSK for Gastric Cancer. 1994;343:1122–6.
113. Ogoshi K, Satou H, Isono K, et al. Immunotherapy for esophageal cancer. A randomized trial in combination with radiotherapy and radiochemotherapy. Cooperative

Study Group for Esophageal Cancer in Japan. Am J Clin Oncol 1995;18:216–22.
114. Torisu M, Hayashi Y, Ishimitsu T, et al. Significant prolongation of disease-free period gained by oral polysaccharide K (PSK) administration after curative surgical operation of colorectal cancer. Cancer Immunol Immunother 1990;31:261–8.
115. Mitomi T, Tsuchiya S, Iijima N, et al. Randomized, controlled study on adjuvant immunochemotherapy with PSK in curatively resected colorectal cancer. The Cooperative Study Group of Surgical Adjuvant Immunochemotherapy for Cancer of Colon and Rectum (Kanagawa). Dis Colon Rectum 1992;35:123–30.
116. Ohwada S, Kawate S, Ikeya T, et al. Adjuvant therapy with protein-bound polysaccharide K and tegafur uracil in patients with stage II or III colorectal cancer: randomized, controlled trial. Dis Colon Rectum 2003;46:1060–8.
117. Ohwada S, Ikeya T, Yokomori T, et al. Adjuvant immunochemotherapy with oral tegafur/uracil plus PSK in patients with stage II or III colorectal cancer: a randomised controlled study. Br J Cancer 2004;90:1003–10.
118. Toi M, Hattori T, Akagi M, et al. Randomized adjuvant trial to evaluate the addition of tamoxifen and PSK to chemotherapy in patients with primary breast cancer. 5-Year results from the Nishi-Nippon Group of the Adjuvant Chemoendocrine Therapy for Breast Cancer Organization. Cancer 1992;70:2475–83.
119. Iino Y, Yokoe T, Maemura M, et al. Immunochemotherapies versus chemotherapy as adjuvant treatment after curative resection of operable breast cancer. Anticancer Res 1995;15:2907–11.
120. Ohno R, Yamada K, Masaoka T, et al. A randomized trial of chemoimmunotherapy of acute nonlymphocytic leukemia in adults using a protein-bound polysaccharide preparation. Cancer Immunol Immunother 1984;18:149–54.
121. Small EJ, Frohlich MW, Bok R, et al. Prospective trial of the herbal supplement PC-SPES in patients with progressive prostate cancer. J Clin Oncol 2000;18:3595–603.
122. Pfeifer BL, Pirani JF, Hamann SR, Klippel KF. PC-SPES, a dietary supplement for the treatment of hormone-refractory prostate cancer. BJU Int 2000;85:481–5.
123. Oh WK, George DJ, Hackmann K, et al. Activity of the herbal combination, PC-SPES, in the treatment of patients with androgen-independent prostate cancer. Urology 2001;57:122–6.
124. Yano H, Mizoguchi A, Fukuda K, et al. The herbal medicine sho-saiko-to inhibits proliferation of cancer cell lines by inducing apoptosis and arrest at the G0/G1 phase. Cancer Res 1994;54:448–54.
125. Oka H, Yamamoto S, Kuroki T, et al. Prospective study of chemoprevention of hepatocellular carcinoma with sho-saiko-to (TJ-9). Cancer 1995;76:743–9.
126. Sun AS, Ostadal O, Ryznar V, et al. Phase I/II study of stage III and IV non-small cell lung cancer patients taking a specific dietary supplement. Nutr Cancer 1999;34:62–9.
127. Drew AK, Myers SP. Safety issues in herbal medicine: implications for the health professions. Med J Aust 1997;166:538–41.
128. Labriola D, Livingston R. Possible interactions between dietary antioxidants and chemotherapy. Oncology (Huntingt) 1999;13:1003–8.
129. Mindbranch. Available at: http://www.mindbranch.com/listing/product/R567-0094.html (accessed Dec 29, 2004).
130. Cooper RA, Henderson T, Dietrich CL. Roles of nonphysician clinicians as autonomous providers of patient care. JAMA 1998;280:795–802.
131. Chiropractic: state of the Art. Arlington (VA): American Chiropractic Association; 1994.
132. Naturopathy Online. Available at: http://www.naturopathy-online.com/ (accessed Dec 29, 2004).
133. State Licensure Information, National Certification Commission For Acupuncture and Oriental Medicine. Available at: http://www.nccaom.org/StateData.htm (accessed May 25, 2005).
134. Council of Colleges of Acupuncture and Oriental Medicine. Available at: http://www.ccaom.org/ (accessed Dec 30, 2004).

RECOMMENDED WEBSITES

Aboutherbs Web Site, Memorial Sloan-Kettering Cancer Center
http://www.mskcc.org/aboutherbs
American Cancer Society
http://www.cancer.org/
Dietary Supplement Fact Sheets
http://ods.od.nih.gov/Health_Information/Information_About_Individual_Dietary_Supplements
Drug Digest, Herbs and Supplements
http://www.drugdigest.org/DD/DVH/Herbs/0,3913,,00.html
FDA/Center for Food Safety & Applied Nutrition – Dietary Supplements
http://www.cfsan.fda.gov/~dms/supplmnt.html
HerbMed - American Herbal Products Association
http://www.ahpa.org/herbmed/
International Bibliographic Information on Dietary Supplements (IBIDS) Database
http://ods.od.nih.gov/Health_Information/IBIDS.aspx
Medline Plus – Herbal Medicine
http://www.nlm.nih.gov/medlineplus/herbalmedicine.html
National Cancer Institute
http://www.nci.nih.gov/cancertopics/treatment/cam
National Center for Complementary and Alternative Medicine (NCCAM)
http://nccam.nih.gov/
Office of Dietary Supplements (ODS)
http://ods.od.nih.gov/
Quackwatch
http://www.quackwatch.org/

Section 21

PAIN AND PALLIATION

66

Palliative Care

Natalie Moryl, MD
Alan C. Carver, MD
Kathleen M. Foley, MD

Palliative care is the term used to describe an interdisciplinary model of care, which is patient and family centered, and that focuses on the management of physical, psychological, and social distress with its major goal being to improve the quality of life of patients. Palliative care is now recognized as one of the four essential aspects of national cancer control programs, along with prevention, early diagnosis, and treatment. In 1982, the World Health Organization, in developing its national cancer control strategies, defined palliative care as "the active total care of patients' whose disease is not responsive to curative treatment."[1] In 2002, the WHO adapted its definition of palliative care to emphasize the importance of symptom control and supportive therapies throughout the continuum of cancer assessment and treatment. Evolution in thinking about the role of palliative care is reflected in the widening of the focus of palliative care in the modern society from treating suffering to prevention of needless suffering. WHO defined palliative care as "an approach which improves the quality of life of patients and families facing life-threatening illness through the prevention and relief of suffering by means of early identification and impeccable assessment and treatment of pain and other problems physical, psychosocial and spiritual."

The WHO's cancer and palliative care unit has developed a series of monographs addressing the principles and practice of palliative care for both adults and children with cancer. These include publications on cancer pain relief, guidelines for opioid availability, symptom relief in terminal illness, and palliative care for both adults and children with cancer.[2–5] The WHO has been the major advocate for palliative care's integration in international strategies for patients with cancer, for care of the elderly, for children, for patients with HIV/AIDS. It has recently published two monographs the "Solid Facts of Palliative Care" and "Better Care of the Elderly" to better inform policy makers who are interested in integrating palliative care in national health strategies.[6,7] These monographs emphasize palliative care as an important aspect of public health strategies for chronic illness.[8]

The availability and implementation of palliative care services need to be balanced with other cancer care services. Symptom control and supportive therapies are necessary throughout the patient's illness, with the proportion of palliative care services varying with the patient's trajectory of illness, and the setting of care. In developing countries where cancer patients present late in their illness and no antitumor therapies are available or effective, palliative care may be the main therapy provided. In developed countries where early diagnosis is possible and disease-specific therapies are available, palliative care services enhance cancer care, addressing symptoms and quality of life concerns.

Palliative medicine is the term used to describe the medical specialty that involves the study and management of patients who have active progressive disease from incurable illness. In line with the aging of the population in the developed countries, increasingly more people die as a result of chronic illness including cancer. After reaching the age of 65, people now live on average another 12 to 22 years, with France and Japan having the highest life expectancies. As of now increased longevity is accompanied by a longer period of disability towards the end of life. In the United States up to 50% of Medicare payments are presently spent in the last six months of the person's life. At the same time, with smaller dispersed families and other changes in social structure the numbers of informal caregivers will be decreasing. Public movements toward increasing patient's autonomy and dignified death fueled by the media coverage of a series of end-of-life controversies brought the issues of the end-of-life care to the attention of the society. Oncologists therefore will find themselves challenged to provide compassionate and cost-effective care for a larger proportion of the advanced cancer patients in their practice. Core competencies of the oncologist are essential for establishing and developing the relationship with the patient and the medical team and for preventing burnout for the oncologist.

There are well-established curricula, masters programs, fellowship programs, and faculty development programs in palliative care both within the United States and internationally. Britain, Sweden, Norway, Australia, and Canada have recognized palliative medicine as a medical specialty and have designated university chairs in palliative medicine. In the United States, there are both physician and nurse certification programs, identifying those trained with special expertise in palliative care.

In the United States, three Institute of Medicine reports have emphasized the importance of palliative care as an integral part of our healthcare delivery system. In 1997, the Institute of Medicine issued the report entitled "Approaching Death," identifying serious barriers to the provision of palliative care in the United States (Table 66-1). The report made seven recommendations, emphasizing the lack of knowledge and competency of health care professionals as major limiting factors in the provision of palliative care to Americans. Two reports from the National Cancer Policy Board of the Institute of Medicine declared the provision of palliative care to be a quality cancer care issue and devoted one entire report, entitled "Improving Palliative Care for Cancer," to the subject to under-

Table 66-1 The Institute of Medicine's Recommendations for Improving End-of-Life Care

Recommendation #1: People with advanced, potentially fatal illnesses and those close to them should be able to expect and receive reliable, skillful, and supportive care.

Recommendation #2: Physicians, nurses, social workers, and other health professionals must commit themselves to improving care for dying patients and to using existing knowledge effectively to prevent and relieve pain and other symptoms.

Recommendation #3: Because many problems in care stem from system problems, policymakers, consumer groups, and purchasers of healthcare should work with healthcare practitioners, organizations, and researchers to:

a. strengthen methods for measuring the quality of life and other outcomes of care for dying patients and those close to them;
b. develop better tools and strategies for improving the quality of care and holding healthcare organizations accountable for care at the end of life;
c. revise mechanisms for financing care so that they encourage rather than impede good end of life care and sustain rather than frustrate coordinated systems of excellent care; and
d. reform drug prescription laws, burdensome regulations, and state medical board policies and practices that impede effective use of opioids to relieve pain and suffering.

Recommendation #4: Educators and other health professionals should initiate changes in undergraduate, graduate, and continuing education to ensure that practitioners have relevant attitudes, knowledge, and skills to care well for dying patients.

Recommendation #5: Palliative care should become, if not a medical specialty, at least a defined area of expertise, education, and research.

Recommendation #6: The nation's research establishment should define and implement priorities for strengthening the knowledge base for end-of-life care.

Recommendation #7: A continuing public discussion is essential to develop a better understanding of the modern experience of dying, the options available to patients and families, and the obligations of communities to those approaching death.

Adapted from Field MJ and Cassel CK, editors.

score the evidence base for advancing palliative care services, research, and education in the United States as a quality care issue for patients with cancer. The report strongly argues that "in our accepting a single-minded focus on research toward cure, we have inadvertently devalued the critical need to care and support patients with advanced disease and their families."[9]

In 2002, *US News and World Report* began including palliative care in its criteria for its annual hospital ranking: "This year, hospice and palliative care were added to certain specialties because of increasingly recognized importance of end-of-life issues and pain management". A growing number of hospital administrators have found that introduction of palliative care services helps their institutions meet JCAHO standards for pain and other quality measures while also meeting clear patient needs.

Concurrent with these national policy documents identifying the need for research and education in palliative care there are growing, broad, nongovernmental efforts to advance professional education for physicians, nurses, social workers, and other health care professionals. Thus, the American Medical Association and the American Board of Internal Medicine have developed initiatives in continuing education for physicians in practice and competency criteria for residents in training.[10,11]

This chapter focuses on the oncologist's role in providing palliative care and the importance of such care as a fundamental aspect of treating patients with cancer.

ROLE OF THE ONCOLOGIST

In 1998, a Task Force of the American Society of Clinical Oncology (ASCO) surveyed its members and issued a statement strongly supporting the need to provide excellent palliative and end of life care: ASCO believes that provision of optimal end-of-life care requires access to and availability of state-of-the-art palliative care rendered by skilled clinicians, buttressed when necessary, by palliative care experts.[7] The survey identified the key barriers, including serious shortcomings, in the training and current practices of a large proportion of oncologists. Most oncologists reported that they have not had formal training in the key skills needed to provide excellent palliative and end-of-life care. Fewer than one-third of oncologists reported their training as very helpful in communicating with dying patients, coordinating their care, shifting to the focus of palliative care, or beginning hospice care. Fewer than 6% felt that they could arrange for their patients to get all of the services that they need and 56% reported that a palliative care team was either not available or not easy to access.

Numerous specific barriers were identified in this survey, including inappropriate attitudes of healthcare professionals and patients toward death, ineffective communication, fragmentation of care, and patients' and their families' unrealistic expectations of treatment options. To remove the barriers, ASCO emphasizes a "humane system of cancer care based on these principles:

1. Cancer care is centered around the long-standing and continuous relationship between the primary oncologist or another physician with training and interest in end-of-life care and the patient;
2. Cancer care is responsive to the patient's wishes and to the parents' wishes if the patient is a child;
3. Cancer care is based on truthful, sensitive, empathic communication with the patient, and in the case of pediatric patients, that care is both family centered as well as child focused; Cancer care optimizes quality of life throughout the course of an illness through meticulous attention to the myriad physical, spiritual, and psychosocial needs of the patient and family.[12]

For most patients, the medical oncologist is the primary provider of cancer treatment and is therefore in a unique position to coordinate the delivery of antitumor therapies as well as a wide range of care, including palliative care. In one prospective survey of a large teaching hospital, 23% of patients admitted to the oncology unit were admitted solely for palliative care issues. In this unit, palliative care activity accounted for 34% (169 bed days) of daily activity, as compared with 32% (163 bed days) for the administration of chemotherapy.

Symptom burden and health-related quality of life deteriorate as disease progresses and may serve as prognostic clues in patients with terminal cancer.[13] It is critical that oncologists develop expertise in palliative care including end-of-life care by mastering a series of skills, including skills in communication, decision making, management of complications of treatment and disease, symptom control, psychological care of the patient and the family, and the care of the dying patient.[12]

COMMUNICATION

Communication regarding treatment options, prognosis, advanced directives, and patient and family support, is vital to the development of a relationship between the oncologist and the patient. A major tenet of palliative medicine is the understanding that the oncologist will remain involved in every aspect of their care up to and including the moment of death. If properly communicated, this promise will assure the patient that the patient's physician will not abandon the patient should antitumor therapies fail, but will provide vigilant attention to symptom control and quality of life for the patient and support for the family for every stage of illness. As previously noted in the ASCO survey, communicating with patients with advanced cancer and their families is hampered by lack of physician training in communication with dying patients. Communicating at the end of life is usually a self-taught skill. Observed by an investigator, physicians discussed DNR with their patients on the average of 5.6 min (0.9 to 15 minutes), out of which physicians spoke for 3.9 minutes and patients spoke for 1.7 minutes.[14]

Fallowfield and colleagues report that among 178 oncologists who attended a recent course on communication skills, fewer than 35% had received any previous communications training. Although time, experience, and seniority alone had not improved their skills prior to the course, 95% of the physicians in attendance reported significant changes in their clinical practice following the seminars. In addition, 75% began to teach what they had learned about communication to other faculty.[11]

ASCO is now developing a series of educational initiatives to enhance oncologist competency.

Breaking Bad News One of the greatest challenges oncologists face is knowing when and how to tell the patient and the patient's family that the treatments are not working or cannot be tolerated. Questions about the prognosis and the patient's life expectancy may need to be answered, and details of the dying process may need to be discussed. This is a stressful task that requires knowledge about prognostic signs, communication skills, and sensitivity. Patients' requirements for knowledge vary greatly.[15,16] For some patients, candid supportive discussion enables participation in the planning of their remaining time until death, whereas for others, the news comes as a crushing blow from which they do not have the coping resources to recover. For the latter patients, truth can be an assault.[17] Buckman outlined a protocol for breaking bad news, which includes the following elements, among others.[18]

1. The setting should be private and quiet. The patient should have the opportunity to invite other significant family members to join in the discussion. The physician should sit at eye level or below that of the patient.
2. Ascertain the patient's current level of knowledge, how much the patient wants to know, and share information consistent with the patient's desire for knowledge. When patients say that they know nothing at all, or if there is a major discrepancy between their impression and the actual facts, this may indicate that they wish to maintain their coping mechanism of denial.
3. Respond to the patient's feelings. Supportive and empathic listening skills are critical in this interaction. The quality of the physician-patient relationship, and whether it will be a supportive one, is largely determined by the way in which the oncologist responds to the patient's feelings in this sort of dialogue.
4. Organize and plan. Buckman suggests reviewing the patient's problem list distinguishing between remediable and nonremediable problems, proposing therapeutic solutions to solvable problems, and identifying and reinforcing the patient's coping resources, as well as identifying other sources of support that can be integrated into the care plan.

It has been increasingly recognized that discontinuation of active antitumor treatment is the most important decision for the majority of patients. Such discussion may be much more threatening than discussion about resuscitation. Shared decision making with the patient and the patient's family may be extremely effective in preserving the sense of control in a patient and at the same time facilitating open dialogue.

Racial and Cultural Barriers to Palliative Care Clinicians should be aware of cultural differences in attitudes toward communications and patient autonomy. In a recent study of 800 patients, 200 in each group were interviewed in 31 senior citizen centers in California about their preferences in sharing information.[19] A series of questions were asked of the elderly patients of different descent and the percent of the patients that answered "yes" included:

1. "The patient should be told the diagnosis of metastatic cancer"
   - Korean Americans 47%
   - Mexican Americans 65%
   - European Americans 87%
   - African Americans 88%
2. "The patient should be told of terminal prognosis"
   - Korean Americans 35%
   - Mexican Americans 48%
   - European Americans 69%
   - African Americans 63%
3. "The patient should make decisions about the use of life-supporting technology"
   - Korean Americans 28%
   - Mexican Americans 41%
   - European Americans 65%
   - African Americans 60%

Recognizing personal cultural preferences of the patients and their families, the physician needs flexibility and expertise in communication to deliver the information to the patient and the caregiver in manner that is legally, ethically, and medically acceptable.

In caring for patients in our diverse society, a full spectrum of the end-of-line treatment preferences should be considered. Differences in the religious preferences, lack of access to health care, greater negative perceptions about quality of hospital care in blacks than whites and other factors should be acknowledged and accepted. Historic racial discrepancies are striking and may be well known to the underserved population. Clinicians providing palliative care should be aware of some of the issues that may influence patient's decisions:

- Hospitals and health facilities were racially segregated before 1960s,
- Studies reveal that African-Americans receive less resource intensive care despite preferences for more life,
- Much evidence that current options for end-of-life care is not a good "fit" for minorities,
- Less than 10% of all hospice patients are African-American,
- Questionable interpretation of the "goals of care" in context of incomplete access to full medical care.

Current access to medical care remains unequal. For example African-Americans are less likely to receive surgery for lung cancer.[20] Current data regarding the lack of access to health care is shaping attitudes about EOL care:

- African-Americans are less likely to opt for discontinuation of life-support measures because of the perception that they may be treated differently and receive inferior care if advanced directives are signed,
- African-Americans are more likely to opt for aggressive treatment interventions (eg, dialysis, artificial nutrition, surgery, etc.) even if in a persistent vegetative state,[21]
- African-Americans want to live as long as possible almost under any circumstances,[22]
- African-Americans physicians placed higher value on length of life than European-American physicians. They are more likely to support CPR, mechanical ventilation, dialysis, and artificial feeding for themselves if they were in a persistent vegetative state. [23]

Influence of the physician's race on the physician's attitudes regarding the end-of-life issues were explored a few years ago.[24] The differences between white and African-American physicians were quite distinct:

- Are tube feedings "heroic" in terminally ill patients? Yes: 58% white MDs; 28% black MDs ($p < .001$), Is MD-assisted suicide an acceptable treatment alternative? Yes: 36% white MDs; 26.5% black MDs ($p < 0.05$)
- Preferences for treatment if in a persistent vegetative state. Black MDs 6 times more likely than white MDs to request aggressive treatment for themselves ($p < .001$).

Understanding the different cultural backgrounds of patients is important. Generalizations, however, should be avoided. If appropriate, family and religious leaders may be asked to help in communications about the end-of-life care. Each patient should be assessed individually and in the context of his or her social group, religious preferences and racial historical and perceived differences.

SYMPTOM MANAGEMENT

Control of pain and other physical and psychological symptoms, and of existential distress are the major goals of palliative care. Cancer patients report at least eight major symptoms that interfere with their quality of life. Multiple surveys of cancer patients have demonstrated a high prevalence of pain, fatigue, weakness, dyspnea, delirium, nausea, vomiting, depression, and anxiety (Table 66-2). Portenoy and colleagues developed a validated tool to assess symptom prevalence, intensity and frequency, and to evaluate their impact on patients' quality of life.[25] By using the Memorial Symptom Assessment Scale, they reported that among 246 patients receiving active treatment, independent of tumor type, 40 to 80% experienced lack of energy, pain, drowsiness, dry mouth, insomnia, or psychological distress. The mean number of symptoms per patient was 11.5.[26–28] The prevalence of symptoms in cancer patients 4 weeks and 1 week before death is shown in Table 66-2.[29]

The management of pain and psychiatric symptoms is thoroughly discussed elsewhere in this textbook.

Dyspnea Dyspnea represents a major symptom that commonly increases in prevalence in dying patients. The prevalence of dyspnea in advanced cancer patients varies between 29 and 74%.[29] It is frequently one of the most difficult symptoms to treat and for many patients, there may be no more frightening sensation than that of air hunger. The causes of dyspnea in cancer patients are outlined in Table 66-3.[30] Both antitumor and palliative thera-

Table 66-2 Prevalence of Symptoms Volunteered by Advanced Cancer Patients 4 Weeks and 1 Week Before Death (*n* = 90)

	n (%)	
Symptom	4 Weeks Before Death	1 Week Before Death
Fatigue	52 (58)	47 (52)
Pain	49 (54)	31 (34)
Generalized weakness	39 (43)	44 (49)
Mental haziness/confusion	22 (24)	51 (57)
Anxiety	19 (21)	16 (18)
Weakness of legs	16 (18)	15 (17)
Shortness of breath	15 (17)	25 (28)
Nausea	11 (12)	12 (13)
Decreased hearing	8 (9)	5 (6)
Depression	7 (8)	4 (4)
Loss of appetite	7 (8)	5 (6)
Inability to sleep	6 (7)	5 (6)
Weakness of upper limb	6 (7)	5 (6)
Cough	5 (6)	6 (7)
Restlessness/irritability	5 (6)	6 (7)
Swollen limb	4 (4)	7 (8)
Constipation	5 (4)	6 (7)
Difficulty swallowing	3 (3)	6 (7)
Pulmonary congestion	1 (1)	5 (6)
Dizziness	1 (1)	5 (6)
Incontinence	3 (3)	5 (6)
Difficulty speaking	5 (6)	5 (6)

Reprinted from Coyle N, Adelhardt J, Foley KM, Portenoy PK, Character of Terminal Illness in the Advanced Cancer Patient: Pain and Other Symptoms During the Last Four Weeks of Life, J Pain Symptom Manage 1990;5:83–93.

pies are available and often need to be combined. Chemotherapy, radiation therapy, or surgery may be the most helpful in providing lasting relief. Radiotherapy may relieve a blocked bronchial passage even after a single treatment and may be useful not only as an antitumor agent but also in the palliation of breathlessness.[31,32] Pleurocentesis and aggressive diuretic therapy are useful in dyspnea caused by pleural effusion. Palliative approaches include bronchodilators, corticosteroids, intravenous, or inhaled morphine.[32] Blood transfusion, widely used during chemotherapy, may become a subject of controversy when given to terminally ill patients. This decision is greatly influenced by the personal views of the medical team. A recent survey of 500 physicians and nurses revealed that dyspnea, worsening congestive heart failure, active bleeding, functional deterioration, and hemoglobin level less than 7 mg/dL usually trigger a consideration of blood transfusion.[33] These agreed-on suggestions for transfusion in terminally ill cancer patients may serve as a reasonable standard for this complex medical and ethical issue.

Oxygen is a commonly used medication that usually provides some improvement. It is indicated in symptomatic hypoxia or hypercarbia presenting as severe fatigue, dyspnea or changes in mental status. Without hypoxia and hypercarbia, oxygen may be helpful by providing a cooling sensation to the face or nasal cavity. Low dose intravenous morphine is the treatment of choice for dyspnea in advanced cancer patients with the goal of striking a balance between a patient's level of comfort and sedation. Nebulized morphine has been reported to be effective in several positive case reports, but results from several small studies do not support its routine use in dyspnea.[34] Morphine reduces excessive respiratory drive and significantly decreases ventilation in response to borderline hypoxia and hypercarbia.[35] Morphine decreases the sensation of air hunger and by slowing respirations makes breathing more efficient. In a patient with high risk of hypercarbia such as in a patient with COPD, morphine can cause CO_2 retention that will not be reversed by naloxone. Intubation may be considered if appropriate. In dying patients, naloxone and intubation for CO_2 retention are contraindicated. Sedation may be necessary to control dyspnea in the imminently dying.[36,37] Anxiolytic medications such as short-acting benzodiazepines may also be helpful to reduce sensation of breathlessness and decrease anxiety associated with it.

Table 66-3 Causes of Dyspnea in Cancer Patients

Dyspnea directly caused by cancer
- Pulmonary parenchymal involvement (primary or metastatic)
- Lymphangitic carcinomatosis
- Intrinsic or extrinsic airways obstruction by tumor
- Pleural tumor
- Pleural effusion
- Pericardial effusion
- Ascites
- Hepatomegaly
- Phrenic nerve paralysis
- Multiple tumor microemboli
- Pulmonary leukostasis
- Superior vena cava syndrome

Dyspnea indirectly caused by cancer
- Cachexia
- Electrolyte abnormalities
- Anemia
- Pneumonia
- Pulmonary aspiration
- Pulmonary emboli
- Neurologic paraneoplastic syndromes

Dyspnea caused by cancer treatment
- Surgery
- Radiation therapy
- Chemotherapy-induced pulmonary disease
- Chemotherapy-induced cardiomyopathy

Dyspnea unrelated to cancer
- Chronic obstructive pulmonary disease
- Asthma
- Congestive heart failure
- Interstitial lung disease
- Pneumothorax
- Anxiety
- Chest wall deformity
- Obesity
- Neuromuscular disorders
- Pulmonary vascular disease
- Fever

Reprinted with modifications from Dudgeon DJ., Rosenthal S., Management of Dyspnea and Cough in Patients with Cancer, In Cherny NI, Foley KM, (eds.) Pain and Palliative care, Hematology/Oncology Clinics of North America, Vol. 10, N0.1 February 1996, pg. 159.

The majority of cases of superior vena cava obstruction are seen in lung cancer patients (80%) although the condition may be seen in patients with lymphoma (15%), breast, testicular, and other carcinomas.[38,39] The onset of superior vena cava (SVC) syndrome may be seen early in the disease, often preceding the tissue diagnosis of cancer. Tissue diagnosis and pathophysiologic treatment, including chemotherapy and radiation therapy, constitute standard approaches. In the case of a medical emergency, such as airway compromise, cerebral dysfunction, spinal cord compression, or decreased cardiac output, aggressive diuresis and high-dose steroids are usually administered, although evidence-based proof of this approach is limited in cases other then neurologic emergencies.[40]

The National Hospice Study found that nausea and vomiting occurred in 62% of cancer patients in the last 6 months of life.[41] The management of these symptoms requires addressing psychological, physiologic, and physical factors.[42] Reduction of anticipatory nausea and anxiety, serving meals in small portions, correction of constipation and of decreased gastric motility, and treatment of mechanical bowel obstruction are commonly needed interventions.[43,44] Intractable nausea and vomiting caused by brain metastases or by radiation therapy to the gastrointestinal (GI) tract or brain may respond to high-dose steroids. Nausea caused by oral thrush and GI tract candidiasis responds to antifungal medications. Metabolic abnormalities such as uremia and hypercalcemia are also likely to cause nausea and should be adjusted as needed.

Identifying the reversible causes of nausea and vomiting and addressing them may include the following:

- Reviewing and discontinuing all nonessential medications (chemotherapeutic agents, antibiotics, iron, carbamazepine, digoxin, and others).
- Reducing the opioid dose when possible, changing the route of opioid administration to parenteral, or changing the opioid itself. Lipid-soluble opioids such as fentanyl and methadone are less likely to cause or worsen nausea than morphine.
- Removing irritating or offensive odors such as perfumes, wound or colostomy smell, or odor of food between meals.
- Correcting electrolyte abnormalities.

Medications such as metoclopramide 10 to 20 mg q6 to 8h, meclizine 25 mg bid, lorazepam 0.5 mg q4h prn, haloperidol 0.5 mg q8h, or scopolamine 1.5 to 3 mg transdermal q3d, may be given as a single agent or in drug combinations targeting the multifactorial nature of nausea and vomiting (Table 66-4). Steroids may be very effective with a rapid onset of therapeutic action (hours), but risks and benefits of high-dose steroid should be considered and discussed with the patient. Ondansetron or granisetron may be effective, but are lacking in proof of their therapeutic advantage over traditional antinausea medications, except in the setting of chemotherapy or radiation therapy. Octreotide decreases the volume of fluids within the intestine

Table 66-4 Common Antiemetics in Palliative Care

Drug	Dosage	Side Effects
Haloperidol	1.6–20 mg/d	Dystonias, akathisia
Metoclopramide	10–30 mg q2–4h	Dystonias, esophageal spasm
Domperidone	10–30 mg PO, 30–90 mg pr q4–8h	Colic if obstructed, esophageal pain
Prochlorperazine	5–20 mg PO, 12–25 mg IM, 25 mg pr, q6–8h	Sedation, hypotension
Cyclizine	25–50 mg PO/SC/pr q8h	Dry mouth, blurred vision, sedation
Ondansetron	8 mg PO/IV q8h	Headache, constipation/diarrhea
Decadron	2–10 mg PO/IV q6h	Hyperglycemia, GI bleed
Scopolamine	1.5–3 mg transdermal q3d	Dry mouth, confusion
Lorazepam	0.5–2 mg PO/IV q3–6h	Sedation
Granisetron	1–2 mg PO/IV/d	Headache
Palonosetron	0.25 mg IV once	Headache
Dronabinol	5–10 mg PO	Psychiatric

GI = gastrointestinal; IM = intramuscularly; NSAID = nonsteroidal anti-inflammatory drug; SC = subcutaneously.
Adapted from Mannix KA[31a] and from Waller A, Caroline NL. Palliative Care in Cancer. 2nd ed. Butterworth-Heinemann; 2000. p. 188–189.

and has been increasingly used for nausea and vomiting caused by bowel obstruction. Cannabinoids, that is, dronabinol, are approved for the treatment of cancer-associated nausea, but their use is limited (see Table 66-3). Corticosteroids are the most potent antiemetics and appetite stimulants and may be advantageous for the end-of-life patients with intractable nausea.

Constipation, Ileus, Bowel Obstruction Constipation is characterized by difficult or painful defecation, infrequent bowel evacuations, and hard, small feces. Most common causes of constipation in cancer patients include medications such as opioids, diuretics, anticholenergics, iron, ondansetron, and nonsteroidal anti-inflammatoryh drugs. Dehydration, immobility and electrolyte disturbances, hypercalcemia in particular can worsen constipation. Constipation caused by spinal cord compression is on of the most challenging to manage. In patients with cancer, opioids are the most common cause of constipation. μ-Agonist induced constipation results from a cascade of changes that opioids cause in the GI tract: diminished or abolished propulsive peristalsis waves in the colon, increased bowel tone to the point of spasm, increased water absorption because of the delayed passage of bowel contents, decreased intestinal secretions, and increased tone of the anal sphincter with reduced response to rectal dilatation. Constipation should be prevented or treated as soon as possible. The most common effective combination is a stool softener and a stimulant, but a variety of laxative combinations may be effective (Table 66-5). Increased fluid intake and increased activity, if possible, are recommended.

Naloxone or its derivatives are μ-opioid antagonists that may be considered in persistent uncontrolled opioid-induced constipation and ileus. In a double-blind, randomized, placebo-controlled study of 4 mg or 2 mg of oral naloxone, or placebo, given three times daily, all the patients who received oral naloxone had some improvement in their bowel frequency, but about 30% of the patients also experienced reversal of analgesia. Subcutaneous methylnaltrexone may reverse the opioid-induced bowel symptoms. It's advantage is the fact that it is unable to cross the blood-brain barrier. This feature makes it effective in eliminating unwanted effects on opiate receptors in gut and skin while retaining the pain relieving activity of opioids in the brain and spinal cord. In more than 90% of patients, relief from constipation came within a few minutes of the first administration. This is promising medication that soon will be available for clinical use.

Ileus Intestinal distention and the slowing or absence of passage of luminal contents without a demonstratable mechanical obstruction. The most common causes of ileus are medications (opioids, psychotropics, anticholinergics), intestinal ischemia or sepsis, spinal cord injury, metabolic and electrolyte abnormalities (hypokalemia, hyponatremia, hypomagnesemia, uremia, uncontrolled diabetes), and surgery or abdominal infection.

Mechanical Bowel Obstruction Mechanical bowel obstruction occurs in 3% of advanced cancer patients, and is seen most frequently with ovarian or colon cancer. It is characterized by rapidly escalating abdominal pain and vomiting. In up to 35% of cases, bowel obstruction results from either benign causes such as adhesions or new primary tumor that may be resected. Mortality can be as high as 55%.[45,46] The possibility of consecutive reobstruction in up to 57% of patients, sepsis, and fistula formation should be considered when weighing the pros and cons of surgical intervention. If the performance status of the patient is significantly impaired or if the patient declines surgical intervention, short-term nasogastric suctioning or use of percutaneous draining gastrostomies may be considered. In those patients who are not candidates for surgical intervention, bowel obstruction may be treated with decreased oral intake, treatment of nausea, correction of electrolyte abnormalities, rehydration, and systemic analgesia. Opioids are the most effective drugs for management of abdominal pain both continuous and colicky. Alternatively the opioid-sparing agents can be used: anticholinergics (effective for colicky pain not controlled with opioids alone), octreotide, ketorolac, steroids, and ketamine. Parenteral administration of fluids and medication is preferred.[47]

Intractable vomiting caused by intestinal obstruction may be diminished by the continuous subcutaneous infusion of octreotide (0.3 to 0.6 mg/24 h).[48] Octreotide, a somatostatin analogue, reduces the volume of gastrointestinal secretions by decreasing the secretion of water, sodium, and chloride, and by stimulating the absorption of water and other electrolytes.[49] The role of corticosteroids in this setting is controversial. A Cochrane Database Systematic Revue analyzed three unpublished, randomized, placebo, double-blind controlled trials and seven pub-

Table 66-5 Common Laxatives in Palliative Care

Category	Mechanism of Action	Time to the Onset of Action
Stimulants (most commonly used)		
Senna	Must transform to active metabolite	8–12 h
	Works only in the large bowel	
	Stimulates peristalsis of the large bowel	
Bisacodyl	Can cause abdominal cramps	10–24 h (oral)
		20–60 min (supps)
Stool softeners (most commonly used)		
Docusate	Reduce stool surface tension	1–3 days
	Increase water penetration into the stool	
	Increases secretion of fluids in small and large bowel	
Osmotic laxatives	Not absorbed from the gut	
Polyethylene glycol	Retain water in the lumen	
Lactulose	Increase stool volume	48 h
	Increase peristalsis	
	Requires high fluid intake to work	
	May cause nausea and abdominal distention	
Suppositories	Avoid in immunocompromised	
	Avoid when thrombocytopenic	
Bisacodyl		20–60 min
Glycerine		1–6 h
Bulk forming agents		
Psyllium	Increases stool bulk	2–4 days of daily use
	Increases water content	
	Requires high fluid intake to work	

lished (prospective and retrospective) trials. The data were suggestive of a trend (not statistically significant) for the resolution of bowel obstruction using corticosteroids without a statistically significant difference in mortality at one month. The morbidity associated with corticosteroids appeared to be very low. Dexamethasone 6 to 16 mg intravenously may bring about the resolution of bowel obstruction.[50]

Delirium Delirium is common in patients with advanced cancer at or near death. In one series, 85% of patients dying of cancer developed delirium.[51] Symptoms include waxing and waning level of consciousness, disturbance in the sleep–wake cycle, disorientation, visual or auditory hallucinations, and memory and language disturbances. Several assessment scales have been developed, including the Delirium Rating Scale, which is a 10-item clinician-rated measurement.[52] Most commonly, delirium is the indirect result of the patient's underlying cancer (eg, metabolic disarrangement, treatment side effect, infection, nutritional deficiencies, and others). Management of delirium generally involves discontinuing all medications that are not absolutely necessary, especially psychoactive drugs. Intravenous or oral haloperidol, starting at 0.5 mg bid is the drug of choice and may be titrated upward safely for clinical effect. Other useful neuroleptic drugs include chlorpromazine (available in intravenous form), risperidone, and olanzapine (now available in transmucosal form). Alternative strategies in the dying patient include the use of benzodiazepine (midazolam) and barbiturate (pentobarbital) infusions,[53,54] although in some instances, even short-acting benzodiazepines, that is, lorazepam, may worsen delirium by further sedating and disinhibiting the patient or by causing a paradoxical agitation.

CANCER FATIGUE

Severe, debilitating fatigue is now recognized as an independent symptom interfering with quality of life and more prevalent than pain. In a recent study among females receiving chemotherapy for gynecologic cancers a mean fatigue score was 6.48 on a scale of 0 to 10. On a 0 to 4 scale, women reported mean fatigue distress of 2.21. A majority (59%) had not communicated with their health care providers about fatigue at their last appointments, and 56% reported never receiving recommendations for managing fatigue.[55] Fatigue can affect performance status or remain a subjective symptom. Numerous causes of fatigue including cachexia, mood disorders, hypogonadism, cognitive impairment, anemia, hypothyroidism, and infections should be looked for and addressed when possible. Pharmacologic treatment of fatigue includes corticosteroids, amphetamines, and megestrol. Considering existence of level 1 clinical evidence, corticosteroids are often the drug of choice. Psychostimulants are commonly used for opioid induced sedation. Megestrol improves quality of life and affects fatigue in ways other than due to weight gain. Methylphenidate's effects on cancer fatigue are related to its effect on mood and cognition and decrease of opioid induced sedation. In patients with hypogonadism testosterone may be used, but more data are needed to incorporate it into the guidelines for fatigue treatment. Other medications used to treat cancer fatigue include thalidomide and selective serotonin reuptake inhibitors. Nonpharmacologic interventions include counseling, physiotherapy, and occupational therapy.

ROLE OF NUTRITION AND HYDRATION

Cancer cachexia has been increasingly recognized as a separate entity difficult to reverse. It is especially common in such malignancies as pancreatic, gastric and esophageal carcinoma. There is no correlation between the tumor bulk and degree of cachexia, except in breast carcinoma. Total parenteral nutrition (TPN) failed to improve survival in any of the patients with cancer who were studied.[56] In fact, even in healthy people, TPN does not offer protein restoration.[57] The provision of artificial nutrition and hydration is a controversial topic. One may consider TPN only for selected patients: support through recovery from surgery, radiation, or bone marrow transplantation, and in patients with ovarian carcinoma with bowel obstruction but otherwise high performance status. After being started, TPN becomes even more of an ethical problem since it is difficult to stop in both adults and children, thus it should be initiated with discretion. If oral enteral feeding is not possible, gastrostomy or jejunostomy tubes may be used. Gastrostomy, however, may be associated with the risks of aspiration, skin erosion, electrolyte disturbances, diarrhea, and abdominal distention. In the terminal cancer patient the goals, risks, and benefits of artificial nutrition and hydration should be weighed and discussed with the family. Loss of appetite, inability to process the food force-fed by the family, and the possibility of its becoming a burden to the patient should be taken into consideration. Hydration in some instances may reduce nausea and temporarily improve mental status, but it does not change xerostomia or thirst. Some authors suggest that the cessation of intravenous fluids decreases pulmonary secretions and coughing, and reduces the need for suctioning.[58]

For some families, there is great symbolic meaning to the provision of food and water and the withholding and withdrawal of such support may be associated with feelings of guilt or abandonment.[59] In the setting of advanced cancer, the request to withhold nutrition and hydration can be made by the patient or the health care proxy. Such a request should be explored, discussed with the other caregivers, including family members and staff, and be granted, unless depression or delirium impairs the patient's understanding of the implications of such decision or a malicious intent is suspected. The current national ethical and legal guidelines support the patient's right to refuse nutrition and hydration, as well as the right of the patient and healthcare proxy to withdraw such support.

Sedation in the Imminently Dying For the vast majority of cancer patients, even in the setting of terminal disease, close adherence to established pain management (see Chapter 67, "Management of Cancer Pain") and other guidelines will provide adequate symptom relief. For refractory symptoms, however, the alternative of induced sedation may be helpful in relieving distress and assuring a dignified death. Ventafridda reported that up to 50% of 120 patients in a home-based palliative care program in Italy required sedation to control intractable symptoms of dyspnea, delirium, nausea, and vomiting. Careful attention to the evaluation of symptoms and the applications of detailed specific algorithms is described in palliative care textbooks.[57,60,61]

In deciding that a symptom is refractory, the clinician must perceive that further invasive and noninvasive interventions are (1) incapable of providing adequate relief, (2) associated with excessive and intolerable acute or chronic morbidity, or (3) unlikely to provide relief within a tolerable time frame.[62] Deciding to accept sedation as an unavoidable side effect in order to optimally manage delirium, severe dyspnea, and intractable pain should occur within the setting of a patient, family, and caregiver team. Inability to continue oral hydration and nutrition during moderate to severe sedation may need to be discussed. Artificial hydration and nutrition may be continued or stopped depending on the patient's wish and clinical situation. Use of a medication targeting the most disturbing symptom and the upward titration to symptom control is preferred. Development of new symptoms such as myoclonus or agitated delirium often necessitates the addition of a second agent. A benzodiazepine with a short half life, such as midazolam or lorazepam, is generally recommended.[63,64] Barbiturates may be used for refractory agitation.[65] Sedation is occasionally required for dying patients with otherwise refractory psychological symptoms of depression and anxiety or existential distress.

The ethical validity of this approach is derived from the principle of "double effect." This principle supports the use of medication that may risk respiratory depression to the point of death if such dose is required for symptomatic relief.[66] The major tenet of the principle of double effect is that there is a critical distinction between a foreseen but unintended outcome and a primarily intended outcome. The primary intention is relief of suffering, although the foreseen but unavoidable consequences may result in sedation or death. In addition, there are data that suggest that terminal patients who are given analgesics or sedatives for pain control do not die sooner than those who are not given such medications.[67]

A recent survey of neurologists in the United States revealed that 37% erroneously think it is illegal to administer analgesics in doses that risk respiratory depression to the point of death, and 39% agreed with the statement that treating dyspnea in a dying amyotrophic lateral sclerosis patient with enough morphine to decrease respiratory drive is equivalent to the practice of euthanasia.[68] These data suggest that there is a sizable gap between well-established medical guidelines that support sedation in the imminently dying when necessary for comfort, and the beliefs and practices of those surveyed. This raises important implications for education and training (see below). Palliative care clinicians should become comfortable with the ethical justification and technical expertise needed to provide sedation with continuous infusions of midazolam, thiopental, and propofol to patients in whom routine PRN (as needed) sedation does not adequately relieve suffering in their final days of life.[69]

Facing Death The role of the oncologist at the bedside of the dying patient is to provide adequate pain relief and other symptom control, as well as to offer support for grieving family and friends. The physician should attend not only to the patient's symptoms to assure comfort at the moment of death, but also to the family's grief and suffering. Many families, having perceived the oncologist as the guarantor of success of therapy throughout the disease progression, continue to identify the oncologist as a key person, directing the care and "delivering the promise" of "good death." Families vary in the degree of professional support and guidance that they require. It is the obligation of the oncologist to understand and be sensitive to the particular needs and dynamics of the patient's family and to provide that level of care that would be most helpful at such a difficult and sad time. Some families may prefer privacy with the knowledge that the physician is available though in the background in accordance with the family's particular needs.

It is important for families to know what to expect when the patient is imminently dying, including understanding agonal respirations and the frequent pooling of pharyngeal secretions often called the "death rattle." Decrease or discontinuation of intravenous fluids at that point may be helpful to decrease the amount of secretions. Transdermal or parenteral scopolamine can be useful in drying up the secretions, which can be a source of significant distress to family members at the bedside. If it is clear that death is imminent, it is often appropriate to indicate this to the family with the reassurance that the patient appears comfortable. The family's concerns should be elicited and explored, since this may help the family to preserve a sense of control. Reinforcing the family's participation in the decision making at this time may minimize the family's frustration and guilt, and may facilitate future bereavement. The clinician should tell the family when death has occurred and offer support and condolences. Some families may need to talk and cry at the bedside of the dead person kissing or hugging him or her. Adequate provision for time and privacy should always be made.

Personal contact with the family who has suffered loss of a loved one is often helpful not only for the family but also for the physician. All members of the care team may require some degree of emotional recuperation and they may benefit from meeting together to review the patient's life, illness, and death, to express emotions, and to address any outstanding issues or concerns. Because the relief of suffering is at the heart of palliative medicine, the opportunity to assure a comfortable and dignified death with sensitivity and kindness toward the grieving family may not only provide permanent meaning for the family but an incomparable sense of usefulness and reward for the care team. If the physician is not present at the time of death, families find great meaning when they receive cards or telephone calls expressing condolences. This may also facilitate closure for the physician.

Table 66-6 List of Factors Contributing to Patient Distress

Physical symptoms
Pain
Lack of energy
Feeling drowsy
Dry mouth
Lack of appetite
Nausea
Feeling bloated
Change in the way food tastes
Numbness/tingling in hands/ feet
Constipation
Cough
Swelling of arms or legs
Itching
Weight loss
Weight gain
Diarrhea
Dizziness
Problem with sexual interest or activity
Shortness of breath
Vomiting
Problems with urination
Difficulty swallowing
Psychological symptoms
Anxiety
Depression
Sleep disturbance
Irritability
Impaired concentration
Nightmares
Delirium
Existential concerns
Disrupted or distorted personal integrity
Changes in body image
Changes in body function
Concern for spouse and family
Changes in social and professional function
Diminished attractiveness as a sexual partner
Increased dependency
Distress from retrospection
Unfulfilled aspirations
Depreciation of the value of previous achievements
Remorse from unresolved guilt
Distress from future concerns
Separation
Hopelessness
Futility
Meaninglessness
Concerns about death
Religious concerns
Illness as a punishment
Fear of divine retribution
Fear of a void

SUFFERING IN THE PATIENT, FAMILY, AND PHYSICIAN

In addition to meticulous attention to symptom assessment and management, an appreciation of the suffering of the cancer patient as distinct from the patient's disease or other distressing symptoms (eg, pain) is of paramount importance. Cherny and colleagues defined suffering as "an aversive emotional experience characterized by the perception of personal distress that is generated by adverse factors undermining the quality of life."[70] They developed a taxonomy of factors that may contribute to distress among patients, families, and physicians. It is beyond the scope of this chapter to discuss these factors at length (Tables 66-6 to 66-9).

Caring for dying patients may be particularly stressful for medical oncologists whose professional goals and intellectual energies have been spent seeking curative therapies (see Table 66-9).[71] A survey of 81 general practitioners in France found that 86% agreed that encounters with death were a cause of physician suffering.[72] In that study, the major causes of physician suffering were ending of the doctor–patient relationship (58%), feelings of uselessness (55%) and failure (38%), increased awareness of the physicians' own mortality (49%), and the presence of "questions without answers" (31%). At the bedside of the dying patient, the most commonly reported feelings noted by the physicians in the study were sadness (94%), helplessness (89%), failure (61%),

Table 66-7 Factors Contributing to Distress in Family Members

Empathic suffering with patient (see Table 66-6)
Physical illness
Family dynamic
Family stability
Intrafamily conflict
Inability to work cohesively
Impending bereavement
Loss
The end of their life as they have known it
Finding a way of living together in anticipation of death
Role changes
Burdens of care
Physical
Psychological
Esthetic
Financial
Conflicts
Adequate relief of distressing symptoms vs preservation of alertness and avoiding the hastening of death
Duty to care for a loved one vs duty to care for oneself and one's other responsibilities
Distress related to health care services
Psychological
Anxiety, depression, etc.
Existential concerns
Distress from retrospection, future concerns, religious concerns

Adapted from Cherny NI, Coyle N, Foley KM, Suffering in the advanced Cancer Patient: A Definition and Taxonomy, J Palliative Care 1994; 10:2, 57–70.

Table 66-8 Factors Contributing to Distress Among Healthcare Providers

Empathic suffering with the patient (see Table 66-6)
Empathic suffering with the family (see Table 66-7)
Burdens of care
Frequent life-and-death decisions
Frequent exposure to death
Frequent exposure to profound emotional distress
High consumer expectations (patient and family)
Severe patient dependency (physical, emotional)
Severe patient disfigurement
Severe patient odor
Inadequate resources
Inadequate training to manage the prevailing patient and family problems
Inadequate assistance
Excessive workload
Conflict
With colleagues (substantive or style)
With patient and/or family (substantive or style)
With decision making for self in ambiguous circumstances
Duty to care for patient vs duty to care for oneself and one's other responsibilities
Psychological
Anxiety
Depression
Sleep disturbance
Substance abuse
Existential concerns
Distress from retrospection
Deprecation of the value of previous achievements
Guilt about limitations of therapeutic efficacy
Distress from future concerns
Futility
Meaningless
Concerns about death

Adapted from Cherny NI, Coyle N, Foley KM, Suffering in the advanced Cancer Patient: A Definition and Taxonomy, J Palliative Care 1994;10:2,57–70.

Table 66-9 Contributing Factors to Physician Distress in the Care of Dying Patients

Uncertainty and fear associated with cancer
High prevalence of side effects from cancer treatments
The palliative rather than curative nature of most interventions
Difficulties of therapeutic decision making
Difficulties in confronting patient and family reactions while continuing to treat the patient
Difficulties in communicating with others outside the workplace about the stresses to which he/she is exposed
Fear of death
Inadequate training in:
Communicating with dying patients
Communicating with the relatives of dying patients
Management of pain
Management of other physical symptoms
Psychological symptoms in dying patients
Collaborative practice with other care disciplines
Conflict regarding the goals of care
With self
With patient
With family
With colleagues
Unrealistic expectations of the clinician, colleagues, patient, or family
Uncertainty in decision making

Adapted from Cherny NI, Coyle RN, Foley KM. Guidelines in the Care of the Dying Cancer Patient. In: Cherny NI, Foley KM, editors Pain and Palliative care, Hematology/Oncology Clinics of North America 1996;10: 262.

disappointment (59%), and loneliness (51%). Eric Cassel explains, "suffering is experienced by persons, not merely by bodies, and has its source in challenges that threaten the intactness of the person as a complex social and psychological entity. Suffering can include physical pain, but is by no means limited to it. The relief of suffering and the cure of disease must be seen as twin obligations of a medical profession that is truly dedicated to the care of the sick."[73]

Barriers and Challenges for the Physician Several challenges have been identified as especially salient to the practicing oncologist who provides care for very sick and dying patients.[74] Care of cancer patients in advanced stages of the disease is time-consuming. Planning discussions of the goals of care in advance, preventing crises by appropriate communication early in the disease progression, preparing the patient and the family to expect symptoms, rather than responding to crises, and involvement of a multidisciplinary team to assess all the possible aspects of the patient's disease may improve care and save time.

1. "Death talk." Both social and medical models of care for the sick are usually devoid of discussion about death and dying, unless death has happened or death is imminent. Talking about dying, health care proxies, advance directives, and treatment preferences with the cancer patient should be incorporated into routine follow-up clinical visits.
2. "Failure." Failure of cancer-specific treatment to achieve cure may be falsely viewed by oncologists as personal physician failure. It is critical to acknowledge that in spite of the best treatment approximately 50% of cancer patients will die from disease progression. Early, open discussions about the possibility of poor outcome, staying involved, and directing palliative care after cancer specific therapy is not effective, may alleviate the burden of treatment failure.

Cross-cultural barriers have been increasingly recognized in palliative care and pain management. Honest, but culturally sensitive discussion about end-of-life care targeted to the particular patient and the patient's cultural background is the cornerstone of successful communication with many patients. The clinician's awareness of the patient's sociocultural history and sensitivity to documented health system inequalities in access and quality of services are essential when discussing end-of-life issues. A patient's family, clergy, and other community can be important contributors to end-of-life discussions and in developing achievable goals of care.

Cassem described nine features required of physicians in the care of dying patients[75]:

1. *Clinical competence:* Adequate training and experience in the management of pain and other symptoms that are widely prevalent in terminally ill cancer patients is critical. Patients have a reasonable right to expect a high level of clinical competence from the medical oncologist in the care of the dying.
2. *Compassion:* Demonstrating compassion acknowledges that what is happening to the patient is of critical importance not only to the patient, but to the physician, and assures the patient that the physician will not abandon the patient in the final hours of life.
3. *Comfort:* Adequate relief of physical and psychological symptoms must be provided.
4. *Communication:* Talking with dying patients reaffirms their ongoing worth as living human beings and provides an opportunity to identify concerns and problems that can and should be addressed. Communication is more than verbal; a hand on the shoulder, a hand to hold, a wave, a smile, and on occasion, an embrace, communicate care, and concern.
5. *Visits from children:* Visits from child relatives reinforce the continuity of the personhood of the dying patient and are a potential source of significant consolation and pleasure.
6. *Family cohesion and integration:* By facilitating the support of family members for one another, feelings of being a burden are mitigated, and the potential for improved relations (when necessary) can be enhanced.
7. *Cheerfulness:* Dying persons have no particular desire for depressed and doleful company. At the other extreme, inappropriate flippancy or frivolity that is insensitive to the mood and situation of the patient can increase a dying person's feeling of isolation. The physician or other visitor should take the cue from the patient.
8. *Consistency and perseverance:* Dying patients have a realistic fear of abandonment and isolation. Regular visits or telephone contact provide reassurance of continued support and concern. Cassem points out that patients are quick to identify those who show interest at first but who gradually disappear from the scene.
9. *Equanimity:* Clinician nervousness undermines patient security. Clinicians who display composure in the presence of a dying person convey reassurance to both the patient and the family.

Factors that may contribute to the distress in the clinicians include the following:

- Frequent life-and-death decisions, exposure to death
- High expectations of the patient and the family
- Severe patient dependency
- Inadequate resources
- Inadequate training in communication
- Excessive workload
- Conflicts with colleagues, patients, families
- Conflict of interests of the patient, caregivers, and self

- Clinicians' anxiety, depression, poor sleep, substance abuse
- Depreciation of the previous achievements
- Guilt of limitations of therapeutic interventions
- Concerns about futility, meaninglessness, death

Physicians' emotions should not be viewed as disorders but do need to be acknowledged and understood to prevent burn-out. The clinician should attempt to self-monitor, reflect and work on preventing burn-out: identify risk factors that predispose to emotions that may affect patient care, monitor for signs (behavior) and emotions, name and accept the emotion, identify possible sources of emotion, step back from the situation to gain perspective, and consult a trusted colleague if needed. Some teams use interdisciplinary rounds to discuss the "difficult" patients and address some of the inner life of clinician issues at these forums.

GUIDELINES IN THE CARE OF THE DYING PATIENT

Algorithm-based clinical guidelines should be generated from the excellent descriptive guidelines that are available. End-of-Life Pathway recommendations, developed at Memorial Sloan-Kettering Cancer Center are an example of such guidelines.

OPTION FOR THE CARE OF THE DYING PATIENT

Many patients and their families prefer that care be delivered at home rather than in an institutional setting.[76] In reality, nearly 80% of United States residents die in hospitals or long-term care facilities, and one-third to one-half of patients are incontinent, bed-bound, and cognitively impaired at the time of death.[77]

In the setting of disease progression and increasing care needs, patient and family attitudes regarding preferred place of death frequently change.[78] Current options of caregivers in the care of the dying include family members at home, home care program, home hospice, inpatient hospice, nursing home, and hospital. Multiple models have been developed for the delivery of care to dying patients. The Memorial Sloan-Kettering Cancer Center Supportive Care Program model is a nurse-centered palliative care model that provides services to dying patients at home.[79] Others have developed an inpatient palliative care unit attached to an out-patient home care and hospice unit or home delivery of chemotherapy, supportive therapy, and palliative care from a mobile van.[80,81] Calvary Hospital in the Bronx, NY, is an acute care hospital for patients with terminal cancer that has developed a network of outpatient hospice and home care programs.

Financial regulations have an enormous impact on the delivery of palliative care, and on end-of-life care in particular. The Medicare hospice benefit is a capitated system of care. The care is home based with a multidisciplinary team of nurses, social workers, chaplains with physician supervision, and with 80% of the care delivered at home. Respite care and inpatient admissions for caregiver support and symptom management are available for limited periods of time. This home-based care model allows patients to die at home and receive expert pain and symptom management, psychosocial support, spiritual care, and provides bereavement support for family members following a patient's death. Patients for the most part must forgo active therapies, for example, chemotherapy. By imposing a restriction of a "prognosis of less than 6 months," enrollment may compel patients to pursue a death-accepting course that might limit technologically advanced interventions. The inadequate reimbursement for professional psychological care is especially problematic. These restrictions translate into some limitations of hospice care. Reimbursement of $100 to 200 USD per day in particular led to no or minimal physician involvement, minimal or no laboratory or radiological tests, and minimal artificial hydration, bisphosphonates or cancer-specific therapy. Poor medical prognostication, well described tendency of clinicians to overestimate the life expectancy superimposed on the "6 months" hospice requirement led to the fact that patients are usually referred to hospice 20 days before death. Although the hospice movement is rapidly growing, availability of hospice services varies widely from state to state in the United States and from country to country.

Contingency plans for inpatient respite care or ongoing care and what would trigger admission to a hospice are critical.[82,83] A study to identify reasons for admitting terminally ill cancer patients to the hospital found that the two major reasons were the requirement of special medical and nursing care unavailable in the home (40%) and the need to provide care for some patients with no family or friend support (27%).

As of 2004, there were over 3,200 hospice programs in the United States providing care for well over 900,000 Americans. Data available estimate that 40% of adult Americans who experience death with a preceding period of dependency, receive hospice care, and up to 50% of United States hospice patients have a non-cancer diagnosis.[84] Depending on the community, 50 to 90% of cancer patients receive hospice care before their death. Whether in a palliative or acute care ward, adequate private provisions must be made and appropriate services offered to the patient and family.

MEDICAL DECISION MAKING

To make appropriate decisions, patients need to know the facts of their illness, yet many are ambivalent about learning such information. In a survey of patients admitted to a palliative care service, many reported a preference to discuss end-of-life care issues with their families rather than with their doctors for fear that their physicians might give up too soon.[85] Chochinov and colleagues, however, reported that knowledge of prognosis did not necessarily have an impact on dying patients' degree of hope.[86] Further research on the impact of information on the patient's coping abilities and quality of life is needed to provide better end-of-life care. Current data suggest that patients' knowledge of their prognosis will directly impact on their medical decision making.[87–89] Increased attention to the care of the dying patient has focused on the need to improve communication about decisions at the end of life. The need for communication guidelines and standards is further substantiated by the degree of distress many clinicians experience when talking to patients about death and dying, especially in the setting of a patient's reluctance to initiate such discussion. Addressing advance care planning, the role of a do-not-resuscitate order, and the understanding and attitude about withholding and withdrawal of care are critical elements in the competent care of cancer patients.

Discussions about end-of-life issues are often delayed even in the face of severe and progressing illness, as was demonstrated by the SUPPORT study (Study to Understand Prognoses and Preferences for Outcomes and Risks for Treatment).[90] This pivotal two phase study of almost 10,000 patients in five major United States hospitals revealed serious limitations in the care of patients with life threatening illness. Patient and family communication with healthcare professionals about care at the end-of-life was poor, the cost of care depleted some family's life savings, and 50% of patients expressed moderate to severe pain in the last three days of life. This study coupled with surveys of public attitudes and beliefs and focus group discussions led to a growing consensus that there were significant barriers—organizational, institutional, educational, and economic—that needed to be addressed to improve end-of-life care.

The difficulty with discussing a poor prognosis may result from uncertainty in the prognosis, or fear of wrong perception by the patient in seeing such a discussion as "giving up." Circumstances urging the physician to discuss death and dying include imminent death, patients wanting or requesting to be assisted to die, and inquiries about hospice care. Such discussions may be driven by the patient or by family thoughts about stopping the burdensome cancer specific treatment, and by fears about physical anguish at the time of death, or fears of being abandoned. Supportive discussion, reviewing the goals of care and discussion about specific fears is usually sufficient.

The Patient Self-Determination Act guarantees the right of patients to determine the kinds of medical care they will and will not accept should they lose the capacity to participate in decision-making by virtue of disease progression or any other cause.[91] If this contingency arises, the presence of the advance directive substantially reduces the burden of decision making for the patient's family and physicians, and it ensures that the patient's preferences are respected. Patients should be encouraged to prepare a written advance directive, and to discuss their wishes with their physician and family. When death is imminent, there is a renewed opportunity to establish the goals of care. This is best accomplished by arranging a family meeting, if appropriate, to set these goals and develop strategies for their implementation.

A LEGAL MANDATE FOR PALLIATIVE CARE

The United States Supreme Court has firmly established the right of patients to have their life-sustaining medical treatment withheld or withdrawn.[92] In 1996, the Court addressed two additional fundamental questions: Is there a constitutional right to assistance in suicide, and is the right to refuse treatment the same as the right to receive assistance in committing suicide?[93] In *Compassion in Dying vs Washington,* the plaintiffs argued that the state's law prohibiting physician-assisted suicide should be overturned based on a violation of the liberty clause of the 14th Amendment to the United States Constitution.[94] The plaintiff claimed that a person has a fundamental right to determine the time and manner of his or her own death and because of this "liberty interest" in securing this right, the state law making physician-assisted suicide illegal was unconstitutional. In *Quill vs Vacco,* in the state of New York, the plaintiff cited the equal rights clause of the 14th Amendment to argue that laws against physician-assisted suicide deny equal protection to all dying patients.[95] Dr Quill, who had publicly acknowledged assisting a patient in suicide, argued that withholding or withdrawing life-sustaining treatment is synonymous with physician-assisted suicide and because the former is legal, the latter must be as well, making New York's law prohibiting physician-assisted suicide unconstitutional.[96]

Regarding the Washington case, the Court ruled that there is no fundamental constitutional right to assisted suicide stating, "We certainly gave no intimation that the right to refuse treatment could be somehow transmuted into a right to assistance in committing suicide."[97] In the New York case, the court upheld the right to refuse care as entirely distinct from the receipt of a lethal prescription. Justice O'Connor wrote, "The parties and amici agree that in these States a patient who is suffering from a terminal illness and who is experiencing great pain has no legal barriers to obtaining medication, from qualified physicians, to alleviate that suffering, even to the point of causing unconsciousness, and hastening death."[98] In the opinion of one constitutional legal scholar, by authoritatively supporting the role of sedation in the imminently dying as distinct from assisted suicide, the Court supported a constitutional right to palliative care.[99]

At the present time, physician-assisted suicide is permitted in Oregon and is illegal in 49 states. A recently published study, regarding the stability of attitudes regarding physician-assisted suicide and voluntary euthanasia among oncologists, oncology patients, and the general public, revealed that up to one-third of the participants overall changed their views over a 6- to 12-month period.[100] Physician opposition to physician-assisted suicide and voluntary euthanasia increased over time, when faced with patients with unremitting pain, suggesting an increasing awareness of the importance of competent pain control and symptom management in dying patients. Although the American Society of Clinical Oncology would neither condemn nor condone physician-assisted suicide in their statement on cancer care at the end of life, the ASCO Task Force noted, "The most important response to the physician-assisted suicide debate is to take every responsible measure to assure that all physicians are well-trained in optimal end-of-life care and to remove all barriers to delivery of such care."

CONCLUSION: THE NEED FOR EDUCATION AND TRAINING IN END-OF-LIFE CARE

The American Medical Association's Graduate Medical Education Report for 1993 noted that only 26% of United States residency programs offered a formal course in end-of-life care. Only five United States medical schools offered a separate required course in the care of dying patients.[101] Despite some notable exceptions, the opportunities for palliative care education are most often hidden in other courses, offered as electives, provided only in lecture format, and frequently provided in the preclinical years.[102] There have been no national standards proposed by accrediting organizations for medical education in end-of-life care. In one study of medical students after completion of their third-year clerkships, 41% were never present when an attending physician talked with a dying person, 35% never discussed with an attending physician how to deal with a patient who is terminally ill, 73% had never been present during a surgical rotation when a surgeon had to tell the family bad news after an operation, and 33% could not identify problems that would be encountered by a family when a dying relative was discharged to home.[103,104] A recent survey of medical school deans revealed that although 89% of medical schools offer some formal teaching, only 11% offer a full-term course on death education. Fifty-two percent offer modules in required courses, and 30% offer one or two lectures as part of another course. In 83% of the courses, the lecture is the primary format.[105]

In a recently published review of end-of-life care in four medical textbooks—*Harrison's Principles of Internal Medicine,* 32nd ed, *The Merck Manual,* 16th ed, *Scientific American Medicine on CD-ROM,* 1994 ed, and *The Washington Manual of Medical Therapeutics,* 28th ed—Carron and colleagues reviewed the chapters on 12 leading causes of death in the United States, paying particular attention to the coverage of end-of-life issues.[106] The authors note, "Throughout the textbooks, frankness about death was strikingly absent.... Sometimes dead persons were termed 'non-survivors.' Often, the physician was vaguely advised that 'supportive care is all that can be offered at this point.'" Of note, the editors of *The Merck Manual* and of *Scientific American Medicine* responded to this study by launching improvement efforts in this area. Reviewers of the end-of-life care content in 50 medical textbooks, including the fourth edition of *Cancer Medicine* among six oncology texts, gave the highest ratings for excellent coverage to texts in family medicine, psychiatry, and geriatrics. The lowest ratings were in textbooks of acquired immunodeficiency syndrome, surgery, neurology, and oncology.[107] The texts were analyzed for the presence of various domains of end-of-life care, including epidemiology, natural history, symptom management, psychological issues, ethics and law, physician responsibilities, and physicians' roles, among others. The World Health Organization has challenged training institutions to ensure that palliative care is:

- compulsory in courses leading to a basic professional qualification;
- accepted as suitable subject testing by examination boards;
- recognized by universities and professional bodies as an appropriate subject for study, dissertations, certificates, diplomas, and advanced degrees;
- included in postgraduate programs of continuing professional education; and
- recognized as an appropriate subject for scholarships, fellowships, and grants by academic institutions and research-funding bodies.[108]

Responding to urgent need for improvement in end-of-life care, The American Board of Internal Medicine has identified core competencies expected of board-certified internists in the care of dying patients (Table 66-10).

The Robert Wood Johnson Foundation has supported public education on this issue through the Last Acts initiatives. ASCO has been developing a curriculum in palliative care, integrating it throughout the entire continuum of cancer care, for the oncology-related professional societies. The latest ASCO curriculum is designed as a comprehensive educational resource consisting of 29 teaching modules that address the best practices in palliative care. Topics include effective communication, creating written care plans, management of pain, depression, dyspnea, and other physical and psychological symptoms. The curriculum is designed for formal oncology training programs as well as for self-education. ASCO has also been conducting sessions on communication and a wide range of palliative care topics at annual meetings and throughout the year, along with encouragement of research in psychosocial support, pain and symptom management, and end-of-life care. The *Journal of Clinical Oncology* began its regular feature, "The Art of Oncology—When the Tumor is Not the Target," by discussing symptom control, ethical decision making, communication, and patient autonomy.

There is increasing attention in medical schools, nursing schools, schools of social work, and pastoral care educational programs to incorporate palliative care as an educational topic.[109]

At the graduate level, a series of consensus documents have outlined the Core Principles of

Table 66-10 ABIM Physician Competencies for the Care of Dying Patients

Components	Core Competencies
Medical knowledge	Palliative care
	Assessment and treatment of pain and psychological distress
Interviewing and counseling skills	Listening
	Truth telling
	Discussing dying as a process
	Giving bad news
	Dealing with families of dying patients
Team approach	Understanding the multidisciplinary nature of end-of-life care
	Promoting collegiality
	Enhancing ability of team to fulfill professional responsibilities
Symptom and pain control	Communication skills
Assessment and management	Comfort
	Use of opioids, sedation, adjuvant analgesics, NSAIDs
	Control of dyspnea, anxiety
	AHCPR and WHO guidelines
Professionalism	Altruism
	Nonabandonment
	Respect for colleagues
	Accountability
	Honoring patient's wishes
	Confidentiality
	Transference and countertransference
Humanistic qualities	Integrity
	Respect
	Compassion
	Courtesy
	Sensitivity to patients' needs for comfort and dignity
Medical ethics	Advance directives
	Do-not-resuscitate or do-not-intubate orders
	Nutrition and hydration
	Conflicts of interest
	Futility
	Double effect
	Surrogate decision making
	Physician-assisted suicide

Adapted from Scott JF, et al. Palliative medicine education. In: Doyle D, Hanks GWC, MacDonald N, editors. Oxford textbook of palliative medicine. 2nd ed. New York: Oxford University Press; 1998. p. 1171. AHCPR = Agency for Health Care Policy Research; NSAIDs = nonsteroidal antiinflammatory drugs; WHO = World Health Organization.

Table 66-11 National Cancer Policy Board Recommendations for Promoting Excellent Palliative Care

Recommendation #1: Centers of excellence in symptom control and palliative care both for adults and children to deliver best care, carry out research, and teaching should be designated by the National Cancer Institute (NCI).

Recommendation #2: NCI should add the requirement of research in palliative care and symptom control for recognition as a "Comprehensive Cancer Center."

Recommendation #3: The Health Care Financing Administration (HCFA) should fund demonstration projects for service delivery and reimbursement that integrate palliative care and potentially life-prolonging treatments throughout the course of disease.

Recommendation #4: Private insurers should provide adequate compensation for end-of-life care. The special circumstances of dying children, including communication with children, parents, and between medical professionals, should be taken into account in setting reimbursement levels and in actually paying claims for these services when providers bill for them.

Recommendation #5: Organizations that provide information about cancer treatment (NCI, the American Cancer Society, health insurers, pharmaceutical companies, and others), should revise their inventories of patient-oriented materials, as appropriate, to provide comprehensive, accurate information about palliative care throughout the course of disease. Patients would also be helped by having reliable information on survival by type and stage of cancer easily accessible. Attention should be paid to cultural relevance and special population (eg, children). Palliative care should become, if not a medical specialty, at least a defined area of expertise, education, and research.

Recommendation #6: Best available practice guidelines should dictate the standard of care for both physical and psychological symptoms. Development, validation, and use of such standards should be encouraged by care systems, payers, standard-setting bodies and professional societies. Leadership and training for nonspecialists, who provide most of care for cancer patients, should be provided.

Recommendation #7: The National Cancer Policy Board recommendations on Enhancing Data Systems to Improve the Quality of Cancer Care should be applied equally to palliative and end-of-life care as to other aspects of cancer treatment. These recommendations include

- developing a core set of cancer care quality measures;
- increasing public and private support for cancer registries;
- supporting research and demonstration projects to identify new mechanisms to organize and finance the collection of data for cancer care quality studies;
- supporting the development of technologies, including computer documentation and intranet-based communication, to optimize availability of clinical data relevant to assessing quality of cancer care;
- expanding support for training in health services research and other disciplines needed to measure quality of care;
- increasing support for health services research aimed toward improved quality of cancer care measures;
- developing models for linkage studies and the release of confidential data for research purposes that protect the confidentiality and privacy of healthcare information; and
- funding demonstration projects to assess the impact of quality monitoring programs within healthcare systems.

Recommendation #8: NCI should convene a State of the Science Meeting on palliative care and symptom control, that would result in a high-profile strategic research agenda that can be pursued by NCI and its research partners over the short- and long-term.

Recommendation #9: NCI should establish the most appropriate institutional locus (or more than one) for palliative care, symptom control, and other end-of-life research, possibly within the Division of Cancer Treatment and Diagnosis.

Recommendation #10: NCI should review the membership of its advisory bodies to ensure representation of experts in cancer pain, symptom management, and palliative care.

Palliative Care that have been adopted by 19 national professional organizations to include in their professional teaching programs for a specific subspecialty.[110] Curricula for various medical and surgical subspecialties as well as for certain diseases and states such as cancer, HIV/AIDS, geriatrics, pediatrics, and surgery are available. The Veterans' Healthcare Administration (VA), where one in seven Americans receive care, has developed an expansive initiative to support and sustain the development of palliative care teams and leaders, making palliative care integral to their health care system.

To date there are more than 2,000 physicians who are certified by the American Board of Hospice and Palliative Care and over 10,000 nurses and nursing assistants are certified by the Hospice and Palliative Care Nursing Association. There are over 42 physician fellowship training programs in palliative care in the United States and 20 are now certified as having met the qualifications to train fellows in clinical competency in palliative care. Similar fellowship programs are developing in nursing and social work. Many national efforts to train physicians in practice, spearheaded by the American Medical Association in its educational initiative entitled EPEC and a nursing curriculum ELNEC to train nursing leaders, as well as a recently published compendium on the role of social worker's in end-of-life care are some examples of the growing postgraduate educational initiatives.

The American Board of Hospice and Palliative Care is in the process of applying for specialty status and has defined its scope of practice, curricula, and certification process.

ASCO brings research findings to a wide audience via its official site, <www.asco.org.> Palliative care in general and end-of-life Internet Web sites have been increasing in number and include

http://www.epec.net
http://www.palliative.org
http://www.lastacts.com
http://www.palcare.org
http://www.abcd-caring.com
http://www.careofdying.org
http://www.americanhospice.org
http://hospicecare.org (IAHPC)
http://palliative.mdanderson.org

and many others.

To date 20% of American hospitals (1,100) have developed palliative care units and/or consultation teams. Increasingly palliative care is identified with quality care. There now appears to be a greater openness to talking about end-of-life issues and options for care facilitating a consumer advocacy movement (Table 66-11).

Good care for the dying requires mastery of the emerging science of palliative medicine, a dedication to further research, and a compassionate concern for patient care at each stage of illness. Palliative care at its best is concerned not about death, but about life until death, and affirms the right of all human beings to live well until they die, cared for and supported by competent clinicians.

REFERENCES

1. Cancer Pain Relief and Palliative Care: Report of a WHO Expert Committee. Geneva, Switzerland: World Health Organization Technical Report Series 1990;804.
2. Klastersky J, Schimpff SC, Senn HJ. Supportive care in cancer, a handbook for oncologists. 2nd ed. New York: Marcel Dekker 1999. p. vi.
3. Institute of Medicine Committee on Care at the End of Life. In: Field MJ, Cassel CK, editors. Approaching death-improving care at the end of life. Washington DC: National Academy Press; 1977.
4. Billings JA, Block S. Palliative care in undergraduate medical education—status report and future directions. JAMA 1997;278:733–8.
5. Hearn J, Higginson IJ. Do specialist palliative care teams improve outcomes for cancer patients? A systematic literature review. Palliat Med 1998;12:317–22.
6. Blank LL. Overview on ABIM End-of-life Patient Care Project: caring for the dying: identification and promotion of physician competency. Hosp J 1998;13:145–50.
7. Cancer care during the late phase of life. ASCO special article. J Clin Oncol 1998:16;1986–96.
8. Davies E, Higginson IJ, editors. In: Davies E, Higginson IJ, editors. Palliative care—the solid facts. World Health Organization Collaboration Project, Geneva, Switzerland 2004. Better care for older people. World Health Organization Collaboration Project. Geneva, Switzerland 2004.
9. Institute of Medicine National Research Council, Foley KM, Gelband H. Improving palliative care for cancer. Washington DC: National Academy Press 2001. p. XI.
10. Education for Physicians on End-of-life Care. Available at: http://www.epec.net (accessed February 2003).
11. Fallowfield L, Lipkin M, Hall A. Teaching senior oncologists communication skills: results from phase 1 of a comprehensive longitudinal program in the United Kingdom. J Clin Oncol 1998;16:1961–8.
12. Cherny NI, Catane R. Palliative medicine and the medical oncologist: defining the purview of care. In: Pain and Palliative Care. Cherny NI, Foley KM, editors, Hematology/Oncology Clinics of North America, February 1996;10:1–20.
13. Vigano A, Donaldson N, Higginson IJ, et al. Quality of life and survival prediction in terminal cancer patients: a multicenter study. Cancer. 2004 Sep 1;101:1090–8.
14. Tulsky, JA, Fischer DS, et al. Opening the black box: how do physicians communicate about advance directives? Ann Intern Med 1998:441–9.
15. Maguire P, Faulkner A. Communicate with cancer patients: 1. Handling bad news and difficult questions. BMJ 1988;297:907–9.
16. Neff P, Lyckholm L, Smith T. Truth or consequences: what to do when the patient doesn't want to know. J Clin Oncol 2002;20:3035–7.
17. Latimer E. Ethical challenges in cancer care. J Palliat Care 1992;8:65–70.
18. Buckman R. Communication in palliative care: a practical guide. In: Doyle D, Hanks GWC, MacDonald N, editors. Oxford textbook of palliative medicine, 2nd ed. New York: Oxford University Press; 1998, p. 141–56.
19. Blackhall LJ, Murphy ST, Frank G, et al. Ethnicity and attitudes toward patient autonomy. JAMA 1995;274:820–5.
20. Bach PB, Cramer LD, Warren JL, Begg CB. Racial differences in the treatment of early-stage lung cancer. N Engl J Med 1999;341:1198–205.
21. Caralis PV, Davis B, Wright K, Marcial E. The influence of ethnicity and race on attitudes toward advance directives, life-prolonging treatments, and euthanasia. J Clin Ethics 1993;4:155–65.
22. Neubauer BJ, Hamilton CL. Racial differences in attitudes toward hospice care. Hosp J 1990;6:37–48.
23. Mebane EW, Oman RF, Kroonen LT, Goldstein MK. The influence of physician race, age, and gender on physician attitudes toward advance care directives and preferences for end-of-life decision-making. J Am Geriatr Soc 1999;47:579–91.
24. McKinley ED, Garrett JM, Evans AT, Danis M. Differences in end-of-life decision making among black and white ambulatory cancer patients. J Gen Intern Med 1996;11:651–6.
25. Portenoy RK, Thaler HT, Kornblith AB, et al. The Memorial Symptom Assessment Scale: an instrument for the evaluation of symptom prevalence, characteristics, and distress. Eur J Cancer 1994;30A:1326–36.
26. Portenoy RK, Thaler HT, Kornblith AB, et al. Symptom prevalence, characteristics and distress in a cancer population. Qual Life Res 1994;3:183–9.
27. Curtis EB, Krech R, Walsh TD. Common symptoms in patients with advanced cancer. J Palliat Care 1991;7:25–9.
28. Donnelly S, Walsh D. The symptoms of advanced cancer. Semin Oncol 1995;22 (Suppl 2):67–72.
29. Ahmedzai S. Palliation of respiratory symptoms. In: Doyle D, Hanks GWC, MacDonald N, editors. Oxford textbook of palliative medicine. 2nd ed. New York: Oxford University Press; 1998. p.583–616.
30. Dudgeon DJ, Rosenthal S. Management of dyspnea and cough in patients with cancer. In: Cherny NI, Foley KM, editors. Pain and palliative care. Hematol/Oncol Clin N Amer 1996;10:157–71.
31. Lung Cancer Working Party. Inoperable non–small-cell lung cancer (NSCLC): a Medical Research Council randomised trial of palliative radiotherapy with two fractions or ten fractions. Br J Cancer 1991;63:265–70.
32. Plataniotis GA, Kouvaris JR, Dardoufas C, et al. A short radiotherapy course for locally advanced non-small cell lung cancer (NSCLC): effective palliation and patients' convenience. Lung Cancer 2002;35:203–7.
33. Leibovitz A, Baumoehl Y, Walach N, et al. Medical staff attitudes: views and positions regarding blood transfusion to terminally ill cancer patients. Am J Clin Oncol 2004;27:542–6.
34. Brown SJ, Eichner SF, Jones JR. Nebulized morphine for relief of dyspnea due to chronic lung disease. Ann Pharmacother 2005;39:1088–92. [Epub 2005 Apr 19.]
35. Ripamonte C. Management of dyspnea in advanced cancer patients. Support Care Cancer 1999;7:233–43.
36. Thomas JR, von Gunten CF. Clinical management of dyspnea. Lancet Oncol 2002;3:222–8.
37. Thomas JR, von Gunten CF. Treatment of dyspnea in cancer patients. Oncology (Huntingt) 2002;16:745–50; discussion 750, 755, 758–60.
38. Jones LA. Superior vena cava syndrome: an oncologic complication. Semin Oncol Nurs 1987;3:211–5.
39. Sculier JP, Field R. Superior vena cava obstruction syndrome: recommendations for management. Cancer Treat Rev 1985;12:209–18.
40. Rowell NP, Gleeson FV. Steroids, radiotherapy, chemotherapy and stents for superior vena caval obstruction in carcinoma of the bronchus. Cochrane Database Syst Rev 2001;4:CD001316.
41. Reuben DB, Mor V. Nausea and vomiting in terminal cancer patients. Arch Intern Med 1986;146:2021–3.
42. Ripamonti C. Management of bowel obstruction in advanced cancer patients. J Pain Symptom Manage 1994;9:193–200.
43. Andrews PL, Naylor RJ, Joss RA. Neuropharmacology of emesis and its relevance to anti-emetic therapy. Consensus and controversies. Support Care Cancer 1998;6:197–203.
44. Mannix KA. Palliation of nausea and vomiting. In: Doyle D, Hanks GWC, MacDonald N, Oxford textbook of palliative medicine 2nd ed. New York: Oxford University Press 1998. p. 491.
45. Miller G, Boman J, Shrier I, Gordon PH. Small-bowel obstruction secondary to malignant disease: an 11-year audit. Can J Surg 2000;43:353–8.
46. Blair SL, Chu DZ, Schwarz RE. Outcome of palliative operations for malignant bowel obstruction in patients with peritoneal carcinomatosis from nongynecological cancer. Ann Surg Oncol 2001;8:632–7.
47. Ripamonti C, Zecca E, De Conno F. Pharmacological treatment of cancer pain: alternative routes of opioid administration. Tumori 1998;84:289–300.
48. Mercandante S. The role of octreotide in palliative care. J Pain Symptom Manage 1994;9:406–11.
49. Mercandante S, Kargar J, Nicolosi G. Octreotide may prevent definitive intestinal obstruction. J Pain Symptom Manage 1997;13:325–6.
50. Feuer DJ, Broadley KE. Corticosteroids for the resolution of malignant bowel obstruction in advanced gynaecological and gastrointestinal cancer. Cochrane Database Syst Rev 2000;2:CD001219.
51. Massie MJ, Holland JC, Glass E. Delirium in terminally ill cancer patients. Am J Psychiatry 1983;140:1048–50.
52. Trzepacz PT, Baker RW, Greenhouse J. A symptom rating scale for delirium. Psychiatry Res 1988 23:89–97.
53. McNamara P, Minton P, Twycross RG. The use of midazolam in palliative care. Palliat Med 1991;5:244–9.
54. Truog RD, Berde CB, Mitchell C, et al. Barbiturates in the care of the terminally ill. N Engl J Med 1992;327:1678–82.
55. Donovan HS, Ward S. Representations of fatigue in women receiving chemotherapy for gynecologic cancers. Oncol Nurs Forum 2005;32:113–6.
56. American College of Physicians. Parental nutrition in patients receiving cancer chemotherapy. Ann Intern Med 1989;110:734–6.
57. Ng EH, Lowry SF. Nutritional support and cancer cachexia. Evolving concepts of mechanisms and adjunctive therapies. Hematol Oncol Clin North Am 1991;5:161–84.
58. Twycross R, Lichter I. The terminal phase. In: Doyle D, Hanks GWC, MacDonald N, editors. Oxford textbook of palliative medicine. 2nd ed. New York: Oxford University Press; 1998. p. 977–92.
59. Hoefler JM. Making decisions about tube feeding for severely demented patients at the end of life: clinical, legal, and ethical considerations. Death Stud 2000;24:233–54.
60. Report of the WHO Expert Committee on Cancer Pain Relief and Active Supportive Care. Cancer pain relief with a guide to opioid availability. 2nd ed., Technical report series 804. Geneva: World Health Organization; 1996.
61. Portenoy RK, Bruera E, editors. Topics in palliative care. Vols. 1–3. New York: Oxford University Press, 1997.
62. Cherny NI, Portenoy RK, Sedation in the treatment of refractory symptoms: guidelines for evaluation and treatment. J Palliat Care 1994;10:31–8.
63. Bottomly DM, Hanks G. Subcutaneous midazolam infusion in palliative care. J Pain Symptom Manage 1990; 5:259–61.
64. Johanson GA. Midazolam in terminal care. Am J Hosp Palliat Care 1993;10:13–4.
65. Stirling LC, Kurowska A, Tookman A. The use of phenobarbitone in the management of agitation and seizures at the end of life. J Pain Symptom Manage 1999;17:363–8.
66. Krakauer EL, Pensen RT, Truog RD, et al. Sedation for intractable distress of a dying patient: acute palliative care and the principle of double effect. Oncologist 2000;5:53–62.
67. Wilson WC, Smedira NG, Fink C, et al. Ordering and administration of sedatives and analgesics during the withholding and withdrawal of life support from critically ill patients. JAMA 1992;267:949–53.
68. Carver AC, Vickrey BG, Bernat JL, et al. End of life care: a survey of US neurologists' attitudes, behavior, and knowledge. Neurology 1999;53:284–93.
69. Levy MH, Cohen SD. Sedation for the relief of refractory symptoms in the imminently dying: a fine intentional line. Semin Oncol 2005;32:237–46.
70. Cherny NI, Coyle N, Foley KM. Suffering in the advanced cancer patient: a definition and taxonomy. J Palliat Care 1994;102:57–70.
71. Cherny NI, Coyle RN, Foley KM. Guidelines in the care of the dying cancer patient. In: Cherny NI, Foley KM, editors. Pain and palliative care, Hematol Oncol Clin North Am 1996;10:261–86.
72. Schaerer R. Suffering of the doctor linked with the death of patients. Palliat Med 1993;7:27–37.
73. Cassell EJ. The nature of suffering and the goals of medicine. N Engl J Med 1982;306:639–45.
74. Gilewski T. The art of medicine: teaching oncology fellows about the end of life. Clin Rev Oncol Hematol 2001;40:105–13.
75. Cassem NH. The dying patient. In: Cassem NH, Stern TA, Rosenbaum JF, Jellinek MS, editors. Massachusetts General Hospital handbook of general hospital psychiatry. 4th ed. St. Louis: Mosby-Year Book Inc; 1997. p. 605–36.
76. Townsend J, Frank AO, Fermont D, et al. Terminal cancer care and patients' preferences for place of death: a prospective study. BMJ 1990;301:415–7.
77. Field MJ, Cassel CK, editors. Approaching death: improving care at the end of life. Washington, DC: National Academy Press; 1997.
78. Hinton J. Can home care maintain an acceptable quality of life for patients with terminal cancer and their relatives? Palliat Med 1994;8:183–96.
79. Coyle N. Supportive care program, pain service. Memorial Sloan-Kettering Cancer Center. Support Care Cancer 1995;3:161–3.
80. Walsh D. The Harry R. Horvitz Center for Palliative Medicine (1987–1999): development of a novel comprehensive integrated program. Am J Hosp Palliat Care 2001;18:239–50.

81. Vinciguerra V. Home oncology medical extension (H.O.M.E.)—an effective alternative to hospital care. Prog Clin Biol Res 1983;120:319–26.
82. Walsh S, Kingston RD. The use of hospital beds for terminally ill cancer patients. Eur J Surg Oncol 1988;14:367–70.
83. Viney LL, Walker BM, Robertson T, et al. Dying in palliative care units and in hospital: a comparison of the quality of life of terminal cancer patients. J Consult Clin Psychol 1994;62:157–64.
84. National Consensus Project. Clinical Practice Guidelines for Quality Palliative Care. National Consensus Project. Brooklyn, NY 2004.
85. Constantini-Ferrando MF, Foley KM, Rapkin BD. Communicating with patients about advanced cancer [letter]. JAMA 1998;280:1403.
86. Chochinov HM, Tataryn DJ, Wilson KG, et al. Prognostic awareness and the terminally ill. Psychosomatics 2000;41:500–4.
87. Weeks JC, Cook EF, O'Day SJ, et al. Relationship between cancer patients' predictions of prognosis and their treatment preferences. JAMA 1998;279:1709–14.
88. Smith TJ, Swisher K. Telling the truth about terminal cancer. JAMA 1998;279:1746–8.
89. Baile WF, Glober GA, Lenzi R, et al. Discussing disease progression and end of life decisions. Oncology 1999;13:1021–8.
90. Covinsky KE, Fuller JD, Yaffe K, et al. Communication and decision-making in seriously ill patients: findings of the SUPPORT project. The Study to Understand Prognoses and Preferences for Outcomes and Risks of Treatments. J Am Geriatr Soc 2000;48 (Suppl 5):187–93.
91. Grant KD. The patient self-determination act: implications for physicians. Hosp Pract 1992;27:44–8.
92. *Cruzan v. Director*, Missouri Dept. of Health, 497 U.S. 261 (1990).
93. Annas GJ. The bell tolls for a constitutional right to physician-assisted suicide. N Engl J Med 1997;337:1098–103.
94. *Compassion in Dying v. Washington*, 79 Fed. 790 (9th Cir. 1996).
95. *Quill v. Vacco,* 80 F.3d 716 (2d Cir. 1996).
96. Quill TE. Death and dignity: a case of individualized decision making. N Engl J Med 1991;324:691–4.
97. *Washington v. Glucksberg,* 117 S. Ct. 2254 (1997).
98. *Vacco v. Quill, 117 S.* Ct. 2293 (1997).
99. Burt RA. The Supreme Court speaks: not assisted suicide but a constitutional right to palliative care. N Engl J Med 1997;337:1234–6.
100. Wolfe J, Fairclough DL, Clarridge BR, et al. Stability of attitudes regarding physician-assisted suicide and euthanasia among oncology patients, physicians, and the general public, J Clin Oncol 1999;17:1274–9.
101. Hill TP. Treating the dying patient: the challenge for medical education. Arch Intern Med 1995;155:1265–69.
102. Weissman DE, Griffie J. Integration of palliative medicine at the Medical College of Wisconsin 1990–1996. J Pain Symptom Manage 1998;15:195–201.
103. Rappaport W, Witzke D. Education about death and dying during clinical years of medical school. Surgery 1993; 113:163–5.
104. Billings JA, Block S. Palliative care in undergraduate medical education: status report and future directions. JAMA 1997;278:733–8.
105. Merman AC, Gunn DB, Dickinson GE. Learning to care for the dying: a survey of medical schools and a model course. Acad Med 1991;66:35–8.
106. Carron AT, Lynn J, Keaney P. End of life care in medical textbooks. Ann Intern Med 1999;130:82–6.
107. Rabow MW, Hardie GE, Fair JM, McPhee SJ. End-of-life care content in 50 textbooks from multiple specialties. JAMA 2000;283:771–8.
108. Report of the WHO Expert Committee on Cancer Pain Relief and Active Supportive Care. Cancer pain relief with a guide to opioid availability. 2nd ed. Technical report series 804. Geneva: World Health Organization; 1996.
109. Aulino F, Foley K. Professional education in end-of-life care. A US Perspective. J Royal Soc Med 2001;95:472–6.
110. Cassel C, Foley K. Principles for care of patients at the end of life: an emerging consensus among the specialties of medicine. Milbank Memorial Fund. New York, NY 1999.

Management of Cancer Pain

Natalie Moryl, MD
Alan C. Carver, MD
Kathleen M. Foley, MD

International Association for the Study of Pain defines pain as "an unpleasant sensory and emotional experience associated with actual or potential tissue damage or described in terms of such damage" (IASP, 1979).

The evaluation and treatment of pain in the patient with cancer have evolved to encompass a series of scientifically based guidelines that define a comprehensive approach to the surveillance and management of this difficult clinical problem. Current knowledge in cancer pain includes a delineation of the common pain syndromes in patients with cancer as well as their postulated neurophysiologic mechanisms,[1,2] the psychological factors that contribute to and alter the pain complaint,[3–5] and methodologies to measure pain, as well as pharmacokinetic and pharmacodynamic data that correlate drug therapy with pain relief.[6–9] These advances have focused attention on the patient with cancer as the clinical model of pain and have led to improved care for this serious symptom.

Pain management for the patient with cancer has as its primary goal effective symptom control improving patient's and caregiver's quality of life and allowing patients to participate in diagnostic and therapeutic interventions.

Scope of the Problem Cancer is a major world health problem.[10]

Every year, about 17 million new cases are diagnosed; half in developing countries, and 5 million patients die from these diseases annually. In Europe alone nearly 2.9 million new cases of cancer and more than 1.7 million cancer deaths were registered in 2004. Prevalence data indicate that there are currently about 14 million people worldwide with cancer. Published reports indicate that between 30 and 50% of such cancer patients are in active therapy, and that 70 to 90% of patients with far-advanced disease suffer significant pain.[10] It is conservatively estimated by the World Health Organization (WHO) that 5 million people are currently suffering from cancer pain with or without satisfactory treatment. The prevalence of pain increases with disease progression and varies according to the primary site. Other factors correlating with pain include the presence of metastases, the proximity of tumor to neural structures, and patient psychosocial characteristics.

Several studies have demonstrated that cancer patients experience more than one type of pain.[11–13] In one survey, 81% of patients reported two or more distinct pain complaints, and 34% of these patients reported more than three types.[13] Pain has an enormous effect on the quality of life of patients with cancer. Several methods have been developed to assess this observation.[14] The public perception of pain has also been studied. Patients' fear of cancer is directly related to their fear of severe pain.[15–17] Sixty-nine percent of patients with cancer who were surveyed, reported that severe pain from cancer might lead them to consider suicide, and 57% perceive death from cancer as painful.

Pain is a common presentation of cancer or its progression and the importance of a comprehensive evaluation cannot be overstated. In a study of 276 consecutive pain consultations at Memorial Sloan-Kettering Cancer Center (MSKCC) the consultation identified a previously undiagnosed etiology for the pain in 64% of patients. New neurological diagnoses were made in 36% of patients, and 18% of patients received radiotherapy, surgery, or chemotherapy, based on the findings of the pain consultation.[18]

Barriers to Cancer Pain Management Despite the publication of numerous national and international guidelines on how to manage cancer pain effectively,[6,10] undertreatment of pain remains a significant problem. Barriers include poor physician's training, inadequate knowledge of pharmacologic and other management strategies, and negative physician and patient attitudes toward opioid use for pain.[15]

The Study to Understand Prognoses and Preferences for Outcomes and Risks of Treatments (SUPPORT) showed that 50% of adults who die in the hospital experience moderate to severe pain in the immediate period prior to death.[19,20] A large multicenter study to address knowledge and attitudes of physicians regarding cancer pain management demonstrated that 86% of physicians felt that the majority of patients were undermedicated.[21] Only 51% believed pain control in their own practice setting was good or very good, and 31% would wait until the patient's prognosis was 6 months or less before they would start maximal analgesia. The study also identified critical barriers to effective pain management (Table 67-1). Poor pain assessment was rated by 76% of physicians as the single most important barrier to adequate pain management. Other barriers included patient reluctance to report pain and to take opioids, physician reluctance to prescribe opioids, and nursing reluctance to give opioids. Physicians expressed dissatisfaction with their training for pain management in medical school and in residency or fellowship.

A study of 4,000 elderly nursing home residents with cancer revealed that 24, 29, and 38% of those over the age of 85, 74 to 84, and 65 to 74 years, respectively, reported daily pain. Twenty-six percent of patients in daily pain did not receive any analgesics, and those over age 85 who reported daily pain were the most likely to receive no analgesia.[22] Sixty percent of all outpatients seen at an oncology clinic in the Netherlands were in pain, and 20% of this group reported a score of 5 or greater on a scale of 1 to 10.[23] These data emphasize the need for broad educational programs that address the fundamental principles of cancer pain management, the barriers, and the importance of institutional commitment to provide improved pain management.[24–26]

Mechanisms of Cancer Pain Pain associated with cancer most commonly results from tumor infiltration of pain-sensitive structures such as bones, soft tissue, nerves, viscera, and blood vessels. Pain may also be caused by surgery, chemotherapy, or radiation therapy. Although the cause of the pain and the type of injury vary, the mechanisms that underlie these different clinical problems are now becoming understood as a constellation of complex neurophysiologic and neuropharmacologic phenomena.[27] Two broad categories of pain have been described and are referred to as nociceptive pain, which include both somatic and visceral pain, and neuropathic pain.

Neurophysiology of Pain There are sensory receptors preferentially sensitive to noxious stimuli. These nociceptors are primary afferent nerves with peripheral terminals that respond differentially to noxious stimuli. These nociceptors serve two major functions, defined as transduction and transmis-

Table 67-1 Barriers to Cancer Pain Management

Inadequate assessment
Patient reluctance to report pain
Patient reluctance to take opioids
Physician reluctance to prescribe opioids
Inadequate staff knowledge about pain management
Nursing staff reluctance to give opioids
Excessive state regulation of analgesics

Adapted from Von Roenn JH et al.[21]

sion. A series of chemical, mechanical, or thermal factors can produce receptor activation, producing an electrochemical nerve impulse in the primary afferent. The information is then transmitted to the central nervous system, where pain perception occurs. Both myelinated and unmyelinated nociceptors convey pain sensation to the central nervous system. The myelinated nociceptor responds to noxious mechanical stimuli almost exclusively and has a rapid conduction over A delta fibers, causing a sharp stinging pain. Unmyelinated nociceptors are polymodal, responding to mechanical, thermal, and chemical stimuli, have a slower rate of conduction in a C fiber range, and are associated with a dull, burning, or aching pain. In general, unmyelinated nociceptors are not spontaneously active but become sensitized with any tissue injury. A variety of substances can mediate this sensitization, including potassium ions, adenosine triphosphate, bradykinin, prostaglandins (especially prostaglandin E2), and leukotrienes. Tumor infiltration and compression may cause both mechanical and chemical activation of nociceptors. Primary hyperalgesia or accentuated pain response to painful stimulus occurs by nociceptor sensitization at the site of tissue injury. Secondary hyperalgesia refers to the expansion of the area of cutaneous hyperalgesia beyond the area of injury.[27] Allodynia is pain resulting from an innocuous stimulus, usually associated with nerve damage. Once activated, pain is transmitted over A delta and C fibers and enters the spinal cord laterally, synapsing in the superficial dorsal horn to activate ascending nociceptive systems. Sensory transmission is mediated through neuropeptides, substance P, calcitonin gene-related peptides, and the excitatory amino acids glutamate and aspartate.[28] Central sensitization occurs as a result of an excitatory amino acid binding to the *N*-methyl-D-aspartate (NMDA) receptor. On binding, influx of calcium intracellularly results in second-messenger activation and the generation of nitric oxide, among other compounds.

The activation of the NMDA receptor and the alpha-amino-3-hydroxy-5-methyl-4-isoxazolepropionic acid (AMPA) receptor contribute to the establishment of central sensitization and neuronal windup that underlie in part secondary hyperalgesia, allodynia, and persistent pain states.

Two physiologically distinct pathways ascend in the anterolateral quadrant of the spinal cord. The neospinothalamic pathway projects to the ventrobasilar thalamic complex, and from there, axons project to the somatosensory cortex in the parietal lobe. This pathway mediates sensory-discriminative aspects of pain perception (stimulus localization and intensity). The paleospinothalamic tract ascends, projecting to the reticular formation, posterior thalamic nucleus, intralaminar thalamic nuclear complex, and to the cortex. This pathway mediates the arousal, emotional, and affective/suffering components of pain.

The existence of a specific nucleus in the posterior thalamus responsible for pain and temperature sensation has recently been elucidated.[29] There is an endogenous pain suppression pathway that arises in the periaqueductal gray (PAG) of the midbrain and descends to the nucleus raphe magnus (NRM) in the medulla. From the NRM, there are projections to the dorsal horn of the spinal cord through the dorsal longitudinal fasciculus. This pathway modulates afferent nociceptive impulses. Electrical stimulation of the PAG, NRM, or dorsal horn or microinjection of morphine at these sites produces analgesia without concomitant motor, sensory, or autonomic blockade. Serotonin and norepinephrine are the putative neurotransmitters in these areas. Endogenous opioid compounds are also involved as modulators in this pain suppression system. Enkephalin, β-endorphin, and dynorphin are the most potent inhibitors of nociceptive activity. These three peptides are derived from three precursor molecules: (1) pro-opiomelanocortin is the common precursor for β-endorphin, (2) proenkephalin A is the common precursor for met-enkephalin and leu-enkephalin, and (3) proenkephalin B is the precursor for dynorphin. Enkephalin is distributed in specific nuclei in the brain stem and spinal cord. β-Endorphin is found in the arcuate nucleus of the hypothalamus and in the pituitary. These endogenous opioid peptides produce analgesia by binding to specific receptors that are found in high concentration in cortical, brain stem, and spinal cord sites. β-endorphin binds to the mu receptor, enkephalin to the delta receptor, and dynorphin to the kappa receptor. Morphine and the commonly used opioids mimic the action of endogenous opioid peptides.

Assessment of Pain Critical to the development of a successful therapeutic strategy is the physician's ability to establish a trusting relationship with the patient (Table 67-2). This requires a complete history of the pain complaint, including the patient's description of pain and intensity; its quality, exacerbating, and relieving factors, its radiation if any; its exact onset and temporal pattern. Impact of pain on the activities of daily living, sleep, mood, and affect should be assessed. Multiple pain complaints, particularly common in patients with advanced disease, need to be prioritized and classified. Careful history, medical, and neurologic examination help to provide the necessary data to substantiate the clinical diagnosis.[30,31] Patient's extent of disease and response to treatment, beliefs, and attitudes about pain medications, goals, and expectations of therapy are important in setting the treatment goals and developing the appropriate treatment plans. Knowledge of characterized pain syndromes and careful pain assessment can direct the examination. For instance, complaints of back pain, the most common symptom for neurological referral at MSKCC, may lead to diagnosis of a number of the neurologic complications of cancer, including epidural spinal cord compression with resultant paraplegia. Another example is postmastectomy or postlumpectomy pain syndrome that is quite characteristic and can be diagnosed by its temporal relationship to the surgery, the site of pain in the distribution of the intercostobrachial nerve, and the pain description.[2]

Table 67-2 Algorithm for the Clinical Assessment of Pain

1. Believe the patient's complaint of pain.
2. Take a careful history of the pain complaint to place it temporally in the patient's cancer history.
3. Assess the characteristics of each pain, including its site, its pattern of referral, and its aggravating and relieving factors.
4. Clarify the temporal aspects of the pain: acute, subacute, chronic, episodic, intermittent, breakthrough, or incident.
5. List and prioritize each pain complaint.
6. Evaluate the response to previous and current analgesic therapies.
7. Evaluate the psychological state of the patient.
8. Ask if the patient has a past history of alcohol or drug dependence.
9. Perform a careful medical and neurologic examination.
10. Order and personally review the appropriate diagnostic procedures.
11. Treat the patient's pain to facilitate the necessary work-up.
12. Design the diagnostic and therapeutic approach to suit the individual.
13. Provide continuity of care from evaluation to treatment, to ensure patient compliance and to reduce patient anxiety.
14. Reassess the patient's response to pain therapy.
15. Discuss advance directives with the patient and the family.

Of greatest importance, no patient should be inadequately evaluated because the patient's inability to cooperate with examination and imaging studies. Early management of the pain while investigating its cause will markedly improve the patient's ability to complete the necessary diagnostic procedures.

Psychological factors accounting for differences in pain experiences in patients with cancer must be recognized.[3,32,33] A series of psychiatric syndromes have been described in patients with cancer, with depression occurring in as many as 25% of patients.[33] Psychiatric symptoms in cancer pain patients without psychiatric history usually is a consequence of uncontrolled pain. This has been documented in both adults and children.[33]

In this group with pain, the psychiatric diagnoses included adjustment disorders with depressed or mixed mood and major depression.[32] As depression is often a treatable disorder, patients may experience significant pain relief if their psychiatric symptoms are promptly recognized and managed appropriately. The National Comprehensive Cancer Network has provided important guidelines for the management of psychiatric symptoms in the cancer population (see Chapter 59, "Principles of Psycho-Oncology").[34]

In a study of the incidence of psychiatric disorders in patients with cancer, 39% of those patients who received a psychiatric diagnosis had significant pain. In contrast, only 19% of patients who did not receive a psychiatric diagnosis had significant pain.

Uncontrolled pain, as well as low family support and depression are major factors in cancer-related suicide.[35,36]

Pain is recognized as one of the patient-related factors that predicts for potential psychiatric morbidity along with disease and treatment-related variables, interactions between patient and illness, and factors relating to the patient's environment.[5] Personality factors that may be quite distorted by the presence of pain often disappear with adequate pain relief. Closely allied to these psychologic factors is the concept of the meaning of pain. It is not uncommon for patients during active therapy to endure significant pain for the promise of a successful outcome. With advanced disease, when active antitumor therapy is no longer effective, it is common for patients and families to request that if nothing else can be done that at least their pain should be adequately managed.[37–39]

The use of several scales such as the Brief Pain Inventory, the McGill Pain Questionnaire, the Memorial Pain Assessment Card (MPAC), and the Memorial Symptom Assessment Scale (MSAS) allows for repetitive valid measurement of pain and mood and clearly facilitates the health care professional in determining the degree of physical pain and emotional distress present in the individual patient.[7,8] We commonly request that patients understand these distinctions to help distinguish physical pain from psychological distress to allow us to direct appropriate therapy. Using the MPAC, pain relief and mood can be evaluated in 20 seconds. The use of such a scale provides a format for communication between the patient and health care professional, which can then be used to choose the appropriate therapy. Recording pain intensity on the daily chart of each inpatient at Memorial Sloan-Kettering Cancer Center not only establishes pain intensity as a fifth vital sign but also underscores a critical institutional commitment to pain management.[40]

Types of Pain **Somatic Pain** Somatic pain is the most common type of pain in patients with cancer and bone metastases are the most prevalent cause. Somatic pain is characterized as well localized, intermittent, or constant and is described as aching, gnawing, throbbing, or cramping. Bone metastases are characterized by bone destruction with concurrent new bone formation. Prostaglandins sensitize nociceptors and produce hyperalgesia and pain as osteolysis and osteoclast formation occur.[30] Other factors, such as osteoclast-activating factor, also sensitize nociceptors and produce increased pain perception.[41] Drugs that interfere with prostaglandin synthesis and osteoclast formation inhibit bone pain by inhibiting this sensitization and may also inhibit tumor growth. This partially explains relatively high potency of non-steroidal analgesics (NSAIDs) in bone pain. The widespread use of bisphosphonates has resulted in improved analgesia and a significant reduction of skeletal complications in patients with malignant bone pain (see "Adjuvant Drugs" section). Steroids and radiopharmaceuticals are the other two groups of analgesics that add to the traditional analgesic regimen in cancer pain management.

Visceral Pain Visceral pain is mediated by discrete nociceptors in the cardiovascular, respiratory, gastrointestinal, and genitourinary systems, is usually described as deep, squeezing, or colicky, and is commonly referred to cutaneous sites, which may be tender. This referral pattern is thought to be related to the fact that somatic and visceral structures have dual innervation by common afferent fibers. These fibers converge in the dorsal horn in the spinal cord. The pain of a visceral site may be misrepresented as a cutaneous one. Shoulder pain, resulting from diaphragmatic irritation from a pleural disease, similarly to left jaw pain with myocardial infarction, is an example of a cutaneous referral of a visceral pain. Visceral pain results from mechanical or chemical activation of nociceptors by tumor compression or visceral distension and responds to a wide variety of pain management approaches including pharmacologic, anesthetic, and neurosurgical procedures.[41–43] Recent experimental data in animals suggest that kappa-opioid receptor agonists may be uniquely efficacious in the treatment of visceral pain.[44–46] The role of such agents in the management of human cancer pain requires further investigation. The only clinically used opioid that in addition to the mu-opioid activity is thought to be a kappa-opioid agonist is oxycodone.

Neuropathic Pain The second category of pain common in cancer patients is neuropathic pain, which results from injury to the peripheral receptor, afferent fiber, or central nervous system. Such injury is associated with spontaneous and ectopic firing in the peripheral nerve, at the level of the dorsal horn or brain, including thalamus. Neuropathic pain is clinically described as a burning, dysesthetic, squeezing sensation with paroxysms of shock-like pain. Chemotherapy-induced peripheral neuropathy is the most common cause of cancer-associated neuropathic pain. Tumor infiltration of the brachial and lumbar plexus are common in cancer patients as well.[47] Neuropathic pain may result from injury to the peripheral nerve as occurs in postmastectomy and post-thoracotomy pain.

Tricyclic antidepressants, selective serotonin reuptake inhibitors, anticonvulsants, local anesthetics, NMDA antagonists, opioids, intrathecal, and epidural opioids with local anesthetics and other adjuvant analgesics, as well as some neurostimulatory procedures have improved the outcome for cancer patients with neuropathic pain (see below).

Common Pain Syndromes in Patients with Cancer Over the last 15 years, a series of well-defined pain syndromes have been described in patients with pain and cancer. Many of these pain syndromes are unique to cancer and are often misdiagnosed because health care professionals are unfamiliar with their clinical presentation.[1,2,48] Knowledge of the common pain syndromes, essential in an oncologist's training, facilitates recognition and improves treatment of cancer pain management. The major categories of pain syndromes are listed in Table 67-3.

Table 67-3 Cancer Pain Syndromes

Pain syndromes associated with tumor infiltration
Headache
Cranial neuralgias
Glossopharyngeal neuralgia
Trigeminal neuralgia
Pain syndromes associated with cancer therapy
Postchemotherapy pain syndromes
Peripheral neuropathy
Perineal pain
Steroid pseudorheumatism
Aseptic necrosis of bone
Headache
Mononeuropathy
Postsurgical pain syndromes
Postmastectomy pain
Postradical neck dissection pain
Post-thoracotomy pain
Phantom limb and stump pain
Postradiation pain syndromes
Radiation fibrosis of brachial plexus
Radiation fibrosis of lumbosacral plexus
Radiation myelopathy
Radiation-induced peripheral nerve tumors
Acute herpetic and postherpetic neuralgia
Pain syndromes unrelated to cancer or cancer therapy
Lumbar disk disease
Osteoporosis

One of the biggest challenges is metastatic bone pain. Rapid escalation of pain escalating with movement may require opioid dose that may be excessive for the patient at rest. Balance between suboptimal analgesia of incident pain and sedation at rest may be a challenge. Vertebral metastases cause up to 90% of cases of spinal cord compression. Most common cancers associated with painful bone metastases are lung, breast, prostate, colon, and renal metastases.

Para vertebral metastases may cause spinal cord compression by tumor extension through neural foramen. They are seen mostly in lymphoproliferative disorders.

Spinal cord compression usually presents with local vertebral pain associated with radicular pain, progressing weakness below the lesion, followed by sensory loss, reflex abnormalities, bladder, and bowel dysfunction.

Multiple new sites of pain with numerous symptoms may be seen in leptomeningeal metastases. Headache, facial pain, back, and radicular pain may be associated with nausea, vomiting, lethargy, seizures, visual and hearing loss, extremities weakness, and bladder and bowel incontinence or pain may be the only presenting symptoms with any physical findings.

Post-thoracotomy and postmastectomy pain, as well as phantom limb pain are neuropathic pain syndromes that may require polypharmacy. Post-thoracotomy pain is usually localized to the area of the incision and is caused by the intercostals nerve injury. Chronic post-thoracotomy pain may be complicated by the adhesive capsulitis if pain in not rapidly controlled. Postmastectomy pain can start up to 6 months after mastectomy or lumpectomy. It is caused by the injury of the intercosto-brachial nerve (T1–T2 distribution) or a neuroma. It may be as prevalent as in up to 15% of all mastectomies. Pain is neuropathic, burning and constricting, associated with severe allodynia of the axillary area and the anterior chest wall. Adhesive capsulitis is a common co-morbidity.

Brachial plexopathy and lumbosacral plexopathy may present with pain in the plexus distribution. It is usually associated with a burning sensation and dysesthesia; pain is usually followed by progressive weakness, and later by atrophy. Predominantly upper brachial plexus involvement and ipsilateral Horner's syndrome are suggestive of epidural tumor extension. Plexopathy may be tumor or radiation related. Chemotherapy may worsen pre-existing plexopathy. Autoimmune plexitis is a self-limiting plexopathy that is clinically almost indistinguishable from the tumor-associated plexopathy, except for a relatively rapid onset of atrophy.

Of painful conditions related to chemotherapy, peripheral neuropathy is most common. Pain and usually burning, may be associated with numbness, paresthesia, and allodynia mostly in the fingers and toes. Decreased vibration sense is the earliest physical finding, followed by absent ankle reflex and weakness in the distal muscle groups.

One of the big challenges in cancer pain management is a postherpetic neuralgia (PHN) that is not uncommon in patients undergoing chemo or radiation therapy. It is important to be aware that acyclovir given for 7 to 10 days reduces pain at 1 to 3 months as compared to placebo. Famcyclovir reduces the prevalence of postherpetic neuralgia at 6 months as compared with acyclovir. Use of steroids in acute herpes has questionable value. Both tricyclic antidepressant drugs and gabapentin are effective in reducing pain in postherpetic neuralgia after 36 weeks as compared to placebo. Being a non-malignant pain syndrome, PHN may significantly affect the cancer patient's quality of life, at times having more adverse effect than cancer itself. Number needed to treat (NNT) is a calculated measure of effectiveness of the analgesic. The NNT indicates the number of patients needed to be treated for one patient to report 50% pain reduction. In neuropathic pain it is relatively high for different groups of analgesics (Table 67-4).

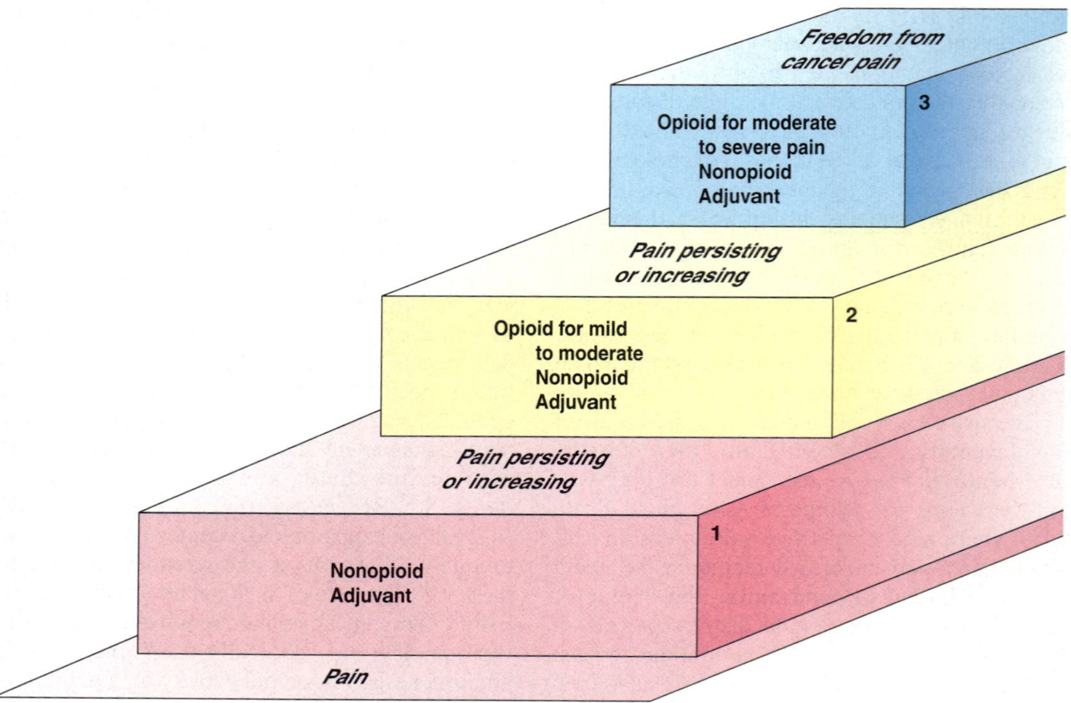

Figure 67-1 The World Health Organization three-step analgesic ladder for cancer pain.

STRATEGY FOR ASSESSMENT AND TREATMENT

In developing a strategy to manage the pain in a cancer patient, establishing the cause of the pain and the specific pain syndrome is paramount. The guiding principles of a therapeutic strategy for cancer pain must include: (1) detailed assessment of the patient's pain, (2) appropriate choice of the therapeutic approach, (3) assurance of available expertise to provide alternative therapeutic strategies to patients, (4) continual reassessment of the degree of pain relief and impact on mood, functional status, patient and family acceptance, and the patient's overall quality of life, (5) ongoing communication between the physician and patient in defining the options for therapy and the potential risk/benefit ratios of any of the therapeutic approaches, and (6) defining the goals of pain and symptom management in dying patients. At the current time, a series of algorithms have been developed for the management of this population of patients.[30,49] A randomized, controlled clinical trial implementing a treatment algorithm based on the Agency for Health Care Policy and Research Guidelines for Cancer Pain Management revealed that patients in the treatment algorithm group experienced a significant reduction in pain intensity compared to the control group.[50] Furthermore, reduction in pain intensity correlated with the patients' adherence to analgesic therapies.

Table 67-4 Number Needed to Treat (NNT) Measurement of Analgesics

Analgesic	NNT
Opioids	2.6 and above
Tramadol	3.4
Gabapentin	3.7–3.2
Amitriptyline	3.5–2.1
Mexiletine	10
Dextromethorphan	1.9
Capsaicin	6–7

THERAPEUTIC APPROACHES TO CANCER PAIN

Pharmacological Approaches Pharmacological approaches are the most commonly used method for managing cancer pain. The World Health Organization has recognized that analgesic drug therapy is the mainstay of pain treatment for cancer patients. The WHO Cancer Pain and Palliative Care Program advocates the three-step approach shown in Figure 67-1.[10,51] Validation studies of the WHO guidelines reveal successful treatment of cancer pain in 69 to 100% of patients.[52–56] Such an approach advocates the use of nonopioid, opioid, and adjuvant analgesics alone and in combination, titrated to the needs of the individual patient.

The Agency for Health Care Policy and Research has developed guidelines for the treatment of cancer pain,[6] and the Joint Commission on Hospital Accreditation has established pain assessment and treatment as an important priority in the delivery of high-quality inpatient care. The effective use of analgesic drugs should be a major part of every physician's armamentarium in managing patients with pain.

The specific guidelines for the use of pharmacologic approaches are detailed in Table 67-5. The fundamental concept that underlies this approach is individualization of pharmacotherapy. The selection of the right analgesic administered in the right dose on a regular schedule to maximize pain relief and minimize adverse effects begins with the use of non-opioids for mild pain. In patients with moderate pain that is not controlled with non-opioids such as acetaminophen, nonsteroidal anti-inflammatory drugs (NSAIDs), and adjuvant medications (WHO step 1), the so-called weak opioid-agonists (codeine, hydrocodone, oxycodone, and tramadol) alone or in combination are prescribed (step 2). In patients with severe pain, a strong opioid (morphine, hydromorphone, fentanyl, methadone, oxycodone, oxymorphone, or levorphanol) is the drug of choice (step 3). At all levels, certain NSAIDs and adjuvant drugs may be used for specific indications.

It is critical that patients presenting in severe pain should generally be treated with a strong opioid immediately.

Non-Opioid Analgesics **Nonsteroidal Anti-Inflammatory Drugs** The non-opioid analgesics include acetaminophen and NSAIDs, of which aspirin is the prototypic agent. The drugs in

Table 67-5 Guidelines for the Use of Analgesic Drugs in Cancer Pain Management

Start with a specific drug for a specific type of pain

1. Clarify the patient's pain, its nature, site, duration, and intensity, and the degree of pain relief from prior non-opioid and opioid drug use.
2. Complete a careful medical and neurologic history and examination.
3. Assess the psychological factors contributing to the pain complaint, and understand the meaning of the pain for the patient.
4. Know the pharmacology of the available drugs, non-opioid, opioid, and adjuvant. Titrate the dose to the individual needs of the patient.
   i. Start with a dose that is at least equivalent or slightly greater than the equianalgesic dose of the previous analgesic used.
   ii. Order the medication on a regular basis (every 3 to 4 hours).
   iii. Instruct the patient to take the medication on a PRN basis if the patient is opioid naive.
   iv. Order "rescue medication" equivalent to 1/2 the standing dose to begin with on a PRN basis.
   v. Inform the patient of options in taking the medication, and request that he or she report side effects of excessive sedation or confusion.
5. Choose the route of administration to fit the needs of the individual patient
   i. Choose the oral route as the simplest approach.
   ii. Consider the buccal or rectal routes for patients who cannot tolerate oral drugs and refuse parenteral routes. Start intravenous intermittent boluses or continuous infusions in patients requiring rapid escalation of opioids for pain control.
   iii. Use intermittent boluses or continuous subcutaneous infusions for patients without venous access or in patients at home.
   iv. Choose the epidural or intrathecal route in patients who develop limiting side effects from systemic opioids.
   v. Instruct patients in the use of PCA, and use PCA pumps for selected patients in hospital and at home.
6. Use a combination of drugs to provide additive analgesia to reduce side effects or to control other symptoms
   i. Know the various adjuvant drugs that provide additive analgesia, eg, hydroxyzine, corticosteroids.
   ii. Use neurostimulants to reduce sedative effects, eg, caffeine, dextroamphetamine, methylphenidate.
   iii. Use tricyclic antidepressants to manage neuropathic pain.
7. Anticipate and treat side effects
   i. Watch for respiratory depression, and use naloxone if needed (in diluted doses to prevent acute withdrawal).
   ii. Counteract sedation with neurostimulants.
   iii. Use antiemetics to suppress the emetic effect of opioids.
   iv. Define an individualized bowel regimen to prevent and manage constipation.
   v. Treat myoclonus by switching to an alternative analgesic, or suppress it with anxiolytic drugs.
8. Watch for the development of tolerance
   i. Distinguish tolerance from progression of tumor.
   ii. Recognize that there is no limit to tolerance.
   iii. Switch to an alternative opioid.
   iv. Use epidural local anesthetics to control localized pain.
   v. Consider cordotomy in a patient with chronic unilateral pain below the waist with stable pulmonary function.
9. Differentiate physical and psychological dependence
   i. Prevent withdrawal by administering 25% of the opioid daily dose and tapering the dose in decrements of 10%.
   ii. Use diluted doses of naloxone to reverse respiratory depression without reversing analgesia.
10. Reassess the patient's pain, mood and quality of life
   i. Re-evaluate the pain symptoms.
   ii. Evaluate the patient's quality of life.
   iii. Assess the patient for suicidal ideation.
   iv. Clarify the patient's DNR status.

DNR = do not resuscitate; PCA = patient-controlled analgesia; PRN = pro re nata (according as circumstances may require).

this group have a higher analgesic potential than aspirin and serve as an important first step in the management of patients with pain and cancer (Table 67-6). Survey data from WHO demonstration projects suggest that between 20 and 40% of patients obtain pain relief with the use of non-opioid analgesics alone.[10,57–59]

NSAIDs differ from each other both in duration of analgesic action and in pharmacokinetic profile. These drugs may have a special role to play in the management of bone pain because numerous studies have shown that aspirin inhibits tumor growth in an animal model of metastatic bone tumors. However, a meta-analysis of NSAIDs in bone pain did not demonstrate them to be more effective than weak opioids.[60,61]

Aspirin and the other NSAIDs have analgesic, antipyretic, anti-inflammatory, and antiplatelet actions. These drugs produce analgesia by inhibiting the arachidonic acid cascade that follows nociceptive tissue injury and serves as a substrate for the cyclo-oxygenase (COX) pathway. Affecting prostaglandin E2 (PGE2) and prostacyclin production, NSAIDs are said to decrease hyperalgesia as well. In addition to this peripheral action, a recent study indicates that they may also interfere with the action of glutamate and substance P in the central nervous system when cyclooxygenase is inhibited.[60] Two isoforms of the cyclooxygenase enzyme have been identified. cyclooxygenase-1 is a normal constituent of blood vessels, stomach, and kidney. Cyclooxegenase-2 (Cox-2) is induced in the setting of peripheral inflammation and acts as an attractant of inflammatory mediators. These compounds are most commonly used orally. Intravenous ketorolac is the only NSAID available in the United States for intravenous (IV) use. Although very useful as an opioid-sparing or opioid-reducing agent in cancer patients who are difficult to manage with morphine alone, its use is limited to a 5-day course due to gastrointestinal toxicity.[63] In clinical experience, some patients respond better to one NSAID than to others, and each patient should therefore be given an adequate trial of one drug on a regular basis before switching to another.

Absence of tolerance and physical dependence with repeated administration of NSAIDs is of great therapeutic value. When used short term their side effects profile compares favorably with opioid analgesics, unless specific contraindications are present.

Limitation of NSAID as a group is a ceiling effect, that is, increasing the dose beyond a certain level (eg, 900–1,300 mg per dose of aspirin and 300–400 mg of acetaminophen) will produce no increase in peak effect. Adverse effects of NSAIDs include gastrointestinal (GI) and renal toxicity. From the standpoint of morbidity and mortality, GI side effects constitute the most important toxicity that includes GI ulceration,

Table 67-6 Non-Opioid Analgesics Commonly Used for Mild to Moderate Pain

Name	Starting Oral Dose Range (mg)	Comments (Precautions)
Aspirin	650	Often used in combination with opioid analgesics (renal dysfunction; avoid during pregnancy, in hemostatic disorders, and in combination with steroids)
Choline magnesium trisalicylate (Trilisate)	1,500	Does not affect platelet function
Acetaminophen (Tylenol)	650	Like aspirin but does not affect platelet function
Ibuprofen (Motrin, Advil)	200–400	Higher analgesic potential than aspirin
Diflunisal (Dolobid)	500–1,000	Longer duration of action than ibuprofen; higher analgesic potential than aspirin
Naproxen (Naprosyn)	250–300	Like diflunisal
Ketorolac (Toradol)	10 (30 IM)	Not to exceed 5 days
Tramadol (Ultram)	50–200	Weak mu agonist and serotonergic and catecholamine reuptake inhibitor
Cox-2 inhibitors		
Celecoxib (Celebrex)	100–200	Contraindicated in sulfa-allergic patients

Table 67-7 Opioid Analgesics Commonly Used for Moderate to Severe Pain Narcotic Agonists

	Parental (mg)	Oral (mg)	Conversion Factor (IV to PO)	Comments
Morphine	10	30	3	Standard of comparison for opioid analgesics; lower dose for aged patients and patients with impaired ventilation, bronchial asthma, increased intracranial pressure, liver failure, renal failure
Hydromorphone (Dilaudid)	1.5	7.5	5	Slightly shorter-acting
Methadone (Dolophine)	10	20	2	Good oral potency, long plasma half-life; like morphine, may accumulate with repetitive dosing, causing excessive sedation
Fentanyl	100 μg = 4 mg morphine IV	—	—	Short half-life; transdermal and transmucosal preparations available
Meperidine (Demerol)	75	300	4	Not recommended in chronic cancer pain due to toxic metabolite, impaired renal function, or if receiving monamine oxidase inhibitors
Levorphanol (Levo-Dromoran)	2	4	2	Like methadone
Codeine	130	200	1.5	Often used in combination with non-opioid analgesics; biotransformed, in part, to morphine
Oxycodone (Roxicodone, Tylox)	—	30	—	Also in combination with non-opioid analgesics, that limit dose escalation
Oxymorphone (Numorphan)	1	—	6 (rectal)	Like methadone; not available orally

perforation and hemorrhage.[64–66] Serious GI toxicity may be seen without any warning sign and can be seen in 2 to 4% of the patients after 1 year of chronic use. The risk of NSAIDs gastropathy are increased in females, patients over the ago of 60, and those with a history of peptic ulcer disease or other morbidity. Concomitant use of NSAIDs and steroids may increase the risk of NSAIDs gastropathy up to 4 times. Ibuprofen in daily doses of 1,600 mg or less was associated with the lowest relative risk of severe GI toxicity. Aspirin and diclofenac are 1.6 to 1.8 times more likely, and ketoprofen is moreover 4 times likely to cause gastropathy with chronic use. Misoprostol, an FDA approved agent to reduce the risk of GI ulceration should be used with caution in childbearing age females due to its teratogenic potential.

NSAIDs can cause small asymptomatic aminotransferase elevation in 1 to 15% of patients taking NSAIDs chronically. Prior to starting chronic NSAIDs treatment aminotransferase should be checked as a baseline and periodically thereafter.

Renal toxicity may be seen in patients with reduced renal blood flow or systemic hypovolemia. In addition, NSAIDs can affect renal tubular function, causing edema, mild hypertension and hyperkalemia.

Nonacetylated salicylates and choline magnesium trisalicylate in particular has the advantage of analgesic effect similar to aspirin although causing substantially less GI toxicity and little or no effect on platelets.

Acetaminophen, which is as potent as aspirin, is an analgesic and antipyretic but is much less effective as an anti-inflammatory agent and does not interfere with platelet function or cause any significant GI toxicity. It also does not cross-react in aspirin-sensitive asthma. Liver toxicity may be encountered with daily doses above 4 grams, especially in patients that are fasting, alcoholics or patients with prior liver injury. Only substantial doses (15–25 grams) will usually produce serious or fatal liver injury, however.

Tramadol Tramadol (Ultram), classified as opioid analgesic in some European countries is not a schedule II analgesic in the United States. Having some opioid-activity it also inhibits serotonin/norepinephrine reuptake. It is generally weaker that other opioids (10-fold less potent in mu receptor binding than codeine) and has a ceiling dose. In some European trials, it was shown to be safe and effective in a double-blind randomized placebo-controlled trial for the treatment of diabetic neuropathic pain.[67,68] The risk of abuse and dependence with tramadol has been found to be very low. It has been shown to produce synergistic analgesic response in preclinical studies at 1:8 mg-to-mg tramadol:acetaminophen ratio. Ultracet, a combination of tramadol 37.5 mg and acetaminophen 325 mg is now available in the United States.

Opioid Analgesics The opioid analgesics as a class consist of heterogeneous compounds whose pharmacologic effects are derived from their interaction with multiple central nervous system opiate receptors.[69] The morphine agonist drugs bind to discrete opiate receptors and produce analgesia. The opioid antagonists block and reverse the effects of opioid receptors. All clinically available opioids are mu opioid agonists and only oxycodone has kappa-opioid agonist activity as well. A number of opioid analgesics is available for clinical use and are listed in Table 67-7.

Codeine is considered to be a weak opioid and has a limited analgesic efficacy. It is used for the management of mild to moderate pain and has been included in step 2 of the analgesic ladder.[70] Codeine is metabolized to morphine that is its main active metabolite. It is about 6 times weaker than morphine. In single dose studies of cancer, dental, and post-operative pain codeine 60 mg was found to be equianalgesic to aspirin 650 mg or acetaminophen 600 to 1,000 mg. Approximately 15% of the population cannot convert codeine to morphine because of the lack of a specific enzyme and thus cannot gain pain relief.[71] At the higher doses required to treat severe pain, codeine is poorly tolerated by patients because it produces significant nausea.

Oxycodone is included in both step 2 and step 3 of the analgesic ladder. Oxycodone is available in combination with acetaminophen (Percocet, Tylox) or alone in tablet form and liquid form. Oxycodone is 10 times more potent than codeine. Oxycodone 5 mg has similar analgesic effect to acetaminophen 500 mg. When used in combination these drugs offer enhanced analgesia, an "opioid-sparing" effect and improved side effect and safety profile.[72]

Bioavailability of oxycodone is about 50%. It's potency compares with oral morphine, ratio being about 3:2.[73,74] Oxycodone is now available as 5 and 10 mg immediate-release preparations, as well as extended release OxyContin. There is 80 mg generic OxyContin sold in the United States that favorably compares in price with the brand name formulation.

Morphine remains the drug of choice for the management of patients with pain and cancer because of its place on the essential drug list of the WHO, its familiarity to physicians, and its wide oral use in the management of cancer pain.[10] Morphine, the prototypic drug, has an oral bioavailability that is about 35% and a plasma half-life of 2 to 3 hours in a young patient with normal renal and liver function. With repeated administration, the pharmacokinetics of morphine and its metabolites, morphine-3-glucuronide (M-3-G, 55%) and morphine-6-glucuronide (M-6-G, 15%) usually remain linear, but may change significantly in elderly patients and in patients with renal or liver insufficiency.[75,76] Conflicting data have been reported on the role of M-3-G and the development of tolerance.[77] Some studies suggest that the accumulation of M-3-G may be associated with the side effects of central nervous system excitation (eg, myoclonus and delirium) whereas M-6-G accumulation may result in the depressive side effects (eg, drowsiness and respiratory depression).[76] Half-life of M-6-G, a potent opioid agonist, in an elderly patient or a patient with significant renal insufficiency may be up to a few days and cause sedation that outlives the normally expected analgesic and sedating effects of morphine.[81,82,84–86] As judged by single-dose studies the relative potency of parenteral to oral morphine is 1:3, that is, 10 mg parenteral morphine produce analgesia equal to 30 mg of oral morphine.[78,79]

Morphine is now available in a wide variety of preparations, including immediate release tablets, oral solutions, controlled-release tablets (for 8, 12, or 24 hours), buccal tablets, rectal suppositories, and parenteral forms (intravenous, subcutaneous, epidural, and intrathecal).[80] Morphine delivered by a new delivery system, Avinza was shown to offer 24 hours pain relief in an arthritis model, providing 10% of the dose as immediate release. Because of the preservative, fumaric acid, its daily dose should not exceed 1,600 mg. It can be sprinkled on food, but should not be dissolved to avoid immediate release of the 24-hour morphine dose. Kadian is another 24-hour formulation of slow-release morphine that can be sprinkled on food and given via percutaneous gastrostomy tube as well.

Hydromorphone (Dilaudid) is a strong opioid (1.5 mg of hydromorphone intravenously is equipotent to 10 mg of intravenous morphine) and a useful alternative to morphine in the treatment of moderate to severe cancer pain. Although myoclonus has been described in the setting of continuous high-dose infusion, possibly due to accumulation of hydromorphone-3-glucuronide,[81] hydromorphone may be a suitable alternative to morphine in the setting of toxicity. Given its water solubility, availability in a high-potency formulation (10 mg/mL), and 87% bioavailability, hydromorphone is the drug of choice for chronic subcutaneous administration. It is also available in a suppository form and a controlled-release formulation, Palladone, administered q 24 hours orally that has recently been approved in the United States. In a double-blind trial comparing morphine and hydromorphone patient-controlled analgesia, no differences were found with respect to analgesia or side effects.[82] It has less histamine-release effects compared to the other morphine cogeners and can be used in patients who develop histamine-induced headache or itch.

Fentanyl is a mu-opioid with shortest half-life that together with the unique transdermal delivery system makes it an opioid of choice for patients with renal or liver insufficiency or those who need to bypass GI tract or are non-compliant due to forgetfulness or other cognitive problems. It is available for intravenous use, in a transdermal patch, and in an oral transmucosal preparation. Fentanyl is about 25 times more potent than morphine.

Transdermal fentanyl patch is contraindicated in opioid-naïve patients. After the patient is started on a fentanyl patch there is a 6 to 12 hour delay in the onset of analgesia, and therefore, patients need to have their pain controlled by the immediate release medication during this titration phase. With transdermal application of fentanyl the patch has to be changed every 72 hours in the majority of patients, but every sixth patient may experience end-of dose failure reporting escalation of pain on day three. Escalation of the dose or changing the fentanyl patch (Duragesic) every 48 hours should be considered then.

Transdermal fentanyl is commonly used for the long-term management of pain in patients with advanced cancer of the GI tract, head and neck, and other malignancies.[80,83] Steady state is generally achieved within 12 to 24 hours following application of the patch. Some studies have suggested that patients who receive transdermal fentanyl may be more satisfied with analgesia and side effect profile when compared with those who receive sustained-release morphine.[84–86] Administration of fentanyl patch may not eliminate or even significantly decrease the need for PRN short-acting opioids in some patients.

Table 67-8 Oral Transmucosal Fentanyl Citrate

	Actiq	Oralet
Indication	Breakthrough pain	Procedure pain (adult and children) Anesthetic premedication (children)
Available doses	200,400,600,800,1,000, 1,600 µg/unit	Discontinued in the USA
Patient population	Opioid-tolerant adults	Opioid-naive adults and children
Color of lozenge	White	Red
Packaging	Child-resistant Requires scissors to open	Non–child-resistant
Flavoring	Lemon	Strawberry/cherry

Oral transmucosal fentanyl citrate (OTFC) is a valuable option for the treatment of highly prevalent cancer-related breakthrough pain, a transient increase in pain over a well-controlled baseline pain.[87,88] Two formulations of OTFC are currently approved for use in the United States (Table 67-8).

Fentanyl Oralet is approved as an anesthetic premedication in children and for procedure-related pain in adults and children. It is available in 100, 200, 300, and 400 µg and is indicated for opioid-naive patients.

Fentanyl Actiq is available in a wider range of dosages (200–1,600 µg) and is indicated for the management of breakthrough pain in opioid-tolerant adults. Twenty-five to 50 percent of both preparations are absorbed transmucosally over a 15-minute period, and an additional 25% is absorbed via the gastrointestinal tract over the following 90 minutes. Onset of relief may occur within 5 minutes.[88] In dose-titration trials, OTFC has been shown to be safe and effective in comparison with other agents used for breakthrough pain.[89,90] In multi-center dose-titration trials, the effective OTFC dose fentanyl was associated with fewer side effects than morphine.

Levorphanol is a second-line drug with the potential drug accumulation associated with its long half-life (12 to 16 hours). The d-isomer of levorphanol (dextrorphan) is relatively devoid of analgesic action but acts as an NMDA receptor antagonist that may offer additional value in pain management.

Methadone is an old opioid that has been increasingly used in cancer pain management over the last few years. Advantages to the use of methadone in cancer pain include 48 to 96% bioavailability, lack of active metabolites, low cost, long half-life resulting in larger intervals between doses, and improved patient compliance. Methadone is a potent opioid with an unpredictable half-life. Half-life varies among patients, ranging from a few hours to a few days. This leads to potential drug accumulation even if the patient continues to take the stable dose that was initially prescribed. This dose accumulation and resulting escalation of blood levels associated with increased analgesia and possible increasing side effects may be seen 1 to 2 days to 7 days after the initiation of methadone treatment. Sedation, confusion, and even death can occur when patients are started on an excessive dose of methadone that initially may be well tolerated. Concerns about safety of methadone have led to its limited use, especially in frail patients.[91,92] The original equianalgesic table was based on single dose studies, which demonstrated morphine: methadone ratio as 1:1. The American Pain Society suggests the parenteral morphine: methadone equianalgesic ratio to be 2:1. However when switching from an initial opioid to methadone in a patient with uncontrolled pain, one may hardly suggest establishing equianalgesic doses because analgesia has not yet been achieved. Thus, rather than searching for the equianalgesic dose ratio, a safe and effective starting methadone dose should be sought. The latest literature suggests starting with 10:1 ratio. That means that when switching from morphine to methadone the initial parenteral dose methadone is equivalent to 10% of a preswitch parenteral morphine dose.[93,94] In addition, numerous reports in the literature suggest that the equianalgesic ratio may be significantly influenced by the previous opioid dose and the length of time the patients were receiving the previous opioid.[95–97] In rotating patients from morphine to methadone, Ripamonti and colleagues used a dose ratio of 4:1 for patients who received 30 to 90 mg of morphine daily, 6:1 for patients who received 90 to 300 mg daily, and 8:1 for patients who received 300 mg or more. Other studies suggest that as little as one-tenth the equianalgesic dose of methadone can provide effective analgesia in patients tolerant to other opioid analgesics.[98] Bruera and colleagues demonstrated that the hydromorphone/methadone ratio is correlated with total opioid dose, and that in switching from hydromorphone to methadone, much lower doses than expected may provide satisfactory analgesia.[98] In patients receiving more than 330 mg of hydromorphone prior to the switch, the dose ratio was 1.6:1 whereas in patients receiving less than 330 mg of hydromorphone daily, the dose ratio was 0.95:1.[98]

Using a conservative starting methadone dose (10:1 ratio), administered in three divided doses (tid), it is essential to have the PRN dose available liberally. Some groups suggest that methadone should be administered at a fixed dose, but patient controlled intervals. Within the first 3 days, the patient self-titrates to the therapeutic dose. Considering the long half-life and dose accumulation of methadone, if excellent analgesia occurs within 24 hours and no PRN medication is needed a 50% reduction of the total dose should be considered.

The safety of methadone has been also demonstrated in the presence of chronic liver and renal disease, common at the end of life.[99] Mercandante and colleagues recently reported that in comparing the use of methadone versus morphine in pain management of advanced cancer at home, those who received methadone required fewer dose escalations, supporting a definite role for methadone in the hands of an experienced clinician.[100]

Meperidine is an opioid with unique properties. Meperidine has been recently shown to block Na+ channels with molecular pharmacologic features of a local anesthetic. Mostly preclinical findings support classification of meperidine as a local anesthetic, but with less overall potency than lidocaine. Repetitive dosing of meperidine in a patient with renal insufficiency can lead to accumulation of a toxic metabolite, normeperidine resulting in central nervous system hyperexcitability. This adverse effect is characterized by subtle mood changes followed by tremors, multifocal myoclonus, and occasionally, seizures. This complication occurs more commonly in patients with renal disease but can occur following repeated administration in patients with normal renal function.[101]

OPIOID AGONIST/ANTAGONISTS AND PARTIAL AGONISTS

Opioid agonist/antagonists have the main advantage of causing less respiratory depression and having less abuse potential. However, the clinical use of these agents in cancer pain management is limited by the undesirable side effects and by ceiling analgesic effects. Pentazocine is a kappa-opioid agonist and a weak mu opioid antagonist or partial agonist. Its analgesic effect is mediated mostly by kappa-opioid receptors. Higher doses (60 to 90 mg) elicit dysphoric and psychotomimetic effects, as well as increased blood pressure and heart rate. When given to a patient who is tolerant to opioids pentazocine may precipitate withdrawal symptoms. Ceiling effect for analgesia and respiratory depression are observed above 50 to 100 mg of pentazocine. Nalbuphine and butorphanol are similar to pentazocine in agonist/antagonist opioid effects. Buprenorphine, partial mu-receptor agonist, is a semisynthetic opioid that is 25 to 50 times more potent than morphine. It is not currently available in the United States for use in analgesia.

The role of opioids in the management of neuropathic pain has been controversial because of concerns about ineffectiveness, the potential for development of tolerance, and limiting side effects. Several recent placebo-controlled trials have studied the use of opioids in the management of neuropathic malignant and nonmalignant pain.[102–106] Opioids appear selectively to reduce spontaneous and touch-evoked allodynia in a trial using quantitative methods for sensory testing.[107] Given lack of data derived from randomized placebo-controlled trials about how to manage neuropathic cancer pain, we must focus urgent attention on the needs of suffering patients. Patients with neuropathic pain should be given a trial of an opioid to assess the degree of opioid responsiveness.[108]

Start with a Specific Drug for a Specific Type of Pain Choosing an analgesic regimen requires knowledge of the pharmacokinetic and pharmacodynamic properties of the opioid analgesics and adjuvant analgesic medications. Each physician should become familiar with several drugs in these groups and adapt them to the needs of his or her clinical practice. Cherny and colleagues have documented the strategies used by pain physicians for the selection of analgesic drugs and routes of administration.

A common approach is to start a patient on a non-opioid, followed by the use of codeine or oxycodone alone or in combination with the non-opioid. If with repeated doses the patient does not obtain effective pain relief, switch him or her to morphine, hydromorphone, fentanyl, levorphanol, or methadone. We commonly choose morphine, but in patients intolerant to morphine, we use hydromorphone as our first line drug. In the elderly patient, to avoid morphine metabolites accumulation, we often choose oxycodone, hydromorphone, or fentanyl before morphine because our clinical empiric data suggest that they may produce fewer central nervous system side effects than morphine.[109] Transdermal fentanyl has a number of advantages in patients with renal and liver insufficiency, patients unable to take oral analgesics and patients with low compliance. Levorphanol and methadone tend to be second-line drugs, particularly in the elderly patient where their long half-lives present a potential risk of dose accumulation. The dose is then titrated to the individual needs of the patient.

Opioid Rotations After tissue injury there is great interindividual variability among patients in the amount of pain experience (pain intensity and duration of pain) and in the degree of pain relief from analgesics.[110–112]

In a prospective study, 80 of 100 patients referred to the Memorial Sloan-Kettering Cancer Center Pain Service required changes in either opioid or route of administration to obtain adequate analgesia with tolerable side effects. Eighty percent of patients required one opioid switch, 44% of patients required two switches and 20% of patients required three or more switches.[113]

These are some of the common reasons to consider an opioid rotation to improve efficacy and avoid toxicity:

- cognitive failure; sedation
- hallucinations; myoclonus
- pruritus
- urinary retention
- nausea; vomiting
- Change route of administration
  - oral to parenteral opioids
  - change to transdermal/transmucosal—fentanyl
- Decrease costs

A study on 273 patients with cancer documented the reasons for rotation to be: (1) insufficient analgesia 43%, (2) side effects 20%, (3) both 15%, and (4) patient choice 18%.[114] Most patients experienced significantly better analgesia and a reduction in side effects with the substitution of one opioid for another.[115]

This process of opioid substitution or rotation is a common clinical practice based on the significant inter-individual variability in analgesia and side effect profile.[115] These variable responses may, in part, be explained by the presence of different opioid receptor subtypes, including the differences mediated by the specific single nucleotide polymorphisms (SNPs) at the mu-opioid receptor gene.[116–118] More than 50 SNPs have been identified in the mu-opioid receptor gene. A118G SNP has been associated with the following opioid responses:

- Increasing dosage requirements of morphine and alfentanil
- Altered efficacy to mu-opioid antagonists
- Altered hypothalamic-pituitary-adrenal axis activation
- Increased adverse effects to morphine-6-glucuronide

Minimal data on the role of genetic polymorphisms in drug transporters and their effects on pain relief in humans is currently available. Opioid rotation for now remains an empiric intervention based on the experience of the clinician.

When a new adverse effect appears in a previously stable patient the clinician should suspect that another process may be interfering with the assessment. Common causes of comorbidity are sepsis, metabolic events such as hypercalcemia, hyponatremia, uremia, and liver failure. Centrally acting medications should be reviewed.

The main advantages of the opioid rotation are minimizing polypharmacy and improving analgesia. Among disadvantages are variable and unpredictable outcomes and potential need for consecutive opioid rotations and possibility of eventual need for a number of adjuvant analgesics.

Choose the Starting Dose During the opioid rotation it is most useful to start with the dose that is equivalent to one-half the equianalgesic dose of the previous drug that provided good analgesia. Anticipating the dose accumulation of methadone within the first few days of stable dose administration should be remembered and a conservative dose of 10% of the previous morphine equivalent should be used if close monitoring for sedation and other side effects is not possible. If the patient has had no prior opioid exposure and presents with severe pain, start the medication on an as needed basis, requesting that the patient ask for medication when he feels his pain beginning to return. This may be every 2 to 3 hours. Depending on the pain control, half-life of the medication, renal and liver function, but usually after achieving steady state, that is, after 5 half-lives of the drug, the around the clock long-acting (sustained release) opioids are started. Rescue medications equivalent to one-half of the standing dose should be made available to patients.[87]

Choose the Route of Administration Recent studies have demonstrated that the majority of cancer patients require at least two routes of administration of analgesic drugs, and that 30% of patients need three routes of administration during the course of their disease.[119]

Oral Route The oral route is convenient and should be preferred unless specific contraindications or problems exist. In general, orally administered drugs have a slower onset of action and a longer duration of effect; drugs administered parenterally have a more rapid onset of action but a shorter duration of effect.

Numerous studies have led to the use of oral opioid analgesics in chronic cancer pain.[75,78] When given orally, the opioids differ substantially with respect to their presystemic elimination, that is, the degree to which they are inactivated as they are absorbed from the gastrointestinal tract and passed through the liver into the systemic circulation. As indicated in Table 67-7, morphine and hydromorphone have parenteral/oral potency ratios of 1:3 and 1:5, respectively, and methadone and levorphanol are subject to less presystemic elimination, resulting in an intravenous/oral potency ratio of at least 1:2. Bioavailability of methadone can fluctuate between 46 and 98% so parenteral to oral ratio may be anywhere from 1:2 to 1:1. Conservative dosing should be used if close monitoring is not possible.

Intranasal, Sublingual, Buccal, Rectal, and Transdermal Routes The intranasal, sublingual, buccal, rectal, and transdermal routes of administration provide alternative approaches for patients who cannot take oral drugs. These routes obviate the need for parenteral administration and offer the advantage of eliminating the first pass effect through the liver because they are rapidly taken up into the systemic circulation.

Intranasal butorphanol, a mixed agonist-antagonist, provides adequate analgesia for patients with acute postoperative pain but is not commonly used for chronic cancer pain management. Sublingual buprenorphine, not used in the United States for pain management, but only for the treatment of drug addiction and thus requiring a special license to be prescribed, is widely used outside of the United States in the second step of the WHO analgesic ladder. Both fentanyl and methadone are well absorbed sublingually, as demonstrated in a study of normal volunteers.[120] An oral transmucosal formulation of fentanyl (see above) has been demonstrated to be efficacious in treating breakthrough pain in cancer patients. Morphine is poorly absorbed sublingually but has been reported anecdotally to be effective.[121]

Oxymorphone, hydromorphone, and morphine are available as rectal suppositories and are effective in managing chronic cancer pain.

Studies of sustained-release morphine rectal suppositories in normal volunteers reported no significant differences in morphine absorption between the oral and rectal methods except that rectal absorption was delayed.[122] The available pharmacokinetic data do not clearly define whether rectal administration of morphine does avoid the first pass effect through the liver.

The transdermal fentanyl patch offers a unique route of opioid administration, when the patch is applied topically, but provides systemic drug administration (see above). In the setting of GI and head and neck malignancy, as well as significant malabsorption, or noncompliance, this route may be especially desirable.

Intravenous Boluses and Infusions The common use of permanent central catheters to provide intravenous access for patients controlled analgesia (PCA) is discussed in the following sections.

Intermittent or Continuous Subcutaneous Infusions This approach, in addition to the continuous intravenous infusions, has been particularly useful in obviating the pain management problems of patients who cannot take oral opioids because of nausea or vomiting, gastrointestinal intolerance, or obstruction.[123–125] In patients with lack of available venous access, with pain requiring continuous treatment, and with adverse effects from bolus injections, the use of continuous subcutaneous infusions obviates these practical problems and allows patients' pain management to be maintained in a hospital or discharged home with adequate pain control. Using a portable infusion pump attached to a butterfly needle, and rotating the subcutaneous sites, this approach has been useful in patients for periods of 24 hours to 12 months in chronic cancer pain management.[123] The infraclavicular and anterior chest sites provide the greatest freedom of movement for patients. The infusion site is changed every 3 to 7 days, and a wide variety of opioid analgesics, including morphine, hydromorphone, levorphanol, oxymorphone, heroin, and fentanyl, have been used safely and effectively by this approach. Methadone use has been complicated by the development of cutaneous rashes and inflammatory lesions thought to be a hypersensitivity response.[91] Limited pharmacokinetic studies have demonstrated that the bioavailability of drug from subcutaneous sites at steady state varies from 78 to 100%.[124,125] Guidelines for the use of this approach have been well described in the literature.[124,125]

Epidural and Intrathecal Infusions Although the vast majority of cancer patients receive adequate analgesia with oral opioids, patients who experience intolerable side effects or who are unable to take medication by mouth may receive significant relief from epidural and intrathecal infusions.[126] Opioid receptor agonists bind to selective sites within the substantia gelatinosa of the spinal cord and produce analgesia.[127] Data suggest that depending on the medical setting up to 10% of cancer patients require this approach to provide adequate analgesia.[128,129] The combination of low doses of local anesthetics with opioids has expanded the usefulness of this technique in patients with neuropathic pain.[130] The use of clonidine alone or in combination has demonstrated efficacy in neuropathic cancer pain, particularly associated with spasticity (see "Adjuvant Drugs" section).

The availability of patient-controlled devices that can be attached to subcutaneous reservoirs to which the epidural catheter is attached has allowed patients to be fully ambulatory using this technique.[131] The pharmacokinetics of epidural opioids suggest that a substantial amount of opioid (10 to 100 times the amount that would be there from a systemic injection) diffuses into cerebrospinal fluid from the epidural space. There is concurrent systemic uptake of the drug comparable to an intramuscular injection that is the highest in lipophilic drugs such as fentanyl. Therefore, the epidural route is associated with both cerebrospinal fluid as well as systemic uptake of the drug. In contrast, intrathecal administration is associated with significantly less systemic uptake of drug.[132,133] The advantage of both these routes of administration is that smaller doses of opioids can be used, and the undesirable central effects (eg, somnolence and respiratory depression) of the opioids can be minimized. However, in a recently published 3-year retrospective outcomes study on the use of epidural catheters in the management of chronic cancer pain, technical problems, and infections, including epidural abscesses, occurred in a significant number of patients, suggesting that the epidural route may be most useful in patients with limited life expectancy.[134] In Cherney and colleagues' study, cited above, of the 12% of patients who received an epidural or intrathecal catheter for cancer pain, the infusion was continued in only 4%.[114]

Epidural clonidine may be useful in cancer patients with severe pain who cannot be optimally managed on opiates, due to side effects.[135] In a randomized placebo-controlled trial in the setting of intractable cancer pain, 45% of patients received analgesia versus 21% in the placebo group.[136] Clonidine was especially useful in patients with neuropathic pain. Given its properties as an alpha-2-adrenergic agonist, blood pressure and heart rate must be continuously monitored.

Patient-Controlled Analgesia This method of opioid administration employs the concept of individualization of analgesic dose, in which the patient can titrate the analgesic doses within the limits set by the clinician to provide adequate relief. This term has been used to describe the use of specifically designed infusion pumps that can deliver a continuous infusion with bolus doses by the intravenous, subcutaneous, or epidural routes. Each pump can be programmed to the needs of the individual patient with a set "lock-out time" to prevent patients from overdosing themselves. This approach is most useful for managing the patient with acute pain, including post-operative or pain crisis, as well as chronic cancer pain who is unable to tolerate drugs by the oral route. Intravenous bolus doses of opioids provide the most rapid onset and shortest duration of analgesia. The time to peak effect correlates with the lipid solubility of the opioid and can range from 2 to 5 minutes for methadone to 10 to 15 minutes for morphine.[137] This mode of administration allows for complete systemic absorption. Intravenous bolus injections are used to titrate opioid doses in the patient with rapidly escalating pain.[138] This approach has been widely used to manage patients with acute postoperative pain as well as chronic cancer pain in the home setting.[139] Continuous infusions provide more stable analgesia without the peak and trough effects seen with repeated boluses. Specific guidelines for the use of continuous infusions have been developed and are summarized in Table 67-9.[138]

In patients requiring frequent repeated intravenous boluses to maintain analgesia, a continuous infusion often is a more practical approach. This approach can be also useful in a patient with far advanced disease in the terminal stages of his or her illness.

In a study of 46 infusions in 36 patients with pain and cancer, continuous IV infusion provided effective pain control in the majority. The goal for intravenous infusions in the dying patient needs to be clearly delineated to both families and staff to avoid any concern that such an approach is a form of "slow euthanasia."[140,141] The intent of continuous intravenous infusions in this setting is to provide patients with continuous relief of pain and suffering. The wide variety of PCA pumps, from simple devices to sophisticated computerized systems, combined with the use of intravenous or subcutaneous administration has been a major advance in cancer pain management for the dying patient.[142] In such patients with intractable nausea and gastrointestinal obstruction, antiemetics can be combined with the opioids to manage bowel obstruction in the terminal phase.

Use Equianalgesic Doses When Switching to Alternative Routes Changing the route of administration is usually associated with the end of the pain crisis and/or intravenous titration period, that is, selecting a route more convenient and practical long term, the need to simplify opioid schedule such as decrease the number of pills or patches, or when the patient is no longer able to take oral medications. When converting a patient from the intramuscular to the intravenous route, we have assumed that the equianalgesic dose is the same for these two routes.

Table 67-9 Guidelines for the Management of Continuous Intravenous Infusion (CII) of Opioids

1. CII should be indicated (bolus effect, nursing considerations, or rapid titration of dose).
2. Select an appropriate drug (consider the efficacy of current analgesic, prior opioid exposure, and pharmacokinetic factors such as half-life).
3. Choose the infusion device. (Flow-calibrated infusion pump should be used.)
4. Convert the current total daily opioid consumption to intramuscular equivalent milligrams.
5. If the current drug is used, infuse this quantity over the next 24 hours.
6. For CII with a drug different from the current one, convert the daily quantity of opioid into intramuscular equivalent mg of the new drug, and infuse one-half this amount over the next 24 hours.
7. Administer a loading bolus at the start and with each increase in infusion rate (10–15 morphine equivalent mg of a short half-life drug if the maintenance rate is between 15–30 morphine equivalent mg per hour and 30 morphine equivalent mg if the maintenance rate is greater than 30 equivalent mg per hour).
8. Increase infusion rate until analgesia is achieved or intolerable side effects develop. (If close monitoring is available, repeat the bolus injection, and increase the infusion rate by 10–20% every few hours. If close monitoring is not available, offer a "rescue dose" [a dose of a short-half-life drug equivalent to the loading dose administered] every 2 hours as needed, and increase the infusion rate after 12–24 hours by either 10–20% or an amount equivalent to the total rescue doses during the preceding period.)
9. Take vital signs every 30 minutes for 4 hours after a loading dose accompanied by an increase in the infusion rate and every 30 minutes for 2 hours after a rescue dose (guidelines vary between the institutions depending on the familiarity of the clinical staff with the continuous opioid administration).
10. If possible, control side effects with adjuvant drugs; if not effective, an alternative method of analgesia, such as CII with a different drug, should be considered.

Adjuvant Drugs There is a series of adjuvant drugs that are used in patients with pain and cancer.[143,144] These drugs have been developed and approved for clinical indications other than analgesia, including nausea, vomiting, anxiety, mania, depression, and seizures. Moreover, there are specific adjuvant drugs for the treatment of neuropathic pain and bone pain. The choice of the drugs must be individualized using the simplest but most potent of combinations.

Antidepressant Drugs This class of drugs appears to be the most useful in the management of patients with neuropathic pain.[145] Their analgesic effects are thought to be mediated in part by serotonergic and noradrenergic activity in the central nervous system. Controlled studies in migraine, postherpetic neuralgia, and diabetic neuropathy have demonstrated their efficacy. They appear to be equally useful in controlling chronic burning pain, continuous dysesthesia, and lancinating or shock-like pain common in patients with peripheral nerve injury.

Amitriptyline is the most commonly used drug, but imipramine, desipramine, and paroxetine have also been reported to be effective.[146,147] For amitriptyline, the suggested dosing schedule is to start at 10 to 25 mg in a single dose at bedtime, with dosing increments of the same amount. Doses can be increased every 1 to 2 days, particularly when using 10-mg tablets. Compliance with the regimen as well as the establishment of a therapeutic level can be facilitated by the assessment of plasma levels. Upward titration should be considered if the levels are below a therapeutic range. However, there is no therapeutic window for analgesia with amitriptyline. The majority of patients will note some response within a week, but it may take 2 to 3 weeks to see an analgesic effect. Paroxetine has demonstrated efficacy in postherpetic neuralgia, with fewer side effects than amitriptyline.[148] One study suggests that it may be particularly helpful in managing pruritus in the advanced-cancer patient.[149]

Post-herpetic neuralgia and diabetic neuropathy require three times as much amitriptyline and selective serotonin reuptake inhibitors as is needed for 50% reduction in pain from other causes.

Recently, Cymbalta (duloxetine hydrochloride) was approved for the management of the pain associated with diabetic peripheral neuropathy. This is the first drug specifically approved for this indication. The safety and effectiveness of Cymbalta were established in two randomized, controlled studies of approximately 1,074 patients. Although the mechanism of action is unknown, patients treated with Cymbalta reported a greater decrease in pain compared to placebo. In these trials, 51 percent of patients treated with duloxetine (Cymbalta) reported at least a 30 percent sustained reduction in pain. In comparison, 31 percent of patients treated with placebo reported this magnitude of sustained pain reduction.

Anticonvulsant Drugs Anticonvulsant drugs have been used in the management of pain since the 1960s. Their clinical use in chronic neuropathic pain is considered when the pain is lancinating or burning. Carbamazepine and gabapentin are anticonvulsant drugs that suppress spontaneous neuronal firing. In patients with cancer, carbamazepine has been used specifically in managing the acute shocklike neuralgic pain in the cranial or the cervical distribution caused by tumor infiltration or surgical injury. This drug has also been effective in patients with stump pain secondary to traumatic neuroma and patients with lumbosacral plexopathy reporting acute lancinating pain. Patients should commonly start at 100 mg at bedtime, slowly titrating up to 400 to 600 mg per day. Three placebo-controlled studies of carbamazepine in trigeminal neuralgia had a combined number needed to treat for 50 % pain relief (NNT) for effectiveness of 2.5. A single placebo-controlled trial of gabapentin in postherpetic neuralgia had an NNT of 3.2. For diabetic neuropathy NNTs for effectiveness were as follows: (one RCT for each drug) carbamazepine 2.3, gabapentin 3.8 and phenytoin 2.1. The minimal effective concentration for analgesia is not known, but evaluation of the plasma levels of carbamazepine is helpful in determining compliance and evaluating drug absorption in the individual patient. Carbamazepine is contraindicated in patients with leukopenia because of its independent ability to produce leukopenia.

Gabapentin is effective in improving analgesia in patients with neuropathic cancer pain already treated with opioids.[150] Its excellent side-effect profile, lack of hepatic metabolism, and lack of any known drug-drug contraindications make it a prime choice. Although small numbers of patients report bothersome gastrointestinal side effects and mental clouding, it is generally well tolerated up to 4,800 mg per day. The dose should be reduced in patients with renal insufficiency.

Both clonazepam and valproic acid have been reported to be effective in a series of anecdotal case reports and may be considered as alternative agents in patients who are unable to benefit from carbamazepine, gabapentin, or phenytoin.[143] Lamotrigine, a new antiseizure medication, has been recently used for pain. Recent trial showed no significant effect of lamotrigine on spontaneous and evoked pain in complete and incomplete spinal cord injury, it reduced spontaneous pain and evoked pain in the area of spontaneous pain.[151] In a prospective survey, out of 20 patients with chronic, neuropathic pain not responding to interventional therapy who received lamotrigine, ten patients did not respond to the drug, 4 were temporary responders, and 6 patients obtained sustained pain relief. Five patients regained opioid responsiveness and the drug combination produced excellent pain relief for more than 5 months.[152]

Phenothiazine Drugs Methotrimeprazine has been shown to have effects equianalgesic to morphine in single-dose studies in patients with postoperative pain and chronic cancer pain.[153,154] This drug is not currently available in the United States.

Haloperidol is the drug of choice in the management of patients with acute psychosis and delirium. Animal studies demonstrate that haloperidol potentiates morphine analgesia and has an independent analgesic effect. The doses of haloperidol in patients with acute delirium or acute psychotic reaction start with 0.5 to 1 mg orally at bedtime to 2 to 3 mg three times a day, depending on the patient's symptomatology and ability to tolerate the drug.[3,145]

Atypical Neuroleptics Evidence-based review of the available studies on the potential effectiveness of the atypical neuroleptics for the treatment of pain reveals that 90% of the published reports indicate that the atypical neuroleptics did have an analgesic effect. The overall strength and consistency of this evidence is variable. There are, however, few double-blind, placebo-controlled studies, and many of the reports/studies have less than 50 patients. As such, this question requires further research.

Risperidone may be useful for treatment of both hyper and hypo-active delirium. It is associated with few parkinsonian side effects. The same is true for olanzapine (Zyprexa), a relatively new atypical neuroleptic that may be quite sedating and in elderly patients may be associated with worsening delirium. It's sedating properties may be of great value under certain circumstances. It also comes as a dissolvable tablet that may be an advantage in dysphagia or if a patient is too sedated or weak to be able to cooperate.

Antihistamine Drugs Hydroxyzine has been shown to have analgesic effects when combined with morphine or meperidine in doses of 100 mg parenterally.[146] Hydroxyzine also has antiemetic and sedative properties, both of which can be desirable in patients with nausea, vomiting, and acute anxiety. Common practice is to use hydroxyzine at doses of 25 mg in combination with opioids to control these other effects. Most published data is derived from the anecdotal reports.

Corticosteroids Corticosteroids are the most widely used general-purpose adjuvant analgesics. Analgesic effects of steroids consist of the anti-inflammatory effect and in cultured dorsal root ganglia were shown to reduce ectopic neural discharge that is thought to be the explanation of their effectiveness in neuropathic pain. They may ameliorate pain and produce beneficial effects on appetite, nausea, and mood. They provide analgesia from pain syndromes associated with raised intracranial pressure, acute spinal cord compression, superior vena cava syndrome, metastatic bone pain, neuropathic pain due to infiltration or compression by tumor, and hepatic capsular distension.[30] Systemic, intra-articular and epidural routes of administration are most common. Patients with advanced cancer who experience pain and other symptoms that may respond to steroids are usually given relatively small doses (dexamethasone, 1 to 2 mg twice daily). In patients with epidural spinal cord compression, high doses (dexamethasone, 24 or 100 mg IV, followed by a slow taper) can be used to manage an acute episode of severe pain.[30]

Eighty-five percent of patients receiving 100 mg of dexamethasone as a part of a radiotherapy protocol reported significant relief associated with marked reduction in analgesic requirements within 24 hours of administration of this dose. Several studies demonstrate prolonged survival times and reduced opioid doses in terminal cancer patients receiving steroids. In patients with prostate cancer, 30 mg of prednisone on a regular basis improves patients' quality of life and reduces their pain symptomatology.[30,147–150] Pain resulting from tumor infiltration of the brachial and lumbosacral plexus is often improved by the use of steroids. Steroids also improve the headache and radicular pain commonly seen in leptomeningeal disease. Corticosteroids may be particularly helpful in the patient who is admitted to the hospital with far-advanced disease and diffuse pain in an acute painful crisis. We often use a large dose of steroids in this setting (10 to 24 mg of dexamethasone IV) to stabilize the patient and provide rapid symptom control.

However, steroid psychosis can complicate steroid use and can occur during dose escalation and withdrawal. Steroid-induced psychosis is treated with dose reduction and neuroleptics.

Neurostimulant Drugs Dextroamphetamine has been demonstrated to provide additive analgesia in patients receiving morphine for postoperative pain.[151] In a controlled repeated-dose trial, oral methylphenidate reversed opioid-induced sedation and provided supplemental analgesia in a population of patients with cancer pain.[152,153]

Recent anecdotal evidence suggests that pemoline in starting doses of 18.5 mg per day may also be useful to counter opioid-induced sedation, but controlled studies are lacking. Pemoline is rarely associated with significant hepatic dysfunction and should be used with appropriate caution. Provigil (modafinil) is a wakefulness-promoting agent for oral administration similar in action to sympathomimetic agents including amphetamine and methylphenidate, although its pharmacologic profile is not identical to that of sympathomimetic amines. Unlike sympathomimetic agents, modafinil has minimal effects on cardiovascular and hemodynamic parameters. The effectiveness of Provigil in reducing the excessive sleepiness (ES) associated with narcolepsy was established in two United States 9-week, multicenter, placebo-controlled, two-dose (200 mg per day and 400 mg per day) parallel-group, double-blind studies of outpatients with American Sleep Disorders Association criteria for narcolepsy.

Topical and Systemic Local Anesthetics Topical drugs, including lidocaine and benzocaine creams are most useful in the management of painful cutaneous and mucosal lesions and as a premedication prior to skin puncture. Controlled studies have demonstrated the effectiveness of a eutectic mixture of 2.5% lidocaine and 2.5% prilocaine (EMLA) in reducing pain associated with venipuncture, lumbar puncture, and arterial puncture.[154,155] Viscous lidocaine is frequently used in the management of oropharyngeal ulceration.[156] Lidoderm patch is a delivery system delivering 5% lidocaine transcutaneously with minimal blood concentration. It is the only topical agent approved for post-herpetic neuralgia. It is applied for 12 hours of every 24 hours to avoid tachyphylaxis. Oral mexiletine in the dose of 100 to 300 mg three times daily have been studied in the management of neuropathic pain. NNT for mexiletine is relatively high and has been reported to be 30 in some studies.[157]

Lidocaine, bupivacaine, and ropivacaine are the most commonly used parenteral local anesthetics for trigger point injections, intercostals, brachial, epidural, and intrathecal infusions. Unfortunately, positive response to lidocaine infusion does not predict mexiletine analgesia. Epidural bupivacaine offers good motor and sensory separation and lasts two to three times longer than lidocaine. That leads to its frequent use in the epidural and intrathecal infusions. Bupivacaine is quite cardiotoxic when given parenterally and caution should be executed if the patient is receiving both epidural and intravenous infusions simultaneously. Special marked tubing delivering bupivacaine should be used to avoid drug errors.

Adjuvants for Bone Pain Bisphosphonate drugs (pamidronate, clodronate, zoledronate, and etidronate) bind to bone hydroxyapatite, inhibiting osteoclast activity, and are highly effective in the management of metastatic disease to the bone and in managing multiple myeloma. Some randomized double-blind studies have demonstrated their efficacy not only in relieving bone pain but also in reducing skeletal complications[158,159] Recent combined analysis of two multicenter, randomized, placebo-controlled studies of pamidronate disodium for the palliation of bone pain in men with metastatic prostate cancer failed to demonstrate a significant overall treatment benefit.[160] In women with advanced breast cancer and clinically evident bone metastases, the use of bisphosphonates (oral or intravenous) in addition to hormone therapy or chemotherapy, when compared with placebo or no bisphosphonates, delays any skeletal event and reduces the risk of developing one. Bisphosphonates may also reduce bone pain in women with advanced breast cancer and clinically evident bone metastases.[161] Pamidronate, given as a 90 mg monthly infusion, has recently been shown to be safe for up to 2 years.[162] Although the currently available bisphosphonates do not appear to affect overall survival, they are very useful palliative agents. Third generation bisphosphonates (zoledronate) are now available for clinical use.[163] Zoledronic acid (4 mg) has been compared to placebo in a randomized phase III trial involving 422 men with hormone-refractory prostate cancer metastatic to bone. Zoledronic acid demonstrated a significant advantage over placebo for median time to first SRE, the proportion of patients with an SRE over 15 months, and mean skeletal morbidity rate. In addition, the effects of zoledronic acid were apparent early, at 3 months whereas 6 months had previously been reported for pamidronate.[164]

Strontium-89, among other radiopharmaceuticals, is an effective treatment of patients with chemotherapy-refractory prostate cancer, but careful and prolonged monitoring of hematologic parameters after therapy is required. In a recent study of the 14 administered treatments, 8 (57%) resulted in improved pain control, with 2 patients able to stop analgesia. The median duration of response was 56 days. There was significant and prolonged bone marrow toxicity, with 6 patients requiring red blood cell transfusion.[165] Strontium-89 is effective and safe in bone pain palliation in breast cancer. In a recent study 25 patients with painful multifocal bone metastases from breast cancer received 148 MBq 89Sr i.v. The global response rate was 84%. The duration of pain relief ranged from 2 months to 14 months (mean of 125 days). A moderate hematological toxicity resolved within 12 weeks after 89Sr administration.[166]

Other Adjuvants Dextromethorphan, an oral antitussive is an NMDA receptor antagonist as well as a calcium channel blocker. In experimental models, dextromethorphan prevents and reverses the development of tolerance.[167,168] In a cancer population, however, dextromethorphan given at 30 mg three times a day was found to be ineffective in providing analgesia when compared with conventional therapies based upon the WHO analgesic ladder.[169]

Octreotide, a somatostatin analogue with analgesic and palliative effects, inhibits pancreatic, gastric, and intestinal secretions and facilitates water and electrolyte absorption.[170,171] It may be useful for pain, particularly in the setting of bowel obstruction.

Nitrous oxide has analgesic properties and has been used in the management of patients with far advanced disease to provide additive analgesia. It is administered with oxygen through a nonrebreathing face mask, with concentrations varying from 25 to 75%. Its role is in the management of patients undergoing procedures that are associated with a significant amount of mechanical pain.[172]

Ketamine has been shown to produce analgesia via infusion in cancer patients in doses much lower than those required for anesthesia (typically 0.1 to 1.5 mg/kg/h). A double-blind cross-over study evaluating the effect of intrathecal ketamine on spinal morphine analgesia revealed that ketamine enhanced the analgesic effect and reduced the amount of morphine required.[173] Ketamine significantly reduced the pain intensity, can improve morphine analgesia in difficult pain syndromes, such as neuropathic pain. However, the occurrence of central adverse effects should be taken into account, especially when using higher doses.[174] Increasing number of good outcomes with oral, subcutaneous, and intravenous ketamine in cancer patients has been reported in non-controlled studies. This observation should be tested in studies of prolonged ketamine administration. Ketamine is usually considered when respiratory depression and extreme uncontrollable sedation pose risks for the opioid and sedating adjuvant analgesics. In a recent study when 12 patients with intractable cancer pain received a test dose of 5 to 10 mg of ketamine in order to determine their response and tolerance to the drug, it allowed a 50% total morphine daily dose reduction (range: 200–1,200 mg). Eight patients were discharged home with a portable pump administering morphine and ketamine for a median 58 days (range: 7–350 days). Side effects were moderate (dizziness) and they were limited to the test phase.[175]

Treatment of Side Effects A number of side effects associated with opioid analgesics can, depending upon the circumstance, be characterized as desirable or undesirable. Sedation, confusion, nausea, vomiting, constipation, multifocal myoclonus, and respiratory depression are the most common side effects encountered in the clinical use of opioids. When evaluating for opioid-related side effects clinician should attempt to establish whether the side effects are due to the opioid, other drugs or the disease progression.

Sedation This side effect is particularly bothersome for patients who are trying to maintain their normal daily work and social activities. Tolerance develops to this effect within several days. In patients who are excessively sedated but who are obtaining adequate analgesia, opioid dose reduction may be tried first. If opioid dose cannot be reduced without compromising analgesia the use of caffeine, modafinil, dextroamphetamine, or methylphenidate as described above may counteract this effect (Table 67-10). Level 1 evidence now exists to support the use of the psychostimulants to treat opioid-induced sedation and fatigue.

Table 67-10 Algorithm for the Management of Persistent Opioid-Induced Sedation

Eliminate non-essential psychoactive medications
If analgesia is satisfactory, reduce opioid dose by 25%
Consider addition of a psychostimulant
Consider:
- addition of a non-opioid or adjuvant drug
- opioid substitution
- use of an anesthetic or neurosurgical approach

Nausea and Vomiting Nausea and vomiting can occur from the action of opioid analgesics on the medullary chemoreceptor trigger zone (CTZ) and direct effect on the gastrointestinal mortality. Opioids may delay gastric emptying by more than 10 hours. The incidence of nausea and vomiting is markedly increased in ambulatory patients, suggesting that the opioid drugs also alter vestibular sensitivity. Opioid-induced nausea and vomiting appears to vary with the drug and the patient, so that some advantage may result from switching to an equianalgesic dose of another opioid. Alternatively, an antiemetic may be used at the initiation of the opioid. Commonly used drugs for control of nausea and vomiting associated with opioids include prokinetic agents prochlorperazine and metoclopramide. Scopolamine may be advantageous in a patient with mostly orthostatic nausea. Lorazepam may be particularly effective in anticipatory nausea, but can be quite sedating. Dexamethasone is a potent antinausea medication associated with significant side effects with long term use. The 5-HT3 antagonists ondansetron, granisetron, and others are well tolerated, but quite expensive, which may decrease patient compliance, especially if they have to pay for the medications. Tolerance to this side effect generally develops within 2 to 3 days.

Constipation Constipation is the most common adverse effect of the opioid analgesics. These drugs act at multiple sites in the gastrointestinal tract and spinal cord to produce a decrease in intestinal secretions and peristalsis, resulting in a dry stool and constipation. Tolerance to constipation develops slowly if at all making laxatives an absolutely necessary component of the opioid therapy. Provision for a regular bowel regimen including cathartics and stool softeners should be instituted. The use of an osmotic cathartic may be the next step. Whatever approach is taken, it should be used regularly and aggressively to prevent fecal impaction and bowel obstruction.

Multifocal Myoclonus In chronic systemic administration of opioids, especially with rapid dose escalation, the corresponding opioid blood levels and metabolites may increase causing multifocal myoclonus.[176] Multifocal myoclonus if untreated may degenerate into a grand mal seizure. Standard approach to this side effect is to switch the patient to an alternative opioid. If myoclonus is observed in a dying patient, the use of benzodiazepines or barbiturates to suppress the myoclonic jerks may be preferred.

Confusion and Hallucinations In chronic systemic administration of opioids, especially with rapid dose escalation, the corresponding metabolites may increase steadily with increased doses and exceed the highest tolerated levels

Table 67-11 Algorithm for the Management of Confusion/Delirium in Cancer Patients Receiving Opioids

Step 1	Evaluate underlying cause of patient's encephalopathy; pay attention to treatable causes
Step 2	Eliminate non-essential psychoactive medications
	If analgesia is satisfactory, reduce opioid by 25%
	Reassess the patient
Step 3	If delirium persists, consider:
	trial of neuroleptic (eg, haloperidol)
	opioid substitution
	use of an invasive anesthetic or neurosurgical technique.

causing delirium. This occurs in 40 to 90% of patients at the end of life, and it is one of the most distressing symptoms for patients and their families (Table 67-11). Uncontrolled pain with delirium is usually managed by an "opioid rotation" to another opioid. Sequential therapeutic trials used to determine the most favorable drug has become a standard strategy in pain management. When switching opioids in the treatment of cancer pain, one should be aware that 80% of patients require one switch, 44% of patients require two switches and 20% of patients require three or more switches.[113] Delirium should be viewed as a medical emergency, evaluated and treated urgently (treatment of delirium is described in Chapter 59, "Principles of Psycho-Oncology").

Respiratory Depression Respiratory depression is potentially the most serious adverse effect. The morphine-like agonists act on brain stem respiratory centers to produce, as a function of dose, increasing respiratory depression to the point of apnea. In man, death from an overdose of a morphine-like agonist is nearly always due to respiratory arrest. Therapeutic doses of morphine may depress all phases of respiratory activity: rate, minute volume, and tidal exchange.

However, as carbon dioxide accumulates, it stimulates central chemoreceptors, resulting in a compensatory increase in respiratory rate, which masks the degree of respiratory depression. At equianalgesic doses, all the morphine-like agonists produce an equivalent degree of respiratory depression. Respiratory depression most commonly occurs in opiate-naive patients after acute administration of an opioid and is typically associated with other signs of central nervous system (CNS) depression, including sedation and mental clouding.

Tolerance develops rapidly to this effect with repeated drug administration, allowing the opioid analgesics to be used in the management of chronic cancer pain without significant risk of respiratory depression. If respiratory depression does occur, it can be rapidly reversed by the administration of the specific opioid antagonist, naloxone. The use of naloxone should be based on the prior opioid exposure of the patient. In patients chronically receiving opioids who develop respiratory depression, the standard naloxone dose, 0.4 mg/mL, should be diluted in 9 cc of saline and slowly titrated in the patient to reverse respiratory depression. This approach prevents the patient from experiencing excruciating pain with reversal of the analgesic effects of the current opioid whereas providing improved respiratory function. If effective, naloxone reverses sedation and respiratory depression within seconds. One should be aware that in a patient with CO_2 narcosis, naloxone may not reverse the opioid-induced respiratory depression even if it blocks the opioid receptors. Intubation if appropriate needs to be considered if the patient has high CO_2 and does not respond to naloxone. Patients with cancer receiving opioids chronically are very sensitive to naloxone's effects, and patients who have been taking drugs with a long half-life, such as methadone or levorphanol, or who have been taking a slow release morphine preparation or using a transdermal patch will require a continuous infusion of naloxone to maintain a stable respiratory pattern.

The dose of naloxone for continuous infusion should be calculated from the initial dose used to reverse depression. Commonly, 1.2 mg of naloxone is diluted in 250 mL of saline and slowly titrated to the needs of the individual patient. Before administering naloxone to a comatose patient, an endotracheal tube should be placed to prevent aspiration given the possibility of respiratory compromise, excessive salivation, and bronchial spasm.

Hypogonadism Profound hypogonadism has been noted in patients receiving intrathecal opioids.[177] It has been increasingly recognized that chronic opioid exposure can cause hypogonadism presenting with severe fatigue and decreased sexual drive. Survivors of cancer who chronically consumed opioids experienced symptomatic hypogonadism with significantly higher levels of depression, fatigue, and sexual dysfunction.[178] With the increasing use of opioids among patients with cancer, monitoring and if appropriate supplementation of testosterone may be needed.

PSYCHOLOGICAL AND BEHAVIORAL APPROACHES

Psychological management of cancer pain includes the use of psychotherapeutic, cognitive-behavioral, and psychopharmacologic interventions. The use of short-term supportive psychotherapy based on a crisis intervention model allows patients to receive emotional support, information, and skills and information to assist in adapting to a pain crisis.[3] Psychiatrists and psychologists trained in psycho-oncology can be pivotal in managing patients who have significant psychological morbidity associated with their cancer pain.[33] Cognitive-behavioral techniques are helpful in promoting an increased sense of control, thus reducing the sense of hopelessness and helplessness common to many cancer pain patients.[179,180] These techniques are most useful in three clinical situations: (1) in the management of patients with intermittent predictable pain (such as pain associated with procedures), (2) in the management of incident pain (eg, in the patient with pain on movement), and (3) in the management of chronic cancer pain. A series of cognitive-behavioral approaches used with cancer patients are listed in Table 67-12. The goal of such interventions is to enhance the sense of personal control of a patient in pain. Some techniques are primarily cognitive, focusing on perceptual, and thought processes, and others are predominantly behavioral, directed at developing modulation of behavior to help patients cope with pain and cancer. These approaches are used concurrently with analgesic drug therapy and anesthetic and neurosurgical approaches.

Table 67-12 Cognitive-Behavioral Techniques for Cancer Pain

- Preparatory information
- Cognitive restructuring
- Focusing
- Controlled mental imagery
- Distraction
    - Controlled attention
    - Mental, behavioral
    - Music therapy
    - Hypnosis
    - Biofeedback

ANESTHETIC APPROACHES

Anesthetic approaches can be divided into six major types: (1) trigger-point injections, (2) peripheral nerve blocks, (3) autonomic nerve blocks, (4) epidural and intrathecal infusions, (5) surgical approaches, and (6) neurostimulatory approaches. The techniques for each of these procedures have been described in detail in standard textbooks.[129]

Short-acting and long-acting anesthetics are used for temporary and diagnostic nerve blocks whereas phenol, alcohol neurolysis, cryo- and radio-frequency lesioning are used for permanent blocks, although it is not uncommon that a permanent nerve block provides analgesia for about 2 to 3 months only. Destruction of neurons with hypertonic solution and ice crystal formation with cryotherapy is partially reversible by regeneration of the affected nerve. Alcohol causes a non-selective tissue destruction by dehydration and extraction of lipids and coagulating mucoproteins and lipoproteins.

Trigger-Point Injections Patients with significant musculoskeletal pain often describe specific tender trigger-point areas and significant pain relief may be achieved when these trigger points are injected with saline, local anesthetic, or Botox.[181] Effective relief, however, is not diagnostic of musculoskeletal pain alone, and evaluation of the cause of pain is still necessary to rule out the specific etiology.

Peripheral Nerve Blocks Peripheral nerve blocks can be used to localize the nerve distribution, and for therapy. The usefulness of this technique is limited to areas of the body in which interruption of both motor and sensory function will not interfere with the patient's functional status. This approach is most commonly used in patients who have pain in the head (gasserian ganglion, glossopharyngeal, trigeminal nerve and its branches, occipital, and other blocks), extremities (interscalene, supraclavicular, infraclavicular and axillary brachial plexus blocks, musculocutaneous, ulnar, median and radial nerve blocks, sciatic, femoral, and other nerve blocks), and chest (intercostals, paraspinal blocks).[182–185] In intercostal and paraspinal nerve blocks multiple nerves usually must be blocked to provide adequate analgesia. The highest blood levels of local anesthetic are seen with multilevel intercostals nerves. Risk of bleeding, infection, and pneumothorax should be considered. Anesthesia dolorosa is a potentially devastating complication of a permanent nerve block when the patient develops painful anesthesia at the site of the block. Thus, neurolytic blocks are most suitable for patients with localized unilateral pain and a short life expectancy.[186] This approach has very limited value in managing upper and lower limb pain associated with brachial and lumbosacral plexopathy because of the high risk of associated motor function loss. Epidural neurolysis, when neurolysis is performed via the epidural catheter carries a somewhat higher risk of spinal cord injury. Permanent nerve blocks and epidural neurolysis may be considered in the following instances: (1) exhaustion of the appropriate antitumor approaches (radiation, surgery), (2) clear clinical and radiologic definition of the cause of pain, (3) failure of pharmacological interventions to produce adequate analgesia without significant side effects, (4) a favorable response to a temporary block with a local anesthetic and (5) magnetic resonance imaging performed before the procedure to rule out epidural tumor infiltration.

NEUROSURGICAL APPROACHES

Laminectomies and vertebral body resection with reconstruction are usually used for pain associated with spinal cord compression or spine instability, usually caused by a pathological collapse (Table 67-13).[187,188] Neuroablative procedures are designed to interrupt pain pathways in either the peripheral or central nervous system. Risk of the loss of function resulting from such procedure is a major concern. Patients will rarely give up neurologic function for improvement in pain, particularly if the neurologic deficit may be associated with incontinence or leg weakness. Chemical *hypophysectomy*, reported to be effective especially in breast and prostate cancer patients, has become a rare procedure.[189] *Dorsal rhizotomy* involves cutting the dorsal roots. It can be performed as an open surgical procedure following laminectomy or by a percutaneous radiofrequency technique through the intervertebral foramina under radiographic control.[188] *Cordotomy* can be performed as an open or percutaneous unilateral or bilateral surgical procedure (Figure 67-2). A unilateral cordotomy remains the neurosurgical treatment of choice for patients with refractory cancer pain, but neurosurgical procedures have become less frequent.[189] The procedure is performed using radiographic visualization. Penetration of the cord by a fine electrode, usually in the C1-C2 interspace is monitored by electrical impedance. The ability to complete the procedure technically varies from 70 to 99% of attempts. This approach is particularly useful in patients with unilateral pain below the T1 region.[190,191] Pain relief reports vary from 70 to 95% and may last from 3 weeks to 6 months.[192]

Table 67-13 Neurosurgical Procedures for Cancer Pain

Antitumor procedures
Anterior vertebral body resection and reconstruction
Decompressive laminectomy
Ventricular shunts for headache due to increased intracranial pressure
Debulking of tumor in brachial and lumbosacral plexus
Analgesic procedures
Peripheral neurectomy
Cranial neurectomy (trigeminal, glossopharyngeal)
Dorsal rhizotomy
Dorsal root entry zone lesion
Cordotomy (unilateral or bilateral)
Chemical hypophysectomy
Neurostimulatory procedures
Transcutaneous electrical nerve stimulation (TENS)
Peripheral nerve or plexus stimulation
Dorsal column stimulation
Thalamic stimulation
Neuropharmacologic procedures
Epidural opioids, local anesthetic and clonidine infusions
Intrathecal opioids, local anesthetic and clonidine infusions
Intraventricular opioids

Dorsal Root Entry Zone Lesion This procedure was developed to manage predominantly neuropathic pain by producing a surgical lesion in the dorsal root entry zone. In a group of patients with Pancoast's tumor infiltration of the brachial plexus, Sindou and Lapras reported that 66% obtained pain relief.[193] In general the practicality of dorsal root entry zone for the management of cancer patients remains undefined.

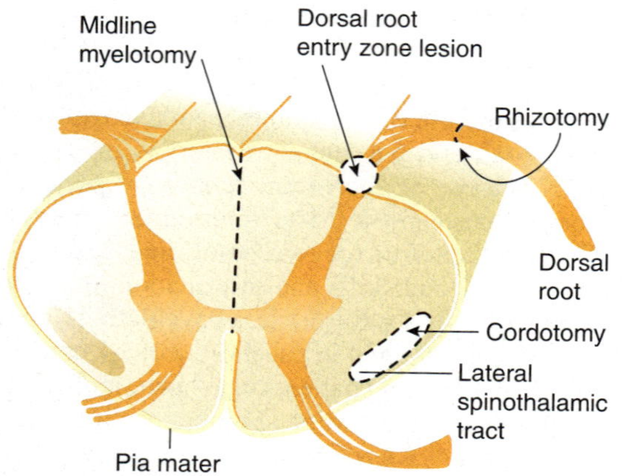

Figure 67-2 Cross-section of the spinal cord showing sites of neuroablative procedures for pain control. (Reprinted with permission from Sundaresan N, et al.[187])

Cingulotomy Cingulotomy has recently received new attention in the treatment of some patients with cancer pain. The development of a stereotactic procedure using magnetic resonance imaging for guidance to place a radiofrequency lesion has led to new interest in this procedure. In a group of patients recently reported by Hassenbusch and colleagues, four patients with pain from widely metastatic diffuse bone disease and who were receiving opioid analgesics reported immediate pain relief with bilateral cingulate lesions.[194] The pain relief persisted in this group of patients until death in 2 to 6 weeks. This procedure has previously been used to treat patients with psychiatric illness.

Neurostimulatory Procedures These procedures are based on the Gate Theory of Pain, which suggests that a neurophysiologic gating mechanism exists in the spinal cord, probably within the substantia gelatinosa. Stimulation of the small fibers tends to promote pain or open the gate whereas stimulation of large fibers tends to inhibit pain or close the gate.

Transcutaneous Electrical Nerve Stimulation (TENS) The use of TENS has developed as a clinical tool in managing patients with mild pain, most typically of a musculoskeletal or neuropathic nature. By using a small battery-operated device with superficial electrodes that can be placed over the painful area, both low- and high-intensity stimulation have been reported in uncontrolled studies to be effective in controlling mild pain in a peripheral nerve distribution.

Peripheral Nerve Stimulation Stimulation of peripheral nerves by implantation of electrodes was proposed on the basis of the concept of selectively activating large nerve fibers to suppress activity in small, presumably pain, fibers.[195] Experience to date suggests up to 30 to 50% incidence of relief, with a general falloff in efficacy within the first 2 years.

Dorsal Column Stimulation As the large nerve fibers ascend in a compact bundle through the dorsal column, they are accessible to selective electrical stimulation. The dorsal column stimulating technique involves introducing an electrode into the epidural or intrathecal space and advancing it to the appropriate level overlying the dorsal columns. The main indication for placement of a dorsal column stimulator is intractable dysesthetic or neuropathic pain of the limbs or trunk, such as occurs in patients with radiation-induced brachial or lumbosacral plexopathy. This procedure is effective in 43 to 75% of patients and carries a low morbidity rate.[196,197] The trial is considered positive if more than 50% improvement is achieved. The most common complication is failure of the device itself, which occurs in approximately 10% of patients annually. Other complications include infections, cerebrospinal fluid (CSF) fistula, allergy or rejection response to the device material, and changes in stimulation over time, which may be related to cellular changes around the electrode or shifts in its position.

Thalamic Stimulation The stereotactic insertion of stimulating electrodes into the medial thalamus has been most commonly used to manage intractable pain characterized by a predominantly neuropathic component described as a steady, tingling, burning element of pain.[198,199] Complications with this procedure include infection in 2 to 15% of patients, electrode migration in 2 to 27%, and worsening neurologic dysfunction in 2 to 15%.

Implantation of intrathecal pumps are the most common neurosurgical procedure today in cancer pain management. Patients with uncontrolled cancer pain and inability to tolerate higher oral opioids and who have a life expectancy of more than 6 months (3 months are paid for by some insurance companies) may be considered. Opioids, clonidine and local anesthetics may be added to the intrathecal solution, a drug combination not available by intravenous route. Magnetic resonance imaging must be performed prior to the procedure to rule out epidural tumor infiltration that may increase the risk of bleeding into the epidural and intrathecal space. Before the implanted pump or permanent epidural catheter is placed it is important to perform an appropriate trial. An epidural catheter allows patient-controlled analgesia (ie, rescue [PRN] drug administration), in addition to the continued infusion not available by the intrathecal route. Drug combinations can be delivered epidurally as well. As a rule, the epidural dose is significantly smaller than the equianalgesic dose of the oral opioid. The dose reduction is even more pronounced when opioid is administered intrathecally. Surgical complications include perioperative bleeding that may lead to pocket hematoma as well as epidural and intrathecal hematomas with neurological injury. This and other complications are rare, but should be watched for.

Specific Autonomic Nerve Blocks Celiac plexus block is commonly used for intolerable upper abdominal and upper back pain associated with localized pancreatic carcinoma. Outcome is generally worse when liver metastases or retroperitoneal lymphadenopathy is present. Patients usually continue to require opioids, but may need less dose or slower dose escalation for up to 2 to 3 months after the celiac plexus block.[173,187] The major side effect of the procedure is transient hypotension and diarrhea. Patients must be well hydrated and monitored during the procedure and for 4 to 6 hours afterward. Significant neurologic complications such as paraparesis and renal hemorrhage occur in less than 1% of patients if proper technique is used. The procedure should only be performed under radiologic guidance to avoid such complications. Splanchnic nerve block may provide relief of pain in patients who fail to obtain relief from celiac plexus block. In patients with cancer it may help to reduce opioid requirements and improve function.

Hypogastric and ganglion of Impar blocks are usually considered for treating intractable pelvic pain. In postsurgical/postradiation pelvic cancer pain results may be limited due to the disturbed anatomy.

SEDATION IN THE IMMINENTLY DYING

Close adherence to established pain management guidelines produces effective and satisfactory analgesia in 70 to 100% of cancer patients. Ventafridda and colleagues reported that up to 50% of patients in his home-care palliative service had uncontrolled symptoms in the last days of life and required sedation for adequate control.[200] In those patients whose pain cannot be relieved without cognitive impairment, the use of sedation is an acceptable strategy when the intent is to relieve suffering. The United States Supreme Court has defined sedation as appropriate care of the dying, different from physician-assisted suicide.[201–203] In patients who are sedated for symptom control, such an approach should include an open discussion with the patient's family, a do-not-resuscitate order, the appropriate use of drugs for symptom control, and dose escalation only to manage clearly defined signs and symptoms. By invoking the principle of double effect, pain medication may be provided in doses that may risk respiratory depression to the point of death if required for symptomatic relief. The primary intention must always be pain relief although the foreseen but unintended result may be sedation or death. Such practices are considered an important part of appropriate and compassionate care of the dying at cancer centers worldwide.[204–206]

TOLERANCE

Tolerance is a pharmacologic effect characterized by the fact that with repeated administration, increasing doses are necessary to provide the same effect. Tolerance develops at different rates for the various opioid effects. Tolerance to respiratory depression, as discussed above, develops rapidly in contrast to no or slow tolerance to the constipating effects. The first sign of analgesic tolerance is the patient's report that the duration of analgesic effect is reduced from its initial interval. The patient who reports the shorter duration of pain relief is often labeled as a clock-watcher, and that patient's report may be misinterpreted by health care professionals as an early sign of addiction. It is common for patients even with stable pain to increase their dose of opioid analgesic during the titration phase until they have reached steady state and are stabilized on a dose. This stabilized dose may be reached over a 2- to 4-week period. Dose escalation in the cancer patient most often is a sign of disease progression and should prompt a thorough medical investigation.[207] It is critical to remember that in patients with increasing pain, the degree of relief of pain and its analgesic effect are based on a log-dose relationship, and doubling the dose may therefore be necessary to provide adequate analgesia.

During opioid titration intolerable side effects occur before adequate analgesia is achieved. Switching to an alternative analgesic, using adjuvant drugs and employing a neurosurgical approach may be used in this instance.

Differentiate Physical Dependence from Psychological Dependence Physical dependence is the term used to describe the phenomenon of withdrawal when an opioid is abruptly discontinued or when an opioid-mixed agonist-antagonist or antagonist (eg, naloxone) is administered. The severity of this withdrawal is a function of the dose and duration of prior opioid administration. Prior exposure to an opioid agonist can greatly increase a patient's sensitivity to an antagonist.

Opioid withdrawal symptoms include:

- Anxiety, irritability, insomnia,
- Sweating, increased salivation, tearing, rhinorrhea
- Hot flashes, chills
- Diarrhea, abdominal cramping, nausea, vomiting.

To prevent acute withdrawal, patients receiving opioids should not be discontinued abruptly, but be tapered off their drug. Twenty-five percent of the previous daily dose will usually prevent signs and symptoms of withdrawal in a majority of patients, but to minimize the withdrawal symptoms downward titration by 25% every 1 to 3 days if commonly preferred.

In contrast to physical dependence, *psychological dependence* is a term used to describe a behavioral pattern of drug use characterized by continued craving for an opioid for effects other than pain relief. An overwhelming involvement with drug use and procurement as compulsive traits are the salient features of this type of dependence. Cancer patients chronically receiving opioids become physically but not psychologically dependent on their drugs. Patients' and physicians' fears of addiction are the major barrier to adequate cancer pain management.[208–210] Patients with poorly managed and/or undertreated pain may mimic the signs of psychological dependence, displaying a behavioral pattern known as *pseudoaddiction*.[211] The prevalence of true psychological dependence among cancer patients without history of addiction is extremely rare.

ADDICTION AND DRUG ABUSE IN CANCER PAIN PATIENTS

The American Academy of Pain Medicine, the American Pain Society, and the American Society of Addiction Medicine (2001) defined addiction as a primary, chronic, neurobiologic disease, with genetic, psychological, and environmental factors influencing its development and manifestations. It is characterized by behaviors that include one or more of the following: impaired control over drug use, compulsive use, use despite harm, and craving.

The World Health Organization characterizes addiction as:

- Usage out of control
- Obsession with obtaining a supply
- Use causes personal and legal difficulties
- Use continues despite problems
- User denies taking the substance
- Quality of life is NOT improved

Known risk factors and prevalence of addiction/chemical coping in the general population correlate with similar rate, 10% (3–18%), of aberrant drug behavior in pain patients.[212–215]

The management of pain in cancer patients with history of chemical dependency requires a comprehensive assessment and requires a treatment approach directed both at pain and the associated problems. Loss of control over the use of opioids, preoccupation with obtaining opioids despite the presence of adequate analgesia and adverse consequences associated with opioid use are suggested by the Consensus Statement of the American Society of Addiction Medicine, American Academy of Pain Medicine and American Pain Society (2001). Personal history of substance abuse, poor social support and substance abuse in the family and friends, and psychiatric history may influence the follow-up and clinical monitoring strategy that needs to be implemented. Psychiatric assessment, social worker assessment, and referral to Pain Management group may be helpful for one time evaluation of support throughout the treatment period. It is hard to overestimate the importance of a team approach, consistent treatment plan and exchange of information between providers participating in care for the cancer pain patient with substance abuse to insure good analgesia and safety. On the other hand, it is important to keep in mind that patients with a history of substance abuse are at high risk of under treatment of pain, both because of the clinician's caution in prescribing opioids at the doses they would be comfortable with in a patient without history of addiction, but also because many of the patients with history of substance abuse are opioid tolerant and need relatively high opioid dose.

When starting opioid analgesics in a high risk patient the clinician should monitor the patient to ensure that the opioids:

- Reduce pain levels
- Improve functionality ("up-time") and mood
- Improve activities of daily living
- May help to return to work
- May lead to reduced consumption of health care resources

After a high-risk patient is identified the following steps may be taken:

- Educate the patient and the family
- Monitor supportive environment
- Prevent unilateral dose escalation
- Rule out psychiatric comorbidity as uncontrolled anxiety, depression or psychosis

A clinician should be aware that a patient with a history of chemical dependency has increased stress during cancer treatment. A worsening of prognosis may precipitate a relapse.

Pseudoaddiction Pseudoaddiction is patient behavior that is reminiscent of addiction, but are driven by under treatment of pain and disappear with adequate analgesia. It is not uncommon for a patient with pseudoaddiction to exhibit anger and demanding behaviors, insisting on a specific drug or specific doses/route of administration.

Adequate analgesia in a patient with pseudoaddiction leads to the resolution of the aberrant behavior.

Urine drug testing in clinical practice is a consensual diagnostic test directed to verification of the compliance with the medications prescribed and abstinence from illicit or non-prescribed substances. In order to perform the urine drug test the clinician has to provide full explanation regarding the nature and purpose of testing to the patient and obtain at least verbal consent from the patient. The clinician ordering the test must be familiar with the reliability of the urine toxicology laboratory chosen. Codeine and heroin are metabolized to morphine and will test positive for morphine in urine. Generally, semi-synthetic and synthetic opioids such as oxycodone and methadone are not detected unless chromatography/mass spectrometry is used. Hydromorphone is partially metabolized to morphine and may test positive for it. Most opioids will reliably test positive for the first 2 days after the last dose; cocaine metabolites test positive for 2 to 4 days, propoxyphene for 6 to 48 hours, and cannabinoids for 5 to 28 days depending on the frequency and the dose. If not familiar with the assays used in the institution the clinician may need to be in close contact with the laboratory to interpret the urine drug test results correctly. If used appropriately, such testing, especially in a high-risk patient, may help to set and enforce boundaries based on mutual trust and honesty.

In summary, most cancer patients presenting with pain have advanced disease and need opioids for analgesia. Concerns about addiction, lack of access and other barriers should not interfere with the availability of opioids and other analgesics to the patient in need.

REFERENCES

1. Cherny NI, Portenoy RK. Practical management of cancer pain. In: Wall PD, Melzack R, editors. Textbook of pain. 3rd ed. Edinburgh: Churchill Livingstone; 1994. p. 1437–68.
2. Elliott K, Foley KM. Neurologic pain syndromes in patients with cancer. In: Portenoy RK, editor. Neurology clinics. Pain: mechanisms and syndromes. Vol 7. Philadelphia: W.B. Saunders; 1989. p. 333.
3. Breitbart W. Psychiatric management of cancer pain. Cancer 1989;63:2336.
4. Foley KM. The treatment of cancer pain. N Engl J Med 1985;313:84.
5. Harrison J, Maguire P. Predictors of psychiatric morbidity in cancer patients. Br J Psychiatry 1994;165:593–8.
6. Agency for Health Care Policy and Research. Management of cancer pain: clinical practice guideline. Rockville (MD): U.S. Public Health Service Agency for Health Care Policy and Research; 1994. Publication No.: 94–0592.
7. Fishman B, Pasternak S, Wallenstein SL, et al. The Memorial pain assessment card: a valid instrument for the evaluation of cancer pain. Cancer 1987;60:1151.
8. Graham C, Bond SS, Gerkocic MM, Cook MR. Use of McGill pain questionnaire in the assessment of cancer pain: replicability and consistency. Pain 1980;8:377.
9. Mather LE. Pharmacokinetic and pharmacodynamic profiles of opioid analgesics: a sameness amongst equals. Pain 1990;43:3.
10. Report of the WHO Expert Committee on Cancer Pain Relief and Active Supportive Care. Cancer pain relief with a guide to opioid availability. 2nd ed. Technical Report Series, 804. Geneva: World Health Organization; 1996.
11. Grond S, Zech D, Diefenbach C, Bischoff A. Prevalence and pattern of symptoms in patients with cancer pain: a prospective evaluation of 1,635 cancer patients referred to a pain clinic. J Pain Symptom Manage 1994;9:372–82.
12. Portenoy RK, Kornblith AB, Wong G, et al. Pain in ovarian cancer patients: prevalence, characteristics, and associated symptoms. Cancer 1994;73:907–14.
13. Twycross RG, Fairfield S. Pain in far-advanced cancer. Pain 1982;14:303.
14. Ferrell BR, Wisdon C, Wenzl C. Quality of life as an outcome variable in management of cancer pain. Cancer 1989;63:2321.
15. Cleeland CS, Gonin R, Hatfield A, et al. Pain and its treatment in outpatients with metastatic cancer. N Engl J Med 1994;330:592–6.
16. Cleeland CS. The impact of pain on patients with cancer. Cancer 1984;54:263.
17. Levin D, Cleeland CS, Dar R. Public attitudes toward cancer pain. Cancer 1985;56:2337.
18. Gonzales GR, Elliott KJ, Portenoy RK, Foley KM. The impact of a comprehensive evaluation in the management of pain. Pain 1991;47:41–4.
19. The SUPPORT principal investigators. A controlled trial to improve care for seriously ill hospitalized patients: the study to understand prognosis and preferences for outcomes and risks of treatments. JAMA 1995;274:1591–8.
20. Desbiens NA, et al. Patient empowerment and feedback do not decrease pain in seriously ill hospitalized adults, Pain 1998;75:237–46.
21. Von Roenn JH, Cleeland CS, Gonin R, et al. Physician attitudes and practice in cancer pain management: a survey from the Eastern Oncology Group. Ann Intern Med 1993;119:121–6.
22. Bernabei R, Cleeland CS, Gonin R, et al. Management of pain in elderly patients with cancer. JAMA 1998;279:1877–82.
23. Schuit KW, et al. Symptoms and functional status of patients with disseminated cancer visiting outpatient departments. J Pain Symptom Manage 1998;16:290–7.
24. Ferrell BR, Dean GE, Grant M, Coluzzi P. An institutional commitment to pain management. J Clin Oncol 1995;13:2158–65.
25. Foley KM. Pain relief into practice: rhetoric without reform. J Clin Oncol 1995;12: 2149–51.
26. Max M, Donovan M, Miaskowski C, et al. American Pain Society quality improvement guidelines for the treatment of acute and chronic pain. JAMA 1995;274:1874–80.
27. Gonzales GR, Payne R. Pathophysiology of pain in cancer and other terminal diseases. In: Doyle D, Hanks GW, MacDonald RN, editors. Oxford textbook of palliative medicine. 2nd ed. New York Oxford University Press; 1998. p. 299–309.
28. Foley KM. Advances in cancer pain. Arch Neurol 1999;56:413–7.
29. Craig AD, Bushnell MC, Zhang ET, Bolmqvist A. A thalamic nucleus specific for pain and temperature sensation. Nature 1994;372:770–3.
30. Posner JB. Neurological complications of cancer. New York: FA Davis; 1995.
31. Clouston P, DeAngelis L, Posner JB. The spectrum of neurological disease in patients with systemic cancer. Ann Neurol 1992;31:268–73.
32. Derogatis LR, Morrow GR, Fetting J, et al. The prevalence of psychiatric disorders among cancer patients. JAMA 1983;249:751.
33. Holland JC. Psycho-oncology. New York: Oxford University Press; 1998.
34. Holland JC. Preliminary guidelines for treatment of distress. Oncology 1997;11:109–14.
35. Breitbart W. Cancer pain and suicide. In: Foley KM, Bonica JJ, Ventafridda V, editors. Advances in pain research and therapy. Second International Congress on Cancer Pain. Vol 16. New York: Raven; 1990. p. 399.
36. Chochinov HM, Wilson KG, Enns M, et al. Desire for death in the terminally ill. Am J Psychiatry 1995;152:1185–91.

37. Cherny NI, Portenoy RK. Sedation in the treatment of refractory symptoms: guidelines for evaluation and treatment. J Palliat Care 1994;10:31–8.
38. Cherny NI, Coyle N, Foley KM. Suffering in the advanced cancer patient. Part I: a definition and taxonomy. J Palliat Care 1994;10:71–9.
39. Truog RD, Berde CB, Mitchell C, Greir HE. Barbiturates in the care of the terminally ill. N Engl J Med 1992;327:1678.
40. Bookbinder M, et al. Improving pain management practices. In: McGuire DB, Yarbo CH, Ferrell BR, editors. Cancer pain management. 2nd ed. Boston: Jones & Bartlett; 1995, 321–361.
41. Mundy PR, Raisz LG, Cooper RA. Evidence for the secretion of an osteoclast stimulating factor in myeloma. N Engl J Med 1974;291:1041.
42. Cherny NI, Foley KM, editors. Pain and palliative care. Hematology/oncology clinics of North America. Vol 10. Philadelphia: W.B. Saunders; 1996.
43. Portenoy RK. Cancer pain: pathophysiology and syndromes. Lancet 1992;339: 1026–31.
44. Mayer EA, Gebhart GF. Basic and clinical aspects of visceral hyperalgesia. Gastroenterology 1994;107:271–93.
45. Sengupta JN, X Su, Gebhart GF. Kappa, but not mu or delta, opioids attenuate responses to distention of afferent fibers innervating the rat colon. Gastroenterology 1996;111:968–80.
46. Burton MB, Gebhart GF. Effects of kappa-opioid receptor agonists on responses to colorectal distension in rats with and without acute colonic inflammation. J Pharmacol Exp Ther 1998;285:707–15.
47. Jaeckle KA, Young DF, Foley KM. The natural history of lumbosacral plexopathy in cancer. Neurology 1985;35:8.
48. Foley KM. Pain assessment and cancer pain. In: Doyle D, Hanks GW, MacDonald RN, editors. Oxford textbook of palliative medicine. 2nd ed. New York: Oxford University Press; 1998. p. 310–30.
49. Portenoy RK, Lipton RB, Foley KM. Back pain in the cancer patient an algorithm for evaluation and management. Neurology 1986;37:134.
50. DuPen SL, DuPenn AR, Polissar N, et al. Implementation of guidelines for cancer pain management results of a randomized controlled clinical trial. J Clin Oncol 1999;17:361–70.
51. Foley KM, Portenoy RK. World Health Organization/International Association for the Study of Pain: joint initiative in cancer pain treatment. J Pain Symptom Manage 1993;8:335–9.
52. Jadad AR, Bowman GP. The WHO analgesic ladder for cancer pain management. Stepping up the quality of its evaluation. JAMA 1996;274:1870–3.
53. Ventafridda V, Tambourini M, Caraceni A, et al. A validation study of the WHO methods for cancer pain relief. Cancer 1987;59:850–6.
54. Zech Detlev FJ, Grond S, Lynch J, et al. Validation of WHO guidelines for cancer pain relief: a 10-year prospective study. Pain 1995;63:65–76.
55. Payne R. Issues pertinent to the revision of national guidelines, NCCN proceedings. Oncology 1998;12:169–75.
56. American Pain Society. Principles of analgesic use in the treatment of acute pain and chronic cancer pain: a concise guide to medical practice. 3rd ed. Skokie (IL): American Pain Society; 1994.
57. Lane NE. Pain management in osteoarthritis: the role of Cox-2 inhibitors. J Rheumatol 1997;24:20–4.
58. Grond S, Zech D, Schug SA, et al. Validation of World Health Organization guidelines for cancer pain relief during the last days and hours of life. J Pain Symptom Manage 1992;6:411–22.
59. Ventafridda V, Caraceni A, Sloanotto AM, et al. Non-steroidal anti-inflammatory drugs as the first step in cancer pain therapy: double-blind, within-patient study comparing nine drugs. J Int Med Res 1990;18:21–9.
60. Ingham JM, Portenoy RK. Drugs in the treatment of pain: NSAIDS and opioids. Curr Opin Anaesthesiol 1993;6:838–44.
61. Eisenberg E, Berkey CS, Carr DB, et al. Efficacy and safety of nonsteroidal antiinflammatory drugs for cancer pain: a meta-analysis. J Clin Oncol 1994;12: 2756–65.
62. Malmberg AB, Yaksh TL. Hyperalgesia mediated by spinal glutamate or substance P receptor blocked by spinal cyclooxygenase inhibition. Science 1992;257:1276–9.
63. Joishy SK, Walsh D. The opioid-sparing effects of intravenous ketorolac as an adjuvant analgesic in cancer pain: application in bone metastases and the opioid bowel syndrome. J Pain Symptom Manage 1998;16:334–9.
64. Kaufman DW, Kelly JP, Sheehan JE, et al. Nonsteroidal anti-inflammatory drug use in relation to major upper gastrointestinal bleeding. Clin Pharmacol Ther 1993;53:485–94.
65. Laporte JR, Carne X, Vidal X, et al. Upper gastrointestinal bleeding in relation to previous use of analgesics and non-steroidal anti-inflammatory drugs. Lancet 1991; 337:85–9.
66. Henry D, Lim LL, Garcia Rodriguez LA, et al. Variability in risk of gastrointestinal complications with individual non-steroid anti-inflammatory drugs: results of a collaborative meta-analysis. BMJ 1996;312:1563–6.
67. Wilder-Smith CH, Schimke J, Osterwalder B, Sann HJ. Oral tramadol, a mu-opioid agonist and monamine reuptake-blocker and morphine for strong cancer-related pain. Ann Oncol 1994;5:141–6.
68. Harati Y, Gooch C, Swensen M, et al. Double-blind randomized trial of tramadol for the treatment of the pain of diabetic neuropathy. Neurology 1998;50:1842–6.
69. Pasternak GW. Morphine and enkephalin receptors and the relief of pain. JAMA 1988;259:1362.
70. Chary S, Goughnour BR, Moulin DE, et al. The dose-response relationship of controlled-release codeine (codeine Contin) in chronic cancer pain. J Pain Symptom Manage 1994;9:363–71.
71. Mikus G, Somogyi AA, Bochner F, Chen ZR. Polymorphic metabolism of opioid narcotic drugs: possible clinical implications. Ann Acad Med Singapore 1991;20:10–11.
72. Gammaitoni A, Galer BS, Bulloch S, et al. Randomized, double-blind, placebo-controlled comparison of the analgesic efficacy of oxycodone 10 mg/acetaminophen 325 mg versus controlled-release oxycodone 20 mg in postsurgical pain. J Clin Pharmacol 2003;43:296–304.
73. Bruera E, Belzile M, Pituskin E, et al. Randomized, double-blinded, cross-over trial comparing safety and efficacy of oral controlled-release oxycodone with controlled-release morphine in patients with cancer pain. J Clin Oncol 1998; 15:3222–9.
74. Parris Winston CV, Johnson BW Jr., Croghan MK, et al. The use of controlled-release oxycodone for the treatment of chronic pain: a randomized, double-blind study. J Pain Symptom Manage 1998;16:205–11.
75. Sawe J, Svensson JO, Rane A. Morphine metabolism in cancer patients on increasing oral doses: no evidence for autoinduction or dose dependence. J Clin Pharmacol 1983;16:85–93.
76. Mercandante S. The role of morphine glucuronides in cancer pain. Palliat Med 1999;13:95–104.
77. Sjögren P. Clinical implications of morphine metabolites. In: Portenoy R, Bruera E, editors. Topics in palliative care. New York: Oxford University Press; 1977. p. 163–76.
78. Twycross RG. Clinical experience with diamorphine in advanced malignant disease. Int J Clin Pharmacol Ther Toxicol 1974;9:184.
79. Kaiko RF. Commentary: equianalgesic dose ratio of intramuscular/oral morphine, 1:6 versus 1:3. In: Foley KM, Inturrisi CE, editors. Advances in pain research and therapy. Vol 8. Opioid analgesics in the management of clinical pain. New York: Raven; 1986. p. 87.
80. Kaiko RF. Controlled-release oral morphine for cancer-related pain. The European and North American experiences. In: Foley KM, Bonica JJ, Ventafridda V, editors. Advances in pain research and therapy. Vol 16. Second International Congress on Cancer Pain. New York: Raven; 1990. p. 171.
81. Babul N, Darke AC, Hagen N. Hydromorphone metabolite accumulation in renal failure. J Pain Symptom Manage 1995;10:184–5.
82. Rapp SE. A multidimensional comparison of morphine and hydromorphone pain controlled analgesia. Anesth Analg 1996;82:1043–8.
83. Donner B, Zenz M, Strumpf M, Raber M. Long-term treatment of cancer pain with transdermal fentanyl. J Pain Symptom Manage 1998;15:168–75.
84. Payne R, Chandler S, Elmhaus M. Guidelines for the clinical use of transdermal fentanyl. Anticancer Drugs 1995;6 Suppl:50–3.
85. Payne R, et al. Quality of life and cancer pain: satisfaction and side effects with transdermal fentanyl versus oral morphine. J Clin Oncol 1998;16:1588–93.
86. Ahmedzai S, Brooks D.The TTS-Fentanyl Cooperative Trial Group. Transdermal fentanyl versus sustained-release oral morphine in cancer pain: preference, efficacy, and quality of life. J Pain Symptom Manage 1997;13:254–61.
87. Portenoy RK, Hagen NA. Breakthrough pain: definition, prevalence, and characteristics. Pain 1990;41:273–81.
88. Farrar JT, Cleary J, Rauck R, et al. Oral transmucosal fentanyl citrate: randomized, double-blinded, placebo-controlled trial for treatment breakthrough pain in cancer patients. J Natl Cancer Inst 1998;90:611–6.
89. Portenoy RK, et al. Oral transmucosal fentanyl citrate (OTFC) for the treatment of breakthrough pain in cancer patients, a controlled dose titration study. Pain 1999;79:303–12.
90. Christie JM, et al. Dose-titration multicenter study of oral transmucosal fentanyl citrate for the treatment of breakthrough pain in cancer patients using transdermal fentanyl for persistent pain. J Clin Oncol 1998;16:3238–45.
91. Fainsinger RB, Schoeller T, Bruera E. Methadone in the management of cancer pain: a review. Pain 1993;52:137–47.
92. Grochow L, Sheidler V, Grossman S, et al. Does intravenous methadone provide longer lasting analgesia than intravenous morphine? A randomized, double-blind study. Pain 1989;38:141.
93. Crews, Sweeney, Denson, Clinical efficacy of methadone in patients refractory to other mu-opioid receptor agonist analgesics for management of terminal cancer pain. Case presentations and discussion of incomplete cross-tolerance among opioid agonist analgesics. Cancer 1993;72:2266–72.
94. Lawlor PG, Turner KS, Hanson J, Bruera ED. Dose ratio between morphine and methadone in patients with cancer pain: a retrospective study. Cancer 1998 Mar 15;82:1167–73.
95. Ripamonti C, Groff L, Brunelli C, et al. Switching from morphine to oral methadone in treating cancer pain: what is the equianalgesic dose ratio? J Clin Oncol 1998;16:3216–21.
96. Foley KM, Houde R. Methadone in cancer pain management: individualize dose and titrate to effect. J Clin Oncol 1998;16:3213–5.
97. Ripamonti C, Zecca E, Bruera E. An update on the clinical use of methadone for cancer pain. Pain 1997;70:109–15.
98. Bruera E, et al. Opioid rotation in patients with cancer pain. A retrospective comparison of dose ratios between methadone, hydromorphone, and morphine. Cancer 1996;78:852–7.
99. Mercadante S. Methadone in cancer pain. Eur J Pain 1997;1:77–85.
100. Mercandante S, et al. Morphine versus methadone in the pain treatment of advanced cancer patients followed up at home. J Clin Oncol 1998;16:3656–61.
101. Kaiko RF, Foley KM, Grabinski PY, et al. Central nervous system excitatory effects of meperidine in cancer patients. Ann Neurol 1983;13:180.
102. Dellernijn PLI, Vanneste JAL. Randomized double-blind active-placebo-controlled crossover trial of intravenous fentanyl in neuropathic pain. Lancet 1997;349: 753–756.
103. Derllernijn PLI, Van Duijn H, Vannesta JAL. Prolonged treatment with transdermal fentanyl in neuropathic pain. J Pain Symptom Manage 1998;16:220–9.
104. Watson C, Peter N, Babul N. Efficacy of oxycodone in neuropathic pain. A randomized trial in postherpetic neuralgia. Neurology 1998;50:1837–41.
105. Cherny NI, et al. Opioid responsiveness of cancer pain syndromes caused by neuropathic pain. A randomized trial in postherpetic neuralgia. Neurology 1994;44:857–61.
106. Rowbotham MC, Twilling L, Davies PS, et al. Oral opioid therapy for chronic peripheral and central neuropathic pain. N Engl J Med. 2003;348:1223-32139.
107. Hegarty A, Portenoy RK. Pharmacotherapy of neuropathic pain. Semin Neurol 1994;14:213–24.
108. Portenoy RK, Foley KM, Inturrisi CE. The nature of opioid responsiveness and its implications for neuropathic pain: new hypothesis derived from studies of opioid infusions. Pain 1990;3:273–86.
109. Kalso E, Vainio A. Morphine and oxycodone hydrochloride in the management of cancer pain. Clin Pharmacol Ther 1990;5:639–46.
110. Mercadante S, Portenoy RK. Opioid poorly responsive cancer pain. Part 1: Clinical considerations. J Pain Symptom Manage 2001;21:144–50.
111. Mercadante S, Portenoy RK. Opioid poorly-responsive cancer pain. Part 2: Basic mechanisms that could shift dose response for analgesia. J Pain and Symptom Management 2001;21:255–64.
112. Mercadante S, Portenoy RK. Opioid poorly responsive cancer pain. Part 3: Clinical strategies to improve opioid responsiveness. J Pain and Symptom Management 2001;21:338–54.
113. Foley KM, Houde RW. Methadone in cancer pain management: individualize dose and titrate to effect. J Clin Oncol 1998;16:3213–5.
114. Cherney NJ, Chang V, Frager G, et al. Opioid pharmacotherapy in the management of cancer pain. Cancer 1998;76:1288–95.

115. Ashby MA, Martin P, Jackson KA. Opioid substitution to reduce adverse effects in cancer pain management. Med J Aust 1999;170:68–71.
116. Wand GS, McCaul M, Yang X, et al. The mu-opioid receptor gene polymorphism (A118G) alters HPA axis activation induced by opioid receptor blockade. Neuropsychopharmacol 2002;26:106–14.
117. Meroz Y, Davidson EM, Shir Y, Caraco Y. 2001. Variable response to alfentanil due to genetic polymorphism. Anesthesiol 95:A1358.
118. Lotsch J, Skarke C, Grosch S, et al. 2002. The polymorphism A118G of the human mu-opioid receptor gene decreases the pupil constrictory effect of morphine-6-glucuronide but not that of morphine. Pharmacogenetics 12:3–9.
119. Coyle N, Adelhardt J, Foley KM, Portenoy RK. Character of terminal illness in the advanced cancer patient: pain and other symptoms during the last four weeks of life. J Pain Symptom Manage 1990;5:83.
120. Weinberg DS, Inturrisi CE, Reidenberg B, et al. Sublingual absorption of selected opioid analgesics. Clin Pharmacol Ther 1988;44:335.
121. Hirsch JD. Sublingual morphine sulfate in chronic pain management. Clin Pharm 1984;3:585.
122. Kaiko RF, Healy N, Pav J. The comparative bioavailability of MS Contin tablets following rectal and oral administration. In: Doyle D, editor. Royal Society of Medicine Service International Congress and Symposium Series N149. Royal Society of Medicine Services Ltd.; 1989.
123. Bruera E, Brenneis C, Chadwick S, et al. Subcutaneous infusion of narcotics using a disposable portable device. Cancer Treat Rep 1987;10:953.
124. Coyle N, Mauskop A, Maggard J. Continuous subcutaneous infusions of opiates in cancer patients with pain. Oncol Nurs Forum 1986;13:53.
125. Ventafridda V, Spoldi E, Caraceni A, et al. The importance of continuous subcutaneous morphine administration for cancer pain control. Pain Clinic 1986;1:47.
126. Gilmer-Hill HS, Boggart JE, Smith K, Wagner FC. Intrathecal morphine delivered via subcutaneous pump for intractable cancer pain. A review of the literature. Surg Neurol 1999;51:12–15.
127. Yaksh TL. Spinal opiate analgesia: characteristics and principles of action. Pain 1981;11:293.
128. Cousins MJ. Anesthetic approaches in cancer pain. In: Foley KM, Bonica JJ, Ventafridda V, editors. Advances in pain research and therapy. Vol 16. Second International Congress on Cancer Pain. New York: Raven; 1990. p. 249.
129. Cousins MJ, Bridenbaugh PO. Neural blockade in clinical anesthesia and management of pain. 2nd ed. Philadelphia: Lippincott; 1988.
130. Nitescu P, Appelgren L, Linder L, et al. Epidural vs. intrathecal morphine-bupivacaine: assessment of consecutive treatments in advanced cancer pain. J Pain Symptom Manage 1990;5:18.
131. Plummer JL, Cherry DA, Cousins MJ, et al. Long term spinal administration of morphine in cancer and non-cancer pain: a retrospective study. Pain 1991;44:212.
132. Van Dongen RT, Crul BJ, De BM. Long-term intrathecal infusion of morphine and morphine/bupivacaine mixtures in the treatment of cancer pain: a retrospective analysis of 51 cases. Pain 1993;55:119.
133. Moulin DE, Inturrisi CE, Foley KM. Epidural and intrathecal opioids: cerebrospinal fluid and plasma pharmacokinetics in cancer pain patients. In: Foley KM, Inturrisi CE, editors. Advances in pain research and therapy. Vol. 8. Opioid analgesics in the management of clinical pain. New York: Raven; 1986. p. 369.
134. Smitt PS, et al. Outcomes and complications of epidural analgesia in patients with chronic cancer pain. Cancer 1998;83:2015–22.
135. Tumber PS, Fitzgibbon DR. The control of severe cancer pain by continuous intrathecal infusion and patient controlled intrathecal analgesia with morphine, bupivacaine and clonidine. Pain 1998;78:217–20.
136. Eisenbach JC, DuPen S, Dubois M, et al. the Epidural Clonidine Study Group. Epidural clonidine analgesia for intractable cancer pain. Pain 1995;61:391–9.
137. Inturrisi CE, Portenoy RK, Max MB, et al. Pharmacokinetic-pharmacodynamic (PKPD) relationships of methadone infusions in patients with cancer pain. Clin Pharmacol Ther 1990;47:565.
138. Portenoy RK, Moulin DE, Rogers AG, et al. Intravenous infusion of opioids in cancer pain: clinical review and guidelines for use. Cancer Treat Rep 1985;70:575.
139. Coyle N. A model of continuity of care for cancer patients with chronic pain. In: Payne R, Foley KM, editors. Medical clinics of North America, cancer pain. Vol. 71. Philadelphia: W.B. Saunders; 1987. p. 259.
140. Billings AJ, Block SD. Slow euthanasia. J Palliat Care 1996;12:21–30.
141. Portenoy RK. Morphine infusions at the end of life: the pitfalls in reasoning from anecdote. J Palliat Care 1996;12:44–6.
142. Citron ML, Johnston-Early A, Boyer M, et al. Patient controlled analgesia for severe cancer pain. Arch Intern Med 1986;146:734.
143. Hegarty A, Portenoy RK. Pharmacotherapy of neuropathic pain. Semin Neurol 1994;14:213–24.
144. Portenoy RK. Adjuvant analgesics. In: Cherny NI, Foley KM, editors. Hematology/oncology clinics of North America: pain and palliative care. Vol 10. Philadelphia: W.B. Saunders; 1996. p.103.
145. Bruera E, Neumann CM. The uses of psychotropics in symptom management in advanced cancer. Psychooncology 1998;7:346–58.
146. Beaver WT. Comparison of analgesic effects of morphine sulfate, hydroxyzine and other combinations in patients with postoperative pain. In: Bonica JJ, Ventafridda V, editors. Advances in pain research and therapy. New York: Raven; 1976. p. 553.
147. Della Cuna GR, Pellegrini A, Piazza M. Effect of methylprednisolone sodium succinate on quality of life in preterminal cancer patients: a placebo-controlled multicenter study. Eur J Cancer Clin Oncol 1989;29:1817.
148. Ettinger AB, Portenoy RK. Use of corticosteroids in the treatment of symptoms associated with cancer. J Pain Symptom Manage 1988;3:99.
149. Tannock I, Gospodarowicz M, Meakin W, et al. Treatment of metastatic prostatic cancer with low-dose prednisone: evaluation of pain and quality of life as pragmatic indices of response. J Clin Oncol 1989;7:590.
150. Bruera E, Roca E, Cedaro L, et al. Action of oral methylprednisolone in terminal cancer patients: a prospective randomized double-blind study. Cancer Treat Rep 1985;69:751.
151. Forrest WH Jr, Brown BW, Brown CR. Dextroamphetamine with morphine for the treatment of postoperative pain. N Engl J Med 1977;296:712.220.
152. Bruera E, Watanabe S. Psychostimulants as adjuvant analgesics. J Pain Symptom Manage 1994;9:412–415.
153. Dalal S, Melzack R. Potentiation of opioid analgesia by psychostimulant drugs: a review. J Pain Symptom Manage 1998;18:245–53.
154. Halperin DL, Koren G, Attias D, et al. Topical skin anesthesia for venous, subcutaneous drug reservoir and lumbar punctures in children. Pediatrics 1989;84:218.
155. Maunuksela EL, Korpela R. Double-blind evaluation of a lignocaine-prilocaine cream (EMLA) in children: effect on the pain associated with venous cannulation. Br J Anaesth 1986;58:1242.
156. Carnel SB, Blakeslee DB, Oswald SG, Barnes M. Treatment of radiation- and chemotherapy-induced stomatitis. Otolaryngol Head Neck Surg 1990;102:326.
157. Sindrup SH, Jensen TS. Pharmacologic treatment of pain in polyneuropathy. Neurology 2000;55:915–20.
158. Theriault RL, et al. Pamidronate reduces skeletal morbidity in women with advanced breast cancer and lytic bone lesions: a randomized, placebo-controlled trial. J Clin Oncol 1999;17:846–54.
159. Body JJ, et al. Current use of bisphosphonates in oncology. J Clin Oncol 1998;16:3890–3899.
160. Small EJ, Smith MR, Seaman JJ, et al. Combined analysis of two multicenter, randomized, placebo-controlled studies of pamidronate disodium for the palliation of bone pain in men with metastatic prostate cancer. J Clin Oncol 2003;21(23):4277–84. Epub 2003 Oct 27.
161. Pavlakis N, Stockler M. Bisphosphonates for breast cancer. Cochrane Database Syst Rev. 2002;(1):CD003474.
162. Hortobagyi GN, et al. Efficacy of pamidrone in reducing skeletal complications in patients with breast cancer and lytic bone metastases. N Engl J Med 1996;335: 1785–91.
163. Berenson JR, Lipton A. Use of bisphosphinates in patients with metastatic bone disease. Oncology 1998;12:1573–80.
164. Lipton A, Small E, Saad F, et al. The new bisphosphonate, Zometa (zoledronic acid), decreases skeletal complications in both osteolytic and osteoblastic lesions: a comparison to pamidronate. Cancer Invest 2002;20(Suppl 2):45–54.
165. Gunawardana DH, Lichtenstein M, Better N, Rosenthal M. Results of strontium-89 therapy in patients with prostate cancer resistant to chemotherapy. Clin Nucl Med 2004;29:81–5.
166. Sciuto R, Festa A, Pasqualoni R, et al. Metastatic bone pain palliation with 89-Sr and 186-Re-HEDP in breast cancer patients. Breast Cancer Res Treat 2001;66:101–9.
167. Elliott K, Hynansky A, Inturrisi CE. Dextromethorphan attenuates and reverses analgesic tolerance to morphine. Pain 1994;59:361–8.
168. Elliott KJ, Brodsky M, Hyanansky A, et al. Dextromethorphan shows efficacy in experimental pain (nociception) and opioid tolerance. Neurology 1995;45(Suppl 8):66–8.
169. Mercandante S, Casuccio A, Genovese G. Ineffectiveness of dextromethorphan in cancer pain. J Pain Symptom Manage 1998;16:317–22.
170. Merrcandante S. The role of octreotide in palliative care. J Pain Symtom Manage 1994;9:406–11.
171. Mercandante S, Kargar J, Nicolosi G. Octreotide may prevent definitive intestinal obstruction. J Pain Symptom Manage 1997;13:325–6.
172. Fosburg NT, Crone RK. Nitrous oxide analgesia for refractory pain in the terminally ill. JAMA 1983;250:511.
173. Yang C-Y, Wong O-S, Chang J-Y, Ho S-T. Intrathecal ketamine-reduced morphine requirements in patients with terminal cancer pain. Can J Anaesth 1996;43: 379–83.
174. Mercadante S, Arcuri E, Tirelli W, Casuccio A. Analgesic effect of intravenous ketamine in cancer patients on morphine therapy: a randomized, controlled, double-blind, crossover, double-dose study. J Pain Symptom Manage 2000;20:246–52.
175. Lossignol DA, Obiols-Portis M, Body JJ. Successful use of ketamine for intractable cancer pain. Support Care Cancer 2005;13:188–93. Epub 2004 Oct 6.
176. Payne R. Pharmacologic management of pain. In: Berger A, et al, editors. Principles and practice of supportive oncology. Philadelphia: Lippincott-Raven Publishers; 1998.
177. Roberts LJ, Finch PM, Pullan PT, et al. Sex hormone suppression by intrathecal opioids: a prospective study. Clin J Pain 2002;18:144–8.
178. Rajagopal A, Vassilopoulou-Sellin R, Palmer JL, Kaur G, Bruera E. Symptomatic hypogonadism in male survivors of cancer with chronic exposure to opioids. Cancer 2004;100:851–8.
179. Fishman B. The treatment of suffering in patients with cancer pain: cognitive-behavioral approaches. In: Foley KM, Bonica JJ, Ventafridda V, editors. Advances in pain research and therapy. Vol. 16. Second International Congress on Cancer Pain. New York: Raven; 1990. p. 301.
180. Loscalzo M, Jacobsen PB. Practical behavioral approaches to the effective management of pain and distress. J Psychosoc Oncol 1990;8:139.
181. Travell JG, Simons DG. Myofascial pain and dysfunction: the trigger point manual. Baltimore: Williams & Wilkins; 1983.
182. Tasker RR. Management of nociceptive, deafferentation and central pain by surgical intervention. In: Fields HL, editor. Pain syndromes in neurology. Boston: Butterworths; 1990. p. 143.
183. Myers DP, Lema MJ, de Leon-Casasola OA, Bacon DR. Intrapleural analgesia for the treatment of severe cancer pain in terminally ill patients. J Pain Symptom Manage 1992;17:166.
184. Cousins MJ, Dwyer B, Gibb D. Chronic pain and neurolytic blockade. In: Cousins MJ, Bridenbaugh PO, editors. Neural blockade in clinical anesthesia and management of pain. 2nd ed. Philadelphia: Lippincott; 1988. p.1053.
185. Plancarte R, Amedcua C, Patt RB, Aldrete JA. Superior hypogastric plexus block for pelvic cancer pain. Anesthesiology 1990;73:236.
186. Brown DL, Bulley CK, Quiel EC. Neurolytic celiac plexus blockage for pancreatic cancer pain. Anesth Analg 1987;66:869.
187. Sundaresan N, Sachdev VP, Krol G. Neurosurgical antitumor approaches for pain relief. In: Foley KM, Bonica JJ, Ventafridda V, editors. Advances in pain research and therapy. Vol. 16. Second International Congress on Cancer Pain. New York: Raven; 1990. p. 275.
188. Arbit E, Galicich JH, Burt M, Mallya K. Modified open thoracic rhizotomy for treatment of intractable chest wall pain of malignant etiology. Ann Thorac Surg 1989;48:820.
189. Tasker RR, Tsuda T, Hawrylyshyn P. Percutaneous cordotomy: the lateral high cervical techniques. In: Schmidek HH, Sweet WH, editors. Operative neurosurgical technique: indications, methods and results. New York: Grune and Stratton; 1988. p. 1191.
190. Ischia S, Ischia A, Luzzani A, et al. Results up to death in the treatment of persistent cervicothoracic (Pancoast) and thoracic malignant pain by unilateral percutaneous cervical cordotomy. Pain 1985;21:339.
191. Ischia S, Luzzani A, Ischia A, Pacini L. Role of percutaneous cervical cordotomy in the treatment of neoplastic vertebral pain. Pain 1984;19:123.

192. Ischia S, Luzzani A, Ischia A, et al. Subarachnoid neurolytic block (L5-S1) and unilateral percutaneous cervical cordotomy in the treatment of pain secondary to pelvic malignant disease. Pain 1984;20:139.
193. Sindou MP, Blondet E, Emery E, Mertens P. Microsurgical lesioning in the dorsal root entry zone for pain due to brachial plexus avulsion: a prospective series of 55 patients. J Neurosurg 2005;102(6):1018–28.
194. Hassenbusch SJ, Pillay PK, Barnett GH. Radiofrequency cingulotomy for intractable cancer pain using stereotaxis guided by magnetic resonance imaging. Neurosurgery 1990;27:220.
195. Picaza JA, Hunter SE, Cannon BW. Pain suppression by peripheral nerve stimulation: chronic effects of implanted devices. Appl Neurophysiol 1977;40:223.
196. Shealy CN, Mortimer JT, Hagfors NR. Dorsal column electroanalgesia. J Neurosurg 1970;32:560.
197. Urban BJ, Nashold BS Jr. Percutaneous epidural stimulation of the spinal cord for relief of pain: long-term results. J Neurosurg 1978;48:323.
198. Turnbull IM, Shulman R, Woodhurst WB. Thalamic stimulation for neuropathic pain. J Neurosurg 1980;52:486.
199. Young RF, Brechner T. Electrical stimulation of the brain for relief of intractable pain due to cancer. Cancer 1986;57:1266.
200. Ventafridda V, Ripamonti C, DeConno F, et al. Symptom prevalence and control during cancer patients' last days of life. J Palliat Care 1990;6:7–11.
201. Compassion in Dying vs. Washing, 79 F.3d 790, 9th Ctr. (1996).
202. Quill vs Vacco 80 F 3d 716, 2d Ctr. (1996).
203. Burt RA. The Supreme Court speaks: not assisted suicide but a constitutional right to palliative care. N Engl J Med 1997;337:1234–6.
204. Cherny NI, Portenoy RK. Sedation in the treatment of refractory symptoms: guidelines for evaluation and treatment. J Palliat Care 1994;10:31–8.
205. Twycross RG, Lichter I. The terminal phase. In: Doyle D, Hanks GWC, MacDonald N, editors. Oxford textbook of palliative medicine. 2nd ed. Oxford: Oxford University Press; 1996.
206. Chater S, Viola R, Paterson J, Jarvis V. Sedation for intractable distress in the dying survey of experts. Palliat Med 1998;12:255–69.
207. Foley KM. Changing concepts of tolerance to opioids: what the cancer patient has taught us. In: Chapman CR, Foley KM, editors. Current and emerging issues in cancer pain: research and practice. New York: Raven; 1993. p. 331–49.
208. Cleeland CS, Cleeland LM, Dar R, Rinehardt LC. Factors influencing physician management of cancer pain. Cancer 1986;58:796.
209. Hill CS. Relationship among cultural, educational, and regulatory agency influences on optimum cancer pain treatment. J Pain Symptom Manage 1990;5(Suppl):37.
210. Hill CS, Fields S. Advances in pain research and therapy. Vol. 11. Drug treatment of cancer pain in a drug-oriented society. New York: Raven; 1989.
211. Weissman DE, Haddox JD. Opioid pseudoaddiction—an iatrogenic syndrome. Pain 1989;36:363–6.
212. Adams NJ, Plane MB, Fleming MF, et al. Opioids and the treatment of chronic pain in a primary care sample. J Pain Symptom Manage 2001;22:791–6.
213. Fishbain DA. Report on the prevalence of drug/alcohol abuse and dependence in chronic pain patients (CPPs). Subst Use Misuse 1996;31:945–6.
214. Passik SD, Kirsh KL. Managing pain in patients with aberrant drug-taking behaviors. J Support Oncol 2005;3:83–6.
215. Fishman SM. Opioid side effects, addiction, and anti-inflammatory medications. J Pain Palliat Care Pharmacother 2005;19:51–5.

Section 22

SOCIETAL ONCOLOGY

68

Ethics in Oncology

Ezekiel J. Emanuel, MD, PhD
Steven Joffe, MD, MPH

Many paradigmatic medical ethical issues have arisen first or presented themselves most forcefully in oncology practice. Several early, important informed consent cases involved cancer patients.[1,2] Oken's famous 1961 study demonstrating that most physicians did not inform patients about their cancer diagnosis highlighted controversies over truth-telling.[3] Similarly, several examples of unethical research cited by Beecher in 1966 involved cancer patients.[4] Much discussion about euthanasia and physician-assisted suicide focuses on cancer patients. Given the prominence of clinical research, the complex medical interventions, the threat to survival, and the high costs, ethical questions pervade the care of patients with cancer. Hence, there is a need for a concise but systematic review of medical ethical issues as they relate to oncology practice.

This chapter focuses on the prevailing ethical and legal standards for seven major issues (1) informed consent, (2) human subjects research, (3) terminating medical care, (4) euthanasia and assisted suicide, (5) financial incentives, (6) confidentiality, and (7) genetics in cancer research and care. Excellent sources are available on other medical ethical issues.[5–9]

INFORMED CONSENT

Historical Perspective The first reported legal decision involving informed consent was the 1767 English case of *Slater v. Baker and Stapelton*.[10,11] A patient sued two surgeons for rebreaking a partially healed fracture, without his consent, to improve its alignment. The court ruled that it is "the usage and law of surgeons" to obtain the patient's consent before embarking on an operation. Although the specifics have evolved, the physician's obligation to obtain patient consent prior to initiating interventions has been recognized over the centuries.[12]

In the United States, the modern era of consent began in the early 20th century.[1] This case involved the resection of a tumor without clear consent and perhaps against the patient's verbal statements. The term "informed consent" entered the legal lexicon with the 1957 case *Salgo v. Leland Stanford Jr. University Board of Trustees*.[13] Salgo began the long effort to specify the precise disclosure and other requirements that constitute informed consent (Table 68-1).

Ethical Standards Regarding Informed Consent The fundamental principle underlying the obligation to seek informed consent is respect for the autonomy of persons.[11,12,14] By obtaining informed consent—or informed refusal—we respect patients' rights to determine the course of their lives. Informed consent constrains paternalism—the tendency to decide for patients in their "best interests." Although other moral principles can occasionally override the need to obtain informed consent, the burden of proof generally falls on those who argue for suspension of respect for autonomy.[5,11,12]

Five criteria together constitute valid informed consent (1) disclosure, (2) capacity, (3) understanding, (4) voluntariness, and (5) decision.[11,12,15] Disclosure, which refers to the information that must be provided to patients prior to requesting consent, includes the nature and purpose of the proposed treatment, the foreseeable risks and discomforts, the potential benefits, and the available alternatives.[11,12,15,16]In clinical research, United States' regulations also require description of which procedures are experimental, the impact of research participation on confidentiality, the plan for compensation of and treatment for research-related injuries, the contact person for questions related to the research, and the right to decline participation or withdraw without prejudice.[17]

The standard for determining which risks to disclose varies from one jurisdiction to another.[11,12] Generally, frequent complications should be disclosed regardless of severity, and serious or irreversible risks should be disclosed regardless of frequency. [11,12,16]

Capacity is a person's ability to make health care decisions.[5] It is a clinical rather than a legal determination. In the absence of specific evidence to the contrary, adults are presumed capable. Capacity might be judged according to several criteria, including the ability to (1) make a choice, (2) understand relevant information, (3) appreciate a situation and its consequences, or (4) rationally manipulate information.[11,18] The stringency of the standard varies with the degree to which the patient's decision seems consistent with her health and well being.[19] For example, the patient who chooses to undergo surgery for a ruptured appendix might be held to a low standard of capacity, whereas the patient who chooses to forego the procedure might need to meet a higher standard before we accept her refusal.

Understanding requires that patients comprehend the information presented and appreciate its relevance for their situations. However, neither the legal nor the ethics literature clarifies what constitutes adequate understanding.[11,12] Courts have not established that failure of understanding invalidates informed consent, preferring instead to rely on evidence of disclosure to determine whether physicians met their obligations.[11,16]

Voluntariness implies that patients must be "free from coercion and from unfair persuasions and inducements."[15] This does not preclude physicians from attempting to influence patients' decisions through a respectful process of dialogue and recommendation.[20] Finally, the patient must make a decision for or against a particular plan, and must authorize the clinician to carry it out.

Table 68-1 Major Legal Cases Regarding Informed Consent

Case	Year	Facts	Decision
Schloendorff v. Society of New York Hospitals 211 N.Y. 125	1914	Woman with an abdominal tumor. Physician advised her that it could not be examined except under anesthesia. She consented to the examination but explicitly stated she did not want the tumor removed. The surgeon removed the tumor without the patient's prior consent and against her explicit wish not to have it removed.	"In the case at hand, the wrong complained of is not merely negligence. It is trespass. Every human being of adult years and sound mind has a right to determine what shall be done with his own body; and a surgeon who performs an operation without his patient's consent commits an assault, for which he is liable in damages."
Salgo v. Leland Stanford Jr Board of Trustees 154 Cal. App. 2d 560	1957	55-year-old male with leg cramping and other symptoms of extensive arterial disease. The patient underwent translumbar aortography by a surgeon. There was no apparent complication to the procedure, although the next morning the patient awoke paralyzed from the waist down. The patient claimed that his physicians had not warned him of the risk of paralysis.	"A physician violates his duty to his patient and subjects himself to liability if he withholds any facts which are necessary to form the basis of an intelligent consent by the patient to the proposed treatment...At the same time, the physician must place the welfare of his patient above all else and [recognize] that the patient's mental and emotional condition is important and in certain cases may be crucial, and that in discussing the element of risk, a certain amount of discretion must be employed consistent with the full disclosure of facts necessary to an informed consent."
Natanson v. Kline 186 Kan. 393	1960	Woman with breast cancer was treated with cobalt radiation therapy after mastectomy. The radiation therapy caused substantial burns including necrosis of the skin, muscles, and ribs. The woman claimed that she received an excessive dosage of radiation and that the physicians failed to inform her of probable consequences of the treatment.	The standard for what information should be disclosed to patients is based on what a competent medical practitioner would disclose. "The rule in effect compels disclosure by the physician in order to assure that an informed consent of the patient is obtained. The duty of the physician to disclose, however, is limited to those disclosures which a reasonable medical practitioner would make under the same or similar circumstances...[Appropriate disclosure is what would be disclosed if] the physician was motivated only by the patient's best therapeutic interests and he proceeded as competent medical men would have done in a similar situation."
Canterbury v. Spence 464 F.2d. 772	1972	19-year-old male with severe back pain. Laminectomy was performed without complications. While voiding, patient slipped off the bed and fell. He developed paralysis from the waist down; surgery to remove pressure on the spinal cord was partially successful in restoring movement of his legs but left him with urinary incontinence. The patient claimed the physician did not disclose any risk of paralysis.	Ruling established that the amount of information to be disclosed is established not by medical practice or standards but by the patient's need to know. "True consent to what happens to one's self is the informed exercise of a choice, and that entails an opportunity to evaluate knowledgeably the options available and the risks attendant upon each...[There is] the need, and in turn the requirement of a reasonable divulgence by physician to patient to make such a decision possible...It seems obviously prohibitive and unrealistic to expect physicians to discuss with their patients every risk of proposed treatment—no matter how small or remote...The scope of the physician's communication to the patient, then, must be measured by the patient's need, and that need is the information material to the decision."
Truman v. Thomas 622 P.2d 902	1980	Dr. Thomas repeatedly advised Ms. Truman about the need to get a Pap smear. She repeatedly refused even though he indicated he would waive his fee. Ms. Thomas died at 30 years of age from cervical cancer. Ms. Thomas' children sued claiming that she had not been told about the risks of refusing a Pap smear.	Established that the duty to disclose risks of refusing a procedure is not different from the duty to disclose risks of undergoing a procedure.
Arato v. Avedon 23 Cal. Rptr. 2d 131	1993	43-year-old male had an operation to remove a nonfunctioning kidney. A tumor in the tail of the pancreas was incidentally discovered and resected. The patient was told about the substantial chance of recurrence and incurability but was never given the precise statistical mortality rate. Experimental therapy with a combination chemotherapy regimen of fluorouracil, doxorubicin, and mitomycin (FAM) and radiation was recommended. About 9 months after the surgery, recurrence was noted, and the patient died within 3 months. Family sued contending the patient would not have undergone the chemotherapy, if he had known the statistical prognosis.	Informed consent does not require disclosure of statistical prognostic data. The court affirmed "the obligation of a treating physician of reasonable disclosure of the available choices with respect to proposed therapy and of the dangers inherently and potentially involved in each...[but argued this does not include] the mandatory disclosure of life expectancy probabilities."

Although signed forms are often used to facilitate and document the informed consent process, they should be considered secondary to the discussions between clinician and patient.

Ideally, informed consent is a process, not an event. Conceptualized as an event, informed consent "...is temporally circumscribed... [it] begins when a physician offers a patient recommendations with accompanying information and ends with the patient's decision."[11] Although convenient, and often suitable for one-time procedures, the event model is inadequate for interactions and therapies that occur over time. The process model "...is based on the assumption that medical decision making is a continuous process, not a discrete event. The exchange of information... should take place throughout the course of the physician–patient relationship."[11]

Incapacity and Surrogate Decision Making Some patients, because of temporary or permanent mental disability, cannot make decisions regarding their care. When determining capacity, there are dual risks. Mistakenly declaring that a person lacks capacity fails to acknowledge his autonomy. Conversely, wrongly deciding that a person retains decision making capacity can fail to protect a vulnerable individual.

When a patient lacks capacity, a surrogate must make health care decisions. Ideally patients, while still competent, will have designated a preferred surrogate using a Health Care Proxy (HCP) form. A HCP legally empowers the surrogate to make decisions for the patient in the event of future incapacity. Adults with cancer should be strongly encouraged to name a surrogate decision maker through a HCP. In the absence of a HCP, a family member generally serves as the surrogate decision–maker. State rules on the order of priority within the family vary. When there is no obvious proxy, or in cases of family conflict, court involvement may be necessary to designate a surrogate.

The two main standards to guide surrogate decision making are the substituted-judgment and the best-interests standards.[5,11] Under substituted judgment, the surrogate must determine what the patient would want were he able to decide. When the patient left specific instructions about future contingencies, application of the substituted-judgment standard is relatively straightforward. In the absence of specific instructions, the standard is more problematic.[11]

The best-interests standard asks the surrogate to determine which course of action is most favorable for the patient. Although it seems objective, and applies equally to patients who left no evidence of their wishes, it too is fraught with difficulty. Reasonable disagreements about a patient's best interests often occur. The procedures for resolving such disputes are unclear.

In practice, the substituted-judgment and best-interests standards can be complementary. Substituted judgment may be viewed as a way of further specifying a patient's best interests from his or her perspective.[11] The more specific the guidance left by a patient, the more one can invoke a substituted-judgment framework and consider the decision from the patient's point of view.

Outside of pediatrics, surrogates' authority to agree to incompetent patients' participation in clinical research is unclear.[21] Federal regulations permit a subject's "legally authorized representative" to agree to research on the subject's behalf, but uncertainty over the precise scope and meaning of this right, as well as variations in relevant state laws, cloud its application.[22] The US National Bioethics Advisory Commission (NBAC) and others have encouraged clarification of these issues, including the extension of HCPs to authorize consent to research.[23,24] These recommendations are controversial and have not been translated into regulation.

Is Informed Consent Always Appropriate? Despite its important and positive role in clinical medicine, rigid insistence on informed consent is sometimes inappropriate.[11,12] For example, differences in cultural assumptions about the relationships between individuals and families may impact expectations about how and with whom to discuss terminal diagnoses.[25,26] In some cultures, decisions about the use of life-sustaining technologies might be felt to reside with family members rather than with the patient. Cultural attitudes about truth telling may also vary, and discussion of bad news may be considered a deep affront.[25,26] Even in the absence of cultural differences, some patients prefer not to be fully informed or to own decision-making responsibility.[27–30] How can we reconcile the obligation to obtain informed consent with the need to respect such patients' desires?

If autonomous persons do not wish certain types of information, or prefer to delegate certain decisions, we respect their autonomy by accepting their wishes. In practice, of course, determining how much information or decision making authority a patient wants can be exquisitely difficult. Family members may insist that a patient not be told about a cancer diagnosis. Without exploring further, the physician might fail to uncover that the patient's desires differ from those of the family.

Freedman describes a sensitive process for "offering truth."[31] The physician asks the patient to describe her understanding of her medical condition. Using gentle questions about what information and decision making role the patient desires, the physician allows her to guide and limit the conversation. In such a nondirective exchange, patients who prefer to delegate decisions will usually make their wishes clear. This approach "...affords a means of satisfying legal and ethical norms of patient autonomy, ameliorating conflicts between families and physicians, and acknowledging the cultural norms that underlie family desires."[31]

HUMAN SUBJECTS RESEARCH

Historical Perspective Experimentation involving human beings is at least 200 years old; awareness of ethical challenges in research dates back almost as long.[32] In the early 20th century, Walter Reed developed a contract—the forerunner to informed consent documents—delineating the risks and compensation to participants in yellow fever experiments.[32] In 1916, Walter Bradford Cannon unsuccessfully proposed amending the American Medical Association code of ethics to specify researchers' obligations to subjects.[32] The 10 principles of the Nuremberg Code responded to abuses by Nazi doctors.[33] In 1966, Henry Beecher described unethical research practiced by prominent researchers and institutions.[4] Beecher's revelations, along with publicity about the Tuskegee Syphilis Study,[34] prompted creation of the National Commission for the Protection of Human Subjects of Biomedical and Behavioral Research. The Commission wrote the Belmont Report, which provides the ethical framework for United States' regulations on human subjects research, which is known as the Common Rule.[17,35] These regulations have largely eliminated gross violations. However, within the last few years controversy about the ethics of clinical research has intensified again.[36]

Therapy versus Research Until recently, the Declaration of Helsinki postulated "a fundamental distinction... between medical research in which the aim is essentially diagnostic or therapeutic for a patient, and medical research, the essential object of which is purely scientific...."[37,38] Clinicians and investigators commonly distinguish between "therapeutic" and "nontherapeutic" research. However, commentators have challenged this distinction, arguing that it is impossible to determine which studies are therapeutic and which are not, and that all studies have nontherapeutic elements and objectives.[39] For example, is an RCT that involves a placebo "therapeutic?" Given these criticisms, the Declaration no longer articulates this distinction.[38]

In considering a research project, it is important to clearly define which activities are research and which are treatment.[40] In pure clinical care, the physician is expected to place the current patient's interests above all else. Conversely, the investigator's primary purpose is to generate knowledge that, directly or through additional research, will improve treatment for future patients. Because the purpose of research is to generate knowledge for others, there is always a threat of exploiting research participants, using them as means for the benefit of others.[39,41] Although most cancer trials succeed in reconciling the tensions between research and care, the potential for these two activities to conflict is inherent in even the best-designed studies. The ethical requirements for clinical research are meant to minimize the chance that research will exploit human subjects.[41]

Ethical Standards for Clinical Research Research with human beings must satisfy eight ethical principles (Table 68-2).[41,42] First, studies must reflect a collaborative partnership between researchers and the community from which participants are drawn. Usually this partnership is embodied in support from advocacy groups and the public, as well as inclusion of subject representatives in research advisory and oversight boards. Such support provides tangible evidence that the community that presumably will benefit from answers to the study questions shares the investigators' objectives. Second, the research must be socially valuable, addressing meaningful gaps in therapy or scientific understanding.[43] Third, the methods must be reliable and valid so that there is a reasonable chance that study will achieve its objectives.[42,43] Research involving invalid or biased methods is unethical because no amount of risk or inconvenience to subjects can be justified.[39,41,43] Fourth, subjects must be selected fairly. Eligibility requirements and recruitment strategies must serve scientific objectives, not social prejudice or vulnerability.[35] It is unreasonable to recruit individuals of a certain group into a study for convenience alone. Conversely, it is not permissible preferentially to enroll privileged individuals in studies of especially promising interventions. Unfair selection is rarely a problem in cancer research, where recruitment is necessarily tied to the disease under study.

Historical inequities have led to efforts to increase participation by women, minorities, and children in clinical research. Such inclusionary practices help ensure that the benefits of medical advances will extend to all.[44] Evidence about the representation of minority groups in clinical trials is conflicting.[45,46] The well-documented under-representation of the elderly may constitute an injustice to that group.[46,47]

Fifth, the research must offer subjects a reasonable balance of risks and benefits.[35,48] Although risks are intrinsic to cancer research, investigators should make every effort to minimize them. Similarly, they should strive to enhance the potential benefits, both to subjects themselves and to future patients. Although weighing risks to participants against the sum of benefits to present and future subjects is difficult, such a calculus is morally and legally required.[17,48]

Sixth, research must undergo independent review by a committee of peers and laypersons.[17,39] Independent review ideally offers both unbiased scientific and ethical oversight and insti-

Table 68-2 Eight Requirements for Making a Research Trial Ethical

Requirement	Explanation	Justifying Ethical Values
Community partnership	Inclusion of patients, representatives of advocacy groups, and other community members in determining research priorities and strategies for studies	Nonexploitation and respect for community's self-determination
Social or scientific value	Evaluation of a treatment, intervention or theory that will improve health and well being or increase knowledge.	Scarce resources and non-exploitation
Scientific validity	Use of accepted scientific principles and methods, including statistical techniques, to produce reliable and valid data.	Scarce resources and non-exploitation
Fair subject selection	Selection of subjects so that stigmatized and vulnerable individuals are not targeted for risky research and favored classes not favored for potentially beneficial research.	Distributive justice
Favorable risk/benefit ratio	Minimization of risks; maximization of potential benefits; risks to the subject are proportionate to the benefits to the subject and society.	Nonmaleficence, beneficence, and non-exploitation
Independent review	Review of the design of the research trial, its proposed subject population and risk-to-benefit ratio by individuals unaffiliated with the research.	Public accountability, minimizing influence of potential conflicts of interest
Informed consent	Provision of information to subjects about purpose of the research, its procedures, potential risks, benefits, and alternatives so that the individual understands this information and can make a voluntary decision whether to enroll and continue to participate.	Respect for subject, autonomy
Respect for potential and enrolled subjects	1. Permitting withdrawal from the research 2. Protecting privacy through confidentiality 3. Informing of newly discovered risks or benefits 4. Informing about results of clinical research 5. Maintaining welfare of subjects	Respect for subject, autonomy, and welfare

tutional and public accountability.[41,42] In the United States, independent review is the responsibility of the Institutional Review Board (IRB). IRBs derive their regulatory authority from federal law, and though they retain considerable discretion they must apply certain standards in deciding whether or not to approve research.[17] There is no ethical requirement for multiple reviews of the same protocol. Indeed if resources are wasted without added protections then multiple reviews are imprudent if not unethical.

Seventh, subjects must offer informed consent.[17,35,38,39,41,42,48] Obtaining consent facilitates respect for autonomy by allowing individuals to decide if they want to assume the risks, contribute to the project, and can fulfill the protocol's requirements. In cases of incapacity, including pediatric cases, permission from a surrogate is generally required. Whenever possible, children with sufficient cognitive maturity should participate in decision making regarding research.[49]

Finally, respect for persons must continue throughout a trial's duration. This includes, but is not limited to, respect for subjects' rights to privacy and to relevant new findings, and recognition of the ongoing voluntary nature of participation.

Informed Consent to Research and the Therapeutic Misconception Obtaining consent for clinical research differs from obtaining consent to routine care. When a patient enters a study, the structure of the trial and the requirements of the scientific method constrain the physician's ability to deliver individualized care. For example, randomization necessarily depersonalizes decision making. It may be difficult for participants to comprehend such differences between physician–patient and investigator–subject relationships.[11] Despite careful efforts to explain the nature of clinical trials, including their necessary role in generating new scientific knowledge and improving treatments for future patients, subjects may persist in the "therapeutic misconception" that clinical trials are designed with participants' individual benefit in mind.[50] Though the data are incomplete, some studies suggest that cancer clinical trial participants may hold therapeutic misconceptions.[51,52] Efforts to address the problem will likely require a greater focus on the conceptual aspects of clinical trials. Discussions should address how being in a trial differs from ordinary clinical care, as well as how the specific trial under consideration differs from available alternatives.

Ethics of Phase I Research The primary objectives of phase I trials, which often, although not always study new agents, are to assess safety and to identify appropriate doses for further research. Their dose-escalation design makes it likely that some participants will receive suboptimal doses whereas others will experience serious toxicity.

The criticisms of phase I research are twofold: unfavorable risk-benefit ratio and inadequate informed consent.[53–55] In response to the first criticism, empirical evidence suggests that the likelihood of benefit from phase I participation, though low, is not zero. Given the heterogeneity of phase I trials, it is difficult to generalize about response rates. The probability of an objective response is 3 to 4.5% among adults participating in classic trials, and higher among those participating in trials that combine new and approved agents.[56–58] Recent studies demonstrate that the nature of Phase I trials has changed, with many dose-escalation trials of FDA-approved agents and combinations as well as biologic agents such as immunomodulators, anti-angiogenesis agents, signal transduction inhibitors, and vaccines. For the whole group the CR + PR rate has increased to over 10%.[57,58] Furthermore, there may be some quality of life benefits.[59] The likelihood of toxic death remains low at 0.5%.[56–58] These tradeoffs may be reasonably viewed as favorable by some patients with advanced cancer, who even outside the context of phase I trials may be more likely than medical professionals or healthy individuals to accept interventions with a limited likelihood of benefit.[60]

The second criticism is that consent from patients with incurable cancer is invalid. Detractors argue that such patients are vulnerable and should be protected from overzealous researchers who exaggerate the benefits, minimize the risks, and coerce patients into participating.[53] The claim that terminally ill patients lack capacity to make decisions about research participation, however, fails to respect their autonomy. In addition, though few data exist, it appears that subjects in phase I research do receive adequate disclosure and consider themselves to be well informed.[51,61,62] Although it seems plausible that some phase I subjects might choose not to participate if they fully understood the low likelihood of benefit and the ways in which phase I designs reconcile clinical and scientific objectives, evidence for this contention is not strong.[54,62]

Some investigators have proposed altering the design of phase I trials to maximize response rates as well as the efficiency with which trials are completed. Novel designs generally strive to minimize the number of subjects enrolled at suboptimal doses. Innovations include intrasubject dose escalation, fewer subjects per cohort, and larger initial dose increments. Ironically, efforts to maximize benefits necessarily increase risk.[63]

Randomized Controlled Trials Randomized Controlled Trials (RCTs) are the gold standard of clinical investigation, providing the best evidence with which to compare a therapy to the alternatives. Yet ethical discomfort with RCTs persists, and some clinicians and patients find it difficult to accept chance assignment.[64,65] First, random assignment requires that physicians and patients set aside their own beliefs about the relative merits of different treatment approaches. Second, it forces both parties to accept limits on individualized care. Finally, the informed consent process may be particularly challenging when describing RCTs.[66,67]

The most widely accepted ethical basis for randomized trials is clinical equipoise.[68] Clinical equipoise requires genuine uncertainty or disagreement about the relative merits of two or more therapies in the expert medical community. An RCT is conducted to resolve this professional uncertainty. This is the ethical equivalent of the statistical dictum that an RCT must begin with an honest null hypothesis.[68] Whereas an individual physician may prefer one arm of the trial, the disagreement in the community legitimizes enrolling patients.

RCTs remove some decisions about treatment from both physician and patient, thereby seeming to threaten the fiduciary nature of the doctor–patient relationship. Some worry that this devalues the doctor's commitment to the best interests of the individual patient in favor of the investigator's commitment to science or to the needs of society.[64] However, advocates of clinical equipoise argue that, when equipoise obtains, entry into a trial by definition is consistent with a patient's best interests.[68–70] Either arm might offer the best chance of the desired outcome.

Discomfort with obtaining informed consent for RCTs may compromise accrual.[66] Some physicians report that requirements for informed consent lead to an overemphasis on the investigator–subject rather than the doctor–patient relationship; may compromise physician autonomy; and force an uncomfortable conversation about the uncertainty that ultimately undermines the therapeutic alliance. However, tenets of informed consent obligate clinicians to present all reasonable alternatives, including RCTs.[70,71] Finally, uncertainty is a constant companion in the practice of medicine. Patients have a right to know the strength of the evidence for or against each potential course of action, whether or not that action involves a trial.

Difficult issues arise as preliminary results from the trial begin to point in one or another direction.[72] Although a trial may begin in equipoise, accumulating data are likely to disturb that equipoise. A priori stopping rules, data monitoring committees, and disclosure to potential subjects of policies on release of preliminary information and early termination buttress the integrity of RCTs.[5]

Some challenge the validity of clinical equipoise in justifying RCTs. Miller and Brody argue that clinical equipoise is founded on a mistaken assumption that physicians' obligations to patients constrain clinical trials.[73] Given the integration of clinical research into cancer medicine, this ongoing controversy is of particular importance for the practice of oncology.[74,75]

Placebo Controls Most commentators agree that placebo controls are ethical when there is no known effective treatment for the condition under study. Over the last decade, however, the use of placebo controls when effective treatments are available has been hotly controversial. Several authors have argued that, in such circumstances, one should not ask a patient to accept randomization to a placebo-only control arm.[76] These authors also claim that the clinically relevant question is not how new therapies compare to placebo, but rather how they compare to existing standards. Defenders of placebo controls argue that when the consequences of non-treatment are minor, offering patients enrollment in a placebo-controlled trial, even when an effective therapy exists, can be ethical because there is no risk of serious or permanent harm. Furthermore, for methodological reasons, there are circumstances when studies without a placebo control may be uninformative.[77,78] The World Medical Association (WMA), in its 2000 revision of the Declaration of Helsinki, initially sided with the critics of placebos. Article 29 of the Declaration states, "The benefits, risks, burdens, and effectiveness of a new method should be tested against those of the best current prophylactic, diagnostic, and therapeutic methods. This does not exclude the use of placebo, or no treatment, in studies where no proven prophylactic, diagnostic or therapeutic method exists."[38] The WMA subsequently clarified this article, however, to permit use of a placebo arm in limited circumstances.[38] Most other guidance endorses use of a placebo arm when the risks are minor and there are compelling scientific reasons.[79]

Research Involving Stored Tissue There are an estimated 280 million stored human biological samples in the United States.[80] Worries about genetic knowledge and technology, as well as the increasing attention to privacy and confidentiality engendered by managed care and the electronic storage of medical information, have contributed to worries about research on tissue samples. Given these samples' promise for understanding the biology of cancer, the increasing constraints on their use are controversial.[80–83]

Two questions face the researcher considering a study that involves stored tissue. First, does the project require IRB review? In the United States, studies involving "identifiable private information" about "a living individual" are human subjects research.[17] Therefore, projects involving samples that can be linked, directly or through a code, to the individual or "source" from whom they came fall within the scope of these regulations and require submission to the IRB. Many of these projects, however, should qualify for expedited review.

Second, should consent from sources be sought prior to proceeding with the research? Some ethicists argue that respect for autonomy requires consent in virtually all circumstances.[84,85] Sometimes sources will have previously given consent that is sufficiently specific to cover the proposed research, but usually a consent requirement would necessitate recontacting the individuals. Such a requirement both increases cost and logistical difficulty and might introduce selection biases.[86] Ultimately, within the constraints imposed by the relevant laws and regulations, researchers and IRBs must weigh these concerns against the interests of individuals in controlling what is done with their tissues. In the United States, IRBs may waive the consent requirement when several conditions are met, including that the research involves no greater than minimal risk and could not "practicably" be carried out without the waiver.[17]

Separate questions arise when considering prospective storage of tissue samples. There is agreement that individuals should be asked to specify what uses they would permit for their tissues whenever samples are obtained.[80–83] Disagreement focuses on what participants should consent to. The NBAC and others have recommended that, in the future, individuals be asked to specify their wishes on 6 different questions, such as what types of research they would permit with their sample, whether on the same disease or a different disease, whether the samples could be sent to another researcher at other institutions.[80,81] Others contend this long list is neither desirable nor ethically necessary. They cite studies in which people who have contributed their biological material simply want to determine whether the material is used for research or not.[87,88] Prudence suggests asking patients and research participants whether they are willing to have their samples used for any future research rather than detailed questions about the type of use they would permit. Unfortunately, the Health Insurance Portability and Accountability Act (HIPAA) appears to rule out obtaining open-ended consent for future research on tissue samples at this time.[89]

TERMINATING MEDICAL CARE

Historical Perspective The first suggestion that physicians withhold medical interventions from terminally ill patients probably dates to Hippocrates' injunction "to refuse to treat those [patients] who are overmastered by their disease, realizing that in such cases medicine is powerless."[90] In 1835, Jacob Bigelow urged members of the Massachusetts Medical Society to withhold "therapies"—such as cathartics and emetics—from hopelessly ill patients.[91] In 1848, John Warren, the surgeon who performed the first operation with ether anesthesia, urged that ether should be used "in mitigating the agonies of death."[92] In 1958, Pope Pius XII, in response to questions about resuscitating patients and maintaining comatose patients on respirators, stated that physicians had no obligation to use such "extraordinary" means to forestall death.[93]

In 1976, however, the *Quinlan* case dramatically changed the nature and content of terminating care discussions, and recognized the right to refuse life-sustaining treatments.[94] Recently, three things have happened. First, seizing on the broad recognition of a right to refuse medical care, some have advocated broadening the right to include euthanasia and physician-assisted suicide. Simultaneously, as highlighted in the *Schiavo* case, some have tried to constrict the right to refuse medical treatments for patients who are mentally incapacitated. Finally, there has been recognition that a right to terminate care is not the ultimate goal, but the mechanism to a goal. This recognition has lead to a de-emphasis of the language of patient's rights, focusing instead on providing optimal end-of-life care. For physicians to understand acceptable practices for the termination of care, it is most useful to consider three topics, (1) legal standards governing the termination of medical care (2), advance-care documents, and (3), end-of-life care practices.

Legal Standards Regarding Terminating Medical Care Prior to 1976, legal cases involving the refusal of life-sustaining medical care usually involved Jehovah's Witnesses and justified the decision by appeal to the First Amendment's right of religious freedom. *Quinlan* changed the focus to the following four fundamental questions: (1) Do patients have a right to refuse medical care? (2) What types of care can be terminated? (3) Who can make terminating care decisions? and (4) What criteria should guide such decisions?

Is There a Right to Refuse Medical Care? In its 1990 *Cruzan* decision, the US Supreme Court agreed that competent patients have a constitutional right to refuse medical care. The Court located this right in the Fourteenth Amendment's guarantee "that no State shall deprive any person of life, liberty, or property, without due process of law."[95] In its 1997 decision regarding euthanasia and physician-assisted suicide, the Supreme Court reaffirmed patients' right to refuse medical treatments.[96] As Chief Justice Rehnquist put it: "[A]lthough *Cruzan* is often described as a 'right to die' case...we were, in fact, more precise: we assumed that the Constitution granted competent persons a 'constitutionally protected right to refuse lifesaving hydration and nutrition.'...[A] liberty interest in refusing unwanted medical treatment may be inferred from our prior decisions."[96] By identifying a constitutional basis for this right, the Supreme Court has made it a national standard, ensuring that it will no longer be subject to the vagaries of individual state laws or court rulings.

The issue is more complicated regarding mentally incapacitated patients. Although they have the same right, how it is exercised is complex. The Supreme Court allowed states to impose restrictions on how explicit and specific the patient's prior wishes had to be.[95,97] Nevertheless, the Supreme Court's consistent refusal to intervene in the *Schiavo* case on behalf of her parents' desire to continue nutrition and hydration is reaffirmation of this right even for mentally incapacitated patients.

Competent patients need not be terminally ill to exercise this right to refuse interventions; they have the right regardless of health status. Moreover, the right applies equally to withholding proposed treatments and to discontinuing initiated treatments. Finally, this right to refuse medical care does not imply a correlative right to demand treatment.[98]

In theory, the right of patients to refuse medical therapy can be limited by four countervailing interests (1) preservation of life, (2) prevention of suicide, (3) protection of third parties such as children, and (4) preserving the integrity of the medical profession.[98] In practice, these interests almost never override the right of competent patients and incompetent patients who have left explicit advance directives.

What Types of Medical Interventions May Be Terminated? *Quinlan* focused on the withdrawal of mechanical respirators.[94] Subsequently, legal cases have sanctioned the withholding or withdrawal of chemotherapy, blood transfusions, hemodialysis, and major surgical operations (Table 68-3).[98] In *Cruzan*, the US Supreme Court definitively stated that artificial nutrition and hydration are medical interventions that can be withheld or withdrawn under the guidelines that apply to other medical treatments.[95] As Justice O'Connor stated, "The liberty guaranteed by the Due Process Clause must protect, if it protects anything, an individual's deeply personal decision to reject medical treatment, including the artificial delivery of food and water."[95]

Who Decides Whether Care Can Be Terminated? Competent patients have the exclusive right to refuse medical care. Even in cases where the patient's wishes may conflict with those of his or her family, the patient's right to refuse care is determinative. For mentally incapacitated patients who left living wills or other advance care documents, the wishes in these directives are determinative.

Recently, who decides whether interventions can be terminated for patients who are mentally incapacitated who did not leave advance care documents or other explicit indications of their views on terminating care has become more problematic. Many have maintained that the incapacitated patient's family is the most appropriate surrogate decision maker.[99] In the 1980s, many courts affirmed this view, recognizing that when patients had explicit but unrecorded conversations with family, friends, and others about their wishes regarding terminating treatments, these conversations should be used as decision making guides (see Table 68-3).

However, there have been objections to this position.[99] For instance, in other areas of medical care, families are not necessarily permitted to make decisions for mentally incapacitated patients. In addition, empirical studies suggest that spouses and other family members generally do not know the preferences of patients regarding the termination of life-sustaining treatments; therefore, they may not reach the same decision that the patient would have reached.[99]

In *Cruzan*, the US Supreme Court addressed the issue of mentally incapacitated patients.[95] After suffering anoxic brain damage in a car accident, Nancy Cruzan remained in a persistent vegetative state maintained by artificial nutrition and hydration (see Table 68-3). Her parents asked that the feedings be discontinued. The state of Missouri agreed that the patient had a right to refuse medical care but argued that without a living will or "clear and convincing" evidence of Nancy Cruzan's views on terminating life-sustaining care, her parents were not entitled to exercise her right to terminate the artificial nutrition and hydration.

The US Supreme Court held that there is no constitutional requirement that families be permitted to exercise the right of mentally incapacitated patients to terminate care when the patients have not left explicit statements of their preferences.[95] Importantly, however, the Court did not delineate uniform national rules regarding who should decide for mentally incapacitated patients. Instead, the Court permitted each individual state to make the rules it deemed best. The Court also endorsed, as legally acceptable but not required, Missouri's contention that the "evidence of the incompetent's wishes as to the withdrawal of treatment be provided by clear and convincing evidence." The "clear and convincing" evidence standard is a technical one, and it requires more than a casual conversation. Ultimately, the Missouri courts terminated Cruzan's artificial nutrition and hydration, relying on the recollection of a conversation with a cousin many years before.

Recently, several state supreme courts have limited the right of families to decide for incompetent patients when there is no advance care directive or formal appointment of the proxy.[100–102] These courts have accepted that when a patient who is mentally incapacitated is in a persistent vegetative state, comatose, or terminally ill, family members, even if not formally appointed as proxy decision makers, can withdraw life-sustaining treatments based on prior conversations with the patient or their understanding of the patient's values. However, although these courts have affirmed the right of patients to refuse all manner of medical interventions, they have refused to permit families not formally appointed as proxies to terminate life-sustaining treatments from mentally incapacitated but conscious patients, patients who can interact minimally. These courts maintain that for family members, even spouses, to terminate care from mentally incapacitated but conscious patients, there must be clear and convincing evidence of the patient's wishes. Explicit statements by the patient that relate to not wanting to be on life support or in a vegetative state, courts have argued, do not meet the standard of "clear and convincing" evidence. For a surrogate, who is not formally appointed, to decide to terminate life sustaining treatments from an incompetent but conscious patient, the patient's statements must (1) address the condition the patient is in, not a closely related one, (2) identify the specific intervention being considered for termination, and (3) indicate that the comments are to be used to guide medical decision making. This level of specificity for guidance of surrogate decision makers is a change. Until recently, this view had limited application—it

Table 68-3 Major Legal Cases Regarding the Termination of Life-Sustaining Medical Care

Case and Citation	Year	State	Facts	Decision
In re Quinlan, 70 N.J. 10	1976	NJ	21-year-old female who ceased breathing for two 15-minute periods at a party. Friends tried to resuscitate her. In the emergency room, her pupils were unreactive and she was unresponsive to deep pain. She was placed on a respirator. Three days later she displayed decorticate posture. A year after the event she was in a persistent vegetative state and was respirator dependent, receiving artificial nutrition and hydration through a nasogastric tube.	The right to privacy includes a right to refuse medical care. This right extends to incompetent patients and Karen Quinlan's guardian—her father—could terminate her respirator. The court recommended that a hospital ethics committee certify the patient's prognosis prior to the decision, but emphasized that in most cases there was no need for prior judicial review.
Superintendent of Belchertown v. Saikewicz, 373. Mass. 728	1977	MA	67-year-old mentally handicapped man with a mental age of 2 years 8 months who had always lived in a state institution developed acute myelomonocytic leukemia. The institution inquired whether providing chemotherapy is required.	All persons including incompetent persons have the right to refuse medical treatment. Using substituted judgment, the court determined that the patient would not want chemotherapy.
In re Eichner(Brother Fox), 52 N.Y. 2d 262	1981	NY	83-year-old priest who had a cardiac arrest during a herniorrhaphy that left him vegetative and respirator dependent. Prior to the event, he had publicly discussed the *Quinlan* case and stated that he would not want to be respirator dependent if he were in a vegetative state.	Patients have the right to determine the course of their own medical care. Brother Fox's wishes were known, even if not expressed in writing, and they should determine whether his respirator is disconnected.
In re Conroy, 98 N.J. 321	1985	NJ	84-year-old bedridden, totally impaired woman with organic brain syndrome living in a nursing home being fed by a nasogastric tube. Her nephew requests removal of the tube.	Nasogastric tube feedings are medical interventions that can be withdrawn. In addition, the court outlines a "pure objective test" for determining when to terminate medical care from incompetent patients who have left no indication of their wishes. According to this test, care can be terminated when it causes "recurring, unavoidable, and severe pain" rendering life "inhumane."
Brophy v. New England Sinai Hospital, 398 Mass. 417	1986	MA	49-year-old man in persistent vegetative state after a ruptured aneurysm maintained by gastric tube feedings. Although he had no written living will, he had explicitly stated that he would never want to live on life support systems. After having rescued a man from a burning truck who lived for some time with severe burns before dying, he stated that he regretted his actions and requested that if he were ever in a similar situation, the plug should be pulled.	Common law and the constitutional right of privacy give a person the right to refuse medical treatment. The patient's wishes are clearly known from explicit conversations. Thus, by using substituted judgment the gastric tube can be withdrawn.
Bouvia v. Superior Court, 225 Cal. Rptr. 297	1986	CA	29-year-old woman with cerebral palsy that left her almost completely immobile and totally unable to care for herself is receiving morphine by pump for painful degenerative arthritis. Physicians insert a nasogastric tube to supplement her inadequate oral intake. She requests that the nasogastric tube be removed.	A competent patient has the "right to refuse any medical treatment, even that which may save or prolong her life."
In re Jobes, 108 N.J. 394	1987	NJ	32-year-old woman who is in a permanent vegetative state and receiving J-tube feedings. Her husband and parents request termination of the feedings. She left no clear written or verbal indication of her wishes on such care.	Incompetent patients have the right to refuse medical care even if they have left no clear indication of their wishes. This right can be exercised by the incompetent patient's family. Using substituted judgment the family is permitted to terminate the J-tube feedings.
Cruzan v. Director of Missouri Department of Health, 110 S. Ct. 2841	1990	MO	33-year-old woman left in a persistent vegetative state after suffering anoxic brain damage in a car accident. She was maintained by gastric tube nutrition and hydration. Her parents requested that these tube feedings be terminated.	By 8 to 1, the US Supreme Court ruled that patients have a constitutional right to refuse medical care and that this applies to artificial nutrition and hydration. The majority argues that states could regulate the family's ability to exercise an incompetent patient's right to refuse treatment if there was no "clear and convincing" written or verbal statement of the patient's wishes. Because the state of Missouri felt that families should not be permitted to terminate care from patients without explicit prior statements by the patient, Cruzan's feedings continued. A cousin recalled a conversation with the patient indicating that she would not want life-sustaining treatments if she were in a persistent vegetative state. Other states could permit families to exercise the incompetent's right to refuse care in the absence of explicit directives or clear and convincing statements.
In re Helga Wangie, 1991 Fourth Judicial District (Dist. Ct., Probate Ct. Div.) PX-91-283. Minnesota (Hennepin County)	1991	MN	85-year-old woman admitted for dyspnea and is emergently intubated. After 5 months on the respirator she was discharged to a chronic care facility. After 1 week at the facility, she had a cardiac arrest but was resuscitated and taken to an intensive care unit. After several weeks, physicians concluded that she was in a persistent vegetative state. Physicians suggested withdrawing life-sustaining treatment because the patient was receiving no benefit. The family refused to have any life-sustaining treatments withdrawn. No other facility would accept the patient in transfer. After 7 months, the hospital went to court hoping to have the respirator discontinued.	A trial court ruled the husband should represent the patient's interests, and he refused to discontinue the respirator.

(Continued)

Table 68-3 Major Legal Cases Regarding the Termination of Life-Sustaining Medical Care *(Continued)*

Case and Citation	Year	State	Facts	Decision
Wendland vs Wendland, 110 Cal. Rptr. 2d 412	2001	CA	42-year-old man conscious with severe cognitive impairments, hemiparesis, and limited communication who required a feeding tube. The feeding tube fell out and needed to be replaced. After authorizing replacement of the feeding tube three times, the wife refused replacement. Ethics committee agreed, but lower court disagreed.	A unanimous California Supreme Court ruled that patients have a right to refuse medical treatments including life-sustaining treatments. This right can be exercised for mentally incapacitated patients through advance care directives. Thus, all interventions including artificial nutrition and hydration can be terminated from competent patients and incapacitated patients who are not terminally ill if they completed an advance care directive stating this preference. For patients who are terminally ill, in persistent vegetative state, or comatose who have not completed an advance care directive, proxies who have not been formally appointed can terminate interventions if these are deemed in the best interest of the patient. However, for mentally incapacitated patients who remain conscious, "clear and convincing" evidence is needed of the patient's wishes before life-sustaining treatment can be stopped. To satisfy this "clear and convincing" evidence requirement, the patient's comments must be very specific referring to the exact type of disability and interventions. Comments about not wanting to be kept as a vegetable or on a respirator will not suffice to indicate a patient's wishes.

was only for mentally incapacitated but conscious patients who did not formally appoint a proxy. But the *Schiavo* case in Florida suggests the possibility that these limitations will be extended to other patients, including terminally ill cancer patients. Indeed, these limits and the controversy over the *Schiavo* case emphasize the value of having patients complete formal advance care directives, specifying their wishes regarding life-sustaining treatments and who they want to be their proxy decision maker.

One problem that seems to be arising with increasing frequency is that families want patients in a coma, in a persistent vegetative state, or with anencephaly maintained with life-sustaining treatments, although the treating physicians object to providing such care. In the *Wanglie* case, for instance, the family of an elderly woman in a persistent vegetative state wanted her respirator continued.[103] Her physicians objected and went to court to have her feedings terminated, arguing that they were not providing a benefit to the patient (see Table 68-3). The court ruled that the family had a right to decide what treatments the patient should receive.

What Criteria Should Guide Decisions to Terminate Care? Competent patients have the right to refuse medical care and can use whatever criteria they deem acceptable; it is their values, whatever they are, that guide the choice. In the words of the California Supreme Court: "The right to refuse medical treatment is basic and fundamental. Its exercise requires no one's approval. It is not merely one vote subject to being overridden by medical opinion... The controlling decision belongs to a competent informed patient... It is a moral and philosophical decision that, being a competent adult, is the [patient's] alone."[104] Similarly, for mentally incapacitated patients who left advance directives that specify the interventions they want or do not want, their values determine their choices.

Regarding mentally incapacitated patients who either appointed a proxy without specific indications of their wishes or who never completed an advance care directive, this question remains controversial. Four guiding criteria have been proposed (1) the ordinary/extraordinary care distinction, (2) futile care, (3) substituted judgment, and (4) best interests.[98] Catholic doctrine, as outlined by Pope Pius XII, advocates a distinction between ordinary and extraordinary care, with ordinary care being mandatory, whereas extraordinary care may be withheld.[93] Many ethicists and courts have concluded that this distinction is too vague and has "too many conflicting meanings" to be helpful in guiding surrogate decision makers and physicians.[97] Thus the ordinary/ extraordinary distinction should not be used to justify decisions about stopping treatment.[98]

In the late 1980s, some argued that physicians could terminate futile treatments.[105–108] Unfortunately, the term futility has been used inconsistently. Physiologic futility means that an intervention will have no physiologic effect. Some have defined a qualitatively futile treatment as that which "fails to end a patient's total dependence on intensive medical care."[105] Quantitative futility occurs "when physicians conclude (either through personal experience, experiences shared with colleagues, or consideration of reported empiric data) that in the last 100 cases, a medical treatment has been useless."[105] In general, it is now agreed that there is no objective standard of futility; the term merely conceals subjective value judgments about when a treatment is "not beneficial."[107,108] Deciding whether to pursue chemotherapy for an additional 6 weeks of life or a 1% survival advantage, depends on patients' preferences and goals. Furthermore, several studies indicate that physicians' predictions of when treatments are futile deviate markedly from the quantitative definition of the less than 1 case in the last 100 cases.[109]

Third, many courts advocate use of the substituted-judgment criterion, which holds that the surrogate should try to imagine what the patient would do if the patient were competent.[98] A problem with this criterion is that most surrogates, even close family members, cannot accurately predict what the patient would have wanted.[99] Therefore, in the absence of specific guidance from the patient when competent, substituted judgment becomes more of a guessing game—or, as some courts have called it, "a legal fiction at best"—than a way of fulfilling the patient's wishes.[98]

Fourth, the best-interests criterion holds that the surrogate should evaluate treatments by balancing their benefits and risks and select those treatments in which the benefits maximally outweigh the burdens of treatment.[97,98] This criterion has been criticized because there is no objective way of determining the balance between benefits and burdens; it depends on a patient's personal values. In *Cruzan*, the US Supreme Court avoided discussing what criteria should help guide surrogate decision makers.[95] As a matter of practice, physicians rely on family members to make decisions that they feel is best and only object if these decisions seem to demand treatments that the physicians consider non-beneficial. Without a perfect solution to the problems raised by proxy decision making, this approach may be the most reasonable one in difficult circumstances.

Advance Care Documents and Durable Powers of Attorney The living will was first proposed in 1967. In 1976, after the *Quinlan* decision, California enacted the first living will law. By 2005, all states but Massachusetts, Michigan, and New York had enacted laws authorizing the use of living wills.[111] However, in these other states, the courts have recognized living will documents as legally enforceable expressions of patient's wishes.

In the *Brother Fox* case, an 83-year-old priest suffered a cardiac arrest during a herniorrhaphy and remained in a persistent vegetative state.[112] Prior to the operation, he had participated in a teaching session on the *Quinlan* case and had clearly stated that he would never want to be maintained by mechanical respirator if he became vegetative. A New York court permitted the withdrawal of the respirator because Brother Fox had clearly expressed his considered opinion, even if

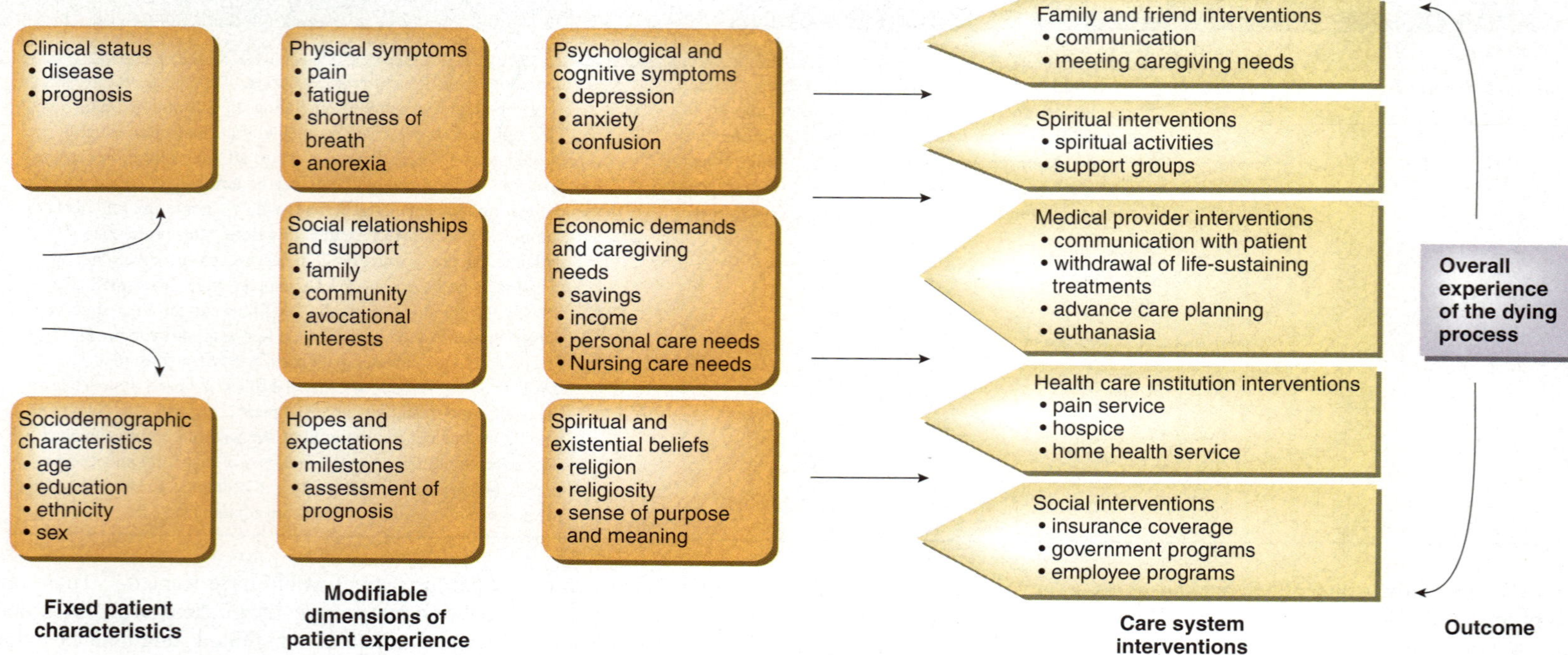

Figure 68-1 Framework for a good death.

only verbally.[112] A similar decision was rendered in Massachusetts in the *Brophy* case.[113] Many states permit clear and explicit verbal statements to be legally binding directives even if not written down (see Table 68-3). But, as noted, many state courts have refused to extend the logic of the *Brother Fox* case to patients who are mentally incompetent but still conscious.[100–102] In the *Wendland,* case a 42-year-old man suffered permanent brain damage and hemiparesis in a car accident.[100] His family wanted his tube feedings discontinued. Wendland was not in a persistent vegetative state; he was conscious, able to draw shapes, and follow very simple commands such as choosing a color block. A few months prior to his accident, he had explicitly stated that he would not want to live like his father-in-law who was dying of gangrene and had his ventilator withdrawn at the family's request. Similarly, he explicitly stated to his brother just days before his accident that his brother should not let him be kept alive in a vegetative state. The California Supreme Court ruled that when the patient is conscious and there is no advance care directive there must be "clear and convincing" evidence of the patient's view. "Clear and convincing" evidence requires prior comments to refer to the specific intervention in the specific circumstances of the patient, not a similar health state.

In 1984, California passed the first law recognizing the appointment of a designated proxy for health care decisions with the power to terminate life-sustaining medical treatment. By 2005, all 50 states and the District of Columbia had enacted statutes recognizing the durable power of attorney for health care decisions.[111] In some cases, the durable power of attorney is limited. For instance, whereas most states permit proxies to terminate life-sustaining treatments, Alaska precludes such decisions by proxies. In other states, orally appointed proxies are limited to a particular hospitalization or episode of illness. Nevertheless, it appears that any properly filled out formal advance care document or durable power of attorney designation, whether it conforms to a state's specific document or not, is protected by the United States Constitution and must be honored.[95]

End-of-Life Care Practices Data on end-of-life care practices indicate that withholding or withdrawing life-sustaining treatment is routine and occurs in over 90% of all deaths. In addition, most physicians, and especially oncologists, have become significantly more comfortable in stopping medical treatments. For instance, approximately a third of patients with cancer in the United States, and more than 50% in some areas, die receiving hospice care—a form of withholding life-sustaining medical interventions.[114] Furthermore, more than 85% of Americans die without cardiopulmonary resuscitation, and the proportion of oncology patients who die without resuscitation may be even higher.[115] Similarly, data from studies of intensive care units indicate that 90% of patients who die in intensive care units (ICUs) do not receive resuscitation efforts, and 90% die after medical interventions are withheld or withdrawn.[116]

Despite widespread legal recognition, passage of the federal Patient Self-Determination Act (PSDA), which requires hospitals and other health care facilities to inform patients about their right to complete an advance care directive, and polling data showing that more than 70% of Americans endorse the use of advance directives, the proportion of Americans who have completed such documents remains at 20%—the same level for the last 15 years. Some data do suggest that oncology patients may complete advance directives at significantly higher rates. Preliminary data suggest more Americans have completed advance directives since the *Schiavo* case. More importantly, even when there are advance care directives, they are frequently not in the patient's medical record, and the patient's physician may not be aware of their existence or content.[117,118] In addition, recent studies suggest that most advance directives are either proxy forms or standard living wills, and that few have any specific directions from the patient.[119] Finally, all studies confirm that proxies and family members do not know patients' wishes regarding end-of-life care and therefore cannot actually makes decisions as the patient would.[99] Thus, despite decades of publicity, and legal support, few patients use advance directives.

The low use of advance care directives and problems with implementing those that exist have made it clear that emphasizing patient's rights and patient control over decision making are ineffective ways to improve care for dying patients. Consequently, people have adopted an entirely different conception about end-of-life care. First, there has been an effort to emphasize integrating symptom management and palliative care with active anticancer treatment prior to the terminal phase of illness. This makes end-of-life care less of a dramatic change and a more routine part of oncology practice. There is evidence that this is already the norm since receiving chemotherapy near the end of life is positively associated with receiving hospice care.[120]

Similarly, efforts have been made to clarify the process of a "good death" and to define the various domains that are necessary for optimal end-of-life care (Figure 68-1).[121,122] These domains—physical symptoms, psychological symptoms, spiritual and existential fulfillment, social supports and care needs—can serve several critical functions. They provide the outcomes for evaluating the care of dying patients. Third, there has been attention to improving physicians' training in end-of-life care. Comprehensive curricula, such as the Educating Physicians in End-of-Life Care (EPEC),[123] have been developed as have curricula devoted to communication and breaking bad news to cancer patients.[124] Such training is essential because oncologists need to have skills to assess symptoms in each domain and to orchestrate the various interventions available—including terminating care—to enhance care in each of these domains.

Table 68-4 Definitions of Assisted Suicide and Euthanasia

Term	Definition
Voluntary active euthanasia	Intentionally administering medications or other interventions to cause the patient's death with the patient's informed consent.
Involuntary active euthanasia	Intentionally administering medications or other interventions to cause the patient's death when the patient was competent to consent but did not—eg, the patient may not have been asked.
Nonvoluntary active euthanasia	Intentionally administering medications or other interventions to cause the patient's death when the patient was incompetent and was mentally incapable of consenting—eg, the patient might have been in a coma.
Passive euthanasia	Withholding or withdrawing life-sustaining medical treatments from a patient to let the patient die (terminating life-sustaining treatments).
Indirect euthanasia	Administering narcotics or other medications to relieve pain with the incidental consequence of causing sufficient respiratory depression to result in the patient's death.
Physician-assisted suicide	A physician provides medications or other interventions to a patient with the understanding that the patient can use them to commit suicide.

ASSISTED SUICIDE AND EUTHANASIA

Historical Perspective The ethics of euthanasia have been a contentious issue since the beginning of medicine.[125] The Hippocratic Oath takes a strong stand against euthanasia, requiring doctors to pledge never to "give a deadly drug to anybody if asked for it, nor…make a suggestion to this effect."[6] In ancient Greece and Rome, this position was the minority view as it was common for physicians to participate in euthanasia and physician-assisted suicide (PAS). The modern debate about euthanasia can be dated from 1870, when a nonphysician, Samuel Williams, argued for euthanasia in front of the Birmingham Speculative Club.[125] The growing acceptance of terminating life-sustaining care, the legalization of euthanasia in the Netherlands and Belgium, the Kevorkian suicide machine, and the publication in 1988 of the article "It's over, Debbie"[126] have all stimulated the contemporary debate about the value of euthanasia and physician-assisted suicide.

Definitions Table 68-4 summarizes the essential definitions. Importantly, so-called passive euthanasia is actually the withdrawal or withholding of life-sustaining medical interventions and is widely accepted as both ethical and legal. So-called indirect euthanasia, increasing narcotics to ease a patient's pain even if this has the consequence of hastening the patient's death, is also a misnomer since it has generally been deemed both ethical and legal for over 100 years.[125] Almost all commentators agree that involuntary, and non-voluntary active euthanasia are unethical because they end the life of a patient without consent. Consequently, the focus of debate is on PAS and voluntary, active euthanasia. To avoid confusion, use of the term euthanasia should be restricted to voluntary, active euthanasia.

Ethical Standards Regarding Euthanasia and Assissted Suicide Proponents typically cite four reasons to justify PAS or euthanasia.[127–129] First, they claim that euthanasia ensures patients' autonomy. Individuals have different values and goals in life; we protect patient autonomy by permitting patients to pursue their goals. A proper death is as essential to a person's goals and values as any other choice. Hence, to respect patients' autonomy, we must respect patients' wishes regarding the manner and timing of their death through euthanasia and PAS. Second, for some patients the dying process inflicts significant pain and suffering; euthanasia or PAS may relieve them of these burdens. Hence, euthanasia or PAS furthers beneficence or the well being of sick patients. Indeed, for some people just knowing there is the possibility of having euthanasia or PAS is reassuring. Third, proponents argue that euthanasia is morally indistinguishable from the accepted practices of withholding and withdrawing life-sustaining care. Ultimately, the peaceful death of a patient is the same in either scenario and because there is no moral difference between acts of omission and acts of commission, euthanasia and terminating life-sustaining treatments are morally equivalent. Finally, potential adverse consequences of legalization are too speculative and hypothetical to determine whether to prohibit euthanasia or PAS.

Opponents of euthanasia and PAS offer four parallel arguments.[127,130–132] First, opponents claim that autonomy does not justify euthanasia or PAS. Autonomy does not mean a person should be permitted to do anything he or she wishes, especially those actions that end the ability to act autonomously. On this basis, we do not permit voluntary dueling or voluntary enslavement. In addition, even if a person wants to commit suicide, it is another issue entirely to permit others to help. Second, beneficence may argue against euthanasia or PAS. Many terminally ill patients experience inadequately treated pain, fatigue, and depression. Treating these symptoms would mean few people would have the pain and suffering to justify euthanasia or PAS. Third, it is argued that there is an ethical distinction between acts of omission and acts of commission. Evaluating the ethics of an act does not only depend on its final result, but we also must evaluate how that result was produced and the intention of the actors. There are ethical and legal differences between cases in which a person was killed by mistake and cases in which the killing was premeditated. Similarly, there is a difference between stopping a medical treatment and letting a patient die and intentionally and actively injecting the patient with a medication to cause his or her death. Finally, opponents note a variety of adverse consequences that might result from legalizing euthanasia or PAS, including disruption of the physician–patient relationship, intrusion of the courts into terminating care decisions, coercion of terminally ill patients to commit euthanasia or PAS, and extension of euthanasia to children, mentally incapacitated patients, and others.

US Supreme Court Ruling on Euthanasia and PAS In June 1997, the US Supreme Court ruled unanimously that there is no constitutional right to euthanasia or PAS.[96] Many of the justices wrote separate opinions and many seemed sympathetic to the notion of PAS and euthanasia, even if they did not deem it a constitutional right. The majority view—written by Chief Justice Rehnquist—drew a distinction between the right to withdraw or withhold life-sustaining treatments as a liberty interest in being free of unwanted bodily invasion versus the right to PAS, which does not contain a liberty interest.[96] The unanimity of the ruling suggests that it is unlikely to be overturned in the future. Importantly, the Supreme Court did not view PAS or euthanasia as inherently unconstitutional, and thus permitted individual states, such as Oregon, to legalize these interventions.

Within weeks of the Supreme Court ruling, Florida's state supreme court ruled also that there is no state constitutional right to PAS.[133] Similarly, other state supreme courts have ruled that PAS is not a fundamental right.[134] Many states have rejected referenda to legalize PAS. Oregon has enacted its Death with Dignity Act and has had 208 cases of PAS since 1998.[135]

Euthanasia and PAS in the Netherlands The Netherlands and Belgium legalized euthanasia and PAS. Several safeguards must be adhered to, including that (1) the patient has unbearable pain and suffering that cannot be medically relieved, (2) the patient is competent and repeatedly makes a request to have his or her life ended, and (3) the physician consults a second physician.[135]

The Dutch government commissioned detailed studies of the practices of euthanasia and PAS in 1990, 1995, and 2001, and individual researchers have conducted many other studies.[136] These studies show that just over 50% of Dutch physicians have participated in euthanasia or PAS at some point in their careers.[136] The proportion of Dutch physicians who would never perform euthanasia has consistently declined since 1990. Indeed, only 1% of Dutch physicians indicated that they would never perform euthanasia or PAS and not refer patients for these interventions.[136]

According to the latest data, approximately 9,700 patients explicitly request euthanasia or PAS each year. Overall, in the Netherlands 2.6% of all deaths are by euthanasia, 0.2% are by PAS, and 0.7% are deaths in which active measures are taken to end the patient's life without the patient's explicit request.[136] Thus, approximately 3.4% of all deaths in the Netherlands, or 4,600 deaths annually, are by euthanasia or PAS. This is higher than in any other European country suggesting that legalization may increase use of these interventions.[137] Importantly, over 80% of the Dutch cases involve patients with cancer. Indeed, 7.4% of cancer patients in the Netherlands died by euthanasia or PAS.[136]). Between 1990 and 2001, the frequency of euthanasia and PAS cases increased from 1.9% to 2.8% of all deaths, although the frequency of intentional deaths without the patient's explicit request remained constant at 0.7 to 0.8% of all deaths.[136]

Empirical Data Regarding Euthanasia and PAS Although the Dutch studies of euthanasia and PAS are the most valid and reliable, data are accumulating on the attitudes and practices of euthanasia and PAS in many countries.[138] Surveys indicate that a majority of the American public is willing to support euthanasia and PAS in hypothetical cases and for terminally ill patients with extreme pain.[139] Support is lower when the question involves euthanasia or PAS for reasons other than pain.[139] Interestingly, this high level of support for euthanasia and PAS has been constant since the mid-1970s and has not increased with the debates over the last 15 years.[138] The American public makes no distinction between euthanasia and PAS; the same proportion support both interventions for the same situation.[138] People who are religious, Catholics, those older than 65 years of age, and African Americans are much less likely to support euthanasia or PAS. Support among American physicians is significantly less than among the public.[138,139] In almost all surveys, less than half of American physicians support euthanasia or PAS; and significantly fewer support euthanasia than support PAS. Furthermore, there is evidence that at least among American oncologists support for both euthanasia and PAS has declined significantly, by as much as 75%.

Surveys in a number of countries in which euthanasia and PAS are illegal indicate that physicians receive requests for these interventions and do perform them. In Britain, it has been reported that 45% of physicians have been asked to hasten death.[140] In Alberta, Canada, 20% of physicians reported receiving requests for active euthanasia. In the United States, many physicians have received requests for euthanasia and PAS, but different studies provide vastly different estimates of the frequency.[138] Among non-oncologists in the United States, it is reported that between 18.3% and 26% have received requests for euthanasia or PAS. Reports among oncologists indicate that between 43% and 62.9% of oncologists have received requests for euthanasia or PAS.

In Britain, 32% of physicians indicated that they have "taken active steps to bring about the death of a patient," although this may include terminating life-sustaining interventions.[140] Again, in the United States, there is a large difference between oncologists and other physicians. Among non-oncologists, it is reported that approximately 1.7 to 4.7% had performed euthanasia and 3.3 to 4.6% had performed PAS in their career.[138] Among oncologists, it is reported that 3.7 to 4% had performed euthanasia, whereas 10.8 to 18% had performed PAS in their career.[138] These data suggest a very low number of cases of euthanasia and PAS in the United States, fewer than 1,000 cases per year, a tiny fraction of the 2.4 million Americans who die annually.

All available data indicate that the vast majority of cases of PAS and euthanasia involve oncology patients. For instance, in Oregon, 79% of all patients who used PAS suffered from cancer.[135] Contrary to expectations, pain is not the main motivating factor behind the desire for euthanasia or PAS. For instance, among the Oregon patients only 22% have pain.[135] Data suggest that shortness of breath or fatigue are the physical symptoms most consistently associated with requests for euthanasia or PAS. More important, depression, psychological distress, and hopelessness appear to be the main symptoms motivating patients' desires for euthanasia or PAS.[135,138,139,141–143]

Finally, the existing data suggest certain problems. One is the failure of cases of PAS. In the Netherlands, approximately 20% of PAS cases do not result in the patient's death.[144] And in the United States, one report indicates that 15% of PAS cases result in failure.[138,145] How these cases are handled is unknown. In 2004, Oregon reported just a 5% complication rate although in a recent case a patient was comatose for 3 days and then woke up.[135] In addition, although the majority of physicians who participate in euthanasia and PAS report satisfaction with their action, between 10% and 20% of physicians report regret at having participated in these interventions.[138] The long-term sequelae for these physicians and the consequences for the families of patients who die by euthanasia or PAS are not known.

Responding to Patient's Request for Euthanasia or Physician-Assisted Suicide When a physician receives a request for euthanasia or PAS, the initial response should be to reassess the patient's circumstances, including physical symptoms, psychological symptoms, social supports, spiritual fulfillment, and caregiving needs (see Figure 68-1). Special attention should be devoted to assessing depression and the extent of caregiving needs, as data suggest that these are strongly associated with patients' interest in euthanasia and PAS. The physician should also reassess whether additional interventions, including palliative care consultations, psychiatric evaluations, skilled or unskilled home health care services, and pastoral services, are required. A psychiatric evaluation can be obtained without necessarily revealing that a request for euthanasia or PAS prompted concern. Obviously, the patient and family should also be reassured that the physician will not abandon the patient and will provide care and attend to the patient's symptoms and needs.

FINANCIAL INCENTIVES

Historical Perspective Financial incentives to physicians are a specific instance of the more general ethical issue of conflict of interest. Debates about physicians' conflicts of interest have not arisen with the rise of stock options from biotechnology companies. In 1899, Lydston studied the issue of fee splitting—the practice in which the physician who referred a patient to a specialist or surgeon would expect a payment.[146] He found that 60% of surgeons would provide a physician with a 50% commission for patient referrals. Other financial incentives, such as physicians receiving payments from diagnostic laboratories based on the number of patients they referred, ophthalmologists selling glasses, or physicians dispensing pharmaceuticals, were recognized and debated for many decades. However, the response of physicians and organized medicine to such financial incentives has been inconsistent, and enforcement of prohibitions on such conflicts has been lax under most circumstances.[147] Given the tremendous increase in money flowing through health care, the financial implications of research results, and the rise of managed care and capitated payments, there has been more attention paid to physician financial incentives.

Ethical Standards for Financial Incentives Financial incentives are inherent in medicine as in any profession. A professional renders a service and must earn an income for rendering the service. In some cases, financial incentives can become conflicts of interest.

What is a conflict of interest? In the context of medicine, it is commonly argued that physicians have three primary interests (1) promoting their patients' well-being and health, (2) advancing biomedical knowledge through research, and (3) training future physicians and other health professionals. There is a hierarchy of these primary interests—promoting patients' health is most important. In addition to these primary medical interests, physicians have other legitimate interests, such as earning a living, raising a family, and pursuing avocational interests. The other interests are not nefarious or wrong. Indeed, they are usually laudable. A conflict of interest occurs when one of these other interests undermines—or appears to undermine—the integrity of a physician's judgment related to a primary interest.[146] Thus, a conflict of interest exists when a financial interest might compromise patient welfare by inclining a physician to provide unnecessary medical services, withhold needed services, or engage in fraud in clinical research.[146]

Broadly speaking, it is possible to distinguish two different types of conflicts of interest. There are conflicts of interest by commission, in which physicians have a financial or other incentive to provide more care than is deemed appropriate or to pursue a certain research project. Conflicts of interest by commission occur when physicians have an investment in medical facilities, refer their patients to those facilities and, thereby, realize a profit when the patients receive medical services from the facilities. Conflicts of interest by omission occur when physicians have financial incentives to withhold tests, consultations, hospitalizations, or otherwise provide less care than is appropriate.

Empirical Data Regarding Financial Conflicts of Interest There are three types of data on financial conflicts of interest. Studies in the late 1980s and early 1990s demonstrated that physician investments or ownership interests in medical facilities affected use, charges, and in some cases, the quality of care delivered. The most extensive studies conducted in Florida revealed that 76% of ambulatory surgical facilities, 78% of radiation therapy centers, and 93% of diagnostic imaging facilities were owned wholly or in part by physicians.[147–149] Physical therapy facilities in which physicians had ownership interests had more visits and higher revenues per patient, but therapists spent about half the time with patients as compared to facilities in which physicians did not have an ownership interest.[147] A national study of diagnostic imaging in physician offices found similar results.[148] When physicians performed the radiologic and other diagnostic imaging examinations in their own offices, studies were performed more frequently and at higher cost. More relevant to clinical oncologists are the results of a study in Florida indicating that when physicians were whole or part owners of radiation-therapy facilities, costs were 40 to 60% higher than other radiation facilities in the United States.[153] More important, radiation physicists at physician-owned radiation-therapy facilities spent on average 18% less time with patients. There were no differences in the cases of cancer or the morality rates that explained these differences.[149]

Studies also show that interaction with pharmaceutical company representatives can significantly influence physicians' attitudes and even prescribing patterns.[150] One study found that after physicians attended an all-expense paid trip to a vacation resort to attend pharmaceutical company-sponsored symposia, there was a significant increase in their prescribing of drugs highlighted at the symposia. Another study showed that physicians were significantly more likely to request specific drugs to be added to a hospital formulary if they had accepted money from the pharmaceutical company to attend or speak at an educational symposium or for research.[151] A meta-analysis of all studies related to physician interactions with pharmaceutical company representatives concluded that these meetings "were associated with requests by physicians for adding the drugs to the hospital formulary and changes in prescribing practices."[150] In addition, attending presentations given by pharmaceutical representatives was associated with "nonrational prescribing behavior" by physicians. Although these data may be less than conclusive for a causal correlation, presumably executives at pharmaceutical companies focused on the "bottom line" would not spend such substantial sums of money on marketing to physicians unless they produced positive attitudes and increased the prescribing of drugs.[150]

Finally, although there are great concerns about the influence of investments and other financial conflicts of interest on clinical research and although it appears that it is fairly common for researchers to have financial interest in their research, there are limited empirical data on this topic. Financial interests have a varied effect on different aspects of the research process. In terms of study design, the data show that industry-sponsored research is no worse and may actually be more methodologically rigorous than research sponsored by non-profit entities.[152,153] However, industry funded clinical research leads to positive results—or results favorable to industry—more frequently than non-industry funded studies. In one study that looked at 136 randomized controlled trials focused on treating multiple myeloma, the studies sponsored by drug companies (74% new treatment vs 26% standard treatment) were more likely than those sponsored by non-profit organizations (47% vs 53%) to favor the new treatment over the standard therapy.[154] These data do not necessarily demonstrate bias or compromised studies—there may be many explanations for this finding—but non-dissemination of negative studies by pharmaceutical companies is a reasonable possibility.

More important are the effects financial ties have on researcher judgment. One study found that 96% of researchers and authors who supported the use of calcium-channel antagonists in the treatment of cardiovascular disease were significantly more likely to have financial relationships—that is, funding to attend a symposium, honorarium, funding for an educational symposium, research support, or consultation—with manufacturers of calcium-channel antagonists than the 37% of researchers and authors who were critical of the use of this class of drugs.[155] Another study examined oncology studies sponsored by drug companies versus those sponsored by non-profit sources, finding that industry-sponsored studies were less likely than non-industry funded studies to report unfavorable outcomes (5% vs 38% of the time), and that overstatements of quantitative results occurred in 30% of industry sponsored studies but in only 13% of non-industry sponsored studies.[156]

Financial interests are most likely to adversely affect dissemination of research findings. Industry-funded clinical research that produces positive results are more likely to be published than government-funded clinical research and financial ties are associated with publication delays and data withholding. The data have been especially apparent in the case of selective serotonin reuptake inhibitors (SSRIs) to treat depression.[157,158] One study examined 42 placebo-controlled trials submitted to Swedish drug regulators. When the experimental drug was found to be more effective than placebo, 19 out of 21 (90.5%) of those studies results were published, whereas when the experimental drug was not more effective than placebo, only 6 out of 21 (28.6%) of those studies were published.[157] In another British study that examined placebo-controlled studies of five SSRIs that were either published in a peer-reviewed journal or unpublished and reviewed by the Committee on the Safety of Medicines, the authors found that when published data alone were considered, it appeared that there was a favorable risk-benefit ratio for all five of the drugs studied. When unpublished data were taken into account, however, the risks outweighed the benefits for four of those drugs.[158] It is unknown whether the results of both of these studies are due to negative publication bias at journals, author delays, or industry withholding of negative data. However, there have been multiple high profile attempts by industry—including the Betty Dong/Boots Pharmaceuticals case and the Nancy Olivieri/Apotex case—to prevent publication of negative data.[159] No systematic data exist that link financial conflicts of interest among clinical researchers to research misconduct or harm to subjects. Nevertheless, there are recent controversies involving claims that research subjects have been adversely impacted by conflicts of interest, and these have prompted changes in institutional conflict-of-interest policies.

Policies Regarding Conflicts of Interest There are three general approaches to regulating conflicts of interest: disclosure, management, and prohibitions.[146] Disclosure may be an effective policy because it gives those affected by the conflict the information that they need to assess its impact. However, disclosure may have limited effectiveness because in many cases those who receive the information may not know how to interpret it and may not be in a position to act on the information.[146] Are patients or research subjects able to understand and respond to revelations that their physician owns stock in the company sponsoring the research trial they are about to enroll in? Furthermore, disclosure can actually undermine trust in physicians, researchers, and the entire medical system. In general, "disclosing a conflict only reveals a problem, without providing any guidance for resolving it."[146] Some conflicts can be managed by having oversight or other methods of mediating the conflict, including data safety and monitoring boards or independent consent monitors in the case of research. Finally, in many cases risks of compromising the integrity of clinical or research judgments and the potential harm that could result may be too great. In such cases, the conflicts have to be prohibited.

Regarding conflicts that arise in clinical care, the American Medical Association and the Pharmaceutical Research and Manufacturers of America have made recommendations regarding gifts from pharmaceutical manufacturers to physicians. The recommendation states that physicians may accept gifts of minimal value but should "refuse substantial gifts from drug companies, such as the costs of travel, lodging, or other personal expenses… for attending conferences or meetings."[160] In addition, under the so-called Stark rules, physicians are prohibited from profiting by sending Medicare patients to facilities in which they have an ownership stake.

There has been much controversy over the regulation of capitation payments for clinical care. Capitation is not inherently unethical, but its ethics depend on how it is designed.[161] Some have argued that to be ethical, capitation arrangements must (1) limit the intensity of the incentives, that is, what range of services are covered, the amount of money involved, and whether there are any "stop-loss" provisions to minimize huge losses, (2) limit the immediacy of the incentives, that is, the number of physicians and patients in the risk pool, (3) target the incentives toward services that are known to be overused, combined with monitoring for overuse, (4) balance the financial stick with carrots for good performance, and (5) risk adjust.[161]

Over the last few years there has been much concern regarding conflicts of interest that arise in clinical research. Medical journals require authors to disclose any financial interests that might affect their research results. In addition, some courts, research centers, and ethical bodies have ruled that researchers need to disclose financial interests when obtaining informed consent.[38,162] The US National Institutes of Health (NIH) and Food and Drug Administration (FDA) have issued temporary guidelines regarding conflicts of interest for NIH-sponsored research and for research seeking regulatory approval. Unfortunately, these rules differ regarding the amounts to be disclosed, to whom disclosure is to be made, and in other aspects.[163]

Many other organizations, such as the American Association of Medical Colleges and the American Society for Clinical Oncology, have proposed stricter rules regarding conflicts of interest for research. In general, these rules require disclosure by researchers and others who have responsibility for the development, conduct, analysis, and dissemination of clinical research and their financially dependent relatives.[164,165] They require disclosure of all equity, stocks, and stock options, as well as leadership positions, such as membership on a board of directors or executive position or scientific advisory board, in sponsors of research, honoraria, gifts, and travel. They propose that institutions establish conflicts of interest committees to collect and review these disclosures and communicate potential conflicts to IRBs. Finally, certain conflicts of interest are prohibited. In general, it is argued that principal investigators are absolutely prohibited from having financial ties to sponsors of research unless there is a compelling countervailing reason.

Others have also adopted certain prohibitions for research. For instance, the Howard Hughes Medical Institute's policy prohibits scientists it funds from both consulting for and collaborating in research with the same company. An even more important type of prohibition occurred in the GUSTO trial, a cardiovascular study comparing tissue plasminogen activator and streptokinase that involved 41,600 patients at 1,500 sites worldwide. "The Steering Committee unanimously voted to prohibit any honoraria for speaking engagements, payment for consultancy or travel or reimbursement of any kind from any of the five corporate sponsors until 1 year after publication of the results" of the trial.[166] These prohibitions applied not just to Steering Committee members, but principal investigators at participating sites were required to provide written documentation "that acknowledges the lack of any equity interest in the sponsors."

PRIVACY AND CONFIDENTIALITY

Historical Perspective Concern about the confidentiality of patient information is as old as medicine.[5,6] The Hippocratic Oath requires physicians to pledge that "things I may see or hear in the course of the treatment… I will keep to myself holding such things shameful to be spoken."[6] More recently, however, the ascent of managed care, the increasing prevalence of electronic health information, and heightened distrust and consumerism among patients have increased attention to privacy and confidentiality in health care.[167,168]

Ethical Standards Regarding Confidentiality Privacy and confidentiality are distinct, if related, concepts. Privacy is the expectation that our personal information (relationships, decisions, etc) will be free from observation and interference by others. Confidentiality is the expectation that, once we have let another into our zone of privacy, he will treat that which we have entrusted to him appropriately. Privacy involves obligations not to intrude, whereas confidentiality involves obligations not to divulge.

There are many reasons why physicians need to protect patient information. First, without assurances of confidentiality, patients are unlikely to share necessary information.[6] Second, breaches of confidentiality can cause harm, subjecting patients to stigmatization, discrimination, and possibly loss of employment or insurance. Third, privacy allows people to develop their own ideas and pursue their own plans. The promise of confidentiality protects this "personal space" and is therefore essential for the exercise of autonomy.[6,167] Finally, confidentiality involves elements of promise-keeping. Patients reveal private information expecting that it will only be used and disclosed appropriately. When we fail to respect these expectations, we violate our patients' trust.

Confidentiality raises difficult ethical issues because it rubs up against other activities and values. Some, such as prescription drug marketing,[169] will rarely justify limitations on confidentiality. However, others constitute important public goods, and then confidentiality must sometimes yield.[170] When it comes to communicable diseases, public safety hazards, violent threats, or knowledge of child abuse, it is often appropriate for physicians to place the interests of third parties over those of their patients. These situations may generate an ethical "duty to warn," and often involve a legal obligation to inform appropriate civil authorities.[171,172] For example, the neuro-oncologist whose patient has cognitive and coordination difficulties might need to notify the Department of Motor Vehicles that he may be an unsafe driver. Public health surveillance, including the submission of data to tumor registries, is usually undertaken without consent.[173,174] The provision of optimum health care requires reasonable sharing of information among health professionals, and third-party payers may require certain information prior to reimbursing for services. Medical education can compromise confidentiality, as when a case is presented at Grand Rounds in a way that permits identification of the individual. Finally, much observational and retrospective health research, as well as most quality improvement activities, have traditionally taken place without explicit patient authorization.[175] Restricting some of these activities in the name of confidentiality might be justified ethically, but it is important to recognize that such restrictions have real costs.

The Privacy Rule, part of HIPAA, took effect in the United States in April 2003.[89] This Rule is the first comprehensive set of regulations in the United States governing the privacy and confidentiality of health information. It permits use and disclosure of "protected health information" (PHI) by "covered entities" (including any health care providers who transmit information in electronic form) for treatment, payment and health care operations, without explicit patient authorization. Use or disclosure of PHI for other purposes requires either patient authorization or a waiver of this requirement by a privacy board or, in the case of research, by an IRB. A complete discussion of HIPAA is beyond the scope of this chapter; reviews of HIPAA overall and as it pertains to research are available.[176]

Just as the events of 2001 remind us that balancing security with civil liberties requires public debate, determining the appropriate equilibrium between medical confidentiality and other important goods demands public deliberation. Given the need for patients' voices to influence policy, the paucity of empirical data on how patients view confidentiality and weigh it against other priorities is remarkable.[177] Without such data, it is difficult to know whether increasing demands for health information privacy reflect the values of a majority of patients, or whether a vocal but effective minority is driving policy. Wherever the pendulum ultimately rests, it seems evident that providers and health care systems should pay greater attention to issues of confidentiality than has traditionally been the case. At a minimum, we need to (1) be transparent about the ways in which patient information will be used, (2) be able to justify those uses of information, and (3) restrict disclosures to the minimum necessary to accomplish legitimate objectives.

ETHICAL ISSUES IN CANCER GENETICS

The heritable cancer predispositions require that oncologists consider ethical issues regarding genetic information.[178] These issues include: (1) appropriate use of genetic tests in high- and average-risk persons, (2) genetic testing of children, (3) familial implications of genetics, (4) protection of genetic privacy, and (5) the problems raised by genetic research.

Genetic Exceptionalism Before addressing specific ethical issues in cancer genetics, we must consider whether genetics raises qualitatively different ethical concerns than other areas of medical and scientific practice. The claim that genetics is unique and requires special handling, such as anti-discrimination or genetic privacy laws, is called *genetic exceptionalism*. This view has been advocated on several grounds, including: (1) our genes constitute a "future diary,"[179,180] (2) genetic information has implications for family members and communities, (3) the risks of genetic information are primarily social and psychological, (4) genetic information is probabilistic and difficult for professionals and laypersons to interpret, (5) few established interventions are available to decrease genetic risk, and (6) genetics carries particular symbolic weight in the public consciousness. Others, however, argue that genetic exceptionalism is mistaken as a guide to policy. These commentators claim that genetic information is similar to other types of health information, and that promulgating special rules for genetic information paradoxically reinforces the stigma and deterministic thinking that proponents of exceptionalism wish to counteract.[181] As genetics becomes more integrated into the routine practice of medicine, the arguments for exceptionalism will lose some force. Nevertheless, the ethical collection and use of genetic information will continue to require attention.

Genetic Tests in High- and Average-Risk Individuals A genetic test may be performed for confirmatory purposes in an individual perceived to be at increased risk, or for screening purposes in a population of average-risk individuals. In the former situation, the purpose of the test is to confirm or refute the diagnosis. Detection of a relevant mutation will presumably lead to consideration of therapeutic or prophylactic intervention, if available. For example, identification of the typical RET mutation in a child with phenotypic features of MEN IIb should lead to early discussion of prophylactic thyroidectomy.[182] More difficult considerations arise when diagnostic tests are available but subsequent interventions are not well established or entail complex tradeoffs. For example, detection of a *BRCA1* mutation in a woman with a family history of early breast cancer may lead to difficult decisions with regard to prophylactic surgery, intensified screening, or chemoprophylaxis.[183–185] Management of the patient with a mutation in the *TP53* gene and a family history consistent with the Li-Fraumeni syndrome is even less clear.[178]

The complex and value-laden judgments implicit in genetic testing require utmost attention to informed consent. The decision to test is rarely urgent. Informed consent should therefore extend over time. Discussions should address the purpose of the test, practical details of its administration, confidentiality issues, and the significance of positive, negative, and indeterminate tests.[186] The availability or lack of therapeutic options for those who test positive should be discussed in advance. Reproductive, family, psychological, and social implications should be considered. Referral to a cancer geneticist or genetic counselor may be appropriate when either the clinician or patient feels the need for additional scientific or counseling expertise. Some groups have urged that testing in the absence of established medical interventions only be conducted as part of a research protocol.[178]

Genetic screening is performed in an average-risk population. Individuals with positive screening tests are considered to be at increased risk and require confirmatory testing.[187] There are no current examples where screening of average-risk individuals for cancer susceptibility mutations has been validated.[188] Such screening should be performed only in the context of IRB-approved research protocols.[187] Like non-genetic screening tests, the use of genetic testing in average-risk individuals may be harmful and should not be adopted before evidence of its effectiveness is available.[189,190]

Genetic Testing for Cancer Predisposition in Children The question of whether or not to test a minor for a genetic predisposition may arise in various situations. Establishing a genetic diagnosis may have direct medical benefits for the child; knowledge of mutation status may occasionally be helpful to the minor with respect to reproductive decisions; testing may be requested by the child or parents in the absence of obvious medical benefit; or testing may be desired by another family member in order to permit linkage analysis.[191] As with adults considering testing, results may carry the potential for social harms to the child. In addition, testing may carry intrafamilial risks, such as limitation of expectations and opportunities for children who test positive for cancer-risk mutations, as well as "survivor guilt" in those who test negative.[191] Finally, testing a child precludes him or her from making an autonomous choice upon reaching adulthood.[192]

There is a broad consensus that genetic testing of minors should be encouraged when positive results would lead to therapeutic or prophylactic interventions of established efficacy.[191–195] Conversely, testing should be discouraged when cancer only arises in adulthood and no interventions are available in childhood to decrease risk. Where the onset of cancer begins in childhood but risk-reducing interventions have not been established, as in Li-Fraumeni syndrome, various guidelines offer conflicting advice, with some permitting and others discouraging testing.[191–195]

Genetic Information and the Family Identification of a cancer risk mutation in an individual implies that family members may also be affected. Two related considerations flow from the familial nature of genetic risk information. First, individuals contemplating a genetic test should understand the implications for family members. Second, identification of a genetically susceptible individual may prompt consideration of whether biologic relatives should be notified of their potential risk. Where notification of family members would permit them to take steps to prevent or ameliorate symptomatic disease, the clinician should encourage the affected person to disclose relevant genetic information to family members.[195] If the patient refuses, some commentators raise the possibility of a duty to warn.[195,196] In oncology, limited circumstances may exist where physicians might justifiably inform family members. Such suspension of confidentiality might be reasonable if "...attempts to encourage disclosure on the part of the patient have failed; where the harm is highly likely to occur and is serious and foreseeable; where the at-risk relatives are identifiable; and where either the disease is preventable/treatable or medically accepted standards indicate that early monitoring will reduce the genetic risk...[and] the harm that may result from failure to disclose should outweigh the harm that may result from disclosure."[195] Situations that meet these criteria are currently rare.

Protection of Genetic Privacy Genetic tests may reveal a predisposition to illness that has the potential to compromise individuals' insurability and employability, though no data suggest that this is a prevalent problem. A consensus exists that, with rare exceptions, genetic susceptibility testing should not be used to exclude workers from employment.[197] Nevertheless, individuals have rarely been denied employment, health insurance, and the right to adopt a child on the basis of genetic risk. It is reasonable to assume that genetic information about an identifiable individual has the potential to seriously harm him or her if inappropriately released. Such data should, therefore, be treated with utmost caution, and issues of confidentiality and the potential for discrimination should be discussed during pretest counseling.[194] In the United States, privacy regulations under HIPAA, although not genetic-specific, constitute the first federal standards for protection of genetic and other health-related information.[89]

Research and Genetic Tests In the context of genetic research, additional considerations arise with respect to informed consent, privacy, disclosure of test results, and implications for affected communities. Informed consent for research involving genetic testing may require discussion of issues not often considered in other types of research. In particular, the possibility of informational harm resulting from disclosure of results to subjects themselves, to family members, or to third parties requires explicit consideration.[198]

Protocols involving genetic susceptibility testing require careful attention to subject confidentiality.[199] In studies in the United States, it might be appropriate to obtain a Certificate of Confidentiality that would immunize data from subpoena or other third-party disclosure.[200]

Investigators and IRBs must also decide whether to share results of tests with subjects or their physicians. On the one hand, disclosure to subjects who desire their results is consistent with respect for autonomy. On the other hand, disclosure carries psychological as well as social risks. There is general agreement that findings with clear clinical relevance should be disclosed to subjects, and that findings that are so premature as to have no clinical impact should not be shared. Disagreement arises when individuals' study results are of uncertain significance.[201] Regardless of the standard of clinical relevance used, it is critical that both subjects and physicians know the study's policy on disclosure of test results in advance. When studies disclose results, adequate pre- and post-test counseling must be built into the protocol.

In genetic predisposition studies in which the clinical syndrome is more prevalent in particular ethnic or other groups, research holds the potential for risks, such as stigma, to communities as well as to individuals. It is ethically appropriate for investigators and IRBs to consider these community risks in their deliberations, often with formal involvement of and input from community representatives.[202] Whereas concern for impact on community should not necessarily prohibit valuable research from going forward, it does argue for careful attention to confidentiality as well as for efforts to develop partnerships with affected groups.

REFERENCES

1. *Schloendorff v. Society of New York Hospitals,* 211 N.Y. 125 (1914).
2. *Natanson v. Kline,* 186 Kan. 393, 350 P.2d 1093, *opinion on denial of motion for rehearing,* 187 Kan. 186, 354 P.2d 670 (1960).
3. Oken D. What to tell cancer patients: a study of medical attitudes. JAMA 1961;175:1120–8.
4. Beecher HK. Ethics and clinical research. N Engl J Med 1966;274:1354–60.
5. Beauchamp TL, Childress JF. Principles of biomedical ethics. 4th ed. New York: Oxford University Press; 1994.
6. Kass LR. Toward a more natural science. New York: The Free Press; 1985.
7. Daniels N. Just health care. Cambridge (UK): Cambridge University Press; 1985.
8. Menzel PT. Strong medicine: the ethical rationing of health care. New York: Oxford University Press; 1990.
9. Callahan D. Setting limits. New York: Simon & Schuster; 1987.
10. *Slater v. Baker and Stapelton,* 95 Eng. Rep. 860 (K.B. 1767).
11. Berg JW, Appelbaum PS, Lidz CW, Parker LS. Informed consent: legal theory and clinical practice, 2nd ed. Oxford: Oxford University Press; 2001.
12. Faden RR, Beauchamp TL. A history and theory of informed consent. New York: Oxford University Press; 1986.
13. *Salgo v. Leland Stanford Jr. Board of Trustees,* 317 P.2d 170(Cal. Ct. App. 1957).
14. National Commission for the Protection of Human Subjects of Biomedical and Behavioral Research. The Belmont report: ethical principles and guidelines for the protection of human subjects of biomedical and behavioral research. Washington, DC: US Government Printing Office; 1978.
15. Meisel A, Roth LH, Lidz CW. Toward a model of the legal doctrine of informed consent. Am J Psychiatry 1977; 134:285–9.
16. *Canterbury v. Spence.* 464 F.2d 772 (D.C. Cir. 1972).
17. The Common Rule, Title 45 Code of Federal Regulations Part 46 (Protection of Human Subjects) Subparts A-D. Available at: http://www.hhs.gov/ohrp/humansubjects/guidance/45cfr46.htm. Accessed June 16, 2005.
18. American Psychiatric Association. Guidelines for assessing the decision-making capacities of potential research subjects with cognitive impairment. Am J Psychiatry 1998;155:1649–50.
19. Drane JF. The many faces of competency. Hastings Cent Rep 1985;15:17–21.
20. Emanuel EJ, Emanuel LL. Four models of the physician-patient relationship. JAMA 1992;267:2221–6.
21. Wendler D, Martinez RA, Fairclough D, et al. Views of potential subjects toward proposed regulations for clinical research with adults unable to consent. Am J Psychiatry 2002;159:585–91.
22. Dresser R. Mentally disabled research subjects. The enduring policy issues. JAMA 1996;276:67–72.
23. National Bioethics Advisory Commission. Research involving persons with mental disorders that may affect decisionmaking capacity. Washington, DC: U.S. Government Printing Office; 1998.
24. Michels R. Are research ethics bad for our mental health? N Engl J Med 1999;340:1427–30.
25. Blackhall LJ, Murphy ST, Frank G, et al. Ethnicity and attitudes toward patient autonomy. JAMA 1995;274:820–5.
26. Carrese JA, Rhodes LA. Western bioethics on the Navajo reservation. Benefit or harm? JAMA 1995;274:826–9.
27. Ende J, Kazis L, Ash A, Moskowitz MA. Measuring patients' desire for autonomy: decision making and information-seeking preferences among medical patients. J Gen Intern Med 1989;4:23–30.
28. Degner LF, Kristjanson LJ, Bowman D, et al. Information needs and decisional preferences in women with breast cancer. JAMA 1997;277:1485–92.
29. Strull WM, Lo B, Charles G. Do patients want to participate in medical decision making? JAMA 1984;252:2990–4.
30. Schneider CE. The practice of autonomy. New York: Oxford University Press; 1998.
31. Freedman B. Offering truth. One ethical approach to the uninformed cancer patient. Arch Intern Med 1993;153:572–6.
32. Lederer SE. Subjected to science: human experimentation in America before World War II. Baltimore (MD): Johns Hopkins University Press; 1995.
33. Annas GJ, Grodin MA. The Nazi doctors and the Nuremberg code: human rights in human experimentation. New York: Oxford University Press; 1992.
34. Jones JH. Bad blood: the Tuskegee syphilis experiment. New York: Simon & Schuster; 1992.
35. National Commission for the Protection of Human Subjects of Biomedical and Behavioral Research. The Belmont report: ethical principles and guidelines for the protection of human subjects of research. Washington DC: U.S. Government Printing Office; 1979. Available at: http://www.hhs.gov/ohrp/humansubjects/guidance/belmont.htm. Accessed June 16, 2005.
36. Steinbrook R. Improving protection for research subjects. N Engl J Med 2002;346:1425–30.
37. World Medical Association. Declaration of Helsinki: JAMA 1997;277:905–6.
38. World Medical Association. Declaration of Helsinki, 5th revision, 2000. Available at: http://www.wma.net/e/policy/b3.htm. Accessed June 16, 2005.
39. Levine RJ. Ethics and regulation of clinical research. 2nd ed. Baltimore (MD): Urban & Schwarzenberg; 1986.
40. Freedman B, Fuks A, Weijer C. Demarcating research and treatment: a systematic approach for the analysis of the ethics of clinical research. Clin Res 1992;40:653–60.
41. Emanuel EJ, Wendler D, Grady C. What makes clinical research ethical? JAMA 2000;283:2701–11.
42. Emanuel EJ, Wendler D, Killen J, Grady C. What makes clinical research in developing countries ethical? The benchmarks of ethical research. J Infect Dis 2004;189:930–7.
43. Freedman B. Scientific value and validity as ethical requirements for research: a proposed explication. IRB 1987;9:7–10.
44. National Institutes of Health. Guidelines on the inclusion of women and minorities as subjects in clinical research. Fed Reg 1994;59:14508–13.
45. Tejeda HA, Green SB, Trimble EL, et al. Representation of African Americans, Hispanics, and whites in National Cancer Institute cancer treatment trials. J Natl Cancer Inst 1996;88:812–6.
46. Murthy VH, Krumholz HM, Gross CP. Participation in cancer clinical trials: race-, sex-, and age-based disparities. JAMA 2004;291:2720–6.
47. Hutchins LF, Unger JM, Crowley JJ, et al. Under representation of patients 65 years of age or older in cancer-treatment trials. N Engl J Med 1999;341:2061–7.
48. The Nuremberg code. JAMA 1996;276:1691.
49. Committee on Bioethics of the American Academy of Pediatrics. Informed consent, parental permission, and assent in pediatric practice. Pediatrics 1995;95:314–7.
50. Appelbaum PS, Roth LH, Lidz CW, et al. False hopes and best data: consent to research and the therapeutic misconception. Hastings Cent Rep 1987;17:20–4.
51. Daugherty C, Ratain MJ, Grochowski E, et al. Perceptions of cancer patients and their physicians involved in phase I trials. J Clin Oncol 1995;13:1062–72.
52. Joffe S, Cook EF, Cleary PD, et al. Quality of informed consent in cancer clinical trials: a cross-sectional survey. Lancet 2001;358:1772–7.
53. Annas GJ. The changing landscape of human experimentation: Nuremberg, Helsinki, and beyond. Health Matrix 1992;2:119–40.
54. Miller M. Phase I cancer trials. A collusion of misunderstanding. Hastings Cent Rep 2000;30:34–43.
55. Agrawal M, Emanuel EJ. Ethics of phase 1 oncology studies: reexamining the arguments and data. JAMA 2003;290:1075–82.
56. Decoster G, Stein G, Holdener EE. Responses and toxic deaths in Phase I clinical trials. Ann Oncol 1990;1:175–81.
57. Roberts TG, Jr., Goulart BH, Squitieri L, et al. Trends in the risks and benefits to patients with cancer participating in phase 1 clinical trials. JAMA 2004;292:2130–40.
58. Horstmann E, McCabe MS, Grochow L, et al. Risks and benefits of phase 1 oncology trials, 1991 through 2002. N Engl J Med 2005;352:895–904.
59. Cheng JD, Hitt J, Koczwara B, et al. Impact of quality of life on patient expectations regarding Phase I clinical trials. J Clin Oncol 2000;18:421–8.
60. Slevin ML, Stubbs L, Plant HJ, et al. Attitudes to chemotherapy: comparing views of patients with cancer with those of doctors, nurses, and general public. BMJ 1990;300:1458–60.
61. Horng S, Emanuel EJ, Wilfond B, et al. Descriptions of benefits and risks in consent forms for phase 1 oncology trials. N Engl J Med 2002;347:2134–40.
62. Meropol NJ, Weinfurt KP, Burnett CB, et al. Perceptions of patients and physicians regarding phase I cancer clinical trials: implications for physician-patient communication. J Clin Onc 2003;21:2589–96.
63. Simon R, Freidlin B, Rubinstein L, et al. Accelerated titration designs for Phase I clinical trials in oncology. J Natl Cancer Inst 1997;89:1138–47.
64. Hellman S, Hellman DS. Of mice but not men. Problems of the randomized clinical trial. N Engl J Med 1991; 324:1585–9.
65. Angell M. Patients' preferences in randomized clinical trials. N Engl J Med 1984;310:1385–7.
66. Taylor KM, Margolese RG, Soskolne CL. Physicians' reasons for not entering eligible patients in a randomized clinical trial of surgery for breast cancer. N Engl J Med 1984;310:1363–7.
67. Kodish E, Eder M, Noll RB, et al. Communication of randomization in childhood leukemia trials. JAMA 2004;291:470–5.
68. Freedman B. Equipoise and the ethics of clinical research. N Engl J Med 1987;317:141–5.
69. Freedman B. A response to a purported ethical difficulty with randomized clinical trials involving cancer patients. J Clin Ethics 1992;3:231–4.
70. Ashcroft R. Giving medicine a fair trial. Trials should not second guess what patients want. BMJ 2000;320:1686.

71. Marquis D. How to resolve an ethical dilemma concerning randomized clinical trials. N Engl J Med 1999;341:691–3.
72. Cannistra SA. The ethics of early stopping rules: who is protecting whom? J Clin Oncol 2004;22:1542–5.
73. Miller FG, Brody H. A critique of clinical equipoise. Therapeutic misconception in the ethics of clinical trials. Hastings Cent Rep 2003;33:19–28.
74. Miller FG, Rosenstein DL. The therapeutic orientation to clinical trials. N Engl J Med 2003;348:1383–6.
75. Grunberg SM, Cefalu WT. The integral role of clinical research in clinical care. N Engl J Med 2003;348:1386–8.
76. Freedman B, Glass KC, Weijer C. Placebo orthodoxy in clinical research I and II. J Law Med Ethics 1996;24:243–59.
77. Temple R, Ellenberg SS. Placebo-controlled trials and active-control trials in the evaluation of new treatments. Part 1: ethical and scientific issues. Ann Intern Med 2000;133:455–63.
78. Emanuel EJ, Miller FG. The ethics of placebo-controlled trials—a middle ground. N Engl J Med 2001;345:915–9.
79. Lie RK, Emanuel EJ, Grady C, Wendler D. The standard of care debate: the Declaration of Helsinki versus the international consensus opinion. J Med Ethics 2004;30:190–3.
80. National Bioethics Advisory Commission. Research involving human biological materials: ethical issues and policy guidance. Rockville, MD: National Bioethics Advisory Commission; 1999.
81. Clayton EW, Steinberg KK, Khoury MJ, et al. Informed consent for genetic research on stored tissue samples. JAMA 1995;274:1786–92.
82. ASHG report. Statement on informed consent for genetic research. The American Society of Human Genetics. Am J Hum Genet 1996;59:471–4.
83. ACMG statement. Statement on storage and use of genetic materials. American College of Medical Genetics Storage of Genetics Materials Committee. Am J Hum Genet 1995;57:1499–500.
84. Annas GJ. Rules for research on human genetic variation—lessons from Iceland. N Engl J Med 2000;342:1830–3.
85. Veatch RM. The patient as partner: a theory of human-experimentation ethics. Bloomington: Indiana University Press; 1987.
86. Tu JV, Willison DJ, Silver FL, et al. Impracticability of informed consent in the Registry of the Canadian Stroke Network. N Engl J Med 2004;350:1414–21.
87. Chen DT, Rosenstein DL, Muthappan P, et al. Research with stored biological samples: what do research participants want? Arch Intern Med 2005;165:652–5.
88. Malone T, Catalano PJ, O'Dwyer PJ, Giantonio B. High rate of consent to bank biologic samples for future research: the Eastern Cooperative Oncology Group experience. J Natl Cancer Inst 2002;94:769–71.
89. National Institutes of Health. HIPAA Privacy Rule: information for researchers. Available at: http://privacyruleandresearch.nih.gov/authorization.asp. (accessed June 16, 2005)
90. Hippocrates. The art. In: Jones WHS, editor. Hippocrates: The Loeb classical library. Cambridge (MA): Harvard University Press; 1923. p.128.
91. Bigelow J. Self-limited disease: address to the Massachusetts Medical Society, May 27, 1835. Nature in disease. Boston: Ticknor and Fields; 1854.
92. Warren J. Etherization, with surgical remarks. Boston: Ticknor & Co; 1848.
93. Pope Pius XII. The prolongation of life. In: Reiser SJ, Dyck AJ, Curran WJ, editors. Ethics in medicine. Cambridge (MA): MIT Press; 1977. p. 501–4.
94. *In re Quinlan,* 70 N.J. 10 (1976).
95. *Cruzan v. Director of Missouri Department of Health,* 110 S. Ct. 2841 (1990).
96. *Washington v. Glucksberg,* 117 S. Ct. 2302 (1997).
97. *In re Conroy,* 98 N.J. 321 (1985).
98. Emanuel EJ. A review of the ethical and legal aspects of terminating medical care. Am J Med 1988;84:291–301.
99. Emanuel EJ, Emanuel LL. Proxy decision making for incompetent patients. An ethical and empirical analysis. JAMA 1992;267:2067–71.
100. *Wendland v. Wendland, 110* Cal. Rptr. 2d 412 (2001).
101. *In re Edna,* MF 563 N.W.2d 485 (Wis. 1997).
102. *In re Martin,* 538 N.W.2d 399 (Mich. 1995).
103. Miles SH. Informed demand for "non-beneficial" medical treatment. N Engl J Med 1991;325:512–5.
104. *Bouvia v. Superior Court, 225* Cal. Rptr. 297 (1986).
105. Schneiderman LJ, Jecker NS, Jonsen AR. Medical futility: its meaning and ethical implications. Ann Intern Med 1990;112:949–54.
106. Truog RD, Brett AS, Frader J. The problem with futility. N Engl J Med 1992;326:1560–4.
107. Veatch RM. Why physicians cannot determine if care is futile. J Am Geriatr Soc 1994;42:871–4.
108. Helft PR, Siegler M, Lantos J. The rise and fall of the futility movement. N Engl J Med 2000;343:293–6.
109. Curtis JR, Park DR, Krone MR, Pearlman RA. Use of the medical futility rationale in do-not-attempt-resuscitation orders. JAMA 1995;273:124–8.
111. Caring Connections. Available at: http://www.partnershipforcaring.org (accessed June 30, 2005).
112. *In re Eichner (Brother Fox),* 52 N.Y.2d 262 (1981).
113. *Brophy v. New England Sinai Hospital,* 398 Mass. 417 (1986).
114. Emanuel EJ, Ash A, Yu W, et al. Managed care, hospice use, site of death and medical expenditures in the last year of life. Arch Intern Med 2002;162:1722–1728.
115. Vitelli CE, Cooper K, Rogatko A, Brennan MF. Cardiopulmonary resuscitation and the patient with cancer. J Clin Oncol 1991;9:111–5.
116. Prendergast TJ, Luce JM. Increasing incidence of withholding and withdrawal of life support from the critically ill. Am J Respir Crit Care Med 1997;155:15–20.
117. Danis M, Southerland LI, Garrett JM, et al. A prospective study of advance directives for life-sustaining care. N Engl J Med 1991;324:882–8.
118. The SUPPORT Principal Investigators. A controlled trial to improve care for seriously ill hospitalized patients. The study to understand prognoses and preferences for outcomes and risks of treatments (SUPPORT). JAMA 1995;274:1591–8.
119. Teno JM, Licks S, Lynn J, et al. Do advance directives provide instructions that direct care? SUPPORT Investigators. Study to Understand Prognoses and Preferences for Outcomes and Risks of Treatment. J Am Geriatr Soc 1997;45:508–12.
120. Emanuel EJ, Young-XU Y, Levinsky NG, et al. Chemotherapy use among Medicare beneficiaries at the end of life. Ann Intern Med 2003;138:639–43.
121. Emanuel EJ, Emanuel LL. The promise of a good death. Lancet 1998;351:S21–9.
122. Field MJ, Cassel CK. Approaching death: improving care at the end of life. Washington, DC: National Academy Press; 1997.
123. Education in Palliative and End of Life Care. Available at: http://www.epec.net. Accessed June 29, 2005.
124. Baile WF, Buckman R, Lenzi R, et al. SPIKES—A six-step protocol for delivering bad news: application to the patient with cancer. Oncologist 2000;5:302–11.
125. Emanuel EJ. The history of euthanasia debates in the United States and Britain. Ann Intern Med 1994;121:793–802.
126. It's over, Debbie. JAMA 1988;259:2094–8.
127. Emanuel EJ. Euthanasia. Historical, ethical, and empiric perspectives. Arch Intern Med 1994;154:1890–901.
128. Rachels J. The end of life: euthanasia and morality. New York: Oxford University Press; 1986.
129. Brock DW. Voluntary active euthanasia. Hastings Cent Rep 1992;22:10–22.
130. Wolf SM. Holding the line on euthanasia. Hastings Cent Rep 1989;19:S13–5.
131. Singer PA, Siegler M. Euthanasia—a critique. N Engl J Med 1990;322:1881–3.
132. Callahan D. When self-determination runs amok. Hastings Cent Rep 1992;22:52–5.
133. *Krischer v. McIver,* 697 So.2d 97 (Fla. 1997).
134. *Sampson et al. v. State of Alaska,* No. 5474, Sept. 21, 2001.
135. Office of Disease Prevention and Epidemiology. Department of Human Services Seventh Annual Report of Oregon's Death With Dignity Act. March 10,2005 Available at: http://egov.oregon.gov/DHS/ph/pas/docs/year7.pdf (accessed June 30, 2005).
136. Onwuteaka-Philipsen BD, van der Heide A, Koper D, et al. Euthanasia and other end-of-life decisions in the Netherlands in 1990, 1995, 2001. Lancet 2003;362:395–9.
137. van der Heide A, Deliens L, Faisst K, et al. End-of-life decision-making in six European countries: descriptive study. Lancet 2003;362:345–50.
138. Emanuel EJ. Euthanasia and physician-assisted suicide: a review of the empirical data from the United States. Arch Intern Med 2002;162:142–52.
139. Emanuel EJ, Fairclough DL, Daniels ER, Clarridge BR. Euthanasia and physician-assisted suicide: attitudes and experiences of oncology patients, oncologists, and the public. Lancet 1996;347:1805–10.
140. Ward BJ, Tate PA. Attitudes among NHS doctors to requests for euthanasia. BMJ 1994;308:1332–4.
141. Breitbart W, Rosenfeld BD, Passik SD. Interest in physician-assisted suicide among ambulatory HIV-infected patients. Am J Psychiatry 1996;153:238–42.
142. Ganzini L, Johnston WS, McFarland BH, et al. Attitudes of patients with amyotrophic lateral sclerosis and their care givers toward assisted suicide. N Engl J Med 1998; 339:967–73.
143. Emanuel EJ, Daniels ER, Fairclough DL, Clarridge BR. The practice of euthanasia and physician-assisted suicide in the United States: adherence to proposed safeguards and effects on physicians. JAMA 1998;280:507–13.
144. Groenewoud JH, van der Heide A, Onwuteaka-Philipsen BD, et al. Clinical problems with the performance of euthanasia and physician-assisted suicide in the Netherlands. N Engl J Med 2000;342:551–6.
145. Emanuel EJ, Fairclough DL, Emanuel LL. Attitudes and desires related to euthanasia and physician-assisted suicide among terminally ill patients and their caregivers. JAMA 2000;284;2460–8.
146. Rodwin MA. Medicine Money & Morals: physicians' conflicts of interest. New York: Oxford University Press 1993. Chapters 1–2.
147. Mitchell JM, Scott E. Physician ownership of physical therapy services. Effects on charges, utilization, profits, and service characteristics. JAMA 1992;268:2055–9.
148. Hillman BJ, Joseph CA, Mabry MR, et al. Frequency and costs of diagnostic imaging in office practice—a comparison of self-referring and radiologist-referring physicians. N Engl J Med 1990;323:1604–8.
149. Mitchell JM, Sunshine JH. Consequences of physicians' ownership of health care facilities—joint ventures in radiation therapy. N Engl J Med 1992;327:1497–501.
150. Wazana A. Physicians and the pharmaceutical industry: is a gift ever just a gift? JAMA 2000;283:373–80.
151. Chren MM, Landefeld CS. Physicians' behavior and their interactions with drug companies. A controlled study of physicians who requested additions to a hospital drug formulary. JAMA 1994;271:684–9.
152. Bekelman JE, Li Y, et al. Scope and impact of financial conflicts of interest in biomedical research: a systematic review. JAMA 2003:289;454–65.
153. Cho MK, Bero LA. The quality of drug studies published in symposium proceedings. Ann Intern Med 1996;124:485–9.
154. Djulbegovic B, Lacevic M, et al. The uncertainty principle and industry-sponsored research. Lancet 2000;356:635–8.
155. Stelfox HT, Chua G, O'Rourke K, Detsky AS. Conflict of interest in the debate over calcium-channel antagonists. N Engl J Med 1998;338:101–6.
156. Friedberg M, Saffran B, et al. Evaluation of conflict of interest in economic analyses of new drugs used in oncology. JAMA 1999;282:1453–7.
157. Melander H, Ahlqvist-Rastad J, et al. Evidence b(i)ased medicine—selective reporting from studies sponsored by pharmaceutical industry: review of studies in new drug applications. BMJ 2003;326:1171–3.
158. Whittington CJ, Kendall T, et al. Selective serotonin reuptake inhibitors in childhood depression: systematic review of published versus unpublished data. Lancet 2004;363:1341–5.
159. Bonetta L. Inquiry into clinical trial scandal at Canadian research hospital. Nat Med 1998;4:109
160. Gifts to physicians from industry. JAMA 1991;266:61–3.
161. Pearson SD, Sabin JE, Emanuel EJ. Ethical guidelines for physician compensation based on capitation. N Engl J Med 1998;339:689–93.
162. McCrary SV, Anderson CB, et al. A national survey of policies on disclosure of conflicts of interest in biomedical research. N Engl J Med 200;343:1621–6.
163. Department of Health and Human Services. Final Guidance Document: Financial Relationships and Interest in Research involving Human Subjects: Guidance for Human Subjects Protections. Available at: http://www.hhs.gov/ohrp/humansubjects/finreltn/fguid.pdf (accessed June 30, 2005).
164. Association of American Medical Colleges. Protecting Subjects, Preserving Trust, Promoting Progress: Policy and Guidelines for the Oversight of Individual Financial Interests in Human Subjects Research Available at: http://www.aamc.org/members/coitf/firstreport.pdf (accessed June 30, 2005).
165. American Society of Clinical Oncology. American society of clinical oncology: revised conflict of interest policy. JCO 2003;21:1–3.
166. Topol EJ, Armstrong P, Van de Werf F, et al. Confronting the issues of patient safety and investigator conflict of interest in an international clinical trial of myocardial reperfusion.

Global Utilization of Streptokinase and Tissue Plasminogen Activator for Occluded Coronary Arteries (GUSTO) Steering Committee. J Am Coll Cardiol 1992;19:1123–8.
167. Gostin LO. National health information privacy: regulations under the Health Insurance Portability and Accountability Act. JAMA 2001;285:3015–21.
168. Al-Shahi R, Warlow C. Using patient-identifiable data for observational research and audit. BMJ 2000;321:1031–2.
169. Lo B, Alpers A. Uses and abuses of prescription drug information in pharmacy benefits management programs. JAMA 2000;283:801–6.
170. Etzioni A. Medical records. Enhancing privacy, preserving the common good. Hastings Cent Rep 1999;29:14–23.
171. Roth LH, Meisel A. Dangerousness, confidentiality, and the duty to warn. Am J Psychiatry 1977;134:508–11.
172. *Tarasoff v. Regents of the University of California,* 17 Cal. 3d. 425 (1976).
173. Verity C, Nicoll A. Consent, confidentiality, and the threat to public health surveillance. BMJ 2002;324:1210–3.
174. Bayer R, Fairchild AL. Public health. Surveillance and privacy. Science 2000;290:1898–9.
175. Melton LJ 3rd. The threat to medical-records research. N Engl J Med 1997;337:1466–70.
176. Gunn PP, Fremont AM, Bottrell M, et al. The Health Insurance Portability and Accountability Act Privacy Rule: a practical guide for researchers. Med Care 2004;42:321–7.
177. The Bolton Research Group. Patients' knowledge and expectations of confidentiality in primary health care: a quantitative study. Br J Gen Pract 2000;50:901–2.
178. Li FP, Garber JE, Friend SH, et al. Recommendations on predictive testing for germ line p53 mutations among cancer-prone individuals. J Natl Cancer Inst 1992;84:1156–60.
179. Annas GJ. Privacy rules for DNA databanks. Protecting coded "future diaries." JAMA 1993;270:2346–50.
180. Roche PA, Annas GJ. Protecting genetic privacy. Nat Rev Genet 2001;2:392–6.
181. Murray TH. Genetic exceptionalism and "future diaries": is genetic information different from other medical information? In: Rothstein MA, editor. Genetic secrets: protecting privacy and confidentiality in the genetic era. New Haven (CT): Yale University Press; 1999. p. 60–76.
182. Eng C, Clayton D, Schuffenecker I, et al. The relationship between specific RET proto-oncogene mutations and disease phenotype in multiple endocrine neoplasia type 2. International RET mutation consortium analysis. JAMA 1996;276:1575–9.
183. Kauff ND, Satagopan JM, Robson ME, et al. Risk-reducing salpingo-oophorectomy in women with *a BRCA1* or *BRCA2* mutation. N Engl J Med 2002;346:1609–15.
184. Meijers-Heijboer H, van Geel B, van Putten WL, et al. Breast cancer after prophylactic bilateral mastectomy in women with *a BRCA1* or *BRCA2* mutation. N Engl J Med 2001;345:159–64.
185. Weber BL, Giusti RM, Liu ET. Developing strategies for intervention and prevention in hereditary breast cancer. J Natl Cancer Inst Monogr 1995;17:99–102.
186. American Society of Clinical Oncology policy statement update: genetic testing for cancer susceptibility. J Clin Oncol 2003;21:2397–406.
187. Glass KC, Weijer C, Lemmens TM, et al. Structuring the review of human genetics protocols: genetic diagnostic and screening studies. IRB 1997;19:1–13.
188. Kodish E, Wiesner GL, Mehlman M, Murray T. Genetic testing for cancer risk: how to reconcile the conflicts. JAMA 1998;279:179–81.
189. Schilling FH, Spix C, Berthold F, et al. Neuroblastoma screening at one year of age. N Engl J Med 2002;346:1047–53.
190. Tannock IF. Eradication of a disease: how we cured symptomless prostate cancer. Lancet 2002;359:1341–2.
191. Wertz DC, Fanos JH, Reilly PR. Genetic testing for children and adolescents. Who decides? JAMA 1994;272:875–81.
192. Nelson RM, Botkin JR, Kodish ED, et al. Ethical issues with genetic testing in pediatrics. Pediatrics 2001;107:1451–5.
193. Points to consider: ethical, legal, and psychosocial implications of genetic testing in children and adolescents. American Society of Human Genetics Board of Directors, American College of Medical Genetics Board of Directors. Am J Hum Genet 1995;57:1233–41.
194. American Society of Clinical Oncology Policy Statement Update: Genetic Testing for Cancer Susceptibility. J Clin Oncol 2003;21:2397–406.
195. ASHG statement. Professional disclosure of familial genetic information. The American Society of Human Genetics Social Issues Subcommittee on Familial Disclosure. Am J Hum Genet 1998;62:474–83.
196. Offit K, Groeger E, Turner S, et al. The "duty to warn" a patient's family members about hereditary disease risks. JAMA 2004;292:1469–73.
197. Council on Ethical and Judicial Affairs of the American Medical Association. Use of genetic testing by employers. JAMA 1991;266:1827–30.
198. Reilly PR, Boshar MF, Holtzman SH. Ethical issues in genetic research: disclosure and informed consent. Nat Genet 1997;15:16–20.
199. Reilly PR. ASHG statement on genetics and privacy: testimony to United States Congress. Am J Hum Genet 1992;50:640–2.
200. Earley CL, Strong LC. Certificates of confidentiality: a valuable tool for protecting genetic data. Am J Hum Genet 1995;57:727–31.
201. Kodish E, Murray TH, Shurin S. Cancer risk research: what should we tell subjects? Clin Res 1994;42:396–402.
202. Weijer C, Goldsand G, Emanuel EJ. Protecting communities in research: current guidelines and limits of extrapolation. Nat Genet 1999;23:275–80.

Legal Aspects of Cancer

Joseph Taraska, JD

Today, the physician who works to diagnose or treat cancer has a difficult dilemma. The patients' expectations regarding the discovery and cure of their disease often are at odds with the realities of cancer.[1] Unfortunately, this may result in legal difficulties for the physician and the patient. This chapter is intended to assist the physician in gaining an understanding of the legal process as it relates to commonly encountered problems in this field. With this understanding, the practitioner will be better able to avoid entanglements in the legal system and so devote himself or herself more fully to the patients.

ELEMENTS OF LIABILITY

In the United States judicial system, the same elements must be proven to establish a right to recovery, regardless of the nature of the claim. These are (1) that a duty existed which was breached, (2) that the breach caused an injury, and (3) that an injury, in fact, resulted. Despite the fact that these elements are the same for all claims, the necessary proof to establish each element in cases involving cancer may vary because of the particular characteristics of this area of medicine.

The Standard of Care The first element, breach of duty, more commonly is referred to as failure to abide by the applicable "standard of care." The first question this raises is: Who establishes the standard of care? Because of the complexity of medicine, it is almost universally held that jurors may not create the standard to which doctors are held; rather, jurors must apply the standard that is recognized by the medical profession. This standard generally is established through expert medical testimony. Unfortunately, litigation is often seen as a battle of experts, wherein the jury is left to measure the credibility of two competing viewpoints. As might be expected, this at times leads to confusion in a juror's mind. Medicine is not static, and the overlap between competing schools of thought or evolution from a prior practice to a more current approach creates a gray zone wherein most litigation of this nature occurs. The only remedy for the physician is to stay informed about developing practice parameters and understand when to refer patients to those with greater expertise. If the physician elects to provide treatment in an area not usually managed by those with his or her training, the physician may be held to the standard of the specialist whose role has been assumed.

The question of who is qualified to act as an expert often creates intense argument at trial. It seems logical that an oncologist should be called to testify against an oncologist or a radiologist against a radiologist; however, this is not always the case. In most jurisdictions, if an expert can demonstrate an understanding of the appropriate standard of care, either through training, practice, or association with those in the field, he or she often is given the latitude to testify. It, then, is up to opposing counsel to assist the jury in weighing the credibility of this testimony by demonstrating any shortfalls that the individual may have in his or her understanding of the relevant medical practice.[2]

In addition to the use of expert testimony, either side may attempt to establish the standard of care by referring to general medical literature and practice parameters. For example, a joint effort by the American Colleges of Radiology, Surgeons, Pathologists, and the Society of Surgical Oncology has resulted in practice guidelines for breast conservation treatment, against which one's actual practice may be measured.[3] Although most jurisdictions currently hold that such literature and guidelines, if established as authoritative, may be introduced as some evidence of the standard of care, they are not considered to be dispositive of that issue. The usual practice is to preclude the introduction of such parameters to establish the standard but to allow it in cross-examination and impeachment of the opposing side's expert. In this fashion, the jury has the benefit of the standards when measuring the testimony of an expert and may consider them as they deem appropriate.[4]

A final point to consider is that the standard of care is clearly a national standard. Originally, standards were measured by the prevalent practice in that physician's locale. However, with the establishment of national board examinations and the sharing of medical information, standards are now more broadly based. One caveat is that if the facilities available in the locale are not the equivalent of those that may be found in larger cities, the physician may be judged by what is available. Once again, however, he must be cautious in determining when the facilities are inadequate and the patient must be transferred to another's care.

Causation To impose liability, not only must there be a breach of the appropriate standard of care, but that breach must be causally related to an injury. In legal terminology, the term *proximate cause* generally is used.

In applying this concept, most jurisdictions now require proof that "but for" the act, the injury would not have occurred. This test is explained most clearly in jury instructions such as the following:

> Negligence is a legal cause of injury if it directly in a natural and continuous sequence produces or contributes substantially to producing such injury, so that it can reasonably be said that but for the negligence, the injury would not have occurred.[5]

When following this instruction, a jury could not impose liability in most instances, unless it determined that the act probably (interpreted as a greater than 50% chance) caused the injury. Cancer cases, however, present a complicating factor. There are patients who when they first present to a physician's office have less than a 50% chance of avoiding an adverse outcome, whether that outcome is death or other injury. As a result, if such were to go to court, it could never be said that "but for" the negligent act of a physician the injury occurred.

The courts have recognized this difficulty, but have split on the manner in which they handle the problem. In fact, two conflicting schools of thought have developed for such cases. Although both express the traditional concept that the plaintiff must prove that it is more likely than not that an injury was caused by the physician's act, they disagree as to the nature of the injury and the evidence required.

The first school of thought focuses on the actual illness and/or death of the patient as the injury. Courts that follow this approach require that it must first be demonstrated by the plaintiff that there was a greater than 50% likelihood of avoiding an adverse outcome when the patient first presented. It must then be proven that, as a result of the physician's negligence, either an adverse outcome has already occurred or the chance of avoiding the injury has been reduced to below 50%. In other words, either the injury has occurred or it is now more likely than not that it will.

Courts that follow the second school of thought hold that the injury that must be proven is not the illness and/or death, but rather the loss of any percentage of opportunity to avoid that adverse outcome.[6] Those who adhere to this standard have determined that regardless of the initial percentage of chance of survival and/or avoiding illness, if that percentage has been reduced, then an injury has occurred and that injury is compensable.

Damages The final element in establishing liability is damages; in other words, if the act fell below the acceptable standard, it must have resulted in an injury or loss. Such damages are uniformly divided into compensatory and punitive. Compensatory damages are those meant to compensate an individual for a loss and are measured by the value of that loss. Punitive damages, however, have no relationship to the loss but are intended simply to punish or deter conduct that society deems to be outrageous. As might be expected, the type of act that is necessary to support this form of compensation is significantly greater than simple negligence, and it generally requires that the act be so wanton or reckless as to be tantamount to an intentional act. Such is seldom seen in these cases.

Generally, compensatory damages include loss of income, therapy, medical expenses and related costs, along with mental anguish. When considering mental anguish there usually must be a related physical injury before a court will allow a claim for it. This helps to discourage fraudulent claims. There have been, however, exceptions to this general rule. Although not universally recognized, one such exception has been noted in some jurisdictions where a diagnosis of cancer was made and no cancer actually existed, thus causing only emotional distress. A case where a dentist observed a lesion on the roof of a patient's mouth is illustrative of this.[7] The dentist performed a biopsy, and although no cancer was noted in the specimen, the dentist referred the patient to an oral surgeon. The oral surgeon advised the patient that there was a 50% chance that she was suffering from lethal midline granuloma, a rapidly growing lesion that may result in death. Ultimately, it was determined that no cancer existed. The patient sought recovery for "cancer phobia." The court noted there had been expert testimony that the dentist deviated from acceptable standards in telling the patient she had cancer when the test results were normal. It was then reasoned that it was foreseeable to expect that a mistaken diagnosis of cancer would result in emotional harm to the patient.

Such cases place the physician in an awkward circumstance. The physician cannot avoid the responsibility of communicating his or her opinion to the patient. If that communication is not based on sufficient information, however, it may be the basis for a cause of action and damages. The lesson is that when imparting the diagnosis of cancer, the physician should take reasonable steps to ensure that the diagnosis has a medical basis and include this in the discussion. Such a reasoned approach is likely to deter adverse legal outcomes.

THE DOCTOR–PATIENT RELATIONSHIP

It is generally acknowledged that a physician has no duty, absent a constitutional or statutory requirement, to render care unless he or she has agreed to do so. A physician may find, however, that he or she has created a doctor–patient relationship, and thus is obligated to care for the patient, even when the physician had not thought that he or she had created such a relationship. As a result, it is necessary to understand which circumstances create a relationship and which end it.

The most common manner in which the doctor–patient relationship is created is by express agreement. The physician simply agrees to render medical care and attention and the patient consents to that relationship. Traditionally, this occurs when the patient presents himself or herself to the physician's office or the physician consults on the patient while in a medical facility. This relationship may also arise where a physician has contracted with an entity that provides medical care to a group of patients. For example, hospital by-laws often provide that a staff physician cover the emergency room on an on-call basis. This often is considered a contract between the physician and the hospital, and patients are considered to be third-party beneficiaries of this contract. As such, a patient who presents to the emergency room may claim the benefit of that contract. In other words, because the on-call physician has been contacted, he or she generally is responsible to make a determination as to whether further evaluation is required and, if so, to provide that evaluation until the patient either is stable or referred to another physician or entity. Without the contractual arrangement (in this instance, the by-laws), the duty does not exist.

Another question that often arises is whether an appointment made by a patient to see a physician in and of itself creates a doctor–patient relationship. Generally, such a call only implies that the doctor has agreed that the patient may come to the office so that he or she can determine whether they will enter into such a relationship. This can be altered, however, depending on the manner in which the appointment is made. Such a circumstance may arise where the patient provides his or her clinical history by phone to the doctor's office and it is apparent he or she has an acute illness that requires urgent care. If an appointment is made in this circumstance, the lines blur as to whether there is an agreement to treat that illness. As such, it is better to go forward and commence the relationship, using a legally sufficient manner to terminate the relationship, when appropriate. Of course, the one exception to this is if the requested therapy is beyond the capabilities of the physician. In this circumstance, there is no obligation to treat, but the physician should assist in arranging for follow-up care with another physician.

Casual encounters are fraught with potential difficulties. Every physician has been in a situation in which a friend or acquaintance asks for medical advice in an informal setting. This may be as innocent as asking the physician to look at an unusual mole or listen to a particularly bothersome cough. Although it is difficult to disengage from such conversations, this is the more prudent course. If one listens to such complaints and gives advice, it may be assumed that a doctor–patient relationship has been created; it is not necessary that compensation change hands. The better course in such circumstances is to advise the patient that perhaps he or she should come to the medical office, or that of another physician, for a full evaluation of the difficulty.

Informal conversations with a patient generally are not considered in the same light as an informal conversation with another physician. Generally, when one physician informally discusses his or her patient with a second physician, and there is no agreement for the second physician to undertake care of the patient or provide a formal consult, no doctor–patient relationship has been created.[8] To hold otherwise would severely hamper the free flow of information between physicians. All physicians must have the opportunity to discuss with peers the conduct of their profession. This same circumstance applies when various cases are presented for educational reasons, whether in a school environment or hospital meeting (eg, tumor boards).[9] This, however, must be clearly distinguished from a formal consultation. Such can occur face to face, through a note on the hospital chart, or by phone. The distinguishing line is that the physician consulted understands that he or she is being engaged to provide a professional opinion for the medical care and attention of a patient.

Another question that often is encountered by those who specialize in cancer therapy is whether the patient who once was seen by the physician can claim the benefit of that doctor–patient relationship for all time. In other words, does a relationship, once started, continue in perpetuity? In most areas of medical practice, the line is fairly clear. Once a patient begins treatment for an acute illness, the relationship between patient and physician continues until the illness subsides or one party withdraws from the arrangement in a legally appropriate manner. This line may not be, however, as clear when treating cancer, which has the potential for long-term therapy, follow-up, and recurrence. For this reason, it is imperative that the physician clarifies his or her expected role with the patient. In the event there has been no understanding with regard to future care and the patient seeks care from the physician, the physician should make a determination as to whether an acute or unstable situation exists. If the patient is unstable, the appropriate course is to assist the patient in stabilizing and then to ensure that the patient is transferred to another physician if one does not wish to continue providing care.

Once the doctor–patient relationship has begun, a physician may not abandon the patient without incurring liability. Terminating the relationship usually requires either a mutual agreement of the parties, the patient deciding to withdraw from the physician's care, or the physician making a unilateral decision to withdraw in a manner that complies with legal requirements.

When making this determination, the circumstance that created the relationship must first be analyzed. If there was a contract to render care, the physician may not be able to withdraw. For example, as noted earlier, hospital staff by-laws create an obligation for an on-call specialist to attend when called by the emergency room physician. Unless the by-laws provide a method in which this relationship may be avoided, the physician may have no choice but to attend. This does not require, however, that he or she continue to care for the patient. In such circumstances, the physician's only obligation generally is to attend during the immediate and unstable condition. The patient then may be referred to another physician for follow-up care. Similarly, in the case of managed care contracts, the physician may not be allowed to terminate the relationship with a patient unless the physician follows the prerequisites of those contracts.

In most circumstances, the physician may elect to terminate for any reason that does not violate federal or state laws (such as those that prohibit discrimination) or his own contract with a health-care entity. In doing so, however, there are general tenets that should be followed:

- The physician should determine whether the patient's condition requires immediate attention. If so, the patient should be stabilized before terminating the relationship.
- The patient should be made aware of the nature of his or her illness and, if required, that follow-up care is necessary.
- The patient should be notified by the physician of his or her intent to withdraw from care as of a specific date.
- The patient should be made aware that the physician will cover the patient for emergencies up to the date set out in the previous tenet.
- If the physician wishes to provide a specific referral, that may be accomplished. He or she is under no obligation to do so, however, and may instead refer the patient to the general medical community. In this circumstance, the physician should make the patient aware of the type of medical specialist to be sought and cover the patient for a reasonable time.
- The patient also should be informed that he or she is entitled to a copy of his or her medical records and that such will be provided to the patient or, if the patient so prefers, to the subsequent treating physician on request.[10]

These instructions may be given orally, but if so, the better practice is to follow up in writing. Perhaps the most practical method of documentation is simply to post a letter to the patient with this information to the patient's last known address. As with all medical communications, the documents should be marked as personal and confidential, and a copy kept with the chart.

CONSENT

It is axiomatic that touching an individual without consent is battery. If battery results, it is actionable. This theory of law generally has been applicable to the medical profession since the early 1900s[11]; however, in the field of cancer, there is increasing confusion with regard to obtaining informed consent. In part, this results from the nature of the diseases, the evolving therapies that are available, and the role of the physician both as a treater and as a researcher. In this regard, questions have arisen, such as how much information patients with incurable diseases really wish to know, and whether it is counterproductive to disclose a dismal prognosis; whether statistical data on morbidity or mortality are irrelevant to the individual patient's course; and whether the physician's personal interest, either through research or otherwise, should be disclosed to the patient. This section discusses these and other questions and will be instructive to the physician in avoiding the pitfalls that have led to increased litigation.

The first question to be addressed by the physician is: Who has the duty to obtain consent? It generally is accepted that the physician who performs the diagnostic procedure or therapy has the duty. Physicians may delegate the work that this responsibility entails to others, but they cannot avoid the responsibility itself. For example, a physician may allow a resident or office personnel to explain a procedure and its risks to the patient; however, if information is incorrectly imparted, the physician will bear the responsibility for failing to obtain informed consent. This does not suggest that physicians should not use assistants in the technical aspects of consent, such as having the forms signed. However, the physician should participate in the direct communications with the patient when the essential information is imparted.

Another area of concern is whether a referring physician or the referred physician has the duty to obtain the party's consent. Courts that have reviewed this issue generally find that the obligation to obtain informed consent rests with the specialist who is to perform the procedure or render the care.[12] This does not suggest that the referring physician should avoid discussion with the patient before referral. Rather, the referring physician should keep in mind that too detailed a discussion may confuse the patient, if conflicting information is provided by the specialist who is to render the care.

The second question in obtaining consent is: Who has the right to give the consent? As a rule, the competent adult whose health is at risk has the right to receive the information and provide consent. If this individual is not competent, however, then the physician must look to another. In those circumstances where a court has declared the individual to be incompetent and appointed another, this process is relatively easy. If the physician is unsure in this regard, he may contact the clerk of the local court, who will determine whether a guardian has been appointed. If the individual has not been declared incompetent, but the physician nonetheless believes this may be the case, the physician has several options. The first, when time is not of the essence, is to advise the family that a judicial determination may need to be made, and have them seek counsel for the appointment of an appropriate guardian. The second is to rely on consent of the next of kin; however, this is not universally accepted in that jurisdictions vary regarding who may consent under various circumstances. As a result, it is appropriate for the physician to consult legal counsel in this circumstance.

A related question is: Who has the authority to consent for a child? Parents generally hold this right, and the physician is justified in relying on them. As with other areas of the law, however, confusion may exist in certain circumstances. This most often occurs when the child (ie, an individual younger than 18 years of age in most states) is mature. With greater frequency, courts are beginning to require that mature minors be involved in the decision-making process.[13] Unfortunately, no bright line exists by which a physician can judge this circumstance. Rather, if he or she believes that the minor is mature enough to understand the nature of the illness, the risks of providing or withholding therapy, and the likely results, then that minor should be involved in the process. Closely related to the circumstance of the mature minor is that of the emancipated minor. This generally is thought of as someone who is below the statutory age of adulthood but who, nonetheless, is living on his or her own and is self-sufficient. These minors usually are thought of as having the right to consent to their own care.

Once it has been determined which physician will obtain the consent and who has the right to give consent, the next concern is what information must be imparted. The consensus in most jurisdictions is that the following information should be included in discussions with the patient:[14]

- Nature of the patient's illness.
- Nature of the proposed therapy.
- Reasonable alternative therapies.
- Chance of success with the proposed therapies.
- Substantial risks inherent in the therapies.
- Risk of failing to undergo therapy for the illness.

When considering the quantum of information to be contained in these categories, courts are divided along two tracks. The first is to measure the quantum of information that reasonable physicians would provide to their patients under the same or similar circumstances. The second is to consider what a reasonable patient would want to know in making his or her determination.[15] Regardless of which test is used, the best rule is for physicians to understand the information generally imparted by their peers and, additionally, to consider what they would like to know if in the patient's position attempting to make the decision. This combination of considerations generally will lead to an appropriate disclosure.

In considering the required disclosure, physicians who work in this area should be aware of a developing line of cases that may expand the quantum of information to be disclosed. This is illustrated by a recent Florida case, in which the question was whether a duty existed on the part of a surgeon to advise a couple that the wife's condition (medullary thyroid carcinoma) could be inherited by her children.[16] Those courts that require such disclosures follow the line of cases imposing on psychiatrists a duty to warn certain individuals about a danger of harm from their patient[17] or to protect others from infectious diseases.[18] Although in the Florida case, the court declined to hold the physician liable for failing to inform the parents, the better rule would be to advise the parents if such risks of inheritability exist. In deciding such questions, courts generally seek to determine whether an injury was foreseeable and the injured person was in the zone of risk. In the case of inheritable diseases, the risk would seem to be foreseeable, and the children certainly would seem to be in the zone of danger.

There are, of course, exceptions to obtaining consent. In the realm of diagnosis and treatment for cancer, however, these are less common. The first is the emergency circumstance. Obviously, the law allows one to act in an emergency, if time would not permit obtaining an appropriate consent; it is presumed that the patient would consent. The second, which occurs in the most rare of circumstances, is the therapeutic privilege. As one court explained:

> ...[P]atients occasionally become so ill or emotionally distraught on disclosure as to foreclose a rational decision, or to complicate or hinder the treatment or perhaps even to pose psychological damage to the patient. Where that is so, the cases have generally held that the physician is armed with a privilege to keep the information from the patient, and we think it clear that portents of that type may justify the physician in action he deems medically warranted.[19]

Even in this circumstance; however, the best rule to follow is that if the patient is not to be provided information for therapeutic reasons, then the patient's next of kin should be given the information and asked to provide consent for therapy.

An issue that has created renewed attention is whether physicians must disclose a personal interest when obtaining informed consent. Such interests may occur with protocols, grants, patents, and relationships established with medical equipment manufacturers and drug companies. The Supreme Court of California addressed this issue in a case in which a patient was undergoing treatment for hairy cell leukemia.[20] Because of the patient's particular disease, the physicians were able, over a period of time, to develop a cell line from his blood that ultimately was patented by them. Unfortunately, they had neglected to tell the patient they were drawing blood from him for this purpose. In reviewing the matter, the court held that a physician must disclose personal interests unrelated to the patient's health, whether for research or economic gain, that may affect the physician's professional judgment; and a physician's failure to disclose such interests may give rise to a cause of action for performing medical procedures without informed consent or breach of a fiduciary duty.[20]

In reaching this conclusion, the court noted that there might be conflicting loyalties under these circumstances. Physicians who add their own economic or research interests to the balance may be tempted to order a scientifically useful procedure or test that offers marginal, or no, benefit to the patient. The possibility that an interest extraneous to the patient's health has affected the physician's judgment is something that a reasonable patient would want to know in deciding whether to consent to a proposed course of treatment. It is material to the patient's decision and thus a prerequisite to informed consent.[20,21]

Finally, a question also has been raised as to the proper role of statistical data in describing to a patient, the risks that are inherent in the patient's disease and the success of proposed therapies. Most recently, this was considered by the Supreme Court of California.[22] In this case, the patient was suffering from pancreatic cancer. Discussions were held with the patient concerning the use of a chemotherapy regimen known as FAM (5-fluorouracil, Adriamycin, and mitomycin C) and radiation therapy. Apparently, this combination had shown some promise in treating pancreatic cancer in experimental trials at that time. (The patient's care was rendered in 1980.) Neither the operating surgeon nor the treating oncologist, however, disclosed to the patient the high statistical mortality rate that was associated with pancreatic cancer. The patient later testified that had he known, he would have chosen to forgo this therapy and, thus, improve the quality of his life over the time remaining. In considering the matter, the court noted that statistics are inherently unreliable in predicting the fate of an individual patient. As such, the court refused to mandate that statistical data regarding the mortality rate of a given cancer be provided to a patient. In doing so, it did not preclude the physician from using this information; rather, it indicated that this question should be decided on a case-by-case basis, which might include statistical data depending on the circumstance.[23] Considering the state of the law, no specific rule can be fashioned. Rather, as noted, the physician must consider this for each patient.

As might be expected, some of the more traditional concepts of informed consent (eg, which physician has the duty to obtain consent and which individual may provide consent) remain relatively static. With the development of new therapies, methods for measuring the success of those therapies, and participation of physicians in research, however, an evolution is occurring in the quantum of information that is expected to be imparted to the patient. As a result, legal counsel should be sought if confusion exists in the mind of the practitioner.

THE PHYSICIAN AS AN EXPERT WITNESS

There is considerable debate today as to whether our current system of judging professional disputes is appropriate. In fact, we may be seeing the beginning of an evolution to a more efficient and beneficial system. However, for the time being we must settle these disagreements in an adversarial system. Each side presents its point of view supported by those with experience in the appropriate medical endeavor. These experts often have opposing views, which are left to a jury to resolve.

As long as this system continues, it is essential that physicians who do qualify as having sufficient training and experience agree to review these matters and provide testimony for the defendant provider or the plaintiff depending on which position the physician believes is correct. If this does not occur, data may be presented to the jury that are not correct with an unjust result. This discussion focuses on the physician's role in this crucible of competing viewpoints.

A common question is whether a treating physician can be compelled to provide testimony. The judicial system allows either side to subpoena treating physicians to render their thoughts regarding the medical aspects of the case. The American Medical Association Council on Ethical and Judicial Affairs has supported this view in its Code of Medical Ethics. In so doing, the Council notes that although a physician should not become an advocate or partisan in legal proceedings; he or she has an ethical obligation to assist in the administration of justice by providing testimony regarding a patient, when requested.[24] This does not, however, open the floodgate to any question an attorney may seek to ask of the treating physician. Rather, physicians generally are allowed to limit their testimony to their own care and treatment as well as their thoughts regarding the prognosis for the patient. In most circumstances, they are not compelled to render expert opinions on hypothetical facts presented by either side, nor are they compelled to render testimony as to whether another physician deviated from the acceptable standard of care. They may elect to participate in this fashion but, as noted, generally are not compelled to do so.

The hypothetical expert is in a different category. This individual usually is retained by one side or the other because of a special expertise to comment on one or more aspects of the litigation (ie, standard of care, proximate cause of injury, injuries suffered by the patient). If a physician elects to participate in this fashion, it should be with the full understanding that absent some advanced limitation, he or she will be expected to review the materials submitted as well as render testimony in discovery depositions and court proceedings.

Once a physician has elected to participate, it is incumbent on him or her to request of the attorney submitting materials those documents that are required for testimony. The treating physician may need no more than his or her own records; however, the hypothetical expert is in a different circumstance. In most instances, the expert's review should consist of the patient's medical records and the deposition testimony of the various treating physicians, the patient, and other experts. Although some physicians elect to forgo the testimony and base their opinions solely on the records, they should nonetheless review this testimony before appearing in court. Failing to do so subjects their opinion to an attack on credibility in that they may not have considered all relevant facts. In addition, an expert should review his or her own medical literature on the subject in question. In today's arena of computer-assisted litigation, both sides may avail themselves of *MEDLINE* searches and often start with a search of all published literature by experts retained in the matter. This does not suggest that a physician's opinions may never change once published. However, the physician should be aware of his or her prior thoughts so that an adequate explanation of his or her current thinking, aside from all of the literature, can be given.

WITHDRAWING LIFE SUPPORT/ PHYSICIAN-ASSISTED SUICIDE AND EUTHANSIA

A clear distinction has been drawn in the law between the withdrawal/withholding of life support, physician-assisted suicide, and euthanasia. The prior is considered to be passive in nature in that it simply allows nature to take its course. The latter two categories, however, are considered to be active, in that they involve the participation of a physician either in prescribing medication or using medical devices to cause death.

Since the early 1970s, there has been a great deal of judicial and legislative attention focused on how to deal with the patient, and those who assist the patient, in the withdrawal and/or withholding of life support. The seminal case was that of the New Jersey Supreme Court involving Karen Quinlan.[25] This started a line of decisions that brought us to the United States Supreme Court decision in *Cruzan*.[26] The effect of these decisions has been to recognize the right of a patient to refuse medical treatment even to the extent of withholding and/or withdrawing life support, including artificial nutrition and hydration. Additionally, the courts that have considered the matter have held that the right should not be diminished upon the incompetence of the individual. As a result, substitute decision makers are allowed to speak for the patient when he or she is no longer able to express their decision.

There has been considerable debate, however, as to how the court determines what the patient's election would have been in those circumstances where they have not made it absolutely clear through writing or otherwise. The case of Terri Schiavo in Florida illustrates the confusion and difficulties this can cause.[27] Fifteen years ago, Mrs. Schiavo became, by most medical evaluations, persistently vegetative. Her husband, who is her surrogate decision maker, attempted to have her hydration and sustenance withheld. Her parents, however, believed that this would not have been their daughter's desire and petitioned the courts to block the withholding of this form of life support. Every court that considered the matter determined that in fact the husband was correct that Mrs. Schiavo would not have wanted to continue this way. Prior to the removal of the feeding tube, however, the Governor of Florida, with the support of the Legislature attempted to reverse all prior court decisions on this matter by enacting a law, which was obviously meant to only address the case of Mrs. Schiavo. In essence, it would have prohibited the withdrawal of her life support.

Although this law was subsequently held unconstitutional by the Florida Supreme Court, the federal legislature then passed a bill, which the President signed into law, allowing Mrs. Schiavo's parents to seek an injunction in federal court against the withdrawal of Mrs. Schiavo's life support.[28] The federal courts denied the parents' motions for a temporary restraining order, and the courts continued to deny all appeals made by Mrs. Schiavo's parents until their daughter's death. These bills attempted to overturn 30 years of practical and compassionate legislation designed to protect the patient and their family. Fortunately, both state and federal courts understood the need to maintain the current state of the law and did not succumb to the pressure of various special interest groups, which could have been devastating to all parties. Hopefully, the publicity this case has generated along with the public's awareness of the need to clearly make these decisions will avoid such protracted litigation in most cases.

Having decided the parameters for the withdrawal/withholding of life support, the United States Supreme Court, in 1997, turned its attention to physician-assisted suicide. It did so by reviewing the laws of Washington and New York, states that prohibited physician-assisted suicide. The question raised was whether this was a right protected by the United States Constitution. The Court ruled that there was no Federal constitutional right to physician-assisted suicide or euthanasia.[29]

These rulings did not end the issue of physician-assisted suicide or euthanasia. Rather, as noted by one of the justices, the court left the matter to the "laboratory" of the states to allow each to address the issue within the context of that state's constitution and legislative enactments. It should be noted that some state constitutions are worded in such a fashion that protection might be afforded in that state for assisted suicide. In addition, there is apparently no prohibition to a state enacting its own laws for or against physician-assisted suicide. One potentially negative effect of these decisions is that we may now have a myriad of laws forming a patchwork quilt across the United States addressing this issue from different perspectives.

The first successful legislation legalizing physician-assisted suicide came in Oregon in 1997.[30] The Oregon initiative was most likely successful because of its limited scope. It applied to patients with less than 6 months to live and was further limited in that it allowed only prescriptions for lethal drugs. The Oregon statute provides:

> An adult who is capable, is a resident of Oregon, and has been determined by the attending physician and consulting physician to be suffering from a terminal disease, and who has voluntarily expressed his or her wish to die, may make a written request for medication for the purpose of ending his or her life in a humane and dignified manner in accordance with this Act.

The statute's safeguards include:

- The initial request for drug prescriptions has to be in writing and witnessed by two individuals concurring that the patient was competent.
- At least two physicians have to concur that the patient is suffering from a terminal illness and is likely to die within 6 months.
- In the event that the patient is thought to be suffering from a psychiatric disorder, the patient must be referred for counseling. Records have to be maintained and submitted annually to the Health Division of the state for review.
- Two oral requests are required, separated by at least 15 days, before a physician can accept the written request. Once accepted, the prescription cannot be filled for 48 hours after the written request.[31]

The constitutionality of the Oregon initiative was challenged, but the statute withstood attack. Following that, it was submitted to the voters a second time and reaffirmed by 60%. It went into effect October 1997.

An analysis of the first 6 years that this act has been in effect provides some, although small, statistical guidance. The number of patients ingesting lethal medication has gone up slightly as follows: 42 in 2003, 38 in 2002, 21 in 2001, 27 in 2000, 27 in 1999, and 16 in 1998. An analysis of their characteristics indicate that patients were also slightly more apt to be older—median age 73 years of age—and slightly more apt to be higher educated. The medical conditions resulting in the greater use of the act included amyotrophic lateral sclerosis, HIV/AIDS, and malignant neoplasms.

Although, as noted, the database available to date is small, it seems to be pointing in a direction that would alleviate two major fears: first, that there would be a rush toward use of this form of physician assistance and second, that it would in some way be disproportionately chosen by or forced on terminally ill patients who are poor, uneducated, uninsured, or fearful of the financial consequences of their illness. There does not seem to be evidence supporting these fears from the data collected.[32] However, as noted, the caveat is that the database is small and the time over which this statute has been in effect is relatively short. These issues will require continuing evaluation.

In addition to surviving early legal challenges[33] there were two separate federal legislative attempts to preempt the act, both of which also failed to pass. (Lethal Drug Abuse and Prevention Act of 1998 was introduced in Congress in 1998 and would have preempted the Oregon Act but failed to reach the floor of either the House or the Senate. The Pain and Relief Promotion Act of 1999 passed the House in 1999 but failed to reach the Senate floor for a vote.) More recently, the United States attorney general's office attempted to circumvent the courts and the legislature by issuing a directive in which Attorney General Ashcroft declared in relevant part that:

- Controlled substances may not be dispensed to assist suicide, thus reversing the position taken by his predecessor Attorney General Janet Reno in June 1998;
- Assisted suicide is not a "legitimate medical purpose" and that prescribing, dispensing or administrating federally controlled substances to assist suicide violates the Comprehensive Drug Abuse Prevention and Control Act;
- Prescribing, dispensing, or administrating federally controlled substances to assist suicide may "render (a physician's) registration...inconsistent with the public interest" and therefore subject to possible suspension or revocation under 21 USC § 824(a)(4); 66 CFR 56608 (Nov. 9, 2001).[34]

Oregon immediately brought the matter to federal district court, which rendered its opinion on April 17, 2002.[35] In that decision the court issued an injunction prohibiting the Ashcroft directive from being placed into effect in Oregon. In doing so, the court noted that the attorney general had determined that assisting a suicide was not a "legitimate medical purpose" within the meaning of federal regulations and that prescribing, dispensing, or administrating federal controlled substances to assist suicide violated the Comprehensive Drug Abuse Prevention and Control Act of 1970 (CSA). However, in examining this issue, the federal court determined that the attorney general could not make the determination as to what constituted a "legitimate medical purpose." It further found that this issue is one best left to each state's determination. In this instance, the court noted that Oregon had made that determination. This matter is currently pending for final decision before the United States Supreme Court.[36]

As is obvious, the issue of physician-assisted suicide and euthanasia remains in flux. The one area that is fixed is a patient's right to refuse care and/or life support. The guidelines for this process can be found in the laws of those states that have addressed the issue.

REFERENCES

1. Spratt J, Spratt S. Medical and legal implications of screening and follow-up procedures for breast cancer. Cancer 1990;66 Suppl 6:1351–62.
2. *Green & Goldberg*, 630 So.2d 606 (Fla. Dist. Ct. App. 1993).
3. Winchester D, Cox J. Standards for breast conservation treatment. CA Cancer J Clin 1992;42:134.
4. Hirschfield E. Should practice parameters be the standard of care in malpractice litigation? JAMA 1991;266:2886.
5. Florida Standard Jury Instructions, 5.1(a), p.1.
6. *Kilpatrick v. Bryant*, 868 S.W.2d 594 (Tenn. 1993).
7. *Rodriguez v. Calman*, NYLJ Sept. 18, 1992 at 22 (N.Y. Cty. Sup. Ct., Sept. 1992).
8. *Oliver v. Brock*, 342 So.2d 1 (Ala. 1977).
9. *Raynor v. Grossman*, 31 Cal. App.3d 539, 107 Cal. Rptr. 469 (1973).
10. Taraska J. Legal guide for physicians. New York: AHAD Press; 1987. p. 2.04(1).
11. *Schloendorff v. Society of New York Hospital*, 211 N.Y. 125, 105 N.E. 92, 93 (1914); Canterbury v. Spence, 464 F.2d 772, 780 (D.C. Cir.), cert. denied, 409 U.S. 1064 (1972).
12. *Johnson v. Whithurst*, 652 S.W.2d 441 (Tex. Civ. App. 1983).
13. *Belcher v. Charleston Area Medical Center*, 188 W. Va. 105, 422 S.E.2d 827 (1992).
14. Taraska JM. Legal guide for physicians. New York: AHAD Press; 1987. p. 6.02.
15. *Culbertson v. Mernitz*, 602 N.E.2d 98 (Ind. 1992).
16. *Pate v. Threlkel*, 640 So.2d 183 (Fla. Dist. Ct. App., 1994).
17. *Tarasoff v. Regents of the University of California*, 141 Cal. Rptr. 14, 551 P.2d 334 (1976).
18. *Hoffman v. Blackman*, 241 So.2d 752 (Fla. Dist. Ct. App. 1970), cert. denied, 245 So. 257 (Fla. 1971).
19. *Canterbury v. Spence*, 464 F.2d 772, 789 (D.C. Cir.), cert. denied, 409 U.S. 1064 (1972); *Nishi v. Hartwell*, 473 P.2d 116 (Haw. 1970).
20. *Moore v. Regents of the University of California*, 271 Cal. Rptr. 146, 793 P.2d 479 (1990).
21. Annas G. Informed consent, cancer and truth in prognosis. N Engl J Med 1994;330:223, but see *Pulvers v. Kaiser Foundation Health Plan*, 99 Cal. App.3rd 650, 160 Cal. Rptr. 392 (1979).
22. *Arato v. Avedum*, 5 Cal.4th 1172, 23 Cal. Rptr.2d 131, 858 P.2d 598 (1993).
23. Annas G. Informed consent, cancer and truth in prognosis. N Engl J Med 1994;330:223.
24. American Medical Association. Council on Ethical and Judicial Affairs, code of medical ethics § 9.07 (2005 ed.)
25. In re Quinlan, 70 N.Y. 10, 355 A.2d 647 (1976), cert. denied, 429 U.S. 992 (1976).
26. *Cruzan v. Director, Missouri Dept. of Health*, 497 U.S. 261 (1990).
27. *Bush v. Schiavo*, 885 So.2d 321 (Fla. 2004).
28. An Act for the relief of the parents of Theresa Marie Schiavo, Pub. L. No. 109-3 (March 21, 2005).
29. *Washington v. Glucksberg*, 177 S. Ct. 2258 (1997); Bacco v. Quill, 117 S. Ct. 2293 (1997).
30. Oregon Death with Dignity Act, Oregon Rev. Stat. 127.800-127.897.
31. Annas G. Death by prescription. N Engl J Med 1993; 331:1240–1.
32. Chin A. Legalized physician-assisted suicide in Oregon—the first year's experience. N Engl J Med 1999; 340:577; see also Oregon v. Ashcroft et al, 192 F. Supp.2d 1077, 1082 (2002).
33. *Lee v. State of Oregon*, 891 F. Supp. 1429 (D. Or. 1995), vacated, 107 F.3rd 1382 (9th Cir. 1997).
34. *Oregon v. Ashcroft et al*, 192 F. Supp.2d at 1078, 1079 (2002).
35. *Oregon v. Ashcroft et al*, 192 F. Supp.2d 1077 (2002)
36. *Ashcroft v. Oregon et al*, 192 F. Supp.2d 1077 (D. Or. 2002), *cert. granted*, 73 U.S.L.W. 3298 (U.S. Feb. 22, 2005) (No. 04-623).

The Government and Cancer Medicine

Anna D. Barker, PhD
Hamilton Jordan

INTRODUCTION

The historical role of the federal government in eradicating cancer has been to provide funds for cancer research, primarily through the National Cancer Institute (NCI). The fact that cancer affects most of our citizens either directly or indirectly and costs the nation countless billions of dollars each year moved the government in 1971 to undertake a serious effort to conquer cancer. In the ensuing years, cancer research, by necessity, focused largely on understanding the differences between normal and cancer cells. This long period of exploration has led to an enormous explosion of data and new knowledge that fueled both the drive to sequence the human genome and the development of the biotechnology industry in America. The past 15 years (especially the last 5 years) have been a period of unrelenting and disruptive change, not just in the blistering pace of scientific discovery and the development of advanced technologies, but perhaps more importantly, also in the emerging opportunities to achieve measurable progress against cancer. Based on this "inflection point" in cancer research, in 2003 the director of the NCI challenged the cancer research community to capitalize on this unprecedented opportunity to accelerate progress against cancer and "eliminate the suffering and death due to cancer by 2015."

Despite steady increases in the survival of patients with many types of cancer, it continues to extract a high toll today in terms of both human and economic costs, but in 10 to 20 years the shifting demographics of America will produce a cancer burden that could swamp the health care system. For more than 30 years, this looming health care crisis has seemed like a distant possibility. Even today, the nation's cancer medicine enterprise has not come together to develop a comprehensive, proactive strategy to address the burden that cancer will inflict on individuals, families, and systems as our nation's population ages. Perhaps the people who most recognize the need for a major national program with the goal of finally defeating cancer are those most affected by the disease—patients and their families, who have stepped in, with a real sense of urgency, to insist that the nation do everything possible to accelerate progress against cancer. Beginning in earnest in the early 1990s, this advocacy movement has proceeded on a cancer-by-cancer basis, beginning with the breast cancer activists and evolving in the late 1990s into efforts designed to pull the disparate factions into a more focused advocacy effort. It is interesting that even in the face of this disease-focused cancer advocacy, the public, overall, remains relatively oblivious to the realities of the aging population and the increased number of cancer cases that will result from this demographic shift in a relatively few years.

Congress and the administration listened to their constituents and undertook a major initiative to invest more resources into biomedical research through a bipartisan initiative that doubled the budget of the National Institutes of Health (NIH) over 5 years. Interestingly, this doubling of the NIH budget spanned the Clinton and Bush (first-term) administrations. They also heard the activists and in the 1990s designed new mechanisms to target funds for specific cancers. In an environment of decreasing budgets for the NIH and the NCI, it is likely that earmarking for specific diseases will decrease and accountability for targeted programs will increase. One thing is certain, the magnitude of the current and future cancer epidemics means that more investment (and leadership) will be required from all of the sectors that comprise the National Cancer Program. Ironically, on the basis of unprecedented progress in cancer research over the past 34 years, we have reached an inflection point in science where progress can be exponential in the next few years, but the end of the doubling years of the NIH budget will likely slow these advances. The inability to capitalize on many of these opportunities will have far-reaching effects because so many aspects of postgenomics science are interrelated.

Finally, the events of September 11, 2001, have forever changed America. The conquest of cancer must now compete with a war to defeat terrorism around the globe. We must of course win both of these wars. It will be up to the cancer community to make the case, but in this age of enormous scientific promise, this responsibility falls more directly on the shoulders of scientists and clinicians than ever before in our history.

CANCER: A MAJOR NATIONAL HEALTH CARE PRIORITY

Thirty-four years after President Richard Nixon declared "war" on cancer and firmly committed the nation to its defeat, cancer remains a disease of staggering human and financial impact. A recent survey[1] found that cancer is the disease that Americans fear most. Although we have made significant progress against several forms of cancer, the sheer numbers of people affected by the disease partially accounts for this finding. In 2004, approximately 1,368,030 Americans will be diagnosed with cancer and 563,700 are expected die from their disease—more than 1,500 individuals every day.[2] Reflecting progress in early detection and treatment, approximately 10 million Americans are alive today who have a personal history of cancer.

As we look forward into the twenty-first century, at current rates, it is projected that one-half of men and one-third of women in America today will be diagnosed with cancer in their lifetime, and 25% of our population will die from cancer. In 2005 cancer surpassed heart disease as the leading cause of death in Americans under 85 years of age. Although cancer is already an epidemic in America, unless we do a great deal more now, it will likely become a major health care crisis as the nation's "baby boomers" age and our demographics change over the next 10 to 20 years. Adding to this burden is the fact that the poor, medically underserved and minority populations of America suffer a disproportionate burden of cancer.

Cancer is primarily a group of diseases of people over the age of 55, and it is especially prevalent in individuals who are 65 to 85 years of age. Approximately 80% of cancers are diagnosed in individuals 55 and older. Therefore, the anticipated increase in America's aging population is expected to have a significant impact on numbers of new cancer cases in the next 10 to 30 years.[3] In only 30 years, the number of Americans over the age of 65 is expected to double and those over 85 to quadruple. America will see the effects on numbers of new cancer cases as early as 2010 to 2020, since the 75 million members of the baby boomer population are turning 50 at the rate of one every seven seconds. A report published from the work of the March Research Task Force[4] predicted that at current rates the number of new cancer cases will increase by 30% in the next 15 to 20 years, and cancer mortality will increase by 25%.

Although we do not have a precise understanding of the annual cost of cancer in the United States, the NCI estimates the total economic burden for 2003 at approximately $189.5 billion.[2] Of this total, approximately $64 billion were spent for direct medical care of cancer patients.[5] The overall economic impact of the morbidity and premature death from cancer is more difficult to derive, but is estimated at $120.4 billion for 2004. The cost of cancer is further compounded by the fact that a large percentage of our population has no or inadequate health insurance, and when patients do not have access to health care services, cancer is often diagnosed and treated at later, more expensive stages. Cancer is often diagnosed at advanced stages in these populations, which results in increased costs to the health care system.

Since the passage of the National Cancer Act in 1971, cancer has grown beyond a national health care problem to become a major sociopolitical issue. The increasing impact of cancer on all Americans is requiring that the federal government through the NCI assume a more aggressive strategy to transfer laboratory advances from cancer research into clinical trials and address the discovery, development, and delivery of new cancer interventions. As a nation, we must be a great deal more realistic in facing the financial and human toll of this epidemic versus our level of investment. In addition to providing appropriate funding to accelerate progress in all areas of cancer research, development, and delivery, we must also become more strategic in terms of leveraging federal funds. The cancer medicine enterprise is a tripartite system comprised of federal, private, and nonprofit sectors. All three must form alliances to remove barriers and optimize distribution and application of finite resources. The reality is that there are infinite needs and finite resources. Fortunately, past investments in cancer research have paid off in improved understanding, prevention, diagnosis, and treatment of cancer. Going forward, if we are bold in our vision and national commitment, the nation can confront cancer with unparalleled new knowledge that will translate into unparalleled progress. Never in our history have we been more prepared to eliminate suffering and death due to cancer by capitalizing on the convergence of molecular oncology and advanced technologies.

Table 70-1 Legislative History of the National Cancer Program

Legislation	Key Points
National Cancer Institute Act – 1937 (P.L. 244)	Established National Cancer Institute (NCI) Established National Advisory Cancer Council
National Cancer Act – 1971 (P.L. 92-218)*	NCI Director – Presidential appointment Set up National Cancer Advisory Board and President's Cancer Panel Bypass budget directly to the president Broad coordination mandate, first cancer centers, cancer control programs
National Cancer Amendments – 1974 (P.L. 93-352)	Broadened information collection, analysis, and dissemination authority Authorized construction grants
Community Mental Health Center – 1978 Extension Act – 1978 (P.L. 95-622)	Expanded program for cancer prevention Expanded mission of cancer centers Expanded cancer control mandate
Health Research Extension Act – 1985 (P.L. 99-158)	Established Assoc. Director, Prevention Research on continuing patient care
Health Omnibus Program Extension – 1988 (P.L.100-607)	Added rehabilitation research Further expanded information dissemination
The NIH Revitalization Amendments of 1993–1993 (P.L. 103-43) **	Expanded research – breast, prostate cancer; Set aside cancer control

*Key formative legislation for the National Cancer Program.
**Initial legislation supporting targeted cancer research.

LEGISLATIVE HISTORY OF THE NATIONAL CANCER PROGRAM

The mission of the National Institutes of Health (NIH), an agency in the Department of Health and Human Services (DHHS), is to develop and apply fundamental knowledge about the nature and behavior of living systems to extend healthy lives and reduce the burden of illness and disability. The NIH, which began as a one-room Laboratory of Hygiene in 1887, today has over 27 institutes and centers and a 2005 budget of more than $28 billion. It stands as an unparalleled national (and international) resource and is the focal point for nearly all federally sponsored health research. It was within this context of improving the health of the nation, through research and application of knowledge, that the National Cancer Act was envisioned in the years between the establishment of the National Cancer Institute (NCI) in 1937 and the development of this unprecedented legislation in 1971.

As shown in Table 70-1, an act of Congress in 1937[6] made the conquest of cancer a national goal and set the stage for the formation of the NCI in 1939 from two existing laboratories.[7] The Office of Cancer Investigations at Harvard merged with a pharmacology division of the NIH, and the NCI was relocated to Bethesda, MD. This legislation also established the National Cancer Advisory Cancer Council, and directed the surgeon general to "provide for, foster, and aid in coordinating research related to cancer within the NCI and among other agencies and organizations." It would be 34 years before President Richard Nixon would sign bold legislation that would elevate the conquest of cancer to a national crusade.

President Nixon signed the National Cancer Act on December 23, 1971, and declared a "war" on cancer. This unprecedented legislation, P.L. 92-218,[8] was the outgrowth of an equally unprecedented research advocacy effort, led by philanthropist Mary Lasker and businessman Benno Schmidt, that prompted the Senate to adopt a resolution in 1970 calling for a study of cancer in America. The subsequent report from the Yarborough Commission, headed by Texas Senator John Yarborough, provided the details for a legislative plan that would become the National Cancer Act. It is interesting that this legislation never fully defined the concept of a National Cancer Program, which remains a topic of individual interpretation to this day.

The major goals of the National Cancer Act were to create a National Cancer Program that significantly expanded the authorities and responsibilities of the NCI, while maintaining it as an institute within the NIH. The most unique aspect of the National Cancer Act was that it provided the NCI director with direct access to the president of the United States. The act specifically mandated that the NCI develop its programs with the advice of a new National Cancer Advisory Board (NCAB) and submit an annual budget, termed the Bypass Budget, directly to the president, bypassing the approval of the NIH director. In addition, the act established a three-member panel, the President's Cancer Panel (PCP), which was specifically required to submit an annual report to the president. The NCI director and members of both the NCAB and PCP became presidential appointees. This sweeping legislation granted the director of the NCI broad authority to plan and develop an expanded, intensified, and coordinated National Cancer Program that included the NCI and related programs, other research institutes, and federal and nonfederal programs. The National Cancer Act also authorized the first 15 cancer centers and mandated cancer control programs. As shown in Table 70-1, the 1971 legislation was amended in 1974 (P.L. 93-352) to further broaden the authorities of the NCI to include the awarding of construction grants and information collection, analysis, and dissemination responsibilities.

Although the Mary Lasker-led advocacy movement of the 1970s led to the National Cancer Act, the broad scientific community voiced concerns about singling out one institute and granting it such sweeping authorities. There were also concerns that the NCI would subsume funding from other institutes and that the increased investment in cancer research would undermine the quality of research across the NIH. The reality is that the national focus on defeating cancer over the past 31 years has only served to attract additional funding for nearly all of the institutes of the NIH. Moreover, the relatively small number of approved individual investigator-initiated grants funded in 2004, approximately 23%, indicates that far too many good ideas still go unfunded. Therefore, the concern expressed in the 1970s that increased support for cancer research would result in "blanket funding" of mediocre science has never emerged as a problem. In fact, the ever-increasing size, scope, and complexity of the National Cancer Program serves to keep the relative level of funding for new ideas and new investigators significantly below where it was in 1971.

Legislation passed in 1978, P.L. 95-622, recodified the National Cancer Act and further consolidated and expanded the authorities of the NCI director (see Table 70-1). Interestingly, the language describing the National Cancer Program dropped the phrase "including other federal and nonfederal programs." This legislation significantly expanded the mission of cancer centers to include basic research and prevention and called for an overall expanded and intensified research program focused in cancer prevention. Perhaps the most important aspect of the changes mandated in this act was the significant emphasis on environmental carcinogenesis and prevention.

Although some additional laws were passed between the ensuing years that further strengthened some aspect of the National Cancer Program, or mandated a specific emphasis area, it was not until 1993 that patient advocacy would once again have a profound effect on the National Cancer Program. In June of 1993, the NIH Revitalization Amendments[9] specifically required the NCI to intensify and expand research on breast and prostate cancer. Further, the legislation mandated a case control study of elevated breast cancer rates on Long Island and mandated a set-aside for cancer control activities at 7%, 9%, and 10% for 1994, 1995, and 1996, respectively. The period of "earmarking" for specific cancers had arrived and continues to the present day.

The legislative history of the NCI and the National Cancer Program parallels the focus and effectiveness of cancer survivors and advocates over the years, beginning in 1971 with the group led by Mary Lasker. Today cancer has evolved beyond a health problem into a sociopolitical issue of enormous scope and impact. Interestingly, another concern expressed by the scientific community at the time of the enactment of the National Cancer Act was well founded—the unrealistic expectation of a quick cure for cancer. Many would argue that the lack of such a dramatic cure during the past 34 years has led to an increasing overall sense of apathy (and/or denial) among the public at large. In 2005 Congress will begin debating the reauthorization of the NIH, which will include renewal of the authorities granted to the NCI in the 1971 landmark legislation, and the outcome of this process is uncertain.

FEDERAL SUPPORT FOR THE NATIONAL CANCER PROGRAM

Cancer research, and medical research overall, are funded primarily by the federal government through the NCI and other agencies such as the Centers for Disease Control and Prevention (CDC) and the National Institute for Environmental Health Sciences (NIEHS). Funds for cancer research also increasingly come from a range of nonprofit organizations and foundations; and, although difficult to estimate, the private sector invests in cancer research at a level that is greater than the overall federal commitment.

The cancer problem is an enormous societal issue, and as previously shown, its overall impact on both the health of our citizens and the economy requires a significant and sustained level of investment that must come from the federal government. When the National Cancer Act was passed in 1971, Congress assumed that providing more money and setting up the national program would allow scientists to virtually eradicate cancer by 1976, in time to commemorate the 200th anniversary of the republic. In retrospect, this resolution seems naïve, but no one could have foreseen the enormous scientific challenge inherent in unraveling the mystery of the cancer cell and the level of commitment that would ultimately be required to understand a disease that is in reality over 200 different diseases.

Cancer Research Funding and the Federal Budget Process Since the NCI and the National Cancer Program were authorized through legislation, funding for the NCI must occur each year through the federal budget process. The Congressional Budget Committees of the House and Senate, established in 1974 by the Congressional Budget and Impoundment Control Act, are responsible for setting the annual fiscal agenda and spending priorities. Each year the president submits a budget to Congress in early February, which triggers the budget committees' efforts to complete their work and submit a joint budget to the House and Senate in April. The president's budget provides the framework for the budget resolution and subsequent appropriations process, which determines funding for specific programs. The Constitution requires that all revenue (tax) and appropriations bills originate in the House and subsequently be referred to the Senate for action. Funding for the NIH (and the NCI) occurs in the Labor, Health and Human Services Subcommittee of the Appropriations Committee. Each year the subcommittee holds hearings at which heads of agencies such as the NCI speak in support of the president's budget request, followed by additional hearings where witnesses speak in support of specific diseases or programs that are funded through these agencies. This process of public witness testimony can potentially affect final appropriations, but this depends almost totally on the extent to which constituents and advocates make contact through letters, faxes, e-mails, phone calls, etc with the members and request their support for a specific funding priority. Advocates also have an opportunity to interject language into the final appropriations bill, which provides direction to agency heads on how funds should be spent. This language is often the source of significant pressure to fund specific programs. Through a series of defined steps, the bill is marked up, taken to the "floor," approved by both the House and Senate, finalized in conference, and sent to the president for action.

NCI Funding 1971 to 2004 As envisioned in the National Cancer Act of 1971, each year the NCI director submits a "professional needs" budget directly to the president, with only comments (not approvals) from the NIH and the DHHS. As shown in Figure 70-1, the first Bypass Budget, totaling $550,790,000 was submitted in 1973. Since the Constitution vests in Congress the requisite powers to establish budgets and determine fiscal policy, the fact that the Bypass Budget is submitted directly to the president only served as an advantage in terms of fully funding the request during the early years of the National Cancer Program. Figure 70-1 illustrates the fact that the budget appropriated by Congress versus the Bypass

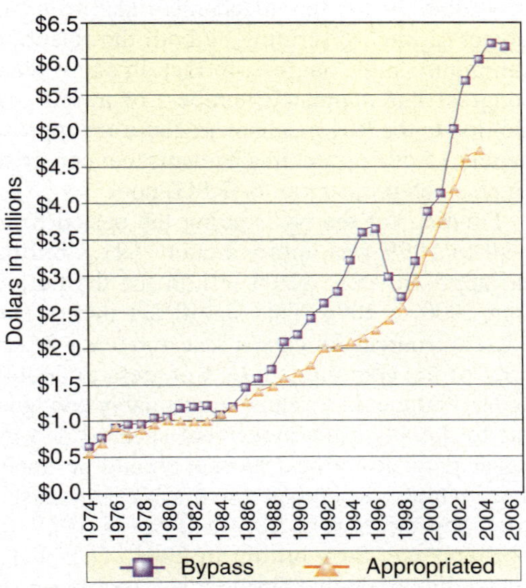

Figure 70-1 Comparison of the NCI Bypass Budget vs Final Appropriation from 1974–2006.

Budget requested were similar only in the early years of the National Cancer Program, which provided the NCI with real purchasing power directly after passage of the act. In the period beginning in 1976 and through the mid-1990s, the apparent steady growth of the NCI's appropriated budget must be considered in light of inflation and purchasing power. This period actually produced very little real budget growth, and when adjusted for inflation, decreased in the early 1980s.[10] The appropriation for the NCI would not see real increases in terms of purchasing power until the late 1990s, as the result of a congressional action to double the budget of the NIH over a 5-year period, beginning in 1999. The Bypass Budget request has continued to increase significantly over the years, with requests of $6.211 billion and $6.170 billion for fiscal years 2002 and 2003,[5] respectively.

Through the first 30 years of the National Cancer Program, the US federal budget totaled approximately $35 trillion and the NCI's budget for the same period totaled about $44 billion. Overall, we have invested at a level of about 1/10 of 1% in the research required to cure and prevent cancer. Looked at another way, in 2004, through the NCI, we invested approximately $4.8 billion in research to cure and prevent cancer, which costs the nation conservatively $190 billion per year. The war on cancer was declared in 1971, but the scope, significance, and resource needs for a full-scale campaign have never really been defined or made available on a national scale. Therefore, in 2005 the "war" metaphor no longer represents the same call to action as it did during the first few years following the signing of the National Cancer Act.

Funding for Research Project Grants (RPGs) The major gold standard through which the NCI distributes funds to the scientific community to pursue research ideas is through the investigator-initiated (R01) grant. Historically, funding for this mechanism has been the subject of intense scrutiny by both the scientific community and Congress. In fact, in some years Congress has mandated numbers of awards. In addition to the R01 mechanism, there are approximately 15 other grant mechanisms that comprise the research project grants (RPG) pool.

Funding for the NCI during the period from 1990 to 1999 was approximately $21.8 billion and approximately $20.6 billion for the period from 2000 to 2004. This significant increase in federal resources for cancer research was a direct result of the commitment by Congress to double the NIH budget in 5 years—presumably owing in part to the advocacy movement spearheaded by cancer patients in the 1990s. It should be noted that, in fact, the budget for the NCI increased from approximately $2.9 billion in 1999 to approximately $4.8 billion in 2004. The NCI's budget did not double during this 5-year period.

As illustrated in Figure 70-2, the numbers of RPGs funded have increased, and as a percentage of the total budget have remained near 50% since 1997. In 2004 the NCI funded 5,467 RPGs, the largest number in its history, for a total of $2.2 billion (Table 70-2). Although the number of RPGs has increased significantly since the 5-year doubling of the NIH began, the increase has generally not met the expectations of the scientific community. The limitation on new approved competing RPGs reflects two important considerations: The average cost of grants has increased significantly since 1999, and the NIH made a decision in the mid 1990s to fund an increased number of 5- and 7-year awards. To accommodate this increased requirement for out-year funding and the increased cost of individual grants, the number of new grants funded by the NCI has not kept pace with the competing applications.

As a consequence of the increased costs for established investigators working on competing renewals, funding for the number of noncompeting grants has remained nearly stable, increasing slightly in 2003 and 2004. Noncompeting grants often come from young scientists seeking their first grant or represent more innovative ideas from established investigators. During the past 10 years, several other opportunities have opened up for new investigators, primarily through the Department of Defense (DoD) programs in breast, prostate, and ovarian cancer. This may well reflect a new order of development for new investigators, where the DoD programs may partially fund the entry of new investigators into cancer research. This should ultimately improve the chances that new investigators will be more competitive for R01 grants through the NCI and other agencies.

During 2004, NCI funded approximately 24% of approved competing grants and all noncompeting grants. When the National Cancer Act was passed in 1971, 45% of approved new grants were funded, as nearly all were competing at this early point. In today's environment of unprecedented opportunities for progress in the postgenomics era of cancer research, many scientists believe that the percentage of grants going to individual investigators should be significantly higher than current levels. However, given the need for the NCI to empower its entire enterprise with new infrastructure in areas such as bioinformatics, proteomics, and genomics, it is unlikely that additional funds will be available to fund the overall portfolio, including individual-initiated grants. Table 70-2 shows that beyond the RPGs, the NCI must also support a range of additional important strategic elements that make up the National Cancer Program, and most of these demands will increase.

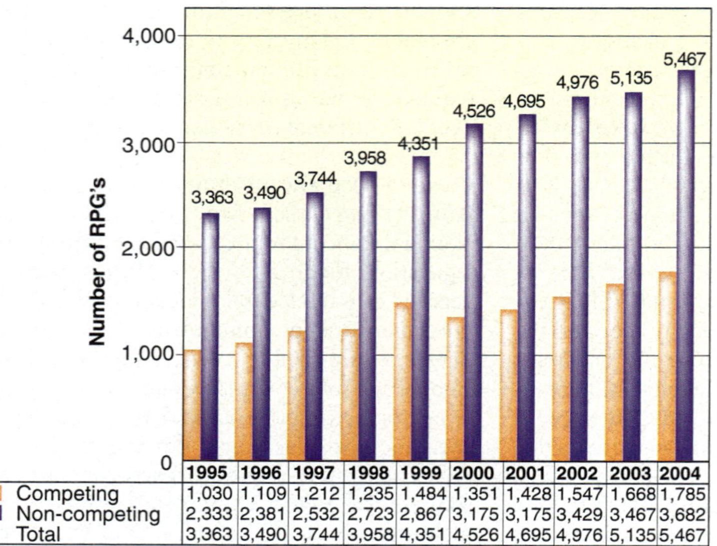

Figure 70-2 Numbers of Competing and Noncompeting Research Project Grants Awarded by the NCI from 1995–2004.

Increased funding is needed for cancer centers, Specialized Programs of Research Excellence (SPOREs), training, cooperative groups, key advanced technologies, common bioinformatics platforms, cancer prevention and control, intramural research, and other mechanisms. The NCI is also attempting to address significant gaps in investment across the overall research continuum, especially in translational and clinical research, and cancer in underserved and minority populations. There are also critical needs that must be addressed in areas such as bioinformatics that will impact all areas of cancer research and development. In the future, support for the National Cancer Program will increasingly depend on leveraging federal funds through partnerships and alliances to address both funding needs and requirements for expertise and know-how in critical areas such as translational research and technology development.

NCI Funding for Specific Cancers Although the NCI has historically focused on nondirected research that is broadly applicable to all cancers, the institute has also extended significant effort in disease-focused research. Although this shift is based somewhat on the sheer volume of data and knowledge available to address specific cancers, there is little doubt that this shift in focus also reflects pressure from cancer advocacy groups. Although budget decreases are clearly impacting the capability of the NCI to pursue organ-specific research, the NCI's Bypass Budget in 2003,[5] "The Nation's Investment in Cancer Research: A Plan and Budget Proposal for Fiscal Year 2003," stated that "the Institute plans, promotes and carries out an ambitious program of disease-specific research." To address this need, the NCI began by using panels of experts termed Progress Review

Table 70-2 NCI Funding Trends by Research Mechanism (in Millions)

	1998	1999	2000	2001	2002	2003	2004
Total NCI	$2,527.5	$2,891.6	$3,311.1	$3,753.7	$4,176.7	$4,592.3	$4,723.9
Research project grants	1,230.8	1,361.8	1,528.0	1,696.4	1,893.2	2,058.7	2,161.4
Intramural research	437.8	448.2	507.8	567.3	637.6	693.1	708.9
Cancer centers	134.0	153.2	169.1	202.9	224.8	255.0	259.9
SPOREs	30.9	42.6	52.3	76.8	94.9	123.1	149.4
Clinical cooperative groups	93.0	120.2	144.6	154.3	163.8	158.7	154.3
Cancer prevention & control	249.9	306.3	389.4	459.5	501.2	533.2	530.0
R&D contracts	171.1	214.1	251.6	284.0	298.2	370.8	361.6
Other mechanisms	180.0	245.2	268.3	312.3	363.0	399.7	398.4

Source: NCI.

Table 70-3 Current NCI Progress Review Groups*

Cancer Site
Breast cancer
Prostate cancer
Colorectal cancer
Brain tumors
Pancreatic cancer
Leukemia-lymphoma-myeloma
Lung cancer
Gynecologic cancers
Kidney/bladder cancer
Stomach/esophageal cancer
Liver/bile duct cancer
Skin cancer

Source: NCI.
*Expert disease-focused groups that deliberate and report on gaps, barriers, and research priorities.

Groups (PRGs) to assess the status of scientific knowledge surrounding a specific cancer and to identify specific needs for future research. It was anticipated that these recommendations, or roadmaps, could be used by the NCI and the community to assess progress against a specific type of cancer. Examples of the PRGs conducted by the NCI are summarized in Table 70-3.

Given the extent of patient advocacy from the breast and prostate cancer groups, it is not surprising that these were the first two PRGs completed. The NCI has done only a few additional PRGs in recent years owing primarily to the evolution of its Specialized Programs of Research Excellence grants that are focused on specific cancer sites. Although the impact of the PRG per se is still difficult to assess, targeted disease-specific research is now an integral part of NCI's portfolio. The NCI now tracks expenditures by disease. The reported funding allocated to specific cancer sites from 1997 to 2004 is shown in Table 70-4.

In addition to the PRGs, the NCI has also initiated disease-focused programs called designated SPOREs. The SPOREs were designed to be centers for translational research to facilitate the translation of findings between the clinic and laboratory in both directions. Today, SPOREs are a major portion of the NCI's portfolio, with over 58 established programs in most major cancers including breast, lung, gastrointestinal, prostate, bladder, ovarian, uterine, pancreatic, head and neck, leukemia, lymphoma, myeloma, and skin.

Recent Legislative Actions and Funding for the NCI During the period from 1993 to 2000, the disease-focused cancer advocacy movement began in earnest in America, and Congress was moved to do more about funding for research on specific cancers and also for the NIH. The ultimate increases for the NIH, NCI, and specific targeted programs occurred in a convoluted manner and involved a series of creative actions by individual members of Congress, including funding specific cancer research programs through the DoD. Perhaps the most unusual scenario that played out during the 8 years of the Clinton presidency was the regular submission of presidential budgets that provided little or no increases for the NIH. Each year, Congress would then "bid up" the appropriation for the NIH through the appropriations process, and a few members of the House and Senate became the champions for increasing funding for the NIH and the NCI. Interestingly, this built a congressional constituency for cancer, and for increased funding for biomedical research, that ultimately led to the doubling of the NIH budget.

In the mid-1990s several true congressional advocates for increasing the nation's investment in medical research emerged, and many offered creative approaches to fund the NIH and the NCI in the face of the Balanced Budget Act of 1997 that produced broad spending caps on domestic programs. Among these congressional leaders, Senators Tom Harkin (D-Iowa), Mark Hatfield (R-Oregon), Connie Mack (R-Florida), Arlen Specter (R-Pennsylvania), and Congressman John Porter (R-Illinois), among others, led a series of initiatives designed to create new sources of funds for medical research. Several of these initiatives garnered significant interest and support from the advocacy community, notably a proposed 1% set-aside on insurance premiums (Harkin and Hatfield), the Health Trust Fund of 1997, and subsequently, the National Fund for Health Research Act (Harkin and Specter). These initiatives, and the cancer advocacy movement of the 1990s, paved the way for a proposal to double the budget of the NIH from 1999 to 2003, which gained wide congressional support.

In the late 1990s, Senator Dianne Feinstein (D-California) took a personal and legislative interest in accelerating the war on cancer, holding hearings on the Report from the March Research Task Force in 1998, becoming vice chairperson of the National Dialogue on Cancer (NDC), and introducing the National Cancer Act of 2002.

Continuing this momentum, in his first and second budget submission to Congress, President George W. Bush fulfilled his campaign promise and proposed to fully fund the NIH at levels that would complete the doubling over the 5 years proposed by the congressional leaders that predated him. Since completion of the doubling of the NIH budget, the tragic events of September 11, 2001, homeland security needs, and the Iraq war have led to significant restraints on domestic spending. In 2005, the NCI is rebalancing its portfolio and stopping programs to find funds for new programs and strategic initiatives that will accelerate progress against cancer and the goal to eliminate suffering and death due to cancer by 2015.

Table 70-4 NCI Funding for Specific Cancers (in Millions)

	1998	1999	2000	2001	2002	2003	2004
Total NCI	$2,551.3	$2,891.0	$3,311.1	$3,753.7	$4,176.7	$4,592.3	$4,732.9
Brain & central nervous system	54.3	63.5	71.9	80.7	95.2	111.5	132.3
Breast cancer	348.7	387.2	438.7	475.2	522.6	548.7	566.2
Cervical cancer	58.0	66.3	67.0	72.6	67.6	79.0	79.0
Colorectal cancer	121.0	152.9	175.8	207.4	245.0	261.6	262.0
Head & neck	41.9	45.9	47.0	50.0	58.9	77.7	88.2
Hodgkin's lymphoma	8.3	8.2	9.4	10.2	11.8	16.5	17.4
Leukemia	103.4	122.2	141.7	154.0	177.2	200.9	214.7
Liver cancer	38.1	39.8	46.2	54.5	62.5	63.7	63.0
Lung cancer	139.8	151.0	175.0	206.5	237.5	273.5	276.5
Melanoma	50.3	60.1	67.9	71.8	82.3	90.7	94.9
Multiple myeloma			18.0	19.7	20.8	26.3	23.9
Non-Hodgkin's lymphoma	57.1	66.2	70.4	79.5	85.6	95.2	99.6
Ovarian cancer	40.8	56.5	65.5	76.9	93.5	99.4	99.5
Pancreatic cancer	14.2	17.3	20.0	21.8	33.1	42.3	52.7
Prostate cancer	86.9	135.7	203.2	258.0	278.4	305.2	308.5
Stomach cancer	8.2	7.6	6.8	9.0	11.4	13.4	11.6
Uterine cancer	12.2	13.8	16.0	18.8	23.1	25.5	27.0

Source: NCI.

RETURN ON INVESTMENT FROM FEDERAL FUNDS

America's investments in medical research through the NIH, NCI, and the overall National Cancer Program have produced unimagined returns. Seminal advances in understanding cancer cells through studies in molecular biology, genetics, cell signaling, cell death, etc, combine to provide a stunning array of possibilities for current and future progress from research to product continuum. Overall, advances in cancer and biomedical research ranging from unprecedented new targeted cancer treatments to advanced molecular technologies for early detection will ultimately lead to more lives saved and significant economic returns.

Through a combination of innovative research, unprecedented developments in technology, and novel partnerships, the sequencing of the human genome was completed well ahead of schedule. This breakthrough did not occur in isolation, but with complementary and synergistic advances in areas such as immunology, chemistry, informatics, computer modeling, etc. As a result, emerging advanced technologies such as genomics, nanotechnology, and proteomics are providing extraordinary opportunities to discover, develop, and commercialize targeted interventions to detect, prevent, and cure cancer.

In 2001, following fast-track review, the Food and Drug Administration (FDA) approved a new drug, STI571 (imatinib),[11] for the treatment of patients with chronic myelogenous leukemia (CML). STI571 (Gleevec) was designed to inhibit the division of CML cells that express a specific molecular defect (*bcr-abl* gene) not found in normal white blood cells. In clinical trials, Gleevec restored normal blood counts in 53 of 54 CML patients, with few side effects. The extraordinary efficacy of Gleevec received a great deal of national attention and set the stage for the discovery and development of a new paradigm in targeted genomics- and proteomics-based cancer drugs (see Chapter 54).

In parallel, complementary advances in areas such as advanced imaging technologies and biomarker-based assays have significantly improved our ability to detect cancer early. For the first time in decades, cancer incidence and mortality for selected types of cancer are falling.[2] In the period from 1974 to 1976, the relative 5-year survival rate for a newly diagnosed cancer patient was 50%, increasing to 64% from 1995 to 2000. Although this reflects real progress in areas such as early detection and more tailored cancer treatment, this is not a reflection of individuals who are cured of their disease.

Turning to the issue of the economic impact of cancer, a recent landmark study supported by the Lasker Charitable Trust and other foundations[12] estimated that reducing the mortality rate of cancer by 20% would be worth $10 trillion in economic value—more than one year's GDP; and eliminating deaths from cancer would be worth about $47 trillion. Although the numbers from this study are "mind-numbing," the message is clear—medical research pays very big dividends.

Although we are poised to make real progress in cancer discovery, development, and delivery of new agents and advanced technologies to patients, we have never faced more competing challenges. There is still a great deal that we must learn about the cancer cell through basic research in the face of a compelling need to translate laboratory advances into the clinic. We must create needed infrastructure for translational research, deploy and integrate advanced technologies, train critically needed personnel, create effective public-private partnerships, build our national bioinformatics capabilities, update and reform the regulatory process, and increase participation in clinical trials, to name some of the key hurdles that today represent barriers to progress. These problems must be solved in parallel with maintaining our emphasis on the basic science that fuels the engine of scientific discovery.

The American public, Congress and the administration expect a return on the federal dollars invested in cancer research. Increasingly, scientists are asked to communicate the relevance of their research and respond to requests for accountability measures. The concept of assessing return on dollars invested in medical research is likely to continue to grow, especially in an environment where investments in cancer research are decreasing. It ultimately falls to the scientific and clinical communities, in partnership with cancer survivors and advocates, to undertake a sustained effort to educate and inform the administration and Congress on research advances that translate to broad patient benefit.

PUBLIC ATTITUDES CONCERNING CANCER

We must endeavor to understand why even in the face of declining incidence and mortality for several cancers, it remains the disease that Americans fear most. There is little doubt that a portion of this fear reflects the fact that, from the standpoint of semantics, the term cancer was historically synonymous with a slow painful death. Fortunately, in the past few years we have made some progress in reducing the public's perception that cancer is a death sentence, and it is finally being discussed openly and publicly.

We can now envision a future where more cancer will be cured or treated as a chronic illness, and prevention of cancer will be possible using rational strategies. Increased relative 5-year survival rates for most cancer means that more patients are surviving, and advances occurring during their remissions offer the promise of eventually treating cancer as a chronic disease. However, there remains a disconnect between this reality and the public's perception of their own personal risk of cancer and what will happen if they fall victim to the disease. Education is obviously the key to changing this situation, but we need to acquire a better understanding of the public's perceptions of the cancer threat overall. We also need a better understanding of the public's ideas about personal risk and the options available today to predict, prevent, diagnose, and treat cancer.

Although recent disease-focused advocacy indicates that awareness is increasing in the context of specific cancers, the public at large remains relatively disconnected from the growing realities of the cancer problem in the United States and around the world. America is facing a potential health care crisis in the next 10 to 20 years because of increasing numbers of people who will suffer from one or more cancers in their later years of life. The problem of understanding how to leverage the power of public opinion for cancer advocacy and a broad commitment to controlling cancer is compounded by a lack of focused and rigorous research on trends in public awareness and attitudes over the past 30 years.

During the summer of 2000, the American Association for Cancer Research (AACR) teamed up with two well-known cancer survivors and advocates, Mr. Hamilton Jordan and Mr. Lance Armstrong, in an attempt to assess the public's attitudes about cancer in the context of the presidential election and the candidates' priorities.[1] (They also repeated this process in late 2003 during the presidential campaign, with essentially the same results.) The product of this working partnership was a survey that focused on assessing the public's knowledge of cancer risk, federal funding for cancer research, and their expectations of a new administration, among other issues. The results of the AACR 2000 survey were presented to both presidential campaigns, in hopes of making the conquest of cancer a top health care priority for both candidates. The surveys were conducted by respected national survey researchers with significant political experience.

The 2000 survey was conducted from among a cross section of 1,002 registered voters nationwide. The attitudes of the voters were surveyed in several focus areas, including fear of cancer versus some other tragic event, risk of being a cancer victim, understanding of federal funding for cancer research, and opinions concerning where cancer falls on the national agenda versus other campaign issues. Briefly, some of the more interesting findings from the survey were as follows:

- The broad and tragic reach of cancer was evident; 73% of responders had a close friend or family member die from cancer, 45% knew someone who had cancer and was cured, and 11% reported having cancer.
- Most Americans are uninformed about the realities of cancer, and were surprised by key facts about the disease; 50% of voters surveyed believed that their risk of developing some form of cancer was 1 in 100 or less, including 24% who felt that their risk was less than 1 in 1000, and only 15% felt that their risk was 20% or greater.
- Respondents did not recognize their cancer risk, and in fact, many (45%) did not believe the real statistics when they were presented; only 46% knew that over half of the patients who develop cancer now survive 5 years or more.
- Cancer was the disease that people feared most; 48% said they feared cancer more than any other illness, and surprisingly, cancer topped the list of Americans' greatest overall fears (32%). Americans also feared cancer (32%) more than any potential catastrophe (eg, violent crime, nuclear attack). (When the survey was repeated post-9/11/01 the response was 30%.)
- Personal experience and fear of cancer made the conquest of cancer a major goal in the minds of voters; 28% of respondents ranked cancer second only to providing health care to all children (38%) as key national agenda goals (eg, environmental protection, nuclear defense, etc).
- Conquering cancer was the overwhelming choice of voters for investment of research dollars, and there was strong support for dramatic federal funding increases to accelerate the conquest of cancer; 70% of those queried felt that federal support for cancer research

should increase, including 46% of voters who would triple current levels.

There are several compelling messages from this important research. First, although cancer has touched most American families, fear of cancer keeps them from recognizing their own cancer risk. There is a call to action in these findings. We must educate Americans on their cancer risk and enlist them as partners in early detection and prevention of cancer. Second, Americans want to remove this threat from their lives and want more done across all of cancer research and clinical care. Third, there is a clear message to political candidates and elected and appointed leaders that defeating cancer should be a national priority. It is interesting to note that soon after then Governor Bush's campaign received these results in 2000, he delivered a speech pledging to make the conquest of cancer a major goal for his administration. He subsequently fulfilled his commitment to complete the 5-year plan to double the budget of the NIH in 2003 ($27.3 billion) and proposed that the budget for the NCI increase from $4.19 billion in 2002 to approximately $4.6 billion in 2003.[5]

As shown in these unprecedented surveys, Americans are concerned about the impact of cancer on their lives, and they want a more proactive national strategy that will accelerate progress and ensure that Americans can live without the fear of dying from cancer. It was this spirit that drove early activists such as Mary Lasker and Benno Schmidt and fueled the emerging, mainly disease-focused, cancer advocacy movement that found its "legs" in the 1990s.

THE CANCER ADVOCACY MOVEMENT

More than 30 years after philanthropist and cancer research advocate Mary Lasker persuaded then President Richard Nixon to declare a national war on cancer, cancer advocacy can be described as a movement, albeit still small considering the human and economic impact of the disease. Unlike other conditions—such as heart disease, diabetes, and AIDS—where advocacy organizations can organize around and focus on a central (and more narrow) research agenda, the highly diverse cancer community organizes around different agendas that reflect the reality that cancer is a family of more than 200 different diseases, each with highly different origins, causes, and treatment options. Consequently, the funding for cancer research must be spread across numerous diseases, notwithstanding the hope that some core mechanisms of cancer causation and progression may produce interventions that will be broadly effective across several forms of cancer.

The survey summarized in the prior section suggests that the advocacy community is increasingly "connecting the dots" between the deep and widespread fear of cancer among our citizens and their desire to achieve success in this long national effort. The fact is that cancer touches almost everyone, and the survey demonstrates that nearly 80% of the American public wants more attention and resources applied to this most feared disease. The early 1990s saw the beginning of an advocacy movement that focused the anger and frustration of cancer victims and their families and friends to do something more about cancer. This movement would shift the way that cancer research is conceived, reviewed, and funded—relevance would take on new meaning. Perhaps the best example of the impact of this cancer advocacy movement was the breast cancer activists who would become a political force in the 1990s.

Breast Cancer Advocacy in the 90s: Targeted Funding for Specific Cancers Taking their lead from the AIDS activists, in the beginning of the 1990s, the National Breast Cancer Coalition (NBCC) led a grassroots movement to increase the nation's attention to breast cancer, and to specifically dedicate more resources to the research necessary to cure and prevent the disease. The "three hundred million more" campaign got a lot of attention from congressional members anxious to show their support for this critical women's issue in an election year. In a now famous interaction between the director of the NCI and the leader of the NBCC, Dr. Samuel Broder informed Ms. Frances Visco that the NCI was a large battleship that could not be "turned on a dime," to which Ms. Visco replied, "then we will build our own battleship." As a result, during 1992, an election year, the NBCC led an effort to lobby Congress to address the breast cancer problem. Congress responded with a directive to the NCI to increase funding not only for breast cancer research, but also for prostate and ovarian cancers collectively by $100 million a year. Because of budget cuts in 1993, the NCI was able to increase its level of funding for breast cancer research to only approximately $196 million, far less than the $365 million that the breast cancer advocates felt was necessary to address the increasing problem of breast cancer in America. However, in the meantime, the breast cancer advocates achieved their goal, as the NCI did increase funding for breast cancer research, presumably by cutting other programs.

The next chapter in this story speaks to the power of patient advocacy. The breast cancer advocates took their case to Senator Tom Harkin (D-Iowa), who introduced an amendment to the Department of Defense (DoD) Appropriations Bill that would add $185 million to increase the DoD's breast cancer appropriation to $210 million in 1993. The "Harkin Amendment for Breast Cancer" passed by a vote of 99 to 4, ultimately leading to the establishment of what would become the Congressionally Directed Medical Research Program (CDMRP). To determine how to invest these funds, the Department of the Army contracted with the Institute of Medicine (IOM) to recommend a process for creating the required infrastructure for the programs and to define areas of potential research focus. Among the many recommendations made by the IOM panel was a two-tiered peer and programmatic review system and an advisory council to (among other things) assess program relevance and suggested areas for investment.

The extraordinary program that derived from this advocacy effort, the DoD Breast Cancer Research Program (BCRP) (and soon thereafter, the prostate, ovarian, and other cancer programs), was an unprecedented partnership among the army, breast cancer consumers, and the scientific community. From the beginning of the program, the partners have been steadfast in their support of the best peer-reviewed science in a context that encourages and welcomes new innovative ideas and fills important gaps in the research continuum. The partners began anew with the way that research is planned, reviewed, and supported, and the advisory council that oversees this process became the Integration Panel (IP). This group of scientists and breast cancer consumers reviews progress on an annual basis in preparation for an unusual process called vision setting, which drives the annual proposal solicitation process. After proposals are received, they are peer reviewed and come to the IP for programmatic review.

Each year the IP undertakes a strategy to fund a balanced portfolio of research that includes a selection of high-risk, high-gain projects and funding for under-represented areas such as behavioral research and programs that address underserved and minority populations. The results of these investments have been presented and publicly reviewed at three national meetings, the "Era of Hope Meetings," the most recent of which was held in 2005.

The BCRP has compiled a list of firsts, including having breast cancer survivors involved in all aspects of the program, and paradigm-shifting programs, such as innovative ideas grants that do not require preliminary data, innovator awards for scientists doing groundbreaking work, and translational awards. Many of the models and new mechanisms developed through the BCRP have been adopted by other agencies and organizations, creating new opportunities for synergy and collaboration to accelerate progress against breast cancer. In 1997 the Institute of Medicine issued a report titled "A Review of the Department of Defense's Program for Breast Cancer Research."[13] Among the conclusions of the report are that the BCRP has "successfully established a fair review system and a broad-based research portfolio," and that the BCRP fills "a unique niche among public and private funding sources for cancer research." Although these programs are now over 10 years old, advocates must rewin the funding each year through their lobbying efforts.

There is little doubt that the efforts of the breast cancer advocates in the 1990s and those who have come after them have changed the way we think about, perform, and evaluate cancer research. Perspectives have changed. Scientists feel a sense of real urgency and are willing to examine old approaches and consider new strategies, while cancer advocates have gained a better understanding of the research process and its inherent complexity. It is a model that optimizes the call for increased accountability of invested research dollars and rapid analysis and communication to the public.

The question of funding targeted research remains an issue, but it is now asked in the context of whether or not it is at the expense of traditional basic research that could theoretically benefit all cancers. In the mid-1990s, the scientific community was not favorably inclined toward targeted research; however, as the years have passed it has become clear that the two are not mutually exclusive. In the past few years, with increasing budget constraints, it has become clear that we must pay careful attention to the balance between targeted and nondirected research. We have learned many lessons in the 90s that will serve us well in the twenty-first century in terms of forging unique partnerships between cancer advocates and scientists. We must now use that experience to design and undertake innovative programs to address scientific and other barriers and capitalize on key opportunities that will accelerate progress against cancer.

The 1998 March, Coming Together to Conquer Cancer Cancer advocacy reached a major milestone in September 1998 when The March, Coming Together to Conquer Cancer was held in the Mall in Washington, DC. Although estimates of attendance vary from 300,000 to 500,000, the numbers are not nearly as important as the precedent. Americans from all walks of life united in activities and marches across the United States, and on the Mall, with a unifying theme: No more cancer. The goal of The March was to visibly demonstrate that Americans are concerned about the increasing human and economic burden of cancer, and to demand that the government commit the resources required to wage a full-scale war on cancer and win it. The major themes of The March were (1) to fully support a national cancer research agenda at the level required to ensure that scientific opportunities can be realized for the benefit of all cancer patients; and (2) that all Americans would have access to quality cancer care, especially the medically underserved and minority populations.

In order to design a specific cancer research agenda, The March Research Task Force was formed and charged with developing a plan that defined the major opportunities for accelerating progress against cancer and defining the barriers that stand in the way of realizing these critical milestones. The March Research Task Force was composed of 180 leading basic and clinical scientists, executives, survivors, and advocates from the leading academic cancer centers and private industry who worked in 13 subcommittees for over a year to develop recommendations that would cover the scope of cancer research from basic and clinical areas to prevention, behavior, and quality-of-life research. The theme of the task force was to think outside the box, determine what could be done if resources for research were made available to fund creative ideas and solutions to long-standing problems. The Report from the March Research Task Force[4] outlined a series of recommendations to realize both the exceptional range of scientific opportunities for progress and specific actions to remove the major barriers.

The Report from the Research Task Force was the first to highlight the potential impact of the changing demographics in America and the aging population on future cancer rates. The Report predicted that at current rates, the number of new cancer cases may increase by 29% and the number of cancer deaths may increase by 25% as early as 2010, and the cost of cancer will increase to over $200 billion a year.[4] It is interesting that 2001 estimates predict that the economic impact of cancer in 2010 will far exceed $200 billion. Finally, the Task Force addressed the issue of accountability, stating that implementation of the recommendations would reduce the incidence of cancer by 20% in 10 years, and as much as 30% in 20 years, and decrease mortality by 25% to 40% over this same period.

Some examples of major recommendations contained in this historic report (The Report from the March Research Task Force) were as follows:

- Double the NCI budget to $5.0 billion in 1999 and increase this budget by 20% per year for the next 4 years to a level of $10 billion by 2004.
- Develop public-private consortia to accelerate the development of new cancer therapies.
- Improve early detection technologies, establish risk profiling-based national programs for early detection programs, and educate the American public on their value.
- Double the nation's current investment in cancer prevention research, fund new Prevention Centers of Excellence and a nationwide tobacco research and control effort, and develop novel public-private partnerships to fund expensive cancer prevention clinical trials.
- Increase quality of life for all cancer patients through increased funding for behavioral and psychosocial, pain, and symptoms management research and improved end-of-life care.
- Increase research on disproportionate cancer rates in certain minority and medically underserved populations and ensure delivery of state-of-the-art care to all populations.
- Fully engage the private sector in cancer research through incentives such as tax credits, market exclusivity, and patent extension.
- Develop a new national cancer clinical trials system and increase patient participation on trials from 2% to 10%.
- Create a training program for clinical investigators through renewable 5-year grants and increase research grants to clinical investigators.
- Fully empower the NCI by reducing bureaucracy and policy constraints.

One of the long-term goals of The March was to create a new successor organization that would mobilize and move the American public in a broad advocacy movement, but such an organization did not emerge. However, The March set the stage for a new forum, the National Dialogue on Cancer, that is focused on establishing communication among a broad range of cancer organizations and on solving common problems. The March stands as the singular example of a national demonstration of the passion that drove the cancer advocacy movement of the 1990s: pain, frustration, and a desire to remove the shadow of cancer from the lives of all Americans—with a sense of urgency.

The National Dialogue on Cancer (Renamed C-Change) Although a successor organization did not emerge following The March, in late 1999, the American Cancer Society convened a small group of leaders from across the spectrum of cancer groups to create a forum that would facilitate information exchange and improve dialogue among the various organizations, sectors, and individuals that comprise the cancer community. This small group became the founding steering committee of the National Dialogue on Cancer (NDC). The organization was subsequently renamed C-Change in 2004. The history of the development of the NDC in many ways reflects the range of interests and agendas that now comprise the nation's cancer establishment. The construct, governance, funding, and the priorities of the NDC evolved into a formal organization in 2004.

Today C-Change is a working group of 160 collaborating partners who share a common mission of eliminating cancer as a major public health problem at the earliest possible time, and a 10-year goal of preventing an additional million new cancer cases and 500,000 cancer deaths.[14] C-Change is cochaired by former President George Bush and Barbara Bush. Senator Dianne Feinstein serves as the vice chairperson of C-Change. Members of the C-Change include heads of federal agencies (including the NCI and the CDC), chief executive officers of major pharmaceutical and other companies, nonprofit organizations, professional societies, elected officials, media personalities, etc. The NDC Web site in 2002[14] described the forum as a virtual town hall, with an opportunity to coalesce around specific problems or interest areas through the formation of issue-driven teams.

Six issue-driven teams in Cancer Research, Clinical Trials, Primary Prevention, Early Detection, State Cancer Plans, and Access to Quality Care currently represent the spectrum of focus areas through which C-Change takes action. The issue-driven teams generally focus on overarching issues and problems that affect all sectors. For example, the Cancer Research Team undertook a project to identify the major barriers to discovering and developing genomics- and proteomics-based cancer drugs. Through an unprecedented meeting in 2002[15] that involved all sectors, the team formed four working groups to pursue strategies for the removal of the top four barriers identified. Each of the other teams undertake similar complex problems that can be best solved through multisector efforts.

The National Cancer Legislative Advisory Committee The National Cancer Legislation Advisory Committee (NCLAC) was formed in late 1999 following a meeting of the then NDC, in which the NDC vice chairperson, Senator

Dianne Feinstein asked the group for a battle plan to conquer cancer. The senator's goal was to build on the success of the National Cancer Act of 1971 through new legislation that would update and extend the original act. She asked that the group (ultimately 21 experts from across the cancer research and advocacy communities) develop comprehensive recommendations that could provide the basis for policy and other government-led actions to re-energize and accelerate the nation's effort to conquer cancer. The NCLAC brought together more than 250 stakeholders from a wide range of communities, including scientists, cancer survivors, patient advocates, health care professionals, pharmaceutical and biotechnology executives, and leaders from federal agencies involved in the National Cancer Program. NCLAC issued its 50-page report[16] and recommendations, "Conquering Cancer: A National Battle Plan to Eradicate Cancer in our Lifetime", in September 2001.

The Committee's recommendations focused on four interdependent areas, including discovery (Goals 1–3), translation (Goals 4–6), access (Goals 7–9), and delivery (Goals 10–12) as follows: (1) Fund the National Cancer Institute (NCI) Bypass Budget in this and future years and provide additional supplemental funding for critical research that is not adequately covered in the Bypass Budget; (2) Increase the pool of talented and well-trained biomedical researchers; (3) Increase National Institute for Environmental Health Science (NIEHS) and NCI funding for cancer research that examines the interaction of genes and the environment; (4) Enhance our cancer research centers (and other cancer-focused efforts) to build a multidisciplinary network of translational centers to move new drugs and technologies forward into clinical trials, and ultimately to develop new methods and products to prevent and cure cancer; (5) Streamline and accelerate the Food and Drug Administration's approval system for cancer drugs, biologics, devices, and technologies; (6) Empower federal agencies to build public-private partnerships across the entire continuum of cancer research to ultimately develop new cancer treatments, preventatives, and technologies; (7) Provide adequate health insurance coverage for all Americans concerned about or diagnosed with cancer; (8) Significantly increase the pool of health care professionals trained to conquer cancer; (9) Launch a National Cancer Screening initiative to substantially increase the early detection of cancer; (10) Implement comprehensive state-based cancer action plans, in collaboration with all relevant experts in the region; (11) Develop, communicate, and use universal guidelines and practice standards to provide quality cancer care to all cancer patients, and monitor progress through improved quality care surveillance systems; and (12) Implement a National Cancer Prevention Initiative that focuses on eliminating tobacco use, increasing physical activity, and improving nutrition.

The NCLAC process and report were similar to the Yarborough Commission of 1971; and indeed, Senator Feinstein did create legislation, based in large part on the Committee's recommendations, and introduced it in early 2002. Unfortunately, the complexity of the legislative agenda in 2002 and lack of cohesive support from the cancer community resulted in the National Cancer Act not passing.

THE NATIONAL CANCER ACT OF 2002

During early 2002, Senator Dianne Feinstein developed and introduced cancer legislation on the basis of recommendations from the National Cancer Legislative Advisory Committee. This legislation was designed to modernize and revitalize the National Cancer Program that was created in 1971 by President Nixon. The scope of the National Cancer Act of 2002[17] was very diverse, including issues ranging from significantly increasing support for basic and translational cancer research to regulation of tobacco. The legislation called for more resources and authorities for the NCI and recommended that translation of laboratory advances be accelerated through the creation of translational cancer research centers, increased enrollment in clinical trials, and support for novel public-private partnerships. The legislation also proposed sweeping changes in the early detection and prevention of cancer through new screening and prevention programs that would require reimbursement by insurance companies. Specific aspects of this comprehensive cancer legislation would provide the following:

- Increased support for approved individual investigator-initiated research grants funded by the NCI to 40%.
- Increased salaries for postdoctoral cancer researchers and debt relief for medical school loans.
- Increased support for an increased number of clinical trials tied to a requirement for insurers to cover routine costs of trials.
- Expanded use of the Orphan Drug Act to provide incentives for the private sector to develop drugs for smaller cancer markets.
- An increase in the nation's workforce of cancer care providers through new recruitment and training programs sponsored by the Health Resources and Services Administration (HRSA).
- Wide availability of early cancer screening and detection with insurers required to cover selected costs.
- Funding for the Centers for Disease Control and Prevention (CDC) to aid states in the preparation of state cancer plans.
- Provide the US Food and Drug Administration (FDA) with the authorities to regulate tobacco products.

Unfortunately, the legislation did not pass and was not enacted.

The Impact of the 1990s Cancer Advocacy Movement One of the themes of cancer advocacy over the past 30 years has been the robust growth of major organizations like the American Cancer Society (ACS) with its broad agenda and mandate and the concomitant proliferation of disease-specific organizations with very narrow, focused, and well-financed agendas built around understanding, preventing, and treating very specific diseases. The best examples of these disease-specific organizations are perhaps among the breast cancer and prostate cancer groups, which have led the way in developing high levels of public recognition of these cancers, raising independent funding for cancer research, and effectively lobbying the legislative and executive branches of government on a variety of issues.

Although some could argue that the growth of these disease-specific organizations has come at the expense of a unified national cancer community and agenda, others would say that a national consensus across so many different diseases is not possible and that the achievements of these groups yielded results not otherwise possible. In point of fact, today there are organizations for nearly every form of cancer, and in some instances multiple organizations with the same disease focus, but with varying agendas. Some are narrowly focused on research, while others address a broad array of survivorship issues.

The bottom line is that there are more and more cancer advocates and organizations today that provide opportunities for focused volunteer activity. The cancer advocacy movement has increased public awareness and enhanced support for more public and private activities aimed at prevention, early detection, and the treatment of cancer. Taken together, the result of this broad movement is a better-informed citizenry who are more proactively demanding that the government take a more active role in defeating cancer with a real sense of urgency.

In turn, the federal government has responded with actions ranging from the doubling of the NIH budget to Senator Feinstein's National Cancer Act of 2002. The history of the cancer advocacy movement tracks closely with increasing resources for cancer research and a slowly evolving understanding of the critical need to capitalize on current opportunities in cancer research to achieve the NCI's 2015 challenge goal. This alliance will become even more important in the future. In the face of declining budgets and indications that the organizational structure of the NIH is likely to change, cancer research and the fate of our national effort to conquer cancer is increasingly in doubt.

FEDERAL POLICIES AND CANCER RESEARCH

In addition to funding for the continuum of cancer medicine research, development, and delivery, the federal government increasingly plays a major role in the process of medical research through the development of new policies and regulations. Although there are a number of areas where federal policy is having a major impact, perhaps the most important is in the critical area of the protection of patient privacy, specifically genetic privacy. A number of other important areas have attracted significant attention from both legislators and regulators, but in the postgenomics era, most take a backseat to the genetic privacy question.

Although Congress attempted to deal with the issue of protecting private health information over several years, they were never able to develop a bill that garnered sufficient bipartisan support for passage. This has been an ongoing area of debate where the parties agree that it is critical to protect a patient's personal health information, especially as we better understand the genetics of disease and all that it portends, while preserving the ability to conduct medical research.

On March 27, 2002, the U.S. Department of Health and Human Services (HHS) published proposed amendments to the privacy regulations that had first been published in December 2000. Subsequently, the final rule, Standards for Privacy of Individually Identifiable Health Information, was finalized and the comment period extended following the election of George W. Bush. Many of the more onerous provisions were removed following extensive feedback from organizations and individuals across the very diverse basic and clinical research communities. The final rule requires that an Institutional Review Board (IRB) review and approve any study that proposes to use medical records without patient consent. Although these studies can proceed if the IRB determines that the research could not be done otherwise, IRBs must now make decisions on whether or not the value of research outweighs the risk of infringing on patient privacy. Institutions are spending significantly more resources on setting up review boards to ensure compliance, and researchers are increasingly challenged to design studies that comply with these privacy regulations. The regulations as originally proposed have had a chilling effect on medical research, and as postgenomics research moves forward toward personalized medicine, the issues of patient privacy protection will become even more important. This area will continue to occupy all of the involved communities, but absent legislation, this rule will govern how medical research is conducted in the future.

Clinical Trials Access to quality cancer care continues to be an area of concern. One of the areas on which there is near uniform agreement is that if we are ever to achieve the nation's goal of preventing and curing cancer, patients must have access to state-of-the-art clinical trials. It is estimated that currently only 3% of adult cancer patients enroll in a cancer clinical trial each year versus being treated with agents that have limited therapeutic potential. Many members of Congress have embraced this issue, primarily because of their own personal experiences in confronting cancer, and historically have undertaken a number of policy initiatives to improve access to clinical trials. In addition, the cancer advocacy community has worked to increase access to clinical trials by lobbying for legislation to force private insurance companies to cover the standard of care associated with these trials.

Increasing participation in cancer clinical trials is an area where patient advocates, payers, scientists, and clinicians must work together with Congress to ensure that trials are conducted in a manner that protects patient privacy and facilitates the availability of safe, more efficacious agents to prevent cancer and cure more cancer patients. Ultimately, for many cancers, clinical trials must become the gold standard for quality cancer care. To accomplish this goal, the reimbursement problem must be solved—presumably through legislative mandate.

THE FUTURE

As we enter the twenty-first century, it is becoming apparent to scientists, politicians, the private sector, cancer advocates, and the American public that cancer is a national problem of staggering current and future human and financial impact that requires a great deal more of our attention and resources. The aging of America's baby boomers will produce unprecedented numbers of new cancer cases in the next 15 to 20 years, and the poor, medically underserved and minority populations of America suffer a disproportionate burden of cancer. In retrospect, if the National Cancer Act of 1971 had not been passed and a war on cancer declared, something similar would have eventually been required to address the human and economic costs of cancer.

Our past investments in cancer and biomedical research have paid huge dividends, and mortality rates for certain cancers are declining. We have entered the golden age of biology and biotechnology. Never have we had greater potential to make real and substantial progress against cancer. The human genome provides unprecedented opportunities for creating new targeted therapeutics and preventives: immunotherapy, gene therapy, and vaccines, which are maturing into clinical practicality, and for the first time we can think rationally about preventing cancer in targeted ways.

As a result of progress across the continuum of cancer research, we now understand cancer as a disease process, which provides clear opportunities for targeted therapies and diagnostics. In addition, advances in enabling technologies are empowering fields such as genomics, nanotechnology, proteomics, and bioinformatics, and they are moving at an unprecedented pace. Fueled by a vision of a world where people no longer die from cancer, but instead live long and productive lives with a chronic and manageable condition, the NCI has challenged the cancer research community to capitalize on this revolution and move strategically to eliminate the suffering and death from cancer in the next decade. As outlined in "The Nation's Investment in Cancer Research,"[17] the director of the NCI has called on the entire cancer research enterprise to rise to this challenge and transform cancer into a manageable chronic disease. Achieving this vision will require that a significant number of strategic enterprise initiatives be successfully implemented, including programs in integrative (systems) cancer biology; advanced technologies, such as advanced imaging and nanotechnology; bioinformatics; integrated clinical trials; and programs in cancer prevention, early detection, and the elimination of health disparities.

Paradoxically, at this time of greatest promise and hope from research, we face unprecedented uncertainty. Federal resources for cancer research are decreasing; managed care leaves little time or money to pursue clinical research, funds for training a new generation of scientists and clinicians are extremely limited, cancer advocacy groups are demanding attention to their disease, and regulatory and profitability pressures combine to decrease the interest of the private sector in developing new cancer therapies and preventives. Clearly, Congress and the administration must empower and fund the NCI and other federal health organizations to take a more proactive leadership role, especially in the areas of strategy development and coordination. We must also optimize and leverage the investment of federal resources and identify new sources of funds to remove barriers and accelerate the pace of translating laboratory advances to patients. As we address new threats that America faces at home and around the world, we must also strengthen our resolve to protect the health of our citizens by rededicating ourselves to eliminating the specter of cancer with a renewed sense of urgency.

REFERENCES

1. American Association for Cancer Research (AACR). Americans' attitudes toward cancer research: a poll commissioned by the AACR. Peter Hart Research Associates, Inc. and Speakout.com; August 2000.
2. American Cancer Society. Cancer Facts and Figures. 2004.
3. Polednak AP. Projected numbers of cancers diagnosed in the US elderly population, 1990 through 2030. Am J Public Health 1994;84:1313–6.
4. Sigal EV, Barker AD. Report from the March Research Task Force. Cancer Res 1998;58:5590–627.
5. National Cancer Institute. The nation's investment in cancer research: a plan and budget proposal for fiscal year 2003. 2002.
6. P.L. 244, 75th Congress. The National Cancer Institute Act of 1937. S. 2607; 1937.
7. National Cancer Institute. Closing in on cancer: solving a 5000-year old mystery. 1998.
8. P.L. 92-218, 92nd Congress. The National Cancer Act of 1971. S. 1828; 1971.
9. P.L. 103-43, 93rd Congress. NIH Revitalization Amendments of 1993. S. 1641; 1993.
10. National Cancer Institute. NCI fact book 2003. 2004.
11. Druker BJ, Talpaz M, Resta DJ, et al. Efficacy and safety of a specific inhibitor of the BCR-ABL tyrosine kinase in chronic myeloid leukemia. N Engl J Med 2001;344:1031–7.
12. Funding First: An Initiative of the Mary Woodward Lasker Charitable Trust. Exceptional returns: the economic value of America's investment in medical research. May 2000.
13. Institute of Medicine. A review of the department of defense's program for breast cancer research. Washington DC: Institute of Medicine, National Academy Press; 1997.
14. National Dialogue on Cancer (Renamed C-Change). The mission and vision of the NDC. www.ndc.org; 2002.
15. National Dialogue on Cancer. Cancer research team, Optimizing the discovery and development of genomics/proteomics based cancer drugs: a forum to explore public private and other partnerships, Washington D.C.; February 28–March 2, 2002.
16. National Cancer Legislative Committee. Conquering cancer: a national battle plan to eradicate cancer in our lifetime. September 2001.
17. S. 1976. 107th Congress, The National Cancer Act of 2002. February 2002.
18. The National Cancer Institute. The nation's investment in cancer research. A plan and proposal for 2006.

Delivering High-Quality Cancer Care in a Changing Health Care Environment

Martin N. Raber, MD
Ronald S. Walters, MD

For more than a decade, the American health care system has been buffeted by successive waves of change. The original mandate for reform was driven in part by large employers, who, along with the government, bear the major costs of health care. These employers believed that uncontrolled increases in health care costs threatened the profitability of American industry in a global economy. Employers also believed that the medical reimbursement system was flawed in that the providers of health care (the physician and the hospital) were rewarded for overuse of resources, whereas the payers (employers and government) had no one acting on their behalf to eliminate waste and control costs. Similarly, the government felt that uncontrolled increases in Medicare and Medicaid costs threatened the economic stability of the country. A third driver of change was the political ideal that all Americans should receive adequate health care and that if we controlled overuse, we could afford to insure everyone.

This political discussion was mirrored by an intellectual discussion driven by a group of health care economists informally referred to as the Jackson Hole group, named after the site of their meetings. This group, heavily influenced by the health maintenance organization (HMO) experience, provided a model for reform.[1,2] Although government reform of the health care system did not emerge from the legislative process, industry adopted the model and initiated a "market-driven" reform of the health care system.[3] In fact, what has been reformed, thus far, has been the health care payment system and not the delivery system itself.[3] Nevertheless, these changes have had a significant impact on the treatment of patients with cancer.

EFFECTS OF HEALTH CARE REFORM

The HMO model on which health care reform was based led to a health care reimbursement methodology referred to as "managed care." At its essence, managed care attempts to control health care costs by linking providers into defined networks that trade price for access to patients controlled by insurers or other risk holders. Costs are controlled through case management and often by passing some of the insurance risk to the providers themselves. Patients are assigned to physician gatekeepers, who are often at financial risk of specialty care referrals. As managed care took hold across America, it forced tremendous consolidation among physician and hospital providers and eventually among insurers, HMOs, and the managed care organizations themselves.

In the short term, income was transferred from providers (hospitals and physicians) to insurers and managed care organizations. Physician and hospital reimbursement decreased significantly. Hospitals reduced their bed capacities and increased efficiency. As reimbursement continued to fall, hospitals remained busy, but profit margins in the industry fell. Physicians are in a similar situation, finding themselves to be working harder and seeing more patients but receiving less reimbursement.

This initial reform effort was followed by a series of efforts led by different groups trying to control health care costs. In successive waves, employers, politicians (through Medicare payment reform), insurers, and Wall Street investors have all tried to "reform health care delivery" by altering the reimbursement system.[4] The savings were passed on to insurers and investors as corporate profits and to employers in the form of stable premiums. Unfortunately, the savings were ephemeral. Although inefficiencies were eliminated, as new pharmaceutical and diagnostic technologies developed and patients demanded open access to physicians, costs rose rapidly, often leaving the insurers with significant losses. Health care went through a series of consolidations of hospitals, physician practices, and insurers. Many of these consolidation attempts have failed. Although it is true that today we have fewer health care insurers, more hospital networks, and fewer solo medical practitioners, one might erroneously conclude that the basic structure of health care delivery has been changed. Throughout most of the country, delivery of health care remains determined by local issues, and, from the physician's perspective, health care remains very much a series of "cottage industries." These unstructured efforts have significantly changed American medicine in ways not predicted by the original architects.

Now, after more than a decade of reform efforts, patients, providers, and insurers all find themselves in many ways in a worse position than when we began yet facing the same problems that started the upheaval. Medical costs, after a short period of control, continue to rise rapidly. Businesses feel that increasing health care costs threaten their profitability and, in the case of small businesses, their very existence. The government is faced with the threat of significant Medicare shortfalls. Hospitals and physicians are continually challenged to provide more service for less reimbursement, and more Americans are uninsured today than ever in recent history, straining the public hospital systems.

Current reform efforts focus on shifting more of the burden to the true consumer of health care, the patient. At the employer level, this is done by increasing copays. At the national level, this is manifested in the move to medical savings accounts. In both cases, the underlying philosophy is that if patients realize that they are, in fact, paying real money for the care given, they will be a better "consumer" of the services. This, in part, has fostered the idea of "consumerism in health care," that is to say viewing health care as a commodity, with the "user" of services seeking to discover those purchasing options that deliver the greatest "value," however that is defined.[5,6]

FACTORS IMPACTING CANCER CARE

Although these changes have implications for all physicians, the unique aspects of oncology suggest that the effects of health care reform may be different for oncology providers and patients than in the case of other illnesses. These unique aspects include the following.

Impact of the Aging of the American Population Although the actual incidence of cancer in the United States in 2001 was estimated to be 469 in 100,000 and has likely fallen since its peak in 1992,[7] worldwide, the World Health Organization predicts a 50% increase in cancer incidence to 15 million new cases in 2020. The incidence of many cancers is age related, and since, with better treatments and supportive care, cancer is becoming a chronic disease, the aging of the population will significantly increase the prevalence of cancer in the United States over the next 20 years. In 2000, about 17% of the population was over 60 years of age; by 2020, it will be about 25%. The National Cancer Institute estimates that in 2001, there were 9.8 million cancer survivors, or about 3.5% of the population, 61% of whom were over 65 years of age. Interestingly enough, 14% of these survivors were diagnosed more than 20 years ago. The average age of the cancer survivor is now 69 years for males and 64 years for females. It is also known that cancer in the elderly population is associated with increased comorbid conditions, complicating therapy. The appropriate management of elderly cancer patients is not entirely clear and is an area currently under intense study.

Against the background of this expected remarkable increase in the prevalence of cancer patients is the issue of medical manpower. When last assessed by the American Society of Clinical Oncologists (ASCO) in the mid-1990s, medical oncology manpower was felt to be adequate. Since then, we have not seen significant increases in the number of oncology training positions. As the population ages and the large cohort of oncologists trained in the late 1970s and early 1980s retires, the country may well find itself lacking enough trained oncologists to provide excellent cancer care.

New Technology As the fruits of the revolution in molecular biology become apparent, the pace of introduction of new anticancer drugs is quickening. There are currently over 150 new agents in active testing, most of which will be part of the routine care of cancer patients in the near future. Agents such as imatinib, gefitinib, bevacizumab, and bortezomib, to name a few, are only the beginning of a new age in chemotherapy. These new drugs tend to be target specific and, although active, probably not curative as single agents. They also tend to be expensive, increasing significantly the cost of cancer care.

New technology is not limited to therapeutics. New diagnostic techniques, both laboratory based and imaging, are changing our diagnostic strategies and increasing the cost of cancer care. The use of positron emission tomography (PET) and combined computed tomography (CT)-PET examinations, three-dimensional conformational imaging, and microarray analysis of tumors will only increase over the coming years, and the pace of newer technology development is increasing.

Another aspect of the problem of increasing numbers of cancer patients relates to the development of successful therapies for previously incurable cancers. As treatment recommendations in common tumors, such as breast and colon cancer, have changed, patients are being followed and treated by oncologists for a longer period of time, adding to the already strained cancer delivery system.

Need for Specialized Treatment Although the training of general internists provides experience with cancer patients, after the diagnosis is made, most primary care physicians feel uncomfortable making therapeutic decisions and administering treatment. Although the role of the general internist and family practitioner in the prevention, screening, and diagnosis of cancer remains paramount, the treatment of cancer patients remains the domain of specialists. In our experience, most primary care physicians prefer that specialists continue to follow-up cancer patients even after the acute treatment phase of the illness is over. With increasing numbers of cancer patients, this may become a luxury that the country cannot afford.

Furthermore, as discussed above, because cancer is becoming a chronic disease with more effective therapy, the length of life and the length of treatment are increasing significantly, requiring longer periods of time being treated by these specialists.

Multidisciplinary Treatment of Cancer Unlike many other illnesses, the treatment of patients with cancer often requires a prospectively designed multidisciplinary treatment plan. This requires the collaboration of a team of specialists. The organization of such a team is beyond the expertise of general practitioners and internists. This is a particularly difficult issue in health care environments in which the provision of care is not well organized because of competitive forces. Reward systems currently favor the individual practitioner's care and not that of the team approach to treatment required by most patients.

Need to Incorporate Clinical Research in the Practice of Oncology Given the overall poor results of systemic therapy for patients with metastatic cancer, it is not surprising that oncologists have always been quick to incorporate new strategies and new therapies into treatment plans. Today, more than ever before, with an increasing number of new compounds entering clinical trials, the participation of all oncologists is needed to speed the process of cancer drug development. In fact, the division between the academic centers, formally the "home" of clinical trials, and the private practitioner disappeared with the development of CCOPs, research networks, and similar arrangements. Unfortunately, regulatory and reimbursement issues remain significant barriers to increasing the numbers of patients entering clinical trials. If we are to be successful, we must develop strategies to facilitate the conduct of our trials and participation at the community level.

Demands of Patients Facing Terminal Illnesses When faced with terminal disease, the American patient is particularly demanding in searching for information and treatment options. Widespread Internet access has significantly increased the information available. This need is met best by specialists broadly knowledgeable in the natural history and therapeutic options available. These specialists must be current in the latest results of clinical trials and must serve as a counselor and a reference standard for patients who wish to pursue alternative treatment. They also must be expert in the ethical and social issues surrounding management of patients with fatal illnesses and the resources required for such care.

Given the changes in demographics and treatment outlined above, it is apparent that cancer is becoming a chronic illness of increasing frequency in the population, with significantly improved treatments available at significantly increased costs, in a health care system that is rapidly changing through the introduction of new technology, increased demands for service and quality, and severe financial constraints.

BARRIERS TO ACHIEVING EFFICIENT, HIGH-QUALITY CANCER CARE

Peculiarities of Cancer Care Reimbursement In a health care system designed in an earlier era, it is not surprising that the reimbursement system currently being used has a number of anomalies when applied to the treatment of cancer patients. Most significant are the regulations that apply to coverage of outpatient cancer therapy treatments. These include regulations relating to coverage of oral anticancer agents by Medicare and the more vexing problem of bundling drug and administration costs together in the price paid for pharmaceuticals. Both of these issues are currently under study by Congress.[8] Cancer care is expensive and getting more so. An example of the constant movement toward progress is the replacement of an older agent, tamoxifen, and its lower cost, with the newer, more effective aromatase inhibitors, at a higher cost.

Lack of Standardized Information Systems In contrast to relatively standardized, defined data sets for other diseases, such as diabetes, asthma, and congestive heart failure, the corresponding data sets do not yet exist for oncology. This is partly related to the complexity of the disease, as well as its breadth. The sheer number of cancer diagnoses, staging implications for each, and patient factors all work to complicate the development of such standardized systems. This directly translates into difficulty reaching widespread concordance regarding an electronic medical record for cancer, a common, workable coding system for billing, and a useable system for making comparisons across populations. The recent CMS initiative to achieve a national health care information technology infrastructure, headed by Dr. David Brailer, is still very much in the early stages of planning.[9]

Government Regulation Certainly, all individuals would want their most private medical information to be held in the utmost privacy and made available only to those who require this information to provide medical care. Arguably, however, the enactment of the Health Insurance Portability and Accountability Act of 1996 has and will continue to impact the delivery of medical care more than any other legislation.[10]

Increasing Demand for the Elusive Definition of "Quality" in Cancer Care With the consumer demanding clear definitions for value-driven health care, and with payers, both private and governmental, indicating that those systems that clearly demonstrate such "quality" will be favorably reimbursed, the need is greater than ever to define exactly what constitutes high-quality cancer care. One of the first problems encountered in arriving at such a definition is to consider from whose perspective it is being defined. It is quite obvious that the perspectives of the patient and family members, private or governmental payers, the oncologist providing the care, the hospital system in which it is being delivered, and all other providers may well differ. In fact, one of the challenging concepts underlying the application of consumerism to health care is that, as in other industries, the "most important" perspective is that of the consumer, that is, the patient. In medicine, that perspective is only one of many, and the consumer is not necessarily as well informed as he or she may be in other marketplaces—thus, the difficulty in prioritizing cost, efficiency, outcomes, quality of life, quantity of life, adherence to standard treatment protocols, and other potential measures.

Nonetheless, although most current definitions of "quality" focus on administrative data weighted toward use ratios, it is quite clear that these represent only one perspective about quality. Certainly, patient satisfaction, performance according to national clinical standards, and more traditional disease-specific outcomes measures are important to such a definition.

Even though the precise definition of quality has not been standardized in relation to cancer care delivery, it is a caveat that there exists a direct correlation between the delivery of high-quality care, improved outcomes, and efficient use of resources. Thus, it would appear to be a truism that the highest quality care will also be the most cost-effective in the long run.

CURRENT STRATEGIES FOR THE DELIVERY OF CANCER CARE

The training and development of a cadre of cancer specialists over the past three decades, coupled with significant scientific advancement, have resulted in the current era of high-quality, multidisciplinary cancer care. Although it can be argued that the system of unrestricted reimbursement resulted in the overuse of medical resources and in some cases the over treatment of some patients, it also allowed physicians to focus on the individual patient's needs and provide the optimum treatment available.

In this period of uncertainty, when many different reimbursement systems are being used simultaneously and there is continued change in reimbursement philosophy, oncologists must develop a comprehensive approach that provides appropriate care for all patients at what the community considers acceptable costs and the physician considers adequate reimbursement. This requires strategies that result in predictable costs and predictable outcomes, in a setting in which evaluation of outcome is feasible. It also requires a plan that allows for multidisciplinary care, broad access to clinical trials, and the incorporation of new, effective therapies as they become available.

In general, the following steps are critical to the delivery of high-quality cancer care:

1. The diagnosis must be accurate.
2. The stage of the patient must be clearly and accurately defined.
3. There should be a multidisciplinary process in the planning of care.
4. An assessment should be made as to the experience of the disciplines involved in the treatment of that disease (volume-outcome relationships).
5. An assessment should be made as to the potential relative contributions of "standard care" to that of a more investigational approach.
6. There should be an attempt to apply the use of nationally adopted guidelines or pathways.
7. There should be an objective, prospective process to obtain outcomes for the unbiased assessment of comparison to national standards ("scorecards").
8. The culture of care should support the "right treatment" being given for the "right diagnosis" at the "right location" and at the "right time."

Getting the Diagnosis Correct It seems a bit obvious, but since all therapeutic decisions are diagnosis based, any discrepancy in the diagnosis could lead to an inappropriate care plan. As recently as 1999, a study by Kronz and colleagues demonstrated that although the overall rate of change of diagnosis was very small, 1.4% in that study, it was site variable, and yet the impact on therapeutic decisions could be great.[11] Although most obvious in the hematologic malignancies and tumors with neuroendocrine differentiation, every disease site specialist can give examples of how subtle differences in pathology impact treatment decisions. In breast cancer, for example, it is not infrequent to have differing opinions regarding invasive, "microinvasive," and noninvasive disease classifications.[12]

Getting the Stage of Disease Correct As critical as the correct diagnosis is to the treatment decision, the same is true for having the patient properly staged, whether it be by surgery, radiology, or both. The Society of Surgical Oncology maintains on its Web page criteria for the proper training of surgical techniques in the diagnosis, staging, and therapy of cancer.[13] As discussed below and in the volume-outcome relationship literature, the effect is not only on surgical expertise in the removal of the cancer but, as stressed by the Society of Surgical Oncology, proper clarification of surgical stage.[14] However, outside an academic medical center, the majority of cancer surgery is performed by general surgeons, or even specialty-based surgeons, for whom only a part of their practice is oncology related.

The advent of newer technologies on stage migration was described in 1985 by Feinstein and colleagues.[15] It is important to bear this in mind as new technologies become incorporated into standard practice, bearing with them the potential for false-positive stage assignments and the resulting treatment decisions. The newer "screening" procedures, such as PET and PET-CT, are capable of demonstrating very minute abnormalities, thus raising the specter of false-positives and yet potentially affecting basic treatment decisions.

Incorporating a Multidisciplinary Planning Process The most important decision, once the diagnosis and the stage have been confirmed, is when, where, and by whom therapy is initiated. In the community, this process is usually quite dependent on referral processes and the communication between practicing physicians. Quite frequently, selected patients are presented at tumor boards with representation of the major specialties present. A more formalized process occurs in many of the academic medical centers, often with patient-specific planning conferences. No one process is superior to another as long as the principle of adequate discussion of the situation is facilitated, with the opportunity to examine the application of evidence-based practices to the individual patient case, prior to the initiation of therapy.[16]

Volume-Outcome Relationship The relationship between volumes of procedures performed and subsequent outcomes has been the subject of much controversy.[17,18] Although probably an intuitive concept, it is perceived to threaten the very existence of much of the practice of oncology in the community. Volume-outcome relationships have been published for a few select cancers. Although a higher volume generally is correlated with better outcomes, it remains to be determined how many is enough, over what time frame, what constitutes superior outcomes, and, more importantly, if all of the foregoing are established, how one achieves the sufficient experience if patients are directed elsewhere for treatments. Nonetheless, this continues to be a relevant question, especially as consumers, payers, and business-driven groups demand this information for the choice of location of care.

Assessment and Incorporation of Clinical Research The cost of patient care in clinical trials is an important issue for patients, physicians, and payers. The recognition that a clinical trial in a cancer patient may be state-of-the-art therapy and not an experiment is clear to patient advocacy groups and professionals but not yet completely accepted by payers and insurers. The actual added costs of clinical trials are much debated, without good data.[19,20] Historically, clinical investigators have cost-shifted their hospital and professional charges to support research. Although the costs of specific investigational drugs and the costs related to data management are often paid by the sponsor of a study, patient care unrelated costs have usually been paid by a third-party payer. In the new reimbursement paradigms, the clinical costs associated with clinical investigations are not always reimbursed. It is felt by insurers and employers that these charges should be paid by the study sponsor. In oncology, where many major advances have been made by academic investigators in unsponsored studies conducted after US Food and Drug Administration (FDA) drug approval, the problem is significant. Since there is no effective therapy for many cancer patients, the pressure to pursue experimental treatments is intense, and the patient and physician may find themselves in a situation in which approved therapies known to be ineffective are reimbursed, whereas promising, investigational treatments will not be paid for.

The resolution of this problem has taken many forms and is an ongoing issue of debate. A number of states have passed laws requiring insurers to pay for costs associated with therapeutic clinical trials. In 2000, the federal government decided to cover the clinical costs associated with "qualified" clinical trials in the Medicare program, setting a reasonable standard.[21]

Although these issues have not been completely resolved, oncologists need to have a responsible approach to the treatment of patients with today's incurable cancers. The concept that care will not be reimbursed if it is given in the context of a clinical trial regardless of the agents used is not tenable. Patients who receive drugs for FDA-approved indications at the approved dose and schedule should have their care reimbursed, regardless of participation in a trial, particularly if the costs are similar to those of conventional therapy. The "off-label" use of anticancer drugs is an important issue because many of our most active drugs are used for indications that are not specifically approved. It is reasonable that patients receiving drugs used for off-label indications in diseases in which their efficacy has been demonstrated should be reimbursed under the same conditions outlined above. Unfortunately, the implementation of this philosophy remains to a great degree in the hands of regional Medicare carriers, and there can be significant geographic variability in coverage decisions.

A more difficult situation arises with drugs that are of unproven benefit. Most current insurance policies exclude investigational therapy, and the use of these agents is often not reimbursed or reimbursable. The federal guidelines require that the trial have a "therapeutic" intent. When the experimental agent is given along with drugs approved for treatment of the disease, insurers should be willing to pay the charges associated with the standard treatment. In those cases in which the experimental drugs are given alone for disease states in which there is no known effective therapy, the investigational nature of the treatment must be acknowledged and a source of support identified.

Application of Appropriate Guidelines and Pathways The ability to deliver high-quality health care in an environment in which cost is a primary consideration depends on broad agreement among specialists about the management of the common cancers. Guidelines are an overview of cancer treatments appropriately sequenced for the management of specific clinical presentations. These guidelines must include the common presentations of cancer patients and detail the multidisciplinary approach. Such a consensus approach allows some uniformity of pretreatment evaluation, treatment planning, and follow-up for patients across the country and allows providers to better estimate the costs of therapy. This approach also has the advantage of protecting providers against accusations of negligence or concerns that the pressures to reduce cost have unreasonably affected treatment planning.

Guidelines as defined above have been developed across the country through large specialty societies, such as the ASCO, the National Cancer Center Network, cancer centers, and groups of providers.[22] They have become standard practices in many communities and are published and available from many sources. In oncology, the concept of the use of guidelines is acceptable to most oncologists and can be effective in decreasing cost and improving outcomes.[23] The success of these guidelines is also apparent in their acceptance by payers and insurers as the standard of care. This has greatly simplified the approval process with insurers, as well as negotiations with governmental agencies.

Clinical pathways provide a more detailed approach to patient management and allow the individual groups of providers to detail their specific resource use (eg, specific chemotherapy regimens, drug doses and schedules, schedules for imaging studies, follow-up parameters). Although there is great uniformity in the guidelines developed to date, there is more diversity in the specifics of the clinical pathways being developed. At the same time that these standardized approaches to care are being developed, providers must also develop case management systems to ensure that the approaches agreed on are being followed and to deal with patients whose clinical situations do not fit a clear pathway. Most case management remains centered on hospitalized patients because the inpatient arena still encompasses a large portion of the expense of treating patients. However, to truly control costs and outcomes, this approach will need to be integrated into the outpatient setting and be extended to the management of the entire course of the disease. Disease management programs in cancer have recently begun to emerge, developed by insurers, "disease management companies," and academic centers. These programs attempt to organize and oversee the delivery of all cancer-related care in a defined population, usually based on inpatient and outpatient case management centered on clinical guidelines. Although interesting, the cost-effectiveness of this approach has not yet been demonstrated.

Application of Prospective, Objective Self-Assessment of Outcomes From an ethical perspective, as well as being demanded more frequently by consumers, it is the responsibility of the individual practitioner to be capable of a self-assessment of his or her individual practice outcomes in relation to those of others. Internalizing the "report card" process can only serve to optimize the "right care, right place, right time" decision in relation to the individual patient. Unfortunately, most practitioners do not have the system infrastructure to support this practice, relying primarily on their memory of the extremes and an internally cultivated viewpoint of "what they feel comfortable" treating. Extending this assessment to their "referred from" and "referred to" associates increases the variability and decreases the amount of actual data available. Nonetheless, consumers are demanding that the individual practitioner be able to answer, in some detail, "how many of what" have they done and what the outcomes have been. This movement is being assimilated into networks of "sanctioned" providers, based on actual patient outcomes. Thus, it behooves each practitioner to formalize the development of such systems.

FUTURE DIRECTIONS IN HEALTH CARE REFORM

Predicting the future of health care reform in America is clearly not possible. If we look back at the objectives enunciated in 1992, the current attempts at reform transiently held health care premiums stable. We are now currently once again experiencing double-digit increases. We have more uninsured Americans than before we began the reform process. Both patients and physicians are unhappy with the current system. The HMO model, which drove the initial process, has been shown to be unacceptable to the public, who continue to demand "choice" of provider and unfettered access to specialists. Economically, this is not viable in our current "for profit" model. In many ways, we have not reformed health care delivery. Rather, we have altered the payment system. If we are to truly accomplish the initial goals of the reform movement, we will need to change the delivery system more fundamentally.

However, one prediction is certainly likely to be true. As in other markets, the public will expect to receive high-quality cancer care in an affordable system while maintaining the ability to choose their providers based on transparent, accessible results.

REFERENCES

1. Enthoven A. A consumer-choice health plan for the 1990s. Universal health insurance in a system designed to promote quality and economy (1) and (2). N Engl J Med 1989;320:29–37.
2. Enthoven A. N Engl J Med 1989;320:94–101.
3. Enthoven A. The Fortune 500 model for health care: is now the time to change? J Health Polit Policy Law 2002;227:37–48.
4. Brown LD. Comparing health systems in four countries: lessons for the United States. Am J Public Health 2003;93:52–6.
5. Crawshaw R. Grass roots participation in health care reform. Ann Intern Med 1994;120:677–81.
6. Rosenthal M, Milstein A. Awakening consumer stewardship of health benefits: prevalence and differentiation of new health plan models. Health Serv Res 2004;39(4 Pt 2):1055–70.
7. National Cancer Institute cancer progress report 2003.
8. Colloquy on Cancer Care Reimbursement, Proceedings and Debates of the 108th Congress, First Session.
9. US Department of Health and Human Services press office release. May 6, 2004.
10. Turner GM. HIPAA and the criminalization of American medicine. Healthcare News 2001; Oct 1.
11. Kronz JD, Westra WH, Epstein JI. Mandatory second opinion surgical pathology at a large referral hospital. Cancer 1999;86:2426–35.
12. Staradub VL, Messenger KA, et al. Changes in breast cancer therapy because of pathology second opinions. Ann Surg Oncol 2002;9:982–7.
13. Training Committee of the Society of Surgical Oncology. Society of Surgical Oncology requirements for surgical oncology training. 2001.
14. Hodgson CD, Zhang W, Zavlasky AM, et al. Relationship of hospital volume to colostomy rates and survival for patients with rectal cancer. J Natl Cancer Inst 2003;95:708–16.
15. Feinstein AR, Sosin DM, Wells CK. The Will Rogers phenomenon. Stage migration and new diagnostic techniques as a source of misleading statistics for survival in cancer. N Engl J Med 1985;312:1604–8.
16. Zorbas H, Barraclough B, Rainbird K, et al. Multidisciplinary care for women with early breast cancer in the Australian context: what does it mean? Med J Aust 2003;179:528–31.
17. Birkmeyer NJ, Goodney PP, Stukel KT, et al. Do cancer centers designated by the National Cancer Institute have better surgical outcomes? Cancer 2004;103:435–41.
18. Panageas KS, Schrag D, Riedel E, et al. Effect of clustering on the association of procedure volume and surgical outcomes. Ann Intern Med 2003;139:658–65.
19. Brown ML. Cancer patient care in clinical trials sponsored by the National Cancer Institute: what does it cost? J Natl Cancer Inst 1999;91:818–9.
20. RAND Corporation. J Clin Oncol 2001;19:105–10.
21. CMS memorandum. National coverage decision June 7, 2000.
22. National Comprehensive Cancer Network. Clinical practice guidelines in oncology.
23. Bahtsevani C, Uden G, Willman A. Outcomes of evidence-based practice guidelines: a systematic review. Int J Technol Assess Health Care 2004;20:427–33.

Part VI
Cancer Management

Section 23

CENTRAL NERVOUS SYSTEM

72

Primary Neoplasms of the Central Nervous System in Adults

Michael D. Prados, MD

Tumors of the central nervous system (CNS) represent a unique, heterogeneous population of both benign and malignant neoplasms. In recent years, there have been significant gains in our understanding of the molecular events associated with the malignant phenotype that will hopefully result in improved survival and quality of life. Over the course of the last several decades, with improved surgical techniques and radiation oncology technology, survival has improved slightly for the most malignant glioma, glioblastoma multiforme (GBM); however, older adults with this disease rarely live longer than 1 year. Much more research is required, both preclinically and in human trials, to finally achieve long-term control, and, ultimately, a cure for primary brain tumors. A multi-disciplinary clinical approach along with constant dialogue with tumor biologists has become more prevalent, and thus the future of neuro-oncology is becoming increasingly hopeful.

EPIDEMIOLOGY

The overall annual incidence rate of primary benign and malignant brain tumors in the United States is estimated at 14.1 cases per 100,000 person-years (CBTRUS Statistical Report 1997–2001).[1] The incidence of primary malignant brain tumors is 6.4 per 100,000 person-years, with a higher incidence in males (7.6 per 100,000 person-years) than in females (5.3 per 100,000 person-years).[1] A very consistent epidemiologic finding is that neuroepithelial tumors occur more frequently in males (GBMs are 1.6 times more common in men), whereas benign meningiomas are almost twice as common in females.[1] An estimated 41,000 new cases of primary brain tumors are expected to be diagnosed each year, with a prevalence rate of 130.8 per 100,000. Primary brain tumors are the second most common cancer in childhood, with an incidence of 4.0 per 100,000 person-years.[2] An estimated 3,200 new cases of childhood primary brain tumors are expected each year, the majority of whom will be less than 15 years of age.

Tumors of neuroepithelial origin account for approximately 49% of CNS tumors (GBMs comprise the majority at 23%), meningiomas account for 26% of CNS tumors, sellar tumors 7%, cranial and spinal nerve tumors 7%, CNS lymphomas 3%, and other brain tumor types 8%.[1] For males between the ages of 15 and 34 years, CNS tumors are the third leading cause of cancer death; for females in this same age group, they are the fourth leading cause of cancer deaths. For boys younger than age 15 years, brain and other CNS tumors are the second leading cause of death after leukemia, whereas for girls younger than age 15 years they are the leading cause of cancer deaths.

The average age of onset for all primary brain tumors is 54 years, although this figure varies depending on the histologic tumor type. The average age of onset for both GBMs and meningiomas is 62 years, whereas for medulloblastomas the mean age of onset is 16 years. The highest incidence for all brain tumors occurs in the 75- to 84-year-old age group, with GBMs occurring most frequently in patients older than age 65 years.[1] In children, the peak incidence occurs in patients younger than 4 years of age. The most common histologies in the pediatric age group are the embryonal tumors (eg, medulloblastoma) and pilocytic (grade I) astrocytomas, which together account for more than 30% of all childhood brain tumors.[1]

An increase in the incidence and mortality of brain tumors in adults has been noted over the past several decades, reaching as high as 300% in developed countries. For children, the incidence of primary malignant brain tumors has increased approximately 35% over the same time period.[3] Some of these increases are certainly a result of better diagnostic imaging and improved access to medical care. However, other causal factors may be important in this trend, and until specific risk factors are identified, the full explanation for these increases is still awaited. Males have a 0.67% lifetime risk of being diagnosed with a primary malignant brain tumor (excluding lymphoma) and a 0.49% lifetime risk of dying from such a diagnosis. For females, the lifetime risk is 0.52% for diagnosis and 0.40% of dying from a primary malignant brain tumor.[1]

The relative 2- and 5-year survival rates for patients with primary malignant brain tumors are 36.2% and 27.6%, respectively. Five-year relative survival rate for patients with pilocytic astrocytomas is 87.2%, but is only 3.2% in GBM patients.[4] Thus, age and tumor histology are very significant prognostic factors, even more so than treatment modality. Other prognostic indicators that may influence survival include extent of disease, extent of resection, and tumor location. For all meningiomas, the 2- and 5-year overall survival rates are 81% and 69%, respectively, whereas the rates for malignant meningiomas are 72% and 54.6%, respectively.[5] For childhood tumors, 5-year survival expectation is 72%,[6] reflecting a higher frequency of lower-grade lesions and tumors that respond better to current therapies (eg, medulloblastomas). In general, survival for children younger than age 3 years is worse than children older than age 3.

Conditional survival probabilities have also been calculated for brain tumor patients. These rates are reported as 5-year conditional probabilities given survival to 2 years after diagnosis, or as the probability of surviving an additional 3 years after surviving 2 years after diagnosis. In their study, Davis and colleagues noted that the conditional 5-year survival for all brain and CNS tumors (76.2%) was significantly higher than the relative 5-year survival (27.6%).[7] It was also noted that the conditional survival probability increased with increasing years after diagnosis (ie, the estimated 3-year survival rate for a patient who has survived 2 years after diagnosis is higher than the 3-year survival rate for a patient with a newly diagnosed brain tumor). These trends are of particular importance to older patients with GBM, who comprise the subgroup with the most dismal prognosis. Conditional 5-year survival for GBM patients (all ages) was 36.4%, as compared to the relative 5-year survival of 3.2% of GBM patients. The most significant gains in conditional survival occurred between patients in the 45- to 64-years old and older than 65 years age groups. For patients in the 45 to 64 years old age group, the conditional 3-year survival after survival to 2 years was 58.6%, as compared to the observed 3-year survival rate of 17.5%. For patients older than age 65 years, the conditional 3-year survival rate was 56%, whereas the observed 3-year survival rate was only 6.1%.[7] Thus, conditional survival rates may be useful and encouraging for brain tumor patients, especially for older GBM patients.

RISK FACTORS

Risk factors are elusive, despite an ever-increasing amount of research in CNS tumors that is ongoing. Definitive identification of risk factors has been problematic as a consequence of a number of factors, including significant heterogeneity of primary brain tumors; retrospective exposure assessments; differences in histologic diagnoses and groupings leading to diagnostic inconsistencies; and undefined latency periods. In addition, methodologic differences between studies have made comparisons of their results complicated. Further carefully designed studies involving large populations will hopefully reveal the environmental risk factors that are significant for CNS tumorigenesis.

The role of high-dose therapeutic ionizing radiation as a significant risk factor for brain tumors has been consistently noted. The low doses used to treat tinea capitis and skin hemangiomas in children is associated with an increased risk of brain tumors.[8] A relative risk of 18, 10, and 3 have been observed for nerve sheath tumors, meningioma, and glioma, respectively, following an average dose of 1.5 Gray (Gy) of radiation for the treatment of tinea capitis. An average dose of 7 centigray (cGy) used to treat skin hemangiomas causes a 40% increased risk of intracranial tumors.[9] In addition, an elevated risk of subsequent primary brain tumors was observed after radiation treatment for childhood tumors other than leukemia.[10] Atomic bomb survivors in Japan have not shown an increased risk of CNS tumors. Although prenatal exposure to radiation (radiation therapy) may be a risk factor for childhood brain tumors, results from several studies are conflicting.[8] Diagnostic radiation therapy (XRT) exposures from medical or dental radiographs do not appear to be significant risk factors in glioma formation, whereas mutagen sensitivity to radiation has been reported to be significantly associated with an increased risk for glioma.[11] Electromagnetic fields (EMF) may be associated with increased risk. A recent meta-analysis suggests a nonsignificant increased risk of childhood brain tumors and leukemia in children living in homes with high EMF exposure, as well as an increased risk of brain cancer in electrical workers.[12] Despite these trends, however, a direct causal effect has not been proven. Although considerable attention and concern has been given recently to the potential association between cellular phone use and brain tumors, several studies have not demonstrated such an association.[13,14] However, further studies should be performed to definitively determine the risks among long-term users and for longer induction periods.

A number of studies have evaluated the risk of certain occupations and industries with development of brain tumors. Unfortunately, studies supporting or refuting the risk within the same industry have suggested that these inconsistencies may be due in part to a lack of an identified causal agent or cofactor(s). Certain industries do show increased risk, including pesticide and fertilization manufacturing, synthetic rubber processing, vinyl chloride industries, and petrochemical and oil refinery workers.[15] Some of the many difficulties encountered with this research include the fact that workers are only rarely exposed to a single suspected carcinogen, and only a small number of such workers are ever diagnosed with a brain tumor. Many chemical, biologic, or infectious agents may be considered to be potential causal agents, including N-nitroso compounds, organochlorides, nitrates and nitrites, and vinyl chloride. Formaldehyde has been proposed as a causal factor in the formation of brain tumors. Significant increased risks of brain tumors were found in embalmers, pathologists, and anatomists. However, an increased incidence of brain tumors was not found among industrial workers exposed to formaldehyde, which seemingly argued against formaldehyde playing a causal role in brain tumorigenesis.[16]

Diet, particularly exposure to N-nitroso compounds, is of interest because of the known association with these compounds and brain tumors in laboratory animals.[17] However, as with the occupational and industrial exposures described above, it is difficult to reliably determine the extent of exposure to these compounds because they are so common with both endogenous digestive processes and exogenous sources, such as tobacco smoke. Some studies support an association of exposure to subsequent development of a brain cancer, whereas others refute the link. Because of the uncertainty of the latency period needed for exposure and development of a brain cancer, as well as the complex interactions of foods to modify formation of these compounds, it is unlikely that a true causal relationship will be shown. Prenatal exposure to certain foods, like those that produce N-nitroso compounds, may increase the risk of childhood or adult brain cancer. Other foods or vitamin supplementation may decrease the risk.

Additional research evaluating the association of head trauma, seizure history, maternal alcohol consumption, cigarette smoking, residential chemical exposure, prior infectious history with viruses, drug and medication use, and others have been inconclusive or have had inconsistent results.[15,18] Numerous case-control and cohort studies have found little association between active smoking and adult primary brain tumors,[8] as well as between maternal smoking (actively before or during pregnancy, and passive smoking during pregnancy) and childhood brain tumors.[19] Maternal alcohol (ethyl alcohol [ETOH]) consumption appears to have a nonsignificant role in childhood brain tumors. Interestingly, beer and wine consumption may be associated with a decreased risk for glioma formation in adults.[8] The potential role of viruses and other infectious agents in brain tumorigenesis has not been adequately studied. Studies of simian virus 40 (SV40)-contaminated polio vaccine, varicella-zoster virus, and *Toxoplasmosis gondii* have not demonstrated convincing associations with brain tumors.[8]

MOLECULAR GENETICS

Malignant transformation of glial or neuronal cells is a complex process that is still incompletely understood in CNS tumor pathogenesis, but is the subject of intense laboratory research. A multistep process of tumor-suppressor gene inactivation and oncogene activation and overexpression plays a major part in this process, along with alterations in cell-cycle progression, abnormalities in signal transduction pathways, glioma cell invasion, and angiogenesis.

In astrocytic tumors, there is evidence that different genetic pathways may lead to GBMs as a common end point. Progression of astrocytomas is associated with sequentially acquired multiple genetic alterations. There appears to be two types of glioblastoma multiforme: primary (de novo) and secondary GBMs.[20] Histologically, the two GBM types are indistinguishable, but each has a different constellation of genetic alterations. Primary GBM occurs in patients in the fifth and sixth decades without a previous history of lower grade astrocytomas, whereas secondary GBM occurs more often in patients in the third and fourth decades as a consequence of progression from lower grade gliomas. Figure 72-1 is a schematic of the kinds of molecular events associated with transformation to primary and secondary GBMs. Amplification of the epidermal growth factor receptor (EGFR) occurs more frequently in primary tumors, whereas mutations of the *TP53* gene are more frequent in secondary tumors. EGFR overexpression and p53 mutations appear to be mutually exclusive genetic events.[21] Other molecular differences exist within the same pathologic type of tumor, emphasizing the heterogeneity of these lesions.[20]

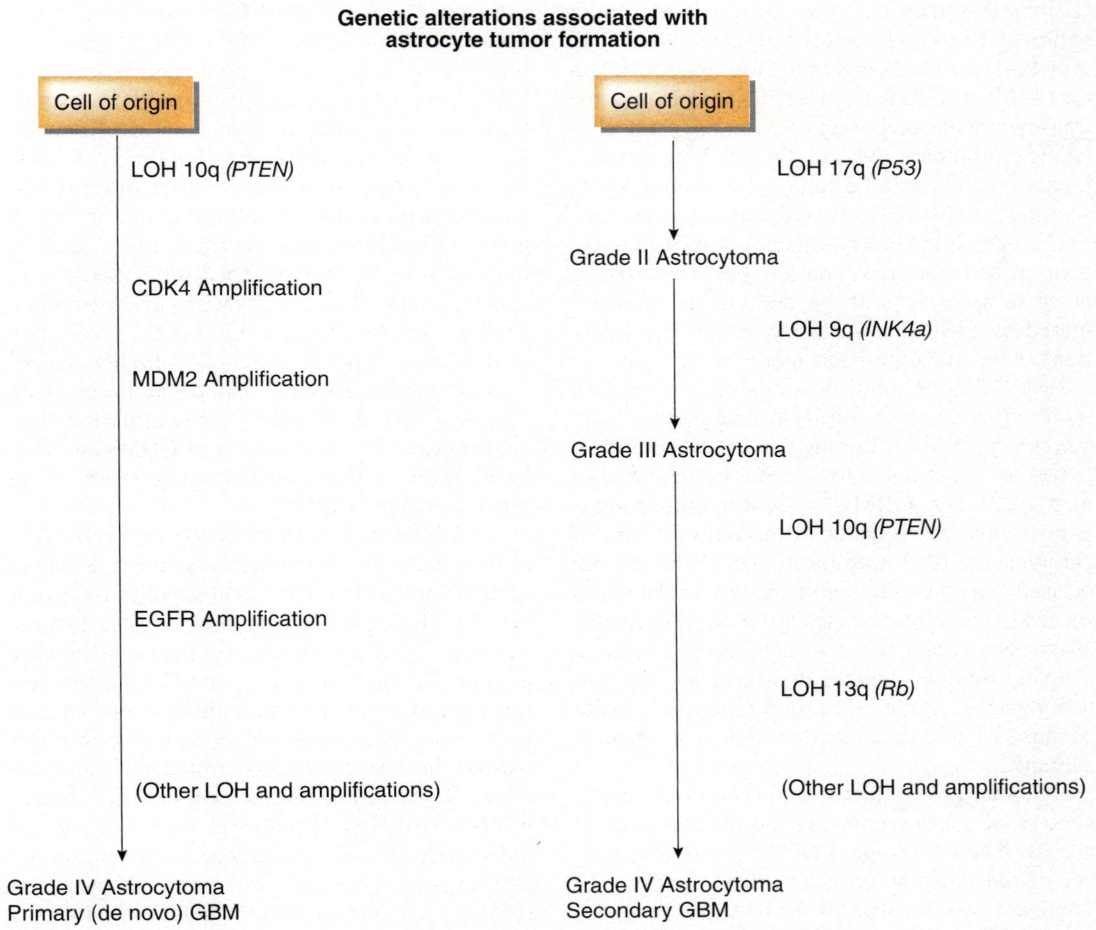

Genetic alterations associated with astrocyte tumor formation

Cell of origin

LOH 10q *(PTEN)*

CDK4 Amplification

MDM2 Amplification

EGFR Amplification

(Other LOH and amplifications)

Grade IV Astrocytoma
Primary (de novo) GBM

Cell of origin

LOH 17q *(P53)*

Grade II Astrocytoma

LOH 9q *(INK4a)*

Grade III Astrocytoma

LOH 10q *(PTEN)*

LOH 13q *(Rb)*

(Other LOH and amplifications)

Grade IV Astrocytoma
Secondary GBM

Figure 72-1 Genetic alterations associated with astrocyte tumor formation. GBM = glioblastoma multiforme; LOH = loss of heterozygosity.

Numerous chromosomal and gene abnormalities have been identified within the various tumor types. The *TP53* gene, located on chromosome 17p13.1, encodes a 53 kilodalton (kDa) protein (p53) which has an integral role in many cellular processes, including upregulation of the expression of the p21 protein and inhibition of cyclin-dependent kinases (CDK).[22,23] Cyclins are important regulators of the cell cycle and are involved in a number of cellular functions. The p53 protein also activates the *bax* gene, which is important in the regulation of the cell cycle, but in this case, via apoptotic cell death. Thus, p53 plays a critical role in cell-cycle regulation in a negative feedback loop. Abnormalities at codon 273 are the most frequent mutation, but many other types of mutation have been described. Inactivation of the p53 locus often involves point mutations on one allele and deletion of the p53 chromosome region on the other allele. Mutations of the *TP53* gene result in prolongation of the half-life of the p53 protein. Thus, p53 mutations demonstrate immunopositivity, whereas lack of p53 immunoreactivity indicates the presence of wild-type *TP53* gene.[24] *TP53* mutations have been reported in approximately 40% of grades I and II astrocytomas, 30% of grade III (anaplastic) astrocytomas, and 30% of GBMs, suggesting that *TP53* mutations are primarily associated with the transformation of normal cells into low-grade astrocytomas, rather than with progression of low-grade to high-grade astrocytomas. Interestingly, although *TP53* mutation is thought to confer radiation resistance in cancer cells, Tada and colleagues reported that GBM patients whose tumors harbored *TP53* mutations had a statistically significant increase in the recurrence-free period after XRT.[25] The reason for this finding is unclear, but one possibility is that wild-type p53 may actually protect GBM cells from radiation-induced apoptosis by imposing a p21-mediated G_1 arrest, and mutations of *TP53* may remove this radiation protection. Unregulated tumor cell growth is one consequence of nonfunctional p53. This laboratory observation supports the hypothesis that restoration of p53 in tumor cells that have nonfunctional or inactive p53 may inhibit cell growth. In fact, transfection experiments with wild-type p53 into human glioma tumor cells with mutations of *TP53* typically result in cell death via apoptotic pathways.[26] Clinical strategies to exploit this fact are ongoing in brain cancer patients.

The *MDM2* (*m*ouse *d*ouble *m*inute 2) gene, located on chromosome 12q14.3-q15, encodes a 54 kDa protein (MDM2). This protein binds to the acidic activation domain of *TP53,* thereby inhibiting its ability to promote transcription, and also promotes *TP53* degradation as well. Approximately 15% of anaplastic astrocytomas (AAs) and GBMs have been reported to have amplification of *MDM2*.[27] MDM2 can function as an oncogene, where its activation leads to increased cellular proliferation. MDM2 has been found to be overexpressed in a high proportion of primary, but not secondary, GBMs. Thus, primary GBMs, which typically do not have mutated p53, will have a "nonfunctional" p53 associated with overexpression of MDM2. The regulation of cell cycle control in these lesions is still being examined, and clearly is a complex, elaborate system even when one looks at just a few components in this process.

The *INK4a* (*In*hibit *cdk4*) gene is located on chromosome 9q21 and encodes two unrelated proteins: p16$^{\text{INK4a}}$ and p19^{ARF}. These proteins are derived from two transcripts (E1-containing transcript encodes p16$^{\text{INK4a}}$, E10-containing transcript encodes p19^{ARF}) resulting from alternative splicing and an alternative reading frame, and are both capable of inducing cell-cycle arrest.[28] Homozygous deletions of *INK4a* occur in approximately 25 to 50% of AAs and 40 to 70% of GBMs. p14^{ARF} (an analog of p19^{ARF}) has a significant role in the p53 pathway for binding specifically to MDM2, which stabilizes both p53 and MDM2.[29] Curiously, ARF expression is negatively regulated by p53. The overexpression of p14^{ARF} leads to cellular apoptosis that is p53-dependent. Inactivation of p14^{ARF} (either by homozygous deletion or hypermethylation of the p14^{ARF} promoter) was noted to occur in 50% of primary and 75% of secondary GBMs (58% of GBMs overall).[30] Because the difference in frequency of p14^{ARF} alterations between primary and secondary GBMs was not statistically significant, the loss of p14^{ARF} expression may be a significant molecular event in the pathways of both primary and secondary GBMs. p16$^{\text{INK4a}}$ functions to inhibit CDK4 by preventing it from forming an active complex with cyclin D proteins, which prevents the phosphorylation of pRb, thus preserving the ability of pRb to inhibit E2F and control cellular proliferation. Lack of expression of either p16$^{\text{INK4a}}$ or pRb, or the overexpression of CDK4 alone, appears to be sufficient to disrupt the cell-cycle regulatory mechanism, thereby leading to tumor formation.[31]

The retinoblastoma gene (*Rb1*) has been mapped to chromosome 13q14 and was one of the first tumor-suppressor genes identified.[32] *Rb1* encodes pRb, a 110 kDa protein that has two globular domains (A and B) that bind to viral oncoproteins (such as SV40 T antigen) in its unphosphorylated state. These domains are also important for binding to transcription factors, such as E2F, which is an important mediator of cellular proliferation. The ability of pRb to regulate cell growth is closely linked to its ability to bind and inhibit E2F. Phosphorylation of the Rb protein (pRb) is one of the key steps that control cell-cycle progression in the G_1 phase. As mentioned earlier, cyclins and CDKs phosphorylate key substrates involved in the activation of the cell cycle, with different CDKs functional at different stages of the cycle.[33] Inhibition of cell cycle progression occurs under the influence of CDK inhibitors (CDKIs). Alteration of the function of these numerous CDKs and CDKIs can result in either cell-cycle progression or inhibition. CDK4, which maps to chromosome 12q13-q14 and encodes a 33 kDa protein, phosphorylates pRb, which inhibits the ability of pRb to bind to transcription factors such as E2F.[22] CDKI p21 mediates p53-induced cell-cycle arrest, an important pathway initiated in response to deoxyribonucleic acid (DNA)-damaging agents. Mutations of any of these protein substrates could abrogate what normally might result in cell-cycle arrest, instead allowing cell proliferation to continue with persistent DNA damage. Alterations in this complex pathway are found in CNS tumors, and include overexpression of CDK4, deletions in p16 and p21, as well as mutations in p53 and Rb. Modification of these abnormal protein factors by drug or gene therapy strategies is currently being developed for clinical trials.

PTEN (also known as *MMAC* or *TEP1*) is a tumor-suppressor gene located on chromosome 10q23. Germ line *PTEN* mutations have been reported in inherited diseases, such as Cowden syndrome and Bannayan–Zonana syndrome, as well as in gliomas and cancers of the prostate, lung, and breast. PTEN is a 55 kDa protein with domains homologous to the catalytic region of protein tyrosine phosphatases, as well as to tensin and auxilin. PTEN possesses lipid phosphatase activity, and preferentially dephosphorylates PIP3 (phosphatidylinositide triphosphate) at the D3 position of the inositol ring. PTEN may be a direct antagonist of PIP and PI3-kinase (phosphatidylinositol 3-kinase).[34] PIP3 plays an important role in stimulating cellular proliferation and inhibiting apoptosis. PTEN decreases cellular PIP3 levels, which decreases the activity of protein kinase B (PKB/Akt). Akt is a major component in cell survival and is a downstream effector of PI3-kinase. Introduction of activated Akt and Ras into glial cells in mouse brain leads to the formation of GBM.[35] Thus, functional PTEN suppresses proliferation and promotes cellular apoptosis mediated by PIP3 and Akt. PTEN mutations occur more frequently in GBM than in AA. Smith and colleagues reported a statistically significant difference in frequency of PTEN alterations in GBM (34%) versus AA (18%).[36] PTEN also appears to have prognostic significance, as PTEN mutations were statistically significantly associated with decreased survival in AA patients,[36] as well as in pediatric AA and GBM patients with PTEN alterations.[37] PTEN may also regulate tumor-induced angiogenesis, suggesting that because angiogenesis is a hallmark of malignant behavior, PTEN may be an important component of tumor progression.[34] Hence, PI3-kinase inhibitors, which have been observed to block angiogenesis in vitro, may have efficacy as antiangiogenic agents to treat malignant gliomas.

Oncogene amplification is another pathway in the development of malignant glioma. One of the first genes found was the *c-erbB* oncogene, which encodes EGFR.[38] The human *EGFR* gene has been localized to chromosome 7p11-p12, and appears to play a role in cell proliferation and transformation. The EGFR protein is a 170 kDa transmembrane receptor that transduces growth signals after interaction with its extracellular ligands, epidermal growth factor (EGF) and transforming growth factor (TGF)-α. EGFR has four major domains: the transmembrane anchoring domain; the extracellular ligand-binding domain; the catalytic tyrosine kinase domain; and the carboxyl terminus, which stimulates ligand-activated endocytosis. The *EGFR* gene is the most frequently amplified oncogene in astrocytomas, and has been reported to occur in up to 62% of AA and GBMs, as determined by FISH (fluorescence in situ hybridization), with the significant majority occurring in GBMs.[39] EGFR amplifications have also been reported to occur in mostly primary rather than secondary GBMs, affirming that EGFR amplification is an important genetic event in the development of de novo GBMs.[40] EGFR amplification is almost always associated with complete loss of chromosome 10.[41] Amplification of EGFR has not been demonstrated to significantly correlate with survival.[40,42] In some cases, gene rearrangements also occur, leading to a truncated receptor without a ligand-binding domain that remains constitutively active. Tumor cell proliferation may occur because of this uncontrolled, autocrine growth stimulus.

Another growth factor important in the pathogenesis of astrocytomas, is the platelet-derived growth factor receptor (PDGFR), another member of the receptor tyrosine kinase family.[43–46] There are two isoforms of the receptor (α and β) with two ligands (α and β). PDGF-α only binds to the α-receptor, whereas PDGF-β can bind to both receptors. Human astrocytomas express high levels of the ligands and receptors, primarily because of overexpression rather than amplification or rearrangements. PDGFR-α overexpression appears to be an early event in tumorigenesis and is present in most tumor grades, whereas PDGFR-β overexpression has been reported in higher-grade tumors.[47] One study noted that PDGFR-α was amplified in 19% of grade IV tumors with oligodendroglioma features, whereas none of the 147 grade IV astrocytomas had this amplification, suggesting that PDGFR-α is associated with the oligodendroglioma phenotype.[48]

Aberrant cellular proliferation and transformation may be consequences of receptor tyrosine kinase genes via abnormal signaling pathways, such as activation of Ras protein and other substrates that control cell growth. Inhibition of Ras may be clinically feasible using farnesyl transferase inhibitors (FTI), which can block post-translational modification of Ras.[49,50] One FTI, SCH6636, substantially inhibits growth of astrocytoma cell lines and xenograft models in mice.[51] Another FTI, R115777, is currently being evaluated in phase II clinical trials.

Protein kinase C (PKC) is another member of the protein kinase family involved in signal transduction, and is often highly expressed in malignant gliomas.[52–54] PKC is believed to function in the regulation of astrocyte growth, differentiation of oligodendrocytes, prolongation of neuron potentiation, and neurotransmitter release. There are several isoforms of PKC, and selective inhibition of these isoforms is of interest, as growth of glial tumor cells can be modulated based upon PKC activity. Specifically, isoform PKCs α and ε have been implicated in glioma cell proliferation and invasion.[55] Nonselective inhibition of PKC has been used as a therapeutic strategy for patients with malignant gliomas, such as treatment with high-dose tamoxifen. More specific inhibitors are being developed, such as UCN-01 and bryostatin. Recent work with gene expression profiling studies shows that IGFBP2 (insulin-like growth factor binding protein 2) is highly overexpressed only in GBMs as opposed to lower-grade gliomas.[56] Thus, IGFBP2 overexpression may contribute to the invasiveness of GBMs and may be involved in the anaplastic progression of an astrocytoma to GBM.[57]

In addition to growth factor and cell-cycle alterations, malignant tumors acquire the ability to invade and develop new blood supplies by angiogenesis. Gliomas are often very invasive tumors, and although local control of tumor is potentially possible for short periods of time by surgery and radiotherapy, the fact that tumor cells invade beyond the macroscopic margins is one of many reasons that cure by local control alone is not possible. Degradation of the extracellular matrix involves secretion of proteases by tumor cells in order to break down the adjacent brain substrate, allowing cells to invade. Matrix metalloproteases (MMPs) are one of several kinds of proteases secreted by glioma cells.[58] Interestingly, inhibitors of MMPs can also be secreted by these same tumor cells, which suggests that an elaborate regulatory process may ultimately control the rate of cell invasion. Clinical trials using MMP inhibitors are ongoing in patients with CNS tumors in an attempt to control at least one aspect of the complex process of tumor growth. A novel matrix metalloproteinase inhibitor, SI-27, has also been noted to significantly suppress vascular endothelial growth factor (VEGF)-mediated angiogenesis in vitro, suggesting an angiosuppressive effect in addition to its inhibitory effect on MMP.[59]

In addition to invasion, angiogenesis is also an important factor in CNS tumor growth. Angiogenesis leads to prominent microvascular proliferation, which is a histopathologic hallmark of GBMs. VEGF is a mitogen that induces angiogenesis and vascular permeability.[60–62] VEGF is the most important regulator of vascular proliferation in glioma-induced angiogenesis. VEGF is typically not expressed in normal brain endothelium, but is upregulated in proliferating tumor vessels. VEGF is a dimeric glycoprotein and binds to VEGF receptor-1 and receptor-2. Overexpression of VEGF and its receptors is found in many tumors, including malignant gliomas, which are highly vascularized and often hypoxic tumors. One hallmark of GBM is the presence of necrosis. Hypoxia is able to induce VEGF expression, and it is likely that tumor cells that become hypoxic increase VEGF secretion in an attempt to survive. VEGF acts specifically on endothelial cells to not only induce angiogenesis, but to also increase vas-

Table 72-1 Characteristic Features of Familial Brain Tumor Syndromes

Syndrome	Characteristic CNS Lesions	Characteristic Skin Lesions	Ophthalmologic Features	Chromosome	Gene	Protein
NF-1	Optic pathway glioma Brainstem glioma Neurofibromatosis bright objects	Café-au-lait spots Axillary freckling	Lisch nodules	17q11	NF1	Neurofibromin
NF-2	Bilateral acoustic schwannomas Multiple meningiomas	HF-2 plaque Subcutaneous schwannomas		22q12	NF2	Merlin
Retinoblastoma	Pineoblastoma (trilateral retinoblastoma)		Leukokoria	13q14	Rb1	Rb1
von Hippel–Lindau	Hemangioblastoma of the cerebellum/spine		Retinal angioma (hemangioblastoma)	3p25	VHL	VHL
Tuberous sclerosis	Subependymal giant cell astrocytoma	Ash-leaf spots	Retinal astrocytoma (mulberry lesion)	9q34	TSC1	Hamartim
	Subependymal nodule Cortical tuber	Adenoma sebaceum Shagreen patch Ungual fibroma		16p13.3	TSC2	Tuberin
Sturge-Weber	Leptomeningeal angiomatosis Cortical calcifications Hemispheric atrophy	Port-wine nevus	Choroidal hemangioma Glaucoma			
Turcot syndrome	Glioblastoma (BTP[a] type 1)				DNA mismatch repair genes	
	Medulloblastoma (BTP type 2)			5q21	APC	
Nevoid basal cell carcinoma (Gorlin) syndrome	Medulloblastoma	Basal cell carcinomas		9q22.3	PTCH	
Lhermitte-Duclos/ Cowden syndrome	Dysplastic gangliocytoma of the cerebellum	Facial trichilemmoma (Cowden syndrome)		10q23.3 (Cowden syndrome)	PTEN	
Li–Fraumeni	Malignant glioma PNET[b]			17q (between exon 5 and 9)	P53	

CNS = central nervous system.
[a]Brain tumor polyposis.
[b]Primitive neuroectodermal tumor.
Reproduced with permission from Pan E et al.

cular permeability. Hence, VEGF may be an important factor not only for microvascular proliferation, but also for the peritumoral edema consistently observed with malignant gliomas. Interestingly, dexamethasone, which is used to decrease cerebral edema, has been noted to down-regulate VEGF expression. Endothelial cells in the tumor vasculature contain the receptors for VEGF, whereas the ligands for these receptors are expressed on the tumor cell, suggesting a paracrine loop supporting tumor growth. Several studies of inhibitors of angiogenesis, including antibodies to VEGF, are now ongoing to treat malignant gliomas, particular GBMs.

FAMILIAL TUMOR SYNDROMES OF THE CENTRAL NERVOUS SYSTEM

The familial brain tumor syndromes are a heterogeneous group of genetic disorders characterized by a combination of systemic manifestations (often dermatologic) and CNS neoplasms. Some of these syndromes include neurofibromatosis types 1 and 2, tuberous sclerosis, von Hippel–Lindau (VHL) disease, and Li–Fraumeni syndrome. Table 72-1 lists some characteristic features of the various familial brain tumor syndromes.

Neurofibromatosis 1 Neurofibromatosis type 1 (NF1), also known as von Recklinghausen disease, is one of the most common genetic syndromes, with a prevalence of 1 in 4,000.[63] It is an autosomal dominant disorder with 100% penetrance and a 50% spontaneous mutation rate.[64] The *NF1* gene has been mapped to chromosome 17q11.2 and encodes the tumor-suppressor protein neurofibromin.[65] Patients with this disorder manifest a number of abnormalities, including café au lait spots, Lisch nodules, axillary freckling, and bony abnormalities. The predominant CNS tumors in NF1 are optic pathway and brainstem gliomas. Pathologically, optic pathway gliomas (OPGs) are pilocytic astrocytomas. Brainstem gliomas (BSGs) in NF1 patients are predominantly astrocytomas, although it has been noted that these tumors are more indolent and have significantly better prognoses than BSGs in non-NF1 patients.[66] The typical peripheral nervous system (PNS) tumor in NF1 is the plexiform neurofibroma, which usually involves the paraspinal and cranial nerves. Most of the CNS and PNS tumors in NF1 follow an indolent course.[67] Curiously, certain lesions, called neurofibromatosis bright objects (NBOs), seen on magnetic resonance imaging (MRI) are specifically associated with NF1. They are found mostly in the globus pallidus and brain-stem (particularly in the midbrain).[68] The exact nature of these NBOs is uncertain, but most follow a benign course with regression by age 20 years.

Neurofibromatosis 2 Neurofibromatosis type 2 (NF2), also called central neurofibromatosis, is an autosomal dominant disorder that was recently recognized as a separate syndrome from NF1. NF2 has a much lower prevalence than NF1 (1 in 50,000[63]) and accounts for only 10% of all neurofibromatosis cases. The *NF2* gene, which is felt to be a tumor-suppressor gene, is located at chromosome 22q12, and encodes a protein called merlin (or schwannomin).[69,70] Both germ line and somatic mutations have been described. Cutaneous features of NF2 are more rare and subtle than in NF1, including intracutaneous plaque-like lesions and occasional café au lait spots. Ophthalmologic features are also prominent in NF2 (particularly cataracts). The predominant CNS tumors in NF2 are the cranial nerve VIII (vestibular) schwannomas, which often occur bilaterally, and cranial meningiomas. Peripheral tumors in NF2 include spinal schwannomas and neurofibromas. Table 72-2 describes the diagnostic criteria for both NF1 and NF2.

von Hippel–Lindau VHL disease is also an autosomal dominant disorder with highly expressive variability and a penetrance of approximately 80 to 90% by age 65 years. The birth incidence in eastern England is 1 in 36,000.[71] The *VHL* gene has been mapped to chromosome 3p25-p26.[72] The protein product (pVHL) forms a protein complex (CBC^{VHL}), which is often mutated in VHL.[71] Mutations in the *VHL* gene lead to the upregulation

Table 72-2 Diagnostic Criteria for Neurofibromatosis Types 1 and 2

Neurofibromatosis Type 1 (2 or more are diagnostic)
1. Six or more café-au-lait spots, greater than 5 mm in diameter in prepubertal and over 15 mm in diameter in postpubertal individuals
2. Two or more neurofibromas of any type, or 1 plexiform neurofibroma
3. Axillary and/or inguinal freckling
4. Optic nerve glioma
5. Osseous lesions, such as dysplasia of the sphenoid wing, thinning of long bone cortex, with or without pseudoarthrosis
6. First-degree relative (parent, sibling, or offspring) with NF1 according to above criteria

Neurofibromatosis Type 2
1. Bilateral vestibular schwannomas; or
2. A first-degree relative with NF2, and either
   a) A unilateral vestibular schwannoma or
   b) Two of the following: meningioma, schwannoma, glioma, neurofibroma, posterior subcapsular lens opacity, or cerebral calcifications; or
3. Two of the following:
   a) Unilateral, vestibular schwannoma
   b) Multiple meningioma
   c) Either schwannoma, glioma, neurofibroma, posterior subcapsular lens opacity, or cerebral calcification

of VEGF, which affirms the observation that angiogenesis is a major factor underlying the pathogenesis of VHL.[73] The main clinical feature of VHL is the hemangioblastoma, which almost always occurs infratentorially to involve the posterior fossa and/or upper cervical spinal cord, and which has been noted to significantly overexpress VEGF. Other VHL lesions include retinal angiomas (hemangioblastomas), renal cell carcinomas, pheochromocytomas, pancreatic and renal cysts, and endolymphatic sac tumors. There are several subtypes of VHL, each with their own associated tumor types and each determined by different types of *VHL* gene mutations (Table 72-3). This interesting genotype–phenotype correlation can be useful in genetic counseling, as well as in further evaluating the genetic mechanisms of cancer in general.

Tuberous Sclerosis Tuberous sclerosis (TS), previously called Bourneville disease, is an autosomal disorder that affects approximately 1 in 10,000 births,[74] and is the second most common neurocutaneous disorder (behind NF1).[75] TS has been linked to two different loci: TS complex-1 (TSC1) is located on chromosome 9q34 and encodes the protein hamartin,[76] whereas TSC2 has been mapped to chromosome 16p13.3 and encodes the protein tuberin.[77] Both proteins have been suggested to be tumor-suppressor genes. Approximately 50% of TS families exhibit genetic linkage to TSC1 and TSC2 each, although they result in essentially identical syndromes.[74] The classic clinical triad of TS (seizures, mental retardation, and facial angiofibromas) occurs only in severe cases of TS. Major systemic features of TS include ash-leaf spots, shagreen patches, periungual fibromas, adenoma sebaceum (facial angiofibromas), retinal hamartomas ("mulberry lesions"), cardiac rhabdomyomas, and renal angiomyolipomas. The hallmark CNS tumor in TS is the subependymal giant cell astrocytoma. They occur in 5 to 10% of TS patients[78] and are pathologically benign (World Health Organization [WHO] grade I). However, they are a major cause of death in TS patients because of their typical location near the foramen of Monro, where they can obstruct cerebrospinal fluid (CSF) ventricular flow and cause brainstem herniation. Other typical CNS lesions in TS include cortical tubers and subependymal glial nodules ("candle gutterings"). Although these lesions are also benign, cortical tubers can cause morbidity by obstructive hydrocephalus and as foci for seizures, whereas a high number of subependymal nodules has been correlated with increased infantile spasms and mental retardation (intelligence quotient [IQ] < 70).[79]

Li–Fraumeni Syndrome Li–Fraumeni syndrome (LFS) is a rare autosomal dominant disorder affecting children and young adults, and is caused by germ line mutations of *TP53*.[80,81] The LFS mutation is located at the area between exons 5 and 9 of the *TP53* gene.[82] A germ line mutation in human checkpoint kinase 2 (*hCHK2*), a possible tumor-suppressor gene associated with LFS, has been found in some members of LFS families.[83] Thus far, more than 100 families with this syndrome have been studied, and the tumors most often observed include breast cancer, soft-tissue sarcomas, osteosarcomas, leukemia, and adrenocortical carcinomas. The CNS tumors associated with LFS are the malignant neuroepithelial tumors (AAs and GBMs), with primitive neuroectodermal tumors (PNETs) less-commonly associated.[84] Although p53 mutations are established causal events in the pathogenesis of LFS, the molecular genetics of LFS are still not completely understood. It is likely that p53 mutation is only one major event, and that LFS involves interactions with multiple cell-cycle regulatory genes and pathways.

HISTOPATHOLOGY OF NEUROEPITHELIAL CENTRAL NERVOUS SYSTEM TUMORS

The World Health Organization has classified CNS tumors into seven categories in its most recent revision of its classification system.[85] Primary CNS tumors comprise approximately 50 to 70% of intracranial tumors, with the majority being neuroepithelial tissue tumors. Neuroepithelial tumors are further subclassified into tumor types described in Table 72-4. In general, children present most frequently with PNETs, low-grade astrocytomas, and ependymomas. These tumors have a predilection toward midline locations, and 70% of childhood tumors are infratentorial. Adults, on the other hand, more frequently present with higher-grade astrocytomas and have fewer PNETs or ependymomas. Of adult CNS tumors, 70% occur supratentorially and tend to occur in non-midline locations. Glioblastoma is a highly cellular tumor with increased nuclear and cellular pleomorphism, endothelial proliferation, mitotic figures, and frequent necrosis. Although necrosis is a hallmark of this tumor, its presence is not absolutely required to designate a tumor as GBM in the WHO classification. Microvascular proliferation is also a histologic hallmark feature of GBM, as it is indicative of the ability of this highly malignant tumor to create its own blood supply for rapid growth and spread. Anaplastic astrocytomas are less cellular, with less pleomorphism and mitoses than GBM, and do not exhibit necrosis. Grade II astrocytomas are composed of a fairly uniform group of proliferating astrocytes in a fibrillary matrix. They exhibit slight nuclear atypia and cellular pleomorphism compared to the higher-grade astrocytomas. Mitoses are rare, and they do not have necrosis or microvascular proliferation. Grade I tumors, or juvenile pilocytic astrocytomas (JPAs), almost exclusively occur in the pediatric population, and are often seen as OPGs in NF1 patients. Histologically, they exhibit low cellularity, often contain Rosenthal fibers, and present with mural nodules. The presence of vascular proliferation, occasional hyperchromatic nuclei, and rare mitoses are common in JPAs, and are not signs of malignancy. They are usually associated with a good prognosis. Of the various neuroepithelial tumor types, perhaps the lower-grade tumors represent the most challenging for pathologists to classify. Numerous subtypes of low-grade glioma exist, including ganglioglioma, mixed tumors, pleomorphic xanthoastrocytoma, dysembryoplastic neuroectodermal tumor (DNET), neurocytoma,

Table 72-3 Clinical and Molecular Classification of von Hippel–Lindau Disease Lesions

Lesion	Type I	Type IIA	Type IIB	Type IIC
Pheochromocytoma	No	Yes	Yes	Yes
CNS hemangioblastoma	Yes	Yes	Yes	No
Retinal hemangioblastoma	Yes	Yes	Yes	No
Endolymphatic sac tumors	Yes	Yes	Yes	No
Renal cell carcinoma	Yes	No	Yes	No
Pancreatic tumors	Yes	No	Yes	No
Molecular Characteristics				
Protein truncation	73–96%	8–31%		
Amino acid substitution	4–27%	100%	69–92%	100%
Mutation loci	Multiple	Codon 98	Codon 167	

Adapted from Richard S et al.

Table 72-4 World Health Organization Classification of Tumors of Neuroepithelial Tissue

I. Astrocytic tumors
 1. Diffuse astrocytoma (fibrillary, protoplasmic, gemistocytic, mixed)
 2. Anaplastic (malignant) astrocytoma
 3. Glioblastoma (giant cell, gliosarcoma variants)
 4. Pilocytic astrocytoma
 5. Pleomorphic xanthoastrocytoma
 6. Subependymal giant cell astrocytoma
II. Oligodendroglial tumors
 1. Oligodendroglioma
 2. Anaplastic (malignant) oligodendroglioma
 3. Ependymal tumors
 4. Ependymoma (cellular, papillary, clear cell, tanycytic)
 5. Anaplastic (malignant) ependymoma
 6. Myxopapillary ependymoma
 7. Subependymoma
III. Mixed tumors
 1. Oligoastrocytoma
 2. Anaplastic (malignant) oligoastrocytoma
IV. Choroid plexus tumors
 1. Choroid Plexus papilloma
 2. Choroid Plexus carcinoma
V. Neuronal and mixed neuronal-glial tumors
 1. Gangliocytoma
 2. Ganglioglioma
 3. Dysembryoplastic neuroepithelial tumor (DNET)
 4. Dysplastic gangliocytoma of the cerebellum (Lhermitte-Duclos)
 5. Desmoplastic infantile astrocytoma/ganglioglioma
 6. Central neurocytoma
 7. Anaplastic ganglioglioma
 8. Cerebellar liponeurocytoma
 9. Paraganglioma of the filum terminale
VI. Pineal tumors
 1. Pineocytoma
 2. Pineoblastoma
 3. Pineal parenchymal tumor of intermediate differentiation
VII. Embryonal tumors
 1. Medulloblastoma (desmoplastic, large cell, melanotic, medullomyoblastoma)
 2. Medulloepithelioma
 3. Supratentorial primitive neuroectodermal tumors (PNETs)
  a. Neuroblastoma
  b. Ganglioneuroblastoma
  c. Ependymoblastoma
  d. Atypical teratoid/rhabdoid tumor
VIII. Neuroblastic tumors
 1. Olfactory (esthesioneuroblastoma)
 2. Olfactory neuroepithelioma
 3. Neuroblastomas of the adrenal gland and sympathetic nervous system
IX. Glial tumors of uncertain etiology
 1. Astroblastoma
 2. Gliomatosis cerebri
 3. Chordoid glioma of the third ventricle

and pineocytoma. These are uncommon tumors with different treatment strategies. Unfortunately, it is also not uncommon that expert neuropathologists disagree with each other in the identification of these tumors.

Another set of tumors that tends to cause discordance among pathologists is oligodendrogliomas. Oligodendrogliomas and mixed oligoastrocytomas correspond to WHO grade II tumors; anaplastic oligodendrogliomas and anaplastic oligoastrocytomas correspond to WHO grade III tumors. Oligodendrogliomas are characterized by uniform round cells with the associated delicate capillary ("chicken-wire") vasculature, frequent calcifications, and artifactual perinuclear halos around the oligodendroglioma cells ("fried-egg" appearance) resulting from formalin fixation of the tumor. Occasionally, some oligodendroglial tumors show sufficient anaplasia, pleomorphism, mitoses, and necrosis that would fulfill the criteria of a WHO grade IV tumor. These unique tumors tend to have a better outcome following therapy than their pure astrocytoma counterparts. A uniform consensus does not exist to help classify these tumors as either pure oligodendrogliomas or mixed tumors, and the degree of anaplasia that constitutes criteria to classify them as grade II or III tumors varies amongst neuropathologists. One common molecular alteration noted in these tumors is loss of genetic material on chromosomes 1p and 19q.[86] Increased sensitivity to chemotherapy is common when these chromosomal alterations are present. However, not all oligodendroglial tumors have these losses, and they cannot be relied upon to make a specific diagnosis.

Of the childhood tumors, PNETs most frequently occur in the cerebellum and are traditionally called medulloblastomas. PNETs of the pineal region are called pineoblastomas, and in the cerebral hemispheres they are referred to as supratentorial PNETs. These tumors are characteristically fast growing and have a high propensity toward dissemination along CSF pathways. Histologically, medulloblastomas are comprised of a predominant population of round to oval undifferentiated small blue cells ("blue-cell tumors"). Occasionally, they contain Homer–Wright rosettes, which are structures of neuroblastic differentiation in PNETs. Astrocytic tumors in childhood tend to occur along the midline axis, including the cerebellum, optic nerve, and chiasm, or hypothalamic regions. Most are low-grade tumors, such as JPAs or fibrillary grade II astrocytomas. Ependymomas in children commonly occur in the posterior fossa, may disseminate to other areas of the brain and spine, and tend to have a worse outcome than in adults, particularly in the younger age group (younger than age 3 years).

As molecular markers become more fully understood, CNS tumors will become better characterized. It is becoming evident that histopathologic diagnosis is insufficient to accurately predict tumor behavior and prognosis, particularly with the problem of interobserver variability with regard to histologic diagnosis. Molecular markers will become a much more objective and accurate measure of tumor behavior, especially for CNS tumors without a consensus regarding histopathologic criteria for diagnosis.

CLINICAL PRESENTATION

Patients with intracranial lesions may present with general, nonfocal signs and symptoms, or with focal manifestations related to the specific area of brain occupied by tumor. General signs include headache, nausea, vomiting, generalized seizures, and/or change in level of consciousness. Few patients with headaches have brain tumors, the presenting symptom in only 20% of cases ultimately diagnosed with a tumor. Seizures in adults, however, are more frequently associated with tumors and a new-onset seizure in an adult should prompt full neurologic evaluation, including neuroimaging. It should be noted that less than 5% of patients with acute stroke have seizure, whereas seizure is the presenting symptom in as high as 15% of brain tumor patients. Headache, nausea and vomiting are common presenting symptoms of raised intracranial pressure, as well as cranial nerve palsies, motor and sensory abnormalities, and changes in level of consciousness. Focal findings include motor and sensory abnormalities (posterior frontal lobe), personality changes including apathy, inattention, impaired intellect, and depression changes (anterior frontal lobes), speech, language, and memory difficulties (dominant temporal lobe), spatial disorientation and problems with taste, hearing, smell, and complex partial seizures (non-dominant temporal lobe), visual abnormalities, visual field defects, visual hallucinations (occipital lobe). Thalamic lesions may cause hemisensory loss, hemiparesis, movement disorders, and pain syndromes. Hypothalamic and pituitary tumors cause endocrine dysfunction including anorexia, acromegaly, Cushing's disease, precocious puberty, infertility, loss of libido, amenorrhea, galactorrhea, and the syndrome of inappropriate antidiuretic hormone secretion (SIADH). Tumors of the cerebellum and posterior fossa may cause ipsilateral ataxia, nystagmus, voluntary coordination abnormalities, unsteady gait, and limb ataxia (among other signs/symptoms).

It is important to be aware that most patients who are ultimately diagnosed as having a malignant brain tumor have had signs and symptoms of their disease for weeks, months, or sometimes years before a histologic diagnosis is made. For any adult who presents with a new-onset seizure, personality changes, or new focal neurologic findings, a brain neoplasm should be considered in the differential diagnosis and should have the appropriate neurologic work-up.

DIAGNOSTIC NEUROIMAGING

Patients with signs and symptoms suggestive of an intracranial mass should undergo neuroimaging studies. The neuroimaging modality of choice for CNS tumors is the MRI.

MRI is the neuroimaging technique most frequently used in the evaluation and follow-up review of patients with malignant brain tumors. MRI has several advantages over contrast-enhanced CT. First, multiple planar images are available. Second, lesions of the spine or posterior fossa are seen in far greater detail than with CT. In addition, patients are not exposed to radiation or to iodinated contrast agents, obviating potential allergic reactions. The paramagnetic agent, gadolinium (Gd) with diethylenetriamine pentaacetic acid (DTPA), allows enhancement in areas of disrupted or abnormal blood–brain barrier with minimal risk of allergic reaction. Hydrogen protons in extracellular H_2O are of low signal intensity on T_1-weighted MRI images (T1WI) and are of high signal intensity on T_2-weighted MRI images (T2WI). Thus, lesions such as tumors, which produce an increase in extracellular H_2O, show decreased T1WI signal and appear hypointense, and show increased T2WI signal, and thus appear hyperintense. However, this observation is by no means absolute.

There are several limitations to MR imaging that must be recognized. Perhaps the most important is a lack of specificity. Multiple pathologic lesions appear hypointense on T1WI and hyperintense on T2WI. The MRI differential diagnosis for intracranial neoplasms includes infarcts, demyelinating lesions, radiation necrosis, infections, and other inflammatory processes. Also, enhancement does not always equate with histologic tumor grade. In general, higher-grade tumors will frequently show enhancement on MRI. However, an exception to this rule is seen in a very slow-growing tumor such as JPA, which will frequently show contrast-enhancing areas within the tumor. Similarly, some higher-grade tumors will not enhance.[87] Thus, although MRI features of a lesion can be very helpful, histologic verification is necessary to establish a diagnosis. MRI is also not able to distinguish the "edge" of a tumor, or determine the full extent of disease. Viable tumor cells are known to exist beyond the borders of abnormal contrast-enhancement or T_2-weighted abnormalities.[88] Finally, imaging abnormalities seen following treatment are often nonspecific. Radiation injury, including radiation necrosis, is virtually indistinguishable from tumor regrowth, and MRI alone cannot be relied upon to determine whether tumor is present or not following such therapy. Despite these limitations, MRI remains the standard imaging technique in neuro-oncology. Specific imaging characteristics of each tumor type will be presented in those discussions.

Magnetic resonance spectroscopic imaging (MRSI)

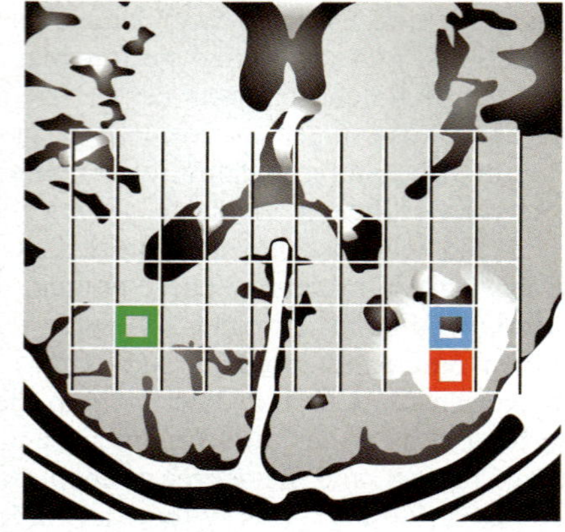

T1-weighted contrast enhanced MRI with PRESS region

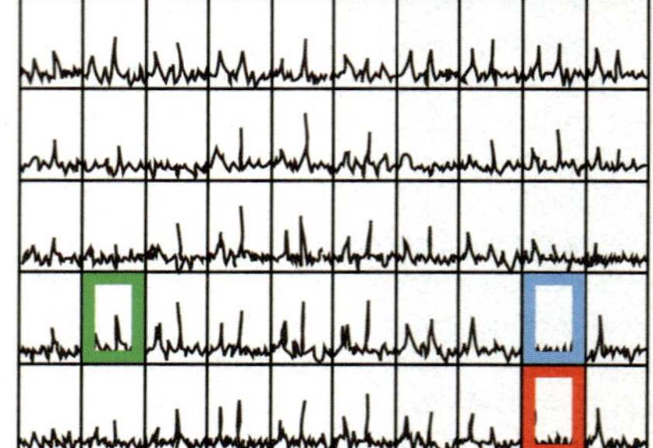

PRESS excited region

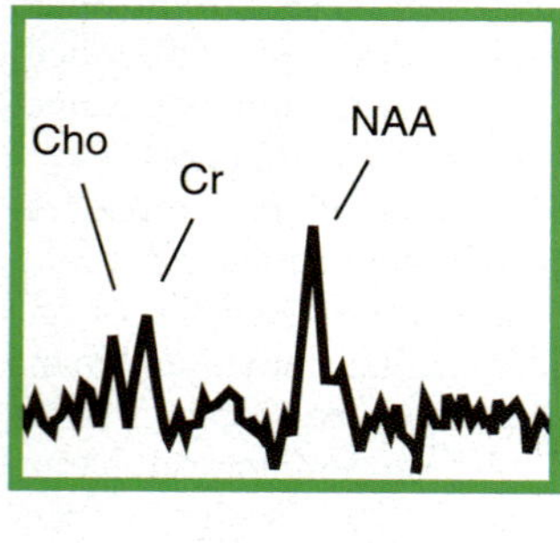

Normal brain

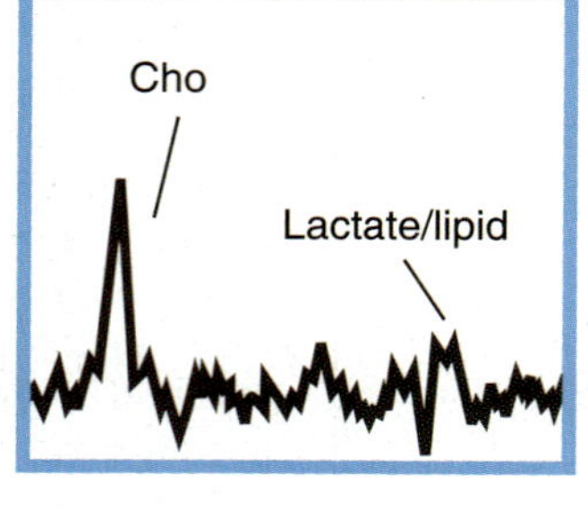

Active tumor

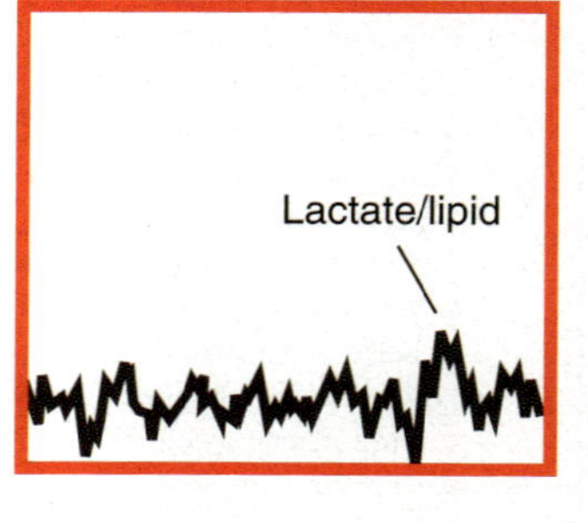

Necrosis

Figure 72-2 Magnetic resonance imaging (MRI) and magnetic resonance spectroscopy (MRS) of tumor compared to radiation necrosis. Point resolve spectroscopy (PRESS) is used to excite a region containing both the enhancing lesion and contralateral normal tissue. Individual voxels are then characterized by the size of the peaks corresponding to choline (Cho), creatine (Cr), *N*-acetyl-aspartate (NAA), and lactate/lipid. The typical patterns for normal white matter, tumor, and necrotic tissue are highlighted above.

Other Imaging Techniques Although proton MRI has significantly improved our ability to detect and follow tumors in the central nervous system, it still lacks diagnostic specificity. New MRI techniques are being developed to investigate the biochemical basis of tumors. Of those techniques, proton MRI spectroscopy (MRS) holds great promise for improving the diagnostic efficiency of MRI.[89–91] MRI spectroscopy is a procedure in which nuclear MRI signals are obtained from nuclei other than water. Thus, MRS measures protons in nuclei from tissue elements other than water. The metabolites of interest for brain tumors include *N*-acetyl-aspartate, choline, and lactate. An increase in choline signal represents increased membrane synthesis and cell turnover rates secondary to increased phospholipid metabolism. An increase in lactate suggests dependence on anaerobic metabolism, such as seen in hypoxic areas of tumor or radiation injury. Absence of lactate would be indicative of necrosis. The role of *N*-acetyl-aspartate is not completely understood, but appears to be involved in lipid synthesis, and is localized to neurons. This metabolite is decreased in tumor-bearing areas of brain, or in areas of necrotic brain. Changes in the patterns of these metabolites, compared to normal brain, can assist in the determination of active tumor growth versus radiation necrosis, which appear similar on routine MRI.[91] In general, necrotic areas of tumor or necrosis related to radiation treatment will exhibit reduced levels of choline, lactate, and *N*-acetyl-aspartate. Tumors will show an increase in choline and a reduction in *N*-acetyl-aspartate; lactate may be increased in hypoxic tumor areas or absent in necrotic areas. Figure 72-2 shows a typical MRS pattern associated with tumor and with radiation necrosis. Perfusion and diffusion MR imaging are two newer techniques that are also being studied to evaluate blood flow and angiogenesis, and movement of water in brain tissue, respectively. The combination of anatomic with metabolic and physiologic imaging holds great promise in understanding tumor biology and response to treatment. Positron emission tomography (PET) using the glucose analog 2-(18F)-fluorodeoxy-D-glucose (18-FDG) has also shown promise in differentiating viable tumor from necrosis related to various forms of radiation therapy.[92,93] High-dose focal irradiation is often associated with changes on MRI that are difficult to interpret. Radiation injury can develop as early as several months after XRT, and typically will be present within 6 to 8 months. MRI shows a contrast-enhancing lesion with surrounding edema, and may show an increase in intracranial pressure (ICP) with a shift of midline structures. These findings are also typical of recurrent tumor, which may follow a similar time course. A patient's MRI scans and clinical history may suggest either tumor recurrence or radiation necrosis, which is impossible to distinguish on MRI alone. The basis of using FDG-PET in glioma recurrence evaluation is predicated on the observation that there is increased glucose metabolism in brain tumors, particularly in the higher-grade tumors, which is thought to be related to the anaerobic glycolysis process in tumors. Thus, tumor lesions will have increased 18-FDG uptake and appear as "hot spots" on PET imaging. Conversely, radiation necrosis would not have an increased 18-FDG uptake and would appear as "cold spots." It is important to note that PET scans should be evaluated as a side-by-side comparison with MRI for anatomic correlation, as normal tissue can be mistaken for recurrent tumor because 18-FDG signal is usually not greater than normal cortex.[90] FDG-PET imaging also has prognostic significance. A statistically significant association was found regarding the ratio of cerebral metabolic rate of 18-FDG metabolism in tumors compared with that of the contralateral normal cortex. Di Chiro noted that patients with a ratio of > 1.4 had a median survival of 5 months, whereas the median survival of brain tumor patients with ratios of < 1.4 was 19 months.[94] FDG-PET also appears to be helpful in distinguishing low versus high-grade gliomas. Low-grade gliomas had a mean uptake of 3.8 µmol/100 g/min, whereas high-grade gliomas had a mean uptake of 6.6 µmol/100 g/min.[94] Delbeke and colleagues used the 18-FDG tumor-to-white matter ratio to evaluate 32 high-grade and 26 low-grade gliomas. Using a cutoff ratio of 1.5, they achieved a 94% sensitivity and 77% specificity in distinguishing low versus high-grade gliomas.[95] This work suggests that PET can be used in follow-up evaluations of patients with low-grade malignancies to correctly diagnose malignant transformation, and thus guide subsequent management.

Functional MRI (fMRI) is a rapidly evolving technique that maps the functional organization of the brain, particularly the primary motor, sensory, and language cortices. The underlying basis for fMRI lies in the fact that increased neuronal activity leads to a regional increase in cerebral blood flow (CBF), and that O_2 delivery exceeds the tissues' ability to extract the increased O_2 content. Thus, there is an increase in oxyhemoglobin with a reciprocal decrease in deoxyhemoglobin.[96] Because deoxyhemoglobin is a paramagnetic substance, decreasing intravascular deoxyhemoglobin leads to a local increase in MRI signal brought upon by neuronal activation. Thus, fMRI can be used as a noninvasive method of determining hemispheric language dominance, and it does not have the significant problems associated with the Wada test. Although fMRI at this point cannot replace direct intra-operative cortical stimulation for mapping eloquent cortex, it will become a more important technique as neurosurgery becomes less invasive.

SURGICAL DIAGNOSIS AND RESECTION

Despite the significant improvements in neuroimaging, a specific diagnosis cannot be established through imaging alone. Tissue analysis is necessary to establish a precise tumor diagnosis and to effectively plan therapy. Neurosurgical morbidity and mortality rates have improved to such a degree over the past several decades that a decision not to operate is rare. For almost every intracranial lesion, tissue can be obtained for histologic diagnosis either by craniotomy and biopsy or resection or by ultrasound-guided or stereotactic-guided biopsy. From a purely oncologic point of view, surgery is still the most rapid method of tumor cell burden reduction. Apart from diagnostic accuracy and tumor debulking, there are several other reasons for a surgical approach to the management of malignant brain tumors. Surgery may be lifesaving in the setting of a rapid increase in intracranial pressure, allowing the patient to survive long enough to receive other therapies. Moreover, surgery reduces the tumor cell population, leaving fewer tumor cells to be eradicated with irradiation and chemotherapy. Surgery also produces partial or complete resolution of symptoms and may delay the onset of new symptoms.

Variables that affect the overall outcome must also be understood in order to plan surgery most effectively. Many slow-growing, low-grade astrocytic lesions are difficult to surgically resect completely, for instance, because they are often large, diffusely infiltrative and have indistinct margins. If extensive tumor removal is virtually certain to improve overall survival, then the potential risk of neurologic deterioration should be discussed with the patient and weighed against the benefit of longer life. For large, diffuse hemispheric lesions, the impact of extensive tumor removal in improving survival is still debatable, a fact the patient must clearly understand. In other situations, the impact of surgery is more definable. A lesion causing severe mass effect with the potential for herniation requires surgery urgently. In a patient older than 50 years of age, the most common tumor causing severe mass effect is a malignant glioma, most likely a GBM. Such cases require more than just a diagnostic biopsy: extensive tumor resection makes the diagnosis, relieves symptoms, improves survival, and affords time to discuss and implement further therapies. The benefit of initial, extensive resection to improve survival in such situations has been documented.[97] The recommended approach is to perform as nearly total a resection as is possible while preserving maximal function.

Patients who are in poor physical health and harbor a deep-seated lesion may be best managed with stereotactic biopsy under local anesthesia to document the tumor histology before more extensive surgery is undertaken. If the histologic diagnosis is primary CNS lymphoma, for instance, attempts at extensive tumor resection are unwarranted because they would not change the prognosis for survival; however, if the lesion is an astrocytoma, then a more definitive surgical resection is indicated. Protection of normal brain is the limiting consideration for aggressive tumor removal, but within that restriction, the possibility of increasing survival has renewed surgeons' interest in pursuing extensive tumor removal, even in the knowledge that total resection is impossible and that further therapy is necessary. As opposed to a large residual tumor burden, which often has hypoxic or poorly vascularized areas that cause the lesion to be less responsive to radiation and chemotherapy, the reduced tumor burden afforded by extensive resection is more easily managed with adjuvant therapies.

CORTICAL MAPPING AND INTERACTIVE IMAGE-GUIDED RESECTIONS

In light of the potential advantages of extensive resection in both children and adults, cerebral cortical mapping with neurophysiologic monitoring is an important surgical adjunct.[98] Intraoperative cortical electrical stimulation is the gold standard for identifying primary motor, sensory, and language cortices.[99] Cortical mapping during surgery allows a more complete resection with a higher probability of retaining function and minimizing neurologic morbidity. It permits a physiologic representation to be drawn in relation to the gross anatomy of the brain, giving the surgeon a more precise knowledge of the probable effects of operating in the area of the tumor. Subcortical stimulation permits more extensive resection of lesions deep within the white matter as well. The technique entails stimulation of excitable cortex. The cortical loci of eloquent faculties, such as language, are variable and particular to each individual patient. Identification of the appropriate cortical loci permits a more extensive resection of intervening tumor while preserving eloquent function. Motor cortex can be defined while the patient is under general anesthesia, but an awake and cooperative patient is required for sensory and speech cortical mapping. Thus, young patients and those with significant preoperative aphasia are not good candidates for intraoperative cortical mapping.

With its other potential benefits, cortical mapping can also provide seizure control via simultaneous resection of the seizure foci, although the focus of seizure activity is often adjacent to, rather than in the area of the tumor.[100]

The operating room of the next millennium will look much different than current operating suites. Stereotactic techniques now allow for new systems for the surgeon to employ to aid in the safe resection of tumors. Currently available in a few specialized centers, these new operating rooms allow a greater likelihood of a complete resection, with real-time analysis of anatomic detail and functional imaging, linked by elaborate computers that coregister images and surgical navigation tools. A key element in this development has been the allowing of MR scanners into the operating room, and, further, allowing surgery to take place within the magnet itself. Newer systems either allow the patient to be moved back and forth into the magnet, or allow the magnet to be moved back and forth around the patient. In either case, using modified instrumentation, surgical procedures can be done with MR image guidance and instantaneous visual feedback is available to the surgeon. Functional, metabolic, and anatomic imaging are linked to the surgical navigation instruments in three-dimensional physical space. Greater precision, smaller incision, decreased operating time, and improvements in resectability are just a few of the benefits of this elaborate technology.

POSTOPERATIVE IMAGING

Contrast enhancement on the postoperative MRI-Gd image may be attributable to residual tumor volume, as well as to events related to surgery, such as gliosis and revascularization. In a study of 78 patients who were followed by using MRI after surgery, nonspecific enhancement in the tumor resection site began to appear as early as the fourth postoperative day.[101] In addition, the use of steroids may influence the interpretation of the scans.[102] For these reasons, postoperative scans should be done within 3 days of surgery to reflect as accurately as possible the extent of residual tumor, and to minimize the postoperative changes in and around the tumor bed which may be confused with tumor recurrence on MRI.

GLIOBLASTOMA MULTIFORME AND ANAPLASTIC ASTROCYTOMA

EPIDEMIOLOGY Patients with GBM (mean age, 54 years) are generally older than patients with AA (mean age, 45 years), with less than 10% of cases occurring in children. Median overall survival in GBM patients can range from 6 to 24 months, depending upon various patient factors, with a median survival of approximately 15 months, whereas median survival for AA patients is 3 to 4 years. The male:female ratio is 1.5:1 for GBMs and 1.2:1 for AAs. GBMs are twice as common in whites than African Americans, and arise most often in the temporal (32%) and frontal lobes (31%), whereas AAs are frequently found in the frontal lobes (40%).[103]

PROGNOSTIC FACTORS Factors that influence survival include patient age at diagnosis, Karnofsky performance score (KPS), and extent of resection (biopsy vs subtotal or gross total resection [GTR]). The Radiation Therapy Oncology Group (RTOG) examined patient factors that influenced survival outcome in 1,578 patients enrolled in 3 clinical trials conducted from 1974 through 1989.[104] A recursive partitioning analysis of prognostic factors resulted in six important subgroups. For patients younger than age 50 years, the most significant factor was histology, with median survival of 49.4 months for patients with anaplastic glioma and 13.7 months for patients with GBM. For patients older than 50 years of age, KPS was highly important. Patients with KPS ≥ 70 lived a median of 10.3 months, as compared to patients with KPS < 70, who lived a median of only 5.3 months. Further subgroups were defined by histology (GBM vs AA), mental status changes, extent of surgery, and radiation dose. This landmark analysis serves as an important baseline when results of phase II studies are compared to historical controls.

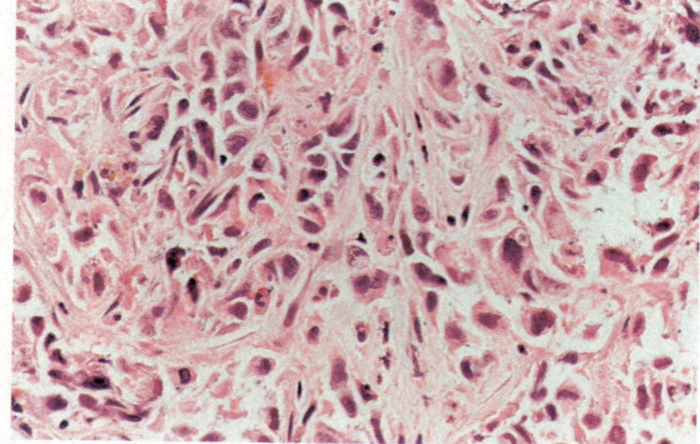

Figure 72-3 Histologic appearance of glioblastoma multiforme.

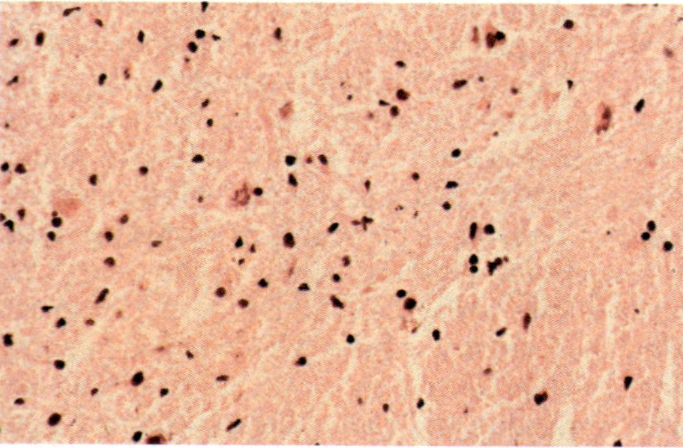

Figure 72-4 Histologic appearance of low-grade glioma.

PATHOLOGY The histopathologic characteristics of AA and GBM were discussed in the section on "Histopathology of Neuroepithelial CNS Tumors." GBMs are microscopically infiltrative lesions with a high labeling index, which is indicative of their highly proliferative nature. AAs are also infiltrative and have high labeling indices, which are usually lower than those of GBMs. Figure 72-3 depicts the typical histologic appearance of a GBM. Note the increased cellularity and pleomorphism of the tumor cells. In contrast, Figure 72-4 shows the appearance of a low-grade lesion, with only a minimal increase in cellularity and more normal-appearing cells.

DIAGNOSTIC NEUROIMAGING The usual appearance of a GBM or AA on MRI is that of a contrast-enhancing lesion causing mass effect. It is often very difficult to distinguish a GBM from a contrast-enhancing AA lesion by MRI alone. GBMs characteristically spread along the white matter tracts of the corpus callosum to invade the contralateral hemisphere ("butterfly" appearance). GBMs usually exhibit heterogeneous signal intensity on both T1WI and T2WI caused by cysts, necrosis, and hemorrhage commonly seen with GBM. Up to 95% of GBMs demonstrate contrast enhancement, and are almost always associated with high signal on T2WI. AAs also exhibit heterogeneous signal intensity on non-contrast T1WI and T2WI, but the frequency of contrast enhancement is less than in GBM. Large GBM lesions may demonstrate prominent areas of central necrosis with peritumor edema. Figure 72-5 shows the appearance of a recurrent GBM just posterior to the original resection cavity. Figure 72-6 shows the typical appearance of an anaplastic astrocytoma in both the axial and coronal planes. In both cases, the lesion is contrast enhancing, and imaging alone cannot distinguish GBM from AA.

SURGICAL DIAGNOSIS AND TREATMENT Surgery for patients with GBM or AA is designed to make the diagnosis, preserve life, alleviate symptoms, and to resect as much tumor as is safely possible. It is impossible to remove all microscopic disease even if there appears to have been a GTR on postoperative images caused by the infiltrative character of these lesions.[105] In patients with GBM, surgery alone will extend life no longer than a few months, as proved in the initial early research trials comparing surgery alone with the combination of surgery and irradiation.

There are no prospective randomized trials that have been conducted with the specific intent to address the impact of extensive resection versus biopsy alone or lesser degrees of resection on patient outcome. Most reported studies have been retrospective, typically single institutional studies based on nonvolumetric analysis of residual tumor volume. However, a retrospective analysis of three RTOG prospective randomized trials evaluated 645 GBM patients and observed a statistically significant difference in median survival between patients who had GTRs (11.3 months) versus those patients who received a biopsy only (6.6 months). There was also a statistically significant difference between the median survivals of partially resected and biopsy-only patients (10.4 months and 6.6 months, respectively).[106] Thus, extent of resection appears to be a significant prognostic factor for GBM, and biopsy alone offers inferior survival for GBM patients compared to more extensive resections. Several conclusions may still be reached about the extent of resection and outcome, however. First, there has been a significant reduction in mortality and morbidity associated with surgery over the last 30 years. Second, patients who undergo aggressive tumor removal usually improve or remain stable neurologically.[107,108] Third, most cooperative group prospective trials using a multimodality approach demonstrate that the extent of resection is one

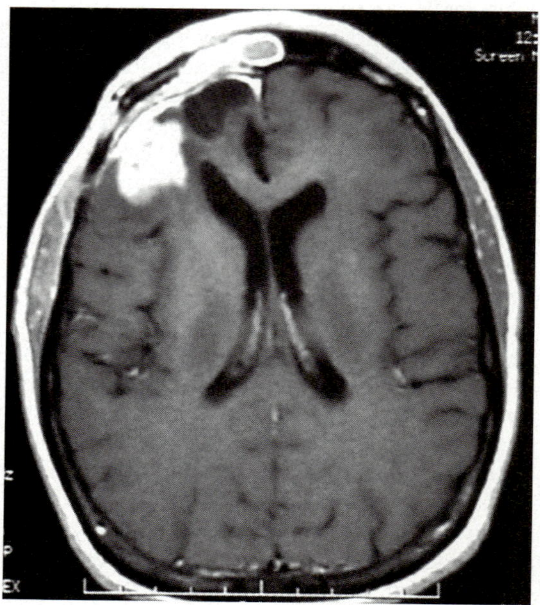

Figure 72-5 Typical magnetic resonance imaging appearance of glioblastoma multiforme.

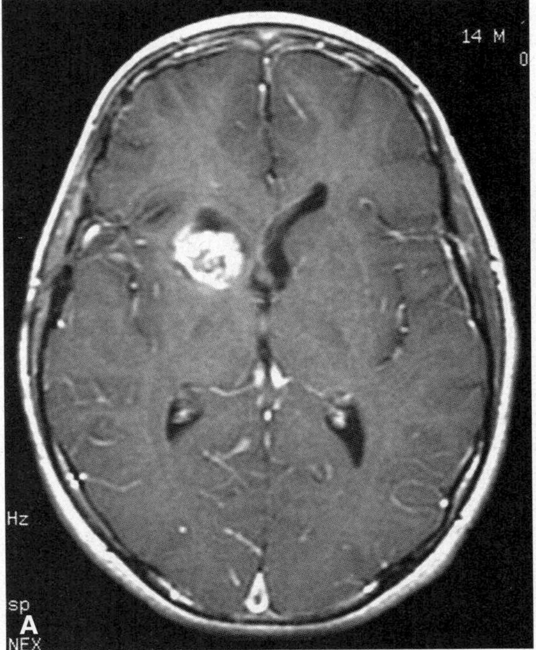

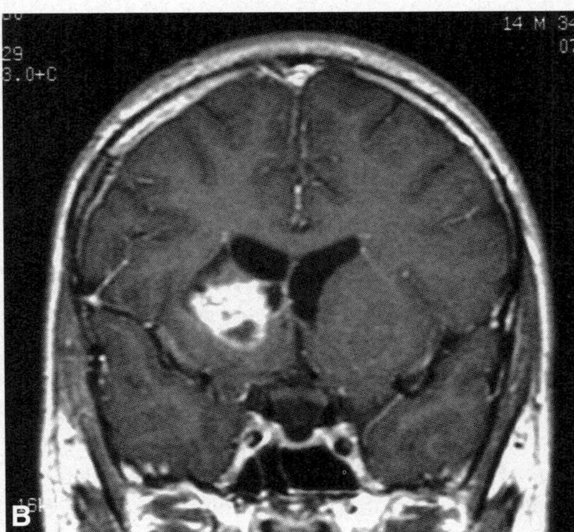

Figure 72-6 Magnetic resonance imaging appearance of an anaplastic astrocytoma. **A**, Lesion in the axial plane. **B**, Lesion in the coronal plane.

factor that influences survival.[97] Fourth, despite aggressive attempts at local control using surgery and local irradiation, the pattern of relapse is within 2 to 4 cm of the original tumor margins in most cases.[109,110] Thus, although there appears to be a compelling rationale to support aggressive resections because of the potential for prolonged quality survival, adjunctive therapy is still needed.

Radiation Therapy and Chemotherapy After surgery, patients with GBM or AA are treated with radiation therapy, and in most cases, with chemotherapy.[97] Irradiation is an effective adjuvant to surgery for malignant gliomas, and in prospective trials has afforded better survival than either surgery alone or surgery plus chemotherapy. Indeed, after surgical resection, radiation therapy is the single most effective treatment for both of these tumor types. Chemotherapy is used adjuvantly with surgery and radiation therapy. The early studies of chemotherapy involved the nitrosoureas, chosen for their lipophilic characteristics and in vitro sensitivity. These drugs include carmustine (BCNU), 1-(2-chloroethyl)-3-cyclohexyl-1-nitrosourea (lomustine, or CCNU), and *N'*-[(4-amino-2-methyl-5-pyrimidinyl)methyl]-*N*-(2-chloroethyl)-*N*-nitrosourea (nimustine, or ACNU). Other agents with antitumor activity include procarbazine, vincristine, cisplatin, carboplatin, tamoxifen, CPT-11, and temozolomide.

The initial studies of irradiation and adjuvant chemotherapy were conducted by the Brain Tumor Study Group (BTSG) in 1969.[111] In this landmark study, patients who had undergone surgery were randomized into four different treatment groups: (1) supportive care only; (2) carmustine (80 mg/m^2) given on three successive days every 6 weeks for 1 year; (3) whole-brain irradiation to a total of 50 to 60 Gy; and (4) whole-brain irradiation to a total of 50 to 60 Gy and carmustine (80 mg/m^2) given on three successive days every 6 weeks for 1 year. Patients with GBM constituted 90% of the treated groups. The median survival periods in the four groups were 14, 19, 36, and 35 weeks, respectively. The 12-month survival rates were 3%, 12%, 24%, and 32%, respectively. Comparison of the survival rates demonstrated that surgery plus radiation therapy offered a significantly improved survival time over that afforded by either surgery alone or surgery plus chemotherapy ($p < .05$), documenting the advantage of adjuvant irradiation in increasing survival for patients with GBM. The 12-month survival rates for patients treated with radiation plus carmustine were only slightly higher than those for patients receiving radiation only.

After this study, a series of trials undertaken by the BTSG reaffirmed the survival advantage afforded by radiation therapy after surgery and suggested a further advantage in some subsets of patients with the addition of adjuvant nitrosourea chemotherapy. One study compared the results of irradiation plus either carmustine or semustine to those of irradiation or semustine alone. Patients receiving carmustine plus radiation had a longer survival than those receiving semustine alone, but the survival rates with carmustine plus radiation were not significantly longer than those for people treated with radiation alone or with radiation plus semustine.[111] A trial conducted jointly by the Radiation Therapy Oncology Group (RTOG) and the Eastern Cooperative Oncology Group (ECOG) compared four treatment groups: (1) whole-brain irradiation to a total dose of 60 Gy; (2) whole-brain irradiation to 60 Gy plus a boost of 10 Gy to the tumor bed; (3) whole-brain irradiation to 60 Gy plus carmustine alone; and (4) whole-brain irradiation to 60 Gy plus semustine and dacarbazine (DTIC).[112] There were no differences in survival between the patients treated with 60-Gy whole-brain irradiation and those receiving whole-brain irradiation to 60 Gy with a 10-Gy boost to the tumor bed. The chemotherapy plus irradiation arms showed longer survival than either irradiation-only arm, but only in patients 40 to 60 years old; no advantage was seen in patients younger than age 40 years or older than age 60 years. More patients survived 2 years or longer in the chemotherapy arms. The DTIC plus semustine combination was more toxic than the carmustine treatment. Salazar and colleagues reviewed patients treated with whole-brain irradiation in increasing doses from 50 Gy to 60 Gy and up to 75 Gy, and noted an increased survival in patients receiving the higher doses; however, the consequence of the highest dose was a steady decline in KPS to a state of general debilitation by 18 to 24 months.[113] Peritumoral necrosis was often seen on CT. It appears from these and subsequent trials that 60 Gy is the optimal dose of XRT when single-dose radiation fractions are used. The Northern California Oncology Group (NCOG) evaluated the results obtained in a three-drug regimen of procarbazine, lomustine, and vincristine (PCV) with results in patients receiving carmustine alone after radiation therapy.[114] Patients with AA had a survival advantage when treated with PCV as compared with carmustine alone, median survivals being 157 weeks versus 82 weeks, respectively ($p = .021$). The three-drug combination offered no survival advantage over that obtained with carmustine alone for patients with GBM. More recently, a retrospective review of a larger group of patients with AA treated with PCV or with BCNU was analyzed, and suggested that there may not be a survival benefit for PCV.[115] Recently, a large, randomized phase III study of 674 patients with newly diagnosed GBM or AA were treated with radiation only, or radiation plus PCV chemotherapy.[116] This study showed no survival benefit for the patients treated with PCV chemotherapy, in either histologic types. Subsequent phase II studies in newly diagnosed GBM suggested that temozolomide added to radiation and given adjuvantly, may increase overall survival.[117] These results led to a phase III study conducted in Canada and Europe that randomized patients with newly diagnosed GBM to radiation plus temozolomide versus radiation only.[118] A total of 573 patients from 85 centers were randomized. At a median follow-up of 28 months, the median survival was 14.6 months with radiotherapy plus temozolomide versus 12.1 months with radiotherapy alone. The two-year survival rate was 26.5% with the combined treatment versus 10.4% with radiotherapy alone. From these and other studies, a role for surgery, irradiation, and in most cases, chemotherapy has been established. The role of adjuvant chemotherapy for GBM patients appears well established particularly in the better prognostic groups (younger patients with minimal residual disease and good performance status). In the special case of AA, more specific survival information is still needed, as there has yet to be a prospective phase III study conducted specifically in this patient population of sufficient size to confirm the role of chemotherapy. Specific therapy other than surgery, focal irradiation, and adjuvant chemotherapy remains investigational.

Many of the more recent attempts at improving survival have focused on radiation strategies, particularly alterations of dose or fractionation, and on newer chemotherapy agents. As mentioned earlier, most patients with malignant glioma will have relapses within 2 to 4 cm of the initial tumor margins. This observation would suggest that strategies to increase the duration of local control might ultimately increase overall survival. One such strategy is to increase the therapeutic index of irradiation.[119] Approaches to this problem have included the use of higher doses of irradiation using altered fractionation techniques and the use of interstitial radiation therapy.

Standard fractionated radiation therapy involves delivering the optimal total radiation dose of 60 Gy in daily fractions of 1.8 to 2.0 Gy over 6 weeks. Fractionated XRT treatments are typically given using high-energy (≥ 4 MeV) photon beams generated by linear accelerators. The dosage for primary brain tumor patients is delivered conformally to the shape of the tumor, rather than giving whole-brain XRT. RTOG has evaluated different fractionation schemes and higher total doses. In hyperfractionated radiation therapy, more than one fraction of the total dose is given each day, generally in smaller doses of radiation per fraction. The rationale for hyper-fractionation is to reduce late effects of radiation, especially necrosis, and to prevent tumor repopulation by using more than one treatment each day.[120] Between 1983 and 1987, phase I and phase II studies evaluated doses of 64.8, 72.0, 76.8, and 81.4 Gy, giving a twice daily dose of 1.2 Gy (RTOG protocol 83-02).[121] All patients received adjuvant BCNU chemotherapy. The dose of 72.0 Gy was chosen as the dose to compare to the standard 60 Gy dose in a phase III study. No benefit has been noted with the higher dose hyperfractionated schema, and based upon these investigations, the dose of 60 Gy still remains the current recommendation for treatment of malignant gliomas. Studies to improve the efficacy of radiation given in the conventional dosage include investigations of hypoxic cell sensitizers. Unfortunately, to date no studies demonstrate any improvement in survival with hypoxic cell sensitizers such as misonidazole and metronidazole. Radiation sensitizers such as the halogenated pyrimidines have been investigated in several studies. 5-Bromo-2'-deoxyuridine (broxuridine, or BUdR) and 5-iodo-2'-deoxyuridine (idoxuridine, or IUdR) are two nonhypoxic cell-sensitizing agents that are incorporated into the DNA of dividing cells in place of thymidine. Nondividing cells, such as those in normal glial and neuronal tissue, do not take up these agents. As with the hypoxic cell sensitizers, encouraging initial results have not been confirmed with phase III testing.[122,123] A phase III study was conduced by the RTOG, randomizing patients to radiation with or without BUdR, with all patients receiving adjuvant chemotherapy. The initial results of that study appeared negative, and the study was stopped prematurely.[124]

Interstitial brachytherapy involves the implantation of temporary high-activity or permanent low-activity radioactive sources ("seeds") within a tumor during the time of resection, and has been used to treat primary and recurrent malignant gliomas. The seeds remain in place within the tumor until the desired dose is delivered. Then, in a simple procedure done in the patient's room, the catheters and sources are removed. The major complications are seizures during source placement and, rarely, infection. Because of its risks and the precision required for proper placement of the radioactive sources, careful selection of patients for brachytherapy is imperative. The most commonly used radiation source is iodine 125 (^{125}I). The literature regarding the prognostic benefit of brachytherapy in the initial management of malignant glioma patients is mixed. One nonrandomized study reported a survival benefit for newly diagnosed GBM patients treated with temporary implants that delivered 40 cGy/h over 7 days.[125] However, a subsequent randomized study did not show benefit in ^{125}I implant patients (median survival for ^{125}I patients was 13.8 months, as compared to 13.2 months in patients without the implants).[126] Studies have not demonstrated any survival advantage of brachytherapy in AA patients.[127,128] Toxicity resulting in clinical deterioration from increasing radiation necrosis lesions may be significant. Hyperthermia has been evaluated in conjunction with brachytherapy in an attempt to increase local control, to reduce the radiation dose because heat enhances the effects of radiation therapy, and to decrease the risk of radiation necrosis. The results of a phase III trial favored the use of hyperthermia, one of the few controlled studies documenting an advantage to hyperthermia.[129] Unfortunately, many patients are not candidates for brachytherapy. The tumor volume that can be safely implanted is generally less than 5 cm in any dimension, and lesions in eloquent areas (corpus callosum, thalamus, and other mid-line deep-seated areas) of the brain are not implantable. The typical treated lesion is small, superficial, and located in an area where necrosis produced by the seeds can be tolerated. Given these limitations, most patients with GBM, AA, or even recurrent tumor, are ineligible for brachytherapy.

Radiosurgery is another technique used in this patient population. Radiosurgery is used to treat malignant glioma patients after conventional XRT either as a boost, or for recurrent tumors that are small (tumor volume < 30 cc) and do not involve critical brain structures. In this procedure, an external beam of radiation is precisely collimated and directed to a small volume in a single large fraction. Several radiation sources have been investigated for use with radiosurgery, including heavy particles, cobalt 60 (^{60}Co), and the conventional linear accelerator. The radiation beam is directed using coordinates on a standard stereotactic head frame or using a gamma unit, a device with a sophisticated head frame that permits precise assignment of coordinates along concentric arcs to cause a convergence of the ^{60}Co source.[130] The objective of radiosurgery is to deliver a finely focused radiation beam precisely to the target. This is based on the principle that a given dose of photon radiation has a much higher radiobiologic effect on tumor tissue than the same dose given over multiple treatment sessions (ie, fractionation). Immediate and delayed side effects appear to be less severe than in brachytherapy. Immediate side effects from radiosurgery include nausea, headache, seizure, dizziness, and are usually mild and transient.[131] In one study, 22% of radiosurgery patients required reoperation to resect radiation necrosis, as compared to 44% of patients treated with brachytherapy.[132] Critical evaluation in recently opened trials must address issues concerning dose and tumor volume, and identify specific criteria for selecting tumors that would benefit from this therapy. Studies have suggested a survival benefit as a boost for malignant glioma patients and at tumor recurrence.[133] One study reported equivalent efficacies for both radio-surgery and brachytherapy in recurrent malignant glioma patients.[132] Ongoing RTOG phase III studies will define the role of radiosurgery in newly diagnosed GBM. Brachytherapy may still have a preferred role in larger lesions, because radiosurgery has a tumor volume limit that is smaller than that of brachytherapy. However, radiosurgery has the advantages of fewer immediate and delayed side effects, as well as the fact that radiosurgery is noninvasive whereas brachytherapy requires a craniotomy.

Recommendation for Initial Therapy From the studies of various combinations of radiation therapy and adjuvant chemotherapy reported thus far, the standard treatment to which other therapies should be compared is single daily fraction irradiation to a total dose of 60 Gy plus adjuvant chemotherapy, typically either temozolomide or a nitrosourea. For patients with GBM, there is no survival advantage in using whole-brain radiation therapy, hyperfractionated XRT, interstitital brachytherapy or radiosurgery. Adjuvant chemotherapy improves 2-year survival rates and median survival in GBM patients and appears to improve median and long-term survival in AA patients, although not proven by prospective phase III studies in AA patients. However, it seems that only a subpopulation of GBM and AA patients benefit from adjuvant chemotherapy. These patients are younger with good KPS and minimal residual tumor burden after resection, which are positive predictors of survival to begin with. Some older GBM patients, who are more susceptible to chemotherapy toxicities, may be better off without adjuvant chemotherapy at initial diagnosis.

Recurrence The diagnosis of tumor recurrence requires, at the minimum, an increase in tumor volume demonstrated on sequential contrast-enhanced MR images. Although seemingly straightforward, neuroimaging studies may be difficult to interpret in light of previous treatment, or the changes seen on MRIs may be only slightly worse in the case of a clinically stable patient. MRI changes seen after interstitial brachytherapy or radiosurgery are, in particular, very difficult to interpret and may represent tumor recurrence, radiation necrosis, or a combination of both. As previously discussed, MRS or PET studies may be very helpful in distinguishing tumor from treatment effects. Once it is determined that a tumor has progressed, further treatment may include palliative care, another surgical resection, brachytherapy, radiosurgery, and/or chemotherapy. Several factors are important in the assessment of further treatment, including the patient's age, KPS, tumor histology, the expected outcome of additional therapies weighed against specific risks, and the needs and expectations of the patient and family. Elderly patients with poor KPS and recurrent GBMs have a poor prognosis and little chance of increasing their survival for more than an additional 2 to 3 months with further therapy. In the clinical situation of a bedridden patient with little remaining cognitive function, even maintenance of the status quo may be undesirable. Conversely, for a younger patient who is neurologically intact and has small tumor regrowth, there is a greater chance of achieving tumor control with little risk of a negative impact on quality of life. In such a case, it may be possible to achieve a median survival time of greater than a year, as measured from recurrence, in selected patient groups. Patients with recurrent malignant gliomas who are treated on research protocol studies generally live longer than those who are not; this reflects both an institutional referral bias and the benefit of further interventions that often occur in sequential treatment regimens. Patients on aggressive treatment programs are often young, strongly motivated, and in relatively good neurologic condition. For these reasons, the individual characteristics of groups tested should be weighed carefully and critically when interpreting the results of trials for patients with tumor recurrence.

When tumor recurrence is diagnosed, often the first decision to be made is whether further surgery should be recommended. Several studies have addressed the impact of reoperation on quality of survival. Ammirati and colleagues reviewed 55 patients with recurrent malignant astrocytoma who underwent a second resection and reported median survival of 36 weeks, which is similar to the reported survival of other groups.[108] Barker and colleagues also reviewed this issue more recently, and reached similar conclusions, emphasizing that some patient factors remain critical, including age and performance status.[134] Appropriate selection of patients for reoperation is important, as is the use of additional therapies following surgery. Interstitial brachytherapy and stereotactic radiosurgery are important salvage techniques for the small group of patients who have a recurrent malignant glioma of sufficiently small size in an appropriate location to permit accurate and safe placement of the interstitial catheters or treatment planning for radiosurgery.[127,128,130,135,136] Unfortunately, most patients with recurrent tumors are not eligible for either procedure, primarily because of the size and location of their recurrence.

For patients who are not eligible for brachytherapy or radiosurgery, treatment with chemotherapy is a reasonable alternative.[137–139] The nitrosoureas remain active agents for the treatment of recurrent tumors. Many trials using carmustine, either alone or in combination with other agents, show median survival times of 20 to 50 weeks, depending on tumor histology, with GBM being more rapidly lethal than AA. Other drugs, either alone or in combination, for malignant glioma treatment includes procarbazine, etoposide, *cis*-retinoic acid, thalidomide, vincristine, and high-dose tamoxifen. Investigation of new agents continues in structured phase I and phase II studies. Drug trials for recurrent tumors are often aimed at identifying new agents, or combinations of agents, that eventually may be used in phase III trials. Temozolomide was recently approved by the US Food and Drug Administration for the treatment of recurrent AA, and is the first such chemotherapy to be approved in more than 20 years. This drug is a cytotoxic methylating agent, orally active, and minimally toxic. Approval for the drug came as a result of a single-arm phase II trial for patients with recurrent AA.[140] Objective responses were noted in 35% of patients and the 6-month progression-free survival was close to 50%. This study was encouraging because of the minimal toxicity noted in patients, as well as the observation that patients who were previously felt to be resistant to nitrosourea therapy still had tumor regression noted. Many new studies are ongoing with this drug, in combination with other cytotoxic or biologic agents. Other drugs under investigation include novel agents that inhibit known growth factor receptors (such as the platelet derived growth factor receptor, the epidermal growth factor receptor, the vascular endothelial growth factor receptor) that influence cell growth. Indeed, a wide range of new agents are entering clinical trials for malignant glioma, and patients with recurrent disease should be encouraged to consider these new studies. Table 72-5 describes several new agents and targets undergoing investigation in malignant glioma at this time.

The outcome of patients treated at the time of recurrence is poor. Wong and colleagues reviewed the outcome of patients with recurrent malignant glioma treated according to eight consecutive phase II studies.[141] Of the 225 cases with recurrent GBM, the median progression-free survival was only 9 weeks, and for the 150 cases of recurrent AA, median progression-free survival was 13 weeks. Overall, the median survival was 30 weeks. The best response noted in the trials was 9%, with median response duration of 44 weeks. In a separate analysis, the same authors noted that the 52-week progression-free survival rate for patients who were progression-free at 13 weeks was 48% for responders versus 28% for nonresponders.[142] The authors concluded that a response to treatment was important in determining progression-free intervals and that agents that produce a response warranted further investigation. As noted, however, the response rate in this patient population is very low when using cytotoxic agents.

Table 72-5 New Agents Being Evaluated in Brain Tumor Therapy and Their Targets

Target	Agent
VEGFR inhibitors	PTK 787
	Bay 43-9006
	AEE 788
PDGFR inhibitors	Imatinib mesylate (STI-571)
	MLN518
	SU101
EGFR inhibitors	Erlotinib (OSI-774)
	AEE788
	Gefitinib (ZD 1839)
	Lapatinib (GW 572016)
MTor inhibitors	CCI-779
	Rapamycin
	RAD001
Histone deacetylase inhibitors	Suberoylanilide hydroxamic acid (SAHA)
	Depsipeptide
	Depakote
PKC inhibitors	Tamoxifen
	Enzastaurin (LY317615)
Farnesyltransferase inhibitors	Lonafarib (SCH 66336)
	Tipifarnib (R115777)

ANAPLASTIC OLIGODENDROGLIOMA

Patients with anaplastic oligodendrogliomas (AO) have shown exceptional chemosensitivity and frequently exhibit a complete response following chemotherapy using PCV.[143] The reason for this unusual response is unknown, but an observation has been made that molecular alterations seen in some of these patients is linked to chemotherapy response and survival. The allelic loss of chromosomes 1p and 19q are a molecular signature of these tumors and occur in 50 to 70% of cases.[86] There is an association between this molecular marker and response to chemotherapy. In a recent study, 100% of AO patients with loss of 1p or combined 1p and 19q loss had an objective response to chemotherapy (24 of 24 and 22 of 22, respectively).[86] In contrast, only 25% and 31% of those patients that retained these alleles responded. The 5-year survival rate for patients with loss of heterozygosity (LOH) at both 1p and 19q is 95%, as opposed to a 25% 5-year survival rate in patients with AOs that retained these alleles. Ino and colleagues stratified AO patients by clinical and molecular parameters into four prognostically relevant subgroups: AO with chromosome 1p and 19q loss (median survival > 123 months); 1p loss with 19q retention or 1p loss plus p53 mutation or other genetic alterations (71 months); 1p retention plus p53 mutation (71 months); and 1p retention with no p53 mutation (16 months).[144] This study suggests that molecular markers may be useful to identify patients who have a greater likelihood of a response to chemotherapy, and that therapeutic decisions at diagnosis may be adapted to the particular AO genetic subtypes. A recently completed phase III trial randomized newly diagnosed AO patients to receive either radiation alone or radiation preceded by PCV chemotherapy. Preliminary results have been presented at the 2004 meeting of the American Society of Clinical Oncology (ASCO). The addition of neoadjuvant PCV chemotherapy to radiation prolonged progression-free survival but did not improve overall survival.[145] Median survival of patients treated with PCV plus radiation was 4.8 years, versus 4.5 years for radiation alone. Independent of treatment regimen, patients who had deletions for 1p and 19q lived longer than other patients; median survival had not been reached in this group, versus 2.8 years in patients without those deletions. Thus, in cases of anaplastic oligodendroglioma, there does not appear to be a survival advantage by adding chemotherapy to radiation, and one of the best predictors of outcome is the presence or absence of 1p and 19q.

LOW-GRADE GLIOMAS

Low-grade gliomas (LGGs) include astrocytomas, oligodendrogliomas, mixed tumors such as oligoastrocytomas, and a variety of more unusual lesions such as gangliogliomas and neurocytomas. Astrocytomas may be further classified as pilocytic, protoplasmic, or fibrillary, based on their histologic appearance. The childhood cerebellar JPA is one of the most common LGGs and is somewhat distinct from the other low-grade lesions. It has a characteristic appearance on MRI and is often curable with surgery alone. However, when it arises from the hypothalamus, complete surgical resection is usually not possible, and other forms of therapy are often needed. Other LGGs, such as DNETs, are rarely treated even with minimal resection. The histologic diversity and biologic behavior of these diseases make generalizations difficult. However, the term *low grade* suggests tumors that are biologically very slow growing, and may not require intervention for many years. Accurate classification must be based on pathologic assessment; neuroimaging alone is not sufficient to make a diagnosis or to predict behavior in many of these tumors. Because of the rarity of LGGs other than astrocytoma, oligodendroglioma, and mixed oligoastrocytoma, discussion is focused on these specific subtypes. Table 72-6 lists the low-grade gliomas included in the current WHO classification system.

Table 72-6 World Health Organization Classification of Low-Grade Gliomas

Tumor	WHO Grade
Astrocytomas	II
Fibrillary	
Gemistocytic	
Protoplasmic	
Pilocytic astrocytoma	I
Pleomorphic xanthoastrocytoma	II
Subependymal giant cell astrocytoma	I
Subependymoma	I
Oligodendrogliomas	II
Mixed tumors	
Oligoastrocytoma	II
Neuronal and mixed glial-neuronal tumors	
Ganglioglioma	I/II
Central neurocytoma	II
Dysembryoplastic neuroepithelial tumors	I

Etiology and Epidemiology Low-grade gliomas may occur in many areas of the brain, including the optic nerve, cerebellum, hypothalamus, cerebral hemispheres, or brainstem. LGGs constitute approximately 10% of primary brain tumors. The mean age at diagnosis for patients with low-grade astrocytoma (excluding JPA) is 37 years, with a mean age ranging from 10 to 66 years; it is 14 years for those with JPA. The male:female ratio for low-grade astrocytomas is 1.4:1. In children, the incidence of glial neoplasms is 2 to 5 cases per 100,000 population per year, and approximately 70% of those neoplasms are LGGs. Patients with NF1 or NF2 are at increased risk for these lesions, especially for low-grade astrocytomas (LGAs) of the optic pathways. Comprising 5 to 10% of the total number of gliomas, oligodendrogliomas (oligos) most often occur in young and middle-aged adults and account for only 5 to 6% of CNS tumors in children. Oligos most often arise in hemispheric white matter but may be located wherever oligodendroglial cells occur in the CNS. Frequent locations include the frontal (more than 40%), parietal (30%), and temporal lobes (20%). They may be pure oligos or mixed oligoastrocytomas.

Prognostic Factors There are a number of significant pretreatment factors associated with prognosis in LGG patients. Table 72-7 lists the survival rates for supratentorial LGGs. As is evident from this table, histology has a significant role in tumor prognosis. Among the LGG subtypes (excluding JPAs), survival rates increase with higher proportions of oligodendroglioma cells in the tumor tissues. Age is another important prognostic factor. The age of 40 years is the most consistent cut-off age for survival prognosis, as patients younger than age 40 years have reported median survivals of 10.8 years, as compared to 8.1 years in patients older than age 40 years.[146] Children with LGAs have mean 5- and 10-year survival rates of 90% and 85%, respectively. Seizures that preceded the diagnosis by 6 months or more in the absence of other neurologic symptoms are associated with improved prognosis. In one series, 5-year survival rate was 64% in LGG patients with seizures, as compared to 14% in those without a seizure history.[147] A recursive partitioning analysis of pretreatment factors for LGG patients noted several statistically significant positive prognostic factors, such as KPS ≥ 70, age < 40 years, a seizure history prior to diagnosis, and the absence of enhancement on MRI or CT.[148] A retrospective study of LGG patients from European Organization for the Research and Treatment of Cancer (EORTC) trials 22844 and 22845 reported that the presence of neurologic deficits (except epilepsy) prior to surgery, tumors crossing the midline, and tumors ≥ 6 cm in greatest diameter were statistically significant negative prognostic factors.[149] With regard to molecular markers, the most common genetic alteration is mutation of *TP53,* which occurs in 30 to 45% of LGAs. Chozick and col-leagues reported an accumulation of abnormal p53 protein in 29% of grade II astrocytoma patients; there was a statistically significant difference in the 4-year survival rate in these patients (25%) versus those patients whose tumors did not accumulate abnormal p53 protein (87%).[150] VEGF expression has also been analyzed as a potential prognostic factor. A significant correlation was noted between median survival of LGA patients whose tumors expressed VEGF (11.2 years), as compared to those who did not (5.3 years). Fibroblastic growth factor (FGF) and EGFR expression did not significantly influence survival.[151] Thus, genetic alterations such as *TP53* mutation and VEGF expression may be used as important prognostic variables to stratify LGG patients in clinical trials.

Pathology The histopathologic characteristics of the main LGG subtypes were previously described. Pathologically, LGAs are infiltrative lesions with a population of uniform cells, a

Table 72-7 Survival Rates of Supratentorial Low-Grade Gliomas

Histologic Subtype	Median Survival (Years)	2-Year (%)	5-Year (%)	10-Year (%)	15-Year (%)
PA	NR	88	85	79	79
A	4.7	80	46	17	7
OA	7.1	89	63	33	17
O	9.8	93	73	49	49

A = astrocytoma; NR = not reached; O = oligodendroglioma; OA = oligoastrocytoma; PA = pilocytic astrocytoma.
Adapted from Shaw EG.

slight increase in cellularity, and minimal pleomorphism.[152] Most often, there is no clear border between the tumor and surrounding normal brain parenchyma. The astrocytes may show a fibrillary or protoplasmic morphology, or they may be mixed with abnormal oligodendrocytes or ependymal cells. JPA lesions in the hypothalamus and optic pathways may appear identical. Biologic growth is slow, both in the infiltrative fibrillary astrocytomas and JPAs. Oligos appear as small, round cells in a monotonous pattern. One of the more perplexing problems in contemporary neuropathology is the designation of a lesion as oligodendroglioma or mixed oligoastrocytoma. A consensus has yet to be reached as to the criteria that should be used to make these diagnoses. Because of this fact, interpretation of clinical outcomes of patients may be difficult to compare between various institutions and groups.

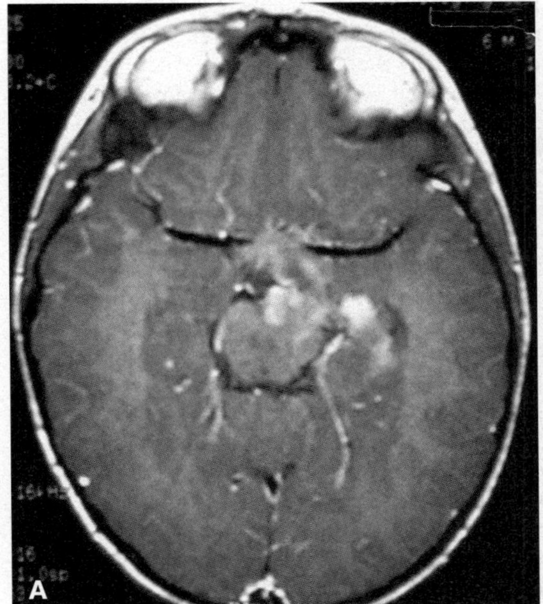

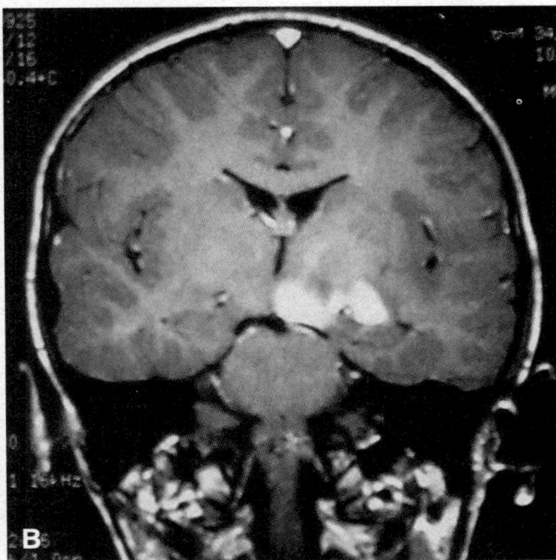

Figure 72-7 Typical magnetic resonance image appearance of a pilocytic lesion in the hypothalamus and optic tracts. **A,** Lesion in the axial plane. **B,** Lesion in the coronal plane.

Clinical Presentation Patients with astrocytoma often present with seizures (more often focal than generalized) that may have been present for many years prior to the diagnosis. In most series, seizures are the most common presenting symptom (67%), followed by headache, and also focal neurologic findings. The most common sign at presentation is a sensory or motor deficit. The median duration from onset of symptoms to diagnosis is 6 to 17 months, and may be as long as 17 years. Cerebellar JPAs in children present with symptoms of clumsiness, ataxia, head tilt, intermittent headaches, and vomiting. JPAs of the optic nerve, chiasm, tract, and hypothalamus may present with eye movement disorders, visual field defects, and in older children, precocious puberty. Cerebral lesions show signs and symptoms associated with the specific location of the lesion.

Diagnostic Neuroimaging In general, CT often shows a cystic or solid tumor of low density and variable amounts of contrast enhancement. Pilocytic astrocytomas appear as cystic masses with intense contrast enhancement. Classically, the cerebellar JPA appears as a large, smooth-walled cyst with a small enhancing mural nodule. In adults, astrocytoma in the cerebrum will often appear diffusely infiltrative, or solid and hypodense. These lesions may or may not enhance. Often the lesion involves an entire lobe (mostly frontal or temporal) but has indistinct margins and causes minimal mass effect. MRI reveals either a hypointense or isointense lesion on T1WI, with a larger area of strong hyperintensity on T2WI. The CT appearance of oligodendroglioma is a hypodense or isodense lesion that may or may not enhance. Many oligodendrogliomas have calcifications scattered within the lesion, reflecting the mineralization seen histologically within blood vessel walls, with little peritumoral edema. MRI reflects the CT lesion, with a hypointense or isointense lesion on T1WIs, a hyperintense appearance on T2WIs, and areas of signal void where calcifications arise. Enhancement with Gd for both LGA and low-grade oligodendrogliomas (LGOs) is variable. Figure 72-7 depicts a typical pilocytic astrocytoma arising from the hypothalamus and extending into the optic radiations in both the axial and coronal plane. A lesion in this location could not be completely resected and would require additional treatment.

Treatment Options The treatment of LGGs depends on several factors, including the location of the tumor, the age of the patient at diagnosis, the extent of resection possible, and evaluations based on an understanding of the biology of these lesions. Options include observation alone, biopsy and/or resection, surgery plus irradiation, chemotherapy alone, or some combination of surgery, irradiation, and chemotherapy. Childhood cerebellar JPA, for instance, are manageable in most cases with surgical resection alone. Only in very rare cases do JPAs recur following GTR, and even the rare patient with recurrence may still have a good outcome with repeat surgical interventions, with or without adjuvant radiation therapy. In contrast, infiltrative astrocytomas in adults often are not amenable to GTR, and usually require additional therapy such as irradiation.

Surgery is necessary in almost all cases to accurately establish the pathologic diagnosis. There are a few instances where neuroimaging alone will support a diagnosis. For instance, children with NF1 and a lesion in the optic nerve or hypothalamus will occasionally be treated based on imaging criteria alone. Beyond this situation, most biopsies of brain lesions should at least be performed. A more extensive resection may also be appropriate, assuming that the procedure can be done safely. In one series by Berger and colleagues, the pre- and postoperative tumor volume was used to analyze the probability of recurrence in patients with low-grade tumors.[153] When the authors reviewed the postoperative volume, they noted that 15% of patients recurred with a median time to tumor progression of 50 months if the volume was less than 10 cm^3. However, in cases with a postoperative tumor volume of greater than 10 cm^3, 46% of patients recurred at a median of 30 months. Other series tend to support the notion that reduction of tumor burden by surgery will lengthen the time to tumor progression.[154–157] However, not all series have demonstrated a significant survival benefit for extensive resection, and there are no prospective randomized studies that have addressed this question. Institutional bias, subsequent treatment beyond surgery, inadequate tissue sampling when biopsy alone is used to make a diagnosis, and the retrospective nature of these reviews need to be considered when one interprets the data concerning surgery in low-grade glioma. Other factors may influence the decision to attempt an extensive resection in these lesions, including patient age, the potential need for subsequent irradiation and its long-term associated risks, and patient preference. Surgery data for LGO patients show significant survival benefit for more extensive resection.[158]

One potential option in the management of LGG patients after histologic diagnosis is observation with serial MRIs, with deferral of further treatment until tumor recurrence is noted. This is not an inherently intuitive concept, as the initial impulse for patients, their families, and physicians is to pursue further aggressive treatment for brain tumors. However, this option has been supported by studies that have not conclusively demonstrated a survival benefit to initiating treatment immediately after diagnosis.[159]

The next question that usually arises in LGGs is the need for and timing of radiation therapy.

The EORTC reported a phase III trial in adults with supratentorial LGGs (excluding JPAs), randomizing them to either observation only or initial treatment with radiation. Although there was a significant improvement in the 5-year progression-free survival rate for patients who initially received radiation versus the observation group (44% versus 37%), the 5-year overall survival rate was similar in the two treatment groups (63% versus 65%).[160] Two-thirds of the cases randomized to the observation arm ultimately received radiation. Thus, observation and deferral of radiation may be justified without negative impact on overall survival. This approach remains controversial, however, and it is probable that certain subsets of patients will benefit from an observation approach and others from an immediate treatment approach. Philippon and colleagues reviewed data from a group of patients with low-grade tumors and concluded that radiation did not improve survival when all patients were considered, except in the subset of patients age 50 years and older who had a subtotal resection or biopsy.[161] In that subset, the 3-year survival with radiation was 50% versus 25% in the older grade II tumor patients who were not irradiated immediately following surgery. The series by Shaw and colleagues also supported this notion of prognostic subgroups.[162] Patients older than age 35 years had longer 5-year survival if they had postoperative irradiation to a dose larger than 53 Gy. Five and 10-year survival rates for patients older than age 35 years who received 53 Gy or more postoperatively were 67% and 45%, respectively, as compared to 37% and 5% for patients who had surgery alone or less than 53 Gy or postoperative XRT. The dose used for radiation has been partially addressed in two prospective randomized studies.[163,164] The EORTC randomized 379 patients to receive low-dose (45 Gy) or high-dose (59.4 Gy) radiation given to a local field, and reported no difference in outcome. The 5-year survival rate was 58% with 45 Gy and 59% with 59.4 Gy. The second study compared doses of 50.4 Gy and 64.8 Gy, and an initial analysis also shows no 5-year survival advantage to the higher dose (73% and 68% respectively). A recently closed, but not yet reported trial of the RTOG uses 54 Gy in the treatment of these patients. In practice, when radiation therapy is used, the most common dose is between 50 and 60 Gy, given conformally to a focal field. The large EORTC study reported a lower level of functioning, higher fatigue, malaise and insomnia in patients treated at the higher doses of radiation, suggesting that a negative impact on quality of life is a potential risk over time when higher doses of radiation are used.[165] One study reported a 46% response rate and an 87% control rate for grade II astrocytomas treated with radiosurgery, with a mean follow-up period of 27.6 months, suggesting that radiosurgery may a viable treatment option for surgically inaccessible LGAs.[166]

Chemotherapy currently is being investigated in the initial management of adults with newly diagnosed low-grade glioma. The role of chemotherapy appears well established in younger children, with an attempt to defer XRT for as long as possible. However, as of this time, there is no conclusive evidence that chemotherapy either used prior to or following radiation improves survival in adults. Thus, currently there is no proven role for chemotherapy in the management of LGGs in adults, particularly for astrocytomas. A randomized trial by the Southwest Oncology Group (SWOG) demonstrated no survival benefit for patients with subtotally resected supratentorial LGAs who received XRT with CCNU versus those who received XRT alone.[167] For LGOs, Mason and colleagues reported a 100% response rate in 9 adult LGO patients treated initially with PCV; only 1 patient who had stable disease after six cycles of PCV had to be given XRT.[168] This is not unexpected, as anaplastic oligos have been well documented to be chemosensitive to PCV.[143] A recently completed phase III trial randomized patients into three arms: low-risk LGG patients (age < 40 years with GTRs) are only observed; high-risk patients (age ≥ 40 years or subtotal resection/biopsy) are randomized into receiving XRT alone (54 Gy) or XRT with six cycles of PCV. The results of this study will not be known for several more years.

Recurrence Various treatment strategies are available for LGG recurrences, including reoperation, chemotherapy, radiation therapy, or some combination of those modalities. Generally, survival following tumor recurrence is poor, but is significantly influenced by histology. In one series, median survival following recurrence of LGGs was 39 months for all LGG patients, 16 months for LGAs and 60 months for recurrent LGOs.[146] Many patients will be candidates for repeat resection and should be considered for those procedures. Symptom control may be one reason to consider surgery, but there is also the benefit of tumor reduction and a more accurate diagnosis of the recurrent disease. Many low-grade tumors will progress to a more malignant phenotype, often with histologic features that are consistent with anaplastic glioma or GBM. In the series reported by Leighton and colleagues, malignant transformation occurred in approximately 50% of patients.[146] Malignant transformation influences subsequent treatment strategies, and surgery should be considered as part of the overall management of these patients. If prior radiation has been used, reirradiation may be possible with either radiosurgery or interstitial brachytherapy. Chemotherapy is also an option, although response rates are variable. Response rates have been noted in 33% of recurrent LGA patients treated with BCNU and interferon-α,[169] and in 90% of recurrent LGO patients treated with PCV. More recent studies have used temozolomide in the setting of recurrent LGG, particularly oligodendroglioma, with response rates as high as 50%.[170]

Management Recommendations Low-grade astrocytomas that can be totally resected may be managed with surgery alone, with the goal being a maximal and safe resection. Incompletely resected tumors may be managed by observation alone or by surgery and irradiation. Adult patients with incompletely resected LGGs who are treated with radiation typically receive 54 Gy using single daily dose fractions to the tumor volume and a surrounding small margin. Chemotherapy is typically reserved for recurrent disease, although more studies are now being conducted to evaluate the role of chemotherapy at the time of initial diagnosis. Despite the optimism associated with the treatment of lower-grade lesions, many patients still die of this disease. New approaches are needed in the management of these tumors, with clinical research trials designed to answer questions concerning the optimal extent of resection, the timing and dose of radiation therapy, and the timing of chemotherapy use.

EPENDYMOMA

Epidemiology Ependymomas constitute approximately 5% of adult intracranial gliomas and up to 10% of childhood CNS tumors. Ependymomas are the third most common childhood brain tumor. There is a peak incidence at age 5 years and then again at age 34 years.

Pathology Ependymomas are tumors that resemble normal ependymal cells and tend to occur along the surfaces of the ventricles. They may also occur in the parenchyma adjacent to the ventricle or anywhere along the entire length of the spinal canal and the filum terminale. More than 60% of ependymomas occur infratentorially, most of which occur in the posterior fossa, and arising predominantly from the fourth ventricle. Most supratentorial ependymomas are parenchymal rather than intraventricular in location, and occur most frequently in the frontal and parietal lobes. Tumor extension may occur along the leptomeninges, around the medulla and upper cervical cord to the conus, and along nerve roots; ependymal cells may be found in the CSF.

Ependymomas are classified as either differentiated (low-grade or grade II) or anaplastic (malignant or grade III) tumors. Most are cellular tumors consisting of uniform polygonal cells in a collagenous background with well-defined cytoplasmic borders. They may also contain areas of cysts, calcifications, and occasional hemorrhage. Some groups of cells form clusters around a circumscribed central space (ependymal rosette). Anaplastic ependymomas have features that resemble GBM. These lesions may have high mitotic activity, endothelial proliferation, and necrosis. A very highly cellular, embryonal form of ependymal tumor occurring in infants and children younger than age 5 years is the ependymoblastoma.[171] This tumor is biologically and pathologically distinct from the other types of ependymomas. The ependymoblastoma often disseminates along the CSF pathways and requires irradiation of the craniospinal axis (CSA). Children with this tumor rarely live more than 2 to 3 years. Ependymoblastomas are most likely a form of PNET with ependymal differentiation, and are treated in the same fashion as medulloblastoma. This variant of ependymoma should be regarded as distinct from malignant (anaplastic) ependymoma in terms of treatment.

Prognostic Factors One of the most important prognostic variables is the amount of residual tumor after resection.[172] Children with low-grade nondisseminated ependymomas that have been completely resected have the best prognosis, whereas incomplete resection or dissemination carries a poor prognosis. The retrospective series by Horn and colleagues evaluated the outcome of 83 children with ependymoma treated at 11 institutions between the years 1987 and 1991.[172] This is an important contemporary review and the data is useful as a baseline from which to compare new trials. In this review, the overall survival at 5 and 7 years was 57% and 46%, respectively; event-free survival for the same periods was 42% and 33%. Patients younger than age 3 years had significantly worse outcome. Univariate analysis revealed that young age, subtotal resection, and grade III histology were important adverse risk factors for event-free survival. Overall survival was negatively influenced by the same factors, with high-grade histology having only borderline significance (p = .05) in a multivariate analysis. Most patients (89%) progressed at the original tumor location. Adjuvant chemotherapy or CSA irradiation did not significantly influence outcome. The authors concluded that improvement of local control is an important goal for future studies.

There are conflicting data concerning the prognostic implications of anaplasia in these tumors.[173,174] Ross and Rubinstein reviewed a series of 15 patients classified as having anaplastic ependymomas (excluding cases of ependymoblastoma) in an attempt to correlate pathology with survival; postoperative survival was not found to correlate with anaplastic histology. The median survival for 10 patients with malignant tumors was 8.8 years; 5 patients who had tumor recurrence died within 13 months to 6 years (median 2.5 years). In their review, Horn and colleagues found WHO grade III histology a significant adverse risk factor for overall survival and event-free survival in univariate analyses, but only of borderline significance in overall survival when correcting for other factors, such as extent of disease.[172]

Clinical Presentation Clinically, patients may present with subtle signs and symptoms for years before the diagnosis is made or may present abruptly with obstructive hydrocephalus or an expanding ependymoma of the spinal cord. Other focal findings include visual field defects, focal seizures, headache, nausea, and vomiting.

Diagnostic Neuroimaging The neuroimaging of ependymomas is nonspecific, but some findings are useful that suggest the diagnosis, including calcification associated with a fourth ventricular tumor. They tend to extend out of the fourth ventricle into the cerebellum, foramen magnum, cerebellopontine angle, and upper cervical arachnoid space. The MRI appearance of ependymomas is heterogeneous. The solid portions are hypointense on T1WI and hyperintense on T2WI. Almost all ependymomas are contrast enhancing, although the enhancement is often irregular and patchy. Intratumoral cysts are more common in supratentorial ependymomas and usually have slightly higher intensity signal than CSF on T1WI. Because many lesions may be confused with ependymomas (such as PNETs), treatment should not proceed without histologic verification of the tumor and an assessment of the degree of anaplasia.

Treatment The goal of surgery for ependymoma should be to achieve a GTR as often and as safely as possible. Unfortunately, extensive resection is often impossible, particularly for lesions of the posterior fossa or for spinal cord ependymomas involving the cauda equina. Supratentorial lesions are more amenable to GTR. In patients older than age 3 years with GTRs of low-grade nondisseminated ependymomas, deferring further adjuvant therapy may be a viable option. In one study, all 5 patients with the above tumor profile were alive after a median follow-up of 44 months, with a median progression-free survival over 38 months.[175] Low-grade ependymoma of the spine may be managed with surgery alone if the resection is complete. Staging is a critical aspect in the management of ependymomas. This involves an MRI of the brain and the entire spinal cord with contrast, as well as CSF cytology to rule out neuraxis dissemination.

Several retrospective series strongly suggest an advantage to the addition of radiation therapy in improving survival.[176–178] In the series by Ernestus and colleagues, patients with supratentorial grade II ependymomas treated with radiation had a median survival 185 months. The benefit of postoperative irradiation was even more striking in patients who underwent only a partial resection: the median disease-free survival was 9 months in patients undergoing surgery only, but was more than 108 months in those who received postoperative radiation therapy. Survival was only 21 months for those with grade III tumors despite irradiation. Other trials have documented the radiosensitivity of ependymomas. The literature does not identify, however, the optimal perimeters of the radiation field for treating ependymomas in specified locations or whether the craniospinal axis should always be included in the field. The risk of spinal subarachnoid metastasis is greatest with infratentorial anaplastic ependymomas (approximately 30%) and is least likely with supratentorial low-grade ependymomas (5 to 10%). There is also a risk of intraventricular and intracranial spread from a malignant supratentorial lesion. For these reasons, the extent of the irradiated field is an important issue. Salazar and colleagues reported a local control rate of 12% using small-volume fields, as compared to 78% control with whole-brain irradiation in a group of patients with low-grade ependymomas.[177] The 5-year survival rate was 12% with partial-brain and 67% with whole-brain treatment. Other series show no benefit to craniospinal irradiation.[172,174,179,180] Because the primary site of recurrence of both low- and high-grade ependymomas is usually within the local radiation field, whole-brain or craniospinal irradiation is probably not indicated. Staging is a critical aspect in the management of ependymomas. The consensus management approach is to give focal irradiation after maximal resection to the resection cavity and to the surrounding tissue area, rather than CSA irradiation if there is no evidence of dissemination.

Chemotherapy unfortunately has only a minor role in these tumors, and may be most useful in the treating of recurrent ependymoma. Adjuvant chemotherapy does not improve over-all survival in ependymoma patients. Despite their frequent posterior fossa location, ependymomas, unlike PNETs, are fairly chemoresistant. These tumors are occasionally sensitive to several agents, including the nitrosoureas and platinum compounds. A CCG study randomized pediatric patients with newly diagnosed posterior fossa ependymomas into two groups: those who received CSA irradiation, and those who received CSA irradiation and an adjuvant chemotherapy regimen of CCNU, vincristine, and prednisone for 1 year. There was no difference in outcome between the two groups, suggesting that this chemotherapy regimen does not improve survival of infratentorial ependymoma patients.[181] Much more research is needed to find new agents to treat ependymoma.

SPINAL CORD TUMORS

Etiology and Epidemiology Primary spinal cord tumors constitute 10 to 15% of all primary CNS lesions. The subtypes of spinal cord tumors are grouped depending on their location, which is often determined by their cell of origin. The most common extradural spinal lesion is a metastatic tumor from another primary site. Intradural lesions are divided into two categories, depending on whether they involve the substance of the spinal cord (intramedullary) or are outside the spinal cord but within the dura (extramedullary). Tumors of glial origin (eg, astrocytomas, ependymomas) are usually intradural intramedullary in location, whereas nerve sheath tumors (eg, neurofibromas and schwannomas) are typically intradural extramedullary lesions. Meningiomas can be either extradural or intradural extramedullary lesions. Like supratentorial meningiomas, they occur most often in females, and account for 25 to 50% of primary intraspinal tumors and 40% of intradural extramedullary tumors. The spectrum of lesions in the adult population differs from that in the pediatric age groups. In children, the most common location of the spinal lesion is intramedullary, with the most frequent tumor being an astrocytoma, whereas in adults, intradural extramedullary tumors are more common. In unusual cases, adult ependymomas and astrocytomas may be exophytic and extramedullary.

Clinical Presentation Clinical symptoms of spinal cord lesions include back pain, motor and sensory disturbances, and bowel, bladder, and sexual dysfunction. The most common presenting symptom is axial back pain at the lesion site, which is worse at night and in the supine position. Symptoms often correlate with tumor growth rate rather than tumor size, as slow-growing tumors may cause little or no neurologic sequelae, whereas rapidly growing tumors may cause significant neurologic deficits at presentation. Intramedullary tumors arising from the central part of the cord, often spare sensation over the sacral region ("sacral sparing"), because of the somatotopic organization of the spinal cord, in which the sacral sensory fibers are at the most peripheral position within the spinal cord. Extramedullary tumors grow in relation to nerve roots and produce radicular pain that frequently is worse at night and is aggravated by maneuvers that increase intracranial pressure, such as straining or coughing. Intramedullary lesions frequently do not present with pain as the initial symptom but rather signs of central cord destruction, including reduced sensation to pain and extreme temperatures, long tract signs, weakness, bowel and bladder incontinence, and sexual dysfunction. Ependymomas are frequently situated at the cauda equina and produce sphincter and peripheral lower extremity weakness.

Diagnostic Neuroimaging MRI is the neuroimaging modality of choice in the evaluation of spinal cord tumors. The ability of MRI to depict the extent of the lesion and its specific location in relation to other structures, as well as its definition of cysts associated with tumors, makes it preferable to other techniques, such as CT myelography. MRI permits an accurate prediction of the histology of the lesion in many cases; for instance, astrocytomas often show heterogeneous enhancement in an asymmetric fashion, whereas ependymomas frequently enhance uniformly with smooth edges. Tumor nodules associated with cysts are easily visualized, providing valuable information for surgical planning. The extent of cysts above or below the lesion defines the level of the laminectomy and the extent of exposure needed. One of the most distinguishing MRI features of intramedullary tumors is spinal cord parenchymal expansion. Other intramedullary lesions, such as transverse myelitis and multiple sclerosis plaques, usually do not expand the cord. To eliminate artifacts caused by cardiac pulsations, respiration, and CSF flow, cardiac gating and other flow-compensatory mechanisms are used. For young children, sedation is often required because the acquisition of data requires that they remain motionless for a long period.

Surgical Treatment The goals of surgery for spinal cord lesions are to make the diagnosis and relieve symptoms. For ependymoma, meningioma, and neurofibroma, GTR is the treatment of choice. Astrocytomas comprise 90% of all intramedullary neoplasms in adults, although they present more frequently in children. Most are grades I or II, with only 10 to 15% of spinal astrocytomas being higher in grade. Five-year overall survival for spinal astrocytomas is 50 to 60%.[182,183] Extent of resection for intramedullary astrocytomas in adults has not been found to influence survival rates.[184] The most significant prognostic factor for survival is histologic grade. Five-year survival rates for grade I spinal astrocytomas is 80%, whereas it only reaches 15% in grades II and III astrocytomas.[182] Median survival was 68 months for grade II and 15 months for grade III spinal astrocytomas.[183] For astrocytoma, especially a diffuse lesion occupying large areas of the spinal cord, only a biopsy and partial removal can be accomplished due to their highly infiltrative nature, although recently, some surgeons have emphasized a more aggressive surgical approach for spinal astrocytomas.

The role of surgery in children with low-grade intramedullary spinal cord tumors may be more significant. A retrospective study of 124 children and patients up to 21 years of age with low-grade intramedullary spinal cord tumors noted a 5-year progression-free survival rate of 78% in patients treated with extensive surgery alone, which was comparable to the rates of patients treated with minimal resection and XRT. The authors concluded that the optimal treatment at initial diagnosis for young patients with low-grade intramedullary tumors is radical resection only, with deferral of XRT and chemotherapy.[185] Radical excision has not been shown to improve outcome in patients with spinal anaplastic astrocytomas.[186]

More frequently than for spinal astrocytomas, spinal ependymomas can be approached with the intention of complete surgical removal. They usually arise in children and young adults, and are intramedullary or in the region of the filum terminale. Most spinal ependymomas are WHO grade II tumors. Myxopapillary ependymomas, which are found exclusively in the filum terminale region, are grade I lesions and are associated with a good prognosis, with a reported 10-year survival rate of 89%.[187] Little is known about the efficacy of chemotherapy in spinal cord tumors. Unsurprisingly, few reports of success with chemotherapy have been reported, as both astrocytomas and ependymomas are generally chemoresistant. For subtotally resected or anaplastic ependymomas, XRT gives effective disease control, with 5- and 10-year overall survival rates of 69% and 62%, respectively.[188] GTR is potentially curative with no need for further therapy. In one series, no evidence of recurrence was noted in any patient during a mean follow-up period of 62 months.[189] Retrospective series have reported 5- and 10-year overall survival rates of 83% and 75%, respectively.[190] Cooper reviewed the results obtained in 51 adults with a variety of intramedullary tumors treated with radical surgical resection.[191] Of the 24 patients with ependymoma, only 2 died (1 a suicide and 1 from a progressive tumor). In comparison, 12 of 18 patients with astrocytomas died. All patients with ependymoma and astrocytoma who had residual tumor after surgery were treated with radiation therapy. The extent of surgery was considered important to outcome in the case of ependymomas, as only 1 of 11 patients believed to have had total removal had recurrence, whereas tumor recurred in 5 of 13 patients who had had incomplete resection. All of the patients with high-grade anaplastic astrocytomas eventually died of their tumor.

Radiation Therapy and Chemotherapy Linstadt and colleagues reviewed the results of 42 patients with primary spinal cord tumors treated at University of California at San Francisco with radiation therapy: 21 patients had ependymoma, 12 had low-grade astrocytoma, 3 had anaplastic astrocytoma, and 6 had tumors of uncertain histology.[192] The radiation dose was in the range of 45 to 54.7 Gy. The projected actuarial 10-year disease-free survival for patients with localized ependymomas was 93%. Three patients had ependymoma diffusely involving the cord, 1 of whom died from a cerebral metastasis; the other 2 are alive and disease free. The corresponding 10-year survival rate for the 12 patients with low-grade astrocytoma was 91%, and no patient who had an anaplastic astrocytoma survived longer than 8 months. In both the ependymoma and low-grade astrocytoma groups, most patients who had a treatment failure had tumor regrowth in the original site of disease.

The prognosis is quite poor in patients with spinal AAs. Most patients die of this disease despite extensive surgical resections and irradiation to the limit of cord tolerance. Other approaches to these lesions are needed.

Chemotherapy only delays the inevitable. Various combinations of chemotherapy, primarily nitrosourea-based, have produced no long-term survivors; other agents, including platinum compounds, thiotepa, and cyclophosphamide, have had only limited and transient benefit. One study analyzed the "8-in-1" chemotherapy regimen for high-grade spinal astrocytoma patients. Despite this aggressive treatment regimen, mean survival was only 6 months.[193]

Recurrence Recurrent spinal cord ependymoma is more amenable to therapy than astrocytoma, including repeat surgical resections, re-irradiation using hyperfractionated techniques (especially for lesions of the conus), and chemotherapy with the nitrosoureas, temozolomide or platinum agents. When an ependymoma recurs in the spinal cord, the entire neuraxis should be imaged to assess the extent of disease, because even a histologically benign ependymoma occasionally disseminates. Using sequential therapies, it is possible to control this lesion for years. Recurrent astrocytoma of the spinal cord should be treated with chemotherapy at relapse, preferably on an investigational protocol. Initial therapy may consist of nitrosourea-based chemotherapy, followed by other agents described previously in the GBM/AA section. For pediatric patients with recurrent intramedullary spinal cord tumors, of which the large majority are LGGs, carboplatin-based chemotherapy regimens have been reported anecdotally to improve survival rates.[194–196]

ADULT MEDULLOBLASTOMAS

Epidemiology Medulloblastoma is a highly malignant CNS tumor that arises from the cerebellum. It is the most common primary malignant intracranial childhood neoplasm, accounting for 25% of all childhood tumors.[197] More than 80% of medulloblastomas are diagnosed in children during the first 15 years of life, the median age at diagnosis being 5 years. In adults (patients ≥ 16 years of age), medulloblastomas are much less common, accounting for < 1% of all adult brain tumors.[198] The incidence of adult medulloblastomas is approximately 0.5 per million per year, and decreases with increasing age.[199] The etiology of medulloblastomas is not known. Given the rarity of adult medulloblastomas, published studies of these patients are retrospective.

Pathology Medulloblastomas are tumors consisting of small round blue cells.[200] Histologically, about half of these tumors have recognizable cell lines combined with undifferentiated components. The two main medulloblastoma variants are the classical and desmoplastic. The latter variant has large amounts of reticulin and collagen. A relationship between prognosis and the degree of cellular differentiation has been proposed, but although some reports suggest that the more undifferentiated tumors are associated with a better outcome than those with predominant astrocytic differentiation, others suggest that differentiation imparts a better prognosis.[200] At present, there is no consensus regarding prognosis as it relates to histology.

Clinical Presentation Because of its posterior fossa location, medulloblastoma often produces hydrocephalus and symptoms of increased ICP, as well as cerebellar signs (eg, truncal and limb ataxia, nystagmus). Papilledema also can be noted on examination. Disease may exist as nodular lesions outside the primary site any-where within the neuraxis, including the spine and supratentorial cerebrum, and may involve the CSF, as detected by positive cytology results. Occasionally, there may be disease beyond the CNS at the time of the original diagnosis, most often in the bone and/or soft tissue structures, including the lymph nodes.

Diagnostic Neuroimaging The imaging modality of choice is MRI. Lesions are usually iso- to hypointense on T1WI, have variable signal on T2WI, and frequently demonstrate contrast enhancement. These tumors tend to be homogenous in appearance, with occasional cystic or necrotic areas. Because of the high rate of neuraxis dissemination, MR imaging of the entire brain and spine in the setting of a posterior fossa lesion is recommended. Figure 72-8 shows the typical appearance of a medulloblastoma arising out of the fourth ventricle in both the axial and coronal planes.

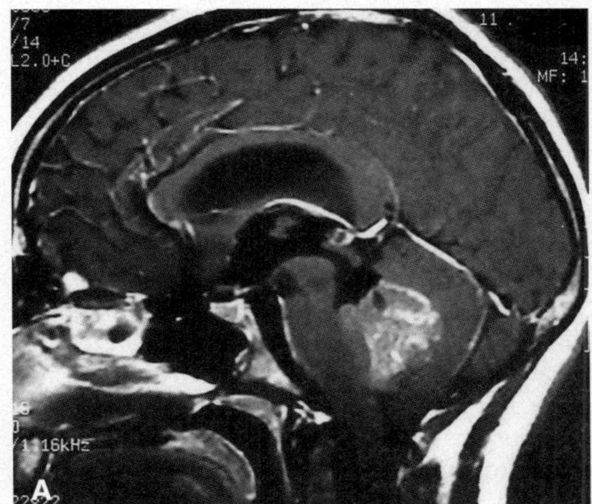

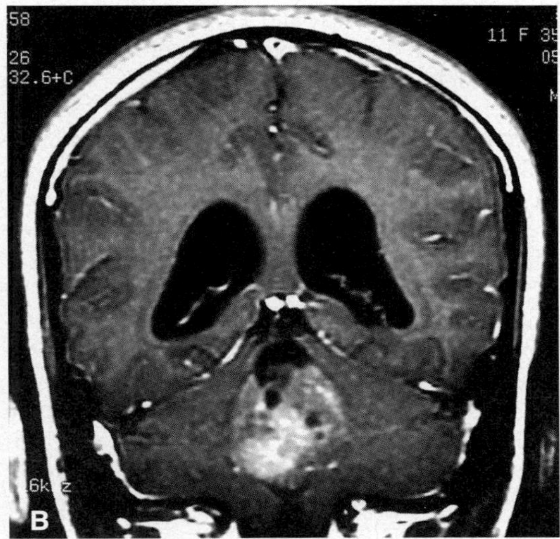

Figure 72-8 Magnetic resonance imaging appearance of a fourth ventricular medulloblastoma. **A,** Lesion in the sagittal plane. **B,** Lesion in the coronal plane.

Prognostic Factors The 5-year overall survival rates range from 58 to 84%,[201–205] which are comparable to those of childhood medulloblastoma patients; 5-year progression-free survival rates range from 40%[201] to approximately 61%.[204,205] Reported median survivals have varied from 6 years[202] to 17.6 years.[199]

For pediatric medulloblastoma patients, therapeutic strategies and survival expectations differ between standard- and poor-risk groups. Poor-risk adult medulloblastoma patients have one or more of the following clinical factors: > 25% of tumor remaining after resection, evidence of brainstem invasion, tumor cells present in the CSF, or evidence of distant metastases. Prados and colleagues retrospectively evaluated 26 poor-risk and 21 standard-risk adult medulloblastoma patients, and found that 5-year over-all survival and disease-free survival rates significantly differed between the risk groups (overall survival: 81% vs 54%; disease-free survival: 58% vs 38%).[201] These findings were comparable to those of childhood medulloblastoma patients, suggesting that treatment decisions may also be modified based on risk groups. Le and colleagues also noted a statistically significant difference in overall survival.[202] Kunschner and colleagues did not find a statistically significant difference in progression-free survival rate or median survival, although only 3 of 16 poor-risk patients had metastatic disease, which may have accounted for the long median survival (approximately 8.2 years) of the poor-risk patient group.[205]

A number of individual prognostic factors have been evaluated in adult medulloblastoma patients, particularly those that are known to be predictive in pediatric medulloblastoma patients, such as patient age at diagnosis, M stage, and extent of resection. In contrast to childhood medulloblastomas, these factors have not been found to be significantly predictive in adults. Age, which is a very important prognostic factor in the pediatric medulloblastoma population, has not been found to be a significant independent prognostic variable for adults. Age may be relevant in subsets of the adult medulloblastoma population, as was noted in one study in which the effect of older age was most pronounced in male patients with localized disease.[202] M0 stage was reported to be highly significantly (p = .0005) associated with improved disease-free survival,[203] but a subsequent study did not find a significant association (p = .68).[206] The results of one study showed GTR to be significantly associated with improved disease-free survival and posterior fossa tumor control.[206] However, other series did not find this association.[202,203,205]

Male gender was reported to be significantly predictive of worse overall survival in one study,[202] but not in subsequent series.[205,206] Unlike tumors arising in childhood, adult medulloblastomas have higher incidences of the desmoplastic compared to the classic histologic variant (30%) and lateral cerebellar location compared to the midline (30 to 40%).[203] However, medulloblastoma location has not been reported to be a significant prognostic variable, and the desmoplastic variant has been noted by most studies to also not have prognostic value. Carrie and colleagues did report a statistically significant trend (p = .03) for improved event-free survival, but central pathologic review was not performed. Other variables noted to be significant positive prognostic factors include higher postoperative functional status[203,204] and the absence of hydrocephalus and ventriculoperitoneal shunt.[201–203] *MDM2* overexpression, but not *TP53* gene mutation, was found in one study to be statistically significantly associated with worse survival in adult medulloblastoma patients.[207] The data concerning molecular markers in adult medulloblastomas is exceedingly scant. Definitive prognostic factors, both clinical and molecular, need to be delineated in order to optimize treatment for adult medulloblastoma patients.

Treatment The goal of surgery is to remove all visible tumor. Survival of adult medulloblastoma patients may be influenced by the extent of residual disease following surgery, particularly for patients without evidence of dissemination. Treatment of associated hydrocephalus can be managed by external drainage with tumor decompression, tumor decompression alone, or by the use of various shunting procedures.

Craniospinal axis radiation therapy is the standard of care for the treatment of adult medulloblastoma patients, as medulloblastomas are quite radiosensitive. Standard radiation doses to the craniospinal axis involve delivering 35 to 45 Gy to the brain and 30 to 40 Gy to the spine, with a dose of 54 Gy to the primary tumor site. Long-term adult medulloblastoma survivors who were previously treated with whole-brain radiation were found to have below-average IQs and notable deficits in memory, visuospatial skills, reasoning, and arithmetic.[208]

In contrast to childhood medulloblastoma, the role of chemotherapy in adult medulloblastoma patients is undetermined. A number of chemotherapy regimens used for pediatric medulloblastoma patients have been evaluated, including the 8-in-1 regimen, vincristine with CCNU, and CCV (cisplatinum, CCNU, and vincristine). In their study, Prados and colleagues found that those patients who received adjuvant chemotherapy (mostly nitrosourea-based regimens) had a statistically significantly longer survival as compared to those who did not receive adjuvant chemotherapy.[201] However, other series did not find any significant survival benefit for adjuvant chemotherapy.[202,204–206] There may be a defined role for chemotherapy in adult medulloblastoma patients, but issues such as timing (when to give chemotherapy), which specific therapeutic agents to use, and who will most benefit from chemotherapy still need to be resolved.

Recurrence The recurrence rate for medulloblastomas in adults is approximately 50 to 60%.[201–206] The median time-to-tumor progression (TTP) is approximately 30 months,[204] and the median survival after recurrence has been reported to be approximately 1.3 years.[203] The most common site of recurrence is the posterior fossa. Other sites of recurrence include the spine, CSF, supratentorial cerebrum, bone, and other extraneural sites. Late recurrences are more common in adults than in children. In one study, 59% of all recurrences occurred more than 2 years after treatment,[206] whereas, in general, 75% of childhood medulloblastoma recurrences occur within the first 2 years after treatment.[209] Recurrences as late as 14 years after treatment have been reported.[198] Thus, long-term monitoring is important for adult medulloblastoma patients.

Conclusion Adult medulloblastoma patients have traditionally been managed with therapies used to treat pediatric medulloblastoma patients based on the assumption that these tumors behave similarly in both populations. However, adult medulloblastomas have notable differences, such as higher frequencies of lateral cerebellar location, desmoplastic histology, and late recurrences. Although the 5-year overall survival rates are comparable between the adult and pediatric population, the prognostic factors that are well defined in childhood medulloblastoma patients have not been definitively established in adult medulloblastoma patients. Currently, the management of adult medulloblastoma patients involves a thorough staging work-up (including brain and whole-spine MRI and CSF cytology analysis), as complete a resection as possible, and postoperative CSA irradiation. Nitrosourea based chemotherapy is reserved for recurrent disease, as adjuvant chemotherapy has not been definitively shown to have significant benefit in adult medulloblastoma patients. Other treatment modalities, such as radiosurgery, may also have a role in certain medulloblastoma patients. Because of its infrequent occurrence, the majority of data about adult medulloblastomas is derived from retrospective studies. Prospective studies are needed to accurately define significant prognostic factors and treatment regimens for adult patients with medulloblastomas.

OTHER PRIMARY TUMORS OF THE CENTRAL NERVOUS SYSTEM

Primary Germ Cell Tumors **Etiology and Epidemiology** Primary intracranial germ cell tumors are a rare group of diverse tumors that account for less than 5% of childhood tumors and less than 1% of adult tumors.[210] In the United States, fewer than 50 cases are diagnosed each year. Most germ cell tumors occur during the first and second decades of life. For unknown reasons, their incidence is higher in Japan. They present as midline tumors, either in the pineal region, where they comprise 60% of all pineal region tumors, or in the suprasellar region. Other areas include the thalamus, basal ganglia, intraventricular areas, and intramedullary spinal cord. Two-thirds of the germ cell tumors in the pineal region occur in male patients, whereas two-thirds of suprasellar tumors affect females. Most nongerminomas arise from the pineal region, whereas germinomas may present in the pineal or suprasellar region, or in both areas; 10% of germ cell tumors arise elsewhere from the pineal region. The most common histologic type is germinoma, which is believed to be the most primitive form. Table 72-8 lists other germ cell tumors. In general, these lesions are grouped together as either germinoma or nongerminoma because the former are very radiation-sensitive, whereas the latter are not. Except for the benign teratoma, all germ cell tumors are malignant neoplasms with the potential to disseminate throughout the entire neuraxis.

Table 72-8 World Health Organization Classification of Germ Cell Tumors

Germinoma
Embryonal carcinoma
Choriocarcinoma
Teratoma (mature, immature, teratoma with malignant transformation)
Yolk sac tumor
Mixed germ cell tumor

Pathology Intracranial germ cell tumors are histologically identical to gonadal germ cell tumors. *Germinoma* is used for intracranial tumors as seminoma is used in the testis or dysgerminoma is used in the ovary. The germ cell tumor may be a mixture of several elements or may exhibit only one element. It has been suggested that germ cell tumors arise from developmental nests of primitive germ cells in midline structures, including the pineal and suprasellar regions of the brain.[211] Germinoma accounts for 65% of CNS germ cell tumors, and teratoma is the next most frequent at 18%, whereas choriocarcinoma is the rarest. Embryonal carcinoma and endodermal sinus tumors are intermediate in frequency. Germinomas consist of two cell populations: large round cells and a lymphocytic infiltrate. In rare cases, syncytiotrophoblasts may be present that stain positively for β-human chorionic gonadotrophin (β-HCG). Germinoma also stains positively for placental alkaline phosphatase (PLAP) and human placental lactogen (HPL). The nongerminomas, including teratomas, usually have mixtures of many cellular elements. Immunoperoxidase staining reveals β-HCG and/or α-fetoprotein in embryonal carcinoma and choriocarcinoma, as well as in endodermal sinus tumors.[211]

Clinical Presentation Patients present with acute findings related to obstructive hydrocephalus and increased ICP. Other findings of germ cell tumors in the pineal region include Parinaud syndrome (impaired vertical gaze, pupillary dilatation, loss of the accommodation reflex) and convergence–retraction nystagmus. For patients with suprasellar lesions, hypothalamic and pituitary dysfunction dominate, including growth failure, precocious puberty, and diabetes insipidus. Neuroimaging studies reveal a contrast-enhancing lesion with occasional calcifications.

Surgical Diagnosis and Treatment Surgery is strongly recommended to determine the histology of a lesion in the pineal region. The differential diagnosis of lesions in this area includes germinoma, nongerminoma, teratoma, pineocytoma, pineoblastoma, astrocytoma, and in rare instances metastatic tumor. The therapeutic options depend on the tumor type. A negative β-HCG or α-fetoprotein finding in the CSF or serum does not exclude a germinoma, although the presence of these markers is indicative of these tumors. Tumor marker profiles for germ cell tumors are determined by measuring the elevated amounts of β-HCG and α-fetoprotein in the serum and CSF. Germinomas and choriocarcinomas have high β-HCG levels but not elevated α-fetoprotein; embryonal cell carcinomas have elevated β-HCG and α-fetoprotein levels; endodermal sinus tumors have high α-fetoprotein but nonelevated β-HCG; teratomas usually do not have increased levels of either β-HCG or α-fetoprotein; whereas malignant teratomas and undifferentiated germ cell tumors may or may not have elevated marker levels. Modern surgical techniques make sampling or partial removal of tumors in this area safe and appropriate. In the past, because of the risks of surgery, such tumors were treated as if they were germinomas without tissue diagnosis. If the lesion disappeared after a short course of irradiation, it was believed to be a germinoma, but if it did not respond, its exact etiology could not be resolved. Differentiating these lesions is critical. A regimen of chemotherapy for pineoblastoma, for instance, might be different from that for a mixed germ cell tumor, as would be the decision to use CSA irradiation.

Radiation Therapy Radiation is directed to localized germinomas using the involved field as well as encompassing the ventricular system; 25 Gy is directed to the larger field, with a boost of an additional 20 to 25 Gy to the tumor bed.[212,213] The field of irradiation and dosage are topics of controversy. Some authors advocate irradiation of the craniospinal axis for all patients with histologically proven germinomas due to the risk of dissemination. The issue of CSA irradiation has not been resolved with germinomas. Currently, if CSF markers are negative and staging of the spine, including cytology and MRI with contrast, is negative, then wide-field irradiation, including the ventricular volume, is used. Germinomas are very radiation sensitive. The survival rate for patients with biopsy-proven germinoma is as high as 80% in some series, and as high as 90% when whole-brain irradiation to at least 50 Gy was used.[214] There is some concern that the 50-Gy dose of radiation is too high, and for this reason lesser doses comparable to those used for testicular seminoma (30 Gy or less) have been suggested.

Chemotherapy Nongerminomas are less responsive to radiation and frequently are treated initially with chemotherapy. The drugs used are similar to those used for gonadal tumors, including cisplatin, etoposide, vinblastine, bleomycin, and cyclophosphamide. As many as six courses of chemotherapy with a combination of agents has been used, followed by restaging. Residual disease is then treated with radiation therapy. There are many reports that document high objective response rates with the two-drug combinations of cisplatin and etoposide or of carboplatin and etoposide.[215] Shorter-course therapy of only four cycles has also been used. Considering the rarity of these tumors, a consensus has not been developed concerning the optimal regimen and duration of therapy. In the case of disseminated germinomas, primary treatment with chemotherapy is also reasonable in order to defer or omit the use of CSA irradiation. All cases are routinely staged before treatment to help define the treatment modality to be used.

MENINGIOMA **Epidemiology** Meningiomas account for about 26% of intracranial brain tumors.[1] They most often occur during the fourth through the sixth decades of life, with a peak incidence at about 45 years of age. There is a well-known association between meningiomas and female gender. Asymptomatic meningiomas occur more frequently in woman, especially during the seventh or eighth decades. Approximately 65% of all meningiomas occur in women, or almost twice as frequently in women than men. This ratio rises to 20:1 with regard to spinal meningiomas. The preponderance of meningiomas in women suggests a role for female sex hormones in the development of meningiomas. Most benign sporadic meningiomas are estrogen receptor negative and progesterone receptor positive.[216] The definitive roles for estrogen and progesterone in meningioma development remain to be elucidated. Interestingly, female predominance is not present in malignant meningiomas, as 64% of such tumors occurred in men.[217] Multiple meningiomas occur in about 10% of patients with sporadic meningiomas, as well as in patients with NF2.

Pathology Meningiomas are thought to originate from arachnoidal cap cells, and not the dura itself. Thus, they are most commonly located in the parasagittal, sphenoid wing, convexity, and falx regions. Meningiomas of the posterior fossa (3 to 16%) and intraventricular (< 10%) areas are uncommon. They are graded as benign (WHO grade I), atypical (WHO grade II), or malignant (WHO grade III). Atypical tumors represent between 5 and 7% of tumors, whereas malignant tumors are found in 1 to 3% of cases. The three classic histopathologic subtypes are meningothelial, transitional, and fibroblastic. In benign meningiomas, cellular whorls and psammoma bodies are frequently noted. Histologically malignant or anaplastic features include the presence of frequent mitotic figures (more than one or two per 10 high-power fields), atypical mitoses, papillary structures, high cellularity, and necrosis. Invasiveness is itself thought to represent malignant potential, as are the variant sub-types of hemangiopericytoma and other forms of angioblastic meningiomas. In the review by Perry and colleagues, 116 patients were reviewed who were classified as malignant as a consequence of brain invasion, frank anaplasia, and/or extracranial metastasis.[218] Survival was variable. In a multivariate analysis, factors associated with poor outcome included anaplasia, partial resection, 20 mitoses per 10 high-power fields, and nuclear atypia. There were 89 cases that invaded brain and were classified as otherwise benign (23%), atypical (61%), or malignant (17%). In this group of invasive tumors, those without anaplasia behaved more like atypical tumors than malignant lesions. These authors concluded that invasion was important as a criterion for atypical tumors, but frank anaplasia is needed to designate a tumor as malignant.

Prognostic Factors McCarthy and colleagues recently reviewed more than 9,000 cases of meningioma to explore factors affecting survival in patients with meningioma.[5] Five-year overall survival rate was 69%, which decreased with age. Benign tumors had a 5-year survival rate of 70%, atypical tumors 75%, and malignant tumors 55%. Patients who had complete removal of a benign lesion had a 5-year recurrence rate of 20.5%. Prognostic factors for benign tumors included age at diagnosis (older patients fared worse), tumor size, extent of resection, and radiation therapy; for malignant tumors, the factors included age at diagnosis, extent of resection and radiation therapy. The 5-year overall survival rate was 81% for patients younger than age 65 years and 56% for patients older than age 65 years. Palma and colleagues reviewed 42 cases of atypical and 29 cases of malignant meningioma.[219] Survival at 5 years was 95% in cases of atypical tumors and 64.3% for malignant tumors. Multivariate analysis indicated that radical resection and histology were significant predictors for survival.

Molecular Genetics The most consistent karyotypic alteration in meningiomas is deletion of the long arm or all of chromosome 22.[220] The tumor-suppressor gene *NF2* is contained within this region, and is mutated in up to 60% of sporadic meningiomas. The next most frequent alteration is deletion of chromosome 1p; LOH of 1p32 in one series occurred in 34% of cases, and was associated with chromosome 22 deletions.[221] Other alterations include losses on chromosomes 6q, 10q, 14q, 17p, and 18q. Certain peptides have stimulatory effects on meningioma cell growth, including EGFR[222] and platelet-derived growth factor receptor p chain.[223] VEGF was found to have 3.4 times the level of messenger ribonucleic acid (mRNA) expression in meningiomas with peritumoral edema versus those tumors without edema.[224] This suggests that VEGF overexpression plays an important role in edema produced by meningiomas. Another study found that corticosteroids and growth factors (eg, EGF and basic fibroblast growth factor [bFGF]), but not sex hormones, induced VEGF secretion by meningioma cells in vitro.[225] Suppression of *ras* proteins has been reported to inhibit the proliferation of meningioma cells in vitro after transfection of Ad-rasN17, a recombinant adenovirus encoding the dominant-negative ras protein, into meningioma cell cultures.[226] Hence, drugs that inhibit *ras* activity may be of benefit in higher-grade meningiomas.

Clinical Presentation Meningioma patients typically present with headache, seizures, personality changes, or progressive focal neurologic deficits. Other signs and symptoms are site-specific. Olfactory groove meningiomas cause frontal lobe signs, anosmia, and visual loss; occasionally, they may produce symptoms of the Foster–Kennedy syndrome (anosmia, unilateral optic atrophy, contralateral papilledema). Meningiomas of the cavernous sinus may compress cranial nerves III to VI, resulting in extraocular muscle palsies, facial numbness, diplopia, and headache. Parasagittal meningiomas may cause headache, focal seizures, and bilateral lower extremity weakness. Because most meningiomas are slow growing, they can grow to enormous sizes before signs and symptoms are noticed. Systemic metastases of malignant meningiomas can occur in up to 24% of malignant meningioma patients, with the most common sites being the lungs, liver, and bone.

Diagnostic Imaging Most meningiomas are iso- or hypointense on T1WI and have variable signal on T2WI. They enhance homogeneously and often have the "dural tail" sign suggestive of a meningioma. Cysts within the walls of meningiomas, which are hypointense on T1WI, have more-aggressive pathology than the tumors themselves.[227] Meningiomas are typically dural based, and hence extraaxial in location. This is an important distinguishing radiographic feature of meningiomas, as most other CNS lesions, such as gliomas, and usually intraaxial in location.

Treatment Observation with serial MRIs is an acceptable treatment plan for asymptomatic patients whose tumors are radiographically consistent with benign meningiomas. In one study, 57 meningioma patients were observed for a mean follow-up period of 32 months, with none becoming symptomatic and only 10 of 45 patients who received imaging had tumor growth noted.[228] Nongrowing meningiomas more likely demonstrate intratumoral calcification and/or hypointensity on T2WI.[229] Thus, many meningioma patients can be observed and have treatment deferred until they exhibit symptomatic progression. When surgery is necessary, most meningiomas are benign tumors and are treated successfully with surgical resection alone. The goal of surgery is to remove the tumor and its dural attachment with any involved bone. Simpson noted that the risk of meningioma recurrence increased with failure to achieve a GTR with coagulation of the dural attachment rather than excision.[230] One series reported that 76% of meningiomas that were totally resected (Simpson grades I to III) had local control rates of 93%, 80%, and 75% at 5, 10, and 15 years, respectively. However, those patients who received subtotal resections (Simpson grade IV) had local control rates of 53%, 40%, and 30%, respectively.[231] In another series, 5- and 10-year progression-free survival rates were 88% and 75%, respectively, for GTR meningioma patients, and 61% and 39%, respectively, for subtotal resection patients.[232] The treatment of malignant meningiomas requires as extensive a resection as possible followed by irradiation to a dose of 60 Gy using single daily fractions. Dziuk and colleagues reviewed the outcome of 38 cases of malignant meningioma treated between 1984 and 1992.[233] Actuarial disease-free survival at 5 years was 39% following total resection versus 0% after subtotal removal. For all of the totally resected tumors, the disease-free survival improved from 28% with surgery alone to 57% with adjuvant radiation therapy. They concluded that extensive resection followed by radiation therapy were important factors that increase the likelihood of longer disease-free survival and overall survival. Most authors would agree that incompletely resected benign or malignant meningioma have improved outcome with radiation therapy.

Radiosurgery has also been explored in this disease. Morita and colleagues reviewed a series of 88 consecutive patients with skull base meningioma treated with the gamma knife radiosurgery between 1990 and 1996.[234] In this series, the 5-year progression-free survival rate was 95%. The risk of radiation injury to cranial nerves was associated with doses higher than 19 Gy. Although long-term follow-up using this technique is short for most series, the use of radiosurgery appears to be safe and effective, and is considered an alternative strategy to standard fractionated radiation in many centers. A prospective randomized study has not been conducted comparing these two methods of radiation.

Recurrence Treatment of recurrent meningioma is problematic. Most of these tumors are malignant lesions that were previously treated with multiple surgeries and radiation therapy. Radiosurgery for recurrent malignant meningiomas has been evaluated. In one trial, the 2- and 5-year overall survival rate after radiosurgery was 75% and 40%, respectively, while 2- and 5-year progression-free survival rates were 32% and 26%, respectively. Statistically significant factors affecting time to progression were age < 50 years and tumor volume < 8 cc.[235] Interstitial brachytherapy may also have a role in the management of recurrent benign or malignant meningiomas, but further evaluation is needed. Chemotherapy has little impact in terms of response or survival. Kaba and colleagues reviewed 6 patients treated with interferon-α.[236] Five of the 6 cases showed stabilization or minor response, lasting from 6 to 14 months. They concluded that interferon has activity in this disease, possible acting as an anti-angiogenesis agent. Schrell and colleagues also reviewed their experience in a small series of patients treated with hydroxyurea.[237] Preclinical laboratory experiments suggested that this agent inhibited growth in vitro and in vivo by apoptotic mechanisms. Four patients were treated, and 3 had evidence of tumor regression. The antiprogestational agent RU-486 (mifepristone) was evaluated in 10 meningioma patients, with 3 having temporary tumor regression, but only 1 patient had a response noted.[238] Goodwin and colleagues reported on a series of 21 patients who were treated with tamoxifen242: 1 patient had a partial response, and 6 remained stable for a median duration of 31 months; 32% of patients had no tumor growth, whereas 53% had tumor progression. Although the results of hormone therapy trials are disappointing thus far, further investigation of hormone receptor antagonists may eventually yield effective and safe treatments for recurrent and high-grade meningiomas.

PRIMARY CENTRAL NERVOUS SYSTEM LYMPHOMA **Epidemiology** Primary CNS lymphoma (PCNSL) is a unique high-grade brain tumor that arises from nonneural tissue. It occurs in both the immunocompetent and immunocompromised (especially males with acquired immunodeficiency syndrome [AIDS]) population. Its incidence has risen to approximately 0.47 cases/1,000,000 person-years (0.28 per 100,000 persons years in immunocompetent individuals, and up to 4.7 per 100,000 in patients with AIDS).[1,239] Mean age of onset is 58 years in the immunocompetent population and 43 years in human immunodeficiency virus (HIV) patients.

Clinical Presentation Most PCNSLs occur in the deep gray and periventricular white matter, with approximately 38% of cases having subependymal spread. They can involve deep structures, such as the basal ganglia. Sixty percent of immunocompetent patients have single lesions, whereas more than 90% of AIDS patients have multiple lesions. Thus, symptoms of cranial PCNSLs include headache, cognitive and personality changes, and focal neurologic deficits. Seizures are less common than in gliomas. The mean duration of symptoms prior to diagnosis is 2.8 months in immunocompetent and 1.8 months in immunocompromised patients. Ocular CNS lymphomas can cause blurred vision, floaters, and decreased visual acuity. Vitrectomy may be needed to make a diagnosis of ocular lymphoma. PCNSLs of the spine can present with back pain, limb motor and sensory loss, radiculopathy, and bowel/bladder dysfunction. Ocular involvement occurs in 12 to 18% of PCNSL patients, and at least 40% have detectable leptomeningeal dissemination at diagnosis. Approximately 15% of patients who undergo lumbar puncture will have positive tumor cells identified.

Pathology PCNSLs are high-grade B cell lymphomas that have an angiocentric pattern that forms collars of tumor cells within concentric perivascular reticulin deposits. Almost all tumors exhibit a diffuse growth pattern, with geographic necrosis occurring when the tumors become confluent. They express immunohistochemical markers such as CD19, CD20, and CD79a, as well as monoclonal surface immunoglobulins (most frequently IgM/1c). Comparative genomic hybridization studies have noted that DNA gains (chromosomes 1, 7, 11, 12, and 18) are more common than losses (chromosomes 6, 18, and 20). Loss of DNA copy number on chromosome 6q has been reported as a statistically significant negative prognostic factor.[240]

Diagnosis The modality of choice is MRI. PCNSLs are usually iso- to hypointense on T1WI and have relatively low signal on T2WI. They enhance intensely with contrast. AIDS-related PCNSL lesions may have hemorrhage or necrosis, and hence produce ring-enhancing lesions on MRI. It is important to note that the administration of corticosteroids prior to a biopsy for diagnosis may cause the PCNSL lesions to disappear on MRI, thereby reducing the chance of obtaining a successful tissue diagnosis. A staging workup is essential to accurately assess the extent of disease and modify the treatment plan to maximize survival and quality of life. In addition to the brain MRI with contrast, ophthalmologic evaluation (including slit lamp exam), LP for CSF cytology, HIV test, and spine MRI (if indicated) are part of the staging process for PCNSL patients. Systemic staging identifies an extra-CNS site in less than 4% of cases. Elevated CSF protein and lactic acid dehydrogenase (LDH) isoenzyme-5 have been found to be significantly associated with leptomeningeal tumor spread in PCNSL.[241]

Treatment Modalities PCNSL is rapidly fatal if untreated, with mean survival of only 3.3 months.[242] Overall 2-year survival rate is only 28%[243] and 5-year overall survival rate is only 3 to 4% with whole-brain radiation alone.[244] AIDS-related PCNSL is more aggressive than in immunocompetent patients, with median survival of 27 days without treatment, with only 20% surviving to 3 months, and none surviving to 6 months and beyond.[245] Resection alone does not improve survival, with median survival reaching only 4.6 months.[242] There is also no significant improvement in survival with more extensive resection versus biopsy alone.[243] Thus, unlike gliomas, there is no role for surgery in PCNSL except for diagnosis with a biopsy, and also when urgent decompression is required to relieve increased ICP.

PCNSL is a very radiosensitive tumor. Whole-brain radiation alone has increased median survival to 12 months.[243] The only prospective trial evaluating XRT dosage for PCNSL treatment found no survival benefit in patients receiving 40 Gy of whole-brain radiation with a 20-Gy boost versus 40 Gy of whole-brain radiation alone.[243] Thus, the recommended XRT dose is 45 Gy of whole-brain radiation without a boost. CSA irradiation has not demonstrated a survival benefit over whole-brain radiation,[246] and thus is not recommended for the initial treatment of PCNSL. XRT for ocular lymphoma involves delivering 40 Gy to the affected eye, including the posterior two-thirds of the globe. Although XRT yields frequent disease control, subsequent relapse within the brain can occur in up to 80% of PCNSL patients.[247] XRT is the mainstay of treatment for AIDS-related PCNSL patients. However, even with whole-brain radiation the median survival for these patients is only 3 months, with fewer than 10% surviving up to 1 year after diagnosis.[248] More recent encouraging results have been noted in patients with AIDS-related PCNSL who are treated with effective antiretroviral therapies to reduce viral load. Patients with low viral load and a high CD4 T-cell count are better able to tolerate radiation and methotrexate-based chemotherapy. In some cases, reconstitution of the immune system can lead to PCNSL regression, and for that reason should be pursued.

Early chemotherapy regimens using CHOP (cyclophosphamide, doxorubicin, vincristine, and prednisone) prior to XRT have not increased survival of PCNSL patients beyond whole-body radiation alone. This regimen is used to treat non-Hodgkin's lymphoma (NHL), of which PCNSL is one example. The RTOG studied the pre-irradiation CHOD (substituting dexamethasone for prednisone) regimen and found that median survival was 16.1 months, with a 2-year survival rate of 42% of PCNSL patients, which was comparable to whole-body radiation alone.[249] The efficacy of methotrexate (MTX) has been demonstrated in multiple clinical trials, with 5-year survival rates of up to 22% when combined with XRT.[250] One study analyzed high-dose MTX (3.5 g/m^2) given to PCNSL patients prior to XRT; overall median survival was 33 months (42.5 months for responders).[251] There was no significant survival difference between patients receiving MTX every 10 days versus every 3 weeks. Blay and colleagues confirmed that MTX-based regimens significantly improved overall survival in PCNSL patients over other chemotherapy regimens; treatment with cytarabine-containing regimens also conferred a significant survival advantage.[252] Other regimens evaluated include PCV,[253] BVAM (BCNU, vincristine, cytarabine, MTX),[254] and MTX with procarbazine and thiotepa.[255] Intrathecal chemotherapy has been reported to increase median survival from 23 to 37 months in PCNSL patients when added to high-dose MTX, cyclophosphamide, and other chemotherapy agents.[246] Another study found that treatment of the CSF with intrathecal chemotherapy provided longer disease-free survival and less-frequent leptomeningeal relapses regardless of CSF cytology results.[241]

Combined modality therapy has been shown to be the most effective way of controlling PCNSL. Typically, chemotherapy is given prior to radiation, particularly when high-dose methotrexate is used, to try and minimize the risk of late neurotoxicity, including leukoencephalopathy and dementia. The late effects of both radiation and methotrexate are synergistic, particularly in older patients; with up to 80% of patients over the age of 60 developing some form of dementia.[256] Thus, several groups are investigating the use of chemotherapy alone in the initial management of this disease.

Responses of ocular lymphoma to chemotherapy are less reliable than in the cerebrum. Both MTX (both intravenous and intrathecal) as well as cytarabine have been used. Valluri and colleagues treated 3 ocular lymphomas with a regimen of intravenous (IV) and intrathecal MTX, ocular XRT, whole-body radiation (2 of the patients also had cerebral lymphoma), and two cycles of high-dose cytarabine. All 3 patients responded, with disease-free periods exceeding 24 months.[257] Intravitreal MTX has also been used, and in one study, 6 of 7 eyes in 4 ocular lymphoma patients responded, with disease-free periods up to 19 months, and no adverse reactions noted.[258]

Neoplastic Meningitis Neoplastic meningitis (NM) is a common clinical problem in neurooncology, affecting approximately 5% of all patients with cancer. Clinical series have estimated NM to occur in 4 to 15% of patients with solid tumors, in 7 to 15% of patients with lymphomas, in 5 to 15% of patients with leukemias, and in 1 to 2% of patients with primary brain tumors.[259–262] Solid tumors are disproportionately represented in clinical series of patients with NM because of their high frequency of occurrence where breast (range of occurrence: 12 to 34%), lung (10 to 26%), melanoma (17 to 25%) and gastrointestinal (4 to 14%) cancers are the most frequently encountered. Autopsy studies of patients with cancer demonstrate a very high incidence of NM exceeding that seen in clinical series. In the Memorial Sloan-Kettering Cancer Center experience of 2,375 patients with cancer and post-mortem CNS analysis, an 8% incidence of NM was noted.[260] In the National Cancer Institute study of small-cell lung cancer, an 11% incidence of NM was seen ante-mortem, as compared to a 25% incidence seen postmortem.[263] The incidence of AIDS-related lymphomatous meningitis is increasing in frequency. Lymphomatous meningitis occurs in 25% of AIDS-related PCNSL patients and in 20% to 22% of AIDS patients with systemic NHL.[264]

Clinical Presentation Neurologic symptomatology may occur, depending on location.[265] The clinical presentation profile of NM patients can be grouped into three CNS sites: cerebral hemispheres, cranial nerves, and spinal cord and roots. In the cerebrum, the most common symptom is headache and the most common sign is mental status change. Other signs and symptoms of cerebral NM include seizures, nausea, vomiting, sensory dysfunction, and hemiparesis. Cranial nerve symptoms most frequently include double vision, as well as hearing loss, facial weakness and numbness, and visual loss. Physical findings may include ophthalmoplegia (with abducens palsies seen more frequently than oculomotor dysfunction, whereas oculomotor palsies are more common than trochlear palsies), trigeminal sensory or motor loss, cochlear dysfunction, and optic neuropathy. Spine symptoms may occur secondary to involvement of either the spinal cord or exiting nerve roots and the spinal meninges. The most common symptoms of spinal NM include lower motor neuron weakness and paresthesias, whereas the most frequent signs are asymmetric reflexes and weakness. They may also include bowel and bladder dysfunction, numbness, and pain (neck, back, or radicular). Common signs of spinal cord dysfunction are extremity weakness and dermatomal or segmental sensory loss.

Survival Median survival for untreated NM patients is 1 month. The expected median survival of treated NM patients is 2 to 6 months. Median survival expectations of treated NM patients do vary depending on the primary tumor site, such as melanoma (4 months), non–small-cell lung carcinoma and AIDS-related lymphoma (6 months), breast cancer (7.5 months), and non–AIDS-related lymphoma (10 months).[266]

Cerebrospinal Fluid Diagnosis The single most useful laboratory test in diagnosing NM is an examination of the CSF.[267] Most patients will have abnormal findings regardless of CSF cytology results, such as high opening pressure (> 150 mm H_2O), elevated CSF protein (> 50 mg/dL) and white blood cell count (> 4 mm^3), and decreased CSF glucose levels (< 60 mg/dL). Not all patients will have positive cytology, however. The yield from CSF cytology increases significantly with serial lumbar punctures. Wasserstrom and colleagues noted that 5% of NM patients had positive cytology results only with CSF obtained from the ventricles or cisterna magna.[261] Thus, there is a subset of NM patients with persistently negative cytologies regardless of the level from which the CSF is withdrawn. In this series, the initial lumbar CSF examination was cytologically positive in 55% and increased to 80% following a second examination. Little benefit was seen in performing multiple lumbar punctures following the initial two lumbar CSF examinations. Kaplan and colleagues also noted a high positive cytologic yield (> 90%) following one or two lumbar punctures.[259] In the largest postmortem analysis of patients with NM, Glass and colleagues demonstrated that 41% of patients undergoing antemortem CSF cytology and autopsy-proven NM had negative premortem CSF cytology.[267] Furthermore, Glass and colleagues demonstrated that patients with pathologically focal NM had negative cytology more than 50% of the time, emphasizing the frequent cooccurrence of patients with NM and negative CSF cytology. Evaluation of DNA by flow cytometry permits an estimation of aneuploidy and the number of cells in S and G_2M phases of the cell cycle.[268] Flow cytometry may be capable of detecting tumor cells not found by conventional CSF cytology, particularly with lymphomatous or leukemic meningitis, where differentiating malignant lymphocytes from background mononuclear cells may be difficult. B-cell marker monoclonal anti-bodies used to differentiate leukemic and lymphomatous meningitis from the normal or reactive T-cell CSF lymphocyte population may also be helpful.[265,269] VEGF in CSF has been noted to be significantly elevated in patients with NM, but not in patients with viral meningitis, multiple sclerosis, paraneoplastic syndromes, or brain metastases without NM. Also, NM patients that responded to therapy had negative CSF cytologies before the clearance of VEGF from the CSF.[270] Thus, VEGF levels in CSF may be a useful biologic marker for NM patients and should be further evaluated.

Diagnostic Neuroimaging MR-Gd appears to have a greater specificity and sensitivity (1.5- to 2.0-fold increase in lesion detection) when compared with CT in the evaluation of NM patients, and is the preferred imaging modality.[271–274] A high incidence of false negatives (30% by MR-Gd) still exists, however, and negative studies do not necessarily exclude a diagnosis of NM. The tumor nodules are typically small enhancing lesions that often coat the dorsal surface of the cord ("drop mets"). Radionuclide CSF flow studies provide a physiological assessment of the functional anatomy of the CSF spaces. However, flow studies are informative only with respect to compartmentalization of CSF and provide no information regarding bulky leptomeningeal disease, an aspect of NM best resolved by spine MRI. Flow studies provide the best radiographic assessment of CSF circulation and are abnormal in 30 to 40% of patients with NM. Failure of radionuclide to appear in a given CSF compartment is defined as CSF flow block. These abnormalities are most commonly seen at the base of brain, in the spinal subarachnoid space (particularly at the level of the conus medullaris or cauda equina), and over the cerebral convexities. Approximately 50% of patients with an intracranial disturbance of CSF flow and 30% of patients with an intraspinal disturbance of CSF flow will have restored normal CSF flow as assessed by flow studies performed after radiotherapy.[275]

The characteristic pattern of tumor growth in NM is diffuse infiltration of the leptomeninges. Tumor growth is prominent along the ventricular surface (especially in the chiasmatic and infundibular cisterns). Ependymal nodules may obstruct CSF outflow channels, particularly at the level of the basal cisterns or fourth ventricle, resulting in hydrocephalus. Tumor infiltration in the spinal cord is more frequent over the dorsal surface of the spinal cord and cauda equina. NM patients also have coexistent CNS metastases, including brain parenchyma (occurrence is approximately 25 to 40%), dural metastases (16 to 37%), leptomeningeal nodular disease (10 to 15%), and epidural spinal cord compression (1 to 5%).[266]

Patients with suspected NM should undergo CSF analysis with at least two lumbar punctures followed by either a ventricular or cisternal CSF examination. MR imaging should also be done to assess bulky disease in the brain or spine, and to evaluate for epidural masses. Radionuclide studies should be considered if treatment is to be given to evaluate CSF flow, as well as compartmentalization or CSF flow block. The diagnosis of NM can be made in a patient with tumor cells documented by CSF cytology, or in patients with proven cancer and negative CSF cytology who have a clinical syndrome consistent with NM. The latter would include a cancer patient with the onset of communicating hydrocephalus, cranial nerve palsies, or cauda equina syndrome.

Radiation Therapy There are no universally accepted treatment regimens for NM patients, as all established treatments are palliative rather than curative. The principle of NM treatment is to encompass the entire subarachnoid space, including the ventricular system, basal cisterns, and spinal subarachnoid space. Deciding whom to treat is not a simple decision, as many NM patients are poor candidates for aggressive therapy. Radiation therapy is the initial modality of treatment. XRT is used to treat bulky disease and compartmentalized NM, as intra-CSF chemotherapy has limited tumor nodule penetration, diffusing only 2 to 3 mm from the tumor–CSF interface,[276] and homogeneous distribution is not possible when bulky NM disease causes blockage of the CSF pathways. XRT is delivered to the involved sites of symptomatic and bulky disease, to sites of CSF outflow obstruction, or as CSA irradiation for diffuse extensive CSF involvement.

Chemotherapy Systemic chemotherapeutic treatment of NM often fails because of poor CSF penetration of nearly all chemotherapeutic agents, and the difficulty in achieving a significant intra-CSF drug exposure interval.[277,278] Exceptions are seen with systemic high-dose intravenous methotrexate, cytarabine, and thiotepa, all of which result in cytotoxic CSF levels and have successfully been used to treat NM. In contrast, intra-CSF chemotherapy spares systemic dose-limiting toxicity and therefore achieves systemic rescue. Only three chemotherapeutic agents are routinely used for intra-CSF drug administration for patients with NM. These include methotrexate, cytosine arabinoside (ara-C, or cytarabine) and thiotepa.[273,279,280] A number of investigational agents are being explored, including DepoFoam encapsulated cytarabine, mafosphamide (a derivative of cyclophosphamide), diaziquinone, 4-hydroperoxycyclophosphamide (another derivative of cyclophosphamide), interferon, monoclonal antibodies, gene therapy, and interleukin-2.[265,273,281] A randomized trial compared an intrathecal sustained-release form of cytarabine, DepoCyt, against standard intrathecal MTX in solid tumor NM patients. The patients who received DepoCyt had a statistically significantly longer median TTP of 58 days, as compared to 30 days for the intrathecal MTX group; however, median overall survival was not statistically significantly different (15 weeks for DepoCyt, 11.1 weeks for intrathecal MTX).[282] The comparable side effect profile to intrathecal MTX and its more convenient dosing schedule makes DepoCyt a potentially viable alternative treatment option for some NM patients. At present, there is no compelling data to suggest an improved response when using multiple agents versus single agent intra-CSF drug therapy, nor when comparing single agent methotrexate to thiotepa in the treatment of NM. One study observed that a subset of NM patients, with primary tumors being lymphoma or breast cancer, may respond to standard dose systemic chemotherapy without intra-CSF chemotherapy.[283] Notwithstanding the pharmacokinetic advantages of intraventricular versus intralumbar CSF drug administration, there are no studies that document if intraventricular administration results in improved patient survival when compared to intralumbar drug administration.

The majority of North American neurooncologists treat patients with NM via the intraventricular route, using an intraventricular catheter and subgaleal reservoir. A variety of drug schedules exist, but most are typically administered as a bolus twice a week.[284,285] Alternatively, a concentration multiplied by time approach based on pharmacokinetic principles may be considered. For instance, methotrexate may be administered at 2 mg per day for 5 consecutive days every other week for 4 treatment weeks (total 8 weeks). Ara-C may be delivered at 25 mg daily for 3 consecutive days weekly for 4 weeks (total 4 weeks), and thiotepa may be administered at 10 mg per day for 3 consecutive days weekly for 4 weeks (total 4 weeks) as induction therapies. Complications of intra-CSF chemotherapy occur as a result of direct neurotoxicity, and include aseptic chemical meningitis, leukoencephalopathy (particularly with MTX), and myelopathy.

FUTURE DIRECTIONS

Neuro-oncology is making significant progress through laboratory investigation into the molecular biology and genetics of CNS neoplasms. Clues to the etiology and pathogenesis of malignant brain tumors are being detected at a rapid pace, and with further knowledge of the nature of these tumors, it is likely that a greater number of rationally designed, specific, nontoxic therapies will be forthcoming. Current clinical research strategies emphasize the inhibition of angiogenesis, invasion, and critical signaling pathways for proliferation. It is extremely critical that a detailed understanding of cell-cycle regulatory controls and pathways is achieved in order to help properly guide the development of innovative and effective treatments for brain tumors. New drugs delivered directly into the tumor by convection-based delivery are rapidly being evaluated in clinical trials. Our hope is that with improved translational strategies and a greater reliance on close clinical-laboratory interaction, the quality-adjusted survival will become markedly enhanced and a cure will be a realistic expectation and outcome.

REFERENCES

1. Central Brain Tumor Registry of the United States. Statistical report: primary brain tumors in the United States, 1997–2001. Chicago: CBTRUS; 2004–2005
2. Surawicz TS, McCarthy BJ, Kupelian V, et al. Descriptive epidemiology of primary brain and CNS tumors: results from the Central Brain Tumor Registry of the United States, 1990–1994. Neurooncol 1999;1:14–25.
3. Black WC. Increasing incidence of childhood primary malignant brain tumors—enigma or no-brainer [editorial; comment; see comments]? J Natl Cancer Inst 1998;90:1249–51.
4. Davis FG, Kupelian V, Freels S, et al. Prevalence estimates for primary brain tumors in the United States by behavior and major histology groups. Neurooncol 2001;3:152–8.
5. McCarthy BJ, Davis FG, Freels S, et al. Factors associated with survival in patients with meningioma. J Neurosurg 1998;88:831–9.
6. Grovas A, Fremgen A, Rauck A, et al. The National Cancer Data Base report on patterns of childhood cancers in the United States. Cancer 1997;80:2321–32.
7. Davis FG, McCarthy BJ, Freels S, et al. The conditional probability of survival of patients with primary malignant brain tumors: surveillance, epidemiology, and end results (SEER) data. Cancer 1999;85:485–91.
8. Wrensch M, Bondy ML, Wiencke J, et al. Environmental risk factors for primary malignant brain tumors: a review. J Neurooncol 1993;17:47–64.
9. Karlsson P, Holmberg E, Lundell M, et al. Intracranial tumors after exposure to ionizing radiation during infancy: a pooled analysis of two Swedish cohorts of 28,008 infants with skin hemangioma. Radiat Res 1998;150:357–64.
10. Little MP, de FVathaire, Shamsaldin A, et al. Risks of brain tumour following treatment for cancer in childhood: modification by genetic factors, radiotherapy and chemotherapy. Int J Cancer 1998;78:269–75.
11. Bondy ML, Wang LE, El-Zein R, et al. Gamma-radiation sensitivity and risk of glioma. J Natl Cancer Inst 2001;93:1553–7.
12. Kheifets LI, Sussman SS, Preston-Martin S. Childhood brain tumors and residential electromagnetic fields (EMF). Rev Environ Contam Toxicol 1999;159:111–29.
13. Muscat JE, Malkin MG, Thompson S, et al. Handheld cellular telephone use and risk of brain cancer. JAMA 2000;284:3001–7.
14. Inskip PD, Tarone RE, Hatch EE, et al. Cellular-telephone use and brain tumors. N Engl J Med 2001;344:79–86.
15. Preston-Martin S. Epidemiology of primary CNS neoplasms. Neurol Clin 1996;14:273–90.
16. Blair A, Saracci R, Stewart PA, et al. Epidemiologic evidence on the relationship between formaldehyde exposure and cancer. Scand J Work Environ Health 1990;16:381–93.
17. Berleur MP, Cordier S. The role of chemical, physical, or viral exposures and health factors in neurocarcinogenesis: implications for epidemiologic studies of brain tumors. Cancer Causes Control 1995;6:240–56.
18. Bondy ML, Wrensch MR. Epidemiology of primary malignant brain tumours. Baillieres Clin Neurol 1996;5:251–70.
19. Norman MA, Holly EA, Preston-Martin S. Childhood brain tumors and exposure to tobacco smoke. Cancer Epidemiol Biomarkers Prev 1996;5:85–91.
20. Kleihues P. Subsets of glioblastoma: clinical and histological vs genetic typing [editorial; comment]. Brain Pathol 1998;8:667–8.
21. Watanabe K, Tachibana O, Sata K, et al. Overexpression of the EGF receptor and p53 mutations are mutually exclusive in the evolution of primary and secondary glioblastomas. Brain Pathol 1996;6:217–23; discussion 23–4.
22. Gomez-Manzano C, Fueyo J, Kyritsis AP, et al. Characterization of p53 and p21 functional interactions in glioma cells en route to apoptosis. J Natl Cancer Inst 1997;89:1036–44.
23. Haas-Kogan DA, Yount G, Haas M, et al. p53-dependent G1 arrest and p53-independent apoptosis influence the radiobiologic response of glioblastoma. Int J Radiat Oncol Biol Phys 1996;36:95–103.
24. Simmons ML, Lamborn KR, Takahashi M, et al. Analysis of complex relationships between age, p53, epidermal growth factor receptor, and survival in glioblastoma patients. Cancer Res 2001;61:1122–8.
25. Tada M, Matsumoto R, Iggo RD, et al. Selective sensitivity to radiation of cerebral glioblastomas harboring p53 mutations. Cancer Res 1998;58:1793–7.
26. Gomez-Manzano C, Fueyo J, Kyritsis AP, et al. Adenovirus-mediated transfer of the *p53* gene produces rapid and generalized death of human glioma cells via apoptosis. Cancer Res 1996;56:694–9.
27. Reifenberger G, Reifenberger J, Ichimura K, et al. Amplification of multiple genes from chromosomal region 12q13–14 in human malignant gliomas: preliminary mapping of the amplicons shows preferential involvement of CDK4, SAS, and MDM2. Cancer Res 1994;54:4299–303.
28. Quelle DE, Zindy F, Ashmun RA, et al. Alternative reading frames of the INK4a tumor suppressor gene encode two unrelated proteins capable of inducing cell cycle arrest. Cell 1995;83:993–1000.
29. Kamijo T, Weber JD, Zambetti G, et al. Functional and physical interactions of the ARF tumor suppressor with p53 and Mdm2. Proc Natl Acad Sci U S A 1998;95:8292–7.
30. Nakamura M, Watanabe T, Klangby U, et al. p14ARF deletion and methylation in genetic pathways to glioblastomas. Brain Pathol 2001;11:159–68.
31. He J, Olson JJ, James CD. Lack of p16INK4 or retinoblastoma protein (pRb), or amplification- associated over-expression of cdk4 is observed in distinct subsets of malignant glial tumors and cell lines. Cancer Res 1995;55:4833–6.
32. Buchkovich K, Duffy LA, Harlow E. The retinoblastoma protein is phosphorylated during specific phases of the cell cycle. Cell 1989;58:1097–105.
33. Morgan DO. Principles of CDK regulation. Nature 1995;374:131–4.
34. Wen S, Stolarov J, Myers MP, et al. PTEN controls tumor-induced angiogenesis. Proc Natl Acad Sci U S A 2001;98:4622–7.
35. Holland EC, Celestino J, Dai C, et al. Combined activation of Ras and Akt in neural progenitors induces glioblastoma formation in mice. Nat Genet 2000;25:55–7.
36. Smith JS, Tachibana I, Passe SM, et al. PTEN mutation, EGFR amplification, and outcome in patients with anaplastic astrocytoma and glioblastoma multiforme. J Natl Cancer Inst 2001;93:1246–56.
37. Raffel C, Frederick L, O'Fallon JR, et al. Analysis of oncogene and tumor suppressor gene alterations in pediatric malignant astrocytomas reveals reduced survival for patients with PTEN mutations. Clin Cancer Res 1999;5:4085–90.
38. Bigner SH, Humphrey PA, Wong AJ, et al. Characterization of the epidermal growth factor receptor in human glioma cell lines and xenografts. Cancer Res 1990;50:8017–22.
39. Sauter G, Maeda T, Waldman FM, et al. Patterns of epidermal growth factor receptor amplification in malignant gliomas. Am J Pathol 1996;148:1047–53.
40. Galanis E, Buckner J, Kimmel D, et al. Gene amplification as a prognostic factor in primary and secondary high-grade malignant gliomas. Int J Oncol 1998;13:717–24.
41. von Deimling A, Louis DN, von Ammon K, et al. Association of epidermal growth factor receptor gene amplification with loss of chromosome 10 in human glioblastoma multiforme. J Neurosurg 1992;77:295–301.
42. Waha A, Baumann A, Wolf HK, et al. Lack of prognostic relevance of alterations in the epidermal growth factor receptor-transforming growth factor-alpha pathway in human astrocytic gliomas. J Neurosurg 1996;85:634–41.
43. Betsholtz C, Nister M, Rorsman F, et al. Structural and functional aspects of platelet-derived growth factor and its role in the pathogenesis of glioblastoma. Mol Chem Neuropathol 1989;10:27–36.
44. Nakayama Y, Sueishi K, Oka K, et al. Stromal angiogenesis in human glioma: a role of platelet-derived endothelial cell growth factor. Surg Neurol 1998;49:181–7; discussion 187–8.
45. Jennings MT, Hart CE, Commers PA, et al. Transforming growth factor beta as a potential tumor progression factor among hyperdiploid glioblastoma cultures: evidence for the role of platelet-derived growth factor. J Neurooncol 1997;31:233–54.
46. Hermanson M, Funa K, Koopmann J, et al. Association of loss of heterozygosity on chromosome 17p with high platelet-derived growth factor alpha receptor expression in human malignant gliomas. Cancer Res 1996;56:164–71.
47. Lafuente JV, Adan B, Alkiza K, et al. Expression of vascular endothelial growth factor (VEGF) and platelet-derived growth factor receptor-beta (PDGFR-beta) in human gliomas. J Mol Neurosci 1999;13:177–85.
48. Smith JS, Wang XY, Qian J, et al. Amplification of the platelet-derived growth factor receptor-A (PDGFRA) gene occurs in oligodendrogliomas with grade IV anaplastic features. J Neuropathol Exp Neurol 2000;59:495–503.
49. Guha A, Feldkamp MM, Lau N, et al. Proliferation of human malignant astrocytomas is dependent on Ras activation. Oncogene 1997;15:2755–65.
50. Guha A. Ras activation in astrocytomas and neurofibromas. Can J Neurol Sci 1998;25:267–81.
51. Feldkamp MM, Lau N, Roncari L, et al. Isotype-specific Ras. GTP-levels predict the efficacy of farnesyl transferase inhibitors against human astrocytomas regardless of Ras mutational status. Cancer Res 2001;61:4425–31.
52. Pollack IF, Randall MS, Kristofik MP, et al. Response of malignant glioma cell lines to activation and inhibition of protein kinase C-mediated pathways. J Neurosurg 1990;73:98–105.
53. Pollack IF, Kawecki S. The efficacy of tamoxifen as an antiproliferative agent in vitro for benign and malignant pediatric glial tumors. Pediatr Neurosurg 1995; 22:281–8.
54. Pollack IF, Kawecki S. The effect of calphostin C, a potent photodependent protein kinase C inhibitor, on the proliferation of glioma cells in vitro. J Neurooncol 1997;31:255–66.
55. da Rocha AB, Mans DR, Regner A, et al. Targeting protein kinase C: new therapeutic opportunities against high-grade malignant gliomas? Oncologist 2002;7:17–33.
56. Fuller GN, Rhee CH, Hess KR, et al. Reactivation of insulin-like growth factor binding protein 2 expression in glioblastoma multiforme: a revelation by parallel gene expression profiling. Cancer Res 1999;59:4228–32.

57. Zhang W, Wang H, Song SW, et al. Insulin-like growth factor binding protein 2: gene expression microarrays and the hypothesis-generation paradigm. Brain Pathol 2002;12:87–94.
58. Pilkington GJ. Tumour cell migration in the central nervous system. Brain Pathol 1994;4:157–66.
59. Yoshida D, Noha M, Watanabe K, et al. SI-27, a novel inhibitor of matrix metalloproteinases with antiangiogenic activity: detection with a variable-pressure scanning electron microscope. Neurosurgery 2002;50:578–86; discussion 586–8.
60. Cheng SY, Huang HJ, Nagane M, et al. Suppression of glioblastoma angiogenicity and tumorigenicity by inhibition of endogenous expression of vascular endothelial growth factor. Proc Natl Acad Sci U S A 1996;93:8502–7.
61. Saleh M, Stacker SA, Wilks AF. Inhibition of growth of C6 glioma cells in vivo by expression of antisense vascular endothelial growth factor sequence. Cancer Res 1996;56:393–401.
62. Im SA, Gomez-Manzano C, Fueyo J, et al. Antiangiogenesis treatment for gliomas: transfer of antisense-vascular endothelial growth factor inhibits tumor growth in vivo. Cancer Res 1999;59:895–900.
63. National Institutes of Health Consensus Development Conference. Neurofibromatosis. Conference statement. Arch Neurol 1988;45:575–8.
64. Romanowski CA, Cavallin LI. Neurofibromatosis types I and II: radiological appearance. Hosp Med 1998;59:134–9.
65. Seizinger BR, Rouleau GA, Ozelius LJ, et al. Genetic linkage of von Recklinghausen neurofibromatosis to the nerve growth factor receptor gene. Cell 1987;49:589–94.
66. Molloy PT, Bilaniuk LT, Vaughan SN, et al. Brainstem tumors in patients with neurofibromatosis type 1: a distinct clinical entity. Neurology 1995;45:1897–902.
67. Pollack IF, Mulvihill JJ. Special issues in the management of gliomas in children with neurofibromatosis 1. J Neurooncol 1996;28:257–68.
68. Mukonoweshuro W, Griffiths PD, Blaser S. Neurofibromatosis type 1: the role of neuroradiology. Neuropediatrics 1999;30:111–9.
69. Trofatter JA, MacCollin MM, Rutter JL, et al. A novel moesin-, ezrin-, radixin-like gene is a candidate for the neurofibromatosis 2 tumor suppressor. Cell 1993;75:826.
70. Rouleau GA, Merel P, Lutchman M, et al. Alteration in a new gene encoding a putative membrane-organizing protein causes neuro-fibromatosis type 2 [see comments]. Nature 1993;363:515–21.
71. Couch V, Lindor NM, Karnes PS, et al. von Hippel–Lindau disease. Mayo Clin Proc 2000;75:265–72.
72. Latif F, Tory K, Gnarra J, et al. Identification of the von Hippel–Lindau disease tumor suppressor gene [see comments]. Science 1993;260:1317–20.
73. Decker HJ, Weidt EJ, Brieger J. The von Hippel–Lindau tumor suppressor gene. A rare and intriguing disease opening new insight into basic mechanisms of carcinogenesis. Cancer Genet Cytogenet 1997;93:74–83.
74. Crino PB, Henske EP. New developments in the neurobiology of the tuberous sclerosis complex. Neurology 1999;53:1384–90.
75. Hurst JS, Wilcoski S. Recognizing an index case of tuberous sclerosis. Am Fam Physician 2000;61:703–8, 710.
76. van Slegtenhorst M, de Hoogt R, Hermans C, et al. Identification of the tuberous sclerosis gene *TSC1* on chromosome 9q34. Science 1997;277(5327):805–8.
77. The European Chromosome 16 Tuberous Sclerosis Consortium. Identification and characterization of the tuberous sclerosis gene on chromosome 16. Cell 1993;75:1305–15.
78. Nabbout R, Santos M, Rolland Y, et al. Early diagnosis of subependymal giant cell astrocytoma in children with tuberous sclerosis. J Neurol Neurosurg Psychiatry 1999;66:370–5.
79. Hosoya M, Naito H, Nihei K. Neurological prognosis correlated with variations over time in the number of subependymal nodules in tuberous sclerosis. Brain Dev 1999;21:544–7.
80. Li FP, Fraumeni JF Jr, Mulvihill JJ, et al. A cancer family syndrome in twenty-four kindreds. Cancer Res 1988;48:5358–62.
81. Garber JE, Goldstein AM, Kantor AF, et al. Follow-up study of twenty-four families with Li–Fraumeni syndrome. Cancer Res 1991;51:6094–7.
82. Brown LT, Sexsmith E, Malkin D. Identification of a novel PTEN intronic deletion in Li–Fraumeni syndrome and its effect on RNA processing. Cancer Genet Cytogenet 2000;123:65–8.
83. Bell DW, Varley JM, Szydlo TE, et al. Heterozygous germ line hCHK2 mutations in Li–Fraumeni syndrome. Science 1999;286:2528–31.
84. Dockhorn-Dworniczak B, Wolff J, Poremba C, et al. A new germline *TP53* gene mutation in a family with Li–Fraumeni syndrome. Eur J Cancer 1996;32A:1359–65.
85. Kleihues P, Cavenee WK, editors. Pathology and genetics. Tumors of the nervous system. World Health Organization classification of tumors. Lyon: International Agency for Research on Cancer (IARC) Press; 2000. p. 6–7.
86. Cairncross JG, Ueki K, Zlatescu MC, et al. Specific genetic predictors of chemotherapeutic response and survival in patients with anaplastic oligodendrogliomas. J Natl Cancer Inst 1998;90:1473–9.
87. McDermott MW, Krouwer HG, Asai A, et al. A comparison of CT contrast enhancement and BUDR labeling indices in moderately and highly anaplastic astrocytomas of the cerebral hemispheres. Can J Neurol Sci 1992;19:34–9.
88. Earnest FT, Kelly PJ, Scheithauer BW, et al. Cerebral astrocytomas: histopathologic correlation of MR and CT contrast enhancement with stereotactic biopsy. Radiology 1988;166:823–7.
89. Wald LL, Nelson SJ, Day MR, et al. Serial proton magnetic resonance spectroscopy imaging of glioblastoma multiforme after brachytherapy. J Neurosurg 1997; 87:525–34.
90. Nelson SJ, Day MR, Buffone PJ, et al. Alignment of volume MR images and high resolution [18F]fluorodeoxyglucose PET images for the evaluation of patients with brain tumors. J Comput Assist Tomogr 1997;21:183–91.
91. Nelson SJ, Huhn S, Vigneron DB, et al. Volume MRI and MRSI techniques for the quantitation of treatment response in brain tumors: presentation of a detailed case study. J Magn Reson Imaging 1997;7:1146–52.
92. Holzer T, Herholz K, Jeske J, et al. FDG-PET as a prognostic indicator in radiochemotherapy of glioblastoma. J Comput Assist Tomogr 1993;17:681–7.
93. Kim CK, Alavi JB, Alavi A, et al. New grading system of cerebral gliomas using positron emission tomography with F-18 fluorodeoxyglucose. J Neurooncol 1991;10: 85–91.
94. Di Chiro G. Positron emission tomography using [18F] fluorodeoxyglucose in brain tumors. A powerful diagnostic and prognostic tool. Invest Radiol 1987;22:360–71.
95. Delbeke D, Meyerowitz C, Lapidus RL, et al. Optimal cutoff levels of F-18 fluorodeoxyglucose uptake in the differentiation of low-grade from high-grade brain tumors with PET. Radiology 1995;195:47–52.
96. Ogawa S, Tank DW, Menon R, et al. Intrinsic signal changes accompanying sensory stimulation: functional brain mapping with magnetic resonance imaging. Proc Natl Acad Sci U S A 1992;89:5951–5.
97. Fine HA. The basis for current treatment recommendations for malignant gliomas. J Neurooncol 1994;20:111–20.
98. Haglund MM, Berger MS, Shamseldin M, et al. Cortical localization of temporal lobe language sites in patients with gliomas. Neurosurgery 1994;34:567–76; discussion 576.
99. Matz PG, Cobbs C, Berger MS. Intraoperative cortical mapping as a guide to the surgical resection of gliomas. J Neurooncol 1999;42:233–45.
100. Berger MS, Kincaid J, Ojemann GA, et al. Brain mapping techniques to maximize resection, safety, and seizure control in children with brain tumors. Neurosurgery 1989;25:786–92.
101. Forsting M, Albert FK, Kunze S, et al. Extirpation of glioblastomas: MR and CT follow-up of residual tumor and regrowth patterns. AJNR Am J Neuroradiol 1993;14:77–87.
102. Cairncross JG, Macdonald DR, Pexman JH, et al. Steroid-induced CT changes in patients with recurrent malignant glioma. Neurology 1988;38:724–6.
103. Enam SA, Rock JP, Rosenblum ML. Malignant gliomas. In: Berger MS, Bernstein M, editors. Neuro-oncology: the essentials. New York: Thieme; 2000. p. 309–18.
104. Curran WJ Jr, Scott CB, Horton J, et al. Recursive partitioning analysis of prognostic factors in three Radiation Therapy Oncology Group malignant glioma trials [see comments]. J Natl Cancer Inst 1993;85:704–10.
105. Kelly PJ, Daumas-Duport C, Kispert DB, et al. Imaging-based stereotaxic serial biopsies in untreated intracranial glial neoplasms. J Neurosurg 1987;66:865–74.
106. Simpson JR, Horton J, Scott C, et al. Influence of location and extent of surgical resection on survival of patients with glioblastoma multiforme: results of three consecutive Radiation Therapy Oncology Group (RTOG) clinical trials. Int J Radiat Oncol Biol Phys 1993;26:239–44.
107. Ciric I, Ammirati M, Vick N, et al. Supratentorial gliomas: surgical considerations and immediate postoperative results. Gross total resection versus partial resection. Neurosurgery 1987;21:21–6.
108. Ammirati M, Vick N, Liao YL, et al. Effect of the extent of surgical resection on survival and quality of life in patients with supratentorial glioblastomas and anaplastic astrocytomas. Neurosurgery 1987;21:201–6.
109. Liang BC, Thornton AF Jr, Sandler HM, et al. Malignant astrocytomas: focal tumor recurrence after focal external beam radiation therapy. J Neurosurg 1991;75:559–63.
110. Gaspar LE, Fisher BJ, Macdonald DR, et al. Supratentorial malignant glioma: patterns of recurrence and implications for external beam local treatment. Int J Radiat Oncol Biol Phys 1992;24:55–7.
111. Walker MD, Alexander E Jr, Hunt WE, et al. Evaluation of BCNU and/or radiotherapy in the treatment of anaplastic gliomas. A cooperative clinical trial. J Neurosurg 1978;49:333–43.
112. Chang CH, Horton J, Schoenfeld D, et al. Comparison of postoperative radiotherapy and combined postoperative radiotherapy and chemotherapy in the multidisciplinary management of malignant gliomas. A joint Radiation Therapy Oncology Group and Eastern Cooperative Oncology Group study. Cancer 1983;52:997–1007.
113. Salazar OM, Rubin P, Feldstein ML, et al. High dose radiation therapy in the treatment of malignant gliomas: final report. Int J Radiat Oncol Biol Phys 1979;5:1733–40.
114. Levin VA, Silver P, Hannigan J, et al. Superiority of post-radiotherapy adjuvant chemotherapy with CCNU, procarbazine, and vincristine (PCV) over BCNU for anaplastic gliomas: NCOG 6G61 final report. Int J Radiat Oncol Biol Phys 1990;18:321–4.
115. Prados MD, Scott C, Curran WJ Jr, et al. Procarbazine, lomustine, and vincristine (PCV) chemotherapy for anaplastic astrocytoma: a retrospective review of radiation therapy oncology group protocols comparing survival with carmustine or PCV adjuvant chemotherapy. J Clin Oncol 1999;17:3389–95.
116. Medical Research Council Brain Tumor Working Party: Randomized trial of procarbazine, lomustine, and vincristine in the adjuvant treatment of high-grade astrocytoma: A Medical Research Council Trial. J Clin Oncol 2001;19: 509–18.
117. Stupp R, Mason WP, van den Bent MJ, et al: Promising survival for patients with newly diagnosed glioblastoma multiforme treated with concomitant radiation plus temozolomide followed by adjuvant temozolomide. J Clin Oncol 2002;20:1375–82.
118. Stupp R, Mason WP, van den Brent MJ, et al: Radiotherapy plus concomitant and adjuvant Temodar for glioblastoma. N Engl J Med 2005;352: 987–96.
119. Leibel SA, Scott CB, Loeffler JS. Contemporary approaches to the treatment of malignant gliomas with radiation therapy. Semin Oncol 1994;21:198–219.
120. Withers HR. Biologic basis for altered fractionation schemes. Cancer 1985;55 (Suppl 9):2086–95.
121. Nelson DF, Curran WJ Jr, Scott C, et al. Hyperfractionated radiation therapy and bis-chlorethyl nitrosourea in the treatment of malignant glioma—possible advantage observed at 72.0 Gy in 1.2 Gy B.I.D. fractions: report of the Radiation Therapy Oncology Group Protocol 8302. Int J Radiat Oncol Biol Phys 1993;25:193–207.
122. Levin VA, Prados MR, Wara WM, et al. Radiation therapy and bromodeoxyuridine chemotherapy followed by procarbazine, lomustine, and vincristine for the treatment of anaplastic gliomas. Int J Radiat Oncol Biol Phys 1995;32:75–83.
123. Phillips TL, Levin VA, Ahn DK, et al. Evaluation of bromodeoxyuridine in glioblastoma multiforme: a Northern California Cancer Center Phase II study [see comments]. Int J Radiat Oncol Biol Phys 1991;21:709–14.
124. Prados MD, Scott C, Sandler H, et al. A Phase 3 randomized study of radiotherapy plus procarbazine, CCNU, and vincristine (PCV) with or without BUdR for the treatment of anaplastic astrocytoma: a preliminary report of RTOG 9404 [see comments]. Int J Radiat Oncol Biol Phys 1999;45:1109–15.
125. Selker RG, Eddy MS, Deutsch M, et al. On the development of an interstitial radiation protocol for a multicenter consortium. Experience with permanent low-dose rate and temporary high-dose rate 125I implants in "failed" and "newly diagnosed" glioblastoma patients: quality assurance methodology and a possible future adjuvant for therapeutic enhancement. J Neurooncol 1995;26:141–55.
126. Laperriere NJ, Leung PM, McKenzie S, et al. Randomized study of brachytherapy in the initial management of patients with malignant astrocytoma. Int J Radiat Oncol Biol Phys 1998;41:1005–11.
127. Scharfen CO, Sneed PK, Wara WM, et al. High activity iodine-125 interstitial implant for gliomas. Int J Radiat Oncol Biol Phys 1992;24:583–91.
128. Sneed PK, Larson DA, Gutin PH. Brachytherapy and hyperthermia for malignant astrocytomas. Semin Oncol 1994;21:186–97.

129. Sneed PK, Stauffer PR, McDermott MW, et al. Survival benefit of hyperthermia in a prospective randomized trial of brachytherapy boost +/– hyperthermia for glioblastoma multiforme. Int J Radiat Oncol Biol Phys 1998;40:287–95.
130. Larson DA, Gutin PH, McDermott M, et al. Gamma knife for glioma: selection factors and survival [see comments]. Int J Radiat Oncol Biol Phys 1996;36:1045–53.
131. Werner-Wasik M, Rudoler S, Preston PE, et al. Immediate side effects of stereotactic radiotherapy and radiosurgery. Int J Radiat Oncol Biol Phys 1999;43:299–304.
132. Shrieve DC, Alexander E 3rd, Wen PY, et al. Comparison of stereotactic radiosurgery and brachytherapy in the treatment of recurrent glioblastoma multiforme. Neurosurgery 1995;36:275–82; discussion 282–4.
133. Shrieve DC, Alexander E 3rd, Black PM, et al. Treatment of patients with primary glioblastoma multiforme with standard postoperative radiotherapy and radiosurgical boost: prognostic factors and long-term outcome. J Neurosurg 1999;90:72–7.
134. Barker FG II, Chang SM, Gutin PH, et al. Survival and functional status after resection of recurrent glioblastoma multiforme. Neurosurgery 1998;42:709–20; discussion 720–3.
135. Halligan JB, Stelzer KJ, Rostomily RC, et al. Operation and permanent low activity 125I brachytherapy for recurrent. Int J Radiat Oncol Biol Phys 1996;35:541–7.
136. Sneed PK, Gutin PH, Prados MD, et al. Brachytherapy of brain tumors. Stereotact Funct Neurosurg 1992;59:157–65.
137. Prados MD, Russo C. Chemotherapy of brain tumors. Semin Surg Oncol 1998;14:88–95.
138. Chang SM, Prados MD. Chemotherapy for gliomas. Curr Opin Oncol 1995;7:207–13.
139. Burton E, Prados M. New chemotherapy options for the treatment of malignant gliomas. Curr Opin Oncol 1999;11:157–61.
140. Yung WK, Prados MD, Yaya-Tur R, et al. Multicenter phase II trial of temozolomide in patients with anaplastic astrocytoma or anaplastic oligoastrocytoma at first relapse. Temodal Brain Tumor Group. J Clin Oncol 1999;17:2762–71.
141. Wong ET, Hess KR, Gleason MJ, et al. Outcomes and prognostic factors in recurrent glioma patients enrolled onto Phase II clinical trials. J Clin Oncol 1999;17:2572–78.
142. Hess CF. [Supratentorial low-grade glioma in adults: the prognostic factors and their effect on the timing of radiotherapy.] Strahlenther Onkol 1998;174:49–50.
143. Cairncross JG. Aggressive oligodendroglioma: a chemosensitive tumor. Recent Results Cancer Res 1994;135: 127–33.
144. Ino Y, Betensky RA, Zlatescu MC, et al. Molecular subtypes of anaplastic oligodendroglioma: implications for patient management at diagnosis. Clin Cancer Res 2001;7:839–45.
145. Cairncross G, Seiferheld W, Shaw E, et al: An Intergroup randomized controlled clinical trial of chemotherapy plus radiation versus radiation alone for pure and mixed anaplastic oligodendrogliomas: Initial report of RTOG 94-02. Proceedings of ASCO 2004;22:107s.
146. Leighton C, Fisher B, Bauman G, et al. Supratentorial low-grade glioma in adults: an analysis of prognostic factors and timing of radiation [see comments]. J Clin Oncol 1997;15:1294–301.
147. Rudoler S, Corn BW, Werner-Wasik M, et al. Patterns of tumor progression after radiotherapy for low-grade gliomas: analysis from the computed tomography/magnetic resonance imaging era. Am J Clin Oncol 1998;21:23–7.
148. Bauman G, Lote K, Larson D, et al. Pretreatment factors predict overall survival for patients with low-grade glioma: a recursive partitioning analysis. Int J Radiat Oncol Biol Phys 1999;45:923–9.
149. Pignatti F, van Den Bent M, Curran D, et al. Prognostic factors for survival in adult patients with cerebral low-grade glioma. J Clin Oncol 2002;20:2076–84.
150. Chozick BS, Pezzullo JC, Epstein MH, et al. Prognostic implications of p53 overexpression in supratentorial astrocytic tumors. Neurosurgery 1994;35:831–7; discussion 837–8.
151. Abdulrauf SI, Edvardsen K, Ho KL, et al. Vascular endothelial growth factor expression and vascular density as prognostic markers of survival in patients with low-grade astrocytoma. J Neurosurg 1998;88:513–20.
152. Kleihues P, Soylemezoglu F, Schauble B, et al. Histopathology, classification, and grading of gliomas. Glia 1995;15:211–21.
153. Berger MS, Deliganis AV, Dobbins J, et al. The effect of extent of resection on recurrence in patients with low grade cerebral hemisphere gliomas [see comments]. Cancer 1994;74:1784–91.
154. Celli P, Nofrone I, Palma L, et al. Cerebral oligodendroglioma: prognostic factors and life history. Neurosurgery 1994;35:1018–34; discussion 1034–5.
155. Bahary JP, Villemure JG, Choi S, et al. Low-grade pure and mixed cerebral astrocytomas treated in the CT scan era. J Neurooncol 1996;27:173–7.
156. Piepmeier J, Christopher S, Spencer D, et al. Variations in the natural history and survival of patients with supratentorial low-grade astrocytomas. Neurosurgery 1996;38:872–8; discussion 878–9.
157. Nicolato A, Gerosa MA, Fina P, et al. Prognostic factors in low-grade supratentorial astrocytomas: a uni- multivariate statistical analysis in 76 surgically treated adult patients. Surg Neurol 1995;44:208–21; discussion 221–3.
158. Shaw EG, Scheithauer BW, O'Fallon JR, et al. Oligodendrogliomas: the Mayo Clinic experience. J Neurosurg 1992;76:428–34.
159. Recht LD, Lew R, Smith TW. Suspected low-grade glioma: is deferring treatment safe? Ann Neurol 1992;31:431–6.
160. Karim AB, Afra D, Cornu P, et al. Randomized trial on the efficacy of radiotherapy for cerebral low-grade glioma in the adult: European Organization for Research and Treatment of Cancer Study 22845 with the Medical Research Council study BRO4: an interim analysis. Int J Radiat Oncol Biol Phys 2002;52:316–24.
161. Philippon JH, Clemenceau SH, Fauchon FH, et al. Supratentorial low-grade astrocytomas in adults. Neurosurgery 1993;32:554–9.
162. Shaw EG, Scheithauer BW, Gilbertson DT, et al. Postoperative radiotherapy of supratentorial low-grade gliomas. Int J Radiat Oncol Biol Phys 1989;16:663–8.
163. Karim AB, Maat B, Hatlevoll R, et al. A randomized trial on dose-response in radiation therapy of low-grade cerebral glioma: European Organization for Research and Treatment of Cancer (EORTC) Study 22844. Int J Radiat Oncol Biol Phys 1996;36:549–56.
164. Shaw E, Arusell R, Scheithauer AR, et al. A prospective randomized trial of low-versus high-dose radiation therapy in adults with supratentorial low-grade glioma: Initial report of a North Central Cancer Treatment Group/Radiation Therapy Oncology Group Eastern Cooperative Oncology Group Study. Clin Oncol 2002;1:2267–76.
165. Kiebert GM, Curran D, Aaronson NK, et al. Quality of life after radiation therapy of cerebral low-grade gliomas of the adult: results of a randomised Phase III trial on dose response (EORTC trial 22844). EORTC Radiotherapy Co-operative Group. Eur J Cancer 1998;34:1902–9.
166. Kida Y, Kobayashi T, Mori Y. Gamma knife radiosurgery for low-grade astrocytomas: results of long- term follow up. J Neurosurg 2000;93 Suppl 3:42–6.
167. Eyre HJ, Crowley JJ, Townsend JJ, et al. A randomized trial of radiotherapy versus radiotherapy plus CCNU for incompletely resected low-grade gliomas: a Southwest Oncology Group study. J Neurosurg 1993;78:909–14.
168. Mason WP, Krol GS, DeAngelis LM. Low-grade oligodendroglioma responds to chemotherapy. Neurology 1996;46:203–7.
169. Buckner JC, Brown LD, Kugler JW, et al. Phase II evaluation of recombinant interferon alpha and BCNU in recurrent glioma. J Neurosurg 1995;82:430–5.
170. van de Bent MJ, Taphoorn MJ, Brandess AA, et al. Phase II study of first-line chemotherapy with temozolomide in recurrent oligodendroglioma: The European Organisation of Research and Treatment of Cancer Brain Tumor Group study 26971. J Clin Oncol 2003;21:2525–8.
171. Mork SJ, Rubinstein LJ. Ependymoblastoma. A reappraisal of a rare embryonal tumor. Cancer 1985;55:1536–42.
172. Horn B, Heideman R, Geyer R, et al. A multi-institutional retrospective study of intracranial ependymoma in children: identification of risk factors. J Pediatr Hematol Oncol 1999;21:203–11.
173. Ross GW, Rubinstein LJ. Lack of histopathological correlation of malignant ependymomas with postoperative survival. J Neurosurg 1989;70:31–6.
174. Robertson PL, Zeltzer PM, Boyett JM, et al. Survival and prognostic factors following radiation therapy and chemotherapy for ependymomas in children: a report of the Children's Cancer Group [see comments]. J Neurosurg 1998;88:695–703.
175. Awaad YM, Allen JC, Miller DC, et al. Deferring adjuvant therapy for totally resected intracranial ependymoma. Pediatr Neurol 1996;14:216–19.
176. Ernestus RI, Wilcke O, Schroder R. Intracranial ependymomas: prognostic aspects. Neurosurg Rev 1989;12:157–63.
177. Salazar OM, Castro-Vita H, VanHoutte P, et al. Improved survival in cases of intracranial ependymoma after radiation therapy. Late report and recommendations. J Neurosurg 1983;59:652–9.
178. Shaw EG, Evans RG, Scheithauer BW, et al. Postoperative radiotherapy of intracranial ependymoma in pediatric and adult patients. Int J Radiat Oncol Biol Phys 1987;13:1457–62.
179. Goldwein JW, Corn BW, Finlay JL, et al. Is craniospinal irradiation required to cure children with malignant (anaplastic) intracranial ependymomas? Cancer 1991;67:2766–71.
180. Pollack IF, Gerszten PC, Martinez AJ, et al. Intracranial ependymomas of childhood: long-term outcome and prognostic factors. Neurosurgery 1995;37:655–66; discussion 666–7.
181. Evans AE, Anderson JR, Lefkowitz-Boudreaux IB, et al. Adjuvant chemotherapy of childhood posterior fossa ependymoma: cranio-spinal irradiation with or without adjuvant CCNU, vincristine, and prednisone: a Children's Cancer Group study. Med Pediatr Oncol 1996;27:8–14.
182. Minehan KJ, Shaw EG, Scheithauer BW, et al. Spinal cord astrocytoma: pathological and treatment considerations. J Neurosurg 1995;83:590–5.
183. Innocenzi G, Salvati M, Cervoni L, et al. Prognostic factors in intramedullary astrocytomas. Clin Neurol Neurosurg 1997;99:1–5.
184. Kim MS, Chung CK, Choe G, et al. Intramedullary spinal cord astrocytoma in adults: postoperative outcome. J Neurooncol 2001;52:85–94.
185. Constantini S, Miller DC, Allen JC, et al. Radical excision of intramedullary spinal cord tumors: surgical morbidity and long-term follow-up evaluation in 164 children and young adults. J Neurosurg 2000;93 Suppl 2:183–93.
186. Epstein FJ, Farmer JP, Freed D. Adult intramedullary astrocytomas of the spinal cord. J Neurosurg 1992;77:355–9.
187. Sgouros S, Malluci CL, Jackowski A. Spinal ependymomas—the value of postoperative radiotherapy for residual disease control. Br J Neurosurg 1996;10:559–66.
188. Whitaker SJ, Bessell EM, Ashley SE, et al. Postoperative radiotherapy in the management of spinal cord ependymoma. J Neurosurg 1991;74:720–8.
189. McCormick PC, Torres R, Post KD, et al. Intramedullary ependymoma of the spinal cord. J Neurosurg 1990;72:523–32.
190. Waldron JN, Laperriere NJ, Jaakkimainen L, et al. Spinal cord ependymomas: a retrospective analysis of 59 cases. Int J Radiat Oncol Biol Phys 1993;27:223–9.
191. Cooper PR. Outcome after operative treatment of intramedullary spinal cord tumors in adults: intermediate and long-term results in 51 patients. Neurosurgery 1989;25:855–9.
192. Linstadt DE, Wara WM, Leibel SA, et al. Postoperative radiotherapy of primary spinal cord tumors. Int J Radiat Oncol Biol Phys 1989;16:1397–403.
193. Cohen AR, Wisoff JH, Allen JC, et al. Malignant astrocytomas of the spinal cord. J Neurosurg 1989;70:50–4.
194. Hassall TE, Mitchell AE, Ashley DM. Carboplatin chemotherapy for progressive intramedullary spinal cord low-grade gliomas in children: three case studies and a review of the literature. Neuro-oncol 2001;3:251–7.
195. Doireau V, Grill J, Zerah M, et al. Chemotherapy for unresectable and recurrent intramedullary glial tumours in children. Brain Tumours Subcommittee of the French Society of Paediatric Oncology (SFOP). Br J Cancer 1999;81:835–40.
196. Bouffet E, Amat D, Devaux Y, et al. Chemotherapy for spinal cord astrocytoma. Med Pediatr Oncol 1997;29:560–2.
197. Rutka JT. Medulloblastoma. Clin Neurosurg 1997;44:571–85.
198. Bloom HJ, Bessell EM. Medulloblastoma in adults: a review of 47 patients treated between 1952 and 1981. Int J Radiat Oncol Biol Phys 1990;18:763–72.
199. Giordana MT, Schiffer P, Lanotte M, et al. Epidemiology of adult medulloblastoma. Int J Cancer 1999;80:689–92.
200. Rorke LB, Trojanowski JQ, Lee VM, et al. Primitive neuroectodermal tumors of the central nervous system. Brain Pathol 1997;7:765–84.
201. Prados MD, Warnick RE, Wara WM, et al. Medulloblastoma in adults. Int J Radiat Oncol Biol Phys 1995;32:1145–52.
202. Le QT, Weil MD, Wara WM, et al. Adult medulloblastoma: an analysis of survival and prognostic factors. Cancer J Sci Am 1997;3:238–45.
203. Frost PJ, Laperriere NJ, Wong CS, et al. Medulloblastoma in adults. Int J Radiat Oncol Biol Phys 1995;32:951–7.
204. Carrie C, Lasset C, Alapetite C, et al. Multivariate analysis of prognostic factors in adult patients with medulloblastoma. Retrospective study of 156 patients. Cancer 1994;74:2352–60.
205. Kunschner LJ, Kuttesch J, Hess K, et al. Survival and recurrence factors in adult medulloblastoma: the M.D. Ander-

son Cancer Center experience from 1978 to 1998. Neurooncol 2001;3:167–73.
206. Chan AW, Tarbell NJ, Black PM, et al. Adult medulloblastoma: prognostic factors and patterns of relapse. Neurosurgery 2000;47:623–31; discussion 631–2.
207. Giordana MT, Duo D, Gasverde S, et al. MDM2 overexpression is associated with short survival in adults with medulloblastoma. Neuro-oncol 2002;4:115–22.
208. Kramer JH, Crowe AB, Larson DA, et al. Neuropsychological sequelae of medulloblastoma in adults. Int J Radiat Oncol Biol Phys 1997;38:21–6.
209. Bloom HJ. Medulloblastoma: prognosis and prospects. Int J Radiat Oncol Biol Phys 1977;2:1031–3.
210. Paulino AC, Wen BC, Mohideen MN. Controversies in the management of intracranial germinomas. Oncology (Huntingt) 1999;13:513–21; discussion 521–2, 528–3.
211. Sano K. Pathogenesis of intracranial germ cell tumors reconsidered. J Neurosurg 1999;90:258–64.
212. Kretschmar CS. Germ cell tumors of the brain in children: a review of current literature and new advances in therapy. Cancer Invest 1997;15:187–98.
213. Wolden SL, Wara WM, Larson DA, et al. Radiation therapy for primary intracranial germ-cell tumors. Int J Radiat Oncol Biol Phys 1995;32:943–9.
214. Shibamoto Y, Takahashi M, Sasai K. Prognosis of intracranial germinoma with syncytiotrophoblastic giant cells treated by radiation therapy. Int J Radiat Oncol Biol Phys 1997;37:505–10.
215. Ushio Y, Kochi M, Kuratsu J, et al. Preliminary observations for a new treatment in children with primary intracranial yolk sac tumor or embryonal carcinoma. Report of five cases. J Neurosurg 1999;90:133–7.
216. Black PM. Hormones, radiosurgery and virtual reality: new aspects of meningioma management. Can J Neurol Sci 1997;24:302–6.
217. Younis GA, Sawaya R, DeMonte F, et al. Aggressive meningeal tumors: review of a series. J Neurosurg 1995;82:17–27.
218. Perry A, Scheithauer BW, Stafford SL, et al. "Malignancy" in meningiomas: a clinicopathologic study of 116 patients, with grading implications. Cancer 1999;85:2046–56.
219. Palma L, Celli P, Franco C, et al. Long-term prognosis for atypical and malignant meningiomas: a study of 71 surgical cases. J Neurosurg 1997;86:793–800.
220. Seizinger BR, de la Monte S, Atkins L, et al. Molecular genetic approach to human meningioma: loss of genes on chromosome 22. Proc Natl Acad Sci U S A 1987;84:5419–23.
221. Sulman EP, Dumanski JP, White PS, et al. Identification of a consistent region of allelic loss on 1p32 in meningiomas: correlation with increased morbidity. Cancer Res 1998;58:3226–30.
222. Carroll RS, Black PM, Zhang J, et al. Expression and activation of epidermal growth factor receptors in meningiomas. J Neurosurg 1997;87:315–23.
223. Black PM, Carroll R, Glowacka D, et al. Platelet-derived growth factor expression and stimulation in human meningiomas. J Neurosurg 1994;81:388–93.
224. Kalkanis SN, Carroll RS, Zhang J, et al. Correlation of vascular endothelial growth factor messenger RNA expression with peritumoral vasogenic cerebral edema in meningiomas. J Neurosurg 1996;85:1095–101.
225. Tsai JC, Hsiao YY, Teng LJ, et al. Regulation of vascular endothelial growth factor secretion in human meningioma cells. J Formos Med Assoc 1999;98:111–7.
226. Shu J, Lee JH, Harwalkar JA, et al. Adenovirus-mediated gene transfer of dominant negative Ha-Ras inhibits proliferation of primary meningioma cells. Neurosurgery 1999;44:579–87; discussion 587–8.
227. Zee CS, Chen T, Hinton DR, et al. Magnetic resonance imaging of cystic meningiomas and its surgical implications. Neurosurgery 1995;36:482–8.
228. Olivero WC, Lister JR, Elwood PW. The natural history and growth rate of asymptomatic meningiomas: a review of 60 patients. J Neurosurg 1995;83:222–4.
229. Kuratsu J, Kochi M, Ushio Y. Incidence and clinical features of asymptomatic meningiomas. J Neurosurg 2000; 92:766–70.
230. Simpson D. The recurrence of intracranial meningioma after surgical treatment. J Neurol Neurosurg Psychiatry 1957;20:22–39.
231. Condra KS, Buatti JM, Mendenhall WM, et al. Benign meningiomas: primary treatment selection affects survival. Int J Radiat Oncol Biol Phys 1997;39:427–36.
232. Stafford SL, Perry A, Suman VJ, et al. Primarily resected meningiomas: outcome and prognostic factors in 581 Mayo Clinic patients, 1978 through 1988. Mayo Clin Proc 1998;73:936–42.
233. Dziuk TW, Woo S, Butler EB, et al. Malignant meningioma: an indication for initial aggressive surgery and adjuvant radiotherapy. J Neurooncol 1998;37:177–88.
234. Morita A, Coffey RJ, Foote RL, et al. Risk of injury to cranial nerves after gamma knife radiosurgery for skull base meningiomas: experience in 88 patients. J Neurosurg 1999;90:42–9.
235. Ojemann SG, Sneed PK, Larson DA, et al. Radiosurgery for malignant meningioma: results in 22 patients. J Neurosurg 2000;93 Suppl 3:62–7.
236. Kaba SE, DeMonte F, Bruner JM, et al. The treatment of recurrent unresectable and malignant meningiomas with interferon alpha-2B. Neurosurgery 1997;40:271–5.
237. Schrell UM, Rittig MG, Anders M, et al. Hydroxyurea for treatment of unresectable and recurrent meningiomas. II. Decrease in the size of meningiomas in patients treated with hydroxyurea [see comments]. J Neurosurg 1997;86:840–4.
238. Lamberts SW, Tanghe HL, Avezaat CJ, et al. Mifepristone (RU 486) treatment of meningiomas. J Neurol Neurosurg Psychiatry 1992;55:486–90.
239. Cote RT, Manns A, Hardy CR, et al: Epidemiology of brain lymphoma among people with or without acquired immune deficiency syndrome. J Natl Cancer Inst 1996;88:675–9.
240. Rickert CH, Dockhorn-Dworniczak B, Simon R, et al. Chromosomal imbalances in primary lymphomas of the central nervous system. Am J Pathol 1999;155:1445–51.
241. Balmaceda C, Gaynor JJ, Sun M, et al. Leptomeningeal tumor in primary central nervous system lymphoma: recognition, significance, and implications. Ann Neurol 1995;38:202–9.
242. Henry JM, Heffner RR Jr, Dillard SH, et al. Primary malignant lymphomas of the central nervous system. Cancer 1974;34:1293–302.
243. Nelson DF, Martz KL, Bonner H, et al. Non-Hodgkin's lymphoma of the brain: can high dose, large volume radiation therapy improve survival? Report on a prospective trial by the Radiation Therapy Oncology Group (RTOG): RTOG 8315. Int J Radiat Oncol Biol Phys 1992;23:9–17.
244. DeAngelis LM, Yahalom J, Thaler HT, et al. Combined modality therapy for primary CNS lymphoma. J Clin Oncol 1992;10:635–43.
245. Baumgartner JE, Rachlin JR, Beckstead JH, et al. Primary central nervous system lymphomas: natural history and response to radiation therapy in 55 patients with acquired immunodeficiency syndrome. J Neurosurg 1990;73:206–11.
246. Reni M, Ferreri AJ, Garancini MP, et al. Therapeutic management of primary central nervous system lymphoma in immunocompetent patients: results of a critical review of the literature. Ann Oncol 1997;8:227–34.
247. Peterson K, Gordon KB, Heinemann MH, et al. The clinical spectrum of ocular lymphoma. Cancer 1993;72:843–9.
248. Sparano JA. Clinical aspects and management of AIDS-related lymphoma. Eur J Cancer 2001;37:1296–305.
249. Schultz C, Scott C, Sherman W, et al. Preirradiation chemotherapy with cyclophosphamide, doxorubicin, vincristine, and dexamethasone for primary CNS lymphomas: initial report of radiation therapy oncology group protocol 88–06. J Clin Oncol 1996;14:556–64.
250. Abrey LE, DeAngelis LM, Yahalom J, Long-term survival in primary CNS lymphoma. J Clin Oncol 1998;16:859–63.
251. Glass J, Gruber ML, Cher L, et al. Preirradiation methotrexate chemotherapy of primary central nervous system lymphoma: long-term outcome. J Neurosurg 1994;81:188–95.
252. Blay JY, Conroy T, Chevreau C, et al. High-dose methotrexate for the treatment of primary cerebral lymphomas: analysis of survival and late neurologic toxicity in a retrospective series. J Clin Oncol 1998;16:864–71.
253. Chamberlain MC, Levin VA. Primary central nervous system lymphoma: a role for adjuvant chemotherapy. J Neurooncol 1992;14:271–5.
254. Bessell EM, Lopez-Guillermo A, Villa S, et al. Importance of radiotherapy in the outcome of patients with primary CNS lymphoma: an analysis of the CHOD/BVAM regimen followed by two different radiotherapy treatments. J Clin Oncol 2002;20:231–6.
255. Sarazin M, Ameri A, Monjour A, et al. Primary central nervous system lymphoma: treatment with chemotherapy and radiotherapy. Eur J Cancer 1995;31A:2003–7.
256. Abrey LE, Yahalon M, DeAngelis LM. Treatment for primary CNS lymphoma: the next step. J Clin Oncol 2000;18: 3144–50.
257. Valluri S, Moorthy RS, Khan A, et al. Combination treatment of intraocular lymphoma. Retina 1995;15:125–9.
258. Fishburne BC, Wilson DJ, Rosenbaum JT, et al. Intravitreal methotrexate as an adjunctive treatment of intraocular lymphoma. Arch Ophthalmol 1997;115:1152–6.
259. Kaplan JG, DeSouza TG, Farkash A, et al. Leptomeningeal metastases: comparison of clinical features and laboratory data of solid tumors, lymphomas and leukemias. J Neurooncol 1990;9:225–9.
260. Posner JB, Chernik NL. Intracranial metastases from systemic cancer. Adv Neurol 1978;19:579–92.
261. Wasserstrom WR, Glass JP, Posner JB. Diagnosis and treatment of leptomeningeal metastases from solid tumors: experience with 90 patients. Cancer 1982;49:759–72.
262. Shapiro WR, Posner JB, Ushio Y, et al. Treatment of meningeal neoplasms. Cancer Treat Rep 1977;61: 733–43.
263. Rosen ST, Aisner J, Makuch RW, et al. Carcinomatous leptomeningitis in small cell lung cancer: a clinicopathologic review of the National Cancer Institute experience. Medicine (Baltimore) 1982;61:45–53.
264. Chamberlain MC, Dirr L. Involved-field radiotherapy and intra-Ommaya methotrexate/cytarabine in patients with AIDS-related lymphomatous meningitis. J Clin Oncol 1993;11:1978–84.
265. Grossman SA, Moynihan TJ. Neoplastic meningitis. Neurol Clin 1991;9:843–56.
266. Chamberlain MC. Diagnosis and treatment of neoplastic meningitis. In: Prados M, editor. Brain cancer. Hamilton [ON]: BC Decker; 2002. p. 391–405.
267. Glass JP, Melamed M, Chernik NL, et al. Malignant cells in cerebrospinal fluid (CSF): the meaning of a positive CSF cytology. Neurology 1979;29:1369–75.
268. Cibas ES, Malkin MG, Posner JB, et al. Detection of DNA abnormalities by flow cytometry in cells from cerebrospinal fluid. Am J Clin Pathol 1987;88:570–7.
269. Recht LD. Neurologic complications of systemic lymphoma. Neurol Clin 1991;9:1001–15.
270. Stockhammer G, Poewe W, Burgstaller S, et al. Vascular endothelial growth factor in CSF: a biological marker for carcinomatous meningitis. Neurology 2000;54:1670–6.
271. Chamberlain MC, Sandy AD, Press GA. Leptomeningeal metastasis: a comparison of gadolinium-enhanced MR and contrast-enhanced CT of the brain. Neurology 1990;40:435–8.
272. Chamberlain MC. Comparative spine imaging in leptomeningeal metastases. J Neurooncol 1995;23:233–8.
273. Chamberlain MC. Leptomeningeal metastases: a review of evaluation and treatment. J Neurooncol 1998;37:271–84.
274. Ascherl GF Jr, Hilal SK, Brisman R. Computed tomography of disseminated meningeal and ependymal malignant neoplasms. Neurology 1981;31:567–74.
275. Chamberlain MC. Radioisotope CSF flow studies in leptomeningeal metastases. J Neurooncol 1998;38:135–40.
276. Blasberg RG, Patlak C, Fenstermacher JD. Intrathecal chemotherapy: brain tissue profiles after ventriculocisternal perfusion. J Pharmacol Exp Ther 1975;195:73–83.
277. Slevin ML, Piall EM, Aherne GW, et al. Effect of dose and schedule on pharmacokinetics of high-dose cytosine arabinoside in plasma and cerebrospinal fluid. J Clin Oncol 1983;1:546–51.
278. Lopez JA, Nassif E, Vannicola P, et al. Central nervous system pharmacokinetics of high-dose cytosine arabinoside. J Neurooncol 1985;3:119–24.
279. Balm M, Hammack J. Leptomeningeal carcinomatosis. Presenting features and prognostic factors [see comments]. Arch Neurol 1996;53:626–32.
280. Bleyer WA. Current status of intrathecal chemotherapy for human meningeal neoplasms. Natl Cancer Inst Monogr 1977;46:171–8.
281. Grossman SA, Finkelstein DM, Ruckdeschel JC, et al. Randomized prospective comparison of intraventricular methotrexate and thiotepa in patients with previously untreated neoplastic meningitis. Eastern Cooperative Oncology Group. J Clin Oncol 1993;11:561–9.
282. Glantz MJ, Jaeckle KA, Chamberlain MC, et al. A randomized controlled trial comparing intrathecal sustained-release cytarabine (DepoCyt) to intrathecal methotrexate in patients with neoplastic meningitis from solid tumors. Clin Cancer Res 1999; 5:3394–402.
283. Siegal T, Lossos A, Pfeffer MR. Leptomeningeal metastases: analysis of 31 patients with sustained off-therapy response following combined-modality therapy. Neurology 1994;44:1463–9.
284. Balis FM, Poplack DG. Central nervous system pharmacology of antileukemic drugs. Am J Pediatr Hematol Oncol 1989;11:74–86.
285. Collins JM. Pharmacokinetics of intraventricular administration. J Neurooncol 1983;1:283–91.

Brain Metastases

Sean Grimm, MD
Lisa M. DeAngelis, MD

Metastasis is the most common tumor affecting the brain. Autopsy studies find intracranial metastases in approximately 25% and brain metastases in 15% of patients who die of cancer.[1] Between two-thirds and three-quarters of such patients had symptoms from the intracranial metastasis during life which approximates the 9.6% incidence of brain metastasis reported in a recent population-based study.[2,3] Thus, approximately 70,000 patients have symptomatic intracranial metastases annually, a number that far exceeds the 17,000 patients with malignant primary brain tumors. Most brain metastases present late during the course of what is usually a widely metastatic cancer. In a smaller percentage of patients (perhaps about 10% of patients with lung cancer), a brain metastasis may be the first evidence that the patient suffers from cancer; alternatively, a patient with cancer believed to be localized may have an asymptomatic brain metastasis found on computed tomography (CT) or magnetic resonance imaging (MRI).[4] In recent years, with more effective systemic therapy, brain metastases are emerging as the only site of relapse in many patients with otherwise controlled cancer.[5–8] Because of the increasing incidence of brain metastasis as the sole site of relapse, prophylactic cranial radiation is often administered to those patients with small-cell lung cancer who achieve a complete remission from initial chemotherapy.[9,10] Some authors have even recommended prophylactic cranial radiation for the treatment of those patients with non–small-cell lung cancer who have achieved control of their systemic tumor.[10]

In adults, the most common sources of brain metastases are lung and breast carcinoma, and melanoma (Table 73-1). However, any malignant neoplasm can metastasize to the brain and it is likely that one will see an increasing number of metastases from what are believed to be uncommon sites, for example, bladder,[6] neuroblastoma in children,[5] or multiple myeloma.[11] In as many as 10% of patients with brain metastases, no primary tumor is found on initial search. On rare occasions, the primary tumor is not identifiable even at autopsy, although immunocytochemical analysis of the brain metastasis may help identify the primary site.[12]

Brain metastases are only one of many neurologic complications of cancer. We discuss the others, both metastatic, and nonmetastatic, in Chapter 127.

PATHOPHYSIOLOGY OF THE METASTATIC PROCESS

To reach the brain, a systemic cancer must develop its own blood supply, invade local tissues, and enter the circulation either by invading venules or lymph channels that eventually reach the venous circulation (Figure 73-1).[1,13,14] Because systemic tumors enter the venous circulation and, ultimately, the right side of the heart, the first capillary bed they encounter is in the lung. Accordingly, the majority of patients with brain metastases have either primary lung tumors or lung metastases at the time the brain lesions become symptomatic. To reach the arterial circulation, the tumor must either (1) grow in the lung and seed the pulmonary venous circulation; (2) traverse the lung capillary bed to enter the left side of the heart; or (3) cross a patent foramen ovale to enter the left heart directly. Some have proposed that tumor reaches the brain via the vertebral venous system (Batson's plexus) to explain the absence of lung metastases.[15]

Two factors promote intracranial metastases: (1) In the resting state, the brain receives 15 to 20% of the body's blood flow, thus making it likely that circulating tumor cells will reach the brain. (2) Certain tumor cells find the brain a propitious place for arrest and growth. This is one of the reasons that the probability of brain metastasis varies among tumor types and that the site of a brain metastasis may vary depending on the histology of the primary tumor. For example, certain primary tumors such as those from the kidney and colon are more likely to metastasize to the cerebellum than are lung cancers or those arising elsewhere in the body.[16] Once in the intracranial cavity, the tumor must arrest within the capillary bed, cross the endothelium and vessel wall, grow within the organ, vascularize itself through the process of angiogenesis, and then grow large enough to cause symptoms. At each step in the metastatic process, the tumor cells may fail, so that probably only 0.01% of cells that reach the circulation ever become metastases.[17]

Tumors may metastasize to virtually any portion of the intracranial cavity, but the overall distribution of brain metastasis is also determined by the size of the region and its vasculature. Thus, about 85% of brain metastases are found in the cerebral hemispheres, usually in the posterior portion of the hemispheres at the watershed between the middle and posterior cerebral arteries. There is also an over-representation in the anterior border zone between the anterior and middle cerebral arteries. Approximately 10 to 15% of metastases are found in the cerebellum, a number somewhat larger than might be expected on the basis of blood supply, and probably represents the predilection for some pelvic tumors to metastasize to the cerebellum. Only approximately 3% of metastases are found in the brainstem.

In patients whose systemic tumor is otherwise controlled, the brain is often a site for isolated metastatic disease. Neither blood flow nor the nature of the central nervous system (CNS) micro-environment fully explains this phenomenon, but the blood–brain barrier may. In the first half of the twentieth century, when no treatment

Table 73-1 Source of Brain Metastases in 729 Patients with Cancer Lesions*

Primary Tumor	Total (%)	Single	Multiple
Lung cancer	288 (39)	137	151
Non–small-cell	178	89	89
Small-cell	110	48	62
Breast	121 (17)	59	62
Melanoma	80 (11)	39	41
Genitourinary	81 (11)	49	32
Renal cell	45	25	20
Bladder	14	9	5
Prostate	11	9	2
Testicular	11	6	5
Gynecologic	52 (7)	28	24
Uterine/vulvar	38	20	18
Ovarian	14	8	6
Gastrointestinal	45 (6)	30	15
Unknown	33 (5)	23	10
Miscellaneous	29 (4)	19	10
Total	729	384	345

*Adapted from Nussbaum ES et al.[59]

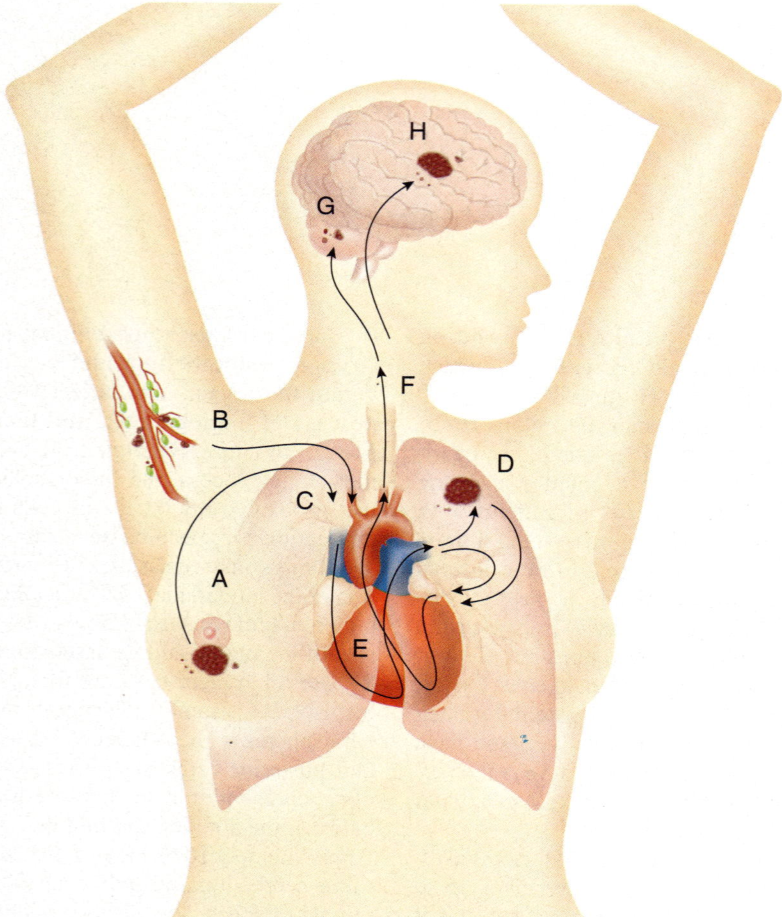

Figure 73-1 Pathophysiology of the metastatic process. Metastasis is a multistep process. In this schematic illustration: **A**, malignant neoplasm arises in an organ distant from the central nervous system and, as it grows, it develops its own vascular supply. **B,** Clone(s) of malignant cells with metastatic potential enter blood or lymph channels and eventually reach the venous circulation. **C,** The malignant cells enter the right heart with the venous circulation and either exit through the pulmonary artery to the lung **D,** or cross a patent foramen ovale **D,** to enter the systemic circulation. Most tumors that enter the lung either arrest in the pulmonary capillary bed, grow as pulmonary metastases and subsequently seed the pulmonary venous circulation, or, alternately, **E,** transverse the pulmonary vascular bed without arresting **E,** to enter the pulmonary venous circulation. Malignant clones in the pulmonary venous circulation then enter the left heart and exit into the systemic circulation **F,** along with those cells that may have crossed a patent foramen ovale **F.** Once in the systemic circulation, the likelihood of entering the cerebral circulation is high because, in the resting state, 15 to 20% of cardiac output supplies the central nervous system. Tumor cells entering the cerebral circulation must then arrest in brain capillaries or venules, cross the vessel wall, and grow within the brain **G, H.** Reproduced with permission from DeAngelis LM et al.[14]

was available for acute leukemia, CNS involvement was rare because patients died from uncontrolled systemic leukemia. As chemotherapeutic agents became effective in controlling systemic disease, the incidence of CNS involvement began to rise to the point where it reached almost 50% in patients with acute lymphoblastic leukemia. The chemotherapeutic agents used to treat leukemia were largely water-soluble and did not cross the blood–brain barrier. The few leukemic cells that reached the CNS were protected from these drugs by the blood–brain barrier, and they could proliferate until they produced neurologic symptoms. "Prophylactic" treatment of the CNS by radiation therapy and/or intrathecal drugs has again decreased the incidence of CNS metastases from leukemia to under 10%.[18] However, once tumor is established in the brain, the blood–brain barrier is disrupted and the CNS becomes accessible to treatment with agents that do not normally cross it. Furthermore, some water-soluble systemic agents can penetrate an intact blood–brain barrier when given in high doses (eg, high-dose methotrexate).

The CNS as a sanctuary site of microscopic disease now appears to apply to breast,[8] small-cell lung, and perhaps other cancers.[6,7,19] When a chemosensitive tumor has relapsed in the CNS, it does not necessarily mean that the CNS disease is resistant to the chemotherapeutic agents that controlled the systemic tumor. The blood–brain barrier may have prevented those tumor cells from ever seeing a significant concentration of the drug, thus preserving the tumor cells' intrinsic chemosensitivity to that agent.[20]

The symptoms and signs of brain metastases are related to the involved brain area (Table 73-2). Focal symptoms include muscle weakness (hemiparesis), gait disturbances, visual field defects, and aphasia. Generalized symptoms usually relate to increased intracranial pressure and include headache, cognitive or behavioral abnormalities, nausea, and vomiting. Often, edema surrounding a brain metastasis increases brain volume, and thus intracranial pressure, much more than the tumor itself. Because brain edema responds to corticosteroids, the initial treatment of brain metastases with steroids (see below) often relieves both generalized and focal signs and symptoms. The tumor itself usually causes symptoms by compressing surrounding brain rather than destroying it. As a result, removing the tumor often returns the patient's neurologic state to normal.

Table 73-2 Signs and Symptoms of Brain Metastases at Presentation

	% of Patients
Headache	24
Hemiparesis	20
Cognitive and behavioral disturbances	14
Seizures (focal or generalized)	12
Ataxia	7
Other	16
No symptoms	7

Symptoms usually evolve over a few weeks; sometimes the symptoms begin acutely, corresponding to a hemorrhage into the metastasis or a seizure with a prolonged postictal state. Any intracranial metastatic tumor can bleed, but certain primary tumors, such as melanoma, thyroid, renal, and choriocarcinoma, have a propensity to bleed. Because the most common source of metastasis is lung cancer, the most common hemorrhagic metastases, overall, are from the lung. When multiple metastases are present, it is common to see simultaneous hemorrhage into many of the lesions; the mechanism for this is unclear. On occasion, focal seizures can cause neurologic signs that do not resolve. The tumor probably causes ischemia in the brain immediately surrounding it by stealing its blood supply, thus causing the seizure.

The only necessary diagnostic test is an MRI. Although the scan cannot unequivocally differentiate metastases from other lesions, certain abnormalities suggest metastases. Metastases are usually spherical and have more regular margins than primary tumors. They are usually found at gray-white matter junctions in watershed areas of the brain.[16,21] When small, they uniformly contrast enhance, and when larger, they may ring enhance. The tumor is usually surrounded by substantial edema. Very small metastases may appear as small dots of contrast enhancement with or without hyperintensity on the T_2-weighted image; they usually lack surrounding edema. Fifty percent of patients have a single identifiable brain metastasis, 20% have two metastases, and 13% have three metastases. The remainder has more than three.[16]

A characteristic MRI in a patient with known cancer usually establishes the diagnosis. However, the diagnosis can be incorrect in approximately 10% of patients, and other considerations

Table 73-3 Treatment of Brain Metastases

Supportive
Corticosteroids (usual dose 8 to 16 mg dexamethasone daily)
Anticonvulsants (not for prophylaxis)
Antibiotics (prophylaxis for pneumocystis)
Anticoagulants (deep vein thrombosis)
Definitive
Surgery (1 to 3 metastases)
Whole-brain radiation therapy (multiple lesions, postoperative)
Stereotactic radiosurgery
Gamma knife
Linear accelerator
Single dose
Fractionated
Chemotherapy (chemosensitive primary)
Radiosurgery (renal cell, melanoma)

include abscesses, primary brain tumors, demyelinating lesions, or inflammation.[22] If there is sufficient uncertainty about the diagnosis, biopsy may be necessary.

Treatment The therapeutic approach to patients with brain metastases depends on the number and location of metastases, on the biology of the primary tumor, and on the extent of systemic disease. Treatment is divided into supportive and definitive measures (Table 73-3).[14]

Supportive Care **Corticosteroids** Supportive care may include corticosteroids, anticonvulsants, psychotropic drugs, antibiotics, and anticoagulants.[1] Corticosteroids are necessary only for symptomatic metastases, where they usually produce a dramatic response, and during the course of definitive treatment with surgery or radiation therapy (RT). Corticosteroids are not required for asymptomatic patients with small metastases unless RT or surgery is imminent. Because of their frequent side effects, the dose of corticosteroids should be tapered to the lowest level that controls neurologic symptoms. In patients expected to be on corticosteroids for more than 6 weeks, prophylactic antibiotics to prevent *Pneumocystis carinii* infection are indicated. However, these drugs often cause side effects, particularly platelet suppression.

Anticonvulsants Anticonvulsants have no prophylactic benefit and are used only if the patient has had a seizure.[23,24] Patients who require anticonvulsants should be placed on agents that do not enhance the hepatic microsomal system. Drugs such as phenytoin, phenobarbital and carbamazepine increase p450 activity, which can reduce the serum level of many chemotherapeutic agents, thus compromising treatment of the underlying malignancy. Some of the newer anticonvulsants, such as topiramate, levetiracetam, or gabapentin are better choices although none can be administered parenterally.

Anticoagulants Thromboembolic disease requiring treatment with anticoagulants is common in patients with cancer. Brain metastases are not a contraindication to the use of anticoagulants provided there is no intracranial hemorrhage. Anticoagulants are more effective than Greenfield filters in these patients and are safe provided that the anticoagulant is maintained in the therapeutic range.[25]

Definitive Treatment **Surgery** Two controlled trials clearly indicate that for patients with a single brain metastasis, surgical removal is superior to whole-brain radiation therapy, both in preventing brain relapse and in improving quality of life.[22,26] A third trial[27] found no benefit. In our opinion, in patients whose systemic disease is quiescent or controllable, surgical removal of a single brain metastasis substantially improves survival. Technological improvements in surgery, including functional magnetic resonance imaging (fMRI) preoperatively to locate eloquent areas of the brain, stereotactic surgical resection, intraoperative ultrasonography, intraoperative MRI, and cortical mapping, have helped assure complete resection with lower surgical morbidity and virtually no mortality.[28] Two-year survivals are 15 to 20%, depending on the primary tumor; 5-year survival rates are approximately 10%, and occasional "cures" are reported. Retrospective analysis supports the resection of two or even three metastases, with the outcome comparable to a surgically treated single brain metastasis.

A randomized controlled trial indicates that patients with a single resected metastasis who receive postoperative RT have fewer recurrences of cancer in the brain and are less likely to die of neurologic causes than are similar patients treated with surgery alone.[29] However, overall survival was comparable between the two groups because patients with controlled cerebral disease died of progressive systemic tumor. These data suggest that an appropriate patient with a single, surgically accessible brain metastasis should have that metastasis removed and receive postoperative whole-brain radiation therapy (WBRT). However, because of the toxicity of WBRT, particularly in the over 60 age group, many physicians do not use it in the immediate postoperative period, but reserve radiation until relapse, even though RT may be less effective once a tumor has recurred.

Radiation Therapy The time-honored treatment of brain metastases has been WBRT, delivering 3,000 cGy in 10 fractions. For patients with extensive systemic disease or multiple brain metastases, this remains the best option. Most patients have at least a transient response to radiation (Figure 73-2); they symptomatically improve with steroids and RT, and are less likely to die of their neurologic disease than are patients who do not receive this treatment. However, survival is short, with a median of 4 to 6 months, because most patients die of uncontrolled systemic tumor. Even those patients who respond to RT and whose tumors are controlled are at risk for reseeding the brain from systemic tumor. In occasional patients, RT actually sterilizes the brain metastases and they do not recur. Because of late-delayed radiation toxicity in those patients whose systemic prognosis is more than a year, we recommend a dose of 4,000 to 5,000 cGy given in 180 to 200 cGy fractions. The lower dose per fraction is believed to diminish radiation toxicity but cognitive dysfunction may occur even with small fractions, especially if the patient has received chemotherapy.[30] Cognitive deficits from RT are more severe in children under 3 years of age and in adults over 60 years of age, and in those who receive extensive chemotherapy. Nevertheless, even young adults often complain of memory loss after WBRT.

Radiosurgery Radiosurgery is increasingly employed instead of surgery for the treatment of single or even multiple brain metastases.[31–34] Radiosurgery can be delivered either using the gamma knife[35] or a linear accelerator,[36] and can be given either as a single dose[37] or can be fractionated.[38] The treatment appears to be most effective against those tumors that are relatively resistant to conventional external beam RT, such as melanoma[37] and renal cell carcinoma.[39] The reason is unclear, but the higher dose per fraction may eliminate otherwise resistant tumor cells. Some report approximately 80% tumor control with < 10% complications.[31] Tumor control is defined as disappearance, decrease in size, or no increase in size of the treated lesion. Post-radiosurgery MRI may show a transient increase in tumor size[40,41] because of radiation injury or tumor necrosis. This can resolve over a few months and, therefore, an increase in lesion size a few weeks to months after stereotactic radiosurgery does not necessarily indicate tumor progression. Local control may be maintained over two years in 60% of patients,[40] but with increasing survival, symptomatic recurrence becomes increasingly likely.[42] Radiosurgery has advantages over surgery in that it is relatively noninvasive, rarely requires hospitalization, and can often reach areas that are surgically inaccessible. Radiosurgery has the disadvantage that it is not useful for tumors larger than 3 to 4 cm.

A recent randomized, prospective trial comparing WBRT and WBRT followed by stereotactic radiosurgery boost in 331 patients with one to three newly diagnosed brain metastases, showed no survival advantage with the addition of radiosurgery.[43] Those with a single brain metastasis had longer survival when radiosurgery was added to WBRT (median 6.5 vs 4.9 months, $p = .0393$), but survival was not improved for those with multiple metastases. There was no significant difference between treatment groups in time to tumor progression or neurologic death rates.

There have been no randomized, prospective studies directly comparing neurosurgery and radiosurgery as treatment of solitary brain metastasis, and retrospective studies have shown conflicting results. Once case-controlled, retrospective trial of the two modalities found that patients lived longer and did better with surgical resection.[44] This was partially attributed to the propensity for radiosurgery to cause brain necrosis that in itself is symptomatic and may require surgery for removal. A more recent retrospective study comparing surgical resection and stereotactic radiosurgery in patients with tumor size less than 35 mm and sim-

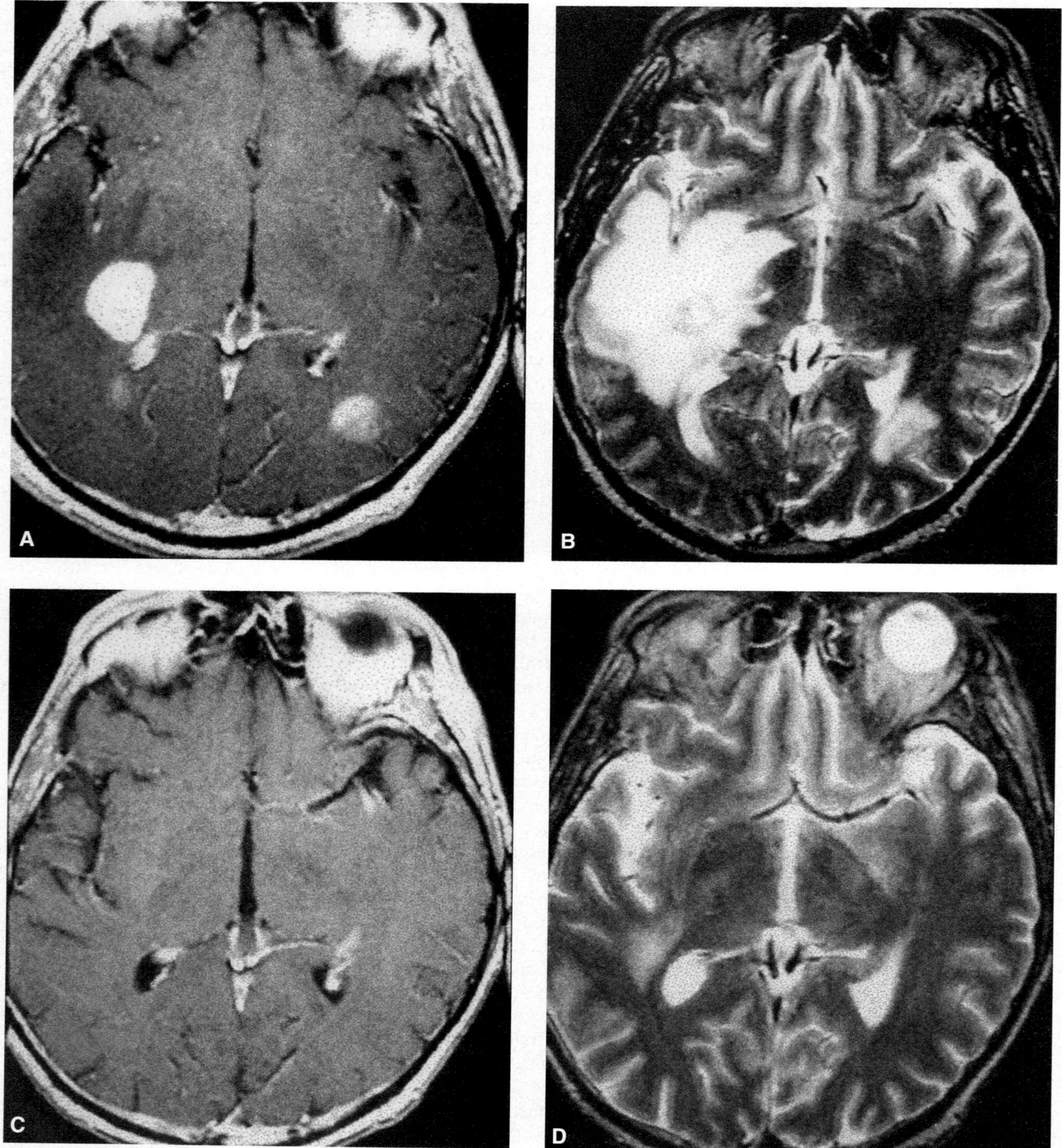

Figure 73-2 Metastatic small-cell lung cancer before and after radiation therapy. **A,** The T_1-weighted image before radiation shows two of the multiple contrast enhancing metastases; the larger one is surrounded by hypointense brain edema. **B,** The T_2-weighted image before radiation shows hyperintense edema surrounding the relatively hypointense tumor. **C,** and **D,** MRI scans after radiation show an excellent response to radiation therapy.

ilar use of post-procedure WBRT (82% vs 96%, respectively) yielded similar survival rates during the first year after the procedure, but the neurosurgical patients survived longer during the second year.[45] However, the difference in overall survival was not statistically significant ($p = .15$). Recurrence rates were similar between the neurosurgical and radiosurgery groups (30% vs 29%), but there were significantly more local recurrences in the neurosurgical group compared with the radiosurgical group ($p = .02$). A retrospective study comparing radiosurgery with surgery plus WBRT yielded similar periprocedure morbidity (7.7% vs 8.9%), mortality (1.6% vs 1.2%), and 1-year survival (53% vs 43%, not statistically significant) rates. Local control rates were also similar at 1 year (75% vs 83%).[46] In contrast to the more recent study, none of the radiosurgery patients received WBRT, suggesting it may be unnecessary. Others agree,[39,47] although this contradicts the controlled trial of RT after surgery.[29] At this time, we use surgery to resect single lesions from accessible locations if they are > 3 to 4 cm, associated with significant vasogenic edema or hemorrhage, or causing obstruction of CSF flow. Radiosurgery is an excellent option for smaller lesions or those in a surgically inaccessible location; we rarely treat more than three lesions in a patient, and usually do not administer WBRT concurrently.

Chemotherapy Chemotherapy is increasingly being recognized as efficacious for brain metastases from chemosensitive systemic cancers. These include germ cell tumors, breast cancer, small-cell lung cancer,[48] and some others.[49,50] Chemotherapy is often reserved for patients whose brain metastases have recurred after surgery or WBRT, but chemotherapy should be considered in patients with brain metastases that have disrupted the blood–brain barrier, ie, contrast enhance, before RT. "Upfront" systemic chemotherapy is indicated for patients who have one or more asymptomatic metastases (usually discovered on a screening MRI), and who have other systemic disease requiring chemotherapy. This implies a primary cancer that is relatively sensitive to chemotherapeutic agents.

In addition, systemic chemotherapy is probably best used in patients who do not require corticosteroids because those drugs restore blood–brain barrier function and decrease the amount of water soluble drug that can reach the tumor. Surprisingly there are several instances of patients who develop brain metastases late in the course of a systemic cancer where chemotherapeutic agents previously successful against the systemic tumor, for example, cyclophosphamide, methotrexate, and 5-fluorouracil (CMF) in breast cancer, may be effective against brain metastases even though the systemic tumor is now resistant.[51] On the other hand, at times, brain metastases either develop during administration of or fail to respond to chemotherapeutic agents that are effective against the primary tumor and other systemic metastases.[52] Whether the lack of response results from intrinsic resistance of the metastases, different from the primary, or from failure of sufficient chemotherapy to reach the tumor as a result of residual blood–brain barrier function is unclear. Newer drugs such as temozolomide have also shown efficacy in some patients with recurrent brain metastases, particularly those with lung cancer, even though this agent is not used to treat the primary disease.[53]

There are several reasons for administering chemotherapy before radiation: (1) It is useful to judge tumor response to chemotherapy before initiating radiation therapy. If the tumor is responsive, the chemotherapy can be continued even after radiation is given. (2) Radiation therapy decreases the blood supply to the tumor and thus may decrease the amount of chemotherapeutic agent that reaches the metastases. (3) Some evidence suggests that chemotherapy delivered before radiation is less neurotoxic than the converse because RT may open the blood–brain barrier and allow entry of potentially toxic agents that are given post-RT. The evidence is best for methotrexate but may apply to other drugs as well. Despite blood–brain barrier disruption, overall blood flow to the tumor is reduced so that drug delivery to the metastases is not necessarily enhanced by radiotherapy.

Prognosis Untreated symptomatic brain metastases usually cause death within 1 or 2 months.[54] Patients treated with corticosteroids survive a little longer with a median of 1.3 months.[54] Patients treated with whole-brain radiotherapy have a median survival of 3.6 months, and those treated by surgery followed by whole-brain radiation have a median survival of 8.9 months. Patients with controlled systemic disease treated by surgery and radiation have a 10 to 15% 5-year survival and an occasional apparent cure. Prolonged survival can also be seen after radiosurgery.[55]

Prognostic factors include mental status, response to steroids, activity of the systemic tumor, and treatment modality. In one series, site of the primary tumor, age, and the number of brain metastases were prognostic factors, although with lesser importance than those indicated above. In patients with lung primaries, male sex was a significant factor. In patients with breast primaries, the interval between the primary tumor and the development of brain metastases was also significant, with a longer interval correlating with better survival. The RTOG performed a recursive partitioning analysis of prognostic factors in 1,200 patients with brain metastases treated with WBRT on three RTOG trials.[56] They segregated patients into three classes based only on KPS, age, and the presence of extracranial metastases. Class 1 patients had a KPS $\geq$ 70, and were < 65 years of age with a controlled primary and no extracranial metastasis; median survival was 7.1 months. Class 3 patients had a KPS < 70 and a median survival of 2.3 months. Class 2 included all other patients and had a median survival of 4.2 months. This classification scheme may apply to patients treated with surgery and radiosurgery.[57,58]

Approach All patients with cancer and neurologic symptoms should undergo contrast-enhanced MRI. Asymptomatic patients at high risk for development of brain metastases (eg, lung cancer, melanoma) should be considered for screening of the brain for occult cerebral metastases. Screening is particularly important if the patient is to undergo a major surgical procedure for treatment of the primary tumor. If a single or, in some cases, two or three surgically accessible lesions are found in a patient with a good performance status and a reasonable systemic prognosis (at least 6 to 12 months), the lesion(s) should be removed surgically. The decision concerning radiation after removal of a single metastasis should be made on an individual basis, depending on the surgeon's view of the success of tumor removal, the patient's general state, and the patient's age. Patients with one to three surgically inaccessible lesions smaller than 4 cm, particularly from radioresistant tumors such as melanoma and renal cell carcinoma, should be considered for radiosurgery. Symptomatic patients with multiple metastases or whose systemic prognosis is poor can be treated with palliative whole-brain radiation therapy. Patients with systemic disease about to undergo systemic chemotherapy, whose brain lesions are small and either asymptomatic or only mildly symptomatic, should be evaluated for their response to chemotherapy prior to radiation or surgery. If it is clinically possible, corticosteroids should be withheld unless they are part of the chemotherapy regimen. Patients who fail surgery and radiation should also be considered for chemotherapy.

REFERENCES

1. Posner JB. Neurologic complications of cancer. Philadelphia: FA Davis; 1995.
2. Cairncross JG, Kim J-H, Posner JB. Radiation therapy of brain metastases. Ann Neurol 1980;7:529–41.
3. Barnholtz-Sloan JS, Sloan AE, Davis FG, et al. Incidence proportions of brain metastases in patients diagnosed (1973 to 2001) in the metropolitan Detroit cancer surveillance system. J Clin Oncol 2004;22:2865–72.
4. Quint LE, Tummala S, Brisson LJ, et al. Distribution of distant metastases from newly diagnosed non–small-cell lung cancer. Ann Thorac Surg 1996;62:246–50.
5. Law A, Karp DD, Dipetrillo T, Daly BT. Emergence of increased cerebral metastasis after high-dose preoperative radiotherapy with chemotherapy in patients with locally advanced non–small-cell lung carcinoma. Cancer 2001;92:160–4.
6. Kramer K, Kushner B, Heller G, Cheung NKV. Neuroblastoma metastatic to the central nervous system—the Memorial Sloan-Kettering Cancer Center experience and a literature review. Cancer 2001;91:1510–9.
7. Dhote R, Beuzeboc P, Thiounn N, et al. High incidence of brain metastases in patients treated with an M- VAC regimen for advanced bladder cancer. Eur Urol 1998;33:392–5.
8. Boogerd W, Hart AAM, Tjahja IS. Treatment and outcome of brain metastasis as first site of distant metastasis from breast cancer. J Neurooncol 1997;35:161–7.
9. Tai THP, Yu E, Dickof P, et al. Prophylactic cranial irradiation revisited: cost-effectiveness and quality of life in small-cell lung cancer. Int J Radiat Oncol Biol Phys 2002;52:68–74.
10. Pottgen C, Stuschke M. The role of prophylactic cranial irradiation in the treatment of lung cancer 1. Lung Cancer 2001;33 Suppl 1:S153–8.
11. Patriarca F, Zaja F, Silvestri F, et al. Meningeal and cerebral involvement in multiple myeloma patients. Ann Hematol 2001;80:758–62.
12. Giordana MT, Cordera S, Boghi A. Cerebral metastases as first symptom of cancer: a clinicopathologic study. J Neurooncol 2000;50:265–73.
13. Puduvalli VK. Brain metastases: biology and the role of the brain microenvironment 2. Curr Oncol Rep 2001; 3:467–75.
14. DeAngelis LM, Gutin PH, Leibel SA, et al. Intracranial tumors: diagnosis and treatment. London: Martin Dunitz; 2002. p. 367–394.
15. Ogawa K, Toita T, Sueyama H, et al. Brain metastases from esophageal carcinoma—natural history, prognostic factors, and outcome. Cancer 2002;94:759–64.
16. Delattre J-Y, Krol G, Thaler HT, Posner JB. Distribution of brain metastases. Arch Neurol 1988;45:741–4.
17. Luzzi KJ, MacDonald IC, Schmidt EE, et al. Multistep nature of metastatic inefficiency—dormancy of solitary cells after successful extravasation and limited survival of early micrometastases. Am J Pathol 1998;153:865–73.
18. Surapaneni UR, Cortes JE, Thomas D, et al. Central nervous system relapse in adults with acute lymphoblastic leukemia. Cancer 2002;94:773–9.
19. Robnett TJ, Machtay M, Stevenson JP, et al. Factors affecting the risk of brain metastases after definitive chemoradiation for locally advanced non–small-cell lung carcinoma. J Clin Oncol 2001;19:1344–9.
20. Castiglione-Gertsch M, Tattersall M, Hacking A, et al. Retreating recurrent breast cancer with the same CMF-containing regimen used as adjuvant therapy. Eur J Cancer 1997;33A:2321–5.
21. Hwang TL, Close TP, Grego JM, et al. Predilection of brain metastasis in gray and white matter junction and vascular border zones. Cancer 1996;77:1551–5.
22. Patchell RA, Tibbs PA, Walsh JW. A randomized trial of surgery in the treatment of single metastases to the brain. N Engl J Med 1990;322:494–500.
23. Forsyth PA, Weaver S, Fulton D, et al. Prophylactic anticonvulsants in patients with brain tumour. Can J Neurol Sci 2003;30:106–112.
24. Glantz MJ, Cole BF, Forsyth PA, et al. Practice parameter: anticonvulsant prophylaxis in patients with newly diagnosed brain tumors—report of the Quality Standards Subcommittee of the American Academy of Neurology. Neurology 2000;54:1886–93.
25. Schiff D, DeAngelis LM. Therapy of venous thromboembolism in patients with brain metastases. Cancer 1994;73:493-498.
26. Vecht CJ, Haaxma-Reiche H, Noordijk EM, et al. Treatment of single brain metastasis: radiotherapy alone or combined with neurosurgery? Ann Neurol 1993;33:583–90.
27. Mintz AH, Kestle J, Rathbone MP, et al. A randomized trial to assess the efficacy of surgery in addition to radiotherapy in patients with a single cerebral metastasis. Cancer 1996;78:1470–6.
28. Weinberg JS, Lang FF, Sawaya R. Surgical management of brain metastases 4. Curr Oncol Rep 2001;3:476–83.
29. Patchell RA, Tibbs PA, Regine WF, et al. Postoperative radiotherapy in the treatment of single metastases to the brain: a randomized trial. JAMA 1998;280:1485–9.

30. Fonseca R, O'Neill BP, Foote RL, et al. Cerebral toxicity in patients treated for small-cell carcinoma of the lung. Mayo Clin Proc 1999;74:461–5.
31. Loeffler JS, Barker FG, Chapman PH. Role of radiosurgery in the management of central nervous system metastases. Cancer Chemother Pharmacol 1999;43:S11–4.
32. Seung SK, Sneed PK, McDermott MW, et al. Gamma knife radiosurgery for malignant melanoma brain metastases. Cancer J Sci Am 1998;4:103–9.
33. Sanghavi SN, Miranpuri SS, Chappell R, et al. Radiosurgery for patients with brain metastases: a multi-institutional analysis, stratified by the RTOG recursive partitioning analysis method. Int J Radiat Oncol Biol Phys 2001;51:426–34.
34. Omuro AM, Abrey LE. Brain metastases. Curr Neurol Neurosci Rep 2004;4:205–10.
35. Kim DG, Chung HT, Gwak HS, et al. Gamma knife radiosurgery for brain metastases: prognostic factors for survival and local control. J Neurosurg 2000;93:23–9.
36. Joseph J, Adler JR, Cox RS, Hancock SL. Linear accelerator-based stereotaxic radiosurgery for brain metastases: the influence of number of lesions on survival. J Clin Oncol 1996;14:1085–92.
37. Mingione V, Oliveira M, Prasad D, et al. Gamma surgery for melanoma metastases in the brain 1. J Neurosurg 2002;96:544–51.
38. Lederman G, Wronski M, Fine M. Fractionated radiosurgery for brain metastases in 43 patients with breast carcinoma. Breast Cancer Res Treat 2001;65:145–54.
39. Muacevic A, Kreth FW, Mack A, et al. Stereotactic radiosurgery without radiation therapy providing high local tumor control of multiple brain metastases from renal cell carcinoma. Minim Invasive Neurosurg 2004;47:203–8.
40. Peterson AM, Meltzer CC, Evanson EJ, et al. MR imaging response of brain metastases after gamma knife stereotactic radiosurgery. Radiology 1999;211:807–14.
41. Huber PE, Hawighorst H, Fuss M, et al. Transient enlargement of contrast uptake on MRI after linear accelerator (LINAC) stereotactic radiosurgery for brain metastases. Int J Radiat Oncol Biol Phys 2001;49:1339–49.
42. Regine WF, Huhn JL, Patchell RA, et al. Risk of symptomatic brain tumor recurrence and neurologic deficit after radiosurgery alone in patients with newly diagnosed brain metastases: results and implications. Int J Radiat Oncol Biol Phys 2002;52:333–8.
43. Andrews DW, Scott CB, Sperduto PW, et al. Whole brain radiation therapy with or without stereotactic radiosurgery boost for patients with one to three brain metastases: phase III results of the RTOG 9508 randomised trial. The Lancet 2004;363:1665–72.
44. Bindal AK, Bindal RK, Hess KR, et al. Surgery versus radiosurgery in the treatment of brain metastasis. J Neurosurg 1996;84:748–54.
45. O'Neill BP, Iturria NJ, Link MJ, et al. A comparison of surgical resection and stereotactic radiosurgery in the treatment of solitary brain metastases. Int J Radiat Oncol Biol Phys 2003;55:1169–76.
46. Muacevic A, Kreth FW, Horstmann GA, et al. Surgery and radiotherapy compared with gamma knife radiosurgery in the treatment of solitary cerebral metastases of small diameter. J Neurosurg 1999;91:35–43.
47. Sneed PK, Lamborn KR, Forstner JM, et al. Radiosurgery for brain metastases: is whole-brain radiotherapy necessary? Int J Radiat Oncol Biol Phys 1999;43:549–58.
48. Grossi F, Scolaro T, Tixi L, et al. The role of systemic chemotherapy in the treatment of brain metastases from small-cell lung cancer. Crit Rev Oncol Hematol 2001;37:61–7.
49. Cormio G, Gabriele A, Maneo A, et al. Complete remission of brain metastases from ovarian carcinoma with carboplatin. Eur J Obstet Gynecol Reprod Biol 1998;78:91–3.
50. Abrey LE, Christodoulou C. Temozolomide for treating brain metastases. Semin Oncol 2001;28:34–42.
51. Rosner D, Nemoto T, Lane WW. Chemotherapy induces regression of brain metastases in breast carcinoma. Cancer 1986;58:832–9.
52. Freilich RJ, Seidman AD, DeAngelis LM. Central nervous system progression of metastatic breast cancer in patients treated with paclitaxel. Cancer 1995;76:232–6.
53. Abrey LE, Olson JD, Raizer JJ, et al. A phase II trial of temozolomide for patients with recurrent or progressive brain metastases. J Neuro-Oncol 2001;53:259–65.
54. Lagerwaard FJ, Levendag PC, Nowak PJ, et al. Identification of prognostic factors in patients with brain metastases: a review of 1,292 patients. Int J Radiat Oncol Biol Phys 1999;43:795–803.
55. Sheehan JP, Sun MH, Kondziolka D, et al. Radiosurgery for non-small cell lung carcinoma metastatic to the brain: long-term outcomes and prognostic factors influencing patient survival time and local tumor control. J Neurosurg 2002;97:1276–81.
56. Gaspar L, Scott C, Rotman M, et al. Recursive partitioning analysis (RPA) of prognostic factors in three Radiation Therapy Oncology Group (RTOG) brain metastases trials. Int J Radiat Oncol Biol Phys 1997;37:745–51.
57. Regine WF, Rogozinska A, Kryscio, et al. Recursive partitioning analysis classifications I and II: applicability evaluated in a randomized trial of resected single brain metastases. Am J Clin Oncol 2004;27:505–9.
58. Sanghavi SN, Miranpuri SS, Chappell R, et al. Radiosurgery for patients with brain metastases: a multi-institutional analysis, stratified by the RTOG recursive partitioning analysis method. Int J Radiat Oncol Biol Phys 2001;51:426–34.
59. Nussbaum ES, Djalilian HR, Cho KH, Hall WA. Brain metastases—histology, multiplicity, surgery, and survival. Cancer 1996;78:1781–8.

Section 24
THE EYE

74

Neoplasms of the Eye

David H. Abramson, MD, FACS
Amy C. Schefler, MD
Ira J. Dunkel, MD
Beryl McCormick, MD

This chapter reviews benign and malignant ocular, orbital, and lid tumors in both children and adults. The most common of these are listed in Table 74-1.

PEDIATRIC OPHTHALMIC ONCOLOGY: OCULAR DISEASES

Benign Disease Benign pediatric ocular lesions are very rare. Choroidal nevi, which are present in more than 10% of the adult population, are rare before puberty and are never seen in the infant. Conjunctival and iris nevi are also extremely rare in prepubertal children. Iris nevi detected in children often represent Lisch nodules, a manifestation of neurofibromatosis type 1.

Benign retinal tumors are also rare. When found they are usually astrocytic hamartomas and are frequently part of the tuberous sclerosis syndrome. When viewed with indirect ophthalmoscopy, astrocytic hamartomas usually have a thin, transparent membrane overlying the retina and typically obscure retinal blood vessels. They may enlarge and calcify with time. They may be confused with myelinated nerve fibers, which are white, follow the distribution of the nerve fiber layer, and obscure retinal vessels.

Hamartomas of the retinal pigment epithelium are rare in children. They are frequently near the optic disc and are pigmented, with distortion of retinal vessels and a slightly opaque appearance. They have no malignant potential.

Primary Malignant Disease (Retinoblastoma) **Introduction to Retinoblastoma** The most common primary ocular malignancy of childhood is retinoblastoma.[1] Retinoblastoma arises from an unidentified retinal progenitor cell. Although retinoblastoma is relatively rare, it has been the subject of great interest because of its well-studied genetic inheritance pattern and molecular biology.[2]

Retinoblastoma has a cumulative lifetime incidence rate of one in 18,000 to 30,000 live births worldwide. Surveys suggest a relatively constant occurrence in this century.[3] The incidence in the United States is relatively low, at 3.58 cases for each million children under the age of 15 years, and decreases with advancing age. The overall median age at diagnosis in the United States is 18 months, with the median age of diagnosis of bilateral cases occurring at 12 months and of unilateral cases at 24 months.[4] In rare instances, retinoblastoma is detected prenatally via ultrasound or during adulthood.[5–7]

Survival rates for retinoblastoma patients in the developed world have increased dramatically over the past century. The mortality of retinoblastoma was reported to be 83% in 1897 in children who were treated with enucleation, and 43% in all children in 1916.[8] In contrast, recent cancer registry reports in Europe and the United States have demonstrated 5-year survival rates of 90 and 98%, respectively.[9,10] The improved survival rate is due to earlier detection of the tumor and improved techniques for local tumor control. In contrast to developed countries, however, developing nations report dramatically low survival rates, since patients in these countries typically present with widespread metastatic disease.

There are no differences in incidence by sex, race, or right versus left eye.[11] Some data suggest geographic clustering, but convincing evidence is lacking. Retinoblastoma does appear to occur more commonly in poor patients worldwide. Preliminary evidence suggests that the reason for this predilection is that the presence of human papilloma virus (HPV) sequences in retinoblastoma tumor tissue may play a role in the development of sporadic retinoblastoma.[12]

Molecular Biology of Retinoblastoma Retinoblastoma occurs in two forms, germinal and nongerminal. The disease results from loss or mutation of both alleles of the retinoblastoma gene (*rb1*). In nongerminal cases, accounting for two-

Table 74-1 Most Common Ophthalmic Neoplasms, Benign and Malignant

	Benign	Malignant	
		Primary	Secondary
Children			
Ocular	—	Retinoblastoma	Leukemia
Orbital	Capillary hemangioma	Rhabdomyosarcoma	Leukemia
Adult			
Ocular	Choroid nevus	Uveal melanoma	Metastasis (lung, breast)
Orbital	Cavernous hemangioma	Lymphoma	Sinus cancer
Lids	Chalazion	Basal cell carcinoma	Lymphoma

thirds of all patients, both *rb1* alleles are inactivated somatically in a single developing retinal progenitor cell. Nongerminal retinoblastoma is always unilateral and unifocal, although the tumor may break apart resulting in hundreds of tiny intraocular seeds.

The remaining one-third of patients have germinal retinoblastoma. These patients carry an inactivated *rb1* allele in their germline, present in all cells in the body, and then suffer a loss of the second allele somatically in a retinal cell or cells. Eighty-five percent of germinal retinoblastoma demonstrates high penetrance (nearly all carriers develop the disease) and high expressivity (multifocal bilateral tumor development).[13] All patients with bilateral disease are presumed to carry a germinal *rb1* mutation, and the mean number of tumors distributed between the two eyes in bilateral cases is five. In 15% of patients with germinal retinoblastoma, the disease demonstrates reduced penetrance and expressivity, often called low-penetrance retinoblastoma. Affected carriers may develop only unilateral retinoblastoma (often multifocal) or spontaneously arrested retinoblastoma (also known as retinoma).

The proposed retinoblastoma gene was localized to chromosome 13q14 through deletion studies and linkage analysis.[14–16] A candidate gene was isolated from this locus in 1986 by Friend and colleagues.[17] Further characterization of the gene revealed that it spans 180 kb and is composed of 27 exons. The gene encodes a 4.8 kb mRNA transcript which is expressed in all adult tissues. The 110 kD nuclear phosphoprotein (pRB) consists of 928 amino acids.

The protein is a regulator at the cell cycle checkpoint between G1 and entry into the S-phase (Figure 74-1). The phosphorylation pattern of pRB varies during the cell cycle, and the current model suggests that the hypophosphorylated normal pRB binds transcriptional regulators that promote entry into the S-phase. This function of pRB is inactivated by phosphorylation or by viral oncoprotein binding of pRB. When phosphorylated, pRB dissociates from the transcription factor E2F, freeing E2F to bind to DNA and stimulate transcription of downstream genes that

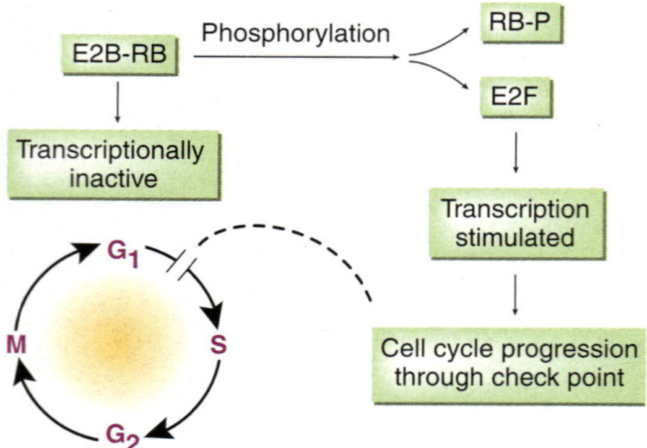

Figure 74-1 Artistic rendition of molecular mechanism of retinoblastoma gene action.

promote progression through the cell cycle. Loss of normal *rb1* function, as in the case of the tumors, allows for uncontrolled entry into the S-phase and more rapid cell division.[18]

Rb1 was the first tumor suppressor gene to be identified. The tumor suppressive function of the *rb1* gene was confirmed in studies that demonstrated the loss of both alleles of the gene in tumor tissue specimens.[19] Later studies showed that a germinal *rb1* mutation was present in virtually all retinoblastoma kindreds and that inheritance of the mutant *rb1* allele predicted disease.[20,21] The tumor suppressive function of the gene has furthermore been demonstrated in transfection studies showing that the introduction of wild-type expression in pRB-defective cell lines partially reverses the malignant phenotype.[22]

Genetic Testing Both population data gathered from families and our current understanding of the molecular mechanisms of inheritance of the disease have enabled us to predict the likelihood that new offspring in families affected by retinoblastoma will develop the disease (Table 74-2). Karyotypic studies, which analyze the morphology of entire chromosomes, are generally not useful for the clinical diagnosis of retinoblastoma because they can identify only deletions spanning 2 to 5 million base-pairs, and only 3 to 5% of retinoblastoma patients carry deletions this large.[23] Instead, more sophisticated indirect and direct techniques that detect smaller mutations are used.[24,25] Direct detection methods are more sensitive than the indirect tests and can be performed on tumor tissue or blood samples of patients with germinal disease. Although these techniques are capable of detecting genetic alterations as small as a single base-pair change, they are costly and time consuming for routine clinical use, and they fail to identify mutations in 17 to 20% of patients with bilateral retinoblastoma.[25] Future research that will further increase the sensitivity of these tests will enable patients and their family members to undergo the analyses in a faster and more economical manner.

Prenatal Intervention Given the shortcomings of the above testing methods, several groups have recently begun to investigate the use of preimplantation genetic testing (PGD) for families who have children with germinal retinoblastoma. Recently, PGD was used in order to produce a healthy newborn whose father had a history of germinal retinoblastoma (Figure 74-2).[26] The prevention of retinoblastoma through the use of PGD is now an important option to consider for select families affected by the germinal form of the disease. Caution should be taken, however, in using in vitro fertilization (IVF) (without PGD) in a couple with subfertility and a family history of retinoblastoma in either parent. A large retrospective study was recently performed in the Netherlands suggesting an increased relative risk of the development of retinoblastoma in patients conceived by IVF.[27]

Presenting Signs and Symptoms of Retinoblastoma The most common presenting signs and symptoms of retinoblastoma vary depending on the socioeconomic conditions in which the patient presents. In developing countries, children have often developed extraocular disease before they are diagnosed and frequently present with proptosis and an orbital mass (Figure 74-3). These children are older at diagnosis (age 4–6 years) than patients in the United States and few survive. Many large retrospective studies over the past quarter century have examined the most common presentations of retinoblastoma in large

Table 74-2 Genetic Counseling for Retinoblastoma

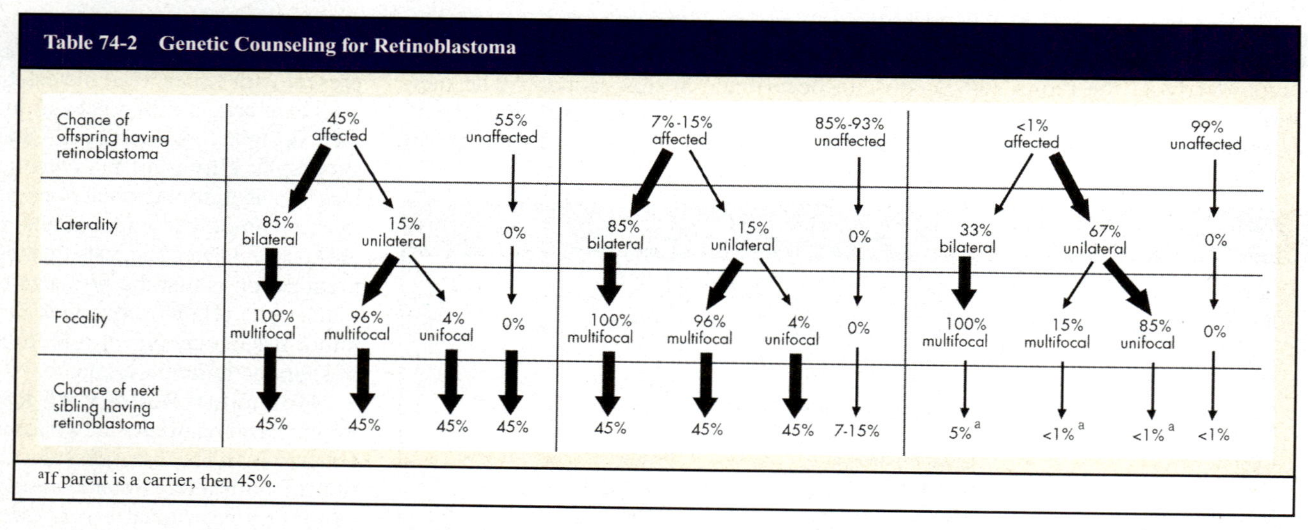

Chance of offspring having retinoblastoma	45% affected			55% unaffected	7%-15% affected			85%-93% unaffected	<1% affected			99% unaffected
Laterality	85% bilateral	15% unilateral		0%	85% bilateral	15% unilateral		0%	33% bilateral	67% unilateral		0%
Focality	100% multifocal	96% multifocal	4% unifocal	0%	100% multifocal	96% multifocal	4% unifocal	0%	100% multifocal	15% multifocal	85% unifocal	0%
Chance of next sibling having retinoblastoma	45%	45%	45%	45%	45%	45%	45%	7-15%	5%[a]	<1%[a]	<1%[a]	<1%

[a]If parent is a carrier, then 45%.

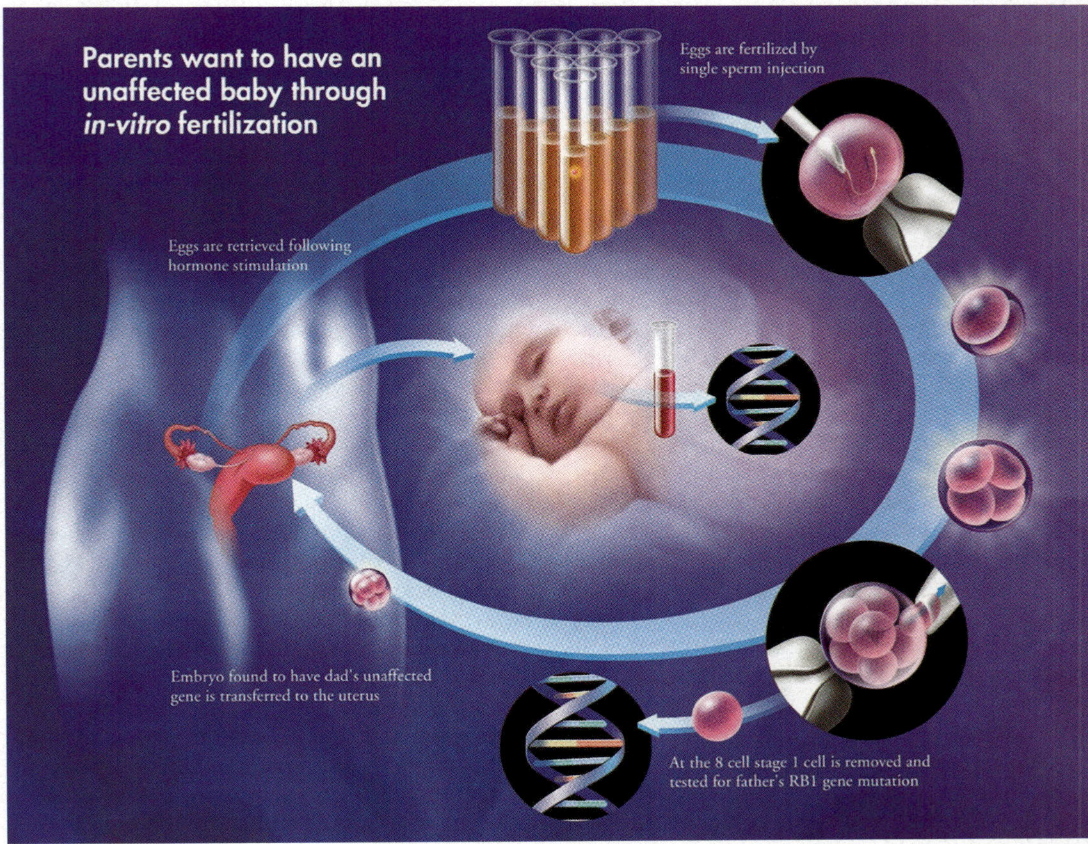

Figure 74-2 Illustration depicting the preimplantation genetic diagnosis procedure (PGD). This procedure was used to enable a successful birth of a retinoblastoma-free child. The father survived germinal retinoblastoma, and the couple's first child was born with a germinal *rb1* retinoblastoma mutation. The first child was examined numerous times during the first 2 years of life and was successfully treated for her retinoblastoma with focal therapy only, but developed a pineoblastoma at 2 years old. The couple's second child was born healthy and free of the *rb1* mutation at 37 weeks after PGD.

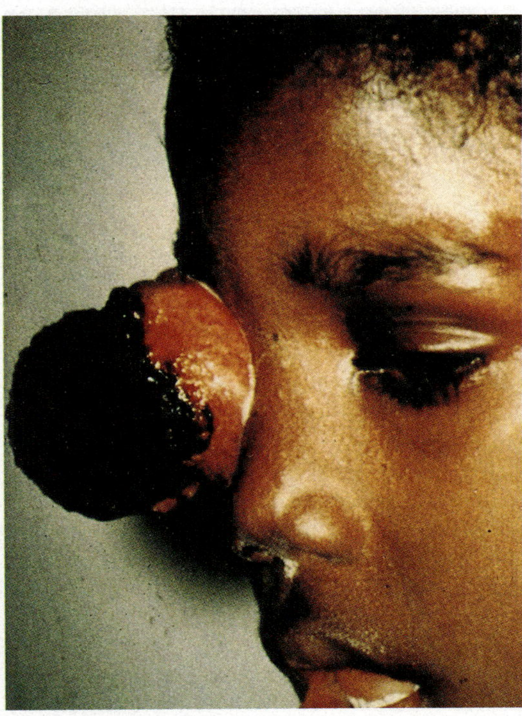

Figure 74-3 Advanced orbital presentation of retinoblastoma. (Courtesy of A. Wachtel, M.D., Lima, Peru.)

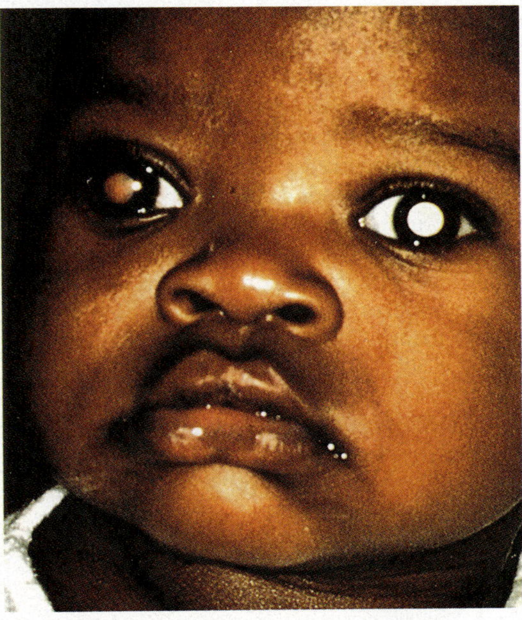

Figure 74-4 Leukocoria (white pupillary reflex) caused by retinoblastoma. The tumor can be seen in the vitreous. There are seeds in the anterior chamber, anterior to the iris.

developed nations.[28-31] In the United States, the most common presenting sign (60% of cases) is leukocoria, a white pupillary reflex (Figure 74-4). The reflex is caused either by the reflection of incoming light off the tumor or by the retinal detachment caused by the underlying tumor.

Presenting signs in the United States that occur less commonly include strabismus, (misalignment of the eyes), inflammatory signs (mimicking orbital cellulitis), anisocoria (different sized pupils), heterochromia (different colored irides), hyphema (blood in the anterior chamber), tumor hypopyon (tumor in the anterior chamber) and nystagmus. Two large retrospective studies on large populations of retinoblastoma patients have recently examined the patterns of detection of retinoblastoma in the United States. The vast majority of patients' disease was discovered by a family member (80%) rather than by a pediatrician (8%) or an ophthalmologist (10%).[29] Furthermore, enucleation was necessary in many of the patients whose retinoblastoma was detected by the pediatrician: 75% of patients with pediatrician-detected leukocoria, 46% of patients with pediatrician-detected strabismus, and 86% of patients with pediatrician-detected red eye, heterochromia, or other symptoms.[28]

Diagnostic Testing The differential diagnosis of retinoblastoma includes lesions that can simulate a solitary ocular tumor such as astrocytic hamartomas and *Toxocara canis*, and lesions that can cause a total retinal detachment such as Coats' disease, retinopathy of prematurity, and persistent hyperplastic primary vitreous (persistent fetal vasculature syndrome) (Table 74-3). Patients suspected of having retinoblastoma should undergo indirect ophthalmoscopy and fundus photography as well as ophthalmic ultrasonography. Ultrasonography is useful since it demonstrates masses with high reflectivity that block sound, causing characteristic shadowing behind the tumor. Needle biopsies are rarely indicated in retinoblastoma, since puncturing the eye can lead to tumor seeding with orbital invasion and even death from metastatic disease.

Staging of Intraocular Retinoblastoma The Reese-Ellsworth Classification scheme is the most commonly used classification system for describing intraocular tumors (Table 74-4).[32] It is not a true staging scheme, for untreated patients do not progress from Group I to higher groups, but it has served as an excellent ocular reference for comparison of different series and treatment schemes. A higher numeric classification signifies that a tumor is more anterior and that there is a decreased success rate in treating the lesion with lateral port external beam radiation. In recent years, its usefulness has been questioned by many ophthalmic oncologists who feel it is no longer appropriate given the current trend away from the use of external beam radiation. Several authors have proposed new classification systems, but no single new scheme has been widely accepted yet among ophthalmologists.

Treatment of Intraocular Retinoblastoma Survival rates in excess of 95% are currently achieved for most patients treated at

Table 74-3 Lesions Simulating Retinoblastoma

Solitary ocular tumor
Astrocytic hamartoma
Toxocara canis
Total retinal detachment
Coats' disease
Retinopathy of prematurity
Persistent hyperplastic primary vitreous (PHPV)

major centers in developed countries with a multimodal treatment approach incorporating enucleation, external beam radiation, brachytherapy, transpupillary thermotherapy, cryotherapy, and chemotherapy. The treatment strategy for each patient depends on several factors: involvement of one or both eyes, heredity of the disease, age of the patient, tumor volume and localization, stage of disease (including Reese-Ellsworth classification), and presence of extraocular disease.[33]

Enucleation Enucleation is surgical removal of the eye without resecting the lids or extraocular muscles. Patients considered for enucleation include those with advanced retinoblastoma in one or both eyes, active tumor in a blind eye, and painful glaucoma from tumor invasion. More than 99% of patients with unilateral retinoblastoma without microscopic or macroscopic extraocular disease are cured with this procedure.[34]

External Beam Radiation External beam radiation, once employed in many patients with intraocular retinoblastoma, has fallen out of favor in recent years because of its association with the development of second nonocular cancers in germinal retinoblastoma patients. Several studies have indicated that radiation given after patients reach 1 year of age does not increase the risk of second cancers, and thus some clinical centers believe that this treatment modality may be used with impunity after this milestone.[35,36] When radiation is given, it is often used as salvage therapy after focal therapies have failed. In cases of bilateral advanced intraocular disease, external beam radiation can be used bilaterally. In these cases, one or both eyes may eventually require salvage enucleation.

Survival of children who undergo external beam radiation in the United States is 85 to 100%, mirroring the excellent survival rates in general of children with this disease.[37–39] Overall local control in the radiated eye, defined as preservation of the eye (avoidance of enucleation), varies in different series from 58 to 95%. Rates of eye preservation are as high as 95% for Reese-Ellsworth groups I to III eyes, and an 83% 3-year eye preservation rate was observed in the most recent large series of group IV and V eyes treated with a standard lateral beam approach.[40] A recent study of Reese-Ellsworth group Vb eyes alone demonstrated an 81% 1-year ocular survival rate and a 53% 10-year ocular survival.[41] Location of the tumor determines the likelihood that it will respond to external beam radiation: Tumors in the posterior pole tend to have the best results with this treatment.

Transpupillary Thermotherapy (TTT) TTT is a newer treatment modality for retinoblastoma that is delivered using modifications to the hardware and software of the infrared diode laser. TTT is used to treat selected small retinoblastomas. A large study of 108 tumors treated with TTT and chemotherapy demonstrated an 86% regression rate with complications including focal iris atrophy and focal paraxial lens opacity[42] A recent study examining the use of TTT as single modality therapy for small tumors found that 92% of tumors 1.5 disc diameters or less in base diameter were successfully cured with TTT alone.[43]

Cryotherapy Cryotherapy is used as a primary treatment of small peripheral retinoblastomas or as secondary treatment of recurrent tumors treated previously with external beam radiation. Rapid freezing (–90°C per minute) results in intracellular ice crystal formation, protein denaturation, pH changes, and finally, cell membrane rupture. All studies examining the use of cryotherapy alone have demonstrated 90 to 100% cure rates in tumors that are less than 3 mm in diameter and less than 1 mm in thickness with minimal complications.[44–46]

Brachytherapy Episcleral brachytherapy was pioneered in 1933 by the British ophthalmologist Henry Stallard.[47] Over the last few years, plaques have been used more commonly as primary therapy in the effort to avoid external beam radiation therapy. Relative indications for radioactive plaques include tumors that are classified as Reese-Ellsworth stage IVa or less and tumors that are between 4 and 10 disc diameters in size. Brachytherapy can also be used as a salvage technique in eyes that have failed other types of therapy, including external beam radiation, photocoagulation, or cryotherapy. ^{125}Iodine is currently the most commonly used isotope in brachytherapy for retinoblastoma. This isotope is advantageous because the radioactive seeds can be placed into a custom-built plaque designed to match the size of the lesion.

A tumor recurrence rate of 12% at 1 year post-treatment has been reported when plaques are used as primary treatment of retinoblastoma.[48] Radioactive plaques can also be successful when used as salvage therapy for eyes that have failed other treatment methods. Merchant and colleagues recently reported a 60% overall eye preservation rate (15 of 25 eyes) for salvage brachytherapy after primary chemotherapy or radiation therapy.[49] Shields and colleagues reported on 148 tumors treated with plaques after failure of other methods.[48] Tumor recurrence at 1 year was detected in 8% of tumors previously treated with chemoreduction and 25% of tumors previously treated with external beam radiotherapy.

Systemic Chemotherapy The indications for chemoreduction are not yet well established. Most commonly, this treatment is used for patients who have visual potential in eyes containing tumors that are too large to treat initially with focal methods. Chemoreduction is used to shrink these tumors so that focal treatments such as cryotherapy, thermotherapy, or radioactive plaques can be administered afterward.

Most studies of chemoreduction for retinoblastoma since 1996 have used vincristine, carboplatin, and an epipodophyllotoxin, either etoposide or teniposide.[50–68] The addition of cyclosporine as a P-glycoprotein inhibitor has also been suggested to decrease the ability of tumor cells to transport antineoplastic drugs out from the intracellular space, thereby allowing the cells to develop multidrug resistance.[50,55] Choice of agents as well as number and frequency of cycles varies currently at different institutions.

The results of recent studies examining the efficacy of chemoreduction followed by focal therapies have been most promising for patients with Reese-Ellsworth groups I to III eyes. For these patients, many authors have demonstrated that enucleation can be successfully avoided almost 100% of the time. Results for patients with Reese-Ellsworth groups 4 and 5 eyes have been more discouraging. In a recent meta-analysis of patients treated with chemoreduction, 37% of eyes avoided *both* external beam radiation and enucleation. Forty-one percent of eyes required radiation but avoided enucleation, and 40% of eyes required enucleation (with or without prior radiation).[69]

There is substantial recent evidence that, despite the dramatic shrinkage observed in tumors during the use of systemic chemotherapy, new tumors can still develop while patients are undergoing a course of chemotherapy. A Kaplan-Meier analysis of 162 eyes treated by Shields and colleagues with vincristine, carboplatin, and etoposide found that new tumor development would

Table 74-4 Intraocular and Extraocular Classification of Retinoblastoma

Reese-Ellsworth Scheme for Intraocular Retinoblastoma
Group I
a. Solitary tumor, less than 4 disc diameters in size, at or behind the equator
b. Multiple tumors, none over 4 disc diameters in size, all at or behind the equator
Group II
a. Solitary tumor, 4 to 10 disc diameters in size, at or behind the equator
b. Multiple tumors, 4 to 10 disc diameters in size, behind the equator
Group III
a. Any lesion anterior to the equator
b. Solitary tumors larger than 10 disc diameters behind the equator
Group IV
a. Multiple tumors, some larger than 10 disc diameters
b. Any lesion extending anteriorly to the ors serrata
Group V
a. Massive tumors involving over half the retina
b. Vitreous seeding

occur in 23% of patients by 1 year of follow-up and 24% of patients by 5 years of follow-up.[70] Lee and colleagues reported on 54 eyes in patients with bilateral familial retinoblastoma treated with carboplatin only and found that 47% of patients developed new tumors during treatment. A greater fraction of patients under 6 months old developed new tumors (60%) than patients over 6 months old (31%).[71]

Treatment of Extraocular Retinoblastoma In most developed nations, extraocular disease occurs only in a small minority of patients. A brief discussion of extraocular disease follows. For more complete information on the treatment of extraocular retinoblastoma, the reader is encouraged to consult more extensive sources.[72–87]

Retinoblastoma can spread beyond the eye via several routes. It may grow contiguously through the choroid and into the sclera and then into the orbit, or it may grow back through the optic nerve and then invade the brain. It may enter the subarachnoid space and then spread throughout the leptomeninges via the cerebrospinal fluid. It may also spread hematogenously, causing metastatic disease in the bone marrow, bone, and organs such as the liver. Rarely retinoblastoma may spread through the lymphatics to produce cervical node disease, but of note, the eye only has lymphatic drainage through the conjunctiva.

Treatment of extraocular disease is implemented based on the extent of metastatic involvement. Different protocols are implemented for patients with the following sites of disease: optic nerve invasion, orbital disease, distant metastases not including the central nervous system (CNS), and CNS involvement. In general, various chemotherapeutic agents have been used for the treatment of patients with optic nerve invasion, although in the past there has been extensive debate as to which pathologic features dictated the need for adjuvant therapy after enucleation.[72–76] Recent studies indicate that only two categories of pathologic findings after enucleation require treatment with chemotherapy: involvement of the surgical margin of the optic nerve and postlaminar optic nerve involvement (not up to the margin) and scleral or choroidal involvement.

Orbital disease has generally been treated with combinations of chemotherapy and radiation therapy.[77–80] Patients with distant metastases have been treated in recent years with intensive chemotherapy with autologous stem cell or bone marrow rescue with success.[80–83] Patients with CNS disease have a very poor prognosis and disappointing results have been observed with various treatment regimens, including combination intravenous and intrathecal chemotherapy and radiation therapy.[77,79,84,85]

Second Malignancies In 1949, it was first recognized that some retinoblastoma patients develop second nonocular neoplasms years after the successful treatment of the eye cancer.[88] Since then the incidence of additional nonocular cancers in survivors of retinoblastoma who carry the *rb1* mutation has been reviewed extensively.[35,36,89–95] Previous analyses have also shown that additional nonocular cancers are the leading cause of death in survivors of germinal retinoblastoma in the United States.[93] Of the survivors of germinal retinoblastoma, cumulative incidence reports of second malignancies vary, but most large studies with adequate long-term follow-up have reported yearly incidence rates of approximately 0.5 to 1% per year.[36,96]

Table 74-5 Risk Factors for Second Nonocular Cancer Development in Retinoblastoma Survivors

Factor	Strength of Association with Incidence of 2nd Cancers
Presence of germinal mutation in *rb1* gene	Definite causation (necessary risk factor)
Dose of external beam radiation	Dose dependent causation
External beam radiation given at < 1 year of age	Very likely association
Presence of lipomas	Definite association
Smoking	Definite association
Chemotherapy	Possible association
Sun exposure	Possible association
Growth hormone	Possible association

Several clinical risk factors and treatment-related exposures have been shown to have an association with the development of second nonocular cancers in retinoblastoma survivors (Table 74-5). All patients with a history of retinoblastoma who develop second nonocular malignancies carry the germinal mutation. External beam radiation definitively increases the risk of development of second cancers in a dose-dependent fashion. The presence of lipomas has been shown to have an association with second cancer development for unclear reasons.[89] Exposure to smoking and sunlight as well as treatment with growth hormone, have been linked to the types of cancers that retinoblastoma survivors develop, although no definite link among retinoblastoma patients has been documented.

Recent clinical data indicate that chemotherapy may also contribute to the development of second neoplasms. Several agents used in current chemoreduction studies for retinoblastoma have been demonstrated to increase the risk of secondary cancers either in retinoblastoma patients or in patients treated with these drugs for other primary malignancies.

Second malignancies observed in retinoblastoma survivors include, in order from most common to least: osteogenic sarcomas of the skull and long bones, soft tissue sarcomas, pineoblastomas, cutaneous melanomas, brain tumors, Hodgkin's disease, lung cancer, breast cancer, and salivary gland and oral cancers.

The location and timing of second cancers which affect survivors of germinal retinoblastoma depend on whether the patients received external beam radiation. In general, patients who never undergo radiation develop approximately two-thirds of their second cancers outside of the theoretical radiation field after a latency period of 15 or more years. Patients who undergo external beam radiation develop approximately two-thirds of their second cancers within the radiation field after a shorter latency period (a mean of 7 years).[35]

Secondary Malignant Disease (Leukemia)

Childhood acute lymphocytic leukemia (ALL) is the most common malignant tumor that involves the eyes of children. Leukemia primarily involves the uveal tract: the iris, ciliary body, and/or choroid. It can also involve the retina, optic nerve, and orbit.

Leukemic iris infiltrates can appear as creamy clusters of cells floating on the surface of the iris. When iris infiltrates are present, they can manifest as heterochromia (different color irides), cells in the anterior chamber (tumor hypopyon mimicking idiopathic iritis), or bleeding in the anterior chamber (hyphema). Hyphema can be associated with glaucoma and a painful, photophobic, red, sensitive eye. In contrast to iris involvement, leukemic infiltration is virtually impossible to detect ophthalmoscopically in the ciliary body or choroid because ALL diffusely invades the choroidal blood vessels. This subtle thickening is often detectable only by B-scan ultrasound.[97] Leukemic infiltration in the choroid has been identified in 90% of eyes at autopsy after death from leukemia. Retinal involvement is rare.

Leukemic infiltration of the eye can present in different time sequences in relation to the overall presentation of the disease. Most commonly, the infiltration presents simultaneously with the initial presentation of the leukemia. The majority of patients with ALL demonstrate ultrasonic ocular findings at presentation. When the leukemia is treated, the choroidal involvement usually disappears within days. Leukemic infiltration of the eye can also present as an isolated site of relapse following induction treatment and CNS radiation prophylaxis. In these children the CNS has often been treated with radiation but the eye has been spared treatment, creating a sanctuary site. Treatment of the eye alone in such cases may be justified. Finally, leukemic infiltration can present as a sign of CNS recurrence with or without evidence of a gross mass in the CNS. These patients frequently have leukemic cells near the posterior pole and in the vitreous. In these cases, the tumor cells enter the eye via the optic nerve, which has been seeded directly from the CNS.[98] In these cases, treatment to the brain with chemotherapy or external beam radiation is generally considered.

PEDIATRIC OPHTHALMIC ONCOLOGY: ORBITAL DISEASES

Benign Disease **Capillary Hemangiomas** Benign tumors of the orbit in children are frequently incidental problems detected on CT scan or observed because of lid or orbital asymmetry. Many require no treatment. The most common benign orbital tumor of childhood is the capillary hemangioma.[99] Capillary hemangiomas are highly cellular, angioblastic, and rarely encapsulated. As many as 25% may not be apparent at birth, but they grow so rapidly and frequently bleed that they may be mistaken for rhabdomyosarcomas. Because rhabdomyosarcomas require biopsy, diagnostic imaging should first be used to distinguish between capillary hemangiomas and rhabdomyosarcomas. On CT, capillary hemangiomas are usually associated with congenitally enlarged orbits while rhabdomyosarcomas are not. Despite growth that may appear explosive, their natural course is to stop growing after 6 to 12 months, when they will slowly involute (over 2–5 years) and largely regress. They may be associated with strawberry hemangiomas of the nearby skin.

These tumors can cause profound and permanent visual loss if left untreated. The mechanism of visual loss can be ptosis or occlusion of the pupil and consequent development of deprivation amblyopia. The mass can press on the eye itself causing significant astigmatism with the development of anisometropic amblyopia. Rarely hemangiomas cause corneal damage by proptosis and exposure, and they may press on the optic nerve and cause optic atrophy. If they sequester platelets they may cause thrombocytopenia. They may also cause high output cardiac failure.

Treatment of these hemangiomas is difficult. Surgery, either conventional or with the KTP (532 nm potassium titanyl phosphate) laser rarely removes enough of the lesion to prevent the ocular complications. The tumors respond to low dose radiation and we have used fractionated doses up to 800 cGy with success. There have been reports of injecting sclerosing solutions into the lesions or even occluding them with interventional radiological techniques, but experience is limited. There have also been several reports of successful treatment with recombinant interferon alpha.[100]

Fortunately these tumors respond to local or systemic steroids. Systemic treatment must continue for months to achieve a permanent response, and with the doses recommended for the young children (20 mg/day), systemic toxicity is common and worrisome. Local injections of short and long-acting steroids are probably the treatment of choice when mandated by visual or overwhelming cosmetic reasons.

Dermoid Cysts Dermoid cysts are among the most common orbital tumors of childhood. They are benign and represent congenital ectodermal rests. They are usually in the anterior portion of the superior orbit and cause a characteristic hollowed-out appearance of the orbital bone. Occasionally the dermoids have calcification and even aberrant tooth formation within the mass. Treatment is surgical, but utmost care must be taken because many have dumbbell-shaped posterior orbital extensions that can extend intracranially. When the cysts rupture, either from trauma or from incomplete surgical removal, a violent orbital inflammation may ensue.

Lymphangioma Despite the fact that lymphatics do not exist in the orbit, benign lymphangiomas do.[101] These tumors are thought to be congenital and have no malignant potential, but in contrast to hemangiomas are rarely present at birth. They are most commonly seen at around age 6 years, with explosive proptosis caused by bleeding of the tumor into the cystic spaces referred to as *chocolate cysts*. These lesions consist of primitive lymphatic channels with lymphoid hyperplasia and may enlarge during upper respiratory infections. Treatment is difficult. They do not respond to steroids or radiation and they are impossible to remove completely by surgery. Surgery with electrocautery, which may have to be repeated many times, with or without the KTP laser, is the treatment of choice. Satisfactory cosmetic results are difficult to attain.

Malignant Disease **Rhabdomyosarcoma** The most common primary malignant orbital tumor of childhood is rhabdomyosarcoma. The average age at diagnosis is 6 to 10 years, with equal incidence in both sexes and both orbits. Although the hallmark presentation of an orbital rhabdomyosarcoma is rapid, progressive, painless proptosis, patients can present with a less dramatic course with slow, progressive proptosis or with ptosis, strabismus, or a subconjunctival fleshy mass.[102] The diagnosis of rhabdomyosarcoma should be considered whenever rapid progressive proptosis occurs in the first 20 years of life. Other conditions must be considered in the differential diagnosis and they are listed in Table 74-6. The most common location in the orbit is superonasal. CT or MRI scans can help define the extent of the tumor.

Urgent biopsy is mandatory. All attempts should be made to biopsy the lesion directly without going through the sinuses or skull because of the possibility of causing metastatic disease by tracking tumor cells along the biopsy path. The most common histologic type is an embryonal rhabdomyosarcoma. When rhabdomyosarcomas present in the inferior orbit, they are usually histologically alveolar type. These malignancies do not originate from extraocular muscles, but from undifferentiated pluripotential mesenchymal elements in the orbital soft tissues.

Table 74-6 Causes of Rapid Proptosis in Childhood

1. Orbital rhabdomyosarcoma
2. Orbital lymphangioma
3. Orbital hemangioma (capillary)
4. Metastatic neuroblastoma
5. Encephalocele
6. Inflammatory disease
   a. Orbital cellulitis (infectious /following rupture of dermoid, teratoma)
   b. Benign reactive lymphoid hyperplasia
7. Leukemia

External beam radiation was first used in the mid-1960's and later combined with chemotherapy, producing excellent local cures and better than 90% long-term survival. The Intergroup Rhabdomyosarcoma studies in the 1980s demonstrated that the most effective combination for disease localized to the orbit was vincristine, actinomycin-D, and radiation.[103] In giving radiation, the eye was not spared or shielded. Long-term follow-up demonstrated that after a median of 7 years, only 14% of such eyes were enucleated, but vision was impaired in 70% of them.[104] A more recent meta-analysis completed by four international collaborative groups found no significant difference in survival for those patients treated with chemotherapy alone versus chemotherapy plus radiation.[105]

ADULT OPHTHALMIC ONCOLOGY: OCULAR DISEASES

Benign Disease Benign tumors of the lid, conjunctiva, iris, and choroid are common, while those of the retina and cornea are rare. Benign tumors of the lens and vitreous do not occur. The most important benign tumors of the eye are choroidal nevi.

Choroidal Nevi Choroidal nevi are never present at birth, but generally present around puberty. In the United States, 10 to 13% of the adult population has choroidal nevi. They are racially related; choroidal nevi in blacks are very rare.

Choroidal nevi are flat, pigmented, benign lesions with edges that can be feathered and irregular or rounded (Figure 74-5). They are usually slate gray to light chocolate in color. Over time (months to years), there can be associated changes visible by ophthalmoscopy. Many demonstrate changes on their surface such as drusen or have associated findings such as subretinal fluid or neovascular membranes. They may also cause visual field defects. Since 10% of the adult population has choroidal nevi and there are only

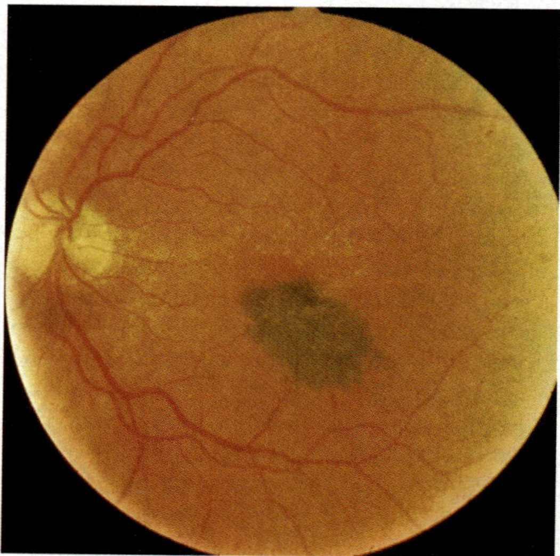

Figure 74-5 Choroidal nevus.

Table 74-7 Predictive Factors: Nevus to Melanoma Transformation

1) Size: The greater the thickness of a choroidal nevus, the greater is the chance of it becoming a melanoma. Of nevi 2.5 mm in thickness, approximately 1% per month become melanomas.
2) Location: Nevi at the posterior portion of the eye more commonly become melanomas than those situated anteriorly.
3) Orange Pigment: When choroidal nevi develop orange pigment on their surface, the chance of a melanoma developing greatly increases.
4) Serous Fluid: Serous fluid in the form of an overlying retinal detachment can be seen with nevi, and such nevi more likely become melanomas.
5) Hot Spots on Fluorescein Angiography
6) Symptoms (decreased vision or visual field defect)

1,500 choroidal melanomas in the United States yearly, it is assumed that the chance of a choroidal nevus becoming a melanoma is less than one in a thousand. A number of studies have now demonstrated which nevi are more likely to undergo malignant transformation. The predictive factors are shown in Table 74-7.

A melanocytoma is a special type of choroidal nevus often observed in darker-skinned whites of Mediterranean origin. Melanocytomas are brown-black lesions that most commonly originate from the optic nerve head, but can evolve from the choroid, ciliary body, or iris. The lesions may be several millimeters high, can grow slowly, and can affect the visual field or visual acuity. Pathologically, the lesion is a magnocellular nevus with jet-black pigmentation. Although the lesions are benign, rare cases of transformation to malignancy have been recorded.

The differential diagnosis of a choroidal nevus includes congenital hyperplasia of the retinal pigment epithelium (CHRPE), hamartomas of the retinal pigment epithelium, and hemorrhages within the retina, especially hemorrhages beneath the retinal pigment epithelium (most commonly associated with age-related macular degeneration). Ophthalmoscopic appearance as well as results of a fluorescein angiogram and ultrasonography are used to distinguish these lesions from each other.

Iris Nevi and Melanomas Iris nevi are benign lesions of the iris that appear on slit lamp examination as pigmented flat areas. They are common, may be multiple, and occur more often in blue-eyed patients. Like choroidal nevi, iris nevi are rarely present at birth and present around puberty. Rarely, they can appear elevated and can grow and shed pigmented cells into the anterior chamber angle, clogging the trabecular meshwork and causing a severe secondary glaucoma that can blind the eye. These lesions have often been referred to as iris melanomas. Widespread metastases, however, are seen rarely if ever. Many clinicians have theorized that the reason for the less aggressive behavior observed in iris melanomas versus choroidal melanomas is simply the smaller size of these lesions. Management of iris melanoma is based on the presence or absence of glaucoma, and should not be guided by a need to prevent metastases. Melanomas that originate in the ciliary body and extend into the iris, however, often demonstrate very aggressive behavior and can metastasize.

Malignant Disease **Introduction to Choroidal Melanoma** The most common primary ocular malignant tumor of adults, choroidal malignant melanoma accounts for about 1,500 new cases per year in the United States. The average age at diagnosis is 55 to 65 years, with men and women equally affected and no predilection for right versus left eye. In the United States, 99% of choroidal melanomas occur in whites. The most common way in which the tumor is detected is on routine examination (41%).[106] Men more often present with symptoms, and when there are symptoms, the right eye is more often found to have the tumor. The most common symptom is a perceived deficit in the peripheral visual field followed by decreased vision. The lesion is not painful, unlike metastatic tumors to the eye in which pain is not unusual.

The visual field defect is characteristic. There is an absolute scotoma overlying the tumor associated with a surrounding relative field defect that does not obey the horizontal meridian (as most ocular defects do) and does not observe the vertical meridian (as many CNS defects do).[107]

Melanomas of the choroid originate in melanocytes that normally lie within the choroid. The choroid, the layer between the sclera and retina is a rich, high-flow syncytium of vascular lobules that not only supply blood to the photoreceptors (rods and cones) of the retina, but also serve as a heat sink to dissipate heat energy liberated by absorbed visible light.

Whether all melanomas of the choroid originate from choroidal nevi is not known, but patients with flat, pigmented, untreated nevi followed for more than 20 years have developed melanomas arising from the previously dormant lesion. The cause of choroidal melanomas is unknown, but predisposing medical conditions include melanosis oculi (Ota's nevus), dysplastic nevus syndrome, pregnancy, and possibly HIV. Medications that have been shown to cause increased growth of the tumors include estrogen replacement therapy, and levodopa. Occupational associations include agriculture and farming work and several industrial operations.[108] We have also seen an increased risk in World War II holocaust survivors.

Diagnosis of Choroidal Melanoma The diagnosis of choroidal melanoma can usually be made on the basis of ophthalmoscopic examination alone. The lesions most often appear as elevated, dome-shaped masses that can rupture Bruch's membrane (Figure 74-6). When Bruch's membrane is ruptured, the tumors are referred to as mushroom-shaped or collar-button because of their characteristic shape. The lesions can also be multilobed or flat and diffuse. Lesion color varies from patient to patient and from area to area within the tumor. As many as 40% of the tumors have no pigment clinically. When pigmented, the tumors are frequently a dusky gray to charcoal in color, but occasionally they are deep brown. Black lesions within the eye are rarely melanomas.

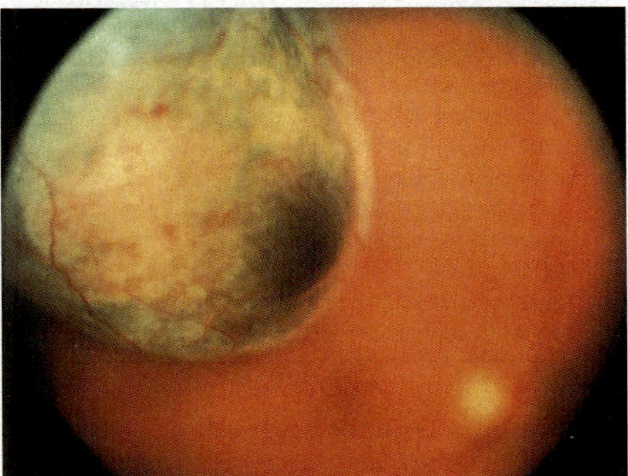

Figure 74-6 Malignant melanoma of the choroid.

Ocular ultrasonography and sometimes fluorescein angiography can also aid in diagnosis. All choroidal melanomas have associated retinal detachments. In some cases it may be difficult to detect the detachments ophthalmoscopically, while in others the retinal detachment may be so extensive that the melanoma is not seen clinically. Typically the B-scan ultrasound demonstrates an elevated solid tumor[109] and the A-scan demonstrates medium to low reflectivity.[110] With the use of rigorous and standardized ophthalmic and systemic examinations, a diagnostic accuracy of 99.7% was reached in the Collaborative Ocular Melanoma Study (COMS).[111] Since clinical accuracy is so high, needle biopsy is rarely needed.

Since there are no lymphatics in the eye or within the orbit, melanomas of the choroid metastasize through vascular channels. More than 75% of such metastases are first identified within the liver. Fewer than 1% of patients with metastasis survive 5 years.

Clinical and Pathologic Risk Factors A number of clinical and pathologic features have been shown to correlate with patient survival.[112] First, larger tumors, measured clinically using the height, and/or greatest base diameter to volume, are more likely to metastasize. Second, location of the melanoma affects prognosis. Patients with melanomas originating in the iris have the best outcome. Ciliary body melanomas have a threefold mortality compared with choroidal melanomas. Third, patients younger than 60 years have better survival than those older than 60 years. Fourth, patients with extraocular extension have higher mortality rates than those who do not. Finally, many pathologic features (only available in cases where the eye has been removed) correlate with survival and are covered extensively elsewhere.[113] The best known of these is cell type. Epithelioid cells, which are larger and more pleomorphic, are more likely to be contained in large tumors, and carry a worse prognosis.

The COMS Group, which included 44 institutions across the United States, has now completed multiple prospective, randomized clinical trials

Table 74-8 Classification of Choroidal Melanomas

Small melanomas
Apical height: 1–2.5 mm
Largest basal diameter: 5 mm or less
Medium melanomas
Apical height: 2.5–10 mm
Largest basal diameter: 5–16 mm
Large melanomas
Apical height: 10 mm or greater
Largest basal diameter: 16 mm or greater

and other reports on the prognosis and treatment of small, medium, and large choroidal melanomas. The COMS size classification scheme is shown in Table 74-8 and the results of the studies are detailed in Table 74-9.

Treatment and Prognosis of Small Melanomas The COMS demonstrated that of choroidal melanomas initially managed by observation, 21% demonstrated growth to medium or large tumors by 2 years and 31% by 5 years.[114] Factors significantly associated with growth were greater initial tumor thickness and diameter, presence of orange pigment, absence of drusen, and absence of areas of retinal pigment epithelial changes adjacent to the tumor. Overall, patients with small melanomas were shown to have a 5-year survival rate of 96%.[115] Clinically, most patients with small melanomas are observed until tumor growth is documented by fundus photography or ultrasonography. Patients with small melanomas have a 100% 5-year survival rate in cases in which serial examinations demonstrate no interval lesion growth.

Treatment and Prognosis of Medium Melanomas In the past, patients with tumors in this group were treated with local excision, enucleation, external beam radiation, proton beam therapy, or brachytherapy. The COMS completed a prospective, randomized clinical trial enrolling 1,317 patients with medium-sized melanomas in which patients were randomly assigned to enucleation or brachytherapy with ^{125}I plaques at a tumor dose of 10,000 cGy.[116] The study concluded mortality rates following brachytherapy (81% 5-year survival) did not differ from mortality rates following enucleation (82% 5-year survival) for up to 12 years after treatment. Given the findings of this study, patients with medium-sized melanomas are now offered both enucleation and brachytherapy as potential treatment options. Brachytherapy with ^{125}I plaques is usually administered at doses of 7,500 cGy to 10,000 cGy. The fractionation schemes vary markedly without an apparent effect on local control, metastasis, or complications. Complications include radiation retinopathy and optic neuropathy.[117]

Treatment and Prognosis of Large Melanomas In the past, patients with large tumors were generally treated with enucleation, with or without preoperative radiation. The COMS prospective, randomized clinical trial for patients with large tumors found that there was no survival difference between patients treated with enucleation alone (57% 5-year survival) and patients treated with pre-enucleation radiation (62% 5-year survival).[118] The patients assigned to the pre-enucleation radiation group in this study were treated with 5 fractions of 200 cGy external beam radiation and enucleation within 72 hours. Patients with large melanomas are now generally treated with enucleation alone.

METASTATIC DISEASE The most common malignant neoplasm in the eye or orbit, in children or adults, is metastatic cancer to the choroid. Although there are only 350 cases of retinoblastoma and 1,500 cases of choroidal melanoma yearly in the United States, it is estimated that 30,000 to 100,000 patients with cancer develop metastases to the eye each year.[119]

Most cancers metastasize to the uveal tract (iris, ciliary body, and choroid), with choroidal metastases occurring most frequently. Metastases to the lids, conjunctiva, optic nerve, orbit, extraocular muscles, and orbital bones are also reported. Metastases to the retina are rare.

Choroidal metastases are usually amelanotic, multiple, bilateral, minimally elevated, and painful when situated around the optic nerve or invading the sclera. In contrast, ocular melanomas are typically pigmented, solitary, unilateral, significantly elevated, and painless. Metastatic tumors, like ocular melanomas, always have an associated serous detachment, but the amount of detachment is proportionally greater with metastases. Ultrasonographically, most metastases have high reflectivity on ultrasound. Most ocular melanomas are detected on routine examinations, whereas ocular metastases are typically identified because of symptoms of decreased visual field and diminished visual acuity due to serous retinal detachments.

Metastasis to the eye most commonly occurs in adults aged 55 to 65, the same age distribution as that for ocular melanomas. Metastases originate most commonly from a primary lung cancer and second most commonly from a primary breast cancer. As many as 34% of patients who present with metastases to the choroid have no previously known history of a primary cancer.[120] Many other cancers metastasize to the eye, including GI, prostate (though more commonly to orbital bones), thyroid, ovarian, cutaneous melanoma, and sweat gland carcinomas. Virtually all cancers have been found to be capable of metastasizing to the eye.

The most striking feature of metastatic ocular lesions is their association with concurrent CNS metastases. Although the true concordance of these two lesions is unknown, it has been our experience that more than 75% of cases of ocular metastasis have concurrent CNS disease, though frequently the CNS disease is initially undetectable with imaging. It has therefore been speculated that some ocular metastases do not arrive through blood borne routes, but that CNS metastases may actually seed the choroid via the subarachnoid space as they do in childhood leukemia.

Treatment of ocular metastasis is considered when symptoms of diminished vision, pain, or diplopia are present. Treating the ocular lesion rarely has an impact on survival, except in carcinoid metastases, but may significantly alter the quality of life. Many ocular metastases respond to chemotherapy the way other systemic metastases respond. Chemotherapy and/or hormonal manipulation may cause rapid regression of the tumor and of subretinal fluid. External beam radiation is also used to palliate symptoms from ocular metastases. Except for carcinoid, breast cancer, and childhood neoplasms, median survival in patients with metastatic choroidal lesions is just over 6 months.

CANCER-ASSOCIATED RETINOPATHY (CAR) Cancer-associated retinopathy (CAR) is a paraneoplastic disorder characterized by visual loss in patients with cancer. Patients report photopsias or entopic phenomenon as well as light sensitivity and night blindness. Examination reveals decreased visual acuity, decreased color vision, and scoto-

Table 74-9 Results of the Collaborative Ocular Melanoma Study (COMS)

	Small	Medium	Large
Reference	Arch Ophthalmol 1997 Dec;115(12):1537–44	Arch Ophthalmol 2001 Jul;119(7):969–82	Am J Ophthalmol 1998 Jun;125(6):779–96
Type of study	Nonrandomized, prospective follow-up study	Prospective randomized clinical trial	Prospective randomized clinical trial
Number of patients in study	204	1317	1003
Size of melanomas included in study	Apical height: 1.0–2.5 mm; Largest basal diameter: 5 mm	Apical height: 2.5–10.0 mm; Largest basal diameter: 5–16 mm	Apical height: 10.0 mm or larger; Largest basal diameter: 16 mm or larger
Objective of study	To describe time to tumor growth and determine baseline characteristics associated with growth of small tumors	I^{125} Brachytherapy vs enucleation for treatment of medium tumors	Pre-enucleation radiation vs enucleation alone for treatment of large tumors
Findings of study	21% grew by 2 years; 31% grew by 5 years; Characteristics associated with growth: initial tumor thickness and diameter, presence of orange pigment, absence of drusen, absence of retinal pigment epithelial changes	No clinically or statistically significant difference in survival rates between the 2 treatments for up to 12 years after treatment	No significant difference in survival rates between the 2 treatments Age and largest basal diameter of the tumor are the only factors that affect prognosis

mas.[121] A CAR antibody, a 23-kDa protein commonly found on blood testing, is known to be specific for a photoreceptor and bipolar cell-specific calcium-binding protein. The underlying tumor is thought to express recoverin and stimulate this antibody response. The circulating antibodies then react with the retina, resulting in photoreceptor degeneration. Although antibodies to recoverin account for the majority of cases, additional antibodies to 46-kDa, 45-kDa, 60-kDa, and 65-kDa proteins have been described.[121] Lung, endometrial sarcoma, lymphoma, and prostate cancer have been associated with the syndrome. Treatment is difficult. Steroids, plasmapheresis, intravenous immunoglobulin (IVIG), and treatment of the underlying tumor have been attempted. Although individual successes have been reported, most patients have little improvement and there is no clear consensus as to the best treatment.[122,123]

Ocular Lymphoid Tumors Non-Hodgkin's lymphomas can occasionally infiltrate the intraocular tissues and become clinically apparent even before identification of the systemic disease. Immunocompromised patients, especially those with viral illness such as those with HIV/AIDS, show an increased incidence of this disease.

Primary malignant lymphomas of the eye have historically been called *reticulum cell sarcoma* or *microgliomatosis* and usually present with cells in the vitreous with associated retinal and optic nerve involvement. Diagnosis is made by vitrectomy or lumbar puncture. Treatment is accomplished with systemic steroids and external beam radiation therapy of 2,400 cGy to the affected eye and/or chemotherapy. These patients frequently have CNS disease but rarely have systemic disease. There is controversy about whether to treat the brain in those cases in which diagnostic lumbar puncture and MRI demonstrate no disease. Median survival is 3.5 years and is usually determined by the extent of brain involvement.

Uveal lymphoid infiltration is a rare disorder characterized by localized or diffuse infiltration of the uveal tract by lymphoid cells. Patients typically present with painless, progressive visual loss. Nodular amelanotic thickening of the choroid or exudative retinal detachment with secondary glaucoma can be present.[124] Biopsy confirmation should be targeted to the most accessible tissue. Management emphasizes globe conservation aimed at visual presentation and generally involves oral steroids and/or external beam radiation. Prognosis for survival is excellent and is generally based on the degree of systemic involvement. Associated CNS involvement is rare.

ADULT OPHTHALMIC ONCOLOGY: ORBITAL DISEASES

Introduction to Orbital Tumors The diagnosis of orbital tumors has undergone a revolution in the past 20 years as a result of the widespread use of ultrasonography, CT scans, and MRI scans. Prior to this revolution, virtually all cases of proptosis required biopsy, and it was not unusual to be unable to find a tumor. The number of orbital lesions that require biopsy has decreased, and the chance of finding the diseased area has become much higher as a result of noninvasive imaging. Fortunately, malignant tumors of the orbit are unusual. Neoplasms account for approximately 20 to 25% of orbital disease and are most common in patients in their sixties or older. Biopsy is rarely needed for definitive diagnosis even in cases of metastatic disease to the orbit. Malignant primary cancers of the orbit that do require biopsy and surgical management include lacrimal gland tumors and orbital lymphoma. The clinical findings suggestive of a malignant orbital tumor are listed in Table 74-10.

Table 74-10 Findings Suspicious of Orbital Tumor

Finding	Explanation
Proptosis/exophthalmos	Anterior displacement of the globe
Globe displacement	Masses in the inferior orbit cause vertical displacement of the globe; masses in the superior orbit cause infra-displacement
Limitation of motility	Globe motility limited by simple mass effect, direct involvement of extraocular muscle(s), direct/indirect effect on the nerves to extraocular muscles, adhesions of tumor to globe
Orbital pain	Especially in rapidly progressing tumors
Increased retropulsion	Digitally pushing back the globe gives more resistance on the side of the tumor
Foreshortened globe	Mass effect flattens globe with increased hyperopia/decreased myopia
Periocular paresthesias/anesthesia	Effect on sensory nerves
Ptosis	Droopy lid caused by proptosis
Palpable mass	Possible in anteriorly placed tumors only
Visual field defect	Defect limited to one eye
Lid edema	May indicate obstruction of venous flow
Papilledema	From mass effect on the retrobulbar optic nerve

All cases of suspected orbital tumor should undergo imaging, including ophthalmic ultrasound, CT scans with or without contrast, and/or MRI with or without contrast in order to define more clearly the location of the tumor. An algorithm for differential diagnosis and treatment of orbital tumors is shown in Figure 74-7.

Benign and Malignant Disease **Well-Delineated Orbital Masses** The most common benign orbital tumor of adults is the cavernous hemangioma. Patients have slowly progressive, painless proptosis with a mass indenting the globe, showing striae in the retina and a flattened globe on imaging studies. Treatment is surgical, and complete removal is possible. Other well-circumscribed lesions include neurofibromas, schwannomas, hemangiopericytomas, meningiomas, and gliomas.

A mucocele or mucopyocele is a cystic, encapsulated mass originating in a paranasal sinus (usually the frontal sinus) that follows repeated bouts of sinusitis, often leading to recurrent orbital cellulitis. It is the most common cause of proptosis in children. The bony wall is not intact on imaging studies. Treatment involves antibiotics. Surgical drainage is necessary if antibiotics fail to achieve resolution of the pyomucocele or if optic nerve compression is present.

Diffuse Orbital Mass Diffuse orbital masses usually require a biopsy and include orbital lymphoma, orbital cellulitis, fibrous histiocytoma (benign and malignant), neurofibromas, and sarcomas. Their management is presented in Figure 74-7.

Lymphoproliferative neoplasms account for greater than 20% of all orbital mass lesions. The incidence of non-Hodgkin's lymphoma of all anatomic sites has been increasing at a rate of 3 to 4% per year, and orbital lymphomas have been increasing at an even greater rate, although the factors responsible for this rise are poorly understood.[124] Historically, lymphoid tumors were classified as either reactive lymphoid hyperplasia or malignant lymphoma. More recently, it has been recognized that lymphoproliferative lesions represent a continuum and that ultimate behavior is difficult to predict. Currently, 70 to 90% of orbital lymphoproliferative lesions are designated as malignant lymphomas on the basis of molecular genetic studies and monoclonal cell-surface markers.

The typical lymphoproliferative lesion presents as a gradually progressive, painless mass. It can be located anteriorly in the orbit or beneath the conjunctiva. Orbital imaging reveals the characteristic molding of the tumor around normal structures, and bony erosion is rare except in high-grade lesions. Up to 50% of all lesions arise in the lacrimal fossa, and up to 17% of lesions occur bilaterally. For all lesions, early biopsy is recommended to establish a diagnosis and characterize the lesions to reflect distinct morphologic, immunologic, cytogenetic, and molecular properties under the Revised European American Lymphoma (REAL) classification.[125,126] This classification has been shown to predict differences in the clinical behavior of these lesions. The classification allocates adnexal lymphomas to one of five categories: marginal zone lymphoma, diffuse lymphoplasmacytoid/lymphoplasmacytic lymphoma, follicle center cell lymphoma, diffuse large B-cell lymphoma, and other rare lymphomas.

Management of adnexal lymphoma involves a metastatic work-up by an oncologist. Ocular disease is generally treated with 2,000 to 3,000 cGy of external beam radiation therapy, which results in local control in virtually all cases and may prevent systemic spread. At least 50% of lesions eventually spread systemically, however, and treatment of sys-

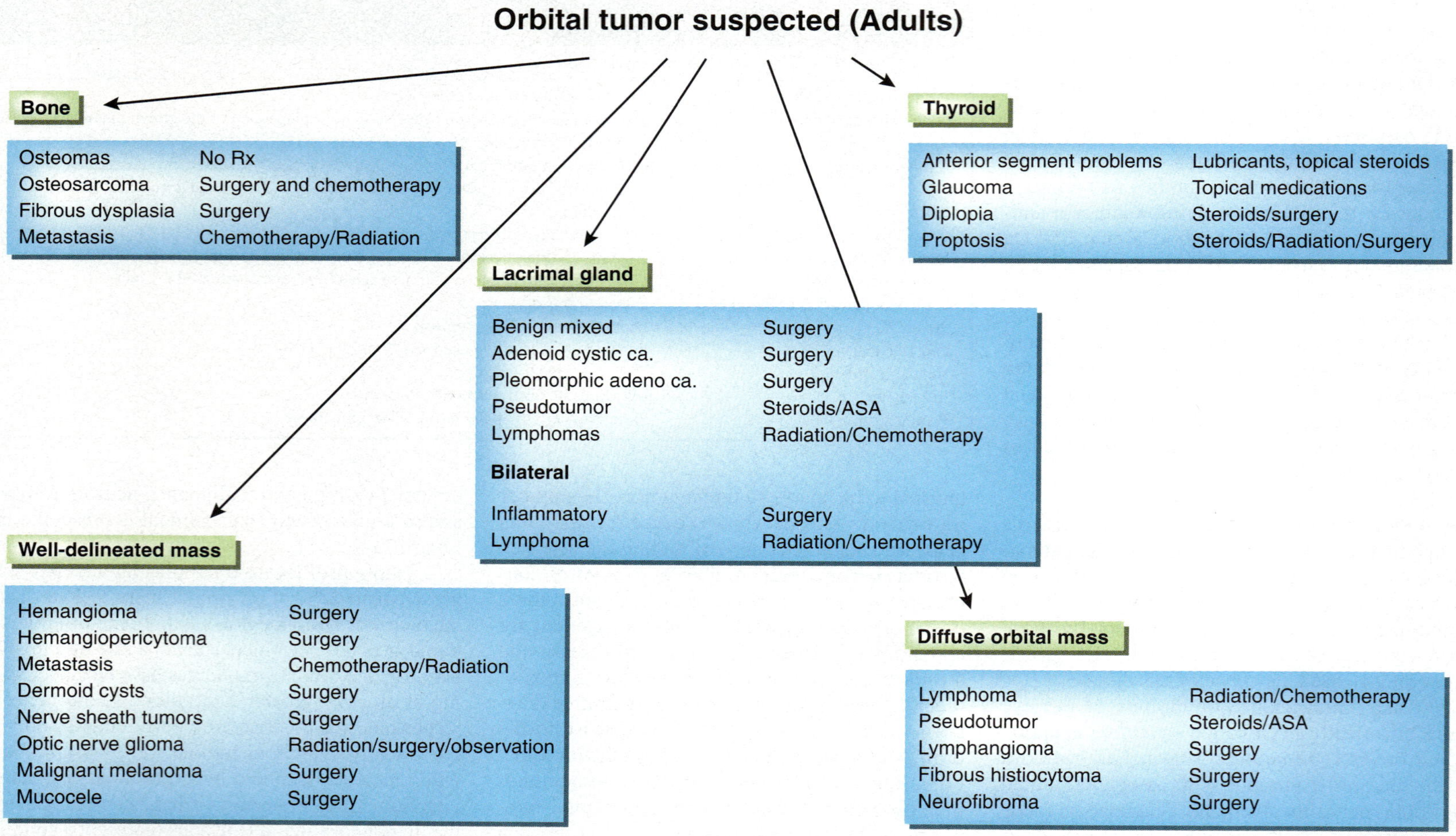

Orbital tumor suspected (Adults)

Bone

Osteomas	No Rx
Osteosarcoma	Surgery and chemotherapy
Fibrous dysplasia	Surgery
Metastasis	Chemotherapy/Radiation

Thyroid

Anterior segment problems	Lubricants, topical steroids
Glaucoma	Topical medications
Diplopia	Steroids/surgery
Proptosis	Steroids/Radiation/Surgery

Lacrimal gland

Benign mixed	Surgery
Adenoid cystic ca.	Surgery
Pleomorphic adeno ca.	Surgery
Pseudotumor	Steroids/ASA
Lymphomas	Radiation/Chemotherapy
Bilateral	
Inflammatory	Surgery
Lymphoma	Radiation/Chemotherapy

Well-delineated mass

Hemangioma	Surgery
Hemangiopericytoma	Surgery
Metastasis	Chemotherapy/Radiation
Dermoid cysts	Surgery
Nerve sheath tumors	Surgery
Optic nerve glioma	Radiation/surgery/observation
Malignant melanoma	Surgery
Mucocele	Surgery

Diffuse orbital mass

Lymphoma	Radiation/Chemotherapy
Pseudotumor	Steroids/ASA
Lymphangioma	Surgery
Fibrous histiocytoma	Surgery
Neurofibroma	Surgery

Figure 74-7 Algorithm for diagnosis and treatment of orbital tumors.

temic dissemination is based on the pathologic grade of the lesion and its characteristic degree of aggressiveness. Some indolent lymphomas are refractory to cure by chemotherapy but are associated with long-term survival, whereas more aggressive lymphomas may be cured with aggressive chemotherapy and/or radiation.

Some studies suggest that patients with bilateral orbital involvement have a poorer prognosis. Conjunctival lesions have the lowest likelihood (20%) of developing systemic disease. Eyelid lymphomas have the highest likelihood (67%), with orbital lesions in between (35%).[127]

Thyroid Ophthalmopathy Proptosis is a presenting sign of many orbital tumors, but thyroid orbitopathy represents the most common cause of both bilateral and of unilateral proptosis. The eye findings may be associated with clinical or laboratory evidence of hyperthyroidism, hypothyroidism, or euthyroidism. The disease is 4 to 5 times more common in women, usually those in middle age. Cigarette smoking is associated with a more fulminant course. The pathogenesis of the disease is complex and involves several mechanisms: a cellular response manifested through fibroblasts and adipocytes, an immunologic response mediated through cytokines, and a mechanical component that results from a discrepancy between the fixed volume of the bony orbit and the increased volume of the swollen retrobulbar tissues.[124] There is controversy regarding guidelines for appropriate treatment, especially regarding the utility of external beam radiation therapy.[128]

Lacrimal Gland Tumors Lacrimal gland tumors can be easily identified with ophthalmic ultrasonography, but a more clear definition of tumor location, especially bony involvement, is best demonstrated with CT scans. When lacrimal gland masses are bilateral on orbital imaging, they generally represent lesions such as sarcoid, orbital pseudotumor, or lymphoma. Of those lacrimal gland masses not presenting with inflammatory signs, the majority represent lymphoproliferative disorders, as fully 50% of orbital lymphomas develop in the lacrimal fossa. Only a minority of lacrimal fossa lesions are primary epithelial neoplasms of the lacrimal gland. Percutaneous biopsy is necessary in suspected cases to establish a pathologic diagnosis.

Approximately 50% of primary epithelial neoplasms of the lacrimal gland are benign mixed tumors (pleomorphic adenomas) and about 50% are carcinomas. Approximately half of the carcinomas are adenoid cystic tumors (Figure 74-8), and the remainder include malignant mixed tumors, primary adenocarcinomas, mucoepidermoid carcinomas, and squamous carcinomas. Treatment of primary malignant lacrimal gland tumors includes steroids, excisional surgery, and radiation therapy. Except for pleomorphic adenomas that undergo successful surgical removal without a preliminary biopsy (with resultant tumor capsule rupture, increasing risk of recurrence), the clinical course for most of these tumors is that of multiple painful recurrences with ultimate mortality from intracranial extension or systemic metastases, often occurring a decade or more after initial presentation.

Bone Lesions CT scans best delineate bony lesions causing proptosis. Primary bony lesions

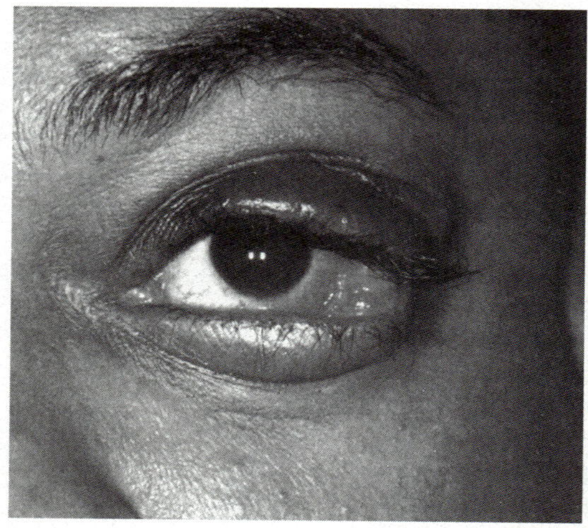

Figure 74-8 Adenoid cystic carcinoma of the lacrimal gland in a patient who underwent 2 biopsies of the mass, both of which were equivocal. The patient developed metastases to the parotid gland and later died.

include osteomas, osteogenic sarcomas, and fibrous dysplasia. Secondary lesions of bone include metastases, especially from prostate, thyroid, lung, breast, kidney, and the nonmetastatic eosinophilic granuloma (histiocytosis X spectrum).

ADULT OPHTHALMIC ONCOLOGY: LID DISEASE

Benign Disease Benign tumors of the lid can be divided into two sub groups: cystic and noncystic. These masses can sometimes masquerade as malignant lesions. Cystic lesions usually arise from the sebaceous (Meibomian) glands. These are known as chalazia and are inflammatory, sterile lipogranulomas. Treatment is varied and depends on severity. Recurrent chalazia require biopsy to rule out sebaceous gland carcinoma (masquerade syndrome).

Noncystic lesions include keratoacanthoma, which can simulate squamous cell carcinoma. The two lesions can be distinguished based on the rapidity of growth and central ulceration present in acanthomas. The histology shows marked atypia and inflammation.

Malignant Disease Lid malignancies can be primary or metastatic with primary tumors accounting for 98% of all cancerous lid growths.[129] The most common primary lid cancer is basal cell carcinoma (BCC), representing over 92% of lid tumors.[129] Less common tumors, in descending order of prevalence, include squamous cell carcinoma (SCC), sebaceous cell carcinoma, melanoma, and lymphoma. BCC, SCC, and cutaneous melanoma arise from the skin, and sebaceous cell carcinomas arise from the Meibomian glands of the upper and lower lids.

BCC occurs most often as the nodular variant, which has no metastatic potential but can invade the orbit if left untreated over a long period of time. Medially located lesions are most likely to invade the orbit. Morpheaform (sclerosing) BCC, which represents 15% of all BCC, has a high rate of recurrence, especially if the tumor extends beyond the clinically suspicious site. The treatment of choice for BCC is surgical excision using frozen section control (Mohs micrographic technique). At least 5 mm margins are ideal for these tumors. Local recurrence rates appear similar to those after surgery if the BCC is treated with external beam radiation.

SCC, like BCC, arises in sun-damaged skin and invades locally, but unlike BCC, SCC has metastatic potential. Metastases occur principally in the regional lymph nodes. Certain histopathologic variations are associated with more aggressive disease: spindle-cell and adenosquamous variants are more often associated with perineural invasion.[130] Tumors with perineural invasion have a 50% chance of recurrence and a 35% risk of metastases if treated with excision alone. External beam radiation following resection offers the best results for lesions with perineural involvement, with a 5-year disease-free rate of 85 to 95% if the tumor is localized. Mohs surgery of both primary and recurrent periocular SCC yields cure rates close to 95%. The Mohs technique cannot be used if the cancer has breached the orbital septum. In these patients, orbital exenteration is necessary. Routine regional dissection is not advised in the treatment of periocular SCC. Lymphoscintigraphy may be useful in deciding if head and neck dissection is necessary. Systemic or intralesional chemotherapy has been shown to result in partial or complete regression. Chemotherapeutic agents used systemically include cisplatin and doxorubicin. Interferon alpha-2b has been used intralesionally with success.[131]

Sebaceous gland carcinoma usually arises in the Meibomian glands or the glands of Zeiss in the lid. Delay in diagnosis is common, as the lesions can be easily confused with chalazia. The tissue specimen should be sent in saline to facilitate oil red O staining. Once the diagnosis of sebaceous gland carcinoma is made, map biopsies of the conjunctival surface are indicated, as this tumor is multicentric and exhibits pagetoid spread. Treatment is surgical via wide excision alone or excision combined with cryotherapy. Radiation is another option if the patient is not a surgical candidate. Exenteration is reserved for cases of spread to the orbit or globe.

REFERENCES

1. Abramson DH. Retinoblastoma. Pediatr Emerg Casebook 1985;3:3–15.
2. Abramson DH. Retinoblastoma: diagnosis and management. CA Cancer J Clin 1982;32:130–40.
3. Tamboli A, Podgor MJ, Horm JW. The incidence of retinoblastoma in the United States: 1974 through 1985. Arch Ophthalmol 1990;108(1):128–32.
4. Augsburger JJ, Oehlschlager U, Manzitti JE. Multinational clinical and pathologic registry of retinoblastoma. Retinoblastoma International Collaborative Study report 2. Graefes Arch Clin Exp Ophthalmol 1995;233(8):469–75.
5. Salim A, Wiknjosastro GH, Danukusumo D, et al. Fetal retinoblastoma. J Ultrasound Med 1998;17(11):717–20.
6. Mietz H, Hutton WL, Font RL. Unilateral retinoblastoma in an adult: report of a case and review of the literature. Ophthalmology 1997;104(1):43–7.
7. Singh AD, Black SH, Shields CL, Shields JA. Prenatal diagnosis of retinoblastoma. J Pediatr Ophthalmol Strabismus 2003;40(4):222–4.
8. Albert DM. Historic review of retinoblastoma. Ophthalmology 1987;94(6):654–62.
9. Sant M, Capocaccia R, Badioni V. Survival for retinoblastoma in Europe. Eur J Cancer 2001;37(6):730–5.
10. Novakovic B. U.S. childhood cancer survival, 1973–1987. Med Pediatr Oncol 1994;23(6):480–6.
11. Abramson DH, Ellsworth RM, Grumbach N, Kitchin FD. Retinoblastoma: survival, age at detection and comparison 1914–1958, 1958–1983. J Pediatr Ophthalmol Strabismus 1985;22(6):246–50.
12. Orjuela M, Castaneda VP, Ridaura C, et al. Presence of human papilloma virus in tumor tissue from children with retinoblastoma: an alternative mechanism for tumor development. Clin Cancer Res 2000;6(10):4010–6.
13. Van Quill KR, O'Brien JM. The Role of the retinoblastoma protein in health, malignancy, and the pathogenesis of retinoblastoma. In: Albert DM, Polans A, editors. Ocular oncology. New York: Marcel Dekker; 2003. p. 103–28.
14. Yunis JJ, Ramsay N. Retinoblastoma and subband deletion of chromosome 13. Am J Dis Child 1978;132(2):161–3.
15. Sparkes RS, Sparkes MC, Wilson MG, et al. Regional assignment of genes for human esterase D and retinoblastoma to chromosome band 13q14. Science 1980;208(4447):1042–4.
16. Connolly MJ, Payne RH, Johnson G, et al. Familial, EsD-linked, retinoblastoma with reduced penetrance and variable expressivity. Hum Genet 1983;65(2):122–4.
17. Friend SH, Bernards R, Rogelj S, et al. A human DNA segment with properties of the gene that predisposes to retinoblastoma and osteosarcoma. Nature 1986;323(6089):643–6.
18. Hernando E, Nahle Z, Juan G, et al. Rb inactivation promotes genomic instability by uncoupling cell cycle progression from mitotic control. Nature 2004;430(7001):797–802.
19. Fung YK, Murphree AL, T'Ang A, et al. Structural evidence for the authenticity of the human retinoblastoma gene. Science 1987;236(4809):1657–61.
20. Dunn JM, Phillips RA, Becker AJ, Gallie BL. Identification of germline and somatic mutations affecting the retinoblastoma gene. Science 1988;241(4874):1797–800.
21. Dunn JM, Phillips RA, Zhu X, et al. Mutations in the RB1 gene and their effects on transcription. Mol Cell Biol 1989;9(11):4596–604.
22. Muncaster MM, Cohen BL, Phillips RA, Gallie BL. Failure of RB1 to reverse the malignant phenotype of human tumor cell lines. Cancer Res 1992;52(3):654–61.
23. Harbour JW. Overview of RB gene mutations in patients with retinoblastoma. Implications for clinical genetic screening. Ophthalmology 1998;105(8):1442–7.
24. Mastrangelo D, Squitieri N, Bruni S, et al. The polymerase chain reaction (PCR) in the routine genetic characterization of retinoblastoma: a tool for the clinical laboratory. Surv Ophthalmol 1997;41(4):331–40.
25. Lohmann DR, Brandt B, Hopping W, et al. The spectrum of RB1 germ-line mutations in hereditary retinoblastoma. Am J Hum Genet 1996;58(5):940–9.
26. Xu K, Rosenwaks Z, Beaverson K, et al. Preimplantation genetic diagnosis for retinoblastoma: the first reported liveborn. Am J Ophthalmol 2004;137(1):18–23.
27. Moll AC, Imhof SM, Cruysberg JR, et al. Incidence of retinoblastoma in children born after in-vitro fertilisation. Lancet 2003;361(9354):309–10.
28. Shields CL, Gorry T, Shields JA. Outcome of eyes with unilateral sporadic retinoblastoma based on the initial external findings by the family and the pediatrician [quiz 72–3]. J Pediatr Ophthalmol Strabismus 2004;41(3):143–9.
29. Abramson DH, Beaverson K, Sangani P, et al. Screening for retinoblastoma: presenting signs as prognosticators of patient and ocular survival. Pediatrics 2003;112(6):1248–55.
30. Bedford MA, Bedotto C, Macfaul PA. Retinoblastoma. A study of 139 cases. Br J Ophthalmol 1971;55(1):19–27.
31. Tarkkanen A, Tuovinen E. Retinoblastoma in Finland 1912–1964. Acta Ophthalmol (Copenh) 1971;49(2):293–300.
32. Reese AB. Tumors of the eye. 3rd ed. New York: Harper and Row; 1976.
33. Schouten-Van Meeteren AY, Moll AC, Imhof SM, Veerman AJ. Overview: chemotherapy for retinoblastoma: an expanding area of clinical research. Med Pediatr Oncol 2002;38(6):428–38.
34. Abramson DH, Ellsworth RM. The surgical management of retinoblastoma. Ophthalmic Surg 1980;11(9):596–8.
35. Abramson DH, Frank CM. Second nonocular tumors in survivors of bilateral retinoblastoma: a possible age effect on radiation-related risk [discussion 9–80]. Ophthalmology 1998;105(4):573–9.
36. Moll AC, Imhof SM, Schouten-Van Meeteren AY, et al. Second primary tumors in hereditary retinoblastoma: a register-based study, 1945–1997: is there an age effect on radiation-related risk? Ophthalmology 2001;108(6):1109–14.
37. Blach LE, McCormick B, Abramson DH. External beam radiation therapy and retinoblastoma: long-term results in the comparison of two techniques. Int J Radiat Oncol Biol Phys 1996;35(1):45–51.
38. Zelter M, Damel A, Gonzalez G, Schwartz L. A prospective study on the treatment of retinoblastoma in 72 patients. Cancer 1991;68(8):1685–90.
39. Hernandez JC, Brady LW, Shields JA, et al. External beam radiation for retinoblastoma: results, patterns of failure, and a proposal for treatment guidelines. Int J Radiat Oncol Biol Phys 1996;35(1):125–32.
40. Scott IU, Murray TG, Feuer WJ, et al. External beam radiotherapy in retinoblastoma: tumor control and comparison of 2 techniques. Arch Ophthalmol 1999;117(6):766–70.
41. Abramson DH, Beaverson KL, Chang ST, et al. Outcome following initial external beam radiotherapy in patients with Reese-Ellsworth group Vb retinoblastoma. Arch Ophthalmol 2004;122(9):1316–23.
42. Shields CL, Santos MC, Diniz W, et al. Thermotherapy for retinoblastoma. Arch Ophthalmol 1999;117(7):885–93.
43. Abramson DH, Schefler AC. Transpupillary thermotherapy as initial treatment for small intraocular retinoblastoma: technique and predictors of success. Ophthalmology 2004;111(5):984–91.
44. Hopping W, Bunke-Schmidt A. Light coagulation and cryotherapy in retinoblastoma. In: Blodi FC, editor. Retinoblastoma. New York: Churchill Livingstone; 1985. p. 95–110.
45. Abramson DH, Ellsworth RM, Rozakis GW. Cryotherapy for retinoblastoma. Arch Ophthalmol 1982;100(8):1253–6.

46. Shields JA, Shields CL, De Potter P. Cryotherapy for retinoblastoma. Int Ophthalmol Clin 1993;33(3):101–5.
47. Stallard HB. The conservative treatment of retinoblastoma. Highlights Ophthalmol 1963;6:129–30.
48. Shields CL, Shields JA, Cater J, et al. Plaque radiotherapy for retinoblastoma: Long-term tumor control and treatment complications in 208 tumors. Ophthalmology 2001;108(11):2116–21.
49. Merchant TE, Gould CJ, Wilson MW, et al. Episcleral plaque brachytherapy for retinoblastoma. Pediatr Blood Cancer 2004;43(2):134–9.
50. Gallie BL, Budning A, DeBoer G, et al. Chemotherapy with focal therapy can cure intraocular retinoblastoma without radiotherapy. Arch Ophthalmol 1996;114(11):1321–8.
51. Kingston JE, Hungerford JL, Madreperla SA, Plowman PN. Results of combined chemotherapy and radiotherapy for advanced intraocular retinoblastoma. Arch Ophthalmol 1996;114(11):1339–43.
52. Murphree AL, Villablanca JG, Deegan WF 3rd, et al. Chemotherapy plus local treatment in the management of intraocular retinoblastoma. Arch Ophthalmol 1996;114(11):1348–56.
53. Shields CL, De Potter P, Himelstein BP, et al. Chemoreduction in the initial management of intraocular retinoblastoma. Arch Ophthalmol 1996;114(11):1330–8.
54. Greenwald MJ, Strauss LC. Treatment of intraocular retinoblastoma with carboplatin and etoposide chemotherapy. Ophthalmology 1996;103(12):1989–97.
55. Chan HS, DeBoer G, Thiessen JJ, et al. Combining cyclosporin with chemotherapy controls intraocular retinoblastoma without requiring radiation. Clin Cancer Res 1996;2(9):1499–508.
56. Shields CL, Shields JA, Needle M, et al. Combined chemoreduction and adjuvant treatment for intraocular retinoblastoma. Ophthalmology 1997;104(12):2101–11.
57. Gunduz K, Shields CL, Shields JA, et al. The outcome of chemoreduction treatment in patients with Reese-Ellsworth group V retinoblastoma. Arch Ophthalmol 1998;116(12):1613–7.
58. Friedman DL, Himelstein B, Shields CL, et al. Chemoreduction and local ophthalmic therapy for intraocular retinoblastoma. J Clin Oncol 2000;18(1):12–7.
59. Beck MN, Balmer A, Dessing C, et al. First-line chemotherapy with local treatment can prevent external-beam irradiation and enucleation in low-stage intraocular retinoblastoma. J Clin Oncol 2000;18(15):2881–7.
60. Vazquez E, Castellote A, Piqueras J, et al. Second malignancies in pediatric patients: imaging findings and differential diagnosis. Radiographics 2003;23(5):1155–72.
61. Wilson MW, Rodriguez-Galindo C, Haik BG, et al. Multiagent chemotherapy as neoadjuvant treatment for multifocal intraocular retinoblastoma [discussion 14–5]. Ophthalmology 2001;108(11):2106–14.
62. Shields CL, Honavar SG, Meadows AT, et al. Chemoreduction plus focal therapy for retinoblastoma: factors predictive of need for treatment with external beam radiotherapy or enucleation. Am J Ophthalmol 2002;133:657–64.
63. Shields CL, Honavar SG, Shields JA, et al. Factors predictive of recurrence of retinal tumors, vitreous seeds, and subretinal seeds following chemoreduction for retinoblastoma. Arch Ophthalmol 2002;120:460–4.
64. Brichard B, De Bruycker JJ, de Potter P, et al. Combined chemotherapy and local treatment in the management of intraocular retinoblastoma. Med Pediatr Oncol 2002;38:411–5.
65. Shields CL, Honavar SG, Meadows AT, et al. Chemoreduction for unilateral retinoblastoma. Arch Ophthalmol 2002;120:1653–8.
66. Rodriguez-Galindo C, Wilson MW, Haik BG, et al. Treatment of intraocular retinoblastoma with vincristine and carboplatin. J Clin Oncol 2003;21:2019–25.
67. Balasubramanya R, Pushker N, Bajaj MS, et al. Visual outcome in macular retinoblastoma treated with primary chemotherapy. Ophthalmologica 2003;217(6):417–21.
68. Sussman DA, Escalona-Benz E, Benz MS, et al. Comparison of retinoblastoma reduction for chemotherapy vs external beam radiotherapy. Arch Ophthalmol 2003;121(7):979–84.
69. Abramson DH, Schefler AC. Update on retinoblastoma. Retina 2004;24(6):828–48.
70. Shields CL, Shelil A, Cater J, et al. Development of new retinoblastomas after 6 cycles of chemoreduction for retinoblastoma in 162 eyes of 106 consecutive patients. Arch Ophthalmol 2003;121(11):1571–6.
71. Lee TC, Hayashi NI, Dunkel IJ, et al. New retinoblastoma tumor formation in children treated initially with systemic carboplatin. Ophthalmology 2003;110:1989–94.
72. Chantada GL, Fandino AC, Raslawski EC, et al. Experience with chemoreduction and focal therapy for intraocular retinoblastoma in a developing country. Pediatr Blood Cancer 2005; 44: 455-460.
73. Chantada G, Fandino A, Davila MT, et al. Results of a prospective study for the treatment of retinoblastoma. Cancer 2004;100(4):834–42.
74. Uusitalo MS, Van Quill KR, Scott IU, et al. Evaluation of chemoprophylaxis in patients with unilateral retinoblastoma with high-risk features on histopathologic examination. Arch Ophthalmol 2001;119(1):41–8.
75. Khelfaoui F, Validire P, Auperin A, et al. Histopathologic risk factors in retinoblastoma: a retrospective study of 172 patients treated in a single institution. Cancer 1996;77(6):1206–13.
76. Shields CL, Shields JA, Baez K, et al. Optic nerve invasion of retinoblastoma. Metastatic potential and clinical risk factors. Cancer 1994;73(3):692–8.
77. Doz F, Neuenschwander S, Plantaz D, et al. Etoposide and carboplatin in extraocular retinoblastoma: a study by the Societe Francaise d'Oncologie Pediatrique. J Clin Oncol 1995;13(4):902–9.
78. Kiratli H, Bilgic S, Ozerdam U. Management of massive orbital involvement of intraocular retinoblastoma. Ophthalmology 1998;105(2):322–6.
79. Chantada GL, Fandino A, Mato G, Casak S. Phase II window of idarubicin in children with extraocular retinoblastoma. J Clin Oncol 1999;17(6):1847–50.
80. Dunkel IJ, Aledo A, Kernan NA, et al. Successful treatment of metastatic retinoblastoma. Cancer 2000;89(10):2117–21.
81. Stram DO, Matthay KK, O'Leary M, et al. Consolidation chemoradiotherapy and autologous bone marrow transplantation versus continued chemotherapy for metastatic neuroblastoma: a report of two concurrent Children's Cancer Group studies. J Clin Oncol 1996;14(9):2417–26.
82. Saarinen UM, Sariola H, Hovi L. Recurrent disseminated retinoblastoma treated by high-dose chemotherapy, total body irradiation, and autologous bone marrow rescue. Am J Pediatr Hematol Oncol 1991;13(3):315–9.
83. Saleh RA, Gross S, Cassano W, Gee A. Metastatic retinoblastoma successfully treated with immunomagnetic purged autologous bone marrow transplantation. Cancer 1988;62(11):2301–3.
84. Namouni F, Doz F, Tanguy ML, et al. High-dose chemotherapy with carboplatin, etoposide and cyclophosphamide followed by a haematopoietic stem cell rescue in patients with high- risk retinoblastoma: a SFOP and SFGM study. Eur J Cancer 1997;33(14):2368–75.
85. Schvartzman E, Chantada G, Fandino A, et al. Results of a stage-based protocol for the treatment of retinoblastoma. J Clin Oncol 1996;14(5):1532–6.
86. White L. Chemotherapy in retinoblastoma. Am J Pediatr Hematol Oncol 1991;13(2):189–201.
87. Puccetti D. Treatment of extraocular retinoblastoma. In: Albert DM, Polans A, editors. Ocular oncology. New York: Marcel Dekker; 2003. p. 489–98.
88. Reese AB, Merriam GR, Martin HE. Treatment of bilateral retinoblastoma by irradiation and surgery. Report on 15-year results. Am J Ophthalmol 1949;32:175–90.
89. Li FP, Abramson DH, Tarone RE, et al. Hereditary retinoblastoma, lipoma, and second primary cancers. J Natl Cancer Inst 1997;89(1):83–4.
90. Abramson DH, Melson MR, Dunkel IJ, Frank CM. Third (fourth and fifth) nonocular tumors in survivors of retinoblastoma. Ophthalmol 2001;108(10):1868–76.
91. Wong FL, Boice JD Jr., Abramson DH, et al. Cancer incidence after retinoblastoma. Radiation dose and sarcoma risk. JAMA 1997;278(15):1262–7.
92. Draper GJ, Sanders BM, Kingston JE. Second primary neoplasms in patients with retinoblastoma. Br J Cancer 1986;53(5):661–71.
93. Eng C, Li FP, Abramson DH, et al. Mortality from second tumors among long-term survivors of retinoblastoma. J Natl Cancer Inst 1993;85(14):1121–8.
94. Derkinderen DJ, Koten JW, Wolterbeek R, et al. Non-ocular cancer in hereditary retinoblastoma survivors and relatives. Ophthalmic Paediatr Genet 1987;8(1):23–5.
95. Moll AC, Imhof SM, Bouter LM, Tan KE. Second primary tumors in patients with retinoblastoma. A review of the literature. Ophthalmic Genet 1997;18(1):27–34.
96. Abramson DH. Second nonocular cancers in retinoblastoma: a unified hypothesis. The Franceschetti Lecture. Ophthalmic Genet 1999;20:193–204.
97. Abramson DH, Jereb B, Wollner N, et al. Leukemic ophthalmopathy detected by ultrasound. J Pediatr Ophthalmol Strabismus 1983;20(3):92–7.
98. Gomez DG, Manzo RP, Fenstermacher JD, Potts DG. Cerebrospinal fluid absorption in the rabbit. Optic pathways. Graefes Arch Clin Exp Ophthalmol 1988;226(1):1–7.
99. Haik BG. Vascular tumors of the orbit. In: Hornblass A, editor. Ophthalmic and orbital plastic reconstructive surgery. Baltimore: Williams and Wilkins; 1989. p. 509–17.
100. Teske S, Ohlrich SJ, Gole G, et al. Treatment of orbital capillary haemangioma with interferon. Aust N Z J Ophthalmol 1994;22(1):13–7.
101. Jones IS. Lymphangiomas of the ocular adnexae: an analysis of 62 cases. Am J Ophthalmol 1961;51:481–509.
102. Abramson DH, Ellsworth RM, Tretter P, et al. The treatment of orbital rhabdomyosarcoma with irradiation and chemotherapy. Ophthalmology 1979;86(7):1330–5.
103. Wharam M, Beltangady M, Hays D, et al. Localized orbital rhabdomyosarcoma. An interim report of the Intergroup Rhabdomyosarcoma Study Committee. Ophthalmology 1987;94(3):251–4.
104. Raney RB, Anderson JR, Kollath J, et al. Late effects of therapy in 94 patients with localized rhabdomyosarcoma of the orbit: Report from the Intergroup Rhabdomyosarcoma Study (IRS) - III, 1984–1991. Med Pediatr Oncol 2000;34(6):413–20.
105. Oberlin O, Rey A, Anderson J, et al. Treatment of orbital rhabdomyosarcoma: survival and late effects of treatment--results of an international workshop. J Clin Oncol 2001;19(1):197–204.
106. Servodidio CA, Abramson DH. Presenting signs and symptoms of choroidal melanoma: what do they mean? Ann Ophthalmol 1992;24(5):190–4.
107. Abramson DH. Computerized visual defects of choroidal melanomas. Glaucoma 1988;10:39–44.
108. Ajani UA, Seddon JM, Hsieh CC, et al. Occupation and risk of uveal melanoma. An exploratory study. Cancer 1992;70(12):2891–900.
109. Coleman DJ, Abramson DH, Jack RL, Franzen LA. Ultrasonic diagnosis of tumors of the choroid. Arch Ophthalmol 1974;91(5):344–54.
110. Byrne SF, Green WL. Ultrasound of the eye and orbit. St. Louis: Mosby; 1992.
111. Accuracy of diagnosis of choroidal melanomas in the Collaborative Ocular Melanoma Study [COMS report no. 1]. Arch Ophthalmol 1990;108(9):1268–73.
112. Shields JA, Shields CL, Donoso LA. Management of posterior uveal melanoma. Surv Ophthalmol 1991;36(3):161–95.
113. Histopathologic characteristics of uveal melanomas in eyes enucleated from the Collaborative Ocular Melanoma Study [COMS report no. 6]. Am J Ophthalmol 1998;125(6):745–66.
114. Factors predictive of growth and treatment of small choroidal melanoma. The Collaborative Ocular Melanoma Study Group [COMS Report No. 5]. Arch Ophthalmol 1997;115(12):1537–44.
115. Mortality in patients with small choroidal melanoma. The Collaborative Ocular Melanoma Study Group [COMS report no. 4]. Arch Ophthalmol 1997;115(7):886–93.
116. Diener-West M, Earle JD, Fine SL, et al. The COMS randomized trial of iodine 125 brachytherapy for choroidal melanoma, III: initial mortality findings [COMS Report No. 18]. Arch Ophthalmol 2001;119(7):969–82.
117. Abramson DH, Servodidio CA. Ocular complications due to cancer treatment. In: Survivors of childhood cancer: assessment and management. St. Louis: Mosby; 1994. p. 111–32.
118. The Collaborative Ocular Melanoma Study (COMS) randomized trial of pre-enucleation radiation of large choroidal melanoma II: initial mortality findings [COMS report no. 10]. Am J Ophthalmol 1998;125(6):779–96.
119. Ophthalmic pathology and intraocular tumors. In: Basic and clinical science course. San Francisco: American Academy of Ophthalmology Publishers; 2004. p. 277–80.
120. Shields CL, Shields JA, Gross NE, et al. Survey of 520 eyes with uveal metastases. Ophthalmol 1997;104(8):1265–76.
121. Cornblath WT. Paraneoplastic disorders of ophthalmic interest. Ophthalmol Clin North Am 2004;17(3):447–54, vii.
122. Guy J, Aptsiauri N. Treatment of paraneoplastic visual loss with intravenous immunoglobulin: report of 3 cases. Arch Ophthalmol 1999;117(4):471–7.
123. Keltner JL, Thirkill CE, Tyler NK, Roth AM. Management and monitoring of cancer-associated retinopathy. Arch Ophthalmol 1992;110(1):48–53.
124. Orbit, eyelids, and lacrimal system. In: Basic and clinical science course. San Francisco: American Academy of Ophthalmology Publishers; 2004. p. 81–9.
125. Coupland SE, Krause L, Delecluse HJ, et al. Lymphoproliferative lesions of the ocular adnexa. Analysis of 112 cases. Ophthalmol 1998;105(8):1430–41.
126. Johnson TE, Tse DT, Byrne GE Jr., et al. Ocular-adnexal lymphoid tumors: a clinicopathologic and molecular genetic study of 77 patients. Ophthal Plast Reconstr Surg 1999;15(3):171–9.

127. Knowles DM, Jakobiec FA, McNally L, Burke JS. Lymphoid hyperplasia and malignant lymphoma occurring in the ocular adnexa (orbit, conjunctiva, and eyelids): a prospective multiparametric analysis of 108 cases during 1977 to 1987. Hum Pathol 1990;21(9):959–73.
128. Kazim M, Goldberg RA, Smith TJ. Insights into the pathogenesis of thyroid-associated orbitopathy: evolving rationale for therapy. Arch Ophthalmol 2002;120(3):380–6.
129. Aurora AL, Blodi FC. Reappraisal of basal cell carcinoma of the eyelids. Am J Ophthalmol 1970;70(3):329–36.
130. Goepfert H, Dichtel WJ, Medina JE, et al. Perineural invasion in squamous cell skin carcinoma of the head and neck. Am J Surg 1984;148(4):542–7.
131. Edwards L, Berman B, Rapini RP, et al. Treatment of cutaneous squamous cell carcinomas by intralesional interferon alfa-2b therapy. Arch Dermatol 1992;128(11):1486–9.

Section 25

ENDOCRINE GLANDS

75

Neoplasms of the Endocrine Glands: Pituitary Neoplasms

Chirag D. Gandhi, MD
Kalmon D. Post, MD

Pituitary adenomas are epithelial tumors arising from the adenohypophysis that can manifest with neurological symptoms from local mass effect such as headaches, visual disturbances, increased intracranial pressure, and cranial nerve palsies, or as a variety of clinical entities depending on the hormones that they secrete. In rare cases, (< 1%) patients can also present with diabetes insipidus. These tumors constitute 10 to 15% of intracranial tumors, although the incidence is as high as 24% in autopsy series. They are most common in the third and fourth decades of life and overall affect both sexes equally. There are, however, differences in frequency between the sexes for certain subtypes, such as Cushing's disease, which is more frequent in women; prolactin (PRL)-secreting adenomas, which are more common in young women; and null-cell adenomas, oncocytomas, and gonadotropin-secreting adenomas, which are more common in men.

The classification of pituitary neoplasms has undergone a variety of modifications since its conception. Classically, they were separated based on the light microscopy characteristics of cell cytoplasm and were divided into acidophilic, basophilic, and chromophobic tumors. Acidophils were thought to produce excess amounts of growth hormone (GH) and were linked to acromegaly and gigantism; basophils were thought to secrete adrenocorticotrophic hormone (ACTH) and cause Cushing's disease; and chromophobes were regarded as hormonally inactive. This system has only limited value since it does not take into consideration either hormone secretion or cellular derivation. It has been well established that both acidophilic and basophilic adenomas may secrete other hormones and that chromophobes can be hormonally active and may secrete GH, PRL, ACTH, thyroid-secreting hormone (TSH), follicle-stimulating hormone (FSH), luteinizing hormone (LH), or α-subunit.[1]

Adenomas are now more commonly classified based on the hormones they secrete.[2,3] Endocrinologically, they are considered either active or inactive and are classified as active only if the amount of hormone they secrete exceeds normal levels in the blood and is clinically evident. Inactive adenomas contain secretory and cellular components necessary for hormone production, but they are not associated with clinical and biochemical evidence of hormone excess. The reason is not well understood, but it is thought that "inactive" cells either produce undetectable levels of hormone or abnormal hormone that is not recognized by the antibody in radioimmunoassay, or that these cells have lost the ability to produce any hormone through some acquired genetic defect.[4] This functional classification is now being further modified to incorporate recent advances in molecular and immunohistochemical advances in pituitary research.

Recent investigations in pituitary tumorigenesis have shown that adenomas are monoclonal proliferations[5–7] and that neoplastic progression is related to oncogenes and to defects in tumor suppressor genes. The only initiating mutation that has been identified so far is in a subset of 10 to 40% of GH-secreting tumors that possess a constitutive activation of the cAMP pathway owing to a point mutation in the α-chain of the GTP binding protein, Gs. This results in elevated cAMP formation and subsequent GH hypersecretion and adenoma proliferation.[8] Although it has been theorized that adenomas with this *gsp* oncogene mutation are smaller and more sensitive to medical therapy, recent studies have failed to demonstrate any phenotypic differences in patients with and without the *gsp* mutation.[9] Extensive research has resulted in a multiplicity of other factors that influence pituitary tumor progression. Other oncogenes that have been linked to adenoma progression include cAMP-responsive nuclear transcription factor, *CREB*, which is also thought to be promoted by the overexpression of Gsα;[9] *ras* oncogene mutations that have been detected in aggressive prolactinomas;[10] and more recently, the pituitary tumor transforming gene, *PTTG*, which may be a new marker for invasiveness in secretory adenomas.[11] Tumor suppressor genes such as *Rb*, *menin*, *TP53*, *p27*, *p16*[12,13] as well as promoting factors such as hypothalamic neurohormones and locally produced growth factors and cytokines are also being studied to aid in the understanding of adenoma growth. Novel therapeutic target receptors are also being investigated. These include galectin-3 (Gal-3), found only in prolactin, and ACTH hormone-secreting tumor lines, as well as the nuclear receptor, peroxisome proliferator-activated receptor gamma (PPAR-γ), which has been isolated in a variety of adenoma lines.[14–16] The exact molecular mechanisms of pituitary adenoma proliferation are still incompletely understood, but once they are better defined, additional treatment options may be available.

Patients presenting with a suspected or known pituitary adenoma need to undergo a complete radiographic and endocrine assessment prior to the initiation of either medical or surgical therapy. Magnetic resonance imaging (MRI) is the modality of choice and should be requested with a localized pituitary protocol that includes thin cuts in the coronal and sagittal planes (Figures 75-1A and B). MRI helps to depict tumor size, extension,

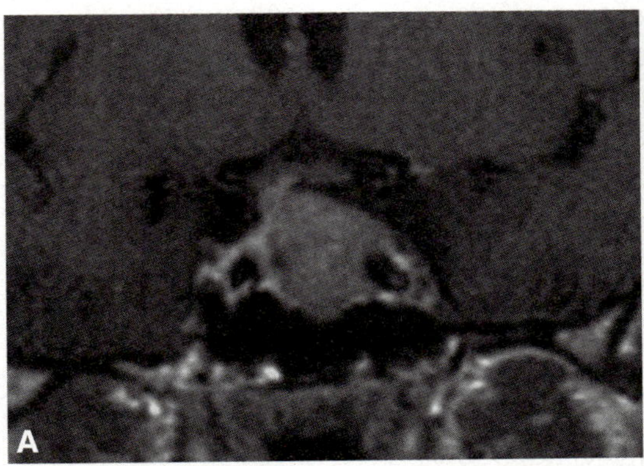

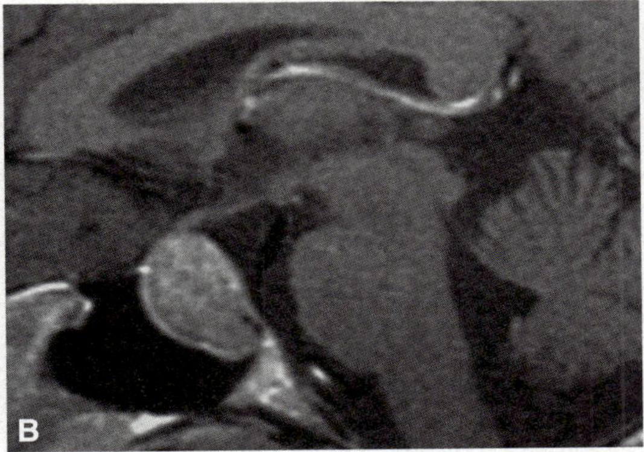

Figure 75-1 A 38-year-old woman with an ACTH-secreting adenoma. **A,** Coronal T1-weighted magnetic resonance with contrast demonstrates a hypointense macroadenoma within the sella that extends into the left cavernous sinus and encases part of the carotid artery. **B,** Sagittal T1-weighted magnetic resonance with contrast demonstrates a hyperintense macroadenoma within the sella.

and characteristics such as hemorrhagic and cystic changes (T2-weighted images). Gadolinium is also essential for increasing the diagnostic yield for microadenomas (< 10 mm) and useful in delineating normal and abnormal tissue in macroadenomas (T1-weighted images pre- and post-gadolinium).[17] In general, a hypointense lesion on a noncontrast MRI that demonstrates less enhancement with gadolinium than normal pituitary tissue raises the suspicion of a pituitary adenoma. This is particularly important in parasellar invasive tumors. Based on radiographic imaging, Jules Hardy first classified pituitary adenomas based on their extent of intrasellar and extrasellar extension as well as their invasiveness (Figure 75-2).[18] In addition to radiographic imaging, the patient's baseline endocrine panel should include serum GH, insulin-like growth factor (IGF-1), TSH, free T4, T3, PRL, ACTH, cortisol, LH, FSH, and testosterone. Following these tests, the determination of further medical or surgical treatments can be made.

With the exception of prolactinomas, which can be medically managed long term with dopamine agonists, and asymptomatic, endocrine-inactive tumors that can be followed with serial imaging; surgery is the preferred definitive treatment of pituitary adenomas. Based on innovative work by Cushing, Guiot, and Hardy the transsphenoidal approach is the preferred surgical technique for most adenomas.[19] The goals of surgery include the reduction of any mass effect created by the tumor, the cessation of endocrine hyperactivity, and the preservation or restoration of pituitary function. These goals can now be achieved quickly with minimal morbidity through the transsphenoidal approach.[20] Postoperatively, based on the type of pituitary adenoma, hormone status, and the degree of extrasellar extension, decisions regarding adjuvant therapy can then be made.

PROLACTIN-SECRETING PITUITARY ADENOMAS

Prolactinomas are the most commonly diagnosed pituitary adenoma, representing approximately 30% of cases.[21] Rarely life threatening, they cause symptoms primarily as a result of hyperprolactinemia, which, in turn, results in alterations in reproductive and sexual function, but may also cause symptoms related to mass effect. This is the only pituitary tumor in which a reliably effective medical treatment is available, and that in most cases is the favored primary therapy (Figure 75-3). Surgical treatment, however, has been proven to provide similar results as in other endocrine-secreting adenomas and is applicable as the primary intervention for prolactinomas in certain cases.

Clinical Presentation Although prolactinomas are distributed evenly between men and women at autopsy, women are four times more likely to become symptomatic than men. With very few exceptions, prolactinomas are slow growing and the clinical presentation differs in men and women. In women of reproductive age, the symptoms are typically oligomenorrhea or secondary amenorrhea, galactorrhea, and sterility followed by decreased libido, dry vaginal mucosa owing to a deficiency in estrogen, weight gain, and psychological symptoms such as depression and anxiety. Approximately 5% of women with primary amenorrhea and 25% of women with secondary amenorrhea (excluding pregnancy) have a prolactinoma.[22] When galactorrhea accompanies amenorrhea, the incidence increased to 70 to 80%.[23] In men and in postmenopausal women the tumors grow to much larger sizes and are only detected once they begin to produce mass effect resulting in headaches, visual disturbances (most commonly a bitemporal hemianopsia from chiasmal compression), hypopituitarism, ophthalmoplegia, and, rarely, hydrocephalus from obstruction of the foramen of Monro. Men may also experience a diminished libido, impotence, gynecomastia, and infertility from decreased androgen production.

There still exists significant debate on the exact mechanism of hypogonadism caused by hyperprolactinemia. The most likely explanation is that prolactin, through dopamine inhibition, alters the hypothalamic release of gonadotropin-releasing hormone (GnRH), causing disruptions in the normal pulsatile secretion of LH.[24] Prolonged periods of hyperprolactinemia have also been linked to bone demineralization, which is the result of hypogonadism and not of the elevated prolactin levels per se, as previously believed, since bone density is normal in eumenorrhic hyperprolactinemic women.[25]

Diagnosis Besides prolactinomas, hyperprolactinemia can be associated with a variety of causes such as pregnancy, hypothyroidism, prolactin-stimulating drugs (eg, phenothiazines, butyrophenones, metoclopramide), and renal failure that need to be considered in the differential diagnosis. In addition, physiological hyperprolactinemia can occur from psychological and physical stresses, such as exercise, surgery, and hypoglycemia, but the prolactin level rarely exceeds 40 ng/mL in these cases.[26] A definitive diagnosis of prolactinoma is difficult and in most cases requires radiographic evidence in addition to elevated PRL levels. In men, a basal PRL value greater than 100 ng/mL is almost always indicative of a prolactinoma. In women, levels over 200 ng/mL are also highly suggestive of prolactinomas and values 100 to 200 ng/mL are also likely to be associated with

Sella Turcica radiological classification	Extrasellar extensions: Suprasellar			Parasellar	
Grade 0 (normal)	A	B	C	D	E
Grade I					
Grade II					
Grade III					
Grade VI	Symmetrical			Asymmetrical	

Figure 75-2 Hardy's classification of pituitary adenomas. Grade I and II are enclosed within the sella. Grades III and IV are invasive. Extrasellar classifications A, B, and C are increasing amounts of direct suprasellar adenomas. D is asymmetric extension, and E is lateral extension into the cavernous sinus. (Adapted from Hardy J and Somma M.[18])

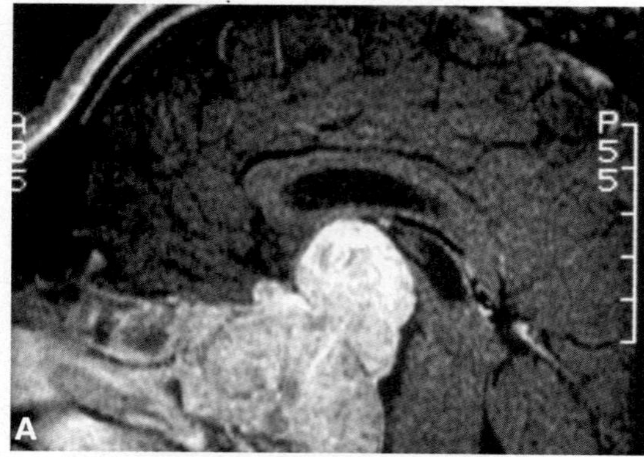

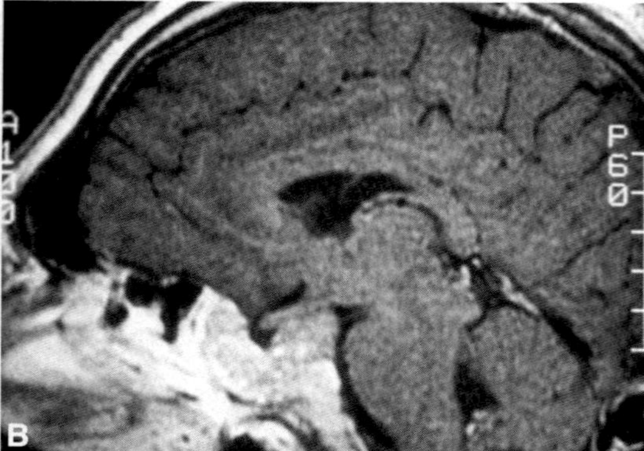

Figure 75-3 A 52-year-old male with diminished libido and a macroprolactinoma. **A,** Sagittal T1-weighted magnetic resonance with contrast demonstrates a large sellar/suprasellar adenoma with compression of the optic chiasm. **B,** Sagittal T1-weighted with contrast demonstrates a significant reduction in tumor volume after being treated medically with bromocriptine.

prolactin-secreting adenomas.[26,27] The greatest diagnostic uncertainty lies in women with PRL values from 50 to 100 ng/mL, which is termed moderate hyperprolactinemia. In these cases the elevated prolactin could be from a prolactin-secreting tumor, but could also be from "stalk effect" caused by a nonsecreting adenoma that interferes with the flow of prolactin-inhibitory factor (PRIF) from the hypothalamus. Although various endocrine stimulation tests to differentiate these two possibilities have been suggested, they have not proven to be reliable.[28]

Serum PRL levels are an index of secretory activity and have been found to be associated with the size of the prolactinoma, excluding any associated cystic or necrotic component. If the PRL is less than 200 ng/mL, 80% of tumors are microadenomas; if PRL is greater than 200 ng/mL, only 20% are microadenomas. This relationship, however, does not hold true for giant prolactinomas (> 4 cm). The PRL may be > 1,000 ng/mL, but falsely low serum prolactin levels (25–150 ng/mL) have also been described despite the existence of giant or invasive prolactinomas; the phenomenon is known as the "hook effect."[29,30] Briefly, the hook effect occurs when during radioimmunoassay the antibody binding sites become saturated and the binding curve is no longer proportional to the prolactin level. This can be resolved by performing serial dilutions.

Treatment The treatment options available to a patient with a prolactinoma include observation, medical therapy, surgical therapy, and radiotherapy. The best treatment depends on tumor size, prolactin level, clinical manifestations, tolerance of medical therapy, and the desire for fertility. Studies have demonstrated that the vast majority of microprolactinomas (< 10 mm) do not increase in size.[31] Additionally, autopsy series have found the frequent occurrence of incidental microprolactinomas. Based on this, if patients have only mildly elevated prolactin, normal pituitary function, no clinical symptoms, and no desire for pregnancy, observation with serial radiographic and endocrine evaluation is reasonable.

Lactotrophs are controlled by a negative dopaminergic effect from the hypothalamus, and based on this, dopamine agonists have become the standard medical therapy. Unlike long-term medical treatment of other endocrine-active pituitary disorders, dopamine agonists have been remarkably effective in both reducing the size of the tumor as well as normalizing serum prolactin levels below the accepted remission level of 25 ng/mL. Bromocriptine was the first of these medications, but more recently, others such as cabergoline, quinagolide, lisuride, pergolide mesylate, and terguride are also used. Biomolecular studies have shown that dopamine agonists selectively activate type D2 dopamine receptors blocking the transcription of the prolactin gene.[32] The shrinkage of prolactin cells results in amyloid deposition in and fibrosis of the tumor.[33] Dopamine agonists have been shown to have a high response rate with reports of normalization of prolactin in 70 to 80%, tumor shrinkage in 80 to 90%, and restoration of ovulation in 80 to 90%.[34] Based on these results, some would argue that medical treatment should be used in all patients except the 10% who have significant side effects.[35] In addition, an important recent study indicates that a majority of patients who respond to cabergoline with normalization of prolactin levels and a reduction in tumor size may experience remission of hyperprolactinemia following discontinuation of the drug.[36] Although the follow-up period has been relatively short, this study suggests the potential for a curative treatment with medical therapy in a select group of patients.

Dopamine agonists do have some significant disadvantages that may temper their use in all patients. The effects are reversible, making the therapy lifelong in most cases, and thus requiring significant compliance. Additionally, there can be significant side effects including nausea, vomiting, postural hypotension, headaches, as well as depression and anxiety that can make long-term compliance even more difficult in some patients. In cases of pituitary apoplexy and in tumors with large cystic components, dopamine agonists are not effective in shrinkage. A group of bromocriptine-resistant prolactinomas with increased aggressiveness and increased incidence in males has also been recently described.[37]

The role of surgery in the treatment of prolactinomas has been under discussion. Some argue that surgery should be the initial treatment, with medical therapy as an adjunct only in cases without remission.[38] The rate of long-term remission varies significantly, however, depending on the size of the tumor and preoperative prolactin levels. The most favorable results have been demonstrated in microadenomas with levels below 200 ng/mL with remission rates ranging from 50 to 84% in long-term follow-up.[34,38–40] The remission rate drops with macroadenomas and with prolactin levels from 200 to 500 ng/mL, even though these tumors are amenable to surgical resection. Surgery has not been shown to be useful in giant adenomas and in tumors with prolactin levels greater than 500 ng/mL, where the remission rate decreases to 0%. These lesions are better treated with medical therapy, possibly in conjunction with surgery and radiation. Overall, the lower the prolactin level, the greater the chance of long-term cure.

Because of the successful long-term control of prolactinomas with medical and surgical options, conventional radiotherapy is generally not considered a primary mode of treatment. It is used in certain invasive tumors, but even that indication is under debate.[41] The use of stereotactic radiosurgery as either a primary treatment modality[42] or as an adjuvant therapy[43] is becoming increasingly common. In various recent studies, in addition to a decrease in the prolactin level, the endocrine cure rates with radiosurgery have been approximately 30%.[44] These results, however, are confounded by variations in the number of patients who are on medical therapy at the time of radiosurgery, making a true assessment of efficacy unclear.

Recommendation Based on the results discussed above, the recommendations for the optimum treatment of prolactinomas needs to be tailored to the tumor size, prolactin level, and the patient's own wishes. Medical therapy is the first option for almost all prolactinomas. Treatment with a dopamine agonist can be considered as the primary treatment with almost all microadenomas, including patients desiring pregnancy or those with primary amenorrhea.

Based on the most current literature, surgical removal with a high remission can be recommended for most macroadenomas with prolactin < 200 ng/mL. For tumors larger than 2 cm and prolactin < 500 ng/mL, patients should be first treated with a dopamine agonist to reduce the tumor volume and then undergo surgical resection. Any residual tumor can then be treated medically. For very large or invasive tumors or for tumors with prolactin greater than 500 ng/mL, medical therapy should be the primary treatment modality.

The subgroup that needs specific discussion comprises patients who are pregnant and harbor prolactinomas. There is a small but serious risk related to the possible rapid expansion of the tumor. Complications occur primarily from macroprolactinomas that have suprasellar extension; they are much less frequent in cases of microprolactinomas.[45] If the patient becomes symptomatic, a dopamine-agonist can be administered. The data regarding the effects of continuous dopamine-agonist therapy on the fetus are limited, however, but suggest no ill effect. During pregnancy, surgery should be undertaken only if the tumor does not respond to medical treatment and if there are progressive neurological symptoms. Patients with macroadenomas who desire pregnancy should undergo a transsphenoidal resection prior to conception.

GROWTH HORMONE-SECRETING PITUITARY ADENOMAS

Growth hormone secretion is under hypothalamic control through somatostatin and growth hormone releasing hormone (GHRH). Upon release, GH causes the production of IGF-1 from the liver, which, in turn, affects bone and tissue growth and also inhibits further release of GH and GHRH. These inhibitory feedback loops are ineffective in acromegaly, and GH release continues autonomously. The clinical manifestations of growth hormone-secreting pituitary tumors have been found to better correlate with IGF-1 levels than with GH levels.

Clinical Presentation These tumors account for about 30% of all endocrine-active pituitary tumors and most patients present in their third to fifth decade with macroadenomas with a long subclinical course ranging from 4 to 10 years.[46] Growth hormone excess classically presents as acromegaly or gigantism, both marked by an insidious coarsening of features with frontal bossing and prognathism, macroglossia, and exaggerated acral growth. Patients are also found to develop organomegaly, hypertension, cardiomyopathy, congestive heart failure, restrictive lung disease, sleep apnea, and arthropathies. Additionally, a very high percentage of acromegalic patients have impaired glucose metabolism and diabetes mellitus. Common symptoms include fatigue, headaches, arthralgias, oily skin, hyperhidrosis, and in patients with a cosecreting prolactin variant, amenorrhea, galactorrhea, and loss of libido. The slow, progressive symptoms are associated with mortalities as high as 50% by the age of 50 in untreated patients, 2 to 3 times that of the general population.[47]

Diagnosis The diagnosis is usually apparent based only on the characteristic physical appearance and the frequent subclinical history. Elevated basal fasting GH levels greater that 2.5 ng/mL or, more accurately, an elevated IGF-1 is suggestive of acromegaly. IGF-1 levels must be corrected for age and sex. These values are more accurate than GH levels because they are more stable throughout the day. Dynamic testing is usually not useful in diagnosis and is usually reserved for monitoring therapeutic efficacy. The most common test is the oral glucose tolerance test (OGTT), which involves the tracking of serial GH levels after a 75- to 100-gram oral glucose load. In normal patients, GH levels should suppress below 1 ng/mL.

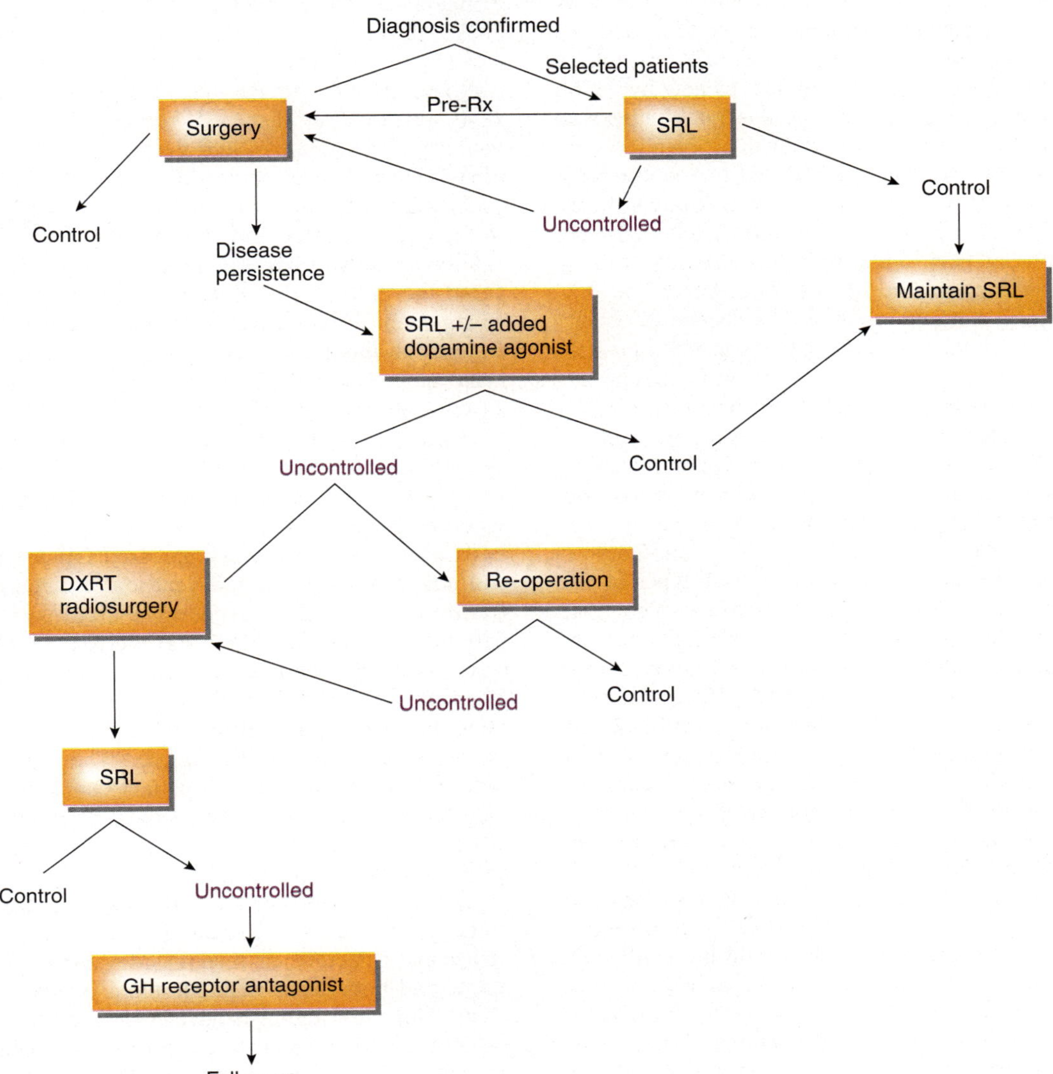

Figure 75-4 The algorithm for the management of acromegaly. Control suggests a glucose-suppressed GH less than 1 ng/mL, a normalized age, and gender matched IGF-1. DXRT = radiation therapy. (From Melmeds et al,[47] with permission.)

A lack of suppression is diagnostic for a growth hormone-secreting tumor. Owing to the improved sensitivity and specificity of the GH assay, there have been questions about whether GH suppression criteria during an OGTT in patients with acromegaly should be modified for gender or age similar to those for IGF-1. A recent study of 92 patients with acromegaly, however, suggests that nadir levels of GH did not vary significantly based on either age or gender.[48]

Once the clinical and biochemical diagnosis is confirmed, an MRI determines the location and size of the tumor. If this fails to demonstrate a pituitary tumor, a possible ectopic GHRH source, occurring in about 1% of cases, should be sought in the chest or abdomen.

Treatment Outcome measures for cure have been modified multiple times since the initial availability of a growth hormone assay in the 1960s. Currently, the biochemical goals of therapy are to reduce basal GH levels to less than 2.5 ng/mL, to normalize IGF-1 levels, and to achieve a nadir GH level of less than 1 ng/mL with an oral glucose tolerance test[49] (Figure 75-4). A complete cure should lead to recovery of normal pituitary function in most cases a slow reversal of both cosmetic and physiological abnormalities.

Transsphenoidal surgery remains the primary treatment of these adenomas.[47] The advantages of surgery include a prompt decrease in GH levels, relief of mass effect, and a tissue diagnosis. At our institution, a 14-year review of 115 patients yielded a biochemical remission in 61% of cases with transsphenoidal surgery alone.[50] The rate was 88% for microadenomas and 53% for macroadenomas. Tumor size and preoperative GH levels were found to correlate negatively with surgical outcome. Immediate postoperative GH levels were found to correlate with long-term outcome. In cases where the postoperative GH level was less than 3 ng/mL, the chance of favorable long-term outcome was 89%. Postoperative radiotherapy was given to 32 patients and 31% of these cases are still in remission. An additional 3 patients are in remission with surgery, radiotherapy, and medical treatment. The overall complication rate was 6.9%, with no CSF leaks, meningitis, permanent diabetes insipidus, or new hypopituitarism. The recurrence rate was 5.4%. Other studies have reported similar results.[51,52]

Both radiotherapy and, more recently, radiosurgery have been used for the treatment of acromegaly. The use of conventional external radiation has been found to reduce GH levels to less than 5 ng/mL in 50 to 70% of cases, but these effects can take as long as a decade to occur.[53] Hypopituitarism has been found in 50% of patients 10 years after irradiation, with an increasing incidence annually thereafter.[54] Radiosurgery has demonstrated that normalization of GH levels can be achieved within 3 to 5 years.[55] A similar rate of hypopituitarism is likely to occur, however. Additionally, damage to the optic chiasm remains a concern, and a safety distance of 4 mm should be respected in the management of all types of pituitary adenomas. In general, radiosurgery continues to be an adjunctive therapy after failed transsphenoidal surgery. Remissions have been demonstrated in an additional 30 to 50% of patients within 2 years.[51,56,57] A recent review found that a significant problem in the interpretation of radiosurgical results was the inconsistent definition of "normal."[44] Endocrine cure rates in a variety of small studies were found to range from 0 to 96% and improvement in 0 to 67%. Out of 20 studies reviewed, 6 did not cite their criteria for cure, and 11 of 14 other studies used different criteria to define cure. These results are further confounded by the inconsistent use of somatostatin analogues in patients undergoing radiosurgery. Current studies on the efficacy of radiosurgery also have limited long-term follow-up. Additional randomized studies are needed.

Medical management as the primary or adjuvant treatment of acromegaly remains a controversial topic. In patients who do not have visual loss, some neuroendocrinologists have advocated treatment with somatostatin analogues as the primary treatment.[58] Most practitioners, however, citing the significant morbidity associated with acromegaly, advocate surgical resection followed by adjuvant medical treatment or radiotherapy if needed. Three classes of drugs are used to treat acromegaly: dopamine agonists, somatostatin analogues, and GH-receptor blockers. Dopamine agonists such as bromocriptine and cabergoline have been shown to provide symptomatic relief in some acromegalic patients. However, these medications rarely reduce the basal GH to less than 2.5 ng/mL and normalize IGF-1 in less than 30% of patients.[59] Their effectiveness is also limited by the side effects. Despite their limited efficacy as compared with other medical options, dopamine agonists remain popular because of their lower cost and ease of oral administration. Somatostatin analogues such as octreotide have been found to be more effective. Octreotide normalizes IGF-1 levels and reduces GH levels to less than 5 ng/mL in approximately 50% of patients.[60] The long-acting analogues such as lanreotide and octreotide LAR can reduce GH below 2.5 ng/mL in 70% of cases and normalize IGF-1 in 88% of patients.[61–63] The newest medication group is the GH-receptor antagonist pegvisomant, which does not act on the pituitary gland, but instead prevents dimerization of the GH-receptor, and thus inhibits the generation of IGF, the primary effector of GH action. A recent study demonstrated 97% of patients treated with pegvisomant had a reduction in their age-adjusted IGF-1 to normal levels.[64] Additional studies, however, have raised concerns about the elevation of liver transaminases and enlargement in tumor size in a small number of patients on this medication.[65] These side effects make interval MRI and liver function testing imperative in patients using this medication.

Medical treatment has been found to provide symptomatic relief of headaches and hyperhidrosis as well as to improve arthropathy and cardiac function. Recent studies have demonstrated that in patients whose glucose-suppressed GH levels and IGF-1 normalized, left-ventricular ejection fraction (LVEF) improved. In a majority of patients with uncontrolled acromegaly, LVEF deteriorated.[66,67] Although current medical therapies are well tolerated and demonstrate good efficacy, they are required lifelong, with recurrence once the medication is discontinued. The significant cost and problems with patient compliance long term continue to make medical treatments more useful as an adjuvant treatment after surgery and radiosurgery have been used.

Between 20 and 30% of GH-secreting adenomas cosecrete PRL. Women often report amenorrhea and galactorrhea, men may develop impotence, and both sexes may complain of loss of libido. Dopamine agonists have been found to be particularly effective in the treatment of acromegalic patients with mixed GH- and PRL-secreting tumors, but transsphenoidal surgery remains the primary treatment.[68]

ADRENOCORTICOTROPHIC HORMONE-SECRETING ADENOMAS

In Cushing's disease, the largest subset of Cushing's syndrome, hypersecretion of ACTH by the pituitary results in adrenal hyperplasia and hypercortisolism. Cushing's disease is considered by many to be the most challenging pituitary endocrinopathy to diagnose and treat. The problems in long-term cure arise from difficulties in detection of minute tumors, even with MRI. Furthermore, aggressive macroadenomas have a high rate of recurrence. The incidence is nine times more frequent in women and usually occurs in the third and fourth decades.

Clinical Presentation Only about 10 to 20% of ACTH-secreting adenomas are large enough to produce mass effect, resulting in visual field deficits, cranial nerve involvement, or hypopituitarism. Over 50% of tumors are less than 5 mm and first become evident because of the endocrine presentation. Patients with Cushing's disease most commonly present with centripetal obesity, moon facies, buffalo hump, hirsutism, purple abdominal striae, and acne. The main signs include hypertension, osteopenia, proximal myopathy, diabetes mellitus, and significant psychiatric disorders. These clinical syndromes not only cause severe morbidity, but also a 5-year mortality rate of 50% among untreated patients.[69]

Diagnosis The accurate diagnosis of Cushing's disease is actually a two-step process once a patient has suggestive clinical signs and symptoms. The first step is to determine that the hypercortisolism is actually the result of a pituitary adenoma and not the result either of an adrenal or another ectopic source. The second step is the accurate localization of the adenoma, which in many cases is not possible by static MRI alone. The algorithm for a complete diagnosis is nearly 100% accurate,[70] but each test alone carries a failure rate of 10 to 30%[71] (Table 75-1).

Hypercortisolism can be quickly verified by an elevation in the 24-hour urinary free cortisol and 17-OH corticosteroids. More recently, a midnight salivary cortisol level has been demonstrated to be a highly sensitive and specific method by which to diagnose hypercortisolism.[72] The diagnosis of Cushing's disease may then be suggested with a low-dose dexamethasone suppression test that does not suppress serum cortisol to less than 10 µg/dL. Adrenal cortisol-producing adenomas can be ruled out if plasma ACTH is more than 5 ng/L.[73] After ACTH-dependent hypercortisolism has been established, the next step is the exclusion of an ectopic ACTH syndrome by a high-dose dexamethasone suppression test. In 95% of Cushing's disease cases, the plasma cortisol levels are reduced to less than 50% of baseline, whereas in ectopic ACTH or adrenal tumors cortisol levels remain unchanged. Corticotropin-releasing hormone (CRH) stimulation is also advocated in conjunction with the dexamethasone suppression test in order to increase sensitivity.[74] In patients where this testing is not compelling, inferior petrosal sinus sampling (IPSS) must be performed to confirm the pituitary etiology.

After the definitive diagnosis of Cushing's disease has been established, the tumor must be localized before treatment can be initiated. If an MRI demonstrates a possible adenoma, treatment can then be initiated. The threshold for most MRI techniques is an adenoma 3 mm in diameter; however, 50% of ACTH-secreting tumors may thus be undetected. In this case IPSS and cavernous sinus sampling to measure the levels of ACTH after CRH stimulation should be performed. A gradient of 2:1 localizes the adenoma within the pituitary gland. The results may suggest laterality in the pituitary gland with this technique, but there is a 25 to 30% error rate in the localization.[75]

Treatment Transsphenoidal surgical resection is the first option for treatment of Cushing's disease. A review of the current surgical literature demonstrates that the remission rates range from

Table 75-1 The Biochemical Evaluation for Cushing's Syndrome

A. Screening for Cushing's syndrome
1. Measurement of 24 hr UFC in 2 or 3 collections. Test is unequivocal for hypercortisolism if the cortisol level is 4-fold that of normal in 2 of 3 screens. If equivocal, proceed to the low-dose DST. Salivary cortisol levels are also highly sensitive and specific.
2. Low-dose DST. 1 mg dexamethasone is administered at 11 pm and serum cortisol is drawn the following day at 8 am. A 2-day test is also commonly performed.
   If < 5 μg/dL: Cushing's syndrome is excluded
   If 5–10 μg/dL: Indeterminate and retesting is necessary
   If > 10 μg/dL: Cushing's syndrome is probably present

B. Tests to distinguish primary Cushing's disease from ectopic or adrenal tumors
1. Serum ACTH is low in adrenal tumors. Plasma ACTH (values > 10 pg/mL are suggestive of ACTH-dependent disease; values < 5 pg/mL are suggestive of ACTH-independent disease).
   Abdominal CT can help identify a unilateral adrenal mass or bilateral adrenal enlargement in ACTH-dependent cases
2. High-dose DST. 8 mg of dexamethasone is administered at 11 pm and serum cortisol is drawn the following day at 8 am. A 2-day test is also commonly performed.
   In 95% of cases of Cushing's disease, plasma cortisol is suppressed by 50%
   No suppression is seen with ectopic or adrenal sources
3. CRH stimulation test. Can be used after an equivocal high-dose DMT.
   Cushing's disease responds to CRH with further increases in plasma cortisol levels
   Ectopic and adrenal tumors do not respond to CRH
4. IPSS is reserved for persistent equivocal testing or in reoperations in which IPSS was not initially performed.
   After CRH administration, an inferior petrosal sinus/plasma cortisol gradient > 3:1 is suggestive of Cushing's disease and aids with lateralization

DST = dexamethasone suppression test; UFC = urinary free cortisol.

76 to 91%, and in microadenomas, ranges from 84 to 94%.[76] Outcomes with the latter group were found to be dependent on the ability to visualize that adenoma on MRI.[77] The outcomes in macroadenomas appear to be dependent on the degree of invasiveness, with a reported 64% cure rate with surgery alone and 83% with adjuvant radiotherapy.[76] During the immediate postoperative period there is a rapid decline in both serum cortisol and ACTH levels, and patients must be monitored closely for symptoms of hypocortisolism (Addisonian crisis). Most patients require replacement therapy for up to 1 year as their own hypothalamic-pituitary axis recovers from the chronic overstimulation by ACTH. Various studies have attempted to assess the predictors of long-term cure.[78,79] Subnormal levels of cortisol and ACTH postoperatively are strong indicators for full remission, but even in these cases a 15 to 25% recurrence rate may occur over time.[16,80] In our experience, even normal cortisol and restoration of normal dexamethasone suppression do not necessarily indicate lasting remission. Because of this, long-term follow-up is essential in these patients.

Both radiotherapy and radiosurgery have been commonly used as adjuvant treatment of patients with recurrent or invasive tumors that are not cured by surgery alone. The cure rates of conventional radiotherapy have been reported to be as high as 90% at 5 years post-treatment. A large proportion of these patients began to experience hypopituitarism in later years, and 5% developed Nelson's syndrome.[81] Conventional radiation is not used as a primary modality because remission cannot be achieved for a long period of time, and patients continue to suffer from the symptoms and morbidities of Cushing's disease. As an alternative, radiosurgery has the advantage of having an effect on ACTH secretion much sooner than conventional radiation. Cure rates of 35 to 90% are reported, and much lower rates of hypopituitarism.[82,83] The reported rates of success, however, are confounded by inconsistent measures of "cure" and limited long-term follow-up. Radiosurgery as a primary treatment modality has limited outcome assessment.

For patients who fail surgical treatment or in whom surgery cannot be tolerated, the most common medical treatment is ketoconazole, which acts by blocking adrenal steroid synthesis. Occasionally, ketoconazole is also used for a few weeks preoperatively to control the severe manifestations of hypercortisolism. Cortisol and ACTH levels can return to normal in up to 90% of patients, but patients must be monitored closely for hepatotoxicity; the effects of ketoconazole stop immediately after discontinuation.[84] Other agents have also been employed, including aminoglutethimide, metyrapone, mitotane, and cyproheptadine. Recent studies are attempting to assess the role of dopamine agonists in the treatment of ACTH-secreting tumors. The administration of cabergoline therapy for 3 months was found to inhibit cortisol secretion in 60% of patients, with a normalization in 40% of patients.[85] This study also demonstrated dopamine receptor (D2) immunostaining in a majority of ACTH-secreting adenomas and requires further study. The PPAR-γ ligand rosiglitazone is also being studied as a possible new treatment option.[86]

Total adrenalectomy can also control hypercortisolism but requires lifelong dependence on exogenous glucocorticoid and mineral corticoid replacement. Additionally it can result in Nelson's syndrome in 10 to 30% of patients and carries a generally unfavorable prognosis. Nelson's syndrome presents as hyperpigmentation from loss of cortisol inhibition and the stimulation of melanocytes by elevated ACTH. Most patients that present with Nelson's syndrome harbor large, invasive pituitary adenomas that are very difficult to cure surgically and often require adjuvant radiotherapy and medical treatment. Studies have demonstrated variable effectiveness of neurosurgical treatment of Nelson's syndrome, ranging from 10 to 70%. These small series, however, have been plagued by lack of uniform definitions of "cure" and limited long-term follow-up.[87,88] More recently, a report on 13 patients with Nelson's syndrome with a median follow-up of 17 years more convincingly demonstrated the efficacy of neurosurgical intervention.[89] Fortunately, the overall incidence has declined significantly since transsphenoidal surgery replaced bilateral adrenalectomy as the primary treatment of Cushing's disease.

In the event of a noncure, a second surgical procedure with a more aggressive exploration of the pituitary gland for tumor is usually effective, since the most common cause of surgical failure is that the adenoma could not be found.[90] If IPSS was not performed prior to the first surgery, it should be before a second surgery. A complete hypophysectomy, even after initial failure, is rarely indicated; it is performed at our institution only for patients with a tenuous condition or in those who insist on it. In the event of surgical failure after a second surgery, medical therapy, radiation, or even bilateral adrenalectomy can be considered. Because of the significant rate of recurrence, even many years after surgery, patients in remission need to be followed with interval endocrine evaluations.

Silent ACTH-Secreting Adenomas A more recently described entity is that of silent ACTH-secreting adenomas in which immunohistochemical staining demonstrates reactivity for ACTH without any preoperative signs or symptoms of hypercortisolism. The exact incidence is unclear but has been reported to be between 6 and 43% in published studies.[91] In addition to the lack of any clinical findings of Cushing's disease, there is also no evidence of hypercortisolism on laboratory testing. This is usually a surprise diagnosis, and the role of the pathologist in accurately determining the entity is critical for the immediate postoperative period as well as for long-term management. Studies have suggested that silent corticotrophic adenomas behave aggressively with a high rate of recurrence, as high as 37%.[92,93] This underscores the reason for long-term follow-up as well as the possibility of postoperative radiation. In addition, studies have also shown that in the immediate postoperative period, a subgroup of silent ACTH-secreting adenomas develop ACTH-cortisol axis dysfunction and require postoperative steroid replacement.[91]

GONADOTROPIN-SECRETING AND NONSECRETING PITUITARY ADENOMAS

Approximately one-third of pituitary tumors are considered nonsecreting adenomas. They are generally associated with an older age population, with a peak in the fifth decade. Patients usually present with signs and symptoms of hypopituitarism, and commonly with associated visual field defects and other ophthalmologic problems. Despite their similar clinical presentation, endocrine-inactive tumors are a heterogeneous group of tumors. Ultrastructural studies have demonstrated that these tumors actually contain secretory granules and that a majority of them synthesize FSH, LH, and the α-subunit with a smaller subset producing other anterior pituitary hormones that do not show clinical manifestations.[94] No clear and consistent difference in treatment or prognosis has emerged among the various subtypes, however.

Clinical Presentation Because endocrine-inactive tumors do not cause hypersecretion syndromes, they usually present with symptoms associated with mass effect. Patients usually complain of headaches, visual changes, and symptoms of pituitary insufficiency. In a majority of cases the tumor is a macroadenoma at the time of diagnosis.

Diagnosis Aside from undergoing a routine endocrine evaluation, patients with a suspected endocrine-inactive tumor should have determination of the FSH, LH, and glycoprotein α- and β-subunits. Elevated levels of FSH and LH may be tentatively suggestive of a gonadotropin-cell adenoma, especially in postmenopausal women. Secretion of uncombined α- or β-subunits has been recognized with increasing frequency in pituitary tumors, suggesting the existence of still unknown defects in the coupling process.[95] In some patients, the tumor mass may interfere with the normal dopamine-modulated suppression within the pituitary stalk and result in a mildly elevated prolactin level.

Treatment Surgery remains the primary treatment of patients with inactive adenomas. The goals are to relieve the mass effect, restore pituitary function, and to obtain a tissue diagnosis. As with other pituitary adenomas, the preferred approach is transsphenoidal, but cases with significant extension outside the sella may require a transcranial approach. The results of surgery for endocrine-inactive tumors are not as clearly described as for other adenomas because there are no clear criteria for cure. Studies have consistently demonstrated that 70 to 80% of patients experience significant improvement in visual function.[96] In addition, nearly 100% of patients report resolution of headaches,[97] and there is an improvement in pituitary function ranging from 15 to 57%, depending on the series and the criteria for hypopituitarism.[96]

Clinical improvement is not suggestive of complete tumor removal. Postoperative imaging a few months after surgery is required to assess the extent of tumor resection. Early imaging may not be as helpful or accurate because of confounding edema, postoperative hemorrhage, and hemostatic material. Studies report that residual tumor is identified in 66 to 86% of patients, but the rate of recurrence with gross resection is highly variable in the literature.[98,99]

Radiotherapy or radiosurgery is rarely used as the primary treatment of inactive adenomas, but rather as an adjuvant in patients found to have residual tumor postoperatively or significant suprasellar or cavernous sinus involvement preoperatively. Because of the significant risks of radiation therapy to the pituitary region, however, many practitioners advocate that residual tumors should be followed with serial imaging and radiated only if the tumors grow.[100,101] A recent study by Tanaka and colleagues focuses on the "natural history" of residual nonfunctioning adenoma by correlating tumor-volume doubling time, patient's age, and a proliferation index (MIB-1).[102] In 40 patients with a mean follow-up of 53 months, they found a significant difference in doubling time in patients below and above 61 years of age. Specifically, doubling time was much longer in older patients, suggesting that age should be taken into consideration when deciding on adjuvant treatment strategies.

A variety of studies have confirmed the limited efficacy of the medical management of nonsecreting adenomas. In a recent evaluation of tumor volume in nine nonfunctioning adenomas after 1 year of cabergoline treatment, expression of D2 dopamine receptors was found in 67% of cases.[103] Tumor shrinkage by MRI was observed in 56% of cases, but was truly notable in only two cases. Various other medical therapies, including bromocriptine, other dopamine-agonists, octreotide, and GnRH agonists and antagonists, have been tried without consistent shrinkage in tumor size and are seldom used.

TSH-SECRETING PITUITARY ADENOMAS

TSH-secreting adenomas are the least common of the pituitary tumors, representing only 1 to 2% of cases.[104]

Clinical Presentation Patients can present with constitutional complaints consistent with long-standing thyroid dysfunction such as heat intolerance, diarrhea, weight-loss, fatigue, and exophthalmos, or complaints from the local mass effect such as headaches, visual changes, and symptoms of hypopituitarism. There is often a delay in diagnosis of these tumors because they are commonly misdiagnosed as Graves' disease and often present when already large and invasive. They can be difficult to cure.[105]

Diagnosis A large proportion of TSH-secreting tumors are associated with elevated levels of TSH, in spite of elevated free T3 and free T4. Additionally, documentation of an elevated α-subunit/TSH ratio increases the sensitivity of the biochemical diagnosis. Ultrasensitive immunometric TSH assays allow a distinction between patients with primary hyperthyroidism and those with central hyperthyroidism or resistance to thyroid hormone.

Treatment Prior to any surgical intervention, the hyperthyroidism should be controlled in order to minimize the risk of cardiac arrhythmias that may occur during induction of anesthesia or intraoperatively. This is commonly done with a preoperative beta blocker. If the surgery is nonemergent, an antithyroid drug (propylthiouracil or methimazole) can also be added. Transsphenoidal surgery is the primary treatment, but is associated with cure rates of only about 35 to 62% with surgery alone and 55 to 81% in conjunction with medical treatment and radiotherapy.[106–108] The criteria for cure in TSH-secreting adenomas have not yet been well defined. External radiation is used if clinical remission is not obtained with surgery alone but not as a primary treatment modality.

Medical treatment of tumors with octreotide has been reported to be effective in 92% of TSH-secreting adenomas, with a normalization of TSH and tumor shrinkage in the vast majority.[109] Octreotide is often useful as an adjuvant therapy, but the long-term costs and problems of compliance preclude octreotide as the primary treatment in most cases. More recent reports have also shown that lanreotide, a long-acting analogue, may have efficacy similar to that of octreotide.

CONCLUSION

Pituitary adenomas are a heterogeneous tumor population that require different management paradigms depending on the individual subtype. Transsphenoidal surgery remains the most common intervention in the treatment of these tumors. Adjuvant medical and radiation therapies continue to play a significant role in long-term control. In addition, recent advances in molecular biology, drug development, and improved radiosurgical outcomes hold significant promise for future treatment improvements.

REFERENCES

1. Melmed S. Pathogenesis of pituitary tumors. Endocrinol Metab Clin North Am 1999;28:1–12.
2. Landolt AM. Ultrastructure of human sella tumors. Correlations of clinical findings and morphology. Acta Neurochir (Wien) 1975;Suppl 22:1–167.
3. Asa SL. Tumors of the pituitary gland. In: Atlas of tumor pathology. 3rd series, fascicle 22. Washington DC: Armed Forces Institute of Pathology; 1998. p. 159–60.
4. Kovacs K, Horvath E, Vidal S. Classification of pituitary adenomas. J Neurooncol 2001;54:121–7.
5. Herman V, Fagin J, Gonsky R, et al. Clonal origin of pituitary adenomas. J Clin Endocrinol Metab 1990;71:1427–33.
6. Lloyd RV. Molecular pathology of pituitary adenomas. J Neurooncol 2001;54:111–9.
7. Yu R, Melmed S. Oncogene activation in pituitary tumors. Brain Pathol 2001;11:328–41.
8. Landis CA, Masters SB, Spada A, et al. GTPase inhibiting mutations activate the alpha chain of Gs and stimulate adenylyl cyclase in human pituitary tumours. Nature 1989;340:692–6.
9. Lania A, Persani L, Ballare E, et al. Constitutively active Gs alpha is associated with an increased phosphodiesterase activity in human growth hormone-secreting adenomas. J Clin Endocrinol Metab 1998;83:1624–8.
10. Cai WY, Alexander JM, Hedley-Whyte ET, et al. ras mutations in human prolactinomas and pituitary carcinomas. J Clin Endocrinol Metab 1994;78:89–93.
11. Pei L, Melmed S. Isolation and characterization of a pituitary tumor-transforming gene (PTTG). Mol Endocrinol 1997;11:433–41.
12. Woloschak, M, Yu, A, and Post, KD, Frequent inactivation of the p16 gene in human pituitary tumors by gene methylation. Mol Carcinog 1997;19:221–4.

13. Woloschak M, Roberts JL, Post KD. Loss of heterozygosity at the retinoblastoma locus in human pituitary tumors. Cancer 1994;74:693–6.
14. Riss D, Jin L, Qian X, et al. Differential expression of galectin-3 in pituitary tumors. Cancer Res 2003;63:2251–5.
15. Heaney AP, Fernando M, Melmed S. PPAR-gamma receptor ligands: novel therapy for pituitary adenomas. J Clin Invest 2003;111:1381–8.
16. Kreutzer J, Fahlbusch R. Diagnosis and treatment of pituitary tumors. Curr Opin Neurol 2004;17:693–703.
17. Naidich MJ, Russell EJ. Current approaches to imaging of the sellar region and pituitary. Endocrinol Metab Clin North Am 1999;28:45–79, vi.
18. Hardy J, Somma M. Acromegaly: surgical treatment by transsphenoidal microsurgical removal of the pituitary adenoma. In: Tindall GT, Collins WS, editors. Clinical management of pituitary disorders. New York: Raven Press; 1979. p. 209–11.
19. Gandhi CD, Post KD. Historical movements in transsphenoidal surgery. Neurosurg Focus 2001;11:1–4.
20. Jane JA Jr, Thapar K, Kaptain GJ, et al. Pituitary surgery: transsphenoidal approach. Neurosurgery 2002;51:435–44.
21. Riedel M, Noldus J, Saeger W, et al. Sellar lesions associated with isolated hyperprolactinaemia. Morphological, immunocytochemical, hormonal and clinical results. Acta Endocrinol (Copenh) 1986;113:196–203.
22. Weiss M, Pituitary tumors: an endocrinological and neurosurgical challenge. Clin Neurosurg 1992;39:114–22.
23. Liu JK, Couldwell WT. Contemporary management of prolactinomas. Neurosurg Focus 2004;16:E2.
24. Park SK, Keenan MW, Selmanoff M. Graded hyperprolactinemia first suppresses LH pulse frequency and then pulse amplitude in castrated male rats. Neuroendocrinology 1993;58:448–53.
25. Klibanski A, Biller BM, Rosenthal DI, et al. Effects of prolactin and estrogen deficiency in amenorrheic bone loss. J Clin Endocrinol Metab 1988;67:124–30.
26. Schlechte JA. Clinical practice. Prolactinoma. N Engl J Med 2003;349:2035–41.
27. Randall RV, Scheithauer BW, Laws ER Jr, et al. Pituitary adenomas associated with hyperprolactinemia: a clinical and immunohistochemical study of 97 patients operated on transsphenoidally. Mayo Clin Proc 1985;60:753–62.
28. Persani L, Beck-Peccoz P, Medri G, et al. Thyrotropin alpha- and beta-subunit responses to thyrotropin-releasing hormone and domperidone in normal subjects and in patients with microprolactinomas. Neuroendocrinology 1991;53:411–5.
29. Shrivastava RK, Arginteanu MS, King WA, et al. Giant prolactinomas: clinical management and long-term follow up. J Neurosurg 2002;97:299–306.
30. Frieze TW, Mong DP, Koops MK. "Hook effect" in prolactinomas: case report and review of literature. Endocr Pract 2002;8:296–303.
31. Schlechte J, Dolan K, Sherman B, et al. The natural history of untreated hyperprolactinemia: a prospective analysis. J Clin Endocrinol Metab 1989;68:412–8.
32. Maurer RA. Dopaminergic inhibition of prolactin synthesis and prolactin messenger RNA accumulation in cultured pituitary cells. J Biol Chem 1980;255:8092–7.
33. Bevan JS, Adams CB, Burke CW, et al. Factors in the outcome of transsphenoidal surgery for prolactinoma and non-functioning pituitary tumour, including pre-operative bromocriptine therapy. Clin Endocrinol (Oxf) 1987;26:541–56.
34. Molitch ME. Disorders of prolactin secretion. Endocrinol Metab Clin North Am 2001;30:585–610.
35. Colao A, Annunziato L, Lombardi G. Treatment of prolactinomas. Ann Med 1998;30:452–9.
36. Colao A, Di Sarno A, Cappabianca P, et al. Withdrawal of long-term cabergoline therapy for tumoral and nontumoral hyperprolactinemia. N Engl J Med 2003;349:2023–33.
37. Delgrange E, Sassolas G, Perrin G, et al. Clinical and histological correlations in prolactinomas, with special reference to bromocriptine resistance. Acta Neurochir (Wien) 2005;147:751–8.
38. Tyrrell JB, Lamborn KR, Hannegan LT, et al. Transsphenoidal microsurgical therapy of prolactinomas: initial outcomes and long-term results. Neurosurgery 1999;44:254–63.
39. Nomikos P, Buchfelder M, Fahlbusch R. Current management of prolactinomas. J Neurooncol 2001;54:139–50.
40. Couldwell WT, Rovit RL, Weiss MH. Role of surgery in the treatment of microprolactinomas. Neurosurg Clin N Am 2003;14:89–92, vii.
41. Ozgen T, Oruckaptan HH, Ozcan OE, et al. Prolactin secreting pituitary adenomas: analysis of 429 surgically treated patients, effect of adjuvant treatment modalities and review of the literature. Acta Neurochir (Wien) 1999; 141:1287–94.
42. Pan L, Zhang N, Wang EM, et al. Gamma knife radiosurgery as a primary treatment for prolactinomas. J Neurosurg 2000;93 Suppl 3:10–3.
43. Landolt AM, Lomax N. Gamma knife radiosurgery for prolactinomas. J Neurosurg 2000;93 Suppl 3:14–8.
44. Witt TC. Stereotactic radiosurgery for pituitary tumors. Neurosurg Focus 2003;14:E10.
45. Molitch ME. Pregnancy and the hyperprolactinemic woman. N Engl J Med 1985;312:1364–70.
46. Jane JA Jr, Thapar K, Laws ER Jr. Acromegaly: historical perspectives and current therapy. J Neurooncol 2001;54:129–37.
47. Melmed S, Casanueva FF, Cavagnini F, et al. Guidelines for acromegaly management. J Clin Endocrinol Metab 2002;87:4054–8.
48. Freda PU, Landman RE, Sundeen RE, et al. Gender and age in the biochemical assessment of cure of acromegaly. Pituitary 2001;4:163–71.
49. Giustina A, Barkan A, Casanueva FF, et al. Criteria for cure of acromegaly: a consensus statement. J Clin Endocrinol Metab 2000;85:526–9.
50. Freda PU, Wardlaw SL, Post KD. Long-term endocrinological follow-up evaluation in 115 patients who underwent transsphenoidal surgery for acromegaly. J Neurosurg 1998;89:353–8.
51. Laws ER, Vance ML, Thapar K. Pituitary surgery for the management of acromegaly. Horm Res 2000;53 Suppl 3:71–5.
52. Trepp R, Stettler C, Zwahlen M, et al. Treatment outcomes and mortality of 94 patients with acromegaly. Acta Neurochir (Wien) 2005;147:243–51.
53. Feek CM, McLelland J, Seth J, et al. How effective is external pituitary irradiation for growth hormone-secreting pituitary tumors? Clin Endocrinol (Oxf) 1984;20:401–8.
54. van der Lely AJ, de Herder WW, Lamberts SW. The role of radiotherapy in acromegaly. J Clin Endocrinol Metab 1997;82:3185–6.
55. Zhang N, Pan L, Wang EM, et al. Radiosurgery for growth hormone-producing pituitary adenomas. J Neurosurg 2000;93 Suppl 3:6–9.
56. Kim SH, Huh R, Chang JW, et al. Gamma Knife radiosurgery for functioning pituitary adenomas. Stereotact Funct Neurosurg 1999;72 Suppl 1:101–10.
57. Kim MS, Lee SI, Sim JH. Gamma Knife radiosurgery for functioning pituitary microadenoma. Stereotact Funct Neurosurg 1999;72 Suppl 1:119–24.
58. Vance ML. Treatment of patients with a pituitary adenoma: one clinician's experience. Neurosurg Focus 2004;16:E1.
59. Cozzi R, Attanasio R, Barausse M, et al. Cabergoline in acromegaly: a renewed role for dopamine agonist treatment? Eur J Endocrinol 1998;139:516–21.
60. Colao A, Lombardi G. Growth-hormone and prolactin excess. Lancet 1998;352:1455–61.
61. Davies PH, Stewart SE, Lancranjan L, et al. Long-term therapy with long-acting octreotide (Sandostatin-LAR) for the management of acromegaly. Clin Endocrinol (Oxf) 1998;48:311–6.
62. Stewart PM, Kane KF, Stewart SE, et al. Depot long-acting somatostatin analog (Sandostatin-LAR) is an effective treatment for acromegaly. J Clin Endocrinol Metab 1995;80:3267–72.
63. Ayuk J, Stewart SE, Stewart PM, et al. Long-term safety and efficacy of depot long-acting somatostatin analogs for the treatment of acromegaly. J Clin Endocrinol Metab 2002;87:4142–6.
64. Stewart PM, Pegvisomant: an advance in clinical efficacy in acromegaly. Eur J Endocrinol 2003;148 Suppl 2:S27–32.
65. van der Lely AJ, Hutson RK, Trainer PJ, et al. Long-term treatment of acromegaly with pegvisomant, a growth hormone receptor antagonist. Lancet 2001;358:1754–9.
66. Colao A, Cuocolo A, Marzullo P, et al. Effects of 1-year treatment with octreotide on cardiac performance in patients with acromegaly. J Clin Endocrinol Metab 1999;84:17–23.
67. Colao A, Cuocolo A, Marzullo P, et al. Is the acromegalic cardiomyopathy reversible? Effect of 5-year normalization of growth hormone and insulin-like growth factor I levels on cardiac performance. J Clin Endocrinol Metab 2001;86:1551–7.
68. Freda PU, Reyes CM, Nuruzzaman AT, et al. Cabergoline therapy of growth hormone & growth hormone/prolactin secreting pituitary tumors. Pituitary 2004;7:21–30.
69. Hentschel SJ, McCutcheon IE. Stereotactic radiosurgery for Cushing disease. Neurosurg Focus 2004;16:E5.
70. Grossman AB, Howlett TA, Perry L, et al. CRF in the differential diagnosis of Cushing's syndrome: a comparison with the dexamethasone suppression test. Clin Endocrinol (Oxf) 1988;29:167–78.
71. Graham KE, Samuels MH, Nesbit GM, et al. Cavernous sinus sampling is highly accurate in distinguishing Cushing's disease from the ectopic adrenocorticotropin syndrome and in predicting intrapituitary tumor location. J Clin Endocrinol Metab 1999;84:1602–10.
72. Trilck M, Flitsch J, Ludecke DK, et al. Salivary cortisol measurement--a reliable method for the diagnosis of Cushing's syndrome. Exp Clin Endocrinol Diabetes 2005;113:225–30.
73. Newell-Price J, Trainer P, Besser M, et al. The diagnosis and differential diagnosis of Cushing's syndrome and pseudo-Cushing's states. Endocr Rev 1998;19:647–72.
74. Yanovski JA, Cutler GB Jr, Chrousos GP, et al. The dexamethasone-suppressed corticotropin-releasing hormone stimulation test differentiates mild Cushing's disease from normal physiology. J Clin Endocrinol Metab 1998;83:348–52.
75. Bonelli FS, Huston J 3rd, Carpenter PC, et al. Adrenocorticotropic hormone-dependent Cushing's syndrome: sensitivity and specificity of inferior petrosal sinus sampling. AJNR Am J Neuroradiol 2000;21:690–6.
76. Ludecke DK, Flitsch J, Knappe UJ, et al. Cushing's disease: a surgical view. J Neurooncol 2001;54:151–66.
77. Semple P, Vance M, Findling J, et al. Transsphenoidal surgery for Cushing's disease: outcome in patients with a normal magnetic resonance imaging scan. Neurosurgery 2000;46:553–9.
78. Chen JC, Amar AP, Choi S, et al. Transsphenoidal microsurgical treatment of Cushing disease: postoperative assessment of surgical efficacy by application of an overnight low-dose dexamethasone suppression test. J Neurosurg 2003;98:967–73.
79. Rollin GA, Ferreira NP, Junges M, et al. Dynamics of serum cortisol levels after transsphenoidal surgery in a cohort of patients with Cushing's disease. J Clin Endocrinol Metab 2004;89:1131–9.
80. Bochicchio D, Losa M, Buchfelder M. Factors influencing the immediate and late outcome of Cushing's disease treated by transsphenoidal surgery: a retrospective study by the European Cushing's Disease Survey Group. J Clin Endocrinol Metab 1995;80:3114–20.
81. Estrada J, Boronat M, Mielgo M, et al. The long-term outcome of pituitary irradiation after unsuccessful transsphenoidal surgery in Cushing's disease. N Engl J Med 1997;336:172–7.
82. Vladyka V, Liscak R, Novotny J Jr, et al. Radiation tolerance of functioning pituitary tissue in gamma knife surgery for pituitary adenomas. Neurosurgery 2003;52:309–17.
83. Sheehan JM, Vance ML, Sheehan JP, et al. Radiosurgery for Cushing's disease after failed transsphenoidal surgery. J Neurosurg 2000;93:738–42.
84. Invitti C, Giraldi FP, de Martin M, et al. Diagnosis and management of Cushing's syndrome: results of an Italian multicentre study. Study Group of the Italian Society of Endocrinology on the Pathophysiology of the Hypothalamic-Pituitary-Adrenal Axis. J Clin Endocrinol Metab 1999;84:440–8.
85. Pivonello R, Ferone D, de Herder WW, et al. Dopamine receptor expression and function in corticotroph pituitary tumors. J Clin Endocrinol Metab 2004;89:2452–62.
86. Ambrosi B, Dall'Asta C, Cannavo S, et al. Effects of chronic administration of PPAR-gamma ligand rosiglitazone in Cushing's disease. Eur J Endocrinol 2004;151:173–8.
87. Pereira MA, Halpern A, Salgado LR, et al. A study of patients with Nelson's syndrome. Clin Endocrinol (Oxf) 1998;49:533–9.
88. Wislawski J, Kasperlik-Zaluska AA, Jeske W, et al. Results of neurosurgical treatment by a transsphenoidal approach in 10 patients with Nelson's syndrome. J Neurosurg 1985;62:68–71.
89. Kelly PA, Samandouras G, Grossman AB, et al. Neurosurgical treatment of Nelson's syndrome. J Clin Endocrinol Metab 2002;87:5465–9.
90. Post KD. Radiosurgery and Cushing's disease. J Neurosurg 2000;93:907–9.
91. Lopez JA, Kleinschmidt-Demasters Bk B, Sze CI, et al. Silent corticotroph adenomas: further clinical and pathological observations. Hum Pathol 2004;35:1137–47.
92. Scheithauer BW, Jaap AJ, Horvath E, et al. Clinically silent corticotroph tumors of the pituitary gland. Neurosurgery 2000;47:723–30.
93. Webb KM, Laurent JJ, Okonkwo DO, et al. Clinical characteristics of silent corticotrophic adenomas and creation

of an internet-accessible database to facilitate their multi-institutional study. Neurosurgery 2003;53:1076–85.

94. Black PM, Hsu DW, Klibanski A, et al. Hormone production in clinically nonfunctioning pituitary adenomas. J Neurosurg 1987;66:244–50.
95. Saccomanno K, Spada A, Bassetti M, et al. Immunodetection of chorionic gonadotropin and its subunits in human nonfunctioning pituitary adenomas. J Clin Endocrinol Metab 1994;78:1103–7.
96. Losa M, Mortini P, Barzaghi R, et al. Endocrine inactive and gonadotroph adenomas: diagnosis and management. J Neurooncol 2001;54:167–77.
97. Ebersold MJ, Quast LM, Laws ER Jr, et al. Long-term results in transsphenoidal removal of nonfunctioning pituitary adenomas. J Neurosurg 1986;64:713–9.
98. Marazuela M, Astigarraga B, Vicente A, et al. Recovery of visual and endocrine function following transsphenoidal surgery of large nonfunctioning pituitary adenomas. J Endocrinol Invest 1994;17:703–7.
99. Colao A, Cerbone G, Cappabianca P, et al. Effect of surgery and radiotherapy on visual and endocrine function in nonfunctioning pituitary adenomas. J Endocrinol Invest 1998;21:284–90.
100. Lillehei KO, Kirschman DL, Kleinschmidt-DeMasters BK, et al. Reassessment of the role of radiation therapy in the treatment of endocrine-inactive pituitary macroadenomas. Neurosurgery 1998;43:432–9.
101. Losa M, Franzin A, Mangili F, et al. Proliferation index of nonfunctioning pituitary adenomas: correlations with clinical characteristics and long-term follow-up results. Neurosurgery 2000;47:1313–9.
102. Tanaka Y, Hongo K, Tada T, et al. Growth pattern and rate in residual nonfunctioning pituitary adenomas: correlations among tumor volume doubling time, patient age, and MIB-1 index. J Neurosurg 2003;98:359–65.
103. Pivonello R, Matrone C, Filippella M, et al. Dopamine receptor expression and function in clinically nonfunctioning pituitary tumors: comparison with the effectiveness of cabergoline treatment. J Clin Endocrinol Metab 2004;89:1674–83.
104. McCutcheon IE, Weintraub BD, Oldfield EH. Surgical treatment of thyrotropin-secreting pituitary adenomas. J Neurosurg 1990;73:674–83.
105. Socin HV, Chanson P, Delemer B, et al. The changing spectrum of TSH-secreting pituitary adenomas: diagnosis and management in 43 patients. Eur J Endocrinol 2003;148:433–42.
106. Brucker-Davis F, Oldfield EH, Skarulis MC, et al. Thyrotropin-secreting pituitary tumors: diagnostic criteria, thyroid hormone sensitivity, and treatment outcome in 25 patients followed at the National Institutes of Health. J Clin Endocrinol Metab 1999;84:476–86.
107. Losa M, Giovanelli M, Persani L, et al. Criteria of cure and follow-up of central hyperthyroidism due to thyrotropin-secreting pituitary adenomas. J Clin Endocrinol Metab 1996;81:3084–90.
108. Sanno N, Teramoto A, Osamura RY. Long-term surgical outcome in 16 patients with thyrotropin pituitary adenoma. J Neurosurg 2000;93:194–200.
109. Beck-Peccoz P, Brucker-Davis F, Persani L, et al. Thyrotropin-secreting pituitary tumors. Endocr Rev 1996;17:610–38.

Neoplasms of the Thyroid

Steven I. Sherman, MD
Ann Marie Gillenwater, MD

It was estimated that nearly 26,000 individuals would be diagnosed in 2005 with carcinoma of the thyroid gland and that about 1,600 patients would die as a consequence of complications of these diseases or their treatments.[1] Now the eighth most commonly diagnosed malignancy in women, the age-adjusted incidence of thyroid carcinoma has risen faster than that of any other cancer, and the age-adjusted mortality is also among the most rapidly increasing.[2] Histologically, 80 and 14%, respectively, are either papillary or follicular carcinomas, differentiated carcinomas that derive from the thyroid hormone producing follicular epithelial cells. Another 4% are medullary carcinoma, a neuroendocrine malignancy, and the remaining 2% are the highly aggressive anaplastic carcinoma. Rates of disease recurrence and cancer-specific mortality are increased in patients with metastases, especially those with extracervical spread. In the Surveillance, Epidemiology, and End Results (SEER) report of 15,700 patients, the overall 10-year age- and gender-corrected survival rates were 98% for papillary, 92% for follicular, 80% for medullary, and 13% for anaplastic carcinoma.[3] Older age at diagnosis and wider spread of disease are associated with a worse prognosis, independent of the type of cancer. Although differentiated carcinomas have a 2:1 female predominance, male gender confers a slightly worse prognosis.

Because of a lack of randomized comparative trials, decisions regarding the selection of treatments for these diseases are based largely on retrospective analyses and consensus recommendations.[4] Therapy routinely involves multiple modalities, including surgery and thyroid hormone, radioiodine (for differentiated tumors), and external radiation and chemotherapy for selected patients with advanced disease. However, the poor response to treatment for metastatic thyroid cancer has recently triggered a spate of clinical trials of newer therapeutic strategies.

DIAGNOSTIC EVALUATION OF THE SOLITARY THYROID NODULE

The most common clinical presentation of a patient with thyroid carcinoma is with a solitary thyroid nodule (Table 76-1).[5] Ultrasonography, however, reveals clinically unsuspected nodules in up to 30% of individuals without palpable lesions, and multiple nodules are frequent. Sonographic criteria that increase the likelihood of malignancy include the presence of microcalcifications, hypoechogenicity, and increased intranodular vascularity.[6] In the setting of an unsuppressed serum thyroid-stimulating hormone (TSH) concentration, thyroid ultrasound followed by cytologic examination of a fine-needle aspirate (FNA) of solitary nodules at least 1 cm in size is the most appropriate diagnostic procedure; in the setting of multiple nodules, those with suspicious sonographic appearances should be preferentially aspirated.[7] Papillary, medullary, and anaplastic carcinomas can be readily diagnosed on the basis of cytologic criteria. However, the distinction between follicular carcinoma and benign follicular adenoma requires histologic demonstration of either invasion through the tumor capsule or vascular invasion. Hence, follicular adenomas and carcinomas are grouped together cytologically as indeterminate or suspicious follicular neoplasms. Up to 25% of aspirations are inadequate or nondiagnostic, largely because of aspiration of cystic, hemorrhagic, or hypocellular colloid nodules.[8] The false-positive and false-negative rates for nodules characterized as "malignant" and "benign," respectively, are less than 5%.[9] For suspicious follicular lesions, the overall rate of carcinoma is approximately 20%, with higher rates associated with larger nodule size, older age, and male gender.[10–12] Intraoperative frozen section evaluation adds little to the evaluation of follicular neoplasms, but may occasionally be helpful to confirm the diagnosis of cytologically suspected papillary carcinoma.[13,14] For nodules in which fine-needle aspiration yields inadequate diagnostic material, repeat aspiration, particularly with ultrasonography guidance, can augment the accuracy of the procedure.[15]

Table 76-1 Differential Diagnosis of a Thyroid Nodule

Benign thyroid disease
Macrofollicular
Colloid adenoma
Adenomatoid hyperplasia
Microfollicular
Follicular adenoma
Hürthle cell adenoma
Toxic adenoma
Hashimoto thyroiditis
Graves disease
Infection
Tuberculosis
Fungal
Pneumocystis
Abscess
Thyroid cyst
Infiltrative and granulomatous disease
Malignant thyroid disease
Differentiated thyroid carcinoma
Papillary thyroid carcinoma
Follicular thyroid carcinoma
Medullary thyroid carcinoma
Anaplastic thyroid carcinoma
Primary thyroid lymphoma
Metastatic
Breast carcinoma
Renal cell carcinoma
Lung carcinoma
Melanoma
Colon carcinoma
Gastric carcinoma
Extrathyroidal disease
Parathyroid adenoma, cyst, or carcinoma
Esophageal diverticulum
Lipoma
Aberrant subclavian artery

By radionuclide scanning, malignant thyroid lesions are usually hypofunctioning or "cold," but this finding is both nonspecific and nondiagnostic. In contrast, a "hot" hyperfunctioning nodule causing thyrotoxicosis is highly likely to be a benign follicular adenoma. Thus, only patients with a suppressed TSH should undergo radioiodine scanning to determine the function of significant nodules, and FNA only performed for nonfunctioning lesions. Other imaging procedures, such as computed tomography (CT), magnetic resonance imaging (MRI), and positron emission tomography (PET) have no role in the routine diagnostic evaluation of thyroid nodules.

DIFFERENTIATED THYROID CARCINOMA

Pathogensis The only well-established risk factor for differentiated thyroid cancer is radiation exposure, especially during infancy. External radiation, delivered therapeutically decades ago for benign conditions, such as thymic and tonsillar enlargement, and currently for malignant diseases, such as Hodgkin lymphoma and before bone marrow transplantation, is associated with an excess relative risk for thyroid malignancy of 3 to 9 per Gy.[16] Exposure to internal sources of radiation after the Chernobyl nuclear accident led to a 3- to 75-fold increase in the incidence of papillary carcinoma, the highest risks seen in younger children.[17] Although nuclear weapon testing and other sources of radiation fallout have affected large areas of the United States, follow-up studies have yet to identify definite evidence of increased rates of thyroid cancer.[18,19]

Differentiated carcinoma is a component of several inherited syndromes, including familial adenomatous polyposis, Gardner syndrome, Cowden disease, Turcot syndrome, and Carney complex. Familial nonmedullary carcinoma, described in families with at least two first-degree relatives with the disease, has been reported in 5% of all papillary carcinoma patients,[20] and may portend a more-aggressive disease course.[21] Putative susceptibility loci have been identified on chromosomes 1q21, 2q21, and 19p13.2.[22]

Follicular cell tumorigenesis may develop along several paths, many of which are also common in other solid tumors. For papillary carcinoma, an early initiating event is usually activation of intracellular signaling upstream from the MAP (mitogen-activated protein) kinase, including (1) the V600E mutation in the BRAF kinase, (2) one of several chromosomal rearrangements forming *ret/PTC* oncogene genes, or (3) activated *ras*.[23,24] BRAF mutations have been associated with more aggressive histologic variants and greater frequency of recurrence.[25] Other factors that may contribute to progression of papillary carcinomas include overexpression of other intracellular kinases, deoxyribonucleic acid (DNA) hypermethylation and histone deacetylation leading to silencing of tumor-suppressor genes, and cell-cycle dysregulation.[26–28] In contrast, follicular carcinomas may rarely arise from benign adenomas as a result of transforming events. Mutations in *ras,* which are also common in follicular adenomas, may lead to greater genomic instability, increased allelic loss, and more risk for transforming chromosomal rearrangements, such as t(2;3)(q13;p25) that fuses the DNA binding domain of a thyroid-specific transcription factor, PAX8, to peroxisome proliferator-activated receptor (PPAR)-gamma-1 in follicular carcinoma but not benign lesions.[29–31]

Pathologic Features Papillary carcinomas are characterized by the presence of papillae consisting of a well-defined fibrovascular core surrounded by one or two layers of tumor cells (Figure 76-1). Follicles and colloid are typically absent. Nuclei tend to be large, oval, and appear crowded and overlapping on microscopic sections. The nuclei contain hypodense powdery chromatin, cytoplasmic pseudoinclusions caused by a redundant nuclear membrane, and nuclear grooves. Individually, these features are not pathognomonic of papillary carcinoma, but in combination they define the disease. About one-half of papillary carcinomas contain calcified psammoma bodies, which are the scarred and calcified remnants of tumor papillae that presumably infarcted.

Of the several histologic subtypes, the follicular variant accounts for approximately 10% of all papillary carcinomas.[32] The cells are organized into follicles rather than papillae, but cytologically, they display the typical nuclear features of papillary carcinomas. Rates of recurrence and survival with the follicular variant are very similar to those of patients with common-type papillary carcinomas. In contrast, the tall-cell variant

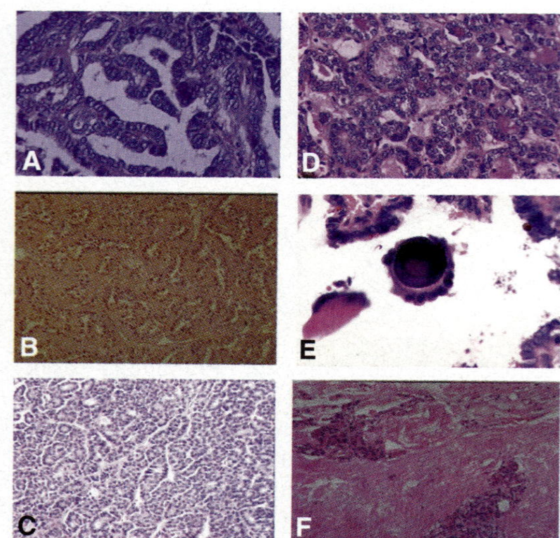

Figure 76-1 Pathologic features of differentiated thyroid carcinoma. **A,** Papillary carcinoma, with characteristic fibrovascular papillary formation, crowded nuclei, and nuclear clearing. **B,** Follicular variant of papillary carcinoma, with typical cells of papillary carcinoma in follicular formations. **C,** Tall cell variant of papillary carcinoma, with cells at least twice as tall as they are wide and eosinophilic cytoplasm. **D,** Psammoma body of papillary carcinoma. **E,** Microfollicular neoplasm, with scant colloid. **F,** Follicular carcinoma, demonstrating invasion across a thick capsule into neighboring thyroid.

of papillary carcinoma is a more aggressive tumor, characterized by tumor cells with eosinophilic cytoplasm that are twice as tall as they are wide.[33] The primary tumors tend to be large, are often invasive, and frequently have both local and distant metastases at the time of diagnosis. The 5-year survival rate is 75 to 85%.

Follicular carcinomas are distinguished from benign follicular lesions on the basis of invasiveness. These tumors are commonly encapsulated, and invasion can commonly be demonstrated in one or more foci along the capsule or across vascular endothelial walls. Semiquantitative assessment of the magnitude of invasion can separate follicular carcinomas into minimally invasive and widely invasive lesions; a minimally invasive follicular carcinoma has only scattered foci of capsular or vascular invasion. Cytologic features do not reliably distinguish benign from malignant follicular lesions.

Hürthle cell neoplasms are formed by cells containing numerous mitochondria, which impart a granular, eosinophilic appearance to their cytoplasm.[34] Most have a follicular architecture and are diagnosed as adenomas or carcinomas by the same criteria applied to other follicular neoplasms. A Hürthle-cell variant of papillary carcinoma is much less common and tends to be more aggressive than typical papillary carcinomas.

Insular carcinomas are often placed in the category of poorly differentiated thyroid carcinomas, which implies a status between that of differentiated and anaplastic carcinomas. Insular carcinomas generally concentrate radioiodine and are therefore treated as differentiated cancers. They are formed by small cells with variable mitotic activity, arranged in nests, with foci of necrosis.

Clinicopathologic Staging Although multiple clinicopathologic staging schemes exist for differentiated thyroid carcinoma,[35–43] the sixth edition of the TNM (tumor, node, metastases) staging approach (Table 76-2) is generally recommended for use, but evidence for a superior value for predicting death caused by thyroid cancer has only been reported for the previous fifth edition.[41,42] Both TNM versions classify patients with distant metastases but who are under the age of 45 years as being at "low risk" for death, one of several significant caveats to clinical use of these schemes. The importance of histologic features such as tumor size and extrathyroidal invasion underscore the need for pathologists to report these data uniformly on thyroidectomy specimens.[44,45]

Primary Surgical Management Total thyroidectomy is the preferred initial surgical procedure for most patients with differentiated thyroid carcinoma, as supported by these arguments: (1) foci of papillary carcinoma are found in both thyroid lobes in 60 to 85% of patients[46]; (2) 5 to 10% of recurrences of papillary carcinoma after unilateral surgery occur in the contralateral lobe, with subsequent high risk of disease-related death[47]; and (3) the efficacy of therapy with radioiodine and the specificity of serum thyroglobulin levels as a tumor marker are maximized by resection of as much thyroid tissue as possible. In contrast, the major argument put forth to support a unilateral procedure is the risk for more complications following bilateral surgery, including hypoparathyroidism and recurrent laryngeal nerve paralysis.[52,53] In a retrospective analysis of the outcomes of 1,685 low-risk patients, the 20-year recurrence rate after lobectomy was 22%, compared with 8% for patients treated with total thyroidectomy.[48] Other retrospective studies (although not all) reported similar results of reduced recurrence.[40,49,50] Most recently, analysis of a multicenter prospective thyroid cancer registry database has demonstrated improved survival associated with total or near-total thyroidectomy in patients with stages II to IV disease (risk ratio for mortality compared with less than near-total thyroidectomy 0.64 for stage II, 0.79 for stages III and IV combined).[51]

In the absence of prospective trials, consensus panels have generally recommended that a near-total or total thyroidectomy should be performed by an experienced thyroid surgeon if the primary papillary carcinoma or Hürthle cell carcinoma is at least 1 cm in diameter, if there is extrathyroidal extension of tumor, or if there are metastases.[4, 54–57] This operation should also be performed in patients with a history of exposure to ionizing radiation of the head and neck, given the high rate of tumor recurrence with lesser operations.[58] In selected patients whose papillary tumor is < 1 cm in diameter and confined to one lobe of the gland, a unilateral lobectomy may be sufficient.[40] For patients with a cytologically suspicious follicular neoplasm, unilateral lobectomy and isthmusectomy should be performed; a complete thyroidectomy is done if there is a diagnosis of malignancy.

Table 76-2 TNM (Tumor, Node, Metastases): The AJCC (American Joint Committee on Cancer) Staging Scheme for Thyroid Carcinomas (Sixth Edition)

T: Tumor status		
T1	< 2 cm	
T2	2–4 cm	
T3	> 4 cm or minimal extraglandular invasion	
T4	Extraglandular invasion	
T4a	Gross invasion	
T4b	Prevertebral, carotid, or mediastinal invasion	
Tx	Tumor status unknown	
N: Regional node status		
N0	No nodes involved	
N1a	Cervical level VI nodes positive	
N1b	Unilateral, contralateral or bilateral cervical levels II-V or mediastinal nodes positive	
Nx	Nodes status unknown	
M: Distant metastases		
M0	No distant metastases	
M1	Distant metastases	
Mx	Metastases status unknown	
Stage assignments		
	Differentiated carcinoma (< 45 years)	Differentiated carcinoma (>45 years) or medullary carcinoma
Stage I	Any T, any N, M0	T1, N0 M0
Stage II	Any T, any N, M1	T2, N0, M0
Stage III		T3–4, N0, M0 Any T, N1a, M0
Stage IV		A: T4a, any N, M0 Any T, N1b, M0 B: T4b, any N, M0 C: Any T, any N, M1
Anaplastic carcinomas		
All are classified as stage IV		

Although microscopic regional nodal metastasis of papillary carcinoma occurs in up to 80% of patients, only about 35% have cervical or mediastinal node metastasis grossly detectable at the time of surgery, most commonly found in lateral cervical compartments.[59] Unlike most other malignancies, the presence of lymph node metastasis is only a minor risk factor for mortality. Whereas resection of central, level VI nodes has been associated with improved survival, a meta-analysis of nine studies demonstrated no relationship between the lateral lymph node status at presentation and survival.[60] Several of the studies analyzed did show an increased risk of tumor recurrence. As a surrogate outcome measure, however, disease recurrence after nodal metastasis of papillary carcinoma may portend a markedly increased risk for mortality.[61] Two of five studies that examined follicular carcinoma demonstrated decreased survival rates in patients with initial nodal disease, although this is an uncommon presentation.[60]

Routine central compartment (level VI) neck dissection should be performed at the time of thyroidectomy, and compartment-oriented modified radical lateral dissections performed if node involvement is identified. In a retrospective analysis of 141 papillary carcinoma patients, 51% who were treated with thyroidectomy alone developed regional recurrence, as compared with 18% who also had lateral and central neck dissection.[62] These results suggest that neck dissections at the time of initial thyroidectomy may decrease the incidence of regional recurrence and support the practice of routine preoperative ultrasonography to evaluate regional lymphatics. In the presence of invasion of aerodigestive tract structures, similar survival rates are achieved from either complete surgical resection or shave excision leaving only microscopic residual disease.[63] In the presence of frank cartilage destruction or intraluminal involvement of the aerodigestive tract structures, a shave excision cannot be performed without leaving gross tumor behind, leading to a 50% death rate within 4 years. Surgery in patients with extensively invasive thyroid carcinoma should, therefore, aim to remove all gross tumor, attempting to retain as much airway, vocal, and digestive function as possible. However, only if the tumor is unresectable or the patient does not agree to a radical resection should gross tumor be left behind in the neck.

Postoperative Adjuvant Therapy **Radioiodine** Adjuvant ablation of residual thyroid tissue following primary surgery has two rationales: (1) to destroy any residual microscopic foci of disease, and (2) to increase the specificity and negative predictive value of subsequent serum thyroglobulin measurements and ^{131}I scanning for detection of recurrent or metastatic disease by eliminating residual normal tissue. Conflicting data have been reported from multiple retrospective studies of the efficacy of radioiodine. In a recent metaanalysis, only one of the seven included studies reported improved survival following adjuvant radioiodine,[40] and improved locoregional disease-free survival was observed in only three.[64] In the more recent multicenter thyroid cancer registry, improved survival was associated with postoperative radioiodine use in stages II to IV disease patients after adjustment for extent of thyroidectomy, and in stage III to IV patients when also adjusted for thyroid hormone suppression therapy.[51] For patients with residual disease following optimal surgery, including extracervical metastases, radioiodine therapy is also recommended. In contrast, ablation may be withheld for patients with small solitary primary tumors without evidence of extrathyroidal invasion or metastasis, particularly if under age 45 at diagnosis.

The efficacy of radioiodine depends on patient preparation, tumor-specific characteristics, sites of disease, and administered radioiodine activity. Iodide uptake by thyroid tissue is stimulated by TSH and is suppressed by increased endogenous iodide stores. Following thyroidectomy, the patient's thyroid hormone levels must decline sufficiently to allow the TSH concentration to rise to above 25 to 30 mU/L.[65] This period of hormone withdrawal typically lasts 4 to 5 weeks. To minimize the resulting symptoms of hypothyroidism, the shorter-acting hormone liothyronine (T3) is often administered at doses of 25 µg two times per day. Lower doses are administered to elderly patients and those with ischemic heart disease. Liothyronine is stopped at least 2 weeks prior to radioiodine dosing. An alternative to thyroid hormone withdrawal may be the use of exogenous recombinant human thyrotropin alfa, which in a recent small randomized study appeared equivalent to thyroid hormone withdrawal for stimulating radioiodine uptake and successful ablation.[66] Patients should avoid foods with high iodine content for at least 2 weeks prior to the scanning.[67] For similar reasons, radioiodine uptake can be iatrogenically suppressed for 1 to 3 months after administration of iodinated intravenous contrast for radiographic procedures. Urinary iodine content can be measured to confirm excessive iodine intake if suspected.

Whole-body radioiodine scans for localization of uptake prior to ablation or therapy are frequently performed 24 to 72 hours after administration of a diagnostic activity of 2 to 5 mCi of ^{131}I. Most patients demonstrate significant uptake of radioiodine within the thyroid bed following thyroidectomy, presumably from normal residual thyroid. Greater sensitivity for the detection of residual or metastatic tumor can be attained with the use of higher amounts of ^{131}I. But larger radioisotope activities can lead to "stunning," in which reduced uptake of the subsequent ablative or therapeutic dose occurs as a consequence of radiation delivered by the diagnostic dose.[68–70] Use of ^{123}I, with a lower radiation dose to thyroid tissue, may prevent stunning of therapeutic uptake after a diagnostic scan without loss of diagnostic accuracy.[71] However, the exact utility of scanning before therapy in the absence of known metastatic disease is undefined, and therefore scanning before ablation may be considered optional for patients who are apparently free from gross metastases.[55,57,71] An alternative approach is to use a low activity of ^{123}I to measure radioiodine uptake in the thyroid bed before treatment, without requiring greater activities necessary for imaging.

With postoperative radioiodine uptake in the thyroid bed, or if no pretherapy scanning or uptake has been performed, an empirically selected activity of ^{131}I is administered for adjuvant ablation, typically 30 to 100 mCi. In general, higher efficacy rates have been reported with larger administered activities. Assuming that the 24-hour radioiodine uptake is less than 5%, this lower activity has a similar efficacy of successful ablation and could be considered for patients with disease entirely confined to the thyroid gland.[72,73] Nonetheless, there is scant information about long-term outcomes, and considerably more study is required before such low doses can be generally recommended.[40] Alternatively, quantitative dosimetry can be applied to estimate the radioiodine activity necessary to deliver an effective radiation dose to the tissue of at least 30,000 cGy.[74] When substantial yet unsuspected locoregional disease or excessive thyroid remnants are detected, strong consideration is given to additional surgery before radioiodine administration.

A post-treatment scan is performed several days after administration of the radioiodine dose, but the diagnostic utility of such scans immediately after treatments is maximal in patients whose thyroid bed activity was previously ablated.[68,75]

Thyroid Hormone Patients require life-long thyroid hormone administration to treat postsurgical hypothyroidism and to minimize TSH stimulation to tumor growth. With TSH-suppressive thyroid hormone therapy, both overall survival and disease-free survival may be improved two- to threefold, particularly in TNM or National Thyroid Cancer Treatment Cooperative Study (NTCTCS) stages III and IV patients.[51,76–78] Lesser degrees of suppression may also improve overall survival in stage I and II patients.[51] However, potential morbidity from overly aggressive thyroid hormone suppression therapy includes acceleration of osteoporosis,[79,80] provocation of atrial fibrillation,[81] and possibly cardiac hypertrophy and dysfunction and impaired quality of life.[82] The clinician must balance the risk for disease recurrence or progression with the risk for thyrotoxic complications in determining the degree of TSH-suppressive therapy. At least during the initial years of follow-up, patients at lower risk for thyroid cancer morbidity and mortality should have their TSH levels maintained between 0.1 and 0.5 mU/L, whereas patients at higher risk should have TSH levels suppressed to less than 0.1 mU/L.[55,56,57] Patients who remain disease-free for 5 to 10 years may potentially have their degree of TSH suppression reduced by lowering their doses of thyroid hormone; other mitigating factors, such as concurrent cardiac disease, may also dictate a need for reduced hormone dosing.

External Beam Radiation External-beam radiotherapy (EBRT) may be an effective adjuvant therapy to prevent locoregional recurrence in older patients with locally invasive papillary carcinoma.[83,84] A review of 282 patients found that postoperative EBRT did not significantly affect the locoregional control or disease-specific survival rates. However, in a subgroup of 155 patients with papillary histology and microscopic residual disease (evidence of disease at or within 2 mm of the resection margin, or tumor that was shaved off cervical structures), EBRT produced a significant improvement in 10-year rates of locoregional control (93% vs 78%) and disease-specific survival (100% vs 95%).[83] Increased freedom from locoregional and distant relapse has been reported in patients older than age 40 years with extrathyroidal extension and lymph node involvement from papillary carcinoma, when treated with adjuvant EBRT in addition to total thyroidectomy, two courses of ^{131}I, and TSH suppression.[84] In neither study was a benefit of adjuvant EBRT demonstrated for patients with follicular carcinoma. Adjuvant EBRT is likely of little benefit to those younger than age 45 years, and esophageal and tracheal side effects may be poorly tolerated by the elderly patient (> 65 years).[85] EBRT, 40 to 50 Gy to the thyroid bed, is recommended in the setting of gross extrathyroidal invasion with presumed microscopic residual disease, as well as following incomplete resection near aerodigestive structures.[55–57]

LONG-TERM FOLLOW-UP Diagnostic Imaging and Serum Thyroglobulin Monitoring The follow-up paradigm for differentiated thyroid carcinomas has undergone significant changes in the past several years, in part due to the improved utility of cervical ultrasound and serum thyroglobulin measurements. Whereas patients following initial radioiodine ablation previously underwent routine radioiodine scanning,[86] this procedure is now being used more selectively.

Ultrasonography of the thyroid bed and cervical node compartments can accurately identify locoregional metastases and recurrence measuring several millimeters in diameter and facilitate confirmatory FNA of such lesions.[87–88] Neither CT nor MRI is as sensitive for detecting such small lesions, although these techniques are more readily standardized and less operator-dependent. Routine chest radiographs are of limited sensitivity, and probably can be avoided in low risk patients.

The synthesis and secretion of thyroglobulin (Tg) is a differentiated characteristic of thyroid follicular cells.[89.90] In the long-term follow-up of patients, measurement of the serum Tg concentration aids the detection of residual, recurrent, or metastatic disease, particularly given the rough correlation between tumor size and Tg level. After thyroid resection and ablation, serum Tg concentrations should approach the limits of assay detectability, but may take several years to decline to an undetectable nadir following primary therapy.[91] An important factor in the interpretation of Tg concentrations is the concurrent level of TSH, given the dependence on TSH for Tg production. The sensitivity for detection of residual cancer is enhanced by elevation of the serum TSH during thyroid hormone withdrawal or by the use of recombinant TSH (thyrotropin alfa).[92] The sensitivity of detecting disease by measurement of Tg following TSH stimulation is 85 to 95% but may be as low as 50% during TSH suppression or with dedifferentiated tumors.[93] The utility of stimulated Tg measurements in the absence of scanning combined with cervical ultrasound has the greatest accuracy in low risk patients, but radioiodine scanning remains valuable for follow-up in high risk patients.[94,95]

In immunometric assays, reported Tg concentrations can be falsely lowered by autoantibodies that bind Tg and prevent antigen interaction with assay's antibodies.[96] For the 25% of the thyroid cancer population with anti-Tg autoantibodies, serum Tg levels must be interpreted with caution. The persistence of anti-Tg autoantibodies following thyroidectomy and radioiodine ablation may in itself indicate the presence of residual thyroid tissue and an increased risk for recurrence.[97]

THERAPY OF METASTATIC DISEASE Surgery Function-preserving compartmental node dissection is preferred, if possible, for patients with nodes > 1 cm in diameter.[60] In the setting of disease invading aerodigestive structures, grossly complete surgical excision can improve survival, but may require more extensive procedures such as tracheal resection and anastomosis or pharyngectomy. Palliative procedures can be employed when curative resection is not feasible, and can include tracheal stents, tracheotomy, and laser ablation, in addition to partial excision. For extracervical metastases, surgical resection can lead to improved survival in selected patients. In one report, nearly 30% of patients who underwent complete resection of their skeletal, pulmonary or intraabdominal metastases remained disease free after an average follow-up of 8 years.[98] Among patients with one or more brain metastases, surgical removal significantly improved median survival from 4 to 22 months.[96] Symptom palliation can also result from surgical treatment, particularly for lesions causing pain or spinal cord compression.

Radioiodine ^{131}I treatment of regional nodal metastases yields a complete response in 80% of patients when at least 8,000 to 10,000 cGy is delivered, but can be suboptimal in patients with bulky disease.[74] Patients with residual postoperative disease in the thyroid bed or in the regional lymph nodes are treated with high activities of ^{131}I. Efficacy has been reported with 150 mCi as an average dose, either as a result of empiric therapy or as determined by dosimetry.

Patients treated for iodine-concentrating pulmonary metastases, which occur in approximately 5% of cases of differentiated cancer, have a 5-year survival rate of 60 to 80%, as compared with a 5-year survival rate of 30% for those whose tumors do not take up iodine.[99–101] Long-term survival is highest in those patients with pulmonary metastases seen on ^{131}I scanning, but not seen on chest radiography or CT. Nevertheless, only a minority of patients with such micronodular disease have a complete remission, perhaps because the delivery of tumoricidal radiation doses is minimized for metastases < 1 mm in size.[102] Patients with macronodular pulmonary follicular cells, metastatic disease can be suspected by the presence of a detectable serum Tg in the absence of radioiodine uptake. Such "false-negative" results occur in up to 15% of diagnostic radioiodine scans in patients with detectable Tg levels following thyroid ablation. Because a high frequency of post-therapy scans demonstrate foci of radioiodine uptake combined with a subsequent decrease in the serum Tg level, it has been proposed that patients with elevated serum Tg and negative diagnostic radioiodine scans should receive empiric 131I therapy with 100 to 300 mCi.[107,108] But, the underlying risk for disease-related morbidity or mortality in patients with scan-negative, Tg positive disease is not well defined, particularly for patients without evidence of tumor mass by other imaging modalities. At present, there is no evidence that either partial reductions in serum Tg levels or elimination of radioiodine uptake visible only on post-therapy scans is associated with improved patient outcome, and Tg levels often decline over a period of years without radioiodine treatment.[109,110] The potential risks of repeated high-dose empiric therapy must be considered as well. Diagnostic imaging should be performed to identify foci of disease that could be surgically resected or treated by other means (Figure 76-3), such as cervical ultrasonography, CT, or MRI.[111–113] PET imaging following injection of FDG can be particularly useful in localizing disease in patients with Tg levels greater than 10 ng/mL and negative radioiodine imaging. Given the propensity of follicular thyroid carcinoma to metastasize to bone, skeletal imaging with ^{99m}technetium pyrophosphate may also be of value. In the absence of surgically resectable disease, only patients with evidence of progressive metastases, rising Tg levels greater than 10 ng/mL, or who are at high risk for disease-related mortality might receive a therapeutic trial of radioiodine before embarking on other sys-

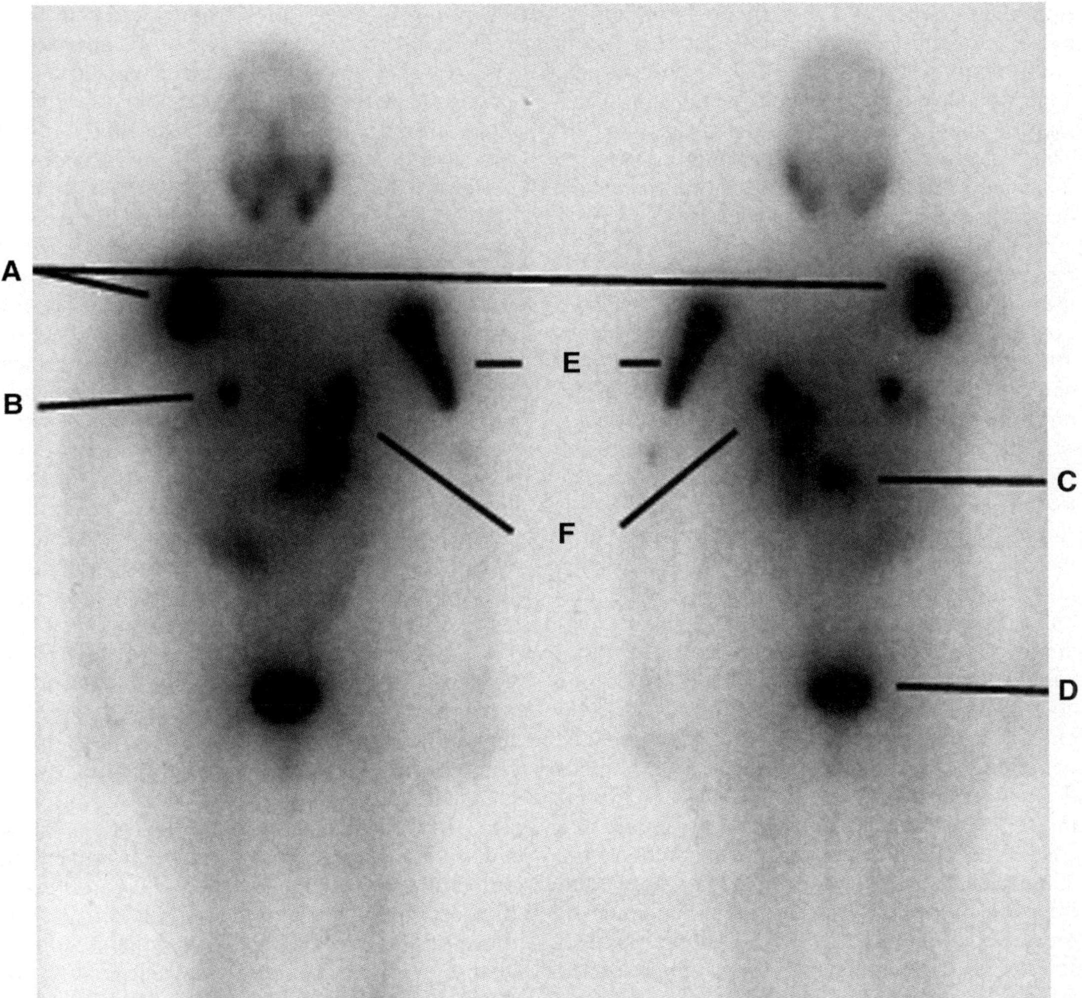

Figure 76-2 Anterior and posterior views of whole-body ^{131}I imaging in a patient with metastatic follicular thyroid carcinoma. Two years after a thyroidectomy and radioiodine ablation, the patient developed back and extremity pains. Following thyroid hormone withdrawal, a radioiodine scan was performed that revealed multiple skeletal and pulmonary metastases. External beam radiotherapy and multiple repeated doses of radioiodine led to resolution of her pain and stabilization of her disease. **A,** Right shoulder metastasis. **B,** Right lung metastasis. **C,** Thoracic vertebra metastasis. **D,** Radioiodine excreted in bladder. **E,** Left humerus metastasis. **F,** Left lung metastases superimposed on physiologic excretion into stomach.

metastases seen on chest radiography but not detected by ^{131}I scanning have the worst prognosis, and only rarely respond to large doses of ^{131}I. Radioiodine activities of 150 to 175 mCi are recommended for empiric treatment of pulmonary metastases. Advocates of dosimetry suggest treatment of distant metastases with the maximum tolerable doses, that is, that dose which delivers no more than 200 cGy to the red marrow and 80 to 120 mCi whole-body retention.[103] Such activities may exceed 300 to 400 mCi, but are calculated to allow the greatest degree of tumor kill without dose-limiting toxicity. Skeletal metastases often do not concentrate ^{131}I; complete resolution of disease occurs in fewer than 10% of treated patients, and partial remission in only 35%.[100] Patients with follicular carcinoma may be more likely to respond (Figure 76-2). Empiric doses of 200 mCi are generally suggested for distant metastases outside the lungs. Following surgical debulking, radioiodine therapy can also be administered to patients with iodine-concentrating intracerebral metastases.[99]

Acute and chronic complications of ^{131}I can limit the usefulness of this treatment. In the short-term, radiation thyroiditis, painless neck edema, sialoadenitis, and tumor hemorrhage or edema occur in 10 to 20% of patients, particularly when higher doses are given. The radioprotectant amifostine may prevent symptomatic reduction in long-term salivary gland function as a result of ^{131}I.[104] Over the long-term, ^{131}I therapy may be associated with development of secondary malignancies, such as acute myelocytic leukemia, usually occurring between 2 and 10 years after therapy. The risk is considerably lower when the total blood dose per treatment is less than 2 Gy, and when repeat treatments are given no more frequently than annually. Increased prevalence of cancers of the bladder, salivary gland, colon, and female breast has also been reported in patients, but with little agreement on the degree of absolute risk.[105,106] Oligospermia and transient ovarian failure also occur, but subsequent infertility is rare, except after high doses. Patients who receive repeated high radiation doses to the lung parenchyma from radioiodine treatment of diffuse pulmonary metastases rarely develop pulmonary fibrosis.

As production of Tg and incorporation of radioiodine represent distinct differentiated functions of

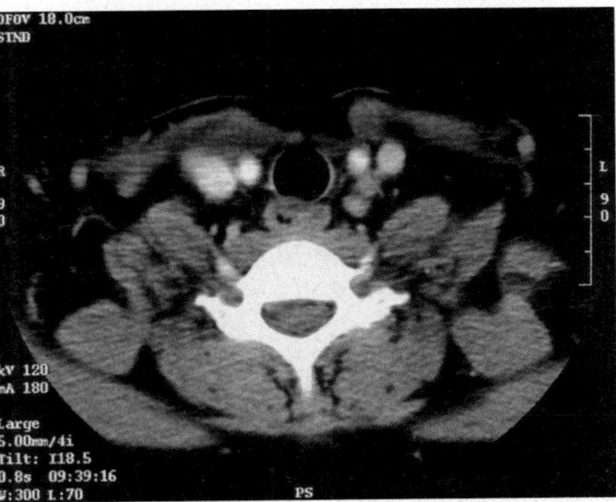

Figure 76-3 Contrast-enhanced CT of the neck in a patient with recurrent papillary thyroid carcinoma. Patient had previously undergone thyroidectomy and radioiodine ablation. Although a diagnostic radioiodine scan performed 1 week previously had shown no pathologic uptake, her serum TSH-stimulated thyroglobulin level was elevated, leading to the radiographic study. Following surgical resection of the two lymph nodes identified posterior to the left internal jugular vein and carotid artery, the serum thyroglobulin level became undetectable.

temic treatment modalities. However, for younger patients with stable or minimally elevated Tg levels and no radiographic evidence of disease, evidence of benefit is insufficient to warrant empiric radioiodine.

Biologic Modifiers of Radioiodine Responsiveness Poor uptake and diminished retention of radioiodine are associated with tumor dedifferentiation and poor response to treatment. Certain histologic subtypes, such as Hürthle cell carcinoma and the tall-cell variant of papillary carcinoma, concentrate ^{131}I less effectively.[34] Older patients and women may also be less likely to have adequate uptake in metastases. Restoration of responsiveness to radioiodine therapy has, therefore, been a major goal of investigation during the past several years. Because lithium can increase iodine retention by thyroid tissue, a recent study examined patients who had diagnostic ^{131}I scans before and after receiving lithium for 1 to 2 days.[114] ^{131}I retention was higher and more prolonged during lithium administration, and the estimated radiation dose to the metastases was 2.3 times higher. This increase was proportionally higher in tumors with lower baseline iodine retention, suggesting a potential approach to poorly responsive metastases. Whether these findings will result in improved eradication of metastases remains to be determined.

Loss of iodide uptake may be related to decreased expression of the sodium-iodide symporter in the tumor cells, which has been partially attributed to epigenetic alterations affecting gene expression. On the basis of the hypothesis that hypermethylation and/or histone deacetylation affecting the promoter region of thyroid-specific transcription factors or the sodium-iodine symporter genes leads to decreased expression and loss of iodide uptake, it could be presumed that hypomethylation might restore iodide uptake. In vitro, a 15-fold increase in iodide uptake was demonstrated in one dedifferentiated papillary thyroid cancer cell line treated with the demethylating agent 5-azacytidine.[115] Similar results have been reported from use of a histone deacetylase inhibitor, depsipeptide, to restore radioiodine uptake in vitro, and clinical trials are now under way with both classes of drugs in patients with iodide-unresponsive thyroid cancers.[116]

External-Beam Radiation Patients with unresectable gross locally invasive or metastatic disease in the neck may also benefit from the addition of EBRT. Of 33 patients with gross residual disease who received postoperative EBRT, the 5-year local control and disease-specific survival rates were approximately 65%.[83] EBRT can also benefit patients with painful skeletal metastases. When surgical resection is not feasible, palliative radiation should be offered to patients with bone lesions that either cause pain or pose a risk for pathologic fracture. Radiation doses of 50 Gy in 25 fractions may be given for solitary lesions, but reduced doses should be administered for vertebral foci.[85]

Chemotherapy Although 10 to 15% of patients with differentiated thyroid cancer die from their disease, and an even higher proportion suffer morbidity from recurrence, two recent authoritative texts devoted to thyroid cancer apportioned only 1% of their content to discussion of chemotherapy for these diseases.[117,118] This reflects the dearth of substantial research in this area. Little progress has been made since the original reports of partial responses to doxorubicin in approximately one-third of patients. The best responses occur in patients with pulmonary metastases and high performance status, in whom doxorubicin probably yields no greater than a 30% response rate for progressive differentiated cancers unresponsive to radioiodine.[119] The recommended dose is 60 to 75 mg/m^2 every 3 weeks, administered as a continuous intravenous infusion for 48 to 72 hours to minimize the risk of cardiac toxicity. Cumulative doses of up to 600 mg/m^2 can be administered in responsive patients. Other single chemotherapeutic agents that have been attempted include paclitaxel, bleomycin, cisplatin, carboplatin, methotrexate, melphalan, mitoxantrone, etoposide, and aclarubicin, without suggestion of improved response rates. In one comparative trial, the combination of doxorubicin, 60 mg/m^2, and cisplatin, 40 mg/m^2, induced complete or partial response in 16%, whereas doxorubicin alone yielded a 31% response rate.[120] Toxicities, including pancytopenia and gastrointestinal side effects, are markedly more common and severe, however, during these combination therapies, without clear evidence of greater benefit. More recently, multiple phase II studies have been initiated with therapies targeted at cellular mechanisms active in thyroid carcinoma, including tyrosine kinase inhibitors against signaling cascades (eg, gefitinib against the EGF receptor, sorafenib against the B-raf kinase, and multiple antagonists of VEGF receptors), proteasome inhibitors to augment levels of key cell cycle regulators such as p27, and epigenetic modifiers. Given the marked increase in availability of such trials, it can now be recommended that patients with metastatic thyroid carcinoma unresponsive to radioiodine should be considered for participation in clinical trials as an alternative to the currently available typical chemotherapeutic agents such as doxorubicin.

Management of Differentiated Carcinoma in Special Populations Thyroid carcinoma in children and adolescents is uncommon, and few large series have evaluated the long-term prognosis and appropriate therapy for young patients with these malignancies. A recent series described the extended follow-up of 112 young patients with differentiated thyroid carcinoma treated at the M.D. Anderson Cancer Center.[121] One-fourth of the 99 living patients had developed recurrent disease, and 6 patients died of thyroid cancer at a mean of 26 years after initial diagnosis. One patient who had lung metastases at the time of diagnosis died of progressive pulmonary disease after 36 years. The other 5 patients developed lung and bone metastases and died after a 2- to 20-year disease-free interval. Three more patients died from complications of radiation therapy, one because of tracheal necrosis 26 years after diagnosis and two because of cervical sarcomas over 20 years after diagnosis. Two died from subsequent breast cancer, although it remains unclear if this was a complication of thyroid cancer therapy.[106] In another series of 61 young patients treated for thyroid cancer, the 20-year survival rate was 97%.[122] Two patients died of progressive metastatic thyroid cancer within 10 years of the initial operations. Three of the 10 patients who had lobectomy or subtotal thyroidectomy developed local recurrence in the residual thyroid gland, whereas none of the 51 patients who had total or near-total thyroidectomy developed a local recurrence, Given the high frequency of multifocal intrathyroidal disease, locoregional spread, and extracervical metastases, total thyroidectomy with nodal dissection and adjuvant radioiodine therapy should be offered to all young patients with differentiated carcinoma. Lifelong close surveillance is warranted because of the risk of late recurrences and disease progression.

Differentiated carcinoma is diagnosed during 0.1% of all pregnancies.[123] There has been some concern that the hormonal factors associated with pregnancy might accelerate the progression of disease and necessitate a more aggressive management strategy. However, the outcomes of 61 pregnant women diagnosed with differentiated carcinoma did not differ from those of 528 age-matched nonpregnant women, despite a delay in definitive treatment in the pregnant women.[124] In most cases, the treatment of thyroid cancer can be safely delayed until the postpartum period.

MEDULLARY THYROID CANCER

Medullary thyroid carcinoma (MTC) derives from the neuroendocrine parafollicular or C cells of the thyroid (Figure 76-4).[125] Sporadic MTC accounts for 80% of all cases of the disease, with the remainder of patients having inherited tumor syndromes, such as multiple endocrine neoplasia (MEN) type 2A, MEN2B, or familial medullary thyroid carcinoma (FMTC). Because the C cells are predominantly located in the upper portion of

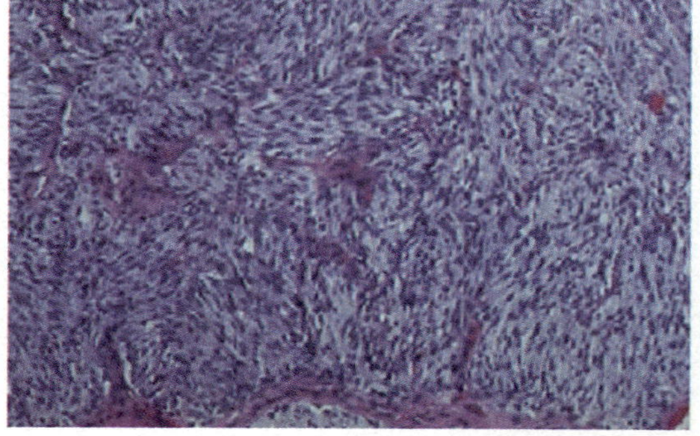

Figure 76-4 Medullary thyroid carcinoma, with nests of spindle-shaped cells. Such nests are often interspersed with clusters of round-to-oval cells, all immunostaining for calcitonin.

each thyroid lobe, patients with sporadic disease typically present with upper pole nodules. Metastatic cervical adenopathy is noted in approximately 50% of patients at initial presentation, and symptoms of upper aerodigestive tract compression or invasion are reported in up to 15% of patients with sporadic disease.[126] Symptoms from distant metastases in the lungs or bones may be elicited from 5 to 10% of patients. The ability of the tumor to oversecrete measurable quantities of calcitonin, occasionally along with other hormonally active peptides, such as adrenocorticotrophic hormone or calcitonin gene-related peptide, leads to unexplained diarrhea, symptoms of Cushing's syndrome, or facial flushing in many patients with advanced disease. Rarely, MTC is suggested by the presence of dense calcifications seen on radiologic imaging of the anterior neck or sites of metastatic disease. The typical age of sporadic presentation is in the fifth or sixth decade, and there may be a slight female preponderance.

The diagnosis of sporadic MTC is usually suspected following FNA of a solitary nodule. Although routine measurement of the serum calcitonin concentration has been suggested as a means of identifying MTC without an FNA, unresolved issues of specificity, assay performance, and cost-effectiveness should limit routine use.[127] However, if the serum calcitonin level has been measured, an unstimulated level greater than 100 pg/mL is associated with a high likelihood of MTC.[125]

In known families with inherited MTC, prospective family screening identified disease carriers long before clinical symptoms or signs were noted.[125] When compared with sporadic disease, the typical age of presentation for familial disease is the third decade, without gender preference; in MEN2A, signs or symptoms of hyperparathyroidism or pheochromocytoma uncommonly present before those of MTC, even in the absence of prospective screening. All familial forms of MTC and MEN2 are inherited in an autosomal dominant fashion. Mutations in *ret,* which codes for a cell membrane-associated tyrosine kinase receptor for glial cell line-derived neurotrophic factor, are found in more than 95% of families with familial forms of MTC.[128,129] Recent evidence suggests that allelic imbalance of overexpressed mutated *ret* genes is responsible for development of MTC in these familial disorders.[130] Mutations associated with MEN2A and FMTC have been primarily identified in several codons of the cysteine-rich extra-cellular domains of exon 10, 11, and 13, whereas MEN2B and some FMTC mutations are found within the intracellular exons 15 and 16 (Table 76-3).[125] Somatic mutations in exons 11, 13, and 16 have also been found in at least 50% of sporadic MTC tumors, particularly the codon 918 mutation that activates the tyrosine kinase function of the receptor and is associated with poorer patient prognosis. Furthermore, approximately 6% of patients with clinically sporadic MTC carry a germ line mutation in *ret,* leading to identification of new families with multiple previously undiagnosed affected individuals.[131] Genetic testing for *ret* proto-oncogene mutations should be offered to all patients newly diagnosed with clinically apparent sporadic MTC, as well as for screening children and adults in known families with inherited forms of MTC.[132] On the basis of the relative frequency of mutations in certain exons, mutational analysis should start with exon 11, followed sequentially by exons 10, 16, 13, 14, and 15.[128] Although common mutations can be identified by broadly available commercial testing sources, only a limited number of sites perform the more thorough analyses that are required to identify the less common mutations. Presently, a 5% error rate is generally reported, underscoring the importance for repeat testing of at least two independently obtained blood samples in more than one laboratory to minimize the likelihood of both false-positive and false-negative results.[132]

Table 76-3 *ret* Protooncogene Mutations in Hereditary Medullary Thyroid Carcinoma

Mutated Codon/Exon	Clinical Syndrome
609/10	FMTC; MEN2A with or without Hirschsprung disease
611/10	FMTC; MEN2A
618/10	FMTC; MEN2A with or without Hirschsprung disease
620/10	FMTC; MEN2A with or without Hirschsprung disease
630/11	FMTC; MEN2A
634/11	FMTC; MEN2A; MEN2A with cutaneous lichen amyloidosis
635/11	MEN2A
637/11	MEN2A
768/13	FMTC
790/13	FMTC; MEN2A
791/13	FMTC
804/13	FMTC; MEN2A
883/15	MEN2B
891/15	FMTC
918/16	MEN2B
922/16	MEN2B

Adapted from Gagel RF and Cote G.[125]

The primary approach to staging of medullary carcinoma is the AJCC-based TNM system.[43] Patients younger than 40 years of age at diagnosis have 5- and 10-year disease-specific survival of approximately 95% and 75%, respectively, as compared with 65% and 50% for those older than age 40 years.[126] Patients with inherited disease appear to have a better prognosis, even after correcting for the early age of diagnosis in familial disease. Despite being typically diagnosed during childhood, patients with MEN2B are more likely than those with either MEN2A or FMTC to have locally aggressive disease.[134] Other factors that may be important for predicting a worse prognosis include the heterogeneity and paucity of calcitonin immunostaining of the tumor, rapidly rising serum carcinoembryonic antigen (CEA), and postoperative residual hypercalcitoninemia.

Initial Surgical Management Unless MEN2 has been ruled out by *ret* testing, serum calcium and plasma metanephrines should be measured to exclude coexistent hyperparathyroidism and pheochromocytoma, respectively. Total thyroidectomy is indicated in all patients with MTC, especially given the high frequency of bilateral disease in both sporadic and familial disease, and has been associated with improved survival.[135] Once an MTC tumor is large enough to be palpated, there is a high frequency of metastasis to adjacent nodal tissue. Even in the absence of clinically detectable nodal metastases, central neck compartment dissection should be performed in all patients, and ipsilateral lateral neck and/or mediastinal dissections should be strongly considered when the primary tumor is > 1 cm or when central compartment disease is present. Disfiguring radical node dissections do not improve prognosis and are not indicated. In the presence of grossly invasive disease, more extended procedures with resection of involved neck structures may be appropriate, but function-preserving approaches are preferred. Post-operative thyroid hormone therapy is indicated, but TSH suppression is not appropriate as C cells lack TSH receptors.

Adjuvant Radiation Therapy EBRT should be considered in patients after maximal surgical therapy who are considered at high risk for regional recurrence. After radiotherapy for microscopic residual disease, extraglandular invasion, or lymph node metastases, the locoregional relapse-free rate at 10 years was 86%, as compared with 52% for those patients who did not receive adjuvant therapy.[136] Typically, 40 Gy is administered in 20 fractions to the cervical, supraclavicular, and upper mediastinal lymph nodes over 4 weeks, with subsequent booster doses of 10 Gy in 5 fractions to the thyroid bed.[137] As for differentiated carcinoma, EBRT can be given to palliate painful bone metastases.

Persistently Elevated Calcitonin Six months postoperatively, serum concentrations of calcitonin and CEA should be measured. Approximately 80% of patients with palpable MTC and 50% of those with nonpalpable but macroscopic MTC who undergo supposedly curative resection will have detectable serum calcitonin values, which is indicative of residual disease. Those with near-normal values can be followed conservatively without intervention, but those with values > 100 pg/mL should be evaluated for either residual resectable disease in the neck or the presence of distant metastases. Patients with serum calcitonin values > 1,000 pg/mL and no obvious MTC in the neck and upper mediastinum probably have distant metastases, most likely in the liver. The prognosis for patients with postoperative hypercalcitoninemia depends primarily on the extent of disease at the time of initial surgery. In a study of 31 patients (10 patients with apparently sporadic disease, 15 with MEN2A, and 6 with MEN2B), the 5- and 10-year survival rates were 90 and 86%, respectively.[138] Two recent studies have reported higher mortality rates for patients with high postoperative serum calcitonin values, with more than half the patients having a recurrence during mean follow-up of 10 years.[139,140]

Given the general failure of routine lymphadenectomy or excision of palpable tumor to normalize the serum calcitonin concentrations in such patients, attention has been directed toward detection and eradication of microscopic deposits of tumor. Of patients undergoing extensive microdissection of the central and bilateral neck compartments, 20 to 40% of patients were biochemically cured, with minimal perioperative morbidity, recurrent hypercalcitoninemia and disease recurrence have been reported.[141–143] In the absence of long-term outcomes, however, application of this approach should probably be limited to those centers experienced in this procedure; only patients with overt disease in the neck and no distant metastases should undergo reoperative neck surgery.

Prophylactic Surgery for Gene Carriers Given the identification of patients with malignant disease as early as age 6 years, prophylactic thyroidectomy by age 5 has been recommended for at-risk family members who are identified as carriers of a familial *ret* mutation.[144] Of 18 patients who underwent prophylactic thyroidectomy at a median age of 14 years, nearly 80% had a histologic diagnosis of MTC, but none had evidence of nodal metastases.[144] In the 13 patients evaluated 3 years after surgery, all had normal levels of stimulated plasma calcitonin. Surveillance with stimulated calcitonin measurements rather than surgery is still suggested by some investigators for young gene carriers without evidence of MTC, although this approach should probably be avoided in children with the more virulent *ret* mutations in exons 10 and 11.[145]

Management of Distant Metastatic Disease Systemic chemotherapy has been reported to yield response in up to 30% of patients with metastases of MTC involving liver, lung or bones. Most regimens in current use combine dacarbazine with other agents including vincristine, 5-fluorouracil, cyclophosphamide, or doxorubicin, without significant advantage of one combination compared with another.[146,147] More recently, therapies targeting key intracellular signaling cascades, particularly *ret* along with other activated tyrosine kinases such as VEGFR, have entered clinical trials.[129,148]

ANAPLASTIC THYROID CARCINOMA

Anaplastic thyroid carcinomas are aggressive undifferentiated tumors, with a disease-specific mortality approaching 100%. Patients with anaplastic carcinoma are older than those with differentiated carcinomas, with a mean age at diagnosis of about 65 years. Fewer than 10% of patients are younger than 50 years, and 60 to 70% are women.[3] Approximately 50% of patients with anaplastic cancer have either a prior or coexistent differentiated carcinoma. Anaplastic carcinoma develops from more differentiated tumors as a result of one or more dedifferentiating steps, particularly loss of the p53 tumor-suppressor protein.[149] No precipitating events have been identified, and the mechanisms leading to anaplastic transformation of differentiated carcinomas are uncertain.

Patients with anaplastic carcinoma present with extensive local invasion, and distant metastases are found at initial disease presentation in 15 to 50% of patients.[150] The lungs and pleura are the most common sites of distant metastases, being seen in up to 90% of patients with distant disease. Approximately 5 to 15% of patients have bone metastases, 5% have brain metastases, and a few have metastases to the skin, liver, kidneys, pancreas, heart, and adrenal glands.

The diagnosis of anaplastic carcinoma is usually established by FNA or surgical biopsy. CT of the neck and mediastinum can accurately determine the extent of the thyroid tumor and identify tumor invasion of the great vessels and upper aerodigestive tract structures.[150] Most pulmonary metastases are nodules that can be detected by routine chest radiography. Bone lesions are usually lytic.

Treatment and Prognosis There is no effective therapy for anaplastic carcinoma, and the disease is uniformly fatal. The median survival from diagnosis ranges from 3 to 7 months, and the 1- and 5-year survival rates are approximately 25 and 5%, respectively.[151] Death is attributable to upper airway obstruction and suffocation (often despite tracheostomy) in half the patients and to a combination of complications of local and distant disease and/or therapy in the remainder. Patients with disease confined to the neck at diagnosis have a mean survival of 8 months, as compared to 3 months if the disease has extended beyond the neck.[152] Other variables that may predict worse prognosis include older age at diagnosis, male gender, and dyspnea as a presenting symptom.

Except for patients whose tumors are small and confined entirely to the thyroid, total thyroidectomy with complete tumor resection does not prolong survival.[153,154] EBRT, administered in conventional doses, also does not prolong survival. Although up to 40% of patients may respond initially to radiation therapy, most have local recurrence. Treatment with single-drug chemotherapy also does not improve survival or control of disease in the neck, although perhaps 20% of patients have some response in distant metastases. The introduction of hyperfractionated radiotherapy, combined with radiosensitizing doses of doxorubicin, may increase the local response rate to about 80%, with subsequent median survival of 1 year; distant metastases then become the leading cause of death.[155] Similar improvement in local disease control has been reported with the combination of hyperfractionated radiotherapy and doxorubicin, followed by debulking surgery in responsive patients. However, the addition of larger doses of other chemotherapeutic drugs has not been associated with improved control of distant disease or improved survival. Paclitaxel has been associated with short-term stabilization in a minority of patients, and may provide some palliative benefit.[156] A report of a recent phase I study of the antiangiogenesis agent combretastatin described one patient with a prolonged complete response despite failure of previous doxorubicin therapy, and is the basis of an ongoing phase II trial.[157]

REFERENCES

1. Jemal A, Murray T, Ward E, et al. Cancer statistics, 2005. CA: Cancer J Clin 2005;55:10–30.
2. . Ries LAG, Eisner MP, Kosary CL, et al, editors. SEER Cancer Statistics Review, 1975–2001, National Cancer Institute. Bethesda, MD. Available at: http://seer.cancer.gov/csr/1975_2001/, 2004.
3. Gilliland FD, Hunt WC, Morris DM, Key CR. Prognostic factors for thyroid carcinoma: a population-based study of 15,698 cases from the Surveillance, Epidemiology and End Results (SEER) program 1973–1991. Cancer 1997;79:564–73.
4. Sherman SI. NCCN practice guidelines for thyroid cancer, version 2005. Vol. 2005. National Comprehensive Cancer Network; 2005. Available at: www.nccn.org.
5. Mandel SJ. A 64-year-old woman with a thyroid nodule. JAMA 2005;292:2632–42.
6. Papini E, Guglielmi R, Bianchini A, et al. Risk of malignancy in nonpalpable thyroid nodules: predictive value of ultrasound and color-Doppler features. J Clin Endocrinol Metab 2002;87:1941–6.
7. Ravetto C, Colombo L, Dottorini ME. Usefulness of fine-needle aspiration in the diagnosis of thyroid carcinoma: a retrospective study in 37,895 patients. Cancer 2000;90:357–63.
8. Cochand-Priollet B, Guillausseau PJ, Chagnon S, et al. The diagnostic value of fine-needle aspiration biopsy under ultrasonography in nonfunctional thyroid nodules: a prospective study comparing cytologic and histologic findings. Am J Med 1994;97:152–7.
9. Gharib H. Fine-needle aspiration biopsy of thyroid nodules: advantages, limitations, and effect. Mayo Clin Proc 1994;69:44–9.
10. Tyler DS, Winchester DJ, Caraway NP, et al. Indeterminate fine-needle aspiration biopsy of the thyroid. Identification of subgroups at high risk for invasive carcinoma. Surgery 1994;116:1054–60.
11. Tuttle RM, Lemar H, Burch HB. Clinical features associated with an increased risk of thyroid malignancy in patients with follicular neoplasia by fine-needle aspiration. Thyroid 1998;8:377–83.
12. Baloch ZW, Fleisher S, LiVolsi VA, Gupta PK. Diagnosis of "follicular neoplasm": a gray zone in thyroid fine-needle aspiration cytology. Diagn Cytopathol 2002;26:41–4.
13. Udelsman R, Westra WH, Donovan PI, et al. Randomized prospective evaluation of frozen-section analysis for follicular neoplasms of the thyroid. Ann Surg 2001; 233:716–22.
14. Roach JC, Heller KS, Dubner S, Sznyter LA. The value of frozen-section examinations in determining the extent of thyroid surgery in patients with indeterminate fine-needle aspiration cytology. Arch Otolaryngol Head Neck Surg 2002;128:263–7.
15. Cramer H. Fine-needle aspiration cytology of the thyroid: an appraisal. Cancer 2000;90:325–9.
16. Figge J, Jennings T, Gerasimov G. Radiation and thyroid cancer. In: Wartofsky L, editor. Thyroid cancer. A comprehensive guide to clinical management. Totowa (NJ): Humana Press; 1999. p. 85–116.
17. Pacini F, Vorontsova T, Demidchik EP, et al. Post-Chernobyl thyroid carcinoma in Belarus children and adolescents: comparison with naturally occurring thyroid carcinoma in Italy and France. J Clin Endocrinol Metab 1997;82:3563–9.
18. Gilbert ES, Tarone R, Bouville A, Ron E. Thyroid cancer rates and ^{131}I doses from Nevada atmospheric nuclear bomb tests. J Natl Cancer Inst 1998;90:1654–60.
19. Hundahl SA. Perspective: National Cancer Institute summary report about estimated exposures and thyroid doses received from iodine-131 in fallout after Nevada atmospheric nuclear bomb tests. CA Cancer J Clin 1998;48:285–98.
20. Musholt TJ, Musholt PB, Petrich T, et al. Familial papillary thyroid carcinoma: genetics, criteria for diagnosis, clinical features, and surgical treatment. World J Surg 2000;24:1409–17.

21. Alsanea O, Wada N, Ain K, et al. Is familial non-medullary thyroid carcinoma more aggressive than sporadic thyroid cancer? A multicenter series. Surgery 2000;128:1043–50.
22. McKay JD, Lesueur F, Jonard L, et al. Localization of a susceptibility gene for familial nonmedullary thyroid carcinoma to chromosome 2q21. Am J Hum Genet 2001; 69:440–6.
23. Cohen Y, Xing M, Mambo E, et al. BRAF mutation in papillary thyroid carcinoma. J Natl Cancer Inst 2003;95:625–7.
24. Nikiforova MN, Stringer JR, Blough R, et al. Proximity of chromosomal loci that participate in radiation-induced rearrangements in human cells. Science 2000; 290:138–41.
25. Xing M. BRAF mutation in thyroid cancer. Endocr Relat Cancer 2005;12:245-62.
26. Elisei R, Shiohara M, Koeffler HP, Fagin JA. Genetic and epigenetic alterations of the cyclin-dependent kinase inhibitors p15INK4b and p16INK4a in human thyroid carcinoma cell lines and primary thyroid carcinomas. Cancer 1998;83:2185–93.
27. Ouyang B, Knauf JA, Ain K, et al. Mechanisms of aneuploidy in thyroid cancer cell lines and tissues: evidence for mitotic checkpoint dysfunction without mutations in BUB1 and BUBR1. Clin Endocrinol (Oxf) 2002; 56:341–50.
28. Specht MC, Barden CB, Fahey TJ 3rd. p44/p42-MAP kinase expression in papillary thyroid carcinomas. Surgery 2001;130:936–40.
29. Saavedra HI, Knauf JA, Shirokawa JM, et al. The RAS oncogene induces genomic instability in thyroid PCCL3 cells via the MAPK pathway. Oncogene 2000;19:3948–54.
30. Kroll TG, Sarraf P, Pecciarini L, et al. PAX8-PPARgamma1 fusion oncogene in human thyroid carcinoma [corrected]. Science 2000;289:1357–60.
31. Fagin JA. Minireview: branded from the start-distinct oncogenic initiating events may determine tumor fate in the thyroid. Mol Endocrinol 2002;16:903–11.
32. Tielens ET, Sherman SI, Hruban RH, Ladenson PW. Follicular variant of papillary thyroid carcinoma. A clinicopathologic study. Cancer 1994;73:424–31.
33. Johnson TL, Lloyd RV, Thompson NW, et al. Prognostic implications of the tall cell variant of papillary thyroid carcinoma. Am J Surg Pathol 1988;12:22–7.
34. Lopez-Penabad L, Chiu AC, Hoff AO, et al. Prognostic factors in Hürthle cell neoplasms of the thyroid. Cancer 2003;97.
35. Byar DP, Green SB, Dor P, et al. A prognostic index for thyroid carcinoma. A study of the E.O.R.T.C. thyroid cancer cooperative group. Eur J Cancer 1979;15:1033–41.
36. Cady B, Rossi R. An expanded view of risk-group definition in differentiated thyroid carcinoma. Surgery 1988; 104:947–53.
37. Hay ID, Grant CS, Taylor WF, McConahey WM. Ipsilateral lobectomy versus bilateral lobar resection in papillary thyroid carcinoma: a retrospective analysis of surgical out-come using a novel prognostic scoring system. Surgery 1987;102:1088–95.
38. Hay ID, Bergstralh EJ, Goellner J, et al. Predicting outcome in papillary carcinoma: development of a reliable prognostic scoring system in a cohort of 1,779 patients treated surgically at one institution during 1940 through 1989. Surgery 1993;114:1050–8.
39. DeGroot LJ, Kaplan EL, McCormick M, Straus FH. Natural history, treatment, and course of papillary thyroid carcinoma. J Clin Endocrinol Metab 1990;71:414–24.
40. Mazzaferri EL, Jhiang SM. Long-term impact of initial surgical and medical therapy on papillary and follicular thyroid cancer. Am J Med 1994;97:418–28.
41. Sherman SI, Brierley JD, Sperling M, et al. Prospective multicenter study of treatment of thyroid carcinoma: initial analysis of staging and outcome. Cancer 1998;83:1012–21.
42. Brierley JD, Panzarella T, Tsang RW, et al. A comparison of different staging systems predictability of patient outcome. Thyroid carcinoma as an example. Cancer 1997;79:2414–23.
43. Greene FL, Page DL, Fleming ID, et al. AJCC cancer staging manual. New York: Springer-Verlag; 2002. p. 421.
44. Sherman SI. Toward a standard clinicopathologic staging approach for differentiated thyroid carcinoma. Semin Surg Oncol 1999;16:12–5.
45. Association of Directors of Anatomic and Surgical Pathology. Recommended reporting format for thyroid carcinoma. Am J Clin Pathol 2000;114:684–6.
46. Katoh R, Sasaki J, Kurihara H, et al. Multiple thyroid involvement (intraglandular metastasis) in papillary thyroid carcinoma. A clinicopathologic study of 105 consecutive patients. Cancer 1992;70:1585–90.
47. Silverberg SG, Hutter RVP, Foote FW Jr. Fatal carcinoma of the thyroid: histology, metastases, and causes of death. Cancer 1970;25:792–802.
48. Hay ID, Grant CS, Bergstralh EJ, et al. Unilateral total lobectomy: is it sufficient surgical treatment for patients with AMES low-risk papillary thyroid carcinoma? Surgery 1998;124:958–64; discussion 964–6.
49. Samaan NA, Schultz PN, Hickey RC, et al. The results of various modalities of treatment of well differentiated thyroid carcinoma: a retrospective review of 1,599 patients. J Clin Endocrinol Metab 1992;75:714–20.
50. DeGroot LJ, Kaplan EL, Straus FH. Does the method of management of papillary thyroid carcinoma make a difference in outcome? World J Surg 1994;18:123–30.
51. Jonklaas J, Sarlis NJ, Litofsky D, et al. Outcomes of patients with differentiated thyroid carcinoma following initial therapy: Results from the National Thyroid Cancer Treatment Cooperative Study Group Registry. Submitted.
52. Cady B. Papillary carcinoma of the thyroid gland: treatment based on risk group definition. Surg Oncol Clin N Am 1998;7:633–44.
53. Sosa JA, Bowman HM, Tielsch JM, et al. The importance of surgeon experience for clinical and economic outcomes from thyroidectomy. Ann Surg 1998;228:320–30.
54. Udelsman R, Lakatos E, Ladenson P. Optimal surgery for papillary thyroid carcinoma. World J Surg 1996; 20:88–93.
55. Cooper DS, et al. American Thyroid Association management guidelines for patients with thyroid nodules and differentiated thyroid carcinoma. Manuscript in preparation.
56. Thyroid Carcinoma Task Force. AACE/AAES medical/surgical guidelines for clinical practice: management of thyroid carcinoma. Endocr Pract 2001;7:203–20.
57. Guidelines for the management of thyroid cancer in adults. London: British Thyroid Association and Royal College of Physicians; 2002.
58. Fogelfeld L, Wiviott MB, Shore-Freedman E, et al. Recurrence of thyroid nodules after surgical removal in patients irradiated in childhood for benign conditions [see comments]. N Engl J Med 1989;320:835–40.
59. Kupferman ME, Patterson M, Mandel SJ, et al. Patterns of lateral neck metastasis in papillary thyroid carcinoma. Arch Otolaryngol Head Neck Surg 2004;130:857–60.
60. Grebe SK, Hay ID. Thyroid cancer nodal metastases: biologic significance and therapeutic considerations. Surg Oncol Clin N Am 1996;5:43–63.
61. Vassilopoulou-Sellin R, Schultz PN, Haynie TP. Clinical outcome of patients with papillary thyroid carcinoma who have recurrence after initial radioactive iodine therapy. Cancer 1996;78:493–501.
62. Simon D, Goretzki PE, Witte J, Roher HD. Incidence of regional recurrence guiding radicality in differentiated thyroid carcinoma. World J Surg 1996;20:860–6.
63. Gillenwater AM, Goepfert H. Surgical management of laryngotracheal and esophageal involvement by locally advanced thyroid cancer. Semin Surg Oncol 1999;16:19–29.
64. Sawka AM, Thephamongkhol K, Brouwers M, et al. A systematic review and metaanalysis of the effectiveness of radioactive iodine remnant ablation for well-differentiated thyroid cancer. J Clin Endocrinol Metab 2004; 89:3668–76.
65. Schlumberger M, Tubiana M, De Vathaire F, et al. Long-term results of treatment of 283 patients with lung and bone metastases from differentiated thyroid carcinoma. J Clin Endocrinol Metab 1986;63:960–7.
66. Pacini F, Ladenson PW, Schlumberger M, et al. Radioiodine ablation of thyroid remnants after preparation with recombinant human thyrotropin in differentiated thyroid carcinoma: results of an international, randomized, controlled study. [Submitted.]
67. Lakshmanan M, Schaffer A, Robbins J, et al. A simplified low iodine diet in I-131 scanning and therapy of thyroid cancer. Clin Nucl Med 1988;13:866–8.
68. Sherman SI, Tielens ET, Sostre S, et al. Clinical utility of posttreatment radioiodine scans in the management of patients with thyroid carcinoma. J Clin Endocrinol Metab 1994;78:629–34.
69. Muratet JP, Daver A, Minier JF, Larra F. Influence of scanning doses of iodine-131 on subsequent first ablative treatment outcome in patients operated on for differentiated thyroid carcinoma. J Nucl Med 1998;39:1546–50.
70. Mandel SJ, Shankar LK, Benard F, et al. Superiority of iodine-123 compared with iodine-131 scanning for thyroid remnants in patients with differentiated thyroid cancer. Clin Nucl Med 2001;26:6–9.
71. Cailleux AF, Baudin E, Travagli JP, et al. Is diagnostic iodine-131 scanning useful after total thyroid ablation for differentiated thyroid cancer? J Clin Endocrinol Metab 2000;85:175–8.
72. Logue JP, Tsang RW, Brierley JD, Simpson WJ. Radioiodine ablation of residual tissue in thyroid cancer: relationship between administered activity, neck uptake and outcome. Br J Radiol 1994;67:1127–31.
73. Bal C, Padhy AK, Jana S, et al. Prospective randomized clinical trial to evaluate the optimal dose of ^{131}I for remnant ablation in patients with differentiated thyroid carcinoma. Cancer 1996;77:2574–80.
74. Maxon HR, Englaro EE, Thomas SR, et al. Radioiodine-131 therapy for well-differentiated thyroid cancer—a quantitative radiation dosimetric approach: outcome and validation in 85 patients. J Nucl Med 1992;33:1132–6.
75. Reynolds JC. Percent ^{131}I uptake and post-therapy ^{131}I scans: their role in the management of thyroid cancer. Thyroid 1997;7:281–4.
76. Pujol P, Daures J-P, Nsakala N, et al. Degree of thyrotropin suppression as a prognostic determinant in differentiated thyroid cancer. J Clin Endocrinol Metab 1996;81:4318–23.
77. Cooper DS, Specker B, Ho M, et al. Thyrotropin suppression and disease progression in patients with differentiated thyroid cancer: results from the National Thyroid Cancer Treatment Cooperative Registry. Thyroid 1998;8:737–44.
78. McGriff NJ, Csako G, Gourgiotis L, et al. Effects of thyroid hormone suppression therapy on adverse clinical outcomes in thyroid cancer. Ann Med 2002; 34:554-64.
79. Stall GM, Harris S, Sokoll LJ, Dawson-Hughes B. Accelerated bone loss in hypothyroid patients overtreated with L-thyroxine. Ann Intern Med 1990;113:265–9.
80. Bauer DC, Ettinger B, Nevitt MC, et al. Risk for fracture in women with low serum levels of thyroid-stimulating hormone. Ann Intern Med 2001;134:561–8.
81. Sawin CT, Geller A, Wolf PA, et al. Low serum thyrotropin concentrations as a risk factor for atrial fibrillation in older persons. N Engl J Med 1994;331:1249–52.
82. Biondi B, Palmieri EA, Fazio S, et al. Endogenous subclinical hyperthyroidism affects quality of life and cardiac morphology and function in young and middle-aged patients. J Clin Endocrinol Metab 2000;85:4701–5.
83. Tsang RW, Brierley JD, Simpson WJ, et al. The effects of surgery, radioiodine, and external radiation therapy on the clinical outcome of patients with differentiated thyroid carcinoma. Cancer 1998;82:375–88.
84. Farahati J, Reiners C, Stuschke M, et al. Differentiated thyroid cancer. Impact of adjuvant external radiotherapy in patients with perithyroidal tumor infiltration (stage pT4). Cancer 1996;77:172–80.
85. Brierley JD, Tsang RW. External-beam radiation therapy in the treatment of differentiated thyroid cancer. Semin Surg Oncol 1999;16:42–9.
86. Grigsby PW, Baglan K, Siegel BA. Surveillance of patients to detect recurrent thyroid carcinoma. Cancer 1999; 85:945–51.
87. Antonelli A, Miccoli P, Fedeghini M, et al. Role of neck ultrasound in the follow-up of patients operated on for thyroid cancer. Thyroid 1995;5:25–8.
88. Krishnamurthy S, Bedi DG, Caraway NP. Ultrasound-guided fine-needle aspiration biopsy of the thyroid bed. Cancer 2001;93:199–205.
89. Franceschi M, Kusic Z, Franceschi D, et al. Thyroglobulin determination, neck ultrasonography and iodine-131 whole-body scintigraphy in differentiated thyroid carcinoma. J Nucl Med 1996;37:446–51.
90. Spencer CA, LoPresti JS, Fatemi S, Nicoloff JT. Detection of residual and recurrent differentiated thyroid carcinoma by serum thyroglobulin measurement. Thyroid 1999;9:435–41.
91. Ozata M, Suzuki S, Miyamoto T, et al. Serum thyroglobulin in the follow-up of patients treated with differentiated thyroid cancer. J Clin Endocrinol Metab 1994;79:98–105.
92. Mazzaferri EL, Robbins RJ, Spencer CA, et al. A consensus report of the role of serum thyroglobulin as a monitoring method for low-risk patients with papillary thyroid carcinoma. J Clin Endocrinol Metab 2003;88:1433-41.
93. Haugen BR, Pacini F, Reiners C, et al. A comparison of recombinant human thyrotropin and thyroid hormone withdrawal for the detection of thyroid remnant or cancer. J Clin Endocrinol Metab 1999;84:3877–85.
94. Robbins RJ, Chon JT, Fleisher M, et al. Is the serum thyroglobulin response to recombinant human thyrotropin suf-

ficient, by itself, to monitor for residual thyroid carcinoma? J Clin Endocrinol Metab 2002;87:3242–7.

95. Pacini F, Molinaro E, Castagna MG, et al. Recombinant human thyrotropin-stimulated serum thyroglobulin combined with neck ultrasonography has the highest sensitivity in monitoring differentiated thyroid carcinoma. J Clin Endocrinol Metab 2003;88:3668–73.
96. Mariotti S, Barbesino G, Caturegli P, et al. Assay of thyroglobulin in serum with thyroglobulin autoantibodies: an unobtainable goal? J Clin Endocrinol Metab 1995;80:468–72.
97. Spencer CA, Takeuchi M, Kazarosyan M, et al. Serum thyroglobulin autoantibodies: prevalence, influence on serum thyroglobulin measurement, and prognostic significance in patients with differentiated thyroid carcinoma. J Clin Endocrinol Metab 1998;83:1121–7.
98. Niederle B, Roka R, Schemper M, et al. Surgical treatment of distant metastases in differentiated thyroid cancer: indication and results. Surgery 1986;100:1088–97.
99. Chiu AC, Delpassand ES, Sherman SI. Prognosis and treatment of brain metastases in thyroid carcinoma. J Clin Endocrinol Metab 1997;82:3637–42.
100. Maxon HR, Smith HS. Radioiodine-131 in the diagnosis and treatment of metastatic well differentiated thyroid cancer. Endocrinol Metab Clin North Am 1990;19:685–718.
101. Ronga G, Filesi M, Montesano T, et al. Lung metastases from differentiated thyroid carcinoma: A 40 years experience. Q J Nucl Med Mol Imaging 2004;48:12-9.
102. Sisson JC, Jamadar DA, Kazerooni EA, et al. Treatment of micronodular lung metastases of papillary thyroid cancer: are the tumors too small for effective irradiation from radioiodine? Thyroid 1998;8:215–21.
103. Furhang EE, Larson SM, Buranapong P, Humm JL. Thyroid cancer dosimetry using clearance fitting. J Nucl Med 1999;40:131–6.
104. Bohuslavizki KH, Klutmann S, Bleckmann C, et al. Salivary gland protection by amifostine in high-dose radioiodine therapy of differentiated thyroid cancer. Strahlenther Onkol 1999;175:57–61.
105. de Vathaire F, Schlumberger M, Delisle MJ, et al. Leukaemias and cancers following iodine-131 administration for thyroid cancer. Br J Cancer 1997;75:734–9.
106. Chen AY, Levy L, Goepfert H, et al. The development of breast carcinoma in women with thyroid carcinoma. Cancer 2001;92:225–31.
107. Pineda JD, Lee T, Ain K, et al. Iodine-131 therapy for thyroid cancer patients with elevated thyroglobulin and negative diagnostic scan. J Clin Endocrinol Metab 1995;80:1488–92.
108. Schlumberger M, Mancusi F, Baudin E, Pacini F. ^{131}I therapy for elevated thyroglobulin levels. Thyroid 1997; 7:273–6.
109. Pacini F, Agate L, Elisei R, et al. Outcome of differentiated thyroid cancer with detectable serum Tg and negative diagnostic ^{131}I whole-body scan: comparison of patients treated with high ^{131}I activities versus untreated patients. J Clin Endocrinol Metab 2001;86:4092–7.
110. Fatourechi V, Hay ID, Javedan H, et al. Lack of impact of radioiodine therapy in Tg-positive, diagnostic whole-body scan-negative patients with follicular cell-derived thyroid cancer. J Clin Endocrinol Metab 2002;87:1521–6.
111. Wartofsky L, Sherman SI, Gopal J, et al. The use of radioactive iodine in patients with papillary and follicular thyroid cancer. J Clin Endocrinol Metab 1998;83:4195–203.
112. Schluter B, Bohuslavizki KH, Beyer W, et al. Impact of FDG-PET on patients with differentiated thyroid cancer who present with elevated thyroglobulin and negative ^{131}I scan. J Nucl Med 2001;42:71–6.
113. Frilling A, Gorges R, Tecklenborg K, et al. Value of preoperative diagnostic modalities in patients with recurrent thyroid carcinoma. Surgery 2000;128:1067–74.
114. Koong SS, Reynolds JC, Movius EG, et al. Lithium as a potential adjuvant to ^{131}I therapy of metastatic, well differentiated thyroid carcinoma. J Clin Endocrinol Metab 1999;84:912–6.
115. Venkataraman GM, Yatin M, Marcinek R, Ain KB. Restoration of iodide uptake in dedifferentiated thyroid carcinoma: relationship to human Na+/I-symporter gene methylation status. J Clin Endocrinol Metab 1999;84:2449–57.
116. Kitazono M, Robey R, Zhan Z, et al. Low concentrations of the histone deacetylase inhibitor, depsipeptide (FR901228), increase expression of the Na(+)/I(-) symporter and iodine accumulation in poorly differentiated thyroid carcinoma cells. J Clin Endocrinol Metab 2001;86:3430–5.
117. Schlumberger M, Pacini F. Thyroid tumors. Gif-sur-Yvette Cedex, France: Nucleon; 1999. p. 317.
118. Wartofsky L. Thyroid cancer: a comprehensive guide to clinical management. Totowa (NJ): Humana Press; 1999. p. 497.
119. Haugen BR. Management of the patient with progressive radioiodine non-responsive disease. Semin Surg Oncol 1999;16:34–41.
120. Shimaoka K, Schoenfeld DA, DeWys WD, et al. A randomized trial of doxorubicin versus doxorubicin plus cisplatin in patients with advanced thyroid carcinoma. Cancer 1985;56:2155–60.
121. Vassilopoulou-Sellin R, Goepfert H, Raney B, Schultz PN. Differentiated thyroid cancer in children and adolescents: clinical outcome and mortality after long-term follow-up. Head Neck 1998;20:549–55.
122. Segal K, Shvero J, Stern Y, et al. Surgery of thyroid cancer in children and adolescents. Head Neck 1998;20:293–7.
123. Akslen LA, Haldorsen T, Thoresen SO, Glattre E. Incidence of thyroid cancer in Norway 1970–1985. Population review on time trend, sex, age, histological type and tumour stage in 2,625 cases. APMIS 1990;98:549–58.
124. Moosa M, Mazzaferri EL. Outcome of differentiated thyroid cancer diagnosed in pregnant women. J Clin Endocrinol Metab 1997;82:2862–6.
125. Gagel RF, Cote GJ. Medullary thyroid carcinoma. In: Braverman LE, Utiger RD, editors. Werner and Ingbar's The Thyroid. Philadelphia: Lippincott Williams & Wilkins; 2004.
126. Saad MF, Ordonez NG, Rashid RK, et al. Medullary carcinoma of the thyroid. Medicine 1984;63:319–42.
127. Horvit PK, Gagel RF. The goitrous patient with an elevated serum calcitonin—what to do [editorial]? J Clin Endocrinol Metab 1997;82:335–7.
128. Gagel RF, Cote GJ. Pathogenesis of medullary thyroid carcinoma. In: Fagin JA, editor. Thyroid cancer. Vol. 2. Boston: Kluwer Academic Publishers; 1998. p. 85–103.
129. Kodama Y, Asai N, Kawai K, et al. The *RET* proto-oncogene: A molecular therapeutic target in thyroid cancer. Cancer Sci 2005;96:143–8.
130. Koch CA, Huang SC, Moley JF, et al. Allelic imbalance of the mutant and wild-type RET allele in MEN 2A-associated medullary thyroid carcinoma. Oncogene 2001;20:7809–11.
131. Wohllk N, Cote GJ, Bugalho MMJ, et al. Relevance of RET proto-oncogene mutations in sporadic medullary thyroid carcinoma. J Clin Endocrinol Metab 1996;81: 3740–5.
132. Brandi ML, Gagel RF, Angeli A, et al. Guidelines for diagnosis and therapy of MEN type 1 and type 2. J Clin Endocrinol Metab 2001;86:5658–71.
133. DeGroot LJ. Thyroid carcinoma. Med Clin North Am 1975;59:1233–46.
134. O'Riordain DS, O'Brien T, Weaver AL, et al. Medullary thyroid carcinoma in multiple endocrine neoplasia types 2A and 2B. Surgery 1994;116:1017–23.
135. Hyer SL, Vini L, A'Hern R, and Harmer C. Medullary thyroid cancer: multivariate analysis of prognostic factors influencing survival. Eur J Surg Oncol 2000;26:686–90.
136. Brierley J, Tsang R, Simpson WJ, et al. Medullary thyroid cancer: analyses of survival and prognostic factors and the role of radiation therapy in local control. Thyroid 1996;6:305–10.
137. Brierley J, Maxon HR. Radioiodine and external radiation therapy in the treatment of thyroid cancer. In: Fagin JA, editor. Thyroid cancer. Vol. 2. Boston: Kluwer Academic Publishers; 1998. p. 285–317.
138. van Heerden JA, Grant CS, Gharib H. Long-term course of patients with persistent hypercalcitoninemia after apparent curative primary surgery for medullary thyroid carcinoma. Ann Surg 1990;212:395–401.
139. Scopsi L, Sampietro G, Boracchi P, et al. Multivariate analysis of prognostic factors in sporadic medullary carcinoma of the thyroid. A retrospective study of 109 consecutive patients. Cancer 1996;78:2173–83.
140. Dottorini ME, Assi A, Sironi M, et al. Multivariate analysis of patients with medullary thyroid carcinoma: prognostic significance and impact on treatment of clinical and pathologic variables. Cancer 1996;77:1556–65.
141. Tisell LE, Hansson G, Jansson S, Salander H. Reoperation in the treatment of asymptomatic metastasizing medullary thyroid carcinoma. Surgery 1986;99:60–6.
142. Moley JF, Debenedetti MK, Dilley WG, et al. Surgical management of patients with persistent or recurrent medullary thyroid cancer. J Intern Med 1998;243:521–6.
143. Fleming JB, Lee JE, Bouvet M, et al. Surgical strategy for the treatment of medullary thyroid carcinoma. Ann Surg 1999;230:697–707.
144. Wells SA Jr, Skinner MA. Prophylactic thyroidectomy, based on direct genetic testing, in patients at risk for the multiple endocrine neoplasia type 2 syndromes. Exp Clin Endocrinol Diabetes 1998;106:29–34.
145. Machens A, Gimm O, Hinze R, et al. Genotype–phenotype correlations in hereditary medullary thyroid carcinoma: oncological features and biochemical properties. J Clin Endocrinol Metab 2001;86:1104–9.
146. Wu LT, Averbuch SD, Ball DW, et al. Treatment of advanced medullary thyroid carcinoma with a combination of cyclophosphamide, vincristine, and dacarbazine. Cancer 1994;73:432–6.
147. Nocera M, Baudin E, Pellegriti G, et al. Treatment of advanced medullary thyroid cancer with an alternating combination of doxorubicin-streptozocin and 5 FU-dacarbazine. Br J Cancer 2000;83:715–8.
148. Carlomagno F, Vitagliano D, Guida T, et al. ZD6474, an orally available inhibitor of KDR tyrosine kinase activity, efficiently blocks oncogenic RET kinases. Cancer Res 2002;62:7284–90.
149. Moretti F, Farsetti A, Soddu S, et al. p53 re-expression inhibits proliferation and restores differentiation of human thyroid anaplastic carcinoma cells. Oncogene 1997;14:729–40.
150. Sherman SI. Anaplastic carcinoma: clinical aspects. In: Wartofsky L, editor. Thyroid cancer. A comprehensive guide to clinical management. Totowa (NJ): Humana Press; 1999. p. 319–25.
151. Takashima S, Morimoto S, Ikezoe J, et al. CT evaluation of anaplastic thyroid carcinoma. AJR Am J Roentgenol 1990;154:1079–85.
152. Venkatesh YSS, Ordonez NG, Schultz PN, et al. Anaplastic carcinoma of the thyroid: a clinicopathologic study of 121 cases. Cancer 1990;66:321–30.
153. Junor EJ, Paul J, Reed NS. Anaplastic thyroid carcinoma: 91 patients treated by surgery and radiotherapy. Eur J Surg Oncol 1992;18:83–8.
154. Haigh PI, Ituarte PHG, Wu HS, et al. Completely resected anaplastic thyroid carcinoma combined with adjuvant chemotherapy and irradiation is associated with prolonged survival. Cancer 2001;91:2335–42.
155. Kim JH, Leeper RD. Treatment of locally advanced thyroid carcinoma with combination doxorubicin and radiation therapy. Cancer 1987;60:2372–5.
156. Ain KB, Egorin MJ, DeSimone PA. Treatment of anaplastic thyroid carcinoma with paclitaxel: Phase 2 trial using 96-hour infusion. Thyroid 2000;10:587–94.
157. Dowlati A, Robertson K, Cooney M, et al. A phase I pharmacokinetic and translational study of the novel vascular targeting agent combretastatin a-4 phosphate on a single-dose intravenous schedule in patients with advanced cancer. Cancer Res 2002;62:3408–16.

Neoplasms of the Adrenal Cortex

David E. Schteingart, MD

Adrenal cortical carcinomas are rare, highly malignant tumors that account for only 0.2% of deaths due to cancer. Their incidence has been estimated at two per million people annually. About half of these tumors produce hormonal and metabolic syndromes that lead to their discovery. The other half are silent and are discovered with metastasis or when the primary tumor becomes large enough to produce abdominal symptoms.

PATHOGENESIS

The etiology of adrenal cancer remains unknown. Although adrenal cancer can occur at any age, most cases occur between ages 30 and 50 years.[1] Risk of developing the disease is increased in men who smoked more than 25 cigarettes daily (odds ratio 2:0; 95% confidence interval [CI] 1.0–4.4) and in women who used oral contraceptives, especially before age 25 (odds ratio 1:8; 95% CI 1.0–3.2).[2]

Clonality studies of adrenal cortical tumors using X-chromosome inactivation analysis indicate monoclonal expansion of a single cell as the origin of adrenocortical carcinoma. Mutations in key genes involved in adrenal cortical cell proliferation may lead to tumor development.[3] Cases of adrenal cancer have been described in families with a hereditary cancer syndrome who exhibit mutations in tumor-suppressor genes. One such condition is the Li-Fraumeni syndrome, a rare autosomal-dominant syndrome caused by germline mutations in the *TP53* tumor-suppressor gene and associated with high susceptibility to a variety of malignancies, including sarcoma, breast cancer, brain tumors, lung cancer, laryngeal carcinoma, leukemia, and adrenal cortical carcinoma. However, adrenal cancer occurs infrequently in this syndrome. The deleterious genotype in these cases is expressed through several generations in both children and adults.[4,5]

Several theories have been put forth to explain tumor development in adrenal cortical carcinoma,[6] including chromosomal gains or losses leading to abnormal regulation of a gene product or chronic stimulation of the gland. In certain populations, chromosomal gains are more frequent than losses because of involvement of a number of oncogenes such as N-*ras*.

Losses have been noted in chromosomal region 2q 22q34, a locus that corresponds to the inhibin A subunit, and in region 17p *TP53*, a tumor-suppressor gene locus. This loss may explain the changes in the *TP53* tumor-suppressor gene and its 53 kDa protein.[7–10] Some of these changes were point mutations in exons 5 through 8 that resulted in a single amino-acid change, leading to synthesis of a protein with an altered half-life. A germline mutation of the *TP53* gene was found in a patient with an incidentally found adrenal cortical carcinoma.[11] This germline mutation resulted in a premature stop codon. However, mutations at the *TP53* loci are found not only in malignant adrenocortical tumors, but also in benign adrenal adenomas and pheochromocytomas.[12] Another study[13] showed alteration in the *TP53* gene product in about 50% of cases of adrenal cortical carcinoma but was unable to show that the *TP53* status had any effect on long-term survival.

Changes in the *Rb* gene have also been reported, but the nature of the changes and the effect on the gene's regulation have not been completely worked out. As with the *TP53* gene, allelic loss at the *Rb* gene locus on chromosome 13q has been described in adrenal cortical carcinoma.[7]

Other genetic markers examined have included the *H19,* the insulin-like growth factor II (IGF-II), and the $p57^{kip2}$ genes. These genes have been mapped to chromosome 11p15.5[13] and appear to be important for fetal growth and development. The levels of expression of the *H19* and IGF-II genes are very high in human fetal adrenal glands,[14] but they subsequently decrease by 50% in adults. The gene product for $p57^{kip2}$, a member of the $p21^{cip1}$ cyclin-dependent kinase family, appears to regulate cell proliferation, exit from the cell cycle, and maintenance of differentiated cells. Loss of activity of the $p57^{kip2}$ gene product has been detected in virilizing adenomas and adrenal cortical carcinomas,[15] suggesting that this gene product plays a role in the normal maintenance of adrenal cortical differentiation and function. *H19* and $p57^{kip2}$ gene expression is adrenocorticotropic hormone (ACTH) dependent, and regulation of the $p57^{kip2}$ gene appears to be related to the cyclic adenosine monophosphate (cAMP)-dependent protein kinase pathway.[15]

The gene product for $p57^{kip2}$ is usually found to be high in most normal human tissues. A markedly reduced expression of the *H19* gene has been found in both nonfunctioning and functioning adrenal cortical carcinomas, especially in tumors that produce cortisol and aldosterone.[15] Reduced expression of the $p57^{KIP2}$ has been found in Beckwith-Wiedemann syndrome, a congenital overgrowth disorder characterized by high risk of development of childhood tumors, including adrenocortical carcinoma.[3] In contrast, IGF-II gene expression has been shown to be high in adrenal cortical carcinomas.

Finally, the c-*myc* gene has been evaluated for a possible role in adrenal tumorigenesis. c-*myc* gene expression is relatively high in neoplasms, and it is often linked to a poor prognosis. However, adrenal cortical carcinomas have low expression of c-*myc*—approximately 10% of that found in normal adrenal tissue,[16] where it is usually localized to the zona fasciculata and zona reticularis. The significance of a low c-*myc* gene expression in adrenal cancer is unknown.

In general, genetic changes increase as the tumor increases its malignancy grade. Some of the genetic changes described are uncovered in the late stages of the disease, and it is likely that a better understanding of early events may lead to a more effective control of the process of tumorigenesis.

DIAGNOSIS

Cushing's syndrome is the most common clinical presentation in adult patients with adrenal cancer. Characteristically, these patients describe rapid development (3–6 months) of the clinical manifestations of cortisol excess, including weight gain, muscle weakness, easy bruising, irritability, and insomnia. In addition, there commonly are manifestations of androgen excess, including hirsutism, acne, and irregular menses or amenorrhea in women. Although virilization frequently accompanies Cushing's syndrome, the predominant clinical manifestations may be those of androgen excess, with only subtle evidence of hypercortisolism. The androgen excess may decrease the severity of the catabolic effect of hypercortisolemia such that skin and muscle atrophy may not be as readily apparent as in those patients with benign tumors. Patients with metastatic disease complain of anorexia and weight loss rather than weight gain. Adrenal cortical carcinomas causing Cushing's syndrome are large, with an average weight of 800 g, but the clinical manifestations of hormone excess may lead to earlier diagnosis and the finding of smaller tumors.

Hormonal findings in patients with clinical manifestations of Cushing's syndrome include high urinary-free cortisol, serum cortisol, dehydroepiandrosterone sulfate (DHEA-S) at baseline, and failure to suppress with a high (8 mg) dose of dexamethasone. ACTH levels are usually suppressed. The steroid profile in serum or urine can help distinguish between benign and malignant adrenal cortical tumors because of the presence of intermediary precursors in the steroid biosynthesis pathway or their metabolites in patients with malignant neoplasms (Figure 77-1).

Sex hormone–producing carcinomas lead to virilization in women and feminization in men. Women with virilizing adrenal cortical carcinomas present with marked androgen-type hirsut-

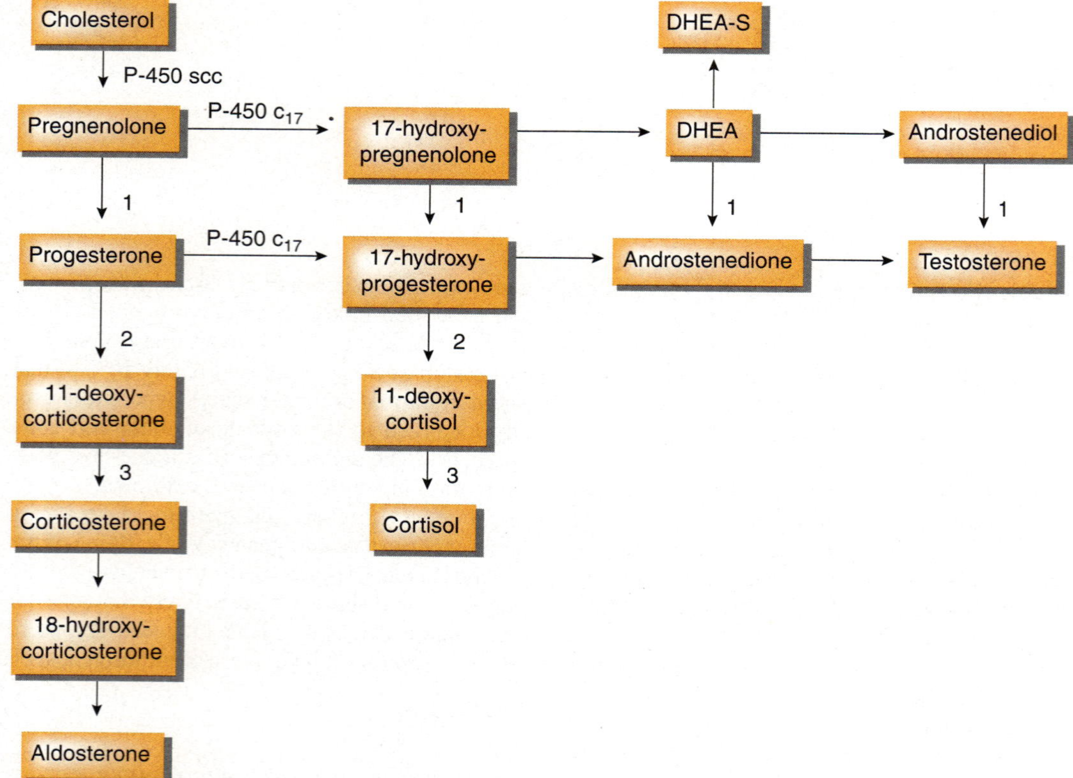

Figure 77-1 Pathways of steroid biosynthesis in the adrenal cortex. Specific enzyme defects in adrenal cortical carcinomas lead to pathway blocks and production of steroid precursors. The numeral 1 represents 38-hydroxysteroid dehydrogenase; 2 represents 21-hydroxylase; and 3 represents118-hydroxylase. C17 = 17-hydroxylase; DHEA = dehydroepiandrosterone; DHEA-S = dehydroepiandrosterone sulfate; SCC = cholesterol side-chain cleavage enzyme.

ism, male-pattern baldness, deepening voice, breast atrophy, clitoral hypertrophy, decreased libido, and oligo- or amenorrhea. In contrast, manifestations of androgen excess are less noticeable in men. Prepubertal boys with androgen excess develop precocious puberty without concomitant testicular enlargement. Feminizing tumors in women cause breast tenderness and dysfunctional uterine bleeding. These tumors in men are associated with gynecomastia, breast tenderness, testicular atrophy, and decreased libido. Prepubertal girls with feminizing tumors experience early breast and uterine development and onset of menarche.

Patients with virilizing tumors demonstrate high serum levels of testosterone, androstenedione, and DHEA-S, whereas patients with feminizing tumors have high serum estradiol levels. Total testosterone levels in virilized women are greater than 2 ng/mL (normal 0.3–0.6 ng/mL).

Aldosterone-producing adrenal cortical carcinomas are extremely rare. Patients present with hypertension and hypokalemia, which are typical clinical manifestations of primary aldosteronism. Compared with patients with benign aldosterone-secreting adenomas, those with carcinoma have larger tumors, higher aldosterone levels, and more severe hypokalemia.[17,18] Evaluation should include measurement of serum electrolytes, aldosterone, and plasma renin levels. Findings include severe hypokalemia with potassium levels below 2.5 mEq/L, hypernatremia, and metabolic alkalosis. Serum aldosterone levels are high, and plasma renin levels are suppressed.

Silent adrenal cortical carcinomas do not present with recognizable symptoms of excessive hormone production, are detected when they attain large size and cause local symptoms, or are detected incidentally in the course of investigation of unrelated abdominal complaints. A hormonal profile on patients with suspected silent adrenal tumors should also be obtained. Some of these tumors produce steroid biosynthesis pathway intermediates, such as progesterone and 11-deoxycortisol.[19] It is important to determine the level of these steroids prior to surgical resection of the tumor because they can be used as biochemical markers in the postoperative follow-up.

DIFFERENTIAL DIAGNOSIS

A major dilemma in the differential diagnosis of adrenal cancer arises with incidentally discovered adrenal masses found in 1% to 3% of patients undergoing abdominal scans by computed tomography (CT). Most of these masses are benign, and adrenal cortical adenomas are 60 times more common than primary carcinoma.[20] Malignant adrenal masses are frequently metastatic from extra-adrenal neoplasms. Age, ethnic background, and comorbidities should be considered when evaluating an incidentally discovered adrenal mass. These masses are uncommon under the age of 30, but their prevalence increases with age. Thus, an incidentally discovered adrenal mass in a young person is of greater concern and should be monitored more closely and for a longer period of time to rule out malignancy. Silent adrenal masses are more common among African-Americans and patients with diabetes mellitus, obesity, and hypertension.

The size of the mass is an important consideration in determining if it is benign or malignant. Masses less than 3 cm in diameter are usually benign[21]; in contrast, the probability that the mass is malignant is generally increased when it measures more than 6 cm. The mean tumor size of adrenocortical carcinomas is 10 cm, and 95 % are larger than 5 cm. The prevalence of carcinoma increases with the larger tumors: 2% in tumors < 2 cm, 6% in tumors 4 to 6 cm, and 25% in tumors > 6 cm. Since early resection of these tumors offers the best chance for cure or long-term survival, an accurate diagnosis of a small tumor is very important. Nonfunctioning small adrenal masses less than 3 cm in diameter usually remain stable for many years. Malignant masses, however, may be initially small but enlarge over time. In contrast, functioning adrenal tumors are associated with significant morbidity that depends on the metabolic effects of the hormones produced in excess.

IMAGING CHARACTERIZATION

A variety of imaging procedures can be useful in the localization and evaluation of the benign or malignant character of an adrenal cortical neoplasm and the extent of disease.

COMPUTED TOMOGRAPHY Unenhanced and contrast-enhanced CT have been used to distinguish benign from malignant adrenal masses on the basis of their lipid content.[22,23] Lipid-rich masses are usually benign, while lipid-poor masses are frequently malignant. Enhancement is measured in Hounsfield units (H). Low-attenuation lesions have low H values. Using unenhanced CT, it was shown that adenomas have values less than +10 H, whereas nonadenomas have values greater than +18 H. These criteria give a sensitivity of 73% for distinguishing adenomas from nonadenomas and a specificity of 96%. CT images obtained 1 hour after the injection of contrast show an enhancement of 11 ± 13 H (< 30) for adenomas and of 49 ± 8.3 H (> 30) for nonadenomas, with a sensitivity of 95% and a specificity of 100%. Adenomas also exhibit a > 60% washout within 15 minutes of contrast injection, whereas nonadenomas exhibit a greater retention of contrast. Malignant adrenal masses are generally larger than 5 cm, have an inhomogeneous pattern because of areas of necrosis within the tumor, and are frequently invasive of the upper pole of the adjoining kidney and of the inferior vena cava (Figure 77-2). The CT procedure also helps determine the presence of involved lymph nodes and hepatic or pulmonary metastases. A definition of metastatic involvement is important in determining the stage of the disease and treatment goals.

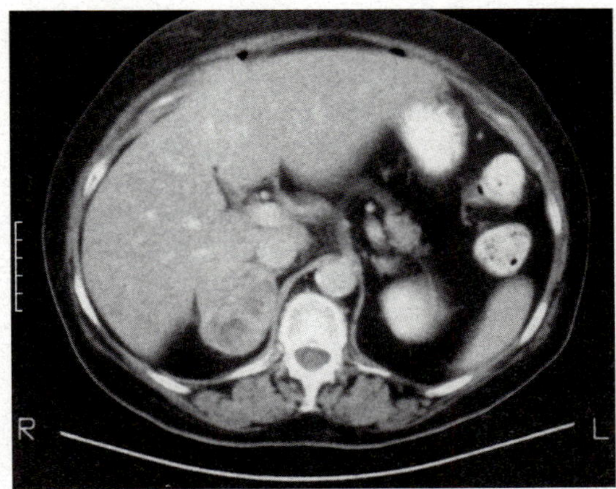

Figure 77-2 Computed tomography appearance of a right adrenal cortical carcinoma. The mass is inhomogeneous, secondary to areas of necrosis within the tumor.

Ultrasonography Malignant lesions vary in echo texture and are heterogeneous in appearance, with focal or scattered echopenic or echogenic zones representing areas of tumor necrosis, hemorrhage, or calcification.[24,25]

Magnetic Resonance Imaging Tumors appear as hypointense masses compared with the liver on T_1-weighted images and hyperintense on T_2-weighted images. Magnetic resonance imaging (MRI) also demonstrates displacement or invasion of adjacent organs as well as liver metastases. Superior blood vessel identification and the multiplanar capabilities of MRI make it the imaging modality of choice in evaluating the extent of disease and planning surgical excision.[26] The distinction between benign and malignant masses on the basis of the presence of lipid can also be determined by chemical shift MRI. Lipid-rich adenomas show a 34% change in relative signal intensity between in-phase and out-of-phase imaging, whereas nonadenomas do not change. This technique gives a specificity of 100% and a sensitivity of 81% in distinguishing these lesions.[27] However, there is no evidence suggesting that MRI is superior to CT in distinguishing between benign and malignant adrenal masses.

^{131}I-6β-Iodomethyl Norcholesterol Scintigraphy Most adrenal cortical carcinomas fail to image with this probe. Because cortisol production suppresses ACTH secretion and the function of the contralateral adrenal gland, patients with cortisol-producing adrenal cortical carcinomas fail to show an image either at the site of the tumor or the contralateral gland. Aldosterone-, androgen-, or estrogen-secreting tumors generally appear as an area of decreased uptake on the side of the tumor mass. The decreased or absent tracer uptake by adrenal cortical carcinomas is in contrast to the increased concentration of radionuclide in benign tumors.[28] This distinction is not absolute. Patients with adrenal cortical carcinoma may occasionally exhibit positive nuclear scans. On the basis of these imaging characteristics, CT and iodomethyl-norcholesterol scintigraphy can be used together in the diagnosis of small (< 4 cm) euadrenal masses. Concordant images (CT image and increased uptake on the same side) are benign in 100% of cases, whereas discordant images (a CT tumor image on one side and increased uptake on the contralateral side) are malignant in 73% of the cases.

Positron Emission Tomography Scanning Positron emission tomography (PET) has been used to image various types of primary tumors and metastatic disease, taking advantage of the increased metabolic activity of neoplastic tissue. Most of these PET studies have used fluorodeoxyglucose (FDG) or ^{11}C-methionine.[29] However, false negative findings were reported in 46% of patients in one series.[30] A better imaging tracer for adrenal tumors may be ^{11}C-metomidate.[31] Although this tracer does not distinguish benign from malignant tumors, the presence of uptake in extra-adrenal sites may indicate recurrence of disease or metastasis in patients who have undergone resection of an adrenocortical carcinoma. Because of limited experience and high cost, FDG-PET is currently not routinely recommended.

STAGING

Adrenal cortical carcinoma can be staged on the basis of the size of the primary tumor and extent of regional or distant tumor involvement, according to the MacFarlane classification,[32] as modified by Sullivan (Table 77-1).[33] Patients in stage I have tumors that measure less than 5 cm in diameter and have no evidence of lymph node involvement or metastases; patients in stage II have tumors larger than 5 cm but are also free of lymph node involvement or metastases. Patients in stage III exhibit tumors of any size with local lymph node invasion or have experienced local recurrence. Patients in stage IV have distant metastases. The sites of tumor spread in stage IV are summarized in Table 77-2. The most frequent sites for metastases are the lung, liver, lymph nodes, and bone. The stage at which an adrenal cortical carcinoma is defined determines the prognosis.[34,35] Whereas 50% of patients in stages I, II, or III are alive 40 months after diagnosis, only 10% of patients in stage IV are alive at that time. The prognosis of patients in stages I and II is not different.

PATHOLOGIC DIAGNOSIS

Pathologic criteria, alone or in combination with clinical features, have been used in the differential diagnosis of benign and malignant adrenal cortical tumors and in assessing their prognosis.[36]

Table 77-2 Sites of Metastasis in Stage IV Adrenal Cortical Carcinoma

Organ	Percent
Lung	45
Liver	42
Lymph nodes	24
Bone	15
Pancreas	12
Spleen	6
Diaphragm	12
Miscellaneous (brain, peritoneum, skin, palate)	12

Adrenal adenomas are usually well encapsulated and homogeneous on cross section (Figure 77-3A) and do not metastasize; in contrast, adrenal carcinomas are large, multilobulated tumors with areas of necrosis and evidence of capsular and vascular invasion (Figure 77-3B).

Various systems of histologic diagnosis have been proposed, but the most commonly used system is the one described by Medeiros and Weiss.[37] Nine histologic findings have been described: (1) high nuclear grade, (2) mitotic grade greater than 5 mitoses/50 high-power fields (HPF), (3) atypical mitosis, (4) low percentage of clear cells, (5) diffuse architecture, (6) necrosis, (7) venous invasion, (8) sinusoidal invasion, and (9) capsular invasion. According to these criteria, a Weiss score (0–9) can be determined for each patient. Malignant tumors meet four or more of these histologic criteria. The three most commonly found are a mitotic rate greater than 5 mitoses/50 HPF, atypical mitosis, and venous invasion.

The mitotic rate is an important criterion not only for distinguishing malignant from benign tumors, but also for predicting the clinical virulence of adrenal cortical carcinomas. Patients with carcinomas having a high mitotic rate (> 20 mitoses/10 HPF) have a shorter disease-free survival period than patients whose carcinomas have a low mitotic rate (< 20 mitoses/10 HPF).

Most adrenal cortical carcinomas are large, but size alone either has no effect on survival time or has minimal effect. Depending on the degree of cell differentiation, adrenal cortical carcinomas have been classified as well-differentiated or anaplastic. Although well-differentiated carcinomas may have a less aggressive course than the anaplastic tumors, cell differentiation may not predict survival independently of the mitotic rate.

Attempts have been made to study adrenal cortical carcinomas by immunohistochemical analysis. Immunohistochemical markers, such as

Table 77-1 MacFarlane Classification of Adrenal Cortical Carcinoma Based on Size and Extent of Disease

Stage	Tumor Size	Lymphadenopathy	Invasion	Metastases	TNM
I	< 5cm	—	—	—	T1-N0-M0
II	> 5cm	—	—	—	T2-N0-M0
III	Any size	+	+	—	T1 or T2-N1-M0
IV	Any size	+	+	+	T1 or T2-N1-M1

TNM = tumor-node-metastasis.

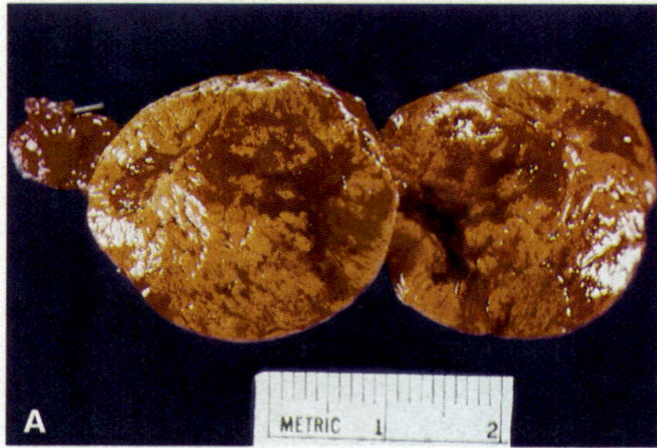

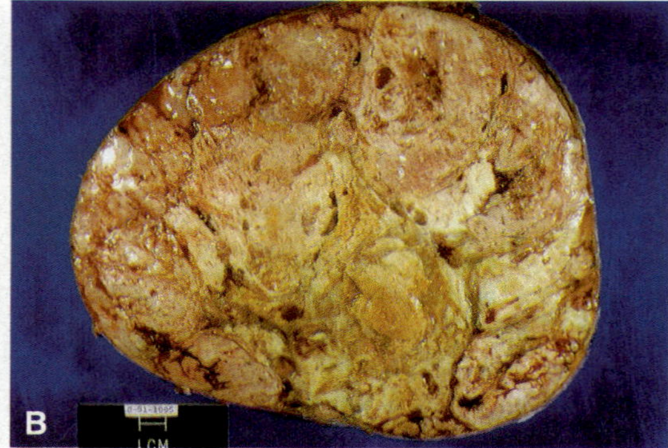

Figure 77-3 Comparison of gross anatomical appearance of benign adrenal adenomas and malignant adrenal cortical carcinomas: **A,** 2.5 cm benign adrenal adenoma causing Cushing's syndrome. The tumor is well encapsulated and of homogeneous appearance. **B,** 25 cm adrenal cortical carcinoma with lobulated appearance and areas of necrosis.

Ki67, are additionally helpful to confirm malignancy and, like D11, Melan-A and chromogranin A to define or exclude the adrenocortical origin of the tumor. In the future, identification of specific gene mutations by gene chip analysis in adrenal cortical carcinomas may be helpful in determining not only diagnosis, but also the malignant grade and prognosis of individual tumors.

CARCINOMA MANAGEMENT

Therapeutic interventions used to treat patients with adrenal cancer include surgery, radiation therapy, cytotoxic chemotherapy, and mitotane.[38] Patients with presumed stages I to III tumors will always be offered surgery. Surgical resection, even if incomplete, should be considered as the initial step in therapy. Because most adrenal carcinomas are large, the surgical approach should be either transabdominal or thoracoabdominal, with an incision of sufficient length to allow adequate exploration and resection of contiguous organs, if necessary, to remove gross tumor. For this reason, laparoscopic surgery is not recommended.[39] The surgical goal should be the resection of the entire tumor mass, whenever possible. Even if this is not possible because of local extension into other structures, tumor debulking should be carried out to the maximum degree possible. It is frequently necessary to remove the adjoining kidney en bloc with the tumor because of invasion of the upper pole. Following tumor removal at first operation, a definite staging should be assessed together with pathological assessment of the tumor (Weiss score). In case of complete resection, the recurrence risk should be assessed and adjuvant therapy should be considered, but its value still needs to be validated. In case of residual tumor, further local radiofrequency ablation or general chemotherapy should be considered.

Surgical resection should be considered for relapses in highly selected patients with excellent performance status and symptomatic (ie, from hormone hypersecretion), limited loco-regional recurrence or isolated distant metastases if complete resection can be achieved. In cases of liver metastases, a partial lobectomy or segmentectomy, with resection of the involved portion of the liver, has led to long-term remission.[40] Adherence to or invasion of the wall of the inferior vena cava may require resection of that portion of the wall and a patch. These aggressive efforts to excise all grossly visible tumors are justified because chemotherapy appears to be most effective when the tumor burden is minimal. Resection of metastases is also recommended when their number is limited and they are surgically accessible (lung, liver). Resection of these lesions should be considered, especially in patients who have had long disease-free intervals after resection of the primary tumor and have favorable tumor biology.[41]

Other approaches to treatment are radiation therapy, chemotherapy, and mitotane. Radiofrequency ablation (RFA) of hepatic lesions and local recurrence has resulted in temporary control of metastatic disease but its utility and value remain to be proven. RFA can be considered in the treatment of lesions less than 6 cm in size that are not near indispensable tissues or large blood vessels. There are very little data in the medical literature documenting the efficacy of radiation therapy in adrenocortical carcinoma. In earlier reports, adrenal cortical carcinomas were reported to be resistant to radiation therapy[42]; however, limited data and anecdotal reports suggest that radiation therapy is likely as effective as in the majority of solid tumors. As with other solid tumors, radiation therapy is recommended in the treatment of bone, brain, and other metastases as well as symptomatic local recurrences. The risk/benefit ratio of this treatment should be individually assessed. Radiation treatment of the adrenal bed can be administered to a patient with an incomplete local resection or after local recurrence. The latter should not replace surgery, especially in patients without evidence of residual disease, but could be used postoperatively as an adjunct to surgery.

The efficacy of first line chemotherapy is very limited. Chemotherapy has resulted in only temporary improvement. Chemotherapeutic protocols used as first line therapy include combinations of etoposide + doxorubicin + cisplatin + mitotane and streptozotocin + mitotane with complete or partial response rates of up to 50% of patients. For second-line therapy, agents are used that have not been used as first line. They include paclitaxel, 5-fluorouracil, vincristine sulfate, cyclophosphamide, and suramin sodium. However, these treatments have not been validated by large, well-controlled studies. The consensus from several series is that systemic chemotherapy is not very effective when given in stage IV; however, several factors contribute to the difficulty of comparing treatment outcomes. These include a relatively small number of patients per series, variability of treatment between and within series, lack of definition of the extent of disease at the time of treatment, and variable grades of malignancy. Some series include patients with low-grade malignancy as well as patients with high-grade malignancy. In addition, treatments are difficult to compare because there is a lack of a uniform definition of response, the duration of response is not always clearly stated, patients within a series frequently receive multiple drugs in variable sequence, and radiation therapy is sometimes combined with chemotherapy.[38,43]

Mitotane has been used in the treatment of patients with metastatic adrenal cortical carcinoma, either as monotherapy or in combination with other chemotherapeutic drugs, but there is no consensus regarding its efficacy.[44,45] Mitotane is an adrenolytic drug with selective action on the adrenal cortex. It belongs to the class of drugs that require transformation into active metabolites for therapeutic action. The active metabolites may covalently combine with specific targets in the cells responsive to the drug and/or induce oxygen activation, leading to toxicity. There is evidence that mitotane is transformed to an acyl chloride by a mitochondrial P-450–mediated hydroxylation and that the acyl chloride covalently combines with specific bionucleophiles within the adrenal cortical cell for the adrenolytic effect to take place. It is possible that adrenal tumors vary in their ability to effect metabolic transformation or initiate free-radical production, thereby expressing variable sensitivity to mitotane. In a series of reports,[46] mitotane has been associated with partial or complete response in 33% of patients with adrenal cancer. The timing of initiation of chemotherapy may influence patient survival. It has been reported[47,48] that adjuvant therapy with mitotane is associated with prolonged survival when initiated immediately after the primary tumor has been surgically excised and before local extension or additional metastases develop. However, prospective studies in which patients were randomly assigned to either adjuvant therapy with mitotane or no therapy failed to show a beneficial effect of mitotane in extending life expectancy.[49]

Mitotane causes significant toxicity in therapeutically effective doses. The adverse effects of mitotane are dose dependent and usually intolerable when doses exceed 6 g daily, a dose that may be required to achieve therapeutic blood levels of 14–20 μg/dL.[50] Treatment begins with doses of 1 g twice daily, and the dose is gradually increased to tolerance. The drug is best administered with fat-containing foods, since its absorption and transport appear coupled to lipoproteins. Patients treated with mitotane should be monitored clinically by measuring urinary-free cortisol, serum electrolytes, serum cholesterol and liver enzymes. Mitotane increases the binding of cortisol to corticosteroid-binding globulin, and serum cortisol levels can be elevated even when the circulating free cortisol level is not.[51] Treatment with mitotane inhibits hormone production and eventually causes necrosis of the contralateral adrenal gland. Patients must receive cortisol replacement of 25 to 35 mg daily. Synthetic glucocorticoids, such as prednisone and dexamethasone, are less desirable because their metabolism may be enhanced by mitotane, making it difficult to determine the optimal replacement dose. In low doses (2–4 g daily), mitotane has less adrenolytic effects on the zona glomerulosa and is less likely to suppress aldosterone production. With larger doses, replacement with fluorocortisol may be necessary. Cholesterol levels may increase during treatment because mitotane is an HMGcoA reductase activator. Treatment with statins reduces these levels.

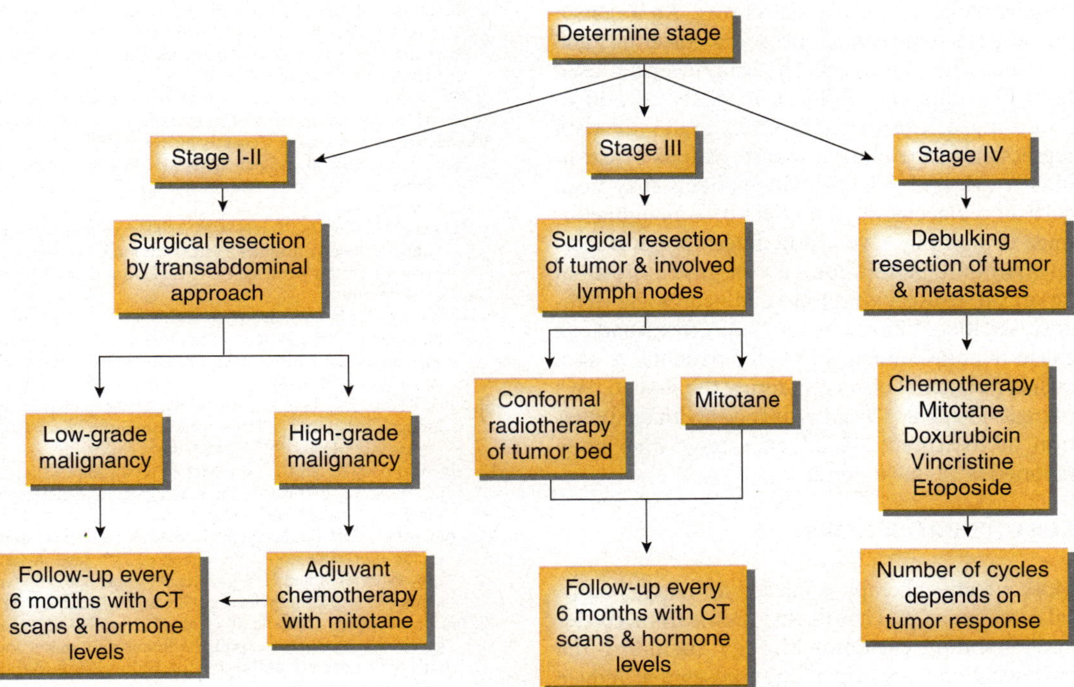

Figure 77-4 Algorithm summarizing the management strategy of adrenal cortical carcinoma based on stage of the disease. Hormone measurements should be followed as tumor markers in patients with functioning adrenal cortical carcinoma.

LONG-TERM TREATMENT OUTCOME

Medical therapy for adrenal cortical carcinoma is of limited effectiveness[52,53]; however, there are a significant number of patients whose life expectancy has been extended with acceptable morbidity. Combined surgical and medical treatment appears to be more effective than medical treatment alone, especially for patients with localized or regional disease (stages I–III). In a comparison of 18 patients treated with mitotane alone and 15 treated with combined surgical resection and mitotane chemotherapy, those who underwent surgical treatment had a more favorable response, with 33% of patients surviving more than 5 years from the time of first recurrence.[41] A study of 49 patients with adrenal carcinoma concluded that surgical excision offered the best chance for prolonged survival. Forty-three percent of patients with a completely resected tumor were alive with no evidence of disease 7.3 years postoperatively.[54] While comparing various types of therapy in 110 patients with adrenal cortical carcinoma, it was noted that 56% of patients responded to surgery for localized and regional disease with a disease-free survival time of at least 2 years. In contrast, abdominal radiation therapy was effective in 15%, systemic chemotherapy in 9%, and mitotane therapy in 29%.[55]

In a review of 82 patients, it was noted that survival of patients with metastatic disease was poor and not improved by treatment with mitotane, cytotoxic chemotherapy, or radiation therapy.[56] In a series of 28 patients with stage IV disease, a combination of etoposide (100 mg/m^2 on days 5–7), doxorubicin (20 mg/m^2 on days 1 and 8), cisplatin (40 mg/m^2 on days 1 and 9), and mitotane (4 g/d) was given. Two patients had a complete response, and 13 had a partial response, for an overall response rate of 53.5%; stable disease was observed in 8 patients. Time to progression was 24.4 months.[57] In another series of 40 patients with adrenocortical carcinoma, a phase II trial was conducted with streptozocin and mitotane. Streptozocin was administered in doses of 1.0 g/d for 5 days, followed by 2 g once every 3 weeks; mitotane was given orally in doses of 1 to 4 g/d. Complete or partial response was obtained in 22 patients with measurable disease. Overall, 2-year survival was 70% and 5-year survival, 32.5%. Significant effect on the disease-free interval (p = .02) and on survival (p = .01) was noted in 17 adjuvantly treated cases, compared with patients without any therapy after complete resection.[58] The combination of streptozocin and mitotane holds promise as adjuvant chemotherapy, but randomized clinical trials are still required.

Thus, survival of patients with adrenal carcinoma with recurrent or metastatic disease is better for those who can receive surgical treatment rather than medical treatment alone. With surgical treatment, 50% of patients survive an average of 70 months, whereas less than 10% of patients are alive for this length of time with medical treatment alone. The surgical treatment involves not only resection of the primary tumor, but also repeated resection of metastases. A management algorithm for each stage of the disease is provided in Figure 77-4.

The prognosis of patients with adrenal cortical carcinoma is poor, but the life expectancy of patients in stages I, II, and III can be significantly extended by a combination of surgical resection and chemotherapy. There are individual cases in which curative resection has been possible and others in which metastatic lesions have regressed on chemotherapy. Early diagnosis is possible in patients with functioning neoplasms, in whom the metabolic manifestations of hormone excess can lead to the discovery of tumors in stages I and II. In contrast, the prognosis of patients in stage IV is poor.

ADRENAL FUNCTION INHIBITORS IN TREATMENT

The metabolic changes associated with excessive hormonal production can cause significant morbidity and shortened life expectancy in patients with residual disease who do not respond to antitumor therapy. Inhibitors of adrenal function have been used to suppress steroid hormone production and improve the clinical manifestations of the disease. The most commonly used inhibitors are ketoconazole and aminoglutethimide.

Ketoconazole is an imidazole derivative that inhibits the synthesis of cortisol by inhibiting mitochondrial cytochrome P-450-dependent enzymes, such as cholesterol side-chain cleavage and 11β-hydroxylase, in rat and mouse adrenal preparations. It is also an important inhibitor of gonadal and adrenal steroidogenesis in vivo when given in doses as low as 200 to 600 mg/d. Ketoconazole has been used to treat patients with Cushing's syndrome and virilization caused by adrenal carcinoma.[59] Clinical improvement occurs frequently, but regression of metastatic disease is rare.[60] When patients are treated with ketoconazole, adrenal insufficiency is avoided by decreasing the dose sufficiently to maintain normal cortisol levels. The most frequent adverse reactions with ketoconazole are nausea and vomiting, abdominal pain, and pruritus in 1% to 3% of patients. Hepatotoxicity, primarily of the hepatocellular type, has been associated with its use.[59]

Aminoglutethimide inhibits cholesterol side-chain cleavage and the conversion of cholesterol to pregnenolone in the adrenal cortex. As a consequence, the synthesis of cortisol, aldosterone, and androgens is suppressed. The drug has been used both in adults and children in doses of 500 to 2,000 mg/d. Cortisol levels fall gradually with regression of the clinical manifestations of Cushing's syndrome.[61] Eventually, patients may need cortisol replacement. The effect of aminoglutethimide is promptly reversed by interruption of therapy. Aminoglutethimide causes gastrointestinal (anorexia, nausea, vomiting) and neurologic (lethargy, sedation, blurred vision) side effects and can cause hypothyroidism in 5% of patients. A skin rash is frequently observed during the first 10 days of treatment, but it usually subsides with continuation of treatment. Headaches have also been reported with the larger doses.

FUTURE PROSPECTS

More effective therapy is needed for adrenal cortical carcinomas, and it is likely to come from a better understanding of tumor biology, including the oncogenic and tumorigenic processes that induce early mutations and drive progression with growth and dissemination of an established tumor. Future approaches to the treatment of adrenal cortical carcinoma are likely to be based on blocking or reversing the biologic mechanisms of tumorigenesis.

Molecular targeted therapy and immunotherapy are still experimental. Tumor immunotherapy with dendritic cells and DNA vaccination are currently being tried in animal models. There are also approaches with adenoviral gene therapy in human adrenocortical cancer cells in vitro and human adrenal cancer xenografts in mice. The adrenals are a preferred target for the adenovirus and the results of preclinical studies are promising. Antiangiogenic strategies have been tested in preclinical studies, but the response in clinical situations has not been validated.[62]

The difficulty in assessing the effectiveness of published treatment protocols stems from the fact that most series are limited in the number of patients studied. There is great variability in the drugs used, the stage and extent of the tumor, and the grade of malignancy. Because adrenal cancer is rare, collaborative, worldwide, multicenter controlled studies will be necessary in order to reach consensus on the efficacy and safety of treatment protocols.[62]

REFERENCES

1. Brennan MF. Adrenocortical carcinoma. CA Cancer J Clin 1987;37:348–65.
2. Hsing AW, Nam JM, Co Chien HT, et al. Risk factors for adrenal cancer: an exploratory study. Int J Cancer 1996;65:432–6.
3. Beuschlein F, Looyenga BD, Reincke M, et al. Clinical impact of recent advances in the biology of adrenocortical cancer. Endocrinologist 2003;13:1–9.
4. Lynch HT, Katz DA, Bogard PJ, et al. The sarcoma, breast cancer, lung cancer and adrenocortical carcinoma syndrome revisited: childhood cancer. Am J Dis Child 1985;139:134–6.
5. Hartley AL, Birch JM, Marsden HB, et al. Adrenal cortical tumors: epidemiological and familial aspects. Arch Dis Child 1987;62:683–9.
6. Stratakis CA. Genetics of adrenocortical tumors: Carney complex. Ann Endocrinol 2001;62:180–4.
7. Stratakis CA, Chrousos GP. Adrenal cancer. Endocrinol Metab Clin North Am 2000;29:15–25.
8. Miyamoto H, Kubota Y, Shuin T, et al. Bilateral adrenocortical carcinoma showing loss of heterozygosity at the p53 and RB gene loci. Cancer Genet Cytogenet 1996;88:181–3.
9. Yano T, Linehan M, Anglard P, et al. Genetic changes in human adrenocortical carcinomas. J Natl Cancer Inst 1989;81:518–23.
10. Reincke M, Karl M, Travis WH, et al. p53 mutations in human adrenocortical neoplasms: immunohistochemical and molecular studies. J Clin Endocrinol Metab 1994;78:790–4.
11. Grayson GH, Moore S, Schneider BG, et al. Novel germline mutation of the p53 tumor suppressor gene in a child with incidentally discovered adrenal cortical carcinoma. Am J Pediatr Hematol Oncol 1994;16:341–7.
12. Lin SR, Lee YJ, Tsai JH. Mutations of the p53 gene in human functional adrenocortical neoplasms. J Clin Endocrinol Metab 1994;78:483–91.
13. McNicol AM, Nolan CE, Struthers AJ, et al. Expression of p53 in adrenocortical tumours: clinicopathological correlations. J Pathol 1997;181:146–52.
14. Liu J, Kahri AI, Heikkila P, et al. Ribonucleic acid expression of the clustered imprinted genes $p57^{kip2}$ insulin-like growth factor-II and H19 in adrenal tumors and cultured adrenal cells. J Clin Endocrinol Metab 1997;82:1766–71.
15. Liu J, Kahri AI, Heikkila P, et al. H19 and insulin-like growth factor-II gene expression in adrenal tumors and cultured adrenal cells. J Clin Endocrinol Metab 1995;80:492–6.
16. Liu J, Voutilainen R, Kahri AI, et al. Expression patterns of the c-myc gene in adrenocortical tumors and pheochromocytomas. J Endocrinol 1997;152:175–81.
17. Farge D, Chatellier G, Pagny JY, et al. Isolated clinical syndrome of primary aldosteronism in four patients with adrenocortical carcinoma. Am J Med 1987;83:635–40.
18. Arteaga E, Biglieri EG, Kater CE, et al. Aldosterone-producing adrenocortical carcinoma. Preoperative recognition and course in three cases. Ann Intern Med 1984;101:316–21.
19. Grondal S, Curstedt T. Steroid profile in serum: increased levels of sulphated pregnenolone and pregn-5-ene-3 beta, 20 alpha-diol in patients with adrenocortical carcinoma. Acta Endocrinol 1991;124:381–5.
20. Copeland PM. The incidentally discovered adrenal masses. Ann Surg 1984;199:116–22.
21. Bencsik Z, Szaboles I, Goth M, et al. Incidentally detected adrenal tumors (incidentalomas): histological heterogeneity and differentiated therapeutic approach. J Intern Med 1995;237:585–9.
22. Korobkin M. CT characterization of the adrenal mass: the time has come [editorial]. Radiology 2000;217:629–32.
23. Caoli EM, Korobkin M, Francis IR, et al. Adrenal mass characterization with combined unenhanced and delayed enhanced CT. Radiology 2002;222:629–33.
24. Korobkin M, Francis IR, Kloos RT, et al. The incidental adrenal mass. Radiol Clin North Am 1996;34:1037–54.
25. Hamper UM, Fishman EK, Hartman DS, et al. Primary adrenocortical carcinoma: sonographic evaluation with clinical and pathologic correlation in 26 patients. Am J Roentgenol 1987;148:915–9.
26. Smith SM, Patel SK, Turner DA, et al. Magnetic resonance imaging of adrenal cortical carcinoma. Urol Radiol 1989;11:1–6.
27. Korobkin M, Lombardi TJ, Aisen AM, et al. Characterization of adrenal masses with chemical shift and gadolinium enhanced imaging. Radiology 1995;197:414–8.
28. Gross MD, Shapiro B, Bouffard J, et al. Distinguishing benign and malignant euadrenal masses. Ann Intern Med 1988;109:613–8.
29. Leskinen-Kallio S. Positron emission tomography in oncology [review]. Clin Physiol 1994;14:329–35.
30. Yasuda S, Ide M, Fujii H, et al. Application of positron emission tomography imaging to cancer screening. Br J Cancer 2000;83:1607–11.
31. Juhlin C, Tornblom S, Rastad J, et al. Differential diagnosis in adrenal gland tumors using PET and ^{11}C-metomidate. Nord Med 1998;113:306–7.
32. MacFarlane DA. Cancer of the adrenal cortex: the natural history, prognosis and treatment in the study of the fifty-five cases. Ann R Coll Surg Engl 1958;23:155–86.
33. Sullivan M. Adrenal cortical carcinoma. Urology 1978;120:660–5.
34. Hogan T. A clinical and pathological study of adrenocortical carcinoma: therapeutic implications. Cancer 1980;45:2880–3.
35. Bradley E. Primary and adjunctive therapy in carcinoma of the adrenal cortex. Surg Gynecol Obstet 1975;141:507–16.
36. Weiss LM. Comparative histologic study of 43 metastasizing and non-metastasizing adrenocortical tumors. Am J Surg Pathol 1984;8:163–9.
37. Medeiros LJ, Weiss LM. New development in the pathologic diagnosis of adrenal cortical neoplasms: a review. Am J Clin Pathol 1991;97:73–83.
38. Schteingart DE. Treating adrenal cancer. Endocrinologist 1992;2:149–57.
39. Gill IS. The case for laparoscopic adrenalectomy. J Urol 2001;166:429–36.
40. Thompson NW. Adrenocortical carcinoma. In: Thompson NW, Vinik AI, editors. Endocrine surgery update. New York: Grune and Stratton; 1983. p. 119–28.
41. Jensen JC, Pass HI, Sindelar WF, Norton JA. Recurrent or metastatic disease in select patients with adrenocortical carcinoma: aggressive resection vs chemotherapy. Arch Surg 1991;126:457–61.
42. Percarpio B, Knowlton AH. Radiation therapy of adrenal cortical carcinoma. Acta Radiol Ther Phys Biol 1976;15:288–92.
43. Schteingart DE. Current perspective in the diagnosis and treatment of adrenocortical carcinoma. Reviews in Endocrine & Metabolic Disorders 2001;2:323–33.
44. Hogan TF, Citrin DL, Johnson BM, et al. o,p'-DDD (mitotane) therapy of adrenal cortical carcinoma: observations on drug dosage, toxicity and steroid replacement. Cancer 1978;42:2177–81.
45. Luton JP, Cerdas S, Billaud L, et al. Clinical features of adrenocortical carcinoma, prognostic factors, and the effect of mitotane therapy. N Engl J Med 1990;263322:1195–201.
46. Wooten MD, King DK. Adrenal cortical carcinoma: epidemiology and treatment with mitotane and a review of the literature. Cancer 1993;72:3145–55.
47. Schteingart DE, Motazedi A, Noonan RA, et al. The treatment of adrenal carcinoma. Arch Surg 1982;117:1142–46.
48. Kasperlik-Zaluska A. Impact of adjuvant mitotane on the clinical course of patients with adrenocortical carcinoma. Cancer 1994;73:1533–4.
49. Vassilopoulou-Sellin R, Guinee VF, Klein MJ, et al. Impact of adjuvant mitotane on the clinical course of patients with adrenocortical cancer. Cancer 1993;71:3119–23.
50. Haak HR, Hermans J, Vande Velde CJH, et al. Optimal treatment of adrenal corticalcarcinoma with mitotane: results in a consecutive series of 96 patients. Br J Cancer 1994;69:947–51.
51. Van Seters AP, Moolenaar AJ. Mitotane increases the blood levels of hormone-binding proteins. Acta Endocrinol 1991;124:526–33.
52. Venkatesh S, Hickey RC, Sellin RV, et al. Adrenal cortical carcinoma. Cancer 1989;64:765–9.
53. Kasperlik-Zaluska A, Migdalska BM, Zgliczynski S, et al. Adrenocortical carcinoma: a clinical study and treatment results of 52 patients. Cancer 1995;75:2587–91.
54. King D, Lack E. Adrenal cortical carcinoma: a clinical and pathological study of 49 cases. Cancer 1979;44:239–44.
55. Bodie B, Novick AC, Pontes JE, et al. The Cleveland Clinic experience with adrenal cortical carcinoma. J Urol 1989;141:257–60.
56. Bradley EL. Primary and adjunctive therapy in carcinoma of the adrenal cortex. Surg Gynecol Obstet 1975;141:507–16.
57. Berruti A, Terzolo M, Pia A, et al. Mitotane associated with etoposide, doxorubicin, and cisplatin in the treatment of advanced adrenocortical carcinoma. Italian Group for the Study of Adrenal Cancer. Cancer 1998;83:2194–200.
58. Khan TS, Imam H, Juhlin C, et al. Streptozocin and o,p'-DDD in the treatment of adrenocortical cancer patients: long term survival in its adjuvant use. Ann Oncol 2000;11:1281–7.
59. Kruimel JW, Smals AG, Beex LU, et al. Favourable response of a virilizing adrenocortical carcinoma to preoperative treatment with ketoconazole and postoperative chemotherapy. Acta Endocrinol 1991;124:492–6.
60. Contreras P, Rojas A, Biagini L, et al. Regression of metastatic adrenal carcinoma during palliative ketoconazole treatment. Lancet 1985;2:151–2.
61. Schteingart DE, Cash R, Conn JW. Aminoglutethimide and metastatic adrenal cancer: maintained reversal (six months) of Cushing's syndrome. JAMA 1966;198:1007–10.
62. Schteingart DE, Doherty GM, Gauger PG, et al. Management of patients with adrenal cancer. Recommendations of an international consensus conference. Endocrine-Related Cancer 2005;12:667–80

Neoplasms of the Diffuse Endocrine System

Evan Vosburgh, MD

INTRODUCTION

Tumors, benign and malignant, derived from cells of the diffuse endocrine system (DES) are, generally speaking, of low incidence; slow growers; often characterized by nonspecific or absent symptoms and signs; and often difficult to detect (< 1 cm in size), even when suspected. In many cases, they have already metastasized at diagnosis and, if not cured surgically, can be managed symptomatically for a period of time. Generally, they are not responsive to traditional chemotherapy agents.

Detailed understanding of somatostatin receptor biology has resulted in improved imaging for diagnosis and follow-up and has resulted in a major advance in control of symptoms through the use of somatostatin analogues. Other advances in biochemical markers and improved imaging techniques for diagnosis and localization, coupled with screening based on specific familial syndromes associated with defined gene mutations, now offer the opportunity for screening and early detection as well as curative surgical treatment of many of these rare tumors. Increased understanding of receptor biology and molecular characteristics of this group of related tumors is beginning to suggest promising therapeutic advances, including development of targeted therapies.

The discussion of tumors of the DES in this chapter will focus on the following:

- Gastroenteropancreatic neuroendocrine tumors (GEP-NET), representing the majority of all tumors of the DES.
- Carcinoid tumors, a group of well-differentiated GEP-NET, representing over one-half of all GEP-NET. A subgroup of these patients will manifest the unique clinical features of the carcinoid syndrome.
- Pancreatic neuroendocrine tumors (PNET), the second highest incidence of GEP-NET, with a variety of unique immunochemical and clinical features related to secretion of specific peptides.
- Multiple endocrine neoplasia (MEN) syndromes 1, 2a, 2b, and medullary thyroid carcinoma (MTC): well-characterized (familial) cancer syndromes involving multiple tissues where cells of the DES are found.
- Pheochromocytoma and parathyroid tumors, both sporadic and associated with MEN syndromes

THE DIFFUSE ENDOCRINE SYSTEM

The diffuse endocrine system (DES) had its descriptive origins in early histology and cell biology that defined a population of normal chromium-avid epithelial cells scattered through the intestinal tract (enterochromaffin cells) and other organs (chromaffin or clear cells).[1] Bayliss and Starling,[2,3] with the identification of secretin and its paracrine effects, established the gut as a source of peptides with local and distant effects ("hormones"). It was hypothesized that the chromaffin cells, scattered throughout many tissues of the body, were responsible for release of secretin along with a variety of peptides and amines, thus the DES. In the 1960s Pearse[4] reported that epithelial cells, classified as part of the DES, had the unifying biochemical properties of storing amines and/or taking up amine precursors and converting to amines via decarboxylation. Grouping these cells and other previously defined cells of the DES, Pearse proposed the APUD (amine precursor uptake and decarboxylation) system.[5] Further investigation of the cells of the APUD system/DES has added to an extensive list of over 100 bioactive peptides, monamines, and eicosanoids.[6]

THE NEUROENDOCRINE CELL

Pearse[5] extended the APUD concept to propose that all cells of the DES had a shared embryologic origin in the neural crest (neuroectoderm). Despite being shown later that the gut endocrine cells actually arise from the gut endoderm,[7,8] it became clear that the cells of the gut DES did in fact share phenotypic and biochemical features with neural cells. Along with the large core dense vesicles (LCDV) of endocrine cells, the DES cells also contain synaptic-like microvesicles (SLMV) characteristic of the synaptic regions of neural cells. The complex and diverse biochemistry and control of secretion from LCDV and SLMV of the DES cells is discussed in detail by Weidenmann and colleagues.[9] Many of the molecules shared by neurons and neuroendocrine cells have been used in studies of neuroendocrine tumors, including the "general markers" of chromogranin A (CgA), synaptophysin, and neuron-specific enolase (NSE) and the "specific markers" found in subtypes of neuroendocrine tumors consisting of the peptide and amine hormones (see below for details of individual markers). Gut DES cells also share a variety of differentiation antigens that have been grouped as "neuroendocrine markers,"[10] giving rise to the synonyms of "endocrine" and "neuroendocrine" when discussing the normal cells of DES and tumors derived from cells of the DES.

A number of peptides originally isolated from gut endocrine tissues, gastrin, cholecystokinin, vasoactive intestinal polypeptide (VIP), and substance P (SP) have been shown to occur in nerves. Peptides that have been found primarily in nervous tissues have now been identified in gut endocrine cells and include somatostatin (somatotropin release-inhibiting factors [SRIF]), enkephalins, neurotensin, and thyrotropin-releasing hormone (TRH).[11–13] Unique to the GEP axis is the ability of the endocrine cell to secrete a variety of peptides and amines. As discussed below, the cosecretion of several hormones and amines and changes of secretion profiles over time within individuals have complicated the use of these peptides and amines in tumor and syndrome characterization.[14]

THE GASTEROENTEROPANCREATIC (GEP) CELLS

Despite the unifying characteristics of this unique set of DES cells with shared endocrine and neural features, a closer look at the accumulated information on the general and specific histologic, morphologic, hormonal content, and tissue distribution characteristics defined a heterogeneous population of distinct cell types. Table 78-1 describes the 15 cell types found in the stomach, pancreas, and intestine of man as outlined by Solcia and colleagues[15] and updated by Rindi and colleagues.[16] Only a limited number of the 15 cell types have been associated with a specific endocrine tumor, and several of the peptides identified in these cells have yet to be identified as being actively secreted by any endocrine tumor. The most important distinguishing feature of each cell type is the specific peptide or bioactive amine hormone content, particularly as it relates to the discussion that follows of the diagnosis and unique clinical features of several tumors of the GEP.

Neuroendocrine Markers Neuroendocrine markers are utilized in histologic and immunohistochemistry of neuroendocrine tumors, and have been utilized to some degree as clinical markers for diagnosis and assessment of response and relapse. The markers are both general and specific, with general markers related to cellular compartments, such as vesicles or the cytosol, and specific markers being related to the individual hormones/amines synthesized and secreted by the various GEP-NET. Comments on a few of the identified markers are included below.

Serotonin and Metabolites The rate-limiting step in GEP-NET (carcinoid tumors) for the synthesis of serotonin is the conversion of tryptophan into 5-HTP, catalyzed by the enzyme tryptophan hydroxylase. In midgut tumors, 5-HTP is rapidly

Table 78-1 Endocrine Cells of the Adult Gastroenteropancreatic System By Cell Type, Hormone Content, Vesicle Markers, and Location

		Vesicle Markers		Gastroenteropancreatic Location						
Cell Type	Hormone Content	LDCV	SLMV	Pan	C/F	A	D	J	I	LI
P/D1	Ghrelin	CgA, VMAT2			+					
EC	5-HT	Cga, VMAT1	Syn		+	+	+	+	+	+
ECL	Histamine	CgA, VMAT2	Syn		+					
A	Glucagon	CgA > CgC VMAT2	Syn	+						
B	Insulin	CgA,VMAT2 NESP55	Syn	+						
CCK	Cholecysto-kinin						+	+		
D	Somatostatin	CgA	Syn	+	+	+	+	+		
G	Gastrin	CgA	Syn			+	+			
GIP	GIP/Xenin	CgA					+	+		
PP	PP	CgA, CgC VMAT2	Syn	+						
L	PYY/GLI	CgC > CgA	Syn					+	+	+
M	Motilin						+	+		
N	Neurotensin	CgA						+	+	
S	Secretin, 5-HT	CgA					+	+		

LDCV = large dense core vesicle; SLMV = synaptic-like microvesicle; pan = pancreas, c/f = corpus/fundus; a = antrum; d = duodenum; j = jejunum; I = ileum; li = large intestine; CgA = chromogranin A; CgC = chromogranin C; VMAT = vesicular monamine transporter; Syn = synaptophysin; 5-HT = 5-Hydroxyhistamine; NESP55 = neuroendocrine secretory protein 55; PP = pancreatic polypeptide; PYY = PP-like peptide; GLP-1 = glucagon-like immunoreactants.
Modified from Rindi G et al.[16]

converted to 5-HT by the enzyme aromatic amino acid decarboxylase (dopa-decarboxylase). 5-HT is either stored in the neurosecretory granules or may be secreted directly into the vascular compartment. Most of the secreted 5-HT is taken up by platelets and stored in their secretory granules. The rest remains free in the plasma, and circulating 5-HT then is largely converted into the urinary metabolite 5-hydroxyindoleacetic acid (5-HIAA) by the enzyme monoamine oxidase and by aldehyde dehydrogenase. These enzymes are abundant in the kidney, and the urine typically contains large amounts of 5-HIAA. The quantification of 5-HIAA in a 24-hour urine collection is perhaps the best characterized and most frequently used clinical assay for diagnosis and follow-up for GEP-NET that synthesize and secrete serotonin.[17] Recently, quantification of plasma metanephrines has been proposed as the preferred test.[18]

In patients with foregut tumors, the urine contains relatively little 5-HIAA, but large amounts of 5-HTP. It is presumed that these tumors are deficient in dopa-decarboxylase, which therefore impairs the conversion of 5-HTP into 5-HT, leading to 5-HTP secretion into the vascular compartment. Some 5-HTP, however, is converted to 5-HT and 5-HIAA, thus the modest increase in these metabolites.[17]

Chromogranin A Chromogranin A (CgA) is a member of the chromogranin family of glycoproteins that are stored along with numerous peptide hormones in the large dense core vesicles (LDCV) of endocrine (and neuroendocrine) cells,[19] and as such is actively secreted from endocrine cells. It therefore can serve as a histologic tumor marker at diagnosis, as well as a plasma marker of tumor mass and secretory activity during treatment. CgA is considered as a "general marker" of neuroendocrine differentiation along with synaptophysin, and the loss of CgA staining correlates with the tumors with more undifferentiated histology. Of the numerous endocrine markers shown to be elevated above normal concentrations in serum/plasma of neuroendocrine patients (see Wilander and colleagues[20]), CgA has been generally accepted as the most useful marker in GEP-NET patients.[21,22] There are three commercially available kits for CgA assay, one ELISA-based (only kit in the United States), and two RIA-based (not available in the United States). Stridsberg and colleagues[23] compared the three assays and found minor differences in sensitivity and specificity, and emphasized the need for an international reference to improve uniformity between assays, centers, and over time, because these patients are often followed for many years.

NESP-55 Neuroendocrine secretory protein-55 (NESP-55) is a member of the chromogranin family, with a less widespread distribution in endocrine and neural tissue than chromogranin A. Srivastava and colleagues[24] studied 63 neuroendocrine tumors for a variety of neuroendocrine markers, and showed that NESP-55 staining was restricted to endocrine tumors of the pancreas and adrenal medulla, and propose that the marker could be used to assign origin to metastatic neuroendocrine tumors.

Synaptophysin Synaptophysin (p38) is a major neuronal protein concentrated in the membrane of small synaptic vesicles of nerve cells.[25] Weidenmann and colleagues[26] demonstrated the presence of synaptophysin in a wide range of normal neuroendocrine cells and neuroendocrine tumors. Buffa and colleagues[27] combined immunohistochemistry and ultrastructural studies on the normal and tumor tissues to localize the synaptophysin to a population of small, clear vesicles distinct from the peptide-containing (CgA-positive) secretory vesicles. The synaptophysin-positive vesicles are now commonly referred to as synaptic-like microvesicles (SLMV). Synaptophysin is frequently used as a histologic general marker of neuroendocrine differentiation.

Neuron-Specific Enolase Neuron-specific enolase (NSE) derives its name from the early observations that the enzyme was restricted to central neurons. It was later found in peripheral autonomic nerves and a number of endocrine cells. Bishop and colleagues[10] demonstrated NSE in all identifiable endocrine and nerve cells of the gastrointestinal tract and pancreas. NSE has replaced earlier histologic argentaffin stains as a cytosolic general marker of normal neuroendocrine cells and tumors.

VMAT1, 2 The vesicular monamine transporter protein has two isoforms, VMAT1 and VMAT2, which serve as amine transporters in the granule/vesicular membrane of a variety of cell types. They differ in cellular distribution, substrate specificity, and drug sensitivity.[28] VMAT1 is expressed primarily in the enterochromaffin cells (EC) of the GI tract and the adrenal chromaffin cells. VMAT2, on the other hand, is expressed in gastric enterochromaffin-like cells (ECL), adrenal chromaffin cells, as well as various central and peripheral neurons (including enteric).[29] Rindi and colleagues[30] proposed VMAT2 as an ECL cell and tumor marker. In a study of 211 gastrointestinal tumors, Jakobsen and colleagues[31] demonstrated differential expression: VMAT1 was expressed primarily on ileal and appendicial carcinoids (EC cell-derived tumors) that synthesize serotonin, and VMAT2 was expressed primarily on gastric carcinoids (ECL cell-derived tumors) that synthesize histamine. There was little or no VMAT1 or VMAT2 expression on the peptide producing PNET and rectal carcinoids and nonendocrine tumors of the GI tract.[31] Based on the differential expression, and relative restriction to GEP-NET, the VMAT have been proposed as therapeutic targets in drug and vaccine development.[32]

Table 78-2 Classification of GEP-NET

A: Broad Histologic Categories			
Group	WHO Nomenclature		Common Synonym
1a	Well-differentiated neuroendocrine tumor		Carcinoid
1b	Well-differentiated neuroendocrine carcinoma		Malignant carcinoid
2	Poorly differentiated neuroendocrine carcinoma		Same
B: Clinical and Pathologic Modifiers Used to Refine Prognosis			
Clinicopathologic Features	Benign	Uncertain	Malignant
Tumor size (cm)	< 2	> 2	> 2
Local spread	No	Yes	Yes
Vascular invasion	No	Yes	Yes
Nuclear atypia	No	Yes	Yes
Tissue invasion	No	No	Yes
Metastases	No	No	Yes

Modified from Rindi G et al[272]; Barakat MT et al.[273]

Tumors of the DES Coincident with the description of the normal cells of the DES, Siegfried Oberndorfer[33] in 1907 separated out a group of monotonous-appearing gastrointestinal tumors labeled "karzinoide" (carcinoid), carcinoma-like, as distinct from the more aggressive adenocarcinomas.[1] Masson[34] then established the relationship between the normal enterochromaffin cells of the gut and the cells of the tumor, forging a relationship between the DES and carcinoid tumors. Carcinoids were soon reported in numerous locations, including the lung, bronchi, pancreas, and throughout the gastrointestinal tract. The term carcinoid has for almost 100 years generally applied to all tumors of the DES that share a similar histological appearance and that, to this day, are described as monotonous small cells with regular, well-rounded nuclei with insular, trabecular, glandular, undifferentiated, and mixed growth patterns.[35] With an increased understanding of the DES, more specifically the GEP cells, and the parallels between normal cell types and specific tumor types, the description and classification of carcinoids evolved and an attempt was made to further classify tumors into more biologically and clinically relevant groups.

Embryologic Classification Williams and Sadler[36] in 1963 proposed a classification based on embryologic division into tumors arising from the foregut, midgut, and hindgut that, in fact, captured certain features of each group. The foregut tumors were perhaps the most diverse group and included two distinct foregut carcinoid tumors: sporadic primary, and tumors secondary to achlorhydria. Sporadic primary included carcinoids of the bronchus, stomach, first portion of the duodenum, and pancreas.

The foregut carcinoids were described as argentaffin negative, most often with a low content of serotonin, and demonstrated an array of clinically distinct behaviors based on the numerous secretory (and nonsecretory) products that included the serotonin precursor 5-hydroxytryptophan (5-HTP), histamine, and various polypeptide hormones (discussed under specific clinical syndromes). The carcinoid syndrome for these tumors is referred to as atypical and tends to be of long duration with a purplish or violaceous rather than pink or red hue, and frequently results in telangiectasia and hypertrophy of the skin of the face and upper neck that may result in a "leonine" facies. It is not unusual for these tumors to metastasize to bone. The cells of origin include the Kulchitsky cells of the bronchus and the enterochromaffin-like cell (ECL) of the stomach and upper GI tract.

Midgut carcinoid tumors were found in locations distal to the second portion of the duodenum, the jejunum, the ileum, and the ascending colon. The midgut carcinoids arise from the argentaffin-positive enterochromaffin (EC) cell and characteristically have high serotonin and low histamine content and often produce other vasoactive compounds, such as kinins, prostaglandins, and substance P. The classic carcinoid syndrome (see below) of flushing and diarrhea with or without wheezing is most closely associated with the midgut tumors. These tumors may produce ACTH on rare occasions and infrequently metastasize to bone.

Hindgut carcinoid tumors were located in the transverse colon, left colon, and rectum. Hindgut carcinoids were argentaffin-negative tumors that rarely stained for or secreted serotonin. These tumors are often silent (hormonal symptoms) in their presentation and more frequently metastasize to bone.

The complex and varied tumors in the foregut group, more than those of the midgut and hindgut, is the reason cited for the classification schema not having been more widely adapted for clinical use.[37]

WHO Classification The first WHO classification solidified the use of term carcinoid by using it to refer to the majority of neuroendocrine tumors (primarily of the gastroenteropancreatic tract), except neuroendocrine tumors of the pancreas and thyroid, paragangliomas, small-cell lung carcinoma, and Merkel cell tumors of the skin. Incorporated into the revised classification were additional histologic characteristics, such as those described by Soga and Tazawa,[35] who described growth patterns such as acinar or trabecular. Kloppel and colleagues[38] attribute the failure of the initial WHO classification to the overuse by pathologists of the term carcinoid at a time when the clinical and biological characterization of these tumors was defined by distinct subtypes, and most clinicians were restricting the use of the term carcinoid to those neuroendocrine tumor patients who demonstrated the carcinoid syndrome.

The revised, and current, WHO classification published in 2000 by Solcia and colleagues[39] adapted the term (neuro)endocrine so as to avoid the varied historical definitions of carcinoid. The gastroenteropancreatic neuroendocrine tumors (GEP-NET) were divided into three broad large groups (Table 78-2A) based on pathology. Additional clinical and pathologic features were then incorporated to provide a better estimate of prognosis (Table 78-2B). In attempts to define clinically meaningful groups, using the three broad histologic groups and additional clinical features, the tumors were then defined in more detail within the categories of stomach, duodenum (and upper jejunum), appendix, ileum (and distal jejunum), colon-rectum, and pancreas, with criteria that included tumor size, differentiation, angioinvasion, proliferative activity, local organ invasion, metastases, hormonal secretion, and association with distinct clinical syndromes (ie, carcinoid syndrome) or diseases (ie, neurofibromatosis)—clearly incorporating more than was seen under the microscope. What has resulted can best be described as a combined pathologic and clinical staging system that appears to better predict clinical behavior, but which has not been fully validated.

There remains no broadly accepted histologic classification system for GEP-NET that provides prognostic information for the individual patient. A tumor grading system has been tentatively developed for pancreatic and gastric tumors.[40] The WHO classification, referred by some as "morphofuntional," demonstrates that even the broad designations of benign or malignant require incorporation of clinical staging information in each patient. The assignment of a histologic diagnosis of "carcinoid" remains common, with most using the term as equivalent to the WHO category of well-differentiated neuroendocrine tumor, with or without clinical evidence of the carcinoid syndrome.

It is increasingly clear that histology of tumors of the DES, particularly those of the GEP-NET, does not vary greatly between tumors and provides a limited range of differentiating characteristics to retrospectively or prospectively define distinct and relevant subtypes that predict the biologic behavior of the tumor and the prognosis of a given patient. As will be discussed below, particularly for the PNET, even the immunohistochemical staining for specific amines and peptides does not predict the clinical features for a given patient. Immunohistochemical staining and serum markers have shown that a tumor may secrete more than one hormone at a time, and over time and in metastatic lesions, can change the hormone profile. In the British National Supra-Regional Survey of National Health Service Hospitals, 58% of 353 patients with neuroendocrine tumors had increased serum levels of two or more hormones at diagnosis. Nine percent of patients had clinical symptoms related to different hormones, and 4 patients developed new symptoms from secretion of a second hormone after diagnosis.[41] Numerous efforts are under way to characterize the phenotype by molecular and genetic techniques that will perhaps add more clinically relevant annotation to the often deceptive histology.

Somatostatin and Somatostatin Receptors The biology of somatostatin and the somatostatin receptors (SSTR) and their expression on GEP-NET has yielded information that remains central to the diagnosis and therapy of this group of tumors. Somatostatin analogues used to control secretory symptoms, served as one of the earlier examples of targeted cancer therapy, and contributed greatly to improve the medical and surgical management and quality of life of these patients. Unfortunately SSTR agonist and antagonists have yet to provide a biologically active target that results in significant tumor cell death. The development of radioconjugated somatostatin analogues as imaging agents provides valuable clinical data, and the further extension of these agents as peptide receptor radiotherapy (PRRT) with measurable responses in refractory patients is nearing clinical approval in the United States and Europe, following closely on the clinical efficacy demonstrated for radioconjugated antibodies for certain lymphomas.

Somatostatin and SSTR Biology Somatostatin is a peptide that inhibits a wide variety of physiologic activities, the most relevant for the treatment of GEP-NET being the inhibition of hormone secretion. Somatostatin is found in the central nervous system, hypothalamic-pituitary system, gastrointestinal tract, exocrine and endocrine pancreas, and immune effector cells. It exists as somatostatin-28 and somatostatin-14.[42] Somatostatin-14 (14 amino acids) is pictured in Figure 78-1 with octreotide and several of the

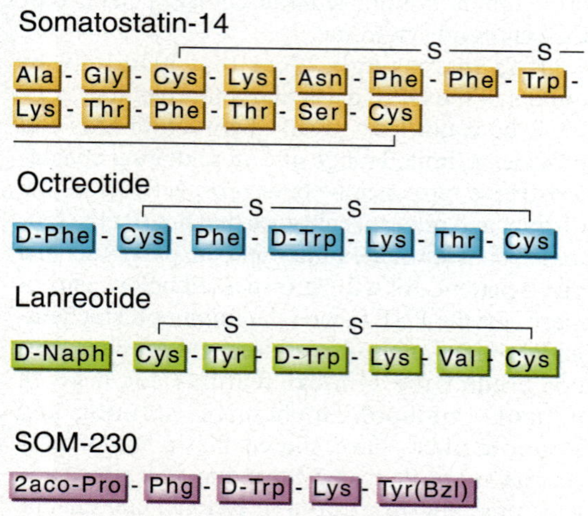

Figure 78-1 SST and analogue structures (including SOM 230).

Table 78-3 Somatostatin Analogue Binding Affinities (IC_{50} [nM]) to SSTR

	sstr1	sstr2	sstr3	sstr4	sstr5
Somatostatin 14	0.93 ± 0.12	0.15 ± 0.02	0.56 ± 0.17	1.5 ± 0.4	0.29 ± 0.04
Octreotide	280 ± 80	0.38 ± 0.08	7.1 ± 1.4	> 1,000	6.3 ± 1.0
Lanreotide	180 ± 20	0.54 ± 0.08	14 ± 9	230 ± 40	17 ± 5

SSTR = somatostatin receptor. Data from Bruns C et al.[274]

somatostatin analogues currently in use or under clinical investigation. Somatostatin, octreotide, and other analogues bind at the plasma membrane with varying affinities to a family of high-affinity somatostatin receptor subtypes, referred to as SSTR 1-5 (Table 78-3). The five subtypes have been cloned, each with a unique chromosomal location, and partially characterized as members of a superfamily of G-protein–coupled receptors (GCPR).[43,44] SSTR isoforms share between 40 and 60% homology, but have different biological effects mediated through activation of these receptors by somatostatin (or analogues). These activities include activation of inhibition of adenyl cyclase, causing a decrease in cAMP levels,[45] reducing Ca^{2+} influx and lowering intracellular calcium levels, stimulating tyrosine phosphatase activity, and activating MAP kinase activity. The increased activation of tyrosine phosphatase occurs via SSTR1 and SSTR2, and activation of adenyl cyclase via SSTR5 can result in decreased cellular proliferation, and the activation of SSTR-3 can increase apoptosis.[42,46,47]

The SSTR1-5 are found in varying distribution on normal tissues in the CNS, anterior pituitary, adrenal gland, and pancreas, where the islets express all five SSTR subtypes. GEP-NET and other neuroendocrine tumors, as well as tumors with neuroendocrine components arising from cells of the DES often express SSTR subtypes—often more than one subtype—in high densities. Several publications by Reubi and colleagues[48–52] and other authors[53,54] have documented the gene expression, translation, and surface distribution of the SSTR1-5 for numerous tumor types and have demonstrated that most SSTR-expressing tumors express more than one SSTR subtype, and that the expression can vary considerably within a given tumor and between tumors of the same histology.

The GEP-NET, particularly the midgut carcinoid and pancreatic islet-cell tumors, with express multiple SSTR subtypes, the most common and highest density being SSTR2 in over 80% of cases, followed by SSTR5.[50,52,55,56] The expression of SSTR2 has been central to the development of somatostatin analogues as therapy to control secretory symptoms, for diagnostic and follow-up nuclear imaging, and for the emerging therapeutic option of peptide receptor radiotherapy (PRRT). Many of the studies of somatostatin analogues as imaging modalities and as therapeutics have by necessity grouped together several types of GEP-NET, and later applied the results to specific GEP-NET in clinical use.

CLINICAL FEATURES OF GEP-NET

Generally speaking, the GEP-NET are difficult to recognize at initial presentation. Pulmonary nodules, pancreatic masses, hepatic metastases, and gastric and rectal lesions at endoscopy often are thought to be more common malignancies prior to pathology reports being issued. The GEP-NET are all rare tumors and, as such, no simple screening program has been developed except in the even rarer familial syndromes. The early symptoms are often nonspecific (ie, abdominal pain and diarrhea), and even when more dramatic or classic secretory symptoms occur, the primary tumors are still often small and difficult to localize. All too often patients have long-standing symptoms and are diagnosed following the development of symptoms related to more advanced local or distant metastatic disease. However, once the diagnosis is considered, advancements in nonspecific (ie, CgA) and specific tumor markers (ie, 5-HIAA, gastrin) along with the imaging capabilities with radiolabeled somatostatin analogues, complemented by ultrasound, CT, MRI, and PET scanning, permit a strong presumptive or confirmed diagnosis to guide medical and surgical management. The variability in the location, secretory status, and biological behavior of these rare tumors has made clinical investigation difficult, resulting in few controlled trials. Despite the lack of comparative trials, consensus based on clinical evidence is available for guiding management of GEP-NET. As an example, the guidelines for neuroendocrine tumors developed by US experts for the National Comprehensive Cancer Network reflect consensus defined as "Category 2A: There is uniform NCCN consensus, based on lower-level evidence including clinical experience, that the recommendation is appropriate."[57]

The initial management of a GEP-NET might involve a patient with biopsy-proven GEP-NET, in whom the challenge is the choice of imaging modalities and other staging procedures toward directing therapy; a patient with classic carcinoid syndrome or other secretory GEP-NET, in whom the challenge is localization of primary and staging; or the rare patient with symptoms only suggestive of, or with laboratory data consistent with, a GEP-NET, in whom the challenge is confirming and localizing the primary and staging before surgery and/or medical therapy. Many GEP-NET share common features of diagnosis, staging, and surgical and medical management, and are best typified and investigated clinically through study of the more common ileal carcinoids and functional PNET. The less common GEP-

NET are partly understood by extension from larger studies of the more common tumors, and partly through detailed investigation in smaller studies of some of the unique features.

EPIDEMIOLOGY One of the challenges facing the classification systems over the past century for carcinoid and related neuroendocrine tumors is that the histology is not particularly informative and tends to be similar from tissue to tissue and for both benign and malignant biologic phenotypes. One distinction that has been maintained with some consistency over time has been the separation of classic carcinoid tumors from the pancreatic islet cell, or pancreatic neuroendocrine tumors (PNET).

The two broad groups of tumors, carcinoid (well-differentiated neuroendocrine tumors) and PNET, are of approximately equal incidence and together comprise over 80% of all tumors of the DES. The carcinoid tumors represent more than 50% of neuroendocrine tumors in clinical practice, most commonly in the small intestine (ileal) and often diagnosed following operative management or found incidentally during endoscopic procedures, and frequently after local or distant metastases are present. The remaining neuroendocrine tumors in clinical practice are divided roughly as follows: 25% "nonfunctional" PNET, and 75% functional PNET consisting of 35% gastrinomas, 25% insulinomas, 10% VIPomas, 5% glucagonomas, and less than 3% neurotensinomas, somatostatinomas, and other rare ectopic hormone-secreting tumors.[58] Many of these "nonfunctional" tumors actually store and secrete pancreatic polypeptide (PP), a hormone, without clinically obvious effects. Other "nonfunctional" PNET stain for specific peptides and amines but do not secrete amounts sufficient to cause a clinical syndrome. The use of the suffix "-oma" in gastrinoma, glucagonoma, insulinoma and VIPoma should be reserved for patients with elevated serum levels of these peptides *and* the associated clinical syndromes. Table 78-4 details the numerous clinical syndromes associated with GEP-NET.

In the most comprehensive epidemiologic report of carcinoid tumors, Modlin and colleagues,[59] in a recent update of Modlin's prior report based on SEER (Surveillance, Epidemiology, and End Results) program data,[60] patterned the analysis to provide continuity with prior reports based on data from the End Results Group (1950–1969) and the Third National Cancer Survey (TNCS) (1969–1971),[61] permitting analysis of incidence data over a half century. The diagnostic codes that form the basis of classification in the SEER database are felt to capture a uniform group of tumors over time, despite the changing classifications. The multidecade analysis of over 13,000 tumors shows, among many interesting observations, that this group of tumors, representing 0.49% of all malignancies, has increased in overall incidence for the past 30 years, with increases and decreases in specific sites. The gastrointestinal tract is the site of over 65% of carcinoids, with an additional 25% occurring in the bronchopulmonary system (Figure 78-2). Within the GI tract, the small bowel remains the most common site with a stable incidence over time, as opposed to the gastric and rectal carcinoids that have increased in recent decades. The changes in gastric and rectal incidence have been attributed to both changes in attribution within TNCS and SEER as well as the increased detection rate with the increasing use of upper and lower endoscopies. Over the same period, the incidence of carcinoids of the appendix decreased, perhaps reflecting the decrease in open abdominal procedures and bystander appendectomies.[59]

The reported overall incidence for carcinoids is about 2 cases per 100,000 (0.002%) in the United States,[60] and just under 1 case per 100,000 population (0.001%) in Scotland and England,[62] Italy,[63] and Japan.[64] These reported incidences are much lower than the reported incidence in autopsy series where Moertel and colleagues[65] from the Mayo Clinic reported carcinoids of the small bowel in 0.65% of unselected autopsies, and Berge and Linell[66] from Sweden reported a 1.2% incidence over a 12-year unselected series of autopsies. A similar large difference in incidence has been seen for PNET where the incidence of diagnosed PNET is about 0.04 per 100,000 and autopsy incidence exceeds 300 per 100,000.[67] It is not known how many of the large number of small bowel carcinoids and PNET found at autopsy would become clinically evident, or even how closely related in biology they are to symptomatic carcinoids. It is of interest that in series of 198 patients who received a gastric bypass operation for morbid obesity at a single center, there were three cases of incidental ileal carcinoids found, for an incidence of about 1.5%.[68]

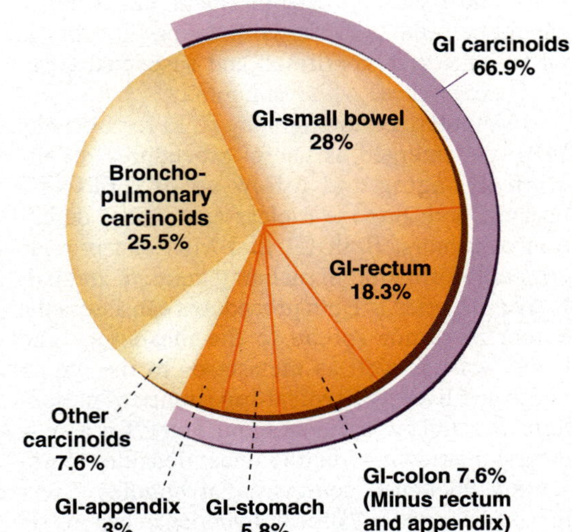

Figure 78-2 Relative incidence of all carcinoid tumors and subgroup of gastrointestinal carcinoids. Data from Modlin IM et al.[59]

Table 78-4 The Clinical Syndromes

Clinical Syndrome	Tumor Type	Site	Hormone(s)
Flushing/diarrhea/wheezing	Carcinoid	Mid foregut Pancreas/foregut Adrenal medulla	Serotonin, substance P NKA, TCT, PP, CGRP, VIP
Ulcer disease	Gastrinoma	Pancreas (85%), duodenum (15%)	Gastrin
Hypoglycemia	Insulinoma sarcomas Hepatoma	Pancreas/uterus Retroperitoneal liver	Insulin/TNF IGF/BP
Dermatitis/dementia Diabetes/DVT	Glucagonoma	Pancreas	Glucagon
Diabetes/steatorrhea	Somatostatinoma	Pancreas	Somatostatin
Cholelithiasis/neurofibromatosis	Somatostatinoma	Duodenum	Somatostatin
Silent/liver mets	PPoma	Pancreas	PP
Acromegaly	GEP	Pancreas	GH (GHRH)
Cushing	GEP	Pancreas	ACTH/CRF
Hypercalcemia	VIPoma	Pancreas	VIP
	GEP	Pancreas	PTHrP
Pigmentation	GEP	Pancreas	MSH

ACTH = adrenocorticotropic hormone, corticotropin; BP = binding protein; CGRP = calcitonin gene, related peptide; CRF = corticotropin releasing factor; DVT = deep venous thrombosis; GEP = gastroenteropancreatic; GH = growth hormone, somatotropin; GHRH = growth hormone-releasing hormone; IGF = insulin-like growth factor; MSH = melanocyte stimulating hormone; NKA = neurokinin A; PP = pancreatic polypeptide; PTHrP = parathyroid hormone related peptide; TCT = thyrocalcitonin; TNF = tumor necrosis factor; VIP = vasoactive intestinal peptide.

IMAGING The GEP-NET are a collection of rare tumors with varied presentations and clinical features. This fact limits the ability to conduct and publish large comparative studies. To date there are very few studies of GEP-NET that fit the criteria for evidence-based clinical decision making. Imaging of GEP-NET is no exception and has been addressed directly by the European Network of Neuroendocrine Tumors[69] (ENET) in a Delphi process that sought to standardize guidelines for diagnostic imaging procedures in neuroendocrine tumors.[70] It was recognized at the outset that there were considerable center-to-center differences, reflecting the lack of controlled studies, but the process was able to yield a series of five workflows. A consensus emerged that somatostatin receptor scintigraphy (SRS) was central to the diagnosis of most cases of GEP-NET, and that CT and MRI provided further definition of SRS-documented disease and were more useful to follow tumor growth than SRS, and that the role of PET scans was still undetermined. Other authors support the opinion that based on the fact that SRS is noninvasive and has high sensitivity for locating both primary and metastatic lesions (including bone), it should be used as the initial imaging modality in all patients with confirmed and suspected GEP-NET, except those with insulinoma.[71–73]

Computerized tomography (CT) remains and MRI has emerged as useful procedures for the clinical staging and follow-up of GEP-NET because both provide a clear anatomical definition of tumors. Both CT and MRI can provide critical information in planning curative and palliative surgeries.[17] Both procedures can assess the extent of tumor spread to the mesentery and bowel wall as well as metastases to the lymph nodes and liver. The typical appearance of mesenteric invasion by carcinoid tumors on CT is a mesenteric mass with radiating linear densities representing thickened neurovascular bundles. Liver metastases appear as focal, hypodense lesions on nonenhanced CT scanning.[74] The advantage of CT is its ability to localize the tumors precisely in relation to the adjacent structure. CT also remains the most useful imaging method for localization of metastatic carcinoid tumors and evaluation of the response of metastatic carcinoid tumors to therapy. GEP-NET (carcinoids) that metastasize to the liver tend to be hypervascular and can appear isodense on CT scan following intravenous contrast. Therefore, suspected and confirmed liver metastases should be evaluated with CT scans before and after the administration of contrast.[75] Magnetic resonance imaging (MRI) may be a very sensitive technique for the detection of liver metastases in some patients whose tumors are not seen well even on three-phase CT, and it may be more sensitive for the diagnosis of skeletal disease than CT. MRI needs further evaluation as a primary modality for the diagnosis and staging of carcinoid tumors because it can be done without the oral contrast used with CT, which usually aggravates carcinoid diarrhea.[76]

Positron emission tomography (PET) has been used to image neuroendocrine gastrointestinal tumors, but experience thus far is limited. Most patients who have been studied had classical midgut tumors and the carcinoid syndrome. Both tryptophan and 5-HTP have been used as tracer substances, but initial studies showed that only ^{11}C-5-HTP was taken up in serotonin-producing tumors. PET has been shown to be capable of identifying midgut carcinoid tumors that have metastasized to a variety of sites.[77]

Scintigraphic Detection with MIBG or Octreotide Scanning The first report of ^{131}I-MIBG for the imaging of a carcinoid tumor was that of Fischer and colleagues in 1984, in which hepatic metastases that were seen as photopenic areas on a ^{99m}Tc-phytate liver scan concentrated ^{131}I-MIBG.[78] Since this initial description, there have been a number of reports of successful imaging of carcinoid tumors using ^{131}I-MIBG.[79] The number studied are far less than those reported for pheochromocytoma or neuroblastoma, however, overall sensitivity is calculated to be 55%. Because MIBG is taken up by a wide variety of neuroendocrine tumors, specificity depends on the certainty of the clinical and biochemical diagnosis, and its use should be reserved for very select cases of GEP-NET where other imaging modalities are not informative.[138]

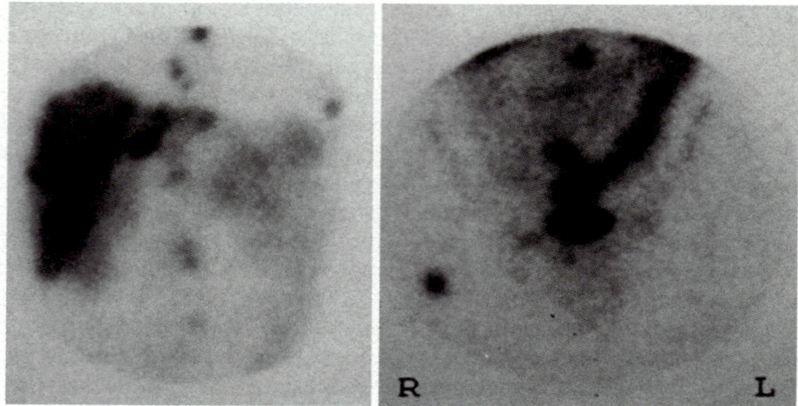

Figure 78-3 Octreotide scan at 24 hours showing liver and pelvic metastases in a patient with malignant carcinoid tumor.

Several octapeptide somatostatin analogues (see Figure 78-1) have been developed that have preferential high affinity binding to SSTR2, SSTR5,[46,47] the SSTR expressed in 70-90% of GEP-NET.[50,52,55,56] The first octapeptide developed for clinical use, octreotide, was also the first analogue used in development for SRS. The first generation incorporated ^{123}I-tyr^{3}-octreotide,[80] but was abandoned for the more convenient, safe, and useful and now most commonly use agent, ^{111}In-pentreotide ([^{111}Indium-DPTA^{0}]octreotide, OctreoScan).[81]

SRS with ^{111}In-DTPA octreotide was evaluated in a European Multicenter Trial (EMT) in 350 patients with a histologically or biochemically proven neuroendocrine gastroenteropancreatic (GEP) tumor.[82] Tumor sites were detected by conventional imaging methods in 88%, whereas SRS was positive in 80%. SRS was positive for most GEP-NET, yielding detection rates of glucagonomas (100%), VIPomas (88%), carcinoids (87%) and non-functioning islet cell tumors (82%). The low detection rate (46%) noted for insulinomas is related to the lower incidence of SSTR2 on insulinoma cells. Not only was SRS able to identify know sites of involvement, but it also revealed another 166 unsuspected lesions; 40% of these unsuspected lesions were later confirmed as true positive findings, leading to management changes in 40% of the 235 patients. This imaging technique is also valuable in identifying metastatic disease to extra-abdominal sites (Figure 78-3).

CARCINOID TUMORS

Carcinoid tumors, or well-differentiated endocrine tumors of the gastroenteropancreatic system, are the most commonly occurring gut endocrine tumors. The (nonautopsy) incidence is estimated to be approximately 1.5 cases per 100,000/year of the general population (ie, approximately 2,500 cases/year in the United States). Nonetheless, they account for 13 to 34% of all tumors of the small bowel and 17 to 46% of all malignant tumors of the small bowel.[65] Carcinoids have been reported as occurring in a multitude of less common locations, and other than the need to recognize that these very rare tumors are often misdiagnosed and managed,[83] most of the practical clinical literature on carcinoids addresses the more common sites of ileal, bronchus, gastric, appendix, and rectal.

Age Distribution Carcinoid tumors have been reported from the first to the tenth decade. Modlin and colleagues[59] report the average age of all carcinoids in their analysis has increased from 59.9 years in the old SEER database, to 61.4 years in the more recent SEER database. The average age for carcinoids of the small intestine, common enough to generate reliable incidence data, shows an average age of 65.4 years, almost the same as the average age for noncarcinoid small intestinal tumors overall.

Natural History In general, except for the small percentage of patients who present with undifferentiated neuroendocrine carcinomas,[84] the tumors at all the sites are slow growing, often remain undiagnosed for many years, and sometimes are recognized only by symptoms related to metastatic spread to lymph nodes, liver, and, less often, bone.

Small Bowel GEP-NET Small bowel GEP-NET (carcinoids) frequently present with small bowel obstruction, abdominal pain, diarrhea, or GI bleeding.[65] Because tumors located in the distal small bowel in most cases have a low intramural profile (Figure 78-4), it is not surprising many of these tumors can grow to larger than 2 cm and remain undiagnosed. The ability of small tumors to cause significant local and distant (cardiac valve fibrosis) symptoms is in part related to the development of events such as ischemia, strangulation, and intussusception from the marked fibrotic reaction that accompanies the tumors. The causes of fibrosis of carcinoids remains poorly understood and of "paramount clinical and scientific importance" to their further understanding and treatment.[85] The likelihood of metastases relates to tumor size. The incidence of metastases

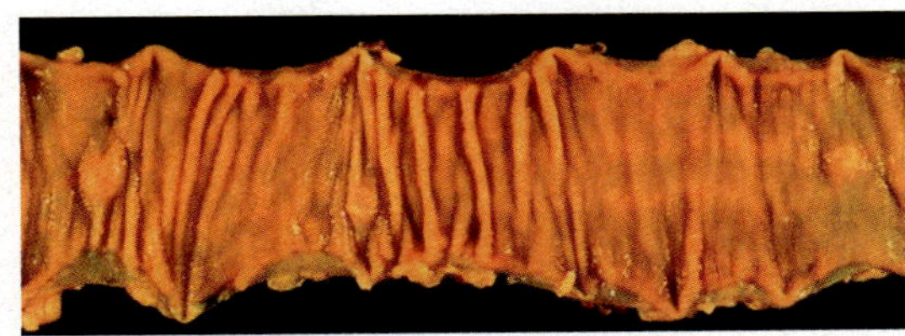

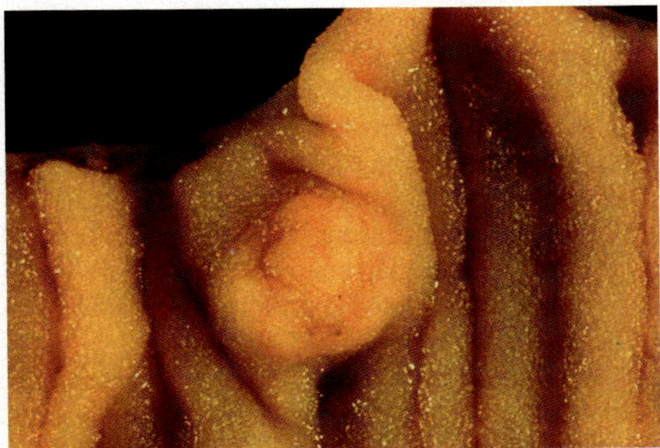

Figure 78-4 Multiple carcinoids of the small bowel (compliments of Ed Uthman, MD). Three small (< 1 cm) intestinal carcinoids found in a young male on inspection of the terminal ileum at colonoscopy.

associated with ileal GEP-NET is less than 15% with a tumor smaller than 1 cm, but rises to 95% with tumors larger than 2 cm. Small bowel GEP-NET account for upwards of 90% of patients with the carcinoid syndrome.[86]

Gastric Carcinoids Gastric carcinoids are divided into three distinct groups based on histology and clinical features. The largest group (~ 75%) involves interesting association between pernicious anemia, atrophic gastritis, chronic thyroiditis, and gastric carcinoid tumors.[87] These tumors arise from the gastric enterochromaffin-like (ECL) cell and usually are small and multiple.[88] Development of these tumors is believed to be secondary to long-standing basal hypergastrinemia, resulting in stimulation of ECL cells and the development of hyperplasia, nodularity, and eventually, carcinoid tumors.[89] The second largest group (~ 20%) are sporadic gastric carcinoids that present with larger lesions than the other gastric carcinoids and tend to metastasize more frequently and have a worse prognosis.[90] The third group (~ 10%) are those gastric carcinoids seen in association with MEN-1 and the Zollinger-Ellison syndrome.[91]

Pulmonary (Tracheobronchial) Carcinoids Pulmonary (tracheobronchial) carcinoids (well-differentiated neuroendocrine tumors) are the more indolent of the spectrum of pulmonary neuroendocrine tumors that includes small-cell lung carcinoma. These tumors comprise about 2% of all lung tumors, present on average in the fifth decade of life, and are associated with the carcinoid syndrome in fewer than 5% of cases. They have been responsible for ectopic hormone secretion leading to Cushing's disease and acromegaly. Overall, they have a favorable prognosis compared with other lung cancers and other carcinoids, with 5-year survivals of about 90%.[84,92] With metastases to the liver, the correct diagnosis generally is arrived at, but unfortunately with a delay of many years.

Diagnosis When not delivered as a surgical or endoscopic diagnosis, the confirmation of carcinoid tumors might be made only after lengthy evaluation of abdominal complaints or iron-deficiency anemia, or astute recognition of a unique clinical syndrome, the carcinoid syndrome, consisting of complaints such as flushing, diarrhea, wheezing, and myopathy. Though not often diagnosed at presentation, patients with longstanding carcinoid syndrome can develop right-sided heart disease, referred to as carcinoid heart disease (discussed below). Clinical suspicion of a neuroendocrine tumor can fortunately be followed by selected biochemical and imaging studies with reasonable sensitivity and specificity for GEP-NET.

No single measurement detects all cases of carcinoid syndrome, although the urine 5-HIAA appears to be the best screening procedure. The normal range for 5-HIAA secretion is 2 to 8 mg per 24 hours, and the quantification of serotonin and all its metabolites usually permits the detection of 84% of patients with carcinoid tumors.[93] False positives can occur with ingestion of serotonin-rich foods, such as nuts, avocados, kiwi, pineapple, and bananas.[94] Chromogranin A has been found to be elevated in 100% of carcinoid patients, but is lacking in specificity because it is elevated in PNET and other neuroendocrine tumors.[95] Other peptides involved include substance P (SP), neuropeptide K, and pancreatic polypeptide (PP). In carcinoids of the GI tract, other peptides are less informative, with neurotensin elevated in 43%, SP in 32%, motilin in 14%, somatostatin in 5%, and VIP rarely.[17]

Carcinoid Syndrome Carcinoid syndrome occurs in less than 10% of patients with carcinoid tumors. Ninety-one percent of cases only occur after metastatic spread to the liver.[96] Principal features include flushing, wheezing, diarrhea, abdominal pain, and after long-standing symptoms, endomyocardial fibrosis with tricuspid and pulmonary valve involvement, and very rarely, pellagra. Diarrhea is found in 83% of cases, flushing in 49%, dyspnea in 20%, and bronchospasm in 6%. Serotonin and its metabolites are thought to be responsible for the majority of carcinoid syndrome symptoms, but other mediators, such as prostaglandins, SP, kallikrein, dopamine, and neuropeptide K, are thought to be involved.[17]

The diarrhea syndrome that occurs with carcinoid tumors usually is of a secretory nature, with diarrhea persisting during fasting or intravenous feeding. Flushing in carcinoid syndrome is of two varieties. First, with midgut carcinoid, the flush usually is of a faint pink to red color and involves the face and upper trunk as far as the nipple line. The flush is initially provoked by alcohol and food containing tyramines (eg, blue cheese, chocolate, red sausage, and red wine). With time, the flush may occur spontaneously and without provocation. It usually is ephemeral, lasting only a few minutes, and may occur many times per day, but generally does not leave permanent discoloration. In contrast, in the second variety with foregut tumors, the flush is often more intense, of longer duration, purplish in hue, frequently followed by telangiectasia, and involves not only the upper trunk but may also affect the limbs. The limbs may become acrocyanotic, and the nose resembles that of rhinophyma. The skin of the face may thicken, with the appearance of a leonine facies resembling that seen in leprosy and acromegaly.[17]

Carcinoid Heart Disease Carcinoid heart disease develops in half to two-thirds of patients with the carcinoid syndrome[97,98] and is characterized by predominantly right-sided valvular lesions described as plaques with proliferation of myofibroblasts and dense extracellular collagen and myxoid deposits.[99] The cardiac disease is a structural disease with thickening and retraction of the valves causing regurgitation (followed later by fusion of fibrous changes to cause stenosis), resulting in right-sided congestive heart failure as the most common cause of death.[100] Moller and colleagues[101] reported on over 100 patients followed with serial echocardiograms or referred for surgery based on initial echocardiograms. Peak 5-HIAA levels and prior chemotherapy were independent predictors of progression of carcinoid heart disease. Evidence for serotonin, and its metabolites, as the primary cause of valvular lesions includes proliferation *in vitro* of cardiac valve fibroblasts that could lead to connective tissue deposition seen on valves in carcinoid heart disease.[102] Indirect evidence includes the histologic similarities to the valvular lesions seen with the diet drugs fenfluramine-phentermine.[103] Studies to date suggest that control of serotonin (5-HIAA) levels *after* carcinoid heart disease has been established does not prevent progression of valvular disease.[101,104]

Prognosis In the recent review of over 13,000 cases of carcinoid tumors, Modlin and colleagues[59] highlight that analysis of over 50 years of data supports that there has been little change in overall survival, and in survival by site and extent of disease (localized, regional, and distant). The conclusion is supported by a lengthy literature showing the lack of success, despite extensive clinical trial efforts, in documenting a clear survival advantage with a long list of chemotherapies (single agent and combined), somatostatin analogues (without and with radionuclides), interferons, aggressive surgical approaches to metastatic lesions, and early trial results with some of the newer targeted agents. Though the general prognosis for neuroendocrine tumors is excellent compared with that of metastatic adenocarcinomas of the colon, stomach, and pancreas, Modlin and colleagues[59] emphasized that combining all tumors, there was documentation of metastatic disease at diagnosis in 12.9%, with an overall 5-year survival of 67.2%—concluding that these data support that carcinoids, and by extension GEP-NET in general, should not be thought of as generally benign tumors.

PANCREATIC NET (PNET) (ISLET-CELL TUMORS)

Most of the noncarcinoid neuroendocrine tumors of the GEP do in fact occur in the pancreas, thus the common use of the classification of PNET (pancreatic neuroendocrine tumors). As a group, they have histologic features that are largely similar to the GEP-NET labeled as carcinoids,[105] and despite efforts to subdivide based on growth patterns and granule ultrastructure, there is not yet a classification scheme that correlates with the type of hormone secreted that is responsible for clinical symptoms, nor a classification that predicts the likelihood of malignant spread for a given patient.[106] The annual incidence is approximately 10 cases per million population, with clinically evident tumors at an incidence of about 3.5 to 4.0 per million. As is often true with neuroendocrine tumors, the incidence at autopsy is much higher; in the case of PNET, the incidence has been reported as high as 10% when particular attention is taken to examine the pancreas in detail.[107] The PNET represent just under half of all neuroendocrine tumors, but represent only a small fraction, 1 to 2%, of all pancreatic tumors. The individual PNET are defined by the clinical syndromes associated with their specific secretory products (see Table 78-4). Nonfunctioning (PPoma) and gastrinoma are the most common malignant PNET, and insulinoma is the most common benign PNET, followed in incidence by a list of rare and interesting tumors. The different PNET have unique biological features relevant to their presentations, diagnostic evaluations, and initial surgical and medical management. Unfortunately, once metastatic neither the surgical nor medical management is curative, but rather, offers palliation of significant symptoms. These therapies will be commented on for all PNET as a group.

Nonfunctioning PNET Nonfunctioning PNET are defined by having no specific associated clinical syndrome, despite staining for one or several peptides and amines or even having quantifiable serum levels of certain neuroendocrine markers. Included in the nonfunctioning pancreatic NET are the PPomas. PP (pancreatic polypeptide) is evident on staining of these tumors and measured in the serum of patients. However, PP has not been found to lead to any identified clinical signs or symptoms. There is no evidence to suggest that the biological characteristics and clinical presentation of PPomas and nonfunctioning PNET without elevated PP are different entities. Upwards of 75% of nonfunctioning PNET will be found to stain positive for PP. These tumors secrete, in addition to PP, markers that include chromogranin A, B, C, α- and β-HCG subunits.[108]

Clinical Presentation and Diagnosis Nonfunctional PNET and PPomas together account for about 15 to 30% of the PNET.[108] Because they have no associated secretory symptoms, they present, based on bulk of disease, with most patients in the fourth or fifth decade, with presenting complaints of abdominal pain in 36%, jaundice in 28%, and incidental finding at surgery in 16%.[109] For the same reason, there is a high reported incidence of metastases at diagnosis that ranges from 60 to 90%. PP is elevated in a variety of NET- and non-NET–related conditions, so cannot be used alone to make the diagnosis of a PPoma. Serum chromogranin A and B are elevated in close to 100% of nonfunctioning PNET.[95] Localization of nonfunctioning PNET is less important than other PNET, given the late presentation with obvious primary tumors. Once diagnosed, CT and MRI along with SRS are used to stage and follow metastatic disease.

Surgery As for most GEP-NET, the treatment of choice and the only therapy that can achieve a cure is surgery. Given the late presentation and high percentage of patients with metastatic disease at presentation, surgical cure is not often possible for nonfunctional PNET/PPomas. However, procedures such as surgical debulking and relief of biliary obstruction can provide significant palliation.

Gastrinoma The gastrinoma syndrome, first named as the Zollinger-Ellison syndrome (ZES), is based on a report of two patients with severe peptic ulcer disease and non-β islet-cell tumors of the pancreas,[110] with later identification of gastrin as the secreted hormone.[111] Gastrinoma patients are characterized by a severe ulcer diathesis and persistent basal gastric acid hypersecretion that is also thought responsible for the frequent symptom of diarrhea resulting from the direct effect of gastric acid on the intestinal mucosa, inactivation of lipase, and precipitation of bile salts. Gastrinomas account for about 25% of all PNET, are found primarily in the duodenum (70%) and pancreas (25%), and demonstrate malignant behavior in approximately 50% of cases. About 20% of gastrinoma patients are found to have MEN-1,[112] and their presentation and course differ from sporadic cases (see the section "MEN-1 Syndrome" below). The incidence of malignant disease exceeds 50% at diagnosis, and increases over time even after surgical resection.[113,114]

Clinical Presentation and Diagnosis The possibility of gastrinoma syndrome should be entertained in all patients with ulcer disease and in those with unexplained secretory diarrhea. Ulcer disease that is recurrent, refractory to therapy, or occurs in unusual locations should all raise suspicion of a gastrinoma. Before development of the radioimmunoassay, 80% of patients with gastrinoma presented with a severe ulcer diathesis, bleeding, intestinal obstruction, or perforation. Today, the diagnosis of gastrinoma should be made even without ulcers, based on diarrhea or mild duodenitis. A history of improvement in the diarrhea with administration of H2-receptor antagonists or proton pump inhibitors is strongly suggestive of the gastrinoma syndrome. Many patients currently present without any abdominal pain, and in fact, diarrhea is perhaps more common than ulcer-related pain and can be the only symptom in upwards of 20% of patients.[112]

The diagnosis requires the demonstration of an elevated fasting serum gastrin (FSG) and elevated basal acid output (BAO). It must be noted that FSG is also elevated in disorders associated with gastric acid hypersecretion, and in those disorders that result in hypo- and achlorhydria. Infection with *Helicobacter pylori* can elevate both FSG and BAO and should be treated and test repeated before considering a diagnosis of ZES. Elevated FSG and low BAO is most often related to antisecretory therapy (ie, omeprazole), and can be seen in chronic gastritis, pernicious anemia, atrophic gastritis, and postvagotomy states.[115] The most sensitive and accurate test remains the secretin stimulation test for gastrin secretion. Secretin, 2 μ/kg, is given intravenously and blood samples for gastrin drawn at 2, 5, 10, 20, and 30 minutes. A rise of more than 100 pg/mL is strongly suggestive of Zollinger-Ellison syndrome.[116]

Gibril and colleagues compared in a prospective study the sensitivity of SRS with that of CT, MRI, ultrasonography, and selective angiography in the detection of primary and metastatic gastrinomas.[117] The SRS scans proved the single most sensitive method for imaging either primary or metastatic liver lesions in patients with Zollinger-Ellison syndrome. The same group studied the effect of SRS on clinical management and found the SRS results altered management of 47% of the patients,[118] concluding that SRS should be the initial imaging modality for patients with gastrinomas.

Improvements in localization (Table 78-5) by imaging, including intraoperative and endoscopic ultrasound, along with more aggressive surgical techniques, have led to a larger percentage of gas-

Table 78-5 Success of Tumor Localization in Gastrinoma

Factor	Ultrasound	Infusion	Computed Tomography	Selective Angiography		PTHVS Local	PTHVS Regional
Sensitivity	21	40	31	60	29	35	94
Specificity	92	100	66	100	100	89	97
Positive predictive value	80	100	83	100	100	—	94
Negative predictive value	40	50	15	60	100	89	—

PTHVS = percutaneous transhepatic portal, pancreatic, and hepatic venous gastrin sampling.
Data from Norton JA and colleagues[119,153,153a] as well as Vinik AI and colleagues.[14,162,162a]

trinomas being localized to the pancreatic head, duodenum, and peripancreatic lymph nodes.[119]

Histology of the primary tumor does not predict for malignancy, only presence of metastatic lesions. Weber and colleagues [114] showed that primary tumor size was the best predictor of malignancy, with liver lesions found in 4% of gastrinomas < 1.0 cm, 28% of tumors > 1.0 cm and < 2.9 cm, and 61% of tumors 3.0 cm or larger. Duodenal gastrinomas have a lower percentage of malignant tumors (5%) compared with pancreatic gastrinomas (52%), but this might simply reflect that pancreatic tumors are generally larger than pancreatic gastrinomas at diagnosis.[114]

Surgery With the ability to control gastric acid hypersecretion over long periods, the quality of life and prognosis of ZES improved significantly, to the point where the long-term survival of patients with very slow growing gastrinomas are now determined largely by the eventual malignant behavior of the tumor.[111,119] Surgery has evolved from gastric resections to control ulcer disease to complex surgery using pre- and intraoperative imaging to localize and resect often small local and regional metastatic disease. The overall survival rate for gastrinomas, excluding patients with MEN-1, at 5 years is between 60 and 80%, and at 10 years is between 45 and 75%.[114,120,121] Norton and colleagues report that in a series of patients operated on with curative intent, the 10-year survival is 94%.[119] Fraker and colleagues report on a study of surgical versus medically managed patients and demonstrate a lower percentage of liver metastases developing in the surgical patients over long-term follow-up.[122]

Medical Therapy Treatment of the gastrinoma syndrome has undergone significant changes since the first case was described in 1955.[110] Until the development of drugs to control excessive acid production, the purpose of operative intervention was to excise the acid-secreting stomach to avoid the excessive morbidity and mortality from massive hemorrhage or perforation. Successive generations of medical therapies including anticholinergics, histamine H2 receptor blockers, and the now more potent and widely used inhibitors of the H^+-K^+ adenosine triphosphatase inhibitors (ie, omeprazole).[108,116,123] Though failure rates in controlling acid hypersecretion with various agents and in different studies over time have varied, failure rates with omeprazole are about 5%, including the fact that the doses required to adequately control acid secretion are often several fold higher than the doses recommended in idiopathic ulcer disease, with average omeprazole dosages of 20 to 80 mg/day.[123]

As stated above for the role of chemotherapy for carcinoids, GEP-NET in general have a low response rate to single and multiagent chemotherapy. This remains true for the gastrinomas, where trials have not shown that this subset of GEP-NET has any higher response. This includes the randomized trials by Moertel and colleagues that explored streptozotocin-based regimens, and the small-cell lung cancer regimen of cisplatin and etoposide.[124–126] The use of chemotherapy remains a decision individualized for each patient, and is generally reserved for patients with metastatic disease, in whom other measures to control symptoms from secretion of hormones and bulk disease have failed. Presence of metastatic disease alone might not require therapy in this slow-growing tumor, noting as Sutliff and colleagues reported that over half of liver lesions in gastrinomas show no or minimal growth over a mean follow-up period of 29 months.[127]

Fifteen gastrinoma patients treated with long acting lanreotide included in a study by Shojamanesh and colleagues[128] demonstrated that only patients classified as slowly progressing before entry in the trial had a clinical or radiological response.[128,129]

Insulinoma Insulinomas were first described by Whipple in a 1938 report of 30 patients with pancreatic adenomas and hypoglycemia.[130] Included in his report were the diagnostic criteria that are still relevant today: symptoms of hypoglycemia, associated blood glucose level of ≤ 50 mg/dL, and immediate relief of symptoms with oral ingestion of glucose. Insulinomas are the second most common functioning PNET, with an incidence of 0.8 to 0.9 cases per million. Overall, the incidence of metastatic disease, about 5 to 15%, is low compared with other PNET. The tumors are often well encapsulated, solitary nodules found evenly distributed throughout the pancreas.[131] The finding of multiple insulinomas should prompt testing for MEN-1, which occurs in about 10% of patients.[132]

Clinical Presentation and Diagnosis Almost all cases of insulinoma present with symptoms of hypoglycemia, with neuroglycopenic symptoms (visual complaints, altered consciousness, weakness) more common than adrenergic symptoms alone (sweating, tremulousness) or in combination with neuroglycopenic symptoms.[131] Diagnosis of suspected cases is made by a supervised fast, where over 90% of patients will develop a serum glucose of < 50 mg/dL during a 48-hour fast, and the corresponding serum insulin level at the time of hypoglycemia will equal or exceed 5 μU/mL.[133] Other true or factious causes of hypoglycemia can be investigated by including proinsulin, C-peptide, and sulfonylurea levels in the supervised fast.

It is generally recommended that in the absence of documented metastases, all insulinoma be surgically removed, even in those with mild symptoms. With surgery, 80 to 90% of all insulinoma patients will be cured.[131,134] The extent of preoperative imaging for insulinomas is still debated. Given the low sensitivity of the SRS for insulinomas in particular,[72] combined with the fact that insulinomas are most often single lesions confined to the pancreas, it is felt that perhaps the only role of preoperative imaging is to rule out obvious liver metastases and prevent unnecessary surgery.[134] This is supported by the increasing role of endoscopic ultrasound (EUS), which has a reported sensitivity of 80%, including tumors less than 1 cm.[135] To avoid blind pancreatic resections; when even EUS cannot localize a lesion, intraoperative ultrasound (IOUS) can be used. Perhaps the most sensitive is selective intra-arterial injection of calcium with hepatic venous sampling, a technique with a reported sensitivity of 94% for insulinomas.[136,137]

Medical Therapy Insulinoma patients not infrequently discover on their own, prior to diagnosis, that they can reduce hypoglycemic symptoms by eating small, frequent meals; this approach can be used effectively short term postdiagnosis. Diet is coupled with medical therapy, including diazoxide and octreotide. Diazoxide, which directly blocks release of insulin from the β-cell, is initiated at a dosage of 150 to 200 mg daily, and increased to a maximum of 600 to 800 mg daily.[138] Octreotide, in dosages from 50 μg to as high as 1,500 μg daily of short-acting formulations, can control symptoms in as high as 60% of patients.[139] Little is known about the long-term control of insulinomas with medical therapy because most patients have surgery soon after diagnosis.

VIPoma The VIPoma (vasoactive intestinal polypeptide) was first described by Verner and Morrison,[140] followed by a review of 55 patients with the syndrome.[141] The diagnostic terms also used include the Verner-Morrison syndrome, as well as the descriptive acronym WDHA syndrome (watery diarrhea, hypokalemia, and achlorhydria), or as proposed by Kvols,[17] the WDHHA syndrome to account for the hypochlorhydria in most cases and the acidosis that results from bicarbonate wasting in some cases. The hormone VIP is thought to be largely responsible for the direct inhibition of gastric acid secretion, stimulation of intestinal secretion, and the resulting electrolyte abnormalities that account for the symptoms of a VIPoma. Unlike other PNET, there are distinct adult and pediatric subsets of patients. VIPoma are rarely seen in patients with an MEN syndrome.[132,142]

Clinical Presentation The VIPomas are quite rare, accounting for only about 5% of the PNET. The mean age of diagnosis in adults is 50 years with a range of 32 to 81 years, distinct from the mean age of diagnosis in children of 2 to 4 years with a range from 10 months to 9 years.[143] In adults, 90% of the tumors are found in the pancreas, most often as solitary nodules. The tumor histology alone cannot distinguish VIPomas from other PNET;[138] however, immunohistochemical detection of tumor VIP is highly suggestive because it is found in very few other neuroendocrine tumors. In adults, upwards of 60% of cases present with or develop metastatic disease. In children, on the other hand, most VIP-secreting tumors are extrapancreatic and are neurogenic in origin, with the most common histology being ganglioneuroblastomas and ganglioneuromas.[144] The diagnosis requires the documentation of elevated plasma VIP concentrations and documentation of large volume secretory diarrhea.[145] The diarrhea generally exceeds 3 L/day and, importantly, does not decrease significantly with oral fasting. Surprisingly, some patients will go months and years prior to diagnosis, partly because the diarrhea is episodic at first and during quiet periods the VIP level may normalize.[17] As the tumor size increases the diarrhea, cramping, and other symptoms become more persistent. The diarrhea could be confused with laxative abuse, other benign secretory diarrheas, and with the diarrhea syndrome caused by another PNET, a gastrinoma (Zollinger-Ellison syndrome). The distinguishing features of gastrinoma and VIPoma (WDHHA) diarrhea are shown in Table 78-6.

The mean fasting plasma VIP levels in VIP patients = 900 pg/mL, far exceeding the normal levels of < 170 pg/mL in most laboratories.[144,145]

Medical Therapy In patients with a suspected VIPoma, the first therapeutic intervention is to correct the hypovolemia, hypokalemia, and acidosis if present. This often requires impressive amounts of intravenous fluid and potassium supplementation. A variety of medications are being used to control the diarrhea,[138] but have largely been replaced with the somatostatin analogue octreotide. Octreotide has been reported to control symptoms in over 80% of patients, corresponding with a drop in the VIP plasma level.[139] The dosages required range from standard octreotide dose of 50 μg 3 times a day to as high as 1,200 μg/day. In patients refractory to even high doses, the addition of a corticosteroid is sometimes successful. Chemotherapy, as discussed below, has shown only occasional responders as seen for carcinoid and other more common GEP-NET.

Surgery Once symptoms are controlled and electrolytes corrected, imaging studies should be done to localize the VIPoma and evaluated for possible surgical resection for cure. Long and colleagues[144] reported that in 52 patients with pancreatic VIPomas, the average lesion was 9 cm in diameter, and thus readily visible by CT or ultrasound. Other studies have shown that some VIPomas require angiography with or without selective venous sampling for VIP levels.[146] The role of SRS, supported by the ENET consensus,[70] is to localize extrapancreatic primary lesions and detect metastatic disease. The finding of an isolated primary VIPoma, or limited metastatic disease should be considered for complete resection. Complete resections have resulted in long-term control of symptoms in 30 to 50% of adult patients.[138,139,147] If metastatic disease is present and not readily resectable, then medical therapy can be maximized prior to considering palliative surgery to help control symptoms.

Table 78-6 Differentiation of Gastrinoma and WDHHA Syndrome

Feature	Gastrinoma	WDHHA
Diarrhea	Acid	Alkaline (HCO_3 loss)
Gastric acid	Increased	Decreased
Gastric volume	Increased	Normal or decreased
Nasogastric suction	Diarrhea improves	Diarrhea unchanged
Motility	Increased[a]	Increased slightly[b]
Abdominal pain	Marked	Rare (initially)
Stool K+ loss	Slight	Marked
Metabolic acidosis	No (alkalosis with gastric suction)	Yes
Lesion location	Primary pancreas (also liver, wall of stomach, and duodenum)	Primary pancreas
Mediator	Gastrin	VIP/other

[a]Motility enhanced secondary to gastric acid stimulation.
[b]Motility may be slightly increased secondary to direct effects of either intraarterial or intraluminal VIP.
VIP = vasoactive intestinal peptide; WDHHA = watery diarrhea, hypokalemia, hypochlorhydria, and acidosis.

Glucagonoma Glucagonoma were first reported in 1966 by McGavran and colleagues, who called attention to a syndrome that included acquired diabetes and glucagon-producing tumors.[148] This rare tumor, estimated to account for 1% of GEP-NET, was later recognized to include a characteristic skin rash, necrolytic migratory erythema (NME) described by Mallinson and colleagues[149] and others.[150,151] The syndrome of diabetes, NME rash, weight loss, diarrhea, stomatitis, and glossitis is thought to be largely due to the direct effects of high circulating levels of glucagon. The tumor occurs almost exclusively in adults over 40 years of age, and is rarely associated with MEN-1.[142]

Clinical Presentation The largest reported single-institution experience was from the Mayo Clinic, which reported on 21 patients seen between 1975 and 1991.[152] The main presenting features of the glucagonoma syndrome included weight loss (71%), the characteristic NME rash (67%) (Figure 78-5), mild diabetes mellitus (38%), diarrhea (29%), and painful glossitis and angular stomatitis (29%). The NME rash can be insidious in onset and typically precedes the diagnosis of the glucagonoma by several years. It usually is widespread, but major sites of involvement are the perioral and perigenital regions along with the fingers, legs, and feet.

The symptoms are largely accounted for by the known effects of glucagon on glycogenolysis, gluconeogenesis, ketogenesis, lipolysis, insulin secretion, intestinal and pancreatic secretion, and intestinal motility. In addition, the amino acid depletion that results from excess glucagon causes, or at least worsens, the NME rash.[153] Amino acid replacement alone has been shown to improve the rash.[138] Another poorly explained feature of the glucagonoma syndrome is that patients have a significant risk of thromboembolic complications, particularly pulmonary embolism.

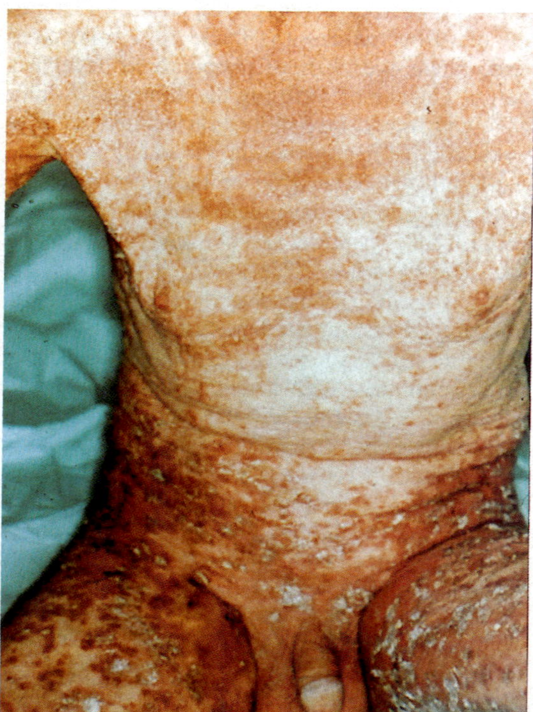

Figure 78-5 Migratory necrolytic erythema of glucagonoma syndrome.

At diagnosis, the glucagonomas are almost all found as single lesions in the pancreas (tail > body), averaging 5 to 10 cm in size, and metastatic disease is already present in over 60% of patients, most often to the liver, as is generally true for all PNET.[138,154] The histology of glucagonomas is similar to other PNET, particularly in that many other PNET stain positive for glucagon. Therefore, the diagnosis requires documentation of increased plasma glucagon levels. Fasting glucagon levels in normal individuals rarely exceed 200 pg/mL. Disorders causing elevated plasma glucagon levels include diabetes mellitus, burn injury, acute trauma, bacteremia, cirrhosis, renal failure, and Cushing's syndrome, and can result in fasting plasma glucagon levels as high as 500 pg/mL. Glucagonoma patients have levels > 500 pg/mL in almost 100% of cases, and > 1,000 pg/mL in over 90% of cases.

If the diagnosis is made while the tumor is still localized, surgical resection can be curative.[155] As in other islet-cell tumors, even when malignant these tumors tend to be extremely slow growing. Almost invariably, the NME rash resolves after successful removal of a glucagon-producing tumor, even if the rash has been present for several years.[156] In addition, in those patients who do not undergo curative resection but are treated with chemotherapeutic agents, the NME rash and other skin manifestations improve as the glucagon levels decrease.[157]

Octreotide has been used to improve the preoperative condition of patients and to treat symptoms related to unresectable and metastatic disease. Both the NME rash and diarrhea, but generally not the glucose intolerance/diabetes, respond in over 50% of the patients, with complete disappearance of symptoms in about 30% treated with somatostatin analogues.[138,139]

Somatostatinoma Somatostatinomas are rare PNET, with about 50 cases reported to date. The first cases were reported in 1977 by Ganda and colleagues[158] and Larsson and colleagues.[159]

Krejs and colleagues[160] reported a series of 8 cases in 1979, and Vinik and colleagues reported the largest review on 48 cases in 1987.[14] The initial papers accurately captured the central clinical features of the somatostatinoma syndrome consisting of diabetes, diarrhea, steatorrhea, gallbladder disease, hypochlorhydria, and weight loss. An elevated plasma level of somatostatin-like immunoreactivity (SLI), an immunoassay that reacts with several forms of somatostatin, is thought to be responsible for the majority of symptoms. The rarity of this tumor and the advanced stage at presentation has not permitted the collection of much information on approaches to diagnosis, imaging, and treatment. Somatostatinomas are rarely seen in association with MEN-1,[142] but an association with MEN-2 and neurofibromatosis is suggested.[14,161]

Diagnosis The accumulated case reports demonstrate that despite a defined clinical syndrome, most cases are diagnosed at laparotomy or laparoscopy, or identified on imaging studies for abdominal complaints or jaundice. Vinik and colleague's report recognized the distinction based on clinical presentations of somatostatinomas presenting in the pancreas, intestine, and extrapancreatic sites.[162] The pancreatic tumors present with symptoms of excess somatostatin, namely diabetes, diarrhea, and steatorrhea. The intestinal tumors, associated with lower tumor content and lower plasma levels of SLI, present more often with cholecystitis, GI bleeding, or an abdominal mass. The tumors tend to present as large masses, reflecting the high levels of somatostatin thought necessary to create symptoms, and not rapid growth. At diagnosis, 85% of the pancreatic and 50% of the intestinal primaries had evidence of metastatic spread.[162] Though the data are minimal, the outlook for those with somatostatinomas is poor, given the high incidence of malignant spread. Close to half of reported patients dying within a year and others surviving variable periods up to as long as 5 years.[162]

GROWTH HORMONE RELEASING FACTOR First described in 1982 by Guillemin and colleagues,[163] growth hormone releasing factor (GRF)omas are perhaps the least common PNET. The clinical features are due to excess plasma growth hormone and are indistinguishable from the acromegaly that results from pituitary tumors. GRFomas have presented with Zollinger-Ellison syndrome or Cushing's diseases as well. The tumors are found in the pancreas, lung, and small intestine and are often greater than 6 cm at diagnosis. The histology is typical of PNET. The diagnosis should be expected in any patient with acromegaly and no pituitary adenoma, or acromegaly and an abdominal mass. Plasma GRF levels confirm the diagnosis.[164]

THERAPY FOR GEP-NET In general, carcinoids and other GEP-NET are slow growing, and symptoms are most often attributable to secretory products. It should be remembered that even patients with extensive metastatic disease could enjoy a normal quality of life as long as the endocrine syndrome is quiescent. For those patients whose tumors are not resectable at diagnosis or who later develop metastatic disease, given the general lack of curative therapies at this stage, the focus is on control of symptoms. The use of the long-acting somatostatin analogs and interferon to decrease secretion of vasoactive and other hormones, combined with bulk-reducing procedures primarily directed at hepatic lesions, the quality of life of GEP-NET patients can be maintained.

SURGERY Primary In general, surgical removal of the primary tumor is the treatment of choice for small and localized tumors as well as for the alleviation of any obstructive symptoms, but surgical cure of GEP-NET tumors is uncommon in the presence of intra-abdominal and hepatic metastases. Gastric and duodenal GEP-NET can, in select cases with tumors < 1 cm, be excised endoscopically.[165] Carcinoids of the small bowel that appear local should be resected en bloc with lymphadenectomy and removal of the mesentery.[166] Carcinoids of the appendix and rectum are both generally treated by appendectomy if < 2 cm, and resection if > 2 cm.[167] Localized low-grade neuroendocrine tumors of the tracheobronchial tree can be successfully treated in a high percentage of cases with segmental or wedge resections.[92]

Hepatic Resections Cytoreductive hepatic surgery can alleviate symptoms associated with pathologically elevated hormones and improve the patient's quality of life. Que and colleagues recently performed a meta-analysis summarizing reports in the medical literature over 26 years.[168] Surgery may involve hemihepatectomy, trisegmentectomy, or wedge resection. The operative mortality after partial hepatectomy for carcinoid tumors in this series was 2.3%. More than 80% had improvement in their carcinoid syndrome and the duration of response ranged from 4 to 120 months.[168]

Hepatic Artery Vaso-Occlusive Therapy Vaso-occlusive therapy to reduce bulk of hepatic lesions to decrease secretory syndromes and mass effects should be attempted after careful consideration given the high risk of complications in the immediate "postembolization" phase as well as longer-term complications and death. No randomized trials of the various modalities have been conducted. Overall, vascular-occlusion therapies have led to biochemical responses as high as 50%, and tumor reduction is as high as 40%, and generally of short duration.[169] Hepatic arterial occlusion combined with sequential chemotherapy has resulted in biochemical responses as high as 80%, with a median duration of 18 months or more.[170,171] Although hepatic artery occlusion may produce subjective and objective responses in the majority of highly selected patients, the toxicity and duration of responses resulting from this therapy generally do not support its routine use.[119]

Hepatic Transplantation The largest series to date on hepatic transplant of neuroendocrine cancers by Le Treut and colleagues included a total of 31 cases, with 15 carcinoid and 16 PNET patients.[172] The 5-year survival was reported as 69%, with 7 of the carcinoid patients alive and disease free.

SOMATOSTATIN ANALOGUES As an agent to improve the quality of life for these patients, somatostatin analogues have had a major impact on the flushing, diarrhea, and wheezing in most patients with metastatic carcinoid and the carcinoid syndrome. Most patients with secretory symptoms related to a GEP-NET are treated first with the long-acting somatostatin analog, octreotide, to at least control the symptoms of diarrhea and flushing.[162,173] The SRS imaging results can also be used in predicting response to octreotide. Janson and colleagues[174] and Kvols and colleagues[175] have shown that patients with carcinoid and other neuroendocrine tumors with positive scans all responded with improvement in symptoms to octreotide, whereas all patients with negative scans failed to respond. There is no question that the somatostatin analogues have provided a major advance in the management of GEP-NET patients with symptomatic secretory syndromes. This simple fact has precluded any clinical evaluation of these agents versus placebo or observation to determine if they have survival advantage in the treatment of newly diagnosed (symptomatic) patients. Also not proven, but clinically accepted, is the fact that the somatostatin analogues have simplified and reduced the risks of surgery, and perhaps allowed many more patients to benefit from more aggressive surgical approaches. As an example, Kvols and colleagues treated a patient, who soon after the induction of anesthesia had a fall in blood pressure that was unresponsive to intravenous fluid, calcium, Neo-Synephrine, or epinephrine administration, and within 1 minute of 100 μg of octreotide given intravenously, blood pressure rose, and the patient made an uneventful recovery.[173]

Of the currently available SST analogues used for treatment of GEP-NET, only octreotide (and its long-acting formulation) is available in the United States at this time.[176] All of the currently available analogues and their long-acting formulations bind with high affinity to SSTR2 and SSTR5 and have *in vitro* antisecretory and antiproliferative activities, and there are reports that binding to SSTR3 occurs with higher doses and can induce apoptosis.[177,178] SOM 230, an analogue in development, binds with high affinity to all SSTR1-5.

Most of the clinical studies over the past three decades with somatostatin and its analogues have included patients with multiple histologies, generally GEP-NET patients diagnosed as carcinoid or pancreatic islet cell, and the vast majority had a defined secretory syndrome (most often carcinoid) or symptomatic bulky disease. As such, the endpoints are varied and most often included symptomatic (SR), biochemical markers (BR), and radiological objective response* (OR), and most reported on stabilization of tumor growth (SD) in groups of patients who were generally highly symptomatic with evidence of progressive tumor growth. Delaunoit and colleagues[179] reviewed the literature for three decades of use of somatostatin analogues in the treatment of GEP-NET. Most studies are single arm with relatively small numbers and a heterogeneous collection of patients. The conclusions that most authors concur with are that complete tumor responses are rare, stabilization of disease can occur in as high as 40% of patients, biochemical responses are commonly in the 70 to 80% range, and symptomatic response is seen in most patients, at least with front-line therapy. An analysis of over 60 published studies by Harris and Redfern[180] showed control of symptoms of diarrhea and flushing in over 80% of patients, and over 70% of those patients showed a decrease in 5-HIAA levels. As is unfortunately typical, octreotide responses were maintained for a median of only 4 months in 40% of patients, with the remainder of patients having sustained control of symptoms from 1 to as long as 2.5 years. The comparative studies of short- and long-acting agents demonstrated similar data, with no significant differences between the agents in terms of response, safety, and efficacy.[181,182] Many of the adverse effects of the agents are mild and resolve with continued use. Though some adverse events are difficult to separate from the secretory symptoms of the tumor itself, the frequency of the same events in acromegaly patients treated with somatostatin analogues lends some clarity. Carcinoid (and acromegaly) patients in clinical trials report nausea, abdominal pain, flatulence (27–38%), constipation (15%), and vomiting (21%). Diarrhea in carcinoid patients is common, but it is not clear if the diarrhea is drug-related. Carcinoid clinical trial patients also report sinus bradycardia in 19%, conduction abnormalities in 9%, and arrhythmias in 3% of those followed with serial EKGs. The most notable of adverse events seen with long-term use of somatostatin analogues relates to the effect on the biliary tree. Of patients treated longer than 18 months, 62% had dilatation, sludge, or stones in the gallbladder. Newly documented stones were documented in 24%; however, only 1% of patients required a cholecystectomy.[179]

High-Dose Somatostatin Analogues Several authors have investigated high doses of both octreotide and lanreotide based on preclinical data that suggested a dose-response relationship, and possible recruitment of the SSTR3 pathway has been implicated in apoptosis of neuroendocrine cells *in vivo* and in animal models.[47] Eriksson and colleagues[183] treated 19 patients with progressive GEP-NET at a lanreotide dosage of 12 mg/day, and Faiss and colleagues[184] treated 30 patients at a lanreotide dosage of 15 mg/day, and all types of responses seem comparable and not particularly better than other lanreotide studies. No systematic study of a dose-response relationship has yet been done for any of the somatostatin analogues.

Biologic Agents **Interferon** Oberg and colleagues pioneered the use of leukocyte interferon in carcinoid GEP-NET[185] and reviewed the early trials in 2000.[186] Most trials investigating interferon in GEP-NET have been conducted in patients who have been previously treated with, and likely failed, a somatostatin analogue. In the majority of these cases, the addition of interferon recovered a symptomatic response in a significant number of patients. Two studies from the Uppsala group[187,188] and a study by Frank and colleagues[189] demonstrated that a biochemical response could be recovered in 63 to 77% of patients, with over 50% reporting stable disease and a rare complete or partial response. These studies and others suggested that the combination of a somatostatin analogue and an interferon as front-line therapy might be more efficacious than either agent alone. Unfortunately, one of the few multicenter, randomized, comparative trials done in the field of GEP-NET to date showed that the objective responses were no higher with the combination as compared with either agent alone.[190] There was a higher symptomatic and biochemical response rate in the combination therapy group, but at the expense of increased toxicity. It remains unanswered whether the combination as front-line therapy, or sequential use of the agents, provides the greatest long-term benefit to the patient.

External Beam Radiotherapy There is no data that supports the routine use of radiation therapy for GEP-NET patients unless they have symptomatic bone metastases, spinal cord compression, bronchial obstruction, or some other symptomatic site of disease.

Peptide Receptor Radiotherapy Despite the lack of demonstrated radiosensitivity, the targeting to overexpressed SSTR provided by somatostatin analogues has led to the development of peptide receptor radiotherapy (PRRT) reagents for GEP-NET. Generally speaking, PRRT is reserved for patients with inoperable primary cancers and those with metastases, and as such, patients have often been previously treated with and failed somatostatin analogues, chemotherapy, and possibly other agents. PRRT also requires that the tumors, including metastases, express the given receptor in high density (and in the case of SSTR-PRRT that the proper isoform is expressed) and as homogeneously as possible.[191] Deciding whether PRRT is an option, therefore, involves evaluating *in vitro* molecular data for a given tumor type, supported by *in vivo* imaging and dosimetry in a selected patient. Currently no radiolabeled somatostatin analogues are approved for general use, and they remain available only through clinical trials or for compassionate use in selected centers.

PRRT is a logical extension of diagnostic imaging with Octreoscan ([^{111}In-diethylenetriaminepentaacetic acid (DTPA)^0]octreotide) for tumor localization, whereby the localization documents the opportunity for selective delivery of a radiopharmaceutical at the site of SSTR2 expressing tumors. The initial trials were in fact performed with high doses of the Octreoscan imaging agent,[192,193] and though a biological response was seen in several patients, objective responses were few, and significant bone marrow and other toxicities occurred. The poor results were felt in large part due to the use of ^{111}Indium and its poor tissue penetration and the relatively low affinity of the agent for SSTR2 and other SSTRs.

Two other radiolabeled somatostatin analogues have undergone phase I and II clinical trial evaluation in GEP-NET. Most of the trials are single arm with a variety of dose-escalation schemes and have various selection criteria for patients. However, they generally involved refractory metastatic patients with SSTR2-expressing tumors, the majority or all of whom had GEP-NET tumors. Five studies involved the compound [^{90}Y-DOTA^0, Tyr^3] octreotide that substituted yttrium for indium with a different coupling agent. Over 180 patients have been evaluated in long term follow-up after treatment, and the studies show overall response rates (CR + PR) ranging from about 10 to 30%, with about 50 to 60% of patients developing stable disease,[194–198] a significant improvement over the [^{111}In-(DTPA)^0]octreotide results. There continued to be grade 3-4 hematologic toxicity in up to 20% of patients as well as several cases of renal and liver toxicity and a few cases of myelodysplasia. Renal toxicity in most of the recent studies has been decreased, even with higher cumulative radiation doses, through the use of amino acid infusions.[199] Another PRRT agent, [^{177}Lu-DOTA^0, Tyr^3] octreotate, incorporates the combined β- and γ-emitting radionuclide ^{177}Luthium, and the use of a modification of the octreotide molecule, octreotate, that has a marked increase in binding affinity to the SSTR2.[200] The most recent follow-up on patients with GEP-NET treated with [^{177}Lu-DOTA^0, Tyr^3] octreotate as PRRT shows less toxicity, with temporary bone marrow suppression, a single case of MDS with a history of prior alkylating agent exposure, and a case of progressive renal insufficiency. The responses included 1 CR (1%), 22 PRs (29%), and stable disease in 30 (40%), and median time to progression not having been reached at 25 months.[201] Predictors of the response to each of these agents have not been studied in detail but it is suggested that bulk of tumor, extent of liver involvement, and other factors might be important. There is animal data to suggest that the ^{90}Y-labeled somatostatin analogues might work better on large tumors, and ^{177}Lu-labeled somatostatin analogues might be better for microscopic tumors, and the combination of the two might give the overall best response.[202] Clearly, though there were clinically significant responses seen with these agents in even refractory patients, there are numerous clinical questions yet to be addressed in clinical trials that await the approval and wider use of these agents.

Chemotherapy for GEP-NET In malignant GEP-NET, chemotherapy has not been shown to be effective for most patients, and this approach

---

*Most of the objective response in these reports would qualify as minimal or partial response, with very few complete responses, according to current clinical response guidelines.

should still be considered investigational. Numerous trials over several decades have been conducted with every class of chemotherapy given by numerous routes including hepatic intra-arterial. This extends to some of the more recently introduced chemotherapeutic agents such as docetaxel.[203] Given the rarity of GEP-NET, and the variety of tumors within this group, many trials could be criticized as being small and including patients with poorly defined criteria, often heavily pretreated, where it may have been difficult to identify drugs with low but appreciable response rates. However, most studies were repeated at more than one institution or in cooperative groups, and still no drug has shown a more significant cytotoxic effect.

Several authors have reviewed the history of treatment of carcinoid, and other GEP-NET, with single-agent and multiagent chemotherapy.[17,204] The single agent most studied in carcinoid tumor is 5-fluorouracil, which accounted for observed response rates of 26% and 18% in single-institution and multi-institutional trials, respectively. Melia and colleagues[205] reported a high complication rate with little benefit when 5-fluorouracil was administered by intra-arterial, portal or peripheral intravenous routes. Other trials showing minimal or no response include single agents intravenous doxorubicin, 60 mg/m^2, every 3 to 4 weeks, and dactinomycin and dacarbazine in metastatic carcinoid tumor,[206,207] and rare objective responses to either cisplatin or etoposide, and no responses to carboplatinum. Activity was seen with pancreatic NET, but not carcinoid using streptozotocin.[17]

Initial experience with combination chemotherapy suggested that this modality might be effective against malignant carcinoid tumor. Early nonrandomized studies of combinations of cyclophosphamide plus methotrexate, streptozotocin plus 5-fluorouracil, or weekly streptozotocin plus doxorubicin reported response rates in excess of 50%; however, rigid criteria for response were not always employed and complete responses were not seen.[17] Based on these observations, the Eastern Cooperative Oncology Group conducted a series of multi-institutional randomized trials of combinations that all contained streptozotocin, despite the low activity of this drug when used alone. In two studies of 170 evaluable patients, the response rates ranged from 23 to 33%. In a prospective trial, the Southwest Oncology Group reported similar response rates of brief duration following a combination of 5-fluorouracil, cyclophosphamide, and streptozotocin with or without doxorubicin.[17]

Thus, in the absence of randomized trials that contain a no-treatment arm, there is no persuasive evidence that single-agent or combination chemotherapy provides any significant impact on disease progression or on survival in patients with malignant carcinoid tumor. Chemotherapy is generally reserved to provide palliation of hormone excess and symptoms related to tumor bulk. There is a serious unmet medical need for effective systemic therapy for advanced GEP-NET.

Adjuvant Therapy Combined modality therapy, such as the use of adjuvant chemotherapy either before or following surgery, remains undefined for metastatic carcinoid. In the absence of well-established activity for chemotherapy in this disease, there is no rationale to support the use of adjuvant chemotherapy.

PARATHYROID CARCINOMA

As discussed below, parathyroid hyperplasia and adenomas are part of both MEN syndromes. Though considered in the diagnosis of hypercalcemia and parathyroid disease, parathyroid carcinomas are not related to MEN syndromes and as such are discussed separately.

Almost all parathyroid tumors are benign and are clinically manifest as producing signs of primary hyperparathyroidism. Parathyroid carcinoma is one of the less common cancers and is not associated with MEN syndromes. On the other hand, the majority of cases of parathyroid hyperplasia are associated with MEN syndromes, either type 1 or type 2.

Epidemiology and Etiology In contrast to benign parathyroid tumors, which have been diagnosed increasingly since the introduction of automated multichannel analyzers in the 1970s, with an annual age-adjusted incidence of 28 per 100,000, parathyroid carcinomas remain rare. In collected cases of hyperparathyroidism, parathyroid carcinomas usually represent < 1% of the cases.[208] Only about 400 cases have been reported, and their etiology is unknown.[209]

Clinical Features Parathyroid carcinomas are usually slow-growing tumors with a tendency to recur locally and metastasize late.[209] The great majority of them (95%) are functioning and produce a more severe picture of primary hyperparathyroidism compared with parathyroid adenomas or hyperplasia (Table 78-7). The major distinguishing features of malignant hyperparathyroidism are younger mean age of onset, presence of a palpable neck mass, and severe hypercalcemia, often > 14 mg/dL.[210] Metastases occur late and are seen most often in the lung (40%), cervical nodes (30%), and the liver (10%).[209] Symptoms are usually severe and include a wide range of classic manifestations such as polyuria, polydipsia, urolithiasis, nephrocalcinosis, bone involvement with classic osteitis fibrosa cystica and/or osteopenia, pathologic fractures, and bone pain; neuromuscular symptoms, gout, pseudogout, chondrocalcinosis, and calcific tendinitis; gastrointestinal symptoms with anorexia, nausea, vomiting, constipation, peptic ulcers, and pancreatitis; cardiovascular manifestations with decreased Q-T interval, arrhythmias, and possibly hypertension; and calcifications of the cornea (classic band keratopathy) and other soft tissue changes in the skin and lungs.[17,211]

Table 78-7 Clinical Features of Primary Hyperparathyroidism Due to Parathyroid Carcinoma and Benign Tumors

	Cancer	Benign
Incidence	2–4%	96–98%
Female:male	1:1	3:1
Age (yrs)		
Mean	45	58
Range	12–84	17–83
Palpable neck mass	42%	Rare
Serum calcium		
Mean mg/dL (mmol/L)	15 (3.75)	11–12 (2.75–3.0)
>14 mg/dL (3.5 mmol/L)	64%	<10%
Renal disease	56%	20%
Lithiasis	49%	20%
Nephrocalcinosis	23%	Rare
Decreased function	51%	14%
Bone disease	63%	6%
Osteitis fibrosa cystica	36%	4%
Renal and bone disease	39%	Rare
Gastrointestinal disease		
Peptic ulcer	11%	8%
Pancreatitis	11%	Rare
Asymptomatic	3%	47%

Laboratory Tests Hypercalcemia, the hallmark of hyperparathyroidism, is usually severe in patients with parathyroid carcinoma. The serum calcium level is above 14 mg/dL in about two-thirds of the patients, compared with less than 10% of patients with benign hyperparathyroidism. By far the most important test to diagnose primary hyperparathyroidism is the serum level of immunoreactive PTH (iPTH). Elevated levels of iPTH are virtually diagnostic and can be very high in cases of functioning parathyroid carcinoma. Ectopic production of PTH is exceptional and has been documented in very few cases of nonparathyroid carcinomas.

Biopsy Biopsy is not necessary in the majority of cases before definitive surgery for either benign or malignant parathyroid tumors and is in fact generally contraindicated.

Imaging Techniques In benign hyperparathyroidism, first-time exploration of the neck by an experienced surgeon will successfully detect the tumor(s) in more than 90% of cases. Imaging techniques are most useful in cases of recurrent or persistent hyperparathyroidism after initial surgery. They are also useful before initial surgery whenever a carcinoma is suspected on clinical grounds, allowing evaluation of the local extent of the tumor.

Noninvasive Techniques Ultrasonography with high-resolution, real-time technology is an excellent noninvasive technique, although its overall results are operator-dependent.[17] In a prospective comparison based on 100 patients with benign parathyroid tumors before surgery, overall sensitivities were as follows: scintigraphy 73%, CT 68%, MRI 57%, sonography 55%, with respective specificities of 94, 92, 87, and 95%.[212] For patients with parathyroid carcinoma, CT scanning appears most useful at this time since it has good sensitivity for detecting the primary tumor and allows evaluation of its local extent and metastases. The diagnosis of primary hyperparathyroidism is clinical and biochemical.

Treatment Surgery is the major and only curative treatment of parathyroid carcinoma.[213] Despite the slow growth of these tumors, the surgery is best performed as early as possible before local and distant spread has occurred. The technique involves removal of the tumor en bloc, with all involved surrounding structures and without violating its capsule. Surgery is the recommended treatment of recurrent tumor as well, offering long-term control of hypercalcemia in the absence of a cure.[214] Parathyroid carcinomas are resistant to radiotherapy, although it can occasionally be useful for palliation of pain from bone metastasis. The experience with chemotherapy is limited to case reports.[215,216] The 5-year survival is about 50% (including 30% without recurrence) and the 10-year survival varies from 13 to 35%, with patients who survive many years despite repeated recurrences and metastasis.[211]

MEN SYNDROMES

The MEN-1 and MEN-2 syndromes describe individuals and families with hyperplasia and/or tumors of multiple endocrine tissues. The MEN-1 and MEN-2 syndromes, however, differ in the type and how often certain endocrine tissues are involved, etiology, clinical presentation, preventive and therapeutic surgery, screening, and follow-up of affected individuals. The neuroendocrine tumors that occur within the MEN syndromes have both similarities and differences to the same tumors when they occur sporadically. Both MEN-1 and MEN-2 involve hyperparathyroidism secondary to hyperplasia or tumors. MEN-1 includes many of the PNET discussed earlier in this chapter. MEN-2 includes medullary carcinoma of the thyroid and pheochromocytoma, which have not been discussed, therefore, both MEN-related, other familial, and sporadic tumors will be discussed below.

Pituitary adenoma/carcinoma, pheochromocytoma, and medullary thyroid carcinoma were each initially identified as independent pathological entities. The clustering of multiple endocrine neoplasia (MEN) syndromes was described later.

MEN-1 Syndrome This syndrome was first referred to as Werner syndrome, after the person who published the observation of groups of individuals with multiple adenomas that appeared to be inherited in an autosomal dominant pattern.[217] In 1968 Steiner and colleagues characterized the collection of multiple endocrine tumors/hyperplasia into two groups referred to as "multiple endocrine adenomatosis [later changed to neoplasia] types 1 and 2."[218] A somewhat unpredictable cluster of neuroendocrine and nonendocrine tumors from a total of about 20 different histologies characterizes MEN-1 syndrome cases and families (Table 78-8). Though there is no "typical" grouping of neuroendocrine tumors for all MEN-1 syndrome families, data from many families show that the most common tumors are parathyroid, including hyperplasia (90%), enteropancreatic (70%), and anterior pituitary (25%).[91] A practical clinical guideline for diagnosis of an MEN-1 individual is to have two of the three principal tumors diagnosed, and a MEN-1 family would involve at least one case as defined above and at least one first-degree relative with at least one of the principal tumors types.

Table 78-8 MEN-1 Tumor Type Distribution and Estimated Penetrance (%) by Age 40 Years

Endocrine Tumors (Common)	Endocrine Tumors (Less Common)	Nonendocrine Features
Parathyroid adenoma (90%)	Thymic carcinoid (2%)	Collagenomas (70%)
Gastrinoma (40%)	Bronchial carcinoid (2%)	Facial angiofibromas (85%)
PP(nonfunctioning)oma (20%)	PNET (VIPoma, glucagonoma, etc) (2%)	Lipomas (30%)
Prolactinoma (20%)	ACTH, GH (2%)	
Insulinoma (10%)	Pheochromocytoma (<1%)	
ECL tumor (10%)	TSH (rare)	

Nonfunctioning adrenal tumors are found in as high as 25% of MEN-1 patients on full evaluation.
Modified from Brandi ML et al.[91]

It is now recognized that about 80% of familial MEN-1 individuals and about 50% of sporadic MEN-1 individuals have a heterozygous germline mutation in the *MEN-1* gene.[219–221] The *MEN-1* gene was first localized to chromosome region 11q13[222] and consists of 10 exons over 7 kilobases (kb), encoding an mRNA of approximately 2.8 kb that codes a protein called MENIN.[219,220] Over 300 mutations have been characterized and they are spread across the coding region of the *MEN-1* gene and include mutations in specific binding regions for the transcription factors, JUN-D, Smad3, and NF-KappaB.[223] MENIN acts as a tumor suppressor and has recently been shown to interact through the lysine-3-histone deactylase,[224] and the various mutations act as loss-of-function mutations. Despite the varied genotypes, no correlation of genotype to predictable clinical phenotype has been determined that could allow a more focused algorithm to justify preventive surgery and a more focused screening of affected family members with specific mutations.[225] This is despite the fact that the gene shows high penetration with over 90% of documented carriers having clinical or biochemical evidence of disease by age 50 years. Similar inactivating somatic mutations are also found to a varying degree in sporadic tumors of the same histology as found in MEN-1 syndromes. MEN-1 mutations remain the most common form of genetic predisposition to neuroendocrine tumors, including those associated with RET, TSC1, TSC2, and VHL.[226] In general, the familial and somatic mutations differ clinically in that the familial cases have an earlier age of onset, affect multiple organs, and often develop multiple tumors within the same organ.[227] Despite these differences, diagnostic and therapeutic decisions often rely on data from studies of the more common non-MEN-1 patients.

MEN-1 and Parathyroid Lesions Most patients first present with symptoms of hyperparathyroidism (HPT), or if in a known MEN-1 family undergoing screening, with biochemical or imaging evidence of parathyroid tumor(s). The average age of onset is 25 to 30 years old, and by age 50, nearly 100% of the MEN-1 patients will have evidence of HPT. The converse is not true, only 2 to 4% of cases of sporadic HPT investigated will be found to have mutations in the *MEN-1* gene,[228] and the average age of onset is 55 to 60 years old.

Although the parathyroid glands are the most frequently involved organs (90%) and hyperparathyroidism is usually the first manifestation of the syndrome, its presence may not be detected until clinical disease of the pituitary or pancreas has brought the patient to medical attention. Hyperparathyroidism is often found during the second decade of life when screening immediate family members of a patient with a proven MEN-1 mutation. In adults first suspected of the MEN-1 syndrome because of manifestations of gastrinoma, hyperparathyroidism is often diagnosed after obtaining serum calcium and parathyroid hormone levels, even though such patients may have had a decade-long history of renal stones.[17]

MEN-1 patients characteristically have multiglandular nodular hyperplasia as the cause of their hyperparathyroidism. Often, the individual gland involvement is variable and is best described as asymmetrical hyperplasia, resulting in enlargement of only one or two glands, particularly in younger patients. This disease usually takes a slow but progressive course, and eventually all glands are involved.

Micro- or macroadenomas of the pituitary gland are commonly detected in MEN-1 patients when biochemical and imaging studies have been performed. Most tumors are functionally active and secrete prolactin. Less frequently, MEN-1 patients may develop tumors that secrete ACTH or growth hormone and present with Cushing's syndrome or acromegaly. In the MEN-1 patient it is especially important to establish that the Cushing's syndrome is pituitary dependent (Cushing's disease) rather than caused by an adrenal adenoma or the ectopic secretion of ACTH or corticotropin-releasing factor (CRF) from islet-cell tumors or a bronchial carcinoid tumor.[17]

MEN-1 and Gastrinoma Gastrinoma, a functioning islet-cell tumor secreting gastrin, is responsible for the Zollinger-Ellison syndrome (ZES), the next most common tumor to follow HPT in MEN-1 patients. Prior to the introduction of potent proton pump inhibitors, ZES was responsible for multiple peptic ulcers and associated high morbidity and mortality.

Approximately 20% of gastrinomas are associated with the MEN-1 syndrome.[112] Gastrinomas diagnosed in association with the MEN-1 syndrome are quite different from those associated with sporadic gastrinomas. Tumors in the MEN-1 syndrome usually present at an earlier age and are multiple, often small or undetectable, and less frequently (7–12%) malignant. Localization of the specific tumors that are secreting gastrin is made difficult by the fact that MEN-1–associated gastrinomas are often multiple and small. The role of surgery for gastrinoma in MEN-1 patients therefore remains poorly defined. Surgery with curative intent might include complete pancreaticoduodenectomy. Given the high biochemical recurrence postsurgery in MEN-1 patients, it is generally recommended to avoid surgery and manage medically, with periodic evaluations for radiological progression of tumors. When there is no evidence of metastatic disease, and venous sampling demonstrates an anatomically localized source of gastrin, enucleation (ie, pancreatic head) or resection (ie, body or tail) may offer excellent palliation, if not cure.[17] Based on the correlation between tumor size and risk of liver metastases, some advocate surgery for those patients with a tumor exceeding 2.5 cm.[114]

MEN-1 Medical and Surgical Management The clinical features of patients with MEN-1 depend entirely upon expression of the natural history of the individual tumor and endocrine hyperfunction. Most patients with MEN-1 pancreatic disease requiring surgical intervention present with a syndrome caused by hypersecretion of a specific hormone such as gastrin, insulin, VIP, or glucagon. Overall, patients with familial MEN-1 neoplasms have long survival, which is significantly better than that for patients with sporadic endocrine pancreatic tumors.[17]

The surgical treatment of the MEN-1 syndrome is dependent on the phenotypic expression in the individual patient. Because components of the syndrome may be metachronous, surgical procedures involving different endocrine organs may be required over a period of many years. Regardless of initial findings, MEN-1 patients must be followed for life for involvement of the pituitary gland, parathyroid glands, endocrine pancreas or duodenum, adrenal glands, thymus, and lungs (bronchial carcinoids).

A lack of predictable genotype-phenotype relationships does not permit preventative surgery and requires a broad sweep of follow-up tests for affected family members. Brandi and colleagues include one of several consensus positions on screening of suspected and confirmed *MEN-1* mutation carriers that include both biochemical and imaging tests.[91] With improved medical management of hypercalcemia and peptic ulcers, more than 30% of MEN-1 patients can be managed successfully for years and now die at later ages of malignancies related to MEN-1.[229,230] The timing (childhood vs adult) and type of operation (total vs partial parathyroidectomy) for prevention of HPT remains controversial, balancing risk of recurrence with adverse effect of possible lifelong hypoparathyroidism.

Table 78-9 Classification of MEN-2 Syndromes

	Percent of MEN-2 Cases	MTC	Pheo	Parathyroid Hyperplasia/Adenoma
MEN-2A	60–90%	95%	50%	20–30%
MEN-2B	5%	100%	50%	Uncommon
FMTC	5–35%	100%	0%	0%

FMTC = familial medullary thyroid carcinoma; MTC = medullary thyroid carcinoma; Pheo = pheochromocytoma.
Data from Hansford JR and Mulligan LM[231]; Ponder BA[232]; Weisner GL and Snow-Bailey K.[253]

MEN-2 Syndromes The MEN-2 syndromes represent several distinct clusters of neuroendocrine tumors with strong association between specific gene mutations of the RET proto-oncogene and phenotype, permitting preventative surgery and focused follow-up and screening of patients and families for specific "at-risk" tumors. MEN-2 has two distinct subtypes, MEN-2A and MEN-2B, and most would also include familial medullary thyroid carcinoma (FMTC) as a MEN-2 syndrome as well (Table 78-9). The syndromes were first recognized by clinical patterns of tumor involvement[218] and later shown to be caused by specific mutations in the RET oncogene. MEN-2A patients as a group are characterized by medullary thyroid carcinoma in 95%, pheochromocytoma(s) in 50%, and hyperplasia/adenoma of the parathyroid glands in 15 to 30% of cases.[230] MEN-2B patients have medullary thyroid carcinoma in 100%, pheochromocytoma(s) in 50%, and varied reported incidences of mucosal neuromas and marfanoid body habitus.[231,232] Both MEN-2 syndromes have defined germline mutations in the RET proto-oncogene, a transmembrane receptor tyrosine kinase. Over 95% of the RET mutations in MEN-2A reported to date involve exons 10 and 11, corresponding to the cysteine-rich extracellular domain of the receptor.[233] About 90% of FMTC have identified RET mutations, including some overlap with mutations at specific codons seen in MEN-2A. Almost every case of MEN-2B reported has the same missense mutation at codon 918 in exon 16, corresponding to the intracellular domain of the receptor.[234] All MEN-2 syndromes have been classified by the American Society of Clinical Oncology policy as Group 1—"a well-defined hereditary cancer syndrome for which genetic testing is considered part of the standard management for at-risk family members,"[235] and the recommendation is to offer genetic counseling and RET gene studies to all affected MEN-2 cases and their at-risk kindred.

Medullary Thyroid Carcinoma Medullary thyroid carcinomas are derived from the thyroid C-cells and are preceded and accompanied by pathologic findings of C-cell hyperplasia (Figure 78-6). C-cell hyperplasia (CCH) is also seen in 5% of the normal population, and therefore can confuse the screening and evaluation of MEN patients.[236]

MTC represents about 5 to 10% of new cases of thyroid cancers, or about 1,000 cases per year in the United States. Of these, about 75% have no family history of MTC (sporadic MTC) and are generally diagnosed around the age of 50 to 60 years.[237] All MEN patients are at high risk of medullary thyroid carcinoma (see Table 78-9). MEN-2A patients often present with MTC before pheochromocytoma or parathyroid disease. In known MEN-2A families, biochemical evidence of early MTC usually occurs between the ages of 5 and 25 years.[238] The MEN-2B patients have an earlier age of onset of cancers, and a more aggressive phenotype of medullary thyroid carcinoma leading to a worse prognosis compared with MEN-2A patients.[239,240] Fortunately, some of these children are recognized prior to the diagnosis of MTC based on the marfanoid body habitus and mucosal neuromas.[241]

MTC and CCH are suspected in the presence of elevated serum calcitonin levels, a sensitive and specific marker for both conditions. In patients at risk, confirmed MTC cases after treatment or MEN-2 family members, the more sensitive calcitonin stimulation test can be performed where calcitonin levels are drawn before and 5 minutes following a calcium infusion. A calcitonin increase threefold greater than baseline, or above a value of 300 ng/L is considered positive.[238] Both MTC and CCH can result in a positive calcitonin stimulation test, and not all cases of CCH will progress to MTC.[236,238] Patients not identified by early screening, about 30% of MTC patients, will present with a (painful) neck mass, and/or diarrhea associated with high calcitonin levels. Unfortunately most of these patients already have local or distant spread of their tumors.[237,242]

Treatment of MTC involves total thyroidectomy and lymph node dissection in almost all cases, with autotransplantation of parathyroid tissue if possible, followed by lifelong thyroid replacement. Of these patients, approximately 50% will develop recurrent disease,[243] so it is recommended that they be screened with a yearly calcitonin stimulation test. Recent data suggest that FDG-PET might be particularly sensitive in detection of MTC metastases.[244] Chemotherapy and radiation therapy have generally been found to result in few responses.[245] Prophylactic thyroidectomy (and autotransplant of parathyroid tissue) is accepted therapy for all patients with documented RET germline mutations. The timing of the surgery, still controversial, can in fact be guided by the specific RET codon affected.[91]

Familial Medullary Thyroid Carcinoma The designation of FMTC, as opposed to MEN-2A, MEN-2B, and sporadic MTC, is defined as

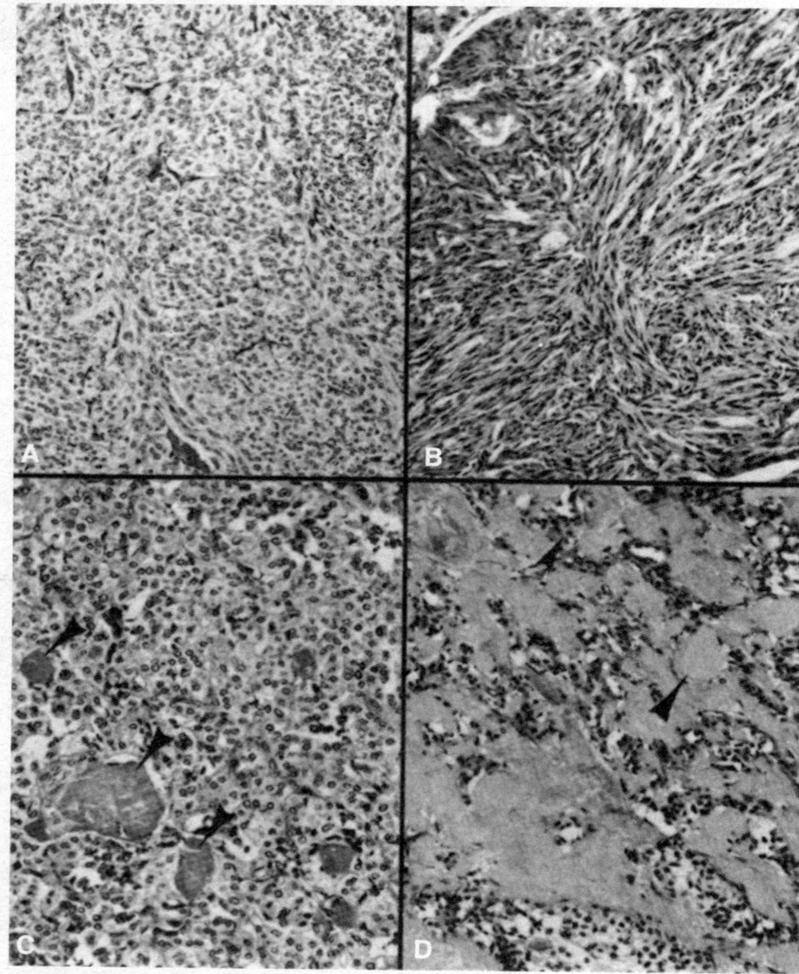

Figure 78-6 Histologic features of medullary thyroid cancer. **A,** Nests of polygonal cells. **B,** Spindle-shaped cells. **C,** Amyloid deposits (*arrows*). **D,** Large amount of fibrous stroma with sparse cells and amyloid nodules (*arrows*).

families with four or more cases of MTC in the absence of a diagnosis of pheochromocytoma or parathyroid hyperplasia/adenoma.[246] Of these cases, almost 90% will be found to have an identifiable RET mutation.[247] It is recommended that all FMTC cases undergo regular screening tests for pheochromocytoma, and parathyroid disease given that some families are later classified as MEN-2A or B.[248] The therapy for FMTC is the same as for MTC in association with MEN-2A, MEN-2B.

Pheochromocytoma Pheochromocytomas arise in the chromaffin cells of the adrenal medulla (Figure 78-7). Paragangliomas arise from tissue of the sympathetic and parasympathetic nervous system. Paragangliomas of the sympathetic nervous system, often called extra-adrenal pheochromocytomas, are most often located in the retroperitoneum. Paragangliomas of the parasympathetic nervous system are often located in the region of the aortic arch, neck, and base of skull (ie, carotid body paragangliomas).[249] Pheochromocytomas are rare. Mayo Clinic data estimate that approximately 800 cases of pheochromocytoma are diagnosed in the US each year.[250] They are found in approximately 0.1 to 0.5% of hypertensive patients.[251]

Clinical Features and Diagnosis Discussions of the diagnosis and management of pheochromocytoma often consider the "rough rule of tens": 10% of neoplasms occur in children, 10% of sporadic cases are bilateral, 10% are extra-adrenal, and 10% are malignant. Previously, this rule included that 10% of pheochromocytomas were familial, but Neumann and colleagues[252] reported on 271 patients without personal or family history of associated endocrine neoplasia, and found that 24% of the screened patients had germline mutations for one of the four susceptibility genes for this disease: *VHL*, *RET*, *SDHD*, or *SDHB*. Overall, including familial and apparent sporadic tumors, about 30% of all pheochromocytoma cases are now thought to have an identifiable germline mutation, leaving over 60% as sporadic tumors. It is now recommended that genetic counseling, and possible gene studies, be considered for all patients diagnosed with pheochromocytoma, particularly those diagnosed under age 50 years with a family history or multifocal disease where the *a priori* risk of identifying a mutation clearly exceeds 10%.[253,254] The documentation of a germline mutation impacts on the medical management of both the patient and family.

Patients may present anywhere in the spectrum from normotensive and asymptomatic to a severe, life-threatening hypertensive crisis.[255] In clinically diagnosed patients, hypertension can be either sustained or episodic, and each occurs in approximately half of patients with pheochromocytoma. Five percent are normotensive. The most common symptoms are headache, sweating, and palpitation; each occurs in about 60% of patients. Almost all patients have at least one or two of these three symptoms.

The fundamental basis for the diagnosis of pheochromocytoma is a high index of clinical suspicion with confirmation by biochemical determinations for catecholamines or catecholamine metabolites in blood or urine. Lenders and colleagues[18] have shown plasma metanephrines to be the single best test for the diagnosis of pheochromocytoma. However, not all laboratories provide plasma metanephrine assays, and one can rely on the more widely available measurements of 24-hour urinary excretion for catecholamines, metanephrines, or vanillylmandelic acid (VMA) (Figure 78-8).[18] In patients with borderline results, a clonidine suppression test can be performed. Plasma catecholamines are sampled before and 3 hours after an oral dose of 0.3 mg of clonidine, and results show that plasma catecholamines will fall below 500 pg/mL in patients with essential hypertension, but not in patients with pheochromocytoma.[256]

CT scanning, as well as MRI, can visualize over 90% of adrenal pheochromocytomas in patients with biochemical evidence of a pheochromocytoma.[257,258] Methyliodobenzylguanidine (MIBG) is a structural analogue of guanethidine and is taken up and stored in secretory granules of the chromaffin cells.[259] ^{131}I-MIBG scans have been shown to have a sensitivity of 87% and a specificity of 97%.[260,261] All patients should have an MIBG scan to confirm that the tumor seen on CT scan/MRI is a pheochromocytoma (Figure 78-9). Because of the risk of catastrophic hemorrhage or hypertensive complications, fine-needle aspiration should not be attempted for cytologic diagnosis.

Surgical Management of Benign or Recurrent Resectable Disease Nearly all benign pheochromocytomas can be cured by surgical resection. Because of its slow growth rate and accompanying significant morbidity, complete resection of local recurrence or limited metastases of malignant pheochromocytoma should be attempted. The value of debulking surgery for patients whose tumor cannot be completely resected is not established, but reports of successful control of symptoms following surgery continue to be reported.[262] The median time for recurrence following primary resection of malignant pheochromocytoma is approximately 6 years and may be as long as 20 years.[17]

Medical Treatment of Recurrent or Metastatic Disease Malignant pheochromocytoma is a rare entity among malignant diseases, with best estimates that about 5 to 25% of all pheochromocytomas are malignant.[263] A review of SEER data for 1973 to 1985 suggests that the yearly age-adjusted rate of malignant pheochromocytoma is

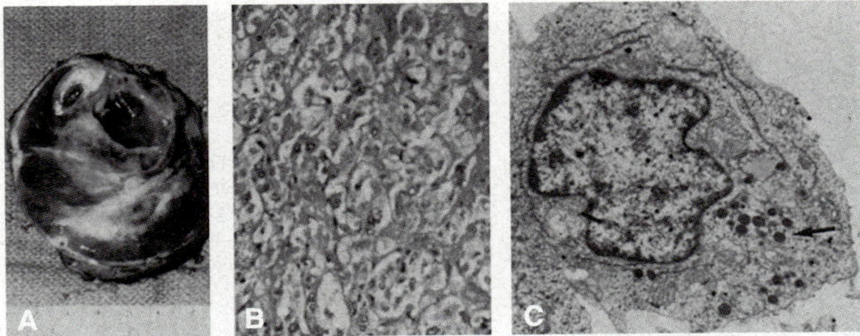

Figure 78-7 Pheochromocytoma. **A,** Gross appearance of a surgically removed hemisected extra-adrenal pheochromocytoma. **B,** Histopathologic appearance of a pheochromocytoma showing typical cords of glandular cells separated by bands of stroma (hematoxylin and eosin, 25 ×). **C.** Ultrastructural appearance of a single pheochromocytoma cell showing dense neurosecretory granules (*arrow*) (6,000 ×).

0.04 per 100,000 population or approximately 100 cases per year in the United States.

The diagnosis of malignant pheochromocytoma can be made only when the tumor is locally invasive and unresectable, recurs after primary extirpation, or is found to be metastatic. Although the natural history of the disease in each of these situations may be variable and somewhat unpredictable, advanced malignant pheochromocytoma is associated with a high morbidity and mortality. The limited data suggest a significant number of patients with disseminated disease may live for long periods without specific antineoplastic therapy.[264]

Targeted radiotherapy using high specific activity MIBG has been evaluated in several small studies, and overall it was found that the majority of patients with malignant pheochromocytoma do not take up and retain sufficient MIBG to deliver an effective radiation dose to the tumor. There is a symptomatic improvement in about 75% of patients, an objective tumor response in about 20%, with few complete responses, and recurrence of symptoms and progression of disease of most cases.[265]

The CVD (cyclophosphamide, vincristine, and dacarbazine) regimen that is effective in children with advanced neuroblastoma was adapted for use in malignant pheochromocytoma. In a study by

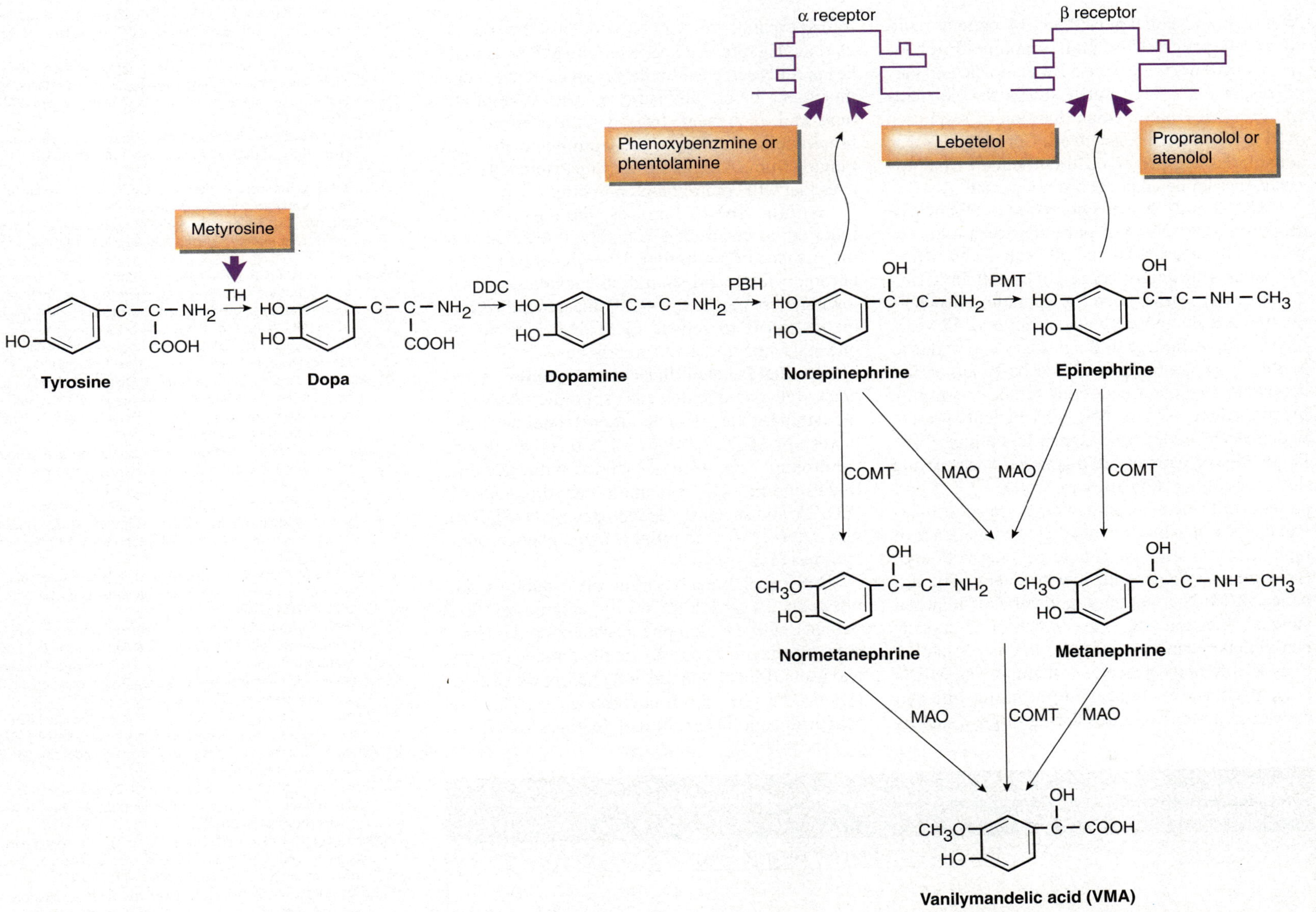

α receptor
β receptor
Phenoxybenzmine or phentolamine
Lebetelol
Propranolol or atenolol
Metyrosine
TH
DDC
PBH
PMT
Tyrosine
Dopa
Dopamine
Norepinephrine
Epinephrine
COMT
MAO
MAO
COMT
Normetanephrine
Metanephrine
MAO
COMT
MAO
Vanilymandelic acid (VMA)

Figure 78-8 Synthetic and metabolic pathways for the catecholamines, norepinephrine and epinephrine, which are stored and secreted by chromaffin cells and pheochromocytomas. *Curved arrows*, physiologic agonist–receptor interaction. *Boxed arrows*, competitive antagonism at the rate-limiting step of synthesis or at receptor sites by therapeutic agents (see text). TH = trosine hydroxylase; DDC = dopa decarboxylase; PBH = phenylamine-β-hydroxylase; PMT = phenylethanolamine-*N*-methyltransferase; COMT = catechol-*O*-methyltransferase; MAO = monoamine oxidase.

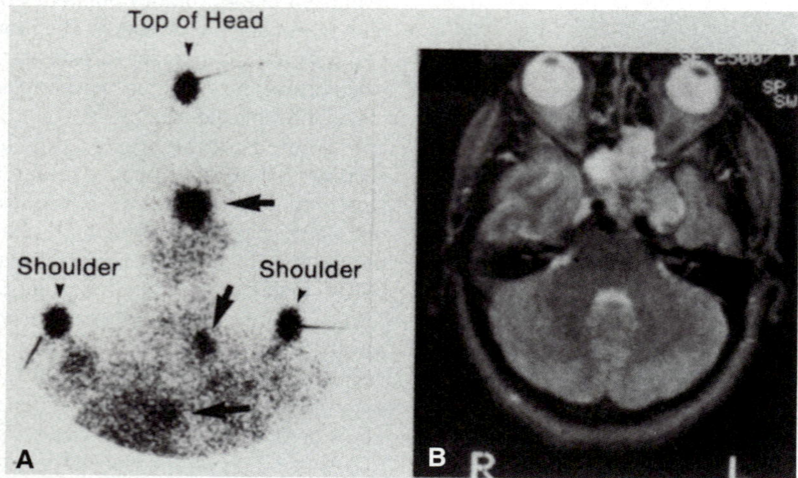

Figure 78-9 Diagnostic imaging in metastatic pheochromocytoma. **A,** Gamma camera image of the upper body of a patient 48 hours following injection of ^{131}I-metaiodobenzylguanidine. Areas of abnormal isotope uptake are noted at the base of the brain, the cervical region, and the mid-thoracic spine (*arrows*). **B,** T_2-weighted magnetic resonance image of the same patient demonstrating a signal-intensive mass encroaching the circle of Willis, the left temporal lobe, and the left optic nerve.

Averbuch and colleagues[266] of 14 patients with advanced, progressive, and symptomatic pheochromocytoma, there were 57% complete and partial responses, 79% complete and partial biochemical responses, and median duration of responses of 21 to 22 months, respectively. Currently, CVD is considered the preferred treatment of symptomatic, disseminated pheochromocytoma.

MEN-2 and Pheochromocytoma Pheochromocytomas in MEN-2 patients are diagnosed between the ages of 20 and 30 years (with MEN-2B patients generally being younger than MEN-2A patients), earlier than the sporadic pheochromocytomas diagnosed between 35 and 45 years old.[267] The earlier age of diagnosis is in part due to MEN-2 patients being screened based on earlier diagnosis of another endocrine tumor or a family history. About 25% of MEN-2A patients present with pheochromocytoma as their first tumor.[268,269] Up to 75% of patients are diagnosed concurrently with medullary thyroid carcinoma.[267] MEN-2 patients with pheochromocytomas develop bilateral tumors and appear to have a lower incidence of malignant transformation than patients with sporadic tumors.[270] Given the low incidence of malignancy in MEN-2 patients, unilateral or bilateral subtotal resection with preservation of adrenocortical function can be considered in this population to avoid lifelong replacement therapy. The MEN-2A patients are often asymptomatic, but can develop hypertensive crises during surgery, such as for hyperparathyroidism or medullary thyroid carcinoma. Therefore, all patients with MEN-2 should be carefully screened for the presence of pheochromocytoma before any surgery or invasive procedure and, if present, treated with α-adrenergic blockade with phenoxybenzamine in dosages ranging from 10 mg twice daily up to tolerable dosages that will control blood pressure.

Within MEN-2 families, the specific RET mutation at codon 634 is highly associated with the presence or eventual development of pheochromocytoma and should be considered in following these patients. Overall, the general recommendation is to screen all MEN-2 patients for pheochromocytoma on a yearly basis.[253]

Familial Isolated Pheochromocytoma It has been well documented that sporadic pheochromocytoma (those without any personal or family history of MEN-2, NF-1, VHL or other genetic syndrome) have been associated with germline mutations in VHL, succinate dehydrogenase B (SDHB) and succinate dehydrogenase D (SDHD), now referred to as familial isolated pheochromocytomas (Table 78-10).

Between 0.1 and 6% of all NF-1 patients, and between 20 and 50% of hypertensive NF-1 patients, will develop pheochromocytoma. However, the diagnosis of NF-1 is often made on clinical grounds in childhood, long before the presentation of a pheochromocytoma in the third or fourth decade. The clinical features of NF-1–associated pheochromocytomas are similar to sporadic cases.[271]

Table 78-10 Germline Mutations Found in Selected Pheochromocytoma Patients without Personal or Family History Suggestive of MEN-2 (Sporadic Cases)

Gene	Number Patients Tested	Number Found to Have a Mutation	Percent with Mutation
VHL	157	9	6
SDHD	37	3	8
SDHB	24	1	4
RET	137	1	< 1
			Total 19

Modified from Bryant J et al.[275]

REFERENCES

1. For a definitive historical discussion on carcinoid tumors, the reader is encouraged to read: Modlin IM, Shapiro MD, Kidd M. Siegfried Oberndorfer: origins and perspectives of carcinoid tumors. Human Pathol 2004;35:1440–51.
2. Bayliss WM, Starling EH. The mechanism of pancreatic secretion. J Physiol 1902;28:325–53.
3. Bayliss WM, Starling EH. On the causation of the so-called peripheral reflex secretion of the pancreas. Proc R Soc Lond B Biol Sci 1902;69:352–3.
4. Pearse AGE. Common cytochemical and ultrastructural characteristics of cells producing polypeptide hormones (the APUD series) and their relevance to thyroid and ultimobranchial C cells and calcitonin. Proc R Soc Lond B Biol Sci 1968;170:71–80.
5. Pearse AGE. The cytochemistry and ultrastructure of polypeptide-hormone producing cells of the APUD series and the embryologic, physiologic and pathologic implications of the concept. J. Histochem Cytochem 1969;17:303–13.
6. Rehfeld JF. The new biology of gastrointestinal hormones. Physiol Rev 1998;78:1087–108.
7. Pictet RL, Rall LB, Phelps P, Rutter WJ. The neural crest and the origin of the insulin-producing and other gastrointestinal hormone-producing cells. Science 1976;191:191–2.
8. Andrew A, Kramer B, Rawdon BB. The origin of gut and pancreatic neuroendocrine (APUD) cells—the last word? J Pathol 1998;186:117–8.
9. Weidenmann B, John M, Ahnert-Hilger G, Riecken EO. Molecular and cell biological aspects of neuroendocrine tumors of the of the gastroenteropancreatic system. J Mol Med 1998;76:637–47.
10. Bishop AE, Power RF, Polak JM. Markers for neuroendocrine differentiation. Pathol Res Prac 1988;183:119–28.
11. Bissette G, Manberg P, Nemeroff CB, et al. Neurotensin, a biologically active peptide. Life Sci 1978;23:2173–82.
12. Blackburn AM, Bloom SR. A radioimmunoassay for neurotensin in human plasma. J Endocrinol 1979;83:175–81.
13. Sundler F, Alumets J, Hakanson R. Peptides in the gut with dual distribution in nerves and endocrine cells. In: Bloom SR, Polak JM, editors. Gut hormones. New York: Churchill-Livingston; 1981. p. 406–13.
14. Vinik AI, Strodel WE, Eckhauser FE, et al. Somatostatinomas, PPomas, neurotensinomas. Semin Oncol 1987;14:263–81.
15. Solcia E, Capella C, Fiooca R, et al. Disorders of the endocrine system. In: Ming SC, Goldman H, editors. Pathology of the gastrointestinal tract. Philadelphia: Williams & Wilkins; 1998. p. 295–322.
16. Rindi G, Leiter AB, Kopin AS, et al. The "normal" endocrine cell of the gut—changing concepts and new evidences. Ann NY Acad Sci 2004;1014;1–12.
17. Kvols LK. Neoplasms of the diffuse endocrine system. In: Kufe DW, Pollack RE, Weichselbaum RR, et al., editors. Cancer medicine. 6th ed. Hamilton (ON): BC Decker; 2003. p. 1288.
18. Lenders JW, Pacak K, Walther MM, et al. Biochemical diagnosis of pheochromocytoma: which test is best? JAMA 2002;287:1427–34.
19. Rindi G, Buffa R, Sessa F, et al. Chromogranin A, B, and C immunoreactivities of mammalian endocrine cells. Distribution, distinction from costored hormones/prohormones and relationship with the argyrophil component of secretory granules. Histochemistry 1986;85:19–28.
20. Wilander E, Lundquist M, Oberg K. Gastrointestinal carcinoid tumours. Prog Histochem Cytochem 1989;19:1–88.
21. Oberg K. Biochemical diagnosis of neuroendocrine GEP tumor. Yale J Biol Med 1997;70:501–8.
22. Tomassetti P, Migori M, Simoni P, et al. Diagnostic value of chromogranin A in neuroendocrine tumours. Eur J Gastroenterol Hepatol 2001;13:55–8.
23. Stridsberg M, Eriksson B, Oberg K, Janson ET. A comparison between three commercial kits for chromogranin A measurements. J Endocrinol 2003;177:337–41.
24. Srivastava A, Padilla O, Fischer-Colbrie R, et al. Neuroendocrine secretory protein-55 (NESP-55 expression discriminates pancreatic endocrine tumors and pheochromocytomas from gastrointestinal and pulmonary carcinoids. Am J Surg 2004;28:1371–8.
25. Jahn R, Schiebler W, Ouimet C, Greengard P. A 38,000-dalton membrane protein (p38) present in synaptic vesicles. Proc Natl Acad Sci U S A 1985;82;4137–41.

26. Weidenmann B, Franke WW, Kuhn C, et al. Synaptophysin: a marker protein for neuroendocrine cells and neoplasms. Proc Natl Acad Sci U S A 1986;83:3500–4.
27. Buffa R, Rindi G, Sessa F, et al. Synaptophysin immunoreactivity and small clear vesicles in neuroendocrine cells and related tumors. Mol Cell Probes 1988;2:367–81.
28. Erikson JD, Schafer MK, Bonner TI, et al. Distinct pharmacological properties and distribution in neurons and endocrine cells of two isoforms of the human vesicular monoamine transporter. Proc Natl Acad Sci USA 1996;93:5166–71.
29. Amara SG, Kuhar MJ. Neurotransmitter transporters: recent progress. Annu Rev Neurosci 1993;16:73–93.
30. Rindi G, Paolotti D, Fiocca R, et al. Vesicular monamine transporter 2 as a marker of gastric enterochromaffin-like cell tumors. Vichows Arch 2000;436;217–23.
31. Jakobsen AM, Andersson P, Saglik G, et al. Differential expression of vesicular monoamine transporter (VMAT) 1 and 2 in gastrointestinal endocrine tumors. J Pathol 2001;195:463–72.
32. Nilsson O, Jakobsen AM, Kolby L, et al. Importance of vesicle proteins in the diagnosis and treatment of neuroendocrine tumors. Ann NY Acad Sci 2004;1014:280–3.
33. Oberndorfer S. Karzinoid Tumoren des Dunndarms. Frankf Z Pathol 1907;1:426–32.
34. Masson P. Carcinoid (argentaffin-cell tumors) and nerve hyperplasia of the appendicular mucosal. Am J Pathol 1928;4:181–212.
35. Soga J, Tazawa K. Pathology analysis of carcinoids: histologic reevaluation of 62 cases. Cancer 1971;28:990–8.
36. Williams ED, Sandler M. The classification of carcinoid tumors. Lancet 1963;1:238–9.
37. Kloppel G, Heitz PU, Capella C, et al. The spectrum and the classification of gastric and duodenal neuroendocrine tumours. Curr Diag Pathol 1995;2:10–4.
38. Kloppel G, Perren A, Heitz PU. The gastroenteropancreatic neuroendocrine cell system and its tumors: the WHO classification. Ann NY Acad Sci 2004;1014:13–27.
39. Solcia E, Kloppel G, Sobin LH, et al. Histologic typing of endocrine tumours. 2nd ed. WHO International Classification of Tumours. Berlin: Springer-Verlag; 2000.
40. Rindi G, Azzoni C, LaRosa S, et al. ECL tumor and poorly differentiated endocrine carcinoma of the stomach: prognostic evaluation by pathological analysis. Gastroenterology 1999;116:532–42.
41. Wynick D, Williams SJ, Bloom RS. Symptomatic secondary hormone syndromes in patients with established malignant pancreatic endocrine tumors. N Engl J Med 1988;319:605–7.
42. Patel Y. Somatostatin and its receptor family. Front Neuroendrinol 1999;20:157–98.
43. Reisine T, Bell GI. Molecular biology of somatostatin receptors. Endocr Rev 1995;16;427–42.
44. Hoyer D, Bell GI, Berelowitz M, et al. Classification and nomenclature of somatostatin receptors. Trends Pharmacol Sci 1995;16:86–8.
45. Patel YC, Greenwood MT, Warszynska A, et al. All five cloned human somatostatin receptors (hSTTR1-5) are functionally coupled to adenyl cyclase. Biochem Biophys Res Comm 1994;198:605–12.
46. Lamberts SW, van der Lely AJ, de Herder WW, et al. Octreotide. N Engl J Med 1996;334:246–54.
47. Bousquest C, Puente E, Buscali L, et al. Antiproliferative effect of somatostatin and analogs. Chemotherapy 2001;4 suppl 2: 30–9.
48. Reubi JC, Krenning E, Lamberts SW, Kvols L. *In vitro* detection of somatostatin receptors in human tumors. Metabolism 1992;41:104–10.
49. Reubi JC, Laissue J, Krenning E, Lamberts SW. Somatostatin receptors in human cancer: incidence, characteristics, functional correlates and clinical implications. J Steroid Biochem Mol Biol 1992;43:27–35.
50. Reubi JC, Laissue J, Waser B, et al. Expression of somatostatin receptors in normal, inflamed, and neoplastic human gastrointestinal tissues. Ann NY Acad Sci 1994;733:122–37.
51. Reubi JC, Schaer JC, Laissue JA, Waser B. Somatostatin receptors and their subtypes in human tumors and in peritumoral vessels. Metabolism 1996;45:49–1.
52. Ruebi JC, Waser B, Schaer JC, Laissue JA. Somatostatin receptor sst1-sst5 expression in normal and neoplastic human tissues using receptor autoradiography with subtype—selective ligands. Eur J Nuc Med 2001;28:836–46.
53. Hofland LJ, Liu Q, van Koetsveld PM, et al. Immunohistochemical detection of somatostatin receptor subtypes sst1 and sst2A in human somatostatin receptor positive tumors. J Clin Endo Metabol 1999;84:775–80.
54. Kimura N, Pilichowska M, Date F, et al. Immunohistochemical expression of somatostatin type 2A receptor in neuroendocrine tumors. Clin Can Res 1999;5:3483–7.
55. Papotti M, Boggiovanni M, Volante M, et al. Expression of somatostatin receptor subtype 1-5 in 81 cases of gastrointestinal and pancreatic endocrine tumors. A correlative immunohistochemical and reverse-transcriptase polymerase chain reaction analysis. Virchows Archiv 2002;440:461–75.
56. Kulaksiz H, Eissele R, Rossler D, et al. Identification of somatostatin receptor subtypes 1, 2A, 3, and 5 in neuroendocrine tumours with subtype specific antibodies. Gut 2002;50:52–60.
57. National Comprehensive Cancer Network Web site: Neuroendocrine tumors: http://www.nccn.org/professionals/physician_gls/PDF/neuroendocrine.pdf (accessed June 22, 2005).
58. Buchanan KD, Johnston CF, O'Hare MMT, et al. Neuroendocrine tumors. A European view. Am J Med 1986;81 suppl 6b:14–22.
59. Modlin IM, Lye KD, Kidd M. A 5-decade analysis of 13,715 carcinoid tumors. Cancer 2003;97:936–59.
60. Modlin IM, Sandor A. An analysis of 8305 cases of carcinoid tumors. Cancer 1997;79:813–29.
61. Godwin J. Carcinoid tumors, an analysis of 2837 cases. Cancer 1975;36:560–9.
62. Newton JN, Swerdlow AJ, dos Santos Silav IM, et al. The epidemiology of carcinoid tumours in England and Scotland. Br J Cancer 1994;70:939–42.
63. Lu Cortez L, Clemente C, Puig V, Mirarda A. Carcinoid tumor. An analysis of 131 cases. Rev Clin Esp 1994;194:291–3.
64. Soga J. Carcinoids of the small intestine: statistical evaluation of 1102 cases collected from the literature. J Exp Clin Cancer Res 1997;16:353–63.
65. Moertel CG, Sauer WG, Docherty MB, Baggenstoss AH. Life history of the carcinoid tumor of the small intestine. Cancer 1961;14:291–3.
66. Berge T, Linell F. Carcinoid tumours. Frequency in a defined population during a 12-year period. Acta Pathol Microbiol Scand [A] 1976;84:322–30.
67. Kimura W, Kuroada A, Morioka Y. Clinical pathology of endocrine tumors of the pancreas. Analysis of autopsy cases. Digest Dis Sci 1991;36:933–42.
68. Keshishian A, Hamilton J, Hwang L, Petrosyan M. Carcinoid tumor and bariatric surgery. Obes Surg 2002;12:874–5.
69. ENETS Web site: http://www.neuroendocrine.net/rel/index.php4 (accessed June 22, 2005).
70. Ricke J, Klose K-J, Mignon M, et al. Standardization of imaging in neuroendocrine tumours: results of a European Delphi process. Eur J Radiol 2001;37:8–17.
71. Gibril F, Jensen RT. Diagnostic uses of radiolabeled somatostatin receptor analogues in gastroenteropancreatic endocrine tumors. Dig Liver Dis 2004;36(S1):106–20.
72. Kwekkeboom D, Krenning EP, de Jong M. Peptide receptor imaging and therapy. J Nucl Med 2000;41:1704–13.
73. Termanini B, Gabril F, Reynolds JC, et al. Value of somatostatin receptor scintigraphy: a prospective study in gastrinoma of its effect on clinical management. Gastroenterology 1997;112:335–47.
74. Gould M, Johnson RJ. Computed tomography of abdominal carcinoid tumor. Br J Radiol 1986;59:881–5.
75. Sugimoto E, Lorelius LE, Eriksson B, Oberg K. Midgut carcinoid tumors: CT appearance. Acta Radiol 1995;36:367–71.
76. Kressel HY, Strategies for magnetic resonance imaging of focal liver disease. Radiol Clin North Am 1988;26:607–15.
77. Eriksson B, Bergstrom M, Lilja A, et al. Positron emission tomography (PET) in neuroendocrine gastrointestinal tumours. Acta Oncologia 1993;32:303–13.
78. Fischer M, Kamanabroo D, Sonderkamp H, Proske T. Scintigraphic imaging of carcinoid tumors with I-131-metaiodobenzylguanidine. Lancet 1984;2:165.
79. Hoefnagel CA, den Hartog Jager FC, Taal BG, et al. The role of I-131-MIBG in the diagnosis and therapy of carcinoids. Eur J Nuc Med 1987;13:187–91.
80. Krenning EP, Bakker WH, Breeman WA, et al. Localization of endocrine-related tumours with radio-iodinated analogue of somatostatin. Lancet 1989;i:242–4.
81. Krenning EP, Kwekkeboom DJ, Bakker WH, et al. Somatostatin receptor scintigraphy with [111In-DTPA-D-Phe1]- and [123I-tyr3]-octreotide: the Rotterdam experience with more than 1000 patients. Eur J Nucl Med 1993;20:716–31.
82. Krenning EP, Kwekkeboom DJ, Pauwels S, et al. Somatostatin receptor scintigraphy. In: Freeman LM, editor. Nuclear medicine annual. New York: Raven Press; 1995. p. 1–50.
83. Modlin IM, Shapiro MD, Kidd M. An analysis of rare carcinoid tumors: clarifying these clinical conundrums. World J Surg 2005;29:92–101.
84. Kulke MH, Mayer RJ. Carcinoid tumors. N Engl J Med 1999;340:858–68.
85. Modlin IM, Shapiro MD, Kidd M. Carcinoid tumors and fibrosis: an association with no explanation. Am J Gastroenterol 2004;99:2466–78.
86. Moertel CG. Treatment of the carcinoid tumor and the malignant carcinoid syndrome. J Clin Oncol 1983;1:727–40.
87. Carney JA, Go VLW, Fairbanks VF, et al. The syndrome of gastric argyrophil carcinoid tumors and nonantral gastric atrophy. Ann Intern Med 1983;99:761–6.
88. Modlin IM, Tang LH. The gastric enterochromaffin-like cell: an enigmatic cellular link. Gastroenterology 1996;111:783–810.
89. Modlin IM, Sandor A, Tang LH, et al. A 40-year analysis of 265 gastric carcinoids. Am J Gastroenterol 1997;92:633–8.
90. Sundler F. Pathogenesis and diagnosis of enterochromaffin-like cell tumors. Ann NY Acad Sci 1994;733:24–35.
91. Brandi ML, Gagel RF, Angeli A, et al. CONSENSUS: Guidelines for diagnosis and therapy of MEN type 1 and type 2. J Clin Endo Metab 2001;86:5658–71.
92. Chugthai TS, Morin JE, Sheiner NM, et al. Bronchial carcinoid—twenty years' experience defines a selective surgical approach. Surgery 1997;122:801–8.
93. Nuttall KL, Pingree SS. The incidence of elevations in urine 5-hydroxyindoleacetic acid. Ann Clin Lab Sci 1998;28:167–74.
94. Feldman J, Lee E. Serotonin content of foods: effect on urinary excretion of 5-hydroxyindoacetic acid. Am J Clin Nutr 1985;42:639–43.
95. Stridberg M, Oberg K, Li Q, et al. Measurements of chromogranin A, chromogranin B (secretogranin I), chromogranin C (secretogranin II) and pancreastatin in plasma and urine from patients with carcinoid tumours and endocrine tumours. J Endocrinol 1995;144:49–59.
96. Soga J, Yakuwa Y, Osaka M. Carcinoid syndrome: a statistical evaluation of 748 reported cases. J Exp Clin Cancer Res 1999;18:133–41.
97. Lundin L, Norheim I, Landelius J, et al. Carcinoid heart disease: relationship of circulating vasoactive substances to ultrasound-detectable cardiac abnormalities. Circulation 1988;77:264–9.
98. Anderson AS, Krauss D, Lang R. Cardiovascular complications of malignant carcinoid disease. Am Heart J 1997;134:693–702.
99. Simula DV, Edwards WD, Tazelaar HD, et al. Surgical pathology of carcinoid heart disease: a study of 139 values from 75 patients spanning over 20 years. Mayo Clin Proc 2002;77:139–47.
100. Connolly HM, Nishimura RA, Smith HC, et al. Outcome of cardiac surgery for carcinoid heart disease. J Am Coll Cardiol 1995;25:410–6.
101. Moller JE, Connolly HM, Rubin J, et al. Factors associated with progression of carcinoid heart disease. N Engl J Med 2003;348:1005–15.
102. Rajamannan NM, Caplice N, Anthikad F, et al. Cell proliferation in carcinoid valve disease: a mechanism for serotonin effects. J Heart Valve Dis 2001;10:827–31.
103. Connolly HM, Crary JL, McGoon MD, et al. Valvular heart disease associated with fenfluramine-phentermine [published erratum appears in N Engl J Med 1997;337:1783]. N Engl J Med 1997;337:581–8.
104. Pellikka PA, Tajik AJ, Khandheria BK, et al. Carcinoid heart disease: clinical and echocardiographic spectrum in 74 patients. Circulation 1993;87:1188–96.
105. Jensen RT. Endocrine tumors of the pancreas. In: Yamada T, editor. Textbook of gastroenterology. New York: Lippincott Williams & Wilkins; 2003.
106. Kloppel G, Schroder S, Heitz PU. Histopathology and immunopathology of pancreatic tumors. In: Mignon M, Jensen RT, editors. Endocrine tumors of the pancreas: recent advances in research and management. Basel, Switzerland: S. Krager; 1995. p. 120.
107. Kimura W, Kuroda A, Morioka Y. Clinical pathology of endocrine tumors of the pancreas. Analysis of autopsy cases. Dig Dis Sci 1991;36:933–42.
108. Eriksson B, Oberg K. PPomas and nonfunctioning endocrine pancreatic tumors: clinical presentation, diagnosis, and advances in management. In: Mignon M, Jensen RT, editors. Endocrine tumors of the pancreas: recent advances in research and management. Basel, Switzerland: S. Karger; 1995. p. 120.
109. Hochwald SN, Conlon KC, Brennan MF. Nonfunctional pancreatic islet cell tumors. In: Doherty GM, Skogseid B,

editors. Surgical endocrinology. Philadelphia: Lippincott Williams and Wilkins; 2001. p. 361.
110. Zollinger RM, Ellison EH. Primary peptic ulceration of the jejunum associated with islet cell tumors of the pancreas. Ann Surg 1955;142;709–23.
111. Gregory RA, Tracy JH, Agarwal KL. Amino acid constitution of the two gastrins isolated from Zollinger-Ellison tumor tissue. Gut 1969;10:603–8.
112. Roy PK, Venzon DJ, Shojamansesh H, et al. Zollinger-Ellison syndrome. Clinical presentation in 261 patients. Medicine (Baltimore) 2000;79:379–411.
113. Hochwald SN, Zee S, Conlon KC, et al. Prognostic factors in pancreatic endocrine neoplasms: an analysis of 136 cases with a proposal for low-grade and intermediate-grade groups. J Clin Oncol 2002;20:2633–42.
114. Weber HC, Venzon DJ, Fishbein VA, et al. Determinants of metastatic rate and survival in patients with Zollinger-Ellison syndrome (ZES): a prospective long-term study. Gastroenterology 1995;108:1637–49.
115. Roy PK, Venzon DJ, Feigenbaum KM, et al. Gastric secretion in Zollinger-Ellison syndrome. Correlation with clinical expression, tumor extent and role in diagnosis—a prospective NIH study of 235 patients and a review of 984 cases in the literature. Medicine (Baltimore) 2001;80:189–222.
116. Jensen RT. Zollinger-Ellison syndrome. In: Doherty GM, Skogseid B, editors. Surgical endocrinology: clinical syndromes. Philadelphia: Lippincott Williams & Wilkins; 2001. p. 291.
117. Gibril F, Reynolds JC, Doppman JL, et al. Somatostatin receptor scintigraphy: its sensitivity compared with that of other imaging methods in detecting primary and metastatic gastrinomas. Ann Intern Med 1996;125:26–34.
118. Termanini B, Gibril F, Reynolds JC, et al. Value of somatostatin receptor scintigraphy: a prospective study in gastrinoma of its effect on clinical management. Gastroenterology 1997;112:335–47.
119. Norton JA, Fraker DL, Alexander HR, et al. Surgery to cure the Zollinger-Ellison syndrome. N Engl J Med 1999;341:635–44.
120. Yu F, Venzon DJ, Serrano J, et al. Prospective study of the clinical course, prognostic factors, causes of death, and survival in patients with long-standing Zollinger-Ellison syndrome. J Clin Oncol 1999;17:615–30.
121. Soga J, Yakuwa Y. The gastrinoma/Zollinger-Ellison syndrome: statistical evaluation of a Japanese series of 359 cases. J Hepatobiliary Pancreat Surg 1998;5:77–85.
122. Fraker, DL, Norton JA, Alexander HR, et al. Surgery in Zollinger-Ellison syndrome alters the natural history of gastrinoma. Ann Surg 1994;220:320–8.
123. Metz DC, Strader DB, Orbuch M, et al. Use of omeprazole in Zollinger-Ellison: a prospective nine-year study of efficacy and safety. Alimnet Pharmacol Ther 1993;7:597–610.
124. Moertel CG, Hanley JA, Johnson LA. Streptozotocin alone compared with streptozotocin plus fluorouracil in the treatment of advanced islet-cell carcinoma. N Engl J Med 1980;303:1189–94.
125. Moertel CG, Lefkopoulo M, Lipsitz S, et al. Streptozotocin-doxorubicin, streptozotocin-fluorouracil, or chlorozotocin in the treatment of advanced islet cell carcinoma. N Engl J Med 1992;326;519–23.
126. Moertel CG, Kvols LK, O'Connell, Rubin J. Treatment of neuroendocrine carcinomas with combined etoposide and cisplatin. Cancer 1991;70 suppl 5:68–71.
127. Sutliff VE, Doppman JL, Gibril F, et al. Growth of newly diagnosed, untreated metastatic gastrinomas and predictors of growth patterns. J Clin Oncol 1997;15:2420–31.
128. Shojamanesh H, Gibril F, Louie A, et al. Prospective study of the antitumor efficacy of long-term octreotide treatment in patients with progressive metastatic gastrinoma. Cancer 2002;94:331–43.
129. Wallace S, Ajani JA, Charnsangavej C, et al. Carcinoid tumours: imaging procedures and interventional radiology. World J Surg 1989;20:147–56.
130. Whipple AO. The surgical therapy of hyperinsulinism. J Int Chir 1938;3:237.
131. Grant CS. Insulinoma. Surg Oncol Clin North Am 1998;7:819–44.
132. Marx S, Spiegel AM, Skarulis MC, et al. Multiple endocrine neoplasia type 1: clinical and genetic topics. Ann Intern Med 1998;129:484–94.
133. Hirshberg B, Livi A, Bartlett DL, et al. Forty-eight hour fast: the diagnostic test for insulinoma. J Clin Endocrinol Metab 2000;85:3222–6.
134. Hashimoto LA, Walsh RM. Preoperative localization of insulinomas is not necessary. J Am Coll Surg 1999;189:368–73.
135. Anderson MA, Carpenter S, Thompson NW, et al. Endoscopic ultrasound is highly accurate and directs management in patients with neuroendocrine tumors of the pancreas. Am J Gastroenterol 2000;95:2271–7.
136. Grama D, Skogseid B, Wilander E, et al. Pancreatic tumors in multiple endocrine neoplasia type I: clinical presentation and surgical treatment. World J Surg 1992;16:611–9.
137. Brown CK, Bartlett DL, Doppman JL, et al. Intraarterial calcium stimulation and intraoperative ultrasonography in the localization and resection of insulinomas. Surgery 1997;122:1189–93.
138. Jensen RT, Norton JA. Pancreatic endocrine tumors. In: Feldman M, Friedman L, Sleisenger MH, editors. Gastrointestinal and liver disease: pathophysiology, diagnosis, and management. Philadelphia: W.B. Saunders; 2002, p. 988.
139. Arnold R, Wied M, Behr TH. Somatostatin analogues in the treatment of endocrine tumors of the gastrointestinal tract. Expert Opin Pharmacother 2002;3:643–56.
140. Verner JV, Morrison AB. Islet cell tumor and a syndrome of refractory watery diarrhea and hypokalemia. Am J Med 1958;25:374–89.
141. Verner JV, Morrison AB. Endocrine pancreatic disease with diarrhea: report of a case due to diffuse hyperplasia of non-beta islet tissue with a review of 54 additional cases. Arch Intern Med 1974;133:492–9.
142. Levy-Bohbot M, Merle C, Goudet P, et al. Prevalence, characteristics and prognosis of MEN-1-associated glucagonomas, VIPomas, and Somatostatinomas: study from the GTE (Groupe des Tumeurs Endocrines) registry. Gastroenterol Clin Biol 2004;28:1075–81.
143. Matuchansky C, Rambuad JC. VIPomas and endocrine cholera: clinical presentation, diagnosis, and advances in management. In: Mignon M, Jensen RT, editors. Endocrine tumors of the pancreas: recent advances in research and management. Basel, Switzerland: S. Krager; 1995.
144. Long RG, Bryant MG, Mitchell SJ, et al. Clinicopathological study of pancreatic and ganglioneuroblastoma tumors secreting vasoactive intestinal polypeptide (VIPomas). BMJ 1981;282:1767–71.
145. Jensen RT. Overview of chronic diarrhea caused by functional neuroendocrine neoplasms. Semin Gastronintest Dis 1999;10:156–72.
146. Mekhjian HS, O'Dorisio TM. VIPoma syndrome. Semin Oncol 1987;14:282–91.
147. Bloom SR, Polak JM. Glucagonomas, VIPomas and somatostatinomas. Clin Endo Metab 1980;9:285–97.
148. McGavran MH, Unger RH, Recant L, et al. A glucagon-secreting alpha-cell carcinoma of the pancreas. N Engl J Med 1966;274:1408–13.
149. Mallinson CN, Bloom SR, Warin AP, et al. A glucagonoma syndrome. Lancet 1974;2:1–5.
150. Sweet RD. A dermatosis specifically associated with a tumour of pancreatic alpha cells. Br J Dermatol 1974;90:301–8.
151. Binnick AN, Spenser SK, Dennison WL. Glucagonoma syndrome. Arch Dermatol 1977;113:749–54.
152. Wermer RA, Fatourechi V, Wynne AG, et al. The glucagonoma syndrome: clinical and pathologic features in 21 patients. Medicine 1996;75:53–63.
153. Norton JA, Kahn CR, Schiebinger R, et al. Amino acid deficiency and the skin rash associated with glucagonoma. Ann Intern Med 1979;91:213–5.
153a. Norton JA. Gastrinoma: advances in localization and treatment. Surg Oncol Clin N Am 1998;7:846–61.
154. Guillausseas PJ, Guillausseas-Scholer C. Glucagonomas: clinical presentation, diagnosis, and advances in management. In: Mignon M, Jensen RT, editors. Endocrine tumors of the pancreas: recent advances in research and management. Basel, Switzerland: S. Krager; 1995. p. 183.
155. Higgins GA, Recent L, Fischman AB. The glucagonoma syndrome: surgical curable diabetes. Am J Surg 1979;137:142–8.
156. Montenegro F, Lawrence GD, Macon W, Pass C. Metastatic glucagonoma: improvement after surgical debulking. Am J. Surg 1980;139:424–7.
157. Marynick SP, Fagadau WR, Duncan LA. Malignant glucagonoma syndrome: response to chemotherapy. Ann Intern Med 1980;93:453–4.
158. Ganda PO, Weir GC, Soeldner JS, et al. Somatostatinoma: a somatostatin-containing tumor of the endocrine pancreas. N Engl J Med 1977;296:963–7.
159. Larsson LI, Hirsch MA, Holst J, et al. Pancreatic somatostatinoma clinical features and physiologic implications. Lancet 1977;1:666–8.
160. Krejs GJ, Orci L, Conlon W, et al. Somatostatinoma syndrome (biochemical, morphological, and clinical features). N Engl J Med 1979;301:285–92.
161. Mao C, Shah A, Hanson DJ, Howard JM. Von Recklinghausen's disease associated with duodenal somatostatinoma: contrast of duodenal versus pancreatic somatostatinomas. J Surg Oncol 1995;59:67–73.
162. Vinik AI, Tsai S, Moattari AR, et al. Somatostatin analogue (SMS-20-995) in the management of gastroenteropancreatic tumors and diarrhea syndromes. Am J Med 1986;81:23–40.
162a. Vinik AI, Moattari AR, Cho K, Thompson N. Transhepatic portal vein catheterization for localization of sporadic and MEN gastrinomas: a ten year experience. Surgery 1990;107:246–55.
163. Guillemin R, Brazeau P, Bohlen P, et al. Growth hormone-releasing factor from a human pancreatic tumor that caused acromegaly. Science 1982;218:585–7.
164. Sano T, Asa SL, Kovacs K. Growth hormone releasing-producing tumors: clinical, biochemical and morphological manifestations. Endocr Rev 1988;9:357–73.
165. Eplinski GR, Norton JA. Gastrointestinal endocrine cancers and nodal metastasis: biologic significance and therapeutic implications. Surg Oncol Clin North Am 1996;5:159–71.
166. Akerstrom G, Makridis C, Johansson H. Abdominal surgery in patients with midgut carcinoid tumors. Acta Oncol 1991;30:547–53.
167. Moertel CG, Weiland LH, Nagorney DM, Dockerty MB. Carcinoid tumor of the appendix: treatment and prognosis. N Engl J Med 1987;317:1699–701.
168. Que FG, Nagnorney DM, Batts KP, et al. Hepatic resection for metastatic neuroendocrine carcinomas. Am J Surg 1995;169:36–43.
169. Eriksson BK, Larson EG, Skogseid BM, et al. Liver embolizations of patients with malignant neuroendocrine gastrointestinal tumors. Cancer 1998;83:2293–302.
170. Drougas JG, Anthony LB, Blair TK, et al. Hepatic artery chemoembolization for management of patients with advanced metastatic carcinoid tumors. Am J Surg 1998;175:408–12.
171. Kim YH, Ajani JA, Carrasco CH, et al. Selective hepatic arterial chemoembolization for liver metastases in patients with carcinoid tumor or islet cell carcinoma. Cancer Invest 1999;17:474–8.
172. Le Treut YP, Delpero JR, Dousset B, et al. Results of liver transplantation in the treatment of metastatic neuroendocrine tumors. A 31-case French multicentric report. Ann Surg 1997;225:355–64.
173. Kvols LK, Martin K, Marsh HM, Moertel CG. Rapid reversal of carcinoid crisis with a somatostatin analogue [letter]. N Engl J Med 1985;313:1229–30.
174. Janson ET, Westlin JE, Eriksson B, et al. [^{111}In-DPTA-d-Phe]octreotide scintigraphy in patients with carcinoid tumors: the predictive value for somatostatin analogue treatment. Eur J Endocrinol 1994;131:577–81.
175. Kvols LK, Reubi JC, Horisberger U, et al. The presence of somatostatin receptors in malignant neuroendocrine tumor tissue predicts responsiveness to octreotide. Yale J Biol Med 1992;65:505–18.
176. FDA approved labeling for octreotide (Novartis Sandostatin®) found at http://www.fda.gov/cder/foi/label/2003/19667scm044_Sandostatin_lbl.pdf (accessed June 22, 2005), and FDA approved labeling for long-acting octreotide (Novartis Sandostatin LAR® Depot) found at http://www.fda.gov/cder/foi/label/2004/21008scs010_sandostatin_lbl.pdf (accessed June 22, 2005).
177. Sharma K, Patel YC, Srikant CB. Subtype-selective induction of wild-type p53 and apoptosis, but not cell cycle arrest, by human somatostatin receptor 3. Mol Endocrinol 1996;10:1688–96.
178. Imam H, Eriksson B, Lukinius A, et al. Induction of apoptosis in neuroendocrine tumors of the digestive system during treatment with somatostatin analogs. Acta Oncol 1997;36:607–14.
179. Delaunoit T, Rubin J, Neczyporenko F, et al. Somatostatin analogues in the treatment of gastroenteropancreatic neuroendocrine tumors. Mayo Clin Proc 2005;80:502–6.
180. Harris AG, Redfern JS. Octreotide treatment of carcinoid syndrome: analysis of published dose-titration data. Aliment Pharmacol Ther 1995;9:387–94.
181. Rubin J, Ajani J, Schirmer W, et al. Octreotide acetate long-acting formulation versus open-label subcutaneous octreotide acetate in malignant carcinoid syndrome. J Clin Oncol 1999;17:600–6.
182. Dogliotti L, Tampellini M, Stivanello M, et al. The clinical management of neuroendocrine tumors with long-acting repeatable (LAR) octreotide: comparison with standard subcutaneous octreotide therapy. Ann Oncol 2001;12 suppl 2;S105–9.
183. Eriksson B, Renstrup J, Imam H, Oberg K. High-dose treatment with lanreotide of patients with advanced neuroen-

docrine gastrointestinal tumors: clinical and biological effects. Ann Oncol 1997;8:1041–4.

184. Faiss S, Rath U, Mansmann U, et al. Ultra-high-dose lanreotide treatment in patients with metastatic neuroendocrine gastroenteropancreatic tumors. Digestion 1999;60:469–76.
185. Oberg K, Funa K, Alm G. Effects of leukocyte interferon on clinical symptoms and hormone levels in patients with mid-gut carcinoid tumors and carcinoid syndromes. N Engl J Med 1983;309:129–33.
186. Oberg K. Interferon in the management of neuroendocrine GEP tumors: a review. Digestion 2000;62 suppl 1:92–7.
187. Tiensuu Janson EM, Ahlstrom H, Andersson T, Oberg KE. Octreotide and interferon alfa: a new combination for the treatment of malignant carcinoid tumours. Eur J Cancer 1992;28A:1647–50.
188. Fjallskog ML, Sundin A, Westlin JE, et al. Treatment of malignant endocrine pancreatic tumors with a combination of alpha-interferon and somatostatin analogs. Med Oncol 2002;19:35–42.
189. Frank M, Klose KJ, Wied M, et al. Combination therapy with octreotide and alpha-interferon: effect on tumor growth in metastatic endocrine gastroenteropancreatic tumors. Am J Gastroenterol 1999;94:1381–7.
190. Faiss S, Pape UF, Bohmig M, et al. Prospective, randomized, multicenter trial on the antiproliferative effect of lanreotide, interferon alfa, and their combination for therapy of metastatic neuroendocrine gastroenteropancreatic tumors—the International Lanreotide and Interferon Alfa Study Group. J Clin Oncol 2003;21:2689–96.
191. Reubi JC. Peptide receptors as molecular targets for cancer diagnosis and therapy. Endocr Rev 2003;24:389–427.
192. Valkema R, deJong M, Bakker WH, et al. Phase I study of peptide receptor radionuclide therapy with [^{111}In-(DTPA)^{0}]octreotide: the Rotterdam experience. Semin Nucl Med 2002;32:110–22.
193. Anthony LB, Woltering EA, Espanan GD, et al. Indium-111-pentetreotide prolongs survival in gastroenteropancreatic malignancies. Semin Nucl Med 2002;32:123–32.
194. Waldherr C, Pless M, Maecke, HR, et al. The clinical value of [^{90}Y-DOTA]-D-Phe^{1}-Tyr^{3}-octreotide (^{90}Y-DOTA-TOC) in the treatment of neuroendocrine tumors: a clinical phase II study. Ann Oncol 2001;12:941–5.
195. Waldheer C, Pless M, Maecke HR, et al. Tumor response and clinical benefit in neuroendocrine tumors after 7.4 GBq ^{90}Y-DOTATOC. J Nuc Med 2002;43:610–6.
196. Waldherr C, Schumacher T, Maecke HR, et al. Does tumor response depend on the number of treatment sessions at constant injected dose using ^{90}Yttrium-DOTATOC in neuroendocrine tumors? Eur J Nucl Med 2002;29:S100.
197. Bodei L, Cremonesi M, Zoboli S, et al. Receptor-mediated radionuclide therapy with ^{90}Y-DOTATOC in association with amino acid infusion: a phase I study. Eur J Nucl Med Mol Imaging 2003;30:207–16.
198. Valkema R, Pauwels S, Kvols L, et al. Long-term follow-up of a phase I study of peptide receptor radionuclide therapy (PRRT) with [^{90}Y-DOTA]-D-Phe^{1}-Tyr^{3}-octreotide in patients with somatostatin receptor positive tumors. J Nucl Med Mol Imaging 2003;30:S232.
199. Valkema R, Stanilas A, Pauwels, et al. Long-term follow-up of renal function after peptide receptor radiation therapy with ^{90}Y-DOTA^{0},Tyr^{3}-octreotide and ^{177}Lu- DOTA^{0}, Tyr^{3}-octreotate. J Nucl Med 2005;46:S83–91.
200. Reubi JC, Scahr JC, Waser B, et al. Affinity profiles for human somatostatin receptor subtypes SST1-SST5 of somatostatin radiotracers selected for scintigraphic and radiotherapeutic use. Eur J Nucl Med 2000;27:273–82.
201. Kwekkeboom DJ, Bakker WH, Kam BL, et al. Treatment with Lu-177 DOTA-Tyr3-octreotate in patients with neuroendocrine tumors: interim results. Eur J Nucl Med Mol Imaging 2003;30:S231.
202. DeJong M, Valkema R, Jamar F, et al. Somatostatin receptor-targeted radionuclide therapy of tumors: preclinical and clinical findings. Semin Nucl Med 2002;32:133–40.
203. Kulke MH, Kim H, Stuart K, et al. A phase II study of docetaxel in patients with metastatic carcinoid tumors. Cancer Invest 2004;22:353–9.
204. Schnirer II, Yao JC, Ajani JA. Carcinoid: a comprehensive review. Acta Oncol 2003;42:672–92.
205. Melia WM, Nunnerley HB, Johnson PJ, Williams R. Use of arterial devascularization and cytotoxic drugs in 30 patients with the carcinoid syndrome. Br J Cancer 1982;46:331–9.
206. van Hazel GA, Moertel CG. Treatment of metastatic carcinoid tumor with dactinomycin or dacarbazine. Cancer Treat Rep 1983;67:583–5.
207. Bukowski RM, Tangen CM, Peterson RF, et al. Phase II trial of dimethyltriazenoimidazole carboxamide in patients with metastatic carcinoid. A Southwest Oncology Group Study. Cancer 1994;73:1505–8.
208. Fraker DL. Update on the management of parathyroid tumors. Curr Opin in Oncol 2000;12:41–8.
209. Shane E. Clinical review 122: parathyroid carcinoma. J Clin Endocrinol Metab 2001;86:485–93.
210. Hakaim AG, Esselstyn CB. Parathyroid carcinoma: 50 year experience at the Cleveland Clinic Foundation. Cleve Clin J Med 1993;60:331–5.
211. Hundahl SA, Fleming ID, Fremgen AM, Menck HR. Two hundred and eighty six cases of parathyroid carcinoma treated in the US between 1985–1995: a National Cancer Data Base Report. The American College of Surgeons Commission on cancer and the American Cancer Society. Cancer 1999;86:538–44.
212. Krubsack AJ, Wilson SD, Lawson TL, et al. Prospective comparison of radionuclide, computed tomographic, sonographic, and magnetic resonance localization of parathyroid tumors. Surgery 1989;106:639–46.
213. Shane E, Bilezikian J. Parathyroid carcinoma: a review of 62 cases. Endocr Rev 1982;3:218–26.
214. Vetto JT, Brennan MF, Woodruf J, Burt M. Parathyroid carcinoma: diagnosis and clinical history. Surgery 1993;114:882–92.
215. Bukowski R, Sheeler L, Cunningham J, Esselstyn C. Successful combination chemotherapy for metastatic parathyroid carcinoma. Arch Int Med 1984;144:399–400.
216. Calandra D, Chejfec G, Foy B, et al. Parathyroid carcinoma: biochemical and pathologic response to DTIC. Surgery 1984;96:1132–7.
217. Werner P. Genetic aspects of adenomatosis of endocrine glands. Am J Med 1954;16:363–71.
218. Steiner AL, Goodman AD, Powers SR. Study of a kindred with pheochromocytoma, medullary thyroid carcinoma, hyperparathyroidism, Cushing's disease: multiple endocrine neoplasia type 2. Medicine 1968;47:371–409.
219. Chandrasekharappa SC, Guru SC, Manickam P, et al. Positional cloning of the gene for multiple endocrine neoplasia-type 1. Science 1997;276:404–7.
220. The European Consotrium on MEN1. Identification of the multiple endocrine neoplasia type 1 (MEN1) gene. Hum Mol Genet 1997;6:1177–83.
221. Tsukada T, Yamaguchi K, Kameya T. The MEN1 gene and associated disease: an update. Endocr Pathol 2001;12:259–73.
222. Bystrom C, Larsson C, Blomberg C, et al. Localization of the MEN1 gene to a small region within chromosome 11q13 by deletion mapping in tumors. Proc Natl Acad Sci U S A 1990;87:1968–72.
223. The Human Gene Mutation Database. MEN1. Available at: http://archive.uwcm.ac.uk/uwcm/mg/search/120173.html (accessed June 22, 2005).
224. Hughes CM, Rozenblatt-Rosen O, Milne TA, et al. Menin associates with a trithorax family histone methyltransferase complex and with the hoxc8 locus. Mol Cell 2004;13:587–97.
225. Wautot V, Vercherat C, Lespinase J, et al. Germline mutation profile of MEN1 in multiple endocrine neoplasia type 1: search for correlation between phenotype and the functional domains of the MEN1 protein. Hum Mutat 2002;20:35–47.
226. Calendar A. Molecular genetics of neuroendocrine tumors. Digestion 2000;62 suppl 1: 3–18.
227. Marx SJ, Agrawal SK, Kester MB, et al. Multiple endocrine neoplasia type I: clinical and genetic features of the hereditary endocrine neoplasia. Recent Prog Hormone Res 1999;54:397–438.
228. Uchino S, Noguchi S, Sato W, et al. Screening of the MEN1 gene and discovery of germline and somatic mutations in apparently sporadic parathyroid tumors. Cancer Res 2000;60:5553–7.
229. Burgess JR, Greenaway TM, Shephers JJ. Expression of the MEN-1 gene in a large kindred with multiple endocrine neoplasia type 1. J Intern Med 1998;243:465–70.
230. Doherty GM, Olson JA, Frisella MM, et al. Lethality of multiple endocrine neoplasia type 1. World J Surg 1998;22:581–5.
231. Hansford JR, Mulligan LM. Multiple endocrine neoplasia type 2 and RET: from neoplasia to neurogenesis. J Med Genet 2003;37:817–27.
232. Ponder BA. The phenotypes associated with ret mutations in the multiple endocrine neoplasia type 2 syndrome. Cancer Res 1999;59:1736s–41s.
233. Mulligan LLM, Kwok JB, Healey CS, et al. Germ-line mutations of the RET proto-oncogene in multiple endocrine neoplasia type 2A. Nature 1993;363:458–60.
234. Eng C, Smith DP, Mulligan LM, et al. Point mutation within the tyrosine kinase domain of the RET protooncogene in multiple endocrine neoplasia type 2B and related sporadic tumours. Hum Mol Genet 1994;3:237–41.
235. ASCO policy statement: genetic testing for cancer susceptibility. Available at: http://www.asco.org/asco/downloads/GeneticTesting.pdf (accessed May 1, 2005).
236. Landsvater RM, Rombouts AG, Meerman GJ, et al. The clinical implications of a positive calcitonin test for C-cell hyperplasia in genetically unaffected members of MEN2A kindred. Am J Hum Genet 1993;52:335–42.
237. Robbins J, Merino MJ, Boice JD, et al. Thyroid cancer: a lethal endocrine neoplasm. Ann Intern Med 1991;115:133–47.
238. Lips CJ, Landsvater RM, Hoppener JW, et al. Clinical screening as compared with DNA analysis in families with multiple endocrine neoplasia type 2A. N Engl J Med 1994;331:828–35.
239. O'Riordain DS, O'Brien T, Weaver AL, et al. Medullary thyroid carcinoma in multiple endocrine neoplasia types 2A and 2B. Surgery 1994;206:1017–23.
240. Skinner MA, DeBenedetti MK, Foley JF, et al. Medullary thyroid carcinoma in children with multiple endocrine neoplasia type 2A and 2B. J Pediatr Surg 1996;31:177–81.
241. Morrison PJ, Nevin NC. Multiple endocrine neoplasia type 2B (mucosal neuromas syndrome, Wagenmann-Froboese syndrome). J Med Genet 1996;33:779–82.
242. Raue F, Frank-Raue K, Grauer A. Multiple endocrine neoplasia type 2. Clinical features and screening. Endocrinol Metab Clin North Am 1994;23:137–56.
243. Cohen MS, Moley JF. Surgical treatment of medullary thyroid carcinoma. J Intern Med 2003;253:616–26.
244. De Groot JW, Links TP, Jager PL, et al. Impact of 18F-flouro-2-deoxy-D-glucose positron emission tomography (FDG-PET) in patients with biochemical evidence of recurrent or residual medullary thyroid cancer. Ann Surg Oncol 2004;11:786–94.
245. Scherubl M, Raue F, Ziegler R. Combination chemotherapy of advanced and differentiated thyroid cancer. Phase II study. J Cancer Res Clin Oncol 1990;116:21–3.
246. Eng C. Seminars in medicine of the Beth Israel Hospital, Boston. The RET proto-oncogene in multiple endocrine neoplasia type 2 and Hirschsprung's disease. N Engl J Med 1996;335:943–51.
247. Mulligan LM, Eng C, Healey CS, et al. Specific mutations in the RET proto-oncogene are related to disease phenotype in MEN 2A and FMTC. Nat Genet 1994;6:70–4.
248. Moers AM, Landsvater RM, Schaap C, et al. Familial medullary carcinoma: not a distinct entity? Am J Med 1996;101:635–41.
249. Baysal BE. Hereditary paragangliomas targets diverse paraganglia. J Med Genet 2002;39:617–22.
250. Sutton MG, Sheps SG, Lie JT. Prevalence of clinically unsuspected pheochromocytoma: review of a 50-year autopsy series. Mayo Clin Proc 1981;56:354–60.
251. Pacak K, Linehan WM, Eisenhofer G, et al. Recent advances in genetics, diagnosis, localization, and treatment of pheochromocytoma. Ann Intern Med 2001;134:315–29.
252. Neumann HP, Bausch B, McWhinney SR, et al. Germ-line mutations in nonsyndromic pheochromocytoma. N Engl J Med 2002;346:1456–66.
253. Weisner GL, Snow-Bailey K. Multiple endocrine neoplasia type 2: Gene-Reviews-GeneTests; 2003. Available at: http://www.geneclinics.org/profiles/men2/ (accessed May 1, 2005).
254. Neumann HP, Reincke M, Eng C. Case 13-2001: genetic testing in pheochromocytoma. N Engl J Med 2001;345:547–8.
255. Manger WM, Gifford RW Jr. Pheochromocytoma. In: Laragh JH, Brenner BM, editors. Hypertension: pathophysiology, diagnosis, and management. New York: Raven Press; 1990. p. 1639.
256. Bravo EL, Tarazi RC, Fouand FM, et al. Clonidine suppression test: a useful aid in the diagnosis of pheochromocytoma. N Engl J Med 1981;305:623–6.
257. Bravo EL, Gifford RW. Current concepts. Pheochromocytoma: diagnosis, localization and management. N Engl J Med 1984;311:1298–303.
258. Egglin TK, Hahn PF, Stark DD. MRI of the adrenal glands. Semin Roentgenol 1988;23:280–7.
259. Shapiro B, Sisson JC, Eyre P, et al. 131I-MIBG-A new agent in diagnosis and treatment of pheochromocytoma. Cardiology 1985;72 Suppl 1:137–42.
260. Shapiro B, Coop JE, Sisson JC, et al. Iodine-131 metaiodobenzylguanidine for the locating of suspected pheochromocytoma: experience in over 400 cases. J Nucl Med 1985;26:576–85.
261. Swensen SJ, Brown MJ, Sheps SG, et al. Use of ^{131}I-MIBG scintigraphy in the evaluation of suspected pheochromocytoma. Mayo Clin Proc 1985;60:299–304.

262. Mishra AK, Agarwal G, Kapoor A, et al. Catecholamine cardiomyopathy in bilateral malignant pheochromocytoma: successful reversal after surgery. Int J Card 2000;76:89–90.
263. Goldstein RE, O'Neil JA, Holcomb GW, et al. Clinical experience over 48 years with pheochromocytoma. Ann Surg 1999;229:755–66.
264. John H, Zeigler WH, Hauri D, Jaeger P. Pheochromocytomas: can malignant potential be predicted? Urology 1999;53:679–83.
265. Eisenhofer G, Bornstein SR, Brouwers FM, et al. Malignant pheochromocytoma: current status and initiatives for future progress. Endocr-related Cancer 2004;11:423–36.
266. Averbuch SD, Steakley CS, Young RC, et al. Malignant pheochromocytoma: effective treatment with a combination of cyclophosphamide, vincristine and dacarbazine. Ann Int Med 1988;109:267–73.
267. Pomares FJ, Canas R, Rodriquez JM, et al. Differences between sporadic and multiple endocrine neoplasia type 2A phaeochromocytoma. Clin Endocrinol (Oxf) 1998;48:195–200.
268. Casanova S, Rosenberg-Bourgin M, Farkas D, et al. Phaeochromocytoma in multiple endocrine neoplasia type 2A: survey of 100 cases. Clin Endocrinol (Oxf) 1993;38:531–7.
269. Neumann HP, Berger DP, Sigmund G, et al. Pheochromocytomas, multiple endocrine neoplasia type 2, and von Hippel-Landau disease. N Engl J Med 1993;329:1531–8.
270. Modigliani E, Vasen HM, Raue K, et al. Pheochromocytoma in multiple endocrine neoplasia type 2: European study. The Euromen Study Group. J Intern Med 1995;238;363–7.
271. Walther MM, Herring J, Enquist E, et al. von Recklinghausen's disease and pheochromocytomas. J Urol 1999;162:1582–6.
272. Rindi G, Capella C, Solcia E. Cell biology, clinicopathological profile, and classification of gastroenteropancreatic endocrine tumors. J Mol Med 1998;76:413–20.
273. Barakat MT, Meeran K, Bloom SR. Neuroendocrine tumours. Endocr-Related Cancer 2004;11:1–18.
274. Bruns C, Lewis I, Briner U, et al. SOM230: a novel somatostatin peptidomimetic with broad somatotropin release inhibiting factor (SRIF) receptor binding and a unique antisecretory profile. Eur J Endocrinol 2002;146:707–16.
275. Bryant J, Farmer J, Kessler LJ, et al. Pheochromocytoma: the expanding genetic differential diagnosis. J Natl Cancer Inst 2003;95:1196–204.

79

Neoplasms of the Head and Neck

Eduardo M. Diaz Jr, MD, FACS
Merrill S. Kies, MD
Erich M. Sturgis, MD, FACS
Lewis Clayman, DMD, MD
George E. Laramore, PhD, MD
Scott M. Lippman, MD
Gary L. Clayman, DMD, MD, FACS

Head and neck cancer poses a serious health risk, with recent projections that over approximately 39,000 new cases of head and neck cancer were diagnosed in the United States and over 11,000 American deaths resulted from head and neck malignancies in 2004.[1] Although head and neck cancer accounts for only 3% of all new cancer cases and 2% of all cancer deaths in the United States annually, it is the fifth most common malignancy worldwide.[1,2] Tobacco and alcohol are the primary etiologic agents in these cancers, suggesting prevention should be a primary public health goal in the field. Emerging evidence suggests that inherited factors and exposure to other agents play important roles, and these may help refine prevention strategies. Nearly identical percentages are reported from Britain, but head and neck cancers have a much greater impact in certain other parts of the world, especially where tobacco and/or betel nut chewing is common, and are the leading causes of cancer mortality worldwide.[3,4] Despite improvements in diagnosis and local management, long-term survival rates in head and neck cancer have not increased significantly over the past 40 years and are among the lowest worldwide of the major cancers. The problem is even worse for select populations, such as African Americans, for whom survival rates have actually decreased. Oropharyngeal cancer, the largest subgroup of head and neck cancers, has a 5-year relative survival rate of only 59% for United States whites and 35% for blacks.[5] Although early-stage head and neck cancers (especially laryngeal and oral cavity) have high cure rates, over 60% of head and neck cancer patients present with advanced disease. Cure rates decrease, of course, in locally advanced cases, whose probability of cure is inversely related to tumor size and even more so to the extent of regional node involvement.

Survival advantages provided by new treatment modalities have been undermined by the significant percentage of patients cured of head and neck squamous cell carcinoma (HNSCC) who subsequently develop second primary tumors.[6,7] Second primaries are a major threat to long-term survival after successful therapy of early-stage HNSCC. HNSCC patients also face tremendous impacts on quality of life after definitive therapy. Despite marked advances in reconstructive surgery and rehabilitation, intensity-modulated radiotherapy (IMRT) and conservation approaches to certain malignancies, patients continue to have significant functional deficits. These compelling problems are responsible for the emerging importance of primary chemotherapy and prevention strategies for HNSCC. HNSCC research, both clinical and basic, is advancing on many fronts and becoming a model for research into other epithelial cancers. Combined-modality approaches involving chemotherapy and radiation are now standards of care for organ preservation and other settings of locally advanced disease. Understanding the biology of head and neck cancer and developing molecular-targeted therapeutic agents (in recurrent disease and other settings) have advanced substantially. Molecular-targeted chemoprevention also is advancing. These new therapeutic and preventive approaches appear to hold great promise for improving the control of head and neck cancer. This chapter reviews both the current status of and future investigative directions for the epidemiology, biology, chemoprevention, diagnosis, and therapy of head and neck cancer.

DESCRIPTIVE EPIDEMIOLOGY

Incidence The United States head and neck cancer estimates for 2004 were 20,010 new cases of oral cavity cancer, 8,250 new cases of pharyngeal cancer, and 10,270 new cases of laryngeal cancer.[1] The absolute incidence of oral cavity and pharyngeal cancer has been approximately 21,000 and 9,000 new cases, respectively, annually since 1985; however, the number of new cases of laryngeal cancer has steadily declined since 1993, when 12,600 new cases were diagnosed.[8,9]

In the United States, approximately 1 in 3 oral cavity/pharyngeal cancers occur in women, while only 1 in 5 laryngeal cancers occur in women.[1] The incidence rates in men are double the rates in women for oral cavity/pharyngeal cancers and triple the rates in women for laryngeal cancer.[10]

Since the mid-1980s, incidence rates (age-adjusted to the 2000 US standard) for both oral cavity/pharyngeal cancer and laryngeal cancer have steadily declined in men to 15.2 of 100,000 and 6.9 of 100,000, respectively, in 1999. However, during the same time period these rates have been relatively stagnant in women.[10] Although black and white women have similar rates of oral cavity/pharyngeal cancer, black men have a 30% higher rate of oral cavity/pharyngeal cancer than white men. Both black men and women have double the rate of laryngeal cancer of white men and women, respectively.[10] Hispanics have the lowest rates of oral cavity/pharyngeal cancer, and Asians have the lowest rates of laryngeal cancer.[10]

The median age at diagnosis for HNSCC is approximately 60 years, but the incidence of these cancers in young adults (age < 40 years) appears to be increasing.[11–15] This increase has not been apparent in blacks, and carcinoma of the tongue appears to account for the majority of this increase in incidence.[5,15]

Head and neck cancer is relatively common in many parts of the world[2,16] and the most common malignancy afflicting men in some parts of the world. For example, in South Central Asia, home to one-fifth of the world's population, head and neck cancer accounted for approximately 155,400 new cases of cancer in 1990 (17% of all cancers and 25% of all cancers occurring in men).[2] Although the 80% of head and neck cancers in South Central Asia are oral cavity and pharyngeal (excluding nasopharyngeal) cancers, in other regions of the world, laryngeal cancers and nasopharyngeal cancers account for a much higher percentage of head and neck malignancies. For example, in the developed world, laryngeal cancer accounts for approximately one-third of head and neck cancers, and in Southern and Eastern Europe, approximately 40% of all head and neck cancers are laryngeal cancers.[2] In China, nasopharyngeal cancer accounts for 55% of all head and neck cancers, and in Southeast Asia, nasopharyngeal cancer accounts for 70% of all head and neck cancers and 5% of all cancers in men.[2]

Prevalence In 1998 in the United States, the prevalence of HNSCC was 313,105, with 219,175 individuals with a history of oral cavity/pharyngeal cancer and 93,930 individuals with laryngeal cancer history.[10] As expected, the sex distribution of these prevalence figures reflects the sex distribution of the incidence of these cancers. However, in 1998 African Americans accounted for only 11.8% of the prevalent population of individuals with a history of laryngeal cancer and only 7.9% of the prevalent population of individuals with oral cavity/pharyngeal cancer. These small percentages of the prevalent populations of these cancers likely reflect the poorer overall survival of African Americans diagnosed with HNSCC. African Americans have demonstrated survival rates approximately 20% worse than whites for oral cavity/pharyngeal cancer and 10% worse than whites for laryngeal cancer over the past 25 years.[1] Not only has the discrepancy in survival between whites and blacks remained relatively constant over the past three decades, but also neither whites nor blacks have seen significant gains in survival over this time period.[1]

Worldwide, head and neck cancer is the third most prevalent cancer after breast and colorectal cancers, accounting for 7% of the 22.4 million individuals with a cancer diagnosis, excluding nonmelanoma skin cancer.[16] Of the approximately 1.6 million individuals with a head and neck cancer diagnosis, 707,100 have a diagnosis of oral cavity cancer, 458,100 have a diagnosis of laryngeal cancer, 248,800 have a diagnosis of oro/hypopharyngeal cancer, and 171,500 have a diagnosis of nasopharyngeal cancer.

Mortality In the United States approximately 11,000 individuals will die from head and neck cancer in 2004, with 5,160 of these deaths due to oral cavity cancer, 2,070 due to pharyngeal cancer, and 3,830 due to laryngeal cancer.[1] However, head and neck cancer accounts for less than 2% of all cancer deaths in the United States annually.[1] Although today pharyngeal cancers account for less than half the number of deaths as they caused in 1985, oral cavity and laryngeal cancers account for approximately the same number of deaths as they did in 1985.[8]

In the United States, the sex distribution for head and neck cancer deaths is similar to the sex distribution for the incidence of these cancers.[1] Although the mortality rates (age-adjusted to the 2000 US Standard Million Population) for oral cavity/pharyngeal cancers has declined steadily over the past two decades, the mortality rate for laryngeal cancer has declined only in white men.[10] Blacks have higher oral cavity/pharyngeal and laryngeal cancer mortality rates than whites.[10] Hispanics have the lowest oral cavity/pharyngeal cancer death rates, while Asians have the lowest laryngeal cancer death rates.[10]

Worldwide, head and neck cancer accounts for 333,400 deaths annually, with 127,900 due to oral cavity cancers, 89,100 due to laryngeal cancers, 78,700 due to oro/hypopharyngeal cancers, and 37,800 of these due to nasopharyngeal cancers.[16] As with other cancer sites, mortality/incidence ratios for head and neck cancers are much higher in developing countries for both men and women as compared with the United States.[16] This likely reflects the better survival for these cancers seen in the United States; however, an opposite trend is seen for nasopharyngeal cancer.

RISK FACTORS

Tobacco Tobacco initiates a linear dose-response carcinogenic effect in which duration is more important than the intensity of exposure. The major carcinogenic activity of cigarette smoke resides in the particulate (tar) fraction, which contains a complex mixture of interacting cancer initiators, promoters, and cocarcinogens. In the late 1950s, a landmark case-control study by Dr. Ernst Wynder established the link between tobacco use and oral cavity cancer.[17] This was followed a year later by a cohort study of over 180,000 men that demonstrated an increased risk of death owing to HNSCC in cigarette smokers as compared with men who never smoked.[18] These studies also demonstrated elevated risks for HNSCC death in cigar and pipe smokers. In 1964, the Advisory Committee to the Surgeon General on Smoking and Health published its report linking smoking to cancer based on many of Hill's classic criteria of disease causality.[19] Because of limitations of sample size and follow-up time, Hill's classic cohort study of over 40,000 British physicians showed only a borderline risk of HNSCC related to smoking.[20] However, his criteria linking HNSCC and tobacco smoking have been clearly demonstrated over the past 40 years in multiple independent studies.[17,18,21–29] Most importantly, the strength and consistency of the association between smoking and HNSCC have been demonstrated in numerous case-control and cohort studies with significant relative risks or odds ratios in the 3- to 12-fold range. Furthermore, a dose-response effect is consistently shown in these studies between the duration and dose of smoking with increasing risk of HNSCC and between the time since quitting and the decreasing risk of HNSCC.[21–27,30] Other mucosal malignancies of the head and neck such as nasopharyngeal carcinoma (NPC) and sinonasal malignancies have a weaker association with tobacco smoking.[31] The specificity of the link between tobacco and HNSCC (and not the non-mucosal/unexposed head and neck malignancies), the coherence and analogy of the explanation of tobacco-induced HNSCC to lung carcinogenesis, and the biologic plausibility of the well-established tobacco-induced carcinogenesis model have all helped establish tobacco as the chief etiologic agent in HNSCC.

Although the risk of bronchogenic carcinoma appears to be less significant for cigar and pipe smokers than for cigarette smokers, these forms of tobacco use are also clearly associated with an increased risk of HNSCC.[17,22,23,25,30,32,33] The pooling of saliva containing carcinogens in gravity-dependent regions may account for the frequent location of oral carcinomas along the lateral and ventral surfaces of the tongue and in the floor of the mouth.[34] Smokeless tobacco use has also demonstrated an association with cancer of the oral cavity.[35–37] Smokeless tobacco users and pipe smokers who have a habitual position for the quid or pipe stem often develop carcinomas and dysplasia of the specific site of use, which suggests that physical and thermal trauma may be contributing factors.

Although smoking rates are declining in the developed world, smoking rates are rising in developing countries, home to four-fifths of the world's population. In the United States, smoking rates have declined since the Surgeon General's warning in 1964.[38] In 1965, 42.4% of the US adult population were current smokers, while in 1999 only 23.5% were current smokers. Although the reduction in cigarette smoking has been much greater in men over the last three decades, the rate of current cigarette use remains higher in men (25.7%) than for women (21.5%), and 40.8% of Native Americans continue to smoke.[39] Other concerns have been the increasing rates of cigarette smoking in high school seniors and the dramatic increase in the number of new cigar users in the last decade.[38] Dramatic increases in smokeless tobacco use have occurred among younger people and have been implicated by some in the rise of oral cancer mortality rates in this group.[11–15,40] Striking variations in head and neck cancer sites and incidence are seen among different regions, cultures, and demographic groups and are due, in large part, to differing patterns of tobacco and other substance abuse.[22,35] Smokeless tobacco and similar products are used greatly in parts of Asia and Africa.[35,37,41,42] In South Central Asia, "pano" (betel leaf, lime, catechu, and areca nut) is commonly chewed and is a strong risk factor independent of tobacco use for carcinoma of the oral cavity, one of the most common cancers in men and women in this region.[41]

Alcohol Alcohol, too, is an important promoter of carcinogenesis and is a contributive factor in at least 75% of HNSCCs.[22] Furthermore, alcohol appears to have an effect on risk of HNSCC independent of tobacco smoking, but these effects are consistently significant only at the highest level of alcohol consumption.[17,22–27] Although studies attempting to correlate the type of alcoholic beverage with specific cancer risks have been conflicting, most investigators believe that ethanol itself is the main causative factor.[22,23,25,27,43] Nevertheless, it appears that the major clinical significance of alcohol consumption is that it potentiates the carcinogenic effect of tobacco at every level of tobacco use. However, this effect is most striking at the highest levels of exposure, and the magnitude of this effect is at least additive, but may be multiplicative, dependent on the subsite of HNSCC and the levels of exposure.[22–27]

Genetic Susceptibility The predominant risk factor for HNSCC is a history of exposure to tobacco and alcohol. However, since only a fraction of smokers develop cancer, variations in genetic susceptibility may be equally important in the disease etiology. A genetic component to this disease is also supported by large family studies demonstrating a three- to eightfold increased risk of HNSCC in first-degree relatives of patients with HNSCC.[44–47] Furthermore, there is molecular epidemiologic evidence supporting the concept of genetic susceptibility in head and neck cancer patients.[48] Emerging data from case-control studies of several phenotypic and genotyping assays support the hypothesis that genetic susceptibility plays an important role in the etiology of HNSCC. According to this hypothesis, inherited differences in the efficiencies of carcinogen metabolizing systems, deoxyribonucleic acid (DNA) repair systems, and/or cell-cycle control/apoptosis systems influence one's risk of tobacco-induced cancers. Identifying such at-risk individuals in the general population by use of these biomarker assays would have a profound impact on primary prevention, early detection, and secondary prevention strategies.

Infectious Agents Although it has been suggested that various infectious agents play a role in head and neck carcinogenesis, only Epstein-Barr virus (EBV) and human papilloma virus (HPV) can be implicated as etiologic agents in head and neck carcinogenesis based on current scientific evidence. EBV appears to be associated with most nasopharyngeal carcinomas, and HPV (most commonly type 16) is associated with approximately 50% of oropharyngeal carcinomas. HPV may also play a role in the etiology of squamous cell carcinomas arising in the sinonasal tract.[49] Although herpes simplex viruses have been suggested as a risk factor for oral cavity cancer,[50] and *Helicobacter pylori* has been suggested as a risk factor for laryngeal cancer,[51] confirmation of these findings is lacking.[52]

Although laboratory evidence supporting the role of HPV as a risk factor for HNSCC is somewhat circumstantial, HPV has been established as an etiologic agent in cervical cancer,[53] and more recently, several investigators have suggested that infection with HPV, especially the high-risk type HPV-16, is a risk factor for oropharyngeal carcinoma.[54–60] The chief oncoproteins of HPV-16 are encoded by the genes *E6* and *E7*. The E6 protein targets the tumor suppressor gene *TP53* for ubiquitination and degradation. In fact, degradation of *TP53* in HPV-positive cells is fully dependent on the presence of E6.[61] The E7 oncoprotein is involved in suppression of pRb function. Reduced pRb expression is common in HPV-positive tonsillar cancers.[62,63] In vitro experiments support the tumorigenicity of HPV-16 in human epithelial cells. Furthermore, numerous studies using methods such as polymerase chain reaction (PCR), Southern blotting, and in situ hybridization have detected HPV DNA in the tumor tissue and sera of oropharyngeal cancer patients.[54–60] Oropharyngeal tumors and tumors in nonsmokers are the most frequent HPV-positive head and neck malignancies.[58,64] However, because they did not include cancer-free controls, most of these studies were unable to estimate the risk of oropharyngeal cancer attributable to HPV-16. Molecular epidemiologic evidence with case-control design supporting the role of HPV-16 in oropharyngeal cancer has been emerging.[50,65–67] These studies have assessed HPV-16 DNA positivity in the mucosa of cancer-free controls. In a study of oral and oropharyngeal cancer patients and cancer-free controls, HPV DNA was identified in 15% of 93 cancer specimens and in only 5% of 205 cancer-free control benign oral specimens (odds ratio [OR] = 3.70; 95% CI, 1.47–9.32).[65] A second study found only a slight difference in high-risk HPV DNA identified in 44 cases with laryngeal cancer and 10 with leukoplakia specimens and 12 cancer-free control benign specimens (18.2%, 20.0%, and 16.7%, respectively).[66] In a third study of 52 patients with tonsillar cancer and 48 age- and sex-matched cancer-free controls undergoing tonsillectomy for benign pathology, 46% of tonsillar carcinomas and only 6.3% of the cancer-free control tonsils were HPV positive.[67] Although these studies were relatively small, a recent nested case-control study of 292 cases and 1,569 controls from a Scandinavian cohort of almost 900,000 subjects (Mork and colleagues) reported that HPV-16 seropositivity was associated with a 2.2-fold increased risk of HNSCC after multivariate adjustment.[68] However, 25% of the cases in that study were not classic HNSCC as 3% were nasopharyngeal cancers, 20% were lip cancers, and 2% were sinus cancers. Because subjects with cancers of these sites were less frequently HPV-16 seropositive, Mork and colleagues may have underestimated the risk of HNSCC associated with HPV-16 exposure. In their subgroup analysis of oropharyngeal cancer, Mork and colleagues reported an estimated risk of 14.4 (95% CI, 3.6–58.1). An additional serologic base study using a population-based case-control study design of 284 subjects with newly diagnosed oral and oropharyngeal carcinoma and 477 cancer-free controls demonstrated a significantly elevated risk associated with HPV-16 seropositivity (adjusted OR = 2.3; 95% CI, 1.6–3.3).[69] Although subgroup risk analysis for oropharyngeal cancer was not performed, the chief effect again appears to be in the oropharyngeal cancer subgroup, where approximately 35% had cancers positive for HPV-16 DNA. Although oropharyngeal cancer patients presenting without the classic tobacco exposures more commonly have HPV-16–associated tumors,[70] it also appears that there may be synergistic interactions between the traditional oropharyngeal risk factors of tobacco and alcohol with HPV-16.[71] The circumstantial, mechanistic, and molecular epidemiologic evidence strongly supports the role of HPV-16 infection in oropharyngeal carcinogenesis. The potential effect of HPV-16 immunizations in the prevention of cervical carcinomas may help prevent oropharyngeal cancers as well.

The epidemiologic link between EBV and nasopharyngeal cancer is quite strong.[72–76] Regardless of histopathologic subtype (World Health Organization [WHO] I to III), geographic or ethnic setting, sporadic or endemic pattern, and premalignant or malignant status, nasopharyngeal carcinoma is an EBV-associated malignancy. Although WHO types II and III are overwhelmingly positive for EBV, EBV is also associated with well-differentiated (WHO type I) nasopharyngeal carcinoma.[77] Both serologic and mucosal swab evidence of EBV infection has been used to enhance the screening for nasopharyngeal carcinoma in endemic areas.[76,78] Evidence of EBV DNA in cervical lymph node metastases of unknown primary origin has been used to identify nasopharyngeal primaries.[74,79] More recently, the detection of EBV DNA in peripheral blood (both cellular and cell-free component) has demonstrated prognostic significance for predicting survival and distant metastases.[80,81] Nasopharyngeal carcinoma may be the best example of a virus-related epithelial carcinoma and has served as a model for the study of virus-induced carcinogenesis elsewhere in the body. The fundamental and early role of EBV in the pathogenesis of NPC is further supported by the identification of EBV DNA in premalignant nasopharyngeal lesions, as well.

Environmental Tobacco Smoke A recent high-profile legal case in Australia has brought significant attention to the risk of HNSCC secondary to environmental tobacco smoke exposure. In May of 2001, the New South Wales Supreme Court found that a 62-year-old nonsmoker's HNSCC was significantly associated with long-term exposure to environmental tobacco smoke in her job as a bar attendant and imposed liability on her employer.[82,83] Two case-control studies supported the court's finding. In a study of 173 cases of HNSCC and 176 cancer-free controls, environmental tobacco smoke was associated with a more than twofold increased risk of HNSCC, and a dose-response relationship was also observed.[84] In a separate study of 44 nonsmokers with HNSCC and 132 cancer-free nonsmoker controls, environmental tobacco smoke was associated with a significantly increased risk of HNSCC (OR = 5.34), and this was particularly true for females (OR = 8.00) and for those reporting exposure at work (OR = 10.16).[85]

Laryngopharyngeal Reflux Observational and anecdotal studies have long suggested that gastroesophageal reflux may be associated with laryngeal cancer.[86,87] Furthermore, multiple studies have objectively documented a high prevalence of gastric reflux into the laryngopharynx via 24-hour pH probe monitoring.[88–90] Recently, a retrospective case-control study of 10,140 hospitalized patients and 12,061 outpatients with laryngeal and pharyngeal cancer and 40,561 hospitalized and 48,244 outpatient controls was performed using computerized hospital and outpatient databases of the US Department of Veterans Affairs.[91] The diagnosis of gastroesophageal reflux disease was associated with a significantly elevated risk of laryngeal cancer (OR = 2.40 [2.15–2.69] and OR = 2.31 [2.10–2.53] for hospitalized and outpatient groups, respectively) and of pharyngeal cancer (OR = 2.38 [1.87–3.02] and OR = 1.92 [1.72–2.15] for hospitalized and outpatient groups, respectively). Furthermore, these risk estimates were adjusted for age, gender, ethnicity, smoking, and alcohol consumption.

Marijuana Marijuana smoke has a four times higher tar burden and a 50% higher concentration of benzopyrene and aromatic hydrocarbons than does tobacco smoke. Although anecdotal evidence has long suggested that marijuana is a risk factor for HNSCC, few reports have found direct evidence of marijuana as an etiologic factor for HNSCC because most users of marijuana are also exposed to tobacco and alcohol.[92,93] A recent case-control study including 173 HNSCC patients and 176 cancer-free controls demonstrated a cigarette-adjusted risk of HNSCC of 2.6 (95% CI, 1.1–6.6) associated with marijuana use, with evidence of a dose-response relationship.[94] Contrarily, a large retrospective cohort of 64,855 health maintenance organization (HMO) members found no association with tobacco-related cancers.[95]

Diet Epidemiologic evidence from traditional case-control study designs suggests that diets high in animal fats and low in fruits and vegetables may be risk factors for HNSCC.[96–99] Winn and colleagues found that the risk of oral and pharyngeal cancer in women was inversely related to the consumption of fresh fruits and vegetables.[96] Similarly, in a study of 871 individuals with oral and pharyngeal cancer and 979 cancer-free controls, McLaughlin and colleagues demonstrated an inverse relationship between fruit intake and oral and pharyngeal cancer risk.[97] In a Chinese population-based case-control study, citrus fruits and dark green/yellow vegetables were associated with a decreased risk of laryngeal cancer, whereas salted fish and meat, as well as deep-fried foods, were associated with an increased risk of pharyngeal and laryngeal cancer.[97] More recently, both European and US studies have confirmed the protective effects of fruits and vegetables and the risk of animal fat consumption, after adjustment for smoking and alcohol use.[99,100] Several studies have used case-control methodology to correlate salted fish consumption with nasopharyngeal carcinoma risk, and this risk may be due to the high content of nitrosamine compounds in preserved foods such as salted fish.[101,102]

Some evidence suggests vitamin A and beta-carotene may be responsible for the protective effect of diets high in fruits and vegetables, and deficiencies of carotenoids appear to be a risk factor for HNSCC and lung cancers.[97] It is not known, however, which of the more than 500 carotenoids are protective, what chemical interactions may occur, or what protective role other micronutrients in carotenoid-rich foods may play. Others have found that total intake of vitamins C and E are also protective.[96,100] Moreover, diets are complex and difficult to assess and validate; in particular, there are often inaccuracies in translating foods into constituent nutrients. Further studies are needed to more precisely define the relationship between dietary intake and serum levels of the various carotenoid components. It may be impossible to determine which of the vast array of compounds is most beneficial, and controlling for other dietary variables and confounding risk factors has remained a difficult methodologic problem. Further confounding this situation, smoking has been associated with reduced dietary intake and serum levels of carotenoids. Despite these many problems, prospective and retrospective nutritional (serum and dietary) epidemiologic studies have provided important clues to the development and prevention of these cancers.

Occupation Although occupational exposures probably play a minor role overall in the development of HNSCC, they are major risk factors for malignancies of the sinonasal region.[103] The most important exposures occur in the metalworking, refining, woodworking, and leather/textile industries.[103–105] Although asbestos has been suggested as a risk factor for laryngeal cancer, most of the evidence does not support this association.[106,107]

Radiation No significant association has been demonstrated between ionizing radiation and the development of HNSCC. However, squamous cell carcinomas of the lip, like skin cancers, are associated with ultraviolet radiation exposure. Furthermore, exposure to gamma radiation is associated with thyroid cancers, sarcomas of the head and neck, and salivary gland malignancies, including paranasal sinus cancers. Although therapeutic irradiation of head and neck malignancies does not appear to induce second primary squamous cell carcinomas of the aerodigestive tract, it is associated with an increased risk of sarcomas of the head and neck.[108] This is a particular concern for children who have received therapeutic irradiation. Furthermore, environmental, medical diagnostic, and therapeutic radiation exposure to the head and neck are all significantly associated with salivary gland malignancies.[109,110] These studies have found a significant dose-response relationship with risk increasing with dose, and mucoepidermoid carcinomas appear to be the most common radiation-induced salivary malignancy.[109,110] In the past, the uses of radium for watch dial painting and thorotrast contrast in sinonasal imaging were both associated with an increased risk of paranasal sinus malignancies; however, these materials are no longer employed.

Ultimately, the public health goal is better prevention and early detection of these malignancies by reducing the use of tobacco and alcohol, discovering and avoiding other causative agents, and identifying the genetically susceptible. Such work will enhance both prevention and screening efforts. Oral cancer screening in the limited number of such studies reported to date has not been effective.[111] Recently reported interim results from a randomized study in India of visual inspection at 3-year intervals indicated no difference in oral cancer mortality between the screened and control groups at 6 years.[112] Current screening efforts include identifying molecular high-risk groups and developing noninvasive molecular genetic screening approaches.

HISTOPATHOLOGY PATHOLOGIC ASSESSMENT

Aside from stating that a particular tumor is squamous cell carcinoma (SSC), additional information reported by the pathologist usually includes tumor grade or differentiation. Traditionally, tumor grading has been based on criteria developed over 50 years ago by Broder.[113,114] Unfortunately, differentiation grade has not been consistently accurate in reflecting the biologic aggressiveness of squamous carcinomas.[114] The difficulty in predicting the behavior of individual tumors is well recognized. Prognosis is influenced by many factors other than grade.[115,116]

These include tumor size; site; vascularity; lymphatic drainage; host immune response; the patient's age, sex, nutritional, and performance status; and other as yet unrecognized variables.

The comprehensive histologic evaluation of squamous cell carcinomas includes characteristics of tumor–host interactions; Jakobsson and colleagues pioneered their incorporation into the determination of tumor grade.[117] Characteristics considered include degree of keratinization, nuclear grade, mitotic rate, inflammatory response, vascular-stromal response, vascular invasion, and pattern of invasion. These characteristics have variably correlated with biologic behavior. Keratinization is the major determinant of Broder grade. Better-differentiated tumors that produce more keratin are thought to be less likely to metastasize. Nuclear grade assesses nuclear pleomorphism. Enlarged, hyperchromatic nuclei are associated with less-differentiated tumors. Nuclear grade accurately predicts the behavior of advanced laryngeal cancers.[118] Enlarged nuclear size and staining presumably reflect chromosomal abnormalities and increased DNA content. Numerous studies of DNA content have demonstrated high rates of aneuploidy in squamous cell cancers that range from 50 to 70%. Aneuploidy has been associated with poor prognosis[119–121] have also importantly shown that ploidy analysis of premalignant squamous lesions is critically important in predicting progression to malignancy as well as death from these cancers. Mitotic rate and labeling index have also been used to reflect proliferative activity, but large-scale studies of head and neck cancers have been lacking.

Features reflecting aggressive disease include lymphatic invasion, perineural invasion, lymph node metastases, and penetration of the tumor through the capsule of involved lymph nodes (extracapsular spread). The presence of regional lymph node metastases is the most important determinant of prognosis in head and neck cancer and is associated with a 50% decrease in survival rates as compared with patients without regional metastases.

More recently, the histologic pattern of invasion of these cancers was systematically studied. Tumors that invade with thin fingerlike projections or single disassociated cells behave more aggressively regardless of differentiation grade and tend to be associated with vascular and neural invasion.[117] The presence of extracapsular spread of tumor in the neck has been directly associated with high rates of distant metastases. These various histologic features play an important role in therapeutic decision making.

Molecular Pathology The head and neck surgical oncologist relies heavily on the pathologist's assessment of surgical margins via frozen section to ensure total excision of the tumor in patients with head and neck cancer. Brennan and colleagues proposed using contemporary molecular techniques to determine whether clonal populations of infiltrating tumor cells harboring mutations of the *TP53* gene could be detected in histopathologically negative surgical margins and cervical lymph nodes of patients with HNSCC.[122] They found that 38% (5 of 13) of patients had molecular positive margins and that approximately 50% had molecular identification of *TP53* mutations in histopathologically negative lymph nodes. Patients with these molecular positive margins had an increased risk of local recurrence. Although advances in molecular techniques are likely to augment enormously what is now considered standard histopathologic assessment, critical studies will be required to determine the meaning and impact of this new pathologic information and appropriate management steps that result.

THE BIOLOGY OF HEAD AND NECK CARCINOGENESIS

Field Cancerization Slaughter and colleagues' classic 1953 report[123] on oral cancer proposed that upper aerodigestive tract (UADT) carcinogenesis is a process of "field cancerization"—the repeated exposure of a region's entire tissue area to carcinogenic insult (eg, tobacco and alcohol), which increases the tissue's risk of developing multiple independent premalignant and malignant foci.[6,124–126] This concept (also called field carcinogenesis or condemned-mucosa syndrome) may explain the clinical occurrence of multiple primary and second primary tumors in HNSCC. The data indicate that second primaries, whether synchronous or metachronous, generally are of squamous histology, develop at a constant rate (4–7% of treated patients per year), are not treatment related, and occur in the aerodigestive field at risk, that is, the head and neck, the upper two-thirds of the esophagus, and the lung.[6,7,124] These characteristics of second primaries support the field cancerization hypothesis. Recent data on *TP53* mutations provide strong molecular support for the field carcinogenesis concept.[127–129] Despite epidemiologic studies having long associated tobacco and alcohol use with the development of HNSCC, the molecular targets of these agents remain to be identified. In studies by Brennan and colleagues,[130] significant tobacco and alcohol use was associated with a high frequency of *TP53* mutations. Their preliminary results suggest these *TP53* mutations occur at nonendogenous mutation sites. These findings suggest a role for tobacco in the molecular progression and field carcinogenesis process in head and neck cancer.

Multistep Carcinogenesis Despite intensive study, much of the complex fundamental biology of HNSCC remains poorly understood. Like other epithelial neoplasms, UADT carcinogenesis appears to evolve through a complex multistep process involving certain biomolecular changes that precede premalignant lesions, which, in turn, precede invasive cancer.[131–133] Much of the cellular and molecular biology supporting the concepts of field and multistep head and neck carcinogenesis in humans was worked out in the translational study of oral intraepithelial neoplasia (IEN).[134]

On the basis of animal studies, epithelial carcinogenesis has been divided into three phases: initiation, promotion, and progression. Although human neoplasia does not fit neatly into this tripartite framework, the framework serves as a useful model for understanding pharmacologic interventions. Pharmacologic interventions at each phase have attendant advantages and disadvantages. Prevention's greatest potential is in the promotion and progression phases of carcinogenesis.

Occurring within the three-phase model described above, multiple subtle steps of UADT carcinogenesis involve genetic alterations, dysregulated epithelial differentiation, abnormal proliferation, and altered regulatory effects. Although the earliest genetic changes precede the relatively simultaneous occurrences of altered differentiation and proliferation, evolving genetic changes occur as carcinogenesis progresses. One important focus of combined clinical and basic research is to establish specific probes and markers for these carcinogenic steps. These probes would help identify individuals at highest risk of UADT cancer and would act as intermediate end-point markers for early evaluations of the efficacy of chemopreventive agents.[135]

Genetic Alterations The degree of genetic damage is a composite of carcinogen exposure and inherent tissue sensitivity. Genomic changes accumulate, presumably in the entire carcinogen-exposed tissue. Clonal malignant foci develop only in specific sites, however, where tumorigenesis is possible. Nonspecific (random) genomic alterations indicated by micronuclei, sister-chromatid exchanges, and aneuploidy can occur in normal, premalignant, and malignant aerodigestive tract tissue.[136–139] Although the fundamental genetic events associated with UADT cancers have not yet been established, several nonrandom chromosomal alterations (eg, alterations in chromosomes 1, 3, 5, 7, 8, 9, 10, 11, 13, and 17) have been detected in HNSCC (fresh-tissue and cell line studies).[136,138,140–142] Short-term cultures of oral premalignant cells may reveal early nonrandom cytogenetic changes.

Carcinogenesis is regulated by the balance between oncogenes and tumor-suppressor genes. This dynamic relationship is under intensive study in HNSCC.[143,144] Aberrant expression (amplifications or mutations) of specific families of cellular oncogenes such as *myc*, *ras*, *neu*, *bcl*, *int*, *ems-1*, *cyclin D1*, and *hst-1* are associated with aerodigestive tract carcinogenesis.[145–149] Up to one-third of cases of primary HNSCC demonstrate amplification of either the *int-2* or *hst-1* gene (both members of the fibroblast growth factor gene family) on chromosome 11q13.[145,150,151] Little is known, however, about when these events take place during the multistep process or what role their gene products play in regulating growth and differentiation. The families of *ras*, *neu*, and n-*myc* oncogenes are amplified in the more advanced stages of oral squamous cell carcinoma (SCC), and activated oncogenes of these families in vitro alter the response to differentiation agents and promote uncontrolled cellular growth, aneuploidy, and tumorigenicity.[146,149]

Differentiation Alterations Dysregulation of differentiation is another hallmark of multistep carcinogenesis. Human oral and esophageal epithelium is stratified squamous in type. Oral mucosa is noncornified except for the mucosa on the gingiva and dorsal surface of the tongue, which undergo keratinization. Cytokeratins, a family of at least 19 intermediate-sized filaments that range from 40 to 68 kDa, are expressed in different complex patterns that correlate with distinct types of epithelial differentiation and with carcinogenic progression.[152–154]

The spatial distribution of several cytokeratins, involucrin, transglutaminase I, and other differentiation antigens is also altered in dysplasia and carcinoma.[152,155–157]

Proliferation Alterations The third major phase of multistep carcinogenesis is dysregulated proliferation. The transition from normal epithelium to hyperplasia and dysplasia is associated with an increased growth fraction and cells proliferating beyond the basal layer. Older histologic assays have correlated this process with increased frequencies of mitotic figures. More recently, DNA flow cytometry and monoclonal-antibody probes to nuclear antigens (eg, Ki-67 and proliferating cell nuclear antigen [PCNA]) have revealed some strong positive correlations in UADT epithelium between abnormal suprabasal proliferation and later carcinogenic stages (severe dysplasia).[135,158,159]

Altered Regulatory Effects Epithelial carcinogenesis is also associated with the abnormal expression of cellular factors that regulate growth and development. The importance of these factors is inferred from their differential expression in normal and malignant tissues. For example, high expression of epidermal growth factor receptor (EGFR) is found in a significant fraction of experimental and human SCCs of the UADT.[160,161] EGFR gene activation occurs early in experimental oral carcinogenesis, and foci of cells expressing EGFR can be found in human premalignant lesions. Similarly, high expression of transforming growth factor-α (TGF-α) has been associated with malignant transformation of a variety of tumors (including oral cancers), and is frequently accompanied by elevated levels of EGFR in SCC.[162,163] The relationship between high TGF-α and high EGFR suggests that an autocrine loop mechanism drives the dysregulation of proliferation.

Molecular Biology As advances in molecular biology and biotechnology continue at a rapid pace, our understanding of the initiation and progression of carcinogenic processes will follow. The most frequent molecular abnormalities in these cancers, to date, are mutations in the tumor-suppressor gene *TP53*, which occur at a rate of approximately 40 to 70%.[164,165] Mutations of *TP53* are present in premalignant areas, including carcinoma in situ or moderate to severe dysplasia, in approximately 20% of cases.[166] No other oncogene or tumor-suppressor gene has been found to be mutated as frequently as *TP53* in head and neck tumor specimens.

Once a head and neck cancer has developed, its phenotypic behavior (the ability to invade, metastasize, respond to radiotherapy, and recur) is dependent on complex microenvironmental and biologic systems. Invasive and metastatic capabilities of a tumor depend on degradative enzymes, including collagenases, plasminogen activators (including urokinase), and cathepsin, as well as angiogenic factors, growth factors, cytokines, receptors, cell surface properties, and motility factors. The tumor milieu is also influenced by nerve fibers, stromal cells, and tumor-associated and tumor-infiltrating lymphocytes. All of these characteristics provide attractive targets for new and more specific therapeutic approaches.

Immunology A variety of immunologic abnormalities occur in HNSCC, but precise cause-and-effect relationships between abnormalities and cancer remain unclear.[167] Both cellular and humoral immunity have important implications for HNSCC prognosis and therapy.

Cell-mediated immunity may be involved in tumor control.[168] Defective cell-mediated immunity as determined by natural killer (NK) cell activity, skin tests, and other measures correlates with advanced disease, early recurrence, and poor survival. Large variations in tumor-infiltrating lymphocyte (TIL) levels in HNSCC have been reported. TILs in HNSCC are primarily CD31 T cells (NK cells are rare), and 30 to 50% of TILs express human leukocyte antigen (HLA)-DR– activation antigens. The prognostic significance of tumor-infiltrating cell subsets is unclear.[169,170]

HNSCC immunology has focused on humoral immune status. A large body of growing evidence suggests that humoral immunity plays a negative role in HNSCC.[171] Increased serum levels of immunoglobulin (Ig) A, IgM, and immune complexes are associated with advanced disease and poor prognosis.[172] Increased IgA can block many aspects of the host cell-mediated immune response, including cytotoxic effects of sensitized lymphocytes, NK cells, and macrophages, and IgG-mediated antibody-dependent cell-mediated cytotoxicity (ADCC). In contrast, increased IgE is associated with a good prognosis in HNSCC. The ratio of IgA to IgE, therefore, may be more predictive of prognosis than either IgA or IgE is individually. Post-treatment patterns of IgA and immune complexes differ; immune complex levels more accurately reflect tumor burden.

Although multiple and prominent immunologic deficits occur in HNSCC, immunologic therapeutic approaches (interferon-α [IFN-α], interleukin-2 [IL-2], plasmapheresis) have yielded only modest response rates and short response durations. The potential for more contemporary approaches including immunization, dendritic cell stimulation, and stem cell approaches are under development and investigation.

Biologic Goals Several nonrandom chromosomal alterations, activated oncogenes, and loss of heterozygosity (LOH) sites likely for tumor-suppressor genes are being actively investigated to develop informative biologic and predictive markers for HNSCC. The recent development of antibody probes for key gene products and molecular probes for gene transcripts should allow future study to identify the timing and sequence of gene alterations during multistep UADT carcinogenesis.

The proposed mechanisms of HNSCC invasion and metastasis are not well established. Recent studies have identified specific membrane proteins, degradative enzymes, and binding sites required for SCC invasion and metastasis (in animal models) and associated with early recurrence (in clinical studies).[155] This work opens the way to novel therapeutic approaches for future use of directed monoclonal antibodies/inhibitors to block key binding sites, thus preventing tumor invasion and metastasis.

Advances in molecular biology and biotechnology are also expanding our concept of the capabilities for molecular (or gene) therapy.[173,174] Novel intervention strategies are being developed that employ contemporary targeting of molecular mechanisms including regulating angiogenesis, invasion, and critical proliferative pathways.

Although agents to attack tumor via their growth factor receptors are of increasing interest to the clinician, it is possible to inadvertently activate these receptors to the detriment of overall outcome. Tumor hypoxia and the effect of low hemoglobin in the head and neck cancer patient has long been a subject of concern to the treating physician. Low hemoglobin may be associated with poor tumor oxygenation, which in turn may decrease the effectiveness of radiation therapy because of the "oxygen effect" on intrinsic radiosensitivity. The development of marrow stimulating agents such as recombinant erythropoietin (EPO) would seem to provide a straightforward way of addressing this problem. However, at least one study has demonstrated a probable deleterious effect with the use of this agent. Henke and colleagues[175] have reported on a randomized radiotherapy trial in which the patient group being treated with EPO fared worse than the group treated without this agent. Patients in this study had tumors of the oral cavity, oropharynx, hypopharynx, or larynx with both definitively treated and postoperative patients being included. For males, the HGB had to be less than 13.0 g/dcl and for females the HGB had to be less than 12.0 g/dcl for entry into the study. Patients were randomized to be treated with either EPO 300 IU/kg given subcutaneously 3 times weekly or a placebo injection given at the same frequency with a total of 351 patients being enrolled. The EPO clearly raised the HGB levels in the treated group, but there was a significant decrease in progression-free survival (at 4 years 28% vs 40%, p = .04). Although the specific reasons for this are still somewhat unclear, it has been hypothesized that tumor growth factor receptors may have been stimulated by the EPO. This prompted an early analysis of the Radiation Therapy Oncology Group (RTOG) 99-03, which also compared radiation + EPO to radiation alone in the head and neck cancer patient population with 135 patients being analyzed. This showed at 2 years a slight but nonsignificant reduction in local control on the radiation + EPO arm (43% vs 49%; $p = .46$) and survival (59% vs 65%; $p = .23$). It was deemed "highly unlikely" that this study would show a positive result if completed, and so it was closed early. Hence, it would seem that unless there are other compelling medical reasons, EPO should not be given to the head and neck cancer patient undergoing radiotherapy.

ANATOMY

The term "cancer of the head and neck" refers to a diverse collection of neoplasms of varying histologies arising from the variety of anatomic sites that make up the UADT.[176] This chapter, however, deals predominantly with squamous cell carcinoma of the UADT as it accounts for approximately 90% of the malignancies of the upper aerodigestive tract.[177] The UADT consists of a complex mucosa-covered conduit for food and air that extends from the vermilion surface of the lips to the cervical esophagus. In common usage, this terminology has been applied primarily to those cancers arising from the mucosal surfaces of the lips, oral cavity, pharynx, larynx, and cervical esophagus. Included in this designation, however, are other important sites, such as the nose and paranasal sinuses, salivary glands (major and minor), thyroid and parathyroid, and skin (both melanoma and nonmelanoma skin cancers). Some cancers arising in this region are typically excluded from the generic designation of head and neck cancer. Examples are tumors of the central nervous system, ocular neoplasms, primary tumors of lymphatic origin, and neural and endocrine malignancies.

Because of the diversity of sites and tissues of origin, the biology of tumor growth, patterns of metastases, natural boundaries for tumor extension, and signs and symptoms of disease are quite varied. The anatomy of the region has also dictated that optimal evaluation, diagnosis, and treatment require specific multidisciplinary expertise, including neurosurgery, otolaryngology, head and neck surgery, oral and maxillofacial surgery, cosmetic and reconstructive disciplines, and specialized radiology, pathology, radiation therapy, and chemotherapy, to name a few. The clinical manifestations of disease are varied and have a significant impact on the cosmetic and functional integrity of the head and neck region. Although the anatomic structures are only millimeters apart, the low metastatic potential and high curability of vocal cord cancers stand in extreme contrast to the early dissemination and grim prognosis of stage-matched pyriform sinus cancers.[178–183] Clinical differences between cancers in different sites are not explained solely by anatomic factors, but also by major biologic differences. Regrettably, the relatively small number of head and neck cancer patients often requires grouping many different types in each HNSCC therapy trial.[5] Associated morbidities of disease and treatment involve all of the special senses to varying degrees, notably speech, swallowing, smelling, breathing, and masticatory functions critically important for social interaction, a good quality of life, and ultimately, survival.

Oral Cavity The oral cavity is defined as starting at the vermilion border of the lips and extends posteriorly to include the lips, buccal mucosa, anterior tongue, floor of the mouth, hard palate, and upper and lower gingiva. The tongue occupies a major portion of the oral cavity and is contiguous with the floor of the mouth. The gingival mucosa overlying the mandibular and maxillary alveolar ridges adheres to the underlying periosteum. The hard palate forms the roof of the oral cavity and consists of mucosa overlying the palatine portion of the maxilla extending from the superior alveolar ridge to the junction with the soft palate, which lies in the oropharynx. Although the delineation between oral cavity and oropharynx might seem artificial, the distinction exists because of different disease patterns, differences in treatment approaches, and numerous functional considerations.

Pharynx The pharynx is a musculomembranous tube suspended from the skull base to the level of the sixth cervical vertebra, supported by overlapping constrictor muscles (superior, middle, and inferior) and other muscles arising from the styloid process and skull base.

This musculomembranous conduit communicates with the oral cavity anteriorly, the nasopharynx superiorly, and the hypopharynx and larynx inferiorly. It is divided into four sites of clinical importance: the tonsillar area, which makes up the major portion of the lateral pharyngeal wall and blends with the tongue base, soft palate, and retromolar trigone; the tongue base; the soft palate; and the posterior pharyngeal wall. Innervation of the pharynx is via the pharyngeal plexus, with contributions from the glossopharyngeal (sensory) and vagus nerves (motor and sensory).

The hypopharynx is divided into three distinct regions: the pyriform sinuses; the posterior surface of the larynx (postcricoid area); and the inferior, posterior, and lateral pharyngeal walls. The pyriform sinuses are paired mucosal pouches wrapped around the larynx, which funnel food around the larynx and into the esophagus. They are bounded superiorly by the pharyngoepiglottic folds and inferiorly by the cricoid cartilage. The sinuses come together at the esophageal introitus and cervical esophagus at the level of C6.

Larynx The larynx consists of a mucosally covered cartilaginous framework (thyroid and cricoid cartilages) suspended from the hyoid bone above by the thyrohyoid membrane and attached below to the trachea. The opening to the larynx is continuous with the pharyngeal airway. Unlike the rest of the pharynx, the mucosa of the larynx consists largely of columnar, ciliated, respiratory-type epithelium. Stratified squamous epithelium is found on the upper posterior epiglottis, aryepiglottic folds, and true vocal folds. It is important to note that although they are lymphatics in the upper larynx, they are sparse in the true vocal folds, or glottis.

The larynx is divided into three anatomic regions: the supraglottic larynx, the glottic larynx, and the subglottic larynx. The supraglottic larynx includes the epiglottis, aryepiglottic folds, laryngeal surface of the arytenoids, false vocal cords, and ventricles. The glottic larynx is derived from the tracheobronchial anlage and consists of both true vocal cords and the mucosa of the anterior and posterior commissures. It extends from the lateral-most apex of the laryngeal ventricle to 1 cm below the free edge of the vocal folds toward the cricoid. It has few, if any lymphatics. The subglottic larynx consists of the region bounded by the glottis above and the inferior border of the cricoid cartilage. Lymphatic supply to the subglottic larynx is extensive and bilateral. The infraglottic lymphatics drain to the cervical nodes through the cricothyroid membrane, while supraglottic lymphatics drain through the thyrohyoid membrane.

Nose and Paranasal Sinuses The term "nose and paranasal sinuses" refers to the region of the upper aerodigestive tract that starts at the vestibule of the nose anteriorly, is covered by squamous epithelium, and extends posteriorly to the posterior choana, where the nasopharynx begins. By definition, paranasal sinus malignancy does not include the nasopharynx unless by extension. It does include the paranasal sinuses, specifically, the maxillary, ethmoid, frontal, and sphenoid sinuses. Although the most common malignancy of the nose and paranasal sinuses is SCC, the nose and paranasal sinuses pose a particular set of problems that deserve separate consideration. As a result, the topic of nose and paranasal sinus malignancy is covered in a later section.

Neck Anatomic considerations in the treatment of cancers of the head and neck must include a thorough understanding of the neural, vascular, and, especially, the lymphatic structures of the neck. Detailed anatomic studies have described the organization of the lymphatic drainage of the UADT. Specific regions of the head and neck and the tumors that arise there have lymphatic drainage that is consistent and predictable. There are 12 major groups of lymph nodes (six each bilaterally) in the head and neck (Figure 79-1),[184] although only levels I to V play a major role in aerodigestive tract squamous cell carcinoma of the head and neck (SCCHN). Primary and secondary echelons of lymph node drainage have been derived for each major region of the head and neck mucosa. A standard rule of thumb is that the lymphatic drainage for any particular region is predicted by the arterial supply of that region. The lip, cheek, and anterior gingiva drain to submandibular and submental lymph node groups. In addition, the cheek and upper lip also drain to inferior parotid and facial nodes, while the posterior gingiva and palate drain to the internal jugular chain and lateral retropharyngeal groups. Lymphatic drainage for the tongue

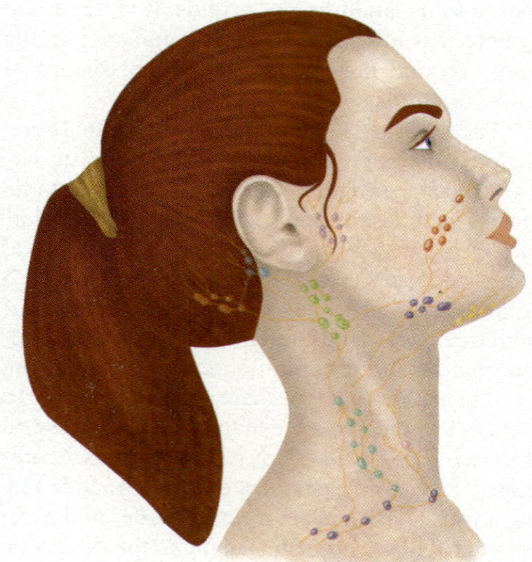

Figure 79-1 Major lymph node groups in the head and neck. These include occipital, mastoid, parotid, submandibular, facial, submental, sublingual, retropharyngeal, anterior cervical, and lateral cervical lymph node groups.

drains to the internal jugular, subdigastric, omohyoid, submandibular, and submental nodal groups. Midline lesions often drain bilaterally. Although metastases to the lower neck nodes are infrequent from the oral cavity, generally the more anterior the tumor location in the tongue, the more likely it is that metastases also will spread to lower jugular nodes. The floor-of-mouth drainage is similar to that of the tongue. The upper portion of the pharynx drains directly to the upper cervical lymph nodes along the internal jugular chain. The oropharynx and tonsil drain through the parapharyngeal space to the midjugular region, particularly to the jugulodigastric nodes. Retro and lateral pharyngeal nodes can also be involved. The regions of the hypopharynx and larynx drain primarily along the routes of their vascular supply to either the deep cervical nodes along the midjugular (upper pharynx, larynx) or the deep nodes along the lower jugular and paratracheal region (lower pharynx, larynx).

For the purposes of local treatment, the various lymph node groups of the neck have been divided into levels. Level I includes the submental group of nodes (IA), located within the triangle bounded by the anterior belly of the digastric muscles and the hyoid bone, and the submandibular group (IB), bounded by both bellies of the digastric muscle and the body of the mandible. Level II nodes consist of the upper jugular lymph nodes located in proximity to the upper third of the internal jugular vein and extending from the skull base to the level of the bifurcation of the carotid artery. The anterior and posterior boundaries are the lateral border of the sternohyoid muscle and the posterior border of the sternocleidomastoid muscle, respectively. Level II is further divided into those lymph nodes located anteroinferior to the vertical plane of the spinal accessory nerve (IIA) and those lymph nodes posterosuperior to the nerve (IIB). Level III nodes include those nodes located adjacent to the middle third of the internal jugular vein from the carotid bifurcation to the plane marked by the omohyoid muscle's crossing over the jugular vein (the level of the cricothyroid notch). Anterior and posterior boundaries are the same as level II. Level IV nodes include the lower jugular group extending from omohyoid muscle above to the clavicle below. Level V nodes are those located along the lower half of the spinal accessory nerve and transverse cervical artery. This level is bounded by the anterior border of the trapezius muscle, the posterior border of the sternocleidomastoid muscle, and the clavicle below. This level, too, is further divided into Va and Vb nodes, with Va nodes being those nodes located above the plane along the inferior edge of the cricoid and including the chain of nodes along the spinal accessory nerve posterior to the sternocleidomastoid muscle. Vb nodes are the nodes below the cricoid plane and include the nodes along the transverse cervical artery and all of the supraclavicular fossa.

DIAGNOSIS AND STAGING

The identification and appropriate management of malignant mucosal lesions in the head and neck are important aspects of patient care that have major impact on overall survival rates. Since stage (extent) of disease at the time of diagnosis is the most important prognostic factor in the treatment of HNSCC, the identification and early treatment of small cancers correlates with excellent survival. Most early premalignant changes or in situ carcinomas of the oral mucosa occur as red (erythroplasia) or white (leukoplakia) patches that may be readily apparent on visual examination. In areas less easily visualized directly, such as the larynx and hypopharynx, early lesions cause such symptoms as chronic hoarseness and sore throat and, later, referred otalgia, or dysphagia. Such symptoms demand visualization of the larynx and hypopharynx usually by fiberoptic approaches.

Appropriate management of leukoplakia and erythroplasia lesions includes a high index of suspicion, particularly in high-risk individuals. The molecular markers aneuploidy and loss of heterozygosity (LOH) indicate high cancer risk in dysplastic oral IEN.[120,185] Although both lesions are considered premalignant, erythroplasia lesions are of greater clinical concern, since approximately half of these lesions contain carcinoma in situ (CIS) or invasive cancer. Additionally, often erythroplasia and leukoplakia may coexist.[131,132] Erythroplasia mandates biopsy to rule out invasive cancer. The management of erythroplasia and leukoplakia depends on the location, extent, and histology. The diffuse field effect and multifocal nature of the epithelial carcinogenic process support the need for effective prevention. White lesions can be confused with mucositis; lichen planus; local tissue irritation from mechanical, thermal, or chemical trauma; histoplasmosis; candidiasis; and other infectious processes. Lesions that persist despite the removal of local irritating factors or that are associated with ulceration, vertical growth, induration, a recent change in size, or pain should be sampled by biopsy and/or excised, although complete surgical resection (as defined by the absence of dysplasia at the margins) does not prevent oral carcinoma development in cases of aneuploid dysplastic leukoplakia,[120] a setting in which molecular-targeted chemoprevention with inhibitors of EGFR and cyclooxygenase-2 shows great promise.[186] Complete resection, however, can reduce the relatively low cancer rate associated with diploid dysplastic leukoplakia. Complete resection of oral IEN stratified by LOH did not statistically significantly reduce the overall risk of cancer, but did significantly reduce the cancer risk associated with molecular high-risk lesions (defined by LOH patterns) when complete resection was confirmed molecularly (versus when not).[187] These findings reflect the critical importance of molecular confirmation of complete resection of oral IEN, in which the surgical margins are often narrow, nonexistent, or not assessed. Future research in this area should evaluate the roles of optimal surgical margin width and complete resection as confirmed by molecular analyses in reducing the cancer risk associated with molecularly defined high-risk oral IEN. Topical supravital staining with toluidine blue of suspicious lesions can be helpful in identifying areas for biopsy and in screening high-risk populations. Toluidine blue staining recently was found to be associated with the presence of LOH in dysplastic, minimally dysplastic, or nondysplastic oral IEN, which suggests the potential of toluidine blue for identifying oral IEN with a molecularly marked high risk of cancer and perhaps for helping guide surgical margin widths.[188,189] Dysphagia, odynophagia, otalgia, hoarseness, mucosal irregularities and ulceration, pain, weight loss, and the presence of an unexplained neck mass are the most common presenting symptoms of invasive HNSCC. The predominant symptoms vary with the site: Chronic dysphagia or odynophagia (for 6 weeks or even less) demands thorough visualization of the oropharynx, hypopharynx, and esophagus; chronic hoarseness demands visualization of the larynx; chronic unilateral serous otitis media in an adult is a result of cancer of the nasopharynx blocking the eustachian tube until proven otherwise; and unilateral nasal polyps, nasal obstruction, or epistaxis is a common presenting sign of nasal cavity or paranasal sinus neoplasms. A firm or hard unilateral neck mass represents cancer until proven otherwise. In persons older than 20 years, such a mass represents neoplasm more than 80% of the time, and 80% of these neoplasms are due to metastatic spread from an UADT primary.

In patients presenting with a suspicious neck mass, a complete head and neck examination usually reveals the primary malignant tumor. If it does not, a thorough search for occult primary cancers both above and below the clavicles is warranted. Technologic advances in fiber optics and in flexible and rigid endoscopes now provide excellent upper airway visualization that previously required special skills in indirect mirror examination. Endoscopic evaluation should include the nasopharynx, oropharynx, hypopharynx, larynx, and upper esophagus. Endoscopic evaluation should be accompanied by chest radiography. If these fail to reveal a primary, then consideration should be given for esophagoscopy as well, since it is much more sensitive for mucosal lesions of the esophagus than is computerized tomography. Most commonly, occult primaries responsible for neck metastases occur in the nasopharynx, tongue base, tonsil, or hypopharynx. In the absence of an identifiable mass, directed biopsies of these sites are indicated during endoscopic evaluation, and, if present, bilateral tonsillectomies should be performed if a primary is not identified. Metastasis to a solitary left supraclavicular lymph node (Virchow's node) is occasionally seen with infraclavicular cancer, especially colon cancer. Generally, isolated metastatic supraclavicular masses (level IV) derive from breast, lung, or infradiaphragmatic neoplasms. Thyroid malignancies may also metastasize to this area.

Three-dimensional imaging with computed tomography (CT) and magnetic resonance imaging (MRI) is frequently used to supplement the clinical evaluation and staging of the primary tumor and regional lymph nodes. More recently, positron emission tomography (PET), especially when combined with tomography (PET-CT), has shown efficacy in the identification of occult primaries and is gaining widespread use. Prior to examination under anesthesia, if no primary is suggested upon comprehensive head and neck physical examination, a PET scan should be considered.

Only after a thorough search for a primary tumor has been completed should a neck mass undergo biopsy. We recommend fine-needle aspiration (FNA) biopsy.[74] If an excisional biopsy is required because FNA is inconclusive or not feasible, then the surgeon and patient should be prepared for definitive neck dissection if the mass should prove to be metastatic squamous cell carcinoma. The potential ramifications of false-negative results on FNA are inherently obvious. Accuracy of the cytologic interpretation of the aspirate is directly dependent on the skill and experience of the pathologist.

Staging criteria for cancers arising in the UADT, paranasal sinuses, and salivary glands have been developed by the American Joint Committee on Cancer (AJCC) (Table 79-1). The criteria undergo regular reevaluation and modification. The stage groupings used for head and neck cancer are based on T (primary tumor), N (regional node), and M (distant metastasis) designations. Because of variations in the growth, behavior, and prognosis of head and neck cancers according to site of origin and extent, differences exist in the staging criteria for each anatomic site. Staging criteria for the primary lesion are site specific. However, except for tumors arising in the nasopharynx and those of the thyroid, there is uniformity in the nodal staging criteria and stage grouping (Table 79-2).

Table 79-2 Clinical Tumor Staging Characteristics for Regional Lymph Nodes and Distant Metastases

Regional Lymph Nodes	
Nx	Regional lymph nodes cannot be assessed
N0	No evidence of regional lymph node metastases
N1	Metastasis in single, ipsilateral regional lymph node < 3 cm in greatest dimension
N2a	Metastasis in single, ipsilateral regional lymph node between 3 and 6 cm in greatest dimension
N2b	Metastasis in multiple ipsilateral regional lymph nodes, none > 6 cm in greatest dimension
N2c	Metastasis in bilateral or contralateral regional lymph nodes, none > 6 cm in greatest dimension
N3	Metastasis to regional lymph node > 6 cm in greatest dimension
Distant Metastases	
Mx	Presence of distant metastasis cannot be assessed
M0	No evidence of distant metastasis
M1	Distant metastases are present in one or more locations

Careful documentation of tumor extent and accurate staging classification are also important for the comparison of the results of different treatment regimens. Accurate evaluation of the results of a given treatment or the efficacy of new treatment strategies requires comparisons with patient groups with tumors of similar extent and behavior. Restaging after treatment or for recurrent cancers must be clearly designated and separate from the primary staging of previously untreated cancers. Postsurgical, or pathologic, staging is gaining importance in the primary treatment of head and neck cancers because of the increasing use of postoperative radiation therapy and/or adjuvant chemotherapy for patients with locally aggressive tumors or extracapsular spread into the soft tissues of the neck.[190]

It should be noted, however, that as good as the widely accepted AJCC staging system is for head and neck cancer, it still falls short in that it too often fails to distinguish between deeply infiltrative tumors and those that are superficial or exophytic. Experience shows that this distinction is an important one and can have a significant impact on survival.

Table 79-1 Clinical Tumor Stage and Groupings for Head and Neck Cancer

Stage 0	Tis	N0	M0
Stage 1	T1	N0	M0
Stage 2	T2	N0	M0
Stage 3	T3	N0	M0
	T1	N1	M0
	T2	N1	M0
	T3	N1	M0
Stage 4	T4	Any N	M0
	Any T	N2 or N3	M0
	Any T	Any N	M1

TREATMENT

General Principles After a histologic diagnosis has been established and tumor extent determined, the selection of appropriate treatment of a specific cancer depends on a complex array of variables, including tumor site, relative morbidity of various treatment options, patient performance and nutritional status, concomitant health problems, social and logistic factors, therapy anticipated for potential recurrences or second primaries, and patient preference. These variables are each considered with respect to the established effectiveness of various treatment regimens available.

The overall management goals in treating patients with head and neck cancer are to achieve the highest cure rates at the lowest cost in terms of functional and cosmetic morbidity. These goals include early diagnosis, effective rehabilitation, and appropriate palliation, when indicated. The achievement of these goals requires the close cooperation of an interdisciplinary team of practitioners representing surgery, radiation, chemotherapy, prosthodontics, dentistry, speech language pathology, social services, dietetics, physical and rehabilitative medicine, pathology, nursing, and often psychiatry.

Effective rehabilitation is an important part of the overall treatment of head and neck cancers. Modern advances in surgical reconstruction, microvascular free-tissue transfer, and prosthodontics have significantly improved post-treatment function.[191] Rehabilitation concerns must be addressed at initial treatment planning and carefully integrated with the various treatment modalities used. Pretreatment dental evaluations and speech and swallowing assessments are routine. Needed dental care and/or extractions should be planned prior to chemotherapy or radiation to reduce the risks of dental-associated sepsis, mucositis, and osteoradionecrosis. The overall impact of treatment and rehabilitation decisions on a patient's quality of life is an important issue that may require specialized social or psychiatric support systems for the patient and family. Furthermore, attention must be paid to nutritional support. Contemporary combined approaches of chemotherapy and radiotherapy place a long-term burden on the patient that must be compensated. Indeed, it is this close attention to nutrition and supplementation that makes possible aggressive treatment regimens. Finally, the prolonged nature of treatment of advanced disease, which may extend over many months, requires consideration of the social and financial impact of treatment decisions on the patient, the family, and the patient's career.

Biopsies of primary tumors need not be excisional unless the biopsy procedure is sufficient for definitive treatment, and the surgeon performing the excision is responsible for providing curative treatment. Oncologic principles of surgical resection must not be compromised by ill-conceived reconstructive efforts or attempts at modi-

Table 79-3 Primary Tumor Staging Characteristics for Oral Cavity Carcinoma

Tx	Primary tumor cannot be assessed (as occurs after excisional biopsy)
T0	No evidence of primary (as in unknown primary tumors)
Tis	Carcinoma in situ
T1	Tumor is 2 cm or less in greatest dimension
T2	Tumor is between 2 and 4 cm in greatest dimension
T3	Tumor is > 4 cm in greatest dimension
T4	Tumor invades adjacent structures (through cortical bone, into maxillary sinus, skin, deep tissue, nerve)
	a: resectable
	b: unresectable

fying the necessary resection in order to minimize functional or cosmetic morbidity. Head and neck cancers are serious threats to life. Temporary preservation of function at the cost of a high risk of recurrence, high morbidity, or death is a poor bargain. Gross residual cancer or positive surgical margins after tumor resection portend inevitable treatment failure. Appropriate management must also include the use of precise modern techniques of conservative surgical resection (eg, partial laryngectomy and functional neck dissection) that, in selected patients, have cure rates similar to those of more radical techniques.[192]

General Overview of Natural History and Treatment by Site: Oral Cavity Both tumor and treatment significantly compromise speech and deglutition, particularly for those patients in whom cancer involves the tongue, the floor of the mouth, or the mandible. Furthermore, the diversity of potential sites of cancer development in the oral cavity and variations of lymphatic drainage and rates of node metastases lend added complexity to treatment planning.[193,194] Despite the fact that this region is readily amenable to visual examination and bimanual palpation, more than 50% of patients are diagnosed in advanced stages. The current T-staging of oral cavity primaries is presented in Table 79-3.

Lips SCCs of the lip are the most common oral cavity cancers. Over 90% occur on the lower lip, usually on the exposed vermilion border, midway between the midline and the oral commissure. Upper lip cancers are most commonly basal cell carcinomas.[195] Well-differentiated and verrucous cancers rarely metastasize. Poorly differentiated and spindle cell varieties tend to grow aggressively and metastasize commonly. Perineural infiltration of large nerves is indicative of aggressive disease and requires aggressive, often combined therapies.

The treatment of lip cancers must consider adequate removal of the disease and yet provide the patient with a lip that functions in speech and chewing and that retains oral competence and adequate cosmesis.[196,197] These goals are achieved equally well with either primary radiation or surgery when the tumors are less than 2 cm in size or are very superficial. Larger lesions, however, are best treated with surgical resection and reconstruction, which allows for greater accuracy in evaluating the extent of tumor and nerve or lymphatic involvement.[198,199] Frequently, adjacent precancerous changes are present that can also be treated with surgery (lip shaving and advancement) to prevent recurrences or the development of second primary tumors.[200,201] For larger lesions, primary reconstruction with local, regional, and sometimes free-tissue flaps avoids defects that result from tissue loss with radiotherapy, provides for future reconstructive and treatment options, and decreases the very real risk of osteoradionecrosis of the mandible. Lesions demonstrating extensive infiltration, bone involvement, or lymphatic metastases should be managed with combined surgery and postoperative radiation.

Radiation therapy techniques for management of lip cancers include external irradiation, interstitial implants, and combinations of both. Local tumor control rates with irradiation exceed 80%,[202–204] with determinant survival at 5 years (including surgical salvage) in excess of 95%. Similar tumor control and survival rates are reported with primary surgical excision.[205] Regional metastasis decreases the survival rates to 36 to 55%.[202,206] Five-year survival rates for patients with carcinomas of the upper lip are lower than for those with similar lower-lip lesions and range from 40 to 60%.[207,208] Involvement of both lips and the lateral commissure is uncommon. The prognosis for commissure lesions is not as good as for cancers of other areas of the lip. Cross reports a 5-year survival rate of 34% for patients with oral commissure carcinoma.[206]

Tongue Tongue cancers account for over 25% of oral cavity SCCs and most commonly arise in the anterior two-thirds of the tongue on the lateral or ventral surface. Squamous cell carcinomas on the dorsum of the tongue are rare. Infiltration of the underlying tongue musculature occurs early. The intrinsic tongue muscles are loosely arranged and endowed with a rich vascular and lymphatic supply, which may explain the high rate of regional metastases and extracapsular spread. Prognosis is directly related to the degree of infiltration and the presence of regional metastases and extracapsular spread. The biologic aggressiveness of small (< 4 cm) tongue cancers is noteworthy and is reflected in higher rates of occult regional metastases than those of similarly staged lesions arising from other oral sites (Table 79-4). Occult nodal metastases are present in 30

Table 79-4 Representative Local Control Rates and Survival for Patients with Squamous Cell Carcinomas of Common Head and Neck Sites Treated with Definitive Radiotherapy

Stage by Site			Local Control	Survival
Oral Cavity	Oral Tongue	T1	80–90	75–80
		T2	60–85	40–60
		T3	30–50	20–30
		T4	25–45	10–15
	Floor of Mouth	T1	75–85	70–85
		T2	60–80	50–60
		T3	30–50	15–40
		T4	5–30	5–20
Oropharynx	Base of Tongue	T1	80–95	65–85
		T2	60–75	40–55
		T3	40–65	15–20
		T4	30–50	5–20
	Tonsil/Tonsillar Pillar	T1	75–95	65–85
		T2	60–80	55–60
		T3	35–70	20–40
		T4	20–30	10–15
	Soft Palate	T1	90–100	90–95
		T2	75–85	65–75
		T3	60–70	25–50
		T4	25–35	5–30
Nasopharynx	Nasopharynx	T1	70–85	60–75
		T2	50–60	50–65
		T3	20–45	25–50
		T4	15–35	5–30
Hypopharynx	Pyriform Sinus	T1	60–70	30–50
		T2	40–50	20–45
		T3	30–40	15–25
		T4	10–25	5–20
Larynx	Supraglottic Larynx	T1	80–90	65–90
		T2	60–80	50–65
		T3	35–70	35–55
		T4	30–60	15–40
	Glottic Larynx	T1	85–95	80–95
		T2	65–75	60–85
		T3	20–35	35–60
		T4	15–0	10–30

Local control rates are for radiation therapy alone. Survival data includes surgical salvage for radiation failures. Overlap in data is due to data coming from different institutions and differences in comorbidities.

to 40% of early lesions.[209–212] Approximately 40% of patients have clinical evidence of node metastases at diagnosis.[213] Primary echelon node drainage is to the upper deep cervical lymphatics; however, involvement of middle and lower neck nodes (levels III and IV) is not uncommon. Bilateral nodal involvement can occur with cancers of the tip or the midline of the tongue. Locoregional recurrence in patients with tongue cancer accounts for 60 to 70% of cancer deaths.[214–216] Distant metastases account for 15% of deaths, and second primaries account for 20 to 40%. The role of lymphatic mapping in oral tongue cancer has been established regarding feasibility but controlled studies evaluating long-term control as compared with planned elective neck dissections are under way.

The management of carcinomas of the tongue has been significantly influenced by a better appreciation of the aggressiveness of small deeply infiltrative lesions, the high rate of occult lymph node metastases, and an interest in improving treatment without unnecessarily compromising oral function. Although surgical excision alone has been the mainstay of treatment, combined surgery and adjuvant radiation therapy to include the primary site and regional nodes is commonly used for most advanced cancers (stages III and IV) and is being used increasingly for small stage II cancers that exhibit pathologic indicators of lymph node metastasis or perineural invasion. Concomitant chemoradiotherapy is used for adverse pathologic findings of perineural invasion and extensive extracapsular lymph node extension.

For stage I cancers, surgical excision is effective and expeditious, with excellent preservation of function. For stage II lesions that are infiltrative, hemiglossectomy or partial glossectomy achieves excellent tumor control rates and should be combined with modified dissection of neck nodes (supraomohyoid dissections) to provide accurate information about staging and determine the need for adjuvant treatment, specifically, postoperative radiotherapy. Hemiglossectomy may result in some functional morbidity in terms of articulation and deglutition. Because of this, radiation therapy may be used in selected cases. Nevertheless, surgery should remain the mainstay of treatment in oral tongue malignancies. Free-tissue transfer reconstruction can significantly offset the morbidity of hemiglossectomy. For radiation to be as effective as surgery in controlling these cancers, interstitial brachytherapy combined with external radiation is essential. Radiation doses of 80 to 85 Gy are generally given via external megavoltage radiation or in combination with brachytherapy. Such high doses, however, are associated with osteoradionecrosis, fibrosis, and impaired function, and as a result, primary treatment of oral cavity SCC with radiation therapy has fallen out of favor. Interstitial treatment requires precise placement and spacing of implants. Accurate dosimetry is enhanced by using afterloading techniques in which the radioactive source is inserted into previously (TD-3) placed hollow tubes. Tracheostomy at the time of implantation is usually needed because of the potential development of tongue edema after implantation. Occult or apparent neck disease is usually treated using external radiation or radiation combined with neck dissection.[209] The complexity and morbidity of these radiation-based therapies has resulted in surgery as the foundation of oral cavity carcinoma therapy.

Extension of cancer to the floor of the mouth or the mandible may necessitate partial mandibulectomy or segmental mandibular resection. Modern reconstructive techniques with vascularized composite bone and soft-tissue free flaps, titanium metal prostheses, and dental implants have improved the functional and cosmetic results of major mandibular resections. An elective neck dissection is recommended for all lesions with greater than 4 mm of invasion owing to the risk of nodal disease. When tumors grossly involve bone, radiation therapy is less effective in these poorly vascularized tissues and requires high doses that are associated with osteoradionecrosis. After local failure of interstitial radiotherapy implants, complication rates for salvage surgical resections are extremely high and are associated with significant morbidity from fistulization, radionecrosis, and failure of primary reconstructive efforts. Although the surgical salvage of radiation failures is often successful in early lesions, success drops to less than 50% in advanced lesions.

For more advanced primary lesions (stages III and IV), surgery and external radiation are generally used. Although radiation has been administered as either planned preoperative or postoperative therapy, currently postoperative treatment is recommended. Although no prospective controlled trials have proved the superiority of combined therapy over surgery alone for disease without nodal metastases, many studies indicate improved locoregional control rates.[7,217–220] These improvements have generally been offset, in part, by an increased frequency of distant metastases and second primaries. Surgical management generally consists of partial glossectomy and neck dissection, with the mandible being spared unless directly involved. In instances with limited periosteal invasion, coronal and other partial mandibular resections can be performed that spare mandibular continuity and maintain function. Where tumors extend to the midline or involve the tongue base, subtotal or total glossectomy may be necessary. Continued improvements in reconstructive techniques have improved the functional results of these aggressive resections. Provision for temporary tracheostomy and prolonged enteral nutrition should be made. Total glossectomy or sacrifice of both hypoglossal nerves frequently necessitates permanent feeding gastrostomy. Current experience indicates that total glossectomy can, in highly select patients, be accomplished without the need for laryngectomy although prolonged or even permanent parenteral feeding will likely be required.[221]

Tumor resection is more difficult after preoperative radiation therapy unless precise tattooing of intended resection margins is accomplished prior to therapy. Likewise, the rates of surgical complications, fistulization, exposed bone, and radionecrosis may be increased with preoperative radiation, although studies have been conflicting. Because of this, most centers have adopted a policy of postoperative radiation; with postoperative radiation, the extent of disease is precisely defined, the histologic status of the lymph nodes is known, and high-risk areas of close margins or residual cancer can be treated to a high dose or concomitant chemoradiotherapy prescribed. For advanced oral cavity cancers, both ipsilateral and contralateral necks are irradiated, with the dosage determined by the extent of disease. Postoperative radiation should begin within 3 to 6 weeks of resection. Interstitial implants are not used. Close surgical margins require high doses (70 Gy) because of the difficulty in eradicating even small amounts of tumor in the tongue after glossectomy.[222] Curative radiation alone with surgical salvage has been shown to be inferior to combined therapy in control of locoregional disease and in the complication rate, even though survival rates are similar with these approaches.[223,224] Even with combined therapy, estimated 2-year disease-free and overall survival rates for advanced disease are only 51% and 53%, respectively.[225] The 5-year survival rates range from 50 to 70% for stages I and II to 15 to 30% for stages III and IV.[214]

The management of the neck is of particular interest in patients with tongue cancer because of the high rate of nodal metastases. For T2 or larger lesions, rates of occult metastases exceed 40%, and some form of neck treatment is generally indicated. When the primary tumor can be adequately excised via a transoral technique, unilateral or bilateral neck dissections should be performed based on the location of the primary disease. Concomitant chemoradiotherapy should be used postoperatively if there is perineural spread or if there is extracapsular spread outside a lymph node. Radiation therapy alone should be considered when there is more than one metastatic lymph node.

Floor of Mouth Floor-of-mouth (FOM) cancers occur with a frequency similar to that of tongue cancer. Early spread to adjacent areas (gingiva and periosteum of the mandible) is common. The periosteum is a natural barrier to invasion. Fixation of the tongue is a sign of deep invasion. The tumor may extend to or through the mylohyoid muscle, which serves as a natural barrier to direct spread below the hyoid bone. Lymph node metastases at presentation are seen in approximately 40% of patients, and an additional 20% have occult lymphatic metastases.[210] The occult metastatic rate increases with the T stage of the primary: T2 tumors have a 40% and T3 tumors a 70% occult metastasis rate.

First-echelon nodes of lymphatic drainage include the submandibular and jugulodigastric lymph nodes (levels I and II). Submental node involvement is comparatively less frequent. Evaluation for early mandibular involvement is facilitated by palpation since fixation to the mandible indicates periosteal involvement and direct bone invasion is present in 50 to 60% of such tumors. This distinction is often aided with bone windows on computed tomography.

Small cancers (T1, T2) are generally treated effectively by wide resection. Lateral floor-of-mouth tumors can often be resected transorally and the resection defect closed with the advancement of adjacent mucosa, skin grafts, or secondary intention. Oftentimes, however, an elective limited neck dissection is performed for even the smallest of these tumors because scarring in the FOM can lead to obstruction of the sublingual and submandibular glands, a painful situation that can even be confused with nodal disease. Elective neck dissection at the time of resection avoids this problem. Plasty of the severed submandibular duct can be performed for superficial lesions. Early cancers involving the mandible are best treated surgically because bone involvement compromises radiation efficacy. Surgery remains the mainstay of treatment of early FOM malignancies, achieving excellent functional and curative results.

Exclusive radiation therapy for small FOM cancers usually involves combinations of external radiation and brachytherapy. Decision making concerning primary therapy takes into consideration the expected functional result, the management of the neck nodes, and the risk of osteoradionecrosis. Radiotherapy for moderate size (T2) anterior FOM lesions and small or deeply invasive cancers must also include treating bilateral first-echelon lymph nodes due to the high rate of occult lymph node metastases.

More advanced FOM cancers (T3, T4) are generally treated with resection combined with similar approaches to that described for oral tongue cancers in the prior section. Again, mandibular continuity-sparing procedures with cortectomies can often be employed. In these instances, we have found fasciocutaneous flaps to offer excellent FOM and tongue reconstructive potential. Large surgical defects are reconstructed with skin grafts, local flaps, myocutaneous pedicled regional flaps, and, frequently, free-tissue transfers. Mandibular reconstruction for segmental defects is performed primarily with composite free-tissue transfers.

Doses of radiation therapy for locoregional tumor control are based on actual tumor volume rather than T stage.[226] Interstitial doses of 65 to 75 Gy are recommended for early lesions (1–3 cm) if brachytherapy alone is used, or external beam radiation of 50 Gy combined with 25 to 30 Gy of interstitial radiation. Postoperative doses are given by external radiation only at doses of 65 Gy over 6 to 7 weeks, or preoperative doses of 50 Gy over 6 weeks. No significant differences in overall survival rates have been shown when comparing preoperative and postoperative radiation regimens.[224]

Treatment results are influenced by the size of the primary tumor, presence of lymph node metastases, degree of mandibular involvement, and adequacy of resection. The 5-year survival rates for localized stage I and II FOM carcinomas range from 60 to 80%. Cancers that cross the midline or involve the tongue or the mandible are associated with 5-year survival rates of 50 to 60%.[227] Survival rates for more advanced lesions (stages III and IV) are less than 50%. Lymph node metastases decrease survival rates to approximately 25%. The major advantage of combined treatment (radiation and surgery) in these patients is improved control of ipsilateral and contralateral neck disease. Because rates of occult nodal disease are high in advanced primary lesions, elective treatment of the neck with radiation or bilateral neck dissections is indicated. Recurrence in the untreated, clinically negative neck is the most frequent site of failure in patients treated only with surgery.[228]

The debate over performing elective neck dissection versus irradiation remains unresolved. If adequate primary tumor margins are uncertain or if multiple histologically positive lymph node metastases are detected, postoperative radiation to the ipsilateral and contralateral neck is administered. The development of second primary cancers is a major cause of morbidity and death. Fu and colleagues reported that 55 of 153 (36%) patients developed second primaries, of whom 30 died of their second cancer.[229] Distant metastases occur in 10 to 15% of patients.[228,229]

Gingival and Buccal Mucosa Gingival cancers occur most commonly (80%) in the lower gingiva, posterior to the bicuspids.[230] For both sites, trismus is an ominous sign indicating extension to the masseter or pterygoid muscles. Clinical staging criteria are similar to those for other oral sites. Overall, regional metastases occur in approximately 15% of gingival cancers.[231] Recently, occult nodal metastases have been documented in as high as 30% of buccal cancers and elective neck dissection recommended in all but the earliest of cancers.[232] Exophytic tumors tend to be papillary or verrucous in appearance and can be confused with benign hyperkeratosis.

Small, superficial gingival cancers can be effectively treated with surgical resection with excellent preservation of function.[233] Generally, the amount of bone resected for small lesions is minimal and resection can be accomplished transorally. Even larger lesions requiring partial maxillectomy or alveolectomy can be resected without external incision. External beam irradiation is not as effective in local tumor control once gross bone involvement has occurred. The intermediate (T2 or larger) lesions are best handled surgically; the risk of osteoradionecrosis is thereby avoided. For larger lesions (T3 and T4), segmental mandibulectomy and/or maxillectomy is required, and adjuvant radiation is frequently recommended. Elective neck dissection is not mandated unless the en bloc resection of a large primary tumor requires neck exposure. Ultrasound or high-resolution CT scanning should be utilized if no therapy is being considered for the neck. Clinically positive neck nodes warrant neck dissection at the time of the resection of the primary tumor.

Buccal carcinomas of early stage (I or II) can be treated equally well with surgery or radiation. Radiation therapy offers the advantage of including the draining lymphatics in the treatment fields, but also risks post-treatment fibrosis and trismus. Large primary tumors or tumors with regional metastases are managed surgically, with the need for adjuvant radiation as previously described.

Overall survival rates for gingival and buccal cancers depend on tumor size, bone involvement, and node metastases. The 5-year survival rates for gingival lesions range from 78% for stage I to 15% for stage IV disease.[234] Surgical results are clearly superior to those of radiation when bone involvement is present. Survival rates (5-year) for stages I and II buccal carcinomas range from 65 to 75%. Determinant survival for stages III and IV disease varies from 20 to 30%.[231] For both gingival and buccal mucosal cancers, overall survival rates have improved over recent years as surgical management has replaced radiation therapy as the primary treatment.

Retromolar Trigone Cancers arising in the retromolar trigone (the narrow band of mucosa that lies behind the mandibular molars and covers the ascending ramus of the mandible) are rarely confined to that gingiva, but involve adjacent buccal mucosa, anterior tonsillar pillar, the floor of the mouth, and/or posterior gingiva. Thus, retromolar trigone cancers that involve the anterior tonsillar pillar behave more like oropharyngeal cancers than like oral cavity primaries. The risk of clinically positive and occult lymph node metastases is higher than with other gingival cancers. The frequent involvement of periosteum mandates partial (rim or marginal) mandibulectomy as part of the surgical management, even for small lesions. Primary radiation therapy is reserved for superficial lesions that cover a large surface area, such as extension to the soft palate or buccal mucosa, and remain mobile. Moderately advanced or deeply invasive lesions are best treated with surgical resection (mandibulectomy and neck dissection), followed by postoperative adjuvant therapy, as indicated.

Oropharynx The clinical staging of oropharyngeal cancers depends primarily on tumor size and is similar to the staging of oral cavity cancers (Table 79-5). Although tumors may arise from any

Table 79-5 Primary Tumor Staging Characteristics for Cancer of the Oropharynx

Tx	Tumor cannot be assessed (as occurs with previous biopsy)
T0	There is no evidence of a primary (as occurs with an unknown primary)
Tis	Carcinoma in situ
T1	Tumor is < 2 cm in greatest dimension
T2	Tumor is between 2 and 4 cm in greatest dimension
T3	Tumor is > 4 cm in greatest dimension
T4	Tumor invades adjacent structures (through cortical bone, muscles of mastication, nerve, deep muscles of tongue, larynx) a: resectable b: unresectable

site in the oropharynx, they arise most commonly from the palatine arch, which includes the tonsillar fossa and base of the tongue. Although traditionally patients with oropharyngeal cancer are in their sixth and seventh decade of life with a significant history of tobacco use, more patients are being seen at a younger age without typical tobacco exposures, and it is likely that the tumors in many such patients are associated with HPV-16.[68,70] Aside from a cervical mass of unknown etiology, the most common presenting symptom is chronic sore throat (often unilateral) and referred otalgia. Change in voice, dysphagia, and trismus are late signs. Regional lymphatic metastases occur frequently and are related to the depth of tumor invasion and tumor size. Upper cervical nodes are generally first involved, but lower nodes can become clinically involved with skipping of the upper first-echelon nodes. Bilateral lymphatic metastases can occur, particularly with cancers of the soft palate, tongue base, and midline pharyngeal wall.

Tonsils The treatment of early tonsillar neoplasms (stages I and II) is usually radiation therapy alone. Transoral wide local excision of small, superficial lesions may be locally effective, but does not address the high potential of occult lymph node metastasis. Deeply invasive cancers require extensive resections of the pharyngeal wall or mandible,[234,235] and contemporary chemoradiotherapy approaches prevail.

Radiation for early tonsillar cancers offers the advantage of treating upper-echelon lymph nodes. Treatment is usually unilateral unless extension to the tongue base or midline soft palate is present that warrants treatment of contralateral lymphatics. Ipsilateral treatment portals allow sparing of the contralateral mucosa and salivary glands. Because much of the tumor may be medial to the mandible, deeper dose calculation with electron beam therapy is used, which can be combined with a small interstitial implant if invasion of adjacent tongue is present. Early cancers of the tonsillar pillar are less effectively treated with radiation alone than are cancers confined to the tonsillar fossa.[236]

Radical radiotherapy to lymph nodes controls approximately 90% of limited nodal disease (N1) if the primary tumor is controlled, but nodal failure increases to more than 20% if failure occurs at the primary tumor site. Overall 5-year survival rates for patients with advanced primary tumors or regional metastases are generally less than 25% with single-modality therapy.[236–239] The combination of chemotherapy and radiotherapy has been shown to be effective in controlling locoregional disease in stage III and IV tonsillar cancers, and thus, surgery is frequently avoided. This is discussed further in the section "Chemotherapy and Radiation for Locally Advanced Disease" below. In general, surgery is rarely recommended for advanced tonsillar carcinoma unless the mandible is grossly invaded. When surgery is planned, postoperative concomitant therapy should be anticipated.

Tongue Base Cancers of the base of the tongue pose a more difficult therapeutic problem than do tonsillar carcinomas. The 5-year survival rates are lower, metastases are more common, early diagnosis is less common, and treatment morbidity is greater. Because of the functional deficits associated with gross total resection of even small tongue-base cancers, most tumors are treated with definitive radiation with or without chemotherapy as described for tonsillar cancer above and expanded in later sections on concomitant therapy. Three-quarters of patients are first seen with stage III or IV disease, primarily because of the early development of regional metastases owing to the rich network of lymphatics present in the base of the tongue. This is true for even T1 or T2 tumors. Understaging of the primary tumor is common because these cancers tend to be diffusely infiltrative beyond their clinical appearance. This may account for similarities in local tumor control rates for both early and advanced lesions. The poor outcome is largely attributable to late diagnosis.[240]

The staging of tongue-base carcinomas is principally dependent on primary tumor size and the extent of regional metastases. Lymph node involvement is present in approximately 60% of patients with small (T1, T2) primaries.[241] Overall 5-year survival rates range from 11 to 45%.[242,243] The 5-year survival rates decrease from over 60% for N0 patients to less than 30% for N1 patients.[241,242,244] The results of radiation therapy alone as definitive treatment of small primary tumors (T1, T2) are better for exophytic than for deeply invasive tumors.[241] Radiation alone is generally reserved for those patients without clinical nodal metastases, but can be combined with planned neck dissection for patients with clinically positive nodes that persist after the completion of radiation-based approaches. Local recurrence is more frequent after radiation alone in most series,[241,242,245] and salvage for local failure is poor. In selected patients, interstitial radiation therapy has been used to treat residual palpable disease after external beam radiation in anticipation of better local control. The use of brachytherapy is associated with higher rates of soft tissue necrosis and osteoradionecrosis, however.[246,247] The results of supplemental interstitial therapy appear to be highly dependent on the dose and technique, with the best results reported with extensive percutaneous lateral cervical loop implants to include treatment of the lateral oropharyngeal wall and pharyngoepiglottic fold.[248] The acute morbidity with implantation techniques is severe and results in massive tongue edema that necessitates at least temporary tracheostomy in all patients. The use of twice daily, hyperfractionated radiotherapy or concomitant chemotherapy and radiotherapy appears to result in improved tumor control without many of the complications associated with implants for larger tumors.[249,250]

Surgical management of early superficial primary tongue-base tumors (T1) achieves results similar to those from radiation alone. In most cases, however, primary tumors are moderately advanced and require transcervical resection via mandibulotomy or lateral pharyngotomy approaches, combined with elective or therapeutic neck dissection. Because of high rates of nodal metastases, most of the patients will still require postoperative radiotherapy. Local tumor control rates are superior to those with radiation alone,[241,242] but regional control is poor if clinically positive nodes are present. Elective neck dissection can serve an important role as a staging procedure, thereby providing a rationale for adjuvant radiation therapy. To date, no prospective randomized trial data are available that compare surgery alone with combined surgery with either pre- or postoperative radiation. Survival rates do not differ substantially by stage of disease for patients with tongue-base cancers, except for those with stage IV disease.

Soft Palate and Pharyngeal Wall Cancers of the soft palate and pharyngeal wall are less common than other oropharyngeal neoplasms. Most soft-palate cancers occur on the anterior surface of the palate and tend to be superficial. Posterior wall lesions tend to be superficial with less tumor bulk than similarly staged lesions elsewhere in the oropharynx. Advanced lesions with deep invasion have ready access to the prevertebral fascia, infratemporal fossa, and skull base and can be associated with extensive submucosal spread with clinical skip areas. Such patients often present with skull base pain and neck stiffness.

Radiation-based approaches as curative treatment are preferred in most cases, even for T3 primary tumors.[251] Resection of all but the smallest soft-palate lesions is associated with severe functional disability. The rates of occult regional metastases are difficult to determine because elective irradiation of bilateral nodal groups is included as part of primary treatment and must include the retropharyngeal lymphatics. Clinically positive lymph nodes at presentation occur in 30% of patients.[252] Small primary tumors with positive nodes can be effectively treated with definitive radiation to the primary tumor and neck. Neck dissections should be performed if disease in the neck persists at 6 to 8 weeks following the completion of external beam therapy. Extensive pharyngeal wall cancers or palate cancers with extension to the tonsil and those cases with advanced regional metastases are usually treated with combined chemoradiotherapy approaches unless gross mandibular involvement is noted. Overall 5-year survival rates for soft-palate and faucial pillar cancers are 60 to 70% and range from 80 to 90% for T1 and T2 lesions to 30 to 60% for stages III and IV lesions.[236] Locoregional recurrence is the most frequent cause of failure.[253]

Hypopharynx The hypopharynx represents one of the most lethal sites for SCC of the head and neck. Lymph node metastases are clinically evident at time of diagnosis in 70 to 80% of patients[178,179,254] and are indicative of advanced disease. Bilateral and contralateral lymph node metastases occur in 10 to 20% of cases, particularly if tumors cross the midline of the hypopharynx. Primary tumor extension beyond the hypopharynx is common.[255,256] Hypopharyngeal cancers are characterized by a propensity to spread submucosally to involve the oropharynx or esophagus. Ulcerated deep infiltration and skip areas are anticipated. This leads to difficulties in adequately assessing the margins of the tumor and contributes to poor local tumor control, even with the addition of adjuvant radiation.[257] The majority (more than 75%) of hypopharyngeal cancers arise in the pyriform sinus, while 20% occur in the posterior pharyngeal wall. Postcricoid cancers are rare (less than 5% of hypopharyngeal cancers). Pyriform cancers spread early to other contiguous structures, such as the larynx, postcricoid area, thyroid gland, and thyroid and cricoid cartilages. Most pyriform sinus cancers arise along the medial wall followed by the lateral wall of the sinus. The postcricoid mucosa is contiguous with the apex of the pyriform and tumor can spread circumferentially to involve the entire lower hypopharynx. Because of the locale of hypopharyngeal cancers and their growth patterns and proximity to the larynx, surgical management often entails total laryngopharyngectomy.[182]

The staging of hypopharyngeal cancer is based on the subsite involved, the size of the tumor, the presence of vocal cord fixation, and the extent of lymph node metastases (Table 79-6). Distant metastases at the time of diagnosis are rare. Staging evaluation is critical for treatment planning and must include endoscopic evaluation to determine the extent including evaluation of adjacent structures and the presence of second primary tumors or skip areas.[258] Determination of the precise site of origin and inferior extent of a tumor can be difficult with large tumors or with those obstructing the esophageal inlet.

Because of the necessity to remove the larynx as part of the surgical treatment of most hypopharyngeal cancers, radiation therapy, for early T1 and T2 and in combination with chemotherapy for T3 has been extensively investigated.[259] Retrospective analyses have consistently demonstrated that survival rates are lower and locoregional failure rates higher with radiation alone as compared with surgery or surgery and radiotherapy.[179,255–257,260,261] Nevertheless, the functional implications of primary surgery for even the earliest of hypopharyngeal cancers has brought about the primary role of radiation-based approaches. However, for small (T1) cancers of the hypopharynx, and particularly for superficial posterior pharyngeal wall lesions, radiation therapy alone has been used effectively, with surgery reserved for salvage.[262,264] Radiation therapy offers the advantage of treating bilateral occult lymph node disease, including that of retropharyngeal nodes, which are frequently involved when cancer arises from the posterior pharyngeal wall.[255] Most patients, however, present with advanced primary tumors (T3 to T4) and positive lymph nodes. In such patients, local control rates with radiation alone decrease to 50% and salvage surgery is rarely successful. Thus, surgical management remains the mainstay of treatment of most advanced hypopharyngeal cancers. This is especially true when function is poor at diagnosis. Specifically, although there is emerging evidence that combinations of chemotherapy and radiotherapy are effective for controlling locoregional disease, one can expect that if a patient's speech and swallowing function are poor at diagnosis as evidenced by weight loss, cord fixation, dysphagia, and/or odynophagia, then function is likely to remain poor even if chemoradiotherapy eradicate disease. In such patients, we recommend surgery followed most commonly by radiotherapy. Resections may entail partial pharyngectomy, pharyngolaryngectomy, or total pharyngectomy combined with neck dissection and the associated difficulties in post-treatment function. Although free-flap reconstructions have improved results, there still remain the difficulties of lack of sensation and dysphagia.

Table 79-6 Primary Tumor Staging Characteristics for Cancer of the Hypopharynx

Tx	Tumor cannot be assessed (as occurs with previous biopsy)
T0	There is no evidence of a primary (as occurs with an unknown primary)
Tis	Carcinoma in situ
T1	Tumor limited to one subsite in the hypopharynx and < 2 cm in greatest dimension
T2	Tumor involves more than one subsite in the hypopharynx or adjacent site, or measures between 2 and 4 cm in greatest dimension and without fixation of the hemilarynx
T3	Tumor measures > 4 cm in greatest dimension or there is fixation of the hemilarynx
T4	Tumor invades adjacent structures (thyroid/cricoid cartilage, carotid artery, soft tissues of the neck, prevertebral fascia/muscles, thyroid, and/or esophagus) a: resectable b: unresectable

Table 79-7 Overall 5-Year Survival Rates (%) in Patients with Squamous Cell Carcinoma of the Hypopharynx

		Stage				
Investigator	n	I	II	III	IV	Overall
Dubois	457	60	47	23	8	16
Bataini	384	36	33	24	10	19
Razack	120	77	63	25	5	28
Carpenter	162	100	66	51	0	47
Pingree	1208		35*		23*	25

*Stages I and II combined and III and IV combined.

Tumors arising in the lower hypopharynx or postcricoid mucosa often spread to involve the esophagus. Distal submucosal spread into the esophagus can be extensive and requires partial or total esophagectomy. Reconstruction with transposition of the stomach (gastric pull-up), jejunal free graft, or tubed fasciocutaneous free flap is currently recommended.[265–267] With improved locoregional control following the advent of total laryngopharyngectomy and postoperative radiation therapy, disease recurrence more commonly occurs in distant sites (ie, the lung). Treatment approaches with combined preoperative or postoperative radiation have dramatically improved the control of locoregional disease, but survival rates have not improved as substantially over those with surgery alone because of the increased rates of distant metastases. Postoperative radiation is currently preferred to preoperative radiation because of its lower local recurrence rates, fewer complications, and less difficulty in accurately assessing tumor margins.[257] The clear superiority of combined surgery and radiation over surgery alone has not been established.[183,256,257,268] Although several studies demonstrate improved survival with combined therapy,[179,260] direct comparisons with surgery alone are difficult because of differences in patient selection factors, tumor extent, and degree of lymph node involvement. Well-designed randomized trials to compare surgery alone with combined therapy have not been performed and likely will never ensue.

The presence of lymph node metastases, extracapsular lymph node involvement, and direct extension of the primary tumor into the soft tissues of the neck are major negative prognostic factors and have ushered in concomitant chemoradiotherapy adjuvant approaches. Overall 5-year survival rates range from 10 to 30% for posterior pharyngeal wall cancers[262,263,269–271] and from 20 to 40% for pyriform sinus cancers (Table 79-7).[178,179,183,255,260,261] Locoregional recurrence continues to account for the greatest number of deaths from disease.[183,272]

Distant metastases are rarely evident at the time of presentation, but may appear many years after primary therapy and seem to correlate with extent of regional lymph node involvement.[179,273] The rates of distant metastases range from 20 to 50%[179,183] and increase with the extent of lymph node disease.

Larynx Because of the prominent role the larynx plays in communication, swallowing, respiration, protection of the lower airway, and, therefore, quality of life, the treatment of cancer of the larynx presents formidable dilemmas regarding the functional consequences of treatment in addition to the intrinsic threat to life posed by these cancers. More so than with any other site of head and neck cancer, quality-of-life issues have been incorporated into treatment decisions and have echoed throughout the management strategy of the other head and neck sites.[274,275] Cancer of the larynx is generally diagnosed at an earlier stage than are other head and neck sites, primarily owing to the early manifestation of symptoms, most commonly hoarseness. As a result, cure rates are generally higher than for other sites.

The larynx is divided into three subsites that form the basis for classifying laryngeal cancers. These separations exist because each site is associated with differences in patterns of local spread, risks of lymphatic metastasis, and control rates. These differences exist as a result of differences in embryologic development and vascular and lymphatic anatomy. The TNM staging for these subsites is listed in Table 79-8.

Table 79-8 Primary Tumor Staging Characteristics for Carcinoma of the Larynx

Supraglottis	T1	Normal vocal cord motility and tumor limited to one laryngeal subsite
	T2	Tumor invades one adjacent site, normal vocal cord motility
	T3	Tumor limited to larynx with arytenoids fixation and/or extends to postcricoid area or preepiglottic tissues
	T4	Tumor extends beyond larynx and/or through thyroid cartilage to soft tissues of neck, thyroid, and/or esophagus
Glottis	T1	Tumor limited to one vocal cord (s) with normal motion T1a: Tumor limited to one cord T1b: Tumor involves both cords
	T2	Tumor extends to supraglottis or subglottis and/or with impaired vocal cord motility without arytenoid fixation
	T3	Tumor limited to larynx but with arytenoid fixation
	T4	Tumor extends beyond larynx and/or through thyroid cartilage to soft tissues of neck, thyroid, and/or esophagus
Subglottis	T1	Tumor limited to subglottis
	T2	Tumor extends to glottis but with normal or impaired motion
	T3	Tumor limited to larynx but with arytenoids fixation
	T4	Tumor extends outside larynx and or trachea

Considerable attention has been devoted to anatomic studies of the vascular and lymphatic compartments of the larynx.[276–279] These studies have defined natural anatomic barriers to cancer spread within the larynx and have contributed to the development of select surgical procedures for partial laryngeal resections of certain cancers.

The true vocal cords present an effective boundary between supraglottic and subglottic lymphatic spread within the larynx. This separation breaks down with tumors involving the anterior or posterior commissures and with deeply invasive tumors that extend vertically across the true and false vocal cords (transglottic cancers). Normally, the inner perichondrium of the thyroid cartilage also presents an effective barrier to cancer spread. However, cancer involvement of the anterior commissure or transglottic extension is associated with invasion of the thyroid cartilage in 40 to 60% of cases.[280,281]

Early diagnosis is critical for achieving high survival rates and larynx preservation.[282] Most cancers that are diagnosed at an early stage of development arise in the glottic larynx. This is because minimal changes in the mass of the vibrating vocal cord from tumor growth result in changes in its vibrating characteristics and presents early as dysphonia or hoarseness. Supraglottic cancers are usually more advanced than glottic cancers at the time of diagnosis because they do not generally produce early symptoms of hoarseness. Rather, the earliest symptoms of a supraglottic cancer are usually sore throat, dysphagia, referred otalgia, or the development of a neck mass representing regional metastasis. Airway compromise may be an early symptom with subglottic cancer.

Modern clinical evaluation of laryngeal cancers includes fiberoptic laryngoscopy, direct laryngoscopy, CT, and MRI of the larynx and neck, as well as videostroboscopic analysis. The radiologic assessments are of value in assessing direct extension to the preepiglottic and paraglottic spaces of the larynx, detecting cartilage invasion and evaluating the soft tissues and lymph nodes of the neck. These studies have completely replaced conventional tomography and contrast laryngography; however, the precise evaluation of tumor extent still requires direct laryngoscopy under anesthesia. With large, obstructive tumors, this may require tracheostomy. In some patients with large obstructive lesions, debulking the tumor mass at the time of direct laryngoscopy can obviate the need for tracheostomy and thereby reduce the potential risk of tumor seeding of the tracheostomy site. Even with precise clinical evaluation, inaccurate estimation of tumor extent (usually underestimation) occurs in 30 to 40% of cases.[283] Most often this involves failure to identify invasion of the laryngeal cartilage framework.

Supraglottic primary tumors account for 25 to 50% of all laryngeal cancers.[284,285] A knowledge of the laryngeal compartments aids in understanding the spread and staging of supraglottic and glottic cancers. The staging of supraglottic cancers is based on the subsite or region of the supraglottis involved in the cancer. Subsites include the false vocal cords, arytenoids, lingual and laryngeal surfaces of the epiglottis, and aryepiglottic folds. The epiglottis itself is also subdivided into the region extending above the plane of the hyoid and that below the hyoid. Suprahyoid epiglottic tumors tend to have a better prognosis than infrahyoid cancers with the exception of those invading the aryepiglottic fold (marginal area) to involve the pyriform sinus. This, again, is due to the richer network of lymphatics in the infrahyoid portion of the epiglottis. Early cancers (T1 and T2) can involve one or more subsites but have normal vocal cord motion. Those cancers that cause fixation of the arytenoid or involve the postcricoid region, medial wall of the pyriform sinus, or preepiglottic space are staged T3. Those that extend beyond the larynx or invade thyroid cartilage are staged T4.

Glottic carcinomas are also staged according to subsites involved. Cancers limited to the true vocal cords are T1 (T1a—one vocal cord involved; T1b—both vocal cords involved), and those with extension to an adjacent site or with impaired cord mobility are staged T2. Impaired vocal cord motion is also staged as T2 and is due to paraglottic disease spread. Whereas, as impaired motion is staged as T2, arytenoid fixation is classified T3. Those tumors with cartilage involvement or extension outside the larynx are T4.

True subglottic cancers that are limited to the subglottic region (T1) or to the subglottis and true vocal cords (T2) are early cancers but, unfortunately, are diagnosed rarely because of a lack of symptoms. Fixation of the vocal cord (T3) and cartilage invasion or extension outside the larynx (T4) is associated with a worse prognosis. The nodal classification for staging is the same as for other HNSCC sites.

Although a great deal of controversy exists regarding the optimal treatment of approach for larynx cancer at The University of Texas M. D. Anderson Cancer Center, curative radiotherapy is generally the treatment of choice for early-stage laryngeal lesions. It is for the moderately advanced lesions that one must consider the trade-offs between definitive radiotherapy with salvage surgery held in reserve versus definitive surgery or, more recently, combined chemotherapy and radiation therapy approaches.

Examination under anesthesia and biopsy make up the gold standard in the assessment of early lesions, combined with radiographic imaging for assessment of the paraglottic space and thyroid cartilage. Radiation therapy remains the management of choice for early glottic cancers. Nevertheless, in some instances, patients may choose conservation laryngeal surgery, including endoscopic laser excision of localized lesions, or partial laryngeal surgery. Both require frozen-section analysis of margins if the patient and tumor factors support such an approach. Additionally, in many instances, conservation laryngeal surgical salvage is effective in those 10 to 20% of cases in which external beam therapy has been unsuccessful for stages I and II cancers (Figure 79-2).

The design of the radiation portals must be tailored to the individual patient, but some general comments can be made. In general, supraglottic tumors have access to a richer lymphatic drainage than do tumors of the glottic larynx, and so radiation fields tend to be larger in order to treat the larger area at risk of metastatic disease.[286] Typically, one treats the primary tumor volume and regions at risk of subclinical metastatic disease to 5,000 cGy, and then reduces the field size to areas of gross disease and delivers an additional 2,000 to 2,400 cGy. The spinal cord is shielded at 4,500 cGy, and megavoltage electron beams are used to treat the posterior cervical nodes to higher doses as required. Because of the V shape of the anterior neck, wedge-compensating filters are often required to ensure uniform radiation dose distributions. If the anterior supraclavicular fossa is at risk of micrometastatic disease, it is treated to 5,000 cGy, using an anterior field suitably matched to the upper-neck fields. Early-stage (T1–2, N0) glottic lesions are generally treated with relatively small fields localized to the primary tumor. Tumors of the subglottic larynx can spread to the upper paratracheal nodes as well

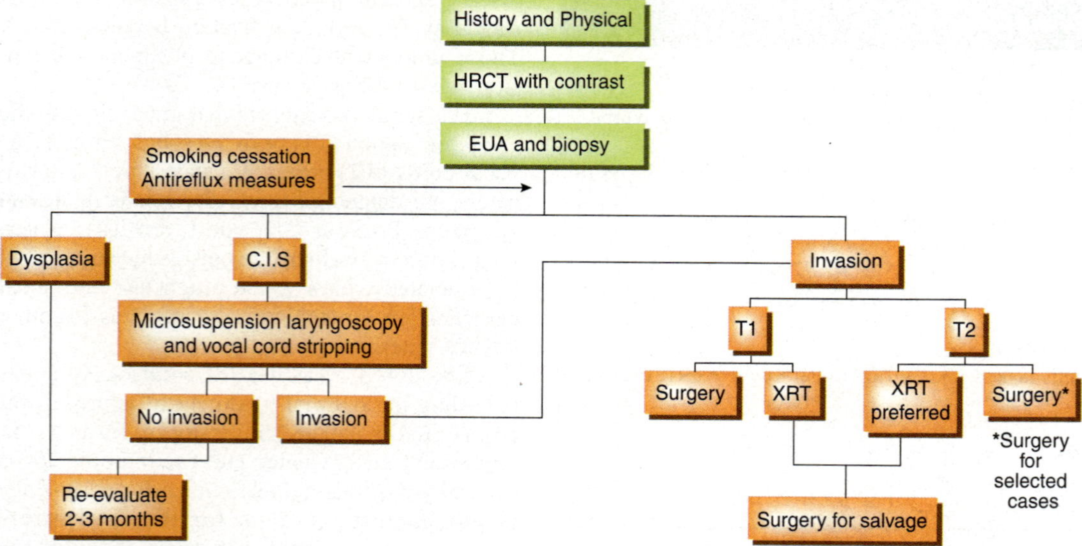

Figure 79-2 Early glottic lesions.

Table 79-9 Risk Factors for Tracheal Stomal Recurrence
Extensive primary lesion (T3 or T4)
Subglottic tumor extension
Preliminary emergency tracheotomy for airway obstruction
Inadequate tumor margins on pathologic review
Tumor involvement of the paratracheal lymphatics
Large, fixed nodes or multiple cervical nodes
Perineural or venous invasion of tumor

as to the nodes in the cervical chain, and radiation fields for this disease must therefore include the upper mediastinum.[287]

The treatment of more advanced laryngeal cancers (T3 and T4) has historically included surgery with or without radiation therapy. Prospective randomized studies have shown convincingly that chemotherapy and radiation therapy (including surgical salvage) are equally effective in the long-term survival of patients with T3 laryngeal cancers as compared with surgery with or without radiation therapy. It is important to note that approximately 60% of patients may preserve their larynx, and thus quality of life has significantly improved.[259,288] Speech communication profiles are clearly better in the group of patients randomized to the larynx preservation arm, but there was no determination of swallowing function.[289] However, local control was poorer for patients with T4 lesions. Current standard of care argues that laryngeal preservation approaches or protocols be considered in treating such patients, with the corollary that patients with poor function at diagnosis will likely have poor laryngeal function after conservation treatment. A treatment algorithm for advanced glottic cancers is shown in Figure 79-3.

Many surgical procedures for laryngeal carcinoma involve the creation of a tracheal stoma. This area is sometimes at significant risk of tumor recurrence, which is most likely associated with peritracheal metastases that erode into the peristomal area. For this reason, bilateral paratracheal dissections should be performed in T4 glottic cancers and radiation therapy provided postoperatively if metastases to this echelon of nodes are found pathologically. Once a stomal recurrence has developed, the prognosis is grave regardless of salvage treatment. Sisson and colleagues reported on a series of 28 patients with stomal recurrences treated with one or more surgical resections.[290] The 5-year survival was only 17%. Schneider and colleagues reported on patients with tracheal recurrences treated with radiotherapy; good palliation of local pain and/or bleeding was achieved, but the 2-year survival rate was only 6%.[291] Given the poor results with salvage therapy, it is clearly better to prevent stomal recurrence in the first place. If risk factors for stomal recurrence are present (Table 79-9), then the tracheal stoma should be irradiated as part of the initial management.

Supraglottic Cancers Important factors in selecting therapy for supraglottic cancers are tumor location, cord fixation and preepiglottic extension. Tumors limited to the suprahyoid epiglottis are amenable to radiation with fields that encompass neck regions at risk of lymphatic metastases. Additionally, some proponents of limited surgical interventions recommend endoscopic laser excision separate from management of the neck. An algorithm for early supraglottic cancers is shown in Figure 79-4. Tumors involving the aryepiglottic folds, pyriform sinuses, or infrahyoid epiglottis tend to be more aggressive, are deeply infiltrative, and frequently involve the preepiglottic space. Radiation alone is less effective than surgery, resulting in more frequent local recurrences that require surgical salvage. Often these recurrences are difficult to detect early enough to allow salvage by laryngeal conservation surgery and therefore require salvage total laryngectomy. Persistent postradiation edema of the supraglottic larynx is not uncommon and contributes to difficulty in detecting recurrence, which occurs in 40 to 50% of cases.[292–294]

Preepiglottic extension of cancer carries a poor prognosis. However, such a situation can be managed effectively with horizontal supraglottic laryngectomy, which allows preservation of the voice. Indeed, even advanced tumors with extension of cancer to the vallecula and tongue base can often be treated by extended supraglottic laryngectomy with results equal to those of total laryngectomy. Very superficial tumors of the suprahyoid epiglottis can also be treated with simple epiglottectomy. Because supraglottic laryngectomy is associated with variable degrees of postoperative aspiration, adequate pulmonary status is a prerequisite for this surgery, as is intact mobility of the true vocal cords.

In any patient undergoing partial laryngectomy, preoperative consent should be obtained for total laryngectomy in case the surgical findings dictate that more extensive surgery is needed. Approximately 20% of patients require prolonged tracheostomy, and this is usually related to edema secondary to postoperative radiation. The rates of persistent swallowing difficulties are low,

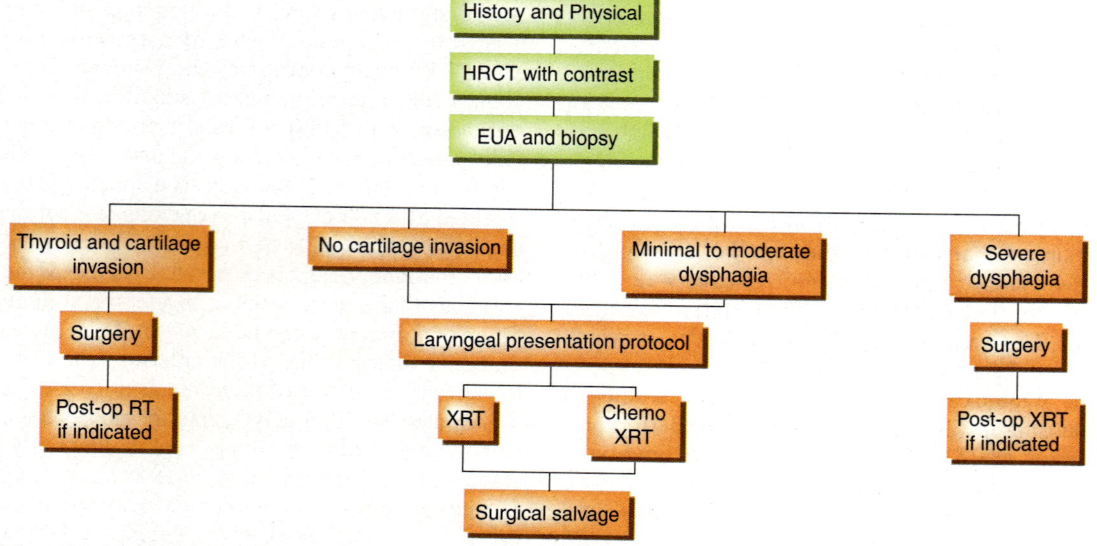

Figure 79-3 Advanced glottic lesions.

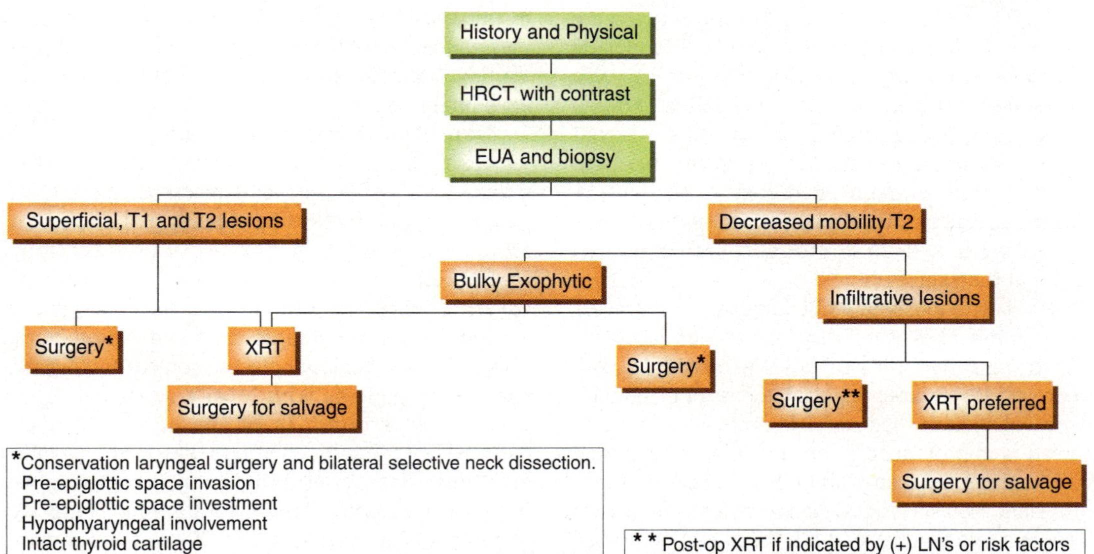

Figure 79-4 Early supraglottic cancers.

however, and the need for completion laryngectomy for persistent aspiration ranges only from 0 to 5%.[295–297]

The frequency of neck node metastases is high with T2 or greater tumors. Treatment of the clinically negative neck may be accomplished with surgery or radiation. Surgical approaches should include removal of bilateral primary nodal groups at risk of occult disease (levels II, III, and IV).[298–300] For T1 and T2 lesions, most authors demonstrate overall cure rates of 68 to 73%[299–302] with determinate 3-year survival rates of 80 to 85%[284,299,301] when elective neck dissection is included. Most recurrences occur in the neck, and this argues for prophylactic neck treatment.[303]

Radiation is also effective for early lesions. Local control rates for patients with supraglottic tumors treated with radiation alone range from 68 to 94%, and survival rates are 50 to 89%. The latter set of survival figures are comparable to those for planned surgery and adjuvant radiotherapy, which range from 46 to 90%. Although the figures are comparable for T1 and T2 lesions, there is a trend favoring the combined approach for larger lesions. Nonrandomized series from different institutions are not strictly comparable since unstated patient selection factors are generally involved. For example, the excellent local control results reported by Goepfert and colleagues for T3 and T4 lesions are for a selected set of tumors that were exophytic in nature.[304]

Survival rates tend to run lower than local control rates for supraglottic tumors because of deaths from second primaries and other intercurrent diseases. Cure rates range from 73 to 75%[305–308] and increase to 80 to 85% with the addition of surgical salvage.[309–311] Most recurrences are local, and preservation of voice is successful in 65 to 70% of patients when salvage surgery is included.[311]

The treatment of more advanced supraglottic cancers (T3, T4) remains controversial, with laryngeal preservation remaining a focus of treatment (Figure 79-5). In cases with clinically evident regional metastases, combined surgery and postoperative radiation is usually recommended since this treatment approach is associated with better local control rates[312] and better control rates for neck disease in both the ipsilateral and contralateral neck.[313] Approximately 50% of patients have clinically palpable lymph nodes at the time of diagnosis, and 20 to 25% have bilateral nodal involvement. In the clinically negative neck, elective neck dissection shows cancer metastases in 15 to 30% of patients. Failure to control disease in the neck is a major cause of mortality in supraglottic cancers. In most reports, radiation alone for the control of supraglottic cancers with N2 or N3 nodes is clearly inferior to combined therapy. Therefore, in instances where T1–T3 lesions of the supraglottis are associated with N2 or N3 disease, neck dissection should be performed when the primaries are treated by radiation therapy. Although the issue of optimal initial management for the patient with N0 disease has not been settled, an individualized approach has been recommended in which bilateral selective node dissections are performed. Postoperative radiation is reserved for patients with proven regional metastases.[296,314]

Overall 5-year survival rates for supraglottic cancers range from 40 to 50%.[310,315] Local failures occur in approximately 10% of patients and regional failures in 15 to 20%. Rates of distant metastases range from 11 to 18%,[286,310,316,317] with rates approaching 30% in patients with stage IV disease.[314] Second primaries (20–25% of failures) are a major cause of death.[310,315] Intercurrent illness accounts for up to 20% of deaths.[314,317,318]

Glottic and Subglottic Cancers The treatment of glottic cancer is greatly influenced by the secondary goal of voice preservation. Mobility of the vocal cords is a critical factor in selecting treatment. For small cancers (T1, T2) with mobile vocal cords, radiation therapy alone for cure achieves excellent local control rates (T1, 85–95%; T2, 65–75%) and overall survival rates similar to those for surgical resection.[319,320] Voice quality, although often impaired by radiation, is generally better than that following surgical resection.[321,322] Local recurrences after definitive radiation can often be salvaged by subsequent surgery. Tumor involvement of the anterior commissure or arytenoids has been associated with higher local recurrence rates for radiation alone, but this may have been related to understaging. As with supraglottic cancers, careful clinical tumor staging is necessary since underestimation of tumor extent is common. The "irradiate-and-watch" treatment strategy is predicated on close follow-up in order to detect recurrences when they are still salvageable by surgery. Delay in the diagnosis of recurrent glottic cancers after radiation is more frequent than with supraglottic cancers[304] and often requires total laryngectomy for cure. Thus, unreliable patients or patients who are difficult to examine may be more suitable for primary surgical management.

Survival figures in radiotherapy series are comparable to local control rates for surgery,

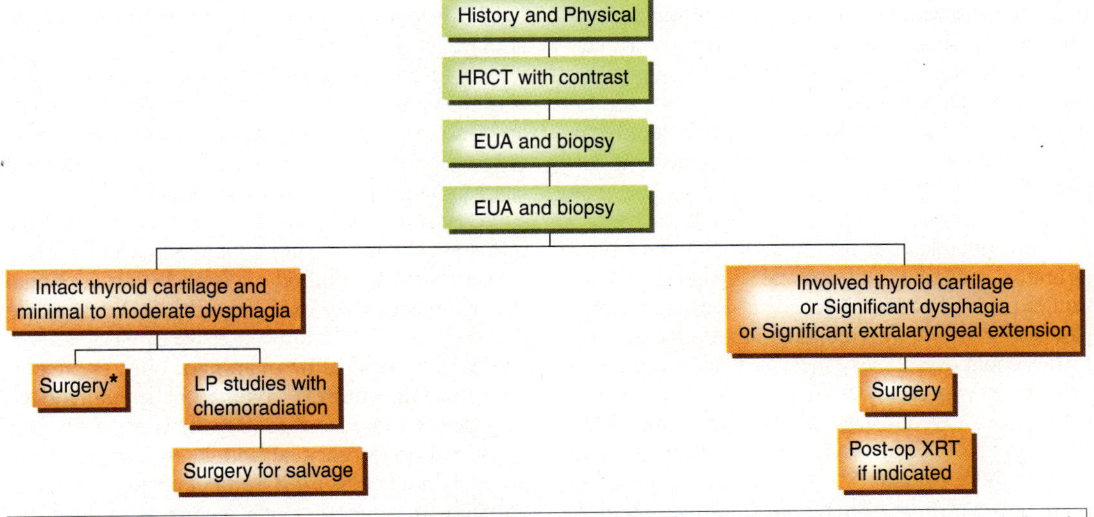

Figure 79-5 Advanced supraglottic cancers.

reflecting the effectives of surgical salvage and the fact that few patients with early-glottic cancer die of their disease. The 5-year survival rates for T1 lesions range from 85 to 95% with either primary surgery or radiation. Rates for T2 lesions are generally in the range of 75 to 85%, but these rates are decreased by 10 to 15% (local control rates by 20–25%) when the mobility of the vocal cords is impaired[323] or transglottic spread is present at presentation.[324] Lesions with impaired mobility owing to muscle invasion behave more like T3 cancers and have a poorer prognosis with radiotherapy alone.[319,325–328] Transglottic cancers and those with subglottic extension have higher rates of regional metastases and more often require total laryngectomy for cure. In selected patients with these more advanced lesions, extended supraglottic laryngectomy or supracricoid partial laryngectomy may effectively salvage the patient and avoid a permanent stoma.[329,330] Voice quality is typically poor with these procedures, and chronic aspiration and permanent tracheostomy may be needed. Additionally, these procedures are technically challenging and experience dependent. However, with proper patient selection, these procedures can be well tolerated and effective.

Management of advanced T3 glottic cancers has historically consisted of total laryngectomy with or without postoperative radiation therapy. Although older series show suboptimal control rates (20–35%) and survival rates (10–50%) for unselected sets of T3 and T4 tumors treated with radiation alone, it is now recognized that with proper selection, radiotherapy control rates for T3 lesions can approach 80%.[331] In patients without regional metastases, local tumor control rates with surgery alone are excellent. Significant increases in local control with the addition of radiation therapy have not been clearly demonstrated. However, in patients with regional metastases, overall prognosis is poor and recurrence in the neck is a major problem when surgery alone is used. Better regional tumor control rates are achieved with the addition of adjuvant radiation therapy.[304] Because rates of occult regional metastases approach 30% in patients with advanced glottic (T3, T4) cancers, elective modified or selective node dissections for staging purposes are recommended when surgery is performed for primary disease. Demonstration of histologically positive nodal metastases has been used as an indication for postoperative radiation. Surgery alone is curative in 50 to 80% of patients without nodal metastases,[306,326,332–334] but this decreases to less than 40% if metastases are present.[326,335,336]

Considerable controversy surrounds the use of definitive radiation with surgical salvage in patients with advanced (T3N0, T4N0) but localized glottic cancers.[332,337,338] The radiation-alone concept presumes equal overall survivorship as compared with primary laryngectomy, with associated low complication rates. Overall survival rates range from 50 to 55%,[335,337,339] with larynx preservation in 60 to 70% of these patients.[324,335,337] High complication rates, however, have been reported with late surgical salvage of radiation failures.[335] The overall patterns are confusing and based entirely on retrospective series. The resolution of this controversy will require carefully designed prospective studies that include assessments not only of survival, but also of voice and quality-of-life issues and complication rates.

A subset of laryngeal cancers that warrant special consideration are those that involve both the glottic and supraglottic regions (transglottic). These cancers are usually advanced and are associated with a high incidence (30–50%) of regional metastases.[324,340]

It was previously thought that distant metastases from laryngeal cancers were uncommon, accounting for less than 10% of failures. However, with improved locoregional control, the recognized incidence of distant metastasis is increasing. Distant spread is approximately four times more common with supraglottic than with glottic cancers.[181] Rates of distant metastases associated with glottic cancer have increased, however, with the use of combined therapy and have been reported in approximately 20% of patients with advanced disease.[339] Rates appear to be directly related to the extent of nodal disease, with reported rates as high as 40 to 50% of failures attributed to distant metastases in patients with N2 or N3 disease.

Subglottic carcinomas are a rare variant of squamous carcinomas of the larynx possessing a high risk for paratracheal metastases, local recurrence, and death from disease.[341–343] Surgery is the preferred therapy except in early superficial diseases of this site.[341–344]

Carcinoma In Situ A special issue relates to the treatment of carcinoma in situ of the vocal cords.[345,346] This disease often can be managed with vocal cord stripping, but if enough serial sections are examined, foci of invasive carcinoma are often found. Pene and Fletcher reported on a series of 79 patients with carcinoma in situ and 7 patients with leukoplakia/atypical hyperplasia who were treated with radiotherapy.[347] Patients were staged as either T1 or T2, using the same criteria as for invasive tumors. Local control rates were the same as for invasive lesions: 89% for T1 and 74% for T2. However, only 2 of 12 failures were on the initially involved cord, suggesting that most were not true recurrences, but rather, multifocal disease developing in dysplastic epithelium. Furthermore, it took about 5 years for 80% of the failures to develop, which further suggests a second neoplastic process. Most of the failures after primary radiotherapy tend to be invasive, whereas failures after vocal cord stripping tend to be equally divided between carcinoma in situ and invasive disease.

Very superficial cancers limited to the free edge of the vocal cord or carcinoma in situ can be effectively treated by limited excision by conventional means or with laser excision, with excellent voice preservation.[348,349] More extensive disease requires cordectomy, vertical hemilaryngectomy, or supracricoid laryngectomy.[350] Numerous methods have been devised for reconstructing the vocal cords after conservation surgery, although, in fact, they are probably not necessary if proper patient selection is pursued. In general, voice results are inferior to those achieved with radiation therapy alone for early lesions. The patient with carcinoma in situ, however, by inference has diffuse premalignant mucosal findings and certainly should be targeted for novel prevention strategies owing to the likelihood of later developing invasive disease.

Nonsurgical Treatment There has been an increasing focus on the use of chemotherapy in the management of laryngeal cancers of all stages. Laccourreye and others have published a series of articles that suggest that exclusive chemotherapy may be effective in select cases.[351–354] Randomized trials have demonstrated that the concomitant administration of chemotherapy and radiotherapy improves local-regional disease control and overall survival in patients with locally advanced squamous cell carcinomas of the head and neck (SCCHN). Induction chemotherapy with cisplatin and fluorouracil has long been recognized as highly active with clinical partial and complete responses observed in 80 to 90% of previously untreated patients.[355–357] It was postulated that a substantial response to initial treatment with chemotherapy would lead to an improvement of therapeutic efficacy for surgery or radiotherapy. This led to the Department of Veterans Affairs Laryngeal Cancer Study,[358] in which 332 patients with stage III or IV squamous cell carcinoma of the larynx were randomized to receive either induction chemotherapy consisting of cisplatin and fluorouracil followed by radiotherapy or surgery and postoperative radiotherapy. Patients who experienced no tumor response to chemotherapy or those who had locally persistent or recurrent cancer underwent salvage laryngectomy. Two-year survival for both treatment groups was 68%, and 41% of patients randomly assigned to the experimental arm were alive with a functional larynx at 2 years. Thus, the efficacy of chemotherapy followed by radiotherapy (with surgical salvage) was similar to that of surgery followed by radiotherapy and established organ preservation as a realistic goal of nonsurgical treatment administered with curative intent. Lefebvre and colleagues[359] later reported similar outcomes in a European trial involving patients with cancers of the hypopharynx.

In the Veterans Affairs study,[358] there were observed trends in patterns of tumor relapse, with 20% of patients in the chemotherapy arm having locoregional recurrence versus 7% in the surgery arm. Distant disease recurrence was more likely in the surgical arm, affecting 17% of patients versus 11% in the chemotherapy/radiotherapy group. Salvage laryngectomy was required more often in patients with glottic cancer than in those with supraglottic primary sites (43% vs 31%), in patients with fixed vocal cords than in those with mobile vocal cords (41% vs 29%), and in patients with gross invasion of thyroid cartilage compared with patients without (41% vs 35%). Salvage laryngectomy was required in 56% of patients with T4 cancers compared with 29% of patients with smaller primary tumors ($p = .001$).

The Veterans Affairs Larynx study prompted further investigations of chemotherapy and radiotherapy in the treatment of intermediate-stage larynx cancer using the sequential administration of induction chemotherapy, consisting of cisplatin and fluorouracil, followed by radiotherapy as the control arm. This was compared with concomitant cisplatin and radiotherapy, and radiotherapy administered as a single treatment modality.[360,361] Patients with stage III and IV disease were eligible, T2/3, N0–3, M0. T1 and most T4 tumors were not allowed. For all groups, totaling 547 patients, surgical salvage was reserved for those patients with persistent or locally recurrent disease. Survival did not seem to be affected by treatment assignment. At a median follow-up of 3.8 years, patients randomly assigned to concomitant cisplatin and radiotherapy achieved a higher rate of laryngeal preservation, 84% versus 72% in patients receiving sequential chemoradiotherapy ($p = .005$) or radiotherapy alone 67% ($p < .001$). At 2 years, 80% of patients on the concomitant chemoradiotherapy arm achieved local control versus 65% of patients receiving sequential chemotherapy and then radiation and 58% of patients treated with radiotherapy alone. As expected, acute toxic effects of treatment were greatest in the patients who received radiotherapy with concomitant cisplatin.

These trials indicate that for patients with intermediate-stage squamous cell carcinoma of the larynx, a combined treatment program with the objectives of tumor eradication and laryngeal preservation is appropriate. It is also important to recognize that patients with locally advanced destructive primary laryngeal cancers were not included in the recent multigroup trial. These patients may require total laryngectomy for optimal tumor control and to preserve swallow function.

NASOPHARYNX

Presentation and Staging In the United States, nasopharyngeal carcinoma (NPC) accounts for 2% of all HNSCC. Its unusual epidemiologic and natural history features include a remarkable tendency toward early regional and distant dissemination. NPC also is extremely sensitive to radiotherapy and cytotoxic chemotherapy.

In the adult, the nasopharynx is a chamber that is approximately cuboidal in shape and 4 cm on an edge. It is bounded anteriorly by the choana of the nasal cavity, superiorly by the clivus, and inferiorly by the soft palate. Its posterior wall is the mucosa that overlies the superior constrictor muscles of the pharynx and the C1 and C2 vertebral bodies. The lateral walls contain the eustachian tube orifices. The epithelium of the superior lateral walls contains pseudostratified columnar cells and occasional goblet cells, while the inferior lateral and posterior walls are stratified squamous in nature. The region is richly endowed with lymphatics that drain to the retropharyngeal and deep cervical nodes.

Malignant neoplasms of the nasopharynx are primarily epithelial, with the presence of keratin associated with a poorer prognosis. The World Health Organization (WHO) recognizes three histopathologic types of NPC: type 1, differentiated SCC (of varying degrees); type 2, nonkeratinizing carcinoma; and type 3, undifferentiated or lymphoepithelial carcinoma.[362] Mixed patterns are common.

About one-third of patients present with a neck mass without other complaints, and about 70 to 75% of patients have enlarged neck nodes at presentation. Other common complaints are epistaxis, nasal stuffiness, headache, and hearing loss (generally unilateral). The tumor can spread laterally and superiorly to cause bony destruction of the base of the skull. Frequently, there are cranial nerve findings, with the sixth nerve being most commonly involved.[363] There are two principal cranial nerve syndromes associated with NPC: (1) the retroparotidian syndrome, involving cranial nerves IX, X, XI, and XII; and (2) the petrosphenoidal syndrome, involving cranial nerves III, IV, V, and VI (and occasionally cranial nerve II via extension through the foramen lacerum into the middle cranial fossa). Evaluation of the nasopharynx should consist of direct visualization with a fiberoptic scope. An MRI scan is important in evaluating base-of-skull involvement and the possible presence of occult-involved lymph nodes.

The most recent revision of the AJCC/Union Internationale Contre le Cancer (UICC) staging system recognizes the uniqueness of nasopharyngeal carcinoma among other head and neck tumors. Both the criteria for T and N staging have been revised, as has the stage grouping. These are summarized in Table 79-10.

Table 79-10 Primary Tumor Staging Characteristics for Carcinoma of the Nasopharynx

T1	Tumor confined to the soft tissues of the nasopharynx
T2	Tumor extends to the soft tissues of the oropharynx and/or nasal fossa
	T2a: Without parapharyngeal extension
	T2b: With parapharyngeal extension
T3	Tumor invades bony structures and/or paranasal sinuses
T4	Tumor exhibits intracranial extension and/or involvement of cranial nerves, infratemporal fossa, hypopharynx, or orbit

Treatment Standard treatment of NPC is radiation therapy or concomitant chemoradiotherapy for early and locally advanced disease, respectively. Surgical resection even for early-stage disease is technically difficult because of the anatomic location of the primary tumor and the frequent bilateral cervical and retropharyngeal node involvement. The role of the surgeon is limited to obtaining tissue for diagnosis, occasionally resecting residual adenopathy after definitive radiotherapy, and surgery for rare non-WHO histologies such as adenoid cystic carcinoma. Fortunately, most nasopharyngeal carcinomas tend to be fairly radiosensitive, and even large lymph nodes often respond to moderate doses of radiotherapy.[364] Prior to initiating therapy, a dental consultation is advised since it is necessary to irradiate the parotid glands bilaterally, and the resulting xerostomia predisposes to serious oral problems.

The initial radiation fields encompass the adjacent base of the skull as well as the nasopharynx itself. The fields are bilaterally directed and include the retropharyngeal drainage and the anterior and posterior cervical chains. A dose of 4,500 cGy is given, using megavoltage photons, and then the fields are reduced to spare the spinal cord and an additional 500 cGy are given. Megavoltage electrons are used to bring the posterior cervical nodes to this same dose. The fields are then reduced in size and an additional 2,000 to 2,200 cGy are given to the nasopharyngeal primary. Regions of positive cervical adenopathy are also boosted with megavoltage photons and/or electrons to total doses of 6,500 to 7,500 cGy, depending on the original size of the node and its response to the first phase of therapy.[365] In selected patients, the boost dose to the nasopharynx itself can be given with an intracavitary implant.[366] Critical normal structures in the treatment region include the cervical cord, the brainstem, the optic nerves, and orbital contents. Proper shielding and limiting the delivered dose to these structures are necessary to avoid untoward complications. An anterior supraclavicular field is generally matched to the initial large lateral fields, and approximately 5,000 cGy are given to treat submicroscopic disease in this area.

Treatment results are related to both stage and histopathology, but many series do not adequately document outcome as a function of these variables. Huang combines the above-listed T1, T2, and T3 stages into his T1/T2 categories.[367] For a clinically negative neck, he reports a 5-year survival of 65%. For groups corresponding to T4N0-N2 and T4N3, he found respective 5-year survivals of 41.3% and 23%. Vikram and colleagues noted a 5-year locoregional control rate for early T-stage N0 patients of 65%.[368] Scanlon and colleagues found a clear worsening of prognosis with increasing cervical adenopathy with 5-year survivals of 67%, 24%, and 14% when the patient had no clinical adenopathy, unilateral adenopathy, or bilateral adenopathy, respectively.[369] It is important to note that these series were treated prior to routine CT/MRI scanning, which would have the tendency to increase the clinical stage of the neck disease.

A clear correlation exists between the degree of cervical adenopathy and the subsequent development of distant metastases, with patients with bilateral adenopathy having a 5-year actuarial risk of approximately 80% of developing distant metastases. Common sites of distant metastases are the lung, bone, and liver. In selected cases, a failure at the primary site alone can be salvaged using a combination of external beam radiotherapy and an intracavitary implant.[370] However, the morbidity associated with this may be substantial. Long-term study has shown that brachytherapy with permanent radioactive gold grain interstitial implantation is an effective salvage treatment in persistent and recurrent NPC patients who have nasopharynx-confined disease.[371] Five-year local control rates were the best for patients with persistent disease (87.2%) versus those with a first recurrence (62.7%) or second recurrence (23.4%, p = .0004). Overall 5-year survival rates for these three patient groups were 79.1%, 53.6%, and 42.9%, respectively. Lesion size was not an independent prognostic factor for local control. Complications of therapy (including headache, palatal fistula, and mucosal radiation necrosis at site of gold grain implantation) of this brachytherapy approach occurred most often in patients with persistent disease (28.3% vs 18.9% and 16% in patients with first and second recurrence, respectively).

Although effective in early stages, standard radiotherapy (despite achieving high complete response rates) produces 5-year survival rates in stage III disease of only 10 to 45% and in stage IV disease of 0 to 30%.[372,373] Despite major differences between NPC and other HNSCC, many chemotherapy studies have included NPC patients, which confounds study results.

The efficacy and toxicity of systemic therapy is presently evaluated in trials that include NPC as a distant entity, and efforts are made to define patient cohorts according to the WHO classification. Including NPC with squamous cancers in studies of other head and neck sites will confound study outcomes in part because of the exquisite sensitivity of NPC to chemotherapy and radiation, but also because of the distinctive patient demographics and patterns of tumor recurrence in NPC.

Reports of phase II trials demonstrate single-agent activity for cisplatin, carboplatin, fluorouracil, bleomycin, methotrexate, anthracycline, vinca alkaloids, and taxanes.[374,375] Response rate ranges from 20 to 60%, with complete responses uncommon. More recent reports of cisplatin-based drug combinations describe tumor responses in 50 to 80% of patients clinically complete in 20 to 25% of these.[376–379] Moreover, Fandi and colleagues[380] have reported durable disease remissions in a cohort of patients followed over a period of years. Chan and colleagues[381] have recently reported that the combination of cetuximab, a chimeric monoclonal antibody directed against the EGFR, and carboplatin has activity (overall disease control rate 60%) even in heavily previously treated NPC patients.

For patients with staging III and IV at diagnosis, chemoradiotherapy has become the standard of care. Concomitant chemotherapy and radiation appears to be the backbone of treatment. In 1995, Chan and colleagues[382] reported no difference in local tumor control or survival in a small study (n = 77) testing the value of chemotherapy with cisplatin/5-FU administered in a sandwich fashion as neoadjuvant and adjuvant treatment with radiotherapy. In the United States, an Intergroup Cooperative Study (IG0099) tested radiotherapy alone versus an experimental arm consisting of concomitant cisplatin given every week during radiotherapy followed by three courses of adjuvant cisplatin and 5-fluorouracil chemotherapy.[383] A total of 147 evaluable patients with stages III and IV tumors were entered onto this study. Notably, approximately one-third of patients in this study were classified WHO 1, unlike most reports from the Pacific Rim in which greater than 95% of patients are WHO 2/3. At 3 years there was improved progression-free survival (69% vs 24%, p = .001), improved overall survival (76% vs 46%, p = .005), and reduced distant metastases (13% vs 35%, p = .002) for the experimental arm. The results of this trial changed the standard of care in the United States. These data were corroborated by another randomized phase III trial, which compared concurrent cisplatin (40 mg/m^2 weekly) and radiotherapy with radiotherapy alone in 350 patients with local and regionally advanced (Ho stage N2 and N3, or N1 with nodal disease ≥ 4 cm) NPC.[384] This study found that treatment with combined chemotherapy plus radiotherapy prolonged progression-free survival (hazard ratio, 1.367; 95% CI, 0.93–2.0). The treatment effect had a notable covariate interaction with tumor stage, and subgroup analysis showed a significant difference in patients with Ho stage T3 disease in favor of the concomitant-therapy arm (p = .0075; hazard ratio, 2.328; 95% CI, 1.26–4.28). The time to first distant failure also was statistically prolonged in patients with T3 tumors of the concomitant-treatment arm versus T3 tumor patients of the radiotherapy-alone arm (p = .016). Treatment in the chemotherapy-plus-radiation arm was well tolerated.[384] An updated report[385] concludes that overall survival benefits after chemoradiotherapy most clearly obtain in patients with T 3/4 staging (p = .013). Lin and colleagues[386] conducted a prospective phase III trial with randomization to radiation therapy (RT) alone or RT with two cycles of concomitant cisplatin and fluorouracil administered during weeks 1 and 5 of RT. Overall survival again favored the combined treatment arm (Table 79-11).

Table 79-11 Selected Concomitant Chemoradiotherapy Trials in Locally Advanced NPC

Study	*n*	Treatment Arms	Outcomes
Al-Sarraf et al[383]	78	cddp 100 mg/m^2 wks 1,4,7-RT + adj cddp/fu	5-yr PFS 58% and OS 67% CM vs 29% and 37% RT
	69	RT	(p < .001)
Lin et al[386]	141	cddp 20mg/m^2/d+fu 400 mg/m^2/d 96 h infusion wks 1 + 5-RT	5-yr PFS 72% and OS 72% CM vs 53% and 54% RT
	143	RT	(p = .001 + .002)
Chan et al[384]	174	cddp 40mg/m^2 wkly-RT	5-yr PFS 60% and OS 70% CM vs 52% and 59% RT
	176	RT	(p = .06 + .05)

cddp = cisplatin; CM = combined modality; fu = fluorouracil; OS = overall survival; PFS = progression-free survival; RT = radiotherapy.

Alternatively, strategies with induction chemotherapy have much appeal because of the high risk of systemic tumor dissemination in patients with NPC. However, a survival advantage for this approach has not been conclusively demonstrated. Chua and colleagues[387] have recently analyzed pooled data from two large phase III trials investigating the role of induction chemotherapy in NPC. In these trials, a total of 784 patients were randomized to receive 2 to 3 cycles of cisplatin-based combination drug therapy then radiotherapy or radiotherapy alone. Five-year relapse-free survival was 50.9% and 42.7%, respectively (p = .014), and disease-specific survival was 63.5% and 58.1% (p = .029). Overall survival was not found to be significantly different between the arms (p = .092). One can conclude that concomitant chemoradiotherapy is the treatment of choice for locally advanced NPC, much in accordance with the Intergroup 0099 trial. However, induction chemotherapy followed by radiotherapy is an option for patients who are not good candidates for concomitant treatment.

The report of Chan and colleagues[381] is notable as data are accumulating to show that the EGFR is a potential therapeutic target in NPC[388,389] and that high surface expression may correlate with poor outcome.[390] Thus, clinical studies of EGFR inhibitors are underway. Small molecule EGFR tyrosine kinase inhibitors are also under study and have demonstrated activity in squamous cell carcinoma of other primary head and neck sites.[391] Surface expression of EGFR, phosphorylated EGFR, MAPK, and Akt are potential molecular markers that may be useful in the future to select patients for treatment with EGFR inhibitor treatment protocols. We anticipate that new molecular treatment regimens will be evaluated in clinical trials of promising induction systemic therapies followed by chemoradiotherapy. This approach uses the induction (neoadjuvant) format as a vehicle to test new drug compounds or regimens in treating naïve patients, while retaining active therapeutic programs administered with curative intent.

SKIN

Although the skin of the head and neck accounts for less than 10% of the body's surface area, 70 to 80% of cutaneous malignancies occur in this region. As a result of greater sun exposure during occupational and recreational activities (with increased ultraviolet-B exposure), the incidence of skin cancer is increasing and the initial age at presentation is decreasing. About 3,000 yearly deaths are attributable to nonmelanoma cutaneous malignancies, and morbidity occurs in a many-fold greater number of people, however, in terms of medical costs, cosmetic deformity, and loss of function. About 1,000,000 new nonmelanoma skin cancers are projected annually in the United States. Treatment is protracted because of the recurrent nature of the disease, the need for repeated reconstructive efforts, and the propensity of second primary skin cancers to occur. Most early lesions are successfully controlled on the first attempt with conservative local therapy.

However, advanced skin cancer of the head and neck is not controlled easily, and its frequently devastating physical consequences can have tremendous influence on a patient's psychological well-being. A recent study ($n = 210$ patients) was conducted to identify nonmelanoma (squamous cell) skin cancer patients at the greatest risk of disease-specific mortality.[392] The individual clinical-pathologic factors most highly associated with adverse disease-specific survival were invasion beyond subcutaneous tissues ($p = .009$), perineural invasion ($p = .002$), and lesion size (≥ 4 cm) ($p = .0003$).

In a phase II study of systemic therapy in advanced SCC of the skin, isotretinoin plus IFN-α had major activity primarily limited to advanced local and regional disease.[393] The second phase II study of systemic therapy plus IFN in SCC produced substantial activity in extensively advanced disease (eg, stages T3 and T4).[394] Smaller series of cytotoxic chemotherapy combinations in similar patient populations reported overall response rates in the 60 to 70% range. (Melanoma of the head and neck region is considered in a separate chapter.)

NOSE AND PARANASAL SINUSES

As mentioned previously, the nose and the paranasal sinuses pose a unique set of problems that deserve separate consideration from SCC of the UADT. For instance, although SCC is still the most common histology found there, it accounts for less than 50% of disease. The four most common malignant histologies of the paranasal sinuses are SCC, sinonasal undifferentiated carcinoma (SNUC), neuroendocrine carcinoma, and esthesioneuroblastoma (often referred to as olfactory neuroblastoma).

Cancer of the nose and paranasal sinuses is relatively rare. When taken as a whole, these malignancies account for only 0.2 to 0.8% of cancers diagnosed annually, or approximately 3% of cancers of the UADT. The incidence is generally reported as 0.3 to 1 per 100,000 population.[395–397] These cancers tend to occur most commonly in the fifth decade of life, although they can occur in the much younger and much older. Cancer of the nose and paranasal sinuses is rare in children except for some sarcomas, such as rhabdomyosarcoma.[398,399] Although there are numerous environmental factors associated with cancer of the nose and paranasal sinuses, as industry has modernized, these have become somewhat less important. There continues to be a relationship between these malignancies and tobacco exposure, however.[400]

Neoplasms of the nose and paranasal sinuses rarely present early. This is because these tumors tend to be asymptomatic and usually contained within either a sinus or the nasal cavity. It is not until the patient develops symptoms from nasal airway obstruction or acute sinusitis that the patient seeks medical attention.[395,400] Early symptoms usually include nasal airway obstruction, rhinorrhea, sinusitis, epistaxis, and, occasionally, dental problems such as dental pain, numbness, and loose teeth. Late symptoms include, cranial nerve deficits, proptosis, facial pain and swelling, ulceration through the palate, and trismus, all of which are ominous signs.

Table 79-12 AJCC Staging for Malignant Primary Tumors of the Maxillary Sinuses

TNM	Staging Characteristics
Tx	Primary tumor cannot be assessed
T0	No evidence of primary tumor
Tis	Carcinoma in situ
T1	Tumor limited to antral mucosa and without invasion or erosion of bone
T2	Tumor casing bone erosion or destruction (except the posterior wall or orbit)
T3	Tumor invades any of the following: posterior wall of the maxillary sinus, subcutaneous tissues, skin of cheek, floor or medial wall of orbit, infratemporal fossa, pterygoid plates, ethmoid sinuses
T4	Tumor invades orbital contents and/or extends to orbital apex, cribriform plate, skull base, nasopharynx, sphenoid or frontal sinuses

The diagnosis of nose and paranasal sinus cancers is made by having a high index of suspicion in a patient who presents with nasal airway obstruction and a nasal mass. Key to this is a thorough endoscopic or fiberoptic examination of the entire nasal cavity to rule out benign disease such as nasal polyposis or uncomplicated acute or chronic sinusitis. Biopsy is indicated when a mass is found. However, great care should be taken as these lesions can hemorrhage, especially neuroendocrine carcinoma and esthesioneuroblastoma, which have a propensity toward epistaxis. In fact, a patient who presents with significant epistaxis with an otherwise smaller, asymptomatic lesion very commonly has neuroendocrine carcinoma. When taking a patient to the operating room for an endoscopic examination and biopsy, a frozen section should be obtained.[395] It is critical to consider minimizing exposure of uninvolved structures, therefore, biopsy only should be performed without Caldwell Luz procedures, septoplasty, or entry into uninvolved sinuses. Although it may be impossible to determine the exact histology of a particular lesion on frozen section, the pathologist is usually able to make a distinction between benign and malignant histology. This allows the surgeon to terminate the procedure if necessary and avoids an unnecessary or contraindicated operation in a patient with a presumed benign diagnosis who actually has a malignant process.

When evaluating the patient with a sinonasal mass, imaging plays an important part in not only the diagnosis and staging of these lesions, but also the surgical planning. CT and MRI both play important roles in the evaluation of sinonasal neoplasms.[395,400] The combination of CT and MRI provides useful information for surgical planning, especially with regard to skull base involvement. Although CT provides more information regarding bony anatomy and helps with surgical planning, MRI is better at assessing perineural involvement and skull base involvement and is better able to distinguish neoplasm from inspissated mucus.

Table 79-13 Primary Tumor Staging Characteristics for Carcinoma of the Ethmoid Sinuses

TNM	Tumor Extent
T1	Tumor confined to the ethmoid sinuses
T2	Tumor extends to the nasal cavity
T3	Tumor extends to the anterior orbit and/or maxillary sinuses
T4	Tumor exhibits extension to the orbital apex, sphenoid or frontal sinuses, or intracranially and/or to external nose

The staging of cancer of the paranasal sinuses is made radiographically.[397,398,401] Because these malignancies rarely present as early stage, the accepted staging systems are not commonly used in clinical practice; however, for completeness, they are provided for the maxillary sinuses and for the ethmoid sinuses (Tables 79-12 and 79-13). Special note is made of "Ohngren's line," or the malignant plane. Ohngren's line was an early attempt at staging of cancers of the paranasal sinuses using plane x-rays. That system divided tumors of the maxillary sinus into favorable and unfavorable, based on their relationship to this plane. The plane is defined on plane x-rays of the sinus and falls between the medial canthus of the orbit and the angle of the mandible. It was considered that tumors above this line (suprastructure) were unfavorable, while those below (infrastructure) were favorable. This is no longer used because we rarely get plane x-ray films. However, the distinction between unfavorable (suprastructure) and favorable (infrastructure) remains true. The distribution of the location of malignant carcinomas of the paranasal sinuses is shown in Table 79-14.

Histology The histology of neoplasms of the nose and paranasal sinuses is varied and can be divided into benign and malignant disease.[395,398,402,403] The most common sinonasal tumor, by far, is benign allergic nasal polyposis. If this is excluded, then the relationship between benign and malignant disease is approximately one to one. The most frequent malignant histologies are listed in Table 79-15. After benign nasal polyposis, inverting papilloma accounts for the majority of noninflammatory pathologies. It is generally felt that inverting papillomas arise from the squamous, or Schneiderian, mucosa. Although inverting papillomas are

Table 79-14 Distribution of Malignant Tumors of the Paranasal Sinuses

Location	%
Maxillary sinuses	55–63
Nasal walls	27–35
Ethmoid sinuses	9–10
Frontal sinuses	2
Sphenoid sinuses	1

Table 79-15 Most Frequent Histologies Found in Malignant Tumors of the Nose and Paranasal Sinuses

Squamous cell carcinoma
Sinonasal undifferentiated carcinoma (SNUC)
Neuroendocrine carcinoma
Melanoma
Adenocarcinoma
Salivary gland neoplasms
Sarcomas
Esthesioneuroblastoma (olfactory neuroblastoma)
Metastases

benign, they can be very aggressive locally, causing destruction of vital structures, invasion of the orbit, diplopia, and significant deformities. Furthermore, these are associated with an approximately 15% incidence of malignancy. As a result of their aggressive nature and risk of malignancy, all inverting papillomas should be excised promptly and completely. Varied approaches exist for the resection of inverting papilloma. These approaches vary in terms of their cosmetic impact on the patient but also in their ability to access different areas of the sinonasal cavities. Although cosmesis is important, the surgeon must maintain complete excision of the inverting papilloma as his primary goal. Despite complete excision, these tumors can recur locally (9%) and degenerate into malignant disease.

As sarcomas and salivary gland malignancies are covered in separate sections, this section will deal only with SCC, SNUC, neuroendocrine carcinoma, and esthesioneuroblastoma.

TREATMENT The treatment of neoplasms of the sinonasal cavity are varied and histology specific.[395,401,404–407] The mainstay of treatment, however, is a multidisciplinary approach to all patients with malignant disease. This includes open communication and cooperation between surgeons, radiotherapists, chemotherapists, speech pathologists, dental practitioners, prosthodontists, and social workers. "Traditional" treatment has been surgery, followed by radiation therapy when indicated.[396,397,400,408] Although very effective for smaller tumors of select histologies, this combination provides poor control in many instances. This is because these tumors usually present with advanced disease. The shortcomings of traditional treatment have led to the incorporation of new approaches, including chemotherapy.

Surgery alone as treatment of sinonasal malignancy is rarely used. It is most commonly associated with postoperative radiation therapy and, more recently, induction or adjuvant chemotherapy. When surgery is indicated, en bloc resection is indicated because piecemeal excision has a higher risk or recurrence and should be avoided. The operation used depends on the location of the tumor, the extent of the tumor, the histology, cosmesis, and patient preference. For each operation of the sinonasal cavities, there usually exists more than one option for incision and access to the lesion. For example, lateral rhinotomy is one option. This incision lies along the side of the nose and extends from the medial canthus to the nasal ala. It can extend around the nasal ala into the nasal vestibule and allows excellent visualization of the nasal cavity. The vertical limb along the side of the nose is best situated halfway between nasal dorsum and the nasomalar crease. It allows excellent exposure for medial maxillectomy. Obviously, however, many are uncomfortable with the scar on the face, and thus a midface degloving is often used. This is performed through a complete transfixion incision of the membranous septum combined with endonasal endocartilagenous incisions bilaterally, which allows the skin of the nose to be elevated completely to the nasion. This incision is then combined with bilateral gingivobuccal incisions that allow the soft tissue of the midface to be elevated from the maxilla, thus exposing the lower two-thirds of the midface. Although this approach allows excellent access to the lower sinonasal cavity, there can be some difficulty in reaching the superior-most aspects of the nasal cavity, ethmoids, and cribriform plate.

For maxillectomies, a variant of the "Weber-Fergusson" incision is often used. Specifically, the Weber-Fergusson incision includes the aforementioned lateral rhinotomy with an extension beneath the eye either through the conjunctiva or in an infraorbital skin crease. There can be an extension lateral to the orbit and the zygoma. This skin incision allows excellent exposure to the maxilla and orbit and allows access to the posterior maxillary tissues, thus facilitating maxillectomy. Cosmesis is a concern, but this incision provides the necessary exposure to the lateral maxilla for performing larger resections.

Endoscopic resection of small tumors, especially inverting papilloma, has gained favor in recent years. Although endoscopic resection is possible in some cases and does provide a valuable tool in biopsy, surveillance and staging, traditional surgical approaches to the midface, are still most commonly used for resection of malignant neoplasms.

The indications for a particular operation are based solely on the extent of the lesion and the surgeon's expertise and experience. Medial maxillectomy is best used for benign disease or those diseases limited to the medial wall of the maxilla or lateral wall of the nasal cavity. It can be performed through a lateral rhinotomy without a lip split or through midface degloving. This is a very effective operation for inverting papilloma and requires no reconstruction. Meticulous closure of the lateral rhinotomy usually leads to a very favorable cosmetic result as well.

Maxillectomy includes removal of the antral walls of the maxillary sinus but leaves the orbital periosteum and the malar strut. It is indicated for T1 and T2 lesions of the maxillary antrum without erosion beyond the sinus. This operation can be tailored to a particular tumor in order to decrease postoperative morbidity. Specifically, when feasible, rather than making a straight midline incision through the palate, the palatal excision can be curved away from the premaxilla, thus saving the incisors and cuspids. This provides a better functional result postoperatively. In addition, the orbital roof can also be preserved if the tumor is located inferiorly. This prevents diplopia, enophthalmos, and helps to prevent contracture of the skin, and avoids ectropion. The reconstruction of this defect is usually limited to a split-thickness skin graft and prosthetic rehabilitation.

When tumor extends beyond the maxillary sinus into the orbit, then total or radical orbital maxillectomy is indicated. Orbital exenteration is indicated when the periorbita is involved. There is much controversy with regard to the need for exenteration when only the orbital periosteum is involved. In instances when orbital fat and especially if extraocular movements are restricted because of muscle involvement, the eye should be sacrificed. Innovations with induction chemotherapy may eventually lead to preservation of the eye in certain situations. Once again, reconstruction is best accomplished through the use of a split-thickness skin graft and prosthesis. Occasionally, a free flap may be required for more extensive resections or to protect the osseous skull base, which frequently will be postoperatively managed by radiation therapy.

Finally, combined craniofacial resections are indicated when tumors extend to the skull base. Although many combined operations can be performed exclusively from below by an experienced head and neck surgeon, combination with neurosurgery allows approach of the tumor from above, and the brain is protected from iatrogenic injury. In this situation, a pericranial flap is usually used to resurface the sinonasal roof and protect intracranial dura and contents. In most cases, a free flap is then used to protect the contents of the cranial vault.

The complications of these operations are varied and depend, obviously, on the particular approach utilized. The most common problem is dysfunction of the lacrimal apparatus. This is especially important for patients who are likely to receive postoperative radiation therapy. As a result, we recommend dacryocystorhinostomy (DCR)[395] in all patients who are having midfacial surgery with disruption of the lacrimal apparatus. In addition, as many as 20% of patients will have postoperative diplopia owing to loss of support from the bony floor. Despite tethering of the medial canthus along the nasal bones and supporting the eye medially, this problem persists. Early intervention by ophthalmology is beneficial. With combined craniofacial resections, pneumocephalus can also occur. It has previously been felt that tracheostomy should be performed in all craniofacial patients to decrease the risk of pneumocephalus. With meticulous closure of the pericranial flap and the use of free flaps as indicated, however, we have not found this to be the case. Rarely do we feel that tracheostomy is indicated for combined craniofacial resections. Pneumocephalus, however, is an indicator of a persistent leak that can often lead to a high likelihood of meningitis and persistent cerebrospinal fluid (CSF) rhinorrhea.

Radiotherapy plays a large role in the management of sinonasal malignancies. It is used both pre- and postoperatively and can be used in select cases as definitive therapy for small T1 and T2 lesions, especially those limited to the nasal vestibule and anterior nasal fossa.[395] In this situation, high locoregional control rates and good cosmetic outcome result. With the increased use of radiotherapy in combination with surgery, ever-improving rates of locoregional control have been achieved. However, this has also lead to higher recognized rates of distant metastasis. Surgery with postoperative radiation therapy remains the standard of care for advanced sinonasal cavity tumors. In select patients who are not felt to be good surgical candidates, or when a tumor is inoperable, radiation therapy alone performs effectively in terms of local control and palliation. Preoperative radiation therapy can also be used for select inoperable tumors.

Essentially all patients who receive radiation therapy either as single agent treatment or in combination with surgery and/or chemotherapy will suffer some negative sequelae from the use of the radiation. Most will resolve over time. Acute complications include skin desquamation, nasal dryness, and mucositis. Chronic side effects include nasal dryness, dry eye, visual impairment, and atrophic rhinitis. Dry eye can range from mild dryness alleviated with over-the-counter drops to significant keratitis, corneal ulceration, and even blindness. Enucleation may even be necessary for significant damage. Although the retina, like most neural structures, is radioresistant, visual impairment can occur as a result of damage to the lens and/or microvasculature that supports both the retina and optic nerve.

Although chemotherapy is covered more extensively in a separate section, some aspects of chemotherapy deserve special consideration and will be mentioned briefly here. Traditionally, chemotherapy has been used for sinonasal tumors in palliative situations or for patients with recurrent tumors. However, an unwillingness to sacrifice the eye has lead to the use of induction chemotherapy in select patients.[409–411] In addition, positive results have led to more widespread and mainstream use of chemotherapy in certain situations.

Finally, regimens previously felt to be too toxic to be used regularly have gained more acceptance as supportive care in these patients has improved. Although the use of chemotherapy remains experimental and should only be administered as part of controlled protocols, recent prospective trials may suggest that control and overall survival are superior with the incorporation of chemotherapy.

In cases of SCC, surgery remains the treatment of choice when sacrifice of vital structures is not required. However, if a surgeon feels, based on clinical examination and imaging findings, that a tumor is not likely to be resectable with negative margins or that surgery would require sacrifice of vital structures, then induction chemotherapy in addition to surgery with postoperative radiation therapy should be considered. Both Choi and colleagues and investigators at the University of Chicago have used induction chemotherapy with combinations of cis-platinum and infusional 5-fluorouracil (5-FU) to achieve improved rates of locoregional control and preserve the eye.[409,412] Many studies using intra-arterial chemotherapy (usually cis-platinum) followed by surgery and/or radiation therapy exist.[413–416] Although these studies have shown some benefit with regard to locoregional control, the morbidity associated with intra-arterial therapy does not appear to justify the intra-arterial approach. Although craniofacial resection has been established as a surgical approach for more advanced disease, Shah and colleagues, published encouraging results of nearly 50% disease control in patients with unresectable skull-based neoplasms managed with concomitant chemoradiotherapy.

SNUC is fortunately rare. It is a lethal cancer typically presenting as advanced disease in elderly patients. Traditional treatment has been surgery followed by postoperative radiation therapy, but this has provided poor long-term control. Scattered reports exist in the literature that describe small series using chemotherapy and/or chemoradiotherapy in association with surgery to achieve some locoregional control.[416–419] SNUC is rare, and existing series are too small and varied to be able to promote one regimen as better than any other. However, in light of the poor locoregional control achieved with traditional surgery and postoperative radiation therapy, most agree that continued exploration for concomitant chemoradiotherapy is the best avenue for these patients.

Neuroendocrine carcinomas, which occur commonly in the larynx as well, have also been traditionally treated with surgery and postoperative radiation therapy. However, the literature suggests that they should be treated much like neuroendocrine carcinoma at other primary sites.[420–423] Specifically, The University of Texas M. D. Anderson Cancer Center advocates the use of induction chemotherapy with cisplatin, carboplatin, and etoposide. If patients achieve a complete response, then they proceed directly to radiotherapy, and surgery is avoided. If, on the other hand, only a partial response is achieved, then surgery followed by radiation therapy is the treatment of choice. This has led to increasing locoregional control rates with decreased morbidity from surgery.

Finally, esthesioneuroblastoma, or olfactory neuroblastoma, is a rare neoplasm of the sinonasal cavity; it emanates from the cribriform plate and early on invades the anterior cranial vault and, often, brain parenchyma.[398] These patients usually present with nasal obstruction and epistaxis. Under the microscope, these tumors present as small blue cell tumors and are often confused with neuroendocrine carcinoma. The distinction between the two is important, however, because although the best approach to treatment of neuroendocrine carcinoma is chemotherapy and/or surgery and radiation therapy, esthesioneuroblastoma is best treated with en bloc resection of the primary and (if indicated) postoperative radiation therapy. Investigators from the University of Virginia reported on 34 consecutively treated patients and the use of preoperative radiation therapy and chemotherapy.[424] They found that patients who responded to induction regimens had decreased disease-specific mortality and had 5- and 10-year survival rates of 81% and 55%, respectively. Finally, a recently published single-institution trial tested carboplatin, lomustine, and vincristine systemically (median 4 cycles) and/or regionally (median 17 cycles) every 2 months in 6 patients with no prior central nervous system involvement with newly identified metastatic esthesioneuroblastoma involving the central nervous system. This study showed that recurrent metastatic disease is treatable with acceptable toxicity and reasonable palliation. Four patients had partial responses; two patients progressed. The median response duration was 9 months (range 2–12 months), and median overall survival was 10.2 months (range 3–13 months).[425]

The management of sinonasal carcinoma differs distinctly from that of malignancies of the remainder of the UADT. This is most likely because traditional approaches using surgery followed by postoperative radiation therapy had significant morbidity and were associated with poor locoregional control. As a result of those unsatisfactory results with traditional therapy, numerous institutions have created differing protocols for the management of these patients. However, one defining principal remains true: Patients suffering from such malignancies require a multidisciplinary approach to their treatment. Our institution advocates that all patients be presented, before treatment, in a multidisciplinary setting with all indicated specialties. Although no one protocol can be advocated over another, we support the continued investigation of chemotherapy in an adjuvant role for the management of these patients, but also feel that surgery will continue to play a large role in the control of this disease. Thus, the surgeon should remain at the core of the interdisciplinary management team.

SALIVARY GLANDS

Anatomy Salivary gland tissue is ubiquitous in the submucosa of the upper gastrointestinal tract and is grouped into three major salivary glands: the parotid, the submaxillary (or submandibular), and the sublingual glands. The most common sites of tumors of minor salivary glands are the palate, the base of the tongue, and the buccal mucosa.[177,426–429]

The majority of salivary gland tumors arise in the parotid glands, and although nearly 80% of these are benign, these glands are the origin of the majority of malignant tumors. Tumors arising in the submandibular, sublingual, or minor salivary glands are more likely to be malignant.

The largest salivary glands are the parotids, which are located on the cheeks anterior to the external auditory canal and pinna. The gland wraps around the mandible, and as the facial nerve passes through the parotid, it divides it into superficial, or lateral, and deep lobes. About 80%

of the gland lies lateral to the facial nerve, and 20% lies deep to this nerve, behind and medial to the mandible. The internal carotid artery, the internal jugular vein, the cervical sympathetic chain, and cranial nerves IX, X, and XI are in close proximity to the deep lobe of the parotid. The lymphatic drainage of parotid tumors is to intraparotid lymph nodes, external jugular chain, and the upper jugular lymph nodes (levels 2 and 3). Additional lymphatic drainage is to adjacent levels, including the posterior triangle or level 5. Depending on histology, many nodes may be involved. The presence of nerves within the parotid gland, especially the facial nerve and the auriculotemporal branch of the trigeminal, can be involved by tumors, especially adenoid cystic carcinoma and SCC, which may exhibit perineural extension. Any parotid mass warrants exploration, and surgical excision is often the only solution since progression of even benign neoplasms may not only cause facial asymmetry, but also place the facial nerve at risk.

The second largest glands are the submandibular glands, located in the triangle formed by the two bellies of the digastric muscle and the mandible. Malignant tumors in this location can spread to the lymph nodes in levels II, III, and IV, as well as grow along the nerves, preferentially the branches of the lingual nerve, the nerve to the mylohyoid, and occasionally the mandibular branch of the facial nerve. Seldom will growth occur along the hypoglossal nerve, in spite of the close proximity of the structure. About half of the tumors in the submandibular glands are benign.

The sublingual glands are the smallest of the major salivary glands and are formed of a conglomeration of glands located underneath the mucosa of the floor of the mouth and surrounding the excretory duct of the submandibular gland, Wharton's duct.

Diagnosis The clinical presentation of malignant salivary gland tumors is variable, depending on the site and histology. The presence of a facial nerve paralysis is uncommon but generally indicates a malignant lesion. Tumors of the deep lobe of the parotid are notorious for producing dysphagia and submucosal deformity of the soft palate. When major invasion of the parapharyngeal space occurs, involvement of cranial nerves IX, X, XI, and even XII can occur. The usual presentation of submandibular gland tumors is a painless swelling below the mandible, and such tumors need to be distinguished from the much more frequent bacterial sialoadenitis of this gland.

On physical examination, a persistent mass without superficial ulceration of either skin or mucosa is the most frequent finding. An important diagnostic procedure to be considered, provided expert cytology opinion is available, is fine-needle aspiration. The objective of this cytologic diagnosis is to rule out neoplasia or confirm the presence of malignancy. This procedure, especially in the parotid and submandibular gland, has gained increasing acceptance and should be considered whenever the information that can be obtained will have an impact on treatment or prognosis. The accurate typing of tumor is often less important and may be deferred to the definitive histologic examination. This has to be applied judiciously in spite of the high accuracy reported by experts (ie, sensitivity, 94%; specificity, 97%; accuracy, 95%).[430]

Table 79-16 Most Common Malignant Tumors of Salivary Glands

Mucoepidermoid carcinoma (low, intermediate, or high grade)
Acinic cell carcinoma
Adenoid cystic carcinoma
Adenocarcinoma
Malignant mixed tumor (carcinoma-expleomorphic adenoma)
Squamous cell carcinoma

Histopathology Benign lesions are the most frequent tumors of the parotid gland. The basic histologic classification of malignant salivary tumors was developed by Foote and Frazzell (Table 79-16).[431] Over the years, this classification has been reviewed and expanded to include some less frequently found malignant tumors, and the present WHO classification is most often quoted.[429,432]

Mucoepidermoid carcinomas constitute about 26%, 21%, and 10% of malignant salivary gland tumors of the palatal, parotid, and submandibular glands, respectively.[431] Mucoepidermoid carcinoma is the most frequent cancer of the parotid gland and is classified into high-grade, intermediate, and low-grade tumors.[433,434] Well-differentiated, low-grade mucoepidermoid carcinoma is characterized by a slow growth rate, a low recurrence rate after complete surgical excision (about 15%), and rare incidence of metastasis. High-grade tumors are more aggressive, and the local recurrence rate after surgery alone approaches 60%.[431] Local recurrences and distant metastases may occur many years after treatment.[177,435] About 50% of patients with high-grade mucoepidermoid carcinomas present with regional metastases, and 30% develop metastases at distant sites.[434,436,437] Acinic cell carcinomas are usually well differentiated and account for approximately 13% of the cancers arising from the parotid glands. Lymph node metastases occur in about 15% of cases. Local recurrence and distant metastases may occur many years after treatment.[177,438] Adenoid cystic carcinomas, once called cylindromas, account for approximately 10% of parotid gland malignancies but 60% of malignant neoplasms of the submandibular or minor salivary glands.[431,439–441] A remarkable feature of this neoplasm is its propensity to invade major nerves and spread along the endoneural and perineural sheaths. This has significant prognostic importance and must be taken into account when deciding treatment and, specifically, when considering postoperative radiotherapy. Although these tumors often follow an indolent course, as many as 40% of patients ultimately develop regional and distant metastases.[439–441]

Adenocarcinomas account for 10% of parotid gland cancers but are more common in the minor salivary glands.[442] The majority of them are high-grade tumors. About 36% of patients either present with or subsequently develop regional lymph node metastases; therefore, the regional lymph nodes need to be addressed in treatment strategies for high-grade adenocarcinomas.[427,443] Distant metastases to lungs and bone are not uncommon.

Carcinoma expleomorphic adenoma arises from preexisting benign pleomorphic adenoma. The risk of malignant transformation increases with time and age of the patient. Of adenomas of less than 5 years' duration, 1.6% can dedifferentiate, and 9.4% of adenomas present for more than 15 years can dedifferentiate.[444] True malignant mixed tumors are very rare, constituting only 2 to 5% of all malignant salivary gland tumors. These are typically aggressive tumors. The neck nodes are involved in 25% of patients.[177] In rare instances, a benign-appearing pleomorphic adenoma may produce distant metastases.

Primary SCC of the salivary gland is rare, accounting for less than 3% of parotid neoplasms. It needs to be distinguished from metastatic SCC to the parotid lymph nodes from cutaneous malignancies or other sites. SCC of the skin of the forehead, temple, or ear may metastasize to this region. Such primary sites must be excluded before the diagnosis of primary squamous carcinoma of the parotid can be made. Primary SCCs of the parotid gland may develop regional lymph node metastases in 50% of patients, and this needs to be considered when patients are treated by surgery and postoperative radiation therapy.

Staging The accepted staging system for salivary gland tumors can be found in the monographs of the AJCC and UICC. Both organizations have agreed to changes bringing the two classifications into agreement.[432,445] The regional lymph node staging and distant metastasis staging criteria are the same as for the common SCC of the UADT (Table 79-17).

The treatment of benign salivary gland tumors is primarily surgical. However, there may be a role

Table 79-17 Primary Tumor Staging Characteristics for Carcinoma of the Salivary Glands

Stage	Tumor Characteristics
Tx	Primary tumor cannot be assessed
T0	No evidence of primary tumor
T1	Tumor limited to gland and < 2 cm in greatest dimension
T2	Tumor limited to gland and between 2 and 4 cm in greatest dimension
T3	Tumor limited to gland and between 4 and 6 cm in greatest dimension
T4	Tumor limited to gland but > 6 cm in greatest dimension

Subdivisions: Each of the above T-stages is divided into (a) local extension or (b) without local extension. Local extension is defined as clinical or macroscopic evidence of tumor invasion of bone, skin, soft tissues of the neck, or nerve.

for postoperative radiation therapy in situations of incomplete removal or recurrences of benign tumor following prior surgical treatment. If microscopic disease remains overlying the facial nerve, postoperative radiation therapy may be effective in preventing subsequent recurrences.[427,446,447]

Surgery is also the primary form of treatment of patients with resectable salivary gland malignancies. Early-stage (T1 or T2) and especially low-grade tumors should be treated with comprehensive excision with free surgical margins. Such tumors arising in the parotid gland are generally treated by parotidectomy with preservation of the facial nerve. Early-stage high-grade tumors of any histology are treated with surgical resection of the primary site, with an attempt to achieve free surgical margins. This often is not possible, and microscopic spread, especially of adenoid cystic carcinoma, may occur along tissue planes, submucosal spaces, and perineural pathways. The dissection of regional lymph nodes should be done judiciously; elective nodal dissection is seldom indicated except in high-grade malignancies, especially salivary duct carcinomas.[448] Salivary glands malignancies were thought to be resistant to conventional photon radiation, but over the years it has become established that postoperative irradiation is highly effective for eradicating subclinical disease.[441,443,446,447,449–451] Postoperative radiotherapy may be indicated for major and minor salivary gland cancers when either of the following exists: (1) the tumor is high grade or is metastatic SCC, regardless of surgical margins; (2) the surgical margins are close or microscopically positive (which also may include tumors arising in the deep lobe of the parotid gland), regardless of grade; (3) a resection has been performed for a recurring cancer, regardless of the histology or margin status; (4) the tumor has invaded beyond the capsule of the gland into skin, bone, nerve, or glandular tissue; (5) regional lymph nodes contain metastatic cancer; or (6) if there is gross residual or unresectable disease.[440] In addition, preoperative radiotherapy prior to planned surgery may actually facilitate parotidectomy in advanced cases and allow preservation of the facial nerve. If the facial nerve is involved at presentation (as evidenced by nerve weakness) then surgery and postoperative radiotherapy is favored.

For T3 and T4 parotid cancer, unless the facial nerve is circumferentially encompassed by tumor or grossly enlarged by cancer, nerve-sparing surgery may be used followed by radiotherapy. Radiation therapy doses to the primary site and involved structures are in the range of 5,511 to 6,500 cGy, depending on tumor type and postsurgical status. Generally, for low-grade mucoepidermoid carcinomas and acinic cell carcinomas, it is not necessary to treat the clinically uninvolved neck. For all other high-grade histologies, the neck nodal drainage is generally treated to doses in the range of 5,000 cGy. In the case of adenoid cystic carcinomas, the radiation fields should include the course of significant major named nerve trunks to the base of the skull.[441] A facial nerve that is involved by cancer but still functional preoperatively should be repaired by appropriate resection and grafting. Postoperative radiotherapy can be given to nerve grafts.

Prognosis The results of treatment depend on both the histologic type and the tumor site. In a series from The University of Texas M. D. Anderson Cancer Center, 5-year survival rates were 100% for patients with acinic cell carcinoma, 95% for patients with adenoid cystic carcinoma, 90% for patients with low-grade mucoepidermoid carcinoma, 80% for patients with high-grade mucoepidermoid carcinoma, 70% for patients with adenocarcinoma, and 59% for patients with malignant mixed tumors.[443,451] At the Princess Margaret Hospital, primary parotid disease was controlled by surgery alone in 24% of cases and by surgery and radiotherapy in 74% of cases.[450]

In the case of submandibular gland tumors, approximately half of treated patients are free of disease after 5 years, compared with a lesser number of patients with high-grade mucoepidermoid histology.[452] Minor salivary gland tumors, especially tumors in the paranasal sinuses, often present with advanced-stage disease. In the M. D. Anderson series, the 2-year local control rate was 47% in patients treated with surgery alone and 76% in patients treated with surgery and postoperative radiation therapy.[442] Results of minor salivary gland tumors are usually more favorable.[451,453–455] In selected instances for minor salivary gland tumors, radiotherapy alone might be an option, but local control is less favorable.[440] T stage affects local control of disease, and the extent of disease is more important than the site itself.

Neutron Radiotherapy For patients with large inoperable salivary gland tumors or for patients who are at high risk of local recurrence after an incomplete resection, fast neutron radiotherapy is an alternative to standard radiotherapy. Fast neutrons have different radiobiologic properties when compared with standard radiation, and in vivo data from Batterman and colleagues on the response of pulmonary metastases to fractionated radiotherapy show a relative biologic effectiveness (RBE) factor in the range of 8.0 for salivary gland tumors, compared with RBEs in the range of 3.0 to 3.5 for late effects in most normal tissues.[456] To put this in perspective, if one were to give a dose of 20 neutron-Gy to a parotid tumor, the biologic effect in terms of the mucosa and temporomandibular joint would be equivalent to 60 to 70 photon-Gy, but the biologic effect on the tumor would be equivalent to 160 photon-Gy—a theoretical therapeutic gain of a factor of 2.3 to 2.6.

The Radiation Therapy Oncology Group (RTOG) in the United States and the Medical Research Council (MRC) in England performed a phase III randomized clinical trial to compare fast-neutron radiotherapy versus conventional photon irradiation for inoperable salivary gland tumors. The fast-neutron group achieved significantly improved tumor clearance at both the primary site and in the regional lymph nodes. At the 2-year endpoint, the local/regional control rates were 67% for the neutron group compared with 17% for the photon group ($p < .005$), and survivals were 62% for the neutron group compared with 25% for the photon group ($p = .1$). Because of the significantly greater locoregional control rate achieved in the fast-neutron group, the study was closed early for ethical reasons. Ten-year data continued to show improved locoregional control on the neutron arm (56% vs 17%, $p = .009$) but no difference in overall survival because of deaths from distant metastases.[457] A summary of single-institution comparative data is consistent with the results of the randomized trial showing a local control rate of 67% for 309 patients treated with fast neutrons compared with 26% for 298 patients treated with conventional photon irradiation.[458]

Modern neutron treatment facilities allow for three-dimensional conformal approaches to treatment, and this has resulted in further improvement of outcome. Douglas and colleagues reviewed the University of Washington experience involving 148 patients with major salivary gland tumors (mixed histologies).[459] Local control was found to be a function of tumor size, with long-term control being achieved in 78% of patients with tumors smaller than 4 cm compared with 40% for patients with tumors larger than 4 cm. The probability of a patient developing distant metastases was found to be strongly dependent on lymph node status being 52% at 5 years for the node-positive group compared with 32% for the node-negative group. It was found that an initial surgical resection was beneficial in terms of reducing the amount of disease present at the time of neutron radiotherapy.

Another analysis by Douglas and colleagues focused strictly on patients with adenoid cystic histologies.[460] This series consisted of 151 patients with tumors arising in both major and minor salivary glands and who had gross tumor at the time of treatment. The overall 5-year local control rate was 59%, with a 5-year actuarial survival rate of 72%. In patients who had undergone an incomplete surgical resection and in whom there was no skull base involvement by tumor, the local control rate was 80%.

Neutron radiotherapy has also been used to treat patients with multiply-recurrent pleomorphic adenomas. The initial treatment of choice for these benign tumors is surgery, with long-term local control rates being in the range of 95%. However, some patients experience multiple recurrences following surgical resection. These cases present a difficult management problem since further surgery may entail a higher than acceptable risk of damage to the facial nerve. In these situations, neutron radiotherapy offers an alternative form of treatment. The number of patients with multiply-recurrent pleomorphic adenomas treated with fast neutrons is small compared with the number of frankly malignant tumors that have been treated, but results appear quite encouraging. Douglas and colleagues reported on 16 patients who were treated with a

Table 79-18 Rates of Distant Metastases in Parotid Carcinoma by Histologic Type

Histology	Rate of Metastasis (%)
Mucoepidermoid	14/84 (8)
Acinic Cell	2/14 (14)
Adenoid Cystic	22/53 (42)
Malignant Mixed Tumor	3/14 (21)
Adenocarcinoma	25/91 (27)
Squamous Cell	2/13 (15)

median time at risk of 96 months.[461] The 15-year actuarial local control was 76% for patients with gross tumors and 100% for those with only positive minimal disease following their last surgical resection.

Systemic therapy for salivary cancer remains an investigational endeavor, with no standard regimen universally accepted. Table 79-18 presents distant metastatic rates of parotid carcinomas based on cystology. Discussed above, all agree that there should continue to be an emphasis on local therapy, most often surgical resection then postoperative radiotherapy dependent on the surgical pathology. Chemotherapy, as a component of primary management, is usually in the setting of a clinical trial.

Previous studies have demonstrated single-agent activity for methotrexate, doxorubicin, cisplatin, 5-fluorouracil, the vinca alkaloids, and, more recently, taxanes. Response rates are in the range of 15 to 20%. Combination therapy provides some increase in response but with no clear survival advantages. A regimen with cyclophosphamide, doxorubicin, and cisplatin (CAP) has produced responses in 40 to 50% of patients treated, with duration 4 to 6 months.[462] Responses are more often observed in patients with adenocarcinomas, and less likely adenoid cystic carcinoma. There has been relatively little demonstrated efficacy for newer targeted compounds and more work is needed.

A decision to proceed with systemic therapy should be considered with attention given to tumor histology, stage, time to disease progression after primary therapy, patient performance status, and the pace of disease progression. Efforts are also underway to identify molecular markers, which may enhance our ability to individualize therapy in determining an applicable treatment plan. Most head and neck oncologists tend to separate patients with adenoid cystic carcinoma from others in developing a treatment strategy. After diagnosis, surgical resection is performed if feasible, and for many patients consideration is given to postoperative radiotherapy. Chemotherapy may be reserved in primary management for patients with locally advanced and unresectable disease. For example, presentation of a nasopharyngeal adenoid cystic primary tumor invading the skull base may not be amenable to surgical resection. Of course, the determination of resectability depends on individual patient characteristics, precise tumor staging and the skill and experience of the attending surgeons. However, for such a patient with bulky disease, radiotherapy can be administered with sensitizing chemotherapy as primary treatment. In this setting, we would consider use of cisplatin 100 mg/m^2 administered on days 1, 22, and 43 of the radiotherapy program.

More often, chemotherapy becomes a treatment option for patients with distant disease recurrence, and common sites of involvement are lung and bone. In this setting, an understanding of the number of metastatic sites, tumor bulk, and the timing of disease progression are important. As metastatic adenoid cystic carcinoma will often be indolent in its growth pattern, a short period of observation is typically indicated, particularly in debilitated or elderly patients. At times, there may be only slow growth over a period of years. However, if serial evaluations show more aggressive cancer, then it would be appropriate to consider an investigational trial or chemotherapy perhaps with a platin-based regimen. Partial response rates of 40 to 50% have been reported in selected patients for CAP and cisplatin-based therapy.[462–466] Airoldi and colleagues[467,468] have combined vinorelbine with cisplatin in a phase II experience with a mix of salivary tumor histologies. They observed moderate activity with occasional complete responses, some long-term survivors, and even activity (CR + PR, 44.4%) in adenoid cystic carcinoma.

In patients with high-grade mucoepidermoid carcinoma or salivary duct adenocarcinoma, traditional cisplatin-based chemotherapy combinations may be more routinely active. In this group of patients, the taxanes are observed to be active as single agents[469] and are being tested in combination chemotherapy regimens. Clinical and pathological data are accumulating, which indicate that the expression of biomarkers such as mutant p53 proteins, expression of vascular endothelial growth factor, and surface EGFR overexpression may predict or identify more aggressive tumor phenotypes, and may also represent potential therapeutic targets. Our group recently reported[470] an early experience with gefitinib, a small molecule, EGFR tyrosine kinase inhibitor, administered in a phase II protocol for patients with advanced salivary tumors. We are observing stabilization of disease in 30 to 40% of patients with adenoid cystic carcinoma. Glisson and colleagues[471] have reported that *HER/2-neu* overexpression is common in salivary duct carcinomas (10 of 12 patients studied). Maruya and colleagues[472] have performed microarray expression analyses of malignant salivary tumors, and have identified a gene set that differentiates adenoid cystic carcinoma from other malignant salivary gland tumors. A high level of c-*kit* expression has also been identified in adenoid cystic carcinoma, but preliminary trials with imatinib mesylate have not demonstrated clinical benefit.[473]

In summary, the emerging molecular biomarker data may have important prognostic implications and hopefully will lead to more active systemic treatment strategies. The observation of HER-2 positivity in salivary duct carcinoma may be the basis for systematic study of chemotherapy and trastuzumab in this uncommon group of patients. However, given the relative rarity of salivary cancers in general, formal trials may require collaboration among multiple, large tertiary centers or implementation through the cooperative oncology group mechanism.

SARCOMAS OF THE HEAD AND NECK

Overview Overall, sarcomas are particularly rare neoplasms as they constitute only 1% of all cancer diagnosed in the United States and 1% of all head and neck primary cancers.[462,474] Furthermore, these tumors do not commonly manifest as primary malignancies in the head and neck region except in the pediatric population, in which as many as 35% of all sarcomas affect head and neck sites.[475] The most commonly encountered sarcomas of the head and neck region are osteogenic sarcoma, malignant fibrous histiocytoma, rhabdomyosarcoma, and angiosarcoma.

The rarity of sarcomas, as well as the multitude of histologic subtypes, can make definitive diagnosis difficult, and an experienced pathologist is key to the initial evaluation. Appropriate pathologic characterization forms the basis for prognosis and subsequent treatment selection. The biology of a neoplasm and its propensity for locally aggressive growth and systemic dissemination are clearly reflected in its histology and grade. Size and location of the lesion, which have become more precisely delineated with improvements in radiographic modalities, also impart reliable prognostic information. All of these factors, along with the complexities of head and neck anatomy (especially regarding function and cosmesis), make optimal treatment difficult to determine in many cases.

Traditionally, surgery has formed the cornerstone of therapy for head and neck sarcomas. However, multimodality treatment of these tumors incorporating a multidisciplinary approach has yielded encouraging results. Data collected by ongoing cooperative studies such as the Intergroup Rhabdomyosarcoma Study Group (IRSG) have demonstrated improved outcomes for those patients treated with surgery along with other nonsurgical modalities. These protocols also serve as a model for the evolving roles of chemotherapy and radiation either as adjuvant treatments or even primary therapy in selected patients. As a result, many patients, particularly children, are now able to avoid surgery in functionally and cosmetically critical areas of the head and neck without compromising their survival.

Osteosarcoma Osteogenic sarcoma is the most common nonhematopoietic malignant neoplasm of bone, usually occurring in the long bones of adolescent patients. However, 10% of these neoplasms arise in the head and neck region and occur in patients who are on average 10 to 15 years older than those patients with osteosarcomas of the long bones.[476] Most of these tumors present as a painless mass of the maxilla or mandible, often accompanied by loose teeth. Surgical resection achieving negative margins remains the crucial element in the treatment of head and neck osteosarcomas. It has been repeatedly shown that surgical margin status correlates significantly with local control and survival. In those cases in which margins were positive following resection, 5-year survival decreased dramatically to 35% from approximately 75% in those individuals with negative margins.[477,478] In one series, positive margins were shown to be uniformly fatal at 4 years after treatment.[476] Most recent experiences with this disease have been with multimodality therapy.[476–480] Several centers have applied external beam irradiation in the postoperative period, particularly in cases of high-grade tumors, large lesions, close or positive margins, or inoperability.[477,479,480] Unfortunately, radiation, whether delivered externally or as brachytherapy, does not appear to significantly improve overall survival in head and neck osteosarcomas.[476,478] The addition of chemotherapy, however, has shown greater promise as an adjuvant modality in the treatment of osteosarcomas for individuals with lesions of the extremities.[476,478,479,481,482] In a meta-analysis of 201 patients with craniofacial osteosarcomas, Smeele and colleagues suggested that chemotherapy increases survival even in those cases of incomplete surgical resection.[482] Nevertheless, other series and meta-analyses have not shown such promising results.[480,483] Five-year survival in larger series is only 42 to 55%, and disease-free survival at 5 years is achieved in only 25 to 30% of all patients.[476–479] Combinations of surgery and chemotherapy, and possibly even radiation, for these aggressive neoplasms may provide better outcomes. Data continue to accrue, and future treatment protocols will be instituted based on these experiences.

Angiosarcoma Angiosarcomas are exceedingly rare vascular sarcomas, but approximately 50% of all angiosarcomas occur in the head and neck region.[484–486] These lesions classically present as bruise-like macules and plaques on the forehead and scalp of elderly white males.[484,486] Because of their innocuous appearance and lack of symptoms, diagnosis is often delayed. Optimal treatment, however, is not clearly defined because of the rarity of angiosarcomas and their almost universally poor prognosis. The ability of these neoplasms to spread subcutaneously over relatively large areas makes local recurrence a defining quality of these malignancies.[485,487,488] Therefore, truly negative surgical margins are unlikely to be achieved, and postoperative wide field radiation therapy has been employed with increasing frequency and success at local control.[484,487,488] With 5-year survival rates ranging from only 12 to 33%, and with death commonly resulting from distant metastases, chemotherapy may have a role in the management of angiosarcomas.[484,485,487]

Rhabdomyosarcoma Rhabdomyosarcoma is a significant disease of childhood and adolescents. It comprises approximately 4 to 8% of all pediatric cancers and is the most common sarcoma of childhood.[489] Approximately 40% of all rhabdomyosarcomas originate in the head and neck region, and of these, 90% affect children.[489] Furthermore, rhabdomyosarcoma accounts for up to a quarter of all head and neck sarcomas.[474,489] Histologically, rhabdomyosarcomas are divided into four subtypes: embryonal, alveolar, botryoidal, and pleomorphic; this classification is clinically relevant as alveolar rhabdomyosarcomas are associated with significantly decreased survival when compared with the other histologic types.[490] Further classification in children is based on the head and neck site, defined as orbital, parameningeal, or nonparameningeal.[491] The orbit is the most common site in children, whereas the sinonasal tract is the most common head and neck site in adults. The particular head and neck site of origin correlates with prognosis and has therefore been incorporated into the tumor-nodes-metastasis (TNM) staging system.[491] Surgicopathologic criteria have also been used by the IRSG to stage rhabdomyosarcomas in pediatric patients according to local extension, regional and distant metastases, and the amount of residual tumor remaining after resection.[491] (The IRSG was founded in 1972 and has since established standard treatment algorithms based on a combination of these staging systems for rhabdomyosarcomas in children and adolescents.)[492] Complete surgical resection remains a critical component of therapy for these patients. However, comprehensive resection is not always possible with sarcomas of the head and neck region because of involvement of vital structures or unacceptable functional or cosmetic morbidity. Consequently, chemotherapy and radiation therapy are used as the primary treatment modalities in many patients with rhabdomyosarcoma of the head and neck region.[492] Advances in the treatment of pediatric patients with rhabdomyosarcoma are reflected in the dramatically improved overall survival rate. Since 1970, the survival rate for all patients diagnosed with rhabdomyosarcoma has increased from approximately 25 to 70%, mostly as a result of the ongoing IRSG studies.[493] Survival data for adult patients are somewhat limited, but overall outcomes are likely significantly worse than those reported for children.[489]

Malignant Fibrous Histiocytoma Malignant fibrous histiocytomas (MFHs) represent the most common variety of soft tissue sarcoma, and it is one of the most common of all head and neck sarcomas.[494–498] As with other sarcomas, MFH usually presents as a painless mass, and other symptoms are highly dependent on the particular structures involved. In the head and neck area, these lesions often occur in the sinonasal tract. Adequate review by experienced pathologists cannot be overemphasized. Fibrous lesions, including MFHs, have a broad spectrum of similar histologic features, but significantly different prognoses.[499] Treatment of MFH of the head and neck is preferably accomplished with wide surgical excision of the primary tumor, obtaining negative margins. Postoperative radiation therapy is recommended for unresectable lesions and in cases of close or positive margins. However, improved local control, especially for MFHs of other anatomic sites, has been achieved in some series using adjuvant radiotherapy regardless of margin status.[495,500] Adjuvant chemotherapy for MFH remains investigational and has so far been used mostly in the setting of metastatic disease.[501] Adjuvant chemotherapy may have a role, based on the report of the Sarcoma Meta-Analysis Collaboration Group, which found improved recurrence-free intervals but not a statistically significant survival advantage.[502] Overall 5-year survival rates following treatment of malignant fibrous histiocytoma of the head and neck region average 40% in larger series.[474,503,504] Local recurrences are seen in approximately 20% of patients, but most disease-related deaths result from distant metastases, usually to the lungs.

ODONTOGENIC TUMORS

Odontogenic tumors constitute a small but interesting subset of lesions of significance in oncology. It is traditional to discuss these entities based on their cell of origin; however, it is much more important from the clinical perspective to analyze their biologic behavior in order to arrive at treatment recommendations. Although many of these odontogenic lesions are of interest predominantly as curiosities to the nonmaxillofacial surgeon, there are several that merit attention. These are the ameloblastoma, the calcifying epithelial odontogenic tumor (CEOT or Pindborg tumor) and the clear cell odontogenic tumor (CCOT). The latter has more recently been accepted as being a carcinoma and most authorities consider it to be a clear cell odontogenic carcinoma. In addition, there are two cysts, the calcifying odontogenic cyst (COC) and the odontogenic keratocyst (OKC) that behave more like a tumor than a cyst. All are unique in their origin from ectodermal components of the dental lamina, or follicle, from which teeth are formed. Their histopathologic appearance is varied and certain members of this class of tumors have the capacity to induce changes in tissues derived from mesoderm, thereby creating highly characteristic mixed histomorphometric patterns.

One group of lesions, the odontomas, formerly regarded as being slow growing noninvasive tumors is now regarded as being hamartomas.

The generally accepted classification of odontogenic tumors is that of the World Health Organization (WHO) listed in Table 79-19.[505] The majority of these are benign. There is also an obscure but deadly group of primary odontogenic malignancies that include intraosseous mucoepidermoid carcinoma, ameloblastic carcinoma, malignant ameloblastoma, clear cell odontogenic carcinoma (also called clear cell odontogenic tumor), and carcinomas arising from the walls of odontogenic cysts or tumors.

Other lesions in the category of odontogenic pathology include the fibro-osseous group consisting of periapical, focal, or florid cemento-osseous dysplasias, ossifying and cemento-ossifying fibromas, and peripheral odontogenic

Table 79-19 World Health Organization Classification of Odontogenic Lesions

Table 79-19 World Health Organization Classification of Odontogenic Lesions
Benign odontogenic tumors
Odontogenic epithelium without odontogenic ectomesenchyme
Ameloblastoma
a) Squamous odontogenic tumor (SOT)
b) Calcifying epithelial odontogenic tumor (CEOT, Pindborg tumor)
Odontogenic epithelium with odontogenic ectomesenchyme, with or without dental hard tissue formation
c) Ameloblastic fibroma (AF), ameloblastic fibrodentinoma (dentinoma), ameloblastic fibro-odontoma
d) Odontoameloblastoma
e) Adenomatoid odontogenic tumor (AOT)
f) Calcifying odontogenic cyst (COC)
g) Odontoma: complex and compound
Odontogenic ectomesenchyme with or without included odontogenic epithelium
h) Odontogenic fibroma
i) Myxoma
j) Cementoblastoma
Malignant odontogenic tumors
Odontogenic carcinomas
k) Malignant ameloblastoma
l) Primary intraosseous carcinoma
m) Malignant variants of other odontogenic epithelial tumors
Malignant changes in odontogenic cysts
Odontogenic sarcomas
n) Ameloblastic fibrosarcoma (ameloblastic sarcoma)
o) Ameloblastic fibrodentinosarcoma and ameloblastic fibro-odontosarcoma
p) Odontogenic carcinosarcoma
Neoplasms and other lesions related to bone
Osteogenic neoplasms
q) Cemento-ossifying fibroma (cementifying fibroma, ossifying fibroma)
• Non-neoplastic bone lesion
• Fibrous dysplasia
• Cemento-osseous dysplasias
r) Periapical cemental dysplasia (periapical fibrous dysplasia)
s) Florid cemento-osseous dysplasia
t) Other cemento-osseous dysplasias
• Cherubism
• Central giant cell granuloma
• Aneurysmal bone cyst
• Solitary bone cyst

fibroma. Adamantinoma of the long bones and craniopharyngioma very closely resemble ameloblastoma histopathologically, but will not be discussed since they do not occur in the jaws.

Although there is significant variation in invasiveness and growth rate of these lesions they are generally slow growing, causing distortion of bone by resorption of the trabeculae of the medullary space and expansion of the cortical bone. Consequently they usually present as painless swellings or as asymptomatic lesions detected during routine dental radiographic assessment of the oral cavity. Pain is uncommon unless the lesion becomes infected, and paresthesia of the lips or tongue is also uncommon. However, large tumors may exhibit a much more aggressive behavior that includes extensive destruction of bone and invasion into the soft tissues. When benign but aggressive tumors like ameloblastoma gain access to the soft tissues, they may become impossible to eradicate successfully.

Odontogenic lesions arise from tissue within the jaws that has the capability of differentiating into the tissue elements found in teeth or periodontal membrane. Therefore, they are found most commonly in the tooth bearing regions of the jaws. Since many of these lesions form tissue that mimics the hard tissues of teeth (enamel, cementum, dentin), the presence of radiodensities in radiographs is not uncommon. Consequently the radiographic appearance of these lesions may range from purely radiolucent to mixed to radiodense. The most common pattern, however, is that of radiolucency caused by resorption of trabeculae. The mixed pattern of calcification may result from inductive interactions between epithelial and mesenchymal tissues.

Some generalizations regarding these odontogenic lesions are the following. They tend to occur in those areas of the jaws where the most common genetic errors in tooth morphology or eruption pattern also occur, namely the third molar, second premolar, and canine regions. Among these cases, the most common sites for tumor occurrence are the mandibular molar and the maxillary canine regions, often in association with the crown of an impacted tooth. These lesions may occur in patients of any sex or age and in any area of the jaws, but there are a few specific patterns that help one to develop a differential diagnosis. These will be discussed with the description of each specific lesion.

The hamartomas consist of odontomas, and these usually occur within cystic cavities, or at least are surrounded by a fibrous capsule that is visible on radiographs as a fine radiolucency surrounding the lesion. The presence of fibrous tissue capsules make enucleation the treatment of choice. True neoplasms like ameloblastoma, calcifying epithelial odontogenic tumor, or odontogenic myxoma infiltrate bone, have high recurrence rates, and require aggressive surgical extirpation with wide margins. The epithelium from which these lesions originate exhibits variability in its degree of differentiation, with malignant change having been detected both in a process of transformation from benign epithelium as well as de novo in odontogenic tumors and cysts. Markers of increased cellular activity, such as increased mitotic figures, increased nuclear content, and pleiomorphism do not affect treatment recommendations unless actual malignant change is present.

The highly controversial odontogenic keratocyst exhibits behavior much more characteristic of tumor than of a cyst. Many believe that resection is the wisest treatment, although others prefer curettage with some form of adjunctive treatment like removal of additional bone with a burr or treatment of the bony cavity with a caustic fluid.

Ectodermal Tumors: Ameloblastoma The ameloblastoma is the most common and important of the odontogenic tumors, representing approximately 1% of all jaw cysts and tumors according to an early definitive report by Small and Waldron.[506] However, a more recent analysis suggests a rate varying from 3 to 19%. When considered as a subset only of odontogenic tumors, the incidence of ameloblastoma is more than 11% based on a review by Reichart whose report was based on literature data from more than 3,000 ameloblastomas. About 70% of all ameloblastomas occur in the molar-ramus region of the mandible. In the maxilla the molar region is also the most common site of occurrence. It is also the most dangerous area, since invasion of the maxillary sinus and nasal cavity is common in large lesions.[507,508] The ameloblastoma is a benign but aggressive epithelial tumor whose cell of origin is derived from remnants of the enamel organ of the dental follicle. Monoclonal antibody and immunofluorescent staining techniques have demonstrated positive staining for CD56 and CD147, confirming that the cell of origin is from the stellate reticulum of the enamel organ and is of neural crest cell origin.[509]

Ameloblastomas have been divided into three groups based on their radiographic appearance and location: unicystic, solid and multicystic, and peripheral.

The unicystic ameloblastoma arises from the odontogenic epithelium within a cyst or de novo as a neoplasm.[510] Radiographically, in its most common form, it resembles a dentigerous cyst, presenting as a radiolytic lesion with a well-defined cortical border surrounding the crown of an unerupted tooth (Figure 79-6).

Simple enucleation and curettage is probably sufficient treatment of the luminal variant. Generally, this diagnosis is rendered as an unwelcome surprise after removal of what appears to have been a dentigerous cyst. After thorough reexami-

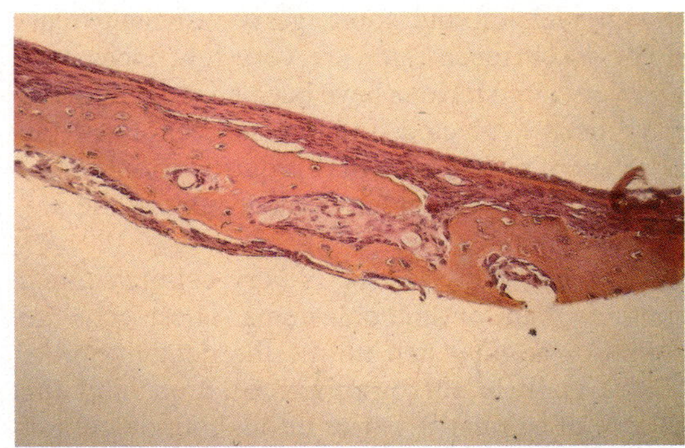

Figure 79-6 Unicystic ameloblastoma demonstrating ameloblastomatous cells in the wall of the "cyst" (hematoxylin and eosin ×100 magnification).

nation of the specimen from the newly established point of view that it is a unicystic ameloblastoma rather than a dentigerous cyst, one must then decide whether to only observe or to curette the bone cavity with hand instruments or a burr. If observation is chosen, there is no time limit to surveillance. The mural variant shows infiltration of the cyst wall and should be treated by peripheral ostectomy or resection, depending on size and location. When treated by simple enucleation and curettage, the recurrence rate has been reported to be between 10 and 33%.[511,512]

Solid Ameloblastoma This solid tumor is also an epithelial tumor whose origin is from the odontogenic rests of Serres and Malassez from the enamel organ and reduced enamel epithelium of the dental follicle. It is the most common subtype of ameloblastoma.

Most frequently the presentation is that of a painless swelling causing expansion of bone in the posterior mandible. When large, the cortical boundaries of the mandible may be breached, resulting in secondary infection of the soft tissue, thereby causing pain. It is most common in the fourth and fifth decades, but may occur at any age. There is no sexual predilection. Either jawbone may be affected, but involvement of the molar region of the mandible is most common. The exception to this pattern is for the desmoplastic variant, which occurs with equal likelihood in either jaw, but with a marked preference for the anterior region. In the mandible, the most likely site is the anterior alveolar process.[508] This is a tumor with a persistently aggressive pattern of growth for which recurrence rates of over 50% have been reported after conservative treatment. Aggressive treatment in the form of marginal mandibulectomy or segmental resection for lower jaw lesions, and partial maxillectomy for upper jaw tumor, has brought the recurrence rate down from 67% in 1937[513] to 33% in 1955[506] to about 20% in 1995. Half of the cases that ultimately recurred did so within 5 years, with the longest recurrence being reported at 33 years.[507] Others have reported a recurrence rate of less than 10%, with recurrences developing more quickly after enucleation and curettage than after resection.[514–517] Therefore, a period of surveillance exceeding 5 years is mandatory for proper management.

Wide excision of the intraosseous ameloblastoma is required. This implies maxillectomy for the maxillary lesion and either marginal or segmental resection of the mandible for mandibular lesions. When the bony confines of the mandible are breached, the soft tissue must also be excised. This must include the periosteum and a reasonable amount of soft tissue beyond it. Particularly in the maxilla, this may be a very difficult maneuver. Bony margins of 1 cm are recommended. A helpful adjunct for determining adequacy of resection in the operating theater is an intraoperative radiograph to assess marginal status, since frozen section control on bone margins is not available. (Illustrated in Figure 79-7, demonstrating the same principle in regard to an odontogenic keratocyst.)

Treatment by enucleation and curettage is unacceptable with recurrence rates of 60 to 90% in the mandible and 100% in the maxilla. Deaths by direct invasion of the skull base have also been reported.[518]

Even with resection, recurrences in the mandible may be expected. There have been many soft tissue recurrences reported in the literature. Our head and neck tumor registry reports one case of a woman who had suffered from persistent, recurring ameloblastoma for nearly 50 years. It was originally treated by maxillectomy with clear margins followed by extra-bony recurrence. Many operations later, she had lost the zygoma, part of the frontal bone, and ultimately died from direct extension along the base of the skull into the brain.

Since most ameloblastomas are located in the molar to ramus area, one must evaluate encroachment on the inferior alveolar nerve to determine whether excision of the nerve as part of the specimen is necessary. For very small unicystic ameloblastomas, the concept of nerve preservation has been suggested by Nakamura in a study showing that tumor did not infiltrate the nerve in unicystic tumors.[519] In multicystic lesions there was consistent infiltration of perineural tissue. In general, since large lesions encroach on the nerve and displace it inferiorly, the nerve should be removed. If nerve reconstruction is chosen, one has to decide whether to reconstruct the nerve with an autogenous sural nerve graft or some other form of nerve conduit. Nerve reconstruction is performed most appropriately at the time of resection.

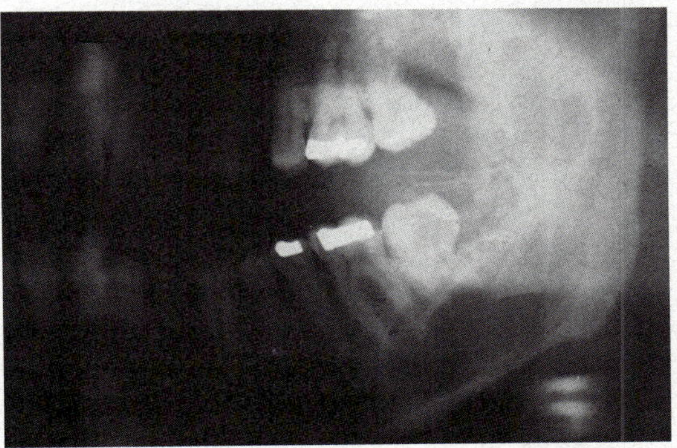

Figure 79-7 Odontogenic keratocyst in dentigerous relationship to unerupted tooth.

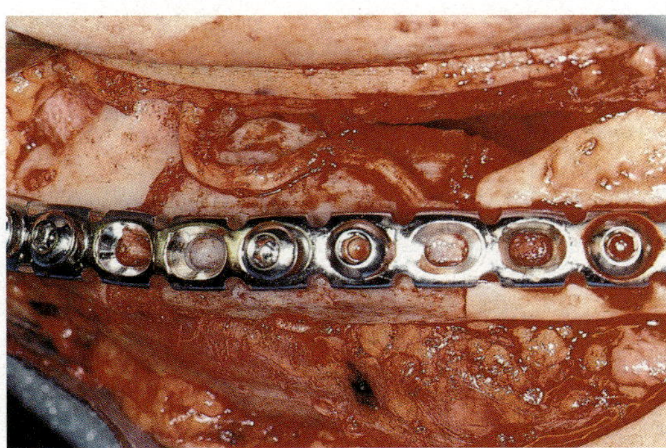

Figure 79-8 Resection-reconstruction for ameloblastoma showing a reconstruction plate to maintain occlusion and autogenous nerve graft to reconstruct inferior alveolar nerve.

Reconstruction of bone may be accomplished either primarily or secondarily. Since the oral mucosa is nearly always violated, the chance for postoperative dehiscence and partial or complete loss of the bone graft is always a threat. However, corticocancellous blocks securely fixed with wire or miniplate osteosynthesis coupled with intermaxillary fixation or a rigid reconstruction plate will usually survive despite dehiscence. Absolute minimization of the risk of dehiscence and/or postoperative infection requires placement of the bone graft on a secondary basis using either corticocancellous blocks or condensed cancellous grafts. A case of resection using a reconstruction plate to maintain the occlusion and primary reconstruction of the inferior alveolar nerve followed by secondary bone grafting is illustrated (Figure 79-8).

Malignant Variant The malignant ameloblastoma is indeed an unusual tumor. It is a tumor histopathologically identical to ameloblastoma, but it metastasizes. Histopathologically there are no features of the nuclei, altered patterns of growth, or dysplastic architecture that would lead one to suspect malignancy. Yet, some ameloblastomas (particularly follicular) recur persistently at the index site along with demonstrated distant metastases. The metastatic lesions themselves have the same histopathologic features as the primary tumor. Lung and lymph nodes have been the two most common sites for metastases in the tumor registry of Sinai Grace Hospital (Detroit), although one case of brain metastasis also occurred. Our observations are consistent with the literature, reporting lymph nodes and lung as the most likely sites for metastases, followed by bone.[506,520,521]

Calcifying Epithelial Odontogenic Tumor (CEOT: Pindborg Tumor) This epithelial odontogenic neoplasm, first described by Jens Pindborg in 1956,[522] closely resembles the ameloblastoma in its clinical and radiographic appearance. It probably arises from neoplastic cells derived from the stratum intermedium of the enamel organ.

There are two variants of this lesion: the central and the peripheral. The central lesion occurs predominantly in middle age, peaking at age 40, with most occurring between age 30 and 50, but may occur at any age with equal distribution between the sexes. There is a predilection for occurrence within the mandible (75%) with the premolar-molar area being most commonly affected. The usual presentation is as a slow-growing and painless swelling of the jaw without an attendant paresthesia. About half of these lesions are associated with impacted teeth.[512,523] Unusual variations include the presence of clear cells that may represent clear cell odontogenic carcinoma.[524] Rarely, malignant transformation to squamous cell carcinoma has been reported.[525]

Case reports do not include any series of significant size with long-term surveillance. However, invasion of marrow spaces does not seem to occur as commonly as is the case for ameloblastoma.[525] The implication frequently drawn from this histopathologic observation is that its behavior is less aggressive than ameloblastoma. On a clinical basis this de-escalation of treatment is not warranted, particularly since recurrence rates after conservative resection have been reported as being in the range of 15%, which is not satisfactory. In addition, recurrences have developed long after resection, in a pattern similar to that of ameloblastoma.[526] A 1 cm bony margin should be obtained, and the reconstruction may be accomplished either primarily or secondarily, according to the conditions found at operation. In contrast to the central CEOT, however, the peripheral CEOT may be treated by simple excision.

Calcifying Odontogenic Cyst (Gorlin Cyst, Keratinizing and Calcifying Odontogenic Cyst) The COC, although named a cyst, is more properly considered to be an odontogenic tumor of ectodermal origin. Both epithelial and mesenchymal components of the tooth germ are present. The distinguishing histologic characteristic of this lesion is its ability to form "ghost" cells. The ghost cells themselves do not impart aggressive biologic behavior to these lesions. Some controversy persists regarding proper treatment. Most lesions are cystic and are associated with either impacted teeth or odontomas, are quite well differentiated, and respond well to enucleation and curettage. Many respond to treatment in a way similar to odontogenic cysts. However, solid varieties that contain a true tumorlike proliferation of epithelial cells, producing both ghost cells and osteoid or dentinoid, may be more aggressive and require limited resection. About 2% of COCs take this solid form.[527] The COC may be found in association with four odontogenic lesions: ameloblastoma, ameloblastic odontoma, ameloblastic fibro-odontoma, and complex odontoma.[528] The traditional maxim that they should be treated like ameloblastomas is still valid.

The COC is usually cystic, although it may present as a solid tumor. The central jaw lesion is much more common than is the peripheral soft tissue variant. In the cystic type, the epithelial lining is usually thin. In the solid, neoplastic type,

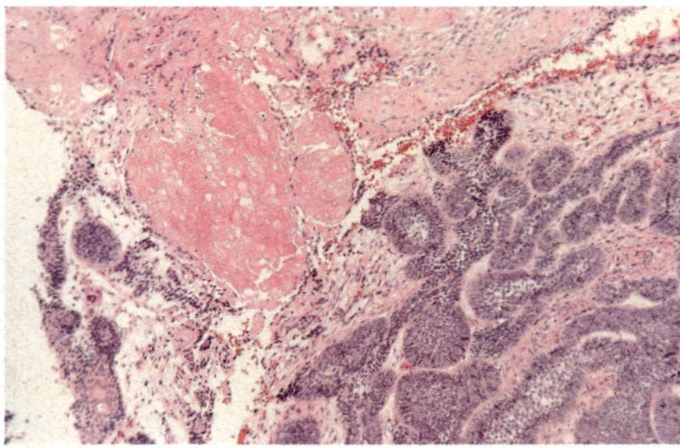

Figure 79-9 Photomicrograph of calcifying odontogenic cyst showing "ghost" cells (hematoxylin and eosin ×100). Courtesy of James Geist, DDS, MS.

there is a proliferation of epithelial cells into the connective tissue capsule and also into the cyst lumen. The epithelial cells may be squamous, cuboidal, or columnar. These cells, arranged in the form of sheets of pale eosinophilic cells, blend with epithelial cells whose nuclei have degenerated, leaving remnant cell outlines. They then become keratinized and calcify, thereby completing the transformation from epithelial to ghost cell (Figure 79-9). These ghost cells are the signature cells of the COC.[529] There may be areas of loose connective tissue resembling the stellate reticulum. These are epithelial cells that lose their nuclei, may keratinize, and then calcify. They are often surrounded by giant cells.

TUMORS ARISING FROM THE PERIODONTAL MEMBRANE

Cemento-Ossifying Fibroma (Ossifying Fibroma, Cementifying Fibroma) In contrast to the radiographically similar but much more common focal cemento-osseous dysplasia, this lesion is a true neoplasm. It belongs to the class of benign fibro-osseous lesions (BFOLs), which are pathophysiologically diverse but microscopically similar.

This tumor occurs in young patients as a slow growing, painless mass, displacing teeth, and expanding the mandible. It occurs with equal frequency in both sexes with the greatest incidence in the third and fourth decades. Although it may occur in either jaw, it affects the mandible much more frequently (Figure 79-10).[530]

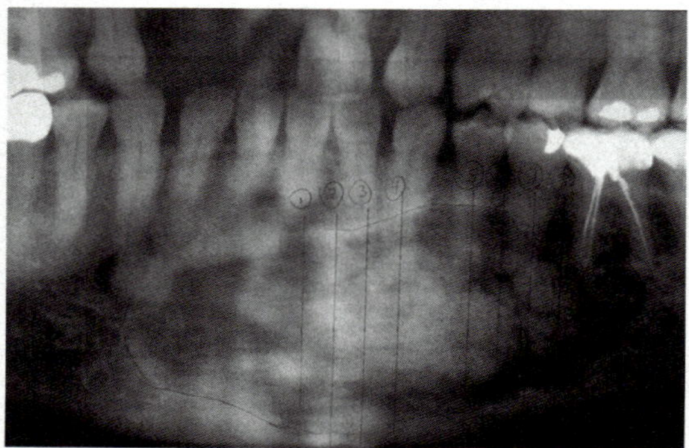

Figure 79-10 Florid cemento-osseous dysplasia with the classic radiographic appearance. Courtesy of Gary Clayman, DMD, MD.

Enucleation and curettage is sufficient treatment. Recurrence rates are very low. Occasionally very large lesions have been encountered that have been neglected by patients because of the absence of pain. These may require formal resection because of complete replacement of the jaw by the tumor.

The connective tissue is very cellular, much more so than for ameloblastoma. These cells are round or angular and mimic the dental papilla. There is little surrounding collagen, and the degree of cellularity varies throughout the tumor. No capsule is present,[531] but the growth pattern is one of expansion rather than infiltration, with a clear border separating the tumor from surrounding tissue.

Cellular markers present in these tumors include proliferating cell nuclear antigen and MIB-1[531] vimentin and cytokeratin.[532]

Treatment is by enucleation and curettage with removal of associated teeth. The recurrence rate is very low. Those that have recurred have generally been associated with incomplete removal of the tumor in an attempt to avoid removing the teeth involved with the tumor.

Ameloblastic Fibro-Odontoma This benign lesion is the second in the group of true mixed odontogenic tumors. The epithelial and connective tissue components resemble ameloblastic fibroma occurring in conjunction with a mineralized component similar to a composite odontoma.[533] This brings up the possibility that this tumor could represent an immature complex odontoma that, if left untreated, would continue to transform itself into an odontoma. Although this controversy has been extant for many years, it is probably unlikely that the AFO represents part of a smooth continuum of differentiation from ameloblastic fibroma to AFO to odontoma.[534] An adequate number of cases of AFO that continue to enlarge indefinitely without "maturing" into odontoma exist to lead one to consider this as a benign tumor that will persist without transforming itself into an odontoma.

The usual presentation is that of a painless, expansile lesion associated with a mass that has the radiodensity of dental hard tissue. It is often associated with an impacted tooth. The maxilla and the mandible are equally affected. Often failed eruption of a tooth is part of the clinical presentation. Most occur in children and young adults without a significant sexual predilection.[535]

Malignant Odontogenic Tumors There is no well-accepted classification of these tumors, most of which are pathological curiosities. Nonetheless, their importance to the unfortunate individuals so afflicted is not to be underestimated. Regrettably, because of their rarity, no well-accepted guidelines exist regarding treatment, particularly of advanced lesions for which combined chemoradiotherapy and surgery might be considered.

Generally these tumors arise de novo within the jawbones from epithelium contained within cyst linings or from malignant transformation of benign odontogenic tumors. Malignant transformation has been reported as occurring within the lining of most odontogenic cysts, although this is definitely a rare event.[537] To further confound histologic classification is the malignant ameloblastoma that has a benign histology, yet kills by metastasizing.

The lesions most commonly thought of are the primary intraosseous carcinomas. These ought to include the mucoepidermoid carcinoma arising within bone and the ameloblastic carcinoma. Another clearly odontogenic malignancy that has finally been classified as such is the clear cell odontogenic tumor (CCOT), more properly named the clear cell odontogenic carcinoma (CCOC), extraordinarily rare but deadly. Arising within the bones but not directly from bone are the malignancies coming from epithelial linings: squamous cell carcinoma ex odontogenic cyst or tumor. I have treated one case of a squamous cell carcinoma arising from a CEOT at an interval of 7 years after treatment of the CEOT by resection and bone graft reconstruction. A case report in 2001 has reported malignant transformation in a CEOT.[525]

The WHO classification is as follows[536]:

Odontogenic Carcinoma:

a. Malignant ameloblastoma

b. Primary intraosseous carcinoma

c. Other carcinoma arising from odontogenic epithelium, including those arising from odontogenic cysts

Malignant ameloblastoma (vs solid ameloblastoma) is most unusual since the histology of the index lesion is that of a benign ameloblastoma. However, the lesion tends to metastasize to lung, pleura, regional and distant lymph nodes, vertebrae, and liver and kidney.[537] The lung is the most common metastatic site, and possibly this is because of aspiration resulting in seeding of the lung.[506] Metastases may occur despite achieving control of the index lesion.

Ameloblastic fibrosarcoma arising from an ameloblastic fibroma, or ameloblastic fibroodontoma, has been reported, presumably with the malignant component being derived from the fibroblastic, mesenchymal component.

The clear cell odontogenic carcinoma (CCOT) has been described as an aggressive tumor of odontogenic origin of which there are 23 cases. Most commonly it is found in the body of the mandible followed in frequency by the anterior and posterior mandible. Pain and paresthesia of the lip have been reported along with mobile teeth. Only 3 of the 23 cases were in the maxilla. It metastasizes to regional nodes and distant organs, particularly lung. The differential diagnosis based on the histopathology includes the clear cell variant of ameloblastoma, the clear cell variant of calcifying epithelial odontogenic tumor (although its amyloid production and calcifications are not characteristic of CCOT), and metastatic renal cell carcinoma. The epithelial pattern is biphasic with sheets and islands of squamoid epithelial cells with distinct desmosomes and a prominent clear cell component. Clear cells are admixed among the squamoid cells and are also arranged in distinct islands. There is mild cellular pleiomorphism and occasional mitotic activity.[538,539] The radiographic presentation is that of an expansile lesion of the posterior mandible that is predominantly radiolucent with some internal opacifications. The borders may be well defined or diffuse, depending on size and growth rate. The computed tomographic scans may show perforation of the cortical bone and expansion into the soft tissues.

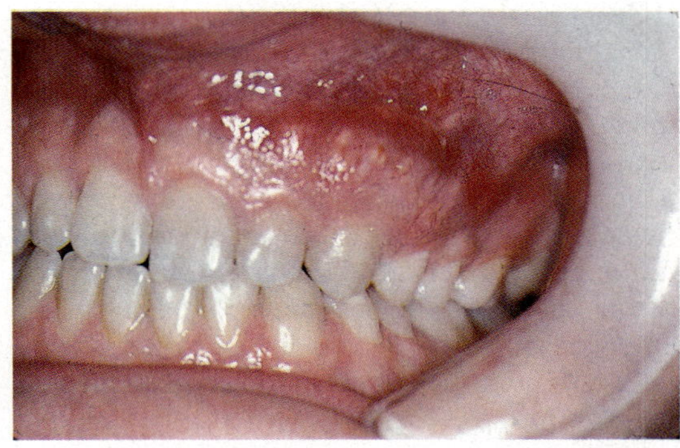

Figure 79-11 Clinical appearance of an ameloblastic carcinoma that presented as a slow-growing mass expanding the maxilla with slight discomfort but no pain.

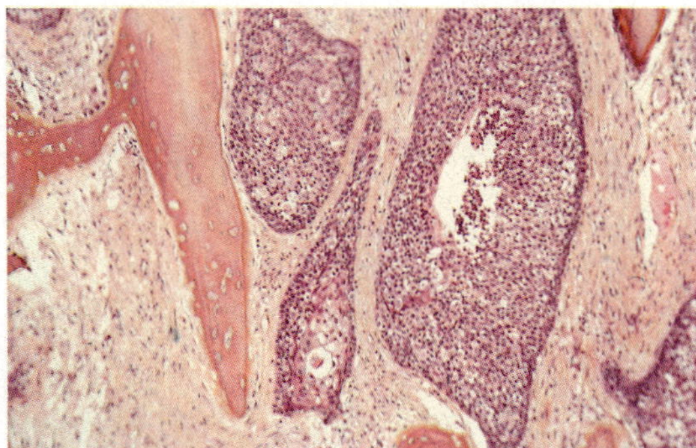

Figure 79-13 Photomicrograph of ameloblastic carcinoma showing hypercellularity, pleomorphism, and atypia (hematoxylin and eosin ×120 magnification).

Treatment is resection, which cured about half of the patients. Ominously, 13% of those with successful resection developed metastasis. Two patients receiving chemotherapy with fluorouracil and platinum did not benefit from the chemotherapy.

The general problem of how to manage odontogenic malignancy is illustrated by the case of a 19-year-old man who presented with a slowly growing, painless mass expanding the left maxilla. Endodontic therapy was performed without success when an area of localized pain developed. The initial biopsy was read as an ameloblastoma with marked cellularity. After review, the diagnosis was changed to ameloblastic carcinoma. The lesion extended into the infratemporal fossa, and it was removed by a combined upper face splitting incision and a bicoronal flap. The left maxilla was removed as was part of the right one. A positive margin was present on the right, and postoperative radiotherapy to 7,000 cGy was given rather than performing a total bilateral maxillectomy. He is alive and well, speaks and swallows normally, has married, and is raising a family 17 years later (Figures 79-11 to 79-14).

The general treatment principle is to treat these odontogenic epithelial carcinomas like squamous cancers with wide excision to a clear margin and postoperative radiation if required for positive margins or extensive local spread. There are no studies that consider simultaneous chemoradiotherapy.

Lastly are the metastatic lesions in the jaws arising from distant sites. A comprehensive review of the English language literature was published in 1994 that culled 390 cases.[540] Of the 384 cases that were usable for analysis, there were 200 women and 184 men with an age range of 6 months to 88 years with a mean of 45.5 years. Eighty-one percent of these lesions were reported in the posterior mandible (Figures 79-15 and 79-16), with 13.6% in the maxilla and 5.4% occurring in both jaws. For all patients, in order of decreasing frequency, the sites were breast (21.8%), lung (12.6%), adrenal (8.7%), kidney (7.9%), bone (7.4%), colorectal (6.6%), and prostate (5.6%). For women the order was breast (42%), adrenal (8.5%), colorectal (8%), genitourinary (7.5%), and thyroid (6%), while for men it was lung (22.3%), prostate (12%), kidney (10.3%), bone (9.2%), and adrenal (9.2%). In the first decade of life the most common site was the adrenal and in the second decade it was bone. In older groups, breast predominated for women and prostate for men. Seventy percent of the tumors were epithelial. In about one-third of the cases, the first presentation of malignant disease was the

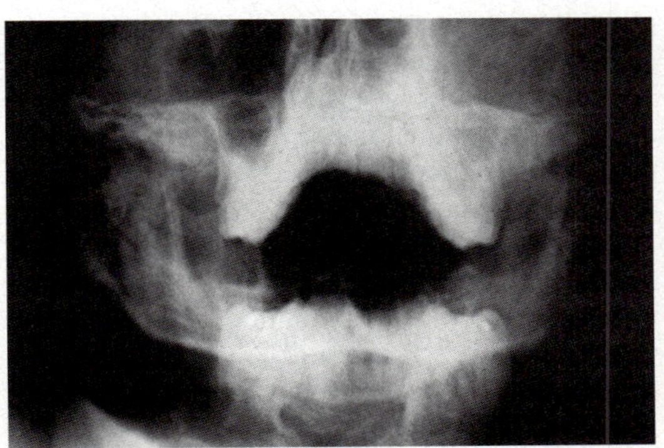

Figure 79-12 Radiograph of the maxilla of a patient with ameloblastic carcinoma showing replacement by tumor and invasion of antrum.

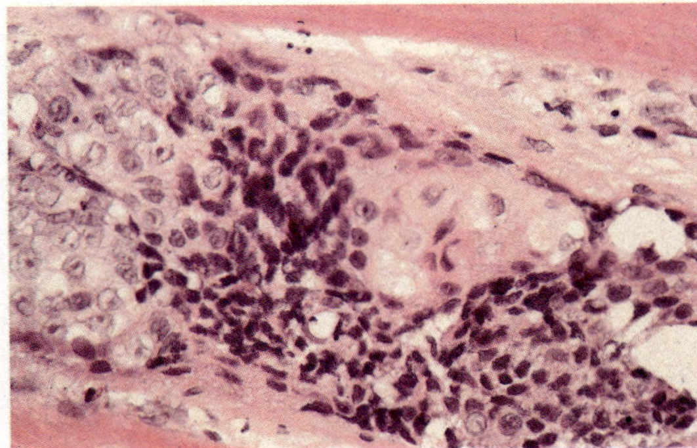

Figure 79-14 High power (×180 magnification) of another area of the ameloblastic carcinoma shown in Figure 79-13.

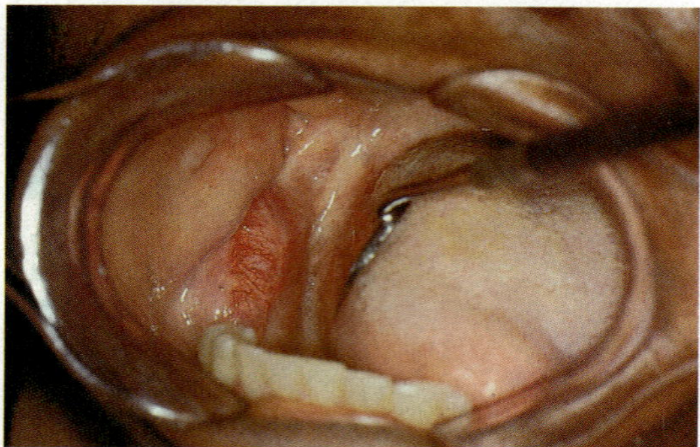

Figure 79-15 Clinical presentation of adenocarcinoma metastatic to the mandible.

metastatic lesion of the jawbones. The most common complaints were swelling (57%), pain (39%), and paresthesia (23%). Radiographically, most of the lesions were radiolytic with ill-defined borders (see Figure 79-16). Prostate was the most likely lesion to demonstrate a pattern of mixed lucency-opacity or predominant opacity. The presence of a metastatic lesion of the jaws indicated a grave prognosis, with the average time from diagnosis of metastasis to death being 7.3 months.[540]

Diagnosis is established by biopsy of the jaw lesion. However, a warning is in order. Prostate and renal cell carcinomas, constituting one-third of all the metastatic lesions in men, both may be associated with impaired hemostasis. Biopsy of either lesion may result in significant bleeding. The definitive treatment is that of the primary disease with expectation of a generally poor outcome.

RADIATION THERAPY

Radiotherapy plays an integral role in the treatment of most head and neck cancers. Used as the sole modality for the treatment of select early-stage disease (T1 and T2), it gives comparable results to a surgical resection, often with less morbidity. For tumors arising in the larynx, it may be preferred to surgery because it may maintain a function and vocal quality. For advanced-sized lesions, it is used as an adjuvant to surgery in order to improve locoregional control. When used as an adjuvant, it is important that there be good communication between the surgeon and the radiation oncologist in order to avoid inadvertent delays that can compromise outcome. For example, Vikram and colleagues[541] have noted that the rate of locoregional tumor recurrence was greater if there was more than a 6-week delay between surgery and the initiation of adjuvant radiotherapy. The adverse impact of a delay in beginning treatment has been confirmed by Mackillop and colleagues,[542] who found an approximate 10% lowering of local control in patients with advanced tonsillar carcinoma per month of delay in beginning radiotherapy. For advanced inoperable lesions and for tumors arising in certain sites, such as the nasopharynx, radiation therapy may be the only potentially curative modality. Its effectiveness has been increased by the concomitant use of chemotherapy and by using more optimal treatment fractionation schemas (discussed below).

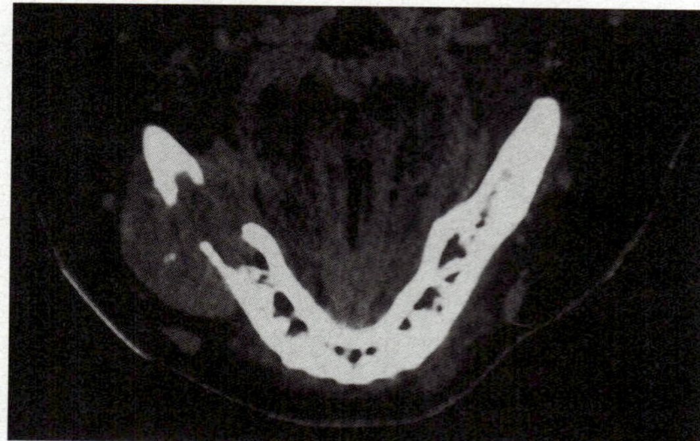

Figure 79-16 Computed tomographic scan of adenocarcinoma metastatic to the mandible presenting as a mass with a pathologic fracture.

Ionizing radiation (high-energy photons, electrons, neutrons, protons, and other charged particles) interacts with matter in subtle ways and should not be thought of as simply a form of cautery.[543] Tumors and normal tissues can vary dramatically in their ability to repair the cellular damage caused by ionizing radiation. This makes it possible to use treatments such as chemotherapy and hyperthermia to reduce the repair capability of tumors and to design fractionation schemes that effectively widen the therapeutic window between tumor control and normal tissue damage. HNSCCs are generally characterized as being "moderately radiosensitive," meaning that fairly large amounts of radiation must be delivered in order to achieve a high probability of tumor control. Fortunately, the required doses are within the tolerance range of most tissues in the head and neck.

The effectiveness of a given dose of radiation depends on how it is given.[542] Over the past 30 years, various "standard" treatment regimens have evolved to treat head and neck cancer. In the United States, the traditional "curative" treatment regimen consists of giving 180 to 200 cGy once a day for 5 days a week to a total dose of 6,500 to 7,400 cGy; in England and Canada, higher daily doses of 220 to 250 cGy are given once a day for 5 days a week to a total dose of 5,000 to 5,500 cGy. These two schemas have evolved empirically, and a review of the literature seems to indicate that they provide comparable tumor control with the main debate relating to differences in complications. Various altered fractionation regimens have been compared with the standard regimens in clinical trials and some of these appear to be evolving into new "standards."

Radiation kills the stem cells in the basal layer of the skin and mucosa, and several weeks later, the cells in the more superficial protective layers are not adequately replaced when they are lost through normal physiologic processes. This denudes the epithelium, giving rise to a mucosal reaction that can greatly inhibit a patient's ability to swallow solids and liquids. This does not occur immediately but is progressive after several weeks of radiotherapy. The use of concomitant chemotherapy and/or altered fractionation treatment regimens can make this reaction occur sooner and be more severe. Patients must be monitored closely to ensure that they maintain adequate nutrition during therapy, and often a feeding tube is required. Placement of such a tube is preferable to giving the patient a break in therapy, which can lower the tumor control probability due to repopulation.[544–546] A similar reaction can occur in the skin in the treatment portals, giving rise to a severe sunburnlike reaction. Amifostine, a radioprotective agent, has been shown to reduce the incidence and severity of these side effects, but is itself associated with nausea as a side effect.[547,548] Thus far, it appears that this agent does not impart any radioprotective effect to patients with HNSCCs.

Radiation to the head and neck area can cause significant changes in salivary gland function and taste perception.[549–551] The severity and duration of these changes are dose dependent. In the absence of amifostine, there is transient loss of saliva and taste after doses of 1,000 to 1,500 cGy; doses of 4,000 to 5,000 cGy cause permanent changes. A University of Michigan study showed substantial reduction in salivary output if the mean dose to the parotid glands was more than 24 Gy. Pilocarpine (Salagen) is effective in maximizing any residual salivary gland output.[552] Both the decrease in the amount of saliva and the changes in its chemical composition allow changes in the distribution of microorganisms inhabiting the mouth, which in turn can markedly increase the risk of dental caries.

Aggressive dental prophylaxis prior to beginning radiotherapy is mandatory in the dentulous patient because the incidence of osteoradionecrosis can be considerably reduced if the necessary repairs and/or extractions are done prior to treatment rather than in heavily irradiated tissues after treatment.[553] If extractions are necessary, a delay of 2 to 3 weeks between the extractions and the initiation of radiotherapy is necessary in order to allow for adequate healing. If extractions or other invasive procedures are required after high-dose radiotherapy, hyperbaric oxygen treatments are helpful in reducing the risk of osteoradionecrosis, particularly if the mandible is involved.[554,555]

Technologic Advances Advances in radiotherapy have been tied to advances in technology. In the early days, low-energy orthovoltage devices and radium 226 sources were used to treat HNSCC. Then came megavoltage beams from linear accelerators and cobalt 60 units and brachytherapy isotopes such as cesium 137, iridium 192, and iodine 125 produced in nuclear reactors. Modern radiotherapy centers use sophisticated linear accelerators producing photon beams of different energies and megavoltage electron beams that can easily treat posterior neck lymph nodes without risk of spinal cord damage. Computer-controlled multileaf collimators facilitate custom blocking techniques to spare uninvolved normal tissues and sequential changes in field geometry as a patient progresses through treatment. CT and MRI are used to locate tumors, with many radiation oncology centers having dedicated scanners used exclusively for simulation and treatment planning. CT, MRI, and PET scans are fused to give the clinician a broader perspective in locating regions at risk of tumor. Noncoplanar field configurations, often using vertex presentations, are standard techniques.

Intensity-Modulated Radiotherapy Intensity-modulated radiotherapy (IMRT) is the next step in the saga to improve dose localization. In this approach, many different treatment fields are used, with each field being divided into multiple segments, and each segment delivering a prescribed amount of radiation.[556] Sophisticated computer programs are used to calculate the doses given by each of these field segments, and the clinician is able to specify normal tissue dose constraints to be used in obtaining the "solution" for a particular patient. Head and neck cancer represents an ideal situation in which to apply this technique because with proper immobilization techniques, organ motion is not a major problem. There often are critical normal structures in close proximity to the tumor, and achieving a sharp dose gradient around the target while limiting the normal tissue dose offers the potential for significant therapeutic gain. Lee and colleagues[557] have reported on the UCSF experience using this approach for nasopharyngeal cancer, which yielded a 97% locoregional recurrence-free survival rate in 67 patients, with a median follow-up time of 31 months. There was less toxicity than would have been expected using concomitant chemotherapy and conventional radiotherapy. The ability to reduce the dose to the parotid glands and to reduce the subsequent xerostomia experienced by the patient is an important advantage of this technique.[558] A comparison between the isodose distributions produced by optimized, three-dimensional conformal radiotherapy and by IMRT for a particularly challenging clinical situation is shown in Figures 79-17 and 79-18. The patient shown has a nasopharyngeal primary with clinically positive cervical and retropharyngeal nodes. Note the ability to spare the parotid glands without sacrificing tumor dose, using the IMRT approach.

Why are these advances important clinically? The advantages of improved tumor imaging are obvious as there should be fewer "marginal misses" than in the past. Another advantage relates to being able to give higher radiation doses to the tumor in a safe manner. Other things being equal, higher doses of radiation lead to a higher tumor control probability. In the case of HNSCC, dose-response curves generally exhibit a steep region, wherein modest increases in radiation dose will give rise to significant improvement in outcome.[543,559,560]

Curative Radiotherapy HNSCC responds to radiation injury through a loss of reproductive capability, resulting in a clonogenic rather than an interphase death. Within the context of a given fractionation schema, the amount of cell killing is essentially an exponential function of this approach is to take advantage of the difference in the shapes of the cell survival curves between tumors and late-responding tissues in order to deliver a higher dose of radiation without increasing the late effects of treatment. A typical example for head and neck cancer would be to give 120 cGy per fraction (Fx) twice daily (bid) to a total dose of 8,160 cGy.[561–563] The interval between fractions must be approximately 4.5 to 6 hours to allow for repair of damage to normal tissues.[564]

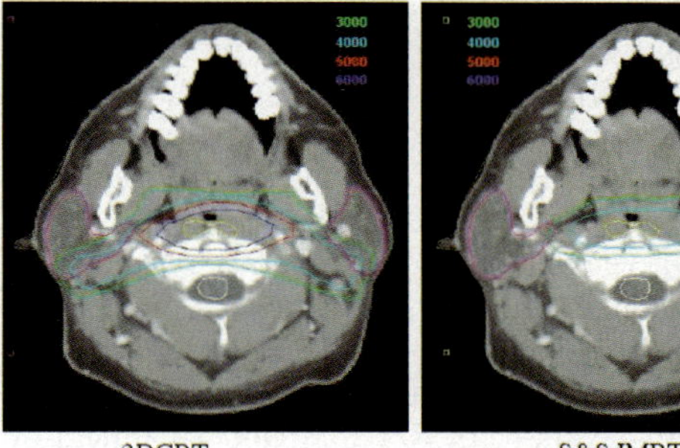

Figure 79-17 A comparison between the isodose distributions produced by optimized, three-dimensional conformal radiotherapy and by IMRT.

Accelerated fractionation refers to using a fraction about the same size (or perhaps slightly smaller) as in conventional fractionation, multiple daily treatments, a shorter overall treatment time, and a total dose about the same as (or perhaps slightly less than) given in the conventional radiation schema. The basic idea with this approach is to overcome the effects of tumor repopulation by shortening the overall time. Theoretically, this should improve tumor control for the same radiation dose without increasing the overall late effects. Following Ang,[565] the various accelerated fractionation schemas can be classified into three categories: (1) a short, intensive course; (2) a split course; and (3) a concomitant boost. The continuous hyperfractionated accelerated radiotherapy (CHART) regimen,[566] which consists of giving 150 cGy/Fx 3 times a day on 12 consecutive days to a total dose of 5,400 cGy, is a prototype regimen in category A. The approach of Wang and colleagues[567,568] (160 cGy/Fx bid to a total dose of 6,720 cGy with a 2-week break after 3,840 cGy) is a prototype regimen in category B. The concomitant-boost approach of Ang and colleagues[565,568] (180 cGy/Fx qd to 5,400 cGy, with an additional daily treatment of 150 cGy/Fx to the final target volume being delivered during the final 12 days of therapy) is a prototype regimen in category C.

Model calculations that show which of these approaches would be expected to produce the best results is critically dependent on the radiobiologic parameters of the tumor (eg, α/β, and the tumor proliferative properties [eg, TD and F1]).[543,569,570] In clinical practice, even tumors arising in a particular site and having the same basic histology can exhibit a wide variation in the valradiation dose. Thus, for a given level of tumor control, the required radiation dose is approximately proportional to the number of clongenic cells in the tumor.[543,571–573] In the context of a once-a-day treatment regimen with daily doses in the range of 180 to 200 cGy, subclinical microscopic disease requires a dose of approximately 5,000 cGy, a 1 cm tumor requires approximately 6,500 cGy, and large T3 or T4 tumors require approximately 7,000 to 7,500 cGy.[573] Patients with head and neck tumors are generally treated with shrinking field techniques, wherein the various regions at risk receive doses commensurate with the amount of tumor they are thought to contain. In the past, doses greater than 7,500 cGy required the use of interstitial radioactive implants to limit the doses received by adjacent normal tissues. Today, however, the use of IMRT and proton beam therapy also allows the clinician to achieve high tumor doses in a safe manner.[556,574] The summary by Laramore describes representative local control rates and survival data for patients with HNSCC treated with definitive radiotherapy delivered in a standard fractionation scheme.[575] Local control rates are excellent for the early-stage tumors, but there is an obvious need for improvement in regard to the more advanced lesions. Hence, altered fractionation approaches and the concomitant use of chemotherapy and radiotherapy are topics of current research interest.

Many factors affect the choice between radiotherapy and surgery as the primary definitive form of treatment. For early lesions of the larynx, the two modalities may yield equivalent locore-

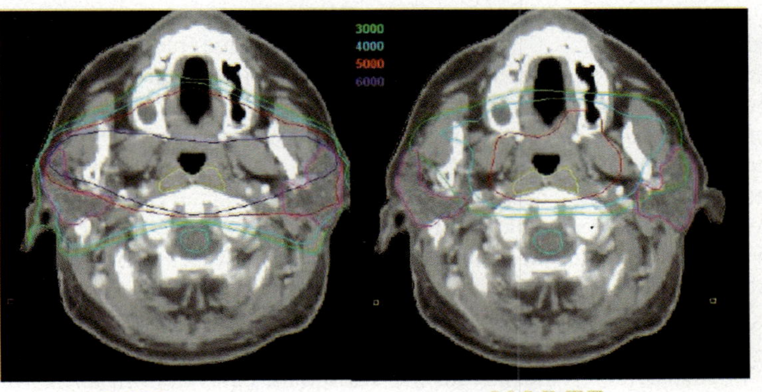

Figure 79-18 A comparison between the isodose distributions produced by optimized, three-dimensional conformal radiotherapy and by IMRT.

gional control and survival, but radiation therapy is perceived to yield a better functional result, making it the treatment of choice. In certain cosmetically sensitive areas, such as the lip or in early lesions of the nose or eyelid, radiation therapy gives a better ultimate result even after reconstructive surgery. For tumors of the nasopharynx, a site that is surgically unapproachable, radiotherapy is the mainstay of treatment. Fortunately, nasopharyngeal tumors tend to be among the more sensitive of the HNSCCs. For early tumors of the tonsil and the base and lateral aspects of the tongue, the overall results between surgery and radiotherapy are approximately equivalent, and informed patient choice should guide the treatment management decision. Radiotherapy is also given following the diagnosis of SCC metastatic to cervical lymph nodes from an unknown primary head and neck site. The treatment fields encompass the probable sites of tumor origin (nasopharynx, tonsillar fossa, tongue base, and hypopharynx), with patient survivals at 2 to 3 years being in the range of 30 to 60%.[576,577]

Accelerated and Hyperfractionated Radiotherapy An area of current interest in the treatment of head and neck cancer is to use "nonstandard" radiation treatment regimens to improve the therapeutic ratio between tumor control and normal tissue damage. Standard once-a-day treatment approaches developed empirically, and although they are convenient from the viewpoint of operating a radiation oncology department, there is no reason to think that they cannot be improved. There are currently two basic approaches that are being investigated in an attempt to find a more optimal radiation treatment fractionation schema.

Hyperfractionation refers to using smaller fraction sizes, multiple daily treatments, a higher total dose of radiation, and a total treatment time that is about the same duration as for conventional radiotherapy. The basic idea with this approach is to take advantage of the difference in the shapes of the cell survival curves between tumors and late-responding tissues in order to deliver a higher dose of radiation without increasing the late effects of treatment. In the absence of predictive assays that would allow the clinician to individualize the treatment of a given patient, large-scale clinical trials are necessary to compare one approach with another for the treatment of specific classes of tumors.

In the United States, early work using hyperfractionation to treat locally advanced head and neck cancer took place at the University of Florida.[578] Doses of up to 8,011 cGy were given, using 120 cGy bid. Compared with historical controls, there was better locoregional control, a greater degree of acute mucositis, and equivalent late effects. The first large phase III trials took place outside the United States. Datta and colleagues[579] reported on 176 patients treated in India who were randomized to standard fractionation to 6,600 cGy versus 120 cGy bid to 7,920 Gy. At 2 years, locoregional control was 63% on the hyperfractionation arm versus 33% on the standard arm ($p < .001$). Pinto and colleagues[580] reported on 98 patients treated in Brazil who were randomized to either 6,600 cGy via standard fractionation or 110 cGy bid to 7,040 cGy. Their patients all had stages III and IV carcinomas of the oropharynx and so represented a reasonably homogeneous population. Locoregional control was 84% on the hyperfractionation arm versus 64% on the standard arm ($p = .02$). Horiot and colleagues[581] reported on a European Organization for Research and Treatment of Cancer (EORTC) study involving 356 patients with oropharyngeal tumors who were randomized to either 7,000 cGy standard fractionation or 115 cGy bid to 8,050 cGy. Locoregional control was 40% on the standard arm versus 59% on the hyperfractionation arm ($p = .02$). In all of these trials, the acute mucositis was more severe on the hyperfractionation arm, but the late effects were similar.

One of the most aggressive of the accelerated treatment regimens is the CHART approach. Doses of 150 cGy/Fx are given 3 times a day on 12 consecutive days to a total dose of 5,400 cGy. An early analysis of a phase I/II study showed more severe early effects and four cases of radiation myelitis in patients whose spinal cords received 4,500 to 4,800 cGy.[566] This high incidence of myelitis cannot be satisfactorily explained on the basis of incomplete repair of nerve tissue between fractions. However, when the regimen was taken into a phase III trial, the cord dose was limited to 4,000 cGy. The randomized trial showed no difference in locoregional control or survival but there were no additional cases of myelitis with this lower dose.[582]

In 1991 the Radiation Therapy Oncology Group (RTOG) began a randomized phase III trial testing four different radiation fractionation schemas for patients with inoperable squamous cell tumors of the head and neck.[563] Standard fractionation at 200 cGy/Fx to 7,000 cGy was the control arm. Another arm was hyperfractionation radiotherapy at 120 cGy/Fx bid to a total dose of 8,160 cGy, which was determined to be an unacceptable dose on a prior dose-searching study.[561,562] The remaining two arms were categories B and C variants of an accelerated fractionation schema. One of these arms was the split-course regimen of Wang and colleagues (described above), and the other was the concomitant boost regimen of Ang and colleagues (also described above). The study closed in 1997 with 1,073 patients being evaluable for analysis.[563]

Analysis of the three altered fractionation regimens was done in comparison with the standard fractionation arm. There was no improvement in locoregional control with the accelerate/split course, but there was a statistically significant benefit with the hyperfractionated ($p = .045$) and concomitant-boost ($p = .05$) regimens. There was also a trend toward improved disease-free survivals, which did not reach statistical significance. As might be expected, with death due to locoregional failure being only about 50% of the total deaths, all the arms were equivalent in terms of absolute survival. The incidence of grade 3 or greater (RTOG/EORTC scoring scheme) acute toxicity was worse on all three altered fractionation arms, with the differences being statistically significant. Only the concomitant-boost regimen had significantly worse late effects when compared with standard fractionation. However, this may be an artifact of the definition of "late effects" as those that are present 90 days or longer following treatment. The "acute effects" on the concomitant-boost arm persisted longer than on the other arms, and hence the difference in scoring. If a longer cutoff time is chosen, then the late effects spectra are the same on all four arms.

The Meta-Analysis of Chemotherapy in Head and Neck Cancer (MACH-NC) Collaborative Group has recently conducted a study that asked the question as to whether there was any evidence that altered fractionation radiation schema could improve patient survival when compared with patients treated with standard fractionation schemas.[583] This analysis was based on individual patient data and included 6,515 patients from 15 different trials. Overall, there was an absolute survival benefit of 3% at 5 years with altered fractionation schemas (39% vs 36%, $p = .04$). There was also a benefit to absolute local control (8%) and nodal control (3%). However, when the analysis was restricted to studies comparing hyperfractionation to standard fractionation (no trials utilizing an accelerated fractionation schema), the absolute improvement in survival was 9%. Hence, it would seem that an increase in total dose rather than a decrease in overall treatment time was a more effective approach.

Fraction size may be important in determining late effects. Jen and colleagues[584] have reported an increased risk of temporal lobe necrosis in patients with nasopharyngeal tumors who were treated with 160 cGy bid instead of 120 cGy bid. In both fractionation schemas, the time interval between same-day fractions was kept at 6 hours. In the 120 cGy fraction group, the total tumor dose was higher at 8,000 cGy, while in the 160 cGy fraction group, the dose was in the range of 6,840 to 7,640 cGy. The portal configuration was the same in each group. None of the 70 patients treated with the 120 cGy fractions developed temporal lobe necrosis, whereas 3 of 11 (27%) of patients treated with 160 cGy fractions developed symptomatic temporal lobe necrosis. The estimated doses to the temporal lobes were, respectively, 6,000 to 7,440 cGy on the 120 cGy bid arm and 4,480 to 6,700 cGy on the 160 cGy bid arm.

Combined Surgery and Radiotherapy Radiotherapy is often given as an adjuvant to surgery for moderately advanced but resectable tumors. For most head and neck sites, giving adjuvant radiotherapy improves local control for T3 or T4 primaries or in situations where there is pathologic involvement of cervical lymph nodes.

Radiotherapy can be given either preoperatively or postoperatively. The aims of preoperative radiotherapy are to sterilize microscopic disease outside the resection field and to shrink the tumor bulk, making surgery more tractable. Theoretically, preoperative radiotherapy should also reduce the risk of disseminating viable tumor cells at the time of surgery. Dosages of 5,000 cGy over 5 to 5.5 weeks are generally given, with no significant wound healing problems occurring at this dosage.[585] Preoperative radiotherapy is rarely indicated today.

In the postoperative setting, the surgical procedure has disrupted the regional blood supply. Conventional wisdom suggests that higher doses of radiation are needed because of the increased likelihood of hypoxic tumor cells, which would be more radioresistant than their well-oxygenated counterparts. Generally, 5,500 to 6,000 cGy in 180 to 200 cGy fractions are given for microscopic residual disease. If the surgical margins are grossly positive or if there is a high likelihood of macroscopic residual disease, then higher doses are used. Peters and colleagues[586] have shown that at least 6,300 cGy should be given if extracapsular nodal extension is found in the operative specimen. Postoperative radiotherapy has the advantage of being given only to those patients thought to be at significant risk of locoregional recurrence based on a review of the pathologic data. It has the additional advantage of not delaying the surgical procedure, which is the most important treatment modality for patients with advanced, operable tumors. Currently, extracapsular extensions and perineural invasion are indications for concomitant chemotherapy and radiation therapy or clinical protocols addressing these adverse pathologic findings.

Although it is generally felt that there is little use for a debulking surgical procedure unless one can achieve microscopic disease levels, there may be situations where a gross total resection followed by high-dose radiotherapy is preferable to treatment with radiotherapy alone. An analysis by the Head and Neck Intergroup (IG0034) showed that excluded patients with positive surgical margins had improved locoregional tumor control compared with matched cohorts from the RTOG databases of patients treated with radiotherapy alone.[587] At 4 years, respective locoregional control rates were 44% versus 24% (p = .007). However, there was no difference in survival. Since this was not a randomized study, the authors do not argue for changing traditional resectability criteria, but, rather, testing this concept in the context of a controlled clinical trial.

SYSTEMIC THERAPY

Chemotherapy and Radiation for Locally Advanced Disease: Induction Chemotherapy It has long been recognized that response rates to cytotoxic chemotherapy administered as the initial or induction treatment ranged from 70 to 90%, with 20 to 30% of patients achieving a clinical complete response.[588,589] Of these, histological confirmation with a negative biopsy is reported in approximately one-third. This has led to induction chemotherapy trials with cisplatin-based drug combinations, confirming marked activity in phase II studies, but with no consistent demonstration of an increase in survival after larger randomized studies.[589] There have been exceptions. Paccagnella and colleagues[590] reported an increase in survival for a subset of patients with unresectable disease randomized to induction chemotherapy with cisplatin/5-FU followed by radiotherapy compared with patients treated with radiotherapy alone. Domenge and colleagues[591] also reported a survival benefit after neoadjuvant chemotherapy for patients with locally advanced oropharyngeal carcinoma. Moreover, a meta-analysis[592] has shown a 5% increase in survival rates for induction chemotherapy with cisplatin-based combinations over local therapy alone (p = .05). However, the well-controlled larynx studies, discussed above, failed to show a survival advantage for induction chemotherapy despite a reduction in distant metastasis as a first site of disease recurrence for patients treated in this fashion.

Recent phase II trials with paclitaxel and carboplatin[593] and paclitaxel, ifosfamide and carboplatin (TIC)[594] have shown impressive antitumor activity, with 80 to 90% of patients achieving partial or complete clinical responses. In both studies, induction chemotherapy was followed by chemoradiation with promising local and distant disease control. An emerging experience at the Dana-Farber Cancer Institute with docetaxel, cisplatin, and infusional 5-FU (TPF)[595] has resulted in histologically confirmed CRs in the primary sites in 89% of patients treated. Presently there are ongoing phase III trials headed by the Boston and Chicago groups with patients randomized to receive TPF induction chemotherapy or not followed by chemoradiation. Eligible patients have stage III or IV squamous cell carcinoma of the oropharynx, hypopharynx, and larynx with N 2/3 M0 staging at diagnosis. Thus, this issue of the potential efficacy of induction chemotherapy is again being put to the test.

Concomitant Chemotherapy and Radiation A sequence of randomized trials[596–606] and meta-analysis[592] demonstrate that the concomitant administration of chemotherapy and radiation leads to improved local control and overall survival in patients with locally advanced squamous cell carcinomas, particularly of the oropharynx. However, most reported trials include patients with invasive squamous cell carcinomas from a mix of primary sites. Scrutiny of these manuscripts is advised as the percentage of patients with oral cavity, pharyngeal, and laryngeal primary sites may vary in reports from different centers, and this may markedly affect study outcomes. Most often, patients with unknown primary head and neck cancers and nasopharyngeal cancers are reported separately.

At The University of Texas M. D. Anderson Cancer Center, oral cavity primary tumors are most often approached surgically if there are no medical contraindications. As discussed in this chapter, cancers of the oral tongue, floor of mouth, and buccal surface are amenable to surgical resection followed by reconstructive procedures. Depending on tumor histology, size, pathologic margins, and the extent of nodal involvement, postoperative radiotherapy is administered. An older French study[607] and recent trials[608,609] have tested the potential value of postoperative chemoradiotherapy with cisplatin administered every 3 weeks in "high-risk" patients. In a review of data from these American and European studies, it appears that patients with positive surgical margins or the presence of extracapsular nodal involvement were most likely to benefit from "combined therapy" rather than with radiotherapy administered as a single modality.[610] Disease-free survival was significantly longer after chemoradiotherapy (hazard ratio for recurrent disease or death 0.78, p = .04), but not overall survival in the RTOG/Intergroup study,[608] while significant advantages for both local control and survival were observed by the EORTC[609] despite use of virtually the same chemoradiotherapy schedule. There were some differences in eligibility criteria. Daily fractionated radiotherapy was given with cisplatin, 100 mg/m^2, administered on days 1, 22, and 43 of the radiotherapy regimen. See Table 79-20 for a comparison of these reports. Notably, acute treatment-related grade 3/4 toxicity, particularly mucocutaneous effects, were greater after chemoradiotherapy relative to radiotherapy alone (77% vs 34%, $p < .001$[608] and 41% vs 21%, p = .001,[609] respectively), although there were no clear differences in late adverse effects in either study.[608,609]

A compilation of prospective, randomized trials that have investigated the potential value of concomitant chemoradiotherapy in patients with locally advanced and often unresectable disease is presented in Table 79-21. A caveat is that although virtually all of the patients entered to these trials had summary stage III or IV disease, there was much variability among the reporting institutions regarding primary site, T and N stages, and the definition of tumor unresectability. Patients were uniformly free of known distant metastases. Little attempt was made to stratify patients according to histologic differentiation or other biomarkers such as surface concentration of epidermal growth factor receptor (EGFR). A variable percentage of patients reported have had salvage therapies, most often surgery or chemotherapy, following tumor recurrence. The effect of such subsequent treatment on mid- and long-term survival is not clear.

With respect to the treatment regimens, there also has been much variability. Cisplatin has been the drug most commonly used in a variety of schedules—daily, weekly, or every 3 weeks—and paired with fluorouracil in some trials. Carboplatin is an agent often used in community practice. Radiotherapy has routinely been administered in a once-daily fractionation sequence, but, alternatively, in a hyperfractionated bid schedule or in a split-course strategy. Most would agree that the use of cisplatin 100 mg/m^2 administered during weeks 1, 4, and 7 of a once-daily RT schedule can be considered a standard program.

Table 79-20 Postoperative Radiotherapy after Definitive Surgical Resection for High-Risk SCCHN with or without Cisplatin: Phase III Trials

Study	Eligibility	Treatment Arms	*n*	Outcomes
Bachaud et al[607]	Stage III/IV and nodal ECS	RT (65–74 Gy, 1.7qd) vs RT + wkly cddp, 50 mg	44 39	LRC 77% CM vs 59% RT (p = .08); 5-yr OS 36% CM vs 13% RT (p < .01)
RTOG 9501[608]	Microsurgically involved surgical margins, ≥ 2 nodal metastases, or ECS	RT (60–66 Gy, 2 Gy qd vs RT + cddp (100 mg/m^2 dL, 22, 43)	231 228	2-yr LRC 82% CM vs 72% RT (p = .04)
EORTC[609]	pT3/4 or any N2/3, ≈ margins, ECS, perineural infiltration, or vascular tumor emboli	RT (54–66 Gy, 2Gy qd) vs RT + cddp (100 mg/m^2 dL, 22, 43)	167 167	5-yr LRC 82% CM vs 69% RT (p = .007); 5-yr OS 53% CM vs 40%RT (p = .02)

cddp = cisplatin; CM = combined modality treatment; ECS = extracapsular spread; LRC = locoregional control; OS = overall survival; RT = radiotherapy; SCCHN = squamous cell carcinoma of the oral cavity, pharynx, or larynx.

As a generalization, the data indicate that concomitant chemotherapy and radiation reduce risk of local or regional tumor recurrence compared with radiotherapy as a single modality. Related to this, overall survival improves. This has also been a finding of the postoperative chemoradiotherapy trials discussed above. There has not been a widely perceived advantage for concomitant chemoradiotherapy with regard to distant disease control or reduction in risk of second primary tumors. However, some investigators have reported that concomitant chemoradiotherapy may have beneficial effects on local and distant disease control.[599]

With regard to toxicity, usually a brisk mucocutaneous reaction occurs with chemoradiation, necessitating the use of oral rinses for hygiene, analgesics, attention to fluid and calorie intake, and involvement of speech and swallowing rehabilitation specialists. Moreover, there is concern that long-term xerostomia, fibrosis, and related swallowing dysfunction may be more likely after concomitant chemoradiotherapy than radiation therapy administered alone. Brizel and others have reported the potential for amifostine, a radioprotector, to reduce acute and chronic xerostomia after radiotherapy.[547] Long-term functional data for most patients have not been routinely reported. In the recent Intergroup larynx trial[596] and the postoperative chemoradiotherapy trials,[607–610] there appeared not to be a high risk of chronic deleterious effects of combined therapy relative to control groups treated with radiotherapy.

In a very exciting recent trial, Bonner and colleagues[611] report a prospectively randomized multi-institutional trial in which previously untreated patients with locally advanced squamous cell carcinoma of the oropharynx, hypopharynx, or larynx received definitive radiotherapy with or without cetuximab. As discussed below in the section "Novel Therapeutics," cetuximab is a chimeric human and murine monoclonal antibody directed against the epidermal growth factor receptor (EGFR) and is under intense study for the treatment of SCCHN. In this phase III trial, 424 patients were entered and median duration of follow-up was 38 months. Notably, there was no increase in severe-grade radiation related mucocutaneous toxicity. Moreover, median survival (28 mo vs 54 mo) and 3-year survival (44% vs 57%) favored the combined therapy arm with a significant advantage in locoregional tumor control.

Thus, the current standard of care for patients with stage III and IV SCCHN, who are not candidates for surgery, is to be treated with concomitant chemoradiotherapy. Most centers agree that cisplatin administered with once-daily radiotherapy is a widely accepted approach. Alternative chemoradiation treatment plans, hyperfractionated radiotherapy with chemotherapy, other drug or multidrug regimens, and sequential chemoradiotherapy (induction or adjuvant drug treatment) should be further studied and may best be administered within the context of a clinical trial.

Furthermore, the promising early results of the radiotherapy and cetuximab trial predict the integration of molecular therapy into multimodal treatment strategies.

Recurrent and Metastatic Disease: Cytotoxics The activity of cytotoxic chemotherapy with single agents has been demonstrated in phase II trials, and expected response rates for multiple drugs are presented in Table 79-22. Treatment responses are generally more likely to be obtained in patients with ECOG performance status 0/1; in patients presenting with distant metastases or with tumor recurrence greater than 6 months from primary therapy; and in patients with sites of involvement such as lung not previously radiated.

Methotrexate, has been a traditional choice of many oncologists for palliation of recurrent or metastatic SCCHN.[375,612,613] The standard dos-

Table 79-21 Prospective Phase III Trials for Locally Advanced SCCHN: Comparing Radiotherapy with Concomitant Chemotherapy and Radiation

Study	Eligibility	Treatment Arms	*n*	Outcomes
Calais et al[598]	Stage III/IV SCC, OP	RT (70 Gy in 35 fx) vs RT + cbdca/fu × 3 cycles	113 109	LRC 66% CM vs 42% RT 3-yr OS 51% CM vs 31% RT (p = .02)
Merlano et al[597]	Unresectable stage III/IV SCCHN	RT (to 70Gy, 2Gy/d) vs alternating cddp/fu × 5 d then RT × 10 fx for 3 full cycles	77 80	CR 42% CM vs 22% RT; 3-yr OS 41% CM vs 23% RT
Brizel et al[600]	Unresectable stage III/IV SCCHN	HFRT (70 Gy) vs HFRT + cddp/fu wks 1+6 then adjuvant cddp/fu × 2	60 56	3-yr LRC 70% CM vs 44% HFRT (p = .01); OS 55% CM vs 34% HFRT (p = .07)
Jeremic et al[599]	Stage III/IV SCCHN	HFRT (77 Gy in 70 fx) vs HFRT + cddp 6 mg/m^2/d	65 65	5-yr LRC + DDC 50% + 86% CM vs 36% + 57% RT (p = .041 + .001, respectively. 5-yr OS 45% CM vs 25% RT (p = .008)
Wendt et al[601]	Unresectable stage III/IV SCCHN	RT (split course to total 70.2 Gy) vs RT + cddp/fu/lv × 3 cycles	135 135	3-yr LRC 36% CM vs 17% RT (p = < .004); 3-yr OS 48% CM vs 24% RT (p < .0003)
Staar et al[602]	Stage III/IV unresectable SCC OP/HP	HF-ACC-RT vs HF-ACC-RT + cbdca/fu d 1–5, 29–33	127 113	2-yr LRC 51% CM vs 45% RT; 1-yr OS+LRC 58% CM vs 44% RT (p = .05); OS + LRC SCC OP 60% CM vs 40% RT (p = .01)
Adelstein et al[603]	Stage III/IV SCCHN	RT (70 Gy in 35 fx) vs RT + cddp 100 mg/m^2 wks 1, 4, and 7 vs RT (split) + cddp/fu	102 97	3-yr OS 37% RT + cddp vs 23% RT (p = .01)
Huguenin et al[604]	Stage II/III/IV SCCHN	HFRT (median 74.4 Gy, 1.2 Gy bid) vs HFRT + cddp 20 mg/m^2 × 5 d, wks 1 + 5	112 112	LRC and DDFS superior CM> RT (p = .039 and .011, respectively, by log rank)
Budach et al[605]	Stage III/IV SCC OC, OP, HP	HF-ACC-RT vs HF-ACC-RT + mmc/fu	194 190	5-yr LRC 49.9% CM vs 37.4% RT (p = .001)

cddp = cisplatin, cbdca-carboplatin; CM = combined modality treatment; DDC = distant disease control; DDFS = distant disease-free survival; fx = fraction; fu = fluorouracil; HF/ACC = hyperfractionated, accelerated; LRC = locoregional control; mmc = mitomycin; OS = overall survival; RT = radiotherapy; SCCHN = squamous cell carcinoma of the oral cavity (OC), oropharynx (OP), hypopharynx (HP), or larynx.

Table 79-22 Single-Agent Activity in Recurrent Head and Neck Cancer

Agent	Approximate Response Percentage
Methotrexate	30
Bleomycin	20
Cisplatin	30
Carboplatin	25
5-Fluorouracil	15
Paclitaxel	30–40
Docetaxel	30–40
Ifosfamide	25

age schedule is 40 mg/m^2/wk intravenously or intramuscularly, with dosage escalation to 60 mg/m^2/wk, until mild toxicity or a tumor response is achieved. This approach is relatively nontoxic, inexpensive, and convenient, features that are critical to palliative therapy.

Cisplatin is an important component of drug therapy for SCCHN and often is administered in an intermittent schedule (80–100 mg/m^2 every 3–4 weeks). The dose response for cisplatin in SCCHN has been studied by several groups but remains uncertain. Driven by the activity and toxicities of cisplatin, analogue development has also been a focus of much activity. Carboplatin is a second-generation platinum complex with substantial activity and less toxicity than cisplatin. Bolus carboplatin has a pharmacokinetic profile similar to continuous-infusion cisplatin but with significantly less renal, otologic, neurologic, and gastrointestinal (nausea/vomiting) toxicity. Reversible myelosuppression (primarily thrombocytopenia) is the dose-limiting toxicity for carboplatin.

Older single-agent studies of carboplatin given monthly in bolus infusion or in fractionated schedules produced objective response rates of 20 to 30% in recurrent and metastatic SCCHN.[613] Bleomycin has been studied extensively as a single agent and in combination regimens in SCCHN.[612] Its spectrum of toxicity is distinctive. Intensive dose scheduling is directly associated with mucositis, and total cumulative dosage is directly associated with skin toxicity and pulmonary fibrosis. Lack of myelosuppression, even with prolonged continuous infusion, promotes use in combinations. Continuous-infusion regimens produce less pulmonary toxicity, but are not clearly more active clinically than intermittent-bolus schedules.[612,613] This drug is no longer in common usage. 5-Fluorouracil has limited single-agent activity in SCCHN. It has been given in varying doses as an intravenous infusion or bolus daily (for 5 days), weekly, or every 3 to 4 weeks. The dose-limiting toxicity of bolus administration is mucositis, diarrhea, and cutaneous erythema. Schedule dependency of 5-FU treatment has received little study in SCCHN, although long-term continuous low-dose infusion (eg, over 6 weeks) is effective palliation for recurrent disease. Continuous-infusion regimens were designed initially to reduce myelosuppression and seem to have enhanced activity. This agent has most commonly been used in combination with cisplatin, as discussed elsewhere in this chapter. Despite modest single-agent activity, preclinical studies indicating synergistic interaction with radiation and enhanced cytotoxicity with chemical modulators (eg, leucovorin) have led to much study of this agent in combination with other principles.

Randomized trials have compared single agents in recurrent SCCHN.[612–615] Phase III studies have directly compared cisplatin and methotrexate (randomized, two-arm design).[613] In one of these studies, Hong and colleagues[614] gave cisplatin at 50 mg/m^2 on days 1 and 8 every month versus methotrexate at 40 to 60 mg/m^2/wk. Response rates were 28.6% and 23.5%, respectively.

Ifosfamide and the taxanes have demonstrated single-agent activity. Ifosfamide has been tested in a wide range of doses and fractionation schedules, producing tumor responses in 25% of patients.[616] The taxanes constitute a distinctive class of established active agents in SCCHN.[617] An early ECOG phase II trial of paclitaxel tested the drug at a high-dose level, 250 mg/m^2 over 24 hours with G-CSF, in 30 patients.[618] There was an impressive 40% major response rate, 9.2-month median survival, and 33% 1-year survival rate. The major high-grade toxicity was neutropenia. Use of docetaxel has produced response rates ranging from 21 to 42% in phase II studies in patients who have not previously received palliative chemotherapy.[619] Gemcitabine, vinorelbine, and camptothecins continue to be under study.[617,620]

General classes of drugs with limited single-agent activity include the anthracyclines, vinca alkaloids, mitomycin (and analogs), and nitrosoureas. The major role for anthracyclines in head and neck cancer appears to be in the therapy of nonsquamous cancers (salivary gland cancer, small-cell carcinoma, and esthesioneuroblastoma).

Combination chemotherapy may produce responses in 30 to 40% of patients, but without significant survival advantages over single-agent therapy, which is usually in the range of 6 to 9 months (Table 79-23).[612–614,617,618,621–627] For patients with disease not amenable to local therapy with curative intent, the goal of chemotherapy is to provide palliation with achievement of a tumor response. For some achieving substantial disease regression, this may lead to increased survival. Nonetheless, in the appropriate context, combination chemotherapy with either cisplatin/FU or a platinum/taxane combination has become the standard of care in good-performance patients with advanced or recurrent SCCHN. A recent report of the Eastern Cooperative Oncology Group is notable. Gibson and colleagues[627] conducted a prospective phase III trial comparing cisplatin and infusional fluorouracil (CF) with cisplatin and paclitaxel (CP). Two hundred eighteen patients were entered. There was no difference in response rate (27% in the CF group and 26% in CP patients) or survival 8.7 months versus 8.1 months, respectively. Toxicity was similar.

It is concluded that survival for patients with recurrent or widely metastatic squamous cell carcinoma of the head and neck remains poor. Approximately 30% of patients survive 1 year. There is a pressing need for new drug development and more efficacious systemic strategies.

Novel Therapeutics Invasive squamous cell cancers emerge after the accumulation of multiple genomic events in a multistep process.[628–630] There appear to be essential molecular alterations that are biologically significant, which confer a survival advantage for cancer cells and which constitute the process of carcinogenesis.[631] As we understand better the underlying cancer biology, potential therapeutic targets have been identified and have led to innovative treatment strategies.

Epidermal Growth Factor Receptor EGFR is a transmembrane glycoprotein activation of which triggers a cascade of "downstream" intracellular signaling events important for regulation of epithelial cell growth. The epidermal growth factor (EGF) and transforming growth factor alpha (TGF-α) are ligands for the receptor. Ligand binding to the extracellular receptor domain prompts intracellular phosphorylation, which, in turn, leads ultimately to transcription of genes that participate in cell growth. Overexpression of EGFR or its principal ligand, TGF-α, has been observed in approximately 90% of SCCHN.[631–636] This increase in both TGF-α and EGFR forms an autocrine loop that results in increased EGFR signaling, which has been linked to cell proliferation, tumor progression, tumor angiogenesis, and increased cell survival.[637–642] Furthermore, surface EGFR and TGF-α expression appears to correlate inversely with overall survival following surgery and RT.[635,643,644] Preclinical studies have demonstrated promise for treatment strategies with monoclonal antibodies (eg, cetuximab) or tyrosine kinase inhibitors (eg, gefitinib) that target the EGFR, most often as a component of a combination regimen. Phase II[645–651] and III trials in humans are well underway, and this represents a relatively advanced area of new drug development.

Gefitinib and erlotinib are small molecules that inhibit phosphorylation of cytoplasmic tyrosine kinases of the EGFR (Table 79-24). Both agents are administered orally and have been tested as single agents in recurrent or metastatic SCCHN.[645,646] Of interest, the Chicago group has observed tumor responses in 12% of patients treated with gefitinib, 500 mg daily,[645] but in a subsequent study the response rate diminished to 3% at the 250 mg dose[652] commonly used for patients with nonsmall-cell lung cancer. Moreover, reports of "gain-of-function" EGFR mutations have not surfaced in SCCHN in contrast to NSCLC, where abnormalities in the exon range 18 to 21 are strong predictors for a response to gefitinib. These oral agents may be administered per gastrostomy feeding tubes, a matter of consequence for many head and neck cancer patients. In these studies, an association between development of skin rash and survival has also been observed.[645,646]

Table 79-23 Selected Randomized Phase III Trials of Chemotherapy in Recurrent or Metastatic Squamous Cell Carcinoma of the Head and Neck

Trial	No. of Patients	Regimen	Response Rate (%)	Survival (*p* Value)
Jacobs et al[622]	79	cddp/fu	32	NS
	83	cddp	17	
	83	fu	13	
Forastiere et al[623]	87	cddp/fu	32	NS
	86	cbdca/fu	21	
	88	mtx	10	
Clavel et al[624]	127	cddp/mtx/bleo/vcr	34	NS
	116	cddp/fu	31	
	122	cddp	15	
Schrijvers et al[625]	122	cddp/fu/ifnα-2b	47	NS
	122	cddp/fu	38	
Forastiere et al[626]	101	cddp/pac (high dose)	35	NS
	98	cddp/pac (low dose)	36	
Gibson et al[627]	104	cddp/fu	22	NS
	100	cddp/pac	28	

bleo = bleomycin; cbdca = carboplatin; cddp = cisplatin; fu = fluorouracil; ifnα-2b = interferon alfa-2b; mtx = methotrexate; NS = not statistically significant; pac = paclitaxel; vcr = vincristine. (Modified from Cohen EE et al.[650])

Cetuximab is a chimeric human/murine monoclonal antibody directed against the extracellular portion of EGFR. Shin and colleagues[653] have reported a phase I experience combining cetuximab and cisplatin, observing tumor responses in 6 of 9 evaluable patients with recurrent SCCHN. Moreover, tumor saturation was achieved at the generally well-tolerated loading dose of 400 mg/m^2 followed by weekly 205 mg/m^2 administrations. Binding of the monoclonal antibody competes with ligand activation and prevents receptor dimerization, with consequent abrogation of multiple downstream signals. In phase II trials (Table 79-24), cetuximab was combined with cisplatin in treating patients refractory to platin-based chemotherapy,[647,648] continuing the administration of the platinating agent after adding cetuximab. Tumor responses were observed in 12 to 14% of patients, a striking result in this very poor prognostic group. Moreover, Trigo and colleagues[649] have more recently reported responses in 12.5% of patients, similarly platin-refractory, with cetuximab administered as a single agent. In aggregate, these trials also demonstrated a relationship between skin rash and activity.

The Eastern Cooperative Oncology Group has completed a randomized placebo controlled trial testing cisplatin with or without cetuximab in recurrent or metastatic SCCHN as first-line therapy.[654] This trial enrolled 123 patients and demonstrated a 26% response rate in the treatment arm versus 10% in the control group ($p = .029$). However, the two cohorts did not differ with respect to the primary end point of progression-free survival (4.1 vs 3.4 months, $p = .27$) or a secondary end point of overall survival (9.2 vs 8 months, $p = .18$). Of signal importance, Bonner and colleagues[655] have also recently reported preliminary results of a prospective randomized phase III trial of radiotherapy, administered with or without cetuximab. As discussed earlier, this study showed that local tumor control and overall survival were significantly improved in the combination therapy arm.

The association of skin toxicity with activity has also been seen in other tumor types[656,657] and needs further exploration. If indeed this relationship exists, it would imply a mechanistic etiology and, since skin rash occurs more frequently at higher doses, possibly a dose-response relationship for these compounds. Furthermore, this would support testing a strategy of escalating dose until rash or dose-limiting toxicities develop.

Intracellular Signaling Newer, targeting compounds that inhibit signal transduction, influence cell cycle activity and apoptosis, regulate transcription, and affect extracellular matrix and angiogenesis are the subjects of intensive study. Most of these compounds are in preclinical or early clinical development and not so far along as the EGFR inhibitors. Cyclin-dependent kinase (CDK) inhibitors are in phase I trials. CDK's phosphorylate crucial intermediates that regulate cell cycling. Cyclin D is commonly overexpressed in SCCHN, and p16, which is a crucial induction inhibitor of CDK4 may be deleted or not transcribed in many tumors. Flavopiridol and another CDK inhibitor, CI-799, which is a structural analog of rapamycin, are under study. Alterations of the *ras* oncogene have been observed in SCCHN,[658] and more frequently in nonsmall-cell lung cancer. Related to this, farnesyl transferase inhibitors were developed to block *ras* recruitment to the cell membrane and subsequent signal transduction.[659] However, recent studies have raised speculation regarding the actual target.[660–662] In a phase Ib trial designed to test the value of the farnesyl transferase inhibitor SCH 66336 in SCCHN, Kies and colleagues[663] administered the drug for 2 weeks preoperatively to 29 patients. Inhibition of farnesylation was reported in all patients tested, despite the short duration of therapy. A phase II trial assessing activity in recurrent or metastatic disease is underway. The phase I study demonstrates the potential for trials with induction systemic therapy as a vehicle wherein new drugs or combinations can be tested with regard to activity, toxicity, and the extent to which there is biochemical inhibition of a molecular target. Are we doing what we think we're doing with a given "targeting agent?"

Angiogenesis New blood vessel formation is a necessary process for tumor growth, and angiogenic molecules are potential therapeutic targets in SCCHN. Interleukin-8 (IL-8) is a major angiogenic factor associated with oral squamous cell carcinoma cell lines[664] and is found in SCCHN tumor samples.[665] Vascular endothelial growth factor (VEGF) is a multifunctional cytokine and a potent stimulator of the growth of endothelial cells. VEGF activates receptor tyrosine kinases, which are located on the surface

Table 79-24 Phase II Trials of EGFR Inhibitors in Recurrent or Metastatic Squamous Cell Carcinoma of the Head and Neck

A. Phase II Trials of EGFR Tyrosine Kinase Inhibitors

	n	Response Rate (%)	Stable Disease (%)	Time to Progression (Mo)	Median Survival (Mo)
Gefitinib (Cohen, 2003[645] and 2004[650])					
250 mg	63	3.3	26.6	NR	NR
500 mg	52	10.6		3.4	8.1
Erlotinib (Soulieres, 2004[646])					
150 mg	115	4.3	38.3	2.5	6.0

B. Cetuximab: Phase II Summary in Platinum-Refractory SCCHN*

Cetuximab	*n*	Response Rate (%)	Median Survival (Mo)
Single agent (Trigo[649])	103	13	5.9
+ a platinum (Baselga[648])	96	11	6.1
+ cisplatin (Kies[647])	131	12	6.1
Historical comparison	151	3	3.4

*After Vermorken.[651]

of endothelial cells, and is critical to the regulation of both normal and cancer-related blood vessel formation. Increased VEGF protein expression is seen in many cancers, including SCCHN,[666–668] and after radiotherapy and may play an important role in the induction of angiogenesis.[669] Experimental evidence has demonstrated that tumor growth can be diminished by inhibiting neovascularization,[664,670–675] making antiangiogenic therapy an attractive potential treatment strategy. SU5416 was tested in a phase II trial in 22 patients with SCCHN, with minimal single-agent activity, a single response.[676] Most reports are of the combination of antiangiogenic compounds with chemotherapy and/or radiotherapy. Bevacizumab is a humanized monoclonal antibody directed against VEGF, preventing binding to receptor tyrosine kinases ($VEGFR_1$ and $VEGFR_2$) with resultant inhibition of tumor cell growth. A phase I trial combining bevacizumab with chemoradiotherapy has demonstrated tolerability and efficacy in poor prognosis patients.[677] Much excitement has recently been generated by the experience with chemotherapy in adenocarcinoma of the lung. In a prospective, randomized study of 444 patients receiving conventional paclitaxel and carboplatin chemotherapy, with or without bevacizumab, there was a response and survival superiority for the experimental arm.[678] Vokes and colleagues[679] combined bevacizumab with gefitinib in a phase I trial in patients with advanced SCCHN and observed tumor responses in 14%, with little toxicity. A solitary patient had grade 4 hemorrhage, although this event was not clearly related to VEGF inhibition.

Tissue Hypoxia Tissue hypoxia is associated with poor outcomes and resistance to treatment in SCCHN, prompting an intense search for agents specifically toxic to this cell population, particularly in combination with RT.[680–683] Mitomycin C is a bioreductive antibiotic with modest single-agent activity and is under study as a radiation sensitizer.[684] Haffty and colleagues[685] have recently conducted a randomized trial of concomitant radiotherapy combined with mitomycin C or porfiromycin with 128 patients. Local tumor control (82% vs 65%) was superior in patients receiving mitomycin. Tirapazamine is a benzotriazine compound that requires reduction to its active free radical form in an hypoxic environment.[686] This agent has demonstrated synergy in vitro with RT[687] and cisplatin.[688] A phase II study with tirapazamine, cisplatin, and radiation demonstrates feasibility and activity, with 3-year locoregional control 84% in previously untreated patients with stage III or IV disease.[689] The addition of tirapazamine to concomitant cisplatin/RT is currently being evaluated in a phase III randomized trial.

Gene Therapy Approaches utilizing adenovirus-mediated wild-type *TP53* gene transfer have generated excitement following the demonstration of tumor responses in some patients.[690] Khuri and colleagues[691] conducted a multicenter phase II trial combining ONYX-015, which is a selective replicating adenovirus, with cisplatin and 5-fluorouracil in treating patients with advanced SCCHN. A response rate of 52% was observed in 30 patients with fully evaluable tumors. In a subset of patients with tumors injectable and not accessible for injection, there was observed a substantial difference with tumor responses observed more often after chemotherapy and ONYX-015 administration ($p = .006$). Ongoing trials with TP53 replacement strategies continue for patients with recurrent SCCHN accessible to injection and as a chemoprevention strategy.

Adjuvant Therapy Adjuvant chemotherapy alone to eradicate micrometastases following definitive local therapy has not been successful. A number of randomized trials have evaluated the impact of adjuvant multiagent chemotherapy with no clear survival impact.[608,613,617] However, concomitant chemoradiotherapy in the adjuvant setting has produced very promising results in phase III trials in "high-risk" patients (see the section "Chemotherapy and Radiation for Locally Advanced Disease" above).

It is critically important to develop effective chemopreventive agents for patients with definitively treated primary cancers of the head and neck because of their high risk of second primary tumors (SPTs). There is an intense research interest in distinguishing, largely through molecular assessments, between recurrences and SPTs,[134] and chemoprevention has evolved, in part, from adjuvant therapy in this setting. A relatively small randomized controlled adjuvant trial of high-dose 13-*cis*-retinoic acid (13cRA) for 1 year in stage I-IV disease was neutral with respect to recurrences, but produced a significant reduction in SPTs.[673] This trial led to a NCI Intergroup trial of low-dose 13cRA for 3 years to prevent SPTs in over 1,000 patients with definitively treated early-stage head and neck cancer. Although better tolerated than the high-dose 13cRA regimen, the low-dose trial had no effect on SPTs, recurrence, or survival.[674] This trial, however, did provide the first definitive proof that the survival rate in former smokers is significantly better than in current smokers, further supporting public health efforts in smoking cessation. Promising phase II data have suggested that a high-dose bioadjuvant regimen of 13cRA, interferon-alpha, and vitamin E can substantially reduce recurrence and SPTs associated with locally advanced head and neck cancer.[675] Based on these data, an ongoing phase III trial (coordinated by ECOG) is testing this regimen for adjuvant therapy in locally advanced disease. These adjuvant/SPT prevention trials evolved largely out of a pioneering program of human chemoprevention involving the translational study of retinoids in oral IEN patients. Details of this study (including the relevant randomized controlled trials) are presented in Chapter 27, "Chemoprevention of Cancer."

New approaches, such as bioadjuvant therapy with 13cRA, interferon-alpha, and vitamin E, must be developed to prevent second primary tumors as well as recurrences, integrating novel agents are necessary second primary tumor chemoprevention in definitively treated head and neck cancer patients also may benefit from molecular-targeted agent combinations in patients identified by molecular markers to have a high SPT risk, such as combinations of EGFR and COX-2 inhibitors that are being tested in cancer therapy and oral cancer prevention in high-risk settings.[186]

Current Directions Systemic therapy is now an integral part of SCCHN treatment. Patients with locally advanced disease are treated with chemotherapy and radiation. Options for the treatment of recurrent disease now include re-irradiation, cytotoxic chemotherapy, and molecularly targeted therapy. We can expect intensive study of more specific targeting compounds aimed at enhancing efficacy and reducing toxicity. Combining targeting agents, as has been demonstrated with bevacizumab and gefitinib, is also anticipated. The recent report of a survival advantage for radiotherapy administered with cetuximab over radiotherapy as a single modality heralds the integration of targeted therapy as a component of primary treatment in SCCHN. Thus, these compounds appear to hold great promise for advancing our therapeutic armamentarium.

REFERENCES

1. Jemal A, Tiwari RC, Murray T, et al. Cancer statistics, 2004. Cancer J Clin 2004;54:8–29.
2. Parkin DM, Pisani P, Ferlay J. Estimates of the worldwide incidence of 25 major cancers in 1990. Int J Cancer 1999;80:827–41.
3. Decker J, Goldstein JC. Risk factors in head and neck cancer. N Engl J Med 1982;306:1151–5.
4. Squier CA. Smokeless tobacco and oral cancer: a cause for concern? CA Cancer J Clin 1984;34:242–7.
5. Ghafoor A, Jemal A, Cokkinides V, et al. Cancer statistics for African-Americans. CA Cancer J Clin 2003;52:326–41.
6. Lippman SM, Hong WK. Retinoid chemoprevention of upper aerodigestive tract carcinogenesis. In: DeVita VT, Hellman S, Rosenberg SA, editors. Important advances in oncology. Philadelphia: Lippincott; 1992. p. 93–109.
7. Vikram B. Changing patterns of failure in advanced head and neck cancer. Arch Otolaryngol 1984;110:564–5.
8. Silverberg E. Cancer statistics, 1985. CA Cancer J Clin 1985;35:19–35.
9. Boring CC, Squires TS, Tong T. Cancer statistics 1993. CA Cancer J Clin 1993;43:7.
10. SEER Cancer Statistics Review 1973–1999.
11. Shemen LJ, Klotz J, Schottenfeld D, Strong EW. Increase of tongue cancer in young men. JAMA 1984;252:1857.
12. Depue RH. Rising mortality from cancer of the tongue in young white males. N Engl J Med 1986;315:647.
13. Schantz SP, Byers RM, Goepfert H. Tobacco and cancer of the tongue in young adults. JAMA 1988;259:1943–4.
14. Myers JN, Elkins T, Roberts D, Byers RM. Squamous cell carcinoma of the tongue in young adults: increasing incidence and factors that predict treatment outcomes. Otolaryngol Head Neck Surg 2000;122:44–51.
15. Schantz SP, Yu GP. Head and neck cancer incidence trends in young Americans, 1973–1997, with a special analysis for tongue cancer. Arch Otolaryngol Head Neck Surg 2002;128:268–74.
16. Parkin DM, Bray F, Ferlay J, Pisani P. Estimating the world cancer burden: Globocan 2000. Int J Cancer 2001;94:153–6.
17. Wynder EL, Bross IJ, Feldman RM. A study of the etiological factors in cancer of the mouth. Cancer 1957;10:1300–23.
18. Hammond EC, Horn D. Smoking and death rates: report on forty-four months of follow-up of 187,783 men. JAMA 1958;166:1294–308.
19. Smoking and health: report of the Advisory Committee to the Surgeon General of the Public Health Service. Washington (DC): US Department of Health, Education, and Welfare; 1964.

20. Doll R, Hill AB. Lung cancer and other causes of death in relation to smoking; a second report on the mortality of British doctors. Br Med J 1956;2:1071–81.
21. Funk GF, Karnell LH, Robinson RA, et al. Presentation, treatment, and outcome of oral cavity cancer: a national cancer data base report. Head Neck 2002;24:165–80.
22. Blot WJ, McLaughlin JK, Winn DM, et al. Smoking and drinking in relation to oral and pharyngeal cancer. Cancer Res 1988;48:3282–7.
23. Franceschi S, Talamini R, Barra S, et al. Smoking and drinking in relation to cancers of the oral cavity, pharynx, larynx, and esophagus in Northern Italy. Cancer Res 1990;50:6502–7.
24. Franceschi S, Levi F, La Vecchia C, et al. Comparison of the effect of smoking and alcohol drinking between oral and pharyngeal cancer. Int J Cancer 1999;83:1–4.
25. Merletti F, Boffetta P, Ciccone G, et al. Role of tobacco and alcoholic beverages in the etiology of cancer of the oral cavity/oropharynx in Torino, Italy. Cancer Res 1989;49:4919–24.
26. Faulk RT, Pickle LW, Brown LM, et al. Effect of smoking and alcohol consumption on laryngeal cancer risk in coastal Texas. Cancer Res 1989;49:4024–9.
27. Schlecht NF, Franco EL, Pintos J, et al. Interaction between tobacco and alcohol consumption and the risk of cancers of the upper aero-digestive tract in Brazil. Am J Epidemiol 1999;150:1129–37.
28. LaVecchia C, Tavani A, Franceschi S, et al. Epidemiology and prevention of oral cancer. Oral Oncol 1997; 33:302–12.
29. Cattaruzza MS, Maisonneuve P, Boyle P. Epidemiology of laryngeal cancer. Eur J Cancer B Oral Oncol 1996;32B:293–305.
30. Schlecht NF, Franco EL, Pintos J, Kowalski LP. Effect of smoking cessation and tobacco type on the risk of cancers of the upper aero-digestive tract in Brazil. Epidemiology 1999;10:412–8.
31. Zhu K, Levine RS, Brann EA, et al. Case-control study evaluating the homogeneity and heterogeneity of risk factors between sinonasal and nasopharyngeal cancers. Int J Cancer 2002;99:119–23.
32. Iribarren C, Tekawa IS, Sidney S, Friedman GD. Effect of cigar smoking on the risk of cardiovascular disease, chronic obstructive pulmonary disease, and cancer in men. N Engl J Med 1999;340:1773–80.
33. Baker F, Ainsworth SR, Dye JT, et al. Health risks associated with cigar smoking. JAMA 2000;284:735–40.
34. Moore C, Catlin D. Anatomic origins and locations of oral cancer. Am J Surg 1967;114:510–3.
35. Scully C, Bedi R. Ethnicity and oral cancer. Lancet 2000;1:37–42.
36. Winn DM. Smokeless tobacco and cancer: the epidemiologic evidence. CA Cancer J Clin 1988;38:236–43.
37. Rao DN, Ganesh B, Rao RS, Desai PB. Risk assessment of tobacco, alcohol and diet in oral cancer—a case-control study. Int J Cancer 1994;58:469–73.
38. Centers for Disease Control and Prevention (CDC). Tobacco use—United States, 1900–1999. MMWR Morb Mortal Wkly Rep 1999;48:986–93.
39. Centers for Disease Control and Prevention (CDC). Cigarette smoking among adults—United States, 1999. MMWR Morb Mortal Wkly Rep 2001;50:869–73.
40. Marwick C. Increasing use of chewing tobacco, especially among younger persons, alarms Surgeon General. JAMA 1993;269:195.
41. Merchant A, Husain SSM, Hosain M, et al. Paan without tobacco: an independent risk factor for oral cancer. Int J Cancer 2000;86:128–31.
42. Idris AM, Ahmed HM, Malik MOA. Toombak dipping and cancer of the oral cavity in the Sudan: a case-control study. Int J Cancer 1995;63:477–80.
43. Kabat GC, Wynder EL. Type of alcoholic beverage and oral cancer. Int J Cancer 1989;43:190–4.
44. Goldgar DG, Easton DF, Cannon-Albright LA, et al. Systematic population-based assessment of cancer risk in first-degree relatives of cancer probands. J Natl Cancer Inst 1994;86:1600–8.
45. Foulkes WD, Brunet JS, Kowalski LP, et al. Family history of cancer is a risk factor for squamous cell carcinoma of the head and neck in Brazil: a case-control study. Int J Cancer 1995;63:769–73.
46. Copper MP, Jovanovic A, Nauta JJP, et al. Role of genetic factors in the etiology of squamous cell carcinoma of the head and neck. Arch Otolaryngol Head Neck Surg 1995;121:157–60.
47. Foulkes WD, Brunet JS, Sieh W, et al. Familial risks of squamous cell carcinoma of the head and neck: retrospective case-control study. BMJ 1996;313:716–21.
48. Sturgis EM, Wei Q. Genetic susceptibility-molecular epidemiology of head and neck cancer. Curr Opin Oncol 2002;14:310–7.
49. Dictor M, Johnson A. Association of inverted sinonasal papilloma with non-sinonasal head-and-neck carcinoma. Int J Cancer 2000;85:811–4.
50. Maden C, Beckmann AM, Thomas DB, et al. Human papillomaviruses, herpes simplex viruses, and the risk of oral cancer in men. Am J Epidemiol 1992;135:1093–102.
51. Aygenc E, Selcuk A, Celikkanat S, et al. The role of *Helicobacter pylori* infection in the cause of squamous cell carcinoma of the larynx. Otolaryngol Head Neck Surg 2001;125:520–1.
52. Grandis JR, Perez–Perez GI, Yu VL, et al. Lack of serologic evidence for *Helicobacter pylori* infection in head and neck cancer. Head Neck 1997;19:216–8.
53. zur Hausen H. Papillomaviruses causing cancer: evasion for host-cell control in early events in carcinogenesis. J Natl Cancer Inst 2000;92:690–8.
54. McKaig RG, Baric RS, Olshan AF. Human papillomavirus and head and neck cancer: epidemiology and molecular biology. Head Neck 1998;20:250–65.
55. Mineta H, Ogino T, Amano HM, et al. Human papillomavirus (HPV) type 16 and 18 detected in head and neck squamous cell carcinoma. Anticancer Res 1998;18:4765–8.
56. Steinberg BM, DiLorenzo TP. A possible role for human papillomaviruses in head and neck cancer. Cancer Metastasis Rev 1996;15:91–112.
57. Snijders P, Cromme FV, van den Brule A, et al. Prevalence and expression of human papillomavirus in tonsillar carcinomas, indicating a possible viral etiology. Int J Cancer 1992;51:845–50.
58. Capone RB, Pai SI, Koch WM, et al. Detection and quantitation of human papillomavirus (HPV) DNA in the sera of patients with HPV-associated head and neck squamous cell carcinoma. Clin Cancer Res 2000;6:4171–5.
59. Gillison ML, Koch WM, Capone RB, et al. Evidence for a causal association between human papillomavirus and a subset of head and neck cancers. J Natl Cancer Inst 2000;92:709–20.
60. Gillison ML, Shah KV. Human papillomavirus-associated head and neck squamous cell carcinoma: mounting evidence for an etiologic role for human papillomavirus in a subset of head and neck cancers. Curr Opin Oncol 2001;13:183–8.
61. Hengstermann A, Linares LK, Ciechanover A, et al. Complete switch from Mdm2 to human papillomavirus E6-mediated degradation of p53 in cervical cancer cells. Proc Natl Acad Sci U S A 2001;98:1218–23.
62. Andl T, Kahn T, Pfuhl A, et al. Etiological involvement of oncogenic human papillomavirus in tonsillar squamous cell carcinomas lacking retinoblastoma cell cycle control. Cancer Res 1998;58:5–13.
63. Munger K, Werness BA, Dyson N, et al. Complex formation of human papillomavirus E7 proteins with the retinoblastoma tumor suppressor gene product. EMBO J 1989;8:4099–105.
64. Fouret P, Monceaux G, Temam S, et al. Human papillomavirus in head and neck squamous cell carcinomas in nonsmokers. Arch Otolaryngol Head Neck Surg 1997;123:513–6.
65. Smith EM, Hoffman HT, Summersgill KS, et al. Human papillomavirus and risk of oral cancer. Laryngoscope 1998;108:1098–103.
66. Smith EM, Summersgill KF, Allen J, et al. Human papillomavirus and risk of laryngeal cancer. Ann Otol Rhinol Laryngol 2000;109:1069–76.
67. Strome SE, Savva A, Brissett AE, et al. Squamous cell carcinoma of the tonsils: a molecular analysis of HPV associations. Clin Cancer Res 2002;8:1093–100.
68. Mork J, Lie AK, Glattre E, et al. Human papilloma virus infection as a risk factor for squamous-cell carcinoma of the head and neck. N Engl J Med 2001;344:1125–31.
69. Schwartz SM, Daling JR, Doody DR, et al. Oral cancer risk in relation to sexual history and evidence of human papillomavirus infection. J Natl Cancer Inst 1998;90:1626–36.
70. Dahlstrom KR, Adler-Storthz K, Etzel CJ, et al. Human papillomavirus type 16 infection and squamous cell carcinoma of the head and neck in never smokers: a matched pair analysis. Clin Cancer Res 2003;9:2620–6.
71. Smith EM, Ritchie JM, Summersgill KF, et al. Human papillomavirus in oral exfoliated cells and risk of head and neck cancer. J Natl Cancer Inst 2004;96:449–55.
72. Henle W, Henle G, Ho HC, et al. Antibodies to Epstein-Barr virus in nasopharyngeal carcinoma, other head and neck neoplasms, and control groups. J Natl Cancer Inst 1970;44:225–31.
73. Pearson GR, Weiland LH, Neel HB, et al. Application of Epstein-Barr virus (EBV) serology to the diagnosis of North American nasopharyngeal carcinoma. Cancer 1983;51:260–8.
74. Feinmesser R, Miyazaki I, Cheung R, et al. Diagnosis of nasopharyngeal carcinoma by DNA amplification of tissue obtained by fine-needle aspiration. N Engl J Med 1992;326:17–21.
75. Yong-Sheng Z, Sham JST, Ng MH, et al. Immunoglobulin A against viral capsid antigen of Epstein-Barr virus and indirect mirror examination of the nasopharynx in the detection of asymptomatic nasopharyngeal carcinoma. Cancer 1992;69:3–7.
76. Chien YC, Chen JY, Liu MY, et al. Serologic markers of Epstein-Barr virus infection and nasopharyngeal carcinoma in Taiwanese men. N Engl J Med 2001;345:1877–82.
77. Raab-Traub N, Flynn K, Pearson G, et al. The differentiated form of nasopharyngeal carcinoma contains Epstein-Barr virus DNA. Int J Cancer 1987;39:25–9.
78. Sheen TS, Ko JY, Chang YL, et al. Nasopharyngeal swab and PCR for the screening of nasopharyngeal carcinoma in the endemic area: a good supplement to the serologic screening. Head Neck 1998;20:732–8.
79. Walter MA, Menarguez-Palanca J, Peiper SC. Epstein-Barr virus detection in neck metastases by polymerase chain reaction. Laryngoscope 1992;102:481–5.
80. Lin JC, Chen KY, Wang WY, et al. Detection of Epstein-Barr virus DNA in the peripheral blood cells of patients with nasopharyngeal carcinoma: relationship to distant metastasis and survival. J Clin Oncol 2001;19:2607–15.
81. Lo YMD, Chan LYS, Lo KW, et al. Quantitative analysis of cell-free Epstein-Barr virus DNA in plasma of patients with nasopharyngeal carcinoma. Cancer Res 1999;59:1188–91.
82. Loff B, Cordner S. Passive smoking test case wins in Australia. Lancet 2001;357:1511.
83. Chapman S. Australian bar worker wins payout in passive smoking case. BMJ 2001;322:1139.
84. Zhang ZF, Morgenstern H, Spitz MR, et al. Environmental tobacco smoking, mutagen sensitivity, and head and neck squamous cell carcinoma. Cancer Epidemiol Biomarkers Prev 2000;9:1043–9.
85. Tan E-H, Adelstein DJ, Droughton MLT, et al. Squamous cell head and neck cancer in nonsmokers. Am J Clin Oncol 1997;20:146–50.
86. Morrison MD. Is chronic gastroesophageal reflux a causative factor in glottic carcinoma? Otolaryngol Head Neck Surg 1988;99:370–3.
87. Ward PH, Hanson DG. Reflux as an etiological factor of carcinoma of the laryngopharynx. Laryngoscope 1988;98:1195–9.
88. Koufman JA. The otolaryngologic manifestations of gastroesophageal reflux disease (GERD): a clinical investigation of 225 patients using ambulatory 24-hour pH monitoring and an experimental investigation of the role of acid and pepsin in the development of laryngeal injury. Laryngoscope 1991;101:1–78.
89. Biacabe B, Gleich LL, Laccourreye O, et al. Silent gastroesophageal reflux disease in patients with pharyngolaryngeal cancer: further results. Head Neck 1998;20:510–4.
90. Copper MP, Smit CF, Stanojcic LD, et al. High incidence of laryngopharyngeal reflux in patients with head and neck cancer. Laryngoscope 2000;110:1007–11.
91. El-Serag HB, Hepworth EJ, Lee P, et al. Gastroesophageal reflux disease is a risk factor for laryngeal and pharyngeal cancer. Am J Gastroenterol 2001;96:2013–8.
92. Donald PJ. Marijuana smoking—possible cause of head and neck carcinoma in young patients. Otolaryngol Head Neck Surg 1986;94:517–21.
93. Caplan GA, Brigham BA. Marijuana smoking and carcinoma of the tongue. Is there an association? Cancer 1990;66:1005–6.
94. Zhang ZF, Morgenstern H, Spitz MR, et al. Marijuana use and increased risk of squamous cell carcinoma of the head and neck. Cancer Epidemiol Biomarkers Prev 1999;8:1071–8.
95. Sidney S, Quesenberry CP, Friedman GD, Tekawa IS. Marijuana use and cancer incidence (California, United States). Cancer Causes Control 1997;8:722–8.
96. Winn DM, Ziegler RG, Pickle LW, et al. Diet in the etiology of oral and pharyngeal cancer among women from the southern United States. Cancer Res 1984;44:1216–22.
97. McLaughlin JK, Gridley G, Block G, et al. Dietary factors in oral and pharyngeal cancer. J Natl Cancer Inst 1988;80:1237–43.
98. Zheng W, Blot WJ, Shu XO, et al. Diet and other risk factors for laryngeal cancer in Shanghai, China. Am J Epidemiol 1992;136:178–91.
99. Levi F, Pasche C, LaVecchia C, et al. Food groups and risk of oral and pharyngeal cancer. Int J Cancer 1998;77:705–9.

100. Schantz SP, Zhang ZF, Spitz MS, et al. Genetic susceptibility to head and neck cancer: interaction between nutrition and mutagen sensitivity. Laryngoscope 1997;107:765–81.
101. Ning JP, Yu MC, Wang QS, Henderson BE. Consumption of salted fish and other risk factors for nasopharyngeal carcinoma (NPC) in Tianjiin, a low-risk region for NPC in the People's Republic of China. J Natl Cancer Inst 1990;82:291–6.
102. Farrow DC, Vaughan TL, Berwick M, et al. Diet and nasopharyngeal cancer in a low-risk population. Int J Cancer 1998;78:675–9.
103. Mannetje A, Kogevinas M, Luce D, et al. Sinonasal cancer, occupation, and tobacco smoking in European women and men. Am J Ind Med 1999;36:101–7.
104. Luce D, Gerin M, Morcet JF, Leclerc A. Sinonasal cancer and occupational exposure to textile dust. Am J Ind Med 1997;32:205–10.
105. Holt GR. Sinonasal neoplasms and inhaled air toxics. Otolaryngol Head Neck Surg 1994;111:12–4.
106. Straif K, Keil U, Taeger D, et al. Exposure to nitrosamines, carbon black, asbestos, and talc and mortality from stomach, lung, and laryngeal cancer in a cohort of rubber workers. Am J Epidemiol 2000;152:297–306.
107. Browne K, Gee JB. Asbestos exposure and laryngeal cancer. Ann Occup Hyg 2000;44:239–50.
108. Ko JY, Chen CL, Lui LT, Hsu MM. Radiation-induced malignant fibrous histiocytoma in patients with nasopharyngeal carcinoma. Arch Otolaryngol Head Neck Surg 1996;122:535–8.
109. Saku T, Hayashi Y, Takahara O, et al. Salivary gland tumors among atomic bomb survivors, 1950–1987. Cancer 1997;79:1465–75.
110. Preston-Martin S, Thomas DC, White SC, Cohen D. Prior exposure to medical and dental X-rays related to tumors of the parotid gland. J Natl Cancer Inst 1988;80:943–9.
111. Allison P. Effectiveness of screening for oral cancer not proven. Evid Based Dent 2004;5:40–1.
112. Ramadas K, Sankaranarayanan R, Jacob BJ, et al. Interim results from a cluster randomized controlled oral cancer screening trial in Kerala, India. Oral Oncol 2003;39:580–8.
113. Broder AC. The microscopic grading of cancer. Surg Clin North Am 1941;21:947.
114. Crissman JD, Liu WY, Gluckman JL, Cummings G. Prognostic value of histopathologic parameters in squamous cell carcinoma of the oropharynx. Cancer 1984;54:2995–3001.
115. Snow GB, Annyas AA, van Slooten EA, et al. Prognostic factors of neck node metastases. Clin Otolaryngol 1982;7:185.
116. Wolf GT, Carey TE, Schmaltz SP, et al. Altered antigen expression predicts outcome in squamous cell carcinoma of the head and neck. J Natl Cancer Inst 1990;82:1566–72.
117. Jakobsson PA, Eneroth DM, Killander D, et al. Histologic classification and grading of malignancy in carcinoma of the larynx. Acta Radiol Ther Phys Biol 1973;12:1–8.
118. Wolf GT, Truelson JM, Beals T, Fisher S. Nuclear area and adjusted DNA index: a new correlate of prognosis in squamous carcinoma of the larynx. Proc Am Assoc Cancer Res 1990;31:189.
119. Ensley JF, Maciorowski Z, Pietraszkiewicz H, et al. Clinical applications of cellular DNA content parameters determined by flow cytometry in squamous cell cancers of the head and neck. In: Jones SE, Salmon SE, editors. Adjuvant therapy of cancer VI. Orlando (FL): Grune and Stratton; 1990. p. 101–8.
120. Kokal WA, Gardive RL, Sheibani K, et al. Tumor DNA content as a prognostic indication in squamous cell carcinoma of the head and neck region. Am J Surg 1988;156:276.
121. Sudbø J, Lippman SM, Lee JJ, et al. The influence of resection and aneuploidy on mortality in oral leukoplakia. N Engl J Med 2004;350:1405–13.
122. Brennan JA, Mao L, Hruban RH, et al. Molecular assessment of histopathological staging in squamous-cell carcinoma of the head and neck. N Engl J Med 1995;332:429–35.
123. Slaughter DP, Southwick HW, Smejkal W. Field cancerization in oral stratified squamous epithelium: clinical implications of multicentric origin. Cancer 1953;6:963–8.
124. Lippman SM, Benner SE, Hong WK. The chemoprevention of cancer. In: Greenwald P, Kramer S, Weed DL, editors. Cancer prevention and control. New York: Marcel Dekker; 1995. p. 329–52.
125. Strong MS, Incze J, Vaughan CW. Field cancerization in the aerodigestive tract—its etiology, manifestation, and significance. J Otolaryngol 1984;13:1–6.
126. Warren S, Gates O. Multiple primary malignant tumors: a survey of the literature and statistical study. Am J Cancer 1932;51:1358–1414.
127. Chung KY, Mukhopadhyay T, Kim J, et al. Discordant p53 gene mutations in primary head and neck cancers and corresponding second primary cancers of the upper aerodigestive tract. Cancer Res 1993;53:1676–83.
128. Shin DM, Kim J, Ro JY, et al. Activation of p53 gene expression in premalignant lesions during head and neck tumorigenesis. Cancer Res 1994;54:321–6.
129. Somers KD, Merrick MA, Lopez ME, et al. Frequent p53 mutations in head and neck cancer. Cancer Res 1992;52:5996–6000.
130. Brennan JA, Boyle JO, Koch WM, et al. Association between cigarette smoking and mutation of the p53 gene in squamous-cell carcinoma of the head and neck. N Engl J Med 1995;332:712–7.
131. Bouquot JE, Kurland LT, Weiland LH. Carcinoma in situ of the upper aerodigestive tract. Incidence, time trends, and follow-up in Rochester, Minnesota, 1935–1984. Cancer 1988;61:1691–8.
132. Bouquot JE, Weiland LH, Kurland LT. Leukoplakia and carcinoma in situ synchronously associated with invasive oral/oropharyngeal carcinoma in Rochester, Minn., 1935–1984. Oral Surg Oral Med Oral Pathol 1988;65:199–207.
133. Einhorn J, Wersall J. Incidence of oral carcinoma in patients with leukoplakia of the oral mucosa. Cancer 1967;20:2189–93.
134. Lippman SM, Sudbø J, Hong WK. Oral cancer prevention and the evolution of molecular targeted drug development. J Clin Oncol 2005;23:346–56.
135. Lippman SM, Lee JS, Lotan R, et al. Biomarkers as intermediate endpoints in chemoprevention trials. J Natl Cancer Inst 1990;82:555–60.
136. Bijman JT, Wagener D, van Rennes H, et al. Flow cytometric evaluation of cell dispersion from human head and neck tumors. Cytometry 1985;6:334–41.
137. Doseva D, Christov K, Kristeva K. DNA content in reactive hyperplasia, precancerosis, and carcinomas of the oral cavity. Acta Histochem 1984;75:113–9.
138. Lee JS, Kim SY, Hong WK, et al. Detection of chromosomal polysomy in oral leukoplakia, a premalignant lesion. J Natl Cancer Inst 1993;85:1951–4.
139. Roa RA, Carey TE, Passamani PP, et al. DNA content of human squamous cell carcinoma cell lines. Analysis by flow cytometry and chromosome enumeration. Arch Otolaryngol 1985;111:565–75.
140. Lester EP, Tharapel SA. Chromosome abnormalities in squamous carcinoma cell lines of head and neck origin. Presented at Third International Head and Neck Oncology Research Conference. Las Vegas; 1990.
141. Voravud N, Shin DM, Ro JY, et al. Increased polysomies of chromosomes 7 and 17 during head neck multistage tumorigenesis. Cancer Res 1993;53:2874–83.
142. Wennerberg J, Heim S, Jin Y, et al. Rearrangements involving chromosome bands 1p22 and 11q13 in squamous cell carcinomas of the head and neck. Presented at Third International Head and Neck Oncology Research Conference. Las Vegas; 1990.
143. Lippman SM, Shin DM, Lee JJ, et al. p53 and retinoid chemoprevention of oral carcinogenesis. Cancer Res 1995;55:16–9.
144. Lippman SM, Hong WK. Chemotherapy and chemoprevention. In: Myers E, Suen JY, editors. Cancer of the head and neck. 3rd ed. Philadelphia: W.B. Saunders; 1995. p. 782–804.
145. Berenson JR, Yang J, Koga H, et al. bcl-1 and Int-2 coamplification in squamous cell carcinomas of the head and neck and lung [abstract 1749]. Proc Am Assoc Cancer Res 1989;30:440.
146. Field JK, Spandidos DA, Stell PM, et al. Elevated expression of the c-myc oncoprotein correlates with poor prognosis in head and neck squamous cell carcinoma. Oncogene 1989;4:1463–8.
147. Gallick GE, Sacks PG, Maxwell SA, et al. Head and neck squamous cell carcinoma cell lines as a model system for the study of oncogene expression during tumor progression and metastasis. Prog Clin Biol Res 1986;212:97–111.
148. Saranath D, Panchal RG, Nair R, et al. Oncogene amplification in squamous cell carcinoma of the oral cavity. Jpn J Cancer Res 1989;80:430–7.
149. Spandidos PA, Lamothe A, Field JK. Multiple transcriptional activation of cellular oncogenes in human head and neck solid tumors. Anticancer Res 1985;5:221–4.
150. Somers KD, Cartwright SL, Schechter GL. Coamplification of int-2 and HST-1 genes in squamous cell carcinoma of the head and neck. Presented at Third International Head and Neck Oncology Research Conference. Las Vegas; 1990.
151. Tsuda T, Tahara E, Kajiyama G, et al. High incidence of coamplification of hst-1 and int-2 genes in human esophageal carcinomas. Cancer Res 1989;49:5505–8.
152. Conti CJ. Markers of keratinocyte differentiation in preneoplastic and neoplastic lesions. In: Russo J, editor. Immunocytochemistry in tumor diagnosis. Proceedings of the Workshop on Immunocytochemistry in Tumor Diagnosis; Detroit (MI). Boston: Martinus Nijhoff; 1984. p. 59–71.
153. Nagle RB, Moll R, Weidauer H, et al. Different patterns of cytokeratin expression in the normal epithelia of the upper respiratory tract. Differentiation 1985;30:130–40.
154. Xu X-C, Lee JS, Lippman SM, et al. Increased expression of cytokeratins CK8 and CK19 is associated with head and neck carcinogenesis. Cancer Epidemiol Biomarkers Prev 1995;4:871–6.
155. Carey TE, Wolf GT, Hsu S, et al. Expression of A9 antigen and loss of blood group antigens as determinants of survival in patients with head and neck squamous carcinoma. Otolaryngol Head Neck Surg 1987;91:221–30.
156. Dabelsteen E, Vedtofte P, Hakomori S, Young WW Jr. Accumulation of a blood group antigen precursor in oral premalignant lesions. Cancer Res 1983;43:1451–4.
157. Lonardo F, Sakr W. Preneoplastic lesions of the upper aerodigestive tract. In: Enley JF, Gutkind JS, Jacobs JR, Lippman SM, editors. Head and neck cancer: emerging perspectives. Elsevier Science, San Diego, CA; 2003. p. 35–53.
158. Coltrera MD, Zarbo RJ, Gown AM, et al. Comparison of two putative markers of premalignant change in the oral cavity: suprabasal expression of CK-19 and proliferating cell nuclear antigen (PCNA). Proceedings of the Third International Head and Neck Oncology Research Conference, Las Vegas; 1990.
159. Shin DM, Voravud N, Ro JY, et al. Sequential increases in proliferating cell nuclear antigen expression in head and neck tumorigenesis: a potential biomarker. J Natl Cancer Inst 1993;85:971–8.
160. Eisbruch A, Blick M, Lee JS, et al. Analysis of the epidermal growth factor receptor gene in fresh human head and neck tumors. Cancer Res 1987;47:3603–5.
161. Wong DT. Amplification of the c-erb B1 oncogene in chemically-induced oral carcinomas. Carcinogenesis 1987;8:1963–5.
162. Grandis JR, Tweardy DJ. Elevated levels of transforming growth factor alpha and epidermal growth factor receptor messenger RNA are early markers of carcinogenesis in head and neck cancer. Cancer Res 1993;53:3579–84.
163. Todd R, Donoff BR, Gertz R, et al. TGF-alpha and EGF-receptor mRNAS in human oral cancer. Carcinogenesis 1989;10:1553–6.
164. Brachman DG, Graves D, Vokes E, et al. Occurrence of p53 gene deletions and human papilloma virus infection in human head and neck cancer. Cancer Res 1992;52:4832–6.
165. Sozzi G, Miozzo M, Donghi R, et al. Deletions of 17p and p53 mutations in preneoplastic lesions of the lung. Cancer Res 1992;52:6079–82.
166. Boyle JO, Hakin J, Koch W, et al. The incidence of p53 mutations increases with progression of head and neck cancer. Cancer Res 1993;53:4477–80.
167. Katz AE. Immunobiologic staging of patients with carcinoma of the head and neck. Laryngoscope 1983;93:445–63.
168. Schantz SP, Guillamondegui OM. Developing perspectives in head and neck tumor immunology. Prob Gen Surg 1988;5:99.
169. Heo DS, Whiteside TL, Johnson JT, et al. Long term interleukin 2 dependent growth and cytotoxic activity of tumor-infiltrating lymphocytes from human squamous cell carcinomas of the head and neck. Cancer Res 1987;47:6353–62.
170. Wolf GT, Hudson JL, Peterson KA, et al. Lymphocyte subpopulation infiltrating squamous carcinomas of the head and neck: correlations with extent of tumor and prognosis. Otolaryngol Head Neck Surg 1986;95:142–52.
171. Strome M, Clark J, Fried M, et al. Prognostic implications of defining natural killer cell function and T-cell sub-sets in patients with squamous cell carcinoma. In: Fee W, Goepfert W, Johns ME, et al, editors. Head and neck. Philadelphia: Marcel Dekker; 1990. p. 89–93.
172. Mukhopadhyaya R, Rao RS, Fakih AR, Gangal SG. Detection of circulating immune complexes in patients with squamous cell carcinoma of the oral cavity. J Clin Lab Immunol 1986;21:189–93.
173. Clayman GL, El-Naggar AK, Roth JA, et al. In vivo therapy with p53 adenovirus for microscopic residual head and neck squamous carcinoma. Cancer Res 1995;55:1–6.
174. Liu TJ, El-Naggar AK, McDonnell TJ, et al. Apoptosis induction mediated by wild-type p53 adenovirus gene

transfer in squamous cell carcinoma of the head and neck. Cancer Res 1995;55:3117–22.
175. Henke M, Laszig R, Rube C, et al. Erythropoietin to treat head and neck cancer patients with anaemia undergoing radiotherapy: radnomized, double-blind, placebo-controlled trial. Lancet 2003;362:1255–60.
176. Crile G. Excision of cancer of the head and neck. JAMA 1906;258:1780–4.
177. Batsakis JG. Tumors of the head and neck: clinical and pathological considerations. 2nd ed. Baltimore: Williams & Wilkins; 1974.
178. Bataini P, Brugere J, Bernier J, et al. Results of radical radiotherapeutic treatment of carcinoma of the pyriform sinus: experience of the Institute Curie. Int J Radiat Oncol Biol Phys 1982;8:1277–86.
179. El Badawi SA, Goepfert H, Fletcher GH, et al. Squamous cell carcinoma of the pyriform sinus. Laryngoscope 1982;92:357–64.
180. Foote RL, Buskirk SJ, Stanley RJ, et al. Patterns of failure after total laryngectomy for glottic carcinoma. Cancer 1989;64:143–9.
181. Probert JC, Thompson RW, Bagshaw MA. Patterns of spread of distant metastases in head and neck cancer. Cancer 1974;33:127–33.
182. Schechter GL, Kalafsky JT. Cancer of the hypopharynx and cervical esophagus: management concepts. Oncology 1988;2:17–24, 34–5.
183. Van den Brouck C, Eschwege F, De La Rochefordiere A, et al. Squamous cell carcinoma of the pyriform sinus: retrospective study of 351 cases treated at the Institute Gustave-Roussy. Head Neck Surg 1987;10:4–13.
184. Robbins KT, editor. Neck dissection and classification and TNM staging of head and neck cancer. 2nd ed. 2001. p. 9.
185. Lippman SM, Hong WK. Molecular markers of the risk of oral cancer. N Engl J Med 2001;344:1323–6.
186. Lippman SM, Gibson N, Subbaramaiah K, Dannenberg AJ. Combined targeting of the EGFR and COX-2 pathways. Clin Cancer Res 2005;11:6097–9.
187. Zhang L, Poh CF, Lam WL, et al. Impact of localized treatment in reducing risk of progression of low-grade oral dysplasia: molecular evidence of incomplete resection. Oral Oncol 2001;37:505–12.
188. Guo Z, Yamaguchi K, Sanchez-Cespedes M, et al. Allelic losses in OraTest-directed biopsies of patients with prior upper aerodigestive tract malignancy. Clin Cancer Res 2001;7:1963–8.
189. Epstein JB, Zhang L, Poh C, et al. Increased allelic loss in toluidine blue-positive oral premalignant lesions. Oral Surg Oral Med Oral Pathol Oral Radiol Endod 2003;95:45–50.
190. Johnson JT, Myers EN, Bedetti CD, et al. Cervical lymph node metastases. Incidence and implications of extracapsular carcinoma. Arch Otolaryngol 1985;111:534–7.
191. Baker SR, Sullivan MJ. Osteocutaneous free scapular flap for one-stage mandibular reconstruction. Arch Otolaryngol 1988;114:267–77.
192. Lee JG, Krause CJ. Radical neck dissection: elective, therapeutic and secondary. Arch Otolaryngol 1975;101:656–9.
193. Kalnins IK, Leonard AG, Sako K, et al. Correlation between prognosis and degree of lymph node involvement in carcinoma of the oral cavity. Am J Surg 1977;134:450–4.
194. Volterrani F, Chiesa F, Molinari R. Argument in favor of precautional treatment of cervical nodes in clinically NO oral cancer. Tumori 1982;68:241–5.
195. Martin H, MacComb WS, Blady JV. Cancer of the lip. Ann Surg 1941;114:226–35.
196. Bailey BJ. Management of carcinoma of the lip. Laryngoscope 1977;87:250–60.
197. Ward GE, Hendrick JW. Results of treatment of carcinoma of the lip. Surgery 1950;27:321.
198. Jesse RH. Extensive cancer of the lip. Surgical therapy. Arch Surg 1967;94:509–16.
199. Schmidseder R, Dick H. Spread of epidermoid carcinoma of the lip along the inferior alveolar nerve. Oral Surg Oral Med Oral Pathol 1977;43:517–20.
200. Mehregan DA, Roenigk RK. Management of superficial squamous cell carcinoma of the lip with Mohs micrographic surgery. Cancer 1990;66:463–8.
201. Wilson JS, Walker EP. Reconstruction of the lower lip. Head Neck Surg 1981;4:29–44.
202. Jorgensen K, Elbrond O, Anderson AP. Carcinoma of the lip. A series of 869 cases. Acta Radiol Ther Phys Biol 1973;12:177–90.
203. Mackay EN, Sellers AH. A statistical review of carcinoma of the lip. Can Med Assoc J 1964;90:670–9.
204. Pigneux J, Richaud PM, Lagarde C. The place of interstitial therapy using 192 indium in the management of carcinoma of the lip. Cancer 1979;43:1073–7.
205. Baker SR, Krause CJ. Carcinoma of the lip. Laryngoscope 1980;90:19–27.
206. Cross JE. Carcinoma of the lip: a review of 563 case records of carcinoma of the lip at the Pondville Hospital. Surg Gynecol Obstet 1948;87:153–68.
207. Molnar L, Ronay P, Tapolcsanyi L. Carcinoma of the lip: analysis of the material of 25 years. Oncology 1974;29:101–21.
208. Schreiner BF, Christy CJ. Results of irradiation treatment of cancer of the lip: analysis of 636 cases from 1926–1936. Radiol 1942;39:293–307.
209. Decroix Y, Ghossein NA. Experience of the Curie Institute in treatment of cancer of the mobile tongue: I. Treatment policies and results. Cancer 1981;47:496–502.
210. DiTroia JF. Nodal metastases and prognosis in carcinoma of the oral cavity. Otolaryngol Clin North Am 1972;5:333–42.
211. Fakih AR, Rao RS, Borges AM, Patel AR. Elective versus therapeutic neck dissection in early carcinoma of the oral tongue. Am J Surg 1989;158:309–13.
212. Spiro RH, Alfonso AE, Farr HW, Strong EW. Cervical node metastases from epidermoid carcinoma of the oral cavity and oropharynx. A critical assessment of current staging. Am J Surg 1974;128:562–7.
213. Spiro RH. Squamous cancer of the tongue. CA Cancer J Clin 1985;35:252–6.
214. Callery CD, Spiro RH, Strong EW. Changing trends in the management of squamous carcinoma of the tongue. Am J Surg 1984;148:449–54.
215. Vermund H, Brennhovd I, Kaalhus O, Poppe E. Incidence and control of occult neck node metastases from squamous cell carcinoma of the anterior two-thirds of the tongue. Int J Radiol Oncol Biol Phys 1984;10:2025–36.
216. Wallner PE, Hanks GE, Kramer S, McLean CJ. Patterns of care study: analysis of outcome survey data-anterior two thirds of tongue and floor of mouth. Am J Clin Oncol 1986;9:50–7.
217. Fletcher GH, Jesse RH. The contribution of supervoltage roentgen therapy to the integration of radiation and surgery in head and neck squamous cell carcinoma. Cancer 1962;15:566.
218. Leipzig B, Cummings CW, Chung CT, et al. Carcinoma of the anterior tongue. Ann Otol Rhinol Laryngol 1982;91:94–7.
219. Leonard JR, Litton WB, Latourette HB, McCube BF. Combined radiation and surgical therapy: tongue, tonsil and floor of mouth. Ann Otol Rhinol Laryngol 1968;77:514–33.
220. Vikram B, Strong EW, Shah JP, Spiro R. Failure at the primary site following multimodality treatment in advanced head and neck cancer. Head Neck Surg 1984;6:720–3.
221. Biller HF, Lawson W, Baek SM. Total glossectomy. A technique of reconstruction eliminating laryngectomy. Arch Otolaryngol 1983;109:69–73.
222. Bamberg M, Schulz U, Scherer E. Postoperative split course radiotherapy of squamous cell carcinoma of the oral tongue. Int J Radiat Oncol Biol Phys 1979;5:515–9.
223. Kramer S. Methotrexate and radiation therapy in the treatment of advanced squamous cell carcinoma of the oral cavity, oropharynx, supraglottic larynx, and hypopharynx: (preliminary report of a controlled clinical trial of the Radiation Therapy Oncology Group). Can J Otolaryngol 1975;4:213–8.
224. Kramer S, Gleber RD, Snow JB, et al. Combined radiation therapy and surgery in the management of advanced head and neck cancer: final report of the study 73-03 of the Radiation Therapy Oncology Group. Head Neck Surg 1987;10:19–30.
225. Wolf GT, Makuch RW, Baker SR. Predictive factors for tumor response to preoperative chemotherapy in patients with squamous carcinoma. The Head and Neck Contracts Group. Cancer 1984;54:2869–77.
226. Mendenhall WM, VanCise WS, Bova FJ, Million RR. Analysis of time-dose factors in squamous cell carcinoma of the oral tongue and floor of mouth treated with radiation therapy alone. Int J Radiol Oncol Biol Phys 1981;7:1005–11.
227. Panje WR, Smith B, McCabe BF. Epidermoid carcinomas of the floor of mouth. Surgical therapy vs combined therapy vs radiation therapy. Otolaryngol Head Neck Surg 1980;88:714–20.
228. Shaha A, Spiro R, Shah J, Strong EW. Squamous carcinomas of the floor of mouth. Am J Surg 1984;148:455–9.
229. Fu KK, Lichter A, Galante M. Carcinoma of the floor of mouth: an analysis of treatment results and the sites and causes and failures. Int J Radiol Oncol Biol Phys 1976;1:829–37.
230. Cady B, Catlin D. Epidermoid carcinoma of the gum. Cancer 1969;23:551–69.
231. Bloom ND, Spiro RH. Carcinoma of the cheek mucosa: a retrospective analysis. Am J Surg 1980;140:556–9.
232. Diaz EM, Sorensen, D, Holsinger FC. Squamous cell carcinoma of the buccal mucosa. Head Neck Surge 2002.
233. Byers RM, Newman R, Russell N, Yue A. Results of treatment of squamous carcinoma of the lower gum. Cancer 1981;47:2236–8.
234. MacComb WS, Fletcher GH. Cancer of the head and neck. Baltimore: Williams & Wilkins; 1967.
235. Petrovich Z, Kuisk H, Jose L, et al. Advanced carcinoma of the tonsil. Treatment results. Acta Radiol Oncol 1980;19:425–31.
236. Remmier D, Medina JE, Byers RM, et al. Treatment of choice for squamous carcinoma of the tonsillar fossa. Head Neck Surg 1985;7:206–11.
237. Chung TS, Stefani S. Distant metastases of carcinoma of tonsillar region: a study of 475 patients. J Surg Oncol 1980;14:5–9.
238. Garrett PG, Beale FA, Cummins BJ, et al. Cancer of the tonsil: results of radical radiation therapy with surgery in reserve. Am J Surg 1983;146:432–5.
239. Terz JJ, Farr HW. Carcinoma of the tonsillar fossa. Surg Gynecol Obstet 1967;125:581–90.
240. Riley RW, Fee WE Jr, Goffinet D, et al. Squamous cell carcinoma of the base of the tongue. Otolaryngol Head Neck Surg 1983;91:143–50.
241. Weber RS, Gidley P, Morrison WH, et al. Treatment selection for carcinoma of the base of the tongue. Am J Surg 1990;160:415–9.
242. Barrs DM, DeSanto LW, O'Fallon WM. Squamous cell carcinoma at the tonsil and tongue-base regions. Arch Otolaryngol 1979;105:479–85.
243. Wawro NW, Babcock A, Ellison L. Cancer of the tongue: experience at the Hartford Hospital from 1931–1963. Am J Surg 1970;119:455–61.
244. Bataini P, Bernier J, Jaulerry C, et al. Impact of cervical disease and its definitive radiotherapeutic management on survival: experience in 2013 patients with squamous cell carcinoma of the oropharynx and pharyngolarynx. Laryngoscope 1990;100:716–23.
245. Rollo J, Rozenbom CV, Thawley S, et al. Squamous carcinoma of the base of the tongue: a clinicopathologic study of 81 cases. Cancer 1981;47:333–42.
246. Gardner KE, Parsons JT, Mendenhall WM, et al. Time dose relationships for local tumor control and complications following irradiation of squamous cell carcinoma of the base of tongue. Int J Radiol Oncol Biol Phys 1987;13:507–10.
247. Hintz BL, Kagan R, Wollin M, et al. Treatment selection for base of tongue carcinoma. J Surg Oncol 1989;41:165–71.
248. Goffinet DR, Fee WE, Wells J, et al. 192Ir pharyngoepiglottic fold interstitial implants: the key to successful treatment of base of tongue carcinoma by radiation therapy. Cancer 1985;55:941–8.
249. Medenhall WM, Stringer SP, Moore-Higgs GJ, Cassisi NJ. Is radiation a preferred alternative to surgery for squamous cell carcinoma of the base of tongue? J Clin Oncol. [In press]
250. Calais G, Alfonsi M, Bardet E, et al. Radiation alone (RT) versus RT with concomitant chemotherapy (CT) in stages III and IV oropharynx. Results of the 94.01 randomized study from the French Group of the Radiation Oncology for head and neck cancer (GORTEC). Int J Radiat Oncol Biol Phys. [In press]
251. Fletcher GH. Squamous cell carcinomas of the oropharynx. Int J Radiol Oncol Biol Phys 1979;5:2073.
252. Lindberg RD, Barkley HT, Jesse RH, Fletcher GH. Evolution of the clinically negative neck in patients with squamous cell carcinoma of the faucial arch. Am J Roentgenol Radium Ther Nucl Med 1971;111:60–5.
253. Weber RS, Peters LJ, Wolf PS, Guillamondegui O. Squamous cell carcinoma of the soft palate, uvula and anterior faucial pillar. Otolaryngol Head Neck Surg 1988;99:16–23.
254. Million RR, Cassisi NJ. Radical irradiation for carcinoma of the pyriform sinus. Laryngoscope 1981;91:439–50.
255. Pingree TF, Davis RK, Reichman O, Derrick L. Treatment of hypopharyngeal carcinoma: a 10 year review of 1362 cases. Laryngoscope 1987;97:901–4.
256. Carpenter RJ, DeSanto LW, Devine KD, Taylor WF. Cancer of the hypopharynx: analysis of treatment and results in 162 patients. Arch Otolaryngol 1976;102:716–21.
257. Eisbach KJ, Krause CJ. Carcinoma of the pyriform sinus: a comparison of treatment modalities. Laryngoscope 1977;87:1904–10.
258. Martin SA, Marks JE, Lee JY, et al. Carcinoma of the pyriform sinus: predictors of TNM relapse and survival. Cancer 1980;46:1974–81.

259. Lefebvre JL, Chevalier D, Luboinski B, et al. Larynx preservation in pyriform sinus cancer: preliminary results of an EORTC phase III trial. J Natl Cancer Inst 1996;88:890–9.
260. Dubois JB, Guerrier B, DiRuggiero JM, Pourquier H. Cancer of the pyriform sinus: treatment by radiation therapy alone and with surgery. Radiology 1986;160:831–6.
261. Razack MS, Sako K, Marchetta FC, et al. Carcinoma of the hypopharynx: success and failure. Am J Surg 1977;134:489–91.
262. Raine CH, Stell PM, Dalby J. Squamous cell carcinoma of the posterior wall of the hypopharynx. J Laryngol Otol 1982;96:997–1004.
263. Spiro RH, Kelly J, Vega AL, et al. Squamous carcinoma of the posterior pharyngeal wall. Am J Surg 1990;160:420–3.
264. Ballantyne AJ. Methods of repair after surgery for cancer of the pharyngeal wall, postcricoid area and cervical esophagus. Am J Surg 1971;122:482–6.
265. Harrison DFN. Surgical management of hypopharyngeal cancer. Arch Otolaryngol Head Neck Surg 1979;105:149–52.
266. Hester TR, McConnel FM, Nahal F, et al. Reconstruction of the cervical esophagus, hypopharynx and oral cavity using free jejunal transfer. Am J Surg 1980;140:487–91.
267. Schechter GL, Baker JW, El-Mahdi AM, Bumata JT. Combined treatment of advanced cancer of the laryngopharynx and cervical esophagus. Laryngoscope 1982;92:11–5.
268. Yates A, Crumley RL. Surgical treatment of pyriform sinus cancer: a retrospective study. Laryngoscope 1984;94:1586–90.
269. Bryce D. The conventional surgical management of carcinoma of the hypopharynx. J Laryngol Otol 1971;85:1221–6.
270. Dalley VM. Cancer of the laryngopharynx. J Laryngol Otol 1968;82:407–19.
271. Wang CC. Radiotherapeutic management of carcinoma of the posterior pharyngeal wall. Cancer 1971;27:894–6.
272. Jacobs C. Adjuvant chemotherapy for head and neck cancer. J Clin Oncol 1989;7:823–6.
273. Jacobs JR, Sessions DG, Ogura JH. Recurrent carcinoma of the larynx and the hypopharynx. Otolaryngol Head Neck Surg 1980;88:425–33.
274. Mirimanoff RO, Wang CC, Doppke KP. Combined surgery and postoperative radiotherapy for advanced laryngeal and hypopharyngeal tumors. Int J Radiat Oncol Biol Phys 1985;11:499–504.
275. McNeil BJ, Weichselbaum R, Parker SG. Speech and survival: tradeoffs between quality and quantity of life in laryngeal cancer. N Engl J Med 1981;305:982–7.
276. Freeland AP, Van Nostrand AW, Jahn AF. Metastasis to the larynx. J Otolaryngol 1979;8:448–56.
277. Kirchner JA, Cornog JL, Holmes RE. Transglottic cancer. Its growth and spread within the larynx. Arch Otolaryngol 1974;99:247–51.
278. Pressman JJ, Dowdy A, Libby M. Further studies upon the submucosal compartments and lymphatics of the larynx by the injection of dye and radioisotopes. Ann Otol Rhinol Laryngol 1956;65:963–80.
279. Welsh LW, Welsh JJ, Rizzo TA Jr. Laryngeal spaces and lymphatics: current anatomic concepts. Ann Otol Rhinol Laryngol Suppl 1983;105:19–31.
280. Kirchner JA. Two hundred laryngeal cancers: patterns of growth and spread as seen in serial sections. Laryngoscope 1977;87:474–82.
281. Laccourreye H, Brasnu DF, Beutter P. Carcinoma of the laryngeal margin. Head Neck Surg 1983;5:500–7.
282. DeSanto LW. The options in early laryngeal carcinoma. N Engl J Med 1982;306:910–2.
283. Pillsbury HR, Kirchner JA. Clinical vs histopathologic staging in laryngeal cancer. Arch Otolaryngol 1979;105:157–9.
284. DeSanto LW. Cancer of the supraglottic larynx: a review of 260 patients. Otolaryngol Head Neck Surg 1985;93:705–11.
285. DeSanto LW, Lillie JC, Devine KD. Cancer of the larynx: supraglottic cancer. Surg Clin North Am 1977;57:505–14.
286. Marks JE, Breaux S, Smith PG, et al. The need for elective irradiation of occult lymphatic metastases from cancer of the larynx and piriform sinus. Head Neck Surg 1985;8:3–8.
287. Fletcher GH, Lindberg RD, Hamberger A, Horiot JC. Reasons for irradiation failure in squamous cell carcinoma of the larynx. Laryngoscope 1975;85:987–1003.
288. Vikram B, Bosl GJ, Pfister D, et al. New strategies for avoiding total laryngectomy in patients with head and neck cancer. Natl Cancer Inst Monogr 1988;6:361–4.
289. Hillman RE, Walsh MJ, Wolf GT, et al. Functional outcomes following treatment for advanced laryngeal cancer. Part I—Voice preservation in advanced laryngeal cancer. Part II—Laryngectomy rehabilitation: the state of the art in the VA System. Ann Otol Rhinol Laryngol Suppl 1998;172:1–27.
290. Sisson GA, Bytell DE, Edison BD, Yeh S. Transsternal radical neck dissection for control of stomal recurrences—end results. Laryngoscope 1975;85:1504–10.
291. Schneider JJ, Lindberg RD, Jesse RH. Prevention of tracheal stoma recurrences after total laryngectomy by postoperative irradiation. J Surg Oncol 1975;7:187–90.
292. Fu KK, Woodhouse RJ, Quivey JM, et al. The significance of laryngeal edema following radiotherapy of carcinoma of the vocal cord. Cancer 1982;49:655–8.
293. Wang CC. Megavoltage radiation therapy for supraglottic carcinoma: results of treatment. Radiology 1973;109:183–6.
294. Ward PH, Calcaterra TC, Kagan AR. The regimen of postradiation edema and recurrent or residual carcinoma of the larynx. Laryngoscope 1975;85:522–9.
295. Bocca E, Pignataro O, Oldini C. Supraglottic laryngectomy: 30 years of experience. Ann Otol Rhinol Laryngol 1983;92:14–8.
296. Lee NK, Goepfert H, Wendt CD. Supraglottic laryngectomy for intermediate-stage cancer: U.T. M.D. Anderson Cancer Center experience with combined therapy. Laryngoscope 1990;100:831–6.
297. Maceri DR, Laupe HB, Makielski KH, et al. Conservation laryngeal surgery. A critical analysis. Arch Otolaryngol 1985;111:361–5.
298. Bocca E. Supraglottic cancer. Laryngoscope 1975;85:1318–26.
299. Bryce DP. The management of laryngeal cancer. J Otolaryngol 1979;8:105–26.
300. DeSanto LW, Lillie JC, Devine KD. Surgical salvage after radiation for laryngeal cancer. Laryngoscope 1976;87:649–57.
301. Coates HL, DeSanto LW, Devine KD, Elveback LR. Carcinoma of the supraglottic larynx. A review of 221 cases. Arch Otolaryngol 1976;102:686–9.
302. Kirchner JA, Som ML. Clinical and histologic observation on supraglottic cancer. Ann Otol Rhinol Laryngol 1971;80:638.
303. Levendag P, Sessions R, Vikran B, et al. The problem of neck relapse in early stage supraglottic larynx cancer. Cancer 1989;63:345–8.
304. Goepfert H, Jesse RH, Fletcher GH, Hamberger A. Optimal treatment for technically resectable squamous cell carcinoma of the supraglottic larynx. Laryngoscope 1975;85:14–32.
305. Harwood AR, Beale FA, Cummings BJ, et al. Supraglottic laryngeal carcinoma: an analysis of dose-time-volume factors in 410 patients. Int J Radiat Oncol Biol Phys 1983;9:311–9.
306. Vermund H. Role of radiotherapy in cancer of the larynx as related to the TNM system of staging. Cancer 1970;25:485–504.
307. Wang CC. Radiation therapy for head and neck neoplasms: indications, techniques and results. Boston: John Wright; 1983.
308. Issa PY. Cancer of the supraglottic larynx treated by radiotherapy exclusively. Int J Radiat Oncol Biol Phys 1985;15:843–50.
309. Mendenhall WM, Parsons JT, Stringer SP, et al. Carcinoma of the supraglottic larynx: a basis for comparing the results of radiotherapy and surgery. Head Neck 1990;12:204–9.
310. Spaulding CA, Krochak RJ, Hahn SS, Constable WC. Radiotherapeutic management of cancer of the supraglottis. Cancer 1986;57:1292–8.
311. Lutz CK, Johnson JT, Wagner RL, Myer EN. Supraglottic carcinoma patterns of recurrence. Ann Otol Rhinol Laryngol 1990;99:12–7.
312. Snow JB, Gelber RD, Kramer S, et al. Comparison of preoperative and postoperative radiation therapy for patients with carcinoma of the head and neck. Interim report. Acta Otolaryngol 1981;91:611–26.
313. Fu KK, Eisenberg L, Dedo HH, Phillips TL. Results of integrated management of supraglottic carcinoma. Cancer 1977;40:2874–81.
314. Soo KC, Shah JP, Gopinath KS, et al. Analysis of prognostic variables and results after supraglottic partial laryngectomy. Am J Surg 1988;156:301–5.
315. Marks JE, Freeman RB, Lee F, Ogua JH. Carcinoma of the supraglottic larynx. AJR Am J Roentgenol 1979;132:255–60.
316. Ghossein NA, Bataini JP, Ennuyen A, et al. Local control and site of failure in radically irradiated supraglottic laryngeal cancer. Radiology 1974;112:187–92.
317. Lustig RA, DeMare PA, Kramer S. Adjuvant methotrexate in the radio-therapeutic management of advanced tumors of the head and neck. Cancer 1976;37:2703–8.
318. Van den Bogaert W, Ostyn F, Van der Schueren E. The differential clinical presentation, behaviour and prognosis of carcinomas originating in the epilarynx and the lower supraglottic. Radiother Oncol 1983;1:117–31.
319. Harwood AR, Hawkins NV, Rider WD, Bryce DP. Radiation therapy of early glottic cancer—I. Int J Radiat Oncol Biol Phys 1979;5:473–6.
320. Karim ABMF, Snow GB, Hasman A, et al. Dose response in radiotherapy for glottic carcinoma. Cancer 1978;41:1728–32.
321. Karim AB, Snow GB, Siek HT, Njo KH. The quality of voice in patient irradiated for laryngeal carcinoma. Cancer 1983;51:47–9.
322. Nass JM, Brady LW, Glassburn JR, et al. Radiation therapy of glottic carcinoma. Int J Radiat Oncol Biol Phys 1976;1:867–72.
323. Harwood AR, Hawkins NV, Keane T, et al. Radiotherapy in early glottic cancer. Laryngoscope 1980;90:465–70.
324. Mittal B, Marks JE, Ogura JH. Transglottic carcinoma. Cancer 1984;53:151–61.
325. Harwood AR, DeBoer G. Prognostic factors in T2 glottic cancer. Cancer 1980;45:991–5.
326. Kaplan MJ, Johns ME, Clark DA, Cantrell RW. Glottic carcinoma: the role of surgery and irradiation. Cancer 1984;53:2641–8.
327. Kelly MD, Hahn SS, Spaulding CA, et al. Definitive radiotherapy in the management of stage I and II carcinomas of the glottis. Laryngoscope 1989;98:235–9.
328. Van den Bogaert W, Ostyn F, Van der Schueren E. The significance of extension and impaired mobility in cancer of the vocal cord. Int J Radiat Oncol Biol Phys 1983;9:181–4.
329. Biller HF, Lawson W. Partial laryngectomy for vocal cord cancer with marked limitations or fixation of the vocal cord. Laryngoscope 1986;96:61–4.
330. Pearson BW, Woods RD II, Hartman DE. Extended hemilaryngectomy of T3 glottic carcinoma with preservation of speech and swallowing. Laryngoscope 1980;90:1950–61.
331. Harwood AR, DeBoer D, Kaxim F. Prognostic factors in T3 glottic cancer. Cancer 1981:47;367–72.
332. DeSanto LW. T3 glottic cancer: options and consequences of the options. Laryngoscope 1984;94:1311–5.
333. Leroux RJ. A statistical study of 620 laryngeal carcinomas of the glottic region personally operated upon more than 5 years ago. Laryngoscope 1985;85:1440–52.
334. Yuen A, Medina JE, Goepfert H, Fletcher G. Management of stage T3 and T4 glottic carcinoma. Am J Surg 1984;148:467–72.
335. Croll GA, Gerritsen GJ, Tiwari RM, Snow GB. Primary radiotherapy with surgery in reserve for advanced laryngeal carcinoma: results and complications. Eur J Surg Oncol 1989;15:350–6.
336. Skolnick EM, Yee KF, Wheatley MA, Martin LO. Carcinoma of the laryngeal glottis therapy and end results. Laryngoscope 1975;85:1453–66.
337. Harwood AR, Bryce DP, Rider WD. Management of T3 glottic cancer. Arch Otolaryngol 1980;106:697–9.
338. Laramore GE. T3NOMO glottic cancer: are more treatment modalities necessarily better? Int J Radiat Oncol Biol Phys 1995;31:423–5.
339. Kazem I, van den Broek P. Planned preoperative radiation therapy vs definitive radiotherapy for advanced laryngeal carcinoma. Laryngoscope 1984;94:1355–8.
340. McGovern MH, Bauer WC, Ogura JH. The incidence of cervical lymph node metastases from epidermoid carcinoma of the larynx and their relationship to certain characteristics of the primary tumor. Cancer 1961;14:55–66.
341. Shaha AR, Shah JP. Carcinoma of the subglottic larynx. Am J Surg 1982;144:456–8.
342. Keim WF, Shapiro MJ, Rosin HD. Study of post laryngectomy stomal recurrence. Arch Otolaryngol 1965;81:183–6.
343. Davis RK, Shapshay SM. Peristomal recurrence. Pathophysiology, prevention and treatment. Otolaryngol Clin North Am 1980;13:499–508.
344. Wiernik G, Bates TD, Bleehen MN, et al. Final report of the general clinical result of the British Institute of Radiology fractionation study of the 3F wk versus 5F wk in radiotherapy of carcinoma of the laryngo-pharynx. Br J Radiol 1990;63:169–80.
345. Crissman JD. Laryngeal keratosis and subsequent carcinoma. Head Neck Surg 1979;1:386–91.
346. Gillis TM, Incze J, Strong MS, et al. Natural history and management of keratosis, atypia carcinoma-in situ, and microinvasive cancer of the larynx. Am J Surg 1983;146:512–6.
347. Pene F, Fletcher GH. Results in irradiation of the in situ carcinomas of the vocal cord. Cancer 1976;37:2586–90.
348. Ossoff RH, Shapshay SM, Sisson GA. Endoscopic management of selected early vocal cord carcinoma. Ann Otol Rhinol Laryngol 1985;94:560–4.
349. Wetmore SJ, Key MJ, Suen JY. Laser therapy for T1 glottic carcinoma of the larynx. Arch Otolaryngol Head Neck Surg 1986;112:853–5.

350. Norris CM. Laryngectomy and neck dissection. Otolaryngol Clin North Am 1969;69:667.
351. Laccourreye O, Veivers D, Hans S, et al. Chemotherapy alone with curative intent in patients with invasive squamous carcinoma of the pharyngolarynx classified as T1–T4N0M0 complete clinical responders. Cancer 2001;92:1504–11.
352. Laccourreye O, Bassot V, Brasnu D, Laccourreye H. Chemotherapy combined with conservation surgery in the treatment of early larynx cancer. Curr Opin Oncol 1999;109:698–704.
353. Laccourreye O, Diaz EM, Bassot V, et al. A multimodal strategy for the treatment of patients with T2 invasive squamous cell carcinoma of the glottis. Cancer 1999;85:40–6.
354. Gillenwater AM, Khuri FR, Diaz EM, et al. An alternative approach to larynx preservation in advanced laryngeal cancer using chemotherapy and surgery: preliminary results. Proceedings of the American Head and Neck Society 5th International Conference on Head and Neck Cancer. San Francisco; 2000.
355. Ensley JF, Jacobs JR, Weaver A, et al. Correlation between response to cisplatinum-combination chemotherapy and subsequent radiotherapy in previously untreated patients with advanced squamous cell cancers of the head and neck. Cancer 1984;54:811–4.
356. Kies MS, Gordon LI, Hauck WW, et al. Analysis of complete responders after initial treatment with chemotherapy in head and neck cancer. Otolaryngol Head Neck Surg 1985;93:199–205.
357. Ervin TJ, Clark JR, Weichselbaum RR, et al. An analysis of induction and adjuvant chemotherapy in the multidisciplinary treatment of squamous-cell carcinoma of the head and neck. J Clin Oncol 1987;5:10–20.
358. The Department of Veterans Affairs Laryngeal Cancer Study Group. Induction chemotherapy plus radiation compared with surgery plus radiation in patients with advanced laryngeal cancer. N Engl J Med 1991;324:1685–90.
359. Lefebvre JL, Chevalier D, Luboinski B, et al. Larynx preservation in pyriform sinus cancer: preliminary results of a European Organization for Research and Treatment of Cancer phase III trial. EORTC Head and Neck Cancer Cooperative Group. J Natl Cancer Inst 1996;88:890–9.
360. Forastiere AA, Goepfert H, Maor M, et al. Concurrent chemotherapy and radiotherapy for organ preservation in advanced laryngeal cancer. N Engl J Med 2003;349:2091–8.
361. Weber RS, Berkey BA, Forastiere A, et al. Outcome of salvage total laryngectomy following organ preservation therapy: the Radiation Therapy Oncology Group trial 91-11. Arch Otolaryngol Head Neck Surg 2003;129:44–9.
362. Peters LJ, Batsakis JG, Goepfert H, Hong WK. The diagnosis and management of nasopharyngeal cancer in Caucasians. In: Williams CJ, Krikorian JG, Green MR, Raghavan D, editors. Textbook of uncommon cancer. Chichester, England: Wiley; 1988. p. 975–1006.
363. Chiang TC, Griem ML. Nasopharyngeal cancer. Surg Clin North Am 1973;53:121–33.
364. Laramore GE, Clubb B, Quick C, et al. Nasopharyngeal carcinoma in Saudi Arabia: a retrospective study of 166 cases treated with curative intent. Int J Radiat Oncol Biol Phys 1988;15:1119–27.
365. Griem ML, Chiang DTC. Nasopharynx. In: Laramore GE, editor. Radiation therapy of head and neck cancer. Berlin: Springer-Verlag; 1989.
366. Wang CC, Busse J, Gitterman M. A simple afterloading application for intracavitary irradiation of the nasopharynx. Radiology 1975;115:737–8.
367. Huang SC. Nasopharyngeal cancer. A review of 1605 patients treated radically with cobalt 60. Int J Radiat Oncol Biol Phys 1980;6:401–7.
368. Vikram B, Mishra UB, Strong EW, Manolatos S. Patterns of failure in carcinoma of the nasopharynx: I. Failure at the primary site. Int J Radiat Oncol Biol Phys 1985;11:1455–9.
369. Scanlon PW, Rhodes RE, Woolner LB, et al. Cancer of the nasopharynx. One hundred forty-two patients treated in the 11-year period 1950–1960. AJR Am J Roentgenol 1967;99:313–25.
370. Wang CC. Re-irradiation of recurrent nasopharyngeal carcinoma—treatment techniques and results. Int J Radiat Oncol Biol Phys 1987;13:953–6.
371. Kwong DL, Wei WI, Cheng AC, et al. Long term results of radioactive gold grain implantation for the treatment of persistent and recurrent nasopharyngeal carcinoma. Cancer 2001;91:1105–13.
372. Hong WK, Choksi A, Dimery IW. Sequential induction chemotherapy and radiotherapy for advanced head and neck cancer: potential impact of treatment in advanced laryngeal and nasopharyngeal carcinomas. In: Head and neck cancer: proceedings of the International Conference. Vol. 2. Toronto: Decker; 1989. p. 282–5.
373. Peters LJ, Harrison ML, Dimery IW, et al. Acute and late toxicity associated with sequential bleomycin-containing chemotherapy regimens and radiation therapy in the treatment of carcinoma of the nasopharynx. Int J Radiat Oncol Biol Phys 1988;14:623–33.
374. Bachouchi M, Cvitkovic E, Azli N, et al. High complete response in advanced nasopharyngeal carcinoma with bleomycin, epirubicin, and cisplatin before radiotherapy. J Natl Cancer Inst 1990;82:616–20.
375. Vokes EE, Weichselbaum RR, Lippman SM, et al. Head and neck cancer. N Engl J Med 1993;328:184–94.
376. Boussen H, Cvitkovic E, Wendling JL, et al. Chemotherapy of metastatic and/or recurrent undifferentiated nasopharyngeal carcinoma with cisplatin, bleomycin, and fluorouracil. J Clin Oncol 1991;9:1675–81.
377. Su WC, Chen TY, Kao RH, et al. Chemotherapy with cisplatin and continuous infusion of 5-fluorouracil and bleomycin for recurrent and metastatic nasopharyngeal carcinoma in Taiwan. Oncology 1993;50:205–8.
378. Au E, Ang PT. A phase II trial of 5-fluorouracil and cisplatinum in recurrent or metastatic nasopharyngeal carcinoma. Ann Oncol 1994;5:87–9.
379. Yeo W, Leung TW, Leung SF, et al. Phase II study of the combination of carboplatin and 5-fluorouracil in metastatic nasopharyngeal carcinoma. Cancer Chemother Pharmacol 1996;38:466–70.
380. Fandi A, Bachouchi M, Azli N, et al. Long-term disease-free survivors in metastatic undifferentiated carcinoma of nasopharyngeal type. J Clin Oncol 2000;18:1324–30.
381. Chan ATC, Hsu MM, Goh BC, et al. Multicenter, phase II study of cetuximab in combination with carboplatin in patients with recurrent or metastatic nasopharyngeal carcinoma. J Clin Oncol 2005;23:3568–76.
382. Chan ATC, Teo PM, Leung TW, et al. A prospective randomized study of chemotherapy adjunctive to definitive radiotherapy in advanced nasopharyngeal carcinoma. Int J Radiat Oncol Biol Phys 1995;33:569–77.
383. Al-Sarraf M, LeBlanc M, Giri PG, et al. Chemoradiotherapy versus radiotherapy in patients with advanced nasopharyngeal cancer: phase III randomized Intergroup study 0099. J Clin Oncol 1998;16:1310–7.
384. Chan ATC, Teo PM, Ngan RK, et al. Concurrent chemotherapy-radiotherapy compared with radiotherapy alone in locoregionally advanced nasopharyngeal carcinoma: progression-free survival analysis of a phase III randomized trial. J Clin Oncol 2002;20:2038–44.
385. Chan ATC, Leung SF, Ngan RK, et al. Overall survival after concurrent cisplatin-radiotherapy compared with radiotherapy alone in locoregionally advanced nasopharyngeal carcinoma. J Natl Cancer Inst 2005;97:536–9.
386. Lin JC, Jan JS, Hsu CY, et al. Phase III study of concurrent chemoradiotherapy versus radiotherapy alone for advanced nasopharyngeal carcinoma: positive effect on overall and progression-free survival. J Clin Oncol 2003;21:631–7.
387. Chua DT, Ma J, Sham JS, et al. Long-term survival after cisplatin-based induction chemotherapy and radiotherapy for nasopharyngeal carcinoma: a pooled data analysis of two phase III trials. J Clin Oncol 2005;23:1118–24.
388. Sheen TS, Huang YT, Chang YL, et al. Epstein-Barr virus-encoded latent membrane protein 1 co-expresses with epidermal growth factor receptor in nasopharyngeal carcinoma. Jpn J Cancer Res 1999;90:1285–92.
389. Leong JL, Loh KS, Putti TC, et al. Epidermal growth factor receptor in undifferentiated carcinoma of the nasopharynx. Laryngoscope 2004;114:153–7.
390. Chua DT, Nicholls JM, Sham JS, et al. Prognostic value of epidermal growth factor receptor expression in patients with advanced stage nasopharyngeal carcinoma treated with induction chemotherapy and radiotherapy. Int J Radiat Oncol Biol Phys 2004;59:11–20.
391. Krause DS, Van Etten RA. Tyrosine kinases as targets for cancer therapy. N Engl J Med 2005;353:172–87.
392. Clayman GL, Lee JJ, Holsinger FC, et al. Mortality risk from squamous cell skin cancer. J Clin Oncol 2005;23:759–65.
393. Lippman SM, Parkinson DR, Itri LM, et al. 13-cis-retinoic acid and interferon alpha-2a: effective combination therapy for advanced squamous cell carcinoma of the skin. J Natl Cancer Inst 1992;84:235–41.
394. Shin DM, Glisson BS, Khuri FR, et al. Phase II and biologic study of interferon alfa, retinoic acid, and cisplatin in advanced squamous skin cancer. J Clin Oncol 2002;20:364–70.
395. Diaz EM Jr. Multidisciplinary approach to head and neck cancer. In: Goepfert H, editor. The multidisciplinary treatment of head and neck cancer. Available at: http://www.headneckcancer.org.
396. Stern SJ, Hanna E. Cancer of the nasal cavity and paranasal sinuses. In: Myers EN, Suen JY, editors. Cancer of the head and neck. Philadelphia: W.B. Saunders; 1996. p. 205–233.
397. Myers EN, Carrau RL. Neoplasms of the nose and paranasal sinuses. In: Bailey BJ, Johnson JT, Kohut RI, et al, editors. Head and neck surgery—otolaryngology. Philadelphia: Lippincott; 1993. p. 1091–109.
398. Batsakis JG. The pathology of head and neck tumors. Nasal cavity and paranasal sinuses, Part 5. Head Neck Surg 1980;2:410–9.
399. Raney RB Jr, Tefft M, Newton WA, et al. Improved prognosis with intensive treatment of children with cranial soft tissue sarcomas arising in nonorbital parameningeal sites. A report form the Intergroup Rhabdomyosarcoma Study. Cancer 1987;59:147–55.
400. Donald PJ. Diagnosis of tumors of the paranasal sinuses and nasal cavity. In: Thawley SE, Panje WR, Batsakis JG, Lindberg RD, editors. Comprehensive management of head and neck tumors. Philadelphia: W.B. Saunders; 1987. p. 304–26.
401. Kadish S, Goodman M, Wine CC. Olfactory neuroblastoma: a clinical analysis of 17 cases. Cancer 1976;37:1571–6.
402. Batsakis JG. Regezi JA, Solomon AR, Rice DH. The pathology of head and neck tumors: mucosal melanomas, part 13. Head Neck Surg 1982;4:404–18.
403. Batsakis JG, Rice DH, Solomon AR. The pathology of head and neck tumors: squamous and mucous-gland carcinomas of the nasal cavity, paranasal sinuses, and larynx, part 6. Head Neck Surg 1980;2:497–508.
404. Jesse RH. Preoperative versus postoperative radiation in the treatment of squamous carcinoma of the paranasal sinuses. Am J Surg 1965;110:552–6.
405. Sisson GA, Toriumi DM, Atiyah RA. Paranasal sinus malignancy. A comprehensive update. Laryngoscope 1989;99:143–50.
406. Lee MM, Vokes EE, Rosen A, et al. Multimodality therapy in advanced paranasal sinus carcinoma: superior long-term results. Cancer J Sci Am 1999;5:219–23.
407. Nishino H, Miyata M, Morita A, et al. Combined therapy with conservative surgery, radiotherapy, and regional chemotherapy for maxillary sinus carcinoma. Cancer 2000;89:1925–32.
408. Collins SL, et al. Head and neck. In: Abeloff MD, Armitage JO, Lichter AS, Niederhuber JE, editors. Clinical oncology. New York: Churchill Livingstone; 1995. p. 996–8.
409. Kies MS, Haraf DJ, Rosen F, et al. Concomitant infusional paclitaxel and fluorouracil, oral hydroxyurea, and hyperfractionated radiation for locally advanced squamous head and neck cancer. J Clin Oncol 2001;19:1961.
410. Brizel DM, Albers ME, Fisher ET, et al. Hyperfractionated irradiation with or without concurrent chemotherapy for locally advanced head and neck cancer. N Engl J Med 1998;338:1798–804.
411. Wendt TG, Grabenbauer GG, Rodel CM, et al. Simultaneous radiochemotherapy versus radiotherapy alone in advanced head and neck cancer: a randomized multi-center study. J Clin Oncol 1998;16:1318–24.
412. Choi KN, Rotman M, Aziz H, et al. Concomitant infusion cisplatin and hyperfractionated radiotherapy for locally advanced nasopharyngeal and paranasal sinus tumors. Int J Radiat Oncol Biol Phys 1997;39:823–9.
413. Papadimitrakopoulou VA, Hong WK. Combined-modality therapy in paranasal sinus cancer. Cancer J 1999;5:208–10.
414. Lee YY, Dimery IW, Van Tassel P, et al. Superselective intra-arterial chemotherapy of advanced paranasal sinus tumors. Arch Otolaryngol Head Neck Surg 1989;115:503–11.
415. Kumar P, Wan J, Wieira F, et al. Five year outcome analyses following treatment of stage III/IV head and neck (H/N) squamous cell carcinoma (SCCa) using supradose intra-arterial targeted cisplatin (SIT-P) and concurrent radiation therapy (RT). Proc Am Soc Clin Oncol 1999:396a.
416. Deutsch BD, Levine PA, Stewart FM, et al. Sinonasal undifferentiated carcinoma: a ray of hope. Otolaryngol Head Neck Surg 1993;108:697–700.
417. Gallo O, Graziani P, Fini-Storchi O. Undifferentiated carcinoma of the nose and paranasal sinuses. An immunohistochemical and clinical study. Ear Nose Throat J 1993;72:588–90, 593–5.
418. Righi PD, Francis F, Aaron BS, et al. Sinonasal undifferentiated carcinoma: a 10-year experience. Am J Otolaryngol 1996;17:167–71.
419. Tufano RP, Mokadam NA, Montone KT, et al. Malignant tumors of the nose and paranasal sinuses: hospital of the University of Pennsylvania experience 1990–1997. Am J Rhinol 1999;13:117–23.

420. Zhen W, Hoffman HT, Mayr NA, et al. Primary neuroendocrine carcinoma of head and neck: the University of Iowa experience. Proc Am Soc Clin Oncol 1999.
421. Raychowdhuri RN. Oat cell carcinoma and paranasal sinuses. J Laryngol Otol 1965;79:253–5.
422. Weiss MD, de Fries HO, Taxy JB, et al. Primary small cell carcinoma of the paranasal sinuses. Arch Otolaryngol 1983;109:341–3.
423. Ordonez NG, Mackay B. Neuroendocrine tumors of the nasal cavity. Pathol Annu 1993;28:77–111.
424. Stewart FM, Lazarus HM, Levine PA, et al. High-dose chemotherapy and autologous marrow transplantation for esthesioneuroblastoma and sinonasal undifferentiated carcinoma. Am J Clin Oncol 1989;12:217–21.
425. Chamberlain MC. Treatment of intracranial metastatic esthesioneuroblastoma. J Clin Oncol 2002;20:357–8.
426. Eneroth CM. Salivary gland tumors in the parotid gland, submandibular gland and the palate region. Cancer 1971;27:1415–8.
427. Guillamondegui OM, Byers RM, duV Tapley. Malignant tumors of the salivary gland. In: Fletcher GH, editor. Textbook of radiotherapy. 3rd ed. Philadelphia: Lea & Febiger; 1980.
428. Spiro RH, Koss LG, Hajdu SI, Strong EW. Tumors of minor salivary gland origin: a clinicopathologic study of 492 cases. Cancer 1973;31:117–29.
429. Seifert G, Sobin LH, editors. WHO international classification of tumors. Histological typing of salivary gland tumors. Berlin: Springer-Verlag; 1991.
430. Klijanienko J, Vielh PH. Salivary gland tumors. Monogr Clin Cytol 2000;15:2–12.
431. Foote FW Jr, Frazell EL. Tumors of the major salivary glands. Cancer 1953;6:1065–133.
432. Sobin LH, Wittekind CH, editors. For the UICC TNM classification of malignant tumors. 5th ed. New York: Wiley Liss; 1997.
433. Goode RK, Auclair PL, Ellis GL. Mucoepidermoid carcinoma of the major salivary glands. Cancer 1998;82:1217–24.
434. Brandwein MS, Ivanov K, Wallace DI, et al. Mucoepidermoid carcinoma. Am J Surg Pathol 2001;25:835–45.
435. Spiro RH, Huvos AG, Strong EW. Cancer of the parotid gland: a clinicopathologic study of 288 primary cases. Am J Surg 1975;130:452–9.
436. McNeese MD, Fletcher GH. Tumors of the major and minor salivary glands. In: Laramore GE. Radiation therapy of head and neck cancer. Berlin: Springer-Verlag; 1988.
437. Johns ME, Goldsmith MM. Incidence, diagnosis, and classification of salivary gland tumors. Oncology 1989;3:47–56.
438. Spiro RH, Huvos AG, Strong EW. Acinic cell carcinoma of salivary origin: a clinicopathologic study of 67 cases. Cancer 1978;41:924–35.
439. Conley J, Dingman DK. Adenoid cystic carcinoma in the head and neck (cylindroma). Arch Otolaryngol Head Neck Surg 1974;100:81–90.
440. Spiro RH, Huvos AG, Strong EW. Adenoid cystic carcinoma: factors influencing survival. Am J Surg 1979;138:579–83.
441. Fordice J, Kershaw C, El-Naggar A, Goepfert H. Adenoid cystic carcinoma of the head and neck. Arch Otolaryngol Head Neck Surg 1999;125:149–52.
442. Goepfert H, Luna M, Lindberg R, White A. Malignant salivary gland tumors of the paranasal sinuses and nasal cavity. Arch Otolaryngol Head Neck Surg 1983;109:662–8.
443. Tapley ND. Irradiation treatment of malignant tumors of the salivary glands. Ear Nose Throat J 1977;56:110–4.
444. Lewis JE, Olsen KD, Sebo TJ. Carcinoma ex-pleomorphic adenoma: pathologic analysis of 73 cases. Hum Pathol 2001;32:596–604.
445. Fleming ID, Cooper JS, Hanson DE, et al. Cancer staging manual. Philadelphia and New York: Lippincott-Raven; 1997.
446. Watson TA. Irradiation in the management of tumors of the head and neck. Am J Surg 1965;110:542–8.
447. Bjorkland A, Eneroth CM. Management of parotid gland neoplasms. Am J Otolaryngol 1980;1:155–67.
448. Medina JE. Neck dissection in the Treatment of cancer of major salivary glands. Otolaryngol Clin North Am 1998;31:815–22.
449. Lampe I, Zatzkin H. Pulmonary metastases of pseudoadenomatous basal cell carcinoma (mucous and salivary gland tumor). Radiology 1949;53:379.
450. Fitzpatrick PJ, Theriault C. Malignant salivary gland tumors. Int J Radiat Oncol Biol Phys 1986;12:1743–7.
451. Garden AS, Weber RS, Ang KK, et al. Postoperative radiation therapy for malignant tumors of minor salivary glands. Cancer 1994;73:2563–9.
452. Conley J, Myers E, Cole R. Analysis of 115 patients with tumors of the submandibular gland. Ann Otol Rhinol Laryngol 1972;81:323–30.
453. Parsons JT, Mendenhall WM, Stringer SP, et al. Int J Radiol Oncol Biol Phys 1996;35:443–54.
454. Vander Poorten VL, Balm AJ, Hilgers FJ, et al. Stages: a major long term outcome predictor in minor salivary gland carcinomas. Cancer 2000;89:1195–204.
455. Lopes MA, Santos GC, Kowalski LB. Multivariate survival analysis of 128 cases of oral cavity minor salivary gland carcinomas. Head Neck 1998;20:699–706.
456. Batterman JJ, Breur K, Hart GAM, et al. Observations on pulmonary metastases in patients after single doses and multiple fractions of fast neutrons and cobalt-60 gamma rays. Eur J Cancer 1981;17:539–48.
457. Laramore GE, Krall JM, Griffin TW, et al. Neutron versus photon irradiation for unresectable salivary gland tumors: final report of an RTOG-MRC randomized study. Int J Radiat Oncol Biol Phys 1993;27:235–40.
458. Laramore GE. Radiotherapy as the primary treatment for malignant salivary gland tumors. In: Johnson JT, Didolkar MS, editors. Head and neck cancer. Vol. III. Amsterdam: Elsevier Press; 1993. p. 599–605.
459. Douglas JG, Lee S, Laramore GE, et al. Neutron radiotherapy for the treatment of locally advanced major salivary gland tumors. Head Neck 1999;21:255–63.
460. Douglas JG, Laramore GE, Austin-Seymour M, et al. Treatment of locally advanced adenoid cystic carcinoma of the head and neck with neutron radiotherapy. Int J Radiat Oncol Biol Phys 2000;46:551–7.
461. Douglas JG, Einck J, Austin-Seymour M, et al. Neutron radiotherapy for recurrent pleomorphic adenomas of major salivary glands. Head Neck 2001;23:1037–42.
462. Agulnik M, Siu LL. An update on the systemic therapy of malignant salivary gland cancers: role of chemotherapy and molecular targeted agents. Curr Med Chem Anticancer Agents 2004;4:543–51.
463. Creagan ET, Woods JE, Schutt AJ, et al. Cyclophosphamide, Adriamycin, and cis-diamminedichloroplatinum (II) in the treatment of advanced nonsquamous cell head and neck cancer. Cancer 1983;52:2007–10.
464. Dreyfuss AI, Clark JR, Fallon BG, et al. Cyclophosphamide, doxorubicin, and cisplatin combination chemotherapy for advanced carcinomas of salivary gland origin. Cancer 1987;60:2869–72.
465. Licitra L, Marchini S, Spinazze S, et al. Cisplatin in advanced salivary gland carcinoma. A phase II study of 25 patients. Cancer 1991;68:1874–7.
466. Airoldi M, Fornari G, Pedani F, et al. Paclitaxel and carboplatin for recurrent salivary gland malignancies. Anticancer Res 2000;20:3781–3.
467. Airoldi M, Pedani F, Succo G, et al. Phase II randomized trial comparing vinorelbine versus vinorelbine plus cisplatin in patients with recurrent salivary gland malignancies. Cancer 2001;91:541–7.
468. Airoldi M, Cortesina G, Giordano C, et al. Update and perspectives on non-surgical treatment of salivary gland malignancies. Acta Otorhinolaryngol Ital 2003;23:368–76.
469. Jennings T, Li Y, Pinto HA, et al. Phase II trial of paclitaxel in advanced or metastatic salivary gland malignancies: an Eastern Cooperative Oncology Group Study. Proc Am Soc Clin Onc 2001;20:236a.
470. Glisson B, Blumenschein G, Francisco M, et al. Phase II trial of gefitinib in patients with incurable salivary gland cancer. Proc Am Soc Clin Onc 2005;23(16S):5532.
471. Glisson B, Colevas AD, Haddad R, et al. HER2 expression in salivary gland carcinomas: dependence on histological subtype. Clin Cancer Res 2004;10:944–6.
472. Maruya S, Kim HW, Weber RS, et al. Gene expression screening of salivary gland neoplasms: molecular markers of potential histogenetic and clinical significance. J Mol Diagn 2004;6:180–90.
473. Hotte SJ, Winquist EW, Lamont E, et al. Imatinib mesylate in patients with adenoid cystic cancers of the salivary glands expressing c-kit: a Princess Margaret Hospital phase II consortium study. J Clin Oncol 2005;23:585–90.
474. Weber RS, Benjamin RS, Peters LJ, et al. Soft tissue sarcomas of the head and neck in adolescents and adults. Am J Surg 1986;152:386–92.
475. Lawrence W Jr, Anderson JR, Gehan EA, et al. Pretreatment TNM staging of childhood rhabdomyosarcoma: a report of the Intergroup Rhabdomyosarcoma Study Group. Children's Cancer Study Group. Pediatric Oncology Group. Cancer 1997;80:1165–70.
476. Goepfert H, Raymond K, Spires JR, et al. Osteosarcoma of the head and neck. Cancer Bull 1990;42:347–54.
477. Daw NC, Mahmoud HH, Meyer WH, et al. Bone sarcomas of the head and neck in children: the St. Jude Children's Research Hospital experience. Cancer 2000;88:2172–80.
478. Ha PK, Eisele DW, Frassica FJ, et al. Osteosarcoma of the head and neck: a review of the Johns Hopkins experience. Laryngoscope 1999;109:964–9.
479. Mark RJ, Sercarz JA, Tran L, et al. Osteogenic sarcoma of the head and neck: the UCLA experience. Arch Otolaryngol Head Neck Surg 1991;117:761–6.
480. Oda D, Bavisotto LM, Schmidt RA, et al. Head and neck osteosarcoma at the University of Washington. Head Neck 1997;19:513–23.
481. Jaffe N, Patel SR, Benjamin RS. Chemotherapy in osteosarcoma: basis for application and antagonism to implementation; early controversies surrounding its implementation. Hematol Oncol Clin North Am 1995;9:825–40.
482. Smeele LE, Kostense PJ, van der Waal I, et al. Effect of chemotherapy on survival of craniofacial osteosarcoma: a systematic review of 201 patients. J Clin Oncol 1997;15:363–7.
483. Kassir RR, Rassekh CH, Kinsella JB, et al. Osteosarcoma of the head and neck: meta-analysis of nonrandomized studies. Laryngoscope 1997;107:56–61.
484. Holden CA, Spittle MF, Jones EW. Angiosarcoma of the face and scalp: prognosis and treatment. Cancer 1987;59:1046–57.
485. Lydiatt WM, Shaha AR, Shah JP. Angiosarcoma of the head and neck. Am J Surg 1994;168:451–4.
486. Maddox JC, Evans HL. Angiosarcoma of skin and soft tissue: a study of forty-four cases. Cancer 1981;48:1907–21.
487. Mark RJ, Tran LM, Sercarz J, et al. Angiosarcoma of the head and neck: the UCLA experience 1955 through 1990. Arch Otolaryngol Head Neck Surg 1993;119:973–8.
488. Morrison WH, Byers RM, Garden AS, et al. Cutaneous angiosarcoma of the head and neck: a therapeutic dilemma. Cancer 1995;76:319–27.
489. Callender TA, Weber RS, Janjan N, et al. Rhabdomyosarcoma of the nose and paranasal sinuses in adults and children. Otolaryngol Head Neck Surg 1995;112:252–7.
490. Raney RB, Anderson JR, Barr FG, et al. Rhabdomyosarcoma and undifferentiated sarcoma in the first two decades of life: a selective review of intergroup rhabdomyosarcoma study group experience and rationale for Intergroup Rhabdomyosarcoma Study V. J Pediatr Hematol Oncol 2001;23:215–20.
491. Dagher R, Helman L. Rhabdomyosarcoma: an overview. Oncologist 1999;4:34–44.
492. Baker KS, Anderson JR, Link MP, et al. Benefit of intensified therapy for patients with local or regional embryonal rhabdomyosarcoma: results from the Intergroup Rhabdomyosarcoma Study IV. J Clin Oncol 2000;18:2427–34.
493. Crist WM, Anderson JR, Meza JL, et al. Intergroup rhabdomyosarcoma study-IV: results for patients with nonmetastatic disease. J Clin Oncol 2001;19:3091–102.
494. Enzinger FM. Malignant fibrous histiocytoma 20 years after Stout. Am J Surg Pathol 1986;10 Suppl 1:43–53.
495. Fagundes HM, Lai PP, Dehner LP, et al. Postoperative radiotherapy for malignant fibrous histiocytoma. Int J Radiat Oncol Biol Phys 1992;23:615–9.
496. Huvos AG, Heilweil M, Bretsky SS. The pathology of malignant fibrous histiocytoma of bone. A study of 130 patients. Am J Surg Pathol 1985;9:853–71.
497. LeVay J, O'Sullivan B, Catton C, et al. Outcome and prognostic factors in soft tissue sarcoma in the adult. Int J Radiat Oncol Biol Phys 1993;27:1091–9.
498. Weiss SW, Enzinger FM. Malignant fibrous histiocytoma: an analysis of 200 cases. Cancer 1978;41:2250–66.
499. Frankenthaler R, Ayala AG, Hartwick RW, et al. Fibrosarcoma of the head and neck. Laryngoscope 1990;100:799–802.
500. Lindberg RD, Martin RG, Romsdahl MM, et al. Conservative surgery and postoperative radiotherapy in 300 adults with soft-tissue sarcomas. Cancer 1981;47:2391–7.
501. Van Glabbeke M, van Oosterom AT, Oosterhuis JW, et al. Prognostic factors for the outcome of chemotherapy in advanced soft tissue sarcoma: an analysis of 2,185 patients treated with anthracycline-containing first-line regimens—a European Organization for Research and Treatment of Cancer Soft Tissue and Bone Sarcoma Group Study. J Clin Oncol 1999;17:150–7.
502. Sarcoma Meta-analysis Collaboration. Adjuvant chemotherapy for localized resectable soft-tissue sarcoma of adults: meta-analysis of individual data. Sarcoma Meta-analysis Collaboration. Lancet 1997;350:1647–54.
503. Freedman AM, Reiman HM, Woods JE. Soft-tissue sarcomas of the head and neck. Am J Surg 1989;158:367–72.
504. Wanebo HJ, Koness RJ, MacFarlane JK, et al. Head and neck sarcoma: report of the Head and Neck Sarcoma

Registry. Society of Head and Neck Surgeons Committee on Research. Head Neck 1992;14:1–7.

505. Kramer IRH, Pindborg JJ, Shear M. Histological typing of odontogenic tumors. Berlin: Springer-Verlag; 1992. p. 24–7.
506. Small IA, Waldron CA. Ameloblastomas of the jaws. Oral Surg 1955;8:282–97.
507. Reichart PA, Philipsen HP, Sonner S. Ameloblastoma: virological profile of 3,677 cases. Oral Oncol, Eur J Cancer 1995;31B:86–99.
508. Kishino M, Murakami S, Fukada Y, Ishida T. Pathology of the desmoplastic ameloblastoma. J Oral Pathol Med 2001;30:35–40.
509. Er N, Dagdeviren A, Tasman F, Zeybek D. Neural cell adhesion molecule and neurothelin expression in human ameloblastoma. J Oral Maxillofac Surg 2001;59:900–3.
510. Kahn MA. Ameloblastoma in young persons. A clinicopathologic analysis and etiologic investigation. Oral Surg Oral Med Oral Pathol 1989;67:706–15.
511. Kim S-G, Jang H-S, Korea K-J. Ameloblastoma. A clinical, radiographic and histopathologic analysis of 71 cases. Oral Surg Oral Med Oral Pathol Oral Radiol Endod 2001;91:649–53.
512. Christian JM, Schmidtke CD, Ydrach AA, Spina AM. Recurrent radiolucent-radiopaque lesion of the mandible. J Oral Maxillofac Surg 2000;58:1289–93.
513. Robinson HBG. Ameloblastoma. A survey of 379 cases from the literature. Arch Pathol 1937;23:831–43 .
514. Mehlisch DR, Dahlin DC, Masson JK. Ameloblastoma: a clinicopathologic report. J Oral Surg 1972;30:9–22.
515. Muller H, Slootweg PJ. The ameloblastoma, the controversial approach to therapy. J Maxillofac Surg 1985;13:79–84.
516. Leider AS, Eversole LR, Barkin ME. Cystic ameloblastoma. A clinicopathologic analysis. Oral Surg Oral Med Oral Pathol 1985;60:624–620.
517. Williams T. The ameloblastoma: a review of the literature. Selected Readings Oral Maxillofac Surg 1992;2:1–17.
518. Sehdev MK, Huvos AG, Strong EW, et al. Proceedings: ameloblastoma of maxilla and mandible. Cancer 1974;33:323–33.
519. Nakamura N, Mitsuyasu T, Higuchi Y, et al. Growth characteristics of ameloblastoma involving the inferior alveolar nerve: a clinical and histopathologic study. Oral Surg Oral Med Oral Pathol Oral Radiol Endod 2001;91:557–62.
520. Lee RE, White WL, Totten RS. Ameloblastoma with distant metastases. Arch Pathol 1959;68:23–9.
521. Batsakis p. 536
522. Pindborg JJ. Calcifying epithelial odontogenic tumors. Acta Pathol Microbiol Scand 1956;111 Suppl:71.
523. Gargiulo EA, Ziter WD, Mastrocola R. Calcifying epithelial odontogenic tumor. Report of case and review of literature. J Oral Surg 1971;29;862–6.
524. Hicks MJ, Flaitz CM, Wong MEK, et al. Clear cell variant of calcifying epithelial odontogenic tumor: Case report and review of the literature. Head Neck 1994;16:272–7.
525. Veness MJ, Morgan G, Collins AP, Walter DM. Calcifying epithelial odontogenic (Pindborg) tumor with malignant transformation and metastatic spread. Head Neck 2001;23:292–6.
526. Lucas RB. Pathology of tumors of the oral tissues. 4th ed. London: Churchill Livingstone; 1984. p.70.
527. Batsakis, p 559.
528. Neville BW, Damm D, Allen CM, Bouquot JE. Oral and maxillofacial pathology. 2nd ed. Philadelphia: Saunders; 2002. p. 33.
529. Praetorius F, Hjorting-Hansen E, Gorlin RJ, Vickers RA. Calcifying odontogenic cyst. Acta Odontol Scand 1981;39:227–40.
530. Regezi JA, Kerr DA, Courtney, RM. Odontogenic tumours: analysis of 706 cases. J Oral Surg 1978;36:771–8.
531. Yamamoto K, Yoneda K, Yamamoto T, et al. An immunohistochemical study of odontogenic mixed tumors. Oral Oncol 1985;32:122–8.
532. Slootweg PJ. An analysis of the interrelationship of the mixed odontogenic tumors-ameloblastic fibroma, ameloblastic fibroodontoma, and the odontomas. Oral Surg Oral Med Oral Pathol Oral Med Endod 1981;52:266–76.
533. Pindborg JJ, Kramer IRH. Histologic typing of odontogenic tumors, jaw cysts and allied lesions. Geneva: World Health Organization; 1971. p. 27.
534. Howell RM, Burke EJ Jr. Malignant transformation of ameloblastic fibroodontoma to ameloblastic fibrosarcoma. J Oral Surg 1977;43:391–401.
535. Okura M, Nakahara H, Matksuya T. Treatment of ameloblastic fibro-odontoma without removal of the associated permanent tooth. Report of cases. J Oral Maxillofac Surg 1992;50:1094–6.
536. Elzay RP. Classification of primary intraosseous carcinoma. Oral Surg Oral Med Oral Pathol 1982;54:299–303.
537. Slootweg PJ, Muller H. Malignant ameloblastoma or ameloblastic carcinoma? Oral Surg Oral Med Oral Pathol 1984;57:168–176.
538. Adamo AK, Boguslaw B, Coomaraswarmy MA, Simos C. Clear cell odontogenic carcinoma of the mandible: case report. J Oral Maxillofac Surg 2002;60:121–6.
539. Kumamoto H, Yamazaki S, Sato A, et al. Clear cell odontogenic tumor in the mandible. Report of a case with duct-like appearances and dentinoid induction. J Oral Pathol Med 2000;29:43–7.
540. Hirshberg A, Leibovich P, Buchner A. Metastatic tumors to the jawbones. analysis of 390 cases. J Oral Pathol Med 1994;23:33–41.
541. Vikram B, Strong EW, Shah J, Spiro RH. Elective postoperative irradiation in stages III and IV epidermoid carcinoma of the head and neck. Am J Surg 1980;140:580–4.
542. Mackillop WJ, Bates JHT, O'Sullivan B, et al. The effect of delay in treatment on local control by radiotherapy. Int J Radiat Oncol Biol Phys 1996;34:243–50.
543. Hall EJ. Radiobiology for the radiologist. 4th ed. Philadelphia: J.B. Lippincott; 1994.
544. Fowler JF, Lindstrom MJ. Loss of local control with prolongation in radiotherapy. Int J Radiat Oncol Biol Phys 1992;23:457–67.
545. Robertson C, Robertson AG, Hendry JH, et al. Similar decreases in local tumor control are calculated for treatment protraction and for interruptions in the radiotherapy of carcinoma of the larynx in four centers. Int J Radiat Oncol Biol Phys 1998;40:319–29.
546. Bhattathiri VN. Cumulative interfraction interval analysis of influence of time and interruptions on radiotherapy results in oral cancers. Int J Radiat Oncol Biol Phys 2002;52:1251–6.
547. Brizel DM, Wasserman HT, Henke M, et al. Phase III randomized trial of amifostine as a radioprotector in head and neck cancer. J Clin Oncol 2000;18:3339–45.
548. Antonadou D, Pepelassi M, Synodinou M, et al. Prophylactic use of amifostine to prevent radiochemotherapy-induced mucositis and xerostomia in head-and-neck cancer. Int J Radiat Oncol Biol Phys 2002;52:739–47.
549. Mossman KL. Quantitative radiation dose response relationships for normal tissues in man. II. Response of the salivary glands during radiotherapy. Radiat Res 1983;95:392–8.
550. Mossman KL, Chencharick JD, Scheedr AC, et al. Radiation induced changes in gustatory function: comparison of effects of neutron and photon irradiation. Int J Radiat Oncol Biol Phys 1979;5:521–8.
551. Mossman KL, Shatzman AR, Chencharick JD. Effects of radiotherapy on human parotid saliva. Radiat Res 1981;88:403–12.
552. Rieke JW, Hafermann MD, Johnson JT, et al. Oral pilocarpine for post-irradiation xerostomia: integrated efficacy and safety results from two prospective randomized clinical trials. Int J Radiat Oncol Biol Phys 1995;31:661–9.
553. Murray CG, Herson J, Daly TE, Zimmerman SO. Radiation necrosis of the mandible: a 10 year study. Part I. Factors influencing the onset of necrosis. Int J Radiat Oncol Biol Phys 1980;6:543–8.
554. Marx RE, Johnson RP. Studies in the radiobiology of osteoradionecrosis and their clinical significance. Oral Surg Oral Med Oral Pathol 1987;64:379–90.
555. NHLBI workshop summary: hyperbaric oxygen therapy. Am Rev Respir Dis 1991;144:1414–21.
556. Leibel SA, Fuks Z, Zelefsky MJ, et al. Intensity-modulated radiotherapy. Cancer J 2002;8:164–76.
557. Lee N, Xia P, Quivey JM, et al. Intensity-modulated radiotherapy in the treatment of nasopharyngeal carcinoma: an update of the UCSF experience. Int J Radiat Oncol Biol Phys 2002;53:12–22.
558. Wu Q, Manning M, Schmidt-Ullrich R, et al. The potential for sparing of parotids and escalation of the biologically effective dose with intensity-modulated radiation treatments of head and neck cancers: a treatment design study. Int J Radiat Oncol Biol Phys 2000;46:195–205.
559. Thames HD, Schultheiss TE, Hendry JH, et al. Can modest escalations of dose be detected as increased tumor control? Int J Radiat Oncol Biol Phys 1991;22:241–6.
560. Withers HR, Peters LJ, Taylor JMG, et al. Local control of carcinoma of the tonsil by radiation therapy: an analysis of patterns of fractionation in nine institutions. Int J Radiat Oncol Biol Phys 1995;33:549–62.
561. Cox JD, Pajak TF, Marcial VA, et al. Dose-response for local control with hyperfractionated radiation therapy in advanced carcinomas of the upper aerodigestive tracts: preliminary report of Radiation Therapy Oncology Group protocol 83-13. Int J Radiat Oncol Biol Phys 1990;18:515–21.
562. Fu KK, Pajak TF, Marcial VA, et al. Late effects of hyperfractionated radiotherapy for advanced head and neck cancer: long-term follow-up results of RTOG 83-13. Int J Radiat Oncol Biol Phys 1995;32:577–88.
563. Fu KK, Pajak TF, Trotti A, et al. A Radiation Therapy Oncology Group (RTOG) phase III randomized study to compare hyperfractionation and two variants of accelerated fractionation to standard fractionation radiotherapy for head and neck squamous cell carcinomas: first report of RTOG 9003. Int J Radiat Oncol Biol Phys 2000;48:7–16.
564. Cox JD, Pajak TF, Marcial VA, et al. ASTRO plenary: interfractionation interval is a major determinant of late effects, with hyperfractionated radiation therapy of carcinomas of the upper respiratory and digestive tracts: results from Radiation Therapy Oncology Group protocol 8313. Int J Radiat Oncol Biol Phys 1991;20:1191–5.
565. Ang KK. Altered fractionation trials in head and neck cancer. Semin Radiat Oncol 1998;8:230–6.
566. Dische S, Saunders MI. Continuous hyperfractionated, accelerated radiotherapy (CHART): an interim report. Radiother Oncol 1989;16:65–72.
567. Wang CC, Blitzer PH, Suit HD. Twice-a-day radiation therapy for cancer of the head and neck. Cancer 1985;55:2100–4.
568. Wang CC, Suit HD, Plitzer PH. Twice-a-day radiation therapy for supraglottic carcinoma. Int J Radiat Oncol Biol Phys 1986;12:3–7.
569. Ang KK, Peters LJ. Principles and practices of oncology. PPO Updates 1994;4:1.
570. Begg AC, Haustermans K, Hart AAM, et al. The value of pretreatment cell kinetic parameters as predictors for radiotherapy outcome in head and neck cancer: a multicenter analysis. Radiother Oncol 1999;50:13–23.
571. Porter EH. The statistics of dose/cure relationships for irradiated tumors. Part I. Br J Radiol 1980;53:210–27.
572. Porter EH. The statistics of dose/cure relationships for irradiated tumors. Part II. Br J Radiol 1980;53:336–45.
573. Peters LJ, Withers HR, Fletcher GH. Alternatives to radical neck dissection: the M.D. Anderson approach. Aust Radiol 1980;24:303–6.
574. Laramore GE, Phillips MH. Particle beam radiotherapy: clinical perspective. In: Brady LW, Perez CA, editors. Principles and practices of radiation oncology. 4th ed. Philadelphia: Lippincott, Williams and Wilkins. [In press]
575. Laramore GE. Radiation therapy of head and neck cancer. Berlin: Springer-Verlag; 1988.
576. Haas JS, Cox JD. Cervical nodal metastases from an unknown primary carcinoma. In: Laramore GE, editor. Radiation therapy of head and neck cancer. Berlin: Springer-Verlag; 1988. p. 211–8.
577. Reddy SP, Marks JE. Metastatic carcinoma in the cervical lymph nodes from an unknown primary site: results of bilateral neck plus mucosal irradiation vs. ipsilateral neck irradiation. Int J Radiat Oncol Biol Phys 1997;37:797–802.
578. Parsons JT, Mendenhall WM, Stringer SP. Twice-a-day radiotherapy for squamous cell carcinoma of the head and neck: the University of Florida experience. Head Neck 1993;15:87–96.
579. Datta NR, Choudhry AD, Gupta S, et al. Twice a day versus once a day radiation therapy in head and neck cancer [abstract]. Int J Radiat Oncol Biol Phys 1989;17S:132–3.
580. Pinto LHJ, Canary PCV, Araujo CMM, et al. Prospective randomized trial comparing hyperfractionated versus conventional radiotherapy in stages III and IV oropharyngeal carcinoma. Int J Radiat Oncol Biol Phys 1991;21:557–62.
581. Horiot JC, LeFur RN, Guyen T, et al. Hyperfractionation versus conventional fractionation in oropharyngeal carcinoma: final analysis of a randomized trial of the EORTC cooperative group of radiotherapy. Radiother Oncol 1993;25:231–41.
582. Saunders MI, Dische S, Barrett A, et al. Randomized multicentre trials of CHART vs. conventional radiotherapy in head and neck and non-small cell lung cancer: an interim report. Br J Cancer 1996;73:1455–62.
583. Bourhis J, Audrey H, Overgaard J, et al. Meta-analysis of conventional versus altered fractionated radiotherapy in head and neck squamous cell carcinoma (HNSCC): final analysis. Int J Radiat Oncol Biol Phys 2004;60:S190–1.
584. Jen Y-M, Hsu W-L, Chen C-Y, et al. Different risks of symptomatic brain necrosis in NPC patients treated with different altered fractionation radiotherapy techniques. Int J Radiat Oncol Biol Phys 2001;51:344–8.
585. Fletcher GH. Lucy Wortham James Lecture: subclinical disease. Cancer 1984;53:1274–84.
586. Peters LJ, Goepfert H, Ang KK, et al. Evaluation of the dose for postoperative radiation therapy of head and neck cancer: first report of a prospective randomized trial. Int J Radiat Oncol Biol Phys 1993;26:3–11.

587. Laramore GE, Scott CB, Schuller DE, et al. Is a surgical resection leaving positive margins of benefit to the patient with locally advanced squamous cell carcinoma of the head and neck? A comparative study using the Intergroup Study 0034 and the Radiation Therapy Oncology Group database. Int J Radiat Oncol Biol Phys 1993;27:1011–6.
588. Khuri FR, Jain SR. Novel agents and incremental advances in the treatment of head and neck. Semin Oncol 2004;31:3–10.
589. Cohen EE, Lingen MW, Vokes EE. The expanding role of systemic therapy in head and neck cancer. J Clin Oncol 2004;22:1743–52.
590. Paccagnella A, Orlando A, Marchiori C, et al. Phase III trial of initial chemotherapy in stage III or IV head and neck cancers: a study by the Gruppo di Studio sui Tumori della Testa e del Collo. J Natl Cancer Inst 1994;86:265–72.
591. Domenge C, Hill C, Lefebvre JL, et al. Randomized trial of neoadjuvant chemotherapy in oropharyngeal carcinoma. French Groupe d'Etude des Tumeurs de la Tete et du Cou (GETTEC). Br J Cancer 2000;83:1594–8.
592. Pignon JP, Bourhis J, Domenge C, et al. Chemotherapy added to locoregional treatment for head and neck squamous-cell carcinoma: three meta-analyses of updated individual data. MACH-NC Collaborative Group. Meta-Analysis of Chemotherapy on Head and Neck Cancer. Lancet 2000;355:949–55.
593. Vokes EE, Stenson K, Rosen FR, et al. Weekly carboplatin and paclitaxel followed by concomitant paclitaxel, fluorouracil, and hydroxyurea chemoradiotherapy: curative and organ-preserving therapy for advanced head and neck cancer. J Clin Oncol 2003;21:320–6.
594. Shin DM, Glisson BS, Khuri FR, et al. Phase II study of induction chemotherapy with paclitaxel, ifosfamide, and carboplatin (TIC) for patients with locally advanced squamous cell carcinoma of the head and neck. Cancer 2002;95:322–30.
595. Haddad RI, Tishler R, Wirth L, et al. Rate of complete pathological responses (pCR) to docetaxel/cisplatin/5-fluorouracil (TPF) induction chemotherapy in patients with newly diagnosed, locally advanced squamous cell carcinoma of the head and neck (SCCHN) [abstract 5511]. Proc Am Soc Clin Oncol 2005.
596. Forastiere AA, Goepfert H, Maor M, et al. Concurrent chemotherapy and radiotherapy for organ preservation in advanced laryngeal cancer. N Engl J Med 2003;349;2091–8.
597. Merlano M, Vitale V, Rosso R, et al. Treatment of advanced squamous-cell carcinoma of the head and neck with alternating chemotherapy and radiotherapy. N Engl J Med 1992;327:1115–21.
598. Calais G, Alfonsi M, Bardet E, et al. Randomized trial of radiation therapy versus concomitant chemotherapy and radiation therapy for advanced-stage oropharynx carcinoma. J Natl Cancer Inst 1999;91:2081–6.
599. Jeremic B, Shibamoto Y, Milicic B, et al. Hyperfractionated radiation therapy with or without concurrent low-dose daily cisplatin in locally advanced squamous cell carcinoma of the head and neck: a prospective randomized trial. J Clin Oncol 2000;18:1458–64.
600. Brizel DM, Albers ME, Fisher SR, et al. Hyperfractionated irradiation with or without concurrent chemotherapy for locally advanced head and neck cancer. N Engl J Med 1998;338:1798–804.
601. Wendt TG, Grabenbauer GG, Rodel CM, et al. Simultaneous radiochemotherapy versus radiotherapy alone in advanced head and neck cancer: a randomized multicenter study. J Clin Oncol 1998;16:1318–24.
602. Staar S, Rudat V, Stuetzer H, et al. Intensified hyperfractionated accelerated radiotherapy limits the additional benefit of simultaneous chemotherapy—results of a multicentric randomized German trial in advanced head-and-neck cancer. Int J Radiat Oncol Biol Phys 2001;50:1161–71.
603. Adelstein DJ, Li Y, Adams GL, et al. An intergroup phase III comparison of standard radiation therapy and two schedules of concurrent chemoradiotherapy in patients with unresectable squamous cell head and neck cancer. J Clin Oncol 2003;21:92–8.
604. Huguenin P, Beer KT, Allal A, et al. Concomitant cisplatin significantly improves locoregional control in advanced head and neck cancers treated with hyperfractionated radiotherapy. J Clin Oncol 2004;22:4665–73.
605. Budach V, Stuschke M, Budach W, et al. Hyperfractionated accelerated chemoradiation with concurrent fluorouracil-mitomycin is more effective than dose-escalated hyperfractionated accelerated radiation therapy alone in locally advanced head and neck cancer: final results of the radiotherapy cooperative clinical trials group of the German Cancer Society 95-06 Prospective Randomized Trial. J Clin Oncol 2005;23:1125–35.
606. Nakamura K, Shioyama Y, Sasaki T, et al. Chemoradiation therapy with or without surgical salvage for early squamous carcinoma of the hypopharynx. Int J Radiat Biol Phys 2005;1:684–9.
607. Bachaud JM, Cohen-Jonathan E, Alzieu C, et al. Combined postoperative radiotherapy and weekly cisplatin infusion for locally advanced head and neck carcinoma: final report of a randomized trial. Int J Radiat Oncol Biol Phys 1996;36:999–1004.
608. Cooper JS, Pajak TF, Forastiere AA, et al. Postoperative concurrent radiotherapy and chemotherapy for high-risk squamous-cell carcinoma of the head and neck. N Engl J Med 2004;350:1937–44.
609. Bernier J, Domenge C, Ozsahin M, et al. Postoperative irradiation with or without concomitant chemotherapy for locally advanced head and neck cancer. N Engl J Med 2004;350:1945–52.
610. Bernier J, Cooper J, van Glabbeke M, et al. Chemo-radiation as adjuvant treatment in locally advanced head and neck squamous cell carcinomas (HNSCC): comparative analysis of selection criteria, disease patterns and treatment outcomes in EORTC 22931 and RTOG 9501/intergroup trials, 6th International Conference on Head and Neck Cancer. Washington (DC): 2004. p 232.
611. Bonner J, Harari P, Giralt J, et al. Cetuximab prolongs survival in patients with locoregionally advanced squamous cell carcinoma of head and neck: a phase III study of high dose radiation therapy with or without cetuximab [abstract 5507]. Proc Amer Soc Clin Oncol 2004;23:438s.
612. Hong WK, Bromer R. Chemotherapy in head and neck cancer. N Engl J Med 1983;308:75–9.
613. Fanucchi M, Khuri FR. Chemotherapy for recurrent or metastatic squamous cell carcinoma of the head and neck. Semin Oncol 2004;31:809–15.
614. Hong WK, Schaefer S, Issell B, et al. A prospective randomized trial of methotrexate versus cisplatin in the treatment of recurrent squamous cell carcinoma of the head and neck. Cancer 1983;52:206–10.
615. Vokes E. Head and neck cancer. In: Perry MC, ed. Chemotherapy source book. Baltimore: Williams & Wilkins; 1992. p. 918–31.
616. Airoldi M, Cortesina G, Giordano C, et al. Ifosfamide in the treatment of head and neck cancer. Oncology 2003;65:37–43.
617. Forastiere A, Koch W, Trotti A, et al. Head and neck cancer. N Engl J Med 2001;345:1890–900.
618. Forastiere AA, Shank D, Neuberg D, et al. Final report of a phase II evaluation of paclitaxel in patients with advanced squamous cell carcinoma of the head and neck: an Eastern Cooperative Oncology Group trial (PA390). Cancer 1998;82:2270–4.
619. Dreyfuss AI, Clark JR, Norris CM, et al. Docetaxel: an active drug for squamous cell carcinoma of the head and neck. J Clin Oncol 1996;14:1672–8.
620. Lamont EB, Vokes EE. Chemotherapy in the management of squamous-cell carcinoma of the head and neck. Lancet Oncol 2001;2:261–9.
621. Shin DM, Glisson BS, Khuri FR, et al. Phase II trial of paclitaxel, ifosfamide, and cisplatin in patients with recurrent head and neck squamous cell carcinoma. J Clin Oncol 1998;16:1325–30.
622. Jacobs C, Lyman G, Velez-Garcia E, et al. A phase III randomized study comparing cisplatin and fluorouracil as single agents and in combination for advanced squamous cell carcinoma of the head and neck. J Clin Oncol 1992;10:257–63.
623. Forastiere AA, Metch B, Schuller DE, et al. Randomized comparison of cisplatin plus fluorouracil and carboplatin plus fluorouracil versus methotrexate in advanced squamous-cell carcinoma of the head and neck: a Southwest Oncology Group study. J Clin Oncol 1992;10:1245–51.
624. Clavel M, Vermorken JB, Cognetti F, et al. Randomized comparison of cisplatin, methotrexate, bleomycin and vincristine (CABO) versus cisplatin and 5-fluorouracil (CF) versus cisplatin (C) in recurrent or metastatic squamous cell carcinoma of the head and neck. A phase III study of the EORTC Head and Neck Cancer Cooperative Group. Ann Oncol 1994;5:521–6.
625. Schrijvers D, Johnson J, Jiminez U, et al. Phase III trial of modulation of cisplatin/fluorouracil chemotherapy by interferon alfa-2b in patients with recurrent or metastatic head and neck cancer. Head and Neck Interferon Cooperative Study Group. J Clin Oncol 1998;16:1054–9.
626. Forastiere AA, Leong T, Rowinsky E, et al. Phase III comparison of high-dose paclitaxel + cisplatin + granulocyte colony-stimulating factor versus low-dose paclitaxel + cisplatin in advanced head and neck cancer: Eastern Cooperative Oncology Group Study E1393. J Clin Oncol 2001;19:1088–95.
627. Gibson MK, Li Y, Murphy B, et al. Randomized phase III evaluation of cisplatin plus fluorouracil versus cisplatin plus paclitaxel in advanced head and neck cancer (E1395): an intergroup trial of the Eastern Cooperative Oncology Group. J Clin Oncol 2005;23:3562–7.
628. Field JK. The role of oncogenes and tumour-suppressor genes in the etiology of oral, head and neck squamous cell carcinoma. J R Soc Med 1995;88:35P–9P.
629. Wong DT, Todd R, Tsuji T, et al. Molecular biology of human oral cancer. Crit Rev Oral Biol Med 1996;7:319–28.
630. Califano J, Westra WH, Meininger G, et al. Genetic progression and clonal relationship of recurrent premalignant head and neck lesions. Clin Cancer Res 2000;6:347–52.
631. Santini J, Formento JL, Francoual M, et al. Characterization, quantification, and potential clinical value of the epidermal growth factor receptor in head and neck squamous cell carcinomas. Head Neck 1991;13:132–9.
632. Salomon DS, Brandt R, Ciardiello F, et al. Epidermal growth factor-related peptides and their receptors in human malignancies. Crit Rev Oncol Hematol 1995;19:183–232.
633. Grandis JR, Tweardy DJ. TGF-alpha and EGFR in head and neck cancer. J Cell Biochem 1993;17F:188–91.
634. Rubin Grandis J, Melhem MF, Barnes EL, et al. Quantitative immunohistochemical analysis of transforming growth factor-alpha and epidermal growth factor receptor in patients with squamous cell carcinoma of the head and neck. Cancer 1996;78:1284–92.
635. Rubin Grandis J, Melhem MF, Gooding WE, et al. Levels of TGF-alpha and EGFR protein in head and neck squamous cell carcinoma and patient survival. J Natl Cancer Inst 1998;90:824–32.
636. Dassonville O, Formento JL, Francoual M, et al. Expression of epidermal growth factor receptor and survival in upper aerodigestive tract cancer. J Clin Oncol 1993;11:1873–8.
637. Oc P, Modjtahedi H, Rhys-Evans P, et al. Epidermal growth factor-like ligands differentially up-regulate matrix metalloproteinase 9 in head and neck squamous carcinoma cells. Cancer Res 2000;60:1121–8.
638. Oc P, Rhys-Evans P, Court WJ, et al. Differential modulation of proliferation, matrix metalloproteinase expression and invasion of human head and neck squamous carcinoma cells by c-erbB ligands. Clin Exp Metastasis 2000;17:631–9.
639. Barrandon Y, Green H. Cell migration is essential for sustained growth of keratinocyte colonies: the roles of transforming growth factor-alpha and epidermal growth factor. Cell 1987;50:1131–7.
640. Chen P, Xie H, Sekar MC, et al. Epidermal growth factor receptor-mediated cell motility: phospholipase C activity is required, but mitogen-activated protein kinase activity is not sufficient for induced cell movement. J Cell Biol 1994;127:847–57.
641. Veikkola T, Karkkainen M, Claesson-Welsh L, et al. Regulation of angiogenesis via vascular endothelial growth factor receptors. Cancer Res 2000;60:203–12.
642. Gille J, Swerlick RA, Caughman SW. Transforming growth factor-alpha-induced transcriptional activation of the vascular permeability factor (VPF/VEGF) gene requires AP-2-dependent DNA binding and transactivation. EMBO J 1997;16:750–9.
643. Ang KK, Berkey BA, Tu X, et al. Impact of epidermal growth factor receptor expression on survival and pattern of relapse in patients with advanced head and neck carcinoma. Cancer Res 2002;62:7350–6.
644. Magne N, Pivot X, Bensadoun RJ, et al. The relationship of epidermal growth factor receptor levels to the prognosis of unresectable pharyngeal cancer patients treated by chemo-radiotherapy. Eur J Cancer 2001;37:2169–77.
645. Cohen EE, Rosen F, Stadler WM, et al. Phase II trial of ZD1839 in recurrent or metastatic squamous cell carcinoma of the head and neck. J Clin Oncol 2003;21:1980–7.
646. Soulieres D, Senzer NN, Vokes EE, et al. Multicenter phase II study of erlotinib, an oral epidermal growth factor receptor tyrosine kinase inhibitor, in patients with recurrent or metastatic squamous cell cancer of the head and neck. J Clin Oncol 2004;22:77–85.
647. Kies M, Arquette M, Nabell L, et al. Final report of the efficacy and safety of the anti-epidermal growth factor antibody Erbitux (IMC-C225), in combination with cisplatin in patients with recurrent squamous cell carcinoma of the head and neck (SCCHN) refractory to cisplatin containing chemotherapy [abstract 925]. Proc Am Soc Clin Oncol 2002;21:226a.

648. Baselga J, Trigo J, Bourhis J, et al. Cetuximab (C225) plus cisplatin/carboplatin is active in patients (pts) with recurrent/metastatic squamous cell carcinoma of the head and neck (SCCHN) progressing on a same dose and schedule platinum-based regimen [abstract 900]. Proc Am Soc Clin Oncol 2002;21:226a.
649. Trigo J, Hitt P, Koralewski E, et al. Cetuximab monotherapy is active in patients (pts) with platinum-refractory recurrent/metastatic squamous cell carcinoma of the head and neck (SSCH): Results of a phase II study [abstract]. Proc Am Soc Clin Oncol 2004;22:5502.
650. Cohen EE, Lingen MW, Vokes EE. The expanding role of systemic therapy in head and neck cancer. J Clin Oncol 2004;22:1743–52.
651. Vermorken JB, Bourhis J, Trigo J, et al. Cetuximab in recurrent/metastatic (R&M) squamous cell carcinoma of the head and neck (SCCHN) refractory to first-line platinum-based therapies [abstract 5505]. Proc Am Soc Clin Oncol 2005;23:16S.
652. Kane M, Cohen EE, List M, et al. Phase II study of 250 mg gefitinib in advanced squamous cell carcinoma of the head and neck (SCCHN) [abstract 5586]. Proc Am Soc Clin Oncol 2004;22:14S.
653. Shin DM, Donato NJ, Perez-Soler R, et al. Epidermal growth factor receptor-targeted therapy with C225 and cisplatin in patients with head and neck cancer. Clin Cancer Res 2001;7:1204–13.
654. Burtness B, Li Y, Flood W, et al. Phase III trial comparing cisplatin (C) + placebo (P) to C + anti-epidermal growth factor antibody (EGFR-R) C225 in patients (pts) with metastatic/recurrent head & neck cancer (HNC) [abstract 901]. Proc Am Soc Clin Oncol 2002;21:226a.
655. Bonner J, Harari P, Giralt J, et al. Cetuximab prolongs survival in patients with locoregionally advanced squamous cell carcinoma of head and neck: a phase III study of high dose radiation therapy with or without cetuximab [abstract 5507]. Proc Amer Soc Clin Oncol 2004;23:438s.
656. Clark G, Perez-Soler R, Siu LL, et al. Rash severity is predictive of increased survival with erlotinib HCI [abstract 786]. Proc Am Soc Clin Oncol 2003;22:196.
657. Saltz L, Kies M, Kearsley JH, et al. The presence and intensity of the cetuximab-induced acne-like rash predicts increased survival in studies across multiple malignancies [abstract 817]. Proc Am Soc Clin Oncol 2003;22:204.
658. Leonard JH, Kearsley JH, Chenevix-Trench G, et al. Analysis of gene amplification in head-and-neck squamous-cell carcinoma. Int J Cancer 1991;48:511–5.
659. Rowinsky EK, Windle JJ, Von Hoff DD. Ras protein farnesyltransferase: a strategic target for anticancer therapeutic development. J Clin Oncol 1999;17:3631–52.
660. Lobell RB, Liu D, Buser CA, et al. Preclinical and clinical pharmacodynamic assessment of L-778,123, a dual inhibitor of farnesyl:protein transferase and geranylgeranyl:protein transferase type-I. Mol Cancer Ther 2002;1:747–58.
661. Kelland LR, Smith V, Valenti M, et al. Preclinical antitumor activity and pharmacodynamic studies with the farnesyl protein transferase inhibitor R115777 in human breast cancer. Clin Cancer Res 2001;7:3544–50.
662. Johnston SR. Farnesyl transferase inhibitors: a novel targeted therapy for cancer. Lancet Oncol 2001;2:18–26.
663. Kies M, Clayman GL, El-Naggar A, et al. Induction therapy with SCH66336, a farnesyltransferase inhibitor, in squamous cell carcinoma (SCC) of the head and neck [abstract]. Proc Am Soc Clin Oncol 2001;20:225a.
664. Lingen MW, Polverini PJ, Bouck NP. Retinoic acid induces cells cultured from oral squamous cell carcinomas to become anti-angiogenic. Am J Pathol 1996;149:247–58.
665. Cohen RF, Contrino J, Spiro JD, et al. Interleukin-8 expression by head and neck squamous cell carcinoma. Arch Otolaryngol Head Neck Surg 1995;121:202–9.
666. Moriyama M, Kumagai S, Kawashiri S, et al. Immunohistochemical study of tumour angiogenesis in oral squamous cell carcinoma. Oral Oncol 1997;33:369–74.
667. Denhart BC, Guidi AJ, Tognazzi K, et al. Vascular permeability factor/vascular endothelial growth factor and its receptors in oral and laryngeal squamous cell carcinoma and dysplasia. Lab Invest 1997;77:659–64.
668. Inoue K, Ozeki Y, Suganuma T, et al. Vascular endothelial growth factor expression in primary esophageal squamous cell carcinoma. Association with angiogenesis and tumor progression. Cancer 1997;79:206–13.
669. Petruzzelli GJ, Benefield J, Taitz AD, et al. Heparin-binding growth factor(s) derived from head and neck squamous cell carcinomas induce endothelial cell proliferations. Head Neck 1997;19:576–82.
670. Kim KJ, Li B, Winer J, et al. Inhibition of vascular endothelial growth factor-induced angiogenesis suppresses tumour growth in vivo. Nature 1993;362:841–4.
671. Hori A, Sasada R, Matsutani E, et al. Suppression of solid tumor growth by immunoneutralizing monoclonal antibody against human basic fibroblast growth factor. Cancer Res 1991;51:6180–4.
672. Millauer B, Shawver LK, Plate KH, et al. Glioblastoma growth inhibited in vivo by a dominant-negative Flk-1 mutant. Nature 1994;367:576–9.
673. Hong WK, Lippman SM, Itri L, et al. Prevention of second primary tumors with isotretinoin in squamous cell carcinoma of the head and neck. N Engl J Med 1990;323:795–801.
674. Khuri F, Lee JJ, Lippman SM, et al. Isotretinoin effects on head and neck cancer recurrence and second primary tumors. Proc Annu Meet Am Soc Clin Oncol 2003;22:90.
675. Seixas-Silva JA Jr, Richards T, Khuri FR, et al. Phase 2 bioadjuvant study of interferon alfa-2a, isotretinoin, and vitamin E in locally advanced squamous cell carcinoma of the head and neck. Arch Otolaryngol Head Neck Surg 2005;131:304–7.
676. Zahalsky A, Wong R, Lis E, et al. Phase II trial of SU5416 in patients with advanced incurable head and neck cancer [abstract 902]. Proc Am Soc Clin Oncol 2002.
677. Winegarden J, Stenson K, Haraf D, et al. Phase I study of bevacizumab and FHX for poor prognosis head and neck cancer. Proc Am Soc Clin Oncol 2002.
678. Sandler A, Gray R, Brahmer J, et al. Randomized phase II/III trial of paclitaxel (P) plus carboplatin (C) with or without bevacizumab (NSC #704865) in patients with advanced non-squamous nonsmall cell lung cancer (NSCLC): an Eastern Cooperative Oncology Group (ECOG) Trial – E4599 [abstract LBA4]. Proc Am Soc Clin Oncol 2005;23:169.
679. Vokes E, Cohen EE, Mauer AM, et al. A phase I study of erlotinib and bevacizumab for recurrent or metastatic squamous cell carcinoma of the head and neck (HNC) [abstract 5504]. Proc Am Soc Clin Oncol 2005;23:501s.
680. Brizel DM, Dodge RK, Clough RW, et al. Oxygenation of head and neck cancer: changes during radiotherapy and impact on treatment outcome. Radiother Oncol 1999;53:113–7.
681. Peters LJ. Targeting hypoxia in head and neck cancer. Acta Oncol 2001;40:937–40.
682. Brizel DM, Sibley OS, Prosnitz LR, et al. Tumor Hypoxia adversely affects the prognosis of carcinoma of the head and neck. Int J Radiat Oncol Biol Phys 1997;38:285–9.
683. Brown JM, Siim BG. Hypoxia-specific cytotoxins in cancer therapy. Semin Radiat Oncol 1996;6:22–36.
684. Yer MJ. Bioeductive agents: a clinical update. Oncol Res 1997;9:392–5.
685. Haffty BG, Wilson LD, Son YH, et al. Concurrent chemoradiotherapy with mitomycin C compared with porfiromycin in squamous cell cancer of the head and neck: final results of a randomized clinical trial. Int J Radiat Oncol Biol Phys 2005;61:119–28.
686. Brown JM. SR 4233 (tirapazamine): a new anticancer drug exploiting hypoxia in solid tumors. Br J Cancer 1993;67:1163–70.
687. Brown JM, Lemmon MJ. Potentiation by the hypoxic cytotoxin SR4233 of cell killing produced by fractionated irradiation of mouse tumors. Cancer Res 1990;50:7745–9.
688. Dorio MJ, Brown JM. Tumor-specific, schedule-dependent interaction between tirapazamine (SR4233) and cisplatin. Cancer Res 1993;53:4633–6.
689. Rischin D, Peters L, Fisher R, et al. Tirapazamine, cisplatin, and radiation versus fluorouracil, cisplatin, and radiation in patients with locally advanced head and neck cancer: a randomized phase II trial of the Trans-Tasman Radiation Oncology Group (TROG 98.02). J Clin Oncol 2005 Jan 1;23(1):79–87.
690. Clayman GL, Frank DK, Bruso PA, et al. Adenovirus-mediated wild-type p53 gene transfer as a surgical adjuvant in advanced head and neck cancers. Clin Cancer Res 1999;5:1715–22.
691. Khuri FR, Nemunaitis J, Ganly I, et al. a controlled trial of intratumoral ONYX-015, a selectively-replicating adenovirus, in combination with cisplatin and 5-fluorouracil in patients with recurrent head and neck cancer. Nat Med 2000;6:879–85.

Section 27
THE THORAX

80

Cancer of the Lung

Amir Onn, MD
Ara A. Vaporciyan, MD
Joe Y. Chang, MD, PhD
Ritsuko Komaki, MD
Jack A. Roth, MD
Roy S. Herbst, MD, PhD

HISTORICAL NOTE

From practically nonexistent malignancy early in the twentieth century, lung cancer has become the most common cancer in the world and, in many countries, the most common cause of cancer-related death. The association between cigarette smoking and lung cancer is well established, and many of the molecular events in lung carcinogenesis have been identified. The long time period between initial exposure to tobacco carcinogens and the development of clinical lung cancer suggests that multiple steps are required for expression of the malignant phenotype, which is characterized by distinct tumor heterogeneity. Between 80 and 90% of all lung cancer cases are nonsmall-cell lung cancer (NSCLC), and most of the others are small-cell lung cancer (SCLC). In contrast to other common solid cancers, lung cancer has no well-established methods for early detection, and most cases are diagnosed in an advanced stage. Although there has been improvement in treatment options, including surgical techniques, chemotherapy, and radiation therapy, the overall 5-year survival rate for patients with lung cancer remains low, at less than 15%.[1] The landscape of lung cancer is beginning to change. In recent years, our understanding of the biology in different subsets of lung cancer has improved significantly, leading to the discovery of several potential molecular targets and the development of novel agents that inhibit their activity. These findings are already translating into improvements in patient survival and quality of life (QOL). Most dramatic has been the introduction of the epidermal growth factor receptor (EGFR) tyrosine kinase inhibitors (TKIs) gefitinib (Iressa, AstraZeneca) and erlotinib (Tarceva, Genentech). Monotherapy with these drugs may prolong survival and improve symptoms in subsets of lung cancer patients. Furthermore, gain-of-function somatic mutations of EGFR have been identified and correlated with response to EGFR inhibitors.[2] Advances have been noted in angiogenesis therapy, and bevacizumab (Avastin, Genentech), a monoclonal antibody to vascular endothelial growth factor (VEGF), has been found to prolong survival in patients with advanced disease when administered in combination with chemotherapy.[3] In addition to advances in molecular targeted therapy, newer and safer strategies for chemotherapy and radiation therapy are being implemented: Adjuvant platinum-based chemotherapy has been introduced to some patients undergoing surgery for early-stage disease,[4] newer chemotherapeutics such as pemetrexed (Alimta, Eli Lilly) have efficacies similar to those of older agents with fewer adverse events (AEs),[5] and newer regimens have shown beneficial efficacy and safety profiles in the elderly.[6] This review provides an overview of the causes, diagnosis, and therapy of lung cancer as we understand it.

ETIOLOGY AND EPIDEMIOLOGY

Worldwide, lung cancer is the most common (1.35 million of 10.9 million new cases) and the deadliest form of cancer (1.18 million of 6.7 million cancer-related deaths).[7] The United States 2005 cancer statistics, published recently, [8] suggest that lung cancer is the second most common cancer for both men and women (13% and 12% of all cases, respectively), but, as in previous years for both sexes, it is the number one cause of cancer death (90,000 men, 31% of all cancer-related deaths, and 73,000 women, 27% of all cancer-related deaths). In fact, more people in the United States die of lung cancer than of the next three causes of cancer-related death—prostate cancer, breast cancer, and colorectal cancer—combined.[8] In 1920, fewer than 1,000 cases of lung cancer were reported, and it was regarded as a rare malignancy. Since the 1950s, however, lung cancer has been recognized as a major public health problem. The incidence of new cases rose first in men and reached a peak in the mid 1980s; a steady decline has been noted since then. The incidence in women increased until the late 1990s and has recently stabilized. These changes occurred in parallel to the widespread adoption of cigarette smoking by both sexes. The decline in lung cancer incidence and mortality among men has been explained by reduction in smoking rates.[9]

SMOKING AND LUNG CANCER

Tobacco is the world's single most avoidable cause of death. The World Health Organization (WHO) has calculated that the 5.6 trillion cigarettes smoked per year at the close of the twentieth century will cause nearly 10 million fatalities per year by 2030. Lung cancer is the most common tobacco-related cause of cancer mortality: One case occurs for every 3 million cigarettes smoked. As described by Proctor, cancers caused by tobacco were among the earliest discovered environmental cancers.[10] First reports on the association between tobacco use and cancer of the oral cavity and lip were published in Europe in the eighteenth and nineteenth centuries. More than 60 years ago, Muller in Germany was the first to recognize the positive association between cigarette smoking and lung cancer. Since then, multiple epidemiological studies have confirmed these observations and elaborated on the molecular mechanisms of smoking carcinogenesis, providing sufficient evidence to establish a strong causal association between cigarette smoking and cancer of the aerodigestive tract (lung, oral cavity, pharynx, larynx, nasal cavities, paranasal sinuses, nasopharynx, esophagus, stomach, liver, and pancreas), urinary bladder, kidney (renal cell carcinoma), and uterine cervix, as well as myeloid leukemia. Other forms of tobacco smoking, such as cigars, pipes, and bidis, also increase risk of cancer, including cancer of the lung and parts of the upper aerodigestive tract. A meta-analysis of over 50 studies on involuntary smoking among never-smokers showed a consistent and statistically significant association between exposure to environmental tobacco smoke and lung cancer risk.[10]

Smoking is currently responsible for a third of all cancer deaths in many Western countries and is a rapidly growing cause of morbidity and mortality in many other countries. It has been estimated that every other smoker will be killed by tobacco.[10,11] To date, smoking accounts for about 85 to 90% of lung cancer deaths in both sexes. The rate at which lung cancer develops is strongly correlated with the duration of tobacco exposure. After 45, 30, and 15 years of cigarette smoking, the annual incidence rates of lung cancer are 0.5%, 0.1%, and under 0.01%, respectively. Thus, a 3-fold increase in the duration of tobacco use can increase the annual incidence of lung cancer by 50-fold. As smoking ceases, the annual risk remains roughly constant thereafter. For instance, after 30 years of smoking, the risk is approximately 0.1%, and if a smoker stops after 30 years, this annual rate will persist indefinitely. Thus, 15 years later, the annual risk is 0.1% instead of 0.5%, which it would have been if smoking had continued. About 80% of the risk is, therefore, avoided by stopping smoking.[12]

In contrast to the decline in smoking rates in men are worrisome reports of increases in cigarette smoking amongst youngsters, and especially on college campuses nationwide, where approximately 40% of students define themselves as active smokers. This is irrespective of the type of college or students' sex, ethnicity, or year in college.[13]

Passive Smoking Smokers are not the only people at increased risk from exposure to tobacco smoke. "Passive smoking" from environmental tobacco smoke also increases the risk of lung cancer death. According to the Environmental Protection Agency, each year about 3,000 nonsmoking adults die of lung cancer as a result of breathing the smoke of others' cigarettes. Analysis has shown that the sidestream smoke emitted from a smoldering cigarette between puffs contains virtually all carcinogenic compounds that have been identified in the mainstream smoke inhaled by smokers. Even though passive smokers are exposed to much lower concentrations of these carcinogens than active smokers, environmental tobacco smoke has become the only agent ever classified by the Environmental Protection Agency as a human carcinogen for which an increased cancer risk has actually been observed at typical environmental levels of exposure.[14] The risk of dying of lung cancer is 30% higher for a nonsmoker living with a smoker than for those living in a totally tobacco-free household.[15]

Cigarette Smoke Composition Dozens of compounds have been identified in cigarette smoke, both particles (solid phase) and gases (vapor phase). More than 60 of these agents have been shown to be carcinogenic in laboratory animals, and some of them are also carcinogenic in humans, including benzo[a]pyrene, a polycyclic aromatic hydrocarbon; aromatic amines; formaldehyde; benzene; and miscellaneous inorganic and organic compounds. Tobacco also contains specific carcinogens related to nicotine, such as 4-(*N*-methyl-*N*-nitrosamino)-1-(3-pyridyl)-1-butanone (NNK), a strong carcinogen in rodents.[16] Following 5 to 20 years of exposure to these agents, certain changes occur in airway epithelium as described in the next sections, leading in some cases to the development of cancer.[10]

LUNG CANCER IN WOMEN

For most of the past 100 years, lung cancer has generally been thought of as a disease affecting primarily men. In the past several decades, however, the incidence of lung cancer has risen among women in the United States and most other parts of the world. Although incidence is still higher among men than women, the gap has narrowed and lung cancer has become the leading cause of cancer death among American women. The rise in rates of lung cancer among women has paralleled the increase in the prevalence of cigarette smoking. Just as in men, the majority (85–90%) of lung cancers among women are considered the result of smoking. There is accumulating evidence suggesting that the development of lung cancer is different in women than in men. For example, women smokers are more likely than men to develop adenocarcinoma of the lung, and women who have never smoked are more likely to develop lung cancer than men who have never smoked. Furthermore, the 5-year survival rate for women who have lung cancer is 15.6%, while it is 12.4% for men; women survive longer after surgical resection of early-stage lung cancer as well as after treatment of metastatic disease; female sex has been associated with longer survival in SCLC as well. Hormonal, genetic, and metabolic differences between the sexes are believed to account for these clinical differences. Indeed, estrogens were found to be involved in lung carcinogenesis, either by acting as estrogen receptor ligands and activating cellular proliferation pathways, or by metabolic activation to reactive intermediates that can produce DNA adducts and cause oxidative damage.[17,18]

Since smoking remains the primary cause of lung cancer, the differences in the clinical profile of the disease between the sexes have been attributed to different response to tobacco carcinogens. Indeed, in the 1990s, several case-control studies indicated that relative risks of lung cancer associated with specific amounts and duration of cigarette smoking may actually be higher among women than among men. Bain and colleagues recently performed a meta-analysis on prospective cohorts to examine this hypothesis and found that women do not appear to have a greater susceptibility to lung cancer than men, given equal smoking exposure.[18] These data are important because they arise from carefully conducted monitoring since 1986 of large cohorts of female nurses (> 60,000) and male health professionals (> 25,000). In total, approximately 1,300 lung cancers were observed in current and former smokers in these cohorts, a sufficient number of cases for the kind of detailed analyses needed to control covariates such as age at start of smoking, age at quitting smoking, height, weight, and diet. The key finding was that the ratio of exposure-standardized lung cancer incidence rates for female current smokers to male current smokers was 1:1. The same ratio of 1:1 was also found for former smokers (95% confidence interval [CI] = 0.95–1.31). In analyses by histologic type of lung cancer, the data confirmed previous findings that female smokers did have a significantly higher rate of adenocarcinoma than male smokers.[18] The equal rates of lung cancer mortality in younger US men and women, corresponding to an era when smoking prevalence in the sexes was equal, also provide evidence against a major sex difference in susceptibility to smoking-induced lung cancer.[19] These data suggest that, although women are not more susceptible than men to smoking-induced lung cancer, the clinical characteristics of their disease differ from those of lung cancer in men.

FAMILIAL PREDISPOSITION

It is interesting that the vast majority of cigarette smokers, including heavy smokers, do not develop lung cancer. This suggests that cancer formation is dependent on an inherited predisposition or cofactors such as additional carcinogens. Studies that have compared risk factors of individuals with histologically confirmed lung cancer and of individuals with other smoking-related cancers found that having relatives with lung cancer did not increase the risk of developing lung cancer, but it did increase the risk of having cancer at some site.[20] This suggests a heritable variation in response to carcinogens. Respiratory diseases also predispose to development of lung cancer. Studies of families predisposed to lung cancer showed that the development of lung cancer in young individuals (aged 50 years or younger) was compatible with Mendelian codominant inheritance or a rare autosomal gene.[21] This gene was involved to a lesser degree in individuals older than 50 years who developed lung cancer, suggesting that the cause of cancer in these noncarriers was long-term exposure to tobacco. Bailey-Wilson and colleagues recently studied the susceptibility genes for familial lung cancer and conducted a genome-wide linkage analysis of 52 extended pedigrees ascertained through probands with lung cancer who had several first-degree relatives with the same disease. The results localized a major susceptibility locus influencing lung cancer risk on chromosome 6q23-25.[22]

Table 80-1 Documented Occupational Lung Carcinogens

Substance	Occupational Exposures
Arsenic	Smelters, pesticide manufacturers
Asbestos	Miners, millers, insulators, railroad and shipyard workers
Chloromethylethers	Ion-exchange resin manufacturers
Chromium	Chromate and pigment manufacturers
Hydrocarbons	Coal-gas workers, roofers
Mustard gas	Poison-gas manufacturers
Nickel	Refiners
Radiation	Miners of uranium and other ores

Adapted from: Frank AL. Epidemiology of lung cancer. In: Roth JA, Ruchdeschel T, Weisenburger T, editors. Thoracic oncology. Philadelphia: WB Saunders; 1989.

Table 80-2 Major Genetic Aberrations in NSCLC and SCLC

		NSCLC	SCLC
MYC	Amplifications	5–20%	20–35%
RAS	Mutations	15–20%	< 1%
EGFR	Mutations	20%	—
INK4a	LOH	70%	50%
p16^{INK4A}	Mutations	20–50%	< 5%
p14^{ARF}	Mutations	20%	65%
TP53	LOH	60%	75–100%
	Mutations	50%	75%
RB	LOH	30%	70%
	Mutations	15–30%	90%
FHIT	Mutations	40%	80%
TSG101	Mutations	—	90%[a]
DMBT1	Mutations	40–50%	100%
LOH in various regions	*3p*	70–80%	90–100%
	4p	10–20%	50%
	4q	30%	80%
	8p	80–100%	80–90%
Promoter hypermethylation			
RASSFIA	30–40%	90–100%	
INK4a	*p16*	25–40%	ND
	p14^{ARF}	8%	ND
RAR		40%	70%
TIMP-3		25%	ND
CDH1		55%	ND
DAPK		19%	ND
GSTP1		1%	ND
MGMT		20–40%	ND

NSCLC = nonsmall-cell lung cancer; SCLC = small-cell lung cancer; LOH = loss of heterozygosity; DMBT1 = deleted in malignant brain tumor; ND = not determined; TIMP-3 = tissue inhibitors of metalloproteinase-3; CDH1 = E-cadherin; DAPK = death-associated protein kinase; GSTP1 = glutathione S transferase P1; MGMT = O6-methylguanine-DNA methyltransferase.
Modified from: Meuwissen R, Berns A. Genes Dev. 2005;19:643–64.

OTHER ENVIRONMENTAL CAUSES

Lung cancer occurs in association with occupational and environmental exposures to carcinogenic agents other than tobacco smoke. Occupational agents classified as Group 1 carcinogens by the International Agency for Research on Cancer include inorganic arsenic, asbestos, bis(chloromethyl)ether, chromium (hexavalent), nickel and nickel compounds, polycyclic aromatic compounds, radon, and vinyl chloride. Group 2A of probable carcinogens include acrylonitrile, beryllium, cadmium, formaldehyde, acetaldehyde, synthetic fibers, silica, and welding fumes. Currently, occupational exposures have been estimated to account for 5 to 15% of all lung cancer cases worldwide (Table 80-1). In areas where shipbuilding was or is a major industry, asbestos exposure appears to be a clear etiologic agent, synergistically with cigarette smoking. Occupational risk for miners traditionally included development of pneumoconioses, chronic obstructive pulmonary disease (COPD), and lung cancer when exposed to radon, uranium, and others compounds. Radon is a gas that accumulates in basements, and indoor radon exposure has been reported to be an important cause of lung cancer in the general population.[23]

MOLECULAR PATHOGENESIS

The rapidly developing technology of molecular biology has allowed the identification of multiple genes responsible for lung carcinogenesis. Interestingly, these genes are altered forms of genes normally present in eukaryotic cells. The plethora of genetic abnormalities and redundancy of altered pathways induced by tobacco and other carcinogens determines lung cancer heterogeneity, which is remarkable in comparison to that of other solid tumors. In this regard, it has to be remembered that individual tumors are characterized by specific genetic alternation(s) and that there is a gradual accumulation of abnormalities in a given tumor, from normal epithelium to invasive carcinoma. This section summarizes areas of recent investigation of molecular events in human lung cancer. Table 80-2 lists genes that have been implicated in lung carcinogenesis.

The gene families implicated in lung carcinogenesis include dominant oncogenes and tumor suppressor genes.[24,25] Proto-oncogenes (normal homologues of the oncogenes) participate in critical cell functions, including signal transduction and transcription. Only a single mutant allele is required for malignant transformation. Primary modifications in the dominant oncogenes that confer gain of transforming function include point mutation, amplification, translocation, and rearrangement. A dynamic interplay exists within the cell between dominant oncogenes and tumor suppressor genes that constrain cell proliferation. Tumor suppressor genes appear to require homozygous loss of function by mutation, deletion, or a combination of these. Tumor suppressor genes appear to play a role in the governance of proliferation by regulating transcription and the cell cycle.

ONCOGENES ***ras* Family** The *ras* family of oncogenes (homologous to the rat sarcoma virus) has three primary members (H-*ras*, K-*ras*, and N-*ras*) that are among the most common activated oncogenes found in human cancer. The *ras* genes encode for proteins located on the inner surface of the plasma membrane, have GTPase activity, and play a role in transducing growth-promoting and survival signals from membrane-bound receptor tyrosine kinases. Hydrolysis of bound GTP to GDP abrogates *ras* signaling, but oncogenic mutations in *ras* impair GTP hydrolysis, causing persistent signaling. The *ras* oncogenes acquire their transforming capacity by point mutations that are detected in 20 to 30% of lung adenocarcinomas and 20% of all NSCLCs. Most point mutations are GT transversions and are correlated with smoking. The mutations are found most frequently in codon 12, followed by mutations in codons 13 and 61. Ninety percent of the mutations are found in K-*ras* in lung adenocarcinomas, whereas no *ras* mutations have been detected in SCLC. The presence of K-*ras* mutations marks a poor prognosis for both early- and late-stage NSCLC.[26] Studies in mice with carcinogen-induced lung cancers implicated genes of the *ras* family in the process of carcinogenesis. Mouse lung tumors induced by tetranitromethane contained mutated K-*ras* genes, and mice harboring the mutated H-*ras* transgene developed tumors exclusively in the lungs within weeks after birth. Lung tumors can be induced in mice with the tobacco-specific nitrosamines NNK or nitrosodimethylamine. Ninety percent of these tumors have transforming genes revealed by the NIH 3T3 assay; the gene was K-*ras* in all lung tumors. The mutations were generally GC to AT transitions, indicating that DNA methylation is the most likely pathway to induction of neoplasia by these carcinogens.[27] Mutations of *ras* can influence the differentiation of tumor cells. For example, infection of SCLC cell lines with the Harvey murine sarcoma virus alters the phenotype of variant but not classic cells. Following infection, the variant SCLC cell line developed features of a large-cell undifferentiated lung carcinoma, including increased carcinoembryonic antigen and keratin expression.

Activation of *ras* has been regarded as sufficient to promote lung cancer progression, but not to induce abnormal cellular proliferation in the absence of cooperating oncogenes. Tuveson and colleagues recently showed, however, that endogenous oncogenic *ras* is sufficient to initiate transformation by stimulating proliferation, while further genetic lesions may be necessary for progression to frank malignancy.[28]

Studies from the laboratory of Dr. J. A. Roth examined antisense technologies to determine the effects of eliminating expression of a mutant K-*ras* oncogene on NSCLC, using in vitro and in vivo models. They showed that reversal of a single genetic abnormality was sufficient to prevent human cancer cells from forming tumors and suggested that it may not be necessary to reverse all the genetic lesions in a cancer cell to achieve a therapeutic effect. These observations raise the intriguing possibility of specific gene therapy for cancer. Gene sequences could be delivered to tumor cells via viral vectors that specifically inhibit expression of the oncogenes activated in the cancer cell. Such constructs would be relatively nontoxic because, as in the example just described, they could target a single gene whose function may be assumed by other redundant genes of the same family. This concept was tested in an orthotopic human lung cancer cell model in nude mice in which a retroviral vector expressing antisense K-*ras*, administered via intratracheal instillation, suppressed tumor growth.[29]

***myc* Family** Ultimate targets of the *ras* signaling pathway are C-*myc*, N-*myc*, and L-*myc*, which are transcription factors that play a role in proliferation and apoptosis. These proto-oncogenes encode basic helix-loop-helix transcription factors that regulate the expression of genes involved in DNA synthesis, RNA metabolism, and cell-cycle regulation. Activation of *myc* genes occurs by amplification or loss of transcriptional control, which results in Myc protein overexpression. In SCLC, C-*myc*, N-*myc*, and L-*myc* are often amplified and aberrantly expressed, whereas in NSCLC, only C-*myc* is found affected and only in a fraction of the tumors. *myc* amplification occurs in 15 to 30% of SCLCs and 5 to 10% of NSCLCs. Increased *myc* mRNA levels were detected in 36% of SCLC cell lines derived from resected metastatic tumors from patients who experienced relapse after chemotherapy. Amplification of *myc* could therefore be indicative of poor prognosis.[30]

GROWTH FACTORS AND AUTOCRINE–PARACRINE GROWTH CONTROL

Tumor cells that produce a growth factor and express its receptor may show self-stimulatory or autocrine growth. Cells that are regulated by an autocrine loop have several features. They secrete a ligand, which is a biologically active growth factor, and demonstrate increased proliferation in response to that factor. Growth factors also may act to stimulate growth in adjacent cells in a paracrine manner. Interaction of ligand and receptor in the cytoplasm of the cell may form an internal autocrine loop.

Autocrine growth factors have been implicated in the stimulation of SCLC tumor cell growth. The majority of SCLC cell lines produce bombesin, a 14-amino acid peptide that is identical to a carboxy-terminal heptapeptide sequence of a mammalian analogue, gastrin-releasing peptide. SCLC cell lines express a single class of high-affinity, saturable binding receptors for bombesin. Bombesin is also a potent stimulator of clonal growth for human NSCLC. Bombesin receptors have not been demonstrated on NSCLC.

Epidermal Growth Factor Receptor (HER1, ErbB) The epidermal growth factor receptor (EGFR) signaling pathway is activated in many tumor cells, but is strictly controlled in normal tissue. The EGFR family comprises EGFR HER1 (or ErbB1), HER2 (ErbB2), HER3 (ErbB3), and HER4 (ErbB4). These receptors share a common molecular structure that consists of an amino-terminal extracellular domain, a single transmembrane-anchoring region, and a carboxyl-terminal intracellular domain that has tyrosine kinase activity. They present in the cell as inactive monomers and, upon ligand binding, form homodimers or heterodimers. This results in autophosphorylation of the intracellular tyrosine kinase domains and activation of signaling pathways that induce several tumorigenic processes. Among the pathways activated by the EGFR are the mitogen-activated protein kinase (MAPK) pathway, which regulates gene transcription and proliferation, and the phosphatidylinositol 3, 4, 5 kinase (PI3K)/protein kinase B (PKB or Akt) signaling pathway, which mediates cell survival. Several molecules have been identified that can specifically bind and activate these receptors. For example, EGF and transforming growth factor-alpha (TGF-α) bind to EGFR, whereas no specific ligand has been identified for HER2.[31] The EGFR is highly expressed in many solid tumors and at all disease stages. The proportion of tumors expressing EGFR varies by tumor type and may be due to different detection methods or because no accepted standards define normal or elevated levels of expression. Forty to 80% of lung cancer tumors express EGFR. High levels of expression have been associated with poor outcome in many solid tumors; however, this is controversial in lung cancer.[32] EGFR signaling may be increased by a number of mechanisms besides high expression levels of EGFR, including receptor mutations, heterodimerization with other members of this receptor family such as HER2 (erbB2), increased expression of (autocrine/paracrine) ligands, and alterations in molecules that control receptor signaling output. Each of these activities could be assessed to give an indication of the magnitude of EGFR signal amplification.[33]

HER2 (ErbB2) HER2 is a member of the EGFR family that lacks ligand activation and exerts its activity via heterodimerization with other members in this family. HER2 acts as a common receptor subunit of other ErbB proteins because it enhances ligand-induced receptor activation, potentiates and prolongs the signal transduction pathways, and increases the affinity of the receptors for their ligands. Indeed, EGFR-HER2 or HER2-HER3 heterodimers have longer and greater proliferative signals than the corresponding homodimers. For example, synchronous overexpression of EGFR and HER2 at the protein level, which probably designates receptor heterodimerization, was detected in 10% of patients with stage I NSCLC, and predicted poor outcome.[34] The role of HER2 in patients with invasive breast cancer is well established and is correlated with shortened disease-free survival and resistance to chemotherapy and endocrine therapy. Its role in lung cancer has not been fully determined. A recent meta-analysis suggested that 31% of patients with lung cancer express HER2, mainly those with adenocarcinoma, and only a few with SCLC. Although most studies correlated HER2 overexpression with poor prognosis, results were not conclusive.[35]

TUMOR SUPPRESSOR GENES

Inactivation of certain genes may contribute to tumor growth. In one scenario, both copies of the gene must be eliminated or inactivated to eradicate the growth-suppressive function of the gene.[25] Because both copies must be eliminated, the tumor suppressor gene is called recessive. This model was developed to explain the inheritance pattern of retinoblastoma. Patients with a familial predisposition to retinoblastoma have a germline inactivation of one copy of the retinoblastoma (*Rb*) gene. The tumor develops when the wild-type allele is either inactivated or deleted. Development of the sporadic form of retinoblastoma requires two somatic mutations. This model has spawned multiple studies searching for consistent chromosomal deletions in human tumors.

One of the earliest known and most consistent chromosomal deletions in lung cancer occurs in chromosome 3 (p14–p23) in SCLC.[36] Allelic loss in this region was documented with polymorphic DNA probes and was seen to occur at a high frequency. Loss of heterozygosity for alleles on chromosomes 3, 11, 13, and 17 occurs in NSCLC as well.[37] The fragile histidine triad (*FHIT*) gene, which is located at the 3p14.2 fragile site, is abnormal in many lung cancers, and its protein product is often not expressed.[38] This suggests that it may be functioning as a tumor suppressor gene. Restoration of expression of *FHIT* in human lung cancer cells that do not express the protein triggered apoptosis and suppression of tumor growth in a xenograft mouse model, confirming the tumor suppressor function of this gene.[39]

The high frequency of chromosomal deletions in both SCLC and NSCLC suggested that loss of specific gene function might be a critical step in the development of lung cancer. Two additional candidate tumor suppressor genes in lung cancer are the genes encoding the nuclear phosphoproteins, *TP53* and *Rb*.

Loss of heterozygosity on chromosome 13q suggests that the R locus, located at 13q14, is deleted. Studies show that up to 60% of SCLC and 75% of carcinoid cell lines do not express *Rb* mRNA. Of 13 SCLC cell lines reviewed in one study, only three expressed more than a trace amount of *Rb* mRNA. The role of *Rb* in NSCLC appears variable. In one study, 90% of NSCLC cell lines expressed *Rb*. In contrast, other studies have shown a significantly higher involvement of altered *Rb* function. One study, for example, found that Rb protein was absent in 10 of 36 immunostained primary NSCLC tumors.

The *TP53* gene encodes a 375-amino-acid phosphoprotein that can form complexes with host proteins such as large T antigen and E1B. Missense mutations that result in loss of suppressor function are common in the *TP53* gene. The *TP53* gene appears multifunctional, with major domains that can transactivate, bind proteins, bind sequence-specific DNA, and oligomerize with *TP53*. Abnormalities in one or more of these functions could contribute to abrogation of the tumor suppressor function of *TP53*. Certain mutations also have a dominant transforming capability. The wild-type *TP53* gene may suppress genes that contribute to uncontrolled cell growth and proliferation or activate genes that suppress uncontrolled cell growth. Thus, either absence or inactivation of wild-type *TP53* may contribute to transformation. Some studies indicate, however, that the presence of the mutant *TP53* may be necessary for full expression of the transforming potential of the gene.

Mutations of *TP53* are common in a wide spectrum of tumors.[40] These mutations occur in both NSCLC and SCLC cell lines and in fresh tumors. The precise role of these mutations in oncogenesis and the mechanisms involved are subjects of active investigation. Mutations in *TP53* positively correlate with lifetime cigarette consumption.[41] Radon exposure, which increases lung cancer risk, is also associated with *TP53* mutations, although the types of mutations differ from those seen in tobacco-associated lung cancer.[42] Insertion of a wild-type *TP53* gene in lung cancer cell lines with a mutant or deleted *TP53* can suppress their growth, even though the cells have multiple genetic lesions.[43] This may occur because of the multiple pathways, including cell cycle and apoptosis, regulated by *TP53*. The TP53 protein may be overexpressed in lung cancer cells, although this is not always associated with the presence of a mutant *TP53* gene. Overexpression of the *TP53* protein has correlated positively, however, with a poor prognosis.[43,44] Deletions in 17p, *TP53* mutations, and 3p deletions have been detected in preneoplastic lesions of the lung, such as severe dysplasia. Mutations in *TP53* and *ras* appear to be independent events. Other candidate tumor suppressor genes include the *APC* and *MCC* genes, first identified in colon cancers.

The therapeutic efficacy of direct administration of a retroviral vector expressing wild-type *TP53* in an orthotopic human lung cancer model has been shown.[45] The wild-type *TP53* retroviral vector suppressed tumor formation in 62 to 100% of the mice, and the effect depended on the amount of virus given.

Development of an adenoviral vector for delivery of wild-type *TP53* has been reported.[46] A high level of expression of exogenous *TP53* was achieved in *TP53*-deleted human lung cancer cells that were infected with the adenovirus-*TP53* vector. Expression lasted for 15 days, which was sufficient for mediating apoptosis of the lung cancer cells. The growth of normal human bronchial epithelial cells taking up the vector was not affected. The efficacy of the adenovirus *TP53* vector in inhibiting tumorigenicity was shown in the mouse model of orthotopic human lung cancer and was similar to that seen with the retrovirus-*TP53* construct.[29]

Clinical trials have begun to assess the feasibility of using gene transfer technology to restore defective tumor suppressor gene function in cancer patients. In the first human clinical trial, nine patients with NSCLC who had tumors with documented *TP53* mutation received a retroviral vector containing the wild-type *TP53* gene under the control of a β-actin promoter.[47] Regression of the injected lesion was seen in three patients, whereas stabilization of disease was seen in three others. One patient had progressive disease, and two were unevaluable (one was intolerant of the general anesthetic and did not complete treatment, and one died within 3 weeks of treatment). These results have been supported by a more recent two-arm study in which a wild-type *TP53* gene was given to 52 patients with NSCLC via an adenoviral vector.[45] Patients received adenovirus-*TP53* (Ad-*TP53*), either alone or preceded by cisplatin. Either bronchoscopically or under computed tomography (CT) guidance, *TP53* treatment was given as a single intratumoral injection once per month for up to 6 months. Both clinical and laboratory evidence of *TP53* expression were observed. PFS interval was longer with Ad-*TP53* and cisplatin as compared with Ad-*TP53* alone. A majority of patients also had evidence of vector DNA upon PCR analysis of post-treatment biopsies. Although antiadenovirus antibodies were detected in all patients after one treatment, subsequent treatments were not accompanied by anaphylaxis or other toxic effects except transient fever. Furthermore, despite high levels of serum antiadenovirus antibody, *TP53* transgene expression occurred in the tumor cells, and clinical responses were maintained.

Even though these studies corrected only one of the many genetic abnormalities present in NSCLC, the evidence suggests an antitumor effect based directly on *TP53*-mediated apoptosis. The two trials provided no evidence for the view that tumor stabilization and regression resulted from a nonspecific immune reaction.

A subsequent study combining Ad-*TP53* with external beam radiation therapy showed a high rate of response with no increase in rates of adverse events.[48] In this study, 19 patients with nonmetastatic NSCLC who were not eligible for chemoradiation or surgery were treated with radiation therapy to 60 Gy over 6 weeks in conjunction with three intratumoral injections of Ad-*TP53*. Seventeen of 19 patients completed all planned therapy. The most common adverse events were grade 1 or 2 fevers (79%) and chills (53%). Complete response was noted in 1 of 19 patients (5%), partial response in 11 cases (58%), stable disease in 3 (16%), progressive disease in 2 (11%), and not evaluable in 2 (11%).

A common theme with many of the genetic lesions occurring in cancers is their relationship to regulation of progression through the cell cycle. Premature entry of cells into the next phase of the cell cycle may prevent completion of important molecular events such as DNA repair and may lead to genetic instability. The cell cycle may pause at both the G_1 and G_2 checkpoints. Phosphorylation of the Rb protein releases the transcription factor E2F and mediates transition across the G_1 checkpoint. Inactivation of *Rb* by mutation or deletion could therefore cause a state of activation. A gene encoding an inhibitor (called variously p21, WAF1, Cip1, or Sdi1) of the proteins that mediate cell-cycle progression (cyclins) is one of the downstream effectors of *TP53* and mediates G_1 arrest. Another inhibitor of the cyclin system is *p16*. This gene is frequently inactivated in many cancers, including lung cancer.

Several other genes (eg, *hSRBC*, *SEMA3B*) are newly identified tumor suppressor gene candidates.[49] Other tumor suppressor genes less frequently involved include *PTEN*, *hOGG1* (DNA repair), and *BAP1* (ubiquination). Many tumor suppressor genes in lung cancer (*APC*, *CDH13*, *RAR*, *FHIT*, *RASSF1A*, *TIMP3*, *p16*, *MGMT*, *SEMA3B*, *DAPK*) appear to be inactivated by promoter hypermethylation.[50] Allelic losses on chromosome arm 3p are the most frequent and earliest genetic abnormalities detected in human lung cancers, indicating the presence of one or more lung cancer tumor suppressor genes in this region. In particular, a 600 kb lung cancer homozygous deletion region at 3p21.3 shows frequent allele loss in tumors and smoking-damaged lung epithelium. A group of candidate tumor suppressor genes in this small region have been identified. Several (*CACNA2D2*, *BLU*, *RASSF1A* isoform, and *SEMA3B*) had their expression extinguished by tumor-acquired promoter DNA methylation. By using a variety of expression vectors, it was found that several of the candidate 3p21.3 tumor suppressor genes (*FUS1*, *101F6*, *NPRL2*, and *SEMA3B*) effectively inhibited tumor cell growth by induction of apoptosis in vitro and in vivo, whereas others (*RASSF1A* and *CACNA2D2*) efficiently inhibited anchorage-independent growth in vitro and xenograft growth in vivo without inducing apoptosis (*RASSF1A*) or inducing apoptosis only in *TP53* wild-type tumors (*CACNA2D2*), strongly suggesting that several of these contiguous 3p21.3 genes function as lung tumor suppressors.[51]

ANGIOGENESIS

Like any other solid tumor, lung cancer growth, progression, invasion, and metastasis depend on adequate vasculature and angiogenesis. Angiogenesis denotes formation of new blood vessels. Small tumors may depend on diffusion of oxygen and nutrients, but to grow to more than 2 to 3 mm^3, tumors must induce angiogenesis. A balance between proangiogenic and antiangiogenic molecules regulates tumor angiogenesis. One of the major regulators in these processes is the VEGF, originally discovered as vascular permeability factor. Increased tumor angiogenesis, which can be identified by overexpression of VEGF, is associated with a worse clinical outcome in NSCLC. Three isoforms of membrane-bound VEGF receptors (VEGFR) have been identified, and their roles in angiogenesis appear to be distinct. VEGFR-1 (also known as fms-like tyrosine kinase-1) has the highest binding affinity for VEGF but is capable of generating relatively little kinase activity. VEGFR-2 (also known as kinase domain region or fetal liver kinase-1) is the isotype most associated with endothelial cell proliferation and chemotaxis. VEGFR-2 has been found in breast, ovarian, and lung tumor tissues and in glioma tissue, indicating that VEGF plays a role in these cancers and leading researchers to identify this receptor as a potential target. VEGFR-3 (also known as fms-like tyrosine kinase-4) appears to regulate primarily lymphangiogenesis. Likewise, other proangiogenic factors, interleukin-8, and basic fibroblast growth factor are considered bad prognostic markers in lung cancer.[52]

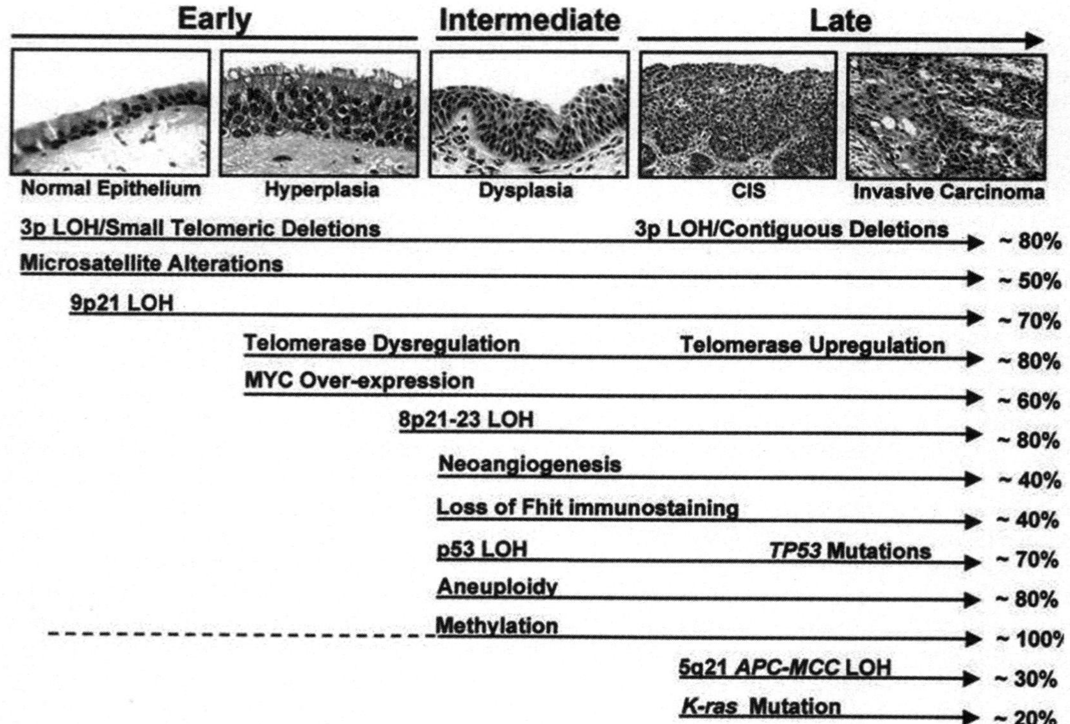

Figure 80-1 Sequential pathogenetic changes involved in lung cancer. Although multiple genetic markers (indicated by the arrows) are abnormal in lung cancers, the timing of their appearance during the lengthy preneoplastic process varies. Several alterations have been described in histologically normal specimens of bronchial epithelium from smokers. Other changes (such as hyperplasia and metaplasia) have been detected in slightly abnormal epithelium and are regarded as early changes. Molecular changes detected frequently in dysplasia are regarded as intermediate in timing, whereas those usually detected in carcinoma in situ or invasive stages are regarded as late changes. Modified from Hirsch FR. Clin Cancer Res 2001;7:5–22, with permission.

MOLECULAR ABNORMALITIES IN PREMALIGNANCY

Structural and genetic epithelial changes occur gradually, and invasive carcinoma develops 5 to 20 years after initial insult to the airways (Figure 80-1). Loss of specific chromosomal regions on a single allele (loss of heterozygosity [LOH]) has been detected frequently in lung cancers and bronchial epithelia exposed to tobacco carcinogens. The regions of earliest and most frequent allelic loss are 3p21, 3p22-24, 3p25, and 9p21.[53] It is noteworthy that many of these changes are seen in histologically normal bronchial epithelium from smokers, but not nonsmokers.[54] However, these changes appear to become more frequent and extensive in terms of chromosome loss with advancing abnormality of premalignancy. In some cases, these molecular changes appear to be clonally independent. Methylated sequences of tumor suppressor gene promoters can be detected in tumors, smoking-damaged normal lung (preneoplastic changes), sputum, and blood. These represent attractive surrogate biomarkers for early detection and monitoring of chemoprevention, smoking cessation, and response to therapy.

SECOND PRIMARY CANCERS

Patients who have had a primary epithelial cancer of the upper aerodigestive tract (head and neck, esophagus, or lungs), have a 10 to 44% risk of developing a simultaneous or subsequent second primary cancer in the region or in distant organs, probably as a result of exposure to the same carcinogen. This effect is called "field cancerization." Many studies have implicated inactivation of *TP53* in both primary and secondary lesions as the cause of this phenomenon. The incidence of second primary tumors is especially high following treatment of laryngeal carcinoma, and up to 25% of these cases develop lung cancer in the first 14 years of follow-up. The most common histologic type of lung cancer in these patients was squamous cell carcinoma, but nonsquamous tumors were noted and occurred more frequently in women.[55] Several series have noted an increased risk of developing a second primary tumor in patients who have had lung cancer, mainly in long-term survivors. Examples are NSCLC as a cause of late mortality in patients with SCLC, and increased risk of developing acute leukemia in SCLC patients treated with chemotherapy. It must be considered that most of these studies reflect therapeutics and diagnostics used in the 1970s and 1980s; changes in therapy since that time may alter these statistics.

Several studies on chemoprevention of lung cancer failed to demonstrate a beneficial effect to any of the agents tested.[56,57]

PATHOLOGY OF LUNG CANCER

The histologic classification of lung tumors and guidelines for their typing were originally pub-

Table 80-3 World Health Organization Lung Cancer Classification

I. Epithelial tumors
- A. Benign
  - 1. Papillomas
  - 2. Adenomas
- B. Dysplasia/carcinoma in situ
- C. Malignant
  - 1. Squamous cell carcinoma
    - a. Spindle-cell variant
  - 2. Small-cell carcinoma
    - a. Oat-cell carcinoma
    - b. Intermediate-cell type
    - c. Combined oat-cell carcinoma
  - 3. Adenocarcinoma
    - a. Adenocarcinoma, mixed subtype
    - b. Acinar adenocarcinoma
    - c. Papillary adenocarcinoma
    - d. Bronchioloalveolar carcinoma
      - Nonmucinous
      - Mucinous
      - Mixed nonmucinous and mucinous or indeterminate
    - e. Solid adenocarcinoma with mucin production
    - f. Fetal adenocarcinoma
    - g. Mucinous (colloid) adenocarcinoma
    - h. Mucinous cystadenocarcinoma
    - i. Signet-ring adenocarcinoma
    - j. Clear-cell adenocarcinoma
  - 4. Large-cell carcinoma
    - a. Giant-cell carcinoma
    - b. Clear-cell carcinoma
  - 5. Adenosquamous carcinoma
  - 6. Carcinoid tumor
  - 7. Bronchial gland carcinoma
  - 8. Others

II. Soft tissue tumors

III. Mesothelial tumors
- A. Benign
- B. Malignant

IV. Miscellaneous tumors
- A. Benign
- B. Malignant

V. Secondary tumors

VI. Unclassified tumors

VII. Tumor-like lesions

Adapted from World Health Organization. Histological typing of lung tumors, 2nd ed. Geneva, Switzerland: WHO; 1981, and Travis WD, et al.[62]

lished by the WHO in 1967 and were revised in 1981, 1999, and again in 2004 (Table 80-3). The histologic types are based on analysis by light microscopy and with standard staining techniques. The four major types are squamous cell carcinoma, adenocarcinoma, large-cell carcinoma (collectively known as NSCLC and reflecting 90% of cases), and small-cell undifferentiated carcinoma.

The relative incidences of the various histologic types change gradually. In past decades, squamous cell carcinoma was the most common type, but in recent years it has decreased in frequency and adenocarcinoma has increased to become the most common type in the United States and Japan. In some parts of the world, and specifically Europe, squamous cell carcinoma is apparently still the most common type. Hypotheses concerning this shift have focused on the potential role of changes in the characteristics of cigarettes and consequent changes in the inhaled doses of carcinogens.[58]

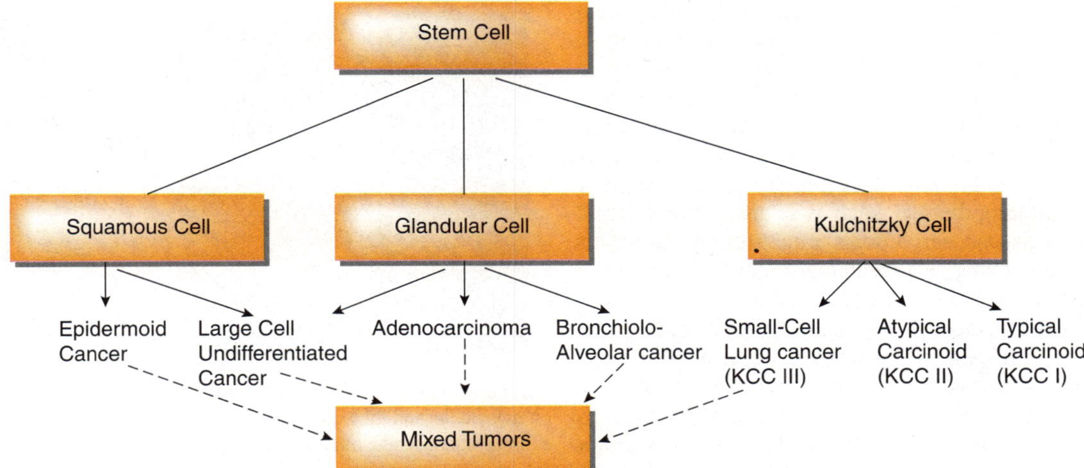

Figure 80-2 The stem cell theory of lung cancer pathogenesis as proposed by Auerbach.

The majority of lung cancers are histologically heterogeneous, a phenomenon that has an immediate impact on the diagnosis because of the potential variation in interobserver and intraobserver interpretation. Histologic heterogeneity is better recognized through evaluation of resected specimens rather than bronchoscopy or imaging-guided biopsy or cytologic studies, which sample only a small portion of the tumor. A study of 100 lung cancer specimens reviewed by five pathologists confirmed the presence of major heterogeneity (adenocarcinoma vs squamous cell carcinoma) in 45% of the cases. Minor (subtype) heterogeneity, with mixtures of acinar and papillary patterns in adenocarcinoma, for example, was found in 21% of the cases.[59]

Lung neoplasms are generally classified by the best-differentiated region of the tumor and graded by its most poorly differentiated portion. For example, a tumor that shows characteristics of squamous differentiation by demonstrating the obvious presence of keratin pearl formation and intercellular bridges would be classified as a squamous cell carcinoma. If most of the cells of the remaining tumor did not show such features, the same tumor would be further labeled as a poorly differentiated squamous cell tumor.

HISTOPATHOGENESIS

The histopathogenesis of lung cancer is not completely understood. Structural alterations include metaplastic changes in bronchial mucosal cells as a result of chronic exposure and repeated injury by inhaled agents, accompanied by a compensatory inflammatory process. Mucosal basal cells proliferate and generate mucus-secreting goblet cells. The columnar epithelium is replaced with stratified squamous epithelium. Further neoplasia results in a cellular atypia and increased mitotic activity leading to mucosal dysplasia. When the process involves the full thickness of the mucosa, carcinoma in situ is present. Invasion of the basement membrane and infiltration of malignant cells into the underlying stroma is the first sign of invasive cancer. The duration of this process may be 5 to 20 years.

The cell of origin for lung cancer has not been identified. Auerbach proposed the pleuripotential stem cell theory, in which a stem cell may differentiate into all types of lung cancer.[60] Yesner advocated the small-cell theory, in which a small-cell neoplasm undergoes transformation and may change into other cell types.[61] Most researchers support the Auerbach theory (Figure 80-2).

Histologic Types **Squamous Cell Carcinomas** Squamous cell carcinomas account for approximately one-third of all lung cancer cases. They usually originate within a central bronchus, and central cavitation from necrosis is a common gross and radiologic finding. Well-differentiated squamous cell cancers generally grow slowly, with less likelihood of distant spread than the poorly differentiated type. Histologically, these tumors show keratin formation, keratin pearl formation, and intercellular bridging between adjacent cells (Figure 80-3).

Adenocarcinomas Adenocarcinomas account for up to approximately 45% of all lung cancers and appear to be increasing in frequency.

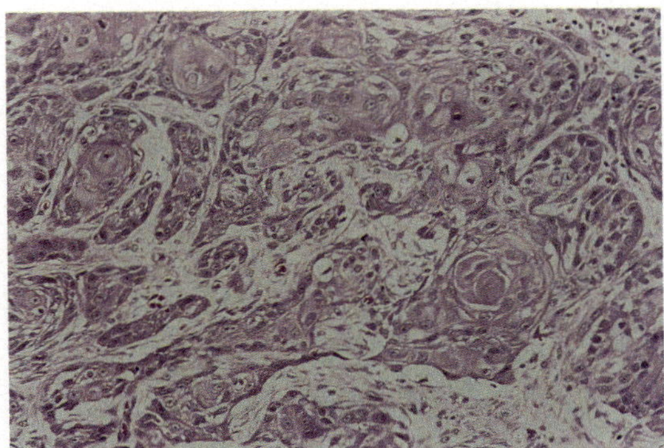

Figure 80-3 Squamous cell carcinoma showing nests and cords of neoplastic cells. Keratin pearl formation is easily identified. Intercellular bridges are also present and are more easily seen at higher magnification.

These tumors usually originate within the periphery of the lung and occur more commonly in women than in men. Central cavitation is uncommon. Adenocarcinoma tends to metastasize early to regional lymph nodes and to distant sites, particularly the brain. Patients with adenocarcinoma may have an associated history of chronic interstitial lung disease, such as scleroderma, rheumatoid disease, sarcoidosis, interstitial pneumonitis, tuberculosis, recurrent pulmonary infections, or other necrotizing pulmonary disease. The term "scar carcinoma" has been used to designate adenocarcinoma in association with a pulmonary scar resulting from chronic disease; possibly the neoplasm results from the long-standing insult of the underlying disease. On histologic examination, these tumors usually demonstrate glandular formation or mucus production in a solid tumor as shown by mucicarmine or periodic acid-Schiff staining. Lung adenocarcinomas typically stain for thyroid transcription factor-1. In the 2004 WHO classification, the only major change was to move adenocarcinoma, mixed type, to the top of the list of subtypes because of its increased frequency (Figure 80-4).

Bronchioloalveolar The bronchioloalveolar (BAC) subtype of adenocarcinoma represents approximately 2 to 4% of all lung cancers. Often, it is associated with previous lung disease leading to fibrosis, such as repeated pneumonias, idiopathic pulmonary fibrosis, granulomata, asbestosis, fibrosing alveolitis, scleroderma, or Hodgkin's disease. Its presence usually is not correlated with smoking. BAC commonly arises in the periphery of the lung and grows in a lepidic fashion along the alveolar septa. The cell of origin is in some dispute, but either Clara cells or type II pneumocytes are the most likely candidates. On gross examination, these tumors may be categorized as solitary, multinodular, or diffuse. Also, the histologic classification may be further subcategorized into well-differentiated and poorly differentiated tumors or into mucin- and nonmucin-containing tumors. Histologically pure BAC is uncommon, accounting for approximately 3% of all invasive lung malignancies. Over half the tumors produce mucin, whereas roughly one-third do not, and the remainder are mixtures. The mucin-producing tumors show gross and microscopic mucin production and tend to be multicentric. The nonmucin-producing tumors are more likely to be solitary. Patients with a solitary well-differentiated BAC have a much better prognosis than patients with the other forms. The diffuse and multinodular forms usually are not amenable to therapy.[62]

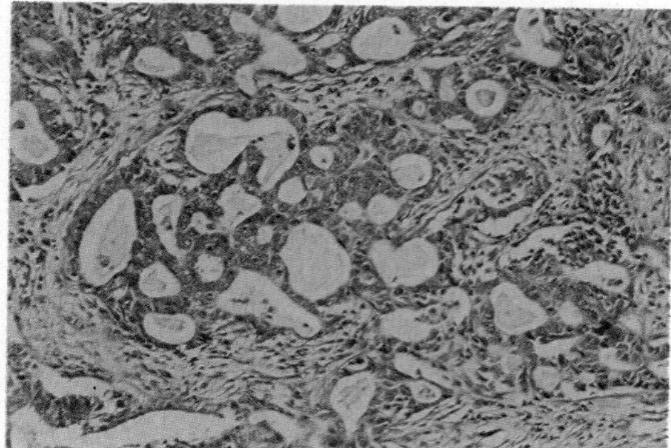

Figure 80-4 Well-differentiated adenocarcinoma showing gland formation by tumor cells.

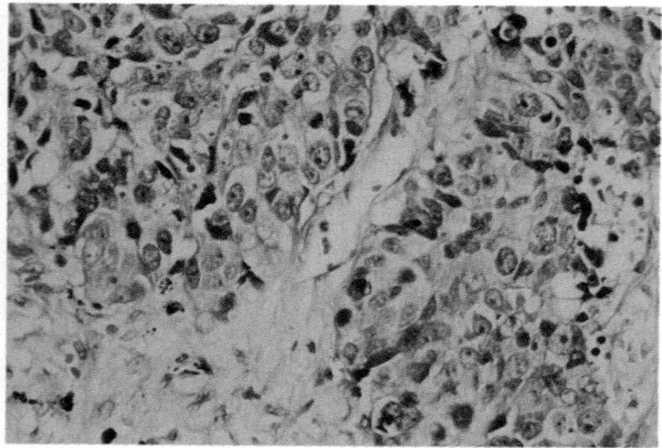

Figure 80-5 Large-cell undifferentiated carcinoma with large nuclei and fairly prominent nucleoli. These tumors lack any glandular, squamous, or neuroendocrine differentiation.

Large-Cell Carcinoma Large-cell carcinoma accounts for approximately 9% of all lung cancers. This tumor is characterized histologically by large cells with large nuclei and prominent nucleoli (Figure 80-5). There is no evidence of squamous or glandular differentiation and no reaction to mucicarmine staining. Large-cell carcinomas often have poor differentiation and no evidence of maturation, and features of adenocarcinoma, squamous carcinoma, or small-cell carcinoma are seen by electron microscopy. Giant- and spindle-cell subtypes have been reported and carry poor prognoses. Giant- and spindle-cell carcinomas account for less than 1% of lung cancers. Giant-cell carcinoma has been classified as a variant of large-cell carcinoma in which large, bizarre, pleomorphic and multinucleated tumor giant cells are found. The tumor cells contain abundant cytoplasm, and the nuclei are particularly large. Over 90% of giant-cell carcinomas are associated with other histologic subtypes such as spindle-cell carcinoma, adenocarcinoma, and large-cell carcinoma.[63]

Spindle-Cell Carcinoma Spindle-cell carcinoma is also regarded as a variant of large-cell carcinoma. Only 9% of spindle-cell carcinomas are associated with squamous cell carcinoma and many cases are associated with mixtures of other histologic types, including giant-cell carcinoma, adenocarcinoma, and large-cell carcinoma. The spindle-cell morphology is often indistinguishable from that of soft tissue sarcomas, and electron microscopy can be helpful in identifying epithelial differentiation. Patients with these tumors often have a poor prognosis, with an overall 5-year survival rate of approximately 10%.[63]

Occasionally, neuroendocrine features are found in association with large-cell carcinoma and justify the subtype referred to as large-cell neuroendocrine carcinoma. Large-cell neuroendocrine tumors have light-microscopic features that are commonly associated with other neuroendocrine tumors, such as palisading and rosette-like growth patterns. These tumors have low nuclear to cytoplasmic ratios, a high mitotic rate, and neuroendocrine features as determined by immunohistochemical studies or electron microscopy.[64] Large-cell neuroendocrine carcinoma is an aggressive malignancy with a prognosis that approaches that of SCLC. Many patients have distant disease at the time of diagnosis. Patients with early-stage disease appear to do much better. The optimal therapy for this type of tumor has not yet been clearly defined because of the small number of reported cases. Most oncologists manage neuroendocrine carcinomas with chemotherapy regimens similar to those used for SCLC.[65]

Adenosquamous Carcinoma Adenosquamous carcinoma (also called "mucoepidermoid carcinoma") accounts for 1 to 2% of lung cancers. Definition requires that at least 5% of the tumor represents each of the two histologic components, adenocarcinoma or squamous cell carcinoma. It has been suggested that adenosquamous carcinoma is associated with poor outcome.[66]

Pulmonary Neuroendocrine Neoplasia Pulmonary neuroendocrine neoplasia includes four major histologic subtypes: SCLC, large-cell neuroendocrine carcinoma, typical carcinoid, and atypical carcinoid. In 10 to 20% of histologically ordinary NSCLCs such as squamous cell carcinoma, adenocarcinoma, or large-cell carcinoma, neuroendocrine differentiation may be identified by immunohistochemical studies or electron microscopy. The term "NSCLC with neuroendocrine differentiation" is sometimes used for these cases.[64]

Typical and Atypical Carcinoid Tumors Typical and atypical carcinoid tumors are characterized by an organoid growth pattern. Histologic features may include spindle-cell, palisading, rosette-like, or papillary patterns. Atypical carcinoid is distinguished from typical carcinoid by the following criteria: (1) increased mitotic activity, with one mitotic figure for 1 to 2 high-power fields; (2) nuclear pleomorphism, hyperchromatism, and an abnormal nuclear to cytoplasmic ratio; (3) areas of increased cellularity with disorganization of the architecture; and (4) tumor necrosis. Typical carcinoid tumors often have cytologic pleomorphism, but necrosis is absent, and mitotic figures are rare.[67]

Carcinoid tumors are low-grade malignant neoplasms, which account for 1 to 2% of all lung tumors. Paraneoplastic processes can occur with carcinoid tumors, but these are rare. Usually, these tumors are asymptomatic, but the most commonly associated clinical manifestations are cough, hemoptysis, and postobstructive pneumonitis. Patients with typical carcinoid have an excellent prognosis and rarely die of the tumor. On the other hand, patients with atypical carcinoid have a higher rate of associated metastatic disease, and survival is significantly reduced.

SCLC SCLC accounts for 10 to 15% of all lung cancers, and approximately 28,000 new cases occur in the United States each year.[68] SCLC has a very aggressive clinical course, with frequent widespread metastases. It is considered a distinct clinical pathologic entity owing to its characteristic aggressive biology, propensity for early metastasis, sensitivity to chemotherapy, and overall poor prognosis. SCLC usually is not amenable to surgical treatment because it is most often diagnosed in an advanced stage. Some difficulties may exist in distinguishing poorly differentiated NSCLC from SCLC. This may occur in up to 5 to 7% of cases. Immunohistochemical analysis for keratin and common leukocyte antigen can be very helpful in such difficult diagnostic circumstances.

SCLCs typically are situated in the peribronchial region and infiltrate the bronchial submucosa and peribronchial parenchyma tissues. Early and extensive metastases are common. Only the minority, less than 5% of cases, present as a localized peripheral parenchymal lesion. In 1981, the WHO proposed that SCLC be subclassified into three subtypes: (1) oat-cell carcinoma, (2) intermediate-cell type, and (3) combined oat-cell carcinoma. This subclassification was not reproducible, however, and significant differences in survival were noted. In 1988, therefore, the International Association for the Study of Lung Cancer (IASLC) proposed that the intermediate-cell type be dropped, and added the category of mixed small-cell/large-cell carcinoma.[69] Examined by microscopy, SCLC is composed of cells that contain a paucity of cytoplasm and have fine, granular nuclear chromatin and indistinct nucleoli (Figure 80-6). Nuclear molding due to "crush" artifact is a consistent finding but is not diagnostic. Mitotic rates are high, and the tumor often grows in sheets with a nonspecific pattern. On occasion, rosettes and peripheral palisading may be present. If necrosis exists, it usually is extensive.

Approximately 4 to 6% of SCLC show a mixture of small-cell and large-cell carcinoma, and approximately 1 to 3% of SCLC may be combined with adenocarcinoma or squamous cell carcinoma.[68]

SOLITARY PULMONARY NODULE

A solitary pulmonary nodule (SPN) is an asymptomatic pulmonary mass measuring less than 3 cm in diameter, surrounded completely by parenchymal tissue with no associated atelectasis, pneumonitis, pneumonia, or adenopathy. The primary concern with any SPN is malignancy. The likelihood of an SPN being malignant directly correlates with the age of the patient, history of smoking, size of the nodule, and history of malignancy. A careful history and physical examination, therefore, are important in considering all benign and extrathoracic malignant possibilities. A history of smoking and age over 40 years are associated with a higher risk of malignancy. A concerted search for previous chest radiographs is imperative. The presence of the nodule on a previous film serves as a mark for comparison. Stability or no growth for at least 2 years are considered good indicators of a benign lesion. SPNs usually grow at a constant rate and are measured by doubling time. A doubling time for malignant nodules is rarely less than 1 month or more than a year.[70]

CT, in particular thin-cut CT in 2 mm slices, is very helpful in determining the specific characteristics of an SPN that suggest malignant potential. CT of the abdomen should be performed in a patient with a previous malignancy. If an SPN is very dense or denser than a phantom reference nodule by CT, the nodule has a high likelihood of being benign. Nodules that are less dense than the phantom nodule are indeterminate, and approximately 25% of these are benign. For malignant nodules, the most important radiographic characteristics are thickness of the cavity wall, spicular edge, and a diameter of more than 3 cm. For benign nodules, the most important radiographic characteristics are benign growth rate and a benign pattern of calcification (diffuse, laminated, dense central, or "popcorn" calcification). Routine preoperative bronchoscopy is usually not helpful in patients with SPN. It should be performed at the time of surgery or reserved for patients in whom operative intervention poses a risk and who need a diagnosis so that method of nonsurgical treatment can be decided. In such circumstances, fine-needle aspiration (FNA; transthoracic or transbronchial) can be performed for diagnosis. Thoracoscopy is a useful technique for removing indeterminate lesions that are peripherally located. It should be used with caution, though, in patients with an SPN that has a high likelihood for malignancy when the patient is a good operative candidate and the probability of thoracotomy for resection is high. The risk of tumor spillage is higher in video-assisted thoracoscopic surgery than open wedge resection, and the morbidity of a limited thoracotomy with wedge resection is minimal. The addition of positron emission tomographic (PET) scanning in the evaluation of SPN has shown great promise in differentiating benign and malignant disease. Its use may help avoid further invasive diagnostic procedures in high-risk individuals.[70]

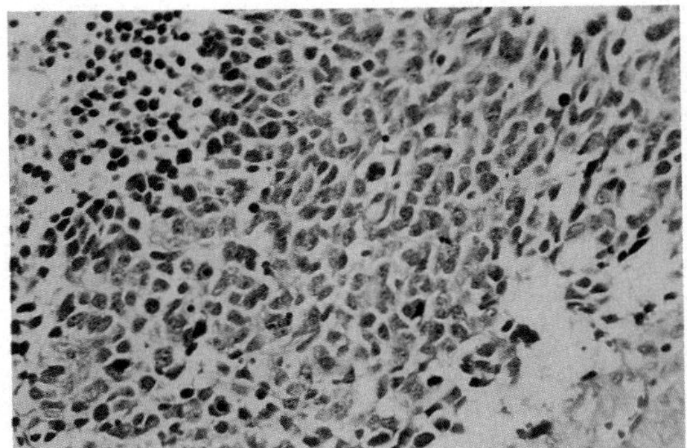

Figure 80-6 Small-cell carcinoma showing cells with high nuclear to cytoplasmic ratios. The cytoplasm is often so discrete that is inconspicuous. The cells show nuclear molding and high mitotic rates.

CLINICAL MANIFESTATIONS

Clinical Presentation Some patients present with an asymptomatic lesion discovered incidentally on chest radiograph. The majority of lung cancers, however, are discovered because of the development of a new or worsening clinical symptom or sign. Although no set of signs or symptoms is pathognomonic for lung cancer, they may be divided into four categories: (1) those due to local tumor growth and intrathoracic spread, (2) those due to distant metastases, (3) nonspecific systemic symptoms, and (4) paraneoplastic syndromes.

Manifestations of Local Tumor Growth and Intrathoracic Spread Signs and symptoms referable to the primary tumor vary depending on location and size of the tumor. Centrally located tumors produce cough, a localized wheeze, hemoptysis, and symptoms and signs of airway obstruction and postobstructive pneumonitis such as dyspnea, fever, and productive cough. Occasionally, large tumor masses, usually of squamous or large-cell histologic type, cavitate and present as malignant lung abscesses. Peripheral tumors are more likely to be asymptomatic when they are small and confined within the lung; occasionally, cough and pleuritic chest pain may be evident.

Intrathoracic spread of lung cancer, either by direct extension or by lymphatic metastasis, is associated with a variety of sign and symptom complexes. The importance of these symptoms and signs is that they generally indicate that the patient is no longer a candidate for curative surgery. Mediastinal invasion may be manifested as vague, poorly localized chest pain in association with other findings of nerve entrapment, vascular obstruction, and/or compression or invasion of the esophagus. One of the most common neurologic disorders arising from mediastinal involvement is hoarseness owing to entrapment of the recurrent laryngeal nerve. Because of its longer intrathoracic course, the left recurrent laryngeal nerve is more likely to be the source of hoarseness than the right recurrent laryngeal nerve. With recurrent laryngeal nerve paralysis, a patient may develop dysphagia for both solids and liquids, resulting in recurrent aspiration. Compression of the esophagus by the tumor also may lead to dysphagia. The formation of a tracheoesophageal or bronchoesophageal fistula, which occurs with a frequency of 0.16%, can be manifested by vigorous cough, especially on swallowing, and recurrent aspiration pneumonia. Involvement of the phrenic nerve is associated with hiccups early, and later leads to paralysis and elevation of the hemidiaphragm with resulting dyspnea.

The principal vascular syndrome associated with the extension of lung cancer into the mediastinum is superior vena cava (SVC) syndrome, most commonly caused by invasion of the vein and extrinsic compression by the tumor, but also by intraluminal thrombosis. Lung cancer accounts for 65 to 90% of all cases of SVC syndrome, and in approximately 85% of these cases the primary lung tumor is on the right, primarily in the right upper lobe or right mainstem bronchus. By cell type, SCLC predominates as the cause of SVC syndrome, followed by squamous cell carcinoma. Establishment of a histologic diagnosis is important before initiating treatment, because the SVC syndrome is no longer considered a radiotherapeutic emergency.

With apical tumors, the classic Pancoast's syndrome (lower brachial plexopathy, Horner's syndrome, and shoulder pain) may become manifest owing to local invasion of the lower brachial plexus (C8 and T1 nerve roots), satellite ganglion, and chest wall. The tumor may cause symptoms through involvement of the first or second rib or vertebrae and other nerve roots. The radiographic signs are those of an asymmetric apical cap or an apical mass. Most superior sulcus tumors are squamous cell carcinomas, although they may be adenocarcinomas, or even in 1 to 2% of cases, SCLC, underscoring the importance of establishing a histologic diagnosis.

Approximately 15% of patients with lung cancer have pleural involvement at initial presentation, and 50% of patients with disseminated lung cancer develop pleural effusion during the course of their illness. A pleural effusion may be asymptomatic when small, but it is usually associated with dyspnea, cough, or chest pain. A number of pathogenic mechanisms have been suggested, but the presence or absence of malignant cells in cytology specimens does not significantly influence survival outcome, although the presence of malignant cells in pleural washings at the time of pulmonary resection for lung cancer has been shown to have a negative impact survival.[71] Rarely, lung cancer can present as an ipsilateral spontaneous pneumothorax, generally attributed to erosion of the visceral pleura by a peripheral tumor, but underlying emphysema also may play a role.

Pericardial involvement arises from direct extension of the tumor or as a result of retrograde spread through mediastinal and epicardial lymphatics. Lung cancer is the single most frequent source of pericardial metastases, accounting for 37% of reported cases. In many cases, the process is not diagnosed before the patient's death. Clinical findings include cardiac dysrhythmias, enlargement of the cardiac silhouette on the chest radiograph, and, infrequently, signs and symptoms of cardiac tamponade (Table 80-4).

Table 80-4 Clinical Manifestations of Lung Cancer Caused by Local Tumor Growth and Intrathoracic Spread at Presentation

	Frequency (%)	
Clinical Manifestation	SCLC	NSCLC
Cough	50–76	40
Dyspnea	34–40	30–40
Chest pain	35–36	25–40
Hemoptysis	15–23	15–35
Pneumonitis	21–25	13–24
Vocal cord paralysis	15	Uncommon
SVC syndrome	12	< 10
Pleural effusion	10–15	15
Pancoast's syndrome	Rare	3
Pericardial effusion	Uncommon	Rare

NSCLC = nonsmall-cell lung cancer; SCLC = small-cell lung cancer; SVC = superior vena cava.

Manifestations of Distant Metastases Approximately 60% of SCLC and 30 to 40% of NSCLC patients present with stage IV metastatic disease. Although lung cancer can metastasize to virtually any organ site, the most common sites of hematogenous spread that are clinically apparent are the central nervous system (CNS), bones, liver, and adrenal glands. Many of these patients do not have symptoms that can be attributed to a specific distant site. Bone pain appears to be common, however, one-third of patients in one large series had "pain other than chest pain" at presentation, and the majority of those episodes were due to bony involvement. Symptoms related to liver involvement (right upper quadrant pain) are less common or nonspecific (nausea, weight loss, anemia). Involvement of the adrenal glands is often asymptomatic, and most adrenal metastases are discovered incidentally during staging evaluation or at autopsy. If symptomatic, it presents with unilateral pain in the flank, abdomen, or costovertebral angle. Much less commonly, signs or symptoms point to brain and CNS involvement. These can range from nonspecific headache or mental status change to focal or generalized seizures and localized weakness. Epidural and intramedullary spinal cord metastases may be the sole neurologic manifestations of lung cancer. Diffuse meningeal involvement is uncommon at the time of initial presentation, but it may be seen later in the course of the disease, particularly with SCLC. The lymphatic spread of lung cancer may manifest with cough and dyspnea, depending on the extent of parenchymal involvement.

Systemic, Nonspecific Signs and Symptoms As shown in Table 80-5, systemic, nonspecific signs and symptoms are common in both SCLC and NSCLC. The 30% rate of anorexia is probably underreported. Weight loss, which is usually but not always accompanied by anorexia, occurs in approximately one-half of the patients and generalized weakness in one-third. Fever and anemia occur less frequently, in fewer than 20% of the patients. Fever is generally not considered paraneoplastic in lung cancer patients; if present, it is usually associated with a documented infection (eg, postobstructive pneumonia) or with liver metastases.

Paraneoplastic Syndromes Table 80-6 lists 21 paraneoplastic syndromes, which induce signs and symptoms away from the primary tumor or its metastasis. The major categories of paraneoplastic syndromes include endocrine, neurologic, cutaneous and musculoskeletal, and cardiovascular and hematological manifestations.[72]

Table 80-5 Clinical Manifestation Caused by Systemic Effect at Presentation

	Frequency (%)	
Clinical Manifestations	SCLC	NSCLC
Anorexia	30	30
Weight loss (≥ 10 lb)	35–52	45–52
Fatigue	23–42	35
Fever	11–15	7–16
Anemia	11–15	16–20

NSCLC = nonsmall-cell lung cancer; SCLC = small-cell lung cancer.

Endocrine Syndromes ***Syndrome of Inappropriate Secretion of Antidiuretic Hormone*** Excess secretion of arginine-vasopressin associated with hyponatremia are the hallmarks of syndrome of inappropriate secretion of antidiuretic hormone (SIADH). The cardinal findings are hyponatremia with corresponding hypo-osmolality of the serum and extracellular fluid; continued renal excretion of sodium; absence of clinical evidence of fluid volume depletion; osmolality of the urine greater than that appropriate for the concomitant osmolality of the plasma, that is, urine less than maximally diluted; and normal function of kidneys, adrenals and thyroid glands. SIADH may be caused by a variety of malignant tumors, and SCLC is the most common (up to 15%, though only one-third of them are symptomatic). Water restriction is usually sufficient to control symptoms until systemic anticancer treatment is initiated, which typically leads to improvement or resolution of the hyponatremia. Saline infusion, furosemide, or demeclocycline is infrequently required. Other conditions associated with SIADH must be considered, such as CNS disorders, pulmonary infections, and positive pressure ventilation. Also, a large number of pharmaceutical agents have been shown to produce SIADH, including a number of cytotoxic drugs such as vincristine, vinblastine, cisplatin, cyclophosphamide, and melphalan. Malignant tumors that cause SIADH are primary brain tumors, hematologic malignancies, intrathoracic nonpulmonary cancers, skin tumors, gastrointestinal cancers, gynecological cancer, breast and prostate cancers, and sarcomas.

Syndrome of Ectopic Adrenocorticotropic Hormone Hyperadrenocorticism in association with ectopic adrenocorticotropic hormone (ACTH) production (> 200 pg/mL) is a frequently observed hormonal syndrome in lung cancer, particularly in SCLC. Serum ACTH levels are elevated in 30 to 72% of SCLC patients, and cortisol secretion is abnormally regulated in 51%, but only 3 to 7% of SCLC patients become symptomatic. Patients with ectopic ACTH syndrome generally fit the demographic characteristics of lung cancer patients and rarely exhibit the classic cushingoid features of centripetal obesity or moon face. Severe weakness and weight loss are universal as are excessive mineralocorticoid effects such as edema (30–40%) and hypertension (30–60%). Hyperpigmentation occurs in 25 to 30% of patients. Distinctive laboratory features of ectopic ACTH syndrome include severe hypokalemic alkalosis (70–90% of patients have a serum potassium level < 3.0 mEq/L), elevated urinary 17-hydroxycorticoid excretion, and high serum ACTH levels (> 200 pg/mL in 65% of patients). The ectopic ACTH syndrome is best managed by effective treatment of the underlying disease, but hypokalemia and hypertension may require appropriate, immediate adjunctive management. Ectopic ACTH syndrome was found to

Table 80-6 Major Paraneoplastic Manifestations of Lung Cancer

Syndrome	Clinical Frequency (%)	Comments
Endocrine		
Inappropriate ADH	5–10	Mainly SCLC
Atrial natriuretic factor	Mainly SCLC	—
Ectopic ACTH	3–7	Most commonly with SCLC
Hypercalcemia of malignancy	10	Most commonly with squamous cell types
Gynecomastia	6	More with large-cell type
Other hormones	—	No significant clinical manifestations
Neurologic		
Eaton-Lambert	6	Mainly SCLC
Subacute sensory neuropathy	Rare	Mainly SCLC
Subacute cerebellar degeneration	Rare	Mainly SCLC
Limbic encephalopathy	Rare	Mainly SCLC
Visual paraneoplastic syndrome	Rare	Mainly SCLC
Subacute necrotic myelopathy	Rare	Mainly SCLC
Cutaneous/Musculoskeletal		
Hypertrophic pulmonary osteoarthropathy	< 10	More with adenocarcinoma
Acanthosis nigricans	Rare	—
Tylosis	Rare	—
Dermatomyositis	Rare	—
Cardiovascular/Hematologic		
Nonbacterial thrombotic endocarditis	Uncommon	More with adenocarcinoma
Migratory thrombophlebitis	Uncommon	More with adenocarcinoma
Hypercoagulable status	10–15	Renal
Glomerulonephritis	Rare	—
Nephrotic syndrome	Rare	—

ACTH = adrenocorticotrophic hormone; ADH = antidiuretic hormone; SCLC = small-cell lung cancer.

be associated with frequent complications from chemotherapy and shortened survival in patients with SCLC.[73]

Other Hormone Production Other hormones elevated in lung cancer, particularly in patients with SCLC, include calcitonin, growth hormone, prolactin, serotonin, insulin, gastrin, and melanocyte-stimulating factors. In most cases, however, these laboratory abnormalities bear minimal clinical significance.

Hypercalcemia of Malignancy It has long been known that cancer patients may have hypercalcemia even without demonstrable bone metastases. Hypercalcemia has been reported to occur in up to 20 to 30% of patients with cancer at some time during the course of their disease. This incidence may be falling owing to the wide use of bisphosphonates in patients with multiple myeloma or breast cancer, although data are lacking. Hypercalcemia leads to progressive mental impairment, including coma, as well as renal failure. These complications are particularly common terminal events among patients with cancer. The detection of hypercalcemia in a patient with cancer signifies a very poor prognosis; approximately 50% of such patients die within 30 days. A parathyroid hormone-related protein, which shares an N-terminal sequence with the parathyroid hormone but has a unique C-terminal portion, has been shown to be responsible for the majority of cases of hypercalcemia of malignancy. Squamous cell carcinoma is the lung cancer mostly associated with hypercalcemia, and SCLC is rarely involved. Hypercalcemia may be completely reversible with effective treatment of the underlying cancer, and bisphosphonates may be used as a specific therapeutic modality.[74]

Neurologic Syndromes Neurologic syndromes associated with lung cancer may occur through autoimmune mechanisms, and they occur mainly in patients with SCLC. Symptoms may precede diagnosis of the cancer by many months or may be the first sign of tumor recurrence. Direct metastatic effects or metabolic or infectious processes must be excluded as contributors to the neurologic findings. The severity of neurologic symptoms is unrelated to tumor bulk, and a primary malignant lesion may be undetected before death, despite disabling symptoms. Most of these conditions are not specific for malignancy.

Eaton-Lambert Syndrome A myasthenia gravis-like disorder that was originally linked to SCLC but was found in other cancers, this syndrome, characterized by proximal limb muscle weakness and fatigue, is caused by the formation of IgG antibodies directed at calcium channels present in both the tumor and the neuromuscular junction. A type 1 antineuronal nuclear autoantibody (ANNA-1, also known as "anti-Hu") has been identified as a marker of neurological autoimmunity that is highly associated with SCLC (97%) and other paraneoplastic neurologic disorders.[75]

Subacute Sensory Neuropathy This is the most characteristic peripheral neuropathy associated with SCLC. Clinical symptoms characterized by progressive impairment of all sensory modalities, with areflexia and marked sensory ataxia followed by stabilization after a period of weeks, may precede the diagnosis of SCLC by several months. It may be accompanied by more widespread evidence of paraneoplastic encephalitis, with cerebellar brainstem dysfunction and dementia.

Cutaneous and Musculoskeletal Syndromes Digital clubbing and hypertrophic pulmonary osteoarthropathy (HPO) are the other major paraneoplastic syndromes associated with lung cancer, most exclusively with NSCLC. Digital clubbing (ie, subungual soft tissue thickening, most commonly involving the fingernails) is more common than HPO, which often resembles rheumatoid arthritis. It is characterized by a symmetric polyarthritis (usually involving the ankles, wrists, and knees), proliferative periostitis of the long bones, and neurovascular changes of the hands and feet, often with little or no evidence of clubbing. Although these conditions are also reported in several disorders not related to cancer and in other tumors metastatic to the chest, lung cancer accounts for more than 80% of cases of HPO in adults.[76] Radionuclide bone scans typically demonstrate increased uptake at the distal ends of the affected long bones, and the results may be confirmed by evidence of new bone formation on plain films; the spine is spared. The onset of HPO is often acute, may precede the diagnosis of cancer by months, and is usually but not invariably associated with inoperability. The cause of HPO is unknown. A variety of underlying mechanisms have been suggested, including the release of platelet-derived growth factor by megakaryocytes or platelet clumps that bypass the pulmonary capillary network. The syndrome may resolve with response of the cancer to therapy. No effective form of treatment is recognized, including aspirin and nonsteroidal anti-inflammatory agents.

Other cutaneous paraneoplastic syndromes include dermatomyositis, acanthosis nigricans, and tylosis or hyperkeratosis of the palms and soles. These conditions are rarely seen in patients with lung cancer.

Cardiovascular and Hematological Manifestations Arterial and, more commonly, venous thrombosis is a frequent complication of cancer and sometimes a harbinger of occult cancer. Moreover, the use of new and aggressive therapy for cancer increases the risk of thrombosis. The two most notable manifestations in lung cancer are nonbacterial thrombotic endocarditis (NBTE) and venous thromboembolism (VTE).

NBTE, also known as marantic endocarditis, has been described most commonly in conjunction with adenocarcinoma and BAC; at autopsy, the incidence of NBTE in each of these cancer subtypes was approximately 7%, and the mitral valve was typically involved. Clinically significant emboli to the CNS, kidneys, and coronary arteries have been found.[77]

Pulmonary embolism and deep venous thrombosis are the two manifestations of VTE. Approximately 20% of VTE in the general population is associated with cancer, and cancer increases the risk of VTE about fivefold. Therapy for cancer, including surgery, chemotherapy, hormonal therapy, growth factors, angiogenesis inhibitors, and central venous catheters, add to the risk of thrombosis. Migratory thrombophlebitis was reported in patients with adenocarcinomas from different origins, mostly gastrointestinal tract (eg, pancreas) and lung.

A hypercoagulable state is noted in 10 to 15% of lung cancer patients. Thrombocytosis (60% of patients), hyperfibrinogenemia (54% of solid tumor patients), and general activation of the clotting system result in thrombosis and occasionally bleeding in lung cancer patients.

Recommended definitive therapy for established VTE includes low-molecular-weight heparin (LMWH) for most patients, unfractionated heparin for patients with renal failure, thrombolysis in cases of massive pulmonary embolism, and inferior vena cava filters when anticoagulation therapy is contraindicated.[78] Most authorities recommend 6 months therapy for secondary prevention. Lee and colleagues suggested that long-term treatment or secondary prophylaxis of VTE in cancer patients should include at least 6 months of LMWH rather than warfarin. (Their data showed probabilities of recurrence of thromboembolism of 17% in the warfarin group and only 9% in the LMWH group at 6 months, without increasing the risk of bleeding).[79]

Miscellaneous Paraneoplastic Associations Renal disorders, such as membranous glomerulonephritis and subsequent nephrotic syndrome, have been reported as paraneoplastic phenomena in patients with lung cancer. The onset frequently precedes the diagnosis of cancer and probably is related to glomerular deposition of circulating antigen–antibody complexes. It is a poor prognostic sign among patients with all types of carcinoma, with a median survival duration of only 12 months from the time of diagnosis of the syndrome and only 3 months from the time of tumor diagnosis. The glomerulonephritis may normalize with appropriate treatment.

DIAGNOSTIC AND STAGING TECHNIQUES

The methods used to establish a diagnosis of lung cancer depend on the individual clinical situation. In some cases, such as a patient who presents with an asymptomatic solitary pulmonary nodule, tissue diagnosis may not be established until the time of definitive surgical resection. In others, the diagnosis may be established at the time of collection of a sputum sample for cytologic studies. In any instance, the evaluation begins with a thorough history and physical examination. Because 30 to 50% of all patients have metastatic disease at the time of presentation, clues to clinical stage will often be evident on examination. Symptoms, signs, and physical findings may suggest a preliminary stage. Particular attention should be directed to these areas. The cervical, supraclavicular, and scalene regions should be examined carefully for possible lymphadenopathy; the skin for cutaneous or subcutaneous nodules; the axillary regions for masses or adenopathy; the chest for signs of bronchial obstruction or pleural effusion; and the abdomen for hepatic enlargement. If the physical examination suggests possible related pathology, these areas should be scrutinized with the use of biopsy or cytologic studies. Moreover, the physical examination should include the breast, rectum, pelvis, and nervous system for areas of concurrent disease, metastatic disease, or primary disease with metastasis to the lung. Neurologic signs or symptoms certainly warrant evaluation with a brain CT scan. An elevated serum alkaline phosphatase level or complaints of bone pain should be followed up with a bone scan. Areas of suspicion identified by bone scan should be evaluated further by site-specific radiography and by biopsy for confirmation should the radiograph so indicate.

Accurate clinical staging includes a combination of noninvasive and invasive procedures. Noninvasive studies include sputum cytology, chest radiography, CT scanning, magnetic resonance imaging (MRI), gallium scanning, and PET scanning. Invasive procedures that directly assess the extent of disease include bronchoscopy, transbronchial or transthoracic FNA biopsy, scalene node biopsy, mediastinoscopy, anterior mediastinotomy, and thoracoscopy. Patients who present with clinical or radiographic evidence of extensive disease usually require the least invasive procedure to establish inoperability. Cytologic or histologic confirmation through FNA biopsy usually is sufficient to confirm suspicion of N3 or M1 disease. Thoracentesis or pericardiocentesis should be performed on associated effusions to assess possible T4 disease. Other patients with less extensive disease often present with subtle radiographic findings that require more invasive techniques for adequate staging, particularly when mediastinal lymph node involvement is suspected.

Noninvasive Studies

Sputum Cytology Cytologic evaluation of sputum, bronchial washings, bronchial brushings, and FNA specimens have high diagnostic value, but the positive and negative predictive values of each and their accuracy of diagnosis certainly are dependent on sampling error, tissue preservation, processing quality, and observer experience. Sputum cytology remains a simple test with a positive predictive value that can approach 100%, but it has a sensitivity rate of only 10 to 15%. If a diagnosis can be established through collective sputum cytology, invasive tests often can be averted. The highest yield occurs in patients with large, centrally located tumors. Small peripheral lesions often require more invasive measures to obtain a diagnosis.

Imaging Lung cancer is generally first imaged by chest radiography. CT scan, PET scan, and occasionally magnetic resonance imaging (MRI) are used to stage a known or suspected lung cancer. The radiographic morphology of lung cancer may be correlated with cell type, with the following generalizations[80]: (1) Adenocarcinoma usually presents as a solitary pulmonary nodule, and most malignant solitary pulmonary nodules are adenocarcinomas. (2) Large central masses are usually squamous cell carcinoma (an endobronchial lesion thus may result in postobstructive changes) or SCLC (may involve mediastinal and hilar lymph nodes, sometimes without an overt parenchymal lesion). (3) A large peripheral mass usually represents large-cell or squamous cell carcinoma. Peripheral squamous cell carcinomas are more prone to central necrosis and formation of a cavity than other histologic types. Lobulated lesions with central masses associated with necrosis and thicker walls than typical for lung abscesses characterize cavitary squamous cell carcinoma. Adenocarcinoma occasionally manifests as a large peripheral mass. (4) Multiple nodules generally occur with BAC, and sometimes with adenocarcinoma. Airspace disease or multiple nodules are late manifestations of BAC. (5) A sclerotic pattern may be identified in adenocarcinomas, as well as areas of chronic scar in association with a long-standing interstitial fibrotic pattern (a finding termed "scar carcinoma").

Chest Radiography Posterior-anterior and lateral chest radiographs remain the simplest method for identifying patients with lung cancer. It is still a preferred initial modality because of its availability, low cost, and low radiation dose. A standard chest radiograph can detect a lesion as small as 3 mm in diameter; however, unsuspected nodules generally are not seen unless larger than 5 mm in diameter. Associated atelectasis, postobstructive pneumonitis, abscess, bronchiolitis, pleural reaction, rib erosion, pleural effusion, or bulky mediastinal lymphadenopathy may be identified on radiographs, raising suspicions of a primary lung malignancy.

Plain chest radiography may identify abnormal pulmonary nodules. There are no absolute criteria to confirm a benign lesion on the basis of its radiographic appearance, but stability of size for 2 years and the presence of specific patterns of calcification (multipunctate foci, a dense central nidus, a popcorn ball, or laminated "bull's eye" appearance) are considered indicators of benignancy. However, some tumors such as BAC and typical carcinoids occasionally appear to be stable for 2 or more years. Since the absence of appreciable growth over a 2-year period had a predictive value of only 65% for a benign lesion, the dictum that 2-year stability on plain-film radiography indicates a benign process should be used with caution.[70]

Computed Tomography As a single comprehensive study, CT scan remains the most effective noninvasive technique for evaluating suspected or known lung cancer and the mediastinum, which may contain associated metastatic disease. Unfortunately, the accuracy of CT scanning in identifying metastatic disease in mediastinal lymph nodes is highly variable; its sensitivity ranges from 51 to 95%. Such a wide range in accuracy is secondary to variations in the criteria for nodal abnormality, which are based on size and shape of a lymph node, CT scanner differences, and nonuniformity in nodal mapping. A lymph node size of 1 cm or more in shortest diameter has been generally accepted as the criterion of abnormal nodal enlargement. Approximately 8 to 15% of patients considered to have a negative CT scan for mediastinal nodal enlargement, with lymph nodes sized 1 cm or less, will ultimately be found to have mediastinal nodal involvement at the time of operation. Mediastinal lymph nodes that are more than 2 cm in diameter contain metastatic disease in over 90% of cases. Lymph nodes that are 1.5 to 2 cm in size contain disease in over 50% of cases. Lymph nodes that are 1 to 1.5 cm in size harbor metastatic disease in 15 to 30% of cases. The negative predictive accuracy of CT scan is 85 to 92% for mediastinal lymph node metastases. Often, patients with unsuspected lymph node metastases that are found at the time of thoracotomy are able to undergo complete resection, including removal of lymph nodes by complete mediastinal dissection. Survival rates are best for this group of patients with N2 disease. Thus, patients with no evidence of mediastinal lymph node enlargement on CT scan usually do not need to undergo invasive staging prior to thoracotomy. Patients who have nodes larger than 1 cm, however, should be considered to have potential N2 disease. An incomplete resection is more likely in this group of patients and does not improve the outcome. Combined-modality therapy is usually indicated. For this reason, these patients warrant further invasive investigation to obtain a cytologic or histologic diagnosis prior to the initiation of therapy.

Magnetic Resonance Imaging (MRI) MRI is not used for the routine evaluation of patients with lung cancer, but it does have specific advantages over CT scan. Because of its heightened ability to discern neurologic and vascular structures, tumors that reside in close proximity to neurovascular structures may be more accurately assessed by MRI than by CT scan. MRI is most useful in evaluating patients with superior sulcus tumors.

Gallium Scintigraphy Gallium scanning is a simple and inexpensive test. Its role in the evaluation of patients with lung carcinoma has met with mixed reviews. If a chest CT scan has been performed, gallium scanning provides very little additional information. Gallium scanning is clearly inferior to CT scan for identification of brain metastases and is less sensitive than bone scans in detecting osseous metastases; therefore, it has few indications for use in evaluating patients with lung carcinoma.

Positron Emission Tomographic Scanning Over the last several years, PET scanning with 2-[18F]fluoro-2-deoxy-D-glucose (FDG-PET) has been increasingly used in the diagnosis and staging of lung cancer. This test identifies areas of increased glucose metabolism, which is a common trait in pulmonary tumors. Since commercial PET scanners provide nominal spatial resolution of 4.5 to 6.0 mm in the center of the axial field of view, even lesions that are less than 1 cm in diameter can be detected on the basis of an increased uptake of FDG. Although initially heralded as a reliable noninvasive method of identifying and staging pulmonary neoplasms, a number of limitations have become apparent. Many inflammatory processes such as abscesses and active granulomatous diseases, as well as hypoxic conditions such as those that exist after radiotherapy, may cause high FDG uptake and lead to false-positive results. Treatment-induced hypermetabolic inflammatory changes also may lead to difficulty differentiating between treatment effects and those of the residual tumor. False-negative results have occurred primarily in tumors with low glucose metabolism (carcinoid and BAC) and in small tumors, owing to the limited spatial resolution of current PET scanners. Slowly, the role of FDG-PET is becoming established. PET is also appealing for assessment of prognosis and treatment. A systematic search of published work shows good evidence that FDG uptake on PET has independent prognostic value in newly diagnosed NSCLC. The role of PET in measuring the biological effects of anticancer therapy and in restaging after induction therapy awaits better standardization and large-scale experience.[81]

Integrated PET-CT PET provides imprecise information on the exact location of focal abnormalities. Thus, even if the results of PET and CT scan are visually correlated, the precise location of lesions is sometimes difficult to determine. To overcome this limitation, integrated PET-CT was recently introduced.[82] Initial results of one study on this emerging technology suggest that integrated PET-CT provided additional information in 20 of 49 patients (41%) beyond that provided by conventional visual correlation of PET and CT scan. Integrated PET-CT had better diagnostic accuracy than the other imaging methods. Tumor staging was significantly more accurate with integrated PET-CT than with CT scan alone ($p = .001$), PET alone ($p < .001$), or visual correlation of PET and CT scan ($p = .013$); node staging was also significantly more accurate with integrated PET-CT than with PET alone ($p = .013$). In metastasis staging, integrated PET-CT increased the diagnostic certainty in two of eight patients. It was concluded that integrated PET-CT improves the diagnostic accuracy of the staging of NSCLC.[82] This technology is currently being tested in many centers in the world.

INVASIVE STUDIES **Bronchoscopy** Fiberoptic bronchoscopy (FOB) is an essential and standard technique for the evaluation of patients with pulmonary neoplasms; it remains the most important procedure for determining the endobronchial extent of disease. FOB permits careful survey of the supraglottic, glottic, tracheal, and bronchial regions to the level of most subsegments. Tumor (T) status can be defined by measuring tumor proximity to the carina and various bronchi and by identifying unsuspected occult lesions that indicate multiplicity of disease. For lesions that are visible by endoscopy, an accurate histologic diagnosis can be achieved in over 90% of cases. For central lesions, cytologic studies via needle aspiration, washings, and brushings, coupled with biopsy, heightens the diagnostic yield to over 95%. Peripheral lesions not visible endoscopically may be approached by cytologic studies of brushings and bronchioloalveolar lavage (BAL), which yield a diagnosis in 50 to 60% of patients. Cytologic studies, coupled with transbronchial FNA (TBNA), greatly enhance diagnostic yield. The efficacy of bronchoscopy in establishing an accurate diagnosis depends on the location of the lesion, the histologic characteristics of the lesion, its accessibility via bronchoscopy, and the level of experience of the cytopathologist.

Fine-Needle Aspiration Biopsy Transthoracic percutaneous FNA biopsy (TPNA) and TBNA for diagnosis and staging of bronchogenic carcinoma have evolved in the United States since the 1970s. The College of American Pathologists Q-Probes Quality Assurance Program studied performance in FNA of pulmonary lesions derived by retrospective analyses of cases performed throughout 1989 by 436 institutions in North America.[83] Diagnostic accuracy was determined from histologically confirmed specimens. In the diagnosis of lung cancer by FNA, results showed the following: 89% sensitivity of procedure, 99% sensitivity of diagnosis, 96% specificity, 99% positive-predictive value, 70% negative-predictive value, 91% efficiency, 0.8% false-positive interpretation, and 8% false-negative rate.

Transthoracic Percutaneous Fine-Needle Aspiration Biopsy TPNA has significantly heightened the ability to diagnose intrathoracic pathologic processes. With fluoroscopic or CT guidance, tissue samples can be obtained from poorly accessible sites in the lung, mediastinum, abdomen, and retroperitoneum. The procedure is performed under local anesthesia using a small-gauge needle. Aspirated material is immediately processed with optimal procedural coordination, using an on-site cytopathologist for interpretation. Should the material be inadequate, a repeat aspiration can be performed. TPNA has been shown to be over 90% effective in establishing a final diagnosis. Diagnostic accuracy rates over 97% have been reported with minimal complication rates. The false-positive rate is low (1%) and the false-negative rate ranges from 23 to 29%. Complications after TPNA include pneumothorax (20–28%), with 5 to 7% requiring chest tube insertion; transient hemoptysis (2–4%); and, rarely, air embolism. Implantation of tumor cells along the needle tract has been reported in isolated cases but, again, is extremely rare.[84]

Transbronchial Fine-Needle Aspiration Biopsy TBNA was first introduced in 1958 by Schieppatti for use with rigid bronchoscopy. In 1983, Wang and Terry reported its usefulness with fiberoptic bronchoscopy in diagnosing and staging carcinoma of the lung.[85] It has been used most widely to sample endobronchial and peripheral lesions, and significantly improves the diagnostic yield when coupled with standard diagnostic measures (washings, brushings, and biopsies). TBNA is best performed in a suite that is equipped with fluoroscopy to enhance localization of the lesion. One of the most important applications of TBNA is the evaluation of mediastinal lymphadenopathy. The true sensitivity and specificity of TBNA appear to range from 14 to 50% and 96 to 100%, respectively. Thus, negative results require definitive operative confirmation, but the risk of a false-positive finding appears to be quite low.[84] The advent of endoscopic sonography (bronchoscopic or esophageal) may improve the yield of TBNA to over 80% and decreases the need for fluoroscopy, which is cumbersome and exposes patients and staff to radiation.[86]

Scalene Lymph Node Biopsy Scalene node biopsy was one of the first invasive techniques used to determine nodal involvement in patients with lung cancer. The procedure is now reserved for patients with potentially resectable N2 disease to rule out scalene or supraclavicular N3 disease, which precludes resection. In over 90% of cases, palpable scalene lymph nodes contain metastatic disease. Nonpalpable nodes contain metastatic disease in only 10% of cases. Anywhere from 3.5 to 22% of nonpalpable ipsilateral scalene and supraclavicular lymph node biopsy specimens are positive; the incidence of positives is highest in patients with nonsquamous tumors and centrally located tumors.

Mediastinoscopy In 1954, Harken and colleagues introduced the use of the Jackson laryngoscope to explore the mediastinum through a supraclavicular incision. They promoted the concept of inoperability of lung tumors with associated mediastinal involvement. For similar purposes, transcervical mediastinoscopy was introduced by Carlens in 1959. Currently it is the best method for invasive evaluation of the middle mediastinum to include the peritracheal and subcarinal lymph nodes. The indication remains preoperative mediastinal nodal assessment in patients with CT scan evidence of cross-sectional lymph node enlargement of more than 1 cm. In such patients who are proven to have lung cancer, the chance that these nodes contain metastasis is over 7%. If the nodes are enlarged to 1.5 to 2 cm or more, the risk of having metastatic involvement is over 30%.

The accuracy of cervical mediastinoscopy ranges from 80 to 90%, and the false-negative rate ranges from 10 to 12%. The lymph node station most commonly missampled is the subcarinal region, which is difficult to access in some patients and challenging to biopsy completely in most patients. The subaortic and aortopulmonary window regions are inaccessible by standard cervical mediastinoscopy, adding to the overall inaccuracy of the procedure.[87] Extended cervical mediastinoscopy, a variation of standard mediastinoscopy, has been useful for staging lesions in the left upper lobe. The standard mediastinoscopy incision is used, with the plane of dissection extending anterior to the innominate artery and aorta, anterolaterally to the level of the aortopulmonary window. Direct tumor invasion into the mediastinum or nodal disease within the prevascular space and aortopulmonary window can be assessed with this technique. Accuracy rates are over 91%. "Anterior mediastinotomy" was originally described by McNeil and Chamberlain. It permits direct visual access to the anterior mediastinum through the second, third, or fourth anterior interspace, with or without removal of a short portion of the adjacent cartilage. For right-sided lesions, the procedure provides access to the proximal pulmonary artery and superior vena cava. The procedure is used on the left side to evaluate disease in the subaortic and lateral aortic regions.

Thoracoscopy Thoracoscopy has been a valuable tool since it was first described by the Swedish internist Jacobaeus in 1910. Although the technique initially was limited primarily to lysing of adhesions to create a pneumothorax for the treatment of tuberculosis, thoracic surgeons retained the procedure as a valuable part of the surgical armamentarium for evaluating pleural diseases.[88] Thoracoscopy permits visualization of the entire visceral, parietal, and mediastinal pleural surfaces. Excisional or incisional biopsies for establishing N and M status can be performed safely under direct vision. Advances in technology and therapy have enabled broader applications for this technique. Thoracoscopy has recently been used both diagnostically and therapeutically in the staging and treatment of lung cancer. With the introduction of video technology and the refinement of endoscopic stapling devices, video-assisted thoracoscopy (VATS) has enabled a broader range of applications, including resectional techniques. Although the role of VATS for the treatment of lung cancer has not been defined, several reports indicate that using such minimally invasive procedures may enhance the accuracy of diagnosis and staging of lung cancer. Thoracoscopy is very helpful for staging lung cancer in the presence of associated pleural disease. Pleural effusions in patients with lung cancer require further evaluation of the pleural surface before thoracotomy. Discontinuous foci of tumor on the pleural surface or positive fluid cytologic findings are indicative of T4 disease and preclude resection. Thoracoscopy affords the potential for more complete staging of disease with suspected mediastinal nodal spread and has become a valuable adjunct to cervical mediastinoscopy and anterior mediastinotomy.

Through separate thoracoscopic incisional sites, the posterior mediastinum as well as the peritracheal, subazygous, hilar, and aortopulmonary window nodal regions can be reached. Precarinal and high subcarinal nodes are usually inaccessible. Low subcarinal nodes can be reached, but they are more easily removed from the right side than the left side. Thoracoscopy can be used to assess contralateral or ipsilateral parenchymal disease remote from the primary tumor, mediastinal masses, and pericardial disease, which may represent T4 or M1 disease.

Operative Staging Operative staging provides the opportunity to verify histologically the extent of gross and microscopic disease. The surgeon is responsible for performing a complete nodal dissection or nodal sampling as an integral part of the thoracotomy. Lymph nodes are removed and labeled according to the location of the station on the regional station map (Figure 80-7). Lymph node maps were introduced in the 1970s when nodal dissection was recognized as an important component of surgical staging. In 1983, the American Thoracic Society (ATS), using transverse section anatomy as defined by CT scan and viewed at thoracotomy, developed a regional lymph node staging map, which was further revised by the Lung Cancer Study Group (LCSG). Another map, which is commonly used, was developed by Naruke, proposed by the Japan Lung Cancer Society (JLCS), and recommended by the American Joint Committee on Cancer (AJCC). The important difference between the two nodal maps is the location of station 10. In the ATS/LCSG map, station 10 represents mediastinal lymph nodes. In the AJCC/JLCS map, station 10 represents hilar lymph nodes. The current staging system places station 10 lymph nodes within the hilar nodes; therefore, they represent N1 nodes. The distinction between station 10 (N1 nodes) and station 4 (N2 nodes) is based on the position of the node relative to the visceral-to-mediastinal pleural reflection. Nodes covered by visceral pleura are level 10.[89] Within the mediastinum, a phantom midline exists to differentiate N2 and N3 nodes. Ipsilateral positive lymph nodes are N2 nodes, and contralateral positive lymph nodes are N3 nodes. If a lymph node straddles the midline and has its major component residing on one side, the nodal station is labeled according to the site of predominant location. Subcarinal nodes always bridge the midline but are classified as N2 nodes. If nodes within the subcarinal region obviously reside on the contralateral side, they should be labeled as N3 nodes. The surgeon ultimately is responsible for determining the boundary of the mediastinal and visceral pleura and for documenting the precise location of all lymph nodes prior to submitting them to the pathologist for examination.

CANCER SCREENING AND EARLY DETECTION

Because symptoms of early-stage localized disease are insidious and nonspecific, they are frequently attributed to the effects of smoking. By the time the patient seeks medical attention, the disease is usually advanced so that complete surgical resection is possible in fewer than 30% of cases, and the overall 5-year survival rate is less than 15%. Clearly, screening and early detection of cancer at a more treatable stage is a desirable goal. Unfortunately, to date there have been no randomized controlled studies that have demonstrated a disease-specific mortality advantage attributable to screening methods of lung cancer.

In the 1970s, the National Cancer Institute (NCI) sponsored three separate randomized trials to assess the efficacy of lung cancer screening in male smokers (aged 45 years or older who smoked at least one pack per day).[90] By 1978, a total of 31,360 patients had been enrolled, and the results of a 5-year follow-up study were published in 1984. The Mayo Lung Project assessed the screening potential of routine chest radiographs versus symptom development, while the other two projects, the Johns Hopkins Lung Project and the Memorial Sloan-Kettering Lung Cancer Screening Program, evaluated the screening potential of routine sputum cytology with chest radiographs versus chest radiographs alone. Chest radiographs detected lung cancer at an ear-

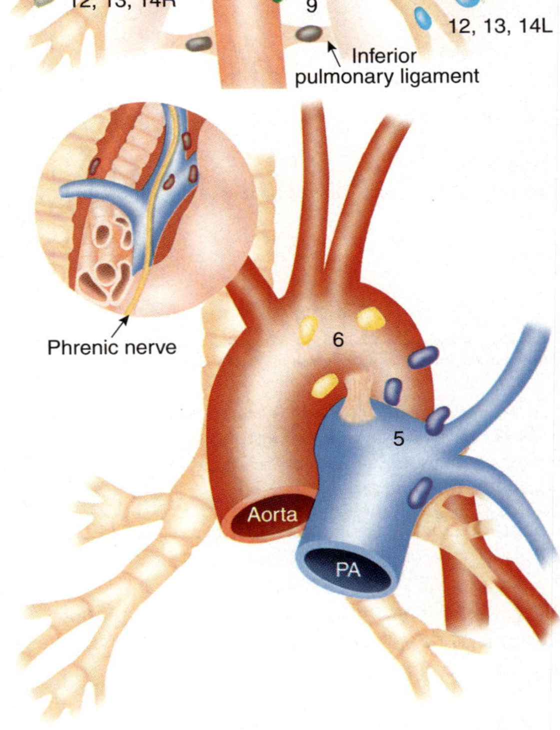

Figure 80-7 Regional lymph node stations for the staging of lung cancer. The location of the lymph nodes and assigned numbers are determined by the surgeon at the time of operation. Adapted from Mountain CF and Dresler CM, with permission.[89]

lier phase, improving resectability rates, whereas sputum cytology had no further impact. Final results of all three studies were unable to demonstrate a disease-specific mortality reduction, and for this reason there is no US policy on standardized screening for lung cancer.[91]

The introduction of low-radiation-dose spiral CT (LDCT) renewed interest in screening high-risk individuals for early lung cancer.[92] Initial data from separate centers suggested that LDCT improves detection of malignant disease by nearly 4- to 10-fold, but at the cost of a significantly high false-positive rate. These false-positive cases require further radiographic and/or invasive evaluation. Though LDCT is still an unproven technique, some medical establishments have been advocating its use for screening for lung cancer in the community at large.

The NCI-sponsored National Lung Screening Trial (NLST) is now conducting a randomized controlled trial to test whether LDCT scanning can reduce lung cancer mortality in asymptomatic individuals. Subjects are randomized to undergo screening with LDCT or chest x-ray. The NLST will enroll 50,000 high-risk heavy smokers (and former heavy smokers who quit within 15 years before randomization), aged 55 to 74 years. Participants will undergo an initial screening and two subsequent annual screenings and will be observed for a minimum of 4.5 years. The trial is powered to detect a modest but clinically relevant reduction of 20% in lung cancer mortality with LDCT screening. Randomization for the NLST began in September 2002 and was closed to further enrollment in 2004. Final analyses are expected in 2009.[93]

The Mayo Clinic recently presented its interim analysis of the NLST data. In a 5-year prospective study of LDCT in 1,520 individuals at high risk of lung cancer, participants (who were aged 50 years or older and had smoked at least 20 pack-years) underwent five annual (one initial and four subsequent) CT scan examinations. Results suggested that CT allowed detection of early-stage lung cancers, and that the benign nodule detection rate was high. However, there was no significant difference in lung cancer mortality rates.[94]

STAGING SYSTEMS

Staging is the determination of the extent of disease, with the intent of grouping patients with similar levels of disease for analytical, therapeutic, and prognostic purposes. The staging of lung cancer provides a scale of relative disease, which can be assigned to all patients with primary lung malignancies. Accurate staging of lung cancer is essential for defining operability, for selecting treatment regimens, for predicting survival, and for reporting comparable end results.

The staging system used in lung cancer has been based primarily on anatomic and morphologic criteria. The tumor-nodes-metastasis (TNM) system developed by Pierre Denoix in 1946 for staging of malignant tumors has remained the fundamental scheme for the classification of primary lung carcinoma. The TNM system has been used as the basis for the staging systems developed by both the AJCC and the International Union Against Cancer (UICC), and more recently for that developed by the International Staging System (ISS), which has replaced the earlier systems.

The accuracy of staging depends on available clinical information and relies on preoperative and subsequent evaluations at different times during the course of the disease: clinical-diagnostic staging (c), surgical-evaluative staging (s), postsurgical resection-pathologic staging (p), retreatment staging (r), and autopsy staging (a). These letters are used as a prefix to the TNM descriptors to identify the point during the course of the disease at which the stage was established (eg, cTNM for clinical-diagnostic staging). Clinical-diagnostic staging is based on the anatomic extent of disease that can be determined by any diagnostic testing short of thoracotomy. Such an evaluation may include findings from the history, physical examination, routine and special radiography, bronchoscopy, esophagoscopy, mediastinoscopy, mediastinotomy, thoracentesis, thoracoscopy, and any other examinations, including those used to demonstrate the presence of extrathoracic metastases. Surgical-evaluative staging, sTNM, is determined by information obtained at the time of exploratory thoracotomy, including biopsy results, but excluding information obtained from complete examination of a therapeutically resected specimen. Surgical-evaluative staging is rarely used today in recognition of the avoidable morbidity associated with thoracotomy. Postsurgical resection-pathologic staging, pTNM, is based on findings at thoracotomy and at pathologic examination of the resected specimen. To ensure accuracy, all other available data are con-

Table 80-7 TNM Descriptors

Primary Tumor (T)	
TX	Primary tumor cannot be assessed, or tumor proven by the presence of malignant cells in sputum or bronchial washings but not visualized by imaging or bronchoscopy
T0	No evidence of primary tumor
Tis	Carcinoma in situ
T1	Tumor ≤ 3 cm in greatest dimension, surrounded by lung or visceral pleura, without bronchoscopic evidence of invasion more proximal than the lobar bronchus* (ie, not in the main bronchus)
T2	Tumor with any of the following features of size or extent: > 3 cm in greatest dimension Involves main bronchus, ≤ 2 cm distal to the carina Invades the visceral pleura Associated with atelectasis or obstructive pneumonitis that extends to the hilar region but does not involve the entire lung
T3	Tumor of any size that directly invades any of the following: chest wall (including superior sulcus tumors), diaphragm, mediastinal pleura, parietal pericardium; or tumor in the main bronchus, ≤ 2 cm distal to the carina but without involvement of the carina; or associated atelectasis or obstructive pneumonitis of the entire lung
T4	Tumor of any size that invades any of the following: mediastinum, heart, great vessels, trachea, esophagus, vertebral body, carina; or tumor with a malignant pleural or pericardial effusion,† or with satellite tumor nodule(s) within the ipsilateral primary-tumor lobe of the lung
Regional Lymph Nodes (N)	
NX	Regional lymph nodes cannot be assessed
N0	No regional lymph node metastasis
N1	Metastasis to ipsilateral peribronchial and/or ipsilateral hilar lymph nodes, and intrapulmonary nodes involved by direct extension of the primary tumor
N2	Metastasis to ipsilateral mediastinal and/or subcarinal lymph node(s)
N3	Metastasis to contralateral mediastinal, contralateral hilar, ipsilateral, or contralateral scalene, or supraclavicular lymph node(s)
Distant Metastasis (M)	
MX	Presence of distant metastasis cannot be assessed
M0	No distant metastasis
M1	Distant metastasis present‡

*The uncommon superficial tumor of any size with its invasive component limited to the bronchial wall, which may extend proximal to the main bronchus, is also classified T1.

†Most pleural effusions associated with lung cancer are due to tumor. However, there are a few patients in whom multiple cytopathologic examinations of pleural fluid show no tumor. In these cases, the fluid is nonbloody and is not an exudate. When these elements and clinical judgment dictate that the effusion is not related to the tumor, the effusion should be excluded as a staging element, and the patient's disease should be staged T1, T2, or T3. Pericardial effusion is classified according to the same rules.

‡Separate metastatic tumor nodule(s) in the ipsilateral nonprimary-tumor lobe(s) of the lung also are classified M1.

Table 80-8 Stage Grouping in Lung Cancer: TNM Subsets*

Stage	TNM Subset
0	Carcinoma in situ
IA	T1 N0 M0
IB	T2 N0 M0
IIA	T1 N1 M0
IIB	T2 N1 M0
	T3 N0 M0
IIIA	T3 N1 M0
	T1 N2 M0
	T2 N2 M0
	T3 N2 M0
IIIB	T4 N0 M0
	T4 N1 M0
	T4 N2 M0
	T1 N3 M0
	T2 N3 M0
	T3 N3 M0
	T4 N3 M0
IV	Any T, Any N, M1

*Staging is not relevant for occult carcinoma, designated TX N0 M0.

sidered as well. Pathologic stage is the most accurate stage achievable, short of autopsy. Retreatment staging, rTNM, refers to the restaging of progressive disease when the primary treatment has failed. Autopsy staging, aTNM, uses data from the postmortem examination and provides an opportunity to assess histologically the extent of disease beyond the confines of the chest and to compare the accuracy of earlier stage evaluations.

Staging of NSCLC The AJCC and UICC lung cancer staging systems served well for approximately 15 years and achieved wide popularity and usage. As time passed, significant differences in survival were noted among certain TNM subsets that had been grouped prospectively into the same clinical stage. To achieve uniformity in the descriptors of the TNM system and to heighten accuracy in predicting stage-specific survival, the AJCC and the UICC in 1985 together developed a single system that has become the primary system used internationally: the International Lung Cancer Staging System or the ISS. This system was revised in 1997 to allow greater specificity in identifying patient groups with similar prognoses and treatment options (Tables 80-7, 80-8, and 80-9).[95] Since its inception, the ISS has gained worldwide acceptance and remains the predominant system for the staging of lung cancer.

TNM Descriptors The primary tumor descriptor T derives its classification on the basis of size, location, and extent of local invasion. T0 indicates no evidence of a primary tumor and is used primarily during retreatment staging. TX describes tumors that are identified cytologically by malignant cells in sputum samples or bronchial washings, but no specific site of origin can be recognized radiographically or bronchoscopically. TX also is used to describe tumors that cannot be adequately assessed during retreatment staging.

Carcinoma in situ can usually be assessed bronchoscopically and represents the earliest stage of disease. Accordingly, those malignancies that are confined to the bronchial mucosa are labeled Tis. T1 tumors are invasive lesions 3.0 cm or less in greatest dimension, surrounded entirely by pulmonary parenchyma or intact visceral pleura, and without evidence of invasion proximal to or including a lobar bronchial orifice. Uncommonly, superficial tumors that are confined to the bronchial wall are classified as T1 tumors; the invasive component is limited to the bronchial submucosa. Such superficial tumors are defined histopathologically, not clinically, and may be located in the main bronchus, within 2 cm from the carina.

T2 tumors are more than 3.0 cm in greatest dimension, or invade the visceral pleura, or have associated atelectasis or pneumonitis extending to the hilum. Associated atelectasis must involve less than the entire lung. The proximal extent of the tumor may include the lobar bronchial orifice, bronchus intermedius, or mainstem bronchus, but must be at least 2 cm distal to the carina.

Tumors that have grown beyond the confines of the pulmonary parenchyma are classified as T3 or T4 lesions. These tumors may be any size. T3 tumors involve structures that are amenable to resection and include the parietal pleura, chest wall, diaphragm, mediastinal pleura, mediastinal fat, pericardium, phrenic nerve, vagus nerve, and sympathetic chain. The T3 descriptor also describes invasive tumors that reside within 2 cm of the carina without involving the carina. Atelectasis of the entire lung is considered consistent with T3 status. T4 includes tumors that invade the structures of the deep mediastinum (including the heart, great vessels, trachea, esophagus, vertebral body, and carina), are associated with a pleural effusion containing malignant cells, or have a satellite tumor nodule(s) in the primary tumor lobe of the lung. The implication of a pleural effusion in conjunction with lung cancer is addressed later in the chapter.

Regional lymph node involvement is classified with the descriptor N. When no demonstrable metastases exist in regional lymph nodes, the N0 descriptor is given. Metastatic disease to the hilar lymph nodes is classified as N1 disease, and metastasis to the ipsilateral mediastinal lymph nodes or subcarinal lymph nodes is classified as N2 disease. The specific locations of involved hilar and mediastinal lymph nodes are important to staging and are discussed later. Metastatic dis-

Table 80-9 Lymph Node Map Definitions

Nodal Station	Anatomic Landmarks
N2 nodes: all N2 nodes lie within the mediastinal pleural envelope.	
1. Highest mediastinal nodes	Nodes lying above a horizontal line at the upper rim of the brachiocephalic (left innominate) vein where it ascends to the left, crossing in front of the trachea at its midline
2. Upper paratracheal nodes	Nodes lying above a horizontal line drawn tangential to the upper margin of the aortic arch and below the inferior boundary of No. 1 nodes
3. Prevascular and retrotracheal nodes	Prevascular and retrotracheal nodes may be designated 3A and 3P; midline nodes are considered to be ipsilateral
4. Lower paratracheal nodes	The lower paratracheal nodes on the right lie to the right of the midline of the trachea between a horizontal line drawn tangential to the upper margin of the aortic arch and a line extending across the right main bronchus at the upper margin of the upper lobe bronchus, and contained within the mediastinal pleural envelope; the lower paratracheal nodes on the left lie to the left of the midline of the trachea between a horizontal line drawn tangential to the upper margin of the aortic arch and a line extending across the left main bronchus at the level of the upper margin of the left upper lobe bronchus, medial to the ligamentum arteriosum and contained within the mediastinal pleural envelope. Researchers may wish to designate the lower paratracheal nodes as No. 4s (superior) and No. 4i (inferior) subsets for study purposes; the No. 4s nodes may be defined by a horizontal line extending across the trachea and drawn tangential to the cephalic border of the azygos vein; the No. 4i nodes may be defined by the lower boundary of No. 4s
5. Subaortic (aortopulmonary window)	Subaortic nodes are lateral to the ligamentum arteriosum or the aorta or left pulmonary artery and proximal to the first branch of the left pulmonary artery and lie within the mediastinal pleural envelope
6. Para-aortic nodes (ascending aorta or phrenic)	Nodes lying anterior and lateral to the ascending aorta and the aortic arch or the innominate artery, beneath a line tangential to the upper margin of the aortic arch
7. Subcarinal nodes	Nodes lying caudal to the carina of the trachea, but not associated with the lower lobe bronchi or arteries within the lung
8. Paraesophageal nodes (below carina)	Nodes lying adjacent to the wall of the esophagus and to the right or left of the midline, excluding subcarinal nodes
9. Pulmonary ligament nodes	Nodes lying within the pulmonary ligament, including those in the posterior wall and lower part of the inferior pulmonary vein
N1 nodes: all N1 nodes lie distal to the mediastinal pleural reflection and within the visceral pleura.	
10. Hilar nodes	The proximal lobar nodes, distal to the mediastinal pleural reflection and the nodes adjacent to the bronchus intermedius on the right; radiographically, the hilar shadow may be created by enlargement of both hilar and interlobar nodes
11. Interlobar nodes	Nodes lying between the lobar bronchi
12. Lobar nodes	Nodes adjacent to the distal lobar bronchi
13. Segmental nodes	Nodes adjacent to the segmental bronchi
14. Subsegmental nodes	Nodes around the subsegmental bronchi

ease located in lymph nodes in the contralateral mediastinum, contralateral hilum, or on either side outside the thorax (scalene or supraclavicular) is classified as N3 disease.

Metastases to distant organs or lymph node sites beyond the N3 sites, or ipsilateral involvement in lobe(s) of the lung other than the site of the primary tumor, chest wall, or pleural nodules discontinuous from the primary tumor, are identified by the M1 descriptor.

Stage 0 includes carcinoma in situ (Tis N0 M0). Stage I comprises T1 or T2 lesions without any lymph node metastases or distant metastases (stage IA, T1 N0; stage IB, T2 N0). Stage II includes T1 or T2 tumors with metastasis to the lymph nodes in the peribronchial or ipsilateral hilar region only, or locally more advanced tumors without any nodal involvement (stage IIA, T1 N1, stage IIB, T2 N1, T3 N0). Stage IIIA disease represents T3 with metastasis limited to the peribronchial or ipsilateral hilar nodes or any metastasis to ipsilateral mediastinal lymph nodes (T3 N1, T1 N2, T2 N2, T3 N2). Stage IIIB disease includes any tumor more extensive than T3, any tumor with supraclavicular or contralateral mediastinal lymph node involvement, or any tumor with a malignant pleural effusion but without evidence of distant metastasis (any T N3, T4, any N). Stage IV disease pertains to distant metastatic spread (any T, any N, M1).

Staging of NSCLC has been modified in recent years with the introduction of FDG-PET. This modality, and more so integrated PET-CT, may provide a combination of anatomical and functional assessment of the primary tumor and suspected areas of metastasis. Guidelines for their use in the preoperative setting are evolving gradually.[82]

Staging of SCLC The AJCC has acknowledged that the TNM system is not applicable to most SCLCs. Only those patients, approximately 5%, with very limited disease appear to benefit from use of detailed staging by the TNM system. In recognition of the difficulty in adequately staging SCLC, and on the basis of the observation that therapy depends on disease that may be encompassed by radiation therapy ports, the Veterans Administration Lung Group (VALG) developed a two-stage system for SCLC.[96] In this classification, patients with inoperable lesions were categorized as having either limited disease (disease confined to one hemithorax including the mediastinal, contralateral hilar, and ipsilateral scalene, or supraclavicular lymph nodes) or extensive disease (disease extending beyond the confines of limited disease). This classification system of the VALG or a slight modification of it, in which tumors with bilateral scalene or supraclavicular lymph node involvement are included in the limited disease category but those with pleural involvement are excluded, is widely used, even now that systemic therapy with combination chemotherapy has emerged as the main modality of treatment of this type of lung cancer.

As in NSCLC, the process of staging of SCLC is key to determining therapy and prognosis. Limited-stage disease usually is treated with a combination of chemotherapy and radiation therapy, whereas extensive-stage disease is usually treated with chemotherapy alone. Outside of a clinical trial setting, only the pertinent tests to confirm the status of the disease extent should be performed. If the mode of treatment is unaffected by stage, only the most simple tests are appropriate. Along these lines, patients' physiologic or functional status should be evaluated to determine their ability to undergo therapy.

A complete history and physical examination are fundamental and often can give clues to the extent of disease. Standard chest radiography with posterior-anterior and lateral views can assess the primary tumor and concurrent parenchymal disease. Mediastinal lymph node involvement often can be suggested by mediastinal widening. CT scan is important in further evaluating the primary tumor and local regional disease. It is often used in planning the ports for administration of radiation therapy.

One of the most common sites of extrathoracic metastatic disease is the bone. Approximately 38% of patients who present with SCLC have bone metastases. For this reason, radionuclide bone scan is important. If bone scan reveals suspect regions that suggest metastatic disease, site-specific bone radiographs are recommended for confirmation. Bone scan is associated with some degree of error because it often highlights areas of benign disease such as osteoarthritis and compression fractures. For this reason, bone scan alone should not be used for therapeutic decision making. Bone marrow examination is indicated in the staging of patients with SCLC when there is no other evidence of extensive disease. The bone marrow is involved with metastatic disease in 17 to 23% of patients. Bone marrow involvement is diagnosed by bone marrow aspiration and biopsy, which are complementary tests. The bone marrow is removed from the iliac crests, and bilateral biopsies increase the yield by approximately 10%. Fewer than 5% of patients present with bone marrow metastases as the only site of extrathoracic disease. MRI of the pelvic and femoral bones has shown promise in identification of metastatic disease to the bone marrow, and in a recent study MRI revealed 40% positivity, whereas biopsy yielded only 10% positivity.

Because the CNS is involved by disease in 5 to 14% of patients at the time of diagnosis, careful attention should be paid to the neurologic review of systems and examination. Metastases to the nervous system have been noted to occur in 30% of patients over the entire course of the disease, and may occur at autopsy in up to 65% of patients.[97] CT scan of the brain documents occult metastases in 5 to 10% of patients. Radionuclide scan of the brain is not accepted as a useful tool for evaluation of brain metastases. MRI of the brain is being used more frequently in the evaluation of patients with potential metastatic disease. On the basis of its apparent higher sensitivity rate, MRI may improve the accuracy of staging. Suspected spinal or leptomeningeal disease with carcinomatous meningitis can be confirmed by MRI coupled with cerebrospinal fluid cytologic studies.

Metastasis to the liver is extremely common in patients with SCLC. Liver function tests usually are not helpful as a screening tool, although patients whose test results are within normal ranges rarely have associated hepatic metastasis. Liver metastases are presented in 22 to 28% of patients at the time of presentation. For this reason, abdominal CT scan is an important addition to staging. Additionally, abdominal CT scanning can identify metastatic disease in other common sites, which include the adrenal glands, kidneys, pancreas, spleen, and intra-abdominal lymph nodes.

Prognostic Factors in SCLC The strongest clinical prognostic factors in patients with SCLC include extent of disease, performance status, sex, and age. Laboratory factors that have implications for prognosis include levels of lactate dehydrogenase (LDH), neuron-specific enolase, and hemoglobin; white cell and platelet counts; and serum sodium, bicarbonate, and alkaline phosphatase levels.[98]

Like NSCLC staging, staging of SCLC has been modified in recent years with the introduction of FDG-PET. This modality, and more so the integrated PET-CT, may provide a combination of anatomical and functional assessment of the primary tumor and suspected areas of metastasis. Guidelines for their use in the preoperative setting continue to develop.[82]

Performance Status In both NSCLC and SCLC, the patient's functional status or performance status (PS) is a key determinant of not only the patient's ability to undergo therapy, but also the patient's prognosis. PS is a general measure of a patient's physiologic status, taking into account the cancer and its associated effects along with other concurrent medical problems, such as cardiac or pulmonary disease. The PS is measured by two scales, the Zubrod and the Karnofsky.

Patients who are fully ambulatory and either asymptomatic (Zubrod PS 0) or mildly symptomatic but fully ambulatory (PS 1) usually tolerate therapy well. Patients who are symptomatic and spend up to 50% of the day in bed (PS 2) do not tolerate therapy as well, are at higher risk of complications of chemoradiotherapy, and usually are not surgical candidates. Patients who are symptomatic and in bed more than 50% of the day, but not bedridden (PS 3), and those patients who are bedridden (PS 4) usually are not candidates for therapy. Introduction of measures to correct medical problems, such as infection, anemia, electrolyte imbalances, malnutrition, and cardiac dysfunction, may improve the PS to permit therapy.

In a study of more than 5,000 patients entered into VALG protocols between 1968 and 1978, 77 prognostic factors were analyzed.[99] The most important prognostic factor was PS at the time of diagnosis. Extent of disease, weight loss greater than 10% in the previous 6 months, and the presence of any systemic symptoms were identified as other key prognostic factors.

General Guidelines for Lung Cancer Staging Patients who present with a new lung lesion and no evidence of metastatic disease by history, physical examination, or chest radiography should undergo CT scanning of the chest, including the liver and adrenal glands. Sputum cytologic studies can provide a diagnosis in about 10% of patients; it is more sensitive in patients with central lesions. A diagnosis also can be obtained by FOB or FNA as already discussed. In some circumstances, when a clinical stage I malignancy is suspected, invasive diagnostic studies can be waived, and the patient can undergo resection for diagnosis and treatment. If a resection beyond a lobectomy is required or if the patient is a high surgical risk, it is best to attempt preoperative diagnosis of the lesion. If the patient requires pneumonectomy, a cancer diagnosis should be made before proceeding with the resection.

Asymptomatic patients who have no abnormal results on physical examination and who are potential surgical candidates with clinical stage I, stage II, or stage IIIA (N0 or N1) disease can undergo resection. Patients with chest CT scan evidence of metastatic disease, particularly N2 or N3 disease, should undergo invasive studies, which may include cervical mediastinoscopy. In some instances, FNA biopsy can be performed. For patients with potentially resectable stage III disease, the status of the mediastinal lymph nodes is the most important factor in determining therapy. If the lymph nodes are radiographically enlarged (> 1 cm in cross-sectional diameter), histologic or cytologic evaluation is necessary prior to proceeding to thoracotomy. Evidence of improved outcome using neoadjuvant chemotherapy in this population has allowed some of these patients to come to resection. Randomized trials and institutional series have sought several different treatment strategies for potentially resectable stage IIIA (N2) disease: preoperative chemotherapy and/or radiation therapy, or chemotherapy and radiation therapy with no surgery. These studies are discussed in more detail later in this chapter. If N3 (stage IIIB) disease is discovered, nonoperative management is appropriate.

The invention of PET significantly changed lung cancer staging. The American College of Surgeons Oncology Group Z0050 studied the utility of PET in staging potentially operable NSCLC. Results suggested that in patients with suspected or proven NSCLC considered resectable by standard staging procedures, PET can prevent nontherapeutic thoracotomy in a significant number of cases. The authors concluded that use of PET for mediastinal staging should not be relied on as a sole staging modality, and positive findings should be confirmed by mediastinoscopy. In addition, they suggested that metastatic disease, especially a single site, identified by PET, required further confirmatory evaluation.[100]

If a diagnosis of SCLC is made, a thorough search for metastatic disease should be undertaken, followed by appropriate treatment in the form of chemotherapy or chemoradiotherapy. In only a small minority of cases (5%), can a patient with SCLC be considered for surgical intervention; these are cases of very early stage disease, that is, disease confined only to the lung without evidence of nodal or metastatic disease.

If the history and physical examination are suggestive of metastatic disease, other noninvasive staging studies directed to the area of concern should be performed. In addition to a chest CT scan, these studies may include a PET scan, a CT scan of the brain, bone scan, and a CT scan of the abdomen if the CT scan of the chest did not include the liver and adrenal glands. FDG-PET is substituted for bone scan in many institutions. The bone scan remains the most sensitive imaging study to detect skeletal metastases, but the apparent false-positive rate is as high as 50%. Bone scan detects metastases in only 3 to 4% of asymptomatic patients, most of whom have other foci of metastases. Bone scanning in asymptomatic patients should generally be reserved for those patients with locally advanced (T3, T4, or N2) or stage IV disease. These scans can be helpful in identifying unsuspected sites of metastases. Should such areas be identified, they should be confirmed radiologically and, if need be, by histologic or cytologic studies.

Upper abdominal CT scan should not be routinely performed for patients with clinical stage I or stage II disease. Extrathoracic metastases are unusual under such circumstances. In one series of patients with potentially resectable disease, 12% had unsuspected hepatic involvement. In the same series, unsuspected adrenal metastases were identified in 8% of patients. In another consecutive series of 172 patients who underwent adrenal CT scanning, 12% had metastatic disease; more than one-half of those patients had no other identifiable site of disease, and metastatic disease was confirmed cytologically by FNA biopsy in all patients. Approximately 10% of all lung cancer patients have CNS metastases at the time of diagnosis. CNS metastases are most common in patients with SCLC. Occult brain metastases are present in approximately 3 to 6% of patients with NSCLC. CT scanning of the brain identified a 13% incidence of metastases in patients being evaluated for resection, although only 21% of these were unsuspected by virtue of unremarkable neurologic examination findings. Because of this low incidence of occult brain metastases, particularly in patients with early clinical stages of disease, routine CT scanning of the brain is not performed.

In patients with locally advanced (T3, T4, or N2) or stage IV disease, a CT scan of the brain and a bone scan are essential. These should be performed, even if extensive disease elsewhere has been confirmed, since the discovery of brain metastases alters the type of therapy. MRI is probably more sensitive than CT scans for identifying and diagnosing asymptomatic metastatic disease to the brain, but its role in routine staging remains to be defined.

THERAPY FOR NSCLC

In patients with NSCLC, the most important prognostic factor is tumor stage, and this factor largely determines treatment.[101] Surgery is the standard mode of treatment of patients with stage I and II tumors and for some patients with stage III tumors; with preoperative or postoperative radiation therapy or chemotherapy (or both) added if the tumor invades the mediastinal lymph nodes. The use of combined-modality therapy in locally advanced stage III NSCLC is an area of intense investigation, as discussed later in this chapter. Patients with stage IV disease are treated with chemotherapy or palliative radiation therapy or with supportive therapy alone. Patients with histologically documented unresectable or inoperable NSCLC are evaluated first for definite therapy "for cure" with a combined chemoradiation therapy approach. If there are pressing symptomatic needs for palliation, such as complete obstruction of a major airway, hemoptysis, SVC obstruction, painful bony metastases in the weight-bearing areas, or symptomatic brain metastases, the initial treatment is radiotherapy with or without chemotherapy. If a patient has evidence of disseminated disease and there is no pressing need for radiotherapy, the approach includes consideration of systemic chemotherapy, or supportive therapy alone if the patient's general condition is not suitable for systemic chemotherapy. Each of the three main disciplines involved in the treatment of lung cancer—surgery, radiotherapy, and chemotherapy—is discussed individually. SCLC, whose treatment is radically different from that of NSCLC, is discussed as a separate section, albeit with similar organization.

Results by Stage **Stages IA and IB** The average 5-year survival rate for patients with stage I NSCLC is approximately 65% (range, 55–90.5%). Within this group, several factors appear to influence survival: T status, tumor size independent of T status, and histology. The more favorable tumors are T1 squamous cell carcinoma and T1 BAC. Focal T1 N0 BAC has been reported to have a 5-year survival rate as high as 90.5%.[102] Significant prognostic factors that adversely affect survival include mucin production by the tumor and diffuse invasion.

Overall survival rates of all patients with T1 N0 disease have been reported to be 82% at 5 years and 74% at 10 years, while those for patients with T2 N0 disease are 68% at 5 years and 60% at 10 years.[103] In this series of 598 patients, the overall incidence of recurrence was 27% (local or regional 7%, systemic 20%). Second primary tumors developed in 206 patients (34%). Of these 206 tumors, 70 (34%) were second primary lung cancers, for an overall incidence of second primary lung cancers of 11.7% (70 of 598). These findings, confirmed by other investigators, prompted division of stage I into two groups, stage IA (TI N0) and IB (T2 N0).

The median survival period for all patients with T1 N0 NSCLC is approximately 8 years. The long-term prognosis for patients with T1 N0 NSCLC has been evaluated by the LCSG, which reported recurrence rates per eligible patient per year of 0.042 for patients with squamous tumors and 0.088 to 0.106 for patients with nonsquamous tumors within the first 5 years after surgery.[104] A later report suggested, however, that the rate of recurrence decreased (from 0.043 to 0.013), whereas the rate of new primary lung cancer increased (from 0.009 to 0.016), with no significant differences between the two histologic subgroups.[103]

Stages IIA and IIB The average 5-year survival rate for patients with stage II disease is 41.2% (range, 29–51%). Several studies have evaluated this group to identify tumor characteristics that affect survival. The LCSG reported significant survival differences between patients with squamous carcinoma and those with adenocarcinoma and between patients with a T1 lesion and those with a T2 lesion.[105] More specifically, patients with T1 squamous carcinoma had a 5-year survival rate of 75%, while those with T2 adenocarcinoma had a 5-year survival rate of 25%. Mountain, in 1986, reported 5-year survival rate in 317 patients: 54% for those with a T1 lesion and 40% for those with a T2 lesion. These persistent differences in survival based on T status led to division of stage II into IIA and IIB.

Patients whose tumor is staged T3 N0 because of chest wall invasion have a favorable 5-year survival rate, as high as 56%. Patients with T3 N2 disease, however, have a 5-year survival rate ranging from 16% to less than 5%. Survival rates are worse in those patients who have incomplete resections. The similarity of the outcomes for T3 N0 and T2 N1 disease supported its reclassification as stage IIB.[71,89]

Adjuvant or Neoadjuvant Chemotherapy Supplementing surgery with chemotherapy has been tested by several studies with promising results.[4] Such an approach in selected patients may prolong survival with reasonable toxicity. This approach is becoming a standard of care in many cases in early-stage disease, and is discussed later in this chapter.

Stage IIIA Approximately 25 to 40% of patients with NSCLC have stage III disease. Of these, approximately one-third present with potentially resectable disease, stage IIIA (T1–3 N2, T3 N1). The median survival duration for all patients with stage IIIA (clinical or surgical stage) disease is 12 months, and the 5-year survival rate is 9 to 15%. Within the stage IIIA subset, however, survival rates vary widely.[71,89]

Burt and colleagues conducted a review of T3 and T4 tumors that involve the mediastinum, but not the mediastinal lymph nodes. The overall 5-year survival rate was 19%, with median survival duration of 18 months. Factors that were found to affect survival were complete resectability and histologic type. The 5-year survival rate with complete resection was 30%, and the 5-year survival rate of patients with adenocarcinoma or large-cell carcinoma was 30%, while that of patients with squamous cell carcinoma was 14%.[106]

Patients with clinical (preoperative) N0 or N1 disease but pathologic (postresection) N2 disease survive longer than patients with clinical N2 disease, and 3- and 5-year survival rates of 47% and 34%, respectively, were reported for such patients.[107] Pearson and colleagues noted that patients with negative mediastinoscopic findings who were found to have N2 disease following resection had a 24% 5-year survival rate; the 5-year survival rate was only 9% for those who underwent resection after positive mediastinoscopy.[108] Patients with "completely resected" pathologic N2 disease have a median 5-year survival rate approaching 22%.

The role of combined-modality treatment remains somewhat unclear. Many trials that included combinations of surgery, radiation therapy, and chemotherapy have been conducted for patients with stage III disease. The various treatment regimens and results are discussed in later sections.

Stage IIIB The median survival duration for stage IIIB patients is 8 months, and the 5-year survival rate is 5% or less.[71,95] The vast majority of these patients receive nonoperative therapy. There is, however, a select group of patients that can be considered for surgical resection: the rare patient with IIIB disease on the basis of a T4 tumor involving the carina and occasionally the superior vena cava (SVC), aorta, or atrium. With increased but acceptable operative morbidity and mortality rates, extended resection and reconstruction techniques can be undertaken. After carinal resection, 3- and 5-year survival rates are directly related to nodal status, and range from 0 to 43%. Extended resections for selected patients with other T3/T4 tumors have been associated with 5-year survival rates that vary from 0 to 18.3%, depending on nodal status.

Stage IV Stage IV disease is beyond the reach of surgical cure, with 5-year survival rate of less than 5%. Treatment of this disease is well outlined in the following sections. On rare occasions, patients with solitary brain metastasis and an otherwise resectable lesion can undergo resection of both tumors. In this select group, surgery seems to prolong life and improve quality of life better than nonsurgical treatment, although no prospective studies have been performed. The 5-year survival rate has been shown to range from 13 to 21%, with median survival duration of 14 months.

Surgical Treatment **Preoperative Assessment** For any patient being considered for pulmonary resection, specific risk factors play an important role in determining operability and the chances of perioperative complications. Factors that are known to be associated with increased perioperative morbidity and mortality are greater age, continued cigarette use, cardiac disease, restricted pulmonary function, and pneumonectomy. In association with these factors, PS is a key general indicator of physiologic function and, as such, is another factor determining risk. With the increasing use of adjuvant and induction therapy, concurrent systemic illnesses (renal or hepatic dysfunction, weight loss, anemia, leukopenia) and a diminished PS score associated with therapy can heighten a patient's intolerance to surgical intervention. Recent reviews of preoperative therapy for patients with stage III lung cancer have noted higher rates of complications than cited in historic reviews, although long-term survival appears to have been positively affected.[109] Several cooperative groups have evaluated the influence of PS on survival in large numbers of patients with inoperable lung cancer.[99] Each study found that a patient's initial PS had a definite impact, not only on prognosis, but also on the ability to tolerate aggressive therapy. A similar observation can be made in the evaluation of patients being considered for aggressive therapy in the form of surgical resection; those with a poor PS are at a higher risk than those with a good PS. Consideration of operability must include careful assessment of a patient's PS in addition to other key risk factors.

Cardiac Function The most common untoward perioperative events are cardiopulmonary ones. For this reason, the cardiopulmonary system must be carefully evaluated and optimally prepared before operative intervention. If there is a history of cardiac or vascular disease or suggestive symptoms, a thorough investigation of the cardiovascular system beyond initial assessment is imperative. Following screening electrocardiography, which should be performed in all patients, further tests to detect cardiac dysfunction or coronary artery disease may be necessary. Stress testing, echocardiography, multigated acquisition (MUGA) scanning, dobutamine echocardiography, or stress/Persantine thallium scanning may give clues to a heightened risk of ischemic disease. Coronary angiography ultimately may be necessary. Au and colleagues reported a postpneumonectomy mortality rate of 21% in patients older than 70 years.[110] The mortality rate was significantly adversely affected if the patient had a history of ischemic heart disease ($p = .001$). Miller and colleagues found that routine thallium scanning identified over 10% of patients with significant asymptomatic coronary artery disease and made a difference in management in half these patients.[111] Their review underscores the importance of careful questioning for possible underlying cardiac pathology. For patients unable to undergo a standard exercise test, Persantine thallium testing is very useful for predicting patients at risk of developing a postoperative cardiac event following major general or vascular procedures (sensitivity 100%, specificity 43%).

If studies reveal significant coronary or valvular disease that should be operatively corrected, angioplasty, coronary artery bypass, or valve repair can be performed prior to or during pulmonary resection. A series of 45 patients who underwent pulmonary resection for lung cancer either at the time of cardiac surgery or within a median of 2 months following surgery revealed operative mortality rates of 6.7% or 0%, respectively.[112] Another study on 11 concomitant cardiac and pulmonary resections for lung cancer revealed no operative deaths. The disadvantage of concomitant surgery is the inability to perform an adequate lymph node dissection for staging.

Patients who have had a recent myocardial infarction (MI) are at a significantly increased perioperative risk of re-infarction or death. Steen and colleagues showed that performance of any operation requiring general anesthesia within 3 months after an MI results in a 27% incidence of re-infarction.[113] The risk dropped to 11% 3 to 6 months after infarction and to 5% thereafter. Wells and colleagues reported no re-infarction in 48 patients who required an operation within 3 months of an MI. Their excellent results may have been secondary to very aggressive perioperative cardiac monitoring and early initiation of medical management. The nature of the procedures and the selection criteria in this study are not well outlined, but the results do suggest that the risk in this group of patients can be reduced with aggressive perioperative measures.[114] The best time to perform a pulmonary resection following an MI is unclear. Certainly, the risk of the operation and possible re-infarction should be weighed against the possibility of growth and spread of the malignancy. Mathisen and Wain postpone resection to at least 4 to 6 weeks after the event.[115] Our approach agrees with that of Mathisen and Wain. If such management is not feasible, alternative treatment should be considered.

Pulmonary Function Most patients with lung cancer have associated chronic lung disease because of many years of smoking. The degree of underlying parenchymal pathology and abnormal chest mechanics may be subtle or subjectively insignificant because of compensatory lifestyle changes. On the other hand, concurrent benign pulmonary disease may be severely, subjectively debilitating for unclear reasons and without objective proof. Various objective studies, noninvasive and invasive, can provide good information in the overall assessment of pulmonary function and can provide the surgeon with a good estimate of risk.

Because pulmonary resection reduces lung volume, precise measurements of pulmonary function and reserve are imperative. Predicted postoperative volumes, based on spirometry, are useful in estimating the amount of lung that can be removed. Spirometric studies measure overall lung capacity, reserve volumes, functional residual capacity, and forced expiratory volumes. These simple tests give a relatively crude but highly useful estimate of lung function and pulmonary mechanics. The presence and extent of underlying disease can be quickly determined, along with any response to therapy (eg, bronchodilators).

Patients with abnormal pulmonary function are known to have an associated increase in perioperative complications. Several spirometric parameters have been analyzed by various authors and are useful in identifying patients at increased risk (Figure 80-8). No single parameter is used alone to select or exclude patients from surgery. The information is always considered collectively, along with other parameters noted below. Patients with limited pulmonary function in the noted risk categories generally are more susceptible to perioperative complications because of limited functional reserve to adapt to postresectional changes and underlying lung disease that is more susceptible to dysfunction caused by inflammation or infection. To optimize pulmonary function, patients are strongly encouraged to stop smoking 2 weeks in advance of surgery to reduce the amount of bronchorrhea and smoking-related bronchitis. Pulmonary physiotherapy is initiated with bronchodilators, incentive spirometry and coughing, appropriate antibiotics, and a walking program. Patients with poor pulmonary function test (PFT) results should have the tests repeated following this 1- to 2-week physiotherapy program. In some instances of severe bronchospasm, a short course of steroid therapy can be helpful.

Arterial Blood Gases Resting hypoxia or hypercapnia is a subtle indicator of chronic pulmonary disease that affects proper gas exchange. A variety of etiologies, both pulmonary and cardiac, can cause blood gas abnormalities. The most common cause in patients with lung cancer is ventilation/perfusion mismatch caused by chronic obstructive pulmonary disease. Areas of pneumonia, atelectasis, or arterial obstruction from a lung tumor only exacerbate a pre-existing mismatch. An arterial oxygen pressure (PO_2) less than 60 mm Hg and a resting partial pressure of carbon dioxide (PCO_2) over 50 mm Hg are indicators of high risk of perioperative complications. Whether because of the tumor, other underlying disease, or both, the presence of abnormal arterial blood gases indicates a problem that can be worsened by resection of an already limited resource of lung.

Xenon Scanning Careful analysis of normally perfused and ventilated lung segments can be helpful in identifying those patients who can safely undergo resection. Split lung function studies using inhaled ^{133}Xenon and injected ^{99m}Tc-labeled macroaggregated albumin give percentages of the total ventilation and perfusion in each lung. The postresectional volumes can be calculated by multiplying the ventilation or perfusion percentage to the remaining lung.

Oxygen Consumption Study The previously mentioned tests are performed primarily with the patient in a resting state without the benefit of exertional stresses. Measurement of a patient's

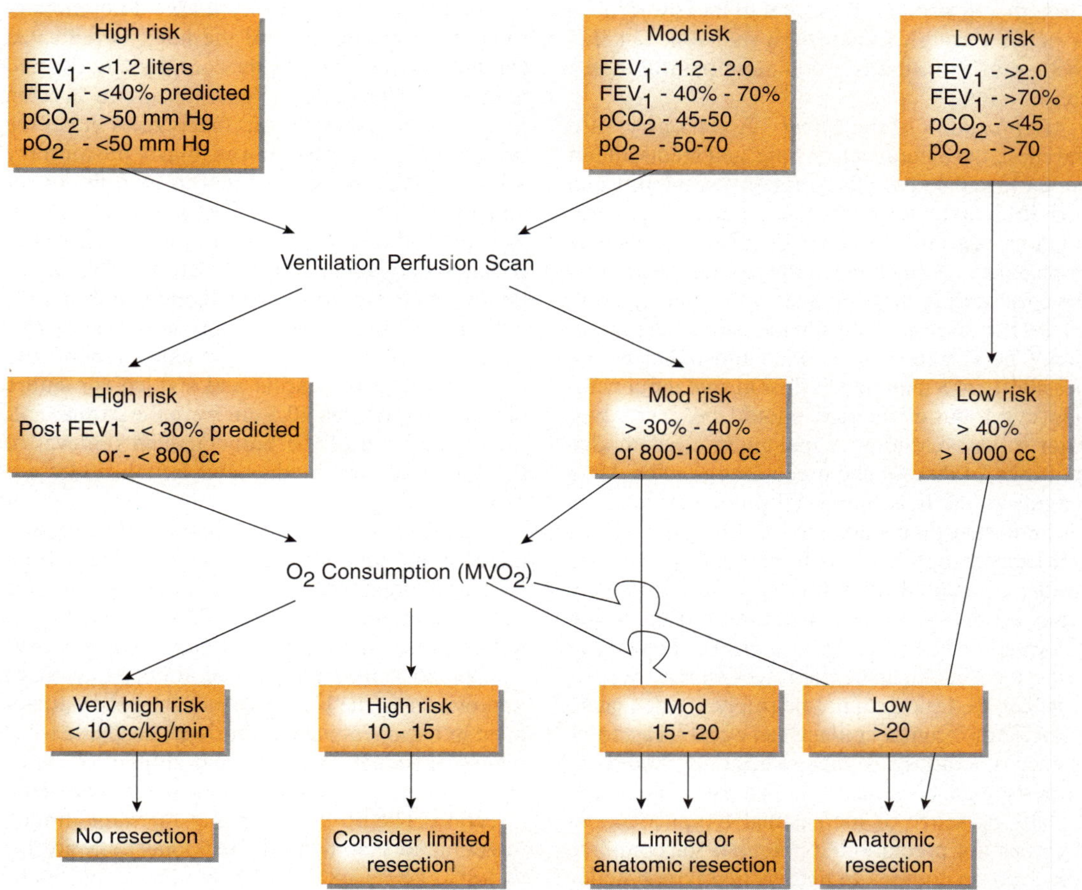

Figure 80-8 Pulmonary risk based on spirometry results, arterial blood gases (ABG), and oxygen consumption studies (MVO_2). CXR = chest radiography; FEV = forced expiratory volume; H & P = history and physical examination.

capacity to exercise may, in fact, be a better predictor of candidacy for surgery. A good measure of exercise capacity is the maximal amount of oxygen that can be consumed during a given period of time. This oxygen consumption study (MVO_2) measures the end product of cardiac and pulmonary interaction in a real-time stress situation that appears to better simulate the physiologic demands of surgery. Several studies have shown the usefulness of MVO_2 in predicting increased risk of perioperative complications.[116] Patients with an MVO_2 higher than 20 mL/kg/min are at low risk of complications, whereas those with an MVO_2 less than 10 mL/kg/min are at a very high risk of complications. Those with values from 10 to 15 are at high risk but may be candidates for limited resection or possibly lobectomy, depending on spirometric results. Patients with values from 15 to 20 have a low to moderate risk and usually can tolerate major resection, including pneumonectomy.

Diffusing Capacity Other parameters of underlying pulmonary disease include abnormal gas diffusion and exchange and an imbalance of ventilation and perfusion. The diffusing capacity for carbon monoxide (DL_{co}) estimates pulmonary capillary surface area and indirectly reflects pulmonary capillary hemoglobin content. DL_{co} also estimates alterations in alveolar microarchitecture, indicating the presence of emphysematous changes. Ferguson and colleagues showed the value of measuring DL_{co} and its usefulness in predicting postoperative pulmonary complications in patients who have underlying parenchymal changes despite having acceptable spirometry results.[117] In their group of patients, as the predicted DL_{co} percent worsened, the prevalence of pulmonary complications and mortality increased, particularly when the DL_{co} was less than 60%. In a more recent, updated study of diffusing capacity, Ferguson and colleagues showed a direct correlation between worsened diffusing capacity and postoperative complications and mortality. They concluded that the predicted postoperative diffusing capacity percentage is the strongest single predictor of risk of complications and mortality after lung resection. They found little relationship between the predicted postoperative diffusing capacity percentage and the predicted postoperative forced expiratory volume in 1 second and suggested that these two values be evaluated independently in estimating operative risk.[117] The usefulness of DL_{co} as a predictor of pulmonary complications has been confirmed by other investigators.

Assessment of Pulmonary Hypertension In patients with chronic lung disease manifested by abnormal arterial blood gas values, reduced diffusing capacity, low values in oxygen consumption studies, or poor spirometric results underlying pulmonary hypertension may be present and often to some degree. Unrecognized pulmonary hypertension can contribute to pulmonary complications and mortality in patients undergoing resection, particularly in those undergoing pneumonectomy. Right ventricular work is already increased in patients with pulmonary hypertension. With resection, further work is imposed and can lead to hemodynamic compromise. Eventually, failure can ensue. The specific values of pulmonary pressures that place a patient at risk of resection are unclear. If marginal spirometry and poor oxygen consumption values coexist with abnormal indicators of right heart function and pulmonary vascular resistance, alternative therapy may need to be considered.

Surgical Technique ***Conduct of Anesthesia*** Pulmonary resections are conducted under general anesthesia. After placement of adequate intravenous access and appropriate monitoring devices, general anesthesia is induced, and the patient is intubated with a single-lumen endotracheal tube. Fiberoptic bronchoscopy is performed if it has not been performed previously by the operating surgeon. Bronchoscopy provides the opportunity to assess the airway, the extent of endobronchial disease, and other possible sites of unsuspected lesions. Following bronchoscopy, in most instances, a double-lumen endotracheal tube is placed to provide selective ventilation. In such a fashion, the operated lung can be deflated, facilitating access to the hilar structures without respiratory activity impeding visualization. In instances of complex resections for which bronchoplastic or vascular reconstruction is required, variations in the conduct of anesthesia may include cross-table ventilation, jet ventilation, or cardiopulmonary bypass. At the completion of the operation, the patient is awakened in the operating room and extubated, depending on the extent of the operation and the condition of the patient. Pain management is key to a smooth recovery. Some accepted modalities for adequate control of post-thoracotomy discomfort are continuous epidural analgesia and continuous intravenous analgesia delivered via a patient-controlled analgesia pump. These methods usually provide satisfactory relief from pain while permitting patients to cough, breathe deeply, and ambulate effectively. Supplemental nonsteroidal agents are used when breakthrough pain occurs. Other methods for pain relief are also used, such as intercostal nerve cryoablation, continuous delivery of local anesthetic agents, and intercostal nerve blocks.

Incisions Several approaches to the chest cavity are used for resection of pulmonary tumors. The most frequently used incision is the posterolateral thoracotomy; it permits the best overall exposure to the pleural space. For this and most other thoracic incisions, the patient is placed in the lateral decubitus position with the table slightly flexed. A "lazy S"-shaped incision is made, passing under the tip of the scapula. The chest cavity is commonly entered through the fifth intercostal space. For resections that must include a portion of the chest wall, the incision is tailored accordingly; in particular, for superior sulcus tumors, the incision is carried posterosuperiorly with division of the trapezius muscle. At the completion of the operation, chest tubes are placed and brought out through separate incisions. Closure is accomplished by reapproximating the ribs and closing the chest wall musculature and subcutaneous tissue in individual layers.

The anterior thoracotomy is used primarily for noncomplex lesions located in the mid, lower, and anterior lung fields. The patient is placed in the supine position. The incision travels in a curvilinear fashion under the border of the pectoralis muscle, although in some instances, some fibers of the pectoralis are divided. In women, the incision is made in the inframammary fold and can be carried laterally or medially as needed. The disadvantage of the anterior thoracotomy is limited exposure of the superior and posterior mediastinum.

The axillary thoracotomy can be used for uncomplicated and straightforward pulmonary resections, primarily for an upper or middle lobectomy. A horizontal or transversed incision can be used to expose the underlying musculature with care to avoid the long thoracic nerve. The only muscle divided is the intercostal muscle, along with splitting of a few fibers of the serratus anterior. The chest cavity is entered through the fourth or fifth intercostal space. The advantages of this approach include better cosmesis, smaller incision length, and quicker opening and closure. Also, the recovery time may be shorter because relatively fewer muscles are divided. Two other types of muscle-sparing thoracotomy are also available: anterior and posterior. In anterior muscle-sparing thoracotomy, the skin incision is placed along the anterior portion of the posterolateral thoracotomy. The latissimus musculature is retracted posteriorly, and the serratus anterior musculature is retracted anteriorly to expose the rib cage. The posterior muscle-sparing thoracotomy is placed along the posterior portion of the posterolateral thoracotomy. The latissimus and underlying serratus are reflected anteriorly, while a small rim of exposed trapezius muscle is retracted posteriorly. The chest cavity is entered through the desired interspace, usually the fifth or sixth. The primary disadvantage of muscle-sparing thoracotomies is their inability to provide adequate access for the opening of an interspace higher than the fifth and a limited ability to spread the ribs for exposure that may be critical in more complex resections.

A median sternotomy or clamshell incision can be used for resections of tumors located in the upper lobes or in cases of bilateral disease when exploration of both thoracic cavities is desired. Sternotomy provides good access to both hemithoraces, facilitates anesthesia by keeping the patient in the supine position, and is a less painful incision than any thoracotomy. The disadvantages of sternotomy are that exposure of the lower lobes is poor, and resection of tumors in this location is difficult. Moreover, mediastinal lymph node dissections are not as complete as those performed through a thoracotomy. Access to the lower lobes is better through a clamshell incision, but this method of exposure is much more painful than a sternotomy.

Exploration of the Chest After entry into the chest, the pleural cavity, lung, and mediastinum are evaluated thoroughly to assess resectability and possible metastatic disease. Parietal pleural implants are indicative of T4 disease, whereas implants extending beyond the parietal pleura into the chest wall or diaphragmatic implants represent metastatic disease. Both situations preclude resection. The presence of pleural fluid indicates the possibility of a malignant effusion, and intraoperative cytologic evaluation should be performed prior to any resection; a malignant effusion also indicates T4 disease and precludes resection. If no diagnosis has been achieved preoperatively, the lesion in question is assessed and biopsied, if this can be accomplished easily and safely. Often, a wedge excisional biopsy is done to completely remove a peripherally located tumor. If the lesion is located centrally, an FNA or Tru-cut biopsy can be performed. An anatomic resection may be necessary if the lesion cannot be safely or adequately biopsied or if tumor spillage can occur as a consequence of a biopsy. A pneumonectomy should not be performed, however, without a tissue diagnosis.

The presence of mediastinal lymphadenopathy does not preclude the potential for complete resection. In contrast to mediastinal lymph nodes that are found to contain metastatic disease prior to thoracotomy, microscopically positive mediastinal lymph nodes (N2) that are discovered at thoracotomy do not carry as poor a prognosis. Patients with clinical (preoperative) N0 or N1 disease but pathologic (postresection) N2 disease survive longer than patients with clinical N2 disease. Tumors that extend deeply into the pulmonary hilum or are densely fixed to the mediastinum or chest wall may require a more extended resection than anticipated. In most instances, resectability can be determined by preoperative noninvasive studies, exploratory thoracotomy revealing unresectable disease in only about 5% of patients. In such circumstances, where unexpected findings occur at thoracotomy, the surgeon decides the feasibility of an extended resection. The first priority remains the safety of the patient and whether an extended resection can be reasonably and completely performed on the basis of the studies that evaluated the patient's cardiac and pulmonary functions. If physiologic evidence indicates an acceptable risk, resectability is then determined, taking into account the factors that differentiate T3 and T4 tumors. The determinants of a T3 tumor usually do not prevent a safe and complete resection; a resection that accomplishes removal of the tumor with negative gross and microscopic margins provides the best opportunity for long-term survival. If the tumor is T4, the likelihood of complete resectability is low except in isolated circumstances in which advanced techniques can be used. These situations are discussed below in the section "Extended Surgical Procedures."

Standard Surgical Procedures Pneumonectomy, the total removal of the lung, is indicated for tumors that cannot be completely resected with a lesser procedure. Pneumonectomy is often indicated for central lesions that involve either the mainstem bronchus or the main pulmonary artery, tumors that are located in both the upper and lower lobes, and locally recurrent tumors. The procedure is most commonly performed through a posterolateral thoracotomy. The vascular structures are mobilized, ligated, and divided within either the thoracic or pericardial cavity (for central tumors). The main bronchus is mobilized to the level of the carina and stapled (or suture closed) no more than 0.5 cm from the carina. Following division of the bronchus and removal of the specimen, the mediastinal lymph nodes are dissected.

Usually, postoperative pleural drainage is unnecessary, unless fluid or blood drainage from the hemithorax needs to be monitored. Aggressive pulmonary toilet and pain control are mandatory to reduce the incidence of pulmonary complications.

Operative mortality and morbidity rates have improved over the last 25 years owing to improvement in perioperative monitoring, anesthetic techniques, postoperative care, and antibiotics. Mortality rates vary depending on the magnitude of the resection. The 30-day mortality rates for limited resection, lobectomy, and pneumonectomy are 1.4 to 3.8%, 1.8 to 3.8%, and 5 to 12%, respectively. Mortality rates for pneumonectomy as high as 21 to 43% have been reported when coupled with aggressive preoperative, concomitant chemotherapy, and radiation therapy. Complications from all causes occur in over one-fourth of all patients. Cardiopulmonary complications (pneumonia, acute respiratory distress syndrome, atelectasis, aspiration, atrial fibrillation, and myocardial infarction) are the most frequent morbidities associated with pulmonary resection and occur in approximately 20 to 30% of patients. Postoperative pneumonia is responsible for the majority of the postoperative deaths. Empyema occurs in approximately 2% of patients undergoing pneumonectomy. Mortality rates for pneumonectomy range from 6 to 12%. For older patients or those undergoing a right pneumonectomy, the mortality rate is higher and can approach 10.6% to as high as 37% for some high-risk patients who have undergone preoperative therapy.[118–121]

Lobectomy is the most common type of resection performed for lung cancer and accounts for approximately 65 to 75% of all resections at our institution. Such anatomic resections provide a method for removing the primary tumor, associated disease, and lymph node-bearing areas while leaving a significant amount of residual functional parenchyma. Cancer survival is equivalent for patients undergoing lobectomy or pneumonectomy for all stages of disease when a complete resection is performed. Lobectomy requires isolation, ligation, and division of the individual segmental arterial and venous branches supplying the lobe. Division of the fissure between the lobes is usually performed with a stapling device to

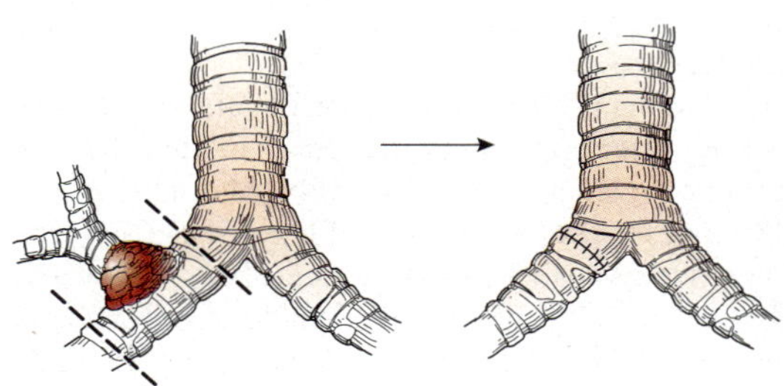

Figure 80-9 A standard right upper lobectomy cannot be performed in this circumstance because residual tumor will remain in the bronchial stump. Rather than performing a pneumonectomy, a sleeve lobectomy is performed to ensure negative margins while still preserving the right middle and lower lobes.

reduce the air leak that occurs from incising the pulmonary parenchyma. The lobar bronchus is closed with a stapler or with sutures. For lesions that are located close to the lobar orifice, an adequate margin of resection often cannot be achieved. In such circumstances, a portion of the main bronchus must be included with the resection. This type of resection is termed a sleeve resection and is performed as a parenchyma-sparing procedure to avoid pneumonectomy (Figure 80-9). It is most commonly performed for lesions located in the right upper lobe, but it may be used for tumors in the left upper lobe, left lower lobe, or bronchus intermedius. The procedure is performed to include a small segment of grossly normal bronchus (5 mm) to ensure an adequate margin. Once frozen section analysis confirms negative margins, the two ends of the bronchus are reapproximated with interrupted sutures, achieving an airtight seal. In selected patients, bronchial sleeve resection has proven to be a safe and effective method for pulmonary preservation, with cancer survival rates comparable with those following pneumonectomy.[122] The overall 5-year survival rate in patients with stage III disease who undergo sleeve lobectomy is 21%. A 5-year survival rate of 38% has been reported following sleeve resection of T3 lesions; the survival rate appears to be directly related to the extent of N2 nodal involvement. As for pneumonectomy, pulmonary complications are the most common event after lobectomy and are the primary cause of postoperative mortality. The overall procedural mortality rate, however, is only 1 to 3%. Sleeve resections also have low operative mortality but carry a 5% risk of anastomotic complications (leak or stricture).[123]

Limited resections include segmentectomy, wedge resection, and lumpectomy. Any segment of lung can be resected, but this form of limited resection requires a bit more tedious dissection through the lung parenchyma than standard lobectomy. A segmentectomy indicates that a distinct anatomic resection was performed. The pulmonary artery and segmental bronchus are individually isolated and divided. The segment is removed from the remaining lobe by stapled excision or blunt dissection, and the segmental pulmonary venous branches are divided as encountered. Wedge excision, in contrast, is performed without identifying the adjacent anatomic landmarks. It is a simple and quick procedure. A stapling device usually is used to remove the lesion, including a rim of grossly normal lung to provide a clear margin. Wedge resections can be used only for peripherally located lesions. Lesions that reside more deeply within the pulmonary tissue often are not amenable to wedge resection and may require precise local excision with laser or electrocautery assistance (lumpectomy). The pulmonary tissue is directly incised and the lesion is removed, with preservation of the surrounding lung. Postoperative air leaks usually are minimal.

Over the past 35 years, lobectomy has been regarded as the procedure of choice for the treatment of early-stage lung cancer. The LCSG completed a prospective phase III trial comparing limited resection (segmentectomy or wedge resection) with lobectomy for patients with small peripheral tumors staged intraoperatively as T1 N0 malignancies.[124] Patients were randomized to undergo standard lobectomy, segmentectomy, or wedge resection. Patients who underwent limited resection had a significantly higher rate of local recurrence. Survival tended to favor patients treated by lobectomy, particularly those with nonsquamous tumors, but the difference was not statistically significant. There was no significant difference in either morbidity or mortality among any of the procedures. The conclusions were that lobectomy should remain the standard procedure for patients with early-stage disease. Nakamura and colleagues recently performed a meta-analysis to compare survival after limited resection and after standard lobectomy for patients with stage I disease. They studied 14 articles, including the sole randomized controlled trial that was reported by the LCSG, and found that survival after limited resection for stage I lung cancer was comparable to that after lobectomy.[125] Most authorities, however, follow the LCSG guidelines and reserve limited procedures for patients with pulmonary function problems or other illnesses that preclude lobectomy.[126] These conclusions are being challenged in an era of earlier detection with high resolution computed tomography. A number of authors have reexamined the role of limited resections for very early (< 1 cm) lesions. In addition, alternative treatment modalities such as radiofrequency ablation and radiosurgery are being examined as well. Additional studies to delineate the role of these treatments and the patients for whom they are suited still need to be done. Ad hoc use of these modalities should be discouraged and enrollment of the patient in a trial designed to evaluate these modalities should be encouraged.

Extended Surgical Procedures Patients with tumors considered T3 N0 because of chest wall invasion who undergo chest wall resection have 5-year survival rates ranging from 26 to 60%. In patients with T3 N2 tumors, on the other hand, the 5-year survival rate is less than 5%, although Martini has reported a 5-year survival rate of 21% for patients with regional lymph node involvement. Other factors adversely influencing survival are incompleteness of resection and depth of invasion of the tumor into the chest wall. Overall 5-year survival rates for patients with surgically resected T3 tumors have ranged from 12 to 40%.[127]

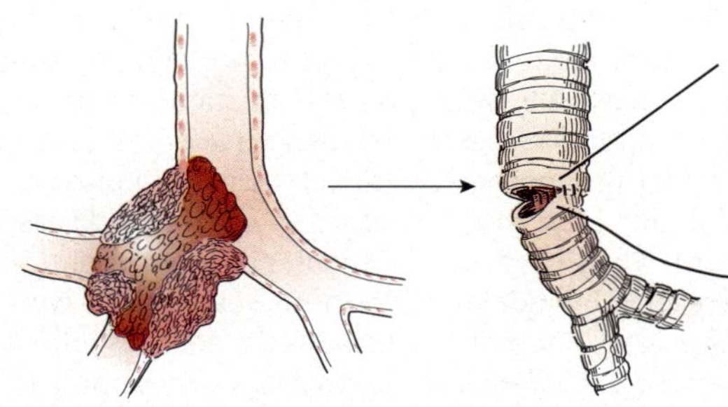

Figure 80-10 A sleeve pneumonectomy. The tracheal carina is resected with a small segment of distal trachea and an anastomosis is made with the proximal left main stem bronchus.

Tumors involving the carina are considered T4 lesions. Most lesions involving the carina are not amenable to surgical resection (Figure 80-10). There are, however, several indications for resection: (1) tumors restricted to the carina, such as rare cases of primary lung cancer arising on the carina, and less common neoplasms such as adenoid cystic carcinoma or mucoepidermoid carcinoma; (2) tumors of the mediastinal trachea that extend to involve the origin of the main bronchus or carina; (3) primary carcinoma of the lung extending proximally to involve the origin of the main bronchus and carina on either the right or left side, which may, in very rare instances, be managed by carinal resection or sleeve pneumonectomy; and (4) rare cases of benign disease involving the carina with local destruction. These are indications that have been defined by F. G. Pearson.[128]

Operative mortality rates for carinal resection and sleeve pneumonectomy are significantly higher than for traditional pulmonary resections and have been reported to range from 10 to 30%. In selected patients with tumors confined to the carina or tracheobronchial angle, sleeve pneumonectomy can achieve a complete resection; however, the significant 30-day mortality risk of 8 to 20.9% indicates that caution must be used in recommending such a procedure. Five-year survival rates for these procedures have been reported as high as 23 to 35%. Survival after resection of T4 tumors that involve the carina is directly related to the extent of nodal disease; 3-year survival rates are 43% for N1 disease, 34% for disease involving only the subcarinal node, and 0% when the upper mediastinal nodes are involved.[129,130]

Tumors that involve the vena cava, aorta, main pulmonary artery, or left atrium are considered T4 tumors. If the vena cava becomes directly involved by the primary pulmonary neoplasm, the effect is compression or wall invasion. Compression or obstruction of the vena cava is manifested by distal venous engorgement, which most frequently compromises the superior vena cava, causing SVC syndrome. Although the more common cause of SVC syndrome is compression from metastatic disease in lymph nodes in the superior mediastinum, direct tumor compression can cause the same process. In most instances, such tumors represent extensive disease and carry a poor prognosis. Treatment is usually nonsurgical, although in a few cases of localized disease with vena cava involvement, the tumor can be resected by including a portion of the vessel wall. Similarly, a tumor that invades the aorta usually is unresectable because the extensive invasion precludes complete extirpation. In rare instances, however, if a tumor locally invades the aorta and is otherwise completely resectable in a low-risk patient, en bloc resection can be performed with reconstruction of the aorta. Intrapericardial extension of the tumor not uncommonly involves the left atrium, precluding resection. In some instances of local invasion of the left atrium, a complete resection can be accomplished without hemodynamic compromise. Tsuchiya and colleagues reported a 5-year survival rate of 22% after resection of the left atrium to achieve a complete resection.[131] Such reports suggest the feasibility of aggressive approaches for selected T4 tumors, and for this reason patients should not be denied a surgical evaluation based on their T status alone.

Synchronous and Metachronous Lung Primaries The presence of synchronous lung lesions raises the suspicion of metastatic disease not only from an extrathoracic site, but also from within the lung. A concerted effort to evaluate all possibilities should be undertaken prior to the initiation of any treatment. The histology is particularly important. If adenocarcinoma is found in the lung, numerous potential extrathoracic sites of origin can exist. A complete examination that includes a thorough evaluation of the gastrointestinal tract, breast, and reproductive system is imperative. If the lung lesion is squamous carcinoma, a systematic inspection of the upper aerodigestive tract and rectum should be performed. This includes panendoscopy (nasopharyngoscopy, laryngoscopy, bronchoscopy, and esophagoscopy), with biopsies of any suspicious lesions. Only after an exhaustive search has been undertaken to rule out nonpulmonary sources should lung primaries be considered. If the lesions are present within the same lobe, these lesions probably originated from the same source. The larger of the two should be considered the primary, while the other represents a satellite lesion, an intraparenchymal metastasis. Satellite lesions are discussed in the next section.

Synchronous primary lung cancers occur in 0.26 to 1.7% of all patients with lung cancer.[132] Practical pathologic and clinical criteria have been proposed as guidelines to distinguish primary and metastatic tumors.[133-135] Probable or definite synchronous lung cancers are physically separate and located in a different segment, lobe, or lung, with no regions of common lymphatic involvement. They have a different histologic type or are proven to arise from different endobronchial lesions by bronchoscopy or from separate foci of carcinoma in situ at pathologic examination. Patients with unilateral tumors and hilar or mediastinal lymph node metastases are not considered to have synchronous tumors. When synchronous tumors are confirmed as individual primaries, they should be staged separately and independently according to standard TNM definitions. The patient's overall tumor stage should be determined by the higher-staged lesion.

Survival rates after complete resection of synchronous lung cancers are worse than for isolated lesions of similar stage. The overall 5-year survival rate for all patients with synchronous lesions ranges from 0 to 44%, and the median survival duration ranges from 11 to 43 months; patients with no hilar or mediastinal node metastases generally survive longer.[135,136]

Metachronous (asynchronous) lesions are distinct tumors that arise in separate anatomic sites and are of different histologic types; they may be of the same histologic type if there was previous complete resection of the initial primary lung cancer without stump involvement, the tumors originated in separate lobes or lungs, there is no cancer in the common lymphatics or extrapulmonary disease at the time of diagnosis, and the site of origin of the second primary can be identified (or, if the original site is unknown, there is an interval of at least 2 to 3 years between the two tumors).[134] As the number of patients successfully treated for lung cancer increases, the incidence of second primaries will also increase. Multiple lung cancers occur in 10 to 25% of patients who survive longer than 3 years.[31] Patients in whom the multiple lesions are metachronous survive significantly longer (10-year survival rates from time of diagnosis of the original tumor reported as 42%) than those in whom the multiple lesions are synchronous. Survival is strongly influenced by the interval to recurrence and the stage of the second primary. The time interval between the development of asynchronous primary lesions may exceed 10 years.

The treatment of these lesions should follow the same pattern of evaluation that has been previously discussed. The only difference pertains to evaluation of the mediastinum. If the chest CT scan does not demonstrate adenopathy and bilateral lesions exist, it has been our practice to perform mediastinoscopy to rule out occult N2 disease prior to performing pulmonary resection. The method for resection depends on the location of the disease and the degree of concomitant pulmonary disease. If both lesions are clinical stage I disease and the patient has normal PFT results, either sternotomy with bilateral resection or staged thoracotomies can be performed. Because lobectomy provides the best opportunity for local control and possible cure, lobectomies are most desirable; such procedures are best performed in a staged fashion. If pulmonary function is limited or sternotomy is performed, limited resections or a lobectomy coupled with a limited resection are probably adequate. If a pneumonectomy is contemplated, staged resections are best to reduce postoperative complications. PFT should be repeated after the first procedure whenever staged resections are performed to ensure adequate pulmonary reserve.

If clinical N1 disease is present and the lesions are unilateral, intraparenchymal metastases are probably present, indicative of higher-stage (stage IV) disease. In the absence of N2 disease, a pneumonectomy can be considered. If both bilateral lesions are clinical stage II disease, the disease is probably beyond the scope of complete resectability, and a nonoperative approach should be considered. If N2 disease is present, the level of suspicion for intraparenchymal metastatic disease should be high, and nonoperative therapy is appropriate. These situations also pertain to metachronous lesions.

Survival rates after treatment of synchronous or metachronous primary lung lesions are better than those for metastatic or locally recurrent disease. Locally recurrent disease has been reported to develop at a median time interval of 13 months and to have a 4-year survival rate of 5 to 23%.[31]

Satellite Lesions Satellite lesions are separate foci of tumor that coexist with the lung primary tumor in the same lobe and represent intraparenchymal metastases. Mountain and colleagues and Deslauriers and colleagues have noted the implications of satellite lesions in their series of patients.[137,138] In the series of Deslauriers and colleagues, patients with a stage I, stage II, or stage III lesion who had an associated satellite tumor had 5-year survival rates of only 32%, 12.5%, and 5.6%, respectively, rates that are clearly worse than expected for early stages of disease. Accordingly, Mountain has recommended that tumors with associated satellite lesions be considered T4 tumors.

Surgery for N2 Disease The frequency of mediastinal lymph node involvement in patients with resectable NSCLC ranges from 22 to 33%.[139] Approximately 33% of patients with stage IIIA disease (based on N2 nodal metastases) present with a single positive node, whereas the remainder present with multiple nodes involved at a single station or at multiple stations. Patients with multiple-station involvement have a significantly worse prognosis than patients with single-node involvement.[140]

In patients with metastases involving a single station, a significant survival difference has not been demonstrated between those with subcarinal metastases and those with metastases to other stations. In patients with multiple-station metastases, the significance of subcarinal involvement is uncertain. The significance of metastases to the highest mediastinal lymph node and the definition of an incomplete resection based on N2 lymph node metastases are unclear.[141] The overall survival rate for patients with completely resected N2 disease is approximately 22%.

Patients with intranodal disease have a significant survival advantage over patients with extranodal extension.[142] Lymph nodes that extend beyond the confines of the nodal capsule have an increased propensity to involve adjacent tissue, reducing the chances of a complete resection. Such gross perinodal spread confers the possibility of microscopic residual disease, which may account for increased local recurrence rates and carry a worse prognosis.[143]

Positive Margins (Bronchial and Parenchymal) At the time of resection, the bronchial margin should be assessed by frozen section to ensure a complete resection. If the margin contains evidence of disease, all reasonable attempts to achieve a negative margin should be undertaken. It can be surmised that the risks of residual disease evolving into gross and potentially metastatic disease are higher in the face of an incomplete resection on the basis of a positive bronchial margin. But several studies have shown that reasonable survival rates can be achieved in the face of a positive bronchial margin. When microscopic disease or carcinoma in situ exists within the mucosa, 5-year survival rate can approach 24%.[144] Shields and colleagues also showed a reasonable survival rate in patients with carcinoma in the bronchial mucosa.[145] In this cohort of patients, however, survival was poor when disease was present outside of the bronchial mucosa or within the peribronchial lymphatics, a finding similar to those of other studies.[144,146]

The role of radiotherapy in patients with positive margins of resection is unclear. Definitive studies that address this issue are difficult to perform. No current evidence indicates that radiation therapy improves rates of survival or local recurrence. Despite this fact, and on the basis of success with radiation therapy in the treatment of gross disease (locally advanced and stage IV), it is assumed that radiation will reduce the increased risk of local recurrence implied by a positive margin. At our institution, the standard of care remains radiation therapy if gross or microscopic disease remains after resection.

Surgery for Metastatic Disease Approximately 25 to 30% of all patients who present with NSCLC have stage IV disease (any T, any N, M1). These patients are usually treated with systemic therapy or palliative radiotherapy; their 5-year survival rate is generally less than 5%.[71] There is one subset of patients who can be considered for surgical intervention: those with resectable lung carcinoma and a resectable solitary brain metastasis. In this select group, surgery seems to prolong life and improve quality of life more effectively than nonsurgical treatment. The 5-year survival rate for the patients who undergo surgery has been shown to range from 13 to 30%, and the median survival duration ranges from 14 to 27 months. It has been suggested that adrenal metastases can be resected in patients with lung cancer, but the benefit, other than local control, is unclear. For lack of evidence to the contrary, conventional therapy for metastatic disease should not typically include the option of surgery except in highly selected cases.[147,148]

Management of Malignant Pleural Effusions Many patients either present with malignant pleural effusion or develop an effusion during or after therapy. Symptomatic effusions should be palliated with the greatest expediency to allow a rapid return of the patient's quality of life. Standard therapy has been thoracoscopy with talc pleuradage or tube thoracostomy with some form of chemical or talc pleurodesis. Both require hospitalization and either a general anesthetic or prolonged placement of an uncomfortable tube thoracostomy. A recent alternative is placement of a chronic indwelling catheter that can be drained by the patient at home and achieves prompt resolution of symptoms and eventual pleural symphysis. This system has the same success rate as tube thoracoscopy when the end point for evaluation is symptomatic relief. Its ease of insertion, minimal patient discomfort, rapid return to an ambulatory status, and reduced cost in this usually preterminal condition makes this system a very attractive option.[149]

Surgery for High-Risk Patients Many patients with potentially resectable disease are excluded from surgery because of severe cardiac or pulmonary limitations. Such high-risk patients are categorized by specific objective criteria. Usual pulmonary measures of high risk include the following: (1) preoperative forced expiratory volume in one second (FEV_1) less than 40% of predicted, (2) predicted postresectional FEV_1 less than 33% of predicted as determined by radioisotopic ventilation–perfusion studies, and (3) resting hypercarbia on arterial blood gas analysis ($PCO_2 > 45$). Cardiac criteria of high risk include (1) MI 3 to 6 months before the anticipated surgery, (2) evidence of class III angina, (3) hemodynamically significant valvular heart disease, (4) atrial fibrillation, (5) age over 75 years, (6) a history of cerebrovascular accident or transient ischemic attack, and (7) an echocardiogram with an ejection fraction of less than 50%. The introduction of improved methods to assess cardiopulmonary function has helped to better assess a patient's candidacy for surgery. The increased operative mortality associated with surgery for these patients can erode the oncologic survival advantage usually achieved with surgery. For most of these patients, radiotherapy carries considerably less risk and achieves similar rates of cure. Highly selected patients with these risk factors can sometimes still be offered surgery. Some examples include resection of a right upper lobe tumor in patients with severe bullous emphysema confined to the upper lobes or correction of cardiac disease immediately before or during pulmonary resection. A surgical evaluation, therefore, should not be denied solely because of cardiac or pulmonary limitations.

Radiotherapy Radiation therapy for lung cancer has changed rapidly in recent years. Our ability to define target volumes and avoid normal structures has been aided by advancements in CT technology and in FDG-PET scanning. It is now possible, moreover, to measure and account for individual variations in respiratory tumor motion. Treatment-planning algorithms can account for tissue heterogeneity, which can improve dose distributions to target volumes. Three-dimensional (3D)-conformal radiotherapy is routinely achieved by using International Commission on Radiation Units and Measurements (ICRU) definitions of volumes and doses. Intensity-modulated radiotherapy (IMRT) is being implemented and proton therapy is becoming a reality. We also look forward to the rational integration of new biologic therapies into standard treatment.

More than 60% of lung cancer patients will receive radiotherapy at some point in their disease, 45% for initial treatment and 17% for palliation.[150] This means that over 100,000 Americans with lung cancer are irradiated yearly. Therefore, it is critical that we aggressively implement the optimal treatment. Experienced teams are required to manage the care of these patients optimally, particularly when combined-modality therapy is used; outcomes are demonstrably better when patients are treated by experienced personnel.[151,152]

Radiation Treatment Techniques and Volumes for Lung Cancer The ICRU has defined several important volumes for the modern treatment of lung cancer:

Gross Tumor Volume Gross tumor volume (GTV) is defined as visible tumor by any imaging modality. The pulmonary extent of lung tumors should be delineated on pulmonary windows, and the mediastinal extent of tumors should be delineated using mediastinal windows. FDG-PET scanning is quite important for radiation treatment planning.[153] It can reduce interobserver differences in GTV contouring,[154] and it can help to categorize suspect mediastinal/hilar lymph adenopathy as either benign or malignant; higher standard uptake values (SUVs) are predictive of metastatic disease. It can also help to identify tumors within an atelectatic lobe, and thereby decrease the amount of normal lung irradiated. Finally, because FDG-PET scans detect distant metastases in about 30% of NSCLC patients (particularly those with otherwise advanced disease), it can help significantly with patient triage.[155]

Clinical Target Volume Clinical target volume (CTV) is defined as the volume that is likely to contain gross and microscopic disease. It has been difficult in the past to determine the extent of microscopic disease, both adjacent to the primary GTV and in the mediastinum. A radiographic–histopathologic comparison of lung tumor size was recently completed.[156] This study demonstrated that to include the tumor within the CTV with 95% accuracy requires GTV to CTV expansions of 6 mm for squamous cancers and 8 mm for adenocarcinomas. Expansions for other histologic types have not been determined, but a conservative approach would be to use 8 mm. Appropriate CTV for the mediastinum has not been rigorously determined. We empirically use 8-mm expansions around involved nodes (either gross involvement or FDG-PET positivity). Obviously, these expansions should not necessarily be applied uniformly along all axes. In the absence of radiographic proof of invasion, CTV for primary tumors should generally not extend into the chest wall or mediastinum. CTV expansions of lymph node disease should not extend into the major airways or lung.

Planning Target Volume Planning target volume (PTV) is defined as CTV with a margin to account for daily set-up error and target motion. PTV is designed to take set-up uncertainty and motion into account, and it is best to separate these two components because the geometries of the expansions are different. Preliminary data at our institution have shown that, when immobilizing patients with a Vac-Loc bag and T-bar, expansion along all axes of 8 mm accounts for 95% of the day-to-day set-up uncertainty. Set-up uncertainty is likely both technique dependent and institution dependent and should be measured individually for each technique.

Accounting for respiratory-dependent tumor motion is similarly challenging and can be approached in several ways. It is clear, however, that two-dimensional (2-D) measurement of tumor motion, such as might be done by fluoroscopy, is inadequate. Such motion is unpredictable and is independent of tumor size, location, and PFT results.[157] Thus, tumor motion is best assessed individually for each patient. Our experience with 3-D measurement of lung tumor motion demonstrates that every tumor moves at least 5 mm with respiration, but the motion from any one angle is less than 5 mm for about one-third of lung cancer patients. For this third of patients, simple expansion along the axis of motion is adequate. For the other two-thirds, the treatment machine can be gated with respiration or the patient can use an assisted breath-hold technique or, possibly, an internal target volume (ITV)-based approach can be used. A commercially available system can be used to gate the linac.[158] This technique uses an externally placed fiducial that is tracked as the patient breathes. The beam can be triggered at a chosen point in the respiratory cycle, typically end-expiration because this is the longest and most reproducible portion of the respiratory cycle. This requires that patients be able to breathe slowly in a regular pattern. Active breathing control and deep inspiration breath hold are two techniques that have been pioneered to help patients hold their breaths at reproducible points in the respiratory cycle.[159,160] The radiation beam is then initiated. These two techniques limit patient respiratory excursion to fixed volumes. They limit diaphragm excursion to about 5 mm instead of 10 to 15 mm.[161] These techniques require very cooperative patients who are able to hold their breath for at least 15 seconds. Unfortunately, patients with poor pulmonary function (who would most benefit from reduction in irradiated lung volumes) are the patients least able to comply with breath-holding techniques. Thus, it is not clear which is the best method to temporally immobilize lung tumors.

Internal Target Volume ITV is an expansion of CTV in which target motion is explicitly measured and taken into account as defined by ICRU62. Using new technologies such as multislice detectors and faster imaging reconstruction, it is now possible to image patients during real-time breathing and assess organ motion using 4-D CT.[162] To determine the ITV from the 4-D CT images, the tumor volume outlined on expiratory phase of the 4-D images is registered on other phases of the images to create a union of target contours enclosing all possible positions of the target. The same principle can be applied to the images acquired with inspiration and expiration breath holds. Attention should be paid to irregular breathing and variation of breathing pattern over the course of the treatment, and the effects of such on the ITV margin. Even with 4-D CT, the free-breathing ITV is only a snapshot and a single stochastic sampling of the patient breathing during the 4-D CT acquisitions. Thus, the true ITV margin should be enlarged on the basis of the uncertainty of patient's breathing during the treatment course.

A more interesting and challenging application for 4-D CT images is 4-D treatment planning in which the actual dose distributions for free-breathing treatment can be calculated. In this process, the dose distributions are calculated for each phase of the breathing cycle and then added together by deformation registration. Such composite dose distribution and DVHs demonstrate the actual dose that the patient is receiving from the treatment if he/she breathes the same way as the 4-D CT images are representing.[163]

Intensity Modulated Radiation Therapy and Proton Radiotherapy Intensity modulated radiation therapy (IMRT) offers the benefit of dose escalation without causing greater toxic effects to surrounding normal tissue for patients with prostate or head and neck cancer.[164] However, the application of IMRT to lung cancer has been delayed owing to general concern and the assumption that IMRT may deliver low yet damaging doses to a larger volume of normal lung tissue. Moreover, the possible movement of a tumor because of respiration introduces another level of complexity to both the IMRT dosimetry and the technique used.

We investigated dosimetric improvement with respect to target dose, tumor conformity, and normal tissue sparing, comparing IMRT with 3-D CT for early and locally advanced NSCLC.[165,166] We found that IMRT may be more suitable than 3-D CT treatment planning for cases of advanced-stage disease with a larger GTV and thus a greater volume of normal lung involvement. Using IMRT, the median absolute reduction in the percentage of lung volume irradiated above 10 and 20 Gy were 7% and 10%, respectively. This corresponded with decreases of more than 2 Gy in the mean total lung dose and 10% in the risk of radiation pneumonitis. The volumes of the heart and esophagus irradiated above 40 to 50 Gy and normal thoracic tissue irradiated above 10 to 40 Gy were reduced using the IMRT plans. In contradiction of the common belief, the integral dose delivered to the patient was also reduced with IMRT in certain cases. There was a marginal increase in the spinal cord maximum dose and lung volume above 5 Gy in the IMRT plans in half of cases, which could have been caused by the significant increase of monitor units and thus leakage dose in IMRT for the sliding window delivery technique used in these studies.

Although IMRT may be effective in reducing normal tissue toxicity and improving tumor coverage, its high-dose gradient and conformity require a high level of precision in dose delivery and tumor localization. In the meantime, the complexity introduced by tumor motion must be recognized when using IMRT. Unlike 3-D conformal radiotherapy (3-D CRT), IMRT treats only a portion of the target volume at a particular time. There is a great deal of concern as whether target motion and collimator motion during IMRT delivery will have significant interplay effect, thus degrading the planned dose distributions. For IMRT to be feasible and more effective in treating NSCLC, motion reduction techniques should be explored further, such as breath holding and tumor tracking. Our preliminary clinical data indicated that IMRT may reduce toxic effects in normal tissue in selected cases, particularly for tumor moves less than 5 mm, and allow further dose escalation.[167] We have recently developed IMRT guidelines for NSCLC using imaging-guided radiotherapy.[168]

The proton is a charged particle that, compared to the photon, possesses a well-defined range of penetration determined by both the beam's energy and the density of the tissue through which it passes. As the proton beam penetrates the body, the particles slow down and deposit the dose sharply near the end of its range, a phenomenon known as the Bragg peak. By modulating the Bragg peak across the target volume, proton beams can deliver a full, localized, uniform dose of energy to the treatment site while sparing the surrounding normal tissues. The physics of the proton beam is ideal for treatments where organ preservation is paramount, such as lung cancer. The preliminary clinical data from Shioyama and colleagues and Bush and colleagues using escalated/accelerated proton radiotherapy showed promising clinical results comparable to those of surgical resection in stage IA cases.[169,170] Again, the accuracy of target delineation and tumor motion consideration are critical for both proton and photon treatment. Proton treatment is more sensitive to anatomical motion, position uncertainties, and tissue inhomogeneity.[168]

In our preclinical study, we found that proton radiotherapy significantly reduced dose to normal lungs, esophagus, spinal cord, and heart in both stage I and stage III NSCLC even with dose escalation (87.5 Gy for stage I, 74 Gy for stage III) compared with standard dose of photon radiotherapy (66 Gy for stage I and 63 Gy for stage III) using either 3-D or IMRT. The improvement was more dramatic in stage I disease and contralateral lung. Further improvement of proton planning, particularly for complicated stage III cases, can be achieved by adding wedges, coordination between beam arrangement, and/or intensity-modulated proton therapy.

We also designed and evaluated several image-guided radiotherapies to study the impact of respiratory motion on dose distributions for 3-D CRT, IMRT, and proton radiotherapy and to assess the potential benefits of accounting for respiratory motion with gating or breath hold. We found that tumor motion has a significant effect on radiation dose distribution. This motion should be considered for both photon and proton radiotherapy. ITV or gated radiotherapy can significantly reduce target missing owing to tumor motion. Compared with photon 3-D CRT and IMRT with gated or nongated radiotherapy, proton radiotherapy (gated or free-breathing with ITV approach) significantly improves normal tissue sparing, especially at low-dose levels.[171] Our data showed that it is possible to have escalated/accelerated proton radiotherapy without significantly increasing toxic effects to normal tissue. This approach may translate to better local control and survival rates for patients with stage I NSCLC. At M. D. Anderson Cancer Center, we are going to conduct phase II clinical trials using imaging-guided proton radiotherapy for stage I and stage III NSCLC. PET/CT studies will be used in all patients for both stage and treatment planning. We plan to deliver a total dose of 87.5 CGE (cobalt gray equivalent): 2.5 CGE per fraction for stage I disease and 74 CGE with concurrent chemotherapy followed by adjuvant chemotherapy for stage III disease. A 4-D CT study will be required to account for tumor motion, and assist in deciding on a treatment delivery technique (free-breath, breath-hold, or gated treatment).

In summary, IMRT and proton treatments represent the most recent technological developments in radiation oncology. These new treatment modalities have the potential to reduce the toxic effects to normal tissue compared with 3-D CRT. However, high-dose conformity and dose sculpting from the IMRT and proton treatments require a greater degree of precision in treatment delivery and careful management of organ motion. Image-guided targeting, and patient positioning will possibly become the standard of practice for future IMRT and proton treatments. The clinical significance of possible increased exposure of low-dose (less than 10) Gy to the chest by IMRT is unknown. IMRT should be used only in selective cases, and target volume motion and low-dose exposure to the lung should be minimized. Proton holds a great potential for sparing normal tissues and may allow further radiation dose escalation/acceleration without significantly increasing normal tissue toxicities.

Primary Radiation Therapy for Stage I and II NSCLC Patients who have surgically resectable NSCLC but are medically inoperable because of their lung function, cardiac function, bleeding tendency, or other comorbid conditions, or patients who refuse surgery, may be considered for conventional fractionated radiotherapy (60–66 Gy 1.8 or 2 Gy/fraction). Observation only is a poor choice for patients with stage I NSCLC, as most will die of their cancer. Primary radiotherapy for early-stage NSCLC is considered reasonable for such patients, with reported 5-year survival rates ranging from 10 to 30% with conventional fractionated radiotherapy.[172,173] Several studies have reported a benefit to dose escalation suggesting a dose-response relationship in both survival and local control in these patients.[172,174–176] Since early-stage NSCLC is not inherently a systemic disease from diagnosis, and since local control is poor after conventional radiotherapy, research measures aimed at improving survival should put significant emphasis on improving local tumor obliteration.

It should be kept in mind that lung cancer in such patients is always staged clinically, which makes comparison with surgically treated patients difficult. Several surgical series demonstrate a 24 to 37% upstaging of cT1-T2 N0 disease, which partially explains the poorer results seen in clinically staged irradiated patients.[124] Small early-stage NSCLC is uncommon in radiation oncology clinics. As we develop better screening tools for early-stage NSCLC, however, the number of patients with small but medically inoperable tumors will increase.[92]

At M. D. Anderson Cancer Center, between 1980 and 1990, 19 patients with clinical T1 N0 disease and 26 patients with clinical T2 N0 disease were treated with curative intent by primary radiotherapy. The median total radiation therapy dose was 6,300 cGy, and 80% of the patients received doses exceeding 60 Gy. Radiographic response was documented at completion of radiation therapy in half the cases, and 60% of the cases showed maximum response within 6 months after completion of radiation therapy. The median follow-up time was 36 months, and the disease-specific survival rates at 3 years by T status were 49% for T1 and 47% for T2. The clinically determined local control rates at 3 years were 89% for T1 lesions and 61% for T2 lesions. The significant prognostic factors for disease-specific survival were Karnofsky PS of 70 or more, tumor size 5 cm or less, and radiation dose of 50 Gy or higher. The important prognostic factors for local control were tumor size 4 cm or less, a radiation therapy dose of 60 Gy or more, and complete response as seen on the chest radiograph by 6 months after completion of radiation therapy. The coverage of nodal drainage areas did not affect survival or local control. No lethal complications were seen with radiation therapy alone, and documented symptomatic radiation pneumonitis occurred in only 7% of cases.

The most important prognostic factor documented in the literature is usually tumor size. Dosoretz and colleagues. reported that rates of distant metastasis were correlated to the size of the primary tumor.[176] The incidence of metastasis in 3 years was 8% in tumors smaller than 3 cm, 27% in tumors measuring 3 to 5 cm, and 50% in tumors larger than 5 cm. They reported that the local control rates in 3 years were 77% for 4 cm lesions and 48% for those larger than 4 cm.

Stereotactic Body Radiation Therapy in Early-Stage NSCLC The development of 3-D conformal radiotherapy (3-D CRT) and stereotactic body radiation therapy (SBRT) has allowed precise targeting and delivery of radiotherapy. SBRT for lung cancer utilizes elements of 3-D CRT and also incorporates a variety of systems for taking tumor motion into consideration and decreasing set-up uncertainty using image-guided radiotherapy techniques. These systems allow reduction of treatment volumes facilitating hypofractionation with markedly increased daily doses (> 10 Gy) and a significantly reduced overall treatment time. The combination of multiple beam angles to achieve sharp dose gradients, high precision localization, and a high dose per fraction in extracranial locations is referred to as SBRT. This approach delivers a high biological effective dose (BED) to the target while minimizing toxic effects to normal tissue; which may translate into improved local control and survival rates.

Dr. Onishi and colleagues reported on the use of SBRT in stage I NSCLC in Japan,[177] retrospectively evaluating results from a Japanese multi-institutional study. Patients with stage I NSCLC (n = 245; median age, 76 years; T1 N0 M0, n = 155; T2 N0 M0, n = 90) were treated with hypofractionated high-dose SBRT in 13 institutions. Stereotactic 3-D treatment was performed using noncoplanar dynamic arcs or multiple static ports. A total dose of 18 to 75 Gy at the isocenter was administered in 1 to 22 fractions. The median calculated BED was 108 Gy (range, 57–180 Gy). During follow-up (median, 24 months; range, 7–78 months), pulmonary complications of National Cancer Institute Common Toxicity Criteria grade 2 or higher were observed in only six patients (2.4%). Local progression occurred in 33 patients (14.5%), and the local recurrence rates were 8.1% for BED ≥ 100 Gy and 26.4% for BED < 100 Gy ($p < .05$). The 3-year overall survival rates of medically operable patients were 88.4% for BED ≥ 100 Gy and 69.4% for < 100 Gy ($p < .05$). Their data showed that hypofractionated high-dose SBRT with BED < 150 Gy was feasible and beneficial for curative treatment of patients with stage I NSCLC. For all treatment methods and schedules, local control and survival rates were better with BED ≥ 100 Gy than with BED < 100 Gy. Survival rates in selected patients (medically operable, BED ≥ 100 Gy) were excellent and were potentially comparable to those of surgery.

In our institution, we have treated about 30 patients using imaging-guided SBRT (4-D CT simulation and daily CT on rail for tumor localization and set-up accuracy) at doses of 40 to 50 Gy (50 Gy for stage I or recurrent NSCLC after surgery and 40 Gy for recurrent NSCLC after radiotherapy) delivered in four fractions (ie, daily treatment for 4 days). Based on preliminary analysis, the local control rate at the primary site is higher than 95%, although the follow-up period is still short (less than 1 year). No clinical significant toxic effects of grade 3 or higher were noted. Long-term follow-up is needed to confirm these data.

Currently, the Radiation Therapy Oncology Group (RTOG) is conducting phase II clinical trials to analyze the efficacy of SBRT in peripheral stage I NSCLC with 60 GY in 3 fractions delivered in 2 weeks. Potential randomized study to compare SBRT with surgery in stage I NSCLC has been proposed by the International Association for the Study of Lung Cancer (IASLC). SBRT may become the future standard radiotherapy for selective peripheral stage I NSCLC.

Preoperative and Postoperative Nodal Irradiation Postoperative radiotherapy (PORT) is currently contraindicated in patients with stage I completely resected disease on the basis of the PORT meta-analysis.[178] Data for stage II and higher-stage disease neither support nor refute the use of PORT (because the hazard ratio error bars include 1.0), although it clearly improves regional control.

The use of PORT for stage II and III NSCLC was first tested in a controlled trial by the LCSG, which randomized 210 patients to receive either 50 Gy in 25 fractions or no treatment. Local recurrence rate was significantly reduced (3% vs 41%), but there was no effect on overall survival or disease-free survival because of the high rate of distant failure. This study and many other similar studies demonstrate that no amount of local therapy can cure most patients with advanced disease. Several approaches have been taken in the treatment of patients with stage III disease to address the issue of systemic failure: combinations of chemotherapy with surgery (which are dealt with elsewhere in this chapter) for patients with resectable disease and combinations of chemotherapy and radiation for those patients with unresectable disease.

In patients with resectable or marginally resectable NSCLC, 5-year survival rates and collective results of surgery alone for stage III (N2) ranged from 14 to 30%. As already discussed, many patients who have clinical N0 disease (even when it is staged by mediastinoscopy) are found to have occult mediastinal lymph node metastases. Approximately 15% of patients with resected T1 tumors have N2 disease, and 40 to 45% of patients with T2-T3 tumors will have N2 disease. Patients with incomplete resection, including positive margins, multiple levels of lymph node involvement, bulky extracapsular extension, and nonsquamous cell carcinoma, usually have a poor prognosis. PORT has been studied for patients with N1 and N2 squamous cell carcinoma and reported to reduce local-regional recurrence for both groups. These patients need PORT with or without chemotherapy.

If N2 disease is bulky and the potential for complete resection is questionable, patients can be treated by neoadjuvant chemotherapy followed by surgery. At M. D. Anderson, 60 patients were randomized to undergo chemotherapy and surgery or surgery alone. Twenty-eight patients received three cycles of cyclophosphamide, etoposide, and cisplatin and then underwent surgery, and they were compared with 32 patients treated with surgery alone. The median survival durations were 64 months versus 11 months, favoring neoadjuvant chemotherapy. The 2-year survival rate was 56% in the neoadjuvant group and 15% in the surgery-only group ($p = .008$). In this study, the patients who had positive margins, multiple levels of positive lymph nodes, or extracapsular extension received PORT between 50 and 60 Gy, and only two patients developed local recurrences. Rosell and colleagues from Barcelona randomized 60 patients treated with or without mitomycin C, ifosfamide, and cisplatin as neoadjuvant chemotherapy.[179] Thirty patients received neoadjuvant chemotherapy followed by surgery, and the other half underwent surgery alone; the median survival duration was 26 months in the neoadjuvant group and 8 months in the surgery-only group. The 2-year survival rate was 29% among the patients who received neoadjuvant chemotherapy and 0% among the patients who received surgery alone, although both groups had PORT of 50 Gy in 5 weeks. The neoadjuvant chemotherapy group had improved 2-year survival rate ($p = .001$).

Increasing numbers of patients with stage III disease are now undergoing induction chemotherapy, followed by surgery, on the basis of the work of Rosell and colleagues and Roth and colleagues.[179,180] To study the issue of surgical resection after induction chemoradiation, the Southwest Oncology Group (SWOG) conducted a phase II trial of concurrent induction chemotherapy, cisplatin, and etoposide, with thoracic radiation therapy in 74 patients with biopsy-proven stage IIIA (N2) NSCLC. Study results suggested that this approach may improve patient survival with reasonable toxicity.[181] After two cycles of chemotherapy, complete responders, partial responders, or patients with stable disease underwent resection. Of 74 patients, 55 (74%) had complete resection. Grade 4 or greater acute toxic effects of induction chemotherapy were reported in 13% of patients, and two patients died of treatment-related causes. Eight patients died postoperatively. Late pulmonary toxicity was reported in 10 patients. Pathologic complete response (CR) was seen in 22% of the resected cases. Median survival duration was 13 months, 2-year survival rate was 37%, and 3-year survival rate was 27%. Median survival duration of patients who had pathologic CR of nodal disease was 30 months, while that of patients with residual nodal disease was 10 months ($p = .0005$). On the basis of the results from this study, the NCI had launched a phase III multicenter trial (Radiation Therapy Oncology Group [RTOG (chair)], SWOG, National Cancer Institute of Canada Clinical Trials Group [NCIC CTG], Eastern Cooperative Oncology Group [ECOG], Cancer and Leukemia Group B [CALGB], North Central Cancer Treatment Group [NCCTG]) for patients with biopsy-proven N2 disease and potentially resectable NSCLC. (NCI Protocol INT 139). Patients were stratified by PS and T status and were randomized to receive induction chemoradiotherapy followed by surgery or chemotherapy with definitive radiotherapy as follows: following randomization, all patients received cisplatin (50 mg/m^2 IV days 1, 8, 29, 36), etoposide (50 mg/m^2 IV days 1–5, 29–33), and thoracic radiotherapy (45 Gy, 1.8 Gy/day, begin day 1) for 5 weeks. Patients in arm 1 who had no local progression or distant metastases at restaging underwent resection approximately 3 to 5 weeks after completion of course 2. Patients in arm 2 without local progression or distant metastases at restaging underwent full-course radiotherapy to 61 Gy. All patients received an additional two courses of chemotherapy. Initial results, presented in 2003, showed better PFS rate in the trimodality arm. Follow-up data, including survival data, were presented at the American Society for Clinical Oncology (annual meeting) (ASCO) 2005 by Albain and colleagues.[181] The study was closed in November 2001 after accrual of 484 patients. At the time the data were presented, all patients had follow-up of more than 2.5 years. Study results confirmed significantly greater PFS for arm 1. Survival curves were superimposed through year 2 and then separated. By year 5, an absolute survival benefit of 7% favored the surgery arm (odds ratio = 0.63 [0.36, 1.10], $p = .10$). Subgroup analysis revealed better survival for patients who underwent a lobectomy ($p = .002$). However, trimodality therapy was not optimal when a pneumonectomy was required owing to the high mortality risk. Finally, N0 status at surgery significantly predicted a higher 5-year survival rate. The authors suggested that surgical resection after chemoradiation can be considered for fit patients if lobectomy is feasible.

Radiation Therapy for Unresectable Stage III NSCLC A radiation dose-escalation trial (RTOG 73-01) was begun in 1973 to determine the optimal radiation dose using single daily fractions. Rates of local control and 3-year relapse-free survival were higher with doses of 60 Gy than with lower doses; however, the incidence of local failure was very high (> 70%), even in this pre-CT era study. In an attempt to increase local control and cure rates, a nonrandomized radiation dose-escalation trial using twice-daily radiotherapy (RTOG 83-11) was performed. This demonstrated that survival and local control were improved with doses of at least 69.6 Gy (delivered at 1.2 Gy per fraction, twice daily), but only about half the patients on each arm had stage III disease. There was no survival advantage with doses higher than 69.6 Gy because of the high rate of systemic failure.

While these studies of radiation alone were underway, several large studies explored different combinations of radiation and chemotherapy. Induction chemotherapy with cisplatin and vinblastine added approximately 4 months to the median survival duration compared with radiation alone (60 Gy in 2 Gy fractions). Although a thorough analysis of intrathoracic control was not performed, 80 to 90% of relapses had an intrathoracic component, with no difference between the treatment arms. A second study compared radiation treatment (65 Gy in 2.5 Gy fractions) with radiation treatment plus concurrent vindesine, cyclophosphamide, cisplatin, and lomustine. Despite very poor compliance in the combined-therapy group (32% did not receive a complete course of radiotherapy), there was a trend toward better survival with combination therapy: the 2-year survival rate was 21% in the combined-therapy arm and 14% in the radiation-alone arm. Again, the local control rate was only 15 to 17% as determined by bronchoscopic biopsy. Treatment modality did not affect local control or the rate of distant metastases. A third study compared split-course radiation (55 Gy delivered as 3 Gy for 10 doses followed by 2.5 Gy for 10 doses with a 4-week break between courses) with the same radiation regimen combined with weekly or daily cisplatin. Overall survival and local control rates were significantly higher in the chemotherapy arms than in the radiation-alone arm: the daily cisplatin arm had a 2-year survival rate of 26% and improved local control. Local failure was still a significant problem; 70 to 80% of patients had some component of local failure. Cisplatin given with this regimen did not affect the rate of distant metastases. A fourth study compared induction chemotherapy (cisplatin and vinblastine) followed by "standard" radiotherapy (60 Gy in 2 Gy fractions) with standard radiotherapy alone or hyperfractionated radiotherapy (69.6 Gy at 1.2 Gy per fraction twice daily). Induction chemotherapy increased median survival duration by 2.4 months over radiation alone. Longer follow-up confirmed the benefits of chemotherapy, but local control was not discussed. Additional analysis of these data showed that outcome depended on tumor histology, such that patients with large-cell carcinoma or adenocarcinoma had more distant (especially brain) metastases, and in these patients, induction chemotherapy followed by irradiation prolonged survival.

These data have been analyzed in several studies. Recent meta-analyses of phase III trials have demonstrated the benefit of combined-modality therapy in the treatment of unresectable NSCLC. Marino and colleagues studied outcomes in 14 trials published between 1980 and 1994 comprising 1,887 patients.[182] Cisplatin-based chemotherapy reduced mortality by 24% and 30%, respectively, 1 and 2 years following treatment. Unfortunately, the risk reduction was not seen beyond 2 years, suggesting that chemotherapy may simply delay progression, not increase cure. Another meta-analysis of combined chemoradiotherapy was performed in 1996.[183] The authors reviewed the same 14 articles and compared survival by treatment category. Their assessment was that radiation (doses from 55–65 Gy) combined with chemotherapy (either concurrent or sequential) resulted in a gain in median survival duration of approximately 2 months over similar radiation without chemotherapy. A third meta-analysis was performed by the Non-Small Cell Lung Cancer Collaborative Group. After analyzing 3,033 patients from 22 randomized trials, the authors concluded that chemotherapy reduced the risk of death (hazard ratio 0.90), corresponding to a benefit of 3% at 2 years and 2% at 5 years, with the bulk of this benefit seen in trials that used cisplatin. Thus, combinations of radiation and chemotherapy seem to offer the best hope of long-term disease-free survival in unresectable stage III NSCLC today,[184] and this is consistent with the ASCO guidelines.[185] It should be noted that the local control rates, when reported, were quite poor in these studies and ranged from 15 to 50%. Despite some improvement in outcome with combined-modality therapy, much better therapy is needed. Toward this end, several combinations of chemoradiation have been tested and are presented in the next section.

Radiation Techniques For many years, the standard of treatment of patients with unresectable stage III NSCLC was high-dose radiation therapy alone. Even now, patients who are ineligible for aggressive combination therapy usually receive a total dose of 60 Gy at 2 Gy per fraction or 63 Gy at 1.8 Gy per fraction in 6 or 7 weeks, respectively; this therapy is delivered to the primary tumor and regional lymph nodes. For upper lobe lesions, the supraclavicular regions are covered by the fields of radiation, and the lower border of the mediastinal radiation fields extends at least 5 cm below the carina. The fields are designed to extend to the diaphragm when the primary tumor arises in the lower lobe. If chemotherapy is given concurrently, the incidence and severity of radiation toxicity (esophagitis and bone marrow suppression) is significantly higher. Consequently, the field of radiation is reduced, and the lower border of the radiation port rarely extends to the diaphragm, even when the primary lesion is in the lower lobe.

In 1998, RTOG pooled the results of its studies on combined chemotherapy–radiotherapy in 461 patients with unresectable stage II-IIIB NSCLC available at that time. These data suggested that concurrent chemoradiotherapy could be tolerated, although it is more toxic than sequential therapy. Three treatment strategies were compared: (1) induction chemotherapy followed by radiotherapy, (2) induction chemotherapy followed by concurrent chemoradiotherapy, and (3) concurrent chemotherapy with hyperfractionated radiotherapy. No clear survival or disease-free survival advantage was seen in any group in this study.

Machtay and colleagues recently presented an update on results of three prospective RTOG trials (RTOG 91-06, 92-04, and 94-10), in which immediate concurrent chemoradiation (cisplatin based) was the primary therapy for patients with good PS stage III (or selected inoperable stage II) NSCLC. A total of 474 patients were analyzed. Median follow-up interval for surviving patients was 6.1 years. Treatment duration was per protocol in 387 (82%), whereas it was prolonged in the remaining 87 patients (18%). Long treatment time was significantly associated with severe acute esophagitis. Median survival duration was slightly longer in patients completing treatment on time (19.5 vs. 14.8 months), but this did not reach statistical significance ($p = .15$) by univariate analysis. In multivariate analysis of treatment duration as a continuous variable, however, prolonged treatment was significantly associated with poorer survival ($p = .02$), indicating a 2% increase in the risk of death for each day of prolongation in therapy. Histology (squamous fared worse) and PS were also significant in the multivariate model. The authors concluded that this retrospective analysis demonstrated a correlation between prolonged overall radiotherapy treatment time and shorter survival in patients with locally advanced NSCLC, even when concurrent chemotherapy was used.[186]

Belani and colleagues recently presented the results of the phase III ECOG 2597 trial, which examined induction chemotherapy followed by either standard thoracic radiotherapy or hyperfractionated accelerated radiotherapy (HART) for patients with unresectable stage IIIA or IIIB NSCLC. The study was conducted to compare once-daily radiation therapy with HART after two cycles of induction chemotherapy (carboplatin plus paclitaxel). Although statistical significance was not achieved and the study closed early, there was a positive statistical trend, suggesting a survival advantage with the HART regimen.[187]

The incidence of severe acute esophagitis (≥ grade 3) in patients treated with standard (once-daily) radiation therapy alone is 1.3%, increasing to 14 to 25% with the addition of concurrent chemotherapy and to 24 to 34% for the combination of hyperfractionated (twice-daily) radiation therapy plus concomitant chemotherapy.[181] Although esophagitis is almost never a cause of death, it results in significant morbidity and may force treatment breaks, which are associated with inferior outcome in NSCLC. The ability of several agents to reduce the rate of esophageal and pulmonary toxicity was tested. The organic thiophosphate compound amifostine (Ethyol) was found to prevent damage to normal tissues resulting from chemotherapy or radiation therapy, based on its broad cytoprotective capability and its selectivity for normal tissues rather than tumors. In the United States, amifostine has been approved for the prevention of cisplatin-induced nephrotoxicity in patients with advanced ovarian carcinoma or NSCLC and for the prevention of xerostomia in patients with head and neck cancer receiving postoperative radiotherapy. RTOG trial 98-01 tested the effect of amifostine in patients with stage II or IIIA/B NSCLC. A total of 243 patients received induction paclitaxel and carboplatin, followed by concurrent paclitaxel and carboplatin and hyperfractionated radiation therapy (69.6 Gy at 1.2 Gy bid). Patients were randomly assigned at registration to receive amifostine 500 mg IV 4 times per week or no amifostine during chemoradiotherapy. Standard toxicity as well as subjective and objective drug effect end points were collected. The data suggested that amifostine did not significantly reduce the incidence of grade 3 or higher esophagitis in these patients. However, patient self-assessments suggested a possible advantage to amifostine.[188] When the Ethyol was used before cisplatin/etoposide and radiotherapy for locally advanced nonsmall cell lung cancer, there was a significant reduction of acute severe esophagitis and pneumonitis in a small randomized trial at the University of Texas M. D. Anderson Cancer Center.[189]

Special Considerations ***Superior Vena Caval Obstruction*** Superior vena caval obstruction (SVCO), also known as SVC syndrome, is a not an uncommon finding in patients with lung cancer and requires prompt recognition and treatment. Approximately 65 to 97% of all cases of SVC syndrome occur secondary to malignancy. Three to five percent of patients with cancer of the lung present with edema of the face, neck, or arms and a prominent venous pattern in the chest wall, indicative of SVCO. Usually, the lung tumors are right-sided lesions. Ten to fifteen percent of patients with right-side malignancies may develop a component of SVCO. Commonly, they have associated shortness of breath, dyspnea, and headache, but rarely is glottic occlusion, laryngeal swelling, airway compromise, or cerebral venous hypertension a problem. Contrary to earlier thinking, SVCO is very rarely an oncologic emergency because few, if any, patients have died of the syndrome. Symptoms usually occur gradually, with accompanying venous collateralization manifested through cutaneous venous engorgement in the upper extremity, neck, and torso. Sometimes, symptoms can occur rather acutely from thrombosis of the major veins. Often the presenting symptoms are compounded by tracheal compression, recurrent nerve paralysis, and airway compromise. Even in such circumstances, treatment should not be initiated without a diagnosis, which usually can be obtained through cytologic or histologic testing. It is usually possible to obtain sputum, bronchial brushings or biopsies, or percutaneous aspirates that will establish the diagnosis. If SCLC is found, standard small-cell treatment protocols are initiated, that is, systemic chemotherapy followed by thoracic irradiation or concurrent chemoradiotherapy. NSCLC causing SVCO is an indication for rapid thoracic irradiation. Large daily doses of 3.5 to 4.0 Gy are delivered for 3 or 4 days; the daily dose is then reduced to 1.8 or 2.0 Gy, and treatment is continued to the usual total doses. Over 80% of patients so treated are relieved of the obstruction. Surgical intervention is rarely indicated, except for highly selected patients with severe symptoms, complete occlusion of the SVC, refractory symptoms after radiotherapy with or without chemotherapy, and thrombosis of venous collaterals. Bypass procedures reroute the venous blood flow of the upper compartment to the right atrium. Other surgical options are en bloc removal of the SVC or stent insertion. The prognosis is slightly worse for patients with SVCO than for patients who do not develop this syndrome because of the volume and extent of the tumor and lower PS. A recent review tested the evidence on the efficacy of different modalities in the treatment of SVCO in lung cancer. The authors suggested that chemotherapy and radiotherapy are effective in relieving SVCO in a proportion of patients, while stent insertion appears to provide relief in a higher proportion and more rapidly. The optimal timing of stent insertion (whether at diagnosis or following failure of other modalities) is currently uncertain. The effectiveness of steroids in SVCO remains uncertain.[190]

Superior Sulcus Tumors Superior sulcus tumors (SST) represent an uncommon presentation of lung cancer, accounting for approximately 3% of all lung cancers. SST with associated Pancoast's syndrome, Horner's syndrome, pain in the C8-T1 distribution, and atrophy of the intrinsic muscles of the hand (usually extrinsic involvement of the brachial plexus) represent a unique subset of these tumors. Irrespective of vertebral body or vascular invasion, tumors with Pancoast's syndrome (true "Pancoast's tumors") carry a poor prognosis and should be classified as T4 lesions. The T3 descriptor is appropriate when the rib, intercostal muscle, sympathetic chain, stellate ganglion, or lowest cord of the brachial plexus is involved. Other poor prognostic findings include N2-3 status, the use of wedge resection instead of lobectomy with en bloc chest wall resection, and incomplete resection. The majority of tumors are of nonsmall-cell histologic types, but occasionally SCLC occurs. The diagnosis can usually be established by FNA. SCLCs are treated with nonoperative therapy by standard small-cell protocols, whereas NSCLCs are usually treated with combined-modality therapy. Magnetic resonance angiography can be helpful in determining the extent of tumor. In many cases, SST can be completely resected, including the lowest chord of the brachial plexus, the sacrifice of which causes minimal neurologic compromise. Tumors that invade the vertebral body, subclavian vessels, or deep aspects of the brachial plexus present difficult surgical problems that may be ameliorated by induction chemotherapy. In some circumstances of limited invasion, however, the subclavian artery can be resected and reconstructed. When the tumor is adherent to the vertebral body, a portion can be removed with an en bloc resection, or the entire vertebral body can be removed and reconstructed.

For patients who have potentially resectable lesions, the best timing for radiotherapy is unknown. Certainly, radiation therapy can diminish the size of the tumor and perhaps improve resectability, particularly in patients who have improvement in their pain during the course of their preoperative radiation therapy. Radiation has its greatest effect when a full and uninterrupted dose can be delivered in the range of 60 to 65 Gy. When radiation therapy is given preoperatively, the usual dosage range is from 30 to 45 Gy. Higher preoperative radiation doses generally increase the perioperative complication rate, although a 5-year survival rate over 60% with full-dose preoperative therapy over 55 Gy, with conventional fractionation of 175 to 200 Gy/day versus high-dose fractionation of 275 to 300 Gy/day, has been reported in association with minimal perioperative morbidity. It should be kept in mind that split-course techniques generally have been found to be inferior to continuous course irradiation. A retrospective analysis at the Massachusetts General Hospital suggested that induction chemoradiation was superior to radiation alone prior to resection, although the radiation dose was 12 Gy higher in the combined group. A prospective phase II intergroup study demonstrated that induction chemoradiation followed by surgery can result in significant complete pathologic responses and very good survival, especially for patients with T2 N0 disease.

At our institution, we feel that the best care for patients with a potentially resectable tumor is immediate thoracotomy followed by PORT. In a retrospective analysis of patients with an SST who received definitive care at M. D. Anderson between January 1977 and December 1987, 85 patients were identified.[191] The male-to-female ratio was 2.7 to 1, and the ages ranged from 35 to 80 (median, 59) years. Karnofsky PS was 80 or higher in 70 of the patients (82%). Thirty patients (35%) had 5% or more loss of body weight. All had histologic or cytologic confirmation of carcinoma: 25% were squamous cell, 2% SCLC, 54% adenocarcinoma, 6% large-cell carcinoma, and 12% unclassified. After complete evaluation, 43 patients were classified as having clinical stage IIIA disease, and 42 as having stage IIIB. One patient with stage IIIA disease underwent surgery; 13, surgery plus radiation therapy; 2, surgery plus radiation therapy plus chemotherapy; 17, radiation therapy plus chemotherapy; and 4, chemotherapy alone. Surgery was a component of therapy more frequently in stage IIIA disease than in stage IIIB disease ($p = < .05$), and systemic treatment was used significantly more often in stage IIIB disease ($p = .0042$). The 1 patient treated with surgery alone lived 2 years. Twenty-three percent (7 of 31) of patients who had radiotherapy alone and none of the 4 patients who had chemotherapy alone lived 2 years. Of the 25 patients who underwent surgery as part of their treatment, 13 (52%) lived over 2 years, while 13 of the 60 (22%) patients who did not undergo surgery lived over 2 years. Of the patients who received radiation therapy as part of their treatment, 31% lived 2 years, and of those who received chemotherapy, 18% lived 2 years. Fifty-two patients (61%) had local control of the tumor; their survival duration was significantly longer ($p \leq .01$) than those who had local failure. In patients with unresectable tumors, total dose of radiotherapy was important ($p \leq .01$) in achieving local control; patients treated with less than 65 Gy had a 38% local control rate, while those treated with more than 65 Gy achieved a 69% local control rate. Ten of 11 patients treated with neutron beam therapy had good local control. Split-course radiotherapy was disadvantageous. High PS, weight loss of less than 5%, and no involvement of the vertebral bodies were significant factors ($p \leq .01$) in prolonging survival. The conclusions of the study were that surgical resection should be used whenever possible for SST. Patients with unresectable disease should receive high-dose photon or neutron radiotherapy, if available.[191] There is a high likelihood of close or positive surgical margins for SST; we have generally preferred induction chemotherapy followed by postoperative radiation to 50 Gy if surgical margins are adequate, 60 Gy for microscopically positive margins, and at least 66 Gy for grossly positive margins (all delivered at 2 Gy per day). This approach was supported by LCSG findings as well as an update by our institution.[192] Others have used preoperative radiation followed by intraoperative brachytherapy in SST. There is no established role for chemotherapy alone for these tumors.

The overall 5-year survival rate for patients with resected SST ranges from 28 to 56%. The presence of nodal disease significantly shortens survival. For patients who receive radiotherapy alone, the 5-year survival rate ranges from 1.6 to 23%.[193]

In summary, combinations of surgery and radiotherapy have been the hallmark of treatment of SST. Aggressive surgery with lobectomy and en bloc chest wall resection and lymphadenectomy is still essential. However, the use of neoadjuvant chemotherapy followed by surgery and radiotherapy has the potential to improve outcome as it has for other stage III NSCLC.

Brachytherapy Endotracheal or endobronchial lesions may cause shortness of breath, postobstructive pneumonitis, and hemoptysis. Endobronchial brachytherapy has been used to achieve high radiation doses to these relatively accessible tumors, either as a component of potentially curative therapy or, more commonly, in the palliative setting after external radiotherapy has failed. High-dose-rate brachytherapy has been shown to accomplish rapid alleviation of symptoms and improve functional status without causing esophagitis, pneumonitis, or the bone marrow suppression seen with external irradiation. High-dose-rate brachytherapy is ideal for patients who need either short-term palliation or quick resolution of symptoms before they undergo definitive treatment. Doses of 35 to 42 Gy in 7 Gy weekly fractions have been delivered to such tumors using high-dose-rate brachytherapy remote afterloading techniques.

Between 1988 and 1993, 81 patients with lung cancer underwent endobronchial brachytherapy at M. D. Anderson.[194] Presenting symptoms were shortness of breath in 65 patients (notably 16 did not have any dyspnea), cough in 53, hemoptysis in 22, wheezing in 31, and chest pain in 11. Squamous cell carcinoma was detected in 46% of cases. Eleven percent (9 of 81) of the patients had endobronchial treatment 3 times at 2-week intervals, and 67% (54 of 81) had treatment twice with 2-week intervals. Ninety-three percent of the patients received 1,500 cGy calculated at a distance of 0.6 cm from the center of sources for mainstem lesions, and the rest of the patients had the same dose calculated at a distance of 0.75 cm from the center of the sources for tracheal lesions. Twenty-six patients (32%) showed improvement, and 25 patients had moderate improvement. Seventeen patients had minimal improvement, and 11 patients showed no change. Five patients became slightly worse and 2 became much worse after the endobronchial brachytherapy. Thus, 85% achieved some response, including 32% of all patients who had an excellent response. The median duration of responses was 4.5 months, and the patients who had an excellent response survived for much longer periods. Median survival duration was 5 months for all patients, ranging from 0.5 to 43 months. There was no significant difference between groups on the basis of histology, although SCLC patients appeared to have less symptom relief and to survive for shorter periods, probably because they were referred to us at their disease's terminal stage and they had a more extrinsic component, that is, mediastinal nodal disease rather than endobronchial lesions.

CHEMOTHERAPY Single Agents The clinical development of chemotherapeutic agents has traditionally been in the setting of stage IV disease. Customarily, drug activity has been reported with respect to response rate, and of the many drugs tested in lung cancer in the early 1980s, six have been found to have predictable and reproducible antitumor activity with response rates in excess of 15%: cisplatin, ifosfamide, mitomycin C, etoposide, vindesine, and vinblastine. Variability in dose and schedule relate to response rates observed, and interpretation of early trial data is further complicated by the heterogeneity of the patient populations tested, especially with regard to major prognostic factors. Nonetheless, these six drugs were considered to be "active" in the early 1990s.

More recently, a new generation of compounds has been demonstrated to possess significant activity against NSCLC. These include topoisomerase I inhibitors, taxanes, and active analogues of previously established chemotherapeutic compounds (ie, gemcitabine, vinorelbine). Irinotecan (CPT-11) is a water-soluble camptothecin shown to achieve response rates in excess of 30% in one phase II trial. When these agents are used in combination with other active agents such as the platinums, response rates have exceeded 50% in pilot studies. Topotecan has shown more mixed results. Of the taxanes, docetaxel has had response rates of approximately 30% in multiple trials, and paclitaxel, rates in excess of 20%. Gemcitabine (deoxyfluorocytidine) is a fluoridated derivative of cytosine arabinoside with a single-agent activity greater than 20% documented in a series of clinical trials. Myelosuppression is not a dose-limiting toxic effect, and therefore this agent has become quite useful when administered in combination with others. Vinorelbine is a synthetic vinca alkaloid with less neurotoxicity than vinblastine but still an active agent. Alimta is a newer multitargeted antifolate, also with demonstrated activity in NSCLC. Response rates in the range of 20% have been observed.[1,5,184,185,193]

Combination Chemotherapy Because single agents have generally modest activity, combination chemotherapy regimens have developed; with the majority including a platinum compound. In summary, these drug combinations consistently produce objective tumor response rates in 20 to 40% of patients with advanced NSCLC and a median survival duration of 6 to 8 months in most randomized trials. A complete tumor response is quite uncommon, however, and no single regimen has emerged as the standard treatment approach. The ECOG recently conducted a randomized phase III study to determine if one of four platinum-based schedules had superior efficacy in patients with advanced NSCLC.[1] This trial involved 1,207 patients randomly assigned to receive the control combination of cisplatin and paclitaxel or cisplatin and gemcitabine, cisplatin and docetaxel, or carboplatin and paclitaxel. The results of this modern trial are notable, because the overall response rate was only 19%, and the median survival duration, 7.9 months. The 1-year survival rate was 33%, and the 2-year survival rate 11%. Neither response rate nor survival duration differed significantly among the treatment arms. Patients with an ECOG PS of 2 had a lower rate of survival than those with a PS of 0 or 1. The carboplatin and paclitaxel treatment arm was associated with less toxicity overall, particularly with respect to febrile neutropenia and nausea. None of these chemotherapy regimens emerged as superior. Several studies have compared cisplatin-based two-drug combination regimens with single agents, and on balance, combination regimens appear to fare better, prolonging survival. Cisplatin and vindesine or vinorelbine prolonged survival over the comparator arms, vinorelbine or vindesine alone. However, other investigators could not confirm these results. Similarly, randomized trials have failed to demonstrate a survival advantage for the combination of cisplatin and etoposide over cisplatin or etoposide given as single agents. Nonetheless, more recent trials have shown that combinations with cisplatin appear to yield consistently higher response rates than cisplatin alone. This improvement is modest but still has translated into a survival advantage, at least for combinations with vinorelbine and gemcitabine. A phase III trial of a combination of cisplatin and tirapazamine has also resulted in beneficial improved response rate and survival duration.[195] In aggregate, these studies indicate that two-drug regimens are significantly more active in the treatment of NSCLC than cisplatin given alone.[1,184,185]

Chemotherapy for Advanced NSCLC ***Chemotherapy versus Best Supportive Care*** A series of trials has demonstrated that treatment with chemotherapy yields superior results to purely supportive care (symptom relief) in patients with advanced NSCLC. The results of earlier studies with long-term alkylating agents were disappointing, but most recent trials using platinum-based combinations with doxorubicin/cyclophosphamide, vindesine, vinorelbine, or gemcitabine have resulted in superior survival for patients receiving active treatment.[196–198] On balance, benefits are modest, with median survival ranging from 20 to 30 weeks versus 10 to 17 weeks. The variability of results is due to differences among studies with small numbers of patients and variable access to care. An estimate of the relative benefit of 27% reduction in the probability of death in the year following diagnosis with cisplatin-based chemotherapy compared with best supportive care alone emerged from a meta-analysis using individual patient data from cisplatin-based trials.[199] For 778 patients, the pooled hazard ratio was 0.73 (95% CI 0.63–0.85, $p = .0007$). Median survival for treated patients was 5.5 months, while that for patients who received supportive care was 4.0 ($p = .001$). In an Italian study, single-agent chemotherapy with vinorelbine prolonged the survival of patients 70 years or older over purely supportive care ($p = .03$).[200] In this trial, median survival duration increased from 21 to 28 weeks. The Canadian multicenter trial has been most comprehensively analyzed.[201] In this study, best supportive care, including radiation therapy, was compared with two chemotherapy regimens: vindesine/cisplatin or cyclophosphamide/doxorubicin/cisplatin. The vindesine/cisplatin regimen was associated with significantly longer survival than supportive care ($p = .01$). A cost-effectiveness analysis concluded that there is no disadvantage to chemotherapy. Indeed, the major part of the cost for each of the treatment arms was associated with hospitalization and not the use of chemotherapy. Moreover, chemotherapy may provide important symptom control in a substantial number of patients; a decrease in cough, dyspnea, pain, and hemoptysis may be obtained in responders.

First-Line Therapy for Advanced NSCLC Although existing data clearly indicate that chemotherapy is warranted in appropriately selected patients with advanced lung cancer, an optimal chemotherapy regimen has not been identified. Until the mid 1990s, regimens of cisplatin in combinations, most often with a vinca alkaloid or etoposide, were most commonly used. More recently, drug regimens with a platinum, either cisplatin or carboplatin, and a second newer drug with known activity are more widely used. That second agent could be a taxane, vinorelbine, gemcitabine, or a camptothecin. Choosing one regimen from among many has been a difficult task, however, since there is no clearly documented survival advantage for one drug program over the others. At times, subtle differences in eligibility criteria (eg, inclusion of patients with stage III tumors or those with poor PS) make it difficult to directly relate the results among trials. Nonetheless, there is a trend indicating that regimens containing platinum with a taxane or gemcitabine probably produce higher response rates and also better survival outcome in some series.[201]

There have been a number of studies of paclitaxel in combination with cisplatin or carboplatin, and other agents. In a three-arm randomized ECOG trial (ECOG 5592), 560 eligible, previously untreated patients were randomized to receive a combination of cisplatin plus etoposide or paclitaxel, either low-dose (135 mg/m^2 over 24 hours) or high-dose (250 mg/m^2 over 24 hours with growth factor) paclitaxel in combination with cisplatin (75 mg/m^2).[202] The response rates for the low-dose and high-dose paclitaxel arms were 26.5% and 32.1%, respectively, significantly better than the cisplatin/etoposide arm. There was also an improvement in overall survival, but it reached statistical significance only when the two paclitaxel arms were combined into a single group and compared with the third arm. In a European trial of similar design, cisplatin plus paclitaxel led to improved response rate and quality of life parameters, but there was no overall survival difference compared with a standard regimen of cisplatin and teniposide.[203]

In a recent survey, paclitaxel plus carboplatin was found to be the most widely favored option for first-line chemotherapy in all stages of NSCLC among United States medical oncologists.[204] This relates to ease of administration on an outpatient basis, manageable toxicity profiles compared with other cisplatin-containing regimens, and promising phase II trial results. Langer and colleagues, in one such phase II trial, reported a response rate of 62% and a 1-year survival rate of 54%.[205] A more recent randomized trial, however, failed to demonstrate a survival advantage over the standard cisplatin plus etoposide regimen, and a SWOG trial showed equivalent survival results in a comparison of paclitaxel and carboplatin with vinorelbine and cisplatin.[206,207] The SWOG investigators concluded that both regimens provide effective palliation in advanced NSCLC, but they favored the paclitaxel plus carboplatin regimen for future studies because of its favorable toxicity profile and better tolerability and compliance.

Like vinorelbine and paclitaxel, gemcitabine is approved by the US Food and Drug Administration (FDA) for use against NSCLC. A series of successful phase II trials of cisplatin plus gemcitabine led to pivotal phase III studies.[208-210] The Hoosier Oncology Group compared gemcitabine plus cisplatin with cisplatin alone and showed that the association yielded a modest improvement in median and 1-year survival rates.[208] On the other hand, the Spanish and Italian trials that compared gemcitabine plus cisplatin with another regimen of cisplatin plus etoposide or mitomycin plus ifosfamide plus cisplatin, respectively, failed to demonstrate survival benefit, although there were significant improvements in overall response rates with the gemcitabine/cisplatin regimens.[209,210] Because gemcitabine is relatively well tolerated without dose-limiting myelosuppression, like vinorelbine, it is being considered for use as a single agent in older or medically compromised patients.[211] Georgoulias and colleagues have compared cisplatin/docetaxel with gemcitabine/docetaxel in a prospective randomized multicenter trial.[212] Four hundred forty-one patients were entered, and there were no apparent differences in overall response rates or median survival durations. The interpretation of the authors was that both drug combinations had comparable activity. Masuda and colleagues compared cisplatin/irinotecan with cisplatin/vindesine and irinotecan alone, finding no significant differences in survival.[213]

Fossella and colleagues have reported a multicenter, multinational study of two docetaxel/platinum regimens for NSCLC.[214] In a three-arm project comparing docetaxel/cisplatin, docetaxel/carboplatin, and vinorelbine/cisplatin (VC), involving 1,218 patients with advanced NSCLC, median survival duration was longest for the docetaxel/cisplatin arm, 11.3 months, with a 1-year survival rate of 46% (vs 41% for VC) and a 2-year survival rate of 21% (vs 14% for VC) ($p = .03$). A recent Japanese trial compared docetaxel/cisplatin with vindesine/cisplatin in 311 patients.[215] Docetaxel/cisplatin produced a significantly higher response rate than vindesine/cisplatin, 37.1% versus 21.2% ($p < .01$), and the duration of response trended longer (13.1 vs 9.3 weeks). Many phase II studies are underway in attempts to identify increasingly active three-drug regimens, nonplatinum-containing combinations, and nonplatinum/nontaxane schedules. To date, a standard "best" regimen has not emerged for the treatment of NSCLC. Still, it seems reasonable to offer therapy to select groups of patients with advanced disease. In the absence of curative therapy, prolongation of survival is a reasonable objective.

Certainly, quality of life concerns should enter the treatment decision-making process, and this area is now receiving increasing scrutiny. With respect to ideal duration of chemotherapy, there are probably no clear guidelines because the nature of treatment itself is rapidly changing. ASCO has recommended that not more than eight cycles of currently accepted chemotherapy regimens be administered to individual patients. Socinski and colleagues recently addressed this issue in a prospective phase III trial comparing a defined duration of therapy with carboplatin/paclitaxel versus continuous treatment in advanced NSCLC.[216] Two hundred thirty patients were randomized. Despite differences in the median number of treatment cycles delivered, there were no significant differences in overall response time or 1-year survival rate. A general consensus is that most conventional chemotherapy regimens should be given for a finite number of cycles and that continuing a maintenance approach is not beneficial. After four to six cycles, chronic treatment-related toxic effects may outweigh benefits.

Second-Line Chemotherapy for Advanced NSCLC With the gradual increase in the efficacy of systemic therapy, NSCLC patients are increasingly demanding thoughtful consideration of alternative chemotherapy programs in the setting of progressive or recurrent disease following first-line treatment. Fossella and colleagues helped to establish the role of docetaxel in second-line chemotherapy. In an early trial, patients with good PS who had previously received cisplatin-containing chemotherapy were treated with this single agent and achieved a partial response rate of 17% and a median survival duration of 39 weeks. The 1-year survival rate was 40%, comparing quite favorably with historic controls (10–15%). The use of paclitaxel in this setting is not so clearly defined because the experience with this compound as a component of first-line therapy is much greater. Experience with other active agents, including vinorelbine and irinotecan, has been disappointing in this setting. Following the early trial, Fossella and colleagues continued to a large trial in which they randomized 373 patients to receive docetaxel (100 or 75 mg/m^2) or a control regimen of vinorelbine or ifosfamide at the choice of the investigators.[217] Treatment groups were well balanced. Response rates in the docetaxel arms were low at 10.8% and 6.7%, respectively (0.8% response with vinorelbine or ifosfamide), but patients who received docetaxel achieved a longer time to tumor progression and a superior 1-year survival rate at the 75 mg/m^2 dose (32%). Previous exposure to paclitaxel did not decrease the likelihood of response to docetaxel, nor did it appear to have an impact on survival. Treatment appeared to be well tolerated. The researchers concluded that the 75 mg/m^2

every-3-week schedule offers meaningful benefit to patients with advanced disease. A second phase III trial was reported by Shepherd and colleagues. In this multicenter international study, patients with advanced NSCLC whose disease had progressed on or after at least one cisplatin-containing chemotherapy regimen were randomly assigned to receive either docetaxel or best supportive care. A total of 204 patients were enrolled. The initial dose of docetaxel was 100 mg/m^2, but it was reduced to 75 mg/m^2 because of toxicity. The overall response rate was only 6%. However, time to progression and survival duration were significantly longer for docetaxel-treated patients. Median survival duration was 7.5 months for patients who received 75 mg/m^2 and 4.6 months for patients who received supportive care (p = .01). A striking finding was that the 1-year survival rate for patients who received docetaxel at 75 mg/m^2 was 37%, while it was 12% for patients in the best supportive care arm (p = .003). Quality of life analyses also have provided evidence favoring treatment with docetaxel in selected patients.[218]

Pemetrexed (Alimta) is a multitargeted antifolate drug that targets the enzymes thymidylate synthase, dihydrofolate reductase, and glycinamide ribonucleotide formyl transferase. The phase III trial of pemetrexed in NSCLC was a survival comparison between pemetrexed and docetaxel in relapsed NSCLC.[5] In this noninferiority study, both pemetrexed and docetaxel were given on day 1 of a 21-day cycle. Patients in both arms were premedicated with dexamethasone. Patients in the pemetrexed arm also received folate and B_{12} supplementation. Seventy-five percent of the patients in both arms had ECOG PS scores of 2. Response rates were 9.1% and 8.8%, and median survival times were 8.3 and 7.9 months in the pemetrexed and docetaxel arms, respectively. The docetaxel arm had higher incidences of grade 3 and 4 neutropenia (40% vs 5%), neutropenic fever (13% vs 2%), and neuropathy (8% vs 3%) than the pemetrexed arm. Thus, pemetrexed produced similar results and was better tolerated than docetaxel in the treatment of patients with pretreated NSCLC, leading to the FDA approval of pemetrexed for relapsed NSCLC.

Supplementation with folic acid and B_{12} has been shown to reduce pemetrexed-related toxic effects without compromising clinical benefit. Hence, supplementation with both vitamin B_{12} and folate is recommended. A useful guideline is to administer folic acid at a dosage of 350 to 1,000 µg/day orally and B_{12} at a dosage of 1,000 µg intramuscularly every 9 weeks. Both supplements should be started 1 to 2 weeks prior to chemotherapy and continued until discontinuation of therapy. This agent had been approved for treatment of mesothelioma, based on a randomized phase III trial that compared cisplatin and a combination of cisplatin and pemetrexed. Additional trials are currently evaluating the effect of pemetrexed in different combinations, including biologic therapy and other chemotherapeutics, and in different lines of therapy.

Despite these advances in treatment, improvements in the survival of patients with NSCLC in recent years have been modest. For patients with advanced disease with good enough PS to tolerate and thus receive third- or fourth-line chemotherapy, a retrospective analysis reported the median overall survival from the start of the last treatment as 4 months.[219]

Combined-Modality Treatment of NSCLC

Advances in Neoadjuvant/Adjuvant Chemotherapy Despite undergoing resection, the vast majority of lung cancer patients experience recurrent and/or metastatic disease; two-thirds of these recurrences and metastases occur systemically and one-third locally. Therefore, supplementing surgery with chemotherapy is a rational treatment strategy.[4] Considerable effort has been directed toward improving therapeutic outcomes (except for the prognostically favorable T1 N0 M0 cancers) with the administration of systemic chemotherapy and/or radiotherapy after surgery. Results from older chemotherapy trials have been disappointing, however, in some cases, resulting in even shorter survival for chemotherapy groups than for controls. Nevertheless there remains much interest in developing effective systemic treatment strategies, because lung cancer is largely a systemic disease.

Neoadjuvant Chemotherapy Pisters and colleagues recently conducted a phase II trial assessing the feasibility of perioperative paclitaxel and carboplatin chemotherapy in patients with early-stage NSCLC.[220] Ninety-four patients with a clinical stage Ib, II, or IIIa lesion were treated with two chemotherapy cycles as initial therapy. Fifty-six percent of patients had a major response, and 94% of enrolled patients proceeded to thoracotomy, 86% to complete resection. Treatment-related toxicity was quite acceptable, with promising 1- and 2-year survival rates of 85% and 56%, respectively. This has led to a phase III North American trial (S9900) comparing primary surgery alone with induction chemotherapy (paclitaxel/carboplatin [PC]) followed by surgery. Preliminary data from this multicenter trial (SWOG [chair], American College of Surgeons Oncology Group [ACOSOG], ECOG, NCCTG, NCIC, and RTOG) were presented at the 2005 ASCO annual meeting by Pisters and colleagues.[221] Consenting patients with clinical stage T2 N0, T1-2 N1, or T3 N0-1 NSCLC (excluding SST) were stratified by clinical stage (IB/IIA vs IIB/IIIA) and randomized to receive preoperative PC (P: 225 mg/m^2 over 3 hours, C: AUC = 6) on day 1, every 3 weeks for three cycles, or surgery alone. Surgery was at least a lobectomy and mediastinal nodal sampling. The planned sample size for this prospective, randomized trial was 600 patients. The median follow-up interval was 28 months. The S9900 closed early to new patient entry in July 2004 following publication of positive data on adjuvant treatment from other studies. A total of 354 patients were accrued: 174 underwent surgery alone, and 180 received preoperative PC. The rate of major response to PC was 40%. The median duration of PFS was 29 months for the PC group and 20 months for the control group. The 1- and 2-year PFS rates were 68% and 54% for the PC group and 47% for the control group (hazard rate, 0.85 [0.63-1.14], p = .26). The median duration of overall survival was 42 months for the PC group and 37 months for control group. Overall survival rates at 1 and 2 years were 82% and 68% for the PC group and 79% and 64% for the control group (hazard rate, 0.88 [0.63-1.23], p = .47). The authors concluded that, although closed early because of data from other studies, this study is one of the largest randomized trials examining preoperative chemotherapy in early-stage lung cancer. As such, it represents a landmark regarding feasibility of this approach. Both PFS and overall trends favored preoperative PC, supporting a role for chemotherapy in early-stage NSCLC.

Adjuvant Chemotherapy The LCSG and the Ludwig Lung Cancer Study Group of Europe have conducted a series of trials investigating the potential benefit of adjuvant chemotherapy in patients with completely resected early-stage lung cancer. The LCSG compared four cycles of cyclophosphamide, doxorubicin, and cisplatin (CAP) with no further treatment in 269 patients.[222] After a mean follow-up duration of 6.4 years, no benefits in disease-free or overall survival rates were apparent. However, critics point out that compliance was poor, because only 80% of patients randomized to receive chemotherapy actually did so, and only 53% of patients completed all four planned treatment cycles. Niiranen and colleagues reported more encouraging results in 110 patients with T1-3 NSCLC (90% of whom had T1-2 N0 staged tumors).[223] Fifty-four patients were randomized to receive six cycles of CAP and 54 to receive no further therapy. Although time to recurrence and overall survival duration were significantly better in the chemotherapy-treated patients, an imbalance in randomization resulted in the assignment of twice as many patients who had undergone pneumonectomy to the no-further-treatment group. After adjustment for this imbalance, results were less impressive.

A more definitive recent trial was conducted by the ECOG.[224] Keller and colleagues reported the results of this prospective randomized study designed to determine whether combination chemotherapy with cisplatin/etoposide and thoracic radiotherapy was superior to thoracic radiotherapy alone for patients with completely resected stage II or IIIa NSCLC. A total of four chemotherapy cycles were administered, the first two given concomitantly with radiotherapy. Radiation was given in a daily fractionation sequence to a total dose of 50.4 Gy and was identical in the two treatment arms. The median duration of follow-up was 44 months for 488 patients entered. Although the combined postoperative treatment was generally well tolerated, there was no decrease in the risk of intrathoracic recurrence for the experimental arm, nor was there evidence of a survival difference between the treatment arms. At this point, we conclude that there is no definitive evidence showing a meaningful clinical benefit for adjuvant chemotherapy after resection of stage II or III NSCLC.

A meta-analysis in 1995 compared surgery alone with surgery followed by cisplatin-based chemotherapy. This study included eight trials and 1,394 patients, and showed a 13% reduction in the risk of death, suggesting that adjuvant chemotherapy afforded an absolute benefit of 5% at 5 years ($p = .08$). This was not affected by patient sex, PS, or age, or by tumor histologic subtype.[225] The International Adjuvant Lung Trial study included 1,867 patients who underwent randomization to receive either three or four cycles of adjuvant cisplatin-based chemotherapy or to undergo observation. The investigators concluded that cisplatin-based adjuvant chemotherapy prolonged survival among patients with completely resected NSCLC.[226] Three studies on adjuvant chemotherapy were presented at the ASCO 2004 annual meeting: two moderate-sized studies showed a significant survival benefit: 15% at 5 years for the NCIC JBR10 study,[227] and 12% at 4 years for the CALGB 9633 study.[228] Furthermore, a Japanese meta-analysis of 2,003 patients randomized in six trials of uracil-tegafur showed a 5% benefit at 7 years,[229] confirming the results of the Japanese Lung Cancer Research Group study.[230] Supplementing surgery for NSCLC with chemotherapy (either adjuvant or neoadjuvant) has not become the standard of care and is still controversial, yet it is expected that standardization, optimization, and individualization of this approach will happen in the near future[231] (Table 80-10).

Table 80-10 Postoperative Adjuvant Chemotherapy in Early-Stage Lung Cancer

Study	Pts	Stage IB %	Chemo	↑ 5 Yr %	HR	95% CI	*p* Value
JBR.10(227)	482	45	VbPac	15	0.70	0.52–0.92	.012
CALGB(228)	344	100	PacCb	12–4 yr	0.62	0.41–0.95	.028

Pts = patients; HR = hazard ratio; CI = confidence interval; Vb = vinorelbine; Pac = paclitaxel, Cb = carboplatin.

Unresectable Stage III NSCLC Thoracic irradiation has been the standard therapy for patients with inoperable IIIa/IIIb NSCLC in the United States for many years. Although chest radiotherapy improves cancer-related symptoms and reduces the frequency of local tumor regrowth, no randomized studies demonstrate that chest radiotherapy increases median survival duration compared with no therapy, and immediate radiation therapy is not associated with greater long-term survival rate. The median survival duration in patients with inoperable disease is only approximately 10 months after chest irradiation, and the 5-year survival rate is less than 5%.

Efforts to improve these results have included altered radiation dose-fractionation schedules and combined chemoradiation approaches. Unfortunately, numerous randomized trials evaluating the benefits of chemotherapy combined with chest irradiation have yielded negative results until recently. With the incorporation of cisplatin-based chemotherapy in combined-modality programs, improved survival results are now reported in the literature and have been further substantiated by randomized trials.

There are theoretical reasons to favor giving chemotherapy early in the treatment course and concurrently with radiation therapy. The mathematical model of Goldie and Coldman suggests that the most effective regimens should be given early to prevent the emergence of resistant clones.[274] Chemotherapy may sensitize the cancer cells to radiation therapy and, with increased cell killing, oxygenation of necrotic/hypoxic tumor fractions may improve. In addition, with a reduction of chemotherapy-resistant cells, radiation therapy may improve vascular access for the delivery of subsequent chemotherapy.

With respect to the issue of sequential versus concomitant chemoradiation, available data indicate that the concurrent approach improves the overall outcome. Recent studies were discussed in the section "Radiotherapy" above.

Chemotherapy in the Elderly Approximately one-third of all patients with NSCLC are aged 70 years or older, and, although these patients are likely to have an increased risk of comorbid conditions and impaired organ function, most studies have suggested that age alone should not be a factor in the decision to treat patients with chemotherapy. Retrospective studies of patients treated for advanced NSCLC found no major differences between patients older than and younger than 65 years of age,[232] and an analysis of age as a risk factor in chemotherapy trials found that the response, toxicity, and survival rates of elderly patients were similar to those of younger patients.[233]

Two important phase III randomized studies of chemotherapy in the elderly have been reported.[234,235] The ELVIS (Elderly Lung Cancer Vinorelbine Italian Study) group performed a multicenter, randomized trial of single-agent vinorelbine as a first-line agent in elderly patients with advanced NSCLC. Results demonstrated that the addition of vinorelbine to best supportive care significantly prolonged survival in this group of patients.[234] Median survival for best supportive care plus vinorelbine was 28 weeks, while it was 21 weeks for best supportive care alone. This benefit was achieved at the cost of some drug-related toxicity, reflected in lower scores on quality-of-life subscales that were directly related to drug toxicity (eg, nausea and constipation). Patients who received vinorelbine scored better than control patients on overall health status and quality-of-life, however, and suffered less from the lung cancer symptoms of shortness of breath, cough, and hemoptysis. Recently, the Multicenter Italian Lung cancer in the Elderly Study (MILES) randomized elderly patients with advanced NSCLC to receive vinorelbine, gemcitabine, or vinorelbine plus gemcitabine. Results demonstrated that the combination of gemcitabine plus vinorelbine does not improve survival or quality-of-life compared with single-agent chemotherapy with vinorelbine or gemcitabine in this patient population. The combination treatment was more toxic than the agents administered alone.[235]

The recommendations of an international expert panel in this controversial field were presented recently.[6] The panel recommended a comprehensive geriatric assessment to better define prognosis and predict tolerance to treatment. They suggested that randomized phase III trials with adequate power are warranted to address unanswered questions regarding the efficacy and tolerability of platinum-based chemotherapy. The panel also reviewed the role of biologic therapy in this age group and suggested that, on the basis of present data, target-based agents as first-line treatment of elderly NSCLC patients are not yet recommended. They concluded that single-agent chemotherapy with a third-generation drug (vinorelbine, gemcitabine, a taxane) should be the recommended option for nonselected elderly patients with advanced NSCLC. Platinum-based chemotherapy is a viable option for fit patients with adequate organ function. Best supportive care remains important, in addition to chemotherapy or as the exclusive option for patients who are unsuitable for more aggressive treatment.[6]

Molecular Targeted Therapy Advances in our understanding of cancer biology have led to the discovery of a number of potential molecular targets and the development of novel agents that, unlike conventional cytotoxic agents, specifically target tumor cells or their blood vessels. This approach has been termed "molecular targeted therapy." Most advanced in clinical research for NSCLC-targeted therapies are EGFR and VEGF inhibitors. Indeed, the first targeted therapies for NSCLC are gefitinib (Iressa, AstraZeneca) and erlotinib (Tarceva, Genentech), EGFR tyrosine kinase inhibitors (TKI) that have been recently approved as monotherapy for advanced NSCLC.

The rationale for EGFR inhibition as a target for cancer therapy was proposed nearly 20 years ago by Mendelsohn and colleagues, who noted that EGFR is frequently overexpressed in human tumors, and in many cases is associated with poor outcome.[32] Several strategies have been developed to target the EGF family of receptors. These include monoclonal antibodies, which either bind the ligand or compete with the ligand for the extracellular domain of the receptor; inhibitors of receptor dimerization; small-molecule inhibitors of the intracellular tyrosine kinase domain; antisense oligonucleotides; and inhibitors of the EGFR downstream signaling network.

Inhibitors of EGFR Tyrsoine Kinase Activity Gefitinib and erlotinib are small molecules that reversibly target EGFR tyrosine kinase. In phase I studies, both have yielded objective responses in heavily pretreated patients with NSCLC when used as single agents.[2,32] They are well absorbed after oral administration and can be given for long periods. The drugs' side effects are usually mild to moderate and consist primarily of dose-dependent skin rash and diarrhea, which are the dose-limiting toxic effects (DLT). The bioavailability of orally administered gefitinib is 59%; it has a terminal half-life of 28 hours and can be administered once daily. A pharmacokinetic analysis in a phase I trial showed that the steady-state concentration of gefitinib was achieved by day 7 of administration. In a phase I study of erlotinib evaluating several administration schedules, a mean half-life of 24.4 hours at the 150 mg/day dosage was documented.

Two randomized phase II multicenter trials (Iressa Dose Evaluation in Advanced Lung Cancer, IDEAL 1 and 2) with two dosages (250 and 500 mg/day) of gefitinib were conducted in over 400 patients with stage III or IV NSCLC whose disease had failed to respond to platinum-based chemotherapy.[236,237] Side effects were generally mild, consisting of skin rash, pruritus, and diarrhea, but they were significantly more common and severe at the higher dosage. In neither trial were there significant differences in efficacy variables between the 250- and 500-mg/day dosages. The researchers showed that, overall, monotherapy with gefitinib induces radiographic response in 12 to 18% and improves symptoms in 40 to 43% of NSCLC patients with advanced disease who experienced chemotherapy failure. Thus, the recommended dosage for patients with NSCLC who have previously undergone platinum-based chemotherapy is 250 mg/day. On the basis of these data, gefitinib received approval in Japan and South Korea in July 2002 as second-line chemotherapy for advanced NSCLC, and in May 2003 in the United States as third-line monotherapy treatment of advanced disease. The recommended dosage was 250 mg/day, since treatment at the higher dosage led to greater toxicity without additional benefit. Gefitinib is currently approved in 35 countries, including Argentina, Australia, Canada, Chile, China, Hong Kong, India, Israel, Russia, Switzerland, and Taiwan. (AstraZeneca Web page: http://www.iressa.com).

Erlotinib was investigated in a phase II trial in 56 patients with advanced NSCLC whose disease had failed to respond to platinum-based chemotherapy. Unlike the gefitinib studies, patients were included only if their tumors overexpressed EGFR (> 10% positive cells). In this study, erlotinib was given continuously at a fixed dosage of 150 mg/day, which produced an acneiform rash in 78% of patients. Twelve percent of patients responded to erlotinib, and 39% of patients had prolonged stable disease during the treatment. Gefitinib and erlotinib do not induce myelosuppression, which makes them appealing for use with chemotherapy. The results of two large, randomized, placebo-controlled, phase III trials (Iressa NSCLC Trial Assessing Combination Treatment [INTACT] trials 1 [gemcitabine and cisplatin] and 2 [paclitaxel and carboplatin]) of gefitinib in chemotherapy-naïve patients with stage IIIB/IV NSCLC have been reported.[238,239] Patients were randomly assigned to receive placebo, gefitinib 250 mg/day, or gefitinib 500 mg/day in addition to chemotherapy. Patients continued with gefitinib or placebo until disease progression. Results showed that gefitinib did not add therapeutic benefits over chemotherapy alone. In two large, randomized similarly designed trials of chemotherapy with or without erlotinib, erlotinib was given concomitantly with a combination of carboplatin and paclitaxel (the TRIBUTE study; n = 1,059) or a combination of cisplatin and gemcitabine (TALENT; n = 1,172).[240,241] Selection of patients for these trials was not based on biologic features. Like the gefitinib phase III trials, these studies showed that erlotinib offered no survival benefit or improvement in response rate over chemotherapy alone. In a randomized, placebo-controlled trial (NCIC BR.21) involving 731 patients, however, single-agent erlotinib was shown to prolong survival in NSCLC patients after first- or second-line chemotherapy.[242] Overall response to erlotinib was 9%, and the overall survival durations were 6.7 months for erlotinib and 4.7 months for placebo (p = .001). On the basis of this study—the first randomized trial to confirm that an EGFR TKI prolongs survival after first- or second-line chemotherapy—erlotinib received approval by the FDA in November 2004.

Interestingly, in a similar study gefitinib did not prolong patient survival. In multicenter study 709, IRESSA Survival Evaluation in Lung cancer (ISEL), 1,692 patients were randomized to receive gefitinib 250 mg/day or placebo. This study demonstrated a difference between gefitinib and placebo in terms of survival, although this did not reach statistical significance in the overall population or in subgroups of patients.[243] The reasons for the differences between BR21 and ISEL results are not clear as of yet. Possible explanations for the discrepancy are that erlotinib was given at a dose closer to its maximal tolerated dose than gefitinib; that the study populations were not comparable (ISEL was almost twice as large), including a higher rate of refractory disease in ISEL; and that these drugs are different after all.

Prediction of EGFR TKI Response Better understanding of the biology of the EGFR system in lung cancer has been the focus of intense research in the last year. Retrospective analyses of gefitinib or erlotinib study data revealed several clinical predictors of response. They repeatedly showed that responses were more frequent among patients who had never smoked, women, patients with adenocarcinomas, and patients of East Asian ethnicity.[2] Two groups from Boston in two pivotal studies examined gain-of-function somatic mutations of EGFR in exons 18-21 and correlated them with response to EGFR inhibitors. Lynch and colleagues[244] and Paez and colleagues[245] found increased sensitivity to gefitinib in patients with these EGFR mutations, and that patients who did not express a mutation had a low probability of responding. The group from Memorial Sloan Kettering Cancer Center extended these data and showed that similar EGFR mutations are also associated with responses to erlotinib.[2] These findings are supported by a report of correlation between these clinical predictors of response and EGFR mutation status.[246] Compiling these data reveals that EGFR mutations are identified in 80% of responders to EGFR small molecule TKI, whereas mutations in K-*ras* (exon 2) are associated with lack of sensitivity to either erlotinib or gefitinib.[2] The role of EGFR or K-*ras* mutation status in prediction of response to EGFR inhibitors in general, and EGFR TKI in particular, is being studied in prospective studies.

Angiogenesis Inhibitors in Lung Cancer
As already discussed, VEGF, which is an endothelial cell survival factor, is essential for tumor angiogenesis. One approach to the modulation of VEGF-mediated angiogenesis is to use antibodies against the VEGF protein itself or VEGFR. Bevacizumab (Avastin, Genentech) is a recombinant humanized monoclonal antibody to VEGF that acts synergistically with chemotherapy in preclinical and clinical models. It is currently the only clinically available antiangiogenic agent and is approved for use in the United States and Europe in combination with 5-fluorouracil–based chemotherapy for first-line treatment of metastatic carcinoma of the colon or rectum. Approval was based on a pivotal study of patients with colorectal cancer who received bevacizumab in combination with chemotherapy, which provided the first clear demonstration of the value of antiangiogenesis over chemotherapy alone in prolonging patient survival.[247]

In a phase I trial, bevacizumab reduced serum VEGF concentrations to undetectable levels when administered at dosages of at least 3 mg/kg/week and showed no pharmacologic interactions when studied in combination with a variety of chemotherapeutic agents. In a phase II study, patients with stage IIIB/IV NSCLC were randomly assigned to undergo standard therapy with carboplatin and paclitaxel alone or with 7.5 mg/kg or 15 mg/kg of bevacizumab.[248] Members of the control group (chemotherapy only) who experienced disease progression were allowed to enter the high-dose bevacizumab arm. Response rates were higher (40.0% vs 21.9%) and time to progression (7.0 vs 3.9 months) and median survival (17.7 vs 11.6 months) were longer in the high-dose arm than in the low-dose arm. An unusual and unexpected toxic effect was the development of life-threatening hemoptysis in six patients, which resulted in four fatalities. This event did not appear to be dose dependent, since all but one of these six cases occurred in the low-dose bevacizumab arm. Bleeding arose from centrally located tumors close to major blood vessels and cavitation or necrosis had occurred in most cases. This adverse event has not been notable in studies of other tumor types.

Because multivariate analysis identified squamous cell histology as a risk factor, an ongoing phase II/III NSCLC study comparing bevacizumab (15 mg/kg) plus carboplatin and paclitaxel with carboplatin and paclitaxel alone includes only patients whose tumors are of nonsquamous histologic type. This trial is being conducted by ECOG (study E4599) and was closed to accrual in June 2004 with approximately 850 patients recruited. A secondary objective of this study is identification of biological surrogate markers of treatment effect. Sandler and colleagues presented preliminary data at the ASCO 2005 annual meeting.[3] Response rate (10% vs 27%, $p < .0001$), PFS duration (4.5 months vs 6.4 months, $p < .0001$), and median survival (10.2 months vs 12.5 months, $p = .0075$) all favored the combination of carboplatin/paclitaxel and bevacizumab. Supplementing chemotherapy with bevacizumab was found to improve survival also in patients with colon cancer, breast cancer, or renal cell carcinomas, and it is expected that this agent will become a part of many standard regimens in the future.

Combination of Treatment Strategies Different combinations of conventional therapy (chemotherapy or radiation therapy) or combinations of targeted therapy are being explored, and some examples are discussed in this section. As already discussed, the mainstay for cancer therapy is still chemotherapy. Concurrent administration of gefitinib or erlotinib with chemotherapy did not improve results of chemotherapy alone.[238–241] Several studies are looking at potential explanations for this phenomenon and studying sequences of combination to elaborate on this issue. Another approach is the combination of growth factor receptor TKI and monoclonal antibodies to improve signaling inhibition. Preliminary preclinical data are encouraging.[249,250]

As alternatives, drugs are now being developed to block several signaling pathways. AEE788 (Novartis) and ZD6474 (Zactima, AstraZeneca) are TKI of VEGFR and EGFR that are currently being tested in the clinic.[52] It has been suggested that, besides complementing chemotherapy regimens, targeted agents could enhance the therapeutic efficacy of radiation therapy.[251] VEGF levels and tumor cell EGFR expression have been shown to increase following exposure to ionizing radiation, and this has been associated with reduced sensitization to radiation therapy. Radiation therapy is a major treatment modality for lung cancer, and there could be potential for increasing its efficacy by concomitant administration of inhibitors of VEGF or EGF activity. This is supported by preclinical studies of ZD6474 and other antiangiogenic agents plus radiation therapy, which demonstrated the additive effects of this approach.[52] The combination of EGFR and VEGFR blockers to improve target inhibition was studied in lung cancer. VEGF inhibition with bevacizumab has been investigated in combination with the EGFR TKI erlotinib in 40 patients with stage IIIB/IV or recurrent NSCLC of nonsquamous cell histology. Treatment with bevacizumab (15 mg/kg IV every 21 days) plus erlotinib (150 mg/day orally) resulted in eight partial responses (20%, CI 7.6–32.4%) and 26 patients with stable disease (65%, CI 50.2–79.8%). The median survival of 34 patients treated in the phase II part of the study was 12.6 months, and 52% of patients were alive at 1 year. No pharmacokinetic interactions were observed between the two agents, and the most common adverse events were mild to moderate rash, diarrhea, and proteinuria. These encouraging data support further evaluation of VEGF/EGF inhibition for the treatment of advanced NSCLC, and a randomized study is currently ongoing.[52] Some of these drugs are listed in Table 80-11.

Table 80-11 Molecular Targeted Therapy for Lung Cancer

Agent	Activity	Comment
Gefitinib, erlotinib	EGFR TKI	Approved as monotherapy third line in advanced NSCLC
Erbitux, panitumumab, EMD732000	Monoclonal antibodies to EGFR	
Bevacizumab	Monoclonal antibody to VEGFR	Approved for first line colon cancer with chemotherapy
ZD6474, AEE788	VEGFR and EGFR TKI	
BAY43-9006 (Sorafenib)	Raf-1, VEGFR, and PDGFR-β TKI	
PTK787	VEGFR TKI	
SU11248	VEGFR, PDGFR, c-Kit, and CSF-1 TKI	

EGFR = epidermal growth factor receptor; TKI = tyrosine kinase inhibitor; NSCLC = nonsmall-cell lung cancer; VEGFR = vascular endothelial growth factor receptor; PDGFR = platelet-derived growth factor receptor; CSF-1 = colony-stimulating factor-1.

Summary of the M. D. Anderson guidelines for diagnosis and therapy of NSCLC are presented in Figure 80-11.

THERAPY FOR SCLC

SCLC differs from other types of lung cancer in its propensity for early systemic spread and relentless progression. Of the patients whose disease is managed without resection of the primary tumor, very few have no evidence of tumor dissemination beyond the thorax after autopsy. Of patients who have had surgery with curative intent and died within 30 days after surgery, 70% have distant metastases at postmortem examination. This aggressive clinical feature is reflected in the short overall survival duration of these patients. Before effective systemic treatment became available, the median survival duration was 12 weeks for those with limited-stage disease and 5 weeks for those with extensive-stage disease. Patients rarely survived longer than 35 weeks.

Locoregional therapy, with either surgery or radiation, prolonged survival only slightly, primarily for a subset of patients with limited-stage disease. An overwhelming majority of patients did not benefit, however, only approximately 20% survived for a year, and 5-year survival was rare. In a landmark trial conducted by the Medical Research Council in England in the 1960s, patients who were considered candidates for surgical resection by the standards of the time were randomized to undergo thoracotomy or definitive irradiation of the primary tumor and regional lymphatics. Radiation therapy resulted in slightly better mean survival duration (6.5 vs 10 months, $p = .04$); 1-, 2-, and 5-year survival rates were 22%, 10%, and 4%, respectively, for radiotherapy and 21%, 4%, and 1%, respectively, for surgery. Notably, the one 5-year survivor in the surgery arm was ultimately unable to undergo surgery and was given radiation therapy instead. This and other experiences led to the abandonment of surgery as a primary modality of treatment of SCLC, with the possible exception of patients with solitary pulmonary nodules. Moreover, chest radiotherapy as a sole treatment would also soon be superseded.

In 1969, Green and colleagues reported the results of a placebo-controlled randomized trial evaluating single-agent alkylating agents in the treatment of lung cancer. Three courses of intravenous cyclophosphamide more than doubled the median survival duration (from 6 to 17 weeks) in patients with extensive-stage SCLC. Randomized trials in most instances have also demonstrated that adjuvant chemotherapy prolongs survival following surgery when compared with no further treatment. Similarly, the addition of concomitant chemotherapy to chest irradiation has prolonged survival in a majority of randomized trials over irradiation as the sole initial treatment, followed by chemotherapy at the time of tumor progression. With the general acceptance of SCLC as a systemic disorder and recognition of the superiority of multimodal regimens over local therapy alone, chemotherapy became the cornerstone of SCLC management.[252]

Surgical Treatment Although it has been established that surgical resection does not customarily play a role in the treatment of SCLC, there are still some clinical settings in which surgery may be of potential benefit. The most accepted role for surgery is in the case of peripheral SCLC. Although two-thirds of patients have extensive disease at the time of presentation, there is a small subset, fewer than 5% of patients with SCLC, who present with the tumor confined to the lung, with or without N1 lymph node metastases. These patients commonly present with a solitary pulmonary nodule on an incidental chest radiograph. Overall 5-year survival rate for patients who have undergone surgery followed by adjuvant therapy has been shown to range from 28 to 60% for patients with stage I disease and 20 to 35% for patients with T1 N1 disease.[253] Isolated reports have described 5-year survival rates as high as 70 to 80% for selected groups of patients with very limited stage disease. The great disparity between the survival rates of these patients and the survival rates of the more common central SCLC has led to several hypotheses. Some investigators believe that these tumors represent a variant of SCLC with altered biology; however, others believe that these tumors are inaccurately diagnosed and may in fact be atypical carcinoids or well-differentiated neuroendocrine carcinomas.[254]

Most patients with peripheral SCLC have the diagnosis made at the time of thoracotomy. A select few, however, have the diagnosis estab-

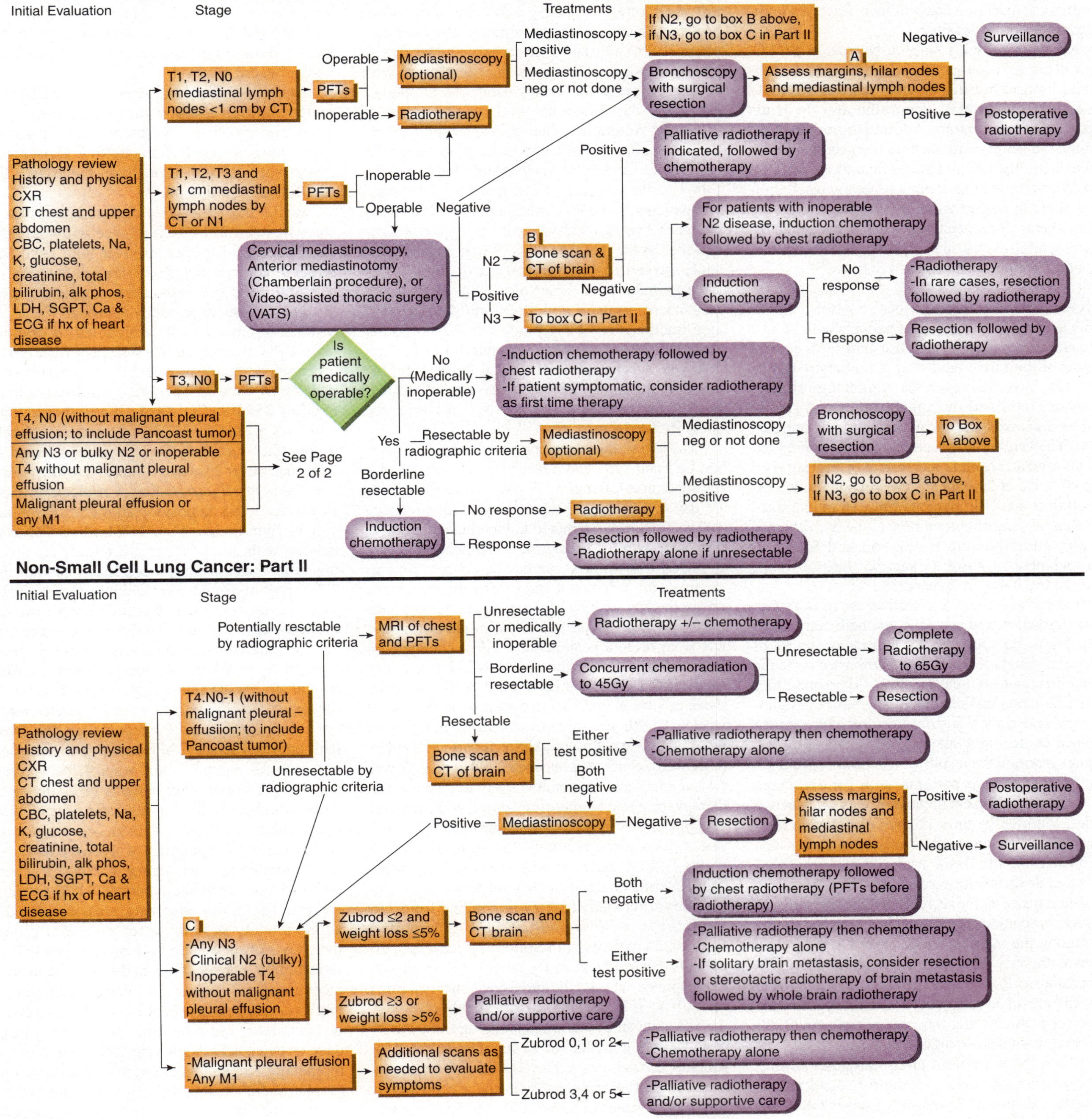

Figure 80-11 Management of nonsmall-cell lung cancer.

lished preoperatively with FNA. The rare but established presentation of SCLC as a peripheral lesion, along with the fact that NSCLC and carcinoids can be misdiagnosed as SCLC on FNA, should prompt the clinician to continue to consider the patient for surgical treatment rather than refer immediately for chemotherapy. In light of this preoperative diagnosis, staging should be even more thorough than usual to reflect the high incidence of occult mediastinal and systemic metastasis associated with SCLC. Thorough radiographic staging, as well as mediastinoscopy and bone marrow aspiration, are employed prior to consideration of surgery. The presence of mediastinal involvement would obviate the role of surgery, but the presence of hilar adenopathy on radiographic staging is not a contraindication to surgery. These patients may still undergo exploration as a means of establishing the presence of disease within the hilar nodes and, in good candidates, resection can still be offered if a complete resection is possible.

All patients with surgically treated SCLC, regardless of whether the diagnosis was established before, during, or after resection, should receive postoperative chemotherapy. In trials reported by the Veterans Administration Surgical Adjuvant Group, patients who received postoperative chemotherapy did better than those who did not. When the timing of chemotherapy was examined, there appeared to be no advantage to giving chemotherapy preoperatively. The agents employed are essentially identical to those recommended for other patients with limited disease.[252]

Radiotherapy Surgical local control is applicable to a very small subset of patients with SCLC. The remainder require some form of local control as part of their treatment, and radiotherapy fulfills this role. Two meta-analyses employing different methods confirmed the value of thoracic irradiation to decrease local recurrence and prolong survival. The first study, based on results from 11 trials, showed an absolute increase in overall survival rate of 5.4% at 2 years.[255] The second study collected data on 2,140 patients from 16 randomized trials comparing chemotherapy alone with chemotherapy plus thoracic irradiation and found an improvement in absolute survival rate of 5.4%, from 15 to 20.4%, at 3 years.[256]

It is obvious that the effectiveness of both thoracic irradiation and systemic chemotherapy needs to be improved. One idea for improving control of local and distant disease is to administer systemic chemotherapy as a radiosensitizer. Alternating thoracic irradiation and chemotherapy has both radiobiologic and clinical justification for improvement of local control and survival. Arriagada and colleagues reported the results of two protocols enrolling 72 consecutive patients with limited-stage SCLC.[257] Induction chemotherapy was given in two cycles, followed by three courses of radiation therapy lasting 2 weeks each. Cisplatin and etoposide were used initially in the trial, but cyclophosphamide and doxorubicin were added. The chemotherapy alternated with the second and the third series of thoracic irradiation. Their long-term survival results are among the most favorable reported: the 2-year survival rate was 40%, and the 5-year rate was 26%. According to their recent report, the disease-free survival rates at 2 years were 28% in the higher-dose group (cisplatin 100 mg/m^2, cyclophosphamide 300 mg/m^2, doxorubicin 40 mg/m^2, etoposide 75 mg/m^2) and 8% in the lower-dose group (cisplatin 80 mg/m^2, cyclophosphamide 225 mg/m^2, doxorubicin 40 mg/m^2, etoposide 75 mg/m^2). Longer follow-up revealed that 2- and 5-year survival rates were 42% and 26%, respectively, in the higher-dose group, and 20% and 8%, respectively, in the lower-dose group. The relative risk of death among those who received higher initial doses of chemotherapy, as compared with those who received lower doses, was 0.63 (95% CI, 0.42–0.96). The results were similar when the analyses were stratified according to center.[257]

Timing of Chemotherapy and Radiotherapy Two strategies of concurrent radiation therapy and chemotherapy have been piloted. McCracken and colleagues reported results from a phase II SWOG trial in which two courses of cisplatin, etoposide, and vincristine were given with concurrent radiation therapy using one fraction of 1.8 Gy per day, 5 days per week, to a total dose of 45 Gy.[258] Additional chemotherapy with vincristine, methotrexate, and etoposide, alternating with doxorubicin and cyclophosphamide for 12 weeks, followed the concurrent therapy. They evaluated 154 patients, and with a minimum period of observation of 3 years, the 2-year survival rate was 42%, and the 4-year rate was 30%. When updated, this study showed a 5-year survival rate of 26%.[259] Turrisi reported a small series of patients treated with concurrent cisplatin and etoposide with accelerated fractionation: 1.5 Gy twice daily, 5 days per week, was given for 3 weeks to a total dose of 45 Gy. Two-year survival rates were 57% and 65% for the Turrisi and Johnson and colleagues studies, respectively. The updated 4-year survival rate from the study by Turrisi was 36%.[260,261]

The two studies were compared at M. D. Anderson between 1987 and 1989.[262] The COPE (cyclophosphamide 750 mg/m^2 IV day 1, vincristine 2 mg IV day 8, cisplatin 20 mg/m^2 days 1–3, etoposide 100 mg/m^2) trial attempted to blend the alternating approach with the accelerated treatment approach, in regard to both dose per day and overall time to complete the radiation therapy. After three cycles of chemotherapy with COPE, patients underwent surgical resection. Those patients who did not have a CR were offered postoperative chemotherapy and interdigitating radiotherapy. Radiotherapy was given at 0.5 Gy twice daily for 1 week, repeated twice at 3-week intervals to a total of 45 Gy over 9 weeks; COPE was given between each cycle of radiotherapy and for an additional two cycles. The other study, conducted between 1990 and 1992, was part of a national cooperative study to give chemotherapy (cisplatin 60 mg/m^2 IV day 1, and etoposide 120 mg /m^2 IV days 1–3 for four cycles, every 3 weeks) with concurrent radiotherapy to 45 Gy in 5 weeks (1.8 Gy daily) or in 3 weeks (1.5 Gy twice daily) starting on day 1 of chemotherapy.

The earlier study (follow-up ranging from 7 to 50 months, with a median of 17.5 months) enrolled 28 patients with limited-stage SCLC; 20 patients achieved CR and 8 patients achieved partial response. The 1-, 2-, and 3-year survival rates were 79%, 39%, and 30%, respectively.

The latter study (follow-up ranging from 1 to 39 months, with a median of 21 months) enrolled 33 patients; 29 patients achieved CR and 4 patients achieved partial response, with the 1-, 2-, and 3-year survival rates of 93%, 70%, and 53%, respectively. Rates of locoregional recurrence and distant metastasis were 44% and 48% in the interdigitating group and 30% and 33% in the concurrent group.

The major toxic effect in both protocols was granulocytopenia. Grade 3 or 4 esophagitis was significantly more common in the concurrent treatment group (five grade 3, two grade 4) than in the interdigitating group (two grade 3, no grade 4). The data suggest that concurrent chemotherapy plus radiation therapy is more effective than induction chemotherapy followed by interdigitating chest radiotherapy and chemotherapy for both local and distant disease control as well as 2- and 3-year overall survival.

The NCIC CTG compared early and late thoracic radiation therapy in a randomized trial. Their trial enrolled 308 patients and showed that early thoracic irradiation yielded significantly longer survival and fewer brain metastases than late thoracic irradiation.[263]

Schild and colleagues conducted a phase III study to determine whether twice-daily radiotherapy resulted in longer survival than once-daily radiotherapy in patients with limited-stage SCLC. The study did not demonstrate an advantage to the split-course, twice-daily approach.[264]

Fractionation The efficacies of standard once-a-day fractionation (1.8 Gy per fraction) and accelerated fractionation (1.5 Gy twice daily) were compared by a cooperative randomized trial (ECOG 3588/RTOG 8815). Radiotherapy consisted of a total of 45 Gy of thoracic radiation, given either once daily over a period of 5 weeks or twice daily over 3 weeks. It was given with concurrent chemotherapy consisting of cisplatin 60 mg/m^2 IV on day 1 and etoposide 120 mg/m^2 IV on days 1–3 in four cycles. Four hundred and nineteen patients with limited-stage SCLC were enrolled in this randomized trial between May 1989 and July 1992, 381 of whom were eligible and evaluable. Twice-daily treatment beginning with the first cycle of chemotherapy significantly prolonged survival compared with concurrent once-daily radiotherapy (p = .04 by the log-rank test). After a median follow-up interval of almost 8 years, the median survival durations were 19 months for the once-daily group and 23 months for the twice-daily group. The survival rates for patients receiving once-daily radiotherapy were 41% at 2 years and 16% at 5 years. For patients receiving twice-daily radiotherapy, the survival rates were 47% at 2 years and 26% at 5 years. Grade 3 esophagitis was significantly more frequent with twice-daily thoracic radiotherapy, occurring in 26% of patients than with once-daily radiotherapy (11%, $p < .001$). Despite the major myelosuppression noted in approximately 90% of patients in both groups, there was only one death from myelotoxicity. There were 11 treatment deaths, 6 in the twice-daily treatment group and 5 in the once-daily group. Overall, four cycles of cisplatin plus etoposide and a course of concurrent radiotherapy, 45 Gy given either once or twice daily beginning with cycle 1 of chemotherapy, resulted in 2- and 5-year survival rates of 44% and 23%, respectively, which are twice as good as they had been a decade earlier. However, sequencing and timing of chemotherapy and thoracic radiotherapy are still controversial.

Total Tolerable Dose Radiation dose to the thorax is another controversial area.[265] The NCIC developed an important study to show dose response in the thorax.[266] A dose response was clearly demonstrated by the results: thoracic PFS was prolonged by giving 37.5 Gy in 15 fractions over 3 weeks rather than 25 Gy in 10 fractions over 2 weeks as consolidation after completion of chemotherapy with cisplatin/etoposide and cyclophosphamide/doxorubicin/vincristine in alternating or sequential regimens. Arriagada and colleagues published a report of 173 patients with limited-stage SCLC treated in three consecutive trials at the Institut Gustave-Roussy, France. The total dose of thoracic radiotherapy increased from 45 Gy (15-15-15) to 55 Gy (20-20-15) to 65 Gy (20-20-20), which was given by split courses interdigitating with chemotherapy. Their 3-year local control rates were 66%, 70%, and 70%, respectively, and 5-year survival rates were 16%, 16%, and 20%, respectively. There was a 10% rate of lethal toxic effects overall with no significant difference by dose. They concluded that there were no significant differences in local control or survival duration with treatment of 45 Gy and 65 Gy when effective chemotherapy was given in this interdigitating manner.[267] Strategies were considered that might increase the local control rate for concurrent chemotherapy and radiation therapy without increasing the esophageal toxicity rate to unacceptable levels. One strategy considered was to increase the total dose by administering daily thoracic radiation therapy at higher levels. This strategy, advocated by Choi, is being studied by the Cancer and Leukemia Group B.[268] Considering the value demonstrated by accelerated fractionation even to a total dose of just 45 Gy in 3 weeks, there was concern that a greater overall duration of thoracic radiation therapy might be disadvantageous. Accelerated fractionation via concomitant boost has been successfully used to treat patients with head and neck cancer without chemotherapy.[269] This strategy uses once-daily irradiation early in the course of treatment and then twice daily irradiation toward the end. Therefore, a strategy that increased the total dose above 45 Gy but also accelerated the delivery of thoracic radiation concurrent with chemotherapy was sought.

The hypothesis was that local failure rate could be reduced without increasing the incidence of acute grade 3 esophagitis, the major nonhematologic toxic effect in the earlier trials. A phase I trial in which the chemotherapy was kept consistent and the thoracic radiation therapy dose was escalated was considered appropriate. Patients would be treated with once-a-day fractionation to a volume initially encompassing both the GTV and a CTV that included sites of suspected metastases to lymph nodes. Toward the end of the 5-week course of treatment, a second fraction would be delivered each day using a concomitant boost technique encompassing only the GTV. Successive increases in the number of fractions delivered by the concomitant boost would constitute the dose escalation. The overall course of treatment would never exceed 5 weeks unless there were interruptions due to toxic effects. Thus, the primary objective of this phase I trial was to determine the maximum tolerated dose (MTD) of increasing doses of thoracic radiation therapy administered by concomitant boost.

RTOG 97-12 was such a trial, a prospective phase I radiation therapy dose escalation study in which radiation was administered concurrent with etoposide and cisplatin. The dose was escalated from 50.4 to 64.8 Gy over 5 weeks. Daily radiation dose was 1.8 Gy to the large field followed by dose escalation to the boost fields to avoid increase in the esophagitis rate. All dose levels were given within 5 weeks to avoid prolongation of the duration of radiotherapy and thus decrease the risk of severe toxic effects. The MTD was 61.2 Gy over 5 weeks.[270] The accrual rate of RTOG 97-12 was 3 or 4 patients per month. It was activated in February 1998 and closed in October 2002 with a total accrual of 64 patients. This study had to be closed for 90 days to evaluate rates of grade 3 or higher acute and sub-acute nonhematologic toxic effects after every 8 to 10 patients were treated on the same radiation dose level. The estimated 18-month survival rate was improved by dose escalation from 50.4 Gy in arm 1 (25% survival) to 61.2 Gy in arm 4 (82% survival).

Cranial Irradiation in SCLC Brain metastases are detected in approximately 10% of SCLC patients at initial presentation, and the likelihood of their development increases with lengthening survival. In the absence of specific therapy to the CNS, the actuarial cumulative probability reached 80% at 28 months of follow-up when the cases of CNS metastasis found at autopsy were included and 58% at 24 months when only clinical brain metastases were counted. At postmortem examination, much higher incidences were reported, ranging up to 65%. With the hope that the CNS would be the only site of residual disease, prophylactic cranial irradiation (PCI) was incorporated as an initial part of treatment of SCLC in the early 1970s.[252]

Since the early 1980s, PCI has been recommended for complete responders on the basis of the findings from a retrospective study from the NCI. Between 1977 and 1995, 11 prospective randomized trials of PCI were published. Although all but two trials reported a significant reduction in the incidence of brain metastasis, none demonstrated an improvement in survival with PCI. Four trials have addressed the issue of PCI in complete responders. All four studies failed to demonstrate any survival benefit of PCI, even among the complete responders, despite significant reduction in the frequency of brain metastases. This lack of survival benefit was attributed to the fact that in most patients the disease progresses at other sites, which is the predominant factor influencing survival. In a most definitive large randomized study of 300 SCLC patients who achieved CR following various chemotherapy regimens, PCI (24 Gy given in eight fractions over 12 days) significantly reduced the rate of brain metastasis as the isolated first site of relapse (45% vs 19% at 2 years, $p < .01$, and overall brain relapse rate at 2 years 67% vs 40%, $p < .01$). The 2-year survival rate of 29% in the PCI group was not significantly different from that of the control group, who did not receive PCI (21.5%, $p = .14$).

Although these trials failed to demonstrate any survival benefit of PCI, a recent meta-analysis concluded that PCI prolongs both overall survival and disease-free survival among SCLC patients in complete remission.[271] This analysis was based on individual data from 987 patients who were enrolled in seven randomized trials to evaluate the role of PCI in complete remission. The relative risk of death in the treatment group, compared with the control group, was 0.84 (95% CI, 0.73–0.97; $p = .01$), which corresponds to a 5.4% increase in the rate of survival at 3 years (15.3% in the control group vs 20.7% in the PCI group). PCI has not been routinely applied, even to patients who achieved CR to thoracic radiotherapy and chemotherapy, because of concern for neurological toxic effects, which were attributed to the PCI, and lack of associated benefit to overall survival. When more fractionated radiotherapy without concurrent PCI was given within optimal timing to patients with a CR, there was reduction of intracranial metastasis without severe neurotoxicity. Furthermore, when patients with limited-stage SCLC were evaluated before and after PCI by an expert neuropsychologist applying detailed neuropsychological testing, 83% (25 of 30 patients) were found to have minor cognitive dysfunction prior to PCI, and no significant differences were found in the comparison of pretreatment and post-treatment neuropsychological results.

The meta-analysis revealed that PCI improved not only overall survival rate, but also disease-free survival rate by 8.8%, from 13.5 to 22.3% ($p = .001$), and reduced cranial recurrence rate by 25.3%, from 58.6 to 33.3% ($p < .001$). There was a trend to reduction of brain metastasis in the subset of PCI patients who received at least 36 Gy in 12 fractions rather than lower doses of PCI.[252]

In summary, the management of limited-stage SCLC has improved median, long-term, and disease-free survival rates in the past 25 years, with some increase in toxicity, although some of the toxic effects could be related to the disease itself and others were never seen because the patients did not live long enough. Patient selection, with consideration of tumor histology, clinical stage, PS, and response to chemotherapy, as well as prompt supportive care with antibiotics, granulocyte-macrophage colony-stimulating factor (GM-CSF), antiemetics, hydration, correction of electrolytes, and aggressive nutritional support, have all contributed to this improvement.

CHEMOTHERAPY The development of active agents has been a high priority in the SCLC treatment program. Numerous chemotherapeutic agents have been found to induce objective tumor responses in newly diagnosed SCLC, and at least four drugs (etoposide, vincristine, mechlorethamine, cyclophosphamide) yield responses in more than 30% of patients, and others (doxorubicin and methotrexate) in more than 25%. More recently, teniposide, carboplatin, ifosfamide, epirubicin, and vindesine have been found to be active in SCLC. Taxanes and camptothecins are also highly active and have been added to the modern drug armamentarium.[252]

Vincristine, cyclophosphamide, doxorubicin, etoposide, cisplatin, paclitaxel, topotecan, and irinotecan are among the most widely used agents in SCLC. Comparison between cisplatin and other agents is not possible because trials using cisplatin in untreated patients are lacking. It can be assumed, however, that cisplatin has significant activity, since it is relatively active in combination regimens for previously treated patients, and the cisplatin plus etoposide combination is a standard for both previously treated and untreated patients with SCLC. Scheduling of etoposide, and probably vincristine, is important in optimizing efficacy. Oral etoposide, given as a sole initial therapy, has yielded promising results. Smit and colleagues reported a 71% overall response rate in 35 elderly patients (aged 70 years or older), despite the fact that the majority of the patients had extensive-stage disease and an ECOG PS of 2 or 3. A more protracted course of daily oral etoposide is also active when given to previously treated patients. But it often is given in combination with other active agents, and this demonstration of the efficacy of a divided dosing schedule is more difficult. In a recent phase III trial in which 21-day oral etoposide was compared with intravenous 3-day etoposide given in combination with cisplatin, the overall and failure-free survival rates were not significantly different. Although these data indicate that oral etoposide is an acceptable initial therapy for selected patients, the optimal frequency and duration of etoposide administration remain unknown. Longer durations of etoposide administration are more attractive on theoretical grounds, and a twice-daily administration schedule is attractive on the basis of pharmacokinetic data.

Rapid acceptance of combination chemotherapy as the standard care of SCLC patients posed significant difficulties for new drug development and raised serious questions about the approach of testing new drugs in previously untreated patients. For all available agents, the response rate is considerably less in previously treated patients than in those who never have been treated with chemotherapy. Thus, new agents are tested in a potentially unfavorable setting. Two of the most active agents, etoposide and carboplatin, yielded greater than 20% response rates in previously treated patients, as did two other active agents, ifosfamide and teniposide. Progressive SCLC during or after initial chemotherapy is usually refractory to further treatment, and the likelihood of disease regression and palliation with subsequent chemotherapy is greater if there is a treatment-free interval of at least a few months.

The identification of newer targeted agents such as STI-571 in recent years heralds still further questions regarding study design, as some compounds may be effective in enhancing the efficacy of known active chemotherapy drugs or radiation. Thus, the practice is increasing of phase I drug testing of the experimental agent in an escalating dose format with other drugs or radiotherapy.

Combination Chemotherapy Only a few prospective randomized trials were conducted in the 1970s to directly compare combination regimens with single-agent regimens. Cyclophosphamide-based combinations yielded better response rates and survival rates than cyclophosphamide alone. Simultaneous administration of four agents yielded a better response rate than sequential single-agent administration of the same agents, but without any survival advantage. The number of drugs in combination regimens has been a subject of study and extensively reviewed. In general, randomized studies demonstrate predictable advantages of combination programs. On the basis of a large number of combination chemotherapy trials, which reported much higher response rates and better survival outcomes than single-agent trials, combination chemotherapy has been accepted as the standard of treatment. Some exceptions exist; elderly or medically compromised patients may be better treated with single agents. During the 1980s, cyclophosphamide-based regimens predominated in SCLC. The cyclophosphamide, doxorubicin, vincristine (CAV) combination was considered to be very active, to yield high response rates, and to be effective in prolonging median and long-term survival. This regimen was considered in the 1980s to be the standard against which newer approaches were compared.

With the discovery of etoposide as an active single agent in SCLC, many randomized trials evaluated whether adding etoposide to or substituting it for one of the components of CAV would be beneficial. Controlled trials compared CAV plus etoposide (CAVE) with CAV alone. In an equitoxic comparison of standard-dose CAV plus etoposide with higher-dose CAV for the initial two cycles of therapy followed by five additional cycles of CAV, there were no differences in response rate or survival rate. When the CAV doses in the CAVE arm were kept identical to those in the CAV arm, multiple studies reported significantly greater response rates with CAVE, but survival was not significantly prolonged. Substituting etoposide for one of the drugs in CAV (either doxorubicin or vincristine) yielded no evident benefit. CEV (cyclophosphamide, etoposide, vincristine) was compared with the same regimen without etoposide, and the three-drug regimen significantly improved response and survival rates in extensive-stage SCLC patients. Similarly, substituting etoposide for methotrexate at two different time points in a 4-week, four-drug regimen of cyclophosphamide, methotrexate, lomustine, and vincristine, prolonged survival when etoposide was given earlier, but not when given later, in the chemotherapy cycle. Therefore, the superiority of the etoposide-containing regimens over regimens without etoposide has not been unequivocally proven in patients with SCLC.

The most widely used regimen in the United States is the combination of cisplatin and etoposide (PE). Both cisplatin and etoposide have only limited single-agent activity in previously treated SCLC patients. Nevertheless, when used together, the PE regimen has generated objective tumor responses in more than 50% of patients with previously treated SCLC. In chemotherapy-naïve patients, the PE regimen yields survival results comparable to those obtained with cyclophosphamide and/or doxorubicin-based regimens. Noda and colleagues recently published the results of an important randomized phase III trial. In patients with extensive-stage disease, cisplatin and irinotecan was compared with cisplatin and etoposide. Two hundred fifty-four patients were entered, and there was a statistically significant difference in overall survival favoring patients treated with irinotecan (12.8 vs 9.4 months, $p = 0.002$). The cisplatin and irinotecan combination was also associated with superior 1-year survival (54% vs 37%) and 2-year survival (20% vs 5%) rates. The experimental arm in this study consisted of cisplatin and irinotecan given at 4-week cycles, with cisplatin 60 mg/m^2 on day 1 and irinotecan 60 mg/m^2 on days 1, 8, and 15.[272] However, Hanna presented the results of a phase III trial at ASCO 2005 (Abstract #7004), which did not show survival benefit for irinotecan/cisplatin regimen as compared with etoposide/cisplatin.

Second-Line Therapy for SCLC The prognosis is poor for patients who receive second-line therapy after relapse. Response is influenced by the time to progression after cessation of first-line therapy. Disease that relapses less than 3 months after first-line therapy is commonly termed refractory, and rates of response to this disease are lower than those for disease that relapses more than 3 months after therapy (which is usually termed sensitive). There is no standard regimen after first-line failure. A number of newer agents have been shown to be active in SCLC. Topotecan is the most extensively studied, and a recent randomized trial demonstrated that topotecan is at least as effective as CAV for SCLC patients whose disease had relapsed at least 60 days after completion of first-line therapy. The response rates were 24.3% in 107 topotecan-treated patients and 18.3% in 104 patients treated with CAV ($p = .285$). There was no difference in median time to progression (13.3 vs 12.3 weeks, $p = .552$) or median survival duration (25.0 vs 24.7 weeks, $p = .795$) between the two groups. However, symptoms improved to a greater degree in the topotecan group than in the CAV group for four of eight symptoms evaluated, including dyspnea, anorexia, hoarseness, and fatigue, as well as interference with daily activity ($p \leq .043$). Grade 4 neutropenia occurred in 38% of topotecan courses and 51% of CAV courses ($p < .001$). Grade 4 thrombocytopenia and grade 3 or 4 anemia occurred more frequently with topotecan, occurring in 10% and 18% of topotecan courses and 1% and 7% of CAV courses, respectively ($p < .001$ for both). These results warrant further study of topotecan in combination with other active agents as a first-line therapy. Irinotecan also has demonstrated activity for chemotherapy-naïve patients and in the second-line setting.

Dose Intensity In preclinical studies, dose escalation has been an important strategy for overcoming drug resistance, yielding higher complete remission rates and increasing curability. Several randomized trials have studied this concept. Cohen and colleagues administered twofold higher doses of the cyclophosphamide, methotrexate, and lomustine (CMC) regimen for an initial 6-week induction.[273] Although there was significant improvement in response rates and median survival duration with higher drug doses, the doses of the "standard" CMC regimen used in comparison might be considered suboptimal. A much larger controlled trial using the CMC regimen with two different cyclophosphamide doses (ie, 700 vs 1,500 mg/m^2) with the same doses of methotrexate (15 mg/m^2) and lomustine (70 mg/m^2) during the first 6 weeks demonstrated significant but modest increases in response and survival rates, particularly in patients with limited-stage disease. However, more recent attempts to build on these early observations have not been successful. In two randomized studies of the CAV regimen, the doses of cyclophosphamide were increased from 20 to 56% and the doses of doxorubicin were increased from 18 to 75% during the first 9 to 12 weeks of chemotherapy. Although the CR rate was higher with the high-dose regimen in one trial in extensive-stage SCLC, there was no difference in either the overall response rate or median survival duration in either study. Life-threatening leukopenia and serious infections requiring hospitalization were more common with high-dose CAV. Moreover, high-dose methotrexate with levamisole rescue offered no advantage over standard-dose methotrexate when added to the CAV regimen. More recently, standard-dose and high-dose regimens involving administration of 67% higher doses of PE over the first 6 weeks of therapy were compared. Despite 68% higher actual doses delivered and 46% higher dose-rate intensity, there was no benefit in terms of CR rate (23% vs 22%, $p = .44$) or median survival duration (10.7 vs 11.4 months, $p = .68$). There was increased myelosuppression with high-dose PE.

A recent French trial randomized patients with limited-stage SCLC to receive a 33% higher dose of cyclophosphamide and a 25% higher dose of cisplatin in the first of six cycles of treatment with cyclophosphamide, cisplatin, doxorubicin, and etoposide. Patients given higher doses of the two drugs survived significantly longer than those who received regular doses. It is possible that benefits of higher doses are of greater magnitude in patients with limited-stage SCLC, but most controlled trials have failed to establish any benefit from higher-than-standard doses of commonly used combination therapy regimens in SCLC.

To obtain greater tumor cell kill, several investigators have used even higher doses of chemotherapy, sometimes with autologous bone marrow transplantation support and often in a protected environment. Although CR rates higher than those achieved with standard regimens have been reported, survival outcomes are similar to those attained with less-intensive standard programs.

Reasoning that only patients with smaller tumor burden would benefit from the intensive treatment approach, several investigators have evaluated high-dose chemotherapy with autologous bone marrow transplantation as a late intensification. Some patients who did not have a CR after standard therapy did achieve a CR to this therapy. The fraction of disease-free long-term survivors has been small, however, and the majority of such patients were those who had achieved excellent responses even before entering the late-intensification program. Overall, there have been no convincing data supporting the benefit of late-intensification therapy with autologous bone marrow transplantation in SCLC. A recent meta-analysis of the dose-rate intensities of 60 published studies, accounting for dose and interval of chemotherapy administration, could not show consistently better therapeutic results with dose-intensification programs of CAV, CAVE, or PE chemotherapy. There are currently no data justifying chemotherapy as a routine initial treatment in doses that cause more than moderately severe myelotoxicity.

Elias and colleagues reported a 2- to 5-year disease-free survival rate of 57% in a small, highly selected group of patients who received late-intensification therapy after achieving CR or near CR with the standard induction regimen. These patients were also given radiation to the chest (50–60 Gy) and the brain. Until a more definitive study confirms the survival benefit of this approach, the use of very high dose chemotherapy with autologous bone marrow transplantation support is recommended only on research protocols. The availability of hematopoietic growth factors has renewed interest in investigating dose escalation in patients with limited-stage SCLC. Given the lack of data supporting the survival advantage of intensive chemotherapy plus marrow transplantation, however, the true benefit of dose escalation that can be achieved with growth factor support remains to be determined.

Another approach to increasing dose intensity is to shorten the intervals between cycles of chemotherapy. Phase II pilot trials of weekly intensive chemotherapy reported higher response rates and survival outcome comparable to those reported for conventional 3-week chemotherapy regimens. However, randomized trials have not established the benefit of weekly intensive chemotherapy over the standard combination regimen. Because of the associated hematologic toxicity, which is similar in most weekly intensive chemotherapy trials, the maximum achievable dose intensities were only 74% of that attempted in one study and 77% of that attempted in the other randomized study. Adding granulocyte colony-stimulating factor (GCSF) to the weekly regimen could mitigate neutropenia, but only a 10% increase in intensity was achieved before other toxic effects became dose limiting.

Alternating Chemotherapy/Maintenance Therapy Goldie and Coldman have provided a mathematical model of the spontaneous development of drug-resistant clones at a mutation rate proportional to the number of actively dividing tumor cells.[274] This model predicts that multiple active agents should be given at full doses to maximize the chance of eradication of the entire tumor cell population; because of overlapping myelosuppressive toxic effects, however, all possible drugs cannot be given simultaneously. An alternative approach is to alternate the administration of two equally effective, noncross-resistant combination regimens. This strategy has been tested in a series of trials.

Most of the recently completed trials compared CAV with CAV alternating with PE. In an early Canadian trial, the alternating schedule of CAV/PE prolonged the overall survival in patients with extensive-stage SCLC compared with six cycles of CAV (9.6 vs 8.0 months, $p = .03$). However, the survival difference did not reach statistical significance when patients with only locoregional disease were excluded from the analysis. Also, because PE alone was not tested in this trial, the possibility could not be eliminated that the superiority of the alternating regimen was due to the better treatment regimen rather than the alternating schedule. Two subsequent studies compared treatment with CAV and PE alone and alternating the two regimens. The Japanese trial showed significant improvement in the overall survival of patients who received the CAV/PE alternating regimen. The median survival duration of that group was 11.8 months, while that of the CAV or PE induction groups was 9.9 months. This survival benefit was seen only in patients with limited-stage SCLC; the median survival duration of the CAV/PE arm was 16.8 months, significantly superior to that of the CAV arm (12.4 months, $p = .014$) or the PE arm (11.7 months, $p = .023$). For the patients with extensive-stage SCLC, there was no difference in overall survival among the three treatment arms. Similar results were obtained for extensive-stage SCLC by the Southeastern Cancer Study Group (SECSG) investigators and others.

In another large randomized trial of 557 patients with extensive-stage SCLC, ECOG investigators reported that alternating induction chemotherapy consisting of CAV and HEC offered a modest but statistically significant improvement in overall survival over induction chemotherapy with CAV (10.7 vs 9.9 months, $p = .002$). These investigators cautioned that this survival benefit must be weighed against the higher incidence of life-threatening toxic effects associated with this alternating induction regimen and did not exclude the possibility that the observed survival prolongation may simply have been an effect of using a new active agent, such as etoposide, early in the treatment course.

For patients with limited-stage SCLC, SWOG investigators conducted a large randomized trial comparing induction with the alternating CAV/PE regimen to that with CAVE. There was no difference in median survival duration between the two arms (16.5 vs 15.1 months, $p = .58$). These data suggest that the simple addition of etoposide to the CAV regimen, rather than the treatment strategy, could account for the improved median survival of the CAV/PE arm. Canadian investigators failed to show an advantage of the alternating CAV/PE strategy in patients with limited-stage SCLC when it was compared with sequential treatment with CAV (three times) followed by PE (three times). German investigators also failed to show the advantage of the alternating chemotherapy treatment strategy over sequential treatment with ifosfamide/etoposide followed by CAV.

Nevertheless, these results do not invalidate the Goldie-Coldman hypothesis, because none of these trials used regimens that were truly noncross-resistant. In addition, many patients whose disease failed to respond to CAV went on to receive the PE regimen. This may have blurred any potential survival advantage of the alternating treatment strategy and should be taken into consideration when designing a similar trial with truly noncross-resistant regimens.

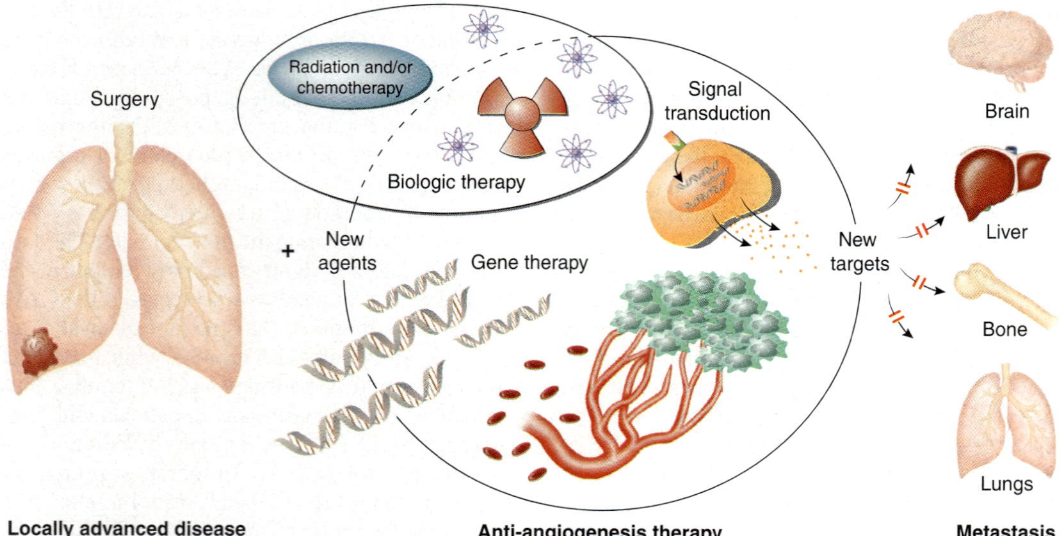

Figure 80-12 Most patients with nonsmall-cell lung cancer die from metastatic disease. Treatment in the locally advanced setting will likely require chemotherapy or radiation therapy in combination with biologic therapy to enhance its effectiveness and prevent metastatic spread of tumor.

Randomized clinical trials have addressed the value of maintenance chemotherapy. These trials fail to show that long-term administration of the same regimen used as an initial treatment prolongs overall survival, although the duration of initial tumor response may be prolonged. Two large British studies compared 6 and 12 cycles and 4 and 8 cycles of chemotherapy, and a study by the European Organization for Research and Treatment of Cancer (EORTC) compared 5 and 12 cycles of chemotherapy. No significant difference in survival was seen when chemotherapy was given at relapse to patients randomized to receive short-term chemotherapy. In patients with limited-stage SCLC, results were quite controversial. Overall, available data indicate that there is no proven benefit to maintenance chemotherapy. The recommended six cycles of initial chemotherapy are adequate, provided that additional chemotherapy is to be given at relapse. This does not completely eliminate the possibility, however, that sequential or alternating applications of more effective regimens would improve the outcome, as exemplified by the SECSG study, in which two additional cycles of PE chemotherapy following six cycles of CAV prolonged the median survival duration by almost 7 months among the responding patients with limited-stage SCLC.

Chemotherapy in Special Clinical Situations For patients with SVC syndrome, acute airway obstruction, or CNS metastases, radiotherapy is a powerful local treatment modality and is widely used. But, as more experience has accumulated with chemotherapy, it is apparent that chemotherapy provides rapid palliation of SVC syndrome in SCLC patients. Therefore, chemotherapy alone is appropriate at least for the initial treatment of SVC syndrome unless chest irradiation is indicated. Similarly, combination chemotherapy alone is also appropriate therapy for airway obstruction at initial presentation.

For brain metastases, systemic chemotherapy was believed to play a limited role until recently because of the widely held view of the brain as a pharmacologic sanctuary. In the 1980s, several groups observed in prospective trials that systemic chemotherapy alone, without brain irradiation, could induce objective regression of the brain lesions. These results clearly indicate that the blood–brain barrier is not the major obstacle for the successful treatment of brain metastases once thought and, in part, explain why patients who present with brain metastases at initial diagnosis of SCLC fare better than those who develop brain metastases later during the disease course. As has been the case with SVC syndrome in SCLC, first-line therapy with cranial irradiation may not be necessary, even though this has not been addressed in a randomized trial setting. For patients with intracranial relapse, however, the available data indicate that the efficacy of second-line chemotherapy is generally much less than in previously untreated patients. Conversely, patients with recurrent brain metastases after previous cranial irradiation should not be denied a trial of systemic chemotherapy solely because of the presence of intracranial lesions.

CONCLUSION AND FUTURE PROSPECTS

Elimination of tobacco consumption is certainly the most effective way to prevent lung cancer. However, this goal remains elusive because of continuing social and economic pressures. In addition, lung cancer is also found in people who have never smoked. Lung cancer will continue well into the twenty-first century to develop in large numbers of persons with long exposure histories. Thus, early detection and new therapeutic options are needed to improve the dismal rate of survival for lung cancer patients. Progress in defining the molecular events involved in the genesis of lung cancer cells has been rapid over the last 15 years, and the potential benefits from this progress for patients may be substantial. The use of molecular profiles to identify persons at high risk of developing lung cancer may enable cost-effective implementation of prevention and early detection programs. For example, low activity of the DNA repair enzyme 8-oxoguanine DNA N-glycosylase has been associated with increased risk of developing lung cancer.[275]

The mainstay of cancer therapy is still surgery, radiotherapy, and chemotherapy, and recent years have shown improvement in patient outcome by their combination and optimization. (Figure 80-12). A large effort has been dedicated to further impact lung cancer outcome by adding biological therapy. Such an approach utilizes alteration of oncogene expression with recombinant gene constructs to allow reversal of the transformed phenotype. In addition, a wealth of biologically active agents that interfere with signal transduction events in the development and progression of lung cancer are now being explored. Rather than targeting the actual genetic errors, these treatments correct or interfere with the sequelae of those genetic changes. For example, genetic mutations that lead to increased expression or activity of a growth factor receptor could be targeted, either by blocking the receptor itself or by interfering with its downstream signal transduction pathways. The first drugs of this kind are the EGFR TKIs recently approved for management of lung cancer. In parallel, monoclonal antibodies to VEGF are combined with conventional chemotherapy to improve survival of patients with lung cancer, colorectal cancer, breast cancer, and renal cell carcinoma among others. The reader is encouraged to follow the literature closely (eg, by using *MEDLINE* searches) and to keep up to date on current protocols (eg, by following the protocol lists via the Physician's Data Query at the NCI Web page: http://cancernet.nci.nih.gov/cancertopics).

In summary, lung cancer therapy efforts in recent years have focused on cancer prevention, early detection and multimodality therapy. Improvements in systemic therapy (chemotherapy and molecular targeted therapy) will certainly have an impact on all stages of disease. Since lung cancer is a heterogeneous disease, it will also be essential to identify and better understand specific molecular targets, and select patients for therapy according to their tumor's biological profile. Progress in these areas will hopefully lead to better control of this disease while minimizing treatment related side effects.

REFERENCES

1. Schiller JH, Harrington D, Belani CP, et al. Comparison of four chemotherapy regimens for advanced non-small-cell lung cancer. N Engl J Med 2002;346:92–8.
2. Pao W, Miller VA. Epidermal growth factor receptor mutations, small-molecule kinase inhibitors, and non-small-cell lung cancer: current knowledge and future directions. J Clin Oncol 2005;23:2556–68.
3. Sandler AB, Gray R, Brahmer J, et al. Randomized phase II/III trial of paclitaxel (P) plus carboplatin (C) with or without bevacizumab (NSC # 704865) in patients with advanced non-squamous non-small cell lung cancer (NSCLC): an Eastern Cooperative Oncology Group (ECOG) Trial - E4599. Proc Am Soc Clin Oncol 2005;23.
4. Pisters KM. Adjuvant chemotherapy for non-small-cell lung cancer—the smoke clears. N Engl J Med 2005;352:2640–2.
5. Hanna N, Shepherd FA, Fossella FV, et al. Randomized phase III trial of pemetrexed versus docetaxel in patients with non-small-cell lung cancer previously treated with chemotherapy. J Clin Oncol 2004;22:1589–97.

6. Gridelli C, Aapro M, Ardizzoni A, et al. Treatment of advanced non-small-cell lung cancer in the elderly: results of an international expert panel. J Clin Oncol 2005;23:3125–37.
7. Parkin DM, Bray F, Ferlay J, Pisani P. Global cancer statistics, 2002. CA Cancer J Clin 2005;55:74–108.
8. Jemal A, Murray T, Ward E, et al. Cancer statistics, 2005. CA: A Cancer Journal for Clinicians 2005;55:10–30.
9. Doll R, Peto R, Boreham J, Sutherland I. Mortality in relation to smoking: 50 years' observations on male British doctors. BMJ 2004;328:1519.
10. Proctor RN. Tobacco and the global lung cancer epidemic. Nat Rev Cancer 2001;1:82–6.
11. Sasco AJ, Secretan MB, Straif K. Tobacco smoking and cancer: a brief review of recent epidemiological evidence. Lung Cancer 2004;45 Suppl 2:S3–S9.
12. Peto, R. Influence of dose and duration of smoking on lung cancer rates. Tobacco: A major international health hazard. Proc IARC 1986;23–24.
13. Patterson F, Lerman C, Kaufmann VG, et al. Cigarette smoking practices among American college students: review and future directions. J Am Coll Health 2004;52:203–10.
14. National Institute of Health. Respiratory health effects of passive smoking: Lung Cancer and other disorders. NCI Monograph 1993;4.
15. American Cancer Society. Cancer facts and figures. Washington, DC: 1995.
16. Hoffmann D, Hoffmann I, El Bayoumy K. The less harmful cigarette: a controversial issue. a tribute to Ernst L. Wynder. Chem Res Toxicol 2001;14:767–90.
17. Patel JD. Lung cancer in women. J Clin Oncol 2005;23:3212–8.
18. Bain C, Feskanich D, Speizer FE, et al. Lung cancer rates in men and women with comparable histories of smoking. J Natl Cancer Inst 2004;96:826–34.
19. Jemal A, Travis WD, Tarone RE, et al. Lung cancer rates convergence in young men and women in the United States: Analysis by birth cohort and histologic type. International Journal of Cancer 2003;105:101–7.
20. Ooi WL, Elston RC, Chen VW, et al. Increased familial risk for lung cancer. J Natl Cancer Inst 1986;76:217–22.
21. Sellers TA, Bailey-Wilson JE, Elston RC, et al. Evidence for mendelian inheritance on the pathogenesis of lung cancer. J Natl Cancer Inst 1990;82:1272–9.
22. Bailey-Wilson JE, Amos CI, Pinney SM, et al. A major lung cancer susceptibility locus maps to chromosome 6q23-25. Am J Hum Genet 2004;75:460–74.
23. Schottenfeld D, Searle JG. The etiology and epidemiology of lung cancer. In: Carbone DP, Johnson DH, Minna JD, Turrisi AT, III. Lung Cancer: Principles and practice, 3rd ed. Philadelphia, PA: Lippincott Williams & Wilkins, 2005:3–24.
24. Bishop JM. Molecular themes in oncogenesis. Cell 1991; 64:235–48.
25. Weinberg RA. Tumor suppressor genes. Science 1991; 254:1138–46.
26. Mascaux C, Iannino N, Martin B, et al. The role of RAS oncogene in survival of patients with lung cancer: a systematic review of the literature with meta-analysis. Br J Cancer 2005;92:131–9.
27. Meuwissen R, Berns A. Mouse models for human lung cancer. Genes and Development 2005;19:643–64.
28. Tuveson DA, Shaw AT, Willis NA, et al. Endogenous oncogenic K-ras(G12D) stimulates proliferation and widespread neoplastic and developmental defects. Cancer Cell 2004;5:375–87.
29. Georges RN, Mukhopadhyay T, Zhang Y, et al. Prevention of orthotopic human lung cancer growth by intratracheal instillation of a retroviral antisense K-ras construct. Cancer Res 1993;53:1743–6.
30. Oster SK, Ho CS, Soucie EL, Penn LZ. The myc oncogene: marvelously complex. Adv Cancer Res 2002;84:81–154.
31. Yarden Y. The EGFR family and its ligands in human cancer. Signalling mechanisms and therapeutic opportunities. Eur J Cancer 2001;37 Suppl 4:53–8.
32. Mendelsohn J, Baselga J. Status of epidermal growth factor receptor antagonists in the biology and treatment of cancer. J Clin Oncol 2003;21:2787–99.
33. Arteaga CL. Epidermal growth factor receptor dependence in human tumors: more than just expression? Oncologist 2002;7 Suppl 4:31–9.
34. Onn A, Correa AM, Gilcrease M, et al. Synchronous overexpression of epidermal growth factor receptor and HER2-neu protein is a predictor of poor outcome in patients with stage I non-small cell lung cancer. Clinical Cancer Research 2004;10:136–43.
35. Meert AP, Martin B, Paesmans M, et al. The role of HER-2/neu expression on the survival of patients with lung cancer: a systematic review of the literature. Br J Cancer 2003;89:959–65.
36. Naylor SL, Johnson BE, Minna JD, Sakaguchi AY. Loss of heterozygosity of chromosome 3p markers in small-cell lung cancer. Nature 1987;329:451–4.
37. Horio Y, Takahashi T, Kuroishi T, et al. Prognostic significance of p53 mutations and 3p deletions in primary resected non-small cell lung cancer. Cancer Res 1993;53:1–4.
38. Sozzi G, Veronese ML, Negrini M, et al. The FHIT gene 3p14.2 is abnormal in lung cancer. Cell 1997;85:17–26.
39. Ji L, Fang B, Yen N, et al. Induction of apoptosis and inhibition of tumorigenicity and tumor growth by adenovirus vector-mediated fragile histidine triad (FHIT) gene overexpression. Cancer Res 1999;59:3333–9.
40. Hollstein M, Sidransky D, Vogelstein B, Harris CC. *p53* mutations in human cancers. Science 1991;253:49–53.
41. Suzuki H, Takahashi T, Kuroishi T, et al. p53 mutations of non-small cell lung cancer in Japan: Association between mutations and smoking. Cancer Res 1992;52:734–6.
42. Vahakangas KH, Samet JM, Metcalf RA, et al. Mutations of p53 and ras genes in radon-associated lung cancer from uranium miners. Lancet 1992;339:576–80.
43. Cajot JF, Anderson MJ, Lehman TA, et al. Growth suppression mediated by transfection of p53 in Hut292DM human lung cancer cells expressing endogenous wild-type p53 protein. Cancer Res 1992;52:6956–60.
44. Quinlan DC, Davidson AG, Summers CL, et al. Accumulation of p53 protein correlates with a poor prognosis in human lung cancer. Cancer Res 1992;52:4828–31.
45. Swisher SG, Roth JA, Nemunaitis J, et al. Adenovirus-mediated p53 gene transfer in advanced non-small cell lung cancer. J Natl Cancer Inst 1999;91:763–71.
46. Zhang WW, Fang X, Mazur W, et al. High-efficiency gene transfer and high-level expression of wild-type p53 in human lung cancer cells mediated by recombinant adenovirus. Cancer Gene Ther 1994;1:5–13.
47. Roth JA, Nguyen D, Lawrence DD, et al. Retrovirus-mediated wild-type p53 gene transfer to tumors of patients with lung cancer. Nature Medicine 1996;2:985–91.
48. Swisher SG, Roth JA, Komaki R, et al. Induction of p53 regulated genes and tumor regression in lung cancer following intratumoral delivery of adenoviral p53 (RPR/INGN 201) and radiation therapy. Clin Cancer Res 2003;9:93–101.
49. Tomizawa Y, Sekido Y, Kondo M, et al. Inhibition of lung cancer cell growth and induction of apoptosis after reexpression of 3p21.3 candidate tumor suppressor gene SEMA3B. Proc Natl Acad Sci U S A 2001;98:13954–9.
50. Zochbauer-Muller S, Fong KM, Virmani AK, et al. Aberrant promoter methylation of multiple genes in non-small cell lung cancers. Cancer Res 2001;61:249–55.
51. Ji L, Nishizaki M, Gao B, et al. Expression of several genes in the human chromosome 3p21.3 homozygous deletion region by an adenovirus vector results in tumor suppressor activities *in vitro* and *in vivo*. Cancer Res 2002;62:2715–20.
52. Herbst RS, Onn A, Sandler A. Angiogenesis and lung cancer: prognostic and therapeutic implications. J Clin Oncol 2005;23:3243–56.
53. Wistuba II, Behrens C, Milchgrub S, et al. Sequential molecular abnormalities are involved in the multistage development of squamous cell lung carcinoma. Oncogene 1999;18:643–50.
54. Mao L, Lee JS, Kurie JM, et al. Clonal genetic alterations in the lungs of current and former smokers. J Natl Cancer Inst 1997;89:857–62.
55. Boice JD Jr, Fraumeni JF Jr. Second cancer following cancer of the respiratory system in Connecticut, 1935-1982. Natl Cancer Inst Monogr 1985;68:83–98.
56. Lippman SM, Lee JJ, Karp DD, et al. Randomized Phase-III intergroup trial of isotretinoin to prevent second primary tumors in stage I non-small-cell lung cancer. J Natl Cancer Inst 2001;93:605–18.
57. Van Zandwijk N, Dalesio O, Pastorino U, et al. EUROSCAN, a randomized trial of vitamin A and N-acetylcysteine in patients with head and neck cancer or lung cancer. For the European Organization for Research and Treatment of Cancer Head and Neck and Lung Cancer Cooperative Groups. J Natl Cancer Inst 2000;92:977–86.
58. Alberg AJ, Brock MV, Samet JM. Epidemiology of lung cancer: looking to the future. J Clin Oncol 2005;23:3175–85.
59. Roggli VL, Vollmer RT, Greenberg SD, et al. Lung cancer heterogeneity: A blinded and randomized study of 100 consecutive cases. Human Pathol 1985;16:569–79.
60. Auerbach O. Natural history of carcinoma of the lung. In: Fishman AP. Pulmonary diseases and disorders. New York: McGraw-Hill, 1990. p. 1388–96.
61. Yesner R. Spectrum of lung cancer and ectopic hormones. Pathol Annu 1978;1:217–40.
62. Travis WD, Garg K, Franklin WA, et al. Evolving concepts in the pathology and computed tomography imaging of lung adenocarcinoma and bronchioloalveolar carcinoma. J Clin Oncol 2005;23:3279–87.
63. Fishback NF, Travis WD, Moran CA, et al. Pleomorphic (spindle and giant cell) carcinomas of the lung: A clinicopathologic study of 78 cases. Cancer 1994;73:2936–45.
64. Travis WD, Linnoila RI, Tsokos MG, et al. Neuroendocrine tumors of the lung with proposed criteria for large cell neuroendocrine carcinoma: An ultrastructural, immunohistochemical and flow cytometric study of 35 cases. Am J Surg Pathol 1991;15:529–53.
65. Gazdar AF, Kadoyama C, Venzon D, et al. Association between histologic type and neuroendocrine differentiation on drug sensitivity on lung cancer cell lines. Monograms NCI 1992;191–6.
66. Ishida T, Kaneko S, Yokoyma H, et al. Adenosquamous carcinoma of the lung. Clinical pathologic and endohistochemical features. Am J Clin Pathol 1992;97:678–85.
67. McCaughan BC, Martini N, Bains MS. Bronchial carcinoids: a review of 124 cases. J Thorac Cardiovasc Surg 1985;89:8–17.
68. Travis WD, Travis LB, Devesa SS. Lung cancer incidence and survival by histologic type. Cancer 1995;75:191–202.
69. Hirsch FR, Matthews MJ, Aisner S, et al. Histopathologic classification of small cell lung cancer. Changing concepts and terminology. Cancer 1988;62:973–7.
70. Ost D, Fein AM, Feinsilver SH. Clinical practice. The solitary pulmonary nodule. N Engl J Med 2003;348:2535–42.
71. Mountain CF. Prognostic implications of the international staging system for lung cancer. Semin Oncol 1988;3:236–41.
72. Beckles MA, Spiro SG, Colice GL, Rudd RM. Initial evaluation of the patient with lung cancer: symptoms, signs, laboratory tests, and paraneoplastic syndromes. Chest 2003;123:97S-104S.
73. Shepherd FA, Laskey J, Evans WK, et al. Cushing's syndrome associated with ectopic corticotropin production and small-cell lung cancer. J Clin Oncol 1992;10:21–5.
74. Stewart AF. Clinical practice. Hypercalcemia associated with cancer. N Engl J Med 2005;352:373–9.
75. Vernino S, Eggenberger ER, Rogers LR, Lennon VA. Paraneoplastic neurological autoimmunity associated with ANNA-1 autoantibody and thymoma. Neurology 2002;59:929–32.
76. Hansen-Flaschen J, Nordberg J. Clubbing and hypertrophic osteoarthropathy. Clin Chest Med 1987;8:287–94.
77. MacDonald RA, Robbins SL. The significance of nonbacterial thrombotic endocarditis: An autopsy and clinical study of 78 cases. Ann Intern Med 1957;46:255–9.
78. Bick RL. Cancer-associated thrombosis. N Engl J Med 2003;349:109–11.
79. Lee AY, Levine MN, Baker RI, et al. Low-molecular-weight heparin versus a coumarin for the prevention of recurrent venous thromboembolism in patients with cancer. N Engl J Med 2003;349:146–53.
80. Kent MS, Port JL, Altorki NK. Current state of imaging for lung cancer staging. Thorac Surg Clin 2004;14:1–13.
81. Vansteenkiste J, Fischer BM, Dooms C, Mortensen J. Positron-emission tomography in prognostic and therapeutic assessment of lung cancer: systematic review. Lancet Oncol 2004;5:531–40.
82. Lardinois D, Weder W, Hany TF, et al. Staging of non-small-cell lung cancer with integrated positron-emission tomography and computed tomography. N Engl J Med 2003;348:2500–7.
83. Zarbo RJ, Fenoglio-Preiser CM. Interinstitutional database for comparison of performance in lung fine-needle aspiration cytology. Arch Pathol Lab Med 1992;116:463–70.
84. Toloza EM, Harpole L, Detterbeck F, McCrory DC. Invasive staging of non-small cell lung cancer: a review of the current evidence. Chest 2003;123:157S-66S.
85. Wang KP, Terry PB. Transbronchial needle aspiration in the diagnosis and staging of bronchogenic carcinoma. Ann Rev Respir Dis 1983;127:344–7.
86. Herth FJ. Mediastinal staging—the role of endobronchial and endo-oesophageal sonographic guided needle aspiration. Lung Cancer 2004;45 Suppl 2:S63–S67.
87. Semik M, Netz B, Schmidt C, Scheld HH. Surgical exploration of the mediastinum: mediastinoscopy and intraoperative staging. Lung Cancer 2004;45 Suppl 2:S55–S61.
88. Landreneau RJ, Hazelrigg SR, Mack MJ, et al. Thoracoscopic mediastinal lymph node sampling: Useful for mediastinal lymph node stations inaccessible by cervical mediastinoscopy. J Thorac Cardiovasc Surg 1993;106:554–8.
89. Mountain CF, Dresler CM. Regional lymph node classification for lung cancer staging. Chest 1997;111:1718–23.

90. Berlin NI, Buncher CR, Fontana RS. The national cancer institute cooperative early launch cancer detection program. Results of the initial screen (prevalence): introduction. Am Rev Respir Dis 1984;130:545–9.
91. Patz EF, Goodman PC, Bepler G. Screening for lung cancer. N Engl J Med 2000;343:1627–33.
92. Henschke CI, McCauley DI, Yankelevitz DF, et al. Early Lung Cancer Action Project: overall design and findings from baseline screening. Lancet 1999;354:99–105.
93. Gohagan J, Marcus P, Fagerstrom R, et al. Baseline findings of a randomized feasibility trial of lung cancer screening with spiral CT scan vs chest radiograph: the Lung Screening Study of the National Cancer Institute. Chest 2004;126:114–21.
94. Swensen SJ, Jett JR, Hartman TE, et al. CT screening for lung cancer: five-year prospective experience. Radiology 2005;235:259–65.
95. Mountain CF. Revisions in the international system for staging lung cancer. Chest 1997;111:1710–7.
96. Yip D, Harper PG. Predictive and prognostic factors in small cell lung cancer: current status. Lung Cancer 2000;28:173–85.
97. Sculier JP, Feld R, Evans WK, et al. Neurologic disorders in patients with small cell lung cancer. Cancer 1987;60:2275–83.
98. Chua YJ, Steer C, Yip D. Recent advances in management of small-cell lung cancer. Cancer Treat Rev 2004;30:521–43.
99. Stanley KE. Prognostic factors for survival in patients with inoperable lung cancer. J Natl Cancer Inst 1980;65:25–32.
100. Reed CE, Harpole DH, Posther KE, et al. Results of the American College of Surgeons Oncology Group Z0050 trial: the utility of positron emission tomography in staging potentially operable non-small cell lung cancer. J Thorac Cardiovasc Surg 2003;126:1943–51.
101. Naruke T, Goya T, Tsuchiya R, Suemasu K. Prognosis and survival in resected lung carcinoma based on the new international staging system. J Thorac Cardiovasc Surg 1988;96:440–7.
102. Daly RC, Trastek VF, Pairolero PC. Bronchoalveolar carcinoma: Factors affecting survival. Ann Thorac Surg 1991;51:368–76.
103. Martini N, Bains MS, Burt ME, et al. Incidence of local recurrence and second primary tumors in resected stage I lung cancer. J Thorac Cardiovasc Surg 1995;109:120–9.
104. Thomas PA, Piantadose S, Lung Cancer Study Group. Postoperative T1 N0 non-small cell lung cancer. J Thorac Cardiovasc Surg 1978;94:349–54.
105. Martini N, Burt ME, Bains MS, et al. Survival after resection of stage II non-small cell lung cancer. Ann Thorac Surg 1992;54:460–6.
106. Burt ME, Pomerantz AH, Bains MS, et al. Results of surgical treatment of stage III lung cancer invading the mediastinum. Surg Clin North Am 1987;67:987–1000.
107. Martini N, Flehinger BJ. The role of surgery in N2 lung cancer. Surg Clin North Am 1987;67(5):1037–49.
108. Pearson FG, Delarue NC, Ilves R, et al. Significance of positive superior mediastinal nodes identified at mediastinoscopy in patients with resectable cancer of the lung. J Thorac Cardiovasc Surg 1982;83(1):1–11.
109. Rusch VW, Albain KS, Crowley JJ, et al. Neoadjuvant therapy: A novel and effective treatment for stage IIIb non-small cell lung cancer. Ann Thorac Surg 1994;58:290–4.
110. Au J, el-Oakley R, Cameron EW. Pneumonectomy for bronchogenic carcinoma in the elderly. European journal of cardio-thoracic surgery : official journal of the European Association for Cardio-thoracic Surgery 1994;8:247–50.
111. Miller JI Jr. Thallium imaging in preoperative evaluation of the pulmonary resection candidate. Ann Thorac Surg 1992;54:249–52.
112. Miller DL, Orszulak TA, Pairolero PC, et al. Combined operation for lung cancer and cardiac disease. Ann Thorac Surg 1994;58:989–94.
113. Steen PA, Tinker JH, Tarhan S. Myocardial infarction after anesthesia and surgery. JAMA 1978;239:2566–70.
114. Wells PH, Kaplan JA. Optimal management of patients with ischemic heart disease for noncardiac surgery by complementary anesthesiologist and cardiologist interaction. Am Heart J 1981;102:1029–37.
115. Mathisen DJ, Wain JC. Cardiac complications following pulmonary resection. Chest Surg Clin North Am 1992;2:793–802.
116. Morice RC, Peters EJ, Rayn MB, et al. Exercise testing in the evaluation of patients at high risk for complications from lung resection. Chest 1992;101:356–63.
117. Ferguson MK, Reeder LB, Mick M. Optimizing selection of patients for major lung resection. Ann Thorac Surg 1995;109:275–83.
118. Ginsberg RJ, Hill LD, Eagan RT, et al. Modern thirty-day operative mortality for surgical resections in lung cancer. J Thorac Cardiovasc Surg 1983;86:654–8.
119. Harpole DH Jr, DeCamp MM Jr, Daley J, et al. Prognostic models of thirty-day mortality and morbidity after major pulmonary resection. J Thorac Cardiovasc Surg 1999;117:969–79.
120. Putnam JB Jr, Lammermeier DE, Colon R, et al. Predicted pulmonary function and survival after pneumonectomy for primary lung carcinoma. Ann Thorac Surg 1990;49:909–14.
121. Walsh GL, O'Connor M, Willis KM, et al. Is follow-up of lung cancer patients after resection medically indicated and cost-effective? Ann Thorac Surg 1995;60:1563–70.
122. Faber LP. Sleeve resections for lung cancer. J Thorac Cardiovasc Surg 1993;5:238–45.
123. Frist WH, Mathisen DJ, Hilgenberg AD, et al. Tracheal sleeve resection with and without pulmonary resection. J Thorac Cardiovasc Surg 1987;93:350–4.
124. Ginsberg RJ, Rubenstein LA. A randomized comparative trial of lobectomy versus limited resection for patients with T1NO non-small cell lung cancer. Lung Cancer 1991;7:83–8.
125. Nakamura H, Kawasaki N, Taguchi M, Kabasawa K. Survival following lobectomy vs limited resection for stage I lung cancer: a meta-analysis. Br J Cancer 2005;92:1033–7.
126. Warren WH, Faber LP. Segmentectomy versus lobectomy in patients with stage I pulmonary carcinoma. J Thorac Cardiovasc Surg 1994;107:1087–94.
127. Paone JF, Spees EK, Newton CG, et al. An appraisal of en bloc resection of peripheral bronchogenic carcinoma involving the thoracic wall. Chest 1982;81:203–10.
128. Pearson FG. Carinal resection: Colon overview. In: Motta G. Staging and treatment. Lung cancer frontiers in science and treatment. Genoa, Italy: Grafica, L.P., 1945. p. 389–92.
129. Watanabe Y, Shimizu N, Oda M, et al. Results in 104 patients undergoing bronchoplastic procedures for bronchial lesions. Ann Thorac Surg 1990;50:607–11.
130. Tsuchiya R, Goya T, Naruke T, Suemasu K. Resection of tracheal carina for lung cancer. J Thorac Cardiovasc Surg 1990;99:779–87.
131. Tsuchiya R, Asamura H, Kondo H, et al. Extended resection of the left atrium, great vessels, or both for lung cancer. Ann Thorac Surg 1994;57:960–5.
132. Ferguson MK. Synchronous primary lung cancers. Chest 1993;103S:398s-401s.
133. Christensen ES. Diagnosis and treatment of bilateral primary bronchogenic carcinoma. J Thorac Cardiovasc Surg 1971;61:501–4.
134. Martini N, Melamed MR. Multiple primary lung cancers. J Thorac Cardiovasc Surg 1975;70:606–11.
135. Deschamps C, Pairolero PC, Trastek VF, Payne WS. Multiple primary lung cancers. Results of surgical treatment. J Thorac Cardiovasc Surg 1990;99:769–78.
136. Ricci C, Rendina EA, Venuta F, et al. Diagnostic imaging and surgical treatment of dumbbell tumors of the mediastinum. Ann Thorac Surg 1990;50:586–9.
137. Mountain CF, Libshitz HI, Hermes KE. Lung cancer: a handbook for staging and imaging. Houston, TX: The University of Texas M. D. Anderson Cancer Center. 1992. p. 37–62.
138. Deslauriers J, Brisson J, Cartier R, et al. Carcinoma of the lung: Evaluation of satellite nodules as a factor influencing prognosis after resection. J Thorac Cardiovasc Surg 1989;97:504–12.
139. Rocmans P. Surgery in non-small cell lung cancer. J Belge Radiol 1985;68:217–20.
140. Martini N, Flehinger BJ, Zaman MB, Beattie Jr. EJ. Prospective study of 445 lung carcinomas with mediastinal lymph node metastases. J Thorac Cardiovasc Surg 1980;80:390–9.
141. Thomas PA, Piantadosi S, Mountain CF. Should subcarinal lymph nodes be routinely examined in patients with non-small cell lung cancer. J Thorac Cardiovasc Surg 1988;95:883–7.
142. Larsson S. Pretreatment classification and staging of bronchogenic carcinoma. Scand J Thorac Cardiovasc Surg 1973;10:1–6.
143. Mountain CF. Expanded possibilities for surgical treatment of lung cancer. Survival in stage III-a disease. Chest 1990;97:1045–51.
144. Soorae AS, Stevenson HM. Survival with residual tumor on a bronchial margin after resection for bronchogenic carcinoma. J Thorac Cardiovasc Surg 1979;78:175–80.
145. Shields TW. The fate of patients after incomplete resection of bronchial carcinoma. Surg Gynecol Obstet 1974;139:569–72.
146. Kaiser LR, Fleshner P, Keller S, Martini N. The significance of extramucosal residual tumor at the bronchial resection margin. Ann Thorac Surg 1989;47:265–9.
147. Macchiarini P, Buonaguidi R, Hardin M, et al. Results and prognostic factors of surgery in the management of non-small cell lung cancer with solitary brain metastases. Cancer 1991;68:300–4.
148. Burt M, Wronski M, Arbit E, et al. Resection of brain metastases from non-small-cell lung carcinoma. results of therapy. J Thorac Cardiovasc Surg 1992;103:399–410.
149. Putnam JB Jr, Walsh GL, Swisher SG, et al. Outpatient management of malignant pleural effusion by a chronic indwelling pleural catheter. Ann Thorac Surg 2000;69:369–75.
150. Tyldesley S, Boyd C, Schulze K, et al. Estimating the need for radiotherapy for lung cancer: An evidence-based, epidemiologic approach. Int J Radiat Oncol Biol Phys 2001;49:973–85.
151. Bach PB, Cramer LD, Schrag D, et al. The influence of hospital volume on survival after resection for lung cancer. N Engl J Med 2001;345:181–8.
152. Lee JS, Scott CB, Komaki R, et al. Impact of institutional experience on survival outcome of patients undergoing combined chemoradiation therapy for inoperable non-small-cell lung cancer. Int J Radiat Oncol Biol Phys 2002;52:362–70.
153. Vanuytsel LJ, Vansteenkiste JF, Stroobants SG, et al. The impact of F-18-fluoro-2-deoxy-D-glucose positron emission tomography (FDG-PET) lymph node staging on the radiation treatment volumes in patients with non-small cell lung cancer. Radiother Oncol 2000;55:317–24.
154. Caldwell CB, Mah K, Ung YC, et al. Observer variation in contouring gross tumor volume in patients with poorly defined non-small-cell lung tumors on CT: The impact of (18)FDG-hybrid PET fusion. Int J Radiat Oncol Biol Phys 2001;51:923–31.
155. MacManus MP, Hicks RJ, Matthews JP, et al. High rate of detection of unsuspected distant metastases by pet in apparent stage III non-small-cell lung cancer: implications for radical therapy. Int J Radiat Oncol Biol Phys 2001;50:287–93.
156. Giraud P, Antoine M, Larrouy A, et al. Evaluation of microscopic tumor extension in non-small-cell lung cancer for three-dimensional conformal radiotherapy planning. Int J Radiat Oncol Biol Phys 2000;48:1015–24.
157. Stevens CW, Munden RF, Forster KM, et al. Respiratory-driven lung tumor motion is independent of tumor size, tumor location, and pulmonary function. Int J Radiat Oncol Biol Phys 2001;51:62–8.
158. Ramsey CR, Scaperoth D, Arwood D, Oliver AL. Clinical efficacy of respiratory gated conformal radiation therapy. Medical Dosimetry 1999;24:115–9.
159. Sixel KE, Aznar MC, Ung YC. Deep inspiration breath hold to reduce irradiated heart volume in breast cancer patients. Int J Radiat Oncol Biol Phys 2001;49:199–204.
160. Rosenzweig KE, Hanley J, Mah D, et al. The deep inspiration breath-hold technique in the treatment of inoperable non-small-cell lung cancer. Int J Radiat Oncol Biol Phys 2000;48:81–7.
161. Akhurst T, Downey RJ, Ginsberg MS, et al. An initial experience with FDG-PET in the imaging of residual disease after induction therapy for lung cancer. Ann Thorac Surg 2002;73:259–64.
162. Nehmeh SA, Erdi YE, Pan T, et al. Four-dimensional (4D) PET/CT imaging of the thorax. Med Phys 2004;31:3179–86.
163. Liu H, Wei X, Jang S, et al. Impact of respiratory motion on dose distributions and DVHs of thoracic structures—evaluation using 4D CT. Med Phys 2005;32:1924.
164. Intensity Modulated Radiation Therapy Collaborative Working Group. Intensity-modulated radiotherapy: current status and issues of interest. Int J Radiat Oncol Biol Phys 2001; 51:880–914.
165. Liu HH, Wang X, Dong L, et al. Feasibility of sparing lung and other thoracic structures with intensity-modulated radiotherapy for non-small-cell lung cancer. Int J Radiat Oncol Biol Phys 2004;58:1268–79.
166. Murshed H, Liu HH, Liao Z, et al. Dose and volume reduction for normal lung using intensity-modulated radiotherapy for advanced-stage non-small-cell lung cancer. Int J Radiat Oncol Biol Phys 2004;58:1258–67.
167. Yom S, Liao Z, Liu H, et al. Analysis of acute toxicity results of intensity modulated radiation therapy in the treatment of non-small cell lung cancer. Lung Cancer 2005;49:S52.
168. Chang JY, Liu HH, Komaki R. Intensity modulated radiation therapy and proton radiotherapy for non-small cell lung cancer. Curr Oncol Rep 2005;7:255–9.
169. Shioyama Y, Tokuuye K, Okumura T, et al. Clinical evaluation of proton radiotherapy for non-small-cell lung cancer. Int J Radiat Oncol Biol Phys 2003;56:7–13.
170. Bush DA, Slater JD, Shin BB, et al. Hypofractionated proton beam radiotherapy for stage I lung cancer. Chest 2004;126:1198–203.

171. Chang JY, Dong L, Mohan R, et al. Image-guided proton radiotherapy for medically inoperable stage I non-small cell lung cancer. Lung Cancer 2005;49:S93.
172. Kaskowitz L, Graham MV, Emami B, et al. Radiation therapy alone for stage I non-small cell lung cancer. Int J Radiat Oncol Biol Phys 1993;27:517–23.
173. Dosoretz DE, Katin MJ, Blitzer PH, et al. Radiation therapy in the management of medically inoperable carcinoma of the lung: results and implications for future treatment strategies. Int J Radiat Oncol Biol Phys 1992;24:3–9.
174. Dosoretz DE, Katin MJ, Blitzer PH, et al. Medically Inoperable Lung Carcinoma: The Role of Radiation Therapy. Semin Radiat Oncol 1996;6:98–104.
175. Sibley GS, Jamieson TA, Marks LB, et al. Radiotherapy alone for medically inoperable stage I non-small-cell lung cancer: the Duke experience. Int J Radiat Oncol Biol Phys 1998;40:149–54.
176. Dosoretz D, Galmarini D, Rubenstein J, et al. Local control in medical inoperable lung cancer: and analysis of its importance in outcome and factors determining the probability of tumor eradication. Int J Radiat Oncol Biol Phys 1993;27:507–16.
177. Onishi H, Araki T, Shirato H, et al. Stereotactic hypofractionated high-dose irradiation for stage I nonsmall cell lung carcinoma: clinical outcomes in 245 subjects in a Japanese multiinstitutional study. Cancer 2004;101:1623–31.
178. Port Meta-analysis Trialists Group. Postoperative radiotherapy in non-small-cell lung cancer: systematic review and meta-analysis of individual patient data from nine randomised controlled trials. The Lancet 1998;352:257–1.
179. Rosell R, Gomez-Condina J, Camps C, et al. A randomized trial comparing preoperative chemotherapy plus surgery with surgery alone in patients with non- small-cell lung cancer. N Engl J Med 1994;330:153–8.
180. Roth JA, Fossella F, Komaki R, et al. A randomized trial comparing perioperative chemotherapy and surgery with surgery alone in resectable stage IIIA non-small-cell lung cancer. J Natl Cancer Inst 1994;86:673–80.
181. Albain KS, Swann S, Rusch V, et al. Phase III study of concurrent chemotherapy and radiotherapy (CT/RT) vs CT/RT followed by surgical resection for stage IIIA (Pn2) non-small cell lung cancer (NSCLC): outcomes update of North American Intergroup 0139 (RTOG 9309). J Clin Oncol 2005;23(16S):624s.
182. Marino P, Preatoni A, Cantoni A. Randomized trials of radiotherapy alone versus combined chemotherapy and radiotherapy in stages IIIa and IIIb nonsmall cell lung cancer. A meta-analysis. Cancer 1995;76:593–601.
183. Pritchard RS, Anthony SP. Chemotherapy plus radiotherapy compared with radiotherapy alone in the treatment of locally advanced, unresectable, non-small- cell lung cancer—a meta-analysis. Ann Intern Med 1996;125:723.
184. Spira A, Ettinger DS. Multidisciplinary management of lung cancer. N Engl J Med 2004;350:379–92.
185. Pfister DG, Johnson DH, Azzoli CG, et al. American Society of Clinical Oncology treatment of unresectable non-small-cell lung cancer guideline: update 2003. J Clin Oncol 2004;22:330–53.
186. Machtay M, Hsu C, Komaki R, et al. Effect of overall treatment time on outcomes after concurrent chemoradiation for locally advanced non-small-cell lung carcinoma: Analysis of the Radiation Therapy Oncology Group (RTOG) experience. Int J Radiat Oncol Biol Phys 2005.
187. Belani CP, Wang W, Johnson DH, et al. Phase III study of the Eastern Cooperative Oncology Group (ECOG 2597): induction chemotherapy followed by either standard thoracic radiotherapy or hyperfractionated accelerated radiotherapy for patients with unresectable stage IIIA and B non-small-cell lung cancer. J Clin Oncol 2005;23:3760–7.
188. Movsas B, Scott C, Langer C, et al. Randomized trial of amifostine in locally advanced non-small-cell lung cancer patients receiving chemotherapy and hyperfractionated radiation: radiation therapy oncology group trial 98-01. J Clin Oncol 2005;23:2145–54.
189. Komaki R, Lee JS, Milas L, et al. Effects of amifostine on acute toxicity from concurrent chemomtherapy and radiation therapy for inoperable non-small cell lung cancer: report of a randomized comparative trial. Int J Radiat Oncol Biol Phys 2004;58:1369–77.
190. Rowell NP, Gleeson FV. Steroids, radiotherapy, chemotherapy and stents for superior vena caval obstruction in carcinoma of the bronchus. Cochrane Database Syst Rev 2001;CD001316.
191. Komaki R, Mountain CF, Holbert JM, et al. Superior sulcus tumors: treatment selection and results for 85 patients without metastasis (MO) at presentation. Int J Radiat Oncol Biol Phys 1990;19:31–6.
192. Komaki R, Roh J, Cox JD, Lopesda-Conceicao A. Superior sulcus tumors: results of irradiation of 36 patients. Cancer 1981;48:1563–9.
193. Farray D, Mirkovic N, Albain KS. Multimodality therapy for stage III non-small-cell lung cancer. J Clin Oncol 2005;23:3257–69.
194. Delclos ME, Komaki R, Morice RC, et al. Endobronchial brachytherapy with high-dose-rate remote afterloading for recurrent endobronchial lesions. Radiology 1996;201:279–82.
195. von Pawel J, von Roemeling R, Gatzemeier U, et al. Tirapazamine plus cisplatin versus cisplatin in advanced non-small-cell lung cancer: A report of the international CATAPULT I study group. Cisplatin and Tirapazamine in Subjects with Advanced Previously Untreated Non-Small-Cell Lung Tumors. J Clin Oncol 2000;18:1351–9.
196. Woods RL, Williams CJ, Levi J, et al. A randomized trial of cisplatin and vindesine versus supportive care only in advanced non-small cell lung cancer. Br J Cancer 1990;61:608–11.
197. Cartei G, Cartei F, Cantone A, et al. Cisplatin-cyclophosphamide-mitomycin combination chemotherapy with supportive care versus supportive care alone for treatment of metastatic non-small-cell lung cancer. J Natl Cancer Inst 1993;85:794–800.
198. Ranson M, Davidson N, Nicolson M, et al. Randomized trial of paclitaxel plus supportive care versus supportive care for patients with advanced non-small-cell lung cancer. J Natl Cancer Inst 2000;92:1074–80.
199. Alberti W, Anderson G, Bartolucci A, et al. Chemotherapy in non-small cell lung cancer: A meta- analysis using updated data on individual patients from 52 randomised clinical trials. Br Med Bull 1995;311:899–909.
200. The Elderly Lung Cancer Vinorelbine Italian Study Group. Effects of vinorelbine on quality of life and survival of elderly patients with advanced non-small-cell lung cancer. J Natl Cancer Inst 1999;91:66–72.
201. Jaakkimainen L, Goodwin P, Pater J, et al. Counting the costs of chemotherapy in a National Cancer Institute randomized trial in non-small cell lung cancer. J Clin Oncol 1990;8:1301–5.
202. Bonomi P, Kim K, Fairclough D, et al. Comparison of survival and quality of life in advanced non-small-cell lung cancer patients treated with two dose levels of paclitaxel combined with cisplatin versus etoposide with cisplatin: results of an Eastern Cooperative Oncology Group trial. J Clin Oncol 2000;18:623–31.
203. Giaccone G, Splinter TAW, Debruyne C, et al. Randomized study of paclitaxel-cisplatin versus cisplatin-teniposide in patients with advanced non-small-cell lung cancer. J Clin Oncol 1998;16:2133–41.
204. Choy H, Shyr Y, Cmelak AJ, Mohr PJ, Johnson DH. Patterns of practice survey for nonsmall cell lung carcinoma in the US. Cancer 2000;88:1336–46.
205. Langer CJ, Leighton JC, Comis RL, et al. Paclitaxel and carboplatin in combination in the treatment of advanced non-small-cell lung cancer: a phase II toxicity, response, and survival analysis. J Clin Oncol 1995;13:1860–70.
206. Belani CP, Natale RB, Lee JS, et al. Randomized phase III trial comparing cisplatin/etoposide versus carboplatin/paclitaxel in advanced and metastatic non-small cell lung cancer (NSCLC). Proc Am Soc Clin Oncol 1998;17:455a.
207. Kelly K, Crowley J, Bunn PA Jr, et al. Randomized phase III trial of paclitaxel plus carboplatin versus vinorelbine plus cisplatin in the treatment of patients with advanced non--small-cell lung cancer: a Southwest Oncology Group trial. J Clin Oncol 2001;19:3210–8.
208. Sandler AB, Nemunaitis J, Denham C, et al. Phase III trial of gemcitabine plus cisplatin versus cisplatin alone in patients with locally advanced or metastatic non-small-cell lung cancer. J Clin Oncol 2000;18:122–30.
209. Crino L, Scagliotti GV, Ricci S, De et al. Gemcitabine and cisplatin versus mitomycin, ifosfamide, and cisplatin in advanced non-small-cell lung cancer: A randomized phase III study of the Italian lung cancer project. J Clin Oncol 1999;17:3522–30.
210. Cardenal F, Lopez-Cabrerizo MP, Anton A, et al. Randomized phase III study of gemcitabine-cisplatin versus etoposide-cisplatin in the treatment of locally advanced or metastatic non-small-cell lung cancer. J Clin Oncol 1999;17:12–8.
211. Thatcher N, Jayson G, Bradley B, et al. Gemcitabine: symptomatic benefit in advanced non-small cell lung cancer. [Review] [37 refs]. Sem Oncol 1997;24:Suppl-S8.
212. Georgoulias V, Papadakis E, Alexopoulos A, et al. Platinum-based and non-platinum-based chemotherapy in advanced non-small-cell lung cancer: a randomised multicentre trial. Lancet 2001;357:1478–84.
213. Masuda N, Fukuoka M, Negoro S, et al. Randomized trial comparing cisplatin (CDDP) and irinotecan (CPT-11) versus CDDP and vindesine (VDS) versus (CPT-11) alone in advanced non-small cell lung cancer (NSCLC). Proc Am Soc Clin Oncol 1999;18(459a):459a.
214. Fossella F, Pereira JR, von Pawel J, et al. Randomized, multinational, phase III study of docetaxel plus platinum combinations versus vinorelbine plus cisplatin for advanced non-small-cell lung cancer: the TAX 326 study group. J Clin Oncol 2003;21:3016–24.
215. Kunitoh H, Nishiwaki Y, Noda K. Phase III randomized trial to compare survival, antitumor response, and tolerability between docetaxel/cisplatin and the standard Japanese regimen (in 1988). Vindesine/cisplatin, in advanced NSCLC. Proc Am Soc Clin Oncol 2001;20:323a.
216. Socinski MA, Schell MJ, Peterman A, et al. Phase III trial comparing a defined duration of therapy versus continuous therapy followed by second-line therapy in advanced-stage IIIB/IV non-small-cell lung cancer. J Clin Oncol 2002;20:1335–43.
217. Fossella FV, DeVore R, Kerr RN. Randomized phase III trial of docetaxel versus vinorelbine or ifosfamide in patients with advanced non-small-cell lung cancer previously treated with platinum-containing chemotherapy regimens: the TAX320 non small cell lung cancer study group. J Clin Oncol 2000;18:2354–62.
218. Shepherd FA, Dancey J, Ramlau R. Prospective randomized trial of docetaxel versus best supportive care in patients with non-small-cell lung cancer previously treated with platinum-based chemotherapy. J Clin Oncol 2000;18:2095–103.
219. Massarelli E, Onn A, Zinner R, et al. New targets for the treatment of advanced non-small cell lung cancer. Cancer Chemother Biol Response Modif 2002;20:717–61.
220. Pisters KMW, Ginsberg RJ, Giroux DJ, et al. Induction chemotherapy before surgery for early-stage lung cancer: a novel approach. J Thorac Cardiovasc Surg 2000;119:429–39.
221. Pisters K, Vallieres E, Bunn P, et al. A phase III trial of surgery alone or surgery plus preoperative (preop) paclitaxel/carboplatin (PC) chemotherapy in early stage non-small cell lung cancer (NSCLC): Preliminary results. Proc Am Soc Clin Oncol 2005;23.
222. Feld R, Rubinstein L, Thomas PA, Lung Cancer Study Group. Adjuvant chemotherapy with cyclophosphamide, doxorubicin, and cisplatin in patients with completely resected stage I non-small-cell lung cancer. J Natl Cancer Inst 1993;85:299–306.
223. Niiranen A, Niitamokorhonen S, Kouri M, et al. Adjuvant chemotherapy after radical surgery for non-small-cell lung cancer: a randomized study. J Clin Oncol 1992;10:1927–32.
224. Keller SM, Adak S, Wagner H, et al. A Randomized Trial of Postoperative Adjuvant Therapy in Patients with Completely Resected Stage II or IIIa Non-Small-Cell Lung Cancer. N Engl J Med 2000;343:1217–22.
225. Non-small Cell Lung Cancer Collaborative Group. Chemotherapy in non-small cell lung cancer: a meta-analysis using updated data on individual patients from 52 randomized trials. BMJ 1995;311:899–909.
226. Arriagada R, Bergman B, Dunant A, et al. Cisplatin-based adjuvant chemotherapy in patients with completely resected non-small-cell lung cancer. N Engl J Med 2004;350:351–60.
227. Winton T, Livingston R, Johnson D, et al. Vinorelbine plus Cisplatin vs. Observation in Resected Non-Small-Cell Lung Cancer. N Engl J Med 2005;352:2589–97.
228. Strauss GM, Herndon J, Maddaus MA, et al. Randomized clinical trial of adjuvant chemotherapy with paclitaxel and carboplatin following resection in Stage IB Non-Small Cell Lung Cancer (NSCLC): Report of Cancer and Leukemia Group B (CALGB) Protocol 9633. J Clin Oncol 22(14S), 7019. 7-15-2004.
229. Hamada C, Ohta M, Wada H, et al. Survival benefit of oral UFT for adjuvant chemotherapy after completely resected non-small-cell lung cancer. J Clin Oncol 22(14S), 7002. 7-15-2004.
230. Kato H, Ichinose Y, Ohta M, et al. A randomized trial of adjuvant chemotherapy with uracil-tegafur for adenocarcinoma of the lung. N Engl J Med 2004;350:1713–21.
231. Le Chevalier T, Arriagada R, Pignon JP, Scagliotti GV. Should adjuvant chemotherapy become standard treatment in all patients with resected non-small-cell lung cancer? Lancet Oncol 2005;6:182–4.
232. Langer CJ. Elderly patients with lung cancer: biases and evidence. Curr Treat Options Oncol 2002;3:85–102.

233. Langer CJ, Manola J, Bernardo P, et al. Cisplatin-based therapy for elderly patients with advanced non-small-cell lung cancer: implications of Eastern Cooperative Oncology Group 5592, a randomized trial. J Natl Cancer Inst 2002;94:173–81.
234. Gridelli C. The ELVIS trial: a phase III study of single-agent vinorelbine as first-line treatment in elderly patients with advanced non-small cell lung cancer. Elderly Lung Cancer Vinorelbine Italian Study. Oncologist 2001;6 Suppl 1:4–7.
235. Gridelli C, Perrone F, Gallo C, et al. Chemotherapy for elderly patients with advanced non-small-cell lung cancer: the Multicenter Italian Lung Cancer in the Elderly Study (MILES) phase III randomized trial. J Natl Cancer Inst 2003;95:362–72.
236. Fukuoka M, Yano S, Giaccone G, et al. Multi-institutional randomized phase II trial of gefitinib for previously treated patients with advanced non-small-cell lung cancer (The IDEAL 1 Trial). J Clin Oncol 2003;21:2237–46.
237. Kris MG, Natale RB, Herbst RS, et al. Efficacy of gefitinib, an inhibitor of the epidermal growth factor receptor tyrosine kinase, in symptomatic patients with non-small cell lung cancer: a randomized trial. JAMA 2003;290:2149–58.
238. Giaccone G, Herbst RS, Manegold C, et al. Gefitinib in combination with gemcitabine and cisplatin in advanced non-small-cell lung cancer: a phase III trial-INTACT1. J Clin Oncol 2004;22:777–84.
239. Herbst RS, Giaccone G, Schiller JH, et al. Gefitinib in combination with paclitaxel and carboplatin in advanced non-small-cell lung cancer: a phase III trial--INTACT 2. J Clin Oncol 2004;22:785–94.
240. Gatzemeier U, Pluzanska A, Szczesna A, et al. Results of a phase III trial of erlotinib (OSI-774) combined with cisplatin and gemcitabine (GC) chemotherapy in advanced non-small cell lung cancer (NSCLC). J Clin Oncol 2004;22(14S):7010.
241. Herbst RS, Prager D, Hermann R, et al. TRIBUTE—a phase III trial of erlotinib HCl (OSI-774) combined with carboplatin and paclitaxel (CP) chemotherapy in advanced non-small cell lung cancer (NSCLC). J Clin Oncol 2004;22(14S):7011.
242. Shepherd FA, Rodrigues PJ, Ciuleanu T, et al. Erlotinib in previously treated non-small-cell lung cancer. N Engl J Med 2005;353:123–32.
243. Thatcher N, Chang A, Parikh P, et al. Results of a phase III placebo-controlled study (ISEL) of gefitinib (IRESSA) plus best supportive care (BSC) in patients with advanced non-small-cell lung cancer (NSCLC) who had received 1 or 2 prior chemotherapy regimens. Proc Am Assoc Cancer Res 2005;46.
244. Lynch TJ, Bell DW, Sordella R, et al. Activating mutations in the epidermal growth factor receptor underlying responsiveness of non-small-cell lung cancer to gefitinib. N Engl J Med 2004;350:2129–39.
245. Paez JG, Janne PA, Lee JC, et al. EGFR mutations in lung cancer: correlation with clinical response to gefitinib therapy. Science 2004;304:1497–500.
246. Shigematsu H, Lin L, Takahashi T, et al. Clinical and biological features associated with epidermal growth factor receptor gene mutations in lung cancers. J Natl Cancer Inst 2005;97:339–46.
247. Hurwitz H, Fehrenbacher L, Novotny W, et al. Bevacizumab plus irinotecan, fluorouracil, and leucovorin for metastatic colorectal cancer. N Engl J Med 2004;350:2335–42.
248. Johnson DH, Fehrenbacher L, Novotny WF, et al. Randomized phase II trial comparing bevacizumab plus carboplatin and paclitaxel with carboplatin and paclitaxel alone in previously untreated locally advanced or metastatic non-small-cell lung cancer. J Clin Oncol 2004;22:2184–91.
249. Matar P, Rojo F, Cassia R, Moreno-et al. Combined epidermal growth factor receptor targeting with the tyrosine kinase inhibitor gefitinib (ZD1839) and the monoclonal antibody cetuximab (IMC-C225): superiority over single-agent receptor targeting. Clin Cancer Res 2004;10:6487–501.
250. Huang SM, Armstrong EA, Benavente S, et al. Dual-agent molecular targeting of the epidermal growth factor receptor (EGFR): Combining anti-EGFR antibody with tyrosine kinase inhibitor. Cancer Res 2004;64:5355–62.
251. Teicher BA, Holden SA, Ara G, et al. Potentiation of cytotoxic cancer therapies by TNP-470 alone and with other anti-angiogenic agents. Int J Cancer 1994;57:920–5.
252. Stupp R, Monnerat C, Turrisi AT III, et al. Small cell lung cancer: state of the art and future perspectives. Lung Cancer 2004;45:105–17.
253. Shepherd FA, Ginsberg RJ, Feld R, et al. Surgical treatment for limited small-cell lung cancer. J Thorac Cardiovasc Surg 1991;101:385–93.
254. Warren WH, Faber LP, Gould VE. Neuro-endocrine neoplasms of the lung—a clinicopathologic update. J Thorac Cardiovasc Surg 1989;98:321–32.
255. Warde P, Payne D. Does thoracic irradiation improve survival and local control in limited-stage small cell carcinoma of the lung? A meta-analysis. J Clin Oncol 1992;10:890–5.
256. Pignon J-P, Arriagada R, Ihde DC, et al. A meta-analysis of thoracic radiotherapy for small cell lung cancer. N Engl J Med 1992;327:1618–24.
257. Arriagada R, Pignon JP, Le Chevalier T. Initial chemotherapeutic doses and long-term survival in limited small-cell lung cancer. N Engl J Med 2001;345:1281–2.
258. McCracken JD, Janaki LM, Crowley JJ, et al. Concurrent chemotherapy/radiotherapy for limited small-cell lung carcinoma: a southwest oncology group study. J Clin Oncol 1990;8(5):892–8.
259. Janaki L, Rector D, Turrisi A, et al. Patterns of failure and second malignancies from SWOG-8629: Concurrent cisplatin, etoposide, vincristine, and once daily radiotherapy for the treatment of limited small cell lung cancer. Proc Am Soc Clin Oncol 1994;13:331–332.
260. Turrisi AT, III. Current perspectives in the treatment of small cell lung cancer. Lung Cancer 1993;9:S109–S117.
261. Johnson BE, Salem C, Nesbitt J, et al. Limited stage small cell lung cancer treated with concurrent hyperfractionated chest radiotherapy and etoposide/cisplatin. Lung Cancer 1993;9:S21–S26.
262. Komaki R, Shin DM, Glisson BS, et al. Interdigitating versus concurrent chemotherapy and radiotherapy for limited small cell lung cancer. Int J Radiat Oncol Biol Phys 1995;31:807–11.
263. Murray N, Coy P, Pater JL, et al. Importance of timing for thoracic irradiation in the combined modality treatment of limited-stage small cell lung cancer. J Clin Oncol 1993;11:336–44.
264. Schild SE, Bonner JA, Shanahan TG, et al. Long-term results of a phase III trial comparing once-daily radiotherapy with twice-daily radiotherapy in limited-stage small-cell lung cancer. Int J Radiat Oncol Biol Phys 2004;59:943–51.
265. Cox JD. Dose response in small cell carcinoma (Editorial). Int J Radiat Oncol Biol Phys 1988;14:393–4.
266. Coy P, Hodson I, Payne DG, et al. The effect of dose of thoracic irradiation on recurrence in patients with limited stage small cell lung cancer. Initial results of a Canadian Multicenter randomized trial. Int J Radiat Oncol Biol Phys 1988;14:219–26.
267. Arriagada R, Le Chevalier T, Ruffie P, et al. Alternating radiotherapy and chemotherapy in 173 consecutive patients with limited small cell lung carcinoma. GROP and the French Cancer Center's Lung Group. Int J Radiat Oncol Biol Phys 1990;19:1135–8.
268. Choi NC, Herndon J, Rosenman J, et al. Phase I study to determine the maximum tolerated dose of radiation in standard fractionated and accelerated twice daily radiation schedules with concurrent chemotherapy for limited stage small cell lung cancer (CALGB 8837). Int J Radiat Oncol Biol Phys 1994;30:179–83.
269. Fu KK, Pajak TF, Trotti A, et al. A Radiation Therapy Oncology Group (RTOG) phase III randomized study to compare hyperfractionation and two variants of accelerated fractionation to standard fractionation radiotherapy for head and neck squamous cell carcinomas: first report of RTOG 9003. Int J Radiat Oncol Biol Phys 2000;48:7–16.
270. Komaki R, Swann RS, Ettinger DS, et al. Phase I study of thoracic radiation dose escalation with concurrent chemotherapy for patients with limited small-cell lung cancer: Report of Radiation Therapy Oncology Group (RTOG) protocol 97-12. Int J Radiat Oncol Biol Phys 2005;62:342–50.
271. Auperin A, Arriagada R, Pignon JP, et al. Prophylactic cranial irradiation for patients with small-cell lung cancer in complete remission. N Engl J Med 1999;341:476–84.
272. Noda K, Nishiwaki Y, Kawahara M. Irinotecan plus cisplatin compared with etoposide plus cisplatin for extensive small-cell lung cancer. N Engl J Med 2002;346:85–91.
273. Cohen MH, Creaven PJ, Fossieck BE Jr. Intensive chemotherapy of small cell bronchogenic carcinoma. Cancer Treat Rep 1977;61:349–54.
274. Goldie JH, Coldman AJ. A mathematical model for relating sensitivity of tumours to their spontaneous mutation rate. Cancer Treat Rep 1979;63:1727–34.
275. Paz-Elizur T, Krupsky M, Blumenstein S, et al. DNA repair activity for oxidative damage and risk of lung cancer. J Natl Cancer Inst 2003;95:1312–9.

Malignant Mesothelioma

Harvey I. Pass, MD
Michele Carbone, MD, PhD
A. Philippe Chahinian, MD

HISTORICAL PERSPECTIVE

The existence of malignant mesothelioma as a primary tumor, as well as its relationship with asbestos had long been controversial. This controversy lasted until 1960, when in a seminal report Wagner and colleagues reported asbestos as the etiologic agent in 32 of 33 cases of mesothelioma, largely by environmental exposure in the "Asbestos Hills" of Cape Province in South Africa.[1] This singular relationship, confirmed in many other countries, including the United States,[2] established the disease as a distinct entity.

INCIDENCE AND EPIDEMIOLOGY

The incidence of mesothelioma has been seriously underestimated in mortality statistics.[3] Cases are clustered in areas of asbestos product plants and shipbuilding facilities, not only in the United States, but also in other industrialized countries, such as England.[4,5] The male to female ratio is approximately 4:1, and 80% arise from the pleura.[6] In autopsy studies, the frequency of malignant mesothelioma varies from 0.02 to 0.7%, with a rate of 0.2% in the largest series.[7] In most hospital series, the pleura is more often involved than the peritoneum, with a predominance of the right side over the left (60:40).[7] In some epidemiologic studies monitoring cohorts of asbestos workers, however, the peritoneal form is more common than the pleural.

The mean age of patients is approximately 60 years,[8] but the disease can occur at any age, including in childhood.[9,10] There are many reports of childhood mesothelioma; on review of the pathology, however, the diagnosis is erroneous in as many as 50% of the cases, and there does not seem to be a relationship in these pediatric cases with asbestos, radiation, or isoniazid.[11]

ETIOLOGY

Epidemiologic and Clinical Evidence of the Role of Asbestos Prior exposure to asbestos is documented in approximately 70 to 80% of all cases of mesothelioma when a careful history was taken.[12,13] Beginning 15 years after onset of exposure, approximately 6 to 10% of asbestos workers older than age 35 years will die of mesothelioma.[14] It is estimated that from 1940 through 1979, approximately 27.5 million workers were occupationally exposed to asbestos in the United States, with a calculated annual death rate from mesothelioma of approximately 2,000 in 1980 up to 3,000 in the late 1990s.[15] Insulation, construction, shipyard industries, and automobile brakes are among the many sources of occupational exposure.[16] The exposure may have been short or minimal, although sometimes a very short exposure may have been intense.[12] The delay between first exposure and onset of the disease, that is, the latency period, is extremely long, averaging 30 to 45 years, with a usual range of 10 to 65 years and a standard deviation of 12 years.[12,17] Because of the long latency and the vastly increased use of asbestos during and after World War II, the incidence of mesothelioma is expected to continue to increase. Although asbestos exposure and cigarette smoking act synergistically to produce lung cancer, smoking is not a factor for mesothelioma, although an association between cigarettes using "micronite" filters has been postulated.[18,19] Exposure can also occur by household contamination of women and children, usually through the work clothes of an asbestos worker.

Asbestos Carcinogenesis Fibers in tissues acquire a proteinaceous iron coating, leading to the formation of ferruginous bodies, which can be detected on pathologic section by using an iron stain.[20] These are not specific and can be called asbestos bodies only if the central core is identified as being asbestos. The asbestos minerals are divided into two major categories: the serpentines (chrysotile), which form long hollow tubes; and the amphiboles, which contain more silica and less magnesium oxide, and which form straight, short, fibers.[21] Among the various types of asbestos associated with mesothelioma, amphiboles (crocidolite in South Africa and amosite in the United States) carry the highest risk.[12,22] Chrysotile, a long, curly fiber with poor pulmonary penetration, which can dissolve in lung tissue, seems to carry a much lower, but finite risk,[12,23] and mesotheliomas occurring in chrysotile-exposed individuals may be related to contamination by tremolite.[24] Tremolite contamination occurs with other substances, including talc or vermiculite.[24] Vermiculite has been used extensively in insulating homes as well as for the constitution of potting soils and has been associated with a greatly increased incidence of mesotheliomas in Libby, Montana, where the substance was mined.[25]

The presence of asbestos fibers in sections of lung tissue is de facto proof of asbestos exposure. Although asbestos fibers can be detected in essentially 100% of the lungs of city dwellers by using special techniques of lung fiber content analysis,[26–28] their number is markedly greater in the lungs of patients with mesothelioma and occupational exposure to asbestos, commonly reaching several million fibers per gram of dry weight. Few lung content analysis studies are available, however, because they require lung tissue. In addition, these studies are not very precise, because of interlaboratory technical differences and because the methods used often cannot detect very thin fibers and fibers less then 5 μm in length. Moreover, chrysotile fibers may also be underestimated since these fibers are cleared from the lungs.[29] Nevertheless, the mean increase of lung fiber burden of mesothelioma patients as compared with controls is 7 times higher for pleural and 16 times higher for peritoneal mesothelioma, but is lower than for patients with asbestosis (48 times higher than controls) or lung cancer with asbestos exposure (32 times higher than controls).[30]

In Vivo Asbestos Carcinogenesis A single intrapleural or intraperitoneal injection of various asbestos fibers (chrysotile or amphibole) produces mesotheliomas in rats, hamsters, and mice, often after a relatively long delay of 7 months or more (Figure 81-1). The most oncogenic fibers are the long, thin ones, with a length of > 8 microns and a diameter of < 0.25 micron, the so-called Stanton hypothesis, whereas shorter fibers may be inactivated by phagocytosis.[31,32] These long, thin fibers may penetrate deep in the lung parenchyma, eventually reaching the subpleural and pleural structures and penetrating cells without killing them, thereby implementing a complex oncogenic process.[33] The effect of gravity on inhaled fibers may explain the predominance of pleural mesothelioma in the lower thorax and on the right side.[34]

The mechanisms of asbestos-induced carcinogenesis are not fully characterized but are the subject of intense scrutiny and study.[35–37] It is thought that when fibers reach the alveoli following inhalation, smaller fibers are phagocytized and efficiently removed from the lung. Larger fibers are not easily engulfed and can usually only be removed if solubilized. However, amphiboles are not soluble, and thus remain in the lung. These fibers may eventually reach the pleura via the lymphatics or direct extension, where they may lead to pleural plaques, fibrosis, and mesothe-

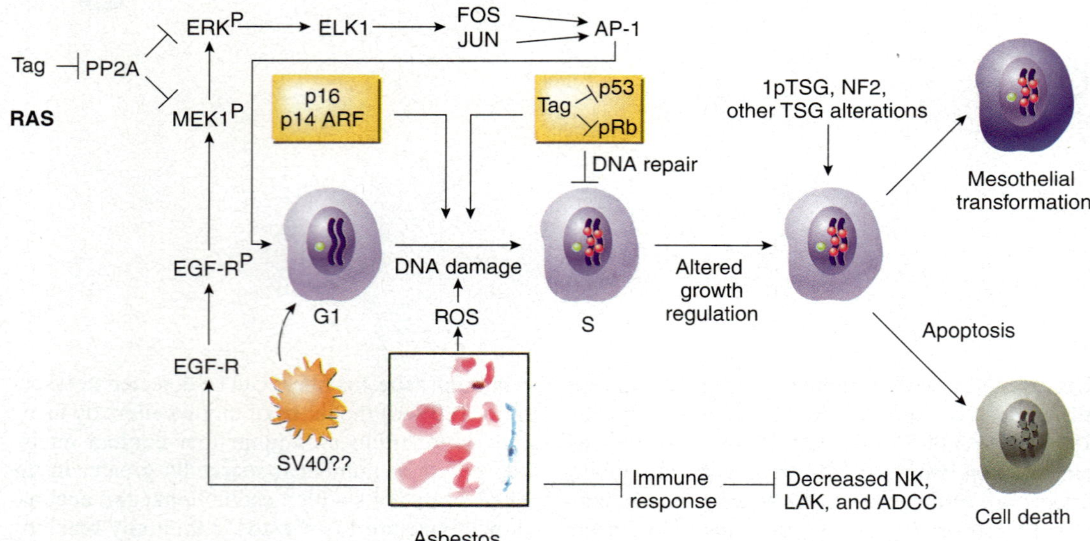

Figure 81-1 Mesothelioma pathogenesis, with known and hypothesized mechanisms possibly linking asbestos and non-asbestos mechanisms of transformation. Increased levels of activator protein 1 (AP-1) stimulate cell division. AP-1 is upregulated through a pathway that involves phosphorylation of the EGF receptor (EGF-R phosphorylated to EGF-RP), activation of ras, and eventual phosphorylation of MEK1 kinase and the extracellular regulated kinases (ERK). Through activation of intermediary kinases including Elk1, and transcription factors such as fos and jun, AP-1 stimulates cell division. Crocidolite asbestos can start this cascade of events since it induces both DNA mutations and phosphorylation of EGF-R. Asbestos can also induce DNA alterations such as p16 loss, and abnormalities of p14 ARF through the production of reactive oxygen species (ROS) that are generated by alveolar macrophages which phagocytize asbestos fibers. Moreover, asbestos is known to have profound effects on the immune system by decreasing natural killer cell (NK) and lymphokine activated killer cell (LAK) number and activity, as well as interfering with antibody dependent cell-mediated cytotoxicity (ADCC). Tag of SV40 could have profound effects in concert with the asbestos including (1) inhibition of phosphatase 2A (PP2A) leading to unregulated AP-1 production, (2) direct DNA damage and (3) binding of p53 and the protein of the retinoblastoma gene (pRB), thus inhibiting cell cycle check points, as well as potential repair of the mutated cells. The mutated cells could then become immortalized through other abnormalities of tumor suppressor genes (TSG), including the neurofibromatosis 2 gene (NF-2), and escape immune surveillance due to the immunomodulatory effects of asbestos. An asbestos body surrounded by alveolar macrophages is depicted in the inset. The green circle represents SV40 DNA that has not integrated into the chromosomes of the mesothelial cell.

lioma. In the pleura, asbestos fibers may cause mutagenic changes through hydroxy radical and superoxide anion production during phagocytosis, leading to DNA strand breaks and deletions. In hamster cells, asbestos fibers can also mechanically interfere with mitotic segregation to alter chromosome morphology and ploidy as well as produce DNA strand breaks. In rat mesothelial cells, crocidolite asbestos was found to cause autophosphorylation of the EGF receptor, leading to stimulation of the extracellular-regulated kinase cascade (ERK), increased AP-1 activity, and mitosis. Finally, it has been suggested that asbestos may also allow tumor development by stimulating macrophages to produce lymphokines and oxyradicals that depress immune function.[38] Neither *ras* or *TP53* mutations are believed to be responsible for asbestos carcinogenesis, although *TP53* may be inactivated by post-translational mechanisms (see the section "Simian Virus 40" below). Growth factors including PDGF,[39] HGF,[40,41] IGF,[42–44] and TGF beta[45,46] are all involved in either autocrine or paracrine pathways in the disease.

OTHER ETIOLOGIC FACTORS

Because approximately 20% of patients do not have an exposure to asbestos, and some mesothelioma patients have an asbestos lung burden similar to that of controls, alternative factors, although rarely proven, are presumably involved.

Simian Virus 40 Simian virus 40 (SV40) is a DNA tumor virus that has been associated with the development of malignant mesothelioma (see Figure 81-1).[38] Although this virus is endogenous in rhesus monkeys, epidemiological studies have shown that it is now widespread among the human population. The modes by which the virus was transferred from monkey to human are uncertain, but it is possible that the bulk of this transfer may have occurred from 1954 to 1963 through SV40-contaminated polio vaccines administered worldwide.[38]

Once inside of its host, SV40 produces two proteins associated with its oncogenesis, the large and small T antigens.[47,48] The large T antigen (Tag) is a 90 kDa protein found predominantly in the nucleus of infected cells, which is capable of inducing structural and numerical chromosomal alterations. It induces insulin-like growth factor expression, inhibits *TP53* and the *pRb* family, and induces c-*met* activity to stimulate cell proliferation.[38,48] The combined activity of both the large Tag and the small tag induces Notch-1 and telomerase activity, which are required for malignant transformation and immortalization.[49,50]

Animal models have shown a clear association between SV40 exposure and mesothelioma development with 60 to 100% developing mesotheliomas within 6 months[51] of virus injection. SV40 sequences were present in 29 of 48 (60%) of the human mesothelioma samples from the initial study that described this relationship. Since this study, several other laboratories as well as a multilaboratory study sponsored by the International Mesothelioma Interest Group confirmed that SV40 sequences were present in human mesotheliomas.[48,52] Although more than 60 laboratories have found SV40 in human mesotheliomas and other tumors, the virus was not detected in Finnish, Austrian, and Turkish mesothelioma specimens,[38,47,48] suggesting that the presence of SV40 in human tumors may be influenced by geographic factors. Three independent panels have reviewed and confirmed the association of SV40 with human tumors, especially mesothelioma.[53,54]

Overall, substantial evidence exists supporting a role for SV40 in mesothelioma pathogenesis. SV40 is present in human mesotheliomas, where it is specifically found in the tumor cells and not in the normal surrounding tissues. Within these tumor cells, SV40 binds and inactivates essential tumor suppressor gene products, including TP53 and pRb, and stimulates *met*, Notch-1, and telomerase activity. Moreover, SV40 causes promoter methylation and thus inactivation of the tumor suppressor RASSF1A, which causes a more aggressive tumor phenotype.[55] It is most likely that asbestos and SV40 act as co-carcinogens in the development of some mesotheliomas, and SV40 and asbestos have been shown to act as co-carcinogens in vitro.[56] The possibility that SV40 and asbestos may also act as co-carcinogens in humans is important, since SV40 is frequently found in mesothelioma patients with a history of asbestos exposure. Additional cofactors such as radiation exposure or genetics may also act in conjunction with SV40, asbestos, or both.

Genetic Predisposition to Mesothelioma Various other fibers, such as zeolites (erionite type) from volcanic rocks, have been incriminated in Turkey,[57] and a few deposits have been found in Oregon in the United States.[58] The potential of zeolites to produce mesotheliomas has been confirmed experimentally after intraperitoneal injection.[59] After inhalation, the mesothelioma yield from zeolites exceeds that of any other fiber.[60] In certain villages in Cappadocia, a region in Central Anatolia, Turkey, 50% or more of deaths are caused by malignant mesothelioma.[61–65] Erionite, commonly found in the stones of the houses of Cappadocian villages,[47,65,66] has been suspected as the causative agent.[63–67] When erionite was injected intrapleurally into animals it caused mesothelioma,[68] and it was concluded that erionite was the cause of mesothelioma in these villages.[65,66,69,70] Closer observation revealed that mesotheliomas only occurred in certain homes and not in others (homes in these areas are inhabited by multiple generations and passed down), even though all homes contained similar amounts of erionite according to recent mineralogical analysis.[47,71] Pedigree analyses of families who lived in homes where mesotheliomas occurred showed that these mesotheliomas appeared to be inherited in an autosomal-dominant pattern. About 50% of descendents of affected parents developed mesotheliomas. When members of unaffected families married into affected families, 50% of their descendents also developed mesotheliomas.[47,71] Whether genetics alone or in conjunction with erionite are responsible for these mesotheliomas remains unknown, but clearly, genetics is a key factor, since mesotheliomas do not develop in nonaffected families regardless of environmental exposure.

Radiation and Mesothelioma Mesotheliomas have occurred within or in proximity to prior radiotherapy fields. In a cumulative review of 23 cases of possible radiation-induced mesothelioma, including two after extravasation of thorium dioxide (Thorotrast), the interval between radiation and mesothelioma ranged from 5 to 41 years (median 13.5 years).[72–74] Mesotheliomas have also developed in young adults who have received radiotherapy because of Wilms' tumor or for mediastinal lymphoma.

PATHOLOGY

Mesothelioma tissues have the singular potential of producing tumors of epithelial or mesenchymal type, or both. Embryologically, the mesothelium is made of a coelomic epithelium developed from the mesoderm, not the mesenchyme, and is supported by mesenchymal tissue. It is not entirely clear whether the malignant cells arise from the mature mesothelial cells or from undifferentiated mesenchymal cells of the submesothelial tissues; however, three major histologic types are recognized: epithelial or tubulopapillary, the most frequent (50–70% of cases); mesenchymal or fibrosarcomatous, the least common (7–20% of cases); and mixed or biphasic, intermediate in frequency (20–35% of cases). The mixed type is the most characteristic, containing both epithelial and mesenchymal elements. Other subtypes of mesothelioma have been described: desmoplastic with prominent fibrosis[75] and lymphohistiocytoid with intense lymphoplasmacytic infiltration,[76] both most often in sarcomatous mesothelioma. To differentiate mesothelioma from such mimics as adenocarcinomas and sarcomas, the diagnosis must be confirmed by immunohistochemistry, which shows that the tumor cells are positive for pankeratin, keratin 5/6, calretinin, and WT-1, and negative for the epithelial markers CEA, LeuM1, B72.3, Ber-EP4, Moc-1, and TTF-1, etc.[77] Usually positive staining for pankeratin and calretinin and negative staining for three epithelial markers is considered sufficient for diagnosis. Occasionally, however, more stainings are required, because some carcinomas are positive for calretinin or are negative for some of the epithelial markers. In these difficult cases, electron microscopy showing the classic long branching microvilli of human mesothelial cells compared with the short nonbranching microvilli of carcinomas can still be considered the gold standard for a correct diagnosis. Another difficult task that may lead to considerable clinical problems is the distinction between malignant mesothelioma, particularly of the desmoplastic type, and benign reactive mesothelial hyperplasia, which can appear atypical in a number of conditions, including pulmonary infarction, cirrhosis of the liver, uremia, and metastatic carcinoma. In such cases, even electron microscopy may not be helpful. Suspicion of malignant mesothelioma should arise in case of invasion of surrounding structures, of focally necrotic and avascular areas, and subtle microscopic features, such as piling and aggregation of mesothelial cells, variability in size, nuclear hyperchromasia, mitotic activity, irregular chromatin pattern, and cytoplasmic vacuolization, or in the presence of any florid mesothelial proliferation. Cytology to diagnose malignant mesothelioma is difficult to differentiate mesothelioma cells from other tumors or from reactive mesothelial cells,[78] so the gold standard remains either pleural biopsy by video-assisted thoracoscopy or by open pleural biopsy, and in a substantial number of cases the histotype of mesothelioma will change compared with either cytologic or needle biopsies performed prior to the definitive procedure.

Mesotheliomas spread by contiguity over the parietal and visceral serosal surfaces. Pleural mesothelioma extends over the diaphragm, mediastinum, pericardium, and, eventually, the peritoneum. It also extends into the interlobar fissures and into the lung itself by contiguity or by interstitial and alveolar spread. Seeding along the track of needle biopsy channels occurs in 10 to 20% of cases.[79] Peritoneal mesothelioma involves mainly the parietal and visceral surfaces, the omentum, and the mesentery with tumor nodules and/or infiltration causing thickening. Involvement of the serosa overlying the small and large bowel, the liver, the spleen, and other organs leads to encasement of these organs in tumor tissue. Lymphatic dissemination is common, and mediastinal nodes are involved in approximately 50% of cases of pleural mesothelioma.[80] Distant blood-borne metastases are more common than was previously thought and are seen at autopsy in 50 to 80% of cases.[81] They can occur in any organ, including the brain.

CLINICAL FEATURES

Pleural Mesothelioma The onset of mesothelioma is usually insidious and is most commonly associated with chest pain, dyspnea, or cough.[81] Progressive invasion of the chest wall often leads to intractable pain. Pleural effusion is present initially in up to 95% of cases. Later, tumor growth usually results in complete obliteration of the pleural space and encasement of the lung. Late symptoms of bulky mesotheliomas include mediastinal invasion with dysphagia, phrenic nerve paralysis, pericardial effusion, and superior vena cava syndrome.

Chest radiographs reveal a variable amount of fluid, with pleural thickening or pleural nodules, often several centimeters in diameter, imposing a scalloped appearance (Figure 81-2). Predominance occurs at the base, and ipsilateral shift of the mediastinum with retraction of the involved hemithorax can occur unless the tumor volume becomes very large. Bilateral pleural involvement or metastasis to the opposite lung is occasionally seen.[81]

Computed tomography (CT) reveals the extent of disease (including chest wall, mediastinum, pericardium, and diaphragm), relative amount of fluid and tumor, involvement of interlobar fissures, and retraction of the involved hemithorax. Stigmata of asbestos exposure, such as contralateral pulmonary fibrosis and/or pleural plaques, are seen in 50% of cases and pleural calcifications are seen in 15%.[12] Whether magnetic resonance imaging (MRI) adds to the workup is debatable, with MRI reported to be superior to CT in showing tumor spread into the fissures, diaphragm, and bony structures, while both procedures are equally effective to detect invasion

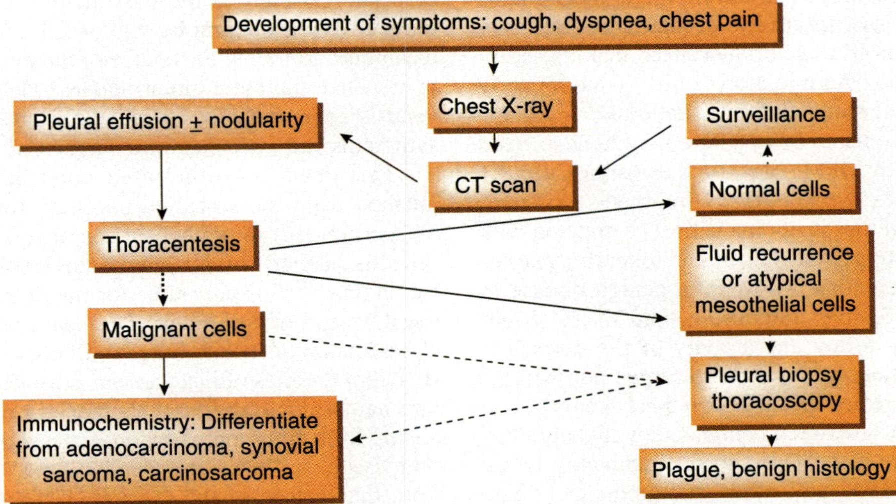

Figure 81-2 Algorithm for the work up of the asbestos exposed individual who presents with new symptoms. Any new pleural effusion must have thoracentesis and immunohistochemical analyses. If atypical mesothelial cells are seen, thoracoscopy should be performed for histologic confirmation of malignancy or inflammatory disease.

into the chest wall, lung, and mediastinum.[82,83] Recently, the role of (18F)-fluorodeoxy-D-glucose (FDG) positron emission tomography (PET) imaging has been examined in a number of studies, and although requiring further validation may hold prognostic importance, depending on the standardized uptake values, and may reveal occult disease preventing an unnecessary thoracotomy.[84,85]

Bronchoscopy is usually normal or reveals only extrinsic pressure. Thoracentesis yields a serous to viscous, gelatinous fluid, which is occasionally frankly bloody. The fluid is an exudate, and pleural fluid glucose can be low, but this finding is nonspecific. Pleural needle biopsy shows malignant disease in 13 to 48% of cases, and a diagnosis of mesothelioma in 10 to 36%. Thoracoscopy is a useful technique in cases where there is an approachable pleural space, and if there is any question of the pathology, open pleural biopsy remains the best diagnostic procedure, yielding the diagnosis in 77 to 100% of patients.[86,87]

Biomarkers for Mesothelioma There have been a number of studies that have attempted to define biomarkers that could predate symptoms in a high-risk-of-mesothelioma population, as well as distinguish MPM from other malignancies. The majority of these studies have very few patients of various stages of MPM and have not been prospectively evaluated. When a battery of serum biomarkers were evaluated for the early detection of malignancy and for distinguishing early stages of mesothelioma and bronchogenic carcinoma, only four markers (tissue polypeptide antigen, carcinoembryonic antigen, hyaluronic acid, and ferritin) were able to distinguish the *late* stages of the two malignancies and asbestosis. Follow-up exploratory studies revealed that hyaluronic acid levels in serum were elevated in MPM patients[88] and were significantly higher than those levels seen in those of healthy volunteers of the same age or in nonmesothelioma malignant tumors.[89,90] Of interest was the finding that patients with asbestosis did not exhibit increased serum hyaluronan. Further studies, however, revealed that during the clinical course of the disease, serum hyaluronate increases only at an advanced stage of the cancer, making serum hyaluronate determination of little value for early detection of malignant mesothelioma.[91]

Measurement of cytokeratins has also been evaluated in MPM. Early studies using Cyfra 21 (which uses cytokeratin 19 fragments) in small numbers of mesothelioma patients compared with controls suggested that this cytokeratin marker could differentiate MPM from benign disease in pleural effusions and serum, and that it could potentially follow the activity of the disease.[92] Later studies, however, with larger numbers of patients revealed that although there seemed to be a cutoff level between benign and malignant effusions, there were really no distinguishing levels between MPM and other malignancies.[93] The value of Cyfra 21-1 was only enhanced when combined with tissue polypeptide antigen (TPA), and in 52 patients with mesothelioma both were highly correlated with survival in a univariate analysis.[94] Unfortunately, however, these data have never been validated prospectively.

CA-125 levels in very limited studies have been reported to be useful in peritoneal mesothelioma diagnosis[95] and may be most useful when combined with other markers (see below). Most recently, TPA, hyaluronan, and CA-125 levels in 11 patients revealed that initial TPA levels reflected prognosis better than corresponding data regarding Hyaluronan and CA-I25.[96]

Mesothelin, originally described by Pastan, is a 40-kDa glycoprotein attached to the cell surface of mesotheliomas, ovarian cancers, and pancreatic cancers, which is thought to have a role in cell adhesion and cell-to-cell recognition and signaling.[97] Mesothelin is synthesized as a precursor 69-kDa protein and forms two proteins, the membrane-bound mesothelin and the soluble protein megakaryocyte potentiating factor.[98] A third member of this family is soluble mesothelin-related protein (SMRP). Robinson and colleagues have reported that determination of SMRP in serum is a marker of mesothelioma with a sensitivity of 83% and specificity of 95% in the first 48 malignant mesothelioma (MM) patients tested. Preliminary work also suggests that the sensitivity and specificity are increased when the marker is combined with CA-125. Changes in serum SMRP levels parallel clinical course/tumor size, and SMRP is elevated in 75% of patients at diagnosis. SMRP may be useful for monitoring disease progression and may prove useful for screening asbestos-exposed individuals for early mesothelioma.[99] Mesothelin assays (MesoMark) are now available in Europe and Australia.

Peritoneal Mesothelioma Pain and abdominal distention with ascites are almost constant in patients with peritoneal mesothelioma. Other clinical findings include nausea and vomiting, bowel obstruction, abdominal and pelvic masses, edema of the lower extremities, fever, hernia, hydrocele, and obstructive uropathy.[100,101] Coexistent pleural effusion may occur. Direct biopsy by laparotomy or peritoneoscopy is the best diagnostic procedure.[102] Ultrasonography and/or CT are useful techniques to follow the course of the disease and to visualize fluid and tumor masses. Median survival is approximately 10 months from onset of symptoms and 7 months from diagnosis.[103]

Peritoneal mesothelioma must be distinguished from the so-called papillary tumors of the peritoneum in women in the absence of an obvious primary tumor such as ovarian serous carcinoma.[104] Special stains for mucin are often negative and of little help. The exact nosologic classification of such tumors is still controversial. Different theories of histogenesis have led to various names, ranging from "papillary carcinoma," arising from embryonic peritoneal nests of müllerian tissue, to "ovarian mesothelioma," arising from the surface of the ovary.[105,106] The tumor can arise in oophorectomized women. Asbestos exposure is uncommonly found. The course of such tumors appears more protracted than the real diffuse peritoneal mesothelioma, and prolonged survival for years after palliative surgery, and sometimes chemotherapy, is another distinguishing feature that makes recognition of this entity clinically important.

DIFFERENTIAL DIAGNOSIS

Some patients with malignant mesothelioma give a history of recurrent pleural effusion for years before the diagnosis is made, and despite thoracenteses and multiple radiologic examinations, the diagnosis is delayed (see Figure 81-2). Effusions are associated with benign asbestos pleurisy in approximately 3 to 5% of asbestos workers.[107] A newly developing pleural effusion in a high-risk cohort of workers should alert the clinician to the possibility of mesothelioma. Almost two-thirds may be asymptomatic, and eventual pleural biopsy may show dense fibrosis with scattered nonmalignant cells. Typically, the fluid resolves spontaneously, but ipsilateral relapses are frequent, and contralateral disease may appear. The frequent difficulties of cytologic diagnosis and differentiation from reactive benign mesothelial proliferation, as discussed above, further compound this important clinical problem. Any suspicion added to a history of asbestos exposure warrants an aggressive diagnostic approach, including thoracoscopy or open biopsy, if necessary. Close follow-up is necessary, because some patients have developed malignant mesothelioma 6 to 12 years after such an episode.[107]

PROGNOSTIC FACTORS

In a multivariate analysis from the European Organization for Research and Treatment of Cancer, poor prognosis was associated with a poor performance status, a high white blood cell count, male gender, and the sarcomatous histologic subtype.[108] The Cancer and Leukemia Group B found that poor performance status, chest pain, dyspnea, platelet count greater than 400,000/μL, weight loss, serum lactate dehydrogenase level greater than 500 IU/L, pleural involvement, low hemoglobin level, high white blood cell count, and increasing age over 75 years were all associated with shortened survival. Several groups have described gene expression patterns using gene chips in order to prognosticate survival and time to progression in surgically treated patients.[109,110]

OTHER TYPES OF MALIGNANT MESOTHELIOMAS

Pericardial mesothelioma[111–114] represents the most frequent primary malignant tumor of the pericardium and can occur at any age with a 3:1 male predominance. The role of asbestos exposure has not been systematically explored. Pericardial effusion leading to cardiac tamponade and superior vena caval syndrome are common symptoms with spread involving the pleura, lung, mediastinum, or distant organs also present in half the cases. Survival time is usually less than 6 months.

Malignant mesothelioma of the tunica vaginalis testis (adenomatoid tumor) presents as a scrotal mass, often associated with a hydrocele.[115–118] Median age is in the mid-sixties, and asbestos exposure can be documented in approximately 25% of the patients.

BENIGN MESOTHELIOMAS

Localized mesothelioma, better referred to as localized fibrous tumor of the pleura (FTP), is thought to originate from the submesothelial cells, but it is unclear what submesothelial cells really are. Solitary fibrous tumor of pleura is usually not related to asbestos exposure and is often pedunculated. These tumors are similar to other fibrous tumors found elsewhere in the body pleural effusion is exceptional. Clubbing and osteoarthropathy are common and are present in 20 to 50% of cases, versus only 6% in malignant mesothelioma.[119] Hyponatremia attributed to inappropriate secretion of antidiuretic hormone and hypoglycemia has been described.[120] Microscopically, these tumors are well-circumscribed fibromas with a variable collagenous matrix containing interweaving bundles of ovoid or spindle cells without atypia.[121] The tumor cells have a benign appearance and are usually immersed in a fibrous and characteristically vascular stroma. FTP cells are characteristically negative for cytokeratin (a marker of mesothelial cells) and positive for CD34, which suggests that these cells are not of mesothelial origin. Surgery for the majority of fibrous tumors is curative, but these tumors can recur locally.

Occasionally, localized fibrous tumors of the pleura are histologically and cytologically malignant,[122,123] and many of these tumors were called hemangiopericytomas, a terminology that has recently been changed. Presently, all these tumors should be called fibrous tumors (of the pleura if in the pleura). The more cellular and histologically aggressive FTP (old hemangiopericytomas) are characterized by multiple recurrences after resection and a poor prognosis. However, the most important predictive factor in the prognosis of FTP is whether the tumor can be completely resected. Thus, pedunculated tumors have a much better prognosis than tumors that grow over a broad pleural area.

Benign multicystic or well-differentiated papillary peritoneal mesothelioma affects mainly young females and produces cysts of variable size.[124–127] Histologically, it is formed by multiple papillary structures covered by cytologically benign mesothelial cells. The lesion is benign, but there have been occasional cases in which several years after diagnosis the patient developed a true mesothelioma.[128,129] The differential with a well-differentiated epithelial malignant mesothelioma, based mostly on the absence of invasion in these benign lesions, may be difficult, and consultation with pathologists who see numerous mesothelial lesions and malignant mesothelioma is highly recommended.[130] The major differential diagnoses are lymphangioma and ovarian cancer of low malignant potential. The disease follows a benign course and is compatible with a normal life expectancy, requiring, occasionally, partial excision or decompression for relief of pain or other symptoms.

Table 81-1 Treatment Options for Mesothelioma

Supportive care	
Effusion control	Talc pleurodesis
	Vats assisted
	Slurry
	Pleurex catheter
	Repeated thoracenteses
Pain control	Narcotics
	Permanent epidural catheter
	Localized radiation
Surgery	Pleurectomy with decortication
	Extrapleural pneumonectomy
Chemotherapy*	Pemetrexed (Alimta) and cisplatin*
	Gemcitabine and cisplatin*
	Vinorelbine (Navelbine)
	Phase I/II trials with targeted agents
Multimodality therapy	Induction chemotherapy, surgery, and postoperative radiotherapy#
	Surgery and postoperative radiotherapy
	Surgery and postoperative chemotherapy
	Surgery and novel cytotoxic/targeted agents#
Novel intrapleural therapies	Hyperthermic chemoperfusion#
	Photodynamic therapy#
	Gene therapy#
Novel radiation techniques at selected centers	Intensity-modulated radiation therapy

*Most commonly used in recent phase II/III trials.
#Under investigation.

TREATMENT

Owing to the small numbers of patients in most clinical trials involving mesothelioma and the lack of uniformity in management, one must conclude that there is no standard approach to the treatment of mesothelioma (Table 81-1). Aggressive approaches generally involve surgery as part of the treatment program, and there have been variations of the type of adjuvant therapies delivered either in the operating room or postoperatively with such multimodal approaches. The nonsurgical candidate usually receives chemotherapy alone, novel agents, or supportive care.

Surgery Surgery is involved in the management of pleural mesothelioma either for diagnosis, palliative therapy, or as part of a multimodal therapeutic plan. The operations involved in this management include thoracoscopy, pleurectomy/decortication, and extrapleural pleuropneumonectomy (EPP). The indications for each of these operations will depend on the extent of disease, performance and functional status of the patient, and the philosophy of the treating institution. Basically, operative intervention in mesothelioma is for primary effusion control, for cytoreduction prior to multimodal therapy, or to deliver and monitor innovative intrapleural therapies.[81] The majority of patients seeking treatment of mesothelioma are middle- to older-aged individuals with a long latency period between asbestos exposure and tumor development. If surgical intervention is to be considered, a detailed physiologic–functional work-up, directed chiefly at the cardiopulmonary axis, must be performed, since operations for mesothelioma are associated with profound blood loss and potentially significant cardiac and respiratory demands.

Staging for Pleural Mesothelioma The Union Internationale Contre le Cancer (UICC) proposed a tumor-nodes-metastasis (TNM) staging system that evolved into the presently described IMIG staging system described by Rusch (Table 81-2). The IMIG staging system has been validated in several large surgical series of mesothelioma.[131–133] Sugarbaker and colleagues have proposed the alternative but complementary Brigham staging system based on tumor, resectability, and nodal status.[134,135]

Surgical candidates include all IMIG clinically staged individuals from stages I-III, for the T3 category of stage III patients, which includes invasion of the endothoracic fascia or mediastinal fat, a solitary focus of tumor invading the soft tissues of the chest wall (ie, at an old thoracoscopy site), and/or nontransmural involvement of the pericardium. The influence of nodal status and eligibility for surgery is less defined since only 30 to 40% of nodes involved from resected mesothelioma patients are in the upper mediastinum, and thus accessible to routine mediastinoscopy.[133] However, it is clear that the involvement of lymph nodes in surgically resected mesothelioma patients is an ominous sign. Therefore, in the absence of routine thoracoscopic sampling of multiple nodal stations in mesothelioma prior to definitive resection, mediastinoscopy may be justified in those patients with obvious (ie, > 1.0 cm) nodal involvement in levels 7, 4R, 4L, 5L, or 6L, or in patients with a suspicion for contralateral nodal involvement on presentation,[136] since it is

Table 81-2 IMIG Staging System for Pleural Mesothelioma

T1	
T1a	Tumor limited to the ipsilateral parietal ± mediastinal ± diaphragmatic pleura, no involvement of the visceral pleura
T1b	Tumor involving the ipsilateral parietal ± mediastinal ± diaphragmatic pleura, tumor also involving the visceral pleura
T2	Tumor involving each of the ipsilateral pleural surfaces (parietal, mediastinal, diaphragmatic, and visceral pleura) with at least one of the following features: • Involvement of diaphragmatic muscle • Extension of tumor from visceral pleura into the underlying pulmonary parenchyma
T3	Describes locally advanced but potentially resectable tumor Tumor involving all of the ipsilateral pleural surfaces (parietal, mediastinal, diaphragmatic, and visceral pleura) with at least one of the following features: • Involvement of the endothoracic fascia • Extension into the mediastinal fat • Solitary, completely resectable focus of tumor extending into the soft tissues of the chest wall • Nontransmural involvement of the pericardium
T4	Describes locally advanced technically unresectable tumor Tumor involving all the ipsilateral pleural surfaces (parietal, mediastinal, diaphragmatic, and visceral pleura) with at least one of the following features: • Diffuse extension or multifocal masses of tumor in the chest wall, with or without associated rib destruction • Direct transdiaphragmatic extension of tumor to the peritoneum • Direct extension of tumor to the contralateral pleura • Direct extension of tumor to mediastinal organs • Direct extension of tumor into the spine • Tumor extending through to the internal surface of the pericardium with or without a pericardial effusion; or tumor involving the myocardium
N–Lymph nodes	
NX	Regional lymph nodes cannot be assessed
N0	No regional lymph node metastases
N1	Metastases in the ipsilateral bronchopulmonar or hilar lymph nodes
N2	Metastases in the subcarinal or the ipsilateral mediastinal lymph nodes including the ipsilateral internal mammary nodes
N3	Metastases in the contralateral mediastinal, contralateral internal mammary, ipsilateral, or contralateral supraclavicular lymph nodes
M–Metastases	
MX	Presence of distant metastases cannot be assessed
M0	No distant metastasis
M1	Distant metastasis present
Stage I	
Ia	T1aN0 M0
Ib	T1bN0 M0
Stage II	T2 N0 M0
Stage III	Any T3 M0 Any N1 M0 Any N2 M0
Stage IV	Any T4 Any N3 Any M1

T = primary tumor; T1 = limited to ipsilateral pleura only (parietal pleura, visceral pleura); T2 = superficial local invasion (diaphragm, endothoracic fascia, ipsilateral lung, fissures); T3 = deep local invasion (chest wall beyond endothoracic fascia); T4 = extensive direct invasion (opposite pleura, peritoneum, retroperitoneum); N = lymph nodes; N0 = no positive lymph node; N1 = positive ipsilateral hilar nodes; N2 = positive mediastinal nodes; N3 = positive contralateral hilar nodes; M = metastases; M0 = no metastases; M1 = metastases; blood-borne or lymphatic.

Adapted from Chahinian.[19,230]

becoming increasingly clear that the median survival of patients with nodal involvement (stage III, IMIG and stage II/III Brigham staging system) is 10 to 12 months after surgery. It is possible that FDG PET scanning will help to at least define those patients with node-involved mesothelioma in the future.[137]

Palliative Surgery In general, the indications for palliative surgery include the control or prevention of effusion that results in disabling dyspnea. Effusion control can be obtained by talc pleurodesis, with or without thoracoscopy, if the lung expands nearly completely after effusion removal. The use of talc or other sclerosants could impact on the suitability for patients to enter innovative trials that incorporate either pleurectomy or EPP and could jeopardize the ability of the surgeon to spare a lung that may not have visceral pleural implants. Hence, the routine use of talc sclerosis at the time of suspected mesothelioma should be discouraged until all treatment options are explained to the patient. The results of video thoracoscopic talc pleurodesis specifically for mesothelioma have shown success rates of 80 to 100% with median survivals ranging from 7 to 9 months, success being defined as no further need for tapping after 1 month.[138–141] Failure of these techniques is usually associated with entrapped lung, a large solid tumor mass, a long history of effusion with multiple thoracenteses leading to loculations, or age > 70 years. For patients whose lung does not expand after thoracenteses, the PleurX catheter, which enables the patient to perform self-drainage, has been widely adapted.[142–144] This device allows the patient to drain him/herself at home. The catheter can be placed under conscious sedation in minutes without the postoperative discomfort frequently associated with talc pleurodesis. It also works well in cases of malignant ascites.[145]

Rationale of Cytoreductive Surgery The majority of diffuse malignant mesotheliomas cannot be surgically removed en bloc with truly negative histologic margins because many of the patients have had a previous biopsy and there is invasion of the endothoracic fascia and intercostal muscles at that site and/or there is pleural effusion that, although cytologically negative, may be breached, leading to local permeation of tumor cells, either into the residual cavity or into the abdomen. In an often-quoted series of EPP performed for mesothelioma from the Boston group, 66 of 183 patients were defined as having negative resection margins after EPP. Patients with this finding who had epithelial mesothelioma were found to have 2- and 5-year survival rates of 68% and 46%, respectively, if the node dissection did not reveal tumor.[135]

The operation of choice, especially for *early* pleural mesothelioma, has yet to be defined. There is no doubt that EPP is a more extensive dissection and may serve to remove more bulk disease than a pleurectomy, chiefly in the diaphragmatic and visceral pleural surfaces. Some surgeons, however, will include diaphragmatic resection and pericardial resection with their pleurectomies to accomplish removal of "all gross disease." For EPP, when performed in patients with bulky disease, it is almost a necessity to include pericardiotomy, with or without resection, since this maneuver aids in the exposure of the vessels and allows intrapericardial control to prevent a surgical catastrophe. There are no real guidelines preoperatively that one can use to assure the patient which operation will be necessary to accomplish tumor removal. The presence of irregular, bulky disease on the CT scan that infiltrates into the fissures probably dictates the necessity for EPP; a large effusion with minimal bulk disease may call for pleurectomy decortication. Moreover, the philosophy of the surgeon regarding the operation may impact on his choice, for some surgeons reserve EPP for those patients with bulky disease that prevents simple pleurectomy, whereas others feel that the greatest chance for complete gross excision will be via EPP performed in the patient with minimal disease. This important factor—preoperative quantitative bulk of disease—may not only influence the choice or resection, but may also be an important preoperative prognostic factor in any patient with mesothelioma.[131]

Pleurectomy When performed by an experienced team, pleurectomy for mesothelioma can be associated with few major complications, and pleurectomy and decortication are very effective in controlling malignant pleural effusion (Figure 81-3).[146–148] In the series that specify postoperative morbidity, the most common complication was prolonged air leak for > 7 days, occurring in 10% of the patients. On average, the chest tubes can be removed in approximately 5.5 days with > 50% of the patients having the chest tube removed within 4 days. Pneumonia and respiratory insufficiency may occur and is usually related to the burden of disease and preoperative functional status. Empyema is a rare occurrence (2%) and is managed by prolonged chest tube drainage and antibiotics. Hemorrhage requiring reexploration is very rare (< 1%).The modern-day mortality from pleurectomy has decreased and is generally considered to be 1.5 to 2%, with death either from respiratory insufficiency or hemorrhage.

Many of the published series using pleurectomy for palliative management have added therapies postoperatively in an uncontrolled, institution-related fashion. The majority have had no sampling of the mediastinal nodes, let alone a mediastinal dissection. Nevertheless, the overall median survival for patients having pleurectomy alone is approximately 13 months. The patients who receive pleurectomy and decortication alone usually have early effusive disease with minimal bulk tumor. If these patients have epithelial mesothelioma and are not found to have nodal involvement, survival rates can be significantly longer than that quoted above.

Extrapleural Pneumonectomy Radical EPP classically has been described for pure epithelial tumor, stage I, that is technically resectable and encapsulated by the parietal pleura (Figure 81-4). In reality, there are few patients who actually qualify for exploration for EPP outside the research setting. In Butchart and colleagues early review, 29 of 46 (63%) of patients were eligible for EPP,[149] and this percentage is similar to DaValle and colleagues', in which 33 of 56 patients over a 27-year period had EPP (59%).[150] Sugarbaker recently reported that 50% of the patients seen at his institution are ineligible for EPP.

In the Lung Cancer Study Group (LCSG) malignant mesothelioma pilot study from 1985 to 1988, only 20 of the 83 evaluated patients were resected with an EPP.[151] The reasons that EPP could not be performed were chiefly extent of disease not allowing complete gross resection (54%), inadequate respiratory reserve (33%), stage IV disease (11%), and concurrent medical illness (10%).

Because of its magnitude, EPP has significantly greater morbidity than pleurectomy. The major complication rate ranges from 20 to 40%, and arrhythmia requiring medical management is the most common complication. In Sugarbaker and colleagues most recent report, major morbidity occurred in 24% of the patients having EPP and minor morbidity in 41%.[152] The rate for bronchopleural fistula is greater with right-sided EPPs with an overall fistula rate of 3 to 20%. The bronchopleural fistula can be handled, for the most part, with open thoracostomy drainage with or without muscle flap interposition.[70]

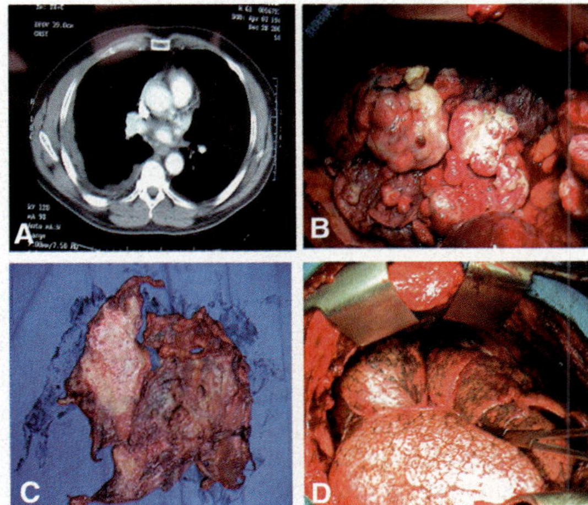

Figure 81-3 Pleurectomy for mesothelioma: **A,** typical computerized tomogram reveals thickened pleura; **B,** operative view reveals disease primarily on the parietal pleura; **C,** operative specimen; **D,** completion of satisfactory cytoreduction with sparing and decortication of the lung.

The mortality rates following EPP were unacceptably high in the 1970s from respiratory failure, myocardial infarction, or pulmonary embolus. Rusch and Venkatraman[133] report a modern-day perioperative mortality of 6% (3 of 50) after EPP, and Sugarbaker and colleagues report a perioperative mortality of 3.8% from myocardial infarction and presumed pulmonary emboli.[152]

There is a higher proportion of local recurrences in the pleurectomy population as compared with the patients having EPP. Sites of first recurrence after EPP are local in 35% of patients, abdominal in 26%, the contralateral thorax in 17%, and other distant sites in 8%.[153]

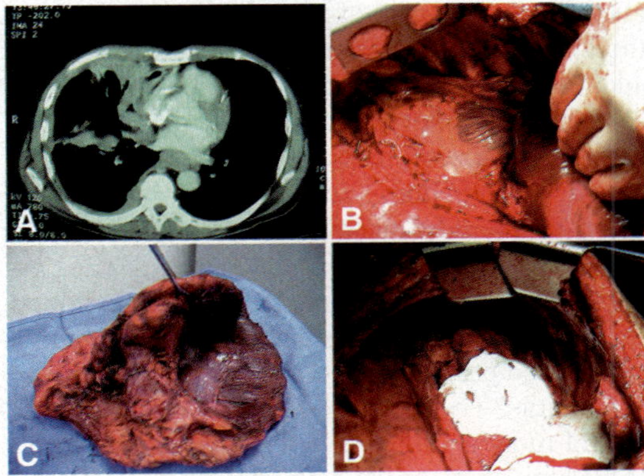

Figure 81-4 Extrapleural pneumonectomy for mesothelioma: **A,** Computerized tomography reveals thickened pleura, pericardium and disease in the fissures. **B,** Intraoperative view after the resection with hand on the liver. Stapled bronchial stump, right atrium, and extent of pericardiotomy is seen. **C,** Operative specimen reveals diaphragmatic resection to the right and thickened pleura encasing the lung. **D,** Reconstruction of the diaphragm and pericardium with Gore-Tex patches.

Long-term survival rates after EPP remain disappointing, with the median survivals ranging from 9.3 to 17 months for the major series but subgroup analyses reveal median survivals of stage I epithelial patients to approach 24 months.[134,154]

Surgery and Multimodality Treatment

Surgery and Intraoperative Radiotherapy The Memorial Sloan-Kettering Cancer Center pioneered the use of surgery and postoperative or intraoperative radiation therapy for mesothelioma. The use of permanent (^{125}I) or temporary (^{192}Ir) implantation techniques for mesothelioma to deliver 3,000 cGy in 3 days as well as radioactive phosphorus 32 (^{32}P), however, have been relegated to historical significance.[155,156]

Surgery and Postoperative Radiatiotherapy Most recently, Rusch and colleagues investigated the role of high-dose hemithoracic radiation after complete resection of malignant pleural mesothelioma to determine feasibility, rates of local recurrence, and survival. Adjuvant radiation, administered to 57 patients at a median dose of 54 Gy, was well tolerated except for one late esophageal fistula. Recurrences were locoregional in 1 (2%), distant in 30 (52.6%) and locoregional + distant in 6 (10%) patients. Median survival was 33.8 months for stages I and II versus 10 months for stages III and IV tumors, implying that postoperative hemithoracic radiation may impact on local control and survival in early-stage mesothelioma.[132]

Intensity modulated radiation therapy (IMRT) offers the potential for administering higher doses of radiotherapy to the hemithorax, while minimizing normal tissue toxicities.[5] Stevens and colleagues at the University of Texas M. D. Anderson Cancer Center have treated 28 patients with IMRT after EPP.[157,158] The hemithorax was treated with doses of 4,500 to 5,000 cGy, and some regions of the hemithorax were boosted to a total dose of 6,000 cGy. Radiation dose homogeneity to the entire hemithorax was excellent. Side effects included nausea, vomiting, dyspnea, and esophagitis. The median follow-up is 9 months and the local control rate is 100%, with a 1-year survival of 65%. These early results are encouraging and worthy of additional study.

Surgery, Chemotherapy, and Radiation Therapy Since 1980, at the Brigham and Women's Hospital in Boston,[134] extrapleural pneumonectomy has been combined with postoperative chemotherapy and targeted postoperative radiotherapy. Over a 19-year period with varying chemotherapy regimens, 183 patients have been treated with a perioperative mortality of 3.8%. The median survival in this group of patients is approximately 17 months, which is a significant improvement over other trials. Favorable subgroups include those with no mediastinal nodal involvement and epithelial histology.[134] These data have been corroborated by a large nonrandomized series from Germany,[159] in which 93 patients chose either best supportive care or multimodal treatment with surgery (pleurectomy decortication or extrapleural pneumonectomy) followed by systemic chemotherapy with doxorubicin, cyclophosphamide, and vindesine. Patients in remission at the end of the chemotherapy (16 of the 57 accrued) received 45 to 60 Gy of radiation therapy to the hemithorax. Median survival was 13 months compared with 7 months for those receiving best supportive care. In a series of 32 patients from Italy,[160–162] EPP followed by adjuvant chemotherapy and concurrent hemithoracic radiation up to a total dose of 55 Gy resulted in a median survival of only 9.5 months, since 50% of the patients were found to be in stage III after the procedure.

Induction Chemotherapy Followed by Surgery Induction or neoadjuvant therapy for pleural mesothelioma followed by surgery has been patterned after similar strategies with nonsmall-cell lung cancer. Results have been disappointing because of the inability of the patients to tolerate both the cytotoxic chemotherapy and the surgery. Anecdotal experiences of increased difficulty in performing the surgical dissection after induction chemotherapy have not been reported. With the improved efficacy of doublet chemotherapy (gemcitabine/cisplatin or pemetrexed/cisplatin), there is renewed interest in investigating a neoadjuvant approach for mesothelioma. A Swiss neoadjuvant study used three cycles of cisplatin 80 mg/m^2 on day 1 and gemcitabine 1,000 mg/m2 on days 1, 8, and 15 every 28 days followed by surgery. Radiation therapy was considered after EPP to areas at risk. In all, 16 of 19 patients had EPP, and 32% had a radiographic response to therapy preoperatively. Median survival was 23 months.[163]

A similar trial was performed by de Perrot, which involved induction chemotherapy, surgery, and postoperative hemithorax radiation therapy with a 6% operative mortality and 74% 1-year survival.[164] A neoadjuvant approach is presently being investigated in the United States as a multicenter trial delivering 4 cycles of pemetrexed and cisplatin followed by extrapleural pneumonectomy and postoperative hemithorax radiation therapy.

Novel Intrapleural Approaches **Intrapleural Photodynamic Therapy** Photodynamic therapy (PDT) involves the light-activated sensitization of malignant cells[165] using a photosensitizer such as Photofrin II, which is retained by malignant tissue in vivo in comparison with normal tissue. The sensitizer is activated by 630 nm light, and then interacts with molecular oxygen to produce an excited reactive oxygen species. A phase III trial of 63 malignant pleural mesothelioma patients randomized to surgery, with or without intraoperative photodynamic therapy revealed no difference in median survival (14.4 vs 14.1 months) or median progression-free time (8.5 vs 7.7 months), and sites of first recurrence were similar. Other phase II trials of photodynamic therapy and mesothelioma have not demonstrated therapeutic efficacy;[166–168] most recently, preliminary results using intrapleural PDT with metaTetraHydroxy-PhenylChlorin after EPP have revealed significant toxicities without survival benefit.[169]

Intrapleural Chemotherapy ± Postoperative Chemotherapy The results of intrapleural chemotherapy after resection for mesothelioma have been modest. Rusch used intrapleural chemotherapy after surgical debulking followed by systemic chemotherapy in 10 patients, and a subsequent report used an even more aggressive regimen of pleurectomy, immediate intracavitary cisplatin and mitomycin C with two cycles of systemic cisplatin and mitomycin C.[170] The most recent trial revealed an overall survival rate of 68% at 1 year and 44% at 2 years in the 27 patients who received the therapy, with a median survival of 17 months[151] with locoregional recurrences predominating. A very similar regimen combining pleurectomy or EPP with cisplatin and mitomycin C resulted in a disappointing median survival of 13 months, and only 50% of the chemotherapy treatments were delivered adjuvantly. In an Italian study of 20 patients, pleurectomy and diaphragmatic or pericardial resection, combined with intrapleural chemotherapy with cisplatin and cytarabine for 4 hours immediately after pleurectomy, followed by systemic chemotherapy with epirubicin and mitomycin C revealed a median time to disease progression of 7.4 months, and median survival of only 11.5 months.[171]

Pleural Perfusion Hyperthermic chemoperfusion of the pleura is an extension of intrapleural cytotoxic therapy and is based on the hypothesis that the treatment will provide increased local control and avoid systemic chemotherapy toxicity. A few phase II studies using cisplatin, or doxorubicin with cisplatin, have recorded morbidity rates of 33 to 65% using temperatures of 40° to 42°C without impacting on survival.[172–174] Chang and Sugarbaker designed a phase I/II trial using hyperthermic cisplatin (42°C) to perfuse both the abdomen and the pleura after pleurectomy/decortication. Operative mortality was 11%, and survival of all patients was 10.5 months; however, in the group of patients surviving surgery who received 225 mg/m^2 of cisplatin, the median survival was 22 months and disease-free survival was 20 months.[175] A trial of bicavitary chemoperfusion after extrapleural pneumonectomy is ongoing.

Novel Gene and Cytokine-Related Therapies A phase I trial of intrapleural suicide gene therapy, which delivered a replication-deficient adenovirus encoding HSV-tk (Ad.HSV-tk) was based on preclinical studies that demonstrated gene transduction and successful treatment of human mesothelioma xenografts in severe combined immunodeficiency (SCID) mice.[176] Gene transfer was demonstrated, and there was one partial response, 3 of the first 18 patients remained stable for up to 2 years following treatment, and 1 early-stage patient was tumor free for more than 31 months. The median survival of all patients was 11 months. Most recently, these investigators at the University of Pennsylvania are now exploring the role of interferon modulation using adenovirus delivery along with inhibitors of the cyclooxygenase pathway.[177,178]

Immunomodulatory gene therapy is also being investigated for mesothelioma by transfecting tumors with cytokine genes that can activate CD4 T cells or stimulate CD8 T cells including intratumoral *IL-2* gene.[179] Preclinical trials of the transfection of interferon β,[180,181] interleukin-4, and p14 (ARF)[182,183] into mesothelioma are ongoing.

The efficacy of interferon-γ by the use of intrapleural cytokine therapy has been documented by Boutin in earlier-stage mesothelioma.[184,185] Eight histologically confirmed complete responses and nine partial responses with at least a 50% reduction in tumor size were obtained. The overall response rate was 20%. The response rate for patients with stage I disease was 45%, with the main side effects being hyperthermia, liver toxicity, neutropenia, and catheter-related infection.

Intrapleural interleukin-2–based regimens have also been exploited in mesothelioma.[186] In 22 patients, there were 11 partial responses and 1 complete response. Stable disease occurred in 3 patients and disease progression in 7 patients. The overall median survival time was 18 months and the 24- and 36-month survival rates for responders were 58% and 41%, respectively. No confirmatory trials of this promising approach have been published.

NOVEL INTRAPLEURAL THERAPIES

Radiotherapy Results of radiotherapy as a primary modality for pleural mesothelioma have been generally disappointing. Conventional doses below 3,000 cGy have produced only temporary relief of symptoms in some cases, and doses in excess of 4,000 cGy are needed to achieve adequate palliation.[187] These doses are difficult to administer in view of the large tumor volume, including the entire hemithorax, diaphragm, and adjacent mediastinum. Elaborate techniques, such as combined photon and electron beams, use of various blocks, and tissue compensators to shield the lung, have not convincingly yielded superior results. Complex treatment plans using CT scans to include the entire pleura down to the base of the diaphragm have been proposed to deliver up to 4,250 cGy by parallel opposed fields with lung and liver blocks, supplemented with electrons up to 3,600 cGy. The fissures that are commonly involved may not be adequately treated, however. One case treated with fast neutron therapy has remained free of recurrence for over 78 months.[188] Present radiotherapy initiatives in mesothelioma are primarily concentrated on postoperative adjuvant treatment and extension of intensity-modulated radiation techniques (see above).

Chemotherapy Chemotherapy in malignant mesothelioma, until recently, has yielded only modest response and survival results, with recent reviews describing no agent or combination of agents that had produced response rates consistently above 20%, and with almost no impact on median survival.[189,190] Of single-agent regimens, the most commonly effective drugs are cisplatin, methotrexate, and trimetrexate. Both cisplatin and carboplatin have been evaluated in the treatment of mesothelioma, as single agents and in combinations. Cisplatin alone resulted in a response rate of 14.3% and a median survival of 7.5 months.[191]

Two phase II studies failed to demonstrate that high-dose cisplatin had an added benefit.[192,193] Cisplatin also has been evaluated in combination with other drugs producing response rates from 12 to 30% and a median survival of about 8 months. The combination of mitomycin (M) and cisplatin (C), which had been discovered to be effective in a nude mouse model, has been active in a randomized phase II trial[194] by the Cancer and Leukemia Group B (CALGB), where it showed a somewhat higher response rate (26%) than doxorubicin with cisplatin (14%), but no survival advantage. Addition of a third drug to the CM combination included agents such as doxorubicin or vinblastine or interferon-α, with no clear-cut benefit. In Japan, the combination of irinotecan (CPT-11) with cisplatin produced a 40% partial response rate in 15 patients. Pharmacokinetic studies of irinotecan and of its active metabolite SN-38 in the pleural fluid showed steady state with plasma levels after 6 hours, except in epithelial mesothelioma, where pleural fluid levels of SN-38 were much higher than in plasma.[195] Interestingly, all responses, except one, were seen in the 10 patients with the epithelial type. Newer phase II trials of cisplatin in combination with gemcitabine have demonstrated response rates from 15 to 47%.

Carboplatin is an analog of cisplatin, which has been developed and utilized in many tumor types owing to its favorable toxicity profile and ease of administration. Carboplatin has modest activity in malignant mesothelioma with response rate of 5 to 16%.[196–198]

Oxaliplatin has also been evaluated in the treatment of mesothelioma. In a recently reported phase II trial from Germany, the combination of gemcitabine and oxaliplatin demonstrated a response rate of 40%.[199]

Gemcitabine (difluorodeoxycytidine) is a prodrug that is metabolized to the triphosphate form intracellularly. The resultant difluorodeoxycytidine triphosphate is incorporated into DNA, which results in chain termination. Three phase II studies of gemcitabine have been conducted in patients with mesothelioma.[200–202] The EORTC Lung Cancer group reported a 7% response rate among 27 chemotherapy naïve mesothelioma patients, while the CALGB did not observe any response in 13 assessable patients.[203] In contrast, Bischoff and colleagues reported an encouraging response rate of 31% among 16 mesothelioma patients.[202] Gemcitabine has also been evaluated in combination with other drugs for mesothelioma using varying schedules, including three studies evaluating the combination of cisplatin and gemcitabine. Two of the studies conducted by Australian investigators reported response rates of 48% and 26%, with median survivals ranging from 7.5 months to 10 months.[204,205] In contrast, a European study conducted by van Haarst and colleagues reported a response rate of only 16%.[206]

Vinorelbine, a microtubule inhibitor, demonstrated an encouraging response rate of 21% among 64 mesothelioma patients in a single phase II study.[207] The patients' quality of life with respect to lung-related symptoms and overall physical well-being also improved. Nevertheless, in a subsequent study performed by the same group oxaliplatin added to vinorelbine demonstrated a response rate of only 10% among 21 patients and was associated with higher toxicity.[208] Other chemotherapy drugs such as docetaxel and capecitabine have been evaluated in patients with mesothelioma and have demonstrated modest benefits.[209,210]

The antimetabolites, particularly antifolates, have the highest response rates in mesothelioma, while platinum compounds and anthracyclines have a slightly lower response rate.[211] Pemetrexed disodium (Alimta, LY231514; Eli Lilly and Company, Indianapolis, IN), is a novel antifolate antimetabolite with multiple enzyme targets involved in both pyrimidine and purine synthesis. Pemetrexed primarily inhibits thymidylate synthase (TS), a folate-dependent enzyme that catalyzes the transformation of deoxyuridine monophosphate (dUMP) to deoxythymidine monophosphate (dTMP),[212] dihydrofolate reductase (DHFR) and glycinamide ribonucleotide formyl transferase (GARFT), a folate dependent enzyme involved in purine synthesis.[212,213] The primary toxicities observed in phase I studies were hematologic, fatigue, diarrhea, mucositis, and cutaneous rash.[214–217] Elevated homocysteine levels at baseline, a sensitive marker of folate deficiency, is highly correlated with severe toxicity, primarily neutropenia accompanied by diarrhea, and a multivariate analysis of adverse events and toxic deaths confirmed the linkage of pemetrexed toxicities to baseline folic acid and Vitamin B_{12} deficiencies.[218] All patients receiving pemetrexed must be supplemented with folic acid (350 μg to 1,000 μg daily) and Vitamin B_{12} (1,000 μg IM every 9 weeks) to prevent associated toxicities. Scagliotti and colleagues evaluated pemetrexed as front line therapy for MPM[219] in 64 patients. The overall response rate was 14.1% and the median survival was 10.7 months. Among the 43 patients who had vitamin supplementation, 7 responded (16.3%) and had a median survival of 13 months as compared with a response rate of 9.5% and a median survival of 8 months among the 21 patients who did not receive vitamin supplementation.

The benefits of the combination of pemetrexed and cisplatin in phase II studies led to the largest phase III study (EMPHACIS trial: Evaluation of Mesothelioma in a phase III study of Alimta and Cisplatin) conducted in MPM patients.[220] A total of 456 patients were randomized to receive either cisplatin 75 mg/m^2 monotherapy or in combination with pemetrexed at 500 mg/m^2. The median survival for the patients who received cisplatin/pemetrexed was 12.1 months, while it was 9.3 months ($p = .02$) for the patients who received cisplatin. Among the patients who received vitamin supplementation the median survival was 13.2 months for the combination arm and 9.4 months ($p = .022$) for the cisplatin arm. Both the response rates (41.3% vs 16.7%; $p < .001$) and median time to progressive disease (5.7 mo vs 3.9 mo; $p = .001$) were significantly better for the patients who received cisplatin/pemetrexed. In a Cox multiple regression analysis, treatment with cisplatin/pemetrexed and vitamin supplementation were associated with prolonged survival.[221] Toxicities were greater in the combination arm than the control arm; however, the toxicities were manageable particularly with vitamin supplementation. Almost all the toxicities in the cisplatin/pemetrexed arm were reduced with vitamin supplementation. Three deaths thought to be possibly study drug-related occurred in the cisplatin/pemetrexed arm among patients who had never received vitamin supplementation. The results of this trial led to FDA approval of the combination of pemetrexed and cisplatinum for mesothelioma in 2004.

Alimta has been combined with other agents for mesothelioma. Hughes and colleagues conducted a phase I study evaluating the combination of carboplatin and pemetrexed in patients with malignant mesothelioma to determine the maximum tolerated dose (MTD) and to evaluate antitumor activity.[222] Patients in this study did not receive folic acid or B_{12} supplementation, since the data regarding vitamin supplementation were not available at the time the study was conducted. The main toxicity observed with the combination was neutropenia. Other toxicities observed were nausea, emesis, rash, and stomatitis. The phase II dose of the combination was determined as carboplatin AUC 5 mg/mL/min and pemetrexed 500 mg/m^2 every 21 days. Among 25 assessable mesothelioma patients, 8 (32%) achieved partial remission and 14 patients experienced stable disease.

Oxaliplatin has been combined with pemetrexed in a phase I trial to evaluate the maximum tolerated dose (MTD) of this combination.[223] The dose-limiting toxicities with the combination were diarrhea, febrile neutropenia, and paresthesia. The MTD was pemetrexed 500 mg/m^2 followed by oxaliplatin at 130 mg/m^2 on day 1, repeated every 21 days.

There is a completed phase II study evaluating the combination of gemcitabine and pemetrexed in patients with malignant mesothelioma. The study is evaluating two different schedules by enrolling patients into two separate cohorts. In the first schedule, patients will receive pemetrexed on day 8, while the patients in second cohort will receive pemetrexed on day 1. Patients in both cohorts receive gemcitabine on days 1 and 8 every 3 weeks. Pemetrexed has also been combined with vinorelbine.[224]

Targeted Therapies Patients with mesothelioma have significantly higher serum levels of vascular endothelial growth factor (VEGF) than patients with any other solid tumors.[225] Various agents targeting VEGF signaling are currently being evaluated in mesothelioma patients, including bevacizumab, an anti-VEGF monoclonal antibody. Other targets that have generated interest in the recent past include the epidermal growth factor receptor (EGFR) and the platelet-derived growth factor (PDGF). Since both these receptors are expressed in mesotheliomas,[226,227] two separate phase II studies evaluating inhibitors of these receptors in mesothelioma patients were recently reported. The response rates, however, with both an EGFR inhibitor and PDGF inhibitor were disappointing.[228,229] Whether or not these or other biologic agents in combination with chemotherapy drugs such as pemetrexed demonstrate benefits in mesothelioma patients remains to be determined.

REFERENCES

1. Wagner JC, Sleggs CA, Marchand P. Diffuse pleural mesothelioma and asbestos exposure in the North Western Cape Province. Br J Ind Med 1960;17:260–71.
2. Selikoff IJ, Churg J, Hammond EC. Relation between exposure to asbestos and mesothelioma. N Engl J Med 1965;272:560–5.
3. Price B, Ware A. Mesothelioma trends in the United States: an update based on Surveillance, Epidemiology, and End Results Program data for 1973 through 2003. Am J Epidemiol 2004;159:107–12.
4. Enterline PE, Henderson VL. Geographic patterns for pleural mesothelioma deaths in the United States, 1968–81. J Natl Cancer Inst 1987;79:31–7.
5. Gardner MJ, Winter PD, Pannett B, et al. Mortality study of workers in the man-made mineral fiber production industry in the United Kingdom. Scand J Work Environ Health 1986;12 Suppl 1:85–93.
6. Connelly RR, Spirtas R, Myers MH, et al. Demographic patterns for mesothelioma in the United States. J Natl Cancer Inst 1987;78:1053–60.
7. Hillerdal G. Malignant mesothelioma 1982: review of 4710 published cases. Br J Dis Chest 1983;77:321–43.
8. Edwards JG, Abrams KR, Leverment JN, et al. Prognostic factors for malignant mesothelioma in 142 patients: validation of CALGB and EORTC prognostic scoring systems. Thorax 2000;55:731–5.
9. Coffin CM, Dehner LP. Mesothelial and related neoplasms in children and adolescents: a clinicopathologic and immunohistochemical analysis of eight cases. Pediatr Pathol 1992;12:333–47.
10. Landrigan PJ. A population of children at risk of exposure to asbestos in place. Ann N Y Acad Sci 1991;643:283–6.
11. Fraire AE, Cooper S, Greenberg SD, et al. Mesothelioma of childhood. Cancer 1988;62:838–47.
12. Cugell DW, Kamp DW. Asbestos and the pleura: a review. Chest 2004;125:1103–17.
13. Ohar J, Sterling DA, Bleecker E, Donohue J. Changing patterns in asbestos-induced lung disease. Chest 2004;125:744–53.
14. LaDou J. The asbestos cancer epidemic. Environ Health Perspect 2004;112:285–90.
15. Nicholson WJ, Perkel G, Selikoff IJ. Occupational exposure to asbestos: population at risk and projected mortality—1980–2030. Am J Ind Med 1982;3:259–311.
16. Roggli VL, Sharma A, Butnor KJ, et al. Malignant mesothelioma and occupational exposure to asbestos: a clinicopathological correlation of 1445 cases. Ultrastruct Pathol 2002;26:55–65.
17. Chahinian AP, Pajak TF, Holland JF, et al. Diffuse malignant mesothelioma. Prospective evaluation of 69 patients. Ann Intern Med 1982;96:746–55.
18. Chapman S, Heidemann A, Woodward S. Were asbestos-filtered Kent cigarettes sold in Australia? Aust NZ J Public Health 1996;20:218–9.
19. Longo WE, Rigler MW, Slade J. Crocidolite asbestos fibers in smoke from original Kent cigarettes. Cancer Res 1995;55:2232–5.
20. King JA, Wong SW. Autopsy evaluation of asbestos exposure: retrospective study of 135 cases with quantitation of ferruginous bodies in digested lung tissue. South Med J 1996;89:380–5.
21. Hawkins R. Types of asbestos fibers and disease-causing potential. Am Fam Physician 1994;50:308.
22. Manning CB, Vallyathan V. Mossman BT. Diseases caused by asbestos: mechanisms of injury and disease development. Int Immunopharmacol 2002;2:191–200.
23. Rogers AJ, Leigh J, Berry G, et al. Relationship between lung asbestos fiber type and concentration and relative risk of mesothelioma. A case-control study. Cancer 2004;67:1912–20.
24. Roggli VL, Vollmer RT, Butnor KJ, Sporn TA. Tremolite and mesothelioma. Ann Occup Hyg 2002;46:447–53.
25. McDonald JC, Harris J, Armstrong B. Mortality in a cohort of vermiculite miners exposed to fibrous amphibole in Libby, Montana. Occup Environ Med 2004;61:363–6.
26. Roggli VL. Malignant mesothelioma and duration of asbestos exposure: correlation with tissue mineral fibre content. Ann Occup Hyg 1995;39:363–74.
27. Nolan RP, Langer AM, Addison J. Lung content analysis of cases occupationally exposed to chrysotile asbestos. Environ Health Perspect 1994;102 Suppl 5:245–50.
28. Roggli VL, Longo WE. Mineral fiber content of lung tissue in patients with environmental exposures: household contacts vs. building occupants. Ann N Y Acad Sci 1991;643:511–8.
29. Smith AH, Wright CC. Chrysotile asbestos is the main cause of pleural mesothelioma. Am J Ind Med 1996;30:252–66.
30. Wagner JC, Newhouse ML, Corrin B, et al. Correlation between fibre content of the lung and disease in east London asbestos factory workers. Br J Ind Med 1988;45:305–8.
31. Harington JS. Fiber carcinogenesis: epidemiologic observations and the Stanton hypothesis. J Natl Cancer Inst 1981;67:977–89.
32. Stanton MF, Layard M, Tegeris A, et al. Relation of particle dimension to carcinogenicity in amphibole asbestoses and other fibrous minerals. J Natl Cancer Inst 1981;67:965–75.
33. Rom WN, Travis WD, Brody AR. Cellular and molecular basis of the asbestos-related diseases. Am Rev Respir Dis 1991;143:408–22.
34. Kannerstein M, Churg J, McCaughey E, Selikoff IJ. Pathogenic effects of asbestos. Arch Pathol Lab Med 1977;101:623–8.
35. Stenton SC. Asbestos, simian virus 40 and malignant mesothelioma. Thorax 1997;52 Suppl 3:S52–7.
36. Mossman BT, Kamp DW, Weitzman SA. Mechanisms of carcinogenesis and clinical features of asbestos-associated cancers. Cancer Invest 1996;14:466–80.
37. Donington JS, Mew DJ, Pass HI. Malignant pleural mesothelioma: newer aspects of carcinogenesis, molecular genetics, and prospects for future therapies. Surg Oncol 1995;4:175–85.
38. Gazdar AF, Butel JS, Carbone M. SV40 and human tumours: myth, association or causality? Nat Rev Cancer 2002;2:957–64.
39. Versnel MA, Claesson-Welsh L, Hammacher A, et al. Human malignant mesothelioma cell lines express PDGF beta-receptors whereas cultured normal mesothelial cells express predominantly PDGF alpha-receptors. Oncogene 1991;6:2005–11.
40. Cacciotti P, Libener R, Betta P, et al. SV40 replication in human mesothelial cells induces HGF/Met receptor activation: a model for viral-related carcinogenesis of human malignant mesothelioma. Proc Natl Acad Sci U S A 2001;98:12032–7.
41. Thirkettle I, Harvey P, Hasleton PS, Ball RY, Warn RM. Immunoreactivity for cadherins, HGF/SF, met, and erbB-2 in pleural malignant mesotheliomas. Histopathology 2000;36:522–8.
42. Pass HI, Mew DJ, Carbone M, et al. The effect of an antisense expression plasmid to the IGF-1 receptor on hamster mesothelioma proliferation. Dev Biol Stand 1998;94:321–8.
43. Hodzic D, Delacroix L, Willemsen P, et al. Characterization of the IGF system and analysis of the possible molecular mechanisms leading to IGF-II overexpression in a mesothelioma. Horm Metab Res 1997;29:549–55.
44. Lee TC, Zhang Y, Aston C, et al. Normal human mesothelial cells and mesothelioma cell lines express insulin-like growth factor I and associated molecules. Cancer Res 1993;53:2858–64.
45. Kumar-Singh S, Weyler J, Martin MJ, et al. Angiogenic cytokines in mesothelioma: a study of VEGF, FGF-1 and -2, and TGF beta expression. J Pathol 1999;189:72–8.
46. Maeda J, Ueki N, Ohkawa T, et al. Transforming growth factor-beta 1 (TGF-beta 1)- and beta 2-like activities in malignant pleural effusions caused by malignant mesothelioma or primary lung cancer. Clin Exp Immunol 1994;98:319–22.
47. Carbone M, Kratzke RA, Testa JR. The pathogenesis of mesothelioma. Semin Oncol 2002;29:2–17.
48. Carbone M, Pass HI, Miele L, Bocchetta M. New developments about the association of SV40 with human mesothelioma. Oncogene 2003;22:5173–80.
49. Gazdar AF, Butel JS, Carbone M. SV40 and human tumours: myth, association or causality? Nat Rev Cancer 2002;2:957–64.
50. Bocchetta M, Miele L, Pass HI, Carbone M. Notch-1 induction, a novel activity of SV40 required for growth of SV40-transformed human mesothelial cells. Oncogene 2003;22:81–9.
51. Foddis R, De Rienzo A, Broccoli D, et al. SV40 infection induces telomerase activity in human mesothelial cells. Oncogene 2002;21:1434–42.
52. Cicala C, Pompetti F, Carbone M. SV40 induces mesotheliomas in hamsters. Am J Pathol 1993;142:1524–33.
53. Gazdar AF, Butel JS, Carbone M. SV40 and human tumours: myth, association or causality? Nat Rev Cancer 2:957–64.
54. Klein G, Powers A, Croce C. Association of SV40 with human tumors. Oncogene 2002;21:1141–9.
55. Wong M, Pagano JS, Schiller JT, et al. New associations of human papillomavirus, simian virus 40, and Epstein-Barr virus with human cancer. J Natl Cancer Inst 2002;94:1832–6.
56. Toyooka S, Carbone M, Toyooka KO, et al. Progressive aberrant methylation of the RASSF1A gene in simian virus 40 infected human mesothelial cells. Oncogene 2002;21:4340–4.
57. Bocchetta M, Di Resta I, Powers A, et al. Human mesothelial cells are unusually susceptible to simian virus 40-mediated transformation and asbestos cocarcinogenicity. Proc Natl Acad Sci U S A 2000;97:10214–9.
58. Emri S, Demir A, Dogan M, et al. Lung diseases due to environmental exposures to erionite and asbestos in Turkey, Toxicol Lett 2002;127:251–7.
59. Wagner JC. Mesothelioma and mineral fibers. Cancer 1986;57:1905–11.
60. Suzuki Y, Kohyama N. Malignant mesothelioma induced by asbestos and zeolite in the mouse peritoneal cavity. Environ Res 1984;35:277–92.
61. Wagner JC. Mesothelioma and mineral fibers. Cancer 57:1986;1905–11.
62. Baris YI, Sahin AA, Ozesmi M, et al. An outbreak of pleural mesothelioma and chronic fibrosing pleurisy in the village of Karain/Urgup in Anatolia. Thorax 1978;33:181–92.
63. Artvinli M, Baris YI. Malignant mesotheliomas in a small village in the Anatolian region of Turkey: an epidemiologic study. J Natl Cancer Inst 1979;63: 17–22.
64. Baris YI, Artvinli M, Sahin AA. Environmental mesothelioma in Turkey. Ann N Y Acad Sci 1979;330:423–32.
65. Baris YI, Saracci R, Simonato L, et al. Malignant mesothelioma and radiological chest abnormalities in two villages in Central Turkey. An epidemiological and environmental investigation. Lancet 1981;1:984–7.
66. Baris I, Simonato L, Artvinli M, et al. Epidemiological and environmental evidence of the health effects of exposure to erionite fibres: a four-year study in the Cappadocian region of Turkey. Int J Cancer 1987;39:10–7.
67. Baris B, Demir AU, Shehu V, et al. Environmental fibrous zeolite (erionite) exposure and malignant tumors other than mesothelioma. J Environ Pathol Toxicol Oncol 1996;15:183–9.
68. Artvinli M, Baris YI. Malignant mesotheliomas in a small village in the Anatolian region of Turkey: an epidemiologic study. J Natl Cancer Inst 1979;63:17–22.
69. Wagner JC, Skidmore JW, Hill RJ, Griffiths DM. Erionite exposure and mesotheliomas in rats. Br J Cancer 1985;51:727–30.
70. Emri S, Demir A, Dogan M, et al. Lung diseases due to environmental exposures to erionite and asbestos in Turkey. Toxicol Lett 2002;127:251–7 .
71. Emri S, Demir A, Dogan M, et al. Lung diseases due to environmental exposures to erionite and asbestos in Turkey. Toxicol Lett 2002;127:251–7.
72. Roushdy-Hammady I, Siegel J, Emri S, et al. Genetic-susceptibility factor and malignant mesothelioma in the Cappadocian region of Turkey. Lancet 2001;357:444–5.
73. Huncharek M. Non-asbestos related diffuse malignant mesothelioma. Tumori 2002;88:1–9.
74. van Kaick G, Dalheimer A, Hornik S, et al. The german thorotrast study: recent results and assessment of risks. Radiat Res 1999;152:S64–71.
75. Neugut AI, Ahsan H, Antman KH. Incidence of malignant pleural mesothelioma after thoracic radiotherapy. Cancer 1997;80:948–50.
76. Hirano H, Maeda H, Sawabata N, et al. Desmoplastic malignant mesothelioma: two cases and a literature review. Med Electron Microsc 2003;36:173–8.
77. Khalidi HS, Medeiros LJ, Battifora H. Lymphohistiocytoid mesothelioma. An often misdiagnosed variant of sarcomatoid malignant mesothelioma. Am J Clin Pathol 2000;113:649–54.
78. Corson JM. Pathology of mesothelioma. Thorac Surg Clin 2004;14:447–60.
79. Fetsch PA, Abati A. Immunocytochemistry in effusion cytology: a contemporary review. Cancer 2001;93:293–308.
80. De Ruysscher D, Slotman B. Treatment of intervention sites of malignant pleural mesothelioma with radiotherapy: a Dutch-Belgian survey. Radiother Oncol 2003;68:299–302.
81. Pass HI, Kranda K, Temeck BK, et al. Surgically debulked malignant pleural mesothelioma: results and prognostic factors. Ann Surg Oncol 1997;4:215–22.

82. Pass HI, Vogelzang N, Hahn S, Carbone M. Malignant pleural mesothelioma. Curr Probl Cancer 2004;28:93–174.
83. Marom EM, Erasmus JJ, Pass HI, Patz EF Jr. The role of imaging in malignant pleural mesothelioma. Semin Oncol 2002;29:26–35.
84. Patz EF Jr, Shaffer K, Piwnica-Worms DR, et al. Malignant pleural mesothelioma: value of CT and MR imaging in predicting respectability. AJR Am J Roentgenol 1992;159:961–6.
85. Nanni C, Castellucci P, Farsad M, et al. Role of 18F-FDG PET for evaluating malignant pleural mesothelioma. Cancer Biother Radiopharm 2004;19:149–54.
86. Wang Z J, Reddy GP, Gotway MB, et al. Malignant pleural mesothelioma: evaluation with CT, MR imaging, and PET. Radiographics 2004;24:105–19.
87. Blanc FX, Atassi K, Bignon J, Housset B. Diagnostic value of medical thoracoscopy in pleural disease: a 6-year retrospective study. Chest 2002;121:1677–83.
88. Boutin C, Frenay C, Astoul P. Endoscopic diagnosis of mesothelioma. Rev Mal Respir 1999;16:1257–62.
89. Roboz J, Chahinian AP, Holland JF, et al. Early diagnosis and monitoring of transplanted human malignant mesothelioma by serum hyaluronic acid. J Natl Cancer Inst 1989;81:924–8.
90. Thylen A, Hjerpe A, Martensson G. Hyaluronan content in pleural fluid as a prognostic factor in patients with malignant pleural mesothelioma. Cancer 2001;92:1224–30.
91. Thylen A, Wallin J, Martensson G. Hyaluronan in serum as an indicator of progressive disease in hyaluronan-producing malignant mesothelioma. Cancer 1999;86:2000–5.
92. Hedman M, Arnberg H, Wernlund J, et al. Tissue polypeptide antigen (TPA), hyaluronan and CA 125 as serum markers in malignant mesothelioma. Anticancer Res 2003;23:531–6.
93. Paganuzzi M, Onetto M, Marroni P, et al. Diagnostic value of CYFRA 21-1 tumor marker and CEA in pleural effusion due to mesothelioma. Chest 2001;119:1138–42.
94. Lee YC, Knox BS, Garrett JE. Use of cytokeratin fragments 19.1 and 19.21 (Cyfra 21-1) in the differentiation of malignant and benign pleural effusions. Aust N Z J Med 1999;29:765–9.
95. Bonfrer JM, Schouwink JH, Korse CM, Baas P. Cyfra 21-1 and TPA as markers in malignant mesothelioma. Anticancer Res 1997;17:2971–3.
96. Almudevar BE, Garcia-Rostan Perez GM, Garcia BF, Jimenez C. Prognostic value of high serum levels of CA-125 in malignant secretory peritoneal mesotheliomas affecting young women. A case report with differential diagnosis and review of the literature. Histopathology 1997;31:267–73.
97. Chang K, Pastan I. Molecular cloning of mesothelin, a differentiation antigen present on mesothelium, mesotheliomas, and ovarian cancers. Proc Natl Acad Sci U S A 1996;93:136–40.
98. Robinson BW, Creaney J, Lake R, et al. Mesothelin-family proteins and diagnosis of mesothelioma. Lancet 2003;362:1612–6.
99. Robinson BW, Creaney J, Lake R, et al. Soluble mesothelin-related protein-A blood test for mesothelioma. Lung Cancer 2005;49 Suppl 1:S109–11.
100. Sugarbaker PH, Welch LS, Mohamed F, Glehen O. A review of peritoneal mesothelioma at the Washington Cancer Institute. Surg Oncol Clin North Am 2003;12:605–21, xi.
101. Acherman YI, Welch LS, Bromley CM, Sugarbaker PH. Clinical presentation of peritoneal mesothelioma. Tumori 2003;89:269–73.
102. Van de WP, Blomme Y, Van OL. Laparoscopy and primary diffuse malignant peritoneal mesothelioma: a diagnostic challenge. Acta Chir Belg 2004;104:114–7.
103. Feldman AL, Libutti SK, Pingpank JF, et al. Analysis of factors associated with outcome in patients with malignant peritoneal mesothelioma undergoing surgical debulking and intraperitoneal chemotherapy. J Clin Oncol 2003;21:4560–7.
104. Koutselini HA, Lazaris AC, Thomopoulou G, et al. Papillary serous carcinoma of peritoneum: case study and review of the literature on the differential diagnosis of malignant peritoneal tumors. Adv Clin Path 2001;5:99–104.
105. Dumke K, Schnoy N, Specht G, Buse H. Comparative light and electron microscopic studies of cystic and papillary tumors of the peritoneum. Virchows Arch A Pathol Anat Histopathol 1983;399:25–39.
106. Kannerstein M, Churg J, McCaughey WT, Hill DP. Papillary tumors of the peritoneum in women: mesothelioma or papillary carcinoma. Am J Obstet Gynecol 1977;127:306–14.
107. Epler GR, McLoud TC, Gaensler EA. Prevalence and incidence of benign asbestos pleural effusion in a working population. JAMA 1982;247:617–22.
108. Curran D, Sahmoud T, Therasse P, et al. Prognostic factors in patients with pleural mesothelioma: the European Organization for Research and Treatment of Cancer experience. J Clin Oncol 1998;16:145–52.
109. Pass HI, Liu Z, Wali A, et al. Gene expression profiles predict survival and progression of pleural mesothelioma. Clin Cancer Res 2004;10:849–59.
110. Gordon GJ, Jensen RV, Hsiao LL, et al. Using gene expression ratios to predict outcome among patients with mesothelioma. J Natl Cancer Inst 2003;95:598–605.
111. Eren NT, Akar AR. Primary pericardial mesothelioma. Curr Treat Options Oncol 2002;3:369–73.
112. Quinn DW, Qureshi F, Mitchell IM. Pericardial mesothelioma: the diagnostic dilemma of misleading images. Ann Thorac Surg 2000;69:1926–7.
113. Warren WH. Malignancies involving the pericardium. Semin Thorac Cardiovasc Surg 2000;12:119–29.
114. Vigneswaran WT, Stefanacci PR. Pericardial mesothelioma. Curr Treat Options Oncol 2000;1:299–302.
115. Garcia de JA, Gil P, zua-Romeo J, et al. Malignant mesothelioma of the tunica vaginalis. Report of a case without risk factors and review of the literature. Int Urol Nephrol 2003;35:59–62.
116. Black PC, Lange PH, Takayama TK. Extensive palliative surgery for advanced mesothelioma of the tunica vaginalis. Urology 2003;62:748.
117. Abe K, Kato N, Miki K, et al. Malignant mesothelioma of testicular tunica vaginalis. Int J Urol 2002;9:602–3.
118. Bruno C, Minniti S, Procacci C. Diagnosis of malignant mesothelioma of the tunica vaginalis testis by ultrasound-guided fine-needle aspiration. J Clin Ultrasound 2002;30:181–3.
119. Mezzetti M, Panigalli T, Giudice FL, et al. Surgical experience of 15 solitary benign fibrous tumor of the pleura. Crit Rev Oncol Hematol 2003;47:29–33.
120. Perks WH, Stanhope R, Green M. Hyponatraemia and mesothelioma. Br J Dis Chest 1979;73:89–91.
121. Chang YL, Lee YC, Wu CT. Thoracic solitary fibrous tumor: clinical and pathological diversity. Lung Cancer 1999;23:53–60.
122. Kanthan R, Torkian B. Recurrent solitary fibrous tumor of the pleura with malignant transformation. Arch Pathol Lab Med 2004;128:460–2.
123. Zhang H, Lucas DR, Pass HI, Che M. Disseminated malignant solitary fibrous tumor of the pleura. Pathol Int 2004;54:111–5.
124. Wong WL, Johns TA, Herlihy WG, Martin HL. Best cases from the AFIP: multicystic mesothelioma. Radiographics 2004;24:247–50.
125. Sethna K, Mohamed F, Marchettini P, et al. Peritoneal cystic mesothelioma: a case series. Tumori 2003;89:31–5.
126. Sawh RN, Malpica A, Deavers MT, et al. Benign cystic mesothelioma of the peritoneum: a clinicopathologic study of 17 cases and immunohistochemical analysis of estrogen and progesterone receptor status. Hum Pathol 2003;34:369–74.
127. Hove KM, Joergensen A, Grove A. Benign multicystic peritoneal mesothelioma. Acta Obstet Gynecol Scand 2002;81:1083–5.
128. Hejmadi R, Ganesan R, Kamal NG. Malignant transformation of a well-differentiated peritoneal papillary mesothelioma. Acta Cytol 2003;47:517–8.
129. Gonzalez-Moreno S, Yan H, Alcorn KW, Sugarbaker PH. Malignant transformation of "benign" cystic mesothelioma of the peritoneum. J Surg Oncol 2002;79:243–51.
130. Usha Kiran TS, Agboola A, Davies R, Stout TV. Benign cystic mesothelioma: a diagnostic dilemma. Aust N Z J Obstet Gynaecol 2002;42:552–4.
131. Pass HI, Temeck BK, Kranda K, et al. Preoperative tumor volume is associated with outcome in malignant pleural mesothelioma. J Thorac Cardiovasc Surg 1998;115:310–7.
132. Rusch VW, Rosenzweig K, Venkatraman E, et al. A phase II trial of surgical resection and adjuvant high-dose hemithoracic radiation for malignant pleural mesothelioma. J Thorac Cardiovasc Surg 2001;122:788–95.
133. Rusch VW, Venkatraman ES. Important prognostic factors in patients with malignant pleural mesothelioma, managed surgically. Ann Thorac Surg 1999;68:1799–804.
134. Zellos LS, Sugarbaker DJ. Diffuse malignant mesothelioma of the pleural space and its management. Oncology (Huntingt) 2002;16:907–13.
135. Sugarbaker DJ, Flores RM, Jaklitsch MT, et al. Resection margins, extrapleural nodal status, and cell type determine postoperative long-term survival in trimodality therapy of malignant pleural mesothelioma: results in 183 patients. J Thorac Cardiovasc Surg 1999;117:54–63.
136. Schouwink JH, Kool LS, Rutgers EJ, et al. The value of chest computer tomography and cervical mediastinoscopy in the preoperative assessment of patients with malignant pleural mesothelioma. Ann Thorac Surg 2003;75:1715–8.
137. Flores RM, Akhurst T, Gonen M, et al. Positron emission tomography defines metastatic disease but not locoregional disease in patients with malignant pleural mesothelioma. J Thorac Cardiovasc Surg 2003;126:11–6.
138. Furedi A, Kecskes L, Geher P, Kiss B. Video-assisted thoracoscopic pleurodesis for malignant pleural effusions. Acta Chir Hung 1999;38:155–7.
139. Charvat JC, Brutsche M, Frey JG, Tschopp JM. Value of thoracoscopy and talc pleurodesis in diagnosis and palliative treatment of malignant pleural mesothelioma. Schweiz Rundsch Med Prax 1998;87:336–40.
140. Canto A, Guijarro R, Arnau A, et al. Videothoracoscopy in the diagnosis and treatment of malignant pleural mesothelioma with associated pleural effusions. Thorac Cardiovasc Surg 1997;45:16–9.
141. Viallat JR, Rey F, Astoul P, Boutin C. Thoracoscopic talc poudrage pleurodesis for malignant effusions. A review of 360 cases. Chest 1996;110:1387–93.
142. Brubacher S, Gobel BH. Use of the Pleurx Pleural Catheter for the management of malignant pleural effusions. Clin J Oncol Nurs 2003;7:35–8.
143. Putnam JB Jr, Walsh GL, Swisher SG, et al. Outpatient management of malignant pleural effusion by a chronic indwelling pleural catheter. Ann Thorac Surg 2000;69:369–75.
144. Pien GW, Gant MJ, Washam CL, Sterman DH. Use of an implantable pleural catheter for trapped lung syndrome in patients with malignant pleural effusion. Chest 2001;119:1641–6.
145. Rosenberg S, Courtney A, Nemcek AA Jr, Omary RA. Comparison of percutaneous management techniques for recurrent malignant ascites. J Vasc Interv Radiol 2004;15:1129–31.
146. Cowan SW, Pechet TT. Pleurectomy and decortication for malignant mesothelioma. Thorac Surg Clin 2004;14:517–21.
147. Rusch VW. Pleurectomy/decortication in the setting of multimodality treatment for diffuse malignant pleural mesothelioma. Semin Thorac Cardiovasc Surg 1997;9:367–72.
148. Soysal O, Karaoglanoglu N, Demiracan S, et al. Pleurectomy/decortication for palliation in malignant pleural mesothelioma: results of surgery. Eur J Cardiothorac Surg 1997;11:210–3.
149. Butchart EG, Ashcroft T, Barnsley WC, Holden MP. Pleuropneumonectomy in the management of diffuse malignant mesothelioma of the pleura. Experience with 29 patients. Thorax 1976;31:15–24.
150. DaValle MJ, Faber LP, Kittle CF, Jensik RJ. Extrapleural pneumonectomy for diffuse, malignant mesothelioma. Ann Thorac Surg 1986;42:612–8.
151. Rusch VW. Trials in malignant mesothelioma. LCSG 851 and 882. Chest 1994;106:359S–62S.
152. Sugarbaker DJ, Jaklitsch MT, Bueno R, et al. Prevention, early detection, and management of complications after 328 consecutive extrapleural pneumonectomies. J Thorac Cardiovasc Surg 2004;128:138–46.
153. Baldini EH, Recht A, Strauss GM, et al. Patterns of failure after trimodality therapy for malignant pleural mesothelioma. Ann Thorac Surg 1997;63:334–8.
154. Kukreja J, Jaklitsch MT, Wiener DC, et al. Malignant pleural mesothelioma: overview of the North American and European experience. Thorac Surg Clin 2004;14:435–45.
155. Hilaris BS, Nori D, Kwong E, et al. Pleurectomy and intraoperative brachytherapy and postoperative radiation in the treatment of malignant pleural mesothelioma. Int J Radiat Oncol Biol Phys 1984;10:325–31.
156. Cain J, Nori D, Huvos A, et al. The role of radioactive colloids in malignant peritoneal mesotheliomas. Gynecol Oncol 1983;16:263–74.
157. Ahamad A, Stevens CW, Smythe WR, et al. Intensity-modulated radiation therapy: a novel approach to the management of malignant pleural mesothelioma. Int J Radiat Oncol Biol Phys 2003;55:768–75.
158. Forster KM, Smythe WR, Starkschall G, et al. Intensity-modulated radiotherapy following extrapleural pneumonectomy for the treatment of malignant mesothelioma: clinical implementation. Int J Radiat Oncol Biol Phys 2003;55:606–16.
159. Calavrezos A, Koschel G, Husselmann H, et al. Malignant mesothelioma of the pleura. A prospective therapeutic

study of 132 patients from 1981–1985. Klin Wochenschr 1988;66:607–13.
160. Maggi G, Casadio C, Giobbe R, Ruffini E. The management of malignant pleural mesothelioma. Eur J Cardiothorac Surg 2003;23:255–6.
161. Maggi G, Giobbe R, Casadio C, Rena O. Palliative surgery for malignant pleural mesothelioma. Eur J Cardiothorac Surg 2002;21:1128–9.
162. Maggi G, Casadio C, Cianci R, et al. Trimodality management of malignant pleural mesothelioma. Eur J Cardiothorac Surg 2001;19:346–50.
163. Weder W, Kestenholz P, Taverna C, et al. Neoadjuvant chemotherapy followed by extrapleural pneumonectomy in malignant pleural mesothelioma. J Clin Oncol 2004;22:3451–7.
164. de Perrot M, Ginsberg R, Payne DA. Phase II Trial of Induction Chemotherapy followed by Extrapleural Pneumonectomy and High Dose Hemithoracic Radiation therapy for malignant pleural mesothelioma [abstract]. Lung Cancer 2003;41:S59.
165. Pass HI, Temeck BK, Kranda K, et al. Phase III randomized trial of surgery with or without intraoperative photodynamic therapy and postoperative immunochemotherapy for malignant pleural mesothelioma. Ann Surg Oncol 1997;4:628–33.
166. Bonnette P, Heckly GB, Villette S, Fragola A. Intraoperative photodynamic therapy after pleuropneumonectomy for malignant pleural mesothelioma. Chest 2002;122:1866–7.
167. Schouwink H, Baas P. Foscan-mediated photodynamic therapy and operation for malignant pleural mesothelioma. Ann Thorac Surg 2004;78:388.
168. Baas P, Murrer L, Zoetmulder FA, et al. Photodynamic therapy as adjuvant therapy in surgically treated pleural malignancies. Br J Cancer 1997;76:819–26.
169. Friedberg JS, Mick R, Stevenson J, et al. A phase I study of Foscan-mediated photodynamic therapy and surgery in patients with mesothelioma. Ann Thorac Surg 2003;75:952–9.
170. Rusch VW, Figlin R, Godwin D, Piantadosi S. Intrapleural cisplatin and cytarabine in the management of malignant pleural effusions: a Lung Cancer Study Group trial. J Clin Oncol 1991;9:313–9.
171. Colleoni M, Liessi G, Avventi C, et al. Response to chemotherapy of brain metastases from malignant pleural mesothelioma. Tumori 1996;82:456–8.
172. Yellin A, Simansky DA, Paley M, Refaely Y. Hyperthermic pleural perfusion with cisplatin: early clinical experience. Cancer 2001;92:2197–203.
173. Hotta T, Taniguchi K, Kobayashi Y, et al. Chemotherapy and serum hyaluronic acid levels in malignant peritoneal mesothelioma. Hepatogastroenterology 2004;51:1073–83.
174. Ratto GB, Civalleri D, Esposito M, et al. Pleural space perfusion with cisplatin in the multimodality treatment of malignant mesothelioma: a feasibility and pharmacokinetic study. J Thorac Cardiovasc Surg 1999;117:759–65.
175. Chang MY, Sugarbaker DJ. Innovative therapies: intraoperative intracavitary chemotherapy. Thorac Surg Clin 2004;14:549–56.
176. Sterman DH, Kaiser LR, Albelda SM. Gene therapy for malignant pleural mesothelioma. Hematol Oncol Clin North Am 1998;12:553–68.
177. Cordier KL, Valeyrie L, Fernandez N, et al. Regression of AK7 malignant mesothelioma established in immunocompetent mice following intratumoral gene transfer of interferon gamma. Cancer Gene Ther 2003;10:481–90.
178. Kruklitis RJ, Singhal S, Delong P, et al. Immuno-gene therapy with interferon-beta before surgical debulking delays recurrence and improves survival in a murine model of malignant mesothelioma. J Thorac Cardiovasc Surg 2004;127:123–30.
179. Mukherjee S, Nelson D, Loh S, et al. The immune antitumor effects of GM-CSF and B7-1 gene transfection are enhanced by surgical debulking of tumor. Cancer Gene Ther 2001;8:580–8.
180. Odaka M, Wiewrodt R, Delong P, et al. Analysis of the immunologic response generated by Ad.IFN-beta during successful intraperitoneal tumor gene therapy. Mol Ther 2002;6:210–8.
181. Odaka M, Sterman DH, Wiewrodt R, et al. Eradication of intraperitoneal and distant tumor by adenovirus-mediated interferon-beta gene therapy is attributable to induction of systemic immunity. Cancer Res 2001;61:6201–2.
182. Yang CT, You L, Lin YC, et al. A comparison analysis of anti-tumor efficacy of adenoviral gene replacement therapy (p14ARF and p16INK4A) in human mesothelioma cells. Anticancer Res 2003;23:33–8.
183. Yang CT, You L, Uematsu K, et al. p14(ARF) modulates the cytolytic effect of ONYX-015 in mesothelioma cells with wild-type p53. Cancer Res 2001;61:5959–63.
184. Boutin C, Nussbaum E, Monnet I, et al. Intrapleural treatment with recombinant gamma-interferon in early stage malignant pleural mesothelioma. Cancer 1994;74:2460–7.
185. Driesen P, Boutin C, Viallat JR, et al. Implantable access system for prolonged intrapleural immunotherapy. Eur Respir J 1994;7:1889–92.
186. Astoul P, Picat-Joossen D, Viallat JR, Boutin C. Intrapleural administration of interleukin-2 for the treatment of patients with malignant pleural mesothelioma: a phase II study. Cancer 1998;83:2099–104.
187. Baldini EH. External beam radiation therapy for the treatment of pleural mesothelioma. Thorac Surg Clin 2004;14:543–8.
188. Blake PR, Catterall M, Emerson PA. Pleural mesothelioma treated by fast neutron therapy. Thorax 1985;40:72–3.
189. Kindler HL. Malignant pleural mesothelioma. Curr Treat Options Oncol 2000;1:313–26.
190. Ong ST, Vogelzang NJ. Chemotherapy in malignant pleural mesothelioma. A review. J Clin Oncol 1996;14:1007–17.
191. Zidar BL, Metch B, Balcerzak SP, et al. A phase II evaluation of ifosfamide and mesna in unresectable diffuse malignant mesothelioma. A Southwest Oncology Group study. Cancer 1992;70:2547–51.
192. Mintzer DM, Kelsen D, Frimmer D, et al. Phase II trial of high-dose cisplatin in patients with malignant mesothelioma. Cancer Treat Rep 1985;69:711–2.
193. Planting AS, van der Burg ME, Goey SH, et al. Phase II study of a short course of weekly high-dose cisplatin combined with long-term oral etoposide in pleural mesothelioma. Ann Oncol 1995;6:613–5.
194. Chahinian AP, Antman K, Goutsou M, et al. Randomized phase II trial of cisplatin with mitomycin or doxorubicin for malignant mesothelioma by the Cancer and Leukemia Group B. J Clin Oncol 1993;11:1559–65.
195. Nakano T, Chahinian AP, Shinjo M, et al. Cisplatin in combination with irinotecan in the treatment of patients with malignant pleural mesothelioma: a pilot phase II clinical trial and pharmacokinetic profile. Cancer 1999;85:2375–84.
196. Mbidde EK, Harland SJ, Calvert AH, Smith IE. Phase II trial of carboplatin (JM8) in treatment of patients with malignant mesothelioma. Cancer Chemother Pharmacol 1986;18:284–5.
197. Raghavan D, Gianoutsos P, Bishop J, et al. Phase II trial of carboplatin in the management of malignant mesothelioma. J Clin Oncol 1990;8:151–4.
198. Vogelzang NJ, Goutsou M, Corson JM, et al. Carboplatin in malignant mesothelioma: a phase II study of the Cancer and Leukemia Group B. Cancer Chemother Pharmacol 1990;27:239–42.
199. Schutte W, Blankenburg T, Lauerwald K, et al. A multicenter phase II study of gemcitabine and oxaliplatin for malignant pleural mesothelioma. Clin Lung Cancer 2003;4:294–7.
200. Van Meerbeeck JP, Baas P, Debruyne C, et al. A phase II study of gemcitabine in patients with malignant pleural mesothelioma. European Organization for Research and Treatment of Cancer Lung Cancer Cooperative Group. Cancer 1999;85:2577–82.
201. Kindler HL, Millard F, Herndon JE, et al. Gemcitabine for malignant mesothelioma: A phase II trial by the Cancer and Leukemia Group B. Lung Cancer 2001;31:311–7.
202. Bischoff HG, Manegold C, Knopp M, et al. Gemcitabine my reduce tumor load and tumor associated symptoms in malignant pleural mesothelioma [abstract]. Proc Am Soc Clin Oncol 1998;17:464a.
203. Van Meerbeeck JP, Baas P, Debruyne C, et al. A phase II study of gemcitabine in patients with malignant pleural mesothelioma. European Organization for Research and Treatment of Cancer Lung Cancer Cooperative Group. Cancer 1999;85:2577–82.
204. Byrne MJ, Davidson JA, Musk W, et al. Cisplatin and gemcitabine treatment for malignant mesothelioma: a phase II study. J Clin Oncol 1999;17:25–30.
205. Nowak AK, Byrne MJ, Williamson R, et al. A multicentre phase II study of cisplatin and gemcitabine for malignant mesothelioma. Br J Cancer 2002;87:491–6.
206. van Haarst JM, Baas P, Manegold C, et al. Multicentre phase II study of gemcitabine and cisplatin in malignant pleural mesothelioma. Br J Cancer 2002;86:342–5,
207. Steele JP, Shamash J, Evans MT, et al. Phase II study of vinorelbine in patients with malignant pleural mesothelioma. J Clin Oncol 2000;8:3912–7.
208. Steele JP, Klabatsa A. Chemotherapy options and new advances in malignant pleural mesothelioma. Ann Oncol 2005;16:345–51.
209. Belani CP, Adak S, Aisner S, et al. Docetaxel for malignant mesothelioma: phase II study of the Eastern Cooperative Oncology Group. Clin Lung Cancer 2004;6:43–7.
210. Otterson GA, Herndon JE, Watson D, et al. Capecitabine in malignant mesothelioma: a phase II trial by the Cancer and Leukemia Group B (39807). Lung Cancer 2004;44:251–9.
211. Ong ST, Vogelzang NJ. Chemotherapy in malignant pleural mesothelioma. A review. J Clin Oncol 1996;14:1007–17.
212. Shih C, Chen VJ, Gossett LS, et al. LY231514, a pyrrolo[2,3-d]pyrimidine-based antifolate that inhibits multiple folate-requiring enzymes. Cancer Res 1997;57:1116–23.
213. Curtin NJ, Hughes AN. Pemetrexed disodium, a novel antifolate with multiple targets. Lancet Oncol 2001;2:298–306.
214. Rinaldi DA. Overview of phase I trials of multitargeted antifolate (MTA, LY231514). Semin Oncol 1999;26:82–8.
215. Rinaldi DA, Kuhn JG, Burris HA, et al. A phase I evaluation of multitargeted antifolate (MTA, LY231514), administered every 21 days, utilizing the modified continual reassessment method for dose escalation. Cancer Chemother Pharmacol 1999;44:372–80.
216. Rinaldi DA, Burris HA, Dorr FA, et al. Initial phase I evaluation of the novel thymidylate synthase inhibitor, LY231514, using the modified continual reassessment method for dose escalation. J Clin Oncol 1995;13:2842–50.
217. McDonald AC, Vasey PA, Adams L, et al. A phase I and pharmacokinetic study of LY231514, the multitargeted antifolate. Clin Cancer Res 1998;4:605–10.
218. Niyikiza C, Baker SD, Seitz DE, et al Homocysteine and methylmalonic acid: markers to predict and avoid toxicity from pemetrexed therapy. Mol Cancer Ther 2002;1:545–52.
219. Scagliotti GV, Shin DM, Kindler HL, et al. Phase II study of pemetrexed with and without folic acid and vitamin B12 as front-line therapy in malignant pleural mesothelioma. J Clin Oncol 2003;21:1556–61.
220. Vogelzang NJ, Rusthoven JJ, Symanowski J, et al. Phase III study of pemetrexed in combination with cisplatin versus cisplatin alone in patients with malignant pleural mesothelioma. J Clin Oncol 2003;21:2636–44.
221. Symanowski J, Rusthoven J, Nguyen B, et al. Multiple regression analysis of prognostic variables for survival from the phase III study of pemetrexed + cisplatin vs. cisplatin in malignant pleural mesothelioma [abstract]. Proc Am Soc Clin Oncol 2003;22.
222. Hughes A, Calvert P, Azzabi A, et al. Phase I clinical and pharmacokinetic study of pemetrexed and carboplatin in patients with malignant pleural mesothelioma. J Clin Oncol 2002;20:3533–44.
223. Misset JL. Bleiberg H, Sutherland W, et al. Oxaliplatin clinical activity: a review. Crit Rev Oncol Hematol 2000;35:75–93.
224. Millward AM, Clarke S, Beale P, et al. Phase I trial of Pemetrexed and Vinorelbine in patients with advanced cancer [abstract]. Proc Am Soc Clin Oncol 2001:20.
225. Linder C, Linder S, Munck-Wikland E, Strander H. Independent expression of serum vascular endothelial growth factor (VEGF) and basic fibroblast growth factor (bFGF) in patients with carcinoma and sarcoma. Anticancer Res 1998;18:2063–8.
226. Morocz IA, Schmitter D, Lauber B, Stahel RA. Autocrine stimulation of a human lung mesothelioma cell line is mediated through the transforming growth factor alpha/epidermal growth factor receptor mitogenic pathway. Br J Cancer 1994;70:850–6.
227. Langerak AW, Van der Linden-Van Beurden CA, Versnel MA. Regulation of differential expression of platelet-derived growth factor alpha- and beta-receptor mRNA in normal and malignant human mesothelial cell lines. Biochim Biophys Acta 1996;1305:63–70.
228. Kratzke RA, Govindan R, Herndon JE. Gefitinib in patients with malignant mesothelioma. A phase II study by the CALGB [abstract]. Proc Am Soc Clin Oncol 2003;22:630.
229. Millward M, Parnis F, Byrne A, et al. A phase II trial of imatinib mesylate in patients with advanced pleural mesothelioma [abstract]. Proc Am Soc Clin Oncol 2003;22:228.

82

Thymomas and Thymic Tumors

A. Philippe Chahinian, MD

The thymus, a key immune system organ, can be the site of many different benign and malignant tumors (Table 82-1). Rosai and Levine emphasized that thymoma is restricted to neoplasms of the thymic epithelial cells.[1] Givel published a detailed historical review of the thymus gland and thymomas.[2] The first description of a thymic tumor is credited to Sir Astley Paston Cooper, a surgeon from London, in 1832. In 1849, the British microscopist Arthur Hill Hassall described the corpuscles unique to the thymus. The first association between myasthenia gravis (MG) and thymoma was discovered in 1899 by the German neurologist Hermann Oppenheim. The first thymectomy for MG was performed in 1911 by Ernst Ferdinand Sauerbruch in Zurich, Switzerland. The thymus showed hyperplasia but no tumor, and myasthenia improved markedly after surgery. Alfred Blalock at Vanderbilt University in Nashville, Tennessee, pioneered the surgical technique of total thymectomy in 1936 (case published in 1939) and advocated it for the treatment of MG.

EPIDEMIOLOGY AND ETIOLOGY

Thymomas are usually slow-growing tumors with about equal incidence in men and women; they occur through a wide age range, with a peak in the forties and fifties.[3–5] Thymomas are rare, and more aggressive, in children.

There are no known etiologic factors for thymomas. Among 23 patients with thymoma, Cohen and colleagues noted that 2 had received radiation for an enlarged thymus in childhood, 17 and 28 years before the diagnosis of thymoma, respectively.[6] In the past, that practice was based on the belief that such physiologic enlargement of the thymus in some infants could cause sudden death (status thymicolymphaticus).[1] Such radiation leads to an increased incidence of cancer, particularly of the thyroid and breast.[1,7] The role of Epstein-Barr virus (EBV) in the etiology of a subtype of thymic carcinoma, the lymphoepithelioma variety, has been documented, as discussed below.

Table 82-1 Thymic Tumors

- Tumors of the thymic epithelium
  - Thymomas (encapsulated or invasive)
  - Thymic carcinomas
    - Lymphoepithelioma
    - Squamous cell
      - Keratinizing
      - Basaloid
    - Clear cell
    - Sarcomatoid
    - Mucoepidermoid
    - Small cell (oat-cell)
- Neuroendocrine tumors
  - Thymic carcinoids
- Lymphoid tumors
  - Hodgkin's disease
  - Burkitt's lymphoma
  - T-Cell lymphoblastic (children)
  - B-Cell (with sclerosis)
  - Other lymphomas
- Germ cell tumors
  - Seminomas
  - Teratomas
  - Carcinomas
    - Embryonal
    - Yolk-sac
    - Choriocarcinoma
    - Teratocarcinoma
- Thymolipoma
- Thymic cysts
- Metastases

ANATOMIC PATHOGENESIS

Embryology and Anatomy The thymus is embryologically derived from the endodermal epithelium of the third pharyngeal pouches (which also give rise to the lower pair of parathyroid glands) and, less constantly, the fourth ones as well.[1,5] The right and left thymic anlagen migrate downward into the anterosuperior mediastinum, joining together without complete fusion to form a bilobate organ.[1] Although most thymic tumors are located in the anterosuperior mediastinum, variations in migration account for the findings of gross or microscopic thymic tissue anywhere between the hyoid bone superiorly and the diaphragm inferiorly.[8] Wide exposure of the mediastinum and even the neck is therefore necessary if surgical removal of the entire thymus is indicated, as in patients with thymoma or those with MG (with or without associated thymoma).[8] The absolute weight of the thymus reaches its peak in the pubertal years (mean 34 ± 15 g between age 10 and 15 years) and then gradually decreases, although this age-related involution normally is never complete.[1]

Histologically, the normal thymus shows distinctive lobules with a sharp demarcation between the cortex, rich in lymphocytes, and the medulla, rich in epithelial cells and characteristic Hassall's corpuscles, formed by concentric layers of mature epithelial cells.

The thymus plays a critical role in the maturation of bone marrow–derived lymphocytes into T cells and, as such, in cell-mediated immunity. It has a rich blood supply but no afferent lymphatics. Efferent lymphatics apparently originate from perivascular spaces and drain into the mediastinal and lower cervical nodes.[1]

Pathology of Thymomas Distinctive features reminiscent of the normal thymus make the pathologic diagnosis of thymoma easy in most cases. A fibrous capsule surrounds the tumor and sends thick, fibrous septa, dividing the tumor into well-demarcated lobules.[1,9–11] Microscopically, there is a distinctive dual-cell population, including lymphocytes (small with dark nuclei) and epithelial cells (larger and lighter) (Plate 19, Figure 82-1). Quantitatively, the lymphocyte to epithelial cell ratio varies widely (average about 2).[12] Even though there is a continuum among the extremes, thymomas are often classified according to the relative ratio of cells between predominantly lymphocytic, mixed epithelial-lymphocytic, and predominantly epithelial. In 4% of cases, only epithelial cells are seen.[1] Because thymomas are defined as neoplasms of thymic epithelial cells, pure lymphocytic tumors are not thymomas and should raise the possibility of lymphoma. The epithelial cells represent the neoplastic component of thymomas.[1] They appear to be cytologically bland; mitosis and cellular atypia are rare. They are typically round or oval but sometimes have a spindle-shaped nucleus, which may represent the predominant cell in approximately 5 to 12% of thymomas, justifying the term *spindle-cell thymoma*, which tends to grow more slowly and to be associated with red cell hypoplasia or hypogammaglobulinemia rather than MG.[1,9] The lymphocytes are not considered neoplastic and, as in the normal thymus, are constituted mainly of T cells in various stages of maturation. They often exhibit mitotic figures. A higher percentage of epithelial cells reportedly has a negative prognostic influence, as seen in cases with recurrent tumor or a more advanced stage.[12–14]

A new histologic classification was recently proposed by the World Health Organization (WHO).[15] Thymic epithelial tumors are classified as follows:

Type A: homogeneous population of neoplastic epithelial cells with a spindle or oval shape

Type AB: type A thymoma admixed with lymphocytes

Type B1: tumor resembles the normal functional thymus

Type B2: plump neoplastic epithelial cells with vesicular nuclei and distinct nucleoli

Type B3: predominantly round or polygonal epithelial cells with mild atypia

Type C: all thymic carcinomas

There are no reliable histologic features of "malignancy" for thymomas. The malignant

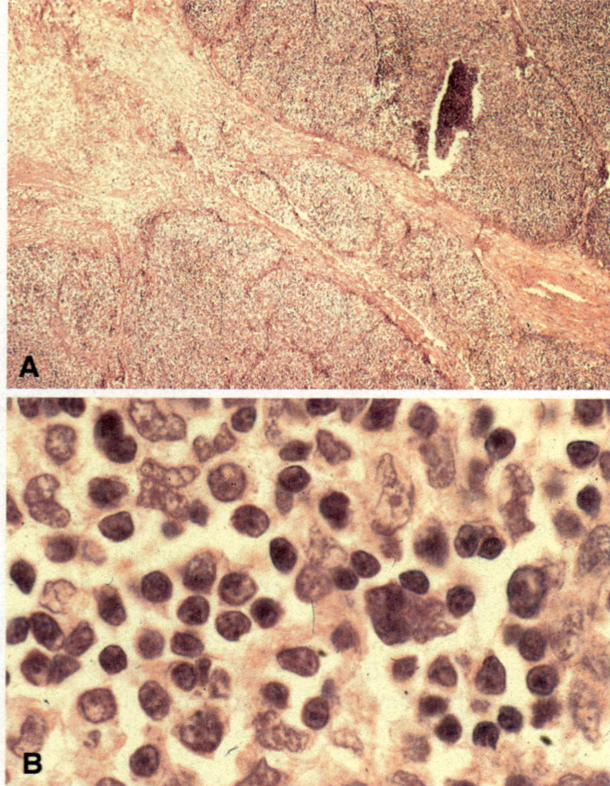

Figure 82-1 Lymphoepithelial thymoma. **A,** Low magnification (×40 original magnification) showing characteristic lobules separated by broad bands of fibrosis. **B,** Higher magnification (×1,000 original magnification) with typical mixture of epithelial cells (large, pale nuclei) and lymphocytes (small, dark nuclei).

behavior of a thymoma is indicated by microscopic or macroscopic invasion of the tumor capsule or of surrounding organs or by the presence of metastasis. Therefore, it is the gross examination of the tumor at surgery that is critical in suspecting or establishing the malignant nature of a thymoma. Approximately 30 to 40% of thymomas are invasive. On the other hand, a well-encapsulated thymoma may, on occasion, recur years after surgical resection. This leads some to suspect that all thymomas are potentially malignant and should be treated as such.[5] Because the term *malignant* can also cause confusion with thymic carcinomas, in which the epithelial cells appear to be cytologically malignant (see the section on thymic carcinoma), it is best to avoid it and divide thymomas into encapsulated and invasive ones. The new WHO classification seems to correlate with invasiveness. The proportion of invasive thymomas was 11.1% for type A, 41.6% for type AB, 47.3% for type B1, 69.1% for type B2, and 84.6% for type B3.[16]

It was also postulated that thymomas may be further subdivided into those with cortical, medullary, and mixed differentiation, reflecting the anatomy of the normal thymus.[17] Cortical thymomas contain large epithelial cells with vesicular chromatin and prominent nucleoli, whereas medullary thymomas show oval- to spindle-shaped epithelial cells with dispersed chromatin and inconspicuous nucleoli.[18] Mixed thymomas contain both cortical and medullary components. Medullary and mixed thymomas appear to follow a more benign course than cortical ones. They show a lower incidence of invasiveness, a lower incidence of MG, a lower recurrence rate, and a better survival rate, even when capsular invasion is present.[18,19] This classification has also been correlated with the size of epithelial cell nuclei by using morphometric analysis.[19] Cortical thymomas have larger epithelial cell nuclei than do medullary ones. The prognostic value of nuclear deoxyribonucleic acid (DNA) content measured by flow cytometry is controversial.[20] Although the percentage of cells in the S phase does not appear to have any prognostic significance, some studies have found that aneuploidy correlates with poorer survival.[20] In one study, the 5-year survival rate was 91% for 11 patients with diploid thymomas and only 23% for 12 patients with aneuploid thymomas.[21]

Other histologic features of thymomas include, in order of frequency,[1] typical perivascular spaces (56%), foci of foamy macrophages (27%), pseudorosette formations of epithelial cells (20%), gland-like structures (20%), Hassall's corpuscles (16%), areas of cystic degeneration that vary in size to produce, occasionally, cystic thymomas (16%), lymphoid follicles with germinal centers (8%), and a variable number of hemorrhagic, necrotic, and/or calcified areas. Occasionally, scattered macrophages among the lymphocytic component can mimic a "starry sky" appearance, not to be confused with Burkitt's lymphoma. Myoid cells, so designated because their cytoplasm contains cross-striations identical to those of skeletal muscle fibers, have also been identified in rare cases.[1] Normal thymic tissue can be found in almost half of the cases at the periphery of the tumor.

In rare cases, special stains may be helpful when the diagnosis is difficult, as in the distinction among thymoma and lymphoma, seminoma, carcinoid, hemangiopericytoma, and sarcoma, or when only a limited amount of tissue is available, such as from needle biopsy or fine-needle aspiration. Epithelial cells in thymomas, even the spindled ones, stain positively with keratin and epithelial membrane antigen and negatively for markers of lymphocytes, such as common leukocyte antigen.[10,11] This pattern rules out a lymphoma or a mesenchymal tumor. The lymphocytes show a predominance of CD1a and terminal deoxynucleotidyltransferase–positive cells, as well as Leu-7 (CD 57)- and/or human leukocyte antigen (HLA)-DR–positive cells.

Finally, electron microscopy can reveal characteristic features of epithelial cells, such as desmosomes, tonofilaments, elongated cell processes, and a lack of dense core granules.[1] Few studies have addressed the genetic changes of thymomas. The most common genetic abnormality was loss of heterozygosity in the region of chromosome 6q23.3-25.3, which occurred in 45.8% of 26 thymomas.[22] Alterations of tp53 were found in 2 of 17 cases of benign thymomas versus 11 of 18 cases of malignant thymomas and 7 of 9 cases of thymic carcinomas.[23] In another study, tp53 protein expression was seen in only 1 of 17 thymomas versus 14 of 19 cases of thymic carcinomas.[24] An inverse correlation between tp53 and bcl-2 protein expression has been described in thymomas.[25]

CLINICAL FEATURES

Most tumor-related symptoms are vague (cough, dyspnea, chest pain) or secondary to local and regional mediastinal spread (pleural effusion, superior vena cava syndrome, or pericardial effusion) and, therefore, often indicate invasiveness. Occasionally, thymomas may present as diffuse pleural tumors and simulate malignant mesothelioma.[26] About half of thymomas occur in asymptomatic persons and are discovered fortuitously on a chest radiograph, which shows a retrosternal mass in the anterosuperior mediastinum forming a bulge in the cardiovascular silhouette. The tumor may be best seen on oblique and lateral views. Computed tomography (CT) is invaluable for detecting small thymomas and assessing possible invasion of surrounding structures, such as the mediastinum, pleura, and pericardium. It can show calcifications in or at the periphery of the tumor in approximately 20% of cases,[5] although they bear no relation to invasiveness. The presence of a fat plane all around the tumor is a good sign of noninvasiveness, but, conversely, fibrous adherence to surrounding structures may simulate invasion.[27] CT can also help differentiate thymomas from vascular structures and tumors, such as aneurysms, particularly when intravenous contrast is used.[27] Thymomas show increased T_1- and T_2-weighted image signal intensity by magnetic resonance imaging, but the role of that technique in detecting possible capsular and vascular invasion, compared with CT, needs further study.[27] The use of positron emission tomography with 18-fluorodeoxyglucose to distinguish malignant from benign mediastinal tumors has been evaluated.[28] Thymic carcinomas and invasive thymomas show high uptake, whereas noninvasive thymomas show low uptake. It should be emphasized, however, that surgical exploration and pathologic evaluation remain the most reliable means to assess the invasiveness of thymomas.

ASSOCIATED PARANEOPLASTIC SYNDROMES

A remarkable number of paraneoplastic syndromes are associated with thymomas. They are mostly related to autoimmune mechanisms and are dominated by three characteristic entities (Table 82-2).

Myasthenia Gravis MG occurs in approximately 33 to 50% of patients with thymoma, and approximately 10% of patients who have MG have a thymoma.[1,29] Such patients are usually older than those with MG without thymoma, although the clinical signs of MG are similar in both groups. Few features distinguish the histologic appearance of thymomas in patients with MG; predominantly spindle cell thymomas are rare in this group, and the surrounding thymic tissue reveals the presence of lymphoid follicles with germinal centers in approximately 50% of the cases (versus only 5 to 8% of cases involving thymomas without MG).[1] MG is an autoimmune disorder that is characterized by the presence of antibodies to the acetylcholine receptors of the neuromuscular junction. Such serum antibodies are found in 90% of patients with generalized MG.[27] The triggering mechanisms are unknown. Myoid cells in the normal thymus raise the possibility of in situ sensitization.[30] Serum striational antibodies directed against elements of the sarcomere, such as titin, are found in 80% of patients with MG and thymoma and in 25% of patients with thymoma but without MG.[27] Total thymectomy rather than thymomectomy is indicated in patients with MG, even in the absence of a thymoma (see "Surgery" below).

Table 82-2 Thymomas: Associated Disorders

Myasthenia gravis	Leukemias
Red cell aplasia	Lymphomas
Hypogammaglobulinemia	Kaposi's sarcoma
Collagen diseases	Eaton-Lambert syndrome
Sjögren's syndrome	Nephrotic syndrome
Pemphigus	Endocrine disorders
Cancer (nonthymic)	

Adapted from Marchevsky AM and Kaneko M.[10]

Red Cell Hypoplasia Also called pure red cell aplasia (PRCA), red cell hypoplasia is an autoimmune disorder that is characterized by an acquired anemia with markedly decreased blood reticulocytes and a virtual absence of erythroblasts in the bone marrow.[1,31] There are often changes (an increase or a decrease) in white blood cell and/or platelet counts. PRCA is seen in approximately 5% of patients with thymoma, but 50% of patients with PRCA have a thymoma, which is of the spindle cell type in two-thirds of these patients.[1] PRCA generally occurs in patients older than 40 years of age who have thymoma, and the incidence of local invasion is not different from other thymomas. The bone marrow is usually quite cellular, and erythropoietin levels are typically high.[31] An immunoglobulin (Ig)G inhibitor of erythroblastic growth has been described in the serum of some patients.[31] Thymectomy produces remission of the anemia in approximately 30% of cases.[31] Corticosteroids and immunosuppressive agents are also effective. Recently, a prolonged complete remission (with tumor regression) was described in one case with the combination of octreotide and prednisone.[32]

Hypogammaglobulinemia First reported by Good in 1954,[33] this acquired syndrome results in extreme susceptibility to recurrent, and often serious, infections.[34] It occurs in approximately 5 to 10% of patients with thymoma, and a thymoma is found in 10% of patients with acquired hypogammaglobulinemia.[1,5] There is a decrease in all major Igs, particularly IgG and IgA, and decreased eosinophils in the blood and bone marrow. A combined deficit in cell-mediated immunity can also be seen. Almost a third of patients also have PRCA. Like those with PRCA, the age group is somewhat older (> 40 years), and the thymoma is of the spindle cell type in 75% of cases.[1] The pathogenesis is obscure. There is a lack of pre-B cells, B cells, and plasma cells in the bone marrow, with decreased peripheral B cells.[34] Thymectomy does not result in any improvement; palliative treatment with Igs is indicated.[34]

A large number of other paraneoplastic syndromes or associated disorders have been described in patients with thymoma (see Table 82-2). It is noteworthy that Cushing's syndrome with ectopic adrenocorticotropin (ACTH) production is a typical feature of thymic carcinoids, not thymomas.[1,35]

DIAGNOSIS

The diagnosis of an anterior mediastinal mass is guided by the clinical suspicion of its etiology. Invasive incisional biopsy techniques, with mediastinoscopy or mediastinotomy for thymoma, carry the risk of violating the tumor capsule and disseminating tumor cells.[36] If typical paraneoplastic syndromes, such as MG, are present, a surgical approach with resection of the tumor en bloc, frozen sections, and definitive surgery (total thymectomy) is justified whenever technically possible. Otherwise, percutaneous fine-needle aspiration or core biopsy under fluoroscopic or CT guidance is generally considered safe and effective. Combined with special stains and electron microscopy, if necessary, it has a sensitivity of 80% and a specificity greater than 90%.[5] It is of prime importance, however, to establish a firm pathologic diagnosis in view of the many other tumor types that may require specific therapies, as discussed below.

DIFFERENTIAL DIAGNOSIS

Extrathymic Tumors Although thymic neoplasms are by far the most common tumors of the anterosuperior mediastinum, other mass lesions in that location include thyroid or parathyroid tumors, nonthymic lymphomas, mediastinal germ cell tumors, aneurysms, myxomas, lipomas, paragangliomas, and bronchogenic cysts.[1,5] Hemangiopericytoma and giant lymph node hyperplasia (Castleman's disease) can resemble thymoma.[1]

Other Thymic Tumors The major differential diagnostic step is to assess the exact nature of a thymic tumor (see Table 82-1).

Thymic Carcinoma Thymic carcinoma is differentiated from thymoma by the epithelial cells appearing to be cytologically malignant.[9,11,37] These are rare tumors; only 16 cases were seen at the Mayo Clinic in 75 years.[11] Several subtypes have been identified. Lymphoepithelioma-like carcinoma bears a strong histologic resemblance to nasopharyngeal carcinoma associated with EBV.[9,37] Indeed, we reported, in 1985, the first case of such a thymic carcinoma associated with EBV.[38] That 19-year-old male patient had a serologic profile similar to that of patients with EBV-associated pharyngeal carcinoma, with elevated antibody titers to the viral capsid antigen (VCA) (IgG and IgA anti-VCA), to the diffuse components of the early antigen (IgG anti-D), and to EBV nuclear antigen. Moreover, hybridization techniques detected an average of 49 EBV genomes per tumor cell. Another such case was reported in 1988 in a 30-year-old woman.[39] The embryologic origin of the thymus from the primitive pharynx further reinforces a possible unified theory about the pathogenesis of lymphoepithelioma-like carcinomas of the pharynx and the thymus.[38] Since then, other investigators have demonstrated the presence of EBV genomes in cases of lymphoepithelioma-like thymic carcinoma, but the role of EBV in other thymic tumors (thymomas and other types of thymic carcinomas) is not established.[40–42]

Other types of thymic carcinomas include keratinizing squamous carcinoma, basaloid squamous carcinoma, clear cell carcinoma, sarcomatoid carcinoma, and mucoepidermoid carcinoma.[11] A unique, and apparently distinctive, chromosome abnormality involving translocation of fragments of chromosomes 15 and 19 has been reported in thymic carcinoma.[43] Primary, small cell (oat cell) carcinoma of the thymus has also been described, and it is histologically similar to the lung variety, which should be excluded as a possible primary neoplasm with thymic metastasis.[35]

The overall 5-year survival rate of 60 cases of thymic carcinoma was 33.3%.[44] Patients with a low-grade histology did much better than those with a high-grade histology.

Lymphomas Lymphomas are, with thymomas, the most common tumors of the thymus. Hodgkin's disease is, as a rule, of the nodular sclerosis type, and it was formerly considered to be a granulomatous thymoma.[4,35] It is frequently confined to the thymus. Although any lymphoma, including Burkitt's lymphoma, may arise in the thymus, the lymphoblastic type in children typically involves the mediastinum in a third of cases and is of T-cell origin.[45] More recently, the occurrence of B-cell lymphomas of the mediastinum with sclerosis and an aggressive course, mainly in young adults, has been emphasized.[45] It is of prime importance to differentiate a lymphoma from a thymoma in view of the different therapeutic approaches. Special stains and electron microscopy may be necessary in difficult cases.

Germ Cell Tumors The thymus is a classic site of extragonadal primary germ cell tumors. This may be explained by the proximity of the urogenital ridge to the primitive pharynx in the embryo.[1,4,35] The most common ones are seminomas (sometimes difficult to differentiate from thymoma) and teratomas (mature or immature). Almost every type of germ cell tumor, however, has been reported in the thymus, either in a pure or mixed form, including embryonal carcinomas, yolk sac tumors, teratocarcinomas, and choriocarcinomas. Most of these tumors occur in men in their twenties or thirties, although mature teratomas occur with equal frequency in males and females.[35] Testicular examination (by palpation and sonography) fails to reveal a tumor, confirming an extragonadal origin.[4,5] It is of prime importance to recognize germ cell tumors of the thymus and to distinguish them from thymomas because of the therapeutic implications. A liberal practice of obtaining serum markers, including alpha-fetoprotein and human chorionic gonadotropin, may help identify a germ cell tumor in patients otherwise diagnosed as having undifferentiated carcinoma of the mediastinum.[46,47] Tissue staining for such markers should also be performed and can be positive even when serum levels are normal. Germ cell tumors are highly responsive to radiotherapy (RT) (seminomas) or chemotherapy, although the overall results and long-term survival are usually inferior to those of corresponding testicular primary tumors.[35]

Thymic Carcinoid Tumors Thymic carcinoid tumors were distinguished from thymomas in 1972.[1,35] They are often aggressive tumors, and extrathoracic metastases are present in 30 to 40% of cases at diagnosis.[35] Cushing's syndrome with ectopic ACTH production in a patient with a thymic tumor should raise this possibility because it occurs in 30% of patients with thymic carcinoid tumor but not in patients with thymoma.[1,35] Other paraneoplastic syndromes, such as osteoarthropathy and Eaton-Lambert syndrome, and an association with multiple endocrine neoplasia (type I or II) have been described.[35] Carcinoid syndrome has not been reported. The microscopic appearance reveals complex organoid patterns, with typical areas of necrosis and calcifications. Special stains show positive argyrophil and negative argentaffin reactions characteristic of foregut neuroendocrine tumors.[35] They may also stain positively for neuron-specific enolase and chromogranin. Characteristic dense neurosecretory-type granules are seen by electron microscopy. Other thymic tumors include thymolipomas, which may become quite large, thymic cysts, and metastases to the thymus.

Table 82-3 Staging of Thymomas

Stage	Extent of Disease	No. of Cases	Survival, % 5 Years	Survival, % 10 Years
I	Totally encapsulated	37	96	67
II	Microscopic or macroscopic capsular invasion into surrounding fat or mediastinal pleura	13	86	60
III	Invasion of surrounding organs (pericardium, lung, great vessels)	32	70	58
IV	(A) Pleural or pericardial implants (B) Embolic metastasis	11	50	0

Adapted from Masaoka A et al.[13]

STAGING

Although there is no standardized staging system for thymoma, the one proposed by Masaoka and colleagues is commonly employed (Table 82-3).[13] Most metastases are intrathoracic (pleura, pericardium) and may represent direct implants from the primary. Extrathoracic and embolic metastases were so rare that only 12 cases were collected from the literature in 1971.[48] In more recent series, however, extrathoracic metastases to the bone, liver, lymph nodes, and other organs were seen in up to 45% of patients, probably as a result of referral selection,[48] a longer survival, or better imaging techniques.

THERAPY

Surgery Because there are no reliable histologic criteria for the malignant nature of thymomas, all such tumors should be considered potentially malignant. Total thymectomy (rather than thymomectomy) is the procedure of choice, even for stage I encapsulated tumors.[4,5] It is also the procedure indicated for patients with MG, with or without thymoma. The usual approach is by median sternotomy, although additional thoracic or cervical incisions may be necessary, and some surgeons advocate maximal thymectomy with exploration of all of the possible areas in which ectopic thymic tissue might be found.[8] There is a need for the surgeon to carefully explore the mediastinum for evidence of local invasion, which is the most reliable indication of malignancy and the most important prognostic factor. The tumor capsule should not be breached. Systematic microscopic examination is necessary to search for capsular invasion and to distinguish it from simple adhesions. Following total thymectomy, the recurrence rate is usually low (about 2%) for stage I encapsulated thymomas.[1] Recently, video thoracoscopic approaches were performed for well-encapsulated small thymomas,[49] but the long-term results are unknown.

In patients with thymoma and MG, remission of MG occurs in approximately 10 to 30% following thymectomy, often after a delay of up to 2 years or more, compared with a remission rate of approximately 40 to 80% after thymectomy for MG without a thymoma.[1,4,5,50,51] An additional fraction of patients show improvement of MG. Early thymectomy (within 1 year) after onset of MG is associated with a higher percentage of less invasive thymomas.[52] Recurrence, and even first occurrence, of MG after apparent total thymectomy has been observed and could be related to tumor regrowth or persistent ectopic thymic tissue.[5] In the past, MG was a poor prognostic sign in patients with thymoma. Most recent surgical series, however, do not show a significant difference in survival for patients with thymoma, with or without MG.[3,4,13,14,53] Such a change is attributed to better surgical and anesthesia techniques, which have largely prevented postoperative deaths from MG.

Local invasion is seen in approximately 30 to 40% of thymomas at surgery,[3,13,14,53] but the slow-growing nature of the tumor and the rarity of distant metastases justify attempts at radical surgery. Identification of the phrenic, recurrent laryngeal and vagus nerves is of major importance.[8] Extended resections—including one lung, one phrenic nerve, pericardium, or even resection and repair of great vessels, such as the innominate vein or superior vena cava—have been performed. They should be undertaken only if they lead to complete tumor resection. RT is indicated in cases of invasive thymoma. With modern techniques of peri- and postsurgical care, surgical mortality is low (0–5%), even in patients with MG.[13,50,53]

In four large series with a total of 744 patients, the 5- and 10-year survival rates were 75 to 85% and 63 to 80%, respectively, for patients with noninvasive encapsulated thymomas.[3,13,14,53] Survival figures for patients with invasive thymomas were 50 to 67% at 5 years and 30 to 53% at 10 years. Whereas invasiveness is the major prognostic factor in patients with thymoma, most series also report a better prognosis for spindle cell thymomas and those with a higher ratio of lymphocytes to epithelial cells.[13,14,53] Local recurrences and/or metastases (often intrathoracic) may also be amenable to surgical resection.

Radiotherapy Thymomas are radiosensitive, and the efficacy of RT has been emphasized in many reports. Following surgical biopsy, or partial excision, survival of more than 10 years after RT has been seen.[48] Most authors do not believe that it is only the lymphocytic component rather than the epithelial one that is sensitive to RT.[48]

The role of RT is best discussed according to stage. For stage I disease following total surgical resection, postoperative RT is not indicated in view of the very low relapse rates. For stage II and III disease, the use of postoperative RT is recommended even after total surgical resection.[4,5,13,14,54] In a review of the literature, as well as their own experience, Curran and colleagues reported a 28% intrathoracic relapse rate after complete surgical resection without RT, as opposed to 5% when postoperative RT was given.[55] The latter figure may be unusual, however, because others have reported no such differences in favor of RT after complete surgical resection.[6] The irradiated volume should include the mediastinum with adjacent areas and probably the supraclavicular areas, which are possible sites of relapse.[48] The total dose is usually about 45 Gy, with appropriate protection of the spinal cord, although doses of 50 Gy and higher have been used.[48,55] Radiation pneumonitis, mediastinitis, pericarditis, coronary artery fibrosis, and hypothyroidism are potential complications, as well as secondary cancers.

RT is also given to patients with residual disease, following biopsy only or incomplete surgical resection for stage III disease. In 20 such cases, Curran and colleagues observed 4 mediastinal recurrences and 5 others outside the mediastinum, whereas no local relapse was seen when RT was given after total surgical resection for stage II or III disease.[55] Partial tumor debulking by surgery prior to RT in patients with stage III or IV disease does not appear to be beneficial.[56] The 5-year survival rate for such patients was 45% overall, including 61% for stage III and 23% for stage IV disease after RT. Collaboration between the surgeon and the radiotherapist is essential to delineate areas of tumor involvement by radiopaque clips and to plan the treatment. Figure 82-2 shows a proposed algorithm for the management of thymoma according to stage.

Chemotherapy Thymomas are relatively chemosensitive. As experience with chemotherapy is increasing, good response rates and sometimes dramatic tumor regressions have been observed.[57]

Single Agents for Thymomas The rarity of thymomas precludes knowledge of the efficacy of many agents.[48,58] The two most commonly used and most active single agents are cisplatin and corticosteroid therapy (Table 82-4).[48,59–70] In the literature, of 28 patients treated with cisplatin at various doses (up to 130 mg/m^2), there were 3 complete and 6 partial responses, for a response rate of 32%. A rather low dose of cisplatin (50 mg/m^2 every 3 weeks) was used in 21 of these patients as part of an Eastern Cooperative Oncology Group trial.[66] Only two partial responses were seen, raising the possibility of a dose-response relationship. The occurrence of complete responses and the long duration of some responses (over 20 months) further indicate that cisplatin is an effective agent.

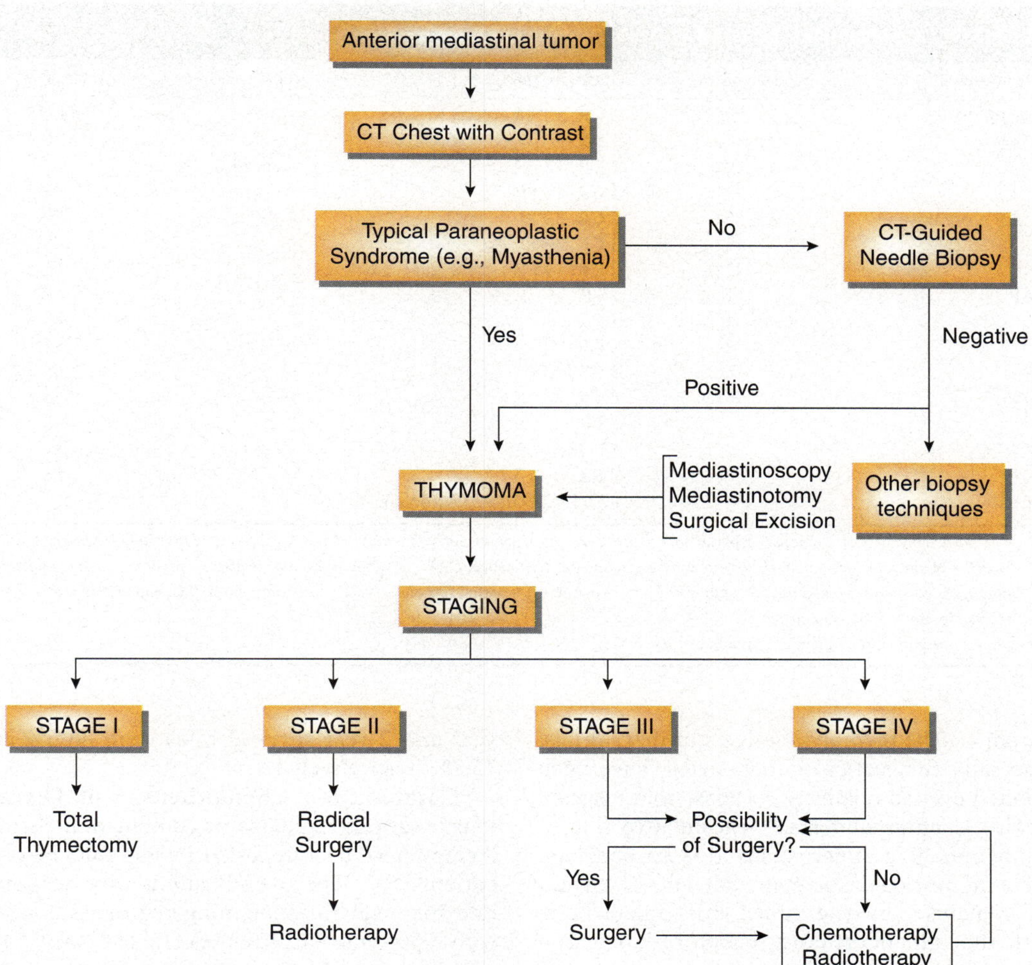

Figure 82-2 Algorithm for the workup and management of thymoma.

Corticosteroid therapy, either as ACTH or glucocorticoids, is effective in inducing tumor regression in patients with invasive or metastatic

Table 82-4 Single Agents in Thymoma

Agent	Patients, *n*	CR	PR	Response Duration, Mo	Survival, Mo	Reference
Cisplatin	1	1	—	13	—	59
	1	1	—	10+	—	60
	1	—	1	4	13	61
	1	—	1	1	—	62
	1	1	—	20+	—	63
	1	1*	—	24	24+	64
	1	—	1	1	—	65
	21	0	2	—	—	66
Total	28	3	6			
Steroids†	12	2	8	—	—	67
	1	—	1	23	—	68
Ifosfamide	13	5	1	66+	—	69
Maytansine	4	0	2	1.5, 4.5	—	48
Doxorubicin	3	0	2	—	—	67
Vincristine	2	0	0	—	—	67
Chlorambucil	2	0	0	—	—	67
Nitrogen mustard	1	0	0	—	—	67
Octreotide	32	0	4	—	—	
+ Prednisone	21	2	6	—	—	70

CR = complete response; PR = partial response.
*With radiotherapy.
†Adrenocorticotropin or corticosteroids.

Table 82-5 Combination Chemotherapy with Cisplatin in Thymoma

Regimen	Patients, *n*	Response Type	Duration, Mo	Reference
BAPP	9*	1 CR, 5 PR*	6–37+	48, 75
CAP	1	1 CR	12+	76
	29	3 CR, 12 PR	Med. 11.8	77
	23	5 CR, 11 PR		78
CAP ± prednisone	6*	2 CR, 3 PR	4–49+	79
	13	3 CR, 8 PR		80
	22	3 CR, 14 PR		81
AP	1	1 PR	6	82
	1	1 PR	3	83
	2	2 CR	4+, 12+	84
EP	16	5 CR, 4 PR	Med. 41	85
PVB	5	2 CR	48+, 72+	86
		2 PR	3, 9	
ADOC	32	15 CR, 14 PR	Med. 11	87
VIP	28	9 PR	Med. 11.9	88
Total	188	42 CR (22%), 87 PR (46%)		

ADOC = Adriamycin (doxorubicin), cisplatin, Oncovin (vincristine), and cyclophosphamide; AP = Adriamycin (doxorubicin) and cisplatin; BAPP = bleomycin, Adriamycin (doxorubicin), cisplatin, and prednisone; CAP = cyclophosphamide, Adriamycin (doxorubicin), and cisplatin; CR = complete response; EP = etoposide and cisplatin; PR = partial response; PVB = cisplatin, vinblastine, and bleomycin; VIP = etoposide, ifosfamide, and cisplatin.

*Includes one patient with thymic carcinoma.

thymoma. The thymolytic effects of these drugs, especially for cortical lymphocytes, have been reported even in relatively corticosteroid-resistant species, such as humans.[48] The relative role of this lympholytic effect versus a direct oncolytic effect on the neoplastic epithelial cells of thymomas remains to be determined. It is of note, however, that glucocorticoid receptors have been found in the cytosol of human thymoma cells,[71] including those with a pure epithelial histology,[72] suggesting a possible direct antineoplastic effect. In 13 reported patients, there were 2 complete and 9 partial responses or improvement from steroid therapy (see Table 82-4). Some of these responses were long-lived (23–36 months) or could be reinduced by resumption of higher daily doses after relapse.[73]

The efficacy of other single agents is largely anecdotal. Ifosfamide, at a dose of 1.5 g/m^2 daily for 5 days every 3 weeks with mesna, has been evaluated in 13 patients, with 5 complete responses (38%) with a median duration of response of 66+ months and 1 partial response.[74] Doxorubicin has produced regressions of short duration in two of three patients. The taxanes have not been evaluated.

Since thymomas express somatostatin receptors, as shown by radiolabeled octreotide scan, a trial of octreotide at a dose of 0.5 mg subcutaneously three times daily was undertaken by the Eastern Cooperative Oncology Group.[70] Patients were evaluated at 2 months, and those who responded continued on octreotide alone for a maximum of 1 year, whereas those who progressed were given prednisone 0.6 mg/kg orally per day in addition to octreotide for a maximum of 1 year. Of 32 evaluable patients with thymoma, there were 2 complete (6%) and 10 partial (31%) objective responses. Of these, 4 partial responses (12.5%) were observed on octreotide alone. None of an additional 6 patients (5 thymic carcinomas and 1 thymic carcinoid) responded. The overall 1-year and 2-year survival rates were 86.6% and 75.7%, respectively.

Combination Chemotherapy of Thymomas Various regimens of combination chemotherapy have been reported in small numbers of patients.[48,58] The overall cumulative response rate for cisplatin-containing regimens is 68%, with 22% complete responses (Table 82-5),[48,75–88] which is not much different from regimens without cisplatin (65% response with 35% complete responses) (Table 82-6).[89–96] In the absence of prospective randomized trials, there is no basis to recommend one regimen over another.

These results are highly encouraging because many patients experienced prolonged responses. Patients with thymoma and severe MG that is resistant to conventional medical therapy can sometimes benefit dramatically from chemotherapy for the relief of myasthenia symptoms. Some patients requiring ventilatory support have been weaned from the respirator just a few days after receiving chemotherapy.[93] Thymic carcinomas also can respond to cisplatin combinations, such as a bleomycin-Adriamycin (doxorubicin)-cisplatin-prednisone[38] or a cisplatin-bleomycin-etoposide combination.[97]

Chemotherapy has also been combined with RT in patients with thymoma.[98,99] This approach has been effective in patients with stage III disease using cyclophosphamide, Adriamycin (doxorubicin), and cisplatin (CAP). In one trial with 23 patients, the response rate was 69.6% and the median survival was 93 months.[59] In another trial, chemotherapy with CAP plus prednisone was followed by surgery and radiotherapy, leading to a 73% disease-free survival at 7 years.[60] Such studies emphasize the importance of combined-modality therapy in patients with advanced thymomas.

An algorithm applicable to the management of the vast majority of patients with thymoma is shown in Figure 82-2. The effectiveness of chemotherapy in thymoma may lead to preoperative use in patients with large or extensively invasive thymomas.[48] The management of such patients requires a combined-modality approach with chemotherapy, surgery, and RT in the most appropriate sequence, according to the individual case. In patients with unresectable thymoma, treatment with RT, chemotherapy, or both can induce tumor regression and allow surgical resection of residual disease, if any. By using this approach, complete tumor eradication was achieved in 5 of 8 patients in one study[61] and in 11 of 16 patients in another study.[62] Thus, the treatment was successful in two-thirds of the patients. This was confirmed more recently in 22 patients with Masaoka stage III or IV thymoma treated with induction chemotherapy (modified CAP regimen plus prednisone), with a

Table 82-6 Combination Chemotherapy without Cisplatin in Thymoma

Regimen	Patients, *n*	Response Type	Duration, Mo	Reference
MVPV	2	2 PR	0.8, 3	89
ACVB	1	1 PR	2	89
COPP	5	4 PR*		90
DC	1	1 CR	13	91
VCC ± prednisone	9	4 CR	31–62	92
		1 PR	2	
CAV	4†	1 CR	12+	93
		3 PR	4–9	
CHOP	1	1 CR	12	94
CHOP ± bleomycin	13	5 CR		95
COP ± procarbazine	6	3 CR, 1 PR		95
PCb	1	1 PR		96
Total	43	15 CR (35%), 13 PR (30%)		

ACVB = Adriamycin (doxorubicin); CAV = cyclophosphamide, Adriamycin (doxorubicin), and vincristine; CCNU = vincristine and bleomycin; CHOP = cyclophosphamide, doxorubicin, vincristine, prednisone; COP = cyclophosphamide, Oncovin (vincristine), and prednisone; COPP = cyclophosphamide, Oncovin (vincristine), prednisone, and procarbazine; CR = complete response; DC = doxorubicin and cyclophosphamide; MVPV = nitrogen mustard, vincristine, procarbazine, and vinblastine; PCb = paclitaxel and carboplatin; PR = partial response; VCC = vincristine, cyclophosphamide, and CCNU.

*Two patients in CR for 33 and 34 months after radiotherapy was added.

†A fifth patient without a measurable tumor had complete remission of myasthenia gravis following chemotherapy.

77% response rate (14% complete response) followed by complete surgical resection in 76% of patients. This was followed by RT and chemotherapy. The overall survival at 5 years was 95%, with 77% progression-free survival.[81] Hence, excellent long-term results are within reach, and it seems justified to add invasive thymoma to the list of neoplasms that are curable even at an advanced stage.

Chemotherapy of Thymic Carcinomas The results of chemotherapy for thymic carcinomas are much less favorable.[99] The efficacy of single agents is virtually unknown. Cisplatin combinations, including cisplatin, etoposide, and bleomycin or cisplatin, etoposide, and ifosfamide, have been evaluated in very small numbers of patients, with response rates of 20 to 60%.[99] Single case reports have shown good results with various regimens, including bleomycin, doxorubicin, cisplatin, and prednisone,[38] or bleomycin, vinblastine and cisplatin, or 5-fluorouracil, methotrexate with cisplatin or doxorubicin and cisplatin, as well as irinotecan alone.

Recently, genetic studies have revealed that *KIT* (CD117), a tyrosine kinase receptor, is frequently overexpressed in thymic carcinomas (86% positivity), whereas it is absent in thymomas or normal thymus.[100] Of interest is the fact that a patient with a poorly differentiated epidermoid thymic carcinoma harboring mutations of *KIT* similar to those seen in gastrointestinal stromal tumors (in-frame deletion in exon 11) experienced a response to imatinib (400 mg/d) for about 6 months.[101] A personal patient also with a poorly differentiated squamous thymic carcinoma positive for *C-KIT* by immunohistochemistry and heavily pretreated with chemotherapy failed to respond to imatinib, however.

REFERENCES

1. Rosai J, Levine GD. Tumors of the thymus. In: Atlas of tumor pathology. 2nd Series. Fascicle 13. Washington (DC): Armed Forces Institute of Pathology; 1976.
2. Givel JC. Historical review. In: Givel JC, Merlini M, Clarke DB, Dusmet M, editors. Surgery of the thymus. Pathology, associated disorders and surgical technique. Berlin: Springer-Verlag; 1990. p. 1.
3. Lewis JE, Wick MR, Scheithauer BW, et al. Thymoma. A clinicopathologic review. Cancer 1987;60:2727.
4. McKenna WG, Bonomi P, Barnes MM, Glatstein E. Malignancies of the thymus. In: Roth JA, Ruckdeschel JC, Weisenburger TH, editors. Thoracic oncology. Philadelphia: Saunders; 1989. p. 466.
5. Rosenberg JC. Neoplasms of the mediastinum. In: DeVita VT Jr, Hellman S, Rosenberg SA, editors. Cancer. Principles and practice of oncology. 4th ed. Philadelphia: Lippincott; 1993. p. 759.
6. Cohen DJ, Ronnigen LD, Graeber GM, et al. Management of patients with malignant thymoma. J Thorac Cardiovasc Surg 1984;87:301.
7. Hildreth NG, Shore RE, Dvoretsky PM. The risk of breast cancer after irradiation of the thymus in infancy. N Engl J Med 1989;321:1281.
8. Jaretzki A III, Wolff M. "Maximal" thymectomy for myasthenia gravis. Surgical anatomy and operative technique. J Thorac Cardiovasc Surg 1988;96:711.
9. Levine GD, Rosai J. Thymic hyperplasia and neoplasia: a review of current concepts. Hum Pathol 1978;9:495.
10. Marchevsky AM, Kaneko M. Surgical pathology of the mediastinum. New York: Raven Press; 1984. p. 58.
11. Wick MR, Rosai J. Epithelial tumors. In: Givel JC, Merlini M, Clarke DB, Dusmet M, editors. Surgery of the thymus. Pathology, associated disorders and surgical technique. Berlin: Springer-Verlag; 1990. p. 79.
12. Masaoka A, Nagaoka Y, Maeda M, et al. Study on the ratio of lymphocytes to epithelial cells in thymoma. Cancer 1977;40:1222.
13. Masaoka A, Monden Y, Nakahara K, Tanioka T. Follow-up study of thymomas with special reference to their clinical stages. Cancer 1981;48:2485.
14. Verley JM, Hollmann KH. Thymoma. A comparative study of clinical stages, histologic features and survival in 200 cases. Cancer 1985;55:1074.
15. Rosai J, Sobin LH. Histological typing of tumors of the thymus. International histologic classification of tumors. 2nd ed. New York: Springer; 1999.
16. Okumura M, Ohta M, Tateyama H, et al. The World Health Organization histologic classification system reflects the oncologic behavior of thymoma. A clinical study of 273 patients. Cancer 2002;94:624.
17. Marino M, Muller-Hermelink HK. Thymoma and thymic carcinoma. Relation of thymoma epithelial cells to the cortical and medullary differentiation of thymus. Virchows Arch (A) Pathol Anat Histopathol 1985;407:119.
18. Quintanilla-Martinez L, Wilkins EW Jr, Choi N, et al. Thymoma. Histologic subclassification is an independent prognostic factor. Cancer 1994;74:606.
19. Nomori H, Ishihara T, Torikata C. Malignant grading of cortical and medullary differentiated thymoma by morphometric analysis. Cancer 1989;64:1694.
20. Pollack A, El-Naggar AK, Cox JD, et al. Thymoma. The prognostic significance of flow cytometric DNA analysis. Cancer 1992;69:1702.
21. Gawrychowski J, Rokicki M, Gabriel A, et al. Thymoma. The usefulness of some prognostic factors for diagnosis and surgical treatment. Eur J Surg Oncol 2000;26:203.
22. Zhou R, Zettl A, Strobel P, et al. Thymic epithelial tumors can develop along two different pathogenic pathways. Am J Pathol 2001;159:1853.
23. Weirich G, Schneider P, Fellbaum C, et al. p53 alterations in thymic epithelial tumours. Virchows Arch 1997;431:17.
24. Hino N, Kondo K, Miyoshi T, et al. High frequency of p53 protein expression in thymic carcinoma but not in thymoma. Br J Cancer 1997;76:1361.
25. Stefanaki K, Rontogianni D, Kouvidou CH, et al. Expression of p53, mdm2, p21/waf1 and bcl-2 proteins in thymomas. Histopathology 1997;30:549.
26. Moran CA, Travis WD, Rosado-de-Christenson M, et al. Thymomas presenting as pleural tumors. Report of eight cases. Am J Surg Pathol 1992;16:138.
27. Morgenthaler TI, Brown LR, Colby TV, et al. Thymoma. Mayo Clin Proc 1993;68:1110.
28. Kubota K, Yamada S, Kondo T, et al. PET imaging of primary mediastinal tumours. Br J Cancer 1996;73:882.
29. Namba T, Brunner NG, Grob D. Myasthenia gravis in patients with thymoma, with particular reference to onset after thymectomy. Medicine (Baltimore) 1978;57:411.
30. Drachman DB. Myasthenia gravis. N Engl J Med 1994;330:1797.
31. Krantz SB. Pure red cell aplasia. In: Givel JC, Merlini M, Clarke DB, Dusmet M, editors. Surgery of the thymus. Pathology, associated disorders and surgical technique. Berlin: Springer-Verlag; 1990. p. 181.
32. Palmieri G, Lastoria S, Colao A, et al. Successful treatment of a patient with a thymoma and pure red-cell aplasia with octreotide and prednisone. N Engl J Med 1997;336:263.
33. Good RA. Agammaglobulinemia: a provocative experiment of nature. Bull Univ Minn Hosp 1954;26:1.
34. Siegal FP. Immunodeficiency diseases and thymoma. In: Givel JC, Merlini M, Clarke DB, Dusmet M, editors. Surgery of the thymus. Pathology, associated disorders and surgical technique. Berlin: Springer-Verlag; 1990. p. 189.
35. Wick MR, Rosai J. Neuroendocrine, germ cell, and nonepithelial tumors. In: Givel JC, Merlini M, Clarke DB, Dusmet M, editors. Surgery of the thymus. Pathology, associated disorders and surgical technique. Berlin: Springer-Verlag; 1990. p. 109.
36. Warren WH, Gould VE. Epithelial neoplasms of the thymus. Chest Surg Clin N Am 1992;2:137.
37. Rosai J. Lymphoepithelioma-like thymic carcinoma: another tumor related to Epstein-Barr virus [editorial]? N Engl J Med 1985;312:1320.
38. Leyvraz S, Henle H, Chahinian AP, et al. Association of Epstein-Barr virus with thymic carcinoma. N Engl J Med 1985;312:1296.
39. Dimery IW, Lee JS, Blick M, et al. Association of the Epstein–Barr virus with lymphoepithelioma of the thymus. Cancer 1988;61:2475.
40. Fujii T, Kawai T, Saito K, et al. EBER-1 expression in thymic carcinoma. Acta Pathol Jpn 1993;43:107.
41. Inghirami G, Chilosi M, Knowles DM. Western thymomas lack Epstein–Barr virus by Southern blotting analysis and by polymerase chain reaction. Am J Pathol 1990;136:1429.
42. Mann RB, MacMahon EM, Ling Y, et al. In situ localization of Epstein–Barr virus in thymic carcinoma. Mod Pathol 1992;5:363.
43. Kubonishi I, Takehara N, Iwata J, et al. Novel t(15;19)(q15;p13) chromosome abnormality in a thymic carcinoma. Cancer Res 1991;51:3327.
44. Suster S, Rosai J. Thymic carcinoma. A clinicopathologic study of 60 cases. Cancer 1991;67:1025.
45. Aisenberg AC. Primary large-cell lymphoma of the mediastinum [editorial]. J Clin Oncol 1993;11:2291.
46. Fox EM, Woods RL, Tattersall MHN, McGovern VJ. Undifferentiated carcinoma in young men: the atypical teratoma syndrome. Lancet 1979;1:1316.
47. Richardson RL, Schoumacher RA, Fer MF, et al. The unrecognized extragonadal germ cell cancer syndrome. Ann Intern Med 1981;94:181.
48. Chahinian AP, Bhardwaj S, Meyer RJ, et al. Treatment of invasive or metastatic thymoma. Report of eleven cases. Cancer 1981;47:1752.
49. Kaiser LR. Thymoma: the use of minimally invasive resection techniques. Chest Surg Clin N Am 1994;4:185.
50. Jaretzki A III, Penn AS, Younger DS, et al. "Maximal" thymectomy for myasthenia gravis. Results. J Thorac Cardiovasc Surg 1988;95:747.
51. Papatestas AE, Albert LI, Osserman KE, et al. Studies in myasthenia gravis: effects of thymectomy. Results on 185 patients with nonthymomatous and thymomatous myasthenia gravis 1941–1969. Am J Med 1971;50:465.
52. Genkins G, Papatestas AE, Horowitz SH, Kornfeld P. Studies in myasthenia gravis: early thymectomy. Electrophysiologic and pathologic correlations. Am J Med 1975;58:517.
53. Maggi G, Giaccone G, Donadio M, et al. Thymomas. A review of 169 cases, with particular reference to results of surgical treatment. Cancer 1986;58:765.
54. Arriagada R, Bretel JJ, Caillaud JM, et al. Invasive carcinoma of the thymus. A multicenter retrospective review of 56 cases. Eur J Cancer Clin Oncol 1984;20:69.
55. Curran WJ, Kornstein MJ, Broks JJ, Turrisi AT III. Invasive thymoma: the role of mediastinal irradiation following complete or incomplete surgical resection. J Clin Oncol 1988;6:1722.
56. Ciernik IF, Meier U, Lutolf UM. Prognostic factors and outcome of incompletely resected invasive thymoma following radiation therapy. J Clin Oncol 1994;12:1484.
57. Holland JF. Karnofsky Memorial Lecture. Breaking the cure barrier. J Clin Oncol 1983;1:75.
58. Bhardwaj S, Chahinian, AP. Chemotherapy for invasive thymomas. In: Givel JC, Merlini M, Clarke DB, Dusmet M, editors. Surgery of the thymus. Pathology, associated disorders, and surgical technique. Berlin: Springer-Verlag; 1990. p. 293.
59. Loehrer PJ, Chen M, Kim K, et al. Cisplatin, doxorubicin, and cyclophosphamide plus thoracic radiation therapy for limited-stage unresectable thymoma. An Intergroup trial. J Clin Oncol 1997;15:3093.
60. Shin DM, Walsh GL, Komaki R, et al. A multidisciplinary approach to therapy for unresectable malignant thymoma. Ann Intern Med 1998;129:100.
61. Kirschner PA. Reoperation for thymoma. Report of 23 cases. Ann Thorac Surg 1990;49:550.
62. Rea F, Sartori F, Loy M, et al. Chemotherapy and operation for invasive thymoma. J Thorac Cardiovasc Surg 1993;106:543.
63. Talley RW, O'Bryan RM, Gutterman JU, et al. Clinical evaluation of toxic effects of *cis*-diamminedichloroplatinum (NSC-119875). Phase I clinical study. Cancer Chemother Rep 1973;57:465.
64. Needles B, Kemeny N, Urmacher C. Malignant thymoma: renal metastases responding to *cis*-platinum. Cancer 1981;48:223.
65. Shetty MR, Arora RK. Invasive thymoma treated with cisplatin. Cancer Treat Rep 1981;65:531.
66. Bonomi P, Aisner S, Ettinger D, Finkelstein D. Phase II trial of cisplatin in recurrent or metastatic malignant thymoma: an ECOG trial. Proc Am Soc Clin Oncol 1988;7:856.
67. Baum ES, Gaynon P, Greenberg L, et al. Phase II trial of cisplatin in refractory childhood cancer: Children's Cancer Study Group report. Cancer Treat Rep 1981;65:815.
68. Cocconi G, Boni B, Cumor A. Long-lasting response to *cis*-platinum in recurrent malignant thymoma. Case report. Cancer 1982;49:1985.
69. Levin L, Sealy R, Barron J. Syndrome of inappropriate antidiuretic hormone secretion following *cis*-dichlorodi-

ammineplatinum II in a patient with malignant thymoma. Cancer 1982;50:2279.
70. Loehrer PJ, Wang W, Johnson DH, Ettinger DS. Octreotide alone or with prednisone in patients with advanced thymoma and thymic carcinoma. An Eastern Cooperative Oncology Group phase II trial. J Clin Oncol 2004;22:293
71. Homo-Delarche F. Glucocorticoid receptors and steroid sensitivity in normal and neoplastic human lymphoid tissue: a review. Cancer Res 1984;44:431.
72. Ranelletti FO, Iacobelli S, Carmignani M, et al. Glucocorticoid receptors and in vitro corticosensitivity in human thymoma. Cancer Res 1980;40:2020.
73. Tandan R, Taylor R, DiCostanzo DP, et al. Metastasizing thymoma and myasthenia gravis. Favorable response to glucocorticoids after failed chemotherapy and radiation therapy. Cancer 1990;65:1286.
74. Highley MS, Underhill CR, Parnis FX, et al. Treatment of invasive thymoma with single-agent ifosfamide. J Clin Oncol 1999;17:2737.
75. Giaccone G, Ardizzoni A, Kirkpatrick A, et al. Cisplatin and etoposide combination chemotherapy for locally advanced or metastatic thymoma. A phase II study of the European Organization for Research and Treatment of Cancer Lung Cancer Cooperative Group. J Clin Oncol 1996;14:814.
76. Hu E, Levine J. Chemotherapy of malignant thymoma. Case report and review of the literature. Cancer 1986;57:1101.
77. Tandan R, Taylor R, DiCostanzo DP, et al. Metastasizing thymoma and myasthenia gravis. Favorable response to glucocorticoids after failed chemotherapy and radiation therapy. Cancer 1990;65:1286.
78. Highley MS, Underhill CR, Parnis FX, et al. Treatment of invasive thymoma with single-agent ifosfamide. J Clin Oncol 1999;17:2737.
79. Chahinian AP, Holland, JF, Bhardwaj S. Chemotherapy for malignant thymoma. Ann Intern Med 1983;99:5.
80. Campbell MG, Pollard R, Al-Sarraf M. Complete response in metastatic malignant thymoma to *cis*-platinum, doxorubicin and cyclophosphamide: a case report. Cancer 1981;48:1315.
81. Kim ES, Putnam JB, Komaki R, et al. Phase II study of a multidisciplinary approach with induction chemotherapy, followed by surgical resection, radiation therapy, and consolidation chemotherapy for unresectable malignant thymomas. Final report. Lung Cancer 2004;44:369.
82. Loehrer PJ, Kim K, Aisner SC, et al. Cisplatin plus doxorubicin plus cyclophosphamide in metastatic or recurrent thymoma. Final results on an Intergroup trial. J Clin Oncol 1994;12:1164.
83. Umsawasdi T, Chiuten DF, Holoye P, et al. Cytoxan + Adriamycin + cisplatin ± prednisone (CAP ± Pr) in treatment of malignant thymic tumors (MTT). Proc Am Soc Clin Oncol 1985;4:149.
84. Shetty MR, Arora RK. Invasive thymoma treated with cisplatin. Cancer Treat Rep 1981;65:531.
85. Thomas J, De Wolf-Peeters C, Tricot G, et al. T-cell lymphocytic leukemia in patient with invasive thymoma in remission with chemotherapy. Cancer 1983;52:313.
86. Klippstein TH, Mitrou PS, Kochendorfer KJ, Bergmann L. High-dose Adriamycin (ADM) and *cis*-platinum (DDP) in advanced soft-tissue sarcomas and invasive thymomas. A pilot study. Cancer Chemother Pharmacol 1984;13:78.
87. Giaccone G, Ardizzoni A, Kirkpatrick A, et al. Cisplatin and etoposide combination chemotherapy for locally advanced or metastatic thymoma. A phase II study of the European Organization for Research and Treatment of Cancer Lung Cancer Cooperative Group. J Clin Oncol 1996;14:814.
88. Dy C, Calvo FA, Mindan JP, et al. Undifferentiated epithelial-rich invasive malignant thymoma: complete response to cisplatin, vinblastine, and bleomycin therapy. J Clin Oncol 1988;6:536.
89. Fornasiero A, Daniele O, Ghiotto C, et al. Chemotherapy of invasive thymoma. J Clin Oncol 1990;8:1419.
90. Loehrer PJ, Jiroutek M, Aisner S, et al. Combined etoposide, ifosfamide and cisplatin in the treatment of patients with advanced thymoma and thymic carcinoma. An Intergroup trial. Cancer 2001;91:2010.
91. Boston B. Chemotherapy of invasive thymoma. Cancer 1976;38:49.
92. Evans WK, Thompson DM, Simpson WJ, et al. Combination chemotherapy in invasive thymoma. Role of COPP. Cancer 1980;46:1523.
93. Kosmidis PA, Iliopoulos E, Pentea S. Combination chemotherapy with cyclophosphamide, Adriamycin, and vincristine in malignant thymoma and myasthenia gravis. Cancer 1988;61:1736.
94. Butler W, Diehl LF, Taylor G, Weltz MD. Metastatic thymoma with myasthenia gravis. Complete remission with combination chemotherapy. Cancer 1982;50:419.
95. Daugaard G, Hansen HH, Rothe M. Combination chemotherapy for malignant thymoma. Ann Intern Med 1983;99:189.
96. Uematsu M, Kondo M. A proposal for treatment of invasive thymoma. Cancer 1986;58:1979.
97. Weide LG, Ulbright TM, Loehrer PJ, Williams SD. Thymic carcinoma. A distinct clinical entity responsive to chemotherapy. Cancer 1993;71:1219.
98. Dziuba SJ, Curran WJ. The radiotherapeutic management of invasive thymomas. Chest Surg Clin N Am 2001;11:457.
99. Chahinian AP. Chemotherapy of thymomas and thymic carcinomas. Chest Surg Clin N Am 2001;11:447.
100. Pan CC, Chen PC, Chiang H. KIT (CD117) is frequently overexpressed in thymic carcinomas but is absent in thymomas. J Pathol 2004;202:375.
101. Strobel P, Hartmann M, Jakob A, et al. Thymic carcinoma with overexpression of mutated *KIT* and the response to imatinib. N Engl J Med 2004;350:2625.

83

Tumors of the Heart and Great Vessels

A. Philippe Chahinian, MD
Andrew J. Einstein, MD, PhD
Valentin Fuster, MD, PhD

CARDIAC TUMORS

The first human primary cardiac tumor was reported by Columbo in 1559,[1] and cardiac myxoma was first described by King in 1845.[2] Since then, a large variety of benign and malignant primary cardiac tumors have been reported.

EPIDEMIOLOGY AND ETIOLOGY

Primary cardiac tumors are rare. In autopsy series, their prevalence varies between 0.0017 and 0.33%.[3] Among over 800 cases of primary tumors of the heart reviewed at the Armed Forces Institute of Pathology, 68% were benign tumors (Table 83-1).[4,5] Among benign tumors, myxomas are by far the most common (approximately 40%). Myxomas affect both sexes about equally and occur in all age groups but more often between the fourth and sixth decades.[5] Although usually sporadic, they can occasionally be familial and multiple.

The primary malignant cardiac tumors are usually sarcomas; angiosarcomas are the most common, accounting for 27% of malignant tumors of the heart, followed by malignant fibrous histiocytoma, which is equated with undifferentiated pleomorphic sarcoma in the current World Health Organization classification (18%), rhabdomyosarcoma (12%), and fibrosarcoma (9%).[4,5] Malignant tumors affect predominantly the right side of the heart, in contrast to benign tumors, which are more common on the left side.[6,7] Cardiac tumors can occur in children and infants, the most common being rhabdomyoma.[8,9] Whereas in adults, cardiac metastases are far more frequent than primary neoplasms by a factor of 20- to 40-fold,[4] metastasis to the heart is rarely observed in the pediatric population.

With the exception of asbestos for pericardial mesothelioma, the etiology of cardiac tumors is largely unknown.[10] Hereditary factors play a role in a few cases of cardiac myxoma. Particles resembling coxsackievirus B4 have been detected in a human cardiac myxoma by electron microscopy and immunofluorescence, but viral cultures were unsuccessful.[11] Rhabdomyoma can occur in patients with tuberous sclerosis, and neurofibroma can occur in patients with von Recklinghausen's disease.[10] Whereas a strong relationship has been established between exposure to arsenic, vinyl chloride, and thorium dioxide and the development of hepatic angiosarcomas, such factors have rarely been implicated in cardiac angiosarcomas.[12]

CLINICAL FEATURES

Benign Primary Cardiac Tumors **Myxomas** Myxomas most commonly occur in the left atrium, but they can also arise in any other cardiac chamber or in both atria. In a meta-analysis of 32 reports encompassing 1,029 patients, 83% of myxomas were found to occur in the left atrium.[13] These tumors occur exclusively on the endocardial surface.[4] In patients with myxoma, a typical clinical triad—systemic symptoms, embolic episodes, and signs of valvular or intracavitary dysfunction—has been described. Presenting symptoms are protean and include dyspnea on exertion, paroxysmal nocturnal dyspnea, fever, weight loss, dizziness, syncope, hemoptysis, and Raynaud's phenomenon. Arrhythmias and sudden death can occur. Physical signs include various murmurs, often mitral systolic or diastolic, which typically vary with respiration or body position. A characteristic "tumor plop" can be heard following the second heart sound. It can be confused with a third heart sound or the opening snap of the mitral valve and is thought to be secondary to tension on the tumor stalk during diastolic prolapse of left atrial myxomas into the left ventricle or by the tumor striking the myocardium.[14]

Histologically, these soft gelatinous tumors are thought to arise from the subendocardial mesenchyme and contain polygonal to stellate myxoma cells ("lepidic cells"), often around vascular channels in an eosinophilic matrix, with various areas of hemorrhage.[5] The cells are positive for factor VIII and can also express neuron-specific enolase and S-100 protein.[14]

Although the majority of myxomas occur sporadically, a sizable fraction of cases may occur in the context of a constellation of conditions, which can include pigmented skin lesions as well as endocrine and peripheral tumors. Dubbed the *Carney complex*, this syndrome is typically familial and inherited in an autosomal dominant fashion. Diagnostic criteria are shown in Table 83-2.[15] For a diagnosis to be made, a patient should exhibit two clinical manifestations of the complex or one manifestation plus one supplemental genetic criterion. Mutations of the *PRKAR1A* gene, located on chromosome 17q22-24, have been identified in roughly half of patients with Carney complex; this gene encodes the type I regulatory subunit of cyclic adenosine monophosphate (cAMP)-dependent protein kinase A. Another responsible gene has been mapped to 2p16, whereas a variant associated with distal arthrogryposis has been shown to be caused by a missense mutation in the myosin heavy-chain gene on 17p12-p13.1.[16–18]

Laboratory studies in myxoma can reveal anemia (possibly hemolytic) or erythrocytosis, leukocytosis, thrombocytopenia, increased serum immunoglobulin levels, and elevated acute-phase reactants, such as sedimentation rate and C-reactive protein. High serum levels of interleukin-6 have been reported, which could explain some of the systemic manifestations of the disease; however, these levels return to normal after surgical resection.[14]

The diagnosis, as for any cardiac tumor, is based on a high index of suspicion. Chest radiographs can reveal cardiomegaly or calcifications within the tumor. More definitive imaging techniques include two-dimensional echocardiography, either transthoracic (TTE), which is useful as a screening method, or transesophageal (TEE), which is more invasive but allows better visualization of the tumor. Although both TTE and TEE are equally effective in detecting cardiac tumors, TEE is superior to TTE in assessing localization and extracardiac spread of tumors.[19] Echocardiographic contrast perfusion imaging may provide additional information in the characterization of cardiac masses,[20] whereas three-dimensional echocardiography can better define their complex geometries.[21] Magnetic resonance imaging (MRI), illustrated in Figure 83-1, provides outstanding tumor localization, tissue characterization, flexibility in the selection of imaging planes, and visualization of the entire mediastinum, enabling demonstration of the effects on adjacent tissue.[22,23] Multislice computed tomography is a rapidly advancing imaging modality that can identify calcification and, like echocardiography and MRI, provide dynamic visualization of tumor motion.[24] Noninvasive imaging using one or more of these complementary modalities[25,26] can obviate the need for angiography, which previously was regarded as the gold standard imaging modality for cardiac tumors but suffers from the risk of tumor embolization.

Treatment is surgical, with complete excision of the tumor and its base. Close follow-up is necessary because recurrence is possible.[27]

Table 83-1 Type and Frequency of Primary Tumors of the Heart and Pericardium in Two Series from the Armed Forces Institute of Pathology

Type	1976–1993 Series *n*	1976–1993 Series %	Pre-1977 Series *n*	Pre-1977 Series %
Benign tumors				
Myxoma	114	27.9	130	29.3
Papillary Fibroelastoma	31	7.6	42	9.5
Rhabdomyoma	20	4.9	36	8.1
Lipoma	2	0.5	45	10.1
Fibroma	20	4.9	17	3.8
Hemangioma	17	4.2	15	3.4
Atrioventricular nodal tumor	10	2.4	12	2.7
Teratoma	4	1.0	14	3.2
Lipomatous hypertrophy, atrial septum	12	2.9	0	0.0
Granular cell tumor	4	1.0	3	0.7
Lymphangioma	2	0.5	2	0.5
Benign fibrous tumor	3	0.7	0	0.0
Neurofibroma	0	0.0	3	0.7
Histiocytoid cardiomyopathy	2	0.5	0	0.0
Inflammatory pseudotumor	2	0.5	0	0.0
Myocytic hamartoma	2	0.5	0	0.0
Paraganglioma	2	0.5	0	0.0
Epithelioid hemangioendothelioma	1	0.2	0	0.0
Total	248	60.6	319	71.8
Malignant tumors				
Angiosarcoma	37	9.0	39	8.8
Unclassified Sarcoma	35	8.6	0	0.0
Rhabdomyosarcoma	6	1.5	26	5.9
Mesothelioma	8	2.0	19	4.3
Fibrosarcoma	9	2.2	14	3.2
Osteosarcoma	13	3.2	5	1.1
Malignant fibrous histiocytoma	16	3.9	0	0.0
Lymphoma	7	1.7	7	1.6
Leiomyosarcoma	12	2.9	1	0.2
Myxosarcoma	8	2.0	0	0.0
Synovial sarcoma	5	1.2	1	0.2
Malignant teratoma	0	0.0	4	0.9
Neurogenic sarcoma	0	0.0	4	0.9
Thymoma*	0	0.0	4	0.9
Liposarcoma	2	0.5	1	0.2
Malignant schwannoma	2	0.5	0	0.0
Yolk sac tumor	1	0.2	0	0.0
Total	161	39.4	125	28.2
Total tumors	409		444	

Adapted from Burke A and Virmani R[4] and McAllister JHA and Fenoglio JJJ.[5] Cysts are excluded.
*From thymic rests in the parietal pericardium.

Table 83-2 Diagnostic Criteria for the Carney Complex

Disease manifestations
- Spotty skin pigmentation, distribution typically involving conjunctiva, lips, canthi, vaginal or penile mucosa
- Cutaneous or mucosal myxoma
- Cardiac myxoma
- Breast myxomatosis (or suggestive magnetic resonance findings)
- Primary pigmented nodular adrenocortical disease or Liddle's test with paradoxical positive response of urinary glucocorticosteroids to administration of dexamethasone
- Acromegaly from growth hormone–producing adenoma
- Large cell calcifying Sertoli cell tumor or characteristic calcification on testicular ultrasonography
- Thyroid carcinoma or multiple ultrasonographically demonstrated nodules in a young patient
- Psammomatous melanotic schwannoma
- Multiple blue nevi
- Multiple ductal adenomas of the breast
- Osteochondromyxoma

Supplemental criteria
- First-degree relative with the Carney complex
- Inactivating mutation of the *PRKAR1A* gene

Adapted from Stratakis CA et al.[15] Included with permission, The Endocrine Society, Copyright 2001.

Other Benign Tumors Papillary fibroelastomas arise usually from the valvular endocardium, most commonly the aortic valve.[28] They resemble a "sea anemone,"[29] being composed of papillary fronds similar to normal chordae tendineae. They can be asymptomatic or can produce anginal symptoms (by obstruction of coronary ostia) as well as embolic phenomena with transient ischemic attacks or stroke.[30,31] Several authorities recommend that papillary fibroelastomas be removed surgically, even if asymptomatic, given the risk of embolic complications from fibroelastomas.[31,32]

Rhabdomyomas occur almost exclusively in children and are often multiple. They are associated with tuberous sclerosis in one-third of patients.[5] Rhabdomyomas tend to regress spontaneously, and surgical excision is usually necessary only in the presence of outflow tract obstruction.[33,34] Lipomas are less common than lipomatous hypertrophy of the atrial septum and can occur anywhere in the heart, like hemangiomas. Fibromas frequently arise from the interventricular septum. Hamartomas of mature cardiac myocytes are very rare.[4] Pericardial cysts are most common in the right costophrenic angle, and bronchogenic cysts can be found in the myocardium.[5]

Malignant Primary Cardiac Tumors Sarcomas, including angiosarcomas, malignant fibrous histiocytomas, rhabdomyosarcomas, and fibrosarcomas, represent the most common malignant tumors of the heart. Whereas angiosarcomas tend to occur in the right atrium, nonvascular sarcomas occur frequently in left-sided chambers.[35]

The peak age for angiosarcomas is between 20 and 50 years, with a two- to threefold male predominance.[5] Like myxomas, they present with a variety of symptoms, including palpitations, dyspnea, and chest pain (pleuritic and/or pericardial). Most commonly, however, primary cardiac tumors present with signs and symptoms related to congestive heart failure or thromboembolism.[3] The electrocardiogram may be normal or may reveal nonspecific findings, such as ST segment or T-wave changes, arrhythmias, or conduction defects. In 10% of patients, the presenting symptoms are systemic, with fever, weight loss, and malaise, without cardiac symptoms. These tumors can spread locally to the pleura or mediastinum. Metastases are common (64% of cases),[36] affecting the lung, liver, bone, adrenal glands, central nervous system, and lymph nodes.[5,10]

The tumors are composed of malignant cells forming vascular channels. Immunoperoxidase stain for factor VIII is positive.[10] The term *hemangiopericytoma* is reserved for rare cases in which more solid areas are seen.[5] The relationship between cardiac angiosarcomas and Kaposi's sarcoma deserves further study. Cardiac involvement has been described in patients with both the African form of Kaposi's sarcoma and that seen in acquired immune deficiency syndrome (AIDS) patients.[10] Whether such involvement can occur without skin lesions is uncertain.

Complete surgical resection of cardiac angiosarcomas, as in other cardiac malignancies, is usually impossible. Orthotopic heart transplantation, at times combined with bilateral lung transplantation, has been described in a few small series and case reports. Although, in most cases, heart transplantation followed by chemotherapy does not affect the long-term outcome,[37] selected patients may have good outcomes with transplantation.[35,38] A survey of the 173 heart transplant centers in the United States and Canada, with a 76% reply rate, revealed only 24 cases of transplantation for primary cardiac malignancy, and an accompanying literature review revealed 104

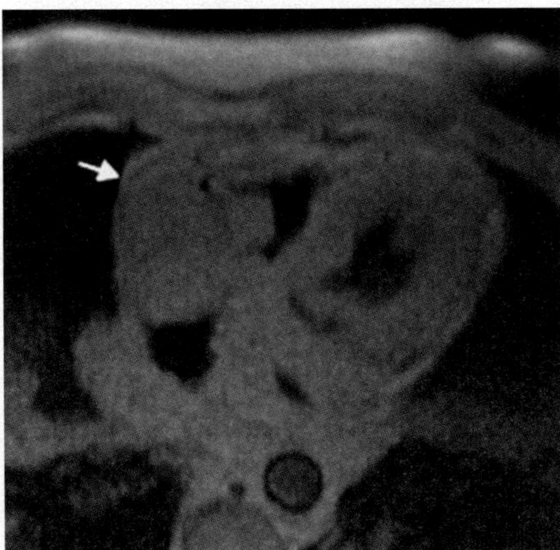

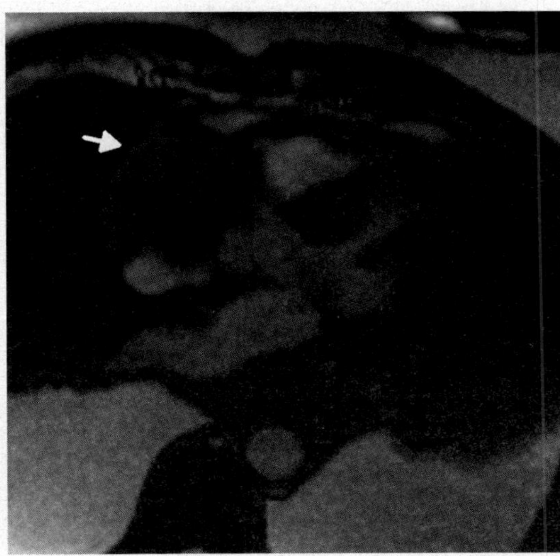

Figure 83-1 Cardiac magnetic resonance images of a 69-year-old man with lymphoma demonstrating a large homogeneous mass (*arrows*) occupying most of the right atrium and extending into the right ventricle and posterior mediastinum. The image on the left is a dark-blood image in the four-chamber view obtained using T_2-weighted half-Fourier acquisition single-shot turbo spin echo. The image on the right is a bright-blood image in the four-chamber view obtained using steady-state free precession; note the large bilateral pleural effusions.

published cases. One-year survival was 54% in the survey and 32% in the review, although at least five patients survived more than 4 years.[39] A novel surgical approach in recurrent atrial malignancies is atrial homograft transplantation using donor atria from a tissue bank.[40]

In other cases, resection has been possible using cardiopulmonary bypass,[23,24] followed by various combinations of radiotherapy and chemotherapy based on doxorubicin. A few patients thus treated have survived to 3 years.[41,42] Regardless of treatment strategy, survival for patients with primary cardiac sarcomas remains poor, with a mean survival of 16.5 months after diagnosis.[43]

Malignant fibrous histiocytomas occur typically in the left atrium, leading to pulmonary congestion, obstruction of pulmonary veins, and mitral stenosis, although these may be preceded by constitutional symptoms. Treatment is surgical palliation. Although adjuvant chemotherapy and/or radiation may be used, an optimal protocol has not been determined. The mean survival is 5 to 18 months.[3]

Rhabdomyosarcomas are seen in all age groups but more commonly in adults. They occur equally commonly in males and females and arise in any cardiac chamber. They are multiple in 60% of the cases. The prognosis is also poor, with a survival of less than a year. Other histologic types of sarcoma may also rarely occur in the heart; some are listed in Table 83-1.

In addition to sarcomas, the other class of primary cardiac malignancies is lymphoma. Primary cardiac lymphomas occur more commonly in patients with human immunodeficiency virus (HIV) infection and may have a good response to chemotherapy if diagnosed early.[44]

Metastatic Tumors to the Heart Most neoplasms of the heart are metastatic, not primary, and the propensity for cardiac or pericardial metastasis varies by tumor type. According to statistics from 6,240 autopsies of cancer patients from two large series, the frequency of heart metastases was, in decreasing order, melanoma (46%), malignant germ cell tumor (38%), leukemia (33%), lung carcinoma (17%), lymphoma (17%), sarcoma (15%), esophageal carcinoma (13%), renal carcinoma (11%), and breast carcinoma (10%).[4] Almost any cancer, however, can metastasize to the heart. Pericardial metastasis occurs most commonly in lung carcinoma (11%).[4] We found a high frequency of cardiac metastasis and/or invasion in patients with malignant pleural mesothelioma.[45] In 19 autopsies, cardiac invasion was found in 14 (74%), with more than half involving the pericardium and more than one-quarter the myocardium.[46]

TUMORS OF THE GREAT VESSELS

Primary tumors involving the aorta, pulmonary artery, and vena cavae are rare, appearing in the literature mainly as case reports or in small retrospective case series.[47–49] As is the case with primary cardiac tumors, risk factors for the development of tumors of the great vessels remain poorly defined. Prior radiation exposure has been postulated as a possible causative factor.[50] Plastic polymers, such as Dacron, are linked to aortic tumors in animal studies. Nonetheless, aortic tumors arising around a Dacron graft in humans, although reported, are extremely rare.[51] The mode of presentation of tumors of the great vessels typically involves thromboembolic events or an obstructive syndrome.[47] MRI and TEE are useful in differentiating tumors of the great vessels from intraluminal thrombus, mediastinal lymphadenopathy, or adjacent lung tumors.[49]

Benign tumors reportedly found in the aorta include endothelial papillary fibroelastomas arising in the aortic sinuses. These tumors may present with emboli to the brain and heart or by intermittent prolapse into a coronary artery.[52] Intra-aortic myxomas have also been detected after presentation with recurrent arterial emboli.[48]

Malignant tumors of the aorta and pulmonary artery are often aggressive, poorly differentiated sarcomas arising from intimal cells and showing myofibroblastic differentiation ("intimal type"). More rarely, they are identified as angiosarcomas or leimyosarcomas.[47] Other tumor types, such as malignant hemangioendothelioma, schwannoma, and fibrous histiocytoma, have also been reported to arise in the great vessels.[53–55] Sarcomas of the inferior vena cava, in contrast to those of the aorta and pulmonary artery, tend to be well-differentiated leiomyosarcomas. Malignant tumors of the great vessels are frequently confined to the lumen on diagnosis.

Sarcomas of the pulmonary artery present at a mean age of 41 years, whereas sarcomas of the aorta present at a mean age of 62 years. In a review of 60 cases, the median age was 52 years, and the male-to-female ratio was 1:2.[56] The median duration of symptoms was 10 months. The clinical picture was suggestive of pulmonary embolism, with dyspnea (70%), chest pain (48%), cough (34%), hemoptysis (30%), and syncope (25%). Metastases to lungs were common (67%), as were lymph node metastases (20%). The cornerstone of therapy for the tumors of the great vessels is complete surgical excision. The use of various grafts has been advocated.[57] Postoperative radiation therapy and chemotherapy, often with an anthracycline-based regimen, are also employed.[47,53] Regression of pulmonary metastases has been observed after a combination of etoposide, vincristine, ifosfamide, and doxorubicin.[57] The average survival is 10 months.[57,58] According to Burke and Virmani, however, the mean survival after diagnosis for sarcomas of the pulmonary artery was 23 months, as opposed to 5 months for aortic sarcomas.[47] Prolonged survival is extremely rare but has been reported.[59] A 75-year-old personal patient remains free of recurrence more than 6 years after surgical resection[60] followed by a course of chemotherapy with doxorubicin, ifosfamide, and mesna. For patients with unresectable disease, endovascular stent grafting may improve quality of life.[61]

REFERENCES

1. Columbo R. De re anatomica libri XV. Venice: Nicolo Bevilacqua; 1559.
2. King TW. On simple vascular growths in the left auricle of the heart. Lancet 1845;2:428–9.
3. Travis WD, Brambilla E, Mueller-Hermelink HK, Harris CC, editors. World Health Organization classification of tumors. Pathology and genetics of tumours of the lung, pleura, thymus, and heart. Lyon (France): IARC Press; 2004.
4. Burke A, Virmani R. Tumors of the heart and great vessels. In: Atlas of tumor pathology. 3rd Series. Fascicle 16. Washington (DC): Armed Forces Institute of Pathology; 1996.
5. McAllister JHA, Fenoglio JJJ. Tumors of the cardiovascular system. In: Atlas of tumor pathology. 2nd Series. Fascicle 15. Washington (DC): Armed Forces Institute of Pathology; 1978.

6. Perchinsky MJ, Lichtenstein SV, Tyers GF. Primary cardiac tumors: forty years' experience with 71 patients. Cancer 1997;79:1809–15.
7. Thomas CR Jr, Johnson GW Jr, Stoddard MF, Clifford S. Primary malignant cardiac tumors: update 1992. Med Pediatr Oncol 1992;20:519–31.
8. Freedom RM, Lee KJ, MacDonald C, Taylor G. Selected aspects of cardiac tumors in infancy and childhood. Pediatr Cardiol 2000;21:299–316.
9. Isaacs H Jr. Fetal and neonatal cardiac tumors. Pediatr Cardiol 2004;25:252–73.
10. Hoch-Ligeti C, Restrepo C, Stewart HL. Comparative pathology of cardiac neoplasms in humans and in laboratory rodents: a review. J Natl Cancer Inst 1986;76:127–42.
11. Burch GE, Shewey LL, Harb JM. Coxsackie B4 viruses and atrial myxoma. Am Heart J 1974;88:634–9.
12. Larbcharoensub N, Singhsnaeh A, Leelachaikul P. Primary cardiac angiosarcoma with systemic metastases; a case report and review of the literature. J Med Assoc Thai 2004;87:1116–22.
13. Kuon E, Kreplin M, Weiss W, Dahm JB. The challenge presented by right atrial myxoma. Herz 2004;29:702–9.
14. Allard MF, Taylor GP, Wilson JE, McManus BM. Primary cardiac tumors. In: Braunwald E, editor. Atlas of heart diseases. Volume III. Cardiopulmonary diseases and cardiac tumors. St. Louis: Mosby; 1995. p. 15.1–6.5.
15. Stratakis CA, Kirschner LS, Carney JA. Clinical and molecular features of the Carney complex: diagnostic criteria and recommendations for patient evaluation. J Clin Endocrinol Metab 2001;86:4041–6.
16. Veugelers M, Bressan M, McDermott DA, et al. Mutation of perinatal myosin heavy chain associated with a Carney complex variant. N Engl J Med 2004;351:460–9.
17. Stratakis CA. Mutations of the gene encoding the protein kinase A type I-alpha regulatory subunit (PRKAR1A) in patients with the "complex of spotty skin pigmentation, myxomas, endocrine overactivity, and schwannomas" (Carney complex). Ann N Y Acad Sci 2002;968:3–21.
18. Basson CT, Aretz HT. Case records of the Massachusetts General Hospital. Weekly clinicopathological exercises. Case 11-2002. A 27-year-old woman with two intracardiac masses and a history of endocrinopathy. N Engl J Med 2002;346:1152–8.
19. Geibel A, Kasper W, Keck A, et al. Diagnosis, localization and evaluation of malignancy of heart and mediastinal tumors by conventional and transesophageal echocardiography. Acta Cardiol 1996;51:395–408.
20. Kirkpatrick JN, Wong T, Bednarz JE, et al. Differential diagnosis of cardiac masses using contrast echocardiographic perfusion imaging. J Am Coll Cardiol 2004;43:1412–9.
21. Lokhandwala J, Liu Z, Jundi M, et al. Three-dimensional echocardiography of intracardiac masses. Echocardiography 2004;21:159–63.
22. Mader MT, Poulton TB, White RD. Malignant tumors of the heart and great vessels: MR imaging appearance. Radiographics 1997;17:145–53.
23. Kaminaga T, Takeshita T, Kimura I. Role of magnetic resonance imaging for evaluation of tumors in the cardiac region. Eur Radiol 2003;13 Suppl 4:L1–10.
24. Feuchtner G, Mueller S, Bonatti J, et al. Images in cardiovascular medicine. Prolapsing atrial myxoma: dynamic visualization with multislice computed tomography. Circulation 2004;109:e165–6.
25. Araoz PA, Mulvagh SL, Tazelaar HD, et al. CT and MR imaging of benign primary cardiac neoplasms with echocardiographic correlation. Radiographics 2000;20:1303–19.
26. Grebenc ML, Rosado de Christenson ML, Burke AP, et al. Primary cardiac and pericardial neoplasms: radiologic-pathologic correlation. Radiographics 2000;20:1073–103; quiz 1110–1, 1112.
27. Attum AA, Johnson GS, Masri Z, et al. Malignant clinical behavior of cardiac myxomas and "myxoid imitators." Ann Thorac Surg 1987;44:217–22.
28. Di Mattia DG, Assaghi A, Mangini A, et al. Mitral valve repair for anterior leaflet papillary fibroelastoma: two case descriptions and a literature review. Eur J Cardiothorac Surg 1999;15:103–7.
29. McAllister HA Jr, Hall RJ, Cooley DA. Tumors of the heart and pericardium. Curr Probl Cardiol 1999;24:57–116.
30. Brown RD Jr, Khandheria BK, Edwards WD. Cardiac papillary fibroelastoma: a treatable cause of transient ischemic attack and ischemic stroke detected by transesophageal echocardiography. Mayo Clin Proc 1995;70:863–8.
31. Giannesini C, Kubis N, N'Guyen A, et al. Cardiac papillary fibroelastoma: a rare cause of ischemic stroke in the young. Cerebrovasc Dis 1999;9:45–9.
32. Carmi D, Touati GD, Roux N, et al. Papillary fibroelastoma. Report of 3 cases. Arch Mal Coeur Vaiss 1999;92:331–5.
33. Beghetti M, Gow RM, Haney I, et al. Pediatric primary benign cardiac tumors: a 15-year review. Am Heart J 1997;134:1107–14.
34. Black MD, Kadletz M, Smallhorn JF, Freedom RM. Cardiac rhabdomyomas and obstructive left heart disease: histologically but not functionally benign. Ann Thorac Surg 1998;65:1388–90.
35. Grandmougin D, Fayad G, Decoene C, et al. Total orthotopic heart transplantation for primary cardiac rhabdomyosarcoma: factors influencing long-term survival. Ann Thorac Surg 2001;71:1438–41.
36. Ogle GD, Bell DR. Angiosarcoma of the heart. Aust N Z J Med 1987;17:74–6.
37. Uberfuhr P, Meiser B, Fuchs A, et al. Heart transplantation: an approach to treating primary cardiac sarcoma? J Heart Lung Transplant. 2002;21:1135–9.
38. Aravot DJ, Banner NR, Madden B, et al. Primary cardiac tumours—is there a place for cardiac transplantation? Eur J Cardiothorac Surg 1989;3:521–4.
39. Rodriguez-Cruz E, Cintron-Maldonado RM, Forbes TJ. Treatment of primary cardiac malignancies with orthotopic heart transplantation. Bol Asoc Med P R. 2000;92:65–71.
40. Stoica SC, Mitchell IM, Foreman J, et al. Atrial transplantation for recurrent cardiac sarcoma. J Heart Lung Transplant 2001;20:1220–3.
41. Percy RF, Perryman RA, Amornmarn R, et al. Prolonged survival in a patient with primary angiosarcoma of the heart. Am Heart J 1987;113:1228–30.
42. Rossi NP, Kioschos JM, Aschenbrener CA, Ehrenhaft JL. Primary angiosarcoma of the heart. Cancer 1976;37:891–4.
43. Donsbeck AV, Ranchere D, Coindre JM, et al. Primary cardiac sarcomas: an immunohistochemical and grading study with long-term follow-up of 24 cases. Histopathology 1999;34:295–304.
44. Kaplan LD, Afridi NA, Holmvang G, Zukerberg LR. Case records of the Massachusetts General Hospital. Weekly clinicopathological exercises. Case 31-2003. A 44-year-old man with HIV infection and a right atrial mass. N Engl J Med 2003;349:1369–77.
45. Chahinian AP, Pajak TF, Holland JF, et al. Diffuse malignant mesothelioma. Prospective evaluation of 69 patients. Ann Intern Med 1982;96:746–55.
46. Wadler S, Chahinian P, Slater W, et al. Cardiac abnormalities in patients with diffuse malignant pleural mesothelioma. Cancer 1986;58:2744–50.
47. Burke AP, Virmani R. Sarcomas of the great vessels. A clinicopathologic study. Cancer 1993;71:1761–73.
48. Das AK, Reddy KS, Suwanjindar P, et al. Primary tumors of the aorta. Ann Thorac Surg 1996;62:1526–8.
49. Parish JM, Rosenow EC III, Swensen SJ, Crotty TB. Pulmonary artery sarcoma. Clinical features. Chest 1996;110:1480–8.
50. Shah IA, Kurtz SM, Simonsen RL. Radiation-induced malignant fibrous histiocytoma of the pulmonary artery. Arch Pathol Lab Med 1991;115:921–5.
51. Weiss WM, Riles TS, Gouge TH, Mizrachi HH. Angiosarcoma at the site of a Dacron vascular prosthesis: a case report and literature review. J Vasc Surg 1991;14:87–91.
52. Boone S, Higginson LA, Walley VM. Endothelial papillary fibroelastomas arising in and around the aortic sinus, filling the ostium of the right coronary artery. Arch Pathol Lab Med 1992;116:135–7.
53. Bacha EA, Wright CD, Grillo HC, et al. Surgical treatment of primary pulmonary sarcomas. Eur J Cardiothorac Surg 1999;15:456–60.
54. Fonseca JL, Fernandez-Valderrama I, Gesto R, et al. Malignant fibrous histiocytoma of the aorta complicated by anuria. Ann Vasc Surg 1992;6:164–7.
55. Shijubo N, Nakata H, Sugaya F, et al. Malignant hemangioendothelioma of the aorta. Intern Med 1995;34:1126–9.
56. Bleisch VR, Kraus FT. Polypoid sarcoma of the pulmonary trunk: analysis of the literature and report of a case with leptomeric organelles and ultrastructural features of rhabdomyosarcoma. Cancer 1980;46:314–24.
57. Zerkowski HR, Hofmann HS, Gybels I, Knolle J. Primary sarcoma of pulmonary artery and valve: multimodality treatment by chemotherapy and homograft replacement. J Thorac Cardiovasc Surg 1996;112:1122–4.
58. Akomea-Agyin C, Dussek JE, Anderson DR, Hartley RB. Pulmonary artery sarcoma mimicking pulmonary embolism: successful surgical intervention. Ann Thorac Surg 1996;61:1536–8.
59. Mattoo A, Fedullo PF, Kapelanski D, Ilowite JS. Pulmonary artery sarcoma: a case report of surgical cure and 5-year follow-up. Chest 2002;122:745–7.
60. Croitoru AG, Klein MJ, Galla JD, Fallon JT. Primary pulmonary artery leiomyosarcoma. Cardiovasc Pathol 2003;12:166–9
61. Totaro M, Miraldi F, Ghiribelli C, Biscosi C. Cardiac angiosarcoma arising from pulmonary artery: endovascular treatment. Ann Thorac Surg 2004;78:1468–70.

84

Primary Germ Cell Tumors of the Thorax

John D. Hainsworth, MD
F. Anthony Greco, MD

The biology and clinical characteristics of mediastinal germ cell tumors have been defined during the last 30 years. These neoplasms, although rare, are of particular interest because they usually affect young males and because curative therapy is now available for many patients. The clinical and pathologic characteristics of benign and malignant germ cell tumors and of poorly differentiated carcinoma of the mediastinum are presented, with special attention focused on the treatment of these neoplasms.

BENIGN TERATOMAS OF THE MEDIASTINUM

Although benign teratomas of the mediastinum (mature cystic teratomas or dermoid tumors) account for only 3 to 12% of mediastinal tumors, they comprise 60 to 70% of all mediastinal germ cell tumors.[1,2] These tumors have been described in patients with ages ranging from 7 months to 65 years; however, most occur in young adults, with an approximately equal incidence in males and females.[2,3] No predisposing conditions or associated abnormalities have been recognized in patients developing these tumors.

Benign mediastinal teratomas have a histologic appearance identical to that of benign teratomas arising in the more common ovarian location. These tumors are usually well encapsulated and are composed either of a single large cystic cavity or of several smaller intercommunicating cystic spaces. On histologic examination, mature tissue from ectodermal, mesodermal, and endodermal germ cell layers is typically present. Mature tissue that recapitulates the histology of any human organ can be found in these tumors. However, the ectodermal component (ie, skin, sebaceous tissue, neural tissue) is usually predominant.[3]

Approximately 95% of benign teratomas arise in the anterior mediastinum; the remainder arise in the posterior mediastinum.[2,3] These tumors are slow growing, and in recent years, 50 to 60% of patients have been asymptomatic at the time of diagnosis by routine chest radiography.[3] When symptoms are present, dyspnea and substernal chest pain are the most common. Cough productive of hair or sebum is pathognomonic of a benign mediastinal tumor. However, this distinctive symptom is extremely rare and occurs late in the natural history of this condition following tumor rupture into the tracheobronchial tree. Superior vena cava syndrome is also rare and is a late manifestation. Most patients with benign mediastinal teratomas appear to be healthy, and physical examination contributes little to the diagnosis. Likewise, laboratory evaluation is usually normal. Serum levels of human chorionic gonadotropin (HCG) and alpha-fetoprotein are always normal in patients with benign teratoma.

The chest radiograph typically reveals a well-circumscribed anterior mediastinal mass that often protrudes into one of the lung fields. These tumors are usually large at the time of diagnosis; in one large series, the median size was $10 \times 8.5 \times 5.4$ cm.[3] Occasionally, chest radiography identifies teeth within the tumor, a pathognomonic finding. Calcification is present in up to 25% of tumors, occurring in fragments of bone, in the tumor wall, or in other areas throughout the tumor, in addition to its occasional occurrence in teeth.

Surgical excision is the treatment of choice for benign teratoma of the mediastinum. Median sternotomy is usually the best surgical approach, although successful resection can also be accomplished by thoracotomy. Surgical removal is sometimes difficult because of the large size of the tumor and the involvement of other structures, such as the pericardium, lung, great vessels, thymus, chest wall, hilar structures, and diaphragm, in decreasing order of frequency. Some 10 to 15% of patients require additional procedures (eg, lobectomy, pericardiectomy) for complete tumor resection. Benign teratomas are resistant to radiation and cytotoxic drugs, and these modalities have no role in their treatment.

Tumor recurrence is rare following complete surgical resection.[2–4] Prolonged survival has also been reported in patients who underwent only subtotal resection owing to the involvement of vital mediastinal structures. The operative mortality rate in recent years has been very low.

MALIGNANT GERM CELL TUMORS

Etiology Malignant mediastinal germ cell tumors of various histologies were first described as a clinical entity approximately 50 years ago.[5,6] Mediastinal and other extragonadal germ cell tumors were initially thought to represent isolated metastases from an inapparent gonadal primary site. However, there is now abundant clinical evidence to substantiate the extragonadal origin of these tumors.[1,7] Extragonadal germ cell tumors, particularly those arising in mediastinal and pineal sites, represent a malignant transformation of germinal elements distributed to these sites and can occur in the absence of a primary focus in the gonad. Some investigators suggest that this distribution arises as a consequence of abnormal migration of germ cells during embryogenesis.[6,8] Others hypothesize a widespread distribution of germ cells to multiple sites during normal embryogenesis, with these cells conveying genetic information or providing regulatory functions at somatic sites.[9]

Epidemiology Malignant germ cell tumors of the mediastinum are uncommon, representing only 3 to 10% of tumors originating in the mediastinum.[10] They are much less common than germinal tumors arising in the testes and account for only 1 to 5% of all germ cell neoplasms.[11] These figures, most of which are derived from retrospective series reported between 1950 and 1975, may underestimate the true occurrence of mediastinal germ cell tumors. The histology of these tumors may be similar to other poorly differentiated mediastinal tumors, including malignant thymoma and high-grade non-Hodgkin's lymphoma. Some patients with poorly differentiated neoplasm or poorly differentiated carcinoma of the mediastinum have the i(12p) chromosomal abnormality diagnostic of germ cell tumor.[12] Other patients with poorly differentiated carcinoma of the mediastinum have clinical characteristics and treatment responses typical of patients with extragonadal germ cell tumors.[13] Although there is no doubt that mediastinal germ cell tumors are uncommon, increasing familiarity with the tumors by both clinicians and pathologists will probably result in their increased recognition.

The great majority of mediastinal malignant germ cell tumors occur in patients between 20 and 35 years of age. For unknown reasons, most are found in males. In the rare occurrences reported in females, mediastinal malignant germ cell tumors have appeared to be histologically and biologically identical to those occurring in males. The relative rarity of extragonadal germ cell tumors in women parallels the lower incidence of female gonadal germ cell tumors compared with their incidence in males. Although the incidence of primary testis tumors is low among racial minorities in the United States, the occurrence of extragonadal germ cell tumors is somewhat more common (7% vs 16% of cases, respectively).[14,15]

Patients with nonseminomatous extragonadal germ cell tumors have a subsequent increased risk of developing testicular cancer, strengthening the concept of a precursor abnormality (the so-called "testicular intraepithelial neoplasm") in the germ cells of these patients.[16]

Histopathology In general, mediastinal germ cell tumors appear to be histologically identical to germ cell tumors arising in the testis, and all histologic subtypes seen in gonadal germ cell neoplasms have also been recognized in the mediastinum. In a recent review of 229 malignant mediastinal germ cell tumors seen between 1960 and 1994 at the Armed Forces Institute of Pathology, pure seminoma was the most common histology, accounting for 52% of cases.[17] Nonseminomatous histologies included teratocarcinoma (20%), yolk sac tumor (17%), choriocarcinoma (3.4%), embryonal carcinoma (2.6%), and mixed nonseminomatous tumors (5.2%).

Clinical Characteristics Unlike benign germ cell tumors of the mediastinum, malignant mediastinal tumors are usually symptomatic at the time of diagnosis. Most mediastinal malignant tumors are large and cause symptoms by compressing or invading adjacent structures, including the lungs, pleura, pericardium, and chest wall. Pure seminomas are somewhat slower growing and have less potential for early metastasis than do tumors with nonseminomatous elements; their initial presentation, therefore, varies somewhat. Pure seminomas and tumors with nonseminomatous elements are discussed separately, although a great deal of overlap exists in their clinical characteristics.

Seminoma Seminomas grow relatively slowly and can become very large before causing symptoms. Tumors 20 to 30 cm in diameter can exist with minimal symptomatology. Approximately 20 to 30% of seminomas are detected by routine chest radiography while still asymptomatic.[18] The most common initial symptom is a sensation of pressure or dull retrosternal chest pain. Additional symptoms include exertional dyspnea, cough, dysphagia, and hoarseness. Superior vena cava syndrome develops in approximately 10% of patients. Systemic symptoms related to metastatic lesions are uncommon.

At the time of diagnosis, only 30 to 40% of patients with mediastinal seminoma have localized disease; the remainder have one or more sites of distant metastases.[19] The regional lymph nodes (cervical, upper abdominal) are the most common metastatic sites; lung and bone are the most common visceral sites.[20] The retroperitoneum is an uncommon site of metastasis in patients with mediastinal seminoma.[1,19,20]

Pure seminoma appears radiographically as a large, noncalcified anterior mediastinal mass that can compress or deviate the trachea or bronchi if of sufficient size. A computed tomographic (CT) scan of the chest typically shows a large homogeneous anterior mediastinal mass that obliterates the fat planes surrounding mediastinal vascular structures.[21] The radiographic findings are not specific enough to allow the distinction of mediastinal seminoma from other mediastinal tumors.

Elevated serum levels of HCG are detected in up to 40% of mediastinal seminomas.[20] However, most of these are low-level elevations (2–10 ng/mL); levels of HCG exceeding 100 ng/mL are unusual and suggest the presence of nonseminomatous elements. The serum alpha-fetoprotein level is always normal in pure mediastinal seminoma, and any elevation of this tumor marker indicates the presence of nonseminomatous elements. Serum lactic dehydrogenase is also elevated in the majority of patients with mediastinal seminoma.[19,20]

Nonseminomatous Germ Cell Tumor Few patients with these rapidly growing neoplasms are asymptomatic at diagnosis. Symptoms caused by compression or invasion of local mediastinal structures are identical to those seen in patients with mediastinal seminoma. However, presenting symptoms caused by metastatic lesions are much more common because 85 to 95% of these patients have at least one metastatic site at the time of diagnosis.[22–24] Common metastatic sites include the lungs, pleura, lymph nodes (particularly supraclavicular and retroperitoneal), and liver. Less frequent sites of involvement include the bone, brain, and kidney. High levels of HCG sometimes are associated with gynecomastia. Neoplasms with elements of choriocarcinoma have a marked hemorrhagic tendency; these patients may have catastrophic events related to uncontrolled hemorrhage at a metastatic site (eg, massive hemoptysis, intracranial hemorrhage).[25] Constitutional symptoms, including weight loss, weakness, and fever, are more common in these patients than in those with pure seminoma.

Chest radiographic features of mediastinal nonseminomatous germ cell tumors are similar to those seen in mediastinal seminomas. The CT scan frequently shows an inhomogeneous mass, with multiple areas of hemorrhage and necrosis, differing from the usually homogeneous appearance of mediastinal seminoma.[21]

The serum tumor markers HCG and alpha-fetoprotein are usually abnormal in patients with mediastinal nonseminomatous germ cell tumors. Alpha-fetoprotein is most frequently abnormal and is elevated either alone or in conjunction with HCG in 80 to 90% of patients, whereas elevation of HCG occurs in only 30 to 35% of patients.[26,27] This pattern of marker elevation differs slightly from that seen in testicular cancer, in which elevations of HCG and alpha-fetoprotein occur with nearly equal frequency and are seen in 50 to 70% of patients with metastatic tumor. As in mediastinal seminoma, elevation of serum lactic dehydrogenase is frequent, occurring in 80 to 90% of patients.[23]

SYNDROMES ASSOCIATED WITH MEDIASTINAL NONSEMINOMATOUS GERM CELL TUMORS

Klinefelter's Syndrome Klinefelter's syndrome is a relatively common chromosomal abnormality characterized by hypogonadism, azoospermia, and elevated gonadotropin levels in association with a 47,XXY karyotype. A slightly increased incidence of breast cancer has been described in these men, but a general predisposition to other cancers has not been observed.[28] The association of Klinefelter's syndrome and mediastinal nonseminomatous germ cell tumors is now well recognized.[29,30] Four of 22 consecutive patients (18%) treated at Indiana University for primary mediastinal germ cell tumors had karyotypic confirmation of Klinefelter's syndrome, and an additional patient had clinical features.[31] The average age of patients with Klinefelter's syndrome who develop extragonadal germ cell tumors is approximately 18 years, 10 years younger than the median age of those developing this tumor in the absence of Klinefelter's syndrome. Testicular germ cell neoplasms have rarely been reported in association with Klinefelter's syndrome; therefore, the association with mediastinal germ cell tumor seems specific.

The explanation for this association is unknown, but it seems reasonable to assume that the chromosomal abnormality plays some role. Increasing evidence indicates that many individuals who develop germ cell tumors have underlying germ cell defects. Many patients with extragonadal germ cell tumors have histories of infertility, and testicular biopsy in these patients shows various abnormalities, including decreased spermatogenesis, peritubular fibrosis, and interstitial edema.[32] In addition, patients who are successfully treated for extragonadal germ cell tumors have a markedly increased risk of developing a subsequent testicular germ cell tumor.[16] These data suggest that either a congenital or an acquired germ cell defect contributes not only to defective spermatogenesis but also to the development of extragonadal germ cell tumors.

Hematologic Neoplasia A unique association between mediastinal nonseminomatous germ cell tumors and a variety of hematologic neoplasms is now well described.[33–39] Hematologic neoplasms have included acute myeloid leukemia, acute nonlymphocytic leukemia, acute lymphocytic leukemia, erythroleukemia, acute megakaryocytic leukemia, myelodysplastic syndrome, and malignant histiocytosis. In a series of 635 patients with extragonadal germ cell tumors, 17 patients developed hematologic malignancies at a median of 6 months after the extragonadal germ cell tumor was diagnosed.[39] All hematologic neoplasms developed in the 287 patients with mediastinal nonseminomatous germ cell tumors, for a 2% incidence in this group. Median survival was only 5 months after the hematologic disorder was diagnosed, and no patient survived for more than 2 years.

Recent evidence indicates that the hematologic neoplasms in this setting are not treatment related but rather arise from clones of malignant lymphoblasts or myeloblasts contained within the mediastinal germ cell tumor. Foci of malignant lymphoblasts have been recognized histologically in several mediastinal germ cell tumors.[35,36] More importantly, several patients have had an identical chromosomal abnormality (an isochromosome of the short arm of chromosome 12) in the neoplastic cells from the mediastinal germ cell tumor and the hematologic neoplasm, providing strong evidence of a common origin.[36–38] However, the specific

Table 84-1 Mediastinal Seminoma: Treatment with Cisplatin-Based Combination Chemotherapy

Study, Year	Number of Patients	Received Previous Radiotherapy	Treatment Regimen	Number of Complete Responses (%)	Number of Long-Term Disease-Free Survivors, Mo
Hainsworth et al, 1982[22]	4	3	PVB	3 (75)	3 (> 24)
Jain et al, 1984[19]	11	0	VAB-6, 8, PVB 1, DDP/CTX 2	10 (91)	10 (19 + –46)
Logothetis et al, 1985[24]	4	Unspecified	DDP/CTX 3, CISCA 21	4 (100)	4 (unspecified)
Loehrer et al, 1987[42]	9	7	PVB ± A or BEP	8 (89)	7 (unspecified)
Bukowski et al, 1993[43]	8	0	PVB/EBAP	5 (63)	4 (> 24)
Delgado et al, 1993[44]	6	0	VAP-6, PVB, BEP	5 (83)	5 (5–103)
Goss et al, 1994[45]	8	0	BEP 6, BEP + RT 1, VAB-6 1	8 (100)	8 (4–132)
Mencel et al, 1994[46]	19	0	VAP-6, EP	19 (100)	18 (> 24)
Gerl et al, 1996[47]	4	1	VIP, EIP	4 (100)	4 (> 24)
Bokemeyer et al, 2001[48]	51	0	Cisplatin based	NA	45 (88%)

A = Adriamycin (doxorubicin); BEP = bleomycin 30 U weekly, etoposide 100 mg/m^2 intravenously (IV) × 5 days, cisplatin 20 mg/m^2 IV × 5 days, cycles repeated q 3 weeks; CISCA = multidrug regimen developed at The University of Texas M. D. Anderson Cancer Center; CISCA2 = multidrug regimen developed at M.D. Anderson; CTX =cyclophosphamide; DDP = cisplatin; EBAP = etoposide, bleomycin, cisplatin; EIP = etoposide, ifosfamide, cisplatin; EP = etoposide, cisplatin; NA = not available; PVB (Einhorn regimen) = cisplatin 20 mg/m^2 IV × 5 days, vinblastine 0.15 mg/kg D 1,2, bleomycin 30 U weekly, cycle repeated VAB-6 = multidrug regimen developed at Memorial Sloan-Kettering Cancer Center; VIP = vinblastine, ifosfamide, cisplatin.

association of leukemias and other hematologic neoplasms with mediastinal nonseminomatous germ cell tumors, rather than with all germ cell tumors, remains unexplained.

In addition to hematologic neoplasia, several cases of idiopathic thrombocytopenia in association with mediastinal nonseminomatous germ cell tumors have been reported.[40,41] These patients had normal numbers of megakaryocytes in the bone marrow; however, immune destruction of platelets could not be demonstrated. Prednisone and splenectomy were unsuccessful in increasing the platelet count; persistent thrombocytopenia caused significant morbidity in all patients and made treatment extremely difficult. At present, the cause of this syndrome is unknown.

PRETREATMENT EVALUATION AND STAGING

The diagnosis of a mediastinal germ cell tumor should be considered in all young males with a mediastinal mass. In addition to physical examination and routine laboratory studies, initial evaluation should include CT of the chest and abdomen and determination of serum levels of HCG and alpha-fetoprotein. Any symptoms suggestive of distant metastases should be appropriately evaluated with radiologic studies.

In patients with suspected mediastinal germ cell tumor, a histologic diagnosis should be made using the least invasive approach because rapid initiation of definitive systemic therapy is important. Because these neoplasms are poorly differentiated, specimens obtained by fine-needle aspiration biopsy are sometimes insufficient for a definitive diagnosis. In such patients, surgical biopsy via median sternotomy or limited thoracotomy is indicated. Attempts at complete surgical resection of these mediastinal neoplasms are not indicated because curative results with other treatment modalities are superior.

TREATMENT OF SEMINOMA

Pure mediastinal seminomas are curable in the large majority of patients, even when metastatic at the time of diagnosis. These tumors are highly sensitive to radiation therapy and to combination chemotherapy, and the selection of treatment therefore depends on the disease stage and the size of the mediastinal tumor.

Highly effective systemic combination chemotherapy now offers the best option for curative treatment for most patients with mediastinal seminoma. When used in advanced testicular seminoma, intensive cisplatin-based regimens are at least as active as they are against nonseminomatous germ cell tumors. Table 84-1 summarizes the experience with modern cisplatin-based combination regimens in the treatment of pure mediastinal seminoma.[19,22,24,42–48] Even with bulky local tumors and frequent metastatic disease, all recent series have shown cure rates of > 80% with initial cisplatin-based chemotherapy. In a large, retrospective analysis of 51 patients treated at 10 centers between 1975 and 1996, 93% of patients treated with cisplatin-based first-line chemotherapy achieved complete remission, with subsequent relapses in only 14%.[48] Therefore, cisplatin-based chemotherapy, using regimens effective in advanced testicular cancer, should be the treatment of choice for all patients with mediastinal seminoma who have bulky (> 6 cm) masses or evidence of metastatic disease.

Radiation therapy is also a potentially curative treatment for mediastinal seminoma.[4,19,49,50] Approximately 60% of patients with localized tumors are cured with radiotherapy; the relapse rate is correlated with tumor size. However, a majority of relapsing patients remain curable with cisplatin-based chemotherapy.[22,42] As a practical approach to treatment, the use of primary radiation therapy for treatment of patients with seminomas < 6 cm in diameter seems reasonable. This approach allows minimization of toxicity by avoiding chemotherapy in a group of patients with a low risk of relapse. These recommendations mirror current recommendations for treatment of patients with stage II testicular seminoma.

Patients with bulky seminoma at any site frequently have residual radiographic abnormalities on CT scan after chemotherapy. In most patients, these masses represent dense scirrhous reactions rather than viable seminoma or benign teratoma.[48,51,52] Residual seminoma is more frequent when residual lesions are > 3 cm in diameter.[52] However, because of dense fibrosis following chemotherapy, surgical exploration and resection of the residual mediastinal mass are technically difficult and are associated with frequent morbidity and mortality. Recently, PET has proved highly sensitive and specific in differentiating residual seminoma from necrotic or fibrotic masses following chemotherapy.[53] In one series, tumor status in all 19 patients with residual lesions > 3 cm and in 95% of patients with lesions ≤ 3 cm was correctly predicted by PET. Based on these new data, patients with residual CT scan abnormalities should have PET 4 to 8 weeks after completion of chemotherapy. Patients with normal PET scans should be followed without further treatment, whereas those with abnormal PET scans should undergo surgical resection. Patients who do not have surgical exploration should have serial CT scans performed every 3 months during the first year following treatment, with biopsy of any enlarging mass on chest CT.

In summary, most patients with mediastinal seminoma can be cured with therapy, and all patients should be approached with this intent. For most patients, initial cisplatin-based chemotherapy is the treatment of choice. Optimal chemotherapy includes four courses of bleomycin, etoposide, and cisplatin, as is recommended for poor-prognosis testicular germ cell tumors.[54] Patients with mediastinal masses < 6 cm in diameter (usually asymptomatic) have the option of radiation therapy as primary therapy, with cisplatin-based chemotherapy available for those who relapse.

TREATMENT OF NONSEMINOMATOUS TUMORS

Prior to the development of effective cisplatin-based chemotherapy, no effective therapy was available for nonseminomatous mediastinal germ cell tumors.[55] Local treatment modalities were ineffective because of the high percentage of patients with metastatic disease and the relative radioresistance of these tumors.

Table 84-2 Results of Initial Treatment with Cisplatin-Based Combination Chemotherapy in Nonseminomatous Mediastinal Germ Cell Tumors

Study, Year	Number of Evaluable Patients	Chemotherapy Regimen	Number of Complete Responders (%)	Number of Long-Term (> 24 Mo) Disease-Free Survivors (%)
Funes et al, 1981[56]	13	PVB	6 (46)	5 (38)
Hainsworth et al, 1982[22]	12	PVB ± A	7 (58)	7 (58)
Logothetis et al, 1985[24]	11	CISCA II CISCA/VBIV	NA	4 (36)
Israel et al, 1985[23]	11*	VAB-6	NA	4 (36)
Kay et al, 1987[57]	11	PVB, BEP	7 (64)	5 (45)
Nichols et al, 1990[26]	31	PVB ± A, BEP	18 (58)	13 (42)
Bukowski et al, 1993[43]	16	PVB/EBAP	9 (56)	9 (56)
Delgado et al, 1993[44]	40	VAB-6, PVB, BEP	15 (38)	14 (35)
Gerl et al, 1996[47]	12	PVB, BEP, ECBC	8 (67)	6 (50)
Hidalgo et al, 1997[58]	27	Cisplatin based	11 (41)	8 (30)
Fizazi et al, 1998[59]	29	VAP-6, PveVB, PVB, BEP	19 (60)	10 (34)
Ganjoo et al, 2000[27]	75	Cisplatin based	49 (65)	36 (48)
Total	288		49 (56)	121 (42)

A = Adriamycin (doxorubicin); BEP = bleomycin 30 units weekly, etoposide 100 mg/m^2 intravenously (IV) × 5 days, cisplatin 20 mg/m^2 IV × 5 days, cycles repeated every 3 weeks; CISCA II, CISCA/VBIV = multidrug regimens developed at The University of Texas M. D. Anderson Cancer Center; EBAP = etoposide, bleomycin, Adriamycin (doxorubicin), cisplatin; ECBC = etoposide, cisplatin, bleomycin, cyclophosphamide; NA = not available; PVB = cisplatin 20 mg/m^2 IV × 5 days, vinblastine 0.15 mg/kg days 1 and 2, bleomycin 30 U weekly; PveVB = cisplatin, etoposide, vinblastine, bleomycin; VAB-6 = multidrug regimen developed at Memorial Sloan-Kettering Cancer Center.
*Includes patients with retroperitoneal tumors.

The use of intensive cisplatin-based chemotherapy developed for the treatment of advanced nonseminomatous testicular neoplasms has improved the previously dismal outlook in patients with mediastinal nonseminomatous germ cell tumors. Although overall cure rates remain lower than those achieved in the treatment of testicular cancer, a compilation of results from reported series containing 10 or more patients and using optimal chemotherapy indicates a 41% long-term survival rate (Table 84-2).[22–24,26,27,43,44,47,56–59] The large bulk of most mediastinal germ cell tumors at the time of diagnosis contributes to these relatively poor results. Comparable long-term survival rates of 40 to 50% have been reported when testicular germ cell tumors with far advanced, bulky metastases are treated with similar cisplatin-based regimens.[60] However, it is now recognized that inherent biologic differences between mediastinal and testicular germ cell tumors also play a role in determining the relatively low cure rate.[61]

At present, treatment for all histologic subtypes of mediastinal nonseminomatous germ cell tumor should follow the same guidelines. Early reports of an unfavorable outcome for patients with pure endodermal sinus tumors have not been confirmed when modern cisplatin-based chemotherapy is used.[62] Pure mediastinal chemocarcinoma probably has a worse prognosis[22]; however, there is currently no rationale for treating these patients differently from other patients with nonseminomatous mediastinal germ cell tumors.

The treatment for mediastinal nonseminomatous germ cell tumors should follow guidelines for poor-prognosis testicular cancer. Initial treatment with four courses of bleomycin, etoposide, and cisplatin is considered standard therapy.[54] As in the treatment of testicular cancer, administration of chemotherapy at full doses and on schedule is important in obtaining optimal results. Following the completion of therapy, patients should be restaged with repeat serum tumor markers and CT scans of the chest and abdomen.

Subsequent management is determined by the response to initial chemotherapy (Figure 84-1). Patients with normal CT scans and tumor marker levels should receive no further therapy. Approximately 20% of these patients subsequently relapse, with almost all relapses occurring during the first 2 years after completion of therapy. Standard follow-up of these patients includes monthly physical examination, chest radiography, and serum tumor marker determinations during the first year and similar evaluations every 2 months during the second year following therapy.

The large majority of patients have residual radiographic abnormalities in the mediastinum after completion of chemotherapy.[27] In these patients, surgical resection of residual masses should be performed if technically feasible. Persistent elevation of serum tumor markers is not a contraindication to surgical resection in this setting because salvage chemotherapy regimens for patients with persistent carcinoma are usually ineffective.[63,64] Pathologic findings in resected specimens have varied widely in different reported series, probably based on differences in patient selection criteria. Residual germ cell carcinoma is found in a substantial proportion of patients (25–66%).[65–67] A small percentage of patients have residual carcinoma of various non–germ cell histologies (eg, sarcoma, adenocarcinoma, neuroendocrine carcinoma).[67] The remainder of patients have either benign teratoma, necrosis, or fibrosis without active carcinoma. Patients with a large component of teratocarcinoma in the original biopsy are more likely to have residual benign teratoma.

Surgical resection of all residual radiographic abnormalities results in curative treatment for a substantial proportion of patients. Patients with no viable tumor remaining have the same low risk of subsequent relapse as do patients achieving complete remission with chemotherapy alone.[65,67] Resection

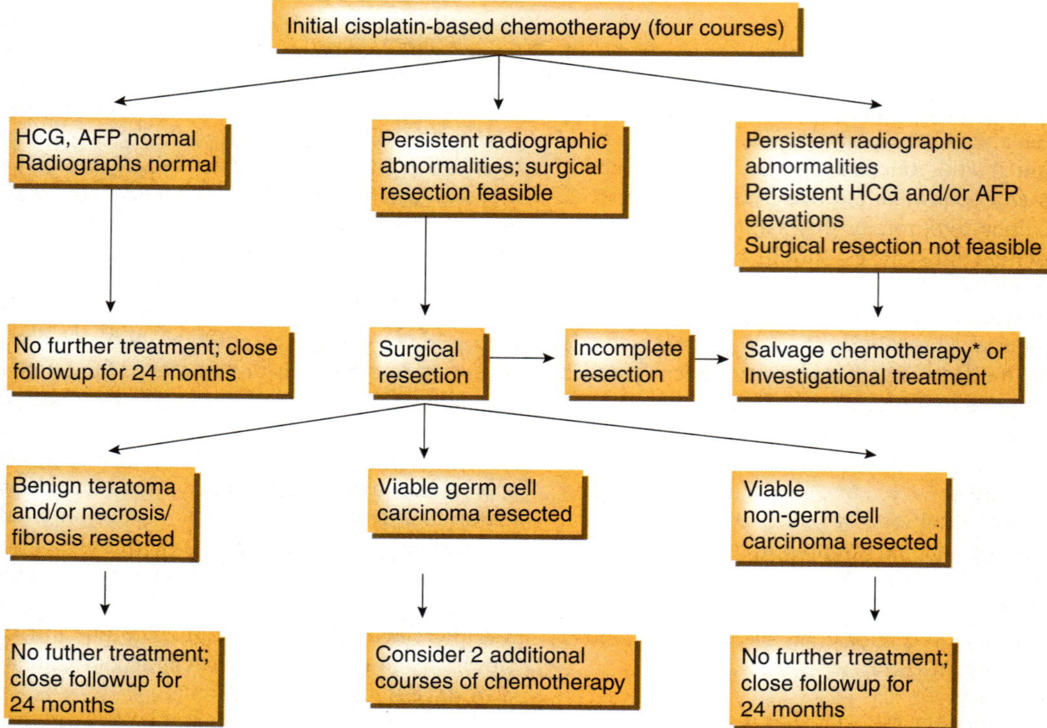

Figure 84-1 Management of mediastinal nonseminomatous germ cell tumors after completion of first-line chemotherapy. AFP = alpha-fetoprotein; HCG = human chorionic gonadotropin. *Salvage regimens used in advanced testicular germ cell tumors are less effective for mediastinal tumors.

of benign teratoma is therapeutic because these can undergo slow local growth or subsequent malignant degeneration if left in place. Patients with resection of residual germ cell carcinoma have a high risk of future relapse; however, surgical resection is curative in 20 to 30%.[66,67] Most patients with residual non–germ cell histologies do poorly even with complete resection, although occasional long-term survivors have been reported.[67] The role of further chemotherapy after resection in patients with residual carcinoma is undefined.

The prognosis is very poor for patients in whom complete surgical resection is not feasible, as well as in those who relapse after surgical resection. Standard second-line cisplatin-based regimens and high-dose chemotherapy regimens are curative in 20 to 50% of patients with recurrent testicular cancer but are effective in only 12% of patients with mediastinal nonseminomatous germ cell tumors.[63,64] These patients should therefore be considered for inclusion in clinical trials evaluating novel approaches.

POORLY DIFFERENTIATED CARCINOMA OF THE MEDIASTINUM

Occasionally, the biopsy diagnosis in a patient with a mediastinal tumor is poorly differentiated carcinoma. This diagnosis poses difficult problems for the clinician because it indicates a tumor with no histopathologic features specific enough to allow identification of the site of origin. Patients with poorly differentiated carcinoma in the mediastinum are sometimes assumed to have metastatic lung cancer with an undetectable primary lesion and are, therefore, assumed to be unresectable and incurable. In this setting, palliative radiation therapy is often administered. However, this approach is no longer adequate because further clinical and pathologic evaluation can establish a definitive diagnosis with specific therapeutic implications in some of these patients. In addition, some patients with poorly differentiated carcinoma involving the mediastinum are curable with intensive cisplatin-based chemotherapy.[13,68]

Pathologic Evaluation Critical pathologic evaluation of mediastinal tumors is essential because a variety of neoplasms with specific therapeutic implications can arise in this location (eg, mediastinal germ cell tumor, lymphoma, thymoma). In addition, effective therapy also exists for some neoplasms that commonly metastasize to the mediastinum (eg, small cell lung cancer). Following light microscopic examination of an adequate biopsy specimen, immunoperoxidase staining and electron microscopy are useful in distinguishing between the various neoplasms occurring in the mediastinum. By using these methods, lymphoma and neuroendocrine tumors (including small cell lung cancer) can be reliably identified, and appropriate therapeutic approaches can be defined. Molecular genetic analysis should also be performed, if possible, because identification of an i(12p) chromosomal abnormality is diagnostic of a germ cell tumor.[12]

Diagnostic Evaluation and Staging Workup All patients should have CT scans of the chest and abdomen, as well as measurement of serum levels of HCG and alpha-fetoprotein. Fiber-optic bronchoscopy should be performed if other studies are nondiagnostic. Small cell lung cancer should be suspected when neuroendocrine features are found in patients with a history of cigarette smoking.

Treatment The diagnostic evaluation defines specific therapy for some patients in this group. Patients with elevated levels of either HCG or alpha-fetoprotein should be treated for a mediastinal nonseminomatous germ cell tumor even if this diagnosis is not made by histologic examination. Patients who have an endobronchial lesion found at bronchoscopy probably have lung cancer, those with neuroendocrine features should receive therapy for small cell lung cancer, and those lacking these features should be treated for non–small cell lung cancer. Patients with poorly differentiated neuroendocrine carcinoma who lack the risk factors and clinical features of small cell lung cancer also have chemotherapy-sensitive tumors and should be treated with platinum and etoposide or paclitaxel, platinum, and etoposide regimens.[69,70]

In a small percentage of patients, no evidence of tumor spread outside the mediastinum is detected. Surgical resection or local radiation therapy should be considered in these patients, usually in conjunction with empiric combination chemotherapy (as described for patients with carcinoma of an unknown primary site; see Chapter 123, "Neoplasms of Unknown Primary Site").

When mediastinal tumors are locally unresectable or have metastasized to distant sites, a trial of combination chemotherapy should be given to all patients with adequate performance status. We treated 43 patients with poorly differentiated carcinoma or poorly differentiated adenocarcinoma located predominantly in the mediastinum.[68] These patients represented 19% of our entire group of patients with poorly differentiated carcinoma of an unknown primary site. The median age was 38 years; 32 patients had other metastatic sites in addition to the mediastinum. Only 5 of 43 patients (12%) had elevated serum levels of HCG or alpha-fetoprotein. All patients received cisplatin-based chemotherapy; 13 patients (30%) had a complete response, and 7 patients (16%) are long-term disease-free survivors. A review of the light microscopic features in these patients failed to reveal any previously unsuspected germ cell tumors or lymphomas.

In summary, patients with mediastinal tumors initially diagnosed as poorly differentiated carcinoma are a heterogeneous group. Some of these patients actually have well-defined tumor types that can be identified with additional pathologic or clinical evaluation. Patients in whom a specific tumor is identified should be treated according to standard guidelines for that tumor type. A trial of platinum and etoposide–based chemotherapy should be given to patients in whom no well-defined tumor type is recognized. Some of these patients have highly responsive neoplasms, and a minority appear to be cured with this treatment.

REFERENCES

1. Luna MA, Valenzuela-Tamariz J. Germ-cell tumors of the mediastinum, postmortem findings. Am J Clin Pathol 1976;65:450–4.
2. Wychulis AR, Payne WS, Clagett OT, Woolner LB. Surgical treatment of mediastinal tumors: a 40-year experience. J Thorac Cardiovasc Surg 1971;62:379–92.
3. Lewis BD, Hurt RD, Payne WS, et al. Benign teratomas of the mediastinum. J Thorac Cardiovasc Surg 1983;86:727–31.
4. Dulmet EM, Macchiarini P, Suc B, Verley JM. Germ cell tumors of the mediastinum: a 30-year experience. Cancer 1993;72:1894–901.
5. Friedman NB. The comparative morphogenesis of extragenital and gonadal teratoid tumors. Cancer 1951; 4:265–76.
6. Schlumberger HG. Teratoma of anterior mediastinum in group of military age: study of 16 cases and review of theories of genesis. Arch Pathol 1946;41:398–444.
7. Johnson DE, Laneri JP, Mountain CF, Luna M. Extragonadal germ cell tumors. Surgery 1973;73:85–90.
8. Willis RA. Borderland of embryology and pathology. 2nd ed. Washington (DC): Butterworth; 1962.
9. Freidman NB. The function of the primordial germ cell in extragonadal tissues. Int J Androl 1987;10:43–9.
10. Boyd DP, Midell AI. Mediastinal cysts and tumors: an analysis of 96 cases. Surg Clin North Am 1968;48:493–505.
11. Collins DH, Pugh RCB. Classification and frequency of testicular tumors. Br J Urol 1984;36:1–11.
12. Motzer RJ, Rodriguez E, Reuter VE, et al. Molecular and cytogenetic studies in the diagnosis of patients with midline carcinomas of unknown primary site. J Clin Oncol 1995;13:274–82.
13. Greco FA, Vaughn WK, Hainsworth JD. Advanced poorly differentiated carcinoma of unknown primary site: recognition of a treatable syndrome. Ann Intern Med 1986;104:547–53.
14. Aliotta PJ, Castilla J, Englander LS, et al. Primary mediastinal germ cell tumors. Histologic patterns of treatment failure at autopsy. Cancer 1988;62:982–4.
15. Einhorn L, Williams S, Loehrer P, et al. Phase III study of cisplatin dose intensity in advanced germ cell tumors. A Southeastern and Southwest Oncology Group protocol. Proc Am Soc Clin Oncol 1990;9:132.
16. Hartmann JT, Fossa SD, Nichols CR, et al. Incidence of metachronous testicular cancer in patients with extragonadal germ cell tumors. J Natl Cancer Inst 2001;93:1733–8.
17. Moran CA, Suster S. Primary germ cell tumors of the mediastinum—I. Analysis of 322 cases with special emphasis on teratomatous lesions and a proposal for histopathologic classification and clinical staging. Cancer 1997;80:681–90.
18. Polansky SM, Barwick KW, Ravin CE. Primary mediastinal seminoma. AJR Am J Roentgenol 1979;132:17–21.
19. Jain KK, Bosl GJ, Bains MS, et al. The treatment of extragonadal seminoma. J Clin Oncol 1984;2:820–7.
20. Bokemeyer C, Droz JP, Horwich A, et al. Extragonadal seminoma: an international multicenter analysis of prognostic factors and long term treatment outcome. Cancer 2001;91:1394–401.
21. Levitt RG, Husband JE, Glazer HS. CT of primary germ cell tumors of the mediastinum. AJR Am J Roentgenol 1984;142:73–8.
22. Hainsworth JD, Einhorn LH, Williams SD, et al. Advanced extragonadal germ cell tumors. Successful treatment with combination chemotherapy. Ann Intern Med 1982;97:7–11.
23. Israel A, Bosl GJ, Golbey RB, et al. The results of chemotherapy for extragonadal germ cell tumors in the cisplatin era: the Memorial Sloan-Kettering Cancer Center experience (1975 to 1982). J Clin Oncol 1985;3:1073–8.
24. Logothetis CJ, Samuels ML, Selig DE, et al. Chemotherapy of extragonadal germ cell tumors. J Clin Oncol 1985;3:316–25.
25. Sickles EA, Belliveau RF, Wiernik PH. Primary mediastinal choriocarcinoma in the male. Cancer 1974;33:1196–203.
26. Nichols CR, Saxman S, Williams SD, et al. Primary mediastinal nonseminomatous germ cell tumors—a modern single institution experience. Cancer 1990;65:1641–6.

27. Ganjoo KN, Rieger KM, Kesler KA, et al. Results of modern therapy for patients with mediastinal nonseminomatous germ cell tumors. Cancer 2000;88:1051–6.
28. Scheike D, Visfeldt J, Petersen B. Male breast cancer. 3. Breast carcinoma in association with the Klinefelter syndrome. Acta Pathol Microbiol Scand 1973;81:352–8.
29. Curry WA, McKay CE, Richardson RL, Greco FA. Klinefelter's syndrome and mediastinal germ cell neoplasms. J Urol 1981;125:127–9.
30. Turner AR, MacDonald RN. Mediastinal germ cell cancers in Klinefelter's syndrome. Ann Intern Med 1981;94:279.
31. Nichols CR, Heerema NA, Palmer C, et al. Klinefelter's syndrome associated with mediastinal germ cell neoplasms. J Clin Oncol 1987;5:1290–4.
32. Carroll PR, Whitmore WF Jr, Richardson M, et al. Testicular failure in patients with extragonadal germ cell tumors. Cancer 1987;60:108–13.
33. Nichols CR, Hoffman R, Einhorn LH, et al. Hematologic malignancies associated with primary mediastinal germ cell tumors. Ann Intern Med 1985;102:603–9.
34. Nichols CR, Roth BJ, Heerema N, et al. Hematologic neoplasia associated with primary mediastinal germ cell tumors. N Engl J Med 1990;322:1425–9.
35. Larsen M, Evans WK, Shephard FA, et al. Acute lymphoblastic leukemia: possible origin from a mediastinal germ cell tumor. Cancer 1984;53:441-4.
36. Orazi A, Neiman RS, Ulbright TM, et al. Hematopoietic precursor cells within the yolk sac tumor component are the source of secondary hematopoietic malignancies in patients with mediastinal germ cell tumors. Cancer 1993;71:3873–81.
37. Chaganti RS, Landanyi M, Samaniego F. Leukemic differentiation of a mediastinal germ cell tumor. Genes Chromosomes Cancer 1989;1:83–7.
38. Landanyi M, Samaniego F, Reuter VE, et al. Cytogenetic and immunohistochemical evidence for the germ cell origin of a subset of acute leukemias associated with mediastinal germ cell tumors. J Natl Cancer Inst 1990;82:221–7.
39. Hartmann JT, Nichols CR, Droz JP, et al. Hematologic disorders associated with primary mediastinal nonseminomatous germ cell tumors. J Natl Cancer Inst 2000;92:54–61.
40. Garnick MB, Griffin JD. Idiopathic thrombocytopenia in association with extragonadal germ cell cancer. Ann Intern Med 1983;98:926–7.
41. Helman LJ, Ozols RF, Longo DL. Thrombocytopenia and extragonadal germ cell neoplasm. Ann Intern Med 1984;101:280.
42. Loehrer PJ, Birch R, Williams SD, et al. Chemotherapy of metastatic seminoma. The Southeastern Cancer Study Group experience. J Clin Oncol 1987;5:1212–20.
43. Bukowski RM, Wolf M, Kulander BG, et al. Alternating combination chemotherapy in patients with extragonadal germ cell tumors. Cancer 1993;71:2631–8.
44. Delgado FG, Tjulandin SA, Gavin AM. Long-term results of treatment in patients with extragonadal germ cell tumors. Eur J Cancer 1993;29A:1002–5.
45. Goss PE, Schwertfeger L, Blackstein ME, et al. Extragonadal germ cell tumors: a 14-year Toronto experience. Cancer 1994;73:1971–9.
46. Mencel PJ, Motzer RJ, Mazumdar M, et al. Advanced seminoma: treatment results, survival, and prognostic factors in 142 patients. J Clin Oncol 1994;12:120–6.
47. Gerl A, Clemm C, Lamerz R, Wilmanns W. Cisplatin-based chemotherapy of primary extragonadal germ cell tumors: a single institution experience. Cancer 1996;77:526–32.
48. Bokemeyer C, Droz JP, Horwich A, et al. Extragonadal seminoma: an international multicenter analysis of prognostic factors and long-term treatment outcome. Cancer 2001;91:1394–401.
49. Hurt RD, Bruckman JE, Farrow GM, et al. Primary anterior mediastinal seminoma. Cancer 1982;49:1658–63.
50. Bush SE, Martinez A, Bagshaw MA. Primary mediastinal seminoma. Cancer 1981;48:1877–92.
51. Schultz SM, Einhorn LH, Conces DJ, et al. Management of postchemotherapy residual mass in patients with advanced seminoma: Indiana University experience. J Clin Oncol 1989;7:1497–503.
52. Puc HS, Heelan R, Mazumdar M, et al. Management of residual mass in advanced seminoma: results and recommendations from the Memorial Sloan-Kettering Cancer Center. J Clin Oncol 1996;14:454–60.
53. DeSantis M, Becherer A, Bokemeyer C, et al. 2-^{18}Fluorodeoxy-D-glucose positron emission tomography is a reliable predictor for viable tumor in postchemotherapy seminoma: an update of the prospective multicentre SEMPET trial. J Clin Oncol 2004;22:1034–9.
54. Williams SD, Birch R, Einhorn LH, et al. Treatment of disseminated germ cell tumors with cisplatin, bleomycin, and either vinblastine or etoposide. N Engl J Med 1987;316:1435–40.
55. Cox JD. Primary malignant germinal tumors of the mediastinum. A study of 24 cases. Cancer 1975;36:1162–8.
56. Funes HC, Mendez M, Alonso E, et al. Mediastinal germ cell tumors treated with cisplatin, bleomycin and vinblastine (PVB) [abstract]. Proc Am Assoc Cancer Res 1981;22:474.
57. Kay PH, Wells FC, Goldstraw P. A multidisciplinary approach to primary nonseminomatous germ cell tumors of the mediastinum. Ann Thorac Surg 1987;44:578–82.
58. Hidalgo M, Paz-Ares L, Rivera F, et al. Mediastinal nonseminomatous germ cell tumors (MNSGCT) treated with cisplatin-based combination chemotherapy. Ann Oncol 1997;8:555–9.
59. Fizazi K, Culine S, Droz JP, et al. Primary mediastinal nonseminomatous germ cell tumors: results of modern therapy including cisplatin-based chemotherapy. J Clin Oncol 1998;16:725–32.
60. International Germ Cell Cancer Collaborative Group. International germ cell consensus classification: a prognostic factor-based staging system for metastatic germ cell cancers. J Clin Oncol 1997;15:594–603.
61. Toner GC, Geller NL, Lin S-Y, Bosl GJ. Extragonadal and poor risk nonseminomatous germ cell tumors: survival and prognostic features. Cancer 1991;67:2049–57.
62. Chong CD, Logothetis CJ, von Eschenbach AC, et al. Successful treatment of pure endodermal sinus tumors in adult men. J Clin Oncol 1988;6:303–7.
63. Saxman SB, Nichols CR, Einhorn LH. Salvage chemotherapy in patients with extragonadal nonseminomatous germ cell tumors: the Indiana University experience. J Clin Oncol 1994;12:1390–3.
64. Hartmann JT, Einhorn L, Nichols CR, et al. Second-line chemotherapy in patients with relapsed extragonadal nonseminomatous germ cell tumors: results of an international multicenter analysis. J Clin Oncol 2001;19:1641–8.
65. Kesler KA, Rieger KM, Ganjoo KN, et al. Primary mediastinal nonseminomatous germ cell tumors: the influence of postchemotherapy pathology on long-term survival after surgery. J Thoracic Cardiovasc Surgery 1999;118:692–9.
66. Vuky J, Bains M, Bacik J, et al. Role of postchemotherapy adjunctive surgery in the management of patients with nonseminoma arising from the mediastinum. J Clin Oncol 2001;19:682–8.
67. Schneider BP, Kesler KA, Brooks JA, et al. Outcome of patients with residual germ cell or non-germ cell malignancy after resection of primary mediastinal nonseminomatous germ cell cancer. J Clin Oncol 2004;22:1195–200.
68. Hainsworth JD, Johnson DH, Greco FA. Cisplatin-based combination chemotherapy in the treatment of poorly differentiated carcinoma and poorly differentiated adenocarcinoma of unknown primary site: results of a twelve-year experience at a single institution. J Clin Oncol 1992;10:912–22.
69. Hainsworth JD, Johnson DH, Greco FA. Poorly differentiated neuroendocrine carcinoma of unknown primary site: a newly recognized clinicopathologic entity. Ann Intern Med 1988;109:364–71.
70. Miranda FT, Spigel DR, Hainsworth JD, et al. Paclitaxel/carboplatin/etoposide (PCE) therapy for advanced poorly differentiated neuroendocrine carcinoma: a Minnie Pearl Cancer Research Network phase II trial [abstract]. Proc Am Soc Clin Oncol 2005;23:322s.

Section 28
GASTROINTESTINAL TRACT

85

Neoplasms of the Esophagus

Stephen G. Swisher, MD
David C. Rice, MD
Jaffer A. Ajani, MD
Ritsuko K. Komaki, MD
Mark K. Ferguson, MD

Neoplasms of the esophagus and gastroesophageal junction are among the most challenging oncologic problems. Management of this disease is plagued by nihilism because of high rates of mortality. Early mortality is common because the majority of the cancers are in an advanced stage at the time of diagnosis and because current therapies are relatively ineffective once the tumor has reached an advanced stage. Esophageal cancer was recognized as early as the twelfth century, and pathologic descriptions were produced in the sixteenth and seventeenth centuries.[1] Initial attempts to treat the tumor included resection of a cervical esophageal cancer in 1877 and intrathoracic cancer in 1913.[2,3] Surgical resection became the mainstay of therapy beginning in the 1940s. Radiotherapy was initially used in the 1920s, but it was not until the development of megavoltage techniques in the 1950s that this modality was used with any frequency. Active chemotherapeutic agents were first identified in the 1960s and have been increasingly incorporated into the treatment of advanced tumors.

ANATOMY AND HISTOLOGY

The esophagus is a muscular organ that extends from the cricopharyngeus muscle at its cephalad margin to the esophagogastric junction. It is divided into regions on the basis of both anatomy and the proclivity for certain neoplasms to develop in specific regions (Figure 85-1). The cervical esophagus extends from the cricopharyngeus muscle to the thoracic inlet (15–18 cm from incisors). The upper third of the thoracic esophagus extends from the thoracic inlet to the tracheal bifurcation, just below the level of the aortic arch (18–24 cm). The middle thoracic esophagus extends from the tracheal bifurcation to a point midway between the carina and the esophagogastric junction (24–32 cm). The lower thoracic esophagus extends from this midway point to the esophagogastric junction (32–40 cm). Tumors of the esophagogastric junction (EGJ) and gastric cardia are often included in discussions of esophageal cancer because of the increasing incidence of adenocarcinomas of this region and their pathophysiologic similarities to adenocarcinomas of the distal esophagus.[4] Classifications of esophagogastric junction tumors have developed that define the different types of tumors according to the epicenter of the mass (ie, type I, > 1 cm above EGJ; type II, 1 cm above to 2 cm below EGJ; type III, > 2–5 cm below EGJ).[5]

The muscle tissues of the esophagus are arranged in an outer longitudinal layer and an inner circular layer. The proximal one-third to one-half of the muscularis propria is derived from the branchial arches, making it principally skeletal (striated) muscle and giving it the potential to develop rhabdomyosarcomas (Table 85-1). The remainder of the esophageal musculature comprises smooth muscle, as does the rest of the foregut, in which leiomyomas or leiomyosarcomas may occur. Fibrous, fatty, and connective tissues interspersed in the wall of the esophagus may also give rise to sarcomas.

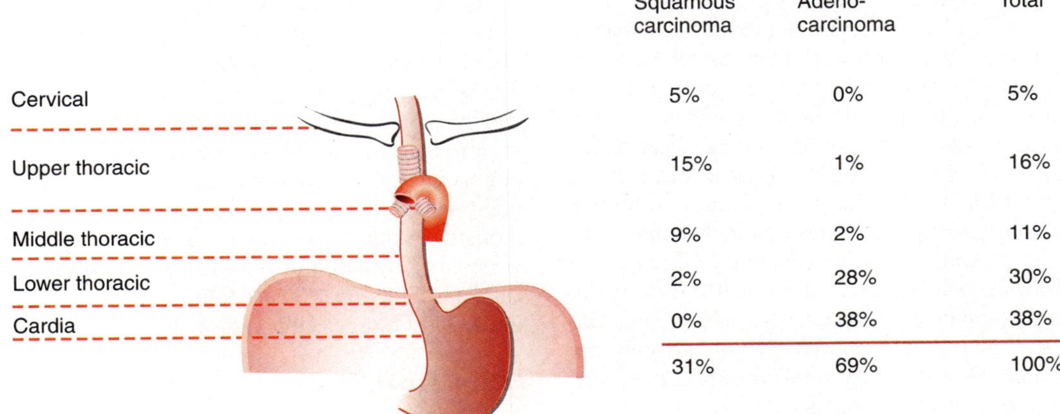

	Squamous carcinoma	Adeno-carcinoma	Total
Cervical	5%	0%	5%
Upper thoracic	15%	1%	16%
Middle thoracic	9%	2%	11%
Lower thoracic	2%	28%	30%
Cardia	0%	38%	38%
	31%	69%	100%

Figure 85-1 The distribution of malignant neoplasms of the esophagus according to cell type and site of occurrence.

Table 85-1 Neoplasms of the Esophagus
Epithelial
Squamous cell carcinoma
Spindle cell carcinoma
Carcinosarcoma
Adenocarcinoma
Adenosquamous carcinoma
Mucoepidermoid carcinoma
Adenoid cystic carcinoma
Small cell carcinoma
Nonepithelial
Leiomyoma
Leiomyosarcoma
Malignant melanoma
Rhabdomyoma
Rhabdomyosarcoma
Granular cell tumors
Malignant lymphoma

The esophagus is lined over most of its length with squamous epithelium, which can give rise to squamous cell carcinoma, the most common neoplasm of the esophagus in most of the world. These cancers occur most often in the cervical esophagus and in the upper and middle thoracic esophagus. Carcinosarcomas and spindle cell carcinomas, which are subtypes of squamous cell cancer, infrequently occur in these regions. The distal 2 to 3 cm of the esophagus and the cardia are lined by columnar epithelium, in which adenocarcinomas may occur.[5] The development of intestinal metaplasia, known as Barrett's esophagus, more proximally because of gastroesophageal reflux and other factors allows the development of adenocarcinomas in the middle and upper thoracic esophagus in isolated instances. Other cellular elements in the mucosa, submucosal glands, and muscularis propria may give rise to unusual neoplasms, such as small cell cancer, malignant melanoma, granular cell tumors, mucoepidermoid carcinoma, and adenoid cystic carcinoma.[6,7] The histologic types of benign and malignant tumors of the esophagus are shown in Table 85-1.

ETIOLOGY

In most of the world, dietary and nutritional factors are the most common etiologic agents and are associated with the development of predominantly squamous cell carcinomas. Among the most frequently cited carcinogens are nitrosamines, which have been found to be in high concentrations in foods in endemic areas of esophageal cancer in northern China.[8] Contamination of food by fungi that reduce nitrate to nitrite may further aggravate this situation. Mechanical factors that have been cited include drinking beverages at excessively high temperatures and consumption of foods containing silica or other substances, such as crushed seeds, that directly irritate the esophagus.[8,9] Deficiencies of folic acid, vitamins A and C, and riboflavin, molybdenum, and selenium also have been implicated in the development of esophageal neoplasms.[10–12]

In the western hemisphere, social factors figure more prominently in the development of esophageal cancer. Heavy alcohol consumption increases the risk of cancer 10 to 25 times, depending on the concentration of alcohol in the beverage.[13] Cigarette smoking has been linked to the development of both squamous cell cancers and adenocarcinomas.[14] The combined exposure to low levels of tobacco and alcohol increases the risk of esophageal cancer by a factor of 10 to 20, whereas the synergistic effect of exposure to high levels of both alcohol and tobacco increases the risk by a factor of over 100.[15] Chronic esophageal injury due to gastroesophageal reflux has also been shown to be a risk factor for the development of adenocarcinoma, with severe, longstanding reflux symptoms increasing the risk of cancer by a factor of 40.[16] Chronic gastroesophageal reflux is believed to be etiologically related to the development of Barrett's esophagus, which occurs primarily in white males and is associated with a 40-fold increase in the risk of adenocarcinoma of the esophagus.[17] A relationship between reflux and the development of squamous cell cancers has also been suggested in patients who consume a diet high in linoleic acid.[18] The lifetime risk of squamous cell cancer of the esophagus is 5 to 10% in patients with esophageal achalasia, a 15-fold increase in incidence that is likely due to chronic irritation from retained food.[19–21]

Race and gender are associated with varying incidences of cancer of the esophagus in the western hemisphere. Men are more commonly affected than are women, blacks develop squamous cell cancers more often than do whites, and white males develop adenocarcinomas more often than do females or individuals of other race groups.[22] However, none of these increased frequencies has yet been linked to genetic factors, and most have been explained by variations in socioeconomic status and the attendant social habits described earlier. The single proven genetic abnormality that is associated with a 25% lifetime incidence of squamous cell cancer of the esophagus is tylosis A, the late-onset, familial form of palmar and plantar hyperkeratosis.[23] A number of genetic alterations are associated with neoplasms of the esophagus, including allelic losses at chromosomes 3p, 5q, 9p, 9q, 13q, 17p, 17q, and 18q. Abnormalities of *TP53*, *Rb*, cyclin D1 and c-*myc* have also been associated with esophageal cancer development.[24]

Infectious agents, including human papillomavirus (HPV), have been implicated in the development of neoplasms of the esophagus. Transforming proteins from high-risk HPV subtypes[16,18] cause loss of function of the tumor suppressor genes *TP53* and *Rb*, resulting in abnormal proliferative states.[25] HPV has been documented in up to 50% of patients with squamous cell cancers of the esophagus and appears to be more common in areas in which esophageal cancer is endemic.[26] These findings have not been universally reproducible, however.[27]

EPIDEMIOLOGY

The most common neoplasm worldwide is squamous cell carcinoma; in the United States and

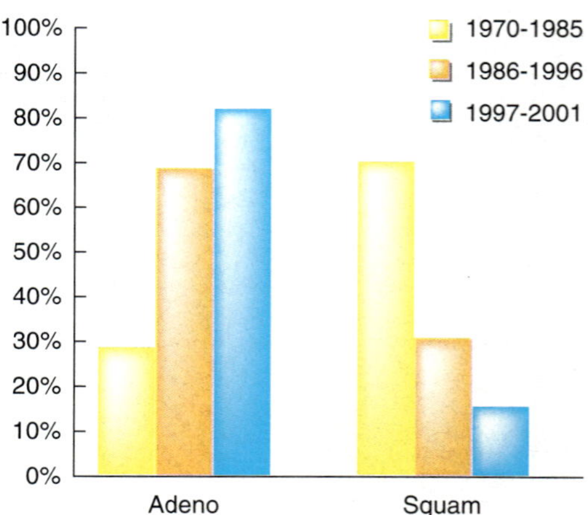

Figure 85-2 The proportion of adenocarcinoma and distal esophageal tumors has increased over time. Adeno = adenocarcinoma; Squam = squamous cell carcinoma. Reproduced with permission from Hofstetter W, et al.[79]

Europe, adenocarcinoma now predominates (Figure 85-2). The incidence of esophageal cancer varies more worldwide than any other cancer. In the United States, the incidence of esophageal cancer is approximately 7 cases per 100,000 people, whereas in high-risk areas in China, Iran, and Russia, it can be more than 100 per 100,000. In rural Linxian, China, esophageal cancer is the leading cause of death.[28,29] These geographical variations imply a strong role for local environmental carcinogens in esophageal carcinogenesis. The long-term survival rate for patients with esophageal cancer, regardless of histology, is less than 10%, which is due, in large part, to the advanced stage at which these cancers are detected. The age-adjusted mortality rate from esophageal cancer in the United States is 4.4 per 100,000 population per year, a figure that increased by 22% between 1973 and 1999.[30] These data translate to an estimated incidence of 13,900 new cases and about 13,000 deaths from esophageal cancer in 2003 (excluding tumors of the esophagogastric junction).[31]

Besides geographical differences, there are other important differences that have been described in the Western hemisphere. Esophageal carcinoma is more common in men than women regardless of the histologic subtype, and squamous cell cancers tend to occur more frequently in blacks than in whites. Additionally, there has been a striking increase in the incidence of adenocarcinoma in the United States and Europe, whereas squamous cell carcinoma has remained stable.[32] Adenocarcinoma of the distal esophagus and cardia have risen by more than 350% among white males since the mid-1970s, increasing at a more rapid rate than any other solid tumor (see Figure 85-2).[22,33–37] The reasons for these dramatic changes in the Western Hemisphere are not clear but may include increased Barrett's, gastroesophageal reflux, obesity, and over-the-counter medications as well as changing smoking and alcohol use.[16] In other areas of the world (outside Europe and North America), squamous cell carcinoma of the esophagus continues to predominate and adenocarcinoma has not increased.

PRESENTATION

Patients usually present because of complaints of dysphagia, which requires either the involvement of the entire circumference of the esophagus by the neoplasm or the growth of a large, polypoid obstructing mass. Dysphagia first develops in response to dense solid foods and progresses to result in difficulties with soft foods and then liquids. Accompanying vomiting and regurgitation are common. Symptoms of heartburn or gastroesophageal reflux (40%) are often associated and occur more frequently in patients with adenocarcinoma.[38] The most common symptom in the absence of dysphagia is pain (25% of cases).[38] It may be related to swallowing (odynophagia) or local extension of the tumor into adjacent structures such as the vertebral bodies, pleura, or mediastinum. In some instances, it may be due to bony metastases from systemic spread. Weight loss is noted in more than 70% of patients and is due to the inability to swallow or to systemic manifestations of the disease.[38] Patients with weight loss have a significantly worse prognosis in many series.[39,40]

The location of the tumor depends in large part on histology. Adenocarcinoma is located predominantly in the lower esophagus, whereas squamous cell carcinoma predominates in the cervical, upper, and middle esophagus (see Figures 85-1 and 85-2). Unfortunately, because of the distensible nature of the esophagus, these symptoms often do not occur until the tumors are quite large and no longer localized to the esophagus.

In contrast to patients who present because of symptoms of dysphagia, a smaller subset of earlier stage adenocarcinoma patients are increasingly being identified in North America and Europe with endoscopic abnormalities noted during endoscopic surveillance for gastroesophageal reflux symptoms or Barrett's esophagus. These patients tend to present with smaller, earlier stage tumors that are more likely to be localized and amenable to treatment. Additionally, in some areas of China where squamous cell cancer is endemic, routine cytologic screening is performed, and if results are diagnostic or suspicious, follow-up endoscopy is performed. These mass screening efforts have led to early diagnosis in many areas of China, with 5-year survivals of more than 90%.[29] The low incidence of esophageal cancer in most areas of the world, however, makes this type of mass screening impractical and cost ineffective from a public health standpoint.

TREATMENT OVERVIEW

Patients who present with suspected esophageal cancer, either because of the above-mentioned symptoms or mass screening efforts, initially require pathologic confirmation of malignancy (see the section "Diagnosis" below). Once the pathologic diagnosis has been obtained, patients are assessed for therapy by determining the clinical stage (see the section "Staging Evaluation" below) of the tumor and the physiologic status of the patient (see the section "Pretreatment Assessment" below). With this information, an informed decision about treatment can be made that optimizes the chance to cure or palliate the disease while minimizing the treatment related morbidity (see the section "Therapy" below) (Figure 85-3).

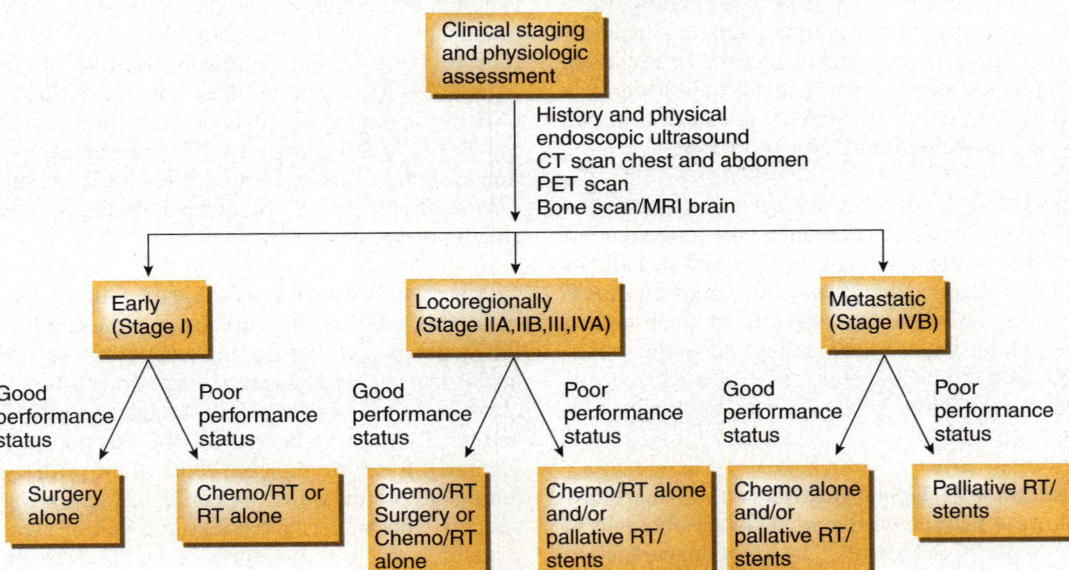

Figure 85-3 Current treatment recommendations for esophageal cancer based on performance status and clinical stage at the University of Texas M.D. Anderson Cancer Center. Chemo = chemotherapy; CT = computed tomography; MRI = magnetic resonance imaging; PET = positron-emission tomography; RT = radiotherapy.

DIAGNOSIS

Symptomatic patients or patients in whom an esophageal mass is diagnosed by screening require endoscopy to enable biopsy for histologic examination and/or brushing for cytologic examination. The overall accuracy of histologic diagnosis of esophageal cancer using flexible endoscopy with biopsy is about 80%.[41,42] Endoscopically directed cytologic brushings have a diagnostic accuracy in excess of 90%. Combining these techniques yields an overall diagnostic accuracy of 98%.[41] If flexible endoscopic diagnostic techniques fail, rigid endoscopy with biopsy, which has a diagnostic accuracy close to 100%, should be considered.[42] In selected patients who have symptoms or findings on physical examination suggestive of metastatic disease, biopsy of the suspected metastatic site provides both a tissue diagnosis and a confirmation of stage.

PRETREATMENT ASSESSMENT

In addition to a careful history and physical examination, the overall assessment of a patient with esophageal cancer focuses on specific concerns. Factors that are associated with treatment-related morbidity and mortality include patient age, a recent history of alcohol or tobacco abuse, body weight, recent weight loss, nutritional status, performance status, hepatic dysfunction, and renal dysfunction. Specific preoperative risk factors have been identified for esophageal resection and are therefore included in the physiologic assessment. Pulmonary complications are predicted by age, preoperative arterial oxygen tension, abnormal chest radiograph, forced expiratory volume in one second (FEV_1).[43] Operative mortality is predicted by age, mid-arm circumference, history of smoking, incentive spirometry, performance status, and the frequency with which the operation is performed in an institution.[43,44] Any symptoms of cardiac disease necessitate careful evaluation with electrocardiography (ECG), echocardiography, stress tests, and coronary arteriography as indicated. Patients with significant coronary artery disease are at increased risk of morbidity and mortality and cardiac intervention may be warranted prior to treatment of the esophageal neoplasm. These physiologic assessments allow patients to be classified as good or poor performance status, which then allows the aggressiveness of treatment to be tailored to their specific risks (see Figure 85-3).

STAGING EVALUATION

Assessment of stage permits medical practitioners to discuss the status of individual patients with accuracy, allows informed recommendations about therapy, and gives patients and their families necessary information about prognosis. The typical assessment for most patients includes upper gastrointestinal endoscopy, contrast radiography of the esophagus, computed tomography (CT) of the chest and abdomen, and possibly endoscopic ultrasonography (EUS) and positron emission tomography (PET). Other examinations are selected on the basis of specific findings in individual patients, such as neurologic symptoms (magnetic resonance imaging [MRI] brain), musculoskeletal symptoms (bone scan), or supraclavicular nodes (neck ultrasonography and biopsy). Staging techniques allow patients to be accurately placed into groups in which risk can be assessed as well as the optimum type of therapy.

Contrast Radiography of the Esophagus A contrast study of the esophagus is often the initial diagnostic examination obtained in patients with dysphagia. It allows confirmation of mucosal irregularity and serves as guide for subsequent endoscopy. It also allows evaluation of the esophagus and stomach distal to the area of stenosis, which cannot also be assessed by endoscopy with tight strictures.

Endoscopy Upper gastrointestinal endoscopy allows a pathologic diagnosis to be obtained in the majority of patients. The gross appearance of the tumor can be categorized as advanced or superficial, and the extent of the tumor can be accurately determined. Additional unsuspected malignancies that may be present in up to 20% of patients with squamous cell cancer may also be identified. Endoscopy also permits assessment of the mobility of a tumor, indicating whether it is fixed within the mediastinum.

Endoscopic Ultrasonography Endoscopic ultrasonography (EUS) was initially introduced to improve the staging accuracy of primary tumors and regional lymph nodes. Subsequent experience has confirmed this initial promise and has demonstrated the additional value of EUS for assessing some nonregional (metastatic) lymph nodes. It has become a critical tool to identify patients with truly early-stage carcinoma who do not need multimodality treatment (see Figure 85-3). EUS depicts the normal esophagus as five alternating hyperechoic and hypoechoic layers representing the mucosa and lamina propria, muscularis mucosa, submucosa, muscularis propria, and adventitia. Depth of tumor invasion is determined by assessing the level to which the tumor extends. EUS is useful for assessing whether there is involvement of the aorta, but airway invasion is not accurately determined because of interference of the ultrasound signal caused by the intratracheal air column. The accuracy of EUS determination of primary tumor stage is related to the pathologic tumor stage, being more accurate for more advanced stages of disease, with an overall accuracy of about 80%.[45–47] EUS is substantially less accurate in staging primary tumors after chemoradiotherapy is administered, primarily because of overstaging. The technique is not able to distinguish between treatment-induced fibrosis and residual tumor, leading to a mean overall accuracy in this setting of 45%.[48]

In assessing lymph nodes with EUS, three criteria are used: size, border characteristics, and internal architecture. Lymph nodes that are enlarged, have a well-defined external border, and are characterized by relatively uniform, hypoechoic internal architecture are more likely to be malignant. Using these criteria, the overall accuracy of lymph node staging by EUS is about 75%.[46,49] After chemoradiotherapy, the accuracy of EUS for staging lymph nodes decreases to just over 50%.[48] Development of fine needle aspiration techniques have allowed pathologic confirmation of enlarged lymph nodes in both regional and nonregional sites.[47–50]

Computed Tomography of the Chest and Abdomen CT has become a standard technique for esophageal cancer staging since its inception in the late 1970s because it has allowed better identification of patients with metastatic (M1b) and locally invasive tumors (T4). CT is not very accurate for determining the depth of the primary tumor (T) status, but it is useful in identifying patients who might have direct invasion of local structures, such as the aorta or major airways, either of which precludes surgical intervention.[45] Aortic invasion is suspected when more than 25% of the aortic circumference is effaced by an esophageal cancer.

CT does not accurately determine lymph node (N) status since normal lymph nodes often vary in size according to their location in the mediastinum and abdomen, and a single size limit for nodes is not possible to establish. In addition, lymph nodes involved by metastatic spread are often not enlarged.[51–54] The sensitivity for CT detection of involved lymph nodes is therefore poor (30–60%), and the overall accuracy of nodal detection by CT is less than 60%.[55–57]

CT is most useful for detecting distant often unsuspected metastatic (M) disease. The most common sites for metastatic spread, aside from nonregional lymph nodes, are (in decreasing order of frequency) the liver, lung, peritoneum, adrenal gland, bone, and kidney. CT of the thorax and abdomen evaluates almost all these regions. Accuracy of the CT detection of liver metastases is in excess of 90%.[51,56,58,59]

Bronchoscopy Bronchoscopy should be performed for all patients who are candidates for surgical therapy and whose tumors are adjacent to the trachea or mainstem bronchi. This permits direct assessment of tumor invasion into the airway lumen or submucosa.

Magnetic Resonance Imaging As a method for routine staging of esophageal neoplasms, MRI offers no advantages compared with CT and is therefore seldom used since it is a more difficult and expensive test to obtain. Both techniques have similar specificities, sensitivities, and overall accuracy for determining resectability with regard to direct invasion of the aorta and airway.[52,53,56] Neither test provides much useful information about regional or metastatic lymph nodes, and MRI offers no improvements over CT in evaluating the liver for metastatic disease. Whether advances in MRI technology will offer improved staging capabilities remains to be seen.

Positron Emission Tomography PET scanning to detect involved lymph nodes and sites of metastatic disease through increased metabolism with 18F-fluorodeoxyglucose was introduced as an investigational staging technique for esophageal cancer in the mid-1990s. The ultimate role of PET for staging esophageal neoplasms remains to be determined, but preliminary data suggest that it will be valuable in the assessment of distant metastatic disease. Another potential role of PET may be in determining response to chemotherapy and radiation therapy although false positives induced by chemotherapy and radiation-induced inflammation remain a problem.[60–62] PET may also have a role in identifying recurrent esophageal cancer by allowing targeting of unsuspected areas of increased metabolic activity.[63]

Bone Scintigraphy Bone scans have been used for decades for staging patients with esophageal neoplasms, although their utility is unproven. In patients without bone pain or other evidence for metastatic disease, the likelihood of identifying skeletal metastases is less than 5%.[64]

Neck Ultrasonography Cervical and supraclavicular lymph nodes are affected by metastatic spread in up to 30% of patients with neoplasms of the thoracic esophagus, and most are not detectable on physical examination. The use of routine ultrasound examination of the neck in patients without palpable lymph nodes yields unsuspected nodal metastases in over 10% of patients.[65] The overall accuracy of cervical and supraclavicular nodal assessment with ultrasonography is about 90%.[66,67] The addition of routine needle aspiration under ultrasound guidance for cytology may improve the yield of this potentially valuable technique.[67] At the present time, however, this is not a commonly used screening technique.

Minimally Invasive Surgical Staging Laparoscopy has been used since the early 1980s, and thoracoscopy has been used since the early 1990s in an effort to improve staging of esophageal neoplasms. Both are used in some centers prior to preresectional therapy. The need for general anesthesia and a separate invasive procedure has limited the popularity of this staging procedure.

Biologic Staging A variety of biologic markers have been investigated for their utility in estimating prognosis in patients with esophageal neoplasms. These include growth factors (epidermal growth factor [EGF], transforming growth factor [TGF]-β, platelet-derived growth factor [PDGF]), oncogenes (c-*myc*, *int-2, hst-1, cyclin D, EGFR, HER-2/neu, h-ras*), tumor suppressor genes (*Rb,TP53, p73, APC, MCC, p27*),

Table 85-2 TNM Staging System for Esophageal Neoplasms

Primary Tumor (T)			
TX		Primary tumor cannot be assessed	
TO		No evidence of primary tumor	
Tis		Carcinoma in situ	
T1		Tumor invades lamina propria or submucosa	
T2		Tumor invades muscularis propria	
T3		Tumor invades adventitia	
T4		Tumor invades adjacent structures	
Regional lymph nodes (N)			
NX		Regional lymph nodes cannot be assessed	
NO		No regional lymph node metastases	
N1		Regional lymph node metastasis	
Distant metastasis (M)			
MX		Distant metastasis cannot be assessed	
MO		No distant metastasis	
M1		Distant metastasis	
		Tumors of the lower thoracic esophagus	
		M1a	Metastasis in celiac lymph nodes
		M1b	Other distant metastasis
		Tumors of the midthoracic esophagus	
		M1a	Not applicable
		M1b	Nonregional lymph nodes and/or other distant metastasis
		Tumors of the upper thoracic esophagus	
		M1a	Metastasis in cervical nodes
		M1b	Other distant metastasis
Stage grouping			
Stage 0	Tis	NO	MO
Stage 1	T1	NO	MO
Stage IIA	T2	NO	MO
	T3	NO	MO
Stage IIB	T1	N1	MO
	T2	N1	MO
Stage III	T3	N1	MO
	T4	Any N	MO
Stage IV	Any T	Any N	M1
Stage IVA	Any T	Any N	M1a
Stage IVB	Any T	Any N	M1b

Regional lymph nodes:
Cervical esophageal tumor: scalene, internal jugular, upper cervical, periesophageal, supraclavicular, cervical not otherwise specified
Intrathoracic esophageal tumor: tracheobronchial, superior mediastinal, peritracheal, carinal, hilar, periesophageal, perigastric, paracardial, mediastinal not otherwise specified
From American Joint Committee on Cancer,[71] with permission.

the cell adhesion molecule E-cadherin, the oncodevelopmental marker CEA, and deoxyribonucleic acid (DNA) content and ploidy.[68–70] To date, none of these techniques have become generally accepted staging techniques except in isolated referral centers.

TNM Staging System These pretreatment staging evaluations allow patients to be clinically staged by a cTNM staging system that can help determine the optimum therapy (see Figure 85-3). The current staging system for esophageal cancer includes epithelial tumors of the cervical, thoracic, and intraabdominal esophagus, as well as of the esophagogastric junction (Table 85-2).[71] Tumors are staged according to clinical findings from noninvasive tests and pathologic findings resulting from any invasive staging procedures. It is useful to specify lymph node locations during biopsy and resection because their location determines whether they are considered regional or metastatic disease if they are involved by tumor (Figure 85-4). The prognosis of patients with esophageal cancer is determined by the depth of penetration of the primary tumor (transmural vs nontransmural), whether there is lymph node involvement, the relative number of lymph nodes involved, and whether distant metastases are present.[71–81,87–92] The long-term survival in patients with esophageal neoplasms correlates well with the pathologic stage (Figure 85-5).[72,78] The ability of the clinical cTNM staging system to accurately predict the pTNM status has improved with time as the use of endoscopic ultrasound, CT of the chest and abdomen, and PET scan has increased.[79]

THERAPY

Standard curative treatment options for esophageal cancer include surgical resection, external beam radiotherapy, chemotherapy, or combinations of two or three of these options. The selection of appropriate therapy is often challenging because few comparisons of these options have been performed in a prospective, randomized fashion with an adequate number of patients. Additionally, these trials have been performed over a long time period during which significant changes in histology and types of treatment have occurred (ie, different radiation equipment, dosages and fields, and different surgical techniques and chemotherapy agents). Clinical staging techniques have also evolved over time, leading to stage migration and poor correlation with pathologic stage, especially from studies prior to CT scan and endoscopic ultrasound.[79] These problems make comparisons between different trials or treatment arms difficult. Treatment strategies have therefore evolved over time based on regional experiences and biases. In an effort, to guide current treatment strategies, we have included an esophageal treatment algorithm that incorporates different treatment strategies based on the physiologic status and clinical stage of the patient (see Figure 85-3). This algorithm reflects the treatment biases of the authors and is meant only to give some guidance in an otherwise confusing therapeutic arena.

In esophageal cancer, local control of the disease, as well as cure, are primary objectives of therapy because of the debilitating effects of dys-

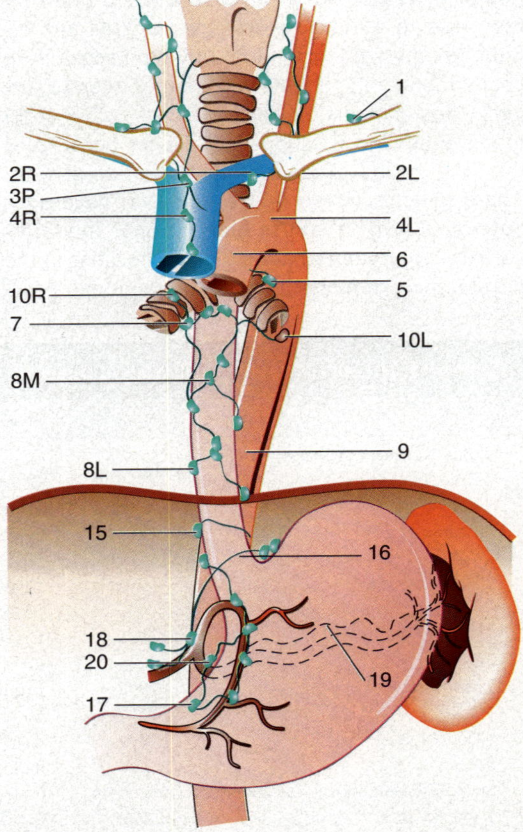

Figure 85-4 Lymph node staging map for neoplasms of the esophagus. Reproduced with permission from Ferguson, MK. Carcinoma of the esophagus and cardia. In: Surgery of the alimentary tract. 5th ed. Vol. 1. The esophagus. 5th ed.

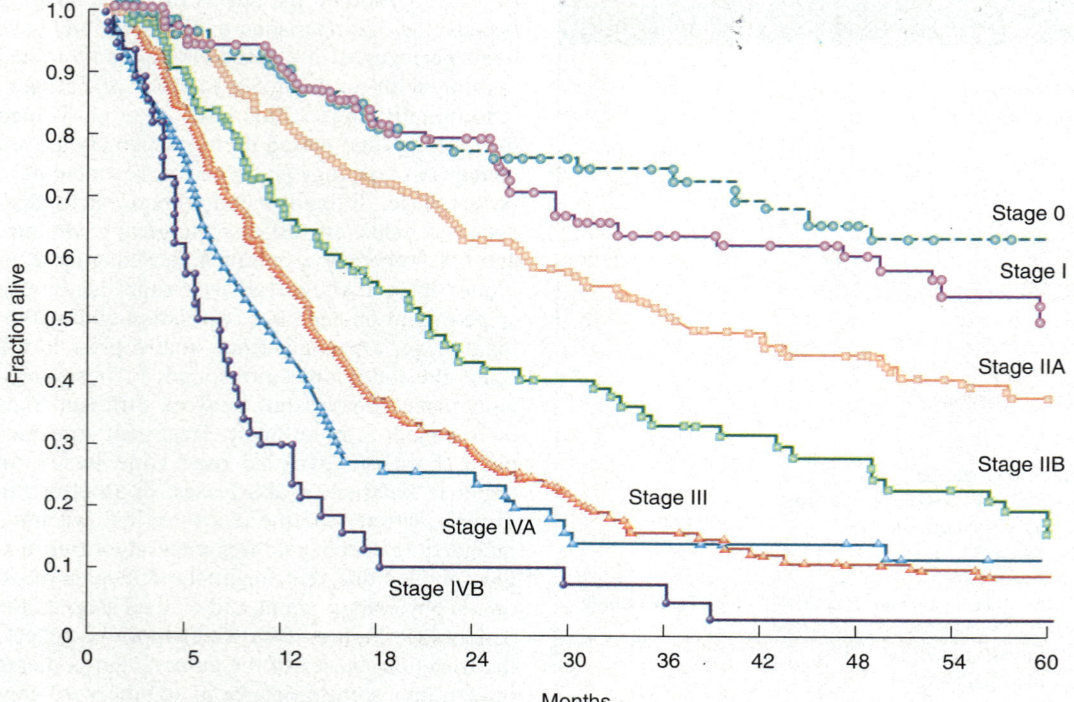

Figure 85-5 Long-term outcome according to pathologic stage of resected esophageal cancers at the University of Texas M.D. Anderson Cancer Center from 1970 to 2000 (*n* = 917).

phagia caused by progressive tumor growth and esophageal obstruction. Early-stage cancers (stage 0, I) traditionally have been treated by resection in good performance patients and by radiotherapy with or without radiation sensitizing chemotherapy in patients who cannot tolerate surgery. Most patients, however, present with locoregionally advanced esophageal cancer because of the long period of asymptomatic tumor growth. These patients (stage II, III, and IVa) have poor outcomes with a single locoregional modality such as surgery or radiation therapy because of the development of metastatic and locoregional recurrences. Attempts have therefore focused on treating these patients with multimodality approaches combining locoregional (surgery/radiation) therapies with systemic (chemotherapy) treatments. Although controversial, many oncologists in North America currently recommend treating these patients with definitive chemoradiation alone or preoperative chemoradiation and surgery. The data to unequivocally support this approach are lacking as demonstrated in the often conflicting randomized trial results (see Table 85-3) and some centers have argued that more aggressive en-bloc resection and 3-field lymphadenectomies are also important. Surgery and chemotherapy are often avoided in poor performance status locoregionally advanced patients because of treatment-related morbidity. In these patients, locoregional palliation can often be achieved with palliative stents and/or radiation. For patients who are initially recognized to be in advanced (metastatic) stages of disease, chemotherapy with or without palliative radiotherapy has been the mainstay of treatment. The development of endoesophageal stents has provided additional locoregional palliation and has limited the need for palliative surgical bypass even in patients with tracheoesophageal fistulas (see Figure 85-3).

Surgery Resection is the mainstay of treatment of neoplasms of the esophagus. It is the best single modality for managing patients with early-stage cancers. Surgery is an integral element in multimodality therapy for regionally advanced cancers because patients who undergo preoperative (neoadjuvant) therapy have a 75% incidence of residual local disease amenable to resection, although this remains controversial since some oncologists argue that surgery should be reserved only for patients who relapse with locoregional disease. Patients with regionally advanced and metastatic disease experience the palliative benefit of resection, which provides local control of disease and eliminates dysphagia although improvements in endoesophageal stenting have allowed patients with metastatic or poor performance locoregionally advanced disease to be palliated in other ways.

Approaches to Resection Surgical approaches to resection include a transthoracic operation, mobilization of the esophagus via a transhiatal route, and thoracoscopic/laparoscopic resection (Table 85-4; Figure 85-6).

Open, transthoracic approaches provide the ability to perform a more complete dissection of the primary tumor and lymph nodes than is possi-

Table 85-3 Results of Randomized Trials of Definitive Chemoradiotherapy for Locoregionally Advanced Esophageal Cancer

Author	Year	Treatment	Technique	Hist.	Pts.	Median Survival	*p*
Chemo/RT vs RT Alone							
Roussel et al[120]	1989	Methotrexate + 56 Gy	C→RT	S	77	9 mo	NS
		56 Gy			73	8 mo	
Araujo et al[116]	1991	5-FU, bleomycin, mito + 50 Gy	C/RT	S	28	18 mo	NS
		50 Gy			31	16 mo	
Hatlevoll et al[121]	1992	Cisplatin, bleomycin + 53 Gy	C→RT	S	46	6 mo	NS
		53 Gy			51	6 mo	
Slabber et al[122]	1998	Cisplatin, 5-FU + 40 Gy	C/RT	S	34	6 mo	NS
		40 Gy			36	5 mo	
Smith et al[117]	1998	Mitomycin, 5-FU + 40 Gy	C/RT	S > A	60	15 mo	.04
		40 Gy			59	9 mo	
Cooper et al[119]	1999	Cisplatin, 5-FU + 50 Gy	C/RT	S > A	61	13 mo	.01
		64 Gy			62	9 mo	
Chemo/RT (high dose) vs Chemo/RT (low dose)							
Minsky et al[114]	2002	Cisplatin, 5-FU + 50 Gy	C/RT	S > A	109	18 mo	NS
		Cisplatin, 5-FU + 64 Gy	C/RT		109	13 mo	
Chemo/RT/Surgery vs Chemo/RT Alone							
Stahl et al[146]	2005	Cis, 5-FU, Etop.→Cis, Etop.+ 40 Gy → Surgery	C→C/RT→S	S	86	16.4 mo	NS
		Cis, 5-FU, Etop.→Cis, Etop.+ 65 Gy	C→C/RT		86	14.9 mo	

A = adenocarcinoma; C = chemotherapy; NS = not significant; RT = radiation therapy; S = squamous cell; 5-FU = 5-fluorouracil.

Table 85-4 Operative Approaches to Resection for Esophageal Cancer

Transthoracic
Ivor Lewis (laparotomy, right thoracotomy, high intrathoracic anastomosis)
McKeown modification of Ivor Lewis (cervical anastomosis)
Left thoracotomy with intrathoracic anastomosis
Left thoracotomy with cervical anastomosis
Thoracoabdominal incision
Transhiatal
Minimally invasive
Thoracoscopically assisted
Laparoscopically assisted
Thoracoscopic/laparoscopic

ble using a transhiatal approach. The transhiatal approach allows the operation to be done more quickly with fewer incisions and potentially less trauma. This latter concept has been expanded with the use of thoracoscopic/laparoscopic techniques, which were introduced in the mid-1990s as a means to perform a thorough esophageal and nodal dissection while theoretically limiting operative morbidity and the duration of postoperative hospital stay.

The selection of an operative approach is dependent, in part, on tumor location and histology. Squamous cell cancers are most often located in the middle and upper thoracic esophagus, a location to which a transhiatal approach is often contraindicated except in the most experienced hands. In contrast, adenocarcinomas, which most often arise in the distal esophagus or cardia, are easily amenable to open transthoracic and transhiatal approaches. Squamous cell cancers are multifocal in nearly 20% of patients, and near-total esophagectomy is recommended to minimize the risk of performing an incomplete resection.[80,81] This usually necessitates a cervical anastomosis for reconstruction. In contrast, adenocarcinomas usually are not multifocal, but tend to spread submucosally. When negative proximal and distal margins are obtained on frozen section at the time of operation, the extent of the esophageal resection is theoretically satisfactory. Recently the performance of esophagectomy using minimally invasive techniques has been described.[82,83] The procedure begins with thoracoscopic mobilization of the thoracic esophagus, followed by laparoscopic creation of the gastric conduit. The specimen is delivered through a cervical incision and the gastric conduit anastomosed to the cervical esophagus. A complete mediastinal and celiac axis lymph node dissection is usually performed without difficulty. The largest series reported to date included 222 patients and documented a very low mortality rate of 1.4% and a major morbidity rate of 32%.[84] Although there have been no prospective comparisons between minimally invasive esophagectomy and open esophagectomy, in a retrospective review, Nguyen and colleagues[85] reported that patients who had minimally invasive esophagectomy had shorter operative times, less blood loss, fewer transfusions, and shortened intensive care unit and hospital courses than patients who underwent open procedures. Recently Horgan and colleagues[86] have described robotic-assisted, minimally invasive esophagectomy. The chief advantage of the surgical robot appears to be enhanced visualization and ability to dissect the thoracic esophagus via a transhiatal approach, which obviates thoracoscopic mobilization.

It is difficult to demonstrate an advantage of any technique over the other. Results from 44 published reports of transthoracic or transhiatal esophagectomy for cancer demonstrate a higher incidence of anastomotic complications in the latter group, but otherwise no important differences in operative morbidity or mortality and similar 5-year survival rates.[88–93] Similarly, the use of a minimally invasive approach, such as thoracoscopic resection, appears to offer little advantage over open approaches. Combined results of the early experiences from a number of centers demonstrate operative morbidity and mortality, as well as postoperative duration of hospital stay, to be similar to results for open procedures.[93–101] Currently, the choice of the approach to esophageal resection depends largely on the training, experience, and personal preference of the surgeon.

Effects of Neoadjuvant Therapy The use of preoperative therapy before surgery has the potential of increasing perioperative morbidity and mortality. One prospective randomized study reported that septic complications, respiratory complications, and operative mortality were higher in patients who underwent preoperative chemotherapy compared with surgery alone.[102] However, several other studies assessing neoadjuvant chemotherapy or chemoradiotherapy have shown no important differences in postoperative complications or operative mortality.[39,103–107] The complexity of esophageal surgery mandates that the procedure be performed at a high volume, referral center to minimize operative morbidity and mortality.[44] Medicare data suggest that high volume centers can perform esophageal resections with a mortality of 3%, whereas less experienced centers have a mortality of 19%.[44] This morbidity and mortality may be even further increased when preoperative therapy is used. At less experienced centers, the morbidity and mortality of the procedure may be greater than the potential benefit, especially when considering the low likelihood of cure in locoregionally advanced patients.

Surgery for Cervical Esophageal Cancer Neoplasms of the cervical esophagus pose special problems with regard to surgical therapy. To

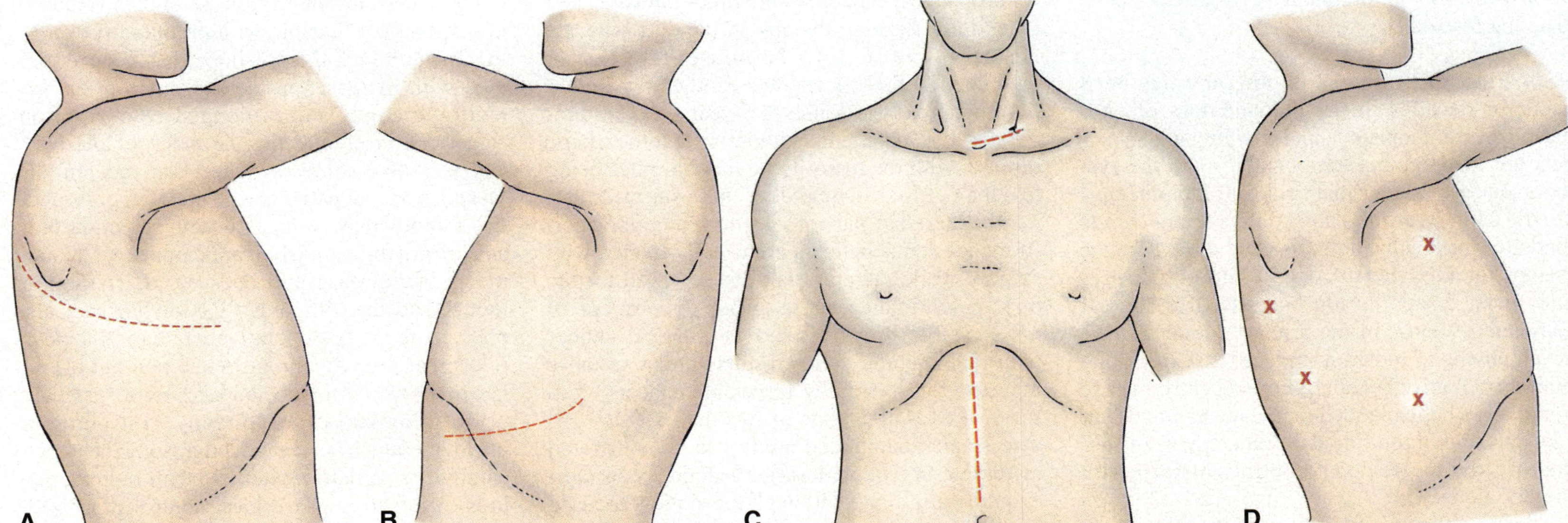

Figure 85-6 Approaches for esophagectomy. **A,** Right thoracotomy and laparotomy with intrathoracic (Ivor Lewis operation) or cervical anastomosis (McKeown modification of Ivor Lewis esophagectomy). **B,** Left thoracotomy, accessing the abdomen through a peripheral incision in the diaphragm, with intrathoracic or cervical anastomosis. **C,** Transhiatal esophagectomy with cervical anastomosis. **D,** Thoracoscopic esophagectomy.

obtain adequate surgical margins in tumors that extend to the cricopharyngeus muscle or invade the proximal trachea, it is necessary to include a laryngectomy as part of the resection, which adds substantial long-term morbidity to what is often a palliative procedure. As a result, a higher percentage of patients with cervical esophageal cancer are treated nonsurgically than is the case for patients with cancers in other locations. Resection provides good palliation for dysphagia but does not appear to substantially influence long-term survival and the morbidity has led most people to recommend chemoradiation in this subset of patients.[108–111]

Reconstruction after Esophagectomy Re-establishing alimentary tract continuity after esophageal resection in a manner that permits ingestion of a normal diet is an important component of surgery for esophageal cancer. Options for reconstruction include using the stomach as a substitute or interposing a segment of colon or jejunum between the proximal esophageal remnant and the stomach (or duodenum after total gastrectomy). The use of the stomach for reconstruction is by far the most common technique because the stomach has the most reliable blood supply among any of the reconstructive options and because only a single anastomosis is required, compared with the three anastomoses necessary for bowel interposition. Cervical anastomoses are favored by some surgeons because they decrease the incidence of acid reflux into the esophageal remnant and because anastomotic leaks are usually easily managed by simple cervical drainage. The disadvantages of cervical anastomoses are a higher incidence of recurrent laryngeal nerve injury and more frequent anastomotic leaks. Whether the additional tumor-free proximal margin provided by a cervical anastomosis offers a survival advantage has not been proven.[112] Use of the posterior mediastinum (esophageal bed) for reconstruction optimizes emptying of the reconstructive organ but may predispose to tumor infiltration if a complete resection is not performed.[113]

Table 85-5 Results of Randomized Trials of Preoperative and Postoperative Radiotherapy for Locoregionally Advanced Esophageal Cancer

Authors	Year	Treatment	Histology	Patients (No.)	5-Year Survival	*p* Value
Preoperative RT vs Surgery Alone						
Launois et al[124]	1981	Surgery alone	S	57	11.5%	NS
		Surgery + 40 Gy		67	7.5%	
Gignoux et al[125]	1988	Surgery alone	S	106	10%	NS
		Surgery + 33 Gy		102	9%	
Wang et al[126]	1989	Surgery alone	S	102	30%	NS
		Surgery + 40 Gy		104	35%	
Arnott et al[130]	1992	Surgery alone	S	86	17%	NS
		Surgery + 20 Gy		90	9%	
Nygaard et al[128]	1992	Surgery alone	S	41	4%	.08
		Surgery + 35 Gy		48	18%	
Postoperative RT vs Surgery Alone						
FUASR[133]	1991	Surgery alone	S	119	18%	NS
		Surgery + 45–55 Gy		102	20%	
Fok et al[131]	1993	Surgery alone	S	65	11% (4yr)	NS
		Surgery + 49–52.5 Gy		65	11% (4yr)	
Ziernan[132]	1995	Surgery alone	S	35	20% (3yr)	NS
		Surgery + 56 Gy		33	23% (3yr)	

Radiation Therapy Radiotherapy has been used for decades in the management of neoplasms of the esophagus and as with surgery targets the locoregional tumor rather than the systemic disease. The primary roles of radiotherapy, as with surgery, are as a potentially curative single modality for localized disease and as a palliative therapy for advanced tumors. Results of both uses have been disappointing because of a lack of complete response of the primary tumor and the development of radiation-induced strictures that limit its palliative benefits. More recently, the use of radiation has expanded to include an important adjuvant role in multimodality therapy to further improve the locoregional control obtained with surgery alone.

Treatment is planned to uniformly irradiate gross tumor and margins suspected of harboring microscopic disease, while minimizing injury to adjacent normal tissues, such as the lung, heart, and spinal cord. Regional nodal basins are usually included, typically cervical and supraclavicular nodes for cervical cancers, supraclavicular and subcarinal lymph nodes for upper thoracic cancers, and celiac axis nodes for lower thoracic and cardiac cancers. Initial treatment is to opposed, anterior-posterior and posterior-anterior fields using high energy (6–24 MV) photons. In patients receiving potentially curative high-dose therapy, the final treatments are delivered at an oblique angle to minimize the total dose to the spinal cord. Daily treatments of 1.8 to 2 Gy to a total of 60 to 70 Gy were formerly used for curative intent, although this has been modified since recent trials have demonstrated equal efficacy and less toxicity with the lower dose (50.4 Gy).[114] Palliative doses tend to be even lower to further reduce this morbidity (30 to 40 Gy).

Radiation as Single Modality Therapy The use of radiation therapy as a single modality for esophageal cancer is sometimes indicated as a potentially curative therapy in patients who are unable to tolerate (or who refuse) resection or combined definitive chemoradiotherapy. Radiation therapy alone achieves 5-year survival rates of 0 to 20% in patients without distant metastatic disease, with the majority of survival rates being less than 10%. Although low, these survival rates may be biased by patient selection since good performance status patients are usually treated with surgery while radiation is often reserved for the poor performance status group. Treatment of unresectable but localized esophageal cancer with radiotherapy yields results similar to those reported for potentially resectable cancers, with survival rates at 5 years of less than 10%.[115–122] One small randomized study has demonstrated increased survival with surgery alone versus radiation therapy alone, although the authors focused more on endpoints of quality of life.[123]

Radiotherapy as an Adjuvant to Resection In an effort to obtain better local control of disease, radiotherapy has been used both preoperatively and postoperatively as an adjunct to resection (Table 85-5).[124–128] The interval between completion of radiotherapy and resection is typically 3 to 5 weeks (1 week/10 Gy), which is felt to minimize perioperative complications from bleeding and radiation-induced fibrosis. In the proper setting, postoperative complication and mortality rates are not increased by the administration of preoperative radiotherapy, although this may be contingent on performing the surgical procedure in a high-volume center.[44] Most randomized, controlled studies have not demonstrated a survival advantage compared with surgery alone although these studies were often performed with outdated radiation therapy techniques.[124–128] Meta-analysis of the combined data from all randomized studies that have been published do not demonstrate improved survival with preoperative radiotherapy.[129]

The use of radiotherapy postoperatively enables the administration of higher radiation doses than are feasible with preoperative radiotherapy although this treatment has been associated with increases in the incidence of anastomotic strictures and prolonged recovery from surgery, adversely affecting the quality of life.[130–132] There is also some evidence that median survival is worse in patients who undergo postoperative radiotherapy, compared with resection only, as a result of an earlier appearance of distant metastatic disease and because of irradiation-induced deaths, although selection bias may also play a role.[131] Postoperative irradiation appears to decrease the local recurrence rate but overall has no proven influence on long-term survival.

Intraluminal Brachytherapy Intraluminal brachytherapy has been added in some centers to curative or palliative external beam radiotherapy in an effort to improve local control of disease. Doses of 10 to 20 Gy are administered after completion of external beam treatment in one or more fractions using Iridium-192. In patients with potentially curable disease, the addition of intraluminal brachytherapy appears to enhance locore-

Table 85-6 Results of Randomized Trials of Preoperative or Postoperative Chemotherapy for Locoregionally Advanced Esophageal Cancer

Author (Ref.)	Year	Treatment	Histology	Patients (No.)	Resectability	Op Mort	Median Survival (Mo)	p Value
Preoperative Chemotherapy								
Roth et al[40]	1988	Cisplatin, bleomycin, vindesine + surgery	S>A	19	—	10%	9	NS
		Surgery Alone		20	—	0%	9	
Nygaard et al[128]	1992	Cisplatin, bleomycin + Surgery	S	50	58%		10	NS
		Surgery Alone		41	69%	13%	7	
Schlag et al[103]	1992	Cisplatin, 5-FU + Surgery	S	21	69%	—	6	NS
		Surgery Alone		24	79%	—	8	
Maipang et al[141]	1994	Cisplatin, bleomycin, vinblastine + Surgery	S	24	—	—	17	NS
		Surgery Alone		22	—	—	17	
Ancona et al[142]	1995	Cisplatin, 5-FU + Surgery	S	35	78%	7%	—	NS
		Surgery Alone		43	86%	5%	—	
Law et al[106]	1997	Cisplatin, 5-FU + Surgery	S	73	95%	9%	13	NS
		Surgery Alone		74	89%	8%	17	
Kelsen et al[107]	1998	Cisplatin, 5-FU + Surgery	A > S	213	76%	7%	15	NS
		Surgery Alone		227	89%	6%	16	
Clarke et al[144]	2002	Cisplatin, 5-FU + Surgery	A > S	400	78%	10%	17	<.05
		Surgery Alone		402	70%	10%	13	
Postoperative Chemotherapy								
Ando et al[129]	1997	Cisplatin, vindesine + Surgery	S	105	—	—	58	NS
		Surgery Alone		100	—	—	47	

A = adenocarcinoma; NS = not significant; S = squamous cell; 5-FU = 5-fluorouracil.

gional control, compared with external beam radiotherapy alone, but is associated with a higher incidence of radiation-induced esophageal strictures.[133–135] Reducing the dose per fraction of intraluminal brachytherapy may in the future limit the incidence and severity of these local complications.[136] The use of brachytherapy in patients with unresectable or recurrent esophageal cancer is still under investigation but may provide better symptomatic relief than other modalities, such as gastric bypass surgery, chemotherapy, laser therapy, and stenting.[137–139]

Chemotherapy and Combination Therapy

Most patients with carcinoma of the esophagus have advanced disease at the time of diagnosis, and long-term survival is dismal even in operable patients. These factors have led to the investigation of systemic chemotherapy in an effort to improve both local and distant control of disease and to prolong survival. Chemotherapy has an emerging role in the treatment of esophageal cancer, either as neoadjuvant or postoperative adjuvant therapy or as part of concomitant chemoradiotherapy.

Single-Agent Chemotherapy A number of agents have been investigated as sole therapy for esophageal cancer, including cisplatin, irinotecan, bleomycin, mitomycin, 5-fluorouracil, paclitaxel, methotrexate, vinorelbine, mitoguazone, vindesine, doxorubicin, and etoposide. Phase II trials have demonstrated responses of 15 to 30% for these agents, with cisplatin, mitomycin, 5-fluorouracil, paclitaxel, and vindesine being the most active.[140] The responses have been short lived and have not led to any meaningful prolongation of survival.

Combination Chemotherapy The observation that single-agent chemotherapy provided modest and short-lived responses has led to the investigation of multidrug therapy for esophageal cancer. The drug combinations, which usually have been cisplatin based, have been evaluated as sole therapy for patients with recurrent or metastatic disease and as preoperative therapy for patients with regionally advanced disease. Responses are better than with single-agent therapy, averaging about 50%, and have become the mainstay of therapy for patients with metastatic esophageal cancer (see Figure 85-3).

In locoregionally advanced esophageal cancer, combination chemotherapy has been investigated in combination with radiation or surgery to try to reduce the high rate of systemic relapse noted when surgery or radiation therapy alone is used. Attempts to use chemotherapy with surgery have included preoperative and postoperative strategies usually with cisplatin-based multiagent regimens. The randomized trials with preoperative chemotherapy usually consist of two or three chemotherapy cycles followed by resection. Some studies have also added postoperative chemotherapy to the regimen. There is no apparent difference in response to chemotherapy based on histology. There is no clear increase in perioperative complications noted with preoperative chemotherapy when the surgery is performed at an experienced center. As Table 85-6 demonstrates, preoperative chemotherapy provides no consistent survival benefit compared with resection alone except in one recent study that enrolled over 800 patients.[40,104,107,108,129,141–144] The reasons for the failure of the majority of trials to demonstrate a clear improvement in survival may be due in part to the small number of patients enrolled or alternatively to the poor locoregional control obtained with standard esophageal resection, negating the small improvement obtained in distant disease control. In Kelsen and colleagues, over 30% of the patients undergoing surgery alone or preoperative chemotherapy demonstrated locoregional relapse within 1 year of completion of therapy, suggesting a need for better locoregional control.[107]

Postoperative chemotherapy (cisplatin, 5-fluorouracil) for patients after esophagectomy has also not demonstrated a clear survival advantage compared with surgery alone and has been associated with increased treatment-related complications (see Table 85-7).[145]

Definitive Chemoradiotherapy Chemotherapy has also been added to radiation therapy alone in an attempt to improve survival in locoregionally advanced esophageal cancer by decreasing metastatic relapse. These studies have used both sequential and concurrent treatment strategies. The concurrent use of chemotherapy and radiotherapy is theoretically appealing because, in addition to the systemic effects of chemotherapy, certain agents behave as radiosensitizers. Whether combined chemoradiotherapy is superior to radiotherapy alone in the management of either squamous cell cancer or adenocarcinoma of the esophagus is difficult to discern from earlier randomized trials, although recent randomized studies with a concurrent strategy appear to demonstrate an advantage to combined treatment (see Table 85-4).[115,117,118,120–123,146] Definitive chemoradiotherapy strategies with surgery used only as salvage appear most effective in squamous cell carcinoma and less effective in adenocarcinoma where long-term survival is much lower.[108]

Chemoradiotherapy has also been investigated in locoregionally advanced esophageal cancer as a preoperative strategy in an attempt to reduce both the high locoregional and systemic relapse rate noted with surgery alone or preoperative chemotherapy and surgery. The theoretical advantages to preoperative as opposed to postoperative chemoradiation therapy include (1) the ability to control subclinical systemic metastases prior to the immune suppression that results from surgery; (2) downstaging locoregional disease to increase the likelihood of a complete resection at surgery; and (3) the ability to administer full doses of chemoradiation that would not be possible to administer postoperatively because of perioperative debility. As Table 85-7 demonstrates, the results are not consistent, although sequential chemoradiation does not appear to be beneficial.[145–150] There have been several trials that

Table 85-7 Results of Randomized Trials of Preoperative Chemoradiotherapy for Locoregionally Advanced Esophageal Cancer

Author (Ref)	Year	Treatment	Histology	Patients (No.)	Technique	Op Mort	Medial Survival (Mo)	*p* Value
LePrise et al[145]	1994	Cisplatin, 5-FU + 20 Gy + Surgery	S	41	Sequential	9%	10	NS
		Surgery Alone		45		7%	10	
Walsh et al[147]	1996	Cisplatin, 5-FU + 40 Gy + Surgery	A	58	Concurrent	12%	17	.01
		Surgery Alone		55		3%	12	
Bosset et al[148]	1997	Cisplatin + 37 Gy + Surgery	S	143	Concurrent	12%	19	NS
		Surgery Alone		139		4%	19	
Urba et al[149]	2001	Cisplatin, 5-FU + 45 Gy + Surgery	A	50	Concurrent	4%	18	.15
		Surgery Alone		50		2%	17	
Burmeister et al[150]	2001	Cisplatin, 5-FU + 35 Gy + Surgery	A,S	128	Concurrent	5%	22	NS
		Surgery Alone		128		5%	19	

A = adenocarcinoma; NS = not significant; S = squamous cell; 5-FU = 5-fluorouracil.

have been encouraging for concurrent preoperative chemoradiation in locoregionally advanced esophageal cancer, but statistical significance may not have been achieved, in part because of an inadequate number of patients. Retrospective trials with larger numbers of patients have suggested that preoperative chemoradiation may offer some survival advantage compared with other strategies, although these studies are limited by different preclinical staging techniques and heterogenous patient populations (Figure 85-7).[80] A survival benefit for combined therapy is evident in most studies in patients who are found to have a complete pathologic response in the surgical specimen and have provided strong incentives to continue the investigations of this strategy. Additionally, since surgery alone or radiation therapy alone has such poor outcomes, many oncologists currently use definitive chemoradiotherapy alone or preoperative chemoradiation and surgery for nonmetastatic, locoregionally advanced esophageal cancer (see Figure 85-3). One randomized trial has been reported comparing definitive chemoradiation versus preoperative chemoradiation and surgery in squamous cell carcinoma. Preliminary results demonstrated improved locoregional control with surgery but no clear survival advantages, although this study was flawed by an inadequate number of patients receiving surgery.[146]

Photodynamic Therapy Photodynamic therapy (PDT) has been investigated in the treatment of patients with carcinoma in situ or superficial cancers who are unable to tolerate or who refuse surgical resection. PDT is performed by first systemically administering a photosensitive compound, and after its uptake in tumor, strong areas of concern are endoscopically treated with low-level laser light to activate the compound, causing selective cell death through release of toxic oxygen metabolites. The complete response rate of 75 to 80% endures for several years, suggesting that some patients may be cured with this therapy although long-term follow-up is still required.[151–154] PDT also is being investigated as one of several techniques, including laser photocoagulation, argon beam cautery, and electrocautery, for ablating Barrett's mucosa as a means of preventing the development of adenocarcinoma, although some authors have expressed concern for this approach since current staging techniques are relatively inaccurate, and up to 50% of patients who undergo resection for high-grade dysplasia in Barrett's esophagus have invasive cancer.[155] Additionally, some authors, have reported development of cancer beneath PDT-ablated mucosa that was more difficult to identify because of the treatment.

Recommendations for Therapy As our treatment algorithm suggests (see Figure 85-3), good performance patients with localized, early-stage disease should undergo surgery, whereas poor performance patients or patients refusing surgery can be treated with definitive chemoradiation or radiation alone. Locoregionally advanced esophageal cancer patients who are good performance are seldom cured with surgery or radiation therapy alone, and may therefore be candidates for investigational trials, definitive chemoradiation, or preoperative chemoradiation and surgery. Poor performance patients with locoregionally advanced esophageal cancer should be treated with chemoradiation or palliative radiation therapy and/or stents. Metastatic esophageal cancer patients who are good performance status may be offered chemotherapy alone with the addition of palliative radiation and/or stents for locoregional control. Chemotherapy should not be used if the patients have a poor performance status since the focus should be on palliation.

PALLIATIVE THERAPY OF ESOPHAGEAL OBSTRUCTION

In patients with advanced esophageal cancer not amenable to potentially curative therapy, a primary goal of treatment is relief of dysphagia.[156] This can be accomplished with palliative resection, but high operative morbidity and mortality rates as well as the prolonged period of recovery that is necessary preclude meaningful palliation and most oncologists currently recommend nonsurgical means for palliation. External beam radiotherapy, as an isolated modality or in combination with chemotherapy, is noninvasive but requires considerable time to complete and results in strictures in up to 30% of patients. Intraluminal brachytherapy is another

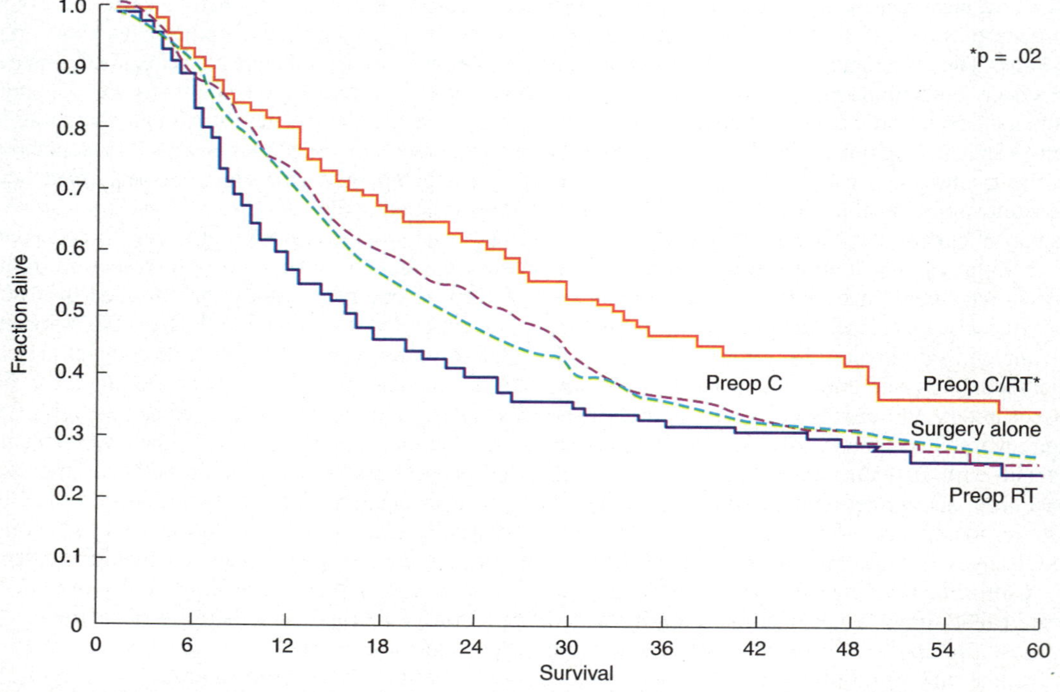

Figure 85-7 Improved long-term survival noted in patients undergoing preoperative chemoradiation (Preop C/RT) prior to surgery (surg) at the University of Texas M.D. Anderson Cancer Center *(n* = 879). Reproduced with permission from Hofstetter W, et al.[79]

options that is considered in some centers.[157,158] Photocoagulative laser therapy is another option and is usually performed with an Nd:YAG laser, with an initial improvement in dysphagia in 85% of patients and a mean duration of response of less than 1 month. PDT offers a similar initial efficacy but provides a more enduring response, although skin photosensitivity is an undesirable side effect.[159]

The development of endoesophageal stents has offered another therapeutic option in these difficult patients. Endoesophageal stent placement has led to rapid and enduring improvement in swallowing for many patients with advanced disease who are obstructed locoregionally. The introduction of self-expanding wire mesh stents has greatly simplified stent placement and associated complications and has improved palliation of dysphagia, compared with plastic prostheses.[160,161] This method of palliation has provided a much less invasive mechanism to palliate these patients and has replaced surgical bypass as the primary modality to relieve dysphagia.

Malignant esophagorespiratory (tracheoesophageal) fistulas pose a special problem in patients with esophageal cancer. These patients were previously treated with surgical bypass although the high morbidity and short life expectancy of these patients was a significant problem.[162] The introduction of coated wire mesh stents offers a better option for the treatment of such fistulas because they palliate dysphagia while occluding the fistula without requiring an extensive surgical procedure in an often debilitated and poor performance status patient.[163,164]

REFERENCES

1. Long ER. A history of pathology. Baltimore (MD): Williams & Wilkins; 1928.
2. Czerny V. Neue Operationen. Vorlaufige Mittheilung Zentralb Cir 1877;4:433–4.
3. Torek F. The first successful case of resection of the thoracic portion of the esophagus for carcinoma. Surg Gynecol Obstet 1913;16:614–7.
4. Dolan K, Sutton R, Walker SJ, et al. New classification of oesophageal and gastric carcinomas derived from changing patterns in epidemiology. Br J Cancer 1999;80:834–42.
5. Siewert JR. Adenocarcinoma of the esophagogastric junction: classification, pathology and extent of resection. Dis Esophagus 1996;9:173–82.
6. Caldwell CB, Bains MS, Burt M. Unusual malignant neoplasms of the esophagus. J Thorac Cardiovasc Surg 1991;101:100–7.
7. Lieberman MD, Franceschi D, Marsan B, et al. Esophageal carcinoma. The unusual variants. J Thorac Cardiovasc Surg 1994;108:1138–46.
8. Craddock VM. Aetiology of oesophageal cancer: some operative factors. Eur J Cancer Prevent 1992;1:89–103.
9. Kinjo Y, Cui Y, Akiba S, et al. Mortality risks of oesophageal cancer associated with hot tea, alcohol, tobacco, and diet in Japan. J Epidemiol 1998;8:235–43.
10. Heimburger DC. Localized deficiencies of folic acid in aerodigestive tissues. Ann NY Acad Sci 1992;669:87–95.
11. Ghadirian P, Vobecky J, Vobecky JS. Factors associated with cancer of the oesophagus: an overview. Cancer Detect Prevent 1988;11:225–34.
12. Jaskiewicz K, Marasas FO, Rossouw JE, et al. Selenium and other mineral elements in populations at risk for esophageal cancer. Cancer 1988;62:2635–9.
13. Kjaerheim K, Gaard M, Andersen A. The role of alcohol, tobacco, and dietary factors in upper aerodigestive tract cancers: a prospective study of 10,900 Norwegian men. Cancer Causes Controls 1998;9:99–108.
14. Yu MC, Garabrant DH, Peters JM, et al. Tobacco, alcohol, diet, occupation, and carcinoma of the esophagus. Cancer Res 1988;48:3843–8.
15. Castellsague X, Munoz N, De Stefani E, et al. Independent and joint effects of tobacco smoking and alcohol drinking on the risk of esophageal cancer in men and women. Int J Cancer 1999;82:657–64.
16. Lagergren J, Bergstrom R, Lindgren A, et al. Symptomatic gastroesophageal reflux as a risk factor for esophageal adenocarcinoma. N Engl J Med 1999;340:825–31.
17. O'Connor JB, Falk GW, Richter JE. The incidence of adenocarcinoma and dysplasia in Barrett's esophagus. Am J Gastroenterol 1999;94:2037–42.
18. Sammon AM, Alderson D. Diet, reflux, and the development of squamous cell carcinoma of the oesophagus in Africa. Br J Surg 1998;85:891–6.
19. Meijssen MAC, Tilanus HW, van Blankenstein M, et al. Achalasia complicated by oesophageal squamous cell carcinoma: a prospective study in 195 patients. Gut 1992;33:155–8.
20. Sandler RS, Nyren O, Ekborn A, et al. The risk of esophageal cancer in patients with achalasia. JAMA 1995;274: 1359–62.
21. Streitz JM Jr, Ellis FH Jr, Gibb SP, et al. Achalasia and squamous cell carcinoma of the esophagus: analysis of 241 patients. Ann Thorac Surg 1995;59:1604–9.
22. Yang PC, Davis S. Incidence of cancer of the esophagus in the U.S. by histologic type. Cancer 1988;61:612–7.
23. Maillefer RH, Greydanus MP. To B or not to B: is tylosis B truly benign? Am J Gastroenterol 1999;94:829–34.
24. Montesano R, Hollstein M, Hainaut P. Genetic alterations in esophageal cancer and their relevance to etiology and pathogenesis: a review. Int J Cancer 1996;69:225–35.
25. Sur M, Cooper K. The role of the human papilloma virus in esophageal cancer. Pathology 1998;30:348–54.
26. Bjorge T, Hakulinen T, Engeland A, et al. A prospective, seroepidemiological study of the role of human papillomavirus in esophageal cancer in Norway. Cancer Res 1997;57:3989–92.
27. Lagergren J, Wang Z, Bergstrom R, et al. Human papillomavirus infection and esophageal cancer: a nationwide seroepidemiologic case-control study in Sweden. J Natl Cancer Inst 1999;91:156–62.
28. Dawsey SM, Shen Q, Nieberg RK, et al. Studies of esophageal balloon cytology in Linxian, China. Cancer Epidemiol Biomarkers Prev 1997; 6:121–30.
29. Yang CS. Research on esophageal cancer in China: a review. J Thorac Cardiovasc Surg 1980;40:2633–44.
30. Ries LAG, Eisner MP, Kosary CL, et al. SEER cancer statistics review, 1973–1999, Bethesda (MD): National Cancer Institute; 2002
31. Jemal A, Murray T, Samuels A, et al. Cancer statistics, 2003. CA cancer J Clin 2003;53:5–26.
32. Pera M, Cameron AJ, Trastek VF, et al. Increasing incidence of adenocarcinoma of the esophagus and esophagogastric junction. Gastroenterology 1993;104:510–3.
33. Maram ES, Kurland LT, Ludwig J, et al. Esophageal carcinoma in Olmsted County, Minnesota, 1935–1971. Mayo Clin Proc 1977;52:24–7.
34. Hesketh PJ, Clapp RW, Doos WG, et al. The increasing frequency of adenocarcinoma of the esophagus. Cancer 1989;64:526–30.
35. Powell J, McConkey CC. Increasing incidence of adenocarcinoma of the gastric cardia and adjacent sites. Br J Cancer 1990;62:440–3.
36. Levi F, LaVecchia C. Adenocarcinoma of the esophagus in Switzerland. JAMA 1991;265:2960.
37. Bytzer P, Christensen PB, Damkier P, et al. Adenocarcinoma of the esophagus and Barrett's esophagus: a population-based study. Am J Gastroenterol 1999; 94:86–91.
38. Swisher SG, Hunt KK, Holmes EC, et al. Changes in the surgical management of esophageal cancer from 1970-1993. Am J Surg 1995;169:609–14.
39. Swisher SG, Holmes EC, Hunt KK, et al. The role of neoadjuvant therapy in surgical resection of esophageal cancer. Arch Surg 1996;131:819–25.
40. Roth JA, Pass HI, Flanagan MM, et al. Randomized clinical trial of preoperative and postoperative adjuvant chemotherapy with cisplatin, vindesine, and bleomycin for carcinoma of the esophagus. J Thorac Cardiovasc Surg 1988;96:242–8.
41. Cusso X, Mones-Xiol J, Vilardell F. Endoscopic cytology of cancer of the esophagus and cardia: a long-term evaluation. Gastrointest Endosc 1989;35:321–3.
42. Ritchie AJ, McGuigan J, McManus, K, et al. Diagnostic rigid and flexible oesophagoscopy in carcinoma of the oesophagus: a comparison. Thorax 1993;48:115–8.
43. Law SYK, Fok M, Wong J. Risk analysis in resection of squamous cell carcinoma of the esophagus. World J Surg 1994;18:339–46.
44. Swisher SG, DeFord L, Merriman KW, et al. Effect of operative volume on morbidity, mortality and hospital use after esophagectomy for cancer. J Thorac Cardiovasc Surg 2000;119:1126–34.
45. Tio TL, Coene PPLO, Luiken GJHM, et al. Endosonography in the clinical staging of esophageal carcinoma [abstract]. Gastrointest Endosc 1990;36:S2–S10.
46. Beseth BD, Bedrod R, Isacoff WH, et al. Endoscopic ultrasound does not accurately assess pathologic stage of esophageal cancer after neoadjuvant chemoradiotherapy. Am Surg 2002;66:827–31.
47. Romagnuolo J, Scott J, Hawes RH, et al. Helical CT versus EUS with fine needle aspiration for celiac nodal assessment in patients with esophageal cancer. Gastrointest Endosc 2002;55:648–54.
48. Peters JH, Hoeft SF, Heimbucher J, et al. Selection of patients for curative or palliative resection of esophageal cancer based on preoperative endoscopic ultrasonography. Arch Surg 1994;129:534–9.
49. Rice TW, Boyce GA, Sivak MV. Esophageal ultrasound and the preoperative staging of carcinoma of the esophagus. J Thorac Cardiovasc Surg 1991;101:536–44.
50. Parmar KS, Zwishcenberger JB, Reevers AL, et al. Clinical impact of endoscopic ultrasound-guided fine needed aspiration of celiac axis lymph nodes (M1a disease) in esophageal cancer. Ann Thorac Surg 2002:73:916–21.
51. Thompson WM, Halvorsen RA, Foster WL Jr, et al. Computed tomography for staging esophageal and gastroesophageal cancer: reevaluation. AJR Am J Roentgenol 1983;141:951–8.
52. Lehr L, Rupp N, Siewert JR. Assessment of resectability of esophageal cancer by computed tomography and magnetic resonance imaging. Surgery 1988;103:344–50.
53. Yasui A, Nimura Y, Hayakawa N. MRI and CT of intrathoracic esophageal carcinoma: radiological, surgical and histopathological correlation. Dis Esoph 1990;3:13–20.
54. Schroder W, Baldus SE, Monig SP, et al. Lymph node staging of esophageal squamous cell carcinoma in patients with and without neoadjuvant radiochemotherapy: histomorphologic analysis. World J Surg 2002;26:584–7.
55. Greenberg J, Durkin M, Van Drunen M, et al. Computed tomography or endoscopic ultrasonography in preoperative staging of gastric and esophageal tumors. Surgery 1994;116:696–702.
56. Quint LE, Glazer GM, Orringer MB. Esophageal imaging by MR and CT: study of normal anatomy and neoplasms. Radiology 1985;156:727–31.
57. Krasna MJ, Reed CE, Jaklitsch MT, et al. Thoracoscopic staging of esophageal cancer: a prospective, multiinstitutional trial. Ann Thorac Surg 1995;60:1337–40.
58. Watt I, Stewart I, Anderson D, et al. Laparoscopy, ultrasound and computed tomography in cancer of the oesophagus and gastric cardia: a prospective comparison for detecting intra-abdominal metastases. Br J Surg 1989;76:1036–9.
59. Block MI, Patterson GA, Sundaresan RS, et al. Improvement in staging of esophageal cancer with the addition of positron emission tomography. Ann Thorac Surg 1997;64:770–7.
60. Riedel M, Hauck RW, Stein HJ, et al. Preoperative bronchoscopic assessment of airway invasion by esophageal cancer. Chest 1998;113:687–95.
61. Flamen P, Lerut A, Van Cutsem E, et al. Utility of positron emission tomography for the staging of patients with potentially operable esophageal carcinoma. J Clin Oncol 2000;18:3202-10.
62. Brucher BLDM, Weber W, Bauer M, et al. Neoadjuvant therapy of esophageal squamous cell carcinoma: response evaluation by positron emission tomography. Ann Surg 2001;233:300–9.
63. Flamen P, Lerut A, Van Cutsem E, et al. The utility of positron emission tomography for the diagnosis and staging of recurrent esophageal cancer. J Thorac Cardiovasc Surg 2000;120:1085–92.
64. Inculet R, Keller SM, Dwyer A, et al. Evaluation of noninvasive tests for the preoperative staging of carcinoma of the esophagus: a prospective study. Ann Thorac Surg 1985;40:561–5.
65. Tachimori Y, Kato H, Watanabe H, et al. Neck ultrasonography for thoracic esophageal carcinoma. Ann Thorac Surg 1994;57:1180–3.
66. Natsugoe S, Yoshinaka H, Shimada M, et al. Assessment of cervical lymph node metastasis in esophageal carcinoma using ultrasonography. Ann Surg 1999;229:62–6.

67. van Overhagen H, Lameris JS, Zonderland HM, et al. Ultrasound and ultrasound-guided fine needle aspiration biopsy of supraclavicular lymph nodes in patients with esophageal carcinoma. Cancer 1991;67:585–7.
68. Mufti SI, Zirvi KA, Garewal HS. Precancerous lesions and biologic markers in esophageal cancer. Cancer Detect Prev 1991;15:291–301.
69. Shimada Y, Imamura M, Shibagaki I, et al. Genetic alterations in patients with esophageal cancer with short-and long-term survival rates after curative esophagectomy. Ann Surg 1997;226:162–8.
70. Wang L-S, Chow K-H, Chi K-H, et al. Prognosis of esophageal squamous cell carcinoma: analysis of clinicopathological and biological factors. Am J Gastroenterol 1999;94:1933–40.
71. American Joint Committee on Cancer. AJCC cancer staging manual. 5th ed. Philadelphia (PA): Lippincott, Williams and Wilkins; 1997. p. 65–9.
72. Korst RJ, Rusch VW, Venkatraman E, et al. Proposed revision of the staging classification for esophageal cancer. J Thorac Cardiovasc Surg 1998;115:660–70.
73. Baba M, Aikou T, Yoshinaka H, et al. Long-term results of subtotal esophagectomy with three-field lymphadenectomy for carcinoma of the thoracic esophagus. Ann Surg 1994;219:310–6.
74. Holscher AH, Bollschweiler E, Bumm R, et al. Prognostic factors of resected adenocarcinoma of the esophagus. Surgery 1995;118:845–55.
75. Nishimaki T, Suzuki T, Suzuki S, et al. Outcomes of extended radical esophagectomy for thoracic esophageal cancer. J Am Coll Surg 1998;186:306–12.
76. Nigro JJ, DeMeester SR, Hagen JA, et al. Node status in transmural esophageal adenocarcinoma and outcome after en bloc esophagectomy. J Thorac Cardiovasc Surg 1999;117:960–8.
77. Tabira Y, Okuma T, Kondo K, et al. Indications for three-field dissection followed by esophagectomy for advanced carcinoma of the thoracic esophagus. J Thorac Cardiovasc Surg 1999;117:239–45.
78. Japanese Committee for Registration of Esophageal Carcinoma. A proposal for a new TNM classification of esophageal carcinoma. Jpn J Clin Oncol 1985;14:625–36.
79. Hofstetter W, Swisher SG, Correa AM, et al. Treatment outcomes of resected esophageal cancer. Ann Surg 2002; 236:376–85.
80. Mizobuchi S, Kato H, Tachimori Y, et al. Multiple primary carcinoma of the oesophagus. Surg Oncol 1993;2:249–253.
81. Pesko P, Rakic S, Milicevic M, et al. Prevalence and clinicopathologic features of multiple squamous cell carcinoma of the esophagus. Cancer 1994;73:2687–90.
82. DePaula, AL, Hashiba, K, Ferreira, EA, et al. Laparoscopic transhiatal esopagectomy with esophagogastroplasty. Surg Laparosc Endosc 1995;1–5.
83. Swanstrom LL, Hansen P. Laparoscopic total esophagectomy. Arch Surg 1997;943–7.
84. Luketich JD, Alvelo-Rivera M, Buenaventura PO, et al. Minimally invasive esophagectomy: outcomes in 222 patients. Ann Surg 2003;486–96.
85. Nguyen NT, Roberts P, Follette DM, et al. Thoracoscopic and laparoscopic esophagectomy for benign and malignant disease: lessons learned from 46 consecutive procedures. J Am Coll Surg 2003;902–13.
86. Horgan S, Berger RA, Elli EF, et al. Robotic-assisted minimally invasive transhiatal esophagectomy. Am Surg 2003;624–6.
87. Jacobi CA, Zieren HU, Muller JM, et al. Surgical therapy of esophageal carcinoma: the influence of surgical approach and esophageal resection on cardiopulmonary function. Eur J Cardio-Thorac Surg 1997;11:32–7.
88. Hulscher JBF, van Sandik JW, De Boer AGEM, et al. Extended transthoracic resection compared with limited transhiatal resection for adenocarcinoma of the esophagus. New Engl J Med 2002;347:1662–9.
89. Pac M, Basoglu A, Kocak H, et al. Transhiatal versus transthoracic esophagectomy for esophageal cancer. J Thorac Cardiovasc Surg 1993;106:205–9.
90. Tilanus HW, Hop WCJ, Langenhorst BLAM, et al. Esophagectomy with or without thoracotomy. J Thorac Cardiovasc Surg 1993;105:898–903.
91. Putnam JB Jr, Suell DM, McMurtry MJ, et al. Comparison of three techniques of esophagectomy within a residency training program. Ann Thorac Surg 1994;57:319–25.
92. Rentz J, Bull D, Harpole D, et al. Transthoracic versus transhiatal esophagectomy: a prospective study of 945 patients; J Thorac Cardiovasc Surg 2003;125:1114–20.
93. Rindani R, Martin CJ, Cox, MR. Transhiatal versus Ivor Lewis oesophagectomy: is there a difference? Aust NZ J Surg 1999;69:187–94.
94. McAnena OJ, Rogers J, Williams NS. Right thoracoscopically assisted oesophagectomy for cancer. Br J Surg 1994;81:236–8.
95. Liu H-P, Chang C-H, Lin PJ, et al. Video-assisted endoscopic esophagectomy with stapled intrathoracic esophagogastric anastomosis. World J Surg 1995;19:745–7.
96. Akaishi T, Kaneda I, Higuchi N, et al. Thoracoscopic en bloc total esophagectomy with radical mediastinal lymphadenectomy. J Thorac Cardiovasc Surg 1996;112:1533–40.
97. Dexter SPL, Martin IG, McMahon MJ. Radical thoracoscopic esophagectomy for cancer. Surg Endosc 1996;10:147–51.
98. Roberston GS, Lloyd DM, Wicks AC, et al. No obvious advantages for thoracoscopic two-stage oesophagectomy. Br J Surg 1996;83:675–8.
99. Law S, Fok M, Chu KM, et al. Thoracoscopic esophagectomy for esophageal cancer. Surgery 1997;122:8–14.
100. Peracchia A, Rosati R, Funagalli U, et al. Thoracoscopic dissection of the esophagus for cancer. Int J Surg 1997;82:1–4.
101. Kawahara K, Maikawa T, Okabayashi K, et al. Video-assisted thoracoscopic esophagectomy for esophageal cancer. Surg Endosc 1999;13:218–23.
102. Lerut T, Coosemans W, De Leyn P, et al. Reflections on three field lymphadenectomy in carcinoma of the esophagus and esophagogastric junction. Hepato-Gastroenterol 1999;46:717–25.
103. Schlag PM, Chirirgische Arbeitsgemeinschaft fuer Onkologie der Deutschen Gesellschaft fuer Chirurgie Study Group. Randomized trial of preoperative chemotherapy for squamous cell cancer of the esophagus. Arch Surg 1992;127:1446–50.
104. Walsh TN, Noonan N, Hollywood D, et al. A comparison of multimodal therapy and surgery for esophageal adenocarcinoma. N Engl J Med 1996;335:462–7.
105. Bosset J-F, Gignoux M, Triboulet J-P, et al. Chemoradiotherapy followed by surgery compared with surgery alone in squamous cell cancer of the esophagus. N Engl J Med 1997;337:161–7.
106. Law S, Fok M, Chow S, et al. Preoperative chemotherapy versus surgical therapy alone for squamous cell carcinoma of the esophagus: a prospective randomized trial. J Thorac Cardiovasc Surg 1997;114:210–7.
107. Kelsen DP, Ginsberg R, Pajak TF, et al. Chemotherapy followed by surgery compared with surgery alone for localized esophageal cancer. N Engl J Med 1998;339:1979–84.
108. Chakkaphak S, Krishnasamy S, Walker SJ, et al. Treatment of carcinoma of the proximal esophagus. Surg Gynecol Obstet 1989;168:307–10.
109. Mansour KA, Picone AL, Coleman JJ III. Surgery for high cervical esophageal carcinoma: experience with 11 patients. Ann Thorac Surg 1990;49:597–602.
110. Kelley DJ, Wolf R, Shaha AR, et al. Impact of clinicopathologic parameters on patient survival in carcinoma of the cervical esophagus. Am J Surg 1995;170:427–31.
111. Marmuse J-P, Koka VN, Guedon C, et al. Surgical treatment of carcinoma of the proximal esophagus. Am J Surg 1995;169:386–90.
112. Ribet M, Debrueres B, Lecomte-Houcke M. Resection for advanced cancer of the thoracic esophagus: cervical or thoracic anastomosis? J Thorac Cardiovasc Surg 1992;103:784–9.
113. Gawad KA, Hosch SB, Bumann D, et al. How important is the route of reconstruction after esophagectomy: a prospective randomized study. Am J Gastroenterol 1999;94:1490–6.
114. Minsky BD, Pajak TF, Ginsberg RJ, et al. INT 0123 (Radiation Therapy Oncology Group 94-05) phase III trial of combined-modality therapy for esophageal cancer: high-dose versus standard-dose radiation therapy. J Clin Oncol 2002;20:1167–74.
115. Schuchmann G, Heydorn W, Hall R, et al. The treatment of esophageal carcinoma. A retrospective review. J Thorac Cardiovasc Surg 1980;79:67–73.
116. Araujo CMM, Souhami L, Gil RA, et al. A randomized trial comparing radiation therapy versus concomitant radiation therapy and chemotherapy in carcinoma of the thoracic esophagus. Cancer 1991;67:2258–61.
117. Smith TJ, Ryan LM, Douglass HO Jr, et al. Combined chemoradiotherapy vs. radiotherapy alone for early stage squamous cell carcinoma of the esophagus: a study of the Eastern Cooperative Oncology Group. Int J Radiat Oncol Biol Phys 1998;42:269–76.
118. Sykes AJ, Burt PA, Slevin NJ, et al. Radical radiotherapy for carcinoma of the oesophagus: an effective alternative to surgery. Radiother Oncol 1998;48:1–21.
119. Cooper JS, Guo MD, Herskovic A, et al. Chemoradiotherapy of locally advanced esophageal cancer. JAMA 1999;281:1623–7.
120. Roussel A, Bleiberg H, Dalesio O, et al. Palliative therapy of inoperable oesophageal carcinoma with radiotherapy and methotrexate: final results of a controlled clinical trial. Int J Radiat Oncol Biol Phys 1989;16:67–72.
121. Hatlevoll R, Hagen S, Hansen HS, et al. Bleomycin/cisplatin as neoadjuvant chemotherapy before radical radiotherapy in localized, inoperable carcinoma of the esophagus. Radiother Oncol 1992;24:114–6.
122. Slabber CF, Nel JS, Schoeman L, et al. A randomized study of radiotherapy alone versus radiotherapy plus 5-fluorouracil and platinum in patients with inoperable, locally advanced squamous cancer of the esophagus. Am J Clin Oncol 1998;21:462–5.
123. Badwe RA, Sharma V, Bhansali MS, et al. The quality of swallowing for patients with operable esophageal carcinoma: a randomized trial comparing surgery with radiotherapy. Cancer 1999;85:763–8.
124. Launois B, Delarue D, Campion JP, Kerbaol M. Preoperative radiotherapy for carcinoma of the esophagus. Surg Gynecol Obstet 1981;153:690–2.
125. Gignoux M, Roussel A, Paillot B, et al. The value of pre-operative radiotherapy in esophageal cancer: results of a study by the EORTC. Recent Rep Cancer Res 1988;110:1–13.
126. Wang M, Gu XZ, Yin WB, et al. Randomized clinical trial on the combination of preoperative irradiation and surgery in the treatment of esophageal carcinoma: report on 206 patients. Int J Radiat Oncol Biol Phys 1989;16:325–7.
127. Arnott SJ, Duncan W, Kerr GR, et al. Low dose preoperative radiotherapy for carcinoma of the oesophagus: results of a randomized clinical trial. Radiother Oncol 1992; 24:108–13.
128. Nygaard K, Hagen S, Hansen HS, et al. Pre-operative radiotherapy prolongs survival in operable esophageal carcinoma: a randomized, multicenter study of pre-operative radiotherapy and chemotherapy. The Second Scandinavian Trial in Esophageal Cancer. World J Surg 1992;16:1104–10.
129. Ando N, Iizuka T, Kakegawa T, et al. A randomized trial of surgery with and without chemotherapy for localized squamous carcinoma of the thoracic esophagus: the Japan Clinical Oncology Group study. J Thorac Cardiovasc Surg 1997;114:205–9.
130. Arnott SJ, Duncan W, Gignoux M, et al. Preoperative radiotherapy in esophageal carcinoma: a meta-analysis using individual patients data (Oesophageal Cancer Collaborative Group). Int J Radiat Oncol Biol Phys 1998;41:579–83.
131. Fok M, Sham JST, Shoy D, et al. Postoperative radiotherapy for carcinoma of the esophagus: a prospective, randomized controlled study. Surgery 1993;113:138–47.
132. Zierens HU, Muller JM, Jacobi CA, et al. Adjuvant postoperative radiation therapy after curative resection of squamous cell carcinoma of the thoracic esophagus: a prospective randomized study. World J Surg 1995;19:444–9.
133. French University Association for Surgical Research, Teniere P, Hay J-M, et al. Postoperative radiation therapy does not increase survival after curative resection for squamous cell carcinoma of the middle and lower esophagus as shown by a multicenter controlled trial. Surg Gynecol Obstet 1991;173:123–30.
134. Sur RK, Singh DP, Sharma SC, et al. Radiation therapy of esophageal cancer: role of high dose rate brachytherapy. Int J Radiat Oncol Biol Phys 1992;22:1043–6.
135. Tanisada K, Techima T, Ikeda H, et al. Prognostic factors for patients with esophageal cancer. Radiat Med 1998;16:461–8.
136. Akagi Y, Hirokawa Y, Kagemoto M, et al. Optimum fractionation for high-dose-rate endoesophageal brachytherapy following external irradiation of early stage esophageal cancer. Int J Radiat Oncol Biol Phys 1999;43:525–30.
137. Smolle-Juettner FM, Smolle J, Pakisch B, et al. Palliation of esophageal cancer in ill, inoperable patients: value of iridium 192 high-dose-rate intracavitary brachytherapy with and without external beam irradiation. Dis Esoph 1990;3:59–65.
138. Iwasa M, Ohmori Y, Iwasa Y, et al. Effect of multidisciplinary treatment with high dose rate intraluminal brachytherapy on survival in patients with unresectable esophageal cancer. Digest Surg 1998;15:227–35.
139. Sur RK, Donde B, Levin VC, Mannell A. Fractionated high dose rate intraluminal brachytherapy in palliation of

advanced esophageal cancer. Int J Radiat Oncol Biol Phys 1998;15:447–53.
140. Kelsen D, Atiq OT. Therapy of upper gastrointestinal tract cancers. Curr Probl Cancer 1991;15:235–94.
141. Maipang T, Vasinanukorn P, Petpichetchian C, et al. Induction chemotherapy in the treatment of patients with carcinoma of the esophagus. J Surg Oncol 1994;56:191–7.
142. Ancona E, Ruol A, Chiarion-Sileni V, et al. Studio prospettico randomizzato di chemioterapia neoadjuvante versus sola chirurgia nel cancro operabile (T2-3, ogni N, M0) dell'esophago. Acta Chirurgia Italiana 1995;51:308–17.
143. Pouliquen X, Levard H, Hay J-M, et al. 5-Fluorouracil and cisplatin therapy after palliative surgical resection of squamous cell carcinoma of the esophagus. Ann Surg 1996;223:127–33.
144. Medical Research Council Oesophageal Cancer Working Party. Surgical resection with or without preoperative chemotherapy in oesophageal cancer: a randomised controlled trial. Lancet 2002;359:1727–33.
145. Le Prise E, Etienne PL, Meunier B, et al. A randomized study of chemotherapy, radiation therapy, and surgery versus surgery for localized squamous cell carcinoma of the esophagus. Cancer 1994;73:1779–84.
146. Stahl M, Stuschke M, Lehmann N, et al. Chemoradiation with and without surgery in patients with locally advanced squamous cell carcinoma of the esophagus. J Clin Oncol. 2005;23:2310–7.
147. Walsh TN, Noonan N, Hollywood D, et al. A comparison of multimodal therapy and surgery for esophageal adenocarcinoma. N Engl J Med 1996;335:462–7.
148. Bosset J-F, Gignoux M, Triboulet J-P, et al. Chemoradiotherapy followed by surgery compared with surgery alone in squamous-cell cancer of the esophagus. N Engl J Med 1997;337:161–7.
149. Urba S, Orringer M, Turrisi A, et al. Randomized preoperative locoregional chemoradiation versus surgery alone in patients with resectable esophageal cancer. J Clin Oncol 2001;19:305–13.
150. Burmeister BH, Smithers BM, Fitzgerald L, et al. Surgery alone versus chemoradiotherapy followed by surgery for resectable cancer of the esophagus: a randomized controlled phase III trial. Lancet Oncology 2005;6:659–68.
151. McCaughan JS Jr, Ellison EC, Guy JT, et al. Photodynamic therapy for esophageal malignancy: a prospective twelve-year study. Ann Thorac Surg 1996;62:1005–10.
152. Gossner L, Stolte M, Sroka R, et al. Photodynamic ablation of high-grade dysplasia and early cancer in Barrett's esophagus by means of 5-aminolevulinic acid. Gastroenterology 1998;114:448–55.
153. Savary JF, Grosjean P, Monnier P, et al. Photodynamic therapy of early squamous cell carcinomas of the esophagus: a review of 31 cases. Endoscopy 1998;30:258–65.
154. Overholt BF, Panjehpour M, Haydek JM. Photodynamic therapy for Barrett's esophagus: follow-up in 100 patients. Gastrointest Endosc 1999;49:1–7.
155. Ferguson MK, Naunheim KS. Resection for Barrett's mucosa with high-grade dysplasia: implications for prophylactic photodynamic therapy. J Thorac Cardiovasc Surg 1997;114:824–9.
156. Reed CE. Comparison of different treatments for unresectable esophageal cancer. World J Surg 1995;19:828–35.
157. Fleischman EH, Kagan AR, Bellotti JE, et al. Effective palliation for inoperable esophageal cancer using intensive intracavitary radiation. J Surg Oncol 1990;44:234–7.
158. Harvey JC, Fleishman EH, Bellotti JE, et al. Intracavitary radiation in the treatment of advanced esophageal carcinoma: a comparison of high dose rate vs low dose rate brachytherapy. J Surg Oncol 1993;52:101–4.
159. Lightdale CJ, Heier SK, Marcon NE, et al. Photodynamic therapy with porfimer sodium versus thermal ablation therapy with Nd:YAG laser for palliation of esophageal cancer: a multicenter randomized trial. Gastrointest Endosc 1995;42:507–12.
160. Lam YH, Chan A, Lau J, et al. Self-expandable metal stents for malignant dysphagia. Aust N Z J Surg 1999;69:668–71.
161. Sanyika C, Corr P, Haffejee A. Palliative treatment of oesophageal carcinoma–efficacy of plastic versus self-expandable stents. S Afr Med J 1999;89:640–3.
162. Meunier B, Stasik C, Raoul J-L, et al. Gastric bypass for malignant esophagotracheal fistula. Eur J Cardio-Thorac Surg 1998;13:184–9.
163. Raijman I, Lynch P. Coated expandable esophageal stents in the treatment of digestive-respiratory fistulas. Am J Gastroenterol 1997;92:2188–91.
164. Low DE, Kozarek RA. Comparison of conventional and wire mesh expandable prostheses and surgical bypass in patients with malignant esophagorespiratory fistulas. Ann Thorac Surg 1998;65:919–23.

86

Carcinoma of the Stomach

James C. Yao, MD
Christopher H. Crane, MD
Paul F. Mansfield, MD

EPIDEMIOLOGY

The incidence of gastric cancer in the United States has dropped dramatically since the 1930s, when it was the leading cause of cancer death in US men. That decline lagged 20 to 30 years after the widespread availability of refrigeration—a factor that has been proposed to account for the phenomenon.[1]

The decline in the incidence of gastric cancer from 1930 to 1976 was also associated with a decline in the incidence of distal lesions. The presenting anatomic location of primary lesions underwent a general shift from noncardial sites to cardial sites. However, since 1976, the incidence of proximal cardial and gastroesophageal (GE) junction adenocarcinoma in the United States and Europe has increased at a rate exceeding that of any other malignancy.[2] This rise in incidence of such lesions suggests a common pathogenesis that is distinct from that of distal gastric lesions, but the causative factor is unclear.

In 2001, the incidence of gastric cancer in the United States was 8.1 per 100,000 population.[3] In 2004, gastric cancer developed in approximately 22,710 people. Gastric cancer is more common in men (Figure 86-1).[4] Currently, blacks, Hispanics, and Native Americans in the United States are 1.5 to 2.5 times more likely than whites to develop gastric cancer.[5] Although gastric cancer is still the second leading cause of cancer death worldwide, its incidence is declining.[6] Gastric cancer is particularly common in China, South America, Eastern Europe, and Japan, where it is the most common malignancy.[7] Of the two general types of gastric cancer,[8] the intestinal type is more common, is more often distal, and predominates in endemic areas as compared with the diffuse type.

Survival in patients with gastric cancer remains poor. Only modest improvements in survival have been observed in the United States (Figure 86-2). According to the Surveillance, Epidemiology, and End Results (SEER) 9 registry, the median survival duration for gastric cancer (all stages) increased from 7 months in 1973–1974 to 9 months in 2000–2001.[3]

ETIOLOGY

Mucosal changes brought about by a variety of environmental insults can eventually lead to atrophic gastritis. Chronic atrophic gastritis and the resulting intestinal metaplasia appear to be precursor conditions for intestinal-type gastric cancer.[9] Host-related, environmental, and infectious causes have been implicated in gastric cancer.

A variety of host-related factors have been associated with gastric cancer. For example, low serum ferritin levels[10] and pernicious anemia have been associated with an increased risk of the disease. Also, although medically treated peptic ulcer disease does not appear to be associated with an increased risk of gastric cancer, patients who have undergone distal gastrectomy for benign peptic ulcer disease have been reported to have as much as a fivefold increase in risk.[11]

Clear evidence shows a heritable risk of gastric cancer in a small number of patients. Familial predisposition has been reported[12] and appears to be independent of environmental factors.[13] This predisposition has also been examined in controlling for dietary risk in patients with hereditary nonpolyposis colorectal cancer (HNPCC) and familial adenomatous polyposis (FAP). Patients with HNPCC have an increased risk of gastric cancer, not shared with those with FAP.[14]

The most compelling evidence for an environmental cause of intestinal-type gastric cancer comes from studies of migrants. Japanese, South American, and Eastern European migrants to the United States have a decreased risk of gastric cancer after two to three generations in a lower-risk environment and eating a lower-risk diet.[15,16] Dietary and environmental factors, particularly early in life, appear to influence the risk of this disease.[15]

The widespread availability of refrigeration has paralleled the reduction in the incidence of intestinal-type gastric carcinoma.[1] Use of refrigeration may have reduced dietary exposure to various carcinogens, such as nitrates and nitrites, by reducing bacterial and fungal contamination of food. However, investigators seeking to correlate nitrate concentrations in drinking water with stomach or esophageal cancer incidence found no such relationship.[17] Another possibility is that increased use of refrigeration led to a reduction in the consumption of smoked, cured, and salted foods. Correlation of those dietary factors with gastric carcinoma rates in epidemiologic studies led to the performance of prospective studies, which found no association with gastric cancer.

Increased consumption of fresh fruit is associated with decreased incidence of gastric cancer,[18] but the reduction does not appear to be related to levels of vitamin C.[19] A diverse diet, especially with regard to fruits and vegetables, has been

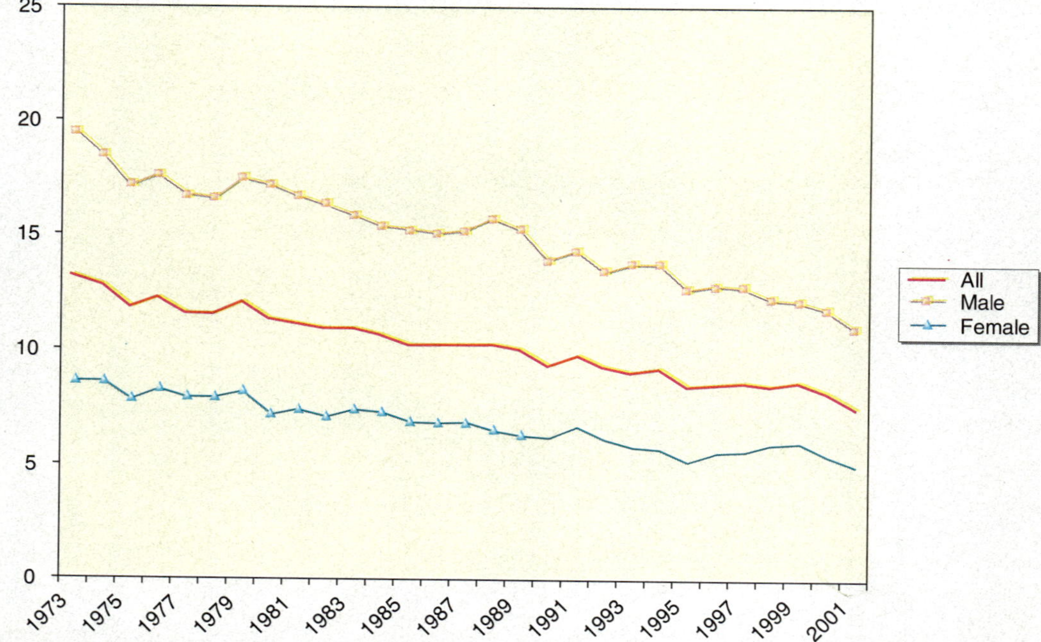

Figure 86-1 Surveillance, Epidemiology, and End Results (SEER) data from 1973 to 2001, showing time changes in the incidence of gastric cancer (per 100,000 population) by sex. Adapted from National Cancer Institute, DCCPS, Surveillance Research Program, Cancer Statistics Branch; released April 2004 based on the November 2003 submission.

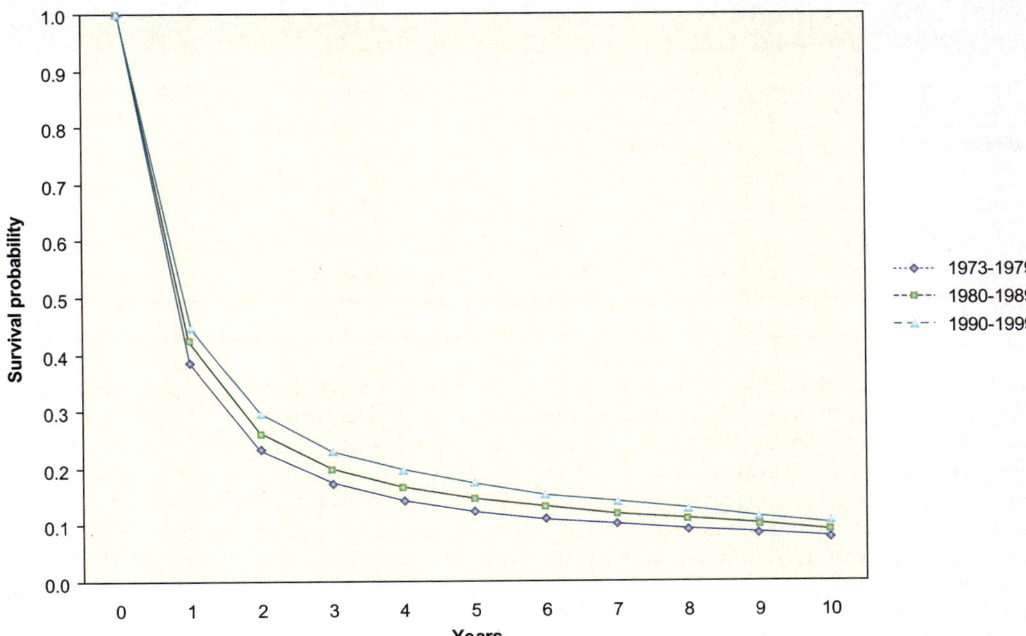

Figure 86-2 Surveillance, Epidemiology, and End Results (SEER) data from 1973 to 2001, showing survival rates in patients with gastric cancer (all stages) by year. Adapted from National Cancer Institute, DCCPS, Surveillance Research Program, Cancer Statistics Branch; released April 2004 based on the November 2003 submission.

reported to be protective.[20] A modest increase in risk has been reported with increased consumption of meat,[21] and a positive correlation between gastric cancer risk and increased meat-cooking time has been reported in retrospective studies of food intake and food preparation preference.[22]

Other environmental factors, such as smoking[18] and industrial dust exposure,[23] may be associated with gastric cancer. A causative role for alcohol has not been established.[24–26]

Infectious factors in gastric cancer, such as *Helicobacter pylori* infection, have been reported in epidemiologic studies,[27] and infection rates have been reported to be high in endemic areas.[28] Prospective serology studies have shown that patients with *H. pylori* infection have a threefold to fivefold increase in risk of noncardial lesions only.[29] Recent evidence identified a specific strain of the species, *CAGA*-positive *H. pylori*, and infection early in life as risk factors for gastric cancer.[30] A reduction in the risk of the disease with treatment of *H. pylori* infection has not been demonstrated, but such treatment has been approved by the Japanese health insurance system. In addition, gastric cancer screening has been determined to be substantially more cost-effective in endemic areas.[31]

A cohort study that looked at stored serum suggested that chronic Epstein–Barr virus infection may play an causative role in a subset of patients.[32] There are undoubtedly additional environmental co-factors that have not yet been identified.

Over the past decade, a number of US investigators have reported a trend of increasing incidence of proximal gastric cancer.[2,33] A similar change in the pattern of gastric cancer localization has been observed in Europe and Asia (Table 86-1).[34–36] In a recent report of the National Cancer Data Base, gastric cancer classified as proximal to distal in orientation was localized in the gastric cardia or fundus in approximately 50% of patients.[37] The cause of this increase in the incidence of proximal gastric cancer is under investigation.

Proximal gastric cancer has a pattern of clinical and biological behavior different from that of distal gastric cancer. Specifically, several investigators have reported a worse prognosis for patients with proximal gastric cancer than for patients whose cancer is located in the mid or distal portions of the stomach.[34,37] Additionally, the incidence of proximal gastric cancer is higher in white patients than in patients of other ethnicities.[22] Furthermore, obesity may play a role in its pathogenesis. Two case-control studies conducted in the United States and one conducted in Sweden found an association between a high body mass index and adenocarcinoma of the gastric cardia.[29,38] Our recent analysis of 1,339 consecutive cases of gastric and GE junction cancer at the University of Texas M.D. Anderson Cancer Center showed that proximal localization was strikingly more frequent in non-Hispanic white men, but that non-Hispanic white women had a pattern of gastric cancer localization similar to that in other ethnic-racial groups.[39,40]

GE junction cancers are classified at the discretion of the treating physician. No distinct morphologic features separate esophageal, GE junction, and gastric cancers. However, when investigators used comparative genomic hybridization to compare distal Barrett's esophageal, GE junction, and gastric cardial cancers, they found that loss of 14q31-32.1 was distinctly more common in patients with distal Barrett's esophageal cancer.[41] That loss was uncommon in patients with gastric cardial cancer and occurred with intermediate frequency in patients with GE junction cancer, implying that the latter is a mixture of cancers arising from the distal esophagus and gastric cardia.

HISTOLOGY

The Lauren and World Health Organization (WHO) classifications are the two major classification systems used for gastric adenocarcinoma.

THE LAUREN CLASSIFICATION The Lauren system simply classifies cancer as intestinal or diffuse.[8] It does recognize that, in some cases, the histology is mixed, with components of both intestinal and diffuse disease. The simplicity of the Lauren system has led to its widespread use.

Intestinal-type gastric cancer is also called epidemic-type gastric cancer. It features a retained

Table 86-1 Gastric Cancer Localization in Selected Countries

	United States[34]		Germany[257]		The Netherlands[35]		Japan[36]		Korea[37]
	Reported	Adjusted*	Reported	Adjusted*	Reported	Adjusted*	Reported	Adjusted*	Reported
Tumor Location	n = 33,085		n = 1,750		n = 711		n = 668		n = 10,783
Proximal	31%	45%	28%	30%	10%	10%	18%	21%	13%
Mid	5%	7%	37%	39%	28%	28%	33%	37%	87%†
Distal	25%	36%	25%	26%	54%	55%	38%	43%	
Diffuse	8%	12%	5%	5%	7%	7%	‡	‡	†
Unknown§	30%		5%		<1%		11%‡		†

* Excludes cases in which the primary tumor location is unknown or cannot be classified in a proximal to distal orientation (greater curve, lesser curve).

† Author reported location only as proximal or distal two-thirds.

‡ Author classified diffuse cases with unknown.

§ Primary tumor location is unknown or cannot be classified in a proximal-to-distal orientation.

glandular structure and cellular polarity. Grossly, it usually has a sharp margin. It arises from the gastric mucosa and is associated with chronic gastritis, gastric atrophy, and intestinal metaplasia. *H. pylori* and environmental factors likely play a major role in its pathogenesis.

The diffuse-type histology is associated with an invasive growth pattern. Scattered clusters of uniformly-sized malignant cells frequently infiltrate the submucosa. However, it has little glandular formation. Mucin production is common. Studies of gastrectomy specimens obtained from patients without clinical disease have shown early diffuse-type gastric cancer arising below normal-appearing epithelium.[42] Tumor cells in this type appear to arise from the superficial layer of the lamina propria.

An infiltrative growth pattern in diffuse-type gastric cancer often results in the absence of a mass. Endoscopically, the cancer may be difficult to identify without the presence of an ulceration or mass. Malignant cells can infiltrate well beyond the apparent tumor margin. In the extreme forms of this cancer, such infiltration leads to linitis plastica (leather-bottle-like stomach).

WHO Classification The WHO scheme classifies gastric cancer into groups that are more detailed than those in the Lauren classification. Specifically, the WHO papillary and tubular groups correspond with the intestinal type of gastric cancer in the Lauren classification, and the mucinous and signet-ring cell groups correspond with the diffuse type. The WHO undifferentiated type lacks features that further identify its origin. Mixed histology, with multiple components, is common. Although the WHO classification divides gastric cancer into more groups than the Lauren system does, it is not uniformly used in Western countries.

CLINICAL MANIFESTATIONS

The symptoms of gastric cancer are often nonspecific, leading to diagnosis at an advanced stage. This nonspecificity is caused in large part by the fact that the stomach and abdominal cavity alike are large and compliant to distention. Early symptoms—such as vague gastrointestinal distress, episodic nausea, vomiting, and anorexia—are common in patients without cancer. Thus, they are often not taken seriously by the patient and the patient's physician unless they persist or progress over a long period of time. Outside of Japan, an industrialized nation in which gastric cancer is common, early detection of gastric cancer is not attempted. In the United States, it is not uncommon for patients to undergo several months of therapy for peptic ulcer disease before a diagnosis of gastric cancer is made.

The most common symptoms of gastric cancer at diagnosis are abdominal pain (50% to 65%) and weight loss (40%). Although anemia is also a frequent finding among patients with gastric cancer, overt upper gastrointestinal bleeding is less common (approximately 17%). Our analyses of more than 1000 cases of gastric cancer at M. D. Anderson Cancer Center have shown that many symptoms vary according to the location of the primary lesion (Table 86-2). Dysphagia occurs predominantly in patients with proximal cancer localization. Nausea and vomiting are more common in patients with nonproximal cancer. Early satiety can be especially prominent in patients with linitis plastica.

Table 86-2 Symptoms at Diagnosis by Gastric Cancer Localization

	Proximal (n = 553)		Nonproximal (n = 689)		
Symptom	(n)	(%)	(n)	(%)	p Value
Abdominal pain	276	50	447	65	<.001
Weight loss	222	40	277	40	NS
Dysphagia	210	38	83	12	<.001
Nausea/vomiting	88	16	182	26	<.001
Early satiety	73	13	132	19	.005
Bleeding	89	16	116	17	NS

NS = nonsignificant.

Physical examination findings are late events that usually indicate advanced, unresectable disease. A palpable epigastric mass indicates a large locally advanced tumor. Jaundice usually indicates hepatic metastasis or metastatic lymphadenopathy in the portal region. Drop metastases into the pelvis can occur as Blumer's shelf nodules or Krukenberg tumors. Also, a periumbilical mass can arise from lymph node metastasis or, more commonly, direct growth through the abdominal wall from peritoneal metastasis. Another site of palpable lymphadenopathy is the left supraclavicular area, the Virchow node. Other, less common dermatologic findings include acanthosis nigricans and multiple seborrheic keratoses.

PATTERN OF SPREAD

Gastric cancer can spread in several ways. Adjacent organs—such as the liver, pancreas, spleen, and colon—are frequently involved by direct extension. Gastric cancer can also spread through the lymphatic system to distant nodes. The liver is frequently hematogenously involved. Finally, as the cancer penetrates the gastric wall, peritoneal metastasis frequently occurs. End-organ failure because of liver or peritoneal metastasis is a frequent cause of death.

Japanese investigators noted that histology and the patient's age may influence the pattern of gastric cancer metastasis. In an autopsy study of 173 cases of gastric cancer, investigators found diffuse histology to be associated with peritoneal metastasis and intestinal histology to be associated with hepatic metastasis.[43] They also found peritoneal metastasis to be more common in younger patients. In a separate surgical study, researchers analyzed the case records of 216 patients who had synchronous hepatic or peritoneal metastasis.[44] Peritoneal metastasis was associated with poorly differentiated histology, and hepatic metastasis was associated with a well to moderately differentiated histology.

On a molecular level, expression of vascular endothelial growth factor (*VEGF*) and its receptor *KDR* (kinase insert domain receptor) has been associated with liver metastasis.[45,46] The role of *VEGF* in angiogenesis is compatible with the presumed hematogenous route of dissemination of gastric cancer to the liver. Expression of VEGF-C, which can cause neogenesis of lymphatic vessels, is associated with lymph-node metastasis.[47,48] Additionally, dysregulation of cellular adhesion is likely central to peritoneal metastasis. An isoform of the CD44 antigen gene (*CD44*H) has been linked with increased adhesion of gastric cancer cells to mesothelial cells and increased peritoneal metastasis in animal models.[49] Amplification of c-*met* has also been linked with peritoneal metastasis.[50,51] Further translational research of the molecular biology of metastasis may improve prediction of failure sites and may refine therapeutic strategies.

MOLECULAR BIOLOGY OF GASTRIC CANCER

Table 86-3 presents molecular markers in gastric cancer and their clinicopathologic correlations.

Hereditary Gastric Cancer Familial clustering has been noted to occur in approximately 1% of gastric cancer cases. Known germline mutations account for only a small portion of these cases. The search for other candidate genes is ongoing. Reaching an understanding of the genetic abnormalities underlying hereditary gastric cancer offers not only opportunity for prevention and surveillance for affected individuals, but also clues regarding the molecular pathology of sporadic gastric cancer.

Hereditary Diffuse Gastric Cancer Syndrome Germline mutations of the E-cadherin gene (*CDH1*) in families with a history of gastric cancer were first reported in three Maori kindreds in 1998.[52] Since then, multiple families with a history of gastric cancer and mutations of this gene have been identified, and the hereditary diffuse gastric cancer syndrome has been established. However, detectable E-cadherin mutation accounts for only a small percentage of families with a history of diffuse gastric cancer. Most detected germline mutations of the E-cadherin gene have resulted in truncated E-cadherin protein. As-yet-undetected mutations of the E-cadherin gene may account for additional cases.

The E-cadherin gene is involved in cellular adhesion. Defects in this gene have been linked with diffuse-type gastric cancer and lobular breast

Table 86-3 Molecular Markers with Clinicopathologic Correlations

Marker	Involvement	Dominant Histology	Clinical Correlation
Epigenetic			
Hypermethylation	Common	Both	—
MSI	31%–39%	Intestinal	Conflicting for survival: favorable or no difference
Tumor suppressor			
TP53	47%–74%	Both (intestinal early event, diffuse late event)	Correlates with stage in diffuse-type cancer
APC	8%–34%	Intestinal	—
MCC	24%–33%	Diffuse	—
DCC	12%–49%	Intestinal	—
FHIT	49%–67%	—	Correlates with stage; conflicting for survival
Adhesion			
E-Cadherin	54%–83%	Diffuse	—
α-Catenin	83%–92%	Diffuse	—
γ-Catenin	91%–100%	Diffuse	—
β-Catenin	—	Intestinal (*GSK3B* region)	Poor survival
CD44	31%–72%	*CD44*v6-intestinal	*CD44*v6 in intestinal-type cancer correlates with inferior survival
Tyrosine kinases			
EGFR	35%–81%	Both	Correlates with stage; conflicting for survival
HER2/neu	10%–38%	Intestinal	Poor survival
PDGFA	42%–45%	Both	Correlates with stage and poor survival
c-*met*	34%–71%	Diffuse	Correlates with stage and peritoneal metastasis
Angiogenesis			
VEGF	—	Intestinal	Correlates with hepatic metastasis
NUDT6	—	Intestinal	Increased recurrence

APC = adenomatosis polyposis coli; *DCC* = deleted in colorectal carcinoma; *EGFR* = epidermal growth factor receptor; *FHIT* = fragile histidine triad; *MCC* = mutated in colorectal cancers; MSI = microsatellite instability; *NUDT6* = nudix-type motif 6; *PDGFA* = platelet-derived growth factor alpha polypeptide; *VEGF* = vascular endothelial growth factor.

cancer.[53,54] Histologically, most cancers in this syndrome have a poorly differentiated, infiltrative, and signet-ring cell histology. A mixed histology with an intestinal component has also been reported.[54]

Affected individuals inherit one copy of the defective E-cadherin gene. Somatic mutation, deletion, or promoter methylation inactivates the other copy. The cancer appears with an autosomal dominant pattern with high penetrance. Moreover, when prophylactic gastrectomy is performed, multifocal early gastric cancers are often found in the resected specimen.[42] Long-term experience with gastrectomy in asymptomatic carriers is lacking, however. Genetic counseling is recommended in suspected cases.

Familial Adenomatous Polyposis Germline mutations of the adenomatosis polyposis coli (*APC*) gene result in FAP. This disorder is inherited in an autonomic dominant pattern with high penetrance. Polyps in such cases frequently undergo malignant transformation. Although the colon is the most common site of polyp formation, gastric polyps occur in 27% to 70% of affected individuals.[55,56] Whereas fundic gastric polyps are usually thought to be hamartomas, foveolar dysplasia and invasive adenocarcinoma have been described by a number of investigators.[55,56]

Hereditary Nonpolyposis Colorectal Cancer HNPCC is a genetic disorder characterized by germline mutations in a group of mismatch repair genes, including mutS homolog 2 (*MSH2*), mutL homolog 1 (*MLH1*), mutS homolog 6 (*MSH6*), postmeiotic segregation increased 1 (*PMS1*), and postmeiotic segregation increased 2 (*PMS2*). Defects in these genes result in genomic instability characterized by microsatellite instability (MSI). Although colorectal and endometrial cancers are the most common manifestations of HNPCC, gastric carcinoma has also been observed. An analysis of the Korean Hereditary Tumor Registry showed a 3.2-fold increase in the relative risk of gastric cancer in families carrying the HNPCC mutation.[57] However, germline mutation of one of the mismatch repair genes accounts for only a small percentage of gastric cancers with MSI.

Li–Fraumeni Syndrome Li–Fraumeni syndrome is characterized by multiple primary malignancies. It is caused by mutations in the tumor protein 53 (*TP53*) tumor suppressor gene. Although gastric cancer has been observed as part of Li–Fraumeni syndrome, it does not significantly contribute to the overall number of cases of familial gastric cancer.[58]

Epigenetic Changes **Hypermethylation** Methylation of CpG islands in the CpG promoter region regulates the expression of various genes. Aberrant methylation of normally unmethylated promoters is now recognized as an alternative pathway for inactivation of various tumor suppressor and tumor-related genes. Promoter methylation of the E-cadherin, *MLH1*, and cyclin-dependent kinase inhibitor 2A (*CDKN2A*) genes has been observed in cases of gastric cancer. Hypermethylation may be involved in the early carcinogenesis of both intestinal-type and diffuse-type gastric cancer.

A defect in the mismatch repair gene *MLH1* has been linked with MSI. Several investigators have examined the relationship between hypermethylation of the *MLH1* gene promoter and MSI. In particular, Japanese investigators found hypermethylation of the *MLH1* promoter in 17 of 18 MSI-positive gastric cancer cases.[59] Furthermore, they observed hypermethylation in the surrounding nonneoplastic tissue in 71% of the cases. In addition, Brazilian investigators searched for mutations and hypermethylation of the *MHL1* gene in patients with MSI-positive gastric cancer.[60] They found bi-allelic *MLH1* promoter hypermethylation in all of the cases, but they did not detect any mutations in the *MLH1* gene.

Germline mutations of the E-cadherin gene lead to diffuse-type gastric cancer. Hypermethylation of the E-cadherin promoter is also commonly observed as an alternative pathway of gene inactivation.[61,62] Aberrant hypermethylation of other genes has also been detected in patients with gastric cancer. These genes include deleted in colorectal carcinoma (*DCC*), *CDKN2A*, O6-methylguanine-DNA methyltransferase, and runt-related transcription factor 3 (*RUNX3*).[63–65] Epigenetic changes resulting from CpG island hypermethylation may lead to development of the replication error (*RER*) phenotype, silencing of tumor suppressor genes, and altered cellular adhesion because of silencing of E-cadherin. These early changes may lead to further accumulation of mutations and progression of cancer.

Microsatellite Instability Microsatellites are monotonous tandem repeats found throughout the human genome. Germline mutations in DNA repair genes *MSH2*, *MLH1*, *MSH6*, *PMS1*, and *PMS2* lead to MSI and the hereditary HNPCC phenotype. Altered lengths of microsatellite markers are the hallmark of the *RER* phenotype; they have been described in a number of human malignancies, including gastric cancer.

Sporadic gastric cancers may be classified as microsatellite-stable, MSI low, or MSI high. The frequency of MSI (high and low) in gastric cancer has been reported to range from 31% to 39%.[66–68] MSI is likely to occur early in gastric carcinogenesis in patients with the *RER* phenotype, leading to inactivation of other tumor suppressor genes. Studies have found MSI in areas of intestinal metaplasia, dysplasia, and gastric adenoma in patients with gastric cancer.[69,70] Also, several presumed downstream mutations have been associated with MSI. Specifically, mutations in the transforming growth factor-β2 gene have been observed in a large percentage of gastric tumors with MSI.[71,72]

Several investigator have reported that MSI is associated with an intestinal histology.[67,70] Also, MSI has been associated with distal gastric cancer.[70] At the present time, whether the MSI status affects outcome in patients with gastric cancer is not clear.

Tumor Suppressor Genes ***TP53*** *TP53*, which is located on chromosome 17q, is a key tumor suppressor gene. Germline mutations of *TP53* lead to multiple malignancies at a high frequency. *TP53* regulates cell replication and apoptosis. Wild-type *TP53* is usually not detected with the use of immunohistochemical techniques. However, mutants are more stable than wild-type *TP53*, accumulate in the nucleus, and lead to so-called *TP53* overexpression, which commonly occurs in gastric cancer.

Studied according to loss of heterozygosity (LOH), allelic deletions involving the *TP53* locus have been detected in up to 64% of gastric cancer cases.[66] Furthermore, studies have shown other *TP53* abnormalities to be involved in 47% to 74% of gastric cancer cases.[66,73]

There are distinct differences in the pattern of *TP53* involvement in the two major types of gastric cancer. Some authors have found mutation of *TP53* to be an early event in the development of intestinal-type gastric cancer not correlated with stage progression.[73,74] With the use of immunohistochemical techniques, mutation of this gene has been detected in 46% to 50% of cases of T1 intestinal-type gastric cancer. *TP53* abnormalities have also been detected in areas of high-grade dysplasia (but not metaplasia).[74] In diffuse-type gastric cancer, mutation of *TP53* is less common in T1 tumors: it has been found in 10% to 20% of cases of early-stage disease.[73,74] However, *TP53* is associated with stage progression in diffuse-type gastric cancer. In one previous study, a *TP53* abnormality was detected in 17% of cases of T1 diffuse-type gastric cancer, but in 50% of cases of T2 or higher disease.[73]

***APC* and Mutated in Colorectal Cancers** The *APC* and mutated in colorectal cancers (*MCC*) genes are both located on chromosome 5q21. Deletion and somatic mutation of the *APC* gene have been described in 8% to 34% of gastric cancer cases.[66,73,75,76] Differences in the frequency of *APC* mutation may vary by histology. Several investigators have reported that mutation of *APC* is more common in well and moderately differentiated cases of intestinal-type gastric cancer.[73,76] Others have failed to observe a difference in frequency by histology.

LOH of the *MCC* locus has been described in two studies. In one, LOH was observed in 33% of the cases without regard to histology.[66] In the other, LOH was present in only 24% of the undifferentiated cases and none of the differentiated cases.[76] The effect of *APC* and *MCC* mutations on clinical outcome remains poorly understood.

DCC The *DCC* gene, which is located on chromosome 18q21, was initially found to correlate with colon cancer progression and metastasis. It has become clear that this gene is also frequently involved in gastric cancer. Methods of *DCC* inactivation include allelic deletion in addition to promoter hypermethylation.[63,73,77] Overall, studies have found loss of *DCC* expression in 12% to 49% of gastric cancer cases.[73,77,78] Two of these studies found *DCC* involvement to be significantly more common in advanced intestinal-type gastric cancer.[73,78] Furthermore, Wu and colleagues[73] examined LOH at the *DCC* locus in gastric cancer cases. Separating cases by histology and stage, they found LOH in none of the T1 cases, 4% of the advanced diffuse-type cases, and 32% of the advanced intestinal-type cases.

Fragile Histidine Triad The fragile histidine triad (*FHIT*) gene is located in a constitutively fragile region of chromosome 3p14. It encodes for a protein with diadenosine triphosphate hydrolase activity. Various techniques have been used to study abnormalities of the *FHIT* gene in gastric cancer, including immunohistochemical, Southern blot, polymerase chain reaction, LOH, and MSI analyses. Mutation and loss of expression of the *FHIT* gene have been described in multiple gastric cancer cell lines.[79] Immunohistochemical analyses of human gastric cancer have shown loss of *FHIT* expression in about half of cases, with reduced expression shown in additional cases.[79–81] Also, LOH analysis has detected deletion of the *FHIT* gene in 16% to 46% of cases.[79,81,82] In one study, LOH of the *FHIT* gene correlated with MSI within the gene, suggesting that a defect in mismatch repair may have resulted in *FHIT* inactivation.[81] In a study involving 55 patients, the investigators found that patients with loss of *FHIT* expression had a higher disease stage, a higher histological grade, and a shorter survival duration as compared with patients retaining *FHIT* expression.[80] However, multivariate analyses were not carried out, and the findings were not confirmed by other investigators.[81,82] Larger studies will be needed to determine the effect of *FHIT* expression on clinical outcome.

RUNX3 *RUNX3* is a recently discovered putative tumor suppressor gene involved in gastric carcinogenesis. This gene is normally expressed in gastric epithelia. In experimental animal models, *RUNX3* knockout mice have been shown to exhibit gastric epithelial hyperplasia with suppression of apoptosis.[65] Examination of human gastric cancer cell lines and tissue has uncovered frequent silencing of *RUNX3* expression by hypermethylation and mutations. Further investigations into the role of *RUNX3* in gastric carcinogenesis are under way.

Cellular Adhesion Loss of normal cellular adhesion is an important feature of human cancer development. Specifically, metastasis is characterized by loss of adhesion that allows cancer cells to invade and leave the site of origin and subsequently to adhere to other sites, such as lymph nodes, the liver, and the peritoneum. Diffuse-type gastric cancer is characterized by aberrant cellular adhesion with a pattern of infiltrative growth by a small cluster of tumor cells (or sometimes a single cell). In conjunction with catenins, the cadherins play a critical role in cell adhesion and polarity.[83] Up to 90% of gastric cancer cases have an abnormality in at least one component of the cadherin–catenin complex.[84]

E-Cadherin E-Cadherin, which is encoded by the *CDH1* gene, is the major cadherin in epithelial cells. Recently, a defect in E-cadherin was recognized as an important feature of diffuse-type gastric cancer. Immunohistochemical analyses have found abnormal E-cadherin staining in more than half of cases of sporadic diffuse-type gastric cancer.[84,85] Examination of nonneoplastic stomach found normal expression in areas of gastritis, intestinal metaplasia, and atrophy.

Using polymerase chain reaction and LOH analyses, investigators found mutations of the E-cadherin gene in approximately 50% of diffuse gastric cancer cases.[86] Others found E-cadherin mutations in 14% of cases of mixed-type gastric cancer.[87] In contrast, they detected only silent mutations in cases of intestinal-type gastric cancer.

Promoter hypermethylation is an alternative pathway of inactivation for E-cadherin.[61,62] Overall, E-cadherin promoter hypermethylation was observed in about half of gastric cancer cases. However, 83% of cases with the diffuse histology had hypermethylation of the E-cadherin promoter. Those results led us to speculate that simultaneous sequencing, LOH, and methylation analyses in a single group of patients with diffuse-type gastric cancer would find E-cadherin abnormalities in most cases.

Catenins When interacting with the cytoplasmic domain of E-cadherin, the α-, β-, and γ-catenin complexes bind the intracellular domain of E-cadherin to actin filaments to maintain cellular adhesion. As with E-cadherin, abnormal expression of α- and γ-catenin is associated with diffuse-type gastric cancer.[85] Immunohistochemical studies have shown abnormal expression of α- and γ-catenin in 83% to 92% and 91% to 100% of diffuse-type gastric cancer cases respectively.[84,85]

In addition, β-catenin interacts with the product of the *APC* gene. Although the expression of β-catenin did not correlate with histology in some studies,[84,88] one group of investigators reported that mutations in the glycogen synthase kinase 3β (*GSK3B*) gene correlated with intestinal histology.[89] In addition, reduction in the membranous expression of β-catenin is associated with poor survival.[84,88]

CD44 The CD44 antigen is a transmembrane glycoprotein involved in cellular adhesion. It has several splice variants that may modulate invasion and metastasis. Silencing of *CD44* by promoter hypermethylation has been reported in human gastric carcinoma cell lines.[90] In animal models, transforming growth factor-β1 has been shown to increase expression of the *CD44*H isoform in patients with diffuse-type gastric cancer, allowing for increased adhesion to mesothelial cells and increased potential for peritoneal metastasis.[49]

The reported frequency of *CD44* expression in human gastric cancer specimens varies widely, ranging from 31% to 72%, which likely reflects differences within the study populations.[91,92] The intensity of *CD44* expression has been found to correlate with the depth of invasion.[91] Specifically, in patients with stage II or IIIa gastric cancer, *CD44* expression correlated with an inferior 5-year survival rate (43% versus 63%; $p = .002$).

Multiple investigators have examined the significance of the *CD44*v6 isoform in gastric cancer. They observed that *CD44*v6 is associated with the intestinal histology.[93–95] Using immunohistochemical techniques, they found that *CD44*v6 was positive in 67% to 92% of cases with the intestinal histology and 17% to 48% of cases with the diffuse histology. Investigators have also reported that *CD44*v6 expression is associated with increased depth of invasion, nodal involvement, and metastasis.[94,95] Among patients with intestinal-type gastric cancer, *CD44*v6 has also been reported to predict inferior survival.[95] However, although the observation about survival was confirmed by other investigators, multivariate survival analysis of this isoform has not been performed.

Tyrosine Kinases **Epidermal Growth Factor Receptor** Epidermal growth factor receptor (*EGFR*) is a transmembrane tyrosine kinase receptor that has been implicated in the pathophysiology of a number of malignancies. It has been reported to be expressed in 35% to 81% of gastric cancer cases.[96,97] Gene amplification has been detected in 9% of gastric cancer cases.[50] *EGFR* does not appear to be associated with any particular histology.[96]

EGFR has been associated with increased depth of invasion in resected gastric cancer specimens.[98] Also, some investigators have reported inferior survival rates in *EGFR*-positive cases.[50] However, these poorer survival rates were not confirmed by other studies. With the recent development of antibodies and small-molecule inhibitors, interest in combining chemotherapy with *EGFR* inhibition has increased.

Erythroblastic Leukemia Viral Oncogene Homolog 2 The erythroblastic leukemia viral oncogene homolog 2 (*HER2/neu* or *ERBB2*) is an oncogene that belongs to the *ERBB* family of membrane tyrosine kinase receptors. It is located on chromosome 17q21 and produces a 185-kDa transmembrane glycoprotein. It forms homodimers and heterodimers with other members of the *ERBB* family, resulting in tyrosine phosphorylation. Amplification of *HER2/neu* has been identified in patients with gastric cancer. Using immunohistochemical, Southern blot, and fluorescence in situ hybridization analyses, investigators have reported *HER2/neu* overexpression in 10% to 38% of gastric cancer cases.[73,96,97] However, the subtypes of gastric cancer have some differences. When grouped by the Lauren histology, *HER2/neu* is more common in cases of intestinal-type gastric cancer (14% to 49%) than in cases of diffuse-type disease (0% to 19%).[73,96] When grouped by primary tumor location in one study, *HER2/neu* overexpression was not found in proximal gastric cancer cases, but was found in 10% of distal gastric cancer cases.

Several investigators have examined the effect of *HER2/neu* status on clinical outcome. When compared with patients with *HER2/neu*-negative tumors, those with *HER2/neu*-positive tumors had a more advanced stage and a higher histologic grade.[96,97,99] In three studies, the median survival duration in patients with *HER2/neu*-positive gastric cancer was half that in patients with *HER2/neu*-negative disease.[96,100]

Platelet-Derived Growth Factor Receptor Platelet-derived growth factor (PDGF) has an α and a β subunit. It thus can form homodimers and heterodimers and activate corresponding PDGF receptor α and β. PDGF may affect an autocrine–paracrine loop that drives proliferation and inhibits apoptosis and may augment angiogenesis by interacting with the stroma. Expression of *PDGFA* has been found in about half of all gastric cancer cases.[101,102] In one study, *PDGFA* expression correlated with nodal involvement in patients with early-stage gastric cancer and with inferior survival in patients with T2 or higher disease.[101] In a subsequent multivariate analysis, *PDGFA* expression was found to be the most reliable molecular predictor of survival in patients with resected gastric cancer.[102]

c-*met* The proto-oncogene c-*met* is the receptor for hepatocyte growth factor. Overexpression of c-*met* has been reported in 34% to 71% of gastric cancer cases.[51,73,103] One study found DNA amplification of the c-*met* gene in 10% of gastric cancer cases. Overexpression of c-*met* is associated with the diffuse histology, an advanced stage, and an infiltrative growth pattern.[50,51,73,103] Investigators have also described an increased tendency toward peritoneal metastasis in patients with c-*met* amplification.[50,51]

Angiogenesis Some data suggest that angiogenesis is essential for the growth of solid tumors. Tumor angiogenesis is governed by a number of proangiogenic and antiangiogenic factors. Recent advances have led to an improved understanding of the mechanism of tumor angiogenesis and to development of antiangiogenesis therapy. Increased angiogenesis in gastric cancer portends an unfavorable prognosis in patients with gastric cancer.[45] *VEGF* and nudix-type motif 6 (*NUDT6*, which used to be called basic fibroblast growth factor) are major regulators of angiogenesis, have prognostic value, and are targets for antiangiogenic therapy in patients with gastric cancer.

VEGF Studies of resected gastric cancer specimens have shown that the level of *VEGF* expression correlates with tumor microvessel density.[45,46] Increased expression of *VEGF* has been linked with increased rates of invasion, metastasis, and disease recurrence.[45,104,105] Also, *VEGFC* expression is involved in the neogenesis of lymphatic vessels. In particular, studies of gastric cancer have linked *VEGFC* expression with increased rates of lymph-node metastasis.[47,48] Furthermore, circulating *VEGF* levels in the blood may predict outcome in patients undergoing surgical resection of gastric cancer.[106]

VEGF expression and tumor vascularity have also been linked with the histology and patterns of metastasis of gastric cancer. In one study, expression of *VEGF* and its receptor *KDR* was observed more frequently in intestinal-type gastric cancer than in diffuse-type disease.[45] Furthermore, primary tumors in patients with synchronous hepatic metastases showed higher vessel counts and *VEGF* expression levels than did tumors in patients with synchronous peritoneal metastases. Similarly, *VEGF* expression has been linked with hepatic relapse of gastric cancer following resection.[46]

NUDT6 *NUDT6* and its receptors are expressed in gastric tumors.[45,107] Also, circulating *NUDT6* can be detected in the blood. When a group of researchers separated gastric cancer cases by histology, they found that *NUDT6*expression was stronger in the intestinal-type cases than in the diffuse-type cases.[45] Groups have also studied the effect of *NUDT6* expression on the sites of gastric cancer metastasis. In one such study, *NUDT6* expression was associated with an increased rate of cancer recurrence after surgery.[107] No significant differences in microvessel density or sites of metastasis were associated with *NUDT6* expression in the study by Takahashi et al.[45]

Transcription Factors Clearly, gastric cancer cells can express multiple growth factors and growth factor receptors. The result is potentially redundant signal transduction pathways. *SP1* is a transcription factor for many genes that regulate multiple aspects of tumor-cell survival, growth, and angiogenesis. We recently reported abnormal expression of *SP1* in cases of human gastric cancer.[108] On the molecular level, the degree of *VEGF* expression correlated highly with *SP1* expression. Clinically, higher *SP1* expression was associated with higher disease stages and nodal involvement. Furthermore, in multivariate analyses, *SP1* expression was superior to *VEGF* expression as a predictor of outcome after gastrectomy.[108]

PATHOLOGICAL AND CLINICAL STAGING

The most widely used staging system for gastric cancer is the American Joint Committee on Cancer (AJCC)/L'Union internationale contre le cancer (UICC) system, which follows a standardized evaluation of the primary tumor (T), regional lymph nodes (N), and distant metastatic disease (M).[109] It is based on an earlier, well-described Japanese system. Table 86-4 shows the current AJCC/UICC system, as revised in 1997. Figure 86-3 shows the correlation between disease stage and survival in a large review of the National Cancer Data Base by Huyndahl and colleagues.[34]1 It also underscores the extremely poor overall survival of gastric cancer in the United States.

In the AJCC/UICC system, the T stage is categorized into one of four levels based on the depth of tumor penetration into the wall of the stomach. T1 tumors are the most superficial, with involvement only as deep as the submucosa. (The Japanese system further separates this group, with the main importance of the separation being to determine which tumors are amenable to endo-

Table 86-4 American Joint Committee on Cancer/L'Union Internationale Contre le Cancer Stage Grouping for Gastric Cancer

	Nodal Stage			
T Stage	N0	N1	N2	N3
T1	Ia	Ib	II	IV
T2a/b	Ib	II	IIIa	IV
T3	II	IIIa	IIIb	IV
T4	IIIa	IIIb	IV	IV

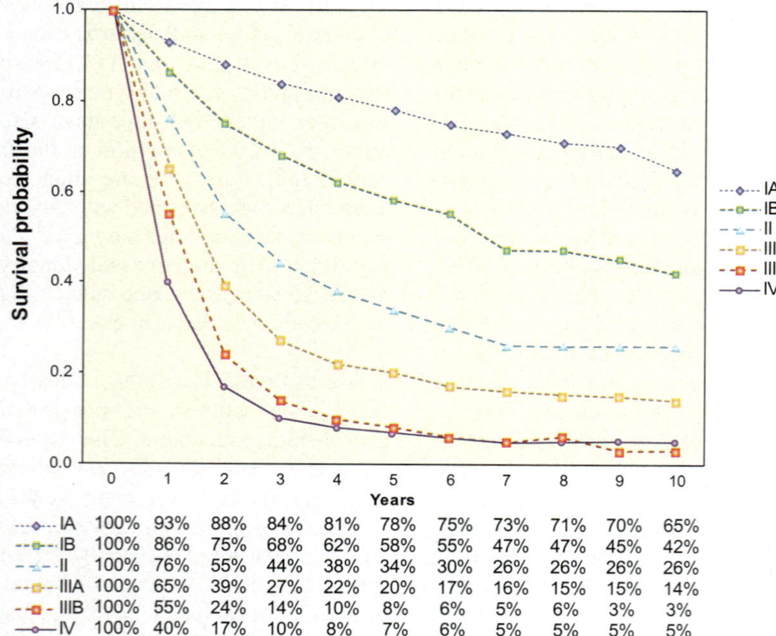

Stage	0	1	2	3	4	5	6	7	8	9	10
IA	100%	93%	88%	84%	81%	78%	75%	73%	71%	70%	65%
IB	100%	86%	75%	68%	62%	58%	55%	47%	47%	45%	42%
II	100%	76%	55%	44%	38%	34%	30%	26%	26%	26%	26%
IIIA	100%	65%	39%	27%	22%	20%	17%	16%	15%	15%	14%
IIIB	100%	55%	24%	14%	10%	8%	6%	5%	6%	3%	3%
IV	100%	40%	17%	10%	8%	7%	6%	5%	5%	5%	5%

Figure 86-3 One-year through 10-year survival rates of patients with gastric cancer after gastrectomy. Adapted from Hundahl and colleagues.[34]

scopic mucosal resection.) T2 tumors invade into the muscularis propria, and T3 tumors invade through the serosa. In the only significant change from the prior staging system, T2 tumors are classified as T2a (invasion of the muscularis propria) or T2b (invasion into the subserosa) tumors, but these additional classifications do not change the stage groupings. Various degrees of serosal involvement are also assessed in the Japanese system, and they have some correlation with the risk of failure in the peritoneal cavity. Finally, T4 tumors directly invade adjacent organs.

The most recent AJCC/UICC staging system reflects the importance of the number of lymph nodes retrieved, resected, and evaluated in a specimen. The more nodes evaluated, the more accurate the staging. However, it is imperative that at least 15 lymph nodes be examined. Nodal staging is divided into four groups:

N0: no positive nodes
N1: 1 to 6 positive lymph nodes with tumor
N2: 7 to 15 positive lymph nodes with tumor
N3: more than 15 positive lymph nodes with tumor

Notably, all patients with N3 disease are classified as having stage IV disease.

The Japanese system on which the previous AJCC/UICC system was based defined nodal stage by anatomic location and proximity to the primary tumor. Although proximity to the primary tumor is not of real prognostic value for nodal staging, the Japanese system of 16 nodal stations does have some value. That system is divided into six perigastric stations (right and left cardia, lesser and greater curvatures, supra- and infrapyloric) and five stations along the named celiac vessels (celiac, hepatic, left gastric, splenic, and hilum of the spleen). Dissecting and sending these specimens separately may increase the total yield of nodes recovered simply by heightening the awareness of the pathologist regarding the task at hand.

To appropriately stage gastric cancer, several clinical procedures should be performed in a stepwise fashion. The steps are physical examination, laboratory studies, computed tomography (CT), endoscopic ultrasound (EUS), and laparoscopy. The role of positron emission tomography for gastric cancer is still evolving; the results of this procedure that we have seen have been mixed.

Physical examination should be directed toward detecting evidence of muscle wasting (particularly around the temples) and spread of the cancer. Palpation for adenopathy in the supraclavicular fossa (Virchow's node), periumbilical area (Sister Mary Joseph's nodule), and the left axilla (Irish's node) is essential.[110] The abdomen is palpated for masses and examined for ascites. Also, a digital rectal exam is performed to assess masses or a Blumer's shelf and to test for the presence of blood.

Laboratory studies include a complete blood count; electrolyte, blood urea nitrogen, and creatinine measurements; and liver function tests (lactate dehydrogenase, alkaline phosphatase, at least one transaminase, and bilirubin). Evaluation of tumor markers such as carcinoembryonic antigen, sialylated Lewis blood group carbohydrate antigen, and cancer antigen 125 may be considered.

CT scanning of the abdomen and pelvis (and the chest for proximal lesions) is performed to detect evidence of the primary tumor (linitis plastica will often have a distinctive appearance, although it must not be confused with a stomach that has not distended), liver metastases, ascites, peritoneal nodules, and nodal metastases beyond the area or areas of resection. EUS is reasonably accurate in assessing the T stage of a tumor and has an accuracy rate slightly better than 50% in evaluating nodal status. It is unusual for an endoscopist to comment on more than a few nodes at the time of EUS. Although the ability to perform needle biopsy analysis of a node endoscopically can be helpful, nodal status can be determined accurately only by pathology assessment of a resected specimen. We believe that EUS should be considered for two purposes: (1) full staging and evaluation of patients entering neoadjuvant therapy trials and (2) assessment of early-stage lesions that might be amenable to endoscopic mucosal resection. A neoadjuvant approach may provide a baseline to aid in the assessment of tumor response, although sonography cannot differentiate between tumor and scar tissue.[111]

Laparoscopy is essential for complete staging of all cases of gastric cancer, with the exception of sonographically detected T1 lesions with a moderately differentiated or well-differentiated histology. Laparoscopy for gastric cancer was first described in 1984. Since then, multiple studies have demonstrated the benefits of laparoscopy in conjunction with other staging modalities for otherwise potentially resectable gastric cancer. In one-fifth to one-fourth of patients, laparoscopy results in upstaging, primarily because of detection of peritoneal metastases not seen on CT scans.[111–113] The detection rate by laparoscopy of liver metastases not seen on high-quality CT scans should be less than 5%.[112] Another benefit of laparoscopy is that, at the time of staging, a feeding jejunostomy tube can be placed with minimal morbidity for nutritional support during neoadjuvant therapy if ascites is identified. However, placing a feeding jejunostomy tube should be carefully weighed against the potential risks. Burke and colleagues[113] demonstrated the cost-effectiveness of laparoscopy.

THERAPY FOR LOCOREGIONAL DISEASE

Endoscopic Mucosal Resection Because gastrectomy can have significant complications and long-term sequelae, and because many patients with very early-stage gastric cancer can expect to have close to a normal life expectancy, better methods of managing the disease have been sought.

In Japan, where nearly half of diagnosed patients have early-stage gastric cancer (owing to significant screening efforts), surgeons have begun to explore the possibility of endoscopically removing early-stage cancers that have little likelihood of nodal involvement. The polyp removal techniques developed for patients with colon cancer provided the rationale for this approach. Fortunately, the wall of the stomach is significantly thicker than that of the colon; excision of mucosa is safer, and the chance of perforation is reduced. Overall, the incidence of nodal positivity with T1 tumors is approximately 10%. However, in this overall favorable prognosis group, numerous features of the primary tumor can help to identify patients who have an extremely low likelihood of nodal metastases and who are thus good candidates for endoscopic resection.

The first of the identifying features is a tumor confined to the mucosa; if a tumor has invaded the submucosa, the incidence of nodal positivity increases to roughly 15% from 1% to 3%.[114] Patients with a Borrmann's classification of the primary tumor (types 1 to 5), with poorly differentiated or signet-ring cell tumors, with evidence of lymphatic invasion, or with a tumor larger in size than 2 cm, and female patients are far more likely than other patients to harbor nodal disease.[115] Thus, patients whose T1 tumor as determined EUS is well-differentiated or has a Borrmann's classification of type I, IIa, or IIb have a very low chance of nodal disease.

In Japan, with its aggressive screening programs, endoscopic resection has gained widespread acceptance for tumors with a low histologic grade.[116] In this technique, the specimen is carefully analyzed: if penetration into the submucosa is identified, the patient undergoes gastrectomy. In a series of 445 patients with 479 cancers at the National Cancer Center Hospital in Tokyo, Ono and colleagues[117] had a great deal of success with endoscopic mucosal resection. They performed the procedure for tumors up to 3 cm in diameter and for depressed but not ulcerated tumors. They found submucosal extension in 74 tumors (15.4%), which was an indication for a more formal resection. They performed a clear resection of 278 (68.6%) of 405 intramucosal tumors. Most importantly, this study had a relatively short follow-up time for patients with early-stage disease, but none of the patients had died of gastric cancer after a median follow-up of 38 months. The major problem with this approach in the United States is a lack of patients who are legitimate candidates for endoscopic mucosal resection. Thus, few endoscopists develop the requisite skills and experience for performing the technique.

An alternative for patients with early-stage tumors with favorable prognostic features is a laparoscopic wedge excision. This procedure was first described in 1994. Since then, several authors have expanded laparoscopic surgery to include formal total gastrectomy.[118,119] Limited procedures can be considered when the risk of nodal metastasis is low; however, the precise role of such procedures in the comprehensive management of gastric cancer is still evolving. The application of laparoscopic gastrectomy is increasing. While its role evolves, the adequacy of nodal dissection in such procedures will remain an important issue.[120]

Surgical Considerations Several factors must be considered when contemplating surgical resection, including organ system function (pulmonary, cardiac, hepatic, and renal) and general performance status. Some patients are so frail or debilitated that surgical resection cannot be considered, because they likely would not recover from the procedure. Patients with evidence of cirrhosis have an increased risk of surgical morbidity and mortality, although a few reports have been published concerning small numbers of patients with even Child class C cirrhosis who have undergone resection. In a study by Isozaki and colleagues,[121] the mortality rate was 10% in cirrhotic patients who underwent gastrectomy and 16% in patients who underwent a D2 dissection, which is significant in a nation such as Japan, where the operative mortality rate for gastrectomy is routinely well under 5%.

The indications for resection of gastric cancer must be carefully considered whether the intervention is being considered for potential cure or for palliation. When palliative resection is being considered, the degree of the patient's symptoms must be very explicitly reviewed. A patient with a true obstruction likely needs operative palliation, but the ability of most patients (≥ 80%) to eat will improve with the use of chemotherapy.[122] Thus, obstruction is a relative, rather than an absolute, indication. Obviously, patients with significant bleeding should at least be considered for palliative resection. These considerations must be kept in mind before the patient is taken to the operating room, because intraoperative findings may change the intent of the planned operation. Awareness that the surgical mortality rate can be quite high with palliative resection is important.[123] Palliative bypass also carries a very high mortality rate and frequently fails to achieve the desired benefit.[123,124] Palliative care in such patients is discussed more thoroughly near the end of this chapter.

Factors to be considered in planning the surgical management of gastric cancer include the type of operation to be performed, the method of reconstruction, and any previous procedures a patient may have undergone. Patients whose stomach is dilated because of outlet obstruction (and who are thus likely candidates for a subtotal gastrectomy) generally should be brought into the hospital 2 to 3 days before a planned resection so that nasogastric (NG) tube suctioning to decompress the stomach can be carried out.[125] That maneuver, and the leaving of a relatively small gastric pouch, will minimize the possibility of delayed postoperative gastric emptying in such patients. Patients who do not have an obstruction generally undergo a bowel prep the day before surgery. That procedure can almost always be accomplished on an outpatient basis.

Surgical Controversies The major surgical issues that have been studied (with varying degrees of success) include (1) the extent of luminal resection, (2) the extent of lymph node dissection, (3) the role of splenectomy, and (4) the method of reconstruction.

The choice of operation for gastric cancer depends on tumor location, histologic type, and disease stage. Gastrectomy is the most widely used approach for the treatment of invasive gastric cancer, and it offers the greatest likelihood of long-term survival. The choices for gastric resection include segmental resection and distal subtotal, total, and proximal subtotal gastrectomy. The gastric and nodal dissection types may both be limited, or they may both be quite extensive, depending on the surgeon's biases and level of experience, the location of the tumor, and the pathologic features of the tumor.

Extent of Luminal Resection Prospective and randomized studies have revealed no survival advantage for total gastrectomy over distal subtotal gastrectomy for tumors of the distal stomach when all of the disease can be removed with adequate margins.[126,127] In particular, Gouzi and colleagues[127] conducted a prospective randomized trial of total versus subtotal gastrectomy in 169 patients with adenocarcinoma of the gastric antrum who underwent resection with curative intent. The postoperative mortality rate was 1.3% for total gastrectomy and 3.2% for subtotal gastrectomy. The complication and 5-year survival rates in the two groups did not differ significantly. The Italian Gastrointestinal Tumor Study Group conducted a similar prospective randomized trial and found 5-year survival rates of 65% and 62% in the subtotal and total gastrectomy groups, respectively.[126]

In most series, the quality of life after a subtotal gastrectomy is superior to that after a total gastrectomy; subtotal gastrectomy should therefore be performed when an adequate margin can be obtained in concert with a reasonably sized gastric remnant.[128,129] Maintaining an adequate blood supply to the remaining stomach should also be a concern. Thus, subtotal gastrectomy with splenectomy can truly be performed safely only with maintenance of the left gastric artery. This maneuver obviously affects the ability to achieve a meaningful nodal dissection. Our technique in performing this operation is described below.

Tumors of the proximal stomach and the GE junction require significantly different considerations for resection and reconstruction. The three types of GE junction tumors described by Professor Siewert from Munich, Germany, constitute the Siewert classification[130,131]:

- Type I: a tumor associated with Barrett's esophagus or a true esophageal carcinoma growing down to the GE junction
- Type II: a tumor at the true GE junction (within 2 cm of the squamocolumnar junction)
- Type III: a tumor at the subcardial region

In patients with an advanced tumor involving the GE junction, the site of origin of the tumor may be unclear. Patients with type I tumors should almost never be considered for a purely transabdominal approach. They are best considered for either a gastric pull-up to the neck (with the stomach, jejunum, or colon) or an Ivor–Lewis procedure. The section on cancer of the esophagus contains a description of and considerations for that procedure.

Type II and III tumors can be treated with either a total gastrectomy or a proximal subtotal gastrectomy (transabdominally, as an Ivor–Lewis procedure, or through a left thoracoabdominal incision [although we try to avoid that approach]), depending on the local extent of the tumor.[132,133] For lesions that do not invade a significant portion of the esophagus, a total gastrectomy may be the more appropriate operation. The two main reasons are that (1) reflux esophagitis is extremely rare after a Roux-en-Y reconstruction (as opposed to the roughly one-third of patients who experience significant reflux after proximal subtotal resection),[128,134,135] and (2) proximal subtotal gastrectomy may fail to fully remove the lymph nodes along the entire lesser curvature, which is the most common site of nodal metastasis. However, not all authors agree that total gastrectomy offers fewer quality-of-life problems than proximal subtotal gastrectomy does, and they therefore champion the latter approach.[133]

For patients whose gastric cancer is associated with Barrett's esophagus, the appropriate operation usually requires removal of more of the esophagus than can be safely achieved abdominally. The relative merits of the Ivor–Lewis procedure and the gastric pull-up to the neck are beyond the scope of this chapter, but the morbidity of an anastomotic leak in the chest is clearly far greater than that of a leak in the neck, even though the risk of a leak is greater with the pull-up procedure.

For poorly differentiated tumors, the general recommendation is to resect a wider margin. Some surgeons have advocated the use of total esophagogastrectomy with colonic interposition for advanced tumors of the GE junction.[136] As may be expected, this operation can carry a significant morbidity and mortality risk. It should therefore be considered under only the most extenuating circumstances. Considerations may include previous surgery or other conditions rendering the stomach unsuitable for reconstruction. In some circumstances, the jejunum can be brought up as high as the carina (without the need for a vascular anastomosis) or neck with supercharging from the carotid and jugular vessels.

Nodal Dissection The extent of lymph node dissection remains the most controversial concern in the surgical management of gastric cancer. Surgeons in Japan, and those in other countries, have for years advocated the use of radical lymph node dissection. That approach often includes removal of periaortic lymph nodes. Over the past decade or so, several investigators have attempted to better define, for a given extent of disease, how radical a dissection should be performed. To that end, they have used both randomized trials, which are discussed below, and a more careful evaluation of the likelihood that a tumor will spread to specific nodal areas.[137,138]

The extent of lymph node dissection is defined by the designation "D." A D1 dissection includes just the perigastric lymph nodes. A classic D2 dissection also includes nodes along the hepatic, left gastric, celiac, and splenic arteries, as well as those in the splenic hilum. A D3 dissection includes nodes along the porta hepatis and in the retropancreatic and periaortic regions.

To more accurately evaluate surgical specimens, the Japanese Research Society for Gastric Cancer created a classification system that divides the draining lymph basins into 16 stations consisting of 6 perigastric stations and 10 stations along the adjacent major vessels, in the splenic hilum, behind the pancreas, and along the aorta. The node content in these nodal stations was elucidated in a study by Wagner and colleagues,[139] who carefully dissected cadavers and assessed each station. They found tremendous variation in the number of nodes recovered from each station, and they observed that the lesser curvature was the only area in which nodes were recovered in every patient.

The number of nodes recovered is affected not only by natural variation among patients and the surgical technique used, but also by the rigor with which the pathologist examines the specimen. Use of a fat-clearing technique can double the number of nodes recovered, which can clearly alter the pathology assessment as a result.[140]

The impact of a lack of staging information was perhaps best demonstrated in the National Cancer Center Data Base study in 1985 by Lawrence and colleagues[141] They found that more than half of patients lacked a stage determination. By 1991, the number of patients had decreased, but nearly one of every four patients still lacked a stage designation.

Retrospective studies from Japan have suggested that extended lymphadenectomy can improve survival, particularly in patients with stage II or III tumors, and can do so with a perioperative mortality rate of 1%.[142] In comparison, the German Gastric Carcinoma Study Group conducted a prospective nonrandomized study of node dissections.[143] In that study, most of the patients were designated to undergo a D2 dissection. However, a significant number of patients were designated to undergo a D1 dissection primarily based on the number of nodes recovered. The study protocol defined a radical dissection as one containing 27 or more nodes in the specimen. In comparing patients who underwent R0 (potentially curative) resections and examination of at least 15 nodes, patients with stage II or IIIA disease had a significant survival advantage. Clearly, based on the percentage of patients with each stage of disease, stage migration may be at least partially responsible for the perceived benefits D2 dissection.

Five prospective randomized trials have examined the extent of lymph node dissection in patients with gastric cancer. In the trial by Dent and colleagues,[144] patients were randomized to undergo a D1 or D2 dissection. The authors evaluated more than 400 patients, but found only 43 who were intraoperative candidates for the study. They found no difference in survival, yet the operative time, blood loss, and hospital stay were all greater in the D2 dissection group. The operative mortality rate was similar in the two groups.

Two large prospective randomized trials of D1 versus D2 dissection in Western patients were also completed and reported.[35,145,146] In the Dutch trial, surgeons who served as reference surgeons for the study were trained in the technique of radical lymph node dissection by a highly experienced senior Japanese surgeon. The surgical quality control in the study was carefully scrutinized. More than 1000 patients were enrolled, 711 of whom underwent an R0 resection, thus making them eligible for evaluation. The operative morbidity and mortality rates were both significantly greater in the D2 group than in the D1 group (43% and 10% versus 25% and 4%, respectively; $p < .01$). The trial failed to show a benefit of extended lymph node dissection over a follow-up duration of more than 10 years. However, a careful review of the data from this study revealed that the increase in the mortality rate was associated either with male patients undergoing D2 dissection or with patients undergoing splenectomy and distal pancreatectomy for complete nodal dissection. Patients who underwent a D2 dissection with preservation of the spleen and tail of the pancreas had a risk of operative mortality quite similar to that of patients who underwent a D1 dissection with preservation of the spleen. However, at 5 years, the rate of recurrence was lower in patients who underwent a D2 dissection than in those who underwent a D1 dissection (37% versus 43%). In the final report of this trial, subset analysis showed that patients with N2 disease fared better with a D2 dissection than with a D1 dissection.

The design of the Dutch trial was based on the assumption that lymph node dissection would increase the survival rate from 20% to 32%. Unexpectedly, 40% of the patients were found to have early-stage gastric cancer. In addition, the investigators may have overestimated the potential benefit of extended lymph node dissection.

The anticipated benefit of extended lymph node dissection may be determined by multiplying the frequency of lymph node metastasis at certain sites by the survival rate of patients with known metastases at those sites. In such a study, Sasako and colleagues[138] found that the incidence of splenic hilar lymph node metastasis was roughly 10% and that the survival rate was 10% in patients with metastasis-positive nodes in that site. Therefore, the potential increase in survival rate with removal of those nodes is only 1%. In patients with metastasis-positive lymph nodes along the common hepatic, celiac, and left gastric sites, the numbers are higher. Specifically, the overall increase in survival rate with extended lymph node dissection may be 5% to 8%, which is less than the additional mortality seen with the use of splenectomy and distal pancreatectomy to achieve D2 dissection in both this trial and one performed by the Medical Research Council (MRC).

The MRC trial examined 200 patients per arm (among 737 registered patients) randomized to undergo D1 or D2 dissection.[146] Thirty-two surgeons participated in the study, which took 7 years to complete. Distal pancreatectomy and splenectomy were liberally applied to achieve D2 dissection. The operative mortality rate was 13% in the D2 group and 7% in the D1 group. The researchers found no survival advantage of the more aggressive procedure. As in the Dutch trial described earlier, the MRC trial found that the increase in the morbidity and mortality rates associated with D2 dissection were almost entirely attributable to the use of splenectomy and distal pancreatectomy. Japanese physicians have routinely used splenectomy to achieve complete nodal dissection and have not discerned any increase in morbidity with the procedure. A large prospective randomized trial in Japan is currently addressing this issue.

Two studies of more aggressive dissections have compared D3 dissection with more conservative procedures. The first of these studies, which was performed by Robertson and colleagues[147] in Hong Kong, compared D3 and D1 dissection. The 55 enrolled patients were randomized as follows: 25 in the D1 group (who also underwent a subtotal gastrectomy) and 30 in the D3 group (who also underwent total gastrectomy, distal pancreatectomy, and splenectomy). The median operative time in the D3 group was nearly twice that in the D1 group; the median hospitalization time in the D3 group was twice as long. The only operative dissection-related death in this relatively small study occurred in the D3 group. The overall survival duration was significantly better in the D3 group.

Most Western surgeons would agree that lymph node metastasis in the periaortic and porta hepatis regions constitutes distant disease; thus, routine removal of nodes in those areas is not recommended. In 2004, Japanese authors reported the initial evaluation of JCOG-9501, a randomized trial comparing D2 and D2+ dissection.[148] Patients were required to have T2 or greater tumors and cancer-negative peritoneal cytology, to undergo an R0 resection, and to be physically fit without significant comorbidities. A total of 523 patients were entered into the study. The overall operative mortality rate was 0.8% in each army. Forty percent of the patients underwent a splenectomy with total gastrectomy.

We believe that only surgeons who have performed aggressive lymph node dissection with extremely low operative morbidity and mortality rates should consider it. One study reported an operative mortality rate of 1.8% for gastrectomy with aggressive lymph node dissection.[149] However, data from the American College of Surgeons found that the mortality rate ranges from 8% to 9% in the United States.[150]

The American College of Surgeons has also conducted large studies of patterns of care for gastric cancer across the United States.[151,152] Data from those studies have demonstrated the need for careful evaluation of resected specimens for proper staging. In one of the studies, lymph nodes in the resected specimen were not reported in one-third of the patients. A similar finding was seen in the Intergroup 0116 trial of adjuvant therapy, in which nodes in the resected specimen were not reported in more than half of the patients.[153] This lack of reporting is likely the product of a less aggressive operation and a reflection of a lack of thoroughness (perhaps reflecting a nihilistic perspective) on the part of the pathologists.

Linitis plastica, an extremely virulent form of gastric cancer, is considered incurable by many clinicians. Some feel that patients with the condition should never undergo gastrectomy.[154] At best, the 5-year survival rates in patients with this disease are in the single digits. We approach patients with linitis plastica from this viewpoint: if a patient is still considered to have potentially resectable disease after a staging laparoscopy, that patient then undergoes neoadjuvant therapy to further select out patients with the most aggressive disease who will never benefit from a gastrectomy. Only patients who remain free of distant disease are then considered for resection. Also, if a patient with linitis plastica has a positive margin, careful consideration should be paid to how far to chase the margin with error on the side of caution if tissues appear grossly normal.

Multivisceral Resections One of the concerns raised by the results of the Dutch and MRC trials described earlier is the role of multivisceral resections in the treatment of gastric cancer. In the two studies, the mortality rate clearly increased to roughly 15% with the application of distal pancreatectomy and splenectomy. That finding prompted a reassessment of such aggressive surgery in Western patients. Piso and colleagues[155] reviewed 33 patients who underwent gastrectomy with pancreatectomy (total, distal, or head) and evaluated operative morbidity and mortality. The overall operative mortality rate was 9%, which is remarkable considering that 9 patients (27%) underwent a palliative resection in the face of known peritoneal or liver metastases. In patients who underwent an R0 resection, the median survival duration was 17 months. The authors also found that only 39% of patients had pathologic confirmation of direct invasion of the pancreas.

A group from Memorial Sloan–Kettering Cancer Center used their prospective database to report on the same issue.[156,157] They found more than 800 patients who underwent an R0 resection over a 15-year period. Roughly one-third of the patients underwent resection of an additional organ, which reflects the referral nature of the institution. Most importantly, the operative mortality rate was only 4%, which is similar to that reported in the Dutch and MRC trials for limited dissection, but is far lower than that for D2 dissection. Interestingly, the likelihood of actual adjacent organ invasion was very low (14%) in the final pathology examination. Nevertheless, the 5-year survival rate in the patients was 32%, although that rate is lower than the rate of 50% in patients who did not need a multivisceral resection to achieve an R0 resection. These data clearly support the appropriate application of multivisceral resection of gastric cancer when required to achieve an R0 resection at centers where the operative mortality rate can be kept low.

Resection Techniques There are many different ways to perform a gastrectomy. This section describes our approach to subtotal and total gastrectomy.

Once a patient is taken to the operating room for a gastrectomy, that patient is placed in the supine position. If the patient has a T2 or greater tumor and has not undergone staging laparoscopy, the gastrectomy is performed at this juncture (if a truly palliative resection is not to be considered).

A midline incision is made from the xiphoid to the umbilicus. Some surgeons use a bilateral subcostal incision; however, we have found that a midline incision provides ample visualization of the upper abdomen and is less painful. Next, the left lateral segment of the liver is mobilized, and the falciform ligament is divided and ligated near the umbilicus. The ligated ligament can be used as a pedicled flap to reinforce either the duodenal stump or the esophagojejunostomy. A self-retaining retractor system is then placed and exploration is again performed to confirm the presence or absence of metastatic disease. The omentum is then dissected off the transverse colon.

Some surgeons prefer to perform an omental bursectomy (resection of the anterior leaf off the transverse mesocolon and the peritoneum off the pancreas) at this time. The rationale is resection of microscopic peritoneal metastases that may be present at this location. A bursectomy is difficult to justify, however, because a subtotal gastrectomy leaves a portion of the lesser sac regardless of the type of resection performed, and, as noted earlier, there is no evidence that total gastrectomy (which would be required to remove the entire omental bursa) is a better oncologic procedure than is subtotal gastrectomy. Also, the belief that removal of microscopic carcinomatosis in and of itself would confer any survival advantage may be overly optimistic. We resect the omentum with the gastrectomy specimen primarily because the blood supply to the omentum is severely compromised by gastrectomy.

Next, the patient is placed in a slight reverse Trendelenburg position to allow gravity to help with exposure. To minimize the risk of injury to the spleen and to improve visualization, the spleen is brought down into the operative site with moist packs placed behind it. With this technique and careful dissection of the left gastroepiploic vessels (and short gastric vessels for a total gastrectomy), the risk of iatrogenic splenectomy should be only about 1%.

With the omentum completely reflected in a cephalad direction, dissection is performed in the left side of the abdomen with identification and ligation of the left gastroepiploic vessels. The omentum is then divided over to the greater curvature of the stomach for a subtotal gastrectomy and, for a total gastrectomy, continues in a cephalad direction, dividing the short gastric vessels. Once the left side of the stomach is fully mobilized, the packs behind the spleen may be removed.

Dissection of the omentum off the colon continues to the right and, at a point near the hepatic flexure, dissection is carried up to the duodenum. The right gastroepiploic vein is then identified entering into the middle colic vein and divided at that point. A packet of lymph nodes is adjacent to the right gastroepiploic artery as it arises off the gastroduodenal artery; those nodes are dissected up with the specimen, and the artery is ligated. The right gastric vessels are then divided near the hepatic artery, and the duodenum is fully mobilized.

With the duodenum elevated, the fatty attachments along the inferior border are ligated with 3-0 silk. Electrocautery should not be used here, because these vessels are fragile and tend to bleed. The duodenum is then transected—typically with a stapler. The gastrohepatic ligament is divided with the use of electrocautery, taking great care to detect an accessory or replaced left hepatic artery, which can almost always be taken with impunity. However, if the artery is extremely large, a test clamping should be performed.

The dissection is next carried over to the esophagus, with incision of the peritoneum along the right crux of the diaphragm. The stomach is retracted in a cephalad direction, and dissection is performed across the superior border of the pancreas, reflecting the nodal bearing tissue in a cephalad direction. Next, the left gastric vein is identified, ligated, and divided. This vein may be located either in front of or behind the hepatic artery. It is quite fragile, and so great care should be taken when dissecting it (Figure 86-4).

The dissection then continues toward the gastroduodenal artery. The node-bearing tissue is reflected in a cephalad direction across the hepatic artery. Dissection continues out of the splenic artery to the posterior gastric artery, arising from the splenic artery and providing blood supply to the upper posterior medial wall of the stomach. The left gastric artery is then identified at its origin, ligated, and divided, and the node-bearing tissue around the celiac axis is dissected back to the crux of the diaphragm. On the left side of the abdomen, the tissue anterior to the adrenal gland is a reasonable plane to work through.

The dissection then returns to the right side of the esophagus. In a subtotal gastrectomy, the node-bearing tissue along the right cardia is dissected off of the GE junction and upper stomach and is swept in a caudal direction. All of the right cardial nodes are resected, even in a subtotal gastrectomy. At this point, for a subtotal gastrectomy, a point at least 5 cm proximal to the upper border of the tumor is selected, and the stomach is transected with a stapler. For a subtotal gastrectomy, the resection is complete at this point, with blood supply coming from the preserved short gastric vessels. For a total gastrectomy, all of the short gastric vessels will already have been divided; thus, the esophagus is divided with the appropriate margin. If greater exposure of the esophagus is needed, the diaphragm may be divided, and if still more exposure is needed, the left phrenic vein is suture-ligated and divided, which usually provides ample exposure of much of the distal esophagus. Stay sutures with 2-0 silk are placed at full thickness in the esophagus before transection. It is important to remember to perform a frozen-section analysis of the resection margins before reconstruction begins.

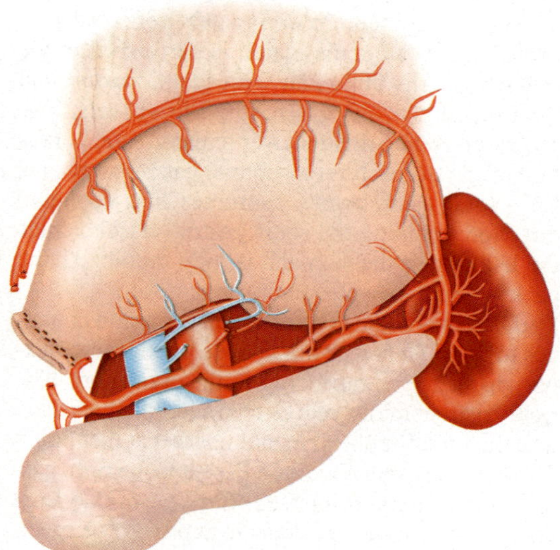

Figure 86-4 Critical area of D2 dissection (spleen-preserving method).

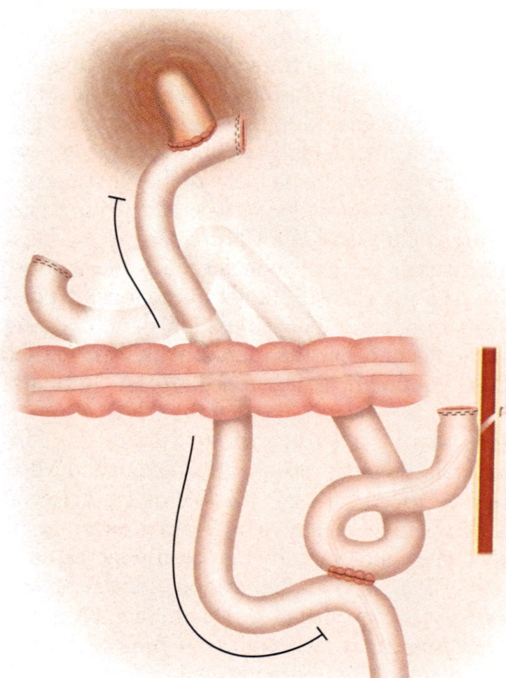

Figure 86-5 Reconstruction after total gastrectomy. A 45 cm Roux limb and defunctionalized short segment for jejunostomy tube placement are used.

Reconstruction Many different methods of reconstruction can be used. For total gastrectomy, the options include the standard Roux-en-Y operation (Figure 86-5), pouch construction, and jejunal interposition (with or without a pouch). Although each of those approaches has its advocates, and numerous small trials have been conducted, no consensus has been reached regarding the best method; various studies support each approach.[134,158–166] The studies have looked at both the nutritional implications and the quality-of-life considerations attending the various reconstruction methods and at the benefits of pouch construction versus standard Roux-en-Y reconstruction, with results both for and against pouch reconstruction.[161,166]

One type of reconstruction that makes sense is jejunal interposition: a 45 cm segment of the small bowel is interposed between the esophagus and duodenum. Studies of this technique have not been conclusive.[165] The biggest drawback of this type of reconstruction is that three anastomoses are performed in series (esophagojejunostomy, duodenojejunostomy, and jejunojejunostomy). However, patients who undergo jejunal interposition tend to lose less body weight and to have a lower incidence of cholelithiasis with food passing through the duodenum. We consider this type of reconstruction for patients who otherwise appear likely to have significant nutritional problems (such as those who have undergone a bowel resection). The most common reconstruction method that we perform for subtotal or total gastrectomy is the Roux-en-Y operation. In the absence of conclusive data, we believe that the simpler the reconstruction method, the better.

Reconstruction options for subtotal gastrectomy include Billroth I gastroduodenostomy, loop reconstruction (Billroth II), jejunal interposition, and Roux-en-Y reconstruction. Loop reconstruction (or Roux-en-Y reconstruction, for that matter) can be performed either at the staple line by removing the line and creating an anastomosis from the end of stomach to the side of the small bowel or on the posterior surface of the stomach (Figure 86-6). Loop reconstruction is typically performed as a two-layer anastomosis, using an inner layer of a running 3-0 absorbable monofilament suture and an outer layer of 3-0 silk Lembert sutures.

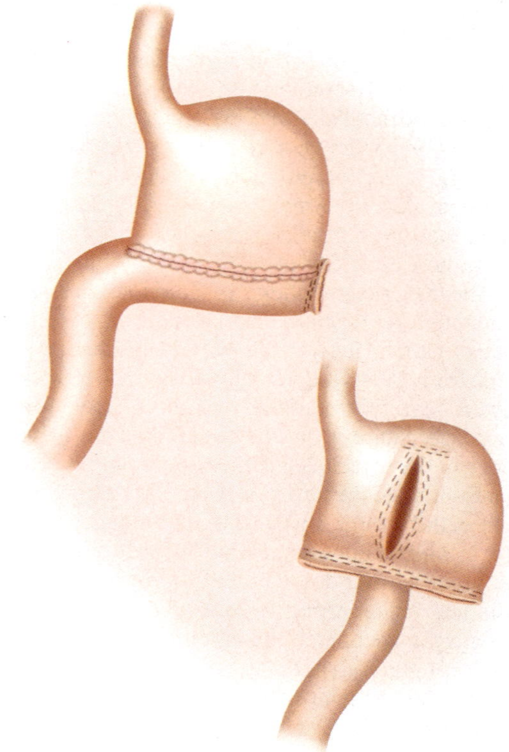

Figure 86-6 Various placement options for gastrojejunostomy after subtotal gastrectomy.

We most frequently perform Roux-en-Y reconstruction by dividing the small bowel roughly 25 cm distal to the ligament of Treitz (or at the site of a previously placed feeding tube used with neoadjuvant therapy). A vascularized limb of the small bowel is then brought up to the posterior wall of the stomach. The limb is aligned in a manner to create a stapled side-to-side anastomosis, with the tip of the small bowel directed toward the left shoulder.

Either anastomosis must be at least 6 cm in length to provide optimal emptying of the gastric remnant.[167] To avoid delayed gastric emptying, it is also important to make sure that the gastric remnant left in place is not too large. Additionally, Roux-en-Y reconstruction prevents the difficult problem of bile reflux, which can occur with Billroth II reconstruction, particularly if the entire lesser curvature has been cleared. The enteroenterostomy is created roughly 45 cm downstream from the gastrojejunostomy in a side-to-side fashion with a short defunctionalized side limb through which a feeding jejunostomy tube can be placed.

Reconstruction after total gastrectomy can be a bit more elaborate than that after subtotal gastrectomy (although it need not be). The most common reconstruction method for total gastrectomy is the Roux-en-Y operation—usually in an end-of-esophagus to side-of-jejunum fashion. The anastomosis can be performed using either a circular or linear stapler technique, or sewing in one or two layers, the latter of which is our preferred approach. The principal reason for using the sewing technique is the lower rate of anastomotic stricture as compared with stapling. In general, there appears to be no substantial difference in the leak rate between sewn and stapled anastomoses. Notably, even surgeons who routinely staple an anastomosis must sew an anastomosis in roughly 10% of cases.

The anastomosis for total gastrectomy is fashioned in a manner similar to that described earlier for subtotal gastrectomy. An exception is that the anastomosis is performed to the esophagus in a single layer with interrupted 3-0 silk sutures. The NG tube is passed across the anastomosis and used to test the anastomosis with air under water before completion of the procedure. If the falciform ligament is long enough, it can be wrapped behind the esophagojejunostomy to bolster the anastomosis.

Postoperatively, we do not routinely perform a contrast study; but, if the patient has unexplained tachycardia or fever, or is slow to regain intestinal function, we do perform a barium swallow. Typically, the NG tube is removed when evidence of bowel function and low output from the NG tube is obtained. Otherwise, the tube is left in, usually for 5 to 7 days. The NG tube is then removed, and the patient begins receiving clear liquids and is advanced to the postgastrectomy diet.

Although some surgeons do not leave an NG tube in place after total gastrectomy, and although pulmonary toilet may be better used without the tube in place, concerns about perforation of a fresh anastomosis when an NG tube is necessary should not be minimized. The nuances of dietary management of patients after gastrectomy in the resumption of oral intake are beyond the scope of this chapter. However, management of dumping and overcoming transient loss of appetite are not trivial difficulties for many patients. Intolerance to fatty food and increased gas are common in such patients.

Finally, the feeding jejunostomy tube is removed when the patient no longer needs it for maintenance of nutrition. It takes from 6 to 12 weeks to reach that point. The feeding jejunostomy tube is an excellent insurance policy when a leak develops and prolonged nothing-by-mouth status is required.

ADJUVANT THERAPY

Surgery remains the only curative option for localized gastric cancer. However, long-term survival rates with surgery alone remain suboptimal for all but the earliest cases of gastric cancer (T1N0M0). This finding is especially true in Western countries. A recent report of the National Cancer Data Base showed that the 5-year survival rates in American patients with stage Ib, II, IIIa, and IIIb gastric cancer were 58%, 34%, 20%, and 8% respectively.[34]

Chemotherapy Over the past four decades, numerous trials of systemic chemotherapy for gastric cancer have been performed in the adjuvant setting. However, the results have often been disappointing. Many of the early trials were underpowered, included improper control groups, or used suboptimal methodologies. Also, the treatment regimens and inclusion criteria were heterogeneous. Those limitations rendered some of the results unreproducible.[168] Meta-analyses of these trials were fraught with difficulties and could not recommend a particular regimen. Nevertheless, two large analyses were performed that yielded conflicting results.[169,170] Each analysis recommended treatment for subgroups such as patients with node-positive disease and Asian patients. A number of trials reporting a benefit for adjuvant therapy had design flaws or were not corroborated in subsequent confirmatory trials.[168] Selected trials that report benefits are described below.

Most of the chemotherapy agents considered to be active against advanced gastric cancer have reported response rates of 15% to 20% when administered alone. Thus, to determine the expected survival benefit, random-assignment trials involving hundreds to thousands of patients would be needed. In particular, the activity of single-agent mitomycin in the adjuvant setting was first reported by Japanese investigators in 1977.[171] They summarized four trials of adjuvant mitomycin. One of the trials showed an improved 5-year survival rate in treated patients as compared with control patients (68% versus 53%; $p = .05$). A subsequent small trial from Spain also reported a survival advantage for patients who received mitomycin as compared with surgery-alone controls (41% versus 26%; $p < .025$).[172] However, the improved survival rate seen in these two trials with single-agent mitomycin must be balanced against the first trial's lack of reproducibility and the second trial's small number of subjects. The numerous trials using mitomycin-containing regimens that demonstrated no survival benefit must also be considered.[168]

More recently, using newer drugs, investigators randomly assigned patients to undergo surgery alone or surgery followed by treatment with epirubicin, 5-fluorouracil (5-FU), and folinic acid; they observed an improved 3-year survival rate in the treated group (25% versus 13%; $p < .01$).[173] However, the trial was a small one, with only 55 patients receiving treatment. Confirmation of the results in a larger trial is needed.

Prolonged continuous administration of an oral 5-FU prodrug has been attractive to a number of investigators. In one trial, 85 patients were randomly assigned to receive treatment with mitomycin alone every 6 weeks for four cycles or with the addition of daily tegafur at the same dosage for 36 consecutive days each cycle. The 5-year survival rate was significantly higher in the group that received mitomycin and tegafur (67% versus 44%; $p = .04$).[174] However, the small number of patients, long accrual time (11 years), and lack of a surgery-alone control group make the results questionable. Larger trials comparing treatment with similar oral fluoropyrimidines and mitomycin with surgery alone need to be performed.[168]

Intraperitoneal Therapy The peritoneal cavity is a frequent site of gastric cancer relapse. Intraperitoneal administration of chemotherapeutic agents may result in improved delivery of those drugs to microscopic residual disease. Several trials have examined the feasibility of such an approach. Two trials compared surgery alone with surgery followed by intraperitoneal delivery of cisplatin.[175,176] No survival differences were observed. However, both trials included patients with metastatic disease and thus were not true trials of adjuvant therapy. Other investigators studied the use of intraperitoneal carbon-adsorbed mitomycin.[177] Compared with patients who underwent surgery alone, 24 patients who received mitomycin had a significantly higher 2-year survival rate (69% versus 27%; $p < .005$). However, the advantage of using this strategy could not be confirmed in a larger trial conducted in Austria; the trial was closed early because of increased postoperative morbidity and mortality in the treated group.[178] Investigators have also studied intraperitoneal delivery of combination chemotherapy. In one such study, the investigators randomly assigned 248 patients to undergo surgery alone or with intraperitoneal mitomycin and 5-FU, but they found no significant difference in overall survival between the two groups.[179]

Continuous hyperthermic peritoneal perfusion was designed to favorably alter the distribution and kinetics of agents used in intraperitoneal chemotherapy.[180] A number of randomized trials of adjuvant continuous hyperthermic peritoneal perfusion have been performed in Japan. As part of a phase I study of intraperitoneal hyperthermic perfusion at our institution, we managed gastric cancer in 12 patients using that approach.[181] In a nonrandomized group of patients with stage IV disease, survival durations were significantly longer for patients who underwent perfusion than for patients who were candidates for perfusion during the same period, but who elected to receive systemic chemotherapy. Unfortunately, two operative deaths (17%) occurred, and all of the patients eventually died of their disease.

Immunotherapy Immunotherapy has been explored in the postoperative setting in hopes of decreasing relapse and improving survival in patients with gastric cancer. However, few immunotherapy trials have had a no-treatment control arm. One that did was a three-arm randomized study that compared surgery followed by observation only, surgery followed by chemotherapy with 5-FU and methyl lomustine (CCNU), and surgery followed by chemotherapy with 5-FU and methyl CCNU plus levamisole.[182] The overall survival rate at 5 years was 50% in all three groups.

The nonspecific immune stimulant picibanil (OK-432) has also been studied in randomized trials. In one such trial, patients were randomly assigned to undergo surgery alone; surgery followed by chemotherapy with mitomycin, 5-FU, and cytarabine; or surgery followed by the same chemotherapy regimen plus OK-432.[183] After a median follow-up duration of 5 years, the investigators found no significant difference in overall survival between the three groups. Korean investigators also studied OK-432 in two randomized trials.[184] In one of the trials, 64 patients underwent surgery alone, and 74 patients underwent surgery followed by chemotherapy with mitomycin, 5-FU, cytosine arabinoside, and OK-432. The 5-year survival rate was higher in the treated group (45% versus 23%; $p < .05$). In the other trial, 159 patients received mitomycin, 5-FU, and OK-432; 77 patients received only mitomycin and 5-FU; and 94 patients underwent surgery alone. The 5-year survival rates were 45%, 30%, and 24% respectively. The results of those trials are encouraging, but must be confirmed in further trials.

CHEMORADIATION FOR GASTRIC CANCER

Chemoradiation for Incompletely Resected Disease Several early trials evaluated the role of chemoradiation in patients with incompletely resected gastric cancer.

Specifically, a randomized trial conducted at Mayo Clinic for a variety of unresected tumors administered radiation at 35 to 40 Gy with and without a bolus of 5-FU for 3 days.[185] The investigators analyzed a small group of patients with gastric cancer and found that the patients who received concurrent 5-FU had a superior 5-year survival as compared with patients who received radiation alone (12% versus 0%), providing evidence of the efficacy of this chemoradiation regimen, which has been used now for three decades.

A subsequent randomized trial conducted by the Gastrointestinal Tumor Study Group in patients with incompletely resected gastric cancer compared chemotherapy alone (using 5-FU and methyl CCNU) with chemoradiation (split course: 5000 cGy with a bolus of 5-FU given at the start of each course of radiotherapy).[186] The trial was stopped early because of six treatment-related deaths and six disease-related deaths within the first 6 months of therapy in the combined-modality arm. Despite those circumstances, the investigators found a statistically significant survival benefit in the combined-modality arm at 5 years (survival rate: 20% versus 6%; $p < .01$). In that study, the gastrointestinal and hematological toxic effects were not optimally managed. Modern supportive care, including jejunostomy tube feeding and cytokine support, might have enhanced the difference in survival in favor of the combined-modality arm.

To confirm their results, the investigators designed a second trial with similar entry criteria. The new trial compared 5-FU, methyl CCNU, and doxorubicin alone with the same regimen followed by chemoradiation (4320 cGy with a bolus of 5-FU) starting on day 57.[187] Unfortunately, this trial was hampered by poor accrual and compliance (of 59 patients, 11 did not receive the prescribed dose of radiation, and 7 did not undergo radiotherapy), which may explain why the trial showed no difference in survival.

Others have investigated postoperative radiotherapy alone for gastric cancer. For example, the British Stomach Cancer Group conducted a phase III trial that stratified 436 patients by age, symptom duration, and disease stage and that then randomized those patients to undergo surgery alone, surgery followed by FAM (5-FU, doxorubicin, and mitomycin) chemotherapy alone, or surgery followed by radiotherapy (45 Gy in 25 fractions with or without a 5.4 Gy boost) alone.[188,189] In spite of the fact that one-third of the patients had residual disease, 18% had positive margins, and one-third received 40 Gy of radiation or less, the researchers found a locoregional control advantage in the radiotherapy arm (90% versus 73% for surgery alone and 81% for surgery followed by chemotherapy; $p < .01$). The cause-specific and overall survival rates were not statistically different. Even though the study did not include a chemoradiation arm, its failure to show a survival impact has influenced the direction of subsequent investigations.

Evidence of the importance of 5-FU administration was demonstrated in a randomized study conducted by the European Organisation for Research and Treatment of Cancer (EORTC).[190] That study showed a survival advantage in patients who underwent chemoradiation as compared with those who received radiation alone (to 55.5 Gy). All patients with gross disease who had no progressive disease received 5-FU concurrently with, and for 18 months after, chemoradiation. Subsequent studies have shown that chemoradiation can be curative in a small percentage of patients with unresectable or partially resected gastric cancer.[185]

Adjuvant Chemoradiation Adjuvant 5-FU–based chemoradiation for gastric cancer was investigated in the postoperative setting as early as three decades ago. A randomized trial was conducted in patients with completely resected gastric cancer. The patients were simply observed or underwent postoperative chemoradiation (37.5 Gy with a bolus of 5-FU at 15 mg/kg for 3 days).[191] By design, the investigators obtained the patients' informed consent after randomization and did not stratify the patients for known prognostic factors. Of 39 patients with favorable prognostic factors, 10 refused to undergo adjuvant therapy after randomization. The locoregional control, overall survival, and relapse-free survival rates were all higher in the adjuvant therapy arm than in the central arm. The overall survival rate was highest in patients who, after randomization, refused to undergo chemoradiation. Upon intent-to-treat analysis, survival was higher in the group that received postoperative chemoradiation, but the difference was not statistically significant (20% versus 12%).

Although the studies described above provided some evidence of the benefit of chemoradiation in patients with gastric cancer, the small patient numbers, inclusion of patients with gross residual disease, use of nonstandardized surgery, administration of suboptimal doses of 5-FU or radiation, or inadequate supportive care prevented definitive conclusions to be drawn. Subsequently, investigators designed an Intergroup trial (INT 0116) to try to minimize those shortcomings.[153] Eligible patients had stage Ib through stage IV gastric cancer that had been treated with curative resection, but most of the 556 evaluable patients had positive lymph nodes (85%) or T3/T4 lesions (68%). Patients were randomly assigned to undergo postoperative chemoradiation (45 Gy with a bolus of 5-FU) or observation after complete surgical resection. At 3 years, patients in the postoperative chemoradiation arm had an 11% absolute (28% relative) survival advantage (50% versus 41%; $p = .0005$) at the cost of significant gastrointestinal (33% grade 3/4) and hematologic (54% grade 3/4) toxic effects. Although CT scanning was not required during follow-up, the available data suggest that the rate of local failure as the first site of failure was significantly reduced (19% versus 29%). Additional improvement in local control could improve outcome further. The importance of the radiotherapy technique is illustrated by the fact that technical radiotherapy errors had to be corrected with a centralized quality assurance effort in 35% of the cases.

Concerns have been raised about the extent of surgery performed in the trial. Specifically, although D2 resection was recommended, only 10% of the patients underwent that procedure, and 54% underwent less than a D1 resection. Because study enrollment and randomization were performed after surgery, the lesser resections probably reflect the pattern of surgical practice in the United States rather than protocol noncompliance. Interestingly, the extent of nodal dissection did not correlate with disease-free or overall survival ($p = .80$)

Table 86-5 Postoperative Chemoradiation with R0 Resection for Stage Ib Through Stage IV Gastric Cancer

Chemotherapy (one 28-day cycle)
5-Fluorouracil (5-FU) 425 mg/m^2 intravenously (IV) daily, days 1 to 5
Folinic acid 20 mg/m^2 IV daily, days 1–5
Chemoradiation (5 weeks)
5-FU 400 mg/m^2 IV daily, days 1 to 4 and on the last 3 days of radiotherapy
Folinic acid 20 mg/m^2 IV daily, days 1 to 4 and on the last 3 days of radiotherapy
External-beam radiation, 45 Gy at 1.8 Gy/day, 5 days per week
One-month recovery period
Chemotherapy (two 28-day cycles)
5-FU 425 mg/m^2 IV daily, days 1 to 5
Folinic acid 20 mg/m^2 IV daily, days 1 to 5

That trial established postoperative adjuvant 5-FU–based chemoradiation as the standard of care for resected gastric cancer. Table 86-5 shows the treatment regimen used in the trial. Several single-institution studies have also reported an advantage with postoperative radiotherapy with or without concurrent chemotherapy.

Intraoperative Radiotherapy A randomized study from Japan showed a survival advantage with intraoperative radiotherapy (IORT) at doses ranging from 28 to 35 Gy for stages II through IV, but not stage I, gastric cancer.[192] Although the study suffered from methodological flaws, it demonstrated proof of principle for the role of IORT in gastric cancer and cancer in general. A smaller study showed a significant local control advantage with IORT.[193]

Irradiation Technique and Supportive Care A comprehensive consensus report on important treatment-planning issues in gastric cancer has been reviewed elsewhere[194] and is summarized here.

During planning for treatment of gastric cancer, all available imaging (CT and barium swallow), endoscopic, pathologic, and operative findings should be reviewed before simulation. Patients should undergo simulation on an empty stomach (nothing by mouth for 3 hours) and should receive treatment in the morning before eating to minimize stomach distention. An oral contrast agent should be given 15 to 30 minutes before simulation, and treatment devices used for arm elevation should be employed. Patients can undergo treatment with either opposed anterior and posterior portals or a multiple-field technique with or without three-dimensional treatment planning. Compared with the use of two fields, the use of four or more radiation fields has been reported to significantly reduce the rate of grade 4 or 5 toxicity.[195] However, lateral fields are not always advisable for patients with an intact stomach, because the gastric fundus frequently extends posteriorly too far. In such instances, the kidneys and spinal cord cannot be shielded without shielding the target.

CT-based treatment planning with dose–volume histograms is helpful in objectively evaluating various technical treatment options in individual patients. For instance, with the use of three-dimensional planning, beam arrangements can be optimized so that the radiation dose delivered to the kidneys and liver is minimized. Using slight right anterior oblique and left posterior oblique beams facilitates coverage of the porta hepatis while avoiding irradiation of the right kidney. Customized blocking should be used to shield the critical structures in the field, including the small bowel, liver, spinal cord, and kidneys.

No uniform agreement has emerged about which lymph node groups should be treated, but treatment volumes should be tailored to the location of each individual tumor. Lymphadenectomy series[196] have provided detailed data regarding risk of nodal involvement that can guide physicians in deciding which nodes are at risk. Depending on the location of the primary tumor in the stomach, perigastric, gastroepiploic, celiac, porta hepatis, subpyloric, gastroduodenal, splenic–suprapancreatic, and retropancreaticoduodenal nodes can be at risk for metastatic spread. The gastric remnant, the perigastric nodes, and the branches of the celiac axis should be treated in all cases. Also, a 5 cm esophageal mucosal margin and the paraesophageal nodes should be included in the cephalad treatment volume for tumors proximal to lesions involving the cardia or GE junction. However, including the duodenal mucosa and periduodenal nodes in the treatment volume for those proximal lesions is not necessary. For distal lesions at or near the gastroduodenal junction, the entire C-loop should be covered to ensure a 5 cm margin of the duodenal mucosa. The suprapancreaticoduodenal nodes should also be treated.

The importance of aggressive supportive care administered by a multidisciplinary care team cannot be overemphasized, as illustrated by the experience of the Gastrointestinal Tumor Study Group,[186] discussed earlier. Nutritional inadequacy can lead to treatment-related death. When performing radiotherapy for gastric cancer, the routine use of prophylactic antiemetics and jejunostomy tube feeding vastly improves treatment tolerance. Nutritionists should monitor patients' calorie intake and weight, provide them with calorie goals, and serve as a resource for other nutrition-related issues.

PREOPERATIVE CHEMOTHERAPY

Despite recent advances in curative gastrectomy followed by postoperative chemoradiation, 5-year survival rates remain below 50% after the procedure.[153] Several potential advantages make preoperative therapy an attractive target of investigation. For example, early initiation of systemic therapy may eliminate micrometastases. Also, the ability to assess tumor response may enable early termination of ineffective therapy. Furthermore, preoperative therapy can downstage the primary tumor and may improve the R0 resection rate. In patients with occult chemoresistant metastasis that manifests during treatment, the delay in energy may prevent the use of nontherapeutic laparotomy. Preoperative therapy also adds prognostic information. An analysis of 83 patients on preoperative chemotherapy protocols at M. D. Anderson showed that response to preoperative chemotherapy was the single most important predictor of survival.[197,198] However, those findings must be balanced with the potential risk of delaying definitive local therapy. Treatment-resistant clones may develop during therapy, and the patient's performance status may decrease, increasing surgical risk.

Accurate clinical staging of gastric cancer is essential in preoperative clinical trials. Because of the potential for downstaging, pretreatment endoscopic sonography and laparoscopy are needed for all enrolled patients for comparison with control groups. A number of chemotherapeutic regimens have been studied in small preoperative trials. The patient selection and treatment plans in those trials were heterogeneous, making the results difficult to compare. However, the trials show that preoperative therapy is feasible and can downstage tumors. A few are summarized in Table 86-6.

More recently, the MRC conducted a phase III random-assignment comparison of pre- and postoperative chemotherapy with surgery alone.[199] In that study, 503 patients with gastric or distal esophageal adenocarcinoma were randomly assigned to surgery alone or to chemotherapy with epirubicin, cisplatin, and 5-FU (ECF) for three cycles both before and after surgery. Investigators reported significant improvements in both progression free (p = .009) and overall (p = .0001) survival. Magnitudes of reported clinic benefits in progression free survival (HR 0.75; 95% CI, 0.60–0.93) and overall survival (HR 0.66; 95% CI, 0.53–0.81) are similar to those reported for post operative chemoradiation in the intergroup 0116 trial.

PREOPERATIVE CHEMORADIATION

Combined-modality chemoradiation in the preoperative setting allows for treatment with the target organ in place. When compared with postoperative radiotherapy, the result may be reduced radiotoxicity in the bowel and other adjacent organs. When using this strategy, feeding gastrostomy tubes should be avoided, because they rarely function well during irradiation, and they increase the risk of subsequent surgery. In comparison, routine placement of feeding jejunostomy tubes enhances tolerance and reduces the need for parenteral support and hospital admission.

In prospective randomized trials, preoperative radiotherapy, both with and without chemotherapy, has been reported to improve outcome.[200–202] These trials, which were conducted in Russia, showed increased resectability and survival without increased morbidity with the use of suboptimal radiation doses without concurrent chemotherapy. Also, in a pilot study conducted in the United States, 24 patients received 45 Gy of external-beam radiation at 1.8 Gy daily, 5 days per week,

Table 86-6 Selected Trials of Preoperative Chemotherapy

Preoperative Treatment	Postoperative Treatment	Patient Selection	Patients (*n*)	R0 Resection (%)	Median Survival	Path CR (*n* [%])	Reference
5-FU + FA + cisplatin ×2	IP FUDR + IP cisplatin ×1	Resectable	59	71	>4 Years	5 (9)	258
FAMTX ×3	5-FU + IP cisplatin + IP 5-FU ×3	T3–4NXM0 T2N1–2M0	56	61	15 Months	Not stated	259
PMUE	PMUE	IV	29	79	Not stated*	0 (0)	
None	PMUE		26	88	Not stated	NA	260
5-FU + 45 Gy	None	M0	24	75	Too early	2 (11)	261
5-FU + FA + cisplatin ×2, 5-FU + 45 Gy	None	M0	33	70	34 Months	8 (30)	198
EFC ×3	EFC ×3	M0	250	79	24 Months	Not stated	199
None	None		253	69	19 Month		

5-FU = 5-fluorouracil; EFC, etoposide, 5-FU, and cisplatin; FA = folinic acid; FAMTX = 5-FU, doxorubicin, and methotrexate; FUDR = fluorodeoxyuridine; IP = intraperitoneal; IV = intravenous; NA = not applicable; Path CR = pathologic complete response; PMUE = cisplatin, mitomycin, etoposide, and uracil–tegafur.

* Overall median survival duration not stated; only subgroup analyses were reported.

concurrent with continuous-infusion 5-FU at 300 mg/m^2 daily on days when irradiation was performed.[203] Surgery was carried out 4 to 6 weeks after completion of the chemoradiation in 19 (79%) of the patients. Intraoperative radiotherapy (10 Gy) was given at resection. A complete pathologic response was observed in 2 patients (8%).

The use of induction chemotherapy followed by chemoradiation is currently under investigation. In a recent small multi-institutional study, patients received two courses of 5-FU, folinic acid, and cisplatin followed by 5-FU–potentiated radiotherapy (45 Gy). A total of 28 patients underwent surgical resection without experiencing excessive complications. Of the treated patients, 30% had a pathologically confirmed complete remission.[198]

Currently, in phase II trials, investigators are studying induction chemotherapy followed by chemoradiation and surgery with the incorporation of newer chemotherapeutic agents. The many theoretical advantages of this preoperative strategy for resectable gastric cancer will have to be proven in large, random-assignment trials.

SYSTEMIC THERAPY FOR ADVANCED DISEASE

In patients with unresectable gastric cancer at the time of diagnosis, or with disease that recurs after primary therapy, the cancer is incurable; thus, therapy is palliative. Despite numerous randomized trials, the survival rates in such patients remain poor. An analysis of the SEER 9 registry showed only modest improvements in overall survival over the past three decades in patients with metastatic disease. The median survival durations reported in clinical trials have ranged from 7 to 10 months. Patients with a poor performance status or multiple sites of metastasis have significantly worse outcomes. The analysis of the SEER 9 registry also showed that the median survival duration in unselected patients with metastatic gastric cancer was 4 months.

Considering this dismal prognosis, several investigators have examined systemic chemotherapy to see whether it has a role in advanced gastric cancer. Four small random-assignment trials assessed the impact of palliative chemotherapy on survival duration and quality of life.[204–207] In all four trials, superior survival durations were reported in patients receiving treatment as compared with patients receiving best supportive care (Table 86-7).

Patients who received best supportive care had median survival durations ranging from 3 to 5 months; those who received chemotherapy had median survival durations ranging from 8 to 12 months. Improvements in symptoms and quality of life were also apparent in the chemotherapy group. Those findings are consistent with the fact that gastric cancer is a relatively chemosensitive disease. Side effects of chemotherapy must be balanced against the potential benefits and the symptoms associated with unchecked cancer growth. Palliative chemotherapy should be considered for most patients with an adequate performance status and nutritional support.

One difficult and controversial area is therapy for nonevaluable disease in asymptomatic patients—for example, those with low-volume abdominal carcinomatosis. Although some clinicians advocate the immediate use of chemotherapy, others advise the use of observation. The rationale for "observation only" lies in the fact that only 30% to 40% of patients will respond to any particular chemotherapeutic regimen. Delaying treatment until the appearance of early symptoms or evaluable disease may spare patients unnecessary toxic effects and may preserve their quality of life. Such patients should be closely observed with a medical history, physical examination, and CT scans, if necessary. Treatment may be initiated when evaluable disease is established or when symptoms appear.

CHEMOTHERAPY Single Agents Numerous commercially available chemotherapeutic agents have been used in single-agent therapy for gastric cancer. With the exception of S-1, which has a reported response rate of 40% to 50%, a response rate of about 20% is required for agents to be considered active in single-agent therapy for gastric cancer (Table 86-8).

Combination Chemotherapy To improve overall survival and response rate, a number of combination chemotherapy programs have been developed based on agents with known activity against gastric cancer. Key randomized trials are summarized in Table 86-9, and selected combination regimens are listed in Table 86-10.

Since the original publication of the use of FAM chemotherapy in 1980, numerous patients have received it.[217] The original study showed a response rate of 42% in patients with advanced gastric cancer. Dose-escalation trials based on FAM or two modified forms of FAM did not improve the response rate.[208,209] Pooled data from all of the FAM and FAM-variant trials showed that the overall response rate for these drug combinations was 30% (95% confidence interval [CI]: 26% to 34%) and that the complete response rate was 2%.

Encouraging phase II study results have not always translated into improved overall survival. A North Central Cancer Therapy Group trial comparing 5-FU alone, 5-FU plus doxorubicin, and FAM

Table 86-7 Trials of Palliative Chemotherapy versus Best Supportive Care (BSC)

Regimen	Patients (*n*)	Median Survival (Months)	*p* Value	Reference
FAMTX versus	30	9.0	.001	205
BSC	10	3.0		
FEMTX versus	17	12.0	.001	206
BSC	19	3.0		
ELF versus	18	7.5	Not stated	207
BSC	19	4.0		
ELF or LF versus	31	8.0	.120	208
BSC	30	5.0		

ELF = etoposide, leucovorin, and 5-FU; FAMTX = 5-FU, doxorubicin, and methotrexate; FEMTX = 5-flourouracil, epirubicin, methotrexate; LF = leucovorin and 5-FU.

Table 86-8 Selected Data from Phase II Trials of Single-Agent Chemotherapy for Advanced Gastric Cancer

Agent	Patients (*n*)	Response Rate (%)	95% CI (%)	Reference
5-FU	51	20	9–30	209
UFT	188	28	22–34	262
S-1	51	49	36–62	263
	51	44	30–59	264
Pemetrexed	27	22	6–38	265
Mitomycin	211	30	24–36	209
Doxorubicin	188	23	17–29	266
	93	13	6–19	267
	34	21	7–35	268
Epirubicin	24	17	2–32	269
	39	8	0–16	270
Etoposide	26	19	3–35	271
	14	21	0–42	272
Irinotecan	66	23	13–34	273
Cisplatin	115	20	13–27	209
Paclitaxel	30	17	6–35	274
	23	5	0–21	275
Docetaxel	33	24	9–39	276
	41	17	8–30	277
	59	24	14–37	278

5-FU = 5-fluorouracil; 95% CI = 95% confidence interval; S-1 = tegafur plus 5-chloro-2,4-dihydropyrimidine; UFT = uracil plus tegafur.

Table 86-10 Selected Combination Chemotherapeutic Regimens for Advanced Gastric Cancer

5-FU, cisplatin (28-day cycle)
- 5-FU 750 mg/m^2 CIV infusion, daily on days 1 to 5
- Cisplatin 20 mg/m^2 IV, daily on days 1 to 5

ECF (21-day cycle)
- 5-FU 200 mg/m^2 CIV infusion, daily on days 1 to 21
- Epirubicin 50 mg/m^2 IV on day 1
- Cisplatin 60 mg/m^2 IV on day 1

5-FU, cisplatin, paclitaxel (28-day cycle)
- 5-FU 750 mg/m^2 CIV infusion, daily on days 1 to 5
- Cisplatin 15 mg/m^2 IV, daily on days 1 to 5
- Paclitaxel 200 mg/m^2 IV over 3 hours on day 1 only

5-FU, cisplatin, docetaxel (21- to 28-day cycle)
- 5-FU 750 mg/m^2 CIV infusion, daily on days 1 to 5
- Cisplatin 75 mg/m^2 IV, daily on day 1 only
- Docetaxel 75 mg/m^2 IV over 1 hour on day 1 only

Irinotecan plus cisplatin (42-day cycle [alternative: 21-day cycle])
- Irinotecan 50–65 mg/m^2 IV on days 1, 8, 15, and 22 (days 1 and 8)
- Cisplatin 25–30 mg/m^2 IV on days 1, 8, 15, and 22 (days 1 and 8)

5-FU = 5-fluorouracil; CIV = continuous intravenous; ECF = epirubicin, cisplatin, and 5-FU; IV = intravenous.

Table 86-9 Selected Randomized Trials of Chemotherapy for Advanced Gastric Cancer

Treatment Group	Patients (*n*)	Response Rate (%)	Median Survival (Months)	*p* Value (Survival Comparison)	Reference
5-FU	51	18	7.0	NS	210
5-FU + Dox	49	27	7.0		
FAM	51	38	7.0		
5-FU	123	16	6.0	NS	211
5-FU + MMC	127	19	5.0		
5-FU	105	11	7.0	NS	279
5-FU + cisplatin	105	34	7.0		
UFT + MMC	70	9	6.0		
FAM	103	9	7.0	.0040	212
FAMTX	105	45	10.5		
5-FU + cisplatin	103	51	9.0	NS	280
FAM	98	25	7.0		
5-FU	94	26	7.0		
EAP	30	20	6.0	NS	213
FAMTX	30	33	7.0		
FAM	52	15	6.0	NS	214
PELF	85	43	8.0		
ECF	111	46	9.0	.0005	215
FAMTX	108	21	6.0		
5-FU + cisplatin	81	20	7.0	NS	216
ELF	79	9	7.0		
FAMTX	85	12	7.0		
5-FU + cisplatin		23	8.5	.0060	281
DCF		39	10.2		

5-FU = 5-fluorouracil; DCF = docetaxel, cisplatin, and 5-FU; Dox = doxorubicin; ECF = epirubicin, cisplatin, and 5-FU; ELF = etoposide, leucovorin, and 5-FU; FAM = 5-FU, doxorubicin, and mitomycin; FAMTX = 5-FU, doxorubicin, and methotrexate; MMC = mitomycin C; NS = nonsignificant; PELF = cisplatin, epirubicin, leucovorin, and 5-FU; UFT = uracil and tegafur.

showed an increasing response rate with the addition of more agents (18%, 27%, and 38% respectively).[210] However, the median survival duration in all three groups was identical. A similar trial comparing 5-FU alone with 5-FU plus mitomycin C also showed no difference in overall survival.[211] Finally, the Japan Clinical Oncology Group Study that compared 5-FU alone with 5-FU and cisplatin or with uracil plus tegafur and mitomycin failed to show survival benefits for the combination therapy, despite improved response rates in the 5-FU and cisplatin group.[218]

To increase the activity of 5-FU–based regimens, investigators combined 5-FU, doxorubicin, and methotrexate (FAMTX).[219] They found that the response rate to FAMTX was 58% and that the complete remission rate was 12%. However, the treatment-related mortality rate was high (3%). Also, the EORTC carried out a multicenter random-assignment trial comparing FAM and FAMTX.[212] The response rate in the FAMTX group was significantly higher than that in the FAM group (45% versus 9%; $p < .0001$). In addition, the median survival duration was longer in the FAMTX group (10.5 months versus 7.0 months).

To explore the possible synergy between etoposide and cisplatin, a phase II trial examining the combination of etoposide, doxorubicin, and cisplatin (EAP) for advanced gastric cancer was performed.[220] In 67 evaluable patients, the response rate was 64% (95% CI: 52% to 76%), and the complete remission rate was 21%; the median survival duration was 8.9 months. However, three subsequent phase II trials of EAP found excessive treatment-related mortality.

Furthermore, a randomized phase II trial compared EAP and FAMTX.[213] The trial was stopped early, however, because of excessive toxic effects and treatment-related deaths (4 of 30 patients [13%]) in the EAP group. The response rate was 33% in the FAMTX group and 20% in the EAP group, with overlapping confidence intervals between the two groups. The median survival rates in the two groups were also similar (6 months in the EAP group, 7 months in the FAMTX group).

Italian investigators compared the combination of cisplatin, epirubicin, leucovorin, and 5-FU (PELF) with FAM.[214] In this random-assignment trial, 85 patients received PELF, and 52 patients received FAM. As compared with patients in the FAM arm, patients in the PELF arm had a higher response rate (43% versus 15%; $p = .001$). In a follow-up trial, 200 patients were randomly assigned to receive PELF or FAMTX.[221] The investigators noted an improved response rate for PELF (39% versus 22%; $p = .009$). However, the differences in the 1- and 2-year survival rate were not statistically significant.

Investigators have also compared ECF with FAMTX. In one phase III trial, 274 patients received treatment.[215] The response rate in the ECF group was 46% (95% CI: 37% to 55%); in the FAMTX group, it was 21% (95% CI: 13% to 28%). Also, the median survival duration was longer in the ECF arm (9 months versus 6 months; $p = .0005$).

Etoposide, leucovorin, and 5-FU (ELF) were combined in an effort to develop an active, less toxic chemotherapy regimen. Etoposide and 5-FU are both active against gastric cancer and do not have any cumulative organ toxicity. In a study of the ELF regimen, 120 mg/m^2 etoposide, 500 mg/m^2 5-FU, and 300 mg/m^2 leucovorin were given daily on days 1 to 3 of a 3- to 4-week cycle.[222] In patients who had heart disease or who were older than 65 years, the response rate was 53%, and the complete remission rate was 12%. Myelosuppression was the only major toxic effect, with 16% of the patients experiencing grade 3 leukopenia and 4% having grade 4 leukopenia. The same ELF regimen given every 3 weeks was studied at M. D. Anderson with granulocyte–macrophage colony-stimulating factor support.[223] Of 29 previously untreated patients, a partial response was observed in 13% of those who were assessable.

To compare these active regimens, the EORTC conducted a three-arm randomized trial of FAMTX, ELF, and 5-FU plus cisplatin. A total of 399 patients were enrolled. In a recent update of the study, the response rate in 245 patients with measurable disease was 12% for FAMTX, 9% for ELF, and 20% for 5-FU plus cisplatin.[216] The median survival duration was 7 months in all three groups.

More recently, 42 patients with advanced gastric cancer were given 60 mg/m^2 cisplatin on day 1, 65 mg/m^2 etoposide on days 1 to 3, and 2,600 mg/m^2 5-FU plus 300 mg/m^2 leucovorin by continuous ambulatory infusion weekly for 21 days of a 28-day cycle starting on day 2 (PE-HDFL).[224] The overall response rate was high (72.5% [95% CI: 56% to 86%]). Of the 40 evaluable patients, 9 (23%) had a complete remission. The toxic effects seen were mainly hematologic: 34% of the patients had grade 3 thrombocytopenia or leukopenia, and 11% had grade 4 hematologic toxic effects. No treatment-related deaths occurred. However, despite the high response rate, the overall median survival duration was only 9 months.

To investigate the role of newer agents in combination chemotherapy programs, three phase II trials examined the combination of irinotecan and cisplatin. In particular, in a phase I/II study using a 4-week cycle, the maximum tolerated dose of irinotecan was 80 mg/m^2 on days 1 and 15 when the cisplatin dose was fixed at 80 mg/m^2 on day 1.[225] Also, the response rate was 42% (95% CI: 22% to 61%). The recommended phase II dose of irinotecan was 70 mg/m^2. In a similar study, 44 Japanese patients received irinotecan at 70 mg/m^2 every 4 weeks on days 1 and 15, and cisplatin at 80 mg/m^2 on day 1.[226] The response rate was 48% (95% CI: 33% to 63%). One complete remission was reported, and the median survival duration was 9 months. At M. D. Anderson, these two drugs were evaluated on a weekly schedule.[227,228] Cisplatin was given at 30 mg/m^2 per week, and irinotecan was given at 50 to 65 mg/m^2 per week (50 mg/m^2 per week for previously treated patients and 65 mg/m^2 per week for previously untreated patients) on days 1, 8, 15, and 22 of a 42-day cycle. The response rates were 58% in previously untreated patients and 31% in previously treated patients.

Building on the 5-FU and cisplatin regimen, Korean investigators tested the combination of 5-FU, cisplatin, and paclitaxel in a phase II trial.[229] Of the 41 patients who received treatment, 51% (95% CI: 37% to 66%) had an objective response. The median survival duration was 6 months.

Docetaxel-based chemotherapy regimens have also been extensively studied in patients with gastric cancer. Several investigators conducted phase II trials with the combination of docetaxel and cisplatin. They administered 75 to 85 mg/m^2 docetaxel and 75 mg/m^2 cisplatin on day 1 of a 21-day cycle.[230–232] The response rates ranged from 33% to 56%, and the median survival durations ranged from 9 to 10 months.

A random-assignment phase III trial compared the combination of docetaxel, cisplatin, and 5-FU (DCF) with 5-FU plus cisplatin.[233] In that trial, the researchers administered 75 mg/m^2 docetaxel on day 1, 75 mg/m^2 cisplatin on day 1, and 750 mg/m^2 5-FU by continuous infusion daily on days 1 to 5. They repeated the cycles every 3 weeks. Use of DCF resulted in a superior response rate (39% versus 23%; $p = .01$) and progression-free survival duration (median: 5.2 months versus 3.7 months; $p < .05$) at the interim analysis. However, the DCF regimen resulted in substantial treatment-related toxic effects. Specifically, 84% of the patients had grade 3/4 neutropenia, and 68% of the patients had at least one grade 3/4 nonhematologic toxic effect.

Recently, Japanese investigators tested the combination of S-1, a new oral fluoropyrimidine, and cisplatin in a phase I/II trial of patients with advanced gastric cancer.[234] They reported a high response rate (76% [95% CI: 55% to 91%]). However, the number of patients was small, and most of the patients had metastasis only in lymph nodes. Numerous trials of combinations containing S-1 are under way.

The trials described here show the median survival duration in patients with advanced gastric cancer to be less than 1 year with standard chemotherapy. Chemotherapy with 5-FU and cisplatin should be considered for patients with an adequate performance status. Single-agent chemotherapy should be considered for patients with a suboptimal performance status who desire systemic therapy. Enrollment of eligible patients into clinical trials should be encouraged.

Despite a number of combination regimens reporting response rates greater then 60%, median survival of treated patients remains at 10 to 11 months. Clearly, novel therapeutic strategies beyond traditional cytotoxic chemotherapy are needed. With the recent approval of imatinib, bevacizumab, gefitinib, cetuximab, and erlotinib, a number of phase II trials combining chemotherapy with agents targeting the *VEGF* or *EGFR* pathway are under way.

SYMPTOM MANAGEMENT

The issue of palliation is perhaps more critical for gastric cancer than for any other disease. This section explores the factors involved in deciding how best to provide palliation and the methods that are best for achieving it. Given the relatively high percentage of patients who present with incurable disease, the issues of quality of life and palliation are particularly germane.

Because of intense screening programs in Japan, 50% of patients may present with early-stage gastric cancer; in the United States, 10% or fewer patients do so.[151] In fact, 40% to 50% of patients are found to have distant metastatic disease upon completion of the initial staging.[112,113] Inconsistencies, discrepancies, and misunderstandings regarding the level of symptoms, the point at which palliation is required, and the conditions that can be palliated further cloud the issue. Moreover, despite R0 resection, some surgeons take a nihilistic approach, classifying all patients with locally advanced tumors in the palliative rather than the potentially curative category, which makes evaluations of survival difficult at best.

Patients with gastric cancer may present with symptoms including bleeding, obstruction, pain, early satiety, and weight loss. A review by Miner and colleagues[235] used a single institution's prospective database to examine 307 patients with gastric cancer who had undergone a noncurative resection. Roughly half of the patients received what the Miner group termed a "truly palliative" resection—most commonly for bleeding (20%), obstruction (43%), or pain (29%). Only 2% of the procedures were performed emergently, which may have been a reflection of the tertiary-care nature of the institution. As might be expected, patients in the palliative group had a much poorer survival duration than did the patients in the nonpalliative group, which contained many patients who had positive-margin resections. Age was also a significant risk factor, with older patients having a worse survival duration.

Kahlke and colleagues[236] found similar results in their review of 169 patients with incurable gastric cancer who underwent surgery. They classified symptoms as major (significant bleeding, confirmed obstruction, or perforation) or minor (all others). They also determined whether patients underwent a resection or simply an exploratory procedure. They found that major symptoms portended poorer survival, but, interestingly, that the type of surgical procedure had no bearing on survival.

In a large review, the American College of Surgeons surveyed more than 18,000 patients with gastric cancer, demonstrating that most patients do not need immediate surgical palliation.[151] Relatively few patients present with complete obstruction; early satiety and dysphagia are much more common. Similarly, patients with gastric cancer do not usually present with massive bleeding; however, many patients are anemic or have guaiac-positive stools at the time of presentation. These differences at presentation permit a broader range of treatment options and provide the time necessary for a complete staging work-up.

Surgery clearly provides the best chance for long-term survival and should be performed for any patient without distant disease unless extenuating circumstances preclude it. However, as noted in the studies described earlier, surgery is not necessarily the best way to obviate symptoms caused by gastric cancer in patients with metastasis. When making decisions about surgical palliation, physicians must keep in mind the expected life span of patients with metastatic disease. Among patients with carcinomatosis, the median survival duration is only about 5 months; 1-year survivors are relatively unusual.[112] Patients with hepatic metastases survive only slightly longer (median survival duration: about 6 to 8 months). Furthermore, in our experience, patients with distant nodal disease have a median survival duration of 8 to 12 months. Patients with ascites may survive for 2 months or less, as may those with lymphangitic spread to the lungs or leptomeningeal disease, both of which are quite rare and usually quickly fatal. Bone marrow metastasis also carries a dismal prognosis. Properly evaluating palliative interventions for gastric cancer requires an understanding of the disease and of the morbidity and time to recovery associated with the planned treatment. The typical presenting symptoms of gastric cancer and the options for alleviating them are described below.

Pain Pain is clearly the most subjective symptom a patient with gastric cancer may have. Pain in a patient can range from no pain at all to pain requiring massive quantities of narcotics. Pain may be caused by invasion of the celiac plexus, by intestinal obstruction, or by bone metastases.

Obstruction can confound the problem of pain management. In the absence of obstruction, long-acting oral narcotics can be easily used. However, if obstruction is present, other methods are required. Until recently, the need for intravenous pain management often required that patients spend their last days in the hospital receiving intravenous medication. However, the development of transdermal fentanyl patches, fentanyl lollipops and sublingual morphine, and anxiolytics have allowed patients to remain at home and keep relatively free from pain at the end of life.

Although celiac axis block has been employed relatively frequently for pancreatic cancer, it is used far less often for gastric cancer. Nevertheless, this technique should be considered for patients with severe intractable pain. Pain may also be caused by raw gastric mucosa; in patients with this problem, sucralfate slurry has been shown to frequently improve the pain. Ablative surgery is rarely indicated purely for the management of pain in such patients.

Several studies have examined pain as an aspect of quality of life. These studies have demonstrated an improvement in quality of life with the use of chemotherapy. For example, Glimelius and colleagues[208] performed a prospective randomized trial of 5-FU and leucovorin (plus etoposide in younger patients or in those with a good performance status) versus best supportive care alone (control). They assessed the quality of life in 61 patients by using the EORTC 30-item quality of life questionnaire. With statistical significance, a greater percentage of patients in the chemotherapy–plus–supportive care arm than in the control arm had improvement in or prolongation of a high quality of life (45% versus 20%; $p < .05$). These results were found with a minimum follow-up duration of 4 months and evaluation by the patients. The physician assessment resulted in a higher perception of improvement in the chemotherapy–plus–supportive care arm (55%; $p < .01$), but mirrored the patient evaluation in the control arm. In addition, the quality-adjusted duration of survival and time to progression were significantly greater in the treatment arm (5 months versus 2 months; $p = .03$), whereas the difference in overall survival was not significant. In an earlier study, the same group found that, among patients with the common gastrointestinal cancers (gastric, pancreatic, and colon), those with gastric cancer were the only group to experience a benefit in terms of survival when receiving palliative chemotherapy versus supportive care alone (10 months versus 4 months; $p < .02$).[208] The researchers also found that, although the average cost of all medical care was about 50% higher in the chemotherapy group, the cost per day was equivalent in the two groups and thus strongly supported the use of chemotherapy in these patients.

Bone metastasis is relatively unusual with gastric cancer, occurring in only about 1% to 2% of patients. However, bone metastasis does appear to be more common in patients with diffuse-type disease and in younger patients (in whom an increased incidence of bone metastasis is seen). In our experience, at least 10% of patients with linitis plastica experience bone metastasis. Bone pain may be best treated with external-beam radiation as described in a study by Yoshikawa and Kitaoka.[237] Those authors evaluated 23 patients with bone metastases seen over a 10-year period. They found that radiotherapy, but not chemotherapy, alleviated the pain, but that patients survived only a few months after the discovery of the bone metastases. Metastases rarely develop in weight-bearing bones; when it happens, orthopedic intervention may be required. Life expectancy is so short in most of these patients that such intervention is often not necessary, but it must be considered carefully.

Bleeding Given the broad spectrum of severity of bleeding, there are perhaps more treatment options for it than for any other symptom of gastric cancer.

Massive bleeding may be treated with arterial embolization or endoscopy; however, resection will usually be required to control the hemorrhage. Only in cases of widely metastatic disease should avoidance of any intervention for bleeding be considered. Telling a patient with newly diagnosed gastric cancer—and that patient's family—about such treatment avoidance is very difficult, but in some instances, it is the right thing to do.

Embolization is a temporizing procedure. As such, it may be used to buy time to complete a work-up or to discuss resuscitation status. Endoscopy with the use of either a heater probe or an argon coagulator can also temporarily control bleeding.

For patients who are experiencing slow oozing and who need a transfusion every 1 to 2 weeks, endoscopy may be successful. Chemotherapy may be risky for patients who are losing blood at such a rate. However, once given, chemotherapy will often further slow blood loss in patients who were losing blood at a slow rate. However, the risk in this case is that the patient may have a major bleeding event at a time when blood counts are low. Savides and colleagues[238] evaluated 42 patients with malignancy and blood loss. In half of these patients, the loss was acute and severe. Patients underwent a combination of cautery and epinephrine injection. One-third of the patients had a recurrence of bleeding, and just over 40% needed an operation. Even with those interventions, the 1-year survival rate was only 11%. Additionally, Loftus and colleagues[239] reported on 15 patients with major upper gastrointestinal bleeding from malignancy that was treated endoscopically. Of those 15 patients, 11 had gastric cancer. The patients underwent epinephrine injections and heater probe or laser coagulation. The bleeding initially stopped in 10 patients. However, 8 of the 10 had a recurrence of bleeding, and one-third of the patients experienced major complications. Two patients died of treatment-related causes.

We have found chemoradiation to be very effective in controlling blood loss in patients who are slowly losing blood. Roughly 80% of patients no longer need transfusions after undergoing chemoradiation. We prefer to use a radiosensitizing dose of 5-FU at 300 mg/m^2 per day, administered by continuous infusion while using external-beam radiation to a dose of 45 Gy over 5 weeks. Several series have indicated that 50% to 75% of patients experience improvement of bleeding, gastric outlet obstruction, and pain with this method.[240,241]

As described earlier, physicians must decide whether patients who are bleeding massively are surgical candidates. They must then either take those patients to the operating room or simply make them comfortable and allow them to die. Endoscopic and embolization maneuvers can occasionally provide the time necessary to make these often difficult discussions.

Obstruction, Dysphagia, and Early Satiety The occurrence of proximal gastrointestinal tract obstruction in patients with gastric cancer is highly dependent on the location of the primary tumor. However, given the high incidence of peritoneal metastasis in these patients, small-bowel and colonic obstructions occur relatively frequently. Aranha and colleagues[242] reviewed 73 patients with small-bowel obstruction secondary to metastatic carcinoma, some of whom had gastric cancer. Those authors found relatively high operative morbidity and mortality rates in those patients. The mortality rate dropped over time; but, even in the most recent period, it exceeded 10%. In general, patients with small-bowel obstruction secondary to metastatic gastric cancer have survival durations that range from a few weeks to a few months.

Dysphagia is typically graded on a scale of 0 to 4, with 0 being no dysphagia, 1 being dysphagia to solid foods, 2 being dysphagia to soft foods, 3 being dysphagia to liquids, and 4 being complete obstruction. Tumors in the body of the stomach are rarely obstructive unless they are of the linitis plastica variety (in which case they are typically functional obstructions rather than mechanical ones). Cardial tumors may be obstructive in a manner that resembles esophageal tumors; prepyloric tumors may be obstructive in a manner that resembles pancreatic cancer.

Many of the evaluations of treatment options for obstruction by a proximal tumor mix patients having those tumors with patients having esophageal tumors. In many instances, the differences are irrelevant. The treatment options for obstruction include laser recanalization, stenting, radiotherapy, bypass, insertion of drainage tubes, and resection. Studies have evaluated interventions ranging from supportive care only to aggressive resection with colonic interposition. However, in the face of metastatic disease, resection should be applied very cautiously. In the absence of large prospective randomized trials, an evaluation of all the studies that discuss resection for palliation suggests that caution should be exercised, considering the inherent bias of not attempting resection in patients with very advanced disease and then attempting to compare patients who have undergone resection with those patients. If a patient's disease is so advanced that the physician will not consider resection, it should not be surprising that the patient fares poorly (as seen in the report by Miner and colleagues[235]).

The technology of expandable stents, such as the Wall stent, has expanded dramatically over the past few years. In a systematic review, Dormann and colleagues[243] reviewed 136 publications reporting the use of self-expanding metal stents for gastroduodenal malignancies in 32 case series. They found that, in 606 patients, stent placement was successful in 97%, and that the placement was technically successful in 87%. They found no procedure-related mortality and a relatively low number of complications. However, in 18% of the cases, the stent became occluded secondary to tumor ingrowth. Fiori and colleagues[244] also conducted a small (18 patients) prospective randomized trial comparing bypass and stenting. They found no differences in morbidity, mortality, emptying, or clinical outcome with the two procedures, indicating that stenting is truly an effective alternative to bypass in patients with gastric cancer.

Endoscopic ablative techniques have also been used to relieve dysphagia. The rate of improvement with these techniques is often rapid, usually requires only one treatment, and shows relatively low complication rates. Success rates are typically high (about 90%), but durability is a potential concern.

Carter and colleagues[245] treated malignant dysphagia in 141 patients with an Nd:YAG laser system and found that 92% of the patients experienced an improvement in swallowing, with 6% suffering a perforation and 3% having a fistula. Mason and colleagues[246] reported a similar rate of initial improvement of symptoms in 189 patients. However, after 6 months, almost 90% of the patients had died. Most of these patients appeared to have had an improvement in their measured quality of life early after treatment. However, as patients near death, their quality of life deteriorates rapidly.[247]

In yet another study, Heindorff and colleagues[248] used argon-beam electrocoagulation in 83 patients. More than half of the patients were able to eat normal food after one treatment, but 16% were never able to eat normal food again. The treatment was repeated every 4 weeks, as needed. The investigators found 7 perforations and were able to manage all but one of them conservatively.

Sargeant and colleagues[249] conducted a prospective randomized trial of the addition of external-beam radiation to laser ablation for the palliation of dysphagia. They randomized 67 patients to receive 30 Gy in 10 fractions or no radiation and then observed the patients. While there was no difference in the immediate improvement of symptoms, the radiotherapy reduced the need for subsequent ablations, doubling the time between treatments. But that benefit did not come without a price, because several of the irradiated patients needed dilatation, which resulted in fistulae and perforations in a few cases.

Spencer and colleagues[250] had a similar intent with the use of brachytherapy in 19 patients. They administered 10 Gy after laser ablation and then observed the patients. One-third of the patients needed no further therapy, and those who did need further ablation did not need a repeat of the procedure for a median of 11 weeks. The median survival duration was approximately 8 months. In addition, Highley and colleagues[251] prospectively evaluated the use of post-treatment systemic chemotherapy (cisplatin, epirubicin, and 5-FU) in 34 patients with malignant dysphagia treated with laser ablation. Almost 60% of the patients had a response to the chemotherapy, with a significant improvement in dysphagia and a reduction in the need for additional laser ablation.

Lo and colleagues[252] examined the use of gastrojejunostomy in 51 patients with gastric cancer and reported an operative mortality rate of 22% and an operative morbidity rate of 55%. The median survival duration was only 14 weeks (2 of which were spent recuperating in the hospital), and more than 20% of the patients suffered delayed gastric emptying. Thus, nearly 50% of the patients (those with delayed gastric emptying plus operative mortality) did not benefit from the procedure. Nevertheless, the authors concluded that gastrojejunostomy is a satisfactory palliative intervention.

Kikuchi and colleagues[124] also examined the use of gastrojejunostomy in 52 patients with antral obstruction, finding a median survival duration of only 5 months and a median palliation duration of less than 3 months. They concluded that justifying this approach in patients with antral obstruction is difficult.

One of the most difficult problems in evaluating the role of resection in palliation is determining the true intent of the operation. Although many surgeons may consider a procedure to be palliative based on their pessimism, the reality may be far different. That concern is at the core of the report by Miner and colleagues[235] One of the most telling examples of this concern is the report by Ekbom and Gleysteen,[253] who reviewed 144 patients with gastric cancer, 55 of whom appeared to have undergone truly palliative resection, and 20 of whom underwent bypass procedures (the remainder underwent potentially curative resections). The survival and symptom relief duration were both markedly better in the resection group than in the bypass group. However, determining whether these groups are truly comparable is difficult. The finding of a long survival duration in patients ostensibly receiving palliative treatment often raises questions as to the intent of the operation, because documentation is often poor.

In comparison, Ouchi and colleagues[254] evaluated 95 patients with peritoneal disease who had undergone palliative procedures—64 resections, 15 bypasses, and 16 explorations alone—in the palliative setting. Of these patients, 94 had stage IV disease. In many of the patients, the stage was based on the presence of disease in sites other than the peritoneum, because the disease was staged as P0 or P1 (no visible peritoneal disease or disease adjacent only to the stomach) in 62 patients and P2 or P3 (scattered metastases to the distant peritoneum or numerous metastases throughout the peritoneum) in 33 patients. Overall, the 3-month hospitalization-free survival rate was 70%. In patients with P2 or P3 disease, the median survival was only 7 months, which (not surprisingly) was less than that in the group with little or no peritoneal disease. Patients who underwent a total gastrectomy with P2 or P3 disease had a median survival of less than 6 months; those who underwent a distal resection had a median survival duration of about 8 months. There were no 2-year survivors in the total gastrectomy group. The authors concluded that neither total gastrectomy or bypass was of benefit in patients with any peritoneal disease away from the stomach.

One of the more aggressive approaches for proximal gastric tumors was reported by Saidi and colleagues.[136] In 70 patients, 49 of whom had stage IV disease, those authors performed a total gastrectomy with mucosectomy of the esophagus and colonic interposition through the deepithelialized esophagus. The operative mortality rate was 10%, and 58 patients had a median survival duration of 17 months. The authors suggested that their approach provided distinct palliation, although that conclusion is debatable. In addition, as described earlier, the median survival duration of 17 months raises suspicion of the likely potential curative aspect in many such patients.

For patients at an advanced age, some authors have suggested that the benefits of potentially curative resection diminish to the point that all such maneuvers are to be considered palliative. Specifically, Ishigami and colleagues[255] found that 1 of every 4 patients over the age of 85 years with gastric cancer was an unfit candidate for surgery and that the patients who did undergo surgery had significantly more complications. We take a highly selective approach to such patients, considering resection based on their physiologic condition. However, in a study of 24 patients over the age of 80 years, Matsushita and colleagues[256] concluded that age alone should not be a reason to avoid the use of potentially curative procedures.

Dysphagia and obstruction are the biggest problem in patients with gastric cancer and have the widest array of management options. Unfortunately, each option has its benefits and risks, such that, in the absence of an institutional protocol, strong consideration must be given to patient comfort and compliance concerns, as well as to the expertise within the institution, before the best treatment approach can be determined.

NUTRITION Roughly half of all patients with gastric cancer have experienced weight loss by the time of presentation. For many patients, maintaining a proper diet is simply a matter of changing to more nutritious foods. Others may need to change to a completely liquid diet with nutritional supplements. The remaining patients are not able to maintain adequate caloric intake regardless of dietary manipulations.

As part of our complete staging of gastric cancer, we routinely perform laparoscopy. In this setting, using a T-fastener kit, we place a feeding jejunostomy tube either for support during planned therapy (preoperative or definitive) or for nutritional support. Patients who later chose to simply let their disease take its course, can have the tube removed after a few weeks. Few actually do so.

Numerous supplements are available, and patients may have to experiment to find the ones that they tolerate best. To help facilitate as normal a lifestyle as possible, we structure feedings so that they take place at night.

The use of total parenteral nutrition for patients with metastatic gastric cancer is very difficult to justify. The rare exception is the patient who would otherwise be a candidate for aggressive systemic therapy.

Good understanding of patients and coherent communication of the pros and cons of the various options for palliative care are essential. There is no best approach to palliation with gastric cancer. However, understanding what can and should be palliated will go a long way to help physicians determine the best method of palliation. We generally encourage consideration of protocol-based chemotherapeutic options for patients with metastatic disease who are able to tolerate chemotherapy. For patients with slow blood loss, we generally use chemoradiation to effectively control the bleeding. Patients with metastatic disease remain the most difficult group to administer treatment to.

CONCLUSIONS

Fortunately, the incidence of gastric cancer is decreasing around the world. However, this decrease is being accompanied by a change in pattern toward more-aggressive variants of the disease. Despite some progress in all areas of management of gastric cancer (surgery, chemotherapy, radiotherapy), most patients in the United States diagnosed with gastric cancer will die of their disease. The ability to define who will develop the disease will lead to the creation of screening and preventive measures.

As the age of targeted molecular therapy begins, agents that target the *VEGF* and *EGFR* systems are entering phase II trials in gastric cancer. Improvements in our understanding of molecular biology and the molecular classification of gastric cancer may lead to rational development of novel therapeutic strategies for the disease.

REFERENCES

1. La Vecchia C, Negri E, D'Avanzo B, Franceschi S. Electric refrigerator use and gastric cancer risk. Br J Cancer 1990;62:136–7.
2. Blot WJ, Devesa SS, Kneller RW, Fraumeni JF Jr. Rising incidence of adenocarcinoma of the esophagus and gastric cardia. JAMA 1991;265:1287–9.
3. Surveillance, Epidemiology, and End Results (SEER) Program. Public-use data (1973–1999). Bethesda, MD: National Cancer Institute, DCCPS, Surveillance Research Program, Cancer Statistics Branch; April 2002. [Electronic resource]
4. Jemal A, Tiwari RC, Murray T, et al. Cancer statistics, 2004. CA Cancer J Clin 2004;54:8–29.
5. Wiggins CL, Becker TM, Key CR, Samet JM. Stomach cancer among New Mexico's American Indians, Hispanic whites, and non-Hispanic whites. Cancer Res 1989;49:1595–9.
6. Pisani P, Parkin DM, Bray F, Ferlay J. Estimates of the worldwide mortality from 25 cancers in 1990. Int J Cancer 1999;83:18–29.
7. Parkin DM, Pisani P, Ferlay J. Global cancer statistics. CA Cancer J Clin 1999;49:33–64.
8. Lauren P. The two histological main types of gastric carcinoma: diffuse and so-called intestinal-type carcinoma. An attempt at a histoclinical classification. Acta Pathol Microbiol Scand 1965;64:31–49.
9. Morson B. Carcinoma arising from areas of intestinal metaplasia in the gastric mucosa. Br J Cancer 1955;9:377–85.
10. Nomura A, Chyou PH, Stemmermann GN. Association of serum ferritin levels with the risk of stomach cancer. Cancer Epidemiol Biomarkers Prev 1992;1:547–50.
11. Dubrow R. Gastric cancer following peptic ulcer surgery [editorial; comment]. J Natl Cancer Inst 1993;85:1268–70.
12. La Vecchia C, Negri E, Franceschi S, Gentile A. Family history and the risk of stomach and colorectal cancer. Cancer 1992;70:50–5.
13. Munoz SE, Ferraroni M, La Vecchia C, Decarli A. Gastric cancer risk factors in subjects with family history. Cancer Epidemiol Biomarkers Prev 1997;6:137–40.
14. Offerhaus GJ, Giardiello FM, Krush AJ, et al. The risk of upper gastrointestinal cancer in familial adenomatous polyposis. Gastroenterology 1992;102:1980–2.
15. Correa P, Cuello C, Duque E, et al. Gastric cancer in Colombia. III. Natural history of precursor lesions. J Natl Cancer Inst 1976;57:1027–35.
16. Haenszel W, Kurihara M, Locke FB, et al. Stomach cancer in Japan. J Natl Cancer Inst 1976;56:265–74.
17. Barrett JH, Parslow RC, McKinney PA, et al. Nitrate in drinking water and the incidence of gastric, esophageal, and brain cancer in Yorkshire, England. Cancer Causes Control 1998;9:153–9.
18. Galanis DJ, Kolonel LN, Lee J, Nomura A. Intakes of selected foods and beverages and the incidence of gastric cancer among the Japanese residents of Hawaii: a prospective study. Int J Epidemiol 1998;27:173–80.
19. Webb PM, Bates CJ, Palli D, Forman D. Gastric cancer, gastritis and plasma vitamin C: results from an international correlation and cross-sectional study. The Eurogast Study Group. Int J Cancer 1997;73:684–9.
20. La Vecchia C, Munoz SE, Braga C, et al. Diet diversity and gastric cancer. Intl J Cancer 1997;72:255–7.
21. De Stefani E, Ronco A, Brennan P, Boffetta P. Meat consumption and risk of stomach cancer in Uruguay: a case-control study. Nutr Cancer 2001;40:103–7.
22. Ward MH, Sinha R, Heineman EF, et al. Risk of adenocarcinoma of the stomach and esophagus with meat cooking method and doneness preference. Int J Cancer 1997;71:14–9.
23. Coggon D, Barker DJ, Cole RB. Stomach cancer and work in dusty industries. Br J Ind Med 1990;47:298–301.
24. Chyou PH, Nomura AM, Hankin JH, Stemmermann GN. A case–cohort study of diet and stomach cancer. Cancer Res 1990;50:7501–4.
25. Kneller R, McLaughlin J, Bjelke E, et al. A cohort study of stomach cancer in a high-risk American population. Cancer 1991;68:672–8.
26. Blot WJ. Alcohol and cancer. Cancer Res 1992;52(7 Suppl):2119s–2123s.
27. Zhang L, Blot WJ, You WC, et al. *Helicobacter pylori* antibodies in relation to precancerous gastric lesions in a high-risk Chinese population. Cancer Epidemiol Biomarkers Prev 1996;5:627–30.
28. Guiraldes E, Pena A, Duarte I, et al. Nature and extent of gastric lesions in symptomatic Chilean children with *Helicobacter pylori*-associated gastritis. Acta Paediatr 2002;91:39–44.
29. Chow WH, Blot WJ, Vaughan TL, et al. Body mass index and risk of adenocarcinomas of the esophagus and gastric cardia. J Natl Cancer Inst 1998;90:150–5.
30. Blaser MJ, Chyou PH, Nomura A. Age at establishment of *Helicobacter pylori* infection and gastric carcinoma, gastric ulcer, and duodenal ulcer risk. Cancer Res 1995;55:562–5.
31. Harris RA, Owens DK, Witherell H, Parsonnet J. *Helicobacter pylori* and gastric cancer: what are the benefits of screening only for the *CAGA* phenotype of *H. pylori*? Helicobacter 1999;4:69–76.
32. Levine PH, Stemmermann G, Lennette ET, et al. Elevated antibody titers to Epstein–Barr virus prior to the diagnosis of Epstein–Barr-virus-associated gastric adenocarcinoma. Int J Cancer 1995;60:642–4.
33. Pera M, Cameron AJ, Trastek VF, et al. Increasing incidence of adenocarcinoma of the esophagus and esophagogastric junction. Gastroenterology 1993;104:510–3.
34. Hundahl SA, Phillips JL, Menck HR. The National Cancer Data Base Report on poor survival of U.S. gastric carcinoma patients treated with gastrectomy: Fifth Edition American Joint Committee on cancer staging, proximal disease, and the "different disease" hypothesis. Cancer 2000;88:921–32.
35. Bonenkamp JJ, Hermans J, Sasako M, van de Velde CJ. Extended lymph-node dissection for gastric cancer. Dutch Gastric Cancer Group. N Engl J Med 1999;340:908–14.
36. Inoue M, Tajima K, Hirose K, et al. Life-style and subsite of gastric cancer—joint effect of smoking and drinking habits. Int J Cancer 1994;56:494–9.
37. Kim JP, Lee JH, Kim SJ, et al. Clinicopathologic characteristics and prognostic factors in 10783 patients with gastric cancer. Gastric Cancer 1998;1:125–33.
38. Powell J, McConkey CC. The rising trend in oesophageal adenocarcinoma and gastric cardia. Eur J Cancer Prev 1992;1:265–9.
39. Lagergren J, Bergstrom R, Nyren O. Association between body mass and adenocarcinoma of the esophagus and gastric cardia. Ann Intern Med 1999;130:883–90.
40. Yao JC, Schnirer II, Reddy S, et al. Effects of sex and racial/ethnic group on the pattern of gastric cancer localization. Gastric Cancer 2002;5:208–12.
41. van Dekken H, Geelen E, Dinjens WN, et al. Comparative genomic hybridization of cancer of the gastroesophageal junction: deletion of 14q31–32.1 discriminates between esophageal (Barrett's) and gastric cardia adenocarcinomas. Cancer Res 1999;59:748–52.

42. Huntsman DG, Carneiro F, Lewis FR, et al. Early gastric cancer in young, asymptomatic carriers of germ-line E-cadherin mutation. N Engl J Med 2001;344:1904–9.
43. Esaki Y, Hirayama R, Hirokawa K. A comparison of patterns of metastasis in gastric cancer by histologic type and age. Cancer 1990;65:2086–90.
44. Maehara Y, Moriguchi S, Kakeji Y, et al. Pertinent risk factors and gastric carcinoma with synchronous peritoneal dissemination or liver metastasis. Surgery 1991;110:820–3.
45. Takahashi Y, Cleary KR, Mai M, et al. Significance of vessel count and vascular endothelial growth factor and its receptor (*KDR*) in intestinal-type gastric cancer. Clin Cancer Res 1996;2:1679–84.
46. Maeda K, Chung YS, Ogawa Y, et al. Prognostic value of vascular endothelial growth factor expression in gastric carcinoma. Cancer 1996;77:858–63.
47. Yonemura Y, Endo Y, Fujita H, et al. Role of vascular endothelial growth factor C expression in the development of lymph node metastasis in gastric cancer. Clin Cancer Res 1999;5:1823–9.
48. Amioka T, Kitadai Y, Tanaka S, et al. Vascular endothelial growth factor-C expression predicts lymph node metastasis of human gastric carcinomas invading the submucosa. Eur J Cancer 2002;38:1413–9.
49. Koyama T, Yashiro M, Inoue T, et al. TGF-beta1 secreted by gastric fibroblasts up-regulates CD44H expression and stimulates the peritoneal metastatic ability of scirrhous gastric cancer cells. Int J Oncol 2000;16:355–62.
50. Tsugawa K, Yonemura Y, Hirono Y, et al. Amplification of the c-*met*, c-*erb*B-2 and epidermal growth factor receptor gene in human gastric cancers: correlation to clinical features. Oncology 1998;55:475–81.
51. Taniguchi K, Yonemura Y, Nojima N, et al. The relation between the growth patterns of gastric carcinoma and the expression of hepatocyte growth factor receptor (c-*met*), autocrine motility factor receptor, and urokinase-type plasminogen activator receptor. Cancer 1998;82:2112–22.
52. Guilford P, Hopkins J, Harraway J, et al. E-Cadherin germline mutations in familial gastric cancer. Nature 1998;392:402–5.
53. Keller G, Vogelsang H, Becker I, et al. Diffuse type gastric and lobular breast carcinoma in a familial gastric cancer patient with an E-cadherin germline mutation. Am J Pathol 1999;155:337–42.
54. Caldas C, Carneiro F, Lynch HT, et al. Familial gastric cancer: overview and guidelines for management. J Med Genet 1999;36:873–80.
55. Abraham SC, Nobukawa B, Giardiello FM, et al. Fundic gland polyps in familial adenomatous polyposis: neoplasms with frequent somatic adenomatous polyposis coli gene alterations. Am J Pathol 2000;157:747–54.
56. Hofgartner WT, Thorp M, Ramus MW, et al. Gastric adenocarcinoma associated with fundic gland polyps in a patient with attenuated familial adenomatous polyposis. Am J Gastroenterol 1999;94:2275–81.
57. Park WS, Oh RR, Kim YS, et al. Absence of mutations in the kinase domain of the *met* gene and frequent expression of Met and Hgf/SF protein in primary gastric carcinomas. APMIS 2000;108:195–200.
58. Shinmura K, Kohno T, Takahashi M, et al. Familial gastric cancer: clinicopathological characteristics, *RER* phenotype and germline *p53* and E-cadherin mutations. Carcinogenesis 1999;20:1127–31.
59. Endoh Y, Tamura G, Ajioka Y, et al. Frequent hypermethylation of the hMLH1 gene promoter in differentiated-type tumors of the stomach with the gastric foveolar phenotype. Am J Pathol 2000;157:717–22.
60. Bevilacqua RA, Simpson AJ. Methylation of the hMLH1 promoter but no hMLH1 mutations in sporadic gastric carcinomas with high-level microsatellite instability. Int J Cancer 2000;87:200–3.
61. Suzuki H, Itoh F, Toyota M, et al. Distinct methylation pattern and microsatellite instability in sporadic gastric cancer. Int J Cancer 1999;83:309–13.
62. Tamura G, Yin J, Wang S, et al. E-Cadherin gene promoter hypermethylation in primary human gastric carcinomas. J Natl Cancer Inst 2000;92:569–73.
63. Sato K, Tamura G, Tsuchiya T, et al. Frequent loss of expression without sequence mutations of the *DCC* gene in primary gastric cancer. Br J Cancer 2001;85:199–203.
64. Jang TJ, Kim DI, Shin YM, et al. $p16^{INK4a}$ Promoter hypermethylation of non-tumorous tissue adjacent to gastric cancer is correlated with glandular atrophy and chronic inflammation. Int J Cancer 2001;93:629–34.
65. Li QL, Ito K, Sakakura C, et al. Causal relationship between the loss of *RUNX3* expression and gastric cancer. Cell 2002;109:113–24.
66. Rhyu MG, Park WS, Jung YJ, et al. Allelic deletions of *MCC/APC* and *p53* are frequent late events in human gastric carcinogenesis. Gastroenterology 1994;106:1584–8.
67. Fang DC, Jass JR, Wang DX, et al. Infrequent loss of heterozygosity of *APC/MCC* and *DCC* genes in gastric cancer showing DNA microsatellite instability. J Clin Pathol 1999;52:504–8.
68. Chong JM, Fukayama M, Hayashi Y, et al. Microsatellite instability in the progression of gastric carcinoma. Cancer Res 1994;54:4595–7.
69. Semba S, Yokozaki H, Yamamoto S, et al. Microsatellite instability in precancerous lesions and adenocarcinomas of the stomach. Cancer 1996;77(8 Suppl):1620–7.
70. Ottini L, Palli D, Falchetti M, et al. Microsatellite instability in gastric cancer is associated with tumor location and family history in a high-risk population from Tuscany. Cancer Res 1997;57:4523–9.
71. Myeroff LL, Parsons R, Kim SJ, et al. A transforming growth factor beta receptor type II gene mutation common in colon and gastric but rare in endometrial cancers with microsatellite instability. Cancer Res 1995;55:5545–7.
72. Guo RJ, Arai H, Kitayama Y, et al. Microsatellite instability of papillary subtype of human gastric adenocarcinoma and hMLH1 promoter hypermethylation in the surrounding mucosa. Pathol Int 2001;51:240–7.
73. Wu MS, Shun CT, Wang HP, et al. Genetic alterations in gastric cancer: relation to histological subtypes, tumor stage, and *Helicobacter pylori* infection. Gastroenterology 1997;112:1457–65.
74. Brito MJ, Williams GT, Thompson H, Filipe MI. Expression of *p53* in early (T1) gastric carcinoma and precancerous adjacent mucosa. Gut 1994;35:1697–700.
75. Horii A, Nakatsuru S, Miyoshi Y, et al. The *APC* gene, responsible for familial adenomatous polyposis, is mutated in human gastric cancer. Cancer Res 1992;52:3231–3.
76. Hsieh LL, Huang YC. Loss of heterozygosity of *APC/MCC* gene in differentiated and undifferentiated gastric carcinomas in Taiwan. Cancer Lett 1995;96:169–74.
77. Fang DC, Jass JR, Wang DX. Loss of heterozygosity and loss of expression of the *DCC* gene in gastric cancer. J Clin Pathol 1998;51:593–6.
78. Graziano F, Cascinu S, Staccioli MP, et al. Potential role and chronology of abnormal expression of the deleted in colon cancer (*DCC*) and the *p53* proteins in the development of gastric cancer. BMC Cancer 2001;1:9.
79. Baffa R, Veronese ML, Santoro R, et al. Loss of *FHIT* expression in gastric carcinoma. Cancer Res 1998;58:4708–14.
80. Capuzzi D, Santoro E, Hauck WW, et al. *FHIT* expression in gastric adenocarcinoma: correlation with disease stage and survival. Cancer 2000;88:24–34.
81. Huiping C, Kristjansdottir S, Bergthorsson JT, et al. High frequency of LOH, MSI and abnormal expression of *FHIT* in gastric cancer. Eur J Cancer 2002;38:728–35.
82. Noguchi T, Muller W, Wirtz HC, et al. *FHIT* gene in gastric cancer: association with tumour progression and prognosis. J Pathol 1999;188:378–81.
83. Hirohashi S. Inactivation of the E-cadherin–mediated cell adhesion system in human cancers. Am J Pathol 1998;153:333–9.
84. Jawhari A, Jordan S, Poole S, et al. Abnormal immunoreactivity of the E-cadherin–catenin complex in gastric carcinoma: relationship with patient survival. Gastroenterology 1997;112:46–54.
85. Shun CT, Wu MS, Lin MT, et al. Immunohistochemical evaluation of cadherin and catenin expression in early gastric carcinomas: correlation with clinicopathologic characteristics and *Helicobacter pylori* infection. Oncology 2001;60:339–45.
86. Tamura G, Sakata K, Nishizuka S, et al. Inactivation of the E-cadherin gene in primary gastric carcinomas and gastric carcinoma cell lines. Jpn J Cancer Res 1996;87:1153–9.
87. Becker K, Atkinson M, Reich U, et al. E-Cadherin gene mutations provide clues to diffuse type gastric carcinomas. Cancer Res 1994;54:3845–52.
88. Ramesh S, Nash J, McCulloch PG. Reduction in membranous expression of beta-catenin and increased cytoplasmic E-cadherin expression predict poor survival in gastric cancer. Br J Cancer 1999;81:1392–7.
89. Park WS, Oh RR, Park JY, et al. Frequent somatic mutations of the beta-catenin gene in intestinal-type gastric cancer. Cancer Res 1999;59:4257–60.
90. Sato S, Yokozaki H, Yasui W, et al. Silencing of the *CD44* gene by CpG methylation in a human gastric carcinoma cell line. Jpn J Cancer Res 1999;90:485–9.
91. Setala L, Lipponen P, Tammi R, et al. Expression of *CD44* and its variant isoform v3 has no prognostic value in gastric cancer. Histopathology 2001;38:13–20.
92. Yoo CH, Noh SH, Kim H, et al. Prognostic significance of *CD44* and *NM23* expression in patients with stage II and stage IIIA gastric carcinoma. J Surg Oncol 1999;71:22–8.
93. Park HS, Won JH, Hong DS, et al. The overexpression of *MDR1*, c-*erbB*-2, and *EGFR* and its clinical relevance in gastric cancer [Abstract]. Proc Am Soc Clin Oncol 1995;14:A1370.
94. Dammrich J, Vollmers HP, Heider KH, Muller-Hermelink HK. Importance of different *CD44*v6 expression in human gastric intestinal and diffuse type cancers for metastatic lymphogenic spreading. J Mol Med 1995;73:395–401.
95. Yamaguchi A, Goi T, Yu J, et al. Expression of *CD44*v6 in advanced gastric cancer and its relationship to hematogenous metastasis and long-term prognosis. J Surg Oncol 2002;79:230–5.
96. Lee EY, Cibull ML, Strodel WE, Haley JV. Expression of *HER-2/neu* oncoprotein and epidermal growth factor receptor and prognosis in gastric carcinoma. Arch Pathol Lab Med 1994;118:235–9.
97. Slesak B, Harlozinska A, Porebska I, et al. Expression of epidermal growth factor receptor family proteins (*EGFR*, c-*erb*B-2 and c-*erb*B-3) in gastric cancer and chronic gastritis. Anticancer Res 1998;18:2727–32.
98. Aoyagi K, Kohfuji K, Yano S, et al. Evaluation of the epidermal growth factor receptor (*EGFR*) and c-*erb*B-2 in superspreading-type and penetrating-type gastric carcinoma. Kurume Med J 2001;48:197–200.
99. Albino AP, Jaehne J, Altorki N, et al. Amplification of *HER-2/neu* gene in human gastric adenocarcinomas: correlation with primary site. Eur J Surg Oncol 1995;21:56–60.
100. Jaehne J, Urmacher C, Thaler HT, et al. Expression of *HER2/neu* oncogene product p185 in correlation to clinicopathological and prognostic factors of gastric carcinoma. J Cancer Res Clin Oncol 1992;118:474–9.
101. Kuwahara A, Katano M, Nakamura M, et al. New therapeutic strategy for gastric carcinoma: a two-step evaluation of malignant potential from its molecular biologic and pathologic characteristics. J Surg Oncol 1999;72:142–9.
102. Katano M, Nakamura M, Fujimoto K, et al. Prognostic value of platelet-derived growth factor-A (PDGF-A) in gastric carcinoma. Ann Surg 1998;227:365–71.
103. Huang TJ, Wang JY, Lin SR, et al. Overexpression of the c-*met* protooncogene in human gastric carcinoma—correlation to clinical features. Acta Oncol 2001;40:638–43.
104. Maeda K, Kang SM, Onoda N, et al. Vascular endothelial growth factor expression in preoperative biopsy specimens correlates with disease recurrence in patients with early gastric carcinoma. Cancer 1999;86:566–71.
105. Maehara Y, Kabashima A, Koga T, et al. Vascular invasion and potential for tumor angiogenesis and metastasis in gastric carcinoma. Surgery 2000;128:408–16.
106. Yoshikawa T, Tsuburaya A, Kobayashi O, et al. Plasma concentrations of VEGF and bFGF in patients with gastric carcinoma. Cancer Lett 2000;153:7–12.
107. Anzai H, Kitadai Y, Bucana CD, et al. Expression of metastasis-related genes in surgical specimens of human gastric cancer can predict disease recurrence. Eur J Cancer 1998;34:558–65.
108. Yao JC, Wang L, Wei D, et al. Association between expression of transcription factor *SP1* and increased vascular endothelial growth factor expression, advanced stage, and poor survival in patients with resected gastric cancer. Clin Cancer Res 2004;10:4109–17.
109. Fleming ID, American Cancer Society, American College of Surgeons, American Joint Committee on Cancer. AJCC cancer staging manual. 5th ed. Philadelphia: Lippincott–Raven; 1997.
110. Davis GR. Neoplasms of the stomach. In: Sleisenger MH, Fordtran JS, editors. Gastrointestinal disease: pathophysiology diagnosis management. 4th ed. Philadelphia, London, Toronto, Montreal, Sydney, Tokyo: W.B. Saunders Company; 1989. p. 754.
111. Feussner H, Omote K, Fink U, et al. Pretherapeutic laparoscopic staging in advanced gastric carcinoma. Endoscopy 1999;31:342–7.
112. Lowy AM, Mansfield PF, Leach SD, Ajani J. Laparoscopic staging for gastric cancer. Surgery 1996;119:611–4.
113. Burke EC, Karpeh MS, Conlon KC, Brennan MF. Laparoscopy in the management of gastric adenocarcinoma. Ann Surg 1997;225:262–7.
114. Adachi Y, Shiraishi N, Kitano S. Modern treatment of early gastric cancer: review of the Japanese experience. Dig Surg 2002;19:333–9.
115. Abe N, Watanabe T, Suzuki K, et al. Risk factors predictive of lymph node metastasis in depressed early gastric cancer. Am J Surg 2002;183:168–72.

116. Maruyama K, Sasako M, Kinoshita T, et al. Surgical treatment for gastric cancer: the Japanese approach. Semin Oncol 1996;23:360–8.
117. Ono H, Kondo H, Gotoda T, et al. Endoscopic mucosal resection for treatment of early gastric cancer. Gut 2001;48:225–9.
118. Ohgami M, Kumai K, Otani Y, et al. Laparoscopic wedge resection of the stomach for early gastric cancer using a lifting-lesion method. Dig Surg 1994;11:64–7.
119. Adachi Y, Kitano S, Sugimachi K. Surgery for gastric cancer: 10-year experience worldwide. Gastric Cancer 2001;4:166–74.
120. Miura S, Kodera Y, Fujiwara M, et al. Laparoscopy-assisted distal gastrectomy with systemic lymph node dissection: a critical reappraisal from the viewpoint of lymph node retrieval. J Am Coll Surg 2004;198:933–8.
121. Isozaki H, Okajima K, Ichinona T, et al. Surgery for gastric cancer in patients with cirrhosis. Jpn J Surg 1997;27:17–21.
122. Ajani JA, Ota DM, Jessup JM, et al. Resectable gastric carcinoma. An evaluation of preoperative and postoperative chemotherapy. Cancer 1991;68:1501–6.
123. Meijer S, De Bakker OJ, Hoitsma HF. Palliative resection in gastric cancer. J Surg Oncol 1983;23:77–80.
124. Kikuchi S, Tsutsumi O, Kobyashi N, et al. Does gastrojejunostomy for unresectable cancer of the gastric antrum offer satisfactory palliation? Hepatogastroenterology 1999;46:584–7.
125. Hocking M, Vogel S. Postoperative delayed gastric emptying. In: Hocking M, Vogel S, editors. Woodward's postgastrectomy syndromes. Philadelphia: W.B. Saunders; 1991. p. 63–77.
126. Bozzetti F, Marubini E, Bonfanti G, et al. Subtotal versus total gastrectomy for gastric cancer. Five year survival rates in a multicenter randomized Italian trial. Ann Surg 1999;230:170–8.
127. Gouzi J, Huguier M, Fagniez P, et al. Total versus subtotal gastrectomy for adenocarcinoma of the gastric antrum. Ann Surg 1989;209:162–6.
128. Bozzetti F. Total versus subtotal gastrectomy in cancer of the distal stomach: facts and fantasy. Eur J Surg Oncol 1992;18:572–9.
129. Davies J, Johnston D, Sue-Ling H, et al. Total or subtotal gastrectomy for gastric carcinoma? A study of quality of life. World J Surg 1998;22:1048–55.
130. Siewert J, Stein H, Sendler A, Fink U. Surgical resection for cancer of the cardia. Semin Surg Oncol 1999;17:125–31.
131. Siewert J, Bottcher K, Stein H, et al. Problem of proximal third gastric carcinoma. World J Surg 1995;19:523–31.
132. Harrison LE, Karpeh MS, Brennan MF. Total gastrectomy is not necessary for proximal gastric cancer. Surgery 1998;123:127–30.
133. Shiraishi N, Adachi Y, Kitano S, et al. Clinical outcome of proximal versus total gastrectomy for proximal gastric cancer. World J Surg 2002;26:1150–4.
134. Buhl K, Schlag P, Herfarth C. Quality of life and functional results following different types of resection for gastric carcinoma. Eur J Surg Oncol 1990;16:404–9.
135. Spector NM, Hicks FD, Pickleman J. Quality of life and symptoms after surgery for gastroesophageal cancer: a pilot study. Gastroenterol Nurs 2002;25:120–5.
136. Saidi F, Keshoofy M, Abbassi-Dezfuli A, et al. A new approach to the palliation of advanced proximal gastric cancer. J Am Coll Surg 1999;189:259–68.
137. Maruyama K, Sasako M, Kinoshita T, et al. Computer assisted surgery for gastric cancer. In: Takahashi T, editor. Recent advances in management of digestive cancers. Berlin: Springer; 1993. p. 109–114.
138. Sasako M, McCulloch P, Kinoshita T, Maruyama K. New method to evaluate the therapeutic value of lymph node dissection for gastric cancer. Br J Surg 1995;82:346–51.
139. Wagner P, Ramaswamy A, Ruschoff J, et al. Lymph node counts in the upper abdomen: anatomical basis for lymphadenectomy in gastric cancer. Br J Surg 1991;78:825–7.
140. Candela FC, Urmacher C, Brennan MF. Comparison of the conventional method of lymph node staging with a comprehensive fat-clearing method for gastric adenocarcinoma. Cancer 1990;66:1828–32.
141. Lawrence W Jr, Menck HR, Steele GD Jr, Winchester DP. The National Cancer Data Base report on gastric cancer. Cancer 1995;75:1734–44.
142. Maruyama K, Okabayashi K, Kinoshita T. Progress in gastric cancer surgery in Japan and its limits of radicality. World J Surg 1987;11:418–25.
143. Roder J, Bottcher K, Siewert J, et al. Prognostic factors in gastric carcinoma: results of the German Gastric Carcinoma Study 1992. Cancer 1993;72:2089–97.
144. Dent DM, Madden MV, Price SK. Randomized comparison of R1 and R2 gastrectomy for gastric carcinoma. Br J Surg 1988;75:110–2.
145. Hartgrink HH, van de Velde CJ, Putter H, et al. Extended lymph node dissection for gastric cancer: who may benefit? Final results of the randomized Dutch Gastric Cancer Group Trial. J Clin Oncol 2004;22:2069–77.
146. Cuschieri A, Weeden S, Fielding J, et al. Patient survival after D1 and D2 resections for gastric cancer: long-term results of the MRC randomized surgical trial. Br J Cancer 1999;79:1522–30.
147. Robertson C, Chung S, Woods S, et al. A prospective randomized trial comparing R1 subtotal gastrectomy with R3 total gastrectomy for antral cancer. Ann Surg 1994;220:176–82.
148. Sano T, Sasako M, Yamamoto S, et al. Gastric cancer surgery: morbidity and mortality results from a prospective randomized controlled trial comparing D2 and extended para-aortic lymphadenectomy—Japan Clinical Oncology Group Study 9501. J Clin Oncol 2004;22:2767–73.
149. Karpeh MS, Leon L, Klimstra D, Brennan MF. Lymph node staging in gastric cancer: is location more important than number? An analysis of 1,038 patients. Ann Surg 2000;232:362–71.
150. Wanebo HJ, Kennedy BJ, Winchester DP, et al. Role of splenectomy in gastric cancer surgery: adverse effect of elective splenectomy on longterm survival. J Am Coll Surg 1997;185:177–84.
151. Wanebo HJ, Kennedy BJ, Chmiel J, et al. Cancer of the stomach. A patient care study by the American College of Surgeons. Ann Surg 1993;218:583–92.
152. Wanebo H, Kennedy B, Winchester D, et al. Gastric carcinoma: does lymph node dissection alter survival. J Am Coll Surg 1996;183:616–24.
153. Macdonald JS, Smalley SR, Benedetti J, et al. Chemoradiotherapy after surgery compared with surgery alone for adenocarcinoma of the stomach or gastroesophageal junction. N Engl J Med 2001;345:725–30.
154. Cady B, Rossi RL, Silverman ML, et al. Gastric adenocarcinoma. A disease in transition. Arch Surg 1989;124:303–8.
155. Piso P, Bellin T, Aselmann H, et al. Results of combined gastrectomy and pancreatic resection in patients with advanced primary gastric carcinoma. Dig Surg 2002;19:281–5.
156. Martin RC 2nd, Jaques DP, Brennan MF, Karpeh M. Achieving R0 resection for locally advanced gastric cancer: is it worth the risk of multiorgan resection? J Am Coll Surg 2002;194:568–77.
157. Martin RC, Jaques DP, Brennan MF, Karpeh M. Extended local resection for advanced gastric cancer: increased survival versus increased morbidity. Ann Surg 2002;236:159–65.
158. Bozzetti F, Bonfanti G, Castellani R, et al. Comparing reconstruction with Roux-en-Y to a pouch following total gastrectomy. J Am Coll Surg 1996;183:243–8.
159. Fuchs KH, Thiede A, Engemann R. Reconstruction of the food passage after total gastrectomy: randomized trial. World J Surg 1995;19:698–705; discussion 705–6.
160. Horvath OP, Kalmar K, Cseke L. Aboral pouch with preserved duodenal passage—new reconstruction method after total gastrectomy. Dig Surg 2002;19:261–4; discussion 264–6.
161. Kalmar K, Cseke L, Zambo K, Horvath OP. Comparison of quality of life and nutritional parameters after total gastrectomy and a new type of pouch construction with simple Roux-en-Y reconstruction: preliminary results of a prospective, randomized, controlled study. Dig Dis Sci 2001;46:1791–6.
162. Liedman B. Symptoms after total gastrectomy on food intake, body composition, bone metabolism, and quality of life in gastric cancer patients—is reconstruction with a reservoir worthwhile? Nutrition 1999;15:677–82.
163. Meyer HJ, Opitz GJ. Stomach carcinoma. Optimizing therapy by stomach replacement or subtotal resection? Zentralbl Chir 1999;124:381–6.
164. Mochiki E, Kamimura H, Haga N, et al. The technique of laparoscopically assisted total gastrectomy with jejunal interposition for early gastric cancer. Surg Endosc 2002;16:540–4.
165. Nakane Y, Michiura T, Inoue K, et al. A randomized clinical trial of pouch reconstruction after total gastrectomy for cancer: which is the better technique, Roux-en-Y or interposition? Hepatogastroenterology 2001;48:903–7.
166. Svedlund J, Sullivan M, Liedman B, et al. Quality of life after gastrectomy for gastric carcinoma: controlled study of reconstructive procedures. World J Surg 1997;21:422–33.
167. Doberneck RC, Berndt GA. Delayed gastric emptying after palliative gastrojejunostomy for carcinoma of the pancreas. Arch Surg 1987;122:827–9.
168. Yao JC, Shimada K, Ajani JA. Adjuvant therapy for gastric carcinoma: closing out the century. Oncology (Huntingt) 1999;13:1485–94; discussion 1497–502.
169. Earle CC, Maroun JA. Adjuvant chemotherapy after curative resection for gastric cancer in non-Asian patients: revisiting a meta-analysis of randomised trials. Eur J Cancer 1999;35:1059–64.
170. Janunger KG, Hafstrom L, Nygren P, Glimelius B. A systematic overview of chemotherapy effects in gastric cancer. Acta Oncol 2001;40:309–26.
171. Imanaga H, Nakazato H. Results of surgery for gastric cancer and effect of adjuvant mitomycin C on cancer recurrence. World J Surg 1977;2:213–21.
172. Grau J, Estape J, Alcobendas F, et al. Positive results of adjuvant mitomycin-C in resected gastric cancer: a randomised trial on 134 patients. Eur J Cancer 1993;29A:340–2.
173. Neri B, de Leonardis V, Romano S, et al. Adjuvant chemotherapy after gastric resection in node-positive cancer patients: a multicentre randomised study. Br J Cancer 1996;73:549–52.
174. Grau JJ, Estape J, Fuster J, et al. Randomized trial of adjuvant chemotherapy with mitomycin plus Ftorafur versus mitomycin alone in resected locally advanced gastric cancer. J Clin Oncol 1998;16:1036–9.
175. Schiessel R, Funovics J, Schick B, et al. Adjuvant intraperitoneal cisplatin therapy in patients with operated gastric carcinoma: results of a randomized trial. Acta Med Austriaca 1989;16:68–9.
176. Sautner T, Hofbauer F, Depisch D, et al. Adjuvant intraperitoneal cisplatin chemotherapy does not improve long-term survival after surgery for advanced gastric cancer. J Clin Oncol 1994;12:970–4.
177. Hagiwara A, Takahashi T, Kojima O, et al. Prophylaxis with carbon-adsorbed mitomycin against peritoneal recurrence of gastric cancer. Lancet 1992;339:629–31.
178. Rosen HR, Jatzko G, Repse S, et al. Adjuvant intraperitoneal chemotherapy with carbon-adsorbed mitomycin in patients with gastric cancer: results of a randomized multicenter trial of the Austrian Working Group for Surgical Oncology. J Clin Oncol 1998;16:2733–8.
179. Yu W, Whang I, Suh I, et al. Prospective randomized trial of early postoperative intraperitoneal chemotherapy as an adjuvant to resectable gastric cancer. Ann Surg 1998;228:347–54.
180. Yonemura Y, Fujimura T, Fushida S, et al. Hyperthermochemotherapy combined with cytoreductive surgery for the treatment of gastric cancer with peritoneal dissemination. World J Surg 1991;15:530–5; discussion 535–6.
181. Mansfield P. Intraperitoneal hyperthermic chemotherapy for gastric cancer. In: Siewert JR, Roder JD, editors. Progress in gastric cancer research 1997. Proceedings of the 2nd International Gastric Cancer Congress; 1997 Apr 27–30; Munich, Germany. Bologna: Monduzzi Editore; 1997. p. 244(76).
182. The Italian Gastrointestinal Tumor Study Group. Adjuvant treatments following curative resection for gastric cancer. Br J Surg 1988;75:1100–4.
183. Jakesz R, Dittrich C, Funovics J, et al. The effect of adjuvant chemotherapy in gastric carcinoma is dependent on tumor histology: 5-year results of a prospective randomized trial. Recent Results Cancer Res 1988;110:44–51.
184. Kim JP, Kwon OJ, Oh ST, Yang HK. Results of surgery on 6589 gastric cancer patients and immunochemosurgery as the best treatment of advanced gastric cancer. Ann Surg 1992;216:269–78; discussion 278–9.
185. Moertel CG, Childs DS Jr, Reitemeier RJ, et al. Combined 5-fluorouracil and supervoltage radiation therapy of locally unresectable gastrointestinal cancer. Lancet 1969;2:865–7.
186. Gastrointestinal Tumor Study Group. A comparison of combination chemotherapy and combined modality therapy for locally advanced gastric carcinoma. Cancer 1982;49:1771–7.
187. Gastrointestinal Tumor Study Group. The concept of locally advanced gastric cancer. Effect of treatment on outcome. Cancer 1990;66:2324–30.
188. Hallissey MT, Dunn JA, Ward LC, Allum WH. The second British Stomach Cancer Group Trial of adjuvant radiotherapy or chemotherapy in resectable gastric cancer: five-year follow-up. Lancet 1994;343:1309–12.
189. Allum WH, Hallissey MT, Ward LC, Hockey MS. A controlled, prospective, randomised trial of adjuvant chemotherapy or radiotherapy in resectable gastric cancer: interim report. British Stomach Cancer Group. Br J Cancer 1989;60:739–44.
190. Bleiberg H, Goffin JC, Dalesio O, et al. Adjuvant radiotherapy and chemotherapy in resectable gastric cancer. A ran-

domized trial of the gastro-intestinal tract cancer cooperative group of the EORTC. Eur J Surg Oncol 1989;15:535–43.

191. Moertel CG, Childs DS, O'Fallon JR, et al. Combined 5-fluorouracil and radiation therapy as a surgical adjuvant for poor prognosis gastric carcinoma. J Clin Oncol 1984;2:1249–54.
192. Takahashi M, Abe M. Intra-operative radiotherapy for carcinoma of the stomach. Eur J Surg Oncol 1986;12:247–50.
193. Sindelar WF, Kinsella TJ, Tepper JE, et al. Randomized trial of intraoperative radiotherapy in carcinoma of the stomach. Am J Surg 1993;165:178–86; discussion 186–7.
194. Smalley SR, Gunderson L, Tepper J, et al. Gastric surgical adjuvant radiotherapy consensus report: rationale and treatment implementation. Int J Radiat Oncol Biol Phys 2002;52:283–93.
195. Henning GT, Schild SE, Stafford SL, et al. Results of irradiation or chemoirradiation for primary unresectable, locally recurrent, or grossly incomplete resection of gastric adenocarcinoma. Int J Radiat Oncol Biol Phys 2000;46:109–18.
196. Maruyama K, Gunven P, Okabayashi K, et al. Lymph node metastases of gastric cancer, general pattern in 1931 patients. Ann Surg 1989;210:596–602.
197. Lowy AM, Mansfield PF, Leach SD, et al. Response to neoadjuvant chemotherapy best predicts survival after curative resection of gastric cancer. Ann Surg 1999;229:303–8.
198. Ajani JA, Mansfield PF, Janjan N, et al. Multi-institutional trial of preoperative chemoradiotherapy in patients with potentially resectable gastric carcinoma. J Clin Oncol 2004;22:2774–80.
199. Cunningham D, Allum WH, Stenning SP. Perioperative chemotherapy in operable gastric and lower oesophageal cancer: Final results of a randomized, controlled trial (the MAGIC trial, ISRCTN 93793971) [Abstract]. J Clin Oncol 2005; 23 (16s):308s.
200. Kosse VA. Combined treatment of gastric cancer using hypoxic radiotherapy [Russian]. Vopr Onkol 1990;36:1349–53.
201. Shchepotin IB, Evans SR, Chorny V, et al. Intensive preoperative radiotherapy with local hyperthermia for the treatment of gastric carcinoma. Surg Oncol 1994;3:37–44.
202. Talaev MI, Starinskii VV, Kovalev BN, et al. Results of combined treatment of cancer of the gastric antrum and gastric body [Russian]. Vopr Onkol 1990;36:1485–8.
203. Lowy AM, Feig BW, Janjan N, et al. A pilot study of preoperative chemoradiotherapy for resectable gastric cancer. Ann Surg Oncol 2001;8:519–24.
204. Glimelius B, Ekstrom K, Hoffman K, et al. Randomized comparison between chemotherapy plus best supportive care with best supportive care with best supportive care in advanced gastric cancer. Gut 1997;40:362–9.
205. Murad AM, Santiago FF, Petroianu A, et al. Modified therapy with 5-fluorouracil, doxorubicin, and methotrexate in advanced gastric cancer. Cancer 1993;72:37–41.
206. Pyrhonen S, Kuitunen T, Nyandoto P, Kouri M. Randomised comparison of fluorouracil, epidoxorubicin and methotrexate (FEMTX) plus supportive care with supportive care alone in patients with non-resectable gastric cancer. Br J Cancer 1995;71:587–91.
207. Scheithauer W, Kornek G, Zeh B, et al. Palliative chemotherapy versus supportive care in patients with metastatic gastric cancer: a randomized trial. In: Proceedings of the International Conference on Biology, Prevention and Treatment of GI Malignancy; 1995; Köln, Germany; 1995. p. 68.
208. Glimelius B, Ekstrom K, Hoffman K, et al. Randomized comparison between chemotherapy plus best supportive care with best supportive care in advanced gastric cancer. Ann Oncol 1997;8:163–8.
209. Preusser P, Achterrath W, Wilke H, et al. Chemotherapy of gastric cancer [Review]. Cancer Treat Rev 1988;15:257–77.
210. Cullinan SA, Moertel CG, Fleming TR, et al. A comparison of three chemotherapeutic regimens in the treatment of advanced pancreatic and gastric carcinoma. Fluorouracil vs fluorouracil and doxorubicin vs fluorouracil, doxorubicin, and mitomycin. JAMA 1985;253:2061–7.
211. Tebbutt NC, Norman A, Cunningham D, et al. A multicentre, randomised phase III trial comparing protracted venous infusion (PVI) 5-fluorouracil (5-FU) with PVI 5-FU plus mitomycin C in patients with inoperable oesophago-gastric cancer. Ann Oncol 2002;13:1568–75.
212. Wils JA, Klein HO, Wagener DJ, et al. Sequential high-dose methotrexate and fluorouracil combined with doxorubicin—a step ahead in the treatment of advanced gastric cancer: a trial of the European Organization for Research and Treatment of Cancer Gastrointestinal Tract Cooperative Group. J Clin Oncol 1991;9:827–31.
213. Kelsen D, Atiq OT, Saltz L, et al. FAMTX versus etoposide, doxorubicin, and cisplatin: a random assignment trial in gastric cancer. J Clin Oncol 1992;10:541–8.
214. Cocconi G, Bella M, Zironi S, et al. Fluorouracil, doxorubicin, and mitomycin combination versus PELF chemotherapy in advanced gastric cancer: a prospective randomized trial of the Italian Oncology Group for Clinical Research. J Clin Oncol 1994;12:2687–93.
215. Waters JS, Norman A, Cunningham D, et al. Long-term survival after epirubicin, cisplatin and fluorouracil for gastric cancer: results of a randomized trial. Br J Cancer 1999;80:269–72.
216. Vanhoefer U, Rougier P, Wilke H, et al. Final results of a randomized phase III trial of sequential high-dose methotrexate, fluorouracil, and doxorubicin versus etoposide, leucovorin, and fluorouracil versus infusional fluorouracil and cisplatin in advanced gastric cancer: a trial of the European Organization for Research and Treatment of Cancer Gastrointestinal Tract Cancer Cooperative Group. J Clin Oncol 2000;18:2648–57.
217. MacDonald JS, Schein PS, Woolley PV, et al. 5-Fluorouracil, doxorubicin, and mitomycin (FAM) combination chemotherapy for advanced gastric cancer. Ann Intern Med 1980;93:533–6.
218. Ohtsu. Selection of the chemotherapy regimen should be based on the results of phase III trials. 2003; :1933.
219. Klein. 1989; :564.
220. Preusser P, Wilke H, Achterrath W, et al. Phase II study with the combination etoposide, doxorubicin, and cisplatin in advanced measurable gastric cancer. J Clin Oncol 1989;7:1310–7.
221. Cocconi G, Carlini P, Gamboni A, et al. Cisplatin, epirubicin, leucovorin and 5-fluorouracil (PELF) is more active than 5-fluorouracil, doxorubicin and methotrexate (FAMTX) in advanced gastric carcinoma. Ann Oncol 2003;14:1258–63.
222. Wilke H, Wils J, Rougier P, et al. Preliminary analysis of a randomized phase III trial of FAMTX versus ELF versus cisplatin/FU in advanced gastric cancer (GC). A trial of the EORTC Gastrointestinal Tract Cancer Cooperative Group and the AIO (Arbeitsgemeinschaft Internistische Onkologie) [Abstract]. Proc Am Soc Clin Oncol 1995;14:A500.
223. Partyka S, Dumas P, Ajani J. Combination chemotherapy with granulocyte–macrophage-colony stimulating factor in patients with locoregional and metastatic gastric adenocarcinoma. Cancer 1999;85:2336–9.
224. Cheng AL, Yeh KH, Lin JT, et al. Cisplatin, etoposide, and weekly high-dose 5-fluorouracil and leucovorin infusion (PE-HDFL)—a very effective regimen with good patients' compliance for advanced gastric cancer. Anticancer Res 1998;18:1267–72.
225. Shirao K, Shimada Y, Kondo H, et al. Phase I–II study of irinotecan hydrochloride combined with cisplatin in patients with advanced gastric cancer. J Clin Oncol 1997;15:921–7.
226. Boku N, Ohtsu A, Shimada Y, et al. Phase II study of a combination of irinotecan and cisplatin against metastatic gastric cancer. J Clin Oncol 1999;17:319–23.
227. Ajani JA, Baker J, Pisters PW, et al. CPT-11 plus cisplatin in patients with advanced, untreated gastric or gastroesophageal junction carcinoma: results of a phase II study. Cancer 2002;94:641–6.
228. Baker J, Ajani J, Ho L,. CPT-11 plus cisplatin as second line therapy of advanced gastric or GE junction adenocarcinoma (AGC-AGEJC) [Abstract]. Proc Am Soc Clinl Oncol 2001;20:163.
229. Kim YH, Shin SW, Kim BS, et al. Paclitaxel, 5-fluorouracil, and cisplatin combination chemotherapy for the treatment of advanced gastric carcinoma. Cancer 1999;85:295–301.
230. Roth AD, Maibach R, Martinelli G, et al. Docetaxel (Taxotere)–cisplatin (TC): an effective drug combination in gastric carcinoma. Swiss Group for Clinical Cancer Research (SAKK), and the European Institute of Oncology (EIO). Ann Oncol 2000;11:301–6.
231. Ridwelski K, Gebauer T, Fahlke J, et al. Combination chemotherapy with docetaxel and cisplatin for locally advanced and metastatic gastric cancer. Ann Oncol 2001;12:47–51.
232. Kettner E, Ridwelski K, Keilholz U, et al. Docetaxel and cisplatin combination chemotherapy for advanced gastric cancer: results of two phase II studies [Abstract]. Proc Am Soc Clin Oncol 2001;20:165.
233. Ajani J, Van Cutsem E, Moiseyenko V, et al. Docetaxel (D), cisplatin, 5-fluorouracil compare to cisplatin (C) and 5-fluorouracil (F) for chemotherapy-naïve patients with metastatic or locally recurrent, unresectable gastric carcinoma (MGC): interim results of a randomized phase III trial (V325) [Abstract]. Proc Am Soc Clin Oncol 2003;22:249.
234. Ohtsu A, Boku N, Nagashima F, et al. A phase I/II study of S-1 plus cisplatin (CDDP) in patients (pts) with advanced gastric cancer (AGC) [Abstract]. Proc Am Soc Clin Oncol 2001;21.
235. Miner TJ, Jaques DP, Karpeh MS, Brennan MF. Defining palliative surgery in patients receiving noncurative resections for gastric cancer. J Am Coll Surg 2004;198:1013–21.
236. Kahlke V, Bestmann B, Schmid A, et al. Palliation of metastatic gastric cancer: impact of preoperative symptoms and the type of operation on survival and quality of life. World J Surg 2004;28:369–75.
237. Yoshikawa K, Kitaoka H. Bone metastasis of gastric cancer. Jpn J Surg 1983;13:173–6.
238. Savides T, Jensen D, Cohen J, et al. Severe upper gastrointestinal tumor bleeding: endoscopic findings, treatment, and outcomes. Endoscopy 1996;2:244–8.
239. Loftus E, Alexander G, Ahlquist D, Balm R. Endoscopic treatment of major bleeding from advanced gastroduodenal malignant lesions. Mayo Clinic Proc 1994;69:736–40.
240. Gunderson LL, Hoskins RB, Cohen AC, et al. Combined modality treatment of gastric cancer. Int J Radiat Oncol Biol Phys 1983;9:965–75.
241. Klaassen DJ, MacIntyre JM, Catton GE, et al. Treatment of locally unresectable cancer of the stomach and pancreas: a randomized comparison of 5-fluorouracil alone with radiation plus concurrent and maintenance 5-fluorouracil—an Eastern Cooperative Oncology Group study. J Clinl Oncol 1985;3:373–8.
242. Aranha GV, Folk FA, Greenlee HB. Surgical palliation of small bowel obstruction due to metastatic carcinoma. Ann Surg 1981;47:99–102.
243. Dormann A, Meisner S, Verin N, Wenk Lang A. Self-expanding metal stents for gastroduodenal malignancies: systematic review of their clinical effectiveness. Endoscopy 2004;36:543–50.
244. Fiori E, Lamazza A, Volpino P, et al. Palliative management of malignant antro-pyloric strictures. Gastroenterostomy vs. endoscopic stenting. A randomized prospective trial. Anticancer Res 2004;24:269–71.
245. Carter R, Smith JS, Anderson JR. Palliation of malignant dysphagia using the Nd:YAG laser. World J Surg 1993;17:608–13.
246. Mason R, Bright N, McColl I. Palliation of malignant dysphagia with laser therapy: predictability of results. Br J Surg 1991;78:1346–7.
247. Loizou L, Rampton D, Atkinson M, et al. A prospective assessment of quality of life after endoscopic intubation and laser therapy for malignant dysphagia. Cancer 1992;70:386–91.
248. Heindorff H, Wajdemann M, Bisgaard T, Svendsen L. Endoscopic palliation of inoperable cancer of the oesophagus or cardia by argon electrocoagulation. Scand J Gastroenterol 1998;33:21–3.
249. Sargeant I, Tobias J, Blackman G, et al. Radiotherapy enhances laser palliation of malignant dysphagia: a randomized study. Gut 1997;40:362–9.
250. Spencer G, Thorpe S, Sargeant I, et al. Laser and brachytherapy in the palliation of adenocarcinoma of the oesophagus and cardia. Gut 1996;39:726–31.
251. Highley M, Parnis F, Trotter G, et al. Combination chemotherapy with epirubicin, cisplatin and 5-fluorouracil for the palliation of advanced gastric and oesophageal adenocarcinoma. Br J Surg 1994;81:1763–5.
252. Lo NN, Kee SG, Nambiar R. Palliative gastrojejunostomy for advanced carcinoma of the stomach. Ann Acad Med Singapore 1991;20:356–8.
253. Ekbom GA, Gleysteen JJ. Gastric malignancy: resection for palliation. Surgery 1980;88:476–81.
254. Ouchi K, Sugawara T, Ono H, et al. Therapeutic significance of palliative operations for gastric cancer for survival and quality of life. J Surg Oncol 1998;69:41–4.
255. Ishigami S, Natsugoe S, Hokita S, et al. Strategy of gastric cancer in patients 85 years old and older. Hepatogastroenterology 1999;46:27:2091–5.
256. Matsushita I, Hanai H, Kajimura M, et al. Should gastric cancer patients more than 80 years of age undergo surgery? Comparison with patients not treated surgically concerning prognosis and quality of life. J Clin Gastroenterol 2002;35:29–34.

257. Siewert JR, Bottcher K, Stein HJ, Roder JD. Relevant prognostic factors in gastric cancer: ten-year results of the German Gastric Cancer Study. Ann Surg 1998;228:449–61.
258. Crookes P, Leichman CG, Leichman L, et al. Systemic chemotherapy for gastric carcinoma followed by postoperative intraperitoneal therapy: a final report. Cancer 1997;79:1767–75.
259. Kelsen D, Karpeh M, Schwartz G, et al. Neoadjuvant therapy of high-risk gastric cancer: a phase II trial of preoperative FAMTX and postoperative intraperitoneal fluorouracil-cisplatin plus intravenous fluorouracil. J Clin Oncol 1996;14:1818–28.
260. Yonemura Y, Sawa T, Kinoshita K, et al. Neoadjuvant chemotherapy for high-grade advanced gastric cancer. World J Surg 1993;17:256–61.
261. Lowy AM, Feig BW, Janjan N, et al. A pilot study of preoperative chemoradiotherapy for resectable gastric cancer. Ann Surg Oncol 2001;8:519–24.
262. Ota K, Taguchi T, Kimura K. Report on nationwide pooled data and cohort investigation in UFT phase II study. Cancer Chemother Pharmacol 1988;22:333–8.
263. Sakata Y, Ohtsu A, Horikoshi N, et al. Late phase II study of novel oral fluoropyrimidine anticancer drug S-1 (1 M tegafur–0.4 M gimestat–1 M otastat potassium) in advanced gastric cancer patients. Eur J Cancer 1998;34:1715–20.
264. Koizumi W, Kurihara M, Nakano S, Hasegawa K. Phase II study of S-1, a novel oral derivative of 5-fluorouracil, in advanced gastric cancer. For the S-1 Cooperative Gastric Cancer Study Group. Oncology 2000;58:191–7.
265. Celio L, Bajetta E, Buzzoni R, et al. Efficacy and toxicity of pemetrexed disodium (Alimta) with folic acid (FA) in gastric cancer [Abstract]. Proc Am Soc Clin Oncol 2001;20:166.
266. Wadler S, Green M, Muggia F. The role of anthracyclines in the treatment of gastric cancer [Review]. Cancer Treat Rev 1985;12:105–32.
267. Levi JA, Fox RM, Tattersall MH, et al. Analysis of a prospectively randomized comparison of doxorubicin versus 5-fluorouracil, doxorubicin, and BCNU in advanced gastric cancer: implications for future studies. J Clin Oncol 1986;4:1348–55.
268. Gastrointestinal Tumor Study Group. Phase II-III chemotherapy studies in advanced gastric cancer. Cancer Treat Rep 1979;63:1871–6.
269. Scarffe JH, Kenny JB, Johnson RJ, et al. Phase II trial of epirubicin in gastric cancer. Cancer Treat Rep 1985;69:1275–7.
270. Coombes RC, Chilvers CE, Amadori D, et al. Randomised trial of epirubicin versus fluorouracil in advanced gastric cancer. An International Collaborative Cancer Group (ICCG) study. Ann Oncol 1994;5:33–6.
271. Ajani JA, Mansfield PF, Dumas P. Oral etoposide for patients with metastatic gastric adenocarcinoma. Cancer J Sci Am 1999;5:112–4.
272. Kelsen DP, Magill G, Cheng E. Phase II trial of etoposide (VP-16) in the treatment of upper gastrointestinal malignancies [Abstract]. Proc Am Soc Clin Oncol 1982;1:96.
273. Kambe M, Wakui A, Nakao I, et al. A late phase II study of irinotecan (CPT-11) in patients with advanced gastric cancers. Proc Am Soc Clin Oncol 1993;12:198.
274. Ajani JA, Fairweather J, Dumas P,. Phase II study of Taxol in patients with advanced gastric carcinoma. Cancer J Sci Am 1998;4:269–74.
275. Einzig AI, Lipsitz S, Wiernik PH, Benson AB 3rd. Phase II trial of Taxol in patients with adenocarcinoma of the upper gastrointestinal tract (UGIT). The Eastern Cooperative Oncology group (ECOG) results. Invest New Drugs 1995;13:223–7.
276. Sulkes A, Smyth J, Sessa C, et al. Docetaxel (Taxotere) in advanced gastric cancer: results of a phase II clinical trial. EORTC Early Clinical Trials Group. Br J Cancer 1994;70:380–3.
277. Einzig AI, Neuberg D, Remick SC, et al. Phase II trial of docetaxel (Taxotere) in patients with adenocarcinoma of the upper gastrointestinal tract previously untreated with cytotoxic chemotherapy: the Eastern Cooperative Oncology Group (ECOG) results of protocol E1293. Med Oncol 1996;13:87–93.
278. Taguchi T, Sakata Y, Kanamaru R, et al. Late phase II clinical study of RP56976 (docetaxel) in patients with advanced/recurrent gastric cancer: a Japanese Cooperative Study Group trial (group A) [Japanese]. Gan To Kagaku Ryoho 1998;25:1915–24.
279. Ohtsu A, Shimada Y, Shirao K, et al. Randomized phase III trial of fluorouracil alone versus fluorouracil plus cisplatin versus uracil and tegafur plus mitomycin in patients with unresectable, advanced gastric cancer: The Japan Clinical Oncology Group Study (JCOG9205). J Clin Oncol 2003;21:54–9.
280. Kim NK, Park YS, Heo DS, et al. A phase III randomized study of 5-fluorouracil and cisplatin versus 5-fluorouracil, doxorubicin, and mitomycin C versus 5-fluorouracil alone in the treatment of advanced gastric cancer. Cancer 1993;71:3813–8.
281. Ajani JA, Fodor M, Van Cutsem E, et al. Multinational randomized phase II trial of docetaxel (T) and cisplatin (C) with or without 5-fluorouracil (FU) in patients (Pts) with advanced gastric or GE junction adenocarcinoma (AGC-AGEJC) [Abstract]. Proc Am Soc Clin Oncol 2000;19:247a.

Primary Neoplasms of the Liver

Paul F. Engstrom, MD
Elin R. Sigurdson, MD, PhD
Alison A. Evans, ScD
Nancy Lewis, MD

INTRODUCTION

The earliest recorded distinction between primary and secondary liver cancer may have been made by Rokitansky in 1849.[1] By the end of the nineteenth century, the first study using epidemiologic methods appeared in von Hansmann's pathologic study of the comparative incidences of primary and secondary liver cancer in Europe.[2] As noted by the author, the incidence of secondary liver cancer far exceeded that of primary liver cancer. It was generally believed that this was the case worldwide, until reports to the contrary appeared in the twentieth century. These reports, originating from South Africa and Asia, indicated that primary liver cancer was a major cause of cancer mortality among the populations of those areas.

EPIDEMIOLOGY

Frequencies and Types of Cancers Population cancer surveillance data usually combine cancers of the liver and intrahepatic bile duct (International Classification of Diseases [ICD]-9 code 155) into one class, which includes hepatocellular carcinoma (HCC), cholangiocarcinoma (CC), angiosarcoma, and hepatoblastoma. Liver cancer is the fifth most common cancer and the third most common cause of cancer mortality worldwide, with approximately 549,000 cases diagnosed per year. Of these, hepatocellular carcinoma is by far the most common worldwide, although the geographic variability of incidence is substantial.[3] In the United States, 70 to 80% of liver cancers are hepatocellular carcinoma and 15% are cancers of the intrahepatic bile ducts[4] (Table 87-1).

Incidence and Mortality The areas of highest liver cancer incidence are in eastern Asia and sub-Saharan Africa, and HCC is often the dominant cause of cancer mortality in these areas. In general, incidence is very low in Western countries, although ethnic subgroups in these populations may be at very high risk because of the high prevalence of chronic hepatitis B virus (HBV) infection.[5] Rates of both HCC and CC appear to be rising in the United States and other developed nations.[6,7] Because survival times for patients with HCC and CC are short, incidence and mortality figures are roughly equivalent. In the United States, there have been slight but statistically significant improvements in 5-year survival rates for liver cancers over the past two decades, but these rates remain at about 5%.[8]

The American Cancer Society estimated that there were 14,270 deaths from liver and intrahepatic bile duct cancers in the United States in 2004, making it the eighth highest cause of cancer mortality in men and the twelfth in women.[8] Surveillance, Epidemiology and End Results (SEER) data from 1992 to 1998 show age-adjusted incidence rates for all liver cancers of 6.6 per 100,000 for males and 2.5 per 100,000 for females in the United States overall.[9]

Age, Sex, Race, and Familial Clusters Aside from the geographical variations in incidence discussed above, there are ethnic and racial differences within populations. In the United States, incidence rates for liver cancer are higher among African Americans than among whites (6.1 vs 2.8 per 100,000), but the highest rates occur among other minorities. In SEER data,[10] 23% of all HCCs occurred among other ethnic groups, such as Hispanics, Asians, Pacific Islanders, and Native Americans. In particular, Alaskan Natives are a high-risk group because of a high frequency of chronic HBV infection among them.[11]

Incidence of HCC increases with age, with the age of peak incidence varying somewhat with population. HCC is seen in childhood in areas where HBV is endemic and infection occurs primarily at birth or early childhood.[5] In all populations worldwide, there is a strong male predominance in HCC incidence. In the United States, the male:female ratio is 2.7:1. Several possible explanations for this have been proposed, including higher rates of chronic viral hepatitis among males, genetic susceptibility, androgenic steroids, higher body iron stores, and higher exposure to other hepatocarcinogenic cofactors (eg, alcohol, aflatoxin). Intrahepatic bile duct cancers also show male predominance, but less pronounced than that seen for HCC.[4]

Familial aggregation of HCC has been reported primarily in families where chronic HBV infection is also present.[12,13] In some studies, however, it has been possible to evaluate the effect of family history independent of HBV status. Evans and colleagues[14] found a relative risk (RR) of 2.3 associated with having a first-degree relative with HCC in a nested case-control study in China. Fernandez and colleagues[15] found an RR of 2.9 for any family history in a case-control study in Spain. Shen and colleagues[16] analyzed pedigrees from Chinese HCC case families and found that familial aggregation could be explained by the interaction of HBV and a major gene. Familial aggregation has also been reported for hepatoblastoma, which occurs in families carrying germline mutations of the APC (adenomatous polyposis coli) gene.[17]

Table 87-1 Relative Frequency of Primary Malignant Tumors of Liver in the US Population

Cancer Type	Frequency (%)
Hepatocellular carcinoma	84
Cholangiocellular and fibrolamellar types	2
Cholangiocarcinoma	13
Angiosarcoma, sarcoma	1

Reproduced with permission from Edmondson HA and Craig JR.[166]

RISK FACTORS

Hepatitis B Virus Chronic HBV infection has been established as a risk factor for development of HCC in numerous studies in human populations, normal liver and tumor cells, and animal models. This relationship was demonstrated for the first time in a prospective epidemiologic study in Taiwan,[18] where male civil servants who were HBV carriers had a 100-fold higher risk than did noncarriers in the same cohort. Numerous studies in other populations have confirmed this relationship. The lifetime risk of HCC among HBV carriers in populations where infection occurs early in life has been estimated at 27% for males and 4% for females. Lifetime risk estimates are more difficult in populations where HBV infection occurs later, but they would be expected to be somewhat lower. The presence of cirrhosis significantly increases the risk of HCC in HBV carriers, with approximately 80% of HCCs occurring on a background of cirrhosis.

Hepatitis C Virus The association of chronic hepatitis C virus (HCV) infection with development of HCC was confirmed shortly after the discovery of this virus, which is responsible for much of what was previously called non-A, non-B hepatitis.[19] That chronic HCV infection increases risk of HCC is well established, but the underlying mechanism is unclear. Unlike HBV, HCV does not integrate into the host genome. HCV-associated HCC without cirrhosis is rare. In HCV patients with cirrhosis, HCC occurs at a rate of 1 to 4% per year.[20–22] Because HCV infection is usually asymptomatic at onset, it has been difficult to study the natural history of this infection outside of clinical populations in which liver disease has already occurred. Based on current knowledge, the proportion of infected persons who develop chronic infection is approximately 80%, and 15 to 20% of those infected will develop serious liver disease although some not until > 30 years after infection. Among those who develop cirrhosis, HCC develops at a rate of 1 to 4% per year. Cofactors that may influence this progression are alcohol intake, age at infection, and co-infection with human immunodeficiency virus (HIV).[21]

Cirrhosis and Alcohol Cirrhosis from both viral and nonviral causes is associated with elevated HCC risk. Patients with primary biliary cirrhosis, for example, have been shown to have a 26-fold increased risk of HCC.[23] At autopsy, the prevalence of undiagnosed HCC in patients with cirrhosis may be as high as 10%.[24] Alcoholic cirrhosis is associated with approximately 15% of HCCs in the United States[25] and is associated with both HCC and cholangiocarcinoma in Denmark.[26] In the absence of cirrhosis, however, alcohol is not carcinogenic in animal studies.[27] Alcohol consumption, even at moderate levels, is associated with increases in levels of circulating HCV RNA in HCV carriers.[28] HCV infection is highly prevalent among alcoholics with chronic liver disease and appears to accelerate the course of alcoholic liver disease.[29] It appears that, in large part, the relationship of alcoholic cirrhosis to liver cancer may be a result of concomitant infection with HCV, although the possibility that alcohol exerts a promoting effect in the absence of HCV remains open.[27]

Aflatoxins Consumption of food contaminated with aflatoxins, toxic metabolites of some species of *Aspergillus* fungi, is associated both with human and animal hepatocellular carcinoma.[30,31] Foods susceptible to *Aspergillus* infection include peanuts/groundnuts, corn/maize, and oil seeds and nuts, such as cottonseed, almonds, and pistachios. Epidemiologic studies have suggested a strong interaction of aflatoxin exposure with HBV carrier status such that combined exposure to both greatly increases risk.[32] In a case-control study in China, McGlynn and colleagues[33] reported an interaction of HBV carrier status and genotypic variation in two loci (glutathione-S transferase M1 [GSTM1] and epoxide hydrolase [EPHX]) possibly involved in the detoxification of aflatoxin exposure. Subjects who were HBV carriers and carried both polymorphisms associated with impaired detoxification had a 135-fold elevated risk as compared to noncarriers with wild-type genotypes. This provides evidence that genetic factors may influence host response to aflatoxin in the presence of HBV infection. Potential interactions of aflatoxin exposure with other HCC risk factors such as HCV infection have not been extensively studied.

Hemochromatosis and Iron Iron overload is associated with a high risk of HCC in patients with untreated hemochromatosis,[34] and this risk can be substantially lowered by iron depletion therapy if cirrhosis has not already occurred.[35] Hereditary hemochromatosis is the most common autosomal recessive disorder among individuals of northern European descent,[34] with the prevalence estimated to be about 5.4 per 1,000 among white Americans.[36] Iron overload in Africans, which may be caused by a genetic mutation, also appears to increase HCC risk.[37] These observations have led many investigators to examine the relationship of dietary iron and HCC in patients without hereditary iron overload.

Steroid Hormones The relationship between oral contraceptive use and benign hepatic adenomas is well established.[38,39] Yu and colleagues,[40,41] in a prospective study in Taiwanese males, reported an association of HCC risk with increased plasma testosterone levels. Risk was also elevated in those with 20 or fewer CAG repeats in the androgen receptor (*AR*) gene and those with the *V* allele of the steroid 5a reductase type II (SRD5A2) V89L polymorphism. In contrast, two studies have shown the opposite effect of *AR* CAG repeat length on HCC risk in women.[42,43] A few studies have focused on the increased risk of HCC with increased parity and/or oral contraceptive use for women in low- to moderate-risk populations.[44–46] Although these findings have been consistent, it is not clear to what extent they apply to higher-risk populations where HBV and/or HCV are endemic. Shimizu and colleagues[47] found that lower hepatocyte estrogen receptor (ER) levels were associated with a 16-fold increase in HCC risk in both males and females. An effect on HCC risk of the antiestrogen tamoxifen has also been hypothesized, but support for this remains weak.[48] The susceptibility of the liver to hepatocellular damage and fibrosis, which usually precede HCC, is also strongly affected by sex hormones through complex mechanisms that are not completely understood. For example, although there is evidence for an androgen effect in HCC etiology in men, cirrhosis itself has feminizing effects through the increased conversion of androgens to estrogens via aromatase (CYP19). Although there is some evidence that estrogens may suppress fibrosis in the damaged liver,[49] hepatocytes are sensitive to estrogen-induced proliferation because of their high concentrations of estrogen receptors.[50] Estrogens may also have more direct genotoxic effects not mediated by ER through the actions of the catechol estrogens;[51] this is an area of new inquiry in the epidemiology of human HCC.

Other Risk Factors Many studies have examined the relationship between tobacco use and HCC in both high- and low-incidence areas.[22] The results are inconsistent. The accumulated body of data does not weigh heavily in favor of smoking being a strong risk factor. If there is an effect, it must either be limited to an as yet undefined subpopulation or be a minor effect that can only be discerned with large sample sizes and in the absence of other major risk factors. Occupational studies show that workers exposed to arsenic[52] or vinyl chloride[53] are at a greatly increased risk of development of angiosarcoma of the liver. High levels of exposure appear to be required for tumor induction, and angiosarcoma of the liver remains an extremely rare diagnosis except in exposed workers.

MOLECULAR PATHOGENESIS

Neither HBV nor HCV immortalizes hepatocytes in vitro.[54] Although HBV integrates into hepatocyte genomes early in infection, the sites of integration found in long-term infections are not clearly conserved. Integrated sequences are generally fragmented and rearranged,[55,56] and the virus carries no known oncogenes of its own. HCV does not integrate into the host genome at all, and it does not appear to carry viral oncogenes. The mechanism by which either virus might act in the etiologic pathway for HCC remains unknown.

If there is a common mechanism of pathogenesis in HCC overall, it is likely to be through chronic liver injury induced by viral and/or environmental factors and the resultant hepatocellular regeneration.[57] Discovery of a specific mechanism or specific genetic mutations that might occur in this process has thus far eluded investigators. Consistent chromosomal changes, however, have been described in HCC tumor tissue. Balsara and colleagues[58] found a high frequency of gains in parts of chromosome 8q and 1q, as well as loss of 16q, consistent with other studies.[59–64] Loss of heterozygosity analysis defined a minimal region of chromosome loss at 16q23.1-24.1, suggesting the presence there of a tumor-suppressor gene important in the etiology of HCC.

In a few geographic locations of high aflatoxin exposure, high frequencies of G-to-T transversions at codon 249 of the *TP53* gene have been detected in HCCs, but low frequencies of this mutation have been observed in HCCs from most locations.[65–67] This suggests a plausible mechanism whereby mutation of *TP53* may be involved in the oncogenic process, but this is by no means a universal mechanism, even in areas where aflatoxin exposure is high. Many researchers have investigated the role of the hepatitis B x antigen (HBxAg) as a viral transactivator. There are suggestions that HBxAg may be capable of functionally inactivating cellular p53 protein, although whether this occurs in vivo is a subject of continued controversy.[68,69] Other potential oncogenic activities have been suggested for HBxAg, including the downregulation of nucleotide excision repair.[70,71]

PREVENTION

Primary Prevention Prevention of HBV and HCV infection are the most effective ways of preventing HCC. A safe, effective vaccine for HBV has been available since 1982. Vaccination in early childhood, particularly in endemic areas, has been the most effective strategy in preventing chronic HBV infection because younger age at infection is associated with a higher probability of chronic infection. In Taiwan, where universal vaccination of newborns has been practiced since 1984, HCC incidence rates have begun to decline in younger age groups, particular among males.[72] Significant obstacles to the implementation of this strategy exist, particularly in the areas of the world where HBV is endemic. In 1991, the Centers for Disease Control and Prevention (CDC) recommended universal infant HBV vaccination in the United States because the previous strategy of targeting high-risk individuals had failed to reduce incidence of HBV infection.[73] In the United States, 36% of chronic infections are acquired before adolescence.[74] The combination of HBV vaccine and hepatitis B immunoglobulin (HBIg) is also recommended for babies of HBV-carrier mothers. Prevention of HCV infection is more difficult because there is no vaccine or effective postexposure prophylaxis available.[75] Because transmission is primarily parenteral, universal precautions against exposure to blood-borne infectious agents will be effective against HCV.[76]

Secondary Prevention Effective secondary prevention is dependent on early detection and resection of small tumors. α-Fetoprotein is a fetal antigen produced by 40 to 75% of HCCs, but not by the normal adult liver. Patients with chronic viral hepatitis or cirrhosis of any etiology are candidates for semiannual or annual screening for α-fetoprotein, with ultrasonographic follow-up of those with α-fetoprotein > 20 ng/mL for early detection of liver tumors.[77] Such screening programs have shown that identification of small, asymptomatic lesions is possible. Shanghai authors reported 50% 5-year survival in a 33-year case series of 391 HCC patients found by screening as compared to 20% in 1,251 patients whose tumors were diagnosed after clinical presentation.[78] The cost-benefit ratio has been questioned, however.[79]

Chemoprevention Because high-risk groups for HCC are clearly defined, this malignancy is an excellent target for chemoprevention regimens. For individuals already infected with HBV or HCV, antiviral treatments have shown promise in the reduction of HCC risk for those whose disease is amenable to such treatment.[80] These agents, however, are most effective in viral carriers with more advanced disease. Chemoprevention strategies that focus on other portions of the etiologic pathways for HCC may be a fruitful avenue for future prevention efforts. The acyclic retinoid, polyprenoic acid, inhibits chemically induced hepatocarcinogenesis in rats[81] and suppresses in vitro human hepatoma cell growth and α-fetoprotein production.[82] The exact mechanism of action of polyprenoic acid is unknown, but research shows in vitro return of cellular function, characteristic of differentiated hepatocytes, in addition to induction of apoptosis via blocking of transforming growth factor-alpha expression.[83] In vivo, a 12-month course of polyprenoic acid is associated with a statistically significant reduction in both recurrent and second primary hepatomas at 38 months; however, follow-up is insufficient to establish an effect on survival.[84]

Other strategies have also been explored for chemoprevention of HCC in specific populations. In areas where aflatoxin exposure is common, agents such as oltipraz for induction of detoxification enzymes and chlorophyllin for reducing aflatoxin bioavailability have been tested with some success.[85] Investigations are continuing in the use of cyclooxygenase-2 (COX-2) inhibitors[86] and natural products such as green tea[87] and traditional herbal medicines.

CLINICAL PRESENTATION

Patients with hepatocellular carcinoma often remain asymptomatic until very late in the course of the disease. As such, HCC is frequently diagnosed in advanced stages when patients seek medical care for symptoms. The most common initial presenting complaints include right upper quadrant abdominal pain and distension owing to a palpable mass, liver enlargement, fever, or ascites. Early satiety, weight loss, and diarrhea are common. Patients may present with symptoms related to their underlying chronic liver disease to include ascites, jaundice, encephalopathy, and variceal bleeding. Bleeding may be complicated by thrombocytopenia, or coagulopathies. Symptoms from distant metastatic disease may include dyspnea or bone pain.

On physical exam, hepatomegaly, splenomegaly, ascites, or superficial collateral venous distension may be evident. Signs of underlying cirrhosis include palmar erythema and gynecomastia. In patients with end-stage liver disease, jaundice, lethargy, and asterixis may be noted. An abdominal bruit may or may not be appreciated. Laboratory findings include thrombocytopenia, hypoalbuminemia, hyperbilirubinemia, elevated alkaline phosphatase, gamma glutamyl transpeptidase (GGT), or elevated transaminases. Frequently, a prolonged prothrombin time (PT) and partial thromboplastin time (PTT) will be measured. Other electrolyte abnormalities and anemia are common.

A number of paraneoplastic syndromes may occur in patients with HCC and include hypoglycemia due to ectopic production of insulin-like growth factor-2 (IGF-2),[88] hypercalcemia,[89] and erythrocytosis due to ectopic erythropoietin production.[90] Cutaneous manifestations include dermatomyositis, seborrheic keratosis, pityriasis rotunde, or porphyria cutanea tarda.[91]

Patients with newly diagnosed HCC should be asked about a history of hepatitis, ethanol use, or a family history of disorders that place patients at high risk of the development of carcinoma, such as hemochromatosis or alpha-1 antitrypsin deficiency.

PATHOLOGIC DIAGNOSIS

Four major gross patterns and two special forms of HCC have been described.[92] (1) The first type is the expanding type, in which the tumor is encapsulated and grows by expanding, compressing, and distorting the surrounding parenchyma of the liver. Late in the course of the disease, satellite nodules or metastases are seen. (2) The second pattern is the spreading type, in which the tumor is poorly defined and occurs in the setting of hepatic cirrhosis. The tumor growth pattern may be nodular, pseudolobular, or invasive (Figure 87-1). (3) A third major type is a multifocal pattern in which several small tumors of similar size are found in multiple sites in the liver and in which a primary to secondary relationship is difficult, if not impossible, to determine. (4) A combination or indeterminate pattern is seen in up to 25% of cases.

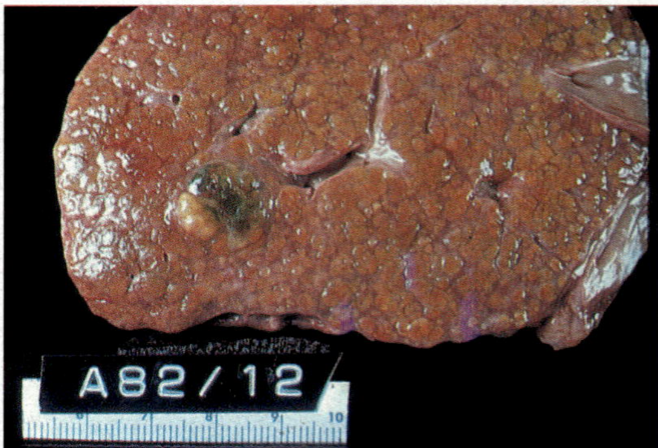

Figure 87-1 Liver with micronodular cirrhosis.

Histopathologically, grades of I to IV are assigned, according to the granularity and acidophilic quality of the cytoplasm, the size and degree of hyperchromatism of the nuclei, the proportion of the cell occupied by the nucleus, the cohesive quality of the tumor cells, and the overall architecture of the tumor (Figure 87-2). A

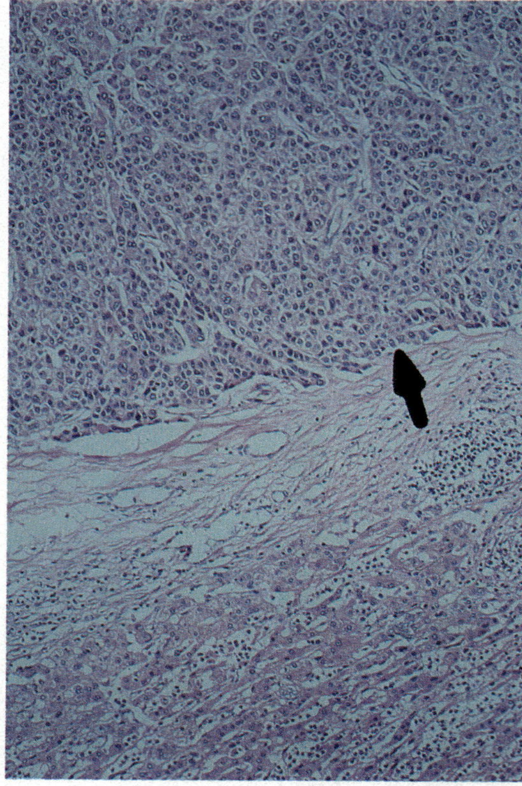
Figure 87-2 Hepatocellular carcinoma composed of tumor cells.

Table 87-2 Immunohistochemical Staining in Cancers of the Liver

	% with Positive Antigen Expression				
Histologic Type	AFP	AAT	CEA	ERY-1	CK-19
Hepatocellular carcinoma	17	41	0[a]	89	0
Cholangiocarcinoma	0	37	75	0	100
Metastatic pancreatic carcinoma	8	50	92	0	100
Metastatic colon carcinoma	0	50	100	0	100

AAT = α-antitrypsin; AFP = α-fetoprotein; CEA = carcinoembryonic antigen; CK-19 = cytokeratin-19; ERY-1 = erythropoiesis-associated antigen-1.
[a]Canalicular membrane staining in 24%.
Data from Ganjei P et al.[167] and Balaton AJ et al.[168]

grade IV hepatocellular carcinoma lacks cohesiveness of cells and shows enough cell spindling to resemble a carcinosarcoma, whereas grade I tumors mimic the normal liver parenchyma.

Two special forms of hepatocellular carcinoma should be distinguished. (1) The fibrolamellar form accounts for no more than 2 to 4% of cases, but is most often seen in young women and is characterized by deeply acidophilic neoplastic hepatocytes with fibrosis arranged in lamellar fashion around the tumor cells. Typically, the unaffected liver is not cirrhotic, and the tumors, which are found predominantly in the right lobe of the liver, are amenable to surgical resection. (2) The other special form, cholangiocellular carcinoma, appears to be a combination of cholangiolar elements as well as hepatocellular elements. These tumors behave more like cholangiocarcinoma and tend to occur in noncirrhotic livers, with a male predominance. The outcome for patients with this form of HCC is uniformly fatal.

A number of immunohistochemical stains distinguish HCC from metastatic adenocarcinoma or cholangiocarcinoma (Table 87-2). Antibodies to α-fetoprotein and α1-antitrypsin are of limited value because they lack sensitivity and specificity. Antibodies to the carcinoembryonic antigen (CEA) may produce a canalicular membrane-staining pattern in well-differentiated hepatomas, but will not produce the intracytoplasmic staining typical of metastatic adenocarcinoma and cholangiocarcinoma.[93] Cytokeratin-19 antibodies stain adenocarcinomas but not neoplastic or normal hepatocytes.[94] Erythropoiesis-associated antigen (Ery-1) is a specific marker for HCC.[93]

STAGING AND PROGNOSIS

The tumor, node, metastases (TNM) staging system for HCC depends on an imaging procedure to demonstrate the size of the largest nodule, number of nodules, and vascular invasion (Table 87-3).[95] The staging system proposed by Okuda and colleagues[96] uses tumor volume and associated liver dysfunction: stage I, not advanced (liver involvement < 50%, no ascites, albumin > 3 g/dL, and bilirubin < 3 mg/dL); stage II, moderately advanced (one or two signs of advanced disease are present); and stage III, very advanced (three or four signs of advanced disease are present). The median survival by stage was 11, 3, and 0.9 months, respectively.

Prognostic indicators include the presence of microscopic vascular invasion[97] and the nuclear and architectural grade.[98] CD34 and E-cadherin expression highlight the presence of vascular invasion.[99] Proteomic and genomic profiling may also be useful.[100]

Serologic Tests of HCC The fetal liver and yolk sac normally produce α-fetoprotein. Serum levels fall progressively after birth and in healthy adults are below 10 ng/mL by sensitive radioimmunoassay. α-Fetoprotein was first noted to be elevated in patients with HCC in 1964 and is raised in 50 to 90% of symptomatic HCC.[101] Interestingly, levels of α-fetoprotein appear to correlate with ethnicity, as 60 to 70% of white Americans and Europeans present with elevated values, while 80 to 90% of Asians with HCC have increased α-fetoprotein. Although the positive predictive value of an elevated α-fetoprotein level > 400 ng/mL exceeds 95%, normal values are not uncommon, particularly in patients with small tumors. A transient, unsustained elevation in α-fetoprotein between 20 and 400 ng/mL may be present in patients with cirrhosis, active hepatitis, or following partial hepatectomy because of hepatocyte regeneration. Recent reports indicate that the lectin-reactive isoenzyme of α-fetoprotein (α-fetoprotein–L3) showed increased sensitivity in the detection of HCC in cirrhotic patients undergoing screening,[102–104] as well as in post-hepatectomy patients undergoing chemoprevention trials for premalignant lesions.[105]

Many additional serologic markers have undergone evaluation as screening mechanisms in high-risk patients, but have failed to be more useful than α-fetoprotein in the detection of early lesions. These tests include the γ-glutamyl-transferase (GGT) isoenzymes, alkaline phosphatase, isoferritins, and monoclonal antibodies against specific tumor antigens.[106] The des-γ-carboxy-prothrombin protein, induced by vitamin K abnormalities, is also widely used and is elevated in up to 91% of patients with HCC. Unfortunately, false-positives can result from metastatic carcinoma, chronic hepatitis, and vitamin K deficiency. At present, α-fetoprotein levels in conjunction with real-time ultrasonography remains the gold standard for screening of high-risk patients.

IMAGING MODALITIES

Imaging plays an important role in the diagnosis, staging, and determination of prognosis in patients with hepatocellular carcinoma. Ultrasonography, triple phase computed tomography, and gadolinium-enhanced magnetic resonance imaging all have a place in the management of HCC. The utility of ^{18}F-FDG-positron emission tomography

Table 87-3 Tumor, Node, Metastases (TNM) Staging System in Hepatocellular Carcinoma

Primary Tumor (T)			
T1	Solitary tumor 2 cm or less in greatest dimension without vascular invasion		
T2	Solitary tumor 2 cm or less in greatest dimension with vascular invasion, or Multiple tumors limited to one lobe, none more than 2 cm in greatest dimension without vascular invasion, or A solitary tumor more than 2 cm in greatest dimension without vascular invasion		
T3	Solitary tumor more than 2 cm in greatest dimension with vascular invasion, or Multiple tumors limited to one lobe, none more than 2 cm in greatest dimension, with vascular invasion, or Multiple tumors limited to one lobe, any more than 2 cm in greatest dimension, with or without vascular invasion		
T4	Multiple tumors in more than one lobe, or Tumor(s) involve(s) a major branch of portal or hepatic vein(s)		
Regional Lymph Nodes (n)			
N0	No regional lymph node metastasis		
N1	Regional lymph node metastasis		
Distant Metastasis (M)			
M0	No distant metastasis		
M1	Distant metastasis		
Stage Grouping			
Stage I	T1	N0	M0
Stage II	T2	N0	M0
Stage IIIA	T3	N0	M0
Stage IIIB	T1	N1	M0
	T2	N1	M0
	T3	N1	M0
Stage IVA	T4	Any N	M0
Stage IVB	Any T	Any N	M1

(PET) scanning is still controversial because the uptake of FDG in HCC is variable with only about 60% of tumors having uptake.[107] However, this modality may prove to be more useful with the development of newer tracer molecules. In addition to initial staging, imaging can identify secondary findings, such as splenomegaly, varices, portal hypertension, thrombosis, and the presence of ascites, which may influence patient management. Imaging can also be used to screen patients at high risk of the development of HCC or for surveillance to monitor for recurrence.

HCC has a variable radiographic appearance and frequently coexists with cirrhotic regenerative and dysplastic nodules, making the interpretation of radiographic studies challenging. The ability to detect lymph node metastasis may be compromised by the presence of reactive lymphadenopathy frequently seen in cirrhosis.

Radiographically, HCC can be massive (a solitary large tumor), nodular (multiple small tumors), or diffuse (infiltrative). The latter can be difficult to distinguish from cirrhotic liver. HCC tends to be a highly vascular tumor and displays a brisk, early enhancement on CT and MRI. Although commonly used, ultrasonography has a limited role in the detection of HCC because of the heterogeneity in cirrhotic livers and has a sensitivity of only 45%.[108] Conventional CT performed during the portal venous phase of enhancement has a sensitivity of 48% and specificity of 70%. Although noncontrast and delayed images may increase detection, the ability to scan during the arterial phase of enhancement with spiral CT provides the best detection method.

There is considerable overlap between the appearance of HCC and regenerative and dysplastic nodules on MRI. HCC demonstrates variable signal intensity on T_1-weighted images and most are hyperintense on T_2-weighted images. Contrast enhancement is a crucial component. With few exceptions, gadolinium-enhanced multiphase (dynamic) MRI is the preferred imaging modality and has been shown to be superior at identifying HCC compared with multiphase contrast-enhanced CT.[109]

The development of spiral CT and dynamic gadolinium-enhanced MRI has largely displaced conventional angiography, although this modality is employed to assist with liver-directed therapy.

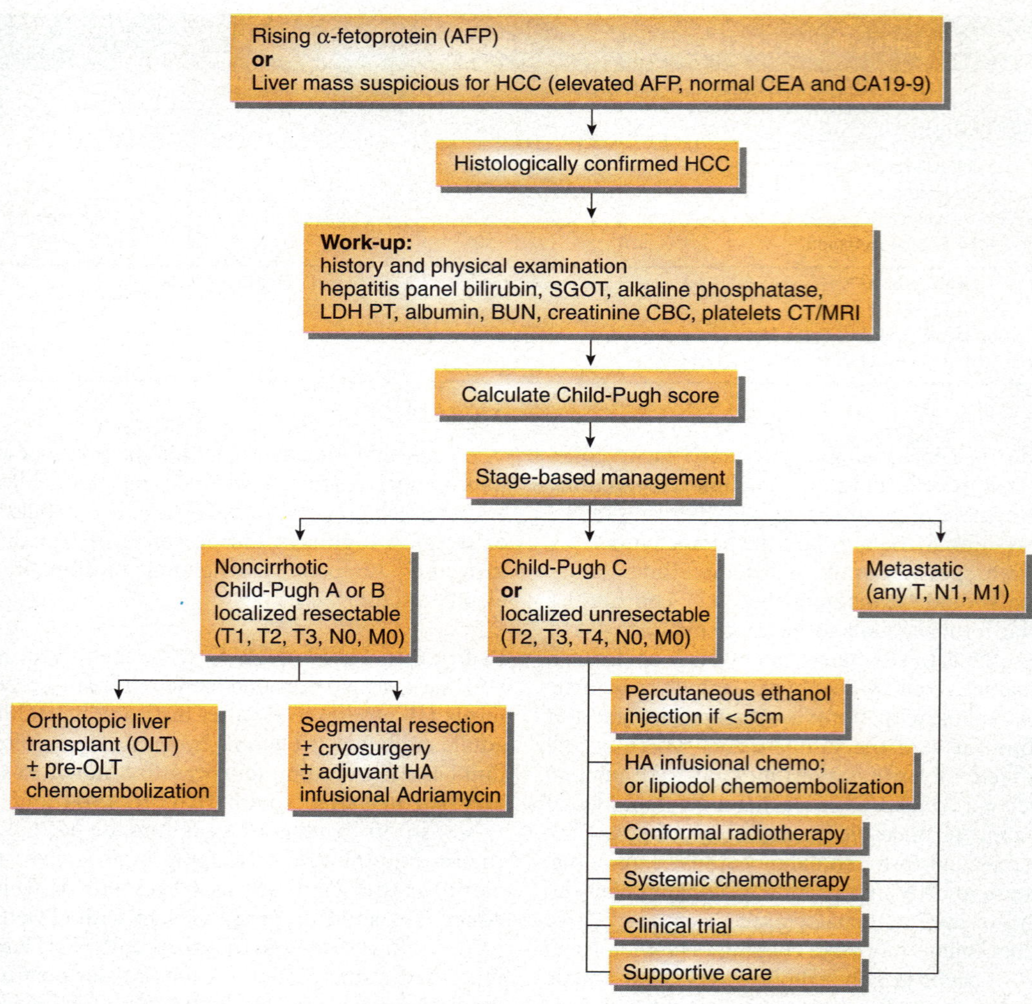

Figure 87-3 Guideline for liver cancer management. BUN = blood urea nitrogen; CEA = carcinoembryonic antigen; CBC = complete blood count; HA = hepatic artery; LDH = lactic acid dehydrogenase; PT = prothrombin time; SGOT = serum glutamic-oxaloacetic transaminase.

MANAGEMENT

Localized, Resectable (T_1, T_2, T_3, N_0, M_0) Surgical management of HCC is limited by cirrhosis, which affects many patients with this malignancy (Figure 87-3). Nevertheless, surgical excision is the most likely therapy to result in long-term survival in patients with cancer.[110–115]

The selection of patients for hepatic resection is primarily governed by the amount and function of liver tissue remaining after removal of the tumor (or tumors) and an adequate margin of surrounding liver tissue.[116,117] Two series found the presence or absence of cirrhosis to be the predominant, nontumor characteristic associated with long-term survival on multivariate analysis.[118,119] In both series, however, the presence of cirrhosis did not affect perioperative mortality, with the vast majority of deaths being attributable to recurrent cancer. Thus, properly selected patients in the hands of experienced surgeons can safely undergo hepatic resection, provided adequate functioning liver is retained.

Liver fibrosis has an impact on outcome following resection, and this information has been incorporated into the AJCC/UICC clinical staging system. Unlike staging systems that predict outcome from diagnosis, the AJCC system has traditionally been used for prognosis following resection or adjuvant therapy. Initially, the AJCC/UICC system used the TNM classification to stratify patients. This included tumor size, number and location, presence of vascular invasion, perforation or penetration into adjacent visceral structures, involvement of regional nodes, and the presence or absence of distant metastases. The newer AJCC/UICC system incorporates tumor grade and fibrosis of the liver[120] This staging system changed the tumor size from 2 to 5 cm. Vascular invasion and multiple tumors over 5 cm remains an important prognostic factor. Severe fibrosis was a negative prognostic indicator in all stages, although the impact of fibrosis on liver recurrence is uncertain.

Tumor resection alone, without pre- or postoperative adjuvant therapy, is the current standard treatment. Fong and colleagues[118] at Memorial Sloan-Kettering Cancer Center reported a series of 412 patients evaluated at a single institution, over a 6-year period beginning in 1991, in which the greatest determinant of long-term outcome was surgical resectability. Additionally, size < 5 cm (RR 0.6) was associated with better survival, while α-fetoprotein > 2,000 mg/mL (RR 1.2) and advanced Child classification (RR 1.3) were associated with worse outcome on multivariate analysis.[118] The presence of vascular invasion was associated with worse outcome on univariate analysis only. Multiple investigators have found the presence of cirrhosis to significantly impact on outcome, both in the patient's ability to tolerate resection and in the recurrence of disease. Additional prognostic factors correlated with recurrence include discovery by screening, satellite nodules, absence of capsule formation, positive resection margins, high nuclear/cytoplasmic ratios, DNA aneuploidy, advanced age, number of tumors, and male sex.[121,122]

Postoperative morbidity and mortality have decreased substantially over the last several years, with three large series reporting perioperative mortality rate of 4.5 to 7.0%.[112,118,123] The lowest operative mortality rate was reported by the Liver Cancer Study Group of Japan, with an operative mortality in 12,118 patients of 0.6%. Of note, they had noticed a decreased incidence of patients with hepatitis in their patient population, while the incidence of hepatitis is increasing in Western Europe and America (Table 87-4).

Preoperative liver function, including the presence of cirrhosis as well as operative blood loss and the occurrence of additional postoperative complications, correlate with hospital mortality. Careful patient selection also impacts on postoperative mortality.

The high hepatic recurrence rate and the frequent association of HCC with cirrhosis have led to the development of total hepatectomy with liver transplantation as an alternative to resection.[124,125] In the United States, approximately 700 transplants are performed each year for HCC or cholangiocarcinoma. No phase III trials comparing resection with total hepatectomy and liver transplantation have been performed, and because of the scarcity of the resources, it is unlikely that such a trial will ever be conducted. There have been three retrospective, nonrandomized comparisons between partial hepatectomy and total resection plus transplantation. In two of the studies, transplantation was superior, and in one study, resection was superior.[126–128] All authors agree that patients with active HBV infection are not candidates for transplantation because of the high risk of recurrent infection and graft loss as a result of hepatitis. A review of the Stanford University transplantation experience points to actuarial survival rates of 73%, and 65.4% at 1 and 3 years, respectively, without any specific clinicopathologic features being associated with survival.[129] Data collected in the United States by the Organ Procurement and Transplantation Network report a 1- and 3-year patient survival of 87% and 80% respectively.[130] Two more-recent series from France[131] and Italy[132] show increasing recurrence-free survival, 76% at 3 years in the former, and 83% at 4 years in the latter, when patient selection is limited to those with tumors < 3 cm, no more than three nodules, and absence of portal venous invasion. Most feel that resection remains the treatment of choice for those with lesions resectable with clean margins and adequate liver reserve. All would agree, however, that the sociopolitical considerations regarding the cost of the procedure and the scarcity of the donated organs carry great weight against transplantation as the primary surgical treatment of HCC. Efforts to increase the number of available donors in the United States have led to the increasing use of living-directed donors (LDLT). Approximately 500 living-directed liver transplants are performed yearly in the United States, with the risk of donor mortality of approximately 0.3%. The ratio at which donor risk to recipient survival is appropriate is a matter of significant medical and ethical debate.[133]

Table 87-4 Selected Surgical Series with Reported 5-Year Survival

Study	No. of Patients	Stage or Size of Tumor	% 5-Year Survival
Liver Cancer Study	918	< 2 cm	50
Group of Japan[169]	2,908	> 2 < 5 cm	40
Tang et al[114]	481	< 5 cm	58.5
	1,261	> 5 cm	18.5
Kawarada et al[170]	25	< 2 cm	57
	40	>2 < 3 cm	54
	41	>3 < 5 cm	35
Nagasue et al[123]	229	2 cm	77.8
		2–5 cm	59.6
		> 5 cm	40.1
Fong et al[118]	154	< 5 cm	57
		> 10 cm	32

Several transplantation programs have been using doxorubicin-based adjuvant chemotherapy regimens, both preoperatively as a temporizing measure and postoperatively in patients undergoing transplantation. The first series, published in 1993, showed an actuarial tumor-free survival rate of 49% at 3 years for patients with tumors > 5 cm in diameter, two of whom had multifocal, bilobar tumors > 15 cm in diameter.[134] More recently, Olthoff and colleagues,[135] from UCLA, reported a 46% overall 3-year survival in patients treated with a 6-month course of postoperative intravenous fluorouracil, doxorubicin, and cisplatin versus 5.8% survival in their historical controls ($p = .0001$). Most of the patients in this study had advanced disease characterized by tumor > 5 cm (56%), multifocal tumors (72%), and stage III or IV disease (80%). Treatment related toxicity was frequent but rarely severe.

Localized, Unresectable (T_2,T_3,T_4, N_0, M_0) Regional or local approaches to patients with unresectable, liver-only disease include direct infusion of chemotherapeutic drugs into the hepatic artery or portal vein, embolization, percutaneous ablation with physical or chemical agents, or the intravascular injection of radioactive agents. Chemoembolization has theoretical advantages. Embolization results in tumoral ischemia, with prolonged exposure of concentrated chemotherapeutic drugs delivered directly to the tumor. Systemic toxicity is minimal. Most US centers mix cisplatin, doxorubicin, and mitomycin-C dissolved in radiographic contrast and embolic agents such as iodized oil, Gelfoam, and polyvinyl alcohol particles. Compromised portal venous flow is a relative contraindication to hepatic embolization, but can be performed safely despite portal vein tumor thrombus if hepatopetal collateral flow is present.[136] Patients with a high risk of acute hepatic failure after hepatic artery chemoembolization include those with > 50% liver volume replaced by tumor, LDH > 425 IU/L, AST > 100 IU/L and total bilirubin ≥ 2 mg/dl.[137] Biliary obstruction, jaundice, or hepatic encephalopathy are absolute contraindications to embolization. Prior biliary bypass surgery and the presence of biliary stents place patients at high risk of liver abscess after chemoembolization despite the prophylactic use of antibiotics.[138] Prior to embolization, diagnostic visceral arteriography should be performed to determine the arterial supply to the liver, confirm portal vein patency, and identify vessels supplying the stomach, gallbladder, and small bowel. Complications of chemoembolization include a syndrome of fever, pain, nausea, and vomiting, which can be managed with supportive care. More serious complications include hepatic insufficiency, infarction, abscess, tumor rupture, cholecystitis, and embolization to other organs.

Two randomized trials demonstrate a survival benefit of chemoembolization in patients with unresectable hepatocellular carcinoma. Lo and colleagues randomized 80 patients to receive either cisplatin/lipiodol/gelatin sponge embolization or supportive care alone. Overall survival at 1, 2, and 3 years was improved in the chemoembolization group (57%, 31%, and 26%, respectively), compared with the control group (32%, 11%, and 3%, respectively, $p = .002$). [139] Llovet and colleagues of the Barcelona Clinic Liver Cancer Group randomized patients to receive embolization with gelatin sponge with or without doxorubicin versus supportive care alone. Those patients undergoing chemoembolization had an improved 1- and 2-year overall survival (82% and 63%) compared with the control group (63% and 27%, $p = .009$).[140]

Other ablative localized therapies that have been used with variable degrees of success include percutaneous ethanol injection, radiofrequency ablation (RFA), microwave coagulation, and cryotherapy. They are generally useful for patients with 1 to 2 tumors with a maximum diameter of 3 cm. The cumulative survival for 319 HCC patients who received RFA as primary treatment was 86% at 2 years and 54% at 5 years.[141]

Metastatic Disease (any T_1N_1 or M_1) The overall prognosis for patients with metastatic HCC is extremely poor and is measured in months. HCC is largely a chemotherapy-resistant tumor with low response rates and short median response duration for single agents or combination regimens (Table 87-5). There are several known mechanisms of resistance to account for this, namely high levels of dihydropyrimidine reductase, overexpression of MDR1/P-glycoprotein, glutathione-S-transferase, and heat shock proteins. No drug or combination has been shown to be better than single agent doxorubicin (response rate 3–28%), which does not improve survival over symptomatic care. Many of the earlier studies suffered from an inability to consistently measure tumors; more recent trials with newer imaging modalities show that the response rates are significantly lower. One of the promising new agents, nolatrexed, is a thymidylate synthase inhibitor. Phase II studies show response rates of only 0 to 8%, with 48 to 54% of patients having stable disease, and median survival rates of about 7 months.[142,143] A phase III trial comparing nolatrexed with single agent doxorubicin is underway. It is generally accepted, however, that there is no standard regimen for the systemic treatment of HCC and that enrollment in phase I or phase II clinical trials should be considered when feasible.

Because up to one-third of HCC tumors express estrogen receptors, there are several reports of tamoxifen therapy in advanced-stage disease patients. A recent meta-analysis totaling 1,709 patients showed that tamoxifen had no effect on median survival (HR 1.05, CI 0.94-1.16, $p = 0.4$) or tumor response rate.[144] Nearly 50% of HCC express somatostatin receptors. However, in a placebo-controlled trial involving 70 patients, there was no antitumor response or improvement in survival.[145] Interferon and antiandrogens have not fulfilled their early promise of improving quality of life in HCC patients either.[146]

Table 87-5 Selected Phase II Chemotherapy Trial Results in Patients with Advanced HCC[146]

Regimen	*n*	RR%	Median Survival (Weeks)
Doxorubicin	20–60	3–28	4–15
Etoposide	22	18	3
Cisplatin	35	6	14
5-Fluorouracil, semustine, doxorubicin	38	21	17
Epirubicin, etoposide	36	39	NS
Gemcitabine, oxaliplatin	21	19	NS

Summary of several studies.
NS = not stated; RR = response rate.

POTENTIAL THERAPEUTIC TARGETS

As our knowledge of cell-cycle regulation and tumorigenesis increases, potential new targets for therapeutic intervention are identified. In hepatocellular carcinoma, potential targets include the vascular endothelial growth factor, epidermal growth factor, or hepatocyte/c-met signaling pathways.[147]

The vascular endothelial growth factor (VEGF) has been shown to be a key proangiogenic protein. VEGF is overexpressed in many solid tumors and results in the development of immature, leaky, twisted blood vessels. VEGF is overexpressed in HCC and correlates with a decrease in disease-free survival (DFS) and overall survival (OS), increased portal vein invasion, and poor tumor encapsulation.[97,148,149] Small molecule tyrosine kinase inhibitors, monoclonal antibodies against VEGF, soluble VEGF traps, and anti-VEGF receptor antibodies are in various stages of development. Bevacizumab led to partial response in 2 patients and stable disease for median survival of 6 months in 9 of 13 patients.[150] The epidermal growth factor receptor has also proven to be a viable target for the treatment of solid tumors. EGFR is overexpressed in 60 to 70% of HCCs. Overexpression is associated with later stage, high grade, and poor prognosis. Targeting this receptor leads to G1 arrest, apoptosis and decreased angiogenesis.[151]

Hepatocyte growth factor (HGF) and its cellular receptor, c-met, activates the Akt/PI3 kinase pathway, which in turn suppresses Fas-mediated cell death in HCC cell lines. HGF stimulates cell growth, promotes cell motility, and can promote invasion by the induction of matrix metalloproteinases.[152–154] HGF induces urokinase-type plasminogen activator (uPA). The expression of plasminogen activators and uPA receptors is associated with HCC growth and invasion.[155] uPA and uPAR play an important role in cell adhesion, migration, and tumor invasion.[156–158] uPA is overexpressed in a number of solid tumors, including HCC, and is associated with tumor recurrence, portal vein invasion, and decreased overall survival.[155,159] Inhibitors of this pathway are in early human clinical trials.

OTHER PRIMARY HEPATIC NEOPLASMS

Cholangiocarcinoma Cholangiocarcinoma is a rare malignancy of the bile ducts with only 2,000 to 3,000 new cases in the United States per year. Patients typically present with symptoms of biliary obstruction with jaundice, pruritus, right upper quadrant pain, weight loss, and fever. Imaging with ultrasound, CT, or MRI/MRCP is helpful, but a tissue diagnosis can frequently be made endoscopically (ERCP) with bile duct brushings and cytology. Palliative bile duct stenting can be performed simultaneously. Tumor markers such as CA 19-9 in conjunction with biopsies can aid in making the diagnosis. Patients with cholangiocarcinoma have a poor prognosis with only 5 to 10% 5-year overall survival. Surgical resection offers the only possibility of a cure with 5-year overall survival between 8 to 44%.[160] Patients with intrahepatic cholangiocarcinoma amenable to hepatic resection have a 3-year survival rate of 22%.[161] The most common site of relapse is local recurrence. The benefit of adjuvant therapy is unproven, but given the overall poor prognosis, postoperative adjuvant radiation therapy with or without 5-FU or gemcitabine-based chemotherapy is frequently offered.

Hepatic Angiosarcoma Hepatic angiosarcoma is a rare tumor of the liver that is associated with long-term exposure to vinyl chloride monomers. Other risk factors include exposure to arsenic and thorium dioxide (Thorotrast). Angiosarcomas do not evolve from hemangiomas. These patients present with fatigue, anorexia, weight loss, and abdominal pain. Hepatomegaly, with or without splenomegaly, is present at the time of diagnosis. Hemorrhagic ascites is common. The serum α-fetoprotein level is normal. Angiography and contrast-enhanced CT of the liver are the best diagnostic tools. Because of the highly vascular substrate of this lesion and the accompanying central hemorrhage, open-liver biopsy is preferred over the percutaneous approach for diagnosis. Unfortunately, the prognosis is extremely poor, and very few patients are candidates for curative resection, owing to multiple lesions or the extensive size and rapid growth of the tumor. These sarcomas are unresponsive to chemotherapy and are relatively radioresistant.

Benign Hepatic Adenomas Hepatic adenomas are benign epithelial tumors seen predominantly in young women. These are often solitary (70–80%), but may grow to be quite large. These lesions are associated with oral contraceptive use, androgen use, and glycogen storage disease. Patients may present with symptoms to include abdominal pain or they may be noted incidentally. Patients should be instructed to discontinue hormones. If patients have large adenomas > 5 cm or are symptomatic, surgical resection is recommended. Small asymptomatic lesions should be followed closely, as malignant transformation has been reported.[162]

Focal Nodular Hyperplasia Focal nodular hyperplasia is a nonmalignant hepatic tumor found predominantly in women. It is most often solitary (80–95%) and > 5 cm in diameter.[163] This lesion must be distinguished from hepatic adenoma, hepatocellular carcinoma, fibrolamellar carcinoma, regenerative nodules, hemangiomas, and malignant metastases. The majority of patients are asymptomatic and the lesions are found incidentally. The alpha fetoprotein (AFP) is normal. Imaging to include ultrasound, CT, MRI, or nuclear scanning with technetium sulfur colloid can be used, as 80% of these lesions will take up the colloid in Kuppfner cells.[164] Patients can usually be managed conservatively.

Hemangiomas Hepatic hemangiomas are the most common benign liver tumors. They can vary in size from a few millimeters to several centimeters and may be solitary or multiple. Most patients are asymptomatic; however, large tumors may cause abdominal pain. The diagnosis can usually be made radiographically. Technetium 99-tagged red blood cell scans have a sensitivity of 69 to 92% and a have an extremely high specificity.[165] The majority remain stable in size, although growth or symptomatic lesions may require resection.

REFERENCES

1. Rokitansky CA. Manual of pathological anatomy. London: Edward; 1849.
2. von Hansmann D. Uber den primaren Krebs der Leber. Berl Klin Wschr 1890;27:353–6.
3. Parkin DM. The global burden of cancer. Semin Cancer Biol 1998;8:219–35.
4. Parkin DM, Ohshima H, Srivatanakul P, Vatanasapf V. Cholangiocarcinoma: epidemiology, mechanisms of carcinogenesis and prevention. Cancer Epidemiol Biomarkers Prev 1993;2:537–44.
5. Parkin D, Whelan S, Ferlay J, Raymond I, editors. Cancer incidence in five continents. IRC Scientific Publications Vol. 7. Lyon, France: Oxford University Press; 1997.
6. McGlynn KA, Tsao L, Hsing AW, et al. International trends and patterns of primary liver cancer. Int J Cancer 2001;94:290–6.
7. Patel T. Increasing incidence and mortality of primary intrahepatic cholangiocarcinoma in the United States. Hepatology 2001;33:1353–7.
8. American Cancer Society. Cancer Facts and Figures. Atlanta: American Cancer Society; 2004.
9. Howe HL, Wingo PA, Thun MJ, et al. Annual report to the nation on the status of cancer (1973 through 1998), featuring cancers with recent increasing trends. Cancer Inst 2001;93:824–42.
10. El-Serag HB, Mason AC. Rising incidence of hepatocellular carcinoma in the United States. N Engl J Med 1999;340:745–50.
11. McMahon BJ, Holck P, Bulkow L, Snowball M. Serologic and clinical outcomes of 1536 Alaska natives chronically infected with hepatitis B virus. Ann Intern Med 2001;135:759–68.
12. Milne A, Moyes CD, Pearce N. Liver disease and hepatitis B infection in a large New England family. N Z Med J 1989;102:318–20.
13. Harvey VJ, Woodfield DG, Probert JC. Maternal transmission of hepatocellular carcinoma. Cancer 1984;54:1360–3.
14. Evans AA, Chen G, Ross EA, et al. Eight-year follow-up of the 90,000 person Haimen City Cohort: I. Hepatocellular carcinoma mortality, risk factors, and gender differences. Cancer Epidemiol Biomarkers Prev 2002;11:369–76.
15. Fernandez E, La Vecchia C, D'Avanzo B, et al. Family history and the risk of liver, gallbladder, and pancreatic cancer. Cancer Epidemiol Biomarkers Prev 1994;3:209–12.
16. Shen F-M, Lee MK, Gong H-M, et al. Complex segregation analysis of primary hepatocellular carcinoma in Chinese families: interaction of inherited susceptibility and hepatitis B viral infection. Am J Hum Genet 1991;49:88–93.
17. Giardiello FM, Petersen GM, Brensinger JD, et al. Hepatoblastoma and APC gene mutation in familial adenomatous polyposis. Gut 1996;39:867–9.
18. Beasley RP, Hwang LY, Lin CC, Chien CS. Hepatocellular carcinoma and hepatitis B virus. A prospective study of 22,707 men in Taiwan. Lancet 1981;2:1129–33.
19. Purcell RH. Does non-A, non-B hepatitis cause hepatocellular carcinoma? Cancer Detect Prev 1989;14:203–7.
20. Ikeda K, Saitoh S, Koida I, et al. A multivariate analysis of risk factors for hepatocellular carcinogenesis: a prospective observation of 795 patients with viral and alcoholic cirrhosis. Hepatology 1993;18:47–53.
21. Lauer GM, Walker BD. Hepatitis C virus infection. N Engl J Med 2001;345:41–52.
22. Tsukuma H, Hiyama T, Tanaka S, et al. Risk factors for hepatocellular carcinoma among patients with chronic liver disease. N Engl J Med 1993;328:1797–801.
23. Di Bisceglie AM. Hepatitis C and hepatocellular carcinoma. Hepatology 1997;26:34S–8S.
24. Chiaramonte M, Stroffolini T, Vian A, et al. Rate of incidence of hepatocellular carcinoma in patients with compensated viral cirrhosis. Cancer 1999;85:2132–7.
25. Austin H. The role of tobacco use and alcohol consumption in the etiology of hepatocellular carcinoma. Houston (TX): Gulf Publishing Company; 1991.
26. Sorensen HT, Friis S, Olsen JH, et al. Risk of liver and other types of cancer in patients with cirrhosis: a nationwide cohort study in Denmark. Hepatology 1998;28:921–5.
27. Farber E. Alcohol and other chemicals in the development of hepatocellular carcinoma. Philadelphia: WB Saunders; 1996.
28. Pessione F, Degos F, Marcellin P, et al. Effect of alcohol consumption on serum hepatitis C virus RNA and histological lesions in chronic hepatitis C. Hepatology 1998;7:1717–22.
29. Fong TL, Kanel GC, Conrad A, et al. Clinical significance of concomitant hepatitis C infection in patients with alcoholic liver disease. Hepatology 1994;19:554–7.
30. Yeh FS, Yu MC, Mo CC, et al. Hepatitis B virus, aflatoxins and hepatocellular carcinoma in southern Guangxi, China. Cancer Res 1989;49:2506–9.
31. van Rensburg SJ, van Schalkwyk GC, van Schalkwyk DJ. Primary liver cancer and aflatoxin intake in Transkei. J Envir Pathol Toxicol Oncol 1990;10:11–6.
32. Qian G, Ross RK, Yu MC, et al. A follow-up study of urinary markers of aflatoxin exposure and liver cancer risk in Shanghai, People's Republic of China. Cancer Epidemiol Biomarkers Prev 1994;3:3–10.
33. McGlynn KA, Rosvold EA, Lustbader ED, et al. Susceptibility to hepatocellular carcinoma is associated with genetic variation in the enzymatic detoxification of aflatoxin B1. Proc Natl Acad Sci U S A 1995;92:2384–7.
34. Fargion S, Mandelli C, Piperno A, et al. Survival and prognostic factors in 212 Italian patients with genetic hemochromatosis. Hepatology 1992;15:655–9.
35. Niederau C, Heintges T, Lange S, et al. Long-term follow-up of HBeAg-positive patients treated with interferon alfa for chronic hepatitis B. N Engl J Med 1996;334:1422–7.
36. Phatak P, Sham R, Raubertas R, et al. Prevalence of hereditary hemochromatosis in 16,031 primary care patients. Ann Intern Med 1988;129:954–61.
37. Mandishona E, MacPhail AP, Gordeuk VR, et al. Dietary iron overload as a risk factor for hepatocellular carcinoma in Black Africans. Hepatology 1998;27:1563–6.
38. Edmondson H, Henderson B, Benton B. Liver cell adenomas associated with the use of the oral contraceptive. N Engl J Med 1976;294:470–72.
39. Mays E, Christopherson W. Hepatic tumors induced by sex steroids. Semin Liver Dis 1984;4:147–57.
40. Yu MW, Yang YC, Yang SY, et al. Hormonal markers and hepatitis B virus-related hepatocellular carcinoma risk: a nested case-control study among men. J Natl Cancer Inst 2001;93:1644–51.
41. Yu M-W, Cheng S-W, Lin M-W, et al. Androgen-receptor gene CAG repeats, plasma testosterone levels, and risk of hepatitis B-related hepatocellular carcinoma. J Natl Cancer Inst 2000;92:2023–8.
42. Yu M-W, Yang Y-C, Yang S-Y, et al. Androgen receptor exon 1 CAG repeat length and risk of hepatocellular carcinoma in women. Hepatology 2002;36:156–63.
43. Yeh S-H, Chang C-F, Shau W-Y, et al. Dominance of functional androgen receptor allele with longer CAG repeat in hepatitis B virus-related female hepatocarcinogenesis. Cancer Res 2002;62:4346–51.
44. Stanford JL, Thomas DB. WHO collaborative study of neoplasia and steroid contraceptives. Cancer Causes Control 1992;3:37–42.
45. Tzonov A, Zavitsanos X, Hsieh C-C, Trichopoulos D. Liveborn children and risk of hepatocellular carcinoma. Cancer Causes Control 1992;3:171–4.
46. Hsing AW, Hoover RN, McLaughlin JK, et al. Parity and primary liver cancer among women. J Natl Cancer Inst 1992;84:1118–9.
47. Shimizu I, Inque H, Yano M, et al. Estrogen receptor levels and lipid peroxidation in hepatocellular carcinoma with hepatitis C virus infection. Liver 2001;21:342–9.
48. Muhlemann K, Cook LS, Weiss NS. The incidence of hepatocellular carcinoma in US white women with breast cancer after the introduction of tamoxifen in 1977. Breast Cancer Res Treat 1994;30:201–4.
49. Yasuda M, Shimizu I, Shiba M, Ito S. Suppressive effects of estradiol on dimethylnitrosamine-induced fibrosis of the liver in rats. Hepatology 1999;29:719–27.
50. Villa E, Colantoni A, Grottola A, et al. Variant estrogen receptors and their role in liver disease. Mol Cell Endocrinol 2002;193:65–9.
51. Chen J, Li Y, Lavigne JA, et al. Increased mitochondrial superoxide production in rat liver mitochondria, rat hepatocytes and HepG2 cells following ethinyl estradiol treatment. Toxicol Sci 1999;51:224–35.
52. Roth F. The sequelae of chronic arsenic poisoning in Moselle Vintners. Deut Med Wochschr 1957;82:211–7.
53. Creech J, Johnson M. Angiosarcoma of the liver in the manufacture of PVC. J Occup Med 1974;16:150–1.
54. Shimotohno K. Hepatitis C virus as a causative agent of hepatocellular carcinoma. Intervirology 1995;38:162–9.
55. Shaul Y, Ziemer M, Garcia PD. Cloning and analysis of integrated hepatitis virus sequences in human hepatocellular carcinomas. Hepatology 1984;51:776–87.
56. Ogston CW, Jonak CJ, Rogler CE, et al. Cloning and structural analysis of integrated woodchuck hepatitis virus sequences from hepatocellular carcinomas of woodchucks. Cell 1982;29:385–94.
57. London W, Blumberg B. A cellular model of the role of hepatitis B virus in the pathogenesis of primary hepatocellular carcinoma. Hepatology 1982;2:10S–4S.
58. Balsara BR, Pei J, De Rienzo A, et al. Human hepatocellular carcinoma is characterized by a highly consistent pattern of genomic imbalances including frequent loss of 16q23.1-24.1. Genes Chromosomes Cancer 2001;30:245–53.
59. Buetow KH, Murray JC, Israel JL, et al. Loss of heterozygosity suggests tumor suppressor gene responsible for primary hepatocellular carcinoma. Proc Natl Acad Sci U S A 1989;86:8852–6.
60. Hammond C, Jeffers L, Carr BI, Simon D. Multiple genetic alterations, 4q28, a new suppressor region, and potential gender differences in human hepatocellular carcinoma. Hepatology 1999;29:1479–85.
61. Kusano N, Shiraishi K, Kubo K, et al. Genetic aberrations detected by comparative genomic hybridization in hepatocellular carcinomas: their relationship to clinicopathological features. Hepatology 1999;29:1858–62.
62. Piao Z, Park C, Park JH, Kim H. Allelotype analysis of hepatocellular carcinoma. Int J Cancer 1998;75:29–33.
63. Pineau P, Nagai H, Prigent S, et al. Identification of three distinct regions of allelic deletions on the short arm of chromosome 8 in hepatocellular carcinoma. Oncogene 1999;18:127–34.
64. Wong N, Lai P, Lee SW, et al. Assessment of genetic changes in hepatocellular carcinoma by comparative genomic hybridization analysis: relationship to disease stage, tumor size, and cirrhosis. Am J Pathol 1999;154:37–43.
65. Bressac B, Kew M, Wands J, Ozturk M. Selective G to T mutations of p53 gene in hepatocellular carcinoma from southern Africa. Nature 1991;350:429-31.
66. Buetow KH, Sheffield VC, Zhu M, et al. Low frequency of p53 mutations observed in a diverse collection of primary hepatocellular carcinomas. Proc Natl Acad Sci U S A 1992;89:9622–6.
67. Hosono S, Chou MJ, Lee CS, Shih C. Infrequent mutation of p53 gene in hepatitis B virus positive primary hepatocellular carcinomas. Oncogene 1993;8:491–6.
68. Greenblatt MS, Feitelson MA, Zhu M, et al. Integrity of p53 in hepatitis B x antigen-positive and negative hepatocellular carcinomas. Cancer Res 1997;57:426–32.
69. Su Q, Schroder CH, Hofmann WJ, et al. Expression of hepatitis B virus X protein in HBV-infected human livers and hepatocellular carcinomas. Hepatology 1998;27:1109–20.
70. Groisman I, Koshy R, Henkler F, et al. Downregulation of DNA excision repair by the hepatitis B virus-x protein occurs in p53-proficient and p53-deficient cells. Carcinogenesis 1999;3:479–83.
71. Jia L, Wang XW, Harris CC. Hepatitis B virus X protein inhibits nucleotide excision repair. Int J Cancer 1999;80:875–9.
72. Chang M-H, Shau W-Y, Chen C-J, et al. Hepatitis B vaccination and hepatocellular carcinoma rates in boys and girls. JAMA 2000;284:3040–2.
73. Centers for Disease Control. Hepatitis B. virus: a comprehensive strategy for eliminating transmission in the United States through universal childhood vaccination. Recommendations of the Immunization Practices Advisory Committee. MMWR Morb Mortal Weekly Rep 1991;40:1–19.
74. Centers for Disease Control. Protection against viral hepatitis. Recommendations of the Immunization Practices Advisory Committee (ACIP). MMWR Morb Mortal Weekly Rep 1990;39:1–26.
75. Ni YH, Chang MH, Huang LM, et al. Hepatitis B virus infection in children and adolescents in a hyperendemic area: 15 years after mass hepatitis B vaccination. Ann Intern Med 2001;135:796–800.
76. Alter MJ. Epidemiology of hepatitis C. Hepatology 1997;26:62S–5S.
77. Colombo M. Screening for cancer in viral hepatitis. Clin Liver Dis 2001;5:109–22.
78. Tang ZY, Yu YQ, Zhou XD, et al. Subclinical hepatocellular carcinoma: an analysis of 391 patients. J Surg Oncol Suppl 1993;3:55–8.
79. Sherman M. Alpha-fetoprotein: an obituary. J Hepatol 2001;34:603–5.
80. Liaw Y-F, Sung JJY, Chow WC, et al. Lamivudine for patients with chronic hepatitis B and advanced liver disease. N Engl J Med 2004;351:1521–31.

81. Moriwaki H, Muto Y, Ninomiya M, et al. Inhibitory effects of synthetic acidic retinoid and polyprenoic acid on the development of hepatoma in rats induced by 3'-methyl-*N,N*-dimethyl-4-aminoazobenzene. J Gastroenterol 1988;23:546–52.
82. Fukutomi Y, Omori M, Muto Y, et al. Inhibitory effects of acyclic retinoid polyprenoic acid and its hydroxy derivative on cell growth and on secretion of alpha-fetoprotein in human hepatoma-derived cell line (PLC/PRF/%). Jpn J Cancer Res 1990;81:1281–5.
83. Nakamura N, Shidoji Y, Yamada Y, et al. Induction of apoptosis by acyclic retinoid in the human hepatoma derived cell line, HH-7. Biochem Biophys Res Comm 1995;207:382–8.
84. Muto Y, Moriwaki H, Ninomiya M, et al. Prevention of second primary tumors by an acyclic retinoid, polyprenoic acid, in patients with hepatocellular carcinoma. N Engl J Med 1996;334:1561–7.
85. Kensler TW, Egner PA, Wang J-B, et al. Chemoprevention of hepatocellular carcinoma in aflatoxin endemic areas. Gastroenterology 2004;127:S310–8.
86. Koga H. Hepatocellular carcinoma: Is there a potential for chemoprevention using cyclooxygenase-2 inhibitors. Cancer 2003;98:661–7.
87. Fujiki H, Suganuma M, Imai K, Nakachi K. Green tea: cancer preventive beverage and/or drug. Cancer Lett 2002;188:9–13.
88. Tietge UJ, Schofl C, Ocran KW, et al. Hepatoma with severe non-islet cell tumor hypoglycemia. Am J Gastroenterol 1998;93:997–1000.
89. Yen TC, Hwang SJ, Wang CC, et al. Hypercalcemia and parathyroid hormone-related protein in hepatocellular carcinoma. Liver 1993;13:311–5.
90. Sakisaka S, Watanabe M, Tateishi H, et al. Erythropoietin production in hepatocellular carcinoma cells associated with polycythemia: immunohistochemical evidence. Hepatology 1993;18:1357–62.
91. Gregory B, Ho VC. Cutaneous manifestations of gastrointestinal disorders. Part I. J Am Acad Dermatol 1992;26:153–66.
92. Hatch MC, Chen C-J, Levin B, et al. Urinary aflatoxin levels, hepatitis-B virus infection and hepatocellular carcinoma in Taiwan. Int J Cancer 1993;54:931–4.
93. Ganjei P, Nadji M, Albores-Saavedra J, Morales AR. Histologic markers in primary and metastatic tumors of the liver. Cancer 1988;62:1994–8.
94. Balaton AJ, Nehama-Sibony M, Gotheil C, et al. Distinction between hepatocellular carcinoma, cholangiocarcinoma, and metastatic carcinoma based on immunohistochemical staining for carcinoembryonic antigen and cytokeratin 19 on paraffin sections. J Pathol 1988;156:305–10.
95. Greene FL, Page DL, Fleming ID, et al. AJCC Cancer Staging Manual. 6th ed. New York: Springer; 2002.
96. Okuda K, Ohtsuki T, Obata H, et al. Natural history of hepatocellular carcinoma. Am J Clin Oncol 1998;21:386–91.
97. Poon RT, Ng IO, Lau C, et al. Tumor microvessel density as a predictor of recurrence after resection of hepatocellular carcinoma: a prospective study. J Clin Oncol 2002;20:1775–85.
98. Tamura S, Kato T, Berho M, et al. Impact of histological grade of hepatocellular carcinoma on the outcome of liver transplantation [discussion 31]. Arch Surg 2001;136:25–30.
99. Salizzoni M, Romagnoli R, Lupo F, et al. Microscopic vascular invasion detected by anti-CD34 immunohistochemistry as a predictor of recurrence of hepatocellular carcinoma after liver transplantation. Transplantation 2003;76:844–8.
100. Kurokawa Y, Matoba R, Takemasa I, et al. Molecular-based prediction of early recurrence in hepatocellular carcinoma. J Hepatol 2004;41:284–91.
101. DiBisceglie AM, Rustgi VK, Hoofnagle JH, et al. NIH conference: hepatocellular carcinoma. Ann Intern Med 1988;108:390–401.
102. Taketa K, Endo Y, Sekiya C, et al. A collaborative study for the evaluation of lectin-reactive α-fetoproteins in early detection of hepatocellular carcinoma. Cancer Res 1993;53:5419–23.
103. Sato Y, Nakata K, Kato Y, et al. Early recognition of hepatocellular carcinoma based on altered profiles of alpha-fetoprotein. N Engl J Med 1993;328:1802–6.
104. Shiraki K, Takase K, Tameda Y, et al. A clinical study of lectin-reactive alpha-fetoprotein as an early indicator of hepatocellular carcinoma in the follow-up of cirrhotic patients. Hepatology 1995;22:802–7.
105. Moriwaki H, Yasuda I, Shiratori Y, et al. Deletion of serum lectin-reactive α-fetoprotein by acyclic retinoid: a potent biomarker in the chemoprevention of second primary hepatoma. Clin Cancer Res 1997;3:727–31.
106. Kew MC, Wolf P, Whittaker D, Rowe P. Tumor-associated isoenzymes of gamma-glutamyl transferase in the serum of patients with hepatocellular carcinoma. Br J Cancer 1984;50:451–5.
107. Wudel LJ, Jr, Delbeke D, Morris D, et al. The role of [18F]fluorodeoxyglucose positron emission tomography imaging in the evaluation of hepatocellular carcinoma [discussion 124–116]. Am Surg 2003;69:117–24.
108. Peterson MS, Baron RL, Marsh JW, Jr., et al. Pretransplantation surveillance for possible hepatocellular carcinoma in patients with cirrhosis: epidemiology and CT-based tumor detection rate in 430 cases with surgical pathologic correlation. Radiology 2000;217:743–9.
109. Noguchi Y, Murakami T, Kim T, et al. Detection of hepatocellular carcinoma: comparison of dynamic MR imaging with dynamic double arterial phase helical CT. AJR Am J Roentgenol 2003;180:455–60.
110. Moran BJ, O'Rourke N, Plant GR, et al. Computed tomographic portography in pre-operative imaging of hepatic neoplasms. Br J Surg 1995;82:669–71.
111. Tang Z-Y, Yu Y-Q, Zhou X-D, et al. Subclinical hepatocellular carcinoma: an analysis of 391 patients. J Surg Oncol 1993;3 Suppl:55–8.
112. Lai EC, Fan ST, Lo CM, et al. Hepatic resection for hepatocellular carcinoma. Ann Surg 1995;221:291–9.
113. Liver Cancer Study Group of Japan. Predictive factors for long term prognosis after partial hepatectomy for patients with hepatocellular carcinoma in Japan. Cancer 1994;74:2772–80.
114. Tang Z-Y, Yu Y-Q, Zhou X-D. Evolution of surgery in the treatment of hepatocellular carcinoma from the 1950s to the 1990s. World J Surg 1993;9:293–7.
115. Kawarada Y, Ito F, Shakurai H, et al. Surgical treatment of hepatocellular carcinoma. Cancer Chemother Pharmacol 1994;33 Suppl:S12–17.
116. Kassianides C, Kew MC. The clinical manifestations and natural history of hepatocellular carcinoma. Gastroenterol Clin North Am 1987;16:553–62.
117. Lai ECS, Ng IOL, You KT, et al. Hepatectomy for large hepatocellular carcinoma: the optimal resection margin. World J Surg 1991;15:141–5.
118. Fong Y, Sun R, Jarnagin W, Blumgart L. An analysis of 412 cases of hepatocellular carcinoma at a western center. Ann Surg 1999;229:790–800.
119. Sasaki Y, Imaoka S, Masutani S, et al. Influence of coexisting cirrhosis on long-term prognosis after surgery in patients with hepatocellular carcinoma. Surgery 1992;112:515–21.
120. AJCC. Cancer Staging Handbook. 6th ed. New York: Springer; 2002.
121. Okada S, Shimada K, Yamamoto J, et al. Predictive factors for postoperative recurrence of hepatocellular carcinoma. Gastroenterology 1994;106:1618–24.
122. Fan S, Lai EC, Lo CM, et al. Hospital mortality of major hepatectomy for hepatocellular carcinoma associated with cirrhosis. Arch Surg 1995;130:198–203.
123. Nagasue N, Kohno H, Chang YC, et al. Liver resection for hepatocellular carcinoma. Ann Surg 1993;217:375–384.
124. Iwatsuki S, Starzi TE. Role of liver transplantation in the treatment of hepatocellular carcinoma. Semin Surg Oncol 1993;9:337–340.
125. Penn I. Hepatic transplantation for primary and metastatic cancers of the liver. Surgery 1991;110;726–34.
126. Bismuth H, Chiche L, Adam R, et al. A liver resection versus transplantation for hepatocellular carcinoma in cirrhotic patients. Ann Surg 1993;218:145–51.
127. Iwatsuki S, Starzl TE, Sheahan DG, et al. Hepatic resection versus transplantation for hepatocellular carcinoma. Ann Surg 1991;214:221–8.
128. Ringe B, Pichlmayr R, Wittekind C, et al. Surgical treatment of hepatocellular carcinoma: experience with liver resection and transplantation in 98 patients. World J Surg 1991;15:270–85.
129. Ojogho ON, So SK, Keefe EB, et al. Orthotopic liver transplantation for hepatocellular carcinoma. Arch Surg 1996;131:935–41.
130. United Network for Organ Sharing. U. S. Transplantation Data. www.unos.org/data/default/asp$displayType=usdata (accessed January 12, 2005)
131. Adam R, Castaing D, Azoulay D, et al. Indications and results of liver transplantation in the treatment of hepatocellular carcinoma in cirrhosis. Ann Chir 1998;52:547–57.
132. Mazzaferro V, Regalia E, Doci R, et al. Liver transplantation for the treatment of small hepatocellular carcinomas in patients with cirrhosis. N Engl J Med 1996;334:693–9.
133. Trotter JF, Wachs M, Everson G, et al. Adult-to-adult transplantation of the right hepatic lobe from a living donor. N Engl J Med 2002;346:1074–82.
134. Stone MJ, Klintmalm GBG, Polter D, et al. Neoadjuvant chemotherapy and liver transplantation for hepatocellular carcinoma: a pilot study in 20 patients. Gastroenterology 1993;104:196–202.
135. Olthoff KM, Rosove MH, Shackleton CR, et al. Adjuvant chemotherapy improves survival after liver transplantation for hepatocellular carcinoma. Ann Surg 1995;221:734–43.
136. Pentecost MJ, Daniels JR, Teitelbaum GP, Stanley P. Hepatic chemoembolization: safety with portal vein thrombosis. J Vasc Interv Radiol 1993;4:347–51.
137. Charnsangavej C. Chemoembolization of liver-tumors. Sem Interv Radiol 1993;10:150–60.
138. Aina R, Oliva VL, Therasse E, et al. Arterial embolotherapy for upper gastrointestinal hemorrhage: outcome assessment. J Vasc Interv Radiol 2001;12:195–200.
139. Lo CM, Ngan H, Tso WK, et al. Randomized controlled trial of transarterial lipiodol chemoembolization for unresectable hepatocellular carcinoma. Hepatology 2002;35:1164–71.
140. Llovet JM, Real MI, Montana X, et al. Arterial embolisation or chemoembolisation versus symptomatic treatment in patients with unresectable hepatocellular carcinoma: a randomised controlled trial. Lancet 2002;359:1734–9.
141. Tateishi R, Shiina S, Teratani T, et al. Percutaneous radiofrequency ablation for hepatocellular carcinoma: an analysis of 1000 cases. Cancer 2005;103:1201–9.
142. Stuart K, Tessitore J, Rudy J, et al. A phase II trial of nolatrexed dihydrochloride in patients with advanced hepatocellular carcinoma. Cancer 1999;86:410–4.
143. Mok TS, Leung TW, Lee SD, et al. A multi-centre randomized phase II study of nolatrexed versus doxorubicin in treatment of Chinese patients with advanced hepatocellular carcinoma. Cancer Chemother Pharmacol 1999;44:307–11.
144. Nowak AK, Stockler MR, Chow PKH, Findlay M. Use of tamoxifen in advanced-stage hepatocellular carcinoma: a systematic review. Cancer 2005;103:1408–14.
145. Yuen MF, Poon RT, Lai CL, et al. A randomized placebo controlled study of long-acting octreotide for the treatment of advanced hepatocellular carcinoma. Hepatology 2002;36:687–91.
146. Burroughs A, Hochhauser D, Meyer T. Systemic treatment and liver transplantation for hepatocellular carcinoma: two ends of the therapeutic spectrum. The Lancet Oncology 2004;5:409–18.
147. Thomas MB, Zhu AX. Hepatocellular carcinoma: the need for progress. J Clin Oncol 2005;23:2892–99.
148. Chao Y, Li CP, Chau GY, et al. Prognostic significance of vascular endothelial growth factor, basic fibroblast growth factor, and angiogenin in patients with resectable hepatocellular carcinoma after surgery. Ann Surg Oncol 2003;10:355–62.
149. Poon RT, Lau CP, Cheung ST, et al. Quantitative correlation of serum levels and tumor expression of vascular endothelial growth factor in patients with hepatocellular carcinoma. Cancer Res 2003;63:3121–6.
150. Schwartz JD, Goldman J, Coll D, et al. Bevacizumab in hepatocellular carcinoma (HCC) in patients without metastasis and without invasion of the portal vein. Proc gastrointestinal cancer symp (ASCO, ASTRO, AGA, SSO), 2004;105:(A128).
151. Huang SM, Harari PM. Modulation of radiation response after epidermal growth factor receptor blockade in squamous cell carcinomas: inhibition of damage repair, cell cycle kinetics, and tumor angiogenesis. Clin Cancer Res 2000;6:2166–74.
152. Suzuki A, Hayashida M, Kawano H, et al. Hepatocyte growth factor promotes cell survival from fas-mediated cell death in hepatocellular carcinoma cells via Akt activation and Fas-death-inducing signaling complex suppression. Hepatology 2000;32:796–802.
153. Daveau M, Scotte M, Francois A, et al. Hepatocyte growth factor, transforming growth factor alpha, and their receptors as combined markers of prognosis in hepatocellular carcinoma. Mol Carcinog 2003;36:130–41.
154. Kamiyama T, Une Y, Uchino J, Hamada J. Hepatocyte growth factor enhances the invasion activity of human hepatocellular carcinoma cell lines. Int J Oncol 1998;12:655–9.
155. De Petro G, Tavian D, Copeta A, et al. Expression of urokinase-type plasminogen activator (u-PA), u-PA receptor, and tissue-type PA messenger RNAs in human hepatocellular carcinoma. Cancer Res 1998;58:2234–9.
156. Tavian D, De Petro G, Benetti A, et al. u-PA and c-MET mRNA expression is co-ordinately enhanced while hepa-

tocyte growth factor mRNA is down-regulated in human hepatocellular carcinoma. Int J Cancer 2000;87:644–9.
157. Dubuisson L, Monvoisin A, Nielsen BS, et al. Expression and cellular localization of the urokinase-type plasminogen activator and its receptor in human hepatocellular carcinoma. J Pathol 2000;190:190–5.
158. Itoh T, Hayashi Y, Kanamaru T, et al. Clinical significance of urokinase-type plasminogen activator activity in hepatocellular carcinoma. J Gastroenterol Hepatol 2000;15:422–30.
159. Zheng Q, Tang ZY, Xue Q, et al. Invasion and metastasis of hepatocellular carcinoma in relation to urokinase-type plasminogen activator, its receptor and inhibitor. J Cancer Res Clin Oncol 2000;126:641–6.
160. Nagorney DM, Donohue JH, Farnell MB, et al. Outcomes after curative resections of cholangiocarcinoma [discussion 877–879]. Arch Surg 1993;128:871–7.
161. Valverde A, Bonhomme N, Farges O, et al. Resection of intrahepatic cholangiocarcinoma: a Western experience. J Hepatobiliary Pancreat Surg 1999;6:122–7.
162. Foster JH, Berman MM. The malignant transformation of liver cell adenomas. Arch Surg 1994;129:712–7.
163. Nguyen BN, Flejou JF, Terris B, et al. Focal nodular hyperplasia of the liver: a comprehensive pathologic study of 305 lesions and recognition of new histologic forms. Am J Surg Pathol 1999;23:1441–54.
164. Boulahdour H, Cherqui D, Charlotte F, et al. The hot spot hepatobiliary scan in focal nodular hyperplasia. J Nucl Med 1993;34:2105–10.
165. Tamm EP, Rabushka LS, Fishman EK, et al. Intrahepatic, extramedullary hematopoiesis mimicking hemangioma on technetium-99m red blood cell SPECT examination. Clin Imaging 1995;19:88–91.
166. Edmondson HA, Craig JR. Disease of the liver. 6th ed. Philadelphia: J.B. Lippincott; 1987.
167. Ganjei P, Nadji M, Albore-Saavedra J, Morales AR. Histologic markers in primary and metastatic tumors of the liver. Cancer 1998;62:1994–8.
168. Balaton AJ, Nehama-Sibony M, Gotheil C, et al. Distinction between hepatocellular carcinoma, cholangiocarcinoma and metastatic carcinoma based on immunohistochemical staining for carcinoembryonic antigen and cytokeratin 19 on paraffin sections. J Pathol 1988;156:305–10.
169. Liver Cancer Study Group of Japan. Primary liver cancer in Japan: clinicopathologic features and results of surgical treatment. Ann Surg 1990;211:277–87.
170. Kawarada Y, Ito F, Shakurai H, et al. Surgical treatment of hepatocellular carcinoma. Cancer chemother pharmacol 1994;33:S12–7.

Treatment of Liver Metastases

Nancy E. Kemeny, MD
Yuman Fong, MD

The liver is a frequent site for metastases from cancers arising at other sites. For cancers that occur in the gastrointestinal tract, the frequency of metastatic disease to the liver is easily explained, since the venous drainage of most gastrointestinal organs is via the portal vein and passes through the liver. It is not surprising, therefore, that for tumors such as colorectal cancer, the liver is the most common and, frequently, the only site of metastatic disease. Extra-abdominal tumors such as bronchogenic carcinoma, breast cancer, and malignant melanoma often spread hematogenously to the liver. In an autopsy series of 10,736 extrahepatic primary tumors, liver metastases with or without metastases to other organs were present in 41%[1] (Table 88-1). Therefore, it is clear that metastatic disease to the liver represents a significant oncologic problem.

Although it is recognized that liver metastases play a major role in the morbidity and mortality associated with many cancers, until recently, the approach to the patient with hepatic metastasis has been nihilistic. In the last two decades, therapies have been developed for hepatic metastases that offer not only effective palliation, but in many cases, cure. Improved imaging modalities such as ultrasonography, computed tomography (CT), magnetic resonance imaging (MRI), and positron emission tomography (PET) have allowed detection of metastases at a sufficiently early stage for effective therapy. Improvements in surgical and anesthetic techniques now permit hepatic resection with perioperative mortality of less than 4%, making these potentially curative resections acceptable from the standpoint of risk. In addition, development of other palliative techniques, such as regional chemotherapy and cryoablation offer effective palliative options in cases where curative resections are not possible. In this chapter, we will discuss the different modalities that can eradicate hepatic metastases and then we will summarize the clinical data supporting the use of various modalities available for the treatment of liver metastases.

IMAGING TECHNIQUES

Imaging modalities have become indispensable to the treatment of the patient with liver metastases. Early, accurate detection of liver metastases permits discovery of tumors at a curable stage, helps in choosing among the alternative therapies, facilitates preoperative planning, and enhances monitoring response in cases when a nonsurgical approach is most reasonable. Modalities that are currently useful are listed below.

COMPUTED TOMOGRAPHY CT is one of the most useful tests to detect liver metastases. A narrow window setting and a lower width (100–150 HU) are the most useful since these settings increase contrast differences between the normal liver parenchyma and abnormal areas. Noncontrast CT is helpful in identifying hypervascular metastases (especially carcinoid, islet cell tumors, and renal cell carcinomas) or visualizing calcifications or hemorrhage. Dynamic CT (where there is a rapid intravenous infusion of contrast) is better for detecting tumors that are hypovascular, such as colorectal carcinomas. One problem with this modality is that lesions may not be distinguishable from liver parenchyma during the equilibrium phase of the contrast injection (when the intravascular and interstitial concentrations equilibrate).[2] CT portography (contrast given via a superior mesenteric vein injection) delivers contrast to the normal parenchyma via the portal vein. Since colorectal metastases are largely nourished by the hepatic artery and derive little blood supply from the portal vein, they appear as filling defects surrounded by liver parenchyma, which is contrast enhanced since the majority of parenchymal blood supply is from the portal vein.[2]

MAGNETIC RESONANCE IMAGING T_1-weighted spin echo images generally show metastases as low intensity lesions, whereas T_2-weighted images of metastases are areas of high-signal intensity (Figure 88-1). At all field strengths, T_2-weighted sequences are generally superior for the detection and characterization of liver masses. Benign cysts and hemangiomas are generally homogeneous and have a bright appearance (termed a "light bulb" sign), whereas metastatic lesions are more heterogeneous and not as bright. On MRI, hemangiomas can be confused with highly vascular tumors and with cysts; however, if dynamic gadolinium injections are given, hemangiomas can be more accurately diagnosed, since they will demonstrate peripheral nodular enhancement. MRI is also useful to distinguish fatty infiltration from metastases (see Figure 88-1).[3] Demonstration of extrahepatic pathology by MRI is inferior to CT.

ULTRASONOGRAPHY: TRANSCUTANEOUS AND INTRAOPERATIVE ULTRASONOGRAPHY Transcutaneous ultrasonic evaluation of the liver for metastases represents the least invasive and least expensive of the diagnostic modalities. However, it is also depends primarily on the expertise and diligence of the operator. In addition, since overlying air may obscure ultrasonic imaging of the liver, overlying bowel and lung tissue may obscure imaging of lesions, particularly at the dome of the liver. Nevertheless, in expert hands, this modality may be as accurate as CT or MRI in determining the number and size of lesions, as well as their relationship to major vessels.[3]

Intraoperative ultrasonography (IOUS) is equally operator dependent but has become indispensable in the surgical treatment of liver tumors. This modality is now being used to increase the ability to detect small and deep hepatic lesions that are not palpable, even by bimanual technique. In two studies of patients with colorectal cancer who underwent colon resection, lesions missed on surgical palpation were detected by IOUS (14 in one study and 7 in the other).[3]

POSITRON EMISSION TOMOGRAPHY It has long been noted that colon cancer cells use glucose at a higher rate than normal tissues. PET exploits this

Table 88-1 Common Primary Site for Cancer Metastatic to the Liver[1]

	Metastatic Site		Percent of MetastaticCases with Liver Involvement
	Liver Only	Liver ± Other	
Lung	602	593	50
Breast	328	643	66
Colon/Rectum	145	383	73
Stomach	123	158	56
Pancreas	32	148	79
Uterus	264	200	43
Ovary	154	177	53
Skin	118	160	58

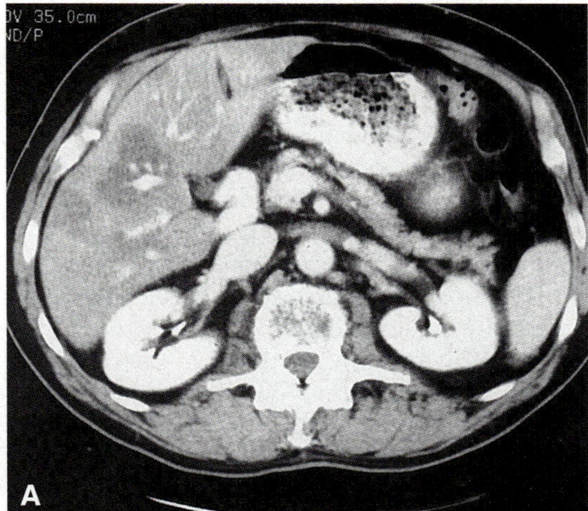

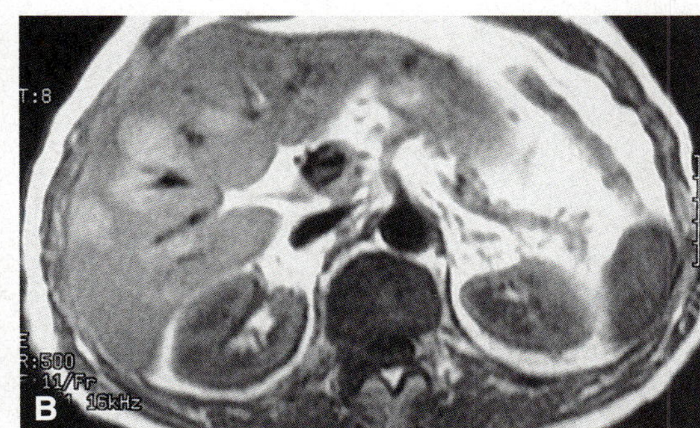

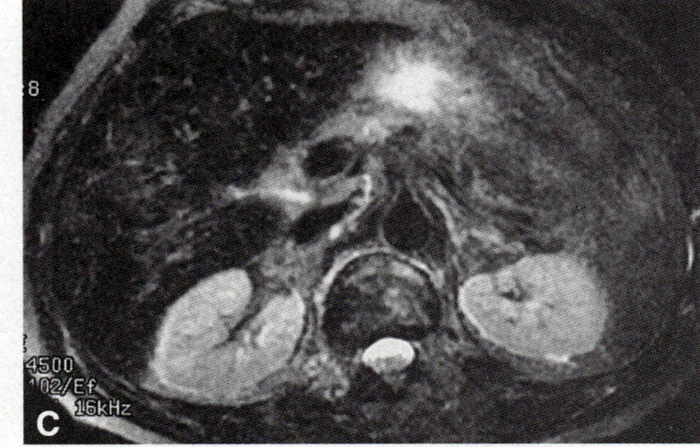

Figure 88-1 A, A CT scan of abdomen showing lesions that were read as metastatic disease. On closer inspection, vessels are seen coursing through the lesions, suggesting fatty infiltrations. **B,** A T_1-weighted spin echo MRI (TR 500, TE111) in which the brightness of the lesions is hyperintense relative to liver, which is a clue that they are fatty infiltrated. **C,** A T_2-weighted fast-spin echo (TR 4500, TE102) with fat saturation. Areas that were bright are now suppressed, indicating fatty liver with vessels coursing through it.

characteristic of tumor cells in order to image tumor sites. When a positron emitting glucose analogue 2-[18F]-fluoro-2-deoxyglucose (18F-FDG) is administered to patients with colorectal cancer, the radiolabeled glucose analogue is transported into tumor cells by the same cell-surface hexose transporters that transport glucose and undergoes phosphorylation to FDG-6-phosphate. 18F-FDG-6-phosphate is not subject to further metabolism in most tumor cells and therefore is selectively retained.[4,5] Imaging by positron detectors allows whole-body staging for cancer.

Four early studies have sought to determine the utility of this modality in the preoperative assessment of patients with liver metastases.[6–9] These preliminary studies suggested that 18F-FDG-PET may detect additional occult disease in up to one-third of patients with metastatic colorectal cancer. Three definitive studies have since further defined the role of FDG-PET in this patient population. In a study examining long-term outcome of patients with hepatic colorectal metastases who were assessed by FDG-PET prior to liver resection, higher resectability, lower recurrence, and improved long-term survival was associated with use of FDG-PET.[10] This study suggests that improved patient selection using this imaging modality may improve ultimate patient outcome. As would be expected, the yield of the FDG-PET is related to the risk of occult disease. A recent study has suggested that a clinical risk score that has been developed for stratification of risk of recurrence can be used to predict yield of FDG-PET scanning.[11] Finally, a study has also shown that although FDG-PET is quite useful in detecting extrahepatic metastases, its utility in detection of small intrahepatic metastases is questionable. This study correlated pathologically assessed liver tumors to preoperative PET scanning and found that subcentimeter tumors in the liver are only detected 20% of the time.[12] In patients undergoing preoperative chemotherapeutic treatments, the record is even worse: only 5% of subcentimeter lesions were detected. From these recent data a few conclusions about FDG-PET can be drawn. It is a useful test in the preoperative staging of patients with metastatic colorectal cancer. Patients with synchronous liver metastases or with high clinical risk scores[13] are particularly good candidates for scanning. FDG-PET should not be used as the sole test in the follow-up of patients after hepatic resection, when liver is the most common site of recurrence.

LIVER RESECTION

Most liver resections for metastatic disease to the liver are performed for cancers that originated from the colon or rectum. These resections are being performed because liver metastases from colorectal cancer are common; the liver is often the only site of metastases, alternative treatments are never curative, and surgical excision can be performed safely and is potentially curative. Of the 150,000 patients presenting each year in the United States with colorectal cancer, over 50,000 will be found during the course of their disease with hepatic metastases.[14–16] If untreated, patients with hepatic colorectal metastases have a median survival of 5 to 10 months; with less than 0.5% surviving 5 years.[14,17–22] Systemic chemotherapy, although it prolongs survival, rarely results in survival over 3 years.[23–31]

On the basis of the hypothesis that metastatic disease may be limited to the liver, and encouraged by autopsy findings that one-third of the patients dying of colorectal cancer have the liver as the only site of metastatic disease, surgeons have resected hepatic metastases in an attempt to cure disease clinically confined to the liver. A number of retrospective studies of resection of metastatic colorectal cancer to the liver provide abundant evidence that major liver resection can be performed safely and provide prolonged disease-free survival and cure (Table 88-2). The reported complication rate in most series is

Table 88-2 Results of Hepatic Resection for Metastatic Colorectal Cancer

	Operative Mortality		Survival			
Study	*n*	%	1 y %	3 y %	5 y %	10 y %
Foster[40]	78	5	—	—	22	—
Thompson[41]	22	11	80	37	31	—
Adson[39]	141	2	82	40	25	—
Fortner[37]	75	7	89	57	35	—
Butler[42]	62	10	—	50	34	21
Iwatsuki[43]	60	0	95	53	45	—
Hughes[44]	607	—	—	—	33	—
Nordlinger[32]	80	5	5	41	25	16
Coburn[45]	56	0	—	—	25	—
Schlag[34]	122	4	85	40	30	—
Doci[35]	100	5	—	—	30	—
Younes[46]	133	—	91	—	—	—
Scheele[52]	219	6	—	—	39	21
Rosen[47]	280	4	84	47	25	—
Gayowski[51]	204	0	91	45	34	—
Scheele[52]	469	4	—	45	38	23
Fong[53]	577	3	88	59	38	—
Nordlinger[54]	1568	2	88	44	28	—
Rees[55]	150	1	94	—	37	—
Jamison[56]	280	4	84	46	27	20
Fong[13]	1001	3	89	57	37	22

Table 88-3 Complications of Liver Resection # (%)

	Scheele[36]	Schlag[34]	Doci[35]	Fortner[37]	Nordlinger[32]
Total	219	122	100	75	80
Liver-Related Complications					
Hemorrhage	7(3)	—	3	1(1)	1(1)
Bile fistula	8(4)	5(4)	4	—	—
Perihepatic abscess	4(2)	11(9)	5	5(7)	2(3)
Liver failure	17(8)	—	3	3(4)	1(1)
Renal failure	3(1)	—	1	—	—
Portal vein thrombosis	—	—	—	1(1)	—
Infections					
Wound	—	7(6)	—	1(1)	—
Sepsis	—	3(2)	2	—	4(5)
General Complications					
Gastrointestinal bleeding	—	M	—	—	1(1)
Deep vein thrombosis	2(1)	M	—	1(1)	—
Pulmonary embolism	4(2)	M	—	1(1)	1(1)
Cardiac/MI	2(1)	6(5)	1	1(1)	1(1)
Pneumonia	0(0)	10(8)	22	3(4)	—
Pleural effusion	—	M	—	6(8)	3(4)

MI = myocarcinoid infarction.

approximately 20% (Table 88-3). The most common complications are pulmonary, with symptomatic pleural effusions occurring in 5 to 10% of the patients,[32,33] pneumonia occurring in 5 to 22%,[34,35] and pulmonary embolism in 1%.[36,37] Hepatic insufficiency occurs in 3 to 8% of all major resections.[34–36,38] Bile leak and biliary fistula occur in approximately 4% of all patients,[34–36] and perihepatic abscess occurs in 2 to 10%.[32,34,36,37] Significant hemorrhage is rare (1–3%) but is a major cause of perioperative mortality. However, the high incidence of complications does not always translate into mortality or prolonged hospital stays. Even for resections of up to 80% of the liver, the mortality associated with elective liver resection for colorectal metastases is less than 5% in the most recent experience (see Table 88-2).[32,34–37,39–47] The reported median hospital stay from centers experienced in liver surgery is less than 2 weeks. In our recent series of 1,001 consecutive resections, including 237 trisegmentectomies, the mortality was 3%; the median hospital stay was 9 days, and ICU admission was required for only 4% of patients.[38]

Long-term results after resection of hepatic colorectal metastases clearly indicate the potentially curative nature of such treatment and justify the risks and costs involved. Representative studies on long-term outcome after liver resection for metastatic colorectal cancer are summarized in Table 88-2.[13,35,43,44,46,48–56] The 3-year survival is above 40%, and the 5-year survival is between 25 and 40%. In series with long enough follow-up, the 10-year survival is reported to be 20%.[32,36,42] The median survival is consistently over 2 years. Such results are superior to any reported for any other treatment modalities, including systemic chemotherapy, intra-arterial chemotherapy, or ablative modalities, and certainly superior to the outcome of untreated cases. Surgical resection must therefore be regarded as the standard of care for resectable colorectal metastases.

Many of the published studies have attempted to identify prognostic factors for poor outcome to refine patient selection criteria (Table 88-4). To date, the only absolute contraindication to resection is extrahepatic disease.[15,37,39,44,47,57] There are other factors associated with poor outcome, such as advanced stage of primary cancer,[35,44] short disease-free interval between primary cancer and hepatic metastases,[36,44,47] multiple tumors,[44,47] bilateral tumors,[15] very high preoperative carcinoembryonic antigen[44,58] and size of tumor.[44,59] However, the presence of any of these factors does not preclude long-term survival. An overwhelming predictor of recurrence, however, is involvement of the resection margin by tumor.[44,58]

Data from many large series have confirmed a potentially curative role for liver resection in the treatment of metastatic colorectal cancer. With improving perioperative outcomes, increasingly aggressive resections are being performed. As a result, there is an increasing need for a simple prognostic scoring system to permit selection of those biologically favorable patients for liver resection. In addition, such a scoring system would be important for stratification of patients for clinical trials. In our recent analysis of 1,001 consecutive liver resections several factors were found to be most influential for poor outcome[13]: (1) size of liver tumors > 5 cm; (2) disease-free interval between colon and liver disease < 12 months; (3) number of liver tumors greater than one; (4) lymph node-positive primary; and (5) preoperative CEA level of greater than 200 ng/mL. However, presence of any one of these characteristics was still associated with a 5-year survival of 24 to 34%, and therefore none can be considered complete contraindications to resection. We now use the clinical risk score based on these five criteria to guide patient selection and stratification. Assigning one point to each of these factors predictive of poor prognosis, the clinical risk score consists of the sum. A score of 2 or less places a patient in a good prognostic group, for whom resection is ideal. For scores of 3 or 4, outcome is less favorable and patients should be considered for aggressive trials of adjuvant therapy. For a score of 5, we have not encountered a long-term survivor, and therefore, resections outside of trials of adjuvant therapy are discouraged. This prognostic scoring system has been verified by independent investigators.[60] This clinical risk score is also now being used to help select the degree of sophistication of

Table 88-4 Predictors of Recurrence after Hepatic Resection for Metastatic Colorectal Cancer

			Metastases							
Study	Patient Age	Primary Stage	Synchronous	Size	Number	Bilobar	Satellite	Chemo	Surgical Margin	CEA
Foster[40]	—	N	N	Y	Y	—	—	—	—	—
Adson[39]	—	Y	N	N	N	N	—	—	—	—
Fortner[37]	N	Y	—	N	N	—	—	N	—	N
Butler[42]	N	Y	N	N	N	—	—	N	N	—
Iwatsuki[43]	N	Y	N	Y	Y	—	—	Y	—	—
Hughes[44]	—	Y	Y	Y	Y	Y	—	Y	Y	Y
Nordlinger[32]	—	N	N	N	N	—	—	—	—	—
Coburn[45]	—	N	N	—	Y	—	N	—	—	—
Schlag[34]	—	—	Y	—	—	—	—	—	—	—
Doci[35]	N	Y	N	N	N	N	—	—	—	Y
Younes[46]	—	N	N	Y	Y	—	—	—	—	Y
Scheele[36]	N	Y	Y	N	N	N	Y	—	Y	—
Rosen[47]	—	N	N	N	N	—	Y	—	N	N
Cady[58]	N	N	N	N	Y	—	—	—	Y	Y

N= no; Y = yes.

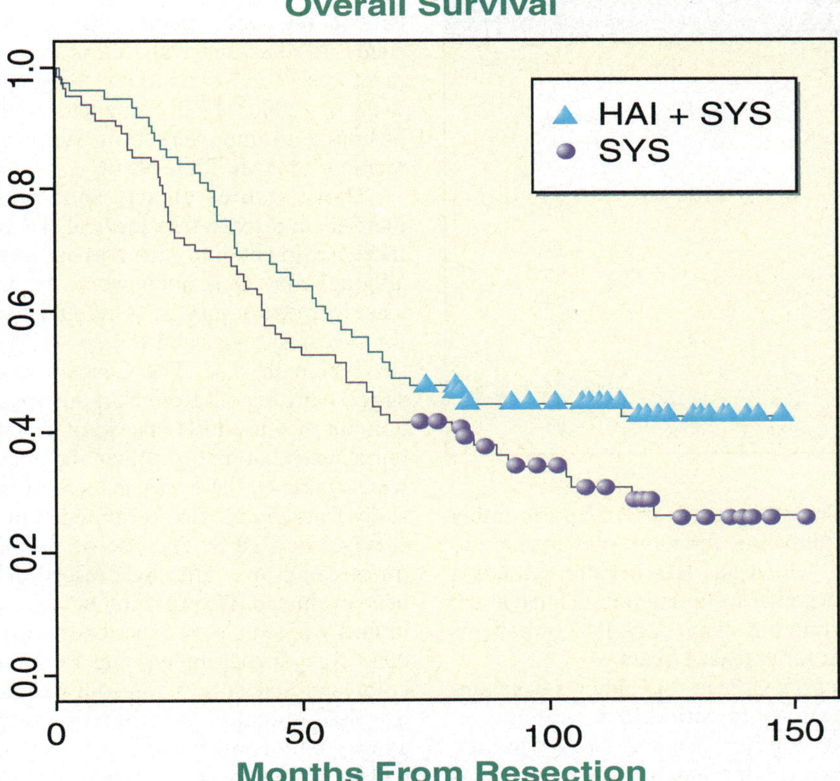

Figure 88-2 Kaplan–Meier estimates of overall survival in the groups assigned to either HAI plus systemic chemotherapy or systemic chemotherapy alone. The estimated median survival was 72.2 months in the combined-therapy group (29 of the 74 patients died) and 59.3 months in the monotherapy group (38 of 82 patients died).

preoperative assessment. A high clinical risk score has been associated with sufficient yield to justify both FDG-pet scanning[11] and laparoscopy[61] in the preoperative staging of patients with hepatic colorectal metastases.

The basis for resection of metastases from cancers other than colorectal adenocarcinoma is much less firm. In general, indications for resecting other metastases can be grouped into four major categories. As with hepatic colorectal metastases, resection of other tumor types is being performed for potential cure.[62–64] Additionally, for tumors such as functional neuroendocrine tumor, resection is carried out for symptomatic relief.[65–68] Hepatic resection for metastatic disease isolated to the liver is also performed when no good alternative therapy exists, such as in cases of metastatic sarcomas, or when all the good alternatives have been exhausted, as in metastatic germ cell cancer or breast cancer after chemotherapy.[69–71] In some tumors that are very sensitive to chemotherapy (such as germ cell tumors), lesions seen on CT scan after chemotherapy may not be viable tumors, and in these situations, hepatic resections may be performed to determine the need for further treatment.[71] At present, however, reports of hepatic resection for these other tumor types are still largely anecdotal. Hepatic colorectal metastases are the only metastatic lesions for which hepatic resection should be considered standard therapy. Resections of all other metastatic tumor types must be considered investigational and ideally should be performed in a research environment where results can be critically analyzed.

ADJUVANT CHEMOTHERAPY AFTER LIVER RESECTION

Nearly two-thirds of patients selected for liver resection of metastatic colorectal cancer will have a recurrence owing to microscopic residual disease undetected at the time of the original liver resection. This provides a rationale for adjuvant chemotherapy.

ADJUVANT SYSTEMIC CHEMOTHERAPY

Few trials have evaluated the role of adjuvant systemic therapy post liver resection. O'Connell and colleagues treated 26 patients with 5-FU and semustine post liver resection and compared them with 26 patients with closely matched prognostic factors treated with liver resection alone. There was no significant survival advantage in the adjuvant chemotherapy group.[72] Portier and colleagues randomized 173 patients to intravenous 5-FU or no chemotherapy post liver resection and demonstrated a 5-year survival of 50% and 40% respectively ($p = .15$).[73] A similar trial by Langer and colleagues reported a 4-year survival of 57% and 47% respectively with a median survival of 53 months and 43 months respectively ($p = .39$).[74]

At present, patients who have not received chemotherapy are usually offered adjuvant oxaliplatin (oxa), 5-fluorouracil (5-FU), and leucovorin (LV) based on an adjuvant chemotherapy trial after primary colon resection.[75] For patients who have had prior chemotherapy, the use of adjuvant systemic therapy has not been studied but because second-line therapy has less activity in the metastatic, it would be reasonable to consider alternate therapies to adjuvant systemic therapy alone.

ADJUVANT HEPATIC ARTERIAL INFUSION

A number of trials have evaluated the use of adjuvant hepatic arterial infusion (HAI) chemotherapy after liver resection. The reason such regional adjuvant treatment was pursued was that in many series the most common site for tumor recurrence after resection of hepatic colorectal metastases is the residual liver.[15,16,32,76]

Five randomized trials examined the role of adjuvant HAI after liver resection. The Memorial Sloan-Kettering Cancer Center (MSKCC) trial[77] was a large, single-institutional study where 156 patients were randomized to systemic 5-FU and LV (SYS) or HAI FUDR and dexamethasone with systemic 5-FU and LV (HAI+SYS).[77] The primary endpoint was 2-year survival. The two treatment groups were stratified by the number of metastases and the type of treatment patients received prior to entry in the study. Approximately 20% of each group had greater than four liver metastases. Baseline characteristics were well matched, including poor prognostic variables (positive hepatic resection margins, synchronous disease), the number receiving large resections (trisegmentectomy or lobectomy), the number with Dukes' C or rectal primaries, and the number of patients with abnormal expression of p53 or high thymidylate synthetase.

Two-year survival was significantly longer for HAI+SYS group (85% and 69% for the HAI+SYS and SYS groups, respectively, $p = .02$). The endpoint of the study was accomplished.[77] When first publicized, the 2-year hepatic disease free survival was significantly longer in the HIA group but progression free survival was not. Now with a median follow-up of 10 years, median overall disease-free survival is significant, 31 months for HAI+SYS and 17 months for SYS-alone group ($p < .02$). Ten-year survival is 41% for HAI+SYS and 27.2% for SYS-alone. (see Figure 88-2) Median survival is 68.4 months and 58.8 months for the HAI+SYS versus SYS alone groups, respectively. Updated median hepatic-free survival has not been reached for the HAI+SYS group and is 32.5 months for the SYS-alone group ($p < .001$). Hepatic toxicity was increased in the HAI+SYS group with increased bilirubin in 11% and 5 patients requiring biliary stents (Table 88-5). If patients are divided into good risk and bad risk patients the 10-year survival is still high for patients who received HAI (Figure 88-3).

Another trial conducted by the Eastern Cooperative Oncology Group randomized patients to observation alone versus a combination of

Table 88-5 Randomized Trial After Liver Resection: HAI + Systemic versus Systemic. Updated Results.

	HAI + Systemic	Systemic	*p*-Value
Median survival (mos.)	68.4	58.8	.1
DFS (mos.)	31.3	17.2	.02
HDFS (mos.)	NR	32.5	< .01
Score 0–2			
Median survival: (mos.)	83.2	82.8	.56
Score 3–5			
Median survival: (mos.)	60	38.3	.13
5-year survival (mos.)	54.9%	48.8%	.86
10-year survival (mos.)	41.1%	29.7%	.74
Score 0–2[13] 10-year survival (mos.):	44.5%	41.9%	.95
Score 3–5[13] 10-year survival (mos.):	37%	16.3%	.60
Median survival (mos.): # mets – 1	117.6	82.8	.86
Median survival (mos.): # mets – 2-4	85.2	44.4	.01
Median survival (mos.): # mets - > 4	48.1	39.6	.99

hepatic arterial FUDR and systemic infusional 5-FU.[78] The study was powered to detect a difference in disease-free survival: 109 patients were randomized, and randomization was done prior to surgery. Twenty-nine patients, though randomized, are not in the study because of extrahepatic disease or unresectable disease. If the patients who actually entered the study are considered, of the 45 patients in the control group, 77.8% had recurrence and 53% in the liver. In the 30 patients in the HAI group, 16 (53%) had recurrence and only 8 (26%) had liver recurrence. The 4-year recurrence-free survival was improved 46% versus 22% in the HAI and control groups, respectively ($p = .04$). The endpoint was recurrence-free survival not overall survival and the endpoint was accomplished. Five-year survival for the patients who actually were in the study was 59% HAI+SYS versus 40% of those in the control group. Median survival was 63.7 months for the HAI+SYS group and 49.4 months for the control group ($p = .6$) (Table 88-6).

A German Cooperative Group performed a randomized trial after hepatic resection of adjuvant HAI of FU and LV versus control.[79] Patients were stratified according to number of liver metastases (one to two versus three to six) and the site of the primary tumor (colon and upper rectum versus mid or lower rectum). Despite the initial randomization, 21% in the HAI arm did not receive the assigned treatment for various reasons, including anatomic variants, extrahepatic disease at time of surgery, technical complications with port placement, and patient refusal after randomization. At the end of the trial, 77% of patients randomized to the HAI+SYS arm actually received this treatment and only 30% finished therapy. At 18-month interim analysis, 33% of patients receiving adjuvant therapy and 36.7% of patients treated with resection alone had relapsed and no survival advantage was seen. When the outcomes were analyzed according to what treatment patients actually received, median survival was 44.8 months in the treated group ($n = 87$) versus 39.7 months in the control group ($n = 114$), respectively. Median time to liver progression doubled in the group receiving HAI: 20 months versus 12.6 months for the control group. The study used arterial ports rather than pumps (allowing for more clot formation) and used FU, which has less hepatic extraction than FUDR. Another troubling point is that at the time of reporting the study, only 38% of patients were followed for at least 2 years.

In a study from Greece, 143 patients were randomized after liver resection to A: mitomycin, FU, LV, and IL-2 given via a port into the hepatic artery and intravenously or B: the same drugs given intravenously only. The survival at 2-years was 92% versus75% and at 5-years 73% versus 60% for group A and B respectively. Median survival was 79 versus 66 months for group A and B, respectively ($p = .04$). Five-year survival was 40% and 34% for A and B, respectively. Three patients in A and 2 patients in B required biliary stents. Median survival free of hepatic involvement was 79 and 44.5 months for A and B, respectively ($p = .0003$).[80] Two smaller studies also demonstrated an improvement in survival with HAI therapy.[81,82] (see Table 88-6).

These studies clearly show a significant increase in disease-free survival. There is also an increase in median survival in some studies, although most were not powered to show a significant increase in survival. One study was powered for 2-year survival and did show an increase in survival with HAI. The German study did not suggest any benefit from HAI therapy after resection but they used FU instead of FUDR and used ports instead of pumps. When the treated patients were examined there was an increase in DFS. The study from Greece demonstrated both increase in survival and DFS. The use of the new agents, irinotecan or oxa, after liver resection has not yet been evaluated. We presently believe that in institutions where there is experience with HAI treatment for patients undergoing liver resection for colorectal metastases, adjuvant treatment should use HAI therapy. Whether the new systemic agents can complement regional therapy or replace it is under ongoing investigation.

NEOADJUVANT CHEMOTHERAPY

Patients with unresectable tumors, who were rendered resectable using systemic chemotherapy,

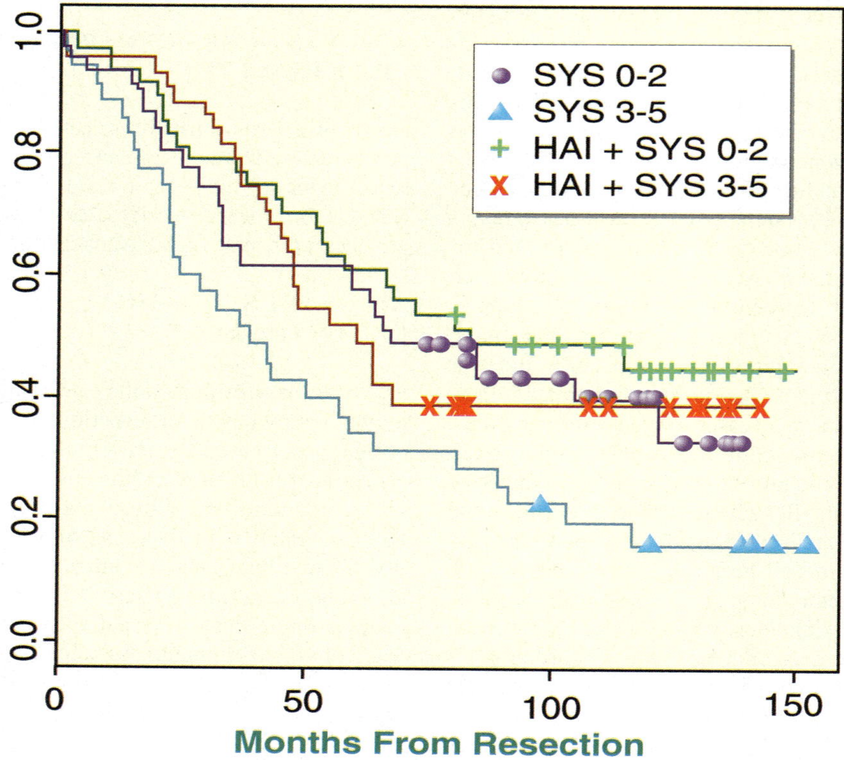

Figure 88-3 Kaplan–Meier estimates of overall survival in the groups assigned to either HAI plus systemic chemotherapy or systemic chemotherapy alone with stratification based on the preoperative clinical risk score. Using the clinical risk score for predicting recurrence after hepatic resection defined by Fong et al.[13] outcomes were significantly better with combined therapy as compared to monotherapy in patients with higher clinical risk scores (3 to 5).

Table 88-6 Randomized Trials of Adjuvant HAI vs SYS Therapy after Liver Resection

	# Patients	Median Survival (Months)		Hepatic Disease Free Survival (Months)		Progression Free (Months)	
		HAI	SYS	HAI	SYS	HAI	SYS
Lorenz M[209]	226	44.8	39.7	44.8	23.3	20	12
Kemeny N[77]	156	69.4	58.8	not reached	32.5	31.3	17.2
Lygidakis NJ [80]	122	76	66	79	44.5	45.5	19
Kemeny M[78]	75	65	50	not reached	20	46	25
Kusunoki M [81]	58	60	30	34.2	18.4	—	—

prompted further investigation of neoadjuvant chemotherapy.[83,84] In a retrospective trial by Bismuth and colleagues, in 330 patients complete macroscopic resection was considered not possible owing to: large lesions, multiple nodules, ill-location or extrahepatic disease. The unresectable patients were treated with chronomodulated oxaliplatin/5-FU/LV and 53 (16%) patients proceeded to liver resection. The 5-year survival following liver resection was 40%. Adam and colleagues, updated these results and identified 701 patients with unresectable liver metastases treated with neoadjuvant chemotherapy, 95 (13.6%) underwent a potentially curative resection.[85] The 5-year survival rate for the resected patients was 34%.

In the retrospective study by Giacchetti, 389 patients with unresectable colorectal metastases, enrolled in 6 trials were evaluated.[86] Unlike the Bismuth and Adam trials, Giacchetti assessed patients with liver only metastases and identified 151 patients who were initially considered unresectable owing to large tumor size (> 5 cm), multinodular (> 4), or ill-located metastases.

Subsequent trials confirmed the ability of neoadjuvant chemotherapy to render patients resectable. Alberts and colleagues reported a 62% response rate in 42 patients using FOLFOX4; resection was possible in 17 (41%) patients.[87] The median survival was 31.4 months. Delaunoit and colleagues evaluated 795 patients treated on the intergroup study N9741.[88] Twenty-two (3.3%) patients were resected, 2 on IFL, 11 on FOLFOX4, and 11 on IROX. Pozzo and colleagues, using FOLFIRI, found 13 of 40 patients were able to undergo resection after neoadjuvant therapy.[89]

Most of the neoadjuvant HAI chemotherapy trials have used HAI alone. Clavien and colleagues, using HAI FUDR and LV, induced resectability in 6 (26%) out of 23 previously treated patients (including 20 previously treated with CPT-11).[90] The actuarial survival at 3 years was 84% for responders to neoadjuvant therapy compared to 40% for non-responders. Elias and colleagues identified 14 (5.8%) out of 239 (contains unspecified number of colorectal and noncolorectal cancer patients) patients that were rendered resectable when treated with 5-FU based HAI.[91] Milandri and colleagues treated 36 patients with 5-FU based HAI (including 13 chemonaive patients who also received systemic therapy) and 4 (11%) patients became resectable.[92] At MSKCC, 21 pretreated patients with very extensive liver metastases received HAI FUDR and dexamethasone plus oxa and irinotecan systemic chemotherapy. The response rate was 90% and though the majority of patients had previous chemotherapy before entry into this trial (many already progressing on systemic therapy) surgical resection of liver metastases was then possible in 7 patients.[93] Neoadjuvant therapy has certain advantages. Some studies suggest that progression of disease on systemic therapy leads to worse survival. Adam and colleagues demonstrated a 5-year survival of 30% in patients who undergo liver resection after a response to chemotherapy and 8% if there was progression on chemotherapy.[94] Allen and colleagues reported an improved survival for patients who did not progress on neoadjuvant therapy versus those who did.[95] However certain chemotherapies can lead to liver toxicity. In one report of preoperative therapy with oxa, 40% of patients developed perisinusoidal and veno-occlusive fibrosis.[96]

SYSTEMIC CHEMOTHERAPY

Responses of liver metastases to systemic chemotherapy are variable and usually reflect the responsiveness of the primary tumor. Most studies of systemic therapy do not differentiate between patients who have only liver metastases and those with generalized metastatic disease. Some tumors are more responsive to chemotherapy. Combination chemotherapy has substantially improved the response rates obtained in treating breast cancer, but liver metastases still have a lower response rate than do soft tissue or pulmonary metastases. In a Southwest Oncology Group study of 262 patients, those with disease sites other than the liver had a 71% response rate (110 of 154) versus only a 47% (41 of 88) response rate for patients with liver metastases only ($p < .001$).[97]

Metastases from gastric carcinoma are more responsive to chemotherapy than are metastases from other gastrointestinal malignancies. With one of the newer regimens using fluorouracil, epirubicin, glutathione, and filgrastim, the response rate was 62% for all metastatic sites, whereas the response rate for those with hepatic metastases was 55% versus 77% for lymph nodes.[98]

In patients with colorectal cancer, the liver is the most common site of dissemination, with up to 70% of patients developing liver metastases during the course of their disease.[29,31,99–103] The overall response with the older regimens was low as was the response rate in the liver (Table 88-7). Recently a number of new agents have become available for the treatment of colorectal cancer. Studies with irinotecan combined with 5-FU and LV have increased response rates and survival over 5-FU/LV alone. The addition of oxa to 5-FU/LV has further improved response rate and survival. In a randomized trial comparing the oxa/5-FU/LV (FOLFOX) to the irinotecan/5-FU/LV (IFL), there was an increase in response rate 45% versus 35% and survival 19.5 months versus 15 months for the FOLFOX group versus the IFL group, respectively. Using an anti-VEGF monoclonal antibody, bevacizumab with IFL versus IFL alone, there was a statistically significant improvement in response rate and survival as well (Table 88-8). None of these new trials separated the response rate for patients with liver metastases from the whole group.

For primary liver cancers, there are a number of trials using gemcitabine either alone or in combination for biliary cancers including cholangiocarcinoma producing response rates generally around 30%[104–106]; however chemotherapy still produces very low response rate for hepatocellular cancers.

SECOND-LINE THERAPY FOR COLORECTAL CANCER

The use of second-line therapy for colorectal cancer is now possible because of the development of new agents. However, with the majority of the new agents the response rate to second-line therapy is anywhere from 9 to 22%. In small studies using HAI therapy, alone or combined with systemic chemotherapy, second-line therapy produced response rates of 52 to 90% and median survival of 13 to 28 months (Table 88-9).

HEPATIC ARTERIAL CHEMOTHERAPY

The rationale for hepatic arterial chemotherapy is based on both anatomic and pharmacologic factors. Liver metastases are perfused almost exclusively by the hepatic artery (once lesions are > 3 cm in diameter), although the normal liver hepatocytes derive their blood supply mostly from the portal vein.[107] Additionally,

Table 88-7 Treatment of Metastatic Colorectal Carcinoma

Drug (Ref)	# Pts	% Response	% Pts with Liver Metastases	% Response in Pts with Liver Mets
FU[24]	31	23	31	23
MeCCNU+FU[23]	152	32	41	31
MeCCNU+FU[26]	133	16	93	18
MOF-Strep[30]	75	32	60	37
FU+Leucovorin[29]	63	33	46	—
CPT-11[210]	41	33	35	28

Table 88-8 Select Randomized Trials of First-Line Chemotherapy for Metastatic Colorectal Cancer

Study	Regimen	% Response	Survival (Mos)	p-Value
Doulliard[12]	5-FU/LV/Irinotecan	41	17.4	< .05
	5-FU/LV(LV5FU2/AIO)	23	14.1	
Saltz[11]	5-FU/LV/Irinotecan	39	14.8	< .05
	5-FU/LV(bolus)	21	12.8	
DeGramont[13]	5-FU/LV/Oxaliplatin	51	16.2	< .05
	5-FU/LV	22	14.7	NS
Goldberg[153]	FOLFOX-4	38	18.6	< .05
	IFL bolus	29	14.1	
	Irinotecan/Oxaliplatin	29	16.5	
Hurwitz[17]	IFL+Avastin	44.8	20.3	.004
	IFL	34.8	15.6	≤ .001

Table 88-9 Second Line IV Chemotherapy for Metastatic Colorectal Cancer

Study	Regimen	Response (%)	Survival (Mos)
Systemic			
Rothenberg[211]	CPT-11	11	9.9
Rothenberg[212]	FOLFOX-4	10	9.8**
Cunningham[213]	C225/CPT-11	23	8.6**
Saltz[214]	C225	9	6.4
HAI			
Kemeny[134]	FUDR/Dex/LV	52	13.5
Kemeny[135]	FUDR/Mito-C	70	19
Kemeny[147]	FUDR/Dex+Sys CPT-11	74	20
Kemeny[93]	FUDR/Dex+Sys Oxal+CPT-11	90	28

certain drugs are largely extracted by the liver during the first pass through the arterial circulation, which results in high local concentrations of the drug with minimal systemic toxicity. Ensminger and colleagues[108] demonstrated that 94 to 99% of FUDR is extracted by the liver during the first pass, compared with 19 to 55% of FU. The pharmacologic advantage of various chemotherapeutic agents for hepatic arterial infusion is summarized in Table 88-10.[108] Drugs with a high total body clearance and short plasma half-life are more useful for hepatic infusion. If a drug is not rapidly cleared, recirculation through the systemic circulation diminishes the advantage of hepatic arterial delivery.[109,110] Newer drugs such as irinotecan have not exhibited increased activity when delivered by HAI.[86]

The liver is often the first and only site of metastatic disease. The theory of the stepwise pattern of metastatic progression proposes that hematogenous spread occurs first via the portal vein to the liver, then from the liver to the lungs, and then to other organs.[111,112] If this theory is valid, aggressive treatment of metastases confined to the liver (resection and/or hepatic infusion) may yield prolonged survival for some patients.

Regional hepatic arterial therapy can be delivered using either a hepatic arterial port or a percutaneously placed intra-arterial catheter connected to an external or a totally implantable pump. Early studies with percutaneously placed hepatic artery catheters produced high response rates, but clotting of the catheters and of the hepatic artery, duodenal ulcers, and bleeding from around the catheters[113] led physicians to abandon this method. The development of a totally implantable pump allowed long-term hepatic artery infusion with good patency of the catheter and the hepatic artery and a low incidence of infection.[114] One study compared three groups: (1) surgical placement of a hepatic artery catheter, (2) percutaneous placement of the catheter, and (3) surgical placement of a reservoir. The reported ability to administer chemotherapy was highest for the reservoir group—115 days—versus 31 and 25 days for groups 1 and 2, respectively.[115] A number of trials using the implantable pump produced high response rates with good survival rates.[116–123]

There are now 10 randomized studies comparing hepatic arterial chemotherapy with systemic chemotherapy (Table 88-11). In a study at the MSKCC, all patients underwent exploratory laparotomy to exclude those with extrahepatic disease. Patients were stratified by percentage of liver involvement and baseline lactate dehydrogenase (LDH) values. Both groups received a 14-day continuous infusion of FUDR, but the dose was lower in the systemic group since the higher dose could not be tolerated as systemic infusion. The response rate was 52% for HAI, and 20% for systemic therapy (p = .001). Crossover from systemic therapy to hepatic infusion was permitted. The median survivals for the HAI and systemic groups as randomized were 17 and 12 months, respectively (p = .424). The patients who did cross over had a median survival of 18 months compared with 8 months for those who did not cross over to HAI (p = .04).[116]

A similar randomized study conducted by the Northern California Oncology Group also used FUDR infusions in both groups.[117] Forty-two percent responded to HAI, and 10% to the systemic therapy ($p < .001$). The median time to progression was 401 and 201 days for the HAI and systemic groups, respectively ($p < .009$), although median survivals were 503 and 484 days, respectively. Forty-three percent of patients on systemic therapy eventually received HAI, which may have obscured survival differences. For the group that crossed over, the median survival was twice as long as for the group that never received HAI. Another flaw in the study was that patients with metastases to hepatic lymph nodes were included.

At the National Cancer Institute, 64 patients were randomized to HAI or systemic FUDR and the response rates were 62% and 17%, respectively ($p < .003$).[118] In the subset of patients without extrahepatic disease, the 2-year survival was 47% in the HAI group versus 13% in the systemic group ($p < .03$).

In another small study conducted by the Mayo Clinic, HAI FUDR was compared to systemic bolus FU for 5 days in 69 patients.[119] Objective tumor response was observed in 48% and 21% (p = .02), and time to hepatic progression was 15.7 and 6 months, respectively (p = .001). Despite the increase in response rate and time to hepatic progression, survival was similar in the two groups (12.6 and 10.5 months, respectively). However, this survival information is difficult to interpret because 48% of the HAI group was either not adequately treated, or had extrahepatic disease.

In a large French trial, patients were randomized to HAI FUDR versus systemic bolus FU.[120] The response rates were 49% and 14%, median time to hepatic progression was 15 and 6 months,

Table 88-10 Drugs for Hepatic Arterial Infusion (HAI)

Drug	Half-Life (Min)	Estimated Increased Exposure by HAI
Fluorouracil (FU)	10	5–10 fold
5-Fluoro-2-deoxyuridine (FUDR)	< 10	100–400 fold
Bischloroethylnitrosourea (BCNU)	< 5	6–7 fold
Mitomycin C	< 10	6–8 fold
Cisplatin	20–30	4–7 fold
Adriamycin (doxorubicin hydrochloride)	60	2–fold

Table 88-11 Randomized Trials of Hepatic Arterial Infusion (HAI) for Unresectable Liver Metastases

Study Group, Date (Ref)	Arms	*n*	No. (%) Receiving Assigned tx	X-Over	Responses (CR+PR)	Med TTP (Mos)	Med TTHP (Mos)	Med Survival (Mos)
MSKCC, 1987 (34)	HAI FUDR	48	45 (94%)	Yes	50%*	9*	NR	17
	IV FUDR	51	48 (94%)		20%	5	NR	12
NCI, 1987 (35)	HAI FUDR	32	21 (66%)	No	62%*	NR	NR	17
	IV FUDR	32	29 (92%)		17%	—	NR	12
NCOG, 1989 (36)	HAI FUDR	67	50 (75%)	Yes	42%*	NR	13*	16.5
	IV FUDR	76	65 (86%)		10%	NR	6.5	15.8
City of Hope, 1990 (37)	HAI FUDR	31	31 (100%)	Yes	55%*	8.8	NR	13.8
	IV FU	10	10 (100%)		20%	7.5	NR	11.6
NCCTG, 1990 (38)	HAI FUDR	39	33 (85%)	No	48%	6.0	15.7*	12.6
	IV FU/LV	35	36 (103%)		12%	5.0	6.0	10.5
French, 1992 (39)	HAI FUDR	81	70 (87%)	No	44%*	NR	14.5*	15*
	IV FU	82	41 (50%)		9%	NR	5.5	11
English, 1994 (40)	HAI FUDR	51	49 (96%)	No	NR	NR	NR	13.5*
	IV FU	49	10 (20%)		NR	NR	NR	7.5
German, 2000 (43)	HAI FUDR	54	37 (69%)	Yes	43%*	5.9	NR	12.7
	HAI FU/LV	57	40 (70%)		45%*	9.2	NR	18.7
	IV FU/LV	57	52 (91%)		20%	6.6	NR	17.6
MRC/EORTC 2003 (44)	HAI FU/LV	145	95 (66%)	No	22%	7.7	NR	14.7
	IV FU/LV	145	126 (87%)		19%	6.7	NR	14.8
CALGB, 2003 (45)	HAI FUDR	68	59 (87%)	No	48%*	5.3	9.8*	24
	IV FU/LV	67	58 (87%)		25%	6.8	7.3	20

* Statistically significant difference ($p < .05$) compared with control group, NR=Not reported. BSC=best supportive care; CR=complete response; FU=5-fluorouracil; FUDR=floxuridine; HAI=hepatic arterial infusion; IV=intravenous; LV=leucovorin; med=median; mos=months; n=number of patients enrolled; no.=number; OS=overall survival; PR=partial response; TTHP=time to hepatic progression; TTP=time to progression; tx=therapy; X-over=crossover to HAI arm.

and median survival was 14 and 10 months for the HAI and systemic therapy groups, respectively. The 2-year survival was 22% for HAI and 10% for the systemic group ($p = .02$). One of the criticisms of this trial is that some patients in the systemic therapy group received chemotherapy late since only symptomatic patients were treated in the systemic group. A British study was designed in a similar manner, (only symptomatic patients treated in the systemic group).[121] The HAI group had a significantly longer survival. Patients in the HAI group had significantly longer normal performance status than did the patients in the systemic therapy group.

A German cooperative group randomized 168 patients to (1) HAI FUDR, (2) HAI FU/LV, or (3) systemic FU/LV.[124] The median time to progression was 5.9, 9.2, and 6.6 months, and median survival times were 12.7, 18.7, and 17.6 months, respectively. In this study, the median survival was better for HAI-FU/LV. Tumor response rates were 43.2%, 45%, and 19.7%, and development of extrahepatic disease was 40.5%, 12.5%, and 18.3%, respectively. Toxicity data indicate that FU/LV therapy was much more toxic than FUDR. The incidence of stomatitis was 8%, 75%, and 64.6%, and of diarrhea was 0%, 11%, and 11% for HAI FUDR, HAI FU/LV and IV FU/LV, respectively. A port instead of a pump was used and dosing for FUDR was different than in the American studies in that FUDR was reduced from 0.2 to 0.15 mg/kg/day after 3 cycles rather than adjusting for patient toxicity. It should be pointed out that although an intention-to-treat analysis was used, only 68.5% randomized to HAI of FUDR were treated but all were included in the survival analysis.

The Medical Research Council/European Organization for the Research and Treatment of Cancer (MRC/EORTC)[101] conducted a randomized trial of IV versus HAI FU/LV in 290 patients. Median and 2-year survival rates were 13.4 months and 23% in the IV arm versus 14.7 months and 20% in the HAI arm. However, 37% of patients allocated to the HAI arm did not receive the treatment and a further 29% had to stop treatment, so approximately 50% of patients in HAI group did not receive treatment or had inadequate treatment and are included in the survival analysis. No breakdown of the treated patients was given.

The Cancer and Leukemia Group B (CALGB) trial differs from others in that it includes the use of dexamethasone and LV in the HAI arm versus 5-FU+LV in the systemic arm with no crossover. The endpoint was survival which was 24.4 months and 20 months in the HAI and systemic groups, respectively, $p = .0034$). The time to hepatic progression was better in the HAI arm (9.8 months vs 7.3 months, $p = .034$) but the time to extrahepatic progression was better in the systemic arm (7.7 months vs 14.8 months, $p < .029$) for the HAI and systemic groups, respectively. Quality of life was improved at 3 and 6 months in the HAI group.

Toxicity of Hepatic Arterial FUDR Infusion The most common problems with HAI are hepatic toxicity and ulceration of the stomach and duodenum. Myelosuppression, nausea, vomiting, and diarrhea do not occur with HAI or FUDR. If diarrhea does occur, shunting to the bowel should be suspected.[125] Clinically, biliary toxicity is manifested as elevations of aspartate transaminase (AST), alkaline phosphatase, and bilirubin. In the early stages of toxicity, hepatic enzyme elevations will return to normal when the drug is withdrawn and the patient is given a rest period, although in more advanced cases, it does not resolve. The bile ducts derive their blood supply almost exclusively from the hepatic artery[126] and thus are undoubtedly perfused with high doses of chemotherapy.

In patients who develop jaundice, an endoscopic retrograde cholangiopancreatogram (ERCP) may demonstrate lesions resembling idiopathic sclerosing cholangitis in 5 to 29% of patients treated by experienced clinicians.[122] Because the ducts are sclerotic and nondilated, sonograms usually do not show dilation. The strictures may be focal and present at the hepatic duct bifurcation, and therefore drainage procedures either by ERCP or by transhepatic cholangiogram may be helpful. Duct obstruction from metastases should first be excluded by CT of the liver.

Close monitoring of liver function tests is necessary to avoid biliary complications. If the serum bilirubin becomes ≥ 3 mg/dL, no further treatment should be given until the bilirubin returns to normal, and then only with a 75% reduction in dose to prevent the development of sclerosing cholangitis.

Ulcer disease results from inadvertent perfusion of the stomach and duodenum with drug via the small collateral branches from the hepatic artery and can be prevented by careful dissection of these collaterals at the time of pump placement.[123] In a large series reviewing 544 patients who received pumps, other toxicities included dislodgement of the catheter (3%), occlusion of catheter (2%), extrahepatic perfusion (3%), and pump infection (2.5%).[127]

New Approaches to Decrease Hepatic Toxicity Three approaches have been tried to decrease hepatic toxicity: (1) HAI dexamethasone (D), (2) circadian modification, and (3) HAI FU alternating with FUDR. The hepatic toxicity induced by hepatic arterial infusion of FUDR may be related to portal triad inflammation which could lead to ischemia of the bile ducts. Hepatic arterial administration of dexamethasone may decrease inflammation and thereby decrease biliary toxicity. In patients with established hepatobiliary toxicity from HAI, dexamethasone promotes resolution of the liver function abnormalities. In a randomized study of FUDR with D versus FUDR alone, there was a trend toward decreased bilirubin elevation in patients receiving FUDR+D compared with the group receiving FUDR alone (9% vs 30%, p = .07).[128] Although the addition of dexamethasone was not associated with the ability to administer a significant increase in the amount of FUDR, the response rate with FUDR+D was 71% versus 40% for FUDR alone (p = .03). Survival was also improved: 23 months for FUDR+D versus 15 months for FUDR alone.

The use of circadian modification of HAI of FUDR is another method to decrease hepatic toxicity. In a nonrandomized study at the University of Minnesota, a comparison of constant (flat) infusion versus circadian-modified (CM) hepatic arterial FUDR, the patients with CM infusion tolerated almost twice the daily dose of FUDR, with a decrease in hepatic toxicity compared with patients receiving flat infusions.[129]

The third approach is to decrease toxicity by alternating drugs such as HAI FUDR with hepatic arterial (HA) FU. Weekly HA bolus of FU does not cause hepatobiliary toxicity; however, it frequently produces treatment-limiting systemic toxicity or arteritis. Stagg and colleagues used alternating HAI followed by HA bolus FU via the pump side port.[130] The response rate was 51%, and median survival was 22.4 months. In contrast to the experience with single-agent HAI of FUDR, no patient has had treatment terminated because of drug toxicity. Metzger and colleagues using an infusion of FU and mitomycin-C, found that median survival was 18 months with a partial response rate of 57%.[131] Sclerosing cholangitis did not occur, but mucositis and leukopenia did. Catheter complications occurred, which led to premature termination of treatment in one-third of the patients. Though the dose of FUDR fits into an implanted pump, the dose of FU requires an external pump for infusion or bolus weekly side port injections. Van Riel and colleagues, using a MediPort to administer FU infusion 1,000 mg/m^2 for 5 days, reported a 34% response rate in 145 patients with a 14.3-month median survival. Arterial thrombosis was seen in 48% and catheter dislocation in 22%.[132] Giving a higher dose of FU 2,200 mg/m^2 over 24 hours weekly with LV, objective responses were seen in 28 out of 50 (56%) patients with a median survival of 23 months.[133]

APPROACHES TO INCREASED RESPONSE RATE

The addition of LV, and mitomycin-C to FUDR have increased response rates but also biliary sclerosis. In previously treated patients FUDR+LV and D produced a 50% response rate and mitomycin side port injection added to HAI FUDR+D produced a 70% response rate,[134,135] both trials, however, increased biliary sclerosis. A large study from Germany used 5-FU, LV, and interferon and degradable starch microspheres via an HAI catheter. In the 95 patients treated, the response rate was 70% and the median survival was 24 months. In patients with less than 25% of their liver involved with tumor, the median survival was 39 months. The major toxicity was diarrhea 58% and there were problems with catheter occlusion in 46%.[136]

Another approach is to use the new agents via the HAI route. Van Riel and colleagues treated 25 patients with a 5-day continuous infusion of HAI irinotecan every 3 weeks.[137] From 22 assessable patients 14% had a partial response and 40% had stable disease. The median survival was 8.1 months. There was lack of hepatic extraction of the drug despite the increased conversion of irinotecan to its active metabolite SN38.[138] Fiorentini treated 12 patients with HAI irinotecan and had a 33% response rate. Similarly Vogl and colleagues noted a partial response of 33% in 9 patients.[139]

A number of trials have evaluated HAI oxa combinations. Kern and colleagues demonstrated an objective response rate of 59% using HAI oxa and 5-FU and folinic acid.[140] Ducreux and colleagues used a similar regimen in a phase II study and found an objective response rate of 79% with 3 of 14 patients undergoing complete resection of their metastases after response to therapy and a 6-month survival of 86%.[141] Other trials have recorded response rates of 13 to 69% for HAI oxa combined with other chemotherapies, given via the intravenous route.[142–145]

Using HAI with concurrent systemic chemotherapy has increased response rates in small phase II trials. Two trials used HAI chemotherapy plus systemic irinotecan. Zelek and colleagues, using HAI pirarubicin plus systemic irinotecan/5FU/LV in 31 patients, demonstrated a response rate of 48% with a median survival of 20.5 months.[146] At MSKCC in a phase I trial using HAI FUDR and systemic irinotecan in previously treated patients, produced a partial response rate of 74%, and the median survival was 20 months.[147] Further work with oxa, irinotecan produced a 90% response rate in previously treated patients (see Table 88-9).

HEPATIC ARTERIAL INFUSION: CONCLUSIONS

There are several advantages to HAI treatment of liver metastases. From a pharmacologic standpoint, HAI is more effective than systemic therapy, because higher drug levels are achieved at the site of metastatic disease.

The high response rates obtained in trials of HAI or FUDR in the treatment of colorectal cancer have not been matched by systemic therapy trials. In seven randomized trials, the response rate was higher with HAI compared with systemic therapy. The time to hepatic progression was significantly longer in the HAI groups versus the systemic groups. The randomized pump studies do not clearly evaluate the issue of survival because (1) in some, a crossover was allowed; (2) in others, patients with positive portal nodes were included in the HAI treated groups; and (3) in some, the number of patients entered was very small.

A meta-analysis[148] of HAI FUDR versus systemic FU or FUDR produced a significant increase in response rate (41% versus 14%) and a significant increase in survival (16 versus 12 months) for HAI and systemic therapy, respectively. The use of HAI therapy after progression or systemic therapy looks promising compared with second-line systemic therapy after progression on first-line (see Table 88-9). The use of HAI for other tumor types has not been studied as extensively. Some of the breast studies using HAI are shown in Table 88-12.[149–155] Most of these studies were conducted with patients whose tumors were failing to respond to systemic therapy, and yet response rates of ≥ 50% were seen in 5 of the 8 studies. For uveal melanoma, the response with HAI fotemustine (40%) was higher than that obtained with other modalities. HAI studies in hepatocellular carcinoma (HCC) and biliary carcinomas are in Tables 88-11 and 88-13.

CRYOSURGERY

It is well known that the freeze/thaw process can bring about cellular destruction. Surgeons have long tried to harness the destructive capacity of the freezing process for the treatment of liver tumors. Advances in the design of cryosurgical instruments and mass marketing of such instruments have generated enthusiasm over the last two decades for use of this modality in the treatment of liver tumors. This modality is particularly attractive for treatment of HCC because of the frequent association of HCC with cirrhosis. Since hepatic resection in cases of cirrhosis has a high risk of complications, including liver failure, cryoablation is a therapeutic modality that allows preservation of liver parenchyma and function in the setting of cirrhosis. The attractiveness of cryoablation in the setting of associated compro-

Table 88-12 Hepatic Arterial Infusion for Breast Cancer*

Ref	No. Patients	Drugs	Partial Response (%)	Median Survival (Mo)
Fraschini[149]	34	Cisplatin + Vinblastine	33	11
Estape[150]	16	VP-16-Cytoxan	50	16
Fraschini[151]	25	Vinblastine	52	11†
Fraschini[152]	26	Cisplatin	19	11
Maral[153]	15	Mitomycin-C + FUDR	53	18‡
Arai[154]	56	FU + Doxo + Mitomycin	81	12.5
Tada[155]	45	Doxorubicin + Mitomycin-C	37	7.5

* = ;† = mean survival only for responders; ‡ = some patients in study also had colon cancer.

mised hepatic function has encouraged extensive investigations of this modality as a treatment for HCC and has resulted in data supporting the use of this modality for HCC.[156]

For metastatic tumors within the liver, however, a role for this modality is less well defined. As treatment for colorectal metastases to the liver, for example, cryoablation should not be considered an alternative to resection because cryoablation is not a proven curative option. Because of the technical limitations of the available instruments, most surgeons will not freeze more than six lesions, and most will not freeze lesions larger than 5 cm. Most lesions that are freezable are therefore likely resectable. Ravikumar and colleagues reported that 18 of 24 patients with colorectal carcinoma were rendered disease free by cryosurgery. Of these 18 patients, 39% were alive and disease free at the time of publication.[157] In 18 patients treated by Onik and colleagues, 14 were not adequately treated and had recurrences, and 4 (22%) had a complete response.[158] Morris and Ross reported less encouraging results.[159] In their hands, 75% of the 67 patients treated by cryosurgery alone had relapse of their preoperative CEA levels within 6 months. Hepatic arterial chemotherapy in conjunction with cryoablation for patients with unresectable colorectal metastases to the liver is now under study. In a series of 85 patients who were judged to have a complete treatment of their tumors, favorable prognosis was associated with liver metastases ≤ 3cm in size, only 3 lesions ablated, and low CEA.[160]

In cases with clearly unresectable metastatic tumors, cryoablation has proven to be a relatively safe option. In most series published to date, no mortality has been encountered.[156–158,161,162] Complications encountered included subphrenic abscess,[157] wound dehiscence, pleural effusions, and myoglobinuria.[162] There were other significant complications including hepatic hemorrhage, biliary fistulation, hepatic abscess formation, and renal impairment.[156–158,161,162]

Cryosurgical methods should be used only by surgeons familiar with liver anatomy and resection, since adequate mobilization of the liver and appreciation of the location of the major intrahepatic blood vessels and bile ducts are essential for the safe application of this treatment modality. Furthermore, the possibility of resection as an alternative should be evaluated by experienced hepatic surgeons. Whether intravenous chemotherapy or intra-arterial chemotherapy should be given after cryoablation is unknown. Formal studies addressing the utility of chemotherapy in this setting are under way. Whether combined resection and ablative therapy should be performed requires further trials.

RADIOFREQUENCY ABLATION

Radiofrequency (RF) ablation is a method that uses heat to kill tumor cells.[163] Using radiofrequency electrodes, which have the appearance of a long needle, electrical energy can be directed from radiofrequency generators to ablate tumors. Such RF electrodes can be guided into position by sonographic, CT, or MRI guidance, and ablation monitored by similar imaging modalities. RF ablation (RFA) can be performed at open laparotomy by laparoscopic surgery, or percutaneously.

The major advantage of RFA over cryoablation is the lower cost of the equipment compared with cryoablation, less time required, and the possibility of performing such ablations percutaneously. The small size of the electrodes permits RFA without laparotomy. The major obstacle to the use of this ablative technique is the limited size of the lesions that can be ablated. As heat is generated within the tumor, charring of tissues occurs, decreasing the conduction of heat. Patients with 1 to 3 lesions located in the periphery of the liver and that are < 3 cm are good candidates for RFA. Much research is also being undertaken to increase the size of the areas that can be ablated. Improvements in technology, such as use of higher power generators, saline-cooled-tip electrodes,[164] and larger arrays may soon allow ablation of lesions up to 5 cm (7 cm zones of ablation). It is important that lesions not be adjacent to bowel, kidney, gallbladder, or diaphragm. Follow-up images may be difficult to interpret since the defect in the liver is larger after ablation with hypoattenuation. Any residual enhancement or increase in size or irregularity should raise concern of recurrence.

For now, the ideal candidates for ablation, either cryo or RF, are those patients with chemotherapy-resistant scattered tumors, patients with chemoresistant tumors and medical contraindications to resection, or patients with hepatic recurrence after previous liver resection.

Studies with relatively long follow-up are beginning to emerge[165,166] indicating that ablations are safe and may be durable treatment. In the largest of these studies, Livrhaghi and his colleagues reported on a 41 center study with 2,320 patients (1,610 with HCC and 501 with metastatic colorectal cancer).[167] In total 3,554 lesions were treated with six deaths (0.3%) and 50 major complications (2.2%). In a recent comprehensive review, Decadt and Siriwardena summarized the known literature published in the English language.[168] Local recurrence rates after RFA are reported to be 1.5 to 28%, with the typical being approximately 10%. Recurrence is clearly related to tumor size and to technique, with surgical ablations associated with better tumor control than percutaneous but with longer recovery.

Compared with other ablative techniques, RFA is simpler than cryotherapy to perform. However, it is easier to assess areas of ablation during cryoablation, where the ice ball generated appears unequivocally as a homogeneous, hypoechoic lesion on ultrasonography. Cryoablation allows ablation of larger lesions and has a longer track record. As instrumentation improves to allow ablation of larger tumors and the record of use of these instruments increases, the indication for RFA will undoubtedly expand. These two ablative techniques will likely remain complementary techniques in our treatment of patients with metastatic colorectal cancer located predominantly within the liver.[169] The most proven uses of ablative techniques for hepatic colorectal metastases are in combination with resection for patients with bilateral metastases.[170] Other indications include ablation after previous liver resection when a re-resection is not technically possible, or as primary local therapy when the patient with small tumors is medically unfit for surgery or unwilling to have surgery. Many ongoing studies are attempting to define the optimal chemotherapy to be administered after such ablative therapies.

The most intriguing line of investigation related to ablative therapies is currently attempt-

Table 88-13 Biliary Tract Carcinoma:HAI Trials

Study	# Patients	HAI Therapy	Response	Median Survival
Warren KW[223]	15	Doxorubicin	60%	NR
Smith GW[225]	11	5-FU/Mito-C	64%	12.5 months
Makela JT[226]	27	Mito-C	48%	14 months
Cantore[227]	26	Epirubicin/Cisplatin Systemic 5-FU IVCI	40%	13.2 months

ing to define the role of such therapies in patients with liver-predominant colorectal metastases. As most patients with liver metastases die of the liver disease, ablative therapies have become very safe and effective at local control. Many patients have only limited extrahepatic disease that may be controllable by systemic therapies, investigators are attempting to determine if ablative therapies can be an additive to effective systemic therapies in improving patient outcome. There is currently a multicenter trial randomizing patients with predominant liver metastases to systemic therapies versus combined liver tumor ablation and systemic therapies.

EMBOLIZATION

Normal liver parenchyma derives its nutrient blood supply from two sources: the hepatic artery and the portal vein. Of the two, the portal vein provides the majority of nourishment for a normal liver, and the hepatic artery can usually be ligated or occluded with little consequence on liver function. Hepatic metastases, however, derive their blood supply from the hepatic artery. Interruption of the hepatic artery may preferentially injure liver tumors, at the same time as preserving liver function. The earliest attempts at arterial interruption involved surgical ligation of the hepatic artery. Although such ligations often produce necrosis and shrinkage of tumor, only a transient effect is usually noted because of the rapid development of collateral vessels. Hepatic arterial ligation has therefore been largely abandoned in favor of transcutaneous embolization.[171] Embolization of oils, gelatin, plastic, collagen, or glass particles (Table 88-14) can be performed to interrupt arterial blood flow to tumors and has the advantage of being nonsurgical. Lipiodol is an ionized oil contrast medium that also can be used. It is taken up preferentially by hepatocellular carcinoma cells and retained for a long time after injection into the hepatic artery. Its main function is to act as a delivery system because of its selective uptake and retention.[172] Furthermore, such embolizations can be repeated to occlude collateral vessels that develop. Such therapy has become standard therapy for nonresectable primary HCC. For metastatic cancers, however, the benefits are less clear except for metastatic neuroendocrine tumors.

A number of studies examining the utility of embolization for metastatic colorectal cancers to the liver have been performed. In a study randomizing 61 individuals with hepatic colorectal metastases to embolization, intraoperative embolization and hepatic artery ligation, or no treatment, median survivals were 9, 13, and 10 months, respectively.[173] In another study that examined 67 patients who were randomized to hepatic artery ligation alone or in conjunction with portal vein infusion of FU, there was only one response.[174] The median survival in both groups was 12 months. These studies suggest that arterial interruption is ineffective for colorectal cancer, not surprising, because hepatic metastases from colorectal cancer are not particularly vascular. Embolization has therefore been largely abandoned as treatment for hepatic metastatic colorectal cancer.

Table 88-14 Agents Used for Embolization

Agents	Particle Size
Ivalon–polyvinyl alcohol foam	150–500 μm
Collagen–angiostat	20–250 μm
Gelfoam–gelatin sponge particles	1–2 μm
Spherex–degradable starch microspheres	45 μm

For highly vascular tumors, such as metastatic neuroendocrine tumors, however, hepatic artery embolization (HAE) has a definite role.[175] Ajani and colleagues treated 22 patients with islet cell carcinoma with HAE using polyvinyl alcohol particles (Ivalon) and gelatin sponge particles (Gelfoam).[176] The median survival in this study was 33 months from initiation of embolization (range 1–72 months); 12 patients had a partial response associated with subjective improvement and decrease in hormone levels. Other studies corroborate these results[175–179] and demonstrate HAE to be effective in symptomatic relief and in reducing circulating levels of secreted hormones. Some rare tumors such as ocular melanoma and gastrointestinal stromal tumors with liver metastases show increased response rates with chemoembolization.[173,180]

Though embolization is relatively safe in patients without associated cirrhosis, many complications have been described. Common systemic symptoms include nausea, vomiting, fever, pain, and changes in liver function tests. Problems less commonly encountered but more ominous include (1) liver necrosis, (2) acute cholecystitis, (3) ischemic necrosis of the bowel by embolization of one of the vessels to the intestinal tract, (4) pancreatic infarction and pancreatitis by embolization of one of the pancreatic vessels, and (5) dyspnea by embolization of the lungs.[175–179] Rapid cell death may also result in tumor lysis syndrome with symptomatic hyperuricemia leading to uric acid nephropathy and oliguria. It is clear that morbidity and mortality are related to pre-embolization liver functional status and amounts of tumor embolized. Patients with cirrhosis, portal vein occlusion, and biliary tract obstruction are usually excluded. When a large tumor burden is present, staged embolizations should be performed. Vigorous hydration and prophylactic allopurinol may also be indicated. In carcinoid tumors, HAE may cause a life-threatening carcinoid crisis from the rapid release of hormones from the tumor cells. Somatostatin analogues may be given, either prior to the procedure or used if a carcinoid crisis occurs.

CHEMOEMBOLIZATION

Chemoembolization is an extension of traditional percutaneous embolization techniques. With chemoembolization, investigators embolize tumors with Gelfoam or Ivalon particles soaked with chemotherapeutic agents. The theoretical advantage is that such embolizations will not only provide vascular occlusion but will bring about sustained therapeutic levels of chemotherapy in the tumor areas. Generalized ischemia would reduce the ability of the cell to protect itself from the toxicity of chemotherapy. In human hepatoma and colon carcinoma cell cultures, hypoxia increased uptake of daunomycin.[180] Despite the widespread usage of such chemoembolization, few randomized studies have demonstrated that the theoretical advantage of adding chemotherapy to embolization translates into a clinical advantage. Llovet randomized 112 patients to (1) chemoembolization with doxorubicin and lipiodol; (2) embolization (Gelfoam particles only); and (3) symptomatic treatment. The 1-, 2-, and 3-year survival rates were 82, 63, and 29% for chemoembolization and 75, 50, and 29% for embolization.[183] Chemoembolization was associated with a reduced incidence of subsequent portal vein invasion.[181] Lin and colleagues,[182] Llovet and colleagues,[183] and Ikeda and colleagues[184] found no advantage to adding chemotherapy to embolization. There were a few meta-analyses looking at chemoembolization or embolization in patients with hepatocellular carcinoma (Table 88-15). In one study, there was an overall benefit to treatment with a *p*-value of .017 and also there was significant 2-year survival saving treatment.[185] One trial showed a significant benefit with embolization with cisplatin and doxorubicin but not with embolization alone.[186] Some studies directly comparing embolization and chemoembolization do not provide evidence of survival advantage.[187,188]

Chemoembolization for liver metastases from colon cancer is less effective. Stagg and colleagues[189] reviewed patients receiving chemoembolization, 19 of 84 (23%) patients with hepatoma responded versus 3 of 38 (9%) patients with colorectal cancer. Some of the other trials using chemoembolization are listed in Table 88-16. Though responses are high in some studies, most report median survivals of 7 to 8 months.

Another form of chemoembolization is to enclose the chemotherapeutic agents in a microsphere. Degradable starch microspheres injected intra-arterially are trapped in an extracapillary network formed in liver metastases.[190,191] The drug dissolved in the microsphere suspension will be retained in the blood vessels of the target organ as long as the blood flow is blocked, and then will gradually release the chemotherapeutic agents, resulting in a longer duration of tumor exposure to the drug. Use of such drug-containing microspheres must also be considered experimental and be performed within the confines of formal prospective investigations.

RADIATION THERAPY

External beam radiation, though effective in the treatment of primary tumors such as colorectal

Table 88-15 Chemoembolization for Hepatocellular Cancer

Investigator	No. Patients	Agent	Partial Response (%)	Median Survival (Mo)
Colleoni[235]	17	LV FU Carboplatin Mitoxantone Ethiodized Oil + Gelatin	62	NS
Kong[236]	38	Lipiodol Doxorubicin Gelatin	29	NS
Clouse[237]	30	Doxorubicin Epinephrine Lipiodol	40	14
Lo[238]	28	Cisplatin Lipiodol + Gelatin	39	18
Llovet[183]	40	Gelatin Doxorubicin	35	28
Groupe d'Etude[239]	50	Cisplatin Lipiodol	18	

cancer, has not been widely used in the treatment of liver metastases. This results from the low tolerance of normal hepatic parenchyma to radiation. Whole liver radiation with doses of more than 3,500 cGy is associated with a significant likelihood of radiation hepatitis and liver failure.[192] External beam radiation is effective in palliating symptoms in approximately 60% of patients. Recently, three different strategies have increased the applicability of external beam radiation to treatment of liver metastases: (1) three-dimensional conformal radiation treatment planning, (2) boost doses to the tumors, and (3) simultaneous administration of radiosensitizing chemotherapeutic agents. Lawrence and colleagues delivered smaller doses of radiation to the normal liver and larger doses to the tumor by conformal three-dimensional treatment planning.[193] Lawrence and colleagues produced a 48% response rate in previously treated patients. In 18 patients with colorectal cancer who had localized hepatic metastases, the median survival was 22 months. Intraoperative interstitial irradiation in a phase I/II study of 22 patients with colorectal cancer produced local control for a median of 8 months (the median number of lesions radiated was 3, range 1–11). In 33 patients treated with irradiation and HAI+FUDR, 48% had an objective response, with a median response duration of 8 months. The palliative role of the combination of well-planned external beam therapy and intra-arterial chemotherapy[194] will have to be determined by comparative trials of systemic or regional chemotherapy alone. Liu, using three-dimensional conformal radiation, treated 37 patients with hepatocellular cancer who had failed or were unsuitable for embolization obtained a 64% response rate with a 2-year survival of 40%.[195]

Other strategies for radioablation of liver tumors have attempted to selectively target tumors, at the same time as minimizing radiation doses to normal parenchyma. The three main strategies that are being explored for specific radioablation of tumors are antibody-directed radioablation, radioembolization, and intraoperative interstitial irradiation using afterloading catheters. In antibody-directed radioablation, a radioisotope such as yttrium-90 or 186Re is attached to an antibody specific for the tumor, such as antibodies to CEA. It is hoped that injection of such radiolabeled antibodies will concentrate the therapeutic radionuclides at the tumor sites.[196] Such an approach is still experimental but has reached the stage of clinical trials for colorectal metastases. Results in the near future should define the utility of radioimmunotherapy.

Attempts at radioembolization have been made to deliver the therapeutic radionuclide physically to the liver tumor. Instillation of glass microspheres containing yttrium-90 into the hepatic artery is one approach. This isotope is a beta emitter with a half-life of 64 hours and a mean energy of disintegration of 0.937. It has a mean tissue penetrance of 2.5 mm and maximum penetrance of 10 mm.[197] With these characteristics, yttrium-90 is well suited for localized internal radiation therapy. Gray and colleagues reported embolization of 10 patients with hepatic colorectal metastases in 1989.[198] The radiation doses administered ranged between 755 and 2,500 MBq and resulted in significant decreases in circulating CEA. No long-term results were reported. Herba and colleagues reported on yttrium-90 embolization of 12 metastatic colorectal cancers, 1 carcinoid, and 1 islet cell tumor.[199] At a follow-up at 7 months, 10 patients had stable disease, and 4 had progression. Andrews and colleagues reported on yttrium-90 embolization of 17 patients with colorectal metastases and of 6 with metastatic neuroendocrine tumors.[200] Although doses of up to 12,500 cGy were relatively well tolerated, partial response was noted in only 5 patients.[200] In a small study (21 patients with colorectal cancer) were randomized to microspheres containing yttrium-90 plus 5FU/LV or 5FU/LV alone. The median survival was 29 and 13 months, respectively.[201] Attempts have also been made to treat metastatic colorectal cancer by embolization with ^{131}I-labeled lipiodol, but with little evidence of effectiveness.[202] The reason that response rates for radioembolization of metastatic tumors are far less than those reported for treatment of primary hepatocellular carcinoma is that most metastatic tumors except for neuroendocrine primaries are far less vascular than HCC. Comparative trials of radioembolization to other treatment modalities need to be performed.

Table 88-16 Chemoembolization for Colon Cancer

Investigator	No. Patients	Agent	Partial Response %	Median Survival (Mo)
Daniels[228]	55	Collagen Cisplatin Doxorubicin Mitomycin-C	34	—
Stuart[229]	20	FU Mitomycin-C Ethiodized Oil Gelatin	59	7
Tellez[230]	30	Angiostat Cisplatin Adriamycin Mitomycin-C	62	8
Link[231]	17	Lipiodol Adriamycin	0	7
Lang[232]	46	Lipidoil Doxorubicin	17 —	
Lorenz	11	Microspheres Mitomycin-C	36 —	
Martinelli[233]	13	Polyvinyl Alcohol FU and Interferone	24 —	
Stagg[189]	12	Gelfoam Doxorubicin Mitomycin-C Cisplatin	0	—

PERCUTANEOUS ETHANOL INJECTION

Direct injection of absolute alcohol into a tumor produces tumor necrosis and death. The first attempts to use this modality to treat hepatic tumors were performed in Japan in 1983.[203] Under ultrasound guidance, up to 30 cc of ethanol can be injected percutaneously with the aim of ablating the tumor. The injections can also be guided by CT. In a report from Italy on 26 patients with metastatic disease, those with lesions of 2 cm had responses in 13 of 15 lesions; those with lesions of 2 to 3 cm had responses in 4 of 5 lesions; whereas in those lesions of 4 cm, there were 0 of 6 responses.[204] Because of this relation of effectiveness to tumor size, most physicians performing percutaneous ethanol injection therapy (PEIT) will only treat less than four lesions, each less than 4 cm in diameter. PEIT is most frequently used for treatment of primary hepatocellular carcinoma,[204–206] since the multifocal nature of the disease and the common association with cirrhosis often make resection of even small amounts of liver prohibitively dangerous. For metastatic disease to the liver, PEIT has been less helpful. Since most cases of liver metastases are not associated with cirrhosis, up to 80% of the liver can be resected with relatively low mortality. Most cases suitable for alcohol injection, therefore, are resectable. Additionally, colorectal metastases, unlike hepatomas, are very hard tumors, making instillation of alcohol difficult. It is not surprising that the reported experience of alcohol injection for metastatic disease to the liver is modest, and no trial comparing PEIT with more accepted therapy has been published. In the largest study to date, Giovannini and Seitz treated 40 patients with metastatic disease to the liver with alcohol injections.[207] These included 32 cases of colorectal cancer, 9 cases of metastatic mammary cancer, 5 carcinoid tumors, 4 undifferentiated tumors, 3 uterine cancers, 1 esophageal cancer, and 1 bronchogenic carcinoma. No major complication was associated with such treatment. For patients with colorectal metastases, the median survival was 28 months, but there were no 4-year survivors. Amin and colleagues recently reported on treatment of 22 patients with colorectal metastases.[208] The median follow-up in this study was only 6.5 months, however, other treatments including interstitial photocoagulation were used in the same patients, precluding any conclusion relating to efficacy of the alcohol treatments. Alcohol injection is a rather safe procedure. However, the simplicity and effectiveness of radiofrequency ablation make that a much more attractive method of local tumor destruction for small tumors, although cryoablation remains the ablative treatment of choice for large tumors.

SUMMARY

Metastatic cancer is frequently found in the liver. For colorectal metastases to this site, resection may be curative and should be considered standard therapy, if the liver is the only site of disease. For other metastatic tumors to the liver, the role of surgical resection remains to be defined. Even when resection cannot be performed with curative intent, cryoablation, intra-arterial chemotherapy, arterial embolization, and radioembolization represent modalities that may bring about effective palliation. The relative merits of each method of therapy in each tumor type remains to be determined by ongoing and future clinical trials.

REFERENCES

1. Pickren JW, Tsukada Y, Lane W. Liver metastases: analysis of autopsy data. In: Weiss E, Gilbert H, editors. Metastases. Boston: GK Medical Publishers; 1982, p. 2.
2. Vassiliades VG, Foley WD, Alarcon J, et al. Hepatic metastases: CT versus MR imaging at 1.5T. Gastrointest Radiol 1991;16:159–63.
3. Castaing D, Emond J, Kunstlinger F, et al. Utility of operative ultrasound in the surgical management of liver tumors. Ann Surg 1986;204:600–5.
4. Yonekura Y, Benua R, Brill A, et al. Increased accumulation of 2-deoxy-2-[18F]fluoro-D-glucose in liver metastases from colon carcinoma. J Nucl Med 1982;23:1133–7.
5. Dimitrakopoulou A, Strauss L, Clorius J, et al. Studies with positron emission tomography after systemic administration of fluorine-18-uracil in patients with liver metastases from colorectal carcinoma. J Nucl Med 1993;34:1075–81.
6. Vitola J, Delbeke D, Meranze S, et al. Positron emission tomography with F-18-fluorodeoxyglucose to evaluate the results of hepatic chemoembolization. Cancer 1996;78:2039–42.
7. Lai D, Fulham M, Stephen M, et al. The role of whole-body positron emission tomography with [18F]fluorodeoxyglucose in identifying operable colorectal cancer metastases to the liver. Archives of Surg 1996;131:703–7.
8. Beets G, Penninck F, Schiepers C, et al. Clinical value of whole body positron emission tomography with [18F]fluorodeoxyglucose in recurrent colorectal cancer. Br J Surg 1994;81:1666–70.
9. Fong Y, Saldinger PF, Akhurst T, et al. Utility of 18F-FDG positron emission tomography scanning on selection of patients for resection of hepatic colorectal metastases. Am J Surg 1999;178:282–7.
10. Strasberg SM, Dehdashti F, Siegel BA, et al. Survival of patients evaluated by FDG-PET before hepatic resection for metastatic colorectal carcinoma: a prospective database study. Ann Surg 2001;233:293–9.
11. Schussler-Fiorenza C, Mahvi D, Niederhuber J, et al. Clinical risk score correlates with yield of PET scan in patients with colorectal hepatic metastases. J Gastrointest Surg 2004;8:150–7.
12. Akhurst T, Kates T, Mazumdar M, et al. Recent chemotherapy reduces the sensitivity of 18F-FDG PET in the detection of colorectal metastases. J Clin Oncol, 2005. [In press]
13. Fong Y, Fortner J, Sun RL, et al. Clinical score for predicting recurrence after hepatic resection for metastatic colorectal cancer: analysis of 1001 consecutive cases. Ann Surg 1999;230:309–18; discussion 318–21.
14. Bengmark S, Hafstrom L. The natural history of primary and secondary malignant tumors of the liver. The prognosis for patients with hepatic metastases from colonic and rectal carcinoma at laparotomy. Cancer 1969;23:1989–202.
15. Ekberg H, Tranberg K, Andersson R, et al. Pattern of recurrence in liver resection for colorectal secondaries. World J Surg 1987;11:541–7.
16. Bozzetti F, Bignami P, Morabito A, et al. Patterns of failure following surgical resection of colorectal cancer liver metastases. Ann Surg 1987;205:264–70.
17. Jaffe B, Donegan W, Watson F. Factors influencing survival in patients with untreated hepatic metastases. Surg Gynecol Obstet 1968;127:1–11.
18. Goslin R, Steele G, Zamcheck N, et al. Factors influencing survival in patients with hepatic metastases from adenocarcinoma of the colon and rectum. Dis Colon Rectum 1982;25:749–54.
19. Bengtsson G, Carlsson G, Hafstrom L. Natural history of patients with untreated liver metastases from colorectal cancer. Am J Surg 1981;141:586–9.
20. Finan P, Marshall R, Cooper E, et al. Factors affecting survival in patients presenting with synchronous hepatic metastases from colorectal cancer: a clinical and computer analysis. Br J Surg 1985;72:373–7.
21. DeBrauw L, DeVelde C, Bouwhuis-Hoogerwerf M. Diagnostic evaluation and survival analysis of colorectal cancer patients with liver metastases. J Surg Oncol 1987;34:81–6.
22. Wood C, Gillis C, Blumgart L. A retrospective study of the natural history of patients with liver metastases from colorectal cancer. Clin Oncol 1976;2:285–8.
23. Baker L, Talley R, Maiter R, et al. Phase III comparison of the treatment of advanced gastrointestinal cancer with bolus weekly 5-FU vs methyl CCNU plus bolus weekly 5-FU. Cancer 1976;38:1.
24. Grage T, Vassilopoulos P, Shingleton W, et al. Results of a prospective randomized study of hepatic artery infusion with 5-fluorouracil vs intravenous 5-fluorourcail in patients with hepatic metastases from colorectal cancer: A Central Oncology Group study. Surgery 1979;86:550–5.
25. Macdonald JS, Kisner DF, Smythe T, et al. 5-Fluorouracil (5-FU), methyl-CCNU, and vincristine in the treatment of advanced colorectal cancer: phase II study utilizing weekly 5-FU. Cancer Treat Rep 1976;60:1597–600.
26. Buroker T, Kim P, Groppe C, et al. 5-FU infusion with methyl-CCNU in the treatment of advanced colon cancer. Cancer 1978;42:1228.
27. Kemeny N, Younes A, Seiter K, et al. Interferon alpha-2a and 5-fluorouracil for advanced colorectal carcinoma. Assessment of activity and toxicity. Cancer 1990;66:2470–5.
28. Nordic GTATG. Superiority of sequential methotrexate, fluorouracil, and leucovorin to fluorouracil alone in advanced symptomatic colorectal carcinoma: a randomized trial. J Clin Oncol 1989;7:1437–46.
29. Ehrlichman C, Fine S, Wong A, et al. Randomized trial of fluorouracil and folinic acid in patients with metastatic colorectal carcinoma. J Clin Oncol 1988;6:469–75.
30. Kemeny N, Yagoda A, Braun DJ, et al. A randomized study of two different schedules of methyl CCNU, 5-FU and vincristine for metastatic colorectal carcinoma. Cancer 1979;43:78–82.
31. Doroshow J, Multhauf P, Leong L, et al. Prospective randomized comparison of fluorouracil versus fluorouracil and high-dose continuous infusion leucovorin calcium for the treatment of advanced measurable colorectal cancer in patients previously unexposed to chemotherapy. J Clin Oncol 1990;8:491–501.
32. Nordlinger B, Quilichini MA, Parc R, et al. Hepatic resection for colorectal liver metastases. Influence on survival of preoperative factors and surgery for recurrences in 80 patients. Ann Surg 1987;205:256–63.
33. Coppa GF, Eng K, Ranson JH, et al. Hepatic resection for metastatic colon and rectal cancer. An evaluation of preoperative and postoperative factors. Ann Surg 1985;202:203–8.
34. Schlag P, Hohenberger P, Herfath C. Resection of liver metastases in colorectal cancer--competitive analysis of treatment results in synchronous versus metachronous metastases. Eur J Surg Oncol 1990;16:360–5.
35. Doci R, Gennari L, Bignami P, et al. One hundred patients with hepatic metastases from colorectal cancer treated by resection: analysis of prognostic determinants. Br J Surg 1991;78:797–801.
36. Scheele J, Stangl R, Altendorf-Hofmann A, et al. Indicators of prognosis after hepatic resection for colorectal secondaries. Surgery 1991;110:13–29.
37. Fortner J, Silva J, Cox E, et al. Multivariate analysis of a personal series of 247 patients with liver metastases from colorectal cancer. Ann Surg 1984;199:317–23.
38. Cunningham JD, Fong Y, Shriver C, et al. One hundred consecutive hepatic resections. Blood loss, transfusion, and operative technique. Arch Surg 1994;129:1050–6.
39. Adson M, Van Heerden J, Adson M, et al. Resection of hepatic metastases from colorectal cancer. Arch Surg 1984;119:647–51.
40. Foster J: Survival after liver resection for secondary tumors. Am J Surg 1978;135:389–94.
41. Thompson HH, Tompkins RK, Longmire WP, Jr. Major hepatic resection. A 25-year experience. Ann Surg 1983;197:375–88.
42. Butler J, Attiyeh F, Daly J. Hepatic resection for metastases of the colon and rectum. Surg Gynecol Obstet 1986;162:109–13.
43. Iwatsuki S, Shaw B, Starzl T. Experience with 150 liver resections. Ann Surg 1983;197:247–53.
44. Hughes KS, Simon R, Songhorabodi S, et al. Resection of the liver for colorectal carcinoma metastases: a multi-

institutional study of patterns of recurrence. Surgery 1986;100:278–84.

45. Cobourn CS, Makowka L, Langer B, et al. Examination of patient selection and outcome for hepatic resection for metastatic disease. Surg Gynecol Obstet 1987;165:239–46.
46. Younes RN, Rogatko A, Brennan MF. The influence of intraoperative hypotension and perioperative blood transfusion on disease-free survival in patients with complete resection of colorectal liver metastases. Ann Surg 1991;214:107–13.
47. Rosen D, Nagorney D, Taswell H, et al. Perioperative blood transfusion and determinants of survival after liver resection for metastatic colorectal carcinoma. Ann Surg 1992;216:493–505.
48. Vogt P, Raab R, Ringe B, et al. Resection of synchronous liver metastases from colorectal cancer. World J Surg 1991;15:62–7.
49. Morrow CE, Grage TB, Sutherland DE, et al. Hepatic resection for secondary neoplasms. Surgery 1982;92:610–4.
50. Logan SE, Meier SJ, Ramming KP, et al. Hepatic resection of metastatic colorectal carcinoma: a ten-year experience. Arch Surg 1982;117:25–8.
51. Gayowski T, Iwatsuki S, Madariaga J, et al. Experience in hepatic resection for metastatic colorectal cancer: analysis of clinical and pathologic risk factors. Surg 1994;116:703–11.
52. Scheele J, Stang R, Altendorf-Hofmann A, et al. Resection of colorectal liver metastases. World J Surg 1995;19:59–71.
53. Fong Y, Cohen AM, Fortner JG, et al. Liver resection for colorectal metastases. J Clin Oncol 1997;15:938–46.
54. Nordlinger B, Guigiet M, Vaillant JC, et al. Surgical resection of colorectal carcinoma metastases to the liver. Cancer 1996;77:1254–62.
55. Rees M, Plant G, Bygrave S. Late results justify resection for multiple hepatic metastases from colorectal cancer. Br J Surg 1997;84:1136–40.
56. Jamison R, Donohur J, Nagorney D, et al. Hepatic resection for metastatic colorectal cancer results in cure for some patients. Arch Surg 1997;132:505–11.
57. Cady B, McDermott WWJ. Major hepatic resection for metachronous metastases from colon cancer. Ann Surg 1985;201:204–9.
58. Cady B, Stone MD, McDermott WWJ, et al. Technical and biological factors in disease-free survival after hepatic resection for colorectal cancer metastases. Arch Surg 1992;127:561–9.
59. Stephenson KR, Steinberg SM, Hughes KS, et al Perioperative blood transfusions are associated with decreased time to recurrence and decreased survival after resection of colorectal liver metastases. Ann Surg 1988;208:679–87.
60. Mala T, Bohler G, Mathisen O, et al. Hepatic resection for colorectal metastases: can preoperative scoring predict patient outcome? World J Surg 2002;26:1348–53.
61. Jarnagin WR, Conlon K, Bodniewicz J, et al. A clinical scoring system predicts the yield of diagnostic laparoscopy in patients with potentially resectable hepatic colorectal metastases. Cancer 2001;91:1121–8.
62. Wolf R, Goodnight J, Krag D, et al. Results of resection and proposed guidelines for patient selection in instances of noncolorectal hepatic metastases. Surg Gynecol Obstet 1991;173:454–60.
63. Kaseki H, Yasui K, Niwa K, et al. Hepatic resection for metastatic squamous cell carcinoma from the uterine cervix. Gynecol Oncol 1992;44:284-7.
64. Bines SD, England G, Deziel DJ, et al. Synchronous, metachronous, and multiple hepatic resections of liver tumors originating from primary gastric tumors. Surgery 1993;114:799–805;discussion 804–5.
65. Akerstrom G, Makridis C, Johansson H. Abdominal surgery in patients with midgut carcinoid tumors. Acta Oncol 1991;30:547–53.
66. Chevinsky AH, Minton JP, Falko JM. Metastatic pheochromocytoma associated with multiple endocrine neoplasia syndrome type II. Arch Surg 1990;125:935–8.
67. Cherner JA, Sawyers JL. Benefit of resection of metastatic gastrinoma in multiple endocrine neoplasia type I. Gastroenterology 1992;102:1049–53.
68. Chiarugi M, Pucciarelli M, Goletti O, et al. Outcome of surgical treatment for extrapancreatic gastrinomas. Surg Gynecol Obstet 1993;177:153–7.
69. Karakousis CP, Blumenson LE, Canavese G, et al. Surgery for disseminated abdominal sarcoma. Am J Surg 1992;163:560–4.
70. Elias D, Lasser P, Spielmann M, et al. Surgical and chemotherapeutic treatment of hepatic metastases from carcinoma of the breast. Surg Gynecol Obstet 1991;172:461–4.
71. Goulet RJ, Jr., Hardacre JM, Einhorn LH, et al. Hepatic resection for disseminated germ cell carcinoma. Ann Surg 1990;212:290–3;discussion 293-4.
72. O'Connell MJ, Adson MA, Schutt AJ, et al: Clinical trial of adjuvant chemotherapy after surgical resection of colorectal cancer metastatic to the liver. Mayo Clin Proc 1985;60:517–20.
73. Portier G, Rougier P, Milan C, et al. Adjuvant systemic chemotherapy using 5-fluorouracil and folinic acid after resection of liver metastases from colorectal origin. Proc Am Soc Clin Oncol 2002.
74. Langer B, Blieberg H, Labianca ea: Fluorouracil (FU) plus l-leucovorin (i-LV) versus observation after potentially curative resection of liver or lung metastases from colorectal cancer (CRC): results of the ENG (EORTC/NCIC CTG/GIVO) randomized trial. Proc Am Soc Clin Oncol 200221:149a.
75. Andre T, Boni C, Mounedji-Boudiaf L, et al. Oxaliplatin, fluorouracil, and leucovorin as adjuvant treatment for colon cancer. N Engl J Med 2004;350:2343–51.
76. Hohenberger P, Schlag P, Schwarz V, et al. Tumor recurrence and options for further treatment after resection of liver metastases in patients with colorectal cancer. J Surg Oncol 1990;44:245–51.
77. Kemeny N, Huang Y, Cohen AM, et al. Hepatic arterial infusion of chemotherapy after resection of hepatic metastases from colorectal cancer. N Engl J Med 1999;341:2039–48.
78. Kemeny MM, Adak S, Gray B, et al. Combined-modality treatment for resectable metastatic colorectal carcinoma to the liver: surgical resection of hepatic metastases in combination with continuous infusion of chemotherapy—an intergroup study. J Clin Oncol 2002;20:1499–1505.
79. Lorenz M, Muller H-H, Schramm H, et al. Randomized trial of surgery versus surgery followed by adjuvant hepatic arterial infusion with 5-fluorouracil and folinic acid for liver metastases of colorectal cancer. Surg 1998;228:756–62.
80. Lygidakis NJ, Sgourakis G, Vlachos L, et al. Metastatic liver disease of colorectal origin: the value of locoregional immunochemotherapy combined with systemic chemotherapy following liver resection. Results of a prospective randomized study. Hepatogastroenterology 2001;48:1685–91.
81. Kusunoki M, Yanagi H, Noda M, et al. Results of pharmacokinetic modulating chemotherapy in combination with hepatic arterial 5-fluorouracil infusion and oral UFT after resection of hepatic colorectal metastases. Cancer 2000;89:1228–35.
82. Rudroff C, Altendorf-Hoffmann A, Stangl R, et al. Prospective randomised trial on adjuvant hepatic-artery infusion chemotherapy after R0 resection of colorectal liver metastases. Langenbecks Arch Surg 1999;384:243–9.
83. Fowler WC, Eisenberg BL, Hoffman JP. Hepatic resection following systemic chemotherapy for metastatic colorectal carcinoma. J Surg Oncol 1992;51:122–5.
84. Shankar A, Leonard P, Renaut AJ, et al. Neo-adjuvant therapy improves resectability rates for colorectal liver metastases. Ann R Coll Surg Engl 2001;83:85–8.
85. Adam R, Avisar E, Ariche A, et al. Five-year survival following hepatic resection after neoadjuvant therapy for nonresectable colorectal. Ann Surg Oncol 2001;8:347–53.
86. Giacchetti S, Itzhaki M, Gruia G, et al. Long-term survival of patients with unresectable colorectal cancer liver metastases following infusional chemotherapy with 5-fluorouracil, leucovorin, oxaliplatin and surgery. Ann Oncol 1999;10:663–9.
87. Alberts S, Donohue J, Mahoney M, et al. Liver resection after 5-fluorouracil and oxaliplatin for patients with metastatic colorectal cancer (MCRC) limited to the liver: A North Central Cancer Treatment Group(NCCTG) phase II study. Proc Am Soc Clin Oncol 2003;22:263.
88. Delaunoit T, Krook J, Sargent D. Chemotherapy allowed resection of metastatic colorectal cancer: A cooperative group experience. Gastrointestinal Cancers Symposium 2003;138.
89. Pozzo C, Basso M, Cassano A, et al. Neoadjuvant treatment of unresectable liver disease with irinotecan and 5-fluorouracil plus folinic acid in colorectal cancer patients. Ann Oncol 2004;15:933–9.
90. Clavien PA, Selzner N, Morse M, et al. Downstaging of hepatocellular carcinoma and liver metastases from colorectal cancer by selective intra-arterial chemotherapy. Surgery 2002;131:433–42.
91. Elias D, Lasser P, Rougier P, et al. Frequency, technical aspects, results, and indications of major hepatectomy after prolonged intra-arterial hepatic chemotherapy for initially unresectable hepatic tumors. J Am Coll Surg 1995;180:213–9.
92. Milandri C, Calzolari F, Giampalma E, et al. [Combined treatment of inoperable liver metastases from colorectal cancer]. Tumori 2003;89:112–4.
93. Kemeny N, Fong Y, Jarnagin W, et al. A phase I trial of systemic oxaliplatin combinations with hepatic arterial infusion in patients with unresectable liver metastases from colorectal cancer. J Clin Oncol 2005;23:4888–96.
94. Adam R, Pascal G, Castaing D, et al: Tumor progression while on chemotherapy: a contraindication to liver resection for multiple colorectal metastases? Ann Surg 2004;240:1052-61; discussion 1061–4.
95. Allen PJ, Kemeny N, Jarnagin W, et al. Importance of response to neoadjuvant chemotherapy in patients undergoing resection of synchronous colorectal liver metastases. J Gastrointest Surg 2003;7:109-15; discussion 116–7.
96. Rubbia-Brandt L, Audard V, Sartoretti P, et al. Severe hepatic sinusoidal obstruction associated with oxaliplatin-based chemotherapy in patients with metastatic colorectal cancer. Ann Oncol 2004;15:460–6.
97. George SL, Hoogstraten B: Prognostic factors in the initial response to therapy by patients with advanced breast cancer. J Natl Cancer Inst 1978;60:731–6.
98. Cascinu S, Labianca R, Alessandroni P, et al. Intensive weekly chemotherapy for advanced gastric cancer using fluorouracil, cisplatin, epi-doxorubicin, 6S-leucovorin, glutathione, and filgrastim: a report from the Italian Group for the Study of Digestive Tract Cancer. J Clin Oncol 1997;15:3313–9.
99. Kemeny N, Yagoda A, Braun D, et al. Therapy for metastatic colorectal carcinoma with combination of methyl-CCNU, 5-fluorouracil, vincristine and streptozotocin (MOF-Strep). Cancer 1980;45:876–81.
100. Kemeny N, Younes A, Seiter K, et al. Combination fluorouracil (FU) and recombinant alpha-interferon (IFN) in advanced colorectal carcinoma: activity but significant toxicity. Cancer 1990;66:2470–5.
101. Wadler S, Schwartz E, Goldman M, et al. Fluorouracil and recombinant alpha-2a-interferon: an active regimen against advanced colorectal carcinoma. J Clin Oncol 1989;7:1769–75.
102. Petrelli N, Douglas H, Herrera L, et al. The modulation of fluorouracil with leucovorin in metastatic colorectal carcinoma: a prospective randomized phase III trial. J Clin Oncol 1989;7:1419–26.
103. Colucci G, Maiello E, Leo S, et al. Biochemical modulation of fluorouracil with high dose methotrexate or folinic acid in advanced colorectal cancer patients. Gruppo Oncologico dell' Italia Meridionale (GOIM). Anticancer Res 1994;14:2157–62.
104. Penz M, Kornek GV, Raderer M, et al. Phase II trial of two-weekly gemcitabine in patients with advanced biliary tract cancer. Ann Oncol 2001;12:183–6.
105. Kubicka S, Rudolph KL, Tietze MK, et al. Phase II study of systemic gemcitabine chemotherapy for advanced unresectable hepatobiliary carcinomas. Hepatogastroenterology 2001;48:783–9.
106. Arroyo G, Gallardo J, Rubio B, et al. Gemcitabine (GEM) in advanced biliary tract cancer (ABTC). Experience from Chile and Argentina in Phase II trials. Proc Am Soc Clin Oncol 2001;20:157a.
107. Breedis C, Young C: The blood supply of neoplasms in the liver. Am J Pathol 1954;30:969–77.
108. Ensminger WD, Rosowsky A, Raso V. A clinical pharmacological evaluation of hepatic arterial infusions of 5-fluoro-2-deoxyuridine and 5-fluorouracil. Cancer Res 1978;38:3789–92.
109. Ensminger WD, Gyves JW. Clinical pharmacology of hepatic arterial chemotherapy. Semin Oncol 1983;10:176–83.
110. Collins JM: Pharmacologic rationale for regional drug delivery. J Clin Oncol 1984;2:498–504.
111. Weiss L: Metastatic inefficiency and regional therapy for liver metastases from colorectal carcinoma. Regul Cancer Treat 1989;2:77–81.
112. Weiss L, Grandmann E, Torhost J, et al. Hematogenous metastatic patterns in colonic carcinoma: an analysis of 1541 necropsies. J Pathol 1986;150:195–203.
113. Tandon R, Bunnell I, Copper R. The treatment of metastatic carcinoma of the liver by percutaneous selective hepatic artery infusion of 5-fluorouracil. Surgery 1973;73:118–21.
114. Ensminger W, Niederhuber J, Dakhil S, et al. Totally implanted drug delivery system for hepatic arterial chemotherapy. Cancer Treat Rep 1981;65:393–400.

115. Yasuda S, Noto T, Ikeda M, et al. Hepatic arterial infusion chemotherapy using implantable reservoir in colorectal liver metastasis. GanTo Kagaku Ryoho 1990;8:1815–9.
116. Kemeny N, Daly J, Reichman B, et al. Intrahepatic or systemic infusion of fluorodeoxyuridine in patients with liver metastases from colorectal carcinoma—a randomized trial. Ann Intern Med 1987;107:459–67.
117. Hohn D, Stagg R, Friedman M, et al. A randomized trial of continuous intravenous versus hepatic intra-arterial floxuridine in patients with colorectal cancer metastatic to the liver: The Northern California Oncology Group Trial. J Clin Oncol 1989;7:1646–54.
118. Chang AE, Schneider PD, Sugarbaker PH. A prospective randomized trial of regional versus systemic continuous 5-flouoroxyuridine chemotherapy in the treatment of colorectal liver metastases. Ann Surg 1987;206:685–93.
119. Martin JKJ, O'Connell MG, Wieland HS, et al: Intra-arterial floxuridine vs systemic fluorouracil for hepatic metastases from colorectal cancer. A randomized trial. Arch Surg 1990;125:1022–7.
120. Rougier P, Laplanche A, Huguier M, et al. Hepatic arterial infusion of floxuridine in patients with liver metastases from colorectal carcinoma: long-term results of a prospective randomized trial. J Clin Oncol 1992;10:1112–8.
121. Allen-Mersh T, Earlam S, Fordy C, et al. Quality of life and survival with continuous hepatic artery floxuridine infusion for colorectal liver metastases. Lancet 1994;344:1255–60.
122. Kemeny M, Battifora H, Flayney D, et al. Sclerosing cholangitis after continuous hepatic artery infusion of FUDR. Ann Surg 1985;202:176–81.
123. Hohn D, Stagg R, Price D, et al. Avoidance of gastroduodenal toxicity in patients receiving hepatic arterial 5-fluoro-2-deoxyuridine. J Clin Oncol 1985;3:1257–60.
124. Lorenz M, Muller HH. Randomized, multicenter trial of fluorouracil plus leucovorin administered either via hepatic arterial or intravenous infusion versus fluorodeoxyuridine administered via hepatic arterial infusion in patients with nonresectable liver metastases from colorectal carcinoma. J Clin Oncol 2000;18:243–54.
125. Gluck W, Akwari O, Kelvin F, et al. A reversible enteropathy complicating continuous hepatic artery infusion chemotherapy with 5-fluoro 2-deoxyuridine. Cancer 1985;56:2424–7.
126. Northover J, Terblance J. A new look at the arterial supply of the bile duct in man and its surgical implications. Br J Surg 1979;66:379–84.
127. Allen P, Nissan A, Picon A, et al. Technical complications and durability of hepatic artery infusion pumps for unresectable colorectal liver metastases: an institutional experience of 544 consecutive cases. J Am Coll Surg 2005;201:57–65.
128. Kemeny N, Steiter K, Niedzweiecki D, et al. A randomized trial of intrahepatic infusion of fluorouridine (FUDR) with dexamethasone versus FUDR alone in the treatment of metastatic colorectal cancer. Cancer 1992;69:327–34.
129. Hrushesky W, Von Roemelling R, Lanning R, et al. Circadian-shaped infusions of floxuridine for progressive metastatic renal cell carcinoma. J Clin Oncol 1990;8:1504–13.
130. Stagg R, Venook A, Chase J, et al. Alternating hepatic intra-arterial floxuridine and fluorouracil: a less toxic regimen for treatment of liver metastases from colorectal cancer. J Natl Cancer Inst 1991;83:423–8.
131. Metzger U, Weder W, Rothlin M, et al: Phase II study of intra-arterial fluorouracil and mitomycin-C for liver metastases of colorectal cancer. Recent Results Cancer Res 1991;121:198–204.
132. van Riel J, van Groeningen C, Albers S, et al. Hepatic arterial 5-fluorouracil in patients with liver metastases of colorectal cancer: single-centre experience in 145 patients. Ann Oncol 2000;11:1563–70.
133. Lorenz M, Mueller HH, Mattes E, et al. Phase II study of weekly 24-hour intra-arterial high-dose infusion of 5-fluorouracil and folinic acid for liver metastases from colorectal carcinomas. Ann Oncol 2001;12:321–5.
134. Kemeny N, Conti JA, Cohen A, et al. Phase II study of hepatic arterial floxuridine, leucovorin, and dexamethasone for unresected liver metastases from colorectal carcinoma. J Clin Oncol 1994;12:2288–95.
135. Kemeny N, Eid A, Stockman J, et al. Hepatic arterial infusion of floxuridine and dexamethasone plus high-dose mitomycin C for patients with unresectable hepatic metastases from colorectal carcinoma. J Surg Oncol 2005;91:97–101.
136. Pohlen U, Mansmann U, Berger G, et al. Multicenter pilot study of 5-fluorouracil, folinic acid, interferon alpha-2b and degradable starch microspheres via hepatic arterial infusion in patients with nonresectable colorectal liver metastases. Anticancer Res 2004;24:3275–82.
137. van Riel JM, van Groeningen CJ, de Greve J, et al. Continuous infusion of hepatic arterial irinotecan in pretreated patients with colorectal cancer metastatic to the liver. Ann Oncol 2004;15:59–63.
138. van Riel J, Van Groeningen C, Kedde M, et al. Continuous administration of irinotecan by hepatic arterial infusion: a phase I and pharmacokinetic study. Clin Cancer Res 2002;8:408–12.
139. Vogl T, Eichler K, Mack M, et al. A phase I study of hepatic arterial infusion (HAI) of irinotecan in patients with inoperable liver metastases of colorectal cancer. Proc Am Soc Clin Oncol 2004;23:298.
140. Kern W, Beckert B, Lang N, et al. Phase I and pharmacokinetic study of hepatic arterial infusion with oxaliplatin in combination with folinic acid and 5-fluorouracil in patients with hepatic metastases from colorectal cancer. Ann Oncol 2001;12:599–603.
141. Ducreux M, Ychou M, Laplanche A, et al. Intra-arterial hepatic chemotherapy (IAHC) with oxaliplatin (O) combined with intravenous treatment with 5FU + folinic acid (FA) in hepatic metastases of colorectal cancer (HMCC). J Clin Oncol 2005;23:4881–7.
142. Pennucci M, Del Freo A, Della Seta R, et al. A feasibility study of hepatic arterial infusion (HAI) with oxaliplatin (Oxa) 5-fluorouracil (FU) and leucovorin (LV) in patients with liver metastases (LM) from colorectal cancer (CRC), 4th National Congress of Medical Oncology, Turin, Italy, 2002, p. 46.
143. Bouchahda M, Tanaka K, Adam R, et al. Hepatic artery chronomodulated infusion of irinotecan, 5-fluorouracil and oxaliplatin against liver metastases in heavily pretreated patients with colorectal cancer. J Clin Oncol 2004;22:3722.
144. Tomirotti M, Pallavicini E, Tacconi F, et al. First-line activity of hepatic arterial infusion (HAI) of oxaliplatin and systemic chemotherapy with leucovorin plus 5-fluorouracil in metastatic colorectal cancer: preliminary data of a multicenter study. Proc Am Soc Clin Oncol 2002;22:135b.
145. Boige V, Lacombe S, De Baere T, et al. Hepatic arterial infusion oxaliplatin combined with intravenous 5-FU and folinic acid in non resectable liver metastasis of colorectal cancer: a promising option for failures to systemic chemotherapy. Proc Am Soc Clin Oncol 2003;22:291.
146. Zelek L, Bugat R, Cherqui D, et al. Multimodal therapy with intravenous biweekly leucovorin, 5-fluorouracil and irinotecan combined with hepatic arterial infusion pirarubicin in non-resectable hepatic metastases from colorectal cancer (a European Association for Research in Oncology trial). Ann Oncol 2003;14:1537–42.
147. Kemeny N, Gonen M, Sullivan D, et al. Phase I study of hepatic arterial infusion of floxuridine and dexamethasone with systemic irinotecan for unresectable hepatic metastases from colorectal cancer. J Clin Oncol 2001;19:2687–95.
148. Meta-Analysis GiC. Reappraisal of HAI in the treatment of nonresectable liver metastases from colorectal carcinoma. J Natl Cancer Inst 1996;88:252–8.
149. Fraschini G, Charngangavej C, Carrasco C, et al. Percutaneous hepatic arterial infusion of cisplatin-vinblastine for refractory cancer metastatic to the liver. Am J Clin Oncol 1988;11:34–8.
150. Estape J, Daniels M, Vinolas N, et al. Combination chemotherapy with oral etoposide plus intravenous cyclophosphamide in liver metastases of breast cancer. Amer J Clin Oncol 1990;13:98–100.
151. Fraschini G, Flesihman G, Charnsangavej C, et al. Continuous 5-day infusion of vinblastine for percutaneous hepatic arterial chemotherapy for metastatic breast cancer. Cancer Treat Rep 1987;71:1001–5.
152. Fraschini G, Fleishman G, Yap H-Y, et al. Percutaneous hepatic arterial infusion of cisplatin for metastatic breast cancer. Cancer Treat Rep 1987;71:313–5.
153. Maral J, Curet P, Baumer R, et al. Intra-arterial chemotherapy for hepatic metastases. Experience of the Pitie-Salpetiere Hospital Group. Ann Gastroenterol Hepatol (Paris) 1985;21:99–101.
154. Arai Y, Sone Y, Inaba Y, et al. Hepatic arterial infusion chemotherapy for liver metastases from breast cancer. Cancer Chemother Pharmacol 1994;33(S):142–4.
155. Tada A, Ogawa M, Ingaki J, et al. Arterial infusion of combination chemotherapy consisting of Adriamycin and mitomycin-C for liver metastases of breast cancer. Gan to Kagaku ryoho (Tokyo) 1986;13:70–74.
156. Ravikumar T, Kane R, Cady B, et al. A 5-year study of cryosurgery in the treatment of liver tumors. Arch Surg 1991;126:1520–4.
157. Ravikumar TS, Steele GJ, Kane R, et al. Experimental and clinical observations on hepatic cryosurgery for colorectal metastases. Cancer Res 1991;51:6233–7.
158. Onik G, Rubinsky B, Zemel R, et al. Ultrasound-guided hepatic cryosurgery in the treatment of metastatic colon carcinoma. Cancer 1991;67:901–7.
159. Morris D, Ross W. Australian experience of cryoablation of liver tumors: metastases. Surg Oncol Clin NA 1996;5:391–7.
160. Seifert JK, Morris DL. Prognostic factors after cryotherapy for hepatic metastases from colorectal cancer. Ann Surg 1998;228:201–8.
161. Morris DL, Horton MD, Dilley AV, et al. Treatment of hepatic metastases by cryotherapy and regional cytotoxic perfusion. Gut 1993;34:1156–7.
162. Charnley RM, Doran J, Morris DL. Cryotherapy for liver metastases: a new approach. Br J Surg 1989;76:1040–1.
163. Solbiati I, SN G, Ierace E, et al. Hepatic metastases: percutaneous radiofrequency ablation with cooled tip electrodes. Radiology 1997;205:367–73.
164. Lencioni R, Goletti O, Armillotta N, et al. Radio-frequency thermal ablation of liver metastases with a cooled-tip electrode needle: results of a pilot clinical trial. Eur Radiol 1998;8:1205–11.
165. Wood TF, Rose DM, Chung M, et al. Radiofrequency ablation of 231 unresectable hepatic tumors: indications, limitations, and complications. Ann Surg Oncol 2000;7:593–600.
166. Solbiati L, Livraghi T, Goldberg SN, et al. Percutaneous radio-frequency ablation of hepatic metastases from colorectal cancer: long-term results in 117 patients. Radiology 2001;221:159–66.
167. Livraghi T, Solbiati L, Meloni MF, et al. Treatment of focal liver tumors with percutaneous radio-frequency ablation: complications encountered in a multicenter study. Radiology 2003;226:441—51.
168. Decadt B, Siriwardena AK. Radiofrequency ablation of liver tumors: systematic review. Lancet Oncol 2004;5:550–60.
169. Bilchik AJ, Wood TF, Allegra D, et al. Cryosurgical ablation and radiofrequency ablation for unresectable hepatic malignant neoplasms: a proposed algorithm. Arch Surg 2000;135:657–62; discussion 662–4.
170. Rivoire M, De Cian F, Meeus P, et al. Combination of neoadjuvant chemotherapy with cryotherapy and surgical resection for the treatment of unresectable liver metastases from colorectal carcinoma. Cancer 2002;95:2283–92.
171. Markowitz J. The hepatic artery. Surg Gynecol Obstet 1952;95:644–6.
172. Konno T. Targeting chemotherapy for hepatoma: arterial administration of anticancer drugs dissolved in Lipiodol. Eur J Cancer 1992;28:403–9.
173. Hunt TM, Flowerdew AD, Birch SJ, et al. Prospective randomized controlled trial of hepatic arterial embolization or infusion chemotherapy with 5-fluorouracil and degradable starch microspheres for colorectal liver metastases. Br J Surg 1990;77:779–82.
174. Gerard A, Buyse M, Pector JC, et al. Hepatic artery ligation with and without portal infusion of 5-FU. A randomized study in patients with unresectable liver metastases from colorectal carcinoma. The E.O.R.T.C. Gastrointestinal Cancer Cooperative Group (G.I. Group). Eur J Surg Oncol 1991;17:289–94.
175. Martenson H, Nobin A, Bengmark S, et al. Embolization of the liver in the management of metastatic carcinoid tumors. J Surg Oncol 1984;27:152–8.
176. Ajani J, Carrasco CH, Charnsanpavej C, et al. Islet cell tumors metastatic to the liver: effective palliation by sequential hepatic artery embolization. Ann Intern Med 1988;108:340–4.
177. Carrasco C, Charnsanparej C, Ajani J, et al. The carcinoid syndrome: palliation by hepatic artery embolization. AJR Am J Roentgenol 1986;147:149–54.
178. Marlink R, Lokich J, Robins J, et al. Hepatic arterial embolization for metastatic hormone-secreting tumors. Cancer 1990;65:2227–32.
179. Moertel C. Treatment of the carcinoid tumor and the malignant carcinoid syndrome. J Clin Oncol 1983;1:727–740.
180. Kruskal JB, Hlatky L, Hahnfeldt P, et al. In vivo and in vitro analysis of the effectiveness of doxorubicin combined with temporary arterial occlusion in liver tumors. J Vasc Interv Radiol 1993;4:741–7.
181. Chang J-M, Tzeng W-S, Pan H-B, et al. Transcatheter arterial embolization with or without cisplatin treatment of hepatocellular carcinoma: a randomized controlled study. Cancer 1994;74:2449–59.
182. Lin DY, Liaw YF, Lee TY, et al. Hepatic arterial embolization in patients with unresectable hepatocellular carci-

noma–a randomized controlled trial. Gastroenterology 1988;94:453–6.

183. Llovet JM, Real MI, Montana X, et al. Arterial embolisation or chemoembolisation versus symptomatic treatment in patients with unresectable hepatocellular carcinoma: a randomised controlled trial. Lancet 2002;359:1734–9.

184. Ikeda M, Maeda S, Shibata J, et al. Transcatheter arterial chemotherapy with and without embolization in patients with hepatocellular carcinoma. Oncology 2004;66:24-31.

185. Llovet JM, Bruix J. Systematic review of randomized trials for unresectable hepatocellular carcinoma: chemoembolization improves survival. Hepatology 2003;37:429–42.

186. Raoul JL, Guyader D, Bretagne JF, et al. Prospective randomized trial of chemoembolization versus intra-arterial injection of 131I-labeled-iodized oil in the treatment of hepatocellular carcinoma. Hepatology 1997;26:1156–61.

187. Kawai S, Okamura J, Ogawa M, et al. Prospective and randomized clinical trial for the treatment of hepatocellular carcinoma--a comparison of lipiodol-transcatheter arterial embolization with and without Adriamycin (first cooperative study). The Cooperative Study Group for Liver Cancer Treatment of Japan. Cancer Chemother Pharmacol 1992;31 Suppl:S1–6.

188. Ikeda K, Saitoh S, Suzuki Y, et al. A prospective randomized administration of 5'-deoxy-5-fluorouridine as adjuvant chemotherapy for hepatocellular carcinoma treated with transcatheter arterial chemoembolization. Am J Clin Oncol 1997;20:202–8.

189. Stagg R, Venook A, Chase J, et al. Chemoembolization of primary and metastatic liver tumors. Reg Cancer Treat 1992;1:53–7.

190. McVie J, Hoefnagel C, Burger J. Tumor targeting of cytostatic compounds using intra-arterial biodegradable microspheres. Ann Rep Netherlands Cancer Inst 1985;:83–4.

191. Aronsen K, Hellekant C, Holmberg J, et al. Controlled blocking of hepatic artery flow with enzymatically degradable microspheres combined with oncolytic drugs. Eur Surg Res 1979;11:99–106.

192. Prasad B, Lee MS, Hendrickson, FR. Irradiation of hepatic metastases. Int J Radiat Oncol Biol Phys 1977;2:129–32.

193. Lawrence TS, Ten Haken RK, Kessler ML, et al. The use of 3-D dose volume analysis to predict radiation hepatitis. Int J Radiat Oncol Biol Phys 1992;23:781–8.

194. Lawrence T, Dworzanin L, Walker-Andrews S, et al. Treatment of cancers involving the liver and porta hepatis with external beam irradiation and intraarterial hepatic fluorodeoxyuridine. Int J Radiat Oncol Biol Physiol 1990;20:555–61.

195. Liu MT, Li SH, Chu TC, et al. Three-dimensional conformal radiation therapy for unresectable hepatocellular carcinoma patients who had failed with or were unsuited for transcatheter arterial chemoembolization. Jpn J Clin Oncol 2004;34:532–9.

196. Goldenberg DM. Imaging and therapy of gastrointestinal cancers with radiolabeled antibodies. Am J Gastroenterol 1991;86:1392–403.

197. Thomas D, Nauta R, Rodgers J, et al. Intraoperative high dose rate interstitial irradiation of hepatic metastases from colorectal carcinoma. Results of a Phase I-II trial. Cancer 1993;71:1977–81.

198. Gray BN, Burton MA, Kelleher DK, et al. Selective internal radiation (SIR) therapy for treatment of liver metastases: measurement of response rate. J Surg Oncol 1989;42:192–6.

199. Herba MJ, Illescas FF, Thirlwell MP, et al. Hepatic malignancies: improved treatment with intraarterial Y-90. Radiology 1988;169:311–4.

200. Andrews J, Walker S, Ackermann R, et al. Hepatic radioembolization with Yttrium-90 containing glass microspheres: preliminary results and clinical followup. J Nucl Med 1994;35:1637–44.

201. Van Hazel G, Blackwell A, Anderson J, et al. Randomised phase 2 trial of SIR-Spheres plus fluorouracil/leucovorin chemotherapy versus fluorouracil/leucovorin chemotherapy alone in advanced colorectal cancer. J Surg Oncol 2004;88:78–85.

202. Bretagne J, Raoul J, Bourguet P, et al. Hepatic artery injection of I-131-labeled lipiodol. Part II. Preliminary results of therapeutic use in patients with hepatocellular carcinoma and liver metastases. Radiology 1988;168:547–50.

203. Livraghi T, Baietta E, Matricardi L, et al. Fine needle percutaneous intratumoral chemotherapy under ultrasound guidance: a feasibility study. Tumori 1986;72:81–87.

204. Livraghi T, Bolondi L, Lazzaroni S, et al. Percutaneous ethanol injection in the treatment of hepatocellular carcinoma in cirrhosis. A study on 207 patients. Cancer 1992;69:925–9.

205. Shiina S, Imamura M, Obi S, et al. Percutaneous ethanol injection therapy for small hepatocellular carcinoma. Gan to Kagaku Ryoho 1996;23:835–9.

206. Sironi S, Livraghi T, DelMaschio A. Small hepatocellular carcinoma treated with percutaneous ethanol injection: MR imaging findings. Radiology 1991;180:333–6.

207. Giovannini M, Seitz JF. Ultrasound-guided percutaneous alcohol injection of small liver metastases. Results in 40 patients. Cancer 1994;73:294–7.

208. Amin Z, Bown SG, Lees WR. Local treatment of colorectal liver metastases: a comparison of interstitial laser photocoagulation (ILP) and percutaneous alcohol injection (PAI). Clin Radiol 1993;48:166–71.

209. Lorenz M, Muller HH, Schramm H, et al. Randomized trial of surgery versus surgery followed by adjuvant hepatic arterial infusion with 5-fluorouracil and folinic acid for liver metastases of colorectal cancer. German Cooperative on Liver Metastases (Arbeitsgruppe Lebermetastasen). Ann Surg 1998;228:756–62.

210. Conti J, Kemeny N, Saltz L, et al. Irinotecan is an active agent in untreated patients with metastatic colorectal cancer. J Clin Oncol 1996;14:709–15.

211. Rothenberg M, Cox JV, DeVore R, et al. A multicentre phase II trial of weekly irinotecan (CPT-11) in patients with previously treated colorectal carcinoma. Cancer 1999;85:786–95.

212. Rothenberg M OA, Bigelow R, Berlin J, et al. Superiority of oxaliplatin and fluorouracil- leucovorin compared with either therapy alone in patients with progressive colorectal cancer after irinotecan and fluorouracil-leucovorin: interim results of a phase III trial. J Clin Oncol 2003;21:2059–69.

213. Cunningham D, Humblet Y, Siena S, et al. Cetuximab monotherapy and cetuximab plus irinotecan in irinotecan-refractory metastatic colorectal cancer. N Engl J Med 2004;351:337–45.

214. Saltz LB, Cox JV, Blanke C, et al. Irinotecan plus fluorouracil and leucovorin for metastatic colorectal cancer. Irinotecan Study Group. N Engl J Med 2000;343:905–14.

215. Kinami Y, Miyazaki I. The superselective and the selective one shot methods for treating inoperable cancer of the liver. Cancer 1978;41:1720–7.

216. Wellwood JM, Cady B, Oberfield RA. Treatment of primary liver cancer: response to regional chemotherapy. Clin Oncol 1979;5:25–31.

217. Cheng E, Watson RC, J F. Regional Intra-arterial infusion of cisplatin in primary liver cancer: a Phase II trial. Proceedings of ASCO 1982;1:179.

218. Atiq OT, Kemeny N, Niedzwiecki D, et al. Treatment of unresectable primary liver cancer with intrahepatic fluorodeoxyuridine and mitomycin C through an implantable pump. Cancer 1992;69:920–4.

219. Patt Y, Charnsangavej C, Yoffe B, et al. Hepatic arterial infusion of floxuridine, leucovorin, doxorubicin, and cisplatin for hepatocellular carcinoma: effects of hepatitis B and C viral infection on drug toxicity and patient survival. J Clin Oncol 1994;12:1204–11.

220. Carr B, Dvorchik I. Effects of cisplatin (DDP) intensity on hepatocellular carcinoma (HCC) responses and survival in 57 patients. Proc Am Soc Clin Oncol 1998;17:288a.

221. Okuda K, Tanaka M, Shibata J et al. Hepatic arterial infusion chemotherapy with continuous low dose administration of cisplatin and 5-fluorouracil for multiple recurrence of hepatocellular carcinoma after surgical treatment. Oncol Rep 1999;6:586–91.

222. Fazio N, Orsi F, S M. Hepatic arterial infusion (HAI) using a percutaneous temporary catheter in patients with advanced primary liver carcinoma. Anticancer Res 2003;23:5023–30.

223. Warren KW, Mountain JC, Lloyd-Jones W. Malignant tumours of the bile-ducts. Br J Surg 1972;59:501–5.

224. Reed ML, Vaitkevicius VK, Al-Sarraf M, et al. The practicality of chronic hepatic artery infusion therapy of primary and metastatic hepatic malignancies: ten-year results of 124 patients in a prospective protocol. Cancer 1981;47:402–9.

225. Smith GW, Bukowski RM, Hewlett JS, et al. Hepatic artery infusion of 5-fluorouracil and mitomycin C in cholangiocarcinoma and gallbladder carcinoma. Cancer 1984;54:1513–6.

226. Makela JT, Kairaluoma MI. Superselective intra-arterial chemotherapy with mitomycin for gallbladder cancer. Br J Surg 1993;80:912–5.

227. Cantore M, Mambrini A, Fiorentini G, et al. Phase II study of hepatic intraarterial epirubicin and cisplatin, with systemic 5-fluorouracil in patients with unresectable biliary tract tumors. Cancer 2005;103:1402–7.

228. Daniels J, Pentecost M, Teitelbaum G, et al. Hepatic artery chemoembolization (HAE) for carcinoma of colon using angiostat collagen and cisplatin, mitomycin, and doxorubicin: response, survival, and serum drug levels. J Vasc Interv Radiol 1993;4:347–51.

229. Stuart K, Huberman M, Posner M, et al. Chemoembolization for colorectal liver metastases. Proc ASCO 1995;14:190.

230. Tellez C, Benson ABI, Lyster M, et al. Chemoembolization for colorectal metastases to the liver. Proc ASCO 1995;14:198.

231. Links M, Ross W, Cliingan P, et al. Treatment of liver metastases with intra-arterial Lipiodol-Adriamycin. Reg Cancer Treat 1993;3:121–4.

232. Lang E, Brown CJ. Colorectal metastases to the liver: selective chemoembolization. Radiology 1993;189:417–22.

233. Martinelli D, Wadler S, Bakal C, et al. Utility of embolization or chemoembolization as second-line treatment in patients with advanced or recurrent colorectal carcinoma. Cancer 1994;74:1706–12.

234. Daniels J, Hanks S, Harrell D, et al. Chemoembolization (HCE) of hepatocellular carcinoma (HCC) with collagen, doxorubicin, cisplatin and mitomycin. Proc Am Soc Clin Oncol 1995;14:196.

235. Colleoni M, Gaion F, Liessi G, et al. Intra-arterial chemotherapy followed by chemoembolization: high objective response rate in unresectable hepatocellular carcinoma (HCC). Proc Am Soc Clin Oncol 1995;14:206.

236. Kong H, Wang T, Wong J, et al. Transcatheter oily chemoembolization (TOCE) in the management of unresectable hepatocellular carcinoma in a Southeast Asian population. Proc Am Soc Clin Oncol 1995;14:207.

237. Clouse ME, Stokes KR, Kruskal JB, et al. Chemoembolization for hepatocellular carcinoma: epinephrine followed by a doxorubicin-ethiodized oil emulsion and gelatin sponge powder. J Vasc Interv Radiol 1993;4:717–25.

238. Lo CM, Ngan H, Tso WK, et al. Randomized controlled trial of transarterial lipiodol chemoembolization for unresectable hepatocellular carcinoma. Hepatology 2002;35:1164–71.

239. A comparison of lipiodol chemoembolization and conservative treatment for unresectable hepatocellular carcinoma. Groupe d'Etude et de Traitement du Carcinome Hepatocellulaire. N Engl J Med 1995;332:1256–61.

Gallbladder and Bile Duct Cancer

Steven A. Curley, MD, FACS

GALLBLADDER CANCER

Adenocarcinoma of the gallbladder is the sixth most common digestive-system malignancy in the United States. In Western countries such as the United States, where there is a low incidence of hepatocellular carcinoma (HCC), gallbladder cancer is relatively more common, with an estimated 6,800 cases of gallbladder and extrahepatic bile duct cancer diagnosed in 2003 compared with 22,000 cases of HCC and intrahepatic bile duct cancer predicted in the same year.[1] During the 1950s, 1960s, and 1970s, there appears to have been a slight increase in the incidence of gallbladder carcinoma in Western countries, but this may be ascribed to more thorough reporting mechanisms rather than to a true increase in incidence.[2] Between 1980 and 1995, mortality rates from gallbladder cancer decreased in the United States, Canada, Australia, and the United Kingdom, while increasing in Japan, Italy, Spain and Chile.[2] Unlike HCC and cholangiocarcinoma, gallbladder carcinoma has a higher incidence in females than males.[2] The preponderance of this cancer in females is even greater in patients less than 40 years old, with a female-to-male ratio of 20:1.[3]

Gallbladder carcinoma is more common in Southwest American Indians than in the general American populace. Incidence rates for US white males, US black males, and American Indian males in New Mexico are 0.4, 0.6, and 3.8 cases per 100,000 per year, respectively. The corresponding rates for females are 1.0, 0.8, and 10.3.[2] Gallbladder carcinoma has been found in 6% of Southwest American Indians undergoing biliary tract surgery.[4] Gallbladder carcinoma is the second most common gastrointestinal malignancy in this population, and the youngest reported case of gallbladder carcinoma occurred in an 11-year-old Navajo girl.[5]

Other human populations also have an increased incidence of gallbladder cancer. In Chile, the incidence of gallbladder cancer is rising, and gallbladder cancer is the number one cause of cancer mortality in Chilean women.[6] The geographic and population-based variations in the incidence of gallbladder cancer suggests that environmental risk factors, including carcinogens, infectious agents like *Salmonella typhi* and *Helicobacter pylori*, and diet have a role in gallbladder tumorigenesis.

Causative Factors There are no apparent associations between gallbladder carcinoma and hepatitis B or C virus infection, cirrhosis, or mycotoxin exposure. Similarly, chemical hepatocarcinogens have not been clearly demonstrated to increase the risk of developing gallbladder carcinoma. However, there are suggestions that workers exposed to carcinogenic substances, such as methylcholanthrene and nitrosamines, have a higher incidence and earlier onset of gallbladder carcinoma when compared with control populations.[7] There is a significant association between gallstones and gallbladder carcinoma, with gallstones present in 74 to 92% of patients with gallbladder carcinoma.[8–10] The risk of developing gallbladder carcinoma increases directly with increasing gallstone size.[11] Patients with gallstones 2.0 to 2.9 cm in diameter have a 2.4 times higher relative risk of developing gallbladder carcinoma, whereas patients with gallstones greater than 3.0 cm in diameter have a 10.1 times higher risk. Patients with long-standing chronic cholecystitis can develop calcification of the gallbladder wall, also known as porcelain gallbladder. It is possible that chronic inflammation and/or infection of the gallbladder increases the risk of developing gallbladder carcinoma because 22% of patients with calcified gallbladders have gallbladder carcinoma.[12,13] Furthermore, pathogenic bacteria are cultured from the gallbladders of patients with gallbladder cancer at a significantly greater frequency than from patients with simple cholelithiasis.[14] Cholelithiasis and cholecystitis are more common in females, which may in part explain the higher incidence of gallbladder carcinoma in females.[15]

Gallstones or other factors that cause chronic inflammation of the gallbladder mucosa may induce a series of premalignant changes. If not treated with a cholecystectomy, patients with these premalignant lesions may progress to invasive gallbladder carcinoma. Epithelial dysplasia, atypical hyperplasia, and carcinoma in situ have been identified in the gallbladder mucosa of 83%, 13.5%, and 3.5%, respectively, of patients undergoing cholecystectomy for cholelithiasis or cholecystitis.[16] Areas of mucosal dysplasia can be observed in more than 90% of patients with invasive gallbladder carcinoma.[17] There also is evidence that adenomatous polyps arising from the gallbladder mucosa are premalignant lesions, because a review of 1,605 cholecystectomies produced 11 benign adenomas, 7 adenomas with areas of malignant transformation, and 79 invasive gallbladder carcinomas.[18] There appears to be an increased expression of epithelial growth factors and protooncogene, particularly *ras*, in the progression from chronic cholecystitis to dysplasia and then to invasive carcinoma.[19] In patients with anomalous pancreaticobiliary ductal union, a condition known to be associated with an increased risk of developing gallbladder cancer, chronic inflammation results in hyperplasia of the gallbladder epithelium.[20] K-*ras* mutations were noted in some of these patients with high-grade dysplasia, suggesting that mutations in this protooncogene may be an early event in gallbladder mucosal proliferation leading to carcinogenesis. Studies performed in patients with invasive gallbladder carcinoma have demonstrated that the majority have abnormal or mutated tumor suppressor (*p53* and *p16*), cell cycle regulation (cyclin E), and apoptosis regulation (Bcl-2) genes, as well as increased expression of angiogenesis factors (VEGF).[21–24]

Pathology The gross appearance of gallbladder carcinoma varies, depending on the stage of the disease and extent of spread. Early-stage lesions that have not infiltrated through all layers of the gallbladder wall may be indistinguishable from chronic cholecystitis. On opening the gallbladder in these early-stage patients, gallstones usually are present, and there may be subtle mucosal abnormalities, such as plaque-like lesions or small ulcerations. Occasionally, a sessile or pedunculated tumor is present and suggests the diagnosis of a gallbladder carcinoma.[25] More advanced gallbladder carcinomas are grossly evident by infiltration into the liver or contiguous organs, such as the duodenum or stomach.[26]

Microscopically, more than 90% of gallbladder carcinomas are adenocarcinomas, with the remaining cases being adenosquamous carcinomas, anaplastic carcinomas, and, rarely, carcinoid tumors or embryonal rhabdomyosarcoma.[8,25] Carcinoma in situ is an early lesion, with the malignant cells involving only the mucosal layer of the gallbladder wall. Gallbladder adenocarcinomas generally have a predominant papillary or tubular arrangement of cells.[25] Papillary adenocarcinoma is characterized by an extended stroma covered by columnar cells. The tubular formations of tubular adenocarcinoma may be lined by tall columnar cells or by cuboidal epithelium. Mucin production and signet-ring cells can be identified frequently in gallbladder adenocarcinomas.[25] More poorly differentiated carcinomas have solid sheets or nests of small, scattered cells infiltrating into the stroma and destroying the normal gallbladder wall architecture. Vascular, lymphatic, and perineural invasion by the carcinoma can be demonstrated frequently.

Advanced locoregional disease usually is present at the time of diagnosis of gallbladder carcinoma. Only 10% of patients with this disease have cancer confined to the gallbladder wall.[8] Direct extension of the carcinoma into the gallbladder fossa of the liver is present in 69 to 83% of patients.[26–28] Direct invasion of the liver usually indicates the presence of other regional disease because fewer than 12% of patients with liver involvement have no other sites of regional disease. Direct invasion of the extrahepatic biliary tract occurs in 57% of cases; the duodenum, stomach, or transverse colon is involved in 40%; and the pancreas is involved in 23%. The hepatic artery or portal vein is encased by tumor in 15% of patients. Regional lymph node metastases in the cystic, choledochal, or pancreaticoduodenal lymphatic drainage basins are present in 42 to 70% of patients.[26] Somewhat more distant lymph node metastases occur along the aorta or inferior vena cava in approximately 25% of cases. Importantly, lymph node metastases can occur in the absence of liver or other contiguous organ involvement by the gallbladder carcinoma.

The pattern of lymph node metastases from gallbladder carcinoma is predictable on the basis of anatomic studies that have identified three pathways of lymphatic drainage of the gallbladder (Figure 89-1).[29] The main pathway is the cholecysto-retropancreatic pathway, with lymphatic vessels on the anterior and posterior surfaces of the gallbladder that converge at a large retroportal lymph node. This principal retroportal lymph node communicates with the choledochal and pancreaticoduodenal lymph nodes. The cholecysto-celiac pathway consists of lymphatics from the anterior and posterior walls of the gallbladder that run to the left in front of the portal vein and then communicate with groups of pancreaticoduodenal lymph nodes or aorticocaval lymph nodes lying near the left renal vein. The final pattern of spread of gallbladder carcinoma is related to vascular invasion. Noncontiguous liver, pulmonary, and bone metastases have been found in 66%, 24%, and 12% of gallbladder carcinoma patients, respectively.[26]

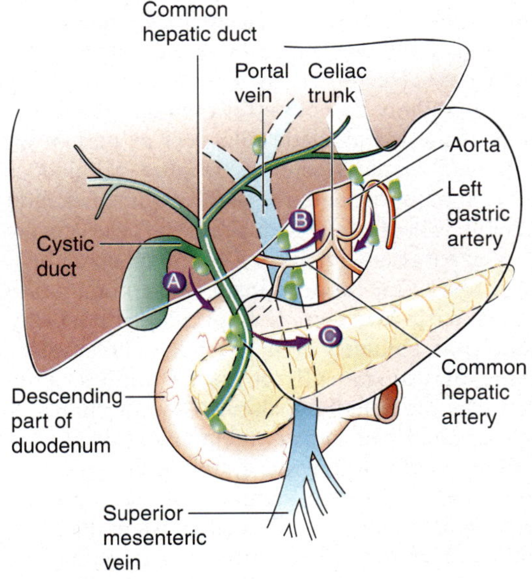

Figure 89-1 Patterns of lymphatic drainage from the gallbladder. ***A,*** The main pathway of lymphatic drainage, and thus, lymph node metastasis from gallbladder cancer is to the cholecysto-retropancreatic nodes. This pathway drains from the gallbladder to nodes along the cystic duct and common bile duct and then to nodes posterior to the duodenum and pancreatic head. ***B,*** The cholecysto-celiac pathway courses from the gallbladder through the gastrohepatic ligament to celiac nodes. ***C,*** The third lymphatic drainage route is the cholecysto-mesenteric pathway, coursing from the gallbladder posterior to the pancreas to aortocaval lymph nodes.

The staging systems used for gallbladder carcinoma are based on the pathologic characteristics of local invasion by the tumor and lymph node metastases. Before the American Joint Cancer Committee (AJCC) developed a tumor-node-metastasis (TNM) staging schema for gallbladder carcinoma, the Nevin and colleagues staging system was used frequently.[30] Studies of gallbladder carcinoma performed in Japan generally apply the staging system of the Japanese Society of Biliary Surgery.[31] Most recent studies stage patients according to the TNM criteria. Carcinoma in situ corresponds to a T1aN0M0 tumor in the AJCC staging system. The characteristics of these three staging systems are outlined in Table 89-1.

Clinical Presentation The most common symptoms and signs in patients with gallbladder carcinoma are nonspecific. Right upper quadrant abdominal pain, which may or may not be exacerbated by eating a fatty meal, is the predominant presenting complaint in 75 to 97% of patients.[2,8,32] Right upper quadrant abdominal tenderness is present in a slightly smaller percentage of patients. These symptoms and signs usually are ascribed to cholelithiasis or cholecystitis. Nausea, vomiting, and anorexia are present in 40 to 64% of patients; clinically evident jaundice is present in 45%; and weight loss of greater than 10% of normal body weight is noted in 37 to 77%.

Although 45% of patients obviously are jaundiced at presentation, 70% of patients present with a serum bilirubin elevated at least 2 times greater than normal.[32] Serum alkaline phosphatase levels are elevated in two-thirds of patients with gallbladder carcinoma. Alanine aminotransferase and aspartate aminotransferase levels are elevated in one-third of patients and are consistent with advanced hepatic invasion and metastases. Serum carcinoembryonic antigen (CEA) levels generally are obtained only in patients diagnosed preoperatively with advanced stages of disease. In these patients with TNM stage III or IV disease, the serum CEA level is elevated in more than 80% of patients.[32] The incidence of elevated serum CEA levels in early-stage disease is not known.

Diagnostic Studies Before ultrasonography and CT became widely available, the preoperative diagnosis rate for gallbladder carcinoma was only 8.6 to 16.3%.[2] Ultrasonography is the primary imaging study for symptomatic patients with presumed cholelithiasis or choledocholithiasis. High-resolution ultrasonography is able to detect early and locally advanced gallbladder carcinoma.[33] An early tumor as small as 5 mm can be recognized as a polypoid mass projecting into the gallbladder lumen or as a focal thickening of the gallbladder wall.[34,35] In patients with locally advanced gallbladder carcinoma, ultrasonography can demonstrate extrahepatic and intrahepatic bile duct obstruction, porta hepatis lymphadenopathy, direct hepatic extension of tumor, and hepatic metastases. Preoperative ultrasonography may suggest the correct diagnosis in up to 75% of patients with gallbladder carcinoma.[34,36,37] However, ultrasonography does not accurately detect celiac or paraortic lymphadenopathy or peritoneal dissemination of tumor.[38] Blood flow studies with color Doppler ultrasonography are also useful because gallbladder cancers have high-velocity arterial flow in 90% of cases, while benign lesions have minimal flow.[39] Recent advances in endoscopic ultrasonography, including the use of contrast-enhancing agents, may improve the diagnostic accuracy in assessing the T stage of the gallbladder cancer.[40]

Computed tomography (CT) scans are performed less frequently in patients with presumed benign biliary tract disease. However, if gallbladder carcinoma is suspected, CT findings can predict correctly the diagnosis in 88 to 95% of patients.[41–43] The CT characteristics of gallbladder carcinoma include diffuse or focal gallbladder wall thickness of greater than 0.5 mm in 95% of patients, gallbladder wall contrast enhancement in 95%, intraluminal mass in 90%, direct liver invasion by tumor in 85% (Figure 89-2), regional lymphadenopathy in 65%, concomitant cholelithiasis in 52%, dilated intrahepatic or extrahepatic bile ducts in 50%, noncontiguous liver metastases in 12%, invasion of contiguous gastrointestinal tract organs in 8%, and intraluminal gallbladder gas in 4%.[42] CT also can demonstrate calcification of the gallbladder wall (Figure 89-3).

Treatment **Resection** The curative resection rates for gallbladder carcinoma range from 10 to 30%.[44–46] The majority of patients are not candidates for curative resection because of extensive locoregional disease, noncontiguous liver metastases, and/or distant metastases. Although it is clear that long-term survival can be achieved in some patients with resectable lesions, the extent of resection remains a controversial issue.

Simple cholecystectomy is an adequate therapy for gallbladder carcinoma confined to the mucosa (T1aN0M0). The 5-year survival rate for patients undergoing simple cholecystectomy for disease confined to the mucosa ranges from 57 to 100%.[47–50] There is not universal agreement on simple cholecystectomy as the sole therapy for patients with T1aN0M0 tumors; some authors recommend that extended cholecystectomy (cholecystectomy, wedge resection of the gallbladder fossa including a 3 to 5 cm margin of normal liver, and a cystic, pericholedochal, gastrohepatic, pancreaticoduodenal, and paraortic lymphadenectomy) be performed to treat patients with these very early stage lesions.[51,52]

Table 89-1 Comparison of the Three Most Commonly Used Staging Systems for Gallbladder Carcinoma

Stage	Nevin	JSBS	AJCC-TNM
I	Cancer confined to the mucosa	Cancer confined to subserosal layers	T1aN0M0, T1bN0M0
II	Cancer involves the mucosa and muscularis	Direct invasion of the liver and/or bile duct, porta hepatis lymph node metastases	T2N0M0
III	Cancer extends through the serosa (all three layers of the gallbladder wall involved)	More extensive liver invasion by cancer, more extensive regional lymph node metastases (gastrohepatic, retropancreatic)	T1N1M0, T2N1M0, T3AnyNM0
IV	Tumor through all three layers of the gallbladder wall with cystic lymph node metastasis	Liver, peritoneal, and/or distant organ metastases	T4AnyNM0, any TAnyNM1
V	Tumor invades the liver by direct extension and/or metastasis to any distant organ	No stage V	No stage V

AJCC = American Joint Committee on Cancer; JSBS = Japanese Society of Biliary Surgery.

T = primary tumor; Tx = primary tumor cannot be assessed; T1 = tumor invades mucosa or muscle layer; T1a = tumor invades mucosa; T1b = tumor invades muscle; T2 = tumor invades perimuscular connective tissue, no extension beyond serosa or into liver; T3 = tumor invades beyond serosa or into one adjacent organ or both (extension < 2 cm into liver); T4 = tumor extends > 2 cm into liver and/or into two or more adjacent organs (stomach, duodenum, colon, pancreas, omentum, extrahepatic bile ducts). N = regional lymph nodes; Nx = regional lymph nodes cannot be assessed; N0 = no regional lymph node metastasis; N1 = regional lymph node metastasis; N1a = metastasis in cystic duct, pericholedochal, and/or gastrohepatic lymph nodes; N1b = metastasis in peripancreatic, periduodenal, periportal, celiac, and/or superior mesenteric artery lymph nodes; M = distant metastasis; Mx = presence of distant metastasis cannot be assessed; M0 = no distant metastasis; M1 = distant metastasis.

These authors recommend that all gallbladders be opened at the time of cholecystectomy for frozen section evaluation of any suspicious areas in the mucosa. If an unsuspected gallbladder carcinoma is diagnosed by frozen section biopsy or if a T1aN0M0 gallbladder carcinoma is diagnosed on final pathology, these authors advocate that an extended cholecystectomy be performed. The bias for this aggressive surgical treatment of T1aN0M0 gallbladder carcinoma is based on the small number of cases of regional lymph node recurrence in patients treated with simple cholecystectomy alone. No rationale is provided for the liver resection because the small number of patients who did fail after simple cholecystectomy developed metastases in the pericholedochal or cystic lymph nodes and not in the liver. Furthermore, the incidence of subsequent lymph node metastases in T1aN0M0 patients was less than 10% in the small groups of 32 and 36 patients, respectively.[51,52] The incidence of lymph node metastases in 201 patients with gallbladder carcinoma confined to the mucosa was only 2.5% in a study of patients who underwent cholecystectomy and regional lymphadenectomy.[48] The mortality rate for extended resection ranges from 2 to 5%, and major postoperative morbidity occurs in 13 to 40%.[47–49,53] Therefore, the morbidity and mortality associated with extended cholecystectomy is excessive compared with the potential survival benefit that would occur in less than 5% of patients with T1aN0M0 lesions.

There is a rationale for performing extended cholecystectomy in patients with T1b tumors or AJCC TNM stage II and III gallbladder carcinomas (Figure 89-4). In 165 patients with T1b gallbladder carcinomas, there was a 15.6% incidence of regional lymph node metastasis.[48] Of 867 patients with a T2 primary lesion, 56.1% had regional lymph node metastases.[48] The 453 patients with T3 tumors had a 74.4% incidence of regional lymph node metastases.[48] The 5-year survival rate following extended cholecystectomy for AJCC stage II and III gallbladder carcinoma ranges from 7.5 to 71%.[46–49,51,53,54] AJCC stage II or III gallbladder carcinoma patients treated with simple cholecystectomy alone had a 5-year survival rate of 0% compared with 29% in those patients treated with extended cholecystectomy.[46] Regional lymph node metastases and/or direct tumor invasion of the hepatic parenchyma are indicators of poor prognosis, with significant reductions in 5-year overall survival rates associated with these pathologic findings.[55–57] Microscopically positive liver resection margins also have a negative impact on survival because these patients had a median survival of 8.9 months compared with 67.2 months for patients with tumor-free margins.[55] Preoperative helical CT scans and intraoperative ultrasonography are used to assess the extent of direct invasion into the hepatic parenchyma, which assists with decision making regarding the extent of liver resection necessary to clear all disease. If adequate tumor-negative resection margins are attained, the radicality of liver resection does not affect survival, as attested by similar long-term survival rates following right lobectomy, extended right lobectomy, right trisegmentectomy, and central bisegmentectomy for gallbladder cancer.[46–49,58–60] T1b patients are classified as stage I in the AJCC system, but, arguably, with a 15.6% incidence of regional lymph node metastases, long-term survival benefit may occur in a significant number of these patients who undergo an extended cholecystectomy (see Figure 89-4).

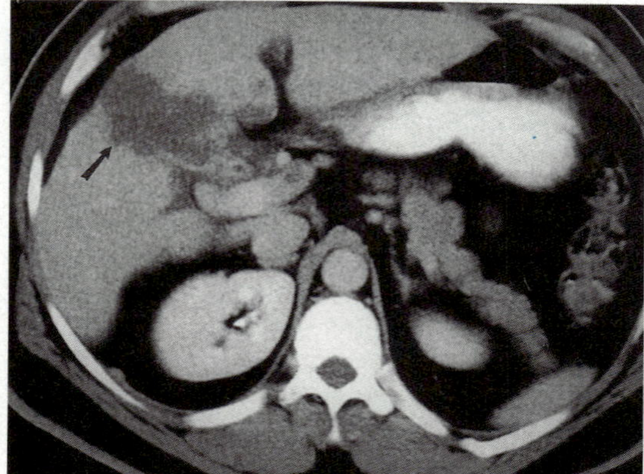

Figure 89-2 High-resolution, helical computed tomography scan in a patient with gallbladder carcinoma. Direct tumor invasion into the hepatic parenchyma is evident (*arrow*).

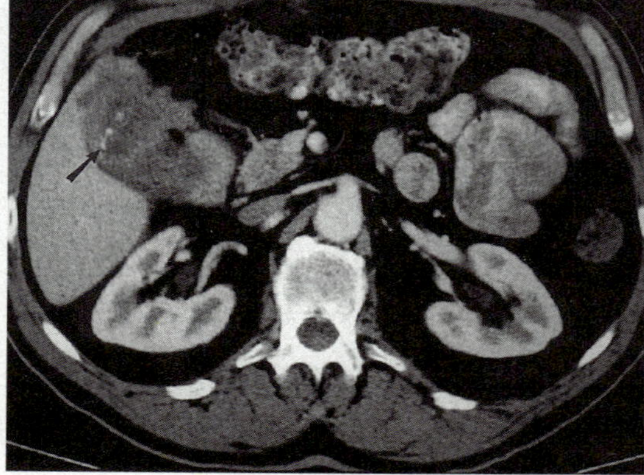

Figure 89-3 A high-resolution, helical computed tomography scan in another patient with gallbladder cancer. A locally invasive tumor is again noted with areas of calcification (*arrow*) noted in the thickened gallbladder wall.

All authors do not perform an en bloc resection of the extrahepatic bile duct as part of an extended cholecystectomy. Because gallbladder carcinoma is found to invade the extrahepatic bile duct in 57% of cases, with almost all cases occurring in patients with T3 or T4 tumors, an en bloc resection of the proper hepatic and common bile ducts with Roux-en-Y hepaticojejunostomy should be included in an extended cholecystectomy of transmurally invasive tumors. This includes those individuals in whom a clinically unsuspected gallbladder carcinoma is diagnosed pathologically following a simple cholecystectomy with a positive margin at the cystic duct. Gallbladder cancer involving the cystic duct and gallbladder neck frequently grows along the proper hepatic and right bile ducts, necessitating a right or extended right hepatic lobectomy and excision of the extrahepatic ducts to remove all disease.[61]

Extremely radical operations have been proposed for patients with extensive T3N1M0 or T4N01M0 tumors. This includes hepatopancreatic duodenectomy and abdominal organ cluster transplantation for locally advanced gallbladder carcinoma.[48,62,63] The operative mortality rate for these radical procedures is at least 15%, with a greater

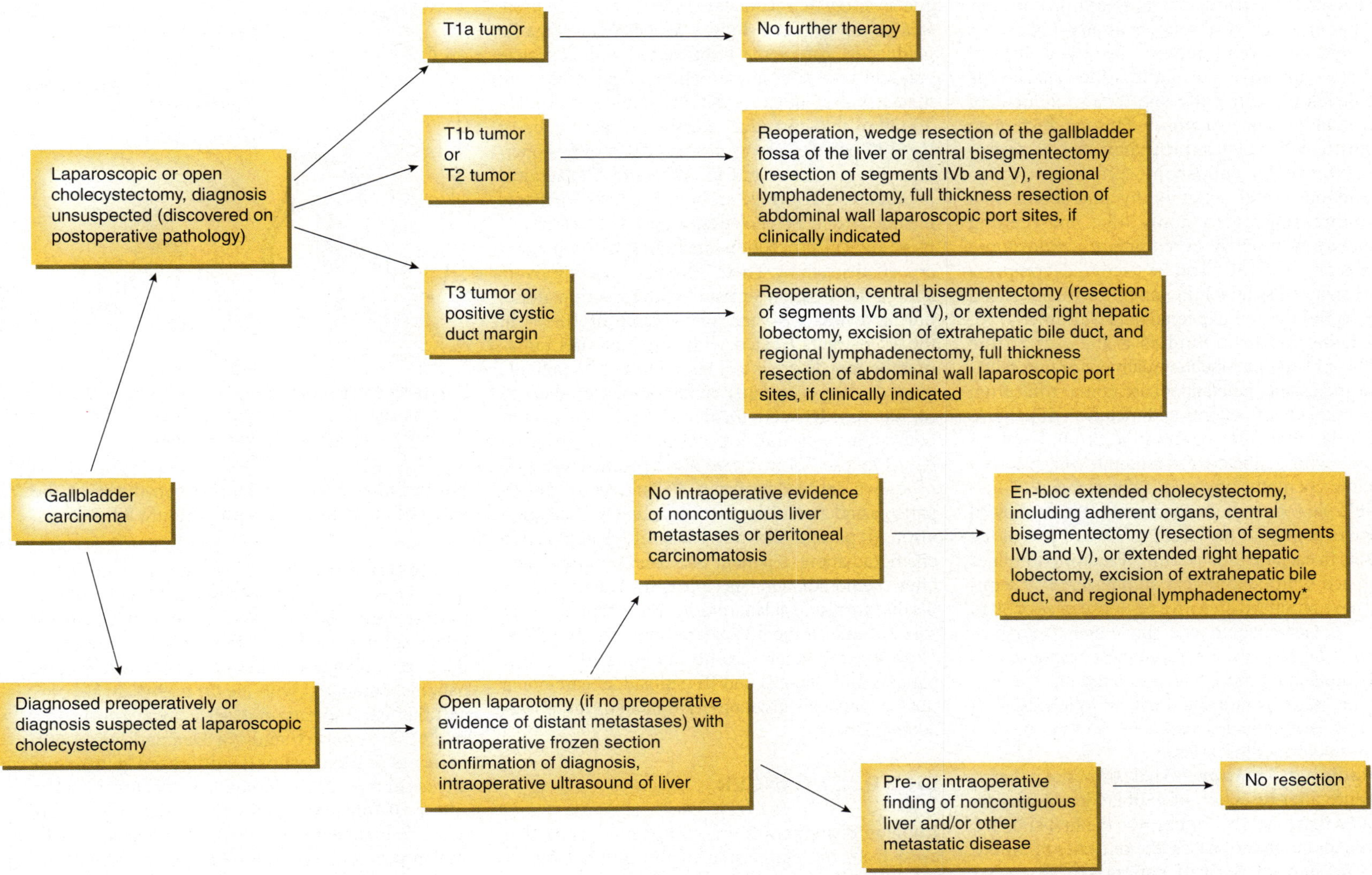

Figure 89-4 Algorithm to guide surgical decision making for patients with gallbladder cancer. *Regional lymphadenectomy includes complete dissection and removal of the cystic, pericholedochal, pancreaticoduodenal, gastrohepatic, and paraortic lymph nodes.

than 90% incidence of major morbidity. Resection of the portal vein and/or hepatic artery with vascular reconstruction frequently is necessary to resect completely all gross malignant disease. The largest report of patients undergoing hepatopancreatic duodenectomy for gallbladder carcinoma is 150 cases from Japan, with a 5-year survival rate of 14%.[48] The patients who did not die from intraoperative or postoperative complications all succumbed to recurrent and/or metastatic carcinoma.

It is estimated that 80,000 laparoscopic cholecystectomies are performed each year in the United States.[64] On average, gallbladder carcinoma is diagnosed in 2% of patients undergoing cholecystectomy for presumed benign biliary tract disease. Thus, approximately 1,600 patients who annually undergo laparoscopic cholecystectomy *could* suffer inadvertent dissemination of gallbladder carcinoma.[64–70] However, the potential laparoscopic dissemination of tumor cells may not significantly alter the natural history of gallbladder cancer in most patients. A review of our experience at the University of Texas M. D. Anderson Cancer Center with diagnostic and therapeutic laparoscopy in patients with gastrointestinal malignancies indicated that port site recurrence is a harbinger of widespread metastasis in more than 95% of patients; thus, it is rarely an isolated site of recurrent malignant disease.[71] Furthermore, a report drawn from the National Cancer Data Base between 1989 and 1995 revealed no change in incidence or survival from gallbladder cancer during the time laparoscopic cholecystectomy supplanted open cholecystectomy as the procedure of choice for gallbladder disease presumed benign.[72] Nonetheless, because of the large number of cholecystectomies being performed laparoscopically and the small but measurable risk of dissemination of tumor cells, it has been recommended that (1) unless the surgeon feels capable of performing a definitive extended cholecystectomy for gallbladder carcinoma, patients in whom gallbladder carcinoma is suspected preoperatively by clinical or radiologic criteria should be referred without laparoscopy, laparotomy, or percutaneous biopsy; and (2) if gallbladder carcinoma is suspected on visual inspection during an attempted laparoscopic cholecystectomy, either an open definitive operation should be performed or the operation should be terminated without biopsy and the patient referred for appropriate surgical therapy.[65] Patients who underwent laparoscopic cholecystectomy and were then found on pathologic analysis to have gallbladder cancer should still be considered for aggressive surgical treatment because long-term disease-free survival will result in a subset of these patients.[46,73]

Palliation The majority of patients with gallbladder carcinoma are diagnosed at an advanced, unresectable stage of disease. As in patients with hilar bile duct cancer, relief of symptomatic jaundice is a consideration. Patients with unresectable gallbladder carcinoma frequently have extensive involvement of the extrahepatic bile duct and may have bulky porta hepatis lymphadenopathy, which makes endoscopic placement of an internal stent difficult. When unresectable gallbladder carcinoma is diagnosed at the time of laparotomy, a surgical biliary bypass, such as an intrahepatic cholangioenteric anastomosis, can be performed and results in significant symptomatic relief in more than 90% of patients.[74] When the diagnosis is made on the basis of radiographic and percutaneous biopsy findings, jaundice can be relieved by placement of percutaneous transhepatic biliary catheters.

In contrast to patients with hilar bile duct carcinoma, in which gastroduodenal obstruction is a relatively rare event, between 30% and 50% of patients with advanced gallbladder carcinoma will develop a clinically significant element of gastroduodenal obstruction.[75] This can be treated surgically with a bypass procedure such as gastrojejunostomy, by endoscopic placement of an expandable metal stent, or by placement of a decompressing gastrostomy tube and feeding jejunostomy tube. A percutaneous endoscopic gastrostomy tube also can be used to decompress the obstructed stomach in patients with advanced disease and limited expected survival time.

Chemotherapy Studies that describe the results of chemotherapeutic treatment of unresectable or metastatic gallbladder carcinoma suffer from small numbers of patients and inclusion of patients with hilar bile duct carcinoma. A study of 53 patients with gallbladder carcinoma who received systemic chemotherapy with 5-fluorouracil (5-FU) or 5-FU plus other chemotherapeutic agents showed objective antitumor responses in 12% or less of the patients in each treatment arm.[76] Fluoropyrimidines combined with doxorubicin administered systemically have produced objective response rates of 30 to 40%.[77,78] Gemcitabine as a single agent may produce similar response rates, but these responses are rarely durable for more than 3 to 6 months.[79] Complete remission is rare and transient following such systemic chemotherapy regimens, and the median survival is 11 months or less.

Radiation Therapy Analysis of the patterns of failure after resection of gallbladder carcinoma revealed that local recurrence was the first and, in a significant number of cases, the only site of failure in more than one-half of patients.[5,80] External beam radiation therapy to a total dose of 45 Gy can produce radiographic evidence of tumor reduction in 20 to 70% of these tumors and provide temporary relief of jaundice in up to 80% of patients.[81–83] In general, external beam radiation therapy is a palliative treatment. The median survival for locally advanced gallbladder carcinoma patients treated with radiation therapy is approximately 10 months.[80–83] Occasional long-term survivors are reported following treatment with higher doses of radiation therapy or with administration of radiation-sensitizing chemotherapeutic agents such as 5-FU during external beam radiation therapy.[80] However, extrahepatic bile duct stricture has been reported in several of the long-term survivors treated with high doses of radiation therapy.[84]

Multidisciplinary Approaches The majority of patients who undergo an extended cholecystectomy or more radical resection for AJCC stage II, III, or IV gallbladder carcinoma develop tumor recurrence and die as a result of their disease. Nonrandomized studies and case reports have suggested that overall survival can be improved by administering adjuvant radiation therapy and/or chemotherapy after resection of stage II, III, or IV tumors.[85,86] Unfortunately, the number of patients who have received postsurgical adjuvant treatment is small, and a variety of treatment regimens have been used. In a nonrandomized study, 9 patients with stage IV gallbladder carcinoma were treated with complete surgical resection alone, while 17 patients were treated with complete resection combined with 20 to 30 Gy of intraoperative radiation therapy.[87] Ten of these 17 patients also received 36.4 Gy of postoperative external beam radiation therapy. The surgical procedures performed in both groups of patients included extended cholecystectomy and a variety of more radical procedures, including hepatopancreatic duodenectomy. There were no 3-year survivors among the 9 patients treated with resection alone, but there was a 3-year survivorship of 10.1% in the 17 patients treated with resection and radiation therapy. There is a single report of 18 patients treated with preoperative chemoradiation therapy (4,500 cGy, 180 cGy/fraction, 5 days/week, continuous intravenous infusion of 5-FU 350 mg/m^2 /d on days 1 to 5 and 21 to 25) prior to a planned resection of known gallbladder cancer.[88] Thirteen of the 18 patients underwent resection; 1 patient refused operation, 1 patient did not complete preoperative chemoradiation, 1 patient had disease progression after chemoradiation, and 2 patients had unresectable disease found at laparotomy. The actuarial 5-year survival rate in the 13 resected patients was 57%. Unfortunately, there are no randomized trials of patients with stage II and III gallbladder carcinoma treated with a coherent program of adjuvant or neoadjuvant therapy.

BILE DUCT CANCER

Cholangiocarcinomas are malignant tumors that arise from the epithelium of the intrahepatic or extrahepatic bile ducts. In the United States, approximately 3,000 patients are diagnosed with cholangiocarcinoma of both the intra- or extrahepatic biliary system annually.[89] There is only a slight male preponderance of cases of cholangiocarcinoma. Cholangiocarcinomas can arise at any site in the intra- or extrahepatic biliary system,

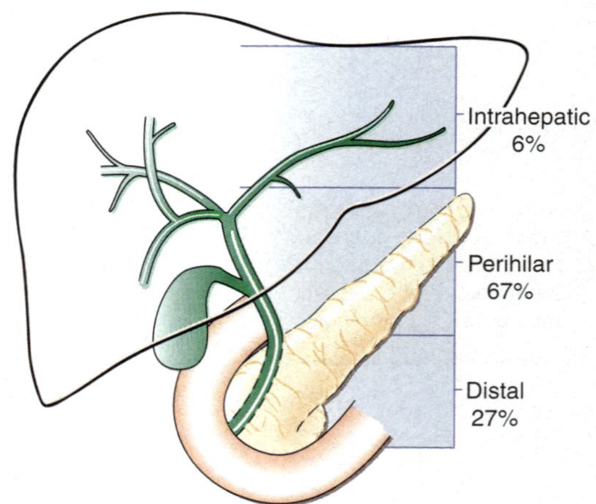

Figure 89-5 The distribution of 294 cholangiocarcinomas into intrahepatic, perihilar, and distal subgroups. Reprinted with permission from Nakeeb A et al.[90]

but perihilar tumors comprise two-thirds of the cases of cholangiocarcinoma (Figure 89-5).[90]

Causative Factors There are distinct differences between the factors associated with cholangiocarcinoma and those associated with hepatocellular carcinoma (HCC) (Table 89-2). Only 10 to 20% of cholangiocarcinomas occur in cirrhotic patients, compared with the 70 to 90% of hepatocellular carcinomas that arise in cirrhotic livers.[89,91,92] A cohort study in Denmark of 11,605 patients with cirrhosis indicated a 60-fold increased risk of developing hepatocellular cancer and a 10-fold increased risk of cholangiocarcinoma.[92] Frequently, the cirrhosis associated with cholangiocarcinomas is a subacute secondary biliary type that results from the neoplastic obstruction of the bile ducts, indicating that, in some cases, cirrhosis in cholangiocarcinoma patients is the result of the tumor rather than its cause.

Cholangiocarcinoma is more prevalent in Southeast Asia than in other parts of the world. The higher incidence in this geographic region is related

Table 89-2 Factors Associated with an Increased Risk to Develop Cholangiocarcinoma Compared with Factors Associated with Hepatocellular Carcinoma

Cholangiocarcinoma	Hepatocellular Carcinoma
Liver fluke infection	Cirrhosis
Ophisthorchis sinensis	Chronic hepatitis B virus infection
Opisthorchis viverrini	Chronic hepatitis C virus infection
Congenital/chronic cystic dilation	Aflatoxin B_1 ingestion of the bile ducts
Choledochal cyst	Chronic ethanol ingestion
Caroli disease	Primary biliary cirrhosis
Hepatolithiasis	Hemachromatosis
Primary sclerosing cholangitis	α-1-antitrypsin deficiency
Ulcerative colitis	Glycogen storage disease
Thorotrast exposure	Hypercitrullinemia
Cholelithiasis	Porphyrias
Asbestos	Hereditary tyrosinemia
Dioxin (Agent Orange)	Wilson disease
Polychlorinated diphenyls	Hepatotoxin exposure
Nitrosamines	Thorotrast
Isoniazid	Polyvinyl chloride
Methyldopa	Carbon tetrachloride

to parasitic infection with the liver flukes *Opisthorchis sinensis* and *Opisthorchis viverrini*.[93,94] Liver flukes induce hyperplasia, fibrosis, and adenomatous proliferation of human biliary epithelium and are associated with hepatolithiasis.[95,96] The fluke infestation suggests a direct etiologic role in the subsequent development of cholangiocarcinoma, but this relationship is not established unequivocally.

Several disorders that can produce chronic inflammation of the bile ducts have been associated with an increased risk of developing cholangiocarcinoma. These include polycystic liver disease, choledochal cysts, congenital dilation of the intrahepatic bile ducts (Caroli syndrome), sclerosing cholangitis (occasionally in association with inflammatory bowel disease), hepatolithiasis, and cholelithiasis.[97–106] Hepatolithiasis is not a common disorder, and only 5 to 7% of patients with documented hepatic stones develop cholangiocarcinoma.[105,106] The reported incidence of cholangiocarcinoma developing in areas of congenital cystic dilation of the bile duct, including choledochal cysts and Caroli disease, ranges from 3 to 30%.[107,108] Patients with primary sclerosing cholangitis are also at increased risk to develop cholangiocarcinoma, with incidence rates ranging from 9 to 40%.[109–111] Patients with ulcerative colitis may also develop sclerosing cholangitis, but cholangiocarcinoma occurs in only 0.4 to 1.4% of individuals with ulcerative colitis.[109] In patients with sclerosing cholangitis, whether associated with ulcerative colitis or not, radiologic distinction between sclerosing cholangitis and cholangiocarcinoma is often impossible. A recent study showed that the serum tumor marker CA19-9 had an 89% sensitivity and 86% specificity in diagnosing cholangiocarcinoma in patients with sclerosing cholangitis.[112] Combining serum CA19-9 levels with serum CEA levels may further increase the diagnostic accuracy to detect cholangiocarcinoma in patients with sclerosing cholangitis.[113]

Patients who underwent diagnostic radiography with intravenous injection of Thorotrast (thorium dioxide) are at high risk of developing hepatocellular carcinoma, angiosarcoma, and cholangiocarcinoma.[114,115] Cholangiocarcinoma is the most frequent hepatic neoplasm reported in patients who have received Thorotrast. Exposure to several drugs or carcinogens has also been linked to an increased risk to develop cholangiocarcinoma (see Table 89-2). Because cholangiocarcinoma is a relatively rare neoplasm, it has been difficult to prove its pathogenesis related to any of these factors, but it is clear that chronic inflammation of the biliary tree by any cause is associated with an increased risk of developing cholangiocarcinoma.

Chronic inflammation of the biliary system or exposure to genotoxic agents concentrated in bile may produce damage to the DNA of biliary epithelial cells, leading to the development of cholangiocarcinoma. Mutations in the *p53* tumor suppressor gene and in the K-*ras* protooncogene have been identified in cholangiocarcinoma patients.[116–118] There may be geographic and population-based differences in the mutation rates of these two genes in cholangiocarcinoma, but alterations in *p53* and K-*ras* are observed in significant proportions of patients with any of the identified factors (see Table 89-2) that increase risk to develop cholangiocarcinoma. Overexpression of c-*erbB-2*, a protooncogene that encodes a transmembrane protein that is highly homologous to epidermal growth factor receptor, has been confirmed in human cholangiocarcinoma cells and in benign proliferative biliary epithelium from patients with hepatolithiasis, primary sclerosing cholangitis, and liver fluke infestation.[119] Alterations in c-*erbB-2* expression may occur early in the chronic inflammation-induced proliferation of biliary epithelium leading to malignant transformation. Chronic inflammation may also produce the overexpression of the *Bcl-2* protooncogene observed in cholangiocarcinomas, which may promote tumorigenesis by inhibiting normal apoptotic processes.[120]

Clinical Presentation The clinical features of cholangiocarcinoma are nonspecific and depend on the location of the tumor. The usual clinical presentation of patients with hilar cholangiocarcinoma is painless jaundice. Patients may also report concomitant onset of fatigue, pruritus, fever, vague abdominal pain, and anorexia. The serum liver function tests in patients with hilar cholangiocarcinoma commonly demonstrate obstructive jaundice, with alkaline phosphatase and total bilirubin levels elevated in greater than 90% of patients.[89] Cholangiocarcinomas that arise in peripheral bile ducts within the hepatic parenchyma usually reach a large size before becoming clinically evident. Patients with these large peripheral hepatic tumors usually present with hepatomegaly and an upper abdominal mass, abdominal and back pain, and weight loss.[89] Jaundice and ascites are late and usually preterminal sequelae in patients with large intrahepatic cholangiocarcinomas. Jaundice associated with a large hepatic cholangiocarcinoma is caused by a combination of extension of the tumor to the bifurcation of the left and right hepatic ducts, and by compression of contralateral bile ducts by the expanding tumor.

Serum alkaline phosphatase levels are elevated in more than 90% of patients with cholangiocarcinoma.[90] Serum bilirubin also is elevated in the majority of cholangiocarcinoma patients, particularly in those with a tumor arising in the central portion of the liver or the extrahepatic hilar bile ducts.[121] In contrast to hepatocellular carcinoma, serum α-fetoprotein levels are abnormal in fewer than 5% of cholangiocarcinoma patients.[90] There is an increase in serum CEA levels in 40 to 60% of cholangiocarcinoma patients.[90,122] Another tumor marker, CA19-9, is elevated in more than 80% of patients with cholangiocarcinoma.[122]

Pathology Cholangiocarcinomas originating in the periphery of the hepatic parenchyma usually are solitary and large, but satellite nodules occasionally are present.[123,124] Gross tumor invasion of the large portal or hepatic veins occurs much less frequently than in hepatocellular carcinoma. The gross and microscopic appearance of intrahepatic cholangiocarcinomas may have prognostic significance because tumors with periductal infiltration have a higher incidence of lymph node and intrahepatic metastasis.[125] Metastases to the regional lymph nodes, lungs, and peritoneal cavity are more common in cholangiocarcinoma than in hepatocellular carcinoma. When the tumor causes longstanding biliary obstruction, the liver may show secondary biliary cirrhosis.

Microscopically, cholangiocarcinoma is characterized by low cuboidal cells that resemble the normal biliary epithelium. Varying degrees of pleomorphism, atypia, mitotic activity, hyperchromatic nuclei, and prominent nucleoli are noted from area to area in the same tumor. Rarely, a clear cell variant of cholangiocarcinoma occurs, which must be distinguished from clear cell renal carcinoma with liver metastasis.[126] Cholangiocarcinomas are mucin-secreting adenocarcinomas, and intracellular and intraluminal mucin often can be demonstrated. The presence of mucin is useful in differentiating cholangiocarcinoma from hepatocellular carcinoma. The absence of bile production by cholangiocarcinoma can also be useful in distinguishing this tumor from a hepatocellular carcinoma. Immunohistochemical staining that is positive for epithelial membrane antigen and tissue polypeptide antigen may be useful in confirming a diagnosis of cholangiocarcinoma.[127,128] Immunohistochemical staining for cytokeratin subtypes can be helpful in differentiating cholangiocarcinoma from metastatic colorectal carcinoma.[129] Cholangiocarcinomas are usually locally invasive, with spread along nerves or in subepithelial layers of the bile ducts.

Diagnostic Studies Peripheral intrahepatic cholangiocarcinoma is often difficult to distinguish pathologically and radiographically from a deposit of metastatic adenocarcinoma within the liver. Although transabdominal ultrasonography can detect an intrahepatic malignant tumor greater than 2 cm in diameter, ultrasound findings do not differ between cholangiocarcinomas, liver metastases from extrahepatic adenocarcinomas, and multinodular hepatocellular carcinoma.[130] Computed tomography (CT) demonstrates a rounded, low attenuation mass with irregular or lobulated margins (Figure 89-6). Satellite lesions

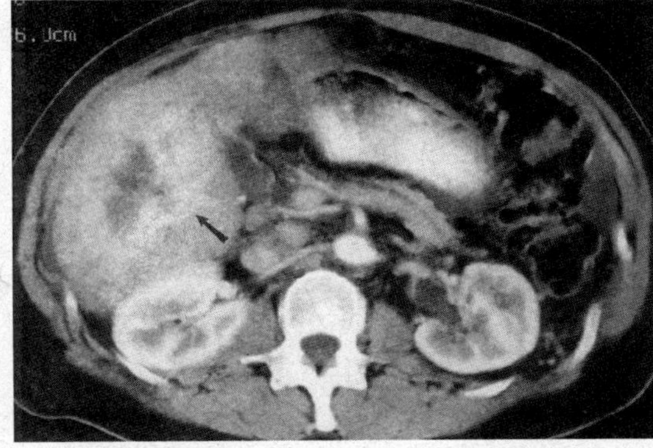

Figure 89-6 High-resolution, helical computed tomography scan during the arterial contrast phase in a patient with an intrahepatic cholangiocarcinoma. The periphery of the tumor (*arrow*) has irregular margins and enhances with contrast. A relatively hypovascular area of scar and tumor necrosis is evident in the center of the tumor.

may be evident, particularly when using helical CT during the optimal period of hepatic contrast enhancement. Calcification within the tumor is present in 25% of cases, and a central scar is observed in 30%.[131] Magnetic resonance imaging (MRI) shows a nonencapsulated mass with irregular margins that is hypointense compared with the normal liver on T_1-weighted and hyperintense on T_2-weighted images. The peripheral rim of the tumor usually enhances following MRI contrast administration. A hyperintense central scar is best seen on T_2-weighted images, but the CT and MRI characteristics of intrahepatic cholangiocarcinomas may be present in other types of hepatic tumors.[131]

A diagnosis of hilar cholangiocarcinoma should be suspected in the patient with painless jaundice whose CT scan demonstrates dilated intrahepatic bile ducts with a normal gallbladder and extrahepatic biliary tree. High-resolution, helical CT scans can provide information on the location of an obstructing biliary tumor and may suggest the extent of involvement of the liver and porta hepatis structures by the tumor (Figure 89-7). Multiphasic helical CT can correctly identify the level of biliary obstruction by a hilar cholangiocarcinoma in 63 to 90% of patients.[132–134] Preoperative helical CT is also useful in demonstrating lobar or segmental liver atrophy caused by bile duct obstruction or portal vein occlusion (Figure 89-8).[134] However, helical CT is not accurate in assessing the resectability of hilar cholangiocarcinomas because of limited resolution in evaluating intraductal tumor spread and significant false-positive and false-negative rates in demonstrating portal vein or hepatic artery involvement by tumor.[132–134]

Like the CT scan, ultrasonography can demonstrate a nondilated gallbladder and common bile duct associated with dilated intrahepatic ducts. In addition, as gray-scale ultrasonography has improved, the diagnosis of cholangiocarcinoma is supported by finding a hilar bile duct mass in 65 to 90% of patients.[135,136] Ultrasonography and CT scan may be used to demonstrate the presence of intrahepatic tumor due to direct extension or noncontiguous metastases and enlarged periportal lymph nodes, suggesting nodal metastases.[136,137] Even intraoperative ultrasonography is suboptimal for detecting intraductal spread by hilar cholangiocarcinoma, correctly demonstrating the extent of tumor spread away from the primary biliary tumor in only 18% of cases.[138] Intraoperative ultrasonography can be used to screen for noncontiguous liver metastases from the primary biliary cancer and can accurately detect direct tumor invasion of the portal vein or hepatic artery in 83.3% and 60% of cases, respectively.[138]

Similar to the intrahepatic variety, hilar cholangiocarcinoma usually shows hypointensity on T_1- and hyperintensity on T_2-weighted MRI. Dilated intrahepatic bile ducts are evident in patients with obstructing tumors, and lobar atrophy is seen in cases of portal venous occlusion. Fast low-angle shot (FLASH) MR with contrast-enhanced coronal imaging has been used to demonstrate intraluminal extension of tumor and to distinguish between blood vessels and bile ducts.[139,140] Magnetic resonance cholangiopancreatography (MRCP) and MR virtual endoscopy can demonstrate hilar bile duct obstruction by tumor with dilated intrahepatic ducts.[139,141] The advantages of MRCP over direct cholangiography include noninvasiveness and possible visualization of isolated bile ducts.

Cholangiography definitively demonstrates a lesion obstructing the left and right hepatic duct at the hilar confluence (Figure 89-9), and percutaneous transhepatic cholangiography (PTC) and endoscopic retrograde cholangiopancreatography (ERCP) are both useful in assessing patients with extrahepatic biliary obstruction. A prospective, randomized comparison of PTC and ERCP in patients with jaundice concluded that the two techniques had similar diagnostic accuracy.[142] PTC was 100% accurate at demonstrating obstruction at the confluence of the left and right hepatic ducts, while ERCP had an accuracy of 92% in demonstrating these lesions. ERCP has the additional benefit of providing a pancreatogram. A normal pancreatogram helps to exclude a small carcinoma of the head of the pancreas as

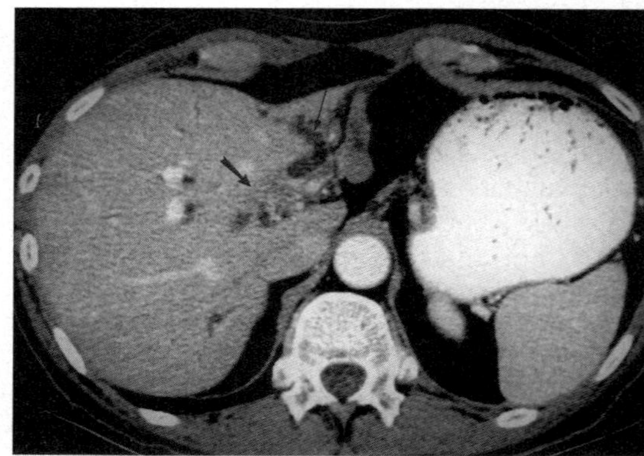

Figure 89-8 High-resolution, helical computed tomography scan in a patient presenting with several months of increasing pruritus followed by the development of clinically evident jaundice. The relatively hypodense hilar cholangiocarcinoma (*large arrow*) is evident. Marked atrophy of the left hepatic lobe is noted with dilated intrahepatic bile ducts (*small arrow*), but little remaining hepatic parenchyma is evident.

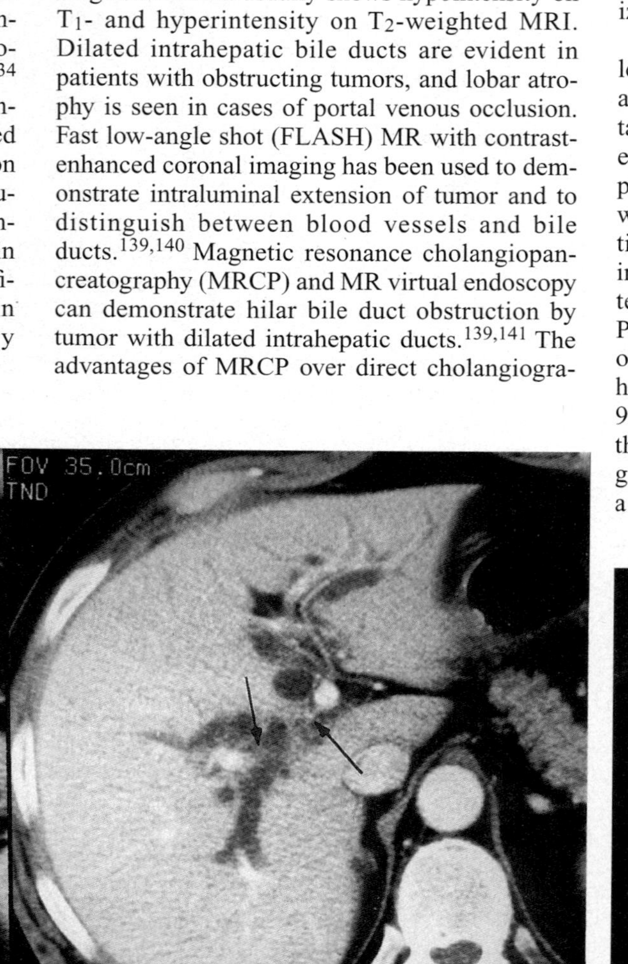

Figure 89-7 High-resolution, helical computed tomography (CT) scan in another patient presenting with obstructive jaundice. The tumor mass (*large arrow, left panel*), producing marked intrahepatic biliary duct dilatation is evident. Areas of tumor invasion of the portal vein (*small arrows, right panel*) suggested on the CT scan were confirmed at the time of operation to be tumor invasion of the portal vein.

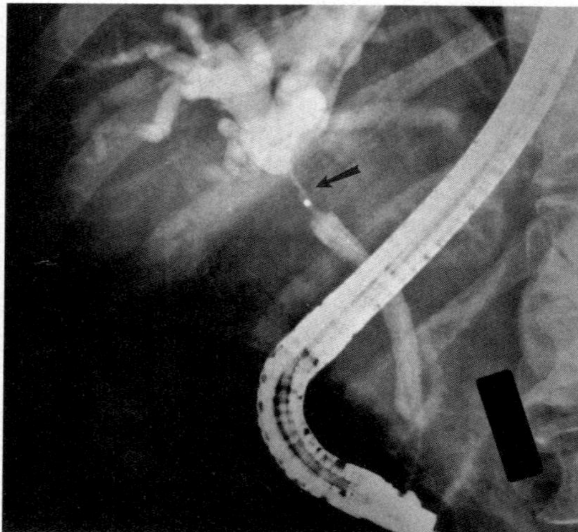

Figure 89-9 Endoscopic retrograde cholangiopancreatography showing a focal stricture of the proper hepatic bile duct (*arrow*) with marked dilatation of the intrahepatic bile ducts. This hilar cholangiocarcinoma was completely resected with Roux-Y hepaticojejunostomy reconstruction of biliary-enteric continuity.

a cause of biliary obstruction. Cytologic specimens can be obtained at the time of PTC and ERCP. The presence of malignant cells in bile or bile duct brushings is confirmed in approximately 50% of patients undergoing PTC or ERCP.[135,142,143,144]

Drainage of the obstructed biliary tree with partial or complete relief of jaundice and associated symptoms can be achieved with PTC. Improvements in catheter technology led to the development of endoprostheses that can be placed across the malignant obstruction into the duodenum to allow internal drainage.[145] It must be emphasized that providing symptomatic relief for patients by decompressing the biliary tract should not be the primary reason to place these catheters. Prospective, randomized studies have failed to demonstrate a benefit in terms of a decrease in hospital morbidity or mortality by preoperative decompression of biliary obstruction.[146,147] However, the catheters are useful in identifying and dissecting the hepatic duct bifurcation at the time of operation and aid in the reconstruction of the biliary tract following extirpation of the tumor.[148,149]

Positron emission tomography (PET) is being evaluated as a diagnostic tool in patients with all types of malignant tumors. PET assesses in vivo metabolism of positron-emitting radiolabeled tracers like [18F] fluoro-2-deoxy-D-glucose (18F-FDG), a glucose analog that accumulates in various malignant tumors because of their high glucose metabolic rates. FDG-PET does not provide anatomic detail to assess resectability of hilar cholangiocarcinomas or intrahepatic malignancies, but it may prove useful in detecting distant metastatic disease that would preclude a curative resection. In patients with primary sclerosing cholangitis, FDG-PET studies may be able to detect small hilar and intrahepatic cholangiocarcinomas and thus may be useful in therapeutic and transplant decision making in these patients.[158] PET has recently been used to aid in the diagnosis and staging of patients with bile duct cancer.[151] PET scan images correctly detected the primary cholangiocarcinoma in 24 of 26 patients (sensitivity 92.3%) and was true negative in 8 patients with benign bile duct disease (adenoma, sclerosing cholangitis, Caroli disease). Distant metastatic disease was diagnosed correctly in 7 of 10 patients with histologically proven metastases, but regional lymph node metastases were identified in only 2 of 15 patients (13.3%).[151]

The role of laparoscopy as part of the diagnostic and staging evaluation of patients with hilar cholangiocarcinoma is being evaluated at our institution. Several patients with seemingly resectable tumors have avoided an exploratory laparotomy when peritoneal tumor implants were found with laparoscopy. In addition, patients at high risk of developing peritoneal carcinomatosis may be identified by positive cytologic specimens obtained from laparoscopic washings. Finally, laparoscopic ultrasonography can be used to exclude the presence of noncontiguous liver metastases or extensive hilar tumor infiltration in patients with extrahepatic bile duct cancers.[152]

Treatment of Intrahepatic Cholangiocarcinomas Intrahepatic cholangiocarcinomas may be detected in 30 to 45% of patients before they metastasize or cause jaundice.[153,154] These patients should be considered for operation because long-term survival has been reported in a proportion of the patients undergoing curative liver resection for intrahepatic cholangiocarcinoma.[91,153–159] A study of 19 patients who underwent resection of intrahepatic cholangiocarcinoma demonstrated that patients with no porta hepatis lymph node metastases had a 3-year survival rate of 64% compared with 0% for patients with nodal metastases.[158] A larger cohort of 32 patients who underwent resection of intrahepatic cholangiocarcinomas confirmed the negative prognostic impact of regional lymph node metastases and large size (> 5 cm diameter) of the primary tumor.[159] The 5-year overall survival rates reported for patients who underwent a margin-negative liver resection for intrahepatic cholangiocarcinoma range from 20 to 48%, with regional lymph node metastases, presence of satellite tumor nodules, portal vein invasion by tumor, and large tumors identified as a poor-prognosis indicator.[153–159] Large size of the primary tumor is a poor-prognosis indicator because of the increased frequency of vascular and lymphatic invasion by the tumor as well as growth along neighboring bile duct walls.[160]

HILAR BILE DUCT CHOLANGIOCARCINOMA

In 1890, Fardel first described a primary malignancy of the extrahepatic biliary tract.[182] A report in 1957 described three patients with small adenocarcinomas involving the confluence of the left and right hepatic ducts.[161] Such primary cholangiocarcinomas arising at the bifurcation of the extrahepatic biliary tree are known commonly as Klatskin tumors, following his report in 1965 of a larger series of patients with these lesions.[162]

Prognostic Factors In contrast to reports the most important factor affecting prognosis is the resectability of the tumor. Patients who undergo curative resection (margin-negative) have 3-year survival rates from 40 to 87% and 5-year survival rates between 10% and 73%.[74,163–165] The wide range of survival rates is explained by variations in the incidence of factors that portend a poor prognosis in the various series. Significant determinants of improved prognosis in patients undergoing curative resection include well-differentiated tumors, absence of lymph node metastases, absence of direct tumor extension into the liver, papillary histology (versus nodular or sclerotic), serum bilirubin at presentation of less than 9 mg/dL, and a near-normal or normal performance status.[77] Palliative resection, surgical bypass procedures, and various types of intubation and drainage procedures are associated with 3-year survival rates of 0 to 4%.[163] Hilar cholangiocarcinomas have a poorer prognosis than do carcinomas arising in the middle or distal thirds of the extrahepatic bile duct, which is related directly to the presentation of hilar tumors at a more locally advanced stage with bilobar liver involvement by tumor and resultant lower rates of curative resection.[166,167] However, like hilar cholangiocarcinoma, the presence of regional lymph node metastases reduces the 5-year overall survival rate following resection of middle or distal third bile duct cancer to 21% compared with the 65% survival rate in patients with node-negative disease.[167]

Pathologic features of the bile duct cancer are predictors of outcome after resection. Prognosis is affected adversely if the tumor infiltrates the serosa of the bile duct, invades directly into the liver, demonstrates vascular invasion, or has metastasized to regional lymph nodes.[168] Histologic type and grade also are important factors. Patients with the relatively unusual papillary bile duct adenocarcinoma have the most favorable prognosis, with 3-year survival rates up to 75%.[163,168,169] Patients with the more common nodular or sclerotic types of hilar cholangiocarcinoma have 3-year survival rates of less than 30%. A pathologic study that correlated gross tumor type with patterns of spread provides evidence that may explain the observed differences in survival outcomes. Papillary and superficial nodular tumors spread predominantly by mucosal extension, rarely invading the deeper layers of the bile duct wall or lymphatic channels, whereas nodular infiltrating or diffuse infiltrating tumors spread by direct or lymphatic extension in the submucosa.[170] The distance of mucosal or submucosal spread away from the gross tumor can be as great as 30 mm, but there were no local or anastomotic recurrences if at least a 5-mm tumor-free margin was attained. Patients with well- or moderately differentiated carcinomas have a 3-year survival rate of up to 51%, whereas no patient with a poorly differentiated carcinoma survived longer than 2 years.[171]

Treatment **Resection** Resection of a hilar cholangiocarcinoma affords the patient the best chance for significant survival; however, 5-year survival rates after resection of hilar cancers are 40% in the most hopeful reports and 10% or less in other accounts. Long-term survival rates after resection of middle or distal common bile duct cholangiocarcinomas, the latter requiring pancreaticoduodenectomy, are generally higher compared with hilar tumors.[90] This is most likely related to higher rates of margin-negative resection with middle or distal extrahepatic bile duct tumors and the absence of direct tumor extension into the liver.

The patterns of failure after curative extrahepatic bile duct resection for hilar cholangiocarci-

Table 89-3 Sites of Tumor Recurrence after Curative Resection of Proximal Hilar Cholangiocarcinomas

Site	Frequency (%)
Liver	62
Tumor bed	42
Regional lymph nodes	20
Peritoneum	16
Lungs	71
Bone	31
Skin	7

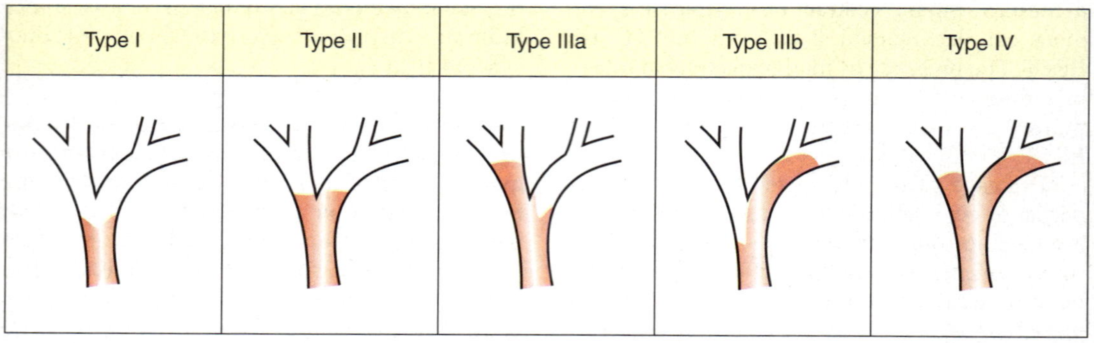

Type I | Type II | Type IIIa | Type IIIb | Type IV

Figure 89-10 Bismuth-Corlette classification of hilar cholangiocarcinoma. Types 1 and 2 can be resected with excision of the extrahepatic bile duct with or without the hilar plate and caudate lobe. Types 3A and 3B can be resected with the addition of an en bloc right or left hepatic lobectomy, respectively. Type 4 is, by definition, unresectable. Reprinted with permission from Bismuth H and Corlette MB.[180]

noma have been described in a few series of patients (Table 89-3).[171] Locoregional tumor recurrence developed in a high percentage of patients, with failure in the liver (62%), tumor bed (42%), and regional lymph nodes (20%). The caudate lobe is the most frequent site of liver recurrence. Regional lymph nodes include porta hepatis, retroduodenal, and perigastric node groups along the gastrohepatic ligament. Distant metastasis develops in the majority of patients who exhibit a locoregional recurrence; however, it was the site of first failure in only 24%.

Detailed anatomic studies have offered an explanation for the high incidence of liver and local recurrence following resection of a hilar cholangiocarcinoma. In a series of 25 patients undergoing surgery for hilar cholangiocarcinoma, direct invasion of hepatic parenchyma at the hilum was noted in 12 patients (46.2%), with 11 patients (42.3%) also having carcinoma extending into the bile ducts draining the caudate lobe or directly invading the caudate lobe parenchyma.[172] A study of 106 adult human cadavers showed that 97.2% had bile ducts draining the caudate lobe that entered directly into the main left hepatic duct, right hepatic duct, or both.[173] These caudate lobe bile ducts frequently enter the main left or right hepatic ducts within 1 cm of the proper hepatic duct. Thus, a carcinoma arising at the confluence of the right and left hepatic ducts need not be large to extend into the bile ducts draining the caudate lobe.

Because cholangiocarcinoma is known to spread along the wall of the bile ducts and because the caudate lobe and hepatic hilum are frequent sites of tumor recurrence following extrahepatic duct resection, a number of authors now recommend more aggressive resections to include the caudate lobe and hepatic hilar parenchyma.[173–179] An understanding of the Bismuth-Corlette classification of hilar cholangiocarcinoma is useful in planning the extent and site of liver resection (Figure 89-10).[180] The median survival associated with a more radical surgical approach has varied from 10 to 37 months, with 5-year survival rates of 20 to 44% and 10-year survival rates as high as 14%.[173–179] Although aggressive surgical resection of hilar cholangiocarcinomas, including hepatic resection, provides the best chance for long-term survival, these operative procedures are associated with significant risk. The operative mortality rate in modern series ranges from 5 to 12%, with postoperative liver failure following an extensive liver resection being the most common cause of death.[173–179] Surgical complications are reported in 25 to 45% of the surviving patients. Infectious complications are the most common postoperative problem, and preoperative placement of biliary stents with resultant contamination of the obstructed biliary tree increases the incidence of infection.[181]

A multimodal approach to reduce locoregional recurrence rates and improve survival after resection has been reported.[182] Of 53 patients who underwent resection of a hilar cholangiocarcinoma, 38 received postoperative external beam radiotherapy to the resection bed at a dose of 50 to 60 Gy. In addition, 27 of these 38 patients received brachytherapy with ^{169}Ir seeds temporarily loaded into their transhepatic biliary stents in the area of the hepatico jejunostomies. These 27 patients received 20 Gy of internal radiation after completion of external beam radiotherapy. There was no significant difference in the 1-, 2-, and 3-year survival rates for patients who underwent resection, with or without radiotherapy, but there were no survivors past 3 years in the group without radiotherapy. The 5- and 10-year survival rates in the group receiving radiotherapy were 11% and 5%, respectively.

We recently reviewed our experience in patients with extrahepatic cholangiocarcinoma treated at the University of Texas M. D. Anderson Cancer Center.[183] Of 91 patients evaluated between 1983 and 1996, 51 (56%) presented with unresectable disease and 40 (44%) underwent resection. The median survival for the resected patients was 22.2 months versus 10.7 months in patients with unresectable disease ($p < .0001$). Nine patients, 5 with hilar and 4 with distal common duct cholangiocarcinoma, were treated with preoperative chemoradiation therapy (continuous intravenous infusion of 5-fluorouracil at 300 mg/m^2/day combined with external beam irradiation). Three of these 9 patients had a pathologic complete response to chemoradiation treatment; the remaining 6 patients had varying degrees of histologic response to treatment. The rate of margin-negative resection was 100% for the preoperative chemoradiation group compared with 54% for the group not receiving preoperative treatment ($p < .01$). The patients treated with preoperative chemoradiation had no operative or postoperative complications related to treatment. Thus, it appears that neoadjuvant chemoradiation for extrahepatic bile duct cancer can be performed safely, produces significant antitumor response, and may improve the ability to achieve tumor-free resection margins.

Liver Transplantation Total hepatectomy with immediate orthotopic liver transplantation (OLT) has been described in patients with hilar cholangiocarcinoma.[159,184–199] The 90-day mortality from hemorrhage, sepsis, and graft rejection was 23.1%. Of the patients who survived more than 3 months following transplantation, the median survival was 11 months in the series prior to 1992 but has improved to 23 months in the recent series. In the older series of patients, the 5-year survival rate was 5.0%. In patients who died later than 3 months after transplantation, death was due to tumor recurrence in 85.4%. The 5-year survival rate following OLT for extrahepatic cholangiocarcinoma in current studies is 25%, and in the highly selected subset of patients with stage I or II disease, 5-year survival is 73%.[197] Nonetheless, because of the poor results in most reports, many transplantation centers no longer perform liver transplantations in patients with hilar cholangiocarcinoma. Liver transplantation for hilar cholangiocarcinoma should probably be considered only as part of a prospective protocol evaluating multimodality treatment.

Palliation In general, curative surgical resection is possible in less than 30% of patients with hilar cholangiocarcinoma.[74,163–165,200] In patients deemed unresectable on the basis of the findings of diagnostic studies, laparotomy can be avoided by placing percutaneous external drains or endoscopically placed endoprostheses.[201,202] Conventional 10- or 12-French polyethylene endoprostheses have a high rate of occlusion and cholangitis.[203] However, new expandable metal wall stents appear to have improved long-term patency rates and may be used to deliver palliative high-dose rate endoluminal brachytherapy.[204,205] When unresectability is determined at the time of laparotomy, a decision must be made on a surgical bypass versus an operative intubation to provide drainage of the obstructed biliary tree. It is clear that techniques for surgical bypass, operative intubation, and percutaneous external drainage are equivalent in partial or complete relief of jaundice in 70 to 100% of patients.[74] Seemingly, the only potential advantage to the patient who undergoes surgical bypass instead of operative intubation is the absence of an external drainage catheter in the former group.

The advantage of not having an external biliary drainage catheter or an internal endoscope is considering the quality-of-life issues related to chemotherapeutic toxicity; systemic chemotherapy has not demonstrated a distinct advantage in patients with hilar cholangiocarcinoma.

Radiotherapy Radiotherapy for bile duct cancer is even more confusing because of the various types, doses, routes of administration, and association with resected and unresected tumors, all in small numbers of patients. Internal radiation with 16 ^{169}Ir wires or seeds may have a palliative role in improving the patency of obstructed bile ducts; however, the number and frequency of episodes of cholangitis were not reduced, so the overall benefit is uncertain.[207] Internal radiation has been associated with prolongation of survival to an average of 16 months, and occasionally patients with unresectable disease survived more than 5 years.[208–210] Although the use of external beam radiotherapy alone to treat patients with unresectable hilar cholangiocarcinoma has not provided significant differences in overall patient survival, rare long-term survivals have been reported.[211] Intraoperative radiotherapy also has been evaluated in association with resectable and unresectable tumors.[212,213] Again, there is a suggestion of a slight prolongation of survival in patients with unresectable tumors, but the most interesting use of intraoperative radiotherapy may be as an immediate surgical adjuvant in the resected high-risk tumor bed.

Chemotherapy Given the high percentage of unresectable hilar cholangiocarcinomas, various chemotherapeutic regimens and radiotherapeutic regimens have been used in the hope of providing improved palliation and prolongation of survival. Adjuvant radiotherapy also has been employed following resection of tumors to reduce locoregional recurrence and potentially to improve survival.[182] Unfortunately, reports describing chemotherapy or radiotherapy for hilar cholangiocarcinoma rarely describe the treatment results in more than 10 to 20 patients.

A 1988 review of systemic chemotherapy for bile duct cancer noted that 97 patients had been treated with nine different treatment programs.[214] Mitomycin-C, doxorubicin, and 5-fluorouracil are the agents that have shown the greatest activity against cholangiocarcinoma. The collective partial response rate in the 97 patients was 29%, with no complete responses. The median survival of these patients receiving systemic chemotherapy ranged between 6 and 11 months. No reports since 1988 have indicated a better response rate with systemic chemotherapy. With no significant increase in survival and coniary drainage tubes, a combination of external beam plus endoluminal boost irradiation is an attractive treatment program. The favored treatment sequence is to start with external beam irradiation to obtain tumor regression, which provides a better dose distribution from the endoluminal boost irradiation to treat any residual tumor. We currently use high-dose rate ^{169}Ir implants in a fractionated treatment schedule of 4 Gy daily for 5 consecutive days. The fractionated high-dose rate treatment, along with the favorable dose distribution obtained with endoluminal therapy, may decrease late-occurring duodenitis. For patients in whom there are technical or medical limitations for fractionated therapy, a single 20 Gy boost with the high-dose technique can be used.

The use of endoluminal ^{169}Ir alone for palliative treatment of patients with unresectable hilar bile duct cancers has been reported.[214] Endoluminal doses ranged from 15 to 35 Gy when combined with external beam irradiation (usually 45–50 Gy), or when endoluminal doses of up to 60 Gy were used alone. The dose reference point may vary from 0.5 to 1.0 cm from the central catheter. The total nominal doses of external beam plus endoluminal boost irradiation are between 60 Gy and 70 Gy to the tumor, and although this range exceeds the liver and small intestine tolerance, the highest doses are confined to a small volume of tissue. The median survival for patients treated by this endoluminal method, with or without external beam irradiation, is 15 to 18 months. Several patients survived for more than 4 years after treatment; however, the majority of patients had local failure.

REFERENCES

1. Jemal A, Murray T, Samuels A, et al. Cancer statistics, 2003. CA Cancer J Clin 2003;53:5–26.
2. Lazcano-Ponce E, Miguel JF, Munoz N, et al. Epidemiology and Molecular pathology of gall bladder cancer. CA Cancer J Clin 2001;51:349–64.
3. De Aretxabala X, Roa I, Araya JC, et al. Gallbladder cancer in patients less than 40 years old. Br J Surg 1994;81:111.
4. Nelson BD, Porvaznik J, Benfield JR. Gallbladder disease in Southwestern American Indians. Arch Surg 1971;103:41–3.
5. Rudolph R, Cohen JJ. Cancer of the gallbladder in an 11-yr-old Navajo girl. J Pediatr Surg 1972;7:66–7.
6. Fox JG, Dewhirst FE, Shen Z, et al. Hepatic Helicobacter species identified in bile and gallbladder tissue from Chileans with chronic cholecystitis. Gastroenterology 1998;114:755–63.
7. Mancuso TF, Brennan MJ. Epidemiological considerations of cancer of the gallbladder, bile ducts and salivary glands in the rubber industry. J Occup Med 1970;12:333–41.
8. Nagorney DM, McPherson GA. Carcinoma of the gallbladder and extrahepatic bile ducts. Semin Oncol 1988;15:106–15.
9. Khan ZR, Neugut AI, Ahsan H, Chabot JA. Risk factors for biliary tract cancers. Am J Gastroenterol 1999;94:149–52.
10. Chow WH, Johansen C, Gridley G, et al. Gallstones, cholecystectomy and risk of cancers of the liver, biliary tract and pancreas. Br J Cancer 1999;79:640–4.
11. Diehl AK. Gallstone size and the risk of gallbladder cancer. JAMA 1983;250:2323–6.
12. Polk HC Jr. Carcinoma and the calcified gall bladder. Gastroenterology 1966;50:582–5.
13. Berk RN, Armbuster TG, Saltzstein SL. Carcinoma in the porcelain gallbladder. Radiology 1973;106:29–31.
14. Csendes A, Becerra M, Burdiles P, et al. Bacteriological studies of bile from the gallbladder in patients with carcinoma of the gallbladder, cholelithiasis, common bile duct stones and no gallstones disease. Eur J Surg 1994;160:363–7.
15. Parkash O. On the relationship of cholelithiasis to carcinoma of the gallbladder and on the sex dependency of the carcinoma of the bile ducts. A study based on the autopsy data from 1928 to 1972. Digestion 1975;12:129–33.
16. Albores-Saavedra J, Alcantra-Vazquez A, Cruz-Ortiz H, Herrera-Goepfert R. The precursor lesions of invasive gallbladder carcinoma. Hyperplasia, atypical hyperplasia and carcinoma in situ. Cancer 1980;45:919–27.
17. Black WE. The morphogenesis of gallbladder carcinoma. In: Fenoglio CM, Wolff M, editors. Progress in surgical pathology. New York: Masson; 1980. p. 207.
18. Kuzuka S, Tsubone M, Yasui A. Relation of adenoma to carcinoma in the gallbladder. Cancer 1982;50:2226–30.
19. Yukawa M, Fujimori T, Hirayama D, et al. Expression of oncogene products and growth factors in early gallbladder cancer, advanced gallbladder cancer, and chronic cholecystitis. Hum Pathol 1993;24:37–40.
20. Tanno S, Obara T, Fujii T, et al. Proliferative potential and K-*ras* mutation in epithelial hyperplasia of the gallbladder in patients with anomalous pancreaticobiliary ductal union. Cancer 1998;83:267–75.
21. Eguchi N, Fujii K, Tsuchida A, et al. Cyclin E overexpression in human gallbladder carcinomas. Oncol Rep 1999;6:93–6.
22. Mikami T, Yanagisawa N, Baba H, et al. Association of Bcl-2 protein expression with gallbladder carcinoma differentiation and progression and its relation to apoptosis. Cancer 1999;85:318–25.
23. Kim YT, Kim J, Jang YH, et al. Genetic alterations in gallbladder adenoma, dysplasia and carcinoma. Cancer Lett 2001;169:59–68.
24. Quan ZW, Wu K, Wang J, et al. Association of p53, p16, and vascular endothelial growth factor protein expressions with the prognosis and metastasis of gallbladder cancer. J Am Coll Surg 2001;193:380–3.
25. Sumiyoshi K, Nagai E, Chijiiwa K, Nakayama F. Pathology of carcinoma of the gallbladder. World J Surg 1991;15:315–21.
26. Fahim RB, McDonald JR, Richards JC, Ferris DO. Carcinoma of the gallbladder. A study of its modes of spread. Ann Surg 1962;156:114–22.
27. Shirai Y, Tsukada K, Ohtani T, et al. Hepatic metastases from carcinoma of the gallbladder. Cancer 1995;75:2063–8.
28. Ohtsuka M, Miyazaki M, Itoh H, et al. Routes of hepatic metastasis of gallbladder carcinoma. Am J Clin Pathol 1998;109:62–8.
29. Ito M, Mishima Y, Sato T. An anatomical study of the lymphatic drainage of the gallbladder. Surg Radiol Anat 1991;13:89–104.
30. Nevin JE, Moran TJ, Kay S, King R. Carcinoma of the gallbladder. Staging, treatment, and prognosis. Cancer 1976;37:141–8.
31. Surgery JSoB. The general rules for surgical and pathological studies on cancer of biliary tract. Tokyo: Kanehara Syuppan; 1986.
32. Perpetuo MD, Valdivieso M, Heilbrun LK, et al. Natural history study of gallbladder cancer. A review of 36 years experience at MD Anderson Hospital and Tumor Institute. Cancer 1978;42:330–5.
33. Koga A, Yamauchi S, Izumi Y, Hamanaka N. Ultrasonographic detection of early and curable carcinoma of the gallbladder. Br J Surg 1985;72:728–30.
34. Kubota K, Bandai Y, Noie T, et al. How should polypoid lesions of the gallbladder be treated in the era of laparoscopic cholecystectomy? Surgery 1995;117:481–7.
35. Okamoto M, Okamoto H, Kitahara F, et al. Ultrasonographic evidence of association of polyps and stones with gallbladder cancer. Am J Gastroenterol 1999;94:446–50.
36. Soiva M, Aro K, Pamilo M, et al. Ultrasonography in carcinoma of the gallbladder. Acta Radiol 1987;28:711–4.
37. Dalla Palma L, Rizzatto G, Pozzi-Mucelli RS, Bazzocchi M. Grey-scale ultrasonography in the evaluation of carcinoma of the gall bladder. Br J Radiol 1980;53:662–7.
38. Bach AM, Loring LA, Hann LE, et al. Gallbladder cancer. Can ultrasonography evaluate extent of disease? J Ultrasound Med 1998;17:303–9.
39. Li D, Dong BW, Wu YL, Yan K. Image-directed and color Doppler studies of gallbladder tumors. J Clin Ultrasound 1994;22:551–5.
40. Hirooka Y, Naitoh Y, Goto H, et al. Contrast-enhanced endoscopic ultrasonography in gallbladder diseases. Gastrointest Endosc 1998;48:406–10.

41. Chijiiwa K, Sumiyoshi K, Nakayama F. Impact of recent advances in hepatobiliary imaging techniques on the preoperative diagnosis of carcinoma of the gallbladder. World J Surg 1991;15:322–7.
42. Thorsen MK, Quiroz F, Lawson TL, et al. Primary biliary carcinoma. CT evaluation. Radiology 1984;152:479–83.
43. Furukawa H, Kosuge T, Shimada K, et al. Small polypoid lesions of the gallbladder. Differential diagnosis and surgical indications by helical computed tomography. Arch Surg 1998;133:735–9.
44. Hamrick RE Jr, Liner FJ, Hastings PR, Cohn I Jr. Primary carcinoma of the gallbladder. Ann Surg 1982;195:270–3.
45. Klamer TW, Max MH. Carcinoma of the gallbladder. Surg Gynecol Obstet 1983;156:641–5.
46. Fong Y, Malhotra S. Gallbladder cancer. Recent advances and current guidelines for surgical therapy. Adv Surg 2001;35:1–20.
47. Gagner M, Rossi RL. Radical operations for carcinoma of the gallbladder. Present status in North America. World J Surg 1991;15:344–7.
48. Ogura Y, Mizumoto R, Isaji S, et al. Radical operations for carcinoma of the gallbladder. Present status in Japan. World J Surg 1991;15:337–43.
49. Wagholikar GD, Behari A, Krishnani N, et al. Early gallbladder cancer. J Am Coll Surg 2002;194:137–41.
50. Kaushik SP. Current perspectives in gallbladder carcinoma. J Gastroenterol Hepatol 2001;16:848–54.
51. Ouchi K, Owada Y, Matsuno S, Sato T. Prognostic factors in the surgical treatment of gallbladder carcinoma. Surgery 1987;101:731–7.
52. Bergdahl L. Gallbladder carcinoma first diagnosed at microscopic examination of gallbladders removed for presumed benign disease. Ann Surg 1980;191:19–22.
53. Chijiiwa K, Nakano K, Ueda J, et al. Surgical treatment of patients with T2 gallbladder carcinoma invading the subserosal layer. J Am Coll Surg 2001;192:600–7.
54. Chijiiwa K, Noshiro H, Nakano K, et al. Role of surgery for gallbladder carcinoma with special reference to lymph node metastasis and stage using Western and Japanese classification systems [discussion 1277]. World J Surg 2000;24:1271–6.
55. North JH Jr, Pack MS, Hong C, Rivera DE. Prognostic factors for adenocarcinoma of the gallbladder. An analysis of 162 cases. Am Surg 1998;64:437–40.
56. Benoist S, Panis Y, Fagniez PL. Long-term results after curative resection for carcinoma of the gallbladder. French University Association for Surgical Research. Am J Surg 1998;175:118–22.
57. Maibenco DC, Smith JL, Nava HR, et al. Carcinoma of the gallbladder. Cancer Invest 1998;16:33–9.
58. Ogura Y, Tabata M, Kawarada Y, Mizumoto R. Effect of hepatic invasion on the choice of hepatic resection for advanced carcinoma of the gallbladder. Histologic analysis of 32 surgical cases [discussion 266–7]. World J Surg 1998;22:262–6.
59. Paquet KJ. Appraisal of surgical resection of gallbladder carcinoma with special reference to hepatic resection. J Hepatobiliary Pancreat Surg 1998;5:200–6.
60. Yoshikawa T, Araida T, Azuma T, Takasaki K. Bisubsegmental liver resection for gallbladder cancer. Hepatogastroenterology 1998;45:14–9.
61. Yamaguchi K, Chijiiwa K, Shimizu S, et al. Anatomical limit of extended cholecystectomy for gallbladder carcinoma involving the neck of the gallbladder. Int Surg 1998;83:21–3.
62. Nimura Y, Hayakawa N, Kamiya J, et al. Hepatopancreatoduodenectomy for advanced carcinoma of the biliary tract. Hepatogastroenterology 1991;38:170–5.
63. Alessiani M, Tzakis A, Todo S, et al. Assessment of five-year experience with abdominal organ cluster transplantation. J Am Coll Surg 1995;180:1–9.
64. Grace PA, Quereshi A, Coleman J, et al. Reduced postoperative hospitalization after laparoscopic cholecystectomy. Br J Surg 1991;78:160–2.
65. Fong Y, Brennan MF, Turnbull A, et al. Gallbladder cancer discovered during laparoscopic surgery. Potential for iatrogenic tumor dissemination. Arch Surg 1993;128:1054–6.
66. Drouard F, Delamarre J, Capron JP. Cutaneous seeding of gallbladder cancer after laparoscopic cholecystectomy. N Engl J Med 1991;325:1316.
67. Pezet D, Fondrinier E, Rotman N, et al. Parietal seeding of carcinoma of the gallbladder after laparoscopic cholecystectomy. Br J Surg 1992;79:230.
68. Clair DG, Lautz DB, Brooks DC. Rapid development of umbilical metastases after laparoscopic cholecystectomy for unsuspected gallbladder carcinoma. Surgery 1993;113:355–8.
69. Kim HJ, Roy T. Unexpected gallbladder cancer with cutaneous seeding after laparoscopic cholecystectomy. South Med J 1994;87:817–20.
70. Contini S, Dalla Valle R, Zinicola R. Unexpected gallbladder cancer after laparoscopic cholecystectomy: an emerging problem? Reflections on four cases. Surg Endosc 1999;13:264–7.
71. Pearlstone DB, Curley SA, Feig BW. The management of gallbladder cancer. Before, during, and after laparoscopic cholecystectomy. Semin Laparosc Surg 1998;5:121–8.
72. Donohue JH, Stewart AK, Menck HR. The National Cancer Data Base report on carcinoma of the gallbladder, 1989–1995. Cancer 1998;83:2618–28.
73. Fong Y, Heffernan N, Blumgart LH. Gallbladder carcinoma discovered during laparoscopic cholecystectomy. Aggressive reresection is beneficial. Cancer 1998;83:423–7.
74. Bismuth H, Castaing D, Traynor O. Resection or palliation. Priority of surgery in the treatment of hilar cancer. World J Surg 1988;12:39–47.
75. Jones RS. Palliative operative procedures for carcinoma of the gallbladder. World J Surg 1991;15:348–51.
76. Falkson G, MacIntyre JM, Moertel CG. Eastern Cooperative Oncology Group experience with chemotherapy for inoperable gallbladder and bile duct cancer. Cancer 1984;54:965–9.
77. Hall SW, Benjamin RS, Murphy WK, et al. Adriamycin, BCNU, Ftorafur chemotherapy of pancreatic and biliary tract cancer. Cancer 1979;44:2008–13.
78. Harvey JH, Smith FP, Schein PS. 5-Fluorouracil, mitomycin, and doxorubicin (FAM) in carcinoma of the biliary tract. J Clin Oncol 1984;2:1245–8.
79. Castro MP. Efficacy of gemcitabine in the treatment of patients with gallbladder carcinoma. A case report. Cancer 1998;82:639–41.
80. Buskirk SJ, Gunderson LL, Adson MA, et al. Analysis of failure following curative irradiation of gallbladder and extrahepatic bile duct carcinoma. Int J Radiat Oncol Biol Phys 1984;10:2013–23.
81. Smoron GL. Radiation therapy of carcinoma of gallbladder and biliary tract. Cancer 1977;40:1422–4.
82. Pilepich MV, Lambert PM. Radiotherapy of carcinomas of the extrahepatic biliary system. Radiology 1978;127:767–70.
83. Kopelson G, Harisiadis L, Tretter P, Chang CH. The role of radiation therapy in cancer of the extra-hepatic biliary system. An analysis of thirteen patients and a review of the literature of the effectiveness of surgery, chemotherapy and radiotherapy. Int J Radiat Oncol Biol Phys 1977;2:883–94.
84. Martenson JA Jr, Gunderson LL, Buskirk SJ, et al. Hepatic duct stricture after radical radiation therapy for biliary cancer. Recurrence or fibrosis? Mayo Clin Proc 1986;61:530–6.
85. Morrow CE, Sutherland DE, Florack G, et al. Primary gallbladder carcinoma. Significance of subserosal lesions and results of aggressive surgical treatment and adjuvant chemotherapy. Surgery 1983;94:709–14.
86. Athlin LE, Domellof LK, Bergman FO. Advanced gallbladder carcinoma. A case report and review of the literature. Eur J Surg Oncol 1987;13:449–53.
87. Todoroki T, Iwasaki Y, Orii K, et al. Resection combined with intraoperative radiation therapy (IORT) for stage IV (TNM) gallbladder carcinoma. World J Surg 1991;15:357–66.
88. Aretxabala X, Roa I, Burgos L. Preoperative chemoradiotherapy in the treatment of gallbladder cancer. Am Surg 1999;65:241–6.
89. Thuluvath PJ, Rai R, Venbrux AC, Yeo CJ. Cholangiocarcinoma. A review. Gastroenterologist 1997;5:306–15.
90. Nakeeb A, Pitt HA, Sohn TA, et al. Cholangiocarcinoma. A spectrum of intrahepatic, perihilar, and distal tumors [discussion 473–5]. Ann Surg 1996;224:463–73,
91. Liver Cancer Study Group of Japan. Primary liver cancer in Japan. Cancer 1984;54:1747–55.
92. Sorensen HT, Friis S, Olsen JH, et al. Risk of liver and other types of cancer in patients with cirrhosis: a nationwide cohort study in Denmark. Hepatology 1998;28:921–5.
93. Schwartz DA. Cholangiocarcinoma associated with liver fluke infection. A preventable source of morbidity in Asian immigrants. Am J Gastroenterol 1986;81:76–9.
94. Kurathong S, Lerdverasirikul P, Wongpaitoon V, et al. Opisthorchis viverrini infection and cholangiocarcinoma. A prospective, case-controlled study. Gastroenterology 1985;89:151–6.
95. Kim KH, Kim CD, Lee HS, et al. Biliary papillary hyperplasia with clonorchiasis resembling cholangiocarcinoma. Am J Gastroenterol 1999;94:514–7.
96. Nakanuma Y, Terada T, Tanaka Y, Ohta G. Are hepatolithiasis and cholangiocarcinoma aetiologically related? A morphological study of 12 cases of hepatolithiasis associated with cholangiocarcinoma. Virchows Archiv A 1985;406:45–58.
97. Landais P, Grunfeld JP, Droz D, et al. Cholangiocellular carcinoma in polycystic kidney and liver disease. Arch Intern Med 1984;144:2274–6.
98. Voyles CR, Smadja C, Shands WC, Blumgart LH. Carcinoma in choledochal cysts. Age-related incidence. Arch Surg 1983;118:986–8.
99. Imamura M, Miyashita T, Tani T, et al. Cholangiocellular carcinoma associated with multiple liver cysts. Am J Gastroenterol 1984;79:790–5.
100. Dayton MT, Longmire WP Jr, Tompkins RK. Caroli's Disease. A premalignant condition? Am J Surg 1983;145:41–8.
101. Wee A, Ludwig J, Coffey RJ Jr, et al. Hepatobiliary carcinoma associated with primary sclerosing cholangitis and chronic ulcerative colitis. Hum Pathol 1985;16:719–26.
102. Chen PH, Lo HW, Wang CS, et al. Cholangiocarcinoma in hepatolithiasis. J Clin Gastroenterol 1984;6:539–47.
103. Koga A, Ichimiya H, Yamaguchi K, et al. Hepatolithiasis associated with cholangiocarcinoma. Possible etiologic significance. Cancer 1985;55:2826–9.
104. Yoshimoto H, Ikeda S, Tanaka M, Matsumoto S. Intrahepatic cholangiocarcinoma associated with hepatolithiasis. Gastrointest Endosc 1985;31:260–3.
105. Chen MF, Jan YY, Wang CS, et al. A reappraisal of cholangiocarcinoma in patient with hepatolithiasis. Cancer 1993;71:2461–5.
106. Chijiiwa K, Ichimiya H, Kuroki S, et al. Late development of cholangiocarcinoma after the treatment of hepatolithiasis. Surg Gynecol Obstet 1993;177:279–82.
107. Robertson JF, Raine PA. Choledochal cyst. A 33-year review. Br J Surg 1988;75:799–801.
108. Lipsett PA, Pitt HA, Colombani PM, et al. Choledochal cyst disease. A changing pattern of presentation. Ann Surg 1994;220:644–52.
109. Cherqui D, Tantawi B, Alon R. Relationships between sclerosing cholangitis, inflammatory bowel disease, and cancer in patients undergoing liver transplantation. Surgery 1995;118:615–9.
110. Kaya M, de Groen PC, Angulo P, et al. Treatment of cholangiocarcinoma complicating primary sclerosing cholangitis. The Mayo Clinic experience. Am J Gastroenterol 2001;96:1164–9.
111. van Laethem JL, Deviere J, Bourgeois N, et al. Cholangiographic findings in deteriorating primary sclerosing cholangitis. Endoscopy 1995;27:223–8.
112. Nichols JC, Gores GJ, LaRusso NF, et al. Diagnostic role of serum CA 19-9 for cholangiocarcinoma in patients with primary sclerosing cholangitis. Mayo Clin Proc 1993;68:874–9.
113. Ramage JK, Donaghy A, Farrant JM, et al. Serum tumor markers for the diagnosis of cholangiocarcinoma in primary sclerosing cholangitis. Gastroenterology 1995;108:865–9.
114. Ito Y, Kojiro M, Nakashima T, Mori T. Pathomorphologic characteristics of 102 cases of thorotrast-related hepatocellular carcinoma, cholangiocarcinoma, and hepatic angiosarcoma. Cancer 1988;62:1153–62.
115. Rubel LR, Ishak KG. Thorotrast-associated cholangiocarcinoma: an epidemiologic and clinicopathologic study. Cancer 1982;50:1408–15.
116. Sturm PD, Baas IO, Clement MJ, et al. Alterations of the p53 tumor-suppressor gene and K-ras oncogene in perihilar cholangiocarcinomas from a high-incidence area. Int J Cancer 1998;78:695–8.
117. Wattanasirichaigoon S, Tasanakhajorn U, Jesadapatarakul S. The incidence of K-ras codon 12 mutations in cholangiocarcinoma detected by polymerase chain reaction technique. J Med Assoc Thai 1998;81:316–23.
118. Ahrendt SA, Rashid A, Chow JT, et al. p53 overexpression and K-ras gene mutations in primary sclerosing cholangitis-associated biliary tract cancer. J Hepatobiliary Pancreat Surg 2000;7:426–31.
119. Terada T, Ashida K, Endo K, et al. c-erbB-2 protein is expressed in hepatolithiasis and cholangiocarcinoma. Histopathology 1998;33:325–31.
120. Celli A, Que FG. Dysregulation of apoptosis in the cholangiopathies and cholangiocarcinoma. Semin Liver Dis 1998;18:177–85.
121. Pitt HA, Dooley WC, Yeo CJ, Cameron JL. Malignancies of the biliary tree. Curr Probl Surg 1995;32:1–90.
122. Jalanko H, Kuusela P, Roberts P, et al. Comparison of a new tumour marker, CA 19-9, with alpha-fetoprotein and carcinoembryonic antigen in patients with upper gastrointestinal diseases. J Clin Pathol 1984;37:218–22.

123. Anthony PP. Tumours and tumour-like lesions of the liver and biliary tract. In: MacSween RNM, Anthony PP, Scheuer PJ, editors. Pathology of the liver. Edinburgh, UK: Churchill Livingston; 1987. p. 574.
124. Weinbren K, Mutum SS. Pathological aspects of cholangiocarcinoma. J Pathol 1983;139:217–38.
125. Aoki K, Takayasu K, Kawano T, et al. Combined hepatocellular carcinoma and cholangiocarcinoma. Clinical features and computed tomographic findings. Hepatology 1993;18:1090–5.
126. Yamamoto M, Takasaki K, Yoshikawa T, et al. Does gross appearance indicate prognosis in intrahepatic cholangiocarcinoma? J Surg Oncol Suppl 1998;69:162–7.
127. Bonetti F, Chilosi M, Pisa R, et al. Epithelial membrane antigen expression in cholangiocarcinoma. An useful immunohistochemical tool for differential diagnosis with hepatocarcinoma. Virchows Archiv A 1983;401: 307–13.
128. Pastolero GC, Wakabayashi T, Oka T, Mori S. Tissue polypeptide antigen—a marker antigen differentiating cholangiolar tumors from other hepatic tumors. Am J Clin Pathol 1987;87:168–73.
129. Sasaki A, Kawano K, Aramaki M, et al. Immunohistochemical expression of cytokeratins in intrahepatic cholangiocarcinoma and metastatic adenocarcinoma of the liver. J Surg Oncol Suppl 1999;70:103–8.
130. Colli A, Cocciolo M, Mumoli N, et al. Peripheral intrahepatic cholangiocarcinoma. Ultrasound findings and differential diagnosis from hepatocellular carcinoma. Eur J Ultrasound 1998;7:93–9.
131. Kuszyk BS, Soyer P, Bluemke DA, Fishman EK. Intrahepatic cholangiocarcinoma. The role of imaging in detection and staging. Crit Rev Diagn Imaging 1997;38:59–88.
132. Feydy A, Vilgrain V, Denys A, et al. Helical CT assessment in hilar cholangiocarcinoma. Correlation with surgical and pathologic findings. AJR Am J Roentgenol 1999;172:73–7.
133. Tillich M, Mischinger HJ, Preisegger KH, et al. Multiphasic helical CT in diagnosis and staging of hilar cholangiocarcinoma. AJR Am J Roentgenol 1998;171:651–8.
134. Han JK, Choi BI, Kim TK, et al. Hilar cholangiocarcinoma. Thin-section spiral CT findings with cholangiographic correlation. Radiographics 1997;17:1475–85.
135. Okuda K, Ohto M, Tsuchiya Y. The role of ultrasound, percutaneous transhepatic cholangiography, computed tomographic scanning, and magnetic resonance imaging in the preoperative assessment of bile duct cancer. World J Surg 1988;12:18–26.
136. Garber SJ, Donald JJ, Lees WR. Cholangiocarcinoma. Ultrasound features and correlation of tumor position with survival. Abdom Imaging 1993;18:66–9.
137. Neumaier CE, Bertolotto M, Perrone R, et al. Staging of hilar cholangiocarcinoma with ultrasound. J Clin Ultrasound 1995;23:173–8.
138. Kusano T, Shimabukuro M, Tamai O, et al. The use of intra-operative ultrasonography for detecting tumor extension in bile duct carcinoma. Int Surg 1997;82:44–8.
139. Lopera JE, Soto JA, Munera F. Malignant hilar and perihilar biliary obstruction. Use of MR cholangiography to define the extent of biliary ductal involvement and plan percutaneous interventions. Radiology 2001;220:90–6.
140. Worawattanakul S, Semelka RC, Noone TC, et al. Cholangiocarcinoma. Spectrum of appearances on MR images using current techniques. Magn Reson Imaging 1998;16:993–1003.
141. Neri E, Boraschi P, Braccini G, et al. MR virtual endoscopy of the pancreaticobiliary tract. Magn Reson Imaging 1999;17:59–67.
142. Elias E, Hamlyn AN, Jain S, et al. A randomized trial of percutaneous transhepatic cholangiography with the Chiba needle versus endoscopic retrograde cholangiography for bile duct visualization in jaundice. Gastroenterology 1976;71:439–43.
143. Fujita N, Noda Y, Kobayashi G, et al. Staging of bile duct carcinoma by EUS and IDUS. Endoscopy 1998;30 Suppl 1:A132–4.
144. Tanaka M, Ogawa Y, Matsumoto S, Nakayama F. The role of endoscopic retrograde cholangiopancreatography in preoperative assessment of bile duct cancer. World J Surg 1988;12:27–32.
145. Yamakawa T, Esguerra RD Jr, Kaneko H, Fukuma E. Percutaneous transhepatic endoprosthesis in malignant obstruction of the bile duct. World J Surg 1988;12:78–84.
146. Pitt HA, Gomes AS, Lois JF, et al. Does preoperative percutaneous biliary drainage reduce operative risk or increase hospital cost? Ann Surg 1985;201:545–53.
147. McPherson GA, Benjamin IS, Hodgson HJ, et al. Pre-operative percutaneous transhepatic biliary drainage. The results of a controlled trial. Br J Surg 1984;71:371–5.
148. Cameron JL, Broe P, Zuidema GD. Proximal bile duct tumors. Surgical management with silastic transhepatic biliary stents. Ann Surg 1982;196:412–9.
149. Crist DW, Kadir S, Cameron JL. The value of preoperatively placed percutaneous biliary catheters in reconstruction of the proximal part of the biliary tract. Surg Gynecol Obstet 1987;165:421–4.
150. Keiding S, Hansen SB, Rasmussen HH, et al. Detection of cholangiocarcinoma in primary sclerosing cholangitis by positron emission tomography. Hepatology 1998;28:700–6.
151. Kluge R, Schmidt F, Caca K, et al. Positron emission tomography with [(18)F]fluoro-2-deoxy-D-glucose for diagnosis and staging of bile duct cancer. Hepatology 2001;33:1029–35.
152. Weber SM, DeMatteo RP, Fong Y, et al. Staging laparoscopy in patients with extrahepatic biliary carcinoma. Analysis of 100 patients. Ann Surg 2002;253:392–9.
153. Roayaie S, Guarrera JV, Ye MQ, et al. Aggressive surgical treatment of intrahepatic cholangiocarcinoma. Predictors of outcomes. J Am Coll Surg 1998;187:365–72.
154. Lieser MJ, Barry MK, Rowland C, et al. Surgical management of intrahepatic cholangiocarcinoma. A 31-year experience. J Hepatobiliary Pancreat Surg 1998;5:41–7.
155. Shirabe K, Shimada M, Harimoto N, et al. Intrahepatic cholangiocarcinoma. Its mode of spreading and therapeutic modalities. Surgery 2002;131:S159–64.
156. Uenishi T, Hirohashi K, Kubo S, et al. Histologic factors affecting prognosis following hepatectomy for intrahepatic cholangiocarcinoma. World J Surg 2001;25:865–9.
157. Harrison LE, Fong Y, Klimstra DS, et al. Surgical treatment of 32 patients with peripheral intrahepatic cholangiocarcinoma. Br J Surg 1998;85:1068–70.
158. Chou FF, Sheen-Chen SM, Chen CL, et al. Prognostic factors of resectable intrahepatic cholangiocarcinoma. J Surg Oncol Suppl 1995;59:40–4.
159. Pichlmayr R, Lamesch P, Weimann A, et al. Surgical treatment of cholangiocellular carcinoma. World J Surg 1995;19:83–8.
160. Sasaki A, Aramaki M, Kawano K, et al. Intrahepatic peripheral cholangiocarcinoma. Mode of spread and choice of surgical treatment. Br J Surg 1998;85:1206–9.
161. Altmeier WA, Gall EA, Zinninger MM. Sclerosing carcinoma of the major intrahepatic bile ducts. Arch Surg 1957;75:450–4.
162. Klatskin G. Adenocarcinoma of the hepatic duct at its bifurcation within the porta hepatis. Am J Med 1965;38:241–8.
163. Nagorney DM, Donohue JH, Farnell MB, et al. Outcomes after curative resections of cholangiocarcinoma [discussion 877–9]. Arch Surg 1993;128:871–7.
164. Nimura Y, Kamiya J, Nagino M, et al. Aggressive surgical treatment of hilar cholangiocarcinoma. J Hepatobiliary Pancreat Surg 1998;5:52–61.
165. Burke EC, Jarnagin WR, Hochwald SN, et al. Hilar cholangiocarcinoma. Patterns of spread, the importance of hepatic resection for curative operation, and a presurgical clinical staging system. Ann Surg 1998;228:385–94.
166. Chung C, Bautista N, O'Connell TX. Prognosis and treatment of bile duct carcinoma. Am Surg 1998;64:921–5.
167. Kayahara M, Nagakawa T, Ohta T, et al. Role of nodal involvement and the periductal soft-tissue margin in middle and distal bile duct cancer. Ann Surg 1999;229:76–83.
168. Tompkins RK, Thomas D, Wile A, Longmire WP Jr. Prognostic factors in bile duct carcinoma. Analysis of 96 cases. Ann Surg 1981;194:447–57.
169. Ouchi K, Suzuki M, Hashimoto L, Sato T. Histologic findings and prognostic factors in carcinoma of the upper bile duct. Am J Surg 1989;157:552–6.
170. Sakamoto E, Nimura Y, Hayakawa N, et al. The pattern of infiltration at the proximal border of hilar bile duct carcinoma. A histologic analysis of 62 resected cases. Ann Surg 1998;227:405–11.
171. Mittal B, Deutsch M, Iwatsuki S. Primary cancers of extrahepatic biliary passages. Int J Radiat Oncol Biol Phys 1985;11:849–54.
172. Mizumoto R, Kawarada Y, Suzuki H. Surgical treatment of hilar carcinoma of the bile duct. Surg Gynecol Obstet 1986;162:153–8.
173. Mizumoto R, Suzuki H. Surgical anatomy of the hepatic hilum with special reference to the caudate lobe. World J Surg 1988;12:2–10.
174. Bengmark S, Ekberg H, Evander A, et al. Major liver resection for hilar cholangiocarcinoma. Ann Surg 1988;207:120–5.
175. Jarnagin WR, Fong Y, DeMatteo RP, et al. Staging, resectability, and outcome in 225 patients with hilar cholangiocarcinoma [discussion 517–9]. Ann Surg 2001;234:507–17.
176. Pinson CW, Rossi RL. Extended right hepatic lobectomy, left hepatic lobectomy, and skeletonization resection for proximal bile duct cancer. World J Surg 1988;12:52–9.
177. Washburn WK, Lewis WD, Jenkins RL. Aggressive surgical resection for cholangiocarcinoma. Arch Surg 1995;130:270–6.
178. Baer HU, Stain SC, Dennison AR, et al. Improvements in survival by aggressive resections of hilar cholangiocarcinoma. Ann Surg 1993;217:20–7.
179. Nagino M, Nimura Y, Kamiya J, et al. Segmental liver resections for hilar cholangiocarcinoma. Hepatogastroenterology 1998;45:7–13.
180. Bismuth H, Corlette MB. Intrahepatic cholangioenteric anastomosis in carcinoma of the hilus of the liver. Surg Gynecol Obstet 1975;140:170–8.
181. Hochwald SN, Burke EC, Jarnagin WR, et al. Association of preoperative biliary stenting with increased postoperative infectious complications in proximal cholangiocarcinoma. Arch Surg 1999;134:261–6.
182. Cameron JL, Pitt HA, Zinner MJ, et al. Management of proximal cholangiocarcinomas by surgical resection and radiotherapy [discussion 97–8]. Am J Surg 1990;159:91–7.
183. McMasters KM, Tuttle TM, Leach SD, et al. Neoadjuvant chemoradiation for extrahepatic cholangiocarcinoma [discussion 608–9]. Am J Surg 1997;174:605–8.
184. Ringe B, Wittekind C, Bechstein WO, et al. The role of liver transplantation in hepatobiliary malignancy. A retrospective analysis of 95 patients with particular regard to tumor stage and recurrence. Ann Surg 1989;209:88–98.
185. O'Grady JG, Polson RJ, Rolles K, et al. Liver transplantation for malignant disease. Results in 93 consecutive patients. Ann Surg 1988;207:373–9.
186. Funovics JM, Fritsch A, Herbst F, et al. Primary hepatic cancer. The role of limited resection and total hepatectomy with orthotopic liver replacement. Hepatogastroenterology 1988;35:316–20.
187. Iwatsuki S, Gordon RD, Shaw BW Jr, Starzl TE. Role of liver transplantation in cancer therapy. Ann Surg 1985;202:401–7.
188. Koneru B, Cassavilla A, Bowman J, et al. Liver transplantation for malignant tumors. Gastroenterol Clin North Am 1988;17:177–93.
189. Yokoyama I, Todo S, Iwatsuki S, Starzl TE. Liver trans-plantation in the treatment of primary liver cancer. Hepatogastroenterology 1990;37:188–93.
190. Yokoyama I, Sheahan DG, Carr B, et al. Clinicopathologic factors affecting patient survival and tumor recurrence after orthotopic liver transplantation for hepatocellular carcinoma. Transplant Proc 1991;23:2194–6.
191. Olthoff KM, Millis JM, Rosove MH, et al. Is liver transplantation justified for the treatment of hepatic malignancies? [Discussion 1266–8]. Arch Surg 1990;125:1261–6.
192. Jenkins RL, Pinson CW, Stone MD. Experience with transplantation in the treatment of liver cancer. Cancer Chemother Pharmacol 1989;23 Suppl:S104–9.
193. Margeiter R. Indications for liver transplantation for primary and secondary liver tumor. Transplant Proc 1986;18:74–80.
194. Arigrisano L, Jurewicz WA, Clements DG. Liver transplantation for liver cancer. Transplant Proc 1986;18:1218–25.
195. Ismail T, Angrisani L, Gunson BK, et al. Primary hepatic malignancy. The role of liver transplantation. Br J Surg 1990;77:983–7.
196. van Thiel DH, Carr B, Iwatsuki S, et al. Liver transplantation for alcoholic liver disease, viral hepatitis, and hepatic neoplasms. Transplant Proc 1991;23:1917–21.
197. Iwatsuki S, Todo S, Marsh JW, et al. Treatment of hilar cholangiocarcinoma (Klatskin tumors) with hepatic resection or transplantation. J Am Coll Surg 1998;187:358–64.
198. Sansalone CV, Colella G, Caccamo L, et al. Orthotopic liver transplantation for primary biliary tumors. Milan multicenter experience. Transplant Proc 1994;26:3561–3.
199. Goldstein RM, Stone M, Tillery GE, et al. Is liver transplantation indicated for cholangiocarcinoma? [Discussion 771–2]. Am J Surg 1993;166:768–71.
200. Langer JC, Langer B, Taylor BR, et al. Carcinoma of the extrahepatic bile ducts. Results of an aggressive surgical approach. Surgery 1985;98:752–9.
201. Lameris JS, Stoker J, Dees J, et al. Non-surgical palliative treatment of patients with malignant biliary obstruc-

tion— the place of endoscopic and percutaneous drainage. Clin Radiol 1987;38:603–8.

202. Huibregtse K, Tytgat GN. Palliative treatment of obstructive jaundice by transpapillary introduction of large bore bile duct endoprosthesis. Gut 1982;23:371–5.
203. O'Brien S, Hatfield AR, Craig PI, Williams SP. A three year follow up of self expanding metal stents in the endoscopic palliation of longterm survivors with malignant biliary obstruction. Gut 1995;36:618–21.
204. McDougall NI, Edmunds SE. An audit of metal stent palliation for malignant biliary obstruction. J Gastroenterol Hepatol 2001;16:1051–4.
205. Kubota Y, Takaoka M, Kin H, et al. Endoscopic irradiation and parallel arrangement of Wallstents for hilar cholangiocarcinoma. Hepatogastroenterology 1998;45:415–9.
206. Mueller PR, van Sonnenberg E, Ferrucci JT Jr. Percutaneous biliary drainage. Technical and catheter-related problems in 200 procedures. AJR Am J Roentgenol 1982;138:17–23.
207. Meyers WC, Jones RS. Internal radiation for bile duct cancer. World J Surg 1988;12:99–104.
208. Karani J, Fletcher M, Brinkley D, et al. Internal biliary drainage and local radiotherapy with iridium-192 wire in treatment of hilar cholangiocarcinoma. Clin Radiol 1985;36:603–6.
209. Johnson DW, Safai C, Goffinet DR. Malignant obstructive jaundice. Treatment with external-beam and intracavitary radiotherapy. Int J Radiat Oncol Biol Phys 1985;11:411–6.
210. Mornex F, Ardiet JM, Bret P, Gerard JP. Radiotherapy of high bile duct carcinoma using intra-catheter iridium 192 wire. Cancer 1984;54:2069–73.
211. Hishikawa Y, Shimada T, Miura T, Imajyo Y. Radiation therapy of carcinoma of the extrahepatic bile ducts. Radiology 1983;146:787–9.
212. Busse PM, Stone MD, Sheldon TA, et al. Intraoperative radiation therapy for biliary tract carcinoma: results of a 5-year experience. Surgery 1989;105:724–33.
213. Iwasaki Y, Todoroki T, Fukao K, et al. The role of intraoperative radiation therapy in the treatment of bile duct cancer. World J Surg 1988;12:91–8.
214. Oberfield RA, Ross RL. The role of chemotherapy in the treatment of bile duct cancer. World J Surg 1988;12:105–8.
215. Nunnerley HB. Interventional radiology and internal radiotherapy for bile duct tumors. In: Preece PE, Cushieri A, Rosin RD, editors. Cancer of the bile ducts and pancreas. Philadelphia: WB Saunders; 1989. p. 93.

90

Neoplasms of the Exocrine Pancreas

Robert A. Wolff, MD
Christopher H. Crane, MD
Donghui Li, PhD
James L. Abbruzzese, MD, FACP
Douglas B. Evans, MD

INTRODUCTION

Pancreatic cancer is the fourth leading cause of cancer-related death for both men and women (following lung, colon, and breast cancer) and is responsible for 5% of all cancer-related deaths.[1] In 2004, adenocarcinoma of the exocrine pancreas accounted for approximately 31,800 deaths in the United States.[1] Because of the frequent inability to diagnose pancreatic cancer when it is still localized and surgically resectable and the very aggressive biologic behavior of this disease, the incidence rates (32,180 in 2004) are virtually the same as the mortality rates. Exocrine pancreatic cancer is characterized by early vascular dissemination and spread to regional lymph nodes; subclinical liver or lung metastases are present in most patients at the time of diagnosis, even when findings from imaging studies are normal.

Survival duration depends on the extent of disease and the patient's performance status at diagnosis. The extent of disease is best categorized as resectable (stage I or II), locally advanced (stage III), or metastatic (stage IV); the AJCC Cancer Staging Manual has been appropriately modified to reflect the emphasis on stage-specific treatment planning and the understanding that most patients are not surgically staged.[2] Patients who undergo surgical resection for localized nonmetastatic adenocarcinoma of the pancreatic head have a long-term survival rate of approximately 20% and a median survival of 18 to 24 months.[3,4] It is common for disease to recur following pancreaticoduodenectomy; in patients who undergo an incomplete surgical resection or surgery without adjuvant therapy, local recurrence may occur in over 50% of patients, peritoneal recurrence in 25%, and liver metastases in 50%.[5–7] Survival duration is superior in patients who receive preoperative or postoperative chemoradiation therapy.[3,4] However, when multimodality therapy is used to maximize local–regional tumor control, distant disease in the liver (and less commonly in lung and bone) becomes the dominant form of tumor recurrence.[3,8]

Patients with locally advanced, nonmetastatic pancreatic cancer have a median survival of 6 to 12 months. A survival advantage has been seen for patients with locally advanced disease treated with chemoradiation therapy compared with no treatment or radiation therapy alone.[9,10] However, because patients with locally advanced pancreatic cancer are a heterogeneous population, it is difficult to complete phase II and phase III studies that utilize survival as a primary endpoint. Patients with metastatic disease have a short survival (3–6 months), the length of which depends on the extent of disease and performance status.

In this chapter, we will review the current literature relevant to the diagnosis and treatment of pancreatic cancer. The diagnostic algorithms emphasize the use of state-of-the-art computed tomography (CT) and the rapidly evolving technique of endoscopic ultrasound (EUS). We will also discuss protocol-based clinical trials, which often involve novel treatments developed as a result of our improved understanding of the molecular mechanisms involved in tumorigenesis.

EPIDEMIOLOGY

The risk of pancreatic cancer is low in the first three to four decades of life but increases sharply after age 50 years, with most patients between the ages of 60 and 80 years at diagnosis.[11] Nonetheless, although pancreatic cancer is uncommon in patients under 40 years of age, apparently, sporadic adenocarcinoma of pancreatic origin does occur in patients younger than 30 years. In the past, pancreatic cancer was more common in men than women, but now the incidence is about the same for both sexes, probably as a result of the increased use of tobacco by women.[1]

Pancreatic cancer incidence and mortality statistics are similar throughout the world. Incidence rates are highest in industrialized societies and western countries. In Europe, rates are highest in the Nordic countries.[11] In the United States, rates are particularly high in native Hawaiians, African Americans, and Korean Americans, with the highest rates in African Americans. The fact that the rates in African Americans are considerably higher than in native Africans suggests an environmental influence. The reasons for the slight regional and ethnic differences in the incidence of pancreatic cancer are unknown, but this may be due to a trend toward a decline in tobacco use in certain groups and regions.[12] Unfortunately, these broad epidemiologic categories do little to identify specific individuals at high risk of pancreatic cancer.

Etiologic Factors An association between diabetes mellitus and pancreatic cancer has long been known, but the precise mechanism has yet to be defined, and not all studies have supported such a relationship.[13] Diabetes mellitus has been implicated both as an early manifestation of pancreatic cancer and as a predisposing factor.[14–19] Related to this is the observation that pancreatic adenocarcinoma of duct cell origin can induce peripheral insulin resistance.[20] In addition, a putative cancer-associated diabetogenic factor has been isolated from the conditioned medium of pancreatic cancer cell lines and from patient serum.[21] From the standpoint of clinical observations, a recent cohort study showed that patients were at increased risk of pancreatic cancer after an initial hospitalization for diabetes, and this risk persisted for more than a decade.[14] Further, the researchers found that the risk of pancreatic cancer in diabetics decreased with the duration of diabetes and was limited to patients who had non-insulin-dependent diabetes or patients whose diabetes was diagnosed at age 40 years or older. In contrast, a meta-analysis of studies published between 1975 and 1994 showed that pancreatic cancer occurred with increased frequency in patients with long-standing diabetes (diabetes diagnosed at least 5 years prior to the diagnosis of pancreatic cancer or death due to pancreatic cancer).[22] Recent cohort studies have shown that abnormal glucose metabolism may be associated with an increased risk of pancreatic cancer.[23,24] Impaired glucose tolerance, insulin resistance, and secondary hyperinsulinism is associated with obesity and inactivity. Positive associations between obesity and pancreatic cancer risk have been reported in several large prospective studies.[24,25] High insulin concentrations in the microenvironment of the pancreatic duct cell may contribute to malignant transformation.[26] In a widely quoted case-control study, the risk of pancreatic cancer was lower in individuals who ate only one meal per day, possibly because of decreased insulin secretion.[27]

Although an association between pancreatitis and an increased risk of pancreatic cancer has also long been suspected, the magnitude of the risk remains uncertain. Older clinical studies suggested that chronic forms of pancreatitis were most closely associated with the development of pancreatic cancer.[28,29] A later retrospective cohort study of 2,015 patients from six countries also demonstrated an increased risk of pancreatic cancer in patients with chronic pancreatitis, with the cumulative incidence of pancreatic cancer increasing with the longer duration of follow-up.[30] Similar observations were made by Talamini and colleagues,[31,32] who studied 715 patients with chronic pancreatitis diagnosed between 1971 and 1995. Chronic pancreatitis patients had a 13- to 18-fold increase in the incidence of pancreatic cancer. Pancreatic cancer was found in 12 patients (1.7%) early (7–42 months) after the diagnosis of chronic pancreatitis and in another 12 patients more than 4 years after the diagnosis of chronic pancreatitis. When the two groups of patients with pancreatic cancer were compared with patients with chronic pancreatitis in whom cancer did not develop, the 12 patients in whom pancreatic cancer developed early after the diagnosis of pancreatitis were older, had a lower percentage of males, infrequently used tobacco and alcohol, and were more likely to be noninsulin-dependent diabetics than were patients in the other two groups. However, patients in whom pancreatic cancer developed late after the diagnosis of chronic pancreatitis could not be distinguished from the patients with chronic pancreatitis without cancer. The authors therefore hypothesized that the cancer causes pancreatitis in some cases (as may be the case with hyperglycemia) and emphasized that, for this reason, cancer should be strongly considered in a patient diagnosed with idiopathic chronic pancreatitis without a history of significant alcohol or tobacco use, especially in the context of hyperglycemia.[31] Somewhat in contrast, however, were the findings of Karlson and colleagues,[33] who identified 230 patients with pancreatic cancer among 29,530 patients in the Swedish national registry discharged 1 year or more after a hospital admission for pancreatitis. Although they found that the standardized incidence ratio (observed/expected) for the development of pancreatic cancer was increased in patients with pancreatitis (2.8; 95% confidence interval, 2.5–3.2), unlike the findings in other studies, after 10 years or more, the excess risk declined and was of borderline significance. The authors concluded that their data thus did not support a causal association between pancreatitis and pancreatic cancer; instead, alcohol consumption and smoking were thought to contribute significantly to the increased cancer risk associated with chronic pancreatitis.

It is also possible, however, that it is the type of pancreatitis that determines the risk of pancreatic cancer. For example, the incidence of pancreatic adenocarcinoma is thought to be increased in patients with hereditary pancreatitis. This type of pancreatitis has an autosomal dominant pattern of transmission with 80% penetrance,[34] and symptoms usually arise by age 40 years, but can occur before age 5 years. To examine the possibility of a connection, Lowenfels and colleagues[35] obtained data on 246 patients with hereditary pancreatitis from pancreatologists in 10 countries. They concluded on the basis of their findings that the estimated cumulative risk of pancreatic cancer developing by age 70 was approximately 40% in this patient population. The mean age at the development of pancreatic cancer was 57 years. Further support for these clinical findings has been provided by recent molecular data strongly suggesting that mutations in the cationic trypsinogen gene play an important role in hereditary and possibly acquired forms of pancreatitis, which would increase the risk of pancreatic cancer.[36] To prevent autodigestion, pancreatic enzymes are secreted as inactive proenzymes. Within the intestinal lumen, trypsinogen is hydrolyzed to (active) trypsin, which then activates the remaining pancreatic enzymes. Multiple defense mechanisms are in place to prevent premature enzyme activation, including the presence of a cationic trypsin cleavage site within the trypsinogen molecule. If trypsin is activated within the pancreatic acinar cell, this feedback mechanism should inactivate wild-type trypsinogen. In hereditary pancreatitis, however, a single amino acid substitution inactivates the cationic trypsin cleavage site, causing uncontrolled trypsin activation and pancreatic autodigestion.

Selected inherited cancer syndromes are also associated with an increased risk of pancreatic cancer.[37] One of these is hereditary breast-ovarian cancer syndrome, which is associated with mutations in *BRCA1* or *BRCA2*. *BRCA2* is a tumor suppressor gene on chromosome 13q12 and its protein product is involved in the repair of DNA strand breaks. Germline mutations in the *BRCA2* gene have been found in 10% of patients with familial pancreatic cancer and in 7% of patients thought to have had sporadic pancreatic cancer.[38,39] Such germline *BRCA2* mutations represent the most common inherited predisposition to pancreatic cancer and are associated with an up to 10 times greater risk of pancreatic cancer than exists in the general population.[40] Another inherited cancer syndrome associated with pancreatic cancer is the Peutz-Jeghers syndrome, which is inherited as an autosomal dominant trait and is caused by mutations in the *LKB1/STK11* tumor suppressor gene on chromosome 19p13. The syndrome is characterized by the presence of hamartomatous gastrointestinal polyps and mucocutaneous pigmentation and is associated with an increased risk of several gastrointestinal cancers. Although patients with Peutz-Jeghers syndrome are at significant risk of pancreatic cancer, the exact magnitude of the risk is unclear. Interestingly, biallelic inactivation of the *LKB1/STK11* gene was also found in 4% of patients with resected sporadic pancreatic cancers.[41] The familial atypical multiple-mole melanoma (FAMMM) syndrome is a rare autosomal dominant disorder with incomplete penetrance caused by germline mutations in the *p16* tumor suppressor gene on chromosome 9p21 and is associated with the development of multiple nevi, including malignant melanoma. FAMM-pancreatic carcinoma (FAMM-PC) is the new term for the form of FAMMM associated with pancreatic cancer.[42] Both early-onset and late-onset pancreatic cancer have been seen in affected families. Hereditary nonpolyposis colon cancer is an autosomal dominant condition caused by germline mutations in mismatch repair genes resulting in an increased risk of both colorectal cancer and other cancers, including cancer of the breast, endometrium, ovary, and pancreas. The magnitude of the increased risk of pancreatic cancer is not clear, however.

Familial pancreatic cancer kindreds have also been identified that are not affected by an inherited cancer syndrome or familial pancreatitis. At-risk patients for familial pancreatic cancer include those with a minimum of two first-degree relatives with pancreatic cancer.[43] A recent report of an ongoing study of a well-known family with familial pancreatic cancer suggests that the susceptibility locus for autosomal dominant pancreatic cancer is on chromosome 4q32-34.[44]

Recent data also suggest an association between *Helicobacter pylori* infection and pancreatic cancer.[45,46] *H. pylori* may result in subclinical pancreatitis (a risk factor of pancreatic cancer as previously discussed) and can increase gastrin levels, which have a trophic effect on the pancreas. In addition, given that the gastric carriage of *H. pylori* is a known risk factor for peptic ulcer formation and gastric cancer, this may explain the association between gastric resection and pancreatic cancer.[47] At variance with this observation is a recent necropsy-based, case-control study performed in Malmo, Sweden, that found no relationship between the development of pancreatic cancer and a remote history of gastric resection.[48] In this study, 439 patients who died of pancreatic cancer and underwent autopsy between 1970 and 1982 were compared with a randomly chosen control group matched for age, gender, and year of death and with 1,337 patients who died of lung cancer. A previous gastric resection had been performed in 3.4% of those who died of pancreatic cancer, in 4.4% of controls, and in 7.6% of those who died of lung cancer. The authors suggested that the relationship between gastric resection and pancreatic cancer is confounded by smoking (a risk factor for peptic ulcer disease, pancreatic cancer, and lung cancer).

Environmental Factors The risk factor most firmly associated with pancreatic cancer is cigarette smoking.[49–52] In animals, pancreatic malignancies can be induced through the long-term administration of tobacco-specific *N*-nitrosamines or the parenteral administration of other *N*-nitroso compounds.[53,54] These carcinogens are metabolized to electrophiles that readily react with DNA, leading to the miscoding and activation of oncogenes. Numerous US and European case-control and cohort studies have shown an increased risk of pancreatic cancer in smokers; indeed, it is currently estimated that approximately 25% of cases of pancreatic cancer are due to cigarette smoking.[55] Recent studies have also shown that the risk of pancreatic cancer increases as the amount and duration of smoking increase and that long-term smoking cessation

(> 10 years) reduces the risk by approximately 30% relative to the risk in current smokers.[51,55] The detection of carcinogen-DNA adducts in human pancreas tissues and tobacco-specific compounds in pancreatic juice further confirm the link between cigarette smoking and pancreatic cancer.[56,57] Recent molecular epidemiological studies have also shown that individual variability in carcinogen metabolism and DNA repair may partially determine the susceptibility to smoking-related pancreatic cancer.[58–60] Information generated from such studies may facilitate the development of chemoprevention strategies.

Various dietary factors have also been implicated in the development of pancreatic cancer. Generally, high intakes of fat or meat increase the risk, whereas high intakes of fruits and vegetables reduce the risk.[61–63] A recent case-control study further suggested that the method of meat preparation as well as the total intake are also important determinants.[64] They focused on well-done, barbecued meat because it contains potential carcinogens such as heterocyclic amines and polycyclic aromatic hydrocarbons, compounds not found in meat prepared in other ways. In that study, Anderson and colleagues studied the association between pancreatic cancer and barbecued meat intake in patients and controls in Minnesota. They found that barbecued meat intake was indeed statistically significant as a predictor of pancreatic cancer risk. Broiled meat and the total amount of meat consumed did not show a statistically significant association with pancreatic cancer risk. Interestingly, however, more patients than controls reported current cigarette smoking and a history of diabetes, which could represent confounding factors.[64] Diets high in salt, dehydrated foods, fried foods, refined sugars, or soybeans may also increase the risk of pancreatic cancer.[11] Decreased pancreatic cancer rates have been associated with the high consumption of vegetables, citrus fruits, fiber, and vitamin C.[63] The protective effects of these food items may have been mediated through folate as indicated by findings from a study of male smokers that the dietary folate intake and serum folate levels were inversely associated with the risk of pancreatic cancer.[65,66] The recent observation that limonene, a natural product found in citrus fruits, is a potent inhibitor of the K-ras oncoprotein[67] makes the association of diets high in citrus fruits with a reduced risk of pancreatic cancer particularly interesting. The data on coffee consumption and excessive alcohol consumption appear conflicting. A few studies have suggested that these factors (coffee, alcohol) are associated with an increased risk of pancreatic cancer, but most studies conducted over the past 15 years have failed to consistently demonstrate such a risk.[63,68,69]

Exposures to some chemicals, usually in a farming or manufacturing setting, have also been associated with an increased risk of pancreatic cancer.[70] Older studies implicated 2-naphthylamine, benzidine, and derivatives of gasoline, but more recent studies have implicated chlorohydrin, aromatic hydrocarbons, and acrylamide.[68] A cohort mortality study of more than 5,000 chemical manufacturing workers suggested that heavy and prolonged exposure to DDT[71] and related compounds[72] also causes pancreatic cancer. Finally, specific occupations (eg, stone miners, cement workers, gardeners, and textile workers) have also been associated with an increased risk of pancreatic cancer, although the specific causative factors or carcinogens responsible for this increase are unclear.[73]

In summary, cigarette smoking may be responsible for causing as many as 25% of the cases of pancreatic cancer, and obesity, inactivity, and diet may be responsible for an additional 15%.[26] Therefore, it is possible that as many as 40% of pancreatic cancer cases are preventable. The exact percentage of pancreatic cancer cases attributable to the inherited pancreatic cancer syndromes discussed above is much smaller, but is unknown at present. However, such high-risk patients are the focus of intense research into the pathophysiology of pancreatic tumorigenesis as well as into ways to prevent the disease. The management of such individuals remains extremely controversial; options range from close observation to aggressive surgical intervention. The optimal surveillance and surgical strategies are rapidly evolving.[74–77]

PATHOLOGY

HISTOPATHOLOGY The normal architecture of the pancreas is typical of the architecture of a secretory gland. A background of acinar cells accounts for approximately 80% of the cell number and volume of the gland; clusters of islet cells account for 1 to 2%; single-layered, cuboidal ductal cells make up 10 to 15%; and there is a sparse interlacing network of blood vessels, lymphatics, nerves, and collagenous stroma. In carcinoma, this architecture is markedly altered: The predominant histologic feature is a dense collagenous stroma with atrophic acini, remarkably preserved islet cell clusters, and a slight-to-moderate increase in the number of ducts, both normal-appearing and cancerous. The diagnosis of ductal adenocarcinoma rests on the identification of mitoses, nuclear and cellular pleomorphism, discontinuity of ductal epithelium, and evidence of perineural, vascular, or lymphatic invasion.[78]

The infiltration of perineural spaces is characteristic of pancreatic adenocarcinoma.[79,80] This is an important consideration because the superior mesenteric artery (SMA) is surrounded by a neural plexus that provides visceral innervation to the small intestine. This neural plexus extends proximally to the celiac ganglion, which surrounds the aorta at and above the level of the celiac artery. Not surprisingly, therefore, infiltration of this mesenteric neural plexus is characteristic of pancreatic adenocarcinoma once it involves the SMA. For this reason, extended pancreatic resection that requires arterial resection typically fails to achieve a negative margin (because the celiac ganglion is commonly infiltrated) and has not been demonstrated to improve survival duration.[81]

Table 90-1 Histologic Classification of Tumors of the Exocrine Pancreas

Malignant
Carcinoma in situ (PanIn III; pancreatic intraepithelial neoplasia)
Ductal adenocarcinoma*
Intraductal papillary mucinous carcinoma (invasive IPMN)
Mucinous cystadenocarcinoma
Acinar cell carcinoma
Pancreatoblastoma
Premalignant
Intraductal papillary-mucinous neoplasm (noninvasive IPMN)†
Mucinous cystadenoma
Uncertain malignant potential
Solid pseudopapillary tumor
Benign
Serous cystadenoma‡

*Variants include adenosquamous carcinoma, mucinous adenocarcinoma, signet ring cell carcinoma, and undifferentiated carcinoma (spindle cell, giant cell, and small cell types).

†Previous names include intraductal mucin-hypersecreting neoplasm, duct ectatic mucinous cystadenoma or carcinoma, and mucinous ductal ectasia.

‡May exhibit uncontrolled local tumor growth, causing the designation "benign" to be questioned.

Almost all malignant neoplasms of pancreatic origin (95%) arise from the exocrine portion of the gland and have light microscopic features consistent with those of adenocarcinomas.[78] Tumors arising from the islets of Langerhans (endocrine) cells of the pancreas are much less common, and primary nonepithelial tumors of the pancreas (eg, lymphomas or sarcomas) are extremely rare. A current view of the histologic classification of exocrine pancreatic neoplasms is presented in Table 90-1. Although the origin of pancreatic adenocarcinomas from the ductal epithelium is generally accepted, identifying the cell of origin of pancreatic adenocarcinoma remains an active area of research.

MOLECULAR PATHOLOGY Studies of archival human pancreatic tumor tissue and human pancreatic cancer cell lines have identified several characteristic genetic abnormalities associated with pancreatic cancer. In particular, specific point mutations have been found at codon 12 of the K-*ras* oncogene, located on chromosome 12p13, in 75 to 90% of pancreatic adenocarcinoma specimens.[82,83] The ras protein is an important signal-transduction mediator for receptor protein tyrosine kinases.[84] Transforming mutations of *ras* are resistant to the GTPase-activating function of GTPase-activating proteins and result in a constitutively active ras protein, unregulated cellular proliferation signals, and susceptibility to transformation. All ras proteins are produced in the cytoplasm as biologically inactive precursor molecules and must undergo post-translational enzymatic modification for them to localize to the membrane, which is necessary for them to exert full biologic activity. The enzyme farnesyl-protein transferase catalyzes the first of a series of steps necessary for the translocation of the ras protein to the cell membrane. Because of the role of this enzyme, inhibitors of farnesyl-protein transferase have been developed and are being studied in patients with pancreatic cancer.[84] Mutations in the K-*ras* oncogene are thought to be an early event in the transformation of normal duct epithelium,[85] and preliminary data suggest that K-*ras* may be the site of action of environmental carcinogens such as cigarette smoke or organochlorine compounds.[86,87] The detection of mutant K-*ras* in body fluids and biopsy specimens is also currently being explored as a technique for the early diagnosis of pancreatic cancer in selected patients.[87,88]

In the progression model of pancreatic cancer proposed by Hruban and colleagues,[85] inactivation of the *p16* tumor suppressor gene is thought to occur after the mutation in K-*ras*. The p16 protein, whose gene is located on chromosome 9p21, belongs to a class of cyclin-dependent kinase (Cdk)-inhibitory proteins (including p21/WAF1/Cip1) and inhibits the cyclin D_1/Cdk-4 complex that normally acts to phosphorylate the retinoblastoma (Rb) protein. Phosphorylation of Rb results in the release of transcription factors that promote the transcription of genes necessary for progression through the G_1 phase of the cell cycle. Therefore, inactivation of *p16* leads to hyperphosphorylated Rb that, in turn, leads to unregulated cell growth. Abrogation of the Rb/p16 pathway can also result from inactivation of the *RB1* gene or the overexpression of cyclin D_1 or Cdk-4. In approximately 95% of pancreatic carcinomas, the Rb/p16 pathway is inactivated when the *p16* gene is inactivated as the result of homozygous deletion, the loss of one allele combined with an intragenic mutation in the other, or hypermethylation of the promotor of the *p16* gene.[89–92] Germline mutations in the *p16* tumor suppressor gene are associated with the newly described FAMM-PC syndrome discussed previously.

Loss of the *TP53*, *DPC4*, and possibly *BRCA2* tumor suppressor genes is thought to occur late in the development of pancreatic cancer.[85] The *TP53* gene is the most commonly mutated gene in human cancer. This tumor suppressor gene, located on chromosome 17p13, regulates progression through the cell cycle and induction of cell death. Following DNA damage, TP53 protein levels increase because of post-translational changes in protein stability. These increased TP53 protein levels lead to the transcriptional activation of $p21^{WAF1/CIP1}$, which inhibits cyclin-dependent kinase activity and prevents cell-cycle progression from the G_1 phase to the S phase.[93] In addition to its effect on the cell cycle, *TP53* also modulates apoptosis in response to DNA damage through the transcriptional activation of additional genes.[94] Seventy percent of pancreatic adenocarcinomas show loss of *TP53* function.[95,96] Inactivation of *TP53* function occurs through the loss of one p53 allele and the mutational inactivation of the other. Mutations in the *TP53* gene are more frequently seen in poorly differentiated tumors.[96]

The *SMAD4/DPC4* tumor suppressor gene on chromosome 18q21 is an important component of the transforming growth factor-β signaling pathway that normally down-regulates the growth of epithelial cells, stimulates differentiation, and promotes apoptosis.[97,98] Loss of this important growth regulatory pathway contributes to unregulated cell growth.[99,100] The *DPC4* gene is inactivated in approximately 55% of human pancreatic tumors as the result of homozygous deletion or the loss of one allele coupled with an intragenic mutation in the second allele.[101] A recent study examined the immunohistochemical features of *SMAD4* expression as a prognostic factor in patients with resected pancreatic adenocarcinoma. The presence of *SMAD4* expression in the tumor was associated with a median survival advantage of 5 months.[102] The ability to restore (and possibly overexpress) *DPC4* function in human pancreatic cancer cells remains an active area of investigation because of its obvious therapeutic implications.[103,104]

Exactly how the known molecular alterations in human pancreatic cancer interact during pancreatic carcinogenesis is still unclear. In addition to these molecular alterations, the metastatic potential of solid tumors has also been shown to correlate with the status of several independent genes that regulate growth factor receptors, angiogenesis, invasion, and multidrug resistance. An increased understanding of these molecular alterations may lead to new treatment strategies that correct these alterations and to an improved knowledge of the relative roles of these changes in pancreatic cancer biology. Although the advances in genomic and proteomic technology are revealing new and exciting targets for therapy, they also are increasingly demonstrating the complex nature of tumorigenesis and metastasis. For additional information on the molecular genetics of pancreatic cancer, the reader is referred to recent comprehensive reviews.[85,105,106]

SYMPTOM PATTERNS

Virtually all patients with periampullary neoplasms and approximately 50% of patients with pancreatic cancer have jaundice at diagnosis as the result of extrahepatic biliary obstruction. Tumors arising in the ampulla of Vater or within the intrapancreatic portion of the common bile duct cause biliary obstruction early in the disease course and, therefore, may be associated with a better prognosis. Small tumors of the pancreatic head strategically located near the intrapancreatic portion of the bile duct also may obstruct the bile duct and cause the patient to seek medical attention while the tumor is still localized and potentially resectable. In contrast, adenocarcinomas arising in the pancreas that do not obstruct the intrapancreatic portion of the bile duct are often not diagnosed until they are locally advanced or metastatic. In the absence of extrahepatic biliary obstruction, few pancreatic cancer patients present with potentially resectable disease.

If jaundice is not present, patient complaints are often nonspecific, as are the clinical signs on physical examination. The pain typical of locally advanced pancreatic cancer is a dull, fairly constant pain of visceral origin localized to the middle and upper back; the pain is due to tumor invasion of the celiac and mesenteric plexus. Some patients have vague, intermittent epigastric pain; its etiology is less clear. Fatigue, weight loss, and anorexia are common even in the absence of mechanical gastric outlet obstruction. Pancreatic exocrine insufficiency, when present, is due to obstruction of the pancreatic duct and commonly results in malabsorption, steatorrhea, and mild changes in stool frequency. Although the pancreatic dust is obstructed in most patients, symptomatic diarrhea (because of the lack of pancreatic enzymes being released into the intestinal lumen) is uncommon. Many patients with pancreatic cancer have hyperglycemia as previously discussed in detail.

Important staging information that has direct implications for therapy can be obtained from the physical examination. This information includes performance status, cardiopulmonary function, and the presence or absence of left supraclavicular adenopathy and ascites.

DIAGNOSTIC EVALUATION

Imaging Biliary obstruction is usually evaluated with abdominal ultrasonography to confirm the mechanical nature of the obstruction and to determine whether the site of obstruction is the intrahepatic or extrahepatic portion of the biliary tree. Obstruction of the intrapancreatic portion of the bile duct is then evaluated with a combination of CT, EUS, and endoscopic retrograde cholangiopancreatography (ERCP). Our diagnostic schema for patients with suspected pancreatic cancer, (Figure 90-1), emphasizes the importance of high-quality CT.

High-quality CT can identify most pancreatic tumors and accurately define the relationship of the tumor to the celiac axis and superior mesenteric vessels.[107,108] The development of multislice or multidetector CT (MDCT) allows imaging of the entire pancreas during the bolus phase of contrast enhancement. In addition, scan data can be processed to display images in three-dimensional and multiplanar formats. Helical CT performed with contrast enhancement and a thin-section technique can accurately assess the relationship of the low-density tumor to the celiac axis, SMA, and superior mesenteric–portal vein (SMPV) confluence. For MDCT scanning at our institution, patients receive 1,000 mL of water or a 2% barium sulfate suspension (Readi-CAT; E-Z-EM, Inc., Westbury, NY) to opacify the stomach and small bowel. Noncontrast-enhanced CT scans are then obtained through the liver and pancreas at a slice thickness of 5 mm, contiguous, to localize the pancreas. Intravenous (IV) contrast enhancement is achieved with nonionic contrast material (300–320 mg iodine/mL) administered by an automatic injector at a rate of 3 to 5 mL/sec for a total of 150 mL. At least two phases of

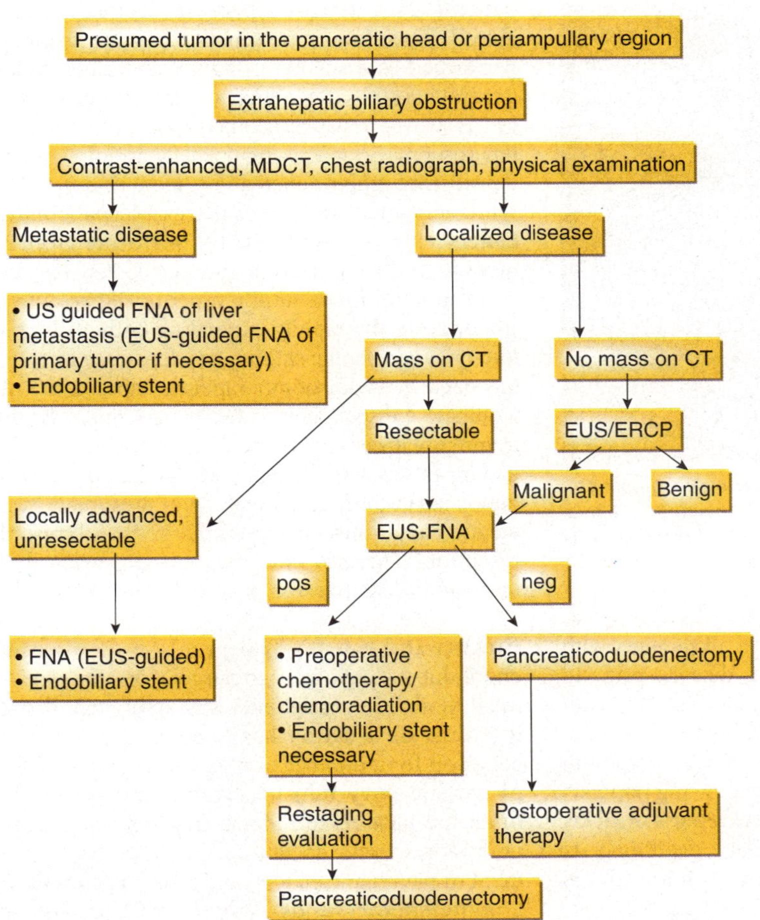

Figure 90-1 Management algorithm employed at our institution for patients with suspected or biopsy-proven adenocarcinoma of the pancreatic head. Accurate radiographic imaging allows patients to be staged as having resectable, locally advanced, or metastatic disease. In patients with locally advanced or metastatic disease, biopsy confirmation of malignancy is mandatory prior to the initiation of specific anticancer therapy. Similarly, before the initiation of neoadjuvant therapy cytologic confirmation of malignancy is required. The development of endoscopic ultrasound (EUS)-guided fine-needle aspiration (FNA) has greatly simplified tissue acquisition for patients with localized, nonmetastatic pancreatic cancer. In patients without cytologic evidence of malignancy (negative biopsy) in whom clinical and radiographic evidence support the diagnosis of a pancreatic or periampullary cancer, we proceed directly to pancreaticoduodenectomy (followed by postoperative adjuvant therapy if indicated). Laparoscopy should be considered prior to opening the abdomen in patients with potentially resectable disease; however, we rarely perform laparoscopy as a separate staging procedure. CT = computed tomography; ERCP = endoscopic retrograde cholangiopancreatography.

contrast-enhanced helical scanning are performed. The first (arterial) phase begins 25 seconds after contrast injection and is performed during a 20-second breathhold, with imaging done from the diaphragm through the horizontal portion of the duodenum at a slice thickness of 2.5 mm contiguous, reconstructed to 1.25 mm slice thickness for multiplanar reconstructions. Imaging during the first phase through the pancreas is done at 35 to 45 seconds after contrast injection, which, at this rate of contrast injection, optimizes the difference in density between the pancreas and tumor. The second (venous) phase, which is done to look for metastases in the liver and abdomen, begins 55 seconds after the start of IV contrast injection and covers the entire liver and upper abdomen at a 5 mm slice thickness, which is then reconstructed to a 2.5 mm slice thickness.

For treatment planning, it is of critical importance to use standardized, objective radiologic criteria for preoperative tumor staging. The CT findings defining a potentially resectable pancreatic cancer (American Joint Committee on Cancer [AJCC] stages I or II) are (1) the absence of extrapancreatic disease, (2) a patent SMPV confluence (assuming it is technically possible to resect isolated involvement of the SMV or SMPV confluence), and (3) no direct tumor extension to the celiac axis or SMA (Figure 90-2). A patient is deemed to have locally advanced, unresectable disease (AJCC stage III) when CT images demonstrate tumor extension to the SMA or celiac axis or occlusion of the SMPV confluence (Figure 90-3). Limited arterial abutment (often referred to as borderline or marginally resectable) may be amenable to a multimodality treatment approach to include eventual surgery. However, in general, tumor extension to the celiac axis, common hepatic artery, or SMA should be considered a contraindication to immediate surgery. The accuracy of CT in predicting such unresectability is well established; it is not necessary to perform

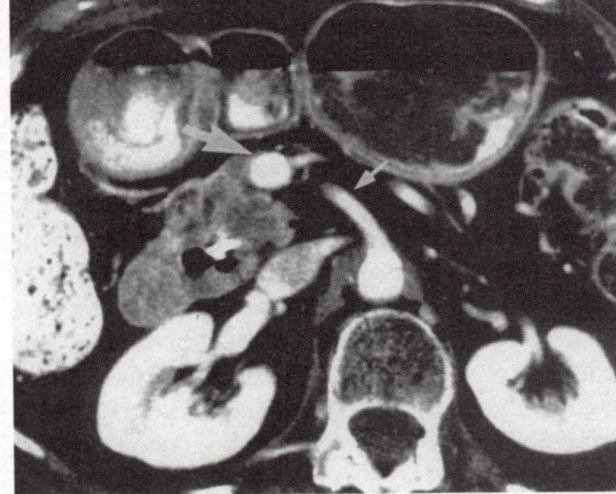

Figure 90-2 Contrast-enhanced computed tomorgraphy scan demonstrating a resectable adenocarcinoma of the pancreatic head. The low-density tumor is easily seen in the pancreatic head. Note the absence of tumor extension to the superior mesenteric artery (*small arrow*); there is a normal fat plane between the low-density tumor and the superior mesenteric artery. However, the tumor (area of low density) does extend to the superior mesenteric vein just inferior to the tip of the large arrow. This patient may require venous resection and reconstruction at the time of pancreaticoduodenectomy. This subtle finding would not be apparent on a lesser quality scan. The intrapancreatic portion of the common bile duct contains a stent that was endoscopically placed for biliary drainage.

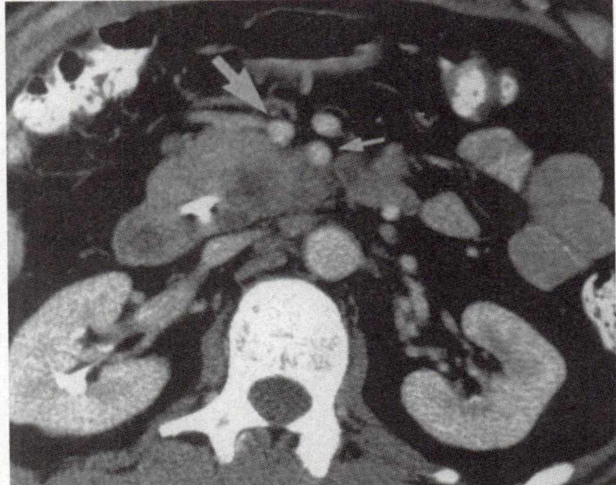

Figure 90-3 Contrast-enhanced computed tomography scan demonstrating an unresectable adenocarcinoma of the pancreatic head and uncinate process. The low-density tumor is inseparable from the posterior wall of the superior mesenteric artery (*small arrow*). Direct intraoperative assessment of the extent of retroperitoneal tumor growth in relation to the superior mesenteric artery is not possible until after gastric and pancreatic transection, at which point the surgeon has committed to resection; accurate preoperative imaging of this vital tumor–vessel relationship is thus critical. The large arrow identifies the superior mesenteric vein.

a laparotomy to assess local tumor respectability when arterial involvement is present.[109–111]

If a low-density mass is not seen on CT scans, patients with suspected pancreatic cancer should undergo upper endoscopy and EUS. Endoscopic evaluation may discover an ampullary tumor or related pathology, and EUS may define a mass in the pancreas or distal bile duct not seen on CT. When possible, upper endoscopy, EUS, and ERCP should always be performed after CT, because if endoscopy (ERCP or EUS-guided biopsy)-induced pancreatitis occurs, it may interfere with accurate assessment of the extent of disease. At the time of ERCP, a malignant obstruction of the intrapancreatic portion of the common bile duct is characterized by the double-duct sign (Figure 90-4), which indicates the proximal obstruction of the common bile and pancreatic ducts. A malignant obstruction can often be accurately differentiated from choledocholithiasis and the long, smooth, tapering bile duct stricture seen in chronic pancreatitis (Figure 90-5). We routinely place endoscopic stents to prevent cholangitis in patients with extrahepatic biliary obstruction who undergo diagnostic ERCP. We also place endoscopic stents in patients with elevated bilirubin levels in whom surgery is expected to be delayed, including those who are enrolled in preoperative chemoradiation therapy protocols. When ERCP is performed for the sole purpose of placing an endobiliary stent (in patients with an easily visible tumor on CT), the risk of complications can probably be reduced by not cannulating the pancreatic duct.

EUS-guided fine-needle aspiration (FNA) is currently the procedure of choice for obtaining a

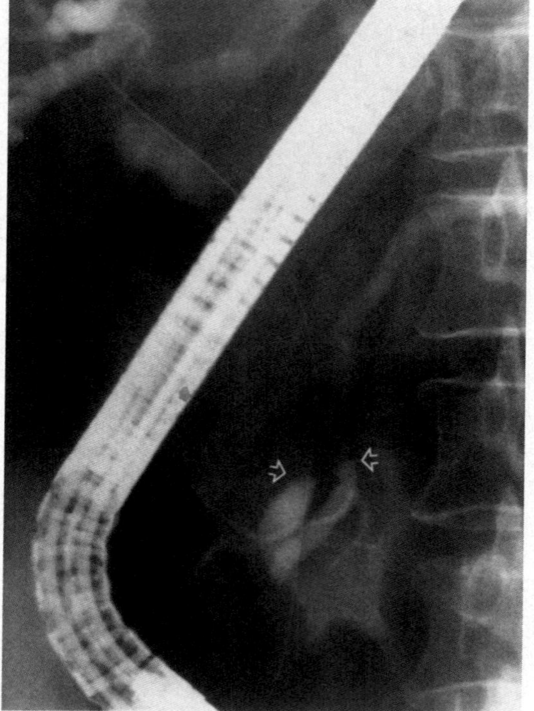

Figure 90-4 Endoscopic retrograde cholangiopancreatography demonstrating the classic double-duct sign seen with adenocarcinoma of the pancreatic head. The open arrows identify the common bile and pancreatic ducts, which are obstructed by the pancreatic cancer.

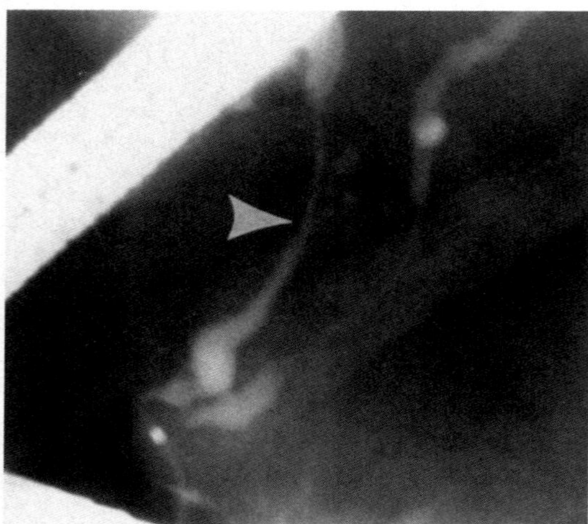

Figure 90-5 Endoscopic retrograde cholangiopancreatography demonstrating the smooth tapering common bile duct stricture (*arrowhead*) seen with biliary obstruction secondary to chronic pancreatitis.

cytologic diagnosis of a malignancy.[112] Confirmation of malignancy is required in all patients with locally advanced or metastatic disease prior to treatment with systemic therapy or external beam radiation therapy (EBRT) and is being done more commonly in patients with localized, potentially resectable disease because of the growing popularity of neoadjuvant therapy. Recent reports of EUS-guided FNA of the pancreas have described its accuracy and safety.[112,113] When FNA material is examined by an experienced cytopathologist, false-positive results should not occur; however, false-negative results may occur, especially when small tumors are involved. Therefore, negative results from EUS-guided FNA should not be considered definite proof that a malignancy does not exist. Further, in a patient who presents with extrahepatic biliary obstruction, a malignant-appearing stricture of the intrapancreatic portion of the common bile duct, and no history of recurrent pancreatitis or alcohol abuse, the absence of a mass on CT or EUS images should not be grounds for ruling out a carcinoma of the pancreas or bile duct. Instead, the results of EUS, with or without FNA, should be considered in the context of the clinical picture and as a complement to CT and ERCP findings. Importantly, as discussed above, high-quality CT imaging should be performed before an FNA is attempted because of the risk of biopsy inducing pancreatitis, which would distort the pancreatic anatomy. Further, FNA biopsy should only be performed if a mass is identified; there is no place for blind biopsy of the pancreas.

For the past decade, laparoscopy has been performed in patients who have radiologic evidence of localized pancreatic cancer to detect extrapancreatic tumor not seen on CT scans, thereby limiting laparotomy to those patients who truly have localized disease.[114,115] However, the favorable initial experience with laparoscopy in the frequent identification of subclinical metastatic disease resulted from laparoscopy being done in the absence of high-quality contrast-enhanced CT. Other, more recent studies have suggested that CT occult extrapancreatic disease is found in only 4 to 13% of patients with tumors otherwise deemed resectable.[116] Therefore, at present, laparoscopy is rarely performed as a separate staging procedure under general anesthesia in patients with pancreatic cancer. However, most surgeons do routinely perform laparoscopy prior to a planned laparotomy when considering major pancreatic resection in patients with presumed localized, resectable pancreatic cancer; laparoscopy can be performed fairly quickly and may prevent the occasional patient from undergoing a nontherapeutic laparotomy. Importantly, the rapidly expanding body of literature on laparoscopic staging has drawn attention to the need to avoid nontherapeutic laparotomy. A fortunate consequence of the recent emphasis on minimally invasive surgery is the realization by clinicians that it is no longer acceptable to perform a major laparotomy in patients with presumed pancreatic cancer just to "explore" the possibility of resection. There is now general consensus that resectability be assessed prior to laparotomy.

Biliary Drainage The practice of placing endobiliary stents prior to surgery or other treatment modalities in patients with malignant distal bile duct obstruction has become increasingly common for a number of reasons. First, the point of patient entry into the health care system is often the gastroenterologist, internist, or family practitioner, who do not specialize in the treatment of pancreatic cancer, and thus, may not have a contemporary understanding of the rapidly expanding stage-specific treatment options for patients with pancreatic cancer. In such situations, placement of a plastic biliary stent is a common way of relieving symptomatic (pruritus, anorexia, etc) jaundice. Second, for patients with potentially resectable disease, surgery is often delayed because of the referral of patients to high-volume centers for primary treatment or for a second opinion. Third, because most patients with pancreatic cancer have extrapancreatic metastatic disease (even if not apparent on imaging studies), there has been a greater emphasis on multidisciplinary treatment, including the delivery of chemotherapy or chemoradiation prior to surgery.

For patients who are believed to have locally advanced or metastatic pancreatic cancer based on the findings from noninvasive imaging studies or laparoscopy, the debate over the merits of surgical bypass versus endoscopic stenting has ended owing to the advent of the expandable metal stent. An endobiliary self-expandable covered metal stent has superior long-term patency compared with plastic stents.[117,118] However, certain groups of patients with symptomatic distal bile duct obstruction should *not* undergo endobiliary metal stent placement. Patients who present a diagnostic dilemma, such as those without an obvious mass in the head of the pancreas or with a history of pancreatitis, should have a plastic stent placed at the first endoscopic intervention in order to permit easy stent removal and additional diagnostic studies as needed. Though covered metal stents can also be removed endoscopically,[119] they should not be used to provide short-term biliary decompression. Therefore, those patients who require endobiliary decompression for only a few weeks prior to surgery, such as those who require detailed medical evaluation to optimize their preparation for major surgery, should undergo plastic stent placement. In addition, those patients with such a significant burden of metastatic disease that they are unlikely to survive beyond 2 months are also appropriate candidates for plastic stent insertion.

In patients who are brought to the operating room for a planned pancreaticoduodenectomy, but are found to have locally advanced or extrapancreatic metastatic disease, we prefer to remove the endobiliary stent and perform a biliary bypass. If an expandable metal stent is in place and the biliary bypass looks to be more difficult than usual, we may not perform an operative biliary bypass. Such situations may include, for example, tumor extension into the porta hepatic, or occlusion of the superior mesenteric or portal vein, resulting in cavernous transformation of the portal vein and extensive dilated collateral veins anterior to the bile duct. When operative biliary bypass is performed, we do not use the gallbladder for biliary decompression, and it should never be used for biliary decompression in the setting of acute or chronic gallbladder disease, cephalad tumor extension, or prolonged stent placement prior to surgery. A further consideration is that hypertrophy and fibrosis of the wall of the bile duct may make the cystic duct–common bile duct junction unsuitable for biliary decompression in patients with a previous endoscopic stent. Therefore, our choice for biliary bypass at the time of surgery is a Roux-en-Y choledochojejunostomy or hepaticojejunostomy. The gallbladder is removed and the common bile duct transected. The endoscopic stent, if present, is removed, the distal bile duct is closed, and an end-to-side choledochojejunostomy is created with a single layer of interrupted monofilament sutures.

At our institution, endoscopic stenting is performed on an outpatient basis in all patients who are not candidates for pancreaticoduodenectomy. In patients who have a life expectancy of less than 3 months (ie, those with a poor performance status or liver or peritoneal metastases), an 11.5-F polyethylene stent is placed. In all other patients a self-expanding covered metal stent is preferred. Patients in whom early stent occlusion or migration develops or who appear clinically to do poorly with endoscopic biliary decompression are quickly referred for operative biliary bypass. A multidisciplinary approach to these patients is critical, and it is essential that the medical oncologist, gastroenterologist, and surgeon communicate and avoid overly dogmatic approaches to palliative care.

TREATMENT OF LOCALIZED, POTENTIALLY RESECTABLE DISEASE

Surgery The accurate preoperative assessment of resectability (local and distant disease) is the most critical aspect of the diagnostic workup in patients with pancreatic cancer. Quality survival time will be greatly improved by avoiding nontherapeutic laparotomy in patients with unresectable pancreatic cancer. Indeed, laparotomy for those who undergo surgical exploration and are found to have unresectable disease is associated with a risk of perioperative morbidity, a hospital stay of at least 1 week, and a median survival after surgery of only 7 to 10 months. If the primary tumor cannot be resected completely (grossly complete resection), surgery for pancreatic cancer (pancreaticoduodenectomy) offers no survival advantage. Patients who undergo a gross incomplete resection have an expected median survival of less than 1 year, which is no different from the survival duration seen in patients with locally advanced, unresectable disease who undergo palliative chemotherapy and irradiation without surgery.[120] Therefore, in contrast to the situation in selected patients with gastric or colorectal cancer, there are no data supporting palliative (incomplete or grossly positive margins) resection for adenocarcinoma of the pancreas.

Owing to recent advances in operative technique, anesthesia, and critical care, the 30-day in-hospital mortality rate is 2% or less in patients who undergo pancreaticoduodenectomy performed by experienced surgeons.[4,121,122] Reported mortality rates from other institutions, including university centers and Department of Veterans Affairs hospitals, range from 7.8% to more than 10%.[123–125] Data from a study conducted by Birkmeyer and colleagues[126] have also demonstrated that higher hospital volume is associated with lower surgery-related mortality. The study population consisted of 10,530 Medicare patients older than 65 years who underwent pancreaticoduodenectomy at 1,868 hospitals from 1994 to 1999. The study population was divided into quintiles according to hospital volume: Very high volume centers were defined as those that performed greater than 16 pancreatic resections per year; high-volume hospitals, 6 to 16 per year; median-volume hospitals, 3 to 5 per year; low-volume hospitals, 1 to 2 per year; and very low volume hospitals, less than 1 per year. Twenty-seven (1.4%) very high volume hospitals performed 2,159 (21%) of the pancreatic resections, and 90 (4.8%) high-volume hospitals performed 2,166 (21%) of the pancreatic resections; 58% of the pancreatic resections were performed at very low, low-, or medium-volume hospitals, where the in-hospital or 30-day mortality was 16.3%, 14.6%, and 11%, respectively. In an analysis of survival duration, after excluding perioperative deaths and adjusting for the case mix, Birkmeyer and colleagues[127] found that patients who underwent surgery at high-volume hospitals were also less likely to experience late mortality. Translating volume-outcome data into public policy has not yet occurred with respect to pancreatic surgery; however, it seems appropriate that this information be made available to patients and that they be given the option of having their surgery at a high-volume center.

Pancreaticoduodenectomy The standard surgical procedure for neoplasms of the pancreatic head and periampullary region is pancreaticoduodenectomy, which involves removal of the pancreatic head, duodenum, gallbladder, and bile duct with or without the gastric antrum. The current technique of pancreaticoduodenectomy has evolved from the procedure first described by Whipple and colleagues[128] in 1935. Their two-stage pancreaticoduodenectomy consisted of biliary diversion and gastrojejunostomy during one operation, followed by resection of the duodenum and pancreatic head after the patient recovered from the earlier procedure (usually about 3 weeks later). By 1941, the world experience totaled 41 cases, with a perioperative mortality rate of 30%.[129] Before 1940, the pancreatic remnant was not reanastomosed to the small bowel, and the high mortality rate was largely because of the development of a pancreatic fistula from the oversewn pancreatic remnant. In 1941, Whipple modified his reconstruction to include a pancreaticojejunostomy, with the entire procedure done in one operation.[129]

Our recommended technique for pancreaticoduodenectomy utilizes a midline or bilateral subcostal incision. The abdomen is first carefully explored to exclude extrapancreatic metastatic disease. The liver and peritoneal surfaces are next examined, and sites of suspected liver or peritoneal metastatic lesions are biopsied, and the material submitted for frozen-section histologic analysis. We do not proceed with tumor resection when biopsy-proven liver or peritoneal metastases are found. In patients who have resectable disease, there is no indication for routine intraoperative pancreatic biopsy. One reason for this is that tumor cells can be disseminated in the peritoneum during surgical manipulation and intraoperative large-needle pancreatic biopsy.[130] In addition, intraoperative pancreatic biopsy may be associated with significant complications, such as pancreatitis, pancreatic fistula formation, and hemorrhage.[131] Nevertheless, because many surgeons perceive that preoperative EUS-FNA is unnecessary, patients who have presumed periampullary or pancreatic neoplasms are often brought to the operating room for a planned intraoperative diagnostic biopsy prior to extirpative surgery. If the frozen-section findings are negative, surgeons may not then proceed with tumor resection because they are concerned about unnecessarily performing such an extensive operation for benign disease.[131] Such situations may be avoided by understanding that the diagnosis of a malignant obstruction of the intrapancreatic portion of the common bile duct should always be accurately established preoperatively by high-quality CT, EUS, and ERCP. Unnecessary and preventable patient morbidity occurs when laparotomy and/or pancreatic biopsy are used as diagnostic studies because of the physician's failure to obtain state-of-the-art pretreatment imaging. Further, if a preoperative or intraoperative FNA result is benign or nondiagnostic, the patient may still have cancer, especially when the clinical presentation and imaging studies suggest a malignant mass or bile duct stricture.

Whether to perform lymph node biopsy for frozen-section analysis remains controversial. The reason for this is that even though positive lymph nodes are a prognostic factor (along with poorly differentiated histology, microscopically positive resection margins, etc.) that predicts decreased survival,[3,4] microscopic metastases are found in regional lymph nodes on permanent-section pathologic evaluation in 60 to 90% of patients who undergo pancreaticoduodenectomy. In a good-risk patient with localized, resectable pancreatic cancer, we do not currently view lymph node metastases as an absolute contraindication to pancreaticoduodenectomy when it is part of a combined-modality treatment approach.[81] Therefore, we do not generally perform random lymph node sampling for frozen-section analysis at the time of pancreaticoduodenectomy. However, each case should be considered individually; for example, when a patient is high-risk because of medical comorbid conditions or when there are oncologic concerns (such as a very high CA19-9 level) or suspicious adenopathy, a positive regional lymph node may be viewed as a contraindication to pancreaticoduodenectomy.

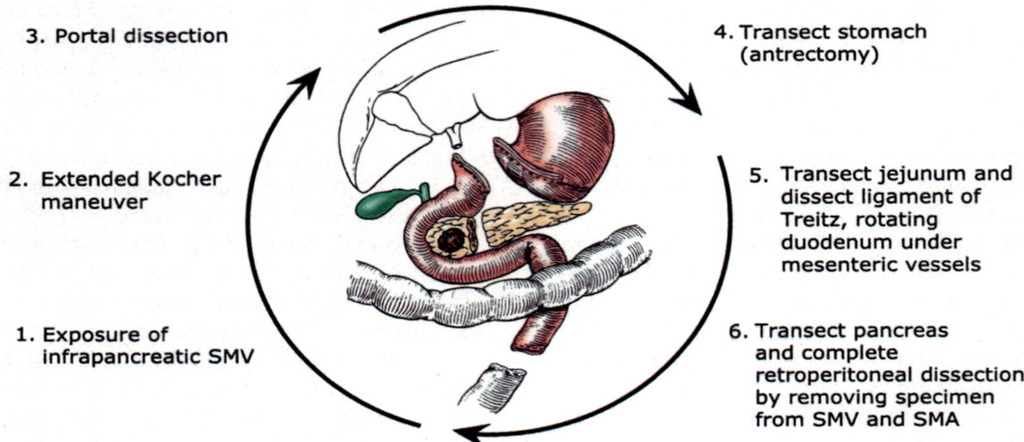

Figure 90-6 Six surgical steps of pancreaticoduodenectomy.

At the time of surgical exploration for a pancreatic head cancer, a Kocher maneuver is traditionally the first maneuver performed so that the tumor's relationship to the SMA can be determined. In this maneuver, by mobilizing the pancreatic head and duodenum from their retroperitoneal attachments, the surgeon attempts to palpate a plane of normal tissue between the firm tumor and the posterior pulsation of the SMA. The relationship of the tumor to the right lateral wall of the SMA is the most critical aspect of the pretreatment staging evaluation. We strongly believe, however, that this critical tumor–vessel relationship should be accurately evaluated by MDCT before the patient is taken to the operating room and that it cannot be accurately assessed intraoperatively following a Kocher maneuver. In the case of larger tumors, tumors with significant peritumoral fibrosis, and reoperation (following a previous unsuccessful attempt at pancreaticoduodenectomy), it is often impossible to determine by palpation the relationship of the primary tumor to the SMA (after mobilization of the duodenum) with any reasonable degree of accuracy. The second maneuver traditionally performed to assess resectability is to develop a plane of dissection between the anterior surface of the SMPV confluence and the posterior surface of the pancreatic neck to exclude tumor involvement of the SMV or SMPV confluence. Such tumor involvement precludes resection, in the opinion of most surgeons. However, the rationale for performing this maneuver early in the operation is also unclear because tumors of the pancreatic head or uncinate process are prone to invade the lateral or posterior wall of the SMPV confluence, but rarely involve the anterior wall when they do not encase of the celiac axis or SMA origin (as seen with locally advanced tumors of the pancreatic neck or body). The relationship of a pancreatic head tumor to the lateral and posterior walls of the SMPV confluence (and the SMA) can be directly seen only after gastric and pancreatic transection, at which point the surgeon has already committed to resection. Again, preoperative imaging using high-quality, contrast-enhanced MDCT can alert the surgeon to the possible need for venous resection and reconstruction.[122]

The technique of pancreaticoduodenectomy currently used in the United States incorporates selected aspects of the traditional Whipple procedure and emphasizes the importance of removing all soft tissue to the right of the SMA. The surgical resection is divided into six clearly defined steps (Figure 90-6); the most oncologically important and difficult part of the operation is step six, during which the pancreas is divided and the specimen is removed from the SMPV confluence and the right lateral border of the SMA. After traction sutures are placed on the superior and inferior borders of the pancreas, the pancreas is transected with electrocautery at the level of the portal vein. If tumor adheres to the portal vein or SMV, the pancreas can be divided more distally in preparation for segmental venous resection. The small venous tributaries to the uncinate process and pancreatic head are then ligated and divided so that the specimen can be separated from the SMPV. Only after full medial mobilization of the SMPV is it possible to identify the SMA (lateral to the SMV). The pancreatic head and all soft tissue to the right of the SMA are then removed by direct ligation of the inferior pancreaticoduodenal artery or arteries. Failure to fully mobilize the SMPV confluence risks injury to the SMA and usually results in a positive resection margin because of incomplete removal of the uncinate process and the mesenteric soft tissue adjacent to the SMA. Furthermore, if the SMPV confluence is not completely mobilized, one cannot expose the SMA, which is necessary for the inferior pancreaticoduodenal arteries to be directly ligated. Mass ligation of this vessel (or vessels) with surrounding mesenteric soft tissue is the major cause of postoperative retroperitoneal hemorrhage, as this vessel can retract from a poorly placed tie or ligature.

The high incidence of local recurrence after standard pancreaticoduodenectomy requires that close attention be paid to the retroperitoneal margin. The retroperitoneal margin (also referred to as the mesenteric margin) is the soft tissue margin along the right lateral border of the proximal SMA (Figure 90-7).[2] It is critical that this margin be identified for the pathologist and assessed histologically; the R status cannot be determined if the retroperitoneal margin is not assessed histologically. Perineural invasion involving the mesenteric plexus at the SMA origin and tumor cell infiltration of lymphatic vessels and connective tissue may extend microscopically beyond the confines of the palpable tumor.[122] During step six of pancreaticoduodenectomy, therefore, the SMPV confluence must be fully mobilized and the SMA exposed so that the specimen can be completely and safely dissected from the right lateral aspect of the proximal SMA.

Vascular Resection Segmental resection of the SMPV confluence is necessary when the tumor cannot be separated from the lateral wall of the SMV or portal vein.[81,122] However, such isolated venous resection should be performed only in patients whose tumors adhere to the SMV or SMPV confluence but who have no evidence of tumor extension to the SMA or celiac axis. Invasion of the SMV or portal vein is not associated with histopathologic variables (positive lymph nodes) that suggest a poor prognosis, and patient survival after pancreaticoduodenectomy is not affected by the need for venous resection.[122] Because the need for venous resection is unexpected in many patients and is discovered only after gastric and pancreatic transection, when nonresectional procedures are no longer an option, surgeons who perform pancreaticoduodenectomies should be familiar with standard vascular techniques for resection and reconstruction of the SMPV confluence.

The standard technique for segmental venous resection involves transection of the splenic vein.[132,133] Division of the splenic vein allows complete exposure of the SMA medial to the

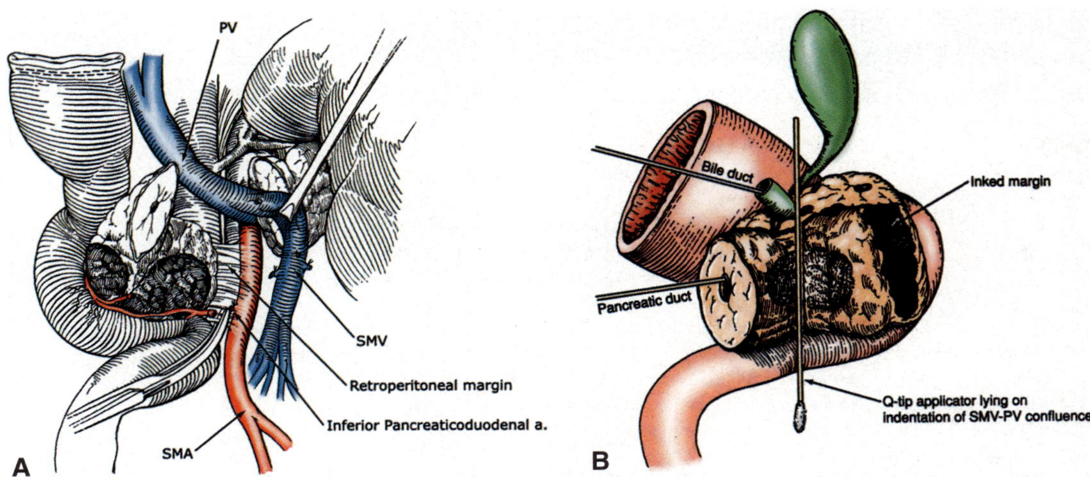

Figure 90-7 Illustration of the retroperitoneal margin as defined at the time of tumor resection **(A)**. Medial retraction of the superior mesenteric vein (SMV) and superior mesenteric–portal vein confluence facilitates dissection of the soft tissues adjacent to the lateral wall of the proximal superior mesenteric artery (SMA); this site represents the retroperitoneal margin. Complete permanent-section analysis of the pancreaticoduodenectomy specimen requires that it be oriented for the pathologist to enable accurate assessment of the retroperitoneal margin of excision and other standard pathologic variables. The retroperitoneal margin must be identified and inked with the pathologist **(B)**; it cannot be assessed retrospectively. As shown here, a probe is in both the pancreatic duct and the bile duct, and a Q-tip applicator lies on the indentation of the SMPV confluence. One can then ink (for final pathologic assessment) the soft-tissue margin adjacent to the proximal SMA; this represents the retroperitoneal (or mesenteric) margin of excision.

SMV and provides increased SMV and portal vein length (since they are no longer tethered by the splenic vein) for a primary venous anastomosis following segmental vein resection. However, we prefer to preserve the splenic vein–portal vein junction whenever possible (Figure 90-8).[122,134] The splenic vein can only be preserved, however, when tumor invasion of the SMV or portal vein does not involve the splenic vein confluence. Preserving the splenic vein–SMPV confluence significantly limits mobilization of the portal vein and prevents primary anastomosis of the SMV (following segmental SMV resection) unless segmental resection is limited to less than 2 cm; therefore, an interposition graft is required in most patients who undergo SMV resection with splenic vein preservation. The internal jugular vein is our preferred conduit for interposition grafting.[134] Preserving the splenic vein adds significant complexity to venous resection because it prevents direct access to the most proximal 3 to 4 cm of the SMA (medial to the SMV).

It is important to emphasize the distinction between regional pancreatectomy and pancreaticoduodenectomy with segmental resection of the SMV or SMPV confluence. Venous resection is not an attempt to improve en-bloc lymphatic and soft tissue clearance, as is performed in regional pancreatectomy. Larger local-regional resections (to the left of the SMA and celiac axis) in poorly selected patients with advanced disease are unlikely to affect survival.[135] Venous resection should be performed only in patients whose tumors adhere to the SMV or SMPV confluence but no evidence of tumor extension to the SMA or celiac axis.

Pylorus Preservation Preservation of the antropyloroduodenal segment during pancreaticoduodenectomy was first described by Traverso and Longmire in 1978.[136] Since then, increasing numbers of pancreatic surgeons have used this modification of the procedure, particularly in patients who have small periampullary lesions or benign disease. Proponents of pylorus preservation argue that preserving the antropyloric pump mechanism improves long-term upper gastrointestinal tract function, has associated nutritional benefits, and improves quality of life.[137–139] In addition, physiologic studies suggest that pylorus preservation decreases intestinal transit time, lessens diarrhea (steatorrhea), normalizes glucose metabolism, and improves postoperative weight gain.[155,156] Detractors of pylorus-preserving pancreaticoduodenectomy counter that the reported improvements in gastrointestinal tract function and nutrition are small, if any, and come at the expense of an increased risk of delayed gastric emptying in the early postoperative period.[140–142] Further, leaving the distal stomach and duodenum may compromise margins of excision and prevent adequate peripyloric lymphadenectomy. In summary, currently available findings from randomized trials suggest no difference in perioperative factors or patient outcome between standard and pylorus-preserving pancreaticoduodenectomy.[142–144] Most investigators would agree that pylorus preservation should not be performed in patients who have bulky tumors of the pancreatic head or duodenal tumors involving the first or second portions of the duodenum.

Pancreatic, Biliary, and Gastrointestinal Reconstruction Pancreatic, biliary and gastrointestinal reconstruction is performed after confirmation by frozen-section analysis that the pancreatic and bile duct margins are histologically negative.[81] The transected jejunum is brought through a small incision in the transverse mesocolon to the left of the middle colic vessels, and a two-layer, end-to-side, duct-to-mucosa pancreaticojejunostomy is performed over a small Silastic stent (if the pancreatic duct is not dilated). If the pancreatic duct is not suitable for a duct-to-

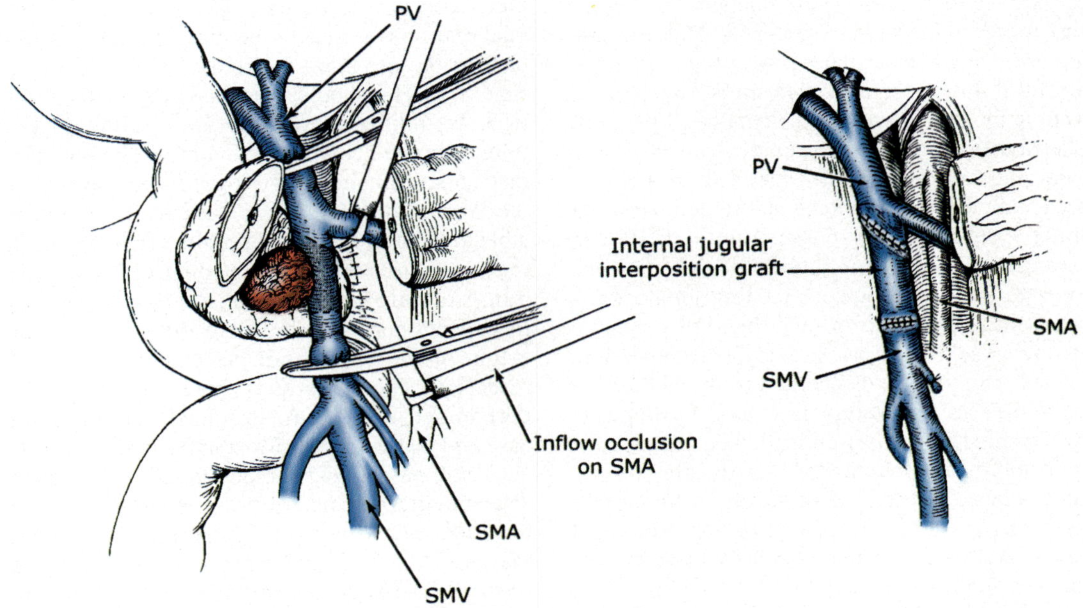

Figure 90-8 Illustration of resection of the superior mesenteric vein (SMV) with splenic vein preservation. The intact splenic vein tethers the portal vein (PV), making a primary anastomosis impossible in most cases. Our preferred method of reconstruction of the SMV is to use an internal jugular vein interposition graft. With the splenic vein intact, exposure is inadequate to separate the specimen from the lateral aspect of the proximal superior mesenteric artery (SMA). Therefore, the graft can be placed prior to specimen removal, thereby allowing medial retraction of the reconstructed superior mesenteric–portal vein confluence, or after separation of the specimen from the SMA posteriorly. Segmental resection of the SMV with splenic vein preservation adds significant complexity to this operation.

mucosa anastomosis, a two-layer anastomosis that invaginates the cut end of the pancreas into the jejunum can be performed. However, we prefer a duct-to-mucosa anastomosis. A single-layer biliary anastomosis is then completed, followed by an anticolic, two-layer, end-to-side gastrojejunostomy or duodenojejunostomy (when pylorus preservation is performed). We are careful to separate the biliary and gastric anastomoses by at least 50 cm to prevent reflux cholangitis. A feeding jejunostomy tube is placed in selected patients using the Witzel technique; we no longer place a drain near the pancreatic anastomosis prior to abdominal closure.

Two complications are associated with gastrointestinal reconstruction after pancreaticoduodenectomy: leak at the pancreaticojejunostomy and delayed gastric emptying. Leaks from the biliary and gastric anastomoses should be rare, however, and were more prevalent in connection with early gastrointestinal reconstruction techniques that involved simple closure of the pancreatic stump. Once the high rate of pancreatic fistula formation was recognized, surgeons quickly switched to implanting the pancreatic remnant into the jejunum.[145] An alternative is to implant the pancreatic remnant into the posterior wall of the stomach.[146–148] Regardless of the technique used, the results seem to depend on the experience of the surgeon: the incidence of complications decreases with greater experience.

Delayed gastric emptying is common after standard pancreaticoduodenectomy and may occur more frequently with pylorus preservation.[140,149] In the absence of an intra-abdominal infection (pancreatic anastomotic leak), delayed gastric emptying is largely related to denervation of the upper gastrointestinal tract during resection of the pancreatic head and attached soft tissues and nerves to the right of the SMA. Delayed gastric emptying causes nausea, vomiting, and postprandial fullness; however, these symptoms resolve in 4 to 12 weeks in virtually all patients. The nutritional consequences of delayed gastric emptying are most significant in those patients with some degree of nutritional depletion preoperatively and in older patients with significant medical comorbid conditions. In such patients, we therefore often place a feeding jejunostomy tube because of the otherwise high cost and inconvenience of intravenous hyperalimentation. Patients can then be discharged from the hospital while they are still receiving enteral feeding (via the jejunostomy tube) and allowed to advance their oral diet as tolerated. A gastrostomy tube is rarely placed at the time of surgery, although in selected patients it effectively avoids prolonged nasogastric tube placement due to temporary gastric emptying dysfunction.

Pathologic (Surgical) Staging The staging system of the AJCC and International Union Against Cancer is given in Table 90-2.[2] The modifications to the TNM staging system in the sixth edition allow the accurate staging of patients even if they do not undergo pancreatic resection. The T4 (and stage III) designation is reserved for locally advanced unresectable primary tumors in the absence of distant metastases.

Table 90-2 TNM Staging System

Definitions	
Primary Tumor (T)	
TX	Primary tumor cannot be assessed
T0	No evidence of primary tumor
Tis	In situ carcinoma
T1	Tumor limited to pancreas and 2 cm or less in greatest dimension
T2	Tumor limited to pancreas and more than 2 cm in greatest dimension
T3	Tumor extends beyond the pancreas but without involvement of the celiac axis or the superior mesenteric artery
T4	Tumor involves the celiac axis or the superior mesenteric artery (unresectable primary tumor)
Regional Lymph Nodes (N)	
NX	Regional lymph nodes cannot be assessed
N0	No regional lymph node metastasis
N1	Regional lymph node metastasis
Distant Metastasis (M)	
MX	Distant metastasis cannot be assessed
M0	No distant metastasis
M1	Distant metastasis

Stage Grouping			
Stage 0	Tis	N0	M0
Stage IA	T1	N0	M0
Stage IB	T2	N0	M0
Stage IIA	T3	N0	M0
Stage IIB	T1-3	N1	M0
Stage III	T4	N0/1	M0
Stage IV	T1-4	N0/1	M1

Adapted from Exocrine pancreas. Greene FL, Page DL, Fleming ID, et al, editors. AJCC Cancer Staging Manual, 6th Edition. New York: Springer; 2002. p. 157–64.

When the pancreaticoduodenectomy specimen is evaluated pathologically, the surgeon and pathologist first evaluate frozen sections of the common bile duct transection margin and the pancreatic transection margin. The retroperitoneal margin (the soft tissue margin directly adjacent to the proximal 3–4 cm of the SMA) (see Figure 90-7) is then evaluated on permanent sections by inking the margin and sectioning the tumor perpendicular to the margin. The pathologist must evaluate the retroperitoneal margin at the time of tumor resection because it is not possible to identify later. Reresection is performed in the event of a positive bile duct or pancreatic transection margin; however, this is not possible in the retroperitoneum, where the aorta and the origin of the SMA limit the extent of surgical resection. The R status of resection cannot be determined if the retroperitoneal margin is not assessed histologically. Most importantly, the surgeon and pathologist should classify this margin after integrating the operative findings and the histologic assessment of this margin. All pancreatic resections should be classified according to residual disease status (termed "R" factor): R0, no gross or microscopic residual disease; R1, microscopic residual disease (microscopically positive surgical margins with no gross residual disease); and R2, grossly evident residual disease. The pathologist cannot usually differentiate an R1 (microscopically positive) from an R2 (grossly positive) retroperitoneal margin in the absence of information regarding the retroperitoneal dissection, which should be included in the operative note. The R designation should appear in the final pathology report (operative note, or other highly visible aspect of the medical record) and should be consistent with the dictated operative note. For example, if the surgeon states that gross tumor was encountered when completing the retroperitoneal dissection, a positive histologic margin should result in the R2 designation in the final pathology report. In the absence of this information being included in the operative report, the proper R designation cannot be determined. The difficulty in differentiating R1 from R2 resections has significant implications for the conduct of clinical trials examining the potential survival advantage of nonsurgical therapies.

Samples from multiple areas of each tumor, including the interface between the tumor and adjacent uninvolved tissue, are also submitted for paraffin-embedded histologic examination (5–10 blocks). In this technique, 4-µm-thick sections are cut and stained with hematoxylin and eosin. The final pathologic evaluation of the permanent sections includes a description of the tumor histology and differentiation; gross and microscopic evaluation of the tissue of origin (pancreas, bile duct, ampulla of Vater, or duodenum); and assessments of the maximum transverse tumor diameter, lymph node status, and the presence or absence of perineural, lymphatic, and vascular invasion. If segmental venous resection has been performed, the area of presumed tumor invasion of the vein wall is serially sectioned and examined to discriminate benign fibrous attachment from direct tumor invasion. If the patient received preoperative chemoradiation therapy, the grade of the treatment effect is assessed using the grading schema developed by Cleary and reported by Evans and colleagues.[150] The Japanese staging system involves an extremely detailed analysis of margins and lymph node groups and is not practical for widespread application.[151] As multimodality treatment strategies for pancreatic cancer become more commonly used, standardized pathologic assessment of tumor specimens will become even more important.

Prognostic Factors Prognostic factors in patients with localized, potentially resectable pancreatic cancer are used to guide treatment recommendations, especially in older patients whose medical comorbid conditions may increase the risks associated with major pancreatic surgery. However, unlike the approach taken with solid tumors, pathologic prognostic variables do not guide the use of adjuvant therapy because, despite a potentially curative pancreaticoduodenectomy, disease recurs in at least 80% of patients. Therefore, in general, adjuvant therapy (as discussed in the next section) is administered to all patients with exocrine pancreatic cancer regardless of the pathologic findings in resected specimens.[152] The prognostic factor of greatest significance for survival, one that is available to the clinician prior to surgery and the pathologic assessment of the resected specimen, is the preoperative radiographic assessment of local tumor extension, because it predicts the eventual resection margin status.[4,120] The margin of greatest importance is the retroperitoneal (or mesenteric) margin along the right lateral border of the SMA as discussed above in detail. When carefully evaluated, 10 to 20% of patients who undergo a grossly complete resection for pancreatic adenocarcinoma will be found to have a microscopically positive retroperitoneal margin (R1 resection). The impact of a truly microscopically positive margin (in the setting of a grossly complete resection) treated with multimodality therapy has not been evaluated outside of experiences of single institutions.[122] An occasional patient will have microscopic extension of tumor cells along the pancreatic duct (positive pancreatic transection margin), but the clinical significance of this is uncertain. Importantly, dysplastic cells secondary to tumor-induced pancreatitis are frequently found at the pancreatic transection margin and should not be cause for further pancreatic resection (in the absence of histologic evidence of invasive adenocarcinoma).

A number of investigators have examined pathologic factors of the resected tumor in an effort to establish reliable prognostic variables associated with decreased survival.[4,139,153,154] Metastatic disease in regional lymph nodes, poorly differentiated histology, and increased size of primary tumors have been associated with decreased survival duration. For example, in a study conducted by Yeo and colleagues,[139] 45 patients with pancreatic adenocarcinoma who underwent complete resection with both negative resection margins and negative regional lymph nodes had a median survival of 32 months and a 5-year survival of 40%. However, in an analysis of 12 5-year survivors (following complete resection) done by Conlon and colleagues,[155] 4 had poorly differentiated histology, 5 had metastatic disease in regional lymph nodes, 9 had histologic evidence of extrapancreatic soft tissue extension of the tumor, and 10 patients had histologic evidence of perineural invasion. Nonetheless, in an otherwise good-risk patient with localized, potentially resectable pancreatic cancer (as shown by objective CT criteria that have already been reviewed), the lymph node status, degree of differentiation of the primary tumor, and other histologic (or molecular) prognostic variables are of little clinical relevance. Regardless of these findings, such a patient should receive multimodality therapy that includes chemotherapy, surgery, and possibly chemoradiation therapy as part of a protocol-based treatment program. However, in elderly patients with comorbid conditions that may increase their risk from pancreaticoduodenectomy, knowledge of poorly differentiated histology and the positive status of regional lymph nodes (information that can now be obtained at major referral centers through the use of EUS-FNA) may be cause to recommend systemic therapy or chemoradiation therapy rather than proceeding directly to major pancreatic surgery.

Lastly, intraoperative variables, such as the perioperative blood loss, the number of red blood cell transfusions, and operative time have also been examined.[4,139] An increase in perioperative blood loss and the need for blood transfusion were both associated with a decrease in survival duration. However, increased tumor size would logically be associated with a more difficult operation, resulting in greater blood loss and the high likelihood of incomplete resection.

Postoperative (Adjuvant) Therapy The Gastrointestinal Tumor Study Group (GITSG) was the first to study whether postoperative adjuvant chemoradiation therapy improved survival in patients with pancreatic adenocarcinoma. In a prospective randomized study of adjuvant chemoradiation (500 mg/m^2/day of 5-FU for 6 days and 40 Gy of radiation) versus observation alone after pancreaticoduodenectomy, a survival advantage was seen for multimodality therapy (20 months vs 11 months with resection alone).[156,157] However, 5 (24%) of the 21 patients assigned to the adjuvant chemoradiation arm could not begin treatment until more than 10 weeks after pancreaticoduodenectomy owing to prolonged recovery from surgery. This was despite the fact that the only patients likely to be considered for protocol entry were those who experienced an uncomplicated recovery following surgery and had a good performance status.

The European Organization for Research and Treatment of Cancer (EORTC) reported their findings for trial 40891 in 1999.[158] Between 1987 and 1995, 218 patients were randomized to receive either chemoradiation (40 Gy in a split course and 5-FU given as a continuous infusion at a dosage of 25 mg/kg/day during EBRT) or no further treatment following pancreaticoduodenectomy for adenocarcinoma of the pancreas or periampullary region. Eleven patients were deemed ineligible for analysis because of extensive local disease with incomplete resection. Of the remaining 207 patients, 114 (55%) had pancreatic cancer. The median survival was 24.5 months for the entire group that received adjuvant therapy and 19 months for the group that received surgery alone (p = .2). For the subset of patients with pancreatic cancer, the median survival was 17.1 months for those who received adjuvant therapy and 12.6 months for those who received surgery alone (p = .099). Although these differences were not significant, the wide confidence interval (relative risk, 0.7; 95% CI, 0.5–1.1) for patients with pancreatic cancer does not exclude the possibility of a clinically meaningful improvement in survival in the chemoradiation arm that may not have been apparent owing to the small sample size. Similar to the GITSG trial, patients were considered for enrollment in the EORTC trial after recovering from pancreaticoduodenectomy; despite this selection bias, 21 (20%) of 104 evaluable patients assigned to receive chemoradiation did not receive the therapy because of patient refusal, medical comorbid conditions, or rapid tumor progression. In addition, the retroperitoneal margin of resection was not assessed, and, therefore, the completeness of surgical resection could not be verified. Although the method of follow-up was not defined (raising a concern about underestimation of the sites of recurrent disease), tumor recurrence in the pancreatic bed was reported as a site of first progression in 20% of patients. This finding combined with the short survival in the observation arm (12 months) raises the possibility that some patients may have undergone an incomplete (R2) resection.

The European Study Group for Pancreatic Cancer (ESPAC)-1 trial was conducted by 83 participating physicians in 61 hospital centers between 1994 and 2000.[5,159] ESPAC-1 enrolled 541 patients following resection for adenocarcinoma of the pancreas. The trial used a four-arm, 2 × 2 factorial design to compare (1) adjuvant chemoradiation (40 Gy in a split course and 5-FU), (2) adjuvant chemotherapy (5-FU and folinic acid), (3) chemoradiation therapy followed by chemotherapy, and (4) observation alone following pancreaticoduodenectomy for pancreatic and periampullary carcinomas. Two-hundred eighty-five patients (53%) were entered into the randomized 2 × 2 factorial design. However, because of the lack of access to EBRT or specific institutional bias, 188 patients were randomized to receive only chemotherapy or no chemotherapy, and 68 patients were randomized to receive either chemoradiation or no chemoradiation therapy. In the latter two nonfactorial groups, patients could receive nonstandardized therapy at the discretion of their treating physicians. For example, patients who were randomized in the nonfactorial design to receive chemotherapy or no chemotherapy could receive EBRT. Importantly, nonrandomized treatments were not standardized. Pooled analysis of all 541 patients enrolled in the ESPAC-1 trial demonstrated no survival advantage for patients receiving chemoradiation compared with those who did not (15.5 months vs 16.1 months, $p = .24$). However, a statistically significant survival benefit was observed in patients who received chemotherapy compared with those who did not (19.7 months versus 14.0 months, $p = .0005$). The median survival durations for the 285 patients randomized in the 2×2 factorial design were 16.9 months (observation), 13.9 months (chemoradiotherapy), 21.6 months (chemotherapy), and 19.9 months (chemoradiation plus chemotherapy). This analysis did not have the statistical power to compare these median survivals directly. However, the median survival among the 145 patients randomized to receive chemoradiotherapy (alone or with chemotherapy) was 15.9 months versus 17.9 months in the patients not assigned to receive chemoradiation (hazard ratio for death, 1.28; 95% confidence interval 0.99–1.66; $p = .05$). Of the 145 patients randomized to receive chemoradiation, only 90 (62%) received the assigned 40 Gy of EBRT and the survival duration of those who did and did not receive intended therapy was not reported. The median survival among the 147 patients randomized to receive chemotherapy (alone or with chemoradiotherapy) was 20.1 months versus 15.5 months among the 142 patients who did not receive chemotherapy (hazard ratio for death, 0.71; 95% confidence interval, 0.55–0.92; $p = .009$). However, only 61 (41%) of the 147 patients received all intended chemotherapy, and the survival duration of those who did and did not receive the intended therapy was not reported. Obvious concerns with this prospective trial included the very low compliance with prescribed therapy (suggesting inadequate central monitoring), the lack of a system for standardized pathologic evaluation of surgical specimens, and the absence of radiation quality control. Again, as seen in the EORTC trial there was concern over the number of patients who may have undergone an incomplete resection prior to enrollment due to the high rate of local failure (62%).

The Radiation Therapy Oncology Group (RTOG) activated the first American phase III cooperative group study of postoperative adjuvant therapy for resected pancreatic adenocarcinoma (RTOG 97-04) since the GITSG trial.[160] Patients were randomly assigned to receive three cycles of weekly gemcitabine or three cycles of infusional 5-FU to be given before and after 5-FU–based chemoradiation therapy. Accrual to this trial is complete, but results are not available at the time of this writing.

Investigators at the Virginia Mason Medical Center have reported their findings from a review of their experience with adjuvant EBRT combined with 5-FU, cisplatin and interferon-α (IFN-α).[161] IFN-α is used in pancreatic cancer because of its ability to function as a radiosensitizer and its use as a systemic agent with possible cytostatic properties. In this study, 33 patients who successfully underwent pancreaticoduodenectomy were then assigned in a nonrandomized fashion to receive either EBRT (45–54 Gy) and concomitant 5-FU or IFN-α–based chemoradiation therapy (45–54 Gy, and concomitant continuous infusions of 5-FU [200 mg/m^2/day], bolus cisplatin [30 mg/m^2/day], and subcutaneous injections of IFN-α [3 million U, qod]). Although the sample size was small, the 17 patients in the IFN-α regimen had a significantly greater actuarial 2-year survival compared with those receiving EBRT and 5-FU alone (84% vs 54%, $p = .04$). The American College of Surgeons Oncology Group is currently conducting a phase II trial to confirm these favorable results.

The largest single-institution experience with postoperative adjuvant chemoradiation has been reported by Sohn and colleagues[4] from Johns Hopkins University. Of 498 evaluable patients who underwent pancreatectomy for adenocarcinoma of the pancreas, 366 (74%) received adjuvant chemoradiation and 132 (26%) declined adjuvant therapy for "various reasons." The number of patients who will not receive adjuvant therapy in 2005 (with the advances made in the surgical treatment of this disease) may be less than the 26% of patients reported from the Hopkins retrospective review; however, the inability to receive postoperative therapy remains a practical concern for the design of postoperative adjuvant trials. In all previously reported and currently ongoing postoperative adjuvant trials (with the exception of the Hopkins data), patient enrollment occurred following recovery from surgery; the number of patients not referred for trial entry (owing to delayed recovery from surgery and other factors) is therefore not known. Adjuvant therapy in the Hopkins study was associated with a statistically significant improvement in survival (19 months vs 11 months, $p < .0001$). However, further reports from Hopkins of the use of an intensified postoperative adjuvant therapy consisting of concurrent 5-FU, leucovorin, dipyridamole, and mitomycin-C, combined with split-course EBRT to 50 Gy indicated that this treatment did not improve survival. Specifically, median survival (16 months) and disease-free survival (12.4 months) were not appreciably improved compared with those in similar patients treated on earlier adjuvant therapy protocols.[162–164] Additional nonrandomized data come from a population-based analysis performed by Lim and colleagues from the Harvard School of Public Health.[165] This study of 396 Medicare-eligible patients residing in 1 of 11 Survival, Epidemiology, and End Results (SEER) registries found that adjuvant chemoradiation was associated with improved survival compared with no adjuvant therapy (29 vs 12.5 months, $p = .0003$).

Preoperative (Neoadjuvant) Therapy There are many practical and theoretical advantages to preoperative treatment of patients with localized pancreatic cancer. Most compelling is the ability to provide immediate systemic therapy for a disease that is systemic at diagnosis in virtually all patients. A second more practical advantage is improved patient selection for pancreatic surgery—an operation associated with significant patient morbidity even when performed in experienced hands. This improved patient selection arises because patients with rapidly progressive systemic disease are identified as part of the restaging evaluation performed following neoadjuvant treatment prior to planned surgery. In prospective trials, approximately 25% of patients who begin a program of preoperative treatment do not undergo successful resection of their primary tumor as a consequence of disease progression or evolution of clinically significant medical comorbidity.[152] These patients are spared the morbidity and prolonged recovery sometimes associated with pancreaticoduodenectomy. In a series of trials performed at our institution, patients who demonstrated disease progression after preoperative chemoradiation had a median survival of only 7 months.[3,8,166] In addition, the high frequency of positive-margin resections supports the concern that the retroperitoneal margin of excision, even when negative, may be only a few millimeters, making surgery alone inadequate local therapy for most patients. Thus, many institutions have begun to investigate the role of chemotherapy and/or chemoradiation given preoperatively, and this overall strategy is becoming more common in the off-protocol setting.

Since 1988, a number of prospective preoperative trials have been completed at our institution.[8,150,166,167] These trials have had identical eligibility criteria using a CT-based definition of resectable disease (as previously described), a uniform surgical technique for the performance of pancreaticoduodenectomy, and a standardized system for pathologic evaluation of surgical specimens, including resection margins. This has maximized the number of variables held constant, while varying only the chemoradiation regimens. All eligible patients were required to have biopsy proven adenocarcinoma of the pancreatic head. In our initial preoperative study reported in 1992, 28 patients received a course of infusional 5-FU (300 mg/m^2/day) in combination with standard-fractionation external beam radiation therapy (EBRT; 50.4 Gy; 180 cGy/fraction for 28 fractions over 5.5 weeks).[150] The gastrointestinal toxic effects (nausea, vomiting, and dehydration) were severe enough to require hospital admission in a third of patients. Preoperative (postchemoradiation) restaging radiographic evaluation 4 to 5 weeks after completing preoperative therapy disclosed evidence of metastatic disease in 25% of patients. Another 15% had intraoperative evidence of metastatic disease at laparotomy for an overall resectability rate of 60%. Median survival for the patients who underwent pancreaticoduodenectomy with curative intent was 18 months. The degree of tumor cell kill was graded using a standardized scoring system, and 40% of the resected specimens had a pathologic partial response to therapy (> 50% of the tumor cells were nonviable). Although the results from this initial trial of preoperative therapy appeared equivalent to those seen with postoperative therapy, the toxicity and hospitalization rate was discouraging. These findings led to a change in the delivery of EBRT in all subsequent preoperative trials performed at our institution.

A rapid-fractionation program of chemoradiation delivered over 2 weeks was designed to avoid the gastrointestinal toxicity associated with standard-fractionation chemoradiation delivered over 5.5 weeks, while maintaining the excellent local tumor control achieved with multimodality therapy.[8] Rapid-fractionation chemoradiation was delivered with 18-MeV photons using a four-field technique to a total dose of 30 Gy (3 Gy/fraction, 10 fractions over 2 weeks). Sequentially performed preoperative chemoradiation trials have evaluated continuous infusion 5-FU, paclitaxel, and gemcitabine, all given as single agents.[3,166–168] Again, restaging with contrast-enhanced CT and chest radiography was performed 4 to 5 weeks after the completion of chemoradiation, in preparation for pancreaticoduodenectomy. In our study of rapid fractionation EBRT with infusional 5-FU, 35 patients were enrolled, 27 were taken to surgery, and 20 (57%) underwent successful pancreaticoduodenectomy.[8] Local tumor control and patient survival were equal to the results with standard-fractionation (5.5 weeks) chemoradiation. Of note, only 2 (10%) of the 20 patients who underwent pancreaticoduodenectomy developed local-regional recurrence, and the median survival for all 20 resected patients was 25 months. Prior to the advent of gemcitabine, paclitaxel was investigated as a preoperative radiosensitizer in a group of patients with resectable pancreatic cancer.[166] Paclitaxel did not provide an advantage over 5-FU–based chemoradiation in terms of resection rate, local treatment effect, or overall survival.

We then moved to gemcitabine-based chemoradiation and performed a phase I study of gemcitabine in combination with EBRT in patients with locally advanced disease.[168] This regimen combined 2 weeks of rapid-fractionation EBRT with 7 weekly infusions of gemcitabine. The maximum tolerated dose of gemcitabine using this treatment schedule was 350 mg/m^2/week, roughly one-third the standard weekly dose. The dose-limiting toxic effects included fatigue, anorexia, nausea, vomiting, and dehydration; febrile neutropenia occurred in only 1 patient. Objective tumor regression was observed in 24% of patients, and 1 patient had a dramatic radiographic response, resulting in eventual surgical resection; the tumor was resected with negative surgical margins and histologically, 95% of the tumor specimen was nonviable. These results were sufficiently encouraging to proceed with a study of gemcitabine-based preoperative chemoradiation in a group of patients with potentially resectable disease.[167] A total of 86 patients were enrolled in this recently completed clinical trial (full manuscript pending). Toxicities were similar to those observed in the initial phase I trial. Despite a longer elapsed time from enrollment to surgery (pancreaticoduodenectomy) compared with previous trials with 5-FU and EBRT (11–12 weeks rather than 7–9 weeks), 74% of patients underwent successful pancreaticoduodenectomy (compared with 60% with 5-FU–based chemoradiation). A pathologic partial response (> 50% of tumor cells nonviable) was seen in over half of the surgical specimens, and there were 2 pathologic complete responses—something not observed in the 5-FU era. Currently, protocol eligible patients with potentially resectable pancreatic cancer seen at our institution are receiving systemic therapy using a combination of gemcitabine and cisplatin, followed by gemcitabine-based chemoradiation prior to planned pancreaticoduodenectomy.

Unfortunately, many reports of neoadjuvant therapy for pancreatic cancer have included heterogeneous patient populations, enrolling patients with locally advanced or marginally resectable pancreatic cancer. Few investigators report clear anatomic definitions of locally advanced disease, and many studies incorporate intraoperative assessment of the extent of local tumor growth, data which are subjective and not reproducible. In general, patients with locally advanced pancreatic cancer should not be included in studies of preoperative therapy because their inclusion confounds reports of resection rates, and complicates comparisons to other studies. Therein lies the importance of using accurate, reproducible anatomic definitions for resectability based on high-quality CT imaging.

Difficulties associated with the delivery of neoadjuvant therapy include the need for a pretreatment pancreatic biopsy and the frequent need for intermediate-term palliation of jaundice using endoscopically placed biliary stents.[112,121,169] In addition, these stents can occlude during preoperative treatment leading to biliary stent-related morbidity. In fact, we have recently used coated metal stents in patients who are planning to receive preoperative therapy, because stent occlusion is more common when the preoperative interval exceeds 2 to 3 months.

Radiotherapy Technique and Dose The standard dose of radiotherapy in the postoperative setting is typically 50.4 Gy in 28 fractions. Field reductions are often made after 45 Gy. Standard fractionation EBRT to 50.4 Gy has also been used in the neoadjuvant setting. As discussed above, 30 Gy in 10 fractions has provided equivalent local tumor control, especially when combined with gemcitabine or the newer targeted agents as radiosensitizers. It is important to remember that patient selection and surgical technique will greatly impact the frequency of local failure; adjuvant therapy with or without radiation can only be effective in preventing local failure if a complete gross resection of the primary tumor has been performed. In contrast to the experience with rectal cancer and other solid tumors, for pancreatic adenocarcinoma, surgical technique and the pathologic assessment of resection margins have not been properly standardized. It therefore is inappropriate to assume that published rates of local failure simply represent inadequate adjuvant (or neoadjuvant) therapy.

It is likely that the majority of the benefit from chemoradiation results from the treatment of the retroperitoneal margin. Although there may not be universal agreement about the size and shape of standard radiation fields, the superior mesenteric artery origin and the celiac axis must be covered with adequate margins. A three- or four-field technique using anterior, posterior, and opposed lateral fields allows critical tissues, such as the liver, kidneys, stomach, spinal cord, and small bowel, to be spared. For tumors located in the pancreatic head, the anterior and posterior fields typically cover the T11-L3 vertebral bodies, although the visceral anatomy is quite variable in relation to the bony anatomy. The porta hepatis should be identified on CT and included in all fields. Inferiorly, the goal is to cover the tumor and duodenal bed with a 2 cm margin. The right border of the anterior and posterior fields and the anterior extent of the lateral fields are defined by the preoperative location of the duodenum. The left border of the anterior and posterior fields is placed 2 cm to the left of the vertebral body edge, as long as there is adequate coverage of the preoperative tumor volume. This usually means that the upper right border of the anterior and posterior fields is located 4 to 5 cm to the right of the vertebral body edge, and the anterior aspect of the lateral field is 5 to 6 cm from the anterior vertebral body edge. Blocking is placed over the inferior pole of the right kidney in the anterior and posterior fields, bisecting the vertebral bodies in the lateral fields. Corner blocks are typically placed in the anterior aspect of the lateral fields as well. Care should be taken not to block the preoperative tumor volume or the porta hepatis in the lateral fields. For lesions of the pancreatic body and tail, similar principles are applied to field location, and the splenic hilum is covered while the porta hepatis and duodenal bed are not; the right field border is typically located 2 cm from the right vertebral body edge.

Similar treatment fields are recommended for patients with an intact pancreas if the goal is neoadjuvant therapy with planned surgical resection. However, if the concurrent chemotherapeutic agent is gemcitabine, we always use conformal fields confined to the gross tumor, grossly enlarged adenopathy, superior mesenteric artery, and celiac axis.

Approach to the Patient with Potentially Resectable Disease There are several factors to consider in the treatment of patients with potentially resectable disease. First, pancreaticoduodenectomy should be performed only in patients whose tumors appear to be resectable based on MDCT and who have a good performance status (ECOG 0-1). Second, pancreaticoduodenectomy should be done as part of a multimodality treatment program that includes preoperative or postoperative chemotherapy with or without EBRT. Current and future treatment programs for patients with resectable pancreatic cancer should emphasize the use of systemic therapy (gemcitabine in combination with other cytotoxics and/or targeted agents), because greater than 80% of patients have regional lymph node or distant organ metastases at the time of diagnosis. Third, because of the modest survival rates seen with previously published treatment programs, the enrollment of all patients into clinical trials of new combinations of surgery, chemotherapy, chemoradiation therapy, and newly developed systemic agents is strongly encouraged. Fourth, published perioperative mortality rates support the referral of patients with potentially resectable disease to centers that frequently perform major pancreatic resections for cancer.[126,170]

TREATMENT OF LOCALLY ADVANCED DISEASE

CHEMORADIATION THERAPY **5-Fluorouracil–Based Chemoradiation Trials** Chemoradiation therapy has been part of the foundation of therapy for locally advanced disease and has been shown to prolong survival compared with radiation alone and chemotherapy alone. In GITSG studies of 5-FU–based chemoradiation therapy in patients with locally advanced pancreatic adenocarcinoma,[9,171] patients were randomly assigned to receive 40 Gy of radiation plus 5-FU, 60 Gy plus 5-FU, or 60 Gy without chemotherapy. Radiation therapy was delivered as a split course, with 20 Gy given over 2 weeks followed by a 2-week rest. 5-FU was delivered IV at a bolus dosage of 500 mg/m^2/day for the first 3 days of each 20-Gy cycle and given weekly (500 mg/m^2) following the completion of chemoradiation therapy. The median survival was 10 months in each of the chemoradiation therapy groups and 6 months for the group that received 60 Gy without 5-FU. In subsequent GITSG studies, neither doxorubicin (Adriamycin)[172] used as a radiation potentiator nor multidrug chemotherapy (streptozocin, mitomycin, and 5-FU [SMF]) alone or continued after chemoradiation therapy[173] was found to be superior to 5-FU-based chemoradiation therapy. Additional chemotherapy after 5-FU–based chemoradiation therapy increased the toxicity without an apparent therapeutic benefit.

In contrast to the results from the GITSG study demonstrating better survival with 5-FU–based chemoradiation therapy than with SMF chemotherapy alone, an ECOG study suggested no benefit to chemoradiation therapy over 5-FU alone.[174] The ECOG study randomly assigned patients with locally advanced or incompletely resected pancreatic adenocarcinoma to receive chemoradiation therapy (40 Gy and 600 mg/m^2/day 5-FU for 3 days) or 5-FU alone (600 mg/m^2/week). The chemoradiation therapy group received weekly bolus administration of 5-FU following chemoradiation therapy until there was evidence of disease progression. Similar to the GITSG studies, all patients were surgically staged and entered in the study within 6 weeks of surgery. Patients with incomplete resections and patients with limited peritoneal involvement were allowed to participate. The median survival was 8.3 months in the group that received chemoradiation therapy and 8.2 months in the group that received 5-FU alone. It was evident both in the GITSG studies and in the ECOG trial that patients with locally advanced, unresectable pancreatic cancer who are symptomatic to the point of not being fully ambulatory do not benefit from anticancer therapy.

More recent trials of chemoradiation for locally advanced pancreatic cancer have investigated continuous-infusion 5-FU in combination with EBRT. The ECOG performed a phase I study to determine the maximal tolerated dose (MTD) of prolonged infusional 5-FU when combined with EBRT to 59.4 Gy in patients with pancreatic or extrahepatic biliary tumors. The MTD of 5-FU was 250 mg/m^2/day, with gastrointestinal toxicity the dose-limiting factor.[10] A subsequent study conducted in Japan demonstrated the feasibility of utilizing low-dose, continuous-infusion 5-FU (200 mg/m^2/day) given over 5.5 weeks combined with a single course of EBRT to 50.4 Gy for patients with locally advanced pancreatic cancer.[175] This was followed by weekly 5-FU treatments until disease progression was documented. Eighty-five percent of patients completed the chemoradiation therapy. The median survival of patients treated was 10 months, similar to the survival of patients treated with bolus 5-FU and EBRT in the GITSG trials.[9,171] Thus, although infusional 5-FU may provide greater radiosensitivity compared with bolus 5-FU, no clear survival advantage has been established for this approach.

Gemcitabine-Based Chemoradiation Trials The introduction of gemcitabine was a modest step forward in the treatment of pancreatic cancer. Its value as a systemic agent in pancreatic cancer and the recognition of its radiosensitizing properties stimulated the study of combinations of gemcitabine with EBRT for patients with localized pancreatic cancer.[168,176–179] Several strategies have been investigated, including seven weekly injections of gemcitabine with short-course EBRT (30 Gy), twice weekly gemcitabine with 50.4 Gy of EBRT, weekly gemcitabine with 50.4 Gy of EBRT, and full dose weekly gemcitabine with escalating doses of radiation. Most of these studies suggested gastrointestinal toxicity as a dose-limiting factor, but hematologic toxicity has also been observed. At the present time, there is no standard approach for combining gemcitabine and radiation, but several variables appear to be important in predicting the MTD. These include variations in the size of the radiation portal, the total radiation dose, possibly the dose of radiation per fraction, and whether gemcitabine is administered once or twice weekly.[180]

Three multi-institutional studies have been completed evaluating gemcitabine-based chemoradiation. In a small study performed in Taiwan, 34 patients with locally advanced pancreatic cancer were randomized to receive 5-FU–based chemoradiation (500 mg/m^2 daily for 3 days, every 14 days with radiation to a total dose of 50.4–61.2 Gy) or gemcitabine and radiation (600 mg/m^2 weekly with equivalent doses of radiation).[181] The objective response rate to gemcitabine and radiation was 50% and only 13% for 5-FU chemoradiation. In addition, median survival was substantially better using gemcitabine compared with 5-FU (14.5 months vs 6.7 months, $p = .027$). The efficacy results must be interpreted with caution because of the limited accrual (34 patients) and the poor results in the control group. Although the authors concluded that there was no increase in toxicity in the gemcitabine arm, therapy was actually poorly tolerated in both arms. Only 75% of patients were able to complete the full dose of radiotherapy and roughly one-third of the patients in both arms were hospitalized for 2 to 6 weeks because of the acute toxicity of treatment. A phase II study conducted in patients with locally advanced pancreatic cancer by the Cancer and Leukemia Group B evaluated gemcitabine given at 40 mg/m^2 twice weekly. In that study, there were 35% and 50% grade 3 or 4 gastrointestinal and hematologic toxicities, respectively, and the median survival was only 8.5 months.[182] Not surprisingly, the Cancer and Leukemia Group B abandoned this approach in locally advanced pancreatic cancer. Both of these studies used regional nodal fields that likely contributed to the significant gastrointestinal toxicity. In contrast, the approach that was developed at the University of Michigan delivers the manufacturer's recommended dose of gemcitabine (1 g/m^2) and a slightly lower radiotherapy dose (36 Gy in 15 fractions over 3 weeks), with conformal radiation fields encompassing the gross tumor volume alone. At that institution, the irradiation of a smaller volume of normal tissue was reported to be well tolerated.[183] Investigators have since embarked on a multi-institutional phase II study evaluating the same regimen. Preliminary results indicate that approximately 25% of patients experience grade 3 or 4 gastrointestinal toxicity.[184]

Several points about gemcitabine-based chemoradiation are worth emphasizing. All chemoradiation regimens that have been studied in patients with locally advanced disease, including regimens that contain gemcitabine, have significant efficacy limitations. Similar to its value as a systemic agent,[185] gemcitabine is probably only modestly better than 5-fluorouracil when it is used with radiotherapy, but it is not tolerated as well.[186] The gastrointestinal toxicity reported in the three multi-institutional studies using gemcitabine calls into question whether the combination of gemcitabine and radiotherapy will be tolerated well enough for future studies that try to build on these experiences. Finally, compared with radiotherapy fields that target the gross tumor only, elective regional nodal irradiation results in increased gastrointestinal toxicity. Because currently available chemoradiation regimens cannot control the primary tumor, it is unlikely that irradiation of microscopic regional nodal metastases contributes anything positive to the outcome of patients with locally advanced pancreatic cancer, regardless of the concurrent chemotherapeutic agent used. Certainly, if gemcitabine is used in combination with irradiation on esophageal, gastric, or duodenal mucosa, the volume of mucosa being treated should be minimized or there will be a significant risk of severe acute toxicity. Because of the significant acute toxicity and limited efficacy that has been reported, the various combinations of gemcitabine and radiotherapy will not likely ever be widely embraced in clinical practice for patients with locally advanced disease. Although it is reasonable for clinicians with experience with any of these

Table 90-3 Selected Ongoing Randomized Trials for Patients with Locally Advanced Pancreatic Cancer

Study	Design	Arms
ECOG 1200	Randomized phase II	Gem 500 mg/m^2 + Cisplatin + 5-FU *followed by* PVI 5-FU + XRT 50.4 Gy + 5.5 weeks Gem 500 mg/m^2 weekly × 5 + XRT 50.4 Gy over 5.5 weeks
ECOG/RTOG 4201	Randomized phase III	Gem 1 gm/m^2 weekly × 3 (max 7 cycles) XRT 50.4 Gy over 5.5 weeks + Gem 600 mg/m^2 *followed by* Gem 1 g/m^2 weekly × 3 (max 5 cycles)
RTOG PA 0411	Phase II	XRT 50.4 Gy over 5.5 weeks + Cape 825 mg/m^2 (PO bid Mon – Fri) + Bev 5 mg/kg every 2 weeks *followed by* Gem 1 g/m^2 weekly × 3 (max 3 cycles) + Bev 5 mg/kg every 2 weeks

Bev = bevacizumab; bid = twice daily; Cape = capecitabine; ECOG = Eastern Cooperative Oncology Group; 5-FU = 5-fluorouracil; Gem = gemcitabine; OS = overall survival; PO = orally; PVI = protracted venous infusion; QOL = quality of life; RFS = relapse-free survival; RR = response rate; RTOG = Radiation Therapy Oncology Group; XRT = radiotherapy.

combinations to use them, it does not appear likely that any of these regimens will be embraced as a standard of care for patients with locally advanced pancreatic cancer.

Capecitabine-Based Chemoradiation The substitution of capecitabine for infusional or bolus 5-FU is less controversial than the use of concurrent gemcitabine, and has similar efficacy to intravenously administered 5-FU.[187] It is an orally administered agent that has a clinical benefit response similar to that of gemcitabine in patients with locally advanced or metastatic pancreatic cancer.[188] Capecitabine has been shown to have a favorable toxicity profile when combined with EBRT for a number of GI tumors to include pancreatic cancer.[189] As demonstrated in a recently completed phase I trial conducted at our institution evaluating bevacizumab-based chemoradiation (discussed below), aggressive adjustment of the capecitabine dose when grade 2 toxicity occurred was sufficient to avoid grade 3 or greater toxicity[190] [manuscript under review, 8/2005]. In contrast to gemcitabine and EBRT, the favorable acute toxicity profile of capecitabine makes it an attractive chemoradiation platform upon which to integrate biologic agents.

Novel Approaches to Chemoradiation Oncology has entered an era of molecular therapy, and details regarding the incorporation of molecular agents into anticancer therapy are discussed throughout this text. In GI tumors, most notably colon cancer, agents such as bevacizumab and cetuximab have begun to change the standard of care for patients with advanced disease, and very recently erlotinib has shown some benefit in pancreatic cancer. Most investigations of these and other drugs have focused on their benefits as components of systemic therapy in patients with advanced disease, although investigation of their benefits in the adjuvant setting are now underway in colon cancer. However, these molecular therapies may play important roles as radiosensitizers. In pancreatic cancer, the anti-VEGF agent bevacizumab has been combined with gemcitabine as a therapy for patients with advanced disease, and the drug's radiosensitizing properties are now being appreciated clinically. The precise mechanism of radiosensitization has not been defined, but possibilities include enhanced lethality of the endothelial cell,[191] the tumor cell,[192] or the improvement in vascular physiology leading to a reduction in tumor hypoxia.[193] The first report of bevacizumab as a radiosensitizer was reported by Willett and colleagues.[194] In the 6 patients treated on this study, bevacizumab was administered prior to the initiation of radiation in a group of patients with rectal cancer. A thoughtful and thorough complement of imaging, serologic, barometric, and histologic correlative studies demonstrated rapid changes in tumor perfusion, interstitial intratumor pressure, and circulating endothelial cells, and were all observed. In a recently completed phase I dose escalation study conducted at our institution, capecitabine and bevacizumab were administered in combination with radiation (50.4 Gy) to 47 patients with locally advanced pancreatic cancer. The study demonstrated that bevacizumab is generally safe when combined with chemoradiation in patients with locally advanced pancreatic cancer. The acute toxicity was minimal and easily managed with dose adjustments of capecitabine, without interruption or attenuation of either the bevacizumab or radiation dose. Even though there was a 43% incidence of grade 2 gastrointestinal toxicity and a 21% incidence of grade 2 hand-and-foot syndrome, adjusting the dose of oral capecitabine in 43% of patients for grade 2 toxicity was sufficient to avoid grade 3 toxicity in the majority of patients. In addition, limiting radiotherapy fields to the gross tumor volume alone was probably a factor that contributed to minimizing the incidence of grade 3 acute toxicity. Bevacizumab did not appear to enhance acute toxicity; however, tumors with invasion of the duodenum appeared to be at higher risk of bleeding or perforation. Overall, the tumors in 9 (20%) of 46 evaluable patients had an objective partial response to initial therapy. This included 6 of 12 tumors treated at a dose of 5 mg/kg of bevacizumab.[190] The Radiation Therapy Oncology Group (RTOG) is conducting a phase II trial to evaluate capecitabine-based chemoradiation with bevacizumab (RTOG PA04-11, Table 90-3), which will be followed by systemic therapy with concurrent gemcitabine and bevacizumab. Patients with tumor invasion of the duodenum are specifically excluded because of the risk of duodenal hemorrhage. The American College of Surgical Oncology Group has proposed a phase II neoadjuvant study (Z5041) in patients who have radiographically resectable tumors. That study will incorporate concurrent bevacizumab and gemcitabine before pancreaticduodenectomy and capecitabine, radiotherapy, and bevacizumab after pancreaticoduodenectomy. The recommended dosage of bevacizumab for further study is 5 mg/kg every two weeks with radiotherapy (50.4 Gy in 28 fractions) and concurrent capecitabine (825 mg/m^2 twice daily Monday through Friday).

Similarly, EGFR inhibitors hold promise as radiosensitizers, although none of the currently available inhibitors (gefitinib, erlotinib, or cetuximab) have been evaluated in multi-institutional trials in combination with radiation. Phase I studies are ongoing at Brown University and Memorial Sloan Kettering evaluating gemcitabine-based chemotherapy in combination with erlotinib. Cetuximab has been shown to improve local tumor control and overall survival in combination with EBRT alone in locally advanced head and neck cancer.[195] A phase II study at our institution is evaluating gemcitabine, oxaliplatin, and cetuximab, followed by capecitabine, radiation therapy (50.4 Gy), and cetuximab, followed by gemcitabine and cetuximab until progression. Trials that combine cetuximab or erlotinib with bevacizumab and EBRT for the treatment of pancreatic cancer are anticipated in the near future.

Radiotherapy Technique for Patients with Locally Advanced Disease Because patients with locally advanced tumors probably do not benefit from regional lymph node irradiation, radiotherapy fields should be confined to the gross tumor. This strategy reduces the gastrointestinal toxicity of chemoradiation. It is important, therefore, to identify the pancreatic tumor correctly. On contrast-enhanced CT, pancreatic tumors are typically hypodense compared with the surrounding pancreatic parenchyma. When there is doubt about the location of the primary tumor, the computed tomographic images should be reviewed with a diagnostic radiologist. Administration of an oral contrast agent at the time of simulation illuminates the duodenal "c-loop." Endobiliary biliary stents can also be visualized, which facilitates identifying the common bile duct.

The pancreas and duodenum move a median of 1 cm with respiratory excursion.[196] If the gross tumor alone is to be treated, respiratory motion must be either controlled or accounted for in radiotherapy planning. The most common way that this is accomplished is by simply adding an additional margin to the planned radiation fields in the cranial and caudal directions. However, because axial tumor motion is negligible, an additional margin for motion in the axial directions is not necessary. Radiation treatment that is gated to the respiratory cycle (respiratory gating)[197] is a necessary component of radiation dose escalation studies that seek to deliver > 60 Gy to the primary tumor while sparing the duodenum. Thus, radiation fields designed to spare the duodenum that are tightly confined to the primary tumor without correction for organ motion could lead to underdosing of the tumor target, or "marginal miss." A four-field technique is recommended with equally weighted anterior, posterior, and opposed lateral fields. A 2 cm block margin is used in the radial directions, and a 3 cm margin is used in the cranial and caudal directions.

Intensity Modulated Radiotherapy (IMRT) or Steriotactic Radiation Therapy (eg, Cyberknife) for Pancreatic Cancer? Intensity Modulated Radiotherapy (IMRT) and stereotactic radiation therapy (CyberKnife) are relatively recent technical innovations in radiotherapy. Both techniques are capable of very precise delivery of radiation to a target that is not moving. If that target is not near a radiosensitive structure, it is possible that the dose could safely be escalated, which may or may not improve outcome. Pancreatic tumors move considerably with respiration and are virtually always surrounded by the duodenum, which is a radiosensitive structure. Finally, dose escalation of radiotherapy beyond 50.4 Gy has never been demonstrated to improve outcome. We abandoned the investigation of IMRT after our phase I trial failed to reduce the toxicity of gemcitabine-based chemoradiation in spite of improved dose precision at the target.[198]

Stereotactic radiation therapy using a radiation delivery system known as the CyberKnife, with very careful control of organ motion using implanted metallic markers at the time of laparoscopy, laparotomy, or percutaneously under CT-guidance, has been evaluated in a phase I dose escalation trial using a single fraction of radiation therapy at Stanford University.[199] The final dose of 25 Gy was well tolerated and has been recommended for further study. The median time to progression was 2 months and there have been no objective responses among an updated experience of 80 patients (Koong, personal communication, 7/05). This study was conducted at a center with very specialized capabilities that are not yet ready for use outside the setting of a clinical trial. Even so, the authors acknowledge that it was "impossible to avoid treating" the duodenum to a high dose in the majority of cases. Given the lack of any convincing prospective data, the constraints of organ motion, and the lack of any evidence that dose escalation in pancreatic cancer improves outcome in any meaningful way, there is no role for either IMRT or stereotactic radiation to be used outside the setting of a clinical trial in pancreatic cancer patients. As discussed in the previous section, treatment of locally advanced pancreatic cancer is well tolerated and a modest median survival benefit is seen when the treatment volumes are confined to the gross tumor and clinically enlarged lymph nodes. This can be accomplished with a standard four-field conformal plan. The dose to the spinal cord, kidneys, and liver can very easily be kept within tolerance using this straightforward approach.

Downstaging Locally Advanced, Unresectable Disease Because surgical resection of the primary tumor remains the only potentially curative treatment of pancreatic cancer, preoperative chemoradiation therapy has been studied for its ability to convert locally unresectable pancreatic cancer to resectable disease.[176,178,200–205] In a study conducted at the New England Deaconess Hospital, 16 patients who had locally advanced, unresectable pancreatic cancer were treated with 45 Gy of EBRT and infusional 5-FU to enhance resectability.[204] However, only 2 (13%) of the patients were able to undergo resection. Similarly, investigators from Duke University reported that only 2 (8%) of 25 patients with locally advanced pancreatic cancer treated with 45 Gy of EBRT and 5-FU (with or without cisplatin or mitomycin C) were able to undergo complete resection with negative margins.[200] Preliminary reports of gemcitabine in combination with radiation have reported sufficient downstaging of locally advanced tumors to occasionally allow for resection with curative intent.[176,178] However, this phenomenon remains uncommon and unlikely to alter the management in the great majority of patients with locally advanced disease. It is also important to remember in interpreting results that, as the definition of locally advanced pancreatic cancer is loosened, results will appear more promising. If one maintains a strict CT definition of locally advanced pancreatic cancer that includes only arterial involvement (low-density tumor inseparable from the SMA or celiac axis on contrast-enhanced CT scans) or SMV or SMPV confluence occlusion, successful downstaging that allows one to proceed to complete surgical resection will be rare with currently available chemotherapy agents and chemoradiation techniques. One reason for this is that patients with locally advanced disease often have complete encasement of the SMA or celiac axis. In this setting, even the most active chemoradiation therapy regimens that cause marked tumor cell killing would not be expected to result in a margin-negative resection. In contrast, there are patients who have marginally resectable disease, in whom the pancreatic tumor abuts or cuffs a portion of the SMA or other vascular structure. As the quality of pancreatic imaging has improved, there is growing recognition that this distinct subset of marginally or borderline respectable tumors exist. For example, the National Comprehensive Cancer Network (NCCN) has defined this subgroup as locally advanced, resectable tumors. In patients with borderline tumors, upfront surgery should be discouraged since positive surgical margins would be expected to occur quite frequently. Rather, preoperative chemotherapy or chemoradiation should be considered since sufficient cytoreduction could render a tumor resectable with curative intent (ie, negative surgical margins).[206] Efforts are now underway to assess the role of preoperative therapy for this distinct group. Mehta and colleagues have reported on the Stanford University experience using preoperative infusional 5-FU and radiation in patients with marginally resectable disease.[207] Fifteen patients received chemoradiation, and of these, 9 (60%) ultimately underwent surgical resection with negative margins. Two patients were reported to have complete pathological responses. Preoperative therapy for borderline resectable tumors is also part of the focus of an ECOG randomized phase II trial in which patients will receive either gemcitabine-based chemoradiation, or a regimen of 5-FU, gemcitabine, and cisplatin, followed by 5-FU-based chemoradiation (see Table 90-3).

As discussed above, the incorporation of biologic agents into preoperative programs for borderline resectable tumors is predicted to be an area of future interest, and selected trials are currently in the design phase.

Intraoperative Radiation Therapy IORT has been used in an attempt to improve local tumor control without increasing normal tissue toxicity in patients with locally advanced disease. In studies conducted at Massachusetts General Hospital and Mayo Clinic of the combination of EBRT and IORT for locally advanced pancreatic cancer, local tumor control was improved; however, the median survival was only approximately 12 months, and the 2-year survival rate remained approximately 20%.[208,209] In an updated review of the results from the Massachusetts General Hospital, the outcomes of 150 patients undergoing IORT were reported. Eight patients were long-term survivors, and there was a significant correlation between smaller tumor size (applicator diameter 5–6 cm), and survival.[194] Not surprisingly, liver metastases, peritoneal seeding, or both developed in most patients. Therefore, although slight gains in survival may be achieved by improving local tumor control, the high incidence of distant metastases precludes significant improvements in long-term survival with IORT.

Management of Gastric Outlet Obstruction Patients with symptomatic gastric outlet obstruction and a reasonable performance status require gastric bypass, which can be performed by laparotomy or laparoscopy. However, the performance of prophylactic gastric bypass at the time of laparotomy in patients found to have unresectable disease remains controversial. Those in favor of prophylactic gastrojejunostomy state that it can be performed safely, is not associated with postoperative delayed gastric emptying, and will prevent subsequent gastric outlet obstruction in 10 to 20% of patients.[210,211] Those who do not recommend prophylactic gastric bypass believe that concomitant gastrojejunostomy (at the time of therapeutic biliary bypass) significantly increases operative morbidity; that the incidence of subsequent gastric outlet obstruction in patients who receive only a biliary bypass is much less than 10%; and that if clinically evident gastric outlet obstruction does occur, it is usually a manifestation of end-stage disease.[212–218] Lillemoe and colleagues[216] reported the results of a prospective randomized trial of prophylactic gastrojejunostomy in patients with adenocarcinoma of the pancreatic head and periampullary region. Patients found to have unresectable disease (and not to have intraoperative evidence of impending gastric outlet obstruction, in which case the patients were excluded from analysis) at the time of laparotomy were randomized to undergo either a prophylactic gastrojejunostomy or no further surgery. Subsequent gastric outlet obstruction developed in 8 (19%) of the 43 patients who did not undergo a gastric bypass and in none of the 44 patients who underwent a gastrojejunostomy. Postoperative delayed gastric emptying (2% of patients) and mean hospital stay (8 days) were not different between groups. Further, there were no perioperative deaths, and the mean survival duration was 8.3 months in both groups. Lillemoe and colleagues therefore concluded that a retrocolic gastrojejunostomy should be performed routinely when a patient with pancreatic or periampullary cancer is found at laparotomy to have unresectable disease.

The opposite conclusion was reached by Espat and colleagues[217] from Memorial Sloan-Kettering Cancer Center, who reported the longitudinal follow-up findings in 155 patients who were found to have unsuspected locally advanced or metastatic disease at the time of staging laparoscopy for presumed localized pancreatic cancer. They found a low incidence of gastric outlet obstruction in patients with advanced pancreatic cancer. Only two patients underwent elective gastric bypass (one was performed laparoscopically). At a median follow-up of 6 months (by which time 81% of patients had died of disease), only 3 (2%) of the 155 patients had undergone a subsequent open palliative surgical procedure, including a gastrojejunostomy for symptomatic gastric outlet obstruction in 2 of these patients. One additional patient required a percutaneous gastrostomy tube to relieve poor gastric emptying during the terminal phase of his disease. The median survival was 6.2 months for those with metastatic disease and 7.8 months for those with locally advanced disease, suggesting that these patients did not have high-volume metastatic disease at the time of laparoscopy. Raikar and colleagues[219] also reported a low incidence of subsequent gastric outlet obstruction in patients with unresectable pancreatic cancer who underwent endoscopic biliary decompression. In that study, only 1 (3%) of 34 patients treated with endoscopic biliary decompression required surgical bypass for gastric outlet obstruction. These two nonrandomized studies therefore do not support the routine practice of prophylactic gastric bypass.

In general, we do not perform prophylactic surgery in patients with pancreatic cancer. If a patient is found to have unresectable disease during a planned pancreaticoduodenectomy, we consider performing a gastrojejunostomy when clinical symptoms or anatomic findings suggest impending obstruction. However, in patients with locally advanced or limited metastatic disease who have a good performance status, the Lillemoe and colleagues data[216] (which come from a prospective randomized trial) would support the creation of a retrocolic gastrojejunostomy.

Tumors of the Pancreatic Body and Tail Because adenocarcinomas of the pancreatic body and tail do not obstruct the intrapancreatic portion of the common bile duct, early diagnosis is rare, and most patients have locally advanced or metastatic disease at the time of diagnosis. The celiac axis or SMA is encased in most patients, except for the anecdotal patient who presents with upper gastrointestinal hemorrhage resulting from sinistral hypertension due to splenic vein occlusion by a small tumor. In the rare patient who appears to have resectable disease on CT scans (no arterial encasement and no extrapancreatic disease), laparoscopy prior to laparotomy is a logical initial step because this frequently reveals peritoneal metastases.[116,218,220] Accurate preoperative imaging and a selective approach to surgical therapy will avoid surgery-related morbidity and mortality in patients who do not have potentially resectable disease.

The scant data on surgical resection confirm the short survival and poor prognosis in this subgroup of patients.[221,222] Further, the 43% 30-day hospital mortality rate seen in a study of 14 patients with pancreatic adenocarcinoma conducted at the Department of Veterans Affairs hospitals suggests that many of the patients who undergo surgery have advanced disease and a poor performance status.[223] Therefore, we routinely use neoadjuvant chemotherapy therapy in patients with apparently localized adenocarcinoma of the pancreatic body or tail. Distal subtotal pancreatectomy is then considered in the rare patient who shows no evidence of disease progression on restaging radiographic studies after chemoradiation therapy and who has a performance status acceptable for major abdominal surgery. In all other patients, enrollment in phase II investigational trials should be considered.

Approach to the Patient with Locally Advanced Disease Published data suggest that survival duration is increased in patients who receive chemoradiation therapy for locally advanced pancreatic cancer, but this is limited largely to patients who have a good performance status. In selected patients, aggressive treatment consisting of EBRT and chemotherapy may result in a median survival of approximately 12 months and a 2-year survival rate of 20%, although long-term survivors are rare. The use of chemoradiation is justified in fully ambulatory patients with locally advanced disease who have pain but otherwise minimal symptoms. Indeed, palliation of pain is a compelling reason to consider chemoradiation in patients with locally advanced disease. The palliative benefit of chemoradiation with or without IORT has not been compared with gemcitabine, which yields a clinical benefit in 23.8% of patients with advanced pancreatic cancer (locally advanced or metastatic).[185] The potential clinical benefit associated with chemoradiation has not been rigorously studied. In one retrospective review of 25 patients with locally advanced disease, Fisher and colleagues[224] observed a clinical benefit in only 24% of patients undergoing chemoradiation, suggesting that the benefit may actually be equivalent to that observed with gemcitabine.

It remains unclear if patients who have received chemoradiation should be treated immediately with further systemic therapy or followed expectantly for clinical and/or radiographic evidence of progressive disease. Progressive disease may take the form of local tumor progression with increasing pain, gastric outlet obstruction, or recurrent biliary obstruction; distant metastatic disease with liver or lung metastases; or peritoneal carcinomatosis. Whenever possible, patients with locally advanced disease having a good performance status should be treated in the context of a clinical trial. This may involve a predefined course of chemotherapy followed by chemoradiation, or alternatively a program of chemoradiation with a targeted agent, followed by further systemic therapy.

Outside of a clinical trial, systemic therapy with gemcitabine alone or in combination also represents a reasonable alternative in patients with locally advanced pancreatic cancer. Systemic therapy alone may improve both pain control and performance status,[185] and avoids the gastrointestinal toxicity associated with chemoradiation.[168] For those patients with stable or responding disease after 4 to 6 months of systemic therapy, chemoradiation can then be used to maximize local-regional tumor control. This treatment sequence has the advantage of avoiding the toxicity of chemoradiation in those patients who show evidence progressive disease following systemic therapy. Chemoradiation is thereby applied only to the patients most likely to benefit as defined by the absence of disease progression during systemic therapy; a similar rationale to the use of neoadjuvant systemic therapy prior to surgery in patients with potentially resectable pancreatic cancer.

The decision regarding the dose of radiation for patients with locally advanced disease outside of a clinical trial depends on the potential for the patient to undergo surgery (see above discussion on downstaging). Based on our experience, the median survival in patients with locally advanced pancreatic cancer treated with concurrent protracted infusion of 5-FU and EBRT to a dose of 30 Gy in 10 fractions over 2 weeks is similar to that achieved with a dose of 50.4 Gy in 28 fractions over 5.5 weeks with the same chemotherapy.[225] Although 50.4 Gy is a more commonly prescribed dose, it does not significantly improve outcome and has a slightly higher risk of acute toxicity. However, patients with minimal arterial abutment ("marginally resectable" cases) should be treated with 50.4 Gy to maximize the possibility of surgical resection. Prospective studies that evaluate novel radiosensitizers should administer 50.4 Gy to maximize the opportunity for radiosensitization.

For patients who have poor performance status, chemoradiation is probably not indicated. Regardless, adequate pain control in these patients—as in all cancer patients—is critically important. Proper pain control improves performance status and quality of life, which may translate into increased survival.[226] The limited therapeutic options available for patients with locally advanced disease and the modest impact of current treatments on survival provide the rationale for the entry of patients with locally advanced pancreatic cancer into trials of novel systemic agents.

TREATMENT OF METASTATIC DISEASE

Progress in the treatment of metastatic pancreatic cancer has been extremely slow for several reasons. First, patients with pancreatic cancer often have rapidly evolving clinical problems. During a course of systemic therapy, biliary obstruction, biliary stent occlusion with cholangitis, significant increases in pain, rapidly accumulating ascites, gastric outlet obstruction, or venous thromboembolism may develop. Given these potential problems, completing a prescribed course of chemotherapy in a timely fashion can be quite challenging for the patient (and physician), even when tumor progression is not the immediate cause. Second, it has taken some time to fully appreciate the resistance of pancreatic cancer to treatment of any kind. Early reports of high response rates to cytotoxic therapy greatly overestimated the activity of chemotherapy in this disease. This misperception had its origins in the inadequate measures used to gauge objective response. Specifically, many early trials of systemic therapy relied heavily on physical examination, liver scan, and ultrasonography to assess response to systemic therapy.[227–230] With the advent of high-quality CT and magnetic resonance imaging (MRI), which provide better cross-sectional imaging,[231] substantially lower response rates have been seen in recent trials of chemotherapy.[185,188,232–246] Moreover, even with improved imaging, interpreting changes in the primary tumor mass is not an accurate measure of response. This is because of the intense desmoplastic reaction to the malignant epithelium within the gland itself.[247] Thus, if some decrease in the primary tumor mass is seen, it may refect the resolution of peritumoral inflammation and desmoplasia rather than malignant cell death. In contrast, the radiographic appearance of a pancreatic mass may remain unchanged, even when significant tumor destruction has occurred.

A third factor hindering the progress of treatment of metastatic disease is that trials of chemotherapy have usually enrolled two groups of patients: those with locally advanced disease and those with metastatic disease. Median survival duration in such patients may vary from 2 months to 12 months depending on tumor burden and performance status. Using such a heterogeneous population, many phase II trials of chemotherapy have reported survival rates that are quite promising compared with standard treatments. However, if the study population consists of a large proportion of patients with locally advanced disease and good performance status, the favorable survival duration may be largely unrelated to the chemotherapy program being studied. Finally, compared with patients with other common malignancies, such as colon cancer or breast cancer, patients with pancreatic cancer are often much more debilitated at the time of diagnosis. This has precluded enrolling large numbers of patients in clinical trials, substantially slowing progress in clinical trial development.

With these factors in mind, the role of systemic therapy in the setting of metastatic pancreatic cancer will be reviewed. As will be discussed, gemcitabine continues to be the standard therapy for patients with metastatic pancreatic cancer. Whether or not the addition of erolitinib to gemcitabine should be considered a new standard regimen for pancreatic cancer is currently being debated, and the basis for this will also be reviewed. In either case, the impact of these treatments has been marginal, and, therefore, all patients with metastatic disease and adequate performance status should be considered for enrollment in well-designed clinical trials.

SYSTEMIC CHEMOTHERAPY FOR PANCREATIC CANCER: A HISTORICAL PERSPECTIVE **Fluorinated Pyrimidines** Thymidylate synthase inhibition with 5-FU has been extensively studied for the treatment of advanced pancreatic cancer.[248–250] In a review of trials dating back to the 1960s and 1970s, the overall response rate to 5-FU was estimated to be 28%.[250] However, these early studies relied on criteria other than CT or MRI findings to define response. With the greater accuracy of CT and MRI, the recent experience with 5-FU has been much more modest.[239,244]

Indeed, the latest trials of 5-FU in advanced pancreatic cancer have shown that it has virtually no activity when given as a bolus injection either weekly or daily for 5 days. For example, in a randomized trial comparing weekly bolus 5-FU with weekly gemcitabine, there were no objective responses observed in 57 patients with bidimensional measurable disease treated with 5-FU.[185] In another trial reported by Ruben and colleagues,[239] a combination of bolus 5-FU with leucovorin given daily for 5 days yielded no objective responses among 31 patients.

Although bolus injections of 5-FU have been ineffective for the treatment of advanced pancreatic cancer, investigations of prolonged infusional 5-FU and orally bioavailable fluorinated pyrimidines delivered over extended time periods suggest some low level activity. In a randomized trial comparing infusional 5-FU with infusional 5-FU plus mitomycin C, 105 patients were randomized to receive infusional 5-FU alone. The response rate among these patients was 8.6% (confidence interval, 3.2–13.7%), which is comparable to the response seen for gemcitabine as a single agent.[244] The oral agents UFT (a fixed combination of tegafur and uracil) and capecitabine have also been studied in pancreatic cancer. In a phase II trial of UFT/leucovorin in which 14 patients with advanced pancreatic cancer were treated, none had an objective tumor response.[242] However, capecitabine, a 5-FU prodrug, appears to have some activity in pancreatic cancer. Cartwright and colleagues[188] treated 42 patients with advanced disease (41 with measurable disease) with the capecitabine and found an objective response rate of 7.3% with 24% of these patients showing a clinical benefit from the drug. Median survival was not reported.

In summary, with over 40 years' experience with 5-FU, widely disparate levels of activity have been reported. Part of this can be explained by inadequate measures of objective response used in early trials. In the era of high-quality cross-sectional imaging, most trials of 5-FU now suggest it is inactive when given as a bolus injection, but when delivered as a continuous infusion, or in the form of capecitabine, response rates range from 7 to 8%. At the present time, these agents continue to be investigated in combination with other drugs, as will be discussed in more detail below.

Drug Combinations Based on 5-FU In general, combination chemotherapy with 5-FU has not proved superior to single-agent 5-FU in the management of pancreatic cancer, with trials dating back over 20 years. For example, the Southwest Oncology Group performed a series of phase II trials comparing single-agent chemotherapy with combinations of 5-FU, doxorubicin, mitomycin C, and streptozocin.[251] The median survival for patients who received single-agent therapy and combination therapy was 3.4 and 4.8 months, respectively, indicating no significant benefit from combination chemotherapy. Other groups have studied combinations of 5-FU, doxorubicin, and mitomycin C (FAM),[228,252] or streptozotocin, mitomycin C, and 5-FU (SMF).[253] In addition, the Mallinson regimen, which consisted of induction therapy with 5-FU, cyclophosphamide, methotrexate, and vincristine, followed by maintenance treatment with 5-FU and mitomycin C has also been tested.[254] After initial enthusiasm for these three regimens in phase II trials, none of them demonstrated any significant advantage over single-agent 5-FU for advanced disease, and some might argue, over best supportive care.[255–257]

More recently, a combination of infusional 5-FU with mitomycin C has been compared with infusional 5-FU alone for patients with advanced pancreatic cancer. Although the response rate to the combination was higher (17.6% vs 8.4%), no survival advantage was seen for the combination (6.5 months versus 5.1 months, $p = .34$). This, despite the fact that a higher proportion of patients treated with the combination had locally advanced disease (44% vs 36%).[244] Lastly, preliminary results using a combination of infusional 5-FU (200 mg/m^2/day), leucovorin (30 mg/m^2/week), mitomycin C (10 mg/m^2 every 6 weeks), and dipyridamole (75 mg/day) were encouraging. In a small pilot trial, this combination produced 12 responses (75%) in 16 patients with locally advanced pancreatic cancer.[258] Five of these were objective complete responses documented by CT and tumor marker measurements. At the time of publication, the median survival had not yet been reached but was projected to be greater than 1 year. Five of the responding patients had received radiotherapy, but this was not believed to have affected overall survival. In a subsequent report from the same group, this regimen was reported to achieve a lower response rate (39%) in 38 patients with locally advanced disease, with CT scans in 6 of the 15 responding patients showing sufficient improvement in their tumor to justify surgical exploration.[201] However, in another phase II trial of this regimen performed by Burch and colleagues,[259] the response rate to this four-drug combination was lower still (22%) among 46 evaluable patients with advanced pancreatic cancer. Moreover, the median survival among the 50 registered patients was only 4.6 months, leading the investigators to believe this regimen was not sufficiently active to justify its investigation in a phase III trial.

In conclusion, a variety of 5-FU based combinations have been tested in pancreatic cancer, with no clear demonstration of superiority of one regimen over another, or over 5-FU alone. Therefore, most modern efforts to improve outcome for patients' metastatic disease have focused on the role of gemcitabine, the camptothecins, and a few other drugs that appear to have either additive or synergistic effects when used together.

Gemcitabine For almost a decade, gemcitabine (2'-deoxy-2'2'-difluorocytidine) has shown modest reproducible activity against advanced pancreatic cancer.[185,232–234] As a prodrug, gemcitabine, which has structural and metabolic similarities to cytarabine, must be phosphorylated to its active metabolites gemcitabine diphosphate (dFdCDP) and gemcitabine triphosphate (dFdCTP). In both preclinical and clinical testing, gemcitabine has demonstrated greater activity against solid tumors than cytarabine.[260] These observations may be explained by gemcitabine's greater lipophilicity, its higher affinity for deoxycytidine kinase, and the greater intracellular retention of dFdCTP than to cytarabine.[261]

Following phase I evaluation,[262] gemcitabine was used in a multicenter trial involving 44 patients with advanced pancreatic cancer.[232] Although only five objective responses (11%) were documented, the investigators noted frequent subjective symptomatic benefits. In another study, gemcitabine again led to few objective responses (2 of 32 patients), but symptomatic improvement was also reported by patients enrolled in the trial.[233] Based on these observations, two subsequent trials of gemcitabine for advanced pancreatic cancer were completed. In one randomized trial, gemcitabine was compared with bolus weekly 5-FU treatment in previously untreated patients.[185] Patients treated with gemcitabine achieved a higher response rate (5.4% vs 0%) and a statistically significant improvement in median survival compared with those treated with 5-FU (5.65 vs 4.41 months, $p = .0025$). The 1-year survival rate for patients treated with gemcitabine was 18%, whereas the rate was only 2% for those treated with 5-FU. Importantly, gemcitabine was found to have more clinically meaningful effects on disease-related symptoms than 5-FU. These clinical benefits were also documented in patients treated with gemcitabine after experiencing disease progression while receiving 5-FU.[263] The clinical benefit and the modest survival advantage associated with gemcitabine as opposed to bolus weekly 5-FU treatment have helped gemcitabine become accepted as first-line therapy for patients with advanced pancreatic adenocarcinoma. In virtually all large phase III trials of frontline chemotherapy for advanced pancreatic cancer, treatment with gemcitabine is usually the control arm.

Further investigations of gemcitabine have been conducted in an attempt to improve its therapeutic index. For example, early phase II trials of weekly, 30-minute infusions of gemcitabine showed that higher doses could be safely administered to chemotherapy-naïve patients than to patients who had received prior chemotherapy. However, cellular pharmacologic studies suggested that simply increasing the dose administered over 30 minutes did not enhance cytotoxicity or improve gemcitabine's therapeutic index. During early clinical trials in patients with solid tumors, measurement of dFdCTP levels in peripheral blood mononuclear cells revealed that the rate of gemcitabine phosphorylation, like that of cytarabine, was subject to saturation kinetics.[262,264] Specifically, the concentration of dFdCTP in the circulating mononuclear cells increased in proportion to a gemcitabine dose of between 35 and 250 mg/m^2, but higher intracellular dFdCTP levels were not observed at higher doses (350–1,000 mg/m^2); instead, the plasma gemcitabine concentrations rose to greater than 20 nmol/L, suggesting a saturation of gemcitabine 5'-phosphate accumulation.[264] The rate of dFdCTP accumulation and the peak cellular concentration were highest at a dose rate of 350 mg/m^2 per 30 minutes (~10 mg/m^2/min), during which steady-state gemcitabine levels of 15 to 20 nmol/L were achieved in plasma. Similar results were found in a pilot trial of gemcitabine in leukemia patients.[265] A more comprehensive phase I trial in leukemia patients showed that a gemcitabine dose rate of 10 mg/m^2/min achieved a mean steady-state gemcitabine level of 26.5 nmol/L and was sufficient to maximize the rate of dFdCTP accumulation in circulating blasts.[266]

The pharmacokinetic relationships documented in the studies just described suggest that increasing the infusion time for gemcitabine while holding the dose rate constant would increase the intracellular levels of the active metabolites dFdCDP and dFdCTP and thus achieve the goal of dose intensification. To establish the feasibility of this approach, a phase I study of gemcitabine was conducted in patients with advanced solid tumors in which doses were escalating by increasing the duration of the weekly gemcitabine infusions while maintaining the fixed dose rate (FDR) at 10 mg/m^2/min.[267,268] A subsequent randomized phase II trial in patients with metastatic pancreatic cancer showed that short infusional schedules of FDR gemcitabine (10 mg/m^2/min) may be more effective than the standard 30-minute bolus technique.[269] Results from this trial further demonstrated that, compared with 2,300 mg/m^2 infused over 30 minutes, FDR gemcitabine dosed at 1,500 mg/m^2 delivered over 150 minutes led to a similar objective response rate, but a trend toward longer survival (8.0 months vs 5.0 months, $p = .13$). Given the limited activity of gemcitabine in pancreatic cancer, optimal drug delivery supported by sound pharmacokinetic principles should continue to be explored and recent clinical studies of gemcitabine have started to investigate FDR gemcitabine.

The Camptothecins Four camptothecins have been evaluated in patients with advanced pancreatic cancer: topotecan, irinotecan, rubitecan, and exatecan mesylate. Topotecan, administered once daily for 5 days or as a 21-day continuous infusion, has been ineffective.[237,270–272] Irinotecan (CPT-11) has been evaluated at a dosage of 350 mg/m^2 every 3 weeks. Objective partial responses were documented in 3 of 34 patients (9%), with a median survival for the group of 5 months.[238] Single-agent irinotecan has not been further pursued, and development of irinotecan as a drug therapy for pancreatic cancer has proceeded in combination with gemcitabine or docetaxel.

The oral topoisomerase I inhibitor, 9-nitrocamptothecin, also known as rubitecan, was initially thought to have significant activity in advanced disease based on results from two phase II trials. In one study involving 107 patients, the drug was given orally (1–1.5 mg/m^2/day, 5 days/week) and the response rate was 32%; 1 patient survived 44 months.[245] However, only 60 of the initial 107 patients enrolled were evaluable for response, which was defined using a panel of parameters, including serum tumor markers, clinical benefit, and objective radiographic response. In another, smaller study with a similar design and dose, rubitecan again demonstrated promising activity, with a response rate of 28.6% in 14 evaluable patients.[246] Of note, 5 patients (26%) enrolled in the study were not considered evaluable for response because of rapid tumor progression during the first 6 weeks of treatment. More recently, rubitecan was compared with "best choice" therapy that included best supportive care or further palliative chemotherapy in 409 patients with refractory disease.[273]

For those patients randomized to best choice, the treating physician made the decision about supportive care or continued chemotherapy. Median survival for patients receiving rubitecan was 108 days, versus 94 days for those randomized to best choice ($p = .626$). Presently, two phase III trials of rubitecan are being conducted. One directly compares gemcitabine to rubitecan as front-line therapy, and the other trial randomizes chemonaïve advanced pancreatic cancer patients to receive either gemcitabine alone or gemcitabine in combination with rubitecan.

Lastly, the camptothecin DX8915f (exatecan mesylate) has been investigated in pancreatic cancer. This drug has been delivered IV once every 21 days and daily for 5 days.[274,275] Unfortunately, preliminary results from a phase III trial directly comparing exatecan mesylate with gemcitabine showed no survival advantage for those patients receiving exatecan mesylate (median survival = 157 days for exatecan mesylate, 197 days for gemcitabine).[276]

Thus far, the preponderance of data suggest that although camptothecins do have some single-agent activity, they offer no meaningful advantage over single-agent gemcitabine. Furthermore, no positive interaction between the camptothecins and gemcitabine have been observed to date. Results of two large phase III trials have failed to demonstrate any survival benefit when either irinotecan or exatecan mesylate has been added to gemcitabine.[277,278] Nevertheless, other camptothecin combinations are currently being investigated in pancreatic cancer. For example, in a phase I study of irinotecan and docetaxel administered to patients with advanced solid tumors, objective responses were observed in 2 patients with pancreatic cancer.[279] This has generated the impetus for a phase II trial of irinotecan/docetaxel in advanced disease conducted through ECOG (www.ecog.org).

Other Agents Tested in Advanced Pancreatic Cancer A large number of other drugs have been tested in pancreatic cancer. Most do not have any significant activity as single agents, including etoposide, trofosphamide, trimetrexate, amonafide, iproplatin, edatrexate, fazarabine, ifosfamide, diaziquone, and mitoguazone.[241,243,251,280–287] A few drugs, most notably cisplatin, oxaliplatin, mitomycin C, and docetaxel appear to have some efficacy, but this is usually seen when they are combined with other agents such as gemcitabine.[244,288–293]

Table 90-4 Selected Phase III Trials of Gemcitabine vs Gemcitabine Doublets for Patients with Advanced Pancreatic Cancer

Author, Year	Number of Patients	Median Survival (Months) Gem-Monotherapy	Gem-Doublet	*p*-Value
Berlin, 2002[234] (Gem ± 5-FU)	322	5.4	6.7	.09
Colucci, 2002[307] (Gem ± CDDP)	107	4.6	7.0	.43
Louvet, 2004[308] (Gem ± Oxaliplatin)	313	7.1	9.0	.13
O'Reilly, 2004[278] (Gem ± Exatecan)	349	6.2	6.7	.52
Herrmann, 2005[309] (Gem ± Capecitabine)	319	7.3	8.4	.314
Moore, 2005[310] (Gem ± Erlotinib)	569	5.91	6.37	.011

Gem = gemcitabine.

Recent Efforts to Improve Systemic Therapy **Gemcitabine Combinations** Given the growing acceptance of gemcitabine as first-line therapy for advanced pancreatic cancer, gemcitabine-based combinations have been under active evaluation for the last several years. In most trials, gemcitabine has been combined with one other agent such as docetaxel, capecitabine, oxaliplatin, 5-FU/leucovorin, cisplatin, UFT, irinotecan, premetrexed, and epirubicin.[288–292,294–303] Generally, response rates to these combinations are higher than those typically reported for gemcitabine alone. In addition, regimens consisting of two to four other drugs with gemcitabine are starting to be described in the literature. These include a combination of gemcitabine, capecitabine, and docetaxel (GTX);[304] gemcitabine, 5-FU, leucovorin, irinotecan, and cisplatin (G-FLIP);[305] and gemcitabine, epirubicin, infusional 5-FU, and cisplatin.[306]

Unfortunately, just as 5-FU based combinations have been disappointing when compared with 5-FU, so too have gemcitabine-based regimens compared with gemcitabine alone. Table 90-4 summarizes the results of a number of phase III trials evaluating gemcitabine against a gemcitabine doublet.[234,278,307–310] Two trials are worth highlighting. The first is a trial conducted by Louvet and colleagues for the French Multidisciplinary Clinical Research Group in Oncology (GERCOR) and the Italian Group for the Study of Gastrointestinal Tract Cancer (GISCAD).[308] In that trial, 313 chemonaïve patients with advanced pancreatic cancer were randomized to receive gemcitabine dosed at 1,000 mg/m^2 delivered over 30 minutes as previously described by Burris, or to GemOx, a regimen of FDR gemcitabine dosed at 1,000 mg/m^2 delivered over 100 minutes on day 1, followed by oxaliplatin 100 mg/m^2 over 2 hours on day 2, repeated every 14 days. The response rate was improved for patients receiving GemOx compared with those randomized to gemcitabine (26.8% vs 17.3%, $p = .04$) as was progression-free survival (5.8 vs 3.7 months, $p = .04$). However, although median survival was also improved from 7.1 months to 9 months with the addition of oxaliplatin, this did not reach statistical significance ($p = .13$). Whether the higher response rate seen with GexOx was attributable to the addition of oxaliplatin or to the delivery of FDR gemcitabine remains debated and is the subject of an ongoing ECOG trial. In that study, patients with advanced pancreatic cancer will be randomized to one of three arms: gemcitabine alone given over the standard 30 minutes, FDR gemcitabine, or FDR gemcitabine with oxaliplatin.[311]

Pending the results of the ECOG trial, the results from the GERCOR/GISCAD trial have been sufficiently compelling to influence recent NCCN guidelines for pancreatic cancer therapy (www.nccn.org). These guidelines allow for the addition of either cisplatin or oxaliplatin to gemcitabine as reasonable alternatives to single-agent gemcitabine in patients with good performance status.

The second noteworthy trial of those summarized in Table 90-4 was performed by the National Cancer Institute of Canada Clinical Trials Group and was designed to investigate whether the addition of the receptor tyrosine kinase inhibitor, erlotinib to gemcitabine provided any survival benefit.[310] This trial has been the first to demonstrate a small survival advantage for a gemcitabine doublet over gemcitabine monotherapy. Although the improvement in survival provided by erlotinib was quite modest, this result has been considered proof of principle in regard to the future promise of molecularly targeted agents and their role in treatment.

Future Approaches to the Treatment of Systemic Disease Although gemcitabine has repeatedly shown modest activity against metastatic pancreatic cancer, the median survival in patients who receive it continues to hover around 6 months. Moreover, although gemcitabine and other agents have been promoted for their palliative benefits, some of these effects may not be substantially different from those achieved with aggressive supportive care alone. Therefore, although the continued development of alternative gemcitabine schedules and combinations is warranted, any documented improvements in patient outcome are predicted to be relatively small. Thus, the investigation of novel cytotoxic and cytostatic agents should be given priority. The recent elucidation of molecular events implicated in pancreatic carcinogenesis and chemoresistance and a greater understanding of the metastatic process, including the role of angiogenesis, provide the foundation for such therapies.

Systemic agents under active clinical investigation are described below, with an emphasis on therapies intended to inhibit specific signals required for cell growth, invasion, and metastasis. Many of the molecular therapies developed to date have been designed to exploit molecular perturbations within the tumor cells. However, there is growing appreciation for the complex interactions between the tumor cells and the host environment, usually referred to as the tumor microenvironment. A variety of factors are involved in fostering this permissive milieu for tumor cells to continue to flourish and disseminate within the body and some drugs now under development are designed to inhibit the interface between the tumor and host. Investigation of any particular agent must recognize what compartment is being targeted for exploitation: the tumor cell, the microenvironment, or both.

Drugs Aimed at the Tumor Cell **Targeting the *Ras* Oncogene: Farnesyl Transferase Inhibitors** Since the *ras* oncogene is mutated and constitutively activated in most pancreatic cancers, inhibiting k-*ras* has been an attractive target for therapy. The protein product of k-*ras* is a guanosine triphosphate GTP-binding protein required to transduce extracellular proliferative signals downstream through the mitogen activated protein (MAP)-kinase cascade. One strategy to inhibit Ras protein function interrupts the post-translational processing (farnesylation) necessary to localize

Ras protein to the cytoplasmic side of the plasma membrane.[312] This approach became feasible with the discovery and synthesis of specific small molecules that inhibit the enzyme farnesyl transferase.[313] The consequence of this prevents Ras oncoprotein localization to the cell membrane and renders it functionally inactive.

A number of farnesyl transferase inhibitors have been tested, including SCH 66336, R115777 (tipifarnib), and BMS 214662. These agents are all orally bioavailable, and phase I clinical testing has been completed.[314–317,376–379] Gastrointestinal toxicity and fatigue are the most common side effects; hematologic toxicity, particularly neutropenia, has also been observed. Early reports of activity in pancreatic cancer initially appeared in abstract form. For example, in a randomized phase II trial, SCH 66336 was compared with gemcitabine in patients with advanced pancreatic cancer.[318] Patients received either gemcitabine at a dosage of 1,000 mg/m^2 weekly for 7 weeks followed by infusions weekly for 3 weeks or SCH 66336 at a dosage of 200 mg twice daily. Two of 33 patients treated with SCH 66336 showed a partial response (6%), which compared favorably with the response to single-agent gemcitabine (3%).

Subsequently, a large phase III trial was conducted to determine if an FTI could improve survival when added to gemcitabine. Van Cutsem and colleagues enrolled 342 subjects with advanced pancreatic cancer to receive either gemcitabine alone or gemcitabine and tipifarnib.[319] The response rates and overall survival were not improved with the addition of the FTI. Although the FTIs as a class continue to be investigated in other malignancies, they are not being developed as treatment of pancreatic cancer. It remains uncertain why these agents, which appeared to hold great promise as targeted therapy for pancreatic cancer, were ineffective. Some have postulated that these drugs inhibit farnesylation of other important intracellular signaling proteins somehow negating any observable antitumor effect caused by mutant Ras inhibition.

Targeting HER2: Traztuzumab The receptor tyrosine kinase HER2 is part of the HER family of receptors that include HER1 (epidermal growth factor receptor-EGFR), and HER3, heregulin. The ligands for HER2 have not been fully elucidated, but binding this protein leads to growth promoting signals and inhibition of apoptosis. In human tumor specimens, HER2 is overexpressed in many, including a subset of breast, ovarian, gastric, colon, and pancreatic cancers. Trastuzumab is a humanized monoclonal antibody to the HER2 receptor that has been intensively studied in breast cancer. In patients with metastatic breast cancer overexpressing HER2 based on immunohistochemical staining, trastuzumab alone can lead to an objective response rate of 11 to 26%.[320,321] When combined with other cytotoxic agents, the response rate is greater. In a randomized trial comparing cytotoxic therapy alone to cytotoxic therapy with trastuzumab, survival was improved for women with metastatic breast cancers overexpressing HER2, particularly when combined with paclitaxel.[322] Furthermore, preliminary results from a recently completed randomized trial have shown that the addition of trastuzumab to adjuvant chemotherapy improves disease-free survival for women with HER2 overexpressing breast cancer compared with the survival for those women receiving adjuvant chemotherapy alone.

Such dramatic results have spurred interest in trastuzumab as a potential weapon against pancreatic cancer, especially since early reports suggested that HER2 was overexpressed in human pancreatic cancer ranging from 20 to 80% of the time.[323,324] Thus, Safran and colleagues investigated the combination of gemcitabine and trastuzumab in a group of patients with advanced pancreatic cancer whose tumors overexpressed HER2 based on immunohistochemistry.[325] Screening tumors for HER2 overexpresson was disappointing with only 16% considered 2+ or 3+ positive for HER2. Of the 34 patients enrolled, only 6% had an objective response rate to the combination. However, median survival for the group was 7 months, suggesting the possibility of a therapeutic benefit with the addition of trastuzumab. Unfortunately, although trastuzumab has been proven to be a potent tumor-directed molecular therapy in breast cancer, the rate of overexpression in pancreatic cancer is too low to consider this strategy as a relevant one for most patients with pancreatic cancer.

Targeting the Tumor Microenvironment

Although the mechanisms underlying tumor invasion, metastasis, and angiogenesis have not been fully elucidated, it is clear these events are complex, interdependent, and tightly regulated. For example, as proliferating tumor cells come into contact with surrounding normal tissues, they secrete degradative enzymes, which act on the basement membrane and other extracellular matrix (ECM) proteins. Locked within the ECM are a number of proangiogenic factors. As the ECM is degraded, these factors are released leading to endothelial migration and proliferation. In addition, other factors may also be unlocked from the ECM promoting tumor cell motility and spurring further growth. Degradation of the basement membrane and ECM also provides access to lymphatic and vasculature channels, permitting tumor embolization to more distant sites where the processes of invasion and angiogenesis continue.

Matrix Metalloproteinase Inhibition: Marimastat Efforts to impede degradation of the ECM have focused on the role of matrix metalloproteinases (MMPs). MMPs are a large family of proteases involved in physiologic tissue remodeling, required for normal wound healing, and in pathologic processes such as arthritis and cancer invasion. In pancreatic cancer, MMP-2 and MMP-9 are highly overexpressed. MMP-2 in particular is thought to play a central role in tumor cell invasion. Although endogenous inhibitors exist to regulate the activity of the MMPs, these are bulky molecules which are unlikely to be clinically relevant given their pharmacologic properties.[326] However, smaller synthetic MMP inhibitors (MMPIs) have been developed, including batimastat, marimastat, BMS-275291, and BAY 12-9566.[327–329] Of these, marimastat, an oral MMP-2 and MMP-9 inhibitor has been the most widely investigated. This drug has been tested as part of treatment of small-cell lung cancer and cancers of the colon, ovary, and pancreas. In pancreatic cancer, three large phase III trials have been completed. In one study, 414 patients with advanced pancreatic cancer were randomized to one of four arms: marimastat at 5 mg, 10 mg, or 25 mg twice daily, or to single-agent gemcitabine.[330] Marimastat at either 5 or 10 mg was inferior to gemcitabine alone, but when marimastat was delivered at a dosage of 25 mg twice daily, survival was not statistically different from survival achieved using gemcitabine. These results suggest a dose response to marimastat's activity. Importantly grade 2 and 3 toxicity was less common using marimastat compared with gemcitabine (15% vs 22%).

In another phase III trial, the combination of gemcitabine with marimastat was compared with treatment using gemcitabine alone. Response and survival times were similar in both arms, implying no added benefit to marimastat.[331]

Antiangiogenic Agents Folkman proposed inhibition of tumor angiogenesis as a potential anticancer therapy 30 years ago.[332] Since then, some important angiogenic factors produced by the tumor cells or released by the ECM have been isolated and characterized. Key among them is vascular endothelial growth factor (VEGF). This protein has been considered critical to endothelial cell survival, proliferation, and migration, but it also has other important functions. A number of drugs have been developed to directly inhibit VEGF binding to its receptors, or to inhibit the activation of VEGF receptors. A number of drugs have entered the clinic, including bevacizumab, a humanized murine monoclonal antibody to VEGF, and several receptor tyrosine kinase inhibitors, SU5416, SU6366, and PTK787/ZK222584.[333–336]

Bevacizumab has already been proven to improve survival in patients with advanced colon cancer when combined with front-line or second chemotherapy. Given its impressive clinical activity in colon cancer, it is now being investigated as a potential agent for the treatment of pancreatic cancer.

Recently Kindler and colleagues combined bevacizumab at a dose of 10 mg/kg with standard dose gemcitabine in a group of 40 patients with metastatic pancreatic cancer. The confirmed partial response rate to this combination was 24%, and although follow-up data remain immature, the estimated 1-year survival rate is 54%.[337] Therefore, a randomized trial comparing gemcitabine monotherapy to gemcitabine with bevacizumab has been launched through the Cancer and Leukemia Group B (CALGB).

Agents That Target Both the Tumor Cell and the Tumor Microenvironment

Pleomorphic Effects of Anti-VEGF Therapy Bevacizumab and other agents designed to inhibit VEGF pathways are generally considered to act through antiangiogenic mechanisms. However, VEGF appears to have broader effects, which may be important to tumor cell proliferation, tumor perfusion, and angiogenesis. For example, one of the first recognized effects of VEGF was the promotion of capillary leakage,[338] which has been thought to explain increases in intratumoral interstitial pressure.[339] When anti-VEGF therapy is introduced in experimental systems, or in patients, interstitial pressures have been shown to decrease, and in some cases result in net increases in regional blood flow.[190,340,341] This effect could potentially allow for improved delivery of cytotoxic chemotherapy within a tumor mass and may explain why bevacizumab increases objective responses to cytotoxic chemotherapy. This may also explain its effect as a radiosensitizer.[190]

In addition, experiments have shown that VEGF receptors are often overexpressed on tumor cells and anti-VEGF therapy may therefore have a direct impact on tumor cell growth inhibition, apoptosis, and motility.[342] These effects may be completely independent from the antiangiogenic effects of anti-VEGF treatment. Therefore, bevacizumab and other drugs that inhibit VEGF signaling may work in two distinct compartments: the tumor cell itself and the tumor microenvironment. This compartmental model may also explain the therapeutic benefits recently observed with the EGFR inhibitors cetuximab and erlotinib.

Epidermal Growth Factor Receptor Antagonism: Cetuximab and Erlotinib For example, antibodies to the epidermal growth factor receptor (EGFR) have been shown to compete with the growth-stimulatory ligands for binding. When bound, antibodies with specificity for EGFR result in growth inhibition and, in some cases, apoptosis. A humanized monoclonal antibody to EGFR, cetuximab, has shown potent competitive binding to the receptor, leading to growth inhibition.[343] In vitro studies suggest an additive effect of C225 when it is given with cytotoxic agents. This supports the postulate that inhibiting EGFR has direct consequences for the tumor cells. Importantly, however, in animal models of metastasis the effects of combining gemcitabine with cetuximab are not simply additive, but synergistic.[344] This implicates other mechanisms for the activity of cetuximab. Emerging data have shown that EGFR is expressed on immature endothelium, and, therefore, EGFR inhibition may also act as an antiangiogenic agent.[345]

Given the encouraging results seen in animal models of pancreatic cancer in which gemcitabine and cetuximab were combined, the combination was investigated in the clinic. Xiong and colleagues have reported the results of a phase II trial of gemcitabine combination with cetuximab.[346] The objective response rate to the combination was 12%, which may be slightly better than previously reported for gemcitabine alone. Moreover, the 1-year survival rate was 32%, which is encouraging when one considers that over 80% of the enrolled patients had metastatic disease at the time of enrollment.[346] These results have been sufficiently provocative to launch a large phase III trial through the Southwest Oncology Group, which is comparing gemcitabine alone with gemcitabine plus cetuximab for the treatment of advanced pancreatic cancer (www.swog.org).

Table 90-5 Summary of Completed Randomized Trials of Gemcitabine Alone (or with Placebo) vs Gemcitabine with a Targeted Agent in the Treatment of Advanced Pancreatic Cancer

Principal Investigator Year Gemcitabine ± Targeted Agent	Number of Patients	Objective Response Rate	Median Survival (Days)	% 1-Year Survival	*p*-Value (Median Survival Comparison)
Van Cutsem, 2004[319]					
Gem + placebo	347	8%	182	24%	
vs					
Gem + tipifarnib	341	6%	193	27%	.75
Bramhall, 2002[331]					
Gem + placebo	119	11%	164	18%	
vs					
Gem + marimastat	120	11%	165.5	17%	.95
Moore, 2005[310]					
Gem	284	8.0%	177	17%	
vs					
Gem + erolotinib	285	8.6%	191	24%	.025

Gem = gemcitabine.

More recently, small-molecule inhibitors of the tyrosine kinase activity of the EGFR have been developed, and their activity is now being investigated in a variety of solid tumors, including pancreatic cancer. One agent worth noting is OSI-774 (erlotinib).[347] This drug is administered orally and its primary toxicities have included rash and diarrhea. Moore and colleagues recently reported on the results of a large phase III trial comparing gemcitabine alone with gemcitabine and erlotinib given at dosages ranging from 100 to 150 mg orally daily (most patients received the 100 mg dose).[310] Over 300 patients were randomized, and no increase in response rate was observed with the addition of erlotinib. However, median survival was improved from 5.91 months to 6.37 months, and although this benefit is quite small, it did reach statistical significance (Table 90-5). In addition, the 1-year survival rate was also improved. Patients randomized to gemcitabine alone had a 1-year survival rate of 17%, whereas it was 24% among patients receiving the combination of erlotinib and gemcitabine.

To date, targeted therapy for pancreatic cancer has not yielded the dramatic clinical benefits that have been observed in other tumor types. Nevertheless the findings with erlotinib provide some encouragement regarding the role of targeted therapy in pancreatic cancer and will certainly foster further investigation. Current conclusions about targeted therapy in pancreatic cancer are fairly clear. Agents that target the tumor cell or the microenvironment have not been able to increase objective response rates, and the survival benefits seen thus far are overall disappointing (see Table 90-5). However, as molecular agents are combined, more meaningful benefits should be anticipated.

Immunotherapy for Pancreatic Cancer

Pancreatic cancer is highly resistant to all conventional cytotoxic agents tested to date. Thus, as with other malignancies refractory to chemotherapy, there has been intense interest in the development of immunologically based therapies to kill pancreatic cancer cells. A variety of approaches have been investigated that utilize both passive and active immunotherapy.[348] Several studies have been conducted in an attempt to demonstrate an enhanced immune response to known tumor cell antigens, such as mutated ras peptides, MUC-1, and heat shock proteins.[349–351]

One approach exploits the ras oncoprotein, which is commonly mutated in pancreatic cancers. Specific mutant ras peptides have been administered to patients with pancreatic adenocarcinoma whose tumors express the corresponding *ras* mutation. This method has yielded enhanced T-cell responsiveness.[349] Another potential immunogen is MUC-1, a glycoprotein commonly present in pancreatic cancer and breast cancer cells. Its expression has been associated with loss of normal adhesion molecules, and it is thought to play a pivotal role in the metastatic process. Efforts are under way to deliver synthetic MUC-1 with adjuvants to generate a more robust response to MUC-1.[352] In addition to this approach, autologous dendritic cells, which are highly efficient antigen-presenting cells, have been modified to express MUC-1 peptides and expanded ex vivo for re-injection. This technique has recently been seen to produce an enhanced immune response to MUC-1.[353]

Although some pancreatic tumor antigens have been identified and are beginning to be exploited, pancreatic tumor cells express a wide array of potential immunogens that are as yet undefined, and, therefore, both autologous and allogeneic whole tumor cells have been administered as vaccines. Of note, it has been well established that the immune response to solid tumors may be attenuated through a variety of mechanisms, including the down-regulation of costimulatory cytokines. Therefore, genetically modified allogeneic tumor cells that express costimulatory cytokines, such as the granulocyte-macrophage colony stimulating factor, (GM-CSF), are being investigated as vaccines. This has been tested clinically, and early results indicate a significant immune response to vaccination with allogeneic tumor cells in a dose-dependent fashion.[354]

At the present time, immunotherapy for pancreatic cancer should be considered investigational, but it is attractive to consider as a component of therapy for this disease. This is based on its relatively high specificity as a cytotoxic intervention with little associated toxicity. Moreover, given that immunotherapy is not expected to worsen the morbidity from surgery, chemotherapy, or radiation therapy, it may become an important adjunct in combination with other modalities.

Approach to the Patient with Metastatic Disease Metastatic pancreatic cancer is a disease characterized by anorexia, cachexia, and pain. Jaundice may result from the primary tumor or intrahepatic metastases. Local tumor progression can lead to worsening pain, gastric outlet obstruction, or gastroparesis, and patients with peritoneal carcinomatosis may suffer from intractable ascites, intestinal dysmotility, or mechanical obstruction; constipation is very common. Patients are also at risk of thrombotic events, including superficial or deep venous thromboses and thromboembolism, but the risk is not clearly higher than that associated with other gastrointestinal tumors.[355] Palliation must always be the primary goal for this group of patients and is facilitated by a multidisciplinary approach. Symptomatic relief of biliary obstruction and pain should be addressed before consideration is given to systemic therapy. If patients with metastatic disease can achieve adequate pain control with the use of long- or short-acting narcotics, without excessive sedation, this approach is preferred.[356,357] However, if pain is not well controlled with oral or transdermal narcotics or if these agents are poorly tolerated, patients should be evaluated by an anesthesiologist or neurologist for celiac plexus or splanchnic plexus ablation.[358] In addition to aggressive pain control efforts, other supportive measures should be considered. Recent studies suggest a benefit to the oral administration of eicosapentaenoic acid in inhibiting and possibly reversing the profound cachexia often seen in patients with advanced disease.[359]

Given the poor prognosis for patients with metastatic disease, biliary obstruction should be relieved through nonsurgical means whenever possible using indwelling endobiliary stents. As previously discussed, studies have suggested improved and more durable patency using expandable metal stents compared with polyethylene biliary stents.[360,361] On occasion, percutaneous biliary drainage may be required to relieve an extrahepatic biliary obstruction. The use of duodenal stents in patients with mechanical gastric outlet obstruction is currently being investigated. For patients with intractable symptomatic ascites, paracentesis is generally perceived as most efficacious,[362] but it is not an intervention with durable benefits. Diuretics may be of some utility, but often lead to intravascular volume contraction with minimal effect on abdominal girth and, therefore, are rarely effective. Shunting procedures for ascites should be reserved for selected patients, but specific indications can not be easily defined and each case must be reviewed on an individual basis.[363]

Systemic therapy for metastatic disease should be actively discouraged in patients with poor performance status (ECOG > 2) or significant metastatic tumor burden. End-of-life discussions and planning are appropriate at the time of diagnosis in patients with metastatic disease. However, if a patient has an adequate performance status, a trial of gemcitabine as first-line therapy is reasonable. The addition of a platinum analog or other cytotoxic drugs should be reserved for those patients who are maintaining excellent performance status. However, for any patient being considered for treatment with gemcitabine monotherapy, the addition of erlotinib is a reasonable alternative; the anticipated benefits of this drug should not be overstated.

The currently recommended dosage of gemcitabine is 1,000 mg/m^2 given IV over 30 minutes each week for 7 weeks. Restaging studies should include CT of the abdomen and pelvis in the eighth week. For patients with an objective response or stable disease, gemcitabine is then given weekly for 3 out of every 4 weeks, with restaging studies generally performed every 8 to 12 weeks.

Whenever possible, patients with good performance status should be treated with systemic therapy in a clinical trial. Most current multicenter trials require that patients have measurable disease, which may include the primary tumor. Survival duration, time to disease progression, objective response, and clinical benefit are all appropriate endpoints of these studies. Patients whose disease progresses during treatment in a clinical trial that does not include gemcitabine may be considered for gemcitabine-based therapy, since some clinical benefit from gemcitabine has been observed for such patients.[263] However, patients who fail to respond to gemcitabine-based therapy are unlikely to receive any meaningful benefit from further conventional chemotherapy and should be offered supportive care. If they maintain an adequate performance status, it may be reasonable for them to participate in a trial of investigational therapy. Second-line treatment with conventional chemotherapy delivered outside of a clinical trial should be discouraged.

In summary, clinically meaningful advances in the treatment of metastatic pancreatic cancer have developed quite slowly. However, with a greater understanding of the underlying genetic and molecular abnormalities involved in pancreatic carcinogenesis, rational chemotherapy, radiation therapy, molecular therapy, and immunotherapy in conjunction with other supportive methods are expected to alter the natural course of this disease in the near future. Continued efforts to enroll patients with advanced pancreatic cancer into well-designed clinical trials should remain a high priority for oncologists across all disciplines.

REFERENCES

1. Jemal A, Murray T, Ward E, et al. Cancer statistics, 2005. CA Cancer J Clin 2005;55:10–30.
2. Exocrine pancreas. In: Greene FL, Page DL, Fleming ID, et al, editors. AJCC cancer staging manual. New York: Springer; 2002. p. 157–64.
3. Breslin TM, Hess KR, Harbison DB, et al. Neoadjuvant chemoradiotherapy for adenocarcinoma of the pancreas: treatment variables and survival duration. Ann Surg 2001;8:123–32.
4. Sohn TA, Yeo CJ, Cameron JL, et al. Resected adenocarcinoma of the pancreas—616 patients: results, outcomes, and prognostic indicators. J Gastrointestinal Surg 2000;4:567–79.
5. Neoptolemos JP, Stocken DD, Friess H, et al. A randomized trial of chemoradiotherapy and chemotherapy after resection of pancreatic cancer. N Engl J Med 2004;350:1200–10.
6. Griffin JF, Smalley SR, Jewell W. Patterns of failure after curative resection of pancreatic carcinoma. Cancer 1990;66:56–61.
7. Willett CG, Lewandrowski K, Warshaw AL, et al. Resection margins in carcinoma of the head of the pancreas: Implications for radiation therapy. Ann Surg 1993;217:144–8.
8. Pisters PWT, Abbruzzese JL, Janjan NA, et al. Rapid-fractionation preoperative chemoradiation, pancreaticoduodenectomy, and intraoperative radiation therapy for resectable pancreatic adenocarcinoma. J Clin Oncol 1998;16:3843–50.
9. Gastrointestinal Tumor Study Group. A multi-institutional comparative trial of radiation therapy alone and in combination with 5-fluorouracil for locally unresectable pancreatic carcinoma. Ann Surg 1979;189:205–8.
10. Whittington R, Neuberg D, Tester WJ, et al. Protracted intravenous fluorouracil infusion with radiation therapy in the management of localized pancreaticobiliary carcinoma: a phase I Eastern Cooperative Oncology Group trial. J Clin Oncol 1995;13:227–32.
11. Gold EB, Goldin SB. Epidemiology of and risk factors for pancreatic cancer. Surg Oncol Clin N Am 1998;7:67–91.
12. Tominaga S, Kuroishi T. Epidemiology of pancreatic cancer. Semin Surg Oncol 1998;15:3–7.
13. Gullo L. Diabetes and the risk of pancreatic cancer. Ann Oncol 1999;10:79–81.
14. Chow WH, Gridley G, Nyrén O, et al. Risk of pancreatic cancer following diabetes mellitus: a nationwide cohort study in Sweden. J Natl Cancer Inst 1995;87:930–1.
15. Fisher WE. Diabetes: risk factor for the development of pancreatic cancer or manifestation of the disease? World J Surg 2001;25:503–8.
16. Gullo L, Pezzilli R, Morselli-Labate AM. Diabetes and the risk of pancreatic cancer. N Engl J Med 1994;331:81–4.
17. La Vecchia C, Negri E, Franceschi S, et al. A case-control study of diabetes mellitus and cancer risk. Br J Cancer 1994;70:950–3.
18. Silverman DT, Schiffman M, Everhart J, et al. Diabetes mellitus, other medical conditions and familial history of cancer as risk factors for pancreatic cancer. Br J Cancer 1999; 80:1830–7.
19. Wideroff L, Gridley G, Mellemkjaer L, et al. Cancer incidence in a population-based cohort of patients hospitalized with diabetes mellitus in Denmark. J Natl Cancer Inst 1997;89:1360–5.
20. Valerio A, Basso D, Brigato L, et al. Glucose metabolic alterations in isolated and perfused rat hepatocytes induced by pancreatic cancer conditioned medium: a low molecular weight factor possibly involved. Biochem Biophys Res Commun 1999;257:622–8.
21. Basso D, Valerio A, Seraglia R, et al. Putative pancreatic cancer-associated diabetogenic factor: 2030 MW peptide. Pancreas 2002;24:8–14.
22. Everhart J, Wright D. Diabetes mellitus as a risk factor for pancreatic cancer. A meta-analysis. JAMA 1995;273:1605–9.
23. Gapstur SM, Gann PH, Lowe W, et al. Abnormal glucose metabolism and pancreatic cancer mortality. JAMA 2000;283:2552–8.
24. Michaud DS, Giovannucci E, Willett WC, et al. Physical activity, obesity, height, and the risk of pancreatic cancer. JAMA 2001;286:921–9.
25. Calle EE, Rodriguez C, Walker-Thurmond K, et al. Overweight, obesity, and mortality from cancer in a prospectively studied cohort of U.S. adults. N Engl J Med 2003;348:1625–38.
26. Gapstur SM, Gann P. Is pancreatic cancer a preventable disease? JAMA 2001;286:967–8.
27. Silverman DT, Swanson CA, Gridley G, et al. Dietary and nutritional factors and pancreatic cancer: a case-control study based on direct interviews. J Natl Cancer Inst 1998;90:1710–9.
28. Ammann RW, Akovbrantz A, Largiader F, et al. Course and outcome of chronic pancreatitis: longitudinal study of a mixed medical-surgical series of 245 patients. Gastroenterology 1984;86:820–8.

29. Lowenfels A. Chronic pancreatitis, pancreatic cancer, alcohol and smoking. Gastroenterology 1984;87:744–5.
30. Longnecker DS, Kuhlmann ET, Freeman DHJ. Characterization of the elastase 1-simian virus 40 T-antigen mouse model of pancreatic carcinoma: effects of sex and diet. Cancer Res 1990;50:7552–4.
31. Talamini G, Bassi C, Falconi M, et al. Early detection of pancreatic cancer following diagnosis of chronic pancreatitis. Digestion 1999;60:554–61.
32. Talamini G, Falconi M, Bassi C, et al. Incidence of cancer in the course of chronic pancreatitis. Am J Gastroenterol 1999;94:1253–60.
33. Karlson BM, Ekbom A, Josefsson S, et al. The risk of pancreatic cancer following pancreatitis: an association due to confounding? Gastroenterology 1997;113:587–92.
34. Gates LK Jr, Ulrich CD 2nd, Whitcomb DC. Hereditary pancreatitis. Gene defects and their implications. Surg Clin North Am 1999;79:711–22.
35. Lowenfels AB, Maisonneuve P, DiMagno EP, et al. Hereditary pancreatitis and the risk of pancreatic cancer. International Hereditary Pancreatitis Study Group. J Natl Cancer Inst 1997;89:442–6.
36. Gorry MC, Gabbaizedeh D, Furey W, et al. Mutations in the cationic trypsinogen gene are associated with recurrent acute and chronic pancreatitis. Gastroenterology 1997;113:1063–8.
37. Berger DH, Fisher WE. Inherited pancreatic cancer syndromes. In: Evans DB, Pisters PWT, Abbruzzese JL, editors. Pancreatic cancer. New York: Springer-Verlag; 2001. p. 73–81.
38. Murphy KM, Brune KA, Griffin DA, et al. Analysis of three candidate genes MKK4, DPC4 and BRCA2 in familial pancreatic cancer [abstract]. 6th Annual Meeting of the Association of Molecular Pathology. 2000.
39. Goggins M, Schutte M, Lu J, et al. Germline BRCA2 gene mutations in patients with apparently sporadic pancreatic carcinomas. Cancer Res 1996;56:5360–4.
40. Klein AP, Hruban RH, Brune KA, et al. Familial pancreatic cancer. Cancer J Clin 2001;7:266–72.
41. Su GH, Hruban RH, Bansal RK, et al. Germline and somatic mutations of the STK11/LBK1 Peutz-Jeghers gene in pancreatic and biliary cancers. Am J Pathol 1999;154:1835–40.
42. Lynch HT, Brand RE, Hogg D, et al. Phenotypic variation in eight extended CDKN2A germline mutation familial atypical multiple mole melanoma-pancreatic carcinoma-prone families. Cancer 2002;94:84–96.
43. Tersmette AC, Petersen GM, Offerhaus GJA, et al. Increased risk of incident pancreatic cancer among first-degree relatives of patients with familial pancreatic cancer. Clin Cancer Res 2001;7:738–44.
44. Eberle MA, Pfutzer R, Pogue-Geile KL, et al. A new susceptibility locus for autosomal dominant pancreatic cancer maps to chromosome 4q32-34. Am J Hum Genet 2002;70:1044–8.
45. Raderer M, Wrba F, Kornek G, et al. Association between Helicobacter pylori infection and pancreatic cancer. Oncology 1998;55:16–9.
46. Stolzenberg-Solomon RZ, Blaser MJ, Limburg PJ, et al. Helicobacter pylori seropositivity as a risk factor for pancreatic cancer. J Nat Cancer Inst 2001;93:927–41.
47. Tersmette AC, Offerhaus GJ, Giardiello FM, et al. Occurrence of non-gastric cancer in the digestive tract after remote partial gastrectomy: analysis of an Amsterdam cohort. Int J Cancer 1990;465:792–5.
48. Hedberg M, Ogren M, Janzon L, et al. Pancreatic carcinoma following gastric resection. Int J Pancreatol 1997;21:219–24.
49. Coughlin SS, Calle EE, Patel AV, et al. Predictors of pancreatic cancer mortality among a large cohort of the United States adults. Cancer Causes Control 2000;11:915–23.
50. Lin Y, Tamakoshi A, Kawamura T, et al. A prospective cohort study of cigarette smoking and pancreatic cancer in Japan. Cancer Causes Control 2002;13:249–54.
51. Talamini G, Bassi C, Falconi M, et al. Alcohol and smoking as risk factors in chronic pancreatitis and pancreatic cancer. Dig Dis Sci 1999;44:1303–11.
52. Mulder I, van Genugten ML, Hoogenveen RT, et al. The impact of smoking on future pancreatic cancer: a computer simulation. Ann Oncol 1999;10:74–8.
53. Hoffman D, Rivenson A, Chung FL, et al. Nicotine-derived N-nitrosamines (TSNA) and their relevance in tobacco carcinogenesis. Crit Rev Toxicol 1991;21:305–11.
54. Rivenson A, Hoffman D, Prokopczyk B, et al. Induction of lung and exocrine pancreas tumors in F344 rats by tobacco-specific and areca-derived N-nitrosamines. Cancer Res 1988;48:6912–7.
55. Silverman DT, Dunn JA, Hoover RN, et al. Cigarette smoking and pancreas cancer: a case-control study based on direct interviews. J Natl Cancer Inst 1994;86:1510–6.
56. Thompson PA, Seyedi F, Lang NP, et al. Comparison of DNA adduct levels associated with exogenous and endogenous exposures in human pancreas in relation to metabolic genotype. Mutat Res 1999;424:263–74.
57. Prokopczyk B, Hoffmann D, Bologna M, et al. Identification of tobacco-derived compounds in human pancreatic juice. Chem Res Toxicol 2002;15:677–85.
58. Duell EJ, Wiencke JK, Cheng T-J, et al. Polymorphisms in the DNA repair genes XRCC1 and ERCC2 and biomarkers of DNA damage in human blood mononuclear cells [published erratum appears in Carcinogenesis (Lond.) 2000;21:1457]. Carcinogenesis 2000;21:965–71.
59. Duell E, Holly EA, Bracci PM, et al. A population-based, case-control study of polymorphisms in carcinogen-metabolizing genes, smoking, and pancreatic adenocarcinoma risk. J Natl Cancer Inst 2002;4:297–306.
60. Li D, Jiao L, Li Y, et al. Polymorphisms of cytochrome P4501A2 and N-acetyltransferase genes, smoking, and risk of pancreatic cancer. Carcinogenesis 2005. (Advanced access published on line at doi:10.1093/carcin/bgi171.)
61. Howe GR, Burch JD. Nutrition and pancreatic cancer. Cancer Causes Control 1996;7:69–82.
62. Woutersen RA, Appel MJ, van Garderen-Hoetmer A, et al. Dietary fat and carcinogenesis. Mutat Res 1999;443:111–27.
63. Li D. Molecular epidemiology. In: Evans DB, Pisters PWT, Abbruzzese JL, editors. Pancreatic cancer. New York: Springer-Verlag; 2001. p. 3–13.
64. Anderson KE, Sinha R, Kulldorff M, et al. Meat intake and cooking techniques: associations with pancreatic cancer. Mutat Res 2002;506–7:225–31.
65. Stolzenberg-Solomon RZ, Pietinen P, Barrett MJ, et al. Dietary and other methyl-group availability factors and pancreatic cancer risk in a cohort of male smokers. Am J Epidemiol 2001;153:680–7.
66. Stolzenberg-Solomon RZ, Albanes D, Nieto FJ, et al. Pancreatic cancer risk and nutrition-related methyl-group availability indicators in male smokers. J Natl Cancer Inst 1999;91:535–41.
67. Gelb MH, Tamanoi F, Yokoyama K, et al. The inhibition of protein prhenyltransferases by oxygenated metabolites of limonine and perillyl alcohol. Cancer Lett 1995;91:169–75.
68. Wolff RA, Abbruzzese JL, Evans DB. Neoplasms of the exocrine pancreas. In: Holland JF, Frei E, Bast RC, et al, editors. Cancer medicine. Ontario: B.C. Decker; 2000. p. 1431–5.
69. Lin Y, Tamakoshi A, Kawamura T, et al. Risk of pancreatic cancer in relation to alcohol drinking, coffee consumption and medical history: findings from the Japan collaborative cohort study for evaluation of cancer risk. Int J Cancer 2002;99:742–6.
70. Bardin JA, Eisen EA, Tolbert PE. Mortality studies of machining fluid exposure in the automobile industry. V. A case-control study of pancreatic cancer. Am J Ind Med 1997;32:240–7.
71. Garabrant DH, Held J, Langholz B, et al. DDT and related compounds and risk of pancreatic cancer. J Natl Cancer Inst 1992;84:764–71.
72. Fryzek JP, Garabrant DH, Harlow SD, et al. A case-control study of self-reported exposures to pesticides and pancreas cancer in southeastern Michigan. Int J Cancer 1997;72:62–7.
73. Partanen T, Kauppinen T, Degerth R, et al. Pancreatic cancer in industrial branches and occupations in Finland. Am J Ind Med 1994;25:851–66.
74. Brentnall TA, Bronner MP, Byrd DR, et al. Early diagnosis and treatment of pancreatic dysplasia in patients with a family history of pancreatic cancer. Ann Intern Med 1999;131:247–55.
75. Rulyak SJ, Brentnal RA. Inherited pancreatic cancer: surveillance and treatment strategies for affected families. Pancreatology 2001;1:477–85.
76. Kern S, Hruban R, Hollingsworth MA, et al. A white paper: the product of a pancreas cancer think tank. Cancer Res 2001;61:4923–32.
77. Ulrich CD. Pancreatic cancer in hereditary pancreatitis: consensus guidelines for prevention, screening and treatment. Pancreatology 2001;1:416–22.
78. Cubilla AL, Fitzgerald PJ. Tumors of the exocrine pancreas. Washington, DC: Armed Forces Institute of Pathology; 1984. p. 118–28.
79. Kayahara M, Nagakawa T, Futagami F, et al. Lymphatic flow and neural plexus invasion associated with carcinoma of the body and tail of the pancreas. Cancer 1996;78:2485–91.
80. Nakai T, Koh K, Kawabe T, et al. Importance of microperineural invasion as a prognostic factor in ampullary carcinoma. Br J Surg 1997;84:1399–401.
81. Evans DB, Lee JE, Pisters PWT. Pancreaticoduodenectomy (Whipple operation) and total pancreatectomy for cancer. In: Baker RJ, Fischer FJ, editors. Mastery of surgery. Philadelphia: Lippincott Williams & Wilkins; 2001. p. 1299–318.
82. Almoguera C, Shibata D, Forrester K, et al. Most human carcinomas of the exocrine pancreas contain mutant c-K-ras genes. Cell 1988;53:549–54.
83. Smit VT, Boot AJ, Smits AM, et al. KRAS codon 12 mutations occur very frequently in pancreatic adenocarcinomas. Nucleic Acids Res 1988;16:7773–82.
84. Midgley RS, Kerr DJ. Ras as a target in cancer therapy. Crit Rev Oncol Hematol 2002;44:109–20.
85. Hruban RH, Goggins M, Parsons J, et al. Progression model for pancreatic cancer. Clin Cancer Res 2000;6:2969–72.
86. Li D, Pirozi PF, Zhang W, et al. DNA adducts, genetic polymorphisms, and K-ras mutation in human pancreatic cancer. Mutat Res 2002;513:37–48.
87. Dianxu F, Shengda Z, Tianquan H, et al. A prospective study of detection of pancreatic carcinoma by combined plasma K-ras mutations and serum CA19-9 analysis. Pancreas 2002;25:336–41.
88. van Heek T, Rader AE, Offerhaus JA, et al. K-ras, p53, and DPC4 (MAD4) alterations in fine-needle aspirates of the pancreas. Am J Clin Pathol 2002;117:755–65.
89. Bartsch D, Shevlin DW, Tung WS, et al. Frequent mutations of CDKN2 in primary pancreatic adenocarcinomas. Genes Chromosomes Cancer 1995;14:189–95.
90. Caldas C, Hahn SA, da Costa LT, et al. Frequent somatic mutations and homozygous deletions of the p16 (MTS1) gene in pancreatic adenocarcinoma. Nat Genet 1994;8:27–32.
91. Naumann M, Savitskaia N, Eilert C, et al. Frequent codeletion of p16/MTS1 and p15/MTS2 and genetic alterations in p16/MTS1 in pancreatic tumors. Gastroenterology 1996;110:1215–24.
92. Schutte M, Hruban RH, Geradts J, et al. Abrogation of the Rb/p16 tumor-suppressive pathway in virtually all pancreatic carcinomas. Cancer Res 1997;57:3126–30.
93. Shimamura A, Fisher DE. p53 in life and death. Clin Cancer Res 1996;2:435–40.
94. Reddy SAG. Signaling pathways in pancreatic cancer. Cancer J 2001;7:274–86.
95. Pellegata NS, Sessa F, Renault B, et al. K-ras and p53 gene mutations in pancreatic cancer: ductal and nonductal tumors progress through different genetic lesions. Cancer Res 1994;54:1556–60.
96. Redston MS, Caldas C, Seymour AB, et al. p53 mutations in pancreatic carcinoma and evidence of common involvement of homocopolymer tracts in DNA microdeletions. Cancer Res 1994;54:3025–33.
97. Lagna G, Hata A, Hemmati-Brivanlou A, et al. Partnership between DPC4 and SMAD proteins in TGF-beta signalling pathways. Nature 1996;383:832–6.
98. Derynck R, Zhang Y, Feng XH. Smads: transcriptional activators of TGF-beta responses. Cell 1998;95:737–40.
99. Grau AM, Zhang L, Wang W, et al. Induction of p21waf1 expression and growth inhibition by transforming growth factor-b is mediated by the tumor suppressor gene DPC-4 in human pancreatic adenocarcinoma cells. Cancer Res 1997;57:3929–34.
100. Hunt KK, Fleming JB, Abramian A, et al. Overexpression of the tumor suppressor gene Smad4/DPC4 induces p21waf1 expression and growth inhibition in human carcinoma cells. Cancer Res 1998;58:5656–61.
101. Hahn SA, Schutte M, Hoque ATMS, et al. DPC4, a candidate tumor suppressor gene at human chromosome 18q21.1. Science 1996;271:350–3.
102. Tascilar M, Skinner HG, Rosty C, et al. The SMAD3 protein and prognosis of pancreatic ductal adenocarcinoma. Clin Cancer Res 2001;4:4115–21.
103. Liu F. SMAD4/DPC4 and pancreatic cancer survival. Clin Cancer Res 2001;7:3853–6.
104. Sohn TA, Su GH, Ryu B. High-throughput drug screening of the DPC4 tumor-suppressor pathway in human pancreatic cancer cells. Ann Surg 2001;233:696–703.
105. Jean ME, Lowy AM, Chiao PJ, et al. The molecular biology of pancreatic cancer. In: Evans DB, Pisters PWT, Abbruzzese JL, editors. Pancreatic cancer. New York: Springer-Verlag; 2001. p. 15–25.
106. van der Heijden MS, Kern SE. Molecular genetic alterations in cancer-associated genes. In: Von Hoff D, Evans DB,

Hruban RH, editors. Pancreatic cancer. Sudbury (MA): Jones and Bartlett; 2005. p. 31–41.
107. Freeny PC. Computed tomography in the diagnosis and staging of cholangiocarcinoma and pancreatic carcinoma. Ann Oncol 1999;10 suppl 4:S12–7.
108. Tamm E, Charnsangavej C. Pancreatic cancer: current concepts in imaging for diagnosis and staging. Cancer J 2001;7:298–311.
109. O'Malley ME, Boland GWL, Wood BJ, et al. Adenocarcinoma of the head of the pancreas: determination of surgical unresectability with thin-section pancreatic-phase helical CT. AJR 1999;173:1510–8.
110. Yeung RS, Weese JL, Hoffman JP, et al. Neoadjuvant chemoradiation in pancreatic and duodenal carcinoma. Cancer 1993;72:2124–33.
111. Warshaw AL, Gu Z, Wittenberg J, et al. Preoperative staging and assessment of resectability of pancreatic cancer. Arch Surg 1990;125:230–3.
112. Raut CP, Grau AM, Staerkel GA, et al. Diagnostic accuracy of endoscopic ultrasound-guided fine-needle aspiration in patients with presumed pancreatic cancer. J Gastrointestinal Surg 2003;7:118–28.
113. Suits J, Frazee R, Erickson RA. Endoscopic ultrasound and fine needle aspiration for the evaluation of pancreatic masses. Arch Surg 1999;134:639–43.
114. Cusheri A. Laparoscopy for pancreatic cancer: does it benefit the patient? Eur J Surg 1988;14:41–4.
115. Warshaw AL, Tepper JE, Shipley WU. Laparoscopy in the staging and planning of therapy for pancreatic cancer. Am J Surg 1985;151:76–80.
116. Pisters PWT, Lee JE, Vauthey JN, et al. Laparoscopy in the staging of pancreatic cancer. Br J Surg 2001;88:325–37.
117. Davids PH, Groen AK, Rauws EA, et al. Randomised trial of self-expanding metal stents versus polyethylene stents for distal malignant biliary obstruction. Lancet 1992;340:1488–92.
118. Kaassis M, Boyer J, Dumas R, et al. Plastic or metal stents for malignant stricture of the common bile duct? Results of a randomized prospective study. Gastrointest Endosc 2003;57:178–82.
119. Kahaleh M, Tokar J, Le T, Yeaton P. Removal of self-expandable metallic Wallstents. Gastrointest Endosc 2004;60:640–4.
120. Neoptolemos JP, Stocken DD, Dunn AJ, et al. Influence of resection margins on survival for patients with pancreatic cancer treated by adjuvant chemoradiation and/or chemotherapy in the ESPAC-1 randomized controlled trial. Ann Surg 2001;234:758–68.
121. Pisters PWT, Hudec WA, Hess KR, et al. Effect of preoperative biliary decompression on pancreaticoduodenectomy-associated morbidity in 300 consecutive patients. Ann Surg 2001;234:47–55.
122. Tseng JF, Raut CP, Lee JE, et al. Pancreaticoduodenectomy with vascular resection: margin status and survival duration. J Gastrointest Surg 2004;8:935–50.
123. Edge SB, Schmieg RE, Rosenlof LK, et al. Pancreas cancer resection outcome in American university centers. Cancer 1993;71:3502–8.
124. Wade TP, Kraybill WG, Virgo KS, et al. Pancreatic cancer treatment in the U.S. veteran from 1987 to 1991: effect of tumor stage on survival. J Surg Oncol 1995;58:104–11.
125. Wade TP, Radford DM, Virgo KS, et al. Complications and outcomes in the treatment of pancreatic adenocarcinoma in the United States veteran. J Am Coll Surg 1994;179:38–48.
126. Birkmeyer JD, Siewers AE, Finlayson EVA, et al. Hospital volume and surgical mortality in the United States. N Engl J Med 2002;346:1128–37.
127. Birkmeyer JD, Warshaw AL, Finlayson SR, et al. Relationship between hospital volume and late survival after pancreaticoduodenectomy. Surgery 1999;126:178–83.
128. Whipple AO, Parsons WB, Mullins CR. Treatment of carcinoma of the ampulla of Vater. Ann Surg 1935;102:763–79.
129. Whipple AO. The rationale of radical surgery for cancer of the pancreas and ampullary region. Ann Surg 1941;114:612.
130. Staley CA, Lee JE, Cleary KA. Preoperative chemoradiation, pancreaticoduodenectomy, and intraoperative radiation therapy for adenocarcinoma of the pancreatic head. Am J Surg 1996;171:118–25.
131. Robinson EK, Lee JE, Lowy AM, et al. Reoperative pancreaticoduodenectomy for periampullary carcinoma. Am J Surg 1996;172:432–8.
132. Fortner J. Technique of regional subtotal and total pancreatectomy. Am J Surg 1985;150:593–600.
133. Ishikawa O, Ohigashi H, Imaoka S, et al. Preoperative indications for extended pancreatectomy for locally advanced pancreas cancer involving the portal vein. Ann Surg 1992;215:231–6.
134. Cusack JC, Fuhrman GM, Lee JE, et al. Management of unsuspected tumor invasion of the superior mesenteric-portal venous confluence at the time of pancreaticoduodenectomy. Am J Surg 1994;168:352–4.
135. Pawlik TM, Abdalla EK, Barnett CC, et al; Feasibility of a randomized trial of extended lymphadenectomy for pancreatic cancer. Arch Surg 2005;140:584–91.
136. Traverso LW, Longmire WP. Preservation of the pylorus in pancreaticoduodenectomy. Surg Gynecol Obstet 1978;146:959–62.
137. Grace PA, Pitt HA, Longmire WP. Pylorus preserving pancreaticoduodenectomy: an overview. Br J Surg 1990;77:968–74.
138. Huang JJ, Yeo CJ, Sohn TA, et al. Quality of life and outcomes after pancreaticoduodenectomy. Ann Surg 2000;231:890–8.
139. Yeo CJ, Cameron JL, Lillemore KD, et al. Pancreaticoduodenectomy for cancer of the head of the pancreas: 201 patients. Ann Surg 1995;221:721–31.
140. Balcom JH, Rattner DW, Warshaw AL, et al. Ten-year experience with 733 resections: changing indications, older patients, and decreasing length of hospitalization. Arch Surg 2001;136:391–8.
141. Patel AG, Toyama MT, Kusske AM, et al. Pylorus-preserving Whipple resection for pancreatic cancer. Is it any better? Arch Surg 1995;130:838–42.
142. Lin PW, Lin YJ. Prospective randomized comparison between pylorus preserving and standard pancreaticoduodenectomy. Br J Surg 1999;86:603–7.
143. Yeo CJ, Cameron JL, Lillemoe KD, et al. Pancreaticoduodenectomy with or without distal gastrectomy and extended retroperitoneal lymphadenectomy for periampullary adenocarcinoma, part 2: randomized controlled trail evaluating survival, morbidity, and mortality. Ann Surg 2002;236:355–68.
144. Seiler CA, Wagner M, Sadowski C. Randomized prospective trial of pylorus-preserving vs. classic duodenopancreatectomy (Whipple procedure): initial clinical results. J Gastrointest Surg 2000;4:443–52.
145. Whipple AO. Observations on radical surgery for lesions of the pancreas. Surg Gynecol Obstet 1946;82:623–31.
146. Mason GR, Freeark RJ. Current experience with pancreatogastrostomy. Am J Surg 1995;169:217–9.
147. Park CD, Mackie JA, Rhoads J. Pancreaticogastrostomy. Am J Surg 1967;113:85–90.
148. Yeo CJ, Cameron JL, Maher MM, et al. A prospective randomized trial of pancreaticogastrostomy versus pancreaticojejunostomy after pancreaticoduodenectomy. Ann Surg 1995;222:580–8.
149. Warshaw AL, Torchiana DL. Delayed gastric emptying after pylorus-preserving pancreaticoduodenectomy. Surg Gynecol Obstet 1985;160:1–4.
150. Evans DB, Rich TA, Byrd DR, et al. Preoperative chemoradiation and pancreaticoduodenectomy for adenocarcinoma of the pancreas. Arch Surg 1992;127:1335–9.
151. International Pancreatic Cancer Study Group. Staging for carcinoma of the pancreas: Japanese stage classification compared to UICC stage classification. In: Pour PM, Konishi Y, Klöppel G, Longnecker DS, editors. Atlas of exocrine pancreatic tumors. Hong Kong: Springer-Verlag Tokyo; 1994. 247–56.
152. Raut CP, Evans DB, Crane CH, et al. Neoadjuvant therapy for resectable pancreatic cancer. Surg Oncol Clin N Am 2004;4:639–61.
153. Nitecki SS, Sar MG, Colby TV, et al. Long-term survival after resection for ductal adenocarcinoma of the pancreas. Is it really improving? Ann Surg 1995;221:59–66.
154. Greer RJ, Brennan MF. Prognostic indicators for survival after resection of pancreatic adenocarcinoma. Am J Surg 1993;165:68–72.
155. Conlon KC, Klimstra DS, Brennan MF. Long-term survival after curative resection for pancreatic ductal adenocarcinoma; clinicopathologic analysis of 5-year survivors. Ann Surg 1996;223:273–9.
156. Gastrointestinal Tumor Study Group. Further evidence of effective adjuvant combined radiation and chemotherapy following curative resection of pancreatic cancer. Cancer 1987;59:2006–10.
157. Kalser MH, Ellenberg SS. Pancreatic cancer: adjuvant combined radiation and chemotherapy following curative resection. Arch Surg 1985;120:899–903.
158. Klinkenbijl JH, Jeekel J, Sahmoud T, et al. Adjuvant radiotherapy and 5-fluorouracil after curative resection for the cancer of the pancreas and peri-ampullary region. Phase III trial of the EORTC Gastrointestinal Tract Cancer Cooperative Group. Ann Surg 1999;230:776–84.
159. Neoptolemos JP, Dunn JA, Stocken DD, et al. Adjuvant chemoradiotherapy and chemotherapy in resectable pancreatic cancer: a randomized controlled trial. Lancet 2001;358:1576–85.
160. Regine WF. Postoperative adjuvant therapy: past, present, and future trial development. In: Evans DB, Pisters PWT, Abbruzzese JL, editors. Pancreatic cancer. New York: Springer-Verlag; 2001. p. 235–42.
161. Nukui Y, Picozzi VJ, Traverso LW. Interferon-based adjuvant chemoradiation therapy improves survival after pancreaticoduodenectomy for pancreatic adenocarcinoma. Am J Surg 2000;179:367–71.
162. Abrams RA, Grochow LB, Chakravarthy A, et al. Intensified adjuvant therapy for pancreatic and periampullary adenocarcinoma: survival results and observations regarding patterns of failure, radiotherapy dose and CA19-9 levels. Int J Radiat Oncol Biol Phys 1999;44:1039–46.
163. Yeo CJ, Abrams RA, Grochow LB, et al. Pancreaticoduodenectomy for pancreatic adenocarcinoma: postoperative adjuvant chemoradiation improves survival. Ann Surg 1997;225:621–36.
164. Chakravarthy A, Abrams RA, Yeo CJ, et al. Intensified adjuvant combined modality therapy for resected periampullary adenocarcinoma: acceptable toxicity and suggestion of improved 1-year disease-free survival. Int J Radiation Oncology Biol Phys 2000;48:1089–96.
165. Lim JE, Chien MW, Earle CC. Prognostic factors following curative resection for pancreatic adenocarcinoma: a population-based, linked database analysis of 396 patients. Ann Surg 2003;237:74–85.
166. Pisters PWT, Wolff RA, Janjan NA, et al. Preoperative paclitaxel and concurrent rapid-fractionation radiation for resectable pancreatic adenocarcinoma: toxicities, histologic response rates, and event-free outcome. J Clin Oncol 2002;20:2537–44.
167. Wolff RA, Evans DB, Crane CH, et al. Initial results of a preoperative gemcitabine (GEM)-based chemoradiation for resectable pancreatic adenocarcinoma [abstract]. Proc Am Soc Clin Oncol 2002;21:130a.
168. Wolff RA, Evans DB, Gravel DM, et al. Phase I trial of gemcitabine combined with radiation for the treatment of locally advanced pancreatic adenocarcinoma. Clin Cancer Res 2001;7:2246–53.
169. Pisters PWT, Hudec WA, Lee JE, et al. Preoperative chemoradiation for patients with pancreatic cancer: toxicity of endobiliary stents. J Clin Oncol 2000;18:860–7.
170. Kotwall CA, Maxwell JG, Brinker CC, et al. National estimates of mortality rates for radical pancreaticoduodenectomy in 25,000 patients. Ann Surg Oncol 2002;9:847–54.
171. Moertel CG, Frytak S, Hahn RG, et al. Therapy of locally unresectable pancreatic carcinoma: a randomized comparison of high dose (6000 rads) radiation alone, moderate dose radiation (4000 rads + 5-fluorouracil), and high dose radiation + 5-fluorouracil. The Gastrointestinal Tumor Study Group. Cancer 1981;48:1705–10.
172. Gastrointestinal Tumor Study Group. Radiation therapy combined with Adriamycin or 5-fluorouracil for the treatment of locally unresectable pancreatic carcinoma. Cancer 1985;56:2563–8.
173. Gastrointestinal Tumor Study Group. Treatment of locally unresectable carcinoma of the pancreas: comparison of combined-modality therapy (chemotherapy plus radiotherapy) to chemotherapy alone. J Natl Cancer Inst 1988;80:751–5.
174. Klaassen DJ, MacIntyre JM, Catton GE, et al. Treatment of locally unresectable cancer of the stomach and pancreas: a randomized comparison of 5-fluorouracil alone with radiation plus concurrent and maintenance 5-fluorouracil-an Eastern Cooperative Oncology Group study. J Clin Oncol 1985;3:373–8.
175. Ishii H, Okada S, Tokuuye K, et al. Protracted 5-fluorouracil infusion with concurrent radiotherapy as a treatment for locally advanced pancreatic carcinoma. Cancer 1997;79:1516–20.
176. Pipas JM, Mitchell SE, Barth RJ, et al. Phase I study of twice-weekly gemcitabine and concomitant external-beam radiotherapy in patients with adenocarcinoma of the pancreas. Int J Radiat Oncol Biol Phys 2001;50:1317–22.
177. McGinn C, Smith D, Szarka C, et al. A phase I study of gemcitabine in combination with radiation therapy in patients with localized, unresectable pancreatic cancer [abstract]. Proc Am Soc Clin Oncol 1998;17:264a.
178. Blackstock AW, Bernard SA, Richards F, et al. Phase I trial of twice-weekly gemcitabine and concurrent radiation in patients with advanced pancreatic cancer. J Clin Oncol 1999;17:2208–12.
179. Ikeda M, Okada S, Tokuuye K, et al. A phase I trial of weekly gemcitabine and concurrent radiotherapy in

patients with locally advanced pancreatic cancer. Br J Cancer 2002;86:1551–4.

180. Crane CH, Wolff RA, Abbruzzese JL, et al. Combining gemcitabine with radiation in pancreatic cancer: understanding important variables influencing the therapeutic index. Semin Oncol 2001;28 suppl 10:1025–33.
181. Li C-P, Chao Y, Chi K-H, et al. Concurrent chemoradiotherapy treatment of locally advanced pancreatic cancer: gemcitabine versus 5-fluorouracil, a randomized controlled study. International J Radiat Oncol Biol Phys 2003;57:98–104.
182. Blackstock AW, Tepper JE, Niedwiecki D, et al. Cancer and leukemia group B (CALGB) 89805: phase II chemoradiation trial using gemcitabine in patients with locoregional adenocarcinoma of the pancreas. Int J Gastrointest Cancer 2003;34:107–16.
183. McGinn CJ, Zalupski MM, Shureiqi I, et al. Phase I trial of radiation dose escalation with concurrent weekly full-dose gemcitabine in patients with advanced pancreatic cancer. J Clin Oncol 2001;19:4202–8.
184. McGinn C, Talamonti M, Small W, et al: A phase II trial of full-dose gemcitabine with concurrent radiation therapy in patients with resectable or unresectable non-metastatic pancreatic cancer. Proc 2004 ASCO GI Symposium, San Francisco, Ca:Pg 89, Abstract #96, 2004.
185. Burris HA 3rd, Moore MJ, Andersen J, et al. Improvements in survival and clinical benefit with gemcitabine as first-line therapy for patients with advanced pancreas cancer: a randomized trial. J Clin Oncol 1997;15:2403–13.
186. Crane CH, Abbruzzese JL, Evans DB, et al. Is the therapeutic index better with gemcitabine-based chemoradiation than with 5-fluorouracil-based chemoradiation in locally advanced pancreatic cancer? Int J Radiat Oncol Biol Phys 2002;52:1293–302.
187. Cassidy J, Scheithauer W, McKendrick J, et al. Capecitabine (X) vs bolus 5-FU/leucovorin (LV) as adjuvant therapy for colon cancer (the X-ACT study): efficacy results of a phase III trial [abstract 3509]. J Clin Oncol 2004;22;14S.
188. Cartwright TH, Cohn A, Varkey JA, et al. Phase II study of oral capecitabine in patients with advanced or metastatic pancreatic cancer. J Clin Oncol 2002;20:160–4.
189. Ben-Josef E, Shields AF, Vaishampayan U, et al. Intensity-modulated radiotherapy (IMRT) and concurrent capecitabine for pancreatic cancer. Int J Radiat Oncol Biol Phys 2004;59:454–9.
190. Crane C, Ellis L, Abbruzzese J, et al. Phase I trial of bevacizumab with concurrent radiotherapy and capecitabine in locally advanced pancreatic adenocarcinoma [abstract 4033]. Proc Am Soc Clin Oncol 2005;23 Supplement 16:316s.
191. Gorski DH, Beckett MA, Jaskowiak NT, et al. Blockage of the vascular endothelial growth factor stress response increases the antitumor effects of ionizing radiation. Cancer Res 1999;59:3374–8.
192. Wey J, Fan F, Gray M, et al. Vascular endothelial growth factor receptor-1 promotes migration and invasion in pancreatic carcinoma cell lines. Cancer 2005;104:427–38.
193. Jain RK. Normalization of tumor vasculature: an emerging concept in antiangiogenic therapy. Science 2005;307:58–62.
194. Willett CG, Fernandez del Castillo C, Shih HA, et al. Long-term results of intraoperative electron beam irradiation (IOERT) for patients with unresectable pancreatic cancer. Ann Surg 2005;241:295–9.
195. Bonner JA, Giralt J, Harari PM, et al. Cetuximab prolongs survival in patients with locoregionally advanced squamous cell carcinoma of head and neck: a phase III study of high dose radiation therapy with or without cetuximab [abstract 5507]. ASCO Annual Meeting 2004.
196. Bussels B, Goethals L, Feron M, et al. Respiration-induced movement of the upper abdominal organs: a pitfall for the three-dimensional conformal radiation treatment of pancreatic cancer. Radiother Oncol 2003;68:69–74.
197. Balter JM, Lam KL, McGinn CJ, et al. Improvement of CT-based treatment-planning models of abdominal targets using static exhale imaging. Int J Radiat Oncol Biol Phys 1998;41:939–43.
198. Crane CH, Antolak JA, Rosen II, et al. Phase I study of concomitant gemcitabine and IMRT for patients with unresectable adenocarcinoma of the pancreatic head. Int J Gastrointest Cancer 2001;30:123–32.
199. Koong AC, Le QT, Ho A, et al. Phase I study of stereotactic radiosurgery in patients with locally advanced pancreatic cancer. Int J Radiat Oncol Biol Phys 2004;58:1017–21.
200. White R, Lee C, Anscher M, et al. Preoperative chemoradiation for patients with locally advanced adenocarcinoma of the pancreas. Ann Surg Oncol 1999;6:38–45.
201. Todd KE, Gloor B, Lane JS, et al. Resection of locally advanced pancreatic cancer after downstaging with continuous-infusion 5-fluorouracil, mitomycin-C, leucovorin, and dipyridamole. J Gastrointest Surg 1998;2:159–66.
202. Kamthan AG, Morris JC, Dalton J, et al. Combined modality therapy for stage II and stage III pancreatic carcinoma. J Clin Oncol 1997;15:2920–7.
203. Safran H, King TP, Choy H, et al. Paclitaxel and concurrent radiation for locally advanced pancreatic and gastric cancer: a phase I study. J Clin Oncol 1997;15:901–7.
204. Jessup JM, Steele G, Mayer RJ, et al. Neoadjuvant therapy for unresectable pancreatic adenocarcinoma. Arch Surg 1993;128:559–64.
205. Jeekel J, Treurniet-Donker AD. Treatment perspectives in locally advanced unresectable pancreatic cancer. Br J Surg 1991;78:1332–4.
206. Wolff RA. Neoadjuvant chemoradiation for localized adenocarcinoma of the pancreas: great logic, grim reality [editorial]. Ann Surg Oncol 2001;8:747–8.
207. Mehta VK, Fisher G, Ford JA, et al. Preoperative chemoradiation for marginally resectable adenocarcinoma of the pancreas. J Gastrointest Surg 2001;5:27–35.
208. Tepper JE, Shipley WU, Warshaw AL, et al. The role of misonidazole combined with intraoperative radiation therapy in the treatment of pancreatic carcinoma. J Clin Oncol 1987;5:579–84.
209. Garton GR, Gunderson LL, Nagorney DM, et al. High-dose preoperative external beam and intraoperative irradiation for locally advanced pancreatic cancer. Int J Radiat Oncol Biol Phys 1993;28:1153–7.
210. Lillemoe KD, Sauter PK, Pitt HA, et al. Current status of surgical palliation of periampullary carcinoma. Surg Gynecol Obstet 1993;176:1–10.
211. Sohn TA, Lillemoe KD, Cameron JL, et al. Surgical palliation of unresectable periampullary adenocarcinoma in the 1990s. J Am Coll Surg 1999;188:658–66.
212. de Rooij PD, Rogatko A, Brennan MF. Evaluation of palliative surgical procedures in unresectable pancreatic cancer. Br J Surg 1991;78:1053–8.
213. Egrari S, O'Connell TX. Role of prophylactic gastroenterostomy for unresectable pancreatic carcinoma. Am Surg 1995;61:862–4.
214. van der Schelling GP, van den Bosch R, Klinkenbij JHG, et al. Is there a place for gastroenterostomy in patients with advanced cancer of the head of the pancreas? World J Surg 1993;17:128–32.
215. Weaver DW, Wiencek RG, Bouwman DL, et al. Gastrojejunostomy: is it helpful for patients with pancreatic cancer? Surgery 1987;102:608–13.
216. Lillemoe KD, Cameron JL, Hardacre JM, et al. Is prophylactic gastrojejunostomy indicated for unresectable periampullary cancer? A prospective randomized trial. Ann Surg 1999;230:322–8.
217. Espat NJ, Brennan MF, Conlon KC. Patients with laparoscopically staged unresectable pancreatic carcinoma do not require subsequent surgical biliary or gastric bypass. J Am Coll Surg 1999;188:649–57.
218. Fernandez-del Castillo C, Warshaw AL. Laparoscopy for staging in pancreatic carcinoma. Surg Oncol 1993;2:25–9.
219. Raikar GV, Melin MM, Ress A, et al. Cost-effective analysis of surgical palliation versus endoscopic stenting in the management of unresectable pancreatic cancer. Ann Surg Oncol 1996;3:470–5.
220. Fernandez-del Castillo C, Warshaw AL. Peritoneal metastases in pancreatic carcinoma. Hepatogastroenterology 1993;40:430–42.
221. Dalton RR, Sarr MG, van Heerden JA, et al. Carcinoma of the body and tail of the pancreas: is curative resection justified? Surgery 1992;111:489–94.
222. Johnson CD, Schwall G, Flechtenmacher J, et al. Resection for adenocarcinoma of the body and tail of the pancreas. Br J Surg 1993;80:1177–9.
223. Wade TP, Virgo KS, Johnson FE. Distal pancreatectomy for cancer: results in US Department of Veterans Affairs Hospitals, 1987–1991. Pancreas 1995;11:341–4.
224. Fisher BJ, Perera FE, Kocha W, et al. Analysis of the clinical benefit of 5-fluorouracil and radiation treatment in locally advanced pancreatic cancer. Int J Radiat Oncol Biol Phys 1999;45:291–5.
225. Wong AA, Delclos ME, Wolff RA, et al. Radiation dose considerations in the palliative treatment of locally advanced adenocarcinoma of the pancreas. Am J Clin Oncol 2005;28:227–33.
226. Lillemoe KD, Cameron JL, Kaufman HS, et al. Chemical splanchnicectomy in patients with unresectable pancreatic cancer. Ann Surg 1993;217:447–55.
227. Bukowski RM, Abderhalden RT, Hewlett JS, et al. Phase II trial of streptozotocin, mitomycin C, and 5-fluorouracil in adenocarcinoma of the pancreas. Cancer Clin Trials 1980:3:321–4.
228. Smith FP, Hoth DF, Levin B, et al. 5-Fluorouracil, Adriamycin, and mitomycin C (FAM) chemotherapy for advanced adenocarcinoma of the pancreas. Cancer 1980;46:2014–8.
229. Bukowski RM, Balcerzak SP, O'Bryan RM, et al. Randomized trial of 5-fluorouracil and mitomycin C with or without streptozotocin for advanced pancreatic cancer: a Southwest Oncology Group Study. Cancer 1983;52:1577–82.
230. Gastrointestinal Tumor Study Group. Phase II trials of hexamethylmelamine, dianhydrogalactitol, razoxane, and b-2'-deoxythioguanosine as single agents against advanced measurable tumors of the pancreas. Cancer Treat Rep 1985;69:713–6.
231. Goldberg HI, Margulis AR. Gastrointestinal radiology in the United States: an overview of the past 50 years. Radiology 2000;216:1–7.
232. Casper ES, Green MR, Kelsen DP, et al. Phase II trial of gemcitabine (2',2'-difluorodeoxycytidine) in patients with adenocarcinoma of the pancreas. Invest New Drugs 1994;12:29–34.
233. Carmichael J, Fink U, Russell RC, et al. Phase II study of gemcitabine in patients with advanced pancreatic cancer. Br J Cancer 1996;73:101–5.
234. Berlin JD, Catalono P, Thomas JP, et al. Phase III study of gemcitabine in combination with fluorouracil versus gemcitabine alone in patients with advanced pancreatic carcinoma: Eastern Cooperative Group Trial E2297. J Clin Oncol 2002;20:3270–5.
235. Rougier P, De Forni M, Adenis A, et al. Phase II study of Taxotere (RP56976, docetaxel) in pancreatic adenocarcinoma [abstract]. Proc Am Soc Clin Oncol 1994;13:200.
236. Okada S, Sakata Y, Matsuno S, et al. Phase II study of docetaxel in patients with metastatic pancreatic cancer: a Japanese cooperative study. Cooperative Group of Docetaxel for Pancreatic Cancer in Japan. Br J Cancer 1999;80:438–43.
237. Sugarman SM, Pazdur R, Daugherty K, et al. A phase II trial of topotecan for the treatment of unresectable pancreatic cancer [abstract]. Proc Am Soc Clin Oncol 1994;13:224.
238. Wagener DJT, Verdonk HER, Dirix LY, et al. Phase II trial of CPT-11 in patients with advanced pancreatic cancer. An EORTC Early Clinical Trials Group study. Ann Oncol 1995;6:129–32.
239. Rubin J, Gallagher JG, Schroeder G, et al. Phase II trials of 5-fluorouracil and leucovorin in patients with metastatic gastric or pancreatic carcinoma. Cancer 1996;78:1888–91.
240. Pazdur R, Meropol NJ, Casper E, et al. Phase II trial of ZD1694 (Tomudex) in patients with advanced pancreatic cancer. Ann Oncol 1996;13:355–8.
241. Thomas E, Dumas P, Ajani JA. Oral etoposide for patients with advanced adenocarcinoma of the pancreas. Invest New Drugs 1999;16:333–5.
242. Mani S, Schiano T, Garcia JC, et al. Phase II trial of uracil/tegafur (UFT) plus leucovorin in patients with advanced pancreatic cancer: a University of Chicago phase II consortium study. Ann Oncol 1998;9:1035–7.
243. Schmidt-Sandte W, Dageforde J, Klapdor R, et al. Trofosfamide in patients with pancreatic cancer. Anticancer Res 1999;19:2485–7.
244. Maisey N, Chau I, Cunningham D, et al. Multicenter randomized phase III trial comparing protracted venous infusion (PVI) fluorouracil (5-FU) with PVI 5-FU plus mitomycin in inoperable pancreatic cancer. J Clin Oncol 2002;20:3130–6.
245. Stehlin JS, Giovanella BC, Natelson EA, et al. A study of 9-nitrocamptothecin (RFS 2000) in patients with advanced pancreatic cancer. Int J Oncol 1999;14:821–31.
246. Konstadoulakis MM, Antonakis PT, Tsibloulis BG, et al. A phase II study of 9-nitrocampthothecin in patients with advanced pancreatic adenocarcinoma. Cancer Chemother Pharmacol 2001;48:417–20.
247. Rothenberg ML, Abbruzzese JL, Moore M, et al. A rationale for expanding the endpoints for clinical trials in advanced pancreatic carcinoma. Cancer 1996;78(3 Suppl):627–32.
248. Kelsen D. The use of chemotherapy in the treatment of advanced gastric and pancreas cancer. Semin Oncol 1994;21:58–66.
249. Bukowski RM. Role of chemotherapy in patients with adenocarcinoma of the pancreas. Adv Oncol 1995;11:25–9.
250. Carter SK, Comis RL. The integration of chemotherapy into a combined modality approach for cancer treatment. VI. Pan-

creatic adenocarcinoma. Cancer Treat Rev 1975;2:193–214.

251. Bukowski RM, Fleming TR, MacDonald JS, et al. Evaluation of combination chemotherapy and phase II agents in pancreatic adenocarcinoma: a Southwest Oncology Group study. Cancer 1993;71:322–5.
252. Bitran JD, Desser RR, Kozloff MF, et al. Treatment of metastatic pancreatic and gastric adenocarcinoma with 5-FU, Adriamycin and mitomycin (FAM). Cancer Treat Rep 1979;63:2049–51.
253. Wiggans RG, Woolley PV, MacDonald JS, et al. Phase II trial of streptozotocin, mitomycin C, and 5-fluorouracil (SMF) in the treatment of advanced pancreatic cancer. Cancer 1978;41:387–91.
254. Mallinson CN, Rake MO, Cocking JB. Chemotherapy in pancreas cancer. BMJ 1980;281:1589–91.
255. Oster MW, Gray R, Panasci L, et al. Chemotherapy for advanced pancreatic cancer. A comparison of 5-fluorouracil, Adriamycin, and mitomycin (FAM) with 5-fluorouracil, streptozotocin, and mitomycin (FSM). Cancer 1986;57:2–33.
256. Gastrointestinal Tumor Study Group. Phase II studies of drug combinations in advanced pancreatic carcinoma: fluorouracil plus doxorubicin plus mitomycin C and two regimens of streptozotocin plus mitomycin C plus fluorouracil. J Clin Oncol 1986;4:1794–8.
257. Cullinan S, Moertel CG, Wieand HS, et al. A phase III trial on the therapy of advanced pancreatic carcinoma. Evaluations of the Mallinson regimen and combined 5-fluorouracil, doxorubicin and cisplatin. Cancer 1990;65:2207–12.
258. Isacoff WH, Botnick L, Rose C, et al. Treatment of patients with locally advanced pancreatic carcinoma with continuous infusion 5-fluorouracil, calcium leucovorin, mitomycin-C and dipyridamole [abstract]. Proc Am Soc Clin Oncol 1993;12:225.
259. Burch PA, Ghosh C, Schroeder G, et al. Phase II evaluation of continuous-infusions 5-fluorouracil, leucovorin, mitomycin-C, and oral dipyridamole in advanced measurable pancreatic cancer: a North Central Cancer Treatment Group trial. Am J Clin Oncol 2000;23:534–7.
260. Hertel LW, Boder GB, Kroin JS, et al. Evaluation of the antitumor activity of gemcitabine (2',2'-difluoro-2'-deoxycytidine). Cancer Res 1990;50:4417–22.
261. Heinemann V, Hertel LW, Grindey GB, et al. Comparison of the cellular pharmacokinetics and toxicity of 2',2'-difluorodeoxycytidine and 1-beta-d-arabinofuranosylcytosine. Cancer Res 1988;48:4024–31.
262. Abbruzzese JL, Grunewald R, Weeks EA, et al. A phase I clinical, plasma, and cellular pharmacology study of gemcitabine. J Clin Oncol 1991;9:491–8.
263. Rothenberg ML, Moore MJ, Cripps MC, et al. A phase II trial of gemcitabine in patients with 5-FU-refractory pancreas cancer. Ann Oncol 1996;7:347–53.
264. Grunewald R, Abbruzzese JL, Tarassoff P, et al. Saturation of 2',2'-difluorodeoxycytidine 5'-triphosphate accumulation by mononuclear cells during a phase I trial of gemcitabine. Cancer Chemother Pharmacol 1991;27:258–62.
265. Grunewald R, Kantarjian H, Keating MJ, et al. Pharmacologically directed design of the dose rate and schedule of 2',2'-difluorodeoxycytidine (gemcitabine) administration in leukemia. Cancer Res 1990;50:6823–6.
266. Grunewald R, Kantarjian H, Du M, et al. Gemcitabine in leukemia: a phase I clinical, plasma, and cellular pharmacology study. J Clin Oncol 1992;10:406–13.
267. Touroutoglou N, Gravel D, Raber MN, et al. Clinical results of a pharmacodynamically based strategy for higher dosing of gemcitabine in patients with solid tumors. Ann Oncol 1998;9:1003–8.
268. Brand R, Capadano M, Tempero M. A phase I trial of weekly gemcitabine administered as a prolonged infusion in patients with pancreatic cancer and other solid tumors. Invest New Drugs 1997;15:331–41.
269. Tempero M, Plunkett W, Ruiz van Haperen V, et al. Randomized phase II comparison of dose-intense gemcitabine: thirty-minute infusion and fixed dose rate infusion in patients with pancreatic adenocarcinoma. J Clin Oncol 2003;21:3402–8.
270. O'Reilly S, Donehower RC, Rowinsky EK, et al. A phase II trial of topotecan in patients with previously untreated pancreatic cancer. Anticancer Drugs 1996;7:410–4.
271. Scher RM, Kosierowski R, Lusch C, et al. Phase II trial of topotecan in advanced or metastatic adenocarcinoma of the pancreas. Invest New Drugs 1996;13:347–54.
272. Stevenson JP, Scher RM, Kosierowski R, et al. Phase II trial of topotecan as a 21-day continuous infusion in patients with advanced or metastatic adenocarcinoma of the pancreas. Eur J Cancer 1998;34:1358–62.
273. Jacobs AJ, Burris HA, Rivkin S, et al. A randomized phase III study of rubitecan vs. best choice in 409 patients with refractory pancreatic cancer. Report from a North-American multi-center study [abstract 4013]. J Clin Oncol 2004;22:14S.
274. Royce ME, Hoff PM, Dumas P, et al. Phase I and pharmacokinetic study of exatecan mesylate (DX-8951f): a novel camptothecin analog. J Clin Oncol 2001;19:1493–500.
275. Sharma S, Kemeny N, Schwartz GK, et al. Phase I study of topoisomerase I inhibitor exatecan mesylate (DX-8951f) given as weekly 24-hour infusions three of every four weeks. Clin Cancer Res 2001;7:3963–70.
276. Cheverton P, Friess H, Andras C, et al. Phase III results of exatecan (DX8951f) versus gemcitabine in chemotherapy-naïve patients with advanced pancreatic cancer [abstract 4005]. J Clin Oncol 2004;22:14S.
277. Rocha Lima CM, Green MR, Rotche R, et al. Irinotecan plus gemcitabine results in no survival advantage compared with gemcitabine monotherapy in patients with locally advanced or metastatic pancreatic cancer despite increased tumor response rate. J Clin Oncol 2004;22:3776–83.
278. O'Reilly EM, Abou-Alfa GK, Letourneau R, et al. A randomized phase III trial of DX-8951f (exatecan mesylate; DX) and gemcitabine vs gemcitabine alone in advanced pancreatic cancer [abstract 4006]. J Clin Oncol 2004;22:14S.
279. Bleickardt E, Argiris A, Rich R, et al. Phase I dose escalation trial of weekly docetaxel plus irinotecan in patients with advanced cancer. Cancer Biol Ther 2002;1:646–51.
280. Carlson RW, Doroshow JH, Odujinrin OO, et al. Trimetrexate in locally advanced or metastatic adenocarcinoma of the pancreas: a phase II study of the Northern California Oncology Group. Invest New Drugs 1990;8:387–9.
281. Linke K, Pazdur R, Abbruzzese J, et al. Phase II study of amonafide in advanced pancreatic adenocarcinoma. Invest New Drugs 1991;9:353–6.
282. Hubbard KP, Pazdur R, Ajani JA, et al. Phase II evaluation of iproplatin in patients with advanced gastric and pancreatic cancer. Am J Clin Oncol 1992;15:524–7.
283. Casper ES, Schwartz GK, Johnson B, et al. Phase II trial of edatrexate in patients with advanced pancreatic cancer. Invest New Drugs 1992;10:313–6.
284. Casper ES, Schwartz GK, Kelsen DP. Phase II trial of fazarabine (arabinofuranosyl-5-azacytidine) in patients with advanced pancreatic adenocarcinoma. Invest New Drugs 1992;10:205–9.
285. Loehrer PJS, Williams SD, Einhorn LH, et al. Ifosfamide: an active drug in treatment of adenocarcinoma of the pancreas. J Clin Oncol 1985;3:367–72.
286. Gastrointestinal Tumor Study Group. Ifosfamide is an inactive substance in the treatment of pancreatic carcinoma. Cancer 1989;64:2010–3.
287. Ajani JA, Abbruzzese JL, Goudeau P, et al. Ifosfamide and mesna: marginally active in patients with advanced carcinoma of the pancreas. J Clin Oncol 1988;6:1703–7.
288. Ryan DP, Kulke MH, Fuchs CS, et al. A phase II study of gemcitabine and docetaxel in patients with metastatic pancreatic carcinoma. Cancer 2002;94:97–103.
289. Louvet C, Andre T, Lledo G, et al. Gemcitabine combined with oxaliplatin in advanced pancreatic adenocarcinoma: final results of a GERCOR multicenter phase II study. J Clin Oncol 2002;20:1512–8.
290. Philip PA, Zalupski MM, Vaitkevicius VK, et al. Phase II study of gemcitabine and cisplatin in the treatment of patients with advanced pancreatic carcinoma. Cancer 2001;92:569–77.
291. Brodowicz T, Wolfram RM, Kostler WJ, et al. Phase II study of gemcitabine in combination with cisplatin in patients with locally advanced and/or metastatic pancreatic cancer. Anti-Cancer Drugs 2000;11:623–8.
292. Heinemann V, Wilke H, Mergenthaler HG, et al. Gemcitabine and cisplatin in the treatment of advanced or metastatic pancreatic cancer. Ann Oncol 2000;11:1399–403.
293. Sherman WH, Fine RL. Combination gemcitabine and docetaxel therapy in advanced adenocarcinoma of the pancreas. Oncology 2001;60:316–21.
294. Stathopoulos GP, Mavroudis D, Tsavaris N, et al. Treatment of pancreatic cancer with a combination of docetaxel, gemcitabine and granulocyte colony-stimulating factor: a phase II study of the Greek Cooperative Group for Pancreatic Cancer. Ann Oncol 2001;12:101–3.
295. Louvet C, Andre T, Hammel P, et al. Phase II trial of bimonthly leucovorin, 5-fluorouracil and gemcitabine for advanced pancreatic adenocarcinoma (FOLFUGEM). Ann Oncol 2001;12:675–9.
296. Oettle H, Arning M, Pelzer U, et al. A phase II trial of gemcitabine in combination with 5-fluorouracil (24-hour) and folinic acid in patients with chemonaive advanced pancreatic cancer. Ann Oncol 2000;11:1267–72.
297. Cascinu S, Silva RR, Barni S, et al. A combination of gemcitabine and 5-fluorouracil in advanced pancreatic cancer, a report from the Italian Group for the Study of Digestive Tract Cancer (GISCAD). Br J Cancer 1999;80:1595–8.
298. Hidalgo M, Castellano D, Paz-Ares L, et al. Phase I-II study of gemcitabine and fluorouracil as a continuous infusion in patients with pancreatic cancer. J Clin Oncol 1999;17:585–92.
299. Feliu J, Lopez Alvarez MP, Jaraiz MA, et al. Phase II trial of gemcitabine and UFT modulated by leucovorin in patients with advanced pancreatic carcinoma. The ONCOPAZ Cooperative Group. Cancer 2000;89:1706–13.
300. Rocha Lima CM, Savarese D, Bruckner H, et al. Irinotecan plus gemcitabine induces both radiographic and CA 19-9 tumor marker responses in patients with previously untreated advanced pancreatic cancer. J Clin Oncol 2002;20:1182–91.
301. Scheithauer W, Kornek GV, Raderer M, et al. Phase II trial of gemcitabine, epirubicin and granulocyte colony-stimulating factor in patients with advanced pancreatic adenocarcinoma. Br J Cancer 1999;80:1797–802.
302. Kindler HL, Dugan J, Hochster H, et al. Clinical outcome in patients with advanced pancreatic cancer treated with premetrexed/gemcitabine [abstract]. Proc Am Soc Clin Oncol 2002;21:125.
303. van Moorsel CJ, Veerman G, Bergman AM, et al. Combination chemotherapy studies with gemcitabine. Semin Oncol 1997;24:17–23.
304. Fine RL, Sherman W, Chabot S, et al. Biochemically synergistic chemotherapy for advanced pancreatic cancer [abstract]. Proc Am Soc Clin Oncol 2002;21:144.
305. Kozuch P, Grossbard ML, Barzdins A, et al. Irinotecan combined with gemcitabine, 5-fluorouracil, leucovorin, and cisplatin (G-FLIP) is an effective and noncrossresistant treatment for refractory metastatic pancreatic cancer. Oncologist 2001;6:488–95.
306. Reni M, Passoni P, Panucci MG, et al. Definitive results of a phase II trial of cisplatin, epirubicin, continuous-infusion fluorouracil, and gemcitabine in stage IV pancreatic adenocarcinoma. J Clin Oncol 2001;19:2679–86.
307. Colucci G, Giuliani F, Gebbia V, et al. Gemcitabine alone or with cisplatin for the treatment of patients with locally advanced and/or metastatic pancreatic carcinoma: a prospective, randomized phase III study of the Gruppo Oncologia dell'Italia Meridionale. Cancer 2002;94:902–10.
308. Louvet C, Labianca R, Hammel P, et al. Gemcitabine in combination with oxaliplatin compared with gemcitabine alone in locally advanced or metastatic pancreatic cancer: results of a GERCOR and GISCAD phase III trial. J Clin Oncol 2005;23:3509–16.
309. Herrmann R, Bodoky G, Ruhstaller T, et al. Gemcitabine plus Capecitabine versus gemcitabine alone in locally advanced or metastatic pancreatic cancer. A randomized phase III study of the Swiss Group for Clinical Cancer Research (SAKK) and the Central European Cooperative Oncology Group (CECOG) [abstract 4010]. J Clin Oncol 2005;23:16S.
310. Moore MJ, Goldstein D, Hamm J, et al. Erlotinib plus gemcitabine compared to gemcitabine alone in patients with advanced pancreatic cancer. A phase III trial of the National Cancer Institute of Canada Clinical Trials Group [abstract 1]. J Clin Oncol 2005;23:16S.
311. Haller DJ. Recent updates in the clinical use of platinum compounds for the treatment of gastrointestinal cancers. Semin Oncol 2004;6 Suppl 14:6–10.
312. Gibbs JB, Oliff A, Kohl NE. Farnesyltransferase inhibitors: ras research yields a potential cancer therapeutic. Cell 1994;77:175–8.
313. Rowinsky EK, Windle JJ, Von Hoff DD. Ras protein farnesyltransferase: a strategic target for anticancer therapeutic development. J Clin Oncol 1999;17:3631–52.
314. Eskens FA, Awada A, Cutler DL, et al. Phase I and pharmacokinetic study of the oral farnesyl transferase inhibitor SCH 66336 given twice daily to patients with advanced solid tumors. European Organization for Research and Treatment of Cancer Early Clinical Studies Group. J Clin Oncol 2001;19:1167–75.
315. Adjei AA, Erlichman C, Davis JN, et al. A phase I trial of the farnesyl transferase inhibitor SCH66336: evidence for biological and clinical activity. Cancer Res 2000;60:1871–7.
316. Zujewski J, Horak ID, Bol CJ, et al. Phase I and pharmacokinetic study of farnesyl protein transferase inhibitor

R115777 in advanced cancer. J Clin Oncol 2000;18:927–41.

317. Papadimitrakopoulou V, Agelaki S, Tran HT, et al. Phase I study of the farnesyltransferase inhibitor BMS-214662 given weekly in patients with solid tumors. Clin Cancer Res 2005;11:4151–9.
318. Lersch C, Van Cutsem E, Amado R, et al. Randomized phase II study of SCH 66336 and gemcitabine in the treatment of metastatic adenocarcinoma of the pancreas [abstract]. Proc Am Soc Clin Oncol 2001;20:153a.
319. Van Cutsem E, van de Velde H, Karasek P, et al. Phase III trial of gemcitabine plus tipifarnib compared with gemcitabine plus placebo in advanced pancreatic cancer. J Clin Oncol 2004;22:1430–8.
320. Vogel CL, Cobleigh MA, Tripathy D, et al. Efficacy and safety of trastuzumab as a single agent in first-line treatment of HER2-overexpressing metastatic breast cancer. J Clin Oncol 2002;20:719–26.
321. Baselga J, Averbuch SD. ZD1839 ('Iressa') as an anticancer agent. Drugs 2000;60 Suppl 1:33–40.
322. Slamon DJ, Leyland-Jones B, Shak S, et al. Use of chemotherapy plus a monoclonal antibody against HER2 for metastatic breast cancer that overexpresses HER2. NEJM 2001;344:783–92.
323. Safran H, Steinhoff M, Mangray S, et al. Overexpression of the HER-2/neu oncogene in pancreatic adenocarcinoma. Am J Clin Oncol 2001;24:496–9.
324. Apple SK, Hecht JR, Lewin DN, et al. Immunohistochemical evaluation of K-ras, p53, and HER-2/neu expression in hyperplastic, dysplastic, and carcinomatous lesions of the pancreas: evidence for multistep carcinogenesis. Hum Pathol 1999;30:123–9.
325. Safran H, Iannitti D, Ramanthan R, et al. Herceptin and gemcitabine for metastatic pancreatic cancers that overexpress HER-2/neu. Cancer Invest 2004;22:706–12.
326. Bramhall SR. The matrix metalloproteinases and their inhibitors in pancreatic cancer. From molecular science to a clinical application. Int J Pancreatol 1997;21:1–12.
327. Nemunaitis J, Poole C, Primrose J, et al. Combined analysis of studies of the effects of the matrix metalloproteinase inhibitor marimastat on serum tumor markers in advanced cancer: selection of a biologically active and tolerable dose for longer-term studies. Clin Cancer Res 1998;4:1101–19.
328. Hurwitz H, Humphrey J, Williams K, et al. A phase I trial of BMS-275291: a novel non-hydrozamate, sheddase-sparing matrix metalloproteinase inhibitor with no dose-limiting arthritis [abstract]. Proc Am Soc Clin Oncol 2001;20:98a.
329. Duievenvoorden WC, Hirte HW, Singh G. Quantification of matrix metalloproteinase activity in plasma of patients enrolled in a BAY 12-9566 phase I study. Int J Cancer 2001;91:857–62.
330. Bramhall SR, Rosemurgy A, Brown PD, et al. Marimastat Pancreatic Cancer Study Group. Marimastat as first-line therapy for patients with unresectable pancreatic cancer: a randomized trial. J Clin Oncol 2001;19:3447–55.
331. Bramhall SR, Schulz J, Nemunaitis J, et al. A double-blind placebo-controlled, randomised study comparing gemcitabine and marimastat with gemcitabine and placebo as first line therapy in patients with advanced pancreatic cancer. Br J Cancer 2002;87:161–7.
332. Raut CP, Ellis LM. Antiangiogenic therapy for pancreatic cancer. In: Von Hoff D, Evans DB, Hruban RH, editors. Pancreatic cancer. Sudbury (MA): Jones and Bartlett; 2005. p. 543–52.
333. Fong TA, Shawver LK, Sun L, et al. SU5416 is a potent and selective inhibitor of the vascular endothelial growth factor receptor (Flk-1/KDR) that inhibits tyrosine kinase catalysis, tumor vascularization, and growth of multiple tumor types. Cancer Res 1999;59:99–106.
334. Laird AD, Vajkoczy P, Shawver LK, et al. SU6668 is a potent antiangiogenic and antitumor agent that induces regression of established tumors. Cancer Res 2000;60:4152–60.
335. Chen HX, Gore-Langton RE, Cheson BD. Clinical trials referral resource: current clinical trials of the anti-VEGF monoclonal antibody bevacizumab. Oncology (Huntington) 2001;15:1017, 1020, 1023–6.
336. Thomas AL, Morgan B, Horsfield MA, et al. Phase I study of the safety, tolerability, pharmacokinetics, and pharmacodynamics of PTK787/ZK 222584 administered twice daily in patients with advanced cancer. J Clin Oncol 2005;23:4162–71.
337. Kindler HL, Friberg G, Stadler WM, et al. Bevacizumab plus gemcitabine is an active combination in patients with advanced pancreatic cancer: interim results of an ongoing phase II trial from the University of Chicago Phase II Consortium [abstract 86]. Proc Gastrointest Cancers Symp (ASCO, AGA, ASTRO, SSO). San Francisco 2004;84a.
338. Brown LF, Berse B, Jackman RW, et al. Expression of vascular permeability factor (vascular endothelial growth factor) and its receptors in adenocarcinomas of the gastrointestinal tract. Cancer Res 1993;53:4727–35.
339. Yang AD, Bauer TW, Camp ER, et al. Improving delivery of antineoplastic agents with anti-vascular endothelial growth factor therapy. Cancer 2005;103:1561–70.
340. Tong RT, Boucher Y, Kozin SV, et al. Vascular normalization by vascular endothelial growth factor receptor 2 blockade induces a pressure gradient across the vasculature and improves drug penetration in tumors. Cancer Res 2004;64:3731–6.
341. Willett CG, Boucher Y, di Tomaso E, et al. Direct evidence that the VEGF-specific antibody bevacizumab has antivascular effects in human rectal cancer. Nat Med 2004;10:145–7.
342. Soker S, Kaefer M, Johnson M, et al. Vascular endothelial growth factor-mediated autocrine stimulation of prostate tumor cells coincides with progression to a malignant phenotype. Am J Pathol 2001;159:651–9.
343. Mendelsohn J. Epidermal growth factor receptor inhibition by a monoclonal antibody as anticancer therapy. Clin Cancer Res 1997;3:2703–7.
344. Bruns CJ, Harbison MT, Davis DW, et al. Epidermal growth factor receptor blockade with C225 plus gemcitabine results in regression of human pancreatic carcinoma growing orthotopically in nude mice by antiangiogenic mechanisms. Clin Cancer Res 2000;6:1936–48.
345. Kim SJ, Uehara H, Karashima T, et al. Blockade of epidermal growth factor receptor signaling in tumor cells and tumor-associated endothelial cells for therapy of androgen-independent human prostate cancer growing in the bone of nude mice. Clin Cancer Res 2003;9:1200–10.
346. Xiong Q, Rosenberg A, LoBuglio A, et al. Cetuximab, a monoclonal antibody targeting the epidermal growth factor receptor, in combination with gemcitabine for advanced pancreatic cancer: a multicenter phase II Trial. J Clin Oncol 2004;22:2610–6.
347. Hidalgo M, Siu LL, Nemunaitis J, et al. Phase I and pharmacologic study of OSI-774, an epidermal growth factor receptor tyrosine kinase inhibitor, in patients with advanced solid malignancies. J Clin Oncol 2001;19:3267–79.
348. Laheru D, Biedrzycki B, Jaffee EM. Immunologic approaches to the management of pancreatic cancer. Cancer J 2001;7:324–37.
349. Gjertsen MK, Bakka A, Breivik J, et al. Vaccination with mutant ras peptides and induction of T-cell responsiveness in pancreatic carcinoma patients carrying the corresponding ras mutation. Lancet 1995;346:1399–400.
350. Finn OJ, Jerome KR, Henderson RA, et al. MUC-1 epithelial tumor mucin-based immunity and vaccines. Immunol Rev 1995;145:61–89.
351. Janetzki S, Palla D, Rosenhauer V, et al. Immunization of cancer patients with autologous cancer-derived heat shock protein gp96 preparations: a pilot study. Int J Cancer 2000;88:232–8.
352. Ramanthan RK, Lee K, Mckolanis J, et al. Phase I study of a MUC-1 synthetic vaccine admixed with SB-AS2 adjuvant in resected and locally advanced pancreatic cancer [abstract]. Proc Am Soc Clin Oncol 2000;19:45.
353. Desai J, Mitchell P, Loveland B, et al. A phase I trial of dendritic cells pulsed with MUC-1 peptide in patients with solid tumors [abstract]. Proc Am Soc Clin Oncol 2002;21:15.
354. Jaffee EM, Hruban RH, Biedrzycki B, et al. Novel allogeneic granulocyte-macrophage colony-stimulating factor-secreting tumor vaccine for pancreatic cancer: a phase I trial of safety and immune activation. J Clin Oncol 2001;19:145–56.
355. Pinzon R, Drewinko B, Trujillo JM, et al. Pancreatic carcinoma and Trousseau's syndrome: experience at a large cancer center. J Clin Oncol 1986;4:509–14.
356. Russell RC. Palliation of pain and jaundice: an overview. Ann Oncol 1999;10 Suppl 4:165–9.
357. Andren-Sandberg A, Viste A, Horn A, et al. Pain management of pancreatic cancer. Ann Oncol 1999;4 suppl 10:265–8.
358. Kawamata M, Ishitani K, Ishikawa K, et al. Comparison between celiac plexus block and morphine treatment on quality of life in patients with pancreatic cancer pain. Pain 1996;64:597–602.
359. Wigmore SJ, Barber MD, Ross JA, et al. Effect of oral eicosapentaenoic acid on weight loss in patients with pancreatic cancer. Nutrition and Cancer 2000;36:177–84.
360. Brugge WR, VanDam J. Pancreatic and biliary endoscopy. N Engl J Med 1999;341:1808–16.
361. Menon K, Romagnuolo J, Barkun AN. Expandable metal biliary stenting in patients with recurrent premature polyethylene stent occlusion. Am J Gastroenterol 2001;96:1429–34.
362. Lee CW, Bociek G, Faught W. A survey of practice in management of malignant ascites. J Pain Symptom Manage 1998;16:96–101.
363. Parsons SL, Watson SA, Steele RJ. Malignant ascites. Br J Surg 1996;83:6–14.

91

Neoplasms of the Small Intestine, Vermiform Appendix, and Peritoneum

Elizabeth G. Grubbs, MD
Douglas S. Tyler, MD

TUMORS OF THE SMALL INTESTINE

The small intestine represents 75% of the total length of the gastrointestinal (GI) tract and comprises 90% of its mucosal surface area, yet rarely does this region develop malignant tumors.[1] Recent figures show that less than 3% of all alimentary tract tumors and 0.4% of all malignancies arise in the small bowel.[2] 5,300 new small bowel malignancies were predicted for 2004 with an estimated 4 stomach tumors and 28 colorectal tumors for every tumor found in the small bowel.

Several mechanisms have been postulated to explain the low incidence of neoplastic transformation within the small intestine. The most important of these are the rapid transit of content through the small bowel, which provides a shorter exposure of its mucosa to carcinogens, increased lymphoid tissue in the small intestine with a high level of immunoglobulin A expression, and a lower bacterial load in the small bowel that results in a decreased conversion of bile acids into potential carcinogens by anaerobic microorganisms.[3,4] In addition, the liquid contents of the small bowel may cause less mucosal irritation than the more solid contents of the large intestine, and there is the presence in the small intestine of mucosal toxifying enzymes such as benzopyrene hydroxylase.[5]

Although 75% of small bowel tumors found at autopsy are benign, most of the symptomatic lesions and tumors discovered during surgery are malignant. Adenocarcinomas comprise 30 to 50% of small bowel malignant tumors, followed by carcinoids (25–30%), lymphomas (15–20%), and, to a lesser extent, sarcomas. Leiomyomas account for 25% of all benign tumors, while others include adenomas and lipomas, and rarer neoplasms such as fibromas, fibromyxomas, neurofibromas, ganglioneuromas, hemangiomas, and lymphangiomas.[6]

Certain conditions are associated with an increased incidence of particular types of small bowel tumors. Familial adenomatous polyposis is known to be a powerful risk factor for adenocarcinoma, with small bowel cancer being the most common cancer after colon cancer itself.[7] The relative risk of small bowel carcinoma in these patients has been described as being > 100.[8] Other hereditary syndromes associated with small bowel tumors include Peutz–Jeghers syndrome (increased incidence of hamartomatous polyps in the jejunum and ileum), Gardner syndrome (adenoma and adenocarcinoma), and von Recklinghausen disease (paraganglioma). Small bowel inflammatory disorders are associated with increased malignancy, including, most notably, Crohn's disease, which may increase the risk of small bowel adenocarcinoma by > 100.[9] Other disorders associated with increased risk of malignancy are celiac disease (lymphoma and adenocarcinoma) and immunoproliferative disease (diffuse intestinal lymphoma and immunoproliferative small intestinal disease).[5]

Clinical Presentation Many small bowel tumors are asymptomatic until late in their course because of their relatively slow growth and the ease with which the liquid contents of the small bowel can pass even a partially obstructing lesion. Half of small bowel cancers are found only at autopsy. The remainder are usually found as a result of the symptoms of partial obstruction: nausea and vomiting if the lesion is proximal, as well as crampy abdominal pain, or other nonspecific findings such as weight loss. Hemorrhage is frequently found in those tumors that penetrate beyond the submucosa, but almost always is occult, presenting as microcytic anemia or stool that is positive on guaiac testing. Certain small bowel tumors have more specific presenting symptoms, such as jaundice (ampullary carcinoma) and fever, diarrhea, and weight loss (lymphoma). Endocrine tumors of the gut, the most common of which are carcinoid tumors, may present with their own set of classic symptoms, such as flushing, diarrhea, cyanosis, and intermittent respiratory distress. Only a small proportion of patients with carcinoid tumors have these symptoms, the vast majority being asymptomatic or having symptoms secondary to mass lesion effects.

Eventually, malignant tumors cause enough symptoms for the ensuing medical work-up to reveal the tumor. Unfortunately, some time may pass between the first symptom and diagnosis. In one series, almost one-third of the patients had had symptoms for 5 years or more prior to definitive diagnosis.[10] A more recent study demonstrated a mean duration of symptoms of 7 months prior to diagnosis.[11] Many patients eventually diagnosed with small bowel tumors present as an emergency with either bowel obstruction or perforation.

Diagnostic Imaging Radiographic studies often aid in the diagnosis of these lesions, especially in advanced disease. However, such studies are often not useful for early diagnosis of curable malignancy. Plain films of the abdomen are unlikely to be of use, except to demonstrate the presence of obstruction or perhaps displacement of the bowel by a mass. The small bowel follow through, although noninvasive and relatively inexpensive, is often insensitive. A more sensitive procedure is the double-contrast modality of enteroclysis, which involves placing a nasogastric tube into the descending duodenum and infusing barium and methylcellulose under pressure. This technique enables better visualization of the intestinal lumen and mucosal surface, and has a 90% sensitivity for small bowel tumors versus only 33% with small bowel follow through.[12] Computed tomographic (CT) scanning with oral contrast has led to nearly 100% recognition of small bowel tumors in some series, although it has limited ability to differentiate among tumor types.[13] This modality appears to be most useful for preoperative staging and metastasis evaluation.[14] In one series, the sensitivity for CT in determining T (tumor) stage was 57%, compared with 61% and 42% for colon and gastric cancer, respectively.[15–17] Angiography and nuclear scanning may be useful in the case of a bleeding tumor or a suspected hemangioma. Endoscopic ultrasonography (EUS) is used to detect and stage small bowel tumors and allows real-time interventional diagnostic procedures, mainly in the periampullary region. EUS has been shown to be superior to CT and MRI (magnetic resonance imaging) in predicting vascular invasion and overall assessment of T stage of ampullary neoplasms.[18,19]

Small bowel endoscopy has become an increasingly used diagnostic tool in the last decade and may be divided into three main categories: push enteroscopy, intraoperative or laparoscopically assisted enteroscopy, and, most recently, double-balloon enteroscopy. Push enteroscopy involves an intestinal intubation of a 220 to 250 cm instrument, usually with fluoroscopic assistance, and can be used to examine the jejunum for mean lengths of 120 cm beyond the ligament of Treitz.[20] In intraoperative endoscopy, the surgeon manually manipulates through the small bowel wall either a push endoscope (anterograde) or a colonoscope (retrograde) to examine the entire small bowel. The surgeon can mark the lesions of interest, usually by suture, and resect at the completion of the enteroscopy. This invasive diagnostic and therapeutic technique is useful in cases of multiple lesions, such as in Peutz–Jeghers syndrome and when other modalities have failed in diagnosis. The recent addition of laparoscopically assisted enteroscopy provides a less invasive technique than interoperative enteroscopy, but still requires general anesthesia and both a surgeon and endoscopist.[21] In double-balloon enteroscopy, an endoscope and a soft flexible overtube, each of which has an inflatable balloon attached to its distal end, are employed together. The two tubes are advanced over one another repeatedly using alternating inflation of the balloons to hold position, allowing deep advancement into the small intestine. The entire small intestine can be examined using this method with less discomfort than experienced with the push method.[22] After receiving FDA approval in 2001, a small, swallowable imaging capsule was introduced by Swain and colleagues that is propelled by peristalsis through the intestinal tract and transmits data to a receiver that captures video images on a regular basis.[23] The clinical indications for the use of this wireless capsule endoscopy are becoming clearer in light of recent studies. One such study shows that capsule endoscopy is superior to push endoscopy in the diagnosis of recurrent small intestinal bleeds after negative gastroscopy and colonoscopy (68% vs 32%).[24] Though capsule endoscopy is a promising technique, several shortcomings still exist, including lack of forward and backward movement to examine an area of interest, inability to use instruments to carry out treatment, and inadequate image resolution.

Treatment The treatment of small bowel tumors is usually surgical, with simple resection for benign lesions and an aggressive approach for malignant lesions. Overall, the survival for adenocarcinomas, carcinoids, lymphomas, and sarcomas was better in 328 cases from a population-based registry than that for all other organs, except the breast, colon, prostate, and uterus.[25] In most cases, the surgical resection must include wide margins, resection of lymph nodes, and removal of the supporting mesentery. In rare cases, radiation or chemotherapy may precede surgery. Duodenal tumors may require pancreaticoduodenectomy if malignant, whereas tumors of the terminal ileum may require right hemicolectomy to ensure complete resection and adequate margins.

Benign Tumors **Leiomyoma** The leiomyoma is the most common symptomatic benign tumor of the small bowel, accounting for approximately 20% of all benign small bowel tumors.[26] They tend to occur in equal numbers in males and females and increase in occurrence with age, with peak incidence at ages 50 to 59 years.[24,27] Microscopically, these tumors are composed of well-differentiated smooth muscle cells arranged into whorls with no evidence of mitosis. Macroscopically, they present most commonly as single, grayish-white, firm, well-defined masses. Four growth patterns have been defined: intraluminal, intramural, extraluminal, and dumbbellshaped.[28] Leiomyomas occur most frequently in the jejunum, followed by the ileum and duodenum. Only 44 to 50% of these tumors are symptomatic, the remainder are discovered at autopsy or during an unrelated surgery.[29] When symptomatic, leiomyomas usually present either with obstruction, as a consequence of their large size encroaching on the lumen, or with bleeding. In the two largest series to date, bleeding was seen in 40 to 67% and obstruction in 25 to 40%.[30,31] Perforation is rare but has been reported.[32] Differentiating between leiomyoma and leiomyosarcoma may be difficult by frozen section owing to nuclear pleomorphism in benign tumors. Thus, treatment should consist of surgical resection with wide margins, generally accepted to be 5 cm.

Adenomas Adenomas are the most common asymptomatic benign small bowel tumors and are usually found at autopsy. Three types of small bowel adenoma have been identified: adenomatous polyps, villous adenomas, and Brunner gland adenomas.[33] Adenomatous polyps are the most common benign tumors of the duodenum.[34] Although usually asymptomatic, they may present with bleeding and obstruction. Often pedunculated, these lesions, when duodenal, may be removed endoscopically. When located in the jejunum and ileum, simple enterotomy and excision may be performed. Villous adenomas occur most frequently in the duodenum. Like adenomas of the colon, large size, atypia, and the villous component of this adenoma increase the risk of malignancy.[5] A study by Sellner, in 1990, illustrated that the presence of the adenoma–carcinoma sequence in the small bowel is similar to the widely accepted sequence that is the root of most cancers in the large bowel.[35] Of 255 symptomatic small bowel adenomas reviewed in this study, 76 (29.8%) showed invasive carcinoma. In another retrospective study of 192 villous adenomas in the duodenum, the incidence of malignant changes at the time of presentation was 42%.[36] Because of this potential for malignancy, these tumors should be removed. The treatment of choice is segmental resection; however, in the duodenum, polypectomy can be performed if the histology of the tumor is benign.

Duodenal adenomas occur in more than 90% of patients with familial adenomatous polyposis (FAP).[37] Proximal small bowel cancer arising from these adenomas is one of the two leading causes of death (the other being desmoid tumors) in FAP patients with previous colectomies.[38] These adenomas may be classified by macroscopic and histologic criteria in five stages (0 to IV) based on Spigelman's criteria.[39] The criteria include a scoring system for number and size of polyps, histology (tubulous, tubulovillous, or villous), and low-grade versus high-grade dysplasia. Management strategies for FAP patients with duodenal polyposis include patients with advanced adenomas (> 1 cm) or high-grade dysplasia undergoing endoscopic treatment, or, alternatively, following these patients until they develop advanced disease (stage IV) or duodenal cancer and treating them with a pancreaticoduodenectomy at that time.[40–43] A more recent study involving a prospective, optimized endoscopic surveillance protocol found a higher duodenal polyposis progression rate and cumulative risk of stage IV disease in FAP patients than in previous, mostly retrospective studies.[38] These findings suggest that current modalities for surveillance and management of these patients need revision.

Brunner's glands "adenomas" are thought to be hyperplastic or hamartomatous lesions and not, as their name implies, true adenomas. Also known as Brunner's glands hamartomas and Brunneromas, they arise from Brunner's glands of the proximal duodenum. When symptomatic, they may be removed by simple excision. There is no potential for malignancy in Brunner's adenomas, and a radical resection should not be performed.

Lipoma The third most common benign tumor of the small bowel is the lipoma.[5] Lipomas consist of masses of adult adipose tissue and may be found anywhere in the small intestine but are most commonly located distally.[44] Most often asymptomatic, lipomas may serve as a point of intussusception, leading to intermittent abdominal obstruction and GI bleeding. Treatment consists of local excision for small tumors and segmental resection for larger tumors.

Hemangioma Hemangiomas represent approximately 10% of benign small bowel tumors in most collected series.[31,45–47] Approximately one-half of the lesions are cavernous, with capillary and mixed types each making up approximately one-quarter of the specimens. Multiple intestinal hemangiomas are much more common than are solitary intestinal lesions. Histologically, these tumors are discrete masses composed of well-developed, thin-walled capillaries and veins and are usually submucosal. Seventy percent of patients present with bleeding, but intussusception and obstruction also occur.[45,48] Treatment consists of resection of the lesion, although in the case of multiple lesions, finding the precise site of bleeding may be difficult. Preoperative angiography may be helpful in localizing briskly bleeding lesions.

Lymphangiomas Lymphangiomas are rare, benign malformations of sequestered lymphatic tissue that fail to communicate with the normal lymphatic system. They most commonly present with symptoms of obstruction as a consequence of their large size, but may also present with GI bleeding.[31,45,49,50] Although it is not known whether these lesions can recur in another segment of intestine, resection with adequate margins and primary anastomosis appears to be sufficient treatment.

Malignant Neoplasms **Adenocarcinoma** Adenocarcinomas are the most common malignant tumors in the small bowel, accounting for approximately 30 to 50% of all malignant small bowel tumors.[51,52] They most commonly arise in the seventh decade of life and are seen slightly more often in men than in women.[53] Primary tumors arise most often in the duodenum (48–52%) and jejunum (23–25%) and less commonly in the ileum (13–16%), the reason for this distribution is unclear.[54,55] Some have postulated that the richness of immunoglobulin A (IgA)-secreting cells in the ileum accounts for its relative sparing from adenocarcinoma by neutralizing luminal carcinogens.[4] Others have noted that the abundance of the enzyme benzopyrene hydroxylase may play a protective role by detoxifying potential carcinogens.[56]

The histogenesis of small bowel adenocarcinoma most likely follows the adenoma–carcinoma sequence described initially for large bowel cancer.[35] As a result, the single most important risk factor for small bowel adenocarcinoma is preexisting adenoma, either single or multiple, as associated with a multiple polyposis syndrome.[57] Small bowel adenocarcinomas have also been associated with alcohol (but not tobacco), nontropical sprue, regional enteritis, celiac disease, and urinary diversion procedures such as ileal conduit.[58–62] Despite the well-known correlation of colonic cancer with ulcerative colitis, much less evidence exists to indict Crohn's disease as a cause of adenocarcinoma of the small bowel.[63] The few reports that are available show a slightly increased risk of tumors associated with Crohn's disease to occur in the terminal ileum and in other sites where Crohn's disease is active.[64–66] The age at diagnosis is usually 10 years younger for the Crohn's patients than for the population at large. As with ulcerative colitis, the diagnosis of Crohn's disease precedes the tumor by about 10 years. Several risk factors have been identified in patients with Crohn's disease who develop adenocarcinoma of the small bowel: duration of Crohn's disease, gender, fistulization, and presence of surgically created blind excluded loops of intestines.[67,68]

Celiac sprue is known to predispose to intestinal lymphoma; it is also associated with adenocarcinoma.[60] The numbers cited in case reports are few, but the presence of disease in otherwise noncharacteristic locations seems to lend credence to the theory that gluten-mediated jejunoileitis is also an independent risk factor for the development of adenocarcinoma of the small bowel as well as lymphomas.[52,60] Adenocarcinoma of the small intestine, often aggressive, can affect children, and is usually associated with degeneration of a Peutz–Jeghers hamartoma.[57]

Symptoms of adenocarcinoma of the small bowel range from obstructive symptoms, such as vomiting and jaundice for those with duodenal tumors, to indistinct abdominal pain, weight loss, and anemia for more distal lesions. The most common complaint is abdominal pain in 30 to 70% of patients. Weight loss is also common, occurring in more than 50% of patients. Obstruction is found in 40 to 70% of patients prior to presentation. In the collected Mayo series, 71% of patients had either overt or clinical evidence of blood loss.[69] Adenocarcinomas, especially duodenal tumors, usually become symptomatic earlier than other small bowel tumors, allowing for earlier diagnosis and intervention. Despite this, 30 to 35% of small bowel adenocarcinomas are metastatic at the time of diagnosis.[54,55] Metastasis can occur via lymphatics, by a hematogenous route (liver, lungs, and bone most commonly), or by direct extension through the serosal surfaces and into the peritoneal cavity. Because of the insidious nature of adenocarcinomas, they tend to present late with either lymph node involvement or distant metastases. One hypothesis for early metastasis is that, unlike large bowel mucosa, small bowel mucosa contains lymphatics that course through the villi extending near the luminal surface, allowing invasion of the mucosal tumor into the lymphatics.

In a recent study conducted by the American College of Surgeons on 5,000 small bowel adenocarcinomas, the overall 5-year disease-free survival was 30.5%.[70] The median survival in this series was 19.7 months. Staging of adenocarcinomas of the small bowel is carried out by the TNM (tumor, node, metastases) classification system. The primary treatment of adenocarcinomas is wide surgical resection, with removal of lymph nodes and the vascular pedicle. Margins of 5 cm are considered acceptable. Recent reports indicate that even this treatment does not yield good survival rates for node-positive patients. In a recent study examining 217 patients with small bowel adenocarcinoma followed over a 10-year period at M.D. Anderson Cancer Center, patients with stage IV disease had a shorter, 5-year overall survival than those with I-III disease (5% vs 36%).[55] The 5-year survival was significantly shorter if the lymph node ratio was greater than 75% versus less than 75% (12% vs 51%). In patients with involvement of the proximal duodenum, pancreatoduodenectomy may be necessary. In those with disease in the terminal ileum, a right hemicolectomy is indicated. In those with jejunal involvement, wide resection is recommended.

All attempts should be made to resect the primary lesion to prevent mucosal bleeding. For patients deemed unresectable intraoperatively, some have advocated the use of intraoperative radiation therapy.[71–73] The lack of clinical trials makes this therapy difficult to recommend in a setting other than centers specialized for it. External beam radiation may be helpful to palliate symptoms, but again, there is a lack of published experience with this treatment. Chemotherapy usually incorporates 5-fluorouracil and nitrosoureas. In some settings, these agents have led to tumor regression and apparently increased lengths of survival.[73]

The genetic mechanisms involved in the carcinogenesis of the small bowel remain unknown, most likely because of the small number of cases. Blaker and colleagues from Germany showed that although small intestinal carcinomas reveal complex genetic changes, a significant number of tumors share karyotypic instability and losses of chromosome 18q21-q22. 18q deletions often target the SMAD4 gene and disrupt tumor suppression through TGFβ-signalling.[74] Svrcek and colleagues, using tissue microarray analysis, determined that inactivation of the SMAD4/DPC4 gene is involved in small intestinal adenocarcinoma tumorigenesis and that over expression of TP53 and abnormal expression of β catenin are two common events in small intestinal adenocarcinoma.[75]

Carcinoid Carcinoid tumors represent approximately 25 to 30% of malignant tumors of the small bowel. They were first described by Lubarsch over 100 years ago.[72,76] The term karzinoide was used by Obendorfer in 1907,[77] but the exact nature of the tumor was not determined until 1928 when Masson described its origin as the chromaffin cell.[78] The most recent population-based review of carcinoid tumors comes from the epidemiologic study by Maggard and colleagues, who analyzed 11,427 cases of carcinoid tumors.[79] The most frequent sites for carcinoids were the GI tract (54.5%) and the bronchopulmonary system (30.1%). Within the GI tract, most occurred in the small bowel (44.7%), rectum (19.6%), and appendix (16.7%). In contradistinction to adenocarcinoma, the carcinoid tends to arise in the distal small intestine rather than in more proximal sites. In the series reported by Moertel, all surgically confirmed, 3% were in the duodenum, 5% in the jejunum, 32% in the proximal ileum, and 60% in the distal ileum.[80] The median age at discovery is 60.9 years, and females constitute 54.2% of patients.[79]

A unique feature of carcinoid tumors is their ability to produce a variety of protein and peptide products, the most characteristic of which is serotonin. Systemic serotonin is thought to cause most of the symptoms of the carcinoid syndrome, including diarrhea, flushing, wheezing, and right-sided heart disease. Carcinoid syndrome is seen in 5 to 7% of patients with large tumor burdens and metastatic disease.[81,82] It is believed that the metastatic component is necessary to ensure drainage of the compounds involved in the syndrome into the systemic circulation and to provide an adequate tumor mass to produce large amounts of peptidergic products.

Carcinoid tumors are traditionally classified according to their embryonic site of origin and their usual histologic type.[83] In 1963, Williams and Sandler reported that those discovered in the foregut (bronchi, stomach, pancreas, biliary tract, and parts one and two of the duodenum) tended to have a histologic pattern of trabeculae and were occasionally associated with the carcinoid syndrome. Those arising from the midgut, the most common site, had a histologic pattern of nests and invading cords and were most commonly associated with the carcinoid syndrome. Finally, those found in the hindgut (descending colon and rectum) had a mixed histologic picture, but were infrequently involved with the carcinoid syndrome.[83]

The clinical manifestations of carcinoid are often vague or absent and the definitive diagnosis is often not made prior to surgery. In a series of 145 patients with gastrointestinal carcinoid tumors, only 12 had a proper diagnosis before surgery and those 12 had definite symptoms of carcinoid syndrome.[80,84] Most often, patients are operated on for signs of bowel obstruction, not by the tumor itself, but by a desmoplastic reaction that leads to shrinking of the mesentery (a result of fibrosis) and kinking of the bowel.[81,85] Standard imaging techniques such as CT, ultrasonography, and even enteroclysis rarely identify the primary tumor, making preoperative diagnosis of small bowel carcinoid very difficult.[82,86] A useful diagnostic tool, if a carcinoid tumor is suspected, is the measurement of carcinoid products and their metabolites including serotonin and 5-hydroxyindoloacetic acid (5-HIAA). A diagnosis of carcinoid syndrome is confirmed if the 24-hour urine 5-HIAA level is more than 10 mg.[83,87] In one study involving primarily patients with metastatic disease, elevated 5-HIAA excretion predicted the presence of carcinoid tumor with a sensitivity of 73% and a specificity of 100%.[84,88] Scintigraphy with radiolabeled octreotide has been successfully used to localize undetected primary and metastatic lesions.[89] Two large European studies show carcinoid lesion detection with a sensitivity of 89% by using this diagnostic tool.[90]

The metastatic potential of a carcinoid tumor correlates closely with its size. In the Moertel series, there were no metastases in tumors less than 0.5 cm in diameter, 15% in tumors 0.5 to 0.9 cm in diameter, 72% in tumors 1.0 to 1.9 cm in diameter, and 95% metastases in tumors larger than 2 cm.[80] Extent of disease, which mainly comprises either lymph node (regional) or liver (metastatic) involvement, is a definite predictor of outcome. In Maggard's analysis of 11,427 carcinoids, 5-year survival for localized, regional, and distant disease of the small intestine was 70.4%, 64.1 %, and 32.4%, respectively.[91] Given these statistics, there is no place for limited resection of small bowel carcinoids. Even with small tumors, an extended resection with relevant lymph node drainage is required. This is the only approach that allows definitive histopathologic staging, resection of occult lymph node metastasis, and prevention of local complications caused by a desmoplastic resection.[83] Careful intraoperative examination is mandatory, because most series report that 30% of these tumors are multicentric.[69] Another reason for meticulous exploration is that associated neoplasms occur with small intestinal carcinoids in 16.6% of cases.[91] In the case of advanced disease, there may be some benefit to debulking procedures, but this remains controversial, because the absolute size of the tumor does not correspond well with the degree of symptoms.[69,92,93] Some authors recommend aggressive treatment even in patients with widely metastatic disease, including resection of all intra-abdominal tumor deposits, segmental liver resection as needed, and hepatic arterial embolization. Cholecystectomy also has been performed to prevent gallbladder necrosis during hepatic embolization. Although it has not been proved whether this aggressive surgical approach increases survival, it has yielded biochemical remission in up to 25% of patients and regression of hepatic metastases for long periods.[91,94] In the M.D. Anderson experience of 81 patients with carcinoid disease metastatic to the liver who underwent hepatic artery embolization or chemoembolization, 67% experienced a partial response with a mean duration of response of 17 months. Overall, 63% of patients had reduction in their tumor-related symptoms and the overall survival time was 31 months.[95]

Medical therapy in the form of somatostatin analogues is effective in relieving symptoms of the carcinoid syndrome, though demonstrated tumor regression is rare. Octreotide is an eight amino-acid, long-acting somatostatin analogue that binds to receptor subtypes 2, 3, and 5 and has been widely used for both detection and treatment of carcinoid tumors.[96] In one study, octreotide was delivered subcutaneously at a dosage of 150 micrograms 3 times a day, showing improved symptoms in 88% of patients and decreased urinary 5-HIAA in 72% of patients.[97]

Prognosis of patients with carcinoid disease varies according to several factors. Size of the primary tumor is an important predictor of metastasis and survival. Carcinoid tumors greater than 2 cm in diameter portend a worse prognosis than those less than 2 cm.[98] This is most likely a result of the propensity to metastasize and not increased biologic aggressiveness of these larger tumors. In the Maggard series, increased tumor size was associated with a greater likelihood of lymph node involvement.[79] In the carcinoid series at Duke University, a direct correlation was found between size of the primary tumor and extent of disease at presentation.[99] In addition, after controlling for stage of disease, region of origin of primary tumor predicted prognosis in this series of patients. In patients with distant metastases at presentation, those with midgut tumors had markedly better prognosis than did patients with foregut or hindgut tumors. The reasons for the relative indolence of metastatic midgut tumors are unclear.

Composite tumors, those that display characteristics of both carcinoid tumors and adenocarcinomas, are well described in the appendix but are less well known in the small intestine. These tumors are relatively rare, with most reports to date encompassing only one or two cases. They are aggressive tumors with a metastatic potential similar to that of adenocarcinoma and should be treated as adenocarcinomas. Lymphatic metastasis appeared histologically to be adenocarcinoma in two cases and carcinoid in one; thus, it seems that these tumors may arise from cells with pluripotential patterns of differentiation.[100]

Gastrointestinal Stromal Tumors Gastrointestinal stromal tumors (GIST) is the current nomenclature for a diverse group of benign or malignant gastrointestinal neoplasms derived from embryonic mesoderm that may have smooth muscle (smooth-muscle GIST), neural differentiation (gastrointestinal autonomic nerve tumor), characteristics of both (mixed GIST), or may appear as undifferentiated spindle cell lesions (GIST not otherwise specified). Malignant GISTs constitute 15 to 20% of the malignant tumors found in the small bowel.[26] GISTs most often classified, until recently, as leiomyomas and leiomyosarcomas, are now known to represent a discrete neoplastic entity. The cellular origin of GIST is proposed to be the interstitial cell of Cajal, an intestinal pacemaker drug.[101] GISTs are characterized by mutations in the protooncogene c-*kit* that lead to constitutive activation of its glycoprotein product KIT and the subsequent tyrosine kinase activity.[102] More than 90% of GISTs express KIT and biochemical evidence of KIT can be found in almost all GISTs.[103] In the majority of these cases, this activation is linked to a somatic mutation KIT, usually involving exon 9 or 11.[102]

Most GISTs present as an abdominal mass causing bowel obstruction evidenced as nausea and vomiting, as pain, or as GI bleeding. GISTs usually grow rapidly, with masses 5 cm in diameter or greater being common.[104] This rapid rate of growth explains the propensity for GI blood loss, because these tumors may outgrow their blood supply, become necrotic, and ulcerate. Blood loss is usually chronic, with laboratory studies revealing a microcytic anemia.[26,34,46,104] Fistulas and abscesses are also caused by tumor necrosis. GISTs usually occur in patients older than age of 50 years, with similar rates of occurrence in both genders.[105] These tumors tend to spread by local extension, growing into the mesentery, surrounding serosal surfaces, or omentum. Vascular metastases are common, but lymphatic spread is unusual. GISTs are usually easy to detect with radiologic examination because of their large size, with CT scanning providing an excellent diagnostic test.

As with other tumors of the small bowel, the primary treatment of GISTs is surgical resection with wide margins. Because lymph node involvement is not common, extensive lymphadenectomy appears to provide no added survival benefit. One study analyzing 200 cases of GISTs over a 16-year period found that in patients with primary disease who underwent complete resection of gross disease, the 5-year actuarial survival rate was 54%.[106] Survival was predicted by tumor size but not microscopic margins of resection. In a study reviewing 50 cases of GISTs specific to the small intestine, Crosby and colleagues identified subgroups with significantly longer overall survival in univariable analysis were those with localized or locally advanced disease (stage I) and those who underwent complete gross resection.[107] Even with complete surgical resection, the majority of tumors will recur, often involving the liver and peritoneal surface. In the largest series of GIST recurrences, the group from Memorial Sloan-Kettering Cancer Center retrospectively analyzed 69 such patients.[106] Local recurrence was seen in 76% of patients, of which half had synchronous liver lesions. Surgical resection for recurrent disease was completed in one-third of cases with median survival of 15 months. Neither complete nor partial resection resulted in significantly improved survival, although the subgroup of patients with isolated, resectable hepatic lesions showed a trend toward longer survival.

With the high recurrence rate after surgery, effective adjuvant therapy is needed. GISTs are resistant to standard chemotherapy and irradiation, with no current role for treatment with these modalities.[108] Because GISTs express a mutated c-*kit* tyrosine kinase, the tyrosine kinase inhibitor imatinib mesylate is currently being evaluated in clinical trials. There are currently two American College of Surgeons Oncology Group trials looking at the role of adjuvant imatinib mesylate after resection for those patients at intermediate or high risk of recurrence. Until the results of these trials are published, the role of imatinib mesylate in the adjuvant setting will remain unclear. In addition, there is an ongoing RTOG trial looking at the role of imatinib mesylate in the neoadjuvant setting. Neoadjuvant imatinib mesylate holds much promise because it can lead to marked shrinkage in tumor size, which can frequently be predicted within 2 to 4 weeks of initiating therapy using PET scans. Whether it will allow surgeons to do smaller operations or will improve survival remains to be determined.

In the metastatic setting, there is much clearer evidence of the effectiveness of imatinib mesylate. In an early report by Joensuu and colleagues, the promise of selectively inhibiting the constitutive activity of mutated KIT in GISTs with imatinib mesylate as an effective therapeutic strategy was realized.[109] In this study, a 50-year-old patient with metastatic GISTs who had undergone resection of multiple recurrent tumors, as well as chemotherapy, continued to have progressive, unresectable disease. After a 2-week trial of imatinib mesylate, magnetic resonance imaging showed a 41% decrease in tumor size; at 14 months there was a greater than 80% decrease. In a European Organization for Research and Treatment of Cancer (EORTC) phase I study, the highest feasible dosage of imatinib was 400 mg twice a day.[110] The dose-limiting side effects at higher doses included severe nausea, vomiting, edema, and rash. A phase II study of 147 patients randomized to receive either 400 mg or 600 mg of imatinib mesylate daily demonstrated a sustained objective response in more than 50% of the patients with advanced unresectable or metastatic GIST with no significant differences in toxic effects or response between the two doses.[111] These favorable results led to rapid development of randomized multicenter phase III trials in the United States and Europe. The EORTC's phase III trial randomized 946 patients to 400 mg of imatinib either once or twice a day and found that if response induction is the only aim of treatment, a daily dose of 400 mg, given for 4 to 6 months, is sufficient. However, in patients with widespread metastatic disease, the prolonged progression-free survival achieved with 400 mg twice a day, would be a more ideal dosage.[112] The US Phase III Sarcoma Group Study S0033 had a similar design and compared the same two daily doses.[113] The major difference in the two studies was the primary endpoint of the S0033 was overall survival whereas the EORTC's was progression-free survival. In the 746-patient S0033 study there was no significant difference in progression-free survival at 2 years between the 400 mg and 800 mg dosages (50% vs 53%).[113]

Lymphoma Lymphoma accounts for 15 to 20% of all malignant small bowel tumors.[114] The stomach is the most common site of GI lymphoma (> 60%), followed by an equal distribution between the large and small intestines.[115] There is a slight male predominance of approximately 1.5:1, and the median age is lower than that of persons with other small bowel tumors (49 years in one large series).[31,34]

Lymphomas are the most frequent malignant neoplasms in transplant recipients.[116] These tumors appear on an average of 20 months after the initiation of cyclosporine. Prognosis is better than for other forms of intestinal lymphomas with two-thirds cured with resection, radiotherapy, acyclovir, and reduction of immunosupression.[117,118]

Small bowel lymphomas also occur in acquired immunodeficiency syndrome (AIDS). Virtually all lesions are B-lymphocyte in origin. Pericecal lymphoma may perforate and simulate acute appendicitis. The prognosis is poor but is dominated by the HIV-related disease such that life expectancy for these patients is not significantly inferior to similar patients without lymphoma.[117]

The clinical presentation of GI lymphoma includes abdominal pain, nausea, vomiting, fatigue, weight loss, and GI bleeding, which may be occult. Perforation may occur in some patients, causing an acute abdomen.[105] Systemic signs of lymphoma, such as lymphadenopathy and fever, may also be present. Radiographic studies, such as a CT scan with oral contrast are of value in making the diagnosis.[105] A mass with bulky adenopathy is highly suggestive of abdominal lymphoma.[119]

Multiple staging systems have been proposed for GI lymphomas, including the Ann Arbor, Musshoff, and newly revised European-American classification system. Each of these major staging systems recognizes four major stages of small bowel lymphoma: stage I for local disease, stage II for regional involvement, and stages III and IV for advanced disease with metastasis. The overall prognosis of the more advanced stages is fair, with a 5-year survival of only 25 to 30 %.[119] In a retrospective analysis of 32 cases of primary small bowel lymphoma treated with either radical surgery (for stages I and II) plus chemotherapy versus chemotherapy alone (for stages III and IV), the overall 5-year survival was 59%, while the relapse-free survival rate among the complete responders was 72%.[120] These results suggest aggressive multimodal therapy may be beneficial.

Resection of small bowel lymphoma is important for local control but rarely eradicates the disease. Disease is often advanced so that fewer than 30% of intestinal tumors are amenable to primary curative resection.[120] Adjuvant therapy is an essential part of the treatment. The surgical resection should always be attempted for localized disease and should involve removal of the bowel segments, with wide margins, and the involved mesenteric lymph nodes, if possible. Margins need to be completely clear of tumor since lymphomas may spread for long distances in the submucosal plane. Adjuvant chemotherapy in patients after potential curative resection is advocated.[121,122] In patients with unresectable lymphoma, radiation therapy and chemotherapy are recommended.[123]

Small bowel lymphoma is particularly common in the Middle East, especially in southern Iran. This Mediterranean lymphoma is found in children and young adults.[124,125] Patients tend to be from lower socioeconomic groups with a background of malnutrition. The tumor progenitor cell is believed to be the perifollicular B cell, which produces IgA. The tumor releases an excess of alpha heavy chains, which are detectable in the serum.[126] Combination chemotherapy is useful in nonresectable disease, although an optimal regimen has not been defined.[127] This lymphoma behaves differently from other small bowel lymphomas and appears to have a worse prognosis.

Metastatic Neoplasms Metastatic neoplastic involvement of the small bowel is more frequent than primary small intestinal neoplasia. Primary tumors of the colon, ovary, uterus, and stomach involve the small bowel, most often by direct invasion or peritoneal spread. Primaries from the breast, lung, and melanoma metastasize to the small intestine hematogenously.[127] Within the GI tract, the small bowel is the most frequent site of metastasis of melanoma, most likely because of its rich blood supply. In one recent series of metastatic melanoma of the intestinal tract, the metastases were the presenting sign that lead to diagnosis of melanoma in 50% of the cases.[128] A retrospective study of 103 cases of malignant melanoma performed by the Armed Forces Institute of Pathology stated that small bowel involvement by melanoma, even in the absence of a known primary, is usually metastatic.[129] Prolonged survival after resection of small bowel melanoma is poor, but aggressive resection in cases without a known primary site may improve quality of life.[130]

TUMORS OF THE APPENDIX

Malignancies of the appendix are rare, making up less than 4% of all intestinal neoplasms.[131] Among 71,000 appendectomy specimens taken over a 40-year period, Collins found 958 malignant tumors, with an overall incidence of 1.35%.[132] In their series of 8,699 appendectomies in a 23-year period at a single institution, Schmutzer and colleagues reported a total of 101 tumors, of which 60 were malignant, for an incidence of 1.2% overall and 0.7% for malignant tumors.[133]

In 1943, Uihlein and McDonald classified appendiceal malignancies into three categories on the basis of morphology: carcinoid tumors, malignant mucoceles, and adenocarcinomas of the colonic type.[134] Although many authors consider the malignant mucocele and adenocarcinoma to be histologically identical and argue that they should be regarded as the same process, others have described significant differences in their clinical features. As a result, despite their microscopic similarity, the natural histories of the two tumors are distinct enough that most consider them different disease processes.[135] In the series by Collins, carcinoids made up 51% of the malignant tumors found, mucoceles accounted for 32%, and 6% were adenocarcinomas.[132] The remainder consisted of a large number of rare tumors, including sarcomas. In addition, Warkel and colleagues described a complex appendiceal tumor distinct clinically and pathologically from carcinoids and adenocarcinomas, but sharing features of both.[136] For this lesion, the term adenocarcinoid is used.

Carcinoids Carcinoids are the most common appendiceal tumor, comprising 32 to 77% of appendiceal neoplasms.[91,137,138] In 1975, Godwin reported a series of 2,837 carcinoid cases identified by the End Results Group (ERG; 1950–1969) and the Third National Cancer Survey (TNCS; 1969–1971) programs of the National Cancer Institute (NCI) between the years 1950 and 1971.[139] This survey reported that the majority of carcinoids were in the appendix (ERG: 43.9%; TNCS: 35.5%). Modlin and Sandor updated this classic study in 1997 by adding to the existing database 5,468 cases collected from 1973 to 1991 through the Surveillance, Epidemiology, and End Results (SEER) program.[91] This study reported a decrease in appendiceal carcinoids from 43.9% (ERG) to 7.6% (SEER) over a 20-year time period. The authors warned that this information should be evaluated cautiously because the ERG file contains both benign and malignant appendiceal carcinoids, whereas the first 14-year period of the SEER program does not. Another explanation offered was the decreased surgical commitment to appendectomy in the past two decades.

The SEER study also revealed a sex predominance for appendiceal carcinoids, with tumors from females comprising 68% of the cases.[91] Similarly, Roggo and colleagues retrospectively analyzed 41 cases of appendiceal carcinomas and reported that 80.5% of the cases occurred in females.[140] This female predominance may reflect the increased number of pelvic procedures performed in women, leading to more incidental findings, including carcinoids of the appendix. Appendiceal carcinoids mostly present at an early age, averaging 32 to 42 years in the literature.[91,140]

Moertel and colleagues, in their evaluation of 150 appendiceal carcinoids over a period of 51 years, noted that 4.7% of the cases metastasized but none of the tumors less than 2 cm exhibited metastatic spread.[141] In general, metastases in appendiceal carcinoids less than 2 cm in diameter are uncommon. Because large carcinoid tumors of the appendix are rare, the overall rate of metastasis in most series is in the range of 1.3 to 4.7%.[142,143] Nonlocalized appendiceal lesions, which in Modlin's ERG registry comprised only 5% of all appendiceal carcinoids, increased significantly to 35.4% in the SEER file. It is unclear whether this increase is due to an elevated awareness of the biology of the lesion and greater sampling of lymph nodes and surrounding tissue, or reflects the inclusion of autopsy data in the SEER group.[91]

The majority of carcinoid tumors of the appendix may be treated with a simple appendectomy.[144] At laparotomy, these tumors appear as small yellow nodules, usually in the distal third of the appendix. Histologically, the cells are small, uniform, and contain a central nucleus with few mitoses. Almost all carcinoids show invasion of the muscular layer of the wall of the appendix and involvement of lymphatic vessels adjacent to the tumor is essentially universal.[144] This being said, few patients have regional or distant dissemination of disease. Malignant carcinoid syndrome is rarely associated with appendiceal carcinoids with only six cases reported, all of which had distant metastases.[91] In view of these observations, the standard recommendation is that tumors < 2 cm require only an appendectomy as adequate treatment, while those > 2 cm require a hemicolectomy. However, because metastases have been found even with primary tumors of 1.5 to 2 cm in diameter, some authors recommend that patients in this group undergo right hemicolectomy. Although hemicolectomy has been advocated for these larger tumors, no prospective studies establish whether aggressive surgery is associated with a better prognosis. Some authors suggest hemicolectomy if mesoappendiceal involvement is found. Given the frequency of invasion of the mesoappendix by carcinoid (16%), mesoappendiceal involvement alone does not warrant right hemicolectomy.[91] In a review of the Danish Cancer Registry, Svendson and Bulow found 10 cases of appendiceal carcinoid tumors involving the mesoappendix. Eight of the 10 cases were associated with primary tumors < 1 cm and were treated with appendectomy without recurrence.[145]

Three series have described experiences with carcinoids of the appendix in the pediatric population. The youngest patient reported was 3 years old. In the most recent of the series, the largest tumor found was 1.2 cm. In 65% of pediatric patients, there was invasion of the muscularis or of the muscularis and serosal layers, which compares with 77 to 90% in other series. In all cases, the tumor was less than 2 cm in diameter, and only appendectomy was performed. There have been no recurrences.[143,145–147] It appears that appendectomy alone is sufficient treatment in children if the initial lesion is less than 2 cm in diameter.

Because most carcinoids are found at the tip of the organ and are small, it has been estimated that only 10% result in acute appendicitis.[148] Distal location was found in 82% of patients in the series reported by Collins[132] and in 71% of patients by Moertel and colleagues.[137] In these series, of appendiceal tumors discovered during appendectomy for appendicitis, only 30% were apparently involved in causing the appendicitis because of obstruction of the appendiceal lumen.[132,137,141]

In Modlin's review of 8,305 carcinoids, the 85.9% 5-year survival for appendiceal carcinoids exceeded that of carcinoids in any other location.[91] This good prognosis is confirmed in reports throughout the literature.[149,150] The reasons for this excellent survival rate may include the anatomic site of the lesion, incidental early discovery, and simple surgical management in the majority of cases.

Mucoceles An appendiceal mucocele is any one of a number of lesions that is characterized by dilation of the appendiceal lumen, alteration of the mucosal lining, hypersecretion of mucus, and occasional extension outside of the appendix.[151] The underlying pathology may be a hyperplastic polyp; a benign neoplasm, such as cystadenoma; or a malignant tumor, such as cystadenocarcinoma. In the original classification system proposed by Uihlein and McDonald, mucoceles make up one of the three major types of appendiceal malignancies. The authors admit the rigid division between malignant mucoceles and adenocarcinoma is not universally accepted.[134] Many authors support the use of a system based on histologic findings, rather than on the presence of a cystic lesion.[151] In this system, mucoceles of the appendix are classified into simple (obstructive) and mucoceles with proliferative epithelial changes.[151] Benign neoplastic proliferative changes may be localized, as in adenoma of colonic type, or diffuse, as in mucinous adenoma or mucinous cystadenoma. Malignant proliferative groups may be classified as colonic-type adenocarcinoma, mucinous cystadenocarcinoma, and mixed carcinoid-adenocarcinoma.[152] The preneoplastic potential of hyperplastic epithelium and the premalignant nature of adenomatous epithelium are seen by the coexistence of hyperplastic, adenomatous, and carcinomatous epithelium all in the same lesion.[152] A consequence of mucoceles of the appendix (cystadenomas and cystadenocarcinomas) is pseudomyxoma peritonei. This lesion, characterized by large quantities of mucus-like material in the peritoneal cavity, is considered to represent dissemination of mucinous cystadenocarcinoma within the peritoneal cavity (see the section "Pseudomyxoma Peritonei" below).[153]

Though the diagnosis of appendiceal mucocele is usually an incidental finding at celiotomy, mucinous cystadenomas and cystadenocarcinomas are among the few appendiceal tumors that may be diagnosed preoperatively.[144] Computed tomography strongly suggests a mucinous tumor if a mass is present in the right lower quadrant with near water density. Ultrasound shows a diagnostic variable sonographic echogenicity because of the combination of mucin with more anechoic fluid. Although both imaging techniques may be helpful in diagnosing a mucocele, other cystic lesions of the peritoneal cavity, such as ovarian cysts, duplication cysts, mesenteric and omental cysts, or an abscess, may have a similar appearance.[154]

Treatment is surgical resection, with the extent of resection dependent on the underlying histology. In the case of hyperplastic polyps or cystadenoma, a simple appendectomy is considered curative. In the series reported by Higa and colleagues, 36 of the 46 patients with mucinous cystadenomas were treated with appendectomy alone with no recurrence.[151] In patients with mucinous cystadenocarcinoma, a substantial number will present with extensive abdominal metastases or pseudomyxoma peritonei. Treatment of the primary lesion includes a formal right hemicolectomy with removal of draining lymph nodes.[155] Stephenson and Brief reviewed 53 appendiceal mucinous cystadenocarcinomas treated by either simple appendectomy or right hemicolectomy. At 10 years, survival was 65% among patients treated with hemicolectomy, in contrast to a 37% rate among patients who had received an appendectomy alone.[156] Surgical debulking of metastatic deposits and evacuation of mucus collections are also recommended.

Adenocarcinoma Primary adenocarcinoma of the appendix is a rare neoplasm, with fewer than 300 total cases described worldwide.[157] Most adenocarcinomas arise from pre-existing adenomas.

The primary adenocarcinoma is a colorectal-type tumor that develops from an adenoma.[151] The mean age of presentation is 50 years and a male predominance is noted of anywhere from 4:1 to 2.8:1.[157–159] The clinical presentation in the majority of patients in the literature is acute appendicitis or an abdominal mass, though the diagnosis is rarely made preoperatively. Perforation may complicate the clinical picture, occurring in up to 40% of cases, but perforation alone has little effect on overall survival.[160]

Histologically, primary adenocarcinoma is distinguished from an adenoma by invasion of the wall of the appendix by the neoplastic tissue. Lymph node metastases are noted in 25% of cases at presentation.[161] Adenocarcinoma of the appendix has a metastatic potential between that of appendiceal carcinoid and colonic adenocarcinoma, with metastases developing in 20% of patients, often to the ovary.[162] The degree of metastatic involvement varies with the histologic grade; about 30% of the well-differentiated tumors are found to have metastasized, whereas nearly 70% of the poorly differentiated tumors are metastatic at the time of laparotomy.[157,158] The overall 5-year survival rate is 55% and varies with Dukes' stage (A 100%, B 67%, C 50%, D 6%).[163]

The extent of tumor invasion is the most important factor when determining treatment of appendiceal adenocarcinoma. Because these tumors behave in a fashion similar to that of colonic adenocarcinomas, they must also be treated with the same aggressive surgical approach. For any lesion with invasion beyond the mucosa, right hemicolectomy with resection of draining lymph nodes is advocated.[164] In the presence of such invasion, the 5-year survival after right hemicolectomy is 60% compared with 20% after appendectomy alone.[163] For lesions truly confined to the mucosa, though there are strong advocates for both hemicolectomy and appendectomy, the consensus is that such a lesion may be treated by appendectomy alone. Any suggestion that the tumor has extended beyond the mucosa is indication for a right hemicolectomy.[165] In one series, a second primary tumor at a distant site (colon, cervix, breast, prostate, esophagus, stomach, ovary, or bladder) was found in 11% of patients;[158] and in the series reported by Chang and Attiyeh, 32% had second tumors. This suggests some genetic role, mutation or loss of a tumor-suppressor gene, or a defect in immunosurveillance.[157]

A rare lesion of the appendix, intermediate between adenocarcinoma and carcinoid, is the adenocarcinoid. This lesion arises from the base of glands and spares the luminal mucosa; it is composed of slender tuboglandular structures, nests of goblet cells, or a mixture of both.[166] The tumor represents, at most, only 5% of all appendiceal neoplasms.[167] Despite their small size when found at celiotomy, adenocarcinoids behave quite energetically, with a propensity to metastasize to the ovaries. They should be treated aggressively with right hemicolectomy, which is considered curative if the margins are clear and there are no involved lymph nodes.

NEOPLASMS OF THE PERITONEUM

Peritoneal surface malignancy may occur as a primary disease, such as peritoneal mesothelioma and primary peritoneal carcinoma, or as a metastatic tumor originating most often from carcinomas of the ovary, stomach, pancreas, and colon. Distant metastases from malignant melanoma, as well as breast and lung cancer, are also common.[168] The pathways of spread of neoplastic disease in the peritoneum include direct invasion, lymphatic paths, intraperitoneal seeding, and hematogenous spread.[169] Peritoneal carcinomatosis may originate from the transparietal diffusion of malignant noninfiltrating tumors.[170] Such tumors involve the peritoneum not because of their aggressive behavior but as a redistribution secondary to gravity, intestinal peristalsis, and peritoneal reabsorption.

Sugarbaker proposed an aggressive treatment approach to peritoneal surface malignancy that uses peritonectomy procedures, perioperative intraperitoneal chemotherapy, and knowledgeable patient selection.[171] Peritonectomy is necessary for complete cytoreduction and is used in areas of visible cancer nodules in an attempt to leave the patient with only microscopic residual disease. Intraperitoneal chemotherapy gives high response rates with microscopic residual disease because the "peritoneal-plasma barrier" provides dose-intensive therapy.[172] A pharmacokinetic advantage to intraperitoneal chemotherapy exists as a result of the barrier effect of the peritoneal lining.[173] Continuous hyperthermic peritoneal perfusion (CHPP) is one such regional strategy designed to deliver high concentrations of cytotoxic agents and hyperthermia directly to the peritoneal tumor while limiting systemic exposure and toxicity.[174] The procedure, performed after the cancer resection is complete, involves heated intraoperative chemotherapy that is siphoned by a roller pump into the abdomen through a Tenckhoff catheter and pulled out through drains. Using the same tubes and drains used for the intraoperative chemotherapy, usually 5 consecutive days of postoperative chemotherapy instillation is recommended.[172]

Mesotheliomas The mesothelium is a simple squamoid epithelium that lines the peritoneal cavity and forms the serosa of organs located within this cavity. Malignant peritoneal mesothelioma is a rare malignancy characterized by primary neoplastic change involving the lining surfaces of the peritoneal cavity. Malignant mesothelioma shows extreme male predominance (93% in one series), and frequently a history of asbestos exposure (83% in this series).[175] The median age at the time of diagnosis is 54 years.[176] The microscopic findings include extensive cell vacuolization, rare psammoma bodies, the presence of hyaluronic acid, and a lack of mucin.[177] Grossly malignant mesotheliomas appear as hard, whitish nodules scattered over the peritoneal surfaces. The nodules coalesce to form plaques, which extend into surrounding tissues. Widespread peritoneal dissemination is common at presentation and the prognosis is poor, with a median survival of 12 to 17 months.[178–181] The disease is usually confined to the peritoneal cavity and the cause of death is related to progression in the peritoneal cavity in the form of encasement and invasion of bowel and intractable ascites. The clinical presentation is usually nonspecific, with the most frequent initial symptom being abdominal pain. Ascites is the most common physical sign, occurring in 90% of patients.[176]

Treatment of malignant peritoneal mesothelioma consists primarily of surgical palliation, including bypassing obstructing lesions or tumor debulking. A study by Park and colleagues examined 18 patients with malignant peritoneal mesothelioma who underwent surgical debulking and CHPP with cisplatin.[182] Overall operative morbidity was 24% with no operative mortality. The median progression-free survival was 26 months and the overall 2-year survival was 80%.

Cystic mesothelioma is a rare benign variant of peritoneal mesothelioma and consists primarily of cysts attached to the peritoneum. No history of asbestos exposure is usually found and the tumor primarily affects young women with a median age of 36 years. Although the disease tends to recur even with aggressive surgical removal, there have been no deaths attributable to this process in the 21 recorded cases.[47] Another benign variant of peritoneal mesothelioma, benign papillary mesothelioma, consists of papillae lined by a single layer of hyperplastic mesothelium. This lesion is thought to require only follow-up care after excisional biopsy, as no malignant potential has been reported.[183,184]

Primary Peritoneal Carcinoma Extraovarian primary peritoneal carcinoma (EOPPC) is a malignancy that spreads widely inside the peritoneal cavity involving mostly the omentum with minimal or no ovarian involvement.[185] Most reported cases of EOPPC are of serous histology (serous surface carcinoma).[186] However, mucinous, endometroid, clear cell, Brenner, and malignant mixed müllerian types are also described in the literature.[187–191] Histopathologic, immunohistochemical, and clinical similarities have been observed between EOPPC and epithelial ovarian cancer (EOC), specifically the serous variety.[192] Epidemiologic differences between EOPPC and EOC include women with EOPPC being significantly older (63.8 vs 55 years of age), having later menarche, and being less likely to use perineal talc powder.[193] A retrospective study of 75 women diagnosed with EOPPC showed the mean overall survival of all patients was 23.5 months with a 5-year survival of 26.5%.[185] Overall survival in patients was affected significantly by primary debulking surgery.

Pseudomyxoma Peritonei Pseudomyxoma peritonei is caused by the rupture of a cystadenocarcinoma of the appendix or colon with seeding of these mucin-producing cells across the peritoneal surface.[10] Even in female patients with synchronous appendiceal and ovarian mucinous tumors, it appears that the appendiceal tumor is often the primary source of the malignancy.[194] Patients with pseudomyxoma peritonei benefit from debulking procedures, and recent work shows the benefits of intraperitoneal chemotherapy.[195] Appendiceal malignancies have unique features that facilitate successful treatment: peritoneal dissemination from appendiceal tumors usually occurs in the absence of lymph node and liver metastasis, and appendix cancer is usually of low biologic aggressiveness with mucinous adenocarcinomas being minimally invasive and layering on the peritoneal surfaces rather than penetrating into the tissues. This characteristic allows complete resection in many cases. In addition, the majority of these tumors are mucinous, a texture that allows greater penetration by intraperitoneal chemotherapy.[171] Sugarbaker and Chang evaluated the results of combined debulking and intra- and postoperative regional chemotherapy in 385 patients with peritoneal surface spread of appendiceal malignancy.[196] Patients with a complete cytoreduction and adenomucinosis by pathology had a 5-year survival of 86%; with hybrid pathology, survival at 5 years was 50%. Incomplete cytoreduction had a survival of 20% at 5 years and 0% at 10 years.

Angiosarcoma Angiosarcoma is a rare tumor of the peritoneum that may histologically resemble benign lesions or other malignancies, such as mesothelioma. The histologic diagnosis is often aided by immunohistochemical methods to demonstrate markers of vascular differentiation. Peritoneal angiosarcoma usually acts aggressively. It may arise following previous radiation treatment to the serous membranes and treatment should be like that of other sarcomas.[197–199]

Malignant Ascites Malignant ascites is a manifestation of advanced malignant disease with patients frequently experiencing a large volume of peritoneal fluid as a cancerous process moves toward its terminal phase. Tumor obstruction of the subdiaphragmatic lymphatics is one pathogenetic mechanism.[200] Malignant ascites can also result from nonobstructive factors including immunomodulators such as interleukin-2, tumor necrosis factor (TNF), and interferon-α, as well as aberrant expression of genes for permeability-inducing factors such as vascular endothelial growth factor.[200] Standard medical treatment options include diuretics and therapeutic paracentesis. Novel pharmacologic treatments being studied include intraperitoneal immunotherapy with interferons and TNF-α. In a study of 29 patients with refractory malignant ascites, 22 responded to intraperitoneal TNF-α administration. Of these 22, 16 had complete and 6 had partial resolution of their ascites.[201] Decreasing permeability of vessels by inhibiting the tyrosine kinase activity of vascular endothelial growth factor receptors inhibits the formation of malignant ascites in animal models.[202] Encouraging results have also been reported with the intraperitoneal installation of the metalloproteinase inhibitor batimastat.[76,203] Metalloproteinases are a family of enzymes overexpressed in colorectal, gastric, and breast cancers that degrade the extracellular matrix and appear to be important in tumor invasion and metastases. Enzyme inhibitors, such as batimastat, can reduce tumor growth, metastatic spread, and malignant ascites formation.[204]

In regards to surgical management, debulking procedures plus intraperitoneal chemotherapy have been successful in eliminating the ascites. The mechanism of action of intraperitoneal chemotherapy on large volume malignant ascites is destruction of surface cancer, which produces a fibrotic layer of tissue that prevents formation of both normal peritoneal fluid and malignant fluids.[171] Usually three to four instillations of intraperitoneal chemotherapy are required after the initial debulking for symptomatic relief. In a preliminary clinical trial combining cytoreductive surgery and CHPP with mitomycin C, 75% (9 of 12) of patients had their malignant ascites controlled with a median follow-up of 7.5 months.[205] It is important to inform patients that CHPP use as a treatment of malignant ascites is for symptomatic relief and should not be considered curative. Surgical management of malignant ascites also includes creation of peritoneovenous shunts (PVS) such as the LeVeen and Denver shunts. Teuche and Pector report the Bordet Institute experience of 24 PVS placed over a 23-year period for malignant ascites.[206] Most patients benefited from the procedure, however, shunt occlusion is a serious problem occurring in 20% of patients. Disseminated intravascular coagulation can be another serious problem that can necessitate ligation of the shunt. Most groups have concluded that shunts should be placed in patients with terminal cancer and recalcitrant ascites selectively to enable a more comfortable quality of life.

REFERENCES

1. Rochlin D, Lingmire W. Primary tumors of the small intestine. Surgery 1961;50:586.
2. Jemal A, Murray T, Bolden S, Thun M. Cancer statistics, 2004. CA Cancer J Clin 2004;54:8–29.
3. Mittal VK, Bodzin JH. Primary malignant tumors of the small bowel. Am J Surg 1980;140:396–9.
4. Williamson RC, Welch CE, Malt RA. Adenocarcinoma and lymphoma of the small intestine. Distribution and etiologic associations. Ann Surg 1983;197:172–8.
5. Gill S, DM DH, Mihas A. Small intestine neoplasms. J Clin Gastroenterol 2001;33(4):267–82.
6. Lee Y. Leiomyosarcoma of the gastrointestinal tract. General pattern of metastasis and recurrence. Cancer Treat Rev 1983;10:91–101.
7. Nadir A, Neugut A, Weinstein B, Holt P. Molecular genetics of small bowel cancer. 1997;6:745–8.
8. Offerhaus G, Gardiello F, Krush A. The risk of upper gastrointestinal cancer in familial adenomatous polyposis. Gastroenterology 1993;102:1982–3.
9. Munkholm P, Langholz E, Davidsen M, Binder V. Intestinal cancer risk and mortality in patients with Crohn's disease. Gastroenterology 1993;105:1716–23.
10. Parsons J, Gray GF, Thorbjarnarson B. Pseudomyxoma peritonei. Arch Surg 1970;101:545–9.
11. O'Riordan B, Vilor M, Herrera L. Small bowel tumors. An overview. Dig Dis Sci 1996;14:245–57.
12. Bender G, Maglinte D, Kloppel V. CT enteroclysis. A superfluous diagnostic procedure or valuable when investigating small bowel disease? AJR 1999;172:373–8.
13. Dudiak KM, Johnson CD, Stephens DH. Primary tumors of the small intestine. CT evaluation. AJR 1989;152:995–8.
14. Buckley J, Jones B, Fishman E. Small bowel cancer. Imaging features and staging. Radiol Clin North Am 1997;35:381–402.
15. Naef M, Buhlmann M, Baer H. Small bowel tumors. Diagnosis, therapy, and prognostic factors. Langenbecks Arch Surg 1999;384:176–80.
16. Halvorsen R, Thompson W. Primary neoplasms of the hollow organs of the gastrointestinal tract. Cancer Treat Rev 1991;61:316–23.
17. Perng DS, Jan CM, Wang WM, et al. Computed tomography, endoscopic ultrasonography and intraoperative assessment in TN staging of gastric carcinoma. J Formos Med Assoc 1996;95:378–85.
18. Shoup M, Hodul P, Aranha GV, et al. Defining a role for endoscopic ultrasound in staging periampullary tumors. Am J Surg 2000;179:453–6.
19. Cannon ME, Carpenter SL, Elta GH, et al. EUS compared with CT, MRI, and angiography and the influence of biliary stenting on staging accuracy of ampullary neoplasms. Gastrointest Endosc 1999;50:27–33.
20. Landi B, Tkoub M, Gaudric M, et al. Diagnostic yield of push-type enteroscopy in relation to indication. Gut 1998;42:421–5.
21. Ingrosso M, Prete F, Pisani A, et al. Laparoscopically assisted total enteroscopy: a new approach to small intestinal diseases. Gastrointest Endosc 1999;49:651–3.
22. Yamamoto H, Kita H, Sunada K, et al. Clinical outcomes of double-balloon endoscopy for the diagnosis and treatment of small intestinal diseases. Clin Gastroenterol H 2004;2:1010–6.
23. Gong F, Swain P, Mill T. Wireless endoscopy. Gastrointest Endosc 2000;51:725–9.
24. Mylonaki M, Fritscher-Ravens A, Swain P. Wireless capsule endoscopy: a comparison with push enteroscopy in patients with colonoscopy and gastroscopy negative gastrointestinal bleeding. Gut 2003;52:1122–6.
25. DiSario J, Burt R, Vargas H, McWhorter W. Small bowel cancer. Epidemiological and clinical characteristics from a population-based registry. Am J Gastroenterol 1994;89:699–701.
26. Skandalakis JE, Gray SW, Shepard D, et al. Smooth muscle tumors of the alimentary tract. A review of 2525 cases. Springfield (IL): Charles C Thomas; 1962. p. 1–468.
27. Blanchard D, Budde J, Hatch GF, et al. Tumors of the small intestine. World J Surg 2000;24:421–9.
28. Starr G, Dockerty M. Leiomyomas and leiomyosarcomas of the small intestine. Cancer Treat Rev 1955;8:101–11.
29. Morgan BK, Compton C, Talbert M, et al. Benign smooth muscle tumors of the gastrointestinal tract. Ann Surg 1990;211:63–6.
30. River L, Silverstein J, Tope JW. Collective review. Benign neoplasms of the small intestine. A critical comprehensive review with reports of 20 new cases. Surg Gynecol Obstet 1956;102:1–38.
31. Wilson JM, Melvin DB, Gray G, Thorbjarnarson B. Benign small bowel tumor. Ann Surg 1975;181:247–50.
32. Perzin KH, Bridge MF. Adenomas of the small intestine: a clinicopathological review of 51 cases and a study of their relationship to carcinoma. Cancer 1981;48:799–819.
33. Ashley SW, Wells SA Jr. Tumors of the small intestine. Semin Oncol 1988; 15:118–28.
34. Darling R, Welch C. Tumors of the small intestine. N Engl J Med 1959;260:397–408.
35. Sellner F. Investigations of the significance of the adenoma-carcinoma sequence in the small bowel. Cancer Treat Rev 1990;66:702–15.
36. Whitteman B, Janssen A, Griffieon G, et al. Villous tumors of the duodenum. An analysis of the literature with emphasis on malignant transformation. Neth J Med 1993;42:5–11.
37. Church J, McGannon E, Hull-Boiner S, et al. Gastroduodenal polyps in patients with familial adenomatous polyposis. Dis Colon Rectum 1992;35:1170–3.
38. Saurin J-C, Gutknecht C, Napoleon B, et al. Surveillance of duodenal adenomas in familial adenomatous polyposis reveals high cumulative risk of advanced disease. J Clin Oncol 2004;22:493–8.
39. Spigelman AD, Williams CB, Talbot IC, et al. Upper gastrointestinal cancer in patients in patients with familial adenomatous polyposis. Lancet 1989;2:783–5.
40. Hirasawa R, Iisgi H, Tatsuta M, et al. Clinicopathologic features and endoscopic resection of duodenal adenocarcinomas and adenomas with the submucosal saline technique. Gastroint Ensosc 1997;46:507–13.
41. Penna C, Bataille N, Balladur P, et al. Surgical treatment of severe duodenal polyposis in familial adenomatous polyposis. Br J Surg 1998;85:665–8.
42. Vasen H, Bulow S, Myrhoj T, et al. Decision analysis in the management of dueodenal adenomatous polyposis. Gut 1997;40:716–9.
43. Groves C, Saunders B, Spigelman AD, et al. Duodenal can-

cer in patients with familial adenomatous polyposis (FAP): results of a 10 year prospective study. Gut 2002;50:636–41.
44. Smith FR, Mayo CW. Submucous lipomas of the small intestine. Am J Surg 1950;80:922–8.
45. Boyle L, Lack EE. Solitary cavernous hemangioma of the small intestine. Arch Pathol Lab Med 1993;117:939–41.
46. Good C. Tumors of the small intestine. Am J Roentgenol 1963;89:685.
47. Miles JM, Hart WR, McMahon JT. Cystic mesothelioma of the peritoneum. Cleve Clin Q 1986;53:109–14.
48. Gentry RW, Dockerty MS, Claggett OT. Vascular malformations and vascular tumors of the gastrointestinal tract. Int Abstr Surg 1949;88:281.
49. Barquist ES, Apple SK, Jensen DM, Ashley SW. Jejunal lymphangioma. An unusual cause of chronic gastrointestinal bleeding. Dig Dis Sci 1997;42:1179–83.
50. Hanagiri T, Baba M, Shimabukuro T, et al. Lymphangioma in the small intestine: report of a case and review of the Japanese literature. Surg Today 1992;22:363–7.
51. Brucher B, Roder J, Fink U, et al. Prognostic factors in resected primary small bowel tumors. Dig Surg 1998;15:42–51.
52. Oija A, Zacherl J, Scheuba C, et al. Primary small bowel malignancies: single center results of three decades. J Clin Gastroenterol 2000;95:2147–8.
53. Neugut A, Marvin M, Rella VA, et al. An overview of adenocarcinoma of the small intestine. Oncology 1997;11:529–36.
54. Chow J, Chen C, Ahsan N, et al. A population-based study of the incidence of malignant small bowel tumors: SEER, 1973–1990. Int J Epidemiol 1996;25:722–8.
55. Dabaja B, Suki D, Pro B. Adenocarcinoma of the small bowel. Cancer 2004;101:518–26.
56. Wattenberg LW. Studies of polycyclic hydrocarbon hydroxylase of the intestine possibly related to cancer. Cancer Treat Rev 1979;28:99–102.
57. Kuttz R, Sternberg S, Miller HH, et al. Upper gastrointestinal neoplasia in familial polyposis. Dig Dis Sci 1987;32:459–65.
58. Kaerlev L, Teglbjaers P, Sabroe S, et al. Is there an association between alcohol intake or smoking and small bowel adenocarcinoma? Results form a European multicenter case-control study. Cancer Causes Control 2000;11:791–7.
59. Petreshock EP, Pessah M, Menachemi E. Adenocarcinoma of the jejunum associated with nontropical sprue. Am J Dig 1975;20:796–802.
60. Straker RJ, Gunasekaran S, Brady PG. Adenocarcinoma of the jejunum in association with celiac sprue. J Clin Gastroenterol 1989;11:320–3.
61. Swinson C, Slavin G, Coles EC, et al. Celiac disease and malignancy. Lancet 1983;1:111–5.
62. Meretyk S, Landau E, Okon E, et al. Adenocarcinoma in an ileal conduit. A late recurrence of urethral adenocarcinoma. J Urol 1987;138:859–60.
63. Bernstein D, Rogers A. Malignancy in Crohn's disease. Am J Gastroenterol 1996;91:434–40.
64. Chen C, Neugut A, Rotterdam H. Risk factors for adenocarcinomas and malignant carcinoids of the small intestine. Pulmonary findings. Cancer Epidemiol Biomarkers Prev 1994;3:205–7.
65. Frank JD, Shorey BA. Adenocarcinoma of the small bowel as a complication of Crohn's disease. Gut 1973;14:120–4.
66. Goldman LI, Bralow SP, Cox W, Peale AR. Adenocarcinoma of the small bowel complicating Crohn's disease. Cancer Causes Control 1970;26:1119–25.
67. Savoca P, Ballantyne G, Cahow C. Gastrointestinal malignancies in Crohn's disease. A 20-year experience. Dis Colon Rectum 1990;33:7–11.
68. Ribiero M, Greenstein A, Heinmann TM, et al. Adenocarcinoma of the small intestine in Crohn's disease. Surg Gynecol Obstet 1991;173:343–9.
69. Moertel C. Small intestine. In: Holland JF, Frei E, editors. Cancer medicine. 2nd ed. Philadelphia: Lea & Febiger; 1982. p. 1808–18.
70. Howe J, Karnell L, Menck HR et al. The American College of Surgeons Commission on Cancer and the American Cancer Society. Adenocarcinoma of the small bowel. Review of the National Cancer Data Base, 1985–1995. Cancer 1999; 86:2693–706.
71. Abe M, Takahashi M, Yabumoto E, et al. Clinical experiences with intraoperative radiotherapy of locally advanced cancers. Cancer 1980;45:40–8.
72. Sindelar WF, Kinsella TJ. Intraoperative radiation therapy for locally advanced cancers. South Med J 1989;82:358–63.
73. Sindelar WF, Hoekstra HJ, Kinsella TJ. Surgical approaches and techniques in intraoperative radiotherapy for intra-abdominal, retroperitoneal, and pelvic neoplasms. Surgery 1988;103:247–56.
74. Blaker H, von Herbay A, Penzel R, et al. Genetics of adenocarcinomas of the small intestine: frequent deletions at chromosome 18q and mutations of the SMAD4 gene. Oncogene 2002;21:158–64.
75. Svrcek M, Jourdan F, Sebbagh N, et al. Immunohistochemical analysis of adenocarcinoma of the small intestine: a tissue microarray study. J Clin Pathol 2003;56:898–903.
76. Lubarsch O. Veber den primaren Krebs des Ileum, nebst bemerkungen uber das gleichzeitige Vorkommen von Krebs und Tuberkulose. Virchows Arch 1888;111:280.
77. Obendorfer S. Uber die Kleinen dunndarm-carcinome. Verh Dtsch Ges Pathol 1907;11:113.
78. Masson P. Carcinoids (argentaffin-cell tumors) and nerve hyperplasia of appendicular mucosa. Am J Pathol 1928;4:181.
79. Maggard M, O'Connell J, Ko C. Updated population-based review of carcinoid tumors. Ann Surgery 2004;240:117–22.
80. Moertel CG. An odyssey in the land of small tumors. J Clin Oncol 1987;5:1502–22.
81. Moertel CG, Sauer WB, Dockerty MB, Baggenstoss AH. Life history of the carcinoid tumor of the small intestine. Cancer 1961;14:901–12.
82. Burke A, Thomas R, Elsayed A, Sobin L. Carcinoids of the jejunum and ileum: an immunohistochemical and clinicopathological study of 167 cases. Cancer 1997;79:1086–93.
83. Williams ED, Sandler M. The classification of carcinoid tumors. Lancet 1963;1:238–9.
84. Thompson GB, van Heerden JA, Martin JK, et al. Carcinoid tumors of the gastrointestinal tract. Presentation, management, and prognosis. Surgery 1998;98:1054–63.
85. Stinner B, Kisker O, Kielke A, Rothmund M. Surgical management for carcinoid tumors of small bowel, appendix, colon, and rectum. World J Surg 1996;20:183–8.
86. Makridis C, Öberg K, Juhlin C, et al. Surgical treatment of midgut carcinoid tumors. World J Surg 1990;14:377–83.
87. Creutzfeldt W, Stockmann F. Carcinoids and carcinoid syndrome. Am J Med 1987;82 Suppl 5B:4–16.
88. Feldman J, O'Dorisio T. Role of neuropeptides and serotonin in the diagnosis of carcinoid tumors. Am J Med 1986;81 Suppl 6B:41–8.
89. Lamberts S, Bakker W, Reubi J, Krenning E. Somatostatin-receptor imaging in the localization of endocrine tumors. N Engl J Med 1990;323:1246–9.
90. Krenning E, Kwekkeboom D, Oei HY, et al. Somatostatin-receptor scintigraphy in gastroenteropancreatic tumors. An overview of European results. Ann N Y Acad Sci 1994;733:416–24.
91. Modlin I, Sandor A. An analysis of 8305 cases of carcinoid tumors. Cancer 1997;79:813–29.
92. Brookes VS, Waterhouse JA, Powell DJ. Malignant lesions of the small intestine. Br J Surg 1968;55:405–10.
93. Chandler JJ, Foster JH. Malignant carcinoid syndrome treated by resection of hepatic metastases. Am J Surg 1965;109:221–2.
94. Ahlman H, Schersten T, Tisell LE. Surgical treatment of patients with the carcinoid syndrome. Acta Oncol 1989;28:403–7.
95. Gupta S, Yao JC, Arhar K, et al. Hepatic artery embolization for treatment of patients with metastatic carcinoid tumors: the M.D. Anderson experience. Cancer Journal 2003;9:261–7.
96. Patel Y, Srikant C. Subtype selectivity of peptide analogs for all five cloned human somatostatin receptors. Endocrinology 1994;135:2814–7.
97. Kvols LK, Moertel CG, O'Connell MJ, et al. Treatment of the malignant carcinoid syndrome: evaluation of a long-acting somatostatin analogue. N Engl J Med 1986;315:663–6.
98. Zeitels J, Naunheim K Kaplan EL, Straus F 2nd. Carcinoid tumors. A 37-year experience. Arch Surg 1982;117:732–7.
99. Onaitis M, Kirshbom P, Hayward TZ, et al. Gastrointestinal carcinoids. A characterization by site of origin and hormone production. Ann Surg 2000;232:542–56.
100. Levendoglu H, Cox CA, Nadimpalli V. Composite (adenocarcinoid) tumors of the gastrointestinal tract. Dig Dis Sci 1990;35:519–25.
101. Kindblom L, Remotti H, Aldenborg F, Meis-Kindblom J. Gastrointestinal pacemaker cell tumor (GIPACT). Gastrointestinal stromal tumors show phenotypic characteristics of the interstitial cells of Cajal. Am J Pathol 1998;152:1259–69.
102. Rubin B, Singer S, Tsao C, et al. KIT activation is a ubiquitous feature of gastrointestinal stromal tumors. Cancer Res 2001;61:8118–21.
103. Druker BJ. Imatinib and cancer therapy. Adv Cancer Res 2004;91:1–30.
104. Pagtalunan RJ, Mayo CW, Dockerty MB. Primary malignant tumors of the small intestine. Am J Surg 1964;108:13–8.
105. Herbsman H, Wetstein L, Rosen Y, et al. Tumors of the small intestine. Curr Probl Surg 1980;17:121–8.
106. DeMatteo RP, Lewis JJ, Leung D, et al. Two hundred gastrointestinal stromal tumors. Recurrence patterns and prognostic factors for survival. Ann Surg 2000;231:51–8.
107. Crosby J, Catton C, Davis A, et al. Malignant GISTs of the small intestine: a review of 50 cases from prospective data. Ann Surg Oncol 2001;8:50–9.
108. Blanke C, Eisenberg B, Heinrich MC, et al. Gastrointestinal stromal tumors. Current treatment options in oncology 2001;2:485–91.
109. Joensuu H, Roberts PJ, Sarloma-Rikala M, et al. Effect of the tyrosine kinase inhibitor STI571 in a patient with a metastatic gastrointestinal stromal tumor. N Engl J Med 2001;344:1052–6.
110. van Oosterom A, Judson I, Verweij J, et al. Safety and efficacy of imatinib (ST1571) in metastatic gastrointestinal stromal tumors: a phase I study. Lancet 2001;358:1421–3.
111. Demetri GD, von Mehren M, Blanke CD, et al. Efficacy and safety of imatinib mesylate in advanced gastrointestinal stromal tumors. N Engl J Med 2002;347:472–80.
112. Verweij J, Casali P, Zalcberg J, et al. Progression-free survival in gastrointestinal stromal tumors with high-dose imatinib: randomised trial. Lancet 2004;364:1127–34.
113. Rankin C, von Mehren M, Blanke C, et al. Dose effect of imatinib in patients with metastatic GIST: phase III sarcoma group study S0033. Proc ASCO 2004;23:815.
114. Crump M, Gospodarowicz M, Shepard F. Lymphoma of the gastrointestinal tract. Semin Oncol 1999;26:324–7.
115. Weingrad D, DeCosse J, Sherlock P, et al. Primary gastrointestinal lymphoma: a thirty year review. Cancer 1982;49:1258–65.
116. Nalesnik M, Jaffe R, Starzl TE, et al. The pathology of post-transplant lymphoproliferative disorders occurring in the setting of cyclosporin A-prednisone immunosuppression. Am J Pathol 1988;133:173–92.
117. Turowski G, Basson M. Primary malignant lymphoma of the intestine. Am J Surg 1995;169:433–41.
118. Penn I. Cancers following cyclosporine therapy. Transplantation 1987;43:32–5.
119. Jacobs EM. Combination chemotherapy of metastatic testicular germinal cell tumors and soft part sarcomas. Cancer 1970;25:324–32.
120. Zinzani P, Magagnoli M, Pagliani G, et al. Primary intestinal lymphoma: clinical and therapeutic features of 32 patients. Haematologica 1997;82:305–8.
121. Dragosics B, Bauer P, Radaszkiewicz T. Primary gastrointestinal non-Hodgkin's lymphomas. A retrospective clinicopathological study of 150 cases. Cancer 1985;55:1060–73.
122. McGovern V. Lymphomas of the gastrointestinal tract. Baltimore: Williams & Wilkins, 1977.
123. Fu K, Stewart JR. Radiotherapeutic management of small intestinal lymphoma with malabsorption. Cancer 1973;31:286–90.
124. Al-Saleem T, Al-Bahrani Z. Malignant lymphoma of the small intestine in Iraq. Cancer 1973;31:291–4.
125. Barekat AA, Saidi F, Dutz W. Cancer survey in south Iran with special reference to gastrointestinal neoplasms. Int J Cancer 1971;7:353–63.
126. Cammoun M, Jaafoura H, Tabbane F, Halphen M. Immunoproliferative small intestinal disease without alpha-chain disease. A pathological study. Gastroenterology 1989;96:750–63.
127. el Saghir NE, Jessen K, Mass RE, et al. Combination chemotherapy for primary small intestinal lymphoma in the Middle East. Eur J Cancer Clin Oncol 1989;25:851–6.
128. Berger A, Cellier C, Daniel C, et al. Small bowel metastasis from primary carcinoma of the lung. Clinical findings and outcome. Am J Gastroenterol 1999;94:1884–7.
129. Blecker D, Abraham S, Furth EE, et al. Melanoma in the gastrointestinal tract. Gastrointestinol 1999;94:3427–33.
130. Elsayled A, Albahra M, Nzeako UC, et al. Malignant melanomas of the small intestine: a study of 103 patients. Am J Gastroenterol 1996;91:1001–6.
131. Hesketh K. The management of primary adenocarcinoma of the vermiform appendix. Gut 1963;4:158–68.
132. Collins DC. 71,000 human appendix specimens. A final report summarizing forty years' study. Am J Proctol 1963;14:265–81.

133. Schmutzer KJ, Bayar M, Zaki AE, et al. Tumors of the appendix. Dis Colon Rectum 1975;18:324–31.
134. Uihlein A, McDonald J. Primary carcinoma of the appendix resembling carcinoma of the colon. Surg Gynecol Obstet 1943;76:711–4.
135. McGregor JK, McGregor DD. Adenocarcinoma of the appendix. Surgery 1960;48:925.
136. Warkel R, Cooper P, Helwig E. Adenocarcinoid, a mucin-producing carcinoid tumor of the appendix. A study of 39 cases. Cancer 1978;42:2781–93.
137. Moertel CG, Dockerty MB, Judd E, et al. Carcinoid tumors of the vermiform appendix. Cancer 1968;21:270–8.
138. Dunn JP. Carcinoid tumors of the appendix. 21 cases with a review of the literature. N Z Med J 1982;95:73–6.
139. Godwin J. Carcinoid tumors. An analysis of 2,837 cases. Cancer 1975;36:560–9.
140. Roggo A, Wood W, Ottinger L. Carcinoid tumors of the appendix. Ann Surg 1993;317:385–90.
141. Moertel CG, Wieland L, Nagorney D, Dockerty MB. Carcinoid tumor of the appendix. Treatment and prognosis. N Engl J Med 1987;317:1699–701.
142. Thirlby RC, Kasper C, Jones RC. Metastatic carcinoid of the appendix. Dis Colon Rectum 1984;27:42–6.
143. Anderson JR, Wilson BG. Carcinoid tumors of the appendix. Br J Surg 1985;72:545–6.
144. Lyss A. Appendiceal malignancies. Semin Oncol 1988;15:129–37.
145. Svendson L, Bulow S. Carcinoid tumors of the appendix in young patients. Acta Chir Scand 1980;146:137–9.
146. Jonsson T, Johannsson JH, Hallgrimsson JG. Carcinoid tumors of the appendix in children younger than 16 years. Acta Chir Scand 1989;155:113–6.
147. Ryden SE, Drake RM, Franciosi RA. Carcinoid tumors of the appendix in children. Cancer 1975;36:1538–42.
148. Antonaides J. Carcinoid tumors of the gastrointestinal tract. New York: Masson; 1982.
149. Saha S, Hoda S, Godfrey R, et al. Carcinoid tumors of the gastrointestinal tract. A 44-year experience. South Med J 1989;82:1501–5.
150. Olney JR, Urdaneta LF,, Al-Jurf AS, et al. Carcinoid tumors of the gastrointestinal tract. Am Surg 1985;51:37–41.
151. Higa E, Rosai J, Pizzimbono C, Wise L. Mucosal hyperplasia, mucinous cystadenoma, and mucinous cystadenocarcinoma of the appendix. A re-evaluation of appendiceal "mucocele." Cancer 1973;32:1525–41.
152. Carr N, McCarthy W, Sobin LH, et al. Epithelial noncarcinoid tumors and tumor-like lesions of the appendix. Cancer 1995;75:757–68.
153. Gibbs NM. Mucinous cystadenoma and cystadenocarcinoma of the vermiform appendix with particular reference to mucocele and pseudomyxoma peritonei. J Clin Pathol 1973;26:413–21.
154. Horgan JG, Chow PP, Richter JO, et al. CT and sonography in the recognition of mucocele of the appendix. AJR Am J Roentgenol 1984;143:959–62.
155. Aranha GV, Reyes CV. Primary epithelial tumors of the appendix and a reappraisal of the appendiceal "mucocele." Dis Colon Rectum 1979;22:472–6.
156. Stephenson J, Brief D. Mucinous appendiceal tumors. Clinical review. J Med Soc NJ 1985;82:381–4.
157. Chang P, Attiyeh FF. Adenocarcinoma of the appendix. Dis Colon Rectum 1981;24:176–80.
158. Ferro M, Anthony PP. Adenocarcinoma of the appendix. Dis Colon Rectum 1985;28:457–9.
159. Hesketh KT. The management of primary adenocarcinoma of the vermiform appendix. Gut 1963;4:158–68.
160. Gilhome RW, Johnston DH, Clark J, Kyle J. Primary adenocarcinoma of the vermiform appendix: report of a series of ten cases and review of the literature. Br J Surg 1984;71:553–5.
161. Deans G, Spencer R. Neoplastic lesions of the appendix. Br J Surg 1995;82:299–306.
162. Rutledge R, Alexander J. Primary appendiceal malignancies. Rare but important. Surgery 1992;11:244–50.
163. Niteeki S, Wolff B, Schlinkert R, et al. The natural history of surgically treated primary adenocarcinoma of the appendix. Ann Surg 1994;21:51–7.
164. Conte CC, Petrelli NJ, Stulc J, et al. Adenocarcinoma of the appendix. Surg Gynecol Obstet 1988;166:451–3.
165. Evans D, Hamid B, Hoare E. Primary adenocarcinoma of the appendix. J R Coll Surg Edinb 1990;35:33–5.
166. Edmonds P, Merino MJ, LiVolsi VA, Duray PH. Adenocarcinoid (mucinous carcinoid) of the appendix. Gastroenterology 1984;86:302–9.
167. Jones RA, MacFarlane A. Carcinomas and carcinoid tumors of the appendix in a district general hospital. J Clin Pathol 1976;29:687–92.
168. Raptopoulos V, Gourtsoyiannas N. Peritoneal carcinomatosis. Eur Radiol 2001;11:2195–206.
169. Meyers MA. Distribution of intraabdominal malignant seeding: dependency on dynamics of flow of ascitic fluid. Am J Roentgenol 1973;119:198–206.
170. Cavaliere F, Perri P, Di Filippo F, et al. Treatment of peritoneal carcinomatosis with intent to cure. J Surg Oncol 2000;74:41–4.
171. Sugarbaker PH. Review of a personal experience in the management of carcinomatosis and sarcomatosis. Jpn J Clin Oncol 2001;31:573–83.
172. Jaquet P, Vidal-Jove J, Zhu BW, et al. Peritoneal carcinomatosis from intraabdominal malignancy. Natural history and new prospects for management. Acta Chir Belg 1994;94:191–7.
173. Dedrik R. Theoretical and experimental bases of intraperitoneal chemotherapy. Semin Oncol 1985;XII:1–6.
174. Alexander H, Fraker D. Continuous hyperthermic peritoneal perfusion with cisplatin in the treatment of peritoneal carcinomatosis. Reg Cancer Treat 1995;8:2–7.
175. Kannerstein M, Churg J. Peritoneal mesothelioma. Hum Pathol 1977;8:83–94.
176. Asensio JA Goldblatt P, Thomford NR. Primary malignant peritoneal mesothelioma. A report of seven cases and a review of the literature. Arch Surg 1990;125:1477–81.
177. Bollinger DJ, Wick MR, Manivel JC, et al. Peritoneal malignant mesothelioma vs serous papillary adenocarcinoma. An immunohistochemical comparison. Lab Invest 1988;58:11A.
178. Moertel CG. Peritoneal mesothelioma. Current clinical concepts. Gastroenterology 1972;63:346–50.
179. Antman KH, Pomfret EA, Aisner J, et al. Peritoneal mesothelioma: natural history and response to chemotherapy. J Clin Oncol 1983;1:386–91.
180. Brenner J, Sordillo PP, Magill GB, Golbey RB. Malignant peritoneal mesothelioma. Review of 25 patients. Am J Gastroenterol 1981;75:311–3.
181. Chang PS, Balfour TW, Bourker JB, Smith PG. Peritoneal mesothelioma. Br J Surg 1975;62:576.
182. Park B, Alexander H, Libutti SK, et al. Treatment of primary peritoneal mesothelioma by continuous hyper-thermic peritoneal perfusion. Ann Surg Onc 1999;6:582–90.
183. Foyle A, Al-Jabi M, McCaughty WT. Papillary peritoneal tumors in women. Am J Surg Pathol 1981;5:241–9.
184. Lindeque BG, Cronje HS, Deale CJ. Prevalence of primary papillary peritoneal neoplasia in patients with ovarian cancer. S Afr Med J 1985;67:1005.
185. Eltabbakh G, Werness B, Piver S, et al. Prognostic factors in extraovarian primary peritoneal carcinoma. Gynecol Oncol 1998;71:230–9.
186. Swerdlow M. Mesothelioma of the pelvic peritoneum resembling papillary cystadenocarcinoma of the ovary: case report. Am J Obstet Gynecol 1959;77:197–200.
187. Banerjee R, Gough F. Cystic mucinous tumors of the mesentery and retroperitoneum. Report of three cases. Histopathology 1988;12:527–32.
188. Clark J, Wood H, Jaffurs WJ, et al. Endometrioid-type cystadenocarcinoma arising in the mesosalpinx. Obstet Gynecol 1979; 54:656–8.
189. Lee K, Verma U, Belinson J. Primary clear cell carcinoma of the peritoneum. Gynecol Oncol 1991;41:259–62.
190. Hampton H, Hufman H, Meeks G. Extraovarian Brenner tumors. Obstet Gynecol 1992;79:844–6.
191. Mirc JL, Fenoglio-Preiser CM, Husseinzadeh N. Malignant mixed müllerian tumor of extraovarian secondary müllerian system: report of two cases and review of the literature. Arch Pathol Lab Med 1995;119:1044–9.
192. Resta L, Maiorano E, Zito FA, et al. Multifocal extraovarian serous carcinoma. A histochemical and immunohistochemical study. Eur J Gynecol Oncol 1988;IX:474–8.
193. Eltabbakh GH, Piver MS, Natarajan N, Mettlin CJ. Epidemiologic differences between women with extraovarian primary peritoneal carcinoma and women with epithelial ovarian cancer. Obstet Gynecol 1998;91:254–9.
194. Ronnett BM, Shmookler BM, Diener-West M, et al. Immunohistochemical evidence supporting the appendiceal origin of pseudomyxoma peritonei in women. Int J Gynecol Pathol 1997;16:1–9.
195. Sugarbaker PH, Landy D, Jaffe G, Pascal R. Histologic changes induced by intraperitoneal chemotherapy with 5-fluorouracil and mitomycin C in patients with peritoneal carcinomatosis from cystadenocarcinoma of the colon or appendix. Cancer 1990;65:1495–501.
196. Sugarbaker PH, Chang D. Results of treatment of 385 patients with peritoneal surface spread of appendiceal malignancy. Ann Surg Oncol 1999;6:727–31.
197. McCaughey WT, Dardick I, Barr JR. Angiosarcoma of serous membranes. Arch Pathol Lab Med 1983;107:304–7.
198. Westenberg A, Wiggers T, Henzen-Logmans SC, et al. Post-irradiation angiosarcoma of the greater omentum. Eur J Surg Oncol 1989;15:175–8.
199. Lin BT, Colby T, Gown AM, et al. Malignant vascular tumors of the serous membranes mimicking mesothelioma. A report of 14 cases. Amer J Surg Pathol 1996;20:1431–9.
200. Aslam N, Marino C. Malignant ascites. Arch Intern Med 2001;161:2733–7.
201. Rath U, Kaufmann M, Schmidd H, et al. Effect of intraperitoneal recombinant human tumor necrosis factor alpha on malignant ascites. Eur J Cancer Clin Oncol 1991;27:121–5.
202. Xu L, Yoneda J, Herrera C, et al. Inhibition of malignant ascites and growth of human ovarian carcinoma by oral administration of a potent inhibitor of the vascular endothelial growth factor receptor tyrosine kinases. Int J Oncol 2000;16:445–54.
203. Beattie G, Smyth J. Phase I study of intraperitoneal metalloproteinase inhibitor BB94 in patients with malignant ascites. Clin Cancer Res 1998;4:1899–902.
204. Parsons SL, Watson SA, Steele RJ. Phase I/II trial of batimastat, a matrix metalloproteinase inhibitor in patients with malignant ascites. Eur J Surg Oncol 1997;23:526–31.
205. Loggie B, Perini M, Fleming RA, et al. Treatment and prevention of malignant ascites associated with disseminated intraperitoneal malignancies by aggressive combined-modality therapy. Am Surg 1997;63:137–43.
206. Teuche S, Pector J. Peritoneovenous shunt in malignant ascites. The Bordet Institute experience from 1975–1998. Hepatogastroenterology 2000;47:1322–4.

Carcinoma of the Colon and Rectum

Miguel A. Rodriguez-Bigas, MD
Paulo Hoff, MD
Christopher H. Crane, MD

CARCINOMA OF THE COLON AND RECTUM

Cancer of the colon and rectum is a public health issue. In the United States alone, over 140,000 new cases are diagnosed annually. With adequate public and physician education the majority of colorectal cancers could be prevented. In the last decade, great strides were made in the fight against this disease. As molecular techniques were developed, a genetic model for colorectal carcinogenesis was proposed.[1] Molecular pathways were proposed, and actual genetic defects in the germline of patients with inherited syndromes predisposing to colorectal cancer were identified. There is a better understanding between genetic interactions and environmental interactions in the etiology of colorectal cancer. However, most of these interactions are not well understood. For the first time in this disease, adjuvant therapy was proved to be effective in decreasing recurrence and improving survival. The new decade will bring advances in chemoprevention, early diagnosis, chemotherapy, and immunotherapy. We are into the twenty-first century, where tumor profiling and molecular targeting of tumors will be exploited. The future is bright; however, there is still a fair amount of work to do.

EPIDEMIOLOGY OF COLORECTAL CANCER

Cancer Statistics Colorectal cancer (CRC) is the third most common malignant tumor and the fourth most common cause of cancer death in the world.[2] In the year 2002, it was estimated that over 1,000,000 new colorectal cancer cases would be diagnosed worldwide, and about 529,000 patients would die from the disease.[2] CRC is more common in developed countries. Environmental and dietary factors, in conjunction with or interacting with genetic factors, may account for the difference in incidence between geographic regions. Studies from migrant populations have demonstrated that individuals migrating from areas of low incidence to areas with high incidence will, over time, acquire the risk of the host country.[3]

Colorectal cancer is most common in the sixth decade of life; however, it can occur at any age. The lifetime risk of developing colorectal cancer in the United States approaches 6%, with males having a slightly higher incidence than females (5.88% vs 5.49%).[4] Up to age 40, the incidence of colorectal cancer is similar among men and women.[4] However, after age 40, men have a slightly higher incidence rate than women.[4]

The incidence of colorectal cancer in the United States has remained stable in almost a decade.[4] Mortality has been declining in both men and women at a rate of approximately 1.7% per year.[4] There are marked differences in colorectal cancer incidence and mortality between races and ethnic groups. African Americans have the highest incidence and mortality rates among all racial and ethnic groups in the United States.[4] Table 92-1 illustrates the incidence and mortality rates from colorectal cancer by race and ethnicity from 1996 to 2000. The reasons for the higher risk in African Americans are unknown. Interactions between the environment, dietary factors, socioeconomic factors, and genetics may play a role in both incidence and mortality. The increase in mortality from colorectal cancer in African Americans may also be in part due to the biology of the tumor, but socioeconomic factors could potentially lead to barriers to early diagnosis and treatment.[5]

Over the last several decades there has been a shift from rectum and left-sided cancers toward more right-sided tumors. It can be speculated that this left to right shift, in part, may be due to better screening. Data collected in the National Cancer Institute Surveillance, Epidemiology and End Results Program (SEER) database between 1975 and 1994 showed that proximal colon cancer rates were higher than distal colon or rectal carcinoma rates, respectively.[6]

RISK FACTORS FOR COLORECTAL CANCER

Age The incidence of colorectal cancer increases after age 50 years. In the Surveillance, Epidemiology and End Results statistics from 1995 to 1999, the incidence of colorectal cancer was 40 per 100,000 for individuals between 40 to 49 years of age, while it was 325 per 100,000 for individuals aged 60 to 69.[7] The incidence increases with each subsequent decade.

Previous Colorectal Neoplasia A personal history of colorectal cancer increases the risk of developing metachronous tumors. The incidence of metachronous colorectal cancer and adenomas in patients with a previous CRC is approximately 6% and 25%, respectively.[8] Similarly, a personal history of adenomas will increase the risk of subsequent adenomas and thus of colorectal cancer. Not all adenomas will become malignant, and several investigators have attempted to outline particular characteristics of polyps that will increase the risk of recurrent adenomas after polypectomy. Among these characteristics are histology, size, and number of adenomas.[9]

Family History Family history of colorectal cancer in a first-degree relative increases the risk of colorectal cancer two- to threefold.[10] The earlier the diagnosis of CRC cancer, the higher the risk. It has been reported that the colon cancer risk of an individual with a first-degree relative is about the same at age 40 as for the general population at age 50.[11] In addition, the more relatives affected, the higher the risk. Second-degree relatives with colorectal cancer also increase an individual risk of CRC, but by about 25 to 50% above the average risk.[12] Family history of adenomas also increases the relative risk of colorectal cancer. In first-degree relatives with adenomas, the relative risk of colorectal cancer was 1.78.[13,14] The younger the affected individual, the higher

Table 92-1 Colorectal Cancer Incidence and Mortality Rates by Race and Ethnicity 1996–2000*

	Incidence		Mortality	
Race/Ethnic Group	Male	Female	Male	Female
African American	72.4	56.2	34.6	24.6
White	64.1	46.2	25.3	17.5
Asian/Pacific Islander	57.2	38.8	15.8	11.0
American Indian/Alaska Native	37.5	32.6	18.5	12.1
Hispanic	49.8	32.9	18.4	11.4

*Rate per 100,000, age-adjusted to the 2000 US standard population.
Source: Ries LAG, Eisner MP, Kosary CP, et al. (eds). SEER Cancer Statistics, Review 1975–2000. Bethesda, MD: National Cancer Institute; http//seer.cancer/gov/csr1975_2000/.

the risk of CRC for the siblings. This was noted in the National Polyp Study especially if the adenoma was diagnosed at age 60 or less.[13,14]

Genetic Syndromes and Inflammatory Bowel Disease Certain genetic syndromes predispose to colorectal cancer. Familial adenomatous polyposis (FAP) is characterized by hundreds to thousands of polyps throughout the large bowel. It is an autosomal-dominant inherited syndrome with a penetrance approaching 100%. If the colorectal adenomas are left untreated, patients with FAP invariably will develop colorectal cancer. The median age of adenoma diagnosis is 15 years.[15] In untreated patients, the mean age of colorectal cancer diagnosis and colorectal cancer death is 39 years and 42 years, respectively.[16] In the milder phenotypic variant, attenuated adenomatous polyposis coli (AAPC), colorectal polyps are less numerous, and colorectal carcinoma in general will occur in the early fifties.

MYH-associated neoplasia has recently been described and is still being characterized. Biallelic mutations in the base excision repair gene *MYH*, most commonly Y165C and G328D, have been identified in individuals with multiple adenomas as well as in patients with classic familial adenomatous polyposis where a germline mutation in the *APC* gene had not been identified.[17–20] In these reports, affected individuals usually had more than 10 adenomas. Colorectal cancer has also been described in some of these patients as well as in patients less than 50 years of age.[20] The phenotype of these individuals appears to be milder than most classic FAP patients, but less severe than the majority of patients with multiple adenomas. *MYH*-associated neoplasia apparently is inherited in an autosomal recessive pattern.[18] The significance of monoalleic mutations in the *MYH* gene is unknown. Germline mutations in *MYH* account for about 8% of classic FAP patients where *APC* mutations have not been detected.[18,19]

Hereditary nonpolyposis colorectal cancer (HNPCC) is an autosomal-dominant syndrome characterized by early-age onset colorectal cancer, right-sided predominance, excess synchronous and metachronous colorectal neoplasms, and extracolonic malignancies such as endometrial cancer, small bowel cancer, renal pelvis and ureter cancer, and skin lesions such as sebaceous adenomas, keratoacanthomas, and sebaceous carcinoma.[21] The median age of onset of CRC is 45 years old. Endometrial cancer can be the index carcinoma in 35% of female patients.[22] Germline mutations in the mismatch repair genes (see mutator pathway) are responsible for the syndrome. MSH6 germline mutations have been associated with later age onset of colorectal cancer onset and with predominant endometrial cancer families.[23] Adenomas do occur in HNPCC. Currently it is believed that once adenomas occur in HNPCC, they progress to carcinoma faster than in sporadic CRC patients.[24]

Peutz-Jeghers (PJ) and Juvenile Polyposis (JP) are the most common hamartomatous polyposis syndromes predisposing to colorectal cancer. PJ patients are also at risk of stomach, pancreas, breast, and uterine carcinoma, as well as ovarian sex cord tumors, Sertoli cell tumors, and adenoma malignum of the cervix.[25–28] In addition to colorectal cancer, JP patients are at risk of gastric, duodenal, and pancreatic cancers.[27,28]

Inflammatory bowel disease is a well-known risk factor for colorectal cancer. The prevalence of CRC in ulcerative colitis (UC) patients has been reported to be 3.7%, increasing to 5.4% for those individuals with pancolitis.[29] The cumulative risk of CRC for any patient with UC was 2% at 10 years, 8% at 20 years, and 18% at 30 years.[29] The incidence and characteristics of colorectal cancer in Crohn's disease has been reported to be similar to ulcerative colitis.[30]

Diet and Lifestyle Epidemiological studies evaluating westernized dietary habits (increased intake of fats and red meat and decreased intake of fruits and vegetables) suggest a relationship between diet and colorectal cancer risk. A high body mass index (BMI) has been shown to be related to increased colon cancer risk in males.[31] In females, results relating colon cancer risk to BMI have been mixed. In cohort and case-control studies stratified for age, a positive association between colon cancer risk and BMI has been reported in younger women.[32,33] It has been postulated that the increased risk of colon cancer and BMI in younger women could be due to menopausal status.[32] Body mass index ≥ 30 kg/m^2 was associated with an almost twofold increase in colorectal cancer risk in women who were premenopausal at baseline, but it was not increased associated in postmenopausal women.[34]

The per capita intake of fat may be related to colorectal cancer incidence and mortality.[35] The type of fat intake may be a more important risk factor than the total fat intake. Increased intake in saturated animal fat appears to be a stronger risk factor than total dietary fat intake.[36] Fish oils, rich in polyunsaturated fat, may have a protective effect.[37] Experimentally it has been demonstrated that feeding rats a western-style mixed-lipid diet increases colon tumorigenesis by fourfold compared with animals fed a diet with a similar amount of total fat containing fish oil or low-fat corn-oil.[38]

The way that food is prepared also influences colorectal cancer risk. Cooking at higher temperatures increases the amounts of heterocyclic amines and carcinogens.[39] Processed meats, which contain nitroso compounds are carcinogens.[40] In the Cancer Prevention Study II (CPSII) Nutrition Cohort study, prolonged high consumption of red and processed meats was associated with colorectal cancer, particularly in the rectum and rectosigmoid, whereas prolonged intake of poultry and fish had no effect on rectal cancer, but marginally decreased the risk of proximal and distal colon cancer.[41] Genetic polymorphisms that alter heterocyclic amines metabolism may also influence colorectal cancer risk.

Lifestyle decisions may influence colorectal cancer risk. Daily alcohol consumption increases the risk of colon cancer. There is a twofold increased risk of colon cancer in individuals who consume greater than two drinks per day.[42] There have been both positive and negative studies with regards to the risk of adenoma and alcohol consumption.[42] A World Cancer Research Fund panel report concluded that the association of colorectal cancer and alcohol was related to the total alcohol intake, not to the type of drink.[43] Cigarette smoking may increase the risk of developing adenomas.[36] There is less clear-cut evidence for an increased risk of colorectal cancer among cigarette smokers. However, the impact of cigarette smoking on colorectal cancer may be related to the cytochrome P-450A1 (CYP1A1) genotype in combination with other polymorphisms.[44] Working in industries such as nonmetallic mineral products, leather goods, meat, poultry and fish products, communications, and petroleum and coal products may increase colon cancer risk.[45] Individuals with sedentary occupations, such as administrators, professionals, and clerical and sales workers, have also been found to have a slightly higher colon cancer risk.[46]

Polymorphisms Variations in normal genes that metabolize or activate cellular pathways can either increase or decrease cancer risk by altering cellular homeostasis and therefore facilitating genomic instability and eventual progression from normal mucosa to cancer. These normal variations in genes are called polymorphisms. GSTT1, *N*-acetyltransferase 2 (NAT2) rapid acetylator phenotype and genotype, and NAT2 rapid acetylator phenotype have been identified in case-control and cohort studies as increasing colorectal cancer risk.[47] Glutathione-S transferases are phase II enzymes involved in the detoxification of mutagenic electrophiles, including polyaromatic hydrocarbons.[48] The *N*-acetyltransferases (NAT1 and NAT2) are phase-II metabolizing enzymes involved in detoxifying aromatic amines.[48] Interactions between polymorphisms may have an impact on CRC risk. CYP1A1 genotype in conjunction with GSTM1 and NAT2 may alter colorectal cancer risk in cigarette smokers.[44] Further studies are needed to identify and evaluate the interactions between these polymorphisms as well as their interactions with lifestyle and the environment.

Polymorphisms in tumor suppressor genes have been associated with increased colorectal cancer in specific populations. The most common polymorphisms reported have been in the adenomatous polyposis coli (*APC*) gene. The I1307K polymorphism, a T→A transition at nucleotide 3920 of the *APC* gene creates a hypermutable region.[49] This polymorphism is only present in the Ashkenazi Jewish population. It has been reported to be present in 6% of controls, 10% of patients with colorectal cancer and 28% of patients with a family history of colorectal cancer.[49] I1307K confers a twofold increase in colorectal cancer risk in the individuals who carry it. Another polymorphism in the *APC* gene that confers an increase in colorectal cancer is the I1317Q.[50] Slattery and colleagues reported the association of diet, lifestyle, and risk of colorectal cancer in a variant in codon 1822 of the *APC* gene.[51] The B1822V allele frequency in the control population was 22.8%.[51] Of these, approximately 5.2% were homozygous for the variant *APC* 1822 valine/valine.[51] There was a reduced risk of colon cancer in individuals with the homozygous variant if they ate a low-fat diet when compared with individuals with the homozygous wild-type variant if they ate a high-fat diet.[51]

PATHOLOGY

Approximately 95% of the malignant colorectal tumors are adenocarcinomas. Table 92-2 illustrates the pathological classification of primary colon and rectal neoplasms. It is accepted that the majority of adenocarcinomas of the large bowel arise from adenomas. It takes several years for an adenoma to progress to a carcinoma. The progression to cancer results from the accumulation of multiple genetic changes.[1] Not all adenomas progress to cancer. In fact, the vast majority of adenomas do not progress to carcinoma. The malignant potential of the adenomas has been correlated to their size, histopathology, and degree of dysplasia.[52]

Macroscopically, colorectal tumors can be described as ulcerative, polypoid, annular, or infiltrative. Histopathologically, adenocarcinomas are classified as well-, moderately, or poorly differentiated, depending on the formation of glandular elements. Well- and moderately differentiated adenocarcinomas have more glandular components than poorly differentiated tumors. Adenocarcinomas of the colon and rectum are also described depending on the histopathological characteristics. Mucin-producing tumors characterized by extracellular mucin pools are semiquantitatively subgrouped according to the amount of mucin present in the tumor. Signet ring cell-type adenocarcinomas characteristically have intracellular mucin pushing the nuclei to give the cell the characteristic signet ring appearance. Adenosquamous carcinomas are composed of both glandular and squamous elements. Medullary carcinomas characteristically are composed of nests or trabeculae of regular small- to medium-sized cells with moderate amounts of eosinophilic cytoplasm.[53] Whenever the clinician encounters the latter histopathology in a colorectal carcinoma, the diagnosis of HNPCC should be considered.[21]

Table 92-2 Pathology of Primary Tumors of the Large Intestine

Adenocarcinoma
Well differentiated
Moderately well differentiated
Poorly differentiated
Mucinous carcinoma
Signet ring cell-type
Medullary
Adenosquamous carcinoma
Carcinoid
Lymphoma
Melanoma
Sarcoma
Small-cell carcinoma
Squamous cell
Undifferentiated carcinoma

In order to adequately manage a patient with colorectal cancer, careful pathology review is mandatory. There must be direct communication between the clinician and the pathologist. It is not unusual to encounter situations where special stains will elucidate the diagnosis of an undifferentiated carcinoma. At times, comparison of the histopathological slides of the primary tumor with metastases will reveal a different histopathology in the metastatic disease, thus altering the management of the patient.

Staging Prognosis in colorectal cancer is related to the stage at diagnosis. Several classifications for staging colorectal cancer have been utilized. The Dukes' classification or its modifications have been the mainstay of colorectal cancer staging.[54] In the last decade, the tumor-node-metastases (TNM) classification has been recommended. Table 92-3 illustrates the correlation of the Dukes' classification, the Astler-Coller[55] modification, and the TNM classification.[56] Currently, the sixth revision of the TNM classification is recommended for staging purposes.

TUMOR MARKERS

Carcinoembryonic Antigen Carcinoembryonic antigen (CEA), a cell membrane glycoprotein, has been useful in prognosis and follow-up of patients with colorectal cancer. Serum CEA levels can be elevated in ovarian, breast, lung, pancreas, and other gastrointestinal tract cancers.[57] Not only do malignant conditions cause an elevation of CEA, but also benign conditions, such as liver dysfunction, hydronephrosis, peptic ulcer disease, pancreatitis, biliary obstruction, bowel obstruction, post 5-fluorouracil (FU)/levamisole chemotherapy, and smoking, can elevate this marker.[58]

In spite of its lack of sensitivity and specificity, CEA is a useful tumor marker in colorectal cancer. It is important to recognize that tumor burden may not correlate with CEA levels.[57] However, in general, CEA correlates with stage of colorectal cancer.[59] Well-differentiated colorectal adenocarcinomas produce more CEA than poorly differentiated adenocarcinomas.[60] CEA is not recommended for screening purposes in colorectal cancer. It is useful as a prognostic indicator after curative resection and during follow-up.[59,61,62] After curative resection, an elevated CEA should drop to normal levels within 4 to 8 weeks.[63] If this decrease to normal does not occur, persistent or recurrent disease is likely. A rising CEA at any time during follow-up should alert the clinician about a possible recurrence. Unfortunately, the lead time in the detection of recurrent disease by CEA monitoring has not been translated to improved survival. In a meta-analysis based on the literature from 1972 to 1996, at a mean 2-years follow-up, Rosen and colleagues reported twice as many resections for recurrent disease and slightly higher cumulative 5-years survival in series with patients who underwent resection for recurrent disease diagnosed by intensive follow-up, which included history and physical exam and CEA levels every 3 months.[64] Approximately 30% of colorectal cancers do not produce CEA and about 40% of patients with a normal preoperative CEA will have an elevated level at recurrence.[65,66] The American Society of Clinical Oncology has recommended that serum CEA levels be performed every 2 to 3 months in patients with stage II or III for ≥ 2 years after diagnosis.[67] CEA levels have also been utilized to monitor response to chemotherapy in metastatic disease. The reader is cautioned that this is not an accepted objective criterion for tumor response.

Table 92-3 Colorectal Cancer Stage Classification

AJCC 2002* (8)	Dukes'**	Modified Astler-Coller***
Stage 0		
Tis N0 M0		
Stage I		
T1 N0 M0	A	A
T2 N0 M0	A	B1
Stage II		
Stage IIA		
T3 N0 M0	B	B2
Stage IIB		
T4 N0 M0	B	B3
Stage III		
Stage IIIA		
T1-T2 N1M0	C	C1
Stage IIIB		
T3-T4 N1 M0	C	C2/C3
Stage IIIC		
Any T, N2 M0	C	C1/C2/C3
Stage IV		
Any T, any N, M1		D

*Tis = carcinoma in situ (intramucosal, intraepithelial)
T1 = tumor confined to mucosa or submucosa
T2 = tumor involves muscularis propria but not beyond
T3 = tumor through the muscularis propria into the subserosa, or into nonperitonealized or perirectal tissues
T4 = tumor directly invades other organs or structures, and/or perforates the visceral peritoneum
N1 = 1–3 metastatic regional lymph nodes
N2 = 4 or more metastatic regional lymph nodes
External iliac or common iliac metastatic lymph nodes are considered M1.
R0 = complete resection with histologically negative margins and no residual tumor left
R1 = incomplete resection with microscopic residual tumor after all gross disease resected
R2 = incomplete resection with macroscopic disease left in place
**A = limited to the bowel wall
B = extends through the bowel wall
C = involvement of regional lymph nodes
***A = limited to the mucosa
B1 = involving the muscularis propria but not beyond
B2 = through the muscularis propria
B3 = invasion into adjacent organs
C1/C2/C3 = similar to B1/B2/B3 except regional lymph nodes involved
D = distant metastases

Monoclonal antibodies against CEA have been developed in an attempt to improve tumor localization in patients with elevated CEA whose conventional testing has not localized the recurrence site. Because of disappointing results, the use of these scans has decreased. It appears that 2-(18F) fluorodeoxy-D-glucose/positron emission tomography (FDG-PET) scans are more useful than monoclonal antibody scans in detecting recurrences. Libutti and colleagues reported a prospective blind study evaluating FDG-PET scans, 99mTc-labeled arcitumomab (CEA-scan), and second-look laparotomy.[68] Twenty-eight patients were explored. Disease was noted in 26 patients. FDG-PET scans predicted unresectable disease in 90% of patients, whereas CEA scans failed to predict unresectable disease in any patient.[68] In patients who were resected, FDG-PET predicted resectability in 81% of the patients, whereas CEA scan predicted resectability in 13%.[68] FDG-PET scan alone has been reported to have an 89% positive-predictive value and 100% negative-predictive value in patients who had a rising CEA and normal conventional radiographic studies.[69]

CEA has also been utilized in the detection of micrometastases in histologically negative lymph nodes. Cutait and colleagues reported on the detection of micrometastases utilizing immunoperoxidase staining of CEA and cytokeratins.[70] At 5-year follow-up, there was no difference in survival between those patients who were upstaged and those whose lymph nodes were free of micrometastases.[70] However, Liefers and colleagues reported that the detection of micrometastases utilizing a CEA-specific RT-PCR was a prognostic tool in stage II colorectal cancer.[71]

CA 19-9 CA 19-9 has been reported elevated in 20 to 40% of colorectal cancers with the highest sensitivity in patients with metastases.[72] It can be elevated in adenocarcinomas of the stomach, pancreas, and large bowel as well as in ovarian, gall bladder, and lung adenocarcinomas.[72] CA 19-9 is not recommended for screening, diagnosis, surveillance, or staging of colorectal cancer patients.[72] However, it may be useful in selecting patients at high risk of recurrence.[72]

Molecular Genetics There are two major genetic pathways responsible for colorectal carcinogenesis. The majority of colorectal cancers progress in an orderly fashion from normal mucosa to adenomas to carcinoma and to metastases. The molecular model for the events was proposed by Fearon and Vogelstein.[1] In their model, a single genetic change was not sufficient to cause cancer, but it was the accumulation of mutations in tumor suppressor genes, oncogenes, as well as other epigenetic changes such as hyper or hypo methylation that drove cells into carcinogenesis. This pathway, known as the suppressor pathway or chromosomal instability (CIN) pathway, is the most common pathway in colorectal carcinogenesis. The majority of sporadic colorectal cancers progress through this pathway.

The other major pathway in colorectal carcinogenesis is the mutator pathway. This pathway was first proposed by Loeb, who hypothesized that the mutation rate in somatic cells was insufficient to account for the high number of mutations noted in human cancer, and thus mutations in genes that maintain the stability of the genome could lead to a "mutator phenotype" that then drove tumor progression.[73] Tumors that develop through this pathway are characterized by somatic mutations (deletions or insertions) in simple repeated sequences leading to microsatellite instability (MSI). This pathway accounts for the majority of HNPCC tumors and approximately 10 to 15% of sporadic cancers. Microsatellite instability occurs in 85 to 90% of CRC from HNPCC tumors.

The most common genes involved in sporadic colorectal cancer are the *APC* gene, k-*ras*, and *TP53*. *APC* is a tumor suppressor gene involved in the regulation of β-catenin, cytoskeleton organization, apoptosis, cell-cycle control, and cell adhesion.[74] It has been reported that mutations in the *APC* gene are sufficient for the early growth of adenomas.[75] *APC* mutations occur in up to 80% of adenomas and up to 80% of carcinomas.[76] Although k-*ras* mutations have been reported in aberrant crypt foci (the earliest abnormality in colorectal carcinogenesis), they are rarely seen in adenomas less than 1 cm, thus suggesting that these mutations occur later in carcinogenesis.[77] *TP53* is a tumor suppressor gene whose protein is a transcription factor involved in cell-cycle progression, apoptosis, and angiogenesis.[78] Approximately 30% of late adenomas and 75 % of carcinomas will have a mutated *TP53*.[78]

Colorectal cancers that develop via the mutator pathway are initiated by either germline or somatic mutations in the mismatch repair genes. These genes are *hMLH1*, *hMSH2*, *hMSH6*, *hPMS1*, *hPMS2*, *hMLH3*, and *hMSH3*.[79] There have been no reported germline mutations in the latter gene. Epigenetic silencing of the *hMLH1* promoter is another mechanism of inactivating *hMLH1*.[80] This mechanism, as well as somatic mutations in *BRAF*, account for microsatellite instability in sporadic colorectal cancers.[81] Mutations in the *TGF β-RII* gene are the most common mutations in the suppressor pathway. Other genes commonly mutated in this pathway include *BAX* and *IGF-2*.[82]

Other pathways proposed for colorectal carcinogenesis include the serrated pathway and the landscaper defect pathway. In the serrated pathway, the initiating step for colorectal carcinogenesis is not through *APC* mutations, but owing to epigenetic silencing of genes involved in DNA repair, cell-cycle control, and differentiation.[83] Morphologically, the precursor lesions are serrated and include hyperplastic, mixed hyperplastic/adenomatous polyps, and serrated adenomas.[83] Tumors originating via this pathway may have any level of microsatellite instability, namely stable, low, or high.[83] In juvenile polyposis and ulcerative colitis, it appears that the defective cells are derived from the stroma and the epithelial tumorigenesis is the result of an abnormal microenvironment.[84] There are still other pathways as of yet not described that will undoubtedly interact with the pathways described, and may even modify these routes to carcinogenesis.

Molecular Markers for Prognosis With the advent of new technologies for molecular diagnosis, there has been an explosion in the literature of studies of molecular markers for prognosis and for response to chemotherapy and radiotherapy. Some of these markers could potentially be utilized to select high-risk patients (especially stage II colon cancer patients) who may benefit from adjuvant therapy. In addition, microarray technology has allowed tumors to be analyzed for up-regulation or down-regulation of thousands of genes at a time, as well as for expression of protein products, and thus, setting the stage for the tumor profiling that will be available in near future. One such example is colon cancer secreting protein-2, a novel transcript expressed 78-fold in stage II, III, and IV colon cancer, but not expressed in normal colon or in other normal body tissues.[85] In this section the most common molecular markers studied in colorectal carcinoma will be discussed.

DNA Ploidy Aneuploid tumors have an abnormal balance of chromosomes and can have additional peaks representing more or less nucleic acids generated on the DNA histogram. Diploid tumors have a single peak in the DNA histogram. Unfortunately, there is no standardized methodology for measuring ploidy; therefore, the studies have to be interpreted with caution.[62] The American Society of Clinical Oncology (ASCO) Tumor Marker Expert Panel reviewed the studies published between 1994 and 1999.[86] The ASCO expert panel concluded that the literature did not support the use of DNA-derived flow cytometry or proliferation analysis to determine prognosis or therapy of operable colorectal cancer.[86]

Ki-*ras* The prognostic significance of Ki-*ras* mutations in colorectal cancer is controversial. The Southwest Oncology Group reported that patients with stage II colon cancer whose tumors had Ki-*ras* mutations had a worse survival compared with those patients whose tumors had wild-type Ki-*ras* (HR = 4.5; 95% CI 1.7–12.1).[87] In that study, there was no benefit in adjuvant chemotherapy for stage II patients irrespective of mutational status. However, stage III patients with wild-type Ki-*ras* benefited from adjuvant chemotherapy.[87]

Ki-*ras* mutations have been correlated with tumor response in patients receiving neoadjuvant chemoradiation for locally advanced rectal cancer.[88] Tumors with specific Ki-*ras* mutations had better response to chemoradiation than those with wild-type Ki-*ras*.[88] At this time, there is not sufficient data to recommend clinical use of Ki-*ras*.

TP53 *TP53* is the most mutated gene in cancer. Similar to Ki-*ras*, there are multiple positive and negative studies with regards to *TP53* mutational status and prognosis in colorectal cancer. The methodology of detection of mutations has been either by overexpression of *TP53* by immunohistochemistry or by direct mutational analysis. There is a concordance of 60 to 85% between immunohistochemistry and molecular analysis with both false positive and false negative staining reported.[89]

TP53 mutational status has also been correlated with response to both preoperative radiation and neoadjuvant chemoradiation in rectal adenocarcinoma. Rectal cancers with *TP53* mutations appear to be more resistant to treatment than those without mutation. In one of the studies, *TP53* overexpression also correlated with an increased likelihood of residual cancer in the lymph nodes in the resected specimen.[90]

18q Deletion It has been reported that patients with stage II colorectal cancer who had an allelic loss at 18q behaved like patients with stage III colorectal cancer.[91] Five-year survival was 93% and 54% in those patients with stage II colorectal cancer whose tumors had no deletion versus those with an 18q deletion, respectively. There was no difference in the frequency of 18q allelic loss between colon and rectal cancers. Survival in stage III patients was not affected by mutational status.[91] The majority of the studies reported have confirmed these findings, but there have been negative studies.

Microsatellite Instability Microsatellite instability (MSI) has been defined as microsatellite instability-high (MSI-H), microsatellite instability low (MSI-L), and microsatellite stable (MSS), depending on the number of unstable loci.[92] Tumors with high microsatellite instability (MSI-H) have been reported to have a better prognosis and to metastasize less often than patients whose tumors are stable. This has been confirmed in both HNPCC patients and in population-based studies of sporadic colorectal cancer patients.[21,93,94] In a population-based study in Ontario, Gryfe and colleagues reported that MSI-H tumors had a significantly better survival independent of other prognostic factors, and that these tumors were less likely to metastasize to regional lymph nodes or to distant sites.[93] Similar results were published in a population-based study in northern California and Utah.[94]

Microsatellite instability status of tumors has also been correlated with response to chemotherapy. Ribic and colleagues reported that patients with stage II or stage III tumors exhibiting low instability (MSI-L) or tumors that were stable (MSS) benefited from adjuvant 5-fluorouracil–based chemotherapy compared with patients with similar stage tumors that were MSI-H.[95] A literature review of 32 published studies where survival was analyzed according to MSI status by genotyping colorectal cancer cases stratified by MSI status confirmed the better prognosis and the suggestion that MSI-H tumors are resistant to 5-FU–based chemotherapy.[96] These findings have not as of yet been evaluated in a prospective randomized fashion.

Other Low Penetrance Alleles Loss of imprinting in normal mucosa and/or in lymphocytes of insulin-like growth factor II (IGF2) has been associated with increased risk of colorectal cancer.[97] A summary of other polymorphisms and their possible association with colorectal cancer has been published.[98]

Thymidylate Synthase, Thymidine Phosphorylase, and Dihydropyrimidine Dehydrogenase Thymidylate synthase (TS), thymidine phosphorylase (TP), and dihydropyrimidine dehydrogenase (DPD) are enzymes involved in the pyrimidine metabolism. Elevated intratumoral levels of thymidylate synthase and thymidine phosphorylase directly correlate with lack of response to 5-FU chemotherapy in the advanced disease setting.[99,100] Intratumoral levels of DPD, the rate-limiting enzyme in 5-FU catabolism, have also been reported to correlate inversely with response to 5-FU–based chemotherapy.[101]

There are other markers not included in the discussion that have been utilized in prognosis of colorectal cancer without consistent results. It is clear that prospective studies need to be done to evaluate prognostic value, and response to therapy whether radiation or chemotherapy alone or in combination. It is with tumor profiling that eventually the correlation between phenotypic, genotypic, and natural history of the tumor will be correlated and new tumor markers and targets for drug therapy will be discovered. The reader is referred to a review article by Iqbal and colleagues where the approach of tailored chemotherapy for colorectal cancer is discussed.[102]

COLORECTAL CANCER MANAGEMENT

Clinical presentation Colorectal cancer symptoms and signs are, in general, nonspecific. Unfortunately, the majority of patients with colorectal cancer are diagnosed because they have symptoms or signs. The most common presenting symptom of colon cancer is vague abdominal pain. In the rectum, patients most frequently complain of blood in the stools. Any patient who presents with either blood in the stools or rectal bleeding should be worked up. Rectal bleeding should not be attributed to hemorrhoids unless a complete evaluation has been performed.

Most of the time, right-sided tumors present less symptomatology than left-sided or rectal tumors. Commonly patients with right-sided tumors present with anemia. Left-sided or rectal cancer patients most commonly present with change in bowel habits or blood in the stools. Other symptoms of colorectal cancer include nausea, vomiting, bloating, diarrhea, tenesmus, constipation, and weight loss.

Partial or complete bowel obstructions as well as perforation, whether localized or free into the abdomen, are not uncommon presentations of colorectal cancer. Both of these situations carry a worse prognosis. In two prospective randomized trials of Dukes' B and C colorectal cancer, the National Surgical Adjuvant Breast and Bowel Project (NSABP) reported that patients with bowel obstruction were at greater risk of treatment failure than those without obstruction.[103] These investigators also reported that the effect of bowel obstruction was influenced by the location of the tumor. The occurrence of bowel obstruction in the right colon was associated with a significantly diminished disease-free survival, whereas obstruction in the left colon demonstrated no such effect.[103]

Perforation occurs most commonly at the site of the tumor itself or in the bowel proximal to the obstruction. These patients can present with localized peritonitis or diffuse peritonitis. In addition, they can be dehydrated, septic, and with electrolyte imbalances. All these factors add to the morbidity of emergent surgery. Perforation can result in adherence to adjacent organs or fistula formation. Concomitant perforation is not uncommon in patients with obstruction. The principles of surgical management are the same as with patients with obstructing carcinomas. Ideally, an attempt at resection should be performed. However, there are times that the inflammatory reaction or patient's condition precludes resection, and thus, it is safer to divert the patient and drain the perforation rather than embark on an unsafe surgical procedure. A downside of this approach is seeding of the drainage tract. The tract must be removed en bloc with the tumor at the time of definitive resection. This potential downside must be weighed with the complications of an unsafe resection through unclear planes in a potentially unstable patient.

Adherence to adjacent organs or fistula formation may be another presentation of colorectal cancer. Any intra-abdominal organ can be adhered to the tumor. These adhesions are malignant in nature in over 40% of the cases. Because clinically it cannot be determined whether the adhesions are inflammatory of malignant in nature, an en bloc resection must be performed. Performing less than an en bloc resection will increase recurrence rate and decrease survival.[104]

Some patients will present with carcinomatosis at the time of diagnosis. Peritoneal carcinomatosis carries a dire prognosis. Cytoreductive surgery combined with intraperitoneal hyperthermic chemotherapy has been shown to improve survival when compared with patients who underwent palliative resection and systemic chemotherapy.[105] Further randomized studies are being planned to confirm the utility of cytoreductive surgery in carcinomatosis.

Approximately 25% of patients with colorectal carcinoma present with metastatic disease. In these patients, symptomatology depends not only on the primary site, but also on the metastases. Usually hepatic and pulmonary metastases do not cause symptoms. However, bulky hepatic metastases may cause right upper quadrant pain. Ascites could be present secondary to carcinomatosis or hepatic metastases. In females, an ovarian or an adnexal mass may be the presenting sign. Fever of unknown origin is an uncommon presentation of metastatic colorectal cancer. Another uncommon presentation of colorectal cancer is *Streptococcus bovis* sepsis.

Preoperative Work-Up Once colorectal cancer has been diagnosed, preoperative evaluation must be performed to assess the best approach for treatment. Surgical resection is the procedure of choice for treatment. However, not all patients will be candidates for surgical resection. Some patients will have comorbidities that will preclude safe surgical resection. Others will have asymptomatic primary tumors with unresectable metastatic disease. The latter patients can be managed selectively with nonoperative therapy.[106] In patients with excessive comorbidities, palliation of the symptoms should be the goal. Endoscopic stents or laser therapy for obstructing tumors may be possible. In patients with bleeding tumors, fulguration, laser therapy, and, at times, radiation therapy may help.

A complete history including a detailed family history and physical examination should be performed on any patient who presents with colorectal adenocarcinoma. The work-up of colorectal cancer includes complete blood count (CBC), electrolytes and liver enzymes, carcinoembryonic antigen (CEA), urinalysis, coagulation profile, electrocardiogram, chest x-ray, and computed tomography (CT) scan of the abdomen and pelvis. If there is a rectal cancer, a transrectal ultrasound should be performed as well as a rigid proctoscopy. The former is useful in determining the pretreatment clinical stage of the tumor. The latter is useful in assessing the distance from the anal verge. Both of these factors are extremely important in the management of rectal adenocarcinoma. The colon should be evaluated for synchronous tumors, not only cancer, but also adenomas, preferably by colonoscopy. If colonoscopy cannot be performed prior to surgery because of obstruction, colonography may be an alternative. Otherwise, careful palpation of the colon should be performed at the time of surgery followed by a colonoscopy 3 to 6 months after recovery. FDG-PET scanning is still investigational in the evaluation of primary colorectal cancer.

SURGICAL MANAGEMENT OF COLORECTAL CANCER

Resection Margins Radical surgery with curative intent is the treatment of choice in the majority of colorectal cancers. The basic surgical principles are removal of the major vascular pedicle feeding the tumor along with its lymphatics, obtaining a tumor-free margin, and en bloc resection of any organs or structures attached to the tumor. True colonic mucosal recurrences are rare. More common are para-anastomotic recurrences reflecting possibly an inadequate lymphadenectomy. In colon cancer, it is recommended that at least a 5 cm margin of normal bowel be obtained on either side of the tumor in order to minimize the possibility of a local recurrence.[107] For right-sided tumors, the length of ileum apparently does not influence the local recurrence rate.[107] In rectal cancer surgery, retrospective studies have demonstrated that inadvertent perforation at the time of surgery occurs in approximately 7 to 25% of the cases and statistically reduces survival and

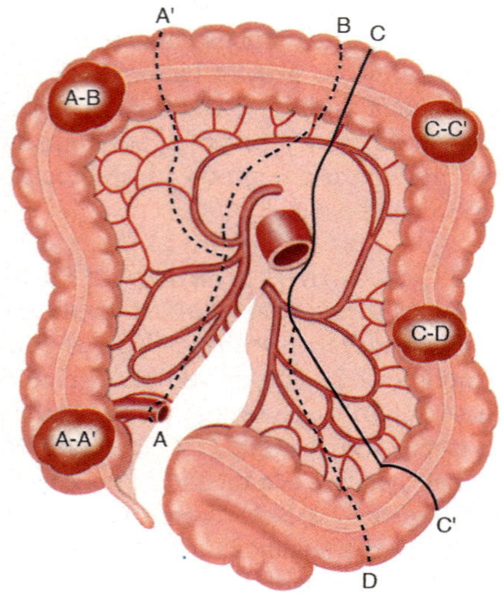

Figure 92-1 Segments of bowel and lymph node containing mesentry to be removed for carcinoma of the cecum (A–A'), hepatic flexure (A–B), splenic flexure (C–C'), and descending colon (C–D).

increases local recurrence.[107] The extent of resections are noted on Figures 92-1 and 92-2.

Curative resections in rectal cancer may require a permanent colostomy. As technology has advanced, so have the efforts to preserve sphincter function without compromising cure. A distal surgical margin of at least 2 cm in the fresh specimen is desired in rectal cancer resections.[107] Rarely, rectal adenocarcinomas will have distal submucosal spread. In patients with distal rectal adenocarcinomas at least a 1 cm margin of resection is desirable. Some authors have reported margins less than 1 cm in patients who received neoadjuvant chemoradiation and underwent sphincter saving procedures without compromising either recurrence or disease-free survival.[108,109]

Lymphadenectomy Performance of an adequate lymphadenectomy cannot be overemphasized. Adequate lymph node resection is imperative for staging and selection of patients for adjuvant treatment. In colon cancer, a minimum of 12 negative lymph nodes should be examined to confirm node-negative disease.[107] In rectal cancer, there is no evidence that high ligation of the inferior mesenteric artery offers any benefit over ligation at the level of the origin of the superior rectal artery. Even though it has been recommended that a minimum of 4 lymph nodes be examined for entry into adjuvant rectal trials, Tepper and colleagues reported that 14 lymph nodes need to be sampled to accurately define nodal status in rectal cancer accurately.[107,110] Four cm of attached distal mesorectum should be obtained with the resected specimen.[107] Routine extended lateral pelvic node dissection is not recommended in rectal cancer surgery. Metastases to these lymph nodes occur in about 10% of patients and imply a dire prognosis. If clinically indicated, an attempt to remove these lymph nodes at the time of surgery is warranted.

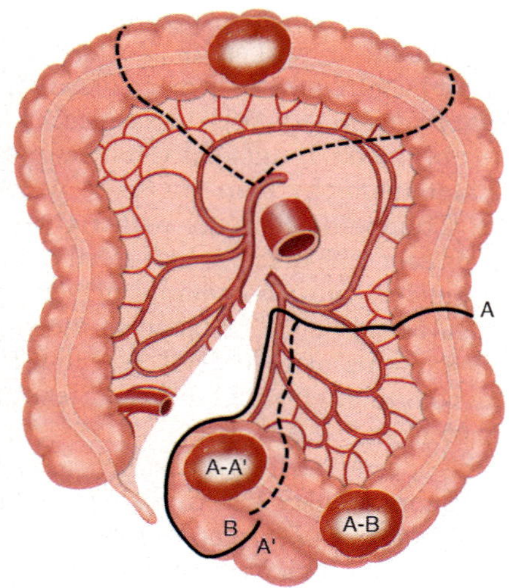

Figure 92-2 Segments of bowel and lymph node containing mesentry to be removed for carcinoma of the transverse colon, the apex of the sigmoid (A–B), and the lower sigmoid or rectosigmoid (A–A').

Sentinel lymph node mapping has changed the management of melanoma and breast cancer. At this time it appears not to have a major effect in altering therapy in colorectal cancer. By identifying the sentinel lymph node(s), immunohistochemical and molecular techniques can be utilized to evaluate for the presence of micrometastases otherwise not diagnosed by conventional pathology. In both single- and multi-institutional studies, it has been shown that lymphatic mapping is feasible in colon cancer patients and indeed may upstage 14 to 18% lymph node negative tumors to node positive status.[111,112] Not all studies have been encouraging. In a multi-institutional trial, Bertagnolli and colleagues reported that the sentinel node evaluated with multilevel sectioning failed to predict nodal status in 54% of patients.[113] The authors concluded that sentinel node examination with multilevel sectioning is unlikely to improve risk stratification for resectable colon cancer.[113] Sentinel lymph node for rectal cancer is more tedious and has not been as extensively evaluated as in colon cancer.

The significance of lymph node micrometastases in colorectal carcinoma is not known. Similar to reports of micrometastases in the bone marrow of patients with colorectal carcinoma undergoing curative resection, a report from the Netherlands suggested that lymphatic micrometastases adversely affected prognosis.[114] Prospective studies are needed to clarify the significance of molecular detection of lymphatic micrometastases.

Laparoscopic Colectomy Laparoscopic-assisted colectomy is a minimally invasive technique that has been gaining popularity in the management of colon and rectal cancer. The procedure consists of mobilization of the colon laparoscopically and performing an extracorporal anastomosis. In some situations, especially in the low sigmoid colon, an intracorporal anastomosis can be performed. In rectal cancer the technique is utilized to mobilize the mesorectum. The main potential benefits from laparoscopic colectomy have been earlier postoperative recovery and less narcotic use. The Clinical Outcomes of Surgical

Therapy Study Group (COST) conducted a multi-institutional prospective randomized trial comparing laparoscopic-assisted colectomy with open colectomy for colorectal cancer in the United States. After 3 years of follow-up, there were no differences in recurrence rates, wound recurrence rates, survival, or complication rates.[115] In that trial, patients undergoing laparoscopically assisted colectomy had a shorter median hospital stay and briefer use of parenteral narcotics and oral analgesics than those undergoing open colectomy.[115] Therefore, the equivalency of laparoscopic-assisted colectomy in experienced surgeons (performing > 20 procedures) to open colectomy has been established by the COST trial. Laparoscopic rectal cancer surgery is being performed, but it has not been evaluated and reported in randomized controlled trials.

Management of Carcinoma in Polyp It is not uncommon for the clinician to be faced with a patient who had an invasive carcinoma in an adenoma. The treatment in these patients has to be individualized. Favorable histopathological characteristics are free margins of resection, well- or moderately well-differentiated adenocarcinoma, and no lymphatic or vascular invasion. In addition, the endoscopist has to be confident that the lesion was completely removed. If these characteristics are met, and the polyp is limited to the submucosa, the incidence of lymph node metastases is less than 5%, but not zero.[116] There are patients who will not tolerate the risk of having lymph node metastases, and therefore will choose surgical resection. Since the majority of the surgical resections will not reveal residual cancer and/or lymph node metastases, it is important to balance the surgical risks with the benefits of the procedure and discuss them clearly with the patient. In patients who choose endoscopic follow-up, colonoscopy should be performed 3 months after endoscopic polypectomy to evaluate the area of excision. If the colonoscopy is normal, then colonoscopy follow-up is repeated in 1 year and, if normal, in 3 years time. Polyps where the cancer has invaded into the muscularis propria should not be treated by endoscopic excision unless surgery resection is contraindicated. The incidence of lymph node metastases in T2 lesions is as high as 20%.

Local Therapy for Rectal Adenocarcinoma Local therapy has been evaluated in selected patients with rectal adenocarcinoma. These therapies include electrofulguration, endocavitary radiation with or without brachytherapy, and local excision with or without external beam radiation or chemoradiation. Of these techniques, local excision has the advantage of providing a specimen for pathological evaluation. Surgical approaches to local excision include transanal, transsacral, or transsphincteric approaches. The latter two procedures are less commonly performed than transanal procedure.

Full thickness transanal local excision has been used for selected small (≤ 4cm) rectal tumors. Patients are staged clinically with history and physical exam, CAT scan of the abdomen and pelvis, and transrectal ultrasound. Patients with clinically enlarged lymph nodes or fixed tumors are not considered good candidates for local excision. Ideally the tumor should be easily palpated during rectal exam, be mobile, and should not involve greater than 40% of the bowel circumference. After full thickness excision, the histopathology is examined. Patients without disease extension to the muscularis propria (T1 tumors) and with favorable histology (moderate or well differentiated) have a local failure risk of < 10%. Because of the low overall risk of recurrence, postoperative chemoradiation is not usually recommended. Patients who have poorly differentiated T1 tumors or T2 tumors with any differentiation have routinely been treated with postoperative chemoradiation in order to reduce the risk of pelvic recurrence. Initial reports with short follow-up were very encouraging and stimulated a significant amount of enthusiasm. Postoperative radiation is recommended among T1 tumors with unfavorable characteristics or T2 tumors because the local disease recurrence risk is about 20%.[117,118]

In the Cancer and Leukemia Group B (CALGB) multi-institutional trial of local excision for T1 tumors and local excision and chemoradiation for T2 tumors, at a median 48 months follow-up, the 6-year actuarial survival and failure-free rates for the eligible T1 and T2 patients were 85% and 78%, respectively.[119] There were 4 failures (2 local only, 1 distant only, and 1 local and distant) in 59 T1 patients. In 51 T2 patients there were 10 recurrences (5 local only, 2 local and distant, and 3 distant only). The salvage rate for local recurrences only was over 50%, but with a short follow-up reported.[119] A retrospective analysis from the University of Minnesota revealed a recurrence rate of 18% and 37% in patients undergoing local excision alone for T1 and T2 tumors, respectively.[120] These investigators subsequently published their results of salvage radical surgery in 29 patients after failed local excision.[121] Twenty-three of 29 patients had surgery with curative intent. At a mean follow-up of 39 months, the disease-free survival was 59%.[121]

Local excision has been used after preoperative (chemo) radiation in medically inoperable patients and patients who refuse abdominal perineal resection and in those patients whose tumors have had a complete or near complete clinical response after neoadjuvant chemoradiation has been reported.[122–124] However, the follow-up in the latter studies is short, and there have been reports of lymph node metastases in specimens of pathologically T0 tumors after neoadjuvant chemoradiation.[125] Another approach has been observation in patients who achieve clinical complete response to chemoradiation. There has been a single report of high local control and survival in such patients without surgery.[126] These results require further validation. Local excision or observation after clinical complete response after neoadjuvant therapy is investigational and should be performed only in the context of a clinical trial.

Endocavitary radiation (contact therapy) is a technique that administers very high doses of radiation that is concentrated in the tumor with minimal radiation dose to surrounding tissues. This treatment is appropriate for medically inoperable patients, or patients who refuse surgery, or early small rectal tumors.

Management of Patients Who Present with Synchronous Distant Metastases The initial management strategy in patients who present with distant metastases from colorectal cancer is controversial. Commonly, patients are treated initially with surgery followed by systemic therapy, and symptomatic patients should be considered for surgical palliation prior to being offered chemotherapy. However, nonsurgical options for asymptomatic patients have gained popularity as the chemotherapy regimens become more effective. Initial chemoradiation has been used with some success instead of nontherapeutic colostomy in rectal cancer patients when systemic options were more limited. Durable symptomatic palliation was achieved in 80% of patients and colostomy was avoided in 90%.[127] The clinical activity and survival improvements for colorectal cancer patients who have been seen with the new chemotherapeutic regimens introduced in recent years makes the use of front-line chemotherapy very appealing in patients with synchronous metastatic and asymptomatic intact primary disease. However, surgery and radiotherapy should be considered for symptomatic patients.

Local Recurrence In contrast to rectal cancer, colon cancer is frequently resected with wide negative margins and local recurrences are less of a problem. In a retrospective analysis, patients with T4 N0 or T4 N1 colon cancer were first shown to have an approximately 30 to 50% local failure rate and a 10% isolated local failure rate.[128] Subsequently, postoperative radiation was used and higher local disease control and disease-free survival rates were seen in these patients.[129,130] The indications for postoperative chemoradiation (50.4 Gy to the tumor bed) are invasion of surrounding organs and tumor perforation of the visceral peritoneum (T4 disease). This therapy is typically given with concurrent continuous infusion of 5-FU and integrated with the adjuvant chemotherapy.[128] The results of the only randomized trial evaluating the role of postoperative chemoradiation in patients with colon cancer who had either T3 N1 or T3 N2 or tumor adherence to or invasion of surrounding structures have been published. Patients were randomized to receive bolus 5-FU and levamisole for one year with or without radiotherapy.[131] There was no detectable difference in overall survival between the two arms, but the authors acknowledge that clinically significant differences in survival could not be excluded because the study was terminated early owing to poor accrual.

Local recurrence after surgery alone for operable rectal cancer has been reported to be between 25 and 50% for stage II and III rectal adenocarcinoma.[132] These high recurrence rates are probably the result of incomplete dissection of the mesorectum. However, with total mesorectal excision, the risk of local recurrence is significantly lower. In the Dutch total mesorectal excision trial, a randomized prospective trial, local recurrence was 8.2% after total mesorectal excision (TME) alone for resectable rectal cancer.[133]

The major risk factors for pelvic tumor recurrence include nodal involvement and tumor penetration beyond the bowel wall (T3 and T4 disease). Extension of tumor into the perirectal fat or adjacent viscera increases the rate of local recurrence to approximately 25 to 50% with surgery alone.[132] The extent of tumor penetration beyond the bowel wall is also a significant factor predicting for recurrence risk. Willet and colleagues examined a group of patients with T3 N0 rectal cancer who underwent resection alone. Surgical specimens were assessed for maximum depth of tumor invasion into perirectal fat, lymphatic or venous involvement, and tumor grade.[134] Local tumor control correlated with increasing extent of tumor penetration beyond the rectal wall. Tumor penetration more than 2 mm led to a > 20% local recurrence rate. In 25 patients with tumors with favorable histological features (well-differentiated or moderately well-differentiated carcinomas invading less than 2 mm into perirectal fat, without lymphatic or venous vessel involvement), the 10-year actuarial rates of local control and recurrence-free survival were 95% and 87%, respectively.[134] The anatomic location of the tumor also correlates with the risk of tumor recurrence. Tumors that are lower in the pelvis are more difficult to resect with wide negative margins because of physical anatomic restrictions. Several clinical experiences bear this out, including the Dutch TME Trial.[133,135,136] Although the factors are probably interrelated, the width of radial margins of resection has also been correlated with the risk of pelvic tumor recurrence in patients who undergo surgery alone. In the Dutch TME Trial, patients who were randomized to total mesorectal excision alone whose resected tumors had at least a 1 cm negative radial margin had 5-year pelvic tumor recurrence risk of less than 5%. A margin of ≤ 2 mm was associated with a local recurrence risk of 16% ($p < .0001$).[137] The radial margin of excision can also serve as an indicator of the quality of the surgery. In the Dutch trial, in a sample of 656 patients who underwent total mesorectal excision alone, 18.3% ($n = 120$) had a positive circumferential margin after curative resection.[137] Patients undergoing abdominoperineal resection (APR) had a higher incidence (28.8%) than those undergoing low anterior resection (LAR) (13.5%).[137] Distant metastases occurred in 37.6% of patients with positive circumferential margins, whereas it was 12.7% in patients with > 1 cm margin.[137] Systematic macroscopic evaluation of the mesorectum was performed in 180 specimens of patients undergoing TME.[138] Almost 24% of the patients had an incomplete mesorectal excision as defined by the pathologist.[138] Even though the follow-up was short, there was a statistically significant difference in survival in patients with a macroscopically incomplete TME.[138] However, there was no statistically significant difference in local recurrence.[138]

In the INT-0114, lower body mass index and female sex correlated with sphincter preservation.[139] Obese men, but not obese women, had significantly worse sphincter preservation and pelvic control.[139] These outcomes are possibly related to the mechanical difficulties associated with adiposity and with operating in the comparatively narrow male pelvis. In summary, the major risk factors for tumor recurrence in patients with resected rectal cancer treated with resection alone include tumor penetration of the muscularis propria (and the extent of penetration), nodal involvement, the number of negative nodes in node-negative patients, and the width of the radial margin. The ability to achieve negative margins and optimize pelvic tumor control is also related to adiposity in male patients. Other favorable factors for local control that are probably not independent include tumor grade and lymphovascular space invasion. Thus a highly selected subgroup of patients with T3 N0 tumors and T1-2 N1 tumors, may have a low risk of tumor recurrence with no further therapy.[140] This concept would be an interesting one to study on a prospective trial.

ADJUVANT THERAPY FOR COLORECTAL CANCER

It is known that not all cancer cells are capable of the complex processes involved in the development of distant metastasis.[141] Experimental studies conducted by collecting blood from the renal vein from patients with renal cell carcinomas clearly demonstrated that the majority of cancer cells that are shed in the circulation cannot survive and die before they are able to establish a new cancer focus at a different site, indicating that the metastatic process is actually quite inefficient.[142] Unfortunately, cancer cells are genetically unstable, and given enough time a clone capable of traveling and metastasizing is likely to develop.[143] Currently, the best indicator whether the cancer cells in a particular colorectal cancer have developed this ability is the pathological staging, which is determined by the depth of tumor penetration and by the presence of metastasis in adjacent lymph nodes.[144] The expected 5-year overall survival rates are now generally over 80% for patients without lymph node involvement, but drops dramatically once they are involved. Moreover, the chance of recurrence is directly related to the number of lymph nodes affected.[144] Unfortunately, although there are available detection methods capable of identifying a few cancer cells in the patient's blood, lymph nodes, and bone marrow, none of these methods are capable of determining if those cells are viable, and they cannot be used to determine which patients should receive treatment. Until better prognostic tools are available, adjuvant chemotherapy will continue to be administered to all patients at risk to address the possible presence of micrometastases, with the understanding that some patients already cured will be unnecessarily exposed to cytotoxic therapy.

When considering adjuvant therapy in any patient, age alone should not be a factor in offering adjuvant chemotherapy. Retrospective studies have consistently shown that chemotherapy not only benefits elderly patients with metastatic colorectal cancer, but also that adjuvant chemotherapy does benefit eligible elderly patients just as well as younger ones.[145] In a pooled analysis of adjuvant chemotherapy in resected elderly patients with stage II and III colon cancer, 5-FU and leucovorin improved the 5-year overall survival from 64 to 71% ($p = .001$), and the 5-year disease-free survival from 58 to 69% compared with surgery alone.[146] Toxicity was not significantly different from that seen among younger patients.

Colon Cancer Numerous adjuvant trials were conducted in the United States and around the world in the early decades of oncology, but all failed to demonstrate a significant improvement over surgery alone until the late 1980s and early 1990s. The major breakthrough came when the North Central Cancer Treatment Group (NCCTG) and the Mayo Clinic first reported that 5-FU and levamisole given for 1 year after curative resection for stage III colon cancer patients decreased recurrence rates and improved survival when compared with surgery alone.[147] These results opened the horizon and offered hope for colorectal cancer patients. There are several agents such as oral fluropyrimidines, oxaliplatin, and irinotecan that have been tested in the adjuvant setting with exciting results.

Adjuvant therapy after curative resection for stage III colon cancer is the standard of care. Its use in stage II colon cancer is controversial. To detect an absolute 4% reduction in deaths at 5 years, with a 90% power, over 4,700 patients with stage II colorectal would be needed, and although many individual trials included stage II colon cancer patients, they were underpowered to yield a definitive result. Three meta-analyses from NSABP, NCCTG, and IMPACT (International Multicenter Pooled Analysis of Colon Cancer Trial) all suggested that adjuvant 5-FU and leucovorin (LV) marginally improved both disease-free survival and overall survival in patients with stage II colon cancer.[148,149] All meta-analyses showed a 2% and 4% increase in disease-free survival and in overall survival associated with 5-FU and LV compared with observation.[148,149]

As previously discussed, there are subsets of patients who are at increased risk of systemic and/or local recurrence. The risk factors include, among others, tumors with perforation or invasion of adjacent organs (T4), bowel obstruction, lymphovascular and perineural invasion, poor differentiation, presence of 18q and possibly microsatellite stability. These tumors are considered high-risk stage II and are usually treated with adjuvant chemotherapy. However, the importance of these molecular markers and other prognostic factors cannot be overemphasized, and they should be evaluated in the context of prospective adjuvant trials. Selection of stage II patients for adjuvant treatment should also take into account the patient's age and life expectancy, performance status, medical comorbidities, and the number of lymph nodes sampled. Ideally, stage II patients should be enrolled in a clinical trial when available.

The results published by Laurie and Moertel on the benefit of 5-FU and levamisole in stage III colon cancer patients were later confirmed in the intergroup 0035 study.[147,150] This study, which was considerably larger, effectively established the role of adjuvant 5-FU and levamisole in resected stage III colon cancer patients.[150] At a median of 3 years after curative resection, adjuvant treatment with 5-FU and levamisole decreased the risk of cancer recurrence by 41% and the overall death rate by 36% compared with surgery alone or surgery and levamisole in patients with stage III colon cancer.[150]

At the same time that 5-FU and levamisole was being developed in the adjuvant setting, the combination of 5-FU and leucovorin (LV) was gaining momentum in the metastatic setting, being used in a number of regimens. In the United States the two most commonly used regimens were the Mayo Clinic regimen using bolus 5-FU 425 mg/m^2/day and leucovorin 20 mg/m^2/day, days 1 to 5 every 28 days, and the Roswell Park regimen using bolus 5-FU 500 mg/m^2 and leucovorin 500 mg/m^2 weekly for 6 weeks every 8 weeks. Considering the activity of 5-FU and leucovorin against metastatic colon cancer, it was not surprising that 5FU/LV was rapidly moved into the adjuvant setting.

The next logical step was the comparison of 6 months of 5-FU and leucovorin versus 1 year of 5-FU and levamisole. Among the several trials that were designed and conducted at the time, at least two deserve to be discussed in greater detail. The first is the NSABP C-04, which compared 5-FU and levamisole for 1 year versus 5-FU and leucovorin or 5-FU, leucovorin, and levamisole for 6 months in patients with Dukes' B and C colon cancer.[151] There were no significant differences in 5-year disease-free survival or mortality among the three different regimens. However, pairwise comparison between 5-FU with leucovorin and 5-FU with levamisole revealed that the patients who received 5-FU and leucovorin had an improvement in disease-free survival (65% vs 60%; p = .04) and a nonstatistical significant trend toward improved overall survival (74% vs 70%; p = .06). There was no added benefit by using the three-drug combination, and levamisole did not add to 5-FU/LV.

The second important trial conducted around the same time was the INT-0089 trial, which with 3,759 patients was designed by the intergroup to be the largest adjuvant trial ever conducted. It basically confirmed the results of the NSABP C-04, showing that patients receiving 6 months of 5-FU, leucovorin, and levamisole had a 5-year survival rate of 67% compared with 63% for those patients who received 5-FU and levamisole for 12 months, and no benefit for the triple regimen.[144]

The combination of studies showing that 6 months of 5-FU and leucovorin was similar to 12 months of 5-FU and levamisole lead to the adoption of 6 months of 5-FU and leucovorin as the preferred adjuvant treatment of stage III colon cancer patients. Since the use of neither the high or the low dose of leucovorin seemed to be superior, both regimens became acceptable. However, there is mounting evidence that the toxicity of the Mayo regimen, particularly mucositis and neutropenia, is more pronounced than that of the weekly Roswell Park regimen, which is associated with more diarrhea, or the protracted regimens of intravenous 5-FU or capecitabine, commonly associated with diarrhea and hand-and-foot syndrome. Table 92-4 illustrates some of the adjuvant trials in stage III colon cancer.

Table 92-4 Recent Adjuvant Trials for Colon Cancer

Study/Author	Patients	Stage	Regimen	Disease-Free Survival (%)	p-Value
X-ACT/Cassidy et al[213]	1987	III	5-FU/LV	60.6	.528
			Capecitabine	64.2	
MOSAIC/Andre et al[152]	2246	II and III	LV5FU2	72.9	.002
			FOLFOX4	78.2	
NSABP-CO7/Wolmark et al[157]	2492	II and III	5-FU/LV	71.6	< .004
			5-FU/LV/Oxaliplatin	76.5	
PETACC 3*/Van Cutsem et al[155]	2094*	III*	LVFU2	60.3	.091
			FOLFIRI	63.3	

*Included 3,005 patients with II and III but results presented for stage III patients only
5-FU/LV: 5-fluorouracil and leucovorin given as a bolus
LV5FU2: 5-fluorouracil and leucovorin given as a protracted infusion
FOLFOX4: 5-fluorouracil and leucovorin given as a protracted infusion with oxaliplatin
FOLFIRI: 5-fluorouracil and leucovorin given as a protracted infusion with irinotecan

In the Multicenter International Study of Oxaliplatin, 5-FU and leucovorin in the Adjuvant Treatment of Colon Cancer (MOSAIC), 2,246 patients with completely resected stage II and III colon cancer were randomly assigned to adjuvant treatment with either the infusional LV5-FU2 regimen of 5-FU and leucovorin, or the FOLFOX4 regimen, which is made up with the same LV5-FU2 regimen plus oxaliplatin 85 mg/m^2 given every 2 weeks for 12 cycles.[152] The results showed that the FOLFOX4 combination was relatively safe, although peripheral neuropathy was quite common among the treated patients. The most severe grade 3 neurotoxicity was observed in 12% of the patients. The primary endpoint of the study was 3-year disease-free survival, and it was significantly better for the FOLFOX4 arm (78.2% vs 72.9%; p = .002), corresponding to a 23% decrease in risk of recurrence in comparison to the 5-FU and leucovorin arm. The benefit was clearer in the stage III setting, with a hazard ratio (HR) of 0.76 (95% CI 0.62–0.92). Patients with stage II disease appeared to benefit from the treatment with a HR of 0.80, but it is important to note that the 95% CI overlapped 1 (0.56–1.15), and the use of this regimen for stage II patients remains a matter of controversy. The positive results from the MOSAIC trial were further confirmed by the almost identical preliminary results of the NSABP C-07 trial, which compared bolus 5-FU and leucovorin following the Roswell-Park regimen versus the same regimen plus oxaliplatin every 2 weeks.[153]

Based on the available data, on November 2004, the US Food and Drug Administration (FDA) approved oxaliplatin in combination with infusional 5-FU (FOLFOX) as an adjuvant treatment of stage III colon cancer. At the present time, the use of FOLFOX in the adjuvant setting is favored in patients with stage III disease unless they are unwilling or unable to tolerate the potential toxicities.

Several studies have been designed and conducted with irinotecan in the adjuvant setting, and two are of particular importance: the Cancer and Leukemia Group B (CALGB) C89803 study and the European PETACC-3. In the CALGB study, 1,260 patients were randomized after resection of stage III colon cancer to receive either weekly 5-FU and leucovorin following the Roswell Park regimen or bolus 5-FU and leucovorin plus irinotecan, following the classic, irinotecan, fluorouracil and leucovorin (IFL) regimen.[154] Increased mortality was observed in the IFL arm compared with the 5-FU and leucovorin arm, with a 60-day mortality of 2.5% in the IFL group and 0.8% in the control group. The excess mortality appeared to be associated with a gastrointestinal syndrome of multiple, often simultaneous, toxicities (diarrhea, vomiting, cramping, dehydration, electrolyte changes) or a vascular syndrome of unexpected thromboembolic events (myocardial infarction, pulmonary embolus, cerebrovascular insult). Although certainly more aggressive, the IFL regimen was not more effective, and there was no added benefit by the addition of irinotecan in this study. The PETACC 3 study was designed using two different schedules of 5-FU by infusion given either alone or with irinotecan for 6 months in the adjuvant setting. Primary endpoint was disease-free survival only for those patients with stage III who received either the LV5FU2 regimen of 5-FU and leucovorin or the same regimen plus irinotecan (FOLFIRI).[155] Patients with stage II disease, or who received a weekly regimen of 5-FU and leucovorin with or without irinotecan were to be included in the secondary analysis. Preliminary results failed to achieve its primary endpoint,[155] and further follow-up is needed for a final conclusion on the role of irinotecan in the adjuvant setting. Until then, this agent cannot be recommended in the adjuvant setting.

Because most patients would appreciate the option of receiving 6 months of treatment with an oral medication instead of an intravenous one, two oral fluoropyrimidines, UFT and capecitabine, have been tested in large, well-designed trials. UFT is a combination of the 5-FU prodrug tegafur with uracil, a natural substrate for dihydropyrimidine dehydrogenase (DPD), the enzyme responsible for the degradation of 5-FU in the human body.[156] The NSABP conducted the C-06 trial comparing the use of 6 months of 5-FU and leucovorin using the Roswell Park regimen versus the oral UFT with leucovorin.[157] The final results showed that there were no significant differences in the disease-free survival or in the overall survival for both groups, and UFT with leucovorin is an acceptable alternative to the use of intravenous 5-FU and leucovorin in the adjuvant setting.[157] Capecitabine is an oral fluoropyrimidine that has been shown to have higher response rates and a better toxicity profile than 5-FU when used in first-line treatment of metastatic colorectal cancer.[158] Capecitabine was investigated as an adjuvant treatment of resected stage III colon cancer in the phase III "X-ACT" trial. A total of 1,987 patients were randomized to receive capecitabine at 1,250 mg/m^2 twice a day for 14 days, followed by 7 days of rest for eight cycles, or to bolus 5-FU and leucovorin following the Mayo Clinic regimen for 6 months after full resection of stage III colon cancer.[159] Capecitabine had a better safety profile than 5-FU/LV, with significantly ($p < .001$) less diarrhea, nausea/vomiting, and stomatitis of any grade. Patients treated with capecitabine also had significantly less grade 3/4 neutropenia, while those treated with 5-FU/LV had significantly less grade 3/4 hand-and-foot syndrome.(all, $p < .001$).[159] Efficacy results from the X-ACT trial confirmed that the disease-free survival and overall survival were at least equivalent for both regimens. In fact, there was a strong trend for better 3-year disease-free interval (DFS) in the capecitabine arm ($p = .04$).[159] Capecitabine offers a very good alternative to 5-FU for patients who may benefit from a fluoropyrimidine-only adjuvant treatment. The combination of capecitabine and oxaliplatin is now being tested against 5-FU and LV.

The role of chemoradiation in locally advanced colon cancer remains unclear, but based on the retrospective data reviewed above, it can be offered to patients with pathologically staged T4 tumors. There is no evidence that patients with T3 tumors should be offered radiotherapy routinely.

Ongoing and Future Adjuvant Colon Trials There are still a sizable number of patients who will develop metastatic disease despite the best available treatment. The advent of effective molecular targeted agents made them obvious targets for future trials in colon cancer. The NSABP has designed and is currently conducting the C-08 trial, comparing the use of 6 months of modified FOLFOX6 regimen with the same regimen for 6 months and bevacizumab for 1 year. Another trial, known as AVANT, is being conducted worldwide with a similar design but with the addition of a third arm, where patients receive 6 months of capecitabine and oxaliplatin and 1 year of bevacizumab. There are no results available for either trial at this point.

The current American intergroup trial (INT-0147) has opted to investigate the impact of a different monoclonal antibody in the adjuvant setting. It has a three by two design; patients are first randomly assigned to receive either modified FOLFOX6 for 6 months, FOLFIRI for 6 months, or a hybrid regimen of modified FOLFOX6 for 3 months followed by FOLFIRI for 3 months. A second randomization assigns patients to receive cetuximab or not. Despite its interesting design, this is a complicated trial and accrual has been slow.

Rectal Cancer Presently, combined-modality therapy reduces, but does not eliminate, the risk of local and distant recurrence and is considered standard care in stage II and III rectal cancer. There is a one-third to two-thirds risk reduction. The major benefit may actually be in the reduced frequency of distant metastases and improvement in survival. Improved local control alone usually does not correspond to improved overall survival. Adequate surgical resection is the mainstay of treatment of rectal adenocarcinoma. The availability of adjuvant and neoadjuvant therapy has encouraged surgeons to be more aggressive in treatment, including treatment of metastatic disease. As the local recurrence rate decreased to the single digits with TME, the practice of adjuvant use of chemoradiation has been, selectively, decreased without proof. The role of chemotherapy alone as a replacement for combined-modality therapy has rarely been tested, and its success or its equivalence to well-tested chemoradiation, is not established.

Preoperative Chemoradiation Several advantages of preoperative chemoradiation over postoperative chemoradiation for rectal cancer have been appreciated. Mobilizing small bowel out of the radiotherapy field can reduce toxicity. This can be accomplished more commonly in patients who have not undergone laparotomy.[160] The use of preoperative chemoradiation can lead to increased sphincter preservation rates.[161–164] Since the irradiated rectum is removed and unirradiated colon can be used to form a reconstructed rectum, the long-term rectal function should be better. However, these points are controversial. Tissue perfusion is uninterrupted in patients who are treated preoperatively. This leads to better drug delivery and better oxygenation. Since oxygen enhances the effects of ionizing radiation, radiotherapy efficacy should increase. Randomized data also indicate that preoperative radiotherapy alone leads to increased local control compared to postoperative chemoradiation.[165] The main disadvantage of preoperative chemoradiation is that since clinical staging has some limitations, some patients may be treated unnecessarily. The number of such patients can be minimized with the use of endoscopic ultrasound. When surgery is performed first, patients can be selected for postoperative chemoradiation based on T-stage, N-stage, margin status, distance from the anal verge, and other prognostic factors. Some clinicians are concerned that the use of preoperative radiotherapy will increase perioperative morbidity. However, it appears that perioperative morbidity is not increased in centers that routinely use preoperative therapy. Surgical experience is an important factor in lowering perioperative morbidity rates in irradiated rectal cancer patients. For example, perioperative complication rates at the University of Texas M. D. Anderson Cancer Center decreased with time after preoperative therapy was introduced.[166] The use of diverting ileostomy while the anastomosis heals is important to reduce perioperative anastomotic leaks, particularly in patients with low rectal anastomosis. Prospective trials have been designed to address this controversy by the Radiation Therapy Oncology Group (RTOG) and NSABP, but the established practice patterns were so rigid that the studies suffered from poor accrual and had to be closed prematurely.

The German CAO/ARO/AIO trial comparing preoperative chemoradiation to postoperative chemoradiation has recently been reported.[164] Patients ($n = 823$) were staged with CT scan and endoscopic ultrasound. Clinical stage T3 or T4 tumors were then randomized to receive either preoperative or postoperative chemoradiation (50.4 Gy in 28 fractions with concurrent high dose infusional 5-FU 1,000 mg/m2/day on days 1–5 and 21–25). Those assigned to the preoperative arm had a lower pelvic recurrence rate (6% vs 13%; $p = .0006$), as well as lower grade III or IV acute (27% vs 40%; $p = .001$) and late toxicity (14% vs 24%; $p = .01$). Overall survival was unchanged. Additional benefits included increased sphincter preservation in patients who were felt to require abdominoperineal resection based on clinical evaluation (39% vs 19%; $p = .004$) and less evidence of anastomotic stricture.[164] This trial has widely been interpreted as having defined the standard of care in the adjuvant treatment of rectal cancer.

Currently, there are different standards of care in some institutions in Europe than in the United States with regard to the dose and schedule of preoperative radiotherapy. In Europe, investigators have established the benefit of preoperative short-course (also known as hypofractionated) radiotherapy (25 Gy/5 fractions/1 week) alone followed by immediate surgery. In the United States, standard preoperative doses range from 45 Gy to 54 Gy at 1.8 Gy/fraction. Concurrent protracted venous infusional 5-FU chemotherapy is routinely administered and surgery is typically delayed for 6 to 8 weeks to allow the tumor to shrink and the patient to recover from the acute toxicities.

Many trials conducted in Europe have demonstrated a pelvic control benefit with the addition of hypofractionated radiotherapy over surgery alone, but only the Swedish Rectal Trial demonstrated a survival benefit. In the Dutch TME Trial patients who received a short course of preoperative radiation (25 Gy/5 fractions in 1 week) and underwent surgical resection with TME had a local recurrence rate of 2.4% compared with 8.2% in those patients who underwent resection with total mesorectal excision alone.[133] In the Swedish trial, preoperative radiotherapy (25 Gy/5 fractions in 1 week) was followed by surgery within 1 week. Improvements were seen in local control (73% vs 89%; $p < .001$), overall survival (58% vs 48%; $p = .004$).[167] This study is the only trial with enough power (1,168 patients) to detect small differences in survival. In addition to being underpowered, previous trials had high perioperative mortality rates in irradiated patients.[168] The perioperative mortality rate has decreased with the use of smaller fields and multiple field techniques.[169] A meta-analysis of 14 randomized trials evaluating preoperative radiotherapy (most using short course) versus surgical resection alone (6,426 patients) was performed.[170] No overall increase in postoperative mortality was reported with radiotherapy except in the trials that failed to use a multiple field technique. Preoperative radiotherapy was found to reduce the 5-year overall mortality rate, cancer-related mortality rate, and local recurrence rate.[170] Furthermore, a detailed analysis by Suwinski and colleagues looked at the effect of time, dose, and fractionation factors using published data from single arm and comparative trials as well as retrospective studies reporting results using preoperative radiotherapy alone. The authors concluded that the percent reduction in pelvic recurrence is comparable in the accelerated hypofractionated schedule (25 Gy/5 fractions/1 week) when compared with the standard schedule (45–50 Gy at 2 Gy/fraction).[171] Thus from an efficacy standpoint, the short-course and standard 5-week approaches are probably similar. However, the potential disadvantages of the short-course approach are that time is not usually allowed for tumor regression prior to surgery, there may be increased perioperative and/or late morbidity and mortality, and radiosensitizing effects of concurrent chemotherapy cannot be fully exploited. Tumor regression with time may contribute to sphincter preservation.[163] This question has been the topic of a randomized trial conducted in Lyon, France. Patients were treated with preoperative radiotherapy alone (39 Gy in 13 fractions) and randomized to a 2-week surgical interval or a 6 to 8 week interval. Pathologic response was significantly increased after the longer interval (26% vs 11%). With regard to toxicity of short-course therapy, the Stockholm trials identified advantages of combined modality therapy, but significant late morbidity and mortality was also observed. Neuropathy, thromboembolism, femoral neck and pelvic fractures, intestinal obstruction, postoperative fistulae, and perioperative death all occurred with a higher frequency than one would expect with standard fractionation.[169] The number of these events to a certain extent were reduced with improved techniques, multiple fields, and dropping the superior border from L2 to the L5/S1 interspace.[167,172] The most recent studies of hypofractionated preoperative radiation (the Swedish Rectal Trial and the Dutch Mesorectal Trial) have reported lower treatment-related morbidity and mortality.[167,173]

In Europe, the use of concurrent chemotherapy with radiotherapy in the preoperative setting had been controversial until recently. The European Organization for the Research and Treatment of Cancer (EORTC) 22921 and the French Federation of Digestive Cancer (FFCD) 9203 trials both evaluated the addition of 5-FU to preoperative standard fractionation radiotherapy.[174,175] The results were consistent between the studies and showed that 5-FU improved pelvic control, but not sphincter preservation or disease-free or overall survival. The use of concurrent 5-FU in the preoperative setting can also be extrapolated from postoperative data.[176]

Postoperative Chemoradiation for Rectal Cancer The use of postoperative chemoradiation (50.4–54 Gy with protracted venous infusion 5-FU 225 mg/m^2/day) and adjuvant chemotherapy (2 months of 5-FU and leucovorin before and 2 months after chemoradiation) in patients with resected stage II and III rectal cancer was established by early randomized trials that evaluated treatment designed to improve the outcome of rectal cancer patients. The Gastrointestinal Tumor Study Group (GITSG) Trial randomized patients to one of four treatment arms: (1) surgery alone, (2) surgery followed by postoperative radiotherapy (40–48 Gy), (3) surgery followed by postoperative chemotherapy (bolus 5-FU and semustine), and (4) surgery followed by postoperative concurrent radiotherapy (40–48 Gy) and chemotherapy (bolus 5-FU and semustine). After an early analysis, the combined modality arm was found to be superior and the trial was discontinued after 227 patients had been accrued. Thus, there was a clear pelvic control and relapse-free survival benefit observed with combined modality therapy compared with surgical resection alone. A survival difference was later reported after more follow-up.[177] Although differences were observed between the other arms, the study did not have enough power to determine the statistical significance of small differences. However, the single modality arms did have different patterns of failure. The addition of radiation therapy decreased the incidence of local failure and the chemotherapy alone arm decreased the incidence of distant disease as the initial forms of disease recurrence. The local failure rate in the chemotherapy alone arm was 27%, which compared with 11% in the combined modality arm and 24% in the control arm.[178] These observations supported the incorporation of an adjuvant chemotherapy component in the design of future studies.

The Mayo/NCCTG subsequently conducted a trial that randomized 204 patients to radiotherapy (45–50.4 Gy in 25–28 fractions) with or without concurrent chemotherapy (bolus 5-FU at 500 mg/m^2 for 3 days at the start of weeks 1 and 5) in resected stage II and III rectal cancer patients. Patients received 1 month of 5-FU and semustine before and after pelvic chemoradiation. Improvements in pelvic disease and distant disease control led to significant disease-free, disease-specific, and overall survival improvements in the combined modality arm.[176] The results of these two trials led to a clinical announcement in 1991 by the National Cancer Institute defining adjuvant chemoradiation as the standard of care for locally advanced rectal cancer patients.[179]

The NSABP R-02 is the only study with enough power to compare postoperative chemoradiation to postoperative chemotherapy alone.[180] In the GITSG study, there were no significant differences in disease-free or overall survival between the chemotherapy alone and combined modality arms of the study, whereas in the NSABP R-01 study, methyl-CCNU or semustine, vincristine, and fluorouracil (MOF) chemotherapy alone was beneficial to male patients and harmful to female patients. Therefore, the NSABP R-02 trial was designed to answer two questions in patients with resected stage II and III rectal cancer. First, was combined modality therapy superior to chemotherapy alone, and second, was MOF chemotherapy better than 5-FU and high dose leucovorin (the Roswell Park regimen) in males? Male patients were therefore subjected to a 2 by 2 randomization and it was recognized that the study could answer the second question only if there were large differences seen. As in previous trials, radiotherapy improved pelvic disease control (13% vs 8%; $p = .02$), but did not improve disease-free or overall survival. In the global test for interactions of covariates that were significant in the multivariate model that was used, subgroups of patients did appear to have a disease-free and/or overall survival benefit from radiotherapy (patients < 60 and those undergoing APR).[180] This finding underscores the notion that probably patients can be selected who have a low pelvic recurrence (and survival) benefit from pelvic radiotherapy. The pelvic recurrence rates in the surgical control arm in this study were lower than in any other randomized trial. Of note is that pelvic imaging was not done in a systematic fashion in follow-up, only first sites of failure were recorded, and diagnostic imaging was not reviewed centrally. Therefore, it is probable that pelvic failure was underestimated in both arms. In spite of its limitations, this is the only randomized trial with enough power to compare chemotherapy alone with combined chemotherapy and radiotherapy in this population, and it can be used to support the use of chemotherapy alone in selected patients with resected stage II and III rectal cancer.

After the role of concurrent chemoradiation was established in the postoperative setting, the gastrointestinal intergroup conducted subsequent trials that evaluated the schedule of administration and biochemical modulation of 5-FU. A phase III trial conducted by the gastrointestinal intergroup compared protracted venous infusion 5-FU with bolus 5-FU with concurrent radiation therapy in a trial that randomized 660 patients with resected stage II and III rectal cancer.[181] Patients received either bolus 5-FU (500 mg/m^2) for 3 consecutive days during weeks 1 and 5 of radiation therapy, or protracted venous infusion 5-FU given at a rate of 225 mg/m^2/day, 7 days per week during pelvic radiation. This trial showed significant improvements in relapse-free and overall survival in the infusional arm. The toxicity profiles were also different; bolus 5-FU had more hematological toxicity and infusional 5-FU had more diarrhea. A meta-analysis was also reported comparing the efficacy of 5-FU in 1,219 patients with advanced colorectal cancer who received 5-FU either by bolus or continuous infusion on clinical trials.[182] Tumor response and overall survival rates were significantly higher in patients who had received protracted venous infusion 5-FU. Hematologic toxicity occurred more frequently with bolus infusion (31% vs 4%; $p < 10^{-16}$) and hand-and-foot syndrome occurred more frequently with infusional 5-FU (34% vs 13%; $p < 10^{-7}$).[182]

A subsequent trial (INT-0114) was conducted that evaluated the role of biochemical modulation of 5-FU. Like in the previous intergroup trial, patients received 2 months of systemic chemotherapy before and after concurrent chemoradiation. However, protracted venous infusion 5-FU was not used with radiotherapy in any of the arms because the results of the prior study were not yet known. In a four-arm study, 1,696 patients with resected rectal cancer were randomized to receive four different chemotherapy regimens: bolus 5-FU alone, 5-FU with leucovorin, 5-FU with levamisole, or 5-FU with leucovorin and levamisole. There was no survival difference between the arms after a median follow-up duration of 48 months, but there was a significantly greater acute gastrointestinal toxicity rate in the 3-drug arm compared with bolus 5-FU alone.[183]

The next intergroup study (INT-0144) has reached its accrual goal and has been presented but not published in manuscript form.[184] This study was designed to compare the current standard postoperative therapy for resected rectal cancer 4 months of 5-FU and leucovorin given on the Mayo Clinic schedule and pelvic radiotherapy with concurrent protracted venous infusion 5-FU (225 mg/m^2/day 7 days per week) to two experimental arms incorporating biochemical modulation and protracted venous infusion of 5-FU throughout, respectively.[184] The results indicate no significant pelvic control, or progression-free or overall survival difference between the arms.[184]

Radiotherapy is traditionally given after 2 months of chemotherapy as in the previous 2 intergroup studies, but this practice is empiric and may not be the best way to sequence therapy. In fact, there are randomized data indicating that delivering radiotherapy during the first 2 months of therapy may have a disease-free survival advantage.[185] It is probably best to assess the relative distant and pelvic failure risks and administer chemotherapy first if the distant risk is more significant (ie, multiple positive nodes) and pelvic radiotherapy if the local therapy risk is more significant (ie, extensive transmural disease, or narrow margin).

Adjuvant Chemotherapy Following Chemoradiation and Surgery The standard postoperative adjuvant chemoradiation regimen includes 4 months of 5-FU–based systemic therapy in addition to pelvic chemoradiotherapy. This standard evolved empirically from pattern of failure observations from the four-arm phase III trial conducted by the GITSG that showed a reduction in the rate of distant metastases with chemotherapy alone and a reduction in pelvic recurrence with radiotherapy alone, and from extrapolations from the results of adjuvant trials in colon cancer (discussed elsewhere in this chapter). Subsequent gastrointestinal intergroup trials have included systemic chemotherapy before and after pelvic chemoradiation.[178,181,183]

There is no uniform agreement regarding the role of postoperative adjuvant chemotherapy in addition to preoperative chemoradiation. The EORTC 22921 study randomized patients to receive either 5-FU–based chemotherapy or no further therapy following preoperative radiation and surgery.[174] There was no benefit with the use of adjuvant chemotherapy.[174] It appears that patients who have an excellent pathologic response to preoperative chemoradiation have an extremely favorable outcome, and therefore stand to benefit less from further chemotherapy.[186,187] Conversely, patients with nodes positive after preoperative chemoradiation have a particularly poor prognosis as reported in an analysis from patients treated in the German Rectal Cancer Trial.[188] It appears that the pathologic response to preoperative chemoradiation can be used as a prognostic factor in the selection of patients for adjuvant chemotherapy, and certainly would be useful as a stratification variable in future trials evaluating adjuvant chemotherapy after chemoradiation and surgery.

Pelvic Recurrence Management Since the use of radiation, chemoradiation, and TME, pelvic recurrences after curative surgery for rectal adenocarcinoma have decreased. Still there are a significant number of patients who present with isolated pelvic or perineal disease in which reresection may be warranted. Surgical approaches for recurrent disease include re-resection with a low anterior resection, abdominoperineal resection, pelvic exenteration (or its modifications), and occasionally extended sacral resections. If chemoradiation was not utilized during the management of the primary tumor, preoperative chemoradiation may be warranted prior to re-resection. In general, these procedures are performed in conjunction with urology, neurosurgery, and plastic surgery. If available, intraoperative radiotherapy should be strongly considered. After re-resection of isolated pelvic recurrences there is a 20% 5-year survival. These procedures carry a significant morbidity and mortality rate and should be performed by experienced surgeons. Other forms of palliation should be considered prior to undertaking an aggressive surgical approach in a patient in whom cure will not be attainable.

Recurrent rectal cancer can vary significantly in its clinical presentation. When local tumor recurrence is identified early and is isolated, curative surgical resection is the mainstay of treatment. If synchronous metastases are present or the tumor is unresectable, then palliative radiotherapy is usually preferred. Preoperative chemoradiation to 50.4 Gy, followed by resection and intraoperative radiotherapy (IORT, 10–20 Gy) is the preferred approach. The goals are to increase resectability and pelvic control. A large experience at the Mayo Clinic indicates that even with this aggressive approach involving preoperative radiotherapy and IORT, the subsequent pelvic recurrence rate in the radiotherapy field was 37% and the distant metastases rate was 54%. The 5-year overall survival was 20%, compared with the 5% expected with surgery alone historical controls.[189] Even with the use of pelvic chemoradiation, aggressive surgery and adjuvant chemotherapy in T4 and locally recurrent rectal cancers, pelvic and distant disease recurrence are significant limitations of therapy. Future investigation of novel radiosensitizers and the development of systemic adjuvant regimens are needed to improve the outcome of T4 and recurrent rectal cancer.

Palliative pelvic radiotherapy can delay progression of recurrent local disease. Investigators from The Princess Margaret Hospital reported a study evaluating 519 patients with locally recurrent rectal cancer who had not been previously irradiated. The median survival time was 14 months after palliative irradiation alone and the median time to local disease progression was 5 months. The pelvic disease progression-free rate was 7% and the 5-year survival was 5%. Multivariate analysis showed that overall survival was correlated to the Eastern Cooperative Oncology Group (ECOG) performance status, absence of extrapelvic metastases, long intervals between the initial surgery and radiotherapy, total radiation dose, and absence of obstructive uropathy.[190]

Classically, patients have not been considered for a second course of radiotherapy to the same site that has previously been irradiated. Because of that, there are very little data evaluating the risk of doing so in patients with recurrent cancer. In general, the risk of late effects (permanent and potentially debilitating or even fatal) of radiotherapy increases with time and has a minimum latency of 6 months. Patients with recurrent rectal cancer have safely undergone repeat irradiation with acceptable toxicity. In a series of 103 patients, patients were treated with a second course of pelvic radiotherapy directed to the tumor alone with margin (median dose 34.8 Gy after a median prior pelvic dose of 50.4 Gy).[191] There was acceptable morbidity, with chronic diarrhea, small bowel obstruction, and fistula being the most significant toxicities. There were surprisingly few bony and neuropathic complications reported. However, the time at risk of complications was limited by the competing risk of disease recurrence (median survival 26 months). There appeared to be fewer complications in patients who had a radiation-to-radiation interval of at least 1 year, suggesting that interval may be necessary for recovery radiotherapy tolerance. It must be emphasized that the risks of repeat irradiation are acceptable in the setting of recurrent rectal cancer because surgery alone is ineffective and symptomatic progression is often debilitating. Therefore, the clinical benefit of reducing the risk of pelvic progression creates a favorable risk-benefit ratio. The risks of symptomatic late radiation effects can be minimized by using three-dimensional treatment, planning, and hyperfractionation. Hyperfractionation is using smaller doses per fraction, and usually two treatments per day separated by a minimum of 6 hours. Smaller doses per fraction leads to a lower risk of late radiation complications. A recommended dose of 39 Gy at 1/5 Gy/fraction given twice daily to the gross tumor with margin while minimizing dose to the femoral heads and intestine takes advantage of important biologic principals of hyperfractionation and acceleration of treatment and rationally addresses the toxicities reported with pelvic reirradiation. IMRT may offer some advantages in selected cases, particularly when the bowel and femoral heads are difficult to exclude with conventional treatment planning.

IMRT Intensity-modulated radiotherapy (IMRT) is a treatment technique that offers increased precision of radiotherapy delivery. Dose distributions can be created with IMRT that cannot be otherwise created. With pelvic radiotherapy, IMRT may improve treatment tolerance in selected patients by reducing the dose to the small bowel. However, the benefits of IMRT are difficult to quantify clinically, particularly in the adjuvant setting. One of the most significant limitations of the application of this technology to gastrointestinal tumors is the challenge posed by organ motion. All of the potential clinical benefits of increased precision of radiotherapy delivery cannot be realized without controlling for organ motion. The tumor could even be missed if organ motion is not accounted for.

METASTATIC COLORECTAL CANCER

Despite intense efforts directed at prevention and early detection, the reality remains that at the time of diagnosis at least 25% of colorectal cancer patients already have metastases. Even more sobering is the fact that half of all patients with colorectal cancer will have distant metastasis at some point in their lives, and most will die from it. The advent of modern chemotherapy associated with more aggressive surgery has improved the chance for cure for a small percentage of those patients with metastatic disease and has doubled the median survival, which now approaches 2 years, for the entire population.

The liver is the most common site of visceral metastases, and it is the only site affected in up to 20% of patients. Other common sites for metastasis include the lung, lymph nodes, and peritoneum. Once thought to be rare, bone and brain metastasis are becoming more common as liver and lung metastasis are better controlled and patients live longer. Ovarian metastases occur in 5 to 8% of all females with colorectal cancer. The knowledge of organs likely to be affected is important for the design of strategies for follow-up of patients without evidence of disease, and of potentially curative surgical strategies for patients with limited metastasis.

Table 92-5 Recent Trials in Frontline Chemotherapy for Metastatic Colorectal Cancer

Author	Patients	Arms	Response Rate (%)	Progression-Free Survival (Mo)	Overall Survival (Mo)
Hoff et al[193]	303	5-FU/LV	15.5*	4.7	13.3
	302	Capecitabine	24.8*	4.3	12.5
Saltz et al[154]	226	5-FU/LV	21*	4.3*	12.6*
	231	IFL	39*	7.0*	14.8*
de Gramont et al[196]	210	LV5FU2	22.3*	6.2*	14.7
	210	FOLFOX4	50.7*	9.0*	16.2
Goldberg et al[307]	264	IFL	31*	6.9*	15.0*
	267	FOLFOX4	45*	8.7*	19.5*
	264	IROX	35	6.5	17.4
Hurwitz et al[198]	412	IFL	34.8*	6.2*	15.6*
	402	IFL + BEV	44.8*	10.6*	20.3*

$^*p < .05$

IFL: Weekly bolus 5-fluorouracil with leucovorin and irinotecan

5-FU/LV: 5-fluorouracil and leucovorin given as a bolus

LV5FU2: 5-fluorouracil and leucovorin given as a protracted infusion

FOLFOX4: 5-fluorouracil and leucovorin given as a protracted infusion with oxaliplatin

IROX: Irinotecan and oxaliplatin

Median survival for metastatic colorectal cancer treated with best supportive care ranges from only 6 to 9 months according to the small series available.[192] With 5-FU and leucovorin the median survival was improved to 10 to 12 months, and the same overall survival is observed with the use of the oral fluoropyrimidines.[158,193,194] With the advent of combinations of 5-FU and leucovorin plus irinotecan or oxaliplatin, median survival was further improved to 14 to 17 months.[195,196]

We now understand that with the availability of multiple new agents with activity in colorectal cancer, the treatment regimens cannot be evaluated solely based on their impact in first line. The benefit of different regimens used in first, second, and possibly third line seem to add to each other to yield the greatest benefit, even with second-line response rates that are disappointing at first glance. For instance, a review of major chemotherapy trials conducted worldwide, just prior to the advent of the molecular targeted agents, determined that the longest median survivals were obtained by those patients who were exposed to all three classes of active cytotoxic agents, with a median survival of around 20 months.[197]

The recent advent of molecular targeted agents is almost certain to increase the median survival for patients with unresectable colorectal cancer even further, but the results available are still preliminary. Bevacizumab and cetuximab are both monoclonal antibodies; the former is humanized antibody directed against the vasculo-endothelial growth factor (VEGF) and the latter is a chimeric antibody directed against the receptor for epidermal growth factor (EGFR). When bevacizumab was combined with bolus 5-FU with leucovorin and irinotecan (IFL), the median survival reached 20 months, despite the use of IFL, which is now considered an inferior regimen, and the fact that only a small percentage of patients were later exposed to oxaliplatin.[198] Cetuximab has been more extensively investigated as a salvage therapy, but there is growing evidence that it will probably also play an important role as part of first-line regimens.[199] In fact, it is conceivable, and even likely, that by adding all the currently available agents, the median survival has already surpassed the 2-year mark, and it is hoped that large ongoing trials will help to confirm that. Table 92-5 shows recent combination trials as front-line therapy for metastatic disease and the median survivals for each regimen.

Fluoropyrimidines Since the late 1950s, 5-FU has played a central role in the treatment of colorectal cancer. The mechanism of action of 5-FU includes inhibiting both DNA and RNA synthesis leading to cell-cycle arrest, and its main target is the thymidylate synthetase (TS) enzyme within the tumor cells. Circulating 5-FU is rapidly metabolized and destroyed by dihydropyrimidine dehydrogenase (DPD).[200] Leucovorin, also known as folinic acid, is a tetrahydrofolic acid derivative that can enhance the therapeutic and toxic effects of fluoropyrimidines such as 5-FU by strengthening the formation of a ternary complex of 5'fluoro2'-deoxyuridine 5''monophosphate (FdUMP), TS, and methylated tetrahydrofolate.[201] Randomized studies have established clear superiority for 5-FU and leucovorin over 5-FU alone in objective response rate and median progression-free survival, with a smaller but apparently real increase in overall survival.[202–204]

Although 5-FU is commonly used as a bolus, its use as a continuous infusion allows for a continuous presence of FdUMP within the target cells, and therefore abrogates the need for extra amounts of leucovorin. An additional benefit of continuous infusion is the low peak plasma levels of 5-FU owing to the constant rate of infusion, with resulting decrease in the incidence of mucositis and neutropenia. A large meta-analysis from 7 randomized studies with 1,219 patients confirmed not only superior response rate for the continuous infusion regimens (22% vs 11%), but also a small but statistically significant survival advantage (12.4 months vs 11.4 months; $p = .02$).[182] The expected differences in toxicity were confirmed, with higher incidence of neutropenia and mucositis among those patients treated with bolus 5-FU and leucovorin, and higher incidence of hand-and-foot syndrome among those who received the continuous infusions.[182] The clear benefit seen when an infusion regimen is used in combination with more modern chemotherapeutic drugs resulted in continuous infusion largely replacing the bolus regimens in most combination regimens used in first- and second-line treatment of colorectal cancer.[205,206]

Oral Fluoropyrimidines The clear benefit of a protracted exposure to 5-FU and the convenience of oral dosing make the use of oral 5-FU extremely attractive. Its oral use was in fact attempted decades ago.[207] However, a relatively large trial comparing oral 5-FU versus intravenous infusions was disappointing, with a significant inferior duration of response for those patients who received the oral agent (11 vs 20 weeks). There was a marked variability in the 5-FU plasma levels among those patients who received the agent orally but not among those who received it intravenously.[207] We now know that the human gastrointestinal tract is rich in DPD, which is the reason for the variability in the absorption of 5-FU.

Despite the early setback, there was continuous interest in the development of an oral fluoropyrimidine. The presence of DPD can be neutralized by the use of a prodrug that could be metabolized into 5-FU after being absorbed, effectively bypassing the DPD, or by the use of a DPD inhibitor.[208] Both strategies have been investigated, alone or in combination, with some success. All the commercially available oral fluoropyrimidines are prodrugs, albeit some also have a DPD inhibitor in their formulation to maximize exposure to 5-FU once the prodrug is activated.

Capecitabine Two large randomized phase III studies compared capecitabine to the Mayo Clinic schedule of 425 mg/m^2/day intravenous 5-FU plus 20 mg/m^2/day leucovorin for 5 days, as first-line therapy in metastatic colorectal cancer.[158,193,209] Both studies reported an improved overall objective tumor response rate with capecitabine, with an equivalent median time to tumor progression and median overall survival.[158,193,209] Patients who received capecitabine had lower incidence of nausea, stomatitis, alopecia, neutropenic fever, and sepsis. The only toxicity more commonly seen among those patients receiving capecitabine was the hand-and-foot syndrome. The only proven effective treatment against hand-and-foot syndrome is a treatment break until the syndrome has improved to grade I, and a subsequent reduction of the dose.[210] Interestingly, although all the randomized trials have been conducted with the dosage of 1,250 mg/m^2/twice daily for 14 days every 21 days, a sizable number of physicians start their patients at a more conservative dosage of 1,000 mg/m^2/twice day instead. There are some small retrospective studies suggesting equal efficacy and better toxicity profile for this lower dose.[211]

Several trials are exploring the use of capecitabine in combination with other agents, including oxaliplatin, irinotecan, and monoclonal antibodies.[212–214] Capecitabine is also being intensively studied in combination with radiotherapy, where it is already considered by many as the preferred radiosensitizing agent for patients receiving radiotherapy to rectal tumors.[206,215] The initial results of these trials seem to confirm that capecitabine could effectively and safely replace the infusion of 5-FU in combination regimens.[206]

Tegafur and UFT Tegafur is a fluorinated pyrimidine that can be used orally because it is absorbed as an intact molecule and is not metabolized by DPD in the gastrointestinal tract. Once tegafur is metabolized to 5-FU, mostly in the liver, it enters the same pathway as intravenous 5-FU and has the same cytotoxic mechanism.[216] Tegafur has been used for decades as a therapy for colorectal cancer.

UFT is a combination of uracil and tegafur in a 4:1 molar ratio. Uracil is naturally metabolized by DPD and competes with 5-FU for the enzyme when the two are administered together, resulting in a significantly prolonged half-life for 5-FU, mimicking a continuous infusion.[156] Leucovorin is occasionally combined with UFT to further potentiate the effect of 5-FU on tumor cells.[200,216]

Two phase III trials in previously untreated patients with metastatic colorectal cancer tested a regimen of 300 mg/m^2/day UFT plus 25 to 30 mg of leucovorin thrice daily for 28 days and repeated every 35 days against the standard Mayo Clinic schedule of 425 mg/m^2/day intravenous 5-FU plus 20 mg/m^2/day leucovorin for 5 days, repeated every 28 days or 35 days.[194,217] Patients receiving UFT and leucovorin experienced less diarrhea and mucositis than those on 5-FU and leucovorin. The incidence of hand-and-foot syndrome with UFT was negligible. Both trials demonstrated that the use of UFT and leucovorin resulted in statistical equivalent response rates, times to progression (TTP), and median survival to those obtained with intravenous 5-FU and leucovorin.[194,217]

S-1 S-1 is the newest member of the tegafur family. It is a combination of tegafur; CDHP, a powerful DPD inhibitor; and potassium oxonate (Oxo), an inhibitor of orotate pyrimidine phosphorybosyl transferase. CDHP is used to maximize exposure to 5-FU, and Oxo is added in an attempt to modulate the gastrointestinal toxicity of 5-FU and its metabolites.[218] In Japan, the main toxicity of the compound is neutropenia, but in the United States and Europe, several phase I trials have been conducted and the dose-limiting toxicity has been consistently diarrhea.[206,219,220] It is unclear exactly why but the maximum tolerated doses are considerably different in Japan and in the West, but pharmacokinetics may be slightly different between both populations.[221,222] S-1 is currently approved as a therapy for gastric cancer in Japan, but has also demonstrated interesting activity against colorectal cancer.

OTHER THYMIDYLATE SYNTHASE INHIBITORS

Raltitrexed Raltitrexed is a quinazoline folate analogue and is capable of directly inhibiting thymidylate synthase, also known as TS, a key enzyme in the de novo synthesis of 2'-deoxythymidine-5'-monophosphate.[223] After the initial phase I and II studies,[223] it was demonstrated that raltitrexed had significant activity in colorectal cancer. Two subsequent international phase III trials have compared raltitrexed 3 mg/m^2 with 5-FU plus low-dose leucovorin using the Mayo regimen and high-dose leucovorin using the Machover regimen.[224,225] A third study done in North America was originally set up to compare two raltitrexed dosage arms (3 and 4 mg/m^2) with 5-FU and low-dose LV, but the 4 mg/m^2 arm was discontinued because of excessive toxicity.[226] Objective response rates were similar for raltitrexed and 5-FU plus leucovorin. Palliative improvements were seen to a similar extent with both treatments in all phase III studies. Survival was statistically similar for raltitrexed and 5-FU plus leucovorin in both international studies[224,225]; however, raltitrexed was associated with inferior survival to 5-FU plus low-dose leucovorin in the North American study.[226] Although the toxicity profile is in general better for patients receiving raltitrexed than for those receiving 5-FU, there is evidence that patients with renal dysfunction have a greater incidence of severe toxicity and should be treated cautiously.[227,228] A randomized study comparing raltitrexed with 5-FU and leucovorin in the adjuvant setting for colon cancer was terminated early because of an increase in mortality among patients receiving the raltitrexed.

Irinotecan Irinotecan is a topoisomerase I inhibitor derived from the camptothecin, a natural compound found in an ornamental tree from China.[229] Topoisomerase I is an enzyme that produces single strand breaks allowing the uncoiling of the super-coiled DNA, a prerequisite for DNA replication or DNA repair. Interruption of this process leads to rapid cell death. Irinotecan, developed under the name CPT-11, is a water-soluble precursor of the SN-38, formed by the action of carboxylesterase, and up to 1,000 times more potent than the parent compound.[230,231]

When used as a single agent, irinotecan can be administered over 30 or 90 minutes, and the dosing can be either every 3 weeks at 350 mg/m^2 or weekly at a dosage ranging from 100 mg/m^2 to 125 mg/m^2 for 4 weeks with 2 weeks rest period.[232–234] The response rate for single agent irinotecan against colorectal cancer ranges from 10% for previously treated patients to as high as 20% for patients who have never been exposed to chemotherapy.[154,235,236]

The effectiveness of irinotecan was initially demonstrated as a second-line therapy for patients with metastatic colorectal cancer refractory to 5-FU. The pivotal trial randomized 287 patients in a 2:1 ratio to irinotecan plus best supportive care versus best supportive care alone as therapy for patients with previously treated metastatic disease.[236] The overall survival was improved from 6.5 months to 9.2 months, a 41% improvement. Since 5-FU given as an infusion was considered an effective second-line treatment, a second trial randomized 256 patients in a 1:1 ratio to receive either irinotecan or 5-FU by protracted infusion. Once more, the median survival was superior for those patients treated with irinotecan, going from 8.5 months to 10.8 months.[237] Those results supported the use of irinotecan as the preferred regimen for the treatment of patients with 5-FU refractory metastatic colorectal cancer.

A randomized phase III trial was conducted to evaluate irinotecan with or without standard bolus 5-FU and leucovorin versus a standard regimen of bolus 5-FU and leucovorin in first line. The combination regimen became known as the IFL regimen and included 5-FU 500 mg/m^2, leucovorin 20 mg/m^2, and irinotecan 125 mg/m^2 given weekly for 4 weeks every 6 weeks.[154] Irinotecan alone was given at 125 mg/m^2 weekly for 4 weeks every 6 weeks, and the 5-FU and leucovorin was given using the standard Mayo Clinic schedule of 425 mg/m^2/day intravenous 5-FU plus 20 mg/m^2/day leucovorin for 5 days, repeated every 28 days.[154] The three-drug regimen was superior to either 5-FU and leucovorin or to irinotecan alone, and the latter produced similar results as the 5-FU and leucovorin regimen. In a comparison of IFL and the Mayo Clinic regimens, the median progression-free survival improved from 4.3 months to 7.0 months, and the median overall survival improved from 12.6 months to 14.8 months.[154] A companion trial conducted in Europe randomized patients to receive a 5-FU and leucovorin by infusion regimen versus the same regimen plus irinotecan.[195] Once more, the median survival improved from 4.4 months to 6.7 months, and the median survival improved from 14.1 months to 17.4 months among those patients who received the three-drug regimen.[195]

There are several variations of the combination of infusional 5-FU, leucovorin, and irinotecan (FOLFIRI) being used around the world, and it would be difficult to determine if one is superior to the others. One of the favored regimens combines 180 mg/m^2 of irinotecan given on day 1 weekly, 400 mg/m^2 bolus leucovorin weekly, 400 mg/m^2 bolus 5-FU leucovorin weekly followed by a 46 hours infusion of 2,400 mg/m^2 of 5-FU. The entire cycle is repeated every 14 days. A European trial compared the use of FOLFIRI versus FOLFOX as a first-line therapy for metastatic colorectal cancer.[238] Although it has been criticized because of its relatively small size, this trial was important because patients not only received the same 5-FU and leucovorin regimen, but were also expected to "cross over" to the other regimen at the time of progression, minimizing potential confounding factors. Both arms had similar response rates and median survivals, making it evident that the availability of all active drugs is more important than the sequence in which they are administered.[238]

Irinotecan can produce an acute cholinergic reaction during or shortly after infusion, consisting of nausea, vomiting, acute salivation, facial flushing, diaphoresis, abdominal cramps, and diarrhea. This acute reaction can be quickly reversed with atropine and discontinuation of the infusion, and there are apparently less acute cholinergic reactions when longer infusions are used. Other side effects include neutropenia, alopecia, asthenia, and hepatic toxicity. However, the most feared irinotecan toxicity is the delayed diarrhea, which usually occurs 7 to 10 days after the irinotecan administration.[235,239] If untreated, the severe diarrhea can lead to severe dehydration with vascular collapse, shock, and death. Although the mechanism of diarrhea is not completely understood, a lot has been learned. The active metabolite SN-38 is conjugated into the inactive SN-38-G by hepatic uridine diphosphate glucuronosyl transferase (UGT1A1). SN-38-G is then excreted into the small intestine, from which it is eliminated with the stools.[239–243] Some studies have shown the ability of intestinal bacteria to produce beta-glucoronidases, and to transform SN-38-G into SN-38, causing direct damage to the intestinal mucosa.[241] Thus, controlling intestinal bacteria may potentially modulate diarrhea caused by irinotecan.[241] Growing evidence shows that the presence of genetic polymorphism for UGT1A1 is largely responsible for the diarrhea, and although the polymorphism cannot be reversed, its determination may identify patients at greater risk who should either be treated with alternative drugs, or if those are not available, should receive lower doses of irinotecan and be treated for diarrhea more aggressively.[240,242,244]

The current recommended treatment of severe irinotecan-induced diarrhea includes a combination of a high-dose loperamide regimen, aggressive supportive measures, treatment break, and subsequent dose reduction.[235,245] Additional measures are being currently investigated.[241,246] Patients with elevated bilirubin, Gilbert's syndrome, and liver dysfunction from any cause seem to have a particularly high risk, and the use of irinotecan on those individuals requires major caution.[247]

Oxaliplatin Oxaliplatin is a diaminocyclohexane platinum derivative that forms DNA adducts causing irreversible DNA replication error and apoptosis.[248,249] When used as a single agent in first line, the response rates have been 20%, in line with the response rates for single agent 5-FU or irinotecan. Oxaliplatin combines well with different chemotherapy drugs, including 5-FU and leucovorin, and most of its development has been done in combination.[197] Oxaliplatin was combined with a regimen of leucovorin and a bolus followed by an infusion of 5-FU, known as FOLFOX. Variations of this regimen are identified by serial numbers.

The first large size, randomized phase III trial comparing 5-FU and leucovorin versus FOLFOX4 included 420 patients.[196] Patients received exactly the same regimen of a 2-hour infusion of 200 mg/m^2 of leucovorin followed by a bolus of 400 mg/m^2 and a 22-hour infusion of 600 mg/m^2 of 5-FU. All drugs were repeated for 2 consecutive days every 2 weeks. Half of the patients were assigned to receive 85 mg/m^2 of oxaliplatin as a 2-hour infusion on day 1 only.[196] Patients allocated to receive FOLFOX4 had significantly longer progression-free survival (median, 9.0 vs 6.2 months; p =.0003) and better response rate (50.7% vs 22.3%; p =.0001) when compared with the control arm. However, although a trend could be seen, the improvement in overall survival did not reach significance (median, 16.2 vs 14.7 months; p =. 12).

Although oxaliplatin had clear activity against colorectal cancer, the lack of survival benefit in the European trials delayed its approval in the United States, which first was obtained for its use in second line. Rothenberg and colleagues randomized 463 patients with metastatic colorectal cancer who had progressed on treatment with IFL to receive single agent oxaliplatin, infusional 5-FU with leucovorin (LV5-FU2), or the FOLFOX4 regimen.[250] Patients who received FOLFOX4 had a response rate 9.9% versus 0% for LV5-FU2 ($p < .0001$). Median TTP was 4.6 months for FOLFOX4 versus 2.7 months for LV5-FU2 ($p < .0001$). Single agent oxaliplatin was not superior to LV5-FU2 in any parameter.[250] This trial not only confirmed the activity of FOLFOX4 in second line, but also demonstrated the lack of significant activity for second-line infusional 5-FU.

At the same time, the NCCTG and the American intergroup conducted the N9741, a phase III trial that started with six arms but eventually was reduced to a three-arm study. The control arm received the IFL regimen, and oxaliplatin was included in the two experimental arms. It was combined at 85 mg/m^2 with 200 mg/m^2 of irinotecan in the irinotecan and oxaliplatin (IROX) regimen, or with 5-FU and leucovorin, following the FOLFOX4 regimen described above.[251] The final results showed a median time to progression of 8.7 months, response rate of 45%, and median survival time of 19.5 months for those patients assigned to FOLFOX4. These results were significantly superior to those observed for IFL (6.9 months, 31%, and 15.0 months, respectively) or for IROX (6.5 months, 35%, and 17.4 months, respectively).[251] FOLFOX4 was generally well tolerated but it was associated with a significantly higher rate of sensory neuropathy. Based on the encouraging results of the N9741 trial, oxaliplatin was approved for first-line use, and several variations of FOLFOX have become quite popular (see Table 92-5).

The main criticisms for the N9741 study are the fact that IFL uses an inferior bolus regimen of 5-FU, while FOLFOX4 used an infusion of 5-FU, and oxaliplatin was not commercially available in the United States at the time of the trial, creating an imbalance in effective second-line treatment availability. Tournigand and colleagues sought to clarify those questions by comparing a simplified version of FOLFOX4, known as FOLFOX6, versus FOL-

FIRI, which in this trial was basically the same FOLFOX6, with irinotecan used instead of oxaliplatin.[238] Both arms had similar response rates and median survivals, making it evident that the availability of all active drugs is more important than the sequence in which they are administered.[238]

Besides the unique spectrum of activity among platinum agents, oxaliplatin also has a very particular toxicity profile. Oxaliplatin usually does not cause renal or hearing problems, nor significant alopecia, and although it can cause severe nausea, vomiting, and diarrhea, those side effects are usually relatively easy to control.[251] Significant marrow suppression in the form of neutropenia can be a problem with oxaliplatin, particularly when the drug is combined with irinotecan and when bolus of 5-FU is used.[196,251,252] Thrombocytopenia is usually a late problem once a significant cumulative amount of oxaliplatin has been given. More recent variations of FOLFOX, such as the FOLFOX6 and 7, have reduced the amount of bolus 5-FU in an attempt to improve toxicity.

The dose-limiting toxicity, however, is peripheral neuropathy, which can be acute, but usually worsens with longer treatment periods, being clearly dose dependent. The peripheral neuropathy is not well understood but seems to be related to direct effect from one of the oxaliplatin metabolites in calcium ion channels at the neuronal level. It usually becomes a significant problem with cumulative doses above 700 to 800 mg/m^2,[196,253] and it may lead to discontinuation of treatment while patients are still having a benefit from the drug. Periodic planned interruptions may allow patients to stay longer on oxaliplatin by allowing patients to recover while oxaliplatin is held.[253] Several medical interventions have been attempted, but the one that seems more promising involves the use of magnesium and calcium infusions 30 minutes prior to and 30 minutes after the oxaliplatin infusion for patients who do not have a contraindication to receiving those agents.[254]

MONOCLONAL ANTIBODIES

Arguably, the most significant recent advance in the treatment of colorectal cancer has come from the use of the immune system against the tumor. This idea is not new but remained elusive until recently. The identification of important targets in the colorectal cancer cells and their environment led to the recent development of a number of newer antibodies, including two that have been recently approved for the treatment of metastatic colorectal cancer.

Anti-EGFR Monoclonal Antibodies The HER growth factor receptor family comprises four structurally related receptor tyrosine kinases: HER1 (EGFR, *erb*B1), HER2 (*neu*, *erb*B2), HER3 (*erb*B3), and HER4 (*erb*B4). The four receptors are composed of an extracellular region, consisting of glycosylated domains; a transmembrane domain containing a single hydrophobic anchor sequence; and an intracellular region containing the catalytic tyrosine kinase domain, with the exception of HER3, which lacks tyrosine kinase activity.[255,256] Most normal cells, particularly those of endothelial origin and many malignant tissues, express epidermal growth factor receptors (EGFR), and known ligands for EGFR include epidermal growth factor (EGF), transforming growth factor-α (TGF-α), amphiregulin, betacellulin, heparin-binding EGF (HB-EGF), and epiregulin. Increased activity of EGFR-mediated signaling appears to confer a proliferative and/or malignant phenotype, possibly by altering signaling pathways involved in cell-cycle progression, proliferation, apoptosis, angiogenesis, and metastasis.[256]

Several monoclonal antibodies directed against EGFR are currently undergoing clinical investigation, including cetuximab, panitumomab, matuzumab, and others. These antibodies are similar in that they all bind to EGFR and competitively inhibit ligand binding. Among these antibodies, cetuximab is the only one currently approved for clinical use.

Cetuximab is a chimeric antibody with a human IgG_1 and a murine variable region against EGFR with activity against colorectal cancer.[199,257] The exact mechanism of anticancer activity remains unclear, but there is strong evidence that the antibody mediates inhibition of tumor cell-cycle progression and proliferation, promotes apoptosis, enhances antibody-dependent cytotoxicity, and inhibits angiogenesis.[258,259]

The pivotal trial for cetuximab was a large randomized phase II trial done in Europe, known as "BOND." A total of 329 patients whose disease had progressed during or within 3 months after treatment with an irinotecan-based regimen were assigned on a 2:1 basis to receive either cetuximab and irinotecan or cetuximab monotherapy.[199] The response rate in the combination group was 22.9% and in the monotherapy group it was 10.8%, with a $p = .007$.[199] The median time to progression and median survival were, respectively, 4.1 months and 8.6 months in the combination group and 1.5 months and 6.9 months in the monotherapy group.[199]

Most anti-EGFR clinical trials have selected patients with any EGFR-positive staining cells, since preclinical models indicated that greater levels of expression of EGFR should correlate with better response to anti-EGFR therapy. However, detailed analysis of the recently published trials fails to demonstrate that the level of EGFR expression has any impact on response rates.[260]

Retrospective studies showed that patients who develop a rash on therapy are more likely to respond than patients who do not. The typical rash resembles an acneiform rash and tends to involve the face as well as the upper trunk. Severe forms of the rash may lead to temporary discontinuation of therapy, but even in those cases, reexposure to the antibody is usually possible. Management of the rash can be challenging, and although unproved, common measures include the use of topical or oral antibiotics. Clindamycin gel and oral doxycycline are usual choices. The use of topical immunosuppressives has been suggested as well. Regardless of treatment, the rash does tend to improve with continuous use of the monoclonal antibody. Less common side effects include nail changes and hypomagnesemia. However, the most feared toxicity is an allergic reaction, which has been described in up to 4% of patients who receive this chimeric antibody for the first time. Currently the recommendation for those patients who have developed a significant allergic event is that they should not be challenged with the antibody a second time.

Anti-VEGF Monoclonal Antibodies The vascular endothelial growth factor (VEGF) family currently comprises six glycoproteins, designated VEGF-A, VEGF-B, VEGF-C, VEGF-D, VEGF-E, and placenta growth factor (PlGF).[261] Its best characterized member is VEGF-A, which is commonly referred simply as VEGF. VEGF receptors have been identified on endothelial cells[262,263] and include a family of specific tyrosine kinase receptors, including VEGFR-1 (Flt-1) and VEGFR-2 (KDR). More recently, several other VEGFRs have been identified, including VEGFR-3, neuropilin-1 (NRP-1), and neuropilin-2 (NRP-2). Studies in various cultured endothelial cell systems have established that VEGFR-2 mediates the majority of the downstream effects of VEGF in angiogenesis, including microvascular permeability.[264]

Bevacizumab is a humanized antibody that targets the circulating VEGF and has a long half-life of around 17 to 21 days. The original phase III randomized trial in previously untreated metastatic colorectal compared what was considered the standard chemotherapy at the time: irinotecan, 5-FU, and leucovorin (IFL) with or without bevacizumab.[198] The response rate with the addition of bevacizumab improved from 35 to 45% ($p = .0029$), the progression-free survival was extended from 7.1 to 10.4 months ($p = .0014$), and more importantly, the overall survival improved from 15.6 to 20.3 months ($p = .00003$). The adverse events in this trial were similar among the treatment groups with some notable exceptions. Patients receiving bevacizumab had an 11% incidence of grade 3 hypertension and a 1.5% incidence of bowel perforations, with one patient dying from related complications. No patients in the IFL arm presented with such problems.[198] Physicians using bevacizumab should be aware of this potentially lethal problem, and abdominal complaints from patients receiving the antibody have to be taken seriously. Later analysis of pooled data from several trials with bevacizumab also demonstrated an increase in the incidence of arterial thromboembolic events, particularly among patients who had prior history of this type of event.

The ECOG 3200 trial compared the use of FOLFOX against single agent bevacizumab or a combination of FOLFOX and bevacizumab as a second-line therapy for metastatic colorectal cancer.[265] In this particular trial, the dose of bevacizumab used was higher, at 10 mg/kg. The survival results have recently become available, and the median survival for the combination was 12.5 months versus 10.7 month for FOLFOX. This result confirmed that bevacizumab does significantly add to FOLFOX, and that this benefit is also seen in second line, provided that bevacizumab was not used in first line.[265] Whether bevacizumab should be continued after progression of first-line treatment is a matter of debate and should be explored in a prospective, randomized trial.

The intergroup is currently conducting a three arm trial, in which patients are first assigned by their physicians to receive either FOLFIRI or modified FOLFOX6 therapy, and subsequently they are randomized to receive cetuximab, bevacizumab, or a combination of both agents.

COLORECTAL CANCER PREVENTION

Colorectal cancer is a preventable disease. Therefore, the general public, government officials, and primary physicians should be proactive in encouraging screening, surveillance, and possible changes in lifestyle that could have an effect on this disease. In this section, screening and surveillance recommendations as well as potential protective factors or interventions will be discussed.

Screening and Surveillance Identification of high-risk groups, such as patients with family history of CRC, adenomas, genetic syndromes, and inflammatory bowel disease is important so that surveillance can be performed at more frequent intervals than the average-risk individual whose only risk factor is age. Screening in the asymptomatic has been estimated to cost between \$15,000 and \$25,000 per year of life saved, a figure comparable to breast cancer screening.[13] The most important aspect is education of patients and health care practitioners.

There are several medical, surgical, and oncology specialty societies that periodically update screening recommendations.[13,266] There are combinations of tests available, such as guaiac-based stool testing, sigmoidoscopy, colonoscopy, and colography. Efficacy in the general population has been demonstrated with a guaiac testing and sigmoidoscopy. Colonoscopy has not been evaluated in a randomized study, but intuitively should be effective in the early detection and prevention of colorectal cancer. Colography or virtual colonoscopy has not been evaluated, and unfortunately most of the time it is being utilized in uncontrolled settings, which preclude gathering of meaningful information.

Screening for colorectal cancer remains a problem. Less than 30% of the individuals in whom screening has been recommended have ever been screened.[267] The present American Cancer Society recommendations for colorectal screening for men and women age 50 or older include a fecal occult blood test (FOBT) every year and a flexible sigmoidoscopy every 5 years or colonoscopy every 10 years or double-contrast barium enema every 5 to 10 years.[266] A digital rectal exam should be performed at the time of sigmoidoscopy, colonoscopy or barium enema.[266] It can be strongly argued that the best method for screening is colonoscopy. The latter procedure allows for direct visualization of the colon, and if necessary, polypectomy. Detractors of colonoscopy as a screening tool argue that the cost to society is too high, that there are not enough qualified endoscopists to perform the procedure, that there are risks and discomfort associated with the procedure, and that flexible sigmoidoscopy will identify patients with significant adenomas allowing the use of colonoscopy in a more efficient way in the patients at high risk of proximal neoplasia. There is no perfect screening test for CRC. Annual fecal occult blood testing has been shown to decrease mortality from colorectal cancer between 15 and 33%. A study evaluating a one-time FOBT with sigmoidoscopy revealed that advanced neoplasia, defined as an adenoma 1 cm or larger, a villous adenoma, an adenoma with high-grade dysplasia, or invasive cancer, would have been missed in 24% of the cases.[268] Two large studies evaluating the risk of advanced proximal neoplasia in patients undergoing evaluation of the distal colon followed by colonoscopy revealed that advanced proximal neoplasia would not have been detected in 50% and 62% of patients since there were no distal neoplasms that would have warranted full colonoscopy.[269,270] In the National Polyp Study, double contrast barium enema failed to detect 48% adenomas greater than 1 cm.[271] Colonoscopy is not perfect. Visualization of the cecum is not always possible. In addition, there is morbidity associated with colonoscopy. The risk of perforation is small after diagnostic colonoscopy, but is higher after polypectomy. Problems with conscious sedation and bleeding after polypectomy have been reported. Two multicenter trials evaluating colonography in asymptomatic individuals (screening) reported discordant results. In the study by Pickhardt and colleagues, colonography had similar or even greater sensitivity for detecting adenomas than colonoscopy.[272] However, in the study by Cotton and colleagues, the sensitivity of colonography for detecting polyps 6 mm and polyps at least 10 mm was 39% and 55%, respectively, much lower than the 88% and 94% reported by Pickhardt for similar size polyps.[273] These contradicting results underscore the need for standardized software, expertise in interpreting results, and a clear definition of the size of the lesion that will be considered significant. Patient acceptance for this procedure may be higher, and therefore in the future this may be a useful screening procedure.

Detection of molecular markers in stool is a reality. This modality is promising and could potentially be utilized for screening asymptomatic patients. A study comparing fecal DNA to fecal occult blood in asymptomatic average-risk individuals undergoing colorectal cancer screening revealed that colonoscopy is still the gold standard for detecting neoplastic lesions.[274] However, the fecal DNA panel detected 18% of adenomas > 1 cm, whereas FOBT was positive in 11% of adenomas > 1 cm.[274] In that study specificity was not compromised. Further studies and refinements in techniques are necessary before this technology can be widely applied.

Screening for colorectal cancer appears to be cost-effective compared with no screening. Each modality discussed above has its advantages and disadvantages. Therefore, screening for colorectal cancer has to be individualized according to the resources available and patient as well as health care provider preferences. A one-time FOBT should not be utilized. FOBT should be used either annually or biennially if it is to be utilized.

The optimal frequency of colonoscopic surveillance after polypectomy is 3 years. In the National Polyp Study, there were no differences in the detection of adenomas with advanced features in patients randomized to a 1-year or a 3-year follow-up after polypectomy.[9] However, this interval should be individualized according to the characteristics, size, and number of polyps detected at index colonoscopy. Colonoscopy has been recommended beginning at age 40 years, or 10 years before the youngest CRC in the immediate family for individuals with a first-degree relative with either colorectal cancer or adenomas diagnosed at age 60 or younger or for any individuals with two first-degree relatives whose family does not have one of the inherited colorectal cancer syndromes.[266] Colonoscopy should be repeated every 5 years. In patients who have undergone colorectal cancer resection, colonoscopy should be performed 1 year after surgery and every 3 years thereafter unless colonoscopic findings warrant a more frequent interval.[111]

Surveillance in individuals with genetic syndromes or inflammatory disease should be more frequent than in sporadic colorectal cancer patients or in patients who had adenomas. In FAP, it should start at age 10 to 12 years. Annual flexible sigmoidoscopy is recommended for all first-degree relatives of affected individuals. Unless adenomas are noted, in which case colonoscopy is the procedure of choice, annual flexible sigmoidoscopy should continue until age 18 to 20 years, at which time colonoscopy should be performed every year. If at age 30 there have been no adenomas, the interval between colonoscopies can be lengthened to between 2 and 3 years. Because *APC* mutations can be detected in the germline of the affected patients, genetic testing is recommended for affected individuals. If a mutation is known in the family, then individuals at risk can be tested for that mutation, and those in whom no mutation is detected can be spared intensive surveillance and fall into the general population risk. It must be noted that genetic testing should be undertaken under an environment where there is genetic counseling and psychological support. Needless to say, informed consent is required.

In HNPCC, colonoscopy should be started at age 20 years in mutation carriers and at-risk family members. Surveillance with colonoscopy at least every 3 years has been shown to decrease colorectal cancer rate by 62% and mortality by 65%. Others have advocated colonoscopy starting at age 21 every 1 to 2 years until age 40, then annually thereafter.[13] Similar principles apply for genetic testing in HNPCC as FAP, except that children are not tested, since the onset of cancer is generally at an older age than the onset of adenomas in FAP. In the Peutz-Jeghers and juvenile polyposis syndromes, there are no evidence-based surveillance recommendations. The recommendations have to be individualized.[26,27] Capsule endoscopy may be useful in these individuals.

Surveillance in UC depends on the extent of the disease and the duration. It is recommended that annual colonoscopy should be performed after 8 years of pancolitis. If the disease is confined to the left side of the colon, then surveillance can be started at a later time.[13] It is imperative to perform random biopsies every 10 cm. If there is severe dysplasia in the specimens, consideration should be given for surgery, as there is a high incidence of occult cancer in the colon. There are no specific recommendations for surveillance in Crohn's disease. However, following the model of ulcerative colitis, recommendations can be made for colonoscopy after 8 years of diagnosis and then every 1 to 2 years.[275] Consideration should be given to random biopsies every 10 cm.[275]

PROTECTIVE FACTORS OR INTERVENTIONS

Fiber Dietary fiber refers to the endogenous components of plant materials in the diet that are resistant to digestion by human enzymes.[276] It is generally accepted that a high-fiber diet has a beneficial effect in decreasing colorectal cancer. However, results from multiple epidemiological, animal, and interventional studies are conflicting regarding the role of fiber in decreasing CRC risk.[276,277]

The exact mechanisms by which fiber may prevent CRC are not completely understood. Burkitt proposed that fiber increased stool bulk, thus diluting stool carcinogens and decreasing transit time between the carcinogens and the bowel mucosa.[278] Binding of mutagens in the stool, such as binding bile acids, preventing the conversion of primary to secondary bile acids, decreasing luminal pH, and fermenting fiber into short-chain fatty acids have been proposed as potential mechanisms.[279–281] By decreasing luminal pH, dietary fiber may reduce the mutagenicity of secondary bile acids.[282] Because the multiple interactions between dietary and lifestyle factors may be more important than individual components in the diet or lifestyle, the American Gastroenterological Association has recommended a diet high in fiber, vegetables, fruits, and cereals, decreasing total intake of animal and saturated fats as well as decreasing red meat intake.[276]

Calcium and Vitamin D There is epidemiologic evidence, although not consistent, of an inverse association with intake of calcium and vitamin D and colorectal cancer risk.[283]

There appears to be a beneficial effect of calcium in the prevention of recurrent adenomas and colorectal cancer in both men and women.[284–286] In a randomized double-blind trial of the effect of calcium carbonate supplementation on the recurrence of colorectal adenomas, Baron and colleagues reported a 15 to 20% risk reduction in the intervention arm compared with the placebo arm.[284] By combining two prospective cohorts, Wu and colleagues examined the association between colon cancer risk and calcium intake in over 100,000 men and women who participated in the Nurses' Health Study and the Health Professionals Follow-up Study.[285] An inverse relation between high calcium intake (> 1,250 mg/day vs ≤ 500 mg/day) and distal colon cancers (descending and sigmoid) was found.[285] No such relationship was noted for proximal colon cancers.[285] In the CPS II prospective cohort study, calcium supplementation was associated with decreased incidence of colorectal cancer.[286] A pooled analysis of 10 cohort studies in five countries assessing dietary intake by questionnaires revealed that higher consumption of milk and calcium was associated with a lower colorectal cancer risk across studies and gender.[287] The effect of milk was limited to the distal colon and rectum.[287]

Multivitamins and Folate The use of multivitamins has been shown to reduce colon cancer risk. In the CPS II study, past use of multivitamins, but not recent use of multivitamins, was associated with decreased colorectal cancer risk.[288] In the Nurses' Health Study, the lowest risk of colon cancer was in subjects who took multivitamin supplements for at least 15 years.[289] In these individuals, colon cancer was reduced by 75%.[289] A subsequent analysis of the same cohort reported on the effect of folate in individuals with a family history of colon cancer.[290] The use of multivitamins containing folate for a period greater than 5 years decreased colon cancer risk by almost 50%.[290] The reduction was greater in subjects with a family history of colorectal cancer than in those without a family history of CRC.[290]

Differences in the activity of 5-10 methylene tetrahydrofolate reductase (MTHFR) may account for differences in CRC risk. This enzyme catalyzes the conversion of 5-10 methylene tetrahydrofolate to 5-methyltetrahydrofolate, a step necessary for methionine synthesis.[48] The polymorphisms C677T and A1298C in the *MTHFR* gene have been the most commonly studied. The variant allele of these polymorphic genes has been associated with reduced MTHFR enzyme activity in vitro.[291] In most of the studies, there is an inverse relationship between the homozygous variant 677TT and 1298CC, and colorectal cancer risk.[291] The studies evaluating the interaction with adenoma risk have been inconsistent.[291]

Carotenoids are precursors for vitamin A. Fruits and vegetables are the major source of dietary carotenoids. Carotenoids have antioxidant properties and potentially could modulate immune response and gene expression.[292] In a case-control study, Slattery and colleagues evaluated the relationship between carotenoid intake and colon cancer with relationship to age at diagnosis, site, and smoking status.[292] They reported that lutein was inversely associated with colon cancer.[292] The greatest inverse association was for individuals diagnosed before age 67 and for tumors located in the proximal colon.[292] There was no significant association with other carotenoids.[292] In a subset analysis of the Polyp Prevention Trial, a protective effect on adenoma recurrence was noted in individuals who were nonsmokers and nondrinkers who took β-carotene supplementation.[293] Similar results with α-carotene and vitamin A were reported in another analysis from this same cohort.[294]

Nonsteroidal Anti-Inflammatory Drugs Nonsteroidal anti-inflammatory drugs (NSAIDs) use is associated with a decreased risk of colorectal cancer. The majority the epidemiological studies in the literature have revealed that there is a decrease in adenoma incidence, carcinoma incidence, and colorectal cancer mortality associated with NSAIDs use. The activity of NSAIDs on colorectal cancer has been observed across different cohorts. It has been reported in the general population, in at-risk individuals, in both sexes, and across continents. Three prospective randomized placebo-controlled studies of aspirin in the prevention of adenomas have been reported.[295–297] Two of these trials were in patients with previous adenomas,[295,297] whereas the other trial was in patients with early-stage colorectal cancer that had been resected.[296] In the study by Baron and colleagues, the dose of aspirin that was effective was 81 mg per day, while in the study by Sandler and colleagues it was 325 mg daily.[295,296]

One of the mechanisms whereby NSAIDs inhibit colorectal neoplasia is through inhibition of cyclooxygenase (COX) required for prostaglandin synthesis. There are two COX enzymes, namely COX-1 and COX-2.[298] COX-1 is present constitutively, whereas COX-2 is inducible in response to inflammation, and its resulting growth factors and cytokines.[299] Sulindac, a nonspecific inhibitor of COX-1 and COX-2, and celecoxib and rofecoxib, specific inhibitors of COX-2, have been shown to decrease the size and number of colorectal adenomas in FAP patients.[300–302] The effect on the adenomas was lost when the therapy was discontinued. However, COX-2 inhibitors have been associated with increased cardiovascular risks.[303]

Hormone Replacement Therapy Hormone replacement therapy (HRT) is discussed in the context of its widespread use not in the context of an intervention. The majority of the studies published have suggested that HRT in postmenopausal women reduces colorectal cancer risk. A meta-analysis of 18 epidemiologic studies of postmenopausal women on HRT and CRC reported a 20% and 19% decrease in colon and rectal cancer risk, respectively.[304] The reduction was noted mainly in current HRT users.[304]

In the Women's Health Initiative Study, a prospective study that randomized patients to placebo versus estrogen plus progestin sponsored by the US National Heart, Lung, and Blood Institute, the risk of colorectal cancer was decreased by 37% in patients receiving HRT.[305] That study was halted because of an increased risk of invasive breast cancer, heart disease, stroke, and pulmonary embolism in study group patients versus placebo.[306]

REFERENCES

1. Fearon ER, Vogelstein B. A genetic model for colorectal tumorigenesis. Cell 1990;61:759–67.
2. Ferlay J, Bray F, Pisani P, Parkin DM. GLOBOCAN 2002: cancer incidence, mortality and prevalence worldwide. IARC CancerBase No. 5, Version 2.0. Lyon: IARCPress; 2004.
3. Elder JP, Castro FG, de Moor C, et al. Differences in cancer-risk-related behaviors in Latino and Anglo adults. Prev Med 1991;20:751–63.
4. Jemal A, Tiwari RC, Murray T, et al. Cancer statistics, 2004. CA Cancer J Clin 2004;54:8–29.
5. American Cancer Society. Cancer facts and figures. Atlanta: American Cancer Society; 2004. p. 1–35.
6. Troisi RJ, Freedman AN, Devesa SS. Incidence of colorectal carcinoma in the U.S.: an update of trends by gender, race, age, subsite, and stage, 1975–1994. Cancer 1999;85:1670–6.
7. National Cancer Institute. SEER cancer statistics review, 1975–2002. Available at: http://seer.cancer.gov/csr?1975_2002/search.pl, 2004. Accessed 9 September 2005.
8. Carlsson G, Petrelli NJ, Nava H, et al. The value of colonoscopic surveillance after curative resection for colorectal cancer or synchronous adenomatous polyps. Arch Surg 1987;122:1261–3.
9. Winawer SJ, Zauber AG, O'Brien MJ, et al. Randomized comparison of surveillance intervals after colonoscopic removal of newly diagnosed adenomatous polyps. The National Polyp Study Workgroup. N Engl J Med 1993;328:901–6.
10. Burt RW. Colon cancer screening. Gastroenterology 2000;119:837–53.
11. Fuchs CS, Giovannucci EL, Colditz GA, et al. A prospective study of family history and the risk of colorectal cancer. N Engl J Med 1994;331:1669–74.
12. Slattery ML, Kerber RA. Family history of cancer and colon cancer risk: the Utah Population Database. J Natl Cancer Inst 1994;86:1618–26.
13. Winawer S, Fletcher R, Rex D, et al. Colorectal cancer screening and surveillance: clinical guidelines and rationale-Update based on new evidence. Gastroenterology 2003;124:544–60.
14. Winawer SJ, Zauber AG, Gerdes H, et al. Risk of colorectal cancer in the families of patients with adenomatous polyps. National Polyp Study Workgroup. N Engl J Med 1996;334:82–7.
15. Campbell WJ, Spence RA, Parks TG. Familial adenomatous polyposis. Br J Surg 1994;81:1722–33.
16. Bussey HJR. Familial polyposis coli: family studies, histopathology, differential diagnosis, and results of treatment. Baltimore: Johns Hopkins University Press; 1975.
17. Al-Tassan N, Chmiel NH, Maynard J, et al. Inherited variants of MYH associated with somatic G:C—>T:A mutations in colorectal tumors. Nat Genet 2002;30:227–32.
18. Sampson JR, Dolwani S, Jones S, et al. Autosomal recessive colorectal adenomatous polyposis due to inherited mutations of MYH. Lancet 2003;362:39–41.
19. Sieber OM, Lipton L, Crabtree M, et al. Multiple colorectal adenomas, classic adenomatous polyposis, and germline mutations in MYH. N Engl J Med 2003;348:791–9.
20. Wang L, Baudhuin LM, Boardman LA, et al. MYH mutations in patients with attenuated and classic polyposis and with young-onset colorectal cancer without polyps. Gastroenterology 2004;127:9–16.
21. Lynch HT, de la Chapelle A. Genetic susceptibility to non-polyposis colorectal cancer. J Med Genet 1999;36:801–18.
22. Aarnio M, Mecklin JP, Aaltonen LA, et al. Life-time risk of different cancers in hereditary non-polyposis colorectal cancer (HNPCC) syndrome. Int J Cancer 1995;64:430–3.
23. Plaschke J, Engel C, Kruger S, et al. Lower incidence of colorectal cancer and later age of disease onset in 27 families with pathogenic MSH6 germline mutations compared with families with MLH1 or MSH2 mutations: the German Hereditary Nonpolyposis Colorectal Cancer Consortium. J Clin Oncol 2004;22:4486–94.
24. Jass JR, Smyrk TC, Stewart SM, et al. Pathology of hereditary non-polyposis colorectal cancer. Anticancer Res 1994;14:1631–4.
25. Giardiello FM, Welsh SB, Hamilton SR, et al. Increased risk of cancer in the Peutz-Jeghers syndrome. N Engl J Med 1987;316:1511–4.
26. Spigelman AD, Murday V, Phillips RK. Cancer and the Peutz-Jeghers syndrome. Gut 1989;30:1588–90.
27. Wirtzfeld DA, Petrelli NJ, Rodriguez-Bigas MA. Hamartomatous polyposis syndromes: molecular genetics, neoplastic risk, and surveillance recommendations. Ann Surg Oncol 2001;8:319–27.
28. Coburn MC, Pricolo VE, DeLuca FG, Bland KI. Malignant potential in intestinal juvenile polyposis syndromes. Ann Surg Oncol 1995;2:386–91.
29. Eaden JA, Abrams KR, Mayberry JF. The risk of colorectal cancer in ulcerative colitis: a meta-analysis. Gut 2001;48:526–35.
30. Ribeiro MB, Greenstein AJ, Sachar DB, et al. Colorectal adenocarcinoma in Crohn's disease. Ann Surg 1996;223:186–93.
31. Giovannucci E. Obesity, gender, and colon cancer. Gut 2002;51:147.
32. Giovannucci E. Insulin, insulin-like growth factors and colon cancer: a review of the evidence. J Nutr 2001;131 (11 Suppl):3109S–20S.
33. Terry P, Giovannucci E, Bergkvist L, et al. Body weight and colorectal cancer risk in a cohort of Swedish women: relation varies by age and cancer site. Br J Cancer 2001;85:346–9.
34. Terry PD, Miller AB, Rohan TE. Obesity and colorectal cancer risk in women. Gut 2002;51:191–4.
35. Rose DP, Boyar AP, Wynder EL. International comparisons of mortality rates for cancer of the breast, ovary, prostate, and colon, and per capita food consumption. Cancer 1986;58:2363–71.
36. Potter JD. Colorectal cancer: molecules and populations. J Natl Cancer Inst 1999;91:916–32.
37. Caygill CP, Charlett A, Hill MJ. Fat, fish, fish oil and cancer. Br J Cancer 1996;74:159–64.
38. Rao CV, Hirose Y, Indranie C, Reddy BS. Modulation of experimental colon tumorigenesis by types and amounts of dietary fatty acids. Cancer Res 2001;61:1927–33.
39. Corpet DE, Stamp D, Medline A, et al. Promotion of colonic microadenoma growth in mice and rats fed cooked sugar or cooked casein and fat. Cancer Res 1990;50:6955–8.
40. Willett WC, Stampfer MJ, Colditz GA, et al. Relation of meat, fat, and fiber intake to the risk of colon cancer in a prospective study among women. N Engl J Med 1990;323:1664–72.
41. Chao A, Thun MJ, Connell CJ, et al. Meat consumption and risk of colorectal cancer. JAMA 2005;293:172–82.
42. Baron JA, Sandler RS, Haile RW, et al. Folate intake, alcohol consumption, cigarette smoking, and risk of colorectal adenomas. J Natl Cancer Inst 1998;90:57–62.
43. World Cancer Research Fund (WCRF) Panel. Diet, nutrition, and the prevention of cancer: a global perspective. Washington, D.C.: WCRF/American Institute of Cancer Research; 1997.
44. Slattery ML, Samowtiz W, Ma K, et al. CYP1A1, cigarette smoking, and colon and rectal cancer. Am J Epidemiol 2004;160:842–52.
45. Goldberg MS, Parent ME, Siemiatycki J, et al. A case-control study of the relationship between the risk of colon cancer in men and exposures to occupational agents. Am J Ind Med 2001;39:531–46.
46. Chow WH, Malker HS, Hsing AW, et al. Occupational risks for colon cancer in Sweden. J Occup Med 1994;36:647–51.
47. Chen K, Jiang QT, He HQ. Relationship between metabolic enzyme polymorphism and colorectal cancer. World J Gastroenterol 2005;11:331–5.
48. Houlston RS, Tomlinson IP. Polymorphisms and colorectal tumor risk. Gastroenterology 2001;121:282–301.
49. Laken SJ, Petersen GM, Gruber SB, et al. Familial colorectal cancer in Ashkenazim due to a hypermutable tract in APC. Nat Genet 1997;17:79–83.
50. Frayling IM, Beck NE, Ilyas M, et al. The APC variants I1307K and E1317Q are associated with colorectal tumors, but not always with a family history. Proc Natl Acad Sci U S A 1998;95:10722–7.
51. Slattery ML, Samowitz W, Ballard L, et al. A molecular variant of the APC gene at codon 1822: its association with diet, lifestyle, and risk of colon cancer. Cancer Res 2001;61:1000–4.
52. Muto T, Bussey HJ, Morson BC. The evolution of cancer of the colon and rectum. Cancer 1975;36:2251–70.
53. Jessurun J, Romero-Guadarrama M, Manivel JC. Medullary adenocarcinoma of the colon: clinicopathologic study of 11 cases. Hum Pathol 1999;30:843–8.
54. Dukes C. The spread of cancer of the rectum. Br J Surg 1929;17:643.
55. Astler VB, Coller FA. The prognostic significance of direct extension of carcinoma of the colon and rectum. Ann Surg 1954;139:846–52.
56. Green FL, Page DL, Fleming ID, et al., editors. AJCC cancer staging handbook. 6th ed. New York: Springer-Verlag; 2002.
57. Mayer RJ, Garnick MB, Steele GD Jr, Zamcheck N. Carcinoembryonic antigen (CEA) as a monitor of chemotherapy in disseminated colorectal cancer. Cancer 1978;42(3 Suppl):1428–33.
58. MacIntosh EL, Rodriguez-Bigas M, Petrelli N. Colorectal carcinoma. In: Johnson FE, Virgo KS, editors. Cancer patient follow-up, 1st ed. St. Louis: Mosby-Yearbook; 1997. p. 118–31.
59. Wanebo HJ, Rao B, Pinsky CM, et al. Preoperative carcinoembryonic antigen level as a prognostic indicator in colorectal cancer. N Engl J Med 1978;299:448–51.
60. Bhatnagar J, Tewari HB, Bhatnagar M, Austin GE. Comparison of carcinoembryonic antigen in tissue and serum with grade and stage of colon cancer. Anticancer Res 1999;19:2181–7.
61. Wagner JL, Tunis S, Brown N. The cost-effectiveness of colorectal cancer screening in average-risk adults. In: Young G, Levin B, Rozen R, editors. Prevention and early detection of colorectal cancer. London: WB Saunders; 1996. p. 321–56.
62. Desch CE, Benson AB 3rd, Smith TJ, et al. Recommended colorectal cancer surveillance guidelines by the American Society of Clinical Oncology. J Clin Oncol 1999;17:1312.
63. Arnaud JP, Koehl C, Adloff M. Carcinoembryonic antigen (CEA) in diagnosis and prognosis of colorectal carcinoma. Dis Colon Rectum 1980;23:141–4.
64. Rosen M, Chan L, Beart RW Jr., Vukasin P, Anthone G. Follow-up of colorectal cancer: a meta-analysis. Dis Colon Rectum 1998;41:1116–26.
65. Safi F, Beyer HG. The value of follow-up after curative surgery of colorectal carcinoma. Cancer Detect Prev 1993;17:417–24.
66. Zeng Z, Cohen AM, Urmacher C. Usefulness of carcinoembryonic antigen monitoring despite normal preoperative values in node-positive colon cancer patients. Dis Colon Rectum 1993;36:1063–8.
67. Clinical practice guidelines for the use of tumor markers in breast and colorectal cancer. Adopted on May 17, 1996 by the American Society of Clinical Oncology. J Clin Oncol 1996;14:2843–77.
68. Libutti SK, Alexander HR Jr, Choyke P, et al. A prospective study of 2-[18F] fluoro-2-deoxy-D-glucose/positron emission tomography scan, 99mTc-labeled arcitumomab (CEA-scan), and blind second-look laparotomy for detecting colon cancer recurrence in patients with increasing carcinoembryonic antigen levels. Ann Surg Oncol 2001;8:779–86.
69. Flanagan FL, Dehdashti F, Ogunbiyi OA, et al. Utility of FDG-PET for investigating unexplained plasma CEA elevation in patients with colorectal cancer. Ann Surg 1998;227:319–23.
70. Cutait R, Alves VA, Lopes LC, et al. Restaging of colorectal cancer based on the identification of lymph node micrometastases through immunoperoxidase staining of CEA and cytokeratins. Dis Colon Rectum 1991;34:917–20.
71. Liefers GJ, Cleton-Jansen AM, van de Velde CJ, et al. Micrometastases and survival in stage II colorectal cancer. N Engl J Med 1998;339:223–8.
72. Filella X, Molina R, Grau JJ, et al. Prognostic value of CA 19.9 levels in colorectal cancer. Ann Surg 1992;216:55–9.
73. Loeb LA. Mutator phenotype may be required for multistage carcinogenesis. Cancer Res 1991;51:3075–9.
74. Sieber OM, Tomlinson IP, Lamlum H. The adenomatous polyposis coli (APC) tumour suppressor—genetics, function and disease. Mol Med Today 2000;6:462–9.
75. Lamlum H, Papadopoulou A, Ilyas M, et al. APC mutations are sufficient for the growth of early colorectal adenomas. Proc Natl Acad Sci U S A 2000;97:2225–8.
76. Powell SM, Zilz N, Beazer-Barclay Y, et al. APC mutations occur early during colorectal tumorigenesis. Nature 1992;359:235–7.
77. Vogelstein B, Fearon ER, Hamilton SR, et al. Genetic alterations during colorectal-tumor development. N Engl J Med 1988;319:525–32.

78. Grady WM, Markowitz SD. Genetic and epigenetic alterations in colon cancer. Annu Rev Genomics Hum Genet 2002;3:101–28.
79. Peltomaki P, Aaltonen LA, Sistonen P, et al. Genetic mapping of a locus predisposing to human colorectal cancer. Science 1993;260:810–2.
80. Veigl ML, Kasturi L, Olechnowicz J, et al. Biallelic inactivation of hMLH1 by epigenetic gene silencing, a novel mechanism causing human MSI cancers. Proc Natl Acad Sci U S A 1998;95:8698–702.
81. Domingo E, Niessen RC, Oliveira C, et al. BRAF-V600E is not involved in the colorectal tumorigenesis of HNPCC in patients with functional MLH1 and MSH2 genes. Oncogene 2005;24:3995–8..
82. Yamamoto H, Sawai H, Weber TK, et al. Somatic frameshift mutations in DNA mismatch repair and proapoptosis genes in hereditary nonpolyposis colorectal cancer. Cancer Res 1998;58:997–1003.
83. Jass JR, Young J, Leggett BA. Evolution of colorectal cancer: change of pace and change of direction. J Gastroenterol Hepatol 2002;17:17–26.
84. Kinzler KW, Vogelstein B. Landscaping the cancer terrain. Science 1998;280:1036–7.
85. Xin B, Platzer P, Fink SP, et al. Colon cancer secreted protein-2 (CCSP-2), a novel candidate serological marker of colon neoplasia. Oncogene 2005;24:724–31.
86. Bast RC Jr, Ravdin P, Hayes DF, et al. 2000 update of recommendations for the use of tumor markers in breast and colorectal cancer: clinical practice guidelines of the American Society of Clinical Oncology. J Clin Oncol 2001;19:1865–78.
87. Ahnen DJ, Feigl P, Quan G, et al. Ki-ras mutation and p53 overexpression predict the clinical behavior of colorectal cancer: a Southwest Oncology Group study. Cancer Res 1998;58:1149–58.
88. Luna-Perez P, Segura J, Alvarado I, et al. Specific c-K-ras gene mutations as a tumor-response marker in locally advanced rectal cancer treated with preoperative chemoradiotherapy. Ann Surg Oncol 2000;7:727–31.
89. McLeod HL, Murray GI. Tumour markers of prognosis in colorectal cancer. Br J Cancer 1999;79:191–203.
90. Spitz FR, Giacco GG, Hess K, et al. p53 immunohistochemical staining predicts residual disease after chemoradiation in patients with high-risk rectal cancer. Clin Cancer Res 1997;3:1685–90.
91. Jen J, Kim H, Piantadosi S, et al. Allelic loss of chromosome 18q and prognosis in colorectal cancer. N Engl J Med 1994;331:213–21.
92. Boland CR, Thibodeau SN, Hamilton SR, et al. A National Cancer Institute Workshop on Microsatellite Instability for cancer detection and familial predisposition: development of international criteria for the determination of microsatellite instability in colorectal cancer. Cancer Res 1998;58:5248–57.
93. Gryfe R, Kim H, Hsieh ET, et al. Tumor microsatellite instability and clinical outcome in young patients with colorectal cancer. N Engl J Med 2000;342:69–77.
94. Samowitz WS, Curtin K, Ma KN, et al. Microsatellite instability in sporadic colon cancer is associated with an improved prognosis at the population level. Cancer Epidemiol Biomarkers Prev 2001;10:917–23.
95. Ribic CM, Sargent DJ, Moore MJ, et al. Tumor microsatellite-instability status as a predictor of benefit from fluorouracil-based adjuvant chemotherapy for colon cancer. N Engl J Med 2003;349:247–57.
96. Popat S, Hubner R, Houlston RS. Systematic review of microsatellite instability and colorectal cancer prognosis. J Clin Oncol 2005;23:609–18.
97. Cui H, Cruz-Correa M, Giardiello FM, et al. Loss of IGF2 imprinting: a potential marker of colorectal cancer risk. Science 2003;299:1753–5.
98. Kemp Z, Thirlwell C, Sieber O, et al. An update on the genetics of colorectal cancer. Hum Mol Genet 2004;13(Suppl 2):R177–85.
99. Leichman CG, Lenz HJ, Leichman L, et al. Quantitation of intratumoral thymidylate synthase expression predicts for disseminated colorectal cancer response and resistance to protracted-infusion fluorouracil and weekly leucovorin. J Clin Oncol 1997;15:3223–9.
100. Metzger R, Danenberg K, Leichman CG, et al. High basal level gene expression of thymidine phosphorylase (platelet-derived endothelial cell growth factor) in colorectal tumors is associated with nonresponse to 5-fluorouracil. Clin Cancer Res 1998;4:2371–6.
101. Salonga D, Danenberg KD, Johnson M, et al. Colorectal tumors responding to 5-fluorouracil have low gene expression levels of dihydropyrimidine dehydrogenase, thymidylate synthase, and thymidine phosphorylase. Clin Cancer Res 2000;6:1322–7.
102. Iqbal S, Stoehlmacher J, Lenz HJ. Tailored chemotherapy for colorectal cancer: a new approach to therapy. Cancer Invest 2004;22:762–73.
103. Wolmark N, Wieand HS, Rockette HE, et al. The prognostic significance of tumor location and bowel obstruction in Dukes B and C colorectal cancer. Findings from the NSABP clinical trials. Ann Surg 1983;198:743–52.
104. Lopez MJ, Monafo WW. Role of extended resection in the initial treatment of locally advanced colorectal carcinoma. Surgery 1993;113:365–72.
105. Verwaal VJ, van Ruth S, de Bree E, et al. Randomized trial of cytoreduction and hyperthermic intraperitoneal chemotherapy versus systemic chemotherapy and palliative surgery in patients with peritoneal carcinomatosis of colorectal cancer. J Clin Oncol 2003;21:3737–43.
106. Scoggins CR, Meszoely IM, Blanke CD, et al. Nonoperative management of primary colorectal cancer in patients with stage IV disease. Ann Surg Oncol 1999;6:651–7.
107. Nelson H, Petrelli N, Carlin A, et al. Guidelines 2000 for colon and rectal cancer surgery. J Natl Cancer Inst 2001;93:583–96.
108. Kuvshinoff B, Maghfoor I, Miedema B, et al. Distal margin requirements after preoperative chemoradiotherapy for distal rectal carcinomas: are < or = 1 cm distal margins sufficient? Ann Surg Oncol 2001;8:163–9.
109. Andreola S, Leo E, Belli F, et al. Adenocarcinoma of the lower third of the rectum surgically treated with a < 10-MM distal clearance: preliminary results in 35 N0 patients. Ann Surg Oncol 2001;8:611–5.
110. Tepper JE, O'Connell MJ, Niedzwiecki D, et al. Impact of number of nodes retrieved on outcome in patients with rectal cancer. J Clin Oncol 2001;19:157–63.
111. Saha S, Wiese D, Badin J, et al. Technical details of sentinel lymph node mapping in colorectal cancer and its impact on staging. Ann Surg Oncol 2000;7:120–4.
112. Saha S, Bilchik A, Wiese D, et al. Ultrastaging of colorectal cancer by sentinel lymph node mapping technique--a multicenter trial. Ann Surg Oncol 2001;8(9 Suppl):94S–8S.
113. Bertagnolli M, Miedema B, Redston M, et al. Sentinel node staging of resectable colon cancer: results of a multicenter study. Ann Surg 2004;240:624–8; discussion 628–30.
114. Lindemann F, Schlimok G, Dirschedl P, et al. Prognostic significance of micrometastatic tumour cells in bone marrow of colorectal cancer patients. Lancet 1992;340:685–9.
115. The Clinical Outcomes of Surgical Therapy Study Group. A comparison of laparoscopically assisted and open colectomy for colon cancer. N Engl J Med 2004;350:2050–9.
116. Gordon MS, Cohen AM. Management of invasive carcinoma in pedunculated colorectal polyps. Oncology (Huntingt) 1989;3:99–104; discussion 104–5.
117. Chakravarti A, Compton CC, Shellito PC, et al. Long-term follow-up of patients with rectal cancer managed by local excision with and without adjuvant irradiation. Ann Surg 1999;230:49–54.
118. Bouvet M, Milas M, Giacco GG, et al. Predictors of recurrence after local excision and postoperative chemoradiation therapy of adenocarcinoma of the rectum. Ann Surg Oncol 1999;6:26–32.
119. Steele GD Jr, Herndon JE, Bleday R, et al. Sphincter-sparing treatment for distal rectal adenocarcinoma. Ann Surg Oncol 1999;6:433–41.
120. Garcia-Aguilar J, Mellgren A, Sirivongs P, et al. Local excision of rectal cancer without adjuvant therapy: a word of caution. Ann Surg 2000;231:345–51.
121. Friel CM, Cromwell JW, Marra C, et al. Salvage radical surgery after failed local excision for early rectal cancer. Dis Colon Rectum 2002;45:875–9.
122. Mohiuddin M, Marks G, Bannon J. High-dose preoperative radiation and full thickness local excision: a new option for selected T3 distal rectal cancers. Int J Radiat Oncol Biol Phys 1994;30:845–9.
123. Kim CJ, Yeatman TJ, Coppola D, et al. Local excision of T2 and T3 rectal cancers after downstaging chemoradiation. Ann Surg 2001;234:352–8; discussion 358–9.
124. Schell SR, Zlotecki RA, Mendenhall WM, et al. Transanal excision of locally advanced rectal cancers downstaged using neoadjuvant chemoradiotherapy. J Am Coll Surg 2002;194:584–90; discussion 590–1.
125. Onaitis MW, Noone RB, Fields R, et al. Complete response to neoadjuvant chemoradiation for rectal cancer does not influence survival. Ann Surg Oncol 2001;8:801–6.
126. Habr-Gama A, Perez RO, Nadalin W, et al. Operative versus nonoperative treatment for stage 0 distal rectal cancer following chemoradiation therapy: long-term results. Ann Surg 2004;240:711–7.
127. Crane CH, Janjan NA, Abbruzzese JL, et al. Effective pelvic symptom control using initial chemoradiation without colostomy in metastatic rectal cancer. Int J Radiat Oncol Biol Phys 2001;49:107–16.
128. Willett CG, Tepper JE, Cohen AM, et al. Failure patterns following curative resection of colonic carcinoma. Ann Surg 1984;200:685–90.
129. Willett CG, Goldberg S, Shellito PC, et al. Does postoperative irradiation play a role in the adjuvant therapy of stage T4 colon cancer? Cancer J Sci Am 1999;5:242–7.
130. Willett CG, Fung CY, Kaufman DS, et al. Postoperative radiation therapy for high-risk colon carcinoma. J Clin Oncol 1993;11:1112–7.
131. Martenson JA Jr, Willett CG, Sargent DJ, et al. Phase III study of adjuvant chemotherapy and radiation therapy compared with chemotherapy alone in the surgical adjuvant treatment of colon cancer: results of intergroup protocol 0130 [comment]. J Clin Oncol 2004;22:3277–83.
132. Rich T, Gunderson LL, Lew R, et al. Patterns of recurrence of rectal cancer after potentially curative surgery. Cancer 1983;52:1317–29.
133. Kapiteijn E, Marijnen CA, Nagtegaal ID, et al. Preoperative radiotherapy combined with total mesorectal excision for resectable rectal cancer. N Engl J Med 2001;345:638–46.
134. Willett CG, Badizadegan K, Ancukiewicz M, Shellito PC. Prognostic factors in stage T3N0 rectal cancer: do all patients require postoperative pelvic irradiation and chemotherapy? Dis Colon Rectum 1999;42:167–73.
135. Tominaga T, Sakabe T, Koyama Y, et al. Prognostic factors for patients with colon or rectal carcinoma treated with resection only. Five-year follow-up report. Cancer 1996;78:403–8.
136. Phillips RK, Hittinger R, Blesovsky L, et al. Large bowel cancer: surgical pathology and its relationship to survival. Br J Surg 1984;71:604–10.
137. Nagtegaal ID, Marijnen CA, Kranenbarg EK, et al. Circumferential margin involvement is still an important predictor of local recurrence in rectal carcinoma: not one millimeter but two millimeters is the limit. Am J Surg Pathol 2002;26:350–7.
138. Nagtegaal ID, van de Velde CJ, van der Worp E, et al. Macroscopic evaluation of rectal cancer resection specimen: clinical significance of the pathologist in quality control. J Clin Oncol 2002;20:1729–34.
139. Meyerhardt JA, Tepper JE, Niedzwiecki D, et al. Impact of body mass index on outcomes and treatment-related toxicity in patients with stage II and III rectal cancer: findings from intergroup trial 0114. J Clin Oncol 2004;22:648–57.
140. Gunderson LL, Sargent DJ, Tepper JE, et al. Impact of T and N stage and treatment on survival and relapse in adjuvant rectal cancer: a pooled analysis. J Clin Oncol 2004;22:1785–96.
141. Fidler IJ, Kripke ML. Metastasis results from preexisting variant cells within a malignant tumor. Science 1977;197:893–5.
142. Glaves D, Huben RP, Weiss L. Haematogenous dissemination of cells from human renal adenocarcinomas. Br J Cancer 1988;57:32–5.
143. Talmadge JE, Wolman SR, Fidler IJ. Evidence for the clonal origin of spontaneous metastases. Science 1982;217:361–3.
144. Le Voyer TE, Sigurdson ER, Hanlon AL, et al. Colon cancer survival is associated with increasing number of lymph nodes analyzed: a secondary survey of intergroup trial INT-0089. J Clin Oncol 2003;21:2912–9.
145. Folprecht G, Cunningham D, Ross P, et al. Efficacy of 5-fluorouracil-based chemotherapy in elderly patients with metastatic colorectal cancer: a pooled analysis of clinical trials. Ann Oncol 2004;15:1330–8.
146. Sargent DJ, Goldberg RM, Jacobson SD, et al. A pooled analysis of adjuvant chemotherapy for resected colon cancer in elderly patients. N Engl J Med 2001;345:1091–7.
147. Laurie JA, Moertel CG, Fleming TR, et al. Surgical adjuvant therapy of large-bowel carcinoma: an evaluation of levamisole and the combination of levamisole and fluorouracil. The North Central Cancer Treatment Group and the Mayo Clinic. [See comment in: SS J Clin Oncol 1990;8:365.] J Clin Oncol 1989;7:1447–56.
148. Mamounas E, Wieand S, Wolmark N, et al. Comparative efficacy of adjuvant chemotherapy in patients with Dukes' B versus Dukes' C colon cancer: results from four National Surgical Adjuvant Breast and Bowel Project adjuvant studies (C-01, C-02, C-03, and C-04). J Clin Oncol 1999;17:1349–55.
149. IMPACT B2 Investigators. Efficacy of adjuvant fluorouracil and folinic acid in B2 colon cancer. International Multi-

centre Pooled Analysis of B2 Colon Cancer Trials. J Clin Oncol 1999;17:1356–63.

150. Moertel CG, Fleming TR, Macdonald JS, et al. Levamisole and fluorouracil for adjuvant therapy of resected colon carcinoma. N Engl J Med 1990;322:352–8.

151. Wolmark N, Rockette H, Mamounas E, et al. Clinical trial to assess the relative efficacy of fluorouracil and leucovorin, fluorouracil and levamisole, and fluorouracil, leucovorin, and levamisole in patients with Dukes' B and C carcinoma of the colon: results from National Surgical Adjuvant Breast and Bowel Project C-04. J Clin Oncol 1999;17:3553–9.

152. Andre T, Boni C, Mounedji-Boudiaf L, et al. Oxaliplatin, fluorouracil, and leucovorin as adjuvant treatment for colon cancer. N Engl J Med 2004;350:2343–51.

153. Wolmark N, Wieand S, Kuebler JP, et al. A phase III trial comparing FULV to FULV + oxaliplatin in stage II or III carcinoma of the colon: results of NSABP protocol C-07. Proc Am Soc Clin Oncol 2005;23:246.

154. Saltz LB, Cox JV, Blanke C, et al. Irinotecan plus fluorouracil and leucovorin for metastatic colorectal cancer. Irinotecan Study Group. N Engl J Med 2000;343:905–14.

155. Van Cutsem E, Labianca R, Hossfeld D, et al. Randomized phase III trial comparing infused irinotecan/5-fluorouracil (5-FU)/folinic acid (IF) versus 5-FU/FA (F) in stage III colon cancer patients (pts). (PETACC 3). Proc Am Soc Clin Oncol 2005;23:3.

156. Hoff PM, Pazdur R, Benner SE, Canetta R. UFT and leucovorin: a review of its clinical development and therapeutic potential in the oral treatment of cancer. Anticancer Drugs 1998;9:479–90.

157. Wolmark N, Wieand HS, Kuebler JP, et al. A phase III trial comparing oral UFT to FULV in stage II and III carcinoma of the colon: results of Protocol C-06 [abstract 3500]. Proc Am Soc Clin Oncol 2005;23.

158. Van Cutsem E, Hoff PM, Harper P, et al. Oral capecitabine vs intravenous 5-fluorouracil and leucovorin: integrated efficacy data and novel analyses from two large, randomised, phase III trials. Br J Cancer 2004;90:1190–7.

159. Twelves C, Wong A, Nowacki M, et al. Updated efficacy findings from the X-ACT phase III trial of capecitabine (X) vs bolus 5-FU/LV as adjuvant therapy for patients (pts) with Dukes' C colon cancer. Proc Am Soc Clin Oncol 2005;23:251.

160. Minsky BD, Conti JA, Huang Y, Knopf K. Relationship of acute gastrointestinal toxicity and the volume of irradiated small bowel in patients receiving combined modality therapy for rectal cancer. J Clin Oncol 1995;13:1409–16.

161. Valentini V, Coco C, Cellini N, et al. Preoperative chemoradiation for extraperitoneal T3 rectal cancer: acute toxicity, tumor response, and sphincter preservation. Int J Radiat Oncol Biol Phys 1998;40:1067–75.

162. Hyams DM, Mamounas EP, Petrelli N, et al. A clinical trial to evaluate the worth of preoperative multimodality therapy in patients with operable carcinoma of the rectum: a progress report of National Surgical Breast and Bowel Project Protocol R-03. Dis Colon Rectum 1997;40:131–9.

163. Crane CH, Skibber JM, Feig BW, et al. Response to preoperative chemoradiation increases the use of sphincter-preserving surgery in patients with locally advanced low rectal carcinoma. Cancer 2003;97:517–24.

164. Sauer R, Becker H, Hohenberger W, et al. Preoperative versus postoperative chemoradiotherapy for rectal cancer.[comment]. N Engl J Med 2004;351:1731–40.

165. Pahlman L, Glimelius B. Pre- or postoperative radiotherapy in rectal and rectosigmoid carcinoma. Report from a randomized multicenter trial. Ann Surg 1990;211:187–95.

166. Janjan NA, Khoo VS, Rich TA, et al. Locally advanced rectal cancer: surgical complications after infusional chemotherapy and radiation therapy. Radiology 1998;206:131–6.

167. Swedish Rectal Cancer Trial. Improved survival with preoperative radiotherapy in resectable rectal cancer. N Engl J Med 1997;336:980–7.

168. Cedermark B, Johansson H, Rutqvist LE, Wilking N. The Stockholm I trial of preoperative short term radiotherapy in operable rectal carcinoma. A prospective randomized trial. Stockholm Colorectal Cancer Study Group. Cancer 1995;75:2269–75.

169. Holm T, Rutqvist LE, Johansson H, Cedermark B. Postoperative mortality in rectal cancer treated with or without preoperative radiotherapy: causes and risk factors. Br J Surg 1996;83:964–8.

170. Camma C, Giunta M, Fiorica F, et al. Preoperative radiotherapy for resectable rectal cancer: a meta-analysis. JAMA 2000;284:1008–15.

171. Suwinski R, Taylor JM, Withers HR. Rapid growth of microscopic rectal cancer as a determinant of response to preoperative radiation therapy. Int J Radiat Oncol Biol Phys 1998;42:943–51.

172. Frykholm GJ, Isacsson U, Nygard K, et al. Preoperative radiotherapy in rectal carcinoma—aspects of acute adverse effects and radiation technique. Int J Radiat Oncol Biol Phys 1996;35:1039–48.

173. Kapiteijn E, Kranenbarg EK, Steup WH, et al. Total mesorectal excision (TME) with or without preoperative radiotherapy in the treatment of primary rectal cancer. Prospective randomised trial with standard operative and histopathological techniques. Dutch ColoRectal Cancer Group. Eur J Surg 1999;165:410–20.

174. Bosset J, Calais G, Mineur L, et al. Preoperative radiation (Preop RT) in rectal cancer: effect and timing of additional chemotherapy (CT) 5-year results of the EORTC 22921 trial [abstract 3505]. J Clin Oncol 2005;23(Suppl 16):247S.

175. Gerard J, Bonnetain F, Conroy T, et al. Preoperative (preop) radiotherapy (RT) + 5 FU/folinic acid (FA) in T3-4 rectal cancers : results of the FFCD 9203 randomized trial [abstract 3504]. J Clin Oncol 2005;23(Suppl 16):S1.

176. Krook JE, Moertel CG, Gunderson LL, et al. Effective surgical adjuvant therapy for high-risk rectal carcinoma. N Engl J Med 1991;324:709–15.

177. Douglass HO Jr, Moertel CG, Mayer RJ, et al. Survival after postoperative combination treatment of rectal cancer. N Engl J Med 1986;315:1294–5.

178. Prolongation of the disease-free interval in surgically treated rectal carcinoma. Gastrointestinal Tumor Study Group. N Engl J Med 1985;312:1465–72.

179. NIH consensus conference. Adjuvant therapy for patients with colon and rectal cancer. JAMA 1990;264:1444–50.

180. Wolmark N, Wieand HS, Hyams DM, et al. Randomized trial of postoperative adjuvant chemotherapy with or without radiotherapy for carcinoma of the rectum: National Surgical Adjuvant Breast and Bowel Project Protocol R-02. J Natl Cancer Inst 2000;92:388–96.

181. O'Connell MJ, Martenson JA, Wieand HS, et al. Improving adjuvant therapy for rectal cancer by combining protracted-infusion fluorouracil with radiation therapy after curative surgery. N Engl J Med 1994;331:502–7.

182. Meta-analysis Group in Cancer. Efficacy of intravenous continuous infusion of fluorouracil compared with bolus administration in advanced colorectal cancer. J Clin Oncol 1998;16:301–8.

183. Tepper JE, O'Connell MJ, Petroni GR, et al. Adjuvant postoperative fluorouracil-modulated chemotherapy combined with pelvic radiation therapy for rectal cancer: initial results of intergroup 0114. J Clin Oncol 1997;15:2030–9.

184. Smalley S, Benedetti J, Williamson S, et al. Intergroup 0144—a phase III trial rectal surgical adjuvant trial of pelvc radiation plus 5-FU based chemotherapy (bolus 5-FU before and after PVI +XRT vs PVI before, during, and after XRT + PVI vs biochemically modulated bolus 5-FU and XRT): Mature outcome results andpelvic failure analysis [abstract 114]. Int J Radiat Oncol Biol Phys 2004;60(Suppl 1):S137.

185. Lee JH, Ahn JH, Bahng H, et al. Randomized trial of postoperative adjuvant therapy in stage II and III rectal cancer to define the optimal sequence of chemotherapy and radiotherapy: a preliminary report. J Clin Oncol 2002;20:1751–8.

186. Janjan NA, Crane C, Feig BW, et al. Improved overall survival among responders to preoperative chemoradiation for locally advanced rectal cancer. Am J Clin Oncol 2001;24:107–12.

187. Mohiuddin M, Regine WF, John WJ, et al. Preoperative chemoradiation in fixed distal rectal cancer: dose time factors for pathological complete response. Int J Radiat Oncol Biol Phys 2000;46:883–8.

188. Sauer R, Roedel C, Martus P, et al. Prognostic factors after neoadjuvant radiochemotherapy for rectal cancer: update of the CAO/ARO/AIO-94 phase III study [abstract 3503]. J Clin Oncol 2005;16:246s

189. Gunderson LL, Nelson H, Martenson JA, et al. Intraoperative electron and external beam irradiation with or without 5-fluorouracil and maximum surgical resection for previously unirradiated, locally recurrent colorectal cancer. Dis Colon Rectum 1996;39:1379–95.

190. Wong CS, Cummings BJ, Brierley JD, et al. Treatment of locally recurrent rectal carcinoma—results and prognostic factors. Int J Radiat Oncol Biol Phys 1998;40:427–35.

191. Mohiuddin M, Marks G, Marks J. Long-term results of reirradiation for patients with recurrent rectal carcinoma. Cancer 2002;95:1144–50.

192. Scheithauer W, Rosen H, Kornek GV, et al. Randomised comparison of combination chemotherapy plus supportive care with supportive care alone in patients with metastatic colorectal cancer. BMJ 1993;306:752–5.

193. Hoff PM, Ansari R, Batist G, et al. Comparison of oral capecitabine versus intravenous fluorouracil plus leucovorin as first-line treatment in 605 patients with metastatic colorectal cancer: results of a randomized phase III study. J Clin Oncol 2001;19:2282–92.

194. Douillard JY, Hoff PM, Skillings JR, et al. Multicenter phase III study of uracil/tegafur and oral leucovorin versus fluorouracil and leucovorin in patients with previously untreated metastatic colorectal cancer. J Clin Oncol 2002;20:3605–16.

195. Douillard JY, Cunningham D, Roth AD, et al. Irinotecan combined with fluorouracil compared with fluorouracil alone as first-line treatment for metastatic colorectal cancer: a multicentre randomised trial. Lancet 2000;355:1041–7.

196. de Gramont A, Figer A, Seymour M, et al. Leucovorin and fluorouracil with or without oxaliplatin as first-line treatment in advanced colorectal cancer. J Clin Oncol 2000;18:2938–47.

197. Grothey A, Goldberg RM. A review of oxaliplatin and its clinical use in colorectal cancer. Expert Opin Pharmacother 2004;5:2159–70.

198. Hurwitz H, Fehrenbacher L, Novotny W, et al. Bevacizumab plus irinotecan, fluorouracil, and leucovorin for metastatic colorectal cancer. N Engl J Med 2004;350:2335–42.

199. Cunningham D, Humblet Y, Siena S, et al. Cetuximab monotherapy and cetuximab plus irinotecan in irinotecan-refractory metastatic colorectal cancer. N Engl J Med 2004;351:337–45.

200. Diasio RB, Lu Z, Zhang R, Shahinian HS. Fluoropyrimidine catabolism. Cancer Treat Res 1995;78:71–93.

201. Tsai CM, Gazdar AF, Allegra C, et al. Enhancement of fluorinated pyrimidine-induced cytotoxicity by leucovorin in human lung cancer cell lines. Int J Cancer 1990;46:101–5.

202. O'Connell MJ. A phase III trial of 5-fluorouracil and leucovorin in the treatment of advanced colorectal cancer. A Mayo Clinic/North Central Cancer Treatment Group study. Cancer 1989;63(6 Suppl):1026–30.

203. Poon MA, O'Connell MJ, Moertel CG, et al. Biochemical modulation of fluorouracil: evidence of significant improvement of survival and quality of life in patients with advanced colorectal carcinoma. J Clin Oncol 1989;7:1407–18.

204. Petrelli N, Douglass HO Jr, Herrera L, et al. The modulation of fluorouracil with leucovorin in metastatic colorectal carcinoma: a prospective randomized phase III trial. Gastrointestinal Tumor Study Group. J Clin Oncol 1989;7:1419–26.

205. Hoff PM, Pazdur R. Progress in the development of novel treatments for colorectal cancer. Oncology (Huntingt) 2004;18:705–8.

206. Hoff PM. New drugs for colorectal cancer. Cancer Chemother Biol Response Modif 2003;21:817–29.

207. Hahn RG, Moertel CG, Schutt AJ, Bruckner HW. A double-blind comparison of intensive course 5-flourouracil by oral vs. intravenous route in the treatment of colorectal carcinoma. Cancer 1975;35:1031–5.

208. Hoff PM, Royce M, Medgyesy D, et al. Oral fluoropoyrimidines. Semin Oncol 1999;26:640–6.

209. Van Cutsem E, Twelves C, Cassidy J, et al. Oral capecitabine compared with intravenous fluorouracil plus leucovorin in patients with metastatic colorectal cancer: results of a large phase III study. J Clin Oncol 2001;19:4097–106.

210. Lassere Y, Hoff P. Management of hand-foot syndrome in patients treated with capecitabine (Xeloda). Eur J Oncol Nurs 2004;8 Suppl 1:S31–40.

211. Bajetta E, Procopio G, Celio L, et al. Safety and efficacy of two different doses of capecitabine in the treatment of advanced breast cancer in older women. J Clin Oncol 2005;23:2155–61.

212. Cassidy J, Tabernero J, Twelves C, et al. XELOX (capecitabine plus oxaliplatin): active first-line therapy for patients with metastatic colorectal cancer. J Clin Oncol 2004;22:2084–91.

213. Jordan K, Kellner O, Kegel T, et al. Phase II trial of capecitabine/irinotecan and capecitabine/oxaliplatin in advanced gastrointestinal cancers. Clin Colorectal Cancer 2004;4:46–50.

214. Borner MM, Bernhard J, Dietrich D, et al. A randomized phase II trial of capecitabine and two different schedules of irinotecan in first-line treatment of metastatic colorectal cancer: efficacy, quality-of-life and toxicity. Ann Oncol 2005;16:282–8.

215. Rich T. Capecitabine and radiation therapy for advanced gastrointestinal malignancies. Oncology (Huntingt) 2002;16(12 Suppl 14):27–30.

216. Hoff PM, Lassere Y, Pazdur R. Tegafur/uracil + calcium folinate in colorectal cancer: double modulation of fluorouracil [review]. Drugs 1999;58 Suppl 3:77–83.
217. Carmichael J, Popiela T, Radstone D, et al. Randomized comparative study of tegafur/uracil and oral leucovorin versus parenteral fluorouracil and leucovorin in patients with previously untreated metastatic colorectal cancer. J Clin Oncol 2002;20:3617–27.
218. Hoff PM. The tegafur-based dihydropyrimidine dehydrogenase inhibitory fluoropyrimidines, UFT/leucovorin (ORZEL) and S-1: a review of their clinical development and therapeutic potential. Invest New Drugs 2000;18:331–42.
219. Taguchi T, Inuyama Y, Kanamaru R, et al. Phase I study of S-1. S-1 Study Group. Gan to Kagaku Ryoho (Jpn J Cancer Chemother) 1997;24:2253–64.
220. Peters GJ, Van Groeningen CJ, Schomage JH, et al. Phase I clinical and pharmacokinetic study of S-1, an oral 5-fluorouracil (5-FU)-based antineoplastic agent [meeting abstract]. Proc Annu Meet Am Soc Clin Oncol 1997.
221. Hoff PM, Saad ED, Ajani JA, et al. Phase I study with pharmacokinetics of s-1 on an oral daily schedule for 28 days in patients with solid tumors. Clin Cancer Res 2003;9:134–42.
222. Comets E, Ikeda K, Hoff P, et al. Comparison of the pharmacokinetics of S-1, an oral anticancer agent, in western and Japanese patients. J Pharmacokinet Pharmacodyn 2003;30:257–83.
223. Judson IR. 'Tomudex' (raltitrexed) development: preclinical, phase I and II studies. Anticancer Drugs 1997;8 Suppl 2:S5–9.
224. Cunningham D, Zalcberg JR, Rath U, et al. Final results of a randomised trial comparing 'Tomudex' (raltitrexed) with 5-fluorouracil plus leucovorin in advanced colorectal cancer. "Tomudex" Colorectal Cancer Study Group [published erratum appears in Ann Oncol 1997;8:407]. Ann Oncol 1996;7:961–5.
225. Cocconi G, Cunningham D, Van Cutsem E, et al. Open, randomized, multicenter trial of raltitrexed versus fluorouracil plus high-dose leucovorin in patients with advanced colorectal cancer. Tomudex Colorectal Cancer Study Group. J Clin Oncol 1998;16:2943–52.
226. Pazdur R, Vincent M. Raltitrexed (Tomudex) versus 5-fluorouracil and leucovorin (5-FU + LV) in patients with advanced colorectal cancer (ACC): results of a randomized, multicenter, North American trial [meeting abstract]. Proc Annu Meet Am Soc Clin Oncol 1997.
227. Cunningham D, Pyrhonen S, James RD, et al. Randomised trial of irinotecan plus supportive care versus supportive care alone after fluorouracil failure for patients with metastatic colorectal cancer. Lancet 1998;352:1413–8.
228. Judson I, Maughan T, Beale P, et al. Effects of impaired renal function on the pharmacokinetics of raltitrexed (Tomudex ZD1694). Br J Cancer 1998;78:1188–93.
229. Atsumi R, Suzuki W, Hakusui H. Identification of the metabolites of irinotecan, a new derivative of camptothecin, in rat bile and its biliary excretion. Xenobiotica 1991;21:1159–69.
230. Kawato Y, Aonuma M, Hirota Y, et al. Intracellular roles of SN-38, a metabolite of the camptothecin derivative CPT-11, in the antitumor effect of CPT-11. Cancer Res 1991;51:4187–91.
231. Kaneda N, Nagata H, Furuta T, Yokokura T. Metabolism and pharmacokinetics of the camptothecin analogue CPT-11 in the mouse [published erratum appears in Cancer Res 1990;50:4451]. Cancer Res 1990;50:1715–20.
232. Abigerges D, Chabot GG, Armand JP, et al. Phase I and pharmacologic studies of the camptothecin analog irinotecan administered every 3 weeks in cancer patients. J Clin Oncol. 1995;13:210–21.
233. Negoro S, Fukuoka M, Masuda N, et al. Phase I study of weekly intravenous infusions of CPT-11, a new derivative of camptothecin, in the treatment of advanced non-small-cell lung cancer. J Natl Cancer Inst 1991;83:1164–8.
234. Von Hoff DD, Burris HA 3rd, Eckardt J, et al. Preclinical and phase I trials of topoisomerase I inhibitors. Cancer Chemother Pharmacol 1994;34 Suppl:S41–5.
235. Rothenberg ML, Eckardt JR, Kuhn JG, et al. Phase II trial of irinotecan in patients with progressive or rapidly recurrent colorectal cancer. J Clin Oncol 1996;14:1128–35.
236. Cunningham D, Pyrhonen S, James RD, et al. Randomised trial of irinotecan plus supportive care versus supportive care alone after fluorouracil failure for patients with metastatic colorectal cancer [comments]. Lancet 1998;352:1413–8.
237. Rougier P, Van Cutsem E, Bajetta E, et al. Randomised trial of irinotecan versus fluorouracil by continuous infusion after fluorouracil failure in patients with metastatic colorectal cancer [comments] [published erratum appears in Lancet 1998;352:1634]. Lancet 1998;352:1407–12.
238. Tournigand C, Andre T, Achille E, et al. FOLFIRI followed by FOLFOX6 or the reverse sequence in advanced colorectal cancer: a randomized GERCOR study. J Clin Oncol 2004;22:229–37.
239. Gupta E, Lestingi TM, Mick R, et al. Metabolic fate of irinotecan in humans: correlation of glucuronidation with diarrhea. Cancer Res 1994;54:3723–5.
240. Marcuello E, Altes A, Menoyo A, et al. UGT1A1 gene variations and irinotecan treatment in patients with metastatic colorectal cancer. Br J Cancer 2004;91:678–82.
241. Alimonti A, Gelibter A, Pavese I, et al. New approaches to prevent intestinal toxicity of irinotecan-based regimens. Cancer Treat Rev 2004;30:555–62.
242. Carlini LE, Meropol NJ, Bever J, et al. UGT1A7 and UGT1A9 polymorphisms predict response and toxicity in colorectal cancer patients treated with capecitabine/irinotecan. Clin Cancer Res 2005;11:1226–36.
243. Ando Y, Ueoka H, Sugiyama T, et al. Polymorphisms of UDP-glucuronosyltransferase and pharmacokinetics of irinotecan. Ther Drug Monit 2002;24:111–116.
244. Iyer L, Das S, Janisch L, et al. UGT1A1*28 polymorphism as a determinant of irinotecan disposition and toxicity. Pharmacogenomics J 2002;2:43–7.
245. Rothenberg ML, Meropol NJ, Poplin EA, et al. Mortality associated with irinotecan plus bolus fluorouracil/leucovorin: summary findings of an independent panel. J Clin Oncol 2001;19:3801–7.
246. Schmittel A, Jahnke K, Thiel E, Keilholz U. Neomycin as secondary prophylaxis for irinotecan-induced diarrhea. Ann Oncol 2004;15:1296.
247. Wasserman E, Myara A, Lokiec F, et al. Severe CPT-11 toxicity in patients with Gilbert's syndrome: two case reports. Ann Oncol 1997;8:1049–51.
248. Bleiberg H. Oxaliplatin (L-OHP): a new reality in colorectal cancer. Br J Cancer 1998;77 Suppl 4:1–3.
249. Raymond E, Faivre S, Woynarowski JM, Chaney SG. Oxaliplatin: mechanism of action and antineoplastic activity. Semin Oncol 1998;25(2 Suppl 5):4–12.
250. Rothenberg ML, Oza AM, Bigelow RH, et al. Superiority of oxaliplatin and fluorouracil-leucovorin compared with either therapy alone in patients with progressive colorectal cancer after irinotecan and fluorouracil-leucovorin: interim results of a phase III trial. J Clin Oncol 2003;21:2059–69.
251. Goldberg RM, Sargent DJ, Morton RF, et al. A randomized controlled trial of fluorouracil plus leucovorin, irinotecan, and oxaliplatin combinations in patients with previously untreated metastatic colorectal cancer. J Clin Oncol 2004;22:23–30.
252. Hoff PM, Saad ED, Pazdur R, et al. Phase I trial of combined irinotecan and oxaliplatin given every three weeks to patients with metastatic colorectal cancer. Invest New Drugs 2004;22:307–13.
253. Grothey A. Oxaliplatin-safety profile: neurotoxicity. Semin Oncol 2003;30(4 Suppl 15):5–13.
254. Gamelin L, Boisdron-Celle M, Delva R, et al. Prevention of oxaliplatin-related neurotoxicity by calcium and magnesium infusions: a retrospective study of 161 patients receiving oxaliplatin combined with 5-Fluorouracil and leucovorin for advanced colorectal cancer. Clin Cancer Res 2004;10(12 Pt 1):4055–61.
255. Citri A, Skaria KB, Yarden Y. The deaf and the dumb: the biology of ErbB-2 and ErbB-3. Exp Cell Res 2003;284:54–65.
256. Yarden Y. The EGFR family and its ligands in human cancer. signalling mechanisms and therapeutic opportunities. Eur J Cancer 2001;37 Suppl 4:S3–8.
257. Saltz LB, Meropol NJ, Loehrer PJ Sr, et al. Phase II trial of cetuximab in patients with refractory colorectal cancer that expresses the epidermal growth factor receptor. J Clin Oncol 2004;22;1201–8.
258. Hoff PM, Ellis LM, Abbruzzese JL. Monoclonal antibodies: the foundation of therapy for colorectal cancer in the 21st century? Oncology (Huntingt) 2004;18:736–41; discussion 742, 745–6.
259. Reynolds NA, Wagstaff AJ. Cetuximab: in the treatment of metastatic colorectal cancer. Drugs 2004;64:109–18; discussion 119–21.
260. Chung KY, Shia J, Kemeny NE, et al. Cetuximab shows activity in colorectal cancer patients with tumors that do not express the epidermal growth factor receptor by immunohistochemistry. J Clin Oncol 2005;23:1803–10.
261. Ferrara N, Gerber HP, LeCouter J. The biology of VEGF and its receptors. Nat Med 2003;9:669–76.
262. Plouet J, Moukadiri H. Specific binding of vasculotropin to bovine brain capillary endothelial cells. Biochimie 1990;72:51–5.
263. Vaisman N, Gospodarowicz D, Neufeld G. Characterization of the receptors for vascular endothelial growth factor. J Biol Chem 1990;265:19461–6.
264. Dvorak HF. Vascular permeability factor/vascular endothelial growth factor: a critical cytokine in tumor angiogenesis and a potential target for diagnosis and therapy. J Clin Oncol 2002;20:4368–80.
265. Giantonio BJ, Catalano PJ, Meropol NJ, et al. High dose bevacizumab improves survival when combined with FOLFOX 4 in previously treated advanced colorectal cancer: results from the Eastern Cooperative Oncology Group (ECOG) study E3200 [abstract 2]. Proc Am Soc Clin Oncol 2005;23:(S16):S247.
266. Byers T, Levin B, Rothenberger D, et al. American Cancer Society guidelines for screening and surveillance for early detection of colorectal polyps and cancer: update 1997. American Cancer Society Detection and Treatment Advisory Group on Colorectal Cancer. CA Cancer J Clin 1997;47:154–60.
267. Tomeo CA, Colditz GA, Willett WC, et al. Harvard report on cancer prevention. Vol 3: prevention of colon cancer in the United States. Cancer Causes Control 1999;10:167–80.
268. Lieberman DA, Weiss DG. One-time screening for colorectal cancer with combined fecal occult-blood testing and examination of the distal colon. N Engl J Med 2001;345:555–60.
269. Lieberman DA, Weiss DG, Bond JH, Aet al. Use of colonoscopy to screen asymptomatic adults for colorectal cancer. Veterans Affairs Cooperative Study Group 380. N Engl J Med 2000;343:162–8.
270. Imperiale TF, Wagner DR, Lin CY, et al. Risk of advanced proximal neoplasms in asymptomatic adults according to the distal colorectal findings. N Engl J Med 2000;343:169–74.
271. Winawer SJ, Stewart ET, Zauber AG, et al. A comparison of colonoscopy and double-contrast barium enema for surveillance after polypectomy. National Polyp Study Work Group. N Engl J Med 2000;342:1766–72.
272. Pickhardt PJ, Choi JR, Hwang I, et al. Computed tomographic virtual colonoscopy to screen for colorectal neoplasia in asymptomatic adults. N Engl J Med 2003;349:2191–200.
273. Cotton PB, Durkalski VL, Pineau BC, et al. Computed tomographic colonography (virtual colonoscopy): a multicenter comparison with standard colonoscopy for detection of colorectal neoplasia. JAMA 2004;291:1713–9.
274. Imperiale TF, Ransohoff DF, Itzkowitz SH, et al. Fecal DNA versus fecal occult blood for colorectal-cancer screening in an average-risk population. N Engl J Med 2004;351:2704–14.
275. Markowitz AJ, Winawer SJ. Screening and surveillance for colorectal carcinoma. Hematol Oncol Clin North Am 1997;11:579–608.
276. American College of Gastroenterology. American Gastroenterological Association medical position statement: impact of dietary fiber on colon cancer occurrence. Gastroenterology 2000;118:1233–4.
277. Sengupta S, Tjandra JJ, Gibson PR. Dietary fiber and colorectal neoplasia. Dis Colon Rectum 2001;44:1016–33.
278. Burkitt DP. Relationship as a clue to causation. Lancet 1970;2:1237–40.
279. Kritchevsky D. Cereal fibres and colorectal cancer: a search for mechanisms. Eur J Cancer Prev 1998;7 Suppl 2:S33–9.
280. Klurfeld DM. Dietary fiber-mediated mechanisms in carcinogenesis. Cancer Res 1992;52(7 Suppl):2055s–9s.
281. Lupton JR, Turner ND. Potential protective mechanisms of wheat bran fiber. Am J Med 1999;106:24S–7S.
282. Bruce WR. Recent hypotheses for the origin of colon cancer. Cancer Res 1987;47:4237–42.
283. Kampman E, Slattery ML, Caan B, Potter JD. Calcium, vitamin D, sunshine exposure, dairy products and colon cancer risk (United States). Cancer Causes Control 2000;11:459–66.
284. Baron JA, Beach M, Mandel JS, et al. Calcium supplements for the prevention of colorectal adenomas. Calcium Polyp Prevention Study Group. N Engl J Med 1999;340:101–7.
285. Wu K, Willett WC, Fuchs CS, et al. Calcium intake and risk of colon cancer in women and men. J Natl Cancer Inst 2002;94:437–46.
286. McCullough ML, Robertson AS, Rodriguez C, et al. Calcium, vitamin D, dairy products, and risk of colorectal cancer in the Cancer Prevention Study II Nutrition Cohort (United States). Cancer Causes Control 2003;14:1–12.
287. Cho E, Smith-Warner SA, Spiegelman D, et al. Dairy foods, calcium, and colorectal cancer: a pooled analysis of 10 cohort studies. J Natl Cancer Inst 2004;96:1015–22.

288. Jacobs EJ, Connell CJ, Chao A, et al. Multivitamin use and colorectal cancer incidence in a US cohort: does timing matter? Am J Epidemiol 2003;158:621–8.
289. Giovannucci E, Stampfer MJ, Colditz GA, et al. Multivitamin use, folate, and colon cancer in women in the Nurses' Health Study. Ann Intern Med 1998;129:517–24.
290. Fuchs CS, Willett WC, Colditz GA, et al. The influence of folate and multivitamin use on the familial risk of colon cancer in women. Cancer Epidemiol Biomarkers Prev 2002;11:227–34.
291. Sharp L, Little J. Polymorphisms in genes involved in folate metabolism and colorectal neoplasia: a HuGE review. Am J Epidemiol 2004;159:423–43.
292. Slattery ML, Benson J, Curtin K, et al. Carotenoids and colon cancer. Am J Clin Nutr 2000;71:575–82.
293. Baron JA, Cole BF, Mott L, et al. Neoplastic and antineoplastic effects of beta-carotene on colorectal adenoma recurrence: results of a randomized trial. J Natl Cancer Inst 2003;95:717–22.
294. Steck-Scott S, Forman MR, Sowell A, et al. Carotenoids, vitamin A and risk of adenomatous polyp recurrence in the polyp prevention trial. Int J Cancer 2004;112:295–305.
295. Baron JA, Cole BF, Sandler RS, et al. A randomized trial of aspirin to prevent colorectal adenomas. N Engl J Med 2003;348:891–9.
296. Sandler RS, Halabi S, Baron JA, et al. A randomized trial of aspirin to prevent colorectal adenomas in patients with previous colorectal cancer. N Engl J Med 2003;348:883–90.
297. Benamouzig R, Deyra J, Martin A, et al. Daily soluble aspirin and prevention of colorectal adenoma recurrence: one-year results of the APACC trial. Gastroenterology 2003;125:328–36.
298. Williams CS, DuBois RN. Prostaglandin endoperoxide synthase: why two isoforms? Am J Physiol 1996;270(3 Pt 1):G393–400.
299. Du BR. COX-2 in large bowel cancer: a one-sided story. Gut 1999;45:636–7.
300. Giardiello FM, Hamilton SR, Krush AJ, et al. Treatment of colonic and rectal adenomas with sulindac in familial adenomatous polyposis. N Engl J Med 1993;328:1313–6.
301. Steinbach G, Lynch PM, Phillips RK, et al. The effect of celecoxib, a cyclooxygenase-2 inhibitor, in familial adenomatous polyposis. N Engl J Med 2000;342:1946–52.
302. Higuchi T, Iwama T, Yoshinaga K, Tet al. A randomized, double-blind, placebo-controlled trial of the effects of rofecoxib, a selective cyclooxygenase-2 inhibitor, on rectal polyps in familial adenomatous polyposis patients. Clin Cancer Res 2003;9:4756–60.
303. Drazen JM. COX-2 inhibitors—a lesson in unexpected problems. N Engl J Med 2005;352:1131–2.
304. Grodstein F, Newcomb PA, Stampfer MJ. Postmenopausal hormone therapy and the risk of colorectal cancer: a review and meta-analysis. Am J Med 1999;106:574–82.
305. Rossouw JE, Anderson GL, Prentice RL, et al. Risks and benefits of estrogen plus progestin in healthy postmenopausal women: principal results from the Women's Health Initiative randomized controlled trial. JAMA 2002;288:321–33.
306. Goldberg RM, Morton D, Sargent J, et al. N9741:oxaliplatin (oxal) or CPT11 plus 5fluorouracil (5FU)/leucovorin (LV) or oxaliplatin + CPT11 in advanced colorectal cancer (CRC), initial toxicity and response data from a GI Intergroup Study. Proc Am Soc Clin Oncol 2002;21:A511.

Neoplasms of the Anus

Brenda Shank, MD, PhD, FACR
Marshall S. Flam, MD, FACP
John Cunningham, MD

Multimodality therapy has been highly successful in the treatment of anal canal carcinoma in that sphincter preservation for even large primary tumors can be achieved, with an excellent long-term disease-free survival. Patients with inguinal node metastases can also have a high cure rate with this approach, without an extensive superficial and deep inguinal node dissection.

Melanoma of the anal canal, in contrast, continues to have a dismal prognosis; only innovative therapies hold any hope for improvement in this disease.

GROSS AND MICROSCOPIC ANATOMY

The pathologic types of tumors that arise in the anal canal are determined by their anatomic location. It is important to be able to distinguish between the anal canal and the anal margin because of the distinct differences in types of tumors and the natural histories of tumors that arise in these two areas. The anal canal commences at the anorectal ring, defined as the junction of the upper portion of the internal sphincter, the distal part of the puborectalis muscle and the deep part of the external sphincter. The anorectal ring, which can be palpated on digital examination, marks the end of the rectum and the beginning of the proximal anal canal. At the anorectal ring, the epithelium is columnar whereas the cuboidal epithelium is just below, extending to the dentate line. The dentate line is defined as the transition from columnar epithelium of the proximal canal to the stratified squamous epithelium of the lower canal. The epithelium in this area changes over a small segment and includes cuboidal and transitional cells. The stratified squamous epithelium then extends to the anal verge that is defined as the junction of the squamous epithelium with the perianal skin, which contains keratinizing squamous epithelium with hair follicles.

The definition of the anal canal and anal margin has been the source of debate and makes interpretation of many papers difficult. The American Joint Committee on Cancer (AJCC) defines the anal canal and its associated tumors as arising from the anorectal ring and going to the anal verge and all tumors arising below this level as anal margin tumors.[1] Others have used the dentate line as the distal cutoff for anal canal tumors. If one accepts the distal margin of the anal canal to be at the anal verge, as mandated by the AJCC, then 85% of tumors arise in the anal canal and 15% in the anal margin. This is an important distinction because the natural history of anal margin tumors is similar to that of the skin tumors that arise from keratinizing squamous epithelium and not like tumors arising in the anal canal.

The arterial supply to the distal rectum and to the anal canal above the dentate line arises from the superior and middle hemorrhoidal vessels; the blood supply to the dentate line and below arises from the middle and inferior hemorrhoidal vessels. The venous outflow from the proximal anal canal drains systemically via the portal system; the venous drainage below the dentate line drains into the inferior hemorrhoidal vein and systemically via the iliac system.

Innervation of the canal also varies at the dentate line. Above the dentate line, visceral autonomic fibers are responsible for neural control; below the line, somatic nerves are responsible. The internal rectal sphincter muscle is controlled by sympathetic fibers, but the sacral parasympathetic nerves mediate the sensation of distention. The external sphincter is innervated by the inferior hemorrhoidal nerve, which arises from the internal pudendal nerve.

The lymphatics of the anal canal drain via the inguinal, pelvic visceral and hypogastric nodes. The lymphatic channels of the anal canal drain upward into the perirectal and superior rectal lymphatics. This flow continues to the inferior mesenteric system and ultimately into the para-aortic nodes. There is also the potential for flow into the obturator and hypogastric nodes. The lymphatic channels of the anal margin, however, drain down and/or laterally to the inguinal or femoral nodes that eventually drain into the iliac system.

EPIDEMIOLOGY

Cancer in the anal region is rare, with only 2 to 3% of large bowel tumors arising in this area.[2] The incidence has been increasing for both men and women; data from the Connecticut Tumor Registry for 1940 to 1988 indicate a 1.9-fold increase among men and a 2.3-fold increase among women since 1960 in that state.[3] In the past, it was most commonly seen in middle age (50 to 60 years), but the age distribution has been shifting to a younger age. In a study from southern California, only 24% of patients were younger than 64 years old in the period 1955 to 1965, but for 1986 to 1995, 75% were younger than 64 years of age.[4] This disease has been more common in females than in males, with a ratio currently of about 4:3.[2] In the United States, there has been an increase in incidence in men younger than 45 years of age.[5] This has reversed the sex ratio in this younger group. Although it had been thought that anal cancers were rare in the Muslim world due to different sanitary habits, a study from Turkey suggested a similar incidence (1.12% of large bowel carcinomas) in a group of 798 patients at two university medical centers.[6]

ETIOLOGY

In the majority of patients with carcinoma of the anus, no etiologic factor has been identified. Male homosexuality does play a role. In a case-control study of 148 patients,[7] a history of anal-receptive intercourse in men (but not in women) was strongly associated with anal cancer (relative risk [RR] = 33.1). A case-control study of women in Denmark and Sweden demonstrated a statistically significant association between anal cancer risk and anal intercourse, young age at first anal intercourse (younger than 30 years), and the number of anal-sex partners.[8] It has been suggested that spermatozoa and seminal fluid may be etiologic agents and/or cofactors.[9] This would imply that sexual behavior, not sexual preference, is a primary factor in anal cancer development.

Strong evidence for human papillomavirus (HPV) as a causative agent has emerged. There is a relationship between this virus and the development of genital warts (condylomata acuminata), which can evolve into anal cancer after 5 to 40 years.[10] In Daling and colleagues' study,[7] squamous cell carcinoma was strongly associated with genital warts (RR = 26.9 in males and 32.5 in females). In addition, 64% of the 14 patients who had tumors that were positive for HPV had a history of genital warts. Deoxyribonucleic acid (DNA) from HPV type 16 has been found most frequently in studies of anal squamous cell carcinoma (Table 93-1).[11–18] The prevalence of type 16 DNA in anal carcinoma varies with geographic area, being significantly lower in India (3%) and South Africa (11%).[19] In a study of 589 men who have sex with men, it was found that the nonprototype-like variant of HPV type 16 had a 3.2 times higher risk of developing in situ anal carcinoma than the prototype-like variant.[20] In another study, women and

Table 93-1 Frequency of HPV DNA Types in Anal Squamous Cell Carcinoma

	HPV DNA Types (%)								
No. Patients	6	11	16	18	31	33	Unclassified	Total	Reference
70	12	0	14	1	—	—	6	33	11
41	0	0	56	5	—	—	—	61	16
18	6	6	22	6	—	6	28	78*	18
99	♂0	0	52	4	0	0	—	56	13
	♀0	0	84	3	5	5	—	89	
13	0	0	0	0	—	—	—	0	12
4	–	–	100	25	—	—	—	100	14
	6/11								
12	8		17	0	0	0	0	25	17
24	15		77	0	23	8	—	85	15

* Includes one patient (6%) with a mixture of three types.

homosexual men were more likely to have tumors that were high risk HPV (hrHPV) positive and to have anal canal tumors rather than perianal tumors when compared with heterosexual men.[21]

In a study of 82 patients who underwent anal epithelial biopsy during endoscopy, 23 with HPV infection by DNA hybridization had evidence of anal intraepithelial neoplasia (AIN), a premalignant condition.[22] In this study, AIN was significantly higher in homosexual men with HPV (17 of 28), as compared with heterosexual men with HPV (1 of 26); in women with anal HPV, AIN was found only when cervical intraepithelial neoplasia (CIN) was also found. In a later study by the same group, 29 (19%) of 152 women with CIN grade III had histologic AIN, in whom 11 were grade III, and 2 had invasive anal squamous cell carcinomas.[23] In this group with high-grade CIN, 18 of 35 (51%) had HPV 16 DNA identified in anal biopsies, whereas only 14% (7 of 50) in a control group with no history of anogenital neoplasia had HPV 16 DNA identified in anal biopsies.

Another study associated type 16 HPV with high-grade AIN and invasive cancer,[15] whereas types 6 and 11 were associated with condyloma and low-grade AIN. Other studies have also correlated abnormal anal cytologic smears and HPV positivity,[24–27] and some have suggested relationships among immunosuppression, HPV infection, and AIN.[26,27] In a Norwegian study, 100% of HPV-infected anal canal carcinoma cases had evidence of viral integration into the host cell DNA, and 67% also had evidence of episomal virus DNA.[13]

The E6 oncoprotein of HPV viruses inactivates the growth-controlling *p53* suppressor gene product,[28] which may play a role in the pathogenesis of anal cancer. Consistent with inactivation of the *p53* gene product is the finding that the presence of HPV in tumor cells is significantly associated with an increased proliferative rate and aneuploidy as compared with HPV-negative tumors.[29] In one study, there was a high level of nuclear *p53* expression (indicative of a mutated *p53* gene) in invasive anal cancer and in high-grade AIN (60 to 75%); only very low concentrations were expressed in low-grade AIN and none were expressed in normal anal squamous epithelium.[30] In another study, mutant *p53* protein was found in a high percentage of anal cancer patients: 42% of squamous carcinomas and 86% of adenocarcinomas.[28]

Anal canal carcinomas are also associated with prior irradiation and many benign conditions, such as fistulas and hemorrhoids, but rigorous studies of relative risk have rarely been reported. A Danish analysis found no evidence of benign anal lesions causing anal cancer, in spite of a strong temporal association between these diagnoses.[31] An analysis of African-American and white American men in Veterans Administration (VA) hospitals supported the conclusion that benign anal lesions do not increase the risk for anal cancer, but instead may represent the early symptoms of these cancers, because the risk of anal cancer is very high in the first year after the benign diagnosis and rapidly declines thereafter.[32]

Immunosuppression clearly plays a role. There is a 100-fold increase in anogenital tumors in kidney transplant patients (who have a high incidence of condylomata and herpes genitalis) when compared with the nontransplanted population.[33]

Smoking has also been pinpointed as a major risk factor.[7,34] In the Daling study, there is an RR of 7.7 in women and 9.4 in men for current cigarette smoking.[7] In a case-control study from Denmark and Sweden, an increased risk of anal cancer associated with smoking was restricted to premenopausal women.[35] The risk was highest in premenopausal women who currently smoked (multivariate odds ratio: 5.6) and increased linearly by 6.7% per pack-year smoked. The authors have proposed an antiestrogenic mechanism of action for smoking in anal carcinogenesis.

Although the human immunodeficiency virus (HIV) as a causative agent has been suggested in homosexual men,[36] a large study of 435 HIV-associated tumors in Italy demonstrated that in intravenous (IV) drug abusers, anal tumors were extremely rare.[37] In homosexual men, high incidence rates of high-grade AIN were associated with HIV positivity as well as lower CD4 levels and HPV infection.[38] One study showed that the prevalence of high-grade dysplasias and carcinoma was higher in HIV-positive patients than in HIV-negative patients, as was relapse of condylomas, presence of oncogenic HPV, and other recurrent anal infections.[39] Another study showed that HIV-positive women had a higher risk of abnormal anal cytology.[40] In these women, abnormal anal cytology was independently associated with anal HPV ribonucleic acid (RNA), HIV viral load, anal intercourse, and concurrent abnormal cervical cytology in a multivariate analysis.

A study using data from acquired immunodeficiency syndrome (AIDS) and cancer registries in seven United States health departments,[41] concluded that there was a strikingly increased risk of anal cancer among both homosexual patients (RR = 84) and nonhomosexual patients (RR = 38) with AIDS. This may reflect the known risk of immunosuppression rather than a risk of HIV directly. However, despite the advent of highly active antiretroviral therapy (HAART), the incidence of anal cancer continued to increase, based on an analysis of Surveillance, Epidemiology, and End Results (SEER) data for three periods: pre-HIV, pre-HAART, and post-HAART.[42]

PATHOLOGY

Various types of tumors arise in the anal canal and anal margin. The primary histologic type is squamous cell carcinoma, which arises from the epithelium of the anal canal and from the keratinizing epithelium of the anal margin (Figure 93-1). The histologic transition zone at the dentate line accounts for the basaloid (cloacogenic) tumors. In addition to squamous tumors, anal margin tumors include basal cell carcinoma, Paget's disease, Bowen's disease, verrucous carcinoma and Kaposi's sarcoma.

Etiologic differences may be apparent in the histologic variation. Of 14 cloacogenic carcinomas, all were negative for HPV, whereas of 21 squamous carcinomas studied, two-thirds were positive for HPV, types 15 or 18 in 12 cases and types 6 or 11 in two of the cases referenced.[43]

The natural history of tumors of the anal canal is to spread locally into adjacent organs and, commonly, to involve the anal musculature. Involvement of the vagina, prostate, bladder, urethra, and seminal vesicles may be seen.[44] Involvement of the inguinal nodes is seen in up to 63% of anal canal tumors, with half presenting in the 12 months after diagnosis.[44–47] Pelvic and mesenteric nodes are

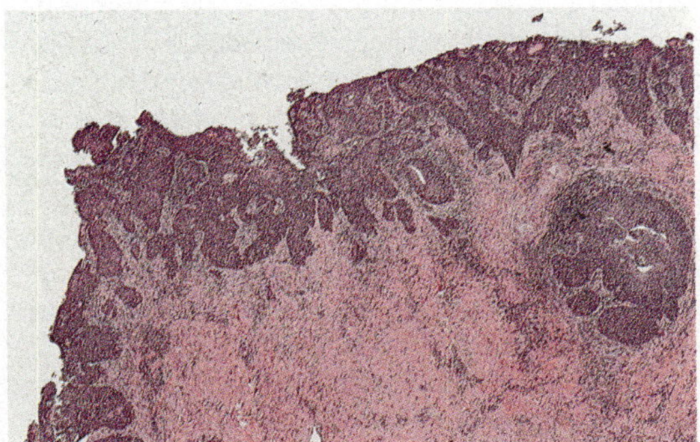

Figure 93-1 In situ and infiltrating epidermoid carcinoma of the anus, with some basaloid features. Courtesy of Stephen S. Sternberg, MD, Memorial Sloan-Kettering Cancer Center.

infrequently involved [44,47] Hematogenous spread of disease is more common in tumors that arise at or above the dentate line because of flow into the systemic circulation via the portal vein. Involvement of liver, lung or bone is seen in about 2 to 5% of cases for each of these organ systems.[44,47] Distant spread is rarely seen with anal margin tumors.

DIAGNOSIS

A differential diagnosis includes many benign conditions. Coexistent conditions (ie, anal fistula, anal fissure, or hemorrhoids) are common. Most commonly, patients notice a palpable mass or bleeding. If pain or spasm is present, a rectal examination may be difficult and physician-related delay may result. A high index of suspicion in the presence of a mass is warranted. Core needle biopsy or incisional biopsy is the definitive method of establishing (1) the initial diagnosis, (2) the effectiveness of anal conservation treatment, and (3) the diagnosis of recurrent disease. Should fear, pain, or any other condition interfere with adequate biopsy, examination and biopsy under anesthesia are warranted. Anal cytology and anoscopy may prove to be useful screening methods for detecting, in high-risk individuals, squamous intraepithelial lesions and other abnormalities related to HPV infection.[48,49]

Treatment is based on an appropriate assessment of the extent of disease. Excision prior to staging is unwarranted, particularly because the majority of patients are not treatable by excision alone. Physical examination should include a search for supraclavicular adenopathy, hepatomegaly, abdominal masses or ascites, inguinal lymphadenopathy, and satellite lesions in the intergluteal folds or leading to the inguinal region, and a careful assessment of the primary lesion itself by digital examination, anoscopy, and proctoscopy. The primary lesion should be evaluated for size, location, depth of invasion, and the presence or absence of inguinal lymphadenopathy.

STAGING

Further workup should include chest radiography, a computed tomographic (CT) scan of the abdomen and pelvis,[50] a complete blood count (CBC), and liver function tests. Transanorectal ultrasonography remains investigational.[51] Two ultrasonographic staging systems have been suggested.[52,53] Tumor-associated antigens are currently under investigation but have not yet proven useful. Fluorodeoxyglucose-PET (FDG-PET) scanning is useful for identifying nodal disease and in radiation treatment planning.[54] The use of sentinel lymph node biopsy for more accurate lymph node staging is currently under evaluation.[55,56] The overall approach to patients with anal carcinoma is diagramed in Figure 93-2.

In a review of multiple studies,[57] tumor size, depth of invasion, location, and the presence or absence of inguinal lymphadenopathy proved to be statistically significant prognostic factors.

AJCC/Union Internationale Contre le Cancer (UICC) staging for anal canal and anal margin reflects these prognostic factors.[1] As the majority of most anal canal cancers are currently treated by nonsurgical methods, the staging system has become more clinical than pathologic.

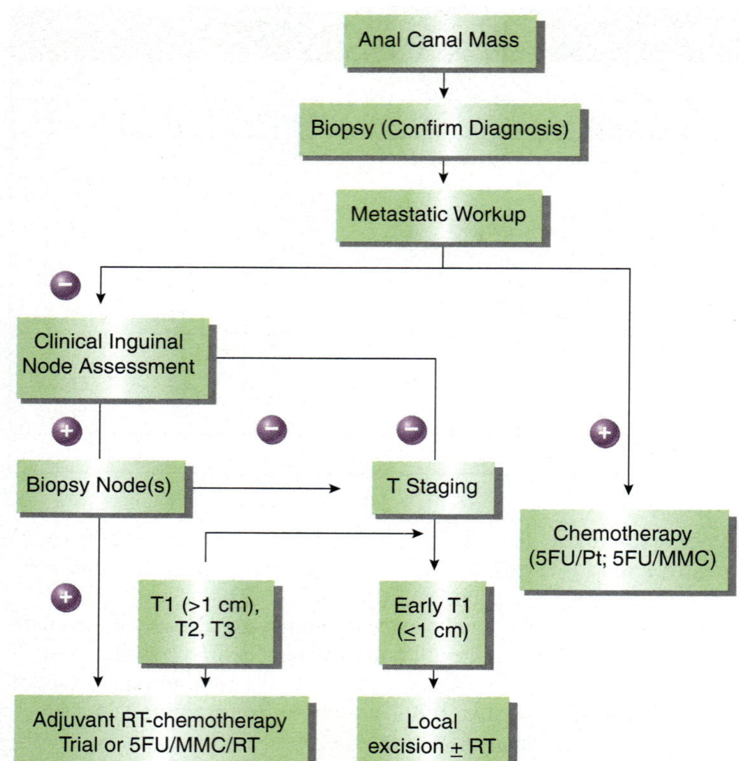

Figure 93-2 Flow diagram of staging and treatment of anal canal carcinoma.

Tumor grade has been reflective of prognosis.[58] DNA ploidy and proliferative indices remain investigational.[58,59] Overexpression of p53 occurs in approximately 50% of tumors and correlates with inferior locoregional control and shorter disease-free survival.[60,61]

A search for perianal premalignant conditions, including Bowen's disease, AIN, HIV positivity, and the presence of HPV should be considered.

TREATMENT

Locoregional Disease **Local Excision** ***Anal Margin Tumors*** Epidermoid tumors of the anal margin have a natural history similar to skin cancers and can be treated by local excision in most instances. An important consideration in the evaluation of a patient for local excision is involvement of the anal sphincter musculature since these muscles are important components of anal continence. Usually, the internal and external muscles can be sacrificed up to one half of the circumference of the anus without loss of anal continence. Local excision results in good local control of disease.[62,63] Local recurrence in patients with anal margin tumors may be treated with repeat local excision. Abdominal-perineal resection (APR) is reserved for locally advanced tumors or tumor recurrence.[62,63]

Anal Canal Tumors Since the advent of multimodality treatment of anal canal tumors, the initial surgery of most of these tumors is limited to a biopsy for diagnosis. Epidermoid tumors of the anal canal can be treated with local excision if the tumor has favorable characteristics. The tumor should be less than 2 cm in size, superficial, and/or well differentiated to be considered for excision alone.[64–66] Of the 19 patients treated at the Mayo Clinic by local excision for tumors less than 2 cm; there was 100% long-term survival.[65] Survival has not been as good with local excision at other institutions with survivals of 60 to 90%.[62,67] Incidental tumors found in hemorrhoidectomy specimens do not need further treatment. Patients who refuse a permanent colostomy, or who are not operative candidates due to associated medical conditions, may also be treated with local excision.

Multimodality Therapy Over the past 30 years, the preferred treatment for most anal tumors evolved from radical surgery to definitive chemoradiation, which is highly effective in achieving cures and preserving anal sphincter function with acceptable toxicity. Surgical intervention is limited to diagnostic biopsy of the primary tumor and suspicious regional lymph nodes, post-treatment biopsy when indicated, and salvage treatment after multimodality treatment failure.

In 1974, Nigro and colleagues first reported a preoperative regimen employing low dose (30 Gy) irradiation (RT) and concomitant chemotherapy with 5-fluorouracil (5-FU) infusion and bolus mitomycin C (MMC).[68] On analysis of the resected specimens from APR, which was performed on six patients 6 weeks after chemoradiation, five patients were pathologically free of tumor. Subsequently, other investigators employed variations of this preoperative regimen in single-arm studies with impressive results.

By 1983, other investigators had extended these observations with studies using chemoradi-

Table 93-2 Multi-Modality Therapy for Loco-Regional Anal Canal Carcinoma

Study	Chemotherapy Regimen	Radiation Regimen	No. Evaluable Patients	No.(%) APR Performed	Treatment-Related Deaths	5-Year Survival (%)
Wayne State[72]	5-FU:1,000 mg/m²/4 d × 2 + MMC: 15 mg/m² d 1	30 Gy/15 fractions (fx)	44	17(39)	0	79
Memorial Sloan-Kettering[73]	5-FU: 750 mg/m²/5 d + MMC: 15 mg/m² d 1	30 Gy/15 fx	42	23(55)	0	82 87*
Kaiser Permanente, Los Angeles[74]	5-FU: 1,000 mg/m²/4 d × 2 + MMC: 10 mg/m² d 1	30 Gy/15 fx	42	7(17)	0	—
Highland Hospital[75]	5-FU:1,000 mg/m²/4 d × 2 +MMC: 10 mg/m² d 2	50–57.5 Gy/25–32 fx	33	4(12)	0	64 70*
Fresno Community Hospital[76]	5-FU: 1,000 mg/m²/4 d × 2 + MMC: 10–15 mg/m² d 2	41–50 Gy/23–28 fx	30	1(3)	0	90
RTOG[77]	5-FU: 1,000 mg/m²/4 d × 2 + MMC: 10 mg/m² d 2	40.8 Gy/24 fx	79	8(10)	0	79†
Instituto Nazionale Tumori, Milan[78]	5-FU: 750 mg/m²/5 d × 2–3 + MMC: 15 mg/m² d 1	54 Gy/30 fx(split)	56	15(27)	1	81
Norwegian Radium Hospital[79]	5-FU: 1,000 mg/m²/4 d + MMC: 10–15 mg/m² d 1	50 Gy/25 fx	94	17(18)	3	72
Princess Margaret[80]	5-FU: 1,000 mg/m²/4 d + MMC: 10 mg/m² d 1	48–50 Gy/24–20 fx (split or continuous)	69	10(14)	0	76†
Massachusetts General Hospital[81]	5-FU: 1,000 mg/m²/4 d + MMC: 10 mg/m² d 1	≤54 Gy/< 30 fx >54 Gy/> 30 fx	14 13	6?‡ (43) 0(0)	1 0	79† 100†
University Hospital Erlangen[82]	5-FU: 1,000 mg/m²/4 d × 1–2 + MMC: 10 mg/m² d 1	50 Gy/25–28 fx	44	8(18)	3	84

RTOG = Radiation Therapy Oncology Group; 5-FU = 5-fluorouracil; MMC = mitomycin-C.
*Cause-specific 5-year survival; † = 3 year survival; ‡? = unclear in abstract.

ation as a definitive nonsurgical treatment.[69–71] Over the next 10 years, many other investigators confirmed the efficacy of this regimen in more than 500 patients in nonrandomized series with 5-year survivals of 65 to 85% and sphincter preservation in 80 to 90% of patients. Table 93-2 shows the results in series with 25 or more patients.[72–82] With higher doses of radiation (45 to 50 Gy), negative biopsies were obtained more frequently, and thus more patients could potentially be spared an APR. The majority of patients received two cycles of 5-FU by continuous infusion and one to two doses of MMC as bolus concomitantly with irradiation during weeks 1 and 5.

The Radiation Therapy Oncology Group (RTOG) later conducted a pilot study with 47 patients (RTOG 9208) employing 5-FU/MMC in standard dosage concomitantly with RT to 59.6 Gy administered over 8.5 weeks, with a 2 week planned therapy break to minimize the anticipated acute local toxicity of the higher RT dose.[83] When compared with patients treated on the 5-FU/MMC + 45 Gy RT arm of the RTOG 8704 trial described below,[84,85] a significant increase in colostomy rates caused by persistent local disease was observed (23% at 1 year and 30% at 2 years in RTOG 9208 vs 6% at 1 year and 7% at 2 years in RTOG 8704). This increased colostomy rate (along with a decreased incidence of dermal toxicity) was thought to be attributable to the split-course delivery of chemoradiation.

Several studies have focused on the possibility of eliminating the break in therapy. Graf and colleagues employed 5-FU/MMC with two RT schedules for a total dose of 45–46 Gy (split course with 2 Gy single fractions and continuous with 1.8 Gy fractions).[86] Local control rates correlated with overall treatment time (OTT) rather than the RT schedule, with local control of 58% for OTT > 41 days compared with 79% for OTT ≤ 41 days. Another study, from Germany, which employed 5-FU/MMC concurrently with external pelvic RT without a planned treatment interruption confirmed the feasibility, efficacy, and lack of increased late toxicity.[87] The use of conformal RT, described by a group from Montreal, also showed the potential of obviating any treatment breaks.[88] With conformal therapy, the ratio of doses to bone marrow, bowel, and skin were less than half that from conventional irradiation volumes (defined by RTOG technique).

Attempts have been made to eliminate MMC from the regimen because of its hematologic toxicity,[89] but in larger studies, inferior local control rates were achieved when MMC was omitted.[80,90,91] In a randomized intergroup study (RTOG 8704), 310 patients received 45-Gy irradiation and two cycles of 5-FU with or without two cycles of MMC.[84,85] Patients with negative post-treatment biopsies received no further treatment. Additional treatment (9 Gy boost RT plus 5-FU and cisplatin) was given to those with positive biopsies. The positive biopsy rate was lower when MMC was given (8 vs 14%), but this was of borderline statistical significance ($p = .135$).[84] At 5 years, the MMC-treated patients demonstrated a highly significant improvement in locoregional failure rates (36% for 5-FU vs 17% for 5-FU/MMC, $p = .014$), colostomy rates (22% 5-FU vs 11% 5-FU/MMC, $p = .019$), and disease-free survival (50% 5-FU vs 67% 5-FU/MMC, $p = .006$).[85] Although colostomy-free survival was significantly different at 4 years, it was not at 5 years (58% 5-FU vs 64% 5-FU/MMC, $p = .17$). Death due to other causes, for example, second malignancies and cardiovascular disease, was the major contributor to the decline in colostomy-free survival in the MMC-treated group. Overall 5-year survivals were not significantly different (65% 5-FU vs 67% 5-FU/MMC, $p = .70$). Grade 4/5 toxicities were higher with MMC than without it (26 vs 7% with $p = .001$).

Because cisplatin as a single agent or in combination with 5-FU has activity in metastatic anal carcinoma, cisplatin/5-FU has been used as neoadjuvant treatment prior to definitive chemoradiation.[92] Of 22 patients treated, 6 (27%) experienced complete remission (CR) and 13 (59%) achieved partial remission (PR), with 20 patients achieving no-evidence-of-disease (NED) status following subsequent chemoradiation. In a randomized study, the M.D. Anderson group treated 92 patients with continuous infusion chemotherapy throughout their radiation course.[93] Both cisplatin (4 mg/m²/day) and 5-FU (250 mg/m²/day) were given as a continuous infusion five days each week concurrent with radiation. At a median follow-up of 44 months, the 5-year overall survival was 85%, disease-free survival was 77%, and colostomy-free survival was 82%. Local recurrences were noted in 17% and distant metastases in 9%. This regimen resulted in RTOG ≥ 4 acute toxicity of 5% and chronic toxicity of 3%. Treatment interruptions were required in < 10% of patients.

Two European prospective nonrandomized trials demonstrated substantial efficacy of 5-FU/cisplatin + RT as definitive treatment.[94,95] Peiffert

Table 93-3 Treatment of Anal Carcinoma with External Radiation Therapy Alone

Investigation	No. of Patients	Primary Site Dose (Gy)	Follow-Up (Years)	Complications Requiring Surgery (%)	5-Year Survival by Size or Stage*		Local Control (%)
Institut Curie[98]	183	60–65	3–14	8	All	59	69
					T ≤ 4 cm	70	
					T > 4 cm, ≤ 6 cm	57	
					T > 6 cm	33	
Institut Gustave Roussy[99]	64	60–65	2–13	14	All	50	81
					T1, T2	72	91
					T3 }	35 (T3, T4)	76
					T4 }		67
St. Francis Memorial. Hosp.[100,101]	39	65	0.5–8.5	10	All	79	80
	35	45–76		6	N0, < 5 cm	92	77
Princess Margaret Hosp.[80]	57	45–60	10–30	8†	All	68§	56
CRLC Val d'Aurelle[120]	28	60–65	5–14	4	T1–3	85	61
					T1	86	71
					T2	92	67
					T3	75	57
Hôpital Tenon[103]	147	60–65	1–17	10	All	61§	71
					T2 (5 cm)‡	71§	77
					T3‡	60§	70
					T4‡	42§	60
Mayo Clinic[104]	18	45–67	2.5–11.2	17	All	94	100
British Columbia Cancer Agency[105]	72	50	2–20	3	All	66	76
					T1	89	
					T2	79	
					T3	75	
					T4	50	

*UICC 1978 stage.
† Two of these refused surgery.
‡ UICC 1987 stage.
§ Cancer-specific survival.

and colleagues treated 80 high-risk patients (T > 4 cm, N+) with two cycles of neoadjuvant 5-FU/cisplatin followed by two concomitant cycles of the same chemotherapy + RT to 45 Gy followed by an RT boost (15 to 20 Gy) 1 to 2 months later.[94] After completion of the entire regimen, 93% of patients achieved a CR. At 3 years, actuarial colostomy-free and disease-free survival were 73% and 67%, respectively. Doci and colleagues treated 35 favorable patients (T1, T2, T3) with two to three cycles of 5-FU/cisplatin with concomitant RT (36 to 38 Gy) followed by a perineal and metastatic inguinal node boost of 18 to 24 Gy.[95] A CR was obtained in 33 patients (94%), including in all 9 patients with lymph node metastases. At a median follow-up of 37 months, 94% were disease-free and 86% were colostomy-free. These nonrandomized trials suggest that 5-FU/cisplatin is at least as effective as 5-FU/MMC in combination with RT.

A final report has recently been presented of the aggressive program studied by the Cancer and Leukemia Group B (CALGB 9281) in 45 poor-prognosis patients (T3/T4 or N2/N3).[96] The induction was 5-FU (1,000 mg/m^2/d continuous infusion (CI) × 5 d) + cisplatin (100 mg/m^2 × 1 d) during weeks 1 and 5, followed by 45 Gy RT during weeks 9 to 17 (19-day break after 30.6 Gy), then concurrent 5-FU (1,000 mg/m^2/d CI × 4 d) + MMC (10 mg/m^2 × 1 d) in weeks 9 and 15. If residual disease persisted, 9 Gy RT with concurrent 5-FU (800 mg/m^2/d CI × 5 d) + cisplatin (100 mg/m^2 × 1 d) was given. After all therapy, in the 44 patients who could be followed (1 patient lost to follow-up, in CR at 1.2 years), there were 37 CRs and 4 PRs. Ten patients (22%) required a colostomy for persistent or recurrent disease and 13 patients died from progressive disease (7 after a CR). In all, 30 of 44 (68%) of these advanced stage patients remained alive, 27 (61%) were disease-free, and 22 (50%) were colostomy- and disease-free at 4 years of follow-up.

An intergroup randomized trial (RTOG 98-11) has been performed that compares 5-FU/MMC + 45 Gy RT with two cycles of 5-FU/cisplatin induction, followed by two cycles of concurrent 5-FU/cisplatin + 45 Gy RT. The RT dose is augmented to 55 to 59 Gy in both arms for high-risk patients (T3, T4, or N+ disease, or T2 lesions), if residual disease is present after 45 Gy. A United Kingdom phase III trial is currently comparing MMC (12 mg/m^2) and cisplatin (60 mg/ m^2) on days 1 + 29 of RT and 5-FU (1,000 mg/ m^2/day) on days 1 to 4 and 29 to 32.[97] This trial is also evaluating the role of consolidative chemotherapy with two cycles of 5-FU/cisplatin versus no further treatment. At present, MMC must be considered an essential component of standard therapy for all but the smallest tumors, in view of the outcome of RTOG 8704. The efficacy and toxicity of 5-FU/cisplatin + higher RT doses for more advanced tumors await the results of the two recent clinical trials cited in this paragraph.

External Irradiation External irradiation alone may be a valid alternative for patients who may not be able to tolerate chemotherapy because of age, poor renal function, AIDS, or some other medical condition. When external RT is used alone, the total dose of radiation required is high (60 to 75 Gy); as a result, complications requiring surgery arise in approximately 5 to 15% of patients treated (Table 93-3).[80,98–105] In the studies shown in Table 93-3, 5-year survival varied from 94 to 50%, with local control rates from 56 to 100%. When lesions were small (T1, T2, or less than 5 cm in diameter), local control and 5-year survival were high (80 to 90%) in many of these series.

In a study of 305 patients treated with radiation therapy alone (303 with external beam irradiation to 45 Gy, then a rest period of 4 to 6 weeks, followed by a boost of 20 Gy, by external beam in 276 or by Iridium-192 in 17 patients), complete clinical responses were seen in 96% of the T1 patients and 87% of the T2 patients.[106] Disease-free survival at 10 years was 74%. Chemoradiation was recommended, however, for tumors ≥ 2 cm in length, and for locally advanced tumors.

A British randomized trial[107] and a European randomized trial[108] comparing multimodality therapy with radiation therapy alone show quite clearly that the addition of chemotherapy is of value for prevention of local recurrence when given with irradiation. Early results of the European Organization for Research and Treatment of Cancer (EORTC) trial for patients with tumors larger than 4 cm, demonstrate an increase in the CR rate from 53 to 77% with the addition of chemotherapy; this resulted in a significant improvement of both locoregional control (by 18%) and colostomy-free rate (by 32%) at 5years (p = .02 and .002, respectively), with a similar overall survival rate in both arms.[108] There was no significant increase in severe side effects between the two arms. The British randomized trial (United Kingdom Coordinating Committee on Cancer Research [UKCCCR]) showed a 46% decrease in local recurrence when chemotherapy with 5-FU/MMC is given during radiation therapy (101 of 283 patients or 36%) compared with irradiation alone (164 of 279 patients or 59%).[107] The relative risk of death from anal cancer was 0.71 in the chemotherapy arm ($p = .02$), but there was no significant advantage in overall survival.

It should be noted that patients with HIV and anal cancer have increased toxic reactions to irradiation, thus requiring treatment interruptions, and often hospitalization.[109] However, combined low-dose RT (30 Gy in 15 fractions) with one cycle of chemotherapy (5-FU/MMC) was well tolerated in one study in eight HIV-positive patients of whom four had AIDS.[110] In a retrospective review of 17 HIV-positive patients, another group demonstrated that morbidity was high in patients with pretreatment CD4 counts < 200 (4 of 8 patients required hospitalization), but acceptable in the nine patients with CD4 counts > 200 (none requiring hospitalization).[111]

Interstitial Irradiation Interstitial irradiation alone, either radium or Ir-192, has been used for early anal cancer.[112,113] The local recurrence rates have been relatively high, however, especially in tumors greater than 5 cm in diameter (77% local recurrence), as one might expect with such localized treatment.[112] Local necrosis has also been high (15 to 25%).[113] Therefore, it is inadvisable to use interstitial irradiation alone as first-line therapy.

Combined Interstitial and External Irradiation Local control was considerably better when interstitial irradiation was combined with external irradiation, but complication rates still were high as a result of the high total dose of irradiation that was necessary.[114,115]

The most extensive series is that of Papillon and colleagues.[116,117] Chemotherapy (5-FU/MMC) was used in approximately one-third of these patients. Ir-192 was used as a boost dose approximately 2 months after external beam therapy to a total dose of 35 Gy. At 5 years, 66% of patients were alive and well; 61% were alive with their sphincters preserved. Even patients with large lesions achieved excellent local control (90% in 89 patients with T3 tumors larger than 4 cm); 78 historical control patients treated with similar irradiation without chemotherapy achieved only 70% local control ($p = .02$).[118] Another French study with interstitial brachytherapy (20 Gy) given about 6 weeks after external irradiation to 40 Gy with some patients also receiving chemotherapy, had a 5-year overall survival of 80% for patients with T1-T2 lesions, but only 53% in patients with T3-T4 lesions.[119] Three other retrospective studies from Europe[115,120–122] and one from the United States[123] used combined external and interstitial Ir-192 irradiation plus chemotherapy. No increase in efficacy was seen.

Boost treatment or additional chemotherapy (possibly 5-FU/cisplatin) with external irradiation may be of value in large lesions; however, in the studies that have been published to date, the use of an interstitial boost has not contributed to any better survival results compared with studies without such a boost.

Radical Surgery Historically, tumors of the anal canal were almost exclusively treated with radical surgery. Surgery included APR, pelvic lymph node dissection, bilateral inguinal node dissections and resection of adjacent organs if involved. Muscle flaps were often needed to close the large surgical defects created by this radical approach. The low yield of positive nodes combined with the high morbidity of the procedure and the 6% survival benefit quickly led to the end of elective lymph node dissections for anal canal tumors.[62,63,124]

The use of APR with node dissection resulted in 5-year survival rates of 55 to 70% with tumor size being the primary determinant of survival.[63,65,66] In patients treated at Memorial Sloan-Kettering Cancer Center (MSKCC) with tumors less than 5 cm in size, the 5-year survival was 60%, but it was only 40% for patients with tumors larger than 5 cm.[66] When preoperative chemotherapy and radiotherapy were given to patients at MSKCC followed by APR, survival improved to 82% at 5 years.[125] In addition to the survival benefit, anal sphincter preservation was possible in the majority of these patients. Now, APR is reserved for tumor recurrence or persistence following multimodality therapy.

Recurrence following radical surgery for anal canal tumors was found in up to 40% of patients; median time to recurrence was 15 months and local recurrence was the predominant type of failure.[45,65,66] Distant metastases were seen less frequently, usually presenting after a local recurrence.

Recurrent Disease **Salvage Treatment** ***Anal Margin Tumors*** Anal margin tumors may recur locally, with regional lymph node disease, or both, with a median time to recurrence of 26 months; these patients are candidates for repeat local excisions with good long-term survival.[62] Patients with regional node recurrence are candidates for dissection with half surviving long term.[62]

Anal Canal Tumors About two months following the completion of multimodality therapy for anal epidermoid tumors, patients should be evaluated endoscopically for response to treatment. Complete response is seen in most patients but up to 15% will have residual disease.[126] Locoregional failure following treatment of anal canal tumors can be treated with repeat chemoradiation, local excision, or salvage APR. Patients with persistent microscopic disease can be treated with local excision whereas patients with gross residual or gross recurrent disease require either repeat chemoradiation or APR. Nigro recommended a second course of chemoradiation for persistent disease, since many patients respond completely, sparing them an APR.[126] Failure following a second course of chemoradiation necessitates an APR.

In the MSKCC series of 38 patients with anal canal squamous tumors treated for their initial local recurrence or persistent disease after chemoradiation by salvage APR, the overall survival rate was 44%.[127] There was a significant rate of distant spread after treatment for local recurrence in this study, suggesting that patients with local recurrence need systemic treatment to enhance their chances of survival.

Inguinal Lymph Node Involvement With surgical resection alone, the prognosis is dismal for synchronous inguinal node involvement, typified by the results reported from MSKCC.[128] Only 2 of 13 patients had their disease controlled after an APR followed by inguinal lymphadenectomy. Radiation alone has been able to control, on average, approximately 65% of inguinal nodes, but with multimodality therapy, more than 90% of synchronous inguinal nodes may be controlled.[129,130] Node involvement is predictive of survival; in one study of 118 patients treated with curative intent, patients with negative inguinal nodes had a 9-year survival of 73%, as compared to only 52% when these nodes were involved.[131] In another study, 5-year overall survival was 54.4% for 27 patients with synchronous inguinal node involvement treated with curative intent, and 41.4% for 19 patients with metachronous involvement, when treatment consisted of inguinal dissection, postoperative irradiation, and, in some patients, concomitant chemotherapy (usually 5-FU/cisplatin).[132] Of interest in that study was the fact that when the primary tumor was clearly located on a single lateral side of the anal canal (36 patients), inguinal node metastases were always homolateral to it.

Multimodality treatment should clearly be the treatment of choice for positive inguinal nodes. Surgery should be for diagnosis, consisting of a limited sampling of the suspected node(s), or for salvage after an isolated inguinal recurrence. Metachronous inguinal node relapse can be treated with a lymph node dissection; disease-free survival at 3 years in one series by Papillon was 64%.[133] Combinations of lesser surgery, radiation, and chemotherapy may also be used successfully, although reports have been only anecdotal.

Metastatic Disease The rarity of anal cancer, its limited propensity for early dissemination, and the success of definitive chemoradiation have resulted in few patients who require systemic chemotherapy without radiation. This topic was reviewed by Flam.[134] Individual case reports suggest some, but limited, activity of 5-FU + MMC against metastatic and recurrent disease when employed without radiation.[117,135–138] Single-agent cisplatin has shown activity in metastatic disease,[139–141] and the combination of 5-FU/cisplatin has shown substantial activity in patients with metastatic disease.[138,142–146] Tanum reported that 3 of 8 patients achieved a CR with 5-FU/cisplatin, of whom 2 were 5-year survivors.[138] Some of these patients had failed 5-FU/MMC/RT, suggesting a lack of cross-resistance between MMC and cisplatin.

Limited activity has been found for a variety of other combinations, often with a price of major toxicity. Sequential MTX/5-FU/leucovorin produced four CRs and four PRs in nine patients.[134] New promising drugs with activity against squamous carcinomas and substantial radiosensitizing properties such as gemcitabine and the taxanes have yet to be evaluated. One author (MSF) has observed excellent responses to Taxol in four patients with metastatic disease.

MELANOMA

Anorectal melanomas are relatively unusual tumors accounting for less than 1% of all melanomas and less than 1% of all anal canal tumors. The presentation of patients with anorectal melanomas is non-specific and often mimics benign conditions of the anus. The diagnosis is seldom made on the initial presentation and the delay in diagnosis may account for the advanced stage at which most anorectal melanomas present.

Due to the late stage at presentation, radical surgery in the management of this disease remains controversial.[147,148] The optimal surgical procedure should provide local control with minimal morbidity and mortality, and preserve anal continence without jeopardizing survival. Since distant recurrence is the rule, surgery needs to be followed by adjuvant therapy if survival is to be maximized. Currently, there is little effective adjuvant therapy to offer, but new treatment modalities have shown promise.

The most common presenting symptom is rectal bleeding, most often attributed to hemorrhoids, which accounts for over 80% of patients being misdiagnosed at the initial evaluation.[149,150] Other symptoms include pain, tenesmus, pruritus, change in bowel habits, and weight loss. On physical examination, a mass may be palpated in the rectum or a lesion may be seen extruding from the rectum that may be pigmented in a third of the cases.[149,150] These tumors arise most commonly at the mucocutaneous junction, but they may arise from the skin of the anal verge or from the transitional epithelium. Inguinal lymph nodes are often palpable at the time of diagnosis. The diagnosis is made by biopsy of the lesion during proctoscopic examination or often it is found incidentally in a hemorrhoid specimen. The histologic findings of anorectal melanoma are identical to those of cutaneous melanoma.

Anorectal melanomas spread by direct extension upward in the submucosal plane of the rectum. Lymphatic spread is most commonly to the mesenteric nodes but it can spread to the inguinal nodes in up to 20% of patients.[147–151] Hematogenous spread is most common to liver, lung, and bone; it may be found in up to 70% of patients.[147–151]

Because of the high rate of systemic failure, radical APR with pelvic and bilateral inguinal node dissections for these melanomas has fallen out of favor. However, early reports of surgical outcomes found that APR in patients with anorectal melanoma resulted in the only long-term survivors.[149,152] Recently, wide local excision of the lesion with 2 cm margins has been advocated as the treatment of choice; long-term survivors have been seen with this approach.[147,150] Comparison trials have shown no survival advantage to APR over local excision for anorectal melanomas but local control is improved following APR.[147,150,151]

Size and depth of invasion are the two tumor characteristics that consistently have been shown to have the most prognostic importance. In one study, the three 5-year survivors all had tumors less than 2 mm in thickness, whereas all the patients with tumors more than 2 mm thick were dead by 5 years, and 85% of those had died by 2 years.[149] The presence of pathologically involved inguinal or mesenteric lymph nodes is uniformly fatal[148,149,151,152] A recent study has shown two favorable prognostic factors: disease found incidentally in a hemorrhoid specimen and female gender.[151]

The effectiveness of radiation therapy, chemotherapy, immunotherapy, or newer novel approaches for treatment of this disease is difficult to ascertain in the adjuvant or metastatic setting because of the small number of patients treated in a uniform manner. Further studies will be needed to elucidate the role of these therapies.

REFERENCES

1. Greene FL, Page DL, Fleming ID, et al, editors. AJCC Cancer Staging Manual, 6th ed. New York: Springer-Verlag, 2002:125–30.
2. Jemal A, Murray T, Bolden S, et al. Cancer statistics, 2002. CA Cancer J Clin 2002;52:23–47.
3. Melbye M, Rabkin C, Frisch M, Biggar RJ. Changing patterns of anal cancer incidence in the United States, 1940–1989. Am J Epidemiol 1994;139:772–80.
4. Tolmos J, Vargas HI, Lim S, Stamos M. A forty-year experience with anal carcinoma: changing trends and impact of multimodality therapy. Am Surg 1997;63:918–22.
5. Peters RK, Mack TM. Patterns of anal carcinoma by gender and marital status in Los Angeles County. Br J Cancer 1983;48:629–636.
6. Cabuk D, Yumuk PF, Abacioglu U, et al. Is the incidence of anal canal cancers different in Moslem societies? [abstract]. J Clin Oncol 2004;22(Suppl):371.
7. Daling JR, Weiss NS, Hislop G, et al. Sexual practices, sexually transmitted diseases, and the incidence of anal cancer. N Engl J Med 1987;317:973–7.
8. Frisch M, Glimelius B, van den Brule AJ, et al. Sexually transmitted infection as a cause of anal cancer. N Engl J Med 1997;337:1350–8.
9. Ablin RJ, Stein-Werblowsky R. Sexual behavior and increased anal cancer. Immunol Cell Biol 1997;75:181–3.
10. Zur Hausen H. Human papillomaviruses and their possible role in squamous cell carcinomas. Curr Top Microbiol Immunol 1977;78:1–30.
11. Beckmann AM, Daling JR, Sherman KJ, et al. Human papillomavirus infection and anal cancer. Int J Cancer 1989;43:1042–9.
12. Duggan MA, Boras VF, Inoue M, et al. Human papillomavirus DNA determination of anal condylomata, dysplasias, and squamous carcinomas with in situ hybridization. Am J Clin Pathol 1989;92:16–21.
13. Holm R, Tanum G, Karlsen F, Nesland JM. Prevalence and physical state of human papillomavirus DNA in anal carcinomas. Mod Pathol 1994;7:449–53.
14. Kiyabu MT, Shibata D, Arnheim N, et al. Detection of human papillomavirus in formalin-fixed, invasive squamous carcinomas using the polymerase chain reaction. Am J Surg Pathol 1989;13:221–4.
15. Palevsky JM, Holly EA, Gonzales J, et al. Detection of human papillomavirus DNA in anal intraepithelial neoplasia and anal cancer. Cancer Res 1991;51:1014–9.
16. Palmer JG, Scholefield JH, Coates PJ, et al. Anal cancer and human papillomaviruses. Dis Colon Rectum 1989;32:1016–22.
17. Taxy JB, Gupta PK, Gupta JW, Shah KV. Anal cancer: microscopic condyloma and tissue demonstration of human papillomavirus capsid antigen and viral DNA. Arch Pathol Lab Med 1989;113:1127–31.
18. Zaki SR, Judd R, Coffield LM, et al. Human papillomavirus infection and anal carcinoma: retrospective analysis by in situ hybridization and the polymerase chain reaction. Am J Pathol 1992;140:1345–55.
19. Scholefield JH, Kerr IB, Shepherd NA, et al. Human papillomavirus type 16 DNA in anal cancers from six different countries. Gut 1991;32:674–6.
20. Xi LF, Critchlow CW, Wheeler CM, et al. Risk of anal carcinoma in situ in relation to human papillomavirus type 16 variants. Cancer Res 1998;58:3839–44.
21. Frisch M, Fenger C, van den Brule AJ, et al. Variants of squamous cell carcinoma of the anal canal and perianal skin and their relation to human papillomaviruses. Cancer Res 1999;59:753–7.
22. Scholefield JH, Sonnex C, Talbot IC, et al. Anal and cervical intraepithelial neoplasia: possible parallel. Lancet 1989;2:765–9.
23. Scholefield JH, Hickson WGE, Smith JHF, et al. Anal intraepithelial neoplasia: part of a multifocal disease process. Lancet 1992;340:1271–3.
24. Kiviat N, Rompalo A, Bowden R, et al. Anal human papillomavirus infection among human immunodeficiency virus-seropositive and -seronegative men. J Infect Dis 1990;162:358–61.
25. Law CM, Qassim M, Thompson CH, et al. Factors associated with clinical and sub-clinical anal human papillomavirus infection in homosexual men. Genitourin Med 1991;67:92–8.
26. Melbye M, Palefsky J, Gonzales J, et al. Immune status as a determinant of human papillomavirus detection and its association with anal epithelial abnormalities. Int J Cancer 1990;46:203–6.
27. Palefsky J, Gonzalez J, Greenblatt R, et al. Anal intraepithelial neoplasia and anal papillomavirus infection among homosexual males with group IV HIV disease. JAMA 1990;263:1911–16.
28. Jakate SM, Saclarides TJ. Immunohistochemical detection of mutant p53 protein and human papillomavirus related E6 protein in anal cancers. Dis Colon Rectum 1993;36:1026–9.
29. Noffsinger AE, Hui Y-Z, Suzuk L, et al. The relationship of human papillomavirus to proliferation and ploidy in carcinoma of the anus. Cancer 1995;75:958–67.
30. Ogunbuyi OA, Scholefield JH, Smith JHF, et al. Immunohistochemical analysis of p53 expression in anal squamous neoplasia. J Clin Pathol 1993;46:507–12.
31. Frisch M, Olsen JH, Bautz A, Melbye M. Benign anal lesions and the risk of anal cancer. N Engl J Med 1994;331:300–2.
32. Lin AY, Gridley G, Tucker M. Benign anal lesions and anal cancer [letter]. N Engl J Med 1995;332:190–1.
33. Penn I. Cancers of the anogenital region in renal transplant recipients. Cancer 1986;58:611–6.
34. Daniell HW. Re: causes of anal carcinoma. JAMA 1985; 254:358.
35. Frisch M, Glimelius B, Wohlfahrt J, et al. Tobacco smoking as a risk factor in anal carcinoma: an antiestrogenic mechanism? J Natl Cancer Inst 1999;91:708–15.
36. Lorenz HP, Wilson W, Leigh B, et al. Squamous cell carcinoma of the anus and HIV infection. Dis Colon Rectum 1991;34:336–8.
37. Monfardini S, Vaccher E, Lazzarin A, et al. Characterization of AIDS-associated tumors in Italy: report of 435 cases of an IVDA-based series. Cancer Detect Prev 1990;14:391–3.
38. Palefsky JM, Holly EA, Ralston ML, et al. High incidence of anal high-grade squamous intra-epithelial lesions among HIV-positive and HIV-negative homosexual and bisexual men. AIDS 1998;12:495–503.
39. Sobhani I, Vuagnat A, Walker F et al. Prevalence of high-grade dysplasia and cancer in the anal canal in human papillomavirus-infected individuals. Gastroenterology 2001;120:857–66.
40. Holly EA, Ralston ML, Darragh TM, et al. Prevalence and risk factors for anal squamous intraepithelial lesions in women. J Natl Cancer Inst 2001;93:843–9.
41. Melbye M, Cote TR, Kessler L, et al. AIDS/Cancer Working Group. High incidence of anal cancer among AIDS patients. Lancet 1994;343:636–9.
42. Chiao EY, Schrag D. Anal cancer incidence in relation to HIV epidemiology [abstract]. J Clin Oncol 2004;22 (Suppl):333.
43. Wolber R, Dupuis B, Thiyagaratnam P, Owen D. Anal cloacogenic and squamous carcinomas. Comparative histologic analysis using in situ hybridization for human papillomavirus DNA. Am J Surg Pathol 1990;14:176–82.

44. Stearns MW Jr, Urmacher C, Sternberg SS, et al. Cancer of the anal canal. Curr Probl Cancer 1980;4:1–44.
45. Clark J, Petrelli N, Herrera L, et al. Epidermoid carcinoma of the anal canal. Cancer 1986;57:400–6.
46. Pyper PC, Parks TG. The results of surgery for epidermoid carcinoma of the anus. Br J Surg 1985;72:712–4.
47. Kuehn PG, Eisenberg H, Reed JF. Epidermoid carcinoma of the perianal skin and anal canal. Cancer 1968;22:932–8.
48. Palefsky JM, Holly EA, Hogeboorn CJ, et al. Anal cytology as a screening tool for anal squamous intraepithelial lesions. J Acquir Immune Defic Syndr 1997;14:415–22.
49. Surawicz CM, Kirby P, Critchlow C, et al. Anal dysplasia in homosexual men: role of anoscopy and biopsy. Gastroenterology 1993;105:658–66.
50. Cohan RH, Silverman PM, Thompson WM, et al. Computed tomography of epithelial neoplasms of the anal canal. Am J Roentgenol 1985;145:569–73.
51. Goldman S, Glimelius B, Norming U, et al. Transanorectal ultrasonography in anal carcinoma: a prospective study of 21 patients. Acta Radiol 1988;29:337–41.
52. Giovannini M, Bardon VJ, Barclay R, et al. Anal carcinoma: prognostic value of endorectal ultrasound (ERUS). Results of a prospective multicenter study. Endoscopy 2001;33:231–6.
53. Tarantino D, Bernstein MA. Endoanal ultrasound in the staging and management of squamous-cell carcinoma of the anal canal: potential implications of a new ultrasound staging system. Dis Colon Rectum 2002;45:16–22.
54. Malayapa RS, Myerson RJ, Dehdashti R, et al. FDG-PET in anal cancer: impact on staging and radiotherapeutic management [abstract]. Int J Radiat Oncol Biol Phys 2004;60:421.
55. Ulmer C, Bembeneck A, Gretschel S, et al. Refined staging by sentinel lymph node biopsy to individualized therapy in anal cancer. Ann Surg Oncol 2004;1(Suppl.3):S259–62.
56. Perera D, Pathma-Nathan N, Rabbitt P, et al. Sentinel node biopsy for squamous cell carcinoma of the anus and anal margin. Dis Colon Rectum 2003;46:1027–31.
57. Enker WE, Heilweil M, Janov AJ, et al. Improved survival in epidermoid carcinoma of the anus in association with pre-operative multi-disciplinary therapy. Arch Surg 1986;121:1386–90.
58. Goldman S, Auer G, Erhardt K, et al. Prognostic significance of clinical stage, histologic grade, and nuclear DNA content in squamous-cell carcinoma of the anus. Dis Colon Rectum 1987;30:444–8.
59. Shepherd NA, Scholefield JH, Love S, et al. Prognostic factors in anal squamous carcinoma: a multivariate analysis of clinical, pathological, and flow cytometric parameters in 235 cases. Histopathology 1990;16:545–55.
60. Bonin SR, Pajak TF, Russell AH, et al. Overexpression of p53 protein and outcome of patients treated with chemoradiation for carcinoma of the anal canal. A report of randomized trial RTOG 87-04. Cancer 1999;85:1226–33.
61. Wong CS, Tsao MS, Sharma V, et al. Prognostic role of p53 protein expression in epidermoid carcinoma of the anal canal. Int J Radiat Oncol Biol Phys 1999;45:309–14.
62. Greenall MJ, Quan SHQ, Stearns MW, et al. Epidermoid cancer of the anal margin. Am J Surg 1985;149:95–101.
63. Beahrs OH, Wilson SM. Carcinoma of the anus. Ann Surg 1976;184:422–8.
64. Al-Jurf AS, Turnbull RB, Fazio VW. Local treatment of squamous cell carcinoma of the anus. Surg Gynecol Obstet 1979;148:576–8.
65. Boman BM, Moertel CG, O'Connell MJ, et al. Carcinoma of the anal canal: a clinical and pathologic study of 188 cases. Cancer 1984;54:114–25.
66. Greenall MJ, Quan SHQ, Urmacher C, et al. Treatment of epidermoid carcinoma of the anal canal. Surg Gynecol Obstet 1985;161:509–17.
67. Welch JP, Malt RA. Appraisal of treatment of carcinoma of the anus and anal canal. Surg Gynecol Obstet 1977;145:837–41.
68. Nigro ND, Vaitkeviceus VK, Considine B Jr. Combined therapy for cancer of the anal canal: a preliminary report. Dis Colon Rectum 1974;17:354–6.
69. Cummings BJ, Rider WD, Harwood AR, et al. Combined radical radiation therapy and chemotherapy for primary squamous cell carcinoma of the anal canal. Cancer Treat Rep 1982;66:489–92.
70. Flam MS, John M, Lovalvo L, et al. Definitive non-surgical therapy of epithelial malignancies of the anal canal. A report of 12 cases. Cancer 1983;51:1378–87.
71. Sischy B, Remington JH, Hinson J, et al. Definitive treatment of anal-canal carcinoma by means of radiation therapy and chemotherapy. Dis Colon Rectum 1982;25:685–8.
72. Nigro ND, Vaitkeviceus VK, Considine B Jr. Dynamic management of squamous cell cancer of the anal canal. Invest New Drugs 1989;7:83–9.
73. Miller EJ, Quan SH, Thaler T. Treatment of squamous cell carcinoma of the anal canal. Cancer 1991;67:2038–41.
74. Smith DE, Shah KH, Rao AR, et al. Cancer of the anal canal: treatment with chemotherapy and low-dose radiation therapy. Radiology 1994;191:569–72.
75. Sischy B. The use of radiation therapy combined with chemotherapy in the management of squamous cell carcinoma of the anus and marginally resectable adenocarcinoma of the rectum. Int J Radiat Oncol Biol Phys 1985;11:1587–93.
76. John MJ, Flam MS, Mowry PA. Clinical potential of synchronous radiotherapy and chemotherapy for advanced squamous cell carcinoma. NCI Monogr 1988;6:375–8.
77. Sischy B, Doggett RLS, Krall JM, et al. Definitive irradiation and chemotherapy for radiosensitization in management of anal carcinoma: interim report on radiation therapy oncology group study no. 8314. J Natl Cancer Inst 1989;81:850–6.
78. Doci R, Zucali R, Bombelli L, et al. Combined chemoradiation therapy for anal cancer: a report of 56 cases. Ann Surg 1992;215:150–6.
79. Tanum G, Tveit K, Karlsen KO, Hauer-Jensen M. Chemotherapy and radiation therapy for anal carcinoma. Cancer 1991;67:2462–6.
80. Cummings BJ, Keane TJ, O'Sullivan B, et al. Epidermoid anal cancer: treatment by radiation alone or by radiation and 5-fluorouracil with and without mitomycin C. Int J Radiat Oncol Biol Phys 1991;21:1115–25.
81. Fung CY, Willett CG, Efird J, et al. Chemoradiotherapy for anal carcinoma: what is the optimal radiation dose? Radiat Oncol Invest 1994;2:152–6.
82. Schneider IHF, Grabenbauer GG, Reck T, et al. Combined radiation and chemotherapy for epidermoid carcinoma of the anal canal. Int J Colorect Dis 1992;7:192–6.
83. John M, Pajak T, Flam M, et al. Dose escalation in chemoradiation for anal cancer-preliminary results of RTOG 92-08. Cancer J Sci Am 1996;2:205–11.
84. Flam M, John M, Pajak TF, et al. Role of mitomycin in combination with fluorouracil and radiotherapy, and of salvage chemoradiation in the definitive nonsurgical treatment of epidermoid carcinoma of the anal canal: results of a phase III randomized intergroup study. J Clin Oncol 1996;14:2527–39.
85. Flam M, John M, Pajak TF, et al. Role of mitomycin in combination with fluorouracil and radiotherapy, and of salvage chemoradiation in the definitive nonsurgical treatment of epidermoid carcinoma of the anal canal: results of a phase III randomized intergroup study—author update. In: Mayer RJ, editor. Classic papers and current comments—highlights of clinical gastrointestinal cancer research. Vol. 3. Philadelphia: Lippincott, Williams and Wilkins 1999:539–52.
86. Graf R, Wust P, Hildebrandt B, et al. Impact of overall treatment time on local control of anal cancer treated with radiochemotherapy. Oncology 2003;65:14–22.
87. Meyer A, Bremer M, Meier zu Eissen J, et al. Organ-preserving radiochemotherapy in patients with anal cancer: is a planned treatment interruption necessary [abstract]. Int J Radiat Oncol Biol Phys 2004;60:423.
88. Vuong T, Devic S, Belliveau P, et al. Contribution of conformal therapy in the treatment of anal canal carcinoma with combined chemotherapy and radiotherapy: results of a phase II study. Int J Radiat Oncol Biol Phys 2003;56:823–31.
89. Byfield JE, Barone RM, Sharp TR, et al. Conservative management without alkylating agents of squamous cell anal cancer using cyclical 5-FU alone and x-ray therapy. Cancer Treat Rep 1985;67:709–12.
90. Hughes LL, Rich TA, Delclos L, et al. Radiotherapy for anal cancer: experience from 1979–1987. Int J Radiat Oncol Biol Phys 1989;17:1153–60.
91. Rich TA, Hughes L, Ajani JA, Brock W. Low dose, continuous infusion 5-fluorouracil plus radiotherapy for anal cancer [letter]. Int J Radiat Oncol Biol Phys 1990;18:710.
92. Brunet R, Sadek H, Vignoud J, et al. Cisplatin (P) and 5-Fluorouracil (5FU) for the neoadjuvant treatment (Tt) of epidermoid anal carcinoma (EACC) [abstract]. Proc Am Soc Clin Oncol 1990;9:114.
93. Hung A, Crane C, Delclos M, et al. Cisplatin-based combined modality therapy for anal carcinoma: a wider therapeutic index. Cancer 2003;97:1195–202.
94. Peiffert D, Giovannini M, Ducreux M, et al. High-dose radiation therapy and neoadjuvant plus concomitant chemotherapy with 5-fluorouracil and cisplatin in patients with locally advanced squamous-cell anal canal cancer: final results of a Phase II study. Ann Oncol 2001;12:397–404.
95. Doci R, Zucali R, LaMonica G, et al. Primary chemoradiation therapy with fluorouracil and cisplatin for cancer of the anus: results in 35 consecutive patients. J Clin Oncol 1996;14:3121–5.
96. Meropol N, Niedzwiecki D, Shank B, et al. Combined-modality therapy of poor prognosis anal canal carcinoma: a Phase II study of the Cancer and Leukemia Group B (CALGB) [abstract]. Am Soc Clin Oncol, 2005 Gastrointestinal Cancers Symposium,; 2005 Jan 27–29. Hollywood FL.
97. James R, Meadows HM. The second UK phase III anal cancer trial of chemoradiation and maintenance therapy (Act II): preliminary results on toxicity and outcome [abstract]. J Clin Oncol 2003;22:287.
98. Salmon RJ, Fenton J, Asselain B, et al. Treatment of epidermoid anal canal cancer. Am J Surg 1984;147:43–8.
99. Eschwege F, Lasser P, Chavy A, et al. Squamous cell carcinoma of the anal canal: treatment by external beam irradiation. Radiother Oncol 1985;3:145–50.
100. Cantril ST, Green JP, Schall GL, et al. Primary radiation therapy in the treatment of anal carcinoma. Int J Radiat Oncol Biol Phys 1983;9:1271–8.
101. Doggett SW, Green JP, Cantril ST. Efficacy of radiation therapy alone for limited squamous cell carcinoma of the anal canal. Int J Radiat Oncol Biol Phys 1988;15:1069–72.
102. Dubois JB, Garrigues JM, Pujol H. Cancer of the anal canal: report on the experience of 61 patients. Int J Radiat Oncol Biol Phys 1991;20:575–80.
103. Touboul E, Schlienger M, Buffat L, et al. Conservative versus nonconservative treatment of epidermoid carcinoma of the anal canal for tumors longer than or equal to 5 centimeters: a retrospective comparison. Cancer 1995;75:786–93.
104. Martenson JA Jr, Gunderson LL. External radiation therapy without chemotherapy in the management of anal cancer. Cancer 1993;71:1736–40.
105. Newman G, Calverley DC, Acker BD. The management of carcinoma of the anal canal by external beam radio-therapy, experience in Vancouver 1971–1988. Radiother Oncol 1992;25:196–202.
106. Deniaud-Alexandre E, Touboul E, Tiret E, et al. Results of definitive irradiation in a series of 305 epidermoid carcinomas of the anal canal. Int J Radiat Oncol Biol Phys 2003;56:1259–73.
107. UKCCCR Anal Cancer Trial Working Party. Epidermoid anal cancer: results from the UKCCCR randomised trial of radiotherapy, 5-fluorouracil, and mitomycin. Lancet 1996;348:1049–54.
108. Bartelink H, Roelofsen F, Eschwege F, et al. Concomitant radiotherapy and chemotherapy is superior to radio-therapy alone in the treatment of locally advanced anal cancer: results of a phase III randomized trial of the European Organization for Research and Treatment of Cancer Radiotherapy and Gastrointestinal Cooperative Groups. J Clin Oncol 1997;15:2040–9.
109. Holland JM, Swift PS. Tolerance of patients with human immunodeficiency virus and anal carcinoma to treatment with combined chemotherapy and radiation therapy. Radiology 1994;193:251–4.
110. Peddada AV, Smith DE, Rao AR, et al. Chemotherapy and low-dose radiotherapy in the treatment of HIV-infected patients with carcinoma of the anal canal. Int J Radiat Oncol Biol Phys 1997;37:1101–5.
111. Hoffman R, Welton ML, Klencke B, et al. The significance of pretreatment CD4 count on the outcome and treatment tolerance of HIV-positive patients with anal cancer. Int J Radiat Oncol Biol Phys 1999;44:127–31.
112. James RD, Pointon RS, Martin S. Local radiotherapy in the management of squamous carcinoma of the anus. Br J Surg 1985;72:282–5.
113. Keiling R, Grunewald JM, Achille E. Radiotherapie des cancers malpighiens de l'anus. J Radiol Electrol Med Nucl 1973;54:634–5.
114. Ng Ying Kin KNY, Pigneux J, Auvray H, et al. Our experience of conservative treatment of anal canal carcinoma combining external irradiation and interstitial implants: 32 cases treated between 1973 and 1982. Int J Radiat Oncol Biol Phys 1988;14:253–9.
115. Wagner J-P, Mahe MA, Romestaing P, et al. Radiation therapy in the conservative treatment of carcinoma of the anal canal. Int J Radiat Oncol Biol Phys 1994;29:17–23.
116. Papillon J, Montbarbon JF. Epidermoid carcinoma of the anal canal: a series of 276 cases. Dis Colon Rectum 1987;30:324–33.

117. Papillon J, Montbarbon JG, Gerard J, et al. Interstitial curietherapy in the conservative treatment of anal and rectal cancers. Int J Radiat Oncol Biol Phys 1989;17:1161–9.
118. Papillon J. Effectiveness of combined radio-chemotherapy in the management of epidermoid carcinoma of the anal canal. Int J Radiat Oncol Biol Phys 1990;19:1217–8.
119. Berger C, Felix-Faure C, Chauvet B, et al. Conservative treatment of anal canal carcinoma with external radio-therapy and interstitial brachytherapy, with or without chemotherapy: long-term results. Cancer Radiother 1999;3:461–7.
120. Allal A, Kurtz JM, Pipard G, et al. Chemoradiotherapy versus radiotherapy alone for anal cancer: a retrospective comparison. Int J Radiat Oncol Biol Phys 1993;27:59–66.
121. Allal AS, Mermillod B, Roth AD, et al. The impact of treatment factors on local control in T2-T3 anal carcinomas treated by radiotherapy with or without chemotherapy. Cancer 1997;79:2329–35.
122. Kapp KS, Geyer E, Gebhart FH, et al. Experience with split-course external beam irradiation ± chemotherapy and integrated Ir-192 high-dose-rate brachytherapy in the treatment of primary carcinomas of the anal canal. Int J Radiat Oncol Biol Phys 2001;49:997–1005.
123. Hwang JM, Rao AR, Cosmatos HA, et al. Treatment of T3 and T4 anal carcinoma with combined chemoradiation and interstitial 192Ir implantation: a 10-year experience. Brachytherapy 2004;3:95–100.
124. Miller EJ, Quan SH, Thaler T. Treatment of squamous cell carcinoma of the anal canal. Cancer 1991;67:2038–41.
125. Greenall MJ, Magill G, Quan S, et al. Recurrent epidermoid cancer of the anus. Cancer 1986;57:1437–41.
126. Nigro ND. Multidisciplinary management of cancer of the anus. World J Surg 1987;11:446–51.
127. Ellenhorn JDI, Enker WE, Quan SHQ. Salvage abdominoperineal resection following combined chemotherapy and radiotherapy for epidermoid carcinoma of the anus. Ann Surg Oncol 1994;1:105–10.
128. Greenall MJ, Quan SHQ, DeCosse J. Epidermoid cancer of the anus. Br J Surg 1985;72(Suppl):97–103.
129. Shank B, Cunningham JD, Kelsen DP. Cancer of the anal region. In: DeVita DT Jr, Hellman S, Rosenberg SA, editors. Cancer: principles and practice of oncology. Philadelphia: Lippincott-Raven; 1997. p. 1234–51.
130. Touboul E, Schlienger M, Buffat L, et al. Epidermoid carcinoma of the anal canal: results of curative-intent radiation therapy in a series of 270 patients. Cancer 1994;73:1569–79.
131. Peiffert D, Bey P, Pernot M, et al. Conservative treatment by irradiation of epidermoid cancers of the anal canal: prognostic factors of tumoral control and complications. Int J Radiat Oncol Biol Phys 1997;37:313–24.
132. Gerard JP, Chapet O, Samiei F, et al. Management of inguinal lymph node metastases in patients with carcinoma of the anal canal: experience in a series of 270 patients treated in Lyon and review of the literature. Cancer 2001;92:77–84.
133. Papillon J. Rectal and anal cancers. New York: Springer-Verlag; 1982.
134. Flam MS. Chemotherapy of persistent, recurrent or metastatic anal cancer. In: Cohen AM, Winawer SJ, Friedman MA, Gunderson LL, editors. Cancer of the colon, rectum, and anus. New York: McGraw-Hill; 1995. p. 1051–60.
135. Newman HK, Quan SHQ. Multimodality therapy for epidermoid carcinoma of the anus. Cancer 1976;37:12–9.
136. Knecht BH. Combined chemotherapy and radiotherapy for carcinomas of the anus. Am J Surg 1990;159:518–21.
137. Greenall MJ, Magill GB, Quan SHQ, et al. Recurrent epidermoid carcinoma of the anus. Cancer 1986;57:1437–41.
138. Tanum G. Treatment of relapsing anal carcinoma. Acta Oncol 1993;32:33–5.
139. Ohzato H, Satomi T, Sakita I. Two cases of cloacogenic carcinoma of the anal canal: chemotherapeutic effect of cis-platinum. Nippon Geka Gakkai Zasshi 1988;89:291–5.
140. Fisher W, Herbst K, Sims J, et al. Metastatic cloacogenic carcinoma of the anus: sequential responses to Adriamycin and cis-dichlorodiamineplatinum (II). Cancer Treat Rep 1978;62:91–7.
141. Salem P, Habboubi N, Naanasissie E, et al. Effectiveness of cisplatin in the treatment of anal squamous cell carcinoma. Cancer Treat Rep 1985;69:891–3.
142. Ajani J, Carrasco H, Jackson D, et al. Combination of cisplatin plus fluoropyrimidine chemotherapy effective against liver metastases from carcinoma of the anal canal. Am J Med 1989;87:221–4.
143. Mahjoubi M, Sadek H, Francois E, et al. Epidermoid anal canal carcinoma (EACC): activity of cisplatin (P) and continuous 5-fluorouracil (5FU) in metastatic (M) and/or local recurrent (LR) disease [abstract]. Proc Am Soc Clin Oncol 1990;9:114.
144. Carey RW. Regression of pulmonary metastases from cloacogenic carcinoma after cis-platinum/5-fluorouracil treatment. J Clin Gastroenterol 1984;6:257–9.
145. Khater R, Frenay M, Bourry J, et al. Cisplatin plus 5-fluorouracil in the treatment of metastatic anal squamous cell carcinoma: a report of two cases. Cancer Treat Rep 1986;70:1345–6.
146. Jaiyesimi IA, Pazdur P. Cisplatin and 5-fluorouracil as salvage therapy for recurrent metastatic squamous cell carcinoma of the anal canal. Am J Clin Oncol 1993;16:536–40.
147. Ross M, Pezzi C, Pezzi T, et al. Patterns of failure in anorectal melanoma: a guide to surgical therapy. Arch Surg 1990;125:313–6.
148. Chiu YS, Unni KK, Beart RW. Malignant melanoma of the anorectum. Dis Colon Rectum 1980;23:122–4.
149. Wanebo HJ, Woodruff JM, Farr GH, et al. Anorectal melanoma. Cancer 1981;47:1891–900.
150. Siegel B, Cohen D, Jacob ET. Surgical treatment of anorectal melanomas. Am J Surg 1983;146:336–8.
151. Brady MS, Kavolius JP, Quan SHW. Anorectal melanoma: a 64-year experience at Memorial Sloan-Kettering Cancer Center. Dis Colon Rectum 1995;38:146–51.
152. Quan SHW, White JE, Deddish MR. Malignant melanoma of the anorectum. Dis Colon Rectum 1959;2:275–83.

94

Renal Cell Carcinoma

Jerome P. Richie, MD
Eric Jonasch, MD
Philip W. Kantoff, MD

Cancers involving the kidney may be primary or secondary. Although the kidney is a relatively common site of metastasis, secondary lesions are usually asymptomatic and are discovered only during postmortem examination.

Renal cell carcinoma (RCC) is the most common malignant lesion of the kidney, accounting for approximately 85% of all renal cancers. The vast majority of these tumors are adenocarcinoma. Nephroblastoma (ie, Wilms' tumor) accounts for 5 to 6% and transitional cell neoplasms of the renal pelvis for 7 to 8%; the remainder are various sarcomas of renal origin.

The diverse presenting signs and symptoms of RCC may challenge even the most astute diagnostician. Previously considered to be "the internist's tumor," perhaps today this tumor should be known as "the radiologist's tumor." More and more renal cancers are now being discovered incidentally during radiographic procedures, such as ultrasonography or computed tomography (CT), for nonurologic problems.

PATHOGENESIS

In 1883, Grawitz observed the resemblance of small, yellow adenomas of the kidney to adrenal tissue and suggested the possibility of adrenal rests.[1] On the basis of this observation, Birch-Hirschfeld and Doederlein introduced the term *hypernephroid tumors* or *hypernephroma*.[2] Since then, the conceptually incorrect term *hypernephroma* has been used to describe renal cell tumors. With the advent of electron microscopy, conclusive demonstration that RCC arises from proximal convoluted tubule cells has emerged. Therefore, *renal cell carcinoma* is the preferred term for this tumor.

Controversy still remains concerning the distinction between renal adenoma and renal cell adenocarcinoma. It is unclear whether RCC is related evolutionarily to renal cortical adenomas.[3] There is a major similarity between renal cortical adenoma and RCC in terms of histogenesis and of features distinguished by light microscopy and by electron microscopy. In the past, all renal cell neoplasms less than 3 cm were often diagnosed as adenomas. Currently, most are thought to represent small RCCs because lesions as small as 1 cm have occasional metastasis. Nonetheless, many pathologists feel that they can separate benign adenoma from renal cell adenocarcinoma based on size less than 5 mm, tubular or papillary (but not solid) architecture, and cell type other than clear or chromophobe.[3]

INCIDENCE

Approximately 36,160 patients in the United States are estimated to be diagnosed with renal cancers in 2005, with an estimated 12,660 deaths.[4,5] The overall incidence of primary RCC seems to have increased slowly over the past 20 years by 2 to 4% per year. The male to female ratio is 2:1.[5] RCC is more common among Scandinavians and North Americans, whereas the incidence is lower among Asians and Africans. Most cases occur in persons between 50 and 70 years of age, but it has been observed even in neonates.[5]

ETIOLOGY

Cigarette smoking and obesity are the main risk factors for RCC. A diet high in fruits and vegetables appears to exert a protective effect.[5] Patients on long-term dialysis have a propensity to develop cysts in their native kidneys, and RCC has been described in such patients.[6] Approximately 30 to 50% of patients on long-term dialysis develop acquired cystic disease, and up to 6% of these patients with acquired cystic disease develop renal cancer.[7]

MOLECULAR BIOLOGY

Over the past decade, an explosion of information has occurred regarding the molecular basis of a variety of cancers, including RCC.

Evaluation of familial RCC syndromes provides valuable insight into the molecular pathogenesis of the corresponding sporadic variants. In the following section, a number of key familial RCC syndromes are discussed in the context of their sporadic counterparts.

von Hippel-Lindau Disease Familial and sporadic forms of clear cell RCC are associated with structural alterations of the short arm of chromosome 3, or 3p.[1–3] von Hippel-Lindau (VHL) disease is a familial disorder characterized by the development of multiple tumors, including bilateral RCC, pheochromocytomas, hemangioblastomas of the central nervous system, retinal angiomas, and pancreatic cysts. The pattern of inheritance is autosomal dominant and occurs in approximately 1 in 35,000 individuals in the United States. There is loss of heterozygosity of the 3p region in RCC and other tumors in patients with VHL disease.[8] Using linkage studies, the *VHL* gene has been localized to the 3p (25–26) region of chromosome 3, and this gene has been cloned and sequenced.[9] The *VHL* gene is an E3 ubiquitin ligase involved in the regulation of hypoxia-inducible factor (HIF)-1α and HIF-2α,[10] transcription factors responsible for increased expression of vascular endothelial growth factor (VEGF) and over 100 other proteins.[11] In a hypoxic environment, HIF cannot be bound and degraded by VHL, and VEGF and other angiogenic factors are transcribed. If *VHL* is mutated, unbridled HIF-dependent transcription occurs regardless of oxygen tension, resulting in increased vascularity and enhanced tumorigenicity.

Molecular genetic analysis of sporadic RCC and cell lines derived from human RCC reveals a loss of heterozygosity of chromosome 3p in approximately 90% of clear cell RCCs. Mutations of the *VHL* gene have been observed in approximately 50% of patients with sporadic clear cell RCC, with hypermethylation of the *VHL* gene seen in another 20 to 30% of cases.[12] Therapies targeting downstream effectors of HIF dysregulation are currently in clinical trials for clear cell RCC, as described below.

Type 1 and Type 2 Hereditary Papillary RCC Type 1 hereditary papillary renal carcinoma syndrome (HPRC) was first described in 1994[13] and is inherited in an autosomal dominant fashion. HPRC is associated with a mutation in the c-*met* gene, found on chromosome 7q31.1-34.[14] Missense mutations in the *met* gene result in constitutive activation of MET, a cell surface receptor tyrosine kinase belonging to the epidermal growth factor (EGF) superfamily. Affected patients demonstrate multiple bilateral renal lesions with up to 3,400 microscopic tumors per kidney.[15] Kidney cancers in HPRC occur in the fourth, fifth, and sixth decades of life. Sporadic papillary RCCs have also been shown to contain *met* mutations in approximately 15% of cases.[16] Sporadic papillary RCCs tend to be unifocal. Studies are under way taking advantage of this knowledge using agents that target the EGF pathway.

Hereditary leiomyomatosis renal cell carcinoma, or type 2 papillary RCC, arises in patients with multiple cutaneous leiomyomas, uterine leiomyomata, and an increased risk of leiomyosarcoma.[17] The affected gene is found on chromosome 1q42.3-q43 and was shown to encode fumarate hydratase, an enzyme of the carboxylic acid cycle.[18] Type 2 renal tumors tend to be solitary RCCs, are aggressive, and tend to metastasize early.

Birt-Hogg-Dubé Syndrome Patients with Birt-Hogg-Dubé (BHD) syndrome have chromophobe RCCs, fibrofolliculomas trichodiscomas, and pulmonary cysts. The cutaneous syndrome was first described in 1977,[19] and in 1993, a patient with bilateral multifocal chromophobe RCC was described.[20] The *BHD* gene, located on chromosome 17, was characterized in 2002 and identified as folliculin.[21] An increased prevalence of multifocal renal neoplasia is seen in individuals with BHD syndrome. Multiple histologies are seen in the renal masses of patients with BHD syndrome. In a National Cancer Institute study, oncocytomas figured prominently, followed by papillary RCC.[22] A separate study demonstrated that 34% of BHD syndrome renal tumors had chromophobe histology, 9% were clear cell tumors, 5% were oncocytomas, and 50% were hybrid oncocytic neoplasms.[21]

As our understanding of the molecular biology of RCC improves, we will be better able to apply the rapidly expanding array of targeted therapies in a rational manner to its distinct molecular subtypes.

Table 94-1 Frequency of Systemic Effects in Patients with Renal Cell Carcinoma

Symptom	Incidence	%
Elevated ESR	362/651	55.6
Anemia	409/991	41.3
Hypertension	89/237	37.6
Cachexia	338/979	34.5
Pyrexia	164/954	17.2
Abnormal liver function tests	60/400	15.0
Elevated alkaline phosphatase	64/434	14.7
Hypercalcemia	33/557	5.7
Polycythemia	33/903	3.7
Neuromyopathy	13/400	3.3
Amyloidosis	12/573	2.1

Adapted from Chisholm GD and Roy RR.[24]
ESR = erythrocyte sedimentation rate.

CLINICAL FEATURES

RCC can present with a multiplicity of clinical manifestations, ranging from the classic presenting triad of hematuria, pain, and palpable renal mass to more obscure symptoms, such as those of paraneoplastic syndromes (Table 94-1). The classic triad usually indicates patients with far-advanced disease and is seen in less than 10% at presentation. More commonly, renal tumors are discovered incidentally during the course of various diagnostic studies.

Hematuria is the most common presenting symptom. It is seen in over 50% of patients with RCC but usually is observed only if the tumor has invaded the collecting system. Microscopic hematuria was found in 63% of patients with proven RCC in a series reported by Gibbons and colleagues.[23] Patients may present with pain if they have clot formation with associated colic. Flank masses are more commonly found in pediatric patients than in adults; tumors of the lower pole of the kidney are more easily palpable. The mass is generally firm and nontender and moves with respiration.

A considerable number of patients with RCC present with systemic symptoms. RCC may masquerade in a variety of symptom patterns that suggest other illnesses. Obscure problems, such as fever of unknown origin, polycythemia, weight loss, or anemia, may occur. The numerous systemic and humoral manifestations of RCC have been known as the *paraneoplastic syndromes*; the frequencies of these systemic effects are listed in Table 94-1.[24] Up to 20% of patients develop fever caused by the production of endogenous pyrogens.[25] The fever usually is intermittent and often abates when the primary tumor has been removed.

Anemia is seen in up to 40% of patients and usually is not explained by blood loss. The anemia usually is a normochromic, normocytic anemia of chronic disease. Anemia generally is associated with a low serum iron and low total iron-binding capacity. Loughlin and colleagues have hypothesized that anemia in patients with RCC relates to an inability to use the iron stores because of problems with lactoferrin.[26]

Erythrocytosis, associated with a hemoglobin greater than 15 g/dL, is seen in almost 5% of patients with RCC. Extracts of such cancer may elaborate erythropoietin. Although increased erythropoietin levels have been hypothesized to be secondary to hypoxia of normal renal parenchyma, human renal cell lines secrete erythropoietin activity, substantiating the production of an erythropoietin-like substance by RCCs.[27]

A reversible hepatic dysfunction, manifested by abnormal results of liver function tests, has been seen in up to 15% of patients. Elevation of the serum alkaline phosphatase, prothrombin time, α_2-globulin, and bilirubin may be noted. The etiology is unknown. In the absence of hepatic metastases, abnormal liver function tests often revert to normal after nephrectomy; the prognosis is ominous if the liver function tests remain elevated. A Budd-Chiari–like syndrome may be seen with venous obstruction secondary to tumor thrombus in the inferior vena cava.

Hypercalcemia is seen in up to 15% of patients. This may be secondary to osseous metastases, but it also may be secondary to ectopic production of parathyroid-like hormone.[28] Immunoreactive parathyroid hormone fragments have been demonstrated in tissue cultures of RCC.[29] In patients with marked hypercalcemia, intensive medical management may include saline diuresis, furosemide, indomethacin, and a bisphosphonate (pamidronate or etidronate).

Secondary amyloidosis is observed in 3 to 5% of patients, and the amyloidosis itself may be responsible for renal failure. The prognosis of patients with amyloidosis secondary to RCC is dismal.[30]

Renin levels are often elevated in patients with RCC. The question remains, however, whether the tumor or compression of adjacent normal parenchyma produces renin.

Immunocytochemical studies have shown that RCCs can produce renin.[31]

Patients may present with a polyneuromyopathy manifested by neurologic complaints. Thrush has postulated an antigen–antibody reaction specifically directed against nerve tissue.[32,33] Elevation of serum human chorionic gonadotropin (HCG) has been seen in patients with RCC and the clinical picture of gynecomastia and diminished libido. Apparently, the production of HCG by RCC is rare; Sufrin and colleagues studied 57 patients with RCC and failed to demonstrate elevation of intact HCG by radioimmunoassay techniques.[33]

RADIOGRAPHIC EVALUATION

A variety of imaging studies are available to delineate whether a space-occupying renal mass is benign or malignant (Figure 94-1). However, even with all available diagnostic modalities, including excretory urography, CT, arteriography,

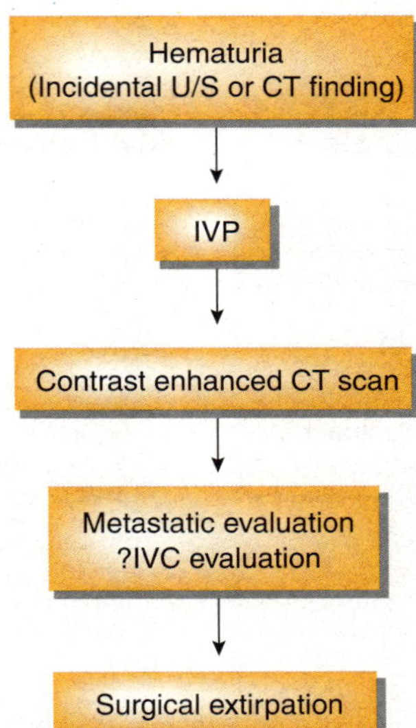

Figure 94-1 Diagnosis of renal cell carcinoma. CT = computed tomography; IVC = inferior vena cava; IVP = intravenous pyelography; U/S = ultrasonography.

venography, ultrasonography, and magnetic resonance imaging (MRI), a certain number of patients still have an indeterminate renal mass. It is important to separate benign renal cysts from solid neoplasms, most of which are malignant. In a series by Lang of over 900 patients, approximately half had benign renal cysts.[34]

Intravenous Urography Excretory urography is commonly used in the initial evaluation of patients with hematuria and generally shows a renal mass lesion if one is present. Moderate-sized tumors, especially on the posterior aspect of the kidney, may be missed, however. The major diagnostic criterion is splaying or distortion of the collecting system. Other subtle signs, such as a lack of visualization of a portion of the collecting system or distortion of the renal outline, may suggest a space-occupying lesion. In many centers, contrast-enhanced CT scan, or CT urography, has replaced excretory urography.

Nephrotomography helps eliminate distortion from bowel gas and can delineate the lateral borders of the kidney more clearly. This examination is helpful in differentiating cystic from solid lesions. A benign cyst on a nephrotomogram should demonstrate a sharp, defined border with the contrast-filled renal parenchyma and have a pencil-thin wall projecting outside the renal parenchyma. The cortical spur or "beak" sign usually indicates a benign subcortical cyst. The mass should be radiographically translucent and uniform in pattern.

Finally, intravenous (IV) urography provides important information regarding the contralateral kidney.

Ultrasonography Ultrasound scanning is a simple, inexpensive modality that has improved our ability to differentiate between a simple benign cyst and a solid tumor.[35] The advent of real-time and grayscale ultrasonography has improved the ability of sonar techniques to delineate homogeneous (ie, sonolucent) from heterogeneous lesions with internal echoes. Smith and Bennett found that ultrasonography alone had a sensitivity of 97%, a specificity of 97%, and a false-negative rate of only 1% in 413 patients.[36] Thus, when nephrotomography and ultrasonography support the diagnosis of a benign cyst, the accuracy rate approaches 97 to 98%. Ultrasonography and radionuclide scanning in combination have been recommended as the definitive modalities for the diagnosis of simple renal cyst.[37] Coexistence of a renal cyst and a tumor is extremely rare.[38] A simple serous cyst and RCC may coexist within the same kidney, but the incidence is less than 1%.[39]

Cyst Puncture If a cystic renal mass does not fit all of the criteria for a benign cyst yet the suspicion for malignancy is still low, percutaneous cyst puncture under ultrasonographic or CT guidance may be considered.[40] This allows evaluation of the cystic fluid and radiographic examination of the interior of the cyst. Cystic fluid may be assayed for fat, protein, lactic acid dehydrogenase, and cytology. After fluid has been aspirated, the cyst may be filled with contrast medium and air and then imaged radiographically. Benign cysts should have homogeneity and regular borders. Bloody aspirate strongly suggests cancer even without abnormal cytology.[41]

The dilemma of whether to aspirate cysts has become increasingly important with the identification of numerous incidental lesions by several imaging techniques. At least 50% of the population over 50 years of age has at least one renal cyst. In asymptomatic patients without hematuria and with a classic benign cyst on ultrasonography, cyst puncture is usually an unnecessary risk. If the clinical suspicion of cancer is high, this procedure can be considered.

Computed Tomography CT has become the imaging procedure of choice for the diagnosis and staging of RCC. It allows visualization of the cross-sectional anatomy and shows the relationship of mass lesions of the kidney to surrounding structures, such as the liver, spleen, and adrenal gland. The results are reproducible, and it is less invasive than arteriography. Use of the Hounsfield attenuation coefficient allows delineation of a water or solid density. In a comparative study of CT and arteriography, Weyman and colleagues confirmed the diagnosis in 59 of 62 patients with CT, whereas arteriography was diagnostic in 44 of 49 patients.[42] In a comparison study at the Brigham and Women's Hospital, CT was more accurate than arteriography in both diagnosis and staging of patients with RCC.[43] CT may give information about the status of the inferior vena cava, but additional studies also may be necessary. With spiral technology, CT allows thin cuts without patient movement and thus three-dimensional reconstruction, an excellent tool for surgical planning.[44,45]

Magnetic Resonance Imaging MRI is a useful modality for evaluating renal vein or inferior vena cava involvement in patients with RCC. The ability to produce a three-dimensional picture of the tumor can be invaluable, with both cross-sectional and parasagittal scans. Most importantly, MRI (especially using new techniques, such as the Grass technique) can visualize flow through the major vessels and accurately depict the presence or absence of thrombus in the inferior vena cava. Although ultrasonography may be able to depict tumor thrombus in the vena cava, MRI has become the procedure of choice for staging renal vein and/or vena cava involvement.[46] MRI, because of its noninvasive nature, has also replaced inferior venacavography as the preferred imaging study.

STAGING AND GRADING

Clinical Staging Once the diagnosis of RCC has been established, attention must be given to delineation of the extent of involvement in both regional and distant sites. Metastases most commonly occur to the regional lymph nodes, lung, skeleton, liver, ipsilateral adrenal gland, and contralateral kidney. CT serves to evaluate many sites of potential metastases. Chest radiography and/or chest CT should be used to evaluate potential sites of pulmonary metastases. In the asymptomatic patient with normal alkaline phosphatase, a bone scan is not necessary.[47] CT of the brain is usually reserved for patients with symptoms of central nervous system involvement.

Pathologic Grading RCC has traditionally been classified by the histologic cell type. However, with the advent of molecular staging, distinct cell types have been identified. These cell types include clear cell carcinoma, accounting for approximately 70% of RCCs; papillary cell type, accounting for 10 to 15%; chromophobe adenocarcinoma; and collecting duct adenocarcinoma. The latter two categories are distinctly uncommon.

The sarcomatoid variant of RCC can be applied to any of the above cell types. These variants are much more anaplastic, with a significantly worse prognosis; only 37% of patients survive 2 years. Nuclear characteristics tend to have some bearing on prognosis, with a higher nuclear grade (Fuhrman classification) associated with a decreased 5-year survival rate.

Pathologic Staging The single most important determinant of prognosis for a patient with RCC is the pathologic stage when the tumor is initially diagnosed and treated. Preoperative studies can give some index of the extent of involvement, especially distant involvement, but accurate staging primarily depends on histologic evaluation of the resected tumor. A pathologic staging system that has been in general use (Table 94-2) was proposed by Flocks and Kadesky[48] and

Table 94-2 Pathologic Staging of Renal Cell Carcinoma

Stage	
I	Tumor is confined within the kidney capsule
II	Tumor invades through the renal capsule but is confined within Gerota's fascia
III	Tumor has invaded the regional lymph nodes, ipsilateral renal vein, or inferior vena cava
IV	Documentation of distant metastases or involvement of adjacent organs other than the ipsilateral adrenal gland

Adapted from Flocks R and Kadesky M[48] and Robson C et al.[52]

Table 94-4 Stage Grouping for Renal Cell Carcinoma

Stage			
I	T1	N0	M0
II	T2	N0	M0
III	T1	N1	M0
	T2	N1	M0
	T3a	N0, N1	M0
	T3b	N0, N1	M0
IV	T4	Any N	M0
	Any T	N2, N3	M0
	Any T	Any N	M1

Adapted from Fleming D et al.[50]

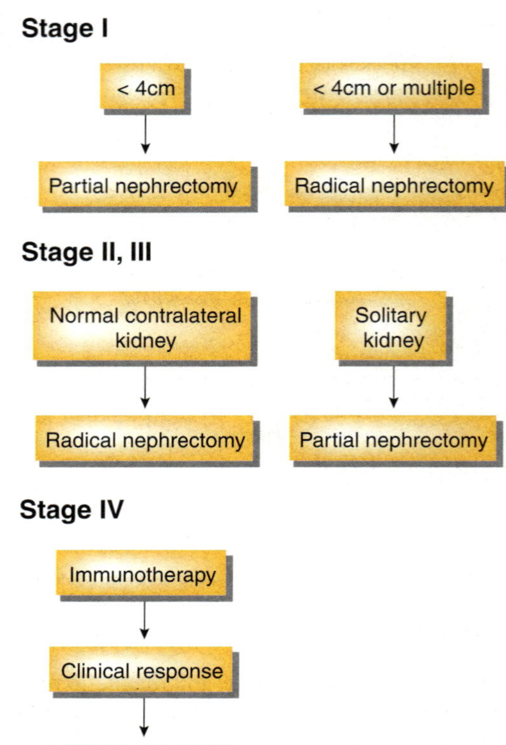

Figure 94-2 Therapy for renal cell carcinoma.

modified by Robson.[49] An international tumor, node, metastases (TNM) classification has been proposed as well (Tables 94-3 and 94-4).[50]

Controversy exists over the effect of renal vein involvement, or even inferior vena cava extension, on prognosis in the absence of regional lymphatic involvement. Waters and Richie showed that renal vein involvement alone carries a prognosis similar to that for stage II tumors, which is a finding that seemingly justifies inclusion of renal vein involvement as a subset of stage II (Table 94-5).[51]

SURGICAL TREATMENTS

The treatment of choice for RCC is surgical removal (Figure 94-2). Radical nephrectomy is accomplished by early ligation of the renal artery, renal vein, and en bloc removal of the kidney with the surrounding Gerota's fascia. The concept of radical nephrectomy with en bloc excision of Gerota's envelope was advocated by Robson and colleagues,[52] who reported a 5-year survival rate of 66% compared with previous cumulative surgical rates of 48% for simple nephrectomy. Thus, radical nephrectomy has become the procedure of choice. The results are comparable with open or laparoscopic radical nephrectomy.

Over the past 5 to 10 years, partial nephrectomy has been used increasingly, especially for smaller tumors (< 4 cm).[53–55] Follow-up after definitive treatment is dependent on tumor size.[56] Various surgical approaches are available for the effective performance of this procedure. The thoracoabdominal approach described by Chute and colleagues offers the advantage of palpation of the ipsilateral lung cavity and mediastinum and the ability to resect solitary pulmonary metastases.[57] Other approaches include an extrapleural supracostal incision or an anterior transabdominal incision. Regardless of which approach is used, the principle of early ligation of the vascular pedicle is important to prevent tumor dissemination at the time of operation.

Laparoscopic partial nephrectomy is being utilized increasingly for renal cell carcinomas < 4 cm. in diameter, especially those that are identified as incidental findings. As more experience has been gained, pure laparoscopic or hand-assisted approaches are gaining equivalency with open partial nephrectomy.[57a,b] The availability of fibrin glues and the ability to clamp the renal vessels via laparoscopy have contributed to the effectiveness of these techniques.[57c-e]

Percutaneous MRI-guided or laparoscopic techniques for ablation of renal cell carcinoma have become increasingly popular as well. Ablative technologies include cryotherapy or radiofrequency ablation.[57f,g] Intermediate follow up with imaging suggests reasonable likelihood of eradication of disease by these techniques for appropriately selected patients.

Regional Lymphadenectomy Involvement of the regional lymphatics and periaortic lymph nodes has been noted in almost 25% of patients with RCC.[58] Hence, a rationale exists for performing regional lymphadenectomy in conjunction with radical nephrectomy. The major value of identifying regional lymph node involvement would seem to be its prognostic import. A rare patient with one or two positive nodes may be a long-term survivor.[59] Nevertheless, this factor may be important in designing trials for adjuvant therapy because the 5-year survival rate in patients with regional node involvement is substantially less than in patients with stage I and stage II tumors. Regional lymphadenectomy adds little in terms of operative time or risk and should be included in conjunction with radical nephrectomy.

Renal Vein and Inferior Vena Cava Involvement Approximately 5% of patients with RCC have renal vein or inferior vena cava involvement. Tumor invasion of the renal vein and inferior vena cava usually occurs as a well-vascularized thrombus covered with its own intimal surface. This has an important bearing on surgical planning and

Table 94-3 Definition of TNM for Renal Cell Carcinoma

Tumor (T)	
TX	Primary tumor cannot be assessed
T0	No evidence of primary tumor
T1	Tumor 7.0 cm or less in greatest dimension limited to the kidney
T2	Tumor more than 7.0 cm in greatest dimension limited to the kidney
T3	Tumor extends into major veins or invades adrenal gland or perinephric tissues but not beyond Gerota's fascia
T3a	Tumor invades adrenal gland or perinephric tissues but not beyond Gerota's fascia
T3b	Tumor grossly extends into renal vein(s) or vena cava
T4	Tumor invades beyond Gerota's fascia
Regional lymph nodes (N)	
NX	Regional lymph nodes cannot be assessed
N0	No regional lymph node metastasis
N1	Metastasis in a single lymph node, 2 cm or less in greatest dimension
N2	Metastasis in a single lymph node, more than 2 cm but not more than 5 cm in greatest dimension, or multiple lymph nodes, none more than 5 cm in greatest dimension
N3	Metastasis in a lymph node more than 5 cm in greatest dimension
Distant metastasis (M)	
MX	Presence of distant metastasis cannot be assessed
M0	No distant metastasis
M1	Distant metastasis

Table 94-5 Correlation of 5-Year Survival Rate with Pathologic Stage in Patients with Renal Cell Carcinoma

Pathologic Stage	No. of Patients	Survival (5 yr %)
I	36	51.0
II	54	58.5
With renal vein involvement	21	64.0
With IVC involvement	7	25.4
III	8	12.3
IV	32	0

Adapted from Waters W and Richie J.[51]
IVC = inferior vena cava.
Previous series have classified patients with renal vein and inferior vena cava involvement as stage III (see text).

approach. In such instances, and in the absence of demonstrable metastases, radical nephrectomy is performed, with early ligation of the renal artery but no manipulation of the renal vein. Vascular control of the inferior vena cava is obtained both above and below the tumor thrombus (occasionally up to the right atrium, if necessary, with cardiopulmonary bypass). The thrombus is resected intact, with subsequent closure of the vena cava.[59] Transesophageal echocardiography can be helpful for real-time intraoperative monitoring of the caval thrombus.[60] Occasionally, a tumor actually may invade the inferior vena cava, thus necessitating inferior vena cava resection, as described by. Survival in patients with actual invasion of the inferior vena cava wall is poor, however, despite aggressive surgical approaches.

Prognosis Five-year survival rates after radical nephrectomy for stage I RCC are approximately 94%, and patients with stage II lesions have a survival rate of 79%.[51,52,61] Patients with renal vein or inferior vena cava involvement have a survival rate of 25 to 50%, and patients with regional lymph node involvement or extracapsular extension have a survival rate of 12 to 25%.

In patients with effective surgical removal of the renal vein or inferior vena cava thrombus, 5-year survival rates of 25 to 50% have been reported.[35,51] The 5-year survival rates for patients with stage IV disease are less than 5%.

Tumors in the Solitary Kidney or Bilateral Simultaneous Tumors Most tumors in solitary kidneys can be managed adequately by in vivo partial nephrectomy techniques, but, occasionally, workbench surgery with autotransplantation is necessary. Laparoscopic partial nephrectomy or percutaneous cryotherapy are acceptable options for treatment in selected patients as well.

Novick and colleagues reviewed 64 patients and found no difference in the overall survival of patients with a tumor in a solitary kidney, whether or not the contralateral kidney was removed owing to carcinoma.[63] The results of intensive therapy by partial nephrectomy in patients with a solitary kidney support the contention that, whenever permitted, a potentially resectable tumor should be excised.

Patients with bilateral synchronous RCC often have evidence of other disseminated disease. Few such patients survive for 2 years, even with radical nephrectomy and partial nephrectomy. Nonetheless, if distant metastases have been excluded, the most reasonable approach would be to treat the contralateral renal involvement as if it were a solitary metastasis and excise it by partial nephrectomy when feasible. Simultaneous surgical management may be achieved through an anterior abdominal (ie, chevron) incision.[64]

The option of complete radical nephrectomy and long-term hemodialysis can be considered in certain patients. The risks of such hemodialysis are considerable, and transplantation with immunosuppression raises the potential risk of tumor recurrence. Satisfactory long-term results can be achieved, however, even though they are infrequent.

Preoperative Arterial Embolization Percutaneous transaortic embolization of the main renal artery has been advocated as a procedure to diminish blood loss, especially in patients with large or locally invasive tumors. This approach helps simplify radical nephrectomy by allowing ligation of the main renal vein initially rather than requiring the more posterior dissection needed to ligate the renal artery first. Several investigators have hypothesized that tumor infarction enhances the immune response. Arterial embolization has been associated with considerable complications, including potential distal emboli, pain, fever, and generalized malaise. Because RCCs attract a neovasculature that parasitizes other circulatory beds, infarction of the tumors is seldom complete. Furthermore, numerous venous collaterals still remain, and blood loss is reduced only minimally. In general, angioinfarction should be reserved for the highly selected patient.

ADJUVANT THERAPY

Adjuvant therapy may include surgical excision of distant metastases, radiation therapy, chemotherapy, and immunotherapy, and it can be divided into prophylactic adjuvant therapy versus definitive treatment for metastatic disease. Surgical excision remains the treatment of choice for patients with RCC. The role of adjuvant radiation therapy remains controversial. RCC tends to be relatively radioresistant. In a randomized study of 141 patients, van der Werf-Messing showed that preoperative radiation therapy did not affect the 5-year survival rate, although it did reduce tumor recurrence in the renal fossa.[65] Randomized studies similarly have shown no improvement in the survival rate of patients who received postoperative radiation therapy.[66] In addition, many patients who received postoperative radiation therapy of up to 5,500 cGy had significant complications.

The question of postoperative adjunctive radiation therapy remains unanswered for patients with deep invasion of Gerota's fascia or adjacent organs or involvement of regional lymph nodes. Several centers have advocated treatment of up to 4,500 cGy in a 5-week course. Although local recurrence may be diminished, survival data have not improved. Such patients, who have a high likelihood of recurrence, may well be candidates for future adjuvant immune manipulation.

There is no established role for systemic adjuvant therapy after nephrectomy. Randomized, controlled trials of medroxyprogesterone acetate, interferon (IFN)-α, and interleukin (IL)-2 after nephrectomy have shown no differences in the time to disease progression or overall survival.[67–74] Future efforts will focus on the application of promising targeted therapies (see below) in high-risk patients.

TREATMENT OF METASTATIC DISEASE

Patients with metastatic RCC constitute an exceedingly difficult group for the disciplines of medical oncology, urology, and radiation oncology. Standard chemotherapy and hormonal approaches have been disappointing. The mainstay of treatment for clear cell RCC in the past 20 years has been immunotherapy, with a modest but clear benefit. A number of new approaches related to defects in VHL disease signaling have shown great promise. The following sections pertain chiefly to tumors with clear cell histology and are not applicable to variant histologies until further study on these entities is performed.

Clear cell RCC is considered to be an immunogenic tumor. A 4% spontaneous regression rate is reported,[75] as well as the presence of tumor-infiltrating lymphocytes. Immunotherapy is considered to be effective in clear cell RCC, but few data exist to support the use of immunotherapy in other histologies. The genes for IL-2 and IFN-α were cloned in 1983 and 1980, respectively,[76,77] and a large number of clinical trials have subsequently been completed using these cytokines as monotherapy, together, and in combination with other agents.

INTERFERON

The IFNs are natural glycoproteins with antiviral, antiproliferative, and immunomodulatory properties. The three major classes are (1) IFN-α, derived from leukocytes; (2) IFN-β, derived from fibroblasts; and (3) IFN-γ, derived from activated lymphocytes. Both natural and recombinant IFNs possess activity in RCC. IFN-α is the most commonly used isoform. There is no well-established dose-response relationship for IFN-α, although the toxicity is dose related.

Two studies have demonstrated the benefit of IFN-α treatment. The Medical Research Council Renal Cancer Collaborators randomized 350 patients with metastatic RCC to receive IFN-α 10 million units (MU) 3×/weekly for 12 weeks or megestrol acetate 300 mg daily for 12 weeks.[78] The primary end point of this trial was overall survival. The median overall survival was 8.5 months in the IFN-α arm and 6.0 months in the megestrol acetate arm, an improvement of 2.5 months (95% confidence interval [CI] 0.5–5.0 months). The 1-year survival rates were 43% for IFN-α and 31% for megestrol acetate, an improvement of 12% (95% CI 3–22%).

In the other study, Pyrhonen and colleagues randomized 160 patients with advanced, progressive RCC to receive either IFN-α 18 MU three times weekly plus vinblastine 0.1 mg/kg IV every 3 weeks or the same dose and schedule of vinblastine alone.[79] The rationale for the use of vinblastine was its modest activity in phase II studies. The primary end point of this trial was overall survival. A significant overall survival advantage was demonstrated with a median overall survival of 15.8 months for the IFN-α arm versus 8.8 months for the vinblastine arm ($p = .0049$). The survival rates favored the IFN-α arm at 1 year (55.7% vs 38.3%). Significant differences in overall response rates (16.5% vs 2.4%; $p = .0025$), complete response rates (8.9% vs 1.2%), and median time to disease progression (3 months vs 2 months; $p = .0001$) were also observed, all favoring the IFN-α arm. Attribution of the survival advantage to IFN-α is also supported by the fact that the addition of vinblastine to IFNs has not been shown to improve survival compared with IFN-α alone. The two largest series randomized 343 patients with metastatic RCC to IFN-α alone or IFN-α in combination with vinblastine. No difference in overall survival was seen in either trial.[80,81]

RCCs express retinoid receptors, and synergism between IFNs and retinoic acid has been observed in preclinical models of human epithelial cancers. Unfortunately, a randomized trial of IFNs with and without retinoic acid failed to show a benefit for the combination.[82]

Interleukin-2 In the 1980s and 1990s, extensive work was performed to optimize the effectiveness of IL-2 therapy in RCC. These efforts started with adoptive cellular immunotherapies using lymphocyte-activated killer or tumor-infiltrating lymphocyte cells plus IL-2. Nearly identical results occurred after IL-2–only infusion, with considerably lower cost, effort, and better patient convenience. High-dose inpatient IL-2 was approved in 1992 for use in metastatic RCC on the basis of a 15% response rate seen in a compilation of 255 patients treated in a series of phase II clinical trials.[83]

Altering the dose and schedule of IL-2 by either continuous infusion or subcutaneous injection appeared to diminish the toxicity and was thought to preserve therapeutic efficacy. The first prospective, randomized trial of high- versus low-dose bolus IL-2 infusion was reported from the National Cancer Institute Surgery Branch; 125 patients with metastatic RCC were randomized to either high-dose (720,000 IU/kg) or low-dose (72,000 IU/kg) IL-2 every 8 hours for a maximum of 15 doses. With a median follow-up of 15 months, there were no statistically significant differences in response rates or the actuarial 1-year survival rate. Low-dose IL-2 was associated, however, with statistically significant lower grades of thrombocytopenia, malaise, and hypotension. These results spurred further investigation of alternate treatment schedules.

Two large phase III clinical trials were recently published comparing high-dose inpatient IL-2 with low-dose inpatient and outpatient cytokine therapy. The first study, published in 2003, contained three arms.[84] Patients were randomized to receive either 720,000 U/kg (high dose) or 72,000 U/kg (low dose), both given by IV bolus every 8 hours. After randomly assigning 117 patients, a third arm of low-dose daily subcutaneous IL-2 was added, and an additional 283 patients were randomly assigned. There was a higher response proportion with high-dose IV IL-2 (21%) versus low-dose IV IL-2 (13%; $p = .048$) but no overall survival difference. The response rate of subcutaneous IL-2 (10%, partial response and complete response) was similar to that of low-dose IV IL-2, differing from high-dose IV IL-2 ($p = .033$). No significant survival advantage was seen in any arm, although complete responders in the high-dose arm enjoyed a high probability of cure. The second trial randomly assigned 192 patients to receive either IL-2 (5 MIU/m^2 subcutaneously every 8 hours for three doses on day 1 and then daily 5 days/wk for 4 weeks) and IFN (5 MIU/m^2 subcutaneously three times per week for 4 weeks) every 6 weeks or high-dose IL-2 (600,000 U/kg/dose IV every 8 hours on days 1 through 5 and 15 to 19 [maximum 28 doses]) every 12 weeks.[85] The response rate was 23.2% (22 of 95 patients) for high-dose IL-2 versus 9.9% (9 of 91 patients) for IL-2 and IFN ($p = .018$). Ten patients receiving high-dose IL-2 were progression free at 3 years versus three patients receiving IL-2 and IFN ($p = .082$). The median response durations were 14 and 7 months ($p = .14$), and the median survival durations were 17.5 and 13 months ($p = .24$). For patients with bone or liver metastases ($p = .001$) or a primary tumor in place ($p = .040$), survival was superior with high-dose IL-2. Although a subset of individuals clearly benefits from IL-2 therapy, the lack of a survival advantage in both studies tempers enthusiasm for wholesale use of IL-2. Vigorous efforts are under way to prospectively define the subset of individuals who benefit from IL-2 therapy.[86]

COMBINATION CYTOKINE THERAPY AND CHEMOIMMUNOTHERAPY

Preclinical models suggested possible synergism between IFNs and IL-2. In a randomized, phase II trial, patients with RCC received high-dose IL-2 or high-dose IL-2 and IFN-α.[87]The response rates were equivalent, and toxicity was higher with the combination therapy. Further work was performed combining cytokine therapy with chemotherapy. Initial studies demonstrated response rates in the 30% range,[88,89] but a subsequent large phase III trial disputes the benefit of combination chemoimmunotherapy in a broader patient population.[90] Toxicity is significantly higher in combination regimens, and, at this point, it is difficult to recommend their use based on cumulative data.

NONMYELOABLATIVE ALLOGENEIC BONE MARROW TRANSPLANTATION

Nonmyeloablative allogeneic bone marrow transplantation has been used in RCC, with initial promising results.[91] The concept herein is to induce a graft-versus-tumor response using chemotherapy to permit allogeneic engraftment. In a small pilot study, 19 patients with metastatic RCC received human leukocyte antigen–matched or single mismatch transplants. Three complete and seven partial responses were elicited, whereas two patients died of transplant-related toxicity. Several other trials have subsequently been published.[92–94] The response rates average 30%, but aggregate treatment-related mortality approaches 20%. Further work is necessary to bring this treatment into the mainstream of therapy options for RCC.

VACCINE THERAPY

Despite compelling preclinical data on the importance of the immune response in the treatment of RCC, published studies on vaccine therapy in metastatic RCC do not show consistent clinical benefit.[95–97] Future efforts may require the combination of vaccine therapy with specific T-cell receptor manipulations to overcome innate tolerance to self-antigens. Candidates include antibodies against cytotoxic T-cell antigen 4,[98] an important negative regulatory T-cell receptor.

THERAPY DIRECTED AT EGF

Epidermal growth factor receptors (EGFRs) are highly expressed on clear cell RCC, and increased expression level is associated with a poorer outcome.[99,100] Based on these and other promising preclinical results, studies were performed employing a number of EGFR blocking agents, including ZD1839 (Iressa). Phase II data from two studies using Iressa did not show evidence of activity.[101,102] Nonetheless, EGFR blockade may augment the potency of other targeted therapies, and this strategy is being investigated in combination with other agents.[103]

THERAPY DIRECTED AT VEGF

The majority of clear cell RCCs harbor *VHL* mutations. Such mutations increase the expression of HIF-1, which, in turn, increases the expression of a variety of growth factors, including VEGF. A variety of agents targeting VEGF or the VEGF receptor have been developed. One such agent, bevacizumab, an antibody directed against VEGF, has been tested in a randomized phase II study.[104] One hundred ten patients with metastatic RCC who had failed or were not eligible for cytokine therapy were randomized to receive either low-dose bevacizumab (3 mg/kg), high-dose bevacizumab (10 m/kg), or placebo treatment. The study was discontinued prematurely because of a significant delay in disease progression associated with high-dose bevacizumab compared with placebo.[105] A 690-patient phase III trial was initiated comparing IFN plus bevacizumab versus IFN alone and will be completed in 2005. A study presented in abstract form assessed the efficacy of combining bevacizumab with erlotinib, an EGFR inhibitor, in 60 patients with previously treated or untreated RCC, demonstrating a 25% response rate.[103]

A small molecule inhibitor of the VEGF receptor, SU5416, did not demonstrate significant activity in RCC patients.[106,107] Another small molecule inhibitor of the type II VEGF receptor, PTK787, was evaluated in a phase I–II study, demonstrating modest tumor shrinkage and longer than expected time to progression. On the basis of that study, phase III studies are planned.

BAY 43-9006 is an oral Raf kinase inhibitor originally anticipated to be an effective agent for tumors with *Ras* mutations, including colorectal and pancreatic cancer. Surprisingly, the agent demonstrated promising activity in patients with clear cell RCC, and further work demonstrated that BAY 43-9006 is also a potent inhibitor of VEGF receptor, platelet-derived growth factor receptor, KIT, and FLT-3. A phase III trial was completed in 2005 randomizing previously treated patients between placebo and BAY 43-9006, demonstrating an improved time to progression in patients receiving the investigational agent.

SU011248 is an oral tyrosine kinase inhibitor that blocks platelet-derived growth factor receptor, VEGF receptor, KIT, and FLT-3. Sixty-three patients with metastatic RCC who failed cytokine therapy were treated with repeated cycles of SU011248 orally at 50 mg daily for 4 weeks followed by a 2-week rest period.[108]

A partial response occurred in 24% of patients, and stable disease was seen in a further 46%. SU011248 demonstrated an acceptable toxicity profile with mostly grade 1 or 2 events, including fatigue or asthenia (78%), nausea (56%), diarrhea (51%), and stomatitis (44%). Grade 3 or 4 toxicities include lymphopenia (30%), elevated lipase (21%), and amylase (8%) without clinical signs of pancreatitis and fatigue or asthenia (8%). Two patients were taken off the study for decreases in left ventricular ejection fraction > 20% without clinical symptoms. A phase III study randomizing previously untreated patients between IFN-α and SU011248 will complete accrual in 2005.

Thalidomide has shown some activity in some forms of cancer. Whether its mechanism of activity is through an immunomodulatory, antiangiogenic, or alternative mechanism is uncertain. Unfortunately, several phase II studies have tested the activity of thalidomide in RCC but have failed to show significant activity.[109–111]

OTHER AGENTS

CCI-779, a mammalian target of rapamycin kinase inhibitor, was found to have activity in patients with previously treated RCC.[112] One hundred eleven patients were randomly assigned to receive 25, 75, or 250 mg CCI-779 weekly as a 30-minute IV infusion. Patients were evaluated for tumor response, time to tumor progression, survival, and adverse events. CCI-779 produced an objective response rate of 7% (one complete response and seven partial responses) and minor responses in 26% of patients. The median time to tumor progression was 5.8 months, and the median survival duration was 15.0 months. The agent was well tolerated, and the most frequently occurring grade 3 or 4 adverse events were hyperglycemia (17%), hypophosphatemia (13%), anemia (9%), and hypertriglyceridemia (6%). A phase III study was completed in 2005, randomizing patients among IFN-α, IFN-α plus CCI-779, and CCI-779 alone.

Until 2000, no chemotherapy was considered consistently effective in metastatic RCC. In 2000, a phase II study of gemcitabine and continuous-infusion 5-fluorouracil was published demonstrating a 17% overall response rate.[113] No data exist documenting the survival rates or the durability of responses with this combination. The combination of gemcitabine and capecitabine, the oral prodrug form of 5-fluorouracil, has been evaluated in a number of studies and may find a role as a salvage regimen in patients with RCC.

FUTURE DIRECTIONS

As the molecular biology of RCC is elucidated, it will become clearer which targets are relevant on both a global and an individual level.[113a] Future efforts will focus on determining which molecules are the most effective targets and which multitargeting strategy provides the best risk-benefit ratio. This is especially true for the non–clear cell tumor histotypes because most treatment strategies to date have either ignored or not specifically addressed their unique biology. The future success of immunotherapy in clear cell RCC will depend on a better understanding of tumor resistance to immunotherapy and the ability to overcome this blockade via rational targeting of critical cofactors.

SURGICAL CONSIDERATIONS FOR METASTATIC DISEASE

Almost 25% of patients with newly diagnosed RCC have evidence of metastases at presentation. In the absence of distant metastatic disease but with locally extensive and invasive tumors, adjacent structures, such as bowel, spleen, or psoas muscle, may be excised en bloc during radical nephrectomy. This radical approach is justified by a reasonable survival after complete resection; survival after incomplete resection is notoriously poor. Response to radiation therapy, percutaneous arterial occlusion, or arterial injection of radioactive seeds is variable but may allow the resolution of symptoms in selected patients. The treatment of patients with disseminated disease is contingent on the location of metastatic involvement, whether the metastasis appears to be solitary or multiple, and whether the patient has symptoms from the primary tumor.

Solitary Metastasis An aggressive surgical approach should be considered for patients with a solitary metastasis from RCC. In a series of 40 patients who underwent removal of a solitary metastatic focus, 33% survived for more than 5 years. The prognosis is more favorable for patients with an isolated pulmonary metastasis. During an evaluation of patients who underwent pulmonary resection for metastatic RCC, Katzenstein and colleagues found that a favorable prognosis was associated with a longer interval from removal of the primary tumor until the appearance of the metastatic focus, evidence of a solitary lesion on radiographic examination (even if multiple nodules were found at operation), and demonstration of extensive necrosis in the resected specimen.[114]

Galicich and colleagues evaluated patients with solitary cerebral metastases from RCC.[115] For those patients in whom a cerebral metastasis appeared more than 1 year following excision of the primary lesion, the 1-year survival rate after local excision and radiation therapy was almost double (36% vs 19%) that of the group in which cerebral metastases appeared less than 1 year after primary tumor excision. The results after excision of isolated metastases (both pulmonary and cerebral) are improved in patients with a longer disease-free interval after resection of the primary tumor. This finding implies that the doubling time of the primary tumor and various host–tumor interactions profoundly affect prognosis in patients with metastases.

Multiple Metastases Individualization is necessary when treating patients with multiple metastases. Palliative nephrectomy has been advocated for relief of syndromes attributable to the primary tumor and for possible induction of spontaneous regression of the metastatic foci. Nephrectomy for symptoms of local pain, hemorrhage, or severe hormonal and paraneoplastic symptoms secondary to the primary tumor is rational in patients with a likelihood of surviving at least several months. Prior to 2002, debulking nephrectomy prior to immunotherapy was not generally considered worthwhile because of the apparent lack of response and the morbidity. Two recent randomized studies, however, suggest a role for cytoreductive nephrectomy in selected cases prior to immunotherapy.[116,117] Both studies (one by the Southwest Oncology Group and the other by the European Organisation for Research and Treatment of Cancer) have shown a significant advantage in response and survival for patients who underwent nephrectomy prior to immunotherapy. The overall increased survival rate, however, was modest. Important caveats include the ability to safely remove the bulk of disease (eg, no inferior vena cava involvement) and good performance status—Karnofsky 1 or 2.

Spontaneous regression of metastatic RCC, often after removal of the primary lesion, has been documented sporadically. Freed and colleagues collected approximately 50 cases of spontaneous regression in the literature.[118] Most patients had pulmonary metastases, and 80% were male. Many of the cases regressed subsequent to radical nephrectomy. Histologic documentation was available in fewer than 20 cases. Furthermore, the term *regression* does not equate with *cure*; most patients with regression relapsed within 1 to 2 years. Nevertheless, that spontaneous regression of metastases has occurred at all (even after radiation therapy for a dominant metastasis) is evidence of a host–tumor interaction in patients with RCC.[119]

SARCOMAS OF RENAL ORIGIN

Sarcomas of primary renal origin are relatively rare, with an estimated incidence of 1 to 3% of all primary malignant tumors of the kidney.[120] The most common histologic type is fibrosarcoma, which usually arises from the renal capsule. The tumor manifests by rapid growth and invades the renal vein in nearly 50% of cases. Presenting symptoms may be a palpable abdominal mass, hematuria, or pain, but these are usually late symptoms. Five-year survival rates are generally poor and have been reported to be as low as 10%.[121] The second most common renal sarcoma is leiomyosarcoma, with approximately 40 patients reported in the literature.[122] These tumors are more common in females than in males. Pain is the usual initial symptom, and metastases are often present at diagnosis. Long-term survival is unusual.

Other rare histologic types include rhabdomyosarcoma, osteogenic sarcoma, and liposarcoma. In general, all of these sarcomas are highly malignant, and they often have local or distant metastatic involvement at diagnosis. Angiographic studies disclose various degrees of vascularity, and CT may allow better imaging of the extent of involvement. Surgical excision with wide margins is the preferred treatment because sarcomas are relatively radioresistant and, in general, respond poorly to various chemotherapeutic regimens.

WILMS' TUMOR (NEPHROBLASTOMA)

Among the most dramatic advances in oncology is the success of combined-modality therapy in Wilms' tumor. This neoplasm is nearly exclusively confined to childhood.

RENAL ONCOCYTOMA

Often classified as well-differentiated renal adenocarcinoma, renal oncocytomas appear to represent a distinct clinical and pathologic entity. Oncocytes, which are large epithelial cells with granular cytoplasm, constitute oncocytomas. Most often, they behave in a benign fashion, but they can present malignant potential. In one series of 90 such patients, 91% of the tumors were confined to the renal capsule without local invasion. Sixty-two patients were grade 1, and 28 patients were grade 2. None of the grade 1 and two of the grade 2 patients developed metastatic disease. The term *renal oncocytoma* probably should be used to characterize a well-differentiated renal tumor with eosinophilic granular cells that behaves in a biologically nonvirulent fashion.[123]

REFERENCES

1. Grawitz P. Die Sogenanneten Lipoma der Niere. Virchows Arch 1883;93:39.
2. Birch-Hirschfeld F, Doederlein A. Zentralbl Krankh Horn Org 1894;3.
3. Grignon A, Eble J. Papillary and metanephric adenomas of the kidney. Semin Diagn Pathol 1998;15:41–53.
4. Jemal A, Murray T, Ward E, et al. Cancer statistics. Cancer J Clin 2005;55:10–30.
5. McLaughlin JK, Lipworth L. Epidemiologic aspects of renal cell cancer. Semin Oncol 2000;27:115–23.
6. Bretan PN Jr, Busch MP, Hricak H, Williams RD. Chronic renal failure: a significant risk factor in the development of acquired renal cysts and renal cell carcinoma. Case reports and review of the literature. Cancer 1986;57:1871–9.
7. MacDougall ML, Welling LW, Wiegmann TB. Renal adenocarcinoma and acquired cystic disease in chronic hemodialysis patients. Am J Kidney Dis 1987;9:166–71.
8. Kaelin WG Jr, Maher ER. The VHL tumour-suppressor gene paradigm. Trends Genet 1998;14:423–6.
9. Gorospe M, Egan JM, Zbar B, et al. Protective function of von Hippel-Lindau protein against impaired protein processing in renal carcinoma cells. Mol Cell Biol 1999;19:1289–300.
10. Lonser RR, Glenn GM, Walther M, et al. von Hippel-Lindau disease. Lancet 2003;361:2059–67.
11. Semenza G.L. Targeting HIF-1 for cancer therapy. Nat Rev Cancer 2003;3:721–32.
12. Kim WY, Kaelin WG. Role of VHL gene mutation in human cancer. J Clin Oncol 2004;22:4991–5004.
13. Zbar B, Tory K, Merino M, et al. Hereditary papillary renal cell carcinoma. J Urol 1994;151:561–6.
14. Schmidt L, Duh FM, Chen F, et al. Germline and somatic mutations in the tyrosine kinase domain of the MET proto-oncogene in papillary renal carcinomas. Nat Genet 1997;16:68–73.
15. Linehan WM, Walther MM, Zbar B. The genetic basis of cancer of the kidney. J Urol 2003;170(6 Pt 1):2163–72.
16. Schmidt L, Junker K, Nakaigawa N, et al. Novel mutations of the MET proto-oncogene in papillary renal carcinomas. Oncogene 1999;18:2343–50.
17. Kiuru M, Launonen V, Hietala M, et al. Familial cutaneous leiomyomatosis is a two-hit condition associated with renal cell cancer of characteristic histopathology. Am J Pathol 2001;159:825–9.
18. Launonen V, Vierimaa O, Kiuru M, et al. Inherited susceptibility to uterine leiomyomas and renal cell cancer. Proc Natl Acad Sci U S A 2001;98:3387–92.
19. Birt AR, Hogg GR, Dube WJ. Hereditary multiple fibrofolliculomas with trichodiscomas and acrochordons. Arch Dermatol 1977;113:1674–7.
20. Roth JS, Rabinowitz AD, Benson M, Grossman ME. Bilateral renal cell carcinoma in the Birt-Hogg-Dubé syndrome. J Am Acad Dermatol 1993;29:1055–6.
21. Nickerson M, Warren M, Toro J, et al. Mutations in a novel gene lead to kidney tumors, lung wall defects, and benign tumors of the hair follicle in patients with the Birt-Hogg-Dubé syndrome. Cancer Cell 2002;2:157.
22. Toro JR, Glenn G, Duray P, et al. Birt-Hogg-Dubé syndrome: a novel marker of kidney neoplasia. Arch Dermatol 1999;135:1195–202.
23. Gibbons RP, Montie JE, Correa J, et al. Manifestations of renal cell carcinoma. Urology 1976;8:201–6.
24. Chisholm GD, Roy RR. The systemic effects of malignant renal tumours. Br J Urol 1971;43:687–700.
25. Cranston WI, Luff RH, Owen D, Rawlins MD. Studies on the pathogenesis of fever in renal carcinoma. Clin Sci Mol Med 1973;45:459–67.
26. Loughlin K, Gittes R, Partridge D, Stelos P. The relationship of lactoferrin to the anemia of renal cell carcinoma. Cancer 1987;59:566–71.
27. Sytkowski A, Richie J, Bicknell K. New human renal carcinoma cell line established from a patient with erythrocytosis. Cancer Res 1983;43:1415–9.
28. Buckle R, McMillan M, Mallinson C. Ectopic secretions of parathyroid hormone by a renal adenocarcinoma in a patient with hypercalcaemia. BMJ 1970;4:724–6.
29. Greenberg A, Martin J, Sutcliff H. Synthesis and release of parathyroid hormone by a renal cell carcinoma in cell culture. Clin Sci Mol Med 1973;45:183.
30. Pras M, Franklin E, Shibolet S, Brangione B. Amyloidosis associated with renal cell carcinoma of the AA type. Am J Med 1982;73:426–8.
31. Lindop G, Fleming S. Renin in renal cell carcinoma: an immunocytochemical study using an antibody to pure human renin. J Clin Pathol 1984;37:27–31.
32. Thrush D. Neuropathy, IgM paraproteinemia, and autoantibodies in hypernephroma. BMJ 1970;4:474.
33. Sufrin G, Mirand EA, Moore RH, et al. Hormones in renal cancer. J Urol 1977;117:433–8.
34. Lang E. Asymptomatic space-occupying lesions of the kidney: a programmed sequential approach and its impact on quality cost of health care. South Med J 1977;70:227–85.
35. Schreck W, Holmes J. Ultrasound as a diagnostic aid for renal cell neoplasms and cysts. J Urol 1970;103:281–5.
36. Smith E, Bennett A. The usefulness of ultrasound in the evaluation of renal masses in adults. J Urol 1975;113:525–9.
37. O'Reilly P, Osborn D, Testa H. Renal imaging: a comparison of radionuclide, ultrasound, and computed tomographic scanning in investigation of renal space-occupying lesions. BMJ 1981;282:943–5.
38. McFarland W, Wallace S, Johnson D. Renal cell carcinoma and polycystic disease. J Urol 1972;107:530–2.
39. Emmett J, Levine S, Woolner L. Co-existence of renal cyst and tumour: incidence in 1,107 cases. Br J Urol 1963;35:403.
40. Wood B, Khan M, McGovern F, et al. Imaging guided biopsy of renal masses: indications, accuracy and impact in clinical management. J Urol 1999;161:1470–4.
41. Harris R, Goergen T, Talner L. The bloody renal cyst aspirate: a diagnostic dilemma. J Urol 1975;114:832–5.
42. Weyman P, McClennan B, Stanley R, et al. Comparison of computed tomography and angiography in the evaluation of renal cell carcinoma. Radiology 1980;137:417–24.
43. Richie J, Garnick M, Seltzer S, Bettman M. Computerized tomography scan for diagnosis and staging of renal cell carcinoma. J Urol 1983;129:1114–6.
44. Chernoff DM, Silverman SG, Kikinis R, et al. Three-dimensional imaging and display of renal tumors using spiral CT a potential aid to partial nephrectomy. Urology 1994;43:125–9.
45. Wirth S, Novick A. 3-Dimensional volume rendered computerized tomography for preoperative evaluation and intraoperative treatment of patients undergoing nephron sparing surgery. J Urol 1999;161:1097–102.
46. Karstaedt N, McCullough D, Wolfman N, Dyer R. Magnetic resonance imaging of the renal mass. J Urol 1986;136:566–70.
47. Staudenharz A, Steiner B, Puig S. Is there a diagnostic role for bone scanning of patients with a high pretest probability for metastatic renal cell carcinoma? Cancer 1999;85:153–5.
48. Flocks R, Kadesky M. Malignant neoplasms of the kidney: an analysis of 353 patients followed five years or more. J Urol 1958;79:196.
49. Robson C. Radial nephrectomy for renal cell carcinoma. J Urol 1963;89:37.
50. Fleming D, Cooper J, Henson D. AJCC cancer staging manual. Philadelphia: Lippincott-Raven; 1997.
51. Waters W, Richie J. Aggressive surgical approach to renal cell carcinoma: review of 130 cases. J Urol 1979;122:306–9.
52. Robson C, Churchill B, Anderson W. The results of radial nephrectomy for renal cell carcinoma. Trans Am Assoc Genitourin Surg 1968;60:122–9.
53. Novick A. Nephron-sparing surgery for renal cell carcinoma. Br J Urol 1998;82:321–4.
54. Herr H. Partial nephrectomy for unilateral renal carcinoma and a normal contralateral kidney: 10-year follow-up. J Urol 1999;161:33–4.
55. Van Poppel H, Barnelis B, Oyen R, Baert L. Partial nephrectomy for renal cell carcinoma can achieve long-term tumor control. J Urol 1998;160:674–8.
56. Levy D, Slaton J, Swanson D, Dinney C. Stage specific guidelines for surveillance after radical nephrectomy for local renal cell carcinoma. J Urol 1998;159:1163–75.
57. Chute R, Soutter L, Kerr W. The value of the thoracoabdominal incision in removal of kidney tumors. N Engl J Med 1949;241:951.

57a. Gill IS, Colombo JR, Frank IM, et al. Laparoscopic Partial Nephrectomy for Hilar Tumors. J Urol 2005;174:850–4.

57b. Wright JL, Porter JR. Laparoscopic Partial nephrectomy: comparison of transperitoneal and retroperitoneal approaches. J Urol 2005;174:841–5.

57c. Margulis V, Matsumoto, ED, Svatek R, et al. Application of novel hemostatic agent during laparoscopic partial nephrectomy. J Urol 2005;174:761–4.

57d. Johnston WK III, Montgomery JS, Seifman BD, et al. Fibrin glue V sutured bolster: lessons learned during 100 laparoscopic partial nephrectomies. J Urol 2005;174:47–52.

57e. Finley DS, Lee DI, Eichel L, et al. Fibrin glue-oxidized cellulose sandwich for laparoscopic wedge resection of small renal lesions. J Urol 2005;173:1477–81.

57f. Varkarakis IM, Allaf ME, Inagaki T, et al. Percutaneous radio frequency ablation of renal masses: results at a 2-year mean follow up. J Urol 2005;174:456–60.

57g. Gill IS, Remer EM, Hasan WA, et al. Renal cryoablation: outcome at 3 years. J Urol 2005;173:1903–7.

58. Skinner D, Colvin R, Vermillion C, et al. Diagnosis and management of renal cell carcinoma: a clinical and pathologic study of 309 cases. Cancer 1971;28:1165–77.
59. Freed S, Gliedman M. The removal of renal cell carcinoma thrombus extending into the right atrium. J Urol 1975;113:163–5.
60. Sigman D, Hasnain J, Del Pizzo J, Sklar G. Real-time transesophageal echocardiography for intraoperative surveillance of patients with renal cell carcinoma and vena caval extension undergoing radial nephrectomy. J Urol 1999;161:36–8.
61. McCullough DL, Gittes RF. Ligation of the renal vein in the solitary kidney: effects on renal function. J Urol 1975;113:163–5
62. Licht M, Novick A, Goormastic M. Nephron-sparing surgery in incidental versus suspected renal cell carcinoma. J Urol 1994;152:39–42.
63. Novick A, Stewart B, Straffon R, Banowsky L. Partial nephrectomy in the treatment of renal adenocarcinoma. J Urol 1977;118:932–6.
64. Finkbeiner A, Moyad R, Herwig K. Bilateral simultaneously occurring adenocarcinoma of the kidney. J Urol 1976;32:26–8.
65. van der Werf-Messing B. Proceedings: carcinoma of the kidney. Cancer 1973;32:1056–61.
66. Kjaer M, Frederiksen P, Engelholm S. Postoperative radiotherapy in stage II and III renal adenocarcinoma: a ran-

domized trial by the Copenhagen Renal Cancer Study Group. Int J Radiat Oncol Biol Phys 1987;13:665–72.

67. Pizzacaro G, Piva L, Di Fronzo G. Adjuvant medroxyprogesterone acetate to radial nephrectomy in renal cancer: 5-year results of a prospective randomized study. J Urol 1997;157:1604–7.
68. Prummer O. Interferon-alpha antibodies in patients with renal cell carcinoma treated with recombinant interferon-alpha-2A in an adjuvant multicenter trial. The Delta-P Study Group. Cancer 1993;71:1828–34.
69. Migliari R, Muscas G, Solinas A, et al. Is there a role for adjuvant immunochemotherapy after radical nephrectomy in pT2-3N0M0 renal cell carcinoma? J Chemother 1995;7:240–5.
70. Messing EM, Manola J, Wilding G, et al. Phase III study of interferon alfa-NL as adjuvant treatment for resectable renal cell carcinoma: an Eastern Cooperative Oncology Group/Intergroup trial. J Clin Oncol 2003;21:1214–22.
71. Basting R, Corvin S, Handel D, et al. Adjuvant immunotherapy in renal cell carcinoma—comparison of interferon alpha treatment with an untreated control. Anticancer Res 1999;19:1545–8.
72. Jeon SH, Chang SG, Kim JI. The role of adjuvant immunotherapy after radical nephrectomy and prognostic factors in pT3N0M0 renal cell carcinoma. Anticancer Res 1999;19:5593–7.
73. Pizzocaro G, Piva L, Colavita M, et al. Interferon adjuvant to radical nephrectomy in Robson stages II and III renal cell carcinoma: a multicentric randomized study. J Clin Oncol 2001;19:425–31.
74. Clark JI, Atkins MB, Urba WJ, et al. Adjuvant high-dose bolus interleukin-2 for patients with high-risk renal cell carcinoma: a Cytokine Working Group randomized trial. J Clin Oncol 2003;21:3133–40.
75. Freed S, Halperin J, Gordon M. Idiopathic regression of metastases from renal cell carcinoma. J Urol 1977;118: 538–42.
76. Degrave W, Tavernier J, Duerinck F, et al. Cloning and structure of the human interleukin 2 chromosomal gene. EMBO J 1983;2:2349–53.
77. Taniguchi T, Fujii-Kuriyama Y, Muramatsu M. Molecular cloning of human interferon cDNA. Proc Natl Acad Sci U S A 1980;77:4003–6.
78. Medical Research Council Renal Cancer Collaborators. Interferon-alpha and survival in metastatic renal carcinoma. early results of randomized controlled trial. Lancet 1999;353:14–7.
79. Pyrhonen S, Salminen E, Ruutu M, et al. Prospective randomized trial of interferon alfa-2a plus vinblastine versus vinblastine alone in patients with advanced renal cell cancer. J Clin Oncol 1999;17:2859–.
80. Neidhart J, Anderson S, Harris J, et al. Vinblastine fails to improve response of renal cancer to interferon alfa-n1: high response rate in patients with pulmonary metastases. J Clin Oncol 1991;9:832–6.
81. Fossa S, Martinelli G, Otto U, et al. Recombinant interferon alfa-2a with or without vinblastine in metastatic renal cell carcinoma: results of a European multi-center phase III study. Ann Oncol 1992;3:301–5.
82. Motzer RJ, Murphy BA, Bacik J, et al. Phase III trial of interferon alfa-2a with or without 13-cis-retinoic acid for patients with advanced renal cell carcinoma. J Clin Oncol 2000;18:2972–80.
83. Fyfe G, Fisher RI, Rosenberg SA, et al. Results of treatment of 255 patients with metastatic renal cell carcinoma who received high-dose recombinant interleukin-2 therapy. J Clin Oncol 1995;13:688–96.
84. Yang JC, et al. Randomized study of high-dose and low-dose interleukin-2 in patients with metastatic renal cancer. J. Clin Oncol 2003; 21: 3127–32.
85. McDermott DF, et al. Randomized phase III trial of high-dose interleukin-2 versus subcutaneous interleukin-2 and interferon in patients with metastatic renal cell carcinoma. J Clin Oncol 2005; 23:133–41.
86. Atkins MB, Regan M, McDermott D. Update on the role of interleukin 2 and other cytokines in the treatment of patients with stage IV renal carcinoma. Clin Cancer Res 2004;10(18 Pt 2):6342S–6S.
87. Bregni M, Dodero A, Peccatori J, et al. Nonmyeloablative conditioning followed by hematopoietic cell allografting and donor lymphocyte infusions for patients with metastatic renal and breast cancer. Blood 2002;99:4234–6.
88. Atzpodien J, Kirchner H, Jonas U, et al. Interleukin-2- and interferon alfa-2a-based immunochemotherapy in advanced renal cell carcinoma: a prospectively randomized trial of the German Cooperative Renal Carcinoma Chemoimmunotherapy Group (DGCIN). J Clin Oncol 2004.
89. Ellerhorst JA, Sella A, Amato RJ, et al. Phase II trial of 5-fluorouracil, interferon-alpha and continuous infusion interleukin-2 for patients with metastatic renal cell carcinoma. Cancer 1997;80:2128–32.
90. Negrier S, Caty A, Lesimple T, et al. Treatment of patients with metastatic renal carcinoma with a combination of subcutaneous interleukin-2 and interferon alfa with or without fluorouracil. J Clin Oncol 2000;18:4009–15.
91. Childs R, Chernoff A, Contentin N, et al. Regression of metastatic renal-cell carcinoma after nonmyeloablative allogeneic peripheral-blood stem-cell transplantation. N Engl J Med 2000;343:750–8.
92. Ueno NT, Cheng YC, Rondon G, et al. Rapid induction of complete donor chimerism by the use of a reduced-intensity conditioning regimen composed of fludarabine and melphalan in allogeneic stem cell transplantation for metastatic solid tumors. Blood 2003;102:3829–36.
93. Rini BI, Zimmerman T, Stadler WM, et al. Allogeneic stem-cell transplantation of renal cell cancer after nonmyeloablative chemotherapy: feasibility, engraftment, and clinical results. J Clin Oncol 2002;20:2017–24.
94. Pedrazzoli P, Da Prada GA, Giorgiani G, et al. Allogeneic blood stem cell transplantation after a reduced-intensity, preparative regimen: a pilot study in patients with refractory malignancies. Cancer 2002;94:2409–15.
95. Marten A, Flieger D, Renoth S, et al. Therapeutic vaccination against metastatic renal cell carcinoma by autologous dendritic cells: preclinical results and outcome of a first clinical phase I/II trial. Cancer Immunol Immunother 2002;51:637–44.
96. Oosterwijk-Wakka JC, Tiemessen DM, Bleumer I, et al. Vaccination of patients with metastatic renal cell carcinoma with autologous dendritic cells pulsed with autologous tumor antigens in combination with interleukin-2: a phase 1 study. J Immunother 2002;25:500–8.
97. Kugler A, Stuhler G, Walden P, et al. Regression of human metastatic renal cell carcinoma after vaccination with tumor cell-dendritic cell hybrids. Nat Med 2000;6:332–6.
98. Abrams SI. Role of anti-CTLA-4 therapies in the treatment of cancer. Curr Opin Mol Ther 2004;6:71–7.
99. Uhlman DL, Nguyen P, Manivel JC, et al. Epidermal growth factor receptor and transforming growth factor alpha expression in papillary and nonpapillary renal cell carcinoma: correlation with metastatic behavior and prognosis. Clin Cancer Res 1995;1:913–20.
100. Langner C, Ratschek M, Rehak P, et al. Are heterogenous results of EGFR immunoreactivity in renal cell carcinoma related to non-standardised criteria for staining evaluation? J Clin Pathol 2004;57:773–5.
101. Druker BJ, Schwartz L, Marion S, Motzer RJ. Phase II trial of ZD 1839 (Iressa), an EGF receptor inhibitor, in patients with renal cell carcinoma. Proc Am Soc Clin Oncol 2002; 2002. 720.
102. Dawson NA, Guo C, Zak R, et al. A phase II trial of gefitinib (Iressa, ZD1839) in stage IV and recurrent renal cell carcinoma. Clin Cancer Res 2004;10:7812–9.
103. Hainsworth JD, Sosman JA, Spigel DR, et al. Phase II trial of bevacizumab and erlotinib in patients with metastatic renal carcinoma (RCC). Am Soc Clin Oncol 2004;2004. 4502.
104. Yang J, Haworth L, Steinberg M, Rosenberg S. A randomized double blind placebo controlled trial of bevacizumab (anti-VEGF antibody) demonstrating a prolongation in time to progression in patients with metastatic renal cell carcinoma. Proc Am Soc Clin Oncol 2002;21: 5a.
105. Yang JC, Haworth L, Sherry RM, et al. A randomized trial of bevacizumab, an anti-vascular endothelial growth factor antibody, for metastatic renal cancer. N Engl J Med 2003;349:427–34.
106. Lara PN Jr, Quinn DI, Margolin K, et al. SU5416 plus interferon alpha in advanced renal cell carcinoma: a phase II California Cancer Consortium Study with biological and imaging correlates of angiogenesis inhibition. Clin Cancer Res 2003;9:4772–81.
107. Kuenen BC, Tabernero J, Baselga J, et al. Efficacy and toxicity of the angiogenesis inhibitor SU5416 as a single agent in patients with advanced renal cell carcinoma, melanoma, and soft tissue sarcoma. Clin Cancer Res 2003;9:1648–55.
108. Motzer RJ, Bacik J, Schwartz, LH, et al. Prognostic factors for survival in previously treated patients with metastatic renal cell carcinoma. J Clin Oncol 2004; 22:454–63.
109. Stebbing J, Benson C, Eisen T, et al. The treatment of advanced renal cell cancer with high-dose oral thalidomide. Br J Cancer 2001;85:953–8.
110. Motzer RJ, Berg W, Ginsberg M, et al. Phase II trial of thalidomide for patients with advanced renal cell carcinoma. J Clin Oncol 2002;20:302–6.
111. Daliani D, Papandreou C, Thall P. A pilot study of thalidomide in patients with progressive metastatic renal cell carcinoma. Cancer 2002;95:758–65.
112. Atkins MB, Hidalgo M, Stadler WM, et al. Randomized phase II study of multiple dose levels of CCI-779, a novel mammalian target of rapamycin kinase inhibitor, in patients with advanced refractory renal cell carcinoma. J Clin Oncol 2004;22:909–18.
113. Rini BI, Vogelzang NJ, Dumas MC, et al. Phase II trial of weekly intravenous gemcitabine with continuous infusion fluorouracil in patients with metastatic renal cell cancer. J Clin Oncol 2000;18:2419–26.
113a. Lam JS, Shvarts O, Leppert JT, et al. Renal cell carcinoma 2005: new frontiers in staging, prognostication and targeted molecular therapy. J Urol 2005;173:1853–62.
114. Katzenstein A, Purvis R, Gmelick J, Askin J. Pulmonary resection for metastatic renal adenocarcinoma. Cancer 1978;41:712–23.
115. Galicich J, Sundaresan N, Arbit E, Passe S. Surgical treatment of single brain metastasis: factors associated with survival. Cancer 1980;45:381–6.
116. Flanigan RC, Salmon SE, Blumenstein BA, et al. Nephrectomy followed by interferon alfa-2b compared with interferon alfa-2b alone for metastatic renal-cell cancer. N Engl J Med 2001;345:1655–9.
117. Mickish G, Garin A, Van Poppel H, et al. Radial nephrectomy plus interferon-alfa-based immunotherapy compared with interferon alfa alone in metastatic renal-cell carcinoma: a randomised trial. Lancet 2001;358:966–70.
118. Freed SZ, Halperin JP, Gordon M. Idiopathic regression of metastases from renal cell carcinoma. J Urol 1977;118:538–42.
119. Fairlamb D. Spontaneous regression of metastases of renal cell cancer: a report of two cases including the first recorded regression following irradiation of a dominant metastasis and a review of the literature. Cancer 1981;47: 2102–6.
120. Gupta O, Dube M. Rare primary renal sarcoma. Br J Urol 1971;43:546–71.
121. Demming C, Harvard B. Tumors of the kidney. Philadelphia: W.B. Saunders; 1970.
122. Loomis R. Primary leiomyosarcoma of the kidney: report of a case and review of literature. J Urol 1972;107:557–60.
123. Lieber M, Tobera K. Renal oncocytoma. J Urol 1981;125:481–5.

Neoplasms of the Renal Pelvis and Ureter

Jerome P. Richie, MD
Philip W. Kantoff, MD

Primary carcinoma of the renal pelvis or ureter is relatively rare, accounting for less than 5% of renal tumors and less than 1% of genitourinary neoplasms. The only exception seems to occur in regions of Balkan endemic familial nephropathy, a condition in which renal pelvic neoplasms account for almost 50% of all renal tumors. Balkan nephropathy is an indolent inflammatory process of the renal interstitium in patients of Balkan or Greek origin and is associated with development of tumors in the renal pelvis and ureter. These tumors generally are superficial and slow growing. The cause of Balkan nephropathy is uncertain.

Transitional cell carcinoma of the upper urinary tract often is a multifocal process; tumors often occur with associated in situ carcinoma in other segments of the upper urinary tract. In addition, synchronous or metachronous tumors can occur elsewhere in the ipsilateral renal pelvis or ureter. The probability of multifocality increases in patients with larger lesions and in those with associated in situ carcinoma. Furthermore, patients with upper tract urothelial tumors have an increased risk of developing transitional cell carcinoma in the bladder. Fortunately, bilateral upper tract tumors are rare, with an incidence of less than 2%.

Tumors of the renal pelvis occur more frequently in men than in women, with a ratio of 2:1. The peak incidence is during the fifth to sixth decades of life, with a progressive increase occurring with advancing age. Ureteral tumors more commonly are seen in the lower third of the ureter, with no predilection for laterality. Ureteral tumors have increased in incidence over the past 23 years.[1]

Most tumors of the renal pelvis and ureter are of urothelial origin, most commonly transitional cell tumors. Squamous cell carcinomas and adenocarcinomas may be associated with chronic infection or stones, but this does not occur frequently. Less than 10% of all tumors in the upper collecting system are squamous cell carcinomas, and adenocarcinomas are extremely rare.

ETIOLOGIC FACTORS

The mucosal surfaces of the collecting tubules, calyces, renal pelvis, ureter, bladder, and urethra have the same embryologic origin; hence, the term *urothelium* has been coined to delineate this mucosal system.[2]

Transitional epithelium that lines the calyceal system and renal pelvis is exposed to various potential carcinogens in urine. Excreted carcinogens may be activated in the urine by hydrolyzing enzymes. Thus, they would be expected to promote oncogenesis throughout the urinary system, resulting in an even higher ratio of bladder-to-urothelial tumors in the upper tract than would be predicted based on surface area alone.

Attention also has been focused on the molecular genetics of transitional cell carcinoma. Restriction fragment length polymorphism analyses of bladder tumors have shown a frequent loss of heterozygosity on chromosome segments 11p, 9q, and 17p of bladder tumors, raising the possibility that tumor-suppressor genes are operative in these tumors. A similar analysis has yet to be performed on tumors of pelvic or ureteral origin. The frequency and role of activated *ras* oncogenes, which sometimes are present in bladder tumors, have not been studied in renal pelvic and ureteral tumors.[3] A reported kindred of familial transitional cell carcinoma has been documented, however, with 22% of affected family members having upper tract tumors, almost 60% having bladder cancer, and 18% having both upper and lower tract tumors.[4] Microsatellite instability has been noted in upper tract tumors.[5] Hopefully, the study of molecular and cellular aspects of the transformation of urothelium will further elucidate the mechanisms of tumor progression and metastasis.

HISTOPATHOLOGY

More than 90% of renal pelvic tumors are classified as transitional cell carcinoma and are virtually identical to those tumors in the ureter and bladder. As such, these tumors can be papillary or solid in configuration and either with or without associated carcinoma in situ. Squamous cell carcinoma, accounting for only 7% of renal pelvic tumors, is usually sessile; this type of cancer is commonly associated with inflammatory processes. These tumors tend to be deeply invasive and thus are associated with a poorer prognosis. Adenocarcinoma of the renal pelvis is exceedingly rare.

DIAGNOSIS

Clinical Presentation Hematuria, either gross or microscopic, is the most common symptom in patients with renal pelvic or ureteral tumors (ie, 70 to 95% occurrence) (Figure 95-1). The appearance of pain is precipitated by ureteral or ureteropelvic junction obstruction secondary to a tumor mass, and it is seen in 8 to 40% of patients. Symptoms of bladder irritation are seen in 5 to 10% of patients, and constitutional symptoms in an additional 5%.

The physical examination usually is not revealing. However, in 10 to 20% of patients, a flank mass secondary to the tumor or associated hydronephrosis has been reported.[6]

Cytology Exfoliative cytologic examination, the value of which has been well documented in tumors of the bladder, has been less reliable in upper urinary tract neoplasms. However, with the use of filter preparations, Cullen and associates reported positive cytologic evidence in 80% of their patients with tumors of the pelvis and ureter.[7]

Voiding specimens for urinary cytologic testing have been noted by numerous investigators to be of questionable value because of the poor yield in low-grade tumors and presence of concomitant bladder tumors.[8–10] Zincke and coworkers found that retrograde collections aided by furosemide diuresis yielded much better results; in 18 patients who underwent both tests, 11 (61%) were noted to have positive cytologic evidence of tumor on retrograde collections, compared with 6 (33%) on voided cytologic specimens.[11] Critical to reliance on cytologic findings is the presence of

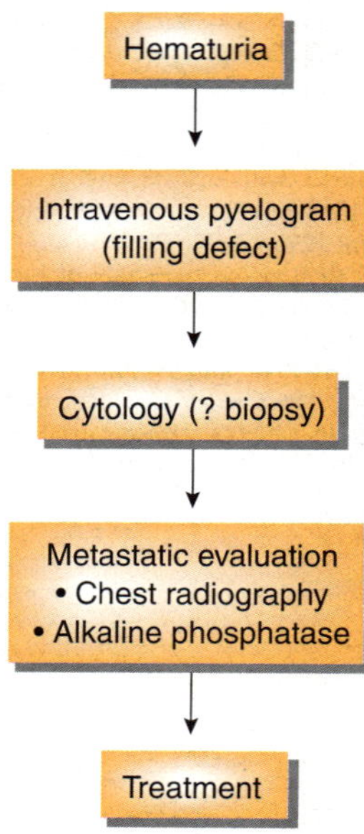

Figure 95-1 Diagnostic algorithm for renal pelvic tumor.

a well-trained pathologist with a substantial interest in cytology.

Nuclear cytologic characteristics indicate the histologic grade of the tumor, but a direct correlation of the cytologic grade with tumor invasiveness is lacking. Eriksson and Johansson studied 43 patients with upper tract urothelial neoplasms; positive cytologic evidence was found in 2 of 5 patients with grade 2 invasive tumors and in 17 of 24 with grade 3 or 4 invasive tumors.[12] Although no cytologic examinations were falsely positive, 35% of the patients with a negative or atypical cytologic result were found to have invasive tumors. In another series, positive cytologic evidence of tumor was demonstrated in only 29% of the patients with proven invasive ureteral carcinoma.[13] Molecular tests for diagnosis of bladder cancer have had limited applicability in upper tract tumor diagnosis.

Intravenous Pyelography The diagnosis of a renal pelvic or ureteral tumor usually is suspected based on an excretory urogram; almost all patients with renal pelvic carcinoma will have an abnormal result on this study. The most common finding is a filling defect in the renal pelvis, which is observed in 50 to 75% of pyelograms.[14] In addition to a solitary filling defect, cancer of the renal pelvis may present with multiple filling defects, ureteral pelvic junction obstruction with hydronephrosis, infundibular stenosis, splaying of the calyces (suggesting a renal mass), and, occasionally, nonvisualization of the renal collecting system. Computerized tomography (CT) urography is rapidly replacing intravenous pyelography.

Williams and Mitchell found intravenous pyelograms to be valuable in 28 of 30 patients in whom disease was discovered that required urgent further investigation.[10] Almgard and associates reported abnormal intravenous pyelographic findings in all 41 patients with ureteric tumor in whom nephrectomy had not been previously performed.[15] In 20 of their patients, a tumor or stricture was suspected, and in the other 21, the ureter could not be evaluated because of the decreased excretion of contrast material. Batata and coworkers reported findings of unilateral nonvisualization in 46% of their patients, hydronephrosis with or without hydroureter in 34%, and ureteral filling defect without obstruction in 19%.[16]

Ureteroscopy The improvement of flexible instruments with small fiberoptic bundles has allowed visualization of the entire collecting system. Initially, 13.5-F, rigid ureteroscopes were used to visualize the entire collecting system. These rigid instruments required dilation of the ureteral orifice and had the potential for perforation. As the state of the art has advanced, smaller rigid ureteroscopes (6 French) now are available, along with flexible ureteroscopes, which allow visualization of the ureter and renal pelvis. Flexible ureteroscopes are steerable, allowing the effective visualization of most of the collecting system. The Mayo Clinic reported 43 patients with upper tract urothelial tumors in whom the diagnosis was confirmed in 86% of renal pelvic tumors and 90% of ureteral tumors; the complication rate was 7% (usually perforation of the ureter.[17] Ureteroscopy allows directed tissue biopsies in many cases.

Table 95-1 Definition of Tumor, Node, Metastases

Stage	Description
Primary tumor (T)	
TX	Primary tumor cannot be assessed
T0	No evidence of primary tumor
Ta	Papillary noninvasive carcinoma
Tis	Carcinoma in situ
T1	Tumor invades subepithelial connective tissue
T2	Tumor invades the muscularis
T3	(For renal pelvis only) Tumor invades beyond muscularis into peripelvic fat or the renal parenchyma
T3	(For ureter only) Tumor invades beyond muscularis into periureteric fat
T4	Tumor invades adjacent organs or through the kidney into the perinephric fat
Regional lymph nodes (N)[a]	
NX	Regional lymph node cannot be assessed
N0	No regional lymph node metastasis
N1	Metastasis in a single lymph node, 2 cm or less in greatest dimension
N2	Metastasis in a single lymph node, more than 2 cm but not more than 5 cm in greatest dimension; or multiple lymph nodes, none more than 5 cm in greatest dimension
N3	Metastasis in a lymph node more than 5 cm in greatest dimension
Distant metastasis (M)	
MX	Distant metastasis cannot be assessed
M0	No distant metastasis
M1	Distant metastasis

[a]Laterality does not affect the N classification.

Source: Greene FL, Balch CM, Page DL, et al, editors. Urethra. In: American Joint Committee on Cancer (AJCC) Cancer Staging Manual. 6th ed. New York: Springer-Verlag, 2002. p. 341–6.

Brush Biopsy Retrograde brushing of the upper urinary tract was described by Gill and associates in 1973.[18] An angiographic catheter is passed transurethrally up the affected ureter and positioned adjacent to a suspicious lesion. A small nylon or steel bristle brush is passed inside its lumen, and material entrapped by the bristles is sent for histologic and cytologic examination. This technique allows diagnosis of moderately differentiated transitional cell carcinoma, but it still produces false-negative results in patients with low-grade lesions. Urine should be collected for cytologic and cell-block preparation after the brush has been removed, because the diagnosis may be more readily made in this fashion. A survey involving 32 patients found brush biopsy to be accurate and confirmed by operative intervention in 84%.[19]

STAGING

Patients with a diagnosis of renal pelvic or ureteral tumor must be carefully evaluated to exclude both multiplicity of tumors and distant metastases. Grabstald and associates reported that approximately 50% of their patients with renal tumors had associated tumors in the bladder, ureter, or both.[20] With the likelihood of multiplicity, it is essential that the entire urinary tract, including the urethra and bladder mucosa, be visualized either radiographically or endoscopically. If the intravenous pyelogram is not adequate to reveal the entire surface, retrograde pyelography should be used.

In addition to assessment of the urothelium, staging procedures should include chest radiographs, a radionuclide bone scan, and a serum multichannel analysis. Liver scans or CT of the liver should not be used in the absence of abnormal liver profile studies. Ultrasonography or CT may have some benefit in assessing the presence or absence of retroperitoneal lymphadenopathy; however, magnetic resonance imaging (MRI) has not proven beneficial.

The difficulty in establishing the diagnosis, as well as the limited accuracy of available staging procedures, precludes the development of a clinical staging system. Instead, the classification of renal pelvic tumors is based on pathologic findings. After studying 70 patients with renal pelvic tumors, Grabstald and associates proposed a classification system based on tumor stage and grade.[20] A modification of this system was proposed by Batata and Grabstald. Similar to the Jewett–Marshall–Strong system for bladder cancer, this system uses letters to indicate the depth of invasion.[13] Stage 0 neoplasms are confined to the mucosa, stage A tumors invade the lamina propria, stage B invade the muscle, stage C extend into the peripelvic fat or renal parenchyma, and stage D represent metastatic disease. The current tumor, node, metastases (TNM) classification is currently used (Table 95-1).

Transitional cell carcinoma may spread by direct extension or by the hematogenous or lymphatic routes. Regional lymph nodes are commonly involved before other sites of metastasis; therefore, surgical therapy should include regional lymphadenectomy. However, almost any organ

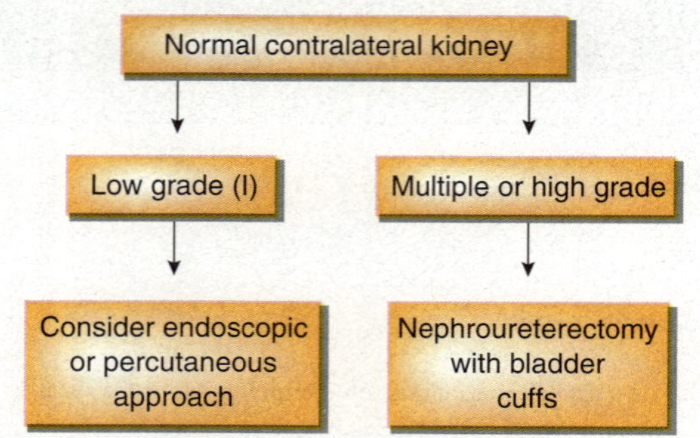

Figure 95-2 Treatment algorithm for renal pelvic tumor.

may receive metastases from transitional cell tumors of the upper urinary tract.

TREATMENT

Operative Therapy The classic management of renal pelvic tumors (Figure 95-2) is nephroureterectomy, with excision of a cuff of the bladder and bladder mucosa. Removal of the entire ureter is recommended because approximately 20% of patients with residual ureteral stumps will develop tumors within them. Although nephroureterectomy traditionally has been considered the treatment of choice, advocates of less radical procedures are increasing in number and now represent a strong minority opinion. Proponents of radical nephroureterectomy with removal of a cuff of bladder emphasize the difficulty in distinguishing the histologic grade of the tumor as well as accurately estimating stage preoperatively.

Of all cases of ureteral tumor, half involve at least the musculature, and they may have lymphatic involvement as well. The high incidence of multiple ipsilateral lesions, both overt and in situ, makes removal of the entire ureteral segment generally preferable to partial ureterectomy for adequate tumor surgery. The well-known phenomenon of recurrence of tumor in the remaining ureteral stump has been reported in more than 30% of patients treated by nephrectomy and partial ureterectomy.[21]

Advocates of conservative surgical intervention for renal pelvic or ureteral tumors stress the poor prognosis that is associated with advanced lesions regardless of the form of surgical therapy and the higher mortality rate occurring with more radical procedures. Articles by Ziegelbaum and coworkers, Gittes, and McCarron and associates illustrate the difficulties in choosing radical versus conservative therapy for patients with tumors of the upper urinary collecting system.[22–24]

To derive a rational recommendation for kidney-sparing versus kidney-sacrificing treatment, several factors should be considered. Recent advances in anesthesia and both pre- and postoperative management have substantially lowered operative mortality rates, so there is very little difference between kidney-conserving and kidney-sacrificing procedures in terms of overall risk. In fact, nephroureterectomy often can be performed more quickly and more easily than some alternative methods of treatment. Therefore, consideration of the morbidity and mortality risks from conservative versus radical procedures should not be a major issue.

The likelihood of implantation, especially with tumors of higher grades, must be considered as an increased risk of kidney-sparing as opposed to kidney-sacrificing procedures. Analogous experiences with open-bladder surgery would indicate a higher likelihood of implantation.

Furthermore, considerations of local recurrence and follow-up problems remain a major problem for patients with kidney-sparing procedures. Because the major site of recurrence in patients undergoing such procedures is in the ipsilateral system, nephroureterectomy obviates the need for follow-up of the initially involved upper system, which is the main thrust of follow-up in patients after a conservative procedure. Nocks and associates reported a high incidence of associated severe dysplasia or carcinoma in situ in association with high-grade, high-stage tumors.[25] They concluded that nephroureterectomy was preferable to conservative procedures in patients with renal pelvic carcinoma.

Based on these considerations, nephroureterectomy with excision of a cuff of bladder seems a preferable procedure for most patients with renal pelvic or ureteral tumors. However, several exceptions are readily apparent. In the patient with a solitary kidney, compromised renal function, bilateral lesions, or Balkan endemic nephropathy, conservation is essential, and preferred treatment would be local excision of a renal pelvic lesion with or without partial nephrectomy or, in the case of ureteral tumor, ureteral excision or ureterectomy with replacement by the ileum. Local excision and reanastomosis should be limited to patients with a localized filling defect, preferably polypoid, and preferably a low-grade and, presumably, low-stage tumor. In such patients, local excision with adequate margins may be the preferred treatment.

For patients with apparently solitary tumors, especially low-grade tumors in the lower third of the ureter, distal ureterectomy with regional lymphadenectomy, and ureter reimplantation with a psoas hitch, represent a reasonable alternative (Figure 95-3). In patients with a lesion of higher grade or stage, the likelihood of coexistent upper tract lesions or compromise to the renal parenchyma would still cause the surgeon to favor nephroureterectomy. Tumors in the middle or upper third of the ureter generally are best treated by nephroureterectomy unless cytologic and brush biopsy specimens demonstrate a low-grade and presumably low-stage tumor. In such an instance, excisional biopsy with ureteroureterostomy can be considered. Laparoscopic nephroureterectomy has increased in popularity and rivals open procedures.[26]

Selected lesions in the renal pelvis and calyceal system also may be considered for conservative treatment provided that the cytologic results show less than a high-grade lesion and brushing specimens demonstrate a low-grade transitional cell tumor. In such an instance, nephroscopy is helpful to make certain the tumor is not of a more extensive nature and that the offending collecting system can be walled off and then removed by partial nephrectomy.

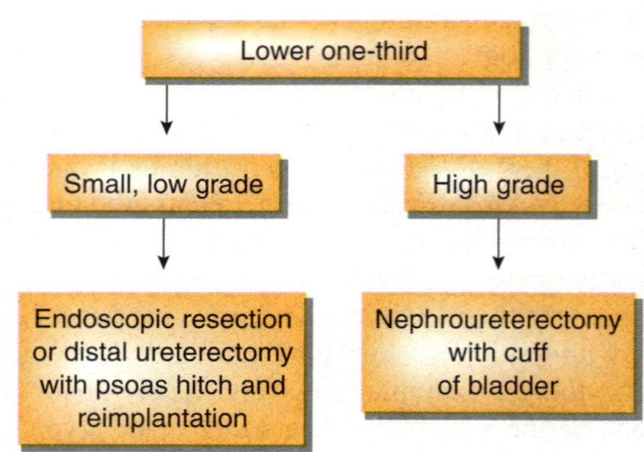

Figure 95-3 Treatment algorithm for ureteral tumor.

Endoscopic Therapy Although the standard treatment of transitional cell carcinomas of the renal pelvis involves open operative approaches (vide supra), certain authors have used endourologic or percutaneous approaches as conservative techniques to manage selected cases of upper tract urothelial tumor.[27] For example, Blute and associates used ureteropyeloscopy with fulguration in 21 patients with a local recurrence rate of 20% for renal pelvic tumors.[17]

A percutaneous approach has been advocated by Smith and colleagues.[28] They reported 9 patients with percutaneous resection of renal pelvic, transitional cell carcinoma for solitary kidney, bilateral synchronous disease, or renal insufficiency. Five of these patients remained free of recurrence with a mean follow-up of 9.5 months. This technique should still be considered experimental, however, because there is a risk of tumor spillage into the perirenal space. A larger series by Jabbour and colleagues showed a 25% recurrence rate.[29]

Prognosis The rate of survival is influenced by both the grade and the stage of the tumor. Overall survival rates are approximately 40%, with a 5-year survival of 56% for a well-differentiated cancer, as opposed to 16% for poorly differentiated lesions. Sixty percent of patients with noninvasive disease survive 5 years, compared with a 25% rate for those with invasive tumors,[17,30,31]

Adjuvant Therapy Radiation therapy remains an unproven adjunct for the control of residual tumor, unresectable disease, or local recurrence. Brady and associates reported 6 patients treated with postoperative radiation therapy, 2 treated for each of the previously mentioned indications.[32] All 6 survived free of disease for 1 year, and of those who were followed for 5 years, 3 of 5 survived that period without evidence of disease. Holtz reported favorably on the use of postoperative radiotherapy,[33] and Batata and associates recommended postoperative, elective irradiation with 6,000 cGy to tumors in stage B, C, or D.[18] A split dose of radiation therapy may render possible resection in some previously unresectable tumors, with the second course of radiotherapy aimed at controlling residual disease.

A study evaluating postoperative irradiation therapy in 41 patients concluded that local recurrence was lower, although distant failure is about the same with postoperative radiation therapy.[34] Anecdotal accounts of long-term survival, however, continue to be reported.[35]

Other investigators have questioned the place of radiotherapy in the management of ureteral carcinoma. Both Scott and Bergman and Hotchkiss recommended radiation therapy in dealing only with symptoms relative to metastatic disease.[36,37] Preoperative radiotherapy has no proven place in the management of ureteral carcinoma, although Abeshouse has conducted a trial of preoperative radiotherapy.[38] The difficulty in establishing an accurate diagnosis—much less accurate staging of the ureteral tumor—is a major deterrent to pre-operative treatment. Moreover, the potential for abdominal complications with the amount of radiation that therapy requires is high. Postoperative radiation therapy in invasive disease is, however, a logical extension of combination therapy in bladder tumors. Radiotherapy should have a place in the eradication of subclinical disease and the control of known residual tumor, and it is hoped that it will improve overall prognosis.

Chemotherapy Urothelial cancers tend to respond to cisplatin-based chemotherapy. Combination chemotherapy with regimens such as MVAC (methotrexate, vinblastine, Adriamycin [doxorubicin], and cisplatin) tends to be more active than single agents. A randomized study of 266 patients with metastatic bladder cancer demonstrated an approximately 4-month survival advantage for those patients treated with MVAC over those treated with single-agent cisplatin.[39] A recent study of 405 patients with bladder cancer comparing MVAC to cisplatin plus gemcitabine, demonstrated no difference in survival and less toxicity with the cisplatin plus gemcitabine combination.[40] Few data exist on the treatment of metastatic renal pelvic and ureteral tumors; in the experience of Sternberg and colleagues, however, metastatic renal pelvic and ureteral tumors tend to be more responsive than transitional cell carcinomas arising in the bladder to MVAC.[40] The role of adjuvant chemotherapy in ureteral and renal pelvic tumors is, however, unproven.

SECONDARY TUMORS OF THE URETER

These uncommon tumors may originate in the upper urinary tract and disperse by seedling metastases from a distant site, spreading by blood or lymphatic channels. When the primary tumor is in proximity to the ureter, spread may occur by direct extension. With the exception of drop metastases, signs and symptoms of urinary tract involvement appear quite late in the course of the disease, and they may be recognized only preterminally or at autopsy.

Drop Metastases These tumors can be difficult to segregate from those arising as separate primary lesions resulting from exposure of the entire urothelium to various carcinogens. Because ureteral tumors frequently can be seen in conjunction with bladder or renal pelvic tumors, the likelihood that cells can flow down from the renal pelvis or reflux up to the ureter and implant with subsequent growth is quite real. Weldon and associates demonstrated implantation of tumor cells in the bladder, especially in previously traumatized areas.[41] In addition, the observation of recurrent bladder tumors clustered around the ureteral orifice of an affected ureter provides strong support for the theory of seedling metastases. Diagnostic features are the same as those for primary carcinoma of the ureter, and the treatment of choice is total nephroureterectomy with a cuff of bladder.

Metastic Ureteral Tumors Carcinoma metastatic to the ureter is rare; only 151 cases have been reported to date. Stow reported the first documented case, and Presman and Ehrlich summarized 35 cases from the literature and established criteria for the diagnosis of metastatic disease to the ureter.[42,43] Symptoms referable to the genitourinary tract were lacking in most patients. Abeloff and Lenhard demonstrated that less than 50% of patients with metastatic tumors were symptomatic,[44] and Cohen and associates found 85% of such patients to be asymptomatic, with tumors discovered only at autopsy.[45]

Richie and associates listed the sites of primary tumors that later involved the ureter in the following order of frequency: breast (10 patients), colon/rectum (7), cervix (6), prostate (6), bladder (6), retroperitoneal lymphoma (5), and miscellaneous (6).[46] Predilection for the lower third of the ureter was evident, and the longest time interval from primary tumor to diagnosis of ureteral obstruction ranged from 8 months (carcinoma of the cervix) to 9 years (bladder carcinoma). In addition, Grabstald and Kaufman described 24 women with periureteral metastases and hydronephrosis from primary breast carcinoma.[9] In their autopsy series of 215 patients with breast carcinoma, 42 (18.3%) were found to have genitourinary metastases (kidney, 9.8%; ureter, 6.4%; bladder, 2.1%). Less than 5% of these patients had symptoms of urinary involvement.

Therapy of ureteral obstruction secondary to metastatic tumor must incorporate ethical, moral, and medical considerations. The relief of ureteral obstruction by indwelling tubes, exteriorized tubes, or ureterolysis (with consequent prevention of terminal uremia) may serve only to prolong suffering, and it should be weighed carefully against the patient's prognosis and the availability of effective alternative treatment for the primary tumor.

Tumor from Direct Extension Ureteral involvement most commonly occurs with carcinoma of the cervix, carcinoma of the colon, or retroperitoneal lymphoma. Most tumors compress rather than invade the ureter. Treatment is directed mainly toward the primary tumor and relief of bilateral ureteral obstruction as noted earlier.

REFERENCES

1. Munoz JJ, Ellison LM. Upper tract urothelial neoplasms. Incidence and survival during the last 2 decades. J Urol 2000;164:1523–5.
2. Melicow MM. Tumors of urinary drainage tract. Urothelial tumors. J Urol 1945;54:186–93.
3. Tsai YC, Nichols PW, Hiti AL, et al. Allelic losses of chromosomes 9, 11, and 17 in human bladder cancer. Cancer Res 1990;50:44.
4. Orphali SLJ, Shols GW, Hagewood J, et al. Familial transitional cell carcinoma of renal pelvis and upper ureter. Urology 1986;27:394.
5. Blaszyk H, Wang L, Dietmaier W, et al. Upper tract urothelial carcinoma. A clinicopathologic study including microsatellite instability analysis. Mod Pathol 2002;15: 790–7.
6. Geerdsen J. Tumours of the renal pelvis and ureter. Symptomatology, diagnosis, treatment and prognosis. Scand J Urol Nephrol 1979;13:287–90.
7. Cullen TH, Popham RR, Voss HJ. Urine cytology and primary carcinoma of the renal pelvis and ureter. Aust N Z J Surg 1972;41:230–6.
8. Cummings KB, Correa RJ Jr, Gibbons RP, et al. Renal pelvic tumors. J Urol 1975;113:158–62.
9. Grabstald H, Kaufman R. Hydronephrosis secondary to ureteral obstruction by metastatic breast cancer. J Urol 1969;102:569–76.
10. Williams CB, Mitchell JP. Carcinoma of the ureter—a review of 54 cases. Br J Urol 1973;45:377–87.
11. Zincke H, Aguilo JJ, Farrow GM, et al. Significance of urinary cytology in the early detection of transitional cell cancer of the upper urinary tract. J Urol 1976;116:781–3.
12. Eriksson O, Johansson S. Urothelial neoplasms of the upper urinary tract. A correlation between cytologic and histologic findings in 43 patients with urothelial neoplasms of the renal pelvis and ureter. Acta Cytol 1976;20:20–5.
13. Batata M, Grabstald H. Upper urinary tract urothelial tumors. Urol Clin North Am 1976;3:79–86.
14. Babaian RJ, Johnson DE. Carcinoma of the renal pelvis. Cancer Bull 1979;31:21.
15. Almgard LE, Freedman D, Ljungqvist A. Carcinoma of the ureter with special reference to malignancy grading and prognosis. Scand J Urol Nephrol 1973;7:165–7.
16. Batata MA, Whitmore WF Jr, Hilaris BS, et al. Primary carcinoma of the ureter. A prognostic study. Cancer 1975;35:1626–32.
17. Blute ML, Segura JW, Patterson DE, et al. Impact of endourology on diagnosis and management of upper urinary tract urothelial cancer. J Urol 1989;141:1298–1301.
18. Gill WB, Lu CT, Thomsen S. Retrograde brushing. A new technique for obtaining histologic and cytologic material from ureteral, renal pelvic, and renal caliceal lesions. J Urol 1973;109:573–8.
19. Blute RD Jr, Gittes RR, Gittes RF. Renal brush biopsy. Survey of indications, techniques and results. J Urol 1981;126:146–9.
20. Grabstald H, Whitmore WF Jr, Melamed MR. Renal pelvic tumors. JAMA 1971;281:845–54.
21. Strong DW, Pearse HD. Recurrent urothelial tumors following surgery for transitional cell carcinoma of the upper urinary tract. Cancer 1976;38:2173–83.
22. Ziegelbaum M, Novick AC, Streem SB, et al. Conservative surgery for transitional cell carcinoma of the renal pelvis. J Urol 1987;138:1146–9.
23. Gittes RF. Management of transitional cell carcinoma of the upper tract. Case for conservative local excision. Urol Clin North Am 1980;7:559–8.
24. McCarron JP, Mills C, Vaughn ED Jr. Tumors of the renal pelvis and ureter: current concepts and management. Semin Urol 1983;1:75–81.
25. Nocks BN, Heney NM, Daly JJ, et al. Transitional cell carcinoma of renal pelvis. Urology 1982;19:472–7.
26. Shalhav AL, Dunn, MD, Portis AJ, et al. Laparoscopic nephroureterectomy for upper tract transitional cell

cancer. The Washington University experience. J Urol 2000;163:1100–4.
27. Chen GL, Bagley, DH. Ureteroscopic management of upper tract transitional cell carcinoma in patients with normal contralateral kidneys. J Urol 2000;164:1173–6.
28. Smith AD, Orihuela E, Crowley AR. Percutaneous management of renal pelvic tumors. The treatment options in selected cases. J Urol 1987;137:852–6.
29. Jabbour ME, Desgrandchamps F, Cazin ST, et al. Percutaneous management of grade II upper urinary tract transitional cell carcinoma. The long-term outcome. J Urol 2000;163;1105–7.
30. Bloom NA, Vidone RA, Lytton B. Primary carcinoma of ureter. A report of 102 new cases. J Urol 1970; 103:590–8.
31. Morioka M, Jo Y, Furukawa Y, et al. Prognostic factors for survival and bladder recurrence in transitional cell carcinoma of the upper urinary tract. Int J Urol 2000;8:366–73.
32. Brady LW, Gislason GJ, Faust DS, et al. Radiation therapy. A valuable adjunct in the management of carcinoma of the ureter. JAMA 1968;206:2871–4.
33. Holtz F. Papillomas and primary carcinoma of the ureter. Report of 20 cases. J Urol 1962;88:380–5.
34. Brookland RK, Richter MP. The postoperative irradiation of transitional cell carcinoma of the renal pelvis and ureter. J Urol 1985;133:952–5
35. Leiber MM, Lupu AN. High-grade invasive ureteral transitional cell carcinoma with a congenital solitary kidney. Long-term survival after ureterectomy and radiation therapy. J Urol 1978;120:368–9.
36. Scott WW. Review of primary carcinoma of ureter, presenting 2 cases. J Urol 1943;50:45–64.
37. Bergman H, Hotchkiss RS. Ureteral tumors. In: Bergman H, editor. The ureter. 2nd ed. New York: Springer Verlag; 1981. p. 271–82.
38. Abeshouse BS. Primary benign and malignant tumors of the ureter. A review of the literature and report of one benign and twelve malignant tumors. Am J Surg 1956;91:237–71.
39. Loehrer PJ, Elson P, Kuebler JP, et al. Advanced bladder cancer. A prospective intergroup trial comparing single agent cisplatin (CDDP) versus M-VAC combination therapy (INT 0078). Proc Am Soc Clin Oncol 1990;9:132.
40. von der Maase H, Hansen SW, Roberts JT, et al. Gemcitabine and cisplatin versus methotrexate, vinblastine, doxorubicin, and cisplatin in advanced or metastatic bladder cancer: results of a large, randomized, multinational, multicenter, phase III study. J Clin Oncol 2000 Sep;18(17):3068-77.
41. Weldon TE, Soloway MS, Persky L. Urothelial susceptibility to neoplastic cellular implantation. Surg Forum 1974;25:547–9.
42. Stow B. Fibrolymphosarcomata of both ureters, metastatic to a primary lymphosarcoma of the anterior mediastinum of the thymus origin. Ann Surg 1909;50:901.
43. Presman D, Ehrlich L. Metastatic tumors of the ureter. J Urol 1948;59:312–25.
44. Abeloff MD, Lenhard RE Jr. Clinical management of ureteral obstruction secondary to malignant lymphoma. Johns Hopkins Med J 1974;134:34–42.
45. Cohen WM, Freed SZ, Hasson J. Metastatic cancer to the ureter. A review of the literature and case presentations. J Urol 1974;112:188–9.
46. Richie JP, Withers G, Ehrlich RM. Ureteral obstruction secondary to metastatic tumors. Surg Gynecol Obstet 1979;148:355–7.

Bladder Cancer

Timothy D. Gilligan, MD
Graeme S. Steele, MD
Anthony L. Zietman, MD
Philip W. Kantoff, MD

Bladder cancer, the second most common genitourinary malignancy in the United States, is largely a preventable disease because most cases result from exposure to environmental carcinogens, the most important of which is cigarette smoke. A large majority of tumors arising in the bladder are transitional cell carcinomas. Bladder cancers are characterized by multifocality and a high recurrence rate. Most tumors diagnosed in the United States are superficial tumors confined to the epithelial or transitional cell layer of the bladder and are easily treated by transurethral resection. These tumors generally are low grade and have low potential for metastatic spread. Tumors that are considered to be high grade and/or invade the deeper layers of the bladder wall have a much greater potential for metastatic spread. Tumors invading into the detrusor muscle are treated with either radical cystectomy or concomitant chemotherapy and radiation. Neoadjuvant chemotherapy prior to cystectomy improves survival rates. The benefit of adjuvant chemotherapy remains unproven. The treatment of metastatic disease is marginal. Although two different cisplatin-based chemotherapy regimens have been shown to prolong survival, only about 5% of patients are long-term survivors and possibly cured.

EPIDEMIOLOGY

In 2005, there will be an estimated 63,210 new cases of bladder cancer diagnosed in the United States and approximately 13,180 deaths.[1] Incidence rises with age, with a median age at diagnosis of 72. Bladder cancer incidence is four times higher among men than women, while mortality is three times higher.[2] Bladder cancers in women tend to be diagnosed at a more advanced stage, and stage-adjusted survival is shorter for women than men.[3,4] In the United States, the lifetime risk of developing bladder cancer is highest among white men, at 3.8%. The lifetime risks among black men, white women, and black women are 1.3, 1.2, and 0.7%, respectively.[5] Whites are almost twice as likely as blacks to be diagnosed with bladder cancer, but only 13% more likely to die from it. Asians, Hispanics, and Native Americans have the lowest incidence and mortality. Bladder cancer incidence increased by over 50% between 1950 and 1987 and has since declined slightly in men, but not in women.[5–7] Bladder cancer mortality declined by 35% over the past 50 years, but the downward trend ended in 1987, except for a very slight subsequent decline among men.

Cigarette smoking is the major risk factor for bladder cancer and accounts for roughly half of all cases in men and one-third of all cases among women.[8–10] Current smokers have a threefold increased risk over nonsmokers, and there appears to be a dose-response relationship between the quantity of cigarettes smoked and risk.[11] Smoking cessation reduces the risk within the first few years, but ex-smokers appear to remain at a persistently elevated risk relative to people who have never smoked.[8,10] Exposure to aromatic amines (including 2-naphthalamine, benzidine, aniline, and toluidine) increases the risk of bladder cancer.[12,13] Studies have supported a strong link between several occupations that involve aromatic amines and the development of bladder cancer, including dyestuff workers, leather workers, rubber workers, painters, dry cleaners, truck drivers, and aluminum workers.[14,15]

Long-term, chronic administration of cyclophosphamide increases the risk of bladder cancer, but whether the cyclophosphamide must first induce a hemorrhagic cystitis for bladder cancer to occur is uncertain. Infection with *Schistosoma haematobium* increases the risk of bladder cancer, probably by inducing chronic inflammation. It is the most common cancer in Egypt and many other African nations.[16,17] Most cancers believed to be attributable to *S. haematobium* infection are squamous cell carcinomas. Smoking appears to increase the risk associated with schistosomiasis.[18]

Preventive measures include abstaining from smoking and avoiding exposure to toxic chemicals and schistosomes. High fluid intake has been associated with a reduced risk of bladder cancer, but this finding has not been adequately confirmed.[19] Diets high in cruciferous vegetables and low in fried meats and fats have also been associated with a lower risk of bladder cancer.[20,21] Coffee does not appear to affect bladder cancer risk.[19,22]

BIOLOGY

The role of environmental factors in urothelial carcinogenesis is not surprising given that the urine exposes the bladder epithelium to chemicals we ingest or inhale, or their metabolites, often in high concentrations and sometimes for extended periods of time.[23] The genetic events that characterize transformation are slowly being defined, and a range of genetic changes have been noted in tumors, and an excellent recent review has been published.[24,25] None of these genetic changes is of proven clinical utility at this time, but overexpression of *TP53* has been used in some studies as a prognostic indicator and there is a growing body of evidence implicating vascular endothelial growth factor and other angiogenesis-related factors in bladder cancer progression and prognosis.[26–28] Cytogenetic analysis of bladder tumors has demonstrated monosomy 9, trisomy 7, and abnormalities of chromosome 17p (the *TP53* locus) as the most common cytogenetic changes. Abnormalities in chromosome 9 have been seen so commonly in all stages and grades of bladder cancer that some investigators believe a critical tumor-suppressor gene resides in this location and that its alteration is an early event in tumor progression. Two regions seem to be involved, one on 9p21 at the cyclin-dependent-kinase inhibitor 2 (*CDKN2*A) tumor suppressor gene locus and the other on 9q. Although several candidate genes have been studied, most notably *TP53*, no single marker has yet been shown to be a powerful enough prognostic indicator to guide treatment decisions.[29] Mutations in *TP53* are common in bladder cancers, occurring in about half of all cases. Some studies also have suggested a critical role for *TP53* in tumor progression and prognosis, but inconsistencies in how *TP53* testing is performed and interpreted has made reconciling the varying results of different reports difficult.[30,31] Altered *TP53* expression has been associated with higher stage and grade disease and, in organ-confined disease, poorer prognosis, but reports have conflicted with regard to whether *TP53* status can be used clinically to predict response to therapy, need for additional therapy, recurrence, or survival following radiation or cystectomy. Mutations affecting the retinoblastoma gene, *BCL-2*, *p16*, *p21*, *MMP-2*, and epithelial growth factor (EGF), and EGF receptors have also been implicated as prognostic markers in bladder cancer. Larger, more definitive studies are awaited.

Two unique aspects of bladder cancer are multifocality and polychronotropism. Although the mechanism by which these phenomena occur has been debated, the most commonly held theories include a genetic "field defect" or a reimplantation of tumor cells. Evidence strongly suggests that tumor reimplantation and/or submucosal migration are operative.[32–34]

PATHOLOGY

Over 90% of cancers arising in the bladder are transitional cell carcinomas (TCCs). Some TCCs show a mixed pattern with squamous features or a glandular component. Less common pathologies are adenocarcinoma, squamous cell carcinoma, and small-cell carcinoma, which comprise approximately 4%, 2%, and less than 1% of bladder tumors, respectively. Adenocarcinomas include carcinomas of the urachal remnant. Sarcomas, sarcomatoid carcinomas, and carcinomasarcomas of the bladder are rare. Two different configurations of TCCs are seen: papillary and solid. Most tumors are papillary and low grade and do not invade the muscularis propria of the bladder wall. Solid tumors typically are high grade and invasive. A significant correlation exists between grade and prognosis.[35] However, although grade 3 disease is associated with a shorter survival than grade 1, the clinical significance of grade 2 disease is less clear.[35] Tumor staging is based on the degree to which the tumor has invaded into or through the bladder wall. Prognosis correlates with stage, but, when controlling for grade, Ta and T1 lesions have similar prognoses.[36] Carcinoma in situ (CIS) of the bladder is used to describe a flat, nonpapillary lesion with cytologic features that are consistent with a high-grade malignancy. By definition, this lesion is confined to the epithelial layer, but it has a high propensity to invade deeper layers, and tumors with associated CIS have a poorer prognosis. The affected mucosa is friable, granular, and red and velvety in appearance.

SIGNS AND SYMPTOMS

Hematuria and irritative symptoms are the most frequent presenting manifestations of bladder cancer. Gross hematuria, which is the presenting sign in 80% of patients with bladder cancer, usually is painless, present through urination, and episodic. Severe bleeding causing clot retention occurs in some patients. Twenty percent of patients experience bladder irritative symptoms, commonly, urinary urgency, frequency, and dysuria, which may suggest CIS or muscle-invasive disease.[37] Most patients are asymptomatic and are diagnosed during evaluation for microscopic hematuria or, less frequently, pyuria. Individuals found to have microscopic or gross hematuria who are over the age of 40 or who have other risk factors for bladder cancer should undergo cystoscopy and urine cytology. A CT urogram or a retrograde or intravenous pyelogram should also be performed to evaluate the upper urinary tract.

Screening for bladder cancer is of uncertain value as it has never been shown to reduce mortality. Potential screening tests include urine dipstick for microscopic hematuria, urine cytology, and cystoscopy. Urine dipstick has a low positive predictive value for bladder cancer, and widespread use in the general population would lead to many healthy people having unnecessary invasive testing.[38,39] Urine cytology has a sensitivity and specificity of about 45% and 95%, respectively,[40] and its main use has been as a surveillance test for patients who have had prior urothelial cancers. Urine cytology has not been evaluated prospectively as a generalized screening test. The cost of the test is generally considered too high for the small number of individuals who might stand to benefit. Cystoscopy is too expensive and uncomfortable to be used as a screening test for the general population. A new generation of potential bladder cancer screening tests is undergoing evaluation, including a telomerase assay,[41,42] human complement factor H–related protein (BTA), and nuclear matrix proteins (specifically NMP22).[43]

Figure 96-1 illustrates the decision-making process for bladder cancer.

DIAGNOSTIC EVALUATION

Cystoscopy Cystoscopy provides direct visualization of the bladder and facilitates biopsy of the bladder. This procedure can be performed on an outpatient basis with minimal patient discomfort using the 17-Fr flexible cystoscope and 2% Xylocaine urethral jelly. During cystoscopy, the endoscopist notes the number, size, shape, and location of tumors as well as the appearance of the surrounding mucosa, urethra, and ureteral orifice. Visualized characteristics with predictive value include size, shape (papillary, sessile, or flat), and nature of the surrounding mucosa. The detection of flat tumors and CIS, which are often difficult to appreciate on plain cystoscopy, can be increased by roughly 20% with fluorescence cystoscopy following intravesical administration of 5-aminolevulinic acid (ALA).[44] A randomized controlled trial enrolling 102 patients who underwent a transurethral resection of bladder tumors (TURBT) with either white-light cystoscopy or AFA fluorescence-assisted cystoscopy reported that 16% of patients undergoing ALA fluorescence-assisted cystoscopy had recurrent tumor 6 weeks after TURBT compared with 39% of those who did not receive ALA ($p = .005$).[45] A significant long-term benefit has not been established.

Urinary Cytology Urinary cytology is less useful than cystoscopy for the diagnosis of most common, low-grade papillary tumors because the individual neoplastic cells comprising grade I TCC appear to be identical cytologically to normal urothelial cells. On the other hand, cytology is extremely valuable for the diagnosis of high-grade TCC—especially CIS—that may be difficult for the endoscopist to visualize. Urine cytology, therefore, should be used to complement the findings of cystoscopy.[46] The presence of high-grade TCC in the cytology specimen from a patient with low-grade papillary TCC suggests either unrecognized CIS or high-grade disease in the upper urinary tracts (ureter or renal pelvis) or urethra.

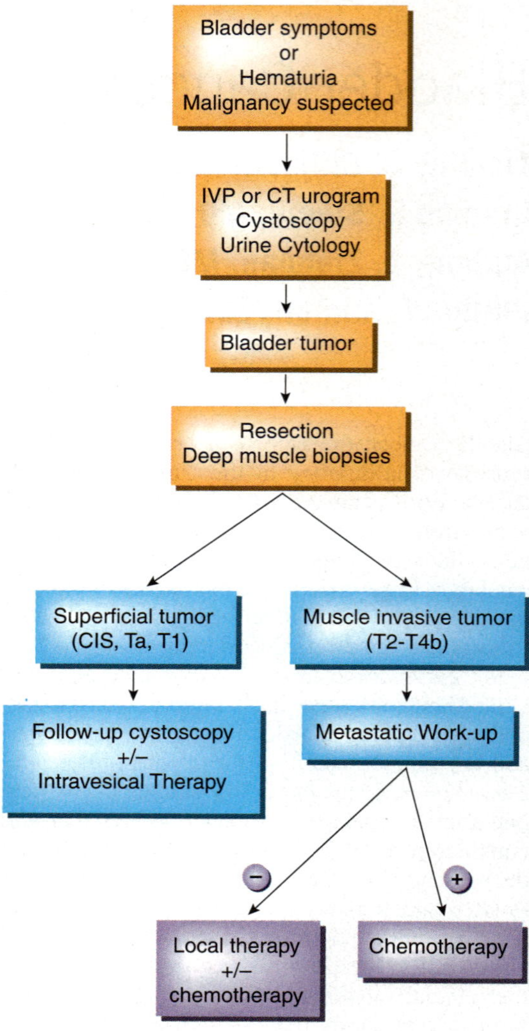

Figure 96-1 Decision tree for suspected bladder cancer. CIS = carcinoma in situ; IVP = intravenous pyelography.

Imaging Urothelial carcinomas are often multifocal and can occur anywhere in the urinary tract from the renal pelvices to the urethra. Patients with bladder cancer should thus undergo radiologic imaging to evaluate the upper urinary tracts using a CT urogram, retrograde pyelogram, or intravenous pyelogram (IVP). Selective cytology from the ureters can also help evaluate for upper tract disease. In patients with bladder cancer, the incidence of concomitant or subsequent upper tract tumors is 2 to 5% overall and 10% for patients with high-grade tumors, CIS, or recurrent tumors following intravesical therapy.[47] The finding of ureteral obstruction or a nonfunctioning kidney in a patient with bladder cancer predicts muscle invasion in 90% of cases.[48] Common sites of metastases include the pelvic and retroperitoneal lymph nodes and the lungs, liver, and bones. Patients with muscle-invasive bladder cancers should undergo a chest radiograph and a CT scan of the abdomen and pelvis.[49] Patients with metastatic disease or an elevated serum alkaline phosphatase should also have a bone scan. CT and MRI scans are not reliable in evaluating

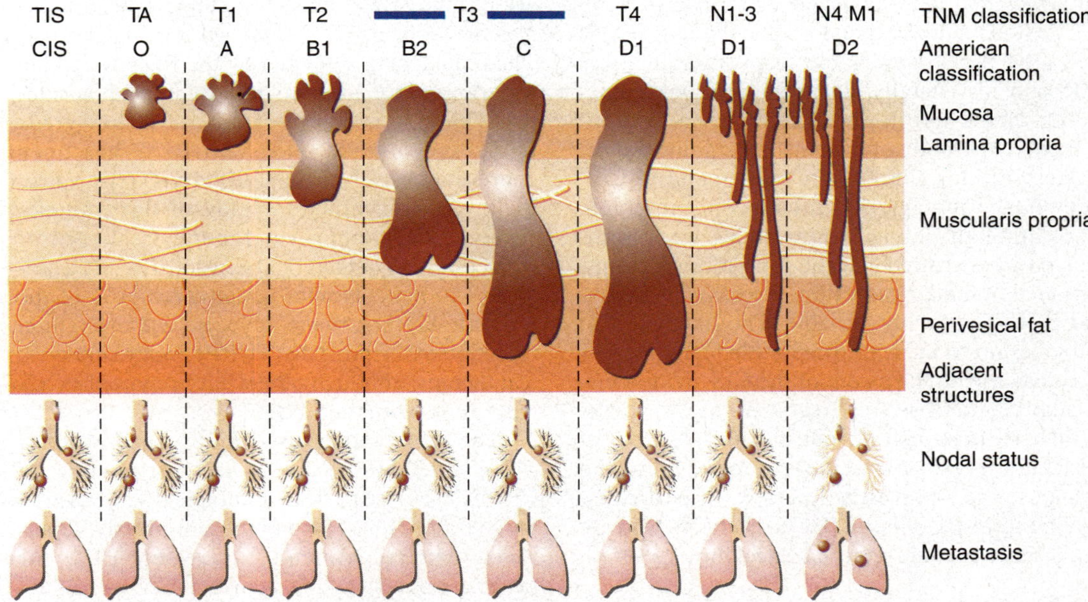

Figure 96-2 TNM staging classification for bladder neoplasms. American classification (Jewett-Marshall) is shown for comparison. Tumors T1 (A) are considered superficial, with tumors T2 (B) or greater being invasive.

the extent of local or regional disease.[50] Both generally tend to overestimate degree of extension through the bladder wall, but underestimate the presence of pelvic lymph node metastasis. Whether MRI offers advantages over CT scans remains unresolved.[51]

Bladder Biopsy and Transurethral Resection of Bladder Tumors TURBT provides tissue for histopathologic diagnosis and staging and may provide definitive therapy for many superficial, as well as some invasive, cancers. The resection must include sufficient muscle to provide adequate pathologic staging. Although an overly aggressive resection may lead to bladder perforation, an inadequate resection may lead to understaging and tumor persistence and regrowth. Although biopsy of normal-appearing bladder mucosa at a distance from overt tumors is controversial,[52–55] such biopsies are frequently performed and detect CIS in 3.5 to 14.5% of patients. When diffuse CIS is present, the prostatic urethra should undergo biopsy because it may contain neoplastic cells in as many as 35% of patients.[56] Additionally, the prostate may be a site of persistent disease after intravesical treatment. Prostatic urethral or ductal involvement should be distinguished from prostatic stromal involvement, as the latter is associated with shorter survival.[57,58] Stromal invasion of prostate may occur by direct extension of tumor (T4a) through the bladder wall or from a prostatic urethral tumor.

Bimanual Examination The assessment of disease extent and resectability is based largely on bimanual palpation of the bladder during anesthesia. By convention, the presence of palpable disease after complete transurethral resection indicates muscle invasion, either within or through the bladder wall.[59] Unfortunately, most invasive cancers are located near the trigone or posterior bladder wall, which cannot reliably be palpated well even under anesthesia, so this crude and inexact technique leads to understaging in 50% of patients. Bimanual examination also allows the urologist to assess whether the bladder is fixed in the pelvis, a finding that indicates an unresectable (T4) tumor.

STAGING

The AJCC clinical staging system divides bladder cancer into the following four categories: superficial (Ta, Tis, and T1), muscle-invasive (T2), locally advanced disease (T3a, T3b, T4a), and unresectable and/or metastatic disease(T4b or N1-3 or M1) (Figure 96-2 and Table 96-1). It is worth remembering that clinical staging underestimates disease extent (judged by pathologic staging) in up to 50% of cases.[60,61]

SUPERFICIAL BLADDER CARCINOMA

Natural History Superficial bladder carcinoma includes a diverse group of lesions, ranging from Ta grade I to T1 grade III tumors and high-

Table 96-1 AJCC Clinical Staging

TNM			
Primary Tumor (T)			
TX	Primary tumor cannot be assessed		
T0	No evidence of primary tumor		
Ta	Noninvasive papillary carcinoma		
Tis	Carcinoma in situ: "flat tumor"		
T1	Tumor invades subepithelial connective tissue		
T2	Tumor invades muscle		
T2a	Tumor invades superficial muscle (inner half)		
T2b	Tumor invades deep muscle (outer half)		
T3	Tumor invades perivesical tissue		
T3a	Microscopically		
T3b	Macroscopically (extravesical mass)		
T4	Tumor invades any of the following: prostate, uterus, vagina, pelvic wall, abdominal wall		
T4a	Tumor invades prostate, uterus, vagina		
T4b	Tumor invades pelvic wall, abdominal wall		
N1	Metastasis in a single lymph node, 2 cm or less in greatest dimension		
N2	Metastasis in a single lymph node, more than 2 cm but not more than 5 cm in greatest dimension, or multiple lymph nodes, none more than 5 cm in greatest dimension		
N3	Metastasis in a lymph node more than 5 cm in greatest dimension		
Distant Metastasis (M)			
MX	Distant metastasis cannot be assessed		
M0	No distant metastasis		
M1	Distant metastasis		
Stage Grouping			
Stage 0a	Ta	N0	M0
Stage Ois	Tis	N0	M0
Stage I	T1	N0	M0
Stage II	T2a	N0	M0
	T2b	N0	M0
Stage III	T3a	N0	M0
	T3b	N0	M0
Stage IV	T4a	N0	M0
	T4b	N0	M0
	Any T	N1	M0
	Any T	N2	M0
	Any T	N3	M0
	Any T	Any N	M1

grade flat CIS.[62,63] Although it is crucial to distinguish the small group of lesions that carry a serious risk of progression to life-threatening muscle-invasive and metastatic disease, the vast majority of superficial tumors have low rates of progression. Rather, they have a significant tendency to recur at multiple sites throughout the urothelium. The natural history of superficial bladder carcinoma has been evaluated in many large studies. The rate of progression to muscle invasion or metastasis is 2 to 4% for grade I, 11 to 20% for grade II, and roughly 20 to 50% for grade III tumors. Although grade tends to correlate with stage, high-grade Ta lesions are not substantially less dangerous than high-grade T1 lesions. Lebret and colleagues reported a 25% rate of progression to muscle-invasive disease and 12% bladder cancer mortality rate among 32 patients with TaG3 disease with 5 years follow-up.[64] Herr reported that among 125 patients with TaG3 lesions treated with TURBT and intravesical BCG, 26% had died of bladder cancer within 15 years of their initial presentation.[65] Anderstrom and colleagues reported that the 5-year survival in 99 patients with T1 tumors was 83% if the grade was II and 63% if III; 7 of 10 patients in whom small-vessel invasion (either lymphatic or vascular) was present in the lamina propria died.[66] A review of large published studies of nonmuscle-invasive bladder cancers identified grade 3 disease and the presence of CIS as the only variables consistently found to be associated with shorter survival, while risk of progression has been associated with grade 3 disease, CIS, T1 disease, multiple tumors, and tumors larger than 3 cm.[35] Although some studies have suggested that lymphovascular invasion and depth of invasion influence prognosis in T1 lesions, it has not been established that these findings contribute additional prognostic information when controlling for stage, grade, and CIS.[66–69]

Prognostic models for superficial TCC exist but remain crude.[70] Millán-Rodríguez and colleagues reported a prognostic scheme dividing patients into low risk (TaG1 or single T1G1 tumor), intermediate risk (multiple T1G1, TaG2, or single T1G2), and high risk (any G3, any CIS, or multiple T1G2).[36] Progression and mortality rates were 0% and 0% in the low-risk group, 1.8% and 0.7% in the intermediate-risk group, and 15% and 10% in the high-risk group, although this may underestimate the risk of progression in high-risk groups. Progression rates have been reported to be as high as 50 to 56% with recurrent T1G3 tumors,[65,71] 25 to 39% with TaG3 tumors,[64,65] and 54% in untreated CIS.[72] In the National Bladder Cancer Group study, the recurrence rate at 3 years was 50% for grade I, 59% for grade II, 80% for grade III, 48% for Ta, and 70% for T1 tumors.[73] Recurrence rates are higher in patients with CIS, multiple tumors, and tumors larger than 3 cm in maximum diameter.[35]

Carcinoma In Situ Defined as noninvasive, high-grade, flat cancer confined to the epithelium, CIS may be localized or diffuse, and it may occur in association with low-stage or muscle-invasive TCC. It is recognized endoscopically as a friable red area indistinguishable from inflammation. CIS spreads laterally, displacing normal epithelium. Urine cytology is positive in 90% of patients. In a study of patients undergoing radical cystectomy for CIS,[40] 34% were found to have previously undiagnosed microscopic invasion, and although pelvic lymph nodes were uninvolved in all patients at the time of cystectomy, 6% died of metastasis within 5 years. The behavior of CIS is highly variable. The likelihood of progression to muscle-invasive bladder cancer is associated with the extent of the CIS. With transurethral surgery as sole treatment, most patients with CIS demonstrate muscle invasion by 10 years. Most patients achieve durable complete responses to intravesical therapy, in particular, bacille Calmette-Guérin (BCG). Patients who are resistant to therapy require cystectomy.

Intravesical Therapy The appeal of intravesical therapy stems from its high therapeutic ratio. Administering agents directly into the bladder results in a high mucosal exposure with little systemic absorption. Intravesical therapy has been used for two general purposes: to eradicate residual tumor in the bladder following resection (particularly diffuse CIS), and to prevent or delay recurrence or progression. Indications for intravesical therapy remain controversial. Prophylaxis has been widely used in patients who demonstrate multiple primary tumors, superficial recurrences, high-grade tumors, invasive tumors (T1), positive urinary cytology postresection, and diffuse CIS.[74] Many intravesical agents commonly used today have never been FDA approved for this purpose. The only agents approved by the FDA for use in superficial TCC are thiotepa, BCG, and valrubicin. Thiotepa is approved for use in low-grade low-stage disease only, and BCG has been approved for use only in patients with CIS. Valrubicin, a semisynthetic analog of doxorubicin, received FDA approval for the treatment of refractory CIS but has not been consistently available.[75] In patients with noninvasive TCC of the prostatic urethra, some advocate a transurethral resection of the prostate (TURP) prior to intravesical therapy, although others have reported excellent results without a TURP.[76,77]

The most widely used intravesical agent is BCG, which has been most useful in eradicating CIS.[78,79] The American Urological Association (AUA) guidelines for nonmuscle-invasive bladder cancer recommend intravesical BCG for treatment of CIS and as adjuvant therapy following TUR of high-grade or T1 tumors.[80] The exact mechanism of action of BCG remains undefined, but this agent provokes an inflammatory reaction and is believed to stimulate a humoral and cellular antitumor immune response.[81] Many controlled trials have studied intravesical BCG for superficial bladder tumors, but they have generally been too small to clearly demonstrate whether or not BCG affects survival or reduces the long-term risk of progression to muscle-invasive disease. Although it has long been clear that BCG reduces the risk of recurrent tumors by about 50%,[79,82] that is not the most important endpoint[65,80] (Table 96-2). A meta-analysis of 24

Table 96-2 Effect of Intravesical Therapy on Recurrence in Controlled Studies

Series	Patients (*n*)	Recurrence (%)		Benefit (%)	*p*
		Control	Treatment		
BCG					
Lamm[280]	57	52	20	32	< .001
Pinsky et al[281]	86	91	63	28	< .001
Pagano et al[282]	133	83	26	57	<.001
Krege et al[283]	224	46	25	21	NS
Melekos et al[284]	94	59	32	27	< .05
Yamamoto et al[285]	44	69	18	51	< .01
Totals	638	64	30	34% Adv	
Mitomycin C					
Huland and Otto[286]	58	40	7	33	.01
Niijima et al[287]	278	62	57	9	NS
Kim and Lee[288]	43	81	81	0	NS
Tolley et al[289]	397	65	42	23	.001
Krege et al[283]	235	46	27	19	.001
Totals	1,011	59	42	17% Adv	
Thiotepa					
Burnand et al[290]	51	97	58	39	.001
Byar and Blackard[291]	88	60	47	13	NS
Nocks et al[292]	42	64	65	–1	NS
Asahi et al[293]	134	41	40	1	NS
Schulman et al[294]	209	69	59	10	NS
Koontz et al[295]	93	66	40	26	.02
Zincke et al[296]	58	71	30	41	.002
Prout et al[297]	90	76	64	12	.05
MRC[298]	243	32	37	–5	NS
Totals	1,008	57	47	10% Adv	

Adv = advantage; NS = not significant.

Table 96-3 Long-Term Follow-Up Following Intravesical BCG

Series	No. Patients	Follow-Up	Recurrence	Progression	Dead	# Dead from TCC
Davis et al[85]	98	10 years (min)	37 (38%)	27 (28%)	71 (72%)	13 (13%)
Herr et al[299]	61	10 years (min)	42 (69%)	25 (41%)	14 (23%)	12 (20%)
Hurle et al[300]	51	5 years (min)	24 (47%)	9 (17%)	15 (29%)	7 (14%)
Losa et al[301]	70	6.2 years (med)	12 (17%)	8 (11%)	11 (16%)	1 (1.4%)
Brake et al[302]	126	4.5 years (med)	37 (29%)	17 (13%)	38 (30%)	9 (7%)
Cheng et al[303]	102	5 years (med)	39%	22%	NA	20%

BCG = bacille Calmette-Guérin; med = median; min = minimum.

controlled BCG trials evaluated data on 2,658 patients on BCG and 2,205 controls and reported that 9.8% of BCG patients progressed compared with 13.8% of controls ($p = .001$).[83] However, the benefit was small in absolute terms (4% absolute risk reduction) and was limited to patients who received maintenance BCG following a standard induction treatment course. On the other hand, in the trials studied in the meta-analysis, fewer than 8% of patients had high-grade tumors (G3), and it is this population that is at high risk of progression. Survival could not be assessed in a meaningful way in this study because most studies did not present survival data and the death rate from bladder cancer is low in patients with low- and intermediate-grade bladder urothelial carcinomas. A follow-up meta-analysis reported specifically that BCG results in a lower rate of progression than intravesical chemotherapy.[84]

There remain important unanswered questions about the role of BCG: Superficial bladder cancers are generally considered curable at the time of diagnosis, but patients whose bladders are not removed retain a long-term risk of recurrence, progression, and death, especially patients with CIS or high-grade tumors[85,86] (Table 96-3). The most definitive therapy is radical cystectomy, but such treatment is unnecessary in those patients who are not destined to progress, and it not only carries risk, but also significantly compromises sexual function and other quality of life parameters for both men and women. The goal of intravesical therapy is to allow patients to keep their bladder without exposing them to an increased risk of dying of progressive disease.

Perhaps the most important use of BCG has been in the treatment of CIS, which carries a roughly 50% risk of progression to invasive disease if untreated.[72] The average complete response rate following intravesical BCG was 72% in over 1,300 patients with CIS treated in 34 studies.[87,88] The durability of response remains poorly defined, however. In a Southwest Oncology Group study comparing BCG with doxorubicin for CIS, 45% of the BCG-treated patients were disease free at 5 years, compared with 18% of the doxorubicin-treated patients. However, 35% of patients who were in remission at 2 years suffered a recurrence over the subsequent decade.[89]

The optimal dose and schedule for BCG have yet to be determined. Maintenance schedules beyond the initial 6 weekly instillations have been shown to reduce the rate of recurrence and progression and increases the complete response rate.[83,90–92] Delivering maintenance therapy was initially reported to be difficult, but more recent studies have reported lower toxicity rates.[93–95]

Cystitis or irritative urinary symptoms occur in 67 to 90% of patients receiving intravesical BCG.[79,80,96] Malaise and low-grade fevers occur in about one in four patients.[96] Approximately 5% of patients treated with BCG experience serious toxicity, including septic reactions (0.4%), pneumonitis or hepatitis (0.7%), fever (2.9%), prostatitis (0.9%), and ureteral obstruction (0.3%).[96] Septic deaths from disseminated BCG infections following intravesical treatment have been described but are extremely rare. Isoniazid, rifampin, and prednisone are currently recommended for the treatment of suspected systemic infection.[97] In order to prevent dissemination of BCG, intravesical administration should not occur until the patient's urothelium has had time to heal from any recent biopsies, TURs, traumatic catheterizations or cystitis. In addition, BCG should not be administered to patients who (1) are pregnant, (2) are HIV positive or immunodeficient, (3) have leukemia or Hodgkin's disease, (4) are transplant recipients, or (5) are suffering from active tuberculosis.[96]

Controlled studies have demonstrated that interferon α-2b, thiotepa, doxorubicin, mitomycin C, epirubicin, valrubicin, and ethoglucid reduce recurrence rates when administered in an intravesical fashion[82,98] (see Table 96-2). Intravesical chemotherapy appears to have no impact on progression or survival.[99] Nor has conclusive documentation of a reduction in long-term recurrence rates been reported.[82] Valrubicin has been approved for BCG-refractory CIS based on a complete response rate of 21% following a 6 week regimen using a weekly intravesical dose of 800 mg.[100] In comparative trials, BCG has been shown to be more effective at reducing recurrences than thiotepa, doxorubicin, epirubicin, and mitomycin.[84,101–104]

Intravesical interferon α-2b as prophylaxis for resected superficial TCC produces recurrence rates of 20 to 60% and has been shown to be less effective than either BCG or mitomycin C in randomized trials.[105–108] One randomized trial found no benefit to interferon dosed at 60 million units when compared with distilled water.[109] A more recent study reported that patients receiving interferon dosed at 100 million units had a 28% relapse rate compared with 64% in patients receiving no intravesical therapy at 21 months follow-up.[110] A third randomized trial in previously untreated patients comparing interferon (80 million units) with no intravesical therapy reported that, with 3 years follow-up, interferon was associated with lower rates of recurrence (22% vs 65%) and progression (4% vs 20%).[111] The durability of responses, however, has not been well established. In patients who had previously failed BCG therapy, the complete response rate is about 20%, and it is in this population that interferon is most frequently used, usually in combination with low-dose BCG. A 231-patient phase II study of combined intravesical interferon plus low-dose BCG in BCG-refractory patients reported a 42% 2-year disease-free rate, a 4.3% progression rate, and metastases in 2.6% of patients. Among 259 BCG-naïve patients enrolled in the same trial, 57% were disease free at 2 years, 5% progressed to muscle-invasive disease and 2.3% developed metastases.[112] Randomized trials of this combined therapy are lacking. There is no published evidence that interferon increases survival.

Photodynamic therapy has some efficacy in diagnosing and treating patients with superficial papillary TCC and CIS, but it is not widely available and its role remains poorly defined, largely because of the absence of randomized trials evaluating whether this approach provides an advantage in terms of survival or freedom from progression.[113,114] Photodynamic therapy has been shown to reduce recurrence rates in patients who have failed conventional intravesical treatment.[115] A review of published studies reported a complete response rate of 66% in carcinoma in situ and 54% in superficial papillary TCC, but complete tumor ablation is generally limited to tumors less than 2 cm in diameter.[114]

In an unfortunate subset of patients, superficial bladder cancer is an aggressive, life-threatening condition. Patients who are most at risk are those with grade 3 tumors, multiple tumors, a tumor greater than 3 cm in diameter, or CIS.[35] Lymphovascular invasion in T1 lesions may also be a risk factor. Patients who recur following two full courses of intravesical BCG should be considered for prompt radical cystectomy.[116] Patients with multifocal tumors and/or CIS should be considered for immediate cystectomy rather than intravesical therapy. However, the absence of prospective randomized trials makes it impossible to issue definitive management guidelines for this challenging patient population.[117–119] It appears in retrospective studies that patients with recurrent high-grade nonmuscle-invasive tumors have superior survival following cystectomy compared with patients with recurrent tumors who only undergo cystectomy once muscle invasion occurs. Herr and Sogani also reported in a retrospective analysis that early cystectomy was associated with longer survival even after controlling for muscle invasion.[116] Nonetheless, a substantial number of patients with recurrent tumors do not ever progress, and cystectomy is unnecessary in such patients. Current prognostic models have only limited power to predict which patients are likely to progress despite TURBT and intravesical therapy and who, therefore, might benefit from immediate cystectomy. Clinicians must balance the competing harms of unnecessary cystectomy and mortality from advanced disease. However, the majority of patients with high-grade T1 disease can initially be managed with transurethral bladder tumor resection and intravesical BCG. In all patients with high-grade bladder tumors, careful follow-up and a high index of suspicion for invasive disease is mandatory.

MUSCLE-INVASIVE BLADDER CANCER

Radical Cystectomy Radical cystectomy is regarded as the standard approach to the treatment of invasive bladder cancer in the United States. This involves the removal of regional pelvic lymph nodes followed by an en bloc resection of the bladder, prostate, and seminal vesicles in men or, in women, an anterior exenteration in which the bladder is removed along with the ovaries, uterus, urethra, and a segment of the anterior wall of the vagina. It is important to note the benefit of an extensive and thorough lymphadenectomy. Several studies have documented a significant, positive correlation between the extent of lymph-node dissection and disease-free survival, and although no randomized trials have addressed this issue, a more extensive lymphadenectomy appears to result in superior outcomes.[120] The major determinant of outcome is the pathological stage, particularly the presence or absence of lymph node metastases at the time of surgery (Table 96-4).[121] Pagano and colleagues reported 5-year actuarial survival rates of 63% and 50% for stages P2 and P3a cancers, respectively.[122] If patients with lymph node metastases are excluded, the figures rise to 68% and 67%. Skinner and colleagues reported on all radical cystectomies performed at the University of Southern California between 1971 and 1997. Five-year recurrence-free survival rates were 62% in 135 with P3bN0 disease, 50% in 79 patients with P4aN0 disease, and 35% in 246 patients with lymph node involvement. Ten-year recurrence-free survival was almost identical to the 5-year figures. The perioperative mortality in this series was 3%.[123] Other recent series have produced similar results.[69,124–127] Local recurrence is seen in less than 10% of cases. It is worth noting that, although lymph node metastases portend a poor prognosis, it is well documented that even patients with N2 nodes discovered at the time of surgery may be cured with cystectomy and lymph node dissection.[128,129]

Numerous reports of experience with laparoscopic cystectomy have been published clearly establishing the feasibility of the procedure in expert hands, but long-term oncologic follow-up is lacking.[130,131] Major benefits from this approach have not been clearly demonstrated and no comparative trials have been published.[132] Centers of excellence report less bleeding and postoperative pain with a laparoscopic approach, but hospital stay does not appear to be shortened. The Montsouris experience including 84 patients reported a median operative time of 4.5 hours, no perioperative mortality, and a relapse rate of 17% with a mean follow-up of 18 months.[130] Nerve-sparing and prostate-sparing cystectomy has also been widely studied and has resulted in potency rates of 85 to 100% in highly selected patients.[133] Both open and laparoscopic operations have been studied.[134] Unresolved issues include optimal patient selection and the impact of sexual-function-preserving cystectomies on oncologic outcomes.

Table 96-4 Relationship between Pathologic Stage and Percent 5-Year Survival

Series	Patients (*n*)	Stage				
		P2	P3A	P3B	P4	N+
Bassi et al[69]	369	63	53	33	28	15
Skinner[123]	1,054	72	58	38	33	31
Pagano et al[122]	261	63	50	15	21	4
Ghoneim et al[127]	1,026	66	47	31	19	23
Madersacher et al[304]	507	63*	40*†		32	26

*Estimated from survival curves.
†Data for stage 3A and 3B combined.

Urinary Diversions The oldest and most common urinary diversion is the ileal conduit, which drains into a urostomy bag. Newer techniques include (1) the formation of a urinary reservoir made of small bowel, which drains via a continent stoma that can be catheterized; and (2) the creation of an orthotopic bladder (neobladder) in which a newly formed urinary reservoir made of small and/or large bowel is anastomosed to the urethra, permitting the patient to void in a relatively normal fashion. These two approaches are used in selected patients for whom quality of life considerations are critical and the increased operative time will not increase perioperative morbidity or mortality.[135] Although many consider prostatic urethral involvement to be an indication for radical urethrectomy or a contraindication for a neobladder, orthotopic neobladders have been associated with a lower rate of urethral recurrence than cutaneous diversions.[136–138] Patients whose cancer involves the female urethra or the penile urethra are generally not considered candidates for neobladders. At present, orthotopic urinary diversion can be performed successfully in both men and women.[139] Neobladders function as a very rough equivalent to the patient's normal bladder. Patients in whom this procedure is performed do have a higher incidence of infection, electrolyte abnormalities, minor to troublesome incontinence, and urinary retention requiring catheterization. Recent attempts at preserving sexual function in men by sparing the nerves controlling erectile function at the time of cystectomy have reported a roughly 40 to 50% postoperative potency rate among men who were potent prior to surgery.[140–142] The magnitude of the impact of radical cystectomy on women's sexual functioning and experience has not been adequately studied.[143]

Preoperative Radiation Therapy The recognition that moderate-dose radiation (20–50 Gy) may reduce the volume of gross disease and eradicate microscopic TCC led to its frequent administration before cystectomy in the 1970s. In nonrandomized studies, these doses were found to reduce the frequency of local recurrence and to increase survival.[144] By the 1980s, however, perhaps owing to improved surgical techniques, a benefit from preoperative radiation was no longer apparent.[145] It has been argued that radiation delays the time to definitive surgery, increases its morbidity, and may compromise the surgeon's ability to perform continent urinary diversions. Furthermore, a number of randomized trials have failed to show any survival advantage with preoperative radiation therapy.[146] These studies were limited in value, however, because of their small size and the inclusion of patients with T2 disease, who have a low probability of extravesical tumor, and T4 disease, who did not stand to benefit from additional local therapy because of an extremely high probability of distant metastases. Parsons and Million[147] demonstrated an apparent survival advantage of preoperative radiotherapy for the T3 subgroup by pooling all studies in the literature. A retrospective review of 133 patients with T3b cancers reported that patients who received preoperative radiation therapy had a pelvic recurrent rate of 10% compared with a rate of 28% among patients who underwent cystectomy without radiation.[148] Others have reported lower rates of pelvic recurrence using cystectomy alone for this subset of patients, and it therefore remains uncertain whether these findings are widely applicable.[145]

The morbidity of preoperative irradiation is small. Whitmore reported comparable rates of wound healing and perioperative mortality for patients who received and those who did not receive irradiation before cystectomy.[149] There is limited experience in the creation of continent urinary diversions after preoperative irradiation, although Housset and colleagues report that it is possible after the delivery of 44 Gy.[150]

Postoperative Radiation Therapy When the cystectomy specimen shows positive surgical margins, the risk of pelvic recurrence is high. Postoperative radiation therapy has been evaluated in only one randomized study. The National Cancer Institute of Egypt[151] reported on 236 patients with T3-4 tumors (68% squamous cell) who received either no adjuvant therapy or postoperative radiation. The incidence of pelvic recurrence was significantly reduced in the latter group (50% vs 10%), but overall survival was not affected. Whether this finding is as applicable to transitional as to squamous cell tumors remains an unanswered question. Patients with T3 tumors are more likely to suffer distant relapses than local relapse,[123,125] and patients with such extensive disease, thus, commonly receive adjuvant chemotherapy, although the ability of this modality to prevent local recurrence or extend survival remains unclear. Radiation rarely cures patients with pelvic wall recurrences following radical cystectomy.[151,152] The morbidity of postoperative irradiation is high because of the large volumes of small bowel that occupy the pelvis after cystectomy.

Bladder Preservation **Partial Cystectomy** Proper patient selection is crucial for a successful partial or segmental cystectomy. Review of the literature reveals that partial cystectomy was considered to be suitable only for 6 to 19% of patients with apparently localized invasive bladder cancers.[153,154] The indications for allowing partial cystectomy are solitary, primary, muscle-invasive cancers that are located in a suitable region of the bladder (typically the dome) that allows for complete excision with a 2 cm tumor-free margin. There should be no associated atypia or CIS in the remaining bladder urothelium, proven by biopsy. Patients with tumor near the bladder neck or trigone in whom ureteral reimplantation would be required to achieve an adequate surgical margin are generally not considered to be good candidates. In elderly, debilitated patients for whom radical cystectomy is not a viable treatment option, partial cystectomy may be the only feasible surgical alternative. Bladder-sparing therapy using TURBT plus chemoradiation should also be considered in such patients. Local recurrence rates of 38 to 78% have been reported following partial cystectomy, with one-half of recurrences appearing in the first year and two-thirds by 2 years. Five-year survival rates are 75 to 100% for grade 1 tumors, 46 to 75% for grade 2, and 22 to 55% for grade 3. Five-year reports of survival rates are 100% for stage Ta, 58 to 80% for T1, 29 to 80% for T2, 14 to 62% for T3a, 0 to 33% for T3b, and 0 to 20% for T4.[155]

Radical Radiation Therapy Radical radiation therapy as the sole treatment modality for muscle-invasive bladder cancer produces a clinical complete response in 40 to 50% of patients[156–159] (Table 96-5). The commonly employed strategy is that those who do not respond completely undergo salvage surgery.[160] Of those who achieve a complete remission, one-quarter to one-third will subsequently experience a local failure. Ultimately, only 30% of patients maintain a tumor-free bladder after radical radiation therapy alone. Several series have shown that prior transurethral resections of gross tumor may improve these rates, and this is a recommended feature in most modern protocols in which bladder preservation is the goal. The likelihood of durable local control with radiation therapy alone is determined by multiple tumor factors, of which size (< 5 cm), stage (T2), morphology, and the absence of ureteral obstruction and coexistent CIS have been found most consistently.[159,161,162] The chance of tumor eradication may be as high as 66% for those with solitary T2 tumors or as low as 9% for those with multiple tumors and hydronephrosis.[159] Because of the high failure rate associated with hydronephrosis, it is now generally considered a contraindication to radical radiation therapy.

Table 96-6 Overall 5-Year Survival and Bladder Preservation: Modern Series

Series	*n*	Treatment	5-Yr Survival (%)	CR (%)	5-Yr Survival with Bladder (%)	Survivors with Tumor-Free Bladder (%)
Erlangen[171]	45	RT + C/5-FU	67	87	54	80
RTOG 1998[169]	123	RT + C ± MCV	49	66	38	78
MGH 2002[176]	190¶	RT + C ± MCV	54	63	—	80
Paris 1997[174]	120§	RT + C/5-FU ± CT	63	77	—	—
Erlangen[173]	115	RT + C	61	85	47	73
Rome 2004[305]	77	RT = C/5-FU	58	90	47	78

C = cisplatin; CT = radical cystectomy.
‡At 3 years.
¶The MGH series includes a considerable number of patients also included in 1998 RTOG series.
§Includes 22 patients who underwent radical cystectomy despite achieving a CR with chemoradiation.

Although two moderate-sized randomized studies compared radical radiation therapy with preoperative radiation therapy followed by cystectomy, both trials were substantially underpowered, and thus left unanswered the question of whether the two approaches result in comparable survival. The first reported a 5-year survival of 39% with preoperative radiation plus cystectomy versus 28% for radical radiation, but this 11% absolute improvement in survival with early cystectomy was not statistically significant.[157] A significant advantage for early cystectomy was seen only in patients under 60 years of age. The Danish Bladder Cancer Group[163] reported 29% 5-year survival in the cystectomy arm compared with 23% in the radiation arm, a statistically insignificant difference. These two trials were thus able neither to confirm nor exclude a clinically meaningful difference in survival; a larger study would be required to do so. An advantage of radical radiation is that only those who prove a need for it by the persistence of tumor undergo cystectomy, thus allowing preservation of the bladder in the remainder. Roughly 40% of patients treated in this way will have a cancer-free bladder 5 years following treatment.

Table 96-5 Complete Responses after Radical Radiation Therapy Alone

Series	Stage	Patients (*n*)	CR (%)
London (1980)	cT2-4	614	28
Inst. Urology (1982)	cT3	81	40
Yorkshire (1983)	cT3	55	51
Edinburgh (1986)	cT3	272	41
London (1988)	cT2-3	182	52
PMH (1989)	cT2-4	121	46
Norway (1991)	cT2-4	146	44
Australia (1995)	cT1-4	342	68

CR = complete response.

Radiation to the bladder can result in fibrosis, low bladder volumes, proctitis, and impaired sexual function. The Danish Bladder Cancer Study Group found that those patients randomized to preoperative irradiation and cystectomy reported the largest reduction in their social and sexual activities 18 to 24 months after treatment.[164] Primarily, this was because all of those undergoing planned cystectomy voided via a urostomy and 100% of men in this arm became impotent. A retrospective analysis in 1996 reported similar findings that quality of life was better following radiation than after cystectomy.[165] With the development of nerve-sparing surgical techniques, which preserve erectile function in roughly half of men, continent diversions and neobladders may be expected to narrow this difference.[140]

Chemoradiation The rationale behind combining chemotherapy with radiation therapy is twofold. First, certain cytotoxic agents, in particular cisplatin and 5-fluorouracil (5-FU), are capable of sensitizing tumor tissue to radiation, thus increasing cell kill in a synergistic fashion. This action enhances both primary tumor control and prospects for bladder preservation. Second, patients with muscle-invading TCC harbor occult metastases in approximately 50% of cases. Chemotherapy, given before, during, or after radiation, addresses this concern early in treatment. Although a number of trials have added either neoadjuvant or adjuvant chemotherapy to simultaneous chemoradiation regimens, neither has ever been shown to offer a benefit.

Results thus far with chemoradiotherapy are comparable to results with cystectomy, but randomized trials are lacking (Table 96-6). Bladder preservation can be achieved in most patients with T2 and T3a tumors. Patients with more advanced disease (T3b and T4) are less likely to achieve local control with this approach, but most ultimately will succumb to systemic disease regardless of the treatment modality. Many phase II studies employing a range of drugs with a variety of radiation doses in differing sequences have been published (see Table 96-6). Overall, there is a clear increase in the complete response rate compared with series employing radiation therapy alone. Three randomized studies have compared radiation alone with simultaneous chemotherapy and radiation, but two used suboptimal chemotherapy regimens: single-agent methotrexate and doxorubicin with 5-FU.[166–168] No survival advantage was seen with combination therapy in any of the studies. In the one trial employing cisplatin given at the same time as the radiation for a sensitizing effect,[168] a significant reduction in local recurrence was associated with combined therapy. Despite the absence of a demonstrated survival benefit, combining chemotherapy with radical radiation has become standard. Single-agent cisplatin typically given at a dose of 100 mg/m^2 for either two cycles 21 days apart[169] or three cycles 14 days apart.[168] Cisplatin plus fluorouracil represents another very promising regimen.[170–172]

The case for a multimodality approach to bladder sparing has been strengthened by four studies from groups at the University of Erlangen[173] and ISSA, University of Paris,[174,175] Massachusetts General Hospital (MGH),[176] and the Radiation Therapy Oncology Group (RTOG).[177] Three employed aggressive transurethral resection with radiation and cisplatin-based chemotherapy, and three also employed selection by initial tumor response. All reported overall survival figures of 45 to 64% at 3 to 5 years. This approach has not yet been compared with cystectomy in a randomized fashion, but these figures are as good as any of the modern, radical cystectomy series, despite a bias in favor of cystectomy that results from reporting by pathologic stage and the inclusion of patients with T1 disease.[178] Two recently reported cystectomy series, one from the University of Southern California and the other from the Memorial Sloan-Kettering Cancer, reported 5- to 10-year disease-specific survival figures very similar to those in all the contemporary chemoradiation series.[123,179] Moreover, a 122-patient Spanish trial that reported results by clinical stage rather than pathological stage, and which is thus easier to compare with chemoradiation series, reported a 5-year survival rate of 42% following radical cystectomy (48% for cT2).[180] These results are inferior to the results of modern bladder-preserving strategies, although patient selection factors are operative. Twice-a-day (accelerated) radiation regimens may be more effective than once-a-day regimens in their ability to induce and maintain a complete response.[181] A pilot study evaluating the use of twice-a-day radiation in conjunction with cisplatin and 5-FU reported a clinical complete response rate of 65%. With a median follow-up of 29 months, the overall survival and survival with a functioning bladder at 3 years were 83% and 66%, respectively.[182]

A critical element of bladder-conserving programs is the recognition that patients at high risk of local failure can be identified early and cystectomy promptly performed. Cystoscopies were carried out 4 to 8 weeks following completion of chemoradiation, and any patient with persistent, invasive tumor was referred for salvage cystectomy. In the MGH and RTOG studies, reevaluation was performed after only 40 Gy of radiation. In the absence of a complete response, cystectomy is then recommended before the bladder has received radical doses. In the Parisian program reported by Housset and colleagues,[150,174] 74% have had complete responses, and only 10% subsequently have failed within the preserved bladder. In the MGH, RTOG, and Erlangen studies, the complete response rates at cystoscopic rebiopsy were 58 to 80%. Of those who had complete responses, 83 to 89% remained free from invasive recurrence.

It has been argued that the radiation is not an essential part of a bladder-conserving approach to invasive cancer and that TURBT alone or in combination with chemotherapy may be equally as effective for smaller tumors amenable to a visibly complete transurethral resection. There is no randomized data to address this issue. Published case series indicate that TURBT followed by MVAC chemotherapy followed by repeat TURBT produces roughly comparable results with TURBT followed by chemoradiation followed by repeat cystoscopy with biopsies.[162,183–185] In both cases, patients with residual tumor should be referred for cystectomy.

Some patients develop subsequent superficial disease following a bladder-sparing approach, but they are still amenable to standard management with transurethral resections and intravesical agents. Zietman and colleagues reported that, with a median follow-up of 6.7 years, 26% of complete responders experienced a superficial relapse.[186] Median time to this failure was 2.1 years. The majority of the superficial failures were carcinoma in situ, and the majority arose at the site of the original invasive tumor. The risk of superficial failure was higher among those who had carcinoma in situ associated with their original muscle-invading tumor. Twenty-seven of these 31 patients were managed conservatively with transurethral resection and intravesical therapy. The 5- and 8-year survival was comparable for those who experienced superficial failure (68% and 54%) and those who had no failure (n = 74, 69% and 61%). There was, however, a substantially lower chance of being alive with the native bladder owing to the need for late salvage cystectomies (34% vs 61%). Cystectomy became necessary in 32% (10 of 31) either because of further superficial recurrence (n = 7) or progression to invasive disease (n = 3). Kachnic and colleagues[187] reported that 15 of 21 patients who developed CIS following chemoradiation have been maintained in remission using BCG with 13 to 97 months of follow-up.

Bladder morbidity for patients receiving chemoradiation after TURBT appears to be comparable with those reports of patients treated by radiation alone. In the Erlangen series, only three cystectomies were necessary for bladder shrinkage among 192 preserved bladders (1.6%).[173] At the MGH, no cystectomies for shrinkage were required, and a recent quality of life study in which patients evaluated their bladder, bowel, and sexual function demonstrated good subjective results. Formal urodynamic studies were also performed on 26 complete responders after a median follow-up greater than 6 years, and 19 (73%) had normally functioning bladders. The remainder showed decreases in compliance or functional capacity. Only two were incontinent, both elderly women.[188] Of note, the Parisian group reported that they were able to create continent diversions in the few patients who recurred locally and requiring salvage cystectomy.[150]

Neoadjuvant and Adjuvant Chemotherapy

Neoadjuvant Chemotherapy Chemotherapy before definitive local therapy has been used in two general settings: before radical cystectomy to enhance local control and decrease the likelihood of systemic relapse, and in conjunction with radiation for bladder preservation. Administering three cycles of MVAC or CMV prior to radical cystectomy has been shown to increase overall survival in two recent meta-analyses.[189,190] Specifically, 5-year overall survival increased from about 50% without neoadjuvant chemotherapy to about 55% with neoadjuvant chemotherapy. Whether it is appropriate to give 100 patients chemotherapy so that 5 or 6 who otherwise would have died will be alive 5 years later is a subjective value judgment, but this small benefit does appear to be real. The chemotherapy mortality rate was reported at 1.1%.

The use of chemotherapy before local therapy offers the potential advantages of providing systemic therapy at the earliest opportunity and sometimes downstaging the primary tumor to allow for complete resection of a tumor that has extended beyond the bladder. The concern of urologists that neoadjuvant chemotherapy will prevent patients from undergoing cystectomy or will increase the rate of perioperative complications has not been borne out in randomized trials.[191] It is established that a favorable response to neoadjuvant chemotherapy selects a group of patients with particularly good survival characteristics.

The relevant randomized neoadjuvant chemotherapy trials used multiagent cisplatin-based regimens. Several small single-agent studies found no benefit, but these represent substandard regimens.[167,180,192,193] Four large trials of neoadjuvant multiagent cisplatin-based chemotherapy have been completed (Table 96-7). The largest randomized study reported 976 patients receiving radical radiation or cystectomy who were randomized either to receive or not to receive three cycles of neoadjuvant MCV.[191] The study was powered to detect an absolute 10% improvement in overall survival because that was the threshold that surveyed physicians identified as the minimum benefit necessary to justify administering neoadjuvant chemotherapy. Only a 7% absolute benefit in survival was reported with 7 years follow-up, but the result was statistically significant.[189] Posthoc subgroup analyses found no association between tumor stage and benefit from chemotherapy, but patients with high grade tumors did appear to benefit. The Nordic Co-Operative Bladder Cancer Study Group performed two randomized studies of neoadjuvant chemotherapy. Each trial showed a statistically nonsignificant trend to longer survival with chemotherapy, but a combined analysis of the data from the two trials reported a significant 8% absolute increase in 5-year survival (p = .049).[194,195] Most recently, a randomized US intergroup study examining the value of neoadjuvant MVAC before cystectomy in 307 patients accrued over 11 years reported a nonsignificant (p = .06)

Table 96-7 Randomized Trials of Neoadjuvant and Adjuvant Chemotherapy for Invasive Cancer

Series	Stage	Patients (*n*)	Primary Therapy	Chemotherapy	Overall Survival (%)	Significance
Neoadjuvant						
MRC/EORTC[191]	cT2 (grade3) N0M0	491	XRT or cystectomy	CMV × 3	55.5 (3 yr)	Yes
	T3-4a N0M0	485		Immediate local therapy	50	
RTOG 89-03[169]	cT2-4 NxM0	61	XRT + cisplatin	CMV × 2	48 (3 yr)	No
		62		Immediate chemoradiation	49	
NCBSG[306]	cT1 (grade 0) NxM0	151	XRT + cystectomy	Cisplatin + doxorubicin	58 (5 yr)	No
	cT2-4 NxM0	160		Immediate local therapy	51	
Nordic 2[307]	cT2-4 NxM0	155	Cystectomy	Cisplatin + Methotrexate × 3	53 (5 yr)	No
		154		Immediate cystectomy	46	
INT-0080[308]	T2-4a N0M0	153	Cystectomy	MVAC × 3	41	No
		154		Immediate cystectomy	35	
GUONE[309,310]		102	Cystectomy	MVAC	62	No
		104		Immediate cystectomy	68	
Adjuvant						
USC[198]	pTany N+M0	44	Cystectomy	CAP × 4	68 (3 yr)	No
	pT3-4 NxM0	47		Observation	47	
Mainz[199]	pT3b-4a N+M0	26	Cystectomy	MVAC or MVEC × 3	42	NR
		23		Observation	17	
Stanford[200]	pT3b-4 N+M0	25	Cystectomy	CMV × 4	NR	No
		25		Observation	NR	

CAP = cyclophosphamide, Adriamycin, and Platinol; CMV = cisplatin, methotrexate, vinblastine; 5-FU = 5-fluorouracil; MVAC = methotrexate, vinblastine, doxorubicin, cisplatin; MVEC = Mtx, VLB, epirubicin; XRT = x-irradiation.

trend toward improved survival in the chemotherapy arm.

Based on the results of the meta-analyses, it appears that neoadjuvant chemotherapy is associated with a modest overall survival benefit. Whether or not there are identifiable high-risk subgroups who stand to receive a larger benefit from such therapy has not been clearly established. Neoadjuvant chemotherapy has also been used to shrink locally advanced tumors to render them operable. Clinical trials have generated abundant evidence that tumor downstaging can be achieved with neoadjuvant chemotherapy. The European trial discussed above reported that 33% of 206 patients randomized to neoadjuvant CMV had no disease detectable in the cystectomy tissue compared with 12% of 211 patients randomized to cystectomy alone.[191] Herr and colleagues reported that among 207 patients with unresectable bladder tumors or pelvic lymph node metastases (stage N2) who underwent cisplatin-based chemotherapy, 92 were deemed to be candidates for radical cystectomy following chemotherapy. Of 60 patients who underwent surgery and were followed for at least 5 years, 19 (32%) were alive.[196] With the realization that sometimes dramatic responses could be achieved with chemotherapy, this modality has been used in conjunction with TURBT or partial cystectomy to spare the bladder. Identifying which patients can safely defer radical surgery, however, remains a challenge. Herr and colleagues reported a series of patients with T2 and T3 tumors who had a pathological complete response when treated with neoadjuvant MVAC followed by either a repeat TUR of the original tumor site ($n = 28$) or partial cystectomy ($n = 15$) rather than radical cystectomy. With a minimum of 10 years follow-up, 32 of 43 patients were alive, 25 of them with a bladder.[185] However, in this highly selected population, 56% developed bladder tumor recurrences, 30% underwent salvage cystectomy, and at least 14% died of metastatic disease.

The RTOG studied the addition of two cycles of neoadjuvant CMV to concomitant cisplatin and radical bladder irradiation in a randomized trial involving 123 patients.[169] The addition of CMV resulted in substantially more toxicity and the trial was closed prematurely because of high rates of febrile neutropenia and three septic deaths. Five-year survival was 48% in the CMV arm and 49% in the control arm. These results have discouraged the use of neoadjuvant chemotherapy prior to radical radiation for bladder cancer.

Adjuvant Chemotherapy The 5-year relapse-free survival rate following radical cystectomy is only 60 to 70%, and for patients with T3bN0, T4N0 tumors or pelvic lymph node involvement, 5-year survival ranges from 22 to 60%.[122,123,125,127,179] Roughly three-quarters of all relapses are distant metastases rather than recurrent disease in the pelvis. Use of chemotherapy following radical cystectomy has thus been studied for patients at high risk of having undetected micromestastic disease at the time of cystectomy. Four randomized trials using multiagent cisplatin-based chemotherapy have been reported (see Table 96-7). Three of these trials reported increased time to progression and nonsignificant trends toward a survival advantage with adjuvant chemotherapy, but each of the trials was profoundly underpowered and had other substantial flaws.[197] Adjuvant chemotherapy thus remains unproven and experimental, but is nonetheless widely utilized. The unanswered question is whether there is an advantage to giving adjuvant chemotherapy to all high-risk patients rather than only giving chemotherapy at the time of relapse. The advantage of adjuvant chemotherapy is that it allows the physician to treat a much smaller volume of disease, but the disadvantage is that a substantial number of people being treated have no residual disease and are thus exposed to the toxicities of chemotherapy unnecessarily.

Skinner and colleagues studied 99 patients with pT3, pT4, or N+ tumors randomized either to observation or to four cycles of CISCA (cisplatin, cyclophosphamide, and doxorubicin) chemotherapy.[198] Although this study was terminated before full accrual and had difficulty delivering chemotherapy as planned, more patients were free of disease at 3 years (70% vs 46%, $p = .001$) in the chemotherapy arm. A statistically nonsignificant trend toward longer survival was seen in the chemotherapy arm, with a 3-year survival rate of 66% versus 50%. Another small randomized study compared three cycles of MVAC (methotrexate, vinblastine, doxorubicin, and cisplatin) or MVEC (epirubicin substituted for doxorubicin) to observation in 49 patients with tumor stages pT3b, pT4a, and/or N1-2.[199] There was a statistically significant difference in relapse-free survival at 4.5 years (58% vs 17%, $p = .0005$), but the trial was severely underpowered and no advantage in overall survival was reported. Moreover, most patients in the observation arm were denied chemotherapy at the time of relapse, meaning that adjuvant chemotherapy was not compared with the current standard of care. Freiha and colleagues[200] conducted a small, randomized study in which 55 patients with pT3b, T4, or N1 bladder cancer following cystectomy were randomized to receive either 4 cycles of CMV (cisplatin, methotrexate, and vinblastine) or observation. With a minimum of 2 years and a median 62 months of follow-up, 12 of 25 treated patients (48%) remained relapse free, compared with 5 of 25 (25%) in the observation group. Although time to progression was superior in the treated groups (37 vs 12 months, $p = .01$), the benefit in median survival was statistically nonsignificant (63 vs 36 months, $p > .05$). No difference was seen in overall survival.

These studies show that adjuvant chemotherapy prolongs relapse-free survival in high-risk

Table 96-8 Randomized Chemotherapy Trials in Patients with Metastatic or Unresectable Bladder Cancer

Arm I	Arm II	No. of Patients Arm I	No. of Patients Arm II	Median Survival (Months) Arm I	Median Survival (Months) Arm II	Significant Survival Difference	Toxic Death Rate Arm I	Toxic Death Rate Arm II	Complete Response Rate Arm I	Complete Response Rate Arm II
MVAC[203]	Cisplatin	133	122	12.5	8.2	Yes	4%	0%	13%	3%
MVAC[204]	CISCA	55	55	11.1	8.3	Yes	0%	2%	35%	25%
MVAC[204]	MV	108	106	7	4.5	Yes	4%	0%	10%	7%
MVAC[222]	FAP	86	83	12.5	12.5	No	7%	8%	24%	10%
MVAC[208]	GC	203	202	14.8	13.8	No	3%	1%	12%	12%
CISCA[311]	Cisplatin	48	45	6.7	4.8	No				
HD-MVAC[201]	MVAC	61	62	15.5	14.1	No	3%	4%	21%	9%
MVAC[221]	M-CAVI	24	23	16	9	Yes	4%	0%	13%	0%
MVAC[312]	DC	109	111	14.2	9.3	Yes	2%	1%	23%	13%
MVAC[222]	FAP	86	86	12.5	12.5	No	7%	8%	24%	10%

TF = survival in months. MVAC = methotrexate, vinblastine, doxorubicin, and cisplatin; HD-MVAC = high-dose intensity MVAC; CISCA = cisplatin, cyclophosphamide, and doxorubicin; FAP = fluorouracil, interferon α-2b, and cisplatin; GC = gemcitabine and cisplatin; M-CAVI = methotrexate, carboplatin, vinblastine. DC = docetaxel, cisplatin; FAP = Interferon β-2b, fluorouracil, cisplatin.

subsets of patients with invasive bladder cancer. An overall survival benefit, however, has not been established. A well powered international randomized trial is currently underway comparing adjuvant chemotherapy (either MVAC or gemcitabine plus cisplatin) to observation in high-risk patients undergoing cystectomy.

Table 96-9 Dose Schedules of Common Bladder Cancer Regimens

Regimen	Dose schedule
MVAC (28-day cycle)[193]	Methotrexate 30 mg/m^2 days 1, 15, 22 Vinblastine 3 mg/m^2 days 2, 15, 22 Doxorubicin 30 mg/m^2 day 2 Cisplatin 70 mg/m^2 day 2
CMV (21-day cycle)[205]	Methotrexate 30 mg/m^2 days 1, 8 Folinic acid 15mg po q6H × 4 days 2, 9 Vinblastine 4 mg/m^2 days 1, 8 Cisplatin 70–100 mg/m^2 day 2
GC (28-day cycle)[208]	Gemcitabine 1,000 mg/m^2 days 1, 8, 15 Cisplatin 70 mg/m^2 day 1
Gemcitabine/paclitaxel (14-day cycle)[234]	Gemcitabine 2,500–3,000 mg/m^2 day 1 Paclitaxel 150 mg/m^2 day 1
Carboplatin/paclitaxel (21-day cycle)[228]	Carboplatin AUC = 6 Paclitaxel 200 mg/m^2

CHEMOTHERAPY FOR METASTATIC DISEASE

Cytotoxic chemotherapy produces high objective response rates in metastatic TCC of the bladder, but has a small impact on survival. Although roughly 4% of patients with metastatic disease can be long-term survivors following the use of chemotherapy, median survival is only about 1 year with the most active regimens.[201–203] MVAC and CMV as first-line therapy are the only regimens that have been shown to provide a survival advantage, and it remains untested whether any second- or third-line chemotherapy extends survival.[203–205] Single-agent chemotherapy and cisplatin-free regimens are sometimes used in frail or heavily pretreated patients, but the benefit of such therapy has never been tested in controlled trials.

Combination Regimens First-line chemotherapy for metastatic or locally advanced, unresectable bladder cancer includes several multiagent cisplatin-based regimens: MVAC,[206] CMV,[205,207] and GC (gemcitabine and cisplatin).[208] However, countless combination regimens have been shown to have activity in the treatment of metastatic bladder cancer. Evaluation of these regimens has been made difficult, however, by variable patient selection and the paucity of comparative trials.

The most widely used regimens have been cisplatin-based (Tables 96-8 and 96-9). Multicenter phase III trials have demonstrated the superiority of multiagent cisplatin-based regimens over single-agent cisplatin and over regimens that exclude cisplatin. The Eastern Cooperative Oncology Group randomized 255 patients to either cisplatin alone or to MVAC, and the combination regimen proved to be superior, with a prolongation of median survival by 4 months (12.6 vs 8.7) (Figure 96-3).[193] Meanwhile, a British Medical Research Council trial randomized 214 patients to either CMV (cisplatin dosed at 70 mg/m^2) or to methotrexate plus vinblastine (MV). Median survival (7 months vs 4.5 months) and 1-year survival (29% vs 16%) were significantly superior in the CMV arm ($p = .0065$), but CMV was also associated with greater toxicity, including five treatment-related deaths compared with none in the MV arm. A third randomized trial comparing MVAC to CISCA (cisplatin, cyclophosphamide, and doxorubicin) in 110 patients with metastatic urothelial carcinomas demonstrated that MVAC resulted in significantly longer survival (median survival 11 months vs 8 months).[204] These trials established MVAC and CMV as first-line therapy. The most encouraging aspect of treatment with combination chemotherapy with MVAC is that a small proportion (< 5%) of patients treated will be long-term survivors. Prognostic factors that predict for prolonged survival with treatment include the absence of lung, liver, or bone metastasis; Karnofsky performance status of 80 or higher; normal hemoglobin level; and transitional cell carcinoma.[202,203] It is worth noting that a small subgroup of patients who undergo resection of residual masses following a partial response to chemotherapy can be long-term survivors, but this represents a highly select subgroup.[206,209]

With the hope of increasing survival and cure rates, intensified MVAC regimens have been studied but have not revealed a compelling advantage.[201,210,211] The one randomized trial compared high-dose-intensity MVAC (methotrexate 30 mg/m^2 day 1; vinblastine 3 mg/m^2 day 2; doxorubicin 30 mg/m^2 day 2; cisplatin 70 mg/m^2 day 2; filgrastim 240 mcg/m^2 days 4–10 in 14-day cycles) with standard MVAC in 263 patients. The high-dose arm had a higher complete response rate (21% vs 9%, $p = .009$) but no significant difference in time to progression or overall survival. Median survival was 15.5 months in the high-dose arm versus 14.1 months in the control arm ($p = .122$). The toxicity profile was more favorable in the high-dose arm, with less myelosuppression and mucositis, likely owing to the

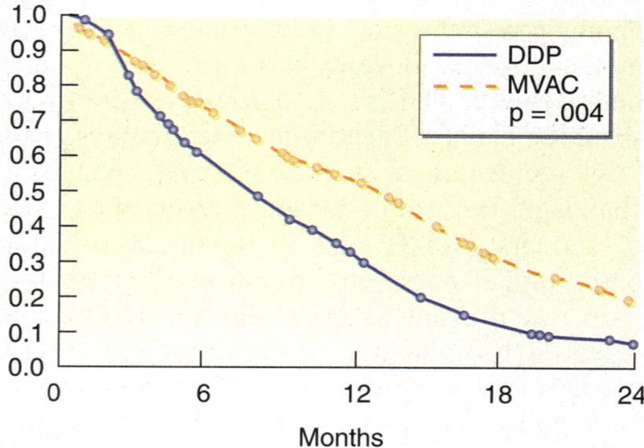

Figure 96-3 INT0078 survival by treatment. DDP = cis-diamminedichloroplatinum; MVAC = methotrexate, vinblastine, doxorubicin, cisplatin.

Table 96-10 Phase II Trials of New Chemotherapy Regimens for Metastatic Bladder Cancer

Regimen	No. Trials	No. Patients	% Who Received Prior Chemotherapy	Response Rates (%)	CR Rates (%)	Median Survival[a]
Paclitaxel, gemcitabine Q 14 days[234]	1	40	100	60	28	14.4
Paclitaxel Q 21 days, weekly gemcitabine[235]	1	54	28	54	7	14.4
Paclitaxel, cisplatin[223,224]	2	87	0	50–70	8–32	10.6–13.4
Paclitaxel, carboplatin[225–228]	4	116	0–18*	21–72	0–31	9– > 13
Paclitaxel, gemcitabine, carboplatin[231]	1	49	12*	65	31	14.7
Paclitaxel, gemcitabine, cisplatin[232]	1	60	8*	75	27	> 12
Paclitaxel, ifosfamide, cisplatin[236]	1	45	0	67	22	20
Gemcitabine, docetaxel, cisplatin[241]	1	35	23*	66	29	15.5
Gemcitabine, carboplatin[229,230]	2	58	0–3	44–56	6–12	10
Docetaxel, cisplatin[237–239]	3	129	0–23	52–60	12–26	8–13.6
Docetaxel, ifosfamide[266]	1	22	100	23	18	4
Docetaxel, epirubicin, cisplatin[240]	1	32	22	63	28	14.5
Ifosfamide, fluorouracil, etoposide, cisplatin[209]	1	29		59	NR	14

[a]Survival in months.

*Adjuvant or neoadjuvant chemotherapy only: no prior chemotherapy for metastatic or recurrent disease.

greater use of GCSF and the lower cumulative dose of methotrexate in the high-dose arm.

CMV and MVAC are aggressive regimens, with toxic death rates of 3 to 4% and febrile neutropenia occurring in 10 to 14% of patients receiving chemotherapy for metastatic disease (less toxicity has been reported in the neoadjuvant and adjuvant settings where fewer cycles of chemotherapy are administered).[193,208,212,213] Less toxic alternatives have been sought. A multicenter, international trial randomized 405 patients to MVAC or GC as first-line chemotherapy. Survival was similar in the two arms (HR = 1.09, 95% CI = 0.88–1.34, p = .66), with median survival times of 15.2 months with MVAC and 14.0 months with GC.[214] However, the trial was powered to demonstrate the superiority of one regimen over the other and was not large enough to establish equivalence according to standard statistical methodology.[215,216] A significant survival advantage with MVAC thus could not be excluded.[217] No quality of life differences were seen between the two arms but fewer GC patients suffered neutropenic sepsis (1% vs 12%, p < .001) or grade 3 or 4 mucositis (1% vs 22%). Although this trial was underpowered and although GC has never been shown to provide a survival advantage, many have interpreted this study as establishing GC as appropriate first-line therapy for metastatic TCC, and it is widely used. In contrast, a trial comparing MVAC to docetaxel plus cisplatin reported longer survival with MVAC.

Several studies have attempted to reduce the toxicity of MVAC by substituting carboplatin for cisplatin[218] and epirubicin or mitoxantrone for doxorubicin.[219] Comparative trials of carboplatin-based versus cisplatin-based regimens, however, although of small size, have reported substantially lower response rates and disease-specific survival in the carboplatin-based regimens.[220,221] A trial randomizing 172 patients to either MVAC or a combination of interferon α-2b, fluorouracil, and cisplatin (FAP)[222] reported that toxicity and survival were comparable but MVAC produced a significantly higher response rate (59% vs 42%). FAP did not appear to offer any advantages over MVAC and may well be less active.

A large variety of other combination regimens have been tested in phase II trials but have never been compared with MVAC, CMV, or GC (Table 96-10). These include cisplatin and paclitaxel[223,224]; carboplatin and paclitaxel[225–228]; carboplatin and gemcitabine[229,230]; paclitaxel, carboplatin, and gemcitabine;[231] paclitaxel, cisplatin, and gemcitabine[232,233]; gemcitabine and paclitaxel[234,235]; ifosfamide, paclitaxel, and cisplatin[236]; docetaxel and cisplatin[237–239]; cisplatin, epirubicin, and docetaxel[240]; and docetaxel, gemcitabine, and cisplatin.[241] Each of these regimens has produced response rates over 50% with acceptable toxicity in previously untreated patients, but the absence of phase III trials makes it impossible to judge their relative utility in treating bladder cancer. An attempt was made to compare MVAC to carboplatin and paclitaxel, but the trial closed because of poor accrual. It is worth noting that the combination of docetaxel and gemcitabine has been associated with severe pulmonary toxicity in several patients.[242]

Single Agents Single-agent chemotherapy has never been shown to provide a survival benefit. Cisplatin has been the most widely used. In phase II studies in which the dose and patient populations differed, response rates have varied from 26 to 65%, with complete responses seen in 0 to 14% among chemotherapy-naïve patients.[243–247] In phase III studies, the response rates generally have been lower, in the range of 12 to 31%, with complete responses seen in fewer than 10% of patients. Carboplatin has also been used in the treatment of bladder cancer because of its more favorable toxicity profile. Overall, the results as a single agent in phase II trials have been roughly comparable with those with cisplatin.[248,249] Comparative studies are lacking.

Three newer agents, paclitaxel, gemcitabine, and docetaxel, have significant activity and are often given as second- or third-line chemotherapy and in patients who are too frail for cisplatin. None of these agents depend on the kidneys for clearance or metabolism.[250,251] Single-agent paclitaxel has one of the highest response rates in phase II trials, with 31 to 56% of patients showing an objective response.[250,252,253] In the largest of these studies, paclitaxel was administered as a single agent to 26 patients with previously untreated bladder cancer at a dosage of 250 mg/m^2 over 24 hours every 3 weeks.[252] Eleven (42%) patients responded, including 7 (26%) complete responders. In contrast, two studies of single-agent paclitaxel in previously treated patients with urothelial cancers reported response rates of only 7 to 10%.[254,255] Studies of single-agent docetaxel have confirmed this agent's activity. Three studies using a dosage of 100 mg/m^2 every 3 weeks reported response rates of 31 to 45% in chemo-naïve patients and 13% in patients who had received cisplatin previously.[251,256,257] Two published studies have tested gemcitabine in previously untreated patients at a dosage of 1,200 mg/m^2 on days 1, 8, and 15 of a 28 day course.[258,259] Response rates were 28% (11 of 39) and 24% (9 of 37), with 10% and 8% of patients achieving a complete response. In one study of weekly gemcitabine in 31 patients who had previously received a platinum-based regimen, a response rate of 22% and a CR rate of 13% were reported.[260]

Other active single-agent drugs in the treatment of bladder cancer include ifosfamide, which has a response rate of 20% (11 of 56 patients)[261]; methotrexate, which has a response rate of 29%; gallium nitrate, which has a response rate of 24% (17 of 81 patients)[262]; doxorubicin, 17% (95% confidence interval [CI], 12–23%); 5-FU, 15% (95% CI, 12–19%)[263]; vinblastine, 16% (95% CI, 4–28%)[263]; and mitomycin, 13% (95% CI, 3–23%).[263]

Second-Line Chemotherapy Optimal second-line chemotherapy for bladder cancer remains poorly defined. Several active regimens have been identified, but no phase III trials have been published, and no survival or palliative benefit has ever been demonstrated relative to best supportive care. Single agents that have produced a response rate greater than 10% in patients who have progressed after receiving cisplatin-based therapy include gemcitabine, ifosfamide, and docetaxel.[251,261,264] Two phase II trials of second-line gemcitabine and paclitaxel administered every 14 days reported response rates of 47 to 67% overall, and 27 to 30% among patients who had received prior chemotherapy for metastatic disease.[234,235] Among patients who had received prior adjuvant or neoadjuvant therapy, the response rate was 80% in both trials. Complete responses were seen in 7 to 28% of patients overall. A phase II trial of paclitaxel, methotrexate, and cisplatin reported partial responses in 10 of 25 patients (40%), including 3 of 7 patients with liver metastases.[265] Two trials have investigated adding a taxane to ifosfamide, but in neither case did the response rate exceed the rate reported with ifosfamide alone.[266,267] The combination of fluorouracil, interferon, and cisplatin produced a response rate of only 13% in a multicenter trial.[268]

Adenocarcinoma of the Bladder Adenocarcinoma of the bladder is categorized into three rare entities: (1) metastatic, (2) primary, and (3) urachal. These tumors comprise less than 2% of all bladder tumors. The most common adenocarcinomas that spread to the bladder, usually by direct extension, are colon, prostate, and tumors of the female reproductive tract. If complete resection is achievable, cure is possible. Primary bladder adenocarcinomas may be papillary, polypoid, or nodular.[269] These tumors arise in patients who have a long history of cystitis; glandular cystitis frequently is associated with this lesion. Histologically, these tumors resemble colonic carcinoma, and most have invaded into muscle at the time of initial diagnosis. These tumors frequently produce mucin, with the signet cell variant being rare and particularly aggressive.[270,271] Primary adenocarcinoma of the bladder is treatable and potentially curable with radical cystectomy or pelvic exenteration. Urachal adenocarcinomas are rare[272] and usually confined to the dome or the anterior wall of the bladder. These are mucin producing as well and may have a signet-cell appearance. On CT scan, these tumors may be cystic or solid and typically are situated in the region of the urachal tract directly behind the anterior abdominal wall.[273] Surgical treatment with either partial or radical cystectomy coupled with umbilectomy generates comparable survival results, with 50% or fewer patients surviving.[272,274,275] Chemotherapy and radiotherapy are of uncertain value for adenocarcinomas of the bladder, but therapeutic successes have been published as case reports.[276]

Squamous Cell Carcinoma Although TCC mixed with squamous metaplasia or frank carcinoma sometimes is seen, pure squamous cell carcinoma of the bladder (SCC) is unusual in the United States, but much more common in areas endemic to *S. haematobium*, such as Egypt. An association also exists between chronic bladder infection and/or long-term indwelling bladder catheterization and the development of these tumors.[277] Patients with SCC in US reports have fared particularly poorly. This is partly due to their tendency to present with more advanced disease, but even among patients with advanced-stage bladder cancers, pure squamous cell tumors are associated with shorter survival.[203] However, a 1997 Egyptian report on SCC representing the largest published experience found that 5-year survival following cystectomy was as high for SCC (50.3%) as for TCC (46.7%). Compared with TCC, squamous cell carcinomas tend to be more locally aggressive and less prone to metastases.[278,279] In general, such patients are treated with aggressive surgical resection because these tumors are less responsive than TCC to radiation and chemotherapy. The locally aggressive nature of this disease has led some to favor preoperative radiation therapy to maximize local control, but there is little data to support or refute this approach.[278,279] Optimal chemotherapy regimens remain poorly defined.

REFERENCES

1. Ries LAG, Eisner MP, Kosary CL, et al, editors. SEER cancer statistics review, 1975–2002. Bethesda (MD): National Cancer Institute; 2005.
2. Hartge P, Harvey EB, Linehan WN, et al. Unexplained excess risk of bladder cancer in men. J Natl Cancer Inst 1990;82:1636–40.
3. Mungan NA, Kiemeney LA, van Dijck JA, et al. Gender differences in stage distribution of bladder cancer. Urology 2000;55:368–71.
4. Mungan NA, Aben KA, Schoenberg MP, et al. Gender differences in stage-adjusted bladder cancer survival. Urology 2000;55:876–80.
5. Ries LAG, Eisner MP, Kosary CL, et al. SEER cancer statistics review, 1973–1999. 2002, Bethesda (MD): National Cancer Institute; 2002.
6. Devesa SS, Silverman DT, Young JL Jr, et al. Cancer incidence and mortality trends among whites in the United States, 1947–84. J Natl Cancer Inst 1987;79:701–70.
7. Greenlee RT, Murray T, Bolden S, Wingo PA. Cancer statistics, 2000. CA Cancer J Clin 2000;50:7–33.
8. Brennan P, Bogillot O, Cordier S, et al. Cigarette smoking and bladder cancer in men: a pooled analysis of 11 case-control studies. Int J Cancer 2000;86:289–94.
9. Engeland A, Andersen A, Haldorsen T, Tretli S. Smoking habits and risk of cancers other than lung cancer: 28 years' follow-up of 26,000 Norwegian men and women. Cancer Causes Control 1996;7:497–506.
10. Zeegers MP, Goldbohm RA, van den Brandt PA. A prospective study on active and environmental tobacco smoking and bladder cancer risk (the Netherlands). Cancer Causes Control 2002;13:83–90.
11. Zeegers MP, Tan FE, Dorant E, van den Brandt PA. The impact of characteristics of cigarette smoking on urinary tract cancer risk: a meta-analysis of epidemiologic studies. Cancer 2000;89:630–9.
12. Case R, Hosker M, Macdonald DB, et al. Tumours of the urinary bladder in workmen engaged in the manufacture and use of certain dyestuff intermediaries in the British chemical industry: part I. Br J Ind Med 1954;11:75–104.
13. Ward E, Carpenter A, Markowitz S, et al. Excess number of bladder cancers in workers exposed to ortho-toluidine and aniline. J Natl Cancer Inst 1991;83:501–6.
14. Silverman DT, Levin LI, Hoover RN. Occupational risks of bladder cancer in the United States: II. Nonwhite men. J Natl Cancer Inst 1989;81:1480–3.
15. Silverman DT, Levin LI, Hoover RN, Hartge P. Occupational risks of bladder cancer in the United States: I. White men. J Natl Cancer Inst 1989;81:1472–80.
16. Tawfik HN. Carcinoma of the urinary bladder associated with schistosomiasis in Egypt: the possible causal relationship. Princess Takamatsu Symp 1987;18:197–209.
17. el-Mawla NG, el-Bolkainy MN, Khaled HM. Bladder cancer in Africa: update. Semin Oncol 2001;28:174–8.
18. Bedwani R, el-Khwsky F, Renganathan E, et al. Epidemiology of bladder cancer in Alexandria, Egypt: tobacco smoking. Int J Cancer 1997;73:64–7.
19. Michaud DS, Spiegelman D, Clinton SK, et al. Fluid intake and the risk of bladder cancer in men. N Engl J Med 1999;340:1390–7.
20. Michaud DS, Spiegelman D, Clinton SK, et al. Fruit and vegetable intake and incidence of bladder cancer in a male prospective cohort. J Natl Cancer Inst 1999;91:605–13.
21. Steineck G, Hagman U, Gerhardsson M, Norell SE. Vitamin A supplements, fried foods, fat and urothelial cancer. A case-referent study in Stockholm in 1985–87. Int J Cancer 1990;45:1006–11.
22. Stensvold I, Jacobsen BK. Coffee and cancer: a prospective study of 43,000 Norwegian men and women. Cancer Causes Control 1994;5:401–8.
23. Braver DJ, Modan M, Chetrit A, et al. Drinking, micturition habits, and urine concentration as potential risk factors in urinary bladder cancer. J Natl Cancer Inst 1987;78:437–40.
24. Bryan RT, Hussain SA, James ND, et al. Molecular pathways in bladder cancer: part 1. BJU Int 2005;95:485–90.
25. Bryan RT, Hussain SA, James ND, et al. Molecular pathways in bladder cancer: part 2. BJU Int 2005;95:491–6.
26. Oka N, Yamamoto Y, Takahashi M, et al. Expression of angiopoietin-1 and -2, and its clinical significance in human bladder cancer. BJU Int 2005;95:660–3.
27. Yang CC, Chu KC, Yeh WM. The expression of vascular endothelial growth factor in transitional cell carcinoma of urinary bladder is correlated with cancer progression. Urol Oncol 2004;22:1–6.
28. Wulfing C, Eltze E, Piechota H, et al. Expression of endothelin-1 and endothelin-A and -B receptors in invasive bladder cancer. Oncol Rep 2005;13:223–8.
29. Knowles MA. What we could do now: molecular pathology of bladder cancer. Mol Pathol 2001;54:215–21.
30. Slaton JW, Benedict WF, Dinney CP. P53 in bladder cancer: mechanism of action, prognostic value, and target for therapy. Urology 2001;57:852–9.
31. Shariat SF, Tokunaga H, Zhou J, et al. p53, p21, pRB, and p16 expression predict clinical outcome in cystectomy with bladder cancer [comments]. J Clin Oncol 2004;22:1014–24.
32. Goto K, Konomoto T, Hayashi K, et al. p53 mutations in multiple urothelial carcinomas: a molecular analysis of the development of multiple carcinomas. Mod Pathol 1997;10:428–37.
33. Sidransky D, Frost P, Von Eschenbach A, et al. Clonal origin bladder cancer. N Engl J Med 1992;326:737–40.
34. Vriesema JL, Aben KA, Witjes JA, et al. Superficial and metachronous invasive bladder carcinomas are clonally related. Int J Cancer 2001;93:699–702.
35. Millan-Rodriguez F, Chechile-Toniolo G, Salvador-Bayarri J, et al. Multivariate analysis of the prognostic factors of primary superficial bladder cancer. J Urol 2000;163:73–8.
36. Millan-Rodriguez F, Chechile-Toniolo G, Salvador-Bayarri J, et al. Primary superficial bladder cancer risk groups according to progression, mortality and recurrence. J Urol 2000;164:680–4.
37. Cummings KB, Barone JG, Ward WS. Diagnosis and staging of bladder cancer. Urol Clin North Am 1992;19:455–65.
38. Britton JP, Dowell AC, Whelan P, Harris CM. A community study of bladder cancer screening by the detection of occult urinary bleeding. J Urol 1992;148:788–90.
39. Logsetty S. Screening for bladder cancer. In: Canadian Task Force on the Periodic Health Examination, editor. Canadian guide to clinical preventive health care. Ottawa: Canadian Government Publishing; 1998. p. 826–36.
40. Farrow GM, Utz DC, Rife CC. Morphological and clinical observations of patients with early bladder cancer treated with total cystectomy. Cancer Res 1976;36:2495–501.
41. Ramakumar S, Bhuiyan J, Besse JA, et al. Comparison of screening methods in the detection of bladder cancer. J Urol 1999;161:388–94.
42. Muller M. Telomerase: its clinical relevance in the diagnosis of bladder cancer. Oncogene 2002;21:650–5.
43. Giannopoulos A, Manousakas T, Gounari A, et al. Comparative evaluation of the diagnostic performance of the BTA stat test, NMP22 and urinary bladder cancer antigen for primary and recurrent bladder tumors. J Urol 2001;166:470–5.
44. Zaak D, Kriegmair M, Stepp H, et al. Endoscopic detection of transitional cell carcinoma with 5-aminolevulinic acid: results of 1012 fluorescence endoscopies. Urology 2001;57:690–4.
45. Riedl CR, Daniltchenko D, Koenig F, et al. Fluorescence endoscopy with 5-aminolevulinic acid reduces early recurrence rate in superficial bladder cancer. J Urol 2001;165:1121–3.
46. Harving N, Wolf H, Melsen F. Positive urinary cytology after tumor resection: an indicator for concomitant carcinoma in situ. J Urol 1988;140:495–7.
47. Hurle R, Losa A, Manzetti A, Lembo A. Upper urinary tract tumors developing after treatment of superficial bladder

cancer: 7-year follow-up of 591 consecutive patients. Urology 1999;53:1144–8.
48. Hatch TR. Barry JM. The value of excretory urography in staging bladder cancer. J Urol 1986;135:49.
49. Montie JE, et al. NCCN practice guidelines in oncology: bladder cancer. National Comprehensive Cancer Network; 2001.
50. Paik ML, Scolieri MJ, Brown SL, et al. Limitations of computerized tomography in staging invasive bladder cancer before radical cystectomy. J Urol 2000;163:1693–6.
51. Tekes A, Kamel I, Imam K, et al. Dynamic MRI of bladder cancer: evaluation of staging accuracy. AJR. Am J Roentgenol 2005;184:121–7.
52. van der Meijden A, Oosterlinck W, Brausi M, et al. Significance of bladder biopsies in Ta,T1 bladder tumors: a report from the EORTC Genito-Urinary Tract Cancer Cooperative Group. EORTC-GU Group Superficial Bladder Committee. Eur Urol 1999;35:267–71.
53. Taguchi I, Gohji K, Hara I, et al. Clinical evaluation of random biopsy of urinary bladder in patients with superficial bladder cancer. Int J Urol 1998;5:30–4.
54. Kiemeney LA, Witjes JA, Heijbroek RP, et al. Should random urothelial biopsies be taken from patients with primary superficial bladder cancer? A decision analysis. Members of the Dutch South-East Co-Operative Urological Group. Br J Urol 1994;73:164–71.
55. Oosterlinck W, Bono AV, Mack D, et al. Frequency of positive biopsies after visual disappearance of superficial bladder cancer marker lesions. Eur Urol 2001;40:515–7.
56. Nixon RG, Chang SS, Lafleur BJ, et al. Carcinoma in situ and tumor multifocality predict the risk of prostatic urethral involvement at radical cystectomy in men with transitional cell carcinoma of the bladder. J Urol 2002;167:502–5.
57. Pagano F, Bassi P, Ferrante GL, et al. Is stage pT4a (D1) reliable in assessing transitional cell carcinoma involvement of the prostate in patients with a concurrent bladder cancer? A necessary distinction for contiguous or noncontiguous involvement. J Urol 1996;155:244–7.
58. Esrig D, Freeman JA, Elmajian DA, et al. Transitional cell carcinoma involving the prostate with a proposed staging classification for stromal invasion. J Urol 1996;156:1071–6.
59. Wijkstrom H, Norming U, Lagerkvist M, et al. Evaluation of clinical staging before cystectomy in transitional cell bladder carcinoma: a long-term follow-up of 276 consecutive patients. Br J Urol 1998;81:686–91.
60. Levy DA, Grossman HB. Staging and prognosis of T3b bladder cancer. Semin Urol Oncol 1996;14:56–61.
61. Dutta SC, Smith JA Jr, Shappell SB, et al. Clinical under staging of high risk nonmuscle invasive urothelial carcinoma treated with radical cystectomy. J Urol 2001;166:490–3.
62. Heney NM. Natural history of superficial bladder cancer. Prognostic features and long-term disease course. Urol Clin North Am 1992;19:429–33.
63. Mostofi M, Davis C, Sesterhenn I. Pathology of tumors of the urinary tract. In: Skinner D, Lieskowsky G, editors. Diagnosis and management of genitourinary cancer. Philadelphia: W.B. Saunders; 1988. p. 83–117.
64. Lebret T, et al. Recurrence, progression and success in stage Ta grade 3 bladder tumors treated with low dose bacillus Calmette-Guérin instillations [comments]. J Urol 2000;163:63–7.
65. Herr HW. Tumor progression and survival of patients with high grade, noninvasive papillary (TaG3) bladder tumors: 15-year outcome. J Urol 2000;163:60–2.
66. Anderstrom C, Johansson S, Nilsson S. The significance of lamina propria invasion on the prognosis of patients with bladder tumors. J Urol 1980;124:23–6.
67. Lopez JI, Angulo JC. The prognostic significance of vascular invasion in stage T1 bladder cancer. Histopathology 1995;27:27–33.
68. Bernardini S, Billerey C, Martin M, et al. The predictive value of muscularis mucosae invasion and p53 over expression on progression of stage T1 bladder carcinoma. J Urol 2001;165:42–46.
69. Bassi P, Ferrante GD, Piazza N, et al. Prognostic factors of outcome after radical cystectomy for bladder cancer: a retrospective study of a homogeneous patient cohort. J Urol 1999;161:1494–7.
70. Kiemeney LA, Witjes JA, Heijbroek RP, et al. Predictability of recurrent and progressive disease in individual patients with primary superficial bladder cancer. J Urol 1993;150:60–4.
71. Cheng L, Weaver AL, Neumann RM, et al. Substaging of T1 bladder carcinoma based on the depth of invasion as measured by micrometer: a new proposal. Cancer 1999;86:1035–43.
72. Lamm DL. Carcinoma in situ. Urol Clin North Am 1992;19:499–508.
73. Heney NM, Ahmed S, Flanagan MJ, et al. Superficial bladder cancer: progression and recurrence. J Urol 1983;130:1083–6.
74. Lamm DL. Long-term results of intravesical therapy for superficial bladder cancer. Urol Clin North Am 1992;19:573–80.
75. Onrust SV, Lamb HM. Valrubicin. Drugs Aging 1999;15:69–76.
76. Palou J, Xavier B, Laguna P, et al. In situ transitional cell carcinoma involvement of prostatic urethra: bacillus Calmette-Guérin therapy without previous transurethral resection of the prostate. Urology 1996;47:482–4.
77. Schellhammer PF, Ladaga LE, Moriarty RP. Intravesical bacillus Calmette-Guérin for the treatment of superficial transitional cell carcinoma of the prostatic urethra in association with carcinoma of the bladder. J Urol 1995;153:53–6.
78. Kim JC, Steinberg GD. The limits of bacillus Calmette-Guérin for carcinoma in situ of the bladder. J Urol 2001;165:745–56.
79. Shelley MD, Kynaston H, Court J, et al. A systematic review of intravesical bacillus Calmette-Guérin plus transurethral resection vs transurethral resection alone in Ta and T1 bladder cancer. BJU Int 2001;88:209–16.
80. Smith JA Jr, Labasky RF, Cockett AT, et al. Bladder cancer clinical guidelines panel summary report on the management of nonmuscle invasive bladder cancer (stages Ta, T1 and TIS). The American Urological Association. J Urol 1999;162:1697–701.
81. Bohle A. BCG's mechanism of action—increasing our understanding. For the EBIN Group. Eur Urol 2000;37 Suppl 1:1–8.
82. Kamat AM, Lamm DL. Intravesical therapy for bladder cancer. Urology 2000;55:161–8.
83. Sylvester RJ, van der Meijden AP, Lamm DL. Intravesical bacillus Calmette-Guérin reduces the risk of progression in patients with superficial bladder cancer: a meta-analysis of the published results of randomized clinical trials. J Urol 2002;168:1964–70.
84. Sylvester RJ, van der Meijden AP, Witjes JA, Kurth K. Bacillus Calmette-Guérin versus chemotherapy for the intravesical treatment of patients with carcinoma in situ of the bladder: a meta-analysis of the published results of randomized clinical trials. J Urol 2005;174:86–92.
85. Davis JW, Sheth SI, Doviak MJ, Schellhammer PF. Superficial bladder carcinoma treated with bacillus Calmette-Guérin: progression-free and disease specific survival with minimum 10-year followup. J Urol 2002;167:494–50l.
86. Cookson MS, Herr HW, Zhang ZF, et al. The treated natural history of high risk superficial bladder cancer: 15-year outcome. J Urol 1997;158:62–7.
87. Sosnowski J, Lamm DL. Immunotherapy of bladder carcinoma. In: Crawford ED, Das S, editors. Current genitourinary cancer surgery. Philadelphia: Lea & Febiger; 1990. p. 480.
88. Lamm DL. BCG immunotherapy for transitional-cell carcinoma in situ of the bladder. Oncology (Huntington) 1995;9:947–52, 955–65.
89. Nadler RB, Catalona WJ, Hudson MA, Ratliff TL. Durability of the tumor-free response for intravesical bacillus Calmette-Guérin therapy. J Urol 1994;152:367–73.
90. Sarosdy MF, Lamm DL. Long-term results of intravesical bacillus Calmette-Guérin therapy for superficial bladder cancer. J Urol 1989;142:719–22.
91. Kavoussi LR, Torrence RJ, Gillen DP, et al. Results of 6 weekly intravesical bacillus Calmette-Guérin instillations on the treatment of superficial bladder tumors. J Urol 1988;139:935–40.
92. Witjes JA, Fransen MP, van der Meijden AP, et al. Use of maintenance intravesical bacillus Calmette-Guérin (BCG), with or without intradermal BCG, in patients with recurrent superficial bladder cancer. Long-term follow-up of a randomized phase 2 study. Urol Int 1993;51:67–72.
93. Lamm DL, Blumenstein BA, Crissman JD, et al. Maintenance bacillus Calmette-Guérin immunotherapy for recurrent TA, T1 and carcinoma in situ transitional cell carcinoma of the bladder: a randomized Southwest Oncology Group Study. J Urol 2000;163:1124–9.
94. Palou J, Laguna P, Millan-Rodriguez F, et al. Control group and maintenance treatment with bacillus Calmette-Guérin for carcinoma in situ and/or high grade bladder tumors. J Urol 2001;165:1488–91.
95. van der Meijden AP, Sylverster RJ, Oosterlinck W, et al. Maintenance bacillus Calmette-Guérin for Ta T1 bladder tumors is not associated with increased toxicity: results from a European Organisation for Research and Treatment of Cancer Genito-Urinary Group phase III trial. Eur Urol 2003;44:429–34.
96. Lamm DL, van der Meijden AP, Morales A, et al. Incidence and treatment of complications of bacillus Calmette-Guérin intravesical therapy in superficial bladder cancer. J Urol 1992;147:596–600.
97. DeHaven JI, Traynellis C, Riggs DR, et al. Antibiotic and steroid therapy of massive systemic bacillus Calmette-Guérin toxicity. J Urol 1992;147:738–42.
98. Kurth K, Tunn U, Ay R, et al. Adjuvant chemotherapy for superficial transitional cell bladder carcinoma: long-term results of a European Organization for Research and Treatment of Cancer randomized trial comparing doxorubicin, ethoglucid and transurethral resection alone. J Urol 1997;158:378–84.
99. Pawinski A, Sylvester R, Kurth KH, et al. A combined analysis of European Organization for Research and Treatment of Cancer, and Medical Research Council randomized clinical trials for the prophylactic treatment of stage TaT1 bladder cancer. European Organization for Research and Treatment of Cancer Genitourinary Tract Cancer Cooperative Group and the Medical Research Council Working Party on Superficial Bladder Cancer. J Urol 1996;156:1934–41.
100. Steinberg G, Bahnson R, Brosman S, et al. Efficacy and safety of valrubicin for the treatment of Bacillus Calmette-Guérin refractory carcinoma in situ of the bladder. The Valrubicin Study Group. J Urol 2000;163:761–7.
101. Witjes JA, van der Meijden AJ, Witjes WP, et al. A randomised prospective study comparing intravesical instillations of mitomycin-C, BCG-Tice, and BCG-RIVM in pTa-pT1 tumours and primary carcinoma in situ of the urinary bladder. Dutch South-East Cooperative Urological Group. Eur J Cancer 1993;29A:1672–6.
102. Martinez-Pineiro JA, Jimenez Leon J, Martinez-Pineiro L Jr, et al. Intravesical therapy comparing BCG, Adriamycin, and thiotepa in 200 patients with superficial bladder cancer: a randomized prospective study. Prog Clin Biol Res 1989;310:237–52.
103. van der Meijden AP, Brausi M, Zambon V, et al. Intravesical instillation of epirubicin, bacillus Calmette-Guérin and bacillus Calmette-Guérin plus isoniazid for intermediate and high risk Ta, T1 papillary carcinoma of the bladder: a European Organization for Research and Treatment of Cancer genito-urinary group randomized phase III trial. J Urol 2001;166:476–81.
104. Melekos MD, Zarakovitis I, Dandinis K, et al. BCG versus epirubicin in the prophylaxis of multiple superficial bladder tumours: results of a prospective randomized study using modified treatment schemes. Int Urol Nephrol 1996;28:499–509.
105. Belldegrun AS, Franklin JR, O'Donnell MA, et al. Superficial bladder cancer: the role of interferon-alpha. J Urol 1998;159:1793–801.
106. Kalble T, Beer M, Mendoza E, et al. [BCG vs interferon A for prevention of recurrence of superficial bladder cancer. A prospective randomized study]. Urologe A 1994;33:133–7.
107. Jimenez-Cruz JF, Vera-Donoso CD, Leiva O, et al. Intravesical immunoprophylaxis in recurrent superficial bladder cancer (stage T1): multicenter trial comparing bacille Calmette-Guérin and interferon-alpha. Urology 1997;50:529–35.
108. Malmstrom PU. A randomized comparative dose-ranging study of interferon-alpha and mitomycin-C as an internal control in primary or recurrent superficial transitional cell carcinoma of the bladder. BJU Int 2002;89:681–6.
109. Portillo J, Martin B, Hernandez R, et al. Results at 43 months' follow-up of a double-blind, randomized, prospective clinical trial using intravesical interferon alpha-2b in the prophylaxis of stage pT1 transitional cell carcinoma of the bladder. Urology 1997;49:187–90.
110. Papatsoris AG, Deliveliotis C, Giannopoulos A, Dimopoulos C. Adjuvant intravesical mitoxantrone versus recombinant interferon-alpha after transurethral resection of superficial bladder cancer: a randomized prospective study. Urol Int 2004;72:284–91.
111. Giannakopoulos S, Gekas A, Alivizatos G, et al. Efficacy of escalating doses of intravesical interferon alpha-2b in reducing recurrence rate and progression in superficial transitional cell carcinoma. Br J Urol 1998;82:829–34.
112. O'Donnell MA, Lilli K, Leopold C, et al. Interim results from a national multicenter phase II trial of combination bacillus Calmette-Guérin plus interferon alfa-2b for superficial bladder cancer. J Urol 2004;172:888–93.
113. Prout GR Jr, Lin CW, Benson R Jr, et al. Photodynamic therapy with hematoporphyrin derivative in the treatment of superficial transitional-cell carcinoma of the bladder. N Engl J Med 1987;317:1251–5.
114. Walther MM. The role of photodynamic therapy in the treatment of recurrent superficial bladder cancer. Urol Clin North Am 2000;27:163–70.

115. Filbeck T, Pichlmeier U, Knuechel R, et al. Clinically relevant improvement of recurrence-free survival with 5-aminolevulinic acid induced fluorescence diagnosis in patients with superficial bladder tumors. J Urol 2002;168:67–71.
116. Herr HW, Sogani PC. Does early cystectomy improve the survival of patients with high risk superficial bladder tumors? J Urol 2001;166:1296–9.
117. Thalmann GN, Markwalder R, Shahin O, et al. Primary T1G3 bladder cancer: organ preserving approach or immediate cystectomy? J Urol 2004;172:70–5.
118. Solsona E, Iborra I, Rubio J, et al. The optimum timing of radical cystectomy for patients with recurrent high-risk superficial bladder tumour. BJU Int 2004;94:1258–62.
119. Masood S, Sriprasad S, Palmer JH, Mufti GR. T1G3 bladder cancer—indications for early cystectomy. Int Urol Nephrol 2004;36:41–4.
120. Ather MH, Fatima S, Sinanoglu O. Extent of lymphadenectomy in radical cystectomy for bladder cancer. World J Surg Oncol 2005;3:43.
121. Whitmore WF Jr, Marshall V. Radical total cystectomy for cancer of the bladder: 230 consecutive cases five years later. J Urol 1962;87:853–68.
122. Pagano F, Bassi P, Galetti TP, et al. Results of contemporary radical cystectomy for invasive bladder cancer: a clinicopathological study with an emphasis on the inadequacy of the tumor, nodes and metastases classification. J Urol 1991;145:45–50.
123. Stein JP, Lieskovsky G, Cote R, et al. Radical cystectomy in the treatment of invasive bladder cancer: long-term results in 1,054 patients. J Clin Oncol 2001;19:666–75.
124. Bassi P. Outcome of radical cystectomy for invasive bladder cancer. Curr Opin Urol 2000;10:459–63.
125. Cheng L, Weaver AL, Leibovich BC, et al. Predicting the survival of bladder carcinoma patients treated with radical cystectomy. Cancer 2000;88:2326–32.
126. Wishnow KI, Tenney DM. Will Rogers and the results of radical cystectomy for invasive bladder cancer. Urol Clin North Am 1991;18:529–37.
127. Ghoneim MA, el-Mekresh MM, el-Baz MA, et al. Radical cystectomy for carcinoma of the bladder: critical evaluation of the results in 1,026 cases. J Urol 1997;158:393–9.
128. Mills RD, Turner WH, Fleischmann A, et al. Pelvic lymph node metastases from bladder cancer: outcome in 83 patients after radical cystectomy and pelvic lymphadenectomy. J Urol 2001;166:19–23.
129. Herr HW, Donat SM. Outcome of patients with grossly node positive bladder cancer after pelvic lymph node dissection and radical cystectomy. J Urol 2001;165:62–4.
130. Cathelineau X, Arroyo C, Rozet F, et al. Laparoscopic assisted radical cystectomy: the Montsouris experience after 84 cases. Eur Urol 2005;47:780–4.
131. DeGer S, Peters R, Roigas J, et al. Laparoscopic radical cystectomy with continent urinary diversion (rectosigmoid pouch) performed completely intracorporeally: an intermediate functional and oncologic analysis. Urology 2004;64:935–9.
132. Ukimura O, Moinzadeh A, Gill IS. Laparoscopic radical cystectomy and urinary diversion. Curr Urol Rep 2005;6:118–21.
133. Tal R, Baniel J. Sexual function-preserving cystectomy. Urology 2005. [In press]
134. Arroyo C, Andrews H, Rozet F, et al. Laparoscopic prostate-sparing radical cystectomy: the Montsouris technique and preliminary results. J Endourol 2005;19:424–8.
135. Malavaud B, Vaessen C, Mouzin M, et al. Complications for radical cystectomy. Impact of the American Society of Anesthesiologists score. Eur Urol 2001;39:79–84.
136. Iselin CE, Robertson CN, Webster GD, et al. Does prostate transitional cell carcinoma preclude orthotopic bladder reconstruction after radical cystoprostatectomy for bladder cancer? J Urol 1997;158:2123–6.
137. Freeman JA, Tarter TA, Esrig D, et al. Urethral recurrence in patients with orthotopic ileal neobladders. J Urol 1996;156:1615–9.
138. Stein JP, Clark P, Miranda G, et al. Urethral tumor recurrence following cystectomy and urinary diversion: clinical and pathological characteristics in 768 male patients. J Urol 2005;173:1163–8.
139. Stein JP, Grossfeld GD, Freeman JA, et al. Orthotopic lower urinary tract reconstruction in women using the Kock ileal neobladder: updated experience in 34 patients [comments]. J Urol 1997;158:400–5.
140. Miyao N, Adachi H, Sato Y, et al. Recovery of sexual function after nerve-sparing radical prostatectomy or cystectomy. Int J Urol 2001;8:158–64.
141. Venn SN, Popert RM, Mundy AR. 'Nerve-sparing' cystectomy and substitution cystoplasty in patients of either sex: limitations and techniques. Br J Urol 1998;82:361–5.
142. Schoenberg MP, Walsh PC, Breazeale DR, et al. Local recurrence and survival following nerve sparing radical cystoprostatectomy for bladder cancer: 10-year followup. J Urol 1996;155:490–4.
143. Zippe CD, Raina R, Shah AD, et al. Female sexual dysfunction after radical cystectomy: a new outcome measure. Urology 2004;63:1153–7.
144. Smith JA Jr, Batata M, Grabstald H, et al. Preoperative irradiation and cystectomy for bladder cancer. Cancer 1982;49:869–73.
145. Skinner DG, Lieskovsky G. Contemporary cystectomy with pelvic node dissection compared to preoperative radiation therapy plus cystectomy in management of invasive bladder cancer. J Urol 1984;131:1069–72.
146. Smith JA Jr, Crawford ED, Paradelo JC, et al. Treatment of advanced bladder cancer with combined preoperative irradiation and radical cystectomy versus radical cystectomy alone: a phase III intergroup study. J Urol 1997;157:805–8.
147. Parsons JT, Million RR. Planned preoperative irradiation in the management of clinical stage B2-C (T3) bladder carcinoma. Int J Radiat Oncol Biol Phys 1988;14:797–810.
148. Cole CJ, Pollack A, Zagars GK, et al. Local control of muscle-invasive bladder cancer: preoperative radiotherapy and cystectomy versus cystectomy alone. Int J Radiat Oncol Biol Phys 1995;32:331–40.
149. Whitmore WF. Integrated irradiation and cystectomy for bladder cancer. Br J Urol 1980;52:1–9.
150. Housset M, Maulard C, Chretien Y, et al. Combined radiation and chemotherapy for invasive transitional-cell carcinoma of the bladder: a prospective study. J Clin Oncol 1993;11:2150–7.
151. Zaghloul MS, Awwad HK, Akoush HH, et al. Postoperative radiotherapy of carcinoma in bilharzial bladder: improved disease free survival through improving local control. Int J Radiat Oncol Biol Phys 1992;23:511–7.
152. Fromenti SC. Management of patients with pelvic recurrence following radical cystectomy. In: Petrovich Z, Baert L, editors. Carcinoma of the urinary bladder: innovation in management. Berlin: Springer-Verlag; 1998. p. 249–58.
153. Reisinger SA, Mohiuddin M, Mulholland SG. Combined pre- and postoperative adjuvant radiation therapy for bladder cancer—a ten year experience. Int J Radiat Oncol Biol Phys 1992;24:463–8.
154. Holzbeierlein JM, Lopez-Corona E, Bochner BH, et al. Partial cystectomy: a contemporary review of the Memorial Sloan-Kettering Cancer Center experience and recommendations for patient selection. J Urol 2004;172:878–81.
155. Sweeney P, Kursh ED, Resnick MI. Partial cystectomy. Urol Clin North Am 1992;19:701–11.
156. Jahnson S, Pedersen J, Westman G. Bladder carcinoma—a 20-year review of radical irradiation therapy. Radiother Oncol 1991;22:111–7.
157. Bloom HJ, Hendry WF, Wallace DM, Skeet RG. Treatment of T3 bladder cancer: controlled trial of pre-operative radiotherapy and radical cystectomy versus radical radiotherapy. Br J Urol 1982;54:136–51.
158. Gospodarowicz MK, Hawkins NV, Rawlings GA, et al. Radical radiotherapy for muscle invasive transitional cell carcinoma of the bladder: failure analysis. J Urol 1989;142:1448–54.
159. Mameghan H, Fisher R, Mameghan J, Brook S. Analysis of failure following definitive radiotherapy for invasive transitional cell carcinoma of the bladder. Int J Radiat Oncol Biol Phys 1995;31:247–54.
160. Blandy JP, England HR, Evans SJ, et al. T3 bladder cancer—the case for salvage cystectomy. Br J Urol 1980;52:506–10.
161. Shipley WU, Rose MA. Bladder cancer. The selection of patients for treatment by full-dose irradiation. Cancer 1985;55:2278–84.
162. Dunst J, Sauer R, Schrott KM, et al. Organ-sparing treatment of advanced bladder cancer: a 10-year experience. Int J Radiat Oncol Biol Phys 1994;30:261–6.
163. Sell A, Jakobsen A, Nerstrom B, et al. Treatment of advanced bladder cancer category T2 T3 and T4a. A randomized multicenter study of preoperative irradiation and cystectomy versus radical irradiation and early salvage cystectomy for residual tumor. DAVECA protocol 8201. Danish Vesical Cancer Group. Scand J Urol Nephrol Suppl 1991;138:193–201.
164. Mommsen S, Jakobsen A, Sell A. Quality of life in patients with advanced bladder cancer. A randomized study comparing cystectomy and irradiation—the Danish Bladder Cancer Study Group (DAVECA protocol 8201). Scand J Urol Nephrol Suppl 1989;125:115–20.
165. Caffo O, Fellin G, Graffer U, Luciani L. Assessment of quality of life after cystectomy or conservative therapy for patients with infiltrating bladder carcinoma. A survey by a self-administered questionnaire. Cancer 1996;78:1089–97.
166. Richards B, Bastable JR, Freedman L, et al. Adjuvant chemotherapy with doxorubicin (Adriamycin) and 5-fluorouracil in T3, NX, MO bladder cancer treated with radiotherapy. Br J Urol 1983;55:386–91.
167. Shearer RJ, Chilvers CF, Bloom HJ, et al. Adjuvant chemotherapy in T3 carcinoma of the bladder. A prospective trial: preliminary report. Br J Urol 1988;62:558–64.
168. Coppin CM, Gospodarowicz MK, James K, et al. Improved local control of invasive bladder cancer by concurrent cisplatin and preoperative or definitive radiation. The National Cancer Institute of Canada Clinical Trials Group. J Clin Oncol 1996;14:2901–7.
169. Shipley WU, Winter KA, Kaufman DS, et al. Phase III trial of neoadjuvant chemotherapy in patients with invasive bladder cancer treated with selective bladder preservation by combined radiation therapy and chemotherapy: initial results of Radiation Therapy Oncology Group 89-03. J Clin Oncol 1998;16:3576–83.
170. Zietman AL, Shipley WU, Kaufman DS, et al. A phase I/II trial of transurethral surgery combined with concurrent cisplatin, 5-fluorouracil and twice daily radiation followed by selective bladder preservation in operable patients with muscle invading bladder cancer. J Urol 1998;160:1673–7.
171. Rodel C, Grabenbauer GG, Kuhn R, et al. Organ preservation in patients with invasive bladder cancer: initial results of an intensified protocol of transurethral surgery and radiation therapy plus concurrent cisplatin and 5-fluorouracil. Int J Radiat Oncol Biol Phys 2002;52:1303–9.
172. Hussain MH, Glass TR, Forman J, et al. Combination cisplatin, 5-fluorouracil and radiation therapy for locally advanced unresectable or medically unfit bladder cancer cases: a Southwest Oncology Group Study. J Urol 2001;165:56–61.
173. Sauer R, Birkenhake S, Kuhn R, et al. Efficacy of radiochemotherapy with platin derivatives compared to radiotherapy alone in organ-sparing treatment of bladder cancer. Int J Radiat Oncol Biol Phys 1998;40:121–7.
174. Housset M, Dufour E, Maulard-Durtux C. Concomitant 5-fluorouracil cisplatin and bifractionated split course radiation therapy for bladder cancer [abstract 1139]. Proc Am Soc Clin Oncol 1997;16:319.
175. Dufour B, Housset M, Chretien Y, et al. [Infiltrating cancer of the bladder. Is concomitant radiochemotherapy an alternative to cystectomy?]. Chirurgie 1996;121:187–92.
176. Shipley WU, Kaufman DS, Zehr E, et al. Selective bladder preservation by combined modality protocol treatment: long-term outcomes for 190 patients with invasive bladder cancer. Urology 2002;60:62–8.
177. Tester W, Porter A, Asbell S, et al. Combined modality program with possible organ preservation for invasive bladder carcinoma: results of RTOG protocol 85-12. Int J Radiat Oncol Biol Phys 1993;25:783–90.
178. Kim HL, Steinberg GD. The current status of bladder preservation in the treatment of muscle invasive bladder cancer. J Urol 2000;164:627–32.
179. Dalbagni G, Genega E, Hashibe M, et al. Cystectomy for bladder cancer: a contemporary series. J Urol 2001;165:1111–6.
180. Martinez-Pineiro JA, Gonzalez Martin M, Arocena F, et al. Neoadjuvant cisplatin chemotherapy before radical cystectomy in invasive transitional cell carcinoma of the bladder: a prospective randomized phase III study. J Urol 1995;153:964–73.
181. Cole DJ, Durrant KR, Roberts JT, et al. A pilot study of accelerated fractionation in the radiotherapy of invasive carcinoma of the bladder. Br J Radiol 1992;65:792–8.
182. Kaufman DS, Winter KA, Shipley WU, et al. The initial results in muscle-invading bladder cancer of RTOG 95-06: phase I/II trial of transurethral surgery plus radiation therapy with concurrent cisplatin and 5-fluorouracil followed by selective bladder preservation or cystectomy depending on the initial response. Oncologist 2000;5:471–6.
183. Herr HW. Transurethral resection of muscle-invasive bladder cancer: 10-year outcome. J Clin Oncol 2001;19:89–93.
184. Sternberg CN, Arena MG, Calabresi F, et al. Neoadjuvant M-VAC (methotrexate, vinblastine, doxorubicin, and cisplatin) for infiltrating transitional cell carcinoma of the bladder. Cancer 1993;72:1975–82.
185. Herr HW, Bajorin DF, Scher HI. Neoadjuvant chemotherapy and bladder-sparing surgery for invasive bladder cancer: ten-year outcome. J Clin Oncol 1998;16:1298–301.
186. Zietman AL, Grocela J, Zehr E, et al. Selective bladder conservation using transurethral resection, chemotherapy,

and radiation: management and consequences of Ta, T1, and Tis recurrence within the retained bladder. Urology 2001;58:380–5.

187. Kachnic LA, Kaufman DS, Heney NM, et al. Bladder preservation by combined modality therapy for invasive bladder cancer. J Clin Oncol 1997;15:1022–9.

188. Zietman AL, et al. Organ conservation as an alternative to radical cystectomy for invasive bladder cancer: urodynamic and quality of life evaluation of patients treated by trimodality therapy. Int J Radiat Oncol Biol Phys 2002. [In press]

189. Advanced Bladder Cancer Meta-Analysis Collaboration. Neoadjuvant chemotherapy in invasive bladder cancer: a systematic review and meta-analysis. Lancet 2003;361:1927–34.

190. Winquist E, Kirchner TS, Segal R, et al. Neoadjuvant chemotherapy for transitional cell carcinoma of the bladder: a systematic review and meta-analysis. J Urol 2004;171:561–9.

191. Anonymous. Neoadjuvant cisplatin, methotrexate, and vinblastine chemotherapy for muscle-invasive bladder cancer: a randomised controlled trial. International collaboration of trialists. Lancet 1999;354:533–40.

192. Wallace DM, Raghavan D, Kelly KA, et al. Neo-adjuvant (pre-emptive) cisplatin therapy in invasive transitional cell carcinoma of the bladder. Br J Urol 1991;67:608–15.

193. Loehrer PJ Sr, Einhorn LH, Elson PJ, et al. A randomized comparison of cisplatin alone or in combination with methotrexate, vinblastine, and doxorubicin in patients with metastatic urothelial carcinoma: a cooperative group study. J Clin Oncol 1992;10:1066–73.

194. Sherif A, Holmberg L, Rintala E, et al. Neoadjuvant cisplatinum based combination chemotherapy in patients with invasive bladder cancer: a combined analysis of two Nordic studies. Eur Urol 2004;45:297–303.

195. Sherif A, Rintala E, Mestad O, et al. Neoadjuvant cisplatin-methotrexate chemotherapy for invasive bladder cancer—Nordic cystectomy trial 2. Scand J Urol Nephrol 2002;36:419–25.

196. Herr HW, Donat SM, Bajorin DF. Post-chemotherapy surgery in patients with unresectable or regionally metastatic bladder cancer. J Urol 2001;165:811–4.

197. Sylvester R, Sternberg C. The role of adjuvant combination chemotherapy after cystectomy in locally advanced bladder cancer: what we do not know and why. Ann Oncol 2000;11:851–6.

198. Skinner DG, et al. The role of adjuvant chemotherapy following cystectomy for invasive bladder cancer: a prospective comparative trial. J Urol 1991;145:459–67.

199. Stockle M, Meyenburg W, Wellek S, et al. Advanced bladder cancer (stages pT3b, pT4a, pN1 and pN2): improved survival after radical cystectomy and 3 adjuvant cycles of chemotherapy. Results of a controlled prospective study. J Urol 1992;148:302–7.

200. Freiha F, Reese J, Torti FM. A randomized trial of radical cystectomy versus radical cystectomy plus cisplatin, vinblastine and methotrexate chemotherapy for muscle invasive bladder cancer. J Urol 1996;155:495–500.

201. Sternberg CN, de Mulder PH, Schornagel JH, et al. Randomized phase III trial of high-dose-intensity methotrexate, vinblastine, doxorubicin, and cisplatin (MVAC) chemotherapy and recombinant human granulocyte colony-stimulating factor versus classic MVAC in advanced urothelial tract tumors: European Organization for Research and Treatment of Cancer Protocol no. 30924. J Clin Oncol 2001; 19:2638–46.

202. Bajorin DF, Dodd PM, Mazumdar M, et al. Long-term survival in metastatic transitional-cell carcinoma and prognostic factors predicting outcome of therapy. J Clin Oncol 1999;17:3173–81.

203. Saxman SB, Propert KJ, Einhorn LH, et al. Long-term follow-up of a phase III intergroup study of cisplatin alone or in combination with methotrexate, vinblastine, and doxorubicin in patients with metastatic urothelial carcinoma: a cooperative group study. J Clin Oncol 1997;15:2564–9.

204. Logothetis CJ, Dexeus FH, Finn L, et al. A prospective randomized trial comparing MVAC and CISCA chemotherapy for patients with metastatic urothelial tumors. J Clin Oncol 1990;8:1050–5.

205. Mead GM, Russell M, Clark P, et al. A randomized trial comparing methotrexate and vinblastine (MV) with cisplatin, methotrexate and vinblastine (CMV) in advanced transitional cell carcinoma: results and a report on prognostic factors in a Medical Research Council study. MRC Advanced Bladder Cancer Working Party. Br J Cancer 1998;78:1067–75.

206. Sternberg CN, Yagoda A, Scher HI, et al. Methotrexate, vinblastine, doxorubicin, and cisplatin for advanced transitional cell carcinoma of the urothelium. Efficacy and patterns of response and relapse. Cancer 1989;64:2448–58.

207. Harker WG, Meyers FJ, Freiha FS, et al. Cisplatin, methotrexate, and vinblastine (CMV): an effective chemotherapy regimen for metastatic transitional cell carcinoma of the urinary tract. A Northern California Oncology Group study. J Clin Oncol 1985;3:1463–70.

208. von der Maase H, Hansen SW, Roberts JT, et al. Gemcitabine and cisplatin versus methotrexate, vinblastine, doxorubicin, and cisplatin in advanced or metastatic bladder cancer: results of a large, randomized, multinational, multicenter, phase III study. J Clin Oncol 2000;18:3068–77.

209. Fukui I, Yonese J, Tsukamoto T, et al. Combination chemotherapy with ifosfamide, 5-fluorouracil, etoposide and cisplatin for metastatic urothelial cancer. Cancer Chemother Pharmacol 2001;48:88–93.

210. Seidman AD, Scher HI, Gabrilove JL, et al. Dose-intensification of MVAC with recombinant granulocyte colony-stimulating factor as initial therapy in advanced urothelial cancer. J Clin Oncol 1993;11:408–14.

211. Loehrer PJ Sr, Elson P, Dreicer R, et al. Escalated dosages of methotrexate, vinblastine, doxorubicin, and cisplatin plus recombinant human granulocyte colony-stimulating factor in advanced urothelial carcinoma: an Eastern Cooperative Oncology Group trial. J Clin Oncol 1994;12:483–8.

212. Tannock I, Gospodarowicz M, Connolly J, Jewett M. M-VAC (methotrexate, vinblastine, doxorubicin and cisplatin) chemotherapy for transitional cell carcinoma: the Princess Margaret Hospital experience. J Urol 1989;142:289–92.

213. Igawa M, Ohkuchi T, Ueki T, et al. Usefulness and limitations of methotrexate, vinblastine, doxorubicin and cisplatin for the treatment of advanced urothelial cancer. J Urol 1990;144:662–5.

214. von der Maase H, Sengelov L, Roberts JT, et al. Long-term survival results of a randomized trial comparing gemcitabine plus cisplatin, with methotrexate, vinblastine, doxorubicin, plus cisplatin in patients with bladder cancer. J Clin Oncol 2005;23:4602–8.

215. Wiens BL. Choosing an equivalence limit for noninferiority or equivalence studies. Control Clin Trials 2002;23:2–14.

216. Jones B, Jarvis P, Lewis JA, Ebbutt AF. Trials to assess equivalence: the importance of rigorous methods. BMJ 1996;313:36–9.

217. Cohen MH, Rothmann M. Gemcitabine and cisplatin for advanced, metastatic bladder cancer. J Clin Oncol 2001;19:1229–31.

218. Boccardo F, et al. Carboplatin, methotrexate, and vinblastine in the treatment of patients with advanced urothelial cancer. A phase II trial. Cancer 1994;73:1932–6.

219. Igawa M, Kadena H, Ueda M, Usui T. M-VEC (methotrexate, vinblastine, epirubicin, and cisplatin) with granulocyte colony-stimulating factor for the treatment of urothelial cancer: an effective and safe chemotherapy regimen. Cancer Chemother Pharmacol 1994;35:S1–.

220. Petrioli R, Frediani B, Manganelli A, et al. Comparison between a cisplatin-containing regimen and a carboplatin-containing regimen for recurrent or metastatic bladder cancer patients. A randomized phase II study. Cancer 1996;77:344–51.

221. Bellmunt J, Ribas A, Fres N, et al. Carboplatin-based versus cisplatin-based chemotherapy in the treatment of surgically incurable advanced bladder carcinoma. Cancer 1997;80:1966–72.

222. Siefker-Radtke AO, Millikan RE, Tu SM, et al. Phase III trial of fluorouracil, interferon alpha-2b, and cisplatin versus methotrexate, vinblastine, doxorubicin, and cisplatin in metastatic or unresectable urothelial cancer. J Clin Oncol 2002;20:1361–7.

223. Dreicer R, Manola J, Roth BJ, et al. Phase II study of cisplatin and paclitaxel in advanced carcinoma of the urothelium: an Eastern Cooperative Oncology Group Study. J Clin Oncol 2000;18:1058–61.

224. Burch PA, Richardson RL, Cha SS, et al. Phase II study of paclitaxel and cisplatin for advanced urothelial cancer. J Urol 2000;164:1538–42.

225. Pycha A, Grbovic M, Posch B, et al. Paclitaxel and carboplatin in patients with metastatic transitional cell cancer of the urinary tract. Urology 1999;53:510–5.

226. Small EJ, Lew D, Redman BG, et al. Southwest Oncology Group Study of paclitaxel and carboplatin for advanced transitional-cell carcinoma: the importance of survival as a clinical trial end point. J Clin Oncol 2000;18:2537–44.

227. Vaughn DJ, Malkowicz SB, Zoltick B, et al. Paclitaxel plus carboplatin in advanced carcinoma of the urothelium: an active and tolerable outpatient regimen. J Clin Oncol 1998;16:255–60.

228. Redman BG, Smith DC, Flaherty L, et al. Phase II trial of paclitaxel and carboplatin in the treatment of advanced urothelial carcinoma. J Clin Oncol 1998;16:1844–8.

229. Carles J, Nogue M. Gemcitabine/carboplatin in advanced urothelial cancer. Semin Oncol 2001;28:19–24.

230. Bellmunt J, de Wit R, Albanell J, Baselga J. A feasibility study of carboplatin with fixed dose of gemcitabine in "unfit" patients with advanced bladder cancer. Eur J Cancer 2001;37:2212–5.

231. Hussain M, Vaishampayan U, Du W, et al. Combination paclitaxel, carboplatin, and gemcitabine is an active treatment for advanced urothelial cancer. J Clin Oncol 2001;19:2527–33.

232. Bellmunt J, Guillem V, Paz-Ares L, et al. Phase I-II study of paclitaxel, cisplatin, and gemcitabine in advanced transitional-cell carcinoma of the urothelium. Spanish Oncology Genitourinary Group. J Clin Oncol 2000;18:3247–55.

233. Lorusso V, Crucitta E, Silvestris N, et al. Randomised, open-label, phase II trial of paclitaxel, gemcitabine and cisplatin versus gemcitabine and cisplatin as first-line chemotherapy in advanced transitional cell carcinoma of the urothelium. Oncol Rep 2005;13:283–7.

234. Sternberg CN, Calabro F, Pizzocaro G, et al. Chemotherapy with an every-2-week regimen of gemcitabine and paclitaxel in patients with transitional cell carcinoma who have received prior cisplatin-based therapy. Cancer 2001;92:2993–8.

235. Meluch AA, Greco FA, Burris HA 3rd, et al. Paclitaxel and gemcitabine chemotherapy for advanced transitional-cell carcinoma of the urothelial tract: a phase II trial of the Minnie Pearl cancer research network. J Clin Oncol 2001;19:3018–24.

236. Bajorin DF, McCaffrey JA, Dodd PM, et al. Ifosfamide, paclitaxel, and cisplatin for patients with advanced transitional cell carcinoma of the urothelial tract: final report of a phase II trial evaluating two dosing schedules. Cancer 2000;88:1671–8.

237. Garcia del Muro X, Marcuello E, Guma J, et al. Phase II multicentre study of docetaxel plus cisplatin in patients with advanced urothelial cancer. Br J Cancer 2002;86:326–30.

238. Dimopoulos MA, Bakoyannis C, Georgoulias V, et al. Docetaxel and cisplatin combination chemotherapy in advanced carcinoma of the urothelium: a multicenter phase II study of the Hellenic Cooperative Oncology Group. Ann Oncol 1999;10:1385–8.

239. Sengelov L, Kamby C, Lund B, Engelholm SA. Docetaxel and cisplatin in metastatic urothelial cancer: a phase II study. J Clin Oncol 1998;16:3392–7.

240. Pectasides D, Visvikis A, Aspropotamitis A, et al. Chemotherapy with cisplatin, epirubicin and docetaxel in transitional cell urothelial cancer. Phase II trial. Eur J Cancer 2000;36:74–9.

241. Pectasides D, Glotsos J, Bountouroglou N, et al. Weekly chemotherapy with docetaxel, gemcitabine and cisplatin in advanced transitional cell urothelial cancer: a phase II trial. Ann Oncol 2002;13:243–50.

242. Dunsford ML, Mead GM, Bateman AC, et al. Severe pulmonary toxicity in patients treated with a combination of docetaxel and gemcitabine for metastatic transitional cell carcinoma. Ann Oncol 1999;10:943–7.

243. Fagg SL, Dawson-Edwards P, Hughes MA, et al. Cis-diamminedichloroplatinum (DDP) as initial treatment of invasive bladder cancer. Br J Urol 1984;56:296–300.

244. Herr HW. Cis-diamminedichloride platinum II in the treatment of advanced bladder cancer. J Urol 1980;123:853–5.

245. Oliver RT, Newlands ES, Wiltshaw E, Malpas JS. A phase 2 study of Cis-platinum in patients with recurrent bladder carcinoma. The London and Oxford Co-operative Urological Cancer Group. Br J Urol 1981;53:444–7.

246. Yagoda A. Phase II trials with cis-dichlorodiammineplatinum(II) in the treatment of urothelial cancer. Cancer Treat Rep 1979;63:1565–72.

247. Soloway MS, Ikard M, Ford K. Cis-diamminedichloroplatinum (II) in locally advanced and metastatic urothelial cancer. Cancer 1981;47:476–80.

248. Barnes J, Calvert A, Freedman LS, et al. A phase II study of carboplatin in metastatic transitional cell carcinoma of the bladder. Eur J Cancer Clin Oncol 1987;23:375–7.

249. Micetich K, et al. A phase II trial of carboplatin in patients with urinary tract malignancy. In: Bunn P, Canetta R, Ozols R, editors. Carboplatin (JM-8): current perspectives and future directions. Philadelphia: W.B. Saunders; 1990. p. 92–7.

250. Dreicer R, Gustin DM, See WA, Williams RD. Paclitaxel in advanced urothelial carcinoma: its role in patients with renal insufficiency and as salvage therapy. J Urol 1996;156:1606–8.
251. McCaffrey JA, Hilton S, Mazumdar M, et al. Phase II trial of docetaxel in patients with advanced or metastatic transitional-cell carcinoma. J Clin Oncol 1997;15:1853–7.
252. Roth BJ, Dreicer R, Einhorn LH, et al. Significant activity of paclitaxel in advanced transitional-cell carcinoma of the urothelium: a phase II trial of the Eastern Cooperative Oncology Group. J Clin Oncol 1994;12:2264–70.
253. Yang MH, Yen CC, Chang YH, et al. Single agent paclitaxel as a first-line therapy in advanced urothelial carcinoma: its efficacy and safety in patients even with pretreatment renal insufficiency. Jpn J Clin Oncol 2000;30:547–52.
254. Papamichael D, Gallagher CJ, Oliver RT, et al. Phase II study of paclitaxel in pretreated patients with locally advanced/metastatic cancer of the bladder and ureter. Br J Cancer 1997;75:606–7.
255. Vaughn DJ, Broome CM, Hussain M, et al. Phase II trial of weekly paclitaxel in patients with previously treated advanced urothelial cancer. J Clin Oncol 2002;20:937–40.
256. de Wit R, Kruit WH, Stoter G, et al. Docetaxel (Taxotere): an active agent in metastatic urothelial cancer; results of a phase II study in non-chemotherapy-pretreated patients. Br J Cancer 1998;78:1342–5.
257. Dimopoulos MA, Deliveliotis C, Moulopoulos LA, et al. Treatment of patients with metastatic urothelial carcinoma and impaired renal function with single-agent docetaxel. Urology 1998;52:56–60.
258. Stadler WM, Kuzel T, Roth B, et al. Phase II study of single-agent gemcitabine in previously untreated patients with metastatic urothelial cancer. J Clin Oncol 1997;15:3394–8.
259. Moore MJ, Tannock IF, Ernst DS, et al. Gemcitabine: a promising new agent in the treatment of advanced urothelial cancer. J Clin Oncol 1997;15:3441–5.
260. Lorusso V, Pollera CF, Antimi M, et al. A phase II study of gemcitabine in patients with transitional cell carcinoma of the urinary tract previously treated with platinum. Italian Co-operative Group on Bladder Cancer. Eur J Cancer 1998;34:1208–12.
261. Witte RS, Elson P, Bono B, et al. Eastern Cooperative Oncology Group phase II trial of ifosfamide in the treatment of previously treated advanced urothelial carcinoma. J Clin Oncol 1997;15:589–93.
262. Seligman PA, Crawford ED. Treatment of advanced transitional cell carcinoma of the bladder with continuous-infusion gallium nitrate. J Natl Cancer Inst 1991;83:1582–4.
263. Steinick G, Cordon-Cardo C, Scher HI. Bladder cancer. In: Schrier RW, Gottschalk CW, editors. Diseases of the kidney. Boston: Little Brown; 1996. p. 803–21.
264. Pollera CF, Cerebelli A, Crecco M, Calabresi F. Weekly gemcitabine in advanced bladder cancer: a preliminary report from a phase I study. Ann Oncol 1994;5:182–4.
265. Tu SM, Hossan E, Amato R, et al. Paclitaxel, cisplatin and methotrexate combination chemotherapy is active in the treatment of refractory urothelial malignancies. J Urol 1995;154:1719–22.
266. Krege S, Rembrink V, Borgermann C, et al. Docetaxel and ifosfamide as second line treatment for patients with advanced or metastatic urothelial cancer after failure of platinum chemotherapy: a phase 2 study. J Urol 2001;165:67–71.
267. Sweeney CJ, Williams SD, Finch DE, et al. A phase II study of paclitaxel and ifosfamide for patients with advanced refractory carcinoma of the urothelium. Cancer 1999;86:514–8.
268. De Mulder PH, Theodore C, Sella A, et al. Phase II EORTC trial with 5-fluorouracil, cisplatin and interferon-alpha as second-line treatment of advanced transitional cell cancer of the urothelial tract. Ann Oncol 2000;11:1391–4.
269. Gill HS, Dhillon HK, Woodhouse CR. Adenocarcinoma of the urinary bladder. Br J Urol 1989;64:138–42.
270. Blute ML, Engen DE, Travis WD, Kvols LK. Primary signet ring cell adenocarcinoma of the bladder. J Urol 1989;141:17–21.
271. Fiter L, Gimeno F, Martin L, Gomez Tejeda L. Signet-ring cell adenocarcinoma of bladder. Urology 1993;41:30–3.
272. Henly DR, Farrow GM, Zincke H. Urachal cancer: role of conservative surgery. Urology 1993;42:635–9.
273. Brick SH, Friedman AC, Pollack HM, et al. Urachal carcinoma: CT findings. Radiology 1988;169:377–81.
274. Kajita Y, Habuchi T, Kamoto T, et al. [Long-term clinical results of 5 cases of urachal carcinoma]. Hinyokika Kiyo 2000;46:711–4.
275. Nakanishi K, Kawai T, Suzuki M, Torikata C. Prognostic factors in urachal adenocarcinoma. A study in 41 specimens of DNA status, proliferating cell-nuclear antigen immunostaining, and argyrophilic nucleolar-organizer region counts. Hum Pathol 1996;27:240–7.
276. Kawakami S, Kageyama Y, Yonese J, et al. Successful treatment of metastatic adenocarcinoma of the urachus: report of 2 cases with more than 10-year survival. Urology 2001;58:462.
277. Bejany DE, Lockhart JL, Rhamy RK. Malignant vesical tumors following spinal cord injury. J Urol 1987;138:1390–2.
278. Serretta V, Pomara G, Piazza F, Gange E. Pure squamous cell carcinoma of the bladder in western countries. Report on 19 consecutive cases. Eur Urol 2000;37:85–9.
279. Wang TM, Chang PL, Huang ST, et al. Squamous cell carcinoma of the bladder: a ten-year retrospective study. Changgeng Yi Xue Za Zhi 1998;21:415–20.
280. Lamm DL. Bacillus Calmette-Guérin immunotherapy for bladder cancer. J Urol 1985;134:40–7.
281. Pinsky CM, Camacho FJ, Kerr D, et al. Intravesical administration of bacillus Calmette-Guérin in patients with recurrent superficial carcinoma of the urinary bladder: report of a prospective, randomized trial. Cancer Treat Rep 1985;69:47–53.
282. Pagano F, Bassi P, Milani C, et al. A low dose bacillus Calmette-Guérin regimen in superficial bladder cancer therapy: is it effective? J Urol 1991;146:32–5.
283. Krege S, Giani G, Meyer R, et al. A randomized multicenter trial of adjuvant therapy in superficial bladder cancer: transurethral resection only versus transurethral resection plus mitomycin C versus transurethral resection plus bacillus Calmette-Guérin. Participating Clinics [comments]. J Urol 1996;156:962–6.
284. Melekos MD, Chionis H, Pantazakos A, et al. Intravesical bacillus Calmette-Guérin immunoprophylaxis of superficial bladder cancer: results of a controlled prospective trial with modified treatment schedule. J Urol 1993;149:744–8.
285. Yamamoto T, Hagiwara M, Nakazono M, Yamamoto H. [Intravesical bacillus Calmette-Guérin (BCG) in the treatment of superficial bladder cancer. Prospective randomized study for prophylactic effect]. Nippon Hinyokika Gakkai Zasshi 1990;81:997–1001.
286. Huland H, Otto U. Mitomycin instillation to prevent recurrence of superficial bladder carcinoma. Results of a controlled, prospective study in 58 patients. Eur Urol 1983;9:84–6.
287. Niijima T, Koiso K, Akaza H. Randomized clinical trial on chemoprophylaxis of recurrence in cases of superficial bladder cancer. Cancer Chemother Pharmacol 1983;11:S79–82.
288. Kim HH, Lee C. Intravesical mitomycin C instillation as a prophylactic treatment of superficial bladder tumor. J Urol 1989;141:1337–40.
289. Tolley DA, Hargreave TB, Smith PH, et al. Effect of intravesical mitomycin C on recurrence of newly diagnosed superficial bladder cancer: interim report from the Medical Research Council Subgroup on Superficial Bladder Cancer (Urological Cancer Working Party). Br Med J (Clin Res Ed) 1988;296:1759–61.
290. Burnand KG, Boyd PJ, Mayo ME, et al. Single dose intravesical thiotepa as an adjuvant to cystodiathermy in the treatment of transitional cell bladder carcinoma. Br J Urol 1976;48:55–9.
291. Byar D, Blackard C. Comparisons of placebo, pyridoxine, and topical thiotepa in preventing recurrence of stage I bladder cancer. Urology 1977;10:556–61.
292. Nocks BN, Nieh PT, Prout GR Jr. A longitudinal study of patients with superficial bladder carcinoma successfully treated with weekly intravesical thio-tepa. J Urol 1979;122:27–9.
293. Asahi T, Matsumura Y, Tanahashi T, et al. The effects of intravesical instillation of Thio-Tepa on the recurrence rate of bladder tumors. Acta Medica Okayama 1980;34:43–9.
294. Schulman CC, Robinson N, Denis L, et al. Prophylactic chemotherapy of superficial transitional cell bladder carcinoma: an EORTC randomized trial comparing thiotepa, an epipodophyllotoxin (VM26) and TUR alone. Eur Urol 1982;8:207–12.
295. Koontz WW Jr, Prout GR Jr, Smith W, et al. The use of intravesical thio-tepa in the management of non-invasive carcinoma of the bladder. J Urol 1981;125:307–12.
296. Zincke H, Utz DC, Taylor WF, et al. Influence of thiotepa and doxorubicin instillation at time of transurethral surgical treatment of bladder cancer on tumor recurrence: a prospective, randomized, double-blind, controlled trial. J Urol 1983;129:505–9.
297. Prout GR Jr, Koontz WW Jr, Coombs LJ, et al. Long-term fate of 90 patients with superficial bladder cancer randomly assigned to receive or not to receive thiotepa. J Urol 1983;130:677–80.
298. MRC Working Party on Urological Cancer. The effect of intravesical thiotepa on the recurrence rate of newly diagnosed superficial bladder cancer. An MRC Study. Br J Urol 1985;57:680–5.
299. Herr HW, Wartinger DD, Fair WR, Oettgen HF. Bacillus Calmette-Guérin therapy for superficial bladder cancer: a 10-year followup. J Urol 1992;147:1020–3.
300. Hurle R, Losa A, Manzetti A, Lembo A. Intravesical bacille Calmette-Guérin in stage T1 grade 3 bladder cancer therapy: a 7-year follow-up. Urology 1999;54:258–63.
301. Losa A, Hurle R, Lembo A. Low dose bacillus Calmette-Guérin for carcinoma in situ of the bladder: long-term results [comments]. J Urol 2000;163:68–72.
302. Brake M, Loertzer H, Horsch R, Keller H. Long-term results of intravesical bacillus Calmette-Guérin therapy for stage T1 superficial bladder cancer. Urology 2000;55:673–8.
303. Cheng CW, Chan SF, Chan LW, et al. Twelve-year follow up of a randomized prospective trial comparing bacillus Calmette-Guérin and epirubicin as adjuvant therapy in superficial bladder cancer. Int J Urol 2005;12:449–55.
304. Madersbacher S, Hochreiter W, Burkhard F, et al. Radical cystectomy for bladder cancer today—a homogeneous series without neoadjuvant therapy. J Clin Oncol 2003;21:690–6.
305. Danesi DT, Arcangeli G, Cruciani E, et al. Conservative treatment of invasive bladder carcinoma by transurethral resection, protracted intravenous infusion chemotherapy, and hyperfractionated radiotherapy: long term results. Cancer 2004;101:2540–8.
306. Malmstrom PU, Rintala E, Wahlqvist R, et al. Five-year followup of a prospective trial of radical cystectomy and neoadjuvant chemotherapy: Nordic Cystectomy Trial I. The Nordic Cooperative Bladder Cancer Study Group. J Urol 1996;155:1903–6.
307. Sherif A, Rintala E, Mestad O, et al. Neoadjuvant cisplatin-methotrexate chemotherapy of invasive bladder cancer. Nordic cystectomy trial 2 [abstract 1030]. Proc Am Urol Assoc 2002.
308. Grossman HB, Natale RB, Tangen CM, et al. Neoadjuvant chemotherapy plus cystectomy compared with cystectomy alone for locally advanced bladder cancer. N Engl J Med 2003;349:859–66.
309. Sternberg CN, Parmar MKB. Neoadjuvant chemotherapy is not (yet) standard treatment for muscle-invasive bladder cancer. J Clin Oncol 2001;19:21s–6s.
310. Bassi P, Pagano F, Pappagallo G, et al. Neo-adjuvant M-VAC in invasive bladder cancer: the GUONE multicenter phase III trial [abstract 567]. Eur Urol 1998;33:142.
311. Troner M, Birch R, Omura GA, Williams S. Phase III comparison of cisplatin alone versus cisplatin, doxorubicin and cyclophosphamide in the treatment of bladder (urothelial) cancer: a Southeastern Cancer Study Group trial. J Urol 1987;137:660–2.
312. Bamias A, Aravantinos G, Deliveliotis C, et al. Docetaxel and cisplatin with granulocyte colony-stimulating factor (G-CSF) versus MVAC with G-CSF in advanced urothelial carcinoma: a multicenter, randomized, phase III study from the Hellenic Cooperative Oncology Group. J Clin Oncol 2004;22:220–8.

Neoplasms of the Prostate

Robert W. Ross, MD
William K. Oh, MD
Mark Hurwitz, MD
Anthony V. D'Amico, MD
Jerome P. Richie, MD
Philip W. Kantoff, MD

INTRODUCTION

Cancer of the prostate is the most commonly diagnosed non-skin neoplasm in men in the United States and the second leading cause of cancer-related mortality. Many controversies exist regarding the diagnosis and management of prostate cancer, especially in the areas of screening and the choice of therapy. The extraordinary biologic heterogeneity that characterizes this disease presents issues unique to its management. One patient may have a low-grade cancer that is unlikely to have any impact on the quality or length of his life, whereas another younger man with a high-grade lesion may die within 5 years of progressive disease. Distinguishing between such patients is a high priority for ongoing research. In addition, new insights into the pathogenesis of prostate cancer are actively sought, which may ultimately lead to better therapies and prevention strategies.

EPIDEMIOLOGY AND RISK FACTORS

In 2004, over 230,000 new cases of prostate cancer were diagnosed in the United States, representing 30% of all new cancer diagnoses in men.[1] One in 6 men will develop prostate cancer at some point in his life. Incidence trends for prostate cancer have reflected an increased detection rate of prevalent cancers with the advent of prostate-specific antigen (PSA) testing (Figure 97-1).[2] In addition, an estimated 29,900 deaths from prostate cancer in 2004 make it the second leading cause of cancer death in men after lung cancer (Figure 97-2).[1] There has been a slow rise in age-adjusted death rates over the past 50 years, although a recent downturn suggests that earlier detection and better therapy may be decreasing mortality.[3,4]

Age is the most important risk factor for prostate cancer (Table 97-1).[5] Data from numerous autopsy studies performed in different countries have shown with remarkable consistency an incidence of occult prostate cancer in 15 to 30% of men over the age of 50.[6–8] By the age of 80 years, as many as 60 to 70% of men have histologic evidence of carcinoma in their prostates.[9,10] Interestingly, in one autopsy series, as many as 27% of men in their thirties and 34% in their forties had histologic evidence of unsuspected cancer, suggesting that the pathogenesis of prostate cancer may take decades. Nine percent of men in their twenties had evidence of prostatic intraepithelial neoplasia.[11] Prostate cancer incidence increases with age faster than any other epithelial malignancy.[12] From 1991 to 1995, age-adjusted incidence rates of prostate cancer for men under age

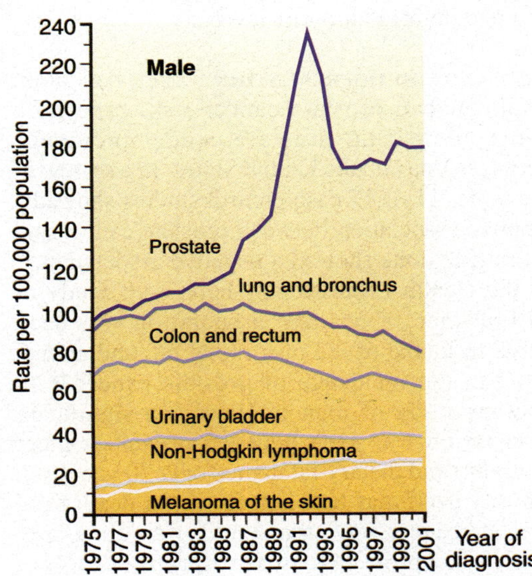

Figure 97-1 Annual age-adjusted cancer incidence rates for men in the United States. Reproduced with permission from Jemal A et al.[1]

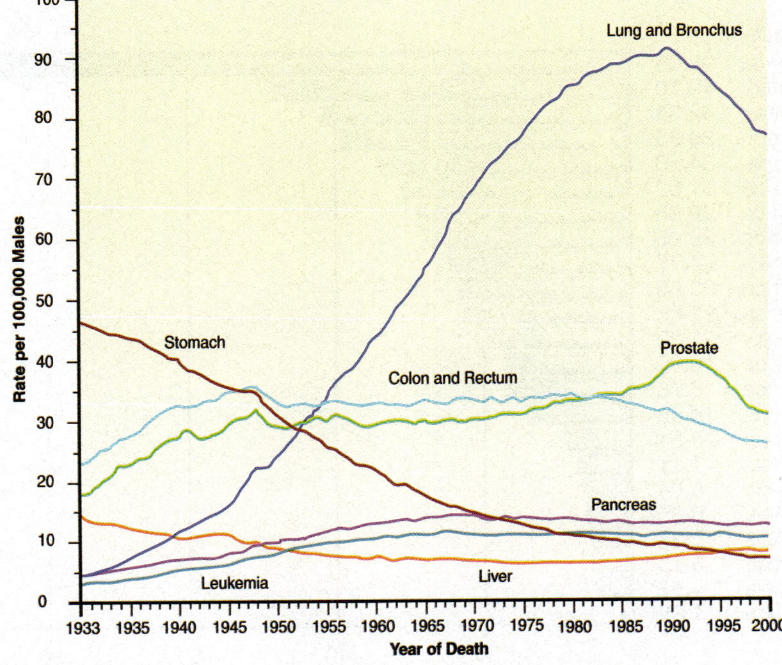

Figure 97-2 Age-adjusted annual cancer death rates among males in the United States. Reproduced with permission from Jemal A et al.[1]

Table 97-1 Risk Factors Associated with Prostate Cancer

Age
Race
Family History
Diet
? Hormone Levels

Table 97-2 Family History and Risk of Prostate Cancer

Number of Affected First-Degree Relatives	Odds Ratio for Development of Prostate Cancer (95% CI)
1	2.2 (1.4–3.5)
2	4.9 (2.0–12.3)
3	10.9 (2.7–43.1)

Adapted from Steinberg GD et al.[23]

65 years was 47.1 per 100,000 men, but was 1,217.8 per 100,000 for men 65 years and older.[13]

Racial and geographic origin confers variable risk. African-American men have the highest incidence of prostate cancer in the world.[14] Surveillance, Epidemiology, and End Results (SEER) program data from 1996 to 2000 demonstrates an age-adjusted incidence rate per 100,000 of 272.1 in African Americans, 164.3 in whites, and 100.0 in Asian Americans.[1] In addition, mortality rates for African Americans was double the rate of whites and five times the rate of Asian Americans. African-American men tend to present with more advanced disease and have a worse prognosis in each stage, but it remains unclear if these differences represent genetic, dietary, socioeconomic, or health care access issues.[15–17] The incidence rates for prostate cancer are highest in North America (92.4 per 100,000) and Western Europe (39.6 per 100,000) (Figure 97-3). In Africa, the incidence rate is moderate (5.1–31.0 per 100,000), whereas in Asia, rates are low (1.1 per 100,000 in China, 8.5 per 100,000 in Japan).[18] Increased rates of prostate cancer are seen in Japanese immigrants to the United States, which suggests that environmental factors play some role in the geographic differences.[19] A family history of prostate cancer remains an important risk of developing the disease.[20] Several studies have suggested an increased risk in male relatives of men with prostate cancer.[21,22] First-degree relatives of men with prostate cancer have a two- to three-fold increased risk of developing prostate cancer compared to the general population. This risk may increase up to 10-fold if three or more relatives are affected (Table 97-2).[23] Families with a strong predisposition to prostate cancer have been described but are uncommon. It has been estimated that about 5 to 10% of all cancers and 40% of early-onset cancers (ie, age at diagnosis less than 50 years old) are hereditary.[24] Genetic linkage studies have implicated several prostate cancer susceptibility loci in families with hereditary prostate cancer, including one on the long arm of chromosome 1 called HPC1.[25] Several candidate genes have been mapped to the critical region of HPC1, including *RNASEL*, which is an enzyme that regulates cell proliferation and apoptosis. Specific germline mutations have been detected in *RNASEL* in HPC1 families, with subsequent loss of heterozygosity and loss of RNase L protein.[25] Macrophage-scavenger receptor-1 (*MSR-1)*, a gene important in macrophage response to inflammation, has also been linked to prostate cancer (Table 97-3).[26]

Although prostate cancer is known to be treatable by manipulation of the hormonal milieu, the role of endogenous steroid hormone levels in contributing to prostate cancer risk is more poorly defined. Prolonged exposure to androgens has been proposed as a mechanism by which prostate cancer may develop. In men with chronic liver disease, rates of prostate cancer are disproportionately low. This phenomena may be due to the elevated levels of plasma estrogens in patients with chronic liver disease that suppress testicular androgen secretion. A number of epidemiologic studies investigating the role of plasma androgens in the etiology of prostate cancer have shown conflicting results.[27–29] The Health Professionals Follow-up Study, a large prospective analysis, did show a direct relationship between prostate cancer risk and the quartile of serum-free testosterone within the normal range.[30] Also, a germline variation in the androgen receptor gene (CAG repeat length) was shown to be a significant predictor for aggressive prostate cancer in a prospective analysis, suggesting that differences in steroid hormone receptors may also play an important role in risk of prostate cancer.[31]

Benign prostatic hypertrophy is often seen in conjunction with cancer, but this association may be incidental rather than causative.[5] Many studies have evaluated vasectomy, with either no added risk[32] or a modest increase (1.5–2.2) in risk of prostate cancer.[33] Detection bias is suspected in such patients, since men seeking vasectomy are also more likely to be screened for cancer. Cigarette smoking also remains an uncertain risk factor for prostate cancer, as data are conflicting. However, two recent studies have suggested approximately a two-fold risk of fatal prostate cancer for those who smoke.[34,35] Higher rates of prostate cancer have been reported in certain occupations, most notably those exposed to cadmium, such as welders.[36] Socioeconomic factors and infections, as well as a host of other risks, have not been associated with prostate cancer.[37] One recent study found a relationship between high ejaculation frequency and decreased prostate cancer risk.[38] Ultraviolet radiation may offer some protective effect,[39] perhaps via vitamin D and parathyroid hormone levels.

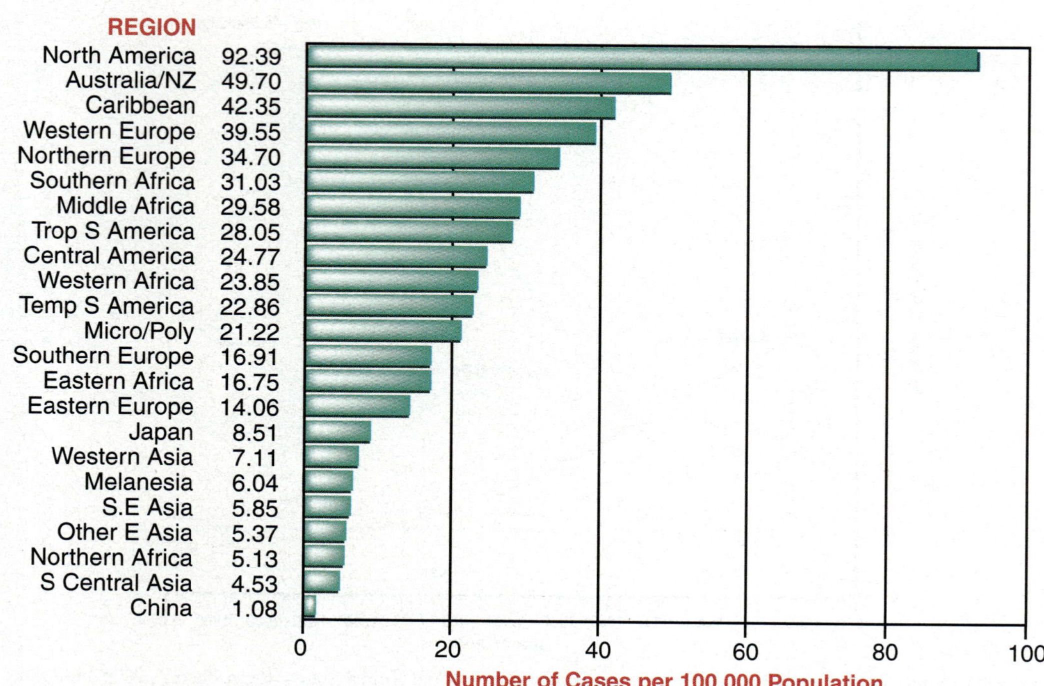

Figure 97-3 Geographic variations in prostate cancer incidence.

Diet and Chemoprevention Diet has been implicated in prostate cancer risk, especially when comparing prostate cancer incidence between Asia and the United States. In a review of the topic, 11 of 17 case-control studies showed a positive association between prostate cancer and fat intake; none showed a negative association.[40] In the Health Professionals Follow-up Study of 51,000 men, a positive association was seen between intake of red meat, total fat, and animal fat, and the incidence of prostate cancer.[41] In another study of men in Hawaii, a significant association was seen between prostate cancer mortality and dietary fat in men over 70 years old. Obesity itself may be a risk factor for death from prostate cancer.[42] On the other hand, eating fatty fish may be protective. In a prospective cohort of more than 6,000 Swedish men, those who ate no fatty fish had a two- to three-fold higher risk of prostate cancer than those who consumed moderate or high amounts.[43]

Table 97-3 Putative Prostate Cancer Susceptibility Gene

Gene	Location	Description
RNASEL	1q24-25	Involved in interferon-induced antiviral activity
ELAC2	17p11	Unknown function
MSR1	8p22	Involved in macrophage response to infections
AR	Xq11-12	Encodes the androgen receptor
CYP17	10q24.3	Encodes an enzyme important in sex-steroid biosynthesis
SRD5A2	2p23	Encodes predominant 5-alpha reductase in the prostate

Adapted from Nelson WG et al.[311]

Another significant difference between Asian and Western diets is the average amount of soy protein consumption, which averages 35 grams/day in Taiwan.[40] The soy isoflavones genistein and daidzein are thought to be the active ingredients responsible for the potential benefits of soy. Genistein inhibits growth of both androgen-dependent and -independent cell lines, although the mechanism of such effects is still unclear. Micronutrients in the diet have also been implicated in the pathogenesis of prostate cancer.[44,45] In the Alpha Tocopherol Beta Carotene Study, the incidence of prostate cancer among men receiving 50 IU per day of vitamin E was only 66% of those on placebo, although these beneficial effects disappeared in long-term follow-up.[46] In the Nutritional Prevention of Skin Cancer Trial, selenium had no effect on skin cancer risk but the incidence of prostate cancer in men given 200 micrograms of selenium per day was only 37% that of the placebo group.[47] Recent studies suggest that higher serum vitamin D levels may reduce the risk of prostate cancer.[48] Others have shown that low serum $1,25(OH)_2$ vitamin D levels correlate with an increased risk of palpable and high-grade tumors. A further link between high dietary calcium intake and prostate cancer risk has been shown, suggesting that chronically high calcium intake might confer risk by causing lower endogenous $1,25(OH)_2$ vitamin D levels.[49]

A higher intake of lycopenes, the agent in tomatoes and beets that gives them their red color, has been shown to decrease risk of prostate cancer.[50] In a large study of food intake and risk of prostate cancer, Giovannucci and colleagues demonstrated an inverse relationship between consumption of lycopenes and the risk of prostate cancer.[51] Several randomized trials are ongoing, evaluating the role of nutrition in preventing prostate cancer progression, but these results will not be available for years. The largest of these is the Selenium and Vitamin E Cancer Prevention Trial (SELECT), sponsored by the National Cancer Institute. In this placebo-controlled trial, 32,000 men without prostate cancer have been randomized in a 2 × 2 factorial design to selenium and/or vitamin E.

The success of tamoxifen in the prevention of breast cancer for women at high risk generated enthusiasm in the area of pharmacologic therapy for prostate cancer prevention. Recently, the Prostate Cancer Prevention Trial reported its results for the first time.[52] This trial randomized 18,882 men 55 years and older with a prostate specific antigen (PSA) ≤ 3.0 ng/mL to finasteride (an inhibitor of 5α-reductase, which converts testosterone to the more potent dihydrotestosterone) or placebo for 7 years. The primary outcome was prostate cancer prevalence. Importantly, the study was designed such that at the end of 7 years men without prostate cancer would undergo a prostate biopsy to determine the true prevalence. The results were unexpected, although there was a statistically significant difference in prostate cancer prevalence favoring the finasteride arm (24.4% vs 18.4%, $p < .001$), tumors of Gleason grade 7, 8, 9, or 10 were more common in the finasteride arm (280 of 757 cancers, 37%, vs 237 of 1,068 cancers, 22.2%, $p < .001$). It is unclear if these upgrades are a result of true increased biologic aggressiveness or simply an artifact of the influence of finasteride on the histologic appearance of tumors. Long-term data will be needed to prove that finasteride prophylaxis actually improves prostate cancer-specific survival. Until then, the use of finasteride to prevent prostate cancer, even in high-risk populations, is still investigational.

BIOLOGY OF PROSTATE CANCER

Normal Histology and Anatomy The prostate sits in the pelvis, surrounded by the rectum posteriorly and the bladder superiorly (Figure 97-4). Its normal function is not well understood; it produces some seminal fluid and may facilitate sperm motility. The prostate is composed of branching glands with ducts that are lined by secretory epithelial cells and basal cells.[53] Scattered neuroendocrine cells are also present, which are thought to provide a paracrine function in the gland.[54] Secretory epithelial cells represent the major cell type in the gland, are androgen-dependent for growth, and produce PSA and prostatic acid phosphatase. The basal cell layer is not dependent on androgen for growth and is thought to contain the stem cell population for the epithelial prostate cells. Surrounding the gland is a stroma that includes fibroblasts, smooth muscle, nerves, and lymphatics. Stromal-epithelial interactions remain poorly understood, but recent insights suggest that the stroma produces multiple growth factors important for growth and development of normal prostate as well as prostate cancer.[55]

Early anatomists suggested that the prostate developed in a lobar pattern, despite the fact that normal adult prostates do not have discernible lobes. More recently, McNeal and colleagues conducted detailed studies of the normal and pathologic anatomy of the prostate and defined a concept of anatomic zones, rather than lobes, to describe the prostate.[56] There are four major zones within the normal prostate: the peripheral zone (70% of glandular tissue), the central zone (20% of glandular tissue), the transition zone (5% of glandular tissue), and the anterior fibromuscular stroma (Figure 97-5). The peripheral zone extends posterolaterally around the gland from the apex to the base and represents the most common site in the prostate for developing prostate carcinomas. The central zone surrounds the ejaculatory duct apparatus and makes up the majority of the prostatic base. The transition zone constitutes two small lobules that abut the prostatic ure-

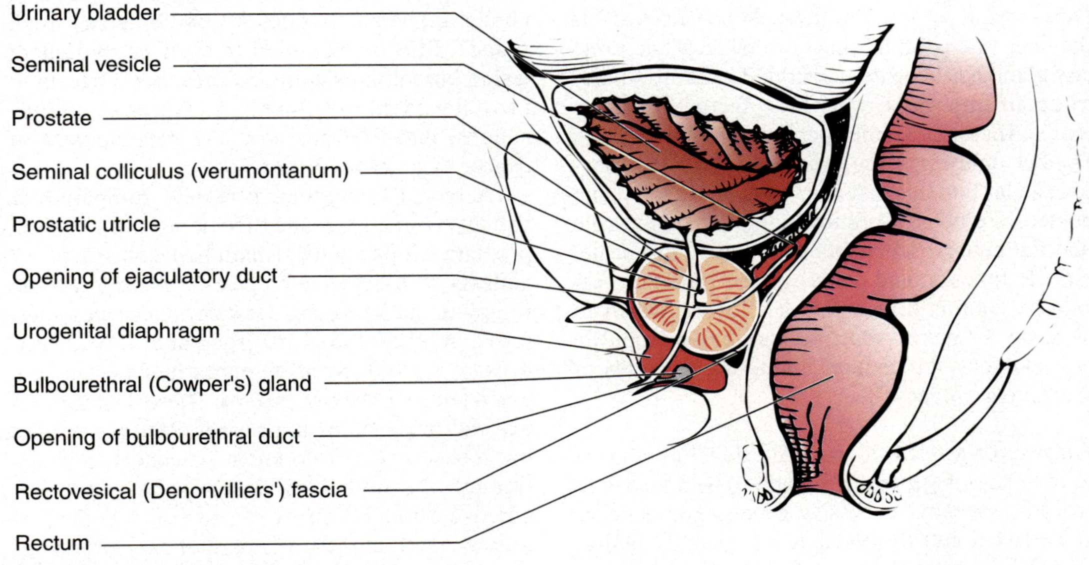

Figure 97-4 Normal prostate anatomy.

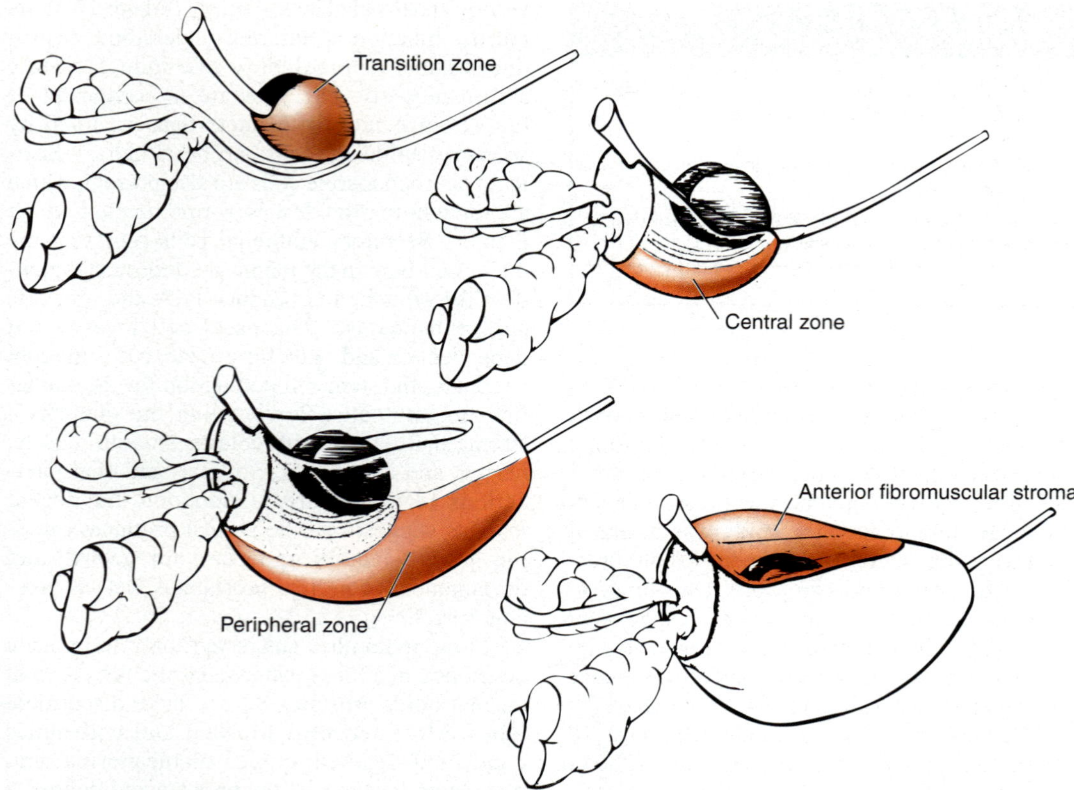

Figure 97-5 Zonal anatomy of the prostate: the three glandular zones of the prostate and the anterior fibromuscular stroma.

thra and represent the region where benign prostatic hypertrophy (BPH) primarily originates. Carcinomas that originate from the transition zone have been suggested to be of lower malignant potential, although other studies have suggested that there is no difference in outcome when controlled for grade and stage compared with peripheral zone cancers.[57,58]

There is no true anatomic capsule that surrounds the prostate. The smooth muscle of the prostatic stroma gradually extends into fibrous tissue that then ends in loose connective and adipose tissue. At the apex and anteriorly, even this minimally distinct border is lost. Although differences exist in how "extracapsular disease" is defined, extension of cancer outside of the prostate gland has been demonstrated in many studies to be an important prognostic factor for recurrence. Anatomic studies performed by Walsh and Donker delineated the presence of the two neurovascular bundles that pass adjacent to the gland posterolaterally.[59] Acknowledgment of the role that the neurovascular bundles played in normal erectile function and defining their presence outside of Denonvillier's fascia allowed Walsh to develop a "nerve-sparing" radical retropubic prostatectomy procedure, improving the odds of preserving potency.[60]

Premalignant Lesions The development of solid tumors is generally thought to be a multistep process, whereby successive genetic events occur in a normal cell to render it increasingly malignant.[61] In prostate cancer, the genetic and epigenetic phenomena that occur that result in cancer are not well understood, but there is evidence that premalignant lesions exist in the prostate that may precede the development of cancer by many years.

Although many terms have been used to describe prostatic epithelial dysplasia or atypia, these heterogeneous morphologic lesions now are considered under the single term "prostatic intraepithelial neoplasia" (PIN) (Figure 97-6).[62] PIN is defined as the presence of cytologically atypical or dysplastic epithelial cells within architecturally benign-appearing glands and acini. Three different grades have been described: grade 1 (mild), grade 2 (moderate), and grade 3 (severe). Grades 2 and 3 PIN often are combined as "high grade." PIN is presumed to be a premalignant lesion based on its common presence adjacent to prostate adenocarcinomas.[63] Autopsy studies suggest that PIN precedes the development of cancer by at least 10 years.

A recent retrospective review compared 61 patients with high-grade PIN alone on their initial prostate biopsy with a matched control of 47 patients with negative biopsies.[64] After a median follow-up of 6.8 years, prostate cancer was diagnosed in 49% of the PIN group and 21% of controls ($p = .003$). No differences in survival were noted between the two groups. These data suggest that the presence of high-grade PIN can predict for subsequent development of cancer, perhaps through the multistep carcinogenesis process noted earlier. However, close routine clinical follow-up remains the standard of care after diagnosis of high-grade PIN alone.

Atypical adenomatous hyperplasia (AAH) is another lesion that may represent a premalignant change, although data for this are more scant than for PIN. The characteristic appearance with AAH is the fulfillment of the architectural criteria for malignancy—with disruption of the basal cell layer, mainly in the transition zone—but without the cytologic changes diagnostic of cancer.[65] Others have suggested that a prostatic lesion composed of focal areas of epithelial atrophy associated with chronic inflammation (called proliferative inflammatory atrophy, or PIA) are precursors to PIN and eventually prostate cancer.[66] Evidence for this hypothesis includes the observation that PIA often occurs adjacent to areas of PIN and prostate cancer,[67] and that somatic genetic abnormalities seen in PIA often resemble those seen in prostate carcinoma.[68]

Histology of Prostate Cancer Over 95% of prostate cancers are adenocarcinomas that arise from prostatic epithelial cells (Figure 97-7).[69] Other rare histologies have been described, including mucinous or signet ring tumors, adenoid cystic carcinomas, carcinoid, large prostatic duct carcinomas (including the endometrial type) adenocarcinomas, and small-cell undifferentiated cancers. It is important to recognize these unusual variants of prostate cancer since standard hormonal therapies may be less effective.[70] Tumors with a neuroendocrine appearance (carcinoid and small-cell undifferentiated) may arise from Kul-

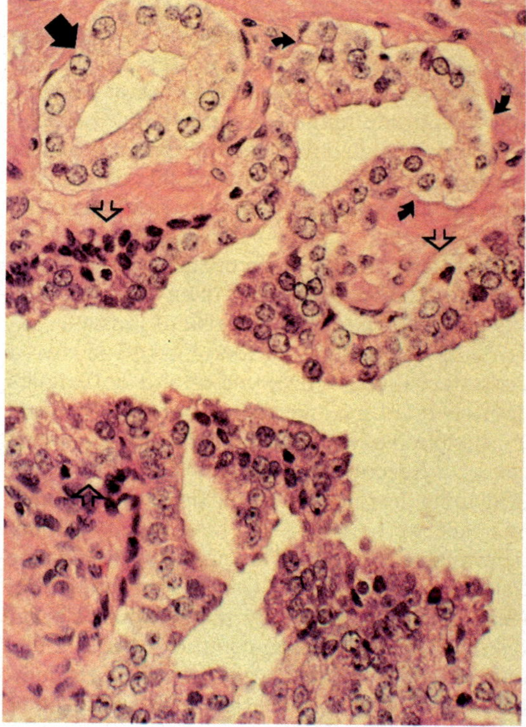

Figure 97-6 Photomicrograph of high-grade prostatic intraepithelial neoplasm (PIN) with basal cell layer (*open arrows*) with budding microacinus lacking basal cells (*curved solid arrows*). A microacinus of invasive Gleason pattern 3 adenocarcinoma is seen in the adjacent stroma (*straight solid arrow*). Hematoxylin and eosin, × 160. (Courtesy of Thomas M. Wheeler, MD.)

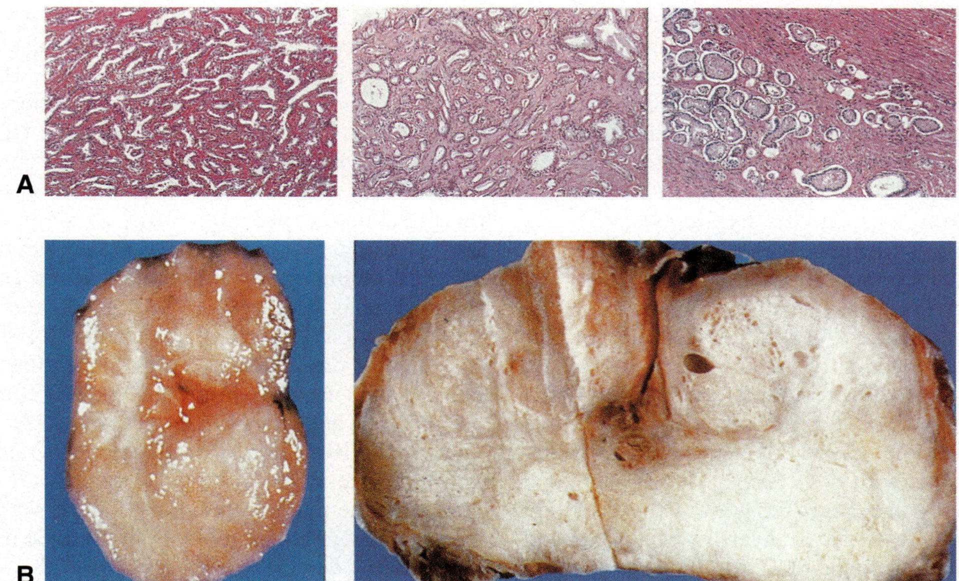

Figure 97-7 **A,** Microscopic histologic appearance of prostate adenocarcinoma. **B,** Gross histologic appearance of prostate adenocarcinoma.

chitsky's cells, which are found in the basal regions of the prostatic epithelium.[54] Small-cell carcinomas of the prostate have similar histologic and clinical features to other extrapulmonary small-cell carcinomas. Transitional-cell carcinomas involving the substance of the prostate may also be mistaken for prostate adenocarcinoma. It may be difficult to distinguish a transitional-cell carcinoma arising in the transitional epithelium of the distal prostatic ducts from a tumor arising from the bladder epithelium and spreading contiguously into the prostatic ducts.

Studies have confirmed the primary prognostic importance of the degree of histologic differentiation of prostate adenocarcinoma. The degree of differentiation is typically graded by patterns of gland formation and, less importantly, by cytologic detail. The most widely accepted grading scheme for adenocarcinoma of the prostate is that developed by Gleason (Figure 97-8).[71] Gleason described a system for classifying prostate tumors based on two levels of scoring, recognizing the heterogeneous differentiation in prostate carcinomas. The primary pattern of differentiation is assigned a Gleason grade of 1 to 5 based on the dominant morphology of the specimen and its departure from normal appearance; the next most common pattern is also assigned a grade. This results in a two-digit score: for example, 3 + 4 = 7. The Gleason system has been criticized for inadequate recognition of the proportion of the tumor that is composed of the secondary pattern as well as a lack of adequate distinction between good and poor prognosis in cancers with Gleason scores of 5 to 7, which represent the majority of patients. However, its reproducibility and reliability between pathologists have been shown consistently to be excellent. Gleason's original work demonstrated a clear association between a higher Gleason score and higher mortality, which others have confirmed.[72] Many other predictors of clinical behavior have been explored, but currently the Gleason score remains the most broadly applicable and prognostically useful histologic grading system.

Molecular Pathogenesis Unlike colorectal cancer, in which a great deal is understood about the progression from normal epithelial cells to invasive adenocarcinoma and the central role of the *APC* gene, a detailed understanding of the stepwise molecular pathogenesis of prostate cancer is lacking.[61] It is clear, though, that prostate cancer cells harbor a large number of somatic mutations, and in advanced disease, additional alterations accumulate. Factors that effect the development and progression of prostate cancer include alterations of the hormonal and growth factor milieu, alterations in hormonal and growth factor receptors, alterations in intracellular signaling pathways and alterations in cell cycle regulation and apoptosis. Although a full discussion is beyond the scope of this chapter, important examples of each factor will be discussed.

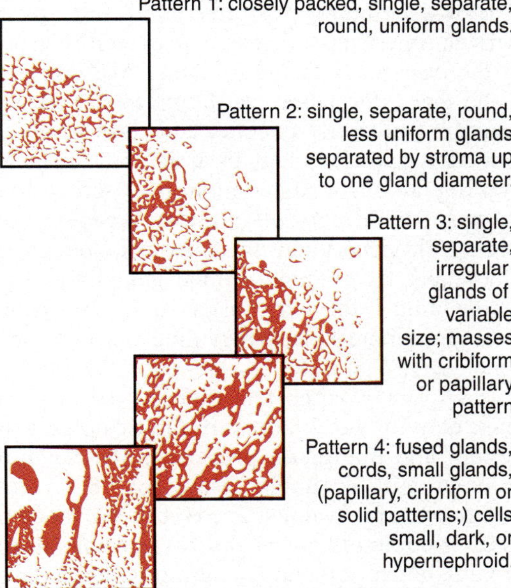

Figure 97-8 Histologic grading scheme for adenocarcinomas of the prostate. Adapted with permission from Gleason DF.[71]

The hormonal and growth factor milieu to which the prostate is exposed has been consistently associated with the pathogenesis of cancer. In population-based studies, two hormones have been implicated: testosterone and insulin-like growth factor (IGF)-I. The association between testosterone and prostate cancer development has been discussed previously. Several lines of evidence suggest that IGF may be important in prostate cancer growth. First, several prostate cancer cell lines and prostate xenograft models express both IGF-I and II and their receptors. Second, Chan and colleagues reported on the relationship between plasma IGF-1 levels and prostate cancer, citing a relative risk of 4.3 for men in the highest quartile compared with men in the lowest quartile.[73] Moreover, Stattin and colleagues found a higher incidence of prostate cancer in patients with higher IGF-I levels in plasma drawn 5 years prior to the cancer diagnosis,[74] supporting the concept that IGF-I may be important early in the development of prostate cancer. Other growth factors, including epidermal growth factor (EGF), vascular endothelial growth factor (VEGF), platelet-derived growth factor (PDGF), and transforming growth factor beta (TGF-β) may also be dysregulated in the development of prostate cancer. (Table 97-4).[75]

Several hormonal and growth factor receptors are altered in prostate cancer cells. Perhaps the best example is alterations in the androgen receptor. Although in early cancer androgen receptor mutations are relatively uncommon,[76] germline variation in the androgen receptor gene (CAG repeats) has been shown to be a predictor of cancer aggressiveness[31] and may play a role in the frequency and aggressiveness of prostate cancer in African Americans.[77] Interestingly, androgen receptor mutations are more commonly seen in androgen-independent prostate cancer,[76,78] arguing

Table 97-4 Growth Factors Implicated in Prostate Cancer
Transforming growth factor beta
Fibroblast growth factor
Epidermal growth factor
Insulin-like growth factor
Platelet-derived growth factor
Vascular endothelial growth factor
Neurotensin
Endothelins
Colony-stimulating factors

that the androgen receptor remains central in the growth and survival of prostate cancer even after the need for the ligand (androgens) has been mitigated. Several theoretical frameworks have been proposed for the development of androgen independence, most of which still postulate a cancer cell that depends on a functional androgen receptor, but that is amplified, oversensitive, promiscuous, or activated by up-regulated coactivators, or down-regulated corepressors.[79] For example, an androgen receptor mutation in LNCaP cells, T877A, results in a substitution of alanine for threonine at position 877 and results in an androgen receptor that is activated by other steroid hormones and by the androgen antagonist flutamide. This mutation was found in 5 of 16 patients who received combined androgen blockade with flutamide,[80] and could help explain the "antiandrogen withdrawal syndrome." This and other observations confirm the centrality of the androgen receptor in the molecular pathogenesis of prostate cancer despite the establishment of androgen independence.

Molecules that alter intracellular signaling pathways also may be important in the pathogenesis and progression of prostate cancer. The clearest example to date is the tumor suppressor gene *PTEN*. The *PTEN* gene encodes for a phosphatase important in the modulation of the signal generated by activated growth factor receptors. There is a high frequency of somatic mutations in *PTEN* in prostate carcinoma cells, suggesting that this may be a frequent target for inactivation. One study documented a 60% rate of *PTEN* mutations; most of these were found in cell lines from metastatic disease, although mutations were also seen in primary cancers.[81] In fact, another group demonstrated higher rates of *PTEN* loss or mutation in advanced stage and grade tumors.[82] Another pathway that may be inappropriately activated in prostate cancer is the hedgehog (HH) pathway. Normal hedgehog signaling is important in early prostate epithelium development and patterning. Recent work by Karhadkar and colleagues demonstrates that the HH pathway activation distinguishes prostate cancer cells from normal prostate and, further, metastatic prostate cancer from localized cancer.[83] Moreover, they demonstrate that HH pathway inhibition results in PC3 xenograft regression. Both the PTEN and HH pathways represent attractive targets for drug development.

Finally, alterations in molecules that regulate the cell cycle and apoptosis offer promising avenues for further investigation. TP53, p27, p21, and Rb have been studied, with variable levels of evidence that they participate in the pathogenesis of prostate cancer. In one study, loss of expression of the tumor suppressor protein p27 was strongly associated with the development of BPH, whereas variable levels of p27 expression were noted in prostate cancers.[84]

SCREENING FOR PROSTATE CANCER

The tools to diagnose prostate cancer have improved dramatically over the past 20 years and, as a result, a greater number of patients are diagnosed at an earlier stage. What remains controversial is whether screening is warranted and in what populations. The success of screening techniques in reducing mortality from breast and cervical cancer suggests that the same can be achieved by screening for prostate cancer. Although prospective, randomized clinical trials are ongoing to test this hypothesis, there is increasing evidence that screening may reduce prostate cancer mortality.

Prostate-Specific Antigen To detect cancer while still potentially curable requires periodic examinations with both digital rectal exam (DRE) and serum PSA. Large screening trials have shown that PSA nearly doubles the rate of detection possible with DRE alone. There has been a significant stage migration toward the detection of lower-stage prostate cancers by using PSA and transrectal ultrasound (TRUS)-guided biopsies in addition to DRE. Before the 1990s, only about 50% of the cancers detected were confined to the prostate clinically (cT1–T2). Today, 90% of cancers detected in screened populations are clinically organ confined. With serial PSA-based screening, the proportion of prostate cancers that are pathologically confined to the prostate is nearly double the proportion in an age-matched group whose cancer was detected in the traditional manner because of abnormal findings on DRE.

Based on these data, PSA testing was approved by the US Food and Drug Administration (FDA) for the screening and early detection of prostate cancer. Both the American Urological Association (AUA) and the American Cancer Society (ACS) recommend that the PSA blood test and DRE be offered annually to healthy men over age 50, who have a life expectancy of at least 10 years. It is recommended that these tests be offered starting at a younger age to men at higher risk of developing prostate cancer, including African Americans and men with a family history of the disease. Both the ACS and AUA recommend that information can be given to patients regarding potential benefits and risks of early detection and treatment to assist each man in making an informed decision. Some other groups, including the American Academy of Family Physicians and the American College of Physicians, have offered similar guidelines, recommending informed consent after discussion with appropriate patients regarding their risks and benefits.

PSA is a glycoprotein that has serine protease activity and is found in the cytoplasm of benign and malignant prostate cells. Several commercially available assays for PSA yield different normal values. The Hybritech Tandem assay is commonly used and has normal values ranging between 0 and 4.0 ng/mL. Other assays (eg, Chiron, Abbott) may give differing results, so patients should be followed serially with the same assay. If ultrasound-guided prostate biopsies are performed in patients with PSA values between 4.0 and 10.0 ng/mL, cancer will be detected in 26% of patients. Serum PSA content is increased in benign prostatic diseases (prostatitis, BPH), as well as in cancer. However, the level of PSA elevation is important. Patients in whom the PSA is more than 10 ng/mL usually have prostate cancer. PSA greater than 10 may occur in 30% of men with disease confined to the prostate (clinical stage T1–2NXM0). There is a clear relationship between serum PSA and stage of prostate cancer. If the PSA value is greater than 10 ng/mL and the gland is palpably normal, the chance for positive biopsy on transrectal ultrasound-directed examination is approximately 50%. The combination of an abnormal DRE, elevated PSA, and abnormal TRUS increases the tumor yield to approximately 75 to 80%. A review of the results of the major screening trials showed an overall cancer detection rate of 4%. Of the prostate cancers detected in these trials, 76% were clinically localized (cT1–T2), and 64% of them were pathologically confined (pT1–T2) to the prostate.[85]

The percentage of organ-confined cancers detected in screening trials (64%) was higher than the frequency of organ-confined cancers in the recently published radical prostatectomy series (48.2%). Catalona and colleagues[85] reported studies on three groups of patients—nonscreened patients, an initial PSA-based screening group, and a serial PSA-based screening group—and showed that the proportion of clinically or pathologically advanced cancers decreased from 57% in the nonscreened group to 29% in the serial PSA-based screening group. They also showed that the proportion of indolent cancers increased from 2.5% in the nonscreened group to 7.8% in the serial PSA-based screening group. PSA values may become elevated following an episode of prostatitis, needle biopsy, or transurethral resection.

Improving the Utility of PSA Testing Serum PSA screening for occult prostate cancer is neither sensitive nor specific. About 20 to 42% of the patients who undergo radical prostatectomy for clinical T1–T2 prostate cancer have PSA levels below 4 ng/mL. Most of these cancers are detected by transurethral prostatic resection (TURP) or DRE, but it is clear that these procedures fail to detect some cancers. In fact, data from the Prostate Cancer Prevention Trial (a trial of finasteride vs placebo to prevent prostate cancer in men ≥ 55 years old) revealed a 15.2% prevalence of prostate cancer in men with a PSA ≤ 4.0 ng/mL.[86] Moreover, 15% of these discovered cancers had a Gleason score of at least 7. These surprising data highlight the poor sensitivity of a serum PSA cutoff of 4.0 ng/mL, but the clinical significance of these incidentally discovered cancers remains unknown. This poor sensitivity is also demonstrated in research by Punglia and colleagues, who note that the overall diagnostic performance of serum PSA becomes significantly worse when corrected for verification bias (bias introduced by the fact that the test itself determines whether the test is confirmed).[87] Their model reveals that a serum PSA cutoff of 4.1 ng/mL potentially misses 82% of cancers in men younger than 60 and 65% of cancers in men older than 60. Others point out that the specificity of serum PSA limits its usefulness at lower ranges. Stamey and colleagues argue that in the era of PSA screening, PSA values less than 10 ng/mL reflect only prostate size (usually a function of BPH), and not the presence of cancer.[88] They reviewed 1,317 radical prostatectomy specimens over 20 years at Stanford University and found that, although there was some correlation between the presence of prostate cancer and serum PSA in the first 5 years of the study, in the most recent 5 years, serum PSA level was only correlated to prostate size. Thus, they argue that in the era of PSA screening, the specificity of a PSA < 10 ng/mL is exceedingly poor.

Several methodologies have been employed to enhance the test characteristics of serum PSA, including PSA density (PSAD), age-specific reference ranges, and percent-free PSA. Since PSA released into the serum is greater per gram of cancer than per gram of BPH tissue, the ratio of PSA to gland volume (PSAD) should help to discriminate cancer from BPH. The results of clinical trials, however, have been variable, and PSAD is used largely to determine whether to repeat a negative biopsy in a patient with a persistently elevated PSA.

Age-specific (and race-specific) reference ranges for PSA have been reported. Based on large samples from a healthy male population, the 95% confidence intervals for men at each decade indicate that the upper limit of normal should be 2.5 for men ages 40 to 49, 3.5 for men ages 50 to 59, 4.5 for men ages 60 to 69, and 6.5 for men ages 70 to 79. The utility of age-specific PSA levels has been challenged in screening trials because sensitivity is lost for a small increase in specificity in older men. In the circulation PSA can be free or complexed with either alpha 1-antichymotrypsin (ACT) or alpha 2-macroglobulin. The percentage of free to total PSA in the serum may help to discriminate patients with cancer from those with BPH. In men with a PSA between 4 and 10 ng/mL, cancer is more likely when free PSA is less than 20 to 25% of the total. The FDA approved the use of percent-free PSA as a diagnostic tool to help distinguish between benign and malignant disease in patients with normal DREs and total PSA tests between 4 and 10 ng/mL. ProPSA, which is the precursor form of PSA, may further add to the ability of free PSA to distinguish cancers from benign processes. In a cohort of 60 patients evaluated recently whose PSA levels were between 2.5 and 4 ng/mL, the ratio of percent proPSA to percent-free PSA had a greater specificity in detecting 75% of cancers compared to percent-free PSA alone.[89]

Latent Prostate Cancer Given the high rate of prostate cancer found incidentally at autopsy in men over 50 years of age, many have questioned the clinical significance of prostate cancer detected through screening. Scardino and colleagues[90] have estimated that the lifetime risk of a 50-year-old man developing a histologically detectable tumor is about 42%, the lifetime risk that he will develop a clinically detectable prostate cancer is about 9.5%, and the risk of death from prostate cancer is 2.9%. Thus, for every 100 men with cancer in their prostates, 23 will be diagnosed with prostate cancer during their lifetime and 7 will die of the disease. Our ultimate strategy must therefore be to detect and cure only those cancers that are clinically significant.

Prostate cancers detected clinically and those found incidentally at autopsy are similar architecturally and cytologically but do differ in several pathologic features. Incidental cancers are usually small, well or moderately differentiated, and confined to the prostate.[91,92] Unsuspected prostate cancers found at the time of cystoprostatectomy for the treatment of bladder cancer are similar to autopsy cancers.[92] Seventy-eight percent of unexpected prostate cancers found in cystoprostatectomy specimens were small, confined to the prostate, and well to moderately differentiated, compared with only 9% of the clinically detected cancers with such features.[91] Twenty-nine percent of the clinical cancers were advanced as compared with none of the cystoprostatectomy cancers.

A recent analysis attempted to quantitate the rate of overdiagnosis as a result of PSA screening in the United States between 1988 and 1998.[93] Overdiagnosis was defined as the detection of prostate cancer through PSA testing that would otherwise not have been diagnosed in the person's lifetime. Using computer modeling, this group reported overdiagnosis rates of approximately 29% for whites and 44% for blacks. They concluded that the majority of PSA-detected cancers would have presented clinically in the patient's lifetime, suggesting again that PSA screening mostly detects cancers that are likely to be of clinical consequence to patients.

Current Recommendations for Screening It will still be many years before the results of larger randomized, controlled clinical trials will determine the impact of screening in the morbidity and mortality of prostate cancer. Despite this lack of conclusive data, Sirovich and colleagues have noted that the prevalence of PSA screening for prostate cancer in the United States is higher than screening for colorectal cancer (75% vs 63%), even though the data supporting the value of screening for colorectal cancer are much stronger.[94] In 1993, the National Cancer Institute (NCI) began a trial designed to evaluate the role of PSA and DRE in reducing morbidity and mortality from prostate cancer. This study is randomizing 165,000 individuals to either yearly screening for prostate, lung, colorectal, and ovarian cancer versus standard care without mandated screening. In the meantime, data available suggest that screening strategies may be having an impact on prostate cancer. The diagnosis of advanced-stage prostate cancer has decreased significantly over the past decade. In addition, there has been a decrease in overall mortality rates in regions where the screening for prostate cancer has become widespread, whereas there is a continuing increase in mortality in countries where screening has been discouraged. Finally, a randomized trial reported by Labrie and colleagues in Canada was the first to report that PSA screening led to decreased mortality from prostate cancer,[4] although serious concerns about the study design have been expressed.

Further studies are needed to define the appropriate interval for screening and to better clarify which populations are at higher risk of death from prostate cancer and are thus most likely to benefit from early detection and treatment. Similarly, improved understanding of the molecular and genetic factors that can lead to aggressive and incurable cancers may provide an impetus to do earlier screening in such patients to reduce mortality from prostate cancer, the second leading cause of cancer death among men in the United States.

DIAGNOSIS AND STAGING OF PROSTATE CANCER

The most common symptom related to prostate disease in men over 50 years of age is bladder outlet obstruction: hesitancy, nocturia, incomplete bladder emptying, diminished urinary stream—signs and symptoms referred to as prostatism. Such signs are much more often related to BPH than to prostate cancer. Nonetheless, these symptoms should prompt an evaluation to include at least a careful DRE, a PSA, and, on occasion, a transrectal ultrasound. Other symptoms associated with prostate cancer include perineal pain, sudden development of impotence, and hematuria.

Diagnosis of prostate cancer requires histologic proof, which is most often obtained by TRUS-guided systematic or targeted needle (18-gauge) biopsies with special spring-driven biopsy devices, or by the unsuspected microscopic appearance of cancer cells in the TURP chips for the treatment of benign prostatic hyperplasia. Because many cancers detected today are neither palpable nor visible by ultrasound, samples are usually obtained systematically from areas (three on each side) in the peripheral zone (sometimes supplemented by two cores from the transition zone).

In 1997, the American Joint Committee on Cancer (AJCC) and the International Union Against Cancer (UICC) updated the TNM classification system that replaced the older Whitmore-Jewett method (Table 97-5).[95] The TNM system has several advantages over the older staging systems: greater detail; separate designations for the primary tumor, regional nodes, and distant metastases; and the inclusion of category T1c for nonpalpable cancers detected by systematic biopsy because of an elevated PSA level. In addition to the DRE, many other studies may be used to evaluate the extent of the disease, including serum PSA, TRUS, computed tomography (CT) of the pelvis and abdomen, and radioisotope bone

Table 97-5 TNM Staging System

Primary Tumor, Clinical (T)	
TX	Primary tumor cannot be assessed
TO	No evidence of primary tumor
T1	Clinically in apparent tumor not palpable or visible by imaging
T1a	Tumor incidental histologic finding in 5% or less of tissue resected
T1b	Tumor incidental histologic finding in more than 5% of tissue resected
T1c	Tumor identified by needle biopsy (eg because of elevated PSA)
T2	Palpable tumor confined within prostate[a]
T2a	Tumor involves half of one lobe or less
T2b	Tumor involves more than half of one lobe, but not both lobes
T2c	Tumor involves both lobes
T3	Tumor extends through the prostatic capsule[b]
T3a	Extracapsular extension (unilateral or bilateral)
T3b	Tumor invades seminal vesicle(s)
T4	Tumor is fixed or invades adjacent structures other than seminal vesicles: bladder neck, external sphincter, rectum, levator muscles, and/or pelvic wall

[a]Tumor found in one or both lobes by needle biopsy, but not palpable or reliably visible by imaging, is classified as T1c.
[b]Invasion into the prostatic apex or into (but not beyond) the prostatic capsule is not classified as T3, but as T2.

Primary Tumor, Pathologic (pT)	
pT2[c]	Organ confined
pT2a	Unilateral, half a lobe or less
pT2b	Unilateral, more than half a lobe
pT2c	Bilateral disease
pT3	Extraprostatic extension
pT3a	Extraprostatic extension
pT3b	Seminal vesicle invasion
pT4	Invasion of bladder, rectum

[c]There is no pathologic T1 classification.

Regional Lymph Nodes (N)	
NX	Regional lymph nodes cannot be assessed
N0	No regional lymph node metastasis
N1	Metastasis in regional lymph node or nodes

Distant Metastasis (M)[d]	
MX	Distant metastasis cannot be assessed
M0	No distant metastasis
M1	Distant metastasis
M1a	Nonregional lymph nodes
M1b	Bone(s)
M1c	Other site(s)

[d]When more than one site of metastasis is present, the most advanced category is used. pM1c is most advanced.

scan. Cancers confined to the prostate pathologically have been reported in patients with very high PSA levels; with rare exception, however, PSA levels greater than 100 ng/mL are associated with metastatic disease. On the other hand, low PSA levels (less than 10 ng/mL) are seldom found in the presence of lymph node metastases, leading some to suggest that a pelvic lymph node dissection is not necessary in select patients. Imaging studies of the prostate have been widely investigated for staging, but their ability to detect microscopic extension of cancer is limited. The results are highly dependent on the imaging protocol and radiologist. CT scans of the abdomen and pelvis rarely provide useful information. Except for patients with signs of advanced cancer, these studies should not be performed. The classic test for metastasis is the bone scan, but even the routine use of bone scans has been questioned in recent series.[96] Although more sensitive than plain films, bone scintigraphy lacks specificity for cancer; false-positive tests are common. In patients with a PSA less than 10 ng/mL, true-positive bone scans are rare (< 1%), and a bone scan is unnecessary. Abnormal bone scans are often followed by plain radiographs, which are useful to document the presence of benign bony abnormalities, such as arthritis, to explain the abnormal scan. Magnetic resonance imaging (MRI) of the bone is the most sensitive and specific technique to confirm or exclude bony metastasis suspected by radionuclide imaging.

Newer Staging Tests Endorectal MRI has been shown by several investigators to be a useful imaging modality to predict pathologic T3 prostate cancer in some clinical stage T1–T2 patients who undergo radical prostatectomy. D'Amico and colleagues have shown that in an intermediate-risk subgroup of patients (PSA between 10 and 20 ng/mL, Gleason score 7 or less, and percent-positive biopsies at least 50%), the erMRI has an accuracy of 78% in predicting extracapsular extension (accuracy = 70%) or seminal vesical invasion (accuracy = 90%).[97] The reproducibility of erMRI interpretations between radiologists is a significant issue, however. MRI using lymphotrophic nanoparticles as a contrast agent represents a new and promising method to evaluate for lymph node metastases. Lymphotrophic nanoparticles have an iron-oxide core surrounded by dextran and cause changes in magnetic properties detectable by MRI. When injected into the circulation, they are slowly transported into lymph nodes by the lymphatic vessels, where they are internalized by macrophages. In lymph nodes partially replaced by cancer, no nanoparticles are visualized because the macrophages in that area have been replaced. In men with high-risk but presumed localized prostate cancer, Harisinghani and colleagues found that this technique was able to accurately identify patients with lymph node involvement (positive predictive value of 94.2%, negative predictive value of 100%).[98]

Reverse transcription of messenger RNA followed by the polymerase chain reaction (RT-PCR) can identify circulating prostate cancer cells that express PSA or prostate-specific membrane antigen (PSMA).[99] Studies in clinically localized patients have shown very variable results, which are at least partly due to significant technical differences. Hematogenous PSA-expressing cells have been identified by RT-PCR in 0 to 81% of patients prior to radical prostatectomy. In patients documented to have metastatic disease, RT-PCR detected circulating cancer cells in 31 to 100% of patients.[100] In a pooled analysis of available data of RT-PCR in peripheral blood, 174 of 757 (23%) patients with pathologic T1 or T2 disease and 151 of 401 (38%) patients with pT3 disease were found to be RT-PCR positive for PSA or PSMA. All but two of the studies evaluated showed no additional advantage to the use of RT-PCR over conventional staging modalities.

A radiolabeled murine monoclonal antibody to PSMA (In-111 Capromab; ProstaScint) has been developed to improve clinical staging, but may be of more value to detect recurrences after local therapy for prostate cancer. In one trial of 32 men who failed radical prostatectomy and received salvage radiotherapy to the pelvis, 70% of the patients who had a normal ProstaScint scan outside the prostatic fossa achieved a durable decrease in PSA to below 0.3 ng/mL, whereas only 22% who had a positive scan outside of the pelvis did so ($p = .02$).[101]

Fluorinated [18F] deoxyglucose positron emission tomography (FDG-PET) has had limited utility in prostate cancer staging to date.[102] Current research is now directed at improved radiotracers for use in prostate cancer, including [18F] fluorocholine, [11C] methionine and [11C] acetate.

PROGNOSTIC FACTORS IN PROSTATE CANCER

Prostate cancer is a heterogenous disease with markedly variable outcomes. Hence, identifying prognostic factors for patients with prostate cancer is an important and fertile area of research.

Table 97-6 8-Year Biochemical Relapse-Free Survival (RFS) after Radical Prostatectomy Based on Pathologic Characteristics

Pathologic Findings	RFS (%)
No extracapsular extension	92
Extracapsular extension	
Margin negative	77
Margin positive	50
Seminal vesicle invasion	34
Lymph node positive	0
Overall	76

Adapted from Clark PE et al.[312]

Countless clinical and pathologic factors (using both routine and novel tests) that have predictive significance have been identified and multiple nomograms have been constructed. Several issues are important to consider when assessing these factors: Is the prognostic factor clinical or pathologic? Is measurement of the factor within routine clinical practice or does it require a novel assay? To what patient population is the factor pertinent (ie, postprostatectomy, postradiation therapy, metastatic androgen independent)? Most importantly, what outcome is being considered? Common outcomes include extent of disease at surgery, PSA recurrence-free survival and prostate cancer-specific survival.

Predicting the extent of disease at surgery is important because disease-free survival from prostate cancer depends in part on surgical findings, especially extracapsular extension, seminal vesicle invasion, and lymph node involvement (Table 97-6). Clinical factors that predict surgical results include biopsy Gleason grade, preoperative serum PSA, and possibly perineural invasion in the biopsy specimen. The Partin score[103] is a validated[104] nomogram that combines summed Gleason grade, PSA, and clinical T stage to predict prostatectomy results—in particular, the probability of organ-confined cancer and the probability of lymph node involvement (Table 97-7).[97]

PSA recurrence (also called biochemical recurrence or PSA control) is a common outcome for studies considering prognostic factors due in part to its ease of measurement and a short time-to-event needed. Importantly, it is of unclear clinical significance, in part because the time from PSA recurrence to the development of metastases can be quite long even without treatment (8 years in a study by Pound and colleagues[105]) and because PSA recurrence does not necessarily imply a worse overall survival.[106] With these caveats, a number of clinical, pathologic factors have been associated with PSA recurrence, including race[107] (although other studies have not[108]), obesity,[107] the number of positive biopsies and the maximum percentage of each core involved.[109] Many other novel, putative prognostic factors have been studied and appear to offer some prognostic value, including loss of p16 expression,[110] transrectal ultrasound results,[111] IL-6 soluble receptor, TGF-β,[112] quantitative nuclear morphometry, DNA ploidy, Ki-67 staining,[113] and microvessel density. Others have con-

Table 97-7 Partin Tables, Percent Likelihood of Pathologic Results, Given Gleason Score, PSA and Clinical Stage

		Gleason Score				
PSA Range (ng/mL)	Pathologic Stage	2–4	5–6	3 + 4 = 7	4 + 3 = 7	8–10
Clinical Stage T1c (nonpalpable, PSA elevated)						
0–2.5	Organ confined	95	90	79	71	66
	Extraprostatic extension	5	9	17	25	28
	Seminal vesicle		0	2	2	4
	Lymph node			1	1	1
2.6–4.0	Organ confined	92	84	68	58	52
	Extraprostatic extension	8	15	27	37	40
	Seminal vesicle	1	4	4	4	6
	Lymph node		1	1	1	
4.1–6.0	Organ confined	90	80	63	52	46
	Extraprostatic extension	10	19	32	42	45
	Seminal vesicle		1	3	3	5
	Lymph node		0	2	3	3
6.1–10.0	Organ confined	87	75	54	43	37
	Extraprostatic extension	13	23	36	47	48
	Seminal vesicle		2	8	8	13
	Lymph node		0	2	2	3
> 10.0	Organ confined	80	62	37	7	22
	Extraprostatic extension	20	33	43	51	50
	Seminal vesicle		4	12	11	17
	Lymph node		2	8	10	11
Clinical Stage T2a (palpable, < 1/2 one lobe)						
0–2.5	Organ confined	91	81	64	53	47
	Extraprostatic extension	9	17	29	40	42
	Seminal vesicle		1	5	4	7
	Lymph node		0	2	3	3
2.6–4.0	Organ confined	85	71	50	39	33
	Extraprostatic extension	15	27	41	52	53
	Seminal vesicle		2	7	6	10
	Lymph node		0	2	2	3
4.1–6.0	Organ confined	81	66	44	33	28
	Extraprostatic extension	19	32	46	56	58
	Seminal vesicle		1	5	5	8
	Lymph node		1	4	6	6
6.1–10.0	Organ confined	76	58	35	25	21
	Extraprostatic extension	24	37	49	58	57
	Seminal vesicle		4	13	11	17
	Lymph node		1	3	5	5
> 10.0	Organ confined	65	42	20	14	11
	Extraprostatic extension	35	47	49	55	52
	Seminal vesicle		6	16	13	19
	Lymph node		4	14	18	17
Clinical Stage T2b (palpable, > 1/2 one lobe, not bilateral)						
0–2.5	Organ confined	88	75	54	43	37
	Extraprostatic extension	12	22	35	45	46
	Seminal vesicle		2	6	5	9
	Lymph node		1	4	6	6
2.6–4.0	Organ confined	80	63	41	30	25
	Extraprostatic extension	20	34	47	57	57
	Seminal vesicle		2	9	7	12
	Lymph node		1	3	4	5
4.1–6.0	Organ confined	75	57	35	25	21
	Extraprostatic extension	25	39	51	60	59
	Seminal vesicle		2	7	5	9
	Lymph node		2	7	10	10
6.1–10.0	Organ confined	69	49	26	19	15
	Extraprostatic extension	31	44	52	60	57
	Seminal vesicle		5	16	13	19
	Lymph node		2	6	8	8
> 10.0	Organ confined	57	33	14	9	7
	Extraprostatic extension	43	52	47	50	46
	Seminal vesicle		8	17	13	19
	Lymph node		8	22	27	27

(Continued)

Table 97-7 Partin Tables, Percent Likelihood of Pathologic Results, Given Gleason Score, PSA and Clinical Stage *(Continued)*

		Gleason Score				
PSA Range (ng/mL)	Pathologic Stage	2–4	5–6	3 + 4 = 7	4 + 3 = 7	8–10
Clinical Stage T2c (palpable, both lobes)						
0–2.5	Organ confined	86	73	51	39	34
	Extraprostatic extension	14	24	36	45	47
	Seminal vesicle		1	5	5	8
	Lymph node		1	6	9	10
2.6–4.0	Organ confined	78	61	38	27	23
	Extraprostatic extension	22	36	48	57	57
	Seminal vesicle		2	8	6	10
	Lymph node		1	5	7	8
4.1–6.0	Organ confined	73	55	31	21	18
	Extraprostatic extension	27	40	50	57	57
	Seminal vesicle		2	6	4	7
	Lymph node		3	12	16	16
6.1–10.0	Organ confined	67	46	24	16	13
	Extraprostatic extension	33	46	52	58	56
	Seminal vesicle		5	13	11	16
	Lymph node		3	10	13	13
> 10.0	Organ confined	54	30	11	7	6
	Extraprostatic extension	46	51	42	43	41
	Seminal vesicle		6	13	10	15
	Lymph node		13	33	38	38

Reproduced with permission from Partin AW, et al.[313]

sidered predictors of PSA recurrence after salvage radiotherapy in patients with a rising PSA after radical prostatectomy.[114,115]

D'Amico and colleagues have defined a methodology using similar preoperative clinical variables to predict PSA recurrence-free survival in patients treated with surgery or radiation therapy.[116] A database of 888 patients treated with radical retropubic prostatectomy and 766 patients treated with external beam radiotherapy were followed for a median of 38 months. Using the three well-defined prognostic factors of PSA, Gleason score, and T stage, the investigators defined three risk groups for PSA failure (Table 97-8). Kattan and colleagues[117] developed a similar nomogram (based on a point system for PSA, Gleason biopsy sum, and clinical T stage), which has recently been validated across a wide spectrum of patient populations.[118,119]

The most clinically useful nomograms would predict prostate cancer-specific survival based on easily accessible pretreatment data (there are no published studies to our knowledge that consider factors predicting survival in patients followed with watchful waiting). Two recent studies considered this issue. In the first, D'Amico and colleagues found that their three risk groups predicting 5-year PSA failure-free survival (see Table 97-8) also predicted prostate cancer-specific mortality after treatment with radical prostatectomy or radiation (Figure 97-9).[120] In fact, those patients in the high-risk groups had a relative risk of prostate cancer-specific mortality of 14.2 (surgery) and 14.3 (radiation) times that of similarly treated patients in the low-risk group.

The second study considered the effect of pretreatment PSA velocity on prostate cancer-specific mortality and overall mortality in patients undergoing radical prostatectomy.[121] Post-treatment PSA doubling time (the time it takes the PSA to double once biochemical recurrence is established) is a known predictor of time to distant failure (positive bone scan) and prostate cancer-specific mortality in patients who experience biochemical recurrence after surgery and radiation.[105,122] This study considered PSA change prior to primary treatment (as opposed to once PSA recurrence was established) as annual PSA velocity (the rate of rise of PSA over the year prior to the diagnosis of prostate cancer). They considered a dataset of 1,091 men who had undergone radical prostatectomy for localized prostate cancer and evaluated annual PSA velocity > 2.0 ng/mL, age at diagnosis, Gleason score, clinical T stage, and PSA at diagnosis. In multivariate analysis, the strongest predictor of death from prostate cancer was annual PSA velocity > 2.0 ng/mL (with a relative risk increase of 9.8 as compared with PSA velocity ≤ 2.0 ng/mL), which was also predictive of death from any cause (relative risk of 1.9) (Figure 97-10). A Gleason score of 8, 9, or 10 and a clinical stage of T2 were also predictive of death from prostate cancer.

Table 97-8 Combined Modality Staging Approach

Risk	Characteristics	5-Year PSA Failure-Free Survival after RP	8-Year CaP-Specific Mortality after RP
Low	T1c, T2a and PSA ≤ 10 ng/mL and Gleason grade ≤ 6	90%	0–1%
Medium	T2b or PSA > 10 and ≤ 20 ng/mL or Gleason grade 7	70%	2–3%
High	T2c or PSA > 20 ng/mL or Gleason grade ≥ 8	45%	7–9%

RP = radical prostatectomy; CaP = prostate cancer.
Adapted from D'Amico AV et al.[120,314]

MANAGEMENT OF LOCALIZED PROSTATE CANCER

The optimal management of prostate cancer that is clinically confined to the prostate remains controversial. Standard treatment options for localized disease include radical prostatectomy, radiation therapy, and expectant management (or "watchful waiting"). There has been a paucity of well-conducted randomized therapeutic trials to help distinguish the comparative risks and benefits of each of these approaches. In addition, rapid improvements have occurred in both the technical aspects of care as well as our understanding of the biology and outcome of therapy for prostate cancer. Nonetheless, there are ample data available to help guide patients toward the most appropriate therapy for their individual circumstances.

Expectant Management When a TURP is done for presumed benign prostatic hypertrophy, approximately 10% of patients are found to have occult cancer. Those with cancer in less than 5% of the pathologic specimen are classified as T1a. Such incidental cancers rarely contain poorly differentiated elements, and long-term survival, with observation alone, approaches that of the normal population. However, T1a cancers may progress locally or metastasize, particularly in younger men followed for more than 10 years. Cancers sampled by transurethral resection are usually transition zone cancers, and such patients often have a separate peripheral zone cancer that can be of a higher grade and stage. Patients with T1a cancer who are considering expectant management should be evaluated with a serum PSA, DRE, and ultrasound, with ultrasound-guided needle biopsies of the peripheral zone 6 to 8 weeks later. Patients with a more extensive (T1b) or high-grade cancer in the resection specimen are more likely to experience progression similar to that of T2 cancers and should be considered for local radical therapy.

The natural history of patients with localized prostate cancer who do not receive definitive local therapy has now been well documented in several large series. Within 10 to 15 years, most patients have cancers that grow locally, fewer patients develop metastases, and, overall, relatively few die from the disease. A pooled analysis of 828 patients from six nonrandomized studies has been reported.[123] Although few men with grade 1 or 2 tumors died of their cancer within 10 years, 19% of the patients with grade 1, 42% with grade 2, and 74% with grade 3 developed metastases within 10 years. Johansson and colleagues have published

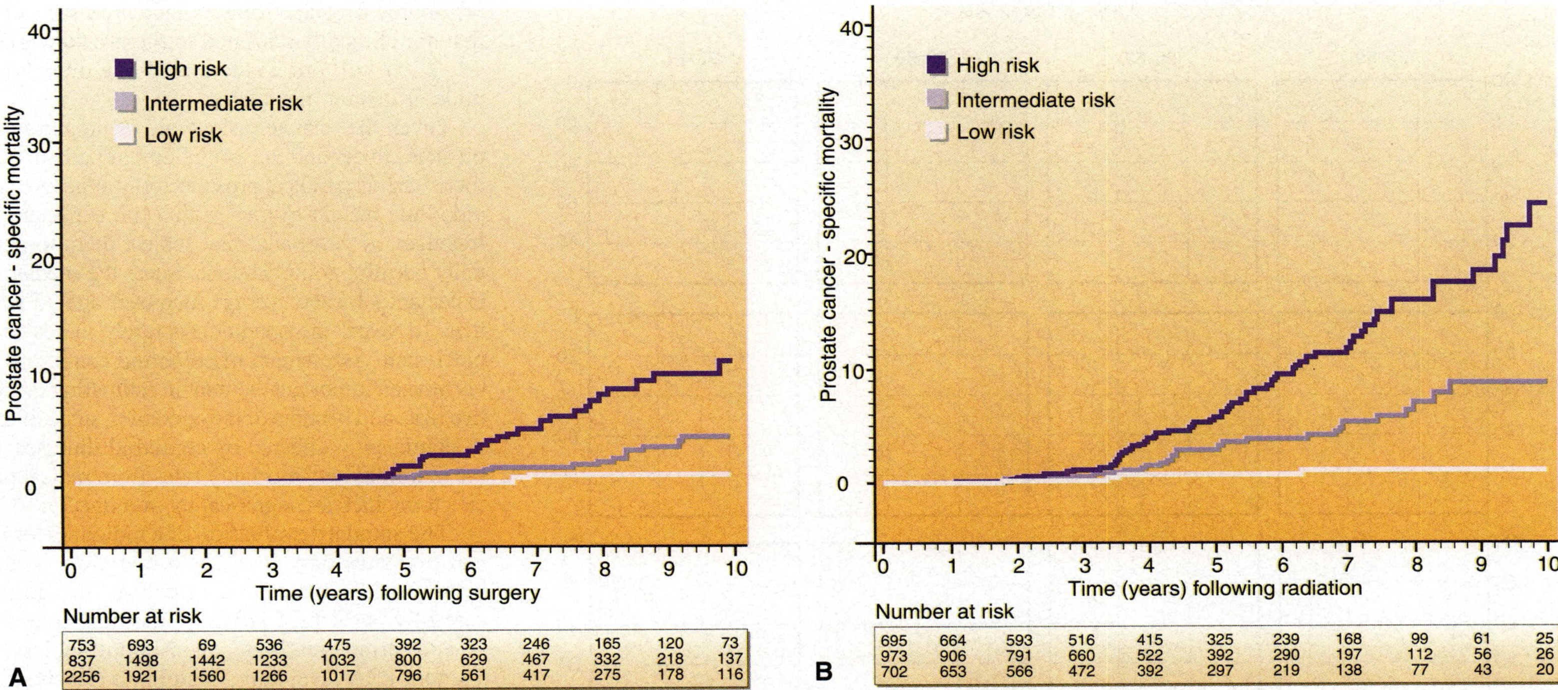

Figure 97-9 Prostate cancer-specific mortality after radical prostatectomy **(A)** and radiation therapy **(B)** stratified by the pretreatment risk group. Pairwise p values (clinical significance defined as $p < .05/3$ or .017). Comparisons of intermediate vs low, high vs low, and high vs intermediate within each treatment modality $p \leq .001$. Reproduced with permission from D'Amico AV et al.[120]

outcomes in a Swedish population-based cohort that demonstrated similar results in patients followed for 15 years (Table 97-9).[124] Interestingly, though, when followed for longer (mean 21 years), substantial decreases in progression-free survival (45–36%), survival without metastases (76.9–61.2%) and prostate cancer-specific mortality (78.7–58.4%) were observed. These data argue that even in this older population with well-differentiated tumors, tumor progression is an important problem in men with a life expectancy greater than 15 years. A large retrospective cohort study reviewed the causes of death of 767 men followed without aggressive local therapy at diagnosis.[125] The Connecticut Tumor Registry was searched for men aged 55 to 74 diagnosed between 1971 and 1984 with localized prostate cancer. None of the patients analyzed had prostate surgery or radiation therapy of any kind, although they could have received hormonal ablation treatment. Results demonstrated a profound impact of Gleason score on prostate cancer-specific mortality at 15 years. The authors concluded that men with prostate biopsies demonstrating Gleason 7 to 10 prostate adenocarcinomas face high rates of death from prostate cancer, even with significant comorbid illnesses or when diagnosed as late as 74 years of age. Conversely, men with Gleason scores of 2 to 6 face minimal to modest risks of prostate cancer death, with slowly increasing risk in the Gleason 5 and 6 tumors over time (Figure 97-11).

Several conclusions can be drawn from these three reports. All demonstrate similar data regarding the impact of histologic grade on cancer-specific survival. Secondly, untreated Gleason 7 tumors behave in an aggressive fashion and should be grouped with higher-grade cancers. Finally, age at diagnosis appears to have little impact on cancer-specific mortality at 15 years in patients with low-grade cancers, although with longer follow-up cancer-specific mortality rises substantially. In summary, expectant management may be considered an option for some patients with low-grade localized prostate cancer and a life expectancy of less than 15 years.

In 2002, a Scandinavian randomized clinical trial of radical prostatectomy versus watchful waiting was published.[126] From 1989 to 1999, 695 men with localized prostate cancer were randomized and observed for a median of 6.2 years. Most of the patients in this trial were detected by an abnormal prostate exam, rather than by PSA screening, and the mean PSA at diagnosis was 12.9 ng/mL. Death from prostate cancer was significantly decreased in the surgery arm compared with watchful waiting (relative hazard 0.50, $p = .02$). However, there was no difference in overall survival between the two

PSA velocity > 200 ng/mL/yr
PSA velocity 101-200 ng/mL/yr
PSA velocity 51-100 ng/mL/yr
PSA velocity < 50 ng/mL/yr
Death from prostate cancer (%)
Years after radical prostatectomy

Number at risk

PSA velocity > 200 ng/mL/yr	262	257	248	226	187	157	123	92	60	36	22
PSA velocity 101-200 ng/mL/yr	288	275	248	229	194	158	131	91	58	36	20
PSA velocity 51-100 ng/mL/yr	289	281	260	227	176	131	94	55	36	18	11
PSA velocity < 50 ng/mL/yr	256	236	200	163	139	108	81	61	34	20	9

Figure 97-10 Kaplan-Meier estimates of cumulative death from prostate cancer after radical prostatectomy, according to quartile of PSA velocity in year before diagnosis. Log rank test $p < .05$ for comparison of PSA velocity > 2.00 ng/mL/yr as compared with each of the three other quartiles. Reproduced with permission from D'Amico AV et al.[121]

Table 97-9 Follow-Up of Conservatively Managed Patients in Sweden

		Progression-Free Survival (%)		Overall Survival (%)		Prostate Cancer–Specific Survival (%)	
		15 Yrs	20 Yrs	15 Yrs	20 Yrs	15 Yrs	20 Yrs
Stage	T01	57.7	52.5	22.2	7.5	81.1	57.9
	T0d	35.9	17.9	14.7	0	69.7	46.4
	T1–2	38.4	33.1	23.1	10.3	80.3	56.9
Grade	1	56.0	46.0	24.3	9.7	88.9	71.8
	2	28.8	24.3	18.2	3.5	64.5	22.1
	3	15.6	0	0	0	28.6	0
All patients		45.0	36.0	21.5	7.5	78.7	54.5

T01 – clinically occult, incidental, cancer < 25% of specimen; T0d – clinically occult, incidental, cancer > 25% of specimen
Grade 1 – highly differentiated; Grade 2 – moderately differentiated; Grade 3 – poorly differentiated

Adapted from Johansson JE et al.[124]

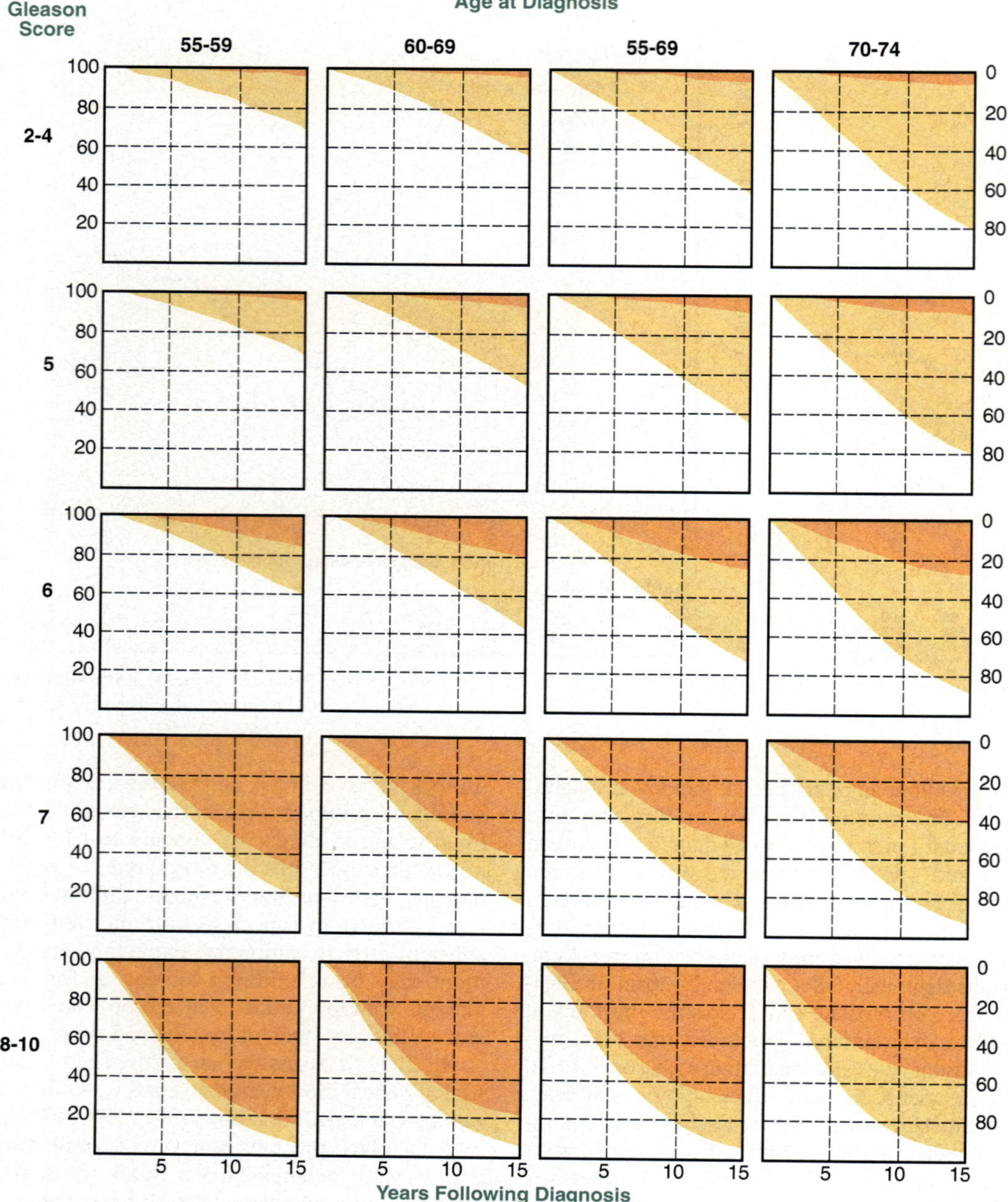

Figure 97-11 Expectant management of clinically localized prostate cancer. Dark shaded area represents mortality from prostate cancer. Light shaded area represents mortality from other causes. Adapted with permission from Albertson PC et al.[125]

groups. Also of significance, however, was that there was a significant increased risk of metastases in the watchful waiting arm. Longer follow-up will be necessary to demonstrate whether a difference in overall survival may be seen.

RADICAL PROSTATECTOMY

Radical prostatectomy has been used to treat prostate cancer for over 100 years. In 1904, Hugh Hampton Young performed the first radical surgery of the prostate in an attempt to cure cancer. For the subsequent 40 years, radical perineal prostatectomy was the surgical treatment of choice for localized prostate cancer. However, in the mid-1940s, Millin introduced the retropubic approach, which has since become the more popular surgical approach, largely because of the technical improvements resulting from delineation of the periprostatic anatomy by Walsh and colleagues in the 1980s. Long-term cancer control has been well documented in patients after radical prostatectomy followed for as many as 30 years. With modern surgical techniques, the morbidity of this procedure is low. The most troubling patient-reported complications are urinary incontinence and loss of erectile function.

Patient Selection The appropriate selection of candidates for radical prostatectomy requires an assessment both of the extent of cancer as well as the age and overall health of the patient. Since radical prostatectomy is curative only if the entire tumor is removed, accurate preoperative staging is essential. Extension of the cancer beyond the immediate periprostatic tissue into the seminal vesicles or pelvic lymph nodes is associated with a high probability of cancer recurrence. Radical retropubic prostatectomy is indicated for cancers that are clinically confined to the prostate (stages T1–T2b) without evidence of regional lymph node or distant metastases.

Given the relatively slow rate of progression of prostate cancer and the availability of palliative hormonal therapy, radical prostatectomy appears to provide little benefit to men with a life expectancy of less than 10 years and may subject them to potentially harmful complications. Since the median life expectancy for the average man over age 75 is less than 10 years, the operation is rarely indicated for older men. Assessment of comorbid conditions has become an important element in estimating the relative risks and benefits of the operation, since lifespan is significantly affected by comorbid illnesses, and the morbidity and mortality rates from radical prostatectomy increase significantly over age 75.

The standard evaluation of candidates for radical prostatectomy includes a complete medical history and physical examination, including a carefully performed DRE. In addition to urinalysis and serum creatinine, other important tests are a serum PSA level and a histologic review of the prostate biopsy specimen. In men with PSA < 10 ng/mL and Gleason score < 7, generally no further staging studies are necessary. In other cases, a bone scan is done to rule out bony metastases. Abdominal-pelvic CT scans are rarely abnormal in patients with clinically localized prostate cancer and need not routinely be performed.

Seminal vesicle invasion is a poor prognostic finding. Patients with palpable extension of cancer to the seminal vesicles (T3c) are not candidates for radical prostatectomy and almost inevitably experience early recurrence of the cancer. Endorectal coil MRI has been used with some success to detect microscopic invasion of the seminal vesicles. Patients with intermediate-risk disease (ie, clinical stage T2b or PSA > 10 and ≤ 20 ng/mL or biopsy Gleason score 7) represent the group that stands to gain the most valuable information from an erMRI. In a study by D'Amico and colleagues,[97] intermediate-risk patients who had at least 50% of their biopsies positive were evaluated by erMRI. Those patients with radiographic T2 disease had a 5-year biochemical freedom from recurrence of 50% compared with only 5% if there was evidence of ECE or seminal vesicle invasion.

Surgical Technique Modern refinements in surgical technique have minimized blood loss such that routine blood transfusions are generally unnecessary. Pain related to the abdominal incision has been ameliorated with the use of smaller incisions, oral anesthetics, and improved nonsteroidal anti-inflammatory drugs. The postoperative hospital stay has decreased to 2 to 3 days with retropubic prostatectomy and 1 to 3 days with perineal prostatectomy. The major advantages of the retropubic approach are a lower risk of positive surgical margins, a greater probability of preservation of potency, and an opportunity to perform a pelvic lymphadenectomy during the same procedure.

Radical retropubic prostatectomy has the advantage that the operation can be modified

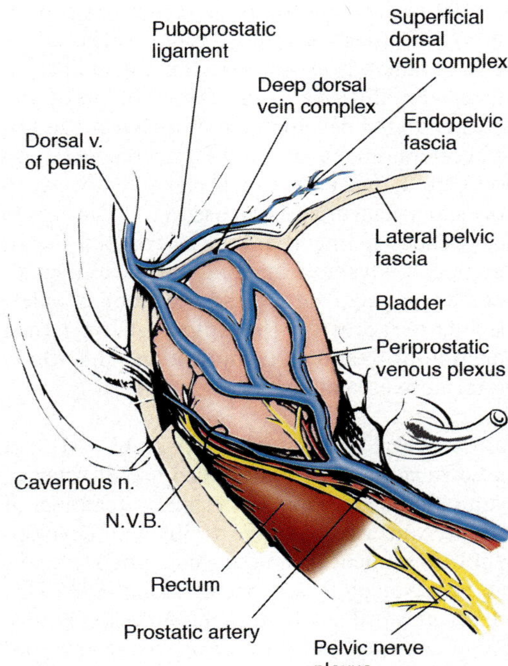

Figure 97-12 Surgical anatomy of the prostate in relationship to the deep dorsal vein complex, neurovascular bundle (NVB), and other surrounding periprostatic structures (lateral view).

depending on the extent of the tumor and the location of the neurovascular bundles in order to ensure wide excision around the cancer (Figure 97-12). It is especially important to dissect widely around the apex of the prostate, where positive surgical margins are reported to be most common. Nerve-sparing prostatectomy is indicated for patients who have preoperative erectile function, organ-confined tumor, serum PSA levels of less than 10 ng/mL, and a DRE that does not indicate tumor at the prostatic apex or posterolateral borders. Depending on the extent of tumor intraoperatively, one or both neurovascular bundles may be preserved by careful anatomic dissection. Further details of surgical technique have been described elsewhere (Figure 97-13).

Cancer Control after Radical Prostatectomy **Pathologic Results** The primary goal of radical prostatectomy is to remove all of the cancer. Treatment failures occur because the cancer had spread to distant sites before the operation or because the local tumor was not completely excised. Positive surgical margins have been reported in 16 to 48% of patients. Several studies have suggested that positive margins are associated with an increased probability of progression, especially local recurrence. Every effort should be made to decrease the rate of positive surgical margins.

In a series reported from Baylor University, positive surgical margins, defined as the presence of cancer cells at the inked margin of resection, were present in 16% of patients.[127] At 5 years, the actuarial progression rate was 17% if the margins were negative, compared with 36% if the margins were positive ($p < .02$). Among patients with positive lymph nodes or seminal vesicle involvement, positive surgical margins had no significant impact on prognosis. Another large series from the Mayo Clinic reported comparable results: 3,170 consecutive patients with clinically localized disease undergoing radical prostatectomy were evaluated, resulting in pathologic organ-confined disease in 47%, capsular penetration and seminal vesicle invasion in 42%, and lymph node involvement in 11%.[128] Positive surgical margins were noted in 24%.

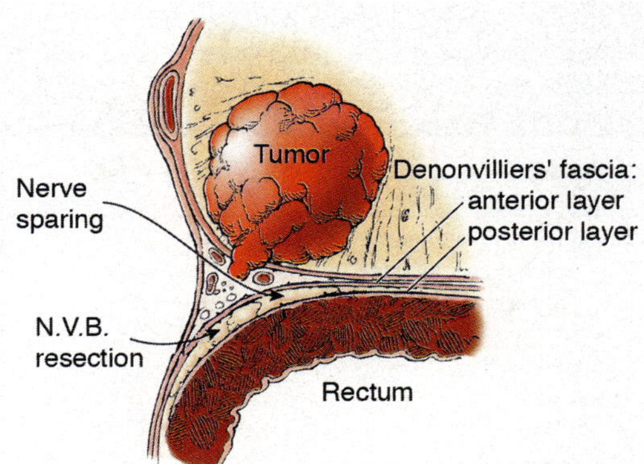

Figure 97-13 Illustration of the relationship of the neurovascular bundle (NVB) to a tumor in the prostate and the rectum. Arrows show the plane of dissection for nerve-sparing radical prostatectomy versus nerve resection.[13]

Overall Recurrence Many different end points have been used to assess the results of radical prostatectomy for clinically localized prostate cancer, including overall survival rates, prostate cancer-specific survival rates, freedom from metastases, freedom from local recurrence, and freedom from biochemical recurrence as documented by serum PSA levels. Serum PSA should normally become undetectable after radical prostatectomy. Rising serum PSA levels generally precede clinical recurrence, detected by DRE or bone scan, by as many as 6 to 8 years.[105] Therefore, biochemical progression rates, defined as time to recurrence documented by PSA levels in patients treated with no other therapy, are the fastest means to assess contemporary results of treatment, although cancer-specific survival remains the gold standard for measuring outcomes of local therapy.

Zincke and colleagues have reported overall survival after radical prostatectomy to be 75% and 60% after 10 and 15 years, respectively.[128] Cancer-specific survival was 90% and 82%, respectively. Gleason grade was the strongest correlate for survival. Ten- and 15-year cancer-specific survival for men with Gleason grades of 4 to 6 were 90% and 82%, respectively, whereas Gleason grades 7 or above were 82% or 71%, respectively. Freedom from PSA recurrence was 52% and 40% at 10 and 15 years, respectively.

In a modern series from the Johns Hopkins Hospital, 2,404 patients with clinically localized prostate cancer underwent nerve-sparing radical prostatectomy with 15-year follow-up. Fifteen year recurrence-free survival rates were 84% for stage T2, 58% for stage T3 (33% if Gleason > 7) and 17% for seminal vesicle involement.[129] No patient with positive lymph nodes was free of PSA recurrence at 15 years. These data make clear that pathologic stage is an important predictor for clinical outcome after radical prostatectomy.

In summary, radical retropubic prostatectomy has been demonstrated to be an effective means to eradicate organ-confined prostate cancer. For men with extracapsular disease, involvement of seminal vesicles, or high-grade cancers, cure is far less likely.

Complications of Radical Retropubic Prostatectomy **Early Complications** The mortality rate from radical prostatectomy ranges from 0.1 to 0.7% in modern series. When stratified by age, however, mortality rates rise. Lu-Yao and colleagues reported men aged 65 to 75 years old with a death rate from prostatectomy of less than 1%, whereas those men over 80 years old had a mortality rate approaching 5%.[130] Traditionally, radical prostatectomy had resulted in substantial blood loss and the frequent need for transfusions. Greater appreciation, however, of the anatomy of the dorsal vein complex and the periprostatic fascia has allowed the development of techniques to control these vessels early in the course of the operation. Mean blood loss during prostatectomy ranges from 600 to over 2,000 mL, and rates of homologous blood transfusion range from 5 to 11.5%.[131] Inadvertent rectal injury is uncommon, occurring in about 1 to 1.2% of patients in most series.[132] This complication can be treated with primary closure or sometimes a temporary diverting colostomy.

With shortened operating times and early ambulation, deep venous thrombosis and pulmonary embolism are seen in only 1 to 2% of patients. In one trial, prophylactic anticoagulation and pneumatic compression stockings were not shown to decrease this rate of thromboembolism.[133] Anastomotic strictures are usually the result of poor apposition of the bladder to the urethra and of tight closure of the bladder neck aperture during reconstruction.[134] Eversion of the bladder neck mucosa has markedly reduced the incidence of this complication. Bladder neck contractures usually necessitate incision, with some patients requiring periodic dilation to maintain an adequate urine flow.

Late Complications Late complications of radical prostatectomy include urinary incontinence and erectile dysfunction. Urinary incontinence remains one of the most troubling side effects. Although the rate of incontinence is lower now than reported 20 years ago, recent series report an incidence of stress urinary incontinence ranging from 5 to 13%.[135] Of 593 patients treated at one institution, 92% had complete continence, 8% had mild or moderate stress urinary incontinence, and 0.3% had severe urinary incontinence at 1 year. The risk of incontinence increases with the age of the patient at the time of the operation. In another series of over 1,300 patients, 92% had complete recovery of urinary continence, which was correlated positively with younger age but not tumor stage or nerve-sparing approach.[136]

When patients are queried by validated questionnaires administered by objective observers, the rate of incontinence is found to be higher. In one

Table 97-10 Urinary Complications of Radical Prostatectomy: Data from Prostate Cancer Outcome Study

Measure	Baseline (%)	24 Months (%)
Level of urinary control		
Total control	78.0	31.9
Occasional leakage	8.5	40.2
Frequent leakage	2.3	6.8
No control	0.7	1.6
Use of pads for incontinence		
None	86.8	58.1
1–2 pads/day	1.3	18.3
≥ 3 pads/day	0.9	3.3
Mean incontinence function score	91.2	75.1*
How big a problem is incontinence?		
No problem	77.8	37.8
Small problem	8.8	33.9
Moderate to big problem	2.7	8.7

* $p < .01$ compared with baseline.
Adapted from Stanford JL et al.[136]

Table 97-11 Sexual Complications of Radical Prostatectomy by Age: Data from Prostate Cancer Outcomes Study

Measure	Baseline (%)	24 Months (%)
Erections firm enough for intercourse, by age in years		
< 60	92.6	39.0
60–64	84.4	21.7
65–74	75.7	15.3
75–79	48.6	19.1
Mean sexual function score	71.5	38.6*
How big a problem is sexual function?		
No problem	50.3	14.0
Small problem	20.2	22.6
Moderate to big problem	17.9	41.9

* $p < .01$ compared with baseline.
Adapted from Stanford JL et al.[136]

such prospective cohort study, Talcott and colleagues evaluated 279 men using self-reported patient symptom questionnaires prior to surgery or radiation therapy and after 3 and 12 months.[137] Urinary problems were uncommon preoperatively. At 3 months, 24% reported some leaking or dribbling, but this decreased to 11% at 12 months. At 3 months, 58% were using pads within the prior week, whereas only 35% were still using this at 1 year. In a large population-based longitudinal cohort study of 1,291 men followed for 18 or more months, 8.4% were incontinent. Age was a strong determinant, with 13.8% of men aged 75 to 79 years developing incontinence but only 0.7 to 3.6% in men younger than 74 years old (Table 97-10). Urodynamic studies of incontinent patients indicate that the functional length of the urethra is an important factor in postprostatectomy incontinence.

Historically, radical prostatectomy caused universal loss of erections. Today, however, a more precise understanding of the anatomy of the neurovascular bundles adjacent to the prostate allows preservation of sexual function in significantly more men. Three major factors are associated with postoperative potency: age, clinical and pathologic stage, and whether the neurovascular bundles were preserved. Walsh and colleagues from Johns Hopkins reported that 342 of 503 patients (68%) were potent with a minimum follow-up of 18 months, and 76% of patients who had both neurovascular bundles preserved were potent compared with 60% who had unilateral neurovascular bundle preservation.[138] Ninety-one percent of men under 50 years of age recovered potency compared with only 25% for men over the age of 70 years. Catalona and colleagues reported a similar outcome of adequate potency in 68% of nearly 800 men in their series who had bilateral nerve-sparing procedures.[139]

Most men of any age experience a substantial decrease in the strength and duration of erections even if they are able to have an unassisted erection satisfactory for intercourse on some occasions (Table 97-11). Fortunately, there are a variety of relatively inexpensive, safe, effective treatments for erectile dysfunction, including new oral agents such as sildenafil (Viagra). There is early evidence that sildenafil may be able to reverse the impotence associated with surgery, although this effect is primarily seen in patients with bilateral nerve-sparing procedures.

RADIATION THERAPY

The first attempt to treat prostate cancer with radiation therapy was undertaken by Hugh Hampton Young and colleagues at Johns Hopkins Hospital in the early twentieth century by intraurethral placement of radium rods.[140] The emergence of radiation as a primary treatment of prostate cancer did not occur, however, until the 1950s, with the development of megavoltage linear accelerators that allowed for deep penetration of radiation, thus providing acceptable toxicity to more superficial organs and tissues.[141] During the past decade, the incorporation of computer technology and advanced imaging has become commonplace in the planning and execution of external beam radiation therapy, resulting in a reduction of treatment complications and allowing for dose escalation.[142]

TREATMENT TECHNIQUE **External Beam Radiotherapy** The widespread use of external beam radiation therapy as a primary treatment of prostate cancer dates to the 1950s with development of treatment techniques using newly available megavoltage linear accelerators.[140,143] This pioneering work led to the common use of a four-field technique using anterior, posterior, and opposed lateral fields. The initial volume, typically including the prostate, seminal vesicles, and, at times, the pelvic lymph nodes, are treated to 4,500 to 5,040 cGy using daily 180 to 200 cGy fractions 5 days per week followed by a boost to the prostate with similar technique to a total dose of 6,600 to 7,000 cGy (Figure 97-14).

The development of more powerful computer-aided treatment planning systems and the direct application of CT for simulation since the late 1980s has led to the use of treatment fields with blocks shaped to conform to the CT-defined prostate and seminal vesicles (so-called conformal three-dimensional planning) (see Figure 97-14). Enhanced visualization of the target volume from

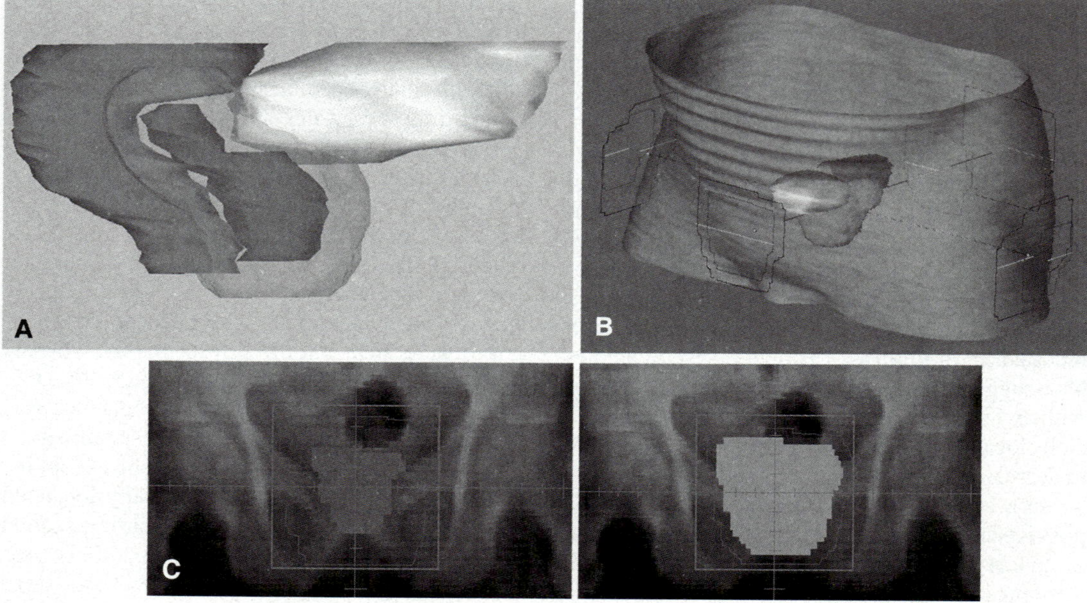

Figure 97-14 **A,** Computed tomography (CT) generated 3-dimensional anatomic definition of the prostate, bladder and rectum. A uniform margin has been projected around the prostate for definition of conformal therapy. **B,** 3-dimensional reconstruction from CT data demonstrating 4 field beam arrangement for conformal therapy. **C,** Beam's eye view of treatment field projected on a digitally reconstructed radiograph (DRR) used to confirm daily treatment set-up.

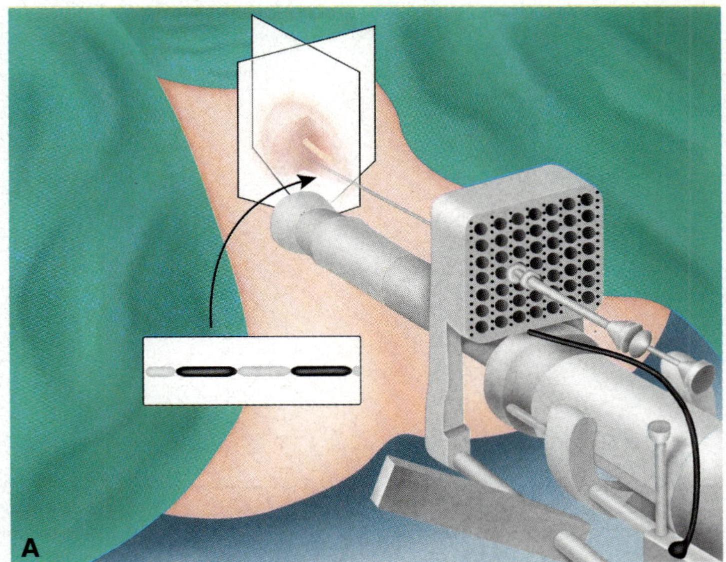

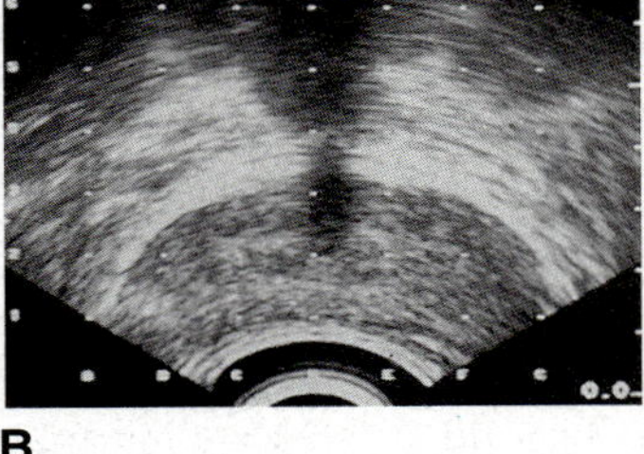

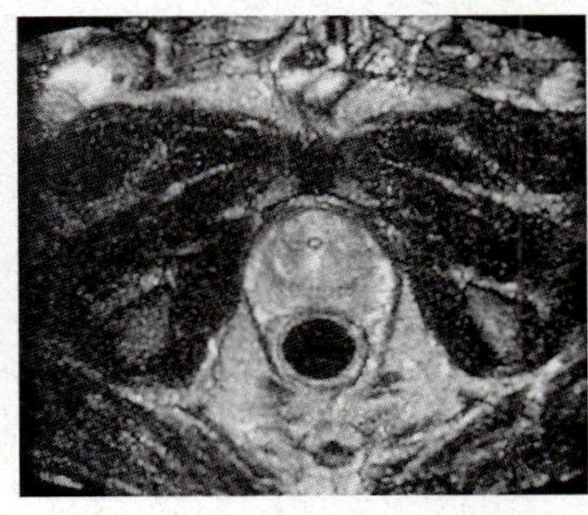

Figure 97-15 **A,** Schematic diagram of stereotactic transperineal prostate brachytherapy using transrectal ultrasound guidance. **B,** Comparison of prostate images obtained by ultrasound (left) and magnetic resonance imaging (MRI) (right) for performance of prostate brachytherapy.

any potential treatment delivery angle, referred to as "beam's eye view," allows for complex three-dimensional field arrangements in place of the four-field box technique. Reduction in complications with complex field arrangement and conformal therapy has allowed for dose escalation beyond 7,000 cGy.

Brachytherapy In the early 1970s, a suprapubic approach for brachytherapy was used, requiring a surgical incision and manual needle guidance by placement of the brachytherapist's hand into the rectum. Although initial reports suggested a favorable disease-free survival,[144] subsequent follow-up yielded higher failure rates attributable to suboptimal dosimetry.[145] In 1983, Holm and colleagues introduced the stereotactic perineal approach using TRUS guidance.[146] Prostate brachytherapy currently is most commonly performed using a low dose rate (LDR) technique but may also be performed as a high dose rate (HDR) procedure. Iodine (I-125) or palladium (Pd-103) are the sources of energy generally used for LDR brachytherapy and involves the permanent placement of seeds into the prostate. Although a preclinical study suggested that Pd-103, with its shorter half-life, might be advantageous for high-grade tumors,[147] subsequent clinical data did not indicate an advantage for either isotope.[148] Iridium-192 is used for HDR brachytherapy.

The procedure is performed under either general or spinal anesthesia with the patient in the dorsal lithotomy position (Figure 97-15). A TRUS probe is placed into the rectum and biplanar ultrasound imaging is used to define the prostate. The ultrasound probe is secured with a stabilizing unit that allows for 5 mm stepping of the probe into or out of the rectum and a stereotactic template is secured against the perineum. Radioactive seeds may then be placed into predetermined positions within the prostate using catheters or an applicator placed through designated coordinate holes in the template. Recent advances in technique include the introduction of real-time three-dimensional MRI-guided brachytherapy,[149] real-time dosimetric feedback including dose-volume histogram analysis, and MR/ultrasound fusion. Alternatively, HDR brachytherapy may be used to place a high activity source temporarily into the prostate. Catheters are prepositioned using a technique similar to LDR brachytherapy and a computerized treatment planning program is used to determine the required dwell time and sequential positioning of the source at each location needed to achieve coverage of the prostate with the prescription dose.

Radiation Therapy and Outcomes **Favorable Prognosis** Favorable prognosis prostate cancer generally includes patients with T1 or T2a disease, PSA < 10 ng/mL, and Gleason grade < 6. Patients in this group have a 5-year freedom from biochemical failure rate of approximately 85%.[116] Radiotherapeutic options for men in this group include external beam radiation therapy or interstitial prostate brachytherapy. The long-term results of external beam radiation therapy in this group are well established.

The Patterns of Care studies performed during the 1970s and 1980s provided long-term survival data for prostate cancer patients treated in a wide range of community practices.[150] These studies, performed before the PSA era, grouped patients by clinical stage alone in reporting their results. Given the older age of most men diagnosed with prostate cancer, particularly prior to PSA screening, survival statistics were reported in comparison with age-matched controls. For men with T1 prostate cancer, there was no or minimal survival decrement at 15 years for men treated in the 1970s.[151] Men with T2 disease had a 30% risk of local failure and 15% decrease in survival compared with age-matched controls. As Gleason grade and PSA were not accounted for in these studies, it is likely that patients with well- or moderately differentiated tumors and low PSAs have significantly better long-term survival than the average of all men presenting with T2 tumors. A single-institution series from Stanford University reported the long-term outcome of treatment of prostate cancer with radiation therapy in 1,245 patients. Fifteen-year overall survival for 377 patients with T1 to T2a disease was 48%, which compares favorably to a 55% 15-year survival expected for age-matched controls.[143]

The introduction of PSA has led to a realization that disease-free survival for prostate cancer is lower than indicated by clinical means of detection regardless of treatment modality. Both radiation and surgical series indicate that 20 to 35% more treatment failures exist by PSA criteria than defined by clinical parameters alone.[150,151] Outcome reporting using a PSA, or biochemical, end point has the advantage of objectivity and greater sensitivity compared with clinical, radiologic, and pathologic determinates of failure. Limitations, however, include the question of impact of PSA failure on survival and the lack of ability to readily differentiate between local and distant failure. Definition of biochemical failure with high sensitivity and specificity postradiation therapy has also been difficult to establish.

In 1996, the American Society of Therapeutic Radiology and Oncology (ASTRO) established a consensus definition of biochemical failure in irradiated patients. ASTRO defines biochemical failure as three consecutive rises in PSA from nadir value post-treatment,[152] with the time to failure defined as the midpoint in time between the nadir and the first rise in PSA. This definition is now used as a benchmark to facilitate comparison of the large number of studies of prostate cancer treated with radiation.

Long-term clinical disease-free survival has been retrospectively correlated in a large number of patients with biochemical relapse-free (bNED) survival. In an assessment of T1b or T2 patients from the Patterns of Care Study and RTOG trials, 65% of men with 10-year clinical disease-free survival were found to have a PSA < 1.5 ng/mL.[151] Series of patients stratified by pretreatment PSA indicate that favorable prognosis patients treated with external beam radiation therapy have 5-year bNED survival rates of approximately 85%.[116] Shipley and colleagues[153] reported results of a multi-institutional pooled analysis of 1,765 men with clinically localized prostate cancer (T1b,

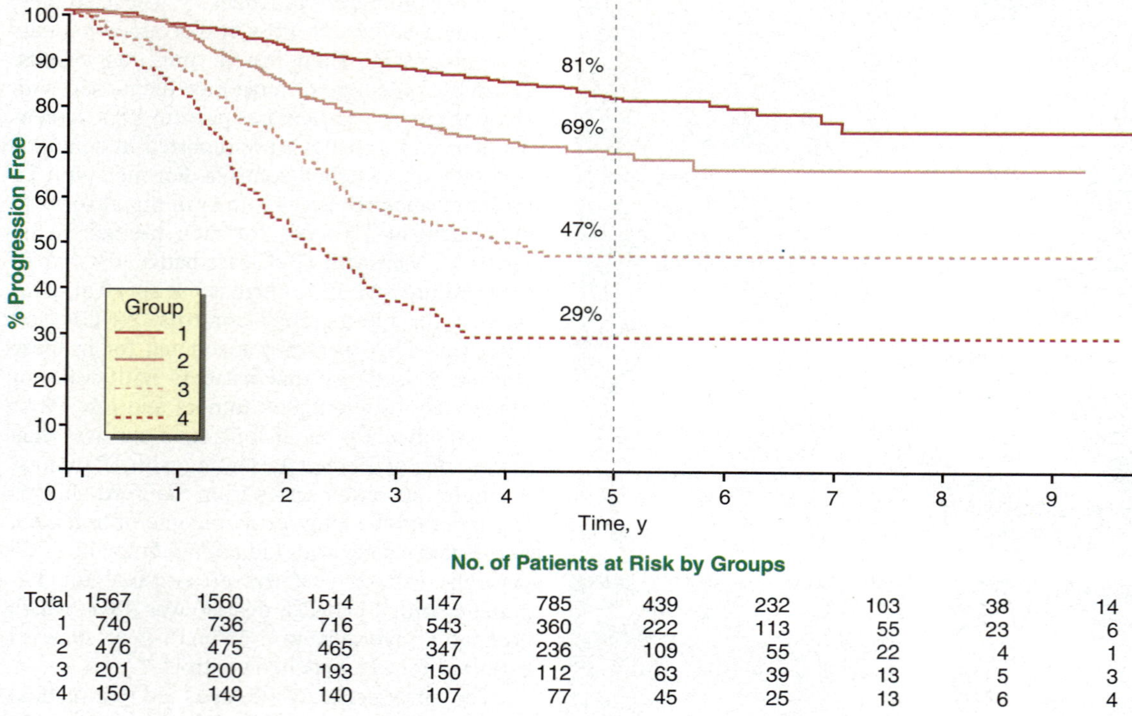

	0	1	2	3	4	5	6	7	8	9
Total	1567	1560	1514	1147	785	439	232	103	38	14
1	740	736	716	543	360	222	113	55	23	6
2	476	475	465	347	236	109	55	22	4	1
3	201	200	193	150	112	63	39	13	5	3
4	150	149	140	107	77	45	25	13	6	4

Figure 97-16 Estimated rates of no biochemical recurrence after external beam radiotherapy for patients grouped into four prognostic factor categories determined by recursive partitioning analysis. (Group 1: Patients with initial PSA < 9.2 ng/mL; Group 2: Patients with PSA 9.2 to < 19.7 ng/dL; Group 3: Patients with PSA of at least 19.7 ng/dL and Gleason score 2- 6; Group 4: Patients with PSA of at least 19.7 ng/dL and Gleason score 7-10. $p < .001$ between all groups. Source: Shipley WU et al.[153]

T1c, and T2) treated with external beam radiation. Twenty-four percent of men had initial PSA values of > 20 ng/mL, placing them in a high-risk group for failure. For all patients, 5-year actuarial estimates of overall survival, disease-specific survival, and bNED survival were 85%, 95%, and 66%, respectively. PSA failure-free rates at 5 and 7 years for men with initial PSA of 10 ng/mL were 78% and 73%. Further analysis yielded four prognostic groups: PSA ≤ 9.2 ng/mL, PSA > 9.2 but < 19.7 ng/mL, PSA ≥ 19.7 ng/mL with Gleason grade 2 to 6, and PSA ≥ 19.7 ng/mL with Gleason grade 7 to 10. Five-year bNED survival rates were 81%, 69%, 47%, and 29%, respectively. Of 302 patients followed beyond 5 years with no evidence of biochemical disease, only 5% relapsed between the fifth and eighth years (Figure 97-16).

Interstitial prostate brachytherapy also has demonstrated promise as treatment of men with favorable prognosis prostate cancer.[154] Recently, Grimm and colleagues reported an 87% 10-year biochemical failure-free rate in 125 consecutive patients with PSA < 10, Gleason 2 to 6 and T1 to T2b treated with brachytherapy alone.[155] Further data on outcome of patients treated with interstitial brachytherapy for favorable prognosis disease are awaited.

Intermediate-Risk Prostate Cancer Intermediate-risk patients include men with bulky clinical T2a or T2b disease, Gleason grade 7, and/or PSA ≥ 10 and < 20 ng/mL. Overall, about 50% of patients with intermediate-risk disease have evidence of biochemical control with conventional radiation or surgery alone at 5 years.[116] Within this broad category, however, are subgroups of men with either much better or worse prognosis than average. Selective use of additional prognostic tests including erMRI and the percentage of positive biopsies has aided treatment selection.[97,109]

Given the significant number of men with intermediate-risk prostate cancer who develop biochemical failure, strategies to improve current outcomes are actively being investigated. Dose escalation is one appealing approach, because higher doses of radiation are required to eradicate greater volumes of disease. Since higher doses will be beneficial only in the absence of distant disease, the intermediate-risk group is well suited for dose escalation since a significant number of these patients have organ-confined disease or only limited extracapsular extension. Clinical studies indicate that dose escalation from 5 to 15% beyond 7,000 cGy may have an important impact on tumor control.[156–158] The ability to take advantage of the steep dose-response curve in this range is dependent on maintaining treatment toxicity at an acceptable level.

In discussion of dose escalation, it is important to understand how dose is reported. The International Commission on Radiation Units and Measurements (ICRU) Report No. 50 recommended that dose be defined at a reference point located at the center of the planning volume on or near the central axis of the beams.[159] For prostate cancer treatment, this point is located centrally within the gland. As treatment is directed at a volume as opposed to a single point, based on institutional preference, dose may be reported as a minimum received by the entire prostate, or clinical target volume (CTV), which is typically 5 to 8% lower than the reference point dose.

Recent reports suggest that the advances in treatment planning discussed previously have resulted in a shift toward fewer complications, allowing for greater dose escalation. At Memorial Sloan-Kettering Cancer Center, a phase I dose escalation trial using three-dimensional conformal radiation therapy yielded improved PSA relapse-free survival at higher dose levels in patients with at least one unfavorable prognostic characteristic (PSA > 10 ng/mL, stage > T2, or Gleason score > 6).[156] PSA relapse-free survival at 4 years was improved for intermediate- and high-risk patients receiving ≥ 7,560 cGy, with the 79% rate achieved in intermediate-risk patients similar to the 85% 4-year relapse-free survival noted in favorable-risk patients.

A retrospective series of 938 men treated at M. D. Anderson Cancer Center yielded 3-year actuarial freedom from failure rates of 61%, 74%, and 96% for doses of ≤ 6,700, > 6,700 to 7,700, and ≥ 7,700 cGy,[158] despite the trend for use of higher doses in patients with adverse risk factors. In a study of dose escalation performed at Fox Chase Cancer Center, patients with pretreatment PSA ≥ 10 ng/mL had improved 5-year bNED survival with higher doses.[157] At 5 years, patients with initial PSAs between 10 and 19.9 ng/mL treated with either 7,600 or 7,000 cGy had bNED survival of 75% or 35%, respectively. High-risk patients with PSA ≥ 20 ng/mL also benefited with 5-year bNED survival of 32% versus 10%, respectively. A subsequent report from this group has indicated improved bNED survival with modest dose escalation in low-risk patients as well. Overall, these data suggest that for each 1 Gy increase in dose, the hazard of bNED failure decreased by 8%. A retrospective matched-pair analysis from Fox Chase indicated a survival advantage with dose escalation above 7,400 cGy, although prospective confirmation is pending.[160] In the only reported randomized study to date addressing the question of dose escalation, 305 patients at M. D. Anderson with T1–T3 disease were randomized to either 7,000 or 7,800 cGy without the use of androgen suppression.[161] For all patients, dose escalation improved biochemical control/freedom from failure at 6 years from 64 to 70%, $p = .03$. In a subgroup analysis, no improvement was seen for men with a PSA ≤ 10 ng/mL, but for patients with a PSA > 10 ng/mL there was a marked difference in biochemical control (43% vs 62%, $p = .01$). The RTOG is now moving forward with the first intergroup study to address the question of dose escalation in the intermediate-risk group.

Combination of external beam radiation therapy and interstitial brachytherapy is an alternative strategy to external beam dose escalation that potentially increases tumor control via provision of enhanced biologic dose. Patients who may most likely benefit from this approach are those with intermediate-risk features; many present with presumed minimal extraprostatic extension that can be addressed by use of external beam therapy while providing a high dose to the bulk of disease within the prostate using brachytherapy. However, there are few long-term reports of outcome with this technique. In a study of 10-year biochemical relapse-free rates on 232 patients treated with external beam and brachytherapy boost, Sylvester and colleagues reported a 90% success rate for patients defined as intermediate-risk, which was similar to results for low-risk patients, as opposed to 48% for high-risk patients.[162] Currently, cooperative group efforts are underway to study this approach under strict quality assurance guidelines. HDR brachytherapy has also been studied as a method of delivery of a high-dose boost. Several single institution studies have yielded promising preliminary results.[163] Multi-institutional prospective trials with adequate follow-up are needed to validate the use of HDR therapy for prostate cancer.

The benefit of androgen deprivation in locally advanced disease has generated interest in the role of hormonal manipulation in patients with intermediate-risk factors. Recently, D'Amico and colleagues reported the results of a randomized trial comparing treatment with 7,000 cGy external beam radiation therapy plus 6 months of adjuvant combined androgen suppression therapy versus external beam radiation therapy alone.[164] Patients had to have intermediate- or high-risk disease at study entry (PSA of at least 10 ng/mL or a Gleason score of at least 7). The investigators found statistically significant improvements in PSA failure, prostate cancer-specific survival and overall survival for the arm that received 6 months of adjuvant androgen suppression, with a 5-year survival rate of 88% in the androgen-suppression arm versus 78% in the radiation-only arm. This study provides the first indication to date that adjuvant hormonal therapy is advantageous in an intermediate-risk patient population, and one of the few studies of either intermediate- or high-risk patients to demonstrate an overall survival benefit.

High-Risk Prostate Cancer High-risk factors include clinical T3 disease, Gleason grade 8 to 10, and/or PSA ≥ 20 ng/mL. The Patterns of Care Studies demonstrated a 15 to 20% decrement in survival at 5 years and 25 to 30% at 10 years as compared with age-matched controls for men with T3 or T4 prostate cancer.[151] Over the past decade, two strategies have shown promise in improving results in these patients: the addition of adjuvant androgen suppression therapy and radiation dose escalation.

Table 97-12 Randomized Phase III Trials Comparing Androgen Deprivation plus Irradiation to Irradiation Alone in Local or Locally Advanced Prostate Cancer

Trial	F/u (Yr)	Stage	*n*	Hormone	Local Relapse (%)	Progression-Free Survival (%)	Overall Survival (%)
RTOG	8	T3 N1	477	LHRHA	23*	32*	49
85–31			468	None	37	8	47
RTOG	8	T2c-T4	226	CAB	30*	16*	53
86–10			230	None	42	3	44
EORTC	5	T1–T2; Grade 3 or	207	LHRHA	NR	74*	78*
		T3–T4, N0–1	208	None	NR	40	62
DFCI	5	T1b-T2b; PSA ≥ 10	102	CAB	NR	82*	88*
		or Gleason ≥ 7	104	None	NR	57	78

* $p < .05$.
CAB = combined androgen blockade; LHRHA = luteinizing hormone releasing hormone analogues; NR = not reported.

Hormonal manipulation in combination with radiation therapy has demonstrated consistent improvement in treatment outcome as compared with standard-dose radiation alone and in some cases overall survival benefit has been observed. There are now six phase III trials reporting advantage in various outcome parameters with the use of androgen deprivation. Four of these trials compared radiation therapy with androgen suppression to radiation therapy alone (Table 97-12). All four have demonstrated improvements in bNED survival, although only two demonstrated an advantage in overall survival. In RTOG 86-10, 456 patients with large (≥ 25 cc) T2B to T4, Nx tumors were randomized to radiation therapy alone or with 4 months of total androgen suppression.[165,166] Five-year progression-free survival and freedom from distant metastases with or without neoadjuvant hormonal therapy was 36% and 66% versus 15% and 59%, respectively. Despite these findings, no difference in overall survival was seen with follow-up of 8 years.[167] In RTOG 85-31, patients with clinical T3 disease < 25 cc, T1/T2 with radiographic or histologic regional lymph node involvement, or postprostatectomy patients with extracapsular extension and positive margin or seminal vesicle involvement were randomized to receive adjuvant goserelin after radiation therapy or no further treatment.[168,169] Five-year bNED survival as defined by PSA < 1.5 ng/mL after at least 1 year was 53% versus 20%, respectively. Despite these improvements, there was no overall survival benefit, although a survival benefit was noted in the subgroup of patients with high-grade disease. In a European Organization for Research and Treatment of Cancer (EORTC) phase III trial, Bolla and colleagues reported an overall survival advantage for patients receiving 3 years of goserelin starting with the initiation of radiation therapy.[170] A majority of patients in this study had stage T3 disease and the remainder were eligible because of high-grade tumors. Actuarial 5-year overall survival with radiation plus goserelin versus radiation alone was 79% and 62%, respectively; disease-free survival was 85% and 48%, respectively. These differences were highly statistically significant. A recent update of this trial with a median follow-up of 61 months sustains these findings.[171] The other randomized trial demonstrating an improvement in overall survival with the addition of androgen suppression is the D'Amico study discussed above, in which both intermediate- and high-risk patients were enrolled. A 5-year overall survival of 88% was seen in the radiation plus 6 months of androgen suppression, while 5-year overall survival in the radiation alone arm was 78%.[164]

Debate continues as to the optimal type, timing, and duration of androgen suppression in combination. In the two studies that demonstrated an overall survival benefit to androgen suppression, one treated with 3 years of an adjuvant LHRH agonist, while the other treated with only 6 months of combined androgen blockade. Two recent phase III intergroup studies have addressed this question. In RTOG 92-02 patients with T2c to T4, N0-1, M0 disease were randomized to a total of 4 months of total androgen suppression with radiation administered after 2 months, or the same regimen followed by an additional 2 years of goserelin.[172] One thousand five hundred fifty-four patients were enrolled. With a median follow-up of 4.8 months, significant differences favoring long-term androgen suppression were noted for biochemical control (46% vs 21%), disease-free survival (54% vs 34%), and disease-specific survival (92% vs 87%). There was no difference in overall survival (78% vs 79%); however a statistically significant difference in overall survival of 80% versus 69% was noted in a subgroup analysis of patients with Gleason 8 disease. RTOG 94-13 was a four-arm study of 1,323 patients with an estimated node positivity risk of > 15% comparing whole-pelvis versus small-field radiation and 4 months of combined androgen suppression, beginning either 2 months prior to radiation therapy or immediately after completing radiation therapy.[173] A difference was seen in progression-free survival (which includes PSA-only recurrences) at 4 years (54% vs 47% for the WP vs PO radiation, $p = .022$), but no difference was seen in overall survival. The best outcomes occurred with a combination of neoadjuvant androgen blockade and whole pelvic radiation, with a 4-year progression-free survival of 60%.

Novel strategies for high-risk patients under investigation include combinations of radiation and androgen deprivation therapy with chemotherapy,[174] hyperthermia, or radiosensitizers as well as use of particle therapy. Hyperthermia is an attractive strategy because cells most resistant to radiation, such as hypoxic cells and those in late S-phase, are most sensitive to hyperthermia.[175] In addition, hyperthermia has been linked directly to apoptosis, increased tissue perfusion, and sensitization of the tumor to radiation via an oxygenation effect. Initial results of use of TRUS hyperthermia indicate good patient tolerance with minimal morbidity.[176]

Both protons and neutrons offer potential advantages over standard photon therapy. Protons have a characteristic Bragg Peak, a region of sharp falloff of dose deposition that can be used to spare adjacent normal tissues. Several trials comparing standard dose-photon radiation with dose escalation with proton beam boost have demonstrated enhanced disease control in high-risk patients. Shipley and colleagues at the Massachusetts General Hospital reported no overall advantage in overall survival or disease-free survival in patients with T3 or T4, Nx-N2 disease receiving a high-dose proton boost versus standard-dose photon radiation.[177] However, patients with poorly differentiated tumors had enhanced local control. Rates of rectal bleeding, however, were significantly higher with proton beam. In an update of the Loma Linda experience with 643 patients treated with either protons alone or in combination with photons, patients in the "early" (T1b–T2b, PSA < 15) and "advanced" (T1b–T2b, PSA > 15 or T2c–T4, PSA < 50) subgroups had bNED survival of 89% and 68%, respectively, at 4.5 years.[178] A phase III dose escalation trial is currently under way.

Neutrons result in less sublethal damage repair and less dependence on oxygen for tumor destruction. Two prospective randomized trials of neutron therapy have been reported. RTOG 77-04 randomized patients with stage C or D1 disease to mixed neutrons and photons versus photons alone.[179] At 10 years, clinically assessed local control was 70% for mixed-beam group versus 58% for the photon-only group. Overall survival was 46% versus 29%, respectively. Both of these differences were significant. The NCI-sponsored Neutron Therapy Collaborative Working Group performed a phase III trial comparing neutron with photon therapy in patients with high-grade T2 or any T3/T4 tumors.[180] There was a decrease with neutrons in 5-year biochemical failure (17% vs 45%) and 10-year local/regional failure (21% vs 47%) but no significant difference in 10-year survival (36% vs 43%). An increase in grade 3 or 4 late complications (24% vs 8%) was noted for patients receiving neutron therapy. A series of prospective trials at Wayne State University has given further support to the use of neutrons in treatment of prostate cancer.[181]

Postprostatectomy Radiation Radiation therapy following prostatectomy has been used in both the adjuvant and salvage settings. In the first instance, radiation therapy is administered in patients without clinical evidence of disease but with adverse finding at the time of prostatectomy. In the latter instance, patients with postoperative evidence of disease, typically a failure to achieve an undetectable PSA level or subsequent rise after nadir, may receive radiation with the goal of eradication of disease remaining after surgery. Several prognostic factors have been identified that may aid in the decision-making process as to when adjuvant or salvage radiation therapy may offer the greatest potential benefit. In the case of adjuvant therapy, two questions help define if radiation is appropriate: first, not all men with adverse factors fail surgery and, second, if subsequent failure is distant, then prostatic bed irradiation will not affect the disease course.

Several authors have identified patients at high risk of recurrence following prostatectomy.[182,183] Disease-free and overall survival rates are lower for men with pT3 disease. The distinction regarding the extent of capsular penetration has been noted to differentiate men at lower versus higher risk of subsequent failure.[184] Positive surgical margins have been linked to increased risk of local recurrence.[185] In a review of 273 patients who underwent prostatectomy, Anscher and Prosnitz identified poorly differentiated histology, positive margins, and elevated acid phosphatase as risk factors that predicted local recurrence on multivariate analysis.[185] Seminal vesicle invasion was associated only with local failure on univariate analysis; however, it was the sole factor associated with increased risk of distant failure on multivariate analysis. Additional factors associated with failure include high preoperative PSA, lymph node involvement, and nondiploid DNA content.[182]

The potential for postprostatectomy radiation therapy to lengthen the biochemical disease-free interval has been demonstrated in several single-institution studies. Investigators at the Mayo Clinic reported advantage of radiation therapy in both the adjuvant and salvage settings.[186] Results of therapy in 288 men with pathologic T3 or T4 prostate cancer who underwent prostatectomy were reviewed. Adjuvant radiotherapy was given to 42 of these men and salvage therapy for detectable PSA was administered in 18 patients. The dose administered was between 5,700 and 6,800 cGy. Freedom from failure rate at 5 years for men receiving adjuvant radiation was 90% compared with 40% for men who did not receive postoperative radiation. When those receiving salvage therapy were included in the analysis, 5-year freedom from failure for patients receiving radiation was 57%. Seminal vesicle invasion was associated with 36% 5-year freedom from failure as opposed to 81% when no seminal vesicle invasion was present. In a series of 146 men, Zietman and colleagues noted a similar 5-year bNED survival of 43% and 73% with adjuvant radiation in men with pT3 disease with and without seminal vesicle involvement, respectively. Prescribed doses were between 6,000 and 6,400 cGy.[187] A Southwest Oncology Group (SWOG) study has completed accrual that randomized patients with pathologic T3 or T4 disease after prostatectomy to either adjuvant radiation or observation and should better clarify the role of adjuvant radiation. In view of recent findings that higher doses may provide better outcome, it is unclear whether the doses used in this study are adequate to definitively answer this question.

Salvage radiation has also been shown to favorably impact on freedom from failure rates. Results from the largest single-institution studies suggest that between 21 and 64% of patients may be salvaged with radiation therapy.[188] Earlier use and higher dose of therapy once PSA failure is established may improve the salvage rate, which will avoid the adjuvant irradiation of patients that do not fail their initial treatment. A PSA of ≥ 0.4 ng/mL following prostatectomy has been shown to be associated with almost universal disease recurrence.[189] A consistent finding has been the impact of time to PSA failure[190] and the PSA level at the time of salvage radiation with greater initial disease-free interval following prostatectomy and lower PSA, preferably ≤ 1 ng/mL, portending a greater likelihood of bNED survival after salvage therapy. A dose response relationship to outcome has also been noted. Schild reported that patients treated to at least 6,400 cGy had improved freedom from failure of approximately 55% compared with 15% for those treated with lower doses.[191] Stephenson and colleagues reported on a retrospective data review of salvage radiation in men with increasing PSAs after radical prostatectomy in five academic centers.[192] Overall, after treatment 4-year progression-free survival was 45%. Predictors of progression after salvage radiation therapy included higher Gleason scores, higher PSA values, faster PSA doubling times, seminal vesicle invasion and negative surgical margins.

The role of hormonal manipulation in post-prostatectomy patients with adverse prognostic factors receiving radiation remains undefined. However, there is a suggestion that androgen deprivation may be beneficial. Eulau and colleagues reported the Stanford experience in 105 men receiving postprostatectomy radiation therapy with or without the use of transient androgen deprivation.[193] Patients received a prostatic fossa dose of 6,000 to 7,000 cGy, and 48 patients also received pelvic nodal irradiation with a median dose of 5,000 cGy. When retrospectively compared at 5 years with patients treated during the same time period with radiation alone, those who received concurrent androgen deprivation had improved freedom from both biochemical (56% vs 27%) and clinical recurrence (100% vs 70%).

A subgroup analysis of 139 patients on RTOG 85-31 receiving postoperative radiation for extracapsular extension and positive margin or seminal vesicle involvement also demonstrated potential advantage to use of androgen deprivation. With median follow-up of 5 years, estimated progression-free survival rates were 65% with and 42% without androgen deprivation. No significant differences were noted, however, in local control, distant failure, or overall survival.[194]

Complications of Radiation Therapy Given the long-term survival experienced by most men with prostate cancer, especially when diagnosed with early-stage disease, the quality of life following definitive treatment is of great importance. Although early treatment offers the greatest opportunity for disease eradication, careful consideration of morbidity must be taken into account, given that most of these patients would enjoy an extended disease-free period with observation alone. When the differences in tumor control among different treatment modalities are difficult to discern, the morbidity profile of each modality weighs heavier on an individual's choice of therapy.

Use of nonconformal external beam therapy to standard doses has yielded an acceptable side-effect profile. One thousand twenty patients with minimum follow-up of 7 years treated on RTOG studies 75-06 and 77-06 had an incidence of grade ≥ 3 intestinal or urinary complications of 3.3% and 7.7%, respectively.[195] The most common grade ≥ 3 intestinal complications included rectal bleeding or ulceration (1.7%) and proctitis (1.6%). The most common urinary sequelae were urethral stricture (4.6%), hematuria (3.1%), and cystitis (2.6%). In a series of 331 patients treated with conventional radiation at Massachusetts General Hospital, similar results were seen.[196] Of note, impotence was noted in 63% at 5 years.

Conformal technique is associated with an improved morbidity profile. Dearnaley and colleagues randomized 225 patients to either conventional or conformal radiation therapy to standard dose (6,400 cGy as normalized to 90%).[197] Significant reduction in rectal toxicity was noted in the conformal group with only 5% of patients experiencing RTOG grade 2 toxicity as opposed to 14% with conventional therapy. Urinary toxicity was not different with 15% and 5% of the conformal group and 19% and 4% of the conventional group experiencing grade 2 or 3 urinary toxicity. The use of a three-field technique including an AP field may have negated potential advantage to conformal technique in reduction of urinary toxicity. Favorable rectal toxicity profile with conformal therapy has also been noted by Sandler and colleagues.[198] In this series of 721 patients, actuarial risk of grade ≥ 3 late rectal toxicity with median dose of 6,840 cGy and some patients receiving up to 8,000 cGy was 3% at 5 years. Notably, 64% of patients were treated with an initial pelvic field.

Improvements in planning and delivery of external beam therapy have led to an improved side effect profile, allowing for dose escalation to be considered. Preliminary findings of a phase I/II dose escalation study by the RTOG 94-06 indicate virtually no grade 3 toxicity with total dose of up to 7,980 cGy. Zelefsky and colleagues reported late intestinal and urinary toxicity in 743 patients treated with three-dimensional conformal technique on a dose escalation trial. Actuarial 5-year grade 2 or 3 intestinal toxicity was 11% and 0.75%, whereas late grade 2 or 3 urinary toxicity was 10% and 3%. Multivariate analysis identified a volumetric dose ≥ 7,560 cGy and corresponding acute symptoms as predictive of late toxicity. In addition, a history of diabetes was also correlated with late intestinal toxicity.[199]

Interstitial prostate brachytherapy has been associated with a favorable morbidity profile. Patients typically return to work or other usual activities within several days of the procedure. Serious complications reported in early series,[200] are now rarely seen with improvements in technique.[201] The use of peripheral loading technique to reduce the urethral dose has had a favorable effect on urinary morbidity with ultrasound technique.[202] Also, a realization of the correlation of significant urinary symptoms prior to treatment with urinary system toxicity following implant has led to better patient selection. Gelblum and colleagues noted in a series of 693 patients that 4.7% required TURP for protracted obstructive symptoms.[202] They further noted that grade 2 acute urinary morbidity as defined by requirement of alpha-blocker therapy for management of frequency occurred in 41%, with 12.8% reporting grade 2 symptoms at 6 months. Further reduction in acute urinary toxicity has been noted with use of magnetic resonance guidance for prostate implants. Acute rectal morbidity is rarely witnessed with prostate brachytherapy because the sources are placed directly into the prostate, avoiding radiation of a larger volume of the rectum as occurs with external beam therapy. Nevertheless, a high dose of radiation is administered to the anterior rectal wall, which may be associated with significant long-term effects on bowel function in a relatively small number of men.[200,203,204]

COMPARISON OF TREATMENT OPTIONS

To date, there is no prospective, randomized, methodologically sound clinical trial comparing the safety and efficacy of radiation therapy with radical prostatectomy in localized prostate cancer (a trial conducted by the Veterans Administration Cooperative Urological Research Group [VACURG] had methodologic problems[205]). The data that do exist are nonrandomized and often single-center and retrospective. Despite this lack of data, practice patterns have been changing, with increased use of brachytherapy and androgen deprivation therapy and corresponding falls in utilization of watchful waiting, external beam radiation therapy, and radical prostatectomy (Figure 97-17).[206] These changes in patterns of treatment have occurred as the percentage of patients presenting with low-risk disease has increased dramatically (29.8% from 1989 to 1992 to 45.3% from 1999 to 2001).

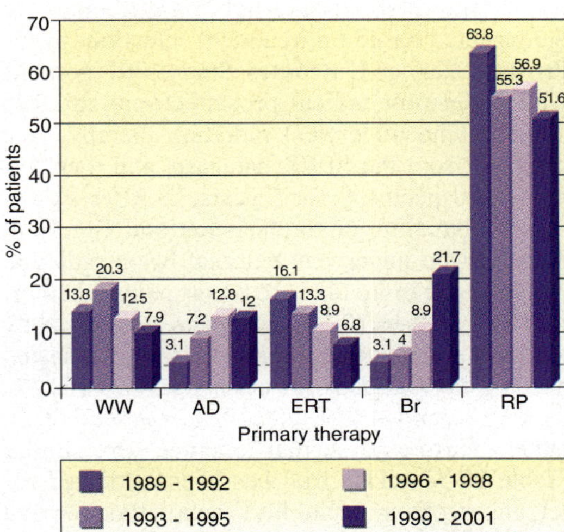

Figure 97-17 Treatment trends among low-risk prostate cancer patients. Trends for each primary treatment alternative are significant at the $p < .0001$ level, with the exception of radical prostatectomy (RP), which is significant with $p = .0019$. WW = watchful waiting; AD = androgen deprivation therapy; ERT = external beam radiotherapy; Br = brachytherapy. Adapted from Cooperberg MR et al.[206]

Without randomization, studies with the greatest validity that compare efficacy between treatments are those that stratify patients by the major pretreatment prognostic criteria. Two large published series examining efficacy have stratified patients in this manner. D'Amico and colleagues reported 5-year treatment results with radical prostatectomy, external beam radiation alone, or permanent interstitial brachytherapy stratified into low-, intermediate-, and high-risk groups as previously described.[116] For low-risk patients, the 5-year actuarial risk of PSA failure was not different between the three groups. There was also no difference for patients with intermediate- or high-risk disease undergoing either prostatectomy or external beam radiation therapy. Patients receiving implant therapy, however, were at greater risk of PSA failure. In the second study, researchers at the Cleveland Clinic compared outcome of 1,682 patients with T1 or T2 disease treated with radiation (628 patients) or prostatectomy (1,054 patients).[207] Median follow-up was 51 months. When controlled for the fact that 51% of patients undergoing radical prostatectomy had favorable tumors (defined as stage T1 to T2A, Gleason scores ≤ 6 and pretreatment PSA ≤ 10 ng/mL), compared with only 34% of radiation therapy patients, there was no impact of treatment modality on biochemical relapse-free survival (bRFS). Of note, there was a difference in bRFS in patients with unfavorable tumors treated with radiotherapy doses to less than 72 Gy as compared with those treated to ≥ 72 Gy or prostatectomy. These studies did not measure the impact of hormonal therapy in combination with radiation.

Studies that consider side effects and quality of life after primary treatment of prostate cancer vary widely in terms of design, patient population, data collection, and length of follow-up. Two recent studies shed some light on differences to be expected based on treatment selection. In the Prostate Cancer Outcomes Study, 901 patients who underwent radical prostatectomy and 286 patients who underwent radiation therapy were sampled from the SEER database, and then followed prospectively for 5 years.[208] After adjusting for baseline characteristics and function, patients who underwent external beam radiation therapy were more likely to report painful hemorrhoids (19.6% vs 10.2%) at 5 years, but less likely to report erections insufficient for intercourse and needing to wear pads for urinary leaking (63.5% vs 79.3% and 4.2% vs 28.6%, respectively). Other measures of sexual function were similar (Table 97-13). This trial has been criticized for relying on patient recall for baseline function and for its use of community data, where treatment expertise may not be ideal. Yet it is the only long-term (5 year) prospective follow-up after primary treatment that attempts to account for baseline function in diverse care settings. Talcott and colleagues added to this literature by highlighting the importance of baseline organ function and time course, as well as primary treatment modality, on side effects at 2 years.[209] Others have considered the differences in direct initial costs between the different treatments.[210]

Helping men choose the best therapy for their localized prostate cancer is a patient-specific process. Other than the Holmberg trial, randomizing patients to radical prostatectomy versus watchful waiting[126] and the methodologically flawed VACURG study, direct comparison data are lacking. A third trial, randomizing patients to watchful waiting versus radical prostatectomy (PIVOT), done through the Veterans Administration Cooperative Clinical Trials Group, will provide helpful data but will take nearly 15 years to complete.[211] Recommendations need to take into account the patient's age; comorbidities; baseline bowel, bladder, and erectile function; and patient preference as well as prognostic factors related to their tumor (T-stage, PSA, Gleason score, percent positive biopsies, and PSA velocity). Helping patients understand the potential side effects of each modality is critical in this process.

Table 97-13 Comparison of 5-Year Prostate Cancer Outcomes Study Survey Results

Domain		RP n = 901	EBRT n = 286	OR (95% CI)
Urinary	No control or frequent leaks vs total control or occasional leaks	14.4 (15.3)	4.9 (4.1)	4.4 (2.2–8.6)
	Leaks ≥ 2 times per day	15.6 (16.1)	4.1 (3.6)	5.3 (2.6–10.8)
	Wears any pads to stay dry	28.6 (28.6)	4.2 (4.2)	9.4 (4.7–18.9)
Bowel	Diarrhea	23.3 (23.9)	28.8 (26.7)	0.84 (0.55–1.26)
	Bowel urgency	17.7 (19.3)	33.4 (28.5)	0.56 (0.36–0.87)
	Painful hemorrhoids	11.0 (10.2)	15.7 (19.6)	0.43 (0.25–0.74)
Sexual	Erection insufficient for intercourse	76.9 (79.3)	73.1 (63.5)	2.5 (1.6–3.8)
	No/little vs some/a lot of interest in sexual activity	46.5 (48.9)	55.2 (47.4)	1.1 (0.73–1.6)
	Bothered by sexual dysfunction	47.4 (46.7)	42.0 (44.6)	1.1 (0.75–1.6)

RP = radical prostatectomy; EBRT = external beam radiation therapy; OR = odds ratio, CI = confidence interval.
Values in columns are unadjusted percentages (adjusted percentages).
Adjustments made for treatment propensity score, age at diagnosis, baseline function, race/ethnicity, comorbidity, and education level.
Adapted from Potsky AL et al.[208]

MANAGEMENT OF LOCALLY ADVANCED PROSTATE CANCER

T3 Disease A national Patterns of Care survey by the American College of Surgeons found that of patients diagnosed in 1990, 15% presented with clinical T3 disease.[212] What is the natural history of clinical T3 prostate cancer? Because of the biologic heterogeneity inherent in all prostate cancers regardless of stage, this remains a difficult question to answer. The longest study of untreated T3 prostate cancer was reported recently in a large prospective population-based study of 642 patients from Sweden. One hundred eighty-three patients with clinical T3 or T4 disease and no evidence of distant metastases were followed without initial local therapy.[124] At 15 years, progression-free survival was 46.6% and disease-specific survival was 56.5%. Notable from these results are the surprisingly high disease-specific survival rates in this cohort in both localized and locally advanced categories of disease.

The management of locally advanced prostate cancer remains controversial.[213] External beam radiation therapy, radical prostatectomy, hormonal therapy, cryosurgery, brachytherapy, observation, and combinations of these modalities have all been advocated and are used to varying degrees. Attempts at curative therapy for clinical T3 prostate cancer are generally unsuccessful since many patients already have occult metastases.[214] When a cancer extends palpably beyond the prostate into the lateral sulci or seminal vesicles, lymph node metastases are common. A multi-institutional pooled analysis was performed of outcomes after surgery for 345 men with T3 prostate cancer.[215] Of 298 evaluable patients, 41% had nodal metastases and/or seminal vesicle invasion. Overall actuarial disease-specific survival and metastasis-free survival rates at 10 years were 57% and 32%, respectively. Well-, moderately, and poorly differentiated tumors had disease-specific survival rates of 73%, 67%, and 29%, respectively. The investigators concluded that radical prostatectomy (RP) might have a role in selected patients with low- and intermediate-grade tumors, but were unlikely alone to result in long-term survival in the patients with high-grade lesions. Neoadjuvant hormonal therapy prior to radical prostatectomy in T3 disease may decrease pathologic stage, but no improvements in progression-free or disease-specific survival have been demonstrated to date in randomized trials.[216]

As noted earlier, the results of the RTOG and EORTC trials have validated the use of hormones and radiation as a better treatment than radiation alone in the treatment of locally advanced prostate cancer. Currently, the combination of neoadjuvant hormones plus external beam radiotherapy can be considered a legitimate standard therapeutic choice in a patient with newly diagnosed T3 disease. New investigational modalities include the use of neoadjuvant chemotherapy prior to surgery or radiation.[213]

Node-Positive Prostate Cancer Clinical detection of pelvic lymph node metastases is not common. In the past, patients with pathologic involvement of lymph nodes may have been detected during staging pelvic lymph node dissection prior to radical prostatectomy or external beam radiation therapy. With improving use of noninvasive staging modalities, the role of staging lymphadenectomy has diminished, and the most common means of detecting pathologic lymph node disease is during a planned retropubic radical prostatectomy. Generally, the presence of involved lymph nodes detected on frozen section analysis will lead to abandonment of the radical prostatectomy.

The probability of lymph node metastases depends on the clinical stage of the cancer, histologic grade, and serum PSA level. In a recent series, positive nodes were found in only 5 to 10% of patients.[184] Prostate cancer is generally not considered to be curable with locoregional therapy alone. There is controversy concerning the role of local therapy and androgen deprivation therapy in these patients. The Mayo Clinic has advocated a combination of radical prostatectomy plus orchiectomy in node-positive patients, with some investigators suggesting that there may be a survival advantage to this strategy.[217] A recent randomized trial has suggested that early hormonal therapy may be of value in men with node-positive cancer. The Eastern Cooperative Oncology Group (ECOG) performed a randomized clinical trial of 98 men who underwent radical prostatectomy and pelvic lymphadenectomy and who were found to have pathologic node involvement to either immediate androgen ablation (goserelin or bilateral orchiectomy) or followed until disease progression.[218] With a median follow-up of 7.1 years, 6% in the immediate hormonal therapy arm versus 31% in the observation arm had died of prostate cancer ($p < .01$). At the time of last follow-up, 77% versus 18% were alive without evidence of recurrent disease in the immediate therapy and observation groups, respectively ($p < .001$).

The role of radiation therapy for patients with established lymph node involvement remains controversial. Given the risk of distant metastases and the limitation of radiation dose to large pelvic fields, treatment with radiation alone has generally yielded disappointing results.[219] Experience with androgen deprivation alone,[220] as well as salvage radiation following failure of hormonal therapy has also been disappointing.[221] Two single-institution studies suggest a benefit to combination of androgen suppression with radiation.[222,223] A follow-up report of the retrospective experience at M. D. Anderson noted 5-year actuarial freedom from relapse or rising PSA of 58% with combined therapy as opposed to 10% with androgen deprivation alone. Although a survival difference was not achieved, divergence of the survival curves suggests that with longer follow-up, a survival advantage might occur. In a subgroup analysis of RTOG 85-31, patients with N+ disease treated with radiation alone had an 11% 5-year bNED survival. When combined with long-term goserelin, however, the 5-year bNED survival was 55%.[224]

MANAGEMENT OF DISSEMINATED CANCER

Disseminated prostate cancer demonstrates a typical pattern of spread involving lymph nodes and bone in over 80% of cases.[225] Osteoblastic bone metastases are seen most commonly, often involving the vertebral bodies, as well as the pelvic bones, sternum, ribs, and femurs. The frequency of bone metastases is much higher than predicted by random dissemination of tumor cells.[226] Recent laboratory insights into the normal differentiation of osteoblasts have provided a better understanding of the molecular changes involved in development of bone metastases. The extracellular matrix, for instance, plays a critical role in prostate tumor growth, adhesion, migration, and metastases.[227] Osteopontin is a noncollagenous bone matrix protein that is overexpressed in human cancers. Thalmann and colleagues showed that human osteopontin stimulated the anchorage-independent growth of the human prostate cancer cell line, LNCaP, and that antibodies to osteopontin could inhibit this effect.[228] Their findings suggest that osteopontin may act as a paracrine and autocrine mediator of prostate cancer growth and progression. Jacob and colleagues found that bone extracts promoted a two- to four-fold increase in chemotaxis by human prostate epithelial cells and a four-fold increase in the invasive ability of human prostate carcinoma cells.[229] The purified active factor was found to be osteonectin, an abundant bone-maturation–associated matrix protein. They conclude that prostate cancer bone metastases are, in part, mediated by the ability of osteonectin to promote migration and invasion. Finally, the similar growth factors needed for both osteoblast and prostate cancer growth have been noted, and the hypothesis has been put forward that prostate cancer cells must be osteomimetic in order to successfully metastasize and grow in the skeleton.[227] The role of basic fibroblast growth factor, insulin-like growth factors, TGF-β, and endothelin-1 interact in such a model to create a selective environment that allows osteoblastic skeletal metastases from prostate cancer to develop.

Metastatic prostate cancer usually presents with symptoms of bone pain. However, other complications of advanced prostate cancer, including cauda equina syndrome, spinal cord compression, leptomeningeal metastases, massive hepatic metastases, and extensive abdominal or thoracic lymph node metastases, have been described. Parenchymal lung metastases are uncommon and not usually clinically significant. Brain metastases are uncommon, although cranial nerve involvement by skull metastases is seen more frequently. Bleeding complications related to disseminated intravascular coagulation may be a presenting sign of advanced prostate cancer.[230] PSA or prostatic acid phosphatase (PAP) immunostaining of tissue may be useful in the differential diagnosis of poorly differentiated carcinoma or adenocarcinomas presenting in unusual sites. As more patients have had cancers detected by PSA, a definite “stage shift” has occurred such that the number of diagnoses of metastatic disease de novo has been decreasing.[231]

Testicular Androgen Suppression Testicular androgen suppression has been the standard therapy for patients with symptomatic metastatic disease for the past 50 years. The original reports of dramatic responses after bilateral orchiectomy by Huggins and colleagues led to the widespread adoption of this procedure in men with advanced prostate cancer. After orchiectomy (or medical castration with LHRH agonists), over 90% of patients experience a significant PSA fall, and 60% report improved pain control. Owing in part to this dramatic response rate and symptom improvement, no trial has ever compared medical or surgical castration with best supportive care.

The psychological resistance of some men to surgical castration led to the development of alternative means to suppress testicular androgen secretion, by inhibiting pituitary release of gonadotropins. The synthetic estrogen, diethylstilbestrol (DES), was the first drug to be compared with surgical castration. Early studies by the VACURG suggested that 5 mg per day of DES was as effective as surgical castration in controlling metastatic prostate cancer.[232,233] However, the benefit of testicular androgen suppression seen at this dose of DES was counteracted by increased cardiovascular morbidity, leading to the evaluation of lower doses.[234] Although 3 mg of DES results in consistent suppression of testosterone to anorchic levels, 1 mg per day achieves castrate testosterone levels in only 70% of men.[235]

Owing to the toxicity of DES (which also includes tender gynecomastia, congestive heart failure, nausea, vomiting, diminished libido, and impotence), other medical methods of castration have been developed. The luteinizing hormone-releasing hormone (LHRH) analogues leuprolide (Lupron) and goserelin (Zoladex) are currently the most popular method to achieve chemical castration. Although both stimulate testosterone secretion for the first 7 to 10 days of administration, with continued treatment, down-regulation of pituitary LHRH receptors occurs as normal pulsatile gonadotropin secretion is blunted, and testosterone levels fall. Anorchic levels of plasma testosterone (generally less than 50) are achieved 14 to 21 days following the initiation of therapy. This initial increase in plasma testosterone has been associated with an increase in bone pain (“flare”) in 5 to 10% of patients treated for metastatic disease. The use of an antiandrogen prior to initiating LHRH agonists effectively blocks this flare reaction. In addition, several LHRH pure antagonists, whose main advantage is an apparent lack of such a flare effect, are currently in clinical trials.

LHRH analogues have been compared with DES or orchiectomy in 10 randomized trials. In patients with symptomatic metastases to bone, the response rate, time to treatment failure, survival, and suppression of plasma testosterone appear to be the same whether one employs orchiectomy or LHRH analogues. The Leuprolide Study Group demonstrated that leuprolide (Lupron) was considerably less toxic than DES (3 mg/d) and appeared equivalent in efficacy.[236] Most studies of LHRH analogues versus DES or orchiectomy did not involve adequate numbers of patients to exclude small but potentially important differences in survival. In addition, LHRH analogues are expensive, and those available in the United States require parenteral administration. Formulations that permit 1-, 3-, and 4-month injections currently are approved for use in the United States.

Antiandrogens and Combined Androgen Blockade Antiandrogens are drugs that compete with circulating androgens for binding to the androgen receptor and thus can inhibit androgen effects. Three nonsteroidal antiandrogens are available in the United States: flutamide (Eulexin), bicalutamide (Casodex), and nilutamide (Nilandron). They have been studied both as monotherapy and in combination with an LHRH analogue in the treatment of advanced prostate cancer. Single agent antiandrogens use is accompanied by an increase in gonadotropins because of competition in the hypothalamus of the antiandrogen with circulating androgens. Sustained gonadotropin increase results in enhanced testosterone secretion, which may override the antiandrogen effect.

Antiandrogen monotherapy has been studied with both flutamide and bicalutamide. Although active as a single agent, flutamide monotherapy was shown to be inferior to DES and should not be considered. High-dose bicalutamide has been compared with combined androgen blockade in at least two large randomized trials in men with locally advanced or metastatic prostate cancer.[237,238] Both studies suggested that high-dose bicalutamide was equivalent to combined androgen blockade for nonmetastatic disease; moreover, one of these trials demonstrated a survival benefit in metastatic disease for combined androgen blockade. There was also evidence that bicalutamide monotherapy was better tolerated, with sustained libido and improved physical capacity. The inability to demonstrate a role for antiandrogens alone, their cost, and their toxicity spectrum have prevented wide acceptance of antiandrogen monotherapy as the initial therapy for advanced prostate cancer.

The rationale for combined androgen blockade (CAB) is based on the theoretical contribution of adrenal androgens to the growth of prostate cancer. The adrenal glands secrete low levels of androgens. Inhibition of adrenal androgen synthesis (eg, with adrenalectomy or hypophysectomy) can result in improvement in some patients with prostate cancer that progresses despite testicular androgen suppression. With CAB, LHRH agonist therapy inhibits testicular androgen secretion and an antiandrogen blocks the effects of adrenal androgens.

One well-accepted advantage of combined LHRH analogue and antiandrogen therapy is that the antiandrogens block the flare reaction that can occur with LHRH analogues alone. Finding a long-term survival benefit to CAB has been more controversial. An NCI intergroup randomized trial comparing leuprolide alone (1 mg/d subcutaneous injection) versus leuprolide plus flutamide (250 mg 3 times a day orally) enrolled 603 patients.[239] A small but significant survival advantage was noted for patients receiving CAB (median survival 28.3 months for leuprolide alone vs 35.6 months for leuprolide plus flutamide, two-sided $p < .035$). Subgroup analysis of individuals indicates the most striking benefit for those patients with "minimal" metastatic disease: only axial skeletal metastases and good performance status. In a randomized trial of the LHRH agonist goserelin (Zoladex) with either flutamide (Eulexin) or bicalutamide (Casodex), the efficacy of both regimens was similar. However, the toxicity profile of flutamide (primarily diarrhea) led to treatment cessation of the antiandrogen in substantially more patients than in those receiving bicalutamide. These data combined with the once-per-day schedule of bicalutamide suggest that this drug may be the antiandrogen of choice in total androgen deprivation approaches.

Multiple other studies have examined the role of CAB in prostate cancer. A meta-analysis performed by the Prostate Cancer Trialists Collaboration evaluated data from over 5,000 patients entered onto randomized trials comparing testicular androgen ablation alone versus CAB.[240] Studies have used different methods or agents to suppress testicular androgen synthesis and different antiandrogens. The meta-analysis failed to demonstrate a significant advantage of total androgen deprivation. A separate meta-analysis using only studies employing a nonsteroidal antiandrogen indeed showed a statistically significant although modest clinical benefit over LHRH monotherapy.[241] Furthermore, in a randomized trial of 1,387 patients with metastatic prostate cancer comparing bilateral orchiectomy with and without flutamide, there was no significant difference between the two groups in overall survival ($p = .14$).[242] The flutamide arm was associated with a slightly increased risk of anemia and diarrhea. Thus, CAB appears to offer at most a modest survival benefit over LHRH agonist therapy alone. It appears to offer no advantage over orchiectomy alone.

Side Effects of Androgen Ablation and Intermittent Therapy The side effects of either orchiectomy or LHRH agonist usage are the side effects of the reduction of serum testosterone levels to castrate levels and include hot flashes, fatigue, gynecomastia, loss of libido, impotence, and weight gain. Potential therapies to ameliorate these issues include antidepressants, megestrol acetate, and acupuncture. More recently, long-term toxicity of testosterone suppression, including osteoporosis, depression, anemia, and loss of muscle mass, is becoming better appreciated. Smith and colleagues reported on a randomized comparison between leuprolide alone and leuprolide plus pamidronate (a bisphosphonate).[243] Over 48 weeks, the men in the leuprolide-alone arm experienced mean falls in bone mineral density (BMD) in the lumbar spine, trochanter and total hip of 3.3%, 2.1% and 1.8%, respectively, while those receiving leuprolide plus pamidronate had no significant changes in BMD. Other studies have shown an improvement in quality of life, muscular fitness, and energy with a resistance exercise program in combination with androgen deprivation.[244] Antiandrogen monotherapy with bicalutamide, with its associated higher levels of serum testosterone and estrogen, has been shown to lessen fat accumulation and improve BMD when compared with leuprolide therapy.[245] Moreover, while gynecomastia was increased, hot flashes, loss of libido, and fatigue were improved in the bicalutamide group.

Another strategy to ameliorate the side effects of androgen deprivation (as well as to potentially improve efficacy) is intermittent hormonal therapy. The original hypothesis proposed that continuous androgen ablation allowed for selection of androgen-independent clones, which then progress more rapidly, whereas periods of treatment cessation allow tumor stem cells to resume androgen-controlled differentiation.[246] In the Shionogi mouse mammary tumor model, castration induces regression almost completely, but tumor growth recurs after about 50 days. With successive transplantation of tumor after only partial regression, progression to androgen independence was seen after approximately 150 days.[247] Several pilot trials with small numbers of patients have been reported that confirm the feasibility of this approach.[246,248,249] One protocol treated patients with combined androgen blockade for an average of 8 months, until serum PSA levels dropped below 4 ng/mL. Treatment was then discontinued and PSA followed monthly until PSA rose above 20 ng/mL for men with metastatic cancer. The average cycle time was 17 months, with 45% of the time off treatment.[248] Randomized clinical trials are ongoing to determine whether the overall duration of hormone sensitivity is the same as continuous treatment.

Early versus Delayed Hormonal Therapy The original VACURG studies noted above were interpreted to suggest that delayed hormonal therapy does not compromise survival compared to immediate hormonal ablation. However, there were significant problems with these trials, including deficiencies in clinical staging and a high crossover rate between treatment arms. More recently, data have suggested that earlier hormonal therapy may delay recurrence and perhaps prolong survival. The Medical Research Council (MRC) performed a recent randomized clinical trial addressing the question of early versus delayed hormonal therapy.[250] Nine hundred thirty-four patients with locally advanced or metastatic prostate cancer were randomized to immediate treatment (orchidectomy or LHRH analogue) or to the same treatment deferred until clinically indicated. Follow-up and management were otherwise according to the participating clinician's normal practice. Progression to metastases, development of bone pain, and urinary obstruction requiring transurethral resection all occurred more rapidly in deferred patients. Complications such as pathologic fracture and spinal cord compression were twice as common in deferred patients. Sixty-seven percent of patient deaths were from prostate cancer: 257 in the deferred arm and 203 in the immediate arm ($p = .001$). Most of the difference was in nonmetastatic patients, with 119 and 81 deaths from prostate cancer, respectively ($p < .001$). The investigators concluded that earlier treatment may be favored, although follow-up remains short. Furthermore, the difference in outcome between the groups may have been a result of excessive delay before starting treatment, because 29 patients in the deferred arm died from prostate cancer before hormonal treatment was started. With the increasing incidence of PSA-only recurrences in the absence of radiographic or symptomatic disease, it remains unclear exactly how early hormonal therapy needs to be started. Current strategies are generally based on PSA doubling times, the presence or absence of metastases, initial tumor characteristics, and patient concerns.

HORMONE-REFRACTORY PROSTATE CANCER

It is clear that prostate cancer, as it progresses to the hormone-refractory state, demonstrates varying levels of hormone sensitivity. Initially, androgen-dependent tumors are similar to normal prostate epithelium and regress in the absence of androgen. Tumors that grow despite initial surgical or chemical castration are considered androgen-independent, even though patients with such tumors may respond to subsequent hormonal maneuvers. Hormone-refractory cancers are truly unresponsive to further hormonal manipulation.

Measuring benefit of therapy in prostate cancer patients similarly has been a topic in evolution. The majority of patients with hormone-refractory prostate cancer do not have measurable disease, making standard phase II criteria seldom useful. Bone metastases remain difficult to quantitate accurately, particularly as a marker of response to treatment. PSA is used in most contemporary studies as a marker of response. Many studies have suggested a correlation between the magnitude of a post-therapy PSA decline and survival. An analysis of 110 patients treated at Memorial Sloan-Kettering Cancer Center demonstrated significant improvement in median survival in patients with 50% or greater decline in PSA compared with less than 50% decline in PSA after treatment (21 vs 8 months, $p = .0002$).[251] The PSA Working Group has recently recommended a standardized method for reporting PSA response in phase II trials.[252] Palliative end points have also proved to be useful in clinical trials of chemotherapy for prostate cancer. As many patients with hormone-refractory prostate cancer experience significant bone pain and cancer-related decreases in quality of life, subjective benefit represents a powerful tool of effectiveness of therapy. The current recommended standard, then, is to report PSA data, palliative end points, and changes in measurable disease independently in each treatment report.

Table 97-14 Secondary Hormonal Therapies for Androgen-Independent Prostate Cancer

Therapy	*n*	PSA Decline > 50%	Measurable Response (CR + PR)
Antiandrogen withdrawal (AAW)			
Flutamide withdrawal	139	15–33	13
Bicalutamide withdrawal	14	29	NR
Either	132	11	2
Second antiandrogen			
Bicalutamide	134	23–24	0
Nilutamide	14	50	NR
Megestrol acetate	193	NR	0–9
	163	12–14	3
Adrenal androgen inhibitors			
Aminoglutemide	583	NR	9
Ketoconazole	204	78–80	16
Low-dose steroids	241	18–22	NR
Estrogenic agents			
DES	405	21–86	NR
	42	24	NR
PC-SPES	114	45–81	NR
	43	40	NR
Combinations			
Ketoconazole after AAW	108	32	7
Ketoconazole with AAW	128	27	20

NR = not reported.
Adapted from Oh WK et al.[258]

Secondary Hormonal Maneuvers The term androgen-independent prostate cancer indicates progressive disease despite castration. Castrate levels of testosterone should be documented in all cases of putative androgen-independent prostate cancer, because bilateral orchiectomy can fail to produce castrate levels of testosterone up to 11% of cases. Discontinuing testicular suppression by stopping estrogen or LHRH agonists can theoretically allow regrowth of the androgen-dependent group of prostate cancer cells. Two retrospective analyses evaluated whether continued testicular androgen suppression affects survival of patients with hormone-refractory prostate cancer. The Eastern Cooperative Oncology Group (ECOG) found a modest survival advantage if patients received continued testicular suppression, but the SWOG could not demonstrate any benefit.[253,254]

In 1993, clinical and PSA responses were reported in men who discontinued the antiandrogen flutamide on developing progressive disease.[255] This "antiandrogen withdrawal syndrome" was a critical discovery in terms of understanding the biology of androgen independence, interpreting clinical trials, and managing patients. About 20 to 30% of patients will experience a significant PSA decline after antiandrogen withdrawal, lasting from 3 to 5 months, although individual responses can last for over 2 years.[256] Such withdrawal responses also have been reported after treatment with bicalutamide and megestrol acetate (Megace).[257] Flutamide can activate specific mutant ARs cloned from prostate cancers, which provides a mechanism to explain antiandrogen withdrawal syndrome.[80]

After antiandrogen withdrawal, other hormonal treatments can be used (Table 97-14), although, unfortunately, it is difficult to predict which patients may respond.[258] The mechanism of action for these further hormonal manipulations depends in part on the fact that approximately 10% of circulating androgen in humans is secreted by the adrenal glands. In androgen-independent (AI) states, some tumor cells must retain sensitivity to androgens since a further decrease in circulating androgen levels by bilateral adrenalectomy or by drugs that inhibit adrenal steroidogenesis can induce a clinical response. Aminoglutethimide (Cytadren), ketoconazole (Nizoral), and corticosteroids act primarily via this mechanism. In a review of 13 clinical trials of aminoglutethimide plus hydrocortisone, there was an overall partial response rate of 9%.[256] Ketoconazole similarly has been noted for many years to be effective in suppressing testicular and adrenal androgen production. A review of 10 studies in AI CaP using high-dose ketoconazole plus replacement hydrocortisone showed measurable responses in approximately 15%.[256] Small and colleagues recently treated 48 evaluable patients with AI CaP and found PSA declines of > 50% in 63%.[259] Toxicity is infrequent and generally mild, including nausea, fatigue, hepatotoxicity, and skin changes. Doses of ketoconazole ranging from 200 to 400 mg 3 times daily may cause adrenal insufficiency, so supplemental corticosteroids are usually administered simultaneously. In a recent phase II study, patients with androgen-independent prostate cancer were randomized to antiandrogen withdraw alone or with ketoconazole 400 mg tid.[260] Crossover to ketoconazole was allowed in the antiandrogen withdraw alone arm. PSA responses and objective responses were increased in the combined arm (27% vs 11% and 20% vs 2%, respectively), although there was no difference in survival and patients crossing over to the delayed ketoconazole had a similarly high PSA response and overall response rate (32% and 7%). Interestingly, adrenal androgen levels, which fell in response to ketoconazole treatment, rose at the time of disease progression, suggesting a possible mechanism of resistance.

Low-dose corticosteroids inhibit adrenocorticotrophic hormone (ACTH) secretion through a negative feedback loop. This, in turn, decreases adrenal androgen production. In two large randomized studies of mitoxantrone plus steroids versus steroids alone, the steroid arm was associated with > 50% PSA declines of 18 to 22% and symptom relief in 8 to 12%.[261,262] Prostate cancers normally express estrogen receptors, which are up-regulated after androgen ablation in animal models. Though antiestrogens have been reported to have measurable response rates in only 0 to 10% of patients, estrogens clearly can induce salvage objective responses. In 10 phase II trials of diethylstilbestrol (DES) or DES diphosphate, PSA declines of > 50% were noted in approximately half of the patients, with means durations of 3 to 7 months.[263] The mechanism for the effect has been postulated to be from either mitotic arrest or direct cytotoxic effects on the cells, perhaps through an apoptotic mechanism. In a randomized study, Oh and colleagues found that the estrogenic herbal therapy, PC-SPES, appeared to have improved PSA response rates and time to progression as compared with DES treatment, although synthetic estrogens were discovered in some of the PC-SPES lots.[264] This product is no longer available because of concerns about contamination.

Other treatments for androgen-independent prostate cancer include the antiandrogens bicalutamide and nilutamide as well as megestrol acetate. Bicalutamide demonstrates a dose response, such that 200 mg, more effectively normalizes PSA than 50 mg in androgen-dependent CaP patients.[265,266] Treatment of AI CaP with bicalutamide 150 to 200 mg results in PSA responses about a quarter of the time, with most seen in those who had received prior flutamide therapy. Nilutamide has also shown modest activity in one study of androgen-independent prostate cancer patients.[267] Megestrol acetate is a steroidal antiandrogen with progestational activity. Its antiandrogenic effects are not promising in treating AI patients, with objective response rates of 0 to 9%. A recent large randomized study reported significant PSA declines only 12 to 14% of the time and rare objective responses.[268] Finally, observation remains a viable choice for asymptomatic patients whose PSAs are rising on androgen ablation therapy as none of the above therapies have been shown to improve survival.

Cytotoxic Chemotherapy Over the past decade, chemotherapy has been used more frequently in men with hormone-refractory prostate cancer. This has been the result of the introduction of more active agents and the results of phase III clinical trials. Such studies in advanced prostate cancer have focused on two areas: pain palliation with mitoxantrone and steroids and survival extension with microtubule inhibition, specifically with the use of docetaxel and (to a lesser extent) estramustine.

Mitoxantrone, an anthracenedione structurally related to the anthracyclines, was the first chemotherapeutic agent approved by the FDA for the treatment of advanced prostate cancer. This approval was based on two trials, both of which demonstrated improvements in pain control without survival extension. In a Canadian trial, 161 symptomatic hormone-refractory prostate cancer patients were randomized to receive mitoxantrone at a median dose of 12 mg/m^2 plus prednisone versus prednisone alone.[261] Nonresponders in the prednisone arm could cross over to receive mitoxantrone. Palliative response, measured on a pain scale, was the primary end point. Patients treated with mitoxantrone plus prednisone had significant pain relief 29% of the time, compared to 12% in the prednisone alone arm ($p = .01$). Palliation also lasted significantly longer in the combination compared to the prednisone alone arm (median 43 vs 18 weeks, $p < .0001$). Overall survival was not different. Additionally, the Cancer and Leukemia Group B (CALGB) randomized 242 patients to mitoxantrone 14 mg/m^2 plus hydrocortisone 40 mg/day versus hydrocortisone alone.[262] Again, overall survival was no different between the two groups (12.3 vs 12.6 months, $p = .77$), although a statistically significant difference in progression-free survival was noted in favor of the mitoxantrone-treated patients (3.7 vs 2.3 months, $p = .025$). Similar to the Canadian trial, improvements in quality of life were noted and toxicity was mild.

Molecules that inhibit microtubule dynamics represent the largest and most diverse class of chemotherapy agents. Three members of this class have been used in advanced prostate cancer with some success. The first, estramustine, is a conjugate of nitrogen mustard and estradiol originally synthesized as an attempt at targeted drug therapy for prostate cancer. However, further experiments revealed that estramustine actually interfered with mitosis by binding to microtubule-binding proteins. Although estramustine alone has modest activity against prostate cancer, it is in the synergy noted when combined with other microtubule inhibitors that promising results have been seen. Estramustine plus vinblastine, an alkaloid that binds to the vinca domain of the polymerizing microtubule, was the first such combination studied. Of 83 patients enrolled in three phase II trials, PSA responses occurred in 42% of patients and objective responses were seen in 6 (31%) of 17 patients with measurable disease.[269] A phase III trial was undertaken to compare vinblastine with vinblastine plus estramustine.[270] Two hundred one patients were randomized to receive either vinblastine 4 mg/m^2 weekly alone or together with estramustine phosphate 600 mg/m^2/day for 6 weeks. There was no difference in the primary end point survival, although a trend favored the combination (11.9 vs 9.2 months, $p = .08$). Estramustine plus vinblastine patients had a small but significant advantage in progression-free survival compared with vinblastine alone (3.7 vs 2.2 months, $p < .001$). Sustained PSA responses of at least 3 months were more common in the arm that included estramustine (25.2% vs 3.2%, $p < .0001$). Although gastrointestinal toxicity was worse with the addition of estramustine, interestingly, there was also significantly less granulocytopenia in the combination arm. The investigators conclude that although survival was not improved with estramustine, improvements in progression-free survival and PSA response warrant continued study of estramustine combinations. Other estramustine drug combinations, including with vinorelbine and etoposide, have similar levels of activity.[271]

Both paclitaxel and docetaxel are isolates from the Pacific Yew tree that bind microtubules and prevent depolymerization. To date, docetaxel is farther along in its development for prostate cancer. After several phase I/II trials established an active dose of docetaxel and safety in combination with estramustine,[272] two phase III trials were undertaken to evaluate the role of docetaxel in advanced hormone-refractory prostate cancer. The first, TAX 327, randomized 1,006 patients to one of three arms: docetaxel 70 mg/m^2 every 3 weeks, docetaxel 30 mg/m^2 weekly 5 of every 6 weeks, or mitoxantrone 12 mg/m^2 q 3 weeks.[273] Each arm also received prednisone 5 mg bid. All patients had chemo-naïve metastatic disease with serum testosterone levels less than 50 ng/mL, and all three arms were equally balanced in terms of Gleason score, primary therapy, number of hormonal manipulations, and baseline PSA. Treatment was planned for 30 weeks. The results revealed a statistically significant improved survival in the every 3-week docetaxel arm as compared with the mitoxantrone arm (median survival 18.9 months vs 16.4 months, $p = .009$), although no improved survival in the weekly docetaxel arm (17.3 months vs 16.4 months, $p = 0.3$). In both docetaxel arms, PSA responses and pain responses were statistically improved as compared with the mitoxantrone arm, although no improvement was seen in the tumor response rates. Toxicity was mild and limited to increased grade 3-4 anemia in the docetaxel arms (5% vs 0% in the mitoxantrone arm), and increased neutropenia in the every 3-week docetaxel arm, with concomitant increases in febrile neutropenia (grade 3-4 neutropenia 35% vs 1.5% in the weekly docetaxel arm, febrile neutropenia of 2.7% versus 0%).

At the same time the Southwest Oncology Group randomized 770 first-line advanced prostate cancer patients to either docetaxel 60 mg/m^2 q 3 weeks plus estramustine 280 mg PO tid versus mitoxantrone 12 mg/m^2 q 3 weeks plus prednisone 5 mg PO bid.[274] The docetaxel dose and the mitoxantrone dose could be increased to 70 mg/m^2 and 14 mg/m^2, respectively, if no grade 3 or 4 toxicities were seen during cycle 1. Warfarin and aspirin were used to prevent vascular complications from the estramustine. Survival was again improved in the docetaxel-containing arm (median survival of 17.5 months versus 15.6 months, $p = .02$). Statistically significant improvements were also seen in progression-free survival and PSA response rates in the docetaxel arm. Toxicity was also increased in the docetaxel plus estramustine arm, including increased rates of grade 3 or 4 infection, hematologic toxicity, GI toxicity, and cardiovascular toxicity.

These two phase III docetaxel trials are the first to show a survival benefit for chemotherapy in advanced prostate cancer (Table 97-15). Taken in combination, they establish docetaxel-based regimens as the first-line chemotherapy of choice. Estramustine clearly adds toxicity and, although no formal docetaxel +/– estramustine study has been reported, is unlikely to add a significant efficacy benefit. Questions also remain about the preferred docetaxel dosing regimen—weekly docetaxel clearly has improved hematologic toxicity, but at the risk of a slight decrease in efficacy. Despite these questions, these two trials are a major step forward in the use of chemotherapy in advanced prostate cancer.

Other taxanes have also been studied in this setting. Initial trials of paclitaxel alone suggested no significant activity, but when combined with estramustine, a PSA response rate of 65% was reported, with measurable responses in 57%.[275] Another phase II trial of estramustine, weekly paclitaxel, and monthly carboplatin showed PSA responses in 67% of patients with a median survival of 19.9 months.[276] In a randomized phase II trial of paclitaxel with or without estramustine, improved activity and improved survival were seen in the combination arm.[277] Epothilone B analogues, another microtubule-active molecule, have also shown interesting phase II results recently.[278] Other chemotherapeutic combinations reported to have activity include oral cyclophosphamide and various triple chemotherapy combinations.[279,280]

Bone-Directed Therapies Radiation is often used for the palliation of bone metastases, which is commonly seen in advanced prostate cancer. Given the excellent initial response to hormonal therapy in most men diagnosed with metastatic prostate cancer, radiation is often reserved for bone pain in the setting of hormone-refractory

Table 97-15 Recent Randomized Trials in First-Line Hormone-Refractory Prostate Cancer

Trial	Arms	*n*	PSA Decline > 50% (%)	Time to Progression (Months)	Median Survival (Months)	Other
TAX 327	Mitoxantrone	337	32		16.5	
	Docetaxel q 3 wks	335	48*		18.9*	
	Docetaxel q wk	334	45*		17.4	
SWOG	Mitoxantrone	336	27	3.2	15.6	
	Estramustine + docetaxel q 3 wks	338	50*	6.3*	17.5*	
Hoosier/Fox Chase	Vinblastine	98	3.2	2.2	9.2	
	Vinblastine + estramustine	95	25.2*	3.7*	11.9	
Canadian	Mitoxantrone + prednisone	130				Significant improvement in palliative response in mitoxantrone arm
	Prednisone	131				
CALGB 9182	Mitoxantrone + hydrocortisone	123	38*	3.7*	12.3	Possible benefit in pain control and QOL
	Hydrocortisone	119	22	2.3	12.6	
US Oncology	Paclitaxel	84	27	4.3	13.1	
	Paclitaxel + estramustine	79	47*	5.5	16.1*	

*$p < .05$.

disease. However, given the gradual onset of response to androgen deprivation, radiation may be initially considered in settings such as spinal cord compression or significant focal bone pain. Palliative external beam radiation typically is administered over a 2-week course to 3,000 cGy in 10 300 cGy fractions. Significant pain relief has been noted in 80 to 90% of patients.[281] Several reports have suggested improved rates of pain relief and bone healing with doses of 4,000 to 4,500 cGy, and this may be considered for men with prolonged life expectancy.[282] Conversely, in men with end-stage disease, a truncated course using higher daily fractions will often suffice.

Hemibody irradiation may be used for men with multiple sites of painful bony metastases, with prompt relief of pain achieved in 60 to 80%, and by 2 weeks, as many as 97% will experience some relief, including 20 to 25% with complete response.[281,283] The unirradiated bone marrow is then allowed to repopulate the lethally irradiated areas. Typical single-fraction doses are 600 cGy for upper body and 800 cGy for lower hemibody radiation. Lung blocks should be used for upper hemibody radiation with electrons used to supplement dose to ribs.

Alternatively, radiopharmaceuticals including Strontium-89 or Samarium-153 may be used for treatment of widespread painful bony metastases. These agents are calcium analog β-particle emitters, which localize to osteoblastic metastases. Overall response rates are between 60% and 80%.[284] The principal toxicities of radioisotope therapy include thrombocytopenia and leukopenia. A multicenter Canadian study of ^{89}Sr versus placebo demonstrated complete pain relief in 17% of the ^{89}Sr group and 2% of the placebo group.[285] Significant improvement in pain relief, freedom from new painful metastases, median time to further radiation therapy, and quality of life were noted. Others have reported similar findings. Several investigators have combined radiopharmaceutical therapy with chemotherapy, consistently finding that the combination of lower-dose chemotherapy and radiopharmaceuticals is superior to either alone in palliating symptoms and possibly in delaying progression of disease in bone.[286–288] Whether this may lead to an improvement in overall survival will require a phase III trial. The introduction of ^{153}Sm with its lower energy profile and shorter half-life has been associated with a favorable rate of hematologic recovery and onset of analgesic response.[289] Other radiopharmaceuticals used for treatment of metastatic prostate cancer include phosphorous-32 and rhenium-188.[290]

Bisphosphonates represent a new therapeutic advance in the management of hormone-refractory prostate cancer. Second and third generation bisphosphonates are increasingly potent at inhibiting osteoclast activity and have demonstrated activity in reducing skeletal complications from metastatic prostate cancer and preventing osteoporosis associated with androgen ablation for prostate cancer. Laboratory data also suggest a direct inhibition of prostate cancer cells by bisphosphonates.[291] A large phase III randomized placebo-controlled trial of zoledronic acid was performed in 643 patients with hormone-refractory prostate cancer patients with at least one bone metastasis.[292] Treatment with zoledronic acid reduced the incidence of skeletal-related events (including fracture and need for radiation to bone) by 25% at 15 months, compared to placebo (p = .021). Results with pamidronate[293] and clodronate[294] have been more disappointing.

Prognosis Prognostic indicators can be important for patients with hormone-refractory prostate cancer, as well as for researchers.[295] Halabi and colleagues developed a model to predict overall survival in men with hormone-refractory prostate cancer using a database of CALBG trials conducted between 1991 and 2001.[296] In this model, lactate dehydrogenase, PSA, hemoglobin, ECOG performance status, Gleason sum, alkaline phosphatase, and the presence of visceral disease contributed to a division of patients into four risk groups (Table 97-16). These risk groups have predicted survivals of 8.8, 13.4, 17.4, and 22.8 months. These factors may help design phase III trials as well as provide prognostic information for patients. Others have conducted nomograms using similar factors.[297]

NEW APPROACHES TO PROSTATE CANCER THERAPY

Although screening and early detection may ultimately prove one day to be a valuable strategy to decrease mortality from prostate cancer, prostate cancer remains the second leading cause of cancer death in the United States. Thus, there is an urgent need to develop new approaches to therapy that can both improve survival and ultimately decrease morbidity. Several areas of research offer the promise of better therapeutics against prostate cancer in the future.

Differentiation Therapy Differentiation is the process by which immature cells develop into the characteristic phenotype of a mature cell. In cancer, differentiation is often characterized by cell-cycle arrest and expression of cellular functions similar to nonmalignant cells and, in some cases, results in programmed cell death, or apoptosis. A number of groups have shown that inducing differentiation of these cancer cells can slow the progression of disease.

Inhibitors of peroxisome proliferator-activated receptor gamma (PPAR gamma) represent a

Table 97-16 Prognostic Factors Predicting Overall Survival for Hormone-Refractory Prostate Cancer in a Multivariate Model

Factor		HR	95% Confidence Interval
Performance status	0	1.00	Referent
	1	1.48	1.31–1.87
	2	2.19	1.94–2.47
Gleason score	< 8	1.00	Referent
	8–10	1.40	1.20–1.62
Log[LDH]		1.37	1.21–1.55
Log[alk phos]		1.23	1.12–1.36
Log[PSA]		1.10	1.05–1.15
Visceral disease	No	1.00	Referent
	Yes	1.17	0.95–1.16
Hemoglobin		0.92	0.87–0.97

LDH = lactate dehydrogenase; alk phos = alkaline phosphatase.
Adapted from Halabi S et al.[296]

promising area for differentiation therapy of prostate cancer.[298] PPAR gamma is a nuclear hormone receptor that plays a key role in the differentiation of adipocytes. Activation of this receptor in vitro can inhibit growth of prostate cancer cell lines. Although initial results with troglitazone, a ligand for PPAR gamma used for treatment of type II diabetes, were promising, a subsequent placebo-controlled trial showed no activity for this agent.[299]

In vitro studies also have demonstrated that 1,25 $(OH)_2$ vitamin D can induce prostate cancer differentiation, as well as decrease proliferation and metastasis. There also may be synergistic effects combining vitamin D or synthetic analogues with other targeted therapies. A phase I study of 1,25 $(OH)_2$ vitamin D was completed at the University of Pittsburgh. Unfortunately, hypercalcemia was seen at all dose levels. For this reason, vitamin D analogues with less hypercalcemic effects are currently under clinical development. More recently, Beer and colleagues demonstrated the feasibility of administering 1,25$(OH)_2$ vitamin D in high doses weekly, without induction of hypercalcemia.[300] This same group performed a subsequent phase II trial of the combination of high-dose calcitriol with weekly docetaxel chemotherapy and reported PSA response rates of 82%.[301]

Induction of Apoptosis One mechanism for developing hormone-refractory disease is thought to involve the bcl-2 oncogene pathway, which belongs to a family of proteins involved in regulating apoptosis (programmed cell death). For instance, overexpression of bcl-2 is seen in hormone-refractory cancers in high levels, compared with patients with hormone-sensitive prostate cancer. Antisense oligonucleotides such as G3139 targeted to bcl-2 mRNA sequences have been shown to decrease bcl-2 protein expression and are being tested in patients in combination with chemotherapy in phase II trials.

Signal Transduction Inhibitors Much of the work leading to the therapeutic development of signal transduction inhibitors is based on molecular studies demonstrating the functional significance of these pathways. As noted earlier, numerous growth factors have been implicated in the growth and progression of prostate cancer. Many inhibitors are being developed against these targets. Although prostate cells are initially regulated by androgen, it is likely that genes encoding one or more of these growth factors become dysregulated from androgen control.

HER-2/neu is an oncogene that encodes for a transmembrane glycoprotein that is structurally related to the epidermal growth factor (EGF) receptor superfamily. Gene amplification of *HER-2/neu* has been detected in various solid tumors and correlates with a poor prognosis. In prostate cancer, the rate of *HER-2/neu* amplification in different studies has varied from 8 to 44% using fluorescence in situ hybridization (FISH) analysis. One study by Signoretti and colleagues suggests that *HER-2/neu* expression in tumors progressively increases after androgen ablation and as tumors become androgen independent.[302] Similarly, Craft and colleagues demonstrated that overexpression of *HER-2/neu* in an otherwise androgen-dependent prostate cancer cell line stimulated androgen-independent growth.[303] This model suggests a novel mechanism for androgen-independent growth of prostate cancer and further points to peptide growth factor pathways as targets for new therapeutics.

Drugs directed at other growth factor receptors, many of which involve inhibition of tyrosine kinases, are actively being tested in the clinic. These include drugs targeting the EGF, endothelin-A,[304] vascular endothelial growth factor, and platelet-derived growth factor receptors.

Vaccine Therapy In theory, it may be possible to repair, replace, or delete a genetic defect and, by doing so, enhance tumor suppression, down-regulate tumor promoters, and amplify the host immune response against a tumor. In practice, knowledge of the genetic defects involved in prostate carcinogenesis and progression is only beginning to be elucidated and, furthermore, delivery of the active gene or element to the appropriate site of action remains a significant hurdle. One promising avenue of gene therapy research has been the use of tumor vaccines to induce cancer-specific immune responses in the host.

Many clinical trials are evaluating PSA- or PSMA-directed vaccine approaches. At Northwest Hospital in Seattle, a phase II trial was conducted to assess the efficacy of infusions of dendritic cells and two HLA-A2-specific PSMA peptides (PSM-P1 and -P2) in 37 patients with local recurrence of prostate cancer after primary treatment failure.[305] One complete and 10 partial responders (30%) were identified based on NPCP criteria by a 50% reduction or by improvement on ProstaScint scan. In another phase I trial at Johns Hopkins, 8 patients were treated with autologous, granulocyte macrophage colony-stimulating factor-secreting, irradiated tumor vaccines prepared from ex vivo retroviral transduction of surgically harvested cells.[306] Vaccination activated new T- and B-cell immune responses against prostate cancer antigens. T-cell responses, evaluated by assessing delayed-type hypersensitivity reactions, were evident in 2 of 8 patients before vaccination and in 7 of 8 patients after treatment. Sera from 3 of 8 vaccinated men contained new antibodies recognizing polypeptides from prostate cells.

Angiogenesis Inhibitors Tumor cells are dependent on the angiogenic growth of new blood vessels.[307] This process is tightly regulated by endogenous molecules that stimulate the process and others that inhibit growth through control of endothelial cell proliferation, migration, and invasion. Endogenous stimulators of angiogenesis include FGFs and VEGFs, and recently described natural inhibitors include endostatin and angiostatin. Prostate tumors are potentially well served by an approach of inhibiting angiogenesis because they are vascular tumors that express high levels of FGF and VEGF as they gain metastatic potential.[308,309] Several phase I and II clinical trials are actively accruing to address this possibility. Of interest, one report suggests that the PSA protein itself has antiangiogenic activity, although the significance of this finding remains unclear.[310]

REFERENCES

1. Jemal A, Tiwari RC, Murray T, et al. Cancer statistics, 2004. CA Cancer J Clin 2004;54(1):8–29.
2. Jacobsen SJ, Katusic SK, Bergstralh EJ, et al. Incidence of prostate cancer diagnosis in the eras before and after serum prostate-specific antigen testing. JAMA 1995;274(18):1445–9.
3. Merrill RM, Stephenson RA. Trends in mortality rates in patients with prostate cancer during the era of prostate specific antigen screening. J Urol 2000;163(2):503–10.
4. Labrie F, Candas B, Dupont A, et al. Screening decreases prostate cancer death: first analysis of the 1988 Quebec prospective randomized controlled trial. Prostate 1999;38(2):83–91.
5. Wynder EL, Mabuchi K, Whitmore WF Jr. Epidemiology of cancer of the prostate. Cancer 1971;28(2):344–60.
6. Guileyardo JM, Johnson WD, Welsh RA, et al. Prevalence of latent prostate carcinoma in two U.S. populations. J Natl Cancer Inst 1980;65(2):311–6.
7. Yatani R, Shiraishi T, Nakakuki K, et al. Trends in frequency of latent prostate carcinoma in Japan from 1965–1979 to 1982–1986. J Natl Cancer Inst 1988;80(9):683–7.
8. Sakr WA, Grignon DJ, Crissman JD, et al. High grade prostatic intraepithelial neoplasia (HGPIN) and prostatic adenocarcinoma between the ages of 20-69: an autopsy study of 249 cases. In Vivo 1994;8(3):439–43.
9. Franks LM. Latent carcinoma of the prostate. J Pathol Bacteriol 1954;68(2):603–16.
10. Edwards CN, Steinthorsson E, Nicholson D. An autopsy study of latent prostatic cancer. Cancer 1953;6(3):531–54.
11. Sakr WA, Haas GP, Cassin BF, et al. The frequency of carcinoma and intraepithelial neoplasia of the prostate in young male patients. J Urol 1993;150(2 Pt 1):379–85.
12. Scott R Jr., Mutchnik DL, Laskowski TZ, Schmalhorst WR. Carcinoma of the prostate in elderly men: incidence, growth characteristics and clinical significance. J Urol 1969;101(4):602–7.
13. Brawley OW, Giovannucci E, Kramer BS. Epidemiology of prostate cancer. In: Vogelzang NJ, Scardino PT, Shipley W, editors. Comprehensive textbook of genitourinary oncology. Philadelphia: Lippincott; 2000. p. 533–44.
14. McDonald CJ. Cancer statistics, 1999: challenges in minority populations. CA Cancer J Clin 1999;49(1):6–7.
15. Danley KL, Richardson JL, Bernstein L, et al. Prostate cancer: trends in mortality and stage-specific incidence rates by racial/ethnic group in Los Angeles County, California (United States). Cancer Causes Control 1995;6(6):492–8.
16. Sohayda CJ, Kupelian PA, Altsman KA, Klein EA. Race as an independent predictor of outcome after treatment for localized prostate cancer. J Urol 1999;162(4):1331–6.
17. Optenberg SA, Thompson IM, Friedrichs P, et al. Race, treatment, and long-term survival from prostate cancer in an equal-access medical care delivery system. JAMA 1995;274(20):1599–605.
18. Hsing AW, Tsao L, Devesa SS. International trends and patterns of prostate cancer incidence and mortality. Int J Cancer 2000;85(1):60–7.
19. Haenszel W, Kurihara M. Studies of Japanese migrants. I. Mortality from cancer and other diseases among Japanese in the United States. J Natl Cancer Inst 1968;40(1):43–68.
20. Lesko SM, Rosenberg L, Shapiro S. Family history and prostate cancer risk. Am J Epidemiol 1996;144(11):1041–7.
21. Bauer JJ, Srivastava S, Connelly RR, et al. Significance of familial history of prostate cancer to traditional prognostic variables, genetic biomarkers, and recurrence after radical prostatectomy. Urology 1998;51(6):970–6.
22. Kupelian PA, Kupelian VA, Witte JS, et al. Family history of prostate cancer in patients with localized prostate cancer: an independent predictor of treatment outcome. J Clin Oncol 1997;15(4):1478–80.
23. Steinberg GD, Carter BS, Beaty TH, et al. Family history and the risk of prostate cancer. Prostate 1990;17(4):337–47.

24. Walsh PC, Partin AW. Family history facilitates the early diagnosis of prostate carcinoma. Cancer 1997;80(9):1871–4.
25. Carpten J, Nupponen N, Isaacs S, et al. Germline mutations in the ribonuclease L gene in families showing linkage with HPC1. Nat Genet 2002;30(2):181–4.
26. Xu J, Meyers D, Freije D, et al. Evidence for a prostate cancer susceptibility locus on the X chromosome. Nat Genet 1998;20(2):175–9.
27. Wu AH, Whittemore AS, Kolonel LN, et al. Serum androgens and sex hormone-binding globulins in relation to lifestyle factors in older African-American, white, and Asian men in the United States and Canada. Cancer Epidemiol Biomarkers Prev 1995;4(7):735–41.
28. Nomura AM, Stemmermann GN, Chyou PH, et al. Serum androgens and prostate cancer. Cancer Epidemiol Biomarkers Prev 1996;5(8):621–5.
29. Garland CF, Friedlander NJ, Barrett-Connor E, Khaw KT. Sex hormones and postmenopausal breast cancer: a prospective study in an adult community. Am J Epidemiol 1992;135(11):1220–30.
30. Gann PH, Hennekens CH, Ma J, et al. Prospective study of sex hormone levels and risk of prostate cancer. J Natl Cancer Inst 1996;88(16):1118–26.
31. Giovannucci E, Stampfer MJ, Krithivas K, et al. The CAG repeat within the androgen receptor gene and its relationship to prostate cancer. Proc Natl Acad Sci U S A 1997;94(7):3320–3.
32. Cox B, Sneyd MJ, Paul C, et al. Vasectomy and risk of prostate cancer. JAMA 2002;287:3110–5.
33. Giovannucci E, Ascherio A, Rimm EB, et al. A prospective cohort study of vasectomy and prostate cancer in US men. JAMA 1993;269(7):873–7.
34. Giovannucci E, Rimm EB, Ascherio A, et al. Smoking and risk of total and fatal prostate cancer in United States health professionals. Cancer Epidemiol Biomarkers Prev 1999;8(4 Pt 1):277–82.
35. Hsing AW, McLaughlin JK, Schuman LM, et al. Diet, tobacco use, and fatal prostate cancer: results from the Lutheran Brotherhood Cohort Study. Cancer Res 1990;50(21):6836–40.
36. Elghany NA, Schumacher MC, Slattery ML, et al. Occupation, cadmium exposure, and prostate cancer. Epidemiology 1990;1(2):107–15.
37. Platz EA, Kantoff PW, Giovannucci E. Epidemiology of and risk factors for prostate cancer. In: Klein EA, ed. Current clinical urology: management of prostate cancer. Totowa (NJ): Humana Press; 1999. p. 19-45.
38. Leitzmann MF, Platz EA, Stampfer MJ, et al. Ejaculation frequency and subsequent risk of prostate cancer. JAMA 2004;291:1578–86.
39. Luscombe CJ, Fryer AA, French ME, et al. Exposure to ultraviolet radiation: association with susceptibility and age at presentation with prostate cancer. Lancet 2001;358(9282):641–2.
40. Yip I, Heber D, Aronson W. Nutrition and prostate cancer. Urol Clin North Am 1999;26(2):403–11, x.
41. Giovannucci E, Rimm EB, Colditz GA, et al. A prospective study of dietary fat and risk of prostate cancer. J Natl Cancer Inst 1993;85(19):1571–9.
42. Calle EE, Rodriguez C, Walker-Thurmond K, Thun MJ. Overweight, obesity, and mortality from cancer in a prospectively studied cohort of U.S. adults. N Engl J Med 2003;348(17):1625–38.
43. Terry P, Lichtenstein P, Feychting M, et al. Fatty fish consumption and risk of prostate cancer. Lancet 2001;357(9270):1764–6.
44. Hsing AW, Comstock GW, Abbey H, Polk BF. Serologic precursors of cancer. Retinol, carotenoids, and tocopherol and risk of prostate cancer. J Natl Cancer Inst 1990;82(11):941–6.
45. Nomura AM, Stemmermann GN, Lee J, Craft NE. Serum micronutrients and prostate cancer in Japanese Americans in Hawaii. Cancer Epidemiol Biomarkers Prev 1997;6(7):487–91.
46. Virtamo J, Pietinen P, Huttunen JK, et al. Incidence of cancer and mortality following alpha-tocopherol and beta-carotene supplementation: a postintervention follow-up. JAMA 2003;290(4):476–85.
47. Clark LC, Combs GF Jr., Turnbull BW, et al. Effects of selenium supplementation for cancer prevention in patients with carcinoma of the skin. A randomized controlled trial. Nutritional Prevention of Cancer Study Group. JAMA 1996;276(24):1957–63.
48. Blutt SE, Weigel NL. Vitamin D and prostate cancer. Proc Soc Exp Biol Med 1999;221(2):89–98.
49. Giovannucci E, Rimm EB, Wolk A, et al. Calcium and fructose intake in relation to risk of prostate cancer. Cancer Res 1998;58(3):442–7.
50. Gann PH, Ma J, Giovannucci E, et al. Lower prostate cancer risk in men with elevated plasma lycopene levels: results of a prospective analysis. Cancer Res 1999;59(6):1225–30.
51. Giovannucci E, Ascherio A, Rimm EB, et al. Intake of carotenoids and retinol in relation to risk of prostate cancer. J Natl Cancer Inst 1995;87(23):1767–76.
52. Thompson IM, Goodman PJ, Tangen CM, et al. The influence of finasteride on the development of prostate cancer. N Engl J Med 2003,349:215–24.
53. McNeal JE. Normal histology of the prostate. Am J Surg Pathol 1988;12(8):619–33.
54. di Sant'Agnese PA. Neuroendocrine cells of the prostate and neuroendocrine differentiation in prostatic carcinoma: a review of morphologic aspects. Urology 1998;51(5A Suppl):121–4.
55. Chung LW. The role of stromal-epithelial interaction in normal and malignant growth. Cancer Surv 1995;23:33–42.
56. McNeal JE, Redwine EA, Freiha FS, Stamey TA. Zonal distribution of prostatic adenocarcinoma. Correlation with histologic pattern and direction of spread. Am J Surg Pathol 1988;12(12):897–906.
57. Greene DR, Wheeler TM, Egawa S, et al. Relationship between clinical stage and histological zone of origin in early prostate cancer: morphometric analysis. Br J Urol 1991;68(5):499–509.
58. Reissigl A, Pointner J, Strasser H, et al. Frequency and clinical significance of transition zone cancer in prostate cancer screening. Prostate 1997;30(2):130–5.
59. Walsh PC, Donker PJ. Impotence following radical prostatectomy: insight into etiology and prevention. J Urol 1982;128(3):492–7.
60. Walsh PC. Anatomic radical prostatectomy: evolution of the surgical technique. J Urol 1998;160(6 Pt 2):2418–24.
61. Vogelstein B, Kinzler KW. The multistep nature of cancer. Trends Genet 1993;9(4):138–41.
62. Haggman MJ, Macoska JA, Wojno KJ, Oesterling JE. The relationship between prostatic intraepithelial neoplasia and prostate cancer: critical issues. J Urol 1997;158(1):12–22.
63. Bostwick DG. Prostatic intraepithelial neoplasia is a risk factor for cancer. Semin Urol Oncol 1999;17(4):187–98.
64. Nauman CJ, Hankins M, Siroky M, Rudders RA. Long term surveillance of men with high grade prostatic intraepithelial neoplasia (PIN) [abstract]. Proc Am Soc Clin Oncol 1999;18:1191.
65. Bostwick DG, Qian J. Atypical adenomatous hyperplasia of the prostate. Relationship with carcinoma in 217 whole-mount radical prostatectomies. Am J Surg Pathol 1995;19(5):506–18.
66. De Marzo AM, Marchi VL, Epstein JI, Nelson WG. Proliferative inflammatory atrophy of the prostate: implications for prostatic carcinogenesis. Am J Pathol 1999;155(6):1985–92.
67. Putzi MJ, De Marzo AM. Morphologic transitions between proliferative inflammatory atrophy and high-grade prostatic intraepithelial neoplasia. Urology 2000;56(5):828–32.
68. Shah R, Mucci NR, Amin A, et al. Postatrophic hyperplasia of the prostate gland: neoplastic precursor or innocent bystander? Am J Pathol 2001;158(5):1767–73.
69. Bostwick DG. The pathology of early prostate cancer. CA Cancer J Clin 1989;39(6):376–93.
70. McWilliam LJ, Manson C, George NJ. Neuroendocrine differentiation and prognosis in prostatic adenocarcinoma. Br J Urol 1997;80(2):287–90.
71. Gleason DF. Classification of prostatic carcinomas. Cancer Chemother Rep 1966;50(3):125–8.
72. Gleason DF, Mellinger GT. Prediction of prognosis for prostatic adenocarcinoma by combined histological grading and clinical staging. J Urol 1974;111(1):58–64.
73. Chan JM, Stampfer MJ, Giovannucci E, et al. Plasma insulin-like growth factor-I and prostate cancer risk: a prospective study. Science 1998;279(5350):563–6.
74. Stattin P, Rinaldi S, Biessy C, et al. High levels of circulating insulin-like growth factor-I increase prostate cancer risk: a prospective study in a population-based non-screened cohort. J Clin Oncol 2004;22:3104–12.
75. Ware JL. Growth factors and their receptors as determinants in the proliferation and metastasis of human prostate cancer. Cancer Metastasis Rev 1993;12(3–4):287–301.
76. Marcelli M, Ittmann M, Mariani S, et al. Androgen receptor mutations in prostate cancer. Cancer Res 2000;60(4):944–9.
77. Bennett CL, Price DK, Kim S, et al. Racial variation in CAG repeat lengths within the androgen receptor gene among prostate cancer patients of lower socioeconomic status. J Clin Oncol 2002;20:3599–604.
78. Taplin ME, Bubley GJ, Shuster TD, et al. Mutation of the androgen-receptor gene in metastatic androgen-independent prostate cancer. N Engl J Med 1995;332(21):1393–8.
79. Feldman BJ, Feldman D. The development of androgen-independent prostate cancer. Nat Rev Cancer 2001;1(1):34–45.
80. Taplin ME, Bubley GJ, Ko YJ, et al. Selection for androgen receptor mutations in prostate cancers treated with androgen antagonist. Cancer Res 1999;59(11):2511–5.
81. Vlietstra RJ, van Alewijk DC, Hermans KG, et al. Frequent inactivation of PTEN in prostate cancer cell lines and xenografts. Cancer Res 1998;58(13):2720–3.
82. McMenamin ME, Soung P, Perera S, et al. Loss of PTEN expression in paraffin-embedded primary prostate cancer correlates with high Gleason score and advanced stage. Cancer Res 1999;59(17):4291–6.
83. Karhadkar SS, Steven Bova G, Abdallah N, et al. Hedgehog signalling in prostate regeneration, neoplasia and metastasis. Nature 2004;431:707–12.
84. Cordon-Cardo C, Koff A, Drobnjak M, et al. Distinct altered patterns of p27KIP1 gene expression in benign prostatic hyperplasia and prostatic carcinoma. J Natl Cancer Inst 1998;90(17):1284–91.
85. Catalona WJ, Smith DS, Ratliff TL, Basler JW. Detection of organ-confined prostate cancer is increased through prostate-specific antigen-based screening. JAMA 1993;270(8):948–54.
86. Thompson IM, Pauler DK, Goodman PJ, et al. Prevalence of prostate cancer among men with a prostate-specific antigen level < or = 4.0 ng per milliliter. N Engl J Med 2004;350(22):2239–46.
87. Punglia RS, D'Amico AV, Catalona WJ, et al. Effect of verification bias on screening for prostate cancer by measurement of prostate-specific antigen. N Engl J Med 2003;349:335–42.
88. Stamey TA, Caldwell M, McNeal JE, et al. The prostate specific antigen era in the United States is over for prostate cancer: what happened in the last 20 years? J Urol 2004;172(4, Pt 1 of 2):1297–301.
89. Sokoll LJ, Chan DW, Mikolajczyk SD, et al. Proenzyme PSA for the early detection of prostate cancer in the 2.5-4.0 ng/ml total PSA range: preliminary analysis. Urology 2003;61(2):274–6.
90. Scardino PT. Early detection of prostate cancer. Urol Clin North Am 1989;16(4):635–55.
91. Ohori M, Wheeler TM, Dunn JK, et al. The pathological features and prognosis of prostate cancer detectable with current diagnostic tests. J Urol 1994;152(5 Pt 2):1714–20.
92. Montie JE, Wood DP Jr., Pontes JE, et al. Adenocarcinoma of the prostate in cystoprostatectomy specimens removed for bladder cancer. Cancer 1989;63(2):381–5.
93. Etzioni R, Penson DF, Legler JM, et al. Overdiagnosis due to prostate-specific antigen screening: lessons from U.S. prostate cancer incidence trends. J Natl Cancer Inst 2002;94(13):981–90.
94. Sirovich BE, Schwartz LM, Woloshin S. Screening men for prostate and colorectal cancer in the United States: does practice reflect the evidence? JAMA 2003;289:1414–20.
95. American Joint Committee on Cancer: Prostate cancer. In: Fleming ID, Cooper JS, Henson DE, Hutter RVP, editors. AJCC cancer staging manual. Philadelphia: Lippincott; 1997. p. 219–24.
96. Lin K, Szabo Z, Chin BB, Civelek AC. The value of a baseline bone scan in patients with newly diagnosed prostate cancer. Clin Nucl Med 1999;24(8):579–82.
97. D'Amico AV, Schnall M, Whittington R, et al. Endorectal coil magnetic resonance imaging identifies locally advanced prostate cancer in select patients with clinically localized disease. Urology 1998;51(3):449–54.
98. Harisinghani MG, Barentsz J, Hahn PF, et al. Noninvasive detection of clinically occult lymph-node metastases in prostate cancer. N Engl J Med 2003;348:2491–9.
99. Seiden MV, Kantoff PW, Krithivas K, et al. Detection of circulating tumor cells in men with localized prostate cancer. J Clin Oncol 1994;12(12):2634–9.
100. Halabi S, Small EJ, Hayes DF, et al. Prognostic significance of reverse transcriptase polymerase chain reaction for prostate-specific antigen in metastatic prostate cancer: a nested study within CALGB 9583. J Clin Oncol 2003;21(3):490–5.
101. Kahn D, Williams RD, Haseman MK, et al. Radioimmunoscintigraphy with In-111-labeled capromab pendetide predicts prostate cancer response to salvage radiotherapy after failed radical prostatectomy. J Clin Oncol 1998;16(1):284–9.

102. Brush JP. Positron emission tomography in urological malignancy. Curr Opin Urol 2001;11(2):175–9.
103. Partin AW, Pound CR, Clemens JQ, et al. Serum PSA after anatomic radical prostatectomy. The Johns Hopkins experience after 10 years. Urol Clin North Am 1993;20(4):713–25.
104. Blute ML, Bergstralh EJ, Partin AW, et al. Validation of Partin tables for predicting pathological stage of clinically localized prostate cancer. J Urol 2000;164(5):1591–5.
105. Pound CR, Partin AW, Eisenberger MA, et al. Natural history of progression after PSA elevation following radical prostatectomy. JAMA 1999;281(17):1591–7.
106. Jhaveri FM, Zippe CD, Klein EA, Kupelian PA. Biochemical failure does not predict overall survival after radical prostatectomy for localized prostate cancer: 10-year results. Urology 1999;54(5):884–90.
107. Amling CL, Riffenburgh RH, Sun L, et al. Pathologic variables and recurrence rates as related to obesity and race in men with prostate cancer undergoing radical prostatectomy. J Clin Oncol 2004,22(3):439–45.
108. Cross CK, Shultz D, Malkowicz SB, et al. Impact of race on prostate-specific antigen outcome after radical prostatectomy for clinically localized adenocarcinoma of the prostate. J Clin Oncol 2002;20(12):2863–8.
109. D'Amico AV, Whittington R, Malkowicz SB, et al. Clinical utility of percent-positive prostate biopsies in predicting biochemical outcome after radical prostatectomy or external-beam radiation therapy for patients with clinically localized prostate cancer [discussion 7]. Mol Urol 2000;4(3):171–5.
110. Chakravarti A, Heydon K, Wu CL, et al. Loss of p16 expression is of prognostic significance in locally advanced prostate cancer: an analysis from the Radiation Therapy Oncology Group protocol 86–10. J Clin Oncol 2003;21(17):3328–34.
111. Augustin H, Graefen M, Palisaar J, et al. Prognostic significance of visible lesions on transrectal ultrasound in impalpable prostate cancers: implications for staging. J Clin Oncol 2003;21(15):2860–8.
112. Kattan MW, Shariat SF, Andrews B, et al. The addition of interleukin-6 soluble receptor and transforming growth factor beta1 improves a preoperative nomogram for predicting biochemical progression in patients with clinically localized prostate cancer. J Clin Oncol 2003;21(19):3573–9.
113. Pollack A, DeSilvio M, Khor LY, et al. Ki-67 staining is a strong predictor of distant metastasis and mortality for men with prostate cancer treated with radiotherapy plus androgen deprivation: Radiation Therapy Oncology Group Trial 92-02. J Clin Oncol 2004;22(11):2133–40.
114. Katz MS, Zelefsky MJ, Venkatraman ES, et al. Predictors of biochemical outcome with salvage conformal radiotherapy after radical prostatectomy for prostate cancer. J Clin Oncol 2003;21(3):483–9.
115. Pollack A, Grignon DJ, Heydon KH, et al. Prostate cancer DNA ploidy and response to salvage hormone therapy after radiotherapy with or without short-term total androgen blockade: an analysis of RTOG 8610. J Clin Oncol 2003;21(7):1238–48.
116. D'Amico AV, Whittington R, Malkowicz SB, et al. Biochemical outcome after radical prostatectomy, external beam radiation therapy, or interstitial radiation therapy for clinically localized prostate cancer. JAMA 1998;280(11):969–74.
117. Kattan MW, Eastham JA, Stapleton AM, et al. A preoperative nomogram for disease recurrence following radical prostatectomy for prostate cancer. J Natl Cancer Inst 1998;90(10):766–71.
118. Graefen M, Karakiewicz PI, Cagiannos I, et al. International validation of a preoperative nomogram for prostate cancer recurrence after radical prostatectomy. J Clin Oncol 2002;20(15):3206–12.
119. Graefen M, Karakiewicz PI, Cagiannos I, et al. Validation study of the accuracy of a postoperative nomogram for recurrence after radical prostatectomy for localized prostate cancer. J Clin Oncol 2002;20(4):951–6.
120. D'Amico AV, Moul J, Carroll PR, et al. Cancer-specific mortality after surgery or radiation for patients with clinically localized prostate cancer managed during the prostate-specific antigen era. J Clin Oncol 2003;21(11):2163–72.
121. D'Amico AV, Chen MH, Roehl KA, Catalona WJ. Preoperative PSA velocity and the risk of death from prostate cancer after radical prostatectomy. N Engl J Med 2004;351:125–35.
122. Lee WR, Hanks GE, Hanlon A. Increasing prostate-specific antigen profile following definitive radiation therapy for localized prostate cancer: clinical observations. J Clin Oncol 1997;15(1):230–8.
123. Chodak GW, Thisted RA, Gerber GS, et al. Results of conservative management of clinically localized prostate cancer. N Engl J Med 1994;330(4):242–8.
124. Johansson JE, Andren O, Andersson SO, et al. Natural history of early, localized prostate cancer. JAMA 2004;291:2713–9.
125. Albertsen PC, Hanley JA, Gleason DF, Barry MJ. Competing risk analysis of men aged 55 to 74 years at diagnosis managed conservatively for clinically localized prostate cancer. JAMA 1998;280(11):975–80.
126. Holmberg L, Bill-Axelson A, Helgesen F, et al. A randomized trial comparing radical prostatectomy with watchful waiting in early prostate cancer. N Engl J Med 2002;347:781–9.
127. Ohori M, Wheeler TM, Kattan MW, et al. Prognostic significance of positive surgical margins in radical prostatectomy specimens. J Urol 1995;154(5):1818–24.
128. Zincke H, Oesterling JE, Blute ML, et al. Long-term (15 years) results after radical prostatectomy for clinically localized (stage T2c or lower) prostate cancer. J Urol 1994;152(5 Pt 2):1850–7.
129. Han M, Partin AW, Piantadosi S, et al. Era specific biochemical recurrence-free survival following radical prostatectomy for clinically localized prostate cancer. J Urol 2001;166(2):416–9.
130. Lu-Yao GL, Albertsen P, Warren J, Yao SL. Effect of age and surgical approach on complications and short-term mortality after radical prostatectomy—a population-based study. Urology 1999;54(2):301–7.
131. Hedican SP, Walsh PC. Postoperative bleeding following radical retropubic prostatectomy. J Urol 1994;152(4):1181–3.
132. McLaren RH, Barrett DM, Zincke H. Rectal injury occurring at radical retropubic prostatectomy for prostate cancer: etiology and treatment. Urology 1993;42(4):401–5.
133. Cisek LJ, Walsh PC. Thromboembolic complications following radical retropubic prostatectomy. Influence of external sequential pneumatic compression devices. Urology 1993;42(4):406–8.
134. Surya BV, Provet J, Johanson KE, Brown J. Anastomotic strictures following radical prostatectomy: risk factors and management. J Urol 1990;143(4):755–8.
135. Haab F, Yamaguchi R, Leach GE. Postprostatectomy incontinence. Urol Clin North Am 1996;23(3):447–57.
136. Stanford JL, Feng Z, Hamilton AS, et al. Urinary and sexual function after radical prostatectomy for clinically localized prostate cancer: the Prostate Cancer Outcomes Study. JAMA 2000;283(3):354–60.
137. Talcott JA, Rieker P, Clark JA, et al. Patient-reported symptoms after primary therapy for early prostate cancer: results of a prospective cohort study. J Clin Oncol 1998;16(1):275–83.
138. Quinlan DM, Epstein JI, Carter BS, Walsh PC. Sexual function following radical prostatectomy: influence of preservation of neurovascular bundles. J Urol 1991;145(5):998–1002.
139. Catalona WJ, Carvalhal GF, Mager DE, Smith DS. Potency, continence and complication rates in 1,870 consecutive radical retropubic prostatectomies. J Urol 1999;162(2):433–8.
140. Barringer B. Radium in the treatment of carcinoma of the bladder and prostate. JAMA 1917;68:1227–30.
141. Bagshaw MA. Definitive radiotherapy in carcinoma of the prostate. JAMA 1969;210(2):326–7.
142. Hanks GE, Hanlon AL, Schultheiss TE, et al. Conformal external beam treatment of prostate cancer. Urology 1997;50(1):87–92.
143. Bagshaw MA, Cox RS, Hancock SL. Control of prostate cancer with radiotherapy: long-term results. J Urol 1994;152(5 Pt 2):1781–5.
144. Grossman HB, Batata M, Hilaris B, Whitmore WF Jr. 125I implantation for carcinoma of prostate. Further follow-up of first 100 cases. Urology 1982;20(6):591–8.
145. Zelefsky MJ, Whitmore WF Jr. Long-term results of retropubic permanent 125iodine implantation of the prostate for clinically localized prostatic cancer [discussion 9–30]. J Urol 1997;158(1):23–9.
146. Holm HH, Juul N, Pedersen JF, et al. Transperineal 125iodine seed implantation in prostatic cancer guided by transrectal ultrasonography. J Urol 1983;130(2):283–6.
147. Ling CC, Li WX, Anderson LL. The relative biological effectiveness of I-125 and Pd-103. Int J Radiat Oncol Biol Phys 1995;32(2):373–8.
148. Cha CM, Potters L, Ashley R, et al. Isotope selection for patients undergoing prostate brachytherapy. Int J Radiat Oncol Biol Phys 1999;45(2):391–5.
149. D'Amico AV, Cormack R, Tempany CM, et al. Real-time magnetic resonance image-guided interstitial brachytherapy in the treatment of select patients with clinically localized prostate cancer. Int J Radiat Oncol Biol Phys 1998;42(3):507–15.
150. Hanks GE, Krall JM, Hanlon AL, et al. Patterns of Care and RTOG studies in prostate cancer: long-term survival, hazard rate observations, and possibilities of cure. Int J Radiat Oncol Biol Phys 1994;28(1):39–45.
151. Hanks GE, Hanlon A, Schultheiss T, et al. Early prostate cancer: the national results of radiation treatment from the Patterns of Care and Radiation Therapy Oncology Group studies with prospects for improvement with conformal radiation and adjuvant androgen deprivation. J Urol 1994;152(5 Pt 2):1775–80.
152. Consensus statement: guidelines for PSA following radiation therapy. American Society for Therapeutic Radiology and Oncology Consensus Panel. Int J Radiat Oncol Biol Phys 1997;37(5):1035–41.
153. Shipley WU, Thames HD, Sandler HM, et al. Radiation therapy for clinically localized prostate cancer: a multi-institutional pooled analysis. JAMA 1999;281(17):1598–604.
154. D'Amico AV, Coleman CN. Role of interstitial radiotherapy in the management of clinically organ-confined prostate cancer: the jury is still out. J Clin Oncol 1996;14(1):304–15.
155. Grimm PD, Blasko JC, Sylvester JE, et al. 10-year biochemical (prostate-specific antigen) control of prostate cancer with (125)I brachytherapy. Int J Radiat Oncol Biol Phys 2001;51(1):31–40.
156. Zelefsky MJ, Leibel SA, Gaudin PB, et al. Dose escalation with three-dimensional conformal radiation therapy affects the outcome in prostate cancer. Int J Radiat Oncol Biol Phys 1998;41(3):491–500.
157. Hanks GE, Hanlon AL, Schultheiss TE, et al. Dose escalation with 3D conformal treatment: five year outcomes, treatment optimization, and future directions. Int J Radiat Oncol Biol Phys 1998;41(3):501–10.
158. Pollack A, Zagars GK. External beam radiotherapy dose response of prostate cancer. Int J Radiat Oncol Biol Phys 1997;39(5):1011–8.
159. Measurements ICoRUa. Prescribing, recording and reporting photon beam therapy. Report Number 601993.
160. Hanks GE, Hanlon AL, Pinover WH, et al. Survival advantage for prostate cancer patients treated with high-dose three-dimensional conformal radiotherapy. Cancer J Sci Am 1999;5(3):152–8.
161. Pollack A, Zagars GK, Starkschall G, et al. Prostate cancer radiation dose response: results of the M. D. Anderson phase III randomized trial. Int J Radiat Oncol Biol Phys 2002;53(5):1097–105.
162. Sylvester JE, Blasko JC, Grimm PD, et al. Ten-year biochemical relapse-free survival after external beam radiation and brachytherapy for localized prostate cancer: the Seattle experience. Int J Radiat Oncol Biol Phys 2003;57(4):944–52.
163. Stromberg JS, Martinez AA, Horwitz EM, et al. Conformal high dose rate iridium-192 boost brachytherapy in locally advanced prostate cancer: superior prostate-specific antigen response compared with external beam treatment. Cancer J Sci Am 1997;3(6):346–52.
164. D'Amico AV, Manola J, Loffredo M, et al. 6-month androgen suppression plus radiation therapy vs radiation therapy alone for patients with clinically localized prostate cancer: a randomized controlled trial. JAMA 2004;292:821–7.
165. Pilepich MV, Krall JM, al-Sarraf M, et al. Androgen deprivation with radiation therapy compared with radiation therapy alone for locally advanced prostatic carcinoma: a randomized comparative trial of the Radiation Therapy Oncology Group. Urology 1995;45(4):616–23.
166. Pilepich MV, Winter K, John MJ, et al. Phase III radiation therapy oncology group (RTOG) trial 86-10 of androgen deprivation adjuvant to definitive radiotherapy in locally advanced carcinoma of the prostate. Int J Radiat Oncol Biol Phys 2001;50(5):1243–52.
167. Horwitz EM, Winter K, Hanks GE, et al. Subset analysis of RTOG 85-31 and 86-10 indicates an advantage for long-term vs. short-term adjuvant hormones for patients with locally advanced nonmetastatic prostate cancer treated with radiation therapy. Int J Radiat Oncol Biol Phys 2001;49(4):947–56.
168. Pilepich MV, Caplan R, Byhardt RW, et al. Phase III trial of androgen suppression using goserelin in unfavorable-prognosis carcinoma of the prostate treated with definitive radiotherapy: report of Radiation Therapy Oncology Group Protocol 85-31. J Clin Oncol 1997;15(3):1013–21.
169. Lawton CA, Winter K, Murray K, et al. Updated results of the phase III Radiation Therapy Oncology Group

(RTOG) trial 85-31 evaluating the potential benefit of androgen suppression following standard radiation therapy for unfavorable prognosis carcinoma of the prostate. Int J Radiat Oncol Biol Phys 2001;49(4):937–46.
170. Bolla M, Gonzalez D, Warde P, et al. Improved survival in patients with locally advanced prostate cancer treated with radiotherapy and goserelin. N Engl J Med 1997;337(5):295–300.
171. Bolla M, Collette L, Blank L, et al. Long-term results with immediate androgen suppression and external irradiation in patients with locally advanced prostate cancer (an EORTC study): a phase III randomised trial. Lancet 2002;360:103–6.
172. Hanks GE, Pajak TF, Porter A, et al. Phase III trial of long-term adjuvant androgen deprivation after neoadjuvant hormonal cytoreduction and radiotherapy in locally advanced carcinoma of the prostate: the Radiation Therapy Oncology Group Protocol 92-02. J Clin Oncol 2003;21(21):3972–8.
173. Roach M 3rd, DeSilvio M, Lawton C, et al. Phase III trial comparing whole-pelvic versus prostate-only radiotherapy and neoadjuvant versus adjuvant combined androgen suppression: Radiation Therapy Oncology Group 9413. J Clin Oncol 2003;21(10):1904–11.
174. Kumar P, Perrotti M, Weiss R, et al. Phase I trial of weekly docetaxel with concurrent three-dimensional conformal radiation therapy in the treatment of unfavorable localized adenocarcinoma of the prostate. J Clin Oncol 2004;22(10):1909–15.
175. Dewey WC, Hopwood LE, Sapareto SA, Gerweck LE. Cellular responses to combinations of hyperthermia and radiation. Radiology 1977;123(2):463–74.
176. Fosmire H, Hynynen K, Drach GW, et al. Feasibility and toxicity of transrectal ultrasound hyperthermia in the treatment of locally advanced adenocarcinoma of the prostate. Int J Radiat Oncol Biol Phys 1993;26(2):253–9.
177. Shipley WU, Verhey LJ, Munzenrider JE, et al. Advanced prostate cancer: the results of a randomized comparative trial of high dose irradiation boosting with conformal protons compared with conventional dose irradiation using photons alone. Int J Radiat Oncol Biol Phys 1995;32(1):3–12.
178. Rossi CJ. Conformal proton beam therapy of prostate cancer—update on the Loma Linda University medical center experience. Strahlenther Onkol 1999;175 Suppl 2:82–4.
179. Laramore GE, Krall JM, Griffin TW, et al. Neutron versus photon irradiation for unresectable salivary gland tumors: final report of an RTOG-MRC randomized clinical trial. Radiation Therapy Oncology Group. Medical Research Council. Int J Radiat Oncol Biol Phys 1993;27(2):235–40.
180. Russell KJ, Caplan RJ, Laramore GE, et al. Photon versus fast neutron external beam radiotherapy in the treatment of locally advanced prostate cancer: results of a randomized prospective trial. Int J Radiat Oncol Biol Phys 1994;28(1):47–54.
181. Forman JD, Warmelink C, Devi S, et al. Alternating conformal neutron and photon irradiation for locally advanced adenocarcinoma of the prostate. Am J Clin Oncol 1995;18(3):231–8.
182. Pound CR, Partin AW, Epstein JI, Walsh PC. Prostate-specific antigen after anatomic radical retropubic prostatectomy. Patterns of recurrence and cancer control. Urol Clin North Am 1997;24(2):395–406.
183. Kupelian P, Katcher J, Levin H, et al. Correlation of clinical and pathologic factors with rising prostate-specific antigen profiles after radical prostatectomy alone for clinically localized prostate cancer. Urology 1996;48(2):249–60.
184. Partin AW, Kattan MW, Subong EN, et al. Combination of prostate-specific antigen, clinical stage, and Gleason score to predict pathological stage of localized prostate cancer. A multi-institutional update. JAMA 1997;277(18):1445–51.
185. Anscher MS, Prosnitz LR. Multivariate analysis of factors predicting local relapse after radical prostatectomy—possible indications for postoperative radiotherapy. Int J Radiat Oncol Biol Phys 1991;21(4):941–7.
186. Schild SE, Buskirk SJ, Wong WW, et al. The use of radiotherapy for patients with isolated elevation of serum prostate specific antigen following radical prostatectomy. J Urol 1996;156(5):1725–9.
187. Zietman AL, Coen JJ, Shipley WU, Althausen AF. Adjuvant irradiation after radical prostatectomy for adenocarcinoma of prostate: analysis of freedom from PSA failure [discussion 8–9]. Urology 1993;42(3):292–8.
188. Tiguert R, Forman JD, Hussain M, Wood DP Jr. Radiation therapy for a rising PSA level after radical prostatectomy. Semin Urol Oncol 1999;17(3):141–7.
189. Lange PH, Lightner DJ, Medini E, et al. The effect of radiation therapy after radical prostatectomy in patients with elevated prostate specific antigen levels [discussion 32–3]. J Urol 1990;144(4):927–32.
190. Patel A, Dorey F, Franklin J, deKernion JB. Recurrence patterns after radical retropubic prostatectomy: clinical usefulness of prostate specific antigen doubling times and log slope prostate specific antigen. J Urol 1997;158(4):1441–5.
191. Schild SE. Radiation therapy after prostatectomy: now or later? Semin Radiat Oncol 1998;8(2):132–9.
192. Stephenson AJ, Shariat SF, Zelefsky MJ, et al. Salvage radiotherapy for recurrent prostate cancer after radical prostatectomy. JAMA 2004;291:1325–32.
193. Eulau SM, Tate DJ, Stamey TA, et al. Effect of combined transient androgen deprivation and irradiation following radical prostatectomy for prostatic cancer. Int J Radiat Oncol Biol Phys 1998;41(4):735–40.
194. Corn BW, Winter K, Pilepich MV. Does androgen suppression enhance the efficacy of postoperative irradiation? A secondary analysis of RTOG 85-31. Radiation Therapy Oncology Group. Urology 1999;54(3):495–502.
195. Lawton CA, Won M, Pilepich MV, et al. Long-term treatment sequelae following external beam irradiation for adenocarcinoma of the prostate: analysis of RTOG studies 7506 and 7706. Int J Radiat Oncol Biol Phys 1991;21(4):935–9.
196. Shipley WU, Prout GR Jr., Coachman NM, et al. Radiation therapy for localized prostate carcinoma: experience at the Massachusetts General Hospital (1973–1981). NCI Monogr 1988;7:67–73.
197. Dearnaley DP, Khoo VS, Norman AR, et al. Comparison of radiation side-effects of conformal and conventional radiotherapy in prostate cancer: a randomised trial. Lancet 1999;353(9149):267–72.
198. Sandler HM, McLaughlin PW, Ten Haken RK, et al. Three dimensional conformal radiotherapy for the treatment of prostate cancer: low risk of chronic rectal morbidity observed in a large series of patients. Int J Radiat Oncol Biol Phys 1995;33(4):797–801.
199. Zelefsky MJ, Cowen D, Fuks Z, et al. Long term tolerance of high dose three-dimensional conformal radiotherapy in patients with localized prostate carcinoma. Cancer 1999;85(11):2460–8.
200. Kleinberg L, Wallner K, Roy J, et al. Treatment-related symptoms during the first year following transperineal 125I prostate implantation. Int J Radiat Oncol Biol Phys 1994;28(4):985–90.
201. Hurwitz MD, Cormack R, Tempany CM, et al. Three-dimensional real-time magnetic resonance-guided interstitial prostate brachytherapy optimizes radiation dose distribution resulting in a favorable acute side effect profile in patients with clinically localized prostate cancer. Tech Urol 2000;6(2):89–94.
202. Gelblum DY, Potters L, Ashley R, et al. Urinary morbidity following ultrasound-guided transperineal prostate seed implantation. Int J Radiat Oncol Biol Phys 1999;45(1):59–67.
203. Wallner K, Roy J, Harrison L. Tumor control and morbidity following transperineal iodine 125 implantation for stage T1/T2 prostatic carcinoma. J Clin Oncol 1996;14(2):449–53.
204. Blasko JC, Wallner KE, Cavanagh W. Radiotherapeutic strategies in the management of clinically localized, "low-risk" prostate cancer: selection, results, and the search for answers. Cancer J Sci Am 1998;4(3):157–8.
205. Hanks GE. More on the Uro-Oncology Research Group report of radical surgery vs. radiotherapy for adenocarcinoma of the prostate. Int J Radiat Oncol Biol Phys 1988;14(5):1053–4.
206. Cooperberg MR, Lubeck DP, Meng MV, et al. The changing face of low-risk prostate cancer: trends in clinical presentation and primary management. J Clin Oncol 2004;22(11):2141–9.
207. Kupelian PA, Elshaikh M, Reddy CA, et al. Comparison of the efficacy of local therapies for localized prostate cancer in the prostate-specific antigen era: a large single-institution experience with radical prostatectomy and external-beam radiotherapy. J Clin Oncol 2002;20:3376–85.
208. Potosky AL, Davis WW, Hoffman RM, et al. Five-year outcomes after prostatectomy or radiotherapy for prostate cancer: the prostate cancer outcomes study. J Natl Cancer Inst 2004;96(18):1358–67.
209. Talcott JA, Manola J, Clark JA, et al. Time course and predictors of symptoms after primary prostate cancer therapy. J Clin Oncol 2003;21(21):3979–86.
210. Burkhardt JH, Litwin MS, Rose CM, et al. Comparing the costs of radiation therapy and radical prostatectomy for the initial treatment of early-stage prostate cancer. J Clin Oncol 2002:2869–75.
211. Wilt TJ, Brawer MK. The Prostate Cancer Intervention Versus Observation Trial: a randomized trial comparing radical prostatectomy versus expectant management for the treatment of clinically localized prostate cancer. J Urol 1994;152(5 Pt 2):1910–4.
212. Jones GW, Mettlin C, Murphy GP, et al. Patterns of care for carcinoma of the prostate gland: results of a national survey of 1984 and 1990. J Am Coll Surg 1995;180(5):545–54.
213. Oh WK, Kantoff PW. Treatment of locally advanced prostate cancer: is chemotherapy the next step? J Clin Oncol 1999;17(11):3664–75.
214. Freeman JA, Esrig D, Grossfeld GD, et al. Incidence of occult lymph node metastases in pathological stage C (pT3N0) prostate cancer. J Urol 1995;154(2 Pt 1):474–8.
215. Gerber GS, Thisted RA, Chodak GW, et al. Results of radical prostatectomy in men with locally advanced prostate cancer: multi-institutional pooled analysis. Eur Urol 1997;32(4):385–90.
216. Bonney WW, Schned AR, Timberlake DS. Neoadjuvant androgen ablation for localized prostatic cancer: pathology methods, surgical end points and meta-analysis of randomized trials. J Urol 1998;160(5):1754–60.
217. Zincke H. Extended experience with surgical treatment of stage D1 adenocarcinoma of prostate. Significant influences of immediate adjuvant hormonal treatment (orchiectomy) on outcome. Urology 1989;33(5 Suppl):27–36.
218. Messing EM, Manola J, Sarosdy M, et al. Immediate hormonal therapy compared with observation after radical prostatectomy and pelvic lymphadenectomy in men with node-positive prostate cancer. N Engl J Med 1999;341(24):1781–8.
219. Hanks GE. The challenge of treating node-positive prostate cancer. An approach to resolving the questions. Cancer 1993;71(3 Suppl):1014–8.
220. Zagars GK, Sands ME, Pollack A, von Eschenbach AC. Early androgen ablation for stage D1 (N1 to N3, M0) prostate cancer: prognostic variables and outcome. J Urol 1994;151(5):1330–3.
221. Lankford SP, Pollack A, Zagars GK. Radiotherapy for regionally localized hormone refractory prostate cancer. Int J Radiat Oncol Biol Phys 1995;33(4):907–12.
222. Sands ME, Pollack A, Zagars GK. Influence of radiotherapy on node-positive prostate cancer treated with androgen ablation. Int J Radiat Oncol Biol Phys 1995;31(1):13–9.
223. Whittington R, Malkowicz SB, Machtay M, et al. The use of combined radiation therapy and hormonal therapy in the management of lymph node-positive prostate cancer. Int J Radiat Oncol Biol Phys 1997;39(3):673–80.
224. Lawton CA, Winter K, Byhardt R, et al. Androgen suppression plus radiation versus radiation alone for patients with D1 (pN+) adenocarcinoma of the prostate (results based on a national prospective randomized trial, RTOG 85-31). Radiation Therapy Oncology Group. Int J Radiat Oncol Biol Phys 1997;38(5):931–9.
225. Garnick MB, Fair WR. Prostate cancer: emerging concepts. Part II. Ann Intern Med 1996;125(3):205–12.
226. Mundy GR. Mechanisms of bone metastasis. Cancer 1997;80(8 Suppl):1546–56.
227. Koeneman KS, Yeung F, Chung LW. Osteomimetic properties of prostate cancer cells: a hypothesis supporting the predilection of prostate cancer metastasis and growth in the bone environment. Prostate 1999;39(4):246–61.
228. Thalmann GN, Sikes RA, Devoll RE, et al. Osteopontin: possible role in prostate cancer progression. Clin Cancer Res 1999;5(8):2271–7.
229. Jacob K, Webber M, Benayahu D, Kleinman HK. Osteonectin promotes prostate cancer cell migration and invasion: a possible mechanism for metastasis to bone. Cancer Res 1999;59(17):4453–7.
230. Goldenberg SL, Fenster HN, Perler Z, McLoughlin MG. Disseminated intravascular coagulation in carcinoma of prostate: role of estrogen therapy. Urology 1983;22(2):130–2.
231. Feuer EJ, Merrill RM, Hankey BF. Cancer surveillance series: interpreting trends in prostate cancer—part II: Cause of death misclassification and the recent rise and fall in prostate cancer mortality. J Natl Cancer Inst 1999;91(12):1025–32.
232. Byar DP. Proceedings: The Veterans Administration Cooperative Urological Research Group's studies of cancer of the prostate. Cancer 1973;32(5):1126–30.

233. Byar DP. Treatment of prostatic cancer: studies by the Veterans Administration cooperative urological research group. Bull N Y Acad Med 1972;48(5):751–66.
234. Bailar JC 3rd, Byar DP. Estrogen treatment for cancer of the prostate. Early results with 3 doses of diethylstilbestrol and placebo. Cancer 1970;26(2):257–61.
235. Kent JR, Bischoff AJ, Arduino LJ, et al. Estrogen dosage and suppression of testosterone levels in patients with prostatic carcinoma. J Urol 1973;109(5):858–60.
236. Leuprolide versus diethylstilbestrol for metastatic prostate cancer. The Leuprolide Study Group. N Engl J Med 1984;311(20):1281–6.
237. Tyrrell CJ, Kaisary AV, Iversen P, et al. A randomised comparison of 'Casodex' (bicalutamide) 150 mg monotherapy versus castration in the treatment of metastatic and locally advanced prostate cancer. Eur Urol 1998;33(5):447–56.
238. Boccardo F, Barichello M, Battaglia M, et al. Bicalutamide monotherapy versus flutamide plus goserelin in prostate cancer: updated results of a multicentric trial. Eur Urol 2002;42(5):481–90.
239. Crawford ED, Eisenberger MA, McLeod DG, et al. A controlled trial of leuprolide with and without flutamide in prostatic carcinoma. N Engl J Med 1989;321(7):419–24.
240. Maximum androgen blockade in advanced prostate cancer: an overview of the randomised trials. Prostate Cancer Trialists' Collaborative Group. Lancet 2000;355(9214):1491–8.
241. Caubet JF, Tosteson TD, Dong EW, et al. Maximum androgen blockade in advanced prostate cancer: a meta-analysis of published randomized controlled trials using nonsteroidal antiandrogens. Urology 1997;49(1):71–8.
242. Eisenberger MA, Blumenstein BA, Crawford ED, et al. Bilateral orchiectomy with or without flutamide for metastatic prostate cancer. N Engl J Med 1998;339(15):1036–42.
243. Smith MR, McGovern FJ, Zietman AL, et al. Pamidronate to prevent bone loss during androgen-deprivation therapy for prostate cancer. N Engl J Med 2001;345(13):948–55.
244. Segal RJ, Reid RD, Courneya KS, et al. Resistance exercise in men receiving androgen deprivation therapy for prostate cancer. J Clin Oncol 2003;21(9):1653–9.
245. Smith MR, Goode M, Zietman AL, et al. Bicalutamide monotherapy versus leuprolide monotherapy for prostate cancer: effects on bone mineral density and body composition. J Clin Oncol 2004;22(13):2546–53.
246. Gleave M, Bruchovsky N, Goldenberg SL, Rennie P. Intermittent androgen suppression for prostate cancer: rationale and clinical experience. Eur Urol 1998;34 Suppl 3:37–41.
247. Akakura K, Bruchovsky N, Goldenberg SL, et al. Effects of intermittent androgen suppression on androgen-dependent tumors. Apoptosis and serum prostate-specific antigen. Cancer 1993;71(9):2782–90.
248. Horwich A, Huddart RA, Gadd J, et al. A pilot study of intermittent androgen deprivation in advanced prostate cancer. Br J Urol 1998;81(1):96–9.
249. Crook JM, Szumacher E, Malone S, et al. Intermittent androgen suppression in the management of prostate cancer. Urology 1999;53(3):530–4.
250. Immediate versus deferred treatment for advanced prostatic cancer: initial results of the Medical Research Council Trial. The Medical Research Council Prostate Cancer Working Party Investigators Group. Br J Urol 1997;79(2):235–46.
251. Kelly WK, Scher HI, Mazumdar M, et al. Prostate-specific antigen as a measure of disease outcome in metastatic hormone-refractory prostate cancer. J Clin Oncol 1993;11(4):607–15.
252. Bubley GJ, Carducci M, Dahut W, et al. Eligibility and response guidelines for phase II clinical trials in androgen-independent prostate cancer: recommendations from the Prostate-Specific Antigen Working Group. J Clin Oncol 1999;17(11):3461–7.
253. Hussain M, Wolf M, Marshall E, et al. Effects of continued androgen-deprivation therapy and other prognostic factors on response and survival in phase II chemotherapy trials for hormone-refractory prostate cancer: a Southwest Oncology Group report. J Clin Oncol 1994;12(9):1868–75.
254. Taylor CD, Elson P, Trump DL. Importance of continued testicular suppression in hormone-refractory prostate cancer. J Clin Oncol 1993;11(11):2167–72.
255. Kelly WK, Scher HI. Prostate specific antigen decline after antiandrogen withdrawal: the flutamide withdrawal syndrome. J Urol 1993;149(3):607–9.
256. Small EJ, Vogelzang NJ. Second-line hormonal therapy for advanced prostate cancer: a shifting paradigm. J Clin Oncol 1997;15(1):382–8.
257. Dawson NA, McLeod DG. Dramatic prostate specific antigen decrease in response to discontinuation of megestrol acetate in advanced prostate cancer: expansion of the antiandrogen withdrawal syndrome. J Urol 1995;153(6):1946–7.
258. Oh WK, Kantoff PW. Management of hormone refractory prostate cancer: current standards and future prospects. J Urol 1998;160(4):1220–9.
259. Small EJ, Baron AD, Fippin L, Apodaca D. Ketoconazole retains activity in advanced prostate cancer patients with progression despite flutamide withdrawal. J Urol 1997;157(4):1204–7.
260. Small EJ, Halabi S, Dawson NA, et al. Antiandrogen withdrawal alone or in combination with ketoconazole in androgen-independent prostate cancer patients: a phase III trial (CALGB 9583). J Clin Oncol 2004:1025–33.
261. Tannock IF, Osoba D, Stockler MR, et al. Chemotherapy with mitoxantrone plus prednisone or prednisone alone for symptomatic hormone-resistant prostate cancer: a Canadian randomized trial with palliative end points. J Clin Oncol 1996;14(6):1756–64.
262. Kantoff PW, Halabi S, Conaway M, et al. Hydrocortisone with or without mitoxantrone in men with hormone-refractory prostate cancer: results of the cancer and leukemia group B 9182 study. J Clin Oncol 1999;17(8):2506–13.
263. Oh WK. The evolving role of estrogen therapy in prostate cancer. Clin Prostate Cancer 2002;1(2):81–9.
264. Oh WK, Kantoff PW, Weinberg V, et al. Prospective, multicenter, randomized phase II trial of the herbal supplement, PC-SPES, and diethylstilbestrol in patients with androgen-independent prostate cancer. J Clin Oncol 2004;22(18):3705–12.
265. Joyce R, Fenton MA, Rode P, et al. High dose bicalutamide for androgen independent prostate cancer: effect of prior hormonal therapy. J Urol 1998;159(1):149–53.
266. Scher HI, Liebertz C, Kelly WK, et al. Bicalutamide for advanced prostate cancer: the natural versus treated history of disease. J Clin Oncol 1997;15(8):2928–38.
267. Desai A, Stadler WM, Vogelzang NJ. Nilutamide: possible utility as a second-line hormonal agent. Urology 2001;58(6):1016–20.
268. Dawson NA, Conaway M, Halabi S, et al. A randomized study comparing standard versus moderately high dose megestrol acetate for patients with advanced prostate carcinoma: cancer and leukemia group B study 9181. Cancer 2000;88(4):825–34.
269. Hudes G. Estramustine-based chemotherapy. Semin Urol Oncol 1997;15(1):13–9.
270. Hudes G, Einhorn L, Ross E, et al. Vinblastine versus vinblastine plus oral estramustine phosphate for patients with hormone-refractory prostate cancer: A Hoosier Oncology Group and Fox Chase Network phase III trial. J Clin Oncol 1999;17(10):3160–6.
271. Kamradt JM, Smith DC, Pienta KJ. Oral chemotherapy for hormone refractory prostate cancer. The University of Michigan experience. Urol Clin North Am 1999;26(2):333–40.
272. Savarese DM, Halabi S, Hars V, et al. Phase II study of docetaxel, estramustine, and low-dose hydrocortisone in men with hormone-refractory prostate cancer: a final report of CALGB 9780. Cancer and Leukemia Group B. J Clin Oncol 2001;19(9):2509–16.
273. Tannock IF, de Wit R, Berry WR, et al. Docetaxel plus prednisone or mitoxantrone plus prednisone for advanced prostate cancer. N Engl J Med 2004;351(15):1502–12.
274. Petrylak DP, Tangen CM, Hussain MH, et al. Docetaxel and estramustine compared with mitoxantrone and prednisone for advanced refractory prostate cancer. N Engl J Med 2004;351(15):1513–20.
275. Hudes GR, Nathan F, Khater C, et al. Phase II trial of 96-hour paclitaxel plus oral estramustine phosphate in metastatic hormone-refractory prostate cancer. J Clin Oncol 1997;15(9):3156–63.
276. Kelly WK, Curley T, Slovin S, et al. Paclitaxel, estramustine phosphate, and carboplatin in patients with advanced prostate cancer. J Clin Oncol 2001;19(1):44–53.
277. Berry WR, Hathorn JW, Dakhil SR, et al. Phase II randomized trial of weekly paclitaxel with or without estramustine phosphate in progressive, metastatic, hormone-refractory prostate cancer. Clin Prostate Cancer 2004;3(2):104–11.
278. Kelly WK, Galsky MD, Small E, et al. Multi-institutional trial of the epothilone B analogue BMS-247550 with ot without estramustine phosphate (EMP) in patients with progressive castrate-metastatic prostate cancer. J Clin Oncol 2004;22(14S):4509.
279. Raghavan D, Cox K, Pearson BS, et al. Oral cyclophosphamide for the management of hormone-refractory prostate cancer. Br J Urol 1993;72(5 Pt 1):625–8.
280. Smith DC, Esper P, Strawderman M, et al. Phase II trial of oral estramustine, oral etoposide, and intravenous paclitaxel in hormone-refractory prostate cancer. J Clin Oncol 1999;17(6):1664–71.
281. Nielsen OS, Munro AJ, Tannock IF. Bone metastases: pathophysiology and management policy. J Clin Oncol 1991;9(3):509–24.
282. Price P, Hoskin PJ, Easton D, et al. Prospective randomised trial of single and multifraction radiotherapy schedules in the treatment of painful bony metastases. Radiother Oncol 1986;6(4):247–55.
283. Poulter CA, Cosmatos D, Rubin P, et al. A report of RTOG 8206: a phase III study of whether the addition of single dose hemibody irradiation to standard fractionated local field irradiation is more effective than local field irradiation alone in the treatment of symptomatic osseous metastases. Int J Radiat Oncol Biol Phys 1992;23(1):207–14.
284. Robinson RG, Preston DF, Schiefelbein M, Baxter KG. Strontium 89 therapy for the palliation of pain due to osseous metastases. JAMA 1995;274(5):420–4.
285. Porter AT, McEwan AJ, Powe JE, et al. Results of a randomized phase-III trial to evaluate the efficacy of strontium-89 adjuvant to local field external beam irradiation in the management of endocrine resistant metastatic prostate cancer. Int J Radiat Oncol Biol Phys 1993;25(5):805–13.
286. Akerley W, Butera J, Wehbe T, et al. A multiinstitutional, concurrent chemoradiation trial of strontium-89, estramustine, and vinblastine for hormone refractory prostate carcinoma involving bone. Cancer 2002;94(6):1654–60.
287. Sciuto R, Festa A, Rea S, et al. Effects of low-dose cisplatin on 89Sr therapy for painful bone metastases from prostate cancer: a randomized clinical trial. J Nucl Med 2002;43(1):79–86.
288. Tu SM, Millikan RE, Mengistu B, et al. Bone-targeted therapy for advanced androgen-independent carcinoma of the prostate: a randomised phase II trial. Lancet 2001;357(9253):336–41.
289. Serafini AN, Houston SJ, Resche I, et al. Palliation of pain associated with metastatic bone cancer using samarium-153 lexidronam: a double-blind placebo-controlled clinical trial. J Clin Oncol 1998;16(4):1574–81.
290. Palmedo H, Manka-Waluch A, Albers P, et al. Repeated bone-targeted therapy for hormone-refractory prostate carcinoma: randomized phase II trial with the new, high-energy radiopharmaceutical rhenium-188 hydroxyethylidene-diphosphonate. J Clin Oncol 2003;21(15):2869–75.
291. Lee MV, Fong EM, Singer FR, Guenette RS. Bisphosphonate treatment inhibits the growth of prostate cancer cells. Cancer Res 2001;61(6):2602–8.
292. Saad F, Gleason DM, Murray R, et al. A randomized, placebo-controlled trial of zoledronic acid in patients with hormone-refractory metastatic prostate carcinoma. J Natl Cancer Inst 2002;94(19):1458–68.
293. Small EJ, Smith MR, Seaman JJ, et al. Combined analysis of two multicenter, randomized, placebo-controlled studies of pamidronate disodium for the palliation of bone pain in men with metastatic prostate cancer. J Clin Oncol 2003;21(23):4277–84.
294. Ernst DS, Tannock IF, Winquist EW, et al. Randomized, double-blind, controlled trial of mitoxantrone/prednisone and clodronate versus mitoxantrone/prednisone and placebo in patients with hormone-refractory prostate cancer and pain. J Clin Oncol 2003;21(17):3335–42.
295. George DJ, Kantoff PW. Prognostic indicators in hormone refractory prostate cancer. Urol Clin North Am 1999;26(2):303–10, viii.
296. Halabi S, Small EJ, Kantoff PW, et al. Prognostic model for predicting survival in men with hormone-refractory metastatic prostate cancer. J Clin Oncol 2003;21:1232–7.
297. Smaletz O, Scher HI, Small EJ, et al. Nomogram for overall survival of patients with progressive metastatic prostate cancer after castration. J Clin Oncol 2002;20(19):3972–82.
298. Smith MR, Kantoff PW. Peroxisome proliferator-activated receptor gamma (PPargamma) as a novel target for prostate cancer. Invest New Drugs 2002;20(2):195–200.
299. Smith MR, Manola J, Kaufman DS, et al. Rosiglitazone versus placebo for men with prostate carcinoma and a rising serum prostate-specific antigen level after radical prostatectomy and/or radiation therapy. Cancer 2004;101(7):1569–74.
300. Beer TM, Lemmon D, Lowe BA, Henner WD. High-dose weekly oral calcitriol in patients with a rising PSA after prostatectomy or radiation for prostate carcinoma. Cancer 2003;97(5):1217–24.
301. Beer TM, Eilers KM, Garzotto M, et al. Weekly high-dose calcitriol and docetaxel in metastatic androgen-independent prostate cancer. J Clin Oncol 2003;21(1):123–8.
302. Signoretti S, Montironi R, Manola J, et al. Her-2-neu expression and progression toward androgen indepen-

dence in human prostate cancer. J Natl Cancer Inst 2000;92(23):1918–25.
303. Craft N, Shostak Y, Carey M, Sawyers CL. A mechanism for hormone-independent prostate cancer through modulation of androgen receptor signaling by the HER-2/neu tyrosine kinase. Nat Med 1999;5(3):280–5.
304. Carducci MA, Padley RJ, Breul J, et al. Effect of endothelin-A receptor blockade with atrasentan on tumor progression in men with hormone-refractory prostate cancer: a randomized, phase II, placebo-controlled trial. J Clin Oncol 2003;21(4):679–89.
305. Murphy GP, Tjoa BA, Simmons SJ, et al. Phase II prostate cancer vaccine trial: report of a study involving 37 patients with disease recurrence following primary treatment. Prostate 1999;39(1):54–9.
306. Simons JW, Mikhak B, Chang JF, et al. Induction of immunity to prostate cancer antigens: results of a clinical trial of vaccination with irradiated autologous prostate tumor cells engineered to secrete granulocyte-macrophage colony-stimulating factor using ex vivo gene transfer. Cancer Res 1999;59(20):5160–8.
307. Folkman J. Tumor angiogenesis: therapeutic implications. N Engl J Med 1971;285(21):1182–6.
308. Ferrer FA, Miller LJ, Andrawis RI, et al. Angiogenesis and prostate cancer: in vivo and in vitro expression of angiogenesis factors by prostate cancer cells. Urology 1998;51(1):161–7.
309. Duque JL, Loughlin KR, Adam RM, et al. Plasma levels of vascular endothelial growth factor are increased in patients with metastatic prostate cancer. Urology 1999;54(3):523–7.
310. Fortier AH, Nelson BJ, Grella DK, Holaday JW. Antiangiogenic activity of prostate-specific antigen. J Natl Cancer Inst 1999;91(19):1635–40.
311. Nelson WG, De Marzo AM, Isaacs WB. Prostate cancer. N Engl J Med 2003:349:366–81.
312. Clark PE, Levin H, Kupelian P. Intermediate-term outcome with radical prostatectomy for localized prostate cancer. The Prostate Journal 2001;3:118.
313. Partin AW, Mangold LA, Lamm DM, et al. Contemporary update of prostate cancer staging nomograms (Partin Tables) for the new millennium. Urology 2001;58(6):843–8.
314. D'Amico AV, Whittington R, Malkowicz SB, et al. Clinical utility of the percentage of positive prostate biopsies in defining biochemical outcome after radical prostatectomy for patients with clinically localized prostate cancer. J Clin Oncol 2000;18(6):1164–72.

Tumors of the Penis and Urethra

Donald F. Lynch Jr, MD

Cancer of the penis is an unusual disease in the United States and Europe, but is a major health problem in parts of South America, Africa, and Asia. Incidence of squamous carcinoma of the penis, by far the most common penile cancer, ranges from 0.4 percent of male genital cancers in the United States to as high as 20–22 percent in China and Uganda. Other cancers involving the penis are epidemic Kaposi's sarcoma, verrucous carcinoma, and transitional cell carcinoma.[1]

Urethral cancer is quite rare, with some 600 reported cases in males and some 1,600 cases in females. It is the only genitourinary malignancy which occurs more frequently in women than in men. Squamous cell carcinoma predominates in both males and females, with transitional cell carcinoma and adenocarcinoma encountered less commonly.

CANCER OF THE PENIS

Histopathology Over 95 percent of penile cancers are squamous cell carcinomas. Verrucous carcinoma, known alternatively as giant condyloma or Buschke-Löwenstein tumor, is a variant of squamous carcinoma which does not metastasize, but which spreads aggressively by local extension and destroys surrounding tissues. Epidemic Kaposi's sarcoma, associated with adult immunodeficiency syndrome (AIDS), is being increasingly encountered. Some 20 percent of male patients with AIDS may be expected to manifest a penile lesion in the course of the disease.[2] Melanoma, sarcoma, and basal cell carcinoma involve the penis infrequently but have been reported.

Bowen's disease is intraepithelial squamous carcinoma-in-situ and is called that when it involves the base of the penis and the scrotum. When it involves the glans penis or prepuce, it is known as erythroplasia of Queyrat. These lesions have the potential to develop into invasive squamous carcinoma.

Paget's disease of the penis is quite rare, but may develop primarily or as the result of an underlying adenocarcinoma of the urethra or periurethral glands. Balanitis xerotica obliterans, leukoplakia, and penile cutaneous horn may occasionally develop into squamous carcinoma. Bowenoid papulosis, a reddish raised lesion resembling erythroplasia of Queyrat but with a benign course may be difficult to distinguish from more problematic lesions. Biopsy is required to establish a diagnosis.

EPIDEMIOLOGY AND ETIOLOGY

In countries where infant circumcision is common, such as Israel and the United States, the incidence of squamous carcinoma of the penis is low. Circumcision later in life does not seem to confer protection.[3] It has been thought that chronic exposure to smegma, a substance secreted by Tyson's glands in the prepuce, might be one mechanism promoting the development of squamous penile cancers. In the uncircumcised penis, proper hygiene may be made more difficult by phimosis, perpetuating chronic inflammation of the glans and preputial tissues. In more developed countries with improved socioeconomic conditions, the incidence of penile cancer has fallen and the stage at presentation has also decreased, suggesting that a combination of improved education coupled with more attentive hygiene has reduced the incidence and severity of the disease.[4]

An association between cervical cancer in women whose spouses have penile cancer has been observed, and there is evidence to suggest that patients infected with human papillomavirus (HPV) types 16, 18, 31, and 33 may have a predisposition to develop squamous carcinoma in both the penis and the cervix.[5,6] Men may develop condyloma accuminata from this infection, may be totally asymptomatic carriers, or may harbor intraurethral lesions—unknown to the patient—which may shed the virus and expose a sexual partner.

Several large studies have shown that smoking is associated with an increased incidence of squamous carcinoma of the penis. Recent studies linking smoking to high-grade lesions of the cervix and vulva suggest an association between HPV, smoking, and cancer, which may also pertain in squamous carcinoma of the penis.[7,8]

Carcinoma-in-Situ Erythroplasia of Queyrat is characterized by a shiny, erythematous maculopapular patch which is slightly raised, velvety in appearance, and typically involves the glans or prepuce. Bowen's disease appears scaly and red, is clearly demarcated, and often involves the scrotum and base of the penis. Histologically, these lesions demonstrate dyskeratosis, vacuolization, and large nuclei with numerous atypical mitotic figures. The full thickness of the epithelium is involved. Clinically, erythroplasia of Queyrat and Bowen's disease are the same disease, with a 10 to 20 percent association with progression to squamous carcinoma of the penis.[9]

Invasive Squamous Carcinoma Early invasive tumors may be small and largely unremarkable, sometimes resembling small abrasions or callused thickenings of penile skin. The initial lesion of squamous carcinoma most commonly presents on the glans or prepuce. It varies from a small, velvety, reddened, raised maculopapule to an ulcer, hyperkeratotic area, or exophytic papillary tumor. Biopsy is required to make the diagnosis, and should include contiguous normal skin for comparison.

More advanced lesions may be exophytic or ulcerated, and very advanced cancers may completely destroy the penile shaft. Metastases to the inguinal lymph nodes may produce large ulcerations in the groins late in the course of the disease. Well-differentiated tumors tend to metastasize infrequently, whereas more poorly differentiated tumors have a high propensity for early metastasis. Several studies have confirmed that higher tumor grade increases the likelihood of inguinal nodal metastases.[10–12]

Verrucous Carcinoma Verrucous carcinoma, or Buschke-Löwenstein tumor of the penis, comprises about 5 percent of all penile cancers and represents a special variant of squamous carcinoma. It is well differentiated and does not metastasize, but spreads aggressively by local extension and may destroy penile tissues entirely if left untreated. These lesions are often associated with HPV types 6 and 11.[13,14]

Other Malignancies Rarely, transitional cell carcinomas of the bladder or urethra may extend to the glans and prepuce. Basal cell carcinoma, melanoma, and primary sarcomas are quite rare.[1] Kaposi's sarcoma, usually the epidemic or AIDS-associated variety, is becoming an increasingly common problem. Local symptomatic management is recommended, although with large tumors surgical intervention may be required. Infiltration of the penile structures with lymphoma or leukemia usually presents as priapism. A thorough search for systemic disease is always indicated. Treatment is with systemic chemotherapy.

Natural History and Course Squamous carcinoma of the penis usually presents as a sore or ulcer of the glans, coronal sulcus, or prepuce. In the uncircumcised male, induration or swelling of the distal penis suggests tumor. Biopsy of the lesion following dorsal slit or circumcision confirms the diagnosis.

Erythroplasia of Queyrat, verrucous carcinoma, and various hyperkeratotic lesions may evolve into squamous carcinoma or may coexist with it. Prompt treatment of these lesions is indicated.

Invasive squamous carcinoma of the penis follows a predictable pattern of metastasis. Lesions of the glans, coronal sulcus, prepuce, and distal shaft spread to the deep inguinal nodes, whereas lesions of the proximal shaft and base of the penis spread to the more lateral and superficial inguinal nodes. Subsequent spread to the external iliac, obturator, and iliac chains follows. Although "skip" metastases to the pelvic nodes have been reported, re-evaluation of old reports and more recent series suggest that pelvic metastases in the absence of inguinal metastases probably do not occur.[15,16] Metastases to distant sites are infrequent and occur late in the course of the disease.

Because primary lesions may be infected or chronically inflamed, secondary inflammation of the inguinal nodes is often present which may be impossible to distinguish from metastatic disease. Careful re-examination of the inguinal nodes following a 4- to 6-week course of broad-spectrum antibiotic therapy may help to differentiate inflammation from cancer.

Tumor Staging Once the diagnosis of squamous carcinoma is established, complete staging is undertaken. Careful palpation of the inguinal nodes is carried out. Additional staging studies should include chest radiography, computed tomography (CT) of the pelvis and inguinal regions, and possibly magnetic resonance scanning (MRI). When patients are obese or when the groins have been subjected to prior surgery, CT or MRI may be superior to palpation in detecting suspicious nodal enlargement. CT and MRI have supplanted lymphangiography as a staging procedure.

The American Joint Committee on Cancer (AJCC) TNM (Tumor, Nodes, Metastases) system of 1997 is the accepted staging system for penile cancer (Table 98-1).[17] The older Jackson system, which is clinically based, is no longer used, but is frequently mentioned in older literature (Table 98-2).[18]

Table 98-1 AJCC (1997) Staging of Penile Cancer [17]

Tumor (T)	
Tx	Primary tumor cannot be assessed
T0	No evidence of cancer
Tis	Carcinoma-in-situ
Ta	Non-invasive verrucous carcinoma
T1	Tumor invades subepithelial connective tissue
T2	Tumor invades corpus spongiosum or cavernosum
T3	Tumor invades urethra or prostate
T4	Tumor invades other adjacent structures
Nodes (N)	
Nx	Regional lymph nodes cannot be assessed
N0	No regional node metastasis
N1	Metastasis to a single, superficial inguinal lymph node
N2	Metastasis in multiple or bilateral superficial inguinal lymph nodes
N3	Metastasis in deep inguinal or pelvic lymph nodes, unilateral or bilateral
Metastasis (M)	
Mx	Presence of distant metastasis cannot be assessed
M0	No distant metastasis
M1	Distant metastasis

Surgical Treatment Treatment of penile cancer is based on the extent of the primary tumor and its tumor grade, established by biopsy of the lesion. Antibiotic therapy is begun prior to biopsy, continued through surgical therapy, and continued for 4 to 6 weeks afterwards. Once the tissue diagnosis is confirmed, small superficial tumors may be successfully treated with local surgical excision, topical chemotherapy, laser surgery, Mohs' micrographic surgery, or superficial radiation therapy.[18–21]

Larger tumors with invasion may sometimes be managed with organ-sparing surgery or radiotherapy, but deeply invasive cancers, particularly those which deform the glans or involve the shaft structures, may not be amenable to conservative measures.

Lesions which involve the distal shaft or glans are usually managed by partial penectomy, providing that a 2 cm margin can be achieved while leaving sufficient penile length to allow the patient to void while standing and to engage in intercourse. More advanced lesions or tumors which involve the base of the penis are best managed by total penectomy with creation of a perineal urethrostomy.[1,22] More extensive lesions, or those involving the base and bulbar urethral portion of the penis, may require cystoprostatectomy or occasionally anterior or total pelvic exenteration with urinary diversion.

Management of the Regional Lymph Nodes Proper management of the inguinal and pelvic lymph nodes in patients with squamous carcinoma of the penis has been one of the most challenging and controversial aspects of penile cancer treatment. Lymphatic drainage of the penile shaft and base is to the superficial inguinal lymph nodes. Drainage from the glans, prepuce, and distal shaft is to the deep inguinal nodes. There is crossover of the lymphatic channels at the base of the penis so that a lesion on one side of the penis may metastasize to the contralateral inguinal nodes. The deep inguinal nodes drain to the external iliac and obturator chains, and subsequently to the common iliac nodes and the retroperitoneal nodes surrounding the aorta and inferior vena cava.

Several clinical studies have shown that in patients with inguinal metastases a meticulous inguinal node dissection will be curative in 40 to 60 percent of cases.[2,17,23] However, the traditional node dissection carries with it a high likelihood of morbidity—flap necrosis, wound infection, chronic lymphangitis, lymphocoele, and chronic lower limb edema. A modified, somewhat less extensive dissection has been adopted by most surgeons which has reduced some of the unpleasant sequelae of groin dissection.[24] Nonetheless, an inguinal node dissection is not to be undertaken lightly, and the indications for a groin dissection in patients with no palpable inguinal nodes are not clear. While some 25 percent of patients with impalpable nodes will have metastatic disease and must undergo a node dissection, others with no metastases, may undergo needless surgery. Determining which patients should have inguinal lymphadenectomy and which may be followed expectantly continues to be a major challenge in the management of this disease. Those patients with metastases to the groins who do not undergo appropriate node dissection will usually die of their disease within 3 years.

Table 98-2 Jackson Staging System for Penile Cancer[62]

I	Tumor confined to glans or prepuce
II	Invasion into shaft or corpora; no nodal or distant metastasis
III	Tumor confined to penis; operable inguinal nodal metastasis
IV	Tumor involves adjacent structures; inoperable inguinal nodes and/or distant metastasis

Clinical staging of the inguinal nodes is highly inaccurate. Several studies have demonstrated that microscopic metastases may be present in impalpable nodes, whereas palpably enlarged nodes are benign half of the time.[21,25–27] Staging techniques using lymphangiography with aspiration of the nodes have proven to be unsatisfactory. The sentinel node biopsy, proposed by Cabanas and colleagues, although initially encouraging, has also proven to be unreliable and has been abandoned.[15,28,29] Patients with negative sentinel nodes have developed inguinal metastases after negative bilateral sentinel node biopsies.[26,28]

TUMOR GRADE

Recent studies have confirmed the importance of tumor grade as well as stage in assessing the risk of nodal metastases, and have helped clarify when node dissection should be performed. Patients with grade I tumors which are limited to the skin and superficial tissues of the penis are unlikely to have tumor spread to inguinal nodes. Patients with grade II or grade III lesions with any degree of invasion of the deeper penile structures have been shown to be at significant risk of groin metastases.[10–12] Although for many years, patients with clinically negative inguinal nodes were followed expectantly and subjected to inguinal node dissection only if palpable node metastases developed, contemporary investigators recommend early surgery if high-grade tumor (grade II or III) and more than superficial invasion is documented on biopsy. At the Eastern

Virginia Medical School, patients are treated with 4 to 6 weeks of broad-spectrum antibiotic therapy. We then perform a modified bilateral inguinal node dissection on any patient with palpably enlarged inguinal nodes, and on patients with impalpable nodes who demonstrate invasion into the penile shaft or show grade II or grade III histopathology on their biopsy.

PELVIC LYMPHADENECTOMY

Patients found to have inguinal node metastases should undergo pelvic lymphadenectomy on the affected side. This can be done extraperitoneally via a midline incision or through a modified Gibson or groin incision. At our institution, pelvic lymphadenectomy is done at the same time inguinal node dissection is performed, although at some centers the procedure is staged several weeks later.[1] Patients found to have fewer than 3 pelvic nodes with metastases, with all nodes below the bifurcation of the internal and external iliac vessels, often will fare well. Metastases above the bifurcation have been almost uniformly lethal.[30,31]

RADIOTHERAPY

Primary radiotherapy of penile cancer is used more widely in Europe than in the United States, but may be appropriate in small, superficial lesions or in selected larger lesions when organ preservation is the goal or when patients refuse surgery.[32–35] In more advanced lesions, however, tissue preservation may not be feasible. Concurrent chemotherapy may enhance the effectiveness of radiation.[36]

Radiotherapy may be administered as teletherapy using cobalt or linear accelerators, or as brachytherapy, with a mold or with Iridium^{192} wires. Iridium^{192} or Cesium^{137} may be used to boost dosages in bulky or extremely cornified tumors. Normally doses of 30 to 50 Gy given over 3 to 5 weeks are used. Boosts to 65 to 70 Gy using various brachytherapy techniques may follow if clinically indicated. Radiation is often the treatment of choice in symptomatic lesions resulting from epidemic (AIDS-related) Kaposi's sarcoma.[37]

Acute radiation reactions—edema and tissue inflammation, with concomitant skin irritation, tenderness, and dysuria—are common accompaniments of both external radiation and brachytherapy. Such symptoms usually subside promptly once therapy is completed. Long-term effects of treatment may include telangiectasia, hyperpigmentation, diminished sensation, scarring, and atrophy of the treated tissues. Fibrotic change and fistulization may occur in large lesions where significant tissue damage has occurred prior to radiotherapy. Late recurrences in radiated sites may occur up to a decade following definitive treatment, affirming that close follow-up is essential.[33]

Radiation of clinically negative groins as a prophylactic measure is controversial as is adjuvant radiation to the groins following inguinal surgery. Although some studies have suggested benefit from such treatment, others show no improvement when compared with studies in which patients are treated with surgery alone.[38,39]

CHEMOTHERAPY

Chemotherapy is used in treating penile cancer as an adjuvant to definitive surgical or radiation therapy or occasionally as a radiopotentiator. Experience with various treatment protocols is limited by the relative rarity of the disease. Multidrug combination chemotherapy programs have shown promise at several institutions. Pizzocaro and Piva of the Milan National Tumor Institute have used combination chemotherapy with vincristine, bleomycin, and methotrexate (VBM) and have been successful at rendering patients with fixed nodal metastases resectable.[40] Dexeus and associates from MD Anderson Cancer Center have used diamino, dichloro, cis-platinum (DDCP)-based chemotherapy as adjuvant therapy following surgery.[41] Similarly, a recently completed multi-institutional Southwest Oncology Group trial using methotrexate, DDCP, and bleomycin to treat advanced, unresectable inguinal metastatic disease demonstrated a 32.5 percent response rate, although toxicity was high.[42] Several combination chemotherapy protocols which have shown effectiveness in treating squamous carcinoma of other sites—anus, esophagus, head, and neck—remain to be tested in squamous carcinoma of the penis. Multi-institutional, multinational trials will be required to enroll sufficient numbers of patients to provide meaningful data.

PROGNOSIS

Left untreated, squamous carcinoma of the penis is invariably lethal, killing most of those afflicted within 3 years. Outcome is directly related to the extent of the disease at diagnosis, and the presence or absence of inguinal metastases.[4,26,27,30]

The National Surveillance, Epidemiology, and End Results (SEER) database (1973–1987; 1,101 patients) shows a relative survival rate of 95 percent for patients with carcinoma-in-situ and 70 percent for all stages. Relative survival for localized tumor was 80 per cent, with survival rates of 52 percent for regional (nodal) disease and 18 percent for distant disease. Horenblas and associates reported 93 percent 5-year survival when nodes were negative versus 50 percent in patients with clinically positive nodes.[39] Srinivas and associates reported a crude 5-year survival rate of 28 percent in patients with proven inguinal metastases. Patients with minimal nodal disease (N1, N2) had 5-year survivals of 50 to 80 percent, whereas those with N3 and N4 disease had a much graver outcome, with survivals of 4 to 12 percent. Patients with no inguinal node metastases had a 74 percent 5-year survival.[30,31] The outcome of patients with pelvic metastases has been very poor.

CONCLUSIONS

Squamous carcinoma of the penis is a preventable disease, and, in fact, incidence has fallen over the past two decades with improved socioeconomic conditions, attention to hygiene, and access to health care. Better understanding of the importance of tumor histology and a more aggressive approach to inguinal disease may provide further improvements in survival. Refinements in surgical and radiotherapeutic techniques have further improved outcome and quality of life. Early recognition of tumor lesions has allowed for effective but less extensive treatment and improvements in organ-sparing procedures.

Further research into combined modality therapies using chemotherapy in conjunction with surgery, radiation therapy, or both, will likely further improve treatment results. Improved understanding of the role of possible causative agents (HPVs and HHVs) should improve both treatment and prevention.

CARCINOMA OF THE URETHRA

Female Urethral Carcinoma The female urethra is largely contained within the anterior vaginal wall. In an adult it is 2 to 4 cm in length. Distally, it is lined with stratified squamous epithelium, changing to stratified or pseudostratified columnar epithelium more proximally. At the bladder neck the mucosa is transitional cell epithelium.

The histopathology of female urethral cancer depends on the tissue of origin. Squamous carcinoma is the most common, comprising about 50 percent of all tumors. Transitional cell carcinoma and adenocarcinoma are next most common and occur with roughly equal frequency.[42] Unlike penile cancers, tumor grade does not appear to influence either propensity for metastasis or prognosis. Female urethral cancers occur more often in white women than in black.[44] Mixed tumors, undifferentiated carcinomas, melanoma, cloacogenic carcinoma, and clear-cell adenocarcinoma have also been reported.[45,46]

Urethral cancers spread first by local extension, and later metastasize via lymphatic channels and bloodborne routes. The lymphatic drainage of the distal urethra and labia is to the superficial and deep inguinal nodes. The proximal urethra drains to the nodes of the iliac, obturator, presacral, and para-aortic lymphatic chains. Palpably abnormal lymph nodes are present in 20 to 50 percent of patients at presentation and almost always represent metastatic cancer. Metastases to distant sites—liver, lung, brain, and bone—occur late and are more common with adenocarcinomas.[43,46,47]

Staging The AJCC/UICC TNM staging system (1997) for urethral carcinoma is shown in Table 98-3.[48] One system is now used for both male and female patients. Older literature commonly refers to tumors involving the distal third of the urethra as "anterior" or "distal" lesions, whereas those involving the proximal two thirds are described as "posterior" or "proximal" tumors.[44,45] These designations are useful in predicting the clinical behavior of urethral cancers and are still often used. Roughly half of tumors involve the entire length of urethra at diagnosis.

A rare variation of urethral cancer is carcinoma arising in a urethral diverticulum. These tumors are usually squamous carcinomas and are usually located in the distal two thirds of the urethra. They have been reported more frequently in black women than in white and likely arise from remnants of wolffian or müllerian ducts or ectopic cloacal epithelium.[49,50]

Surgical Management In the female, most tumors present with bleeding or distal urethral mass. Distal urethral or "anterior" lesions usually present early and are diagnosed while at low stage. These tumors have been successfully managed with local excision, transurethral resection, partial urethrectomy, and fulguration or ablation with either neodymium:yttrium-aluminum-garnet (YAG) or CO_2 laser techniques.[51–53] In rare instances, higher stage local lesions may be managed with total urethrectomy and preservation of the bladder with interposition of a catheterizable segment or with the Mitrofanoff procedure.

More proximal lesions present later and at higher stage than distal lesions. Progressive obstructive symptoms are the hallmark of proximal or "posterior" urethral lesions. For superficial tumors, transurethral resection or laser surgery may be appropriate.[54–56] Advanced or extensive lesions, and those which involve the bladder or vagina, may necessitate cystectomy or anterior exenteration with urinary diversion.[44] Local recurrence in such high stage disease occurs frequently.

In advanced disease, metastases to the lymph nodes are present in 50 percent of cases. Inguinal node dissection should be performed in the presence of palpably enlarged nodes, and pelvic node dissection should be performed when proximal involvement of the urethra is identified. There does not appear to be any therapeutic advantage to prophylactic node dissection when the inguinal nodes are not enlarged.

Radiation Therapy Radiation therapy, administered as both external beam radiation and brachytherapy, has been used for definitive treatment of both localized and advanced tumors. It has also been used to downsize tumors before definitive surgical intervention. Results have been mixed: 5-year survivals averaging about 35 percent in advanced disease.[44,49,54] Side effects and complications, including edema, fistulae, and damage to the bowel, are commonplace.

Chemotherapy and Combined Therapy The rarity of these tumors has precluded much meaningful clinical research in chemotherapeutic treatment, or in chemotherapy combined with radiation or surgery. Combination chemotherapy in conjunction with radiation and surgery has produced promising outcomes in squamous carcinomas of the head and neck, anus, and penis, and may be expected to demonstrate similar benefit in squamous cancers of the urethra.[53,55] However, multinational, multi-institutional trials will be required to provide clinical data to assess the efficacy of any such treatment regimens.

Table 98-3 AJCC (1997) Staging System for Male and Female Carcinoma of the Urethra[47]

Tumor (T)	
Tx	Tumor cannot be assessed
T0	No evidence of primary tumor
Tis	Carcinoma-in-situ
Ta	Non-invasive papillary, polypoid, or verrucous carcinoma
T1	Invades subepithelial connective tissue
T2	Invades any of the following: prostatic stroma, corpus spongiosum, or periurethral musculature
T3	Invades any of the following: corpus cavernosum, beyond prostatic capsule, anterior vagina, or bladder neck (extraprostatic extension)
T4	Invades other adjacent organs [Transitional cell carcinoma of the prostate (prostatic urethra)]
Tis pu	CIS, involvement of prostatic urethra
Tis pd	CIS, involvement of prostatic ducts
T1	Invades subepithelial connective tissue
T2	Invades prostatic stroma, corpus spongiosum, or periurethral musculature
T3	Invades corpus cavernosum, beyond prostatic capsule, or bladder neck (extraprostatic extension)
T4	Invades other adjacent organs (invasion of bladder)
Nodes (N)	
Nx	Regional lymph nodes cannot be assessed
N0	No regional lymph node metastasis
N1	Metastasis to a single lymph node ≤ 2 cm
N2	Metastasis to a single node > 2 cm
Metastasis (M)	
Mx	Metastasis cannot be assessed
M0	No distant metastasis
M1	Distant metastasis

Prognosis Long term survival is related to the stage of the tumor at the time of diagnosis and appears to be independent of tumor histology or grade. Bracken and associates, in one of the few large series, reported an overall 5-year survival of 32 percent in 81 patients.[44] Patients having tumors less than 2 cm in diameter did significantly better than those with tumors larger than 5 cm diameter. Patients having tumors of the anterior or distal urethra have better survival than those with more proximal lesions, apparently because their tumors present earlier in their clinical course. Patients having tumors involving the entire urethra fare the worst, with 5-year survival of only 11 percent. Tumor recurrence rates of 66 to 100 percent have been noted.

MALE URETHRAL CARCINOMA

The male urethra averages some 18 cm in length, and is subdivided into the penile urethra, the membranous urethra, and the prostatic urethra. Beginning distally, the penile urethra is composed of the meatus and fossa navicularis which is lined with stratified squamous epithelium. The pendulous urethra extends from the proximal fossa navicularis to the suspensory ligament of the penis, where it then becomes the bulbar urethra between the ligament and the urogenital membrane. These areas are lined with stratified or pseudo stratified columnar epithelium, as is the short (1.5 cm) membranous urethra. This contains the external sphincter which is composed of striated muscle fibers. The prostatic urethra passes through the prostate and is lined with transitional cell epithelium.

Fifty to 75 percent of male urethral cancers arise in the bulbar urethra. The remainder occur predominantly in the fossa navicularis. Some 90 percent of male tumors demonstrate squamous cell carcinoma histology.[43,47,56] Often, there is an association with stricture of the urethra. Infrequently, transitional cell carcinoma or undifferentiated tumor may predominate at the bladder neck or within the prostatic urethra. Poorly differentiated transitional cell cancers may show some squamous characteristics. Rarely adenocarcinoma may arise in the glands of Littre or the prostatic utricle. Metastases from distant tumor sites to the penis also occur infrequently.

Obstructive symptoms are common in more proximal lesions, while urethral bleeding and palpation of a mass herald more distal lesions. In general, the more proximal a tumor, the later is its development and the higher its stage at diagnosis.

The urethral segment which is retained following cystectomy is a special case. Tumors which arise in this area are almost exclusively transitional cell carcinomas. The retained urethra must be monitored closely with urethroscopy and urethral washings as part of the follow-up of the patient who has had a cystectomy.[57,58] When the urethra is excised, either in conjunction with cystectomy or as a secondary procedure, the entire urethra, including the fossa navicularis, must be excised.

Lymphatic drainage of the distal male urethra is similar to that of penile tumors. Tumors of the fossa and pendulous urethra drain to the superficial inguinal lymph nodes, whereas tumors of the bulbar, membranous, and prostatic urethral segments drain to the iliac, obturator, and presacral node groups. There may be crossover at the prepubic lymphatic plexus.

Staging The AJCC/UICC Staging System for urethral carcinoma (1997) is shown in Table 98-3.[48] A special provision is now made for the staging of transitional cell carcinoma of the prostatic urethra and ducts. The terminology of distal or anterior tumors—those distal to the suspensory ligament—and proximal or posterior tumors—involving the bulbar, membranous, and prostatic segments—may be encountered.

Surgical Management Low-grade, low-stage tumors of the urethra may lend themselves to transurethral resection or laser fulguration, but such lesions are rare. Excisional biopsy may be feasible, and biopsy prior to laser fulguration is essential to assess histopathology and tumor depth.

Selected lesions of the distal urethra may lend themselves to partial penectomy. Tumors must not involve the corpus spongiosum or the corpora cavernosa, and must be amenable to a 2 cm margin. More advanced, or more proximal, lesions may require a total penectomy with creation of a perineal urethrostomy. Proximal cancers may necessitate an anterior exenteration with radical cystoprostatourethrectomy and urinary diversion.[59]

Inguinal and pelvic lymphadenopathy portends metastatic disease. Careful serial examinations of the groins, as well as interval pelvic CT evaluations, are essential in the follow-up of definitive treatment of a urethral primary. Inguinal node dissection should be performed in the presence of clinically positive groin nodes. This has been curative in many cases. In several small series, 5-year survival following inguinal node dissection ranged from 12 to 66 percent.[60,61] Pelvic node dissection has also proven curative in an occasional case and is worthwhile, although the prognosis in pelvic nodal disease is much poorer than with inguinal node dissection.[60] In the absence of inguinal adenopathy, inguinal lymphadenectomy is probably not warranted.

Radiation, Chemotherapy, Combined Therapy Experience with these modalities is limited, although some success in treating superficial, low-grade lesions with external beam radiotherapy in both males and females has been achieved.[54,55] Brachytherapy implants and molds have also been used.[32,55] Successful management of urethral cancer with partial urethrectomy and combination chemotherapy has also been reported.[62]

The infrequency with which these tumors are encountered has made it impossible to amass much experience with chemotherapy, but it might be anticipated that combination chemotherapy with drugs similar to those used in squamous carcinoma of other sites or with transitional cell carcinoma of the bladder and penis, may be similarly effective in urethral lesions of similar pathology. Again, the use of these treatment modalities as well as the employment of combined therapy programs will require large, international, multi-institutional studies to acquire data sufficient for meaningful interpretation.

SUMMARY

Cancers of both the male and the female urethra are quite rare, but the disease may be devastating if not recognized and treated as early as possible. Early surgical or radiotherapeutic intervention may cure these tumors. Advanced disease, at least for the present, carries a grim prognosis. Reliably effective programs of surgery or radiotherapy combined with chemotherapy have not yet been developed, although such programs—based on experience with tumors of similar histopathology in other systems—have the potential for improving outcome. With further refinements in treatment, and with increased availability of modern diagnostic techniques, combination chemotherapy, and worldwide communications and data transmission, there is hope that multinational, multi-institutional programs of treatment may provide effective therapy for those suffering from these cancers while expanding our effectiveness in managing them.

REFERENCES

1. Lynch DF, Pettaway CA . Tumors of the Penis. In: Walsh PC, Retik AB, Vaughan ED, Wein AJ (eds). Campbell's Urology, 8th ed, Philadelphia, WB Saunders Co, 2002. p. 2945–81.
2. D'Ancona CA, de Lucena RG, Querne FA, Martins MH, Denardi F, Netto NR Jr. Long-term followup of penile carcinoma treated with penectomy and bilateral modified inguinal lymphadenectomy. J Urol 2004; 174: 498–501.
3. Schmauz R, Jain DF. Geographical variation of carcinoma of the penis in Uganda. Br J Urol 1971;25:25–9.
4. Gilliland F, Key CR. Male genital cancer. Cancer 1995;75: 295–315.
5. Martinez I. Relationship of squamous cell carcinoma of the cervix uteri to squamous cell carcinoma of the penis among Puerto Rican women married to men with penile cancer. Cancer 1969;24:777–80.
6. Gross G, Pfister H. Role of human papillomavirus in penile cancer, penile intraepithelial squamous cell neoplasias and in genital warts. Med Microbiol Immunol (Berlin). 2004;193:35–44.
7. Moore TO, Moore AY, Carrasco D, et al. Human papillomavirus, smoking, and cancer. J Cutaneous Med Surg 2001;5:323–328.
8. Tsen HF, Morgenstern H, Mack T, et al. Risk factors for penile cancer: results of population-based case-control study in Los Angeles County (United States). Cancer Causes Control. 2001;12:267–77.
9. Schwartz RA. Squamous cell carcinoma. In: Skin Cancer – recognition and management. New York, Springer-Verlag; 1988. p. 174–5.
10. Fraley EE, Zhang G, Manivel C Niehans GA. The role of ilioinguinal lymphadenectomy and significance of histological differentiation in treatment of carcinoma of the penis. J Urol 1989;142:1478–82.
11. McDougal WS. Kirchner FK Jr, Edwards RH, Killion LT. Treatment of carcinoma of the penis: The case of primary lymphadenectomy. J Urol 1986;136:38–41.
12. Theodorescu D, Russo P, Zhang ZF. Outcomes of initial surveillance of invasive squamous cell carcinoma of the penis and negative nodes. J Urol 1996;155:1626–1631.
13. Sherman RN, Fung HK, Flynn KJ. Verrucous carcinoma (Buschke-Lowenstein tumor). Int J Dermatol 1991;30:730–733.
14. Boshart M, zur Hausen H. Human papillomavirus (HPV) in Buschke-Lowenstein tumors: Physical state of the DNA and identification of a tandem duplication in the non-coding region of a HPV-6 subtype. J Virol 1986;58:963.
15. Fowler JE. Sentinel node biopsy for staging of penile cancer. Urology 1984;23:352–3.
16. Ekstrom T, Edsmyr F. Cancer of the penis: A clinical study of 229 cases. Acta Chir Scand 1958;115:25–45.
17. Fleming ID, Cooper JS, Henson DE, et al (eds): Penis. In AJCC Cancer Staging Manual. American Joint Committee on Cancer, 5th ed. Philadelphia: Lippincott-Raven Publishers, 1997. p. 167–9.
18. Jackson SM: The treatment of carcinoma of the penis. Br J Surg 1966;53:33–35.
19. Hanash KA, Furlow WL, Utz DC, Harrison EG Jr. Carcinoma of the penis: A clinicopathologic study. J Urol 1970;104:291–7.
20. Mohs FE, Snow SN, Messing EM, Kuglitsch MG. Microscopically controlled surgery in the treatment of carcinoma of the penis. J Urol 1985;133:961–966.
21. Blastein LM, Finklestein LH. Laser surgery for treatment of squamous cell carcinoma of the penis. J Am Osteopathic Assoc 1990;90:338–42.
22. deKernion JB, Tynbery P, Persky L, Fegen JP. Carcinoma of the penis. Cancer 1973;32:1256–62.
23. Bevan-Thomas R, Slayton JW, Pettaway CA. Contemporary morbidity from lymphadenectomy for penile squamous cell carcinoma.: the MD Anderson experience. J Urol. 2002;167:1638–42.
24. Catalona WJ. Modified inguinal lymphadenectomy for carcinoma of the penis with preservation of saphenous veins: Technique and preliminary results. J Urol 1988;140:306–10.
25. Hardner GJ, Bhanalaph T, Murphy GP, et al. Carcinoma of the penis: Analysis of therapy in 100 consecutive cases. J Urol 1972;108:428–30.
26. Stancik I, Holtl W. Penile cancer: review of the recent literature. Curr Opin Urol 2003;13:467–72.
27. Ornellas AA, Correia AL, Marota A, Seixas ALC. Surgical treatment of invasive squamous cell carcinoma of the penis: Retrospective analysis of 350 cases. J Urol 1994;151:1244–1247.
28. Cabanas RM. An approach for the treatment of penile carcinoma. Cancer 1977;39:456–66.
29. Perinetti EP, Crane DB, Catalona WJ. Unreliability of sentinel node biopsy for staging penile cancer. J Urol 1980;124:734–5.
30. Srinivas V, Morse MJ, Herr HW, Sogani PC, Whitmore WF Jr. Penile cancer: Relation of extent of nodal metastasis to survival. J Urol 1987;137:880–2.
31. Lynch DF. Commentary on: Srinivas SV. Relation of extent of nodal metastasis to Survival. Sem Urol Oncol 15;1997:136–139.
32. Gerbaulet A, Lambin P. Radiation therapy of cancer of the penis. Urol Cl North Am 1992;19:325–332.
33. Pointon RCS. External beam therapy. Proc Soc Med 1975;68:682–93.
34. Kelley CD, Arthur K, Rogolf F, Grabstald H. Radiation therapy of penile cancer. Urology 1974;4:57–73.
35. Delannes M, Malavaud B, Douchez J, et al. Iridium[192] interstitial therapy for squamous cell carcinoma of the penis. Int J Rad Oncol Biol Phys 1992;24:479–483.
36. Culkin DJ, Beer TM. Advanced penile carcinoma. J Urol 2003;170:359–365.
37. Lebourgeois JP, Frikha H, Piedbos P, LePechoux C. Radiotherapy in the management of epidemic Kaposi's sarcoma of the oral cavity, eyelid, and the genitalia. Radiother Oncol 1994;30:263–266.
38. Ravi R. Correlation between the extent of nodal involvement and survival following groin dissection for carcinoma of the penis. Br J Urol 1993;72:817–819.
39. Horenblas S, Van Tinteren H. Squamous cell carcinoma of the penis IV: Prognostic factors of survival, analysis of tumor, nodes, and metastasis classification system. J Urol 1994;147:153–158.
40. Pizzocaro G, Piva L, Bandieramonte G, Tana S. Up-to-date management of carcinoma of the penis. Eur Urology 1997;32:5–15.
41. Dexeus FH, Logothetis CJ, Sella A, Amato R, Kilbourn R, Fitz K, Striegel A. Combination chemotherapy with methotrexate, bleomycin, and cisplatin for advanced squamous cell carcinoma of the male genital tract. J Urol 1991;146:1284–1287.
42. Haas GP, Blumenstein BA, Gaggiano RG et al. Cisplatin, methotrexate, and bleomycin for the treatment of carcinoma of the penis: A Southwest Oncology Group study. J Urol 1999;161:1823–1825.
43. Mostofi FK, Davis CJ Jr, Sesterhenn IA. Carcinoma of the male and female urethra. Urol Clin North Am 1992;19:347–358.
44. Bracken RB, Johnson DE, Miller LS, et al. Primary carcinoma of the female urethra. J Urol 1976;116:188–192.
45. Chu AM. Female urethral carcinoma. Radiology 1973;107: 627–630.
46. Narayan P, Konety B. Surgical treatment of female urethral carcinoma. Urol Clin North Am 1992;19:373–382.
47. Eng TY, Naguib M, Galang T, Fuller CD. Retrospective study of the treatment of urethral cancer. Am J Clin Oncol 2003;26:558–62.
48. Fleming ID, Cooper JS, Henson DE, et al (eds): Urethra. In AJCC Cancer Staging Manual. American Joint Committee on Cancer, 5th ed. Philadelphia: Lippincott-Raven Publishers, 1997. p. 191–40.
49. Tines SC, Bigongiari LR, Weigel JW. Carcinoma in diverticulum of female urethra. AJR 1982;138:582–4.
50. Tesluk H. Primary adenocarcinoma of the female urethra. Urology 1981;17:197–9.
51. Staeler C, Chaussy C, Jocham D, et al. The use of neodymium:YAG lasers in urology: Indication, technique, and critical assessment. J Urol 1985;134:1155–60.

52. Schaeffer AJ. Use of the CO_2 laser in urology. Urol Clin North Am 1986;13:393–404.
53. Dimarco DS, Dimarco CS, Zincke H, Webb MJ, Slezak JM. Surgical treatment for local control of female urethral carcinoma. Urol Oncol 2004;22:404–9.
54. Weghaupt K, Gerstner GJ, Kucera H. Radiation therapy for primary carcinoma of the female urethra: A survey of over 25 years. Gynecol Oncol 1984;17:58–64.
55. Dalbagni G, Donat SM, Eschwege P, Herr HW, Zelefsky MJ. Results of high dose rate brachytherapy, anterior pelvic exenteration, and external beam radiotherapy for carcinoma of the female urethra. Int J Urol 2001;166:1759–61.
56. Ray B, Canto AR, Whitmore WF Jr. Experience with primary carcinoma of the male urethra. J Urol 1977;117:591–594.
57. Schellhammer PF, Whitmore WJ Jr. Transitional cell carcinoma of the urethra in men having cystectomy for bladder cancer. J Urol 1976;115:56–60.
58. Varol C, Thalmann GN, Burkhard FC, Studer UE. Treatment of urethral recurrence following radical cystectomy and ileal bladder substitution. J Urol 2004;172:937–42.
59. Zeidman EJ, Desmond P, Thompson IM. Surgical treatment of carcinoma of the male urethra. Urol Clin North Am 1992;19:359–372.
60. Hoppman HJ, Fraley EE. Squamous cell carcinoma of the penis. J Urol 1978;120:393–398.
61. Marshall VF. Radical excision of locally extensive carcinoma of the deep male urethra. J Urol 1957;78;252–265.
62. Franke HJ, Froehner M, Wirth MP. The treatment of primary urethral carcinoma—the dilemmas of a rare condition: experience with partial urethrectomy and adjuvant chemotherapy. Onkologie 2001;24:48–52.

Testis Cancer

Craig R. Nichols, MD
Arthur Hung, MD
Christopher L. Corless, MD, PhD
Richard S. Foster, MD
Bruce J. Roth, MD
Lawrence H. Einhorn, MD

Cancer of the testis is a relatively uncommon disease, accounting for approximately 1% of all cancers in males. However, it is an important disease in the field of oncology, as it represents a highly curable neoplasm, and the incidence of which is focused on young patients at their peak of productivity. Curative treatment of disseminated nonseminomatous germ cell tumors often combines surgery and chemotherapy. The goal of initial therapy is never palliation nor prolongation of survival, but cure.[1]

EPIDEMIOLOGY

Incidence An age-related incidence curve of testicular cancer reveals a bimodal distribution. The major peak occurs between ages 15 and 35 years, owing almost exclusively to tumors of germ cell origin, which account for approximately 95% of all testicular cancer. Embryonal carcinoma represents the predominant histopathologic diagnosis up to the age of 35 years, after which seminoma is more common up to the age of 75 years. Overall, lymphoma is the most common testicular tumor in older adults.

The incidence of testicular cancer varies markedly based on geographic distribution. The incidence is highest in northern Europe and North America and lowest in Asia and Africa.

There is also a striking influence of race, with the incidence among black and Hispanic males worldwide far less than that for their white counterparts.[2,3] In the US, estimates of the incidence ratio between white and African-American patients ranges from 4 to 5:1 to 40:1.

Testicular cancer appears to be increasing among young white males in the Scandinavian countries, the United Kingdom, and the United States.[4] Age-standardized incidence rates increased annually 2 to 5%, with marginal differences between seminomas and nonseminomas. The trend may be attenuating in some countries, such as Denmark, and there appears to be large geographic differences in the changing incidence. It is estimated that 7,500 cases of testicular cancer were diagnosed in the United States in 2003, with approximately 400 persons dying of the disease.[5]

Risk Factors Cryptorchidism is the major identifiable risk factor associated with the development of testicular cancer, with a risk ratio variably reported between 2.5 and 14 in case-control studies.[6] The location of the maldescended testicle appears to be an important cofactor in the subsequent development of cancer, because those patients with intra-abdominal retention have a fourfold higher incidence of malignancy than those with the testicle retained in the inguinal canal. For a number of reasons, it seems unlikely that maldescent, in and of itself, represents the initiating event in the development of germ cell tumors: Only 10% of testicular tumors are associated with cryptorchidism, whereas 10 to 20% of the malignancies in patients with cryptorchidism occur in the contralateral, normally descended testicle; prepubertal orchiopexy fails to prevent the subsequent development of malignancy in the undescended testicle; and first-degree male relatives of patients with testicular cancer exhibit an increased incidence of cryptorchidism, hydroceles, and inguinal hernias, as well as testicular cancer.[7,8] These data suggest that some genetic predisposition and/or in utero environmental event may result in several genitourinary developmental abnormalities, including maldescent and germ cell neoplasia. Interestingly, an increase in the frequency of cryptorchidism has been observed and appears to parallel the timing and magnitude of the increase in incidence of testicular cancer.

Brothers of men with testicular germ cell tumors (TGCTs) have an 8- to 10-fold risk of developing TGCT, whereas the relative risk to fathers and sons is approximately fourfold. This familial relative risk is much higher than that for most other types of cancer. A genome-wide linkage search yielded evidence for a testicular cancer susceptibility gene on chromosome Xq27 that may also predispose to undescended testes.[9]

Testicular germ cell tumors occur at increased frequency in men with human immunodeficiency virus (HIV). One multicenter study addresses the characteristics of these tumors. Thirty-five patients with HIV-related germ cell tumors (GCTs) were identified. The median age at germ cell tumor diagnosis was 34 years (range, 27–64 years). The median CD4 cell count was 315/mm^3 (range, 90–960/mm^3) at this time. The histologic classification was seminoma in 26 patients (74%) and nonseminomatous germ cell tumor in 9 patients (26%). Twenty-one patients (60%) had stage I disease and 14 patients had metastatic disease. Overall, 6 patients relapsed, 3 died from germ cell tumor, and 7 died from HIV disease, resulting in a 2-year overall survival rate of 81%. HIV-related seminoma occurred more frequently than in the age- and sex-matched HIV-negative population, with a relative risk of 5.4 (95% confidence interval [CI] = 3.35–8.10); however, nonseminomatous germ cell tumor did not occur more frequently, and there was no change in the incidence of gem cell tumor since the introduction of highly active antiretroviral therapy. The conclusions of the authors were that testicular seminoma occurs significantly more frequently in HIV-positive men than in the matched control population. Patients with HIV-related GCTs present and should be treated in a similar manner to those in the HIV-negative population. Most of the mortality relates to HIV infection.[10]

An additional predisposition is the association of mediastinal nonseminomatous germ cell tumors with Klinefelter's syndrome. Approximately 10% of all patients with mediastinal nonseminoma have Klinefelter's syndrome, and there does not appear to be an increased incidence in patients with testicular or retroperitoneal primary tumors.[11]

An association of dysplastic nevus syndrome and testicular cancer has been observed.[12] A twofold higher incidence of multiple atypical nevi, and the attendant risk of melanoma, has been noted.

Patients with a history of unilateral testicular cancer are at risk of developing cancer in the other testicle. In a large Danish series, 2.7% of 2,338 patients developed a contralateral testicular tumor during the period of follow-up.[13–15] Investigators at the Royal Marsden Hospital reported a similar rate of 2.75% for developing contralateral tumors among 760 men in an interval as long as 15 years.[16]

In the United States, the largest series is reported from Memorial Sloan-Kettering. Between 1950 and 2001, 3,984 patients with testicular cancer were treated for germ cell tumor. A total of 58 patients with bilateral testicular germ cell tumors were identified. Median follow-up was 60 months. Ten of the 58 patients (17%) had synchronous tumors, while the other 48 (83%) had metachronous tumors. Overall, seminoma was the most common histology of the synchronous and metachronous tumors. Most patients in the synchronous and metachronous tumor groups presented with low-stage disease. Of the 58 patients, 52 (89%) had no evidence of disease, and 6 (11%) were dead of disease at the last follow-up. Treatment of the second tumor appeared to be influenced by therapy for the first tumor in 16.7% of cases.[17]

Although risk estimates for synchronous and metachronous contralateral testicular cancers vary widely, many clinicians recommend routine biopsy of the contralateral testis for patients diagnosed with unilateral testicular cancer. Fossa and colleagues evaluated the risk of contralateral testicular cancer and survival in a large population-based cohort of men diagnosed with testicular cancer before age 55 years using Surveillance, Epidemiology and End Results (SEER) data. From 29, 515 testicular cancer cases reported to the National Cancer Institute's SEER Program from 1973 through 2001, estimates of prevalence of synchronous contralateral testicular cancer, the observed-to-expected ratio (O/E) and 15-year cumulative risk of metachronous contralateral testicular cancer, and the 10-year overall survival rate of both synchronous and metachronous contralateral testicular cancer were made. A total of 175 men presented with synchronous contralateral testicular cancer; 287 men developed metachronous contralateral testicular cancer (O/E = 12.4 [95% CI[1] = 11.0–13.9%]; 15-year cumulative risk = 1.9% [95% CI = 1.7–2.1%]). In the multivariable analysis, only nonseminomatous histology of the first testicular cancer was associated with a statistically significantly decreased risk of metachronous contralateral testicular cancer (hazard ratio [HR] = 0.60; 95% CI = 0.46–0.79%; $p < .001$). Increasing age at first testicular cancer diagnosis was associated with decreasing risk of nonseminomatous metachronous contralateral testicular cancer (odds ratio = 0.90; 95% CI = 0.86–0.94%). The 10-year overall survival rate after metachronous contralateral testicular cancer diagnosis was 93% (95% CI = 88–96%), and that after synchronous contralateral testicular cancer was 85% (95% CI = 78–90%). The low cumulative risk of metachronous contralateral testicular cancer and favorable overall survival of patients diagnosed with metachronous contralateral testicular cancer is in accordance with the current US approach of not performing a biopsy on the contralateral testis.

These observations underscore the importance of continued long-term follow-up of patients with testicular germ cell tumors.

PATHOLOGY

Origin and Molecular Genetics Testicular tumors fall into several broad groups, as listed in Table 99-1. Classification of the germ cell tumors has historically been based on morphology, but recent molecular studies have yielded a more ontological scheme consisting of five distinct subtypes that differ in their proposed cell of origin.[18] According to this scheme, teratomas and yolk sac tumors arising in neonates and young children derive from primordial germ cells or very early gonocytes distributed along the gonadal ridge or in the testis/ovary. These tumors retain most of the genomic imprinting from both parental genomes. The teratomas remain diploid, while the yolk sac tumors show gains of chromosomes 1q, 12p13-14, and 20q, and losses of 1p, 4, and 6q.[18]

Table 99-1 Germ Cell Tumors

Type	Relative Frequency	Genotype/Comments
Infants and children	~1% of all testis tumors	
Yolk sac tumor	65–80% of prepubertal	Aneuploid
Teratoma	20–35% of prepubertal	Diploid; mature elements; benign
Adolescents and adults	95% of all testis tumors	
ITGCNU	> 90% of postpubertal	Aneuploid (near triploid)
Seminoma	~45% of postpubertal	Aneuploid (near triploid); iso12p

Spermatocytic seminoma is a second, distinct subtype of germ cell tumor thought to derive from postpubertal spermatogonia/spermatocytes. Accordingly, these tumors have a paternal pattern of genomic imprinting and show variable ploidy, sometimes with a gain of chromosome 9.

Two of the other five proposed subtypes of germ cell tumor do not occur in the testis. Dermoid cysts of the ovary, which are thought to arise from oogonia/oocytes, are diploid/tetraploid and show maternal genomic imprinting. Hydatidiform mole (gestational trophoblastic disease) is a placental-derived neoplasm that contains a purely paternal genome as a result of fertilization of an empty ovum.

The fifth subtype of germ cell tumor consists of seminoma and the nonseminomatous germ cell tumor (NSGCT) patterns that, together, account for 95% of primary testicular neoplasms (see Table 99-1). Variants of this germ cell tumor subtype also occur in the ovary (dysgerminoma), anterior mediastinum, and midline brain (germinoma). It is suggested that seminoma and NSGCT are derived from gonocytes that have lost their genomic imprinting as a result of being later in their development than those that give rise to infantile teratomas and yolk sac tumors. Moreover, these gonocytes are polypoid (tri- or tetraploid), probably because of meiotic arrest. Depending on exactly when this arrest occurs during fetal development, the affected cells may be distributed to one or both testes, accounting for the bilateral germ cell tumors observed in 2 to 3% of patients.

Seminomas and NSGCT share a common precursor lesion called intratubular germ cell neoplasia, unclassified (ITGCNU). Growing in situ within seminiferous tubules, ITGCNU cells resemble seminoma cells and express similar markers (Table 99-2), including the transcription factor OCT3/4. This factor is essential to the development of embryonic stem cells in mice, but it is not expressed in normal spermatogonia in mice or humans. Its presence in ITGCNU supports the theory that a pluripotent gonocyte is the cell of origin for both seminoma and NSGCT. In addition, OCT3/4 serves as a highly specific immunohistochemical marker in the diagnosis of extratesticular germ cell tumors.[19,20]

Progression of ITGCNU to an invasive germ cell tumor is accompanied by a number of common events.[21] One is the acquisition of excess genetic material from the short arm of chromosome 12. In 80% of cases, this is accomplished through loss of 12q and reduplication of 12p (isochromosome 12p), while in the remaining 20%, the additional 12p sequences are distributed among other derivative chromosomes. As excess 12p is a nearly universal feature in seminoma and NSGCT, efforts to identify the critical genes represented on this arm are ongoing. Fluorescence in situ hybridization (FISH) for 12p has already come into clinical use on paraffin sections as a diagnostic marker for germ cell tumors of all types and also for nongerm cell derivatives thereof.

Additional events associated with malignant progression of ITGCNU include loss of expression of the homeobox gene *NKX3.1*,[22] loss of the

Table 99-2 Markers of Testicular Germ Cell Tumors

Morphologic Subtype	Serum	Immunohistochemistry	FISH
ITGNCU		PLAP, KIT, OCT3/4	
Seminoma	HCG (low)	PLAP, KIT, OCT3/4	Excess 12p
Embryonal carcinoma	HCG (low)	CD30, OCT3/4, PLAP	Excess 12p
Yolk sac tumor	AFP	AFP, PLAP	Excess 12p
Choriocarcinoma	HCG (high)	HCG	Excess 12p
Teratoma			Excess 12p

AFP = α-fetoprotein; FISH = fluorescence in situ hybridization; HCG = human choriogonadotropin; PLAP = placental/germ cell alkaline phosphatase.

tumor suppressor PTEN,[23] and decreased expression of the cell cycle regulator p21.[24] *MDM2* overexpression is also associated with this transition and appears to be more common than *TP53* mutations.[24]

Although seminoma and NSGCT share a common origin, they are clinicopathologically distinct cancers. Little is known of what determines their differences, but one interesting observation is that oncogenic mutations in KIT (a receptor tyrosine kinase) are found in 25% of seminomas and are essentially absent in NSGCT. These mutations may occur very early in seminoma tumorigenesis, as they are present in ITGCNU[25] and they have also been identified in dysgerminoma/germinoma of the ovary, mediastinum, and brain. Based on studies in mice, *KIT* gene function is essential to the development of primordial germ cells and to normal spermatogenesis; therefore, constitutive activation of this kinase may favor the seminoma pathway. It has also been suggested that *KIT* mutations are more common in patients who develop bilateral disease. Unfortunately, the KIT kinase inhibitor imatinib is not likely to be of benefit to seminoma patients harboring *KIT*-mutant tumors, because most of the published mutations are inherently resistant to this drug.

Seminoma Approximately 45% of all postpubertal testicular germ cell tumors are pure seminoma ("classic" seminoma). The incidence is increased in cryptorchid testes, where it accounts for more than 60% of neoplasms. On gross examination, such tumors are generally homogeneous and well demarcated. Distinct lobulation may be apparent, with the nodules separated by dense fibrous bands. Areas of necrosis and hemorrhage may also be observed but are usually discrete.

Microscopically, there is a monotonous distribution of uniform, rounded cells with large, centralized nuclei and nucleoli. The cytoplasm may be either clear or granular and will frequently stain positively for glycogen, lipid, and/or placental/germ cell alkaline phosphatase (PLAP). Stromal elements are equally characteristic, with an infiltrate rich in T-lymphocytes and containing occasional granulomas (Figure 99-1). These features may predominate histologically and mimic granulomatous orchitis. Approximately 7% of seminomas contain syncytiotrophoblastic giant cells that stain positively for human chorionic gonadotropin (HCG).

Seminoma presents most commonly in the fourth and fifth decades, usually as an enlarging, painless testicular mass. Approximately 70% of patients present with stage I disease (confined to testis), 20% with stage II (enlarged retroperitoneal lymph nodes), and only rarely with disease above the diaphragm. Lymphatic spread is to the para-aortic (PA) lymph nodes, then to the mediastinal or supraclavicular lymph nodes. Hematogenous dissemination to the lung, liver, bone, or adrenal is a late occurrence. Low-level HCG elevation is seen in 5 to 10% of patients with pure seminoma and likely reflects syncytiotrophoblastic elements present within the tumor (see Table 99-2). Seminoma does not secrete α-fetoprotein.

Nonseminomatous Germ Cell Tumors The most common postpubertal germ cell tumors of the testis are composed of one or more elements that are collectively known as "nonseminomatous." Four morphologic patterns are recognized among this group, as detailed below. In the great majority of cases, these patterns are intermixed in varying proportions, often subtly merging from one to the next. Areas of seminoma may be included (termed "mixed germ cell tumors" by some authors), but the prognosis is determined by the presence of the other elements and is less favorable, overall, than for pure seminomas.

Embryonal Carcinoma Embryonal carcinoma is present in up to 90% of NSGCT cases. Macroscopically, it forms a soft, fleshy, inhomogeneous mass with areas of necrosis and hemorrhage. Direct invasion of the spermatic cord, epididymis, and tunica albuginea is not uncommon.

The microscopic appearance is extremely variable and may include papillary, solid, tubular, and glandular patterns, frequently interrupted by geographic necrosis (Figure 99-2). Large polygonal cells with indistinct cytoplasmic borders (unlike seminoma) are the rule, with pale granular cytoplasm, large nuclei, and one or more centrally placed nucleoli. Mitotic figures and multinucleated cells are common. Clinically, these are aggressive tumors with lymph node metastases present in two-thirds of patients.

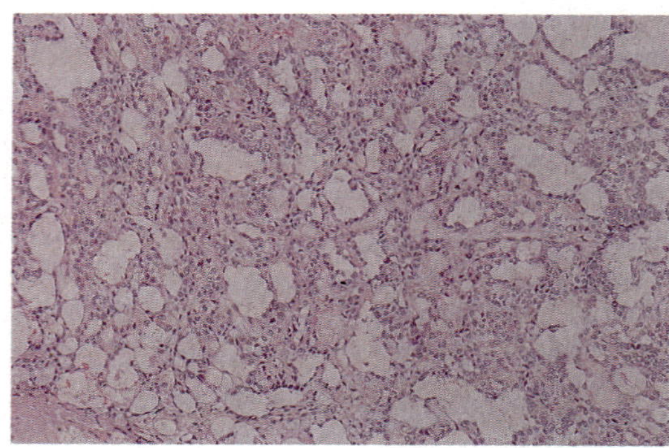

Figure 99-3 Yolk sac tumor. Numerous microcysts occur in the most common pattern of yolk sac tumor.

Yolk Sac Tumor Yolk sac tumor, formerly called endodermal sinus tumor, is present in approximately half of NSGCT cases, but is rare in pure form in the postpubertal patient.[26] The most readily recognized pattern consists of a cluster of tumor cells surrounding a small central blood vessel, a structure referred to as a Schiller-Duval body (Figure 99-3). The morphologic spectrum is quite broad, however, including microcystic (lace-like), micropapillary, solid, and hepatoid patterns. The tumor cell nuclei are somewhat smaller than those of embryonal carcinoma. Cytoplasmic globules are common and stain positively for α-fetoprotein, which accounts for the serum elevations in this marker characteristically present in patients with this tumor (see Table 99-2).

It should be noted that in its pure form, yolk sac tumor is the most common testicular neoplasm in infants and young children (see Table 99-1). Despite morphologic similarity to the subtype observed in postpubertal NSGCT, the pediatric tumor is an oncogenetically distinct entity and carries a better prognosis.

Choriocarcinoma Choriocarcinoma is an uncommon element in NSGCT (15%) and is very rare as a pure tumor. On gross examination, areas of choriocarcinoma are characteristically hemorrhagic. Microscopically, the diagnosis requires a combination of cytotrophoblasts and syncytiotrophoblasts (Figure 99-4). Stroma is sparse, but tends to be highly vascular. Choriocarcinoma of the testis represents the most aggressive subtype of NSGCT, often presenting with large-volume visceral metastases and/or brain metastases.

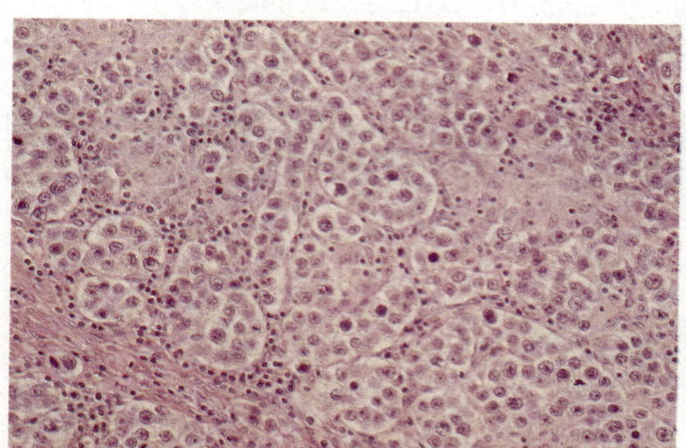

Figure 99-1 Small nests of seminoma are separated by a lymphoid infiltrate and a focal granulomatous reaction.

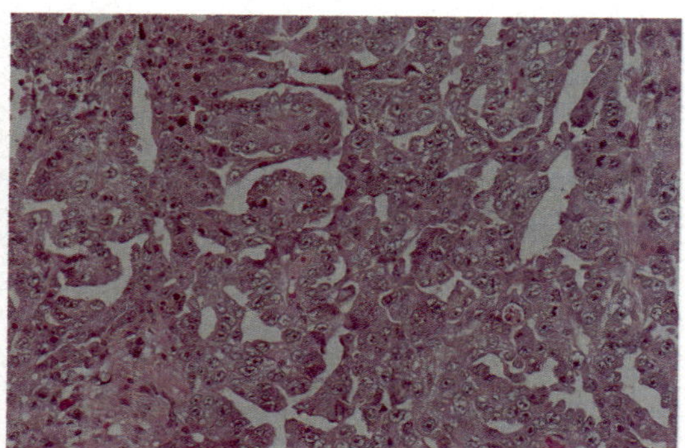

Figure 99-2 Embryonal carcinoma. Irregularly shaped glands and papillae are lined by pleomorphic cells with vesicular, crowded nuclei and poorly defined cytoplasmic membranes.

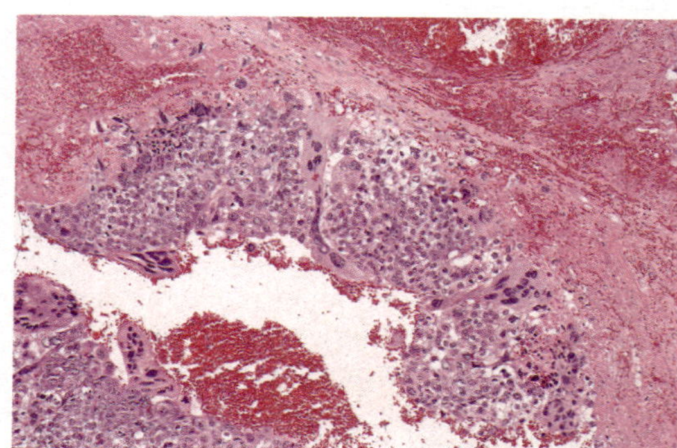

Figure 99-4 Choriocarcinoma. Syncytiotrophoblastic cells "cap" islands of mononucleated cytotrophoblast. Note the hemorrhagic background.

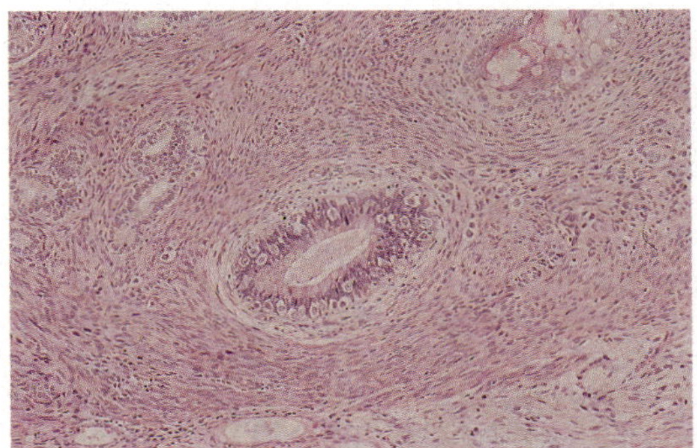

Figure 99-5 Mature teratoma. There are mature-appearing small glands, a portion of a pilosebaceous unit, and bundles of smooth muscle.

Extreme elevations of serum HCG levels are characteristic.

Teratoma Teratoma is defined as a tumor that contains elements of all three germ layers (endoderm, mesoderm, and ectoderm), present with varying degrees of differentiation. Teratomatous elements are recognized in approximately half of NSGCT cases, but are not usually pure. Macroscopically, teratomas tend to be large and have multiloculated cysts containing serosanguineous fluid as well as cartilaginous solid areas. Microscopically, all manner of tissue elements may be present, including cysts with squamous, respiratory or intestinal-type linings, mature cartilage, muscle, and fibroblastic stroma (Figure 99-5). Areas that are less well differentiated ("immature teratoma") are often intermixed (Figure 99-6). Regardless of the degree of differentiation, all teratomas in the postpubertal setting are regarded as malignant. In postchemotherapy specimens (typically from retroperitoneal lymph node dissection) teratoma is the most common residual element. The presence of nonteratomatous NSGCT may be an indication for additional therapy.

A pure form of mature teratoma is common among pediatric patients under the age of four years. Although morphologically similar to mature areas of teratoma within NSGCT, these lesions arise through a different pathway and are essentially benign[27] (see Table 99-1). Rarely, a nonteratomatous element is identified and may give rise to metastases.

Nongerm Cell Cancers Arising from Germ Cell Tumors Given the pluripotent nature of the gonocytes from which seminomas and NSGCT are thought to arise, it is perhaps not surprising that in advanced cases of postpubertal testicular cancer, a nongerm cell element may emerge and become the dominant pattern. Among these are cancers morphologically resembling embryonal rhabdomyosarcoma, adenosquamous carcinoma, leiomyosarcoma, Wilms' tumor, glioblastoma multiforme, and primitive neuroectodermal tumor (PNET), all of which are associated with resistance to chemotherapy.[28] Myelodysplasia and leukemia may also evolve from NSGCT.[29]

Spermatocytic Seminoma Spermatocytic seminoma accounts for only 1 to 2% of testicular germ cell tumors. On gross examination, it has a grayish appearance and tends to be softer than classic seminoma. Microscopically, these tumors tend to form tubular clusters and are composed of round cells of highly variable size that bear resemblance to the cellular stages of normal spermatogenesis (Figure 99-7). In contrast to classic seminoma, stromal lymphocytic infiltration is not a feature of spermatocytic seminoma. This tumor tends to occur over the age of 50, with a median age of 65 years. The prognosis following surgery is excellent, as there are only anecdotal reports of metastases.

Sex Cord–Stromal Tumors Tumors arising from stromal tissue account for only 4% of all adult testicular tumors, but represent almost 20% of childhood testicular tumors. These tumors are thought to arise from primitive gonadal mesenchyme and are subcategorized as Leydig cell tumor, Sertoli cell tumor, gonadoblastoma, granulosa cell tumor and mixed/indeterminate types (see Table 99-1).

Leydig Cell Tumor Leydig cell tumor represents about 3% of all testicular tumors, and although they may be seen in children, the median age of appearance is 60 years. Histologically, they are typified by cells with abundant oncocytic cytoplasm and round, regular nuclei. Clinical symptoms are usually related to the production of both androgens and estrogens by tumor cells, leading to precocious puberty in a child and gynecomastia in the adult. Approximately 10% of Leydig cell tumors metastasize, but this occurs only in the postpubertal patient. In patients with distant metastatic disease, treatment with radiation therapy or standard chemotherapeutic agents has generally been ineffective. Retroperitoneal lymph node dissection (RPLND) is an important staging procedure for these tumors. The therapeutic role of RPLND in low-volume metastatic retroperitoneal disease is unclear, but waiting to resect higher-volume tumor is ineffective. A prophylactic RPLND should, therefore, be considered in patients with clinical stage I tumors.

Sertoli Cell Tumor Sertoli cell tumor shows no age predilection, presenting as a testicular mass that may be accompanied by gynecomastia or impotence secondary to tumor estrogen production. Microscopically, these lesions are composed of rounded cells with distinct cytoplasmic borders growing in cords and sheets in a fibrous background. As with other stromal tumors, therapy is primarily directed at resection of the primary lesion, with a staging work-up to include abdominal computed tomography (CT) scan and chest radiography. It is controversial as to whether an RPLND should be performed with clinical stage I disease. Large primary tumors with frequent mitoses or necrosis may prompt an RPLND. Unlike Leydig cell tumors, Sertoli cell tumors can respond to platinum combination chemotherapy.

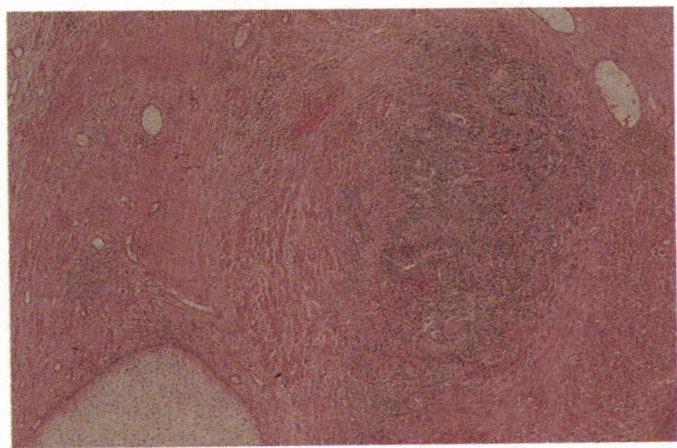

Figure 99-6 Immature teratoma. An island of immature neuroepithelium is present adjacent to a nodule of hyaline cartilage.

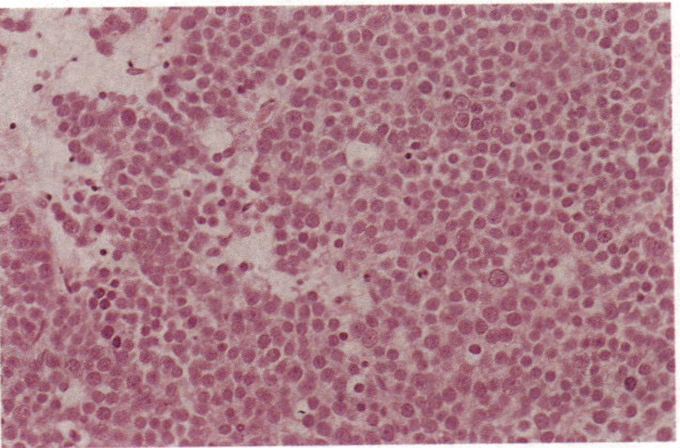

Figure 99-7 Spermatocytic seminoma. There is a diffuse sheet-like arrangement of neoplastic cells that vary in size.

CLINICAL PRESENTATION

Most patients with testicular cancer seek medical attention because of the development of a swollen testis. Accompanying symptoms include a sensation of heaviness or aching in the affected gonad. Severe pain is quite rare, unless there is associated epididymitis or bleeding in the tumor. On occasion, because testicular cancer is commonly associated with low sperm counts, patients may present during the course of an infertility work-up.

Approximately 25% of patients with disseminated disease present with symptoms arising from metastatic disease.[30] Severe back pain from metastasis to the retroperitoneum is the most frequent symptom from metastatic disease of the testis and is the presenting symptom in patients with primary retroperitoneal germ cell tumors. Pulmonary complaints, such as shortness of breath, chest pain, or hemoptysis, are usually manifestations of far-advanced lung metastases. Primary mediastinal germ cell tumors are an exception, in that these tumors (if malignant) present with symptoms of mediastinal compression with pain, dysphagia, shortness of breath, and superior vena cava syndrome. Benign teratomas of the mediastinum produce few symptoms and are commonly discovered on routine chest film obtained for minor chest complaints. Other rare primary sites usually present with symptoms of local mass effect, for example, pineal, sacral presentations.

Diagnosis Understanding the diagnosis and staging of testicular germ cell tumors depends on understanding the anatomy of the vascular and lymphatic drainage of the testis as well as the likely sites of metastatic spread of the disease. The spermatic cord contains the lymphatic and vascular supply of the testis. The lymphatic and vascular supply diverges medially when the spermatic vessels cross ventral to the ureter. The landing zones for the lymphatic drainage of the right testis is the interaortocaval nodes below the renal vasculature and the ipsilateral distribution of nodes, especially the paracaval and preaortic nodes. The primary landing zone for a left-sided primary tumor includes in the PA nodes below the left renal vessels and the PA and preaortic nodes. Ipsilateral common iliac nodes are uncommonly involved unless large-volume disease is present.

Unusual patterns of disease can be seen (or created) in patients who have had prior pelvic surgeries including herniorrhaphy, abdominal orchiopexy, or scrotal violations.[31] It is important to emphasize here that the proper and only diagnostic procedure in this setting should be a radical inguinal orchiectomy. Transscrotal procedures can disrupt predictable patterns of lymphatic metastases and should not be done.

The evaluation for testicular cancer begins with a careful history and physical examination. The examination of the testis is performed by grasping the gonad between the thumb and first two fingers and carefully palpating the testis, epididymis, and cord. Tumors of the testis can present with a discrete nodular density or as diffuse infiltration of the entire testis (particularly seminoma and lymphoma). The other testis serves as a useful reference standard to make comparisons. If a testicular mass is suspected, transscrotal ultrasonography should be performed. The presence of a hypoechoic mass represents a testicular neoplasm, and a radical inguinal orchiectomy is required to make a definitive pathologic diagnosis, as well as to ensure local control of a primary testicular cancer.

Extragonadal germ cell tumors arising within the retroperitoneum or mediastinum require specialized management. A diagnosis may be made on the basis of significantly elevated tumor marker levels in a patient with a mass in the anterior mediastinum or retroperitoneum. If there is no marker elevation, tissue confirmation is required. For mediastinal germ cell tumors, an anterior median sternotomy is favored for diagnosis. Because chemotherapy is the primary modality of treatment, attempts at debulking or total removal of mediastinal germ cell tumors as initial management are inappropriate. Primary retroperitoneal germ cell tumors may be associated with an occult testicular primary. Such patients should have a thorough evaluation of the gonads, including the use of testicular ultrasonography. If a previously unsuspected testicular tumor is found, orchiectomy can serve as the diagnostic procedure. Otherwise, fine-needle aspiration of the abdominal mass or exploratory laparotomy is required to provide tissue for diagnosis. In addition, an i(12p) chromosomal abnormality is diagnostic for germ cell tumor in a patient who presents with undifferentiated cancer.

A transscrotal biopsy should never be performed as this could seed the scrotal contents and, with disruption of regional lymphatics, lead to inguinal lymph node metastasis. Management of patients who have had a scrotal violation depends on the procedure performed and the anticipated treatment of the malignancy. If, at the time of scrotal orchiectomy, the surgeon identified the tumor and removed the testis in toto, then the only additional procedure that need be accomplished is removal of the inguinal portion of the spermatic cord. This can be done at the time of the retroperitoneal lymphadenectomy or through a separate inguinal incision. If a testicular biopsy was performed, management of the hemiscrotum depends on the primary treatment modality. Patients who are receiving primary chemotherapy do not need hemiscrotectomy. Inguinal lymphadenectomy is reserved for patients with palpable inguinal lymphadenopathy. For patients with early-stage seminoma who have had a scrotal violation, approximately 5 to 10% will experience local failure. Extending the field to include the groin and scrotum diminishes these prospects, but is associated with increased infertility. Such patients should be managed on a case-by-case basis, dependent on the desire to have a family and compliance with follow-up.

Tumor Markers Serum HCG and α-fetoprotein represent the quintessential serum markers in oncology. They have significant value in the diagnosis, prognosis, and management of patients with germ cell tumors. α-Fetoprotein is a glycoprotein normally produced by the fetal yolk sac and is derived from the yolk sac or embryonal carcinoma elements of germ cell cancers. Elevated levels of α-fetoprotein are not seen in normal adults. The half-life of this protein in the serum is approximately 5 days. HCG is a smaller glycoprotein that is normally produced by trophoblastic tissues. In germ cell cancers, syncytiotrophoblastic components elaborate HCG. The protein comprises an alpha subunit and a beta subunit, each of which is antigenically distinct. The serum half-life of the entire protein is 18 to 30 hours.

Serum HCG and/or α-fetoprotein are elevated in 85% of patients with disseminated nonseminomatous germ cell tumors. α-Fetoprotein alone is elevated in 40% of patients, and HCG alone is elevated in 50 to 60% of patients with disseminated nonseminomatous testicular cancer. Elevated lactic acid dehydrogenase (LDH) is a less specific marker and is mainly a correlate of disease bulk. Mediastinal nonseminomatous germ cell tumors more commonly have elevation of α-fetoprotein (80%), because of frequent presence of yolk sac tumor, as compared with HCG (40%).

Pure seminoma is most frequently associated with normal α-fetoprotein and HCG, but approximately 10% of all cases, and up to 30% of patients with advanced disease, may have low-level elevation of HCG (usually < 100 mIU/mL).[32] Any elevation of α-fetoprotein in patients with seminoma must be viewed as evidence of nonseminomatous disease, and management should proceed as such.

α-Fetoprotein and HCG should be determined before and after orchiectomy, but the absence of marker elevation should not influence the decision to undertake the procedure. Likewise, normalization of serum markers after orchiectomy does not ensure that all disease has been removed, although persistence of marker elevation implies residual disease.

The rate of disappearance of elevated tumor markers is very useful in determining response to chemotherapy. HCG is the most useful in this regard; the most clinically helpful guideline is that a 10-fold decrease in the HCG level over a 3-week period is consistent with potentially curative chemotherapy. Less steep declines of HCG levels may correlate with the emergence of drug-resistant disease. Likewise, the reappearance of marker elevation often predates the radiographic appearance of recurrent disease and, as such, is an invaluable method of detecting early relapse.

Although the presence of tumor markers and their accurate determination serve as a luxury in the management of patients with germ cell cancer, the presence of these markers also can lead to errors in clinical management if not interpreted with caution. First, HCG determination can be nonspecific, and there is some cross-reactivity in the radioimmunoassay with luteinizing hormone. Also, HCG can be falsely elevated in patients who use marijuana. Low levels of HCG elevation, consequently, are difficult to interpret. A conservative approach to this dilemma is to repeat the HCG determination to ensure that the elevation is not a laboratory error. If the level is still high, the patient should be queried regarding drug usage. Testosterone should be given in a dose of 300 mg intramuscularly to ensure that a hypogonadal state with resultant high levels of luteinizing hormone is not interfering with the determination of HCG. If the level remains increased, restaging procedures and investigation of sanctuary sites (brain and contralateral testis) are in order.

A retrospective review by Zon and colleagues at Indiana University evaluated management problems in patients with very high HCG levels.[33] Forty-one patients with an HCG greater than 50,000 mIU/mL were included. All patients received cisplatin-based chemotherapy. Two of these 41 patients had normal HCG levels at the time of the fourth course of chemotherapy. Eight additional patients had normalized the HCG within 1 month of completion of the fourth course of therapy. Of these 10 patients, 7 remain continuously free of disease, and 3 are currently disease free with salvage therapy. Thirty-one patients still had an abnormal HCG more than 1 month after completing the fourth course of primary chemotherapy. Fifteen of these patients are continuously disease free, despite no further treatment. This review highlights a subset of patients with very high HCG levels who do not have a consistent predictable decline of HCG with treatment. Absolute dependence on predicted patterns of decline in these patients would have resulted in overtreatment or inappropriate initiation of salvage therapy. Our strategy has been to wait for a rising serum HCG before considering salvage therapy.

Table 99-3 Memorial Sloan-Kettering Staging System for Nonseminomatous Germ Cell Tumors

Stage I:	Tumor confined to the testis
Stage II:	Minimal nodal spread, microscopic only and with fewer than six nodes involved, none more than 2 cm
Stage II2:	Grossly positive nodes, or more than six nodes positive in the retroperitoneum
Stage II3:	Bulky retroperitoneal involvement, unresectable
Stage III:	Metastases above the diaphragm or involvement of the solid visceral organs, brain, or bone

Table 99-4 AJCC Staging

TNM Clinical Classification	
T:	Primary tumor
	The extent of the primary tumor is classified after radical orchiectomy (see pT). If no radical orchiectomy has been performed, TX is used.
N:	Regional lymph nodes
NX	Regional lymph nodes cannot be assessed
N0	No regional lymph node metastasis
N1	Metastasis with a lymph node mass ≤ 2 cm in greatest dimension or multiple lymph nodes, not > 2 cm in greatest dimension
N2	Metastasis with a lymph node mass > 2 cm but not > 5 cm in greatest dimension, or multiple lymph nodes, any one mass > 2 cm but not > 5 cm in greatest dimension
N3	Metastasis with a lymph node mass > 5 cm in greatest dimension
M:	Distant metastasis
MX	Distant metastasis cannot be assessed
M0	No distant metastasis
M1	Distant metastasis
M1a	Nonregional lymph node or pulmonary metastasis
M1b	Distant metastasis other than to nonregional lymph node and lungs
pTNM Pathologic Classification	
pT:	Primary tumor
pTX	Primary tumor cannot be assessed (if no radical orchiectomy has been performed TX is used)
pT0	No evidence of primary tumor (eg, histologic scar in testis)
pTis	Intratubular germ cell neoplasia (carcinoma in situ)
pT1	Tumor limited to testis and epididymis without vascular/lymphatic invasion, tumor may invade tunica albuginea, but not tunica vaginalis
pT2	Tumor limited to testis and epididymis with vascular/lymphatic invasion, or tumor extending through tunica albuginea with involvement of tunica vaginalis
pT3	Tumor invades spermatic cord with or without vascular/lymphatic invasion
pT4	Tumor invades scrotum with or without vascular/lymphatic invasion
pN:	Regional lymph nodes
pNX	Regional lymph nodes cannot be assessed
pN0	No regional lymph node metastasis
pN1	Metastasis with a lymph node mass ≤ 2cm in greatest dimension and ≤ 5 positive nodes, none > 2 cm in greatest dimension
pN2	Metastasis with a lymph node mass > 2 cm but not > 5 cm in greatest dimension; or > 5 nodes positive, non > 5 cm; or evidence of extranodal extension of tumor
pN3	Metastasis with a lymph node mass > 5 cm in greatest dimension
pM:	Distant metastasis
	The pM category corresponds to the M category
S:	Serum tumor markers
SX	Serum marker studies not available or not performed
S0	Serum marker study levels within normal limits LDH HCG α-fetoprotein
S1	< 1.5. N and < 5,000 and 1,000
S2	1.5–10. N or 5,000–50,000 or 1,000–10,000
S3	> 10. N or > 50,000 or > 10,000

N = the upper limit of normal for the lactate dehydrogenase assay.

False-positive elevation of α-fetoprotein is quite rare. Differential considerations include laboratory error, other tumor types (such as hepatocellular carcinoma), and liver inflammation from cirrhosis or hepatitis. An occasional patient may have baseline elevation of α-fetoprotein (usually < 100 ng/mL) that remains static over time and does not reflect active disease.[34]

STAGING

Germ cell tumors are typically categorized as stage I, referring to tumors confined to the testis; stage II, indicating metastatic disease to the nodes of the periaortic or vena caval zone without pulmonary or visceral involvement; and stage III, which denotes metastasis above the diaphragm or involving other viscera (Table 99-3). The American Joint Committee on Cancer (AJCC) has refined the classification system and included the important aspect of elevated tumor markers into the classification system. This TNM (tumor-nodes-metastasis)-based system adds important local prognostic parameters, such as vascular invasion; more regional nodal information, including size; and visceral versus nonvisceral metastasis and markers levels. This AJCC and World Health Organization (WHO) classification is the international standard (Table 99-4).[35]

Standard procedures to establish clinical stage include physical examination, abdominal and chest CT scans, and serum levels of α-fetoprotein, βHCG, and LDH. Brain imaging and bone scans should be performed only when clinically indicated. The role of positron emission tomography (PET) remains investigational in the initial staging of patients with germ cell tumors. However, in one series, PET imaging had a positive predictive value of 96% and negative predictive value of 90% when evaluating residual masses following chemotherapy.[36] PET scan will not reliably detect teratoma or microscopic carcinoma. PET scan has been investigated in patients with residual masses after chemotherapy for seminoma, and the persistence of PET avidity is associated with risk of recurrence.[37]

THERAPY

Carcinoma in Situ Carcinoma in situ (CIS) or tubular intraepithelial neoplasia (TIN) is a true premalignant condition leading to both seminomatous and nonseminomatous invasive germ cell tumors in up to 50% of untreated cases (Figures 99-8 and 99-9).[38] Management is controversial. Evaluated approaches for management include close observation, low-dose radiotherapy, and total orchiectomy. Observation after diagnosis of TIN offers the best chance of retained fertility, but requires a compliant patient and risks the possible requirement for more intensive treatment of invasive disease. Low-dose radiotherapy (18–20 Gy in 1.5–2.0 Gy fractions) will eradicate the TIN with high probability at the cost of decreased or eliminated fertility. These dose levels will not, however, usually affect potency, as Leydig cell function is preserved.[38,39] Total orchiectomy will obviously eliminate TIN in the effected testicle, as well as all germ cells and Leydig cells within that testicle. It may be the favored option in some patients with TIN in one testicle and a normal contralateral testicle. Partial orchiectomy alone is ill advised because TIN is typically a diffuse process within the effected testicle. Chemotherapy is not a valid therapy for TIN, as the process recurs with high probability, likely because of the "sanctuary" from chemotherapy aspects of the testicular architecture.[40]

Nonseminoma: Early Stage Knowledge of the natural history of testicular primary lesions and their lymphatic drainage patterns is key to understanding the therapeutic options available for the management of early-stage nonseminoma. Testicular lymphatics arise in proximity to the embryonic origin of the testicle, in the genital ridge in the high lumbar region. Although the afferent lymphatic channels accompany testicular descent into the scrotum, draining lymph nodes remain in the retroperitoneum, including first-echelon lumbar nodes and second-echelon iliac chain nodes.

Treatment of seminoma
Radical inguinal orchiectomy
Clinical stage I*
• Radiation therapy or
• Surveillance only (option for highly selected pts)
* Spermatocytic seminoma pts do not receive further therapy
Clinical stage II
Treatment options vary depending on node size:
Clinical stage III
Cisplatin-based combination chemotherapy
• BEP x 3 cycles or
• EP x 4 cycles
Bulky (LAD ≥ 5 cm):
Cisplatin-based combination chemotherapy
• BEP x 3 cycles or
• EP x 4 cycles
Non-bulky (LAD < 5 cm):
• radiation therapy

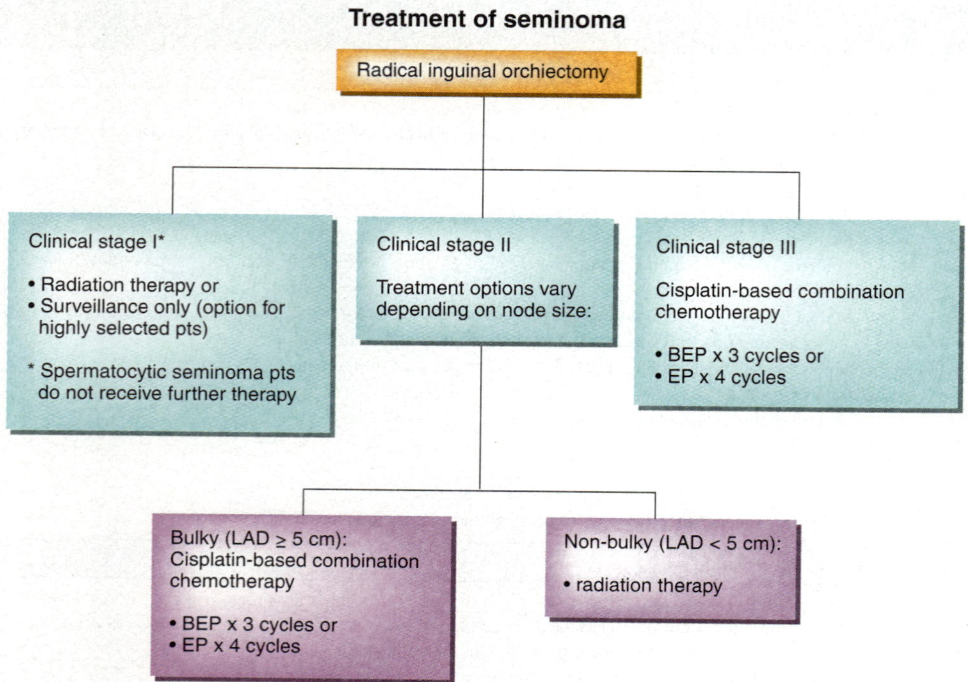

Figure 99-8 Treatment of seminoma.

The specific patterns of lymphatic drainage for testicular tumors have been known for more than 90 years. In 1910, Jamieson and Dobson demonstrated that the drainage pattern differed according to the side of the primary lesion, with right-sided lesions draining to the paracaval, interaortocaval, and preaortic nodes, and left-sided lesions to the PA and preaortic nodes.[41]

There is an ongoing controversy regarding the management of patients with clinical stage I nonseminoma. The three treatment options are RPLND, surveillance, and chemotherapy, each with advantages and disadvantages. Each is discussed below.

Retroperitoneal Lymph Node Dissection On the basis of the knowledge of a predictable pattern of spread of testicular tumors, multiple reports of RPLND surfaced from 1907 through 1950,[42–44] with a significant improvement in the 5-year survival to 46%. A number of surgical techniques have been described to expose and resect retroperitoneal lymph nodes. Radical lymphadenectomy via a thoracoabdominal (extraperitoneal) approach was described in 1950,[45] while reports of pure abdominal (anterior) approaches dominated the 1970s,[46,47] with each approach having intrinsic

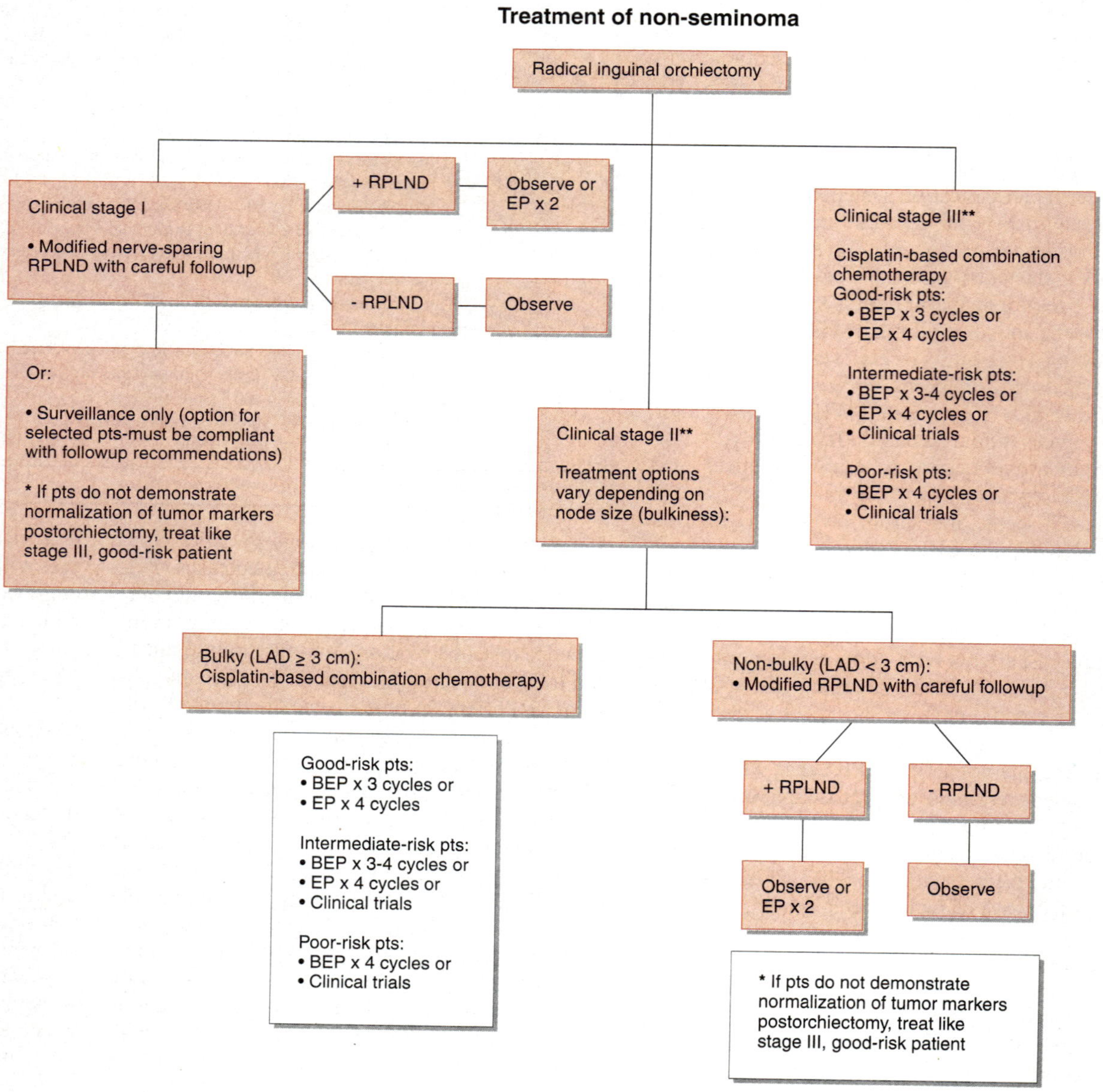

Treatment of non-seminoma
Radical inguinal orchiectomy
Clinical stage I
• Modified nerve-sparing RPLND with careful followup
+ RPLND
Observe or EP x 2
- RPLND
Observe
Or:
• Surveillance only (option for selected pts-must be compliant with followup recommendations)
* If pts do not demonstrate normalization of tumor markers postorchiectomy, treat like stage III, good-risk patient
Clinical stage II**
Treatment options vary depending on node size (bulkiness):
Clinical stage III**
Cisplatin-based combination chemotherapy
Good-risk pts:
• BEP x 3 cycles or
• EP x 4 cycles
Intermediate-risk pts:
• BEP x 3-4 cycles or
• EP x 4 cycles or
• Clinical trials
Poor-risk pts:
• BEP x 4 cycles or
• Clinical trials
Bulky (LAD ≥ 3 cm):
Cisplatin-based combination chemotherapy
Good-risk pts:
• BEP x 3 cycles or
• EP x 4 cycles
Intermediate-risk pts:
• BEP x 3-4 cycles or
• EP x 4 cycles or
• Clinical trials
Poor-risk pts:
• BEP x 4 cycles or
• Clinical trials
Non-bulky (LAD < 3 cm):
• Modified RPLND with careful followup
+ RPLND
Observe or EP x 2
- RPLND
Observe
* If pts do not demonstrate normalization of tumor markers postorchiectomy, treat like stage III, good-risk patient

Figure 99-9 Treatment of nonseminoma.

advantages. The extraperitoneal approach allows easy exposure on the ipsilateral side, whereas the anterior approach is preferable when bilateral dissections are undertaken. An extension of the anterior approach, which included bilateral renal suprahilar dissection, was pioneered by Donohue and colleagues.[48]

In experienced hands, the classic, bilateral RPLND, as described, is associated with minimal perioperative morbidity and virtually no mortality.[49] A major side effect of this approach, however, is the loss of antegrade ejaculation, with resultant infertility in over 90% of patients, a significant factor in young men in the 15- to 34-year age group. Several "nerve-sparing" modifications of the classic node dissection have been described in an attempt to minimize ejaculatory dysfunction and maintain the staging and/or therapeutic benefit of the procedure. An anatomic basis for such modified procedures has been provided by several meticulous mapping studies of retroperitoneal node involvement in early-stage disease.[50,51] In the study by Donohue and colleagues, patients with grossly negative, microscopically involved nodes (stage II1) were analyzed separately.[50] In right-sided primary lesions, no patient had involvement of the suprahilar regions, and only 4% had left PA (contralateral) node involvement. Similarly, in left-sided stage B1 disease, no patient exhibited right paracaval or precaval involvement. These studies suggested that full bilateral dissection is unnecessary in patients with grossly negative nodes at the time of surgery.

Unilateral lymph node dissections have, therefore, become popular for treating early-stage disease, both in the United States[52] and in Europe.[53] Modifications to the classic dissection have generally involved complete dissection of lymph nodes on the same side as the primary lesion, with limited (if any) intervention on the contralateral side, thus preserving the contralateral sympathetic efferents and ejaculatory function in 75 to 90% of patients. Particular emphasis is given to avoidance of the region anterior to the aortic bifurcation, as nerves exiting the thoracolumbar sympathetic trunk cross this region and become the hypogastric plexus. Preservation of these fibers appears to be particularly important in the maintenance of ejaculatory function. In a procedure by Donohue and colleagues, postganglionic sympathetic fibers from lumbar ganglia are prospectively identified and preserved prior to lymphadenectomy.[54] Of 75 patients treated in this manner, all were alive and disease free at 2 years, and 100% have preservation of antegrade ejaculation. Retroperitoneal recurrences occurred in 3 of 14 stage II patients, and in none of the 61 pathologic stage I patients. An updated experience with clinical stage I patients (and nerve-sparing RPLND) has confirmed the early results with the procedure. Ejaculation is reliably maintained, retroperitoneal recurrence is rare, and more than 99% of patients ultimately are cured.[48] Thus, it appears that the majority of patients can have their ejaculatory function preserved following retroperitoneal node dissection for early-stage disease, without a sacrifice in terms of retroperitoneal relapse or survival. Hospitalization times now average 4 to 5 days, as opposed to 7 to 10 days formerly. In addition, only a rare patient requires an intensive care unit (ICU) admission postoperatively.

Radiotherapy Although RPLND has been a mainstay of therapy for early-stage nonseminomatous germ cell tumors in the United States for the past 40 years, radiation therapy had been used in similar clinical situations in Europe, particularly in the United Kingdom and Denmark. However, today the use of radiotherapy in this clinical situation is limited, on the basis of both the success of cisplatin-based combination chemotherapy in distant metastatic disease and the prevalence of "surveillance" as a treatment option in clinical stage I disease.

CLINICAL STAGE I: SURVEILLANCE VERSUS RPLND

As the vast majority of testicular cancer patients are cured today even in the presence of minimal to moderate distant metastatic disease, attention has been focused on a reduction in the toxicity of curative therapy. For nonseminomatous disease clinically limited to the testicle, this has resulted in a reconsideration of the need for RPLND and its attendant morbidity. This type of surveillance policy has been quickly accepted but must be considered in the context of its effect on the natural history of the disease, the implications for patient follow-up, fertility, the potential need for chemotherapy, and, ultimately, patient survival. Therefore, the decision to choose surveillance or RPLND should be individualized.

The accurate diagnosis of clinical stage I disease is critical to the consideration of less interventional therapy. Following inguinal orchiectomy and the diagnosis of nonseminoma, serum levels of βHCG and α-fetoprotein must return to normal (if elevated before orchiectomy), and abdominal CT, chest radiography, and chest CT must all be negative for metastatic disease before a patient can be labeled as having clinical stage I disease. In this clinical setting, approximately 30% of patients will suffer a relapse if no other therapy is administered, with the retroperitoneum remaining as the area at highest risk.

There are now reports of almost 1,000 patients worldwide with clinical stage I disease who have had no other therapy administered following orchiectomy with relapse rates and survival remarkably similar between trials, regardless of the size of the study or country of origin.[55–57] These studies confirm a relapse rate of almost 30% despite optimal clinical staging. Of 236 relapsing patients in these trials, in whom current disease status is available, 94% were alive and disease free at the time of the reports. This survival figure is competitive with that of pathologic stage I disease, confirming that this is a reasonable therapeutic alternative in experienced hands. A reasonable policy for surveillance includes monthly tumor markers, physical examination and chest radiographs, and a regimen of abdominal/pelvic CTs every 2 months for the first year, every 4 months for the second year, and every 6 months for years 3 to 5. Surveillance appears to give equivalent survival results to RPLND in compliant patients. The advantages of RPLND include the lack of necessity for abdominal CTs, surgical staging of the patients, and a reduction in the need for subsequent chemotherapy.

Prognostic factors have been identified to select a group of patients at higher risk of disease recurrence with clinical stage I disease. These include vascular invasion, lymphatic invasion, pathologic T stage higher than 1, the presence of components of embryonal carcinoma, percent of the primary tumor occupied by teratoma, and the presence or absence of yolk sac elements.[55–58] Freedman and colleagues developed a mathematical model on the basis of the four identified prognostic factors in the Medical Research Council (MRC) study in the United Kingdom and were able to identify a subset of patients with a 58% relapse rate at 2 years.[57]

The efficacy and safety of chemotherapy for good-risk metastatic disease and the near-perfect results of two cycles of chemotherapy in the setting of fully resected stage II disease has prompted investigators to consider the use of primary chemotherapy in high-risk stage I disease. Primary chemotherapy achieves a near-universal cure with two cycles of chemotherapy in patients with poor-risk early-stage disease. However, even for high-risk clinical stage I, approximately 50% of these patients will be cured with orchiectomy alone, and the rest would have probably been cured with three cycles of bleomycin, etoposide, and cisplatin chemotherapy. In our opinion, there is minimal difference in toxicity between two and three courses of chemotherapy. However, there is a major difference between no chemotherapy and two courses. Therefore, we do not advocate adjuvant chemotherapy for patients with clinical stage I disease.

Pathologic Stage I Patients with disease clinically limited to the testicle who undergo staging RPLND for nonseminomatous germ cell tumor and are found to have pathologically negative lymph nodes are classified as pathologic stage I. The overall relapse rate for these patients is approximately 10%, with the great majority of relapses occurring in the lungs, since the surgical procedure has effectively removed the retroperitoneum as a significant site of relapse. However, with a significant improvement in the therapy for distant metastatic disease and clinical staging techniques over that same period, 5-year survival rates improved from 77% in 1969 to almost 98% in 1987.[49,59]

In the largest prospective study of observation in pathologic stage I nonseminomatous disease, the Testicular Cancer Intergroup Study enrolled 264 patients after RPLND.[59] With a median follow-up of 45 months, 28 patients (10.5%) had recurred, 25 of whom developed a first relapse within 24 months of node dissection. Six patients (2.3%) died, although only 2 of the 6 died of drug-resistant cancer. At the time of the report, 97.7% of patients were alive and disease free.

The current recommendation for patients with pathologic stage I nonseminomatous disease is for no further therapy to be administered following RPLND. This recommendation is based on the high surgical cure rate with orchiectomy and RPLND alone (90%), the favorable relapse pattern in patients who recur (lung only), and the effectiveness of chemotherapy for small-volume metastatic disease in relapsing patients. Orchiectomy histology is important in the probability of relapse in pathologic stage I disease. In a series reported by Sweeney and colleagues, 18 of 85 (21%) of patients with pathologic stage I disease with predominately embryonal carcinoma relapsed, as compared with only 5 of 141 (3%) in which embryonal carcinoma was not the predominant cell type.[60]

Clinical Stage I The presence of large-volume abdominal disease (> 3 cm on abdominal CT) should be treated with primary chemotherapy. After achievement of a serologic complete remission (normalization of serum βHCG and α-fetoprotein), restaging with abdominal CT should be done. Persistent retroperitoneal disease should be resected postchemotherapy.

Pathologic Stage II Approximately 50% of patients with nodal involvement at RPLND relapse if no additional therapy is given, with lower rates for microscopically positive disease in < 5 nodes. In light of the effectiveness of chemotherapy in disseminated disease, investigators have logically addressed the possibility of using it as a postoperative adjuvant in resected stage II patients or even as a substitute for surgery in clinical stage II disease.

The Testicular Cancer Intergroup Study randomized 195 pathologic stage II patients to no further therapy after RPLND, or to two immediate postoperative courses of adjuvant chemotherapy, either PVB (cisplatin, vinblastine, bleomycin) or VAB-6 (cisplatin, vinblastine, bleomycin, actinomycin D, cyclophosphamide).[59] With a median follow-up of 4 years, there was a significant difference in relapse-free survival, with 49% of the observation group relapsing, as compared with 6% of patients assigned to receive adjuvant chemotherapy. However, the difference is even more striking, as only 1 of the 6 relapsing patients in the adjuvant arm actually received his assigned therapy, and 1 patient on retrospective analysis had an inadequate RPLND. Thus, two courses of cisplatin-based therapy in completely resected stage II patients effectively eliminated the possibility of relapse. In terms of survival, there was no significant difference between the two groups, indicating that either approach should result in a greater than 95% cure rate, provided that complete surgical resection is undertaken and meticulous follow-up observed if adjuvant chemotherapy is not used.

Motzer and colleagues investigated the use of two cycles of etoposide and cisplatin at 3-week intervals in the setting of pathologic stage II nonseminomatous germ cell tumors.[61] Fifty patients were treated. All remain alive and disease free. Behnia and colleagues at Indiana University reviewed 86 patients treated with two cycles of bleomycin, etoposide, and cisplatin at 4-week intervals.[62] Only 1 relapse (teratoma) of 82 evaluable patients has occurred in long-term follow-up, and this patient is disease free after resection of his supraclavicular teratoma.

Seminoma Early Stage Orchiectomy and postoperative radiation therapy constituted the standard of care for early-stage seminoma patients during most of the twentieth century.[63–65] A properly performed radical orchiectomy by an inguinal approach is highly effective therapy for controlling disease at the primary tumor site. Occult or gross PA lymphatic tumor deposits can be eradicated with high probability after low doses of radiation therapy, owing to the extreme radiosensitivity of seminoma. More recently, success in surveillance trials in stage I nonseminomatous testicular cancers has naturally led to similar investigations for seminoma. With a large majority of patients experiencing prolonged disease-free survival in early-stage seminoma, long-term quality-of-life end points will assume increasing significance in evaluating treatment strategies.

Stage I Seminoma: Primary and Adjuvant Therapy Stage I disease comprises 85% of all seminoma cases diagnosed.[66] Stage I disease is where the most experience has been gained and the most evolution in treatment has occurred. Surveillance studies have demonstrated that a proper orchiectomy is curative approximately 80% of the time. Chemotherapy and/or radiation can be given as salvage therapy or as prophylaxis adjuvantly. Regardless of the elected management method, disease-specific survival at 5 years is over 99%.[67–71] The treatment of relapsed treatment-naïve disease appears to be as curable as it is at first presentation.

Four major series, the Princess Margaret Hospital, Danish Testicular Cancer Study Group, Royal Marsden Hospital, and Royal London Hospital, have demonstrated that surveillance is a viable option for treatment.[67,68,70,72–75] Their combined experience was pooled in an attempt to better identify candidates for treatment or surveillance.[67] In the entire group of 638 patients, 6 patients (0.9%) died of disease or complications of treatment of relapse. The overall 5-year and 10-year relapse-free rates were 82.3% and 78.7%, respectively. The majority (68.6%) of relapses occurred within 2 years, but still 7% of recurrences occur after 6 years. In an analysis of potential prognostic factors, the two most important were tumor size and rete testis invasion. Patients with tumors greater than 4 cm in diameter were twice as likely to relapse as those with smaller tumors. The rete testis is a communicating network of seminal channels traversing the mediastinum (or hilum) of the testis. Rete testis invasion was seen in 37% of the reported cases and defined as extension of the tumor into the testicular mediastinum without necessarily involving the tubular lumens. For patients with both factors of large tumor size and rete testis invasion, the rates of recurrence were as high as 33%. Although for patients without these factors, the recurrence rates were as low as 13%. Thus, although surveillance is a very attractive option, the frequency of follow-up imaging and tests cannot be reduced in any given patient. The patients who elect surveillance need to be compliant and reliable. The current recommendation for surveillance is to perform a history and physical, tumor markers including LDH, a chest X-ray, and a CT of the abdomen and pelvis every 4 months for the first 3 years. The interval is reduced to 6 months through year 7, and then annually through year 10.

Patients with stage I seminoma have been successfully treated with orchiectomy and adjuvant radiation for over 60 years with overall survival rates now above 99%. Adjuvant PA radiation results in a 3 to 4% rate of relapse with most of those being salvageable with additional radiation and/or chemotherapy. Analogous to the movement for no initial therapy is a simultaneous drive to reduce the toxicity of initial adjuvant therapy by reducing radiation doses and volumes.

The current practice is to deliver PA radiation from the Top of T11 or Top of T12 to the bottom of L5, and the radiation doses have been gradually reduced. The MRC TE18/EORTC 30942 trial addressed whether the radiation dose could be safely lowered to 20 Gy.[68] Most patients received only radiation to the PA nodes and were randomized to 30 Gy in 15 fractions versus 20 Gy in 10 fractions. The absolute difference in relapse rates was 0.7% and statistically insignificant.[76] A previous MRC trial tested whether an ipsilateral pelvic lymph node field was a necessary addition to the PA node field.[77,78] Ipsilateral pelvic lymph node irradiation did not significantly improve the 96% relapse-free survival at 3 years obtained with PA node field only radiation. But a significant number of the patients who had been treated with PA node radiation had pelvic node involvement as a component of their relapse. Thus, the patients who receive PA node radiation alone must still be followed routinely with CT scans of the pelvis. Ipsilateral pelvic lymph node irradiation is still recommended for patients who have had prior pelvic or inguinal surgery. But because of the less morbidity and better quality of life, PA node radiation alone is sufficient for patients with an undisturbed testicular lymphatic drainage.

Postorchiectomy Chemotherapy Based on pilot studies of adjuvant carboplatin in patients with stage I seminoma and results of carboplatin-based treatment in disseminated seminoma, a large randomized trial was conducted by the EORTC/MRC in which patients with well-staged clinical stage I seminoma were randomly allocated to standard prophylactic radiation therapy (primarily PA radiation at 20–30 Gy) or treatment with single-course, single-agent, carboplatin (AUC 7).[78] This trial was designed as a noninferiority trial powered to exclude an absolute increase in relapse at 2 years of 3%. Twelve hundred patients were required to have a 90% power with a 5% significance (one sided). In a 1:2 randomization scheme, 574 patients were assigned to single-agent carboplatin and 904 were assigned to standard radiation therapy. Clinician-reported toxicity suggested slightly higher rates of thrombocytopenia and neutropenia in the carboplatin arm and higher fatigue and missed work in the radiation-treated patients. There were 27 of 574 (4.7%) relapses in the carboplatin patients and 32 of 904 (3.5%) in patients treated with standard radiation with a median follow-up of 4 years. There was a substantial difference in the pattern of relapse, with the majority of relapses on the carboplatin arm occurring in the abdomen, and almost all of the recurrences in the radiation arm occurring outside the radiation portal. The authors' conclusions were that single-agent carboplatin was a safe and effective adjuvant treatment of clinical stage I seminoma, but longer follow-up was necessary. Criticisms of the study were that the pattern of abdominal relapse with the carboplatin-treated patients may necessitate abdominal imaging in follow-up and that short follow-up may underestimate the true incidence of relapse. In the United States, adjuvant carboplatin has not been adopted as standard at any of the major centers for treatment of testicular cancer.

Stage II Seminoma Several different staging systems have defined stage II seminoma, depending on how the distinctions are made for nodal size. Regardless of the specific staging system used, the potential for supradiaphragmatic involvement increases with the size of the subdiaphragmatic disease. At most centers, the arbitrary cutoff for systemic chemotherapy is 5 cm, while patients with nodal masses < 5 cm can be treated with radiation alone. Unlike with stage I, surveillance is not an option, and the expected 5-year relapse-free survival drops to 89 to 95% for patients treated with radiation alone.[79–82] The overall survival still remains around 97 to 99% because of the effectiveness of salvage therapy. For patients with stage II seminoma, the standard radiation field incorporates the ipsilateral pelvic lymph nodes because of the possibility of retrograde lymphatic flow. The treatment of stage II seminoma with radiation has also evolved to less toxic treatment regimens by incorporating chemotherapy and reducing the volume and dose of radiation. Historically for a patient with stage II seminoma, radiation was delivered to the PA nodes, pelvic lymph nodes, and prophylactically to the mediastinum. This practice, although effective at limiting supradiaphragmatic failures, became associated with late cardiac morbidity. Chemotherapy is now favored for patients who are at risk of supradiaphragmatic involvement.[80]

THERAPY FOR DISSEMINATED DISEASE

Chemotherapy: Precisplatin A broad spectrum of chemotherapeutic agents were tested from 1952 to 1972 in disseminated germ cell tumors, and many were found to have some degree of activity in chemotherapy-naïve patients. In the early 1960s, the vinca alkaloids were tested. Vinblastine, as a single agent, was able to induce complete remissions in 4 of 30 treated patients.[81] Although these were of short duration, they provided investigators with a rational component of subsequent combination regimens.

Several antitumor antibiotics were also found to have single-agent activity, including actinomycin D. Bleomycin was reported in 1970 to have significant activity, including the ability to induce complete remissions.[83,84]

An early combination regimen reported by Li and colleagues in 1960, which contained methotrexate, actinomycin D, and chlorambucil, remained popular throughout the rest of the decade.[85] Li reported an objective response rate of 52%, with more than half of those being complete responses. More importantly, they represented the first durable remissions, with 5 patients alive at 9 to 39 months after treatment at the time of the report.

A further advance in the development of effective chemotherapy for metastatic disease occurred when vinblastine and bleomycin were used in combination, as reported by Samuels and colleagues at the University of Texas M. D. Anderson Cancer Center.[86] This regimen resulted in 65% of patients achieving a complete remission, including some durable responses.

The most important event in the development of curative therapy for disseminated disease was the 1965 report by Rosenberg and colleagues of the antibacterial effect of platinum coordination compounds.[87] One of these compounds, *cis*-diamminedichloroplatinum (II) (cisplatin), was found also to have significant antitumor activity. Preclinical studies revealed testicular atrophy as a side effect in the dog model, prompting some investigators to predict activity for this compound against human testicular malignancies in the clinical setting. Cisplatin was soon reported to be the single most active agent against testicular germ cell tumors, with response rates of 70% and complete remission rates of 50%.[87] Thirty years later, it remains the most active drug in germ cell tumors.

Indiana University Studies In 1974, investigators at Indiana University began studies using PVB in patients with disseminated testicular cancer. The initial study remains a landmark study in modern oncology.[88] This study incorporated principles of combination chemotherapy, as well as the concept of surgically resecting residual disease after the completion of chemotherapy. Induction chemotherapy was brief (three to four courses), and maintenance chemotherapy was given for 2 years after induction therapy. Thirty-three of 47 patients (70%) obtained a complete remission with chemotherapy. Of the remaining 14 patients, 5 obtained a complete remission with resection of residual disease after the completion of chemotherapy. Six of the patients attaining remission relapsed.

The initial study proved that PVB was remarkably effective, and yet there was substantial toxicity. The next study was designed to compare the original PVB program with a similar regimen with a lower dose of vinblastine (0.4 mg/kg vs 0.3 mg/kg).[89] Seventy-eight patients were entered into this study, with 70% of all patients remaining continuously free of disease with equivalent results with the different vinblastine dosages. As expected, however, the reduction in the vinblastine dose was associated with fewer episodes of sepsis and granulocytopenic fever. Thus, on the basis of equivalent therapeutic results with lesser toxicity, the lower dose of vinblastine, along with cisplatin and bleomycin, became the standard regimen for PVB.

Confirmation of the results of these trials at Indiana University was obtained in a large European Organization for the Research and Treatment of Cancer (EORTC) trial of chemotherapy for disseminated testicular cancer.[90] This trial tested the contribution of high-dose vinblastine (0.4 mg/kg) versus lower-dose vinblastine (0.3 mg/kg) and the value of maintenance vinblastine. The trial of 214 patients failed to demonstrate any advantage for patients assigned to high-dose vinblastine therapy or for those assigned to maintenance vinblastine.

A third-generation study was begun at Indiana University in 1978 in conjunction with the Southeastern Cancer Study Group (SECSG).[91] The previous studies had used maintenance therapy with monthly vinblastine for 2 years after the completion of induction therapy. This trial tested the contribution of maintenance chemotherapy. In this study, patients with disseminated testicular cancer were given four courses of induction chemotherapy with PVB. Patients obtaining a complete remission with chemotherapy, or after resection of teratoma, were randomized to receive maintenance vinblastine or no further therapy. This study failed to demonstrate an advantage for those patients randomized to the maintenance therapy arm, with a relapse rate of 12% for those receiving treatment versus 7% for patients receiving induction therapy only.

In the next study, Indiana University, in conjunction with the SECSG, designed a randomized trial comparing cisplatin plus bleomycin and either vinblastine (PVB) or etoposide (BEP).[92] Two hundred sixty-one patients with disseminated germ cell cancer were entered, and 244 were evaluable for response. Of these, 123 were randomly allocated to receive BEP, and 83% achieved a disease-free status. One hundred twenty-one patients were assigned to receive PVB, and 74% attained a disease-free status. In the combined subgroups of patients with minimal or moderate disease by the Indiana classification system, 90% achieved a disease-free status, with no difference between the two treatment arms. Whereas PVB and BEP gave equally good therapeutic results, there was a marked difference in neuromuscular toxicity, with the PVB patients experiencing significantly more paresthesias, myalgias, and abdominal cramping. Because BEP had substantially less neuromuscular toxicity with equal or superior therapeutic results, cisplatin, etoposide, and bleomycin became and remains a standard regimen.

Prognostic Classifications An international consortium collected clinical data on patients receiving platinum-based therapy for metastatic germ cell tumor to develop a new prognostic model for disseminated disease.[93] Data on 5,202 patients with nonseminomatous germ cell tumor and 660 patients with seminoma were analyzed. Independent predictors of outcome in univariate analysis were mediastinal primary site for nonseminoma-

Table 99-5 International Germ Cell Consensus Classification

Good Prognosis
Nonseminoma testis or retroperitoneal primary and no nonpulmonary visceral metastases and α-fetoprotein < 1,000 ng/mL, βHCG < 5,000 IU/L and LDH < 1.5 upper limit of normal
Seminoma of any primary site and no nonpulmonary visceral metastases and normal α-fetoprotein, any βHCG, any LDH
Intermediate Prognosis
Nonseminoma testis or retroperitoneal primary and no nonpulmonary visceral metastases and α-fetoprotein > 1,000 ng/mL and < 10,000 ng/mL or βHCG > 5,000 IU/L and < 50,000 IU/L or LDH > 1.5 normal and < 10 normal
Seminoma of any primary site and nonpulmonary visceral metastases and normal α-fetoprotein, any βHCG, any LDH
Poor Prognosis
Nonseminoma with mediastinal primary, nonpulmonary visceral metastases or α-fetoprotein > 10,000 ng/mL or βHCG > 50,000 IU/L or LDH > 10 upper limit of normal

LDH = lactate dehydrogenase; βHCG = β human chorionic gonadotropin.

tous tumors, degree of α-fetoprotein, HCG, and LDH elevation, and the presence of nonpulmonary visceral metastasis. Using these factors, prognostic categories were derived. Good-risk patients with nonseminomatous disease were those with a testicular or retroperitoneal primary, favorable markers, and no nonpulmonary visceral metastases (anticipated progression-free survival 90%). Poor prognosis included those patients with mediastinal primary nonseminoma, patients with nonpulmonary visceral metastases, or those with unfavorable elevation of tumor markers (anticipated progression-free survival 40%). An intermediate group had an anticipated progression-free survival rate of 75%. For seminoma, only good- and intermediate-risk groups were identified, with good and intermediate risks being discriminated by the absence or presence of nonpulmonary visceral metastases (Table 99-5). This classification should be the standard classification system for comparing results of clinical studies done at various institutions.

TREATMENT OF GOOD-RISK DISSEMINATED GERM CELL TUMORS

Patients with good-risk disease constitute approximately 56% of patients presenting with disseminated disease. The International Germ Cell Consensus Classification (IGCCC) for good-risk disease suggests that more than 90% of patients in this category enjoy long-term disease-free survival.

In the mid-1980s, several clinical trials were designed specifically for this group of patients. Because virtually all these patients achieve complete remission with standard chemotherapy, the trials addressed the possibility of reducing the amount of chemotherapy administered (thus decreasing acute and chronic toxicity), while maintaining the excellent cure rate. Several approaches to this reduction in therapy have been employed, including a shortening of the duration of therapy, use of chemotherapeutic agents with less single-agent toxicity, and a reduction in the number of agents used.

The SECSG performed a trial in which patients with good-risk disease were randomized to receive either three or four courses of BEP.[94] There was no difference in the percent of patients achieving complete remission with either arm, and 92% of patients on both arms were disease free with a median follow-up of 19 months. On the basis of the results of this study, three courses of BEP (cisplatin 20 mg/m^2 plus etoposide 100 mg/m^2 intravenously [IV] days 1 to 5, repeated every 3 weeks, with bleomycin 30 units IV weekly) is standard therapy at Indiana University for patients with good-risk disease.

The Eastern Cooperative Oncology Group (ECOG) completed a trial randomizing patients with minimal or moderate disease to receive three courses of either BEP or etoposide and cisplatin (EP) alone in an attempt to eliminate the inconvenience (and possible pulmonary toxicity) of weekly bleomycin.[95] However, patients receiving bleomycin had superior survival. The EORTC has conducted a trial comparing four cycles of EP with or without bleomycin in patients with good-risk nonseminomatous germ cell tumor.[96] Complete remission rate (95% vs 89%) favored the bleomycin-containing arm, but relapse rates were similar. A trial at the Memorial Sloan-Kettering Cancer Center randomized good-risk patients to receive VP-16 (etoposide), combined with either cisplatin for four cycles (standard arm) or the platinum analog carboplatin.[97] In addition, the Medical Research Council/EORTC compared etoposide and bleomycin with either cisplatin or carboplatin in good-risk patients.[98,99] The advantages of carboplatin in this setting are its relative lack of nephrotoxicity and neurotoxicity and the ability to administer this compound on an outpatient basis without aggressive prehydration. Inferior survival was seen in the patients receiving carboplatin in these trials. Toner and colleagues reported inferior survival with four cycles of a dose-reduced version of BEP in comparison with standard BEP for three cycles.[100] In summary, analysis of all these trials attempting to further reduce toxicity by the elimination of bleomycin or the substitution of carboplatin for cisplatin has shown therapeutic inferiority for the experimental arm.

More recently, Culine and colleagues randomized 250 patients with good risk nonseminomatous tumors to either four courses of EP or three courses of BEP, concluding that both regimens were equivalent in efficacy and toxicity.[101] The current standard therapy of four courses of EP or three courses of BEP in this patient population has minimal acute toxicity, and probably even less long-term toxicity, on the basis of results with more aggressive therapy. Further reductions in the amount of therapy given are, therefore, unlikely to reduce toxicity significantly, but certainly have the potential to reduce the cure rate in this stage of disease. However, alternative schedules of BEP have also been reported. De Wit and colleagues report the results of a study from the EORTC and the Medical Research Council (MRC) in which patients received either three cycles of BEP with etoposide given as 100 mg/m^2 days 1 to 5 or 165 mg/m^2 days 1 to 3, cisplatin given as either 20 mg/m^2 days 1 to 5 or 50 mg/m^2 on days 1 and 2 only, and weekly bleomycin. These two versions of the BEP regimen yielded no significant difference in 2-year overall survival, with a 98% cure rate in patients with HCG < 1,000.[102]

In conclusion, for patients with good-risk disseminated disease, BEP for three cycles is standard therapy. Carboplatin should not be substituted for cisplatin, and EP alone for 3 cycles should also not be used.

TREATMENT OF PATIENTS WITH "POOR-RISK" DISSEMINATED DISEASE

Patients with disseminated testicular cancer who present with poor prognostic features remain a therapeutic challenge. One approach for the initial treatment of these poor-risk patients is the exploration of chemotherapy dose intensification.

Preclinical models, as well as dose-intensity analysis of clinical trials, suggest a steep dose-response relationship for cisplatin. This relationship has been tested in the design of several clinical trials of intensive cisplatin therapy in patients with poor-prognosis germ cell cancer. Ozols and colleagues at the National Cancer Institute (NCI) reported the results of a randomized trial of aggressive, high-dose cisplatin therapy versus PVB in poor-risk testicular cancer patients.[103] In this trial, there was a 2:1 randomization of 52 poor-risk patients to receive an aggressive arm with cisplatin, 40 mg/m^2 (double the standard dose) on days 1 to 5 with vinblastine, bleomycin, and etoposide in standard doses versus classic PVB with cisplatin given at 20 mg/m^2 on days 1 to 5. Of the patients receiving the aggressive arm, 88% had a complete response, as compared with 67% of the patients receiving PVB. The PVB arm had a high incidence of relapse, with 41% of the patients having disease recurrence, as compared with 17% of the patients receiving high-dose cisplatin, bleomycin, and VP-16 (PVeBV). Overall, 68% of the group randomized to the aggressive treatment remained disease free, as compared with only 33% of the patients receiving standard therapy. Unfortunately, accompanying this apparent improvement in outcome was a substantial increase in toxicity. There was significantly more myelosuppression and hearing loss in the patients receiving the high-dose cisplatin therapy. Whether the apparent superiority of the high-dose regimen in this trial was attributable to the high-dose cisplatin, the inclusion of etoposide, or other factors, was not clear from the study design.

Rigid testing of the impact of high-dose cisplatin therapy in disseminated germ cell cancer was accomplished in a trial of the SECSG and the Southwest Oncology Group (SWOG) in advanced germ cell cancer.[104] This trial enrolled only patients with advanced disease by the Indiana classification system. Patients were assigned at random to receive standard doses of etoposide and bleomycin and either standard-dose cisplatin (20 mg/m^2 daily for 5 days) or high-dose cisplatin (40 mg/m^2 daily for 5 days). Between 1984 and 1989, 159 patients with advanced disseminated germ cell cancer were enrolled. Of these, 153 were evaluable for toxicity and response. Among 76 patients assigned to high-dose therapy, 52 (68%) became disease free with chemotherapy alone or subsequent surgery. Among 77 patients on the standard-dose arm, 56 (73%) became disease free with chemotherapy alone or surgical resection of residual disease. Overall, 74% of the patients receiving the high-dose cisplatin are alive, and 63% are continuously free of disease, as compared with 74% alive and 61% continuously free of disease on the standard-dose arm. In addition, the high-dose arm was associated with significantly more ototoxicity, neurotoxicity, gastrointestinal toxicity, and myelosuppression. In contrast to the NCI study, this large randomized trial found no therapeutic benefit of dose escalation of cisplatin beyond standard doses.

In a follow-up to the SECSG trial of cisplatin dose intensity, the ECOG conducted a trial testing the substitution of ifosfamide for bleomycin.[104] From 1987 to 1992, 304 patients with advanced-stage disseminated germ cell cancer by the Indiana classification system were entered into this trial, which randomized patients to either four standard courses of BEP or to four courses of VIP with etoposide (75 mg/m^2 daily for 5 days), ifosfamide (1.2 g/m^2 daily for 5 days), and cisplatin (20 mg/m^2 daily for 5 days). Two hundred ninety patients were fully evaluable for toxicity and 286 were evaluable for response. The rates for complete remission (VIP 37%, BEP 31%), favorable response (VIP 63%, BEP 60%), failure-free at 2 years (VIP 64%, VIP 60%), and 2-year survival (VIP 74%, BEP 71%) were not statistically different between the two treatments. Grade III or greater toxicity, primarily hematologic, was significantly greater on the VIP arm ($p < .0001$). There were five therapy-related deaths on each arm. This analysis failed to demonstrate benefit for the experimental arm, VIP, relative to standard therapy with BEP, as a treatment of poor-risk germ cell tumor.

A similar trial evaluating the role of ifosfamide in poor-risk patients with germ cell tumor was reported by the EORTC and MRC.[105] In this trial, patients were randomized to BEP/EP or intensively scheduled bleomycin, vincristine, and cisplatin followed by VIP-B. There were no differences in time to progression or overall survival. Grade III or IV myelosuppression and weight loss were more pronounced in the bleomycin, Oncovin (vincristine), and prednisone (BOP)/VIP-B arm. The authors concluded that the intensive BOP/VIP-B therapy was more toxic, but without therapeutic advantage in treatment of poor-risk germ cell tumors.

High-Dose Chemotherapy as Primary Treatment of Poor-Risk Disease Investigators in Hanover and at other institutions in Germany have attempted to intensify therapy for poor-risk patients by incorporating growth factors and peripheral blood progenitor cell support to give high-dose, repetitive chemotherapy cycles. In the most recent update of this phase I/II trial, patients with poor-risk disseminated germ cell tumors were given repetitive cycles of cisplatin 25 to 30 mg/m^2 on days 1 to 5, etoposide 100 to 250 mg/m^2 on days 1 to 5, and ifosfamide 2 g/m^2 on days 1 to 5 every 22 days for four cycles.[106] At the highest dose levels, support with growth factors and peripheral blood progenitor cells was required. With these supportive care techniques, this high-dose therapy was tolerated with no dose-limiting myelosuppression, mucositis, renal toxicity, or neurotoxicity. Three of the 32 patients at the highest dose levels died of causes related to therapy. Of the 23 evaluable for response, 20 (87%) attained disease-free status, and 3 patients relapsed.

A randomized trial of 115 patients from the Institut Gustave Roussey has been reported, wherein poor-risk patients were randomized to receive conventional therapy with cisplatin, vinblastine, etoposide, and bleomycin versus similar therapy followed by a single cycle of high-dose cisplatin, etoposide, and cyclophosphamide.[107] Unfortunately, this trial failed to demonstrate any advantage for the high-dose arm.

A large-scale trial has been conducted on poor-risk patients as defined by the International Staging System that compared two courses of standard therapy (BEP) followed by two cycles of very high dose carboplatin, etoposide, and cyclophosphamide versus BEP × 4. The trial was conducted jointly by the Memorial Sloan-Kettering Cancer Center, the SWOG, ECOG, and the Cancer and Leukemia Group B (CALGB), and accrual finished in 2003. Analysis is pending. It is hoped that it will ascertain definitively the role of high-dose chemotherapy as primary therapy for poor-risk disease.

A European trial comparing high-dose VIP to standard therapy in poor-risk germ cell tumors is underway. This trial is based on the promising phase I/II trial reported by Schmoll and colleagues.[109] Between July 1993 and November 1999, 221 patients with either Indiana "advanced-disease" ($n = 39$) or IGCCCG "poor-prognosis" criteria ($n = 182$) received one cycle of VIP followed by three to four sequential cycles of high-dose VIP chemotherapy plus stem cell support every 3 weeks, at six consecutive dose levels. After 4-year median follow-up, progression-free survival and disease-specific survival rates in the poor-prognosis subgroup were 69% and 79% at 2 years and 68% and 73% at 5 years, with 76% for gonadal/retroperitoneal versus 67% for mediastinal primaries. Severe toxicity included treatment-related death (4%), treatment-related acute myeloid leukemia (1%), long-term impaired renal function (3%), chronic renal failure (1%), and persistent grade 2–3 neuropathy (5%).

Postchemotherapy Surgery Depending on the stage at diagnosis, 20 to 50% of patients who undergo induction chemotherapy for disseminated germ cell tumor have significant residual radiographic abnormalities. In this subset of patients, postchemotherapy resection of residual disease is often performed to remove residual teratoma or viable cancer. Several points bear emphasis in this setting. First, postchemotherapy surgery should be considered only if serum α-fetoprotein and HCG have normalized. Patients with persistently elevated serum markers should usually be considered for salvage chemotherapy rather than surgical extirpation. Second, postchemotherapy resection of residual abnormalities is rarely urgent, and sufficient time should be taken to allow the patient to recover from the effects of induction chemotherapy. Typically, patients are taken to surgery 6 weeks after the last round of treatment. Third, repeat imaging of the areas of abnormality should be performed prior to surgery. In occasional patients, continued involution of residual masses occurs after the completion of therapy, and surgical resection is not necessary.

Patients with persistent retroperitoneal disease undergo resection using either a midline or thoracoabdominal approach. Patients with unilateral disease in the pulmonary parenchyma or mediastinum can have resection of this supradiaphragmatic disease performed through a thoracotomy incision. Patients who have received bleomycin as part of induction chemotherapy require specialized management. These patients may have subtle restrictive pulmonary disease and diminished diffusing capacity of lung for carbon monoxide (DLCO). Care should be taken during anesthesia to avoid overhydration and to use colloid fluid replacement rather than crystalloid. Of most importance, inspired oxygen concentration should not exceed 25% in either the intraoperative or postoperative recovery period.

Resection of residual radiographic abdominal abnormalities after induction chemotherapy for disseminated nonseminomatous germ cell cancer has a complication rate significantly different from that of RPLND done for low-stage disease.[109,110] The only significant morbidity of the nerve-sparing RPLND in low-stage disease is a 1% chance of a subsequent small bowel obstruction secondary to postoperative adhesions. On the other hand, RPLND after chemotherapy is associated with a complication rate of 20% and a mortality of 0.8%. The most significant source of morbidity in this postchemotherapy group is pulmonary toxicity related to prior chemotherapy, especially bleomycin. In addition, RPLND is technically demanding, requiring frequent use of the techniques of vascular surgery, vena caval resection/repair, and varied incisions and approaches.

Overall, significant morbidity is rare and operative mortality almost nonexistent. However, the majority of patients undergoing bilateral radical retroperitoneal lymphadenectomy will be rendered infertile as a result of retrograde ejaculation. Recent developments in urologic surgery have allowed for the preservation of the sympathetic fibers that control ejaculation, while maintaining the therapeutic template of the cancer surgery. Depending on the extent of residual disease, some patients can retain ejaculatory function after undergoing resection of residual disease after chemotherapy.

The histopathologic findings in postchemotherapy surgical specimens help define the need for further treatment. In earlier reports, approximately 40% of cases revealed teratoma, 40% showed fibrous necrotic debris, and 20% had residual viable germ cell cancer. Analysis of recent series suggests that the incidence of persistent cancer is decreasing. In a study of optimal duration of chemotherapy in minimal-extent disseminated germ cell cancer, 14 of 107 patients had residual teratoma in the postchemotherapy specimen, and no patient had viable carcinoma.[111] In the same study, 19 of 77 patients with moderate-volume disease had teratoma, whereas only 6 had residual cancer. In a separate study of 153 advanced-disease patients, 30 patients had residual teratoma, and only 6 had persistent germ cell cancer.[95] This apparent decrease in the incidence of residual cancer has been reported by others and is, in part, a result of a better selection of patients for surgery and improvements in primary chemotherapy with incorporation of etoposide.

Those patients with persistent cancer that is identified and totally removed at postchemotherapy surgery require special management. If the surgical margins are free of tumor, all sites of known disease are removed, and the serum tumor markers remain normal, patients should usually receive two postoperative cycles of cisplatin-based therapy similar to induction therapy, but without further bleomycin.[104] Some authors, however, advocate observation only in such cases. Those patients with unresectable disease, positive surgical margins, or elevated tumor markers should be considered for full salvage therapy using new agents and more prolonged courses of therapy. Approximately two-thirds of patients receiving additional postoperative cisplatin-based chemotherapy after total resection of residual viable cancer will remain free of disease.[112]

Chemotherapy of Seminoma Modern chemotherapy series involving patients with bulky stage II or stage III disseminated seminoma report cure rates of more than 90%.[50] When compared with earlier studies of radiotherapy in this setting where cure rates ranged from 20 to 60%, cisplatin-based chemotherapy is clearly the treatment of choice in this clinical presentation. The role of single-agent carboplatin in patients with advanced seminoma has also been explored, but standard initial therapy remains cisplatin combinations.

Patients with nonpulmonary visceral involvement with seminoma do less well and are classified as intermediate risk.[97] Good-risk patients usually receive EP × 4 or BEP × 3 and intermediate-risk patients receive BEP × 4.

An additional area of controversy is the management of patients with residual radiographic abnormalities after completion of cisplatin-based combination chemotherapy. Motzer and colleagues report results of 41 patients with bulky stage II, stage III, or stage IV disease treated with cisplatin-based combination chemotherapy.[113] At the completion of therapy, 23 patients had significant residual radiographic abnormalities, including 14 patients with masses ≥ 3 cm in size. Of these 23 patients, 19 underwent surgical exploration, and 5 were found to have significant findings other than fibrosis (4 viable seminoma and 1 teratoma). The authors recommend biopsy of residual radiographic abnormalities after chemotherapy for seminoma if the residual disease measures ≥ 3 cm.

At Indiana University and other centers, a different policy has been adopted. Surgery in this setting is extremely difficult because the surgeon commonly encounters a dense desmoplastic reaction. Also, these patients are older, sometimes have had abdominal radiotherapy as well as chemotherapy, and, as in several series, are prone to operative mortalities.[113] A review of seminoma from Indiana reports only a 10% incidence of relapse in the setting of residual radiographic disease greater than 3 cm postchemotherapy.[114] There was no evidence in this series that risk of recurrence was related to the diameter of the residual mass. At Indiana University, close observation is the recommended approach in this setting. PET scans may be a useful predictor of viable tumor in postchemotherapy residuals of patients with pure seminoma greater than 3 cm.[115]

In the past, radiation therapy for postchemotherapy residual masses had been considered; however, very few of these masses contain seminoma. Furthermore, the curability with radiation is questionable if chemotherapy does not cure the patient. In addition, the risk of long-term complications, including leukemia, is increased when both chemotherapy and radiation are employed. Therefore, radiation for residual masses should not be performed.[37]

Salvage Chemotherapy Despite the dramatic successes of chemotherapy in disseminated germ cell tumors, 20 to 30% of all such patients will fail to achieve durable complete remission with first-line therapy.[116] These individuals, as well as those who relapse from complete remission, are candidates for salvage chemotherapy. Because of the decreased efficacy and increased toxicity of second-line chemotherapy, this represents an important decision in the treatment of such patients and requires the expertise of individuals well versed in the intricacies of careful assessment of patients with germ cell tumors and of therapeutic options for this stage of testicular cancer.

Patient Selection There are several clinical situations that may mimic persistent, progressive, or recurrent disease. One such situation involves the appearance of nodular lesions on the chest radiograph or chest CT scan at the end of chemotherapy or soon after completion of such therapy.[1] These nodules usually represent bleomycin-induced pulmonary injury and are characteristically located in a subpleural region. This possibility should be considered in a patient who is otherwise responding serologically or radiographically and has new abnormalities in the lungs in separate sites from the original disease.

Another clinical situation frequently mistaken for progressive disease is the syndrome of growing teratoma.[117] Radiographically enlarging metastatic lesions during chemotherapy concurrently with normal serologic markers often represent teratoma. Appropriate management of such a patient is surgical resection of residual radiographic abnormalities rather than administration of salvage chemotherapy. The causes of misinterpretation of tumor markings are detailed earlier in this chapter in the section "Tumor Markers" under the section "Clinical Presentation."

In general, a conservative policy is to reserve the initiation of salvage therapy until there is a demonstration of rising markers on serial determinations. The vagaries of interpretation of low-level marker elevation makes such a policy necessary to ensure that patients are not treated with intensive salvage chemotherapy on the basis of a false-positive marker elevation.

The possibility of occult central nervous system (CNS) metastasis should be considered in the setting of systemic sustained remission and elevation of serum tumor markers. In this situation, CT scans or magnetic resonance imaging (MRI) of the brain should be performed, along with evaluations for a testicular sanctuary site. The CNS evaluation should proceed even in the absence of clinical signs or symptoms if the only evidence of progressive disease is a rising marker.

The other important sanctuary site from chemotherapy in germ cell cancer is the testis. In most settings, the primary in the testis has been removed in the initial diagnostic process. However, in some patients presenting with advanced disease, chemotherapy is initiated without a tissue diagnosis. In such cases, the testis must be removed at the completion of chemotherapy, even if the primary tumor is no longer evident. The possibility of a metachronous testicular primary or an occult testicular primary should also be entertained.

Standard Salvage Therapy The therapeutic results with salvage chemotherapy have not been as dramatic as those for initial therapy, primarily because of the paucity of active single agents in patients refractory to cisplatin. During the three decades since the introduction of cisplatin, several agents, etoposide (VP-16), ifosfamide, paclitaxel, and gemcitabine have demonstrated activity in platinum-refractory patients.

The salvage chemotherapy regimen that serves as a basis for comparison is the regimen of vinblastine, ifosfamide, and cisplatin (VeIP) reported at Indiana University.[118] One hundred thirty-five patients who had not progressed during cisplatin-based therapy received VeIP as initial salvage chemotherapy. Toxicity of the regimen in this pretreated population was significant, with 71% developing granulocytopenic fever. Transfusions of platelets (27%) and red blood cells (49%) were common. Renal insufficiency (serum creatinine > 4 mg%) was observed in 7% of patients. Three patients died of causes related to treatment. Despite the formidable toxicity, the therapeutic results were gratifying. Fifty-six patients (45%) achieved a disease-free status with either chemotherapy alone (34 patients, 25%), or by resection of teratoma (15 patients, 12%), or of viable carcinoma (7 patients, 6%). Twenty-nine (21%) of these patients are continuously disease free, and 37 (30%) are currently disease free (minimum follow-up, 5 years). Among the patients with extragonadal primaries, only 6 of

31 attained disease-free status, and only 1 is continuously disease free. These results have been confirmed by other investigators.[119]

Investigators from Memorial Sloan-Kettering Cancer Center have evaluated a regimen consisting of paclitaxel plus ifosfamide plus cisplatin (TIP) as second-line therapy for patients with favorable prognostic features, but relapsed testicular cancers.[120] In that study 23 of 30 patients (77%) achieved a complete response to chemotherapy alone, and an additional patient achieved a durable partial remission with normal markers. Only 2 patients relapsed. This study underscores the importance of patient selection to favorable responses with standard salvage chemotherapy.

Separate information suggests that recurrent seminoma may be uniquely sensitive to salvage chemotherapy. Miller and colleagues at Indiana University reported the results of VeIP in patients with seminoma recurring after primary cisplatin/etoposide-based treatment.[122] Of these 23 patients, 19 (83%) achieved disease-free status, and 13 (56%) are continuously free of disease.

HIGH-DOSE CHEMOTHERAPY AS INITIAL SALVAGE THERAPY

High-dose chemotherapy has been studied as initial salvage chemotherapy. One of the first reports of such an approach is from Barnett and colleagues at the Cancer Control Agency of British Columbia.[123] They reported the results of 18 patients with recurrent or persistent germ cell cancer after cisplatin-based primary therapy who were given conventional induction chemotherapy with cisplatin, etoposide, vincristine, and bleomycin on a weekly schedule or vinblastine, ifosfamide, cisplatin combinations. At the completion of conventional salvage chemotherapy, consolidation with high-dose chemotherapy was given with autologous bone marrow support. Patients received high-dose carboplatin, etoposide, and either cyclophosphamide or ifosfamide. There were 2 toxic deaths, it was too early to evaluate 2 patients, and 8 of 14 patients remained free of progression of germ cell cancer.

Investigators from Germany have evaluated 80 patients treated with three cycles of TIP with high-dose carboplatin, etoposide, and thiotepa followed by autologous stem cell rescue in patients with relapsed or refractory germ cell tumors and report a response rate of 69% and a 3-year overall survival of 30%.[123] This regimen was associated with significant toxicity and survival results that were not superior to VeIP for four cycles.

Siegert and colleagues in Germany reported the results of high-dose carboplatin, etoposide, and ifosfamide in the treatment of recurrent testicular cancer.[125] Patients received two induction courses of conventional-dose cisplatin, etoposide, and ifosfamide prior to receiving escalated therapy. Seventy-four patients received treatment with conventional therapy, followed by carboplatin 1,500 to 2,000 mg/m^2, etoposide 1,200 to 2,400 mg/m^2, and ifosfamide 0 to 10 g/m^2. Two patients (3%) died of causes related to treatment. Responses included 21 patients (28%) with complete remission with chemotherapy alone or with adjunctive surgery and 14 (19%) patients with marker-negative partial remission. Twenty-five of these patients (34%) maintained their response from 31 to 261 months.

At Indiana University, 65 patients with relapsed testicular cancer were treated with high-dose carboplatin plus etoposide followed by tandem peripheral blood stem cell transplant or autologous bone marrow transplant on a phase II trial.[125] Fifty-seven percent of patients remain continuously disease free at a median follow-up of 39 months. Three additional patients were rendered disease free following salvage surgery.

From these data, we conclude that such an approach is safe and compares favorably with historical data using VeIP as salvage therapy. Our current approach is to give a single cycle of VeIP followed by tandem high-dose cycles of carboplatin 2,100 mg/m^2 and etoposide 2,250 mg/m^2. An additional "wrinkle" to this protocol is the use of maintenance oral etoposide for patients obtaining a complete remission.[126]

TREATMENT OF MULTIPLY RECURRENT GERM CELL CANCER

High-Dose Chemotherapy for Multiply Recurrent Germ Cell Cancer Investigations into the use of high-dose carboplatin (CBCDA) and etoposide (VP-16) with autologous bone marrow support began at Indiana University in 1986. Initial investigations were on patients who were heavily pretreated and for whom no other curative therapeutic options existed.

The initial phase I/II dose escalation study examined the use of two courses of high-dose CBDCA and VP-16 in patients with germ cell tumors refractory to cisplatin (defined as progression after or within 4 weeks of the last cisplatin dose) or recurrent after primary therapy with cisplatin-based therapy and a salvage therapy with an ifosfamide-cisplatin combination.[127] Thirty-three patients were entered into the trial. Overall, 7 (21%) of the patients died as a consequence of treatment. Deaths were primarily caused by infection, although one patient died of veno-occlusive disease of the liver. Of note, this was a very heavily pretreated patient population with more than half the patients having received three or more prior chemotherapy regimens, and 67% of patients were cisplatin refractory. Eight patients obtained a complete remission and 6 had a partial remission, for an overall response rate of 44% (95% confidence interval, 27–63%). Of the eight patients attaining complete remission, 3 are long-term disease-free survivors, and a fourth patient died at 22 months, free of germ cell cancer, from a therapy-related acute myeloid leukemia.[128] An overview of the experience at Indiana University with the first 40 patients with multiply relapsed and refractory germ cell cancer treated with double autologous transplantation demonstrated a 15% long-term disease-free survival.[129] These results have been confirmed in a similar multi-institutional trial performed by the ECOG.[130]

Other Investigations Other investigators have reported similar results using high-dose chemotherapy in patients with multiply relapsed testicular cancer. Taken as a whole, several conclusions can be drawn. First, high-dose chemotherapy can cure 15 to 20% of patients experiencing multiple relapses of germ cell cancer. Patients with germ cell cancer who are overtly cisplatin refractory have a significantly diminished chance of permanent disease control (less than 5%). Second, therapy-related mortality in this heavily treated patient population is now < 5%. Third, there is no standard high-dose salvage regimen. Last, in all these studies, patients with mediastinal nonseminomatous primary tumors fared particularly poorly and represent a group of patients who do not benefit from high-dose chemotherapy.

Salvage Surgery Some patients in the salvage setting are best approached with salvage surgery rather than chemotherapy. This is especially true for late relapsers or patients with relapsed disease confined to a single anatomic site. Indiana University has performed a retrospective review of all patients who were felt to have chemotherapy-refractory disease and were submitted to surgery for attempts at curative resection.[131] All patients had serologic or other evidence of progressive cancer. A total of 48 patients were reviewed, the majority of whom underwent isolated retroperitoneal lymphadenectomy (33 patients). Of these patients, 38 (79%) were rendered free of gross disease by surgery, and 29 (60%) attained a serologic remission. Ten patients (21%) remain continuously free of disease with follow-up ranging from 31 to 89 months. Six additional patients are currently disease free, with additional surgery (4 patients) or high-dose chemotherapy with autologous bone marrow transplantation. Clinical benefit was obtained only in that group of patients with a solitary site of disease at the time of surgery. Patients with multiple sites of metastasis, although resectable, were not cured. In carefully selected patients with chemotherapy-incurable disease, salvage surgery does offer a significant prospect of long-term disease-free survival. Such decisions about surgeries should be made at centers with significant experience in germ cell tumor management.

New Agents The development of new active compounds offers the best hope of truly changing the prospect for cure in recurrent or resistant germ cell tumors, as well as better therapy for patients presenting with poor-risk features. Several classes of drugs are being investigated, including oxaliplatin,[132] the taxanes, and gemcitabine. A phase II study from ECOG evaluated the combination of paclitaxel and gemcitabine in 30 patients with refractory germ cell tumors.[133] The overall response rate was 21.4%, including 3 patients with complete remission CRs. Two patients remain continuously disease free for 15+ and 25+ months.

SPECIAL SITUATIONS

Late Relapse Of patients with disseminated testicular cancer who relapse after achieving a complete remission, most will suffer a recurrence within the first year following therapy, and the overwhelming majority within 2 years. A late relapse in this disease is generally accepted to be one that appears after a disease-free interval of more than 24 months. Late relapses following complete remission occur in 2 to 3% of cases, with recurrences as late as 32 years following complete remission. Those patients who have had recurrences with isolated mature teratoma in general have done well following excision, whereas those with marker-positive carcinoma have tended to recur with large-volume disease and have had less favorable responses to additional chemotherapy and/or surgery.

At Indiana University, 81 patients were analyzed retrospectively who had recurrence of germ cell tumor after 2 or more years of being disease free.[134] Sixty percent of these patients had recurrences after > 5 years (maximum was 32 years). Serum marker elevation was seen, with 56% of patients having an elevated α-fetoprotein and 27% of patients an elevated HCG. Fifteen patients (19%) had a recurrence of teratoma, 8 are continuously free of disease, and 4 patients are currently free of disease after further surgery (271–1,021 months). Seven patients experienced recurrence with sarcomatous elements (with or without teratoma); 4 are currently disease free. Fifty-nine patients had germ cell carcinoma as their initial late recurrence. Only 10 of these patients (17%) are continuously disease free (101–781 months). Nine other patients are currently disease free. Aggressive surgery was required in almost all these patients. Overall, 65 patients received cisplatin-based chemotherapy, and 17 (26%) achieved a disease-free status with chemotherapy with or without adjunctive surgery. Twelve of the 17 have relapsed. Only 2 patients treated with chemotherapy alone are continuously free of disease (neither of these patients had received previous chemotherapy). A second series at Indiana University of 77 additional patients demonstrate similar findings.[135] Based on these data, surgical resection for late relapse remains our preferred approach.

Although the appearance of late relapses is relatively rare, these data support current recommendations for continued lifetime follow-up. We recommend follow-up every 6 months for 2 to 5 years and then annually. If postchemotherapy surgery was done with bulky teratoma resection, abdominal CTs should also be included during the next 5 years of follow-up.

LONG-TERM TOXICITY OF CHEMOTHERAPY

Since the mid-1970s, the majority of testicular cancer patients with disseminated disease have been cured with combination chemotherapy. Late complications of curative therapy have been seen in other malignancies, most notably Hodgkin's disease (eg, sterility, therapy-related second malignancies). Concerns about similar late effects of cisplatin-based therapy have been raised, and information is now available on a significant number of patients with follow-up of more than 10 years.

Nephrotoxicity The acute effects of cisplatin on both renal glomerular and tubular functions are well documented, with decreases in both glomerular filtration rate (GFR) and effective renal plasma flow (ERPF) accompanied by magnesium wasting and elevated levels of 02-microglobulin, indicative of proximal tubule dysfunction. Most investigators have reported that the acute decreases in GFR and ERPF do not deteriorate further during the months to years following completion of chemotherapy; however, long-term subclinical impairment is frequently found.[136–138]

Vascular Toxicity Raynaud's phenomenon is the most common vascular toxicity seen in patients following chemotherapy for testicular cancer. Although anecdotally reported after therapy with single-agent bleomycin, it is much more common following combination therapy. Vogelzang and colleagues reported a 21% incidence of this phenomenon in patients treated with vinblastine plus bleomycin, as compared with 41% when cisplatin was added to these two drugs.[140] Studies employing provocative testing suggest that even asymptomatic individuals may exhibit an exaggerated vasospastic response to cold stimuli.[140] The onset of the phenomenon tends to be delayed, with a median time to appearance of symptoms of 10 months. Symptoms persist indefinitely, with 49% of patients in one series reporting continued symptoms at a median of 8.5 years from completion of therapy. The vasospasm has, in general, been refractory to therapy, although some success has been reported with the calcium channel blocker nifedipine.[141] The replacement of vinblastine by VP-16 in combination therapy with cisplatin and bleomycin has not reduced the incidence of Raynaud's phenomenon.[142]

The relationship of cisplatin-based chemotherapy to large-vessel ischemic events is less clear. There are case reports of myocardial ischemia and infarction, as well as cerebrovascular accidents, following vinblastine administration as a single agent or combined with bleomycin. Several anecdotal reports of major cardiovascular events in young men receiving chemotherapy for testicular cancer suggested a causal association between chemotherapeutic treatments and these events.[93,143,144] Weijl and colleagues identified patients with liver metastases or those receiving high-dose corticosteroids to be at high risk of developing thromboembolic complications.[146] To evaluate the true risk of acute vascular events in patients receiving cisplatin-based chemotherapy for testicular cancer, questionnaires to assess cardiovascular toxicity were distributed to all participants in the Testicular Cancer Intergroup Study, and toxicity reviews from the chemotherapy flow sheets were conducted.[146] Patients with pathologic stage I testicular cancer were registered in the study and observed after retroperitoneal lymphadenectomy. Patients with pathologic stage II disease were randomized to receiving two postoperative courses of adjuvant cisplatin-based chemotherapy or observation. Any patient who experienced a recurrence after observation or adjuvant therapy was given four cycles of cisplatin-based chemotherapy.

A review of toxicity of treatment in those patients receiving adjuvant chemotherapy (n = 97) or chemotherapy for recurrent disease (n = 83) revealed no cases of acute cardiovascular toxicity. When the median follow-up after study enrollment was 5.1 years, 459 questionnaires were mailed, and 270 were returned. The percentage of returns was equal among the observed, adjuvant, and recurrent groups (59%, 54%, and 64%, respectively). There was a significant increase in the incidence of extremity paresthesias in the two groups receiving chemotherapy. Fatal myocardial infarction was reported in two patients in the observation group, and one nonfatal infarct was reported in the adjuvant treatment group. No patient in any group reported stroke. Three patients in the observation group and one patient in the recurrent group experienced a thromboembolic event. Despite sporadic case reports suggesting a causal association between chemotherapy for testicular cancer and acute vascular events, this retrospective analysis provides no evidence of an increased risk of subsequent cardiovascular disease in this patient population. However, longer follow-up may reveal hypertension, unfavorable lipid profiles, and vascular events.[147] All patients should be followed indefinitely for evidence of late relapse. Also, they need good medical management with weight reduction, smoking cessation, lipid profile monitoring, and appropriate blood pressure management. Patients and their treating physicians should remain cognizant of a persisting unfavorable cardiovascular risk profile in long-term survivors.[148,149]

Neurotoxicity The peripheral neuropathy and ototoxicity observed in treated testicular cancer patients are attributable primarily to cisplatin, with a somewhat lesser contribution in older studies by vinblastine. The peripheral effects became manifest clinically as a distal sensory neuropathy, with paresthesias and dysesthesias, disturbances of position and vibratory sensation, and relative sparing of motor units.[150] Subjectively, these symptoms may be present for prolonged periods, with 43% of patients in one study reporting persistent symptoms 6 to 12 years after completion of therapy.[151] Objective studies confirm in 1984 the irreversibility of the neuropathy and suggest that the dorsal root ganglion represents the primary target of cisplatin-induced damage.

The ototoxicity associated with cisplatin administration is represented primarily by high-frequency hearing loss and is related to the cumulative dose of cisplatin.[152,153] Other risk factors for the development of ototoxicity include a serum creatinine level higher than 1.5 mg/dL, increased age, and preexisting hearing impairment.

Second Malignancies Case reports and clinical alerts suggest that treatment with high-dose etoposide can result in the development of a unique secondary leukemia. To estimate the risk of developing leukemia in the more common clinical setting of patients receiving conventional doses of etoposide along with cisplatin and bleomycin, we reviewed records of patients with germ cell cancer entering clinical protocols using etoposide at Indiana University.[154] Between 1982 and 1991, 538 patients entered serial clinical trials, with planned etoposide doses from 1,500 mg/m^2 to 2,000 mg/m^2 in combination with cisplatin plus either ifosfamide or bleomycin. Of these, 348 patients received an etoposide combination as initial chemotherapy, and 190 patients received etoposide as part of salvage treatment. In all, 315 patients are alive, and 337 patients have been followed up beyond 2 years. The median follow-up for patients still alive is 4.9 years. Two patients (0.37%) developed leukemia. One patient developed acute undifferentiated leukemia with a t(4:11)(q21:q23) cytogenetic abnormality 2.3 years after starting etoposide-based therapy, and one patient developed acute myelomonoblastic leukemia with normal chromosome studies 2 years after beginning chemotherapy. During this period, a number of patients were seen outside clinical trials, and we are aware of several hematologic abnormalities in this group, including one patient with acute monoblastic leukemia with a t(11:19)(q13:p13) abnormality. Secondary leukemia after treatment with chemotherapy including conventional-dose etoposide does occur. However, this low incidence of secondary leukemia does not alter the risk-benefit ratio of etoposide-based chemotherapy for germ cell cancer.[129] No significantly elevated risk of secondary solid tumors was observed after chemotherapy in a large series by Bokemeyer and Schmoll.[156]

Fertility Before the effects of therapy on fertility are examined, it must be recognized that up to 80% of testicular cancer patients will be oligospermic at diagnosis, prior to the initiation of any therapy.[156] Although the etiology of this oligospermia is unknown, several mechanisms have been proposed, including an autoimmune process or a primary endocrine dysfunction resulting in impaired spermatogenesis.[157,158]

The chemotherapy administered for testicular cancer has acute effects on both spermatogenesis and Leydig cell function; most patients remain azoospermic with elevated serum gonadotropins for the first 12 months following therapy. These toxic effects are reversible in a significant number of patients, however, as approximately 50% will see a return of both spermatogenesis and Leydig cell function during the second year after completion of therapy.[159,160] Several factors decrease the likelihood of the return of spermatogenesis, including age over 30 years, treatment duration of more than 6 months, and prior abdominal radiotherapy.[161,162] In the Indiana University experience, at least one-third of patients treated with chemotherapy alone have been able to father children without congenital anomalies, confirming previous data. Bohlen and colleagues reported that two cycles of adjuvant cisplatin-based chemotherapy given to patients with high-risk stage I germ cell tumors does not adversely affect fertility or sexual activity.[164] Lampe and colleagues, in an analysis of 170 patients, report that the probability of spermatogenesis increased after orchiectomy and cisplatin-based chemotherapy to 48% by 2 years and to 80% by 5 years.[165]

Pulmonary Toxicity Bleomycin is solely responsible for the pulmonary toxicity observed in chemotherapy-treated testicular cancer patients. Pulmonary fibrosis develops in approximately 5% of individuals and can be fatal.[165] This toxicity is directly related to cumulative dose, with a significant increase above 450 units. The earliest physical finding of bleomycin-induced pulmonary injury is an inspiratory lag and should prompt immediate discontinuation of the drug. Subsequent signs and symptoms include bibasilar rales, nonproductive cough, and exertional dyspnea. Laboratory abnormalities include decreases in DLCO and late changes, including hypoxia and hypercapnia. Radiographic abnormalities include the appearance of subpleural-based nodules, visible on the chest radiograph or chest CT scan.

The risk of developing symptomatic bleomycin-induced lung disease increases with age > 70 years, prior or concomitant chest radiotherapy,[84,166] decreased renal function,[167] and high concentrations of inspired oxygen. Because the mortality for this condition approaches 50% and therapeutic interventions, such as corticosteroids, are ineffective, early diagnosis of asymptomatic patients and subsequent discontinuation of the drug are particularly important. The incidence of clinically significant bleomycin toxicity is negligible, however, with three cycles of BEP.

LONG-TERM TOXICITY OF RADIATION THERAPY

Toxicity of Radiation **Acute** Acute radiation toxicity is dependent on what anatomical organs are irradiated, the radiation dose, and the volume. Two MRC trials have prospectively recorded the acute toxicity of radiation and demonstrate specifically how volume and dose contribute to toxicity. MRC TE10 trial randomized patients to PA only or PA with an ipsilateral pelvic field (dog-leg [DL]).[168] The acute toxicity of nausea/vomiting was similar but slightly higher in the DL arm. As expected the DL field would not include much more small bowel than the PA area (p = .08). Nevertheless, both groups experienced nausea requiring medication in 25 to 30% of patients treated. For leukopenia where the DL treats much more bone marrow, the rates of mild leucopenia were almost twice as high when compared with the PA field alone. Nineteen percent experienced clinically detectable leucopenia for the PA arm versus 42% for the ipsilateral pelvic field arm ($p < .0001$). Additionally, diarrhea was reported in only 7% of the PA arm only, but 14% in the ipsilateral pelvic field arm (p = .013).

In the recently reported MRC TE18 trial comparing 30 Gy with 20 Gy, patients were asked to complete a daily symptom diary in addition to their physician-recorded symptoms. The patients who received 20 Gy appeared to have less nausea than the patients who received the higher dose (p = .06). Leukopenia was also less (p = .02). Significantly more patients receiving 30 Gy reported moderate or severe lethargy (20% vs 5%) and an inability to carry out their normal work (46% vs 28%). But by 12 weeks, the two groups were similar. The lower doses and smaller fields reduce the acute toxicity without compromising treatment and, additionally, should lower the chronic and late sequelae of radiation.

The initial potentially permanent side effect patients and their physicians deal with is infertility. The threshold for temporary sterility for temporary aspermia is around 0.40 Gy for repeated exposures.[59,78] For a single dose, a dose as low as 0.15 Gy may cause temporary aspermia. Permanent sterility occurs after 2 to 3.5 Gy. Hormonal changes require much higher doses and are not detectable based on testosterone. Subtle Leydig cell dysfunction, as measured by serum FSH and LH concentrations, occur at exposures greater than 2 Gy.[155] For a DL field, the incidental amount of radiation to the remaining testicle averages 0.78 Gy over the course of treatment.[8,169] For a PA field, the dose is even lower, around 0.20 Gy.[59] The difference in testicular dose depending on the treated field is illustrated by the MRC TE10 trial comparing the DL and PA with the PA field alone. The median time to the first "normal" post-treatment sperm count was 13 months for PA patients and 20 months for DL patients, despite the fact that scrotal shielding was used in 63% of the DL patients and only 3% of the PA patients.[170] Testicular shielding with a clam shell reduces the dose to the testes by a 3- to 10-fold reduction.[78] For a patient who is concerned about fertility, the radiation dose can easily be lowered to below the threshold where permanent spermatogenesis is affected. But because the majority of patients with seminoma tend to have a lower sperm count at baseline, before adjuvant radiation, appropriate counseling and semen cryopreservation should be considered in patients who wish to preserve fertility.[171,172]

Chronic The avoidance of chronic toxicity or permanent late effects has raised the profile of surveillance as a preferred treatment option. The two major sources of morbidity and mortality are cardiac toxicity and second malignancies. Because radiation for seminoma used to incorporate a mediastinal field, cardiac toxicity developed in many patients. A recent review of patients registered in the United Kingdom from 1982 through 1992 demonstrated that survivors were at a twofold or greater risk of developing cardiovascular disease. Only 8% of patients received mediastinal radiation. A small study was performed to determine whether the PA fields included cardiac tissue. On average, 14% of the cardiac volume received only a dose of 0.9 Gy. Whether the increased cardiac toxicity can be attributed to PA radiation is in doubt because the increased risk of cardiovascular disease was seen in patients treated with chemotherapy alone.[169] Zagars reviewed the M. D. Anderson experience of all 477 men with stage I or II testicular seminoma treated between 1951 and 1999.[173,174] After a median follow-up of 13.3 years, the cardiac-specific standardized mortality ratio was 1.61, while the cancer-specific standardized mortality ratio was 1.91. Both toxicities were only evident after 15 years of follow-up. Fifteen years may represent the latency period for chronic toxicity to develop, but it may also demonstrate that radiation treatment doses and fields prior to 1990 are much more toxic relative to more modern practices.

The risk of second malignancies for patients treated with historical methods around the advent of platinum-based chemotherapy was quantified in a large international population-based cancer registry study.[174] Almost 29,000 survivors of testicular cancer were identified, having been diagnosed from as early as 1935 up to 1993.[175] For patients with seminomas, the observed-to-expected ratio of cancers overall was 1.43. Leukemias were seen as much as 5.2 times the expected rate, and the rate for developing solid tumors was 1.54 times that expected. The increased risk of solid tumors began at 10 years after the diagnosis, whereas the increased risk of leukemias was seen within the first 20 years after the diagnosis. These results are instructive, but difficult to extrapolate to current practices given the majority of the patients were treated at a time when a cure was much more difficult to obtain. Nonetheless, these results dictate our primary objectives of maintaining our high cure rates, while further reducing the long-term impact of our therapies.

Sanctuary Sites and CNS Metastases It is quite uncommon for patients to present with CNS metastasis as an initial manifestation of metastatic testicular cancer. In a study of patients with advanced disease, only 6 of 159 (4%) patients had CNS involvement at the time of the original diagnosis.[176] The rarity of this presentation makes CNS prophylaxis inappropriate for any subset of patients with advanced germ cell cancer. In patients with advanced hematogenous metastases or large-volume choriocarcinoma, however, clinical suspicion should be heightened and careful investigation of even minor CNS symptoms is warranted.

Patients with CNS involvement, either as a part of the initial presentation or as a manifestation of relapse, should be approached with curative intent. Patients with CNS disease accompanying other systemic involvement should receive whole-brain radiotherapy (4,000–5,000 cGy in 5–6 weeks) along with appropriate systemic chemotherapy.[176] Patients relapsing with a solitary CNS metastasis without involvement of other sites undergo resection followed by CNS radiotherapy and two postoperative courses of "adjuvant" cisplatin-based chemotherapy.

The other important sanctuary site from chemotherapy in germ cell cancer is the testis. In most settings, the testicular primary was removed in the initial diagnostic process. However, in some patients presenting with advanced disease, chemotherapy is initiated without a tissue diagnosis. In such cases, the testis must be removed at the completion of chemotherapy even if the primary tumor is no longer evident.

The possibility of a metachronous contralateral testis primary must, at times, be entertained. In the setting of complete radiographic remission of systemic disease and a persistent or new elevation of serum tumor markers, the remaining testicle should be carefully examined and testicular ultrasonography be performed to rule out an occult primary in the remaining testis. For patients with a metachronous contralateral testis, organ-sparing surgery is now a viable option to preserve fertility.[177]

EXTRAGONADAL GERM CELL TUMORS

Germ cell tumors arise predominantly from within the testis, but an important subset of germ cell tumors are extragonadal in origin. Overall, approximately 5 to 10% of all germ cell cancers arise in nongonadal sites, particularly in the mediastinum and retroperitoneum. The initial theory regarding the genesis of these tumors was that they represented metastasis from an occult gonadal primary. Luna and colleagues reported the results of autopsy findings in 20 patients with extragonadal mediastinal germ cell tumors and found only one case of a testicular primary and one patient with a testicular scar.[178] Both these cases were associated with clinically occult lower retroperitoneal involvement. Primary retroperitoneal germ cell tumors are more commonly associated with an occult testicular primary site, especially when the tumor is not midline in origin.

There is now general acceptance that extragonadal germ cell tumors represent malignant transformation of germinal elements distributed to these sites without a testicular focus. Some investigators suggest that this distribution is a consequence of abnormal cell migration during embryogenesis, while others have suggested that there is widespread distribution of germ cells to the liver, thymus, bone marrow, and brain, and that these cells provide important regulatory functions at these sites or convey important genetic hematologic or immunologic information.

In adults, the mediastinum is the most common extragonadal site for the development of germ cell tumors.[179,180] The most common tumor in this site is mature teratoma.[181] This diagnosis can be suggested by the presence of a large circumscribed anterior mediastinal mass with normal serum HCG and α-fetoprotein. Management of mature teratoma is surgical, and there is no role for chemotherapy or radiotherapy. Although these tumors histologically are benign, removal is often difficult. The tumors are commonly adherent to adjacent structures, such as the pericardium, lung, and great vessels. Nonetheless, in this era of modern thoracic surgery, excellent outcome is the rule.[182] In a series from the Mayo Clinic, 64 of 69 patients were long-term survivors. Four of the remaining patients died as the result of surgical complications.

The principles of management of extragonadal nonseminomatous germ cell tumors parallel those of testicular germ cell cancer. The diagnosis should be considered in any young person with a poorly differentiated cancer arising in midline structures. Serum tumor markers should be obtained and, if the clinical condition is stable, a biopsy also should be obtained. In most settings, heroic efforts at surgical debulking should not be considered part of primary management. Cisplatin-based chemotherapy should be given as with testicular germ cell cancer. However, cure rates for nonseminomatous germ cell tumors of mediastinal origin are significantly inferior compared with those of testicular origin. An international analysis of 635 patients with extragonadal germ cell tumors demonstrated an almost 90% change of cure with pure seminoma irrespective of the primary site, but only 45% survival at 5 years for patients with mediastinal nonseminomatous tumors.[183]

Patients with residual radiographic abnormalities after completing chemotherapy should be considered for surgical extirpation of residual disease if elevated tumor markers have normalized. Vuky and colleagues report the surgical results of 32 patients with nonseminoma germ cell tumors arising from the mediastinum who underwent adjunctive surgery following chemotherapy.[184] Viable tumor was discovered in 66% of patients and teratoma in 22%.

Several important biologic associations with mediastinal nonseminomatous germ cell tumors have been described. There is a very high frequency of Klinefelter syndrome in patients with mediastinal nonseminomatous germ cell tumors. Two large series report an association in up to 20% of patients with Klinefelter syndrome.[11,185]

Approximately 10% of patients with mediastinal nonseminomatous germ cell tumors develop associated malignant hematologic dyscrasias. Between 1976 and 1989, of the 40 patients with mediastinal nonseminomatous germ cell tumors at Indiana University, 6 developed a hematologic malignancy.[29] In addition, 11 other patients were referred to Indiana University or case material was forwarded for evaluation of this association. Of this group of patients, 6 developed acute megakaryoblastic leukemia, 5 had acute nonlymphocytic leukemia (not M-7), 2 developed a virulent myelodysplastic syndrome, 2 were found to have extramedullary megakaryocytic myelosis, and 2 presented with massively elevated platelet counts and cytogenetic abnormalities or excess blasts in the marrow. The median time to the development of the hematologic abnormalities was 6 months, with 5 of the patients having simultaneous presentations of the two disorders. Thirty-three similar patients have been reported in the literature. The median interval between the two diagnoses in this review was 5 months, with 13 cases presenting simultaneously. A retrospective review of 287 patients with nonseminomatous mediastinal germ cell tumors revealed 17 patients with hematologic disorders with a median time of onset occurring 6 months after the diagnosis of germ cell tumor and a median survival of only 5 months after the diagnosis of the hematologic disorder.[186]

Careful clinical and cytogenetic analyses of these cases suggest that these tumors do not arise as a consequence of therapy for germ cell tumors, but represent a unique and biologically important association between these disorders. Similar cases are not found among those patients with testicular or retroperitoneal germ cell cancer treated with identical chemotherapy. Most compelling, however, is the finding of the most common karyotypic abnormality of germ cell cancer, isochromosome 12p, in a mediastinal germ cell tumor and in the leukemic blasts of one of these patients.[187] This implies that the mediastinal germ cell tumor and the hematologic malignancy arose from a common progenitor cell.

There are associations of mediastinal nonseminomatous germ cell tumors with other nonhematologic, nongerm cell tumors. In a review of germ cell tumor specimens seen at Indiana University from 1974 to 1982, Ulbright and colleagues found 269 cases of teratoma-containing material, including 209 testicular, 28 retroperitoneal, and 32 mediastinal primary sites.[188] Among this group of patients, 11 were identified who demonstrated malignant nongerm cell elements, including such variants as embryonal rhabdomyosarcoma, adenosquamous carcinoma, leiomyosarcoma, Wilms' tumor, and glioblastoma multiforme. They were identified prior to the initiation of therapy in 10 of the 11 cases. In patients with multiple samples available, histologic progression was often identified, moving from atypical features to overt nongerm cell elements. The authors suggest that these malignant nongerm cell elements are derived from the teratomatous elements within the tumor. Of particular interest, 3 of the 11 cases were patients with mediastinal primaries (27%), whereas mediastinal primaries made up only 12% of cases reviewed.

UNRECOGNIZED GERM CELL TUMOR SYNDROME

On occasion, a patient will present with a clinical picture compatible with an extragonadal germ cell tumor, but without corroborating serologic or histopathologic evidence of a germ cell tumor. Work done at Vanderbilt University by Greco and colleagues suggests that such patients should undergo a very thorough histopathologic evaluation and, in some cases, receive empiric cisplatin-based chemotherapy.[189] The clinical features of the "unrecognized germ cell tumor syndrome" include patients younger than 50 years of age; tumor primarily involving the midline (mediastinum or retroperitoneum), lungs (in the form of multiple pulmonary nodules), or lymph nodes; an elevated βHCG or α-fetoprotein; or clinical evidence of rapid tumor growth. Seventy-one prospectively identified patients fitting this description were classified as having poorly differentiated carcinoma or poorly differentiated adenocarcinoma, and one or more of the above clinical features. Results of serologic investigation in this patient population revealed normal α-fetoprotein and HCG in 51 of these patients. Thirteen patients had elevation of one marker, and 5 had elevation of both markers. Light microscopy revealed poorly differentiated carcinoma in 48 patients (68%), poorly differentiated adenocarcinoma in 18 patients (25%), and poorly differentiated large-cell carcinoma in 5 patients (7%). Electron microscopy resulted in a change in the histologic diagnosis in 17 (52%) of the 33 patients with poorly differentiated carcinoma undergoing this procedure, with neuroendocrine tumors being the most frequent new diagnosis. Sixty-eight of the patients were given some form of therapy, with 62 patients receiving cisplatin-based treatment. In this group, 15 patients (23%) had complete responses, and 18 patients (29%) had partial responses. Patients obtaining a response were generally young, male, and had midline involvement of the retroperitoneum, mediastinum, or cervical lymph nodes. All 15 had the light microscopic diagnosis of poorly differentiated carcinoma. A series of 41 patients with poorly differentiated carcinoma of unknown primary were evaluated by Motzer and colleagues at Memorial Sloan-Kettering Cancer Center.[61] Thirty percent of these patients were found to have tumors containing i(12p), increased copies of 12p, or a deletion of the long arm of chromosome 12. Seventy-five percent of patients demonstrating chromosomal structural abnormalities responded to cisplatin-based chemotherapy versus only an 18% response rate in patients for whom no diagnosis could be made.

These results suggest that poorly differentiated carcinomas of unknown primary are responsive to chemotherapy and may even be chemotherapy curable. A subset of these patients probably represents histologically and serologically atypical germ cell cancers. As such, patients with metastatic poorly differentiated carcinoma should be investigated to identify a primary site. Serum HCG and α-fetoprotein should be measured. Patients with a dominant pulmonary or mediastinal mass should have fiberoptic bronchoscopy. Thorough investigations with light microscopy, immunoperoxidase staining, and cytogenetics should be carried out to further characterize the tumor. Patients should receive a trial of cisplatin and etoposide-based chemotherapy.

REFERENCES

1. Einhorn LH. Treatment of testicular cancer: a new and improved model. J Clin Oncol 1990;8:1777–81.
2. Tulinius H, Day N, Muir CS. Rarity of testis cancer in Negroes. Lancet 1973;1:35–6.
3. Spitz MR, Sider JG, Pollack ES, et al. Incidence and descriptive features of testicular cancer among United States whites, blacks, and Hispanics, 1973–1982. Cancer 1986;58:1785–90.
4. Richiardi L, Bellocco R, Adami HO, et al. Testicular cancer incidence in eight northern European countries: secular and recent trends. Canc Epidemiol Biomarkers Prev 2004;13:2157–66.
5. Jemal A, Thomas A, Murray T, Thun M. Cancer statistics, 2002. CA Cancer J Clin 2002;52:23–47.
6. Swerdlow A, Higgins C, Pike M. Risk of testicular cancer in cohort of boys with cryptorchidism. BMJ 1997;314:1507–12.
7. Dow JA, Mostofi FK. Testicular tumors following orchiopexy. South Med J 1967;60:193–5.
8. Tollerud DJ, Blattner WA, Fraser MC, et al. Familial testicular cancer and urogenital developmental anomalies. Cancer 1985;55:1849–54.
9. Rapley EA, Crockford GP, Teare D, et al. Localization to Xq27 of a susceptibility gene for testicular germ-cell tumours. Nat Genet 2000;24:197–200.
10. Powles T, Bower M, Daugaard G, et al. Multicenter study of human immunodeficiency virus-related germ cell tumors. J Clin Oncol 2003;21:1922–7.
11. Nichols CR, Heerema MA, Palmer C, et al. Klinefelter's syndrome associated with mediastinal germ cell neoplasms. J Clin Oncol 1987;5:1290–4.
12. Raghavan D, Zalcberg JR, Grygiel JJ, et al. Multiple atypical nevi: a cutaneous marker of germ cell tumors. J Clin Oncol 1994;12:2284–7.
13. Berthelsen JG, Skakkebaek NE, von der Maase H, et al. Screening for carcinoma in situ of the contralateral testis in patients with germinal testicular cancer. Br Med J (Clin Res Ed) 1982;285:1683–6.
14. von der Maase H, Rorth M, Walbom-Jorgensen S, et al. Carcinoma in situ of contralateral testis in patients with testicular germ cell cancer: study of 27 cases in 500 patients. Br Med J (Clin Res Ed) 1986;293:1398–401.
15. Osterlind A, Berthelsen JG, Abildgaard N, et al. Incidence of bilateral testicular germ cell cancer in Denmark, 1960–84: preliminary findings. Int J Androl 1987;10:203–8.
16. Sokal M, Peckham MJ, Hendry WF. Bilateral germ cell tumours of the testis. Br J Urol 1980;52:158–62.
17. Holzbeirlein J, Sogani P, Sheinfeld J. Histology and clinical outcomes in patients with bilateral testicular germ cell tumors: the Memorial Sloan Kettering Cancer Center experience 1950 to 2001. J Urol 2003;169:2122–5.
18. Oosterhuis J, Looigenga L. Testicular germ-cell tumours in a broader perspective. Nature Rev Cancer 2005;5:210–22.
19. Jones TD, Ulbright TM, Eble JN, et al. OCT4 Staining in testicular tumors: a sensitive and specific marker for seminoma and embryonal carcinoma. Am J Surg Path 2004;28:935–40.
20. Cheng L. Establishing a germ cell origin for metastatic tumors using OCT4 immunohistochemistry. Cancer 2004;101:2006–10.
21. Reuter V. Origins and molecular biology of testicular germ cell tumors. Mod Pathol 2005;18:51–60.
22. Skotheim R, Korkmaz KS, Klokk TI, et al. NKX3.1 Expression is lost in testicular germ cell tumors. Am J Pathol 2003;163:2149–54.
23. Di Vizio D, Cito L, Boccia A, et al. Loss of the tumor suppressor gene PTEN marks the transition from intratubular germ cell neoplasias (ITGCN) to invasive germ cell tumors. Oncogene 2005;10:1882–94.
24. Datta MW, Macri E, Signoretti S, et al. Transition from in situ to invasive testicular germ cell neoplasia is associated with the loss of p21 and gain of mdm-2 expression. Mod Pathol 2001; 14:437–42.
25. Looijenga LH, de Leeuw H, van Oorschot M, et al. Stem cell factor receptor (c-KIT) codon 816 mutations predict development of bilateral testicular germ-cell tumors. Cancer Res 2003;63:7674–8.
26. Talerman A. The incidence of yolk sac tumor (endodermal sinus tumor) elements in germ cell tumor of the testis in adults. Cancer 1980;36:211–5.
27. Brosman S. Testicular tumors in prepubertal children. Urology 1979;13:581–8.
28. Ulbright TM, Loehrer PJ, Roth LM, et al. The development of non-germ cell malignancies within germ cell tumors. A clinicopathologic study of 11 cases. Cancer 1984;54:1824–33.
29. Nichols CR, Roth BJ, Heerema N, et al. Hematologic neoplasia associated with primary mediastinal germ-cell tumors. N Engl J Med 1990;322:1425–9.
30. Bosl GJ, Vogelzang NJ, Goldman A, et al. Impact of delay in diagnosis on clinical stage of testicular cancer. Lancet 1981;2:970–3.
31. Capelouto CC, Clark PE, Ransil BJ, Loughlin KR. A review of scrotal violation in testicular cancer: is adjuvant local therapy necessary? J Urol 1995;153(3 Pt 2):981–5.
32. Loehrer PJ Sr, Birch R, Williams SD, et al. Chemotherapy of metastatic seminoma: the Southeastern Cancer Study Group experience. J Clin Oncol 1987;5:1212–20.
33. Zon RT, Nichols C, Einhorn LH. Management strategies and outcomes of germ cell tumor patients with very high human chorionic gonadotropin levels. J Clin Oncol 1998;16:1294–7.
34. Morris MJ, Bosl GJ. Recognizing abnormal marker results that do not reflect disease in patients with germ cell tumors. J Urol 2000;163:796–801.
35. American Joint Committee on Cancer. Testis, In: Fleming ID, Cooper JS, Henson DE, et al, editors. AJCC cancer staging manual. 5th ed. Philadelphia: Lippincott-Raven; 1997. p. 225–30.
36. Hain SF, O'Doherty MJ, Timothy AR, et al. Fluorodeoxyglucose positron emission tomography in the evaluation of germ cell tumours at relapse. Br J Cancer 2000;83:863–9.
37. De Santis M, Becherer A, Bokemeyer C, et al. FDG-PET as prognostic indicator for seminoma residuals: an update from the multicenter SEMPET study [abstract 1535]. Proc Am Soc Clin Oncol 2003;22:382.
38. Dieckmann KP, Skakkebaek NE. Carcinoma in situ of the testis: review of biological and clinical features. Int J Cancer 1999;83:815–22.
39. Classen J, Souchon R, Herrmann E, Bamberg M. Value of radiotherapy in interdisciplinary management of testicular germ cell tumors. Urologe A 2000;39:126–32.
40. Christensen TB, Daugaard G, Geertsen PF, von der Maase H. Effect of chemotherapy on carcinoma in situ of the testis. Ann Oncol 1998;9:657–60.

41. Jamieson JK, Dobson JF. The lymphatics of the testicle. Lancet 1910;1:493–5.
42. Hinman F. The operative treatment of tumors of the testicle: with the report of thirty cases treated by orchidectomy. JAMA 1914;63:2009–15.
43. Howard R. Malignant disease of the testis. Practitioner 1907;79:794–810.
44. Lewis S. Radioresistant testis tumors: results in 133 cases; five-year follow-up. J Urol 1953;69:841–4.
45. Cooper J, Leadbetter W, Chute R. The thoracoabdominal approach for retroperitoneal gland resection: its application to testis tumors. Surg Gynecol Obstet 1950;90:486–96.
46. Donohue JP. Retroperitoneal lymphadenectomy: the anterior approach including bilateral suprarenal-hilar dissection. Urol Clin North Am 1977;4:509–21.
47. Whitmore WF. Germinal testis tumors in adults. Seventh National Cancer Conference. Philadelphia: JB Lippincott; 1973. p. 793–801.
48. Donohue JP, Thornhill JA, Foster RS, et al. Retroperitoneal lymphadenectomy for clinical stage A testis cancer (1965 to 1989): modifications of technique and impact on ejaculation. J Urol 1993;149:237–43.
49. Donohue JP, Rowland RG. Complications of retroperitoneal lymph node dissection. J Urol 1981;125:338–40.
50. Donohue JP, Zachary JM, Maynard BR. Distribution of nodal metastases in nonseminomatous testis cancer. J Urol 1982;128:315–20.
51. Raghavan D, Vogelzang NJ, Bosl GJ, et al. Tumor classification and size in germ-cell testicular cancer: influence on the occurrence of metastases. Cancer 1982;50:1591–5.
52. Lange PH, Narayan P, Fraley EE. Fertility issues following therapy for testicular cancer. Semin Urol 1984;2:264–74.
53. Fossa SD, Klepp O, Ous S, et al. Unilateral retroperitoneal lymph node dissection in patients with non-seminomatous testicular tumor in clinical stage I. Eur Urol 1984;10:17–23.
54. Donohue JP, Foster RS, Rowland RG, et al. Nerve-sparing retroperitoneal lymphadenectomy with preservation of ejaculation. J Urol 1990;144:287–92.
55. Hoskin P, Dilly S, Easton D, et al. Prognostic factors in stage I non-seminomatous germ-cell testicular tumors managed by orchiectomy and surveillance: implications for adjuvant chemotherapy. J Clin Oncol 1986;4:1031–6.
56. Javadpour N, Canning DA, O'Connell KJ, Young JD. Predictors of recurrent clinical stage I nonseminomatous testicular cancer. A prospective clinicopathologic study. Urology 1986;27:508–11.
57. Freedman LS, Parkinson MC, Jones WG, et al. Histopathology in the prediction of relapse of patients with stage I testicular teratoma treated by orchidectomy alone. Lancet 1987;2:294–8.
58. Rorth M, Kragh Jacobson G, Lindegaard Madsen E, et al. Prediction of relapse in stage I non-seminomatous testicular cancer. Proc Am Soc Clin Oncol 1990;131.
59. Williams S, Stablein D, Muggia F, et al. Early state testis cancer: the Testicular Cancer Intergroup Studies. In: Jones S, Salmon S, editors. Adjuvant therapy of cancer. 5th ed. Orlando (GA): Grune & Stratton; 1987. p. 587–92.
60. Sweeney CJ, Hermans BP, Heilman DK, et al. Results and outcome of retroperitoneal lymph node dissection for clinical stage I embryonal carcinoma—predominant testis cancer. J Clin Oncol 2000;18:358–62.
61. Motzer RJ, Sheinfeld J, Mazumdar M, et al. Etoposide and cisplatin adjuvant therapy for patients with pathologic stage II germ cell tumors. J Clin Oncol 1995;13:2700–4.
62. Behnia M, Foster R, Einhorn LH, et al. Adjuvant bleomycin, etoposide and cisplatin in pathological stage II non-seminomatous testicular cancer: the Indiana University experience. Eur J Cancer 2000;36:472–5.
63. Boden G, Gibb R. Radiotherapy and testicular neoplasms. Lancet 1951;2:1195–6.
64. Calman FM, Peckman MJ, Hendry WF. The pattern of spread and treatment of metastases in testicular seminoma. Br J Urol 1979;51:154–60.
65. Desjardins AU, Squire FH, Morton SA. Radiotherapy for tumors of the testis. Am J Roentgenol 1929;22:137–46.
66. Steele GS, Richie JP, Stewart AK, Menck HR. The National Cancer Data Base report on patterns of care for testicular carcinoma, 1985–1996. Cancer 1996;86:2171–83.
67. Warde PR, Gospodarowicz MK, Goodman PJ, et al. Results of a policy of surveillance in stage I testicular seminoma. Int J Radiat Oncol Biol Phys 1993;27:11–5.
68. Warde P, Specht L, Horwich A, et al. Prognostic factors for relapse in stage I seminoma managed by surveillance: a pooled analysis. J Clin Oncol 2002;22:4448–52.
69. Singh D, Yi WS, Brasacchio RA, et al. Is there a favorable subset of patients with prostate cancer who develop oligometastases? Int J Radiat Oncol Biol Phys 2004;58(1):3–10.
70. Schmoll H-J, Souchon G, Bokemeyer C. European consensus on diagnosis and treatment of germ cell cancer: a report of the European Germ Cell Cancer Consensus Group (EGCCCG). Ann Oncol 2004;15:1377–99.
71. Zagars GK. Management of stage I seminoma: radiotherapy. In: Horwich A, editor. Testicular cancer: investigation and management. London: Chapman and Hall Medical; 1991. p. 83–107.
72. Horwich A, Alsanjari N, A'Hern R, et al. Surveillance following orchidectomy for stage I testicular seminoma. Br J Cancer 1992;65:775–8.
73. von der Maase H, Specht L, Jacobsen GK, et al. Surveillance following orchidectomy for stage I seminoma of the testis. Eur J Cancer 1993;29A:1931–4.
74. von der Maase H, Specht L, Jackobsen GK, et al. Surveillance following orchidectomy for stage I seminoma of the testis [comment]. Eur J Cancer 1993;29A:1923–4.
75. Warde P, Gospodarowicz MK, Banerjee D, et al. Prognostic factors for relapse in stage I testicular seminoma treated with surveillance. J Urol 1997;157:1705–10.
76. Jones WG, Fossa SD, Mead GM, et al. Randomized trial of 30 versus 20 Gy in the adjuvant treatment of stage I testicular seminoma: a report on Medical Research Council Trial TE18, European Organisation for the Research and Treatment of Cancer Trial 30942 (ISRCTN18525328). J Clin Oncol 2005;23:1200–8.
77. Logue JP, Harris MA, Livsey JE, et al. Short course para-aortic radiation for stage I seminoma of the testis. Int J Radiat Oncol Biol Phys 2003;57:1304–9.
78. Fossa SD, Horwich A, Russell JM, et al. Optimal planning target volume for stage I testicular seminoma: a Medical Research Council randomized trial. J Clin Oncol 1999;17:1146–54.
79. Oliver R, et al. A randomised trial of radiotherapy vs carboplatin in adjuvant treatment of stage I seminoma. Proc Am Soc Clin Oncol 2004.
80. Warde P, Gospodarowicz M, Panzarella T, et al. Management of stage II seminoma. J Clin Oncol 1998;16:290–4.
81. Chung P, Gospodarowicz M, Panzarella T, et al. Stage II testicular seminoma: patterns of recurrence and outcome of treatment. Eur Urol 2004;45:754–60.
82. Zagars GK, Pollack A. Radiotherapy for stage II testicular seminoma. Int J Radiat Oncol Biol Phys 2001;51:643–9.
83. Warwick OH, Alison RE, Darte JM. Clinical experience with vinblastine sulfate. Can Med Assoc J 1961;85:579–83.
84. Samuels ML, Johnson DE, Holoye PY, Lanzotti VJ. Large-dose bleomycin therapy and pulmonary toxicity: a possible role of prior radiotherapy. JAMA 1976;235:1117–20.
85. Li MC, Whitmore WF Jr, Golbey R, Grabstald H. Effects of combined drug therapy on metastatic cancer of the testis. JAMA 1960;174:1291–9.
86. Samuels ML, Lanzotti VJ, Holoye PY, et al. Combination chemotherapy in germinal cell tumors. Cancer Treat Rev 1976;3:185–204.
87. Rosenberg B, Camp LV, Krigas T. Inhibition of cell division in *Escherichia coli* by electrolysis products from a platinum electrode. Nature 1965;205:698–9.
88. Higby DJ, et al. Diamminedichloroplatinum: a phase I study showing responses in testicular and other tumors. Cancer 1974;33:1219–5.
89. Einhorn L, Donahue J. Cis-diamminedichloroplatinum, vinblastine, and bleomycin combination chemotherapy in disseminated testicular cancer. Ann Intern Med 1977;87:293–8.
90. Einhorn LH. Testicular cancer as a model for a curable neoplasm: the Richard and Hinda Rosenthal Foundation Award Lecture. Cancer Res 1981;41(9 Pt 1):3275–80.
91. Stoter G, et al. High-dose versus low-dose vinblastine in cisplatin-vinblastine-bleomycin combination chemotherapy of non-seminomatous testicular cancer: a randomized study of the EORTC Genitourinary Tract Cancer Cooperative Group. J Clin Oncol 1986;4:1199–206.
92. Einhorn L, et al. The role of maintenance therapy in disseminated testicular cancer. N Engl J Med 1981;305:727–31.
93. Williams S, et al. Treatment of disseminated germ-cell tumors with cisplatin, bleomycin, and either vinblastine or etoposide. N Engl J Med 1987;316:1435–40.
94. International Germ Cell Cancer Collaborative Group. International Germ Cell Consensus Classification: a prognostic factor-based staging system for metastatic germ cell cancers. J Clin Oncol 1997;15:594–603.
95. Einhorn LH, Williams SD, Loehrer PJ, et al. Evaluation of optimal duration of chemotherapy in favorable-prognosis disseminated germ cell tumors: a Southeastern Cancer Study Group protocol. J Clin Oncol 1989;7:387–91.
96. Loehrer PJ Sr, Johnson D, Elson P, et al. Importance of bleomycin in favorable-prognosis disseminated germ cell tumors: an Eastern Cooperative Oncology Group trial. J Clin Oncol 1995;13:470–6.
97. de Wit R, Stoter G, Kaye SB, et al. Importance of bleomycin in combination chemotherapy for good-prognosis testicular nonseminoma: a randomized study of the European Organization for Research and Treatment of Cancer Genitourinary Tract Cancer Cooperative Group. J Clin Oncol 1997;15:1837–43.
98. Bajorin DF, Sarosdy MF, Pfister DG, et al. Randomized trial of etoposide and cisplatin versus etoposide and carboplatin in patients with good-risk germ cell tumors: a multi-institutional study. J Clin Oncol 1993;11:598–606.
99. Horwich A, Sleijfer DT, Fossa SD, et al. Randomized trial of bleomycin, etoposide, and cisplatin compared with bleomycin, etoposide, and carboplatin in good-prognosis metastatic nonseminomatous germ cell cancer: a Multi-institutional Medical Research Council/European Organization for Research and Treatment of Cancer Trial. J Clin Oncol 1997;15:1844–52.
100. Toner GC, Stockler MR, Boyer MJ, et al. Comparison of two standard chemotherapy regimens for good-prognosis germ-cell tumours: a randomised trial. Australian and New Zealand Germ Cell Trial Group. Lancet 2001;357:739–45.
101. Culine S, Kerbrat P, Bouzy J, et al. Are 3 cycles of bleomycin, etoposide and cisplatin (3BEP) or 4 cycles of etoposide and cisplatin (4EP) equivalent regimens for patients (pts) with good-risk metastatic non-seminomatous germ cell tumors (NSGCT)? Preliminary results of a randomized trial [abstract 1188]. ASCO Ann Meeting 1999.
102. de Wit R, Roberts JT, Wilkinson PM, et al. Equivalence of three or four cycles of bleomycin, etoposide, and cisplatin chemotherapy and of a 3- or 5-day schedule in good-prognosis germ cell cancer: a randomized study of the European Organization for Research and Treatment of Cancer Genitourinary Tract Cancer Cooperative Group and the Medical Research Council. J Clin Oncol 2001;19:1629–40.
103. Ozols RF, Ihde DC, Linehan WM, et al. A randomized trial of standard chemotherapy v a high-dose chemotherapy regimen in the treatment of poor prognosis nonseminomatous germ-cell tumors. J Clin Oncol 1988;6:1031–40.
104. Nichols CR, Williams SD, Loehrer PJ, et al. Randomized study of cisplatin dose intensity in poor-risk germ cell tumors: a Southeastern Cancer Study Group and Southwest Oncology Group protocol. J Clin Oncol 1991;9:1163–72.
105. Nichols CR, Catalano PJ, Crawford ED, et al. Randomized comparison of cisplatin and etoposide and either bleomycin or ifosfamide in treatment of advanced disseminated germ cell tumors: an Eastern Cooperative Oncology Group, Southwest Oncology Group, and Cancer and Leukemia Group B Study. J Clin Oncol 1998;16:1287–93.
106. Kaye SB, Mead GM, Fossa S, et al. Intensive induction-sequential chemotherapy with BOP/VIP-B compared with treatment with BEP/EP for poor-prognosis metastatic nonseminomatous germ cell tumor: a Randomized Medical Research Council/European Organization for Research and Treatment of Cancer study. J Clin Oncol 1998;16:692–701.
107. Kollmannsberger C, Nichols C, Bamberg M, et al. First-line high-dose chemotherapy +/– radiation therapy in patients with metastatic germ-cell cancer and brain metastases. Ann Oncol 2000;11:553–9.
108. Chevreau C, Droz JP, Pico JL, et al. Early intensified chemotherapy with autologous bone marrow transplantation in first line treatment of poor risk non-seminomatous germ cell tumours. Preliminary results of a French randomized trial. Eur Urol 1993;23:213–7.
109. Schmoll H-J, Kollmannsberger C, Metzner B, et al. Long-term results of first-line sequential high-dose etoposide, ifosfamide, and cisplatin chemotherapy plus autologous stem cell support for patients with advanced metastatic germ cell cancer: an extended phase I/II study of the German Testicular Cancer Study Group. J Clin Oncol 2003;21:4083–91.
110. Baniel J, Foster RS, Rowland RG, et al. Complications of primary retroperitoneal lymph node dissection. J Urol 1994;152(2 Pt 1):424–7.
111. Baniel J, Foster RS, Rowland RG, et al. Complications of post-chemotherapy retroperitoneal lymph node dissection. J Urol 1995;153(3 Pt 2):976–80.
112. Fox EP, Weathers TD, Williams SD, et al. Outcome analysis for patients with persistent nonteratomatous germ cell tumor in postchemotherapy retroperitoneal lymph node dissections. J Clin Oncol 1993;11:1294–9.
113. Motzer R, Bosl G, Heelan R, et al. Residual mass: an indication for further therapy in patients with advanced seminoma following systemic chemotherapy. J Clin Oncol 1987;5:1064–70.

114. Friedman EL, Garnick MB, Stomper PC, et al. Therapeutic guidelines and results in advanced seminoma. J Clin Oncol 1985;3:1325–32.
115. Schultz SM, Einhorn LH, Conces DJ Jr, et al. Management of postchemotherapy residual mass in patients with advanced seminoma: Indiana University experience. J Clin Oncol 1989;7:1497–503.
116. Horwich A, Paluchowska B, Norman A, et al. Residual mass following chemotherapy of seminoma. Ann Oncol 1997;8:37–40.
117. Bellamy EA, Husband JE, Blaquiere RM, Law MR. Bleomycin-related lung damage: CT evidence. Radiology 1985;156:155–8.
118. Samuels ML, Samuels ML, Trindade A, Johnson DE. The growing teratoma syndrome. Cancer 1982;50:1629–35.
119. Loehrer PJ Sr, Gonin R, Nichols CR, et al. Vinblastine plus ifosfamide plus cisplatin as initial salvage therapy in recurrent germ cell tumor. J Clin Oncol 1998;16:2500–4.
120. Motzer RJ, Cooper K, Geller NL, et al. The role of ifosfamide plus cisplatin-based chemotherapy as salvage therapy for patients with refractory germ cell tumors. Cancer 1990;66:2476–81.
121. Motzer RJ, Sheinfeld J, Mazumdar M, et al. Paclitaxel, ifosfamide, and cisplatin second-line therapy for patients with relapsed testicular germ cell cancer. J Clin Oncol 2000;18:2413–8.
122. Miller KD, Loehrer PJ, Gonin R, Einhorn LH. Salvage chemotherapy with vinblastine, ifosfamide, and cisplatin in recurrent seminoma. J Clin Oncol 1997;15:1427–31.
123. Barnett MJ, Coppin CM, Murray N, et al. High-dose chemotherapy and autologous bone marrow transplantation for patients with poor prognosis nonseminomatous germ cell tumours. Br J Cancer 1993;68:594–8.
124. Rick O, Bokemeyer C, Beyer J, et al. Salvage treatment with paclitaxel, ifosfamide, and cisplatin plus high-dose carboplatin, etoposide, and thiotepa followed by autologous stem-cell rescue in patients with relapsed or refractory germ cell cancer. J Clin Oncol 2001;19:81–8.
125. Siegert W, Beyer J, Strohscheer I, et al. High-dose treatment with carboplatin, etoposide, and ifosfamide followed by autologous stem-cell transplantation in relapsed or refractory germ cell cancer: a phase I/II study. The German Testicular Cancer Cooperative Study Group. J Clin Oncol 1994;12:1223–31.
126. Bhatia S, Abonour R, Porcu P, et al. High-dose chemotherapy as initial salvage chemotherapy in patients with relapsed testicular cancer. J Clin Oncol 2000;18:3346–51.
127. Cooper MA, Einhorn LH. Maintenance chemotherapy with daily oral etoposide following salvage therapy in patients with germ cell tumors. J Clin Oncol 1995;13:1167–9.
128. Nichols CR, Tricot G, Williams SD, et al. Dose-intensive chemotherapy in refractory germ cell cancer—a phase I/II trial of high-dose carboplatin and etoposide with autologous bone marrow transplantation. J Clin Oncol 1989;7:932–9.
129. Nichols CR, Breeden ES, Loehrer PJ, et al. Secondary leukemia associated with a conventional dose of etoposide: review of serial germ cell tumor protocols. J Natl Cancer Inst 1993;85:36–40.
130. Broun ER, Nichols CR, Kneebone P, et al. Long-term outcome of patients with relapsed and refractory germ cell tumors treated with high-dose chemotherapy and autologous bone marrow rescue. Ann Intern Med 1992;117:124–8.
131. Nichols CR, Andersen J, Lazarus HM, et al. High-dose carboplatin and etoposide with autologous bone marrow transplantation in refractory germ cell cancer: an Eastern Cooperative Oncology Group protocol. J Clin Oncol 1992;10:558–63.
132. Murphy BR, Breeden ES, Donohue JP, et al. Surgical salvage of chemorefractory germ cell tumors. J Clin Oncol 1993;11:324–9.
133. Kollmannsberger C, Rick O, Beyer J, et al. Oxaliplatin in patients (pts) with cisplatin-refractory germ-cell cancer (GCT) [abstract 770]. ASCO Ann Meeting 2001.
134. Hinton S, Catalano P, Einhorn LH, et al. Phase II study of paclitaxel plus gemcitabine in refractory germ cell tumors (E9897): a trial of the Eastern Cooperative Oncology Group. J Clin Oncol 2002;20:1859–63.
135. Baniel J, Foster RS, Gonin R, et al. Late relapse of testicular cancer. J Clin Oncol 1995;13:1170–6.
136. George D, Foster R, Hromas R, et al. Update on late relapse (LR) of germ cell tumors (GCT): a clinical and molecular analysis [abstract 689]. ASCO Ann Meeting 2001.
137. Dentino M, Luft FC, Yum MN, et al. Long term effect of cis-diamminedichloride platinum (CDDP) on renal function and structure in man. Cancer 1978;41:1274–81.
138. Meijer S, Mulder NH, Sleijfer DT, et al. Influence of combination chemotherapy with cis-diamminedichloroplatinum on renal function: long-term effects. Oncology 1983;40:170–3.
139. Fossa SD, Aass N, Winderen M, et al. Long-term renal function after treatment for malignant germ-cell tumours. Ann Oncol 2002;13:222–8.
140. Vogelzang NJ, Bosl GJ, Johnson K, Kennedy BJ. Raynaud's phenomenon: a common toxicity after combination chemotherapy for testicular cancer. Lancet 1981;2:970–3.
141. Hansen SW, Olsen N. Raynaud's phenomenon in patients treated with cisplatin, vinblastine, and bleomycin for germ cell cancer: measurement of vasoconstrictor response to cold. J Clin Oncol 1989;7:940–2.
142. Hantel A, Rowinsky EK, Donehower RC. Nifedipine and oncologic Raynaud phenomenon. Ann Intern Med 1988;108:767.
143. Cantwell BMJ, Mannix KA, Roberts JT, et al. Thromboembolic events during combination chemotherapy for germ cell malignancy. Lancet 1988;2:1086–7.
144. Doll DC, List AF, Greco FA, et al. Acute vascular ischemic events after cisplatin-based combination chemotherapy for germ-cell tumors of the testis. Ann Intern Med 1986;105:48–51.
145. Vogelzang NJ, Frenning DH, Kennedy BJ. Coronary artery disease after treatment with bleomycin and vinblastine. Cancer Treat Rep 1980;64:1159–60.
146. Weijl NI, Rutten MF, Zwinderman AH, et al. Thromboembolic events during chemotherapy for germ cell cancer: a cohort study and review of the literature. J Clin Oncol 2000;18:2169–78.
147. Nichols CR, Roth BJ, Williams SD, et al. No evidence of acute cardiovascular complications of chemotherapy for testicular cancer: an analysis of the Testicular Cancer Intergroup Study. J Clin Oncol 1992;10:760–5.
148. Vaughn DJ, Gignac GA, Meadows AT. Long-term medical care of testicular cancer survivors. Ann Intern Med 2002;136:463–70.
149. Strumberg D, Brugge S, Korn MW, et al. Evaluation of long-term toxicity in patients after cisplatin-based chemotherapy for non-seminomatous testicular cancer. Ann Oncol 2002;13:229–36.
150. Meinardi MT, Gietema GA, van der Graaf WT, et al. Cardiovascular morbidity in long-term survivors of metastatic testicular cancer. J Clin Oncol 2000;18:1725–32.
151. Thompson SW, Davis LE, Kornfeld M, et al. Cisplatin neuropathy. Clinical, electrophysiologic, morphologic, and toxicologic studies. Cancer 1984;54:1269–75.
152. Roth BJ, Greist A, Kubilis PS, et al. Cisplatin-based combination chemotherapy for disseminated germ cell tumors: long-term follow-up. J Clin Oncol 1988;6:1239–47.
153. Aguilar-Markulis NV, Beckley S, Priore R, Mettlin C. Auditory toxicity effects of long-term cis-dichlorodiammine-platinum II therapy in genitourinary cancer patients. J Surg Oncol 1981;16:111–23.
154. Reddel RR, Kefford RF, Grant JM, et al. Ototoxicity in patients receiving cisplatin: importance of dose and method of drug administration. Cancer Treat Rep 1982;66:19–23.
155. Travis LB, Andersson M, Gospodarowicz M, et al. Treatment-associated leukemia following testicular cancer. J Natl Cancer Inst 2000;92:1165–71.
156. Bokemeyer C, Schmoll HJ. Treatment of testicular cancer and the development of secondary malignancies. J Clin Oncol 1995;13:283–92.
157. Hendry WF, Stedronksa J, Jones CR, et al. Semen analysis in testicular cancer and Hodgkin's disease: pre- and post-treatment findings and implications for cryopreservation. Br J Urol 1983;55:769–73.
158. Guazzieri S, Lembo A, Ferro G, et al. Sperm antibodies and infertility in patients with testicular cancer. Urology 1985;26:139–42.
159. Morrish DW, Venner PM, Siy O, et al. Mechanisms of endocrine dysfunction in patients with testicular cancer. J Natl Cancer Inst 1990;82:412–8.
160. Drasga RE, Einhorn LH, Williams SD, et al. Fertility after chemotherapy for testicular cancer. J Clin Oncol 1983;1:179–83.
161. Lange PH, Narayan P, Vogelzang NJ, et al. Return of fertility after treatment for nonseminomatous testicular cancer: changing concepts. J Urol 1983;129:1131–5.
162. Rustin G, Pekasidis D, Newland E, et al. Fertility and second tumours after treatment of germ cell tumours. In: Jones W, Ward A, Anderson C, editors. Germ cell tumours II. New York: Pergamon Press; 1986. p. 483–7.
163. Senturia YD, Peckham CS, Peckham MJ. Children fathered by men treated for testicular cancer. Lancet 1985;2:766–9.
164. Bohlen D, Burkhard FC, Mills R, et al. Fertility and sexual function after orchiectomy and two cycles of chemotherapy for stage I high-risk nonseminomatous germ cell cancer. J Urol 2001;165:141–4.
165. Lampe H, Horwich A, Norman A, et al. Fertility after chemotherapy for testicular germ cell cancers. J Clin Oncol 1997;15:239–45.
166. Yagoda A, Mukherji B, Young C, et al. Bleomycin, an antitumor antibiotic: clinical experience in 274 patients. Ann Intern Med 1972;77:861–70.
167. Einhorn LH, Krause M, Hornback N, Furnas B. Enhanced pulmonary toxicity with bleomycin and radiotherapy in oat cell lung cancer. Cancer 1976;37:2414–6.
168. Omura G. Enhanced bleomycin toxicity during acute renal failure. Cancer Treat Rep 1981;65:592–3.
169. Gordon W Jr, Siegmund K, Stanisic TH, et al. A study of reproductive function in patients with seminoma treated with radiotherapy and orchidectomy: (SWOG-8711). Southwest Oncology Group. Int J Radiat Oncol Biol Phys 1997;38:83–94.
170. Jacobsen KD, Olsen DR, Fossa K, Fossa SD. External beam abdominal radiotherapy in patients with seminoma stage I: field type, testicular dose, and spermatogenesis. Int J Radiat Oncol Biol Phys 1997;38:95–102.
171. Fraass BA, Kinsella TJ, Harrington FS, Glatstein E. Peripheral dose to the testes: the design and clinical use of a practical and effective gonadal shield. Int J Radiat Oncol Biol Phys 1985;11:609–15.
172. Fossa SD, Kravdal O. Fertility in Norwegian testicular cancer patients. Br J Cancer 2000;82:737–41.
173. Huddart R, et al. Cardiovascular disease as a long-term complication of treatment for testicular cancer. J Clin Oncol 2003;21:1513–23.
174. Zagars GK, et al. Mortality after cure of testicular seminoma. J Clin Oncol 2004;22:640–7.
175. Travis LB, Curtis RE, Storm H, et al. Risk of second malignant neoplasms among long-term survivors of testicular cancer. J Natl Cancer Inst 1997;89:1429–39.
176. Spears T, Franco I, Reda EF, et al. Accessory and ectopic scrotum with VATER association. Urology 1992;40:343–5.
177. Heidenreich A, Weissbach L, Holtl W, et al. Organ sparing surgery for malignant germ cell tumor of the testis. J Urol 2001;166:2161–5.
178. Luna MA, Valenzuela-Tamariz J. Germ-cell tumors of the mediastinum, postmortem findings. Am J Clin Pathol 1976;65:450–4.
179. Feun LG, Samson MK, Stephens RL. Vinblastine (VLB), bleomycin (BLEO), cis-diamminedichloroplatinum (DDP) in disseminated extragonadal germ cell tumors. A Southwest Oncology Group Study. Cancer 1980;45:2543–9.
180. Hainsworth IR, McAllister EJ, Weston R. False-positive markers in testicular tumours. Lancet 1982;2:1346.
181. Logothetis CJ, Samuels ML, Selig DE, et al. Primary chemotherapy followed by a selective retroperitoneal lymphadenectomy in the management of clinical stage II testicular carcinoma: a preliminary report. J Urol 1985;134:1127–30.
182. Lewis IJ, Weeden S, Machin D, et al. Received dose and dose-intensity of chemotherapy and outcome in nonmetastatic extremity osteosarcoma. European Osteosarcoma Intergroup. J Clin Oncol 2000;18:4028–37.
183. Bokemeyer C, Oechsle K, Hartmann JT, et al. Treatment-induced anaemia and its potential clinical impact in patients receiving sequential high dose chemotherapy for metastatic testicular cancer. Br J Cancer 2002;87:1066–71.
184. Vuky J, Bains M, Bacik J, et al. Role of postchemotherapy adjunctive surgery in the management of patients with nonseminoma arising from the mediastinum. J Clin Oncol 2001;19:682–8.
185. Dexeus FH, Logothetis CJ, Chong C, et al. Genetic abnormalities in men with germ cell tumors. J Urol 1988;140:80–4.
186. Hartmann JT, Fels LM, Franzke A, et al. Comparative study of the acute nephrotoxicity from standard dose cisplatin +/– ifosfamide and high-dose chemotherapy with carboplatin and ifosfamide. Anticancer Res 2000;20:3767–73.
187. Ladanyi M, Samaniego F, Reuter VE, et al. Cytogenetic and immunohistochemical evidence for the germ cell origin of a subset of acute leukemias associated with mediastinal germ cell tumors. J Natl Cancer Inst 1990;82:221–7.
188. Ulbright TM, Loehrer PJ, Roth LM, et al. The development of non-germ cell malignancies within germ cell tumors. A clinicopathologic study of 11 cases. Cancer 1984;54:1824–33.
189. Greco A, Leung AW, Zwi LJ, et al. Ileocolic intussusception in large cell lymphoma of the terminal ileum. Report of a case. Acta Radiol Diagn (Stockh) 1986;27:687–90.

Section 30

FEMALE REPRODUCTIVE ORGANS

100

Neoplasms of the Vulva and Vagina

Jacob H. Rotmensch, MD

CANCER OF THE VULVA

Vulvar cancer accounts for about 4% of cancers in the female reproductive organs and 0.6% of all cancers in women. The American Cancer Society estimates that in 2005, about 3,870 cancers of the vulva will be diagnosed in the United States and about 870 women will die of this cancer. Cancer of the vulva accounts for 4.7% of malignant neoplasms in the genital tract. It is the fourth most frequent gynecologic cancer.[1]

Most vulvar carcinomas occur in older women, with more than 50% of the patients being 60 to 79 years of age. Invasive vulvar carcinomas are being seen with increasing frequency in younger patients, however, with 15% of vulvar cancers arising in women under the age of 40 years (Figure 100-1).[2] This increased frequency in younger patients may be attributed to an increase in the number of sexual partners or venereal viral infections within the population.

Several epidemiologic studies suggest a sexually transmitted origin for carcinoma of the vulva. Condyloma acuminatum associated with human papillomavirus (HPV) has been noted in many patients with premalignant and malignant vulvar disease. It has been estimated that in the United States, over 1 million women each year develop perineal warts and that as many as 10% are infected with HPV.[3] Currently, HPV types 6 and 11 are most frequently found in benign vulvar warts, and HPV types 16, 18, 31, 33, and 45 are more frequently associated with intraepithelial neoplasia or invasive carcinoma.[3–5] HPV can be found in approximately 50% of vulvar carcinomas; the tumors are often multifocal and associated with vulvar dysplasias. HPV-negative tumors are often found in older women.[6]

Although epidemiologic evidence strongly suggests a viral cause, other associations have been implied as well. Factors such as granulomatous diseases of the vulva, diabetes, hypertension,

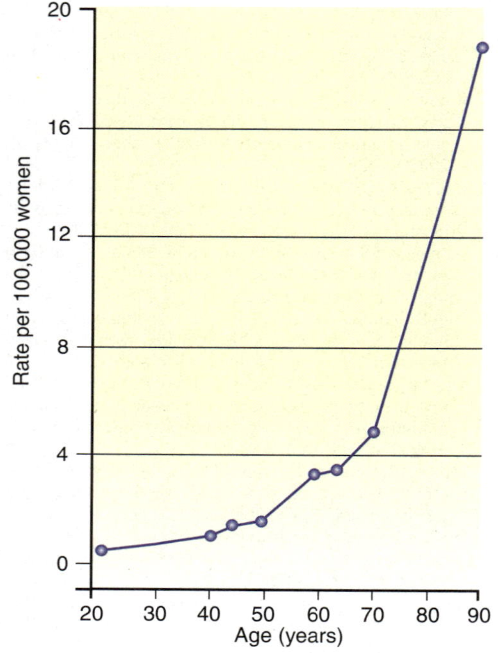

Figure 100-1 Age incidence curve for cancer of the vulva in white women in the United States.

and obesity also have been associated with vulvar carcinoma, but perhaps this is because of the usually advanced age of patients. A case-control study by Mabuchi and colleagues found that domestic servants, or those working in laundry or cleaning plants, have an increased risk of vulvar carcinoma, thus suggesting an environmental component.[7]

The association of carcinoma in situ with invasive carcinoma of the vulva indicates a continuum from preinvasive to invasive carcinoma. The progression of vulvar intraepithelial neoplasia to invasive carcinoma has been estimated to be on the order of 6%.[8,9] Progression, however, may differ between younger and older patients. Some authors suggest that the multifocal carcinoma in situ of women in their thirties or forties may not be as likely to progress as that seen in older women.[10–12]

Vulvar Atypias There has been a lack of uniformity in defining vulvar atypias. There are minimal data to support vulvar dystrophies being a cause of cancer. The International Society for the Study of Vulvar Disease has provided a standard nomenclature for these lesions, and this has been adopted by the International Society for Gynecologic Pathology (Table 100-1).[13] In 1985, the nomenclature was replaced by the terms *carcinoma in situ* or *vulvar intraepithelial neoplasia* (VIN). In addition, the nonpremalignant squamous changes previously termed hyperplastic dystrophy are now considered under the classification of squamous hyperplasia.

Vulvar atypias can present with a variety of symptoms. The most common is irritation or itching; however, 20% of patients are asymptomatic.[14]

Grossly, the lesions can be flat, raised (maculopapular), or verrucous. In color, they may be brown (hyperpigmented), red (erythroplastic), white, or discolored.

Table 100-1 Classification of Vulvar Atypias

Pre-1985 classification
Hyperplastic dystrophy
Without atypia
With atypia (mild, moderate, severe)
Lichen sclerosus
Mixed dystrophy
Without atypia
With atypia
Current classification
Intraepithelial atypias
Mild dysplasia (VIN I)
Moderate dysplasia (VIN II)
Severe dysplasia—CIS (VIN III)
Lichen sclerosus
Miscellaneous

CIS = carcinoma in situ; VIN = vulvar intraepithelial neoplasia.

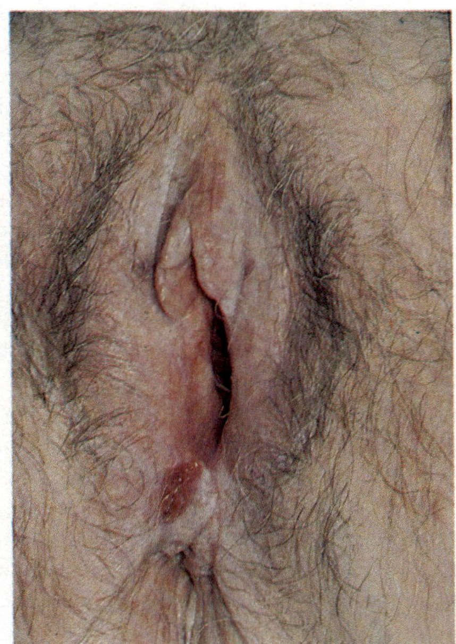

Figure 100-2 Reproduced with permission from Menczer J, Voliovitch Y, Modan B, et al. Some epidemiologic aspects of carcinoma of the vulva in Israel. Am J Obstet Gynecol 1982;143:893.

White lesions can appear to have a whitish, thickened keratin layer (leukoplakia) or a diffuse, white, brittle, paperlike appearance (lichen sclerosus) (Figure 100-2). Areas of squamous hyperplasia (hyperplastic dystrophy) and dysplasia can also have a white appearance. Unlike lichen sclerosus, however, the tissue often is thickened, and the process tends to be focal or multifocal rather than diffuse.[13]

Microscopically, atypical changes in the vulvar epithelium consistent with preinvasive lesions usually are marked by loss of maturation of the squamous epithelium. There is increased mitotic activity and an increase in the nuclear cytoplasmic ratio. Mild dysplasia (VIN I) is diagnosed if changes involve the lower third of the epithelium. If there is moderate dysplasia (VIN II), then half to two-thirds of the epithelium is affected. If there is severe dysplasia (VIN III), then two-thirds of the epithelium is affected. For carcinoma in situ (also classified as VIN III) of the vulva, the full thickness of the epithelium usually is abnormal.

It often is difficult to distinguish between benign squamous hyperplasia and intraepithelial neoplasia. Crum and colleagues suggested that nuclear size may be helpful in diagnosis because intraepithelial neoplasia of the vulva almost always contains nuclei that are fourfold or greater in size compared with benign condyloma or nonneoplastic epithelium.[15,16]

The best method of establishing a diagnosis is a high index of suspicion and early biopsy.

Several methods also can be used to help assess these lesions. Cytology, colposcopy, and toluidine blue O can be used cautiously before biopsy. In general, however, cytologic evaluation of the vulva has not been helpful as a screening examination because the vulvar skin often is thickened and keratinized. Colposcopic examination of the vulva is difficult because unlike cervical lesions, the changes are difficult to recognize. Therefore, colposcopic examination is not used for routine vulvar examination; rather, it is primarily employed for patients who are being evaluated or followed for vulvar atypia or intraepithelial malignancies. The toluidine blue O test is nonspecific and stains nuclei in the superficial part of the epithelium. Colposcopy is performed after applying a 1% aqueous solution of toluidine blue O to the vulva for 1 minute and decolorizing the tissue with 1% acetic acid. Areas that retain the stain are biopsied. A positive test, however, does not always indicate a premalignant condition because 20% of benign areas on the vulva stain positively.[16]

To obtain the entire thickness of the skin for a definitive diagnosis, a biopsy of the vulva usually is done with a Keyes dermal punch. Occasionally, a larger biopsy is needed, in which case, a larger field can be locally anesthetized with lidocaine and a small scalpel or cervical biopsy punch used to obtain a specimen.

Once the correct diagnosis has been established by biopsy, appropriate therapy can be undertaken. For lichen sclerosus, 2% topical testosterone propionate in petrolatum, used twice daily, is an effective preparation to overcome the epithelial atrophy. The medication should be given continuously or the atrophy returns. Side effects such as clitoral hypertrophy and increased hair growth can occur.

Local measures, for example, wearing cotton underclothes and avoiding strong soaps and detergents, often are used to diminish irritation. Topical fluorinated corticosteroids applied twice daily for 1 to 2 weeks are helpful in controlling pruritus, but prolonged use of these steroid preparations can lead to vulvar atrophy or contracture. If long-term therapy is needed, a nonfluorinated compound such as 1% hydrocortisone is used. Some patients with lichen sclerosus have severe contracture in the area of the posterior fourchette. Treating these areas surgically with plastic repair of the fourchette has been suggested.[17,18]

VIN can be treated by a variety of methods, and many authors have reported successful control of the disease by wide local excision.[8,17] Buscema and colleagues reported that 68% of 62 patients had no evidence of recurrence when treated by wide excision.[8] Adequate margins must be obtained with wide excision; however, this often may be difficult because of the multifocal nature of the disease. Friedrich and colleagues reported a 50% risk of recurrence if the margins were involved with neoplasia.[12]

Other modalities also have been reported in the treatment of VIN.

Carbon dioxide laser vaporization of the vulva to a depth of 3 mm has been used, and current evidence indicates that laser therapy is as effective as surgical excision for the control of this disease. Before lasering the vulva, however, it is necessary to ascertain by histologic confirmation that invasive disease does not exist. Leuchter and colleagues treated 142 patients with carcinoma in situ of the vulva.[19] Of those treated by laser, 17% had a recurrence, a result that is similar to that in lesions treated by local excision.

5-Fluorouracil (5-FU) cream has been used successfully to treat carcinoma in situ of the vulva, and application of this has been reported to be successful in 75% of cases. With continuous application, however, this treatment causes edema and pain.

Paget's Disease Paget's disease is a rare intraepithelial disorder of the vulvar skin that is seen in postmenopausal women.[20–22] Unlike VIN, the intraepithelial neoplastic cells are glandular rather than squamous. The lesion primarily occurs in whites of an average age of 65 years. Grossly, it appears as a reddish, eczematoid lesion. Microscopically, this type of lesion is characterized by large pale cells that often occur in nests and infiltrate the epithelium. Once the diagnosis is made, it is important to rule out the presence of an underlying cancer. A review by Lee and colleagues reported a total of 75 cases of Paget's disease of the vulva: 16 (22%) of the patients had underlying invasive carcinoma of the adnexal structures and 7 (9%) had adnexal carcinoma in situ.[21]

Paget's disease of the vulva often spreads in an occult fashion, with margins extending beyond the normal appearance of the lesion.[22] If there is no evidence of an underlying malignant neoplasm, a wide local excision or total vulvectomy usually is performed.[23] If a wide local excision is performed, a slightly deeper excision is needed to remove the epidermis down to the level of the underlying fat to ensure removal of adnexal skin structures. Because this lesion extends subepithelially, a frozen section in the operating room may assist in ensuring complete removal.

Bergen and colleagues evaluated 14 patients with Paget's disease of the vulva that was treated by vulvectomy, skinning vulvectomy with a graft, or hemivulvectomy.[23] With a median follow-up of 50 months, all patients were free of disease; however, three patients had had locally recurrent disease.

Other modalities (topical 5-FU cream, laser) have not been used for treatment of this disease. Because both local and distant recurrence is a major risk, close follow-up is required.

Invasive Vulvar Carcinomas The International Federation of Gynecology and Obstetrics (FIGO) has defined four clinical stages of vulvar carcinoma.[24] In addition, many centers use the tumor, node, metastasis (TNM) classification. In 1988, the FIGO staging was modified to reflect lymph node status and the location of the tumor (Table 100-2). In this classification, a tumor that is located on the perineum is no longer considered to be stage III. In 1995, FIGO instituted a subclassification of stage I into IA and IB, based on whether there is stromal invasion greater than 1 mm.

Squamous Cell Carcinoma Squamous cell carcinomas comprise approximately 90% of primary vulvar malignancies. Grossly, these carci-

Table 100-2 Classification and Staging of Vulvar Carcinoma

TNM Classification		
T	Primary tumor	
Tis	Preinvasive carcinoma (carcinoma in situ)	
T1	Tumor confined to the vulva and/or perineum; 2 cm or less in diameter	
T2	Tumor confined to the vulva and/or perineum; more than 2 cm in diameter	
T3	Tumor of any size with adjacent spread to the urethra, vagina, or anus	
T4	Tumor of any size infiltrating the bladder mucosa, the rectal mucosa, or both, including the upper part of the urethral mucosa, or fixed to the anus	
N	Regional lymph nodes	
N0	No nodes palpable	
N1	Unilateral regional lymph node metastases	
N2	Bilateral regional lymph node metastases	
M	Distant metastases	
M0	No clinical metastases	
M1	Distant metastases (including pelvic lymph node metastases)	
FIGO Staging (1988)		
0	Tis	Carcinoma in situ Intraepithelial carcinoma
I	T1N0M0	Tumor confined to the vulva and/or perineum; 2 cm or less in greatest dimension. No nodal metastasis.
II	T2N0	Tumor confined to the vulva and/or perineum; more than 2 cm in greatest dimension. No nodal metastasis.
III	T3N0M0 T1N1M0 T2N1M0 T3N1M0	Tumor of any size with (1) adjacent spread to the lower urethra and/or the vagina and/or the anus and/or (2) unilateral regional lymph node metastasis
IVA	T1N2M0 T2N2M0 T3N2M0 T4, any N, M0	Tumor invades any of the following: upper urethra, bladder mucosa, rectal mucosa, pelvic bone, and/or bilateral regional node metastasis.
IVB	Any T, any N, M1	Any distant metastasis including pelvic lymph nodes

Adapted from Creasman WT.[24]
FIGO = International Federation of Gynecology and Obstetrics; TNM = tumor, node, metastasis.

nomas usually appear as ulcerated or polyploid masses on the vulva. Biopsy reveals the characteristic histologic appearance: the tumor appears in nests and cords of squamous cells infiltrating the stroma, often with islands of keratin.

The pattern of spread for this carcinoma relates to the intricate lymphatic drainage of the vulva (Figure 100-3).[5] Tumors located in the middle of either labium initially drain to the ipsilateral inguinal femoral nodes, whereas midline perineal tumors can spread either to the left or right side. Using technetium 99m colloid, Iversen and Aas showed that when radioactivity was injected to one side of the vulva, 98% of it localized in the ipsilateral nodes and less than 2% in the contralateral nodes.[25] Tumors along the midline in the clitoral or urethral areas may spread to either groin. From the inguinal-femoral nodes, lymphatic spread continues to the deep pelvic iliac and obturator nodes. Although there has been concern in the past that tumors in the clitoral-urethral area could spread directly to the deep pelvic nodes, current evidence indicates that this is rare.

Stage I Microinvasive Carcinoma There is no uniformly accepted definition regarding microinvasive carcinoma of the vulva, and this may result from confusion in measuring the depth of invasion. Microinvasion has been defined by some as a small lesion of the vulva less than 2 cm in diameter and invading less than 3 mm.[26] The International Society for the Study of Vulvar Diseases has recommended that the term *microinvasive* be dropped and that *stage IA* be used for tumors less than 2 cm in diameter and invading less than 1 mm from the epidermal-stromal junction, the basement membrane.

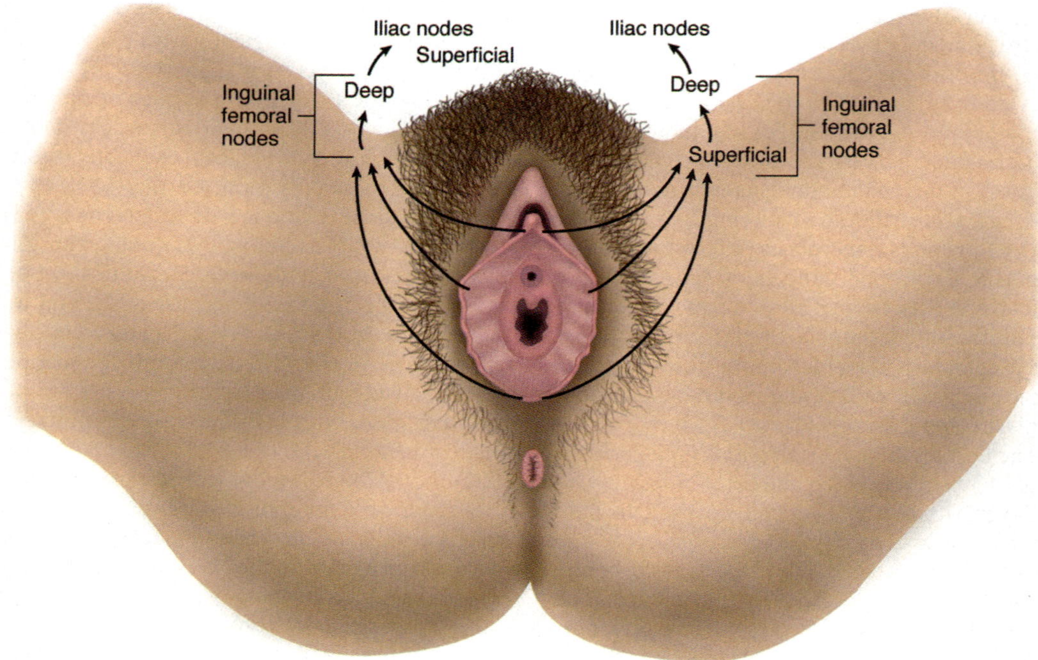

Figure 100-3 Lymphatic drainage of the vulva.

Different clinical results have been reported with this definition. Spread to regional lymph nodes has varied from 0 to 10% in tumors with less than a 5 mm depth of invasion.[27–31] For example, Hoffman and colleagues reported no nodal metastases in 43 patients whose tumor invaded less than 2 mm.[29] Lesions that were at risk of spreading to inguinal nodes included tumors with confluent tongues rather than those with individual tongues merely extending into the stroma. Hacker and colleagues, however, reported that six of seven patients with invasion of less than 3 mm had regional node involvement.[28]

The risk of nodal involvement may be decreased when carcinoma in situ is present in the lesion. Rowley and colleagues noted that only 1 of 35 cases with adjacent carcinoma in situ had nodal metastases.[30] By contrast, 5 of 27 had positive lymph nodes when superficial stage I lesions penetrating 2.1 to 5.0 mm did not have adjacent carcinoma in situ.

For stage IA lesions, therapy may be less extensive than with invasive vulvar carcinoma. Different treatments have been reported, including wide local excision with or without ipsilateral node dissection, simple vulvectomy without node dissection, and radical vulvectomy without node dissection.[31–33] In younger patients, especially those with tumors located at a distance from the clitoris, an operation that spares the clitoris should be considered. DiSaia and colleagues recommended an operative procedure in which the superficial inguinal lymph nodes are removed and sent for frozen section.[32] If positive nodes are found, bilateral complete groin dissection and complete radical vulvectomy are performed; if the nodes are negative, wide local excision of the primary cancer is performed.

Iversen and colleagues reported an alternative approach, recommending a hemivulvectomy with ipsilateral groin dissection for lesions involving the labia.[33] For medial lesions, they suggest conventional radical vulvectomy with bilateral groin dissection. Boyce and colleagues recommended that conservative therapy can be used with minimal risk.[34] This recommendation appears to be advisable if invasion is greater than 1 mm and the tumor diameter is greater than 2 cm.

To identify patients who can be treated more conservatively, investigators have used intraoperative lymphatic mapping and sentinel node identification for squamous cell carcinoma. Investigators have improved the rate of identification of the sentinel node by combining blue dye with radiolocalization.[35,36]

The feasibility of intraoperative lymphatic mapping with vulvar cancer has been demonstrated in 21 patients. In this series, the sentinel node was found in a variety of locations at the femoral vessels and at the medial border of Scarpa fascia. In no patients were the nonsentinel nodes positive if the sentinel nodes were negative.[36–38]

Stage I, II, and III Invasive Carcinoma The prognosis of a patient with vulvar carcinoma relates to the stage of disease (Figure 100-4) and to the nodal status.[39] The presence of carcinoma in the regional lymph nodes correlates with the size and thickness of the primary lesion, the degree of tumor differentiation, and the involvement of vascular spaces by the tumor (Table 100-3). In 272 women with invasive vulvar carcinoma reported by the Gynecologic Oncology Group (GOG), regional nodes were involved in 8.9% of stage I, 25.3% of stage II, and 31.1% of stage III lesions.[40] If a lesion was less than 1 mm thick, there was a 3.1% incidence of positive nodes. With larger lesions, 4 mm or greater in thickness, 31% of nodes were positive. Hacker and colleagues reported an actuarial 5-year survival rate of 96% in those with negative nodes.[41] Survival decreased to 94% with one positive node, 80% with two positive nodes, and 12% with three or more nodes involved by tumor.

Not only is the number of nodes important, but there also appears to be a correlation with the size of the metastases. Hoffman and colleagues noted that 14 of 15 patients with inguinal lymph node metastases measuring less than 36 mm survived free of disease for 5 years compared with 12 of 29 patients whose tumor metastases measured greater than 100 mm.[42]

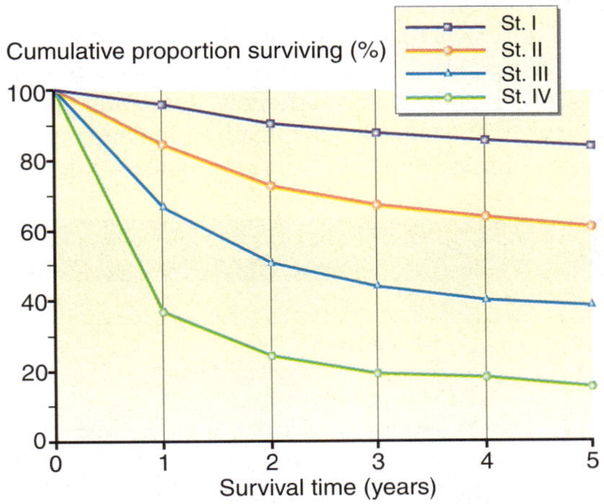

Figure 100-4 Survival of patients with carcinoma of the vulva. Adapted from the 20th report on end results of therapy of gynecologic malignancies. Stockholm: International Federation of Gynecology and Obstetrics; 1988.

Table 100-3 Prognostic Factors of Stage, Grade, and Tumor Thickness Associated with Positive Regional Nodes

Stage	Positive Nodes, %	Grade	Positive Nodes, %	Tumor Thickness, mm	Positive Nodes, %
I	8.9	1	0	< 1	3.1
II	25.3	2	8.0	2	8.9
III	31.1	3	24.6	3	18.6
IV	62.5	4	47.7	> 4	31.0

Adapted from Sedlis A, Homesly H, Bundy BN, et al. Positive groin lymph nodes in superficial squamous vulvar cancer. Am J Obstet Gynecol 1987;156:1159.

The grade of tumor related to the percentage of positive nodes in the GOG study. Patients with grade 1 lesions did not have positive nodes, yet in patients with grade 4 lesions, 47.7% of nodes were positive.

Vascular space involvement also was prognostic because 72% with vascular invasion showed tumor in regional nodes compared with 34% of those without vascular invasion. Nodal involvement also correlated with the location of the primary lesion.[43] Lesions on the labia are associated with 7.4% positive nodes, whereas clitoral lesions have a higher incidence of positive nodes (27.4%).[44] Boyce and colleagues reported that six tumors under 1 cm in diameter had no metastases to regional nodes but that the fraction of tumors with positive nodes rose to 55% for 29 cases with lesions over 4 cm.[34]

Therapy for stage I and II and early stage III vulvar carcinoma is accomplished with radical vulvectomy and bilateral inguinal femoral node dissection. The deep pelvic nodes are rarely removed unless the inguinal nodes are involved. Most oncologists now remove only the inguinal and femoral nodes at the time of operation and treat the deep pelvic nodes with external radiation if superficial nodes are involved with tumor.

A wide variety of management options of the primary lesion have been proposed. In a unilateral lesion less than 1 cm from the midline, radical wide local excision with possible postoperative radiation has been used. This approach has been used for risk factors such as large tumor sites, positive capillary-lymphatic space invasion, or surgical margins that are less than 8 mm. For midline lesions, standard management has varied from use of surgery as primary treatment to use of radiation with possible chemotherapy.

Different surgical approaches to invasive vulvar carcinoma have been evaluated. Classically, an en bloc dissection has been performed. Radical vulvectomy and groin dissection have been carried out through a single suprapubic incision that extends between the left and right anterior iliac spines (Figure 100-5). This operation removed the entire vulva, including the clitoris, subcutaneous tissue, and inguinal femoral nodes. If the lesion involved the distal urethra, this has often been removed without the loss of urinary continence. In this procedure, the major complication has been wound breakdown and infection (occurring in 50% of the patients). Recently, modifications have been introduced to decrease the incidence of wound breakdown. These modifications include performing the inguinal femoral node dissection through separate inguinal incisions and then completing the radical vulvectomy. Tumor recurrences rarely occur in the skin bridge when separate groin incisions are used.[45]

Less mutilating procedures also have been reported in stage I disease. Rowley and colleagues reported using wide local excision and superficial inguinal node dissection in 20 patients with stage I lesions invading to a depth of less than 5 mm.[30] The superficial and contralateral inguinal femoral nodes were removed only if the superficial nodes contained tumor. This approach seems to be reasonable if a unilateral lesion is present; however, with a midline lesion, bilateral inguinal node dissection seems to be appropriate. In a recent update of a series of 50 patients initially reported by DiSaia and colleagues, only 1 patient died because of recurrent carcinoma treated with the latter conservative approach.[32] Six patients had only recurrent carcinoma in situ or minimally invasive carcinoma. Modifying the approach for these early-stage lesions appears to be effective and is associated with less morbidity than the standard radical vulvectomy. If the nodes are free from tumor in stage I and II carcinomas of the vulva, no further therapy is required. If the nodes (especially the femoral nodes) are involved, pelvic irradiation is required. From a randomized study, Homesley and colleagues reported an improved survival rate in 118 patients with positive lymph nodes who received 4,500 to 5,000 cGy of radiation (Figure 100-6).[40]

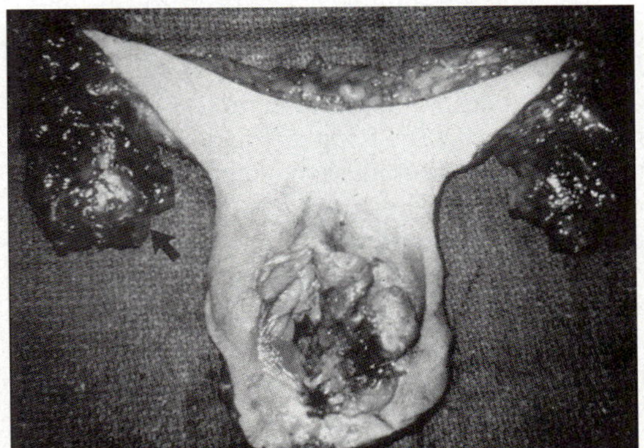

Figure 100-5 Gross vulvectomy specimen showing a vulvar carcinoma.

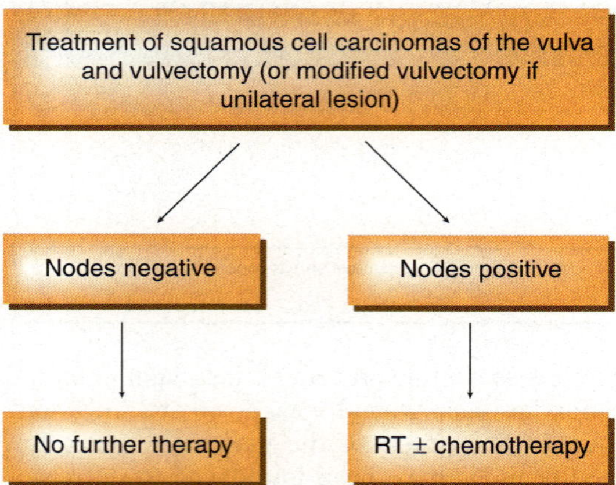

Figure 100-6 Treatment of squamous cell carcinomas of the vulva. RT = radiation therapy.

Advanced Vulvar Tumor Large tumors of the vulva encroaching on the anorectal area and the urethra require more extensive treatment than a radical vulvectomy. In addition to a radical vulvectomy, it is usually necessary to perform a diversion of the urinary or fecal stream. If the nodes are negative, a 5-year survival rate of 50% has been reported.

However, newer approaches that involve a combination of preoperative radiation and surgery have been reported in treating these lesions. External radiation often is given to reduce the size of the tumor before surgical removal by radical vulvectomy, with or without regional lymph node dissection. Approximately 4,000 to 4,500 cGy is delivered to the pelvis and inguinal nodes, the operation being performed 5 weeks after the completion of radiation. This approach may obviate a urinary or fecal diversion. Boronow and colleagues reported a 5-year survival rate of 80% in 26 patients with primary carcinoma of the vagina and vulva who were treated with this technique.[46,47] Rotmensch and colleagues recently reported on 16 patients with advanced vulvar lesions who were treated with preoperative radiation to the vulva and achieved an overall 5-year survival rate of 45%.[48] Recurrences were more likely if the resection margins were within 1 cm of the tumor. Complications have included stenosis of the introitus and urethra as well as rectovaginal fistula.

Recently, an approach has been to not only administer preoperative radiation for advanced lesions but also to add chemotherapy. Commonly, agents such as 5-FU, cisplatin, and mitomycin C have been used, producing up to 46% reduction in tumor with chemoradiation. The most common toxicities were acute cutaneous and wound complications.[49] Investigators have suggested that radiation-sensitive chemotherapeutic drugs, such as *cis*-platinum, may enhance the response to radiation. The GOG has attempted to expedite this; however, the study was terminated owing to a lack of sufficient patients.

Because the vulvar skin is prone to radiation dermatitis, fibrosis, and ulceration, radiation as the sole therapy has been less than desirable. If the patient is inoperable because of medical conditions, however, radiation can be used as the primary treatment of a vulvar carcinoma.[50] Recurrences may be local or distant. More than 80% of recurrences occur in the first 2 years after therapy. The risk of recurrence of vulva carcinoma increases as the stage of disease increases. In an analysis of 224 patients with vulvar carcinoma, Podratz and colleagues reported a recurrence rate of 14% in stage I and 71% in stage IV disease.[51] Local recurrences were the most common. Local recurrences often occur in the skin bridge remaining after a radical vulvectomy.[52]

Different modalities have been used to treat local recurrences. Both radiation therapy and resection of local vulvar recurrence provide effective control and a 5-year survival rate of approximately 50%.

The combination of chemotherapy and radiation therapy has been used to treat recurrent disease and some large primary vulvar carcinomas. Thomas and colleagues reported the use of 5-FU (1 g/m^2) as a continuous intravenous infusion for 4 to 5 days every 4 weeks during radiation.[53] This combined approach was the sole treatment in nine patients, and six patients had a complete remission. Disseminated disease requires chemotherapy, but, unfortunately, no chemotherapy has been successful in this situation.

Bartholin Gland Carcinoma Primary carcinoma of Bartholin's gland accounts for 5% of all vulvar cancers, and over 200 cases have been reported.[54] Only approximately 50% of those tumors are nonepidermoid in nature. Bartholin gland carcinomas can be squamous if they originate near the orifice of the duct or papillary if they arise from the transitional epithelium of the duct, or they can be adenocarcinomas if they arise from the gland itself. An enlargement of Bartholin's gland in a postmenopausal female should raise the suspicion of malignancy. These tumors are treated similarly to primary squamous cell carcinomas of the vulva, by radical vulvectomy and bilateral inguinal femoral lymphadenectomy. The overall 5-year survival rate of approximately 70% is below that reported for all carcinomas of the vulva and probably relates to a delay in diagnosis.

The adenoid cystic variety of Bartholin gland carcinoma invades locally and rarely metastasizes. It usually requires only wide local excision for adequate therapy. Rosenberg and colleagues reported five cases of adenocystic carcinoma of Bartholin's gland, with four patients alive and free of disease 28 to 57 months after treatment.[55]

Basal Cell Carcinoma Basal cell carcinoma is rarely encountered in the female genital tract. Such lesions are usually locally invasive, nonmetastatic tumors that are commonly found on the labium majus. Therapy consists of wide local excision of the lesion. If the surgical margins are free of tumor, the disease is cured.

Verrucous Carcinoma Verrucous carcinoma of the vulva is a variant of epidermoid carcinoma. Clinically, it appears as large, condylomatous lesions. They are locally aggressive, nonmetastatic, fungating tumors that gradually increase in size, pushing into rather than invading the underlying structures. Histologically, they consist of mature squamous cells with extensive keratinization. To establish the diagnosis, adequate biopsy is important because biopsy of a large verrucous carcinoma often can lead to an incorrect diagnosis of condyloma acuminatum.

These tumors tend to grow slowly and invade locally, rarely spreading to regional lymph nodes. In 24 cases of verrucous carcinoma, Japaze and colleagues found no lymph node metastases.[56] Depending on the size and location of the tumor, a wide local excision or simple vulvectomy is effective therapy; radical vulvectomy with inguinal node dissection or radiation therapy is not indicated as treatment for this entity. Radiation therapy is ineffective and can even worsen the prognosis, causing malignant changes within the tumor. The 17 cases treated surgically by Japaze and colleagues had an excellent 5-year survival rate of 94%. Close long-term follow-up is needed because disease can recur locally, especially if the tumor is large. If concurrent squamous cell carcinoma is found within the verrucous carcinoma, local excision is an inadequate therapy.[57]

Melanoma Melanoma is the most frequent nonsquamous cell malignancy of the vulva and comprises approximately 5% of primary carcinomas of the vulva. Approximately 400 cases of melanoma of the vulva have been reported, with an overall 5-year survival rate of approximately 33%, irrespective of the therapeutic modality used. Patients with malignant melanoma of the vulva vary widely in age, ranging from 10 to 96 years, with an average age of approximately 60 years. These lesions most often affect the labia minora or the clitoris.[58]

For vulvar melanomas, the FIGO classification usually has been used. This classification is not, however, as good a prognostic indicator as is the depth of invasion. A system for vulvar melanoma analogous to that used by Clark for cutaneous melanoma has been adopted (Table 100-4). Levels I to V have been identified, based on the Clark classification. The level of invasion correlates with survival, which varies from 100% for level II to 83% for level IV and 28% for level V.[59]

Two varieties of melanoma have been described: nodular and superficial spreading melanoma.[60] The superficial spreading melanoma is more common and has a better prognosis, with a

Table 100-4 Classification of Melanomas of the Vulva

Clark level	
I	Intraepithelial
II	Extension to papillary dermes
III	Filling the dermal papillae
IV	Invasive of collagen in reticular dermis
V	Extension into subcutaneous fat
Breslow depth of invasion	
I	< 0.75 mm from skin surface
II	0.76–1.4 mm from skin surface
III	> 1.5 mm from skin surface

5-year survival rate of 71%. Nodular melanoma has a worse prognosis, and this directly relates to its potential for vertical growth. The 5-year survival rate for nodular melanoma, which is more invasive, is only 38%.

The thickness of the tumor also may be useful in evaluating this lesion. Breslow reported a classification using depth of invasion as measured from the skin surface.[61] In his classification, Breslow reported the overall prognosis as excellent and the spread to regional nodes as unlikely for melanomas with a thickness of less than 0.76 mm, measured from the surface to the deepest point of penetration.

Wide local excision has been recommended for Clark level I and II disease when no palpable regional nodes are present.[62] In a report of 36 melanoma cases, Rose and colleagues noted that wide excision was as effective as radical vulvectomy.[63] Prognosis was better for younger patients, presumably because most had superficial spreading rather than nodular melanomas.

A reasonable approach is to excise a melanoma with a 2 cm margin and without node dissection for cases that are less than 2 mm thick. An excision with a 2 to 3 cm margin combined with node dissection could be performed for more advanced melanomas. An alternative approach for lesions that have extended to Clark levels III, IV, and V is radical vulvectomy with groin and pelvic lymphadenectomy.

It has been reported that melanoma of the vulva can metastasize to pelvic nodes, bypassing the inguinal femoral nodes, but current evidence indicates that pelvic node involvement does not occur without prior inguinal node involvement. A further therapeutic consideration is that patients with melanoma whose pelvic nodes are involved with tumor usually do not survive their disease.

Long-term results generally are not available for large series of melanomas. Most series of malignant melanoma report an overall survival rate of approximately 50%.[64] For lesions that correspond to Clark level I or II (lesions 0.76 mm thick) and are treated by wide local excision, the 5-year survival rate is in the vicinity of 100%. Prognosis becomes poorer with melanomas more than 3 mm thick. If the regional nodes are negative, the survival rate is approximately 60%; if the regional nodes are involved with tumor, survival is only 30%.

The role of chemotherapy for distant metastasis has not been well established. Regressions, but not cures, have been reported with various multiagent cytotoxic programs, including chemotherapy and/or immunotherapy.

Sarcoma Sarcomas of the vulva are rare. Leiomyosarcomas appear to be the most frequently encountered sarcomas in this group of patients,[65] and surgical removal by wide local excision is the recommended initial treatment of choice. The 5-year survival rate is reported to be approximately 100%. Locally recurrent lesions are similarly treated. Chemotherapeutic considerations are the same as for those sarcomas in other sites of the female genital tract.[66]

CANCER OF THE VAGINA

Primary vaginal cancers are rare, constituting less than 2% of all gynecologic malignancies.[1,67,68] Carcinoma of the vagina is defined as a primary carcinoma arising in the vagina and not involving the external os of the cervix superiorly or the vulva inferiorly.

Vaginal cancer is rare and accounts for only about 3% of cancers of the female reproductive system. The American Cancer Society estimates that in 2005, about 2,140 new cases of vaginal cancer will be diagnosed in the United States and 810 women will die of this cancer.

The most common symptom of vaginal carcinoma is abnormal bleeding or discharge. With advanced tumors, pain or urinary frequency occasionally occurs, especially in cases of anterior wall tumors. Constipation or tenesmus has been seen with tumors involving the posterior vaginal wall. These tumors usually are diagnosed by direct biopsy of the tumor mass, and abnormal cytologic findings often will lead to diagnosis of a vaginal cancer.

The staging criteria for vaginal carcinomas according to the FIGO are given in Table 100-5.

Premalignant Vaginal Disease Premalignant disease of the vagina is generally detected on cytologic screening. Once an abnormal cytology is obtained, a biopsy directed by colposcopic examination is required to verify the severity of the changes. Because vaginal intraepithelial neoplasia is often multifocal, it is necessary to inspect the entire vaginal canal.

Most lesions occur at the vaginal apex. Audet-Lapointe and colleagues noted that 61 of 66 cases of vaginal intraepithelial neoplasia occurred in the upper third of the vagina.[69] These lesions usually can be excised locally. Other modalities often are preferred, however, because of the multifocal nature of this disease or the necessity of excising large areas, requiring skin grafting.[70]

Nonsurgical approaches for treating these lesions include laser ablation and 5-FU cream for widespread multifocal disease. Carbon dioxide laser frequently has been used and, if carried to a depth of 2 to 4 mm, allows for vaporization of abnormal tissue. Preliminary results reported by Petrilli and colleagues with this modality have shown a success rate of approximately 90%.[71] Radiation currently is not recommended for the treatment of noninvasive disease because of the proximity of the bladder and rectum and the availability of newer modalities.

Table 100-5 FIGO Staging Classification for Vaginal Carcinoma

Stage	
0	Carcinoma in situ
I	Carcinoma limited to vaginal wall
II	Carcinoma involves subvaginal tissue but has not extended to pelvic wall
III	Carcinoma extends to pelvic wall
IV	Carcinoma extends beyond true pelvis or involves mucosa of bladder or rectum

FIGO = International Federation of Gynecology and Obstetrics.

Another approach to treating vaginal intraepithelial neoplasia is the use of 5% 5-FU cream for approximately 7 days, repeated every 3 to 4 weeks if the vaginal intraepithelial neoplasia persists. Hyperkeratotic lesions appear to be less sensitive to treatment because of their thickness and parakeratosis. Krebs reported on the use of 5% 5-FU daily for 10 days and noted that 17 of 20 patients with vaginal condylomas responded to this therapy.[72] Petrilli and colleagues and Ballon and colleagues reported success rates of 80 to 90% for vaginal intraepithelial neoplasia after multiple cycles of therapy.[71,73]

INVASIVE CARCINOMAS OF THE VAGINA

Squamous cell carcinomas of the vagina may appear grossly as either ulcerated or fungating tumors, or they may be exophytic and protrude through the vaginal canal. They are the most common vaginal malignancy and account for 90% of primary vaginal cancers. The disease occurs primarily in women over 50 years of age. Most squamous cell carcinomas occur in the upper third of the vagina. In examining the patient, it is important to visualize the entire vagina because lesions on the posterior wall can be concealed by the speculum.

Microscopically, these tumors have the classic findings of invasive squamous cell carcinoma. They have pleomorphic squamous cells with occasional keratin pearls.

The location of the tumor determines the areas of lymphatic spread (Figure 100-7).[74] The lymphatics of the middle and upper vagina communicate superiorly with the lymphatics of the cervix and drain into the pelvic nodes of the obturator, internal, and external iliac chains. The lymphatics of the distal third of the vagina drain to the inguinal and pelvic nodes, with a pattern of drainage similar to that of the vulva. The posterior wall lymphatics drain to the rectal lymphatic system.

Depending on the location, both radiation and surgery have been used effectively in treating these lesions (Table 100-6). Treatment is often individualized, depending on the size, stage, and location of the tumor.[73]

If the tumor is less than 2 cm thick, some investigators advocate using only local radiation.[75,76] If the carcinoma is less than 0.5 cm thick, intracavitary irradiation with a vaginal cylinder to deliver 8,000 cGy to the mucosa will give over 90% tumor control.[77] Spirtos and colleagues studied 23 stage I patients and noted only two local recurrences, and both of these had tumor doses of less than 7,500 cGy.[78] For larger lesions, external radiation is used, with a concomitant reduction in the local vaginal component of primary tumor treatment.[79] Implants, however, often cannot be used in patients with larger stage III or IV carcinomas. If such is the case, only external beam radiation is used, and a central boost is

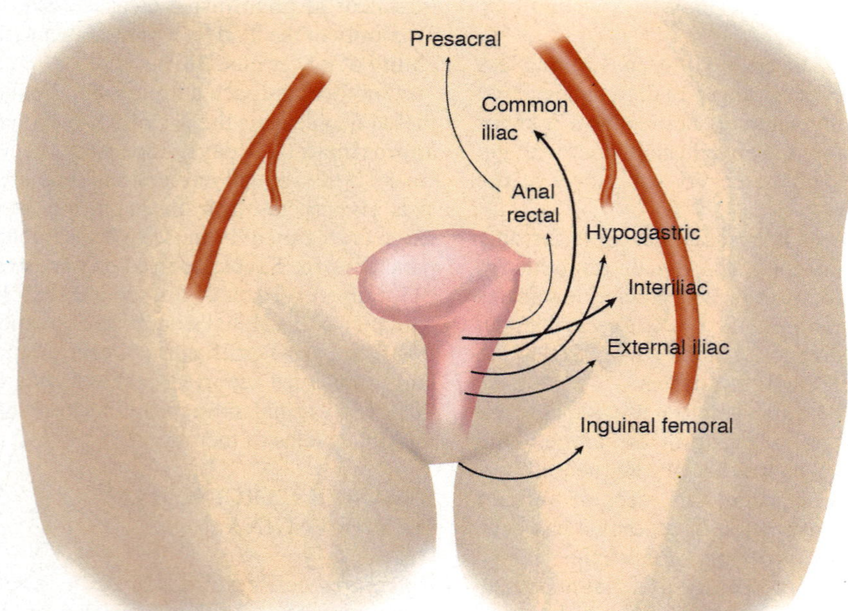

Figure 100-7 Lymphatic drainage of the vagina.

Table 100-6 Treatment Scheme for Vaginal Carcinoma

Stage	External Therapy (cGy)	Implant (Interstitial), cGy
I		
Σ, small tumors (< 2 cm)	—	6,000–7,000
Σ, all others	Whole pelvis (4,000)	3,000–4,000 cGy
II	Whole pelvis (4,000–5,000)	3,000–4,000 cGy
III	Whole pelvis (5,000)	2,000
IV	Whole pelvis (5,000; an additional 1,000–2,000 through reduced field if implant not possible)	2,000 (if possible)

Adapted from Nori D et al.[77]
1 cGy = 1 rad.

given after an initial whole-pelvis dose of 5,000 cGy radiation.[80]

Small tumors located in the upper third of the vagina often can be excised.[81] In patients with these, a radical hysterectomy, partial vaginectomy, or pelvic lymphadenectomy usually is effective. Surgery has been preferred in younger patients.

If distant metastasis occurs, effective chemotherapy for recurrent squamous cell carcinoma of the vagina has not been developed. For squamous cell carcinoma, a variety of regimens using multiagent chemotherapy similar to those for cervical carcinoma have been employed.

The overall survival rate for patients with primary carcinoma of the vagina has been reported as approximately 45% and is related to the stage of the disease (Table 100-7).

CLEAR CELL ADENOCARCINOMA OF THE VAGINA

Clear cell adenocarcinomas have been seen more frequently in young women since 1970 because of the association with intrauterine exposure to diethylstilbestrol.[82,83] Three predominant histologic patterns are found with clear cell carcinoma; they have been described as tubulocystic, solid, and papillary patterns.[84,85] Most clear cell carcinomas of the vagina are polypoid or nodular, with a reddish color.

Clear cell carcinomas can spread locally and by the lymphatic and hematogenous routes. Metastases to regional pelvic nodes have been found in approximately one-sixth of stage I cases. Spread to regional pelvic nodes becomes more frequent in higher-stage tumors.

Clear cell adenocarcinomas are staged as other carcinomas of the vagina are by the FIGO. Some 80% have been diagnosed as stage I or II.

Several prognostic factors have been identified. Older patients (ie, > 19 years of age) have a more favorable prognosis than younger patients.[86] This difference has been associated with the presence of a more favorable tubulocystic pattern of clear cell adenocarcinoma, which is the most frequent histologic pattern found in older patients. In addition, smaller tumor diameter and superficial depth of invasion correlate with improved patient survival.

Table 100-7 Stage and Survival of Squamous Cell Carcinoma of the Vagina

Stage	Survival Rate (%)
I	71
II	47
III	25
IV	8
Overall	45

Adapted from Benedet JL, Murphy KS, Fairey RN, et al. Primary invasive carcinoma of the vagina. Obstet Gynecol 1983;62:715.

Table 100-8 Survival at 5 and 10 Years for 547 Patients with Clear Cell Adenocarcinoma of the Vagina and Cervix

	Survival, %	
Stage	5 Years	10 Years
I	93	87
IIA	80	66
IIB	58	49
II (vagina)	83	67
III	37	12
IV	0	0

Survival also depends on the stage of the disease. In 547 patients treated for clear cell adenocarcinoma of the vagina, the 5-year survival rate for those in stages I, II, III, and IV has been 93%, 83%, 37%, and 0%, respectively (Table 100-8).[86]

Because of the young age of these patients, surgery often is the primary therapy. For stage I and early stage II disease (Figure 100-8), radical hysterectomy, partial or complete vaginectomy, pelvic lymphadenectomy, and replacement of the vagina with a split-thickness skin graft have been the approaches most frequently used.[87]

In patients with small stage I tumors of the vagina, efforts have been made to preserve fertility. The tumor has been excised with retroperitoneal lymph node dissection, followed by local radiation. Senekjian and colleagues reported that the survival rate of patients with small vaginal tumors treated with such an approach compares favorably with that of patients treated with conventional therapy.[87] In their series, eight pregnancies were reported in five patients who were treated locally.

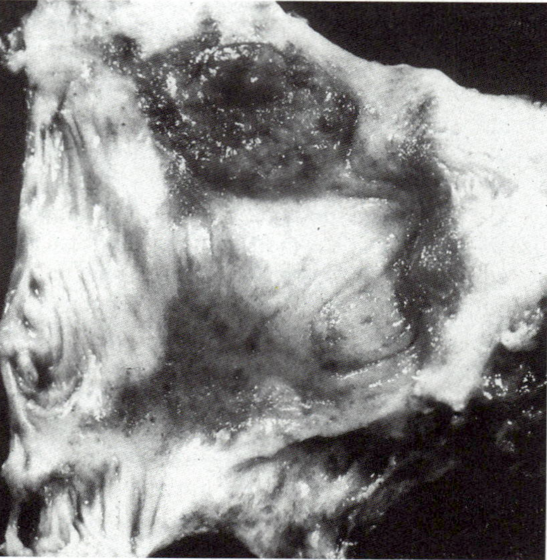

Figure 100-8 Clear cell adenocarcinoma of the anterior wall, with vaginal adenosis on the posterior wall at the edge of the tumor.

Larger tumors have been treated with whole-pelvis radiation in addition to intracavitary implant. For tumors greater than 2 cm, whole-pelvis radiation of 4,000 to 5,000 cGy has been given, with an additional implant of 3,000 to 4,000 cGy.[88] In a few instances, exenterative surgery has been performed for larger tumors; however, this procedure usually has been applied to central recurrences following primary radiation therapy.[89]

If there is a recurrence, therapy consists of additional radical surgery, often requiring exenteration or extensive radiation localized to the pelvis. Systemic chemotherapy has been used in cases of metastatic disease. Cisplatin (75–100 mg/m^2) with a continuous infusion of 5-FU (1 g/m^2 for 3 to 5 days every 3 to 4 weeks) is currently recommended. However, no single agent or combination of chemotherapeutic agents has emerged as the most effective. Prolonged follow-up is necessary because recurrences, especially in the lungs and supraclavicular areas, have been reported as long as 19 years after primary therapy.

Vaginal Melanomas Malignant melanomas of the vagina are rare; they constitute fewer than 1% of all melanomas occurring in females. The age distribution of the neoplasm has ranged from 26 to 98 years,[58] with a median age of 70 years. Most patients are postmenopausal and present with vaginal bleeding, discharge, or a mass. Tumors may vary from 0.5 to 7.5 cm in diameter, with approximately 30% being 2 cm or less in diameter. Most of these tumors develop in the distal third of the vagina, commonly on the anterior wall. Primary vaginal melanomas presumably arise from vaginal melanocytes that are present in approximately 3% of normal females. Histologically, this neoplasm is similar to other melanomas found elsewhere and tends to be deeply invasive in the vagina.

The prognosis is worse than that of vulvar melanomas. Chung and colleagues reported a 5-year survival rate of only 21% in a series of 19 patients.[90] Reid and colleagues reported a 5-year survival rate of 17.4% in 15 cases, but the prognosis was improved for those tumors that were small and less than 3 cm in diameter.[91] More recently, Borazjani and colleagues reported improved survival for cases in which there were fewer than six mitoses/10 high-power fields.[92]

Optimal treatment has not been established. Treatment usually consists of radical surgery or wide excision of the vagina and dissection of the regional lymph nodes, depending on the location of the lesion. Because of the poor prognosis, adjunctive radiation and chemotherapy have been used as local recurrences, and distant metastases with this disease are common.

RARE VAGINAL TUMORS IN YOUNG FEMALES

Endodermal sinus tumor is a rare germ cell malignancy that is usually found in the ovary.[93] This tumor secretes alpha-fetoprotein, which often is a useful tumor marker for monitoring patients with this neoplasm. It is usually found in infants and children, and approximately 20 cases have been reported as occurring in the vaginas of infants who were under 2 years of age.[94,95] Patients generally present with complaints of bleeding or spotting from the vagina. On physical examination, there is a friable red to pinkish-white polypoid tumor. This tumor is aggressive, and most patients have died. Therapy has involved surgery, radiation, and chemotherapy. Young and Scully reported six patients who were disease free from 2 to 9 years after local therapy with operation, irradiation, or both, followed by systemic chemotherapy with vincristine, actinomycin D, and cyclophosphamide (VAC).[96] Copeland and colleagues reported similar results using the combination of chemotherapy and excision,[97] and Collins and colleagues recently noted the regression of tumor with chemotherapy alone.[98] In this report, a 5-month-old patient had regression of the tumor after VAC therapy.

Another rare tumor found in the vaginas of young females is sarcoma botryoides, or embryonal rhabdomyosarcoma.[99] This tumor is usually found in children under 8 years of age. As with endodermal sinus tumor, the most common symptom has been vaginal bleeding. In 58 cases reviewed by Hilgers, the average age at onset of symptoms was 38.3 months.[44] This tumor resembles clusters of grapes and forms multiple polypoid masses that are believed to begin in the subepithelial layers of the vagina and to rapidly expand, filling the vagina. Histologically, these tumors are identified by the presence of rhabdomyoblasts that may contain cross-striations. Because of infiltration of the tumor under the vaginal epithelium, there is often a distinct subepithelial zone, called the cambium layer. The 5-year survival rate of these tumors in the past has ranged from 10 to 35%, and exenterative procedures have often been used.[100] Hilgers reviewed the literature on pelvic exenterations in 21 cases of embryonal rhabdomyosarcoma and found that this form of therapy was ineffective in curing these patients.[44] Effective control with less radical surgery has been achieved using multimodal treatment consisting of multiagent chemotherapy, VAC, combined with operation or radiation.

Hayes and colleagues recently reported 21 patients with vaginal rhabdomyosarcoma who received chemotherapy.[101] In their series, 7 relapsed, with 5 of these 7 having had residual disease following incomplete resection. In 17 of 21 patients who received chemotherapy before surgery, a subsequent delayed excision could be performed. Data regarding the long-term survival of a large number of patients are not available, but such a combined approach appears to result in effective therapy with less mutilating surgery.

A rare, benign, fibroepithelial vaginal polyp that resembles sarcoma botryoides can be found in the vaginas of infants or pregnant women.[60,102,103] Although large atypical cells are present microscopically, epithelial infiltration, a cambium layer, and strap cells are absent. Grossly, these polyps do not resemble the grape-like appearance of sarcoma botryoides. These hormonally stimulated hyperplastic lesions are called pseudosarcoma botryoides, and treatment by local excision is effective.

REFERENCES

1. Landis SH, Murray T, Bolden S, Wingo P. Cancer statistics 1999. CA Cancer J Clin 1999;49:8.
2. Franklin EW III, Rutledge F. Epidemiology of epidermoid carcinoma of the vulva. Obstet Gynecol 1972;39:165.
3. Sutton GP, Stehman FB, Ehrlich CE, Roman A. Human papilloma virus deoxyribonucleic acid in lesions of the female genital tract: evidence for types 6/11 in squamous carcinoma of the vulva. Obstet Gynecol 1987;70:564.
4. Crum CP. Vulvar intraepithelial neoplasia: histology and associated viral changes. In: Wilkinson EJ, editor. Pathology of the vulva and vagina. New York: Churchill Livingstone; 1987.
5. Planner RS, Hobbs JB. Intraepithelial and invasive neoplasia of the vulva in association with human papillomavirus infection. J Reprod Med 1988;33:503.
6. Basta A, Adamek K, Pitynski K. Intraepithelial neoplasia and early stage vulvar cancer: epidemiological, clinical and virological observations. Eur J Gynaecol Oncol 1999;20:111–4.
7. Mabuchi K, Bross DS, Kessler II. Epidemiology of cancer of the vulva: a case control study. Cancer 1985;55:1843–8.
8. Buscema J, Woodruff JD, Parmley TH, Genadry R. Carcinoma in situ of the vulva. Obstet Gynecol 1980;55:225.
9. Skinner MS, Sternberg WH, Inchinose H, et al. Spontaneous regression of bowenoid atypia of the vulva. Obstet Gynecol 1973;42:40.
10. Chafe W, Richards A, Morgan L, Wilkinson E. Unrecognized invasive carcinoma in vulvar epithelial neoplasia (VIN). Gynecol Oncol 1988;31:154.
11. Friedrich EG. Vulvar disease. 2nd ed. Philadelphia: W.B. Saunders; 1983.
12. Fredrich EF, Wilkinson EJ, Fu YS. Carcinoma in situ of the vulva: a continuing challenge. Am J Obstet Gynecol 1980;136:830.
13. International Society for the Study of Vulvar Disease new nomenclature for vulvar disease. Obstet Gynecol 1976;47:122.
14. Hart WR, Norris HJ, Helwig ED. Relation of lichen sclerosus et atrophicus of the vulva to development of carcinoma. Obstet Gynecol 1975;45:369.
15. Crum PC, Liskow A, Petras P, et al. Vulvar intraepithelial neoplasia (severe atypia and carcinoma in situ). Cancer 1984;54:1429.
16. Fu YS, Reagan JW, Townsend DE, et al. Nuclear DNA study of vulvar intraepithelial and invasive squamous neoplasms. Obstet Gynecol 1981;57:643.
17. Rutledge F, Sinclair M. Treatment of intraepithelial neoplasia of the vulva by skin excision and graft. Obstet Gynecol 1968;102:806.
18. Woodruff JD, Genadry R, Poliakoff S. Treatment of dyspareunia and vaginal outlet distortions by perineoplasty. Obstet Gynecol 1981;57:750.
19. Leuchter RS, Hacker NF, Voet RL, et al. Primary carcinoma of the Bartholin gland: a report of 14 cases and review of the literature. Obstet Gynecol 1982;60:361.
20. Helwig EP, Graham JH. Anogenital (extramammary) Paget's disease. Cancer 1963;16:387.
21. Lee SC, Roth LM, Ehrlich C, Hall JA. Extramammary Paget's disease of the vulva—a clinicopathologic study of 13 cases. Cancer 1977;39:2540.
22. Friedrich EG Jr, Wilkinson EJ, Steingraeber PH, Lewis JD. Paget's disease of the vulva and carcinoma of the breast. Obstet Gynecol 1975;46:130.
23. Bergen S, DiSaia PJ, Liao SY, Berman ML. Conservative management of extramammary Paget's disease of the vulva. Gynecol Oncol 1989;33:151.
24. Creasman WT. New gynecologic cancer staging. Obstet Gynecol 1990;75:287.
25. Iversen T, Aas M. Lymph drainage from the vulva. Gynecol Oncol 1983;16:179.
26. Chu J, Tamimi HK, Ek M, Figge DC. Stage I vulvar cancer criteria for microinvasion. Obstet Gynecol 1982;59:716.
27. Dvoretsky PM, Bonfiglio TA, Helkamp BF, et al. The pathology of superficially invasive thin vulva squamous cell carcinoma. Int J Gynecol Pathol 1984;3:331.
28. Hacker NF, Nieburg RK, Berek JS, et al. Superficially invasive vulvar cancer with nodal metastases. Gynecol Oncol 1983;15:65.

29. Hoffman JS, Kumar NB, Morley GW. Microinvasive squamous cell carcinoma of the vulva: a search for definition. Obstet Gynecol 1983;61:615.
30. Rowley KC, Gallion HH, Donalson ES, et al. Prognostic factors in early vulvar cancer. Gynecol Oncol 1988;31:43.
31. Berman ML, Soper JT, Creasman WT, et al. Conservative surgical management in superficially invasive stage I vulvar carcinoma. Gynecol Oncol 1989;35:352.
32. DiSaia PJ, Creasman WT, Rich WM. An alternate approach to early cancer of the vulva. Am J Obstet Gynecol 1979;133:825.
33. Iversen T, Abler V, Aalders J. Individual treatment of stage I carcinoma of the vulva. Obstet Gynecol 1981;57:85.
34. Boyce J, Fruchter RG, Kasambilides E, et al. Prognostic factors in carcinoma of the vulva. Gynecol Oncol 1985;20:364.
35. Levenback C, Burke TW, Morris M, et al. Potential applications of intraoperative lymphatic mapping in vulvar cancer. Gynecol Oncol 1995.
36. Thomas GM, Dembo AJ, Bryson P. et al. Changing concepts in the management of vulvar cancer. Gynecol Oncol 1991;42:9–1.
37. Iversen T, Tretli S. Intraepithelial and invasive squamous cell neoplasia of the vulva: trends in incidence, recurrence, and survival rate in Norway. Obstet Gynecol 1998;91:969–72.
38. Louis-Sylvestre C, Evangelista E, Leonard F. Sentinal node localization should be interpreted with caution in midline vulvar cancer. Gynecol Oncol 2005;1:151–4.
39. Donaldson ES, Powell DE, Hanson MB, Van Nagell JR Jr. Prognostic parameters in invasive vulvar cancer. Gynecol Oncol 1981;11:184.
40. Homesley HD, Bundy BN, Sedlis A, Adcock L. A randomized study of radiation therapy versus pelvic node resection for patients with invasive squamous cell carcinoma of the vulva having positive groin nodes. Gynecologic Oncology Study Group. Obstet Gynecol 1986;68:733.
41. Hacker NF, Berek JS, Lagasse LD, et al. Management of regional lymph nodes and their prognostic influence in vulvar cancer. Obstet Gynecol 1983;61:408.
42. Hoffman JS, Kumar NB, Morley GW. Prognostic significance of groin lymph node metastases of squamous carcinoma of the vulva. Obstet Gynecol 1985;66:402.
43. Figge DC, Tamimi HK, Greer BE. Lymphatic spread in carcinoma of the vulva. Am J Obstet Gynecol 1985;152:387.
44. Hilgers RD. Pelvic exenteration for vaginal embryonal rhabdomyosarcoma: a review. Obstet Gynecol 1975;45:175.
45. Christopherson W, Buchsbaum HJ, Voet R, Lifschitz S. Radical vulvectomy and bilateral groin lymphadenectomy utilizing separate groin incisions: report of a case with recurrence in the intervening skin bridge. Gynecol Oncol 1985;21:247.
46. Boronow RC. Combined therapy as an alternative to exenteration of locally advanced vulvar vaginal cancer. Cancer 1982;49:1085.
47. Boronow RC, Hickman BT, Reagan MT, et al. Combined therapy as an alternative to exenteration for locally advanced vulvovaginal cancer. Am J Clin Oncol 1987;10:1711.
48. Rotmensch J, Rubin SJ, Sutton HG, et al. Preoperative radiotherapy followed by radical vulvectomy with inguinal lymphadenectomy for advanced vulvar cancer. Gynecol Oncol 1990;36:181.
49. Moore DH, Thomas GM, Montana GS, et al. Preoperative chemoradiation for advanced vulvar cancer: a phase II study of the Gynecologic Oncology Group. Int J Radiat Oncol Biol Phys 1998;42:1317–23.
50. Farey RN, McKay PA, Benedet JL. Radiation treatment of carcinoma of the vulva 1950–1980. Am J Obstet Gynecol 1985;151:591.
51. Podratz KC, Symmonds RE, Taylor WF. Carcinoma of the vulva and vagina. In: Coppelson M, editor. Gynecologic oncology. New York: Churchill Livingstone; 1981.
52. Rouzier R, Haddad B, Plantier F, et al. Local relapse in patients treated for squamous cell vulvar carcinoma: incidence and prognostic value. Obstet Gynecol 2002;100:1159–67.
53. Thomas G, Dembo A, DePetrillo A. Concurrent radiation and chemotherapy in vulvar carcinoma. Gynecol Oncol 1989;34:263.
54. Leuchter RS, Hacker NF, Voet RL, et al. Primary carcinoma of the Bartholin gland: a report of 14 cases and review of the literature. Obstet Gynecol 1982;60:361.
55. Rosenberg P, Simonsen E, Risberg B. Adenoid cystic carcinoma of Bartholin's gland: a report of 5 new cases treated with surgery and radiotherapy. Gynecol Oncol 1989;34:145.
56. Japaze H, Dinh TV, Woodruff JD. Verrucous carcinoma of the vulva: study of 24 cases. Obstet Gynecol 1982;60:462.
57. Crowther ME, Lowe DG, Shepherd JH. Verrucous carcinoma of the female genital tract: a review. Obstet Gynecol Surv 1988;43:263.
58. Weinstock MA. Malignant melanoma of the vulva and vagina in the United States: patterns of incidence and population-based estimates of survival. Am J Obstet Gynecol 1994;171:1225–30.
59. Phillips GL, Twiggs LB, Okagaki T. Vulvar melanoma: a microstaging study. Gynecol Oncol 1982;14:80.
60. Mitchell M, Talerman A, Sholl JS, et al. Pseudosarcoma botryoides in pregnancy: report of a case with ultra-structural observations. Obstet Gynecol 1987;70:522.
61. Breslow A. Thickness, cross-sectional areas, and depth of invasion in the prognosis of cutaneous melanoma. Ann Surg 1970;172:908.
62. Veronesi V, Cascinelli N, Adams J, et al. Thin stage I primary cutaneous malignant melanomas, comparison of excision with margins of 1 or 3 cm. N Engl J Med 1988;318:1159.
63. Rose PG, Piver S, Tsukada Y, Lau T. Conservative therapy for melanoma of the vulva. Am J Obstet Gynecol 1988;159:57.
64. Podratz KC, Gaffey TA, Symmonds RE, et al. Melanoma of the vulva: an update. Gynecol Oncol 1983;16:153.
65. DiSaia PJ, Rutledge F, Smith JP. Sarcoma of the vulva—report of 12 patients. Obstet Gynecol 1971;38:180.
66. Lieb SM, Gallousis S, Greedman H. Granular cell myoblastoma of the vulva. Gynecol Oncol 1979;8:12.
67. Friedrich EG. Reversible vulvar atypia: a case report. Obstet Gynecol 1972;39:713.
68. Pride GL, Schultz AE, Chuprevich TW, Buchler DA. Primary invasive squamous carcinoma of the vagina. Obstet Gynecol 1979;53:218.
69. Audet-Lapointe P, Body G, Vauclair R, et al. Vaginal intraepithelial neoplasia. Gynecol Oncol 1990;36:232.
70. Gallup DG, Morley GW. Carcinoma in situ of the vagina: a study and review. Obstet Gynecol 1975;46:334.
71. Petrilli ES, Townsend DE, Morrow CP, Nakao CY. Vaginal intraepithelial neoplasm: biologic aspects and treatment with topical 5-fluorouracil and the carbon dioxide laser. Am J Obstet Gynecol 1980;38:321.
72. Krebs HB. Treatment of vaginal condylomata acuminata by weekly topical application of 5-fluorouracil. Obstet Gynecol 1987;70:68.
73. Ballon SC, Roberts JA, Lagasse LD. Topical 5-fluorouracil in the treatment of intraepithelial neoplasia of the vagina. Obstet Gynecol 1979;54:163.
74. Plentl AA, Friedman EA. Lymphatic system of the female genitalia. Philadelphia: W.B. Saunders; 1971.
75. Andersen ES. Primary carcinoma of the vagina: a study of 29 cases. Gynecol Oncol 1989;33:317.
76. Otton GR, Nicklin JL, Dickie GJ, et al. Early-stage vaginal carcinoma—an analysis of 70 patients. Int J Gynecol Cancer 2004;14:304–10.
77. Nori D, Hilaris BS, Stanimir G, Lewis JL Jr. Radiation therapy of primary vaginal carcinoma. Int J Radiat Oncol Biol Phys 1983;9:1471.
78. Spirtos NM, Doshi BP, Kapp DS, Teng N. Radiation therapy for primary squamous cell carcinoma of the vagina: Stanford University experience. Gynecol Oncol 1989;35:20.
79. Wharton JT, Fletcher GH, Delclos L. Invasive tumors of the vagina. In: Coppleson M, editor. Gynecologic oncology. New York: Churchill Livingstone; 1981.
80. Prempree T, Viravathana T, Slawson RG, et al. Radiation management of primary carcinoma of the vagina. Cancer 1977;40:109.
81. Benedet JL, Murphy KS, Fairey RN, Boyes DA. Primary invasive carcinoma of the vagina. Obstet Gynecol 1983;62:715.
82. Herbst AL, Scully RE. Adenocarcinoma of the vagina in adolescence. Cancer 1970;25:745.
83. Herbst AL, Ulfelder H, Poskanzer DC. Adenocarcinoma of the vagina. N Engl J Med 1971;284:878.
84. Scully RE, Robboy SJ, Herbst AL. Vaginal and cervical abnormalities, including clear cell adenocarcinoma related to prenatal exposure to stilbestrol. Ann Clin Lab Sci 1974;4:22.
85. Scully RE, Welch WR. Pathology of the female genital tract after prenatal exposure to diethylstilbestrol. In: Herbst AL, Bern HA, editors. Developmental effects of diethylstilbestrol (DES) in pregnancy. New York: Thieme-Stratton; 1981.
86. Herbst AL, Anderson D. Recent advances in clear cell adenocarcinoma of the vagina and cervix secondary to intrauterine exposure to DES. In: Piver MS, editor. Seminars in surgical oncology. New York: John Wiley & Sons.
87. Senekjian EK, Frey KW, Anderson D, Herbst AL. Local therapy in stage I clear cell adenocarcinoma of the vagina. Cancer 1987;60:1319.
88. Senekjian EK, Frey KW, Herbst AL. Pelvic exenteration in clear cell adenocarcinoma of the vagina and cervix. Gynecol Oncol 1989;34:413.
89. Senekjian EK, Frey KW, Stone C, Herbst AL. An evaluation of stage II vaginal clear cell adenocarcinoma according to substages. Gynecol Oncol 1988;31:56.
90. Chung AF, Casey MJ, Flannery JT, et al. Malignant melanoma of the vagina: report of 19 cases. Obstet Gynecol 1980;55:720.
91. Reid GC, Schmidt RW, Roberts JA, et al. Primary melanoma of the vagina: a clinicopathologic analysis. Obstet Gynecol 1989;74:190.
92. Borazjani G, Prem KA, Okagaki T, et al. Primary malignant melanoma of the vagina: a clinicopathological analysis of 10 cases. Gynecol Oncol 1990;37:264.
93. Dewhurst J. Genital malignancies in the prepubertal child. In: Coppleson M, editor. Gynecologic oncology. New York: Churchill Livingstone; 1981.
94. Allyn DL, Silverberg SG, Salzberg AM. Endodermal sinus tumor of the vagina: report of a case with 7-year survival and literature review of so-called "mesonephromas." Cancer 1971;27:1231.
95. Andersen WA, Sabio H, Durso N, et al. Endodermal sinus tumor of the vagina. Cancer 1985;56:1025.
96. Young RH, Scully RE. Endodermal sinus tumor of the vagina: a report of nine cases and review of the literature. Gynecol Oncol 1984;18:380.
97. Copeland LJ, Sneige N, Ordonez NG, et al. Endodermal sinus tumor of the vagina and cervix. Cancer 1985;55:2558.
98. Collins HS, Burke TW, Heller PB, et al. Endodermal sinus tumor of the infant vagina treated exclusively by chemotherapy. Obstet Gynecol 1989;73:507.
99. Copeland LJ, Gershenson DM, Saul PB, et al. Sarcoma botryoides of the female genital tract. Obstet Gynecol 1985;66:262.
100. Pivers MS, Rose PG. Long-term follow-up and complications of infants with vulvovaginal embryonal rhabdomyosarcoma treated with surgery, radiation therapy, and chemotherapy. Obstet Gynecol 1988;71:435.
101. Hayes DM, Shimada H, Raney RB, et al. Clinical staging and treatment results in rhabdomyosarcoma of the female genital tract among children and adolescents. Cancer 1988;61:1893.
102. Elliott GB, Reynolds HA, Fidler HK. Pseudosarcoma botryoides of cervix and vagina in pregnancy. J Obstet Gynecol Br Comm 1967;74:728.
103. Miettinen M, Wahlstrom T, Vesterinen E, Saksela E. Vaginal polyps with pseudosarcomatous features: a clinicopathologic study of seven cases. Cancer 1983;51:1148.

Neoplasms of the Cervix

Anuja Jhingran, MD
Patricia J. Eifel, MD
J. Taylor Wharton, MD
Guillermo Tortolero-Luna, MD, PhD

EPIDEMIOLOGY

INCIDENCE AND MORTALITY Cervical cancer is the second most common cancer among women worldwide, with an estimated 493,000 new cases and 274,000 deaths in the year 2002.[1] It is more common in developing countries, where 83% of cases occur and where cervical cancer accounts for 15% of female cancers. The highest incidence rates are observed in sub-Saharan Africa, Melanesia, Latin America, the Caribbean, south-central Asia, and southeast Asia.[1]

In developed countries, cervical cancer accounts for only 3.6% of all new cancers.[1] In the United States, it is estimated that there will be 10,370 new cases of cervical cancer in 2005, with 3,710 related deaths.[2] It is the second leading cause of cancer-related deaths in females between 20 and 39 years of age in the United States.[2] It is more frequently seen in the Hispanic population (16% of all cases of cervical cancer) followed by the African American population (11.8%), Pacific Islanders/Asian (9.5%), whites (8.9%), and American Indians (6%).[2]

In the last 40 years, primarily because of the introduction of screening with the Pap smear, incidence and mortality rates for cervical cancer have declined in most developed countries.[3] In the United States, incidence rates have declined by approximately 70% during this period. Larger declines have been observed among women aged 50 and older (50.5%) than among younger women (36.4%) and among African-American (60.2%) than among Caucasian women (44.5%).[4] In developing countries, however, cervical cancer continues to be a significant health problem because of the lack of effective screening programs and the lack of therapy for precancerous conditions. Furthermore, the decline in incidence and mortality observed in the United States and other developed countries since the mid-1980s seems to be leveling off or reversing.[4] Presently in the United States, the risk of developing cervical cancer is 1 in 130 with overall 5 years. Five-year survival is 74% in whites and 66% in African Americans.[5]

There are no reliable data on the prevalence and incidence of precancerous cervical lesions. In the United States, the National Cancer Institute estimates that each year approximately 300,000 women are found to have premalignant cervical lesions, whereas the American Cancer Society reported that in 2001, an estimated 65,000 women were found to have carcinoma in situ of the cervix. From the SEER data, the overall incidence of squamous cell carcinoma in situ among whites is 41.4 per 100,000 woman-years from 1991 to 1995.[6]

RISK FACTORS FOR CERVICAL NEOPLASIA **Human Papillomavirus and Other Sexually Transmitted Agents** Epidemiologic evidence has long suggested a sexually transmitted etiology for cervical neoplasia. Supporting this hypothesis, several measures of sexual behavior (including multiple sexual partners, early age at first sexual intercourse, and sexual habits of male partners) have consistently been associated with an increased risk of cervical neoplasia.[7] Over the years, several sexually transmitted infectious agents have been the focus of research, including herpes simplex virus type 2 (HSV-2), *Chlamydia trachomatis*, *Trichomonas vaginalis*, cytomegalovirus, *Neisseria gonorrhoeae*, and *Treponema pallidum*.[8] In the mid-1970s, the hypothesis of a causal relationship between human papillomavirus (HPV) and cervical neoplasia was first proposed.[9] Since then, a large body of experimental, clinical, and epidemiologic research has accumulated supporting an etiologic role for some types of HPV.[10]

Of more than 78 types of HPV that have been described, more than 35 are associated with anogenital disease, and 30 or more are associated with cancer.[11] In an international study, HPV DNA was detected in 93% (range 75–100%) of cancer specimens collected in 22 countries and analyzed by the polymerase chain reaction (PCR) technique.[12] Similarly, HPV DNA has been detected by PCR in up to 94% of women with preinvasive lesions (CIN) and in up to 46% of women with cytologically normal tissue.[10,13]

HPV types classified as intermediate and high risk have been identified in about 77% of high-grade squamous intraepithelial lesions (HGSILs) (CIN 2 and 3) and in 84% of invasive lesions.[14] In the series studied by Bosch and colleagues, HPV types 16, 18, 31, and 45 were detected in approximately 80% of the cases.[12] HPV 16 is by far the most prevalent HPV type in women with cervical neoplasia, present in up to 50% of HGSILs and invasive lesions, and it is the most common HPV type identified in cytologically normal women.[14,16,18]

The association between cervical neoplasia and HPV is independent of study population, study design, and HPV detection method.[10,13] Higher risk has been associated with specific HPV types (16, 18, 31, 33, 35, and 45), increasing viral load, and concurrent infection with multiple HPV types.[15,16] An increased risk of high-grade CIN ranging from 16- to 122-fold has been reported among women whose test results were positive for HPV of any type.[17] The percentage of cases of CIN attributed to HPV has been estimated to range from 60 to 92%.[13] In addition, adjustment for HPV status appears to account for most of the associations between cervical neoplasia and number of sexual partners and other characteristics of sexual behavior.[13,15,17]

Although a strong and consistent association between HPV and cervical neoplasia has been clearly established, the discrepancy between HPV prevalence and the incidence of cervical neoplasia suggests that other cofactors are necessary for the development and progression of the disease. The role of sexual and reproductive history, smoking habits, and hormonal and dietary factors, as well as their interaction with HPV, has been assessed in recent studies. Future research will need to assess the effect of recent changes in these factors on the occurrence of cervical cancer.[7]

Numerous studies have addressed the association between human immunodeficiency virus (HIV) and cervical neoplasia.[8] The Centers for Disease Control and Prevention added invasive cervical cancer to the list of acquired immunodeficiency syndrome-related conditions in 1993.[18] HIV-positive women have been reported to have higher rates of cervical abnormalities, larger lesions, higher-grade lesions, and higher recurrence rates than HIV-negative women. In addition, HIV-positive women have been reported to have higher HPV prevalence and HPV persistence rates than HIV-negative women. A meta-analysis by Mandelblatt and colleagues concluded that HIV is a cofactor in the association between HPV and cervical neoplasia, and this association seems to vary with the level of immune function.[19] Results from Ruche and colleagues in Africa support the theory of interaction between HIV-1 and HPV.[20] Although the biologic mechanism for this interaction is not as well understood, it could be explained by the effect of HIV infection on the immune system or by the existence of a molecular interaction between HIV and HPV. Studies are needed to confirm these observations and to assess the role of viral factors for both HPV and HIV in the development of cervical neoplasia.

HSV was the focus of intensive study during the 1960s and 1970s. Serologic studies showed a higher prevalence of HSV-2 antibodies among women with cervical neoplasia than among controls. Two potential mechanisms of action have been suggested: a "hit-and-run" effect and a synergistic effect between HSV-2 and HPV.[21] A statistically significant interaction between HSV-2 and HPV 16/18 was detected by Hildesheim and colleagues and Baldauf and colleagues; however, several recent studies continue to provide evidence against such an interaction.[19,22] An association between the presence of antibodies for *Chlamydia trachomatis* and cervical neoplasia that persists after controlling for HPV status and other potential factors has been reported.[23,24] However, others have failed to show an association with *Chlamydia trachomatis* using antibody determinations or other measures of exposure, including a self-reported history of *Chlamydia trachomatis* infection, culture for *Chlamydia trachomatis*,[23–25] and PCR detection of *Chlamydia trachomatis*.[25]

Cytomegalovirus has been suspected as a risk factor for cervical neoplasia in previous studies. Higher levels of antibodies to cytomegalovirus have been reported among women with cervical neoplasia than among controls; however, some other studies have failed to identify an increased risk of cervical neoplasia associated with cytomegalovirus infection. The evidence remains conflicting, and the role of cytomegalovirus as an etiologic factor or cofactor is unclear[22–25] Inconclusive evidence for other genital infectious agents, including *Trichomonas vaginalis*, Epstein-Barr virus, hepatitis B virus, hepatitis C virus, *Neisseria gonorrhoeae*, *Gardnerella vaginalis*, and *Treponema pallidum*, has been reported.[8]

Other Molecular Markers Other specific genetic abnormalities may also play an important role in carcinogenesis and the aggressiveness of cervical tumors, although, to date, the role of most of these genetic abnormalities in cervical cancer do not appear as important as the role of HPV. The c-*myc* oncogene is expressed in almost all differentiated cell types. It acts as a heterodimer with MAX (a related protein), binds DNA in a sequence-specific way, and acts as a transcriptional activator for genes critical in the regulation of cell growth.[26] The c-*myc* gene also plays a role in apoptosis; by binding MAX, it interacts with TP53, BAX, and BCLX. It induces apoptosis in cells deprived of growth factors.[27] Amplification of c-*myc* is the predominant route of activation in cervical cancer. Most studies report a 32 to 34% incidence of c-*myc* activation in cervical cancers. Amplication may be related to tumor size and nodal status or may be a risk factor for relapse.[28] The *ras* family of genes is also frequently mutated in cancers. Mutations have been reported in the K-*ras* and H-*ras* genes in cervical cancer at a rate of only 10 to 15%.[29] One report found that increased *ras* p21 expression correlated with risk of lymph node metastasis.[30]

In addition to overexpression of *myc* and mutation of *ras*, amplification or overexpression of several different growth factor receptors has been implicated in carcinogenesis. In cervical cancer, epidermal growth factor receptor (EGF-R) and related *HER2/neu* have been studied. Overexpression of the EGF-R is usually related to amplification of the gene, and overexpression seems to confer a growth advantage to cells. EGF-R is expressed not only in a large proportion of cervical carcinomas, but also in normal and premalignant epithelia. Investigators have found a strong correlation between the expression of EGF-R and *HER2/neu*. The prognostic role of EGF-R in cervical carcinoma remains controversial, although two studies found EGF-R prognostic for overall survival and disease-specific survival in patients with invasive cervical cancer.[31,32]

Tumor suppressor genes may also play a role. The most widely investigated gene in cervical cancer is the apoptosis inhibitor gene *BCL2*. As BLC2 protein inhibits apoptosis, overexpression of this gene leads to extension of the cell's survival. Two studies have shown that *BCL2* is overexpressed in 61 to 63% of all cervical cancer and correlates with overall survival,[33,34] whereas other studies have found no correlation with survival.[35]

Angiogenesis is critical for the progression of most cancers. Hockel and colleagues have reported an association between tumor hypoxia and progression of cervical cancer, and this would seem to correlate with the angiogenic potential of the tumor. However, attempts to correlate progression with actual vessel counts or angiogenic factors have proven more difficult. One angiogenic factor, VEGF, has recently been associated with cervical cancer,[36,37] but the precise role that angiogenic factors play in the development and progression of cervical cancer requires further elucidation.

Sexual Behavior Although previous studies report a strong and consistent association between cervical neoplasia and some characteristics of sexual behavior of women and their male sexual partners, a weaker association has been found in more recent studies in which HPV infection has been taken into account.[15,38] The decrease in the magnitude of these associations after controlling for HPV status supports the notion that characteristics of sexual behavior may be only a proxy measurement for infection with HPV and other infectious agents causally related to cervical neoplasia.

In most studies of preinvasive disease, the effect of the number of sexual partners is substantially reduced after adjustment for HPV, but in studies of invasive lesions, the association with the number of sexual partners remained statistically significant or at the border of significance.[15,39] Interestingly, no association is observed between number of sexual partners and cervical neoplasia among HPV-positive women, whereas a positive association remains among HPV-negative women.[15,40] Misclassification of HPV status, the effect of unmeasured cofactors, or a different etiology for the disease among HPV-negative women could explain the latter finding.

The association between early age at first sexual intercourse and increased risk has been less consistent. After controlling for HPV and other risk factors, a statistically significant association between age at first sexual intercourse and cervical neoplasia has remained in some studies, but in others, no association has been observed.[15,17,41] The association between cervical neoplasia and early age at sexual intercourse may indicate a period of higher susceptibility of the cervical tissue, a higher likelihood of exposure, or a longer period of exposure to carcinogenic factors. Whatever the mechanism underlying the association, establishing age at first sexual intercourse as an independent effect is difficult because of its high correlation with number of sexual partners.

An association between factors related to male sexual partners and an increased risk of cervical neoplasia has also been suggested.[42] High rates of cervical cancer in developing countries in which women are traditionally monogamous or have few sexual partners might be explained by the fact that males have large numbers of sexual partners and frequent contact with prostitutes. Penile HPV DNA prevalence is higher in husbands of women with cervical neoplasia than in husbands of women without cervical neoplasia.[13] Among men, the prevalence of HPV has been associated with the number of sexual partners and sexual contact with prostitutes.[43] In addition, higher HPV prevalence has been reported among males in geographic areas with higher rates of cervical cancer incidence than among males in geographic areas with lower rates, which supports a possible contribution of male partners to cervical carcinogenesis in their female sex partners.[43] Male circumcision has been associated with a reduced risk of penile HPV infection and, in the case of men with a history of multiple sexual partners, a reduced risk of cervical cancer in their current female partners.[44]

Reproductive Factors No consistent relationships have been established between cervical neoplasia and menstrual or reproductive characteristics, including age at menarche or menopause; parity; number of spontaneous or induced abortions; age at first pregnancy, first live birth, or last birth; and number of vaginal deliveries or Cesarean sections. An association between higher parity and higher number of live births and increased risk of cervical neoplasia has been reported in six case-control studies after controlling for HPV status.[15,17,39,40]

There is also a strong association between invasive cervical cancer and early age at first birth reported by Bosch and colleagues,[45] coupled with the absence of an association with parity. A 70% increased risk of high-grade dysplasia (CIN 2 and 3) has been found among women with one or more vaginal deliveries. Becker and colleagues[46] found that an association also persisted after adjustment for ethnicity, HPV status, and other sexual and reproductive characteristics. Although there is no clear biologic mechanism to support this association, repeated trauma to the cervix during childbirth has been suggested as an etiologic factor.

Smoking Habits Several epidemiologic studies have provided evidence supporting an association between cigarette smoking and cervical neoplasia. Most studies have shown a twofold increased risk among smokers and a dose-response relationship with duration and intensity of smoking.[47,48] Results from most recent studies controlling for HPV status have been inconsistent. Some support an independent effect of smoking, whereas others do not.[15,17,49] Although a possible interaction between HPV and smoking has been proposed, few studies have examined this joint effect.[21] Results from these studies have also been inconsistent.[39,50,51] In addition to the epidemiologic research, several studies have provided biologic plausibility for this association. Reports have been published of high levels of nicotine and cotinine and tobacco-specific *N*-nitrosamines in the cervical mucus of active and passive smokers, DNA damage in cervical tissue and exfoliated cells of women smokers, and impairment of the local cell-mediated immune response in smokers. Furthermore, reduction of cervical lesion size has been documented among women participating in smoking cessation intervention.[52] In summary, although the mechanism of smoking-induced carcinogenesis in cervical tissue is not fully understood, current biologic, epidemiologic, and clinical studies suggest that cigarette smoking may be a risk factor for cervical neoplasia.

Oral Contraceptives The role of oral contraceptives in cervical neoplasia development remains unclear, despite evidence in support of a biologic mechanism. Early studies showed a weak but statistically significant association, particularly for long-term users.[53] Interpretation of the results, however, is confounded by the correlation between oral contraceptive use, sexual behavior, and patterns of screening for cervical neoplasia; potential surveillance bias and selection of comparison groups; and lack of control for HPV in earlier studies.[53] Results from epidemiologic studies in which control for HPV status has been attained are conflicting.[15,17,39,41] Most of these studies failed to show an association between cervical neoplasia and different measures of oral contraceptive exposure.[15,17,39] An interaction between oral contraceptive use and HPV infection has been suggested; however, epidemiologic evidence of interaction is conflicting.[39] The analysis of an interaction effect is based on a very small number of cases, and results need to be interpreted with caution.

Dietary Factors Several lines of evidence suggest that some nutrients may have a protective effect against cervical neoplasia, particularly vitamin A, carotenoids, vitamin C, vitamin E, and folic acid. The hypothesis that there is an inverse association between vitamin A intake and cervical neoplasia is based on the relationship between vitamin A and other epithelial tumors, mainly squamous cell carcinomas. Vitamin A is capable of reversing metaplastic changes in bronchial epithelium, providing a biologic basis for the association with cervical neoplasia.[54] Vitamin C plays a role in the maintenance of the normal epithelium and the protection of the normal epithelium against carcinogens. Folic acid functions as a coenzyme in the metabolism of single-carbon compounds, such as nucleic acid synthesis and amino acid metabolism.[54] It has been hypothesized that a subclinical folate deficiency may act as a cofactor in the integration of the HPV genome into host DNA.[55]

Despite these findings, epidemiologic studies on the association between vitamin A, carotenoids, vitamin C, and folic acid and cervical neoplasia have provided conflicting results.[7,56] Different methods of nutrient measurement, variation in selection of case and comparison groups, and differences in control for confounding factors make the comparison of these studies difficult. In addition, the correlation between nutrients makes the interpretation of the results a difficult task. In some studies in which control of confounding factors has been better, findings regarding an association between dietary or serum/plasma levels of nutrients and cervical neoplasia remain inconclusive.[50,57] An interaction between red blood cell folate levels and HPV 16–positive status, cigarette smoking, and parity has been suggested.[55] This interaction is consistent with current knowledge on the role of folate in carcinogenesis.

Risk Factors for Cervical Adenocarcinoma Adenocarcinoma of the cervix accounts for more than 20% of all cervical cancers. However, in most developing countries the incidence is increasing, particularly among younger women. Between the early 1970s and mid-1980s, the incidence of adenocarcinoma more than doubled among women under 35 years of age.[58] Several investigators have reported a correlation between cervical adenocarcinoma and prolonged oral contraceptive use, but confounding issues need to be studied.[59–80] Alternatively, the increased incidence of cervical adenocarcinoma may be related to changes in the prevalence of HPV infection or to increased reporting of this histology.[60,61]

Summary Cervical neoplasia continues to be a major health problem worldwide. Higher incidence and mortality rates are observed in developing countries. Among more developed countries, a significant decline in incidence and mortality has been observed in the last 50 years, which has been attributed to the introduction of screening programs. Current epidemiologic data support a strong role for HPV infection in the etiology of cervical neoplasia. This association satisfies all criteria for causality in epidemiologic research: strength, consistency, and specificity of the association; dose-response and temporal relationship; and biologic plausibility.[13] HPV infection appears to explain many of the established risk factors for cervical neoplasia, including sexual behavior and cigarette smoking. Nonetheless, the high prevalence of HPV infection in young healthy women compared with the low incidence of cervical neoplasia and the low progression rate of untreated CIN lesions support the existence of other cofactors in cervical carcinogenesis.[62] Future epidemiologic studies will need to further assess the role of these cofactors and their interaction with HPV. In addition, the role of viral factors such as HPV persistence and HPV variants in the progression of cervical neoplasia as well as of the determinant factors of HPV persistence will require further evaluation.[63] Similarly, the impact of recent trends in such environmental factors as smoking, exogenous hormones, and dietary factors deserves further attention.[7]

HISTOLOGIC CLASSIFICATION OF EPITHELIAL TUMORS

The histologic classification of epithelial tumors of the uterine cervix by the World Health Organization (WHO) separates them into three main groups: squamous cell carcinomas, adenocarcinomas, and other epithelial tumors (Table 101-1).[64,65]

Squamous Cell Carcinoma The majority of cervical carcinomas are squamous cell carcinomas, which are classified as either large-cell nonkeratinizing or large-cell keratinizing. Nonkeratinizing carcinoma is characterized by squamous cells with somewhat hyperchromatic nuclei and a

Table 101-1 Modification of the WHO Histologic Classification of Epithelial Tumors of the Uterine Cervix

Squamous Cell Carcinoma
Microinvasive squamous cell carcinoma
Invasive squamous cell carcinoma
Verrucous carcinoma
Warty (condylomatous) carcinoma
Papillary squamous cell (transitional) carcinoma
Lymphoepithelioma-like carcinoma
Adenocarcinoma
Mucinous adenocarcinoma
Endocervical type
Intestinal type
Signet-ring type
Endometrioid adenocarcinoma
Endometrioid adenocarcinoma with squamous metaplasia
Clear cell adenocarcinoma
Minimal deviation adenocarcinoma
Endocervical type (adenoma malignum)
Endometrioid type
Serous adenocarcinoma
Mesonephric carcinoma
Well-differentiated villoglandular adenocarcinoma
Other Epithelial Tumors
Adenosquamous carcinoma
Glassy-cell carcinoma
Mucoepidermoid carcinoma
Adenoid cystic carcinoma
Adenoid basal carcinoma
Carcinoid-like tumor
Small-cell carcinoma
Undifferentiated carcinoma

Reproduced with permission from Carcinoma and other tumors of the cervix. In Blausteine's Pathology of the Female Genital Tract. 4th ed.

WHO = World Health Organization.

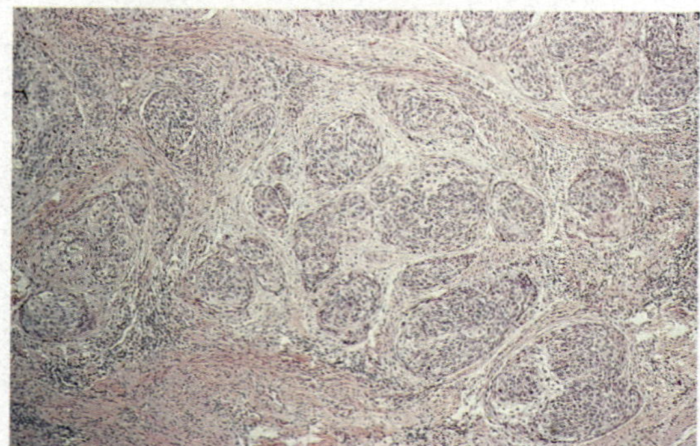

Figure 101-1 Squamous cell carcinoma, nonkeratinizing.

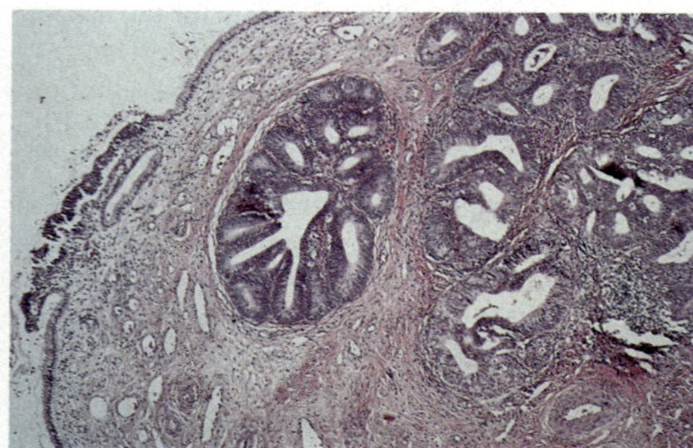

Figure 101-3 Lymphoepithelioma-like carcinoma.

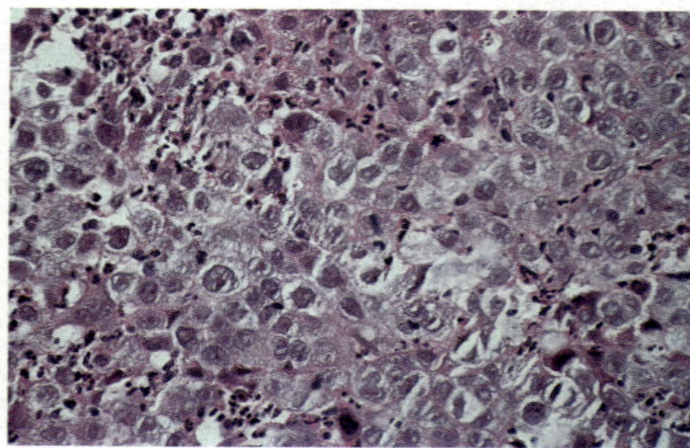

Figure 101-4 Mucinous adenocarcinoma, endocervical type.

moderate amount of cytoplasm growing in discrete nests separated by stroma (Figure 101-1). In the center of some of the nests, the squamous cells appear to differentiate and degenerate. Keratinizing carcinoma is characterized by cells with very hyperchromatic nuclei and densely eosinophilic cytoplasm growing in irregular invasive nests. Many of these nests have central "pearls" that contain abundant keratin. The average age of patients with squamous cell carcinoma is 51.4 years. Selected variants of squamous cell carcinoma are described in the following paragraphs.

Verrucous Carcinoma Verrucous carcinomas are exophytic with frondlike papillae and macroscopically resemble condylomas. They rarely metastasize, but local invasion can be extensive. Death usually occurs because of ureteral obstruction, infection, or hemorrhage. Histologically, the epithelium lacks cytologic atypia and mitotic activity, and the epithelial papillae lack a central fibroconnective tissue core. Mitotic activity may be evident in cells at the base of the tumor, and invasive nests of epithelium are observed along with well-circumscribed nests with a clearly visible or defined tumor-stroma interface. The inflammatory reaction at the epithelial stromal junction is marked.

This tumor rarely goes to the nodes, therefore, for early-stage disease, the treatment of choice is a type II modified radical hysterectomy without lymphadenectomy.

Papillary Squamous Cell Carcinoma Papillary squamous cell carcinomas of the uterine cervix with transitional or squamous differentiation often resemble transitional cell carcinomas of the urinary tract (Figure 101-2). Tumors with transitional cell differentiation have been described in every site in

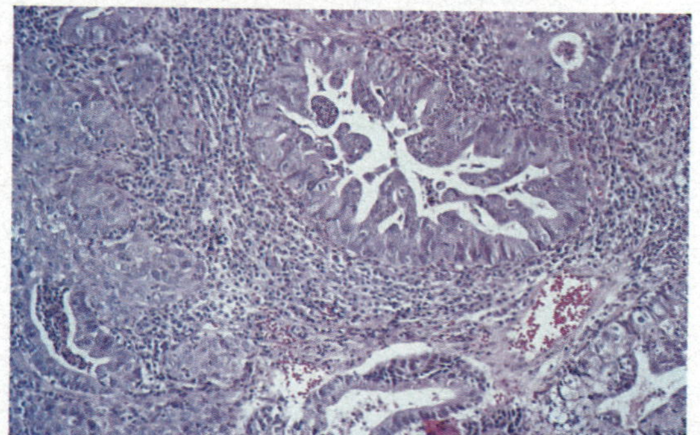

Figure 101-2 Papillary squamous cell (transitional) carcinoma.

the female genital tract. Immunochemical tests identifying cytokeratin polypeptides cytokeratin 7 and cytokeratin 20 are useful in differentiating primary genital tract transitional cell carcinoma from urinary tract transitional tumors.[66] Urinary tract transitional cell carcinomas have a cytokeratin profile strongly positive for cytokeratin 20, whereas primary genital tract transitional cell carcinomas stain positive for cytokeratin 7. Invasive papillary transitional cell carcinomas of the uterine cervix are potentially aggressive carcinomas. It is important to distinguish these carcinomas from benign squamous papillomas and condyloma acuminata.[67] Biopsy material must include the underlying stroma to permit identification of invasion.

Lymphoepithelioma-Like Carcinoma Lymphoepithelioma-like carcinomas are histologically similar to lymphoepitheliomas arising in the nasopharynx and salivary glands (Figure 101-3). These carcinomas are usually well circumscribed and composed of undifferentiated cells. The cells are surrounded by inflammatory infiltrates composed of lymphocytes, plasma cells, and eosinophils.[68] Hasumi and colleagues reported 39 cases from the Cancer Institute Hospital in Tokyo. Their patients, 72% of whom were younger than 50 years of age, were treated with radical hysterectomy and pelvic lymphadenectomy. Two patients had positive lymph nodes. At the time of the report, 38 of the 39 patients were alive. The single death occurred 5 months after surgery and was due to serum hepatitis.

Adenocarcinoma Adenocarcinomas represent 20 to 25% of cervical carcinomas today, whereas from 1950 to 1960 they represented only 5%.[69] This change in prevalence is a worldwide phenomenon.[70] The mean age at diagnosis for patients with invasive adenocarcinoma is between 47 and 53 years. Selected variants of adenocarcinoma are described in the following paragraphs.

Mucinous Adenocarcinoma Mucinous adenocarcinoma is the most common type of cervical adenocarcinoma.[71] In the WHO classification, the first type of mucinous adenocarcinoma is composed of cells that resemble the columnar cells of the normal endocervical mucosa and is referred to as the endocervical type (Figure 101-4). The second type is termed the intestinal type because it is composed of cells similar to those present in adenocarcinomas of the large intestine. A third type is composed of signet-ring cells and designated the signet-ring type. Frequently, mucinous adenocarcinomas are a mixture of these cell types.

Endometrioid Adenocarcinoma Endometrioid adenocarcinoma is the second most common type of primary endocervical tumor, accounting for 30% of all primary endocervical tumors. Endometrioid adenocarcinomas resemble typical endometrioid adenocarcinoma arising from the endometrial cavity (Figure 101-5). Identification of the site of origin (ie, whether the primary tumor is in the endocervix or endometrium) may be difficult, but proper identification is important as the site or origin significantly influences therapy.

Adenoma Malignum It is difficult to distinguish cytologically between adenoma malignum and normal endocervical glands (Figure 101-6). Thus adenoma malignum is also referred to as minimal-deviation adenocarcinoma. A distinguishing feature of adenoma malignum is a bizarre and irregular glandular branching pattern. These irregular glands invade deeply into the stroma, and diagnosis requires a large tissue specimen (ie, one obtained with a cone biopsy). Diagnosis is frequently made on the basis of the hysterectomy specimen. Adenoma malignum is an extremely rare type of cancer and is sometimes associated with Peutz-Jeghers syndrome.[72] The survival rate is poor if the well-differentiated pattern leads to undertreatment.

Other Epithelial Tumors **Adenosquamous Carcinoma** Adenosquamous carcinomas are defined as tumors that contain an admixture of histologically malignant squamous and glandular cells.[73] Adenosquamous carcinomas account for 5 to 25% of the cervical carcinomas in some series.[74,75] These carcinomas are similar in their clinical presentation, epidemiology, and pattern

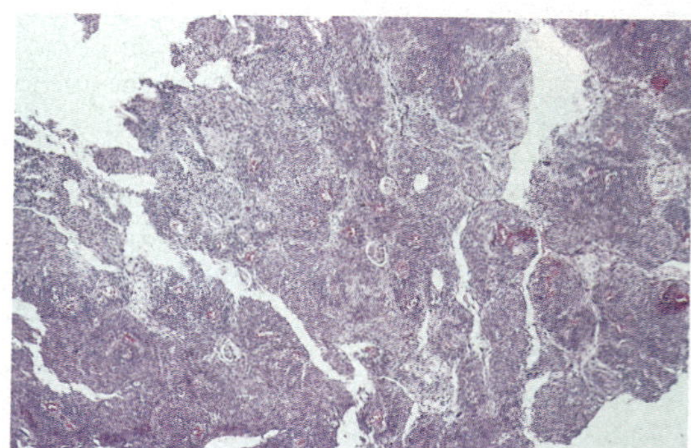

Figure 101-5 Endometrioid adenocarcinoma.

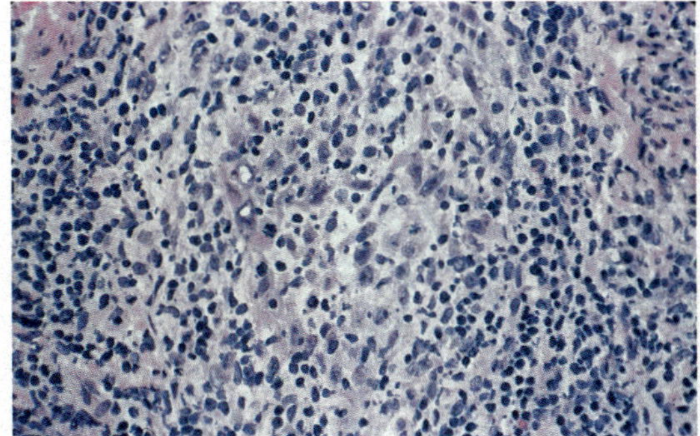

Figure 101-6 Mucinous adenocarcinoma, endocervical type (adenoma malignum).

of spread to squamous cell carcinomas and adenocarcinomas.[102,103] The poorly differentiated form of adenosquamous carcinoma has been referred to as glassy-cell carcinoma. These carcinomas are made up of large uniform polygonal cells with a finely granular cytoplasm of the ground-glass type, hence the term "glassy-cells" (Figure 101-7). Similar to other undifferentiated tumors, glassy-cell carcinomas spread early and are aggressive.[76] The mucoepidermoid carcinoma, also placed in this category, contains large-cell nonkeratinizing or focally keratinizing squamous carcinoma, which stains positive for mucin but lacks recognizable glands. The mucinous component includes goblet or signet ring–type cells localized in a nest of squamous cells. These carcinomas represent 20% of the carcinomas in some series if mucin is measured.

Small-Cell Neuroendocrine Carcinoma Small-cell carcinomas, well defined in the WHO classification of cervical tumors, contain small anaplastic cells with scant cytoplasm (Figure 101-8). These highly aggressive cancers diffusely infiltrate the cervical stroma.[77] Staining reveals neuroendocrine markers in most cases. Women with small-cell carcinoma are likely to be 10 years younger than those with squamous cell carcinoma. Small-cell carcinomas tend to behave very aggressively and are frequently associated with widespread metastasis to multiple sites, including bone, liver, skin, and brain. These tumors should not be confused with small squamous cell carcinomas, which are associated with a better prognosis. Usually, there will be some areas showing squamous or glandular differentiation in the nonkeratinizing squamous cell carcinoma with small cells. Efforts to treat these cancers with approaches typically used for small-cell carcinomas of the lung have had mixed results. Small-cell carcinomas are different and more aggressive than nonkeratinizing squamous carcinoma with small cells.[78]

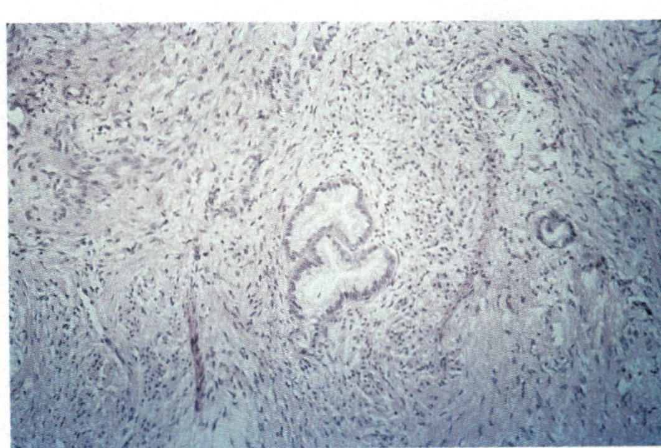

Figure 101-7 Glassy-cell carcinoma.

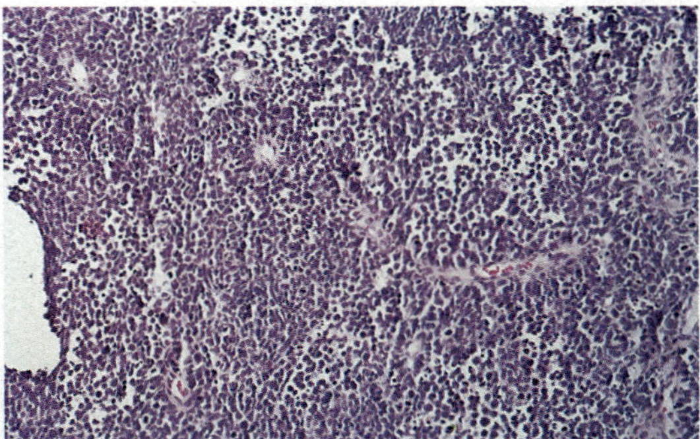

Figure 101-8 Small-cell carcinoma.

Nonsmall-Cell Neuroendocrine Carcinoma Nonsmall-cell neuroendocrine carcinomas of the cervix have been reported, but they are not listed in the current WHO classification of cervical tumors.[79] The tumors contain intermediate to large cells, high-grade nuclei, and eosinophilic cytoplasmic granules of the type seen in neuroendocrine cells. A trabecular pattern is frequently evident, with or without glandular differentiation (Figure 101-9). Tumors are usually immunoreactive for chromogranin. Reported survival rates for patients with these aggressive carcinomas are similar to those for patients with small-cell carcinoma.

Terminology for cervical neuroendocrine tumors is confusing, and many pathologists are recommending application of the classification system used for the more common pulmonary neuroendocrine tumors (ie, typical carcinoid tumor, atypical carcinoid tumor, large-cell neuroendocrine carcinoma, and small [oat]-cell carcinoma).[80]

NATURAL HISTORY OF CARCINOMAS OF THE UTERINE CERVIX

Cullen described carcinoma in situ (CIS), a precursor lesion for invasive cervical carcinoma, at the turn of the twentieth century. Broder reintroduced the term in the 1930s, and a relationship between CIS and invasive cervical carcinoma was described by a number of investigators. During the 1930s, cervical cancer detection programs based on cytologic screening to detect precursor lesions were being created. The identification of a spectrum of precursor lesions followed, and terminology was defined in the 1940s and 1950s. Reagan and Harmonic introduced the term dysplasia to refer to the spectrum of cervical abnormalities that featured cells whose abnormalities were fewer or less severe than those found in CIS.[81] Dysplastic cells resembled cells of the basal layer but had nuclear atypia and other cytoplasmic and nuclear abnormalities. The degree of dysplasia was classified on the basis of the relative thickness of the process in relationship to the thickness of the epithelium. By definition, in dysplasia, atypical cells did not occupy the full thickness of the epithelium, nor did they penetrate the basement membrane.[82] Mild or moderate dysplasia was thought to have a lower potential than severe dysplasia for progression to invasive carcinoma. The term "carcinoma in situ" (CIS) was reserved for atypical cells involving the full thickness of the epithelium. This division of noninvasive cervical lesions into two groups, dysplasia and CIS, was confusing. Clinicians considered dysplasia to be a potentially reversible lesion, whereas they thought of CIS as potentially dangerous and treated it with hysterectomy. Among pathologists, variability in distinguishing severe dysplasia from CIS was common, making a precise definition that had clinical application a necessity.

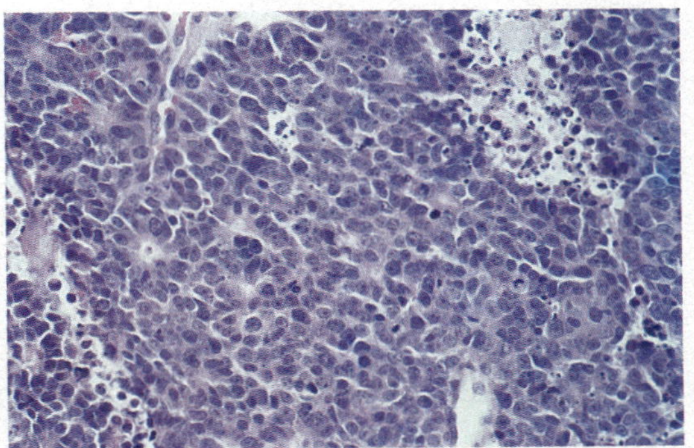

Figure 101-9 Nonsmall-cell neuroendocrine carcinoma.

DNA ploidy studies had demonstrated a similarity between severe dysplasia and CIS. Both entities were found to consist of monoclonal proliferations of abnormal squamous epithelial cells with an aneuploid nuclear DNA content. These findings suggested that dysplasia and invasive carcinoma actually represented different points along the same disease spectrum. Richart introduced the term cervical intraepithelial neoplasia in the late 1960s.[83] The CIN terminology assumed that all types of lesions, from precursor lesions to invasive squamous cell carcinoma, represented a single disease process. Furthermore, because the CIN terminology represented a spectrum of histologic changes that shared a common etiology, its use fit nicely into a clinical treatment plan. When these lesions were diagnosed and adequately treated or destroyed, invasive carcinoma could be prevented.

The 1988 Bethesda System for Reporting Cervical/Vaginal Cytological Diagnoses and its most recent revision classifies precursor lesions as squamous intraepithelial lesions (SILs).[83] Generally, low-grade SILs (LGSILs) have cellular changes that are associated with a heterogeneous group of HPV types and are equivalent to mild dysplasia (CIN I). These lesions are usually diploid or polyploid. HGSILs are usually associated with intermediate-risk (31, 33, 35, 51, 58) or high-risk (16, 18, 56) HPV types. This category includes moderate dysplasia (CIN II), severe dysplasia (CIN III), and CIS. The high-grade lesions are typically aneuploid and are more likely to progress to invasive carcinoma, which makes the HGSILs the most important clinically. A significant percentage of these lesions will progress to invasive cancer if followed long term.[84] LGSILs usually behave in the opposite manner. One-half will regress spontaneously, and only 16% will progress to HGSILs.[85] Pathologists use a variety of terms for these precursor lesions. The written pathology report may use the new Bethesda system for both histologic and cytologic diagnoses, or it may use the new terminology only for the cytologic diagnosis. The older terminology for the histologic diagnosis remains popular. Mild dysplasia is CIN I, moderate dysplasia is CIN II, and severe dysplasia is CIN III or CIS.

The precursors of invasive adenocarcinoma of the cervix were recognized in the 1950s.[86] The best-defined precursor, if one exists, is adenocarcinoma in situ, which occurs infrequently in comparison with HGSILs. A large proportion of adenocarcinomas in situ occur in conjunction with SILs.[87] Adenocarcinoma in situ is associated with HPV DNA, mostly HPV 18, in contrast with SILs, which are associated with HPV 16. Adenocarcinoma in situ is less likely to be detected by Pap smear than SILs.[87] In the majority of cases, adenocarcinoma in situ involves the transformation zone and is unifocal.[88] The transition between normal glands and adenocarcinoma in situ is sharp. The cell type is usually endocervical and consists of atypical columnar glands.[89] Other types of adenocarcinoma in situ may contain colonic-type epithelium and endometrioid or clear cells.[90] The diagnosis of adenocarcinoma in situ is sometimes difficult and may pose a challenge to the experienced pathologist. Tissue specimens that are intact and properly oriented on arrival to the laboratory, of adequate size, and accompanied by the appropriate clinical history are extremely helpful in obtaining the correct diagnosis.

DIAGNOSIS AND TREATMENT OF PRECANCEROUS LESIONS

The most recent guidelines for screening for cervical cancer are listed in Figure 101-10. CIN is an increasingly common finding among sexually active young women. Since the introduction of the Bethesda system, the proportion of Pap smears identified as having low-grade cytologic abnormalities, minimal or ambiguous cytologic changes classified as atypical squamous cells of undetermined significance (ASCUS), or LGSILs has increased.[91] Approximately 50 million Pap smears are done yearly in the United States, and 5 to 10% of these smears are reported as having low-grade cytologic abnormalities. Although near consensus exists regarding the evaluation and management of HGSILs and carcinoma detected on Pap smears, controversy continues regarding appropriate management of ASCUS and low-grade abnormalities.[92] Issues include the risk of progression of the disease, the anxiety caused to the patient, the risk of overtreating patients with minor disease, and, more recently, the financial implications of prompt intervention and treatment.[93]

Management of Low-Grade Cytologic Abnormalities Previously, low-grade cytologic abnormalities were usually considered

- Screening should begin approximately three years after a woman begins having vaginal intercourse, but no later than 21 years of age.
- Screening should be done every year with regular pap tests or every two years using liquid-based tests.
- At or after age 30, women who have had three normal test results in a row may be screened every 2-3 years. However, doctors may suggest a woman be screened more if she has certain risk factors, such as HIV infection or a weakened immune system.
- Women 70 and older who have had three or more consecutive pap tests in the last 10 years may choose to stop cervical cancer screening.
- Screening after a total hysterectomy (with removal of the cervix) is not necessary unless the surgery was done as a treatment for cervical cancer.

Figure 101-10 Screening guidelines for the early detection of cervical cancer.

benign and attributed to an underlying infection.[94] The common practice was to disregard the cytologic findings and repeat the Pap smear the following year.[94] In the 1970s, it was suggested that a more aggressive approach to mildly atypical Pap smear findings might be warranted. Stafl and Mattingly reported that approximately 25% of women with a colposcopic diagnosis of HGSILs (CIN II, III, and CIS) had been referred with an initial diagnosis of a mildly atypical Pap smear.[95] Similarly, Figge and colleagues reported that 15% of women with invasive cervical cancer had initially been referred because of a mildly atypical Pap smear.[96] Following these reports, most clinicians started treating any underlying vulvovaginal infection with antibiotics and repeating the smear several months later. If the smear result regressed to normal, the patient was scheduled for an annual Pap smear screening, whereas patients whose smears remained abnormal were referred for colposcopic evaluation.

As more studies of women with mildly atypical Pap smears were published, data showed that 5 to 20% of women presenting with a single mildly atypical Pap smear were at risk of HGSILs or other more severe lesions.[97] In addition, it has recently been estimated that more than one-third of the HGSIL cases in a routine screening population are proceeded by a cytologic diagnosis of ASCUS.[98] This has led some clinicians to suggest that it is safer and more expeditious to perform colposcopy in women with a finding of ASCUS.[99] However, given the relatively high frequency of low-grade cytologic abnormalities in the absence of significant disease and the high financial and emotional cost of colposcopy, some have argued that these women should be evaluated by repeat cytology rather than colposcopy. The American College of Obstetricians and Gynecologists and a National Cancer Institute (NCI) consensus panel have acknowledged that managing a single mildly atypical Pap smear by repeating the test is an acceptable practice.[92,100]

The main goal in managing ASCUS and low-grade cytologic abnormalities is to identify those women at higher risk of HGSILs, primarily women more than 25 years old who cannot be relied on to return for long-term follow-up, who are suspected of having or known to have a history of abnormal cytologic findings or treatment of cervical neoplasia, who may be promiscuous, and who have no history of adequate screening.[101] Currently, two strategies are recommended for managing these lesions: The physician may repeat the Pap smear and perform a colposcopic evaluation, or, for patients with an ASCUS cytologic diagnosis or LGSILs without clinical evidence of cervical disease and without risk factors, the physician may repeat the Pap smear without performing colposcopy (Figure 101-11).[92,101] Patients should be monitored by

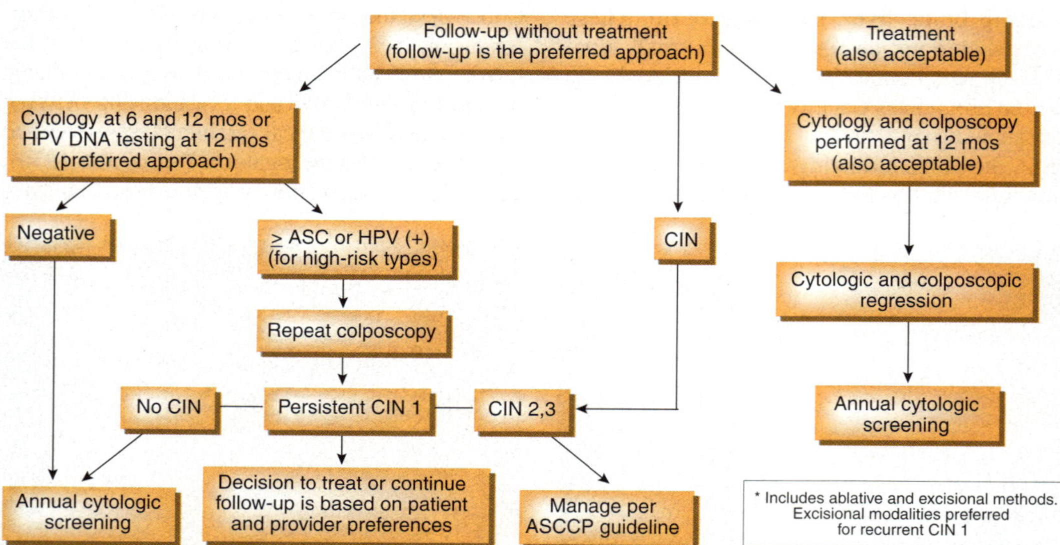

Figure 101-11 Management of women with biopsy-confirmed cervical intraepithelial neoplasia-grade 1 (CIN 1) and satisfactory colposcopy.

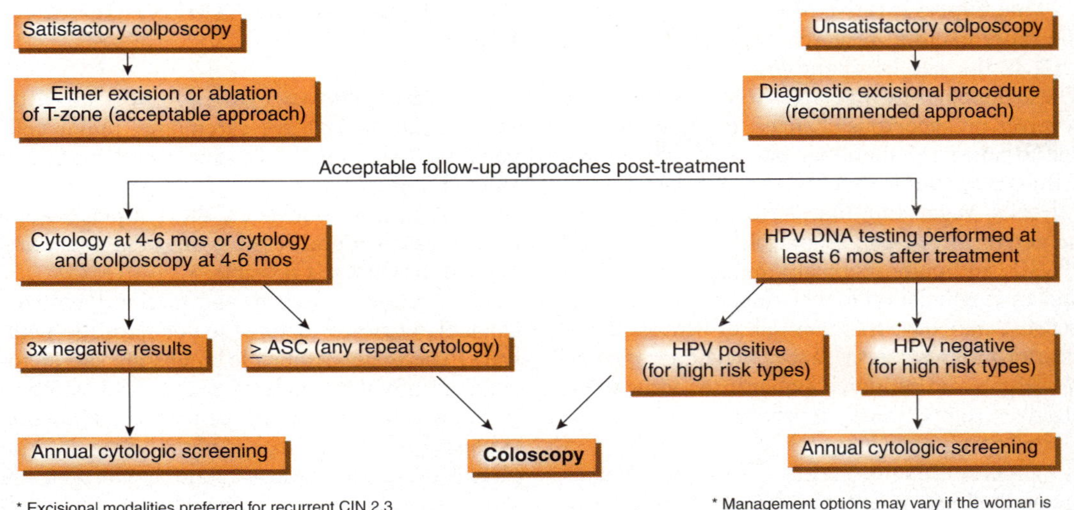

Figure 101-12 Management of women with biopsy-confirmed cervical intraepithelial neoplasia-grade 2 and 3 (CIN 2.3).

Pap test every 4 to 6 months for 2 years. After three consecutive negative smears in the 2-year follow-up period, patients can be monitored using a routine cervical cancer screening protocol. For patients with clinical suspicion of cancer or persistent abnormal Pap smears during the 2-year follow-up, colposcopic evaluation is recommended. Depending on reliability for follow-up and the risk factor profile, women with persistent LGSILs can be treated with such ablative therapies as cryotherapy or loop electrosurgical excision procedure (LEEP). Patients undergoing treatment of LGSILs should be monitored every 4 to 6 months for up to 2 years by cytologic examination and colposcopic and histologic examination if required (Figure 101-12).

Because of the costs, both emotional and economic, associated with evaluating women with low-grade cytologic abnormalities, considerable interest has arisen in developing novel cost-effective triage strategies for these patients. HPV DNA testing, automated cytology screening, and cervicography are being evaluated as adjunct methods in the assessment and triage of patients with low-grade cytologic abnormalities. Most research has focused on the assessment of HPV testing.

In 1996, the NCI initiated a large multi-institutional study to establish the optimal management of mildly abnormal Pap smears With ASCUS or LGSIL.[102,103] Early available data reveal that a very high percentage of women (82.9%) with an LGSIL diagnosis from a Pap smear are positive for HPV DNA by the Hybrid Capture assay (Digene Diagnostics). As a result, it looks as though the potential for HPV testing to direct decisions about the clinical management of women with LGSIL is limited. On the other hand, testing for high-risk HPV DNA might be helpful in women with ASCUS. Preliminary analysis shows that the Hybrid Capture II assay has greater sensitivity in the detection of severe dysplasia or more severe lesions than a single additional cytologic test indicating ASCUS or a more advanced lesion. However, the specificity of the Hybrid Capture II assay was similar to that of repeat cytology. Future analyses and longer follow-up will hopefully help us determine the exact role of HPV testing in screening for cervical neoplasia.

Several researchers have assessed the value of HPV DNA testing as a specific and economical alternative for triage of low-grade cytologic abnormalities and as an adjunct to cervical cytology in primary screening.[104–107] With second-generation HPV DNA detection methods, including PCR-based methods and the Hybrid Capture HPV DNA assay, both of which have a higher sensitivity and detect a broader range of HPV types with high oncogenic risk than earlier methods, results have been more consistent, supporting the role of HPV typing in the triage of patients with low-grade cytologic abnormalities and as an adjunct to cytology in primary screening.[104–107] Cox and colleagues reported that HPV testing had a sensitivity of 86% in the detection of CIN (any grade) and of 93% in the detection of HGSILs.[104] Repeating the Pap smear alone had a sensitivity of only 60% in the detection of any grade of CIN.[104] In addition, they estimated that HPV testing could reduce the colposcopy rate by 58% if only women with a cytologic diagnosis of ASCUS and HPV-positive tests were referred and could reduce the cost of detection of each case of CIN by 38% despite the added cost of HPV testing.[108]

The preferences of clinician and patient and cost considerations should dictate the choice of treatment of CIN; however, proper management of LGSILs is expected to remain a fiercely debated question. Although management guidelines have increasingly included nontreatment of LGSILs as an option for patients who may be reliable for long-term follow-up, concerns over legal responsibility for progressive lesions continue to drive intensive follow-up protocols, particularly in the United States, that may not be cost-efficient.[109] Guidelines recently published may be helpful to follow.

Management of High-Grade Cytologic Abnormalities No dispute exists regarding the optimal management of HGSILs. These cases require colposcopic evaluation and biopsy. The consensus is that HGSILs should be treated once diagnosed.[110] For biopsy-proven HGSILs with negative findings on endocervical curettage (ECC), a satisfactory colposcopy examination, and congruent Pap smear and biopsy results, ablation of the transformation zone has been the standard of care for several decades. Three outpatient therapies are used in the United States for treating these lesions: cryotherapy, laser ablation, and LEEP. For patients with unsatisfactory colposcopic examination findings, a Pap smear result more severe than the biopsy findings, presence of an adenomatous component, suspicion of invasive cancer, or positive findings on ECC, a cone biopsy is indicated. Cone biopsies (talked about later in the chapter) remove tissue to a depth of 20 to 30 mm and up to 30 mm in diameter, including the transformation zone.

The three outpatient therapies of cryotherapy, laser vaporization, and LEEP have been the focus of controversy. Safety, efficacy, and cost issues have dominated the debate. Cryotherapy, introduced in 1972, was the first outpatient treatment of CIN and remains a dependable treatment because of its reliability, low complication rate, ease of use, and low cost.[111] Another advantage of cryotherapy is that leaving a large dead viral HPV load within disrupted cells may improve the immune response to the causative agent of CIN. Major disadvantages include lack of ability to tailor treatment to the size of the lesion, lack of a tissue specimen, and the risk of treatment of undetected invasive lesions. Eligible for cryotherapy are patients with satisfactory findings on colposcopic examination, negative findings on ECC, and small lesions (2.5–3.0 cm in diameter) that allow the entire lesion and transformation zone to be covered by the cryotherapy probe.

Laser vaporization was introduced in 1977. It has the advantage of being easily tailored to lesion size, but the cost of the equipment and the lack of a tissue specimen are major disadvantages.[111] In addition, laser vaporization requires more training and skills than the other two procedures and is associated with more serious safety issues (eye injuries and inadvertent burns). Candidates for this procedure are patients with large CIN lesions, young women with suspicious or invasive lesions or adenocarcinoma in situ in whom preservation of fertility is desired, and patients unwilling to undergo LEEP under local anesthesia.

LEEP was introduced in 1989, and it is currently the technique of choice for the treatment of HGSILs. LEEP is reliable and easy to use. It can be tailored to lesion size and provides a tissue specimen.[111] The advantage of this last characteristic is underscored by the finding of unsuspected adenocarcinoma in situ and microinvasive squamous cell carcinoma in 2 to 4% of LEEP specimens.[101,111] LEEP, however, has the potential to result in unintentional removal of excessive cervical stroma and removal of disease-free tissue (more frequent when LGSILs are treated). Other disadvantages include its high cost and the increased risk of bleeding and infection. Bleeding after LEEP has been reported in 2 to 7% of cases.[111] The high rates of overtreatment observed with LEEP have been related to misdiagnosis of abnormality and multiple punch biopsies of small lesions prior to treatment.[101] The use of LEEP in see-and-treat protocols has been shown to improve patient compliance with treatment when patient selection is adequate. This strategy has been suggested as having the greatest potential benefit for populations with poor treatment compliance.[101]

No statistically significant differences in success rates (based on recurrence and persistence) between cryotherapy and laser vaporization have been reported, but variability in these rates from study to study is striking. In nonrandomized clinical studies, reported success rates range from 86 to 91% for cryotherapy and 89 to 97% for laser vaporization.[112] Similar success rates have been reported for LEEP (range, 84–95%). All these studies have shown an association between persistent or recurrent disease and high histologic grade, disease affecting endocervical gland crypts, and size of lesion. The only randomized controlled trial comparing the efficacy of all three treatment options reported no statistically significant difference in varying success rates: cryotherapy, 24%; laser vaporization, 17%; and LEEP, 16%.[111] Similarly, no statistically significant differences in complication rates were observed between groups. Only lesion size was statistically associated with persistent disease, but risk of recurrence was associated with age more than 30 years, positivity for HPV 16 or 18, and previous treatment of CIN. Cold cone biopsy increases the risk of second-trimester abortions, preterm labor, and having infants of low birth weight. The amount of tissue removed by laser, cryotherapy, and LEEP is small, so these techniques have no adverse effect on pregnancy. Electrocoagulation diathermy also has no adverse effect on pregnancy.

New Concepts in Diagnosis and Prevention **Fluorescence Spectroscopy** The University of Texas M. D. Anderson Cancer Center and the University of Texas Optics Division have developed fluorescence spectroscopy, a very promising new technique. Fluorescence spectroscopy is completely noninvasive and involves the application of white light at different wavelengths to the surface of the cervix. It is a near real-time measurement that is fully automated and does not require the expertise needed for colposcopy. The higher the grade of the dysplasia, the more the absorption, the less the emitted fluorescence, and, therefore, the lower the signal from the tissue.[113] Preliminary data and cost analysis of this technique show that fluorescence spectroscopy of the cervix has a higher sensitivity than the Pap smear test and a higher specificity than colposcopy in differentiating squamous epithelial lesions from normal cervix and in differentiating LGSIL from HGSIL. Patients with an abnormal optical spectrum can be further evaluated with colposcopy, potentially on the same office visit.

Chemopreventative Management One of the more exciting research areas in therapy for CIN is the use of chemopreventative agents. These therapies involve ingestion of an agent that reverses precancerous changes, returning the tissue to normal. Laboratory data have shown that retinoids can induce apoptosis in dysplastic cervical cells, suggesting that these compounds may be active in cell-cycle control.[114] Women with HGSIL and colposcopically evident lesions are the target population for chemoprevention studies because they have a higher risk of persistent disease or progression to cancer. α-Difluoromethylornithine and retinoids (vitamin A derivatives) are two drugs currently receiving attention in the United States and China.[115,116]

Vaccine Development Papillomaviruses are epitheliotropic agents that induce benign papillomas of the skin and mucous membranes. In contrast to hepatitis B virus (HBV), there are more than 100 HPV genotypes (types). A subset of HPV types that are almost always transmitted sexually is the main cause of human cervical cancer. Infection with these HPV types is a strong risk factor for cervical cancer, and HPV DNA from one or more of these types is found in virtually all cervical tumors.[117,118] The virus encodes oncoproteins that appear to be required both for the induction and the maintenance of the cancer.

Because papillomaviruses contain oncogenes, and a prophylactic vaccine would be directed toward healthy young individuals, efforts to develop a prophylactic vaccine have emphasized a subunit approach, analogous to that used for HBV vaccine. Indeed, constitutive high-level expression of the L1 major structural viral protein, even in nonmammalian cells, leads to its efficient self-assembly into virus like particles (VLPs) that resemble authentic viral capsids structurally and antigenically. Preparative amounts of VLPs can be synthesized in insect cells or yeast. Such VLPs are suitable immunogens that, as is true of authentic virions, possess the immunodominant conformational epitopes capable of raising high titers of neutralizing antibodies.

In a placebo-controlled study, a yeast-produced HPV-16 L1 VLP vaccine was 100% efficacious in prevention of CIN caused by HPV-16 infection 17 months after vaccination in women who were HPV-16 naïve at the time of vaccination.[119] Another randomized trial recently published[120] showed that a bivalent HPV vaccine was efficacious in prevention of incident and persistent cervical infections with HPV-16 and HPV-18, and associated cytological abnormalities and lesions. Merrick just published a trial this year looking at quadrivalent HPV vaccine (HPV-16, -11, and -18) and found it to reduce 90% infection or disease compared with placebo.[121] All of these studies conclude that universal HPV vaccination might be most effect when implemented in 10- to 13-year-olds, who are likely to be HPV negative, and hopefully will reduce the incidence of cervical cancer worldwide as well as reduce the burden of full-scale cervical screening that can be quite expensive. Large-scale studies are underway.

DIAGNOSIS AND TREATMENT OF INVASIVE LESIONS

Patterns of Spread During the transition from in situ to invasive carcinoma, tumor cells penetrate the epithelial basement membrane and enter the underlying cervical stroma. Once the cervical stroma is invaded, the lymphatics and blood vessels are accessible, and dissemination beyond the cervix is possible.

The cervical, vaginal, and uterine lymphatic channels coalesce to form major drainage pathways. The major lymphatic trunks are the utero-ovarian (infundibulopelvic), parametrial, and presacral, which drain into the paracervical, obturator, hypogastric, external iliac, common iliac, inferior gluteal, presacral, and lower aortic lymph nodes. A series studying the incidence and distribution pattern of retroperitoneal lymph node metastases in 208 patients with stages 1B, IIA, and IIB cervical carcinomas who underwent radical hysterectomy and systemic pelvic node dissection reported that 53 patients (25%) had node metastasis.[122] The obturator lymph nodes were the most frequently involved, with a rate of 19% (39 of 208), and the authors proposed them as sentinel nodes for cervical cancers. In fact, finding negative obturator nodes may be an indication that the pelvic lymph node dissection can be limited.

Lymph node status and the size and extent of the primary tumor are the most important prognostic factors in patients with cervical cancers. Among patients with early disease, the 5-year survival rate is only 60% in patients with three or more positive nodes and only 25 to 30% in patients with positive para-aortic nodes. Cervical cancers of similar size may have very different metastatic potentials, depending on their intrinsic aggressiveness and histologic cell type. Cervical carcinomas also invade directly. As the cancer grows, disease may extend to the lateral pelvic walls, into the bladder or rectum, or into the vagina.

The incidence of lymph node metastasis at diagnosis for each of the squamous cell carcinoma stages designated by the International Federation of Gynecology and Obstetrics (FIGO) has been well defined by surgical series.[123–125] Pelvic node involvement occurs in 10 to 25% of stage I carcinomas, 25 to 30% of stage II carcinomas, and 30 to 45% of stage III and IV carcinomas. Stage I carcinomas are more likely to metastasize to nodes once they reach 3 cm.[126,127] Because most patients with large bulky adenocarcinomas are treated with radiation therapy, the incidence of positive nodes by tumor size is not as well defined for adenocarcinoma as it is for squamous cell carcinoma. The incidence of positive nodes for poorly differentiated squamous cell carcinoma and for poorly differentiated adenocarcinoma is higher than that for the better differentiated carcinomas.

Carcinoma of the cervix spreads in an orderly manner. Nodes adjacent to the cervix are usually the first to be involved, and "skip" metastases are uncommon. Patients with positive para-aortic nodes usually have positive pelvic nodes. The incidence of positive para-aortic nodes in 978 patients with stage IB and IIA carcinoma whose aortic nodes were sampled prior to radical hysterectomy was 4.7% and 8.4%, respectively. The incidence of positive nodes in patients with adenocarcinomas is probably equal to that in patients with squamous cell carcinomas when cancer size, histologic differentiation, and extent of tumor or FIGO stage are similar. Many large series report poorer survival rates for patients with adenocarcinomas than for patients with squamous cell carcinomas, especially those who have bulky lesions.[128,129] Small-cell carcinoma and some of the carcinomas classified as other epithelial tumors are particularly aggressive. Carcinomas of the cervix, regardless of histology and size of the primary tumor, may contain highly malignant clones of cells that can prove unpredictable and spread extensively.

Clinical Symptoms The clinical symptoms of carcinoma of the cervix are vaginal bleeding, discharge, and pain. The growth pattern of the carcinoma plays a role in the development of symptoms. Exophytic carcinomas bleed earlier in a sexually active patient (because of contact) than lesions that expand the cervix. Lesions that expand the endocervix in a barrel-shaped configuration may leave the squamous epithelium of the exocervix intact until the lesions exceed 5 or 6 cm in transverse diameter; therefore, carcinomas with this growth pattern may be silent and grow large before the patient bleeds. Cytologic findings may be negative unless the endocervix is sampled with a brush device. Ulcerative lesions that destroy the exocervix bleed early, and necrosis and infection induced by the cancer's outgrowing its blood supply result in a foul-smelling vaginal discharge.

Severe pelvic pain experienced during the pelvic examination may indicate salpingitis. Tubal infections require management before radiation therapy. Patients with an adnexal mass need surgical treatment before radiation therapy is started.

Paracervical extension of a carcinoma may remain silent until fixation to the pelvic wall occurs. Fixation with or without nodal involvement may obstruct a ureter. Ureteral encroachment is usually a silent process. Patients may present with bilateral ureteral obstruction with impending renal failure and report no history of urinary system complaints. Direct invasion of branches of the sciatic nerve roots causes back pain, and encroachment on the pelvic wall veins and lymphatics causes edema of a lower extremity. The triad of back pain, leg edema, and a nonfunctioning kidney is evidence of an advanced carcinoma with extensive pelvic wall involvement.

The anatomic position of the bladder, so closely adjacent to the cervix, favors contiguous spread from the cervix to the bladder. Urinary frequency and urgency are early manifestations of such spread; patients with advanced disease may present with hematuria or incontinence, suggesting direct extension of tumor to the bladder. Cystoscopy and biopsy should confirm the cause of hematuria or incontinence.

In contrast, posterior extension to the rectum and disruption of the rectal mucosa is an unusual pattern of disease spread in untreated patients. The deep cul-de-sac provides anatomic separation of the rectum and cervix. In patients who present with rectal mucosal involvement, there is usually extensive involvement of the posterior vaginal wall with direct extension to the rectum. For staging and treatment planning, cystoscopy and sigmoidoscopy are essential.

Metastatic carcinoma in para-aortic nodes may extend through the node capsule and directly invade the vertebrae and adjacent nerve roots. Back pain owing to involvement of the lumbar vertebrae and psoas muscles may be a manifestation of massive nodal disease; however, hematogenous spread to the lumbar vertebrae and involvement of the psoas muscle without significant nodal disease may occur.

Diagnosis The diagnosis of cervical carcinoma is made by pathologic examination of a tissue specimen. A biopsy sample taken from the periphery of a tumor is more likely to contain morphologically intact neoplastic cells that are best able to represent the tumor pathologically. A biopsy specimen taken from the center of a tumor mass may include necrotic tumor debris, the result of hypoxia induced by the tumor's outgrowing its blood supply. Therefore, to rely on these dead and distorted cells is to compromise the accuracy of the histologic interpretation.

The endocervix should be curetted if no lesion is visible or if the cervix is enlarged, nodular, or hard. Older patients with adenocarcinoma require an endometrial biopsy. It may be difficult to distinguish an endocervical primary tumor from an endometrial primary tumor involving the lower uterine segment.

Patients with an abnormal Pap smear and no visible lesion require colposcopy and biopsy. The tissue specimen may be a simple colposcopy-directed biopsy specimen, an endocervical specimen obtained with a curette, or a conization specimen.

It is the current recommendation of FIGO to classify as stage IA any invasive cancer that can be identified only with a microscope. All gross lesions, even with superficial invasion, are at least stage IB cancers. Lesions with invasion of the stroma up to 3 mm in depth and no greater than 7 mm in width are classified as stage IA1. Lesions with invasion of stroma greater than 3 mm and no greater than 5 mm in depth and no wider than 7 mm are classified as stage IA2. For a lesion to be classified as IA2, the depth of invasion should not be more than 5 mm, measured from the base of the epithelium, either squamous or glandular, from which it originates. Vascular space involvement, either venous or lymphatic, should not alter staging.

Many clinicians prefer to use the term microinvasion and use criteria recommended by the Society of Gynecologic Oncologists instead of using the FIGO staging system. Microinvasion is invasion limited to 3 mm in depth, is measured from the base of the squamous or glandular epithelium of origin, and does not encompass lymphatic or vascular space involvement. A simple punch biopsy is inadequate for making the diagnosis of microinvasion: A conization specimen, containing the entire neoplastic process, is necessary. Additional tissue is required from patients with positive cone margins because an occult, frankly invasive carcinoma may lie adjacent to a positive margin.

Table 101-2 Relapse Rates for Patients with Stage IIB or III Cervical Cancer

Hemoglobin (gm/dL)	Patients (No.)	Relapse Rate (%)		
		Local	Distant	Total
< 10	29	46	18	49
10–11.9	319	29	24	47
12–13.9	578	20	16	33
≥ 14	129	20	18	33

Reproduced with permission from Bush R.[130] Relapse rates for patients with stage IIB or III cancer of the cervix according to average hemoglobin level during radiation therapy.
p Values: $p = .002$ (local), $p = .1$ (distant), $p = .0007$ (total).

Evaluation and Staging Successful therapy planning requires detailed evaluation of the patient's general medical condition and the size and extent of the carcinoma. Medical illness must be stabilized and anemia must be corrected before treatment commences. Patients with anemia, which has been extensively studied, have a higher local relapse rate than patients with a normal hemoglobin count (Table 101-2).[130,131] The patient's surgical history is important, and operative notes may describe the status of the abdominal organs as well as report abdominal and pelvic operations. Diagnoses of importance to therapy planning include ulcerative bowel disease, diverticulitis, and pelvic inflammatory disease. Such inflammatory conditions induce adhesions and fix loops of the intestines to each other, to adjacent organs, and to peritoneal surfaces.

Patients with small stage I carcinomas should undergo chest radiography, intravenous pyelography, a complete blood count, urinalysis, and blood chemistry analysis before treatment. Patients with advanced carcinomas require cystoscopy and proctoscopy. It is important to apply the FIGO rules for clinical staging (Table 101-3).[132] FIGO guidelines clearly state that for staging purposes, the following examinations are permitted: cystoscopy, inspection, colposcopy, ECC, hysteroscopy, proctoscopy, intravenous pyelography, chest radiography, and skeletal radiography.[133] Findings from such examinations as lymphangiography, laparotomy, laparoscopy, computed tomography (CT), magnetic resonance imaging (MRI), and other examinations unnamed by FIGO should not be the basis for changing the clinical stage, despite the fact that such examinations or procedures can provide valuable information for planning therapy. The tumor-nodes-metastasis (TNM) staging categories have also been accepted by FIGO.[134] Lymph node status is not addressed in the FIGO staging system for carcinoma of the cervix, but three radiologic imaging techniques are available

Table 101-3 Modified FIGO Staging

Stage	Description
0	Carcinoma in situ, intraepithelial carcinoma. Cases of stage 0 should not be included in any therapeutic statistics for invasive carcinoma.
I	The carcinoma is strictly confined to the cervix (extension to the corpus should be disregarded).
IA	Invasive cancer identified only microscopically. All gross lesions, even with superficial invasion, are stage IB cancers. Invasion is limited to measured stromal invasion with a maximum depth of 5 mm and a width no greater than 7 mm.
IA1	Measured invasion of stroma ≤ 3 mm in depth and ≤ 7 mm in width
IA2	Measured invasion of stroma > 3 mm and ≤ 5 mm in depth and ≤ 7 mm in width
IB	Clinical lesions confined to the cervix or preclinical lesions larger than stage IA
IB1	Clinical lesions ≤ 4 cm
IB2	Clinical lesions > 4 cm
II	The carcinoma extends beyond the cervix but has not extended onto the pelvic wall. Involves the vagina but does not extend as far as the lower third of the vagina
IIA	No obvious parametrial involvement
IIB	Obvious parametrial involvement
III	The carcinoma has extended onto the pelvic wall. On rectal examination, there is no cancer-free space between the tumor and the pelvic wall. The tumor involves the lower third of the vagina. All cases with hydronephrosis or a nonfunctioning kidney should be included unless they are known to result from another cause.
IIIA	No extension onto the pelvic wall but involvement of the lower third of the vagina
IIIB	Extension onto the pelvic wall or hydronephrosis or nonfunctioning kidney
IV	The carcinoma has extended beyond the true pelvis or has clinically involved the mucosa of the bladder or rectum.
IVA	Spread to adjacent organs
IVB	Spread to distant organs

Reproduced with permission from Shepperd.[182] FIGO = International Federation of Gynecology and Obstetrics.

to evaluate lymph node status: CT, MRI, and lymphangiography.

The best radiologic imaging technique for detecting lymph node metastases is unclear. CT and MRI are good in identifying enlarged nodes; however, the accuracy of these techniques in the detection of positive nodes is compromised by their failure to detect small metastases, and many enlarged nodes are due not to metastases but to inflammation associated with advanced disease. The accuracy of MRI in the detection of lymph node metastases (72–93%) is similar to that of CT; however, when compared with surgical findings, MRI is superior to CT, clinical examination, and sonography in the evaluation of tumor location, tumor size, depth of stromal invasion, vaginal extension, and parametrial extension of cervical cancer.[135–138] Furthermore, studies suggest that MRI is a cost-effective method of evaluating cervical cancers.[138] Figure 101-13 shows an MRI of a patient with a cervical tumor.

Positron emission tomography (PET) is a new and rapidly expanding modality in oncologic imaging (Figure 101-14). In a study of 101 patients with carcinoma of the cervix, Grigsby and colleagues reported that CT demonstrated enlarged pelvic lymph nodes in 20% and enlarged para-aortic lymph nodes in 7%, while PET demonstrated abnormal fluorodeoxyglucose (FDG) uptake in pelvic lymph nodes in 67%, abnormal FDG uptake in para-aortic lymph nodes in 21%, and abnormal FDG uptake in supraclavicular lymph nodes in 8%.[139] The 2-year progression-free survival rate, based solely on para-aortic lymph node status, was 64% in CT-normal and PET-normal patients, 18% in CT-normal and PET-abnormal patients, and 14% in CT-abnormal and PET-abnormal patients. The authors concluded that FDG-PET detects abnormal lymph nodes more often than CT and that the findings on PET are a better predictor of survival than those on CT in patients with carcinoma of the cervix. Further studies are needed to confirm these results.

In some patients, surgical examination of the lymph nodes is warranted. The risk of occult para-aortic metastases is highest in patients with grossly involved pelvic nodes, and these patients may be the best candidates for operative exploration. These patients also may benefit from removal of the grossly enlarged nodes, which may be difficult to control with radiation alone.[140] When lymph node metastases are sought surgically, the extraperitoneal approach is currently the preferred technique.[141] It is preferred because high complication rates resulted from using a transperitoneal approach followed by radiation therapy.[142] Lymph node exploration and dissection may also be performed using a laparoscopic approach, which is associated with a shorter post-operative recovery time and probably less late radiation morbidity than open transperitoneal staging.[143] Intraoperative lymphatic mapping may someday improve the accuracy of surgical staging of cervical cancer, and the Gynecologic Oncology Group (GOG) is currently opening a trial evaluating this approach.[144]

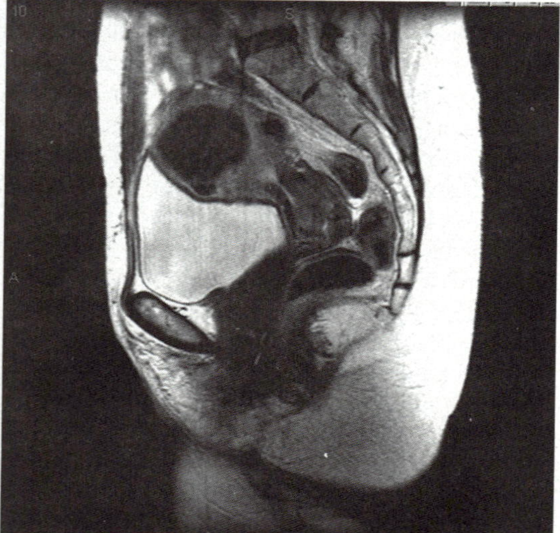

Figure 101-13 Magnetic resonance image of a patient with cervical tumor.

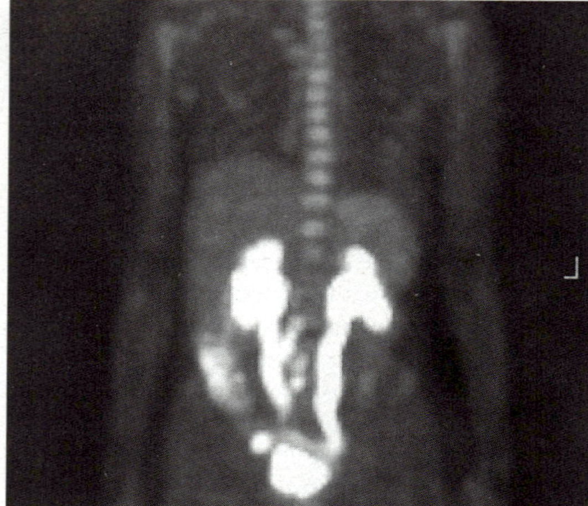

Figure 101-14 Positron emission tomography scan of a patient with cervical tumor showing positive nodes.

Prognostic Factors FIGO stage correlates with survival and control of pelvic disease in patients with cervical cancer; however, prognosis is also influenced by other factors, including tumor characteristics and patient characteristics that are not included in the FIGO staging system.

Tumor Size and Local Extent Tumor size is one of the most important predictors of local recurrence and death in patients with cervical cancer treated with surgery or radiation therapy (Figure 101-15). The FIGO staging classification for stage I disease was recently modified to include tumor diameter (ie, ≤ 4 cm, stage IB1; > 4 cm, stage IB2).[145] For patients with more advanced disease, other estimates of tumor bulk that correlate with prognosis include presence of medial versus lateral parametrial involvement in FIGO stage IIB disease and unilateral versus bilateral pelvic wall involvement in FIGO stage IIIB disease.[146,147]

In patients who have had a radical hysterectomy, histologic evidence of extracervical spread (≥ 10 mm) and deep stromal invasion (> 70% invasion) are associated with a poorer prognosis, as is parametrial extension, which is associated with higher rates of lymph node involvement, local recurrence, and death from cancer.[125,148–150] Uterine body involvement is associated with an increased rate of distant metastases in patients treated with radiation or surgery.[151]

Lymph Node Involvement Lymph node metastasis is another important prognostic factor for survival that is not part of the FIGO staging system. In several surgical series, after a radical hysterec-

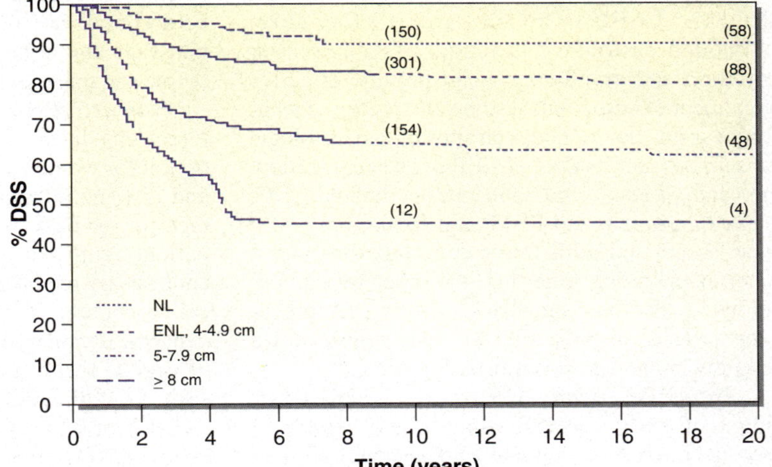

Figure 101-15 Reproduced with permission from Eifel, et al.[207] Disease-specific survival (DSS) is indicated for patients grouped according to size of cervix (NL = cervix of normal size; ENL = enlarged cervix, 4–4.9 cm).

tomy, patients with positive pelvic lymph nodes had a 35 to 40% lower 5-year survival rate than patients with negative nodes.[123,125] However, recent studies suggest that postoperative chemoradiation improves these results.[152] Several authors have reported a correlation between size of the largest node involved or higher number of nodes involved and decreased survival rates. Patients with positive para-aortic nodes have a survival rate that is about half that of patients with similar-stage disease and negative para-aortic nodes.[123,125,149,153,154] With extended-field radiation therapy, patients with early-stage disease and positive para-aortic nodes have a cure rate of approximately 40 to 50%.

There is a strong correlation between positive lymph nodes in patients with cervical neoplasms and positive lymph-vascular space invasion (LVSI) in the tumor specimen. However, LVSI may be an independent predictor of prognosis, as a number of large series of patients treated with radical hysterectomy have demonstrated.[148,149,155,156] Roman and colleagues reported a correlation between the percentage of histopathologic sections containing LVSI and the incidence of lymph node metastasis.[157] In patients with adenocarcinoma of the cervix, there is a strong correlation between LVSI and outcome.[158,159]

Histologic Type There is controversy regarding whether adenocarcinomas of the cervix are associated with outcome similar to that seen with squamous carcinomas of the cervix. In several retrospective studies, investigators found that patients with adenocarcinomas of the cervix had outcome similar to that of patients with squamous carcinoma of the cervix treated with radiation therapy.[160,161] However, other investigators have come to an opposite conclusion. Among patients treated surgically, they found that patients with adenocarcinoma had unusually high relapse rates compared with the rates in patients with squamous cell carcinoma, and among patients treated with surgery or irradiation, they found that patients with adenocarcinoma had poorer survival rates than the rates seen in patients with squamous cell carcinoma.[162–164] Eifel and colleagues, in an analysis of 1,767 patients treated with radiation for FIGO stage IB disease, reported that patients with adenocarcinoma had a significantly higher risk of recurrence and death from disease.[162] This finding was independent of age, tumor size, and tumor morphology. There was no difference in the rate of pelvic recurrence between patients with bulky adenocarcinoma (≥ 4 cm) and patients with squamous cell carcinoma; however, the rate of distant metastasis was almost twice as high in patients with adenocarcinoma as in patients with squamous cell carcinoma. Although the prognostic significance of histologic grade for squamous carcinomas has been disputed, there is a clear correlation between the degree of differentiation and the clinical behavior of adenocarcinomas.[159,165,166]

Other Tumor Factors Baseline pretreatment serum squamous cell carcinoma antigen (SCC-Ag) level correlates well with stage of disease: 30 to 40% of stage I patients, 60 to 70% of stage II patients, and 80 to 90% of stage III and IV patients have elevated values.[167,168] The only exception to this trend is patients with bulky stage IB2 disease, in whom levels are more consistent with advanced-stage disease, suggesting that SCC-Ag level correlates with tumor bulk.[169] Pretreatment SCC-Ag levels have also been shown to correlate with tumor histology, grade, type of tumor (ie, exophytic vs infiltrative), microscopic depth of invasion, and risk of lymph node metastases in patients with early-stage disease.[170] The most important property of the pretreatment SCC-Ag level, however, is its ability to predict clinical outcome. Several authors have reported significantly lower survival rates in patients with very elevated values compared with patients with normal baseline levels, independent of stage.[170–173] Duk and colleagues reported a 70% 5-year survival rate in stage IB patients with elevated pretreatment SCC-Ag levels, compared with 96% in patients with normal values.[173] SCC-Ag testing also provides a marker for monitoring the course of disease and response to treatment in patients with cervical cancer. Correlations of tumor response and SCC-Ag values have ranged from 72 to 95%.[174] For the detection of tumor recurrence, serial SCC-Ag testing has been proven to be more specific than sensitive, with specificities ranging from 90 to 100% and sensitivities ranging from 60 to 90%.[175] Monitoring of tumor response using SCC-Ag needs further investigation, especially studies designed to determine how often SCC-Ag measurement should be done, the level of SCC-Ag that is significant, which patients would benefit from this monitoring and the cost-effectiveness of using SCC-Ag as a tool for monitoring patients after treatment.[176]

Several authors have reported a correlation between HPV subtype and prognosis.[177–179] In two studies of patients with histologically negative lymph nodes, investigators reported higher rates of disease recurrence when findings on PCR assay of the lymph nodes were strongly positive for HPV DNA.[180,181] Other authors have correlated poor prognosis with the presence of HPV mRNA or HPV-related proteins in the peripheral blood of cervical cancer patients.[280,281]

Other molecular markers that have recently been evaluated for predictive power in cervical carcinoma are epidermal growth factor receptor and cyclooxygenase-2. Several studies have reported that overexpression of epidermal growth factor receptor in cervical carcinomas correlates with clinical predictors of poor prognosis such as large tumor size and lymph node involvement; however, this association is controversial, and study populations have generally been too small and heterogeneous to permit establishment of an independent association between epidermal growth factor receptor and prognosis. A preliminary study in patients with cervical cancer suggested that cyclooxygenase-2 overexpression was also correlated with poor prognosis, but, because of the small sample size, the study was not able to establish independent predictive value of this molecular marker.[182]

Other biologic features that have been investigated for their predictive power, with variable results, include inflammatory response in cervical stroma, peritoneal cytology, tumor vascularity and DNA ploidy or S-phase fraction.[183,184]

Patient Factors Several investigators have reported correlations between low hemoglobin level before or during treatment and poor prognosis.[146,185] It has been speculated that the poor prognosis of anemic patients is caused in part by hypoxia-induced radiation resistance. The strongest evidence that this may be true comes from a randomized study of 1,978 patients at Princess Margaret Hospital. In one group, patients' hemoglobin levels were maintained, through the use of transfusions, at least 12 gm%; in the other group, hemoglobin levels were allowed to drop to as little as 10 gm%. The locoregional recurrence rate was significantly higher for the 25 anemic patients in the control arm than it was for the patients who received transfusions.[130] A recent retrospective study from Canada also found that hemoglobin levels of at least 12 gm% during radiation therapy were a significant predictor of successful radiation therapy and disease-free survival.[185] Subsequent studies investigating various techniques aimed at overcoming the theoretical radiobiological consequences of intratumoral hypoxia (use of hypoxic cell sensitizers, hyperbaric oxygen breathing, and neutron therapy) have not been successful.[298–304] The GOG has recently started a study evaluating the effects of hemoglobin on prognosis. Accrual is slow at present, but if the trial is completed, it may help clarify the relationship between anemia and prognosis in patients with cervical carcinoma. Several investigators have correlated low intratumoral oxygen tension levels with poor survival and a high rate of lymph node metastases.[305–307]

Other patient-related factors that have been shown to correlate with prognosis include age, platelet count, socioeconomic status, and smoking.[127,186–188] Kucera and colleagues reported that smokers with cervical cancer had a poorer 5-year survival rate than nonsmokers, and this relationship was statistically significant in patients with stage III disease (5-year survival rate 20.3% vs 33.9%, $p < .01$).[189] A recent study by Eifel and colleagues found that smokers had a significantly higher rate of grade 3 or 4 gastrointestinal complications than did nonsmokers in a group of patients with cervical carcinoma treated with definitive radiation therapy.[190]

Surgical Treatment Options **Cervical Conization** Cervical conization is a procedure that removes or destroys the transformation zone and can be diagnostic, therapeutic, or both. A conization specimen is conical, as the name implies, and its size varies according to the area in question. The cone is shallow when an exocervical lesion is removed. The cone is deeper when the endocervix is being investigated. Patients requiring conization usually have one of the following: normal colposcopy findings and an abnormal Pap smear or positive ECC specimens; abnormal colposcopy findings in the form of failure to visualize the entire squamocolumnar junction or failure to define the extent of the lesion; microinvasive carcinoma in a biopsy specimen; adenocarcinoma in situ in a biopsy or ECC specimen; or a lack of correlation between cytologic (Pap smear), colposcopic, and histologic interpretations.

Technique Conization is typically performed as an outpatient procedure with ECC done at the same time to permit detection of extension of disease into the endocervical canal. A variety of techniques are available for conization, including cold knife conization (CKC), laser conization, and LEEP. Laser conization became popular with the increased use of the laser as an ablative and surgical tool. Laser conization has no advantage in comparison with CKC, is technically more difficult, and requires more costly equipment. For these reasons, this technique is not frequently used. Laser ablation is still used by some, but its primary use remains ablation of vaginal and/or vulvar intraepithelial neoplasms.

Cone biopsy is designed to completely remove the squamocolumnar junction and the lower portion of the endocervical canal in women with very small cervical cancers. The surgical specimen should include the entire lesion, as this permits measurement of both depth of invasion and extent of lateral spread.

Another surgical technique that can be used for conization is LEEP. In LEEP, a thin wire loop electrode is used to excise the lesion in patients with HGSIL. LEEP is an outpatient procedure. Although destructive techniques (such as laser ablation and cryotherapy) can provide effective treatment of suspicious lesions; the preferred technique is one that provides an appropriate histologic specimen, such as CKC, LEEP, or laser conization. Recently, Linares and colleagues compared CKC, laser conization, and LEEP and found that LEEP was associated with fewer complications and a shorter operating time then the other two procedures.[191] The only drawback of the LEEP procedure was a slightly shorter cone depth and a slightly higher risk of lesion recurrence.[191]

Patient Selection Conization as sole treatment of early cervical cancers is a relatively recent concept. For women who have very limited risk of lymph node spread and who have a strong desire to maintain fertility, conization may be an option.[192,193] M. D. Anderson Cancer Center recommends that conization be considered only for patients with squamous cell lesions that invade less than 3 mm, have no LVSI, and have uninvolved resection margins.[194] There is very little information on which to base a recommendation regarding the use of conization as therapy for women with nonsquamous cervical cancer.[195]

Complications Complications of CKC include hemorrhage, pelvic cellulitis, cervical stenosis, and incompetent cervix.[196] In addition, because this procedure requires general anesthesia, there is the additional burden of possible complications and cost of anesthesia.

Complications of LEEP are similar to but not the same as those of CKC: infection, bleeding, burns to the vagina, cervical stenosis, cervical incompetence, and recurrence of dysplasia. With LEEP, however, stenosis is rare (occurring in 1% of patients) and is seen primarily in nulliparous, perimenopausal, or postmenopausal patients. Cervical incompetence is usually only a complication of multiple procedures. The other advantage of LEEP is that it does not require general anesthesia. As mentioned above, when three conization techniques (CKC, laser conization, and LEEP) were compared, LEEP was associated with fewer complication as well as decreased operative time.[191]

Extrafascial Hysterectomy ***Technique*** Characterizing the extrafascial hysterectomy are the following: (1) the uterine vessels are skeletonized (to lessen the need to slide the tip of the clamp off the cervix) and are clamped and cut to allow the ligated vessels to fall away from the cervix, (2) the pubovesicocervical fascia is not separated from the cervix and is excised with the specimen, (3) the plane for bladder separation from the cervix is created with sharp dissection because blunt dissection is more often associated with accidental entry into the bladder, and (4) the uterosacral ligaments are transected separately near their insertion into the cervix. This frees the uterus and cervix posteriorly and gains mobility for the specimen. This facilitates amputation of the vagina in front of the cervix, securing at least a 1 cm vaginal cuff. The extrafascial technique permits removal of the intact uterine fundus and cervix, leaving the parametrial soft tissues or a portion of the upper vagina. Extrafascial hysterectomy can be accomplished through an abdominal incision, transvaginally, or by using a combination of laparoscopic and transvaginal techniques.

Patient Selection Simple extrafascial hysterectomy is the standard definitive treatment option for women with stage IA1 cervical cancers and is sometimes performed following radiation therapy for bulky endocervical carcinomas. For patients with stage IA2 disease, there is some controversy regarding the most appropriate surgical procedure. These patients have 3 to 5% incidence of lymph node metastases and a higher rate of vaginal recurrence than patients with IA1 disease. So, although some data suggest that these IA2 lesions can be effectively resected with extrafascial hysterectomy, many American gynecologic oncologists limit this operation to women with IA1 tumors.[197,198] There is uniform consensus that conization-only therapy should not be offered to women with stage IA2 disease.

Radical Hysterectomy Radical hysterectomy involves the en bloc removal of the uterus, cervix, parametrial tissues, and upper vagina. In the early twentieth century, Wertheim of Vienna described the radical hysterectomy for the treatment of cervical cancer. In the 1940s, Meigs of the United States championed the procedure, to which he added a pelvic lymphadenectomy. Today, radical hysterectomy with pelvic lymphadenectomy is the standard treatment in the management of stage IA2-IIA Tumors.

Technique for Type II (Modified Radical) Hysterectomy The type II (modified radical) hysterectomy is a less extensive version of the type III (radical) hysterectomy. The primary indication for type II hysterectomy is early invasive carcinoma. The type II operation is applicable when invasion is present, yet the tissue orientation or preparation is not optimal for precise interpretation by the pathologist. The type II operation ensures an adequate paracervical specimen and a vaginal cuff of 2 to 3 cm.

In the type II operation, the medial half of the parametrium and upper one-third of the vagina are included in the surgical specimen. This is accomplished by exposing the ureters and taking the medial half of the cardinal and uterosacral ligaments instead of taking these ligaments where they attach to the pelvic wall and pelvic floor. The posterior approach is the surgeon's choice. The incidence of bladder and ureteral complications is lower with the type II operation than with a type III procedure.

The type II hysterectomy can be performed with a modified or complete pelvic lymphadenectomy. The modified lymphadenectomy includes removal of the following node groups: the obturator, the medial chain of the external iliac node group, and the nodes at the bifurcation of the common iliac artery. The nodes and lymphatic channels superior and lateral to the external iliac artery and vein are retained to lessen the risk of lymphocyst and edema of the lower extremities.

Technique for Type III (Radical) Hysterectomy The type III (radical) hysterectomy is the classic Wertheim-Meigs radical hysterectomy.

This operation is reserved for patients with stage IB and selected stage IIA carcinomas. The vaginal extension for stage IIA patients should be limited to no more than 1 cm. The parametrium, cardinal, and uterosacral ligaments are severed at the pelvic wall, and half of the vagina is removed. The uterine vessels are taken at their origin from the internal iliac vessels. The ureters are taken out of their tunnel and reflected laterally. This dissection of the distal ureters sacrifices the blood supply from the uterine and superior vesicle arteries. Reflection of the ureters clears the way for applying instruments across the parametrium along the pelvic wall. Complete removal of the cardinal ligaments and the rectal pillars and uterosacral ligaments at their base results in a greater risk of bladder atony, and loss of the distal-ureter blood supply results in a greater risk of fistulae. This operation produces an excellent cure rate in properly selected patients. In young patients, the ovaries are spared.

Technique for Radical Trachelectomy Recently, for early-stage disease, several groups have tried to preserve the uterus and child-bearing capability by treating patients with a radical vaginal trachelectomy. This technique involves a laparoscopic pelvic lymphadenectomy followed by vaginal resection of the cervix, the upper 1 to 2 cm of the vaginal cuff, and the medial portions of the cardinal and uterosacral ligaments. The cervix is transected at the lower uterine segment, and a prophylactic cerclage is placed at the time of surgery. Several investigators recommend that this procedure be limited to patients with a tumor not exceeding 2 cm.[199,200]

Patient Selection Criteria for selecting patients who are appropriate candidates for radical hysterectomy include factors affecting the patient's suitability for major surgery as well as tumor characteristics, including tumor volume and lymphatic involvement. Patient factors play a very important role in the selection of primary radical surgery versus primary radiation therapy in patients with early-stage disease. The ability to preserve ovarian function as well as a more pliable vagina is important to young women facing this decision. Just as important, for women with significant medical problems, including obesity, primary radiation therapy may be the better treatment option.

In patients with early-stage (IA-IB1) disease, tumor characteristics play a very important role in treatment selection. Patients with high-risk factors may benefit from up-front definitive radiation therapy plus possible chemotherapy. Multiple studies have found that morbidity increases in patients who receive both radical surgery and radiation therapy.[201] High-risk tumor characteristics include large tumor size, which is associated with lymph node spread, increased chance of recurrence, and decreased survival rates. Eifel and colleagues found that disease-specific survival decreased significantly in patients with stage IB carcinoma if the tumor diameter was greater than 5 cm (88% vs 69%, $p < .0001$).[202] Other high-risk factors include lymph node metastases, parametrial involvement, and positive surgical margins.

Table 101-4 5-Year Survival Rates for Stage IB–IIA Cervical Cancer Patients after Radical Hysterectomy and Bilateral Pelvic Lymphadenectomy

First Author (Ref)	Stage	Year	*n*	Survival (%)
Morley[303]	IB	1976	156	87.2
Sall[215]	IB–IIA	1979	219	90.0
Kenter[213]	IB–IIA	1989	213	87.3
Lee[212]	IB–IIA	1989	343	87.2
Ayhan[124]	IB–IIA	1991	270	80.7
Hopkins[165]	IB	1991	213	92.5
Alvarez[208]	IB	1991	401	85
Burghardt[304]	IB	1992	443	83
Averette[123]	IIB–IIA	1993	726	90.1
Landoni[201]	IB--IIA	1997	172	83

n = No. of patients.

Complications Intraoperative and immediate postoperative complications of radical hysterectomy include blood loss (average, 0.8 liters), ureterovaginal fistula (occurring in 1–2% of patients), vesicovaginal fistula (< 1%), pulmonary embolus (1–2%), small-bowel obstruction (1–2%) and postoperative fever secondary to deep vein thrombosis, pulmonary infection, pelvic cellulitis, urinary tract infection, or wound infection (25–50%).[203] Subacute complications include lymphocyst formation and lower-extremity edema, the risk of which is related to the extent of the node dissection. Lymphocysts may obstruct a ureter, but hydronephrosis usually improves with drainage of the lymphocyst.[204] The risk of complications may be increased in patients who undergo preoperative or postoperative irradiation.

Although most patients have transient decreased bladder sensation after radical hysterectomy, with appropriate management severe long-term bladder complications are infrequent. However, chronic bladder hypotonia or atony occurs in approximately 3 to 5% of patients despite careful postoperative bladder drainage.[205] Bladder atony probably results from damage to the bladder's innervation and may be related to the extent of the parametrial and paravaginal dissection.[206] Radical hysterectomy may be complicated by stress incontinence, but reported incidences vary widely and may be influenced by the addition of postoperative radiation therapy.[207] Patients may also experience constipation and, rarely, chronic obstipation after radical hysterectomy.

Outcomes after Surgical Treatment Reported 5-year survival rates for women with stage IB cervical cancer treated with radical hysterectomy and pelvic lymphadenectomy are approximately 80 to 90% (Table 101-4).[123–125,201,208–215] Patients with positive surgical margins or positive lymph nodes are at the highest risk of recurrence and poor outcome. Delgado and colleagues, in a large prospective study, reported 3-year disease-specific survival rates of 85.6% in patients with negative nodes and 50 to 74% in patients with positive nodes.[125] In the group with positive nodes, increasing number of positive nodes and involvement of common iliac nodes correlated with decreased survival. A recent randomized study showed that postoperative chemoradiation improved survival in patients with positive lymph nodes, positive surgical margins, or tumor present in the endometrium.[152]

RADIATION THERAPY

The management of invasive carcinoma of the cervix with primary radiation therapy involves a combination of external beam radiation therapy (EBRT) plus either low-dose-rate (LDR) or high-dose-rate (HDR) intracavitary irradiation. The goal of treatment is to balance these two elements in a way that optimizes the ratio of tumor control to treatment complications. The required dose varies according to the tumor burden in the cervix, paracervical sites, and regional nodes. Factors that influence the tolerable dose of radiation include the patient's vaginal and uterine anatomy, the degree of tumor-related tissue destruction and infection, and patient characteristics (eg, body habitus, comorbid illnesses, and smoking habits).

Treatment Options **EBRT** EBRT is used as initial treatment in patients with bulky tumors. The usual plan is to give 40 to 45 Gy to the whole pelvis. This gives a homogeneous distribution to the central mass plus the regional lymph nodes. Such treatment reduces the primary tumor and any regional lymph nodes harboring disease, and it destroys microscopic foci in lymph-vascular spaces adjacent to the tumor. The shrinkage of the primary tumor allows better dose distribution from intracavitary irradiation.

High-energy photons (15–18 MV) are usually preferred for pelvic treatment because they spare superficial tissues that are unlikely to be involved with tumor. At these energies, the pelvis can be treated either with four fields (anterior, posterior, and two lateral fields) or with anterior and posterior fields alone. When high-energy beams are not available, four fields are usually used because less-penetrating 4- to 6-MV photons often deliver an unacceptably high dose to superficial tissues when only two fields are used.

Simulation films, as well as CT, MRI, PET scan, and lymphangiography, guide the radiation oncologist in selecting boundaries for the portals. The lower boundary of the anterior-posterior–posterior-anterior field is midpubis or 4 cm below

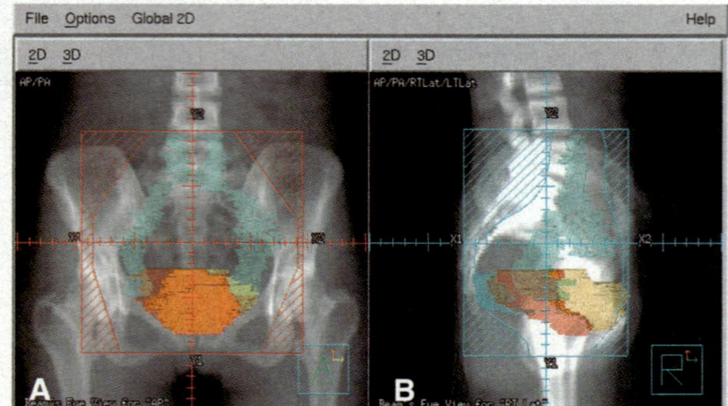

Figure 101-16 Typical radiation fields for a patient with cervical cancer. **A,** Anterior field. **B,** Lateral field.

the lowest extent of vaginal or cervical disease. The lowest extent of the disease can be determined by placing radiopaque seeds in the cervix or at the lowest extent of vaginal disease. The upper border is the L4-L5 interspace or at the bificuration of the aorta. In most patients, this interspace includes the external iliac nodes and a portion of the common iliac nodes.[216] The lateral margins extend 1.5 to 2 cm lateral to the pelvic margins. If a four-field technique is used, selection of the lateral margins usually encompasses S3 posteriorly and the pubic symphysis anteriorly. A standard course of 40 to 45 Gy whole-pelvis EBRT plus two 48-hour or equivalent intracavitary irradiation systems usually delivers at least 85 Gy to point A (a reference location 2 cm lateral and 2 cm superior to the cervical os) and 50 to 56 Gy to the lateral pelvic wall structures. Patients with grossly positive pelvic nodes within the 40- to 45-Gy field require a boost with a small field (Figures 101-16, 101-17).[217] The dose to the boost area is 8 to 10 Gy. The total dose to the positive nodes, including a 1 to 2 cm margin, is 60 to 62 Gy, which includes the contributions from two brachytherapy intracavitary systems. Intensity-modulated radiation therapy may be used to boost the dose to large pelvic nodes (up to approximately 70 Gy) in a very tightly defined volume.

Intracavitary Radiation Therapy (ICRT) The importance of ICRT for cervical cancer should not be underestimated, because, although external beam radiation therapy plays a critical role in sterilizing pelvic wall disease and improving tumor geometry, too much reliance on external beam irradiation will compromise the chance for central disease control and increase the risk of complications.

Brachytherapy is usually delivered using afterloading applicators that are placed in the uterine cavity and vagina. The most popular systems in the United States are variations of the Fletcher-Suit-Delclos low-dose system.[218] In this system, the intrauterine tandem and vaginal applicators are carefully positioned, usually with the patient under anesthesia, to provide an optimal relationship between the system and the adjacent tumor and normal tissues. Vaginal packing is used to hold the tandem and colpostats in place and to maximize the distance between the sources and the bladder and rectum. Radiographs should always be obtained in the operation room at the time of the insertions; the system should be repositioned and repacked if it is suboptimal. Sonography in the operating room may be helpful in determining the position of the tandem in the uterine cavity as well as the position of the tandem in relation to the bladder and the rectum.

Ideal placement of the intrauterine tandem and vaginal ovoids produces a pear-shaped radiation distribution, delivering a high radiation dose to the cervix and paracervical tissues and a reduced dose to the rectum and bladder. Several systems have been used throughout the world to determine dose rates and doses for cervical cancer. In the United States, the paracentral doses are most frequently expressed at a single point, point A, which is defined above. Point A bears no consistent relationship with the tumor or target volume but lies approximately at the crossing of the ureter and uterine artery. Other systems of dose specifications include the International Commission on Radiation Units and Measurements (ICRU) reference points based on ICRU Report 38 (International Commission on Radiation Units and Measurements, 1985) and the milligram-hours system. Whichever system of dose specification is used, emphasis should always be placed on optimizing the relationship between the intracavitary applicators and the cervical tumor and other pelvic tissues. Source, strength, and position should be carefully chosen to provide optimal tumor coverage with exceeding safe doses to normal tissue. In patients with bulky central disease, an effort should always be made to deliver at least 85 Gy (using low-dose-rate brachytherapy) to point A. If the intracavitary placement has been optimized, this can usually be accomplished by not exceeding a dose of 70 to 75 Gy to the bladder reference point or 60 to 65 to the rectal reference point, doses that are usually associated with acceptably low risks of major complications. In addition, the dose delivered to the surface of the lateral wall of the apical vagina should not exceed 120 to 140 Gy.

In the past, clinicians regarded the radiobiological advantages of LDR intracavitary treatment (usually delivery of 40–60 cGy/h to point A) as a major factor contributing to the success of cervical cancer treatment. These low dose rates permit repair of sublethal cellular injury, preferentially sparing normal tissues and optimizing the therapeutic ratio. During the past two decades, computer technology has made it possible to deliver brachytherapy at very high dose rates (< 100 cGy/min) using a high-activity cobalt 60 or iridium 192 source and remote afterloading. HDR therapy is slowly replacing conventional LDR therapy, primarily because of radiation safety. HDR intracavitary therapy is now being used for radical treatment of cervical cancer by a number of groups, including several in Japan, Canada, and Europe and, more recently, in the United States. Clinicians have found this approach attractive because it does not require that patients be hospitalized and may be more convenient for the patient and the physician.

Multiple randomized and nonrandomized studies have suggested that survival rates and complications rates with high-dose-rate treatment are similar to those with traditional low-dose-rate treatment. At least two studies from the United States have shown similar results with high-dose-rate and low-dose-rate therapy in early-stage disease; however, in stage IIIB disease, the survival rate was lower with high-dose-rate than with low-dose-rate therapy.[219,220]

HDR brachytherapy is gaining increasing acceptance in the community and is considered standard therapy for patients with an intact cervix, and in 2000,[221] the American Brachytherapy

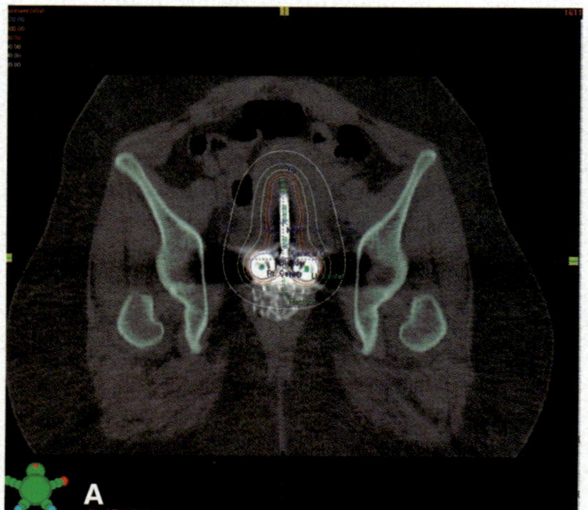

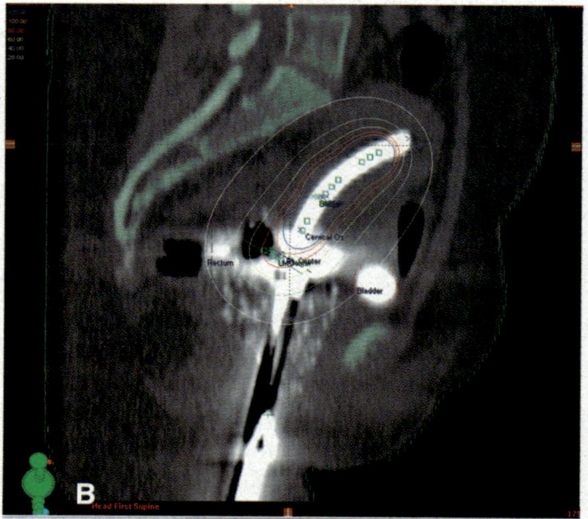

Figure 101-17 Dose distribution of a typical intracavitary system; it is important to note how quickly the dose falls off the further one gets from the system. **A,** Anterior view. **B,** Lateral view.

Society suggested guidelines for the use of HDR brachytherapy for carcinoma of the cervix. The group emphasized the importance of factors that were already considered critical to successful LDR treatment—optimized applicator position, balanced use of external beam therapy and brachytherapy, compact overall treatment duration, and delivery of an adequate dose to tumor while respecting normal tissue tolerance limits.

Interstitial Brachytherapy Several groups have advocated the use of interstitial perineal-template brachytherapy in patients with poor anatomy or parametrial or pelvic sidewall disease. These implants are usually placed transperineally, with placement guided by a Lucite template that encourages parallel placement of hollow needles that penetrate the cervix and paracervical spaces and are usually loaded with iridium 192. Advocates state that the advantages of this method are the ease of inserting implants in patients whose uterus is difficult to probe, the ability to place sources directly into the parametrium, and the relatively homogeneous dose. Recent updates report poor survival rates and higher rates of major complications for patients with stage IIB and IIIB disease.[222,223] Outside of an investigational setting, interstitial treatment of primary cervical cancers should probably be limited to patients who cannot accommodate intrauterine brachytherapy and patients with distal vaginal disease that requires a boost with interstitial brachytherapy.

PATIENT SELECTION For patients with IB1 tumors, the choice between surgery and radiation therapy is based primarily on patient preference, anesthetic and surgical risks, physician preference, and understanding of the nature and incidence of complications of radiation therapy and hysterectomy. In general, surgery is often chosen for younger patients in the hope of preserving ovarian function and hopefully reducing vaginal shortening, while radiation therapy is often selected for older postmenopausal women to avoid the morbidity of a major surgical procedure. Patients with stage IB2 disease can be treated with either surgery followed by radiation therapy or definitive radiation therapy. The biases are so large that the GOG could not complete a trial randomizing patients with stage IB2 disease between surgery followed by chemoradiation therapy and definitive radiation therapy. Radiation therapy is the primary local therapy for most patients with stage IIB–IVA disease.

OUTCOMES **Stage IB–IIA Disease** Radical radiation therapy achieves excellent survival and pelvic disease control rates in patients with stage IB–IIA cervical cancer. Eifel and colleagues reported 5-year disease-specific survival rates of 90%, 86%, and 67% in patients with stage IB tumors with cervical diameters of less than 4 cm, 4 to 4.9 cm, and greater than 5 cm, respectively.[202] The 5-year survival rates of patients with stage IIA disease range from 70 to 85% and, like survival rates in patients with stage IB disease, are strongly correlated with tumor size.[147,224,225] Recent studies suggest that results for patients with bulky tumors may be improved further by concurrent administration of chemotherapy.[226,227]

Table 101-5 Pelvic Disease Control and Survival Rates*

FIGO Stage	Patients (*n*)	Control Rate (%)	Survival Rate (%)
I	229	93	89
IIA	315	88	85
IIB	314	80	62
IIIA	266	63	62
IIIB	216	57	50
IV	43	18	20

Reproduced with permission from Horiot JC, et al.[305]

*Pelvic disease control rates and survival rates of 1,383 patients with carcinoma of the intact uterine cervix treated with irradiation alone, according to the Fletcher guidelines: a French cooperative study.

Stage IIB–IVA Disease Five-year survival rates of 65 to 75%, 35 to 50%, and 15 to 20% have been reported in patients who received radiation therapy alone for stage IIB, IIIB, and IV tumors, respectively (Table 101-5).[146,147,225,228] The addition of cisplatin-containing regimens may further improve local control and survival.[227,229,230]

COMPLICATIONS **Acute Side Effects** Acute side effects of pelvic irradiation include symptoms related to the bowel, bladder, rectum, and vagina. Most patients experience mild fatigue and mild to moderate diarrhea that usually is controllable with antidiarrheal medication and dietary modifications. Less frequently, patients may complain of bladder or urethral irritation. These symptoms may be treated with Pyridium or antispasmodics after urinalysis and urine culture have ruled out a urinary tract infection. Patients treated with extended-field radiation may have nausea, gastric irritation, and mild depression of peripheral blood cell counts. Acute symptoms may be increased in patients receiving concurrent chemotherapy. Unless the ovaries have been transposed, all premenopausal patients who receive pelvic radiotherapy experience ovarian failure by the completion of treatment.

Fatal or life-threatening complications of intracavitary radiation therapy are rare. Among 4,042 patients who received 7,662 LDR intracavitary treatments at M. D. Anderson between 1960 and 1992, there were 11 (0.3%) documented or suspected thromboembolic events resulting in four deaths (0.1%).[231] All four deaths were in patients who had extensive pelvic wall disease that may have obstructed flow in the pelvic vessels. Today, patients receive low-dose heparin during intracavitary radiation therapy to reduce the risk of thromboembolism. Uterine perforation, fever, vaginal laceration, and the usual risk of anesthesia are other less serious complications associated with intracavitary radiation therapy.

Problems after Therapy For patients with cervical cancer, overall estimates of the risk of major complications of radiation therapy usually range between 5 and 15%.[232,233] The risk of experiencing a late complication is greatest within the first 3 years after treatment; however, major complications have been reported as late as 30 years or more after treatment. Lanciano and colleagues reported an overall actuarial rate of major complications of 14% at 5 years in a 1992 review of 1,558 patients with cervical cancer treated in more than 100 facilities randomly selected for survey in the 1972 and 1978 Patterns of Care studies.[232,233] Eifel and colleagues reported an overall actuarial risk of major complications of 14.4% at 20 years in 1,700 patients treated with radiation therapy for stage IB cervical cancer between 1960 and 1989.[232] At 5 years, the incidence was approximately 9.3%. Most complications occurring after radiation involve the rectum, bladder, or small bowel. During the first 3 years after treatment, rectal complications are most common and include bleeding, stricture, ulceration and fistula. In a study by Eifel and colleagues, the risk of major rectosigmoid complications was 2.3% at 5 years.[232] The average onset of major urinary tract complications tend to be somewhat later than that of intestinal complication, with an actuarial risk of hematuria requiring transfusion of 2.6% at 5 years.[232] The overall risk of developing a gastrointestinal or urinary tract fistula was 1.7% at 5 years with an increased risk of patients who underwent adjuvant hysterectomy or pretreatment transperitoneal lymphadenectomy.

The risk of small bowel obstruction is strongly correlated with a number of patient characteristics and treatment factors. Several studies have demonstrated three- to fourfold increases in risk of patients who had transperitoneal lymphadenectomy before radiation.[232,233] However, there appears to be little added risk if the operation is performed with a retroperitoneal approach.[141] The risk of small bowel obstruction is also greater for patients who are very thin, have history of pelvic infection, or who smoke. A recent study from M. D. Anderson revealed a sixfold increase in the risk of small bowel complications for patients who smoked more than one pack of cigarettes per day (12% vs 2% for nonsmokers).[190]

Patients who are treated with radiation for cervical cancer tend to have varying degrees of atrophy, telangiectasia, or scarring of the upper third of the vagina. Bruner and colleagues reported an average reduction in vaginal length of approximately 1 cm during the first 2 years after treatment.[234] However, more severe shortening can occur. Changes may be greater in patients with very extensive tumors and in patients who are elderly, sexually inactive, or hypoestrogenic.[232,234] Regular intercourse and use of vaginal dilators may help prevent vaginal shortening.

CURRENT PRACTICE BY DISEASE STAGE

CARCINOMA IN SITU AND STAGE IA1 DISEASE Treatment of HGSILs is rapidly changing. LEEP is one effective therapy for HGSILs. Other techniques such as cryosurgery and laser ablation have also proven effective. Regardless of the technique used, HGSILs should be entirely visible by colposcopy, the entire transformation zone should be visualized, and the ECC specimen should be negative. Conization with a knife is preferred when the ECC specimen is positive. All margins must be clear of intraepithelial lesions.

Stage IA1 (microinvasive) squamous cell carcinomas that invade the stroma less than 3 mm and have no LVSI are usually not visible to the unaided eye, and cytology is abnormal. The diagnosis requires cone biopsy, which yields a specimen adequate for diagnostic purposes. Conization alone is also potentially a low-risk therapy for patients who wish to retain fertility and who have invasion less than 3 mm in depth with no LVSI. It is important to remember that the margins of a cone specimen must be negative. When the conization specimen has a positive margin, a second tissue specimen must be obtained because foci of frankly invasive carcinoma may lie adjacent to the positive margin. Patients should be informed that the conservative approach carries a small risk. There is very little current information on which to base a recommendation regarding the use of conization as therapy for women with nonsquamous cervical cancers.[195] Patients who elect conization therapy must be willing to be monitored closely for the development of residual or recurrent cervical neoplasia.

The most conventional treatment of stage IA1 disease is a type 1 (simple extrafascial) hysterectomy. If the patient is young, the ovaries are left in place. Patients can also be treated with radiation therapy alone, usually consisting of intracavitary therapy alone. The 10-year disease control rate with radiation therapy alone is 95 to 100%.[235]

Stage IA2 Disease Small lesions that invade 3 to 5 mm have an average risk of lymph node metastasis of about 5%. The standard treatment of patients with this stage of disease is type II (modified radical) hysterectomy and pelvic node dissection. However, if a patient wishes to preserve fertility, vaginal or abdominal radical trachelectomy is a viable option. In a review of 72 cases of stage IA,[236] IB, and IIA cervical cancer, with mean follow-up of 60 months, the recurrence-free survival was 95%. The recommendation from this study and others is that radical trachelectomy is a safe option for patients with tumor size less than 2 cm. This same group reported their rate of pregnancy after the procedure,[237] and there were a total of 50 pregnancies that occurred in 31 women. The majority (66%) had only one pregnancy, 19% had 2 pregnancies, and 16% had 3 pregnancies or more. A total of 36 pregnancies reached the third trimester, of which 3 (8%) ended prematurely. Based on their experience, they feel that the obstetrical results following radical trachelectomy are very encouraging and larger trials are needed.

If surgery is contraindicated, these patients can be treated with radiation alone, usually with pelvic radiation therapy plus brachytherapy. However, in special situations, brachytherapy alone may be sufficient in controlling disease. Hamberger and colleagues reported that all patients with stage IA disease and 96% of patients (89 of 93) with small stage IB disease (< 1 cervical quadrant involved) were disease free 5 years after treatment using intracavitary irradiation alone.[238]

Stage IB1 and Small Stage IIA Disease Treatment of invasive carcinoma or carcinoma of FIGO stage IB or greater is determined on the basis of tumor size and the presence or absence of lymph node metastases (see Figure 101-5).

Stage IB1 tumors, which are less than 4 cm in size, are considered small; however, they are associated with a significant risk of microscopic paracervical extension or lymph node metastasis. In a prospective study in patients treated with radical hysterectomy who had clinically estimated maximum tumor diameter less than 3 cm, the GOG reported that 16% of the patients (42 of 261) had lymph node metastases.[239] Landoni and colleagues found a 25% incidence of positive nodes (28 of 114 patients) in patients treated with radical hysterectomy for stage IB–IIA tumors that measured 4 cm or less on initial clinical examination.[201] Therefore, for patients with stage IB1 or small IIA (< 4 cm diameter) disease, the treatment is either type III (radical) hysterectomy plus bilateral pelvic lymphadenectomy or radical radiation therapy. The goal of both of these treatment options is to destroy malignant cells in the cervix, paracervical tissues, and regional lymph nodes.

Overall survival rates for patients with stage IB1 or small IIA disease treated with either surgery or radiation therapy are usually in the range of 80 to 90%, suggesting that the two treatments are equally effective. However, only one prospective randomized trial has compared the two treatments directly.[201] In this study, patients with IB or IIA disease were randomized to receive either radical hysterectomy or radical radiation therapy. In the surgery arm, patients who had parametrial involvement, positive margins, deep stromal invasion, or positive nodes in the surgical specimen received postoperative pelvic radiation therapy. There were no significant differences in the rates of relapse or survival between the two arms, but the overall rate of grade 2–3 complications was greater for patients treated with hysterectomy. The dose of radiation therapy received by patients in the radiation therapy arms (76 Gy at point A) was low by conventional standards.

For patients with stage IB1 squamous carcinomas, the choice of treatment is based primarily on patient preference, anesthetic and surgical risks, physician preference, and an understanding of the nature and incidence of complications with radiation therapy and hysterectomy. For patients with similar tumors, the overall rate of major complications is similar with surgery and radiation therapy, although urinary tract complications tend to be more frequent after surgical treatment, and bowel complications are more common after radiation therapy. Surgical treatment tends to be preferred for young women with small tumors because it permits preservation of ovarian function and may cause less vaginal shortening. Radiation therapy is often selected for older, postmenopausal women to avoid the morbidity of a major surgical procedure.

The role of pelvic radiation therapy after radical hysterectomy is still being defined. The GOG, in a prospective trial, randomized patients with intermediate risk of recurrence after radical hysterectomy for stage IB carcinoma to pelvic irradiation or no further treatment.[240] Patients were eligible if they had at least two of the following risk factors: greater than one-third stromal invasion, LVSI, or clinical tumor diameter of at least 4 cm. Patients with positive pelvic nodes were excluded. The authors reported a 47% reduction in the risk of recurrence when postoperative pelvic irradiation was given (15% vs 28%, $p = .008$). In this preliminary analysis, follow-up was too immature for a significance level to be assigned to the overall survival comparison, but there were 18 deaths (13%) in the radiation therapy arm versus 30 deaths (21%) in the no-further-therapy arm. Recently, the Southwest Oncology Group reported the results of a randomized trial of patients treated with radical hysterectomy followed by radiation therapy versus radiation therapy plus cisplatin-based chemotherapy. To be eligible, patients had to have pelvic lymph node metastases, parametrial involvement, or involved surgical margins. The authors found that patients who received radiation therapy plus chemotherapy had a significant improvement in survival compared with the survival of patients treated with radiation alone.[152]

Most practitioners agree that patients who have more than one positive lymph node, parametrial involvement, or positive margins require postoperative radiation therapy; however, the risk of late side effects is much higher with combined therapy (surgery plus radiation therapy) than with radiation therapy alone. A National Institutes of Health panel in 1996 concluded that "to minimize morbidity, primary therapy should avoid the routine use of both radical surgery and radiation therapy." However, if radiation therapy needs to be given after surgery, intensive modulated radiation therapy (IMRT) may help minimize the dose to small bowel and, therefore, hopefully reduce late complication (Figure 101-18). Therefore, if a patient's initial work-up suggests that there is a high likelihood of parametrial invasion, deep stromal invasion, or lymph node metastases, strong consideration should be given to treating the patient with radiation therapy alone or with chemoradiation in select cases.

Stage IB2 Disease Patients with tumors greater than 4 cm in diameter whose para-aortic lymph nodes are found to be free of disease have excellent survival rates when treated with whole-pelvis EBRT plus brachytherapy. However, these tumors appear on clinical examination to be technically resectable, and the ideal management of these tumors is a subject of considerable controversy. The approach to these tumors differs widely between centers, and the biases are so large that the GOG closed a trial early owing to a lack of accrual that compared surgery plus chemoradiation versus chemoradiation alone.

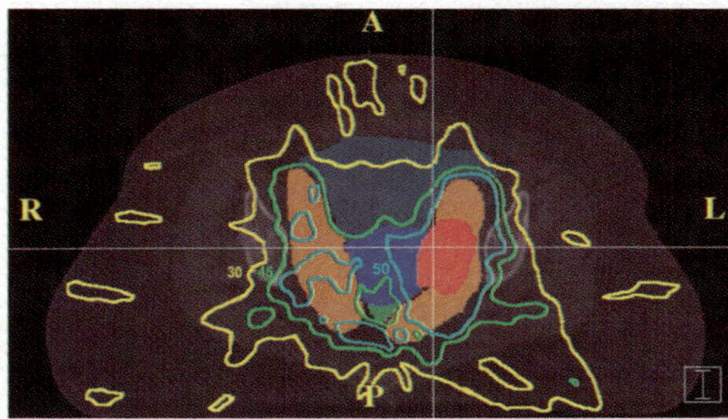

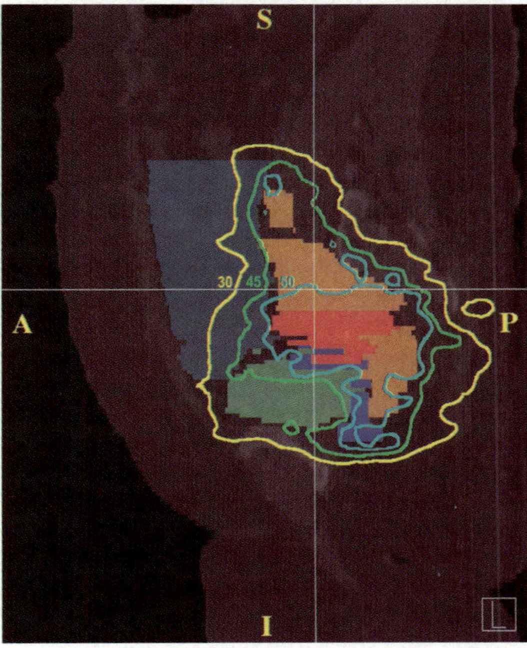

Figure 101-18 This figure shows a patient with cervical cancer being treated with radiation therapy after a hysterectomy. The areas that need to be covered are the nodes and vagina. This is an IMRT (intensity modulated radiation therapy) plan that conforms to the area that needs to be covered while sparing small bowel. With this plan, most of the small bowel receives less than 30 Gy.

Although radiation therapy is effective for many patients with stage IB2 disease, central disease recurrences occur in at least 8 to 10% of patients with bulky endocervical cancers.[202,224,225] The literature contains numerous reports on the use of an adjunctive hysterectomy for patients with bulky endocervical carcinomas treated with primary radiation therapy. In 1991, Mendenhall and colleagues reported on the outcome of patients treated at the University of Florida before or after clinicians began to add adjuvant hysterectomy to the treatment of bulky (> 6 cm) endocervical tumors.[241] They found no difference in pelvic disease control or survival rates with the two treatment policies, but they reported higher complication rates for patients who underwent adjuvant hysterectomy (18% vs 6%, $p = .027$). The GOG completed a trial in 1990 that compared using radiation alone versus radiation plus extrafascial hysterectomy in patients with stage IB cancers measuring 4 cm or more in diameter. In a 1997 abstract about this trial, Keys and colleagues reported no difference in overall survival rates between the two arms, but the final report of this trial has not yet been published.[242] At M. D. Anderson, at this time, extrafascial hysterectomy is used only if the optimal brachytherapy dose cannot be obtained because of multiple large fibroids in the uterus.

Several investigators recommend treating these tumors with initial surgery followed by postoperative radiation therapy or chemoradiation depending on the pathology findings. In a randomized trial by Landoni and colleagues, patients with stage IB2 tumors were randomized to initial surgery versus definitive radiation therapy.[201] In this trial, 84% of the patients treated with initial surgery required postoperative radiation therapy, which contributed to a higher complication rate in that arm. The overall survival rates were similar for patients treated with initial surgery or radiation, but the patients in the radiation arm received more protracted, lower-dose treatments than those recommended by most current experts in the field. A study recently published by Peters and colleagues suggested that chemoradiation should be considered standard therapy for patients with stage IB2 disease following initial surgery.[152]

Recently, several trials have been initiated to study the role of induction chemotherapy before surgical exploration in patients with bulky lesions who would otherwise be poor candidates for radical hysterectomy. In one trial, 205 patients with stage IB cervical cancer underwent surgery with or without an initial course of chemotherapy (cisplatin, vincristine, and bleomycin); all patients also received postoperative radiation therapy.[243] The authors reported that tumors treated with chemotherapy were more often resectable and that the 5-year survival rate of patients who had received neoadjuvant chemotherapy was better (81% vs 66%, $p < .05$). The GOG has recently closed a study also looking at neoadjuvant chemotherapy prior to surgery. The results have not yet been analyzed. A recent meta-analysis[244] collected individual patient data from 21 randomized trials of neoadjuvant chemotherapy in locally advanced cervical cancer. This analysis included data from comparison of the benefits of neoadjuvant chemotherapy followed by radical radiotherapy versus radical radiotherapy alone (2,074), and for comparison of neoadjuvant chemotherapy followed by surgery (± radiotherapy) versus radical radiotherapy alone (872 patients). The first comparison was hindered by heterogeneity between trials and gave conflicting results depending on how trials were grouped by chemotherapy cycle length or dose-intensity. The second comparison showed that patients treated with neoadjuvant chemotherapy had a highly significant 35% reduction in the risk of death ($p = .0004$) that translated into a 14% absolute increase in 5-year overall survival. Unfortunately, this meta-analysis only included trials prior to 1999, when radiotherapy alone was still the standard treatment. Ultimately, however, this approach may need to be compared with optimized chemoradiation to determine the most effective, least toxic therapy for these patients. The EORTC (European Organisation for Research and Treatment of Cancer) is currently running a trial addressing this specific question. Patients with IB2 cancers are being randomized to neoadjuvant chemotherapy followed by radiation or current chemotherapy and radiation (Table 101-6).

Two prospective randomized trials[226,227] indicate that patients who are treated with radiation for bulky central disease benefit from concurrent administration of cisplatin-containing chemotherapy. A third study suggests that patients who require postoperative radiotherapy because of findings of lymph node metastasis or involved surgical margins also benefit from concurrent chemoradiation.[245] These studies are discussed in more detail in the section "Concurrent Chemoradiation," later in this chapter. Patients who have stage IB1 cancers without evidence of regional involvement have excellent pelvic control rates (approximately 97% at 5 years) with radiotherapy alone and probably do not require chemotherapy when they are treated with primary radiotherapy.[202,225]

Stage IIB–IVA Disease Radiation therapy is the primary local treatment of most patients with locoregionally advanced (stage IIIB–IVA) cervical carcinoma. The success of treatment depends on a careful balance between EBRT and brachytherapy that optimizes the dose to tumor and normal tissues and on the overall duration of treatment. Five-year survival rates of 65 to 75%, 35 to 50%, and 15 to 20% are reported for patients treated with radiation therapy alone for stage IIB, IIIB, and IV tumors, respectively.[146,147,228] In the French Cooperative Group study of 1,875 patients treated with radiation therapy according to Fletcher guidelines, Barillot and colleagues reported 5-year survival rates of 70%, 45%, and 10% for patients with stage IIB, IIIB, and IVA tumors, respectively (Table 101-7).[147]

Local and distant disease recurrences continue to be a problem for patients with locally advanced disease. Neoadjuvant chemotherapy has produced excellent tumor responses; however, randomized trials have failed to demonstrate improvements in survival. In fact, in two trials, the survival rates were actually poorer when neoadjuvant chemotherapy was added to radiation therapy. Other approaches that have been used to try to improve outcome in these patients, including neutrons, hyperbaric oxygen, and hypoxic cell sensitizers, have also produced disappointing results.

Concurrent Chemoradiation During the past 5 years, prospective randomized trials involving patients with locoregionally advanced cervical cancer[226,227,230,245,246] have provided compelling evidence that the addition of concurrent cisplatin-containing chemotherapy to standard radiotherapy reduces the risk of disease recurrence by as much as 50%, and thereby improves the rates of pelvic disease control and survival (Table 101-8).

In two studies,[229,230] the GOG randomly assigned patients with stage IIB to IVA disease to receive either hydroxyurea or cisplatin-containing chemotherapy during external beam irradiation. All three of the cisplatin containing regimens in these trials produced local control and survival

Table 101-6 Prospective Randomized Trials: Role of Concurrent Radiotherapy and Cisplatin-Containing Chemotherapy*

First Author (Ref)	Eligibility	Patients (No.)	CT: Investigational Arm	CT: Control Arm	Relative Risk of Recurrence (90% CI)	*p* Values
Rose[229]	FIGO IIB–IVA	526	Cisplatin 40 mg/m^2/wk (up to 6 cycles)	HU 3 g/m^2 (2×/wk)	0.57 (0.42–0.78)	< .001
			Cisplatin 50 mg/m^2; 5-FU 4 g/m^2/96 h; HU 2 g/m^2 (2×/wk) (2 cycles)	HU 3 g/m^2 (2×/wk)	0.55 (0.40–0.75)	< .001
Morris[227]	FIGO IB–IIA (≥ 5 cm); IIB–IVA or pelvic nodes involved	403	Cisplatin 75 mg/m^2; 5-FU 4 g/m^2/96 h (3 cycles)	None*	0.48 (0.35–0.66)	< .001
Keys[226]	FIGO IB (≥4 cm)	369	Cisplatin 40 mg/m^2/wk (up to 6 cycles)	None†	0.51 (0.34–0.75)	.001
Whitney[230]	FIGO IIB–IVA	368	Cisplatin 50 mg/m^2; 5-FU 4 g/m^2/96 h (2 cycles)	HU 3 g/m^2 (2×/wk)	0.79 (0.62–0.99)	.03
Peters[152]	FIGO I–IIA after radical hysterectomy with nodes, margins, or parametrium positive	268	Cisplatin 50 mg/m^2; 5-FU 4 g/m^2/96 h (2 cycles)	None	0.50 (0.29–0.84)	.01
Pearcey[248]	FIGO IB–IIA (≥ 5 cm), IIB–IVA or pelvic nodes involved	259	Cisplatin 40 mg/m^2/wk (up to 6 cycles)	None	0.91 (0.62–1.35)‡	.43
Wong[250]	FIGO IB–IIA (> 4 cm), IIB–III	220	Epirubicin 60 mg/m^2, then 90 mg/m^2 q4 wks for 5 more cycles§	None	~0.65	.02
Thomas[312]	FIGO IB-IIA	234	5-FU 4 g/m^2 over 96 h ×2	None	NS	
Lorvidhaya·[251]	FIGO IB-IVA	926	Mitomycin C 10 mg/m^2 day 1 and 29 Oral 5-FU 300 mg/day days 1–14 and 29–42	None	0.001	

Results from prospective randomized trials that investigate the role of concurrent radiotherapy and cisplatin-containing chemotherapy for patients with locoregionally advanced cervical cancer.
CI = confidence interval; FU = Follow-up; HU = hydroxyurea; PA = para-aortic; RT = radiotherapy.
*Patients in control arm had prophylactic para-aortic irradiation.
†All patients had extrafascial hysterectomy after radiotherapy.
‡Survival.
§Chemotherapy was begun on day 1 and continued every 4 weeks throughout and after radiation therapy.
·This study had four arms: arm 1, conventional radiation therapy (RT); arm 2, conventional RT with adjuvant chemotherapy consisting of 5-FU orally at 200 mg/day given for 3 courses of 4 weeks, with a 2-week rest every 6 weeks; arm 3, conventional RT with concurrent chemotherapy; and arm 4, conventional RT with concurrent and adjuvant chemotherapy. The addition of adjuvant therapy did not affect recurrence, but here was a significant difference in the recurrence rate between the conventional RT and the conventional RT plus concurrent chemotherapy arms.

rates superior to those for the control (hydroxyurea and radiation). In a third study,[226] patients with stage IB tumors measuring at least 4 cm in diameter were randomly assigned to receive radiation alone or radiation plus weekly cisplatin before an extrafascial hysterectomy. Patients who received cisplatin were more likely to have a complete histologic response and were more likely to be disease free at the time of preliminary analysis. A fourth study, sponsored by the Southwest Oncology Group and the GOG,[245] included patients who were treated with radical hysterectomy and were found to have pelvic lymph node metastases, positive margins, or parametrial involvement. Patients were randomly assigned to receive postoperative pelvic irradiation, alone or combined with cisplatin and 5-FU. In a preliminary analysis, patients who received chemotherapy in this study also had a better disease-free survival rate.

During the same interval, the Radiation Therapy Oncology Group (RTOG)[227] conducted a trial in which radiotherapy alone was compared with pelvic irradiation (including prophylactic para-aortic irradiation) plus concurrent cisplatin and 5-FU. This study demonstrated a significant improvement in outcome for patients with stage III or IV disease as well as for patients with stage IB2 or II cervical cancer with concurrent chemotherapy. There was no significant difference in the incidence of late treatment-related complications.[247] Only one large randomized trial has failed to demonstrate a significant advantage from concurrent cisplatin-based chemotherapy in cervical cancer patients. This trial was published by Pearcey and colleagues in 2002.[248] The authors suggest that difference in technique could explain the difference between their results and the results of the five earlier trials, although the survival rate in their control arm indicated that the margin for improvement was smaller than that in the earlier trials. This trial was also the smallest of the six trials.

Taken together, the randomized trials provide strong evidence that the addition of concurrent cisplatin-containing chemotherapy to pelvic radiotherapy benefits selected patients with locally advanced cervical cancer. In fact, in a recent meta-analysis of 18 trials[249] with concurrent chemotherapy and radiation (4,580 patients) in patients with cervical cancer, concomitant chemotherapy and radiotherapy improved overall and progression-free survival and reduced local and distant recurrence in selected patients with cervical cancer. In the future, clinicians will be challenged to determine how these favorable results can be generalized to patients with cervical cancer who may not have been included in the prospective trials because of severe medical or social problems and to the developing nations where invasive cervical cancer is epidemic.

These studies raise other interesting questions that will undoubtedly be the subjects of future studies. Although North American studies have emphasized cisplatin-containing regimens, investigators in Southeast Asia have reported improved

Table 101-7 5-Year Survival Rates after Pelvic Exenteration: A Review of the Literature

Source	Patients (*n*)	5-Year Survival (%)
Bricker[306]	153	34.6
Symmonds[271]	198	32.0
Rutledge[269]	448	41.0
Ketcham[307]	162	38.0
Orr[270]	104	45.3
Morley[308]	100	61
Shingleton[309]	143	50
Magrina[310]	133	41

Table 101-8 Single-Agent Chemotherapy for Cervical Cancer

Agent	Response (%)
Alkylating Agents	
Cyclophosphamide	38/251 (15)
Chlorambucil	11/44 (25)
Melphalan	4/20 (20)
Ifosfamide	35/157 (22)
Mitolactol	16/55 (29)
Heavy Metal Complexes	
Cisplatin	190/815 (23)
Carboplatin	27/175 (15)
Antitumor Antibiotics	
Doxorubicin	45/266 (17)
Bleomycin	19/176 (11)
Mitomycin	5/23 (22)
Antimetabolites	
Fluorouracil	29/142 (20)
Methotrexate	17/96 (18)
Hydroxyurea	0/14 (0)
Plant Alkaloids	
Vincristine	10/55 (18)
Vinblastine	2/20 (10)
Etoposide	0/31 (0)
Miscellaneous Agents	
Altretamine	12/64 (19)
Irinotecan (CPT-11)	36/192 (19)
Paclitaxel	14/74 (19)
Docetaxel	1/13 (8)
Topotecan	8/43 (19)
Hexamethylmelamine	12/64 (19)
Razoxane	5/28 (18)

Data from refs.[313–317]

outcome when radiation was combined with epirubicin[250] or mitomycin and 5-FU.[251] Other drugs that are being studied for their radiosensitizing effects in patients with advanced disease are paclitaxel,[252] carboplatin,[253] and multiple biologic response modifiers. The RTOG has just completed a phase II trial evaluating cisplatin with cerebrex in patients with locally advance cervical cancer—results are pending.

Metastatic Disease Metastatic cancer in the para-aortic lymph nodes can be confirmed with fine-needle aspiration, laparoscopy, or extraperitoneal laparotomy. Laparoscopy and laparotomy, using the extraperitoneal approach, allows the removal of positive nodes and sampling of other para-aortic nodes, which may enhance control with radiation therapy and help design the treatment field.

The superior boundary of the extended EBRT portal provides a margin of 3 cm above the most cephalad of the positive nodes. The superior boundary limit is the T12 vertebra. Currently, patients with positive pelvic nodes or low common iliac nodes may have the field extended to the L1–L2 interspace.

Patients with para-aortic lymph node involvement can be treated effectively with extended-field irradiation. Five-year survival rates range from 25 to 50%.[254–256] The value of prophylactic extended-field irradiation was tested in two randomized trials. The RTOG studied 367 patients with stages 1B and IIA cancers greater than 4 cm in diameter or stage IIB disease in a randomized study. These patients received standard pelvic irradiation or extended-field radiation therapy prior to brachytherapy.[257] Patients treated with extended-field radiation therapy (45 Gy up to L1–L2) had a better absolute survival rate than did those treated with standard pelvic irradiation (67% vs 55% at 5 years), but there was no significant difference in the disease-free survival rates. Para-aortic recurrences were not analyzed separately, and there was no standard method of assessing initial node status.[81]

Another trial from the European Organization for Research and Treatment of Cancer involved a similar randomization of patients between pelvic irradiation and extended-field irradiation (45 Gy up to L1–T12).[258] Twelve centers entered 441 patients. Two hundred twenty-eight patients underwent irradiation of the pelvis, and 213 underwent irradiation of the pelvis and para-aortic nodes. There was no statistically significant difference between the two treatment arms in terms of local control, overall distant metastases, and survival. The subset that received pelvic irradiation alone, which controlled the pelvic disease, had a higher incidence of subsequent para-aortic and distant disease. The incidence of enteric complications in this study was high, and the authors concluded that routine para-aortic irradiation for all high-risk patients with cervical carcinoma is of limited value.

The role of concurrent chemotherapy with extended-field irradiation has been evaluated in several phase II studies. Although side effects are greater when treatment fields are enlarged, combined therapy may be tolerable if careful consideration is given to the chemotherapy regimen, volume of tissue irradiated, and other factors that might increase the risk of serious toxicity. The RTOG studied the efficacy of twice-daily external irradiation to the pelvis and para-aortic field with concurrent chemotherapy consisting of cisplatin and fluorouracil. They concluded that this regimen had an unacceptably high rate (17%, 5 of 29) of grade 4 late side effects, and survival estimates were no better than with standard-fractionation irradiation without chemotherapy.[259] The GOG did a study combining once-daily extended-field irradiation with cisplatin and fluorouracil. Their treatment was better tolerated than that of the RTOG; however, their treatment time was more protracted, toxicity was still significant (18.6% grade 3 to 4 gastrointestinal toxicity, and 7 of 86 patients with late rectal toxicity), and there were numerous protocol deviations. However, the authors concluded that extended-field irradiation can be given safely with concurrent chemotherapy.[260] Malfetano and colleagues reported results of a combination of extended-field irradiation with weekly cisplatin (1 mg/kg, not to exceed 60 mg) in patients with negative para-aortic nodes.[261] The dose used in their regimen was similar to the 40 mg/m^2 used in the GOG with pelvic radiation and appeared to be well tolerated. In conclusion, it is tempting to extrapolate from the results achieved with combinations of pelvic radiation and chemotherapy; however, patients need to be informed that the cost-benefit ratio of concurrent chemotherapy and extended-field irradiation has not been formally tested.

Unsuspected Invasive Cancer Discovered after Simple Hysterectomy Sometimes the pathologist discovers unsuspected invasive cervical carcinoma in the tissue specimen in patients who undergo hysterectomy for what is presumed to be a benign pelvic condition. Many factors can lead to such an event.[262] A false-negative Pap smear provides little opportunity for the gynecologist to avoid such events; however, the following oversights are avoidable: failure to evaluate an abnormal Pap smear, failure to perform a conization when indicated, and proceeding with a hysterectomy when there is a positive cone margin.

Patients with unsuspected invasive cervical carcinoma detected after simple hysterectomy have been classified in five groups according to the amount of disease and presentation: (1) microinvasive cancer, (2) tumor confined to the cervix with negative surgical margins, (3) positive surgical margins but no gross residual tumor, (4) gross residual tumor by clinical examination documented by biopsy, and (5) patients referred for treatment more than 6 months after hysterectomy (usually for recurrent disease).[263] The therapy plan is based on the amount of residual disease. Patients with minimal invasion and no residual disease require at most brachytherapy to the vaginal apex; patients with gross disease at the specimen margin require full-intensity therapy. Patients with minimal or no known gross residual disease (groups 1 to 3) have excellent 5-year survival rates (59–79%), whereas rates for patients with gross residual disease (groups 4 and 5) are poorer (in the range of only 41%).[264] The value of chemoradiation is unproven in this setting; however, in patients with gross disease, it is probably reasonable to add chemotherapy because of the relatively high local recurrence rates after radiation therapy alone.

Recurrent Disease **Prognostic Factors** Various clinicopathologic features have been associated with adverse outcomes in patients with recurrent cervical carcinoma in the pelvis; however, the relatively small numbers of patients and the heterogeneity of clinical and treatment parameters in most series preclude detailed statistical analysis of these factors. Two clinical factors commonly correlated with the probability of the success of salvage therapy are the location (central versus side wall involvement) and the size of the recurrent pelvic tumor.[265] The presence of nodal disease in conjunction with pelvic relapse portends a dismal outcome; other unfavorable clinical variables include nonsquamous histologies (particularly adenocarcinomas) and a higher FIGO stage at the time of diagnosis of the primary tumor.[266] Controversial factors include the interval between primary therapy and relapse and symptomatic versus asymptomatic pelvic failures.[210,266,267]

Radical Hysterectomy In rare, carefully selected patients initially treated with primary radiation therapy, radical hysterectomy for salvage may be a feasible alternative to exenterative surgery. Coleman and colleagues reported on 50 patients who underwent radical hysterectomy for persistent or recurrent disease after definitive radiation therapy.[268] The 5- and 10-year survival rates were 72% and 60%, respectively. Severe complications were noted in 64% of patients, and 42% of patients had permanent complications. The authors concluded that radical hysterectomy was an alternative to exenteration in patients with small, centrally recurrent cervical cancer, but that it should be used only in carefully selected patients.[268]

Pelvic Exenteration Pelvic exenteration is a potentially curative procedure for patients who, following radiation therapy, have a central pelvic recurrence or a new primary tumor in the irradiated field.[269–271] Advances in surgical technique, anesthesia, and postoperative care have decreased intraoperative and postoperative complications, and thus have greatly reduced operative mortality.[262,270,271] Advances in ostomy appliances and care have given patients the opportunity to live a nearly normal life and to be able to meet their personal needs and responsibilities after surgery. The type of exenteration is determined by the anatomical site of the cancer (Figure 101-19).

Anterior Exenteration Anterior exenteration encompasses the removal of the uterus, adnexa, bladder, urethra, and vagina. Patients selected for this operation have cancers that are sufficiently anterior to allow clearance of the rectum and do not extend to involve the vaginal apex

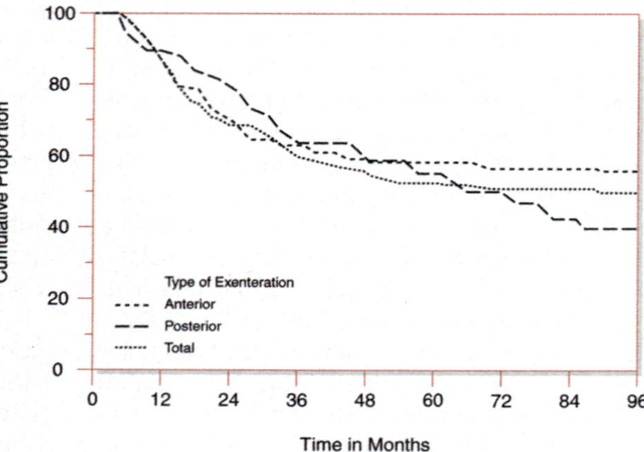

Figure 101-19 Reproduced with permission from Rutledge.[269] Survival curves are shown to compare the three types of exenterations performed in an M. D. Anderson series (1955–1984). Although the curves are similar, it should be noted that posterior exenteration is performed more frequently than the other procedures for vulvar and anorectal cancer and is associated with more local cancer recurrences.

or the posterior vaginal wall. Vaginal reconstruction is performed as indicated.

Posterior Exenteration In posterior exenteration, the uterus, adnexa, anus, rectosigmoid colon, levator muscles, and vagina are removed. Many gynecologic oncologists leave a portion of the anterior vaginal wall to support the urethra, and this can lessen postoperative urinary incontinence. This procedure is performed in patients with lesions confined to the posterior vaginal wall and rectovaginal septum.

Total Pelvic Exenteration In total pelvic exenteration, the uterus, adnexa, bladder and urethra, vagina, rectosigmoid colon, levatores, and anus are all removed. Patients treated with this procedure usually have lesions that are central or involve the upper half of the vagina. Contiguous extension to the base of the bladder and rectovaginal septum leaves no opportunity to perform a less extensive operation. Vaginal reconstruction is performed for functional purposes and to aid in the reconstruction of the pelvic floor. An omental pedicled graft is required to aid in reconstruction of the pelvic floor, and this technique for bringing in a new blood supply has been a major factor in reducing postoperative complications.[272] In both anterior and total pelvic exenteration, a continent urinary conduit can be constructed.

Total pelvic exenteration is widely used, and 5-year survival rates of 40 to 50% can be expected (see Table 101-7). At M. D. Anderson, a total of 448 exenterations were done from 1955 to 1984 and reported by Rutledge.[269] The 5-year survival rates for patients treated with exenteration are shown in Figure 101-19.

Radiation Therapy Patients who have an isolated pelvic recurrence after initially being treated with a radical hysterectomy should be treated with radical radiation therapy. A literature review by Lanciano found disease-free survival rates ranging from 20 to 50% following radiation therapy for locoregional failures. More favorable outcomes were reported in patients with small-volume disease and a central pelvic relapse location.[265] In most patients, treatment consisted of EBRT with or without brachytherapy. Patients who have isolated central recurrences without pelvic wall fixation or regional metastasis can be cured in up to 60 to 70% of cases.[267] The prognosis is much poorer when the pelvic wall is involved (usually 10–20% of patients survive 5 years after radiation therapy). Several authors have reported significantly lower salvage rates in patients with recurrent adenocarcinoma of the cervix.[267,273] Insufficient data are available to permit determination of the benefit of concurrent administration of chemotherapy in this situation; however, in patients without contraindications to chemotherapy, chemoradiation may be a reasonable consideration given the overall poor prognosis in this population.[266,273,274]

Chemotherapy ***Single-Agent Chemotherapy*** Using chemotherapy to treat metastatic or recurrent carcinoma of the cervix is relatively ineffective. Median survival ranges between 4 and 8 months. Cisplatin is regarded as the most active agent in cancer of the cervix. The response rate is 17 to 21%.[275,276] Doses used range from 50 mg/m^2 to 100 mg/m^2. Bonomi and colleagues[276] compared 50 mg/m^2 to 100 mg/m^2 and noted that the higher dose was associated with a better partial response rate (31% vs 21%) and a slightly better complete response rate (13% vs 10%). Response duration, progression-free survival, and survival measures failed to improve with the higher dose.[276] Carboplatin given at 340 to 400 mg/m^2 every 28 days to 175 patients induced a complete response in 10 (5.7%).[277] The total response rate for carboplatin from a number of studies is 19%.[260]

Ifosfamide has been studied as a single agent in patients with recurrent cervical cancer in at least five phase II trials.[278–282] Response rates ranged between 33 and 50% in three studies that were conducted in patients who had received no previous chemotherapy.[280–283] However, the response rates were much lower in two phase II trials that included patients who had received prior systemic chemotherapy, with only three partial responses (8%) seen in 36 patients.[278,279]

Combination Chemotherapy Nineteen single agents have activity against cervical cancer, defined as the ability to induce a 15% response rate when used as a single agent (see Table 101-8), but survival rates have not been improved by adding other drugs to cisplatin. Numerous reports describe a higher response rate with combination therapies (Table 101-9), accompanied by an increase in toxicity. Ifosfamide has received the most interest until recently. Several small phase II studies evaluated treatment with combinations of ifosfamide and either cisplatin or carboplatin in patients who had not received radiotherapy. Response rates for these combinations ranged between 50 and 62%.[284–287] A number of investigators have combined bleomycin with ifosfamide and a platinum compound. Three studies that included patients who had not received radiotherapy reported response rates of 65 to 100%.[288–290] Reports of treatment with these drugs in previously irradiated patients have yielded mixed but generally lower response rates of between 13 and 72%.[289–292]

Combinations of cisplatin and continuous infusion 5-FU,[293–295] cisplatin and paclitaxel,[246,296,297] cisplatin and vinorelbine,[298] and cisplatin and gemcitabine[299,300] also produce high response in previously untreated patients. The combination of carboplatin and liposomal doxorubicin has shown modest activity in this clinical setting.[301] Again, response rates decrease significantly if patients have had previous irradiation.[294,300,302]

A recent GOG randomized phase III trial reported that combining topotecan with cisplatin had a better response rate to cisplatin alone.[291] The response rate was 13% in the cisplatin arm and 27% in the combination arm. There was also an improvement in median survival by 3 months as well as a slight improvement in quality of life as determined by the FACT-CX. They found the previous radiosensitizing chemotherapy and interval from diagnosis predicted for response. Response was more frequent in nonirradiated

Table 101-9 Combination Chemotherapy for Advanced or Recurrent Cervical Cancer

Chemotherapy Regimen (Ref)	Patients (No.)	Previous Radiation Therapy (%)	Response (%)
Cisplatin/ifosfamide[318]	146	90	32
Cisplatin/ifosfamide/bleomycin[318]	141	87	31.2
Cisplatin/paclitaxel[246]	41	90	46.3
Cisplatin/paclitaxel/ifosfamide[319]	60	75	46
Cisplatin/gemcitabine[300]	19	53	41
Cisplatin/mitomycin-C[320]	33	96	42
Cisplatin/topotecan[321]	32	94	28
Cisplatin/topotecan[291]	294	47	27
Cisplatin/5-Fluorouracil[293]	55	90	22

sites (70% vs 23%). This has led the GOG to their new prospective trial for primary stage IVB or recurrent/persistent carcinoma of the cervix. In this trial patients were randomized between four arms: arm 1, paclitaxel and cisplatin; arm 2, vinorelbine and cisplatin; arm 3, gemcitabine and cisplatin; and arm 4, topotecan and cisplatin. This study should help in determining which combination is superior as well as the toxicity and quality of life of each combination.

A number of barriers have impeded drug evaluations in patients with cervical cancer. Most patients have had high-dose EBRT to the pelvis and lower vertebrae. The dose range of 40 to 55 Gy destroys the stem cell population of the bone marrow included within the treatment field. Because myelosuppression is the dose-limiting toxic effect of most drugs used for this disease, the reduced bone marrow reserve limits the amount of drug that can be given. In addition, patients with advanced carcinoma frequently have renal impairment because of ureteral obstruction and loss of a kidney. Marginal renal function prompts dose reductions for drugs requiring renal clearance. Cervical cancer often recurs in irradiated areas that are fibrotic and poorly vascularized. Such hostile environments repress drug deliverability. Tumor regression is difficult to measure by both physical examination and imaging techniques. Cellular mechanisms for chemotherapy and radiation therapy resistance need to be defined in patients with cervical cancer. Despite these obstacles, single-agent and combination chemotherapies have induced complete responses in patients with biopsy-proven carcinomas and hopefully combination chemotherapy will be better. Biological agents as well are being evaluated in phase I and II trials by the GOG as well as around the world.

Summary In patients with recurrent cervical cancer, it is important first to determine if the patient is a candidate for definitive surgery or radiation therapy. Five-year survival rates range from 20 to 50% if one of these therapies can be administered. Systemic chemotherapy should be cautiously used for treatment of both recurrent and metastatic disease. Careful attention should be paid to toxicity. Further research is needed to determine the impact of chemotherapy on quality of life and the sensitivity to chemotherapy of patients who received prior chemotherapy as part of chemoradiation therapy.

FUTURE OPPORTUNITIES

New technologies that would define the aggressiveness of cervical cancers are an interesting future research opportunity. The value of combining such biologic therapeutic agents as the interleukins, specific monoclonal antibodies, vaccines, and interferons with chemotherapy has received little attention in patients with cervical cancer.

Adenocarcinomas of the cervix represent a heterogenous group of carcinomas. Their heterogeneity plus their lower frequency of occurrence (20%) in comparison with squamous cell carcinomas (80%) limits opportunities for randomized trials. Primary papillary serous carcinomas of the cervix may have features in common with their look-alike tumors in the endometrium and ovary. Further research may tell us whether primary endometrioid carcinomas of the endocervix have features and therapy responses similar to those of endometrioid carcinomas of the endometrium. Finally, neuroendocrine (small-cell and nonsmall-cell) carcinomas need standardization of terminology and definitions of histologic features that allow an opportunity for the pathologist and oncologist to diagnose and apply research-driven clinical therapies for these carcinomas. Large national groups have a unique opportunity to lead the way in finding active single agents and combination therapies for these very aggressive cancers.

REFERENCES

1. Parkin DM, Bray F, Ferlay J, et al. Global cancer statistics, 2002. CA Cancer J Clin 2005;55:74–108.
2. Jemal A, Murray T, Ward E, et al. Cancer statistics, 2005. CA Cancer J Clin 2005;55:10–30.
3. Coleman MP, Esteve J, Damiecki P, et al, editors. Trends in cancer incidence and mortality. IARC Sci Publ 1993;121:1–86.
4. Reis LAG, Hankey BF, Miller BA, et al. SEER cancer statistics review, 1973–1996. Bethseda (MD): National Cancer Institute; 1999.
5. American Cancer Society Statistics 2005. Available at: www.americancancersociety.org (accessed August 22, 2005).
6. Wang SS, Sherman ME, Hildesheim A, et al. Cervical adenocarcinoma and squamous cell carcinoma incidence trends among white women and black women in the United States for 1976-2000. Cancer 2004;100:1035–44.
7. Brinton LA. Epidemiology of cervical cancer- overview. In: N. Munoz FB, Bosch FX, Shah KV, Meheus A, editors. The epidemiology of human papillomavirus and cervical cancer. Oxford (UK): Oxford University Press; 1992. p 3–23.
8. Boyle DC, Smith JR. Infection and cervical intraepithelial neoplasia. Int J Gynecol Cancer 1999;9:177–86.
9. Zur Hausen H. Human papillomaviruses and their possible role in squamous cell carcinomas. Curr Top Micorbiol Immunol 1977;78:1–30.
10. International Agency for Research on Cancer Working Group on the Evaluation of Carcinogenic Risks to Humans. Human papillomaviruses. IARC Monogr. Vol 64. Lyon: IARC; 1995.
11. Alamos National Laboratory. Theoretical biology and biophysics. HPV Sequence Database. Vol October 18, 1999.
12. Bosch FX, Manos MM, Munoz N, et al. Prevalence of human papillomavirus in cervical cancer: a worldwide perspective. International biological study on cervical cancer (IBSCC) study group [comments]. J Natl Cancer Inst 1995;87:796–802.
13. Munoz N, Bosch FX. Cervical cancer and papillomavirus: epidemiological evidence and perspective for prevention. Salud Publica Mex 1997;39:274–82.
14. Schneider A, Koutsky LA. Natural history and epidemiological features of genital HPV infection. In: Munoz N, Bosch F, Shah KV, et al, editors. The epidemiology of human papillomavirus and cervical cancer.: Lyon: International Agency for Research on Cancer; 1992. p 25–52.
15. Kjaer S. Risk factors for cervical neoplasma in Denmark. APMIS 1998;116:5–42.
16. Tortolero-Luna G, Mitchell MF, Swan DC, et al. A case-control study of human papillomavirus and cervical squamous intraepithelial lesions (SIL) in Harris County, Texas: differences among racial/ethnic groups. Cad Saude Publica 1998;14 Suppl 3:149–59.
17. Yoshikawa H, Negata C, Noda K, et al. Human papillomavirus infection and other risk factors for cervical neoplasma. Br J Cancer 1999;80:621–624.
18. Centers for Disease Control. Revised classification system for HIV infection and expanded surveillance definition for AIDS among adolescents and adults. MMWR Morb Mortal Wkly Rep 1993;41:1–15.
19. Mandelblatt J, Kanetsky P, Eggert L, et al. Is HIV infection a cofactor for cervical squamous cell neoplasm? Cancer Epidemiol Biomarkers Prev 1999;8:97–106.
20. Ruche G, You B, Leroy V, et al. Is HIV infection a cofactor for cervical squamous cell neoplasm? Cancer Epidemiol Biomarkers Prev 1999;8:729–30.
21. zur Hausen H. Human genital cancer: synergism between two virus infections or synergism between a virus infection and initiating events? Lancet 1982;2:1370–2.
22. Ferrera A, Baay MF, Herbrink P, et al. A sero-epidemiological study of the relationship between sexually transmitted agents and cervical cancer in Honduras. Int J Cancer 1997;73:781–5.
23. Sanjose S, Munoz N, Bosch FX, et al. Sexually transmitted agents and cervical neoplasia in Columbia and Spain. Int J Cancer 1994;56:358–63.
24. Dillner J, Lenner P, Lehtinen M, et al. A population-based seroepidemiological study of cervical cancer. Cancer Res 1994;54:134–41.
25. Hakama M, Lehtinen M, Knekt P, et al. Serum antibodies and subsequent cervical neoplasms: a prospective study with 12 years of follow-up. Am J Epidemiol 1993;137:166–70.
26. Vastrick I, Makela T, Koskinen P, et al. Myc protein: partners and antagonists. Crit Rev Oncol 1994:59–68.
27. Evan G, Harrington E, Fanidi A, et al. Integrated control of cell proliferation and cell death by the c-myc oncogene. Philos Trans R Soc Lond B Biol Sci 1994;345:269–75.
28. Bourhis J, Le MG, Barrois M, et al. Prognostic value of c-myc proto-oncogene overexpression in early invasive carcinoma of the cervix. J Clin Oncol 1990;8:1789–96.
29. Dokianakis DN, Sourvinos G, Sakkas S, et al. Detection of HPV and ras gene mutations in cervical smears from female genital lesions. Oncol Rep 1998;5:1195–8.
30. Garzetti GG, Ciavattini A, Lucarini G, et al. Ras p21 immunostaining in early stage squamous cervical carcinoma: relationship with lymph nodal involvement and 72 kDa-metalloproteinase index. Anticancer Res 1998;18:609–13.
31. Kim YT, Park SW, Kim JW. Correlation between expression of EGFR and the prognosis of patients with cervical carcinoma. Gynecol Oncol 2002;87:84–9.
32. Lee CM, Lee RJ, Hammond E, et al. Expression of HER2neu (c-erbB-2) and epidermal growth factor receptor in cervical cancer: prognostic correlation with clinical characteristics, and comparison of manual and automated imaging analysis. Gynecol Oncol 2004;93:209–14.
33. Tjalma W, Weyler J, Goovaerts G, et al. Prognostic value of bcl-2 expression in patients with operable carcinoma of the uterine cervix. J Clin Pathol 1997;50:33–6.
34. Tjalma W, De Cuyper E, Weyler J, et al. Expression of bcl-2 in invasive and in situ carcinoma of the uterine cervix. Am J Obstet Gynecol 1998;178:113–7.
35. Ozalp SS, Yalcin OT, Tanir HM, et al. Bcl-2 expression in preinvasive and invasive cervical lesions. Eur J Gynaecol Oncol 2002;23:419–22.
36. Soufla G, Sifakis S, Baritaki S, et al. VEGF, FGF2, TGFB1 and TGFBR1 mRNA expression levels correlate with the malignant transformation of the uterine cervix. Cancer Lett 2005;221:105–18.
37. Kanda K, Ueda M, Futakuchi H, et al. Transcriptional expression of the genes implicated in angiogenesis and tumor invasion in cervical carcinomas. Gynecol Oncol 2005. [In press]
38. Morris M, Tortolero-Luna G, Malpica A, et al. Cervical intraepithelial neoplasia and cervical cancer. Obstet Gynecol Clin North Am 1996;23:347–410.
39. Eluf-Neto J, Booth M, Munoz N. Human papillomavirus and invasive cervical cancer. Br J Cancer 1994;69:114–9.
40. Munoz N, Bosch F, de Sanjose S. Risk factors for cervical intraepithelial neoplasia III/carcinoma in situ in Spain and Columbia. Cancer Epidemiol Biomarkers Prev 1993;2:423–31.
41. Olsen AO, Gjoen K, Sauer T, et al. Human papillomavirus and cervical intraepithelial neoplasia grade II-III: a population-based case-control study. Int J Cancer 1995;61:312–5.
42. Barrasso R. HPV-related genital lesions in men. IARC Sci Publ 1992:85–92.
43. Castellsague X, Ghaffari A, Daniel RW, et al. Prevalence of penile human papillomavirus DNA in husbands of women with and without cervical neoplasia: a study in Spain and Colombia. J Infect Dis 1997;176:353–61.
44. Castellsague X, Bosch FX, Munoz N, et al. Male circumcision, penile human papillomavirus infection, and cervical cancer in female partners. N Engl J Med 2002;346:1105–12.

45. Bosch FX, Munoz N, de Sanjose S, et al. Human papillomavirus and cervical intraepithelial neoplasia grade III/carcinoma in situ: a case-control study in Spain and Colombia. Cancer Epidemiol Biomarkers Prev 1993;2:415–22.
46. Becker TM, Wheeler CM, McGough NS, et al. Sexually transmitted diseases and other risk factors for cervical dysplasia among southwestern Hispanic and non-Hispanic white women. JAMA 1994;271:1181–8.
47. Wilkenstein W. Smoking and cervical cancer—current status: a review. Am J Epidemiol 1990;131:945–57.
48. Phillips AN, Smith G. Cigarette smoking as a potential cause of cervical cancer: has confounding been controlled? [Comments]. Int J Epidemiol 1994;23:42–9.
49. Parazzini F, Chatenoud L, La Vecchia C, et al. Determinants of risk of invasive cervical cancer in young women. Br J Cancer 1998;77:838–41.
50. Kanetsky PA, Gammon MD, Mandelblatt J, et al. Dietary intake and blood levels of lycopene: association with cervical dysplasia among non-Hispanic black women. Nutr Cancer 1998;31:31–40.
51. Olsen AO, Dillner J, Skrondal A, et al. Combined effect of smoking and human papillomavirus type 16 infection in cervical carcinogenesis. Epidemiology 1998;9:346–9.
52. Szarewski A. Effect of smoking cessation on cervical lesion size [comments]. Lancet 1996;347:941–3.
53. Negrini BP, Schiffman MH, Kurman RJ, et al. Oral contraceptive use, human papillomavirus infection, and risk of early cytological abnormalities of the cervix. Cancer Res 1990;50:4670–5.
54. Schneider A, Shah K. The role of vitamins in the etiology of cervical neoplasia, an epidemiological review. Arch Gynecol Obstet 1989;246:1–13.
55. Butterworth CE. Effect of folate on cervical cancer. Ann N Y Acad Sci 1992;669:293–9.
56. Potischman N. Nutritional epidemiology of cervical neoplasia. J Nutr 1993;123:424–9.
57. Wideroff L, Potischman N, Glass AG, et al. A nested case-control study of dietary factors and the risk of incident cytological abnormalities. Nutr Cancer 1998;30:130–6.
58. Boffetta P, Parkin DM. Cancer in developing countries. CA Cancer J Clin 1994;44:81–90.
59. Stubblefield PG. Oral contraceptives and neoplasia. J Reprod Med 1984;29:524–9.
60. Herrero R. Epidemiology of cervical cancer. J Natl Cancer Inst Monogr 1996;21:1–6.
61. Ursin G, Peters RK, Henderson BE, et al. Oral contraceptive use and adenocarcinoma of cervix. Lancet 1994;344:1390–4.
62. Southern SA, Herrington CS. Molecular events in uterine cervical cancer. Sex Transm Infect 1998;74:101–9.
63. Franco EL. The sexually transmitted disease model for cervical cancer: incoherent epidemiologic findings and the role of misclassification of human papillomavirus infection. Epidemiology 1991;2:98–106.
64. Scully RE, Bonfiglio TA, Kurman RJ, et al. Histological typing of female genital tract tumours. New York: Springer-Verlag; 1994.
65. Wright TCJ, Ferenczy A, Kurman RJ. Carcinoma and other tumors of the cervix. 4th ed. New York: Springer-Verlag; 1994.
66. Moll R, Lowe A, Laufer J, et al. Cytokeratin 20 in human carcinomas. A new histodiagnostic marker detected by monoclonal antibodies. Am J Pathol 1992;140:427–47.
67. Randall ME, Andersen WA, Mills SE, et al. Papillary squamous cell carcinoma of the uterine cervix: a clinicopathologic study of nine cases. Int J Gynecol Pathol 1986;5:1–10.
68. Mills SE, Austin MB, Randall ME. Lymphoepithelioma-like carcinoma of the uterine cervix. A distinctive, undifferentiated carcinoma with inflammatory stroma. Am J Surg Pathol 1985;9:883–9.
69. Mikuta JJ, Celebre JA. Adenocarcinoma of the cervix. Obstet Gynecol 1969;33:753–6.
70. Eide TJ. Cancer of the uterine cervix in Norway by histologic type, 1970–1984. J Natl Cancer Inst 1987;79:199–205.
71. Saigo PE, Cain JM, Kim WS, et al. Prognostic factors in adenocarcinoma of the uterine cervix. Cancer 1986;57:1584–93.
72. Gilks CB, Young RH, Aguirre P, et al. Adenoma malignum (minimal deviation adenocarcinoma) of the uterine cervix. A clinicopathological and immunohistochemical analysis of 26 cases. Am J Surg Pathol 1989;13:717–29.
73. Cherry CP, Glucksmann A. Incidence, histology, and response to radiation of mixed carcinomas (adenoacanthomas) of the uterine cervix. Cancer 1956;9:971–9.
74. Hale RJ, Wilcox FL, Buckley CH, et al. Prognostic factors in uterine cervical carcinoma: a clinicopathological analysis. Int J Cancer 1991;1:19–23.
75. Yazigi R, Sandstad J, Munoz AK, et al. Adenosquamous carcinoma of the cervix: prognosis in stage IB. Obstet Gynecol 1990;75:1012–5.
76. Gallup DG, Talledo OE, Shah KJ, et al. Invasive squamous cell carcinoma of the vagina: a 14-year study. Obstet Gynecol 1987;69:782–5.
77. Silva EG, Gershenson DM, Sneige N, et al. Small cell carcinoma of the uterine cervix: pathology and prognostic factors. Surg Pathol 1989;2:105.
78. Abeler VM, Holm R, Nesland JM, et al. Small cell carcinoma of the cervix. A clinicopathologic study of 26 patients. Cancer 1994;73:672–7.
79. Gilks CB, Young RH, Gersell DJ, et al. Large cell neuroendocrine [corrected]carcinoma of the uterine cervix: a clinicopathologic study of 12 cases [published erratum appears in Am J Surg Pathol 1997;21:1260.]. Am J Surg Pathol 1997;21:905–14.
80. Albores-Saavedra J, Gersell D, Gilks CB, et al. Terminology of endocrine tumors of the uterine cervix: results of a workshop sponsored by the College of American Pathologists and the National Cancer Institute. Arch Pathol Lab Med 1997;121:34–9.
81. Reagan JW, Harmonic MJ. The cellular pathology in carcinoma in situ: a cyto-histopathological correlation. Cancer 1956;9:385–402.
82. Reagan JW, Ng ABP. The cellular manifestations of uterine carcinogenesis. In: Norris NJ, Hertig AT, Abell MR, editors. The uterus. Baltimore: Williams and Wilkins; 1973. p. 320.
83. Richart RM. Natural history of cervical intraepithelial neoplasia. Clin Obstet Gynecol 1968;5:748–84.
84. McIndoe WA, McLean MR, Jones RW, et al. The invasive potential of carcinoma in situ of the cervix. Obstet Gynecol 1984;64:451–8.
85. Nasiell K, Roger V, Nasiell M. Behavior of mild cervical dysplasia during long-term follow-up. Obstet Gynecol 1986;67:665–9.
86. Friedell GH, McKay DG. Adenocarcinoma in situ of endocervix. Cancer 1953;6:887–97.
87. Cullimore JE, Leusley DM, Rollason TP, et al. A prospective study of conization of the cervix in the management of cervical intraepithelial glandular neoplasia (CIGN): a preliminary report. Br J Obstet Gynecol 1992;99:314–8.
88. Andersen ES, Arffmann E. Adenocarcinoma in situ of the uterine cervix: a clinico-pathologic of 36 cases. Gynecol Oncol 1989;35:1–7.
89. Ostor AG, Pagano R, Davoren RA, et al. Adenocarcinoma in situ of the cervix. Int J Gynecol Pathol 1984;3:179–90.
90. Jaworski RD, Pacey NF, Greenberg ML, et al. The histologic diagnosis of adeno-carcinoma in situ and related lesions of the cervix uteri: adeno-carcinoma in situ. Cancer 1988;61:1171–81.
91. Kaufman RH. Atypical squamous cells of undetermined significance and low-grade squamous intraepithelial lesion: diagnostic criteria and management. Am J Obstet Gynecol 1996;175:1120–8.
92. Kurman RJ, Henson DE, Herbst AL, et al. Interim guidelines for management of abnormal cervical cytology: the 1992 National Cancer Institute workshop. JAMA 1994;271:1866–9.
93. Jones MH. The management dilemma of the mildly abnormal smear: fact or fiction? Ann Acad Med Singapore 1998;27:666–70.
94. Nelson JH Jr, Hall JE. Detection, diagnostic evaluation, and treatment of dysplasia and early carcinoma of the cervix. CA Cancer J Clin 1970;20:150–63.
95. Stafl A, Mattingly RF. Colposcopic diagnosis of cervical neoplasia. Obstet Gynecol 1973;41:168–76.
96. Figge DC, Bennington JL, Schweid AI. Cervical cancer after initial negative and atypical vaginal cytology. Am J Obstet Gynecol 1970;108:422–8.
97. Lindheim SR, Smith-Nguyen G. Aggressive evaluation for atypical squamous cells in Papanicolaou smears. J Reprod Med 1990;35:971–3.
98. Kinney WK, Manos MM, Hurley LB, et al. Where's the high-grade cervical neoplasia? The importance of minimally abnormal Papanicolaou diagnoses. Obstet Gynecol 1998;91:973–6.
99. Richart RM, Wright TCJ. Controversies in the management of low grade cervical intraepithelial neoplasia. Cancer 1993;71:1413–21.
100. American College of Obstetricians and Gynecologists. Cervical cytology: evaluation and management of abnormalities. Washington, DC: ACOG; 1993.
101. Ferenczy C. Optimal management of cervical cancer precursors: low-grade squamous intraepithelial lesions. In: Franco E, Monsonego J, editors. New developments of cervical cancer screening and prevention. Cambridge: Blackwell Science; 1997. p 109–15.
102. The Atypical Squamous Cells of Undetermined Significance/Low-Grade Squamous Intraepithelial Lesions Triage Study (ALTS) Group. Human papillomavirus testing for triage of women with cytologic evidence of low-grade squamous intraepithelial lesions: baseline data from a randomized trial. J Natl Cancer Inst 2000;92:397–402.
103. Solomon D, Schiffman M, Tarone R. Comparison of three management strategies for patients with atypical squamous cells of undetermined significance: baseline results from a randomized trial. J Natl Cancer Inst 2001;93:293–9.
104. Cox JT, Lorincz AT, Schiffman MH, et al. Human papillomavirus testing by hybrid capture appears to be useful in triaging women with a cytologic diagnosis of atypical squamous cells of undetermined significance. Am J Obstet Gynecol 1995;172:946–54.
105. Cuzick J, Szarewski A, Terry G, et al. Human papillomavirus testing in primary cervical screening [comments]. Lancet 1995;345:1533–6.
106. Wright TCJ, Sun XW, Koulos J. Comparison of management algorithms for the evaluation of women with low-grade cytologic abnormalities. Obstet Gynecol 1995;85:202–10.
107. Manos MM, Kinney WK, Hurley LB, et al. Identifying women with cervical neoplasia: using human papillomavirus DNA testing for equivocal Papanicolaou results [comments]. JAMA 1999;281:1605–10.
108. Cox TJ. Evaluating the role of HPV testing for women with equivocal Papanicolaou test findings [editorial]. JAMA 1999;281:1645–7.
109. Cullen AP, Reid R, Campion M, et al. Analysis of the physical state of different human papillomavirus DNA's in intraepithelial and invasive cervical neoplasm. J Virol 1999;65:606–12.
110. Shafti MI, Leusley DM. Management of low grade lesions: follow-up or treat? Baillieres Clin Obstet Gynaecol 1995;9:121–31.
111. Mitchell MF, Tortolero-Luna G, Cook E, et al. A randomized clinical trial of cryotherapy, laser vaporization, and loop electrosurgical excision for treatment of squamous intraepithelial lesions of the cervix. Obstet Gynecol 1998;92:737–44.
112. Cox JT. Management of cervical intraepithelial neoplasia [comments]. Lancet 1999;353:857–9.
113. Ramanujam N. Fluorescence spectroscopy of neoplastic and non-neoplastic tissues. Neoplasia 2000;2:89–117.
114. Oridate N, Suzuki S, Higuchi M, et al. Involvement of reactive oxygen species in N-(4-hydroxyphenyl)retinamide-induced apoptosis in cervical carcinoma cells. J Natl Cancer Inst 1997;89:1191–8.
115. Mitchell MF, Tortolero-Luna G, Lee JJ, et al. Phase I dose de-escalation trial of alpha-difluoromethylornithine in patients with grade 3 cervical intraepithelial neoplasia. Clin Cancer Res 1998;4:303–10.
116. Rui H. Research and development of cancer chemopreventive agents in China. J Cell Biochem Suppl 1997;27:7–11.
117. Walboomers JM, Jacobs MV, Manos MM, et al. Human papillomavirus is a necessary cause of invasive cervical cancer worldwide. J Pathol 1999;189:12–9.
118. Bosch FX, Lorincz A, Munoz N, et al. The causal relation between human papillomavirus and cervical cancer. J Clin Pathol 2002;55:244–65.
119. Koutsky LA, Ault KA, Wheeler CM, et al. A controlled trial of a human papillomavirus type 16 vaccine. N Engl J Med 2002;347:1645–51.
120. Harper DM, Franco EL, Wheeler C, et al. Efficacy of a bivalent L1 virus-like particle vaccine in prevention of infection with human papillomavirus types 16 and 18 in young women: a randomised controlled trial. Lancet 2004;364:1757–65.
121. Villa LL, Costa RL, Petta CA, et al. Prophylactic quadrivalent human papillomavirus (types 6, 11, 16, and 18) L1 virus-like particle vaccine in young women: a randomised double-blind placebo-controlled multicentre phase II efficacy trial. Lancet Oncol 2005;6:271–8.
122. Sakuragi N, Satoh C, Takeda N, et al. Incidence and distribution pattern of pelvic and paraaortic lymph node metastasis in patients with stages IB, IIA, and IIB cervical carcinoma treated with radical hysterectomy. Cancer 1999;85:1547–54.
123. Averette HE, Nguyen HN, Donato DM, et al. Radical hysterectomy for invasive cervical cancer. A 25-year prospective experience with the Miami technique. Cancer 1993;71:1422–37.

124. Ayhan A, Tuncer ZS. Radical hysterectomy with lymphadenectomy for treatment of early stage cervical cancer: clinical experience of 278 cases. J Surg Oncol 1991;47:175–7.
125. Delgado G, Bundy B, Zaino R, et al. Prospective surgical-pathological study of disease-free interval in patients with stage IB squamous cell carcinoma of the cervix: a Gynecologic Oncology Group study. Gynecol Oncol 1990;38:352–7.
126. Piver MS, Chung WS. Prognostic significance of cervical lesion size and pelvic node metastases in cervical carcinoma. Obstet Gynecol 1975;46:507–10.
127. Mitchell PA, Waggoner S, Rotmensch J, et al. Cervical cancer in the elderly treated with radiation therapy. Gynecol Oncol 1998;71:291–8.
128. Eifel PJ, Morris M, Oswald MJ, et al. Adenocarcinoma of the uterine cervix. Prognosis and patterns of failure in 367 cases. Cancer 1990;65:2507–14.
129. Moberg PJ, Einhorn N, Silfverswärd C, et al. Adenocarcinoma of the uterine cervix. Cancer 1986;57:407–10.
130. Bush R. The significance of anemia in clinical radiation therapy. Int J Radiat Oncol Biol Phys 1986;12:2047–50.
131. Hirst D. Anemia: A problem or an opportunity in radiotherapy? Int J Radiat Oncol Biol Phys 1986;12:2009–17.
132. Shepperd JH. Staging announcement: FIGO staging of gynecologic cancers; cervical and vulva. Int J Gynecol Cancer 1995;5:319.
133. Pettersson F. Annual report on the results of treatment in gynecologic cancer. Stockholm: International Federation of Gynecologic Oncology; 1988.
134. American Joint Committee on Cancer. Manual for staging of cancer. Cervix uteri. 3rd ed. Philadelphia: Lippincott; 1988.
135. Kim MJ, Chung JJ, Lee YH, et al. Comparison of the use of the transrectal surface coil and the pelvic phased-array coil in MR imaging for preoperative evaluation of uterine cervical carcinoma. AJR Am J Roentgenol 1997;168:1215–21.
136. Hawighorst H, Schoenberg SO, Knapstein PG, et al. Staging of invasive cervical carcinoma and of pelvic lymph nodes by high resolution MRI with a phased-array coil in comparison with pathological findings. J Comput Assist Tomogr 1998;22:75–81.
137. Yu KK, Hricak H, Subak LL, et al. Preoperative staging of cervical carcinoma: phased array coil fast spin-echo versus body coil spin-echo T2-weighted MR imaging. AJR Am J Roentgenol 1998;171:707–11.
138. Hricak H, Powell CB, Yu KK, et al. Invasive cervical carcinoma: role of MR imaging in pretreatment work-up - cost minimization and diagnostic efficacy analysis. Radiology 1996;198:403–9.
139. Grigsby PW, Siegel BA, Dehdashti F. Lymph node staging by positron emission tomography in patients with carcinoma of the cervix. J Clin Oncol 2001;19:3745–9.
140. Hacker NF, Wain GV, Nicklin JL. Resection of bulky positive lymph nodes in patients with cervical carcinoma. Int J Gynecol Cancer 1995;5:250–6.
141. Weiser EB, Bundy BN, Hoskins WJ, et al. Extraperitoneal versus transperitoneal selective paraaortic lymphadenectomy in the pretreatment surgical staging of advanced cervical carcinoma (a Gynecologic Oncology Group study). Gynecol Oncol 1989;33:283–9.
142. Wharton JT, Jones HW 3rd, Day TG Jr, et al. Preirradiation celiotomy and extended field irradiation for invasive carcinoma of the cervix. Obstet Gynecol 1977;49:333–8.
143. Possover M, Krause N, Plaul K, et al. Laparoscopic para-aortic and pelvic lymphadenectomy: experience with 150 patients and review of the literature. Gynecol Oncol 1998;71:19–28.
144. Levenback C, Coleman RL, Burke TW, et al. Lymphatic mapping and sentinel node identification in patients with cervix cancer undergoing radical hysterectomy and pelvic lymphadenectomy. J Clin Oncol 2002;20:688–93.
145. Shepherd JH. Staging announcement: FIGO staging of gynecologic cancers; cervical and vulva. Int J Gynecol Cancer 1995;5:319.
146. Logsdon MD, Eifel PJ. Figo IIIB squamous cell carcinoma of the cervix: an analysis of prognostic factors emphasizing the balance between external beam and intracavitary radiation therapy. Int J Radiat Oncol Biol Phys 1999;43:763–75.
147. Barillot I, Horiot JC, Pigneux J, et al. Carcinoma of the intact uterine cervix treated with radiotherapy alone: a French cooperative study: update and multivariate analysis of prognostics factors. Int J Radiat Oncol Biol Phys 1997;38:969–78.
148. Sevin BU, Method MW, Nadji M, et al. Efficacy of radical hysterectomy as treatment for patients with small cell carcinoma of the cervix. Cancer 1996;77:1489–93.
149. Kristensen GB, Abeler VM, Risberg B, et al. Tumor size, depth of invasion, and grading of the invasive tumor front are the main prognostic factors in early squamous cell cervical carcinoma. Gynecol Oncol 1999;74:245–51.
150. Zreik TG, Chambers JT, Chambers SK. Parametrial involvement, regardless of nodal status: a poor prognostic factor for cervical cancer. Obstet Gynecol 1996;87:741–6.
151. Noguchi H, Shiozawa I, Kitahara T, et al. Uterine body invasion of carcinoma of the uterine cervix as seen from surgical specimens. Gynecol Oncol 1988;30:173–82.
152. Peters WAI, Liu PY, Barrett R, et al. Cisplatin, 5-fluorouracil plus radiation therapy are superior to radiation therapy as adjunctive therapy in high-risk, early-stage carcinoma of the cervix after radical hysterectomy and pelvic lymphadenectomy. Report of a phase III intergroup study. Gynecol Oncol 1999;72:443.
153. Inoue T, Morita K. The prognostic significance of number of positive nodes in cervical carcinoma stages IB, IIA, and IIB. Cancer 1990;65:1923–7.
154. Kim PY, Monk BJ, Chabra S, et al. Cervical cancer with paraaortic metastases: significance of residual paraaortic disease after surgical staging. Gynecol Oncol 1998;69:243–7.
155. Comerci G, Bolger BS, Flannelly G, et al. Prognostic factors in surgically treated stage IB-IIB carcinoma of the cervix with negative lymph nodes. Int J Gynecol Cancer 1998;8:23–6.
156. Pickel H, Haas J, Lahousen M. Prognostic factors in cervical cancer. Eur J Obstet Gynecol Reprod Biol 1997;71:209–13.
157. Roman LD, Felix JC, Muderspach LI, et al. Influence of quantity of lymph-vascular space invasion on the risk of nodal metastases in women with early-stage squamous cancer of the cervix [comments]. Gynecol Oncol 1998;68:220–5.
158. Eifel PJ, Burke TW, Delclos L, et al. Early stage I adenocarcinoma of the uterine cervix: treatment results in patients with tumors less than or equal to 4 cm in diameter. Gynecol Oncol 1991;41:199–205.
159. Matthews CM, Burke TW, Tornos C, et al. Stage I cervical adenocarcinoma: prognostic evaluation of surgically treated patients. Gynecol Oncol 1993;49:19–23.
160. Waldenstrom AC, Horvath G. Survival of patients with adenocarcinoma of the uterine cervix in western Sweden. Int J Gynecol Cancer 1999;9:18–23.
161. Miller BE, Flax SD, Arheart K, et al. The presentation of adenocarcinoma of the uterine cervix. Cancer 1993;72:1281–5.
162. Eifel PJ, Burke TW, Morris M, et al. Adenocarcinoma as an independent risk factor for disease recurrence in patients with stage IB cervical carcinoma. Gynecol Oncol 1995;59:38–44.
163. Chen RJ, Lin YH, Chen CA, et al. Influence of histologic type and age on survival rates for invasive cervical carcinoma in Taiwan. Gynecol Oncol 1999;73:184–90.
164. Lai C-H, Hsueh S, Hong J-H, et al. Are adenocarcinomas and adenosquamous carcinomas different from squamous carcinomas in stage IB and II cervical cancer patients undergoing primary radical surgery? Int J Gynecol Cancer 1999;9:28–36.
165. Hopkins MP, Morley GW. Radical hysterectomy versus radiation therapy for stage IB squamous cell cancer of the cervix. Cancer 1991;68:272–7.
166. Eifel PJ, Burke TW, Delclos L, et al. Early stage I adenocarcinoma of the uterine cervix: treatment results in patients with tumors greater less than or equal to 4 cm in diameter. Gynecol Oncol 1991;41:199–205.
167. Neunteufel W, Tatra G, Bieglmayer C. Serum squamous cell carcinoma antigen levels in women with neoplasms of the lower genital tract and in healthy controls. Arch Gynecol Obstet 1989;246:243–50.
168. Brioschi PA, Bischof P, Delafosse C, et al. Squamous-cell carcinoma antigen (SCC-A) values related to clinical outcome of pre-invasive and invasive cervical carcinoma. Int J Cancer 1991;47:376–9.
169. Maiman M, Feuer G, Fruchter RG, et al. Value of squamous cell carcinoma antigen levels in invasive cervical carcinoma. Gynecol Oncol 1989;34:312–6.
170. Lin H, ChangChien CC, Huang EY, et al. The role of pretreatment squamous cell carcinoma antigen in predicting nodal metastasis in early stage cervical cancer. Acta Obstet Gynecol Scand 2000;79:140–4.
171. Hong JH, Tsai CS, Chang JT, et al. The prognostic significance of pre- and posttreatment SCC levels in patients with squamous cell carcinoma of the cervix treated by radiotherapy. Int J Radiat Oncol Biol Phys 1998;41:823–30.
172. Massuger LF, Koper NP, Thomas CM, et al. Improvement of clinical staging in cervical cancer with serum squamous cell carcinoma antigen and CA 125 determinations. Gynecol Oncol 1997;64:473–6.
173. Duk JM, Groenier KH, de Bruijn HWA, et al. Pretreatment serum squamous cell carcinoma antigen: a newly identified prognostic factor in early-stage cervical carcinoma. J Clin Oncol 1996;14:111–8.
174. Scambia G, Panici PB, Baiocchi G, et al. The value of squamous cell carcinoma antigen in patients with locally advanced cervical cancer undergoing neoadjuvant chemotherapy. Am J Obstet Gynecol 1991;164:631–6.
175. Holloway RW, To A, Moradi M, et al. Monitoring the course of cervical carcinoma with the squamous cell carcinoma serum radioimmunoassay. Obstet Gynecol 1989;74:944–9.
176. Chan YM, Ng TY, Ngan HY, et al. Monitoring of serum squamous cell carcinoma antigen levels in invasive cervical cancer: is it cost-effective? Gynecol Oncol 2002;84:7–11.
177. Duggan MA, McGregor SE, Benoit JL, et al. The human papillomavirus status of invasive cervical adenocarcinoma: a clinicopathological and outcome analysis. Hum Pathol 1995;26:319–25.
178. Burger RA, Monk BJ, Kurosaki T, et al. Human papillomavirus type 18: association with poor prognosis in early stage cervical cancer [comments]. J Natl Cancer Inst 1996;88:1361–8.
179. Lombard I, Vincent-Salomon A, Validire P, et al. Human papillomavirus genotype as a major determinant of the course of cervical cancer. J Clin Oncol 1998;16:2613–9.
180. Ikenberg H, Wiegering I, Pfisterer J, et al. Human papillomavirus DNA in tumor-free regional lymph nodes: a potential prognostic marker in cervical cancer. Cancer J Sci Am 1996;2:28–34.
181. Kobayashi Y, Yoshinouchi M, Tianqi G, et al. Presence of human papilloma virus DNA in pelvic lymph nodes can predict unexpected recurrence of cervical cancer in patients with histologically negative lymph nodes. Clin Cancer Res 1998;4:979–83.
182. Gaffney DK, Holden J, Davis M, et al. Elevated cyclooxygenase-2 expression correlates with diminished survival in carcinoma of the cervix treated with radiotherapy. Int J Radiat Oncol Biol Phys 2001;49:1213–7.
183. Kristensen GB, Kaern J, Abeler VM, et al. No prognostic impact of flow-cytometric measured DNA ploidy and S-phase fraction in cancer of the uterine cervix: a prospective study of 465 patients. Gynecol Oncol 1995;57:79–85.
184. Gasinska A, Urbanski K, Jakubowicz J, et al. Tumour cell kinetics as a prognostic factor in squamous cell carcinoma of the cervix treated with radiotherapy. Radiother Oncol 1999;50:77–84.
185. Thomas G. The effect of hemoglobin level on radiotherapy outcomes: the Canadian experience. Semin Oncol 2001;28:60–5.
186. Hopkins MP, Morley GW. Squamous cell cancer of the cervix: prognostic factors related to survival. Int J Gynecol Cancer 1991;1:173–7.
187. Lanciano RM, Won M, Coia L, et al. Pretreatment and treatment factors associated with improved outcome in squamous cell carcinoma of the uterine cervix: a final report of the 1973 and 1978 Patterns of Care Studies. Int J Radiat Oncol Biol Phys 1991;20:667–76.
188. Sigurdsson K. Effect of organized screening on the risk of cervical cancer. Evaluation of screening activity in Iceland, 1964–1991. Int J Cancer 1993;54:563–70.
189. Kucera H, Enzelsberger H, Eppel W, et al. The influence of nicotine abuse and diabetes mellitus on the results of primary irradiation in the treatment of carcinoma of the cervix. Cancer 1987;60:1–4.
190. Eifel PJ, Jhingran A, Bodurka DC, et al. Correlation of smoking history and other patient characteristics with major complications of pelvic radiation therapy for cervical cancer. J Clin Oncol 2002;20:3651–7.
191. Linares AC, Storment J, Rhodes-Morris H, et al. A comparison of three cone biopsy techniques for evaluation and treatment of squamous intraepithelial lesions. J Gynecol Tech 1997:151–6.
192. Tseng CJ, Horng SG, Soong YK, et al. Conservative conization for microinvasive carcinoma of the cervix. Am J Obstet Gynecol 1997;176:1009–10.
193. Andersen ES, Nielsen K., Pedersen B. Combination laser conization as treatment of microinvasive carcinoma of the uterine cervix. Eur J Gynaecol Oncol 1998;19:352–5.
194. Burke TW, Lu K. Surgical treatment of invasive cervical cancer. In: Steele GD, Phillips TL, Chabner BA, editors.

American Cancer Society atlas of clinical oncology. Hamilton (ON): BC Decker; 2001. p 133–46.
195. Schorge JO, Lee KR, Sheets EE. Prospective management of stage IA(1) cervical adenocarcinoma by conization alone to preserve fertility: a preliminary report. Gynecol Oncol 2000;78:217–20.
196. Villasanta U, Durkan JP. Indications and complications of cold conization of the cervix. Observations on 200 consecutive cases. Obstet Gynecol 1966;27:717–23.
197. Lohe KJ, Burghardt E, Hillemanns HG, et al. Early squamous cell carcinoma of the uterine cervix. II. Clinical results of a cooperative study in the management of 419 patients with early stromal invasion and microcarcinoma. Gynecol Oncol 1978;6:31–50.
198. Kolstad P. Follow-up study of 232 patients with stage Ia1 and 411 patients with stage Ia2 squamous cell carcinoma of the cervix (microinvasive carcinoma). Gynecol Oncol 1989;33:265–72.
199. Roy M, Plante M. Pregnancies after radical vaginal trachelectomy for early-stage cervical cancer. Am J Obstet Gynecol 1998;179:1491–6.
200. Covens A, Shaw P, Murphy J, et al. Is radical trachelectomy a safe alternative to radical hysterectomy for patients with stage IA-B carcinoma of the cervix? Cancer 1999;86:2273–9.
201. Landoni F, Maneo A, Colombo A, et al. Randomised study of radical surgery versus radiotherapy for stage Ib–IIa cervical cancer. Lancet 1997;350:535–40.
202. Eifel PJ, Morris M, Wharton JT, et al. The influence of tumor size and morphology on the outcome of patients with FIGO stage IB squamous cell carcinoma of the uterine cervix. Int J Radiat Oncol Biol Phys 1994;29:9–16.
203. Orr JW, Shingleton HM, Hatch KD, et al. Correlation of perioperative morbidity and conization-radical hysterectomy interval. Obstet Gynecol 1982;59:726–31.
204. Hatch KD, Parham G, Shingleton H, et al. Ureteral strictures and fistulae following radical hysterectomy. Gynecol Oncol 1984;19:17–23.
205. Mann WJ Jr, Orr JW Jr, Shingleton HM, et al. Perioperative influences on infectious morbidity in radical hysterectomy. Gynecol Oncol 1981;11:207–12.
206. Sasaki H, Yoshida T, Noda K, et al. Urethral pressure profiles following radical hysterectomy. Obstet Gynecol 1982;59:101–4.
207. Ralph G, Tamussino K, Lichtenegger W. Urological complications after radical hysterectomy with or without radiotherapy for cervical cancer. Arch Gynecol Obstet 1990;248:61–5.
208. Alvarez RD, Potter ME, Soong SJ, et al. Rationale for using pathologic tumor dimensions and nodal status to subclassify surgically treated stage IB cervical cancer patients. Gynecol Oncol 1991;43:108–12.
209. Fuller AF, Elliott N, Kosloff C, et al. Determinants of increased risk for recurrence in patients undergoing radical hysterectomy for stage IB and IIA carcinoma of the cervix. Gynecol Oncol 1989;33:34–9.
210. Larson DM, Copeland LJ, Stringer CA, et al. Recurrent cervical carcinoma after radical hysterectomy. Gynecol Oncol 1988;30:381–7.
211. Hopkins MP, Morley GW. Stage IB squamous cell cancer of the cervix: clinicopathologic features related to survival. Am J Obstet Gynecol 1991;164:1520–7.
212. Lee Y-N, Wang KL, Lin M-H, et al. Radical hysterectomy with pelvic lymph node dissection for treatment of cervical cancer: a clinical review of 954 cases. Gynecol Oncol 1989;32:135–42.
213. Kenter GG, Ansink AC, Heintz APM, et al. Carcinoma of the uterine cervix stage I and IIA: results of surgical treatment: complications, recurrence, and survival. Eur J Surg Oncol 1989;15:55–60.
214. Powell JL, Burrell MO, Franklin EW 3rd. Radical hysterectomy and pelvic lymphadenectomy. South Med J 1984;77:596–600.
215. Sall S, Pineda AA, Calanog A, et al. Surgical treatment of stages IB and IIA invasive carcinoma of the cervix by radical abdominal hysterectomy. Am J Obstet Gynecol 1979;135:442–6.
216. Durrance FY, Fletcher GH. Computer calculation of dose contribution to regional lymphatics from gynecological radium insertions. Radiology 1968;91:140–8.
217. Fletcher GH, Hamberger AD. Squamous cell carcinoma of the uterine cervix. Treatment technique according to size of the cervical lesion and extension. In: Fletcher GH, editor. Textbook of radiotherapy. 3rd ed. Philadelphia: Lea & Febiger; 1980. p. 720.
218. Eifel PJ, Moughan J, Owen JB, et al. Patterns of radiotherapy practice for patients with squamous carcinoma of the uterine cervix. A Patterns of Care study. Int J Radiat Oncol Biol Phys 1999;43:351–8.
219. Petereit DG, Sarkaria JN, Potter DM, et al. High-dose-rate versus low-dose-rate brachytherapy in the treatment of cervical cancer: analysis of tumor recurrence—the University of Wisconsin experience. Int J Radiat Oncol Biol Phys 1999;45:1267–74.
220. Kapp KS, Stuecklschweiger GF, Kapp DS, et al. Prognostic factors in patients with carcinoma of the uterine cervix treated with external beam irradiation and IR-192 high-dose-rate brachytherapy. Int J Radiat Oncol Biol Phys 1998;42:531–40.
221. Nag S, Erickson B, Thomadsen B, et al. The American Brachytherapy Society recommendations for high-dose-rate brachytherapy for carcinoma of the cervix. Int J Radiat Oncol Biol Phys 2000;48:201–11.
222. Hughes-Davies L, Silver B, Kapp D. Parametrial interstitial brachytherapy for advanced or recurrent pelvic malignancy: the Harvard/Stanford experience. Gynecol Oncol 1995;58:24–7.
223. Syed AM, Puthawala AA, Abdelaziz NN, et al. Long-term results of low-dose-rate interstitial-intracavitary brachytherapy in the treatment of carcinoma of the cervix. Int J Radiat Oncol Biol Phys 2002;54:67–78.
224. Lowrey GC, Mendenhall WM, Million RR. Stage IB or IIA-B carcinoma of the intact uterine cervix treated with irradiation: a multivariate analysis. Int J Radiat Oncol Biol Phys 1992;24:205–10.
225. Perez CA, Grigsby PW, Nene SM, et al. Effect of tumor size on the prognosis of carcinoma of the uterine cervix treated with irradiation alone. Cancer 1992;69:2796–806.
226. Keys HM, Bundy BN, Stehman FB, et al. Cisplatin, radiation, and adjuvant hysterectomy for bulky stage IB cervical carcinoma. New Engl J Med 1999;340:1154–61.
227. Morris M, Eifel PJ, Lu J, et al. Pelvic radiation with concurrent chemotherapy compared with pelvic and paraaortic radiation for high-risk cervical cancer. New Engl J Med 1999;340:1137–43.
228. Benedet J, Odicino F, Maisonneuve P, et al. Carcinoma of the cervix uteri. J Epidemiol Biostat 1998;3:5–34.
229. Rose PG, Bundy BN, Watkins J, et al. Concurrent cisplatin-based chemotherapy and radiotherapy for locally advanced cervical cancer. New Engl J Med 1999;340:1144–53.
230. Whitney CW, Sause W, Bundy BN, et al. A randomized comparison of fluorouracil plus cisplatin versus hydroxyurea as an adjunct to radiation therapy in stages IIB–IVA carcinoma of the cervix with negative para-aortic lymph nodes: a Gynecologic Oncology Group and Southwest Oncology Group study. J Clin Oncol 1999;17:1339–48.
231. Jhingran A, Eifel PJ. Perioperative and postoperative complications of intracavitary radiation for FIGO stage I–III carcinoma of the cervix. Int J Radiat Oncol Biol Phys 2000;46:1177–83.
232. Eifel PJ, Levenback C, Wharton JT, et al. Time course and incidence of late complications in patients treated with radiation therapy for FIGO stage IB carcinoma of the uterine cervix. Int J Radiat Oncol Biol Phys 1995;32:1289–300.
233. Lanciano RM, Martz D, Montana GS, Hanks GE. Influence of age, prior abdominal surgery, fraction size, and dose on complications after radiation therapy for squamous cell cancer of the uterine cervix. A Patterns of Care study. Cancer 1992;69:2124–30.
234. Bruner DW, Lanciano R, Keegan M, et al. Vaginal stenosis and sexual function following intracavitary radiation for the treatment of cervical and endometrial carcinoma. Int J Radiat Oncol Biol Phys 1993;27:825–30.
235. Grigsby PW, Perez CA. Radiotherapy alone for medically inoperable carcinoma of the cervix: stage IA and carcinoma in situ. Int J Radiat Oncol Biol Phys 1991;21:375–8.
236. Plante M, Renaud MC, Francois H, et al. Vaginal radical trachelectomy: an oncologically safe fertility-preserving surgery. An updated series of 72 cases and review of the literature. Gynecol Oncol 2004;94:614–23.
237. Plante M, Renaud MC, Hoskins IA, et al. Vaginal radical trachelectomy: a valuable fertility-preserving option in the management of early-stage cervical cancer. A series of 50 pregnancies and review of the literature. Gynecol Oncol 2005;98:3–10.
238. Hamberger AD, Fletcher GH, Wharton JT. Results of treatment of early stage I carcinoma of the uterine cervix with intracavitary radium alone. Cancer 1978;41:980–5.
239. Delgado G, Bundy BN, Fowler WC, et al. A prospective surgical pathological study of stage I squamous carcinoma of the cervix: a Gynecologic Oncology Group study. Gynecol Oncol 1989;36:314–20.
240. Sedlis A, Bundy BN, Rotman MZ, et al. A randomized trial of pelvic radiation therapy versus No further therapy in selected patients with stage IB carcinoma of the cervix after radical hysterectomy and pelvic lymphadenectomy: a Gynecologic Oncology Group study. Gynecol Oncol 1999;73:177–83.
241. Mendenhall WM, McCarty PJ, Morgan LS, et al. Stage IB-IIA-B carcinoma of the intact uterine cervix greater than or equal to 6 cm in diameter: Is adjuvant extrafascial hysterectomy beneficial? Int J Radiat Oncol Biol Phys 1991;21:899–904.
242. Keys H, Bundy B, Stehman F, et al. Adjuvant hysterectomy after radiation therapy reduces detection of local recurrence in "bulky" stage IB cervical cancer without improving survival: results of a prospective randomized GOG trial. Cancer J Sci Am 1997;3:117.
243. Sardi JE, Giaroli A, Sananes C, et al. Long-term follow-up of the first randomized trial using neoadjuvant chemotherapy in stage Ib squamous carcinoma of the cervix: the final results. Gynecol Oncol 1997;67:61–9.
244. Neoadjuvant Chemotherapy for Cervical Cancer Meta-Analysis Collaboration. Neoadjuvant chemotherapy locally advanced cervical cancer: a systematic review and meta-analysis of individual patient data from 21 randomised trials. Eur J Cancer 2003;39:2470–86.
245. Peters WA 3rd, Liu PY, Barrett RJ 2nd, et al. Concurrent chemotherapy and pelvic radiation therapy compared with pelvic radiation therapy alone as adjuvant therapy after radical surgery in high-risk early-stage cancer of the cervix. J Clin Oncol 2000;18:1606–13.
246. Rose PG, Blessing JA, Gershenson DM, et al. Paclitaxel and cisplatin as first-line therapy in recurrent or advanced squamous cell carcinoma of the cervix: a gynecologic oncology group study. J Clin Oncol 1999;17:2676–80.
247. Eifel PJ, Winter K, Morris M, et al. Pelvic irradiation with concurrent chemotherapy versus pelvic and para-aortic irradiation for high-risk cervical cancer: an update of radiation therapy oncology group trial (RTOG) 90-01. J Clin Oncol 2004;22:872–80.
248. Pearcey R, Brundage M, Drouin P, et al. Phase III trial comparing radical radiotherapy with and without cisplatin chemotherapy in patients with advanced squamous cell cancer of the cervix. J Clin Oncol 2002;20:966–72.
249. Green JA, Kirwan JM, Tierney JF, et al. Survival and recurrence after concomitant chemotherapy and radiotherapy for cancer of the uterine cervix: a systematic review and meta-analysis. Lancet 2001;358:781–6.
250. Wong LC, Ngan HY, Cheung AN, et al. Chemoradiation and adjuvant chemotherapy in cervical cancer. J Clin Oncol 1999;17:2055–60.
251. Lorvidhaya V, Chitapanarux I, Sangruchi S, et al. Concurrent mitomycin C, 5-fluorouracil, and radiotherapy in the treatment of locally advanced carcinoma of the cervix: a randomized trial. Int J Radiat Oncol Biol Phys 2003;55:1226–32.
252. Chen MD, Paley PJ, Potish RA, et al. Phase I trial of Taxol as a radiation sensitizer with cisplatin in advanced cervical cancer. Gynecol Oncol 1997;67:131–6.
253. Muderspach LI, Curtin JP, Roman LD, et al. Carboplatin as a radiation sensitizer in locally advanced cervical cancer: a pilot study. Gynecol Oncol 1997;65:336–42.
254. Cunningham MJ, Dunton CJ, Corn B, et al. Extended-field radiation therapy in early-stage cervical carcinoma: survival and complications. Gynecol Oncol 1991;43:51–4.
255. Podczaski E, Stryker JA, Kaminski P, et al. Extended-field radiation therapy for carcinoma of the cervix. Cancer 1990;66:251–8.
256. Rubin SC, Brookland R, Mikuta JJ, et al. Para-aortic nodal metastases in early cervical carcinoma: long-term survival following extended-field radiotherapy. Gynecol Oncol 1984;18:213–7.
257. Rotman M, Pajak TF, Choi K, et al. Prophylactic extended-field irradiation of para-aortic lymph nodes in stages IIB and bulky IB and IIA cervical carcinomas. Ten-year treatment results of RTOG 79-20 [comments]. JAMA 1995;274:387–93.
258. Haie C, Pejovic MH, Gerbaulet A, et al. Is prophylactic para-aortic irradiation worthwhile in the treatment of advanced cervical carcinoma? Results of a controlled clinical trial of the EORTC radiotherapy group. Radiother Oncol 1988;11:101–12.
259. Grigsby PW, Heydon K, Mutch DG, et al. Long-term follow-up of RTOG 92-10: cervical cancer with positive para-aortic lymph nodes. Int J Radiat Oncol Biol Phys 2001;51:982–7.
260. Varia MA, Bundy BN, Deppe G, et al. Cervical carcinoma metastatic to para-aortic nodes: extended field radiation

therapy with concomitant 5-fluorouracil and cisplatin chemotherapy: a Gynecologic Oncology Group study. Int J Radiat Oncol Biol Phys 1998;42:1015–23.

261. Malfetano JH, Keys H, Cunningham MJ, et al. Extended field radiation and cisplatin for stage IIB and IIIB cervical carcinoma. Gynecol Oncol 1997;67:203–7.
262. Roman L, Morris M, Eifel P, et al. Reasons for inappropriate simple hysterectomy in the presence of invasive cancer of the cervix. Obstet Gynecol 1992;79:485–9.
263. Andras EJ, Fletcher G, Rutledge F. Radiotherapy of carcinoma of the cervix following simple hysterectomy. Am J Obstet Gynecol 1973;115:647–55.
264. Roman LD, Morris M, Mitchell MF, et al. Prognostic factors for patients undergoing simple hysterectomy in the presence of invasive cancer of the cervix. Gynecol Oncol 1993;50:179–84.
265. Lanciano R. Radiotherapy for the treatment of locally recurrent cervical cancer. J Natl Cancer Inst Monogr 1996;21:113–5.
266. Maneo A, Landoni F, Cormio G, et al. Concurrent carboplatin/5-fluorouracil and radiotherapy for recurrent cervical carcinoma. Ann Oncol 1999;10:803–7.
267. Ijaz T, Eifel PJ, Burke T, et al. Radiation therapy of pelvic recurrence after radical hysterectomy for cervical carcinoma. Gynecol Oncol 1998;70:241–6.
268. Coleman RL, Keeney ED, Freedman RA, et al. Radical hysterectomy after radiotherapy for recurrent carcinoma of the uterine cervix. Gynecol Oncol 1994;55:29–35.
269. Rutledge FN. Pelvic exenteration: an update of the U. T. M. D. Anderson Hospital experience and review of the literature. In: Rutledge FN, Freedman RS, Gershenson DM, editors. Gynecologic cancer: diagnosis and treatment strategies. Austin (TX): University of Texas Press; 1987. p. 7.
270. Orr JWJ, Shingleton HM, Hatch KD, et al. Gastrointestinal complications associated with pelvic exenteration. Am J Obstet Gynecol 1983;145:325–32.
271. Symmonds RE, Pratt JH, Webb MJ. Exenterative operations: experience with 198 patients. Am J Obstet Gynecol 1975;121:907–18.
272. Rutledge RN, Smith JP, Wharton JT, O'Quinn AG. Pelvic exenteration: an analysis of 296 patients. Am J Obstet Gynecol 1977;129:881–92.
273. Wang CJ, Lai CH, Huang HJ, et al. Recurrent cervical carcinoma after primary radical surgery. Am J Obstet Gynecol 1999;181:518–24.
274. Thomas GM, Dembo AJ, Myhr T, et al. Long-term results of concurrent radiation and chemotherapy for carcinoma of the cervix recurrent after surgery. Int J Gynecol Cancer 1993;3:193–8.
275. Thigpen JT, Blessing JA, DiSaia PJ, et al. A randomized comparison of a rapid versus prolonged (24 hr) infusion of cisplatin in therapy of squamous cell carcinoma of the uterine cervix: a Gynecologic Oncology Group study. Gynecol Oncol 1989;32:198–202.
276. Bonomi P, Blessing J, Stehman F, et al. Randomized trial of three cisplatin dose schedules in squamous-cell carcinoma of the cervix: a Gynecologic Oncology Group study. J Clin Oncol 1985;3:1079–85.
277. McGuire WP, Arseneau J, Blessing JA, et al. A randomized comparative trial of carboplatin and iproplatin in advanced squamous carcinoma of the uterine cervix: Gynecologic Oncology Group study. J Clin Oncol 1989;7:1462–8.
278. Sutton GP, Blessing JA, Adcock L, et al. Phase II study of ifosfamide and mesna in patients with previously-treated carcinoma of the cervix: a Gynecologic Oncology Group study. Invest New Drugs 1989;7:341–3.
279. Stehman FB, Perez CA, Kurman RJ. Uterine cervix. In: Hoskins WJ, Perez CA, Young RH, editors. Principles and practice of gynecologic oncology. Philadelphia: Lippincott; 2000. p. 591.
280. Meanwell C, Mould J, Blackledge G, et al. Phase II study of ifosfamide in cervical cancer. Cancer Treat Rep 1986;70:727–30.
281. Cervellino J, Araujo C, Pirisi C, et al. Ifosfamide and mesna at high doses for the treatment of cancer of the cervix: a GETLAC study. Cancer Chemother Pharmacol 1990;26 Suppl:S1–3.
282. Hannigan EV, Dinh TV, Doherty MG. Ifosfamide with mesna in squamous carcinoma of the cervix: phase II results in patients with advanced or recurrent disease. Gynecol Oncol 1991;43:123–8.
283. Sutton GP, Blessing JA, Photopoulos G, et al. Phase II experience with ifosphamide/mesna in gynecologic malignancies: preliminary report of Gynecologic Oncology Group studies. Semin Oncol 1989;15:381–90.
284. Cervellino JC, Araujo CE, Sanchez O, et al. Cisplatin and ifosfamide in patients with advanced squamous cell carcinoma of the uterine cervix. Acta Oncol 1995;34:257–9.
285. Chiara S, Consoli R, Falcone A, et al. Cisplatin and 5-fluorouracil in advanced and recurrent cervical cancer. Tumori 1988;74:471–4.
286. Kuhnle H, Meerpohl HG, Eiermann W, et al. Phase II study of carboplatin/ifosfamide in untreated advanced cervical cancer. Cancer Chemother Pharmacol 1990;26 Suppl:S33–5.
287. Ramm K, Vergote I, Kaem J, et al. Bleomycin-ifosfamide-cisplatinum (BIP) in pelvic recurrence of previously irradiated cervical carcinoma: a second look. Gynecol Oncol 1992;46:203–7.
288. Buxton EJ, Meanwell CA, Hilton C, et al. Combination bleomycin, ifosfamide, and cisplatin chemotherapy in cervical cancer. J Natl Cancer Inst 1989;81:359–61.
289. Kumar L, Bhargava V. Chemotherapy in recurrent and advanced cervical cancer. Gynecol Oncol 1991;40:107–11.
290. Murad AM, Triginelli SA, Ribalta JCL. Phase II trial of bleomycin, ifosfamide, and carboplatin in metastatic cervical cancer. J Clin Oncol 1994;12:55–9.
291. Long HJ 3rd, Bundy BN, Grendys EC Jr, et al. Randomized phase III trial of cisplatin (P) vs. cisplatin plus topotecan (T) vs. MVAC in stage IVB, recurrent or persistent carcinoma of the uterine cervix: a Gynecologic Oncology Group study [abstract 9]. Gynecol Oncol 2004;92:397.
292. Tay SK, Lai FM, Soh LT, et al. Combined chemotherapy using cisplatin ifosfamide and bleomycin (PIB) in the treatment of advanced and recurrent cervical carcinoma. Aust N Z J Obstet Gynecol 1993;32:263–6.
293. Bonomi P, Blessing J, Ball H, et al. A phase II evaluation of cisplatin and 5-fluorouracil in patients with advanced squamous cell carcinoma of the cervix: a Gynecologic Oncology Group study. Gynecol Oncol 1989;37:354–8.
294. Kaern J, Trope C, Kjorstad KE, et al. A phase II study of 5-fluorouracil/cisplatin in recurrent cervical cancer. Tidsskr Nor Laegeforen 1990;110:2759–62.
295. Weiss G, Green S, Hannigan E, et al. A phase II trial of cisplatin and 5-fluorouracil with allopurinol for recurrent or metastatic carcinoma of the uterine cervix: a Southwest Oncology Group trial. Gynecol Oncol 1990;37:354–8.
296. Piver MS, Ghamande SA, Eltabbakh GH, et al. First-line chemotherapy with paclitaxel and platinum for advanced and recurrent cancer of the cervix--a phase II study. Gynecol Oncol 1999;75:334–7.
297. Papadimitriou CA, Sarris K, Moulopoulos LA, et al. Phase II trial of paclitaxel and cisplatin in metastatic and recurrent carcinoma of the uterine cervix. J Clin Oncol 1999;17:761–6.
298. Pignata S, Silvestro G, Ferrari E, et al. Phase II study of cisplatin and vinorelbine as first-line chemotherapy in patients with carcinoma of the uterine cervix. J Clin Oncol 1999;17:756–60.
299. Duenas-Gonzalez A, Lopez-Graniel C, Gonzalez A, et al. A phase II study of gemcitabine and cisplatin combination as induction chemotherapy for untreated locally advanced cervical carcinoma. Ann Oncol 2001;12:541–7.
300. Burnett AF, Roman LD, Garcia AA, et al. A phase II study of gemcitabine and cisplatin in patients with advanced, persistent, or recurrent squamous cell carcinoma of the cervix. Gynecol Oncol 2000;76:63–6.
301. Verschraegen CF, Kavanagh JJ, Loyer E, et al. Phase II study of carboplatin and liposomal doxorubicin in patients with recurrent squamous cell carcinoma of the cervix. Cancer 2001;92:2327–33.
302. Brader KR, Morris M, Levenback C, et al. Chemotherapy for cervical carcinoma: factors determining response and implications for clinical trial design. J Clin Oncol 1998;16:1879–84.
303. Morley GW, Seski JC. Radical pelvic surgery versus radiation therapy for stage I carcinoma of the cervix (exclusive of microinvasion). Am J Obstet Gynecol 1976;126:785–98.
304. Burghardt E, Hofmann HMH, Ebner F, et al. Results of surgical treatment of 1028 cervical cancers studied with volumetry. Cancer 1992;70:648–55.
305. Horiot JC, Pigneux J, Pourquier H, et al. Radiotherapy alone in carcinoma of the intact uterine cervix according to G. H. Fletcher guidelines: a French cooperative study of 1383 cases. Int J Radiat Oncol Biol Phys 1988;14:605–11.
306. Bricker EM. Pelvic exenteration. Adv Surg 1970;4:13–72.
307. Ketcham AS, Deckers PJ, Sugarbaker EV, et al. Pelvic exenteration for carcinoma of the uterine cervix. A 15-year experience. Cancer 1970;26:513–21.
308. Morley GW, Hopkins MP, Lindenauer SM, et al. Pelvic exenteration, University of Michigan: 100 patients at 5 years. Obstet Gynecol 1989;74:934–43.
309. Shingleton HM, Soong SJ, Gelder MS, et al. Clinical and histopathologic factors predicting recurrence and survival after pelvic exenteration for cancer of the cervix. Obstet Gynecol 1989;73:1027–34.
310. Magrina JF, Stanhope CR, Weaver AL. Pelvic exenterations: supralevator, infralevator, and with vulvectomy. Gynecol Oncol 1997;64:130–5.
311. Anderson P, Dische S. Local tumor control and the subsequent incidence of distant metastatic disease. Int J Radiat Oncol Biol Phys 1981;7:1645–8.
312. Thomas G, Dembo A, Ackerman I, et al. A phase III study of concurrent 5-fluorouracil and/or partially hyperfractionated radiation in advanced cancer of the cervix. Proc Soc Gynecol Oncol 1997.
313. Bloss JD, Thigpen T. Chemotherapy of gynecologic cancer. In: Perry MC, editor. The chemotherapy source book. Philadelphia: Lippincott Williams & Wilkins; 2001. p. 732.
314. Look KY, Blessing JA, Levenback C, et al. A phase II trial of CPT-11 in recurrent squamous carcinoma of the cervix: a gynecologic oncology group study. Gynecol Oncol 1998;70:334–8.
315. Takeuchi S, Dobashi K, Fujimoto S, et al. A late phase II study of CPT-11 on uterine cervical cancer and ovarian cancer. Research Groups of CPT-11 in Gynecologic Cancers. Gan To Kagaku Ryoho 1991;18:1681–9.
316. Verschraegen CF, Levy T, Kudelka AP, et al. Phase II study of irinotecan in prior chemotherapy-treated squamous cell carcinoma of the cervix. J Clin Oncol 1997;15:625–31.
317. Kudelka AP, Winn R, Edwards CL, et al. Activity of paclitaxel in advanced or recurrent squamous cell cancer of the cervix. Clin Cancer Res 1996;2:1285–8.
318. Bloss JD, Blessing JA, Behrens BC, et al. Randomized trial of cisplatin and ifosfamide with or without bleomycin in squamous carcinoma of the cervix: a gynecologic oncology group study. J Clin Oncol 2002;20:1832–7.
319. Dimopoulos MA, Papadimitriou CA, Sarris K, et al. Combination of ifosfamide, paclitaxel, and cisplatin for the treatment of metastatic and recurrent carcinoma of the uterine cervix: a phase II study of the Hellenic Cooperative Oncology Group. Gynecol Oncol 2002;85:476–82.
320. Wagenaar HC, Pecorelli S, Mangioni C, et al. Phase II study of mitomycin-C and cisplatin in disseminated, squamous cell carcinoma of the uterine cervix. A European Organization for Research and Treatment of Cancer (EORTC) Gynecological Cancer Group study. Eur J Cancer 2001;37:1624–8.
321. Fiorica J, Holloway R, Ndubisi B, et al. Phase II trial of topotecan and cisplatin in persistent or recurrent squamous and nonsquamous carcinomas of the cervix. Gynecol Oncol 2002;85:89–94.

Endometrial Cancer

Jamal Rahaman, MD
Carmel J. Cohen, MD

It has been predicted that 40,880 new cases of uterine corpus cancer (the vast majority of which are endometrial cancer) will occur in the United States in 2005 and that the disease will result in 7,310 deaths.[1] In 1991, the number of deaths from endometrial cancer in the United States began to exceed the number attributable to cervical cancer, which is the most prevalent gynecologic cancer in the populous, less developed areas of the world and the one that causes the most deaths.[1,2] After declining between the mid-1980s and 1990s, the incidence rates for endometrial cancer increased by about 0.6% per year from 1988 to 1999. Norway, Czechoslovakia, and other northern European countries also reported significant increases in the incidence of endometrial cancer. Five-year survival rates in the United States were estimated to be 84% overall for 1995 to 2000.[1] Table 102-1 shows international survival figures as published in the *Annual Report on the Results of Treatment in Gynecologic Cancer*.[2]

Although the incidence of endometrial carcinoma is lower among black women than among white women, the mortality rates are higher in the former group of patients.[1,3] In their review of the National Cancer Data Base, Hicks and colleagues observed that black women were diagnosed with less favorable histologies, more advanced stages of disease, and poorly differentiated tumors than were white women.[3] Black women were less frequently treated surgically, and the surgically treated patients with advanced-stage disease received adjuvant radiotherapy (RT) less often and chemotherapy more often than did white patients. Most significantly, 5-year survival was poorer for black women, even for those with stage I disease who were treated surgically.[1,3]

Table 102-1 Carcinoma of the Corpus Uteri*

Volume	Year	Number	5-Year Survival, %
16	1962–1968	14,506	63.0
17	1969–1972	10,720	65.4
18	1973–1975	11,501	66.6
19	1976–1978	13,581	67.7
20	1979–1981	14,906	65.1
21	1982–1986	19,402	69.7
22	1987–1989	13,040	72.7
23	1990–1992	7,350	73.4
24	1993–1995	6,260	76.5
25	1996–1998	7,496	77.6
Total		118,762	

*Review of the 5-year survival rate reported in volumes 16 to 25 of the *Annual Report on the Results of Treatment in Gynecologic Cancer*.[2]

RISK FACTORS

The list of conditions thought to increase the risk of endometrial cancer has included body size, obesity, hypertension, diabetes, nulliparity, a history of colon and/or breast carcinoma, syndromes of ovulation failure, syndromes of increased endogenous estrogen exposure, and exposure to exogenous estrogen. Recently, the list was refined and focused, on the basis of an improved understanding of the underlying pathophysiology. Multivariate analysis, controlled for age and obesity, verified the association between endometrial cancer and diabetes but not hypertension. The obesity observed in the typical phenotype associated with the endometrial cancer patient is related to a higher level of circulating estrogen than in cohorts of thinner patients. This results from peripheral aromatization in the fat of estrogen precursors. Data from a recent population-based case-control study contradict earlier reports and suggest that diabetes confers no additional risk of endometrial carcinoma in women who are not overweight (body mass index [BMI] < 29.1) or who are mildly overweight (BMI 29.1–31.9) but are restricted only to those who are obese (BMI > 31.9).[4] Nulliparity, compared with multiparity of five or more births, menopause after age 53 years, and 50 pounds of excess weight are all important risk factors that can increase a woman's probability for endometrial cancer by 5 to 10 times compared with patients without these risk factors.

There are pathologic conditions that are associated with an increased risk of endometrial cancer, and these features have in common the production of increased levels of estrogen or the requirements for exogenous estrogen supplementation. It is known that patients with granulosa theca cell tumors of the ovary have clinical manifestations of increased estrogen exposure.[5] Gusberg and Kardon reviewed the endometrial histology from 115 patients with these ovarian tumors and found that 21% developed endometrial carcinoma and 43% had benign changes that were thought to be precancerous, such as adenomatous hyperplasia.[5] Others have not found the same incidence of adenocarcinoma but have identified a high incidence of atypical hyperplasias.[6,7] Patients with polycystic ovary syndrome usually do not ovulate and, thus, are exposed to continuous estrogen production. When endometrial carcinoma occurs in women younger than 45 years of age, it is usually in patients with polycystic ovary syndrome[8,9] and is most frequently surrounded by atypical hyperplasia histologically. These lesions are usually well-differentiated cancers, suggesting the influence of estrogen exposure. Finally, patients who are treated for ovarian dysgenesis and oophorectomy with unopposed estrogen replacement develop endometrial carcinoma in the residual uterus.[10]

Extrapolating from the observed association between hyperestrogen states and the development of endometrial cancer, clinicians became wary of the theoretic risk of exogenously administered estrogen highlighted by Gusberg's suggestion that the glandular atypicalities originally described by Cullen in 1900 were related to estrogen and were, in fact, precursors of endometrial adenocarcinoma.[11,12] In 1975, Smith and colleagues, in a retrospective case-control study of 317 women with endometrial carcinoma, noted a 4.5-fold relative risk among those women who had been treated with unopposed estrogen compared with 317 controls who had gynecologic cancers other than endometrial cancers.[13] A series of retrospective analyses followed describing the relative risk of endometrial cancer in estrogen users as ranging from 1.7 to 8.0, with some subsets of patients experiencing a risk as high as 14-fold.[14–17] Critics found each of the many studies deficient in some feature, but there was no common deficit among the studies, and a relative risk of four- to sevenfold was consistently found by each investigator.

In 1993, mindful of the defects of the earlier studies, Brinton and Hoover, representing the Endometrial Cancer Collaborative Group, completed a hospital-based case-control study analyzing 300 menopausal women with new diagnoses of endometrial carcinoma and 207 matched-population controls.[18] These investigators identified a relative risk of 3.0 for all users, although the risks were higher for recent use, thin habitus, or cigarette smoking. No clear dose relationship was observed, but women who used low-dose preparations exclusively were found to be at lowest risk, although when low-dose use continued beyond 5 years, this advantage was lost. Although only 4% of the women used progestogens simultaneously with estrogen, there seemed to be a partial protective effect, but the risk was not eliminated. Some investigators have described an immediate decline in risk after cessation of estrogen use,[19] but Brinton and Hoover's study confirms the observation made by others that the excess risk can persist beyond 5 years after discontinuation, especially when there has been long-term exposure.[18]

The Centers for Disease Control and Prevention reported that oral contraceptive use for at least 12 months diminished the risk of endometrial cancer by 50% compared with the risk for women who had never used oral contraception. Nulliparous women seemed to benefit most, and the protection lasted for a decade following the discontinuation of oral contraceptive use.[20] Brinton and Hoover's study observed that previous oral contraceptive use did not protect women from increased relative risk of endometrial cancer when they employed unopposed estrogen in postmenopausal hormone replacement therapy, suggesting that the role of the progestogen in the combination oral contraceptive pills is essential in protecting against endometrial carcinoma.[18]

For more than 20 years, tamoxifen has been used to treat breast cancer, following the observation that it causes regression of metastatic tumor, diminishes the incidence of cancer in the contralateral breast, delays time to recurrence, and improves survival in subsets of patients. Several competitive inhibitors (antihormones) of steroid hormone receptors have been developed. These drugs are currently used for treatment of a variety of endocrine-related disorders and as selective tools allowing the dissection of the receptor transduction pathway. Most antihormones bind competitively to the receptor and induce a conformational change in the ligand binding domain of the steroid hormone receptor. This altered conformation of the receptor promotes the dissociation of the receptor-heat shock protein (HSP) complex, allowing the receptor to interact with deoxyribonucleic acid (DNA), but does not allow a productive association of the receptor and the transcriptional apparatus. Our understanding of the mechanism of action of antiestrogens is the most evolved. Estrogen receptor (ER) contains two distinct transactivation domains: transactivation function 1 (TAF1) at the amino terminus of the receptor and TAF2, contained within the hormone binding domain. In the presence of estrogen, these domains cooperate to produce a productive association of ER with the transcription apparatus. Antihormones are thought to function by disrupting TAF1 or TAF2 cooperativity by inhibiting TAF2 transcriptional activity.[21] Clinically, tamoxifen diminishes serum cholesterol, increases sex hormone–binding globulin,[22] preserves bone density in the lumbar spine,[23] thickens the vaginal epithelium in some patients,[24] and is associated with the enlargement of uterine fibroids, the growth of endometrial polyps, and the development of endometrial neoplastic change. These are all estrogen-like functions. Paradoxically, the same drug is associated with the production of vaginal atrophy, the onset of vasomotor symptoms, and the development of clinical dyspareunia. These are features of estrogen deprivation.

The action of tamoxifen may be organ specific, just as it is known to be species specific in its association with hepatic neoplasia in laboratory animals. When immortalized breast cancer and endometrial cancer cell lines were implanted in athymic mice, both cancers grew well in the same animal. When tamoxifen treatment was given, the breast cancers were inhibited and the endometrial cancers continued to grow.[25] Several investigators have described an increase in the incidence of endometrial cancers among patients with breast cancer who were treated with tamoxifen.[26–28] Killackey and colleagues were the first to report endometrial carcinoma occurring in three breast cancer patients receiving antiestrogens.[28] The strongest initial data implicating tamoxifen use in the subsequent development of endometrial carcinoma were reported by Fornander and colleagues, who reviewed the frequency of new primary cancers in the Swedish Cancer Registry for a group of 1,846 postmenopausal women with early breast cancer.[26] There was a 6.4-fold increase in the relative risk of endometrial cancer in the 931 tamoxifen-treated patients compared with controls. The dose of tamoxifen in this study was 40 mg/d. At doses of 20 mg/d, several investigators with small series have not observed an increased incidence of endometrial cancer. The National Surgical Adjuvant Breast and Bowel Project (NSABP) described observations on 3,863 patients prospectively studied.[27] In the B-14 protocol, 2,843 patients with node-negative, ER-positive breast cancer received either tamoxifen (20 mg/d) or placebo. An additional 1,020 patients taking tamoxifen were registered in this project. The average time in the study was 8 years for the randomized patients and 5 years for the registered patients. Originally, 25 endometrial cancers were reported, but on review, 1 was found to be a sarcoma, and 2 of the cancers developed in women originally assigned to the placebo group, who were ultimately treated with tamoxifen before the discovery of their endometrial cancers. None of the patients who did not receive tamoxifen developed endometrial cancer. This is surprising because the relative risk for endometrial cancer in breast cancer patients is 1.4. The relative risk calculated for the tamoxifen-treated group compared with the placebo group was 7.5, with an annual hazard rate of 0.2 per 1,000 for the placebo group and 1.6 per 1,000 for the randomized tamoxifen-treated group. The distribution of pathologies among the 24 adenocarcinomas was the same as that reported in the National Cancer Institute's Surveillance, Epidemiology, and End Results (SEER) Program data for the years 1983 to 1987.

More recently, in the Breast Cancer Prevention Trial (P-1) of the NSABP, 13,388 women were randomly assigned to receive placebo (6,707) or 20 mg/d of tamoxifen (6,681) for 5 years.[29] Tamoxifen reduced the risk of invasive breast cancer by 49% and of noninvasive breast cancer by 50%. The rate of endometrial carcinoma was increased in the tamoxifen group (risk ratio = 2.53); this increase occurred primarily in women aged 50 years or older. All endometrial carcinomas in the tamoxifen group were stage I, and no endometrial cancer deaths have occurred in this group.

In one report of 15 patients who developed endometrial cancer while exposed to tamoxifen, two-thirds of the patients had histologically virulent tumors. The patients with these tumors were significantly older than the general endometrial cancer patient population, however, and fell into an age group in which sarcomas and nonendometrioid carcinomas are likely to occur more frequently.[30] In several other series of similar size, the distribution of pathology among such patients was no different from that observed in endometrial cancer patients who have not been exposed to tamoxifen.[31] Similarly, Barakat and colleagues, in a retrospective review of 73 patients with a history of breast cancer who subsequently developed endometrial carcinoma, found no significant difference in stage, grade, or histologic subtype.[32]

More recently, studies have focused on the surveillance of breast cancer patients using tamoxifen. Runowicz and colleagues, in a summary analysis of the transvaginal ultrasound and endometrial biopsy data from NSABP (P-1), observed that ultrasonography had a sensitivity of 27% and a specificity of 70%.[33] Of 13 significant biopsies, only 1 showed invasive cancer; the other 12 revealed simple hyperplasia without atypia (9 patients) or complex hyperplasia without atypia (3 patients). The authors did not recommend the substitution of ultrasonography for endometrial biopsy for the assessment of endometrial hyperplasia or carcinoma in this group of patients. A similar prospective longitudinal study in Canada on 304 women with breast cancer receiving tamoxifen found that routine surveillance with ultrasonography was not useful in asymptomatic patients.[34] In another study, Barakat and colleagues evaluated 159 tamoxifen-treated patients by serial office endometrial biopsies obtained at the start of tamoxifen therapy and at 6-month intervals for 2 years, followed by three additional annual biopsies.[35] Although the procedure was feasible, significant pathology requiring hysterectomy was observed in only three patients, and the authors concluded that the utility of routine endometrial biopsy for screening in tamoxifen-treated women is limited. None of these studies provide strong support for screening with ultrasonography or endometrial biopsy. Serial pelvic examinations and prompt evaluation of vaginal bleeding are, given the current data, the reasonable management approach for these patients.

Although a large cohort of women with endometrial carcinoma is noted to have one or more risk factors, the background of hormonal aberration stemming from inappropriate estrogen exposure, either endogenous or exogenous, with all of the attendant typical phenotypes, accounts for no more than 30% of endometrial cancer patients. Historically, this figure was thought to be much higher, and conventional wisdom suggested that women of high parity, lean phenotype, and an unremarkable family history who had not had estrogen replacement therapy and had little intercurrent disease were relatively immune to endometrial cancer. Unfortunately, this is not the case, and many centers are reporting increasing numbers of patients with endometrial cancer who have no recognized risk factors. Such women frequently have more virulent disease (type II) histologically, with implied diminished survival, than do traditional endometrial cancer patients.[36,37]

PATHOLOGY

Endometrial Hyperplasia When Gusberg and colleagues introduced the term "adenomatous hyperplasia" to describe the pattern of hyperplastic glands noted in association with, and often prior to, the development of endometrial adenocarcinoma, they included all of the variants of precursor histology. These ranged from a mild arrangement of densely crowded glands with eosinophilic cytoplasm through the spectrum of more disordered arrangements, with intraluminal tufting, and an increase in mitosis, pseudopalisading, and bizarre nuclei.[38] Hertig and Sommers similarly studied preinvasive changes in the endometrium and described three intensities of abnormality, which they called "adenomatous hyperplasia," "atypical hyperplasia," and "carcinoma in situ."[39] Clinicians were confused because Hertig and Sommers' adenomatous hyperplasia implied a small risk of subsequent transition to cancer, whereas Gusberg and colleagues' adenomatous hyperplasia carried a 15 to 30% risk over time if it was not reversed by therapy.

Kurman and colleagues followed 170 patients with endometrial hyperplasia for a minimum of 1 year; the mean follow-up time was 13.4 years.[40] They established criteria for distinguishing lesions on the basis of architectural abnormalities and cytologic abnormalities. Only 1.6% of patients without cytologic atypia progressed to cancer compared with 23% of those with atypical cytology. Architectural abnormalities were not prognostically important. Table 102-2 presents the details of Kurman and colleagues' classification and observations. Their classification of simple or complex hyperplasia, with or without atypia, is now accepted for describing these lesions.

Table 102-2 Comparison of Follow-Up of 170 Patients with Simple and Complex Hyperplasia and Simple and Complex Atypical Hyperplasia

	No. of Patients	Regressed *n* (%)	Persisted *n* (%)	Progressed to Carcinoma *n* (%)
Simple hyperplasia	93	74 (80)	18 (19)	1 (1)
Complex hyperplasia	29	23 (80)	5 (17)	1 (3)
Simple atypical hyperplasia	13	9 (69)	3 (23)	1 (8)
Complex atypical hyperplasia	35	20 (57)	5 (14)	10 (29)

Adapted from Kurman RJ et al.[40]

Endometrioid Adenocarcinoma Endometrioid adenocarcinoma is the most common of the endometrial cancer histologies. It is characterized by the disappearance of stroma between abnormal glands that have infoldings of their linings into the lumens, disordered nuclear chromatin distribution, nuclear enlargement, and a variable degree of mitosis, necrosis, and hemorrhage. This classic variety accounts for 80 to 95% of the adenocarcinomas.

Adenosquamous Carcinoma Adenosquamous cancer has malignant elements from both its squamous component and its adenomatous component. It usually accounts for 7% or less of the adenocarcinomas of the endometrium. However, in 1974, Reagan described a rising incidence of this entity in the University Hospitals of Cleveland, with adenosquamous cancer making up 20% of the endometrial cancers; these patients had a very poor prognosis.[41] Apparently, this change in the ratio of histologies has not been universal in the United States. The staging convention, now published in the twenty-fifth volume of the *Annual Report*, requires grading of this tumor on the basis of its glandular component and not its squamous component.[2] Although data are still maturing, it is suggested that when this convention is followed, adenosquamous cancer will not behave differently from endometrioid adenocarcinomas of the same stage and grade.

Uterine Papillary Serous Carcinoma Described by Hendrickson and colleagues in 1982, uterine papillary serous carcinoma (UPSC) comprises 5 to 10% of stage I endometrial carcinomas and is characterized by an expansive papillary architecture with a fibrovascular matrix, marked cytologic atypia, bizarre nuclei, and widespread nuclear pleomorphism (Figure 102-1).[42] The features are suggestive of papillary serous cystadenocarcinoma of the ovary. The lesion is highly virulent, usually found with deep myometrial penetration at the time of diagnosis, often extrauterine in location in patients with clinical early-stage disease, and almost always incurable when the disease has spread beyond the uterus. In one series, observations on 15 patients with UPSC were compared with 76 adenocarcinomas and 26 adenocarcinomas with papillary features, all treated in the same institution.[43] At 3 years, 75% of the adenocarcinoma group were alive without disease. For the adenocarcinomas with papillary features, the progression-free interval was 33 months, and for the UPSC group, it was 9 months. In a study of recurrent disease, Lee and Belinson identified 28 recurrences in a series of 227 patients with clinical stage I endometrial carcinoma.[44] Of the 28 patients, 7 had no invasion of the endometrium at the time of diagnosis. Five of these seven patients had histologic characteristics of UPSC, and all died of the disease.

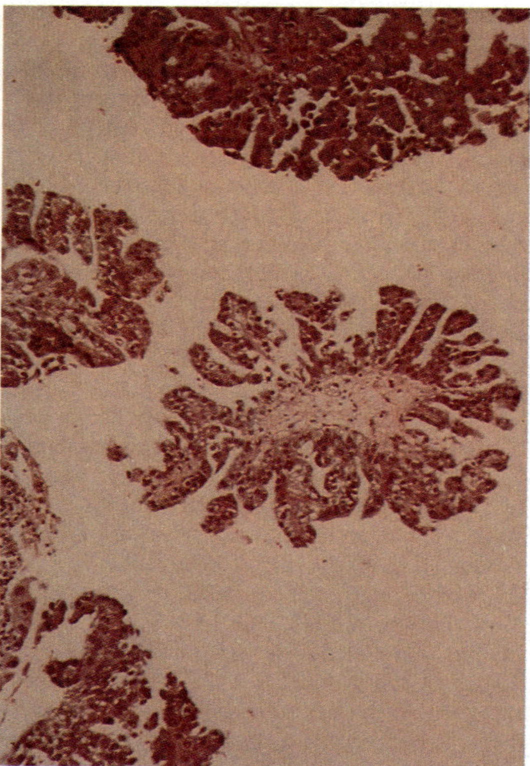

Figure 102-1 Uterine papillary serous carcinoma. Broad stalks supporting papillary fronds, appearing like papillary ovarian carcinoma. Courtesy of Diane Deligdisch, MD, Mount Sinai School of Medicine. A four-color version of the figure is available on the CD-ROM.) [a]Correlation of the Federation Internationale de Gynecologie d'Obstetrique (FIGO), Unio Internationale Contre Cancrum (UICC), and American Joint Committee on Cancer (AJCC) nomenclatures.

Endometrial Papillary Adenocarcinoma Endometrial papillary adenocarcinomas must be distinguished from UPSC because of their different behavior. They are characterized histologically as being usually well-differentiated endometrioid adenocarcinomas composed of very slender papillations, orderly neoplastic epithelial cells, few mitoses, and less cellular disorder than UPSC. The distinction between these two groups has been carefully detailed by Chen and colleagues.[45] The endometrial carcinomas with papillary features behave identically to the endometrioid adenocarcinomas.

Clear Cell Carcinoma Kurman and Scully described clear cell cancers in detail.[46] Histologically, although there are a variety of patterns, a presentation of polygonal or flattened cells with clear cytoplasm accounts for more than half of the cells. This group constitutes approximately 6% of endometrial carcinomas and occurs more frequently in older women. The 5-year overall survival rate is approximately 40%,[47] but this may be a result of the older age of the patients and the fact that clear cell carcinomas are generally found in patients with higher stages of cancer. Clear cells often appear in histologic mixtures when tumors are assigned to a different category on the basis of the prevalent cell type, and their presence usually confers a diminished prognosis.

DIAGNOSIS

The median age for patients with adenocarcinoma of the endometrium is 61 years, with the largest number of women developing their cancers during the sixth decade. Only 5% develop adenocarcinomas before the age of 40 years, and these are usually women with the abnormal syndromes previously discussed. Eighty percent of patients have experienced menopause, and only 20% are diagnosed before they stop menstruating. Irregular or postmenopausal bleeding is the presenting symptom in at least 75% of patients, and at the time of diagnosis, 75% of patients have disease confined to the uterus. Thus, it is obvious that irregular bleeding is a critical symptom, and by explaining it histologically, one has an opportunity to identify endometrial cancer when it is highly curable by relatively uncomplicated therapy.

The traditional technique for diagnosis has been fractional dilation and curettage of the uterus, with careful sampling of both the endometrial cavity and the endocervical canal. Once a procedure for the hospital operating room, this is now performed as an office procedure with greater than 95% accuracy.[48,49] There will always be patients who require general anesthesia in a hospital setting, however, either because of very low pain thresholds, cervical stenosis, or other intercurrent ailments.

Hysteroscopy, either by direct observation or with video-camera amplification, allows direct assessment of the topography of the endometrial cavity with the possibility for more selective sampling and the assurance of not missing any occult lesions. Many reserve this procedure as an accompaniment to formal dilation and curettage under anesthesia. However, caution should be exercised because hysteroscopic dissemination of malignant cells has been described in the literature.[50,51]

Noninvasive radiographic imaging techniques, such as magnetic resonance imaging[52] and ultrasonography,[53] are not cost-effective for screening. However, these techniques can achieve an accuracy rate above 80%, accurately measure disease volume, and, on the basis of grade of tumor and volume of disease, predict probabilities of extrauterine spread of tumor.

Table 102-3 Definitions of the Clinical Stages in Carcinoma of the Corpus Uteri*

Stage 0	Atypical endometrial hyperplasia, carcinoma in situ. Histologic findings are suspicious of malignancy. Cases of stage 0 should not be included in any therapeutic statistics.
Stage I	The carcinoma is confined to the corpus.
Stage IA	The length of the uterine cavity is 8 cm or less.
Stage IB	The length of the uterine cavity is more than 8 cm.
Stage II	The carcinoma has involved the corpus and the cervix, but has not extended outside the uterus.

*Correlation of the Federation Internationale de Gynecologie d'Obstetrique (FIGO), Unio Internationale Contre Cancrum (UICC), and American Joint Committee on Cancer (AJCC) nomenclatures.

STAGING

Historically, endometrial cancer staging was a clinical exercise, based on physical examination, noninvasive radiographic testing, and measurement of the depth of the uterine cavity. One can see from Table 102-3 that clinical staging for those with a large uterus very likely would be inaccurate and would lead to understaging, and possibly undertreating, a significant proportion of the stage I cancers. When tumor grade was identified as an important prognostic feature, many therapists argued for a staging system that would permit consideration of the histologic prognostic variables because a biopsy or curettage was required even to make the diagnosis. In 1971, tumor grade was officially incorporated into the staging system. During this same era, the Gynecologic Oncology Group (GOG) inaugurated a pilot study to perform staging laparotomy in the course of initial surgical treatment of patients with clinical stage I endometrial carcinoma.[54] This study noted that 16 of 140 patients evaluated had cancer in their lymph nodes, despite the fact that they had early-stage disease by preoperative clinical evaluation. In a subsequent expansion of this pilot study, it was noted that 9.6% of 843 patients in clinical stage I had lymph node metastasis.[55] In addition, extensive surgical staging detects extrauterine disease in 23.2% of patients with apparent preoperative clinical stage I disease.[56] These observations strengthened the impetus for more precise staging, and in 1988, the International Federation of Gynecology and Obstetrics (FIGO) introduced the requirement for surgical staging of patients with endometrial carcinoma.

Tables 102-4 and 102-5 present the latest modifications of the surgical staging system, which were promulgated in 1994 and 1995. This system requires the performance of total abdominal hysterectomy, bilateral salpingo-oophorectomy, washings for cytologic examination, lymph node sampling from the pelvic and para-aortic lymph nodes for those patients whose histology and depth of myometrial penetration (determined during the operation) are other than well-differentiated tumors with minimal myometrial penetration, and biopsies of any suspicious areas. Employing the updated FIGO staging system, a recent report described disease-free survival as 90% for stage I, 83% for stage II, and 43% for stage III.[57] When surgical staging is completed, it becomes the strongest predictor of survival. Univariate analysis reveals that the 5-year survival rate for patients in surgical stage IA is 93.8%; in stage IB, 95.4%; and in stage IC, 75%.[58]

The adoption of a surgical staging system has created controversy regarding what constitutes an adequate staging procedure, which patients should be surgically staged, and whether extensive staging or lymphadenectomy has therapeutic value.[56] Recent studies have helped provide answers to these questions. Current data indicate that retroperitoneal palpation contributes little toward accurate retroperitoneal evaluation, particularly in obese patients.[55,59] Also, selective sampling on the basis of nodal enlargement does not appear to be effective, given that nearly half of the diagnosed lymph node metastases in one study occurred in nodes that were less than 1 cm.[60] Selective pelvic and para-aortic lymphadenectomy refers to removal or biopsy of some but not all lymph nodes within the external iliac, internal iliac, obturator, hypogastric, and common iliac groups, as well as the para-aortic groups.[61] Adverse risk factors necessitating lymph node dissection include grade 2 or 3 lesions with > 50% myoinvasion; clear cell, papillary serous, squamous, and undifferentiated cell types; adnexal metastasis; lymph–vascular space invasion and/or cervical invasion; > 50% of uterine cavity involved; and suspicious nodes.[62]

Several investigators have described the therapeutic benefit of node dissection.[59,63,64] Most recently, Trimble and colleagues reported on the impact of pelvic node sampling in 10,066 women with stage I and II endometrioid adenocarcinomas from the SEER Program.[65] They found an improved 5-year relative survival only in patients

Table 102-4 Staging for Corpus Uteri Carcinoma

FIGO Stage*	
I	Tumor confined to corpus uteri.
IA	Tumor limited to endometrium.
IB	Tumor invades up to or less than one half of the myometrium.
IC	Tumor invades to more than one half of the myometrium.
II	Tumor invades cervix, but does not extend beyond uterus.
IIA	Endocervical glandular involvement only.
IIB	Cervical stromal invasion.
III	Local and/or regional spread as specified in T3a, T3b, N1, and FIGO IIIA, IIIB, and IIIC below.
IIIA	Tumor involves serosa and/or adnexa (direct extension or metastasis) and/or cancer cells in ascites or peritoneal washings.
IIIB	Vaginal involvement (direct extension or metastasis).
IIIC	Metastasis to the pelvic and/or paraaortic lymph nodes.
IVA	Tumor invades bladder mucosa and/or bowel mucosa.
IVB	Distant metastasis. (*Excluding* metastasis to vagina, pelvic serosa, or adnexa. *Including* metastasis to intraabdominal lymph nodes other than paraaortic and/or inguinal lymph nodes.)

*Each staging category is subdivided into histologic grade 1, 2, or 3.

Table 102-5 Histopathology: Degree of Differentiation

G1:	5% or less of a nonsquamous or nonmorular solid growth pattern.
G2:	6% to 50% of a nonsquamous or nonmorular solid growth pattern.
G3:	More than 50% of a nonsquamous or nonmorular solid growth pattern.

with stage I, grade 3 tumors. However, data on adjuvant postsurgical treatment were not available in this population. Some centers routinely perform pelvic lymphadenectomy in all patients with endometrial cancer.[66,67]

PROGNOSTIC FACTORS

In a GOG study, 1,180 patients with clinical stage I or II endometrial carcinomas were studied by surgical-pathologic staging.[68] Of this group, 895 patients were evaluable for all of the parameters derived from surgical staging, as well as for follow-up from postoperative treatment to recurrence, with documentation of recurrence site. From this experience and the other previously cited interim GOG reports of surgical staging outcome, one can appreciate those factors that are predictive of extrauterine spread of disease at the time of initial diagnosis and those factors that correlate with ultimate survival.

Surgical stage and age are highly significant prognostic features that maintain their significance in each of the analyses performed in the various reports.

Histologic Type Whereas 80 to 95% of endometrial cancers are classic endometrioid adenocarcinomas, the remainder constitute a series of histologic types with a more unfavorable prognosis. These include serous papillary adenocarcinoma and clear cell, undifferentiated, and squamous cancers. These cell types confer an unfavorable prognosis, independent of other known prognostic factors.[69]

Tumor Grade Within classic endometrioid adenocarcinomas, tumor grade is highly significant as an independent prognostic factor. Additionally, numerous studies have demonstrated that, in general, there is a greater tendency for the less differentiated tumors to be associated with other poor prognostic factors, including deep myometrial penetration, vascular space invasion, and increasing stage.[68,70,71] Recently, Salvesen and colleagues showed that morphometric nuclear grade was a stronger prognostic factor than subjective histologic grade.[72] Further studies are needed to confirm the significance of these findings.

Myometrial Invasion The depth of myometrial penetration is a very important independent prognostic factor for outcome in stage I disease. Deeper penetration is associated with higher probabilities of tumor recurrence and death.[68,70,73] Although increasing depth of invasion correlates with increasing grade of tumor, depth appears to be a more significant prognostic factor and predicts for the presence of extrauterine disease as detected at surgical staging procedures.[55] Regardless of grade, however, only 1% of patients with disease confined to the endometrium have extrauterine disease compared with patients with deep muscle invasion, for which the incidence of pelvic node invasion rises to 17% and para-aortic nodal involvement rises to 25%.[55] DiSaia and colleagues found that patients with only endometrial involvement had an 8% recurrence rate compared with 12% if there was superficial or intermediate myometrial invasion versus 46% if there was involvement of the outer third of the myometrium.[73]

Both relative and absolute measures of the degree of myometrial invasion have been used. Although it is clear from a number of studies that involvement of the uterine serosa is an extremely bad prognostic sign,[74] some difficulties arise in attempting to compare reports with absolute distances from the serosa versus those with relative degrees of penetration into muscle because the thickness of the myometrium varies from patient to patient. The current FIGO staging classification requires uterine thickness to be measured as less than or greater than invasion of 50% of the myometrial thickness.

Capillary–Lymphatic Space Invasion Vascular space invasion is a significant risk factor for recurrence, but it is not as important as the grade and depth of myometrial penetration. Approximately 15% of endometrial adenocarcinomas invade capillary-like spaces.[55,75] There is a significantly increased probability of pelvic and para-aortic lymph node invasion when this happens. Where the capillary-like spaces are involved, pelvic and para-aortic lymph nodes are also involved in 27 and 19% of cases, respectively, representing about a fivefold increase over those without such involvement.[55]

Positive Peritoneal Cytology The presence of positive peritoneal cytology in washings is associated with an increased risk of relapse.[68] Approximately 15% of patients have positive peritoneal cytology,[68] and this is often related to other poor prognostic factors, such as high grade or deep myometrial penetration. Thus, it is not surprising that it is also associated with an increased risk of metastases to pelvic and para-aortic lymph nodes. Opinions and data in the literature conflict with respect to interpreting the independent prognostic significance of peritoneal cytology. Approximately 5% of patients with positive peritoneal cytology have no evidence of extrauterine disease,[55] but approximately one-third of patients with extrauterine disease do have positive cytology.

Unfortunately, no study has correlated the sites of relapse with the presence or absence of positive peritoneal cytology. That positive cytology, independent of other negative prognostic features, conferred a worse prognosis would be more convincing if one could associate an increased risk of peritoneal and upper abdominal relapse in patients with positive cytology compared with those without. Three large series suggest that positive peritoneal cytology may be a poor independent prognostic factor,[76–78] but several small series and one review reported that there are no outcome differences between those with positive peritoneal cytology and those without.[79–81]

Race Liu and colleagues reviewed the treatment patterns, risk factors, and survival of 219 patients treated surgically for endometrial cancer between 1990 and 1993.[82] In this study, black women, when compared with white women, had a higher incidence of unfavorable histology (38% vs 12%), advanced-stage disease (51% vs 19%), poor differentiation (49% vs 18%), and poor survival. There was no difference between the onset of bleeding and hysterectomy in the two groups. Even when corrected for hormone use, these differences persisted. From this study, it may be concluded that black women face a poorer prognosis for survival from endometrial cancer than do their white counterparts.

Hormone Receptor Status The presence of cytoplasmic ER- and progesterone receptor (PR)-binding proteins has been quantitatively associated with better histologic differentiation,[83] favorable histologic subtype, and response to therapy.[84–86]

Ligand binding to ER and PR was higher in well-differentiated lesions and was significantly lower in grade 3 lesions and the nonendometrioid carcinomas.[86] Alterations in receptor expression, receptor assembly and activation, response element recognition, and/or receptor degradation are among the possible explanations for loss of hormone binding. In addition, recent evidence suggests that promoter site hypermethylation might account in part for the loss of ER.[87] Likewise, differential expression of the PR-alpha (PRA) and PR-beta (PRB) have been reported.[88] PRA appears to down-regulate ER action and PRB is the primary activator of the progesterone responsive gene, and the loss of either would theoretically result in an unopposed estrogen effect. Clinically, reduced levels of ligand interaction with the ER, PR, or both in endometrial cancer samples significantly ($p < .01$) correlate with recurrence and death from disease.[85,86]

Tumor Ploidy and Kinetics Although tumor ploidy in endometrial cancer has been widely studied, the results are conflicting. Approximately 65% of these cancers are determined to be diploid by flow cytometry. In general, diploid patterns occur in the better differentiated tumors. In one study, flow cytometry measurements of ribonucleic acid, S-phase fraction, DNA index, and proliferative index were conducted on the tissues from 140 specimens.[89] Only in 19% of patients was advanced disease predicted on the basis of clinical evaluation. However, 40% of patients with advanced disease were found to be aneuploid, 69% had a high S-phase fraction, and 69% had a proliferative index greater than 14%.[89]

The nuclear Ki-67 antigen, which is expressed in all stages of the cell cycle except G_0, may be detected by immunohistochemistry to estimate the proliferative activity in tumors. Salvesen and colleagues observed that Ki-67 expression was significantly higher among patients with FIGO stage III or IV disease, clear cell or serous papillary histology types, and poor histologic grade.[90] Ki-67 expression was significantly related to survival.

Refinements of this approach may hold great promise for prognostic assessment.

ONCOGENE ACTIVATION AND LOSS OF TUMOR SUPPRESSOR FUNCTION

The molecular events involved in the pathogenesis of endometrial carcinoma are poorly defined; however, several aspects of the molecular pathology of this disease were recently elucidated. Mutations in the *TP53* tumor suppressor gene leading to overexpression of mutant TP53 protein are the most common molecular alterations described in human cancers to date.[91] Between 4 and 49% of endometrioid carcinomas[91–102] and between 71.4 and 100% of serous carcinomas[95,97,100,103–105] overexpress TP53 protein. Of note, TP53 protein overexpression has been demonstrated in 10 to 15% of early-stage disease[91,104,106] and in 40 to 50% of advanced-stage disease[91,94] but does not occur in endometrial hyperplasia.[91,97,98] This suggests that *TP53* mutation may be a late event in the histogenesis of endometrial carcinoma[91,97,98] or that acquisition of a *TP53* mutation leads to the development of a virulent endometrial cancer that does not pass through a phase of hyperplasia, as postulated by Berchuck and colleagues.[107] Several studies demonstrated a positive association between TP53 overexpression and high nuclear grade[93,95,108–110] and FIGO stage,[94] although these have not been universal findings.[102,108,110] In addition, overexpression of TP53 is independently associated with poor survival.[94,95,111] For example, Kohler and colleagues observed a median survival of 6.1 years in patients whose tumors did not overexpress TP53 in comparison with a median survival of 1.4 years in patients whose tumors overexpressed TP53.[94]

The ras family of G proteins (N, H, K-ras) plays a critical role in the regulation of cellular proliferation.[107] The most frequent site of mutation of the K-*ras* oncogene in endometrial carcinoma is codon 12. K-*ras* mutations have been identified in both complex atypical hyperplasia[112] and invasive carcinoma. However, there does not appear to be a significant relationship between K-*ras* mutation and survival in endometrial cancer.[113–116]

The *HER2/neu* gene encodes for a tyrosine kinase receptor that forms heterodimers with HER3 or HER4 and is then activated following binding of the ligand heregulin.[117] Several studies suggest that this oncogene product is overexpressed in 10 to 15% of endometrial cancers.[117–122] Hetzel and colleagues, in an immunohistochemical analysis of 247 patients with endometrial cancer, observed strong staining in 37 patients (15%), mild staining in 144 (58%), and no staining in 66 (27%) patients.[119] The 5-year progression-free survival rate was 56% for the strong staining, 83% for the mild staining, and 95% for the nonstaining groups. Strong overexpression was associated with a poor (51%) overall survival. Likewise, Lukes and colleagues found high expression in 12% of patients.[118] Overexpression was more common in stage III and IV patients (24%) than in stage I or II patients (6%) and was associated with poor progression-free survival in univariate analysis. However, in multivariate analysis, *HER2/neu* was found to be an independent variable only if DNA ploidy was excluded from the statistical model.

PTEN (phosphate and tensin homolog deleted on chromosome 10) is a candidate tumor suppressor gene that has been isolated from the 10q23-24 region, possesses growth inhibitory functions, and appears to be differentially expressed in endometrial cancers.[92,123] In fact, the frequency of *PTEN* mutations described by several investigators is several-fold higher than that described for any other gene mutated in endometrial cancers, including K-*ras* and *TP53,* making the *PTEN* mutation the most common defined genetic alteration identified to date in endometrial cancers.[123,124] *PTEN* mutations are infrequent in nonendometrioid endometrial cancers but appear to be relatively common in the endometrioid subtype and are associated with early-stage, nonmetastatic disease and more favorable survival.[124] Furthermore, although *PTEN* mutations were not detected in normal endometrium, Mutter and colleagues identified mutations in 55% of precursor lesions and 87% of endometrioid carcinomas.[123] These observations suggest that *PTEN* mutations may play an early role in carcinogenesis, at least in type I endometrioid endometrial carcinomas.

Microsatellite instability is one of the major mechanisms of cancer susceptibility and has been identified in 17 to 43% of endometrial carcinomas.[92,103,125,126] Microsatellite instability was initially noted in colorectal patients with hereditary nonpolyposis colorectal cancer (HNPCC). Risinger and colleagues observed microsatellite instability in 17% of sporadic endometrial carcinomas and in 75% of those associated with HNPCC.[125] Of note, the sporadic endometrial carcinomas displaying microsatellite instability were all stage I adenocarcinomas with diploid or near-diploid DNA content, indicating that these tumors are from clinical type I patients.[117,125]

Table 102-6 Clinical and Molecular Features of Endometrial Carcinoma

Features	Type I	Type II
Clinical[37]		
Risk factors	Unopposed estrogen	Age
Race	White > black	White = black
Degree of differentiation	Well differentiated	Poorly differentiated
Histology	Endometrioid	Nonendometrioid
Stage	I/II	III/IV
Prognosis	Favorable	Unfavorable
Molecular[107]		
Ploidy	Diploid	Aneuploid
K-*ras* overexpression	Yes	Yes
HER2/neu overexpression	No	Yes
TP53 overexpression	No	Yes
PTEN mutations	Yes	No
Microsatellite instability	Yes	No

In a case-control study by Prasad and colleagues, tamoxifen and non–tamoxifen-associated endometrial carcinomas arising in women with breast cancer demonstrated genetic alterations (*PTEN*, K-*ras*, *TP53*, *CTNNB1*, and microsatellite instability) similar to those of sporadic endometrial carcinomas.[127]

Deligdisch and Holinka classified endometrial carcinoma into type 1, which is associated with unopposed estrogen, good differentiation, endometrioid histology, early stage, and favorable prognosis, and type II, which is associated with older age, poor differentiation, nonendometrioid histology, advanced stage, and an unfavorable prognosis.[36,37] The studies discussed above suggest that this clinical classification can be expanded to include molecular features associated with type 1 and type II endometrial carcinomas. Table 102-6 illustrates these molecular features.

TREATMENT OF PRIMARY DISEASE

Surgery The initial surgical staging procedure, outlined earlier (see Table 102-4), is the standard therapeutic procedure as well. When there is disease outside the uterus and in the retroperitoneal nodes, there is no reason to believe that aggressive cytoreductive efforts might not help in presenting a reduced tumor burden during adjunctive therapy, despite the absence of a clinical trial suggesting efficacy.

There are occasions when, at the time of staging laparotomy, cervical or parametrial invasion is detected and a radical (Wertheim) hysterectomy with pelvic and aortic lymphadenectomy is performed to achieve clearance of all disease. However, the addition of tailored external beam RT following surgery has largely eliminated the routine performance of such procedures.

Surgery for recurrent disease is generally confined to those patients who have symptoms of intestinal or urinary tract obstruction, isolated regional recurrence, or isolated lung metastases that have not responded to cytotoxic or hormonal therapy. For such patients, surgery may be useful to correct functional deficits or to excise isolated recurrences or resistant metastatic deposits.

The first reports of surgical staging of endometrial carcinoma with the use of laparoscopy-assisted vaginal hysterectomy and laparoscopic lymphadenectomy were in 1992.[128,129] Since then, several reports have included laparoscopic bilateral para-aortic lymph node dissections.[130] However, no randomized clinical trials have been completed that compare laparoscopic management of endometrial carcinoma with traditional surgical therapy. The GOG is currently conducting a prospective phase III study comparing laparoscopy-assisted surgical staging with traditional total abdominal hysterectomy and staging. In addition to assessing variables such as completeness of surgical staging, complications, operating room time, and hospital stay, this study will also evaluate expanded outcome variables, including patient-reported measures of quality of life. Single-institution retrospective data have demonstrated that laparoscopic lymphadenectomy and vaginal or laparoscopic hysterectomy with bilateral salpingo-oophorectomy provided 5-year survival and recurrence rates similar to those of the traditional abdominal approach.[131–133]

Figure 102-2 presents an algorithm for the surgical management of endometrial carcinoma.

Radiation Therapy Although surgery, where possible, constitutes the definitive treatment for most patients with endometrial carcinoma, it is clear that RT is the second most effective modality in its management. An understanding of the patterns of failure following surgery alone and knowing the sites of occult extrauterine disease with clinical stage I and stage II endometrial cancer have provided a better understanding of the settings in which adjuvant treatment, such as RT, hormone therapy, or chemotherapy, should be tested in future clinical trials.

Definitive Irradiation for Inoperable Patients Modern surgical techniques and improved postoperative care have diminished the number of patients considered inoperable. Nevertheless, because endometrial cancer is frequently a disease of the elderly (over 65 years of age), who are often obese and sometimes diabetic, with other intercurrent ailments, surgery is not always possible. Table 102-7 shows five relatively large series in which patients received pelvic RT as their definitive management without initial surgery.[134–139]

Table 102-7 Primary Radiotherapy as Definitive Management of Inoperable Clinical Stage I Cancer of the Endometrium

Study	Patients	Complication, %	3-Year DFS %	5-Year DFS, %	5-Year Survival
Abayomi et al, 1982[136]	39	15	*	—	—
Varia et al, 1987[134]	41†	10	72	57*†‡	—
Grisby et al, 1987[135]	69	16	—	88	77
Rose et al, 1993[137]	17	—	71		—
Fishman et al, 1996[138]	39	—	20	§	80

DFS = disease-free survival.
*3-year survival rate of stage I and II cancer = 78%.
†Results by grade: 1, 72%; 2, 59%; 3, 31%.
‡Significant number (12 of 28) died of unrelated causes.
§Median disease-free interval = 36 months.

The proportion surviving depends on tumor grade, just as for patients treated surgically; those with grade 1 tumors have better survival rates than do those with grade 3.[134] Significant numbers of patients die of causes unrelated to their primary carcinoma. In the case-control series (2 controls per case matched for age, stage, and grade) from Yale University, more deaths from intercurrent disease occurred within the inoperable stage I group than with the operable group (28 of 32 vs 3 of 15; $p < .0001$). Inoperable patients had a significantly shorter overall survival and more deaths owing to intercurrent disease than operable patients ($p < .0001$). However, inoperable patients who did not die from intercurrent disease had a median 5-year survival rate that approached that of operable patients.[138]

Some patients with small uteri may have their disease adequately irradiated by intracavitary radiation only, but, usually, definitive management consists of both external beam and intracavitary irradiation because of more favorable radiation dosimetry. Complication rates are acceptable (usually less than 10%). After definitive irradiation, the pattern of failure, in contrast to that following surgery, consists mainly of central failure in the uterus. This observation is important for developing treatment strategies for patients with stage II disease. Removal of the uterus at some point in treatment provides better overall central control than that achieved by radiation alone. Three series indicate 5-year survival rates of approximately 50%.[134,140,141]

Recently, Kucera and colleagues reported their experience with high-dose iridium 192 intracavitary brachytherapy without additional external beam radiation in 228 patients.[142] At 5 years, the overall survival rate was 59.7%. In clinical stage IA disease, the survival rate was 88.6% at 5 years and 82.7% at 10 years—significantly different in comparison with 80.2% and 63.4%, respectively, in stage IB disease. Intrauterine recurrence was 17.5%, but extrauterine pelvic relapse occurred in only 0.4% of patients. Others have also reported high–dose-rate brachytherapy with or without external beam radiation,[143,144] and the American Brachytherapy Society published guidelines and recommendations in 2000.[145]

Adjuvant RT for Clinical Stage I Disease For the majority of patients who are medically operable, RT plays an adjuvant role. It is important to distinguish between patients with clinical stage I disease, for whom decisions for postoperative adjuvant therapy are made on the probability of extrauterine diseases being present, and those with FIGO stage I or surgical stage I cancer, in whom surgery and pathology have excluded extrauterine disease.

Adjuvant RT has been used in the past in clinical stage I disease for patients believed to be at high risk of relapse following bilateral salpingo-oophorectomy and hysterectomy. Historically, most patients with endometrial cancer received preoperative intracavitary irradiation or postoperative vault irradiation, but the use of external beam irradiation was reserved for those considered at high risk.

The present recommendation to give postoperative RT in clinical stage I is dependent on prognosis as defined by the histologic features of the primary tumor within the endometrium. Extensive staging studies have identified that several of the aforementioned factors predict for the presence of clinically occult extrauterine disease.[68]

Although patients considered to be at high risk of recurrence (eg, those with grade 2 or 3 disease with penetration of the outer 50% of the myometrium) have generally been treated with postoperative adjuvant RT, only two randomized trials have examined its contribution to outcome.

Aalders and colleagues reported that 540 patients with clinical stage I endometrial cancer were treated by total abdominal hysterectomy and bilateral salpingo-oophorectomy (TAH-BSO) and 60 Gy to the vaginal vault postoperatively.[70] Patients were then randomized to either no further therapy or external beam pelvic radiation at a dose of 40 Gy in 20 fractions over 4 weeks. The dose to the midline was minimized with a midline block introduced at a tumor dose of 20 Gy. Approximately half of the patients (261) were considered to be in the high-risk category, with greater than 50% myometrial penetration of any

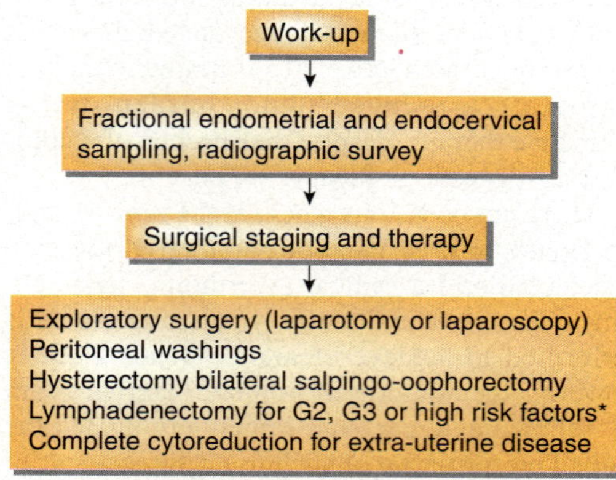

Figure 102-2 Surgical management of endometrial carcinoma.

grade or grade 3 tumors with any degree of invasion. The study showed no improvement in overall survival, death, or recurrence rates for the whole group. Pelvic relapse rates were reduced by approximately 60% in the high-risk group, however. A separate subset analysis of the high-risk patients suggested a survival benefit of approximately 12%.

Recently, the Post Operative Radiation Therapy in Endometrial Carcinoma (PORTEC) trial reported on 741 patients with clinical stage IB, grade 2 to 3 cancer and stage IC, grade 1 to 2 cancer who were randomized to pelvic RT versus no additional treatment (NAT) after TAH-BSO but no lymph node assessment.[146] There was a significant reduction in locoregional recurrence in the RT cohort (4% vs 14%; $p < .001$) but no improvement in overall survival (81% vs 85%; $p = .31$). Treatment-related complications occurred in 25% of RT patients and in 6% of the controls ($p < .0001$).

The majority of patients with clinical stage I endometrial cancer have low-grade tumors with less than 50% myometrial penetration (stage IA and B, grade 1 and 2). Estimates from careful GOG clinical pathologic staging studies suggest that the risk of extrauterine disease in these low-risk patients is probably less than 7% and that overall outcome is unlikely to be improved by the addition of pelvic irradiation.[55] Thus, there would appear to be no data to support the use of any adjuvant irradiation in patients with low-risk clinical stage I disease.

For intermediate-risk disease (stage IB, grade 3; stage IC, grade 1 and 2), omitting RT would leave the patients with a significant risk of vaginal and pelvic relapse. Recent data suggest that vaginal brachytherapy might reduce the risk of vaginal relapse with less morbidity and a better quality of life. This is the rationale for the currently undergoing PORTEC-2 trial randomizing between pelvic RT and vaginal brachytherapy.[146]

Indications for Adjuvant Therapy for Patients with Surgical Stage I Within the sensitivity of the surgical staging procedure, patients with pathologically proven stage I disease have no evidence of extrauterine disease. The indications for adjuvant RT in this circumstance are not settled, and the best data come from the only randomized study, which was conducted by the GOG. Patients with negative extrauterine findings but high-risk factors in the uterus have been designated by the GOG as at intermediate risk based on the surgical staging study GOG 33 as stage IB, IC, IIA, and IIB (occult).[68] The GOG recently reported the results of a phase III randomized trial (GOG 99) of NAT versus 5,040 cGy of pelvic RT in patients with intermediate-risk endometrial cancer defined by the GOG 33. A high–intermediate-risk (HIR) subgroup of patients was defined (as an increased recurrent rate of 25% at 5 years based on GOG 33) as those with (1) moderately to poorly differentiated tumor, the presence of lymphovascular invasion, and outer third myometrial invasion; (2) age 50 years or greater with any two of the risk factors listed above; or (3) age of at least 70 years with any risk factor listed above. All other eligible participants were considered to be in the low–intermediate-risk (LIR) subgroup. The median follow-up for the study was 69 months. Three hundred ninety-two women met all eligibility requirements (202 NAT, 190 RT). The median follow-up was 69 months. In the entire study population, there were 44 recurrences and 66 deaths (32 disease or treatment-related deaths), and the estimated 2-year cumulative incidence of recurrence was 12% in the NAT arm and 3% in the RT arm (relative hazard [RH]: 0.42; $p = .007$). The treatment difference was particularly evident among the HIR subgroup (2-year cumulative incidence of recurrence in NAT vs RT: 26% vs 6%; RH = 0.42). Overall, radiation had a substantial impact on pelvic and vaginal recurrences (18 in NAT and 3 in RT). The estimated 4-year survival rate was 86% in the NAT arm and 92% for the RT arm, which is not significantly different (RH: 0.86; $p = .557$). This HIR subgroup represented about one-third of the patients (132 of 392) and accounted for nearly two-thirds of the recurrences (28) and two-thirds of the cancer-related deaths. The conclusions were that adjunctive RT in early-stage intermediate-risk endometrial carcinoma decreases the risk of recurrence but should be limited to patients whose risk factors fit a high–intermediate-risk definition.[147]

Vault Irradiation The rationale for administering pelvic RT in GOG 99 was to prevent vaginal vault recurrences and to sterilize occult pelvic side wall disease, presumably not excised at surgery. Other occult pelvis side wall disease not found at surgery, such as in the lymphatic channels in the parametrium or in parametrial lymph nodes, occurs infrequently and is an unlikely source of recurrence. Thus, on a theoretic basis, the patient who undergoes thorough staging, ideally with a bilateral pelvic and lower para-aortic lymphadenectomy, might be at low risk of a pelvic side wall recurrence in the absence of lymph node metastasis. This side wall disease, when undetected and untreated, likely would contribute to preventable mortality for this patient population. The major site for possible recurrence within the pelvis for these patients would be the vaginal vault, which is amenable to irradiation with either low– or high–dose-rate applicators with a high probability of local control and, presumably, cure.[148] Growing support of this hypothesis has been published in retrospective studies, which have demonstrated rare pelvic recurrences in high-risk patients (stage IB, grade 3 and stage IC) who undergo therapeutic pelvic lymphadenectomy and either no RT[149] or vault brachytherapy[66] alone in the absence of lymph node metastasis.

In the study from Manitoba, a cohort of 53 surgical stage IC patients were treated with high–dose-rate vaginal brachytherapy after 1995 and compared with a historical cohort of 69 surgical stage IC patients treated at the same center prior to 1995 with pelvic RT and low–dose-rate vaginal brachytherapy. The recurrence rate in the substage IC group spared whole-pelvis RT was 5.7% (3 of 53) compared with 7.2% (5 of 69) for stage IC patients treated with pelvic RT and vault brachytherapy. The authors suggested that whole-pelvis RT can be safely omitted in patients with FIGO stage IC endometrial cancer if nodal status is known.[67]

In another series from Cleveland, Mohan and colleagues reported on a cohort of 28 surgical stage IC patients treated with low-dose brachytherapy after complete surgical staging, including therapeutic pelvic lymphadenectomy, with a median follow-up of 8 years.[66] The 10-year disease-free survival rate was 92%, and the 10-year overall survival was 96%.

Chadha and colleagues reported on the therapeutic efficacy of high–dose-rate vaginal vault brachytherapy alone for 38 surgical stage I patients with high-risk features (12 patients had stage IB, grade 3; 14 had stage IC, grade 1; 9 had stage IC, grade 2; and 3 had stage IC, grade 3).[150] The median follow-up was 30 months. No patient has developed a vaginal or pelvic recurrence. Three patients developed tumor recurrence in the upper abdomen at 11, 18, and 37 months. The 5-year actuarial overall survival and disease-free survival rates are 93 and 87%, respectively. No treatment-related grade 3 or 4 morbidity was observed. The conclusion was that patients with surgical stage IB, grade 3 and stage IC cancer achieved excellent local control and minimal morbidity with the selective use of vaginal brachytherapy alone. Other data have been published on the use of vault irradiation without full staging in patients with low-risk disease.[151]

Stage III The 1988 FIGO surgical staging for endometrial cancer now includes patients with metastases to pelvic and/or para-aortic lymph nodes as stage IIIC. The current staging classification covers a broad spectrum of prognostic groups that have diverse outcomes after standard surgery with or without adjuvant pelvic irradiation. Unfortunately, many of the published series include patients with microscopic extension to the adnexa (stage IIIA), those with malignant ascites (stage IIIA), and those with gross pelvic side wall disease (stage IIIA or IIIC) without distinction, resulting in widely variable survival data. In a series reported by Grigsby and colleagues, the 5-year progression-free survival rate for 22 patients treated with radiation alone was 42%.[152] Aalders and colleagues reported a 5-year survival rate of 40% for patients with surgical or pathologic stage III disease compared with 16% for patients with clinical stage III disease.[153] Similarly, Bruckman and colleagues and Mackillop and Pringle reported 5-year survival rates of 80 to 85% when only the ovary and/or fallopian tube was involved compared with 15% when other extrauterine pelvic structures were affected.[154,155] Because patients with occult adnexal involvement as the only site of extrauterine disease were often treated with pelvic irradiation, it is impossible to know whether and in what proportion patients with adnexal spread were cured with surgery alone and whether they have a propensity for upper abdominal disease, such as primary ovarian cancers, and could benefit from wider-field irradiation.

It is impossible to conclude from the literature what the optimal therapy is for various sites of

Table 102-8 Results of Para-Aortic Radiotherapy in Endometrial Cancer

Study	Complication, %	*n*	NED, %	RT Dose, Gy
Hicks et al, 1993[159]	11*	4	36	45
Rose et al, 1992[63]	26	9	35	45
Komaki et al, 1983[160]	—	7	60	50
Feuer and Calanog, 1987[161]	18	8	44	50
Corn et al, 1992[162]		50†	46	48
Potish et al, 1985[163]	—	48	52	48
Morrow et al, 1991[68]	—	48	20	40

NED = no evidence of disease; RT = radiation therapy.
*Three of 17 with macroscopic disease.
†Twenty-four of 50 para-aortic nodes diagnosed on radiography.

disease within stage III. Different observers have employed surgery and radiation, alone or in combination. Greven and colleagues reported the results of therapy for 52 patients with clinical stage III disease with protracted median survival rates for those undergoing both radiation and surgery compared with those treated with radiation alone.[156] Survival rates of approximately 27% have been reported in small groups of patients with stage III disease.[157,158]

Treatment recommendations at this time for patients with stage III disease must be made on an ad hoc basis. Those in whom appropriate surgical staging has been completed without evidence of disease beyond the ovaries should be considered for adjuvant postoperative pelvic irradiation, although the importance of microscopic adnexal invasion in patients without other risk factors is unclear. For those who have had surgical staging and who have pelvic but not para-aortic nodal involvement, it may be appropriate to offer postoperative adjuvant irradiation confined to the pelvis. Disease-free survival rates between 35 and 60% have been reported for patients receiving 45 to 50 Gy of external beam irradiation to the para-aortic nodes, usually with pelvic irradiation. In almost no case is macroscopic para-aortic nodal disease curable with RT without complete cytoreduction first.[63,68,159–163] Retrospective data from Johns Hopkins Hospital suggest that in patients with stage IIIC endometrial carcinoma, complete resection of macroscopic nodal disease and the administration of adjuvant chemotherapy, in addition to directed RT, are associated with improved survival (Table 102-8).[164]

For patients with gross parametrial or side wall disease at presentation, cure rates are usually less than 10 to 15%.[153,165] These patients are usually treated with RT alone, and if disease shrinkage is total or the residuum is only in the uterus, it may be worthwhile to complete a hysterectomy if residual disease can be removed completely. However, in a series of 101 patients with clinical stage III disease treated at the Norwegian Radium Hospital, 66 received radiation alone and 35 received combined surgery and irradiation.[153] The overall 5-year survival rate was 16%, and no apparent differences were detected between those receiving irradiation and those receiving combined therapy, although the groups may have had different prognostic factors.

Figure 102-3 presents an algorithm for the postoperative management of endometrial carcinoma.

TREATMENT OF RECURRENT DISEASE

Although most patients with recurrence after primary therapy are incurable, a subset treated only with surgery has recurrence confined to the pelvis that may be cured with appropriate radical pelvic irradiation. Several series have documented a substantial fraction of patients surviving disease free when so treated. In general, the probability of long-term disease-free survival depends on the extent of pelvic disease at the time of relapse and also probably on the dose of radiation employed. In a series from Toronto, 54 patients with recurrent endometrial carcinoma were identified from a retrospective review of 304 endometrial cancer patients treated between 1983 and 1989.[166] Forty percent of the entire recurrent population are long-term survivors. Of the 54 relapsing patients, 32 had surgery alone initially and 22 had surgery and adjuvant RT. Isolated pelvic recurrence was the predominant relapse site in those treated by surgery alone (23 of 32; 72%). Distant relapse predominated in those who received adjuvant RT (17 of 22; 77%). Twenty-eight (54%) failed in the pelvis alone, and 26 (46%) had a component of distant failure. Of the 28 with isolated pelvic relapse, 16 had vaginal mucosal disease involvement only and 12 had disease in the parametrium and/or the pelvic side wall. With a minimum follow-up of 5 years for the survivors, 21 of the 28 with isolated pelvic relapse received radical RT, and 14 (67%) had maintained pelvic control until death or last follow-up. Eleven of 14 (79%) with disease confined to the mucosa had pelvic control, whereas only 3 of 7 (43%) with extramucosal disease were controlled. No patient experienced major treatment-related toxicity. In an analysis of prognostic factors, only the anatomic extent of pelvic recurrence showed a nonstatistically significant trend as a predictor for control with $p = .08$. The authors concluded that a significant fraction of patients with disease recurrence confined to the pelvis can be rendered disease free in the long term with maintained pelvic control.

Other retrospective reviews substantiate the curability of patients with isolated vaginal recurrence. In the report from the Mallinckrodt Institute, the 5-year progression-free survival rate for patients with isolated vaginal recurrence was 40% compared with a 20% survival rate for those with more extensive pelvic disease.[167] Similarly, Poulsen and Roberts demonstrated a 10-year survival rate of 45% in those with vaginal disease only compared with 24% for those with more extensive pelvic disease.[168]

In the patient who has had initial adjuvant postoperative pelvic irradiation, there may rarely be a role for interstitial therapy at relapse if there is isolated central pelvic failure. For patients with

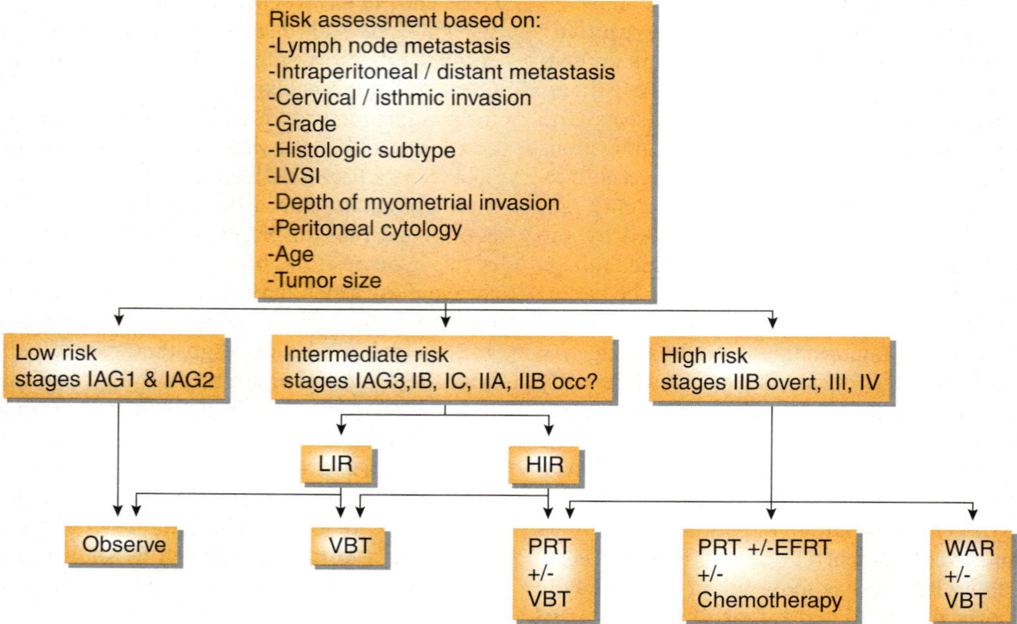

Figure 102-3 Postoperative management of endometrial carcinoma. EFRT = extended field radiation therapy; PRT = pelvic radiation therapy; VBT = vaginal brachytherapy; WAR = whole abdominopelvic radiotherapy; LIR = low intermediate risk; HIR = high intermediate risk based on Gynecologic Oncology Group 99: age < 50, 50–70, > 70, LVSI = lymph–vascular space invasion, outer third invasion, grade 2 or 3 (see text).

other sites of disease or bony, cerebral, or nodal metastases, short courses of palliative irradiation may be useful in relieving the symptoms of disease. Similarly, palliative irradiation may be used for the uncommon patient (approximately 3% of those at presentation) who has stage IV disease.

Unlike ovarian carcinoma, little is known regarding the role of secondary cytoreduction in recurrent endometrial carcinoma. In a report from an Italian group, 20 women with recurrent endometrial adenocarcinoma were treated with maximal cytoreductive surgery.[169] Sixty-five percent of patients had complete resection of their tumor. Women with no residual tumor had a significantly increased progression-free and overall survival compared with women with residual tumor; however, there was a 10% perioperative death rate in this series. The role of pelvic exenteration was examined in a four-institution retrospective review of 31 patients.[170] Twenty patients underwent exenteration with curative intent, all of whom had previously received pelvic irradiation. The 5-year disease-free survival rate was 45%.

CYTOTOXIC CHEMOTHERAPY

Cytotoxic chemotherapy for patients with endometrial cancer was rarely administered before 1980. In his 1974 literature review, Donovan reported only 126 patients who had been treated with 16 different agents.[171] A combination of complete and partial responses was identified in 34 of 126 patients (27%).

In 1977, Muggia and colleagues reported that doxorubicin (Adriamycin, 37.5 mg/m^2) in combination with cyclophosphamide (500 mg/m^2) intravenously (IV) every 21 days in 11 patients with recurrent endometrial cancer resulted in five objective responses.[172] The GOG studied single-agent doxorubicin at a dose rate of 60 mg/m^2 IV every 3 weeks and reported a 37% response rate in 43 patients.[173] Although the most frequent adverse effect was on the hematopoietic system, cardiac toxicity occurred in 12%, and there was one cardiotoxic death in a patient who had received more than 500 mg/m^2 of drug. This study was important because it clearly established the value of doxorubicin as a single agent in the chemotherapy of endometrial cancer. Furthermore it suggested a wider applicability of cytotoxic agents, unrelated to locus of recurrence, and provided a model for the evaluation of other agents. The Eastern Cooperative Oncology Group tested doxorubicin versus cyclophosphamide in patients with advanced or recurrent endometrial adenocarcinoma. The group found no activity for cyclophosphamide when administered at a dose of 660 mg/m^2 IV every 3 weeks.[174] The GOG then tested doxorubicin with or without cyclophosphamide and found no advantage for the combination over doxorubicin alone.[175]

As these studies were being conducted, the activity of cisplatin was demonstrated in patients with advanced endometrial cancer and in those who had failed conventional therapy. In the GOG experience, 23 patients were treated with cisplatin at a dose of 50 mg/m^2 every 3 weeks with only one response, but 20 of these 23 had previously been treated with doxorubicin or an alkylating agent.[176] Trope and colleagues produced four responses (36%) by treating 11 chemotherapy-naive patients with cisplatin at a dose rate of 50 mg/m^2.[177]

A combination of cisplatin and doxorubicin had been used to treat patients with advanced or recurrent ovarian cancer. Extending this approach to patients with endometrial carcinoma, the range of response to these platinum-based combinations in advanced or recurrent disease was 33 to 80%, depending on the proportion of patients previously treated with either chemotherapy or radiation.[178,179]

The demonstrated utility of cytotoxic agents in the treatment of endometrial carcinoma provoked numerous phase II drug trials evaluating over 29 single agents over the last 25 years.[180] If one selects only drugs that have achieved at least a 20% response rate in studies including at least 20 patients, the list is small (Table 102-9). Of note, paclitaxel has emerged as an active drug in recurrent endometrial adenocarcinoma. The GOG studied paclitaxel in patients with advanced or recurrent adenocarcinoma of the endometrium.[181] Among 28 evaluable patients, four complete responses and six partial responses were observed, for an overall response rate of 35.7%. Similarly, Lissoni and colleagues evaluated paclitaxel in 19 patients with advanced endometrial adenocarcinoma previously treated with cisplatin, doxorubicin, and cyclophosphamide.[182] Two complete responses and five partial responses were achieved, for an overall response rate of 37%.

Although there have been many attempts to evaluate combination chemotherapy, most series have been small, with no control arm and hence no opportunity to assess the relative merits of the combination to single-agent therapy. Therefore, our best information on combination chemotherapy comes from the randomized phase III trials listed in Table 102-10. The randomized trials that have included hormonal therapy are listed in Table 102-11.

Table 102-10 lists the randomized trials that compared single agents with one or two different combinations. Thigpen and colleagues reported the GOG experience comparing doxorubicin (A) with doxorubicin and cisplatin (P) in patients with advanced or recurrent endometrial carcinoma.[180] The combination had a higher overall response rate (42% vs 25%) and complete response rate (19% vs 8%) than did doxorubicin as a single agent, but no survival advantage was demonstrated. However, in the European Organisation for Research and Treatment of Cancer (EORTC) study reported by Aapro and col-

Table 102-9 Single-Agent Cytotoxic Chemotherapy for Endometrial Cancer

Agent	Reference	*n*	Prior Treatment	No CR + PR	%
Paclitaxel	181	28	No	4 + 6	36
Paclitaxel	182	19	Yes	2 + 5	37
Cisplatin	212, 213	75	No	3 + 18	28
Carboplatin	214–216	76	No	5 + 18	28
Doxorubicin	173, 180, 183	280	No	31 + 49	29
Epirubicin	217	27	No	2 + 5	26
Fluorouracil	218	34	NS	7	21
HMM	219	30	No	10	33

Adapted from Muss HB[221] and Thigpen JT.[180]
CR = complete response; HMM = Hexamethylmelamine ; NS = not stated; PR = partial response.
Reported series with at least 20 patients with a response rate of at least 20%.

Table 102-10 Randomized Trials of Combination Chemotherapy Regimens for Endometrial Cancer

Study	Regimen	Number Evaluable	RR, %	Median PFS, Mo	Median Overall Survival, Mo
Thigpen et al, 1994[175]	A	132	22	3.2	6.7
	AC	144	30	3.9	7.3
Thigpen et al, 2004[180]	A	150	25	3.8	9.2
	AP	131	42*	5.7*	9.0
Aapro et al, 2003[183]	A	87	17	7.0	7.0
	AP	90	43*	8.0	9.0*
Gallion et al, 2003[184]	AP standard	169	46	6.5	11.2
	AP circadian	173	49	5.9	13.2
Fleming et al, 2004[185]	AP	157	40	7.2	12.6
	AT	160	43	6.0	13.6
Fleming et al, 2004[222]	AP	129	34	5.3	12.3
	TAP	134	57*	8.3*	15.3*

A = Adriamycin (doxorubicin); C = cyclophosphamide; F = 5-fluorouracil; P = Platinol (cisplatin); PFS = progression-free survival; RR = response rate = complete response + partial response; T = Taxol (paclitaxel).
*Significant difference.

Table 102-11 Randomized Trials of Combination Chemotherapy + Hormonal Therapy for Endometrial Cancer

Study	Regimen	Number Evaluable	RR, %
Horton et al, 1982[223]	CA + MA	55	27
	CAF + MA	56	16
Cohen et al, 1984[224]	F-Mel + MA	126	38
	CAF + MA	131	36
Ayoub et al, 1988[206]	CAF	20	15
	CAF + MPA/TAM	23	43*
Cornelison et al, 1995[225]	APE + MA	50	54
	F-Mel + MPA	50	48

A = Adriamycin (doxorubicin); C = cyclophosphamide; F = 5-fluorouracil; MA = megestrol acetate; Mel = melphalan; MPA = medroxyprogesterone acetate; P = Platinol (cisplatin); RR = response rate = complete response + partial response; TAM = tamoxifen.
*Significant difference.

leagues, a survival advantage was demonstrated with a response rate of 43% for the doxorubicin and cisplatin combination versus 17% for single-agent doxorubicin ($p < .001$).[183] The GOG found no difference when doxorubicin and cisplatin were administered in a circadian fashion compared with a standard fashion.[184]

In view of the activity of paclitaxel in endometrial adenocarcinoma, the GOG initiated a phase III study of doxorubicin plus cisplatin versus doxorubicin plus 24-hour paclitaxel in primary stage III or IV or recurrent endometrial carcinoma. This study found no difference in response rate, progression-free survival, or overall survival.[185]

The most recent phase III prospective randomized GOG study (Protocol 177) compared standard doxorubicin (60 mg/m^2) and cisplatin (50 mg/m^2), that is, AP against TAP with paclitaxel (Taxol 160 mg/m^2/3 h), doxorubicin (45 mg/m^2), and cisplatin (50 mg/m^2).[169] Two hundred sixty-six patients were randomized, and the preliminary results indicated that TAP produced a significant improvement in response rate (57% vs 34%; $p < .01$) and progression-free survival (median 8.3 vs 5.3 months; $p < .01$) and overall survival (median 15.3 vs 12.3 months; $p = .037$).[186] The GOG is currently randomly assigning patients with advanced (stage IVB) or recurrent disease to either TAP or paclitaxel and carboplatin to determine whether it is possible to drop doxorubicin from the regimen and substitute carboplatin for cisplatin without loss of efficacy and with a marked improvement in toxicity profile (GOG Protocol 209).[180]

In patients with surgical bulk reduction (to residual < 2 cm) for stage III to IVA disease, the GOG in Protocol 122 (a randomized phase III trial) demonstrated that chemotherapy with doxorubicin (60 mg/m^2) and cisplatin (50 mg/m^2) had superior progression-free survival (0.68; 95% confidence interval [CI] = 0.52–0.89; $p < .01$) and overall survival (0.67; 95% CI = 0.51–0.89; $p < .01$) compared with whole-abdomen radiation.[187]

ADJUVANT CHEMOTHERAPY FOR HIGH-RISK EARLY-STAGE DISEASE

Because of the common adjuvant use of RT for patients with FIGO stage I and stage II endometrial cancer, there has been little impetus for the administration of adjuvant cytotoxic chemotherapy, even when such prognostic features as depth of myometrial invasion and histologic grade have suggested the possibility of recurrence. Three studies are available, from which information may be drawn inferentially.

Stringer and colleagues studied 31 patients with stage I endometrial cancer and 2 patients with occult stage II disease who had the poor prognostic features of deep myometrial invasion, grade III tumors, nonendometrioid histology, or extrauterine disease that was completely resected.[188] Some of these patients were entered into the trial before the introduction of the new surgical staging system. Postoperatively, the patients were treated with cisplatin, 50 mg/m^2, doxorubicin, 50 mg/m^2, and cyclophosphamide, 500 mg/m^2, every 4 weeks for six cycles. The 2-year progression-free interval rate was 79%, and the 2-year survival was 83%. The median survival time for patients with disease confined to the uterus was not reached at 45 months. These results were considered superior to those of historical controls from the same institution.

The GOG treated patients with clinical stage I and stage II disease who had poor prognostic features with postoperative whole-pelvis irradiation with or without doxorubicin.[189] Those patients randomized to receive doxorubicin were treated with 45 to 60 mg/m^2 every 3 weeks to a cumulative dose of 500 mg/m^2 after their RT was completed. No differences were noted in progression-free interval or survival. Patients with disease limited to the uterus had a 63% survival rate with RT only and a 72% survival rate when doxorubicin was added. This difference was not statistically significant because the sample size (181 patients) was too small.

More recently, Burke and colleagues prospectively treated 62 patients at high risk of systemic failure with six courses of cisplatin, doxorubicin, and cyclophosphamide.[190] Although this regimen did not prevent distant failures in women with extrauterine disease, it was effective in patients with disease confined to the uterus, with an actuarial 3-year survival rate of 82%.

HORMONE THERAPY

Progestins Kelly and Baker, in 1961, noticing a profound effect of progesterone on the normal endometrium, treated patients with advanced endometrial cancer with a progestational agent. Their original report describes six objective responses in 21 patients that lasted from 9 months to 4½ years.[191] Since then, there have been numerous reports describing treatment with a variety of progestational drugs: the most commonly employed are 17-hydroxyprogesterone caproate, medroxyprogesterone acetate (MPA), and megestrol acetate (MA). The notion of treating a hormone-dependent tumor with a hormone antagonist without important adverse effects is very attractive when confronting a patient who may be aged, obese, and suffering from imperfect cardiovascular function and who has failed surgical remedy with or without subsequent RT and possible cytotoxic chemotherapy. At the other end of the spectrum, it is also attractive to employ hormonal therapy as a fertility-preserving option in the younger patient or in the medically infirm, who are at very high risk of surgical complications. In an effort to demonstrate efficacy, therapists first applied progestational regimens to the most advanced or recurrent disease.

Reifenstein analyzed 992 patients treated with hydroxyprogesterone caproate by 113 investigators.[192] He studied the records of 314 patients in detail and found that there was little response before 7 weeks of treatment, that the longest remissions were achieved with a minimum of 12 weeks of initial therapy, and that there was no relationship between clinical response and patient age when correction was made for tumor differentiation. Kauppila reviewed 1,068 patients treated in 17 different trials with either MPA (Provera), MA, or hydroxyprogesterone caproate and found an overall response rate of 34%.[193] The duration of response was approximately 20 months, and the average survival time was approximately 25 months.

The optimum dose for progestational treatment has not been determined. Kohorn's early survey of the members of the Society of Gynecologic Oncology identified 15 different dose schedules for the use of MPA.[194] The GOG, employing MPA, 50 mg orally three times a day, in heavily pretreated patients with advanced or recurrent endometrial carcinoma noted a 14% objective response rate. The median survival duration was 10.4 months. The GOG completed a subsequent dose-seeking study comparing oral MPA at doses of 200 mg/d with doses of 1,000 mg/d and found that the lower dose resulted in a response rate of 25% compared with 15% with the higher dose.[195] The GOG also studied high-dose MA (800 mg/d) in advanced or recurrent endometrial carcinoma and concluded that this regimen had no advantage over lower-dose progestins.[196] Of 54 evaluable patients, six complete responses and seven partial responses were observed, for an overall response rate of 24%. Three deaths secondary to cardiovascular events were possibly related to therapy.

Podratz and colleagues noted an objective overall response rate of 11.2% and a 5-year survival rate of only 8% when treating patients with progestational agents.[197] This study group found no difference in response rates among MA, hydroxyprogesterone, and medrogestone.

Several investigators compared oral and parenteral routes of administration employing a variety of progestational agents and found no advantage for the parenteral route.[193,198] Milligram equivalents of progestational agents frequently do not translate into biologic equivalence, and the dose of a particular progestogen required for tumor control may have to be empirically derived.

Ramirez and colleagues, in reviewing the literature, found that the majority of patients reported with well-differentiated endometrial adenocarcinoma who undergo conservative treatment for primary uterine cancer (in lieu of hysterectomy) with a progestational agent respond to treatment (62 of 81 = 76%).[199] When an initial response is not achieved or when disease recurs after an initial response (15 of 62 = 24%), carcinoma extending beyond the uterus is rare.[199] In addition, Montz and colleagues described the feasibility of using a progesterone-containing intrauterine device to treat presumed FIGO stage IA, grade 1 endometrioid cancer in women at high risk of perioperative complications.[200]

In summary, the following generalizations can be made concerning progestational therapy: (1) the response rate for patients with advanced or recurrent endometrial carcinoma ranges from 10 to 30%, probably relating to the receptor level in the tumor; (2) well-differentiated cancers respond best; (3) the PR level diminishes sharply as the grade of the tumor increases; (4) clinical responses may not occur before 7 to 12 weeks of therapy; (5) two-thirds of patients will not respond; (6) there is no published evidence that progestational agents employed in an adjuvant mode offer any benefit; (7) appropriate oral doses are 160 mg/d of megestrol or 200 mg/d of MPA; and (8) oral progestins and the progesterone-containing intrauterine device are alternatives to consider for primary treatment of selected cases of early-stage, low-grade endometrial cancer.

Tamoxifen Hormonal therapy by agents other than progestogens has been studied by many researchers. Extrapolating from the experience with breast cancer, investigators employed tamoxifen in doses of 20 to 40 mg daily for patients with advanced or recurrent endometrial carcinoma. In a review of eight published studies, Moore and colleagues described an overall response rate of 22%.[201] As one might predict, there is a wide spectrum of reported responses, ranging from 0 to 53%.[202] This variation may be explained by the report of Edmonson and colleagues, who found a 21% response rate in patients naive to hormone therapy and no response in patients who had failed progesterone treatment.[203] Not unlike the progestin experience, it would seem that tamoxifen is more likely to be effective in patients with low-grade tumors, receptor positivity, and either no previous hormone therapy or a previous response to progestin therapy.

Because progestins ultimately down-regulate PRs, and because tamoxifen induces these receptors in target tissues, the notion of the combined administration of these hormones has been examined by the GOG with two different strategies. In Whitney and colleagues' report, tamoxifen citrate 40 mg/d combined with alternating weekly cycles of MPA 200 mg/d in 58 patients with recurrent or measurable advanced endometrial carcinoma resulted in a 33% response rate (10.3% complete response and 23.4% partial response), with a median progression-free interval of 3 months and a median overall survival of 13 months.[204] In the Fiorica study, alternating 3-week courses of MA (160 mg/d) and tamoxifen citrate (40 mg/d) in 56 patients with recurrent or measurable advanced endometrial carcinoma produced a 27% response rate (21.4% complete response and 5.4% partial response), with a median progression-free interval of 2.7 months and a median overall survival of 14.0 months.[205]

The combination of tamoxifen, progestin, and chemotherapy has also been tested. Ayoub and colleagues studied 46 patients with metastatic endometrial cancer, randomly assigning them to receive monthly cycles of cyclophosphamide, Adriamycin (doxorubicin), and 5-fluorouracil (CAF) or CAF plus MPA, 200 mg daily for 3 weeks, followed cyclically by tamoxifen, 20 mg daily for 3 weeks.[206] Objective responses of 15 and 43% were seen, respectively, with CAF and CAF plus hormonal therapy (p = .05). Because progestational agents have not improved the response to chemotherapy in previously cited studies,[207] it is reasonable to attribute this difference to the addition of tamoxifen. Recently, Pinelli and colleagues evaluated sequential cyclical hormone therapy (MA and tamoxifen citrate) plus the single agent carboplatin.[208] Of 13 evaluable patients, 4 patients had a complete response and 6 had partial responses, for an overall response rate of 77%. The median progression-free interval was 14 months for complete responders. The median survival was 11 months for all patients and 33 months for complete responders.

Other Hormones Gonadotropin-releasing hormone analogues have been tested in small phase II trials of patients with recurrent endometrial carcinoma, with response rates varying from 0 to 35%.[209–211] Aromatase inhibitors have been tested in a limited fashion. The GOG phase II trial had a 9% response rate (2 partial responses of 23) with anastrozole,[211] whereas the Canadian National Cancer Institute study reported a 9.4% response rate (2 partial responses of 28) with letrozole.[212] A GOG trial of danazol showed hepatic toxicity in four patients but no responses among the 25 patients.[212]

THE FUTURE

Efforts must continue to expand information about oncogene expression to better define risk groups. From a surgical standpoint, the results of randomized studies examining the role of laparoscopy-assisted vaginal hysterectomy and staging are needed to better define the future role of these procedures. For patients with early disease and poor prognostic features, studies with extended fields for RT should be undertaken and can be tested against adjuvant cytotoxic chemotherapy. For patients with advanced or recurrent disease, better cytotoxic agents must be identified. The integration of sequential hormonal and cytotoxic therapy is rational and should be pursued. More randomized trials for chemotherapy combinations must be undertaken and measured against sequenced single-agent therapy. It is obvious that with a cure rate in the United States of approximately 80%, it will be essential that patients with poor prognostic features or recurrent or metastatic disease be entered into collaborative trials to maximize the opportunities for improving survival.

REFERENCES

1. Jemal A, Murray T, Ward E, et al. Cancer statistics, 2005. CA Cancer J Clin 2005;55:10–30.
2. Creasman WT, Odicino F, Maisonneuve P, et al. Carcinoma of the corpus uteri. Int J Gynaecol Obstet 2003;83 Suppl 1:79–118.
3. Hicks ML, Phillips JL, Parham G, et al. The National Cancer Data Base report on endometrial carcinoma in African-American women. Cancer 1998;83:2629–37.
4. Parazzini F, La Vecchia C, Negri E, et al. Diabetes and endometrial cancer: an Italian case-control study. Int J Cancer 1999;81:539–42.
5. Gusberg SB, Kardon P. Proliferative endometrial response to theca-granulosa cell tumors. Am J Obstet Gynecol 1971;111:633–43.
6. Norris HJ, Taylor HB. Prognosis of granulosa-theca tumors of the ovary. Cancer 1968;21:255–63.
7. Mansell H, Hertig AT. Granulosa-theca cell tumor and endometrial carcinoma: a study of their relationship and survey of 50 cases. Obstet Gynecol 1955;6:385–94.
8. Jackson RL, Dockerty MB. The Stein-Leventhal syndrome. Analysis of 43 cases with special reference to endometrial carcinoma. Am J Obstet Gynecol 1957;73:161–73.
9. Gallup DG, Stock RJ. Adenocarcinoma of the endometrium in women 40 years of age or younger. Obstet Gynecol 1984;64:417–20.
10. Sirota DK, Marinoff SC. Endometrial carcinoma in Turner's syndrome following prolonged treatment with diethylstilbestrol. Mt Sinai J Med 1975;42:596–90.
11. Gusberg SB. Precursors of corpus carcinoma, estrogen and adenomatous hyperplasia. Am J Obstet Gynecol 1947;54:905–27.
12. Cullen TH. Cancer of the uterus. Philadelphia: W.B. Saunders; 1900.
13. Smith DC, Prentice R, Thompson DJ, et al. Association of exogenous estrogen and endometrial carcinoma. N Engl J Med 1975;293:1164–7.
14. Ziel HK, Finkle WD. Increased risk of endometrial carcinoma among users of conjugated estrogens. N Engl J Med 1975;293:1167–70.
15. Mack TM, Pike MC, Henderson BE, et al. Estrogens and endometrial cancer in a retirement community. N Engl J Med 1976;294:1262–7.
16. Antunes CM, Strolley PD, Rosenshein NB, et al. Endometrial cancer and estrogen use. Report of a large case-control study. N Engl J Med 1979;300:9–13.
17. Horwitz RI, Feinstein AR. Alternative analytic methods for case-control studies of estrogens and endometrial cancer. N Engl J Med 1978;299:1089–94.
18. Brinton LA, Hoover RN. Estrogen replacement therapy and endometrial cancer risk: unresolved issues. The Endometrial Cancer Collaborative Group. Obstet Gynecol 1993;81:265–71.
19. Hulka BS, Fowler WC Jr, Kaufman DG, et al. Estrogen and endometrial cancer: cases and two control groups from North Carolina. Am J Obstet Gynecol 1980;137:92–101.
20. Combination oral contraceptive use and the risk of endometrial cancer. The Cancer and Steroid Hormone Study of

the Centers for Disease Control and the National Institute of Child Health and Human Development. JAMA 1987;257:796–800.
21. Jordan VC. Estrogens and anti-estrogens. In: Bast RC, Kufe DW, Pollock RE, editors. Cancer medicine. Vol 5. Hamilton (ON): BC Decker; 2000. p. 743–50.
22. Love RR, Newcomb PA, Wiebe DA, et al. Effects of tamoxifen therapy on lipid and lipoprotein levels in postmenopausal patients with node-negative breast cancer. J Natl Cancer Inst 1990;82:1327–32.
23. Love RR, Mazess RB, Barden HS, et al. Effects of tamoxifen on bone mineral density in postmenopausal women with breast cancer. N Engl J Med 1992;326:852–6.
24. Boccardo F, Bruzzi P, Rubagotti A, et al. Estrogen-like action of tamoxifen on vaginal epithelium in breast cancer patients. Oncology 1981;38:281–5.
25. Gottardis MM, Robinson SP, Satyaswaroop PG, et al. Contrasting actions of tamoxifen on endometrial and breast tumor growth in the athymic mouse. Cancer Res 1988;48:812–5.
26. Fornander T, Rutqvist LE, Cedermark B, et al. Adjuvant tamoxifen in early breast cancer: occurrence of new primary cancers. Lancet 1989;1:117–20.
27. Fisher B, Costantino JP, Redmond CK, et al. Endometrial cancer in tamoxifen-treated breast cancer patients: findings from the National Surgical Adjuvant Breast and Bowel Project (NSABP) B-14. J Natl Cancer Inst 1994;86:527–37.
28. Killackey MA, Hakes TB, Pierce VK. Endometrial adenocarcinoma in breast cancer patients receiving antiestrogens. Cancer Treat Rep 1985;69:237–8.
29. Fisher B, Costantino JP, Wickerham DL, et al. Tamoxifen for prevention of breast cancer: report of the National Surgical Adjuvant Breast and Bowel Project P-1 Study. J Natl Cancer Inst 1998;90:1371–88.
30. Magriples U, Naftolin F, Schwartz PE, et al. High-grade endometrial carcinoma in tamoxifen-treated breast cancer patients. J Clin Oncol 1993;11:485–90.
31. Cohen CJ, Rahaman J. Endometrial cancer. Management of high risk and recurrence including the tamoxifen controversy. Cancer 1995;76(10 Suppl):2044–52.
32. Barakat RR, Wong G, Curtin JP, et al. Tamoxifen use in breast cancer patients who subsequently develop corpus cancer is not associated with a higher incidence of adverse histologic features. Gynecol Oncol 1994;55:164–8.
33. Runowicz CD, Costantino MT, Kavanah M, et al. National Surgical Adjuvant Breast and Bowel Project Breast Cancer Prevention Trial summary analysis of transvaginal sonography and endometrial biopsy in detecting endometrial pathology. J Clin Oncol 1999;18:358a.
34. Fung MF, Reid A, Faught W, et al. Prospective longitudinal study of ultrasound screening for endometrial abnormalities in women with breast cancer receiving tamoxifen. Gynecol Oncol 2003;91:154–9.
35. Barakat RR, Gilewski TA, Almadrones L, et al. Effect of adjuvant tamoxifen on the endometrium in women with breast cancer: a prospective study using office endometrial biopsy. J Clin Oncol 2000;18:3459–63.
36. Bokhman JV. Two pathogenetic types of endometrial carcinoma. Gynecol Oncol 1983;15:10–7.
37. Deligdisch L, Holinka CF. Endometrial carcinoma: two diseases? Cancer Detect Prev 1987;10:237–46.
38. Gusberg SB, Moore DM, Martin F. Precursors of corpus cancer II, a clinical and pathologic study of adenomatous hyperplasia. Am J Obstet Gynecol 1954;68:1472–81.
39. Hertig AT, Sommers SC. Genesis of endometrial carcinoma: study of prior biopsy. Cancer 1949;68:964–71.
40. Kurman RJ, Kaminski PF, Norris HJ. The behavior of endometrial hyperplasia. A long-term study of "untreated" hyperplasia in 170 patients. Cancer 1985;56:403–12.
41. Reagan JW. The changing nature of endometrial cancer. Gynecol Oncol 1974;2:144–51.
42. Hendrickson M, Ross J, Eifel P, et al. Uterine papillary serous carcinoma: a highly malignant form of endometrial adenocarcinoma. Am J Surg Pathol 1982;6:93–108.
43. O'Hanlan KA, Levine PA, Harbatkin D, et al. Virulence of papillary endometrial carcinoma. Gynecol Oncol 1990;37:112–9.
44. Lee KR, Belinson JL. Recurrence in noninvasive endometrial carcinoma. Relationship to uterine papillary serous carcinoma. Am J Surg Pathol 1991;15:965–73.
45. Chen JL, Trost DC,. Wilkinson EJ. Endometrial papillary adenocarcinomas: two clinicopathological types. Int J Gynecol Pathol 1985;4:279–88.
46. Kurman RJ, Scully RE. Clear cell carcinoma of the endometrium: an analysis of 21 cases. Cancer 1976;37:872–82.
47. Christopherson WM, Alberhasky RC, Connelly PJ. Glassy cell carcinoma of the endometrium. Hum Pathol 1982;13:418–21.
48. Cohen CJ, Gusberg SB, Koffler D. Histologic screening for endometrial cancer. Gynecol Oncol 1974;2:279–86.
49. Walters D, Robinson D, Park RC, et al. Diagnostic outpatient aspiration curettage. Obstet Gynecol 1975;46:160–4.
50. Romano S, Shimoni Y, Muralee D, et al. Retrograde seeding of endometrial carcinoma during hysteroscopy. Gynecol Oncol 1992;44:116–8.
51. Rose PG, Mendelsohn G, Kornbluth I. Hysteroscopic dissemination of endometrial carcinoma. Gynecol Oncol 1998;71:145–6.
52. Yazigi R, Cohen J, Munoz AK, et al. Magnetic resonance imaging determination of myometrial invasion in endometrial carcinoma. Gynecol Oncol 1989;34:94–7.
53. Cruickshank DJ, Randall JM, Miller ID. Vaginal endosonography in endometrial cancer. Lancet 1989;1:445–6.
54. Creasman WT, Boronow RC, Morrow CP, et al. Adenocarcinoma of the endometrium: its metastatic lymph node potential. A preliminary report. Gynecol Oncol 1976;4:239–43.
55. Creasman WT, Morrow CP, Bundy BN, et al. Surgical pathologic spread patterns of endometrial cancer. A Gynecologic Oncology Group study. Cancer 1987;60(8 Suppl):2035–41.
56. Orr JW. Surgical staging of endometrial cancer: does the patient benefit? Gynecol Oncol 1998;71:335–9.
57. Maneschi M, Maneschi F, Geraci P, et al. Surgical pathological staging of endometrial carcinoma and results of treatment. Eur J Gynaecol Oncol 1992;13(1 Suppl):30–5.
58. Wolfson AH,. Sightler SE, Markoe AM, et al. The prognostic significance of surgical staging for carcinoma of the endometrium. Gynecol Oncol 1992;45:142–6.
59. Chuang L, Burke TW, Tornos C, et al. Staging laparotomy for endometrial carcinoma: assessment of retroperitoneal lymph nodes. Gynecol Oncol 1995;58:189–93.
60. Girardi F, Petru E, Heydarfadai M, et al. Pelvic lymphadenectomy in the surgical treatment of endometrial cancer. Gynecol Oncol 1993;49:177–80.
61. Burke TW. Selective pelvic and para-aortic lymphadenectomy. Oper Tech Gynecol Surg 1996;1:17–21.
62. Morrow CP, Curtin JP. Gynecologic cancer surgery. New York: Churchill Livingstone; 1996.
63. Rose PG, Cha SD, Tak WK, et al. Radiation therapy for surgically proven para-aortic node metastasis in endometrial carcinoma. Int J Radiat Oncol Biol Phys 1992;24:229–33.
64. Kilgore LC, Partridge EE, Alvarez RD, et al. Adenocarcinoma of the endometrium: survival comparisons of patients with and without pelvic node sampling. Gynecol Oncol 1995;56:29–33.
65. Trimble EL, Kosary C, Park C. Lymph node sampling and survival in endometrial cancer. Gynecol Oncol 1998;71:340–3.
66. Mohan DS, Samuels MA, Selim MA, et al. Long-term outcomes of therapeutic pelvic lymphadenectomy for stage I endometrial adenocarcinoma. Gynecol Oncol 1998;70:165–71.
67. Rittenberg PV, Lotocki RJ, Heywood MS, et al. High-risk surgical stage 1 endometrial cancer: outcomes with vault brachytherapy alone. Gynecol Oncol 2003;89:288–94.
68. Morrow CP, Bundy BN, Kurman RJ, et al. Relationship between surgical-pathological risk factors and outcome in clinical stage I and II carcinoma of the endometrium: a Gynecologic Oncology Group study. Gynecol Oncol 1991;40:55–65.
69. Wilson TO, Podratz KC, Gaffey TA, et al. Evaluation of unfavorable histologic subtypes in endometrial adenocarcinoma. Am J Obstet Gynecol 1990;162:418–23; discussion 423–6.
70. Aalders J, Abeler V, Kolstad P, et al. Postoperative external irradiation and prognostic parameters in stage I endometrial carcinoma: clinical and histopathologic study of 540 patients. Obstet Gynecol 1980;56:419–27.
71. Sutton GP, Geisler HE, Stehman FB, et al. Features associated with survival and disease-free survival in early endometrial cancer. Am J Obstet Gynecol 1989;160:1385–91; discussion 1391–3.
72. Salvesen HB, Iversen OE, Akslen LA. Prognostic impact of morphometric nuclear grade of endometrial carcinoma. Cancer 1998;83:956–64.
73. DiSaia PJ, Creasman WT, Boronow RC, et al. Risk factors and recurrent patterns in stage I endometrial cancer. Am J Obstet Gynecol 1985;151:1009–15.
74. Lutz MH, Underwood PB Jr, Kreutner A Jr, et al. Endometrial carcinoma: a new method of classification of therapeutic and prognostic significance. Gynecol Oncol 1978;6:83–94.
75. Hanson MB, van Nagell JR Jr, Powell DE, et al. The prognostic significance of lymph-vascular space invasion in stage I endometrial cancer. Cancer 1985;55:1753–7.
76. Creasman WT, Rutledge F. The prognostic value of peritoneal cytology in gynecologic malignant disease. Am J Obstet Gynecol 1971;110:773–81.
77. Turner DA, Gershenson DM, Atkinson N, et al. The prognostic significance of peritoneal cytology for stage I endometrial cancer. Obstet Gynecol 1989;74:775–80.
78. Sutton GP. The significance of positive peritoneal cytology in endometrial cancer. Oncology (Huntingt) 1990;4:21–6; discussion 30–2.
79. Konski A, Poulter C, Keys H, et al. Absence of prognostic significance, peritoneal dissemination and treatment advantage in endometrial cancer patients with positive peritoneal cytology. Int J Radiat Oncol Biol Phys 1988;14:49–55.
80. Lurain JR, Rumsey NK, Schink JC, et al. Prognostic significance of positive peritoneal cytology in clinical stage I adenocarcinoma of the endometrium. Obstet Gynecol 1989;74:175–9.
81. Milosevic M, Dembo A, Thomas GM. The clinical significance of positive peritoneal cytology in stage I endometrial carcinoma. Int J Gynecol Cancer 1992;2:225–35.
82. Liu JR, Conaway M, Rodriguez GC, et al. Relationship between race and interval to treatment in endometrial cancer. Obstet Gynecol 1995;86(4 Pt 1):486–90.
83. Creasman WT, McCarty KS Sr, Barton TK, et al. Clinical correlates of estrogen- and progesterone-binding proteins in human endometrial adenocarcinoma. Obstet Gynecol 1980;55:363–70.
84. Ehrlich CE, Young PC, Cleary RE. Cytoplasmic progesterone and estradiol receptors in normal, hyperplastic, and carcinomatous endometria: therapeutic implications. Am J Obstet Gynecol 1981;141:539–46.
85. Creasman WT, Soper JT, McCarty KS Jr, et al. Influence of cytoplasmic steroid receptor content on prognosis of early stage endometrial carcinoma. Am J Obstet Gynecol 1985;151:922–32.
86. Mariani A, Sebo TJ, Webb MJ, et al. Molecular and histopathologic predictors of distant failure in endometrial cancer. Cancer Detect Prev 2003;27:434–41.
87. Sasaki M, Kotcherguina L, Dharia A, et al. Cytosine-phosphoguanine methylation of estrogen receptors in endometrial cancer. Cancer Res 2001;61:3262–6.
88. Leslie KK, Kumar NS, Richer J, et al. Differential expression of the A and B isoforms of progesterone receptor in human endometrial cancer cells. Only progesterone receptor B is induced by estrogen and associated with strong transcriptional activation. Ann N Y Acad Sci 1997;828:17–26.
89. Kohler U, Taubert G, Bilek K, et al. The relation between the results of cytophotometric examination of endometrial carcinoma and clinical course of these disease. Arch Gynecol Obstet 1992;252:93–7.
90. Salvesen HB, Iversen OE, Akslen LA. Prognostic significance of angiogenesis and Ki-67, p53, and p21 expression: a population-based endometrial carcinoma study. J Clin Oncol 1999;17:1382–90.
91. Berchuck A, Kohler MF, Marks JR, et al. The p53 tumor suppressor gene frequently is altered in gynecologic cancers. Am J Obstet Gynecol 1994;170(1 Pt 1):246–52.
92. Burton JL, Wells M. Recent advances in the histopathology and molecular pathology of carcinoma of the endometrium. Histopathology 1998;33:297–303.
93. Esteller M, Garcia A, Martinez-Palones JM, et al. Susceptibility to endometrial cancer: influence of allelism at p53, glutathione S-transferase (GSTM1 and GSTT1) and cytochrome P-450 (CYP1A1) loci. Br J Cancer 1997;75:1385–8.
94. Kohler MF, Carney P, Dodge R, et al. p53 overexpression in advanced-stage endometrial adenocarcinoma. Am J Obstet Gynecol 1996;175:1246–52.
95. Inoue M, Fujita M, Enomoto T, et al. Immunohistochemical analysis of p53 in gynecologic tumors. Am J Clin Pathol 1994;102:665–70.
96. Taskin M, Lallas TA, Shevchuk M, et al. P53 expression in adenomyosis in endometrial carcinoma patients. Gynecol Oncol 1996;62:241–6.
97. Kohler MF, Nishii H, Humphrey PA, et al. Mutation of the p53 tumor-suppressor gene is not a feature of endometrial hyperplasias. Am J Obstet Gynecol 1993;169:690–4.

98. Sherman ME, Bur ME,. Kurman RJ. p53 in endometrial cancer and its putative precursors: evidence for diverse pathways of tumorigenesis. Hum Pathol 1995;26:1268–74.
99. Yu CC, Wilkinson N, Brito MJ, et al. Patterns of immunohistochemical staining for proliferating cell nuclear antigen and p53 in benign and neoplastic human endometrium. Histopathology 1993;23:367–71.
100. Zheng W, Cao P, Zheng M, et al. p53 overexpression and bcl-2 persistence in endometrial carcinoma: comparison of papillary serous and endometrioid subtypes. Gynecol Oncol 1996;61:167–74.
101. Soong R, Knowles S, Williams KE, et al. Overexpression of p53 protein is an independent prognostic indicator in human endometrial carcinoma. Br J Cancer 1996;74:562–7.
102. Ito K, Sasano H, Matsunaga G, et al. Correlations between p21 expression and clinicopathological findings, p53 gene and protein alterations, and survival in patients with endometrial carcinoma. J Pathol 1997;183:318–24.
103. Caduff RF, Johnston CM, Svoboda-Newman SM, et al. Clinical and pathological significance of microsatellite instability in sporadic endometrial carcinoma. Am J Pathol 1996;148:1671–8.
104. Tashiro H, Isacson C, Levine R, et al. p53 gene mutations are common in uterine serous carcinoma and occur early in their pathogenesis. Am J Pathol 1997;150:177–85.
105. Manek S, Wells M. The significance of alterations in p53 expression in gynecologic neoplasms. Curr Opin Obstet Gynecol 1996;8:52–5.
106. Kohlberger P, Gitsch G, Loesch A, et al. p53 protein overexpression in early stage endometrial cancer. Gynecol Oncol 1996;62:213–7.
107. Berchuck A, Maxwell Gl, Risinger JI. Genetic alterations in endometrial cancer. Hung J Gynecol Oncol 1997;2:153–7.
108. Ito K, Watanabe K, Nasim S, et al. Prognostic significance of p53 overexpression in endometrial cancer. Cancer Res 1994;54:4667–70.
109. Shiozawa T, Xin L, Nikaido T, et al. Immunohistochemical detection of cyclin A with reference to p53 expression in endometrial endometrioid carcinomas. Int J Gynecol Pathol 1997;16:348–53.
110. Nielsen AL, Nyholm HC. p53 protein and c-erbB-2 protein (p185) expression in endometrial adenocarcinoma of endometrioid type. An immunohistochemical examination on paraffin sections. Am J Clin Pathol 1994;102:76–9.
111. Save V, Nylander K, Hall PA. Why is p53 protein stabilized in neoplasia? Some answers but many more questions? J Pathol 1998;184:348–50.
112. Mutter GL, Wada H, Faquin WC, et al. K-ras mutations appear in the premalignant phase of both microsatellite stable and unstable endometrial carcinogenesis. Mol Pathol 1999;52:257–62.
113. Enomoto T, Fujita M, Inoue M, et al. Alterations of the p53 tumor suppressor gene and its association with activation of the c-K-ras-2 protooncogene in premalignant and malignant lesions of the human uterine endometrium. Cancer Res 1993;53:1883–8.
114. Mizuuchi H, Nasim S, Kudo R, et al. Clinical implications of K-ras mutations in malignant epithelial tumors of the endometrium. Cancer Res 1992;52:2777–81.
115. Duggan BD, Felix JC, Muderspach LI, et al. Early mutational activation of the c-Ki-ras oncogene in endometrial carcinoma. Cancer Res 1994;54:1604–7.
116. Sasaki H, Nishii H, Takahashi H, et al. Mutation of the Ki-ras protooncogene in human endometrial hyperplasia and carcinoma. Cancer Res 1993;53:1906–10.
117. Berchuck A, Rodriguez G, Kinney RB, et al. Overexpression of HER-2/neu in endometrial cancer is associated with advanced stage disease. Am J Obstet Gynecol 1991;164(1 Pt 1):15–21.
118. Lukes AS, Kohler MF, Pieper CF, et al. Multivariable analysis of DNA ploidy, p53, and HER-2/neu as prognostic factors in endometrial cancer. Cancer 1994;73:2380–5.
119. Hetzel DJ, Wilson TO, Keeney GL, et al. HER-2/neu expression: a major prognostic factor in endometrial cancer. Gynecol Oncol 1992;47:179–85.
120. Monk BJ, Chapman JA, Johnson GA, et al. Correlation of C-myc and HER-2/neu amplification and expression with histopathologic variables in uterine corpus cancer. Am J Obstet Gynecol 1994;171:1193–8.
121. Khalifa MA, Mannel RS, Haraway SD, et al. Expression of EGFR, HER-2/neu, P53, and PCNA in endometrioid, serous papillary, and clear cell endometrial adenocarcinomas. Gynecol Oncol 1994;53:84–92.
122. Wang D, Konishi I, Koshiyama M, et al. Expression of c-erbB-2 protein and epidermal growth receptor in endometrial carcinomas. Correlation with clinicopathologic and sex steroid receptor status. Cancer 1993;72:2628–37.
123. Mutter GL, Lin MC, Fitzgerald JT, et al. Altered PTEN expression as a diagnostic marker for the earliest endometrial precancers. J Natl Cancer Inst 2000;92:924–30.
124. Risinger JI, Hayes K, Maxwell GL, et al. PTEN mutation in endometrial cancers is associated with favorable clinical and pathologic characteristics. Clin Cancer Res 1998;4:3005–10.
125. Risinger JI, Berchuck A, Kohler MF, et al. Genetic instability of microsatellites in endometrial carcinoma. Cancer Res 1993;53:5100–3.
126. Suzuki A, Fukushige S, Nagase S, et al. Frequent gains on chromosome arms 1q and/or 8q in human endometrial cancer. Hum Genet 1997;100:629–36.
127. Prasad M, Wang H, Douglas W, et al. Molecular genetic characterization of tamoxifen-associated endometrial cancer. Gynecol Oncol 2005;96:25–31.
128. Childers JM, Surwit EA. Combined laparoscopic and vaginal surgery for the management of two cases of stage I endometrial cancer. Gynecol Oncol 1992;45:46–51.
129. Childers JM, Brzechffa PR, Hatch KD, et al. Laparoscopically assisted surgical staging (LASS) of endometrial cancer. Gynecol Oncol 1993;51:33–8.
130. Boike GM, Elfstrand EP, DelPriore G, et al. Laparoscopically assisted vaginal hysterectomy in a university hospital: report of 82 cases and comparison with abdominal and vaginal hysterectomy. Am J Obstet Gynecol 1993;168(6 Pt 1):1690–7; discussion 1697–701.
131. Magrina JF, Weaver AL. Laparoscopic treatment of endometrial cancer: five-year recurrence and survival rates. Eur J Gynaecol Oncol 2004;25:439–41.
132. Obermair A, Manolitsas TP, Leung Y, et al. Total laparoscopic hysterectomy for endometrial cancer: patterns of recurrence and survival. Gynecol Oncol 2004;92:789–93.
133. Eltabbakh GH. Analysis of survival after laparoscopy in women with endometrial carcinoma. Cancer 2002;95:1894–901.
134. Varia M, Rosenman J, Halle J, et al. Primary radiation therapy for medically inoperable patients with endometrial carcinoma—stages I-II. Int J Radiat Oncol Biol Phys 1987;13:11–5.
135. Grigsby PW, Kuske RR, Perez CA, et al. Medically inoperable stage I adenocarcinoma of the endometrium treated with radiotherapy alone. Int J Radiat Oncol Biol Phys 1987;13:483–8.
136. Abayomi O, Tak W, Emami B, et al. Treatment of endometrial carcinoma with radiation therapy alone. Cancer 1982;49:2466–9.
137. Rose PG, Baker S, Kern M, et al. Primary radiation therapy for endometrial carcinoma: a case controlled study. Int J Radiat Oncol Biol Phys 1993;27:585–90.
138. Fishman DA, Roberts KB, Chambers JT, et al. Radiation therapy as exclusive treatment for medically inoperable patients with stage I and II endometrioid carcinoma with endometrium. Gynecol Oncol 1996;61:189–96.
139. Churn M, Jones B. Primary radiotherapy for carcinoma of the endometrium using external beam radiotherapy and single line source brachytherapy. Clin Oncol (R Coll Radiol) 1999;11:255–62.
140. Grigsby PW, Perez CA, Camel HM, et al. Stage II carcinoma of the endometrium: results of therapy and prognostic factors. Int J Radiat Oncol Biol Phys 1985;11:1915–23.
141. Jones DA, Stout R. Results of intracavitary radium treatment for adenocarcinoma of the body of the uterus. Clin Radiol 1986;37:169–71.
142. Kucera H, Knocke TH, Kucera E, et al. Treatment of endometrial carcinoma with high-dose-rate brachytherapy alone in medically inoperable stage I patients. Acta Obstet Gynecol Scand 1998;77:1008–12.
143. Knocke TH, Kucera H, Weidinger B, et al. [The results of primary HDR-afterloading brachytherapy in corpus carcinoma]. Strahlenther Onkol 1995;171:195–201.
144. Nguyen C, Souhami L, Roman TN, et al. High-dose-rate brachytherapy as the primary treatment of medically inoperable stage I-II endometrial carcinoma. Gynecol Oncol 1995;59:370–5.
145. Nag S, Erickson B, Parikh S, et al. The American Brachytherapy Society recommendations for high-dose-rate brachytherapy for carcinoma of the endometrium. Int J Radiat Oncol Biol Phys 2000;48:779–90.
146. Creutzberg CL, van Putten WL, Koper PC, et al. Surgery and postoperative radiotherapy versus surgery alone for patients with stage-1 endometrial carcinoma: multicentre randomised trial. PORTEC Study Group. Post Operative Radiation Therapy in Endometrial Carcinoma. Lancet 2000;355:1404–11.
147. Keys HM, Roberts JA, Brunetto VL, et al. A phase III trial of surgery with or without adjunctive external pelvic radiation therapy in intermediate risk endometrial adenocarcinoma: a Gynecologic Oncology Group study. Gynecol Oncol 2004;92:744–51.
148. Berman ML. Adjuvant radiotherapy following properly staged endometrial cancer: what role? Gynecol Oncol 2004;92:737–9.
149. Larson DM, Broste SK, Krawisz BR. Surgery without radiotherapy for primary treatment of endometrial cancer. Obstet Gynecol 1998;91:355–9.
150. Chadha M, Nanavati PJ, Liu P, et al. Patterns of failure in endometrial carcinoma stage IB grade 3 and IC patients treated with postoperative vaginal vault brachytherapy. Gynecol Oncol 1999;75:103–7.
151. Eltabbakh GH, Piver MS, Hempling RE, et al. Excellent long-term survival and absence of vaginal recurrences in 332 patients with low-risk stage I endometrial adenocarcinoma treated with hysterectomy and vaginal brachytherapy without formal staging lymph node sampling: report of a prospective trial. Int J Radiat Oncol Biol Phys 1997;38:373–80.
152. Grigsby PW, Perez CA, Kuske RR, et al. Results of therapy, analysis of failures, and prognostic factors for clinical and pathologic stage III adenocarcinoma of the endometrium. Gynecol Oncol 1987;27:44–57.
153. Aalders JG, Abeler V, Kolstad P. Clinical (stage III) as compared to subclinical intrapelvic extrauterine tumor spread in endometrial carcinoma: a clinical and histopathological study of 175 patients. Gynecol Oncol 1984;17:64–74.
154. Bruckman JE, Bloomer WD, Marck A, et al. Stage III adenocarcinoma of the endometrium: two prognostic groups. Gynecol Oncol 1980;9:12–7.
155. Mackillop WJ, Pringle JF. Stage III endometrial carcinoma. A review of 90 cases. Cancer 1985;56:2519–23.
156. Greven KM,. Curran WJ Jr, Whittington R, et al. Analysis of failure patterns in stage III endometrial carcinoma and therapeutic implications. Int J Radiat Oncol Biol Phys 1989;17:35–9.
157. Burke TW, Heller PB, Woodward JE, et al. Treatment failure in endometrial carcinoma. Obstet Gynecol 1990;75:96–101.
158. Pliskow S, Penalver M, Averette ME. Stage III and stage IV endometrial carcinoma: a review of 41 cases. Gynecol Oncol 1990;38:210–5.
159. Hicks ML, Piver MS, Puretz JL, et al. Survival in patients with paraaortic lymph node metastases from endometrial adenocarcinoma clinically limited to the uterus. Int J Radiat Oncol Biol Phys 1993;26:607–11.
160. Komaki R, Mattingly RF, Hoffman RG, et al. Irradiation of para-aortic lymph node metastases from carcinoma of the cervix or endometrium. Preliminary results. Radiology 1983;147:245–8.
161. Feuer GA, Calanog A. Endometrial carcinoma: treatment of positive paraaortic nodes. Gynecol Oncol 1987;27:104–9.
162. Corn BW, Lanciano RM, Greven KM, et al. Endometrial cancer with para-aortic adenopathy: patterns of failure and opportunities for cure. Int J Radiat Oncol Biol Phys 1992;24:223–7.
163. Potish RA, Twiggs LB, Adcock LL, et al. Paraaortic lymph node radiotherapy in cancer of the uterine corpus. Obstet Gynecol 1985;65:251–6.
164. Bristow RE, Zahurak ML, Alexander CJ, et al. FIGO stage IIIC endometrial carcinoma: resection of macroscopic nodal disease and other determinants of survival. Int J Gynecol Cancer 2003;13:664–72.
165. Genest P, Drouin P, Girard A, et al. Stage III carcinoma of the endometrium: a review of 41 cases. Gynecol Oncol 1987;26:77–86.
166. Ackerman I, Malone S, Thomas G, et al. Endometrial carcinoma—relative effectiveness of adjuvant irradiation vs therapy reserved for relapse. Gynecol Oncol 1996;60:177–83.
167. Kuten A, Grigsby PW, Perez CA, et al. Results of radiotherapy in recurrent endometrial carcinoma: a retrospective analysis of 51 patients. Int J Radiat Oncol Biol Phys 1989;17:29–34.
168. Poulsen MG, Roberts SJ. The salvage of recurrent endometrial carcinoma in the vagina and pelvis. Int J Radiat Oncol Biol Phys 1988;15:809–13.
169. Scarabelli C, Campagnutta E, Giorda G, et al. Maximal cytoreductive surgery as a reasonable therapeutic alternative for recurrent endometrial carcinoma. Gynecol Oncol 1998;70:90–3.

170. Morris M, Alvarez RD, Kinney WK, et al. Treatment of recurrent adenocarcinoma of the endometrium with pelvic exenteration. Gynecol Oncol 1996;60:288–91.
171. Donovan JF. Nonhormonal chemotherapy of endometrial adenocarcinoma: a review. Cancer 1974;34:1587–92.
172. Muggia FM, Chia G, Reed LJ, et al. Doxorubicin-cyclophosphamide: effective chemotherapy for advanced endometrial adenocarcinoma. Am J Obstet Gynecol 1977;128:314–9.
173. Thigpen JT, Buchsbaum HJ, Mangan C, et al. Phase II trial of Adriamycin in the treatment of advanced or recurrent endometrial carcinoma: a Gynecologic Oncology Group study. Cancer Treat Rep 1979;63:21–7.
174. Horton J, Begg CB, Arseneault J, et al. Comparison of Adriamycin with cyclophosphamide in patients with advanced endometrial cancer. Cancer Treat Rep 1978;62:159–61.
175. Thigpen JT, Blessing JA, DiSaia PJ, et al. A randomized comparison of doxorubicin alone versus doxorubicin plus cyclophosphamide in the management of advanced or recurrent endometrial carcinoma: a Gynecologic Oncology Group study. J Clin Oncol 1994;12:1408–14.
176. Thigpen JT, Blessing JA, Lagasse LD, et al. Phase II trial of cisplatin as second-line chemotherapy in patients with advanced or recurrent endometrial carcinoma. A Gynecologic Oncology Group study. Am J Clin Oncol 1984;7:253–6.
177. Trope C, Grundsell H, Johnsson JE, et al. A phase II study of cis-platinum for recurrent corpus cancer. Eur J Cancer 1980;16:1025–6.
178. Seltzer V, Vogl SE, Kaplan BH. Adriamycin and cis-diamminedichloroplatinum in the treatment of metastatic endometrial adenocarcinoma. Gynecol Oncol 1984;19:308–13.
179. Pasmantier MW, Coleman M, Silver RT, et al. Treatment of advanced endometrial carcinoma with doxorubicin and cisplatin: effects on both untreated and previously treated patients. Cancer Treat Rep 1985;69:539–42.
180. Thigpen JT, Brady MF, Homesley HD, et al. Phase III trial of doxorubicin with or without cisplatin in advanced endometrial carcinoma: a Gynecologic Oncology Group study. J Clin Oncol 2004;22:3902–8.
181. Ball HG, Blessing JA, Lentz SS, et al. A phase II trial of paclitaxel in patients with advanced or recurrent adenocarcinoma of the endometrium: a Gynecologic Oncology Group study. Gynecol Oncol 1996;62:278–81.
182. Lissoni A, Zanetta G, Losa G, et al. Phase II study of paclitaxel as salvage treatment in advanced endometrial cancer. Ann Oncol 1996;7:861–3.
183. Aapro MS, van Wijk FH, Bolis G, et al. Doxorubicin versus doxorubicin and cisplatin in endometrial carcinoma: definitive results of a randomised study (55872) by the EORTC Gynaecological Cancer Group. Ann Oncol 2003;14:441–8.
184. Gallion HH, Brunetto VL, Cibull M, et al. Randomized phase III trial of standard timed doxorubicin plus cisplatin versus circadian timed doxorubicin plus cisplatin in stage III and IV or recurrent endometrial carcinoma: a Gynecologic Oncology Group Study. J Clin Oncol 2003;21:3808–13.
185. Fleming GF, Filiaci VL, Bentley RC, et al. Phase III randomized trial of doxorubicin + cisplatin versus doxorubicin + 24-h paclitaxel + filgrastim in endometrial carcinoma: a Gynecologic Oncology Group study. Ann Oncol 2004;15:1173–8.
186. Flemming GF, Brunetto AJ, Mundt RT, et al. Randomized trial of doxorubicin (DOX) plus cisplatin (CIS) versus DOX plus CIS plus paclitaxel (TAX) in patients with advanced or recurrent endometrial carcinoma: a Gynecologic Oncology Group (GOG) study [abstract]. J Clin Oncol 2002;21:2029.
187. Randall ME, Brunetto G, Muss HB, et al. Whole abdominal radiotherapy versus combination doxorubicin-cisplatin chemotherapy in advanced endometrial carcinoma: a randomized phase III trial of the Gynecologic Oncology Group. Proc Am Soc Clin Oncol 2003.
188. Stringer CA, Gershenson DM, Burke TW, et al. Adjuvant chemotherapy with cisplatin, doxorubicin, and cyclophosphamide (PAC) for early-stage high-risk endometrial cancer: a preliminary analysis. Gynecol Oncol 1990;38:305–8.
189. Morrow CP, Bundy BN, Homesley HD, et al. Doxorubicin as an adjuvant following surgery and radiation therapy in patients with high-risk endometrial carcinoma, stage I and occult stage II: a Gynecologic Oncology Group study. Gynecol Oncol 1990;36:166–71.
190. Burke TW, Gershenson DM, Morris M, et al. Postoperative adjuvant cisplatin, doxorubicin, and cyclophosphamide (PAC) chemotherapy in women with high-risk endometrial carcinoma. Gynecol Oncol 1994;55:47–50.
191. Kelly RM, Baker WH. Progestational agents in the measurement of carcinoma of the endometrium. N Engl J Med 1961;264:215–22.
192. Reifenstein EC Jr. The treatment of advanced endometrial cancer with hydroxyprogesterone caproate. Gynecol Oncol 1974;2:377–414.
193. Kauppila A. Progestin therapy of endometrial, breast and ovarian carcinoma. A review of clinical observations. Acta Obstet Gynecol Scand 1984;63:441–50.
194. Kohorn EI. Gestagens and endometrial carcinoma. Gynecol Oncol 1976;4:398–411.
195. Thigpen JT, Brady MF, Alvarez RD, et al. Oral medroxyprogesterone acetate in the treatment of advanced or recurrent endometrial carcinoma: a dose-response study by the Gynecologic Oncology Group. J Clin Oncol 1999;17:1736–44.
196. Lentz SS, Brady MF, Major FJ, et al. High-dose megestrol acetate in advanced or recurrent endometrial carcinoma: a Gynecologic Oncology Group study. J Clin Oncol 1996;14:357–61.
197. Podratz KC, O'Brien PC, Malkasian GD Jr, et al. Effects of progestational agents in treatment of endometrial carcinoma. Obstet Gynecol 1985;66:106–10.
198. Sall S, DiSaia P, Morrow CP, et al. A comparison of medroxyprogesterone serum concentrations by the oral or intramuscular route in patients with persistent or recurrent endometrial carcinoma. Am J Obstet Gynecol 1979;135:647–50.
199. Ramirez PT, Frumovitz M, Bodurka DC, et al. Hormonal therapy for the management of grade 1 endometrial adenocarcinoma: a literature review. Gynecol Oncol 2004;95:133–8.
200. Montz FJ, Bristow RE, Bovicelli A, et al. Intrauterine progesterone treatment of early endometrial cancer. Am J Obstet Gynecol 2002;186:651–7.
201. Moore TD, Phillips PH, Nerenstone SR, et al. Systemic treatment of advanced and recurrent endometrial carcinoma: current status and future directions. J Clin Oncol 1991;9:1071–88.
202. Slavik M, Petty WM, Blessing JA, et al. Phase II clinical study of tamoxifen in advanced endometrial adenocarcinoma: a Gynecologic Oncology Group study. Cancer Treat Rep 1984;68:809–11.
203. Edmonson JH, Krook JE, Hilton JF, et al. Ineffectiveness of tamoxifen in advanced endometrial carcinoma after failure of progestin treatment. Cancer Treat Rep 1986;70:1019–20.
204. Whitney CW, Brunetto VL, Zaino RJ, et al. Phase II study of medroxyprogesterone acetate plus tamoxifen in advanced endometrial carcinoma: a Gynecologic Oncology Group study. Gynecol Oncol 2004;92:4–9.
205. Fiorica JV, Brunetto VL, Hanjani P, et al. Phase II trial of alternating courses of megestrol acetate and tamoxifen in advanced endometrial carcinoma: a Gynecologic Oncology Group study. Gynecol Oncol 2004; 92:10–4.
206. Ayoub J, Audet-Lapointe P, Methot Y, et al. Efficacy of sequential cyclical hormonal therapy in endometrial cancer and its correlation with steroid hormone receptor status. Gynecol Oncol 1988;31:327–37.
207. Cohen CJ, Deppe G, Bruckner HW. Treatment of advanced adenocarcinoma of the endometrium with melphalan, 5-fluorouracil, and medroxyprogesterone acetate: a preliminary study. Obstet Gynecol 1977;50:415–7.
208. Pinelli DM, Fiorica JV, Roberts WS, et al. Chemotherapy plus sequential hormonal therapy for advanced and recurrent endometrial carcinoma: a phase II study. Gynecol Oncol 1996;60:462–7.
209. Asbury RF, Brunetto VL, Lee RB, et al. Goserelin acetate as treatment for recurrent endometrial carcinoma: a Gynecologic Oncology Group study. Am J Clin Oncol 2002;25:557–60.
210. Gallagher CJ, Oliver RT, Oram DH, et al. A new treatment for endometrial cancer with gonadotrophin releasing-hormone analogue. Br J Obstet Gynaecol 1991;98:1037–41.
211. Covens A, Thomas G, Shaw P, et al. A phase II study of leuprolide in advanced/recurrent endometrial cancer. Gynecol Oncol 1997;64:126–9.
212. Ma BB, Oza A, Eisenhauer E, et al. The activity of letrozole in patients with advanced or recurrent endometrial cancer and correlation with biological markers—a study of the National Cancer Institute of Canada Clinical Trials Group. Int J Gynecol Cancer 2004;14:650–8.
213. Thigpen JT, Blessing JA, Homesley H, et al. Phase II trial of cisplatin as first-line chemotherapy in patients with advanced or recurrent endometrial carcinoma: a Gynecologic Oncology Group study. Gynecol Oncol 1989;33:68–70.
214. Seski JC, Edwards CL, Herson J, et al. Cisplatin chemotherapy for disseminated endometrial cancer. Obstet Gynecol 1982;59:225–8.
215. Burke TW, Munkarah A, Kavanagh JJ, et al. Treatment of advanced or recurrent endometrial carcinoma with single-agent carboplatin. Gynecol Oncol 1993;51:397–400.
216. Green JB III, Green S, Alberts DS, et al. Carboplatin therapy in advanced endometrial cancer. Obstet Gynecol 1990;75:696–700.
217. Long HJ, Pfeifle DM, Wieand HS, et al. Phase II evaluation of carboplatin in advanced endometrial carcinoma. J Natl Cancer Inst 1988;80:276–8.
218. Calero F, Asins-Codoner E, Jimeno J, et al. Epirubicin in advanced endometrial adenocarcinoma: a phase II study of the Grupo Ginecologico Espanol para el Tratamiento Oncologico (GGETO). Eur J Cancer 1991;27:864–6.
219. Carbone PP, Carter SK. Endometrial cancer: approach to development of effective chemotherapy. Gynecol Oncol 1974;2:348–53.
220. Seski JC, Edwards CL, Copeland LJ, et al. Hexamethylmelamine chemotherapy for disseminated endometrial cancer. Obstet Gynecol 1981;58:361–3.
221. Muss HB. Chemotherapy of metastatic endometrial cancer. Semin Oncol 1994;21:107–13.
222. Fleming GF, Brunetto VL, Cella D, et al. Phase III trial of doxorubicin plus cisplatin with or without paclitaxel plus filgrastim in advanced endometrial carcinoma: a Gynecologic Oncology Group study. J Clin Oncol 2004;22:2159–66.
223. Horton J, Elson P, Gordon P, et al. Combination chemotherapy for advanced endometrial cancer. An evaluation of three regimens. Cancer 1982;49:2441–5.
224. Cohen CJ, Bruckner HW, Deppe G, et al. Multidrug treatment of advanced and recurrent endometrial carcinoma: a Gynecologic Oncology Group study. Obstet Gynecol 1984;63:719–26.
225. Cornelison TL, Baker TR, Piver MS, et al. Cisplatin, Adriamycin, etoposide, megestrol acetate versus melphalan, 5-fluorouracil, medroxyprogesterone acetate in the treatment of endometrial carcinoma. Gynecol Oncol 1995;59:243–8.

Neoplasms of the Fallopian Tube

Carmel J. Cohen, MD
Jamal Rahaman, MD

Malignant neoplasms of the fallopian tube are the rarest of the gynecologic cancers. Although cancers metastatic to the tube occur frequently from ovarian cancer, endometrial cancer, or other sources, and although there are reports of transitional cell carcinomas, adenosquamous carcinomas, and sarcomas, almost all of the primary cancers of the fallopian tube are papillary adenocarcinomas.

The first gross description of fallopian tube cancer was attributed to Renaud in 1847. Rokitansky recorded the first microscopic description in 1861, and Orthman is generally credited with the first case report in 1886.[1] Since that time, fewer than 2,000 patients with fallopian tube carcinomas have been reported, and the vast majority of these reports included less than 50 patients analyzed retrospectively over a period of more than 10 years in individual institutions. Only recently have collaborative groups or multi-institutional investigators begun to report their data. For example, Rosen and colleagues reported on 143 women treated from 1980 to 1995 by the Austrian Cooperative Study Group for Fallopian Tube Carcinoma.[2,3] In addition to reports from single institutions with experience in treating 40 or more patients,[4–8] from which conclusions concerning pathophysiology, clinical presentation and course, and treatment patterns can be drawn, several attempts have been made at definitive literature reviews.[9–12]

EPIDEMIOLOGY

Primary fallopian tube carcinoma comprises approximately 0.31 to 1.11% of cancers of the female genital tract.[9,13,14] The primary epidemiologic study of fallopian tube carcinoma was conducted in 1989 by Rosenblatt and colleagues, who reviewed the records of nine population-based cancer registries from the National Cancer Institute's Surveillance, Epidemiology, and End Results (SEER) Program.[14] The annual incidence rate of epithelial fallopian tube carcinoma was 3.6 per million women per year, and this figure remained constant from 1973 to 1984. Peak incidence occurred between the ages of 60 and 64 years; after age 65 years, the incidence plateaued at an age of 84 years. The incidence is significantly higher in white women (including Hispanics) than in black women. Etiologic factors for the development of primary fallopian tube carcinoma have not been clearly defined. Chronic tubal inflammation commonly coexists in fallopian tubes that contain carcinoma.[10,15] Whether there is an etiologic relationship remains unclear.

The increased risk of fallopian tube carcinoma among *BRCA*-positive patients was described in recent reports, indicating a need to remove completely the fallopian tube when performing prophylactic surgery in these patients.[16–22] Some cases of occult primary fallopian tube carcinoma have been detected at prophylactic bilateral oophorectomy in *BRCA1* mutation carriers, and this risk should not be ignored.[16,18,19,23] In addition, cases of fallopian tube carcinoma have been described following prophylactic salpingo-oophorectomy in known *BRCA* carriers.[22] As a result, several centers have established surgical-pathologic protocols to increase the ability to detect occult fallopian tube cancers by mandating peritoneal cytologic evaluation and employing serial sectioning of the fallopian tubes.[18,24]

CLINICAL PRESENTATION

The most frequently occurring symptoms are vaginal bleeding, unexplained vaginal discharge, and pelvic pain. The discharge may often be serosanguineous, is usually unexplained by microbiologic studies, and is unresponsive to antimicrobial therapy. The uterine bleeding is obviously pathologic because the majority of patients are postmenopausal, and it is almost invariably unexplained by uterine curettage. Thus, primary fallopian tube carcinoma must be considered in the differential diagnosis when postmenopausal bleeding persists after a negative curettage.

The presence of pain is highly significant because cancers of the ovary, endometrium, and cervix do not cause pain until their diagnosis is all too obvious. The syndrome of "hydrops tubae profluens," described by Latzko,[1] in which a patient presents with a pelvic mass, profuse watery or honey-colored vaginal discharge, and pelvic pain that is greatly relieved by the sudden disappearance of the mass, is rarely encountered but is almost pathognomonic. The pain is attributed to distention of the fallopian tube by trapped fluid, and when the fluid is emptied by traversing the tubal-uterine-vaginal channel, the patient is immediately relieved. Pelvic mass is the most common physical finding, occurring in approximately 65% of patients.[12] Ascites accompanies a mass in only 15% of cases, and a variety of less frequent physical findings are attributable to widely metastatic disease at presentation.

PREOPERATIVE DIAGNOSIS

Because of the rarity of this disease, with the resultant low level of suspicion by the medical community, a preoperative diagnosis is made in fewer than 3%[8] of the patients described. The presence of a pelvic mass is rarely attributed to tubal carcinoma by the examining physician, and radiography of the urinary and gastrointestinal tracts is useless in making the diagnosis.

The effectiveness of cytologic diagnosis from cervical and/or vaginal pool samples is widely variable and has been reported as positive in 40 to 60% of women with tubal carcinoma.[10,25] Of greater importance is the presence of adenocarcinoma in cervical or vaginal pool samples in the face of negative fractional dilatation and curettage of the uterus and absent palpable pathology. These patients may have early tubal carcinomas.

During the last decade, there have been increasing numbers of reports of successful diagnosis of fallopian tube carcinoma by ultrasonography.[26,27] The usual ultrasonography findings included a sausage-shaped mass with internal projections into a fluid-filled lumen, giving a characteristic "cogwheel" appearance. The successful preoperative diagnosis of primary fallopian tube carcinoma using transvaginal color and pulsed Doppler ultrasonography was reported by Kurjak and colleagues.[28] Computed tomographic and magnetic resonance imaging features have also been described.[29–31]

In 1984, Niloff and colleagues demonstrated the value of elevated cancer antigen (CA) 125 levels in monitoring four patients with recurrent fallopian tube carcinoma.[32] More recently, Rosen and colleagues determined pre- and postoperative CA 125 values in 13 patients with fallopian tube carcinoma.[33] The median preoperative value was 1,220 IU/mL, significantly higher in comparison with postoperative levels (median 194 IU/mL). Correlation analysis with stage and grading failed to achieve statistical significance; however, a trend for a positive correlation with stage and preoperative value could be observed.

Although it is well established that serum levels of CA 125 can be significantly elevated in patients with pelvic inflammatory disease, endometriosis, and early pregnancy, and although neither CA 125 nor CA 19-9 is highly specific, the presence of an adnexal mass in a postmenopausal woman is an indication for serum marker studies preoperatively, at least to establish reference values for measuring therapeutic response.

CLINICOPATHOLOGIC CLASSIFICATION AND STAGING

Although more than 90% of the fallopian tube cancers are papillary adenocarcinomas, the syn-

Table 103-1 Diagnostic Criteria for Carcinoma of the Fallopian Tube

1. Grossly: the main tumor is in the tube and arises from the endosalpinx
2. Histologically: the pattern reproduces the epithelium of tubal mucosa (papillary pattern)
3. Transition from benign to malignant tubal epithelium should be demonstrated
4. The ovaries and endometrium are normal or have a much smaller tumor volume than that of the tube

Adapted from Hu CY et al[34] and Sedlis A.[35]

chronous presentation of the same histology in multiple pelvic sites recommends the establishment of diagnostic criteria that will identify primary fallopian tube cancer. The criteria established by Hu and colleagues[34] and later modified slightly by Sedlis[35] have been widely accepted (Table 103-1). Hu and colleagues accepted the histologic classification originally proposed by Sanger and Barth in which three grades of tumor were observed (papillary, papillary-alveolar, or alveolar-medullary).[34] This classification is no longer used by many pathologists, and histologic grade is usually simply designated as well, moderately, or poorly differentiated. The degree of differentiation of fallopian tube carcinomas has generally not been related to prognosis.[5,7,36,37]

Until 1991, there was no universally accepted staging system for patients with tubal carcinoma. In 1967, Erez and colleagues proposed a clinical staging system based on prognostic observations.[38] This was modified in 1970 by Dodson and colleagues to conform with the International Federation of Gynecology and Obstetrics (FIGO) surgical staging system for ovarian cancer.[39]The following year, Schiller and Silverberg modified Dodson and colleagues' system to emphasize the importance of disease confined to the tubal lumen and the prognostic importance of invasion through the tubal wall to spread beyond the serosa.[10] These staging systems were prevalent in most of the reports during the last 20 years, and in 1991, FIGO officially promulgated a staging system for tubal carcinoma (Table 103-2).[40]

The new staging system takes into account the hollow viscus observations, the importance of ascites, and the impact of lymphatic spread. However, recently, Alvarado-Cabrero and colleagues proposed expanding the staging system to permit staging of noninvasive tubal carcinomas and fimbrial carcinomas and that substaging based on depth of invasion merits exploration in future studies.[41] Their recommendations are based on the observation that there was a significant difference in the length of recurrence-free survival of patients with no invasion beyond the epithelium or invasion of the lamina propria versus invasion into the muscularis.

PATTERNS OF SPREAD

Studies from the literature indicate that the pattern of spread of fallopian tube carcinoma is similar to ovarian carcinoma, with both intraperitoneal and lymphatic spread commonly encountered.[5,35] However, because older staging systems did not mandate lymphadenectomy, there are few data on the incidence of lymph node metastases at the time of presentation.

Tamimi and Figge reviewed 15 patients treated over a 12-year period in their institution.[15] Lymph node sampling was not routine at the time of initial surgery, yet four of their patients had positive para-aortic nodes at the time of presentation and, overall, eight of their patients had lymph node involvement, either at the time of presentation or at the time of recurrence shortly after treatment. Semrad and colleagues, studying patterns of recurrent disease, noted a 71% incidence of extraperitoneal metastases, suggesting a strong probability of unrecognized lymphatic invasion at the time of initial therapy.[42] This observation is strengthened by reports of other investigators.[4,5,36] More recently, di Re and colleagues, studying the lymphatic spread of fallopian tube carcinoma in 17 patients undergoing surgical staging, observed an increase in the rates of nodal metastases with stage of disease and grade.[43] Of note, the percentage of patients with positive nodes was 33%, 66%, and 80% for stage I, II, and III–IV disease, respectively. Overall, patients with negative nodes had a median survival of 76 months compared with only 33 months if nodal metastases were found.

PROGNOSTIC FACTORS

In view of the inherent difficulties in studying such a rare disease, the role of prognostic factors assumes a greater importance. Stage is the most consistent prognostic factor associated with survival.[2,3,5,36,44] Although the initial tumor burden does not have predictive significance regarding survival, residual disease after cytoreduction is a strong prognostic factor of survival.[4,5,44,45] Other clinical prognostic factors include the presence of ascites.[5] More recently, Rosen and colleagues reported on prognostic factors in 143 women with primary fallopian tube carcinoma.[2] FIGO stage, histologic grade, and the presence of residual tumor had an independent prognostic impact in multivariate analysis. Several histologic factors are prognostic of survival, most notably the extent of tubal invasion. The observation that the extent of tubal invasion was associated with a poorer prognosis was first reported by Schiller and Silverberg.[10] Peters and colleagues, analyzing stage I disease, observed a statistically significant increase in the risk of death with invasion of more than 50% of the tubal muscularis.[44] No association between grade and survival was observed by several investigators.[5,7,36]

TREATMENT

Initial management of carcinoma of the fallopian tube is surgical. No consensus exists regarding the best adjunctive therapy or whether adjuvant therapy has any value. The absence of surgical staging has probably inflated the number of patients assigned to stage I, thereby obscuring the subset that might not require adjuvant treatment. However, by analogy with ovarian cancer, it is possible that patients with grade 1 and stage I tumors require no further therapy. For the remainder, with 5-year survival rates for patients with stage II disease in the range of 50 to 60% and for patients with stage III and stage IV disease in the range of 10 to 20%,[4,5,35,36,46] consideration and investigation of postsurgical therapy are warranted.

Recently, the combined analysis of two large international multicenter trials has demonstrated that platinum-based therapy significantly improves the disease-free interval and overall survival of patients with early-stage high-risk ovarian cancer, with an 8% survival advantage in the chemotherapy treatment arm.[47] By extrapolation, such adjuvant therapy could also be of benefit to early-stage high-risk fallopian tube carcinoma (Figure 103-1).[13]

Table 103-2 Staging of Carcinoma of Fallopian Tube

Stage	Description
Stage 0	Carcinoma in situ (limited to tubal mucosa).
Stage I	Growth limited to the fallopian tubes.
Stage IA	Growth limited to one tube with extension into the submucosa and/or muscularis but not penetrating the serosal surface, no ascites.
Stage IB	Growth limited to both tubes with extension into the submucosa and/or muscularis but not penetrating the serosal surface, no ascites
Stage IC	Tumor either stage IA or IB with tumor extension through or onto the tubal serosa or with ascites present containing malignant cells or with positive washings.
Stage II	Growth involving one or both fallopian tubes with pelvic extension.
Stage IIA	Extension and/or metastasis to the uterus and/or ovaries.
Stage IIB	Extension to other pelvic tissues.
Stage IIC	Tumor either stage IIA or IIB and with ascites present containing malignant cells or with positive peritoneal washings.
Stage III	Tumor involving one or both fallopian tubes with peritoneal implants outside of the pelvis and/or retroperitoneal or inguinal nodes. Superficial liver metastases equals stage III. Tumor seems limited to the true pelvis with negative nodes but with histologically proven malignant extension to the small bowel or omentum.
Stage IIIA	Tumor grossly limited to the true pelvis with negative nodes but with histologically confirmed microscopic seeding of abdominal peritoneal surfaces.
Stage IIIB	Tumor involving one or both tubes with histologically confirmed implants of abdominal peritoneal surfaces, none exceeding 2 cm in diameter. Lymph nodes negative.
Stage IIIC	Abdominal implants greater than 2 cm in diameter and/or positive retroperitoneal or inguinal nodes.
Stage IV	Growth invading one or both fallopian tubes with distant metastases. If pleural effusion is present, there must be positive cytology to be stage IV. Parenchymal liver metastases equals stage IV.

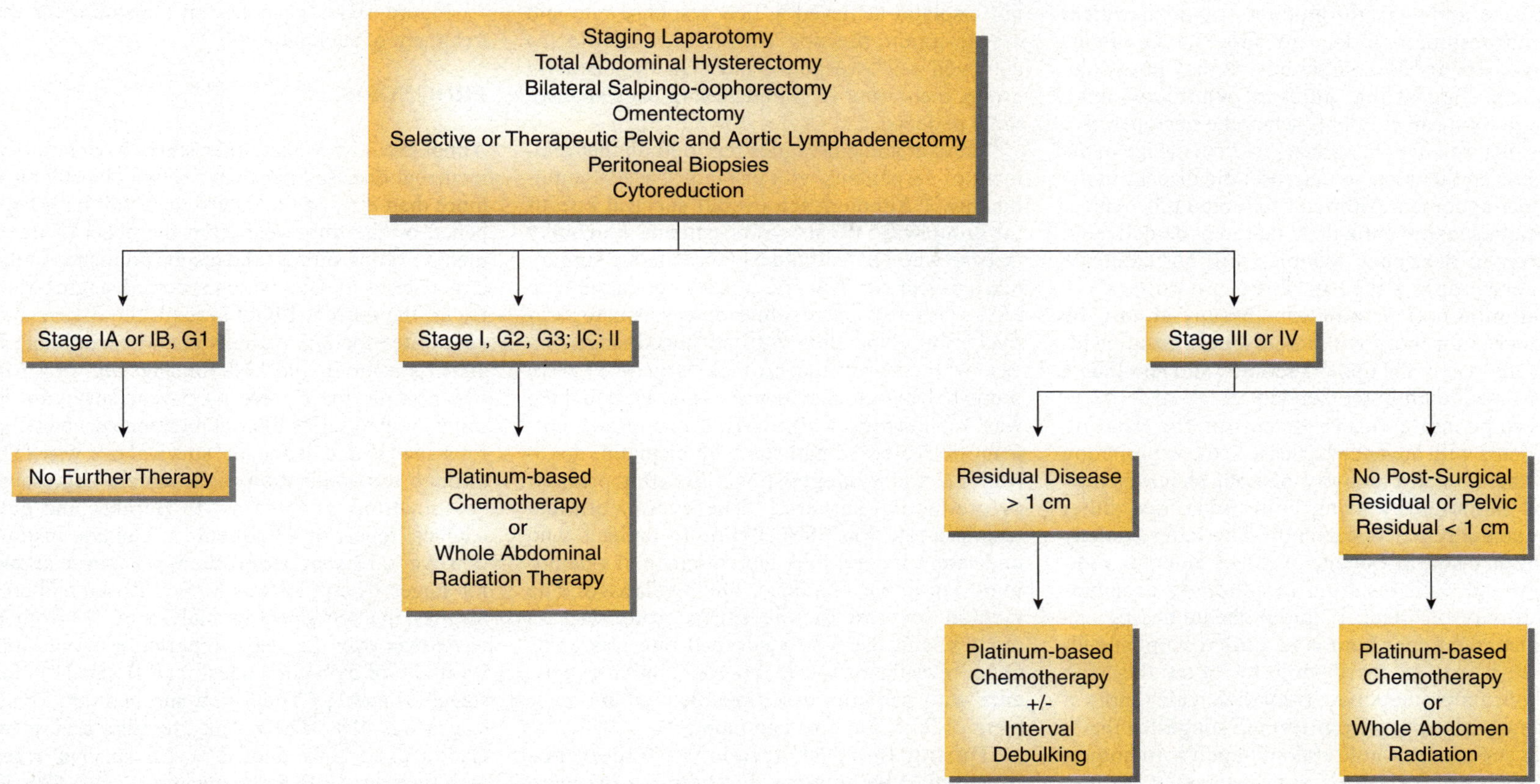

Figure 103-1 Treatment algorithm of primary fallopian tube carcinoma.

SURGICAL THERAPY

Because fallopian tube cancer is rarely diagnosed preoperatively, the surgeon is usually confronted with the diagnosis intraoperatively. The new FIGO staging system requires a surgical exercise similar to that mandated for ovarian carcinoma. This includes cytologic analysis of either ascitic fluid or pelvic and abdominal washings, abdominal hysterectomy and bilateral salpingo-oophorectomy, omentectomy, and selective (or therapeutic) pelvic and para-aortic lymphadenectomy with selective peritoneal biopsies. In apparent early-stage disease, there may be up to a 33% incidence of nodal metastases,[43] highlighting the importance of performing a selective pelvic and para-aortic lymphadenectomy. For advanced disease, the same principles of cytoreductive surgery for ovarian carcinoma apply to fallopian tube carcinoma as well. The importance of cytoreductive surgery is supported by the observations of Eddy and colleagues, who found that the median survival of patients with no gross residual disease was 30 months, significantly longer than the survival of patients whose largest tumor diameter was greater than 2 cm (17 months).[4]

Several studies examining the role of second-look laparotomy in fallopian tube carcinoma have been performed.[4,7,8,45] Barakat and colleagues reported the largest series of patients undergoing second-look laparotomy.[45] Only 19% of patients whom they observed had a recurrence after negative second-look laparotomy, with a mean follow-up of 50 months. This contrasts with advanced-stage ovarian carcinoma patients who are treated with platinum-based chemotherapy, among whom approximately 50% will experience recurrence following a negative second-look procedure, with a median interval of 14 months to recurrence.[48] However, more recently, Cormio and colleagues observed that 31% of patients with a negative second look had recurrences, with a mean follow-up of 49 months.[49]

A recent randomized trial in Europe demonstrated a survival benefit for interval cytoreductive surgery in ovarian cancer patients initially left with residual disease > 1 cm,[50,51] and we would advocate consideration for interval surgery in the same cohort of patients with fallopian tube cancer as illustrated in Figure 103-1. In addition, analogous to the paradigm employed in ovarian cancer, we would consider secondary cytoreductive surgery in highly selected patients who develop recurrences with long disease-free intervals and initial optimal cytoreduction and in whom there is good likelihood of an optimal secondary surgery (residual disease < 1 cm).[52,53]

RADIATION THERAPY

Because of the transcelomic pattern of dissemination, the use of whole abdominopelvic irradiation, as employed for intermediate-risk ovarian cancer, has been explored as postoperative treatment for patients with fallopian tube carcinoma.[5,6,36] This approach has produced better survival rates than radiation therapy confined to the pelvis.[27,40]

There are no data from randomized trials comparing the efficacy of abdominopelvic radiotherapy and cisplatin-containing chemotherapy for the adjuvant treatment of early fallopian tube cancer. A nationwide retrospective cohort analysis comparing irradiation with chemotherapy as adjuvant therapy in primary stage I and II carcinoma of the fallopian tube was conducted in Austria.[54] Ninety-five cases of fallopian tube cancer, including 66 stage I cases and 29 stage II cases, were identified. Group I ($n = 32$) patients underwent complete irradiation with cobalt or photon energies of 23 MV (administering a daily dose of 2 Gy resulted in a total of 45 to 52 Gy in the pelvic areas). Group II ($n = 31$) patients received postoperative platinum-based chemotherapy. The median survival time was 57 months in group I patients compared with 73 months in the chemotherapy-treated group II. This difference was not statistically significant. However, patients in this study were assigned nonrandomly to treatment and there was no stratification for the amount of residual disease among the two groups of patients. The authors concluded that chemotherapy and irradiation were two adjuvant therapies that are similarly effective in stage I and II fallopian tube cancer, with chemotherapy being preferred at the present time. Primary surgical treatment, however, had a crucial impact on the prognosis of fallopian tube cancer.

Although abdominal irradiation has been used in treating patients with more advanced disease and varying amounts of postsurgical tumor residuum, it does not appear to be of curative benefit.[5,55] Comparable studies in ovarian cancer suggest that adjuvant whole-abdomen irradiation can cure only when the postoperative residual tumor is less than 1 to 2 cm in size in the pelvis and there is no macroscopic disease in the upper abdomen. Although fallopian tube cancer is radiosensitive, the dose that may be delivered safely to the upper abdomen will not eradicate macroscopic disease. Thus, postoperative abdominopelvic radiation therapy should be reserved for those with microscopic or no residual disease in the upper abdomen and less than a 1 cm residuum in the pelvis.

A possible future direction for treating patients with advanced disease is the exploitation of the cytotoxic activity of both chemotherapy and radiation by using both modalities either sequentially or concurrently. The latter strategy may also take advantage of enhancement of radiation cell kill, resulting in additivity or supra-additivity of effect. If initial chemotherapy can reduce the tumor burden to a microscopic residuum, it may be worthwhile to follow this with whole abdominopelvic irradiation. One report of sequential therapy from Toronto suggested that it was superior to whole abdominopelvic radiotherapy alone.[56] Overall survival rates for the sequential therapy were 54% for stage I, 68% for stage II, 28% for stage III, and 25% for stage IV disease. The overall survival was significantly influenced by treatment, with a 5-year survival rate of 84% following sequential therapy compared with 37% for the historical cohort treated with radiation alone (p = .0006). The patient groups were comparable with respect to at least two recognized prognostic factors: stage and residual disease. The overall toxicity was deemed acceptable. The authors concluded that a policy of platinum-based chemotherapy followed by abdominopelvic irradiation led to an improvement in overall survival and recommended sequential treatment as their current postoperative management.

CHEMOTHERAPY

Because of similarities in the appearance of papillary carcinomas of the tube and ovary, it was logical to apply to patients with tubal carcinoma the cytotoxic agents known to be active against ovarian carcinoma. Cyclophosphamide, melphalan, doxorubicin, and thiotepa were among the frequently used single agents in the early cytotoxic treatment of tubal carcinoma.[7,8,57,58] Response rates to single alkylating agents were generally less than 20% in small series of patients with disparate stages and prognostic features. With the introduction of cisplatin-containing regimens,[58] complete clinical responses were noted in patients with advanced disease and were confirmed by second-look surgery. Peters and colleagues demonstrated that multiagent chemotherapy with cisplatin achieved an 81% objective response rate, whereas multiagent therapy without cisplatin achieved a 29% response rate and single-agent therapy (other than cisplatin) achieved a 9% response rate.[8] In the cisplatin group, there were 12 complete surgical responses in 20 patients.

Barakat and colleagues reported on the treatment of 38 patients with cisplatin-based chemotherapy.[59] Although the overall survival rate of the group was 51% at 5 years, patients with bulky disease who had complete cytoreductive surgery had a 5-year survival rate of 83% compared with 28% if there was residual disease postoperatively. Of 21 patients with advanced-stage disease who came to second-look surgery, 11 were found to be without evidence of disease and there was 1 recurrence. Similarly, Cormio and colleagues treated 32 patients with cisplatin, doxorubicin, and cyclophosphamide after primary cytoreductive surgery.[60] The overall clinical response rate was 80%. Ten of 14 patients who underwent second-look laparotomy had a pathologic complete response, but 3 relapsed. The median survival for the entire group was 38 months, and the 5-year survival rate was 35%. Other investigators have reported similar experience with platinum-based regimens in the treatment of fallopian tube carcinoma.[61]

During the past decade, as experience increased, it became obvious from the literature that fallopian tube carcinoma responds well to cytotoxic chemotherapy; multidrug regimens containing cisplatin seem to be more active than nonplatinum single agents or multidrug regimens without cisplatin. The platinum-paclitaxel combination is now employed analogous to its standard application in ovarian cancer, as reflected in a report by Gemignani and colleagues in 23 patients treated from 1993 to 1998.[62] Paclitaxel was administered at 135 to 175 mg/m^2 in combination with carboplatin in 17 patients and cisplatin in 6 patients.

The European Organisation for Research and Treatment of Cancer (EORTC) reported a phase II study of a combination of cyclophosphamide, Adriamycin (doxorubicin), and cisplatin (CAP) in 24 eligible patients with advanced fallopian tube carcinoma (FIGO stage III–IV). The CAP regimen consisted of cyclophosphamide 600 mg/m^2, doxorubicin 45 mg/m^2, and cisplatin 50 mg/m^2 administered intravenously every 28 days. Ten patients had a complete and six patients had a partial response (response rate 67%). The median overall survival was 24 months, and the 1-, 3-, and 5-year survival rates were 73%, 25%, and 19%, respectively.[63]

Second-line and salvage therapy currently uses the same agents employed in ovarian cancer,[13,64] including liposomal doxorubicin,[65] topotecan,[66,67] docetaxel,[68,69] and gemcitabine.[70]

The role of hormonal therapy in the treatment of tubal carcinoma is unclear; however, medroxyprogesterone acetate and megestrol acetate have been employed, usually in combination with cytotoxic agents.[5,7,58] There is no evidence that progestational therapy alone is effective in this disease.

Figure 103-1 proposes an algorithm for the treatment of such patients.

PROGNOSIS

Although most of the larger series have reported recurrent disease later than 5 years after therapy, more than 80% of the recurrences will have happened by the third year from the onset of treatment.[42] If one surveys the results published in the larger series to date, which reported staging similar to the current FIGO system, the 5-year survival rates for 228 patients are 61% for stage I, 40% for stage II, and 17% for stage III.[5,8,36,71] In two reports, there were no 5-year survivors in stage IV; two series did not mention survivorship for stage IV; and in one, the survival rate was 25% through the application of extremely aggressive combinations of therapy.[5] In Barakat and colleagues' report of 43 patients at a single institution over a 10-year period, the 5-year survival rate for stages III and IV was 51%.[59] Rosen and colleagues, in a retrospective analysis of 143 women in Austria over 15 years, reported a 5-year survival rate of 59% for stages I and II and 19% for stages III and IV.[2] The 5-year survival rate for all stages was 43%. The recent literature review by Gadducci in 2002 quoted 5-year survival rates ranging from 32 to 80% in stage I, 16 to 58% in stage II, and 0 to 29% in stages III–IV.[13] Using the National Cancer Institute's SEER Program, Kosary and Trimble identified 416 women with fallopian tube carcinoma diagnosed between 1990 and 1997.[72] Almost half of those diagnosed with stage I or II disease did not undergo surgical evaluation of lymph nodes. Most women with stage I or II disease were treated with surgery alone, whereas most women with stage III or IV disease were treated with surgery and chemotherapy. The 5-year relative survival rates by FIGO stage were as follows: stage I (n = 102), 95%; stage II (n = 29), 75%; stage III (n = 52), 69%; stage IV (n = 151), 45%.

In an attempt to identify prognostic features, the Austrian Cooperative Study Group for Fallopian Tube Carcinoma analyzed the 66 patients treated in Austria between 1980 and 1990.[37] The group studied the role of inflammatory reaction, nuclear anaplasia, mitotic activity, and progesterone and estrogen receptor concentrations. The distribution of patients was 35% stage I, 20% stage II, 29% stage III, and 16% stage IV. Ascites was found in 24% of patients but only in FIGO stages III and IV. The overall 5-year survival rate for stages I and II was 50%, and for stages III and IV, it was 14%. The authors found no prognostic impact of degree of differentiation or the presence, absence, or concentration of estrogen and progesterone receptors. Lymphocyte infiltration in the tumor was confirmed as a prognostic factor by multivariate analysis, as was stage of disease. In a separate review of the Austrian experience, 61 specimens of fallopian tube carcinoma were examined by image cytometry for ploidy determination.[3] Forty-eight of the tumors showed an aneuploid pattern. Although patients with a euploid pattern had a median survival of 33.8 months compared with 24.5 months for patients with aneuploid tumors, significance was not reached, nor was there a correlation between ploidy status and the stage or grade of the tumor.

A study was performed of the pathology specimens and clinical case records from 151 patients with fallopian tube carcinoma who were treated consecutively in Norway.[73] In a multivariate analysis, disease stage, the presence of residual tumor, and a hydrosalpinx-like appearance of the fallopian tube were of independent prognostic significance for the whole cohort. For patients with stage I disease, the depth of infiltration in the tubal wall and intraoperative tumor rupture were of independent prognostic significance. Prognostic factors in patients with early-stage (stages 0 and I) fallopian tube carcinoma seem to differ from those in patients with early-stage ovarian carcinoma. For patients with more advanced-stage disease, owing to the striking similarities in prognostic and clinical characteristics between the two diseases, the authors recommended that the treatment and follow-up strategies for patients with ovarian carcinoma be adopted in the management of patients with fallopian tube carcinoma.

OTHER MALIGNANT FALLOPIAN TUBE NEOPLASMS

Fewer than 150 other fallopian tube cancers have been reported, including less than 50 malignant müllerian mixed tumors of the fallopian tube,[74,75] as well as rare primary leiomyosarcomas,[76] rare examples of immature teratomas, and occurrences of trophoblastic disease, primarily choriocarcinomas.[77] The diagnostic approach for any of these tumors is the same as that for primary adenocarcinoma of the fallopian tube, except that in the case of trophoblastic disease, human chorionic gonadotropin serum levels and, in the case of malignant teratoma, alpha fetoprotein levels, are useful. Surgical therapy should be followed by individualized treatment with cytotoxic chemotherapy appropriate to the histology or radiation therapy to postoperative fields according to the primary tumor classification and stage of disease.

REFERENCES

1. Benedet JL, White GW. Malignant tumors of fallopian tube. In Gynecologic oncology: fundamental principles and clinical practice. Edited by Malcolm Coppleson. Churchill Livingston. New York,1981: 621–9.
2. Rosen AC, Klein M, Hafner E, et al. Management and prognosis of primary fallopian tube carcinoma. Austrian Cooperative Study Group for Fallopian Tube Carcinoma. Gynecol Obstet Invest 1999;47:45–51.
3. Rosen AC, Graf AH, Klein M, et al. DNA ploidy in primary fallopian-tube carcinoma using image cytometry. Int J Cancer 1994;58:362–5.
4. Eddy GL,. Copeland LJ, Gershenson DM, et al. Fallopian tube carcinoma. Obstet Gynecol 1984;64:546–52.
5. Podratz KC, Podczaski ES, Gaffey TA, et al. Primary carcinoma of the fallopian tube. Am J Obstet Gynecol 1986;154:1319–26.
6. Benedet JL, White GW, Fairey RN, et al. Adenocarcinoma of the fallopian tube. Experience with 41 patients. Obstet Gynecol 1977;50:654–7.
7. Rose PG, Piver MS, Tsukada Y. Fallopian tube cancer. The Roswell Park experience. Cancer 1990;66:2661–7.
8. Peters WA III, Andersen WA, Hopkins MP. Results of chemotherapy in advanced carcinoma of the fallopian tube. Cancer 1989;63:836–8.
9. Sedlis A. Carcinoma of the fallopian tube. Surg Clin North Am 1978;58:121–9.
10. Schiller HM, Silverberg SG. Staging and prognosis in primary carcinoma of the fallopian tube. Cancer 1971;28:389–95.
11. Schneider C, Wight E, Perucchini D, et al. Primary carcinoma of the fallopian tube. A report of 19 cases with literature review. Eur J Gynaecol Oncol 2000;21:578–82.
12. Nordin AJ. Primary carcinoma of the fallopian tube: a 20-year literature review. Obstet Gynecol Surv 1994;49:349–61.
13. Gadducci A. Current management of fallopian tube carcinoma. Curr Opin Obstet Gynecol 2002;14:27–32.
14. Rosenblatt KA, Weiss NS, Schwartz SM. Incidence of malignant fallopian tube tumors. Gynecol Oncol 1989;35:236–9.
15. Tamimi HK, Figge DC. Adenocarcinoma of the uterine tube: potential for lymph node metastases. Am J Obstet Gynecol 1981;141:132–7.
16. Paley PJ, Swisher EM, Garcia RL, et al. Occult cancer of the fallopian tube in BRCA-1 germline mutation carriers at prophylactic oophorectomy: a case for recommending hysterectomy at surgical prophylaxis. Gynecol Oncol 2001;80:176–80.
17. Aziz S, Kuperstein G, Rosen B, et al. A genetic epidemiological study of carcinoma of the fallopian tube. Gynecol Oncol 2001;80:341–5.
18. Colgan TJ, Murphy J, Cole DE, et al. Occult carcinoma in prophylactic oophorectomy specimens: prevalence and association with BRCA germline mutation status. Am J Surg Pathol 2001;25:1283–9.
19. Hartley A, Rollason T, Spooner D. Clear cell carcinoma of the fimbria of the fallopian tube in a BRCA1 carrier undergoing prophylactic surgery. Clin Oncol (R Coll Radiol) 2000;12:58–9.
20. Tong D, Stimpfl M, Reinthaller A, et al. BRCA1 gene mutations in sporadic ovarian carcinomas: detection by PCR and reverse allele-specific oligonucleotide hybridization. Clin Chem 1999;45:976–81.
21. Levine DA, Argenta PA, Yee CJ, et al. Fallopian tube and primary peritoneal carcinomas associated with BRCA mutations. J Clin Oncol 2003;21:4222–7.
22. Dijkhuizen FP, Huisman A, Boonstra H, et al. [Carcinoma of the fallopian tube after prophylactic laparoscopic ovariectomy in a patient with a BRCAI mutation]. Ned Tijdschr Geneeskd 2003;147:877–9.
23. Agoff SN, Mendelin JE, Grieco VS, et al. Unexpected gynecologic neoplasms in patients with proven or suspected BRCA-1 or -2 mutations: implications for gross examination, cytology, and clinical follow-up. Am J Surg Pathol 2002;26:171–8.
24. Powell CB, Kenley E, Chen LM, et al. Risk-reducing salpingo-oophorectomy in BRCA mutation carriers: role of serial sectioning in the detection of occult malignancy. J Clin Oncol 2005;23:127–32.
25. Johnston GA Jr. Primary malignancy of the fallopian tube: a clinical review of 13 cases. J Surg Oncol 1983;24:304–9.
26. Ajjimakorn S, Bhamarapravati Y. Transvaginal ultrasound and the diagnosis of fallopian tubal carcinoma. J Clin Ultrasound 1991;19:116–9.
27. Ekici E, Vicdan K, Danisman N, et al. Ultrasonographic appearance of fallopian tube carcinoma. Int J Gynaecol Obstet 1995;49:325–9.
28. Kurjak A, Kupesic S, Ilijas M, et al. Preoperative diagnosis of primary fallopian tube carcinoma. Gynecol Oncol 1998;68:29–34.
29. Takagi H, Matsunami K, Noda K, et al. Primary fallopian tube carcinoma: a case of successful preoperative evaluation with magnetic resonance imaging. J Obstet Gynaecol 2003;23:455–6.
30. Mikami M, Tei C, Kurahashi T, et al. Preoperative diagnosis of fallopian tube cancer by imaging. Abdom Imaging 2003;28:743–7.
31. Santana P, Desser TS, Teng N. Preoperative CT diagnosis of primary fallopian tube carcinoma in a patient with a history of total abdominal hysterectomy. J Comput Assist Tomogr 2003;27:361–3.
32. Niloff JM, Klug TL, Schaetzl E, et al. Elevation of serum CA125 in carcinomas of the fallopian tube, endometrium, and endocervix. Am J Obstet Gynecol 1984;148:1057–8.
33. Rosen AC, Klein M, Rosen HR, et al. Preoperative and postoperative CA-125 serum levels in primary fallopian tube carcinoma. Arch Gynecol Obstet 1994;255:65–8.
34. Hu CY, Taylor ML, Hertig AT. Primary carcinoma of the fallopian tube. Am J Obstet Gynecol 1950;59:58–67.
35. Sedlis A. Primary carcinoma of the fallopian tube. Obstet Gynecol Surv 1961;16:209–26.
36. McMurray EH, Jacobs AJ, Perez CA, et al. Carcinoma of the fallopian tube. Management and sites of failure. Cancer 1986;58:2070–5.
37. Rosen A, Klein M, Lahousen M, et al. Primary carcinoma of the fallopian tube—a retrospective analysis of 115 patients. Austrian Cooperative Study Group for Fallopian Tube Carcinoma. Br J Cancer 1993;68:605–9.
38. Erez S, Kaplan AL, Wall JA. Clinical staging of carcinoma of the uterine tube. Obstet Gynecol 1967;30:547–50.
39. Dodson MG, Ford JH Jr, Averette HE. Clinical aspects of fallopian tube carcinoma. Obstet Gynecol 1970;36:935–9.
40. Petterson F. Staging rules for gestational trophoblastic tumors and fallopian tube cancer. Acta Obstet Gynecol Scand 1992;71:244–5.
41. Alvarado-Cabrero I, Young RH, Vamvakas EC, et al. Carcinoma of the fallopian tube: a clinicopathological study of 105 cases with observations on staging and prognostic factors. Gynecol Oncol 1999;72:367–79.
42. Semrad N, Watring W, Fu YS, et al. Fallopian tube adenocarcinoma: common extraperitoneal recurrence. Gynecol Oncol 1986;24:230–5.
43. di Re E, Grosso G, Raspagliesi F, et al. Fallopian tube cancer: incidence and role of lymphatic spread. Gynecol Oncol 1996;62:199–202.
44. Peters WA III, Andersen WA, Hopkins MP, et al. Prognostic features of carcinoma of the fallopian tube. Obstet Gynecol 1988;71:757–62.
45. Barakat RR, Rubin SC, Saigo PE, et al. Second-look laparotomy in carcinoma of the fallopian tube. Obstet Gynecol 1993;82:748–51.
46. Heintz AP, Odicino F, Maisonneuve P, et al. Carcinoma of the fallopian tube. Int J Gynaecol Obstet 2003;83 Suppl 1:119–33.
47. Trimbos JB, Parmar M, Vergote I, et al. International Collaborative Ovarian Neoplasm trial 1 and Adjuvant ChemoTherapy In Ovarian Neoplasm trial: two parallel randomized phase III trials of adjuvant chemotherapy in patients with early-stage ovarian carcinoma. J Natl Cancer Inst 2003;95:105–12.
48. Rubin SC, Hoskins WJ, Saigo PE, et al. Prognostic factors for recurrence following negative second-look laparotomy in ovarian cancer patients treated with platinum-based chemotherapy. Gynecol Oncol 1991;42:137–41.
49. Cormio G, Gabriele A, Maneo A, et al. Second-look laparotomy in the management of fallopian tube carcinoma. Acta Obstet Gynecol Scand 1997;76:369–72.
50. van der Burg ME, van Lent M, Buyse M, et al. The effect of debulking surgery after induction chemotherapy on the prognosis in advanced epithelial ovarian cancer. Gynecological Cancer Cooperative Group of the European Organization for Research and Treatment of Cancer. N Engl J Med 1995;332:629–34.
51. van der Burg ME. Advanced ovarian cancer. Curr Treat Options Oncol 2001;2:109–18.
52. Bristow RE, Lagasse LD, Karlan BY. Secondary surgical cytoreduction for advanced epithelial ovarian cancer. Patient selection and review of the literature. Cancer 1996;78:2049–62.
53. Segna RA, Dottino PR, Mandeli JP, et al. Secondary cytoreduction for ovarian cancer following cisplatin therapy. J Clin Oncol 1993;11:434–9.
54. Klein M, Rosen A, Lahousen M, et al. The relevance of adjuvant therapy in primary carcinoma of the fallopian tube, stages I and II: irradiation vs. chemotherapy. Int J Radiat Oncol Biol Phys 2000;48:1427–31.
55. Schray MF, Podratz KC, Malkasian GD. Fallopian tube cancer: .the role of radiation therapy. Radiother Oncol 1987;10:267–75.
56. Rawlings G, Bush R, Dembo A. Fallopian tube cancer: survival following radiation and chemotherapy. In: Proceedings of the International Gynecologic Cancer Society 3rd Biennial Meeting; Cairns, Australia1991.
57. Boronow RC. Chemotherapy for disseminated tubal cancer. Obstet Gynecol 1973;42:62–6.
58. Deppe G, Bruckner HW,. Cohen CJ. Combination chemotherapy for advanced carcinoma of the fallopian tube. Obstet Gynecol 1980;56:530–2.
59. Barakat RR, Rubin SC, Saigo PE, et al. Cisplatin-based combination chemotherapy in carcinoma of the fallopian tube. Gynecol Oncol 1991;42:156–60.
60. Cormio G, Maneo A, Gabriele A, et al. Treatment of fallopian tube carcinoma with cyclophosphamide, Adriamycin, and cisplatin. Am J Clin Oncol 1997;20:143–5.

61. Jacobs AJ, McMurray EH, Parham J, et al. Treatment of carcinoma of the fallopian tube using cisplatin, doxorubicin, and cyclophosphamide. Am J Clin Oncol 1986;9:436–9.
62. Gemignani ML, Hensley ML, Cohen R, et al. Paclitaxel-based chemotherapy in carcinoma of the fallopian tube. Gynecol Oncol 2001;80:16–20.
63. Wagenaar HC, Pecorelli S, Vergote I, et al. Phase II study of a combination of cyclophosphamide, Adriamycin and cisplatin in advanced fallopian tube carcinoma. An EORTC gynecological cancer group study. European Organization for Research and Treatment of Cancer. Eur J Gynaecol Oncol 2001;22:187–93.
64. Markman M, Bookman MA. Second-line treatment of ovarian cancer. Oncologist 2000;5:26–35.
65. Markman M, Kennedy A, Webster K, et al. Phase 2 trial of liposomal doxorubicin (40 mg/m(2)) in platinum/paclitaxel-refractory ovarian and fallopian tube cancers and primary carcinoma of the peritoneum. Gynecol Oncol 2000;78(3 Pt 1):369–72.
66. Dunton CJ, Neufeld J. Complete response to topotecan of recurrent fallopian tube carcinoma. Gynecol Oncol 2000;76:128–9.
67. Brown JV III, Peters WA III, Rettenmaier MA, et al. A phase I trial of a 3-day topotecan q 21 days for recurrent epithelial cancers of the ovary, fallopian tube, and peritoneum. Gynecol Oncol 2000;79:495–8.
68. Verschraegen CF, Sittisomwong T, Kudelka AP, et al. Docetaxel for patients with paclitaxel-resistant müllerian carcinoma. J Clin Oncol 2000;18:2733–9.
69. Markman M, Kennedy A, Webster K, et al. Combination chemotherapy with carboplatin and docetaxel in the treatment of cancers of the ovary and fallopian tube and primary carcinoma of the peritoneum. J Clin Oncol 2001;19:1901–5.
70. Silver DF, Piver MS. Gemcitabine salvage chemotherapy for patients with gynecologic malignancies of the ovary, fallopian tube, and peritoneum. Am J Clin Oncol 1999;22:450–2.
71. Brown MD,. Kohorn EI, Kapp DS, et al. Fallopian tube carcinoma. Int J Radiat Oncol Biol Phys 1985;11:583–90.
72. Kosary C, Trimble EL. Treatment and survival for women with fallopian tube carcinoma: a population-based study. Gynecol Oncol 2002;86:190–1.
73. Baekelandt M, Jorunn Nesbakken A, Kristensen GB, et al. Carcinoma of the fallopian tube. Cancer 2000;89:2076–84.
74. Horn LC, Werschnik C, Bilek K, et al. Diagnosis and clinical management in malignant müllerian tumors of the fallopian tube. A report of four cases and review of recent literature. Arch Gynecol Obstet 1996;258:47–53.
75. Chang HC, Hsueh S, Soong YK. Malignant mixed müllerian tumor of the fallopian tube. Case report and review of the literature. Changgeng Yi Xue Za Zhi 1991;14:259–63.
76. Jacoby AF, Fuller AF Jr, Thor AD, et al. Primary leiomyosarcoma of the fallopian tube. Gynecol Oncol 1993;51:404–7.
77. Young RH, Scully RE. Pathology of tumors of fallopian tube and broad ligament. In: Coppelson M, editor. Gynecologic oncology. Melbourne: Churchill Livingstone; 1992. p. 843–52.

Ovarian Cancer

Jonathan S. Berek, MD, MMSc
Robert C. Bast Jr, MD

EPITHELIAL OVARIAN CANCER

Ovarian cancer is one of the most treatable solid tumors, as the majority will respond temporarily to surgery and cytotoxic agents. The disease, however, frequently persists and recurs, having the highest fatality-to-case ratio of all the gynecologic cancers. Ovarian cancer represents one-fourth of the malignancies of the female genital tract, but it is the most common cause of death among women who develop cancers of gynecologic origin. Ovarian carcinomas account for 4% of the total cancers in women in the United States, ranked behind malignant neoplasms of the lung, breast, colon and uterus. In 2005, over 22,000 new cases and more than 16,000 deaths are expected.[1] Despite these discouraging statistics, improvement in 5-year survival has occurred steadily over the last three decades with more aggressive surgical management and the development of more effective chemotherapy. Five-year survival for all stages and histologies combined in the United States has improved significantly ($p < .05$) from 37% in 1974–76 to 52% in 1992–1998.[1]

Ovarian cancer is a disease of post-menopausal women, with only 10 to 15% discovered in premenopausal patients.[2] The median age for diagnosis of epithelial ovarian cancer, the most common histologic type, is between 60 and 65 years.[2] Less than 1% of epithelial ovarian cancers are found in women less than 30 years of age, and most ovarian malignancies in these younger patients are germ cell tumors.[2–3] Ovarian cancer occurs sporadically in the population. A strong hereditary component contributes to development of the disease in 10% of cases, but 90% are sporadic. Ovarian cancer is neither a common nor a rare disease. The prevalence of ovarian cancer among postmenopausal women in the United States is 40 per 100,000 or 1 in 2,500. The lifetime risk for a woman to develop ovarian cancer is approximately 1 in 70 (1.4%), compared to 1 in 8 or 9 for breast cancer.[4] The prevalence of ovarian cancer in the general population impacts substantially on strategies for prevention and early detection. In the absence of better markers for increased risk, strategies for prevention must have few serious side effects and screening strategies must be highly specific.

Etiology and Epidemiology The cause of ovarian cancer is unknown.[5] Some have speculated that an etiologic agent or a potentiator of oncogenesis could enter the peritoneal cavity through the lower genital canal and spread through the uterus and the fallopian tubes.[3] Possible carcinogens, such as infectious agents and chemical carcinogens have been studied, and although case-control studies have failed to document a specific agent, some studies have linked environmental exposure to asbestos-contaminated talc in douches and contraceptives with the development of epithelial tumors.[3,4] Cigarette smoking has been linked to mucinous ovarian cancers, but not to the more common serous carcinomas.[5] Case control studies have also pointed to an association of white race, high-fat diet and galactose consumption with a higher incidence of the disease.[4,6]

Among the epidemiologic variables, however, prior reproductive history and the number of ovulatory cycles appear to have the greatest impact on development of the disease, with low parity, infertility, early menarche and late menopause increasing the risk.[6,7] Fertility enhancing drugs, such as clomiphene citrate and gonadotropins used for ovulation induction have been thought to increase the risk of ovarian cancer, but the data have not been consistent and have not adequately distinguished the influence of infertility *per se* from the use of fertility stimulating agents.[8–12] A pooled analysis of eight case-control studies that included 5,207 cases and 7,705 controls found an association of fertility stimulating drugs with serous borderline tumors, but not with invasive ovarian cancers.[10–12] The increased incidence of ovarian cancer in single women, nuns, and nulliparous women suggests that continual ovulation, uninterrupted by pregnancy, may predispose women to develop this malignancy.[13] Over many cycles of ovulation, the ovarian surface epithelium undergoes repetitive disruption and repair. Epithelial cells covering the ovarian surface are stimulated to proliferate, increasing the probability of spontaneous mutations in tumor suppressor or proto-oncogenes that might contribute to oncogenesis. Alternatively, trapping of epithelial cells within the stroma following ovulation can lead to the formation of inclusion cysts where epithelial cells are subjected to a unique microenvironment.

Most case control and cohort studies have failed to link hormone replacement therapy to an increased risk of epithelial ovarian cancer.[14] A large cohort study has recently reopened controversy regarding this issue.[15] Among 44,241 postmenopausal women in the Breast Cancer Detection Demonstration Project, 329 developed ovarian cancer. Women who had received estrogen replacement therapy only, without progestin, for more than 10 years were at increased risk of developing ovarian cancer. By 20 years the relative risk was 3.2-fold.

The incidence of ovarian cancer varies in different geographic locations throughout the world. Western countries, including the United States and the United Kingdom, have an incidence of ovarian cancer that is three to seven times greater than in Japan, where epithelial ovarian tumors are considered rare.[2,3] In Asia, the incidence of germ cell tumors of the ovary appears to be somewhat higher than in the West. Japanese immigrants to the United States, however, have a significant increase in the incidence of epithelial ovarian cancer at a rate approaching that of white women from the United States. The incidence of epithelial tumors is about 1½ times greater in whites than in blacks.

Prevention As parity is inversely related to the risk of ovarian cancer, having at least one child is protective of the disease with a risk reduction of 0.3 to 0.4. Remarkably, use of oral contraceptives for 5 or more years reduces the relative risk to 0.5 (ie there is a 50% reduction in the likelihood of developing ovarian cancer).[9] Women who have had two children and have used oral contraceptives for 5 or more years have a relative risk of ovarian cancer as low as 0.3, or a 70% reduction. Therefore, the oral contraceptive pill is the only documented method of chemoprevention for ovarian cancer, and it should be recommended to women for this purpose. When counseling patients regarding birth control options, this important benefit of oral contraceptive use should be emphasized. This is also important for women with a strong family history of ovarian cancer.[16]

Fenretinide Fenretinide (4-hydroxyphenyl-all-trans-retinoic acid amide), a vitamin A derivative, has been given to women with unilateral breast cancer in an effort to reduce the risk of contralateral breast cancer. In a prospective, randomized, placebo-controlled trial conducted in Italy, women with unilateral breast cancer were given either oral fenretinide or a placebo for five years.[17] In the treatment group, no ovarian cancers developed during the five years on study, whereas there were 6 cases of ovarian cancer in the control group ($p < .01$). When participants were followed long-term, however, the protective effect disappeared after discontinuing the drug.[18] In cell culture, fenretinide can induce apoptosis in ovarian cancer cells and in normal ovarian surface epithelial cells. Trials are ongoing to determine the effect of fenretinide on the ovaries of women at high risk for developing ovarian cancer who will receive the drug prior to prophylactic oophorectomy.

Oophorectomy The performance of a prophylactic oophorectomy will reduce, but not eliminate, the excess risk of cancer in women at high risk for developing ovarian cancer.[19,20] Because the entire peritoneum is at risk, peritoneal carcinomas can occur even after prophylactic oophorectomy in less than 5% of cases. Because the ovaries provide protection from cardiovascular disease and osteoporosis, prophylactic oophorectomy should not be routinely performed in premenopausal women at average risk for ovarian cancer.

Genetic Risk for Epithelial Ovarian Cancer Most epithelial ovarian cancer is sporadic, with familial or hereditary patterns accounting for 5–10% of all malignancies.[21] The risk of ovarian cancer is higher than that of the general population in women with certain family histories.[22–30] Most familial ovarian cancer is associated with mutations in *BRCA1, BRCA2* or DNA mismatch repair genes in the human nonpolyposis colon cancer (HNPCC, Lynch Type II) syndrome.[26–29] There have also been reportable cases of ovarian cancer associated with Li-Fraumeni syndrome that occurs due to TP53 mutations in the germ line.[29] In the past, it had been thought that there were two distinct syndromes associated with a genetic risk, site-specific hereditary ovarian cancer, and hereditary breast/ovarian cancer syndrome. However, it is now believed that these groups essentially represent a continuum of mutations with different degrees of penetrance within a given family.

BRCA1* and *BRCA2 The majority of ovarian cancer families have mutations in the *BRCA1* gene that is located on chromosome 17.[26] A small fraction of inherited disease has been traced to another gene, *BRCA2,* located on chromosome 13.[27] Discovered through linkage analyses, these two genes are associated with the genetic predisposition to both ovarian and breast cancer.

BRCA1/2 mutations are passed via autosomal dominant inheritance, and a full pedigree analysis (ie, both maternal and paternal sides of the family) must be carefully evaluated. There are numerous distinct mutations that have been identified on each of these genes, and the mutations have different degrees of penetrance which may account for the preponderance of either breast cancer, ovarian cancer, or both, in any given family. Based on analysis of women who have a mutation in the *BRCA1* gene and are from high-risk families, the lifetime risk of ovarian cancer may be as high as 28 to 44% and the risk has been calculated to be as high as 27% for those women with a *BRCA2* mutation.[23–25] The risk of breast cancer in women with a *BRCA1* or *BRCA2* mutation may be as high as 56 to 87%.

Hereditary ovarian cancers generally occur in women about 10 years younger than those with nonhereditary tumors.[25] As the median age of epithelial ovarian cancer is in the mid- to late 50s, a woman with a first- or second-degree relative who had premenopausal ovarian cancer may have a higher probability of carrying an affected gene.

Within a given family, a combination of epithelial ovarian and breast cancers can affect a mixture of first- and second-degree relatives. Women with this syndrome tend to develop cancers at a young age, and breast cancers may be bilateral. If two first-degree relatives are affected, this pedigree is consistent with an autosomal dominant mode of inheritance.[23]

Founder Effect More than 100 different mutations of *BRCA1* and *BRCA2* have been cataloged in different families with ovarian and breast cancer. A particularly high carrier rate of *BRCA1* and *BRCA2* mutations has been found in women of Ashkenazi Jewish descent and in Islandic women.[24,28] Three specific mutations occur repeatedly in the Ashkenazi population and are associated with many of the breast and ovarian cancer families: 185delAG and 5382insC in *BRCA1,* and 6174delT in *BRCA2.* One in 40 or 2.5% of all Ashkenazi Jewish women carry at least one of these three mutations. The prevalence of these specific mutations in the Ashkenazi population is thought to have resulted from a "founder effect," where the mutations can be traced to particular families within a defined geographic area.

Pedigree Analysis The risk of ovarian cancer depends on the number of first- and/or second-degree relatives with a history of epithelial ovarian carcinoma and/or breast cancer, and on the number of malignancies that occur at an early age. The degree of risk is difficult to determine precisely unless one performs a full pedigree analysis.

In families with two first-degree relatives (ie, mother, sister, or daughter) with documented premenopausal epithelial ovarian cancer, the risk that a female first-degree relative will have an affected gene could be as high as 35 to 40%.[23] In families with a single first-degree relative and a single second-degree relative (ie, grandmother, aunt, first cousin, or granddaughter) with epithelial ovarian cancer, the risk that a woman will have an affected gene also may be increased. The risk may be two- to ten-fold higher than in those without a familial history of the disease.[23,25,30] In families with a single post-menopausal first-degree relative with epithelial ovarian carcinoma, a woman may not have an increased risk of having an affected gene because the case is most likely to be sporadic. However, if the ovarian cancer occurred in a premenopausal relative, this could be significant, and a full pedigree analysis should be undertaken. Women with a primary history of breast cancer have twice the expected incidence of subsequent ovarian cancer.

Lynch Type II Syndrome The hereditary nonpolyposis colorectal cancer (HNPCC) syndrome includes multiple adenocarcinomas, including familial colon, ovarian, endometrial, and breast cancers, as well as other malignancies of the gastrointestinal and genitourinary systems.[31] Mutations of DNA mismatch repair genes have been associated with this syndrome including mutations of *MSH2, MLH1, PMS1* and *PMS2.* The risk that a woman who is a member of a Lynch type II family will develop epithelial ovarian cancer depends on the frequency of this disease in her first- and second-degree relatives, although these women appear to have at least three times the relative risk of the general population.

Management of Women at High-Risk for Ovarian Cancer Current recommendations for management of women with high-risk for ovarian cancer are summarized in many reports.[29,30,32–34] Women who appear to be at high-risk for ovarian and or breast cancer should undergo genetic counseling and, if the risk appears to be substantial, may be offered genetic testing for *BRCA1* and *BRCA2.* Women who wish to preserve their reproductive capacity can undergo periodic screening by transvaginal ultrasonography and CA 125 every 6 months, although the efficacy of this approach is not clearly established. Prophylactic surgery (bilateral salpingo-oophorectomy with or without a hysterectomy) is the treatment of choice for women who have completed their childbearing. Oral contraceptives should be recommended to young women before undertaking a planned family. Women who do not wish to maintain their fertility, or who have completed their family, may undergo prophylactic bilateral salpingo-oophorectomy. The risk should be clearly documented, preferably established by *BRCA1* and *BRCA2* testing, before salpingo-oophorectomy. These women should be counseled that this operation does not offer absolute protection, as peritoneal carcinomas occasionally can occur after bilateral oophorectomy. In women who also have a strong family history of breast cancer, annual mammographic screening should be performed commencing at age 30 years. Women with a documented HNPCC syndrome should be treated as above, and in addition, should undergo periodic screening mammography, colonoscopy, and endometrial biopsy.[29]

In a recent study, Markov modeling was performed in a simulated cohort of 30-year-old women who tested positive for *BRCA1*/2 mutations.[34] Quality adjustment of survival estimates were obtained from a survey of women aged 33 to 50 years. A 30-year-old woman could prolong her survival beyond that associated with surveillance alone by 1.8 years with tamoxifen, 2.6 years with prophylactic oophorectomy, 4.6 years with both tamoxifen and prophylactic oophorectomy, 3.5 years with prophylactic mastectomy and 4.9 years with both surgeries. Quality adjusted survival could be prolonged by 2.8 years with tamoxifen, 4.4 years with prophylactic oophorectomy, 6.3 years with tamoxifen and oophorectomy and 2.6 years with mastectomy or both operations. Benefits would decrease if institution of these preventive measures were delayed beyond age 30.

Biology and Prognosis of Ovarian Neoplasms The prognosis of ovarian cancer can be correlated with numerous clinical and biologic factors. Tumor stage, grade, and size of metastatic disease after resection correlate best with outcome.[35,36] As discussed below, among patients with low stage disease, tumor grade correlates with prognosis (ie, patients with stage I high-grade lesions have a shorter survival than do those of low-grade).[36] In patients with advanced stage disease, the size of residual disease after surgery correlates most clearly with survival.[37] The rapidity with which disease regresses during chemotherapy also correlates with survival. A short apparent half-life of the serum tumor marker CA 125 has correlated with improved survival in more than a dozen studies.[38] Normalization of CA 125 by the third course of chemotherapy has been associated with a favorable prognosis.[38]

Several biologic factors have been correlated with prognosis in epithelial ovarian cancer. Using flow cytometry, Friedlander and others have shown that ovarian cancers are commonly aneuploid and that a correlation exists between FIGO stage and ploidy, (low-stage cancers tend to be diploid and high-stage tumors tend to be aneuploid).[39,40] Patients with diploid tumors have a significantly longer median survival than those with aneuploid tumors: 5 years versus 1 year, respectively.[40] Multivariate analyses have demonstrated that ploidy is an independent prognostic variable and one of the most significant predictors of survival.[40] Flow cytometric analysis also provides data on the cell cycle, and the proliferation fraction (S-phase) determined by this technique has correlated with prognosis in some studies.[39] More recent reports utilizing comparative genomic hybridization suggest that copy number abnormalities for chromosome segments also have prognostic significance.[41]

Most sporadic ovarian carcinomas evolve from a single clone of cells. When primary cancers and metastases have been compared, more than 90% share the same patterns of loss of heterozygosity, inactivation of the same X chromosome and, when present, the same mutations in *TP53*.[42–43] Ovarian cancers can metastasize by multiple routes. Like other epithelial neoplasms, ovarian cancers can spread through lymphatics to the level of the renal hilus and can also spread hematogenously. Most frequently, however, ovarian cancer spreads over the surface of the peritoneum, studding the serosal surface of the bowel and abdominal wall and ultimately producing intestinal obstruction. Ascites formation results from increased leakage of proteinaceous fluid from capillaries under the influence of VEGF/VPF produced by ovarian cancers and from inhibition of fluid outflow through diaphragmatic lymphatics that have been blocked by metastatic disease.[44] Studies of the immunobiology of the peritoneal cavity suggest that it may function as an immunoprivileged site, with elevated levels of suppressive molecules and growth factors.

Epithelial ovarian cancers are thought to arise from a single layer of cells that covers the ovary or that lines cysts immediately beneath the ovarian surface. These cells are generally quiescent, but proliferate following ovulation to repair the defect created by rupture of a follicle. A distinctive profile of genetic and epigenetic alterations has been observed in early and late stage ovarian cancers.[43] A number of oncogenes have been overexpressed and/or activated (Table 104-1) and the function of several tumor suppressor genes has been lost (Table 104-2).[45–72] Among the oncogenes activated, particular attention has been given to the HER family of transmembrane tyrosine kinase growth factor receptors, including the epidermal growth factor receptor (EGFR) and *c-erbB-2* (*HER-2*). EGFR is expressed by normal ovarian surface epithelial cells and EGFR expression is lost in approximately 30% of ovarian cancers, associated with an improved prognosis.[45] *HER-2* is overexpressed in approximately 12 to 15% of ovarian cancers and, in some studies, has been associated with a poor prognosis.[45] The *ras* oncogene is mutated and activated in less than 20% of serous ovarian cancers, but is more frequently mutated in mucinous and borderline and papillary serous low-grade neoplasms.[46,47] In addition, ras may be physiologically activated in a larger fraction of cancers.[49] Myc is amplified and overexpressed in approximately 33% of cases.[44] More frequent and consistent abnormalities have been found in the PI3 kinase signaling pathway. The p110 catalytic subunit of the PI3 kinase is amplified, overexpressed, and activated in more than half of ovarian cancers.[51] Downstream within the PI3 kinase signaling pathway, AKT is also amplified, overexpressed, and activated in 20% of cases.[52] PTEN is mutated in endometrioid ovarian cancers.[53] Overall, abnormalities of the PI3 kinase pathway have been found in more than 70% of ovarian cancers.[51] A majority of tumors contain mutations of TP53 or loss of ARHI. *TP53* is mutated in as much as 70% of ovarian cancers, and although it is not clearly of prognostic value, it is more likely mutated in high grade, as opposed to low-grade lesions.[48,56,57] When *TP53* is mutated in borderline tumors, their prognosis is worse than the majority of lesions of this histology.[48] Mutation of *TP53* may also be a marker for metastasis, in that mutations are less frequent in stage I. Expression of at least two imprinted genes has been downregulated in ovarian cancers: *LOT1* and *ARH1*. Downregulation of *ARHI* in 50% of ovarian cancers has been associated with decreased disease-free survival.[50,62]

Table 104-1 Oncogenes in Epithelial Ovarian Cancer

Receptor kinases
Overexpression of *HER2*
Continued expression of *EGFR*
Novel expression of *FMS*
Non-receptor kinases
Amplification of *PI3* kinase
Amplification of *AKT* kinase
SRC kinase activated physiologically
Ras rarely mutated but frequently activated physiologically
Overexpression of *MYC*
Activation of *STAT3*

Recently, a murine model has been developed that mimics human ovarian cancer and that permits the introduction of multiple genes using an avian retroviral gene delivery technique.[54] When the ovarian target cells were derived from transgenic mice deficient for p53, the addition of any two of the oncogenes c-*myc*, K-*ras* and *AKT* were sufficient to induce ovarian tumor formation when infected cells were injected at intraperitoneal, subcutaneous or ovarian sites. Another model has been developed from normal human ovarian surface epithelial cells that have also been immortalized with telomerase and with viral T antigen which neutralizes *TP53* and *RB* function. Introduction of activated human H-*ras* or K-*ras* genes transforms these immortalized cells and permits them to grow in immunosuppressed mice with a nodular or papillary histology that resembles human ovarian cancer.[55]

LPA is a ubiquitous growth factor in ovarian cancer. Normal ovarian cells have very little LPA, but the majority of malignant epithelial ovarian tumors express LPA.[69] IL-8, bFGF, and VEGF are all angiogenic factors, which are frequently found in the ascitic fluid of patients.[73,74] In particular, VEGF, a vascular permeability factor, is often found in very high levels in ascites.[59]

Upregulation and aberrant glycosylation of extracellular mucins have provided targets for therapy and markers for monitoring disease. MUC-1 is a mucin expressed by more than 80% of ovarian cancers.[75] In transformed cells, aberrant glycosylation exposes peptide determinants recognized by murine monoclonal antibodies that have been used for serotherapy. CA 125 is also a mucin (MUC-16)

Table 104-2 Putative Tumor Suppressor Genes in Epithelial Ovarian Cancer

Gene	Chromosome Location	Function
SPARC	5q31	matrix
Dab2	5p13	binds GRB2
PTEN (MMAC-1)	10q23	phosphatase
AHRI (*NOEY2*)	1p31	induces p21, inhibits cyclin D1
P53	17p13	DNA stability, apoptosis
LOT-1	6q25	zinc finger
OVCA1	17p13	unknown
BRCA1[a]	17q21	DNA repair
BRCA2[a]	13q12	DNA repair

[a]Predominantly in hereditary ovarian cancer.

Table 104-3 Epithelial Ovarian Tumors

Histologic Type	Cellular Type
I. Serous	Endosalpingeal
A. Benign	
B. Borderline	
C. Malignant	
II Mucinous	Endocervical
A. Benign	
B. Borderline	
C. Malignant	
III. Endometrioid	Endometrial
A. Benign	
B. Borderline	
C. Malignant	
IV. Clear cell "mesonephroid"	Müllerian
A. Benign	
B. Borderline	
C. Malignant	
V. Brenner	Transitional
A. Benign	
B. Borderline ("proliferating")	
C. Malignant	
VI. Mixed epithelial	Mixed
A. Benign	
B. Borderline	
C. Malignant	
VII. Undifferentiated	
Anaplastic	
VIII. Unclassified	
Mesothelioma	
Other	

associated with cells that line the coelomic cavity during embryonic development. CA 125 is shed from 80% of epithelial ovarian cancers[76,77] and can be measured using the murine monoclonal antibody OC125. Regression and progression of disease tend to correlate well with falling or rising CA 125 levels.[77] The precise function of the glycoprotein is unknown.[78,79]

Classification and Pathology Primary ovarian cancers are classified according to the structures of the ovary from which they are derived.[2,80] Most develop from the epithelial cells that cover the ovarian surface or that line inclusion cysts. These cells are ultimately derived from the coelomic epithelium of mesodermal origin and share cytologic markers with mesothelium. Germ cell malignancies constitute the next most common group and the least common tumors are derived from ovarian stromal cells.

Epithelial malignancies account for 85 to 90% of ovarian cancers. The majority of epithelial lesions are seen in patients who are 40 years or older. Under the age of 40 years, epithelial malignancies are uncommon, and most malignancies seen in women under the age of 30 years are of germ cell origin.[2] The histologic types of the epithelial tumors are listed in Table 104-3. The majority of lesions, about 75%, are of the serous type, followed by the mucinous, endometrioid, clear cell, mixed, Brenner, and undifferentiated histologies.[2,80] The cellular patterns of different histotypes resemble different derivatives of the Müllerian duct in different portions of the female

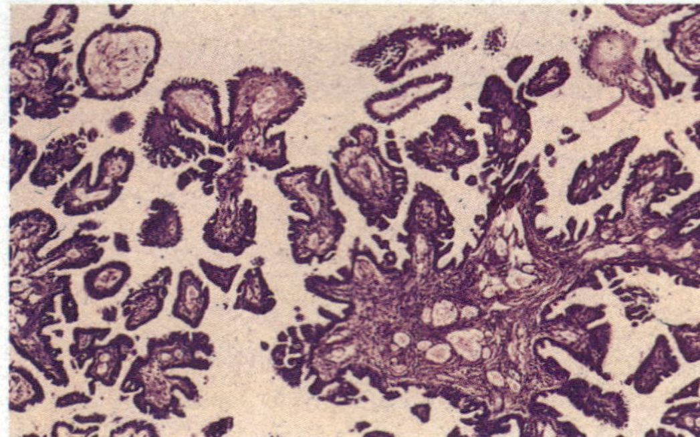

Figure 104-1 Serous cystadenocarcinoma gross with omentum.

reproductive tract. For example, serous epithelial cells resemble cells that line the Fallopian tube, endometrioid epithelial cells resemble the endometrium, and mucinous epithelial cells resemble the uterine endocervix.

Invasive Histologies Serous carcinomas may have a complex admixture of cystic and solid areas with extensive papillations, or they may contain a predominantly solid mass with areas of necrosis and hemorrhage (Figure 104-1) The poorly differentiated tumors may have some areas with a papillary pattern, but other portions may be indistinguishable from the other histologic patterns described below (Figure 104-2). Stage I or II lesions are most frequently unilateral, with about 10 to 20% involving both ovaries. Conversely, about 50 to 70% of stage III serous carcinomas are bilateral.[2]

Mucinous tumors tend to be large, with many masses over 20 cm in diameter (Figure 104-3). The histologic pattern resembles uterine endocervical glands. The lesions frequently contain areas of hemorrhage, necrosis, and various quantities of mucin. These tumors are bilateral in 10 to 20% of cases.[2] Occasionally, mucin is secreted into the peritoneal cavity and produces a condition known as pseudomyxoma or myxoma peritonei. A mucocele of the appendix may also be seen in conjunction with this tumor.

Endometrioid carcinomas of the ovary resemble typical carcinomas of the endometrium. These tumors may be seen with synchronous endometrial carcinoma, and when they are, both lesions may be of low stage.[2] Rarely, endometrioid carcinomas arise in conjunction with pelvic endometriosis,

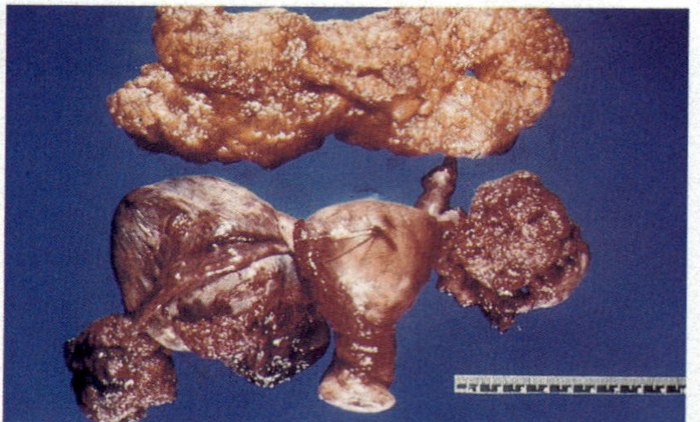

Figure 104-2 Poorly differentiated papillary serous carcinoma of ovary.

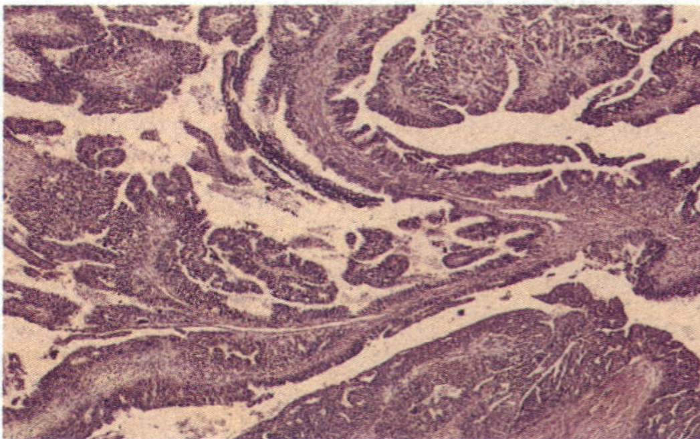

Figure 104-3 Mucinous cystadenocarcinoma.

resulting from malignant transformation of a benign process (Figure 104-4). Bilaterality is seen in 10 to 15% of stage I and II disease, and in about 30% of stage III.[2]

Clear cell carcinomas were formerly called mesonephromas, a term that has been abandoned because clear cell tumors are derived from tissues that are embryologically distinct from mesonephros. About one fourth of clear cell tumors are associated with endometriosis. Clear cell tumors are only rarely bilateral.[2]

Brenner tumors are uncommon, representing less than 1% of all epithelial malignancies. Mixed epithelial tumors may contain small areas of Brenner tumor histology, which have a histologic pattern similar to that of transitional cell. Malignant Brenner tumors are unilateral.[2]

Borderline Tumors Borderline tumors, or those of low malignant potential, are important to differentiate from those that are frankly invasive. The treatment and prognosis for borderline lesions are considerably different from those for invasive malignancies. Borderline tumors tend to remain confined to a single ovary at the time of diagnosis, and also tend to occur in younger, premenopausal women (Figure 104-5). They may be confused with a well-differentiated invasive ovarian cancer, and the treatment for the two may be different. Thus, in a young patient who has a lesion confined to the ovary, which is suspected of being an epithelial ovarian cystadenocarcinoma, a borderline tumor must be excluded, because bilateral oophorectomy, hysterectomy, and chemotherapy are unnecessary in these patients. In women under the age of 40 years, about 60 to 70% of non-benign ovarian neoplasms are borderline, whereas in women over 40 years, only

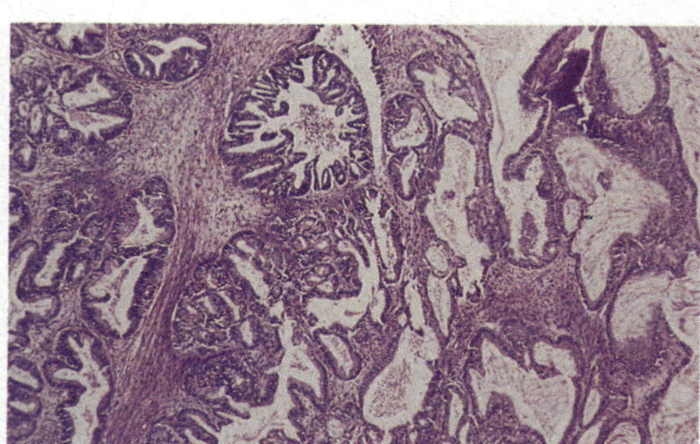

Figure 104-4 Endometrioid carcinoma.

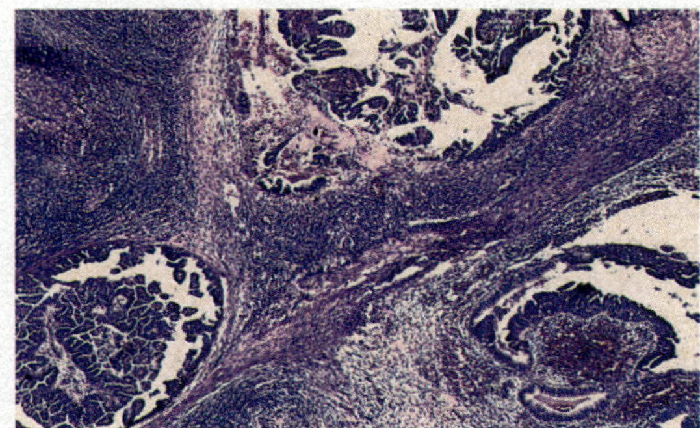

Figure 104-5 Borderline papillary serous tumor.

10% are borderline.[2,81,82] Histologic criteria for borderline tumors include (1) the presence of epithelial cell proliferation with a "piling up" of cells, so-called pseudostratification; (2) cytologic atypia, but with rare mitoses; and (3) no evidence of stromal invasion. Borderline tumors tend to remain confined to the ovary, but may be associated with peritoneal disease, which represents either dissemination or the multifocal evolution of the disease. In those rare patients with peritoneal involvement, death can occur by progressive intestinal obstruction.[81,82]

Primary Peritoneal Carcinomas Malignancy that arises primarily from the peritoneal cells is referred to as peritoneal carcinoma or primary peritoneal (papillary) adenocarcinoma.[19,83] There is some debate as to whether these should all be classified as peritoneal mesotheliomas, or whether this latter group is a specialized variety of a poorly differentiated peritoneal tumor.[84] Some of the lesions appear identical to those tumors that arise from the surface epithelium of the ovaries, and the cells of the peritoneum have the ability to recapitulate any of the histologic patterns seen in ovarian cancer. Thus, the most common pattern of a peritoneal carcinoma is a papillary serous carcinoma.

Knowledge of primary peritoneal carcinomas is important. This lesion explains many instances of unknown primary when no clear explanation for peritoneal carcinomatosis can be documented. Also, the existence of this phenomenon explains the occurrence of ovarian cancer after oophorectomy.[85] In these patients, the presence of carcinomatosis that involves the surface of the ovaries but without ovarian enlargement, represents peritoneal carcinoma with secondary or concomitant involvement of the ovarian surfaces. In this manner, the ovaries are the "innocent bystanders" of the process. Therapeutically, primary peritoneal malignancy should be treated as one would manage an epithelial ovarian cancer.

Patterns of Spread Ovarian epithelial tumors spread primarily by direct exfoliation of cells throughout the peritoneal cavity, but they also spread via the lymphatic and hematogenous routes. Germ cell tumors have a greater predilection for spread via the retroperitoneal lymphatics, which must be evaluated carefully when staging those tumors that appear to be confined to the ovary.[2,86]

The most common and earliest mode of dissemination of epithelial tumors is by the exfoliation of cells along the peritoneal surfaces.[80] The cells spread directly to the pelvic and abdominal peritoneal surfaces, and tend to follow the path of circulation of peritoneal fluid from the right pericolic gutter cephalad to the right hemidiaphragm.[3] The intestinal mesenteries become involved by peritoneal metastases. Adhesions form between loops of intestine producing mechanical obstruction, even though involvement of the lumen of the intestine by direct extension is uncommon. The intestinal dysfunction can also result from involvement by tumor of the myenteric plexus, the autonomic innervation of the intestine that is found in the mesentery. This condition has been referred to as "carcinomatous ileus."[2]

Spread via the lymphatics is common in epithelial ovarian cancer. Apparent stage I and II tumors have retroperitoneal lymphatic dissemination in about 5 to 10% in most series, whereas lymphatic dissemination in stage III has been reported to be as high as 42 to 78% in carefully explored patients.[86,87] Most of these lymph nodes are not enlarged, but are microscopically positive for malignant cells. Spread through the retroperitoneal and diaphragmatic lymphatics can result in metastasis to the supraclavicular lymph nodes.

Blood-borne metastasis of ovarian cancer is uncommon at diagnosis and is often a late finding in the disease. Hematogenous dissemination at the time of diagnosis to the parenchyma of the liver or lung is seen in only 2 to 3% of patients. Indeed, most patients who have disease dissemination cephalad to the diaphragm at the time of presentation have a right pleural effusion. Metastasis to the central nervous system is rare and spread to the bone is very rare, except for the clear cell histologic type.[2,3] However, in patients who survive many months and years with their disease, involvement of distant sites is more common. Distant metastases consistent with stage IV findings were documented in almost two-fifths of patients who died of ovarian cancer originally thought confined to the peritoneal cavity.[3]

Clinical Features Traditionally, ovarian cancer has been considered a "silent killer" that does not produce symptoms until far advanced. Some patients with ovarian cancers confined to the ovary are asymptomatic, but the majority will have nonspecific symptoms that do not necessarily suggest an origin in the ovary. In one survey of 1,725 women with ovarian cancer, 95% recalled symptoms prior to diagnosis, including 89% with stage I/II disease and 97% with stage III/IV disease.[88] Seventy percent had abdominal or gastrointestinal symptoms, 58% pain, 34% urinary symptoms, and 26% pelvic discomfort. At least some of these symptoms could have reflected pressure on the pelvic viscera from the enlarging ovary.

Metastatic ovarian cancer is rarely asymptomatic. In addition to the gastrointestinal and urinary symptoms noted in early stage disease, formation of ascites can produce an increase in abdominal girth. Pleural effusion may lead to dyspnea as the first complaint. Acute symptoms, such as those of adnexal rupture or torsion, are uncommon. Vaginal bleeding is also an uncommon symptom in postmenopausal women, although premenopausal patients may present with irregular or heavy menses.[3] Detection of an adnexal mass by pelvic examination can permit the early diagnosis of ovarian cancer. Since malignancy is rare and the majority of palpable adnexal masses are benign, an enlarged ovary discovered on pelvic examination is not likely to be an ovarian malignancy. In premenopausal women, ovarian cancer is uncommon and represents less than 7% of all adnexal masses. Even in postmenopausal women, 70 to 80% of adnexal tumors are benign. In some patients who complain primarily of abdominal symptoms, a pelvic examination frequently is omitted and the tumor missed. Signs of advanced disease include abdominal distention and a fluid wave consistent with ascites. These signs are nonspecific and can be associated with many conditions arising in the abdominal cavity, especially malignancies of other primary sites or carcinomatosis from metastatic tumors of the gastrointestinal tract and breast.

Diagnosis The diagnosis of ovarian cancer is usually made at laparotomy, but occasionally at laparoscopy. If a pelvic mass is suspicious and the most likely diagnosis is ovarian cancer, surgery should not be unnecessarily delayed. In premenopausal patients, however, predominantly cystic pelvic masses can be observed over a period of 1 to 2 months. Lesions that are essentially mobile, are unilateral, and have a smooth contour are much less likely to be neoplastic, and are unlikely to be malignant. In premenopausal patients with cystic lesions of less than 8 cm, attempted suppression with oral contraceptives is indicated. In women who are definitely post-menopausal, cystic masses larger than 5 cm should be removed unless they represent a chronic finding. Those masses that regress in size can be managed with continued observation, whereas those that persist or enlarge must be evaluated surgically. Conversely, patients whose lesions are irregular, predominantly solid, and somewhat immobile should undergo an exploratory laparotomy.[35]

The preoperative evaluation of patients can be aided by the use of CA 125. Elevated CA 125 levels are most frequently associated with malignant adnexal masses in postmenopausal women. In women over 50 years of age whose serum CA 125 level is greater than 35 U/mL the adnexal mass is malignant in about 80% of cases. A CA 125 of more than 95 U/mL is associated with a positive predictive value of 96% in this setting. Conversely, the majority of premenopausal women with serum CA 125 levels greater than 35 U/mL have benign conditions, such as uterine myomata, endometriosis, and benign ovarian tumors.[3,89] Elevation of serum CA 125 in a postmenopausal patient with a pelvic mass should prompt exploration by surgeons prepared to undertake complete staging and, if necessary, cytoreductive operations.

Ultrasonographic signs of malignancy include an adnexal pelvic mass with areas of complexity, such as irregular borders; multiple echogenic patterns within the mass; and dense, multiple irregular septae. Bilateral tumors are more likely to be malignant, although the individual characteristics of the lesions are of greater significance. Transvaginal ultrasonography may have a somewhat better resolution than transabdominal ultrasonography for adnexal neoplasms.[90,91] Newer techniques using Doppler color flow imaging may enhance the specificity of ultrasonography for demonstrating findings consistent with malignancy.[92]

Radiographic techniques, including abdominal radiographs, computed tomography (CT) scans, and nuclear magnetic resonance imaging (MRI), are not useful prior to the surgical diagnosis of ovarian cancer.[93] The preoperative evaluation of patients who have a suspicious pelvic mass can omit these studies when blood chemistries and enzymes suggest normal hepatic and pancreatic function.[90] In patients with ascites and no pelvic mass, however, a CT or MRI may be useful in identifying other potential sites of origin. Paracentesis is not recommended because of the frequency of metastatic implantation and growth in the needle tract. Liver–spleen scans, brain scans, and bone scans are unnecessary unless specific symptoms suggest metastasis to these sites.

In premenopausal women, radiographic studies of the intestines are not required unless there is the finding of occult blood in the rectum or there are symptoms indicating upper or lower intestinal obstruction. A barium enema or endoscopy is appropriate in postmenopausal patients. Mammography should be performed to exclude primary breast cancer, which can coexist with ovarian cancer or spread to the ovaries. Cervical cytology should be performed, although ovarian cancer cells are unlikely to exfoliate through the uterus to the cervix. In patients with irregular or heavy menses, an endometrial biopsy should be performed to exclude primary endometrial pathology.[35]

The differential diagnosis of an adnexal mass includes a variety of functional changes of the ovary, benign neoplasms of the reproductive tract, and inflammatory lesions of these organs. A hydrosalpinx, endometriosis, and pedunculated uterine leiomyomata can simulate an ovarian neoplasm. Nongynecologic diseases, such as inflammatory processes of the colon and rectum, must be excluded.

Screening There is no well-established strategy for early detection of ovarian cancer. Discovery of a pelvic mass on routine physical examination can lead to surgery prior to the dissemination of a malignancy, but conventional diagnosis detects only 20% of patients in stage I. Given the prevalence of ovarian cancer in the postmenopausal population, any screening strategy must be highly specific (> 99.6%) as well as highly sensitive for early stage disease (> 75%) to achieve a positive predictive value of 10% (ie, 10 laparotomies for each case of ovarian cancer detected). Two approaches have been evaluated for early detection of ovarian cancer: ultrasonography and serum tests such as CA 125.

Ultrasound Transvaginal Sonography Ultrasound transvaginal sonography (TVS) has proven superior to transabdominal sonography (TAU) for the detection of a pelvic mass. In three large studies that screened 66,620 women with TVS, 565 operations were performed to detect 45 ovarian cancers, 34 of which were invasive.[91–95] Overall, the sensitivity for early stage disease was 78%, but the specificity fell just short of that required for a positive predictive value of 10% with 12 operations per case of ovarian cancer detected. The most promising single study achieved a positive predictive value of 9.9%.[94] Confirmatory tests with Doppler ultrasound have not proven consistent, but additional studies with 3-D power Doppler are underway to improve specificity in distinguishing malignant from benign ovarian abnormalities.

CA 125 CA 125 is elevated in 50 to 60% of patients with stage I and in 90% with stage II ovarian cancer.[96] CA 125 levels can rise 10 to 60 months prior to diagnosis with an average estimated lead time of 1.9 years prior to diagnosis of disease in all stages.[99,100] Specificity for a single determination of CA 125 is not adequate to screen a population at average risk, but specificity can be improved with a two-stage strategy that utilizes CA 125 followed by ultrasound in a subset of women with elevated CA 125. Use of CA 125 to trigger ultrasound has been evaluated in trials in Sweden and in the United Kingdom.[99,100] The latter randomized 22,000 women to conventional surveillance or to annual CA 125 with TAU if the value were elevated.[100] When TAU was abnormal, surgery was undertaken. Among 10,985 women screened, 29 operations were performed to detect 6 cancers, providing a positive predictive value of 21%. During 7 years follow-up, 10 more cancers were diagnosed in the screened group. Over the same intervals, 21 ovarian cancers were diagnosed in the control group. Median survival in the screened group (72.9 months) was significantly greater ($p = .0112$) than that in the control group (41.8 months).

Risk of Ovarian Cancer (ROC) Algorithm Analyzing serum samples stored from screening studies in Stockholm and in the United Kingdom with an improved CA 125II assay, it has been possible to improve the specificity of CA 125 as a screening tool by following the values of an individual over time.[101,102] Elevated CA 125 levels in women without ovarian cancer remain static or decrease with time, whereas levels associated with ovarian malignancy tend to rise. This finding has been incorporated into an algorithm that uses age, rate of change of CA 125 and absolute levels of CA 125 to calculate an individual's "risk of ovarian cancer" (ROC). Patients at sufficient risk undergo TVS. Some 10,000 volunteers greater than 50 years of age have been randomized in the United Kingdom to a screening group (5,046) or to a control group (4,954).[101] Using the ROC algorithm, 101 patients were found to be at sufficiently high risk to undergo TVS. Seventeen patients had abnormal findings prompting operations that detected 4 cases of ovarian cancer, yielding a positive predictive value of 20%.

Currently, a trial has begun in the United Kingdom that will include 200,000 post menopausal women who will be randomized to a control group (100,000) who will be followed with conventional pelvic examinations; a second group (50,000) who will have annual TVS; and a third group (50,000) who will have CA 125 determined at least annually. Based on the ROC algorithm, patients in the third group will be referred for TVS and/or surgery. Women will be screened for 3 years and followed for 7 years. This trial may demonstrate more definitively the feasibility of screening for ovarian cancer as well as the impact of early detection on survival.

Complementary Markers Whatever the outcome of the current trial in the United Kingdom or of the Prostate, Lung, Colon, and Ovary (PLCO) screening trial with CA 125 and TVS in the United States, strategies based on CA 125 alone are not likely to exceed a sensitivity of 80%, as CA 125 is not expressed by 20% of epithelial ovarian cancers. Greater sensitivity might be attained through the use of multiple serum markers in combination, provided that specificity was not compromised. From a recent review, 27 serum markers have been evaluated for their ability to complement CA 125 and to improve sensitivity for detection of ovarian cancer.[98] Use of markers 2 to 3 at a time increased sensitivity 5 to 15%, generally at the expense of a substantial decrease in specificity. For example, use of CA 125 in combination with OVX1, a Lewis X determinant on mucin, and M-CSF, a cytokine, increased sensitivity for stage I disease from 69% with CA 125 alone to 84% with the combination, but specificity declined from 99 to 84%.[97,98,103]

A number of novel markers for ovarian cancer have been identified in recent years including mesothelin, a 110 kD fragment of EGFR, lysophosphatidic acid, HE4, prostasin, osteopontin, and human kallikreins 6 and 10.[104–111] Use of surface laser desorption and ionization (SELDI) with subsequent resolution by mass spectroscopy has demonstrated a pattern of low molecular weight moieties that has been reported to distinguish sera from ovarian cancer patients from those of healthy individuals with 100% sensitivity and 95% specificity.[112] Prospective replication of these results and determination of sensitivity for stage I disease should be available in the near future. Methodological issues have been raised regarding these data.[113] SELDI may also identify a limited number of protein peaks that could be assayed by more conventional techniques.[114] Mathematical techniques to combine markers, enhancing their sensitivity without sacrificing specificity, have also been developed. Both artificial neural networks and mixtures of multivariate normal distributions have been used to combine values for four serum markers (CA 125 II, CA 72-4, CA 15-3 and M-CSF) from patients with stage I ovarian cancer and from healthy individuals.[114] Using either technique, sensitivity could be increased from 48% using CA 125II alone to 72 to 75% using the combination, while maintaining specificity at 98%. In a two-stage strategy, an initial stage with 98% specificity would require ultrasounds to be performed in only 2% of women screened.

Current Recommendations for Women at Average Risk The application of screening techniques other than pelvic examination for ovarian cancer in the entire female population is unwarranted at this time. The sensitivity and specificity of ultrasound and CA 125 are low in premenopausal women, making it unlikely that this approach will be useful in this group. However, with refinements of the transvaginal and flow techniques, as well as the addition of other serum markers, screening could become a reality in the future. There is a need for critical studies to define the potential of different screening strategies and to determine whether their application can decrease mortality from the disease.

Current Recommendations for Screening Women at High-Risk In women with strong evidence of a hereditary predisposition for ovarian cancer, screening has been frequently advocated, although the efficacy of such surveillance to reduce risk is unknown. Screening can be problematic because this high-risk population often includes premenopausal women who have a higher incidence of false positive CA 125 elevations and ultrasound abnormalities. In these high-risk populations, initial screening trials using ultrasound alone or in combination with color-flow Doppler were associated with high false-positive rates (2.5–4.9%). The current trend is to combine ultrasound with CA 125.

There are 5 prospective studies where combined screening has been undertaken in high-risk populations.[115–119] In three screening programs involving a total of 1,228 women with a family history of ovarian cancer, no invasive ovarian cancer was detected and false-positive rates have ranged from 0.4 to 3.9%.[115–117] In one of the remaining two studies, one case of ovarian cancer was detected on screening 137 high risk women with a false positive rate of 0.7%; in the other study 9 ovarian cancers were detected in screening 180 women with a false positive rate of 3.9%.[118,119]

Women in the high-risk population who request screening should be counseled about the current lack of evidence for the efficacy for either CA 125 or for sonography as well as the associated false-positive rates. Many will still opt for screening despite the risks and limitations of the available strategies. Screening is best carried out in clinical trials such as those conducted by the Cancer Genetics Network or by several university centers. Screening with TVS every 6 to 12 months and with CA 125 every 3 to 6 months is currently being evaluated.

Table 104-4 FIGO Stages for Primary Carcinoma of the Ovary

Stage	Description
Stage I	Growth limited to the ovaries
Stage IA	Growth limited to the ovary; no ascites. No tumor on the external surface; capsule intact
Stage IB	Growth limited to both ovaries; no ascites. No tumor on the external surfaces; capsule intact
Stage IC	Tumor either stage IA or IB but with tumor on the surface of one or both ovaries; or with capsule ruptured; or with ascites present containing malignant cells or with positive peritoneal washings
Stage II	Growth involving one or both ovaries with pelvic extension
Stage IIA	Extension and/or metastases to the uterus and/or tubes
Stage IIB	Extension to other pelvic tissues
Stage IIC	Tumor either stage IIA or IIB with tumor on the surface of one or both ovaries; or with capsule(s) ruptured; or with ascites present containing malignant cells or with positive peritoneal washings
Stage III	Tumor involving one or both ovaries and/or positive retroperitoneal or inguinal nodes. Superficial liver metastasis equals stage III. Tumor is limited to the true pelvis, but with histologically proven malignant extension to small bowel or omentum
Stage IIIA	Tumor grossly limited to the true pelvis with negative nodes but with histologically confirmed implants of abdominal peritoneal surfaces, none exceeding 2 cm in diameter. Nodes negative
Stage IIIB	Tumor of one or both ovaries with histologically confirmed implants of abdominal peritoneal surfaces, none exceeding 2 cm in diameter. Nodes negative
Stage IIIC	Abdominal implants more than 2 cm in diameter and/or positive retroperitoneal or inguinal nodes
Stage IV	Growth involving one or both ovaries with distant metastasis. If pleural effusion is present, there must be positive cytologic test results to allot a case to stage IV. Parenchymal liver metastasis equals stage IV.

These categories are based on findings at clinical examination and/or surgical exploration. The histologic characteristics are to be considered in the staging, as are results of cytologic testing as far as effusions are concerned. It is desirable that a biopsy be performed on suspicious areas outside the pelvis. In order to evaluate the impact on prognosis of the different criteria for allotting cases to stage IC or IIC, it would be of value to know if rupture of the capsule was (1) spontaneous or (2) caused by the surgeon, and if the source of malignant cells detected was (1) peritoneal washings or (2) ascites.

Staging of Ovarian Cancer Ovarian malignancies are staged according to the International Federation of Gynecology and Obstetrics (FIGO) system. The FIGO staging system of 1987 (Table 104-4) is based on the findings at surgical exploration. A preoperative evaluation should exclude the presence of extraperitoneal metastases. A thorough surgical exploration is important because subsequent treatment will be determined by the stage of disease. In patients whose exploratory laparotomy does not reveal any macroscopic evidence of disease by inspection and palpation of the entire intraabdominal space, a careful search for microscopic spread must be undertaken.[35,87] In an earlier series in which patients did not undergo careful surgical staging, the overall 5-year survival for patients with apparent stage I epithelial ovarian cancer was only about 60%.[1,35] Survival rates of 90 to 100% have been reported for properly staged patients found to have stage IA or IB disease.[35,36]

Metastases in apparent stage I or II epithelial ovarian cancer are common. About 30% of patients whose ovarian epithelial cancers appear to be confined to the pelvis have occult metastatic disease in the upper abdomen or in the retroperitoneal lymph nodes.[35] The importance of a comprehensive initial surgical staging is emphasized by the findings of a cooperative national study in which 100 patients with apparent stage I or II disease who were referred for subsequent therapy underwent additional surgical staging.[120] In this series, 28% of patients initially thought to have stage I disease were upstaged, and 43% of patients thought to have stage II disease had more advanced disease. Thus, 31% of patients were upstaged as a result of additional surgery, and 77% were reclassified as stage III. Histologic grade was a significant predictor of occult metastasis, that is, 16% of patients with grade 1 lesions were upstaged, compared to 34% with grade 2 and to 46% with grade 3 disease.

Although the literature has emphasized the importance of thorough surgical exploration in patients with disease apparently localized to the ovaries, scant recognition is made of the semantic difficulty presented by the concept of extension to other pelvic (ie, stage II) or abdominal (ie, stage III) organs. No problem exists when the surgeon encounters discrete implants, or seeds, separate from the primary tumor, or when solid tumor is found growing into adjacent structures. A more common situation, however, is the apparently benign adherence of the tumor to adjacent structures in the absence of metastatic implants or obvious direct tumor extension. There is a considerable body of evidence that such benign adherence, when it is dense, is associated with a relapse risk equivalent to stage II, and that these patients should not be included in stage I, but rather in stage II.[121–123] Adherence is considered dense when sharp dissection is required to mobilize the tumor, when a raw area is left at the site of adherence, or when cyst rupture results from dissecting free the adhesions. It is the practice at most North American centers to advance the stage of densely adherent tumors to stage II, and this was done in a recent multicenter study of stage I and II disease.[120]

After a comprehensive staging laparotomy, only a minority of women has local or regional disease (FIGO stages I and II). Of the 26,600 women diagnosed yearly with epithelial ovarian cancer in the United States, approximately 2,000 to 3,000 have the disease confined to pelvic structures.[35] The prognosis for these patients depends on clinical-pathologic features, as summarized below.[35,36,120–123]

Although accounting for only 15 to 20% of all cases, approximately one-third to one-half of all cured patients are derived from stage I, highlighting its importance.[123] An in-depth understanding of the management of stage I is hampered by the small fraction of patients with limited disease, as well as by their excellent long-term prognosis (over an 80% 5-year relapse-free rate). Consequently, Phase III randomized trials are difficult to conduct with this group due to their small numbers and low rate of recurrence and death. No controlled study to date has been able to establish a curative advantage to postoperative adjuvant therapy.

The most recent FIGO staging classification of stage I, in practice, is descriptive rather than prognostic. The classification recognizes nine subcategories of stage I. Subclasses A (unilateral), B (bilateral), and C (capsular penetration, tumor spillage, or positive peritoneal cytology) are each further subdivided according to differentiation into three grades.[53]

Within each grade, it is incorrect to assume that the factors that assign patients to substages B and C necessarily carry a worse prognosis than substage A, or that rupture, capsular penetration, and positive peritoneal cytology all worsen prognosis to the same degree, or that ascites in the absence of positive cytology is not prognostic. Indeed, several studies have failed to show that bilaterality or iatrogenic intraoperative rupture had any influence on outcome.[120–123] Data on the prognostic significance of positive peritoneal cytology in ovarian cancer are scarce and inadequate.

Treatment of Early Stage Ovarian Cancer The treatment of early stage epithelial ovarian cancer must be individualized. Thorough surgical exploration and staging are indicated for all patients with early stage disease. Adjuvant treatment with chemotherapy or radiotherapy is appropriate for those women at highest risk of recurrence.

Surgery Properly staged early disease can be managed conservatively. The primary treatment for invasive stage I epithelial ovarian cancer is surgical, that is, the performance of a total abdominal hysterectomy, bilateral salpingo-oophorectomy, and surgical staging.[52] In certain circumstances, a unilateral oophorectomy may suffice, as discussed below.

Radiotherapy There have been randomized studies of external beam radiotherapy in stage I epithelial ovarian cancer comparing pelvic radiotherapy with no postoperative treatment. These data suggest that pelvic irradiation reduced the rate of pelvic relapses, but because relapses occurred throughout the peritoneal cavity, this was of no therapeutic benefit. Abdominopelvic radiotherapy has not been studied in a phase III trial in stage I, but was compared with pelvic radiotherapy or to no treatment. No benefit was found in grade 1, where the risk of relapse was under 5% overall. In grades 2 and 3, a nonsignificant reduction in relapse risk was observed. A significant reduction in relapse risk was seen in patients whose tumors were densely adherent, but these patients are more correctly classified in stage II.[123]

Chemotherapy Based on experience in treating patients with advanced ovarian cancer, cisplatin, carboplatin, cyclophosphamide, and paclitaxel have been administered, individually and in combination, to patients with early stage disease. Several series reported outcomes when cisplatin and/or cyclophosphamide have been used to treat patients with stage I disease.[124–126] In a GOG trial that compared 3 cycles of cisplatin and cyclophosphamide to intraperitoneal ^{32}P in patients with stage IB and IC disease, the progression-free survival of women receiving the platinum-based chemotherapy was 31% higher than that of women who received the radiocolloid.[125] The Gruppo Italiano Collaborativo Oncologica Ginecologica (GICOG) has reported two studies that evaluated treatment with cisplatin for women with early stage disease.[126] The first study included patients who had stage I cancers of grades 1 and 2, without ascites, positive cytology, rupture, or capsular penetration. When observation was compared to six cycles of cisplatin, the 4-year disease-free rates were 70% and 71% respectively. In the second study, patients with all other classes of stage I were randomized to intraperitoneal ^{32}P or six cycles of cisplatin. The 4-year disease-free survival rate with cisplatin was 79% compared to 69% with i.p. radiocolloid, but this difference did not achieve statistical significance. The GOG has subsequently completed an additional trial in which high-risk patients were randomized to three or six cycles of carboplatin and paclitaxel. The results of this trial are currently not available. The current GOG trial provides all patients at high risk of recurrence with 3 cycles of carboplatin and paclitaxel and participants are then randomized to observation or 6 months of weekly low-dose (40 mg/m^2) paclitaxel.

Two large parallel randomized phase III clinical trials were conducted on women with early-stage disease: the International Collaborative Ovarian Neoplasm Trial 1 (ICON1) and the Adjuvant Chemotherapy Trial in Ovarian Neoplasia (ACTION).[127,128] When the data from the two trials were combined and analyzed,[129] a total of 465 patients were randomized to receive platinum-based adjuvant chemotherapy and 460 to observation until disease progression. After a median follow-up of more than 4 years, the overall survival was 82% in the chemotherapy arm and 74% in the observation arm (HR = 0.67, p = .001). Recurrence-free survival was also better in the chemotherapy arm: 76% versus 65% (HR = 0.64, p = .001). The results of this analysis must be interpreted with caution, because most of the patients did not undergo thorough surgical staging, but the findings suggest that platinum-based chemotherapy should be given to patients who have not been optimally staged.

Management of Invasive Early Stage Low Risk Disease (Stage IA and IB, Low Grade) In patients who have undergone a thorough staging laparotomy where there is no evidence of spread beyond the ovary, the performance of an abdominal hysterectomy and bilateral salpingo-oophorectomy is appropriate therapy. The uterus and contralateral ovary can be preserved in women with stage IA diploid lesions who wish to preserve fertility. These women should be followed carefully with periodic pelvic examinations and CA 125 titers. Generally, the other ovary and uterus are removed at the completion of childbearing. In a recent report by Guthrie and colleagues, the outcome of 656 patients with early-stage epithelial ovarian cancer was studied.[130] No patients who had a properly documented stage I, grade 1 cancer died of their disease; that is, there was a 100% survival in this condition when patients were surgically staged, and thus adjuvant chemotherapy is unnecessary in patients with low-risk low stage ovarian cancer.

Management of Invasive Early Stage High-Risk Disease (Stage IA and IB, High Grade, Stage IC and Stage II) High-risk stage I is defined as stages IA or IB, grade 3, stage IC, or clear cell carcinomas. In patients whose disease is more poorly differentiated or in whom there are malignant cells either in ascitic fluid or peritoneal washings, additional therapy is indicated. Patients with grade 2 and grade 3 tumors, with densely adherent tumors, with large-volume ascites, and/or with positive peritoneal cytology, have a relapse risk of 20 to 45%, and postoperative treatment is warranted. Regrettably, it would appear that thorough staging with negative findings, including random peritoneal biopsies and lymph node sampling, does not eliminate the risk of relapse in patients with these characteristics.[202] Chemotherapy for patients with early stage high-risk epithelial ovarian cancer can be either single agent carboplatin or a combination of carboplatin and a taxane for 3 to 6 courses. Melphalan is not recommended due to its leukemogenic properties, its long-term compromise of marrow reserve, and its variable oral absorption, despite its ease of administration.[131] We recommend that 4 to 6 cycles of chemotherapy with carboplatin or carboplatin and paclitaxel be given to patients with high-risk low stage ovarian cancer.

Management of Early Stage Borderline Tumors The principal treatment for borderline ovarian tumors is the surgical resection of the primary tumor. There is no evidence that either subsequent chemotherapy or radiation therapy improves survival. After performing a frozen section and determining that the histology is borderline, premenopausal patients who desire preservation of ovarian function may be managed with a conservative operation, such as a unilateral salpingo-oophorectomy.[35] Thus, hormonal function and fertility can be maintained. In patients in whom an ovarian cystectomy has been performed and a borderline tumor is documented in the permanent pathology, no additional surgery is warranted.

There has been considerable controversy regarding the optimum treatment of patients with localized borderline ovarian tumors. This has been due, in part, to lack of unanimity regarding the histopathologic criteria for borderline tumors. For all stages of ovarian cancer, borderline tumors have a more favorable natural history than have invasive tumors.[36] There have been conflicting reports regarding the efficacy and necessity of adjuvant chemotherapy for patients with localized stage I or stage II borderline tumors. In the large GOG trial described above, a total of 51 patients were reclassified as having borderline tumors. In these carefully staged patients, there have been no deaths directly attributable to cancer. While a substantial number of patients did receive adjuvant chemotherapy in these trials, there is no evidence that it was necessary or beneficial. If, after careful histologic review of multiple slides sectioned at 1-cm intervals, no evidence of stromal invasion is found, patients with localized borderline tumors should not routinely receive adjuvant therapy.

TREATMENT OF ADVANCED STAGE EPITHELIAL OVARIAN CANCER

A scheme for the management of patients with advanced-stage epithelial ovarian cancer is presented in Figure 104-6. The components of this approach are discussed below.

Cytoreductive Surgery in Ovarian Cancer Patients who have advanced-stage epithelial ovarian cancer documented at initial exploratory laparotomy should undergo cytoreductive surgery to remove as much of the tumor and its metastases as possible in order to facilitate the effectiveness of subsequent therapies.[132–141] The operation usually includes the performance of a total abdominal hysterectomy and bilateral salpingo-oophorectomy, a complete omentectomy, and resection of metastatic lesions on the peritoneal surfaces or from the intestines. In addition, the pelvic tumor may directly involve the rectosigmoid colon, the terminal ileum, and the cecum. In some patients, most or all of their disease is confined to the pelvic viscera and the omentum, so that removal of these organs results in the extirpation of all gross tumor, a situation that is associated with a reasonable chance of complete response.

The rationale for cytoreductive surgery relates to three general theoretical considerations: (1) potential physiologic benefits from excising the tumor; (2) improved tumor perfusion and increased growth fraction, that may increase the likelihood of a response to chemotherapy or radiation therapy; and (3) enhanced immunologic competence of the patient.[135,138]

The principal goal of cytoreductive surgery is to remove all of the primary cancer and, if possible, its metastases. If resection of all metastases is not feasible, the goal is to reduce the tumor burden by resection of all individual tumors to an optimal status.[54,119,120] The definition of "optimal" was initially proposed by Griffiths, who found that the survival of patients whose metastatic disease was resected to less than 1.5 cm in maximum dimension was significantly longer than the survival of those whose residual lesions were larger than 1.5 cm.[132] The optimal category of patients had a higher subsequent response rate to chemotherapy and longer disease-progression-free interval. Subsequently, Hacker and colleagues[133] showed that patients whose largest residual lesions were less than 5 mm (defined as minimal residual disease, MRD) survived much longer than did those with larger non-resectable tumor deposits. The median survival of patients in this category was 40 months, compared with 18 months for patients whose disease was greater than 1.5 cm. It has been suggested that the performance of a complete retroperitoneal lymphadenectomy might also improve the survival of patients with advanced stage disease, but this has not been proven in prospective studies.[136] Resectability of the metastatic tumor is often determined by the size of nodules, the extent of carcinomatosis, and the location of the disease.[141]

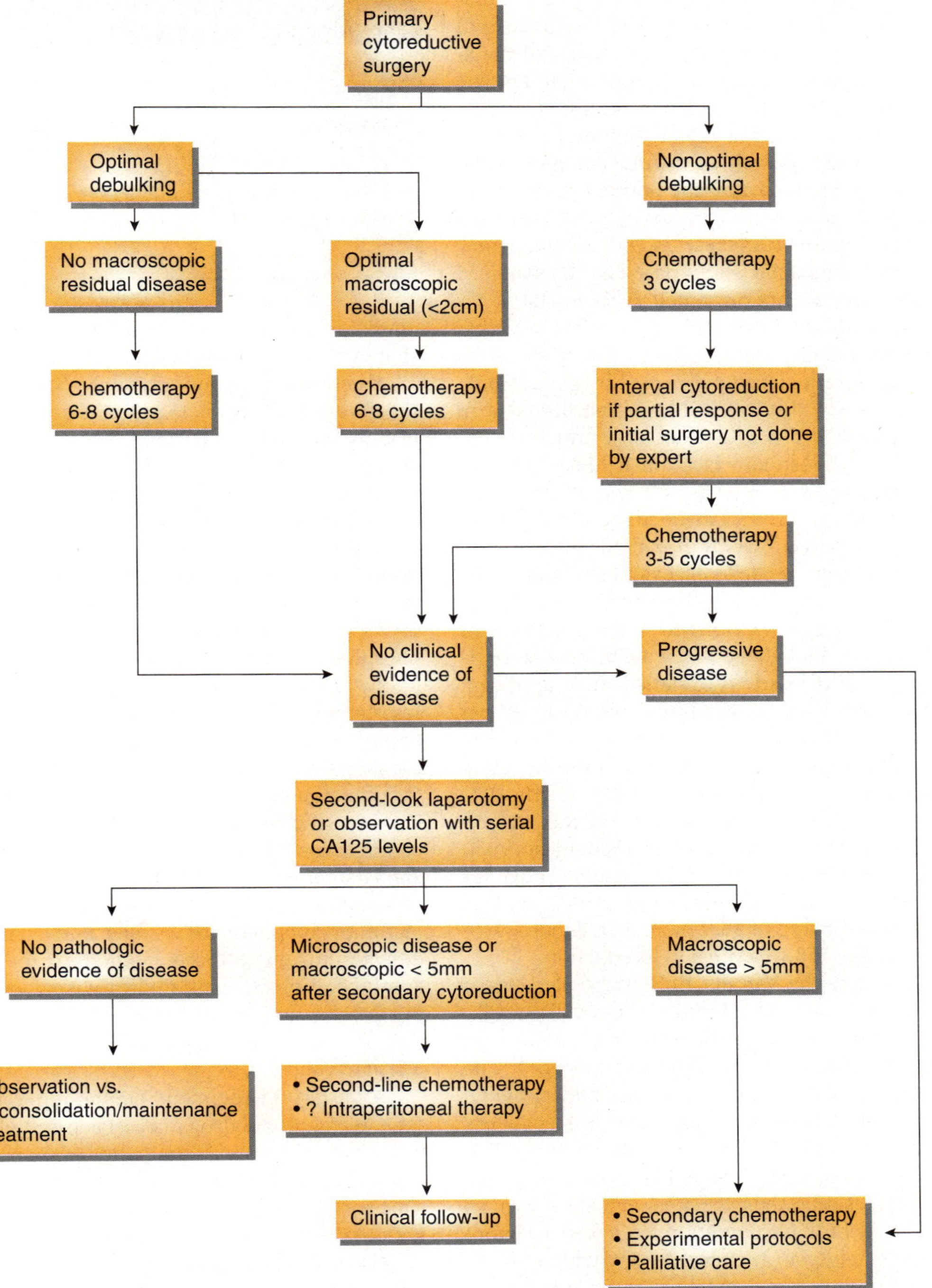

Figure 104-6 Treatment scheme for patients with advanced-stage ovarian cancer.* Do in a research setting where treatment will be based on outcome. Reprinted with permission, from Berek JS, Hacker NF. Practical gynecologic oncology. 4th ed. Baltimore, MD: Lippincott Williams & Wilkins; 2005, p 460.

The ability of cytoreductive surgery to influence survival is limited by the size, extent, and location of metastases prior to cytoreduction, and presumably by the presence of drug-resistant cells.[139–144] For example, in patients whose metastatic disease was very large (ie, greater than 10 cm before cytoreductive surgery), survival was shorter than when less bulky disease was resected. Thus, the value of cytoreductive surgery seems to be more limited in patients with very large metastases, regardless of the extent of tumor removal.[133] This may result from the presence of resistant clones among large masses of tumor cells.[138] Patients with gross ascites also seem to do less well, regardless of the extent of surgical resection.[141] In some patients, very extensive upper abdominal masses, particularly on the diaphragm or in the parenchyma of the liver, will preclude an adequate surgical excision of metastatic disease. Extensive disease involving the base of the small bowel mesentery, the large bowel mesentery, the lesser omentum, and the porta hepatis, as well as diffuse extraperitoneal metastasis, may prevent the optimal resection of tumor.[140] Thus, the efficacy of cytoreductive surgery is limited. From these and other data, definitions of the patients' status based on the extent of residual disease are presented in Table 104-5.

Table 104-5 Nomenclature for Patient Status–Residual Ovarian Cancer

Residual Disease		Status
None	Pathologic	Complete remission
Microscopic disease	Only	Microscopic
Macroscopic disease	<5 mm	Minimal residual
Macroscopic disease	<1–2 cm	Optimal residual
Macroscopic residual disease	>1–2 cm	Suboptimal
Macroscopic disease	>2–3 cm	Bulky residual

Nomenclature for status of patient based on the extent of residual ovarian cancer prior to treatment.

An analysis of the retrospective data available suggests that these operations are feasible in 70 to 90% of patients when performed by gynecologic oncologists[133–137,139–144] Major morbidity is in the range of 5% and operative mortality is 1%.[134,139] Intestinal resection in these patients does not appear to increase the overall morbidity of the operation.[143] The median survival and progression-free interval of patients after cytoreductive surgery relate to the extent of residual disease at the completion of the laparotomy. A meta-analysis has been performed with 81 cohorts of patients that included 6,885 women with stage III or stage IV disease.[144] A statistically significant positive correlation was found between percent maximal cytoreduction and log median survival time that remained significant after controlling for all other variables ($p < .001$). Each 10% increase in maximal cytoreduction was associated with a 5.5% increase in median survival time. Cohorts with 25% or less maximal cytoreduction had a median survival time of 22.7 months compared to 33.9 months in cohorts with greater than 75% maximal cytoreduction.

In a study by Van der Burg and colleagues, a prospective randomized trial of "interval" debulking operations was performed on patients with advanced-stage epithelial ovarian cancer.[145] The patients were referred after having undergone an exploratory laparotomy during which the patient's tumor was not debulked. The patients were then randomized to receive either (1) chemotherapy for three cycles followed by another operation, then an interval debulking operation, followed by more chemotherapy; or (2) chemotherapy with no interval debulking. The patients who underwent the interval debulking had a longer disease-free and overall survival as compared with those patients who did not. These data support the role of debulking surgery in advanced-stage epithelial ovarian cancer and suggest that the sooner the operation can be performed during the course of treatment, the more likely it is that the surgery will improve the survival. In a GOG study of interval cytoreductive surgery, the study design was different because the patients entered on the trial had already undergone a maximal attempt at tumor resection at their initial surgery.[146] The randomized findings showed no difference between the group who had an additional attempt at debulking after three cycles of chemotherapy compared with those who did not (32 vs 33 months). Therefore, primary cytoreductive should be the standard of care in patients with advanced epithelial ovarian cancer. If the primary operation was not attempted, interval debulking should be performed whenever possible.

Chemotherapy for Advanced Stage Epithelial Ovarian Cancer Systemic chemotherapy is the standard treatment for metastatic epithelial ovarian cancer.[147–170] Cisplatin was initially used in combination with cyclophosphamide and doxorubicin, but the modest contribution of doxorubicin to the efficacy of the combination prompted simplification of the standard regimen to cyclophosphamide and cisplatin. By the early 1990s a combination of carboplatin and cyclophosphamide was found to be as effective as cisplatin and cyclophosphamide, but substantially less toxic, with less nausea, renal toxicity and neurotoxicity. Paclitaxel was incorporated into combination chemotherapy in the 1990s.[147–151] Over the last decade, a substantial amount of clinical investigation has centered on (1) whether a combination of a platinum compound and a taxane is superior to an optimal dose of a platinum compound alone, (2) the choice of the optimal platinum compound and taxane, and (3) the most convenient and effective schedule for taxane administration. Recent studies have focused on the introduction of other compounds into a "triplet" or a "sequential doublet" to eliminate drug resistant cancer cells.

A variety of regimens containing combinations of cytotoxic drugs have been tested in the treatment of advanced epithelial ovarian cancer. Combination chemotherapy has been shown to be superior to single-agent therapy in most patients with advanced epithelial ovarian cancer.

Platinum Compounds For the last two decades, platinum compounds have been the most active agents against ovarian cancer. In early studies from England, cisplatin was found superior to cyclophosphamide as a single agent. Concurrently, cisplatin was tested in combination with a variety of different drugs. Platinum-containing regimens have proven superior to regimens that lacked platinum compounds.[153] In a meta-analysis performed on 37 randomized studies involving 5,667 patients with advanced-stage disease, those patients given cisplatin-containing combination chemotherapy were compared with those treated with regimens that did not include cisplatin.[154,160] Platinum based chemotherapy was superior to non-platinum based chemotherapy. A trend favored platinum combinations over single agent platinum. In studies of cisplatin containing regimens, several trials have compared cyclophosphamide and cisplatin (CP) with cisplatin, doxorubicin, and cyclophosphamide (PAC).[155–159] No study showed a significant difference in survival between treatment arms. The GOG's randomized prospective comparison of equitoxic doses of PAC versus PC showed no benefit to the inclusion of doxorubicin in the combination.[155] While a meta-analysis of the combined data from these four trials showed a 7% survival advantage at 6 years for those patients treated with the doxorubicin-containing regimen, the survival curves converge at 8 years. Consequently, in recent years doxorubicin has not been incorporated in regimens for epithelial ovarian cancer in the United States. It is, however, possible that a small subset of ovarian cancer patients benefit substantially from treatment with anthracyclines. In the future, new technologies may permit the identification of those patients and permit individualization of their treatment.

In the 1980s, the second-generation platinum analogue carboplatin became available, exhibiting greater myelotoxicity, but substantially less nephrotoxicity, ototoxicity, peripheral neurotoxicity, and emetogenic potential than did cisplatin. Initial studies showed that carboplatin and cisplatin had approximately a 4:1 ratio of potency. Thus a standard single-agent dose of about 400 mg/M^2 has been used in most phase II trials. The dose is best calculated by using the probable area under the curve (AUC) based on the glomerular filtration rate (GFR) according to the Calvert formula.[166] When used as a single agent, a target AUC of 7 may be appropriate for untreated patients with ovarian cancer. When used in combination with other myelotoxic drugs, AUCs of 5 to 6 have been used more frequently.

Meta-analysis has suggested that cisplatin and carboplatin are equally effective against epithelial ovarian cancer.[167] Direct comparison of cisplatin and cyclophosphamide to carboplatin and cyclophosphamide demonstrated comparable response rates and survival, but significantly less toxicity for the carboplatin containing regimen.[161,162]

Paclitaxel Paclitaxel was shown to be a very active agent against ovarian cancer.[147–151] The overall response rates for paclitaxel in phase II trials was 36% in previously treated patients, which is a higher rate than was seen for cisplatin when it was first tested.[147]

Three large concurrently controlled randomized trials in previously untreated patients with ovarian cancer have compared paclitaxel and a platinum compound to different platinum containing regimens that did not contain paclitaxel.[149,150,163] The Gynecologic Oncology Group randomized 410 women with suboptimally cytoreduced stage III–IV ovarian cancer to six cycles of chemotherapy with a combination of cisplatin (75 mg/M^2) and paclitaxel (135 mg/M^2 over 24 hours) or with cisplatin (75 mg/M^2) and cyclophosphamide (750 mg/M^2) (GOG-111).[149] Patients who received the paclitaxel combination had a superior overall response rate (73% vs 60%), clinical complete response rate (51% vs 31%), prolongation of disease-free survival (18 months vs 14 months), and prolongation of overall survival (36 months vs 24 months).

The superiority of paclitaxel-cisplatin was confirmed in a trial (OV-10) conducted jointly by the European Organization for the Research and Treatment of Cancer (EORTC), the Nordic Ovarian Cancer Study Group (NOCOVA), and the National Cancer Institute of Canada (NCIC) in which 680 women with both optimal and suboptimal disease in stages IIB–IV were treated.[150] Patients were randomized to six cycles of cisplatin (75 mg/M^2) and cyclophosphamide (750 mg/M^2) or to six cycles of cisplatin (75 mg/M^2) with a slightly higher dose of paclitaxel (175 mg/M^2) over a shorter interval (3 hours) than in GOG-111. In this study, the paclitaxel-containing arm produced a significant improvement in median progression-free interval (15.5 vs 11.5 months) and overall median overall survival (35.6 vs 25.8 months) that extended to both optimal and suboptimal groups. Greater neurotoxicity was observed with the combination of paclitaxel and cisplatin when the paclitaxel was infused over 3 hours in OV-10 compared to infusion over 24 hours in GOG-111.

A third study, the International Collaborative Ovarian Neoplasm-3 (ICON-3), was conducted as 4 parallel trials across 130 centers in eight countries in Europe to compare carboplatin (AUC 5) and paclitaxel (175 mg/M^2 over 3 hours) to regimens that did not contain paclitaxel.[163] Prior to randomization, each patient and physician could choose a control arm that included either carboplatin (AUC 5) alone or a combination of cisplatin (50 mg/M^2), doxorubicin (50 mg/M^2) and cyclophosphamide (500 mg/M^2). Of the women on the control arm, 69% received carboplatin. Dose escalation was permitted and occurred in approximately half of patients. Overall, 2,074 women participated with ovarian cancer of all stages, including 20% of women with stage I–II disease. A central review of pathology, surgical staging, cytoreduction, or protocol adherence was not performed. No significant difference was found in overall median survival between the paclitaxel-carboplatin group (36.1 months) and the control group (35.4 months). In comparing the three trials, the outcome was no worse in the paclitaxel-carboplatin arm of ICON-3 than in the paclitaxel-cisplatin arms of GOG-111 and OV-10, but the control group in ICON-3 enjoyed a better outcome. The better survival of controls in ICON-3 might relate to the fraction of early stage patients or possibly to the optimization of carboplatin dosage permitted by dose escalation. A trend (p = .22) was noted toward a benefit of paclitaxel-carboplatin in patients who had > 2 cm residual disease, patients comparable to those entered in GOG-111.

The GOG had undertaken a comparison of sequential and simultaneous paclitaxel-cisplatin (GOG-132).[151] A three-arm comparison of equitoxic doses of paclitaxel (200 mg/M^2 over 24 hours) versus cisplatin (100 mg/M^2) versus a combination of paclitaxel (135 mg/M^2 over 24 hours) and cisplatin (75 mg/M^2) was carried out in 648 suboptimal stage III and IV patients. Crossover was permitted and the three groups exhibited similar median overall survival of 26 to 30 months. The simultaneous regimen was better tolerated than the sequential use of agents at these optimized doses. The overall response rate to cisplatin alone or to the paclitaxel-cisplatin combination was 67%, whereas the response to paclitaxel alone was 42% (p < .001). This observation suggests that more than half of patients who are treated arbitrarily with the combination of paclitaxel and a platinum derivative may not benefit from the taxane. To date, laboratory studies do not support any super-additive interaction of platinum compounds and taxanes, arguing against synergy in the clinic. In the future, using molecular markers it may be possible to identify those patients who would respond or not respond to paclitaxel, providing another opportunity to individualize therapy.

Two randomized, prospective clinical studies have compared the combination of paclitaxel and carboplatin to that of paclitaxel and cisplatin.[161,162] In both studies, response rates and duration of survival are similar, but the carboplatin-containing regimens have more acceptable toxicity. In the first trial conducted by the GOG (GOG-158), patients were randomized to carboplatin (AUC 7.5) and paclitaxel (175 mg/M^2) over 3 hours versus the previous standard of cisplatin (75 mg/M^2) and paclitaxel (135 mg/M^2 over 24 h). Progression-free survival of the carboplatin-containing arm was 22 months versus 21.7 months for the control arm.[161] The gastrointestinal and neurotoxicity of the carboplatin arm were appreciably lower than that of the cisplatin arm. In addition, paclitaxel administration over 3 hours is substantially more convenient than administration over 24 hours. A similar result was obtained in a large randomized trial in Germany, in which carboplatin (AUC 6) and paclitaxel (185 mg/M^2 over 3 hours) were compared to paclitaxel (135 mg/M^2 over 24 hours) and cisplatin (75 mg/M^2).[162] Thus, the best established regimen in patients with advanced stage disease is a combination of carboplatin and paclitaxel over 3 h.

Docetaxel Docetaxel is a semi-synthetic second generation taxane with properties that differ from paclitaxel. Docetaxel is a more potent promoter of microtubule assembly and stabilization than paclitaxel.[169] Docetaxel is taken up, bound, and retained more effectively by cancer cells than paclitaxel. Docetaxel has produced a 23 to 28% overall response rate in platinum resistant ovarian cancer, and a combination of docetaxel and cisplatin or carboplatin has achieved a 66 to 81% overall response rate in phase II trials.[169] Consequently, a combination of docetaxel (75 mg/M^2 over 1 h) and carboplatin (AUC 5) has been compared to paclitaxel (175 mg/M^2) and carboplatin (AUC 5) in the SCOTROC trial.[170] Similar efficacy was observed, but docetaxel-carboplatin was associated with significantly less neurotoxicity. Consequently, a combination of carboplatin and docetaxel should be considered for treatment of ovarian cancer in patients with significant neuropathy.

Other Doublets and Triplets Use of platinum compounds and taxanes has improved median and overall survival, but the outcome in patients with advanced ovarian cancer is still disappointing. Drug resistance ultimately develops in the majority. A number of drugs have exhibited activity against recurrent disease including liposomal doxorubicin, topotecan and gemcitabine. The GOG has conducted a series of phase I pilot studies in previously untreated patients to define combinations that are suitable for a group wide phase III trial. A five-arm study has now been initiated, administering 8 cycles of chemotherapy to women with newly diagnosed stage III/IV ovarian cancer. The control arm consists of paclitaxel (175 mg/M^2 over 3h on day 1) and carboplatin (AUC 6 on day 1). Two additional arms contain triplets. The gemcitabine triplet includes paclitaxel (175 mg/M^2 over 3 hours on day 1), carboplatin (AUC 5 on day 1) and gemcitabine (800 mg/M^2/day on day1 and 8). The Doxil triplet administers paclitaxel (175 mg/M^2 over 3 hours on day 1), carboplatin (AUC 5 on day 1) and Doxil (30 mg/M^2 on day 1 every other cycle). Two arms contain sequential doublets. The topotecan doublet includes 4 cycles of carboplatin (AUC 5 on day 3) with topotecan (1.25 mg/M^2/day on day1 to 3) followed by 4 cycles of paclitaxel and carboplatin. Finally, a gemcitabine doublet includes 4 cycles of carboplatin (AUC 6 on day 8) with gemcitabine (1,000 mg/M^2/day on days 1 and 8) followed by 4 cycles of paclitaxel and carboplatin.

Dose Intensification with Intravenous Chemotherapy Higher or more frequent doses of chemotherapy might be more effective, if tolerated. The issue of dose-intensification of cisplatin was examined in a prospective trial conducted by the GOG. In this study, 243 patients with suboptimal ovarian cancer were randomized to receive either 50 mg/M^2 or 100 mg/M^2 cisplatin plus 500 mg/M^2 cyclophosphamide.[164] There was no difference in response rates in those patients with measurable disease and the overall survival was identical. As one might anticipate, there was greater toxicity associated with the high-dose regimen. A group in Scotland performed a similar study and found that patients who received 100 mg/M^2 cisplatin plus 750 mg/M^2 cyclophosphamide had a significantly longer median survival compared with those who received 50 mg/M^2 cisplatin plus the same dose of cyclophosphamide. The overall median survival time was 114 weeks in the high-dose group and 69 weeks in the low-dose group (p = .0008), but this difference disappeared with longer follow-up.[165] Thus, doubling the dose of cisplatin does not improve long term survival. Dose escalation of paclitaxel and carboplatin require G-CSF because of their combined myelosuppressive effects, but there is no evidence to support more intensive administration of either agent.[161,165]

Intraperitoneal Chemotherapy As ovarian cancer spreads over the surface of the peritoneum and often recurs at this site; investigators have evaluated intraperitoneal (IP) administration of chemotherapy that can achieve high local concentrations of drug. A randomized, prospective trial performed by the Southwest Oncology Group (SWOG) and the GOG compared IP cisplatin (100 mg/M^2) to IV cisplatin (100 mg/M^2), each given with II cyclophosphamide (600mg/M^2), in patients with disease less than 2 cm in diameter.[171] The intraperitoneal cisplatin arm had a significantly longer overall median survival than the intravenous arm, 49 versus 41 months ($p = .03$). In the patients with the least residual disease (< 0.5 cm maximum residual), however, there was not a statistically significant difference in median survival between the two treatments, 51 versus 46 months ($p = .08$).

Results of this randomized trial became available as paclitaxel was being incorporated into clinical practice. In a follow-up trial conducted by the GOG, a standard regimen of IV cisplatin (75 mg/M^2) and IV paclitaxel (135 mg/M over 24 hours) was compared to a dose-intense regimen that was initiated by giving moderately high-dose carboplatin (AUC=9) for two induction cycles followed by IP cisplatin 100 mg/M^2 and IV paclitaxel (135 mg/M^2 over 24 hours).[173] The dose-intense arm produced slightly better progression-free median survival (27.6 months vs 22.5 months, $p = .02$), but there was not a statistically significant difference in overall survival (52.9 months vs 47.6 months, $p = .056$).

A randomized prospective GOG study compared IP cisplatin and paclitaxel to IV cisplatin and paclitaxel.[173] The results of this study suggest that the IP cisplatin and IP paclitaxel result in a longer disease progression-free survival and overall survival compared with the IV administration of these drugs. Because that standard of care is to use carboplatin instead of cisplatin, subsequent studies will compare these findings to carboplatin and paclitaxel given IP and IV. While there is a modest survival advantage for IP therapy using cisplatin and paclitaxel, the IP approach is more cumbersome because it requires the placement and use of intraperitoneal catheters and cisplatin is more toxic than carboplatin. Therefore, based on results of currently available studies, the use of this regimen of IP chemotherapy for the primary treatment of optimally resected stage III ovarian cancer must be individualized.

Neoadjuvant Chemotherapy Some authors have suggested that, for patients with suboptimal stage III and stage IV disease, chemotherapy may be given in lieu of cytoreductive surgery. A series performed at Yale by Schwartz and colleagues suggested that the survival of patients treated with "neoadjuvant" or cytoreductive chemotherapy was comparable to those patients historically treated with cytoreductive surgery followed by conventional chemotherapy in the same institution.[174] As other authors have shown a benefit to debulking patients prior to chemotherapy, the issue would need to be resolved by a prospective clinical trial. However, two or three cycles of chemotherapy prior to cytoreductive surgery may be helpful in patients with massive ascites or large pleural effusions. Chemotherapy may eliminate the effusions, improve the patient's performance status, and decrease postoperative morbidity, particularly within the chest.

RADIOTHERAPY IN ADVANCED INVASIVE DISEASE In the past decade, several studies have refined our knowledge of the possible benefits of radiation therapy in ovarian cancer. In particular, subgroups of patients have been identified who are most likely to have a curative benefit when radiation therapy is used as the sole postoperative treatment. In addition, the technical aspects of whole abdominal radiation (WAR) have been worked out, permitting therapy to be delivered with acceptable late toxicity (Table 104-6).[175] Despite this knowledge, WAR is not used widely. The results of these studies are concordant in showing long-term failure-free survivors determined both by the stage at presentation and by the volume of residual disease, as expressed by the largest diameter of the largest remaining lesion. Between 38 and 62% of patients with identified residual disease less than 2 cm in diameter were cured after whole abdominal and pelvic irradiation. Most of the long-term survivors had stage II disease, in which the postoperative tumor residuum was confined to the pelvis and was encompassed in the boost volume, where radiation doses are significantly higher than can be delivered to the upper abdomen. For patients with larger residual lesions, the probability of cure is small, in the neighborhood of 5 to 15%. Although there is evidence that whole abdominal irradiation is therapeutic for patients with small-volume residual ovarian cancer, questions have been raised about the interpretation of these results in the context of more modern surgical techniques and more effective chemotherapy.

Table 104-6 Whole Abdominal Radiation in Patients with Residual Disease

Study End Point (Ref. No.)	Volume of Residual Disease Prior to Radiation <2 cm	>2 cm
Percent 10-yr RFR[170]	38%	6%
Percent 15-yr FFR[171]	50%	14%
Percent 10-yr RFS[172]	62%	0%
Percent 10-yr survival[173]	42%	10%
Surviving fraction at 6 yrs[174]	41%	—
Percent 9-yr RFR[175]	62%	8%

FFR = failure-free rate; RFR = relapse-free rate; RFS = relapse-free survival.

Management of Advanced Invasive Ovarian Cancer At present, the treatment of choice for patients with advanced invasive epithelial ovarian cancer is cytoreductive surgery followed by six to eight cycles of chemotherapy with a combination of carboplatin (AUC 5-6) and paclitaxel (175 mg/M^2 over 3 hours) every 3 weeks (Table 104-7). Paclitaxel is administered before the carboplatin. In patients at risk for severe neuropathy, for example, diabetics, a combination of docetaxel (75 mg/M^2) and carboplatin (AUC 5) provides an alternative that is less neurotoxic. As data confirming the SCOTROC trial are obtained, the latter regimen may become a standard option for all patients. In women who cannot tolerate the toxicity of taxanes, carboplatin alone (AUC 6-7) can be given. For the rare patient who cannot tolerate IV chemotherapy, an oral alkylating agent can be used for palliation.

Management of Advanced Borderline Tumors The effectiveness of chemotherapy in patients with advanced-stage borderline tumors has not been established. The GOG is evaluating the use of chemotherapy in patients with advanced-stage borderline tumors who have recurrent disease after initial surgery. Until the results of this trial are known, the current approach to treatment is primarily surgical. Patients should undergo cytoreductive surgery and observation. Borderline tumors, even in advanced stage, have a favorable prognosis. The first symptomatic recurrence may be several years after diagnosis. In contrast to the 20 to 25% survival rates for advanced epithelial invasive carcinoma of the ovary, the survival rate for patients with stage III borderline tumors is over 60%.[35,36] Consequently, secondary cytoreductive surgery frequently will lead to another prolonged interval of symptom free survival. Chemotherapy can be administered to the patients in whom cytoreductive surgery is no longer feasible, although its efficacy is uncertain.

ASSESSMENT OF RESPONSE IN PATIENTS WHO ARE CLINICALLY FREE OF DISEASE Many patients who have undergone optimal cytoreductive surgery and subsequent therapy for epithelial ovarian cancer will have no evidence of disease at the completion of treatment. Tumor markers and radiologic assessments have proven to be too insensitive to exclude accurately the presence of subclinical disease.[176–178] Therefore, a technique used to evaluate residual disease has been the second-look operation.[179,180]

A second-look operation is one performed on a patient who has no clinical evidence of disease after a prescribed course of chemotherapy, in order to determine the response to therapy. Most often, patients have undergone a formal reassessment laparotomy. The laparoscope also has been used in some of these cases but there is a 35% false-negative rate if laparoscopy is used as a second-look procedure.[179]

If a second-look operation is performed, the proper surgery should be carried out to maximize the likelihood of detecting any microscopic resid-

Table 104-7 Combination Chemotherapy for Advanced Epithelial Ovarian Cancer: Recommended Regimens

Drugs	Dose	Administration (Hours)	Interval	Number of Treatments
Paclitaxel	175 mg/m^2	3	Every 3 wk	6–8 cycles
Carboplatin	AUC = 5–6			
Docetaxel	75 mg/m^2	1	Every 3 wk	6–8 cycles
Carboplatin	AUC = 5			

Drugs that can be substituted for Taxol, if hypersensitivity to that drug occurs. Standard regimens are given. AUC = "area under the curve" dose by Calvert formula.[260]

ual disease. The technique of the second-look laparotomy is essentially identical to that of the staging laparotomy.[35] The ability to obtain a complete remission with a platinum-based therapy is dependent on the extent of residual disease at the time chemotherapy is initiated. Clinical trials have uniformly demonstrated that patients who have bulky disease (any tumor nodule greater than 2 to 3 cm in diameter) have less than a 10% likelihood of achieving a complete remission with induction chemotherapy with a platinum-based regimen. In contrast, patients who have small-volume disease after the initial laparotomy have a three to four times higher likelihood of achieving a complete remission.[180] There is no evidence that prolonging the number of cycles of induction chemotherapy will increase the complete remission rate.

The levels of CA 125 have been correlated with the findings at second-look surgery. Positive levels are useful in predicting the presence of disease, but negative titers are an insensitive marker for the absence of disease. In studies performed to date, the predictive value of a positive test has been 96%, that is, if the level of CA 125 was positive (> 35 U/mL), disease was almost always detectable in patients at the second-look.[177] In one such prospective analysis, the predictive value of a negative test was only 56%, that is, if the level was less than 35 U/mL, disease was present in 44% of the patients at the time of the second-look.[177] Therefore, the CA 125 is not sensitive enough to exclude subclinical disease in many patients. Serum CA 125 levels can be used to follow those patients during chemotherapy whose level was positive at the initiation of therapy.[178] Changes in CA 125 level (ie, falling, rising, or plateauing) generally correlates with response. Those patients with persistently elevated levels of CA 125 after 3 months of treatment most likely have resistant tumors. Persistently elevated or rising titers on treatment usually indicate treatment failure and suggest that continuation of the current regimen is unlikely to be of value.

Because second-look laparotomies have not been shown to influence patient survival, they should be done only in a research setting, as second-line or salvage therapies in patients with persistent cancer have not yet demonstrated a clear improvement in the overall survival.[35] The findings at a second-look procedure do, however, correlate with subsequent outcome and survival. Patients who have no histologic evidence of disease have a significantly longer survival compared with those who have microscopic or macroscopic disease documented at laparotomy.[180] About 50 to 70% of patients with negative second-look examinations remain free of disease at 5 years, whereas the median survival of patients with any disease (microscopic and macroscopic) is 12 to 18 months. The extent of residual disease documented at the second-look procedure also correlates with patient survival.[35] Patients with microscopic disease only have a 5-year survival of 40 to 50% (median of more than 36 months), compared with 12 months for patients with any evidence of macroscopic disease. Clearly, it is not possible to sample every potential site of disease. In addition, disease can become clinically apparent at sites that are impossible to examine, such as the liver parenchyma. The majority of recurrences after a negative second-look procedure are in patients with poorly differentiated cancers.

Consolidation Chemotherapy and Immunotherapy The optimal management of patients who do achieve a clinical complete remission after induction chemotherapy remains to be determined. Even patients who achieve a surgically confirmed complete remission have a 30 to 50% recurrence rate.[35,180] Some investigators have suggested that second-look laparotomy should be performed to identify patients who may be candidates for intraperitoneal therapy. There is, however, currently no evidence that the routine sequential administration of intraperitoneal chemotherapy after intravenous induction chemotherapy leads to a prolongation of survival.

Clinical trials are in progress to determine whether consolidation therapies are of benefit in patients who achieve a surgically confirmed clinical complete remission. A recent study conducted by the GOG and SWOG compared 3 and 12 monthly cycles of "consolidation" chemotherapy with paclitaxel (135–175 mg/m^2 IV over 3 hours) for patients who had achieved a clinical remission following primary paclitaxel and carboplatin chemotherapy.[181] Progression free survival was 21 and 28 months in the 3-cycle and 12-cycle paclitaxel arms (p = .035). Consequently, 9 months of additional chemotherapy provided an additional 7 months of progression free survival. To date, there is no difference in overall survival between the two arms. Two placebo-controlled randomized trials have been performed in Europe using consolidation with 4 cycles topotecan given to patients in clinical remission following chemotherapy with carboplatin and paclitaxel, and in both trials there was no improvement in survival compared with placebo.[182,183]

A number of experimental regimens are being tested including IP chemotherapy, high dose IV chemotherapy with stem cell support, and immunotherapy with interferon. A randomized trial of IP administration of ^{90}Y-labelled anti-MUC1 antibody showed no survival advantage.[184] The therapeutic potential of an anti-idiotypic response to an anti-CA 125 antibody was discovered in a retrospective analysis of a diagnostic study with MAb-B43.13, where a large group of patients who had been imaged enjoyed unexpectedly long survival. Vaccine trials are ongoing with OvaRex, in an attempt to utilize anti-idiotypic immunity against antibodies reactive with CA 125. A randomized placebo-controlled trial of OvaRex was performed in patients who were in clinical remission after platinum and paclitaxel chemotherapy was performed.[185] While there was no difference in survival in the overall group, the subset of optimal chemosensitive patients had a median relapse-free survival of 24 months compared with 10.5 months for those receiving a placebo (p = .06). Based on these results, a large phase III trial is being conducted in the optimal patients only. Outside of a clinical research setting, a standard approach is to follow patients carefully after the achievement of a clinical complete remission until recurrence.

Consolidation or Salvage Radiotherapy Salvage radiotherapy is inappropriate for most patients with any macroscopic disease after chemotherapy.[186–190] When consolidative radiotherapy has been used, there does not appear to be any curative benefit.

Follow-Up Examinations The optimal frequency of follow-up examinations is unknown, but in those patients who have completed chemotherapy and who are in clinical remission it is reasonable to perform a pelvic examination and to obtain a CA 125 every 3 months for 1 to 2 years. An elevated CA 125 (> 35 U/mL) can provide lead-time of approximately 3 months in detecting recurrent disease. A rising CA 125 can prompt the performance of a CT scan. The role of PET scanning in this setting has not been defined. A rising CA 125 in the absence of changes on physical examination or CT scan in a patient in initial remission poses a dilemma. At present, additional cytotoxic therapy is not recommended based on a rising CA 125 alone. Treatment with tamoxifen has sometimes been given, but the value is uncertain. The GOG is currently comparing tamoxifen to thalidomide in patients with a rising CA 125 without other evidence of disease recurrence. This trial may permit a paradigm for the evaluation of novel cytostatic targeted drugs. As more effective salvage therapy becomes available, serum markers such as CA 125 may have greater utility. In patients whose disease was never found to be metastatic to the chest or who never had a pleural effusion, chest radiograph surveillance is not mandatory. In the absence of a rising CA 125, follow-up CT or MRI scans should be used with discretion, perhaps 6 to 12 months after the completion of chemotherapy, and then again a year later.[35]

Intravenous Second-Line Therapy in Patients with Recurrent or Persistent Advanced Epithelial Ovarian Cancer The overall prognosis is unfavorable for patients who do not achieve a complete remission with induction chemotherapy or who relapse after an initial response. Responses to second-line therapy can, however, be clinically beneficial. The frequency of a response to second-line therapy depends on both the nature of the prior response to initial therapy and the duration of remission. In patients who achieve a complete remission on a platinum-based induction regimen and have a disease-free interval of greater than 6 months, second-line treatment with a platinum compound has approximately a 30% response rate.[191,192] Patients can be retreated with either cisplatin or carboplatin. However, because of its more favorable toxicity profile, carboplatin is the drug of choice for patients who relapse after responding to a platinum-based induction regimen. In contrast, if patients do not achieve a remission on a platinum-based regimen or have a very short response duration, retreatment with a platinum-based regimen is unlikely to be beneficial, and such patients should be encouraged to enter experimental clinical trials.

As noted above, the current treatment of choice for patients with previously untreated ovarian cancer is the combination of carboplatin plus paclitaxel. Successful retreatment with paclitaxel is similar to that described above for platinum compounds. Patients who have responded to initial paclitaxel-based chemotherapy have a significant probability of responding to paclitaxel that is dependent upon the length of response. There is no evidence that retreatment with a combination of paclitaxel plus carboplatin is superior to using these agents sequentially in patients with recurrent disease. However, many investigators do recommend that combination chemotherapy be used as part of reinduction for patients who have a disease-free interval that extends beyond 18 months.[192] In patients who become resistant to paclitaxel and platinum compounds, a wide variety of second-line agents have been shown to have activity, including topotecan, gemcitabine, liposome-encapsulated doxorubicin, oral etoposide, and vinorelbine.[193–202] All of these second-line agents have a comparable degree of activity with partial response rates of approximately 20%. Few formal comparisons have been performed among these drugs. Pegylated liposomal doxorubicin (PLD) has been compared to topotecan in a phase III study.[199,200] Similar response rates (19.7% vs 17.0%) and overall survival times (60 weeks vs 57 weeks) were observed for the entire group of patients with recurrent disease.[199] PLD was more active than topotecan in the subset of women with platinum-sensitive disease, producing improved progression-free survival (29 weeks vs 23 weeks, $p = .037$) and overall survival (108 vs 71 weeks, $p = .008$).[200] Selection of the appropriate agent for an individual patient is based on prior toxicity, expected toxicities of the second-line agent, patient preference for intravenous versus oral administration, and quality of life considerations. It appears the older second-line agents, such as ifosfamide and hexamethylmelamine, have less clinical activity than do newer agents in patients whose tumors have become resistant to paclitaxel and platinum-based chemotherapy. Traditionally, second line agents have been used individually and sequentially, but two recent studies suggest that a combination of cisplatin and gemcitabine may exert synergistic effects, producing response rates of 38% and 70% with responses that have been maintained for 3–5 months.[201,202]

High-Dose Chemotherapy and Stem Cell Transplantation The use of high-dose chemotherapy and either autologous bone marrow transplantation (ABMT) or peripheral stem cell support is being tested in patients with advanced ovarian cancer.[203,204] In one trial of high-dose mitoxantrone, carboplatin, and cyclophosphamide with stem cell support, 89% of patients responded with clinical complete responses in 88% of platinum-sensitive and 47% of platinum-resistant cases.[203] Median progression free survival was 10.1 months for platinum sensitive disease and 5.1 months for platinum resistant disease. In another retrospective analysis of 35 patients treated with high-dose melphalan and stem cell support, 9 of 12 patients with evaluable residual disease had a measurable response. The morbidity of this approach is high, and the survival after this approach in a phase II trial has been similar to the survival following second-line paclitaxel. Transplantation earlier in the course of disease may have a greater impact. One recent study of 96 patients, many of whom were in clinical CR (43%) or PR (34%), produced 6-year survival of 37%. For patients who received transplantation for remission consolidation, the 6-year survival was 53% and the progression free survival was 29%.[204]

Immunotherapy The use of intravenous or subcutaneous immunostimulants in addition to chemotherapy has not improved the response rate or survival of ovarian cancer patients. Based on the response seen with regional nonspecific immunotherapy, several trials of intraperitoneal cytokines have been performed.[205–218] In a phase II trial conducted by the GOG, there was a 28% surgically-documented response rate in 25 patients with platinum-sensitive minimal residual tumors.[209] Overall, 53 surgically evaluated patients have been treated in three trials, with 40% responses and 25% complete responses.[207–209] All of the responding patients had microscopic or small macroscopic residual disease. Thus, the use of high-dose IP recombinant IFN-a given frequently can result in the regional control of very small-volume disease confined to the peritoneal cavity. Whether survival is affected is not known. Other cytokines have been evaluated. A phase I-II trial of intraperitoneal interferon-γ also yielded a 30% response rate.[210] Another phase I trial with intraperitoneal IL-2 has been performed, and the optimal dose was defined.[211,217]

Preclinical studies have examined the interaction of cytokines, such as IFN-α, tumor necrosis factor, and IL-2, with various cytotoxic agents, including cisplatin and doxorubicin.[212,213,217] In a phase II study of IFN-alpha alternating with cisplatin in patients with platinum-sensitive minimal residual disease, the surgically-documented response rate was 28%.[216] In a randomized phase III trial, Windbichler and colleagues have demonstrated that the use of subcutaneous interferon-γ in women receiving first-line platinum-based chemotherapy in ovarian cancer was well-tolerated.[216] A higher complete clinical response rate (68% vs 56%) and longer disease progression-free survival (48 months vs 17 months, $p = .031$) were observed in women receiving the interferon-γ plus chemotherapy than in women who were treated with chemotherapy alone. Improved progression-free survival was seen in patients with residual disease greater than 2 cm, as well as in those with optimal resection.

Monoclonal antibodies raised against antigens on the surface of the epithelial ovarian cells have been used in clinical trials. In a phase II trial of intraperitoneal ^{90}Y-labeled anti-HMFG monoclonal antibody reactive with MUC-1 human milk fat globulin protein (HMFG).[184,219] the i.p. administration of radionuclide conjugate significantly prolonged survival relative to historical controls.[219] However, in a multicenter randomized controlled study comparing IP treatment with ^{90}Y-labeled antibodies to no additional therapy in patients without evidence of disease following second-look laparoscopy, no difference in survival was noted.[184] Trastuzumab (Herceptin) has been studied in a phase II trial by the GOG in ovarian cancers that overexpress *HER-2*. Only 11% of ovarian cancers overexpressed *HER-2* and the response rate was only 4%.[220] Thus, trastuzumab alone is not likely to be useful in ovarian cancer patients. As noted above, there is experience with OvaRex, the anti-CA 125 monoclonal antibody in the setting of consolidation; however, there are no data regarding its potential usefulness in relapsed patients.[185,221] Given the importance of VEGF/VPF in angiogenesis and the production of ascites, anti-VEGF antibodies have been evaluated in preclinical xenograft models and found to be active. A phase II trial of bevacizumab (Avastin) has been completed in recurrent ovarian cancer. In the 40 patients entered on the trial, several responses were noted.[222] Based on these data, a randomized trial of primary therapy in suboptimally debulked ovarian cancer is being undertaken by the GOG. The patients will receive carboplatin and paclitaxel chemotherapy with or without bevacizumab, and a third arm will include a 6-month maintenance therapy with bevacizumab.

Hormonal Therapy Epithelial ovarian tumors frequently contain elevated levels of estrogen and androgen receptors. Some patients with epithelial ovarian tumors have had responses to endocrine therapy, although it appears that the overall response rate is approximately 10 to 20%. Progestational agents and estrogen antagonists, such as tamoxifen, have been used either alone or in combination with cytotoxic chemotherapy in patients with advanced disease, and other studies have used gonadotropin agonists, for example, leuprolide acetate alone or with tamoxifen, or aromatase inhibitors.[223–226] In a study patients with advanced epithelial ovarian cancer were treated with tamoxifen and a 13% partial response rate was reported, but disease progression was delayed in 30%.[225] There is a lack of correlative studies comparing the response to endocrine manipulations and the presence of hormone receptors. Hormonal therapy for patients with advanced ovarian cancer should primarily be reserved for those who have failed chemotherapeutic regimens and who are not candidates for aggressive salvage drug regimens or investigative approaches. These agents are well tolerated and in circumstances where quality of life issues are paramount, such therapies can be employed.

Palliative Radiotherapy in Ovarian Cancer Radiotherapy as a palliative modality in ovarian cancer may be very useful if the sole dominant symptomatic problem for the patient is localized to a site and volume that may be safely encompassed in a limited radiation field. For example, a fixed pelvic mass eroding the vaginal mucosa causing bleeding, pain, or bowel or bladder dysfunction may occur without obvious disseminated symptomatic peritoneal disease. Localized masses in the retroperitoneal nodes or in extra abdominal sites such as the supraclavicular or inguinal node regions or bony or brain metastases may benefit from palliative irradiation as would painful hepatomegaly from hepatic capsular distention.

An objective and subjective response rate of patients treated with radiation for recurrent ovarian cancer after resistance to available chemotherapeutic agents has been reported. A study from Memorial Sloan-Kettering Cancer Center documented subjective or objective responses in 70% of patients who had platinum-refractory disease who had not previously received paclitaxel.[227] While the optimal dose for palliation has not been established, it is clear that durable palliation may be achieved with local radiotherapy for ovarian cancer recurring after chemotherapy even in the presence of chemoresistant disease. Palliative whole brain irradiation is indicated for documented cerebral metastases in those whose life expectancy is several weeks to months.

Survival of Patients with Advanced Ovarian Cancer Cisplatin-based combination chemotherapy regimens have clearly produced higher response rates, complete remission rates, and an improvement in the median survival of patients with advanced ovarian cancer. The impact on long-term survival has been modest, and the majority of patients with advanced ovarian cancer still die of their disease. Five-year survival rates for patients treated with cisplatin-based regimens for advanced disease are approximately 20 to 25%.[228–232] Although this is a substantial improvement over the 5 to 10% survival rate reported for patients with advanced disease in the pre-platinum era, it is obvious that ovarian cancer still remains a formidable challenge and that new treatment approaches are needed.

The prognosis for patients with epithelial ovarian cancer is related to several clinical variables. Survival analyses based on the most commonly used prognostic variables are presented below. Including patients at all stages, patients less than 50 years of age have a 5-year survival rate of about 40%, compared with about 15% for patients older than 50 years.[35,36,232]

The 5-year survival rate for carefully and properly staged patients with stage I disease is 76 to 93%, depending on the tumor grade.[36,125,126] The 5-year survival for stage II is 60 to 74%.[36] The 5-year survival rate for stage IIIa is 41%, for stage IIIB about 25%, for stage IIIC 23% and for stage IV disease 11%.[36] An analysis of the National Cancer Institute's Surveillance, Epidemiology and End Results (SEER) database reveals a trend toward improved survival for ovarian cancer in the United States during the last period of analysis (1988–1994). In this cohort, the survival for stage I was 93%, for stage II 70%, for stage III 37% and for stage IV 25%.[232] Compared with the interval 1983 to 1987, there was a statistically significant improvement in survival for stages I, III and IV disease.

Survival of patients with borderline tumors is excellent, with stage I lesions having a 98% 15-year survival.[36] When all stages of borderline tumors are included, the 5-year survival rate is about 86 to 90%.

For invasive cancers grade affects the prognosis. For invasive stage I disease, the 5-year survival rate for grade 1 epithelial ovarian cancers is about 91%, compared with about 74% for grade 2 and 75% for grade 3.[53] For stage II disease, the survivals are 69%, 60% and 51%, respectively, for grades 1, 2, and 3. Examining stage III–IV patients, the 5-year survivals for grades 1, 2, and 3, respectively, are 38%, 25%, and 19%. Patients with stage III disease with microscopic residual disease at the start of treatment have a 5-year survival rate of about 40 to 75%, compared with about 30 to 40% for those with optimal disease and only 5% for those with non-optimal disease.[138] Patients whose Karnofsky index (KI) is low (< 70) have a significantly shorter survival than those with a KI > 70.[233]

NONEPITHELIAL OVARIAN CANCER

Nonepithelial cancers of the ovary are uncommon. They include malignancies of germ cell origin, sex cord–stromal cell origin, metastatic carcinomas to the ovary, and a variety of extremely rare ovarian cancers, such as sarcomas and lipoid cell tumors (Figure 104-7). Nonepithelial malignancies account for about 10% of all ovarian cancers.[2,3] Although there are many similarities in the presentation, evaluation, and management of these patients, there are also many unique qualities of these tumors that require a special approach. This is particularly true because many more nonepithelial lesions are germ cell in origin, and they are usually found in young patients.

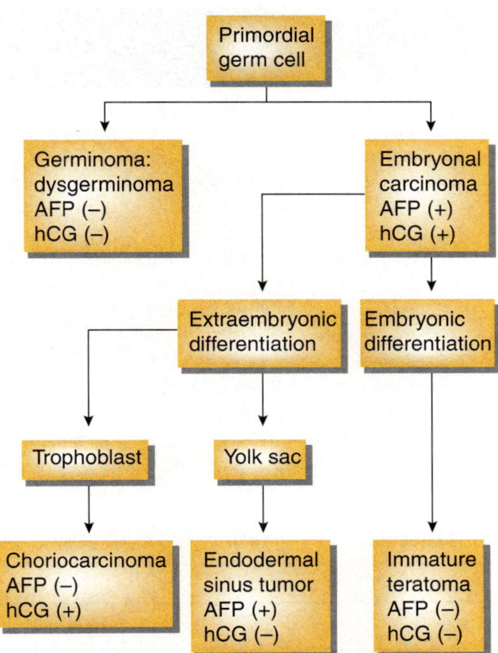

Figure 104-7 Relationship between examples of pure malignant germ cell tumors and their secreted substances. AFP = α-fetoprotein; HCG = human chorionic gonadotropin. Reprinted with permission from Berek JS, Hacker NF. Nonepithelial ovarian cancer. In: Berek JS, Hacker NF, editors. Practical gynecologic oncology. 4th ed. Baltimore, MD: Williams & Wilkins; 2005. p. 513.

GERM CELL MALIGNANCIES

Germ cell tumors are derived from the primordial germ cells of the ovary. Whereas malignant germ cell tumors can arise in extragonadal sites, such as the mediastinum and the retroperitoneum, the majority of germ cell tumors arise in the gonad from the undifferentiated germ cells. The variation in the sites of these cancers is explained by the embryonic migration of the germ cells from the caudal part of the yolk sac to the dorsal mesentery, prior to their incorporation into the sex cords of the developing gonads.[234]

Classification A histologic classification of ovarian germ cell tumors is presented in Table 104-8.[234–236] Alpha-fetoprotein (AFP) and human chorionic gonadotropin (HCG) are both secreted by some germ cell malignancies and, therefore, the presence of circulating hormones can be clinically useful in the diagnosis of a pelvic mass and in monitoring the course of a patient after surgery. Alpha-1-antitrypsin (AAT) can be detected rarely in association with germ cell tumors. By correlating the histologic and immunohistologic identification of these substances in tumors, a classification of germ cell tumors can be made. In this classification, embryonal carcinoma, which is composed of undifferentiated cells, synthesizes both HCG and AFP, and this tumor is the progenitor of several other germ cell malignancies. More

Table 104-8 Histologic Typing of Ovarian Germ Cell Tumors

I. Dysgerminoma
II. Teratoma
  A. Immature
  B. Mature
    1. solid
    2. cystic
      a. dermoid cyst (mature cystic teratoma)
      b. dermoid cyst with malignant transformation
  C. Monodermal and highly specialized
    1. struma ovarii
    2. carcinoid
    3. struma ovarii and carcinoid
    4. others
III. Endodermal sinus tumor
IV. Embryonal carcinoma
V. Polyembryoma
VI. Choriocarcinoma
VII. Mixed forms

Adapted from Scully RE, et al.[2]

differentiated germ cell tumors, such as the endodermal sinus tumor, which secretes AFP, and the choriocarcinoma, which secretes HCG, are derived from the extra-embryonic tissues, whereas the immature teratomas are derived from the embryonic cells that have lost the ability to secrete these substances.[2] Pure germinomas do not secrete these markers.

Epidemiology Although 20 to 25% of all benign and malignant ovarian neoplasms are of germ cell origin, only about 3% of these tumors are malignant.[2] Germ cell malignancies account for less than 5% of all ovarian cancers in Western countries but they represent up to 15% of ovarian cancers in Asian and black societies, where epithelial ovarian cancers are much less common.[5]

In the first 2 decades of life, almost 70% of ovarian tumors are of germ cell origin, and one-third of these are malignant.[2] Germ cell tumors account for two-thirds of the ovarian malignancies in this age group. Germ cell cancers also are seen in the third decade, but thereafter become quite rare.

Clinical Features The most common symptoms in young patients with a germ cell tumor of the ovary are a pelvic fullness, urinary frequency, and dysuria. Rectal pressure, menstrual irregularities in postmenarchal patients, and lower abdominal pain or pressure may be present. Some young patients may misinterpret the early symptoms of a neoplasm as those of pregnancy, and this can lead to a further delay in the diagnosis of the cancer. Acute symptoms associated with the torsion or rupture of the adnexa can develop. These symptoms may be confused with acute appendicitis. In more advanced cases, ascites may develop and the patient can present with extensive abdominal distention.[2,236]

In patients with a palpable adnexal mass, the evaluation should proceed expeditiously. Some patients with germ cell tumors will be premenarchal and may require examination under anesthesia. If the lesions are principally solid or a combination of solid and cystic, as might be noted on an ultrasonographic evaluation, a neoplasm is probable and a malignancy is possible. The rest of the physical examination should search for signs of ascites, pleural effusion, and organomegaly.[235]

Diagnosis When an adnexal mass is 2 cm or larger in a premenarchal female, or 8 cm or larger in other premenopausal females, surgical exploration is frequently required. In young patients, blood tests should include serum HCG and AFP levels, a complete blood count, and liver function tests. A chest radiograph should be performed because germ cell tumors can metastasize to the lung or mediastinum. A karyotype should be obtained preoperatively on all premenarchal females, because of the propensity for these tumors to arise in dysgenetic gonads.[237] A preoperative CT scan may document the presence and extent of retroperitoneal lymphadenopathy or liver metastases, but because these patients require surgical exploration, a more extensive and time-consuming preoperative evaluation is unnecessary. If postmenarchal patients have predominantly cystic lesions up to 8 cm in diameter, they may undergo a trial of hormonal suppression for two menstrual cycles.

Dysgerminomas Dysgerminomas are the most common malignant germ cell tumors, accounting for about 30 to 40% of all ovarian cancers of germ cell origin.[2,236–238] The tumor represents only 1 to 3% of all ovarian cancers, but as much as 5 to 10% of ovarian cancer in patients younger than 20 years of age. Seventy-five percent of dysgerminomas occur between the ages of 10 and 30 years, 5% under the age of 10 years, and rarely over the age of 50 years.[2,236] Because these malignancies occur in young women, 20 to 30% of ovarian malignancies associated with pregnancy are dysgerminomas.

Much has been, and continues to be learned about the management of dysgerminoma by analogy with its male counterpart, testicular seminoma (Figure 104-8).[235] The dominant route of spread in both is nodal, via the gonadal lymphatics to the renal hilar and para-aortic nodes. Both are exquisitely radiosensitive and curable with modest doses of radiotherapy, 2,500 to 3,500 cGy, even when bulk disease up to 5 cm is being treated. For this reason, excellent long-term survival rates are obtained when surgical removal, using oophorectomy or hysterectomy/bilateral salpingo-oophorectomy, is followed by radiotherapy to para-aortic and pelvic nodes.[235,238]

About 75% of dysgerminomas are stage I at diagnosis that is, confined to one or both ovaries. About 85 to 90% of stage I tumors are confined to one ovary; 10 to 15% are bilateral. In fact, dysgerminoma is the only germ cell malignancy that has this significant rate of bilaterality, other germ cell tumors rarely being bilateral.

Dysgerminomas affect younger women (85% are under 29 years of age) and are present in two-thirds of cases as stage IA. Dysgenetic gonads tend to develop dysgerminoma.[236,238] Therapeutic concepts have changed dramatically over the past few years, largely because of (1) the recogni-

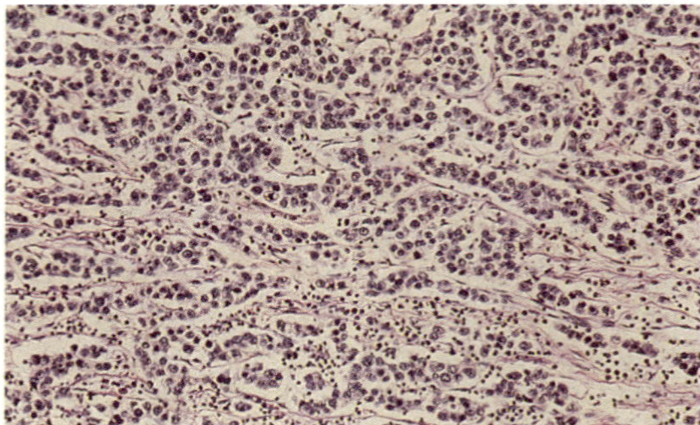
Figure 104-8 Dysgerminoma.

tion of dysgerminomas' chemosensitivity, allowing cure without ovarian ablation by surgery or radiotherapy in many cases; (2) the advent of improved techniques of imaging the retroperitoneum, with lymphography, and CT and MRI scanning that allow detection of disease under 3 to 5 cm in diameter when it is eminently curable; (3) tumor markers, AFP and the beta subunit of human chorionic gonadotrophin (beta-HCG), which distinguish pure dysgerminoma from the mixed germ-cell tumors; and (4) the emerging emphasis in treatment on preservation of childbearing capacity, presumably without compromising cure.

Many aspects of management are controversial, such as the need for complete surgical staging; the extent of the primary operative procedure in unilateral, bilateral, and metastatic disease; the role of postoperative observation in stage IA; the choice between radiotherapy and chemotherapy; the decision as to which chemotherapy drugs should be used; and the need for a second-look operation. The subject was recently reviewed in greater depth than is possible here.

In the 25% of patients who present with metastatic disease, the tumor most commonly spreads via the lymphatics.[2] It also can spread hematogenously, or by direct extension through the capsule of the ovary, with exfoliation and dissemination of cells over the peritoneal surfaces. Metastases to the contralateral ovary occur and may be present when there is no other evidence of spread. An uncommon site of metastatic disease is bone, and when it does occur here, the lesions are seen principally in the lower vertebrae. Metastases to the lungs, liver, and brain are seen most often in patients whose disease is longstanding or recurrent. Metastatic disease to the mediastinum and supraclavicular lymph nodes is usually a late manifestation of disease.

Dysgenetic Gonads Approximately 5% of dysgerminomas are discovered in phenotypic females with abnormal gonads.[2,236] This malignancy can be associated with patients who have pure gonadal dysgenesis (46XY, bilateral streak gonads), mixed gonadal dysgenesis (45X/46XY, unilateral streak gonad, contralateral testis), or the androgen insensitivity syndrome (46XY, testicular feminization). Therefore, premenarchal patients with a pelvic mass should have their karyotype determined. In most patients with gonadal dysgenesis, dysgerminomas arise in gonadoblastomas, which are benign ovarian tumors that are composed of germ cells and sex cord–stroma. If gonadoblastomas are left in place in patients with gonadal dysgenesis, more than 50% will develop into ovarian malignancies.[237] Also, dysgerminomas that contain significant numbers of syncytiotrophoblastic cells can be hormonally active, producing isosexual precocious pseudopuberty in premenarchal females and menstrual irregularities in older women.[234,236,237]

Surgery The treatment of patients with dysgerminoma is primarily surgical, including the resection of the primary lesion and proper surgical staging. If necessary, radiation or chemotherapy is administered to selected patients. Because the disease principally affects young females, special consideration must be given to the preservation of fertility whenever possible.[2,236]

Ideally, the initial operation should include exploration of the abdominal contents, with careful palpation of the retroperitoneal node-bearing areas, sampling of enlarged nodes, and cytologic examination of peritoneal washings. If these steps were omitted in what was apparently stage I disease, the need for reexploration for restaging purposes is questionable, simply because noninvasive imaging techniques are capable of detecting disease of less than 5 cm, which is highly curable, unlike the cystadenocarcinomas. For the same reason, biopsy of nonpalpable lymph nodes is probably unnecessary. A benefit of cytoreductive surgery has not been shown in this disease.

The minimum operation for ovarian dysgerminoma is a unilateral oophorectomy or salpingo-oophorectomy.[236] If there is a desire to preserve fertility, the contralateral ovary, fallopian tube, and uterus should be conserved. This is probably true even in the presence of metastatic disease, because of the sensitivity of the tumor to chemotherapy. In patients whose fertility need not be preserved, it is appropriate to perform a total abdominal hysterectomy and bilateral salpingo-oophorectomy. In patients whose karyotype analysis reveals a Y chromosome, both ovaries should be removed, although the uterus might be conserved for possible future embryo transfer.[237] Dysgerminoma is the only germ cell tumor that tends to be bilateral, and not all of the bilateral lesions have obvious ovarian enlargement. Therefore, excisional biopsy of any suspicious lesion is desirable.[238]

Postoperative workup should include the serum markers AFP and β-HCG, a chest radiograph, and an abdominopelvic CT or MRI scan. In premenarchal females with an ovarian mass, preoperative karyotyping should be performed, as detection of a Y chromosome is an indication for bilateral oophorectomy, as discussed below. Even with a histologic diagnosis of pure dysgerminoma, the presence of an elevated AFP value or a markedly elevated β-HCG level (over approximately 100 IU/L), indicates the presence of nondysgerminomatous elements, and is reason enough to base treatment on these more aggressive elements. As with seminoma, lower β-HCG levels are sometimes found in the pure form of the disease, produced by syncytial-like giant interstitial cells. Lymphography can be useful, both in detecting nodal involvement and in localizing the nodal chains for radiation treatment.

Management of Stage IA The extent of the initial extirpative surgery can be quite conservative. Long-term survival results in concurrent series reported for a policy of unilateral salpingo-oophorectomy with subsequent treatment withheld until relapse (91% in 145 cases) are not inferior to results of hysterectomy, bilateral adnexectomy, and routine postoperative radiotherapy (85% in 53 cases).[236,238] This is so because, in these older series, two-thirds of relapses were salvaged by reexcision or radiotherapy. Better results would be expected today: because marker studies would show that some of the patients included did not have pure dysgerminoma from the outset; because relapse would be detected earlier by modern imaging techniques, when tumor bulk was lower; and because chemotherapy and megavoltage radiotherapy would be expected to salvage nearly all first relapses. However, a conservative approach requires frequent patient monitoring: clinical and tumor marker checks every 2 months, and CT scans every 3 months in the first 2 to 3 years. In patients whose contralateral ovary has been preserved, disease can develop in 5 to 15% of the retained gonads over the next 2 years.[236] This figure includes those not treated with additional therapy, as well as patients with gonadal dysgenesis.

The reasons for a conservative initial approach are (1) to avoid ablative surgery and radiotherapy in the majority of cases (probably 80 to 85% of properly evaluated stage IA patients are cured by oophorectomy), and (2) to preserve fertility. Because the morbidity of low-dose radiotherapy is small, and the dollar cost of close surveillance of conservatively managed patients is appreciable, the strongest justification for conservatism is the desire to preserve fertility. This requires a highly compliant patient and a knowledgeable, attentive physician.

Management of Relapsed Stage I The choice of salvage therapy depends on the site and size of the relapse when it is detected, and the desire to maintain fertility. In general, treatment of relapse need not imply loss of fertility if chemotherapy or pelvis-sparing radiotherapy is used.

There is argument as to whether a tumor size over 10 cm at diagnosis is a contraindication to conservative therapy, since a higher relapse rate is associated with larger tumors.[339] The literature does not resolve this issue, but in the opinion of the authors a large tumor size per se does not preclude a conservative approach.

Stages IB, II, III, and IV About 6% of patients present with bilateral ovarian involvement, and a similar number of stage IA patients experience recurrence in the opposite ovary. In general, bilateral oophorectomy is advised for stage IB, possibly with uterus conservation for future embryo transfer. The choice of postoperative therapy in stage IB–III is as described above for disease that recurs after primary management of stage IA. When radiation is used, the portals should include the pelvic nodes on the affected side(s) and the renal hilar and para-aortic nodes up to the diaphragm. Because a small fraction (10 to 20%) of abdominal spread is transperitoneal, abdominopelvic radiotherapy can also be used as in the epithelial tumors. Prophylactic mediastinal/supraclavicular irradiation is not advised, since its value is questionable, and it may compromise subsequent chemotherapy because of marrow ablation.

The most frequently used chemotherapeutic regimens for germ cell tumors are BEP (bleomycin, etoposide, and cisplatin), VBP (vinblastine, bleomycin, and cisplatin), and VAC (vincristine, actinomycin, and Cytoxan) (Table 104-9).[239–248] Encouraging results (long-term disease-free status over 90% in previously untreated patients, and in about 70% of recurrent cases) have been reported in a number of series using cisplatin, vinblastine, bleomycin (PVB), VAC, or variants.

Unlike the nondysgermanomatous ovarian germ-cell tumors, whose chemoresponsiveness is not as great as for the nonseminomatous testicular tumors, dysgerminoma may be even more chemosensitive than the testicular tumors. For example, one report cites a sustained complete response in 7 of 10 patients with residual disease

Table 104-9 Combination Chemotherapy for Germ Cell Tumors of the Ovary

Regimens and Drugs	Dosage and Schedule[a]
BEP	
Bleomycin	15 U/m²/wk × 5; then on day 1 of course 4
Etoposide	100 mg/m²/d × 5 days every 3 wk
Cisplatin	20 mg/m²/d × 5 days, or 100 mg/m²/d × 1 day every 3 wk
VBP	
Vinblastine	0.15 mg/kg/days 1 and 2 every 3 wk
Bleomycin	15 U/m²/wk × 5; then on day 1 of course 4
Cisplatin	100 mg/m² on day 1 every 3 wk
VAC	
Vincristine	1–1.5 mg/m² on day 1 every 4 wk, not to exceed 2 mg total dose
Actinomycin D	0.5 mg × 5 days every 4 weeks
Cytoxan	150 mg/m²/d × 5 days every 4 weeks

[a]All doses given intravenously.

Table 104-10 POMB/ACE Chemotherapy for Germ Cell Tumors of the Ovary

POMB	
Day 1	Vincristine 1 mg/m^2 IV; methotrexate 300 mg/m^2 as a 12-h infusion
Day 2	Bleomycin 15 mg by 24-h infusion, folinic acid rescue started 24 h after the start of methotrexate in a dose of 15 mg every 12 h for 4 doses
Day 3	Bleomycin 15 mg by 24-h infusion
Day 4	Cisplatin 120 mg/m^2 as a 12-h infusion, given together with hydration and 3 mg magnesium sulfate supplementation
ACE	
Days 1–5	Etoposide (VP16) 100 mg/m^2, days 1 to 5
Days 3–5	Actinomycin D 0.5 mg IV, days 3, 4, and 5
Day 5	Cyclophosphamide 500 mg/m^2 IV, day 5
OMB	
Day 1	Vincristine 1 mg/m^2 IV; methotrexate 300 mg/m^2 as a 12-h infusion
Day 2	Bleomycin 15 mg by 24-h infusion; folinic acid rescue started at 24 h
Day 3	Bleomycin 15 mg by 24-h infusion

The sequence of treatment schedules is two courses of POMB followed by ACE. POMB is then alternated with ACE until patients are in biochemical remission as measured by hCG and AFP, PLAP and LDH. The usual number of courses of POMB is three to five. Following biochemical remission, patients alternate ACE with OMB until remission has been maintained for approximately 12 weeks. The interval between courses of treatment is kept to the minimum (usually 9 to 11 days). If delays are caused by myelosuppression after courses of ACE, the first 2 days of etoposide are omitted from subsequent courses of ACE.

treated with a doxorubicin/cyclophosphamide (AC) combination (two of the three relapses were salvaged with PVB).[244] The same report describes an additional eight patients treated with PVB; all eight are alive without disease, although one patient whose disease relapsed in the brain was salvaged by radiotherapy. Of some note is that four patients had residual ovarian or uterine disease; all are disease-free, and one, treated with AC, has subsequently borne a child.

There have been numerous reports of successful control of metastatic dysgerminomas with systemic chemotherapy, and this should now be regarded as the treatment of choice.[242–248] The obvious advantage is the preservation of fertility.[239]The most frequently used chemotherapeutic regimens for germ cell tumors are BEP, VBP, and VAC. The Gynecologic Oncology Group (GOG) studied 3 cycles of (EC) etoposide (120 mg/M^2 intravenously on days 1, 2, and 3 every 4 weeks) carboplatin (400 mg/M^2 intravenously on day 1 every 4 weeks) for patients with completely resected ovarian dysgerminoma, stages IB, IC, II, or III.[246] The results showed a sustained disease-free remission rate of 100%.

For patients with advanced, incompletely resected germ cell tumors, the GOG studied cisplatin-based chemotherapy on two consecutive protocols.[245,246] In the first study, patients received 4 cycles of vinblastine, bleomycin, and cisplatin. Patients with persistent or progressive disease at second-look laparotomy were treated with 6 cycles of VAC. In the second trial, patients received 3 cycles of BEP initially, followed by consolidation with VAC, which was later discontinued in patients with dysgerminomas. The VAC consolidation after BEP in patients with tumors other than dysgerminoma is still being investigated, but VAC does not appear to improve the outcome of the BEP regimen. A total of 20 evaluable patients with stage III and IV dysgerminoma were treated in these two protocols, and 19 are alive and free of disease after 6 to 68 months (median 26 months). Fourteen of these patients had a second-look laparotomy, and all findings were negative. Another study at M.D. Anderson Hospital used BEP in 14 patients with residual disease, and all patients were free of disease with long-term follow-up.[244] These results suggest that patients with advanced-stage, incompletely resected dysgerminoma have an excellent prognosis when treated with cisplatin based combination chemotherapy. The best regimen is 4 cycles of BEP, based on the data from testes cancers.[249,250]

Recurrent Disease About 75% of recurrences occur within the first year after initial treatment, the most common sites being the peritoneal cavity and the retroperitoneal lymph nodes.[2,236] These patients should be treated with either radiation or chemotherapy, depending on their primary treatment. Patients with recurrent disease who have had no therapy other than surgery should be treated with chemotherapy. If prior chemotherapy with BEP has been given, POMB-ACE may be used (Table 104-10), and consideration should be given to the use of high-dose chemotherapy (eg, with carboplatin and etoposide) and autologous bone marrow transplantation. Alternatively, radiation therapy is effective for this disease, with the major disadvantage being loss of fertility if pelvic and abdominal radiation is required.

These results suggest that patients with advanced-stage, incompletely resected dysgerminoma have an excellent prognosis when treated with cisplatin-based combination chemotherapy. The optimal regimen is unknown, but three to four cycles of BEP seem sufficient.[251–256]

Our recommendations, like the regimens themselves, are based on the literature regarding testicular cancer. In brief, the testicular cancer experience has shown that PVB is more effective than VAC, and that the substitution of etoposide for vinblastine in PVB (ie, BEP) improves the therapeutic ratio by reducing toxicity and improving response rates.[255] It has been demonstrated that dysgerminomas are very sensitive to platinum-based chemotherapy. Williams and colleagues reported treatment of patients with advanced dysgerminomas using platinum-based chemotherapy.[256] At an overall follow-up of 9 to 96 months (median 26 months), 17 of 18 patients with advanced dysgerminoma were disease-free. These excellent results in patients with advanced disease have implications for the treatment of patients with early-stage dysgerminoma.

Second-Look Laparotomy There appears to be no need to perform a second-look laparotomy in patients with dysgerminoma whose macroscopic disease was all resected at the primary operation.[255] In patients with macroscopic residual disease at the start of chemotherapy, we prefer to perform a second-look operation because second-line therapy is available and the earlier persistent disease is identified, the better the prognosis should be.

Coexistent with Pregnancy Because dysgerminomas tend to occur in young patients, they may coexist with pregnancy. When a stage IA cancer is found, the tumor can be removed intact and the pregnancy continued. In patients with more advanced disease, continuation of the pregnancy will depend on gestational age, but chemotherapy can be given in the second half of pregnancy in the same dosages as given for the nonpregnant patient.[239]

Prognosis In patients whose initial disease is stage IA (ie, a unilateral encapsulated dysgerminoma), the conservative approach outlined above results in 5-year disease-free survivals of greater than 95%. The 5-year survival for patients with all stages of dysgerminoma is 85%.[252–256] The features that have been associated with a higher tendency to recur include lesions larger than 10 to 15 cm in diameter, age younger than 20 years, and microscopic characteristics that include numerous mitoses, anaplasia, and a medullary pattern.[2,256]

With current staging methods, the proportion of relapsing patients should be no more than 15 to 20%.[244] The theoretic cure rate of this group is 98%. Although in the past, surgery for advanced disease followed by pelvic and abdominal radiation produced a 5-year survival of 63 to 83%, cure rates of 85 to 90% for this same group of patients are being seen now with combination chemotherapy.[244,252]

Many patients with a dysgerminoma will have a tumor that is apparently confined to one ovary and will be referred after unilateral salpingo-oophorectomy without surgical staging.[252] The options for such patients are repeat laparotomy for surgical staging, regular pelvic and abdominal surveillance with CT scans, and adjuvant chemotherapy. As these are rapidly growing tumors, our preference is to perform regular CT surveillance. Tumor markers (AFP and βHCG) should also be monitored in case occult mixed germ cell elements are present.

Immature Teratomas Immature teratomas contain elements resembling tissues derived from the embryo. Immature teratomatous elements may occur in combination with other germ cell tumors as mixed germ cell tumors. The pure immature teratoma accounts for less than 1% of all ovarian cancers, but it is the second most common germ cell malignancy. This lesion represents 10 to 20% of all ovarian malignancies seen in females under 20 years of age and 30% of the deaths from ovarian cancer in this age group.[2,236] About 50% of pure immature teratomas of the ovary occur between the ages of 10 and 20 years, and they rarely are seen in postmenopausal women. Immature teratomas are classified according to a grading system (grades 1 to 3) that is based on the degree of differentiation and the quantity of immature tissue.[2,236,257–260]

The preoperative evaluation and differential diagnosis are the same as for patients with other germ cell tumors. Some of these lesions will contain calcifications similar to mature teratomas, and these can be detected by a radiograph of the abdomen or by ultrasonography. Rarely, they are associated with the production of steroid hormones and can present with sexual pseudoprecosity.[256] Patients may present with abnormal bleeding, but most frequently the symptoms and signs are nonspecific, usually those of a pelvic mass with or without pelvic pressure or pain. The lesions may be growing rapidly, and thus the symptoms and signs often have a subacute onset. Tumor markers are negative unless a mixed germ cell tumor is present.

Surgery As with the dysgerminoma in a young patient whose lesion appears confined to a single ovary, a unilateral oophorectomy or salpingo-oophorectomy and surgical staging should be performed. In older patients who do not desire preservation of fertility, a total abdominal hysterectomy and bilateral salpingo-oophorectomy should be carried out. Contralateral involvement is rare, and in patients whose contralateral ovary reveals no evidence of gross involvement, routine resection or wedge biopsy is unnecessary.[236] Any lesions on the peritoneal surfaces should be sampled carefully and submitted for histologic evaluation. The most frequent site of dissemination is the peritoneum and, much less commonly, the retroperitoneal lymph nodes. Blood-borne metastases to organ parenchyma, such as the lungs, liver, or brain, are uncommon. When present, they are usually seen in patients with late or recurrent disease, and most often in tumors that are poorly differentiated.

Chemotherapy The results of therapy for patients with germ cell tumors other than dysgerminomas (eg, immature teratomas and endodermal sinus tumors of the ovary) have improved with cisplatin-based chemotherapy. The primary prognostic factor in patients with immature teratoma is the tumor grade. In patients whose tumors are stage IA, grades 2 and 3, chemotherapy should be used.[258,259] There is no evidence that chemotherapy will improve the outcome of patients with stage IA, grade 1 lesions. In patients who have ascites and ruptured tumors, chemotherapy is indicated, regardless of tumor grade. While patients with stage I, grade 1 immature teratoma rarely suffer a relapse, most patients with grades 2 and 3 tumors will not be cured by surgery alone. Similarly, most patients with endodermal sinus tumors will not be cured by surgery alone, as discussed below. Adjuvant chemotherapy is recommended for all patients other than those with stage I, grade 1 immature teratomas. Although nonplatinum-based chemotherapy regimens, such as vincristine, actinomycin, and cyclophosphamide (VAC)[261] have been somewhat successful when administered in the adjuvant situation, they have been replaced by platinum-based regimens.[261] Standard therapy in this situation is now the BEP regimen. In the most recent GOG trial, 50 of 52 stage I, stage II, and stage III patients with completely resected tumor remain disease-free after three courses of BEP.[246]

Patients with stage IA, grade 1 tumors have an excellent prognosis, and no adjuvant therapy is required. In patients whose tumors are stage IA, grade 2 or 3, adjuvant chemotherapy should be used.[261–263] Chemotherapy is also indicated in patients who have ascites, regardless of tumor grade. The most frequently used combination chemotherapeutic regimen has been VAC. However, in a GOG study, the relapse-free survival rate in patients with incompletely resected disease was 75%.[241] The newer approach has been to incorporate cisplatin into the primary treatment of these tumors, and most of the experience has been with the VBP and BEP regimens.[261–263] No direct comparison of these regimens with VAC has been reported, but the BEP combination can save some patients who have persistent or recurrent disease after VAC.

The GOG has been prospectively studying three courses of BEP therapy in patients with completely resected stage I, II, and III ovarian germ cell tumors.[255] Overall, the toxicity has been acceptable, and 91 of 93 patients with nondysgerminomatous tumors treated are clinically free of disease. Thus the BEP regimen, which is used more extensively for testicular cancer, appears to be superior to the VAC regimen in the treatment of completely resected nondysgerminomatous germ cell tumors of the ovary. Because some patients can progress rapidly, treatment should be initiated as soon as possible after surgery, preferably within 7 to 10 days.

The switch from VBP to BEP has been prompted by the experience in patients with testicular cancer, where the replacement of vinblastine with etoposide has been associated with a better therapeutic index (ie, equivalent efficacy and lower morbidity), especially less neurologic and gastrointestinal toxicity. Furthermore, the use of bleomycin appears to be important in this group of patients. In a randomized study of three cycles of etoposide plus cisplatin with or without bleomycin (EP versus BEP) in 166 patients with germ cell tumors of the testes, the BEP regimen had a relapse-free survival rate of 84% compared with 69% for the EP regimen ($p = .03$).[250] In addition, cisplatin may be slightly better than carboplatin in the setting of metastatic germ cell tumors. One hundred ninety-two patients with germ cell tumors of the testes were entered into a study of 4 cycles of etoposide plus cisplatin (EP) versus 4 cycles of etoposide plus carboplatin (EC). There have been three relapses with the EP regimen versus seven with the EC regimen, although the overall survival of the two groups is identical thus far.[249] In view of these results, BEP is the preferred treatment regimen for patients with gross residual disease and has replaced the VAC regimen for patients with completely resected disease.

Immature teratomas with malignant squamous elements appear to have a poorer prognosis than those tumors without these elements.[254] The treatment in these patients is also the BEP regimen.

Second-Look Procedures A second look is not necessary in most patients who have received chemotherapy, particularly those who were treated in an adjuvant setting (ie, stage IA, grades 2 and 3 disease) because chemotherapy in these patients is so effective.[255] An enlarged contralateral ovary may contain a benign cyst or a mature cystic teratoma, which may be managed with an ovarian cystectomy.[236]

Prognosis The most important prognostic feature of the immature teratoma is the grade of the lesion.[2,260] The 5-year survivals have been reported to be 82%, 62%, and 30% for patients with grade 1, 2, and 3 lesions respectively.[260] Occasionally, these tumors are associated with mature or low-grade glial elements that have become implanted throughout the peritoneum, and such patients typically have a favorable long-term survival. In addition, the stage of disease and the extent of tumor at the initiation of treatment also affect the curability of the lesion. Patients whose tumors have been incompletely resected prior to treatment have a significantly lower 5-year survival than do those patients whose lesions have been completely resected (94% versus 50%).[257] In young women with conserved contralateral ovaries and a uterus, normal reproductive function and pregnancy have been reported in a significant fraction of successfully treated patients.[239] Overall, the 5-year survival of patients with all stages of pure immature teratomas is 70 to 80%, whereas it is 90 to 95% for patients with surgical stage I lesions.[2]

Endodermal Sinus Tumors Endodermal sinus tumors (EST) have also been referred to as yolk sac carcinomas, because they are derived from the primitive yolk sac.[2,236,264–271] These lesions are the third most frequent malignant germ cell tumor of the ovary. Endodermal sinus tumors occur at a median age of 18 years, and about one-third of the patients are premenarchal at the time of presentation. Like the other nondysgerminomatous ovarian malignancies, abdominal or pelvic pain is the most frequent presenting symptom, occurring in about 75% of patients. An asymptomatic pelvic mass is documented in about 10% of patients.[2,236]

Most EST lesions secrete AFP and rarely they may produce detectable AAT. There is a good correlation with the extent of disease and the AFP level, although discordance has been observed. The serum level of AFP is particularly useful in monitoring the patient during and after treatment.[236]

Surgery The treatment of EST includes a surgical exploration, a unilateral oophorectomy, and a frozen section for diagnosis. Any gross metastases should be removed if possible, but a thorough surgical staging is not necessary because all patients need chemotherapy. The tumors tend to be solid and large, ranging in size from 7 to 28 cm (median is 15 cm).[2,236] The EST is thought never to be bilateral, and the other ovary will have metastasis only when there are other metastases in the peritoneal cavity. Most patients have early-stage disease: 71% have stage I, 6% have stage II, and 23% have stage III. The performance of a hysterectomy and contralateral salpingo-oophorectomy does not alter outcome.[236]

Chemotherapy Endodermal sinus tumors are treated in all patients, regardless of stage, with either adjuvant or therapeutic chemotherapy.[262–270] Prior to the routine use of combination chemotherapy for this disease, the 2-year survival was only about 25%. With conservative surgery and adjuvant chemotherapy, fertility can be preserved as with other germ cell tumors.

As with other nondysgerminomatous germ-cell tumors, a cisplatin-containing combination chemotherapy regimen, either BEP or VBP, is most effective in the treatment of EST, particularly in the treatment of measurable or incompletely resected tumors.[261–263] In the GOG series, only about 20% of patients with residual metastatic disease responded completely to the VAC regimen, whereas about 60% of those treated with VBP had a complete response.[246] In addition, this regimen might salvage some failures of V therapy. As with patients with immature teratomas, BEP probably is the best current primary chemotherapy for this disease. The optimal number of treatment cycles has not been established. The GOG protocols have used nine treatment cycles of VBP given every 4 weeks.[256] but four to six cycles may be equally effective.[240]

Embryonal Carcinoma Embryonal carcinoma of the ovary is an extremely rare tumor. It can be distinguished from a choriocarcinoma by the absence of syncytiotrophoblastic and cytotrophoblastic cells. Embryonal carcinomas may be hormonally active, with some patients developing precocious pseudopuberty or irregular bleeding. The presentation is similar to that of the EST. The patient's ages ranged between 4 and 28 years (median was 14 years) in one series.[271] The primary lesions tend to be larger than 15 cm in diameter, and about two-thirds are confined to one ovary at the time of presentation. As with the pure EST, these lesions often secrete AFP and HCG, and these markers are useful for following the response to subsequent therapy. The treatment of embryonal carcinomas is the same as for the EST, that is, the performance of a unilateral oophorectomy or salpingo-oophorectomy followed by combination chemotherapy with BEP.[256]

Choriocarcinoma of the Ovary Pure nongestational choriocarcinoma of the ovary is an extremely rare tumor.[272] The majority of patients with this cancer are younger than 20 years. Isosexual precocity has been documented in about 50% of patients whose lesions arise prior to menarche. The presence of HCG can be useful in monitoring the patient during and after treatment. Because of its rarity, there are only a few series of reports in which chemotherapy was used for these nongestational choriocarcinomas, but there have been complete responses reported to the MAC regimen (methotrexate, actinomycin D, and cyclophosphamide).[236] However, as the BEP or EP is active in gestational choriocarcinoma, these regimens are also a reasonable approach for the nongestational lesions. The prognosis for ovarian choriocarcinoma has been poor, with the majority of patients having metastatic disease to organ parenchyma at the time of initial diagnosis.[2,236]

Mixed Germ Cell Tumors Mixed germ cell malignancies of the ovary contain two or more elements of the lesions described above. In one series, the most common component of a mixed malignancy was dysgerminoma, which occurred in 80%, followed by EST in 70%, immature teratoma in 53%, choriocarcinoma in 20%, and embryonal carcinoma in 16%.[244,270] The most frequent combination was a dysgerminoma and an EST. The mixed lesion may secrete either AFP or HCG, or both or neither, depending on the components.

Because most of these lesions contain poorly differentiated elements, mixed germ cell malignancies should be treated with combination chemotherapy, probably BEP or VBP.[270] The serum marker, if positive initially, may become negative during chemotherapy, but this may reflect the regression of only a particular component of the mixed lesion. Therefore, in patients with advanced-stage mixed germ cell malignancies, a second-look laparotomy may be useful to determine the response to therapy, unless the tumor was confined initially to the ovary.

The most important prognostic features are the size of the primary tumor and the relative amount of its most malignant component.[270] In stage IA lesions smaller than 10 cm, survival is 100%. Tumors composed of less than one-third EST, choriocarcinoma, or grade 3 immature teratoma also have an excellent prognosis, but it is less favorable when these components make up the majority of the mixed lesions.

Sex Cord–Stromal Tumors Sex cord–stromal tumors of the ovary account for about 5 to 8% of all ovarian malignancies.[2,236] This group of ovarian neoplasms is derived from the sex cords and the ovarian stroma or mesenchyme. The tumors usually are composed of various combinations of elements, including the "female" cells (granulosa and theca cells) and "male" cells (Sertoli and Leydig cells), as well as morphologically indifferent cells. A classification of this group of tumors is presented (Table 104-11).

Granulosa-Stromal Cell Tumors This group of tumors includes granulosa cell tumors, thecomas, and fibromas. The granulosa cell tumor is a low-grade malignancy, and rarely thecomas and fibromas become malignant and are called fibrosarcomas.[2]

Table 104-11 Sex Cord-Stromal Tumors

A. Granulosa stomal cell tumors
  1. Granulosa cell tumor
  2. Tumors in the thecoma-fibroma group
    a. thecoma
    b. fibroma
    c. unclassified
B. Androblastomas: Sertoli-Leydig cell tumors
  1. Well differentiated
    a. Sertoli cell tumor
    b. Sertoli-Leydig cell tumor
    c. Leydig cell tumor; hilus cell tumor
  2. Moderately differentiated
  3. Poorly differentiated (sarcomatoid)
  4. With heterologous elements
C. Gynandroblastoma
D. Unclassified

Adapted from Scully RE, Young RH, Clement PB.[2]

Granulosa cell tumors, which are estrogen secreting, are seen in women of all ages (Figure 104-9). They are found in prepubertal females in 5% of cases, and the rest throughout the reproductive and postmenopausal years.[236] They are bilateral in 2% of patients. In the rare prepubertal lesion, three fourths are associated with sexual pseudoprecocity because of the estrogen secretion. In the reproductive age group, most patients present with menstrual irregularities or secondary amenorrhea, and cystic hyperplasia of the endometrium may accompany these lesions. In postmenopausal women, abnormal uterine bleeding is frequently the presenting symptom. Indeed, the estrogen secretion in these patients can be sufficient to stimulate the development of endometrial cancer. Endometrial cancer occurs in association with granulosa cell tumors in about 5% of cases; 25% are associated with endometrial hyperplasia.[2,236] The other symptoms and signs of granulosa cell tumors are nonspecific and are the same as for most ovarian malignancies. Ascites is present in about 10% of cases, and, rarely, a pleural effusion is present.[2] Granulosa tumors tend to be hemorrhagic, and occasionally rupture and produce a hemoperitoneum.[2] Inhibin is secreted by granulosa cell tumors and is a useful marker for the disease.[274–276]

Granulosa cell tumors are usually stage I at diagnosis, but they may recur 5 to 30 years after initial diagnosis.[236] The tumors also may spread hematogenously, and patients can develop metastases years

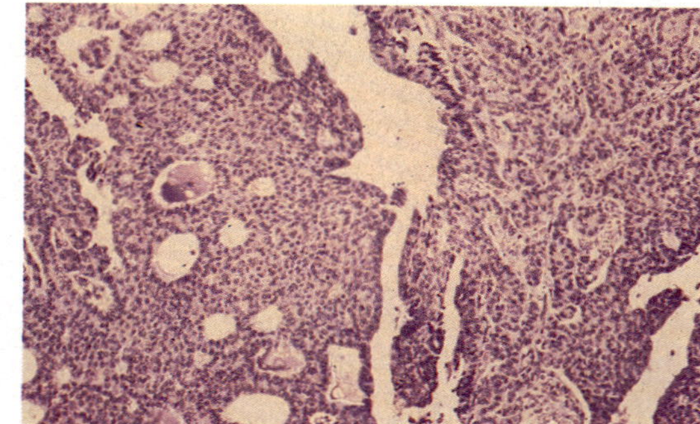

Figure 104-9 Granulosa cell tumor.

after initial diagnosis in the lungs, liver, and brain. When they do recur, they can progress rapidly. Malignant thecomas are extremely rare, and their presentation, management, and outcome are similar to those of the granulosa cell tumors.[2]

Surgery The treatment of a granulosa cell tumor depends on the age of the patient and the extent of disease. For most patients, surgery alone is sufficient primary therapy. The performance of a unilateral oophorectomy or salpingo-oophorectomy is appropriate therapy for stage IA tumors in children or in women of reproductive age.[236] If a granulosa cell tumor is identified by frozen section at laparotomy, a staging operation is performed, including an assessment of the contralateral ovary. If the opposite ovary appears enlarged, it should be biopsied. In perimenopausal and postmenopausal women for whom ovarian preservation is not important, a hysterectomy and bilateral salpingo-oophorectomy should be performed. In premenopausal patients in whom the uterus is not removed, a dilation and curettage of the uterus should be carried out because of a possible coexistent adenocarcinoma of the endometrium.

Radiotherapy and Chemotherapy There is no evidence to support the use of adjuvant radiation therapy for granulosa cell tumors, although pelvic radiation may help to palliate isolated pelvic recurrences.[278] Furthermore, it is unclear that adjuvant chemotherapy will prevent recurrence of disease.[279] However, metastatic lesions and recurrences have been treated with a variety of different antineoplastic drugs. There is no consistently effective regimen in these patients, although complete responses have been reported anecdotally in patients treated with a single alkylating agent, cyclophosphamide or melphalan, as well as those treated with combinations, VAC (vincristine, doxorubicin, cyclophosphamide) and PAC (cisplatin, doxorubicin, cyclophosphamide).[280] The AcFuCy regimen (actinomycin D, 5-fluorouracil, and cyclophosphamide) has been used by the GOG and has been associated with approximately a 20% response rate.[277,278] Response rates of about 30% have been shown with paclitaxel as a single agent and the combination of bleomycin, etoposide and platinum produced responses in 45%.[278] The use of hormonal agents, such as progestins or antiestrogens, has been suggested, but there are no data available.

Prognosis Granulosa cell tumors have a prolonged natural history and a tendency for late relapse, reflecting their low grade. As such, 10-year survivals of about 90% have been reported, with 20-year survivals of 75%.[2,236,278] Most histologic types have the same prognosis, but the more poorly differentiated diffuse or sarcomatoid type tends to do worse.[281]

SERTOLI-LEYDIG CELL TUMORS This group of tumors occurs most frequently in the third and fourth decades, with 75% of the lesions seen in women younger than 40 years. They are rare, representing less than 0.2% of ovarian cancers.[2,282] Sertoli-Leydig cell tumors are usually low-grade malignancies, although a poorly differentiated variety may behave more aggressively.

The tumors typically produce androgens, and clinical virilization is noted in 70 to 85% of patients.[236] Signs of virilization include oligomenorrhea, amenorrhea, breast atrophy, acne, hirsutism, clitoromegaly, a deepening voice, and a receding hairline. Measurement of plasma androgens may reveal an elevated testosterone and androstenedione, with normal or slightly elevated dehydroepiandrosterone sulfate.[2] Rarely, the Sertoli-Leydig tumor can be associated with manifestations of estrogenization, such as, isosexual precocity or irregular or postmenopausal bleeding.

Because these low-grade lesions are only rarely bilateral (under 1%), the usual treatment for patients in their reproductive years is a unilateral oophorectomy or salpingo-oophorectomy and evaluation of the contralateral ovary.[282] In older patients for whom fertility is not an issue, the performance of a hysterectomy and bilateral salpingo-oophorectomy is appropriate. There are insufficient data to document the value of radiation or chemotherapy in patients with persistent disease. The 5-year survival is 70 to 90%, and recurrences thereafter are uncommon. Poorly differentiated lesions account for the majority of fatalities.

UNCOMMON OVARIAN TUMORS

There are several types of rare malignant ovarian tumors that together compose about 0.1% of ovarian malignancies.[2] These lesions include small cell carcinomas, lipoid cell tumors and primary ovarian sarcomas.

SMALL-CELL CARCINOMAS This rare tumor occurs at an average of 24 years (range 2 to 46 years).[283] The tumors are all bilateral. Approximately two-thirds of the tumors are accompanied by paraendocrine hypercalcemia. This tumor accounts for one-half of all of the cases of hypercalcemia associated with ovarian tumors. About 50% of the tumors have spread beyond the ovaries when they are diagnosed.

The management of these malignancies consists of surgery followed by platinum-based chemotherapy and/or radiation therapy. In addition to the primary treatment of the disease, control of the hypercalcemia may require aggressive hydration, loop diuretics and the use of phosphates. The prognosis tends to be poor, with most patients dying within two years of diagnosis in spite of treatment.

LIPOID CELL TUMOR The lipoid cell tumor is thought to arise in adrenal cortical rests that reside near the ovary. Over 100 cases have been reported, and bilaterality in only a few.[2] Most are associated with virilization, and occasionally with obesity, hypertension, and glucose intolerance, reflecting glucocorticoid secretion. Rare cases of hyperestrogenism and isosexual precocity occur.

The majority of lipoid cell tumors have a benign or low-grade behavior, but about 20%, most of which are initially larger than 8 cm in diameter, develop metastatic lesions. Metastases are usually within the peritoneal cavity, and rarely to distant sites.[236] The primary treatment is the surgical extirpation of the primary lesion, and there are no reports of effective radiation or chemotherapy.

SARCOMAS Malignant mixed mesodermal sarcomas of the ovary are rare, and only about 100 cases have been reported.[283–285] Most are heterologous, and 80% occur in postmenopausal women. The presentation is similar to that of most ovarian malignancies, although these tumors are biologically aggressive, and the majority of patients have metastases to organ parenchyma, such as the liver and lung, and to the retroperitoneal lymph nodes.

Adriamycin (doxorubicin), with or without cyclophosphamide, has produced an occasional partial response, and cisplatin is currently undergoing clinical trials.[285] Ifosfamide with mesna has been reported to be useful in metastatic sarcomas of the female genital tract, and this combination might be appropriate for the treatment of ovarian sarcomas. Long-term survivors are uncommon, although some stage I patients have survived for 5 years.

METASTATIC TUMORS

About 5 to 6% of ovarian tumors are metastatic from other organs, most frequently from the female genital tract, the breast, or the gastrointestinal tract.[286–290] The metastasis may occur from direct extension of another pelvic neoplasm, by hematogenous spread, by lymphatic spread, or by transcoelomic spread, that is, by surface implantation of the peritoneal cavity.

Gynecologic Nonovarian cancers of the genital tract can spread by direct extension or metastasize to the ovaries. Tubal carcinomas involve the ovaries secondarily in 13% of cases usually by direct extension. Under some circumstances, it is difficult to ascertain whether the tumor originates in the tube or in the ovary when both are involved. Cervical cancer spreads to the ovary only in rare cases (less than 1%), and most of these are of advanced clinical stage or of adenocarcinoma histotype.[236] Although adenocarcinoma of the endometrium can spread and implant directly onto the surface of the ovaries in as many as 5% of cases, two synchronous primaries probably occur with greater frequency. In these cases, there is usually an endometrioid carcinoma of the ovary associated with the adenocarcinoma of the endometrium. Malignant melanoma rarely can metastasize to the ovaries.[289]

Non-Gynecologic The reported frequency of metastatic breast carcinoma to the ovaries varies, but the phenomenon is common.[289] In autopsy data of women who die of metastatic breast cancer, the ovaries are involved in 24% of cases and 80% of the involvement is bilateral.[290] Similarly, when ovaries are removed to palliate advanced breast cancer, about 20 to 30% of cases reveal ovarian involvement, 60% bilaterally. The involvement of ovaries in early-stage breast cancer appears to be considerably lower, but precise figures are not available. In almost all cases, ovarian involvement either is occult or a pelvic mass is discovered after other metastatic disease becomes apparent.

Krukenberg The Krukenberg tumor accounts for 30 to 40% of metastatic cancers to the ovaries and for 1 to 2% of all malignant ovarian tumors reported at some institutions.[286] It involves the ovarian stroma and has characteristic mucin-filled, signet ring cells.[2] The primary tumor is most often from the stomach, but less commonly from the colon, breast, or biliary tract, and rarely, from the cervix or bladder. Most are bilateral. The lesions may not be discovered until the primary disease is advanced, and most patients die of their disease within a year. In some cases, a primary tumor is not found.

In other cases of metastasis from the gastrointestinal tract to the ovary, the tumor does not have the classic histologic appearance of Krukenberg tumor, and most of these are from the colon and, less commonly, the small intestine. As many as 1 to 2% of women with intestinal carcinomas will develop metastases to the ovaries during the course of their disease.[287] Prior to exploration for an adnexal tumor in a woman older than 40 years, a barium enema is indicated to exclude a primary gastrointestinal carcinoma with metastases to the ovaries. Metastatic colon cancer can mimic a mucinous cystadenocarcinoma of the ovary.[2,287]

Carcinoid Metastatic carcinoid tumors are rare, representing less than 2% of metastatic lesions to the ovaries.[291] Conversely, only about 2% of primary carcinoids have evidence of ovarian metastasis, and only 40% of these patients have the carcinoid syndrome at the time of discovery of the metastatic carcinoid. Therefore, in perimenopausal and postmenopausal women with an intestinal carcinoid, it is reasonable to remove the ovaries to prevent subsequent metastasis. The discovery of an ovarian carcinoid should prompt a careful search for a primary intestinal lesion.

Lymphoma and Leukemia Lymphoma and leukemia can involve the ovary, and when they do, the involvement is usually bilateral.[292] Less than 5% of patients with Hodgkin disease develop lymphomatous involvement of the ovaries, and then typically only with advanced-stage disease. With Burkitt lymphoma, ovarian involvement is very common. Other types of non-Hodgkin lymphoma involve the ovaries more frequently than Hodgkin disease, but leukemic infiltration of the ovaries is uncommon. Sometimes the ovaries can be the only apparent sites of involvement of the abdominal or pelvic viscera with non-Hodgkin lymphoma, and if this circumstance is found, a careful surgical staging is necessary. If a frozen section of a solid ovarian mass reveals a lymphoma, the patient needs a careful operative evaluation, including a palpation of the entire intra-abdominal contents. Treatment for the lymphoma or leukemia involves the use of chemotherapy and/or radiotherapy appropriate for the specific type of primary lesion. Consideration should be given to removal of significantly enlarged ovarian disease to palliate symptoms and possibly to facilitate a response to treatment.

REFERENCES

1. Jemal A, Murray T, Ward E, et al. Cancer statistics, 2005. Cancer J Clin 2005;55:10–30.
2. Scully RE, Young RH, Clement PB. Tumors of the ovary, maldeveloped gonads, fallopian tube, and broad ligament. Third Series, Fascicle 23. Washington, DC: Armed Forces Institute of Pathology;1998.
3. Chen LM, Berek JS. Ovarian and fallopian tubes. In: Haskell CM, editor. Cancer treatment. 5th ed. Philadelphia, PA: WB Saunders; 2000.
4. Cramer DW. Epidemiology and biostatistics. In: Berek JS, Hacker NF, editors. Practical gynecologic oncology. 4th ed. Philadelphia, Lippincott Williams & Wilkins; 2005, p. 243–62.
5. Schildkraut JM, Halabi S, Bastos E, , et al. Obstet Gynecol 2000;95:119–27.
6. Cramer DW, Welch WR. Determinants of ovarian cancer risk. II. Inferences regarding pathogenesis. J Natl Cancer Inst 1983;71:717–24.
7. Cramer DW, Hutchison GB, Welch WR, et al. Determinants of ovarian cancer risk 1. Reproductive experiences and family history. J Natl Cancer Inst 1983;71:711–6.
8. Franceschi S, La Vecchia C, Booth M, et al. Pooled analysis of three European case-control studies of epithelial ovarian cancer: II. Age at menarche and menopause. Int J Cancer 1991;49:57–60.
9. Negri E, Franceschi S, Tzonou A, et al. Pooled analysis of three European case-control studies of epithelial ovarian cancer: I. Reproductive factors and risk of epithelial ovarian cancer. Int J Cancer 1991;49:50–6.
10. Rossing MA, Dalling JR, Weiss NS, et al. Ovarian tumors in a cohort of infertile women. New Engl J Med 1994;331:771–6.
11. Potashnik G, Lerner-Geva L, Genkin L, et al. Fertility drugs and the risk of breast and ovarian cancers: results of a long-term follow-up study. Fertil Steril 1999;71:853–9.
12. Ness RB, Cramer DW, Goodman MT, et al. Infertility, fertility drugs and ovarian cancer: a pooled analysis of case control studies. Am J Epidemiol 2002;155:217–24.
13. Fathalla MF. Incessant ovulation—a factor in ovarian neoplasia? Lancet 1983;71:717.
14. Sit AS, Modugno F, Weissfeld JL, et al. Hormone replacement therapy and formulations and risk of epithelial ovarian carcinoma. Gynecol Oncol 2002;86:118–23.
15. Lacey JV Jr, Mink PJ, Lubin JH, et al. Menopausal hormone replacement therapy and risk of ovarian cancer. J Am Med Assoc 2002;288:334–41.
16. Centers for Disease Control Cancer and Steroid Hormone Study. Oral contraceptives and the risk of ovarian cancer. 1983;249:1596–607.
17. De Palo G, Vceronesi U, Camerini T, et al. Can fenretinide protect women against ovarian cancer. J Natl Cancer Inst 1995;87:146–7.
18. De Palo G, Mariani L, Camerini T. Effect of fenretinide on ovarian carcinoma recurrence. Gynecol Oncol 2002;86:24–7.
19. Fowler JM, Nieberg RK, Schooler TA, Berek JS. Peritoneal adenocarcinoma (serous) of müllerian type: a subgroup of women presenting with peritoneal carcinomatosis. Int J Gynecol Cancer 1994;4:43–51.
20. Kauff ND, Satagopan JM, Robson ME, et al. Risk-reducing salpingo-oophorectomy in women with a BRCA1 or BRCA2 mutation. New Engl J Med 2002;346:1609–15.
21. Rebbeck TR, Lynch HT, Neuhausen SL, Narod SA, et al. Prophylactic oophorectomy in carriers of BRCA1 or BRCA2 mutations. New Engl J Med 2002; 346:1616–22.
22. Ponder B, Genetic testing for cancer risk. Science 1997;278:1050–8.
23. Frank TS, Manley SA, Olopade OI, et al. Sequence analysis of BRCA1 and BRCA2: correlation of mutations with family history and ovarian cancer risk. J Clin Oncol 1998;16:2417–25.
24. Beller U, Halle D, Catane R, et al. High frequency of BRCA1 and BRCA2 germline mutations in Ashkenazi Jewish ovarian cancer patients, regardless of family history. Gynecol Oncol 1997;67:123–6.
25. Burke W, Daly M, Garber J, et al. Recommendations for follow-up care of individuals with an inherited predisposition to cancer. II. BRCA1 and BRCA2. Cancer Genetics Studies Consortium. 1997;277:997–1003.
26. Miki Y, Swensen J, Shattuck-Eidens D, et al. A strong candidate for the breast and ovarian cancer susceptibility gene BRCA1. Science 1994;266:66–8.
27. Wooster R, Bignell G, Lancaster J, et al. Identification of the breast cancer susceptibility gene BRCA2. Nature 1995;378:789–92.
28. Struewing JP, Hartge P, Wacholder S, et al. The risk of cancer associated with specific mutations of BRCA1 and BRCA2 among Ashkenazi Jews. N Engl J Med 1997;336:1401–8.
29. Statement of the American Society of Clinical Oncology. Genetic testing for cancer susceptibility. J Clin Oncol 1996;14:1730–6.
30. NIH Consensus Development Panel on Ovarian Cancer. Ovarian cancer. Screening, treatment and follow-up. 1995;273:491–7.
31. Lynch HT, Cavalieri RJ, Lynch JF, Casey MJ. Gynecologic cancer clues to Lynch syndrome II diagnosis: a family report. Gynecol Oncol 1992;44:198–203.
32. Narod SA, Risch H, Moslehi R, et al. Oral contraceptives and the risk of hereditary ovarian cancer. N Engl J Med 1998;339:424–8.
33. Paley PJ, Swisher EM, Garcia RL, et al. Occult cancer of the fallopian tube in BRCA-1 germline mutation carriers at prophylactic oophorectomy: a case for recommending hysterectomy at surgical prophylaxis. Gynecol Oncol 2001;80:176–80.
34. Grann VR, Jacobson JS, Thomason D, et al. Effect of prevention strategies on survival and quality adjusted survival of women with BRCA1/2 mutations: an updated decision analysis. J Clin Oncol 2002;20:2520–9.
35. Berek JS. Epithelial ovarian cancer. In: Berek JS, Hacker NF, editors. Practical gynecologic oncology. 4th ed. Philadelphia: Lippincott Williams & Wilkins; 2005.
36. Heintz APM, Odicino F, Maisonneuve P, et al. Carcinoma of the ovary. 25th Annual report on the results of treatment of gynaecological cancer, International Federation of Gynecology and Obstetrics. Int J Gynecol Obstet 2003;83:135–66.
37. Hoskins WJ, McGuire WP, Brady MF, et al. The effect of diameter of largest residual disease on survival after primary cytoreductive surgery in patients with suboptimal residual epithelial ovarian carcinoma. Am J Obstet Gynecol 1994;170:974–9.
38. Yedema CA, Kenemans P, Voorhorst F, et al. CA 125 half-life in ovarian cancer: a multivariate survival analysis. Br J Cancer 1993;67:1361–7.
39. Reles AE, Conway G, Schellerschmidt I, et al. Prognostic significance of DNA content and S-phase fraction in epithelial ovarian carcinomas analyzed by image cytometry. Gynecol Oncol 1998;71:3–13.
40. Rice LW, Mark SD, Berkowitz RS, et al. Clinicopathologic variables, operative characteristics, and DNA ploidy in predicting outcome in epithelial ovarian carcinoma. Obstet Gynecol 1995;86:379–85.
41. Suzuki S, Moore DH II, Ginzinger DG, et al. An approach to analysis of large-scale correlations between genome changes and clinical endpoints in ovarian cancer. Cancer Res 2000;60:5382–5.
42. Jacobs IJ, Kohler MF, Wiseman R, et al. Clonal origin of epithelial ovarian cancer: analysis by loss of heterozygosity, p53 mutation and X chromosome inactivation. J Natl Cancer Inst 1992;84:1793.
43. Mok CH, Tsao WW, Knapp RC, et al. Unifocal origin of advanced human epithelial ovarian cancer. Cancer Res 1992;52:5119.
44. Yoneda J, Kuniyasu H, Crispens MA, et al. Expression of angiogenesis-related genes and progression of human ovarian carcinomas in nude mice. J Natl Cancer Inst 1998;90:447–54.
45. Rubin SC, Finstad CL, Federici MG, et al. Prevalence and significance of HER-2/neu expression in early epithelial ovarian cancer. Cancer 1994;73:1456–9.
46. Enomoto T, Inoue M, Perantoni AO, et al. K-ras activation in neoplasms of the human female reproductive tract. Cancer Res 1990;50:6139–45.
47. Mok SC, Bell DA, Knapp RC et al. Mutation of K-*ras* protooncogene in human ovarian epithelial tumors of borderline malignancy. Cancer Res 1993;3:1489–92.
48. Singer G, Stohr R, Cope L, et al. Patterns of p53 mutations separate ovarian serous borderline tumors and low- and high-grade carcinomas and provide support for a new model of ovarian carcinogenesis: a mutational analysis with immunohistochemical correlation. Am J Surg Pathol 2005;29:218–24.
49. Patton SE, Martin ML, Nelson LL, et al. Activation of the Ras-MAP pathway and phosphorylation of ets-2 at posi-

tion threonine 72 in human ovarian cancer cell lines. Cancer Res 1998;58:2253–9.

50. Rosen DG, Wang L, Jain AN, et al. Expression of the tumor suppressor gene ARHI in epithelial ovarian cancer is associated with increased expression of p21 WAF1/CIP1 and prolonged progression-free survival. Clin Cancer Res 2004;10:6559–66.
51. Shayesteh L, Lu Y, Ku WL, et al. P1K3CA is implicated as an oncogene in ovarian cancer. [In press]
52. Bellacosa A, de Feo D, Godwin AK, et al. Molecular alterations of the AKT2 oncogene in ovarian and breast carcinomas. Intl J Cancer 1995;64:280–5.
53. Mills GB, Lu Y, Fang X, et al. The role of genetic abnormalities of PTEN and the phosphatidylinositol 3-kinase pathway in breast and ovarian tumorigenesis, prognosis, and therapy. Semin Oncol 2001;125–41.
54. Orsulic S, Li Y, Soslow RA, Witale-Cross LA, et al. Induction of ovarian cancer by defined multiple genetic changes in a mouse model system. Cancer Cell 2002;:53–62.
55. Dong Y, Walsh MD, McGuckin MA, et al. Reduced expression of retinoblastoma gene product (pRB) and high expression of p53 are associated with poor prognosis in ovarian cancer. Intl J Cancer 1997;74:407–15.
56. Gershenson DM, Deavers M, Diaz S, et al. The prognostic significance of p53 expression in advanced stage ovarian serous borderline tumors. Clin Cancer Res 1999;5:4053–8.
57. Berchuck, A, Kohler MF, Hopkins MP, et al. Overexpression of p53 is not a feature of benign and early-stage borderline epithelial ovarian tumors. Gyn Onc 1994;52:232–6.
58. Mok SC, Chan WY, Wong KK, et al. SPARC, an extracellular matrix protein with tumor-suppressing activity in human ovarian epithelial cells. Oncogene 1996;12:1895–901.
59. Ferero S, Ragni N. Vascular endothelial growth factor, persistent disease, and survival in ovarian cancer. Gynecol Oncol 2005;96:265–6.
60. Mok SC, Wong KK, Chan RK, et al. Molecular cloning of differentially expressed genes in human epithelial ovarian cancer. Gyn Onc 1994;52:247–52.
61. Yu YH, Xu FJ, Fang XJ, et al. Identification of a novel ras-related, tumor suppressor gene in ovarian carcinomas. Proc Natl Acad Sci U S A 1999;96:214–9.
62. Bao J, Le XF, Wang RY, et al. Re-expression of the tumor suppressor gene ARHI induces apoptosis in ovarian and breast cancer cells through a caspase-independent calpain-dependent pathway. Cancer Res 2002;62:7264–72.
63. Stromberg K, Johnson GR, O'Connor DM, et al. Frequent immunohistochemical detection of EGF supergene family members in ovarian carcinogenesis. Intl J Gyn Path 1994;13:342–7.
64. Stromberg K, Collins TJ, Gordon AW, et al. Transforming growth factor-a acts as an autocrine growth factor in ovarian cancer cell lines. Cancer Res 1992;52:341–7.
65. Wu S, Boyer CM, Whitaker RS, et al. Tumor necrosis factor-a as an autocrine and paracrine growth factor for ovarian cancer: monokine induction of tumor cell proliferation and tumor necrosis factor alpha expression. Cancer Res 1993;53:1939–44.
66. Wu S, Meeker WA, Wiener JR, et al. Transfection of ovarian cancer cells with tumor necrosis factor-a (TNF-a) antisense mRNA abolishes the proliferative response to interleukin-1 (IL-1) but not TNF. Gynecol Oncol 1994;53:59–63.
67. Watson JM, Sensintaffar JL, Berek JS, Martinez-Maza O. Constitutive production of interleukin 6 by ovarian cancer cell lines and by primary ovarian tumor cultures. Can Res 1990;50:6959–65.
68. Kacinski BM, Carter D, Mittal K et al. Ovarian adenocarcinomas express fms-complementary transcripts and fms antigen, often with coexpression of CSF-1. Am J Path 1990;137:135–47.
69. Mills GB, Eder A, Fang X, et al. Critical role of lysophospholipids in the pathophysiology, diagnosis, and management of ovarian cancer. Can Treat Res 2002;107:259–83.
70. Havrilesky LJ, Hurteau JA, Whitaker RS, et al. Regulation of apoptosis in normal and malignant ovarian epithelial cells by transforming growth factor-(3. Cancer Res 1995;55:944–8.
71. Wu S, Rodabaugh K, Martinez-Maza O, et al. Stimulation of ovarian cancer tumor cells proliferation with monocyte products including interleukin-1, interleukin-6, and tumor necrosis factor-a. Am J Obstet Gyn 1992;166:997–1007.
72. Strobel T, Swanson L, Cannistra SA. In vivo inhibition of CD44 limits intra-abdominal spread of a human ovarian cancer xenograft in nude mice: a novel role for CD44 in the process of peritoneal implantation. Cancer Res 1997;57:1228–32.
73. Young TN, Rodriguez GC, Moser TL, et al. Coordinate expression of urinary-type plasminogen activator and its receptor accompanies malignant transformation of the ovarian surface epithelium. Am J Obstet Gynecol 1994;170: 1285–96.
74. Yoneda J, Juniyasu H, Crispens MA, et al. Expression of angiogenesis-related genes and progression of human ovarian carcinomas in nude mice. Natl Can Inst 1998;90:447–54.
75. Taylor-Papadimitriou J, Burchell J, Miles DW, Dalziel M. MUC1 and cancer. Biochim Biophys Acta 1999; 1455:301–13.
76. Bast RC Jr, Klug TL, St. John E, et al. A radioimmunoassay using a monoclonal antibody to monitor the course of epithelial ovarian cancer. N Engl J Med 1983; 309:883–7.
77. Bast RC Jr, Feeney M, Lazarus H, et al. Reactivity of a monoclonal antibody with human ovarian carcinoma. J Clin Invest 1981;68:1331–7.
78. Yin BW, Lloyd KO. Molecular cloning of the CA125 ovarian cancer antigen: identification as a new mucin, MUC16. J Biol Chem 2001:27371–5.
79. O'Brien TJ, Beard JB, Underwood LJ, et al. The CA125 gene: an extracellular superstructure dominated by repeat sequences. Tumour Biol 2001:348–66.
80. Serov SF, Scully RE, Robin IH. Histological typing of ovarian tumors: international histological classification of tumors, no. 9. Geneva, Switzerland: World Health Organization; 1973.
81. Barnhill DR, Kurman RJ, Brady MF, et al. Preliminary analysis of the behavior of stage I ovarian serous tumors of low malignant potential: a Gynecologic Oncology Group study. J Clin Oncol 1995;13:2752–6.
82. Seidman JD, Kurman RJ. Subclassification of serous borderline tumors of the ovary into benign and malignant types. A clinicopathologic study of 65 advanced stage cases. Am J Surg Pathol 1996;20:1331–45.
83. Tobacman JK, Greene MH, Tucker MA, et al. Intra-abdominal carcinomatosis after prophylactic oophorectomy in ovarian cancer-prone families. Lancet 1982;2:795.
84. Parmley TH, Woodruff JD. The ovarian mesothelioma. Am J Obstet Gynecol 1974;120:234–9.
85. Chen KT, Schooley JL, Flam MS. Peritoneal carcinomatosis after prophylactic oophorectomy in familial ovarian cancer syndrome. Obstet Gynecol 1985;6(Suppl 3):93s.
86. Benedetti-Panici P, Greggi S, Maneschi F, et al. Anatomical and pathological study of retroperitoneal nodes in epithelial ovarian cancer. Gynecol Oncol 1993;51:150–4.
87. Berek JS, Hacker NF, Lagasse LD, et al. Second-look laparotomy in stage III epithelial ovarian cancer: clinical variables associated with disease status. Obstet Gynecol 1984;64:207–14.
88. Goff BA, Mandel L, Muntz HG, Melancon CH. Ovarian carcinoma diagnosis. Cancer 2000;2068–75.
89. Malkasian GD Jr, Knapp RC, Lavin PI, et al. Preoperative evaluation at serum CA125 in premenopausal and postmenopausal patients with pelvic masses: discrimination of benign from malignant disease. Am J Obstet Gynecol 1988;159:341–8.
90. De Rosa V, Mangioni di Stefano ML, Brunetti A, et al. Computed tomography and second-look surgery in ovarian cancer patients: correlation, actual role and limitations of CT scan. Eur J Gynaecol Oncol 1995;16:123–9.
91. Bast RC Jr, Urban N, Shridhar V, et al. Early detection of ovarian cancer: promise and reality. In: Stack MS, Fishman DA, editors. Ovarian cancer. Boston, MA: Kluwer Publishers; 2002. p. 61–97. (Cancer Treat Res 2002;107:61–97).
92. Bast RC Jr. Status of tumor markers in ovarian cancer screening. J Clin Oncol 2003; 21:200–5s.
93. Bourne TH, Campbell S, Reynolds KM, et al. Screening for early familial ovarian cancer with transvaginal ultrasonography and colour blood flow imaging, Br Med J 1993;306:1025–9.
94. Van Nagell JR, Depriest PD, Reedy MB, et al. The efficacy of transvaginal sonographic screening in asymptomatic women at risk for ovarian cancer. Gynecol Oncol 2000;77:350–6.
95. Sato S, Yokoyama Y, Sakamota T, et al. Usefulness of mass screening for ovarian carcinoma using transvaginal ultrasonography, Cancer 2001;89:582–8.
96. Jacobs I, Bast RC Jr. CA125 tumour-associated antigen: a review of the literature. Hum Reprod 1989;4:1–12.
97. Woolas RP, Xu FJ, Jacobs IJ, et al. Elevation of multiple serum markers in patients with stage I ovarian cancer. J Natl Cancer Inst 1993;85:1748–51.
98. Van Haaften-Day C, Xu F, Yu Y, et al. OVX1, CA 125 and M-CSF as tumor markers for surface epithelial-stromal tumors of the ovary—a critical appraisal. Cancer 2001;92:2837–44.
99. Einhorn N, Sjovall K, Knapp RC, et al. Prospective evaluation of serum CA 125 levels for early detection of ovarian cancer. Obstet Gynecol 1992;80:14–8.
100. Jacobs IJ, Skates S, Davies AP, et al. Risk of diagnosis of ovarian cancer after raised serum CA 125 concentration: a prospective cohort study. Br Med J 1996;313:1355–8.
101. Jacobs IJ, Skates SJ, MacDonald N, et al. Screening for ovarian cancer: a pilot randomized controlled trial. Lancet 1999:1207–10.
102. Skates SJ, Xu F-J, Yu Y-H, et al. Toward an optimal algorithm for ovarian cancer screening with longitudinal tumor markers. Cancer 1995;76:2004–10.
103. Rosenthal AN, Jacobs IJ. The role of CA 125 in screening for ovarian cancer. Int J Biol Makers 1998;13:216–20.
104. Scholler N, Fu N, Yang Y, et al. Soluble member(s) of the mesothelin/megakaryocyte potentiating factor family are detectable in sera from patients with ovarian carcinoma. Proc Natl Acad Sci U S A 1999;96:11531–6.
105. Baron AT, Lafky JM, Boardman CH, et al. Serum sErbB1 and epidermal growth factor levels as tumor biomarkers in women with stage III or IV epithelial ovarian cancer. Cancer Epidemiol Biomarkers 1999;8:129–37.
106. Xu Y, Shen Z, Wiper DW, et al. Lysophosphatidic acid as a potential biomarker for ovarian and other gynecologic cancers. JAMA, 1998;280:719–23.
107. Schummer M, Ng WV, Bumgarner RE, et al. Comparative hybridization of an array of 21,500 ovarian cDNAs for the discovery of genes overexpressed in ovarian carcinomas. Gene 1999;375–85.
108. Mok SC, Chao J, Skates S, et al. Prostasin, a potential serum marker for ovarian cancer: identification through microarray technology. J Natl Cancer Inst 2001;93:1458–64.
109. Kim JH, Skates SJ, Uede T, et al. Osteopontin as a potential diagnostic for ovarian cancer. JAMA 2002;282:1671–9.
110. Diamandis EP, Yousef GM, Soosaipillai AR, Bunting P. Human kallikrein 6 (zyme/protease M/neurosin): a new serum biomarker of ovarian carcinoma. Clin Biochem 2000;33:579–83.
111. Luo LY, Bunting P, Scorilas A, Diamandis EP. Human kallikrein 10: a novel tumor marker for ovarian carcinoma? Clin Chim Acta 2001;111–8.
112. Petricoin EF, Ardekani AM, Hitt BA, et al. Use of proteomic patterns in serum to identify ovarian cancers. Lancet 2002;359:572–7.
113. Zhang Z, Barnhill SD, Baggerly KA, Morris JS, Coombes KR. Reproducibility of SELDI-TOF protein patterns in serum: comparing datasets from different experiments. Bioinformatics 2004;20:777–85.
114. Zhang Z, Bast RC Jr, Fung E, et al A panel of serum biomarkers identified through proteomic profiling for the detection of early stage ovarian cancer. Cancer Res 2004; 64:5882–90.
115. Burke W, Daly M, Garber J, et al. Recommendations for follow-up care of individuals with an inherited predisposition to cancer. II. BRCA1 and BRCA2. Cancer Genetics Studies Consortium. JAMA 1997;277:997–1003.
116. Bourne TH, Whitehead MI, Campbell S, et al. Ultrasound screening for familial ovarian cancer. Gynecol Oncol 1991;43:92–7.
117. Muto MG, Cramer DW, Brown DL, et al. Screening for ovarian cancer: the preliminary experience of a familial ovarian cancer center. Gynecol Oncol 1993;51:12–20.
118. Karlan BY, Raffel LJ, Crvenkovic G, et al. A multidisciplinary approach to the early detection of ovarian carcinoma: rationale, protocol design, and early results. AM J Obstet Gynecol 1993;169:494–501.
119. Schwartz PE, Chambers JT, Taylor KJ. Early detection and screening for ovarian cancer. J Cell Biochem 1995;23:233–7.
120. Young RC, Decker DG, Wharton JT, et al. Staging laparotomy in early ovarian cancer. JAMA 1983;250:3072–8.
121. Sevelda P, Vavra N, Schemper M, Salzer H. Prognostic factors for survival in stage I epithelial ovarian carcinoma. Cancer 1990;65:2349–52.
122. Sjovall K, Nilsson B, Einhorn N. Different types of rupture of the tumour capsule and the impact on survival in early ovarian cancer. Int J Gynecol Cancer 1994;4:333–6.
123. Dembo AJ, Bush RS, Beale FA, et al. A randomized clinical trial of moving-strip versus open-field whole abdominal irradiation in patients with invasive epithelial cancer of

ovary [abstract]. Int J Radiat Oncol Biol Phys 1983;9:97–103.

124. Young RC, Brady MF, Nieberg RM, et al. Adjuvant treatment for early epithelial ovarian cancer: a randomized phase III trial of intraperitoneal ^{32}P or intravenous cyclophosphamide and cisplatin: a Gynecologic Oncology Group study. J Clin Oncol 2003;21:4350–5.
125. Young RC, Walton LA, Ellenberg SS, et al. Adjuvant therapy in stage I and stage II epithelial ovarian cancer. N Engl J Med 1990;322:1021–4.
126. Gadducci A, Sartori E, Maggino T, et al. Analysis of failure in patients with stage I ovarian cancer: an Italian multicenter study. Int J Gynecol Cancer 1997;7:445–50.
127. Trimbos JB, Vergote I, Bolis G, et al. Impact of adjuvant chemotherapy and surgical staging in early-stage ovarian carcinoma: European Organisation for Research and Treatment of Cancer—Adjuvant Chemotherapy in Ovarian Neoplasm Trial. J Natl Cancer Inst 2003;95:113–125.
128. International Collaborative Ovarian Neoplasm (ICON1) Collaborators. International collaborative ovarian neoplasm trial 1: a randomized trial of adjuvant chemotherapy in women with early-stage ovarian cancer. J Natl Cancer Inst 2003;95:125–32.
129. Trimbos JB, Parmar M, Vergote I, et al. International Collaborative Ovarian Neoplasm Trail 1 and Adjuvant Chemotherapy In: Ovarian Neoplasm Trial: two parallel randomized phase III trials of adjuvant chemotherapy in patients with early-stage ovarian carcinoma. JNCI 2003;95:105–12.
130. Guthrie D, Davy MLJ, Phillips PR. Study of 656 patients with "early" ovarian cancer. Gynecol Oncol 1983;17:363–7.
131. Kaldor JM, Day NE, Pettersson F, et al. Leukemia following chemotherapy for ovarian cancer. N Engl J Med 1990;322:1–7.
132. Griffiths CT. Surgical resection of tumor bulk in the primary treatment of ovarian carcinoma. Natl Cancer Inst Monogr 1975;42:101–9.
133. Hacker NF, Berek JS, Lagasse LD, et al. Primary cytoreductive surgery for epithelial ovarian cancer. Obstet Gynecol 1983;61:413–8.
134. Heintz AP, Hacker NF, Berek JS, et al. Cytoreductive surgery in ovarian carcinoma: feasibility and morbidity. Obstet Gynecol 1986;67:783–8.
135. Berek JS. Complete debulking of advanced ovarian cancer. Cancer J 1996;2:134–5.
136. Scarbelli C, Gallo A, Zarrelli A, et al. Systematic pelvic and para-aortic lymphadenectomy during cytoreductive surgery in advanced ovarian cancer: potential benefit on survival. Gynecol Oncol 1995;56:328–37.
137. Bristow R, Montz FJ, Lagasse LD, et al. Survival impact of surgical cytoreduction in stage IV epithelial ovarian cancer. Gynecol Oncol 1999;72:278–87.
138. Goldie JH, Coldman AJ. A mathematical model for relating the drug sensitivity of tumors to their spontaneous mutation rate. Cancer Treat Rep 1979;63:1727–33.
139. Hacker NF. Cytoreduction for advanced ovarian cancer in perspective. Int J Gynecol Cancer 1996;6:159–60.
140. Farias-Eisner R, Kim YB, Berek JS. Surgical management of ovarian cancer. Semin Surg Oncol 1994; 10:268–75.
141. Farias-Eisner R, Teng F, Oliveira M, et al. The influence of tumor grade, distribution and extent of carcinomatosis in minimal residual epithelial ovarian cancer after optimal primary cytoreductive surgery. Gynecol Oncol 1994;55:108–10.
142. Berek JS, Hacker NF, Lagasse LD. Lower urinary tract resection as part of cytoreductive surgery for ovarian cancer. Gynecol Oncol 1983;13:87–92.
143. Berek JS, Hacker NF, Lagasse LD. Rectosigmoid colectomy and reanastomosis to facilitate resection of primary and recurrent gynecologic cancer. Obstet Gynecol 1984;64:715–22.
144. Bristow RE, Tomacruz RS, Armstrong DK, et al. Survival effect of maximal cytoreductive surgery for advanced ovarian carcinoma during the platinum era: a meta-analysis. J Clin Oncol 2002;20:1248–59.
145. van der Burg MEL, van Lent M, Buyse M, et al. The effect of debulking surgery after induction chemotherapy on the prognosis in advanced epithelial ovarian cancer. N Engl J Med 1995;332:629–34.
146. Rose PG, Nerenstone S, Brady MF, et al. Secondary cytoreduction for advanced stage ovarian carcinoma: a Gynecologic Oncology Group study. N Engl J Med 2004;351:2489–97.
147. Eisenhauer EA, ten Bokkel Huinink WW, Swenerton KD, et al. European—Canadian randomized trial of paclitaxel in relapsed ovarian cancer: high-dose versus low-dose and long versus short infusion. J Clin Oncol 1994;12:2654–66.
148. Bookman MA, McGuire WP, Kilpatrick D, et al. Carboplatin and paclitaxel in ovarian carcinoma: a phase I study of the Gynecologic Oncology Group. J Clin Oncol 1996;14:1895–902.
149. McGuire WP, Hoskins WJ, Brady MF, et al. Cyclophosphamide and cisplatin compared with paclitaxel and cisplatin in patients with stage III and stage IV ovarian cancer. N Engl J Med 1996;334:1–6.
150. Piccart MJ, Bertelsen K, James K, et al. Randomized intergroup trial of cisplatin–paclitaxel versus cisplatin–cyclophosphamide in women with advanced epithelial ovarian cancer: three year results. J Natl Cancer Inst 2000;92:699–708.
151. Muggia F, Braly PS, Brady MF, et al. Phase III randomized study of cisplatin versus paclitaxel versus cisplatin and paclitaxel in patients with suboptimal stage III or IV ovarian cancer: a Gynecologic Oncology Group study. J Clin Oncol 2000;18:106–15.
152. Markman M, Rothman R, Hakes J, et al. Second-line platinum therapy in patients with ovarian cancer previously treated with cisplatin. J Clin Oncol 1991;9:389–93.
153. Advanced Ovarian Cancer Trialists Group. Chemotherapy in advanced ovarian cancer: an overview of randomized clinical trials. Br Med J 1991;303:884–93.
154. Young RC, Chabner BA, Hubbard SP, et al. Advanced ovarian adenocarcinoma: a prospective clinical trial of melphalan (L-PAM) versus combination chemotherapy. N Engl J Med 1978;299:1261–6.
155. Omura G, Bundy B, Berek JS, et al. Randomized trial of cyclophosphamide plus cisplatin with or without doxorubicin in ovarian carcinoma: a Gynecologic Oncology Group study. J Clin Oncol 1989;7:457–65.
156. Bertelsen K, Jakobsen A, Andersen JE, et al. A randomized study of cyclophosphamide and cisplatin with or without doxorubicin in advanced ovarian cancer. Gynecol Oncol 1987;28:161–9.
157. Conte PF, Bruzzone M, Chiara S, et al. A randomized trial comparing cisplatin plus cyclophosphamide versus cisplatin, doxorubicin and cyclophosphamide in advanced ovarian cancer. J Clin Oncol 1986;4:965–71.
158. Gruppo Interegionale Cooperativo Oncologico Ginecologia. Randomized comparison of cisplatin with cyclophosphamide/cisplatin with cyclophosphamide/doxorubicin/cisplatin in advanced ovarian cancer. Lancet 1987;2:353–9.
159. Ovarian Cancer Meta-Analysis Project. Cyclophosphamide plus cisplatin versus cyclophosphamide, doxorubicin, and cisplatin chemotherapy of ovarian carcinoma: a meta-analysis. J Clin Oncol 1991;9:1668–74.
160. Swenerton K, Jeffrey J, Stuart G, et al. Cisplatin-cyclophosphamide versus carboplatin-cyclophosphamide in advanced ovarian cancer: a randomized phase III study of the National Cancer Institute of Canada Clinical Trials Group. J Clin Oncol 1992;10:718–26.
161. Ozols RF, Bundy BN, Greer B, et al. Phase III trial of carboplatin and paclitaxel compared with cisplatin and paclitaxel in patients with optimally resected stage III ovarian cancer. J Clin Oncol 2003;21:3194–200.
162. Du Bois A, Lueck HJ, Meier W, et al. A randomized clinical trial of cisplatin/paclitaxel versus carboplatin/paclitaxel as first-line treatment of ovarian cancer. J Natl Cancer Inst 2003;95:1320–30.
163. The International Collaborative Ovarian Neoplasm (ICON) Group. Paclitaxel plus carboplatin versus standard chemotherapy with either single agent carboplatin or cyclophosphamide, doxorubicin and cisplatin: in women with ovarian cancer: the ICON3 randomised trial. Lancet 2002;360:505–15.
164. McGuire WP, Hoskins WJ; Brady MS, et al. An assessment of dose—intensive therapy in suboptimally debulked ovarian cancer: a Gynecologic Oncology Group study. J Clin Oncol 1995;13:1589–99.
165. Kaye SB, Paul J, Cassidy J, et al. Mature results of a randomized trial of two doses of cisplatin for the treatment of ovarian cancer. J Clin Oncol 1996;14:2113–9.
166. Calvert AH, Newell DR, Gumbrell LA, et al. Carboplatin dosage: prospective evaluation of a simple formula based on renal function. J Clin Oncol 1989;7:1748–56.
167. Aabo K, Adams M, Adnitt P, et al. Chemotherapy in advanced ovarian cancer: four systematic meta—analyses of individual patient data from 37 randomized trials. Advanced Ovarian Cancer Trialists' Group. Br J Cancer 1998;78:1479–87.
168. Ozols RF, Markman M, Thigpen JT. ICON3 and chemotherapy for ovarian cancer. Lancet, 2002;360:2086.
169. Kaye SB, Vasey PA. Docetaxel in ovarian cancer: Phase III perspectives and future development. Semin Oncol 2002;29:22–7.
170. Vasey PA, Paul J, Birt A, et al. Docetaxel and cisplatin in combination as first-line chemotherapy for advanced epithelial ovarian cancer. Scottish Gynaecological Cancer Trials Group. J Clin Oncol 1999;17:2069–80.
171. Alberts DS, Liu PY, Hannigan EV, et al. Intraperitoneal cisplatin plus intravenous cyclophosphamide versus intravenous cisplatin plus intravenous cyclophosphamide for stage III ovarian cancer. N Engl J Med 1996;335:1950–5.
172. Markman M, Bundy B, Benda J, et al. Randomized phase III study of intravenous cisplatin/paclitaxel versus moderately high dose intravenous carboplatin followed by intraperitoneal paclitaxel and intraperitoneal cisplatin in optimal residual ovarian cancer: an Intergroup trial (GOG, SWOG, ECOG). J Clin Oncol 2001;19:921–3.
173. Armstrong D, et al. Intraperitoneal cisplatin and paclitaxel versus intravenous cisplatin and paclitaxel in women with optimal ovarian cancer: a Gynecologic Oncology Group Study. Proc Am Soc Clin Oncol 2002.
174. Schwartz PE, Rutherford TJ, Chambers JT, et al. Neoadjuvant chemotherapy for advanced ovarian cancer: long-term survival. Gynecol Oncol 1999;72:93–9.
175. Hruby G, Bull CA, Langlands AO, Gebski V. WART revisited: the treatment of epithelial ovarian cancer by whole abdominal radiotherapy. Australasian Radiol 1997;41:276.
176. Lund B, Jacobson K, Rasch L, et al. Correlation of abdominal ultrasound and computed tomography scans with second- or third-look laparotomy in patients with ovarian carcinoma. Gynecol Oncol 1990;37:279–83.
177. Berek JS, Knapp RC, Malkasian GD, et al. CA125 serum levels correlated with second-look operations among ovarian cancer patients. Obstet Gynecol 1986;67:685–9.
178. Lavin PT, Knapp RC, Malkasian GD, et al. CA125 for the monitoring of ovarian carcinoma during primary therapy. Obstet Gynecol 1989;69:223–8.
179. Berek JS, Griffiths CT, Leventhal JM. Laparoscopy for second-look evaluation in ovarian cancer. Obstet Gynecol 1981;58:192–7.
180. Podczaski E, Manetta A, Kaminski P, et al. Survival of patients with ovarian epithelial carcinoma after second-look laparotomy. Gynecol Oncol 1990;36:43–7.
181. Markman M, Liu PY, Wilczynski S, et al. Phase III randomized trial of 12 versus. 3 months of maintenance paclitaxel in patients with advanced ovarian cancer after complete response to platinum and paclitaxel-based chemotherapy: a Southwest Oncology Group and Gynecologic Oncology Group trial. J Clin Oncol 2003;21:2460–5.
182. DePlacido S, Scambia G, DiVagno G, et al. Topotecan compared with no therapy after response to surgery and carboplatin/paclitaxel in patients with ovarian cancer: multicenter Italian trials in ovarian cancer (MITO-1) randomized study. J Clin Oncol 2004;22:2635–42.
183. Pfisterer J, Lortholary A, Kimmig R, et al. Paclitaxel/carboplatin vs. paclitaxel/carboplatin followed by topotecan in first-line treatment of ovarian cancer FIGO stages IIb-IV: interim results of a Gynecologic Cancer Intergroup phase II trial of the AGO Ovarian Cancer Study Group and GINECO. Proc Am Soc Clin Oncol 2003;22:1793a.
184. Seiden MV, Benigno BB, Verheijen RH, et al. A pivotal phase II trial to evaluate the efficacy and safety of adjuvant treatment with R1549 (yttrium-90-labeled HMFG1 murine monoclonal antibody) in epithelial ovarian cancer. Proc Am Soc Clin Oncol 2004;23:5008a.
185. Berek JS, Taylor PT, Gordon A, et al. Randomized placebo-controlled study of oregovomab for consolidation of clinical remission in patients with advanced ovarian cancer. J Clin Oncol 2004;22:3507–16.
186. Fuks Z, Rizel S, Biran S. Chemotherapeutic and surgical induction of pathological complete remission and whole abdominal irradiation for consolidation does not enhance the cure of stage III ovarian carcinoma. J Clin Oncol 1988;6:509–13.
187. Hacker NF, Berek JS, Burnison CM, et al. Whole abdominal radiation as salvage therapy for epithelial ovarian cancer. Obstet Gynecol 1985;65:60–6.
188. Lawton F, Luesley D, Blackledge G, et al. A randomized trial comparing whole abdominal radiotherapy with chemotherapy following cisplatinum cytoreduction in epithelial ovarian cancer. West Midlands Ovarian Group Trial II. Clin Oncol 1990;2:4–11.
189. Lederman JA, Dembo AJ, Sturgeon JFG, et al. Outcome of patients with unfavorable optimally cytoreduced ovarian cancer treated with chemotherapy and whole abdominal radiation. Gynecol Oncol 2000;37:367–73.
190. Thomas GM. Is there a role for consolidation or salvage

radiotherapy after chemotherapy in advanced epithelial ovarian cancer? Gynecol Oncol 1993;51:97–8.

191. Gore ME, Fryatt I, Wiltshaw E, Dawson T. Treatment of relapsed carcinoma of the ovary with cisplatin or carboplatin following initial treatment with these compounds. Gynecol Oncol 1990;36:207–10.
192. Parmar MK, Ledermann JA, Columbo N, et al. Paclitaxel plus platinum-based chemotherapy versus conventional platinum-based chemotherapy in women with relapsed ovarian cancer: the ICON4/AGO-OVAR-2.2 trial. Lancet 2003;361:2099–106.
193. Bookman MA, Malmstrom H, Bolis G, et al. Topotecan for the treatment of advanced epithelial ovarian cancer: an open-label phase II study in patients treated after prior chemotherapy that contained cisplatin or carboplatin and paclitaxel. J Clin Oncol 1998;16:3345–9.
194. ten Bokkel Huinink WW, Gore M, Carmichael J, et al. Topotecan versus paclitaxel for the treatment of recurrent epithelial ovarian cancer. J Clin Oncol 1997;15: 2183–9.
195. Lund B, Hansen OP, Theilade K, et al. Phase II study of gemcitabine (2x,2x-Difluorodeoxycytidine) in previously treated ovarian cancer patients. J Natl Cancer Inst 1994;86:2530–3.
196. Muggia FM, Hainsworth JD, Jeffers S, et al. Phase II study of liposomal doxorubicin in refractory ovarian cancer: antitumor activity and toxicity modification by liposomal encapsulation. J Clin Oncol 1997;25:987–91.
197. Rose PG, Blessing JA, Mayer AR, et al. Prolonged oral etoposide as second-line therapy for platinum-resistant and platinum-sensitive ovarian carcinoma: a Gynecologic Oncology Group Study. J Clin Oncol 1998;16:405–8.
198. Manetta A, MacNeill C, Lyter JA, et al. Hexamethylmelamine as a second-line agent in ovarian cancer. Gynecol Oncol 1990;36:93–6.
199. Gordon AN, Fleagle JT, Guthrie D, et al. Recurrent epithelial ovarian carcinoma: a randomized phase III study of pegylated liposomal doxorubicin versus topotecan. J Clin Oncol 2001;19:3312–22.
200. Gordon AN, Tonda M, Sun S, et al. Long-term survival advantage for women treated with pegylated liposomal doxorubicin compared with topotecan in a phase III randomized study of recurrent and refractory epithelial ovarian cancer. Gynecol Oncol 2004;95:1–8.
201. Rose PA, Mossbruger K, Fusco N, et al. Gemcitabine reverses cisplatin resistance: demonstration of activity in platinum and multi-drug resistant ovarian and peritoneal carcinoma. Gynecol Oncol 2002;88:17–21.
202. Nagourney RA, Brewer CA, Sommers B, et al. Phase II Trial of gemcitabine plus cisplatin repeating doublet therapy in previously treated, relapsed ovarian cancer patients. Gynecol Oncol 2003;88:35–9.
203. Stiff P, Bayer R, Camarda M, et al. A phase II trial of high-dose mitoxantrone, carboplatin, and cyclophosphamide with autologous bone marrow rescue for recurrent epithelial ovarian carcinoma: analysis of risk factors for clinical outcome. Gyn Oncol 1995;57:278–85.
204. Donato ML, Aleman A, Champlin RE, et al. Analysis of 96 patients with advanced ovarian carcinoma treated with high-dose chemotherapy and autologous stem cell transplantation. Bone Marrow Transplant. 2004; 33:1219–24.
205. Berek JS, Hacker NF, Lichtenstein A, et al. Intraperitoneal recombinant alpha-interferon for "salvage" immunotherapy in stage III epithelial ovarian cancer: a Gynecologic Oncology Group study. Cancer Res 1985;45:4447–53.
206. Berek JS, Markman M, Blessing JA, et al. Intraperitoneal—alpha-interferon alternating with cisplatin in residual ovarian cancer: a phase II Gynecologic Oncology Group study. Gynecol Oncol 1999;74:48–52.
207. Willemse PH, DeVries EG, Mulder NH, et al. Intraperitoneal human recombinant interferon-alpha in minimal residual ovarian cancer. Eur J Cancer 1990;26:353–7.
208. Berek JS, Welander C, Schink J, et al. A phase I-II trial of intraperitoneal cisplatin and alpha interferon in epithelial ovarian cancer. Gynecol Oncol 1991;40:237–42.
209. Berek JS, Markman M, Stonebraker B, et al. Intraperitoneal alpha-interferon in residual ovarian cancer: a phase II Gynecologic Oncology Group study. Gynecol Oncol 1999;75:10–4.
210. Pujade-Lauraine E, Guastella JP, Colombo N, et al. Intraperitoneal administration of interferon-y: an efficient adjuvant to chemotherapy of ovarian cancers. Apropos of a European study of 108 patients. Bull Cancer 1993;80:163–70.
211. Chapman PB, Kolitz JE, Hakes TB, et al. A phase I trial of intraperitoneal recombinant interleukin-2 in patients with ovarian cancer. Invest New Drugs 1988;6:179–84.
212. Bonavida B, Tsuchitani T, Zighelboim J, Berek JS. Synergy is documented in vitro with low-dose recombinant tumor necrosis factor, cisplatin, and doxorubicin in ovarian cancer cells. Gynecol Oncol 1990;38:333–9.
213. Nio Y, Zighelboim J, Berek JS, Bonavida B. Augmentation of cytotoxicity of lymphokine-activated killer cells on ovarian tumor cells by various biological response modifiers. Anticancer Res 1990;10:441–5.
214. Nardi M, Cognetti F, Pollera CF, et al. Intraperitoneal recombinant a-2-interferon alternating with cisplatin as salvage therapy for minimal residual disease ovarian cancer. A phase II study. J Clin Oncol 1990;8:1036–41.
215. Markman M, Berek JS, Blessing JA, et al. Characteristics of patients with small-volume residual ovarian cancer unresponsive to cisplatin-based IP chemotherapy: lessons learned from a Gynecologic Oncology Group phase II trial of IP cisplatin and recombinant a-interferon. Gynecol Oncol 1992;45:3–8.
216. Windbichler GH, Hausmaninger H, Stummvoll W, et al. Interferon-gamma in the first-line therapy of ovarian cancer: a randomized phase III trial. Br J Cancer 2000;82: 1138–44.
217. Boyer P, Berek JS, Zighelboim J. Lymphocyte activation by recombinant interleukin-2 in patients with ovarian cancer. Obstet Gynecol 1989;73:793–8.
218. Steis RG, Urba WJ, VanderMolen LA, et al. Intraperitoneal lymphokine-activated killer cell and interleukin-2 therapy for malignancies limited to the peritoneal cavity. J Clin Oncol 1990;8:1618–23.
219. Hird V, Maraveyas A, Snook D, et al. Adjuvant therapy of ovarian cancer with radioactive monoclonal antibody. Br J Cancer 1993;68:403–6.
220. Bookman MA, Darcy KM, Clarke-Pearson D, et al. Evaluation of monoclonal humanized anti-HER2 antibody, trastuzumab, in patients with recurrent or refractory ovarian or primary peritoneal carcinoma with overexpression of HER2: a phase II trial of the Gynecologic Oncology Group. J Clin Oncol 2003;21:283–90.
221. Schultes BC, Baum RP, Niesen A, et al. Anti-idiotype induction therapy: anti-CA125 antibody (Ab3) mediated tumor killing in patients treated with OvaRex MAb-B43.13 (Ab1). Cancer Immunol Immunother 1998;46:201–12.
222. Berger RA, Sill M, Monk BJ, et al. Phase II trial of bevacizumab in persistent or recurrent epithelial ovarian cancer or primary peritoneal cancer: A Gynecologic Group Study. Proc Am Soc Clin Oncol 2005; Abstract No. 5009.
223. Miller DS, Brady MF, Barrett RJ. A phase II trial of leuprolide acetate in patients with advanced epithelial ovarian cancer. J Clin Oncol 1992;15:125–8.
224. Lopez A, Tessadrelli A, Kudelka AP, et al. Combination therapy with leuprolide acetate and tamoxifen in refractory ovarian cancer. Int J Gynecol Cancer 1996;6:15–9.
225. Hatch KD, Beecham JB, Blessing JA, Creasman WT. Responsiveness of patients with advanced ovarian carcinoma to tamoxifen: a Gynecologic Oncology Group study of second-line therapy in 105 patients. Cancer 1991;68:269–71.
226. Van den Bossche HV, Moereels H, Koymans LM. Aromatase inhibitors–mechanisms for nonsteroidal inhibitors. Breast Cancer Res Treat 1994;30:43–55.
227. Gelblum D, Mychalczak B, Almadrones L, et al. Palliative benefit of external-beam radiation in the management of platinum refractory epithelial ovarian carcinoma. Gynecol Oncol 1998;69:36–41
228. Voest EE, van Houwelingen JC, Neijt JP. A meta-analysis of prognostic factors in advanced ovarian cancer with median survival and overall survival measured with log (relative risk) as main objectives. Eur J Cancer Clin Oncol 1989;25:711–5.
229. Omura GA, Brady MF, Homesley HD, et al. Long-term follow-up and prognostic factor analysis in advanced ovarian carcinoma: the Gynecologic Oncology Group experience. J Clin Oncol 1991;9:1138–50.
230. Sharp F, Blackett AD, Berek JS, Bast RC Jr. Conclusions and recommendations from the Helene Harris Memorial Trust sixth biennial international forum on ovarian cancer. Int J Gynecol Cancer 1997;7:416–24.
231. van Houwelingen JC, ten Bokkel Huinink WW, van der Burg ATM, et al. Predictability of the survival of patients with ovarian cancer. J Clin Oncol 1989;7:769–73.
232. Heintz AP, Odicino F, Maisonneuve P, et al. Carcinoma of the ovary. Int J Gynaecol Obstet 2003;83 Suppl 1:135–66.
233. McGuire WP, Ozols RF. Chemotherapy of advanced ovarian cancer. Semin Oncol 1998;25:340–8.
234. Abu-Rustum NR, Aghajanian C. Management of malignant germ cell tumors of the ovary. Semin Oncol 1998;25:235–42.
235. Bjorkholm E, Lundell M, Gyftodimos A, Silfversward C. Dysgerminoma. The Radiumhemmet series 1927–1984. Cancer 1990;65:38–43.
236. Berek JS, Hacker NF. Nonepithelial ovarian and tubal cancers. In: Berek JS, Hacker, editors. Practical gynecologic oncology. 4th ed. Philadelphia MD: Lippincott, Williams & Wilkins; 2005. p. 511–41.
237. Obata NH, Nakashima N, Kawai M, et al. Gonadoblastoma with dysgerminoma in one ovary and gonadoblastoma with dysgerminoma and yolk sac tumor in the contralateral ovary in a girl with 46XX karyotype. Gynecol Oncol 1995;58:124–8.
238. Gordon A, Lipton D, Woodruff JD. Dysgerminoma: a review of 158 cases from the Emil Novak Ovarian Tumor Registry. Obstet Gynecol 1981;58:497–452.
239. Gershenson DM. Menstrual and reproductive function after treatment with combination chemotherapy for malignant ovarian germ cell tumors. J Clin Oncol 1988;6:270–4.
240. Gershenson DM, Morris M, Cangir A, et al. Treatment of malignant germ cell tumors of the ovary with bleomycin, etoposide, and cisplatin. J Clin Oncol 1990;8:715–9.
241. Williams SD, Blessing JA, Slayton, et al. Ovarian germ cell tumors: adjuvant trials of the Gynecologic Oncology Group. J Clin Oncol 1994;12:701–6.
242. Williams SD, Blessing JA, Moore DH, et al. Cisplatin, vinblastine, and bleomycin in advanced and recurrent ovarian germ cell tumors. Ann Intern Med 1989;111:22.
243. Kurtz JE, Jaeck D, Maloisel F, et al. Combined modality treatment for malignant transformation of a benign ovarian teratoma. Gynecol Oncol 1999;73:319–21.
244. Gershenson DM. Update on malignant ovarian germ cell tumors. Cancer 1993;71:1581–90.
245. Williams SD, Blessing JA, Hatch K, Homesley HD. Chemotherapy of advanced ovarian dysgerminoma: trials of the Gynecologic Oncology Group. J Clin Oncol 1991;9:1950–5.
246. Williams SD, Blessing JA, Liao S, et al. Adjuvant therapy of ovarian germ cell tumors with cisplatin, etoposide, and bleomycin: a trial of the Gynecologic Oncology Group. J Clin Oncol 1994;12:701–6.
247. Williams SD, Brady M, Burnett A, et al. Adjuvant therapy of resected dysgerminoma with carboplatin and etoposide [abstract]. Proc Soc Gyn Oncol 1999;114.
248. Williams SD, Birch R, Einhorn LH, et al. Treatment of disseminated germ cell tumors with cisplatin, bleomycin and either vinblastine or etoposide. N Engl J Med 1987;316:1435–40.
249. Bajorin DF, Sarosdy MF, Bosl GJ, et al. A randomized trial of etoposide plus carboplatin versus etoposide plus cisplatin in patients with metastatic germ cell tumors. J Clin Oncol 1993;11:598–603.
250. Loehrer PJ, Johnson D, Elson P, et al. Importance of bleomycin in favorable-prognosis disseminated germ cell tumors: an Eastern Cooperative Oncology Group trial. J Clin Oncol 1995;13:470–6.
251. Culine S, Lhomme C, Michel G, et al. Is there a role for second-look laparotomy in the management of malignant germ cell tumors of the ovary? Experience at Institute Gustave Roussy. J Surg Oncol 1996;62:40–5.
252. Schwartz PE, Chambers SK, Chambers JT, et al. Ovarian germ cell malignancies: the Yale University experience. Gynecol Oncol 1992;45:26–31.
253. Imai A, Furui T, Tamaya T. Gynecologic tumors and symptoms in childhood and adolescence: 10-years' experience. Int J Gynaecol Obstet 1994;45:227–34.
254. Bekaii-Saab T, Einhorn LH, Williams SD. Late relapse of ovarian dysgerminoma: case report and literature review. Gynecol Oncol 1999;72:111–2.
255. Williams SD, Blessing JA, DiSaia PJ, et al. Second-look laparotomy in ovarian germ cell tumors. Gynecol Oncol 1994;52:287–91.
256. Williams SD, Wong LC, Ngan HYS. Management of ovarian germ cell tumors. In: Gershenson DM, McGuire WP, editors. Ovarian cancer. New York, NY: Churchill-Livingston; 1998. p. 399–415.
257. Gershenson DM. Management of early ovarian cancer: germ cell and sex-cord stromal tumors. Gynecol Oncol 1994;55:S62–72.
258. Wong LC, Ngan HYS, Ma HK. Primary treatment with vincristine, dactinomycin, and cyclophosphamide in nondysgerminomatous germ cell tumour of the ovary. Gynecol Oncol 1989;34:155–8.
259. De Palo G, Zambetti M, Pilotti S, et al. Non-dysgerminomatous tumors of the ovary treated with cisplatin, vinblastine, and bleomycin: long-term results. Gynecol Oncol 1992;47:239–46.
260. O'Conner DM, Norris HJ. The influence of grade on the outcome of stage I ovarian immature (malignant) teratomas and the reproducibility of grading. Int J Gynecol Pathol 1994;13:283–9.
261. Culine S, Kattan J, Lhomme C, et al. A phase II study of

high-dose cisplatin, vinblastine, bleomycin, and etoposide (PVeBV regimen) in malignant non-dysgerminomatous germ-cell tumors of the ovary. Gynecol Oncol 1994;54:47–53.
262. Talerman A. Germ cell tumors of the ovary. Curr Opin Obstet Gynecol 1997;9:44–7.
263. Culine S, Lhomme C, Kattan J, et al. Cisplatin-based chemotherapy in the management of germ cell tumors of the ovary: the Institute Gustave Roussy experience. Gynecol Oncol 1997;64:160–5.
264. Fujita M, Inoue M, Tanizawa O, et al. Retrospective review of 41 patients with endodermal sinus tumor of the ovary. Int J Gynecol Cancer 1993;3:329–35.
265. Sasaki H, Furusata M, Teshima S, et al. Prognostic significance of histopathological subtypes in stage I pure yolk sac tumour of the ovary. Br J Cancer 1994;69:529–36.
266. Cangir A, Smith J, VanEys J. Improved prognosis in children with ovarian cancers following modified VAC (vincristine sulfate, dactinomycin, and cyclophosphamide) chemotherapy. Cancer 1978;42:1234–8.
267. Kurman RJ, Norris HJ. Endodermal sinus tumor of the ovary: a clinical and pathological analysis of 71 cases. Cancer 1976;38:2404–9.
268. Gershenson DM, Wharton JT, Kline RC, et al. Chemotherapeutic complete remission in patients with metastatic ovarian dysgerminoma. Cancer 1986;58:2594–8.
269. Slayton RE, Park RC, Silverberg SC, et al. Vincristine, dactinomycin, and cyclophosphamide (VAC) in the treatment of malignant germ cell tumors of the ovary: a Gynecologic Oncology Group study (a final report). Cancer 1985;56:243–8.
270. Gershenson DM, Del Junco G, Copeland LJ, Rutledge FN. Mixed germ cell tumors of the ovary. Obstet Gynecol 1984;64:200–6.
271. Kurman RJ, Norris HJ. Embryonal carcinoma of the ovary. A clinicopathologic entity distinct from endodermal sinus tumor resembling embryonal carcinoma of the adult testis. Cancer 1976;38:2420–7.
272. Oliva E, Andrada E, Pezzica E, Prat J. Ovarian carcinomas with choriocarcinomatous differentiation. Cancer 1993;72:2441–6.
273. Simosek T, Trak B, Tunoc M, et al. Primary pure choriocarcinoma of the ovary in reproductive ages. Eur J Gynaecol Oncol 1998;19:284–6.
274. Hildebrandt RH, Rouse RV, Longacre TA. Value of inhibin in the identification of granulosa cell tumors of the ovary. Human Pathol 1997;28:1387–95.
275. Lappohn RE, Burger HG, Bouma J, et al. Inhibin as a marker for granulosa-cell tumors. N Engl J Med 1989;321:790–3.
276. Richi M, Howard LN, Bratthauae GL, Tavassoli FA. Use of monoclonal antibody against human inhibin as a marker for sex–cord-stromal tumors of the ovary. Am J Surg Pathol 1997:21:583–9.
277. Malmstrom H, Hogberg T, Bjorn R, Simonson E. Granulosa cell tumors of the ovary: prognostic factors and outcome. Gynecol Oncol 1994;52:50–5.
278. Schumer ST, Cannistra SA. Granulosa cell tumor of the ovary. J Clin Oncol 2003;21:1180–9.
279. Gershenson DM, Copeland LJ, Kavanagh JJ, et al. Treatment of metastatic stromal tumors of the ovary with cisplatin, doxorubicin, and cyclophosphamide. Obstet Gynecol 1987;5:765–9.
280. Miller BE, Barron BA, Wan JY, et al. Prognostic factors in adult granulosa cell tumor of the ovary. Cancer 1997;79:1951–5.
281. Holland DR, Le Riche J, Swenerton KD, et al. Flow cytometric assessment of DNA ploidy is a useful prognostic factor for patients with granulosa cell ovarian tumors. Int J Gynecol Cancer 1991;1:227–32.
282. Young RH, Scully RE. Ovarian sex–cord-stromal tumors: problems in differential diagnosis. Pathol Ann 1988;23:237–96.
283. Young RH, Oliva E, Scully RE. Small cell sarcoma of the ovary, hypercalcemic type: a clinicopathological analysis of 150 cases. Am J Surg Pathol 1994;18:1102–16.
284. Barakat RR, Rubin SC, Wong G, et al. Mixed mesodermal tumor of the ovary: analysis of prognostic factors in 31 cases. Obstet Gynecol 1992;80:660–4.
285. Fowler JM, Nathan L, Nieberg RK, Berek JS. Mixed mesodermal sarcoma of the ovary in a young patient. Eur J Obstet Gynecol Reprod Biol 1996;65:249–53.
286. Woodruff JD, Novak ER. The Krukenberg tumor. Study of 48 cases from the Emil Novak Ovarian Tumor Registry. Obstet Gynecol 1960;15:351 center 9103. J Clin Oncol 1993;11:2405–11.
287. Young RH, Scully RE. Metastatic tumors in the ovary: a problem-oriented approach and review of the recent literature. Semin Diagn Pathol 1991;8:250–76.
288. Young RH, Scully RE. Malignant melanoma metastatic to the ovary: a clinicopathologic analysis of 20 cases. Am J Surg Pathol 1991;15:849–60.
289. Petru E, Pickel H, Heydarfadai M, et al. Non-genital cancers metastatic to the ovary. Gynecol Oncol 1992;44:83–6.
290. Curtin JP, Barakat RR, Hoskins WJ. Ovarian disease in women with breast cancer. Obstet Gynecol 1994;84:449–52.
291. Motoyama T, Katayama Y, Watanabe H, et al. Functioning ovarian carcinoids induce severe constipation. Cancer 1991;70:513–8.
292. Monterroso V, Jaffe ES, Merino MJ, Medeiros LJ. Malignant lymphomas involving the ovary: a clinicopathologic analysis of 39 cases. Am J Surg Pathol 1993;17:154–70.

105

Gestational Trophoblastic Disease

Ross S. Berkowitz, MD
Donald P. Goldstein, MD

Gestational trophoblastic disease (GTD) comprises a group of interrelated diseases that includes complete and partial molar pregnancy, invasive mole, placental site trophoblastic tumor (PSTT), and choriocarcinoma, which have varying propensities for invasion and spread. Gestational trophoblastic tumors (GTTs) are one of the rare human malignancies that are highly curable, even with widespread metastases.[1,2] Although GTTs most commonly follow a molar pregnancy, they may ensue after any gestation. This chapter discusses basic principles of management and recent advances in the diagnosis and treatment of GTDs.

HISTORICAL PERSPECTIVE

In 1956, Li, Hertz, and Spencer inaugurated a new era in the management of GTT when they reported complete regression of metastatic choriocarcinoma in three women treated with methotrexate (MTX).[3] Hertz and colleagues then reviewed the initial 5-year experience with MTX therapy at the National Cancer Institute and reported complete remission in 28 (47%) of 63 patients with metastatic choriocarcinoma.[4] While MTX was a highly effective therapy, it became apparent that it was necessary to identify other active agents. Ross and colleagues first employed actinomycin D (Act-D) in 13 patients with MTX resistance, and 6 patients achieved complete remission.[5] Act-D then joined MTX as the primary single agents in the treatment of GTT.

During the late 1960s, it became increasingly apparent that certain patients with metastatic GTT were relatively resistant to single-agent chemotherapy and experienced a high mortality rate. Ross and colleagues reported that patients with high human chorionic gonadotropin (hCG) levels, delays in diagnosis, and cerebral and hepatic metastases commonly did not attain remission with single-agent treatment.[6] These authors advised that primary combination chemotherapy should be administered in patients with high-risk metastatic GTT.

Etoposide (VP-16) was identified as a highly active agent in GTT in the 1980s. Wong and colleagues reported that primary etoposide induced complete remission in 56 (93%) of 60 patients with GTT.[7] Bagshawe reported that including etoposide with MTX and Act-D resulted in 83% complete remission in high-risk metastatic GTT.[8]

Most patients with GTT can now anticipate a high cure rate with appropriate therapy and follow-up. Because remission can often be achieved while retaining fertility, many patients later have normal pregnancies. However, patients with protracted delays in diagnosis, particularly after nonmolar pregnancies, still present with extensive tumor burdens and are at substantial risk for treatment failure. Efforts are still needed to improve early diagnosis and to develop new effective chemotherapy regimens.

EPIDEMIOLOGY

The reported incidence of GTD varies substantially in different regions of the world. The frequency of molar pregnancy in Asian countries is 3 to 10 times greater than the reported incidence in North America or Europe.[9] Variations in the incidence rates of molar pregnancy partly result from differences between reporting hospital-based versus population-based data. The incidence of complete and partial mole has been determined in Ireland by studying all products of conception from spontaneous abortions.[10] Based upon a thorough pathologic review, the incidence of complete and partial mole was found to be 1 in 1,945 and 1 in 695 pregnancies, respectively.

The high incidence of molar pregnancy in some populations has been attributed to socioeconomic and nutritional factors. Case-control studies have observed that the risk for complete molar pregnancy progressively increased with decreasing levels of consumption of dietary carotene (vitamin A precursor) and animal fat.[11,12] Global regions with a high incidence of vitamin A deficiency correspond to areas with a high frequency of molar pregnancy. Dietary factors such as carotene may therefore partly explain the regional variations in the incidence of molar pregnancy.

The risk of having a complete molar pregnancy also increases with advanced maternal age. Parazzini and colleagues noted that the risk for complete mole was increased two-fold for women older than age 35 years and 7.5-fold for women older than age 40 years.[13] Ova from older women may be more susceptible to abnormal fertilizations. However, the risk for partial mole has not been associated with maternal age.

Etiology Complete moles usually have a 46,XX karyotype and all molar chromosomes are derived from paternal origin.[14] Most complete moles arise from an anuclear ovum that is fertilized by a haploid sperm, which then duplicates its own chromosomes.[15] While most complete moles have a 46,XX karyotype, approximately 10% of complete moles have a 46,XY chromosomal pattern.[16] The 46,XY complete mole arises from fertilization of an anuclear ovum by two spermatozoa. While the chromosomes in the complete mole are entirely of paternal origin, the mitochondrial deoxyribonucleic acid (DNA) is of maternal origin.[17]

Partial moles generally have a triploid karyotype resulting from fertilization of an apparently normal ovum by two spermatozoa.[18] Lage and colleagues[19] and Lawler and colleagues[20] reported that 93% and 90%, respectively, of partial moles were triploid. When fetuses are identified with partial moles, they generally have the stigmata of triploidy, including multiple congenital anomalies and growth retardation. Both complete and partial moles are therefore characterized by an excessive amount of paternal chromosomes, which may induce trophoblastic hyperplasia.

Because GTTs contain paternal genetic material, these tumors are at least a partial allograft. It has been suggested that the regression of GTT following chemotherapy may be partly attributable to host immunologic defenses. Survival with choriocarcinoma has been reported to be more favorable in the presence of a marked lymphocytic infiltrate at the tumor–host interface.[21] Cytokines from activated immune cells have been shown in vitro to inhibit proliferation of choriocarcinoma cells and to enhance human leukocyte antigen (HLA) expression of these cells, thereby increasing their potential immunogenicity.[22,23] Furthermore, Tomoda and colleagues reported HLA compatibility between patients and their partners in drug-resistant choriocarcinoma.[24] The HLA system may therefore influence the natural history of rapidly progressive and fatal choriocarcinoma. However, histocompatibility between patients and their partners does not appear to be a prerequisite for the development and persistence of choriocarcinoma.[25]

HISTOPATHOLOGIC CLASSIFICATION OF GTD

Hydatidiform mole may be categorized as either complete or partial on the basis of gross morphology, histopathology, and karyotype.[26] Complete moles have diffuse swelling of the chorionic villi and diffuse trophoblastic hyperplasia. Embryonic or fetal tissues are not identifiable (Figures 105-1 and 105-2). Partial moles are characterized by the presence of two populations of chorionic villi.

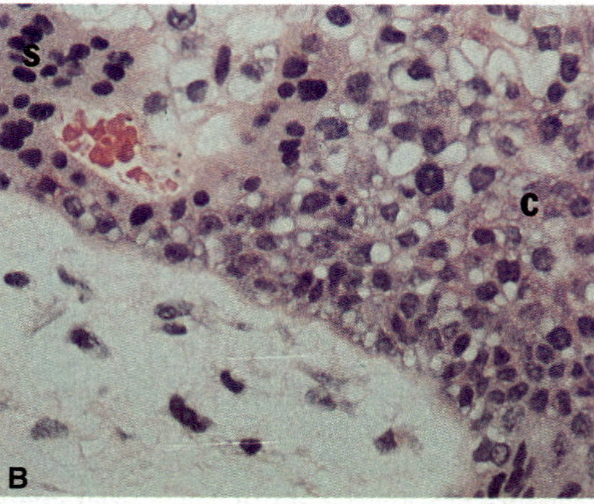

Figure 105-1 First trimester abortion. **A,** Chorionic villi containing fetal blood vessels *(arrows)* in edematous stroma, lined by two layers of trophoblastic cells. Note unipolar trophoblastic proliferation. (Hematoxylin and eosin, ×100.) **B,** Polar trophoblastic proliferation of cytotrophoblast *(c)* and syncytiotrophoblast *(s)*. (Hematoxylin and eosin, ×400.) (Courtesy of Liane Deligdisch, MD, Mount Sinai Medical Center, New York.)

Some chorionic villi exhibit focal swelling and focal trophoblastic hyperplasia as well as villous scalloping and stromal trophoblastic inclusions. Fetal and embryonic tissues are commonly present.

Following both complete and partial mole, patients may develop persistent GTT with either local uterine invasion or metastasis. Postmolar GTT may have the histologic features of either molar tissue or choriocarcinoma.

Choriocarcinoma does not contain chorionic villi but is composed of sheets of both anaplastic cyto- and syncytiotrophoblasts (Figure 105-3). Although choriocarcinoma is most commonly preceded by a molar pregnancy, it may develop after any gestational event. After a nonmolar pregnancy, persistent GTT always has the histologic pattern of choriocarcinoma.

PSTT is an uncommon variant of choriocarcinoma.[27] PSTT is composed almost entirely of mononuclear intermediate trophoblast and does not contain chorionic villi.

MOLECULAR PATHOGENESIS

While the precise molecular pathogenesis of molar pregnancy and choriocarcinoma has not been determined, various growth factors and oncogenes have been studied in these tissues.[28,29] Complete mole and choriocarcinoma are characterized by overexpression of c-*myc*, c-*erbB-2*, *bcl-2*, *TP53*, and Rb, and these oncoproteins may be important in the pathogenesis of GTD.[30,31] Strong immunostaining of epidermal growth factor receptor and c-erb B-3 in the extravillous trophoblast of complete mole was found to be significantly correlated with the development of postmolar tumor.[32]

Familial recurrent molar pregnancy is an infrequent occurrence, but may provide important insights into the molecular biology and genetic pathogenesis of molar pregnancy.[33] Twelve families have been reported in which at least two close relatives have had molar pregnancies and consanguinity was observed in about half of the families. Affected women have had 152 pregnancies resulting in 113 (74 %) complete moles, 26 (17 %) spontaneous abortions, 6 (4 %) partial moles, and only 7 (5%) normal pregnancies. Strikingly, the complete moles in these patients were biparental with one haploid set of both maternal and paternal chromosomes. In normal gestations, certain genes are parentally imprinted such that they are normally expressed only on the maternal or paternal alleles. Although these moles were biparental, the molar tissue did not express maternally transcribed genes like $p57^{KIP2}$ similar to the more usual androgenetic complete moles. Dysregulation of normal parental imprinting of genes with the loss of maternally transcribed genes is likely to be an important event in the pathogenesis of complete mole. Linkage and homozygosity mapping in a large consanguineous family enabled the gene for familial recurrent mole to be mapped to a 1.1 Mb region on chromosome 19 q 13.4.[34] Mutation in this gene or genes likely result in dysregulation of genetic imprinting in the female germ line with abnormal development of extraembryonic and embryonic tissues.

NATURAL HISTORY

Presentation of Complete Molar Pregnancy Vaginal bleeding is the most common presenting symptom in patients with complete mole, occurring in 97% of our patients.[35] Because of earlier diagnosis, patients now less-commonly present with signs of marked trophoblastic proliferation, including excessive uterine enlargement, theca lutein ovarian cysts, and toxemia.[36] Theca lutein cysts result from ovarian hyperstimulation by high serum levels of hCG.

Patients with complete mole and excessive uterine enlargement and high hCG values are at increased risk for such medical complications as toxemia, hyperthyroidism, and respiratory insuf-

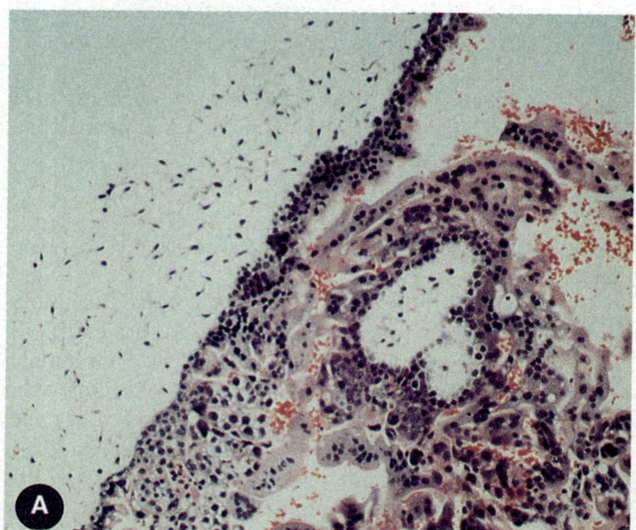

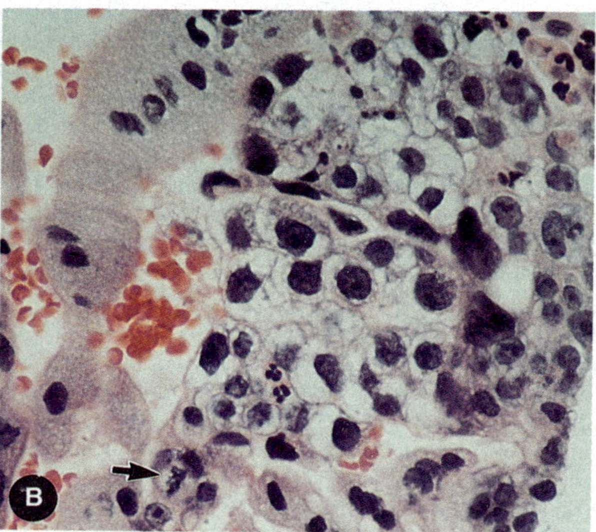

Figure 105-2 Hydatidiform mole. **A,** Chorionic villi with edema and hydropic degeneration (central cistern *top left*). Trophoblastic proliferation is circumferential rather than polar. (Hematoxylin and eosin, ×100.) **B,** Marked proliferation of cytotrophoblastic and syncytiotrophoblast showing nuclear atypia and mitotic activity *(arrows)*. (Hematoxylin and eosin, ×400.) (Courtesy of Liane Deligdisch, MD, Mount Sinai Medical Center, New York.)

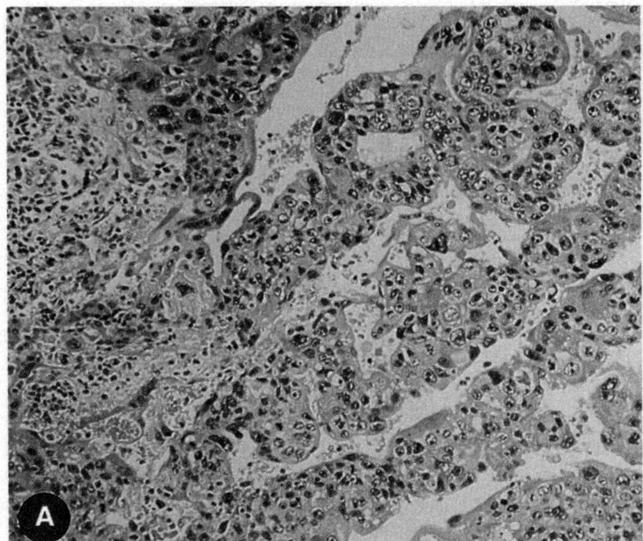

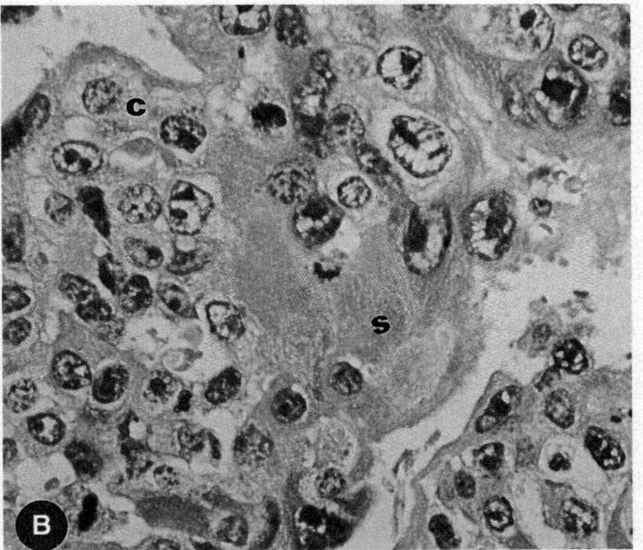

Figure 105-3 Choriocarcinoma. **A,** No villous structure is present. Tumor shows necrosis and hemorrhage at left. (Hematoxylin and eosin, ×100.) **B,** Biphasic tumor pattern composed of severely atypical cytotrophoblasts *(c)* and syncytiotrophoblastic *(s)* cells with high mitotic activity. (Hematoxylin and eosin, ×400.) (Courtesy of Liane Deligdisch, MD, Mount Sinai Medical Center, New York.)

ficiency. While hCG has been proposed as a thyroid stimulator, data concerning hCG levels and thyroid function tests are conflicting.[37] The cause of respiratory insufficiency is usually multifactorial, including trophoblastic embolization as well as the cardiopulmonary effects of toxemia, hyperthyroidism, and vigorous transfusion therapy.

Presentation of Partial Molar Pregnancy Patients with partial mole usually present with the signs and symptoms of missed or incomplete abortion. Excessive uterine enlargement is noted in only 4 to 11% of patients with partial mole.[38,39] We reviewed 81 consecutive patients with partial mole and none of our patients had respiratory insufficiency, hyperthyroidism, or prominent ovarian theca lutein cysts, and only two presented with toxemia.[38] The diagnosis of partial mole is generally considered only after histologic review of the curettage specimens.

Postmolar GTT Complete moles develop uterine invasion or metastasis in 15% and 4% of patients, respectively.[40] The risk for postmolar tumor is substantially increased in complete moles with signs of marked trophoblastic proliferation such as excessive uterine size, high serum hCG levels (> 100,000 mIU/mL), and theca lutein ovarian cysts.[40] Following evacuation, 31% of these patients developed uterine invasion and 9% developed metastases. The risk for postmolar tumor is considerably less for patients who do not present with signs of marked trophoblastic growth. After evacuation, only 3.4% of these patients developed invasion and 0.6% developed metastases. Therefore, patients with complete moles with excessive uterine size and markedly elevated hCG values are categorized as high risk.

Older patients with complete moles are also at increased risk of developing postmolar tumor. Tow[41] and Tsukamoto and colleagues[42] reported that 37% of women older than age 40 years and 56% of women older than age 50 years, respectively, developed persistent tumor after a complete mole.

Approximately 4% of patients with partial mole develop persistent tumor, which is generally nonmetastatic.[43] Patients who developed persistent GTT following partial mole did not have distinguishing clinical or pathologic characteristics.[44]

Presentation of Nonmetastatic GTT Locally invasive GTT occurs in approximately 15% of patients after complete mole and infrequently after other pregnancies.[40] These patients may present with persistently elevated hCG levels, irregular vaginal bleeding, uterine subinvolution or asymmetric enlargement, and/or theca lutein ovarian cysts. Trophoblastic tumor may erode into uterine vessels, causing vaginal hemorrhage, or may perforate through the myometrium, producing intraabdominal bleeding. Bulky necrotic tumor may also be a nidus for uterine sepsis, causing pelvic pain and purulent discharge.

Presentation of Metastatic GTT Metastatic tumor develops in approximately 4% of patients after complete mole and infrequently after other gestations.[40] Metastases are commonly choriocarcinoma, which has a propensity for early vascular invasion and dissemination. Patients may present with signs and symptoms of bleeding from metastases such as hemoptysis, hepatic rupture, or acute neurologic deficits.

The most common site of metastasis is the lungs. Eighty percent of patients with metastatic GTT have pulmonary involvement on chest radiographs. Because respiratory symptoms and radiographic findings may be striking, the patient may be thought to have a primary pulmonary process. Pulmonary hypertension may develop as a result of pulmonary arterial occlusion by trophoblastic emboli. The development of early respiratory failure requiring intubation is associated with a dismal outcome.[45] Importantly, gynecologic symptoms may be minimal or absent. The diagnosis of GTT should be considered in any woman in the reproductive age group with unexplained pulmonary or systemic symptoms.

Vaginal metastases are present in 30% of patients with metastatic GTT. Because these lesions are highly vascular, they may bleed vigorously if biopsied.

Hepatic and cerebral metastases occur in approximately 10% of patients with metastatic GTT. Hepatic and cerebral lesions are generally choriocarcinoma and usually follow a nonmolar pregnancy. These patients generally have protracted delays in diagnosis and extensive tumor burdens. Virtually all patients with hepatic and cerebral metastases have concurrent pulmonary or vaginal involvement.[46,47]

DIAGNOSIS

Complete and Partial Molar Pregnancy Complete molar pregnancy is reliably diagnosed by ultrasonography. Complete moles have a characteristic vesicular sonographic pattern because of the diffuse hydropic swelling of the chorionic villi. Ultrasonography may also contribute to the diagnosis of partial mole by demonstrating focal cystic spaces in the placenta or an increase in the transverse diameter of the gestational sac.[48]

Persistent GTT Following molar pregnancy, the diagnosis of GTT is generally made by the presence of a plateau in the hCG level for at least 3 weeks or a rising hCG level. A persistently elevated hCG measurement without evidence of either intrauterine or ectopic pregnancy is also strongly suggestive of the diagnosis of GTT in any woman in the reproductive age group. These patients may present with gynecologic and/or systemic symptoms. Biopsy of metastatic lesions for diagnosis should be avoided because it may result in exsanguinating hemorrhage. Patients with elevated hCG values should also be considered potentially to have a pregnancy, germ cell tumor of the ovary or other site, a nontrophoblastic gonadotropin-producing tumor, or phantom hCG caused by heterophilic antibody.[49]

STAGING

An anatomic staging system for GTT has been adopted by the International Federation of Gynecology and Obstetrics (FIGO):

Stage I: Lesion confined to uterus
Stage II: Lesion outside uterus but confined to vagina and pelvis
Stage III: Lung metastases
Stage IV: Other metastatic sites (brain, liver)

In addition to anatomic staging, it is useful to consider other prognostic variables that predict the likelihood of drug resistance and assist in selecting chemotherapy. The World Health Organization (WHO) has proposed a prognostic scoring system, which is listed in Table 105-1.[50] When the prognostic score is greater than 7, the patient is categorized as high risk and requires intensive combination chemotherapy to attain remission. Patients with stage I GTT usually have a low-risk score, and those with stage IV GTT generally have a high-risk score. Therefore, the distinction between low and high risk mainly applies to patients with stages II and III disease.

THERAPY

MOLAR PREGNANCY **Surgical Evacuation** When a molar pregnancy is diagnosed, the patient should be evaluated for possible medical complications such as anemia, toxemia, or hyperthyroidism. If the patient desires surgical sterilization, a hysterectomy may be performed. However, suction curettage is the preferred method of evacuation, regardless of uterine size, in patients who desire to preserve fertility.[35]

Prophylactic Chemotherapy Several investigators have reported that prophylactic chemotherapy at the time of molar evacuation reduces the frequency of postmolar tumor.[51,52] Kim and colleagues and Limpongsanurak reported in prospective randomized trials that prophylactic MTX and Act-D, respectively, reduced the incidence of postmolar tumor from 47 to 14% and from 5 to 14%, respectively, in patients with high-risk complete mole.[53,54] Prophylactic chemotherapy may be particularly beneficial in patients with high-risk complete moles when hormonal follow-up is either unavailable or unreliable.

Hormonal Follow-Up All patients should be followed after molar evacuation with hCG measurements to assure remission. Patients are followed with weekly hCG values until undetectable for 3 weeks, and then monthly until undetectable for 6 months.

Patients are encouraged to use reliable contraception during the entire interval of hormonal follow-up. While the incidence of postmolar tumor has been reported to be increased in patients using oral contraceptives, data from the Gynecologic Oncology Group and our center indicate that oral contraceptives do not affect the risk for postmolar GTT.[55–57]

GTT The optimal management of GTT requires a thorough evaluation of the extent of the disease prior to treatment (Figure 105-4). Metastatic work-up should include a chest roentgenogram, ultrasonography of the abdomen and pelvis, and head computed tomography (CT) or magnetic resonance imaging (MRI) scans. While measurement of hCG in the cerebrospinal fluid (CSF) may suggest cerebral involvement, a single plasma to CSF hCG ratio may be misleading because rapid changes in plasma hCG levels may not be promptly reflected in the CSF.[47]

Table 105-1 Scoring System for Gestational Trophoblastic Tumors Based on Prognostic Factors

	Score[a]			
	0	1	2	4
Age (years)	<- 39	> 39		
Antecedent pregnancy	Mole	Abortion	Term	
Interval[b]	< 4	4–6	7–12	
hCG (IU/L)	$< 10^3$	10^3–10^4	10^4–10^5	
ABO groups		O × A	B	
(female × male)		A × O	AB	
Largest tumor, including uterine tumor		3–5 cm	5 cm	
Site of metastases		Spleen, kidney	Gastrointestinal tract, liver	Brain
No. of metastases identified		1–4	4–8	> 8
Prior chemotherapy			Single drug	2 or more drug

[a]Interval is the time (months) between end of antecedent pregnancy and start of chemotherapy.
[b]The total score for a patient is obtained by adding the individual scores for each prognostic factor. Total score: < 4 = low risk; 5–7 = intermediate risk; >- 8 = high risk.
Data from World Health Organization.[50]

STAGE I THERAPY **Primary Therapy of Stage I GTT** The selection of primary therapy of stage I GTT is based upon the patient's desire to preserve fertility. If the patient no longer wishes to retain fertility, hysterectomy with adjuvant single-agent chemotherapy may be performed as

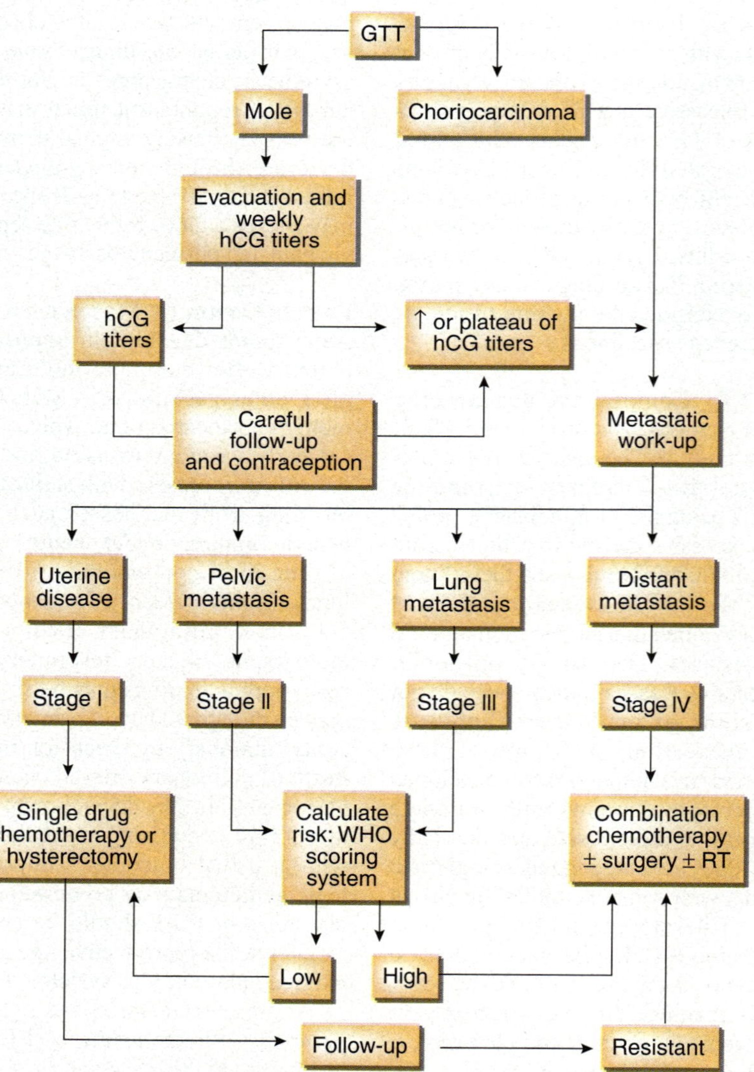

Figure 105-4 Algorithm for the management of gestational trophoblastic disease.

primary treatment. Adjuvant chemotherapy is administered to treat any occult metastases that may already be present. Occult pulmonary metastases are detected by CT scan in 40% patients with presumed nonmetastatic disease.[58] Single-agent chemotherapy with either MTX or Act-D is the preferred treatment in patients with stage I GTT who desire to retain fertility.

Nonmetastatic PSTT should be treated with hysterectomy because of its poor response to chemotherapy.[27] Patients with metastatic PSTT may still achieve remission with intensive combination chemotherapy and surgical intervention.[59]

Secondary Therapy of Stage I GTT Patients with resistance to single-agent chemotherapy are treated with combination chemotherapy with MTX, Act-D, and cyclophosphamide (MAC)[60] (Table 105-2); or etoposide, MTX, Act-D, cyclophosphamide, and Oncovin (EMA-CO) (Table 105-3); or surgical therapy (hysterectomy or local resection). MAC is preferred as the initial combination chemotherapy in these patients because etoposide is associated with an increased risk for second tumors.[61] If the disease is resistant to both single-agent and combination chemotherapy, and if the patient wants to preserve fertility, local uterine resection may be considered. Ultrasonography, MRI scan, and/or arteriography may identify the site of resistant uterine tumor when local resection is planned.

Stages II and III Therapy While patients with low-risk stages II and III GTT (prognostic score ≤7) are treated with primary single-agent chemotherapy with MTX or Act-D, patients with high-risk disease are managed with primary combination chemotherapy with EMA-CO. Patients with disease resistant to single-agent chemotherapy are then treated with EMA-CO. Patients with disease resistant to EMA-CO may be treated by modifying that regimen by substituting cisplatin and etoposide on day 8, and escalating the dose of MTX infusion to 1 g/m^2 (EMA-CE) (Table 105-4).[62]

Stage IV Therapy All patients with stage IV GTT are managed with primary combination chemotherapy with EMA-CO. In the presence of cerebral metastases, the MTX dosage in the infusion is increased to 1 g/m^2.[8] Patients with disease resistant to EMA-CO may then be treated with EMA-CE.

Follow-Up of GTT All patients with stages I, II, and III GTT are followed with weekly hCG values until undetectable for 3 weeks, and then monthly until undetectable for 12 months. Patients with stage IV GTT are followed monthly for 24 months because they are at greater risk for late relapse. All patients must be encouraged to use effective contraception during the entire interval of monitoring.

Surgical Therapy in GTT Surgery is performed to either treat complications of disease or to excise sites of resistant tumor.[63] Hysterectomy may be performed to control uterine hemorrhage or sepsis or to reduce the tumor burden and thereby limit the need for chemotherapy. Bleeding from vaginal metastases may be managed by packing, wide local excision, or arteriographic embolization of the hypogastric arteries. Thoracotomy may be performed to excise persistent viable tumor despite intensive chemotherapy. However, fibrotic nodules may persist indefinitely on chest roentgenograms after complete gonadotropin remission is attained. Hepatic resection may be required to manage hepatic rupture and craniotomy may be necessary to provide acute decompression or to control bleeding.[63]

Radiation Therapy in GTT If cerebral metastases are detected, whole-brain irradiation is promptly instituted at most centers in the United States. The risk of spontaneous cerebral hemorrhage may be reduced by the concurrent use of brain irradiation and chemotherapy. Yordan and colleagues reported that deaths as a result of cerebral involvement occurred in 11 (44%) of 25 patients treated with chemotherapy alone, but in none of 18 patients treated with brain irradiation and chemotherapy.[64]

Administration of Chemotherapy ***Single-Agent Chemotherapy*** Single-agent chemotherapy with either MTX or Act-D has achieved excellent and comparable remission rates in both nonmetastatic and low-risk metastatic GTT.[65] Several protocols using MTX and Act-D have been effectively used in the treatment of GTT, but no study has compared all of these regimens (Tables 105-5 and 105-6).[66–70] Single-agent chemotherapy is administered either at a fixed time interval or on the basis of the hCG regression

Table 105-2 MAC Regimen

Day/Time	Therapy
1	MTX, 1.0 mg/kg, IM Act-D, 12 μg/kg, IV push cyclophosphamide, 3 mg/kg IV bolus
2	FA, 0.1 mg/kg, IM or po Act-D, 12 μg/kg, IV push cyclophosphamide, 3 mg/kg IV bolus
3	MTX, 1.0 mg/kg, IM Act-D, 12 μg/kg, IV push cyclophosphamide, 3 mg/kg IV bolus
4	FA, 0.1 mg/kg, IM or po Act-D, 12 μg/kg, IV push cyclophosphamide, 3 mg/kg IV bolus
5	MTX, 1.0 mg/kg, IM Act-D, 12 μg/kg, IV push cyclophosphamide, 3 mg/kg IV bolus
6	FA, 0.1 mg/kg, IM or po
7	MTX, 1.0 mg/kg, IM
8	FA, 1.0 mg/kg, IM or po

Act-D = actinomycin D; FA = folinic acid; IM = intramuscular; IV = intravenous; MTX = methotrexate; po = per os (by mouth).

Table 105-3 EMA-CO Regimen

Time	Treatment
Day 1	Etoposide 100 mg/m^2 by IV infusion in 200 mL of saline over 30 min Act-D 0.5 mg IV push MTX 100 mg/m^2 IV push MTX 200 mg/m^2 by IV infusion over 12 h
Day 2	Etoposide 100 mg/m^2 by IV infusion in 200 mL of saline over 30 min Act-D 0.5 mg IV push FA 15 mg IM or po every 12 h for 4 doses beginning 24 h after starting MTX
Day 8	Cyclophosphamide 600 mg/m^2 IV in saline Oncovin (vincristine) 1.0 mg/m^2 IV push

Act-D = actinomycin D; FA = folinic acid; IM = intramuscular; IV = intravenous; MTX = methotrexate; po = per os (by mouth).

Table 105-4 EMA-CE Regimen

Time	Treatment
Day 1	Etoposide 100 mg/m^2 by IV infusion in 200 mL of saline over 30 min Act-D 0.5 mg IV push MTX 100 mg/m^2 IV push MTX 1,000 mg/m^2 by IV infusion over 12 h
Day 2	Etoposide 100 mg/m^2 by IV infusion in 200 mL of saline over 30 min Act-D 0.5 mg IV push FA 30 mg IM or po every 12 h for 6 doses beginning 32 h after starting MTX
Day 8	Cisplatin 60 mg/m^2 IV with prehydration etoposide 100 mg/m^2 by IV infusion in 200 mL of saline over 30 min

Act-D = actinomycin D; FA = folinic acid; IM = intramuscular; IV = intravenous; MTX = methotrexate; po = per os (by mouth).
Reproduced with permission from Bagshawe.[8]

Table 105-5 Single-Agent Regimens

Methotrexate Treatments
MTX-FA MTX 1.0 mg/kg IM on days 1, 3, 5, and 7 FA 0.1 mg/kg IM or po on days 2, 4, 6, and 8
5-day MTX MTX 0.4 mg/kg/d IV or IM daily for 5 days
Pulse MTX MTX 50 mg/m^2 IM weekly
Actinomycin D Treatments
5-day Act-D Act-D 12 μg/kg/d IV for 5 days
Pulse Act-D Act-D 1.25 mg/m^2 IV every 2 weeks

FA = folinic acid; IM = intramuscular; IV = intravenous.

Table 105-6 Results of Single-Agent Regimens in Nonmetastatic GTT

Regimen	Number of Patients	Rate of Remission (%)
MTX–FA[66]	163	90.2
5-Day MTX[67]	58	93.0
Pulse MTX[68]	63	81.0
5-day Act-D[69]	31	94.0
Pulse Act-D[70]	31	94.0

curve. At our center, after the first course of single-agent chemotherapy, further chemotherapy is withheld as long as the hCG level is falling progressively. A second course of chemotherapy is administered under the following conditions: the hCG level plateaus for more than 3 consecutive weeks or reelevates, or the hCG level does not decline by 1 log within 18 days after completing the first treatment.

MTX with folinic acid (MTX-FA) has been the preferred single-agent regimen at our center.[66] MTX-FA induced complete remission in 147 (90.2%) of 163 patients with stage I GTT and in 15 (68.2%) of 22 patients with low-risk stages II and III GTT. One course of MTX-FA induced remission in 132 (81.5%) of these patients. Thrombocytopenia (platelets < 100,000/mm^3), granulocytopenia (white blood cell count < 1,500/mm^3), and hepatotoxicity (serum glutamic-oxaloacetic transaminase > 50 units) developed in only 3 (1.6%), 11 (5.9%), and 26 (14.1%) patients, respectively.

Combination Chemotherapy Triple therapy with MTX, Act-D, and cyclophosphamide is inadequate as primary treatment for patients with metastatic GTT and a high-risk score. Triple therapy induced remission in only half of patients with metastases and a high-risk score.[71,72] Bower and colleagues[73] and Bolis and colleagues[74] reported that EMA-CO induced complete remission in 86% and 76%, respectively, of patients with metastases and a high-risk score. The optimal combination drug regimen will most likely include etoposide, MTX, Act-D, and perhaps other agents administered in the most dose-intensive manner.

Combination chemotherapy is administered as soon as toxicity permits until the patient attains three consecutive undetectable hCG levels. After undetectable hCG values are achieved, at least two additional courses of chemotherapy are administered to reduce the risk of relapse.

RESULTS OF THERAPY

Stage I GTT Between July 1965 and December 2002, 534 patients with stage I GTT were treated at the New England Trophoblastic Disease Center and all attained remission. Thirty-one patients were managed with primary hysterectomy and adjuvant single-agent chemotherapy, and all achieved remission with no further treatment. Primary single-agent chemotherapy induced complete remission in 92% of patients. All patients with disease resistant to single-agent chemotherapy attained remission with either combination chemotherapy or surgical intervention.

Stages II and III GTT Complete remission was achieved at our center in all 28 patients with stage II GTT, and in 152 (99.3%) of 153 patients with stage III GTT. Single-agent chemotherapy induced remission in 16 (80%) of 20 patients with low-risk stage II disease, and in 85 (81.7%) of 104 patients with low-risk stage III disease. All patients with disease resistant to single-agent chemotherapy attained remission with combination chemotherapy.

STAGE IV GTT Prior to 1975, only 6 (30%) of 20 patients with stage IV GTT achieved remission at our center. However, after 1975, 15 (78.9%) of 19 patients with stage IV disease attained remission. This dramatic improvement in survival resulted from the use of intensive multimodal therapy early in the course of treatment. While brain irradiation is commonly employed in the United States for cerebral metastases, excellent remission rates have been reported in patients with cerebral metastases who were treated with chemotherapy alone. Thirty of 35 (86%) patients with cerebral lesions attained remission with intensive combination chemotherapy, including high-dose intravenous and intrathecal MTX.[46]

SUBSEQUENT PREGNANCIES

Patients with complete and partial mole can anticipate normal reproduction in the future.[75] However, these patients are at increased risk of developing molar pregnancy in later conceptions. Thirty-four (1 in 150) of our patients had at least two molar pregnancies. Following two episodes of molar pregnancy, the risk of mole in a later gestation is 20%.

Patients with GTT successfully treated with chemotherapy can also expect normal reproduction in the future.[75] Importantly, the frequency of later major and minor congenital malformations is not increased.

SECOND CANCERS

The use of etoposide in GTT has been reported to increase the risk of later secondary tumors, including myeloid leukemia, melanoma, colon cancer, and breast cancer. Among all patients treated with etoposide, 1.5% subsequently developed leukemia.[61]

REFERENCES

1. Bagshawe KD. Risks and prognostic factors in trophoblastic neoplasia. Cancer 1976;38:1373–85.
2. Goldstein DP, Berkowitz RS. Gestational trophoblastic neoplasms: clinical principles of diagnosis and management. In: Philadelphia: WB Saunders;1982. p. 1–301.
3. Li MC, Hertz R, Spencer DB. Effect of methotrexate on choriocarcinoma and chorioadenoma. Proc Soc Exp Biol Med 1956;93:361–6.
4. Hertz R, Lewis JL Jr, Lipsett MB. Five years' experience with chemotherapy of metastatic choriocarcinoma and related trophoblastic tumors in women. Am J Obstet Gynecol 1961;82:631–7.
5. Ross GT, Stolbach LL, Hertz R. Actinomycin D in the treatment of methotrexate-resistant trophoblastic disease in women. Cancer Res 1962;22:1015–7.
6. Ross GT, Goldstein DP, Hertz R, et al. Sequential use of methotrexate and actinomycin D in the treatment of metastatic choriocarcinoma and related trophoblastic diseases in women. Am J Obstet Gynecol 1965;93: 223–9.
7. Wong LC, Choo YC, Ma HK. Primary oral etoposide therapy in gestational trophoblastic disease, an update. Cancer 1986;58:14–7.
8. Bagshawe KD. Treatment of high-risk choriocarcinoma. J Reprod Med 1984;29:813–20.
9. Palmer JR. Advances in the epidemiology of gestational trophoblastic disease. J Reprod Med 1994; 39:155–62.
10. Jeffers MD, O'Dwyer P, Curran B, et al. Partial hydatidiform mole: a common but underdiagnosed condition. Int J Gynecol Pathol 1993;12:315–23.
11. Berkowitz RS, Cramer DW, Bernstein MR, et al. Risk factors for complete molar pregnancy from a case-control study. Am J Obstet Gynecol 1985;152:1016–20.
12. Parazzini F, LaVecchia C, Mangili G, et al. Dietary factors and risk of trophoblastic disease. Am J Obstet Gynecol 1988;158:93–100.
13. Parazzini F, La Vecchia C, Pampallona S. Parental age and risk of complete and partial hydatidiform mole. Br J Obstet Gynecol 1986;93:582–5.
14. Kajii T, Ohama K. Androgenetic origin of hydatidiform mole. Nature 1977;268:633–4.
15. Yamashita K, Wake N, Araki T, et al. Human lymphocyte antigen expression in hydatidiform mole: androgenesis following fertilization by a haploid sperm. Am J Obstet Gynecol 1979;135:597–600.
16. Pattillo RA, Sasaki S, Katayama KP, et al. Genesis of 46,XY hydatidiform mole. Am J Obstet Gynecol 1981;141:104–5.
17. Azuma C, Saji F, Tokugawa Y, et al. Application of gene amplification by polymerase chain reaction to genetic analysis of molar mitochondrial DNA: the detection of anuclear empty ovum as the cause of complete mole. Gynecol Oncol 1991;40:29–33.
18. Szulman AE, Surti U. The syndromes of hydatidiform mole. I. Cytogenetic and morphologic correlations. Am J Obstet Gynecol 1978;131:665–771.
19. Lage JM, Mark SD, Roberts D, et al. A flow cytometric study of 137 fresh hydropic placentas: correlation between types of hydatidiform moles and nuclear DNA ploidy. Obstet Gynecol 1992;79:403–10.
20. Lawler SD, Fisher RA, Dent J. A prospective genetic study of complete and partial hydatidiform moles. Am J Obstet Gynecol 1991;164:1270–7.
21. Elston CW, Bagshawe KD. Cellular reaction in trophoblastic tumors. Br J Cancer 1973;28:245–56.
22. Anderson DJ, Berkowitz RS. Gamma-interferon enhances expression of class I MHC antigens in the weakly HLA+ human choriocarcinoma cell line BeWo but does not induce MHC expression in the HLA-choriocarcinoma cell line Jar. J Immunol 1985;135: 2498–501.
23. Berkowitz RS, Hill JA, Kurtz CB, et al. Effects of products of activated leukocytes (lymphokines and monokines) on the growth of malignant trophoblast cells in vitro. Am J Obstet Gynecol 1988;158:199–203.
24. Tomoda Y, Fuma M, Saiki N, et al. Immunologic studies in patients with trophoblastic neoplasia. Am J Obstet Gynecol 1976;126:661–7.
25. Berkowitz RS, Hornig-Rohan J, Martin-Alosco S, et al. HLA antigen frequency distribution in patients with gestational choriocarcinoma and their husbands. Placenta 1981;3 Suppl:263–7.
26. Szulman AE, Surti U. The syndromes of hydatidiform mole: II. Morphologic evolution of the complete and partial mole. Am J Obstet Gynecol 1978;132:20–7.
27. Feltmate C, Genest DR, Wise L. et al. Placental site trophoblastic tumor: a 17-year experience at the New England Trophoblastic Disease Center. Gynecol Oncol 2001;82:415–9.
28. Cheung AN, Srivastava G, Chung LP, et al. Expression of the *p53* gene in trophoblastic cells in hydatidiform moles and normal human placentas. J Reprod Med 1994;39:223–7.
29. Cheung AN, Srivastava G, Pittaluga S, et al. Expression of *c-myc* and *c-fms* oncogenes in hydatidiform mole and normal human placenta. J Clin Pathol 1993;46:204–7.
30. Fulop V, Mok SC, Genest DR, et al. *p53*, p21, Rb, and mdm2 oncoproteins: expression in normal placenta, partial and complete mole and choriocarcinoma. J Reprod Med 1998;43:119–27.
31. Fulop V, Mok SC, Berkowitz RS. Molecular biology of gestational trophoblastic neoplasia:[Review]. J Reprod Med 2004;49:415–22.
32. Tuncer ZS, Vegh GL, Fulop V, et al. Expression of epidermal growth factor receptor-related family products in gestational trophoblastic disease and normal placenta and its relationship to development of post-molar tumor. Gynecol Oncol 2000;77:389–93.

33. Fisher RA, Hodges MD, Newlands ES. Familial recurrent hydatidiform mole—a review. J Reprod Med 2004; 49:595–601
34. Hodges MD, Rees HC, Seckl MJ et al. Genetic refinement and physical mapping of a biparental complete mole locus on chromosome 19q 13.4 J Med Genet 2003;40:95.
35. Goldstein DP, Berkowitz RS. Current management of complete and partial molar pregnancy. J Reprod Med 1994;39:139–46.
36. Soto-Wright V, Bernstein MR, Goldstein DP, Berkowitz RS. The changing clinical presentation of complete molar pregnancy. Obstet Gynecol 1995;86:775–9.
37. Amir SM, Osathanondh R, Berkowitz RS, Goldstein DP. Human chorionic gonadotropin and thyroid function in patients with hydatidiform mole. Am J Obstet Gynecol 1984;150:723–8.
38. Berkowitz RS, Goldstein DP, Bernstein MR. Natural history of partial molar pregnancy. Obstet Gynecol 1986;66:677–81.
39. Szulman AE, Surti U. The clinicopathologic profile of the partial hydatidiform mole. Obstet Gynecol 1982;59:597–602.
40. Berkowitz RS, Goldstein DP. Chorionic tumors. N Engl J Med 1996;335:1740–8.
41. Tow WSH. The influence of the primary treatment of hydatidiform mole on its subsequent course. J Obstet Gynaecol Br Commonw 1966;73:545–52.
42. Tsukamoto N, Iwasaka T, Kashimura Y, et al. Gestational trophoblastic diseases in women aged 50 or more. Gynecol Oncol 1985;20:53–61.
43. Berkowitz RS, Goldstein DP. Presentation and management of molar pregnancy. In: Hancock BW, Newlands ES, Berkowitz RS, editors. Gestational trophoblastic disease. London: Chapman and Hall; 1997. p. 127–42.
44. Rice LW, Berkowitz RS, Lage JM, et al. Persistent gestational trophoblastic tumor after partial hydatidiform mole. Gynecol Oncol 1990;36:358–62.
45. Bakri YN, Berkowitz RS, Khan J, et al. Pulmonary metastases of gestational trophoblastic tumor: risk factors for early respiratory failure. J Reprod Med 1994;39:175–8.
46. Newlands ES, Holden L, Seckl MJ, et al. Management of brain metastases in patients with high risk gestational trophoblastic tumours (GTT). J Reprod Med 2002;47:465–71.
47. Bakri YN, Berkowitz RS, Goldstein DP, et al. Brain metastases of gestational trophoblastic tumor. J Reprod Med 1994;39:179–84.
48. Fine C, Bundy AL, Berkowitz RS, et al. Sonographic diagnosis of partial hydatidiform mole. Obstet Gynecol 1989;73:414–8.
49. Cole LA, Khanlian SA. Inappropriate management of women with persistent low hCG results. J Reprod Med 2004; 49:423–32.
50. World Health Organization. Trophoblastic diseases: technical report series 692. Geneva: WHO, 1983.
51. Goldstein DP, Berkowitz RS. Prophylactic chemotherapy of complete molar pregnancy. Semin Oncol 1995;22:157–60.
52. Holland JF, Hreschchyshyn MM, Glidewell O. Controlled clinical trials of methotrexate in treatment and prophylaxis of trophoblastic neoplasia. In: Clark RL, Curnley RW, McKay JE, Copeland MM, editors. Tenth international cancer congress abstracts. Houston: Medical Arts Publishing; 1970. p. 461–2.
53. Kim DS, Moon H, Kim KT, et al. Effects of prophylactic chemotherapy for persistent trophoblastic disease in patients with complete hydatidiform mole. Obstet Gynecol 1986;67:690–4.
54. Limpongsanurak, S. Prophylactic actinomycin D for high-risk complete hydatidiform mole. J Reprod Med 2001;46:110–6.
55. Berkowitz RS, Goldstein DP, Marean AR, Bernstein MR. Oral contraceptives and postmolar trophoblastic disease. Obstet Gynecol 1981;58:474–8.
56. Curry SL, Schlaerth JB, Kohorn EI, et al. Hormonal contraception and trophoblastic sequelae after hydatidiform mole (a Gynecologic Oncology Group Study). Am J Obstet Gynecol 1989;160:805–11.
57. Stone M, Dent J, Kardana A, Bagshawe KD. Relationship of oral contraception to development of trophoblastic tumor after evacuation of a hydatidiform mole. Br J Obstet Gynaecol 1976;83:913–6.
58. Garner EIO, Garrett A, Goldstein DP, Berkowitz RS. Significance of chest computed tomography findings in the evaluation and treatment of persistent gestational trophoblastic neoplasia. J Reprod Med 2004; 49:411–14.
59. Papadopoulos AJ, Foskett M, Seckl MJ, et al. Twenty-five years clinical experience of placental site trophoblastic tumors. J Reprod Med 2002;47:460–4.
60. Berkowitz RS, Goldstein DP, Bernstein MR. Modified triple chemotherapy in the management of high-risk metastatic gestational trophoblastic tumors. Gynecol Oncol 1984;19:173–81.
61. Rustin GJS, Newlands ES, Lutz JM, et al. Combination but not single–agent methotrexate chemotherapy for gestational trophoblastic tumors increases the incidence of second tumors. J Clin Oncol 1996;14:2769–73.
62. Newlands ES, Bower M, Holden L, et al. Management of resistant gestational trophoblastic tumors. J Reprod Med 1998;43:111–8.
63. Soper JT. Surgical therapy for gestational trophoblastic disease. J Reprod Med 1994;39:168–74.
64. Yordan EL Jr, Schlaerth J, Gaddis O, Morrow CP. Radiation therapy in the management of gestational choriocarcinoma metastatic to the central nervous system. Obstet Gynecol 1987;69:627–30.
65. Osborne R, Gerulath A. What is the best regimen for low-risk gestational trophoblastic neoplasia? [Review] J Reprod Med 2004; 49:602–16.
66. Berkowitz RS, Goldstein DP, Bernstein MR. Ten years experience with methotrexate and folinic acid as primary therapy for gestational trophoblastic disease. Gynecol Oncol 1986;23:111–8.
67. Hammond CB, Hertz R, Ross GT, et al. Primary chemotherapy for nonmetastatic gestational trophoblastic neoplasms. Am J Obstet Gynecol 1967;98:71–8.
68. Homesley HD, Blessing JA, Rettenmaier M, et al. Weekly intramuscular methotrexate for nonmetastatic gestational trophoblastic tumor. Obstet Gynecol 1998;72:413–8.
69. Osathanondh R, Goldstein DP, Pastorfide GB. Actinomycin D as the primary agent for gestational trophoblastic disease. Cancer 1973;36:863–6.
70. Petrilli ES, Twiggs LB, Blessing JA, et al. Single-dose actinomycin D treatment for nonmetastatic gestational trophoblastic disease. Cancer 1987;60:2173–6.
71. DuBeshter B, Berkowitz RS, Goldstein DP, et al. Metastatic gestational trophoblastic disease: experience at the New England Trophoblastic Disease Center, 1965–1985. Obstet Gynecol 1987;69:390–5.
72. Gordon AN, Gershenson DM, Copeland LJ, et al. High-risk metastatic gestational trophoblastic disease: further stratification into clinical entities. Gynecol Oncol 1989;34:54–6.
73. Bower M, Newlands ES, Holden L, et al. EMA/CO for high-risk gestational trophoblastic tumors: results from a cohort of 272 patients. J Clin Oncol 1997;15:2636–42.
74. Bolis G, Bonazzi C, Landoni F, et al. EMA/CO regimen in high-risk gestational trophoblastic tumor (GTT). Gynecol Oncol 1988;31:439–44.
75. Garner EIO, Lipson E, Bernstein MR, et al. Subsequent pregnancy experience in patients with molar pregnancy and gestational trophoblastic tumors. J Reprod Med 2002;47:380–6.

Gynecologic Sarcomas

Jamal Rahaman, MD
Carmel J. Cohen, MD

Even though the female pelvis is richly endowed with blood vessels, connective tissue, and müllerian elements, sarcomas (including mesenchymal and mixed epithelial-mesenchymal malignancies) of the vulva, vagina, cervix, uterus, and ovaries account for less than 1.5% of the cancers of these organs. The most common site for sarcoma in the female pelvis is the uterus, but only 3% of uterine cancers are sarcomas.[1] Because of the infrequent occurrence of sarcomas, classification of these cancers was a taxonomic dilemma until Ober, in 1959,[2] proposed a classification that became the basis from which modern modifications have been derived. Table 106-1 presents a detailed classification, adapted from Kempson and Bari,[3] and a functional classification developed by the Gynecologic Oncology Group (GOG).

The most widely referenced epidemiologic study on uterine sarcomas was conducted by Harlow and colleagues, who analyzed the population-based registries comprising the Surveillance, Epidemiology, and End Results (SEER) Program of the National Cancer Institute from 1973 to 1981.[1] The incidence rate per million women per year was 8.2 for malignant mixed müllerian tumors (MMMTs), 6.4 for leiomyosarcomas (LMSs), 1.8 for endometrial stromal sarcomas (ESSs), and 0.7 for unclassified sarcomas. The risk of sarcoma is higher in black women than in white women, and the risk of MMMT increases sharply with age.

Epidemiologic risk factors for uterine sarcoma have not been clearly defined, except for previous radiation exposure. An association has been observed between exposure to radiation and development of uterine sarcomas, most of which are MMMTs. Although the relative risk is estimated at 5.4,[4] the percentage of patients with uterine sarcomas who have previously undergone radiation therapy ranges from 12 to 30%.[5] No other epidemiologic factors examined in the literature have consistently demonstrated an effect on the risk of developing uterine sarcoma.

The uterus is the most common site of gynecologic sarcomas. Uterine sarcomas can be assigned to two general categories with an origin from either the endometrial or the myometrial compartment. ESSs are derived only from the endometrial compartment, whereas LMSs arise solely from the myometrial compartment, and the MMMTs have contributions from both derivatives.[3] The homologous tumors include carcinoma plus a sarcoma differentiating toward tissues indigenous to the uterus, and the heterologous tumors include carcinoma plus sarcoma resembling tissue from some extrauterine source (bone, cartilage, striated muscle) with or without homologous elements. Traditionally, authors have reported that MMMT and LMS each account for 35 to 40% of uterine sarcomas, with ESS accounting for 10 to 15% and other sarcomas comprising 5%. However, in one of the most detailed clinicopathologic evaluations of clinical stage I and II uterine sarcomas prospectively performed, the GOG, in an analysis of 453 patients, found that 66% had MMMT, 13% had LMS, and the remaining 21% were predominantly adenosarcoma and ESS.[6]

The reason for this apparent change in the ratio of the two most frequently diagnosed uterine sarcomas is unclear; however, several smaller series reported in the past decade have noticed this trend in the histologic analysis performed. The significance of the GOG studies is that a single group of referee pathologists reviewed all of the pathologic material, and surgeons followed common surgical guidelines so that all patients met strict criteria for the acceptability of both the surgical procedure and the adequacy of pathologic specimens submitted.

Table 106-1 Classification of Uterine Sarcomas

Classification of Kempson and Bari
- I. Pure sarcomas
  - A. Pure sarcomas
    - 1. Leiomyosarcoma
    - 2. Stromal sarcoma
    - 3. Stromal endometriosis (endometrial stromatosis, endolymphatic stromal myosis)
    - 4. Angiosarcoma
    - 5. Fibrosarcoma
  - B. Pure heterologous
    - 1. Rhabdomyosarcoma (includes sarcoma botryoides)
    - 2. Chondrosarcoma
    - 3. Osteosarcoma
    - 4. Liposarcoma
- II. Mixed sarcomas
  - A. Mixed homologous
  - B. Mixed heterologous with or without homologous elements
- III. Malignant mixed müllerian tumors (mixed mesodermal tumors)
  - A Malignant mixed müllerian tumors, homologous type – carcinoma plus one sarcoma or mixture of sarcomas in IA, 1 through 5, above (carcinosarcoma)
  - B. Malignant mixed müllerian tumors, heterologous type – carcinoma plus heterologous sarcoma with or without homologous sarcoma
- IV. Sarcoma unclassified
- V. Malignant lymphoma

Gynecologic Oncology Group Classification
- I. Leiomyosarcomas
- II. Endometrial stromal sarcomas
- III. Mixed homologous müllerian sarcomas (carcinosarcoma)
- IV. Other uterine sarcomas

Adapted from Kempson and Bari.[3]

One of the pitfalls in diagnosing sarcomas is the variability in threshold for distinguishing between atypical benign lesions and clearly malignant ones. In general, it is reasonable to conclude that if a mesenchymal tumor of the uterus has 1 to 4 mitoses per 10 high-power fields, the metastatic potential is virtually nil. If there are 10 or more mitoses per 10 high-power fields, the risk of recurrence is high, irrespective of the presence of atypia. If there are 5 to 9 mitoses per 10 high-power fields without atypia, the risk of recurrence or metastasis is moderate, but if atypia is also present, the patient should be considered to have a sarcoma.

It is important to realize, however, that there are important exceptions to these generalizations. For example, mitotically active smooth muscle tumors without atypia occurring in young women usually behave in a benign manner. Conversely, myxoid LMSs often have deceptively low mitotic counts.

CLINICAL PROFILE

Uterine Endometrial Stromal Tumors

Patients with endometrial stromal tumors tend to be perimenopausal and ordinarily present with irregular vaginal bleeding. If the lesion is small, pain may be absent, but on pelvic examination, tumor tissue may be seen protruding through the cervical os because the tumor originates in the endometrium and may grow large without penetrating through the uterine wall. The diagnosis is made by endometrial sampling, which should be done liberally to explain vaginal bleeding. Among the endometrial stromal tumors is the endometrial stromal nodule, usually an expansile, noninfiltrating, unifocal lesion with low mitotic activity and low virulence. Removal of the nodule has resulted in cure, without further therapy. Endolymphatic stromal miosis is a low-grade stromal sarcoma with a worm-like infiltrative pattern that extends beyond the uterus in approximately 40% of patients. It recurs in approximately 50% after surgical removal but is indolent in its course and is often treated by repeated excisions over a long course of months or years. There is evidence of radiosensitivity and hormone sensitivity,[7] with the observation that oophorectomy alone can control the disease in a subset of patients. High-grade ESSs, on the other hand, are more aggressive cancers. Patients survive well when the tumors are small and confined to the uterus at the time of initial treatment; however, poorly differentiated lesions or those with extrauterine extension are usually lethal.

Mixed Tumors The incidence of MMMT begins to increase at approximately 50 years of age and does not plateau until after age 75 years. The presenting complaints may include vaginal bleeding, heavy discharge, abdominal pain, and sometimes an increase in abdominal girth. The diagnosis is made more frequently by endometrial sampling than in the case of LMS because the latter disease often does not involve the endometrial cavity. Other than previous exposure to ionizing radiation, there is no unusual risk factor for patients with uterine sarcomas.

Uterine Myometrial Tumors LMS commonly occurs during the fourth and fifth decades of life, with a peak incidence at 45 years of age, after which there is a gradual decline in incidence until the eighth decade. The lesion is frequently associated with benign leiomyomas, although among leiomyomas, sarcoma is found less than 1% of the time.[8] There is considerable debate over whether the lesion "develops" from a benign leiomyoma or occurs independently. Ferenczy and colleagues were unable to demonstrate a developmental relationship,[9] whereas Spiro and Koss found intermediate changes in leiomyomas and indicted[10] these benign lesions in 50% of the cases of LMS they studied. Often LMSs are discovered by chance at the time of myomectomy or hysterectomy. Davids, who removed five sarcomas in a series of 1,150 myomectomies, observed that the five patients were well after 5 years and that three of them subsequently became pregnant.[11] No mention was made of virulence indices in the pathologic examination of these tumors.

DIAGNOSIS

Of patients with uterine sarcomas, 75 to 95% present with abnormal vaginal bleeding.[12,13] Pelvic pain, discharge, and aborting tissue occur frequently. Endometrial biopsy usually confirms MMMT; however, LMS and ESS are missed in at least 40 and 20% of cases, respectively.[7,14,15]

Radiography may be useful in diagnosing uterine sarcomas. Computed tomography will identify extrauterine spread, and magnetic resonance imaging can assess the depth of myometrial invasion. Several investigators are currently studying ultrasonography.[16] Kurjak and colleagues evaluated the role of transvaginal color Doppler ultrasonography in differentiating uterine sarcomas from leiomyomas.[16]

SARCOMA-LIKE VARIANTS

Four pathologic entities are abnormal forms of leiomyoma and should be distinguished from uterine sarcomas.

Benign metastasizing leiomyoma is a rare entity in which histologically benign uterine smooth muscle is found in extrauterine deposits, often distant from the uterus, especially in lymph nodes and lungs.[17] Whether the nodules are metastatic or multifocal remains to be resolved. Several observers have noted the hormone dependence of these deposits. After hysterectomy with bilateral salpingo-oophorectomy, the nodules often regress, and if they interfere with performance, they can be individually resected.

Intravenous leiomyomatosis is the growth of histologically benign smooth muscle into venous lumina. Although the pattern is often worm-like, it should not be confused with endolymphatic stromal miosis, which is located primarily extravascularly. Although intravenous leiomyomatosis is histologically benign, deaths have been reported from very long tumor extensions occupying the vena cava and the heart.[18] In this condition, the extension of tumor is contiguous, unlike the widely disparate deposits in benign metastasizing leiomyoma.

Leiomyomatosis peritonealis disseminata is a rare condition in which nodules composed of benign smooth muscle are densely distributed throughout the peritoneal cavity. Much of the peritoneal surface may be occupied by nodules ranging in size from a few millimeters to several centimeters. Treatment requires removal of as much disease as possible and reversal of any estrogenic stimulation, either by removing the ovaries or by treatment with antiestrogen regimens.

Epithelioid leiomyoma or leiomyoblastoma denotes a rare group of benign smooth muscle tumors that are formed by round cells with clear cytoplasm. They are less well circumscribed than a typical leiomyoma and occasionally lack the whorled, cut surface and the discrete borders of a typical leiomyoma. Usually, their mitotic rate is less than three mitoses per 10 high-power fields, and the rate of recurrence or metastasis is low.[19]

PATTERNS OF SPREAD

Uterine sarcomas can spread by lymphatic and hematogenous routes,[20] as well as by local extension and peritoneal spread.[21] Several studies have addressed the metastatic pattern of uterine sarcomas. Chen examined nodal metastases in 20 patients with clinical stage I uterine sarcomas.[22] Fourteen patients had MMMT, four had LMS, and two had ESS. Of nine patients (45%) with lymph node metastases, six had both para-aortic and pelvic node involvement, and three had only pelvic node involvement. Among ESS and MMMT patients, a high frequency of association was observed between nodal spread and deep myometrial invasion. Other sites of extrauterine spread were the ovary (two patients) and the serosa of the uterus (one patient). DiSaia and colleagues reported on 28 patients with clinical stage I and II carcinosarcoma who underwent total abdominal hysterectomy, bilateral salpingo-oophorectomy, and pelvic and para-aortic lymph node sampling.[23] Ten (35%) of the 28 patients had positive pelvic nodes; 4 of these 10 patients also had para-aortic node metastasis (14.5%). In every instance of nodal involvement, the myometrial invasion was to the middle or outer third.

Rose and colleagues studied the autopsy findings of 73 patients with uterine sarcoma, including 43 patients with MMMT, 19 with LMS, 9 with ESS, and 2 with ESM.[20] The peritoneal cavity and omentum were the most frequently involved sites (59%), followed by the lung (52%), pelvic (41%) and para-aortic (38%) lymph nodes, and liver parenchyma (34%). Of note, the presence of lung metastasis was not associated with pelvic or para-aortic nodal metastasis or intraperitoneal disease. In another review of autopsy findings, Fleming and colleagues reviewed the records of 22 patients treated for uterine sarcoma, including 11 MMMTs, 6 ESSs, and 5 LMSs.[21] Fifty-nine percent had lymph node involvement, and 45% died with disease limited to the pelvis and abdomen. The most common site of disease above the diaphragm was the lung. The authors reviewed the autopsy findings of 58 patients from previous reports in the literature and found a similar incidence of nodal involvement (57%) and disease limited to the pelvis and abdomen (31%). In addition, 65.5% of patients had abdominal and distant metastases.

Goff and colleagues examined nodal metastases from uterine LMS and ESS.[14] Retroperitoneal lymph node sampling revealed lymph node metastases in 4 of 15 women with LMS, and in each instance, there was also disseminated intraperitoneal disease. Seven of 10 women with ESS had lymphadenectomies, and none had positive nodes.

PROGNOSTIC FACTORS AND PROGNOSIS

Prognostic factors differ for the three major types of uterine sarcomas. Major and colleagues reported the GOG clinicopathologic study of clinical stage I and II uterine sarcoma, which included 59 patients with LMS and 301 patients with MMMT.[6] Of the 453 patients eligible for analysis, 430 underwent complete surgical staging that included lymphadenectomy. The median survival was 62.6 months for homologous MMMT, 22.7 months for heterologous MMMT, and 20.6 months for LMS. The overall recurrence rate for homologous MMMT was 56%.

In patients with LMS, lymph vascular space involvement and involvement of the cervix and isthmus were common, whereas lymph node metastases, adnexal metastases, and positive peritoneal cytology were infrequent findings. The only surgicopathologic finding that correlated with progression-free interval was the mitotic index. Whereas there were no treatment failures among the three women who had less than 10 mitoses per 10 high-power fields, 61% of women with 10 to 20 mitoses per 10 high-power fields and 79% of women with greater than 20 mitoses per 10 high-power fields developed recurrences. Fewer mitoses were also associated with longer survival. Other investigators have confirmed these results.[24,25]

In contrast to patients with LMS, surgicopathologic factors of MMMT that related to pro-

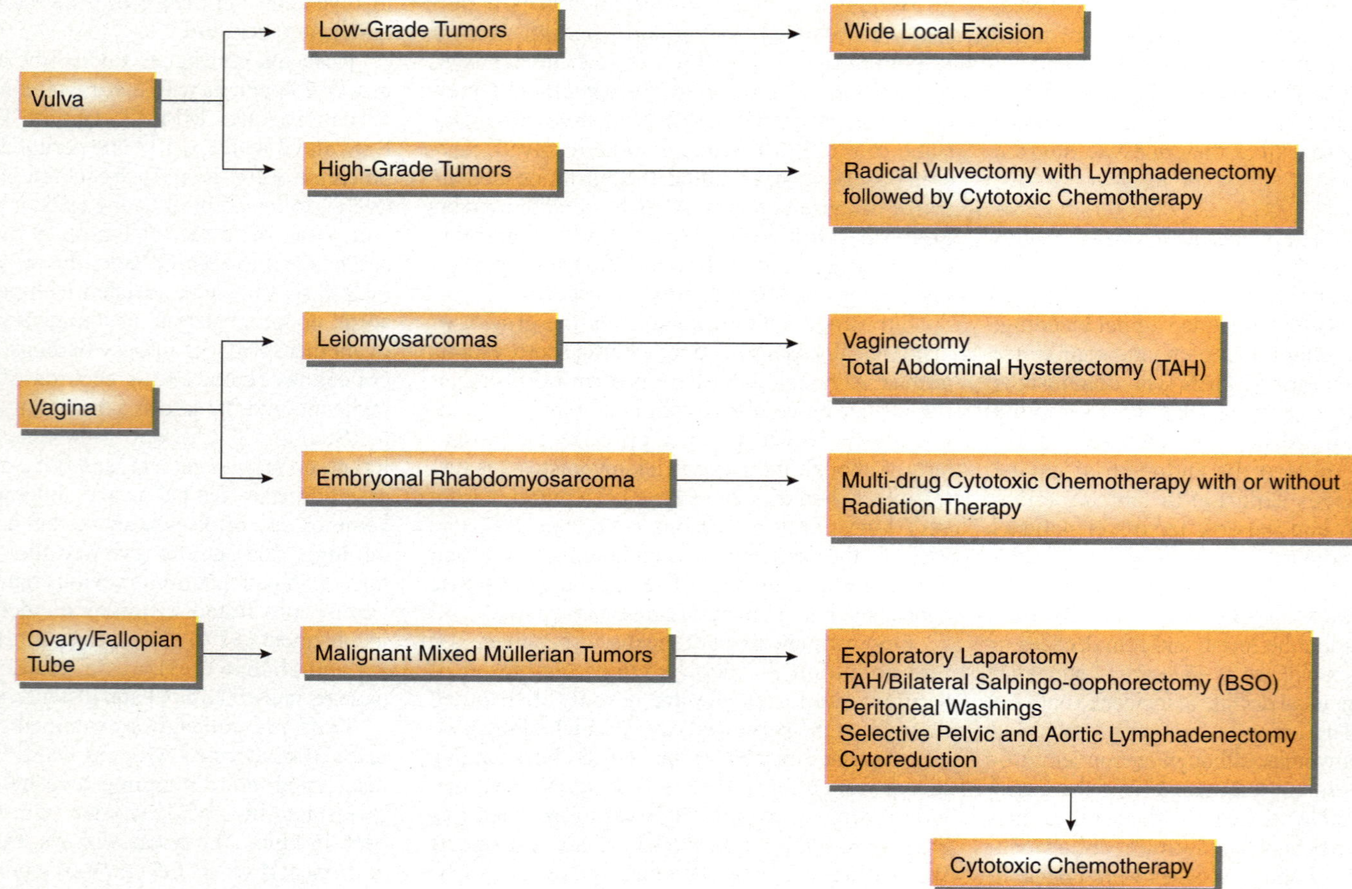

Figure 106-1 Management of nonuterine gynecologic sarcomas.

gression-free interval included adnexal spread, lymph node metastasis, histologic cell type (heterologous versus homologous), and the grade of sarcoma. Of note, patients with MMMT had high rates of nodal and adnexal metastases and positive peritoneal cytology. Pelvic nodes were involved twice as often as aortic nodes (15 vs 7.8%), and both nodal groups were involved in 5% of the patients.

NONUTERINE GYNECOLOGIC SARCOMAS

The Vulva Fewer than 300 patients with vulvar sarcoma have been described in the literature. LMS, rhabdomyosarcoma, and fibrosarcoma are the most frequently diagnosed vulvar tumors. The clinical behavior of these tumors is related to their grade, mitotic count, histology, and stage. For the lowest-grade tumors, wide local excision should suffice. However, for the more aggressive histologic patterns, radical vulvectomy with lymphadenectomy followed by cytotoxic chemotherapy should be considered, although the role of adjuvant chemotherapy has not been studied in these tumors.

The Vagina LMS of the vagina occurs in the same age groups as does LMS of the uterus. Although this tumor is highly virulent, survivors are among those treated by hysterectomy, oophorectomy, and vaginectomy. Embryonal rhabdomyosarcomas, formerly termed sarcoma botryoides, occur most frequently in children and have a typical grape cluster–like appearance. The disease was once uniformly fatal, provoking radical extirpative surgery that resulted in exenteration for young girls. Various multidrug cytotoxic chemotherapy regimens with or without radiation therapy have replaced primary exenteration, and a cure is now expected. Radical surgery is reserved for failures of nonsurgical treatment.

The Ovary Most types of sarcomas described in the vagina, vulva, or uterus have been found in the ovary as well. The diagnosis of ovarian sarcoma is infrequently made prior to laparotomy. The surgical treatment is identical to that for epithelial ovarian cancers. During the past decade, MMMT of the ovary has been described with increasing frequency.[26,27] Survival is better for patients with early-stage disease and those whose tumors have homologous stromal elements. In one group of patients treated between 1977 and 1988, the median survival time for patients receiving doxorubicin and cisplatin chemotherapy after cytoreductive surgery was 16 months.[27] Sixty-two percent were alive at 12 months and 31% at 24 months. Although responses were noted in 85% of treated patients, treatment failed in half of these. Serum cancer antigen 125 levels accurately reflected tumor presence in 82% of the tested patients. Although the cytotoxic chemotherapy employed produced a response, survival from these virulent tumors was poor.

Fallopian Tube The fallopian tube is the least frequent site of primary sarcomas in the gynecologic tract. From reports in the literature, it would seem that carcinoma of the fallopian tube, itself an unusual entity, is more than 20 times more common than fallopian tube sarcoma. The most common histologic type is MMMT.[28,29] In Imachi and colleagues' 1992 review, there were 39 patients with MMMT of the fallopian tube.[28] Clinical features and difficulty in diagnosis are identical to those for patients with adenocarcinoma of the fallopian tube. Half of the patients had homologous elements and half had heterologous components. The surgical approach is the same as that used for ovarian or fallopian tube epithelial carcinoma, and postoperative treatment has usually included cytotoxic chemotherapy. Combinations of cyclophosphamide, doxorubicin, and cisplatin have been effectively applied, as has the combination of vincristine, doxorubicin, and cyclophosphamide.[29,30] More recently, ifosfamide and cisplatin combination chemotherapy, as well as paclitaxel, has been employed. Long-term survivors have been reported but are uncommon.[31]

Figure 106-1 illustrates a summary of the management of the nonuterine gynecologic sarcomas.

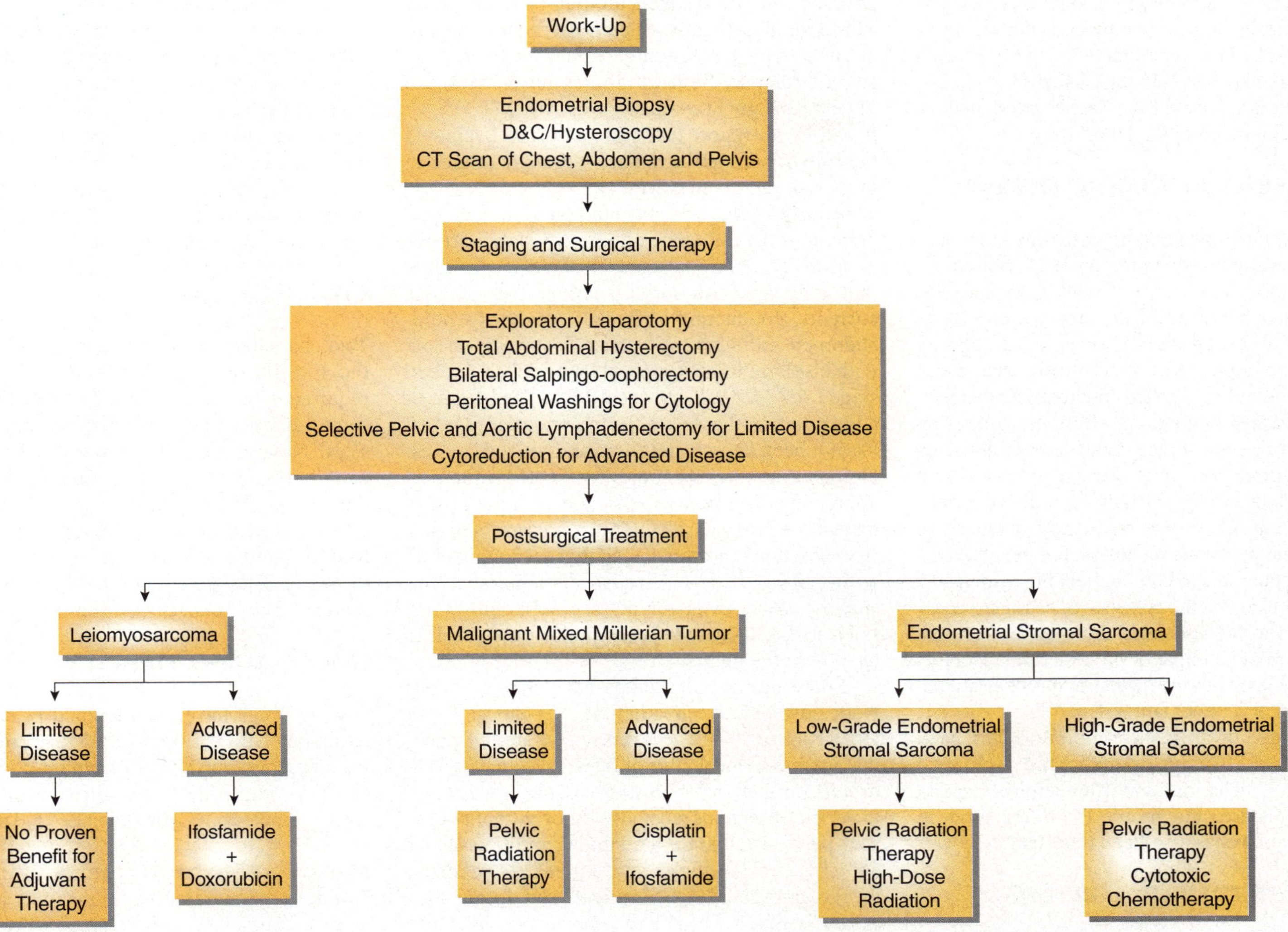

Figure 106-2 Management of uterine sarcomas.

SURGICAL TREATMENT

The initial therapy for sarcomas of the gynecologic tract is surgical except for embryonal rhabdomyosarcomas (Figure 106-2). Patients with uterine sarcoma require total abdominal hysterectomy and careful staging. In patients with MMMT limited to the uterus by pathologic staging, the cytologic presence of malignant cells in the peritoneal washings is a poor prognostic factor.[31]

The ovaries should be retained in premenopausal patients with LMS because this appears to improve their prognosis.[15,32,33] However, a bilateral salpingo-oophorectomy should be performed in all other patients, including those with low-grade ESS, because these tumors may be hormone dependent or responsive and have a propensity for extension into the parametria, broad ligament, and adnexal structures.

For MMMT, a high percentage of patients with clinical stage I or II disease are upstaged at the time of laparotomy[34,35]; thus it appears reasonable to surgically stage these patients. There is a paucity of data regarding the role of lymph node sampling in patients with LMS and ESS, but it appears that almost all patients with these sarcomas who have lymph node metastases also have evidence of intraperitoneal disease spread.[8]

Unlike other gynecologic malignancies, there is a role for thoracotomy or video-assisted thorascopy in patients with uterine sarcoma metastatic to the lung. Levenback and colleagues reviewed 45 patients whose pulmonary metastases from uterine sarcoma were resected at Memorial Sloan-Kettering Cancer Center, the majority of which were LMS (84%).[36] Most lesions were unilateral (71%), 70% were greater than 2 cm, and half were isolated lesions. The mean survival of patients with unilateral disease (39 months) was significantly greater than that of patients with bilateral disease (27 months). No single risk factor was identified that could exclude an individual patient from consideration for pulmonary resection. There is also a role for surgery in the treatment of local and regional recurrences of uterine sarcomas. In The University of Texas M. D. Anderson Cancer Center series of 120 patients with MMMT reported by Spanos and colleagues, 67 patients developed recurrent disease.[37] In the six patients with lesions deemed suitable for resection (one locoregional, two pulmonary, and three abdominal), five complete responses and partial responses occurred, for an overall response rate of 83%. Recurrent or metastatic low-grade ESS may also be amenable to surgical excision of pelvic disease or pulmonary metastases.

The International Federation of Gynecology and Obstetrics (FIGO) staging criteria for corpus cancer is commonly used for uterine sarcomas.[38] This is a surgical staging system.

POSTSURGICAL THERAPY FOR GYNECOLOGIC SARCOMAS

Although complete surgical removal is the ideal initial therapy for patients with sarcoma of the gynecologic tract, there is no randomized study proving that surgical cytoreduction influences overall survival for patients with advanced or recurrent disease. Similarly, the therapeutic benefit of lymphadenectomy has not been proven but is rational. For patients with sarcoma of the uterus or ovary, no formal trial has evaluated the role of lymphadenectomy in addition to hysterectomy and bilateral salpingo-oophorectomy.

For patients with uterine sarcoma, there is no definitive evidence from prospective trials that adjuvant therapy of any type leads to overall improvement in survival. To review the currently understood role of radiotherapy and chemotherapy in sarcomas, LMS is separated from the remaining homologous and heterologous MMMTs because the patterns of relapse for the former are somewhat different from those of the latter group.

HORMONE AND BIOLOGIC THERAPY

Receptors for estrogen and progesterone are identified in patients with uterine sarcoma.[39,40] Sutton and colleagues studied 43 patients with various uterine sarcomas and found estrogen receptors in 55% of the tumors and progesterone receptors in 55%.[39] The median values were much lower than those found in consecutively tested endometrial adenocarcinomas and breast carcinomas from the same laboratory. The presence of receptors was not influenced by stage or grade, but levels were much higher and more prevalent in patients with ESS of low grade, and this group of tumors frequently responds to progestational hormone treatment. For the other sarcomas, receptor status did not affect the response to cytotoxic agents, but the presence of estrogen receptors seemed to be associated with longer survival. The presence of estrogen or progesterone receptors did not correlate with the response to progestational therapy with or without tamoxifen.

Recent use of aromatase inhibitors has been described in ESS, with dramatic and prolonged responses.[41–43] The immunohistochemical expression of aromatase cytochrome P-450 receptors in uterine sarcomas has also been reported.[44]

RADIATION THERAPY FOR LMS

In contrast to other sarcomas, patients with LMS confined to the uterus appear to have a dominant pattern of failure outside the pelvis and abdominal cavity. In three series in which the site of first recurrence was documented, 14 (28%) of 49 patients developed pelvic or abdominal recurrence compared with 32 (65%) of 49 patients whose first recurrence had some component of distant disease.[45–47] Thus, in LMS, although the rate of failure in the pelvis is not insubstantial, little is to be potentially gained by delivering pelvic irradiation as a postoperative adjuvant treatment insofar as two-thirds of patients have some component of distant disease at first recurrence.

Although pelvic radiation has been used historically as an adjunct to surgery, many therapists have abandoned its use in patients with LMS because of the dominant pattern of distant failure, and they reserve radiation treatment for isolated pelvic relapse only. It is unlikely that adjuvant pelvic irradiation contributes significantly to overall survival from LMS.

RADIATION THERAPY FOR MMMT

Historically, pre- or postoperative pelvic irradiation has been used as an adjunct to surgery for MMMT. Many retrospective reviews illustrate this common use.[12,37, 48–52] Often the criteria for selecting patients for pelvic irradiation after surgery have not been stated, although they probably reflect an investigator bias toward the use of radiation therapy for patients deemed to be at high risk of relapse. Several studies have identified adverse prognostic factors for MMMT[12,35,53]; however, no report has systematically evaluated the role of adjunctive radiation therapy related to these risk factors in MMMTs.

Similarly, there has been no randomized comparison of the influence of adjuvant pelvic irradiation on locoregional control or survival versus that achieved with surgery alone. The GOG is currently conducting a phase III study of whole-abdomen radiotherapy versus ifosfamide-mesna with cisplatin in patients with optimally debulked stage I–IV MMMT (Protocol 150). The benefit of adjuvant radiotherapy in the treatment of MMMT has not been demonstrated in randomized studies. However, in several reports for MMMT, the pelvic recurrence rate was 56%, whereas the distant metastasis rate was 45%. This represents a higher risk of pelvic recurrence than that seen in patients with LMS.[12,37,48,49,53] It also demonstrates that surgery alone, even for disease apparently confined to the uterus, is inadequate for control of disease in the pelvis.

Some but not all studies have shown benefit from postoperative irradiation,[54,55] especially in local control.[51,56–60] However, few studies show that increased local control rates have an effect on overall survival.[12,60,61] Rates of distant metastases in series of patients treated with or without adjuvant pelvic irradiation are similar, in the order of 35%.[12,48,51,53] Knocke and colleagues reported local control in 83.4% of patients and distant control in 70.8%.[62] The disease-specific survival rate was 57.7%, which is high when compared with the majority of reports in the literature.

In a study of the GOG conducted between 1973 and 1982, patients with stage I or II uterine sarcomas, including LMS (48 patients), MMMT (95 patients), ESS (10 patients), and unclassified tumors (4 patients), were randomly assigned to receive adjuvant doxorubicin or no chemotherapy following surgery.[51] The use of adjuvant pelvic radiation therapy was not controlled but was left to investigator discretion, and the study was not stratified for the use of radiation therapy. A subset analysis of this study was conducted by Hornback and colleagues and demonstrated a reduction in pelvic recurrence rates attributable to the use of adjunctive pelvic irradiation.[51] The data must be interpreted with some caution, however, because this was a nonrandomized comparison.

The morbidity associated with pelvic recurrence in uterine sarcomas may be substantial; therefore, it is reasonable to offer adjuvant pelvic irradiation to patients with MMMT to improve locoregional control rates. The doses of radiation have not been standardized; however, it is probable that doses should be at least 50 Gy, fractionated over 5 weeks.

Primary pelvic irradiation has been employed rarely in patients with sarcoma deemed inoperable. The possible additional utility of intracavitary irradiation must be evaluated because radiation dose distribution may be inadequate if the uterus is bulky. Literature reports suggest that in approximately half or two-thirds of patients, pelvic disease could be controlled with standard fractionated irradiation; a small proportion of patients are cured with such treatment.[12,37,48,49]

Finally, radiation may be useful as a palliative measure for recurrent or uncontrolled pelvic tumor causing pain or bleeding.

CHEMOTHERAPY

Two characteristics of uterine sarcomas increase the likelihood that systemic therapy will be required: a recurrence rate of at least 50% even in stage I disease and a tendency to recur at distant sites. Nevertheless, the amount of meaningful data on the use of systemic therapy is limited by the low incidence of these lesions. Studies by the GOG first identified the differential sensitivity of MMMT and LMS to drug therapy.[63] Because these two cell types respond differently to chemotherapy, they are discussed separately.

SINGLE-AGENT THERAPY

Several drugs have been studied in advanced or recurrent MMMT and/or LMS (Table 106-2), including cisplatin,[64–67] ifosfamide,[68–70] doxorubicin,[63,71] etoposide,[72–74] mitoxantrone,[75] paclitaxel,[76] topotecan,[77] gemcitabine,[78]and docetaxel.[79]

Malignant Mixed Müllerian Tumor Ifosfamide is the most active single agent in the treatment of advanced or recurrent MMMT of the uterus. Sutton and colleagues conducted a phase II study of ifosfamide (1.5 g/m^2/d for 5 days every 4 weeks) and mesna in 30 patients with advanced or recurrent MMMT who had no previous chemotherapy.[68] Of 28 evaluable patients, 2 complete responses and 3 partial responses were observed. However, the response duration ranged from 1.4 to 8.6 months, with a median response duration of only 3.8 months (see Table 106-2).

Cisplatin also appears to have significant activity.[64] In patients who had previously received chemotherapy, cisplatin 50 mg/m^2 produced an 18% response rate. Of 28 patients available for evaluation, 2 complete responses and 3 partial responses were observed. The duration of the two complete responses was 14 and 16 months, and the median duration of the partial responses was 3 months. Within this population, 42.9% had received radiation therapy and 89.3% had received therapy with doxorubicin or a doxorubicin-containing combination. In patients who had not previously received chemotherapy, the same response rate of 19% was observed among a larger group of 63 patients treated with the same dose and schedule.[65] The median duration of response was 6.6 months; the median survival was 16.8 months for complete responders (five patients) and 9.3 months for partial responders (seven patients). In a separate phase II trial, a higher dose, ranging from 75 to 100 mg/m^2 every

Table 106-2 Single-Agent Activity in Uterine Sarcomas

Drug	Prior Chemotherapy	Schedule	Response, *n* (%)			Reference
			MMMT	LMS	ESS	
Ifosfamide	No	1.5 g/m²/d + mesna, 0.3 g/m²/d, d 1–5 q 4 wk	9/28 (32)	6/35 (17)	7/21 (33)	68–70
Cisplatin	No	50 mg/m² q 3 wk	12/63 (19)	1/33 (3)		64
	Yes	50 mg/m² q 3 wk	5/28 (18)	1/19 (5)		65, 67
	No	75–100 mg/m² q 3 wk	5/12 (42)			66
Doxorubicin	No	60 mg/m² q 3 wk	4/41 (10)	7/28 (25)		63
	No	50–90 mg/m² q 3 wk	0/9 (0)			71
Etoposide	Yes	100 mg/m²/d, d 1–3 q 4 wk	2/31 (6)	3/28 (11)		72, 74
	Yes	50 mg/m²/d, d 1–21 q 4 wk		2/29 (7)		73
	No	100 mg/m²/d, d 1–3 q 3 wk		0/28 (0)		74
Mitoxantrone	Yes	12 mg/m² q 3 wk	0/17 (0)	0/12 (0)		75
Paclitaxel	No	175 mg/m² q 3 wk		3/34 (9)		76
Topotecan	No	1.5 mg/m²/d, d 1–5 q 3 wk		3/36 (8)		77
Gemcitabine	Yes	1,000 mg/m² d 1, 8, 15 q 4 wk		9/44 (20.5)		78
Docetaxel	Yes	100 mg/m² q 3 wk		1/17 (5.9)		79

ESS = endometrial stromal sarcoma; LMS = leiomyosarcoma; MMMT = malignant mixed müllerian tumor.

3 weeks, produced one complete response and four partial responses among 12 patients (42%) who had not received chemotherapy.[66] The small number of cases and the lack of a randomized trial permit no conclusions to be drawn about the merits of the higher dose.

Leiomyosarcoma Of the single agents that have been tested in patients with LMS (see Table 106-2), doxorubicin is the most active. In the two GOG phase III trials comparing doxorubicin-based chemotherapy in combination with dimethyltriazenoimidazole carboxamide (DTIC)[63] or cyclophosphamide[80] in advanced uterine sarcomas, response rates of 25% and 13%, respectively, were observed in patients with LMS treated with doxorubicin alone. Patients with LMS also had a significantly longer survival time than the other histologic cell types studied (12.1 vs 6.0 months). Ifosfamide, 1.5 g/m²/d for 5 days every 3 to 4 weeks, exhibited moderate activity (17.2%), with 6 responses among 35 patients.[69]

Endometrial Stromal Sarcoma There are few data in the gynecologic literature regarding the use of chemotherapy for ESS. The GOG conducted a phase II study of ifosfamide as initial chemotherapy in women with metastatic ESS.[70] Of 21 evaluable patients, there were 3 complete responses and 4 partial responses, for an overall response rate of 33.3%. Other agents have also been found to be active in the treatment of ESS, including doxorubicin[7,14]; the combination of vincristine, actinomycin D, and cyclophosphamide[7]; the combination of mitomycin and vinblastine[7]; chlorambucil[81]; and the combination of cyclophosphamide, vincristine, doxorubicin, and dacarbazine.[81]

In summary, two agents active against MMMT of the uterus have been identified: ifosfamide and cisplatin. In LMS, doxorubicin and ifosfamide appear to have significant activity.

COMBINATION THERAPY

Randomized Trials Three randomized trials evaluating combination chemotherapy have been completed to date and form the basis for current conclusions regarding the role of chemotherapy.

In the first, patients with advanced (stage III or IV or recurrent) uterine sarcoma received either doxorubicin or doxorubicin plus DTIC (Table 106-3).[63] Although no significant differences between the two regimens were observed, conclusions from the trial were limited by an insufficient number of each histologic type to permit subset analysis.

The second randomized trial studied doxorubicin with or without cyclophosphamide (see Table 106-3) and was closed prior to completion of original accrual goals because, on the basis of early data, the likelihood of identifying a difference in the two treatment regimens was extremely small.[80] The overall response rate was the same for doxorubicin with or without cyclophosphamide (19.2% total response rate). When the data were analyzed by cell type, 3 of the 20 patients with MMMT had complete responses.

With recognition of the difference in response between LMS and MMMT, randomized trials had to consider the two major histologic types as distinct entities requiring separate studies. A third phase III trial (GOG Protocol 108), completed in July 1996, compared ifosfamide with and without cisplatin in patients with advanced or recurrent MMMT.[82] Ifosfamide was given in a dose of 1.5 g/m²/d for 5 days every 3 weeks for eight courses, with mesna uroprotection. In the combination arm, cisplatin was added at 20 mg/m² for 5 days. Early in the study, the dose of the combination regimen was decreased by 20% because of toxicity. Overall, 54% of patients treated with the combination regimen and 36% of patients treated with ifosfamide alone responded to therapy. This combination offered a slight prolongation of progression-free survival (relative risk 0.73; 95% upper confidence limit 0.94; $p = .02$, one-tailed test) but no significant survival benefit (relative risk 0.80; 95% upper confidence limit 1.03; $p = .071$, one-tailed test).

Phase II Trials for LMS Studies of LMS continue to focus on the identification of active drugs in phase II trials.

As discussed previously, the GOG demonstrated no benefit to the addition of either cyclophosphamide or DTIC to doxorubicin in advanced uterine sarcomas.[63,80] The GOG conducted a phase II study of doxorubicin in combination with ifosfamide-mesna in previously untreated patients with advanced or recurrent uterine LMS.[83] Of 33 patients, there was 1 complete response and 10 partial responses. Although the overall response rate was 33.3%, the toxicity was severe, with 13 patients developing grade 4 neutropenia and 2 patients developing grade 4 cardiotoxicity. Leyvraz and colleagues reported much higher response rates with a higher dose intensity with the same combination.[84] At the 1998 meeting of the American Society of Clinical Oncology, they presented data on 17 patients with uterine LMS with a 55% response rate using ifosfamide 2 to 2.4 g/m²/d on days 1 to 5, with doxorubicin 20 to 30 mg/m²/d on days 1 to 3. Granu-

Table 106-3 Randomized Trials of Chemotherapy in Advanced or Recurrent Uterine Sarcomas

Study	Regimen, *n* (%)		
	Doxorubicin	Doxorubicin + DTIC	Doxorubicin + Cytoxan
GOG Protocol 2161	13/80 (16)	16/66 (24)	
Leiomyosarcoma	7/28 (25)	6/20 (30)	
Mixed mesodermal sarcoma	4/41 (10)	7/31 (23)	
Other sarcomas	2/11 (18)	3/15 (20)	
GOG Protocol 4278	5/26 (19)		5/26 (19)

DTIC = dimethyltriazenoimidazole carboxamide; GOG = Gynecologic Oncology Group.

Table 106-4 Randomized Trials of Doxorubicin versus No Further Therapy in Completely Resected Stages I and II Uterine Sarcoma

Cell Type	Recurrences		
	Doxorubicin	No Therapy	Total
Leiomyosarcoma	11/25 (44%)	14/23 (61%)	25/48 (52%)
Mixed mesodermal sarcoma	17/44 (39%)	25/49 (51%)	42/93 (45%)
Other sarcomas	3/6 (50%)	4/9 (44%)	7/15 (47%)
Total	31/75 (41%)	43/81 (53%)	74/156 (47%)

From Omura et al.[86]

locyte colony-stimulating factor was used for 10 days and toxicity was still significant, with 63% febrile episodes and 40% grade 2 to 3 mucositis.

The GOG also reported on the results of a phase II trial of hydroxyurea, DTIC, and etoposide in the treatment of advanced or recurrent uterine LMS.[82] Of 38 evaluable patients, there were 2 complete responses and 5 partial responses, for an overall response rate of 18.4%; 6 of the 7 responders had disease outside the pelvis. The response duration was 12.1 months. Thus, this combination had moderate activity in the treatment of advanced or recurrent uterine LMS.

Hensley and colleagues recently reported a phase II trial in patients with unresectable, measurable LMS of the uterus ($n = 29$) or another ($n = 5$) primary site who had failed zero to two previous chemotherapy regimens.[85] Patients received gemcitabine 900 mg/m^2 intravenously days 1 and 8 plus docetaxel 100 mg/m^2 intravenously day 8, with granulocyte colony-stimulating factor subcutaneously days 9 to 15. Cycles were repeated every 21 days. Patients with prior pelvic radiation received 25% lower doses of both agents. Gemcitabine was delivered over 30 or 90 minutes in cycles 1 and 2 and by 90-minute infusion in all subsequent cycles. Responses were measured after cycles 3 and 6 by computed tomography. Sixteen of 34 patients had progressed after doxorubicin-based chemotherapy; 18 had no previous chemotherapy. Among 34 patients, a complete response was observed in 3 patients and a partial response in 15, for an overall response rate of 53% (95% confidence interval 35–70%). Seven patients had stable disease. Fifty percent of patients previously treated with doxorubicin responded. Hematologic toxicity was common (neutropenia: grade 3, 15%; grade 4, 6%; thrombocytopenia: grade 3, 26%; grade 4, 3%), but neutropenic fever (6%) and bleeding events (0%) were rare. The median time to progression was 5.6 months (range 4–10 months). The authors concluded that gemcitabine plus docetaxel is tolerable and highly active in treated and untreated patients with LMS.[85] The GOG is currently evaluating this combination in a larger phase II study.

ADJUVANT THERAPY FOR LIMITED DISEASE

The only randomized trial (GOG Protocol 20) of adjuvant chemotherapy in uterine sarcomas to date assigned patients to either doxorubicin 60 mg/m^2 every 3 weeks for eight cycles or no further therapy (Table 106-4).[86] For the overall patient population, there were no significant differences in recurrence rate, progression-free interval, or survival between those who received no further treatment and those who received adjuvant doxorubicin. Although each of the two major histologic subsets contained too few patients for proper analysis, in each subset, a 12% or greater difference in recurrence rate was noted, favoring the group receiving doxorubicin. The overall median survival was 73.7 months for patients given doxorubicin and 55.0 months for those given no further therapy. The major deficiency in this study—its failure to take into account the difference in response of the two major histologic subsets—is the result of a lack of understanding of this distinction when the trial was conducted.

The GOG also reported a study (GOG Protocol 117) of adjuvant ifosfamide, mesna, and cisplatin in patients with completely resected stage I or II MMMT of the uterus in which no postoperative radiotherapy was allowed. Ifosfamide was given in a dose of 1.5 g/m^2 and cisplatin 20 mg/m^2 daily for 5 days every 3 weeks for three cycles, with mesna uroprotection.[87] Early in the study, the regimen was reduced to 4 days because of myelotoxicity. Of the 65 evaluable patients, the median age was 65 years; 50 patients (77%) were stage I and 15 (23%) were stage II. Progression-free survival and overall survival rates, respectively, were 69% and 82% at 24 months and 54% and 52% at 84 months. The overall 5-year survival rate was 62%. Leukopenia was the most commonly reported, but manageable, toxicity.

REFERENCES

1. Harlow BL, Weiss NS, Lofton S. The epidemiology of sarcomas of the uterus. J Natl Cancer Inst 1986;76:399–402.
2. Ober WB. Uterine sarcomas: Histogenesis and taxonomy. Ann NY Acad Sci 1959. 75:568
3. Kempson RL, Bari W. Uterine sarcomas. Classification, diagnosis, and prognosis. Hum Pathol 1970;1:331–49.
4. Czesnin K, Wronkowski Z. Second malignancies of the irradiated area in patients treated for uterine cervix cancer. Gynecol Oncol 1978;6:309–15.
5. Norris HJ, Taylor HB. Postirradiation sarcomas of the uterus. Obstet Gynecol 1965;26:689–94.
6. Major FJ, Blessing JA, Silverberg SG, et al. Prognostic factors in early-stage uterine sarcoma. A Gynecologic Oncology Group study. Cancer 1993;71(4 Suppl):1702–9.
7. Berchuck A, Rubin SC, Hoskins WJ, et al. Treatment of endometrial stromal tumors. Gynecol Oncol 1990;36:60–5.
8. Leibsohn S, d'Ablaing G, Mishell DR Jr, et al. Leiomyosarcoma in a series of hysterectomies performed for presumed uterine leiomyomas. Am J Obstet Gynecol 1990;162:968–74; discussion 974–6.
9. Ferenczy A, Richart RM, Okagaki T. A comparative ultrastructural study of leiomyosarcoma, cellular leiomyoma, and leiomyoma of the uterus. Cancer 1971;28:1004–18.
10. Spiro RH, Koss LG. Myosarcoma of the uterus. Cancer 1965;18:571–88.
11. Davids AM. Myomectomy surgical technique and results in a series of 1150 cases. Am J Obstet Gynecol 1952;63:592–604.
12. Larson B, Silfverswärd C, Nilsson B, et al. Mixed müllerian tumours of the uterus—prognostic factors: a clinical and histopathologic study of 147 cases. Radiother Oncol 1990;17:123–32.
13. Wen, BC, Tewfik FA, Tewfick HH et al., Uterine sarcoma: a retrospective study. J Surg Oncol 1987;34(2):104–8.
14. Goff BA, Rice LW, Fleischhacker D, et al. Uterine leiomyosarcoma and endometrial stromal sarcoma: lymph node metastases and sites of recurrence. Gynecol Oncol 1993;50:105–9.
15. Berchuck A, Rubin SC, Hoskins WJ, et al. Treatment of uterine leiomyosarcoma. Obstet Gynecol 1988;71(6 Pt 1):845–50.
16. Kurjak A, Kupesic S, Shalan H, et al. Uterine sarcoma: a report of 10 cases studied by transvaginal color and pulsed Doppler sonography. Gynecol Oncol 1995;59:342–6.
17. Cramer SF, Meyer JS, Kraner JF, et al. Metastasizing leiomyoma of the uterus. S-phase fraction, estrogen receptor, and ultrastructure. Cancer 1980;45:932–7.
18. Evans AT III, Symmonds RE, Gaffey TA. Recurrent pelvic intravenous leiomyomatosis. Obstet Gynecol 1981;57:260–4.
19. Kurman RJ, Norris HJ. Mesenchymal tumors of the uterus. VI. Epithelioid smooth muscle tumors including leiomyoblastoma and clear-cell leiomyoma: a clinical and pathologic analysis of 26 cases. Cancer 1976;7:1853–65.
20. Rose PG, Piver MS, Tsukada Y, et al. Patterns of metastasis in uterine sarcoma. An autopsy study. Cancer 1989;63:935–8.
21. Fleming WP, Peters WA III, Kumar NB, et al. Autopsy findings in patients with uterine sarcoma. Gynecol Oncol 1984;19:168–72.
22. Chen SS. Propensity of retroperitoneal lymph node metastasis in patients with stage I sarcoma of the uterus. Gynecol Oncol 1989;32:215–7.
23. DiSaia PJ, Morrow CP, Boronow R, et al. Endometrial sarcoma: lymphatic spread pattern. Am J Obstet Gynecol 1978;130:104–5.
24. Mayerhofer K, Obermair A, Windbichler G, et al. Leiomyosarcoma of the uterus: a clinicopathologic multicenter study of 71 cases. Gynecol Oncol 1999;74:196–201.
25. Gadducci A, Fabrini MG, Bonuccelli A, et al. Analysis of treatment failures in patients with early-stage uterine leiomyosarcoma. Anticancer Res 1995;15:485–8.
26. Barakat RR, Rubin SC, Wong G, et al. Mixed mesodermal tumor of the ovary: analysis of prognostic factors in 31 cases. Obstet Gynecol 1992;80:660–4.
27. Plaxe SC, Dottino PR, Goodman HM, et al. Clinical features of advanced ovarian mixed mesodermal tumors and treatment with doxorubicin- and cis-platinum-based chemotherapy. Gynecol Oncol 1990;37:244–9.
28. Imachi M, Tsukamoto N, Shigematsu T, et al. Malignant mixed müllerian tumor of the fallopian tube: report of two cases and review of literature. Gynecol Oncol 1992;47:114–24.
29. Horn LC, Werschnik C, Bilek K, et al. Diagnosis and clinical management in malignant müllerian tumors of the fallopian tube. A report of four cases and review of recent literature. Arch Gynecol Obstet 1996;258:47–53.
30. Jacobs AJ, McMurray EH, Parham J, et al. Treatment of carcinoma of the fallopian tube using cisplatin, doxorubicin, and cyclophosphamide. Am J Clin Oncol 1986;9:436–9.
31. Ebert AD, Perez-Canto A, Schaller G, et al. Stage I primary malignant mixed müllerian tumor of the fallopian tube. Report of a case with five-year survival after minimal surgery without adjuvant treatment. J Reprod Med 1998;43:598–600.
32. Taylor HB, Norris HJ. Mesenchymal tumors of the uterus. IV. Diagnosis and prognosis of leiomyosarcomas. Arch Pathol 1966;82:40–4.
33. Aaro LA, Symmonds RE, Dockerty ME. Sarcoma of the uterus. A clinical and pathologic study of 177 cases. Am J Obstet Gynecol 1966;94:101–9.
34. Peters WA III, Kumar NB, Fleming WP, et al. Prognostic features of sarcomas and mixed tumors of the endometrium. Obstet Gynecol 1984;63:550–6.

35. Silverberg SG, Major FJ, Blessing JA, et al. Carcinosarcoma (malignant mixed mesodermal tumor) of the uterus. A Gynecologic Oncology Group pathologic study of 203 cases. Int J Gynecol Pathol 1990;9:1–19.
36. Levenback C, Rubin SC, McCormack PM, et al. Resection of pulmonary metastases from uterine sarcomas. Gynecol Oncol 1992;45:202–5.
37. Spanos WJ Jr, Peters LJ, Oswald MJ. Patterns of recurrence in malignant mixed müllerian tumor of the uterus. Cancer 1986;57:155–9.
38. Creasman WT. New gynecologic cancer staging. Obstet Gynecol 1990;75:287–8.
39. Sutton GP, Stehman FB, Michael H, et al. Estrogen and progesterone receptors in uterine sarcomas. Obstet Gynecol 1986;68:709–14.
40. Katz L, Merino MJ, Sakamoto H, et al. Endometrial stromal sarcoma: a clinicopathologic study of 11 cases with determination of estrogen and progestin receptor levels in three tumors. Gynecol Oncol 1987;26:87–97.
41. Spano JP, Soria JC, Kambouchner M, et al. Long-term survival of patients given hormonal therapy for metastatic endometrial stromal sarcoma. Med Oncol 2003;20:87–93.
42. Leiser AL, Hamid AM, Blanchard R. Recurrence of prolactin-producing endometrial stromal sarcoma with sex-cord stromal component treated with progestin and aromatase inhibitor. Gynecol Oncol 2004;94:567–71.
43. Leunen M, Breugelmans M, De Sutter P, et al. Low-grade endometrial stromal sarcoma treated with the aromatase inhibitor letrozole. Gynecol Oncol 2004;95:769–71.
44. Kitaoka Y, Kitawaki J, Koshiba H, et al. Aromatase cytochrome P450 and estrogen and progesterone receptors in uterine sarcomas: correlation with clinical parameters. J Steroid Biochem Mol Biol 2004;88:183–9.
45. Barter JF, Smith EB, Szpak CA, et al. Leiomyosarcoma of the uterus: clinicopathologic study of 21 cases. Gynecol Oncol 1985;21:220–7.
46. Punnonen R, Lauslahti K, Pystynen P, et al. Uterine sarcomas. Ann Chir Gynaecol Suppl 1985;197:11–4.
47. Yu KJ, Ho DM, Ng HT, et al. Leiomyosarcoma of uterus: a review of 14 cases. Zhonghua Yi Xue Za Zhi (Taipei) 1989;44:109–14.
48. Salazar OM, Bonfiglio TA, Patten SF, et al. Uterine sarcomas: analysis of failures with special emphasis on the use of adjuvant radiation therapy. Cancer 1978;42:1161–70.
49. Perez CA, Askin F, Baglan RJ, et al. Effects of irradiation on mixed müllerian tumors of the uterus. Cancer 1979;43:1274–84.
50. Kohorn EI, Schwartz PE, Chambers JT, et al. Adjuvant therapy in mixed müllerian tumors of the uterus. Gynecol Oncol 1986;23:212–21.
51. Hornback NB, Omura G, Major FJ. Observations on the use of adjuvant radiation therapy in patients with stage I and II uterine sarcoma. Int J Radiat Oncol Biol Phys 1986;12:2127–30.
52. Nordal RR, Kristensen GB, Stenwig AE, et al. An evaluation of prognostic factors in uterine carcinosarcoma. Gynecol Oncol 1997;67:316–21.
53. George M, Pejovic MH, Kramar A. Uterine sarcomas: prognostic factors and treatment modalities—study on 209 patients. Gynecol Oncol 1986;24:58–67.
54. Lotocki R, Rosenshein NB, Grumbine F, et al. Mixed müllerian tumors of the uterus: clinical and pathologic correlations. Int J Gynaecol Obstet 1982;20:237–43.
55. Chuang JT, Van Velden DJ, Graham JB. Carcinosarcoma and mixed mesodermal tumor of the uterine corpus. Review of 49 cases. Obstet Gynecol 1970;35:769–80.
56. Rose PG, Boutselis JG, Sachs L. Adjuvant therapy for stage I uterine sarcoma. Am J Obstet Gynecol 1987;156:660–2.
57. Wheelock JB, Krebs HB, Schneider V, et al. Uterine sarcoma: analysis of prognostic variables in 71 cases. Am J Obstet Gynecol 1985;151:1016–22.
58. Tinkler SD, Cowie VJ. Uterine sarcomas: a review of the Edinburgh experience from 1974 to 1992. Br J Radiol 1993;66:998–1001.
59. Sartori E, Bazzurini L, Gadducci A, et al. Carcinosarcoma of the uterus: a clinicopathological multicenter CTF study. Gynecol Oncol 1997;67:70–5.
60. Gerszten K, Faul C, Kounelis S, et al. The impact of adjuvant radiotherapy on carcinosarcoma of the uterus. Gynecol Oncol 1998;68:8–13.
61. Moskovic E, MacSweeney E, Law M, et al. Survival, patterns of spread and prognostic factors in uterine sarcoma: a study of 76 patients. Br J Radiol 1993;66:1009–15.
62. Knocke TH, Kucera H, Dorfler D, et al. Results of postoperative radiotherapy in the treatment of sarcoma of the corpus uteri. Cancer 1998;83:1972–9.
63. Omura GA, Major FJ, Blessing JA, et al. A randomized study of Adriamycin with and without dimethyl triazenoimidazole carboxamide in advanced uterine sarcomas. Cancer 1983;52:626–32.
64. Thigpen JT, Blessing JA, Orr JW Jr, et al. Phase II trial of cisplatin in the treatment of patients with advanced or recurrent mixed mesodermal sarcomas of the uterus: a Gynecologic Oncology Group study. Cancer Treat Rep 1986;70:271–4.
65. Thigpen JT, Blessing JA, Beecham JA, et al. Phase II trial of cisplatin as first-line chemotherapy in patients with advanced or recurrent uterine sarcomas: a Gynecologic Oncology Group study. J Clin Oncol 1991;9:1962–6.
66. Gershenson DM, Kavanagh JJ, Copeland LJ, et al. Cisplatin therapy for disseminated mixed mesodermal sarcoma of the uterus. J Clin Oncol 1987;5:618–21.
67. Thigpen JT, Blessing JA, Wilbanks GD. Cisplatin as second-line chemotherapy in the treatment of advanced or recurrent leiomyosarcoma of the uterus. A phase II trial of the Gynecologic Oncology Group. Am J Clin Oncol 1986;9:18–20.
68. Sutton GP, Blessing JA, Rosenshein N, et al. Phase II trial of ifosfamide and mesna in mixed mesodermal tumors of the uterus (a Gynecologic Oncology Group study). Am J Obstet Gynecol 1989;161:309–12.
69. Sutton GP, Blessing JA, Barrett RJ, et al. Phase II trial of ifosfamide and mesna in leiomyosarcoma of the uterus: a Gynecologic Oncology Group study. Am J Obstet Gynecol 1992;166:556–9.
70. Sutton G, Blessing JA, Park R, et al. Ifosfamide treatment of recurrent or metastatic endometrial stromal sarcomas previously unexposed to chemotherapy: a study of the Gynecologic Oncology Group. Obstet Gynecol 1996;87(5 Pt 1):747–50.
71. Gershenson DM, Kavanagh JJ, Copeland LJ, et al. High-dose doxorubicin infusion therapy for disseminated mixed mesodermal sarcoma of the uterus. Cancer 1987;59:1264–7.
72. Slayton RE, Blessing JA, Angel C, et al. Phase II trial of etoposide in the management of advanced and recurrent leiomyosarcoma of the uterus: a Gynecologic Oncology Group Study. Cancer Treat Rep 1987;71:1303–4.
73. Rose PG, Blessing JA, Soper JT, et al. Prolonged oral etoposide in recurrent or advanced leiomyosarcoma of the uterus: a Gynecologic Oncology Group study. Gynecol Oncol 1998;70:267–71.
74. Thigpen T, Blessing JA, Yordan E, et al. Phase II trial of etoposide in leiomyosarcoma of the uterus: a Gynecologic Oncology Group study. Gynecol Oncol 1996;63:120–2.
75. Muss HB, Bundy BN, Adcock L, et al. Mitoxantrone in the treatment of advanced uterine sarcoma. A phase II trial of the Gynecologic Oncology Group. Am J Clin Oncol 1990;13:32–4.
76. Sutton G, Blessing JA, Ball H. Phase II trial of paclitaxel in leiomyosarcoma of the uterus: a Gynecologic Oncology Group study. Gynecol Oncol 1999;74:346–9.
77. Miller DS, Blessing JA, Kilgore LC, et al. Phase II trial of topotecan in patients with advanced, persistent, or recurrent uterine leiomyosarcomas: a Gynecologic Oncology Group study. Am J Clin Oncol 2000;23:355–7.
78. Look KY, Sandler A, Blessing JA, et al. Phase II trial of gemcitabine as second-line chemotherapy of uterine leiomyosarcoma: a Gynecologic Oncology Group (GOG) Study. Gynecol Oncol 2004;92:644–7.
79. Edmonson JH, Ebbert LP, Nascimento AG, et al. Phase II study of docetaxel in advanced soft tissue sarcomas. Am J Clin Oncol 1996;19:574–6.
80. Muss HB, Bundy B, DiSaia PJ, et al. Treatment of recurrent or advanced uterine sarcoma. A randomized trial of doxorubicin versus doxorubicin and cyclophosphamide (a phase III trial of the Gynecologic Oncology Group). Cancer 1985;55:1648–53.
81. Mansi JL, Ramachandra S, Wiltshaw E, et al. Endometrial stromal sarcomas. Gynecol Oncol 1990;36:113–8.
82. Sutton G, Brunetto VL, Kilgore L, et al. A phase III trial of ifosfamide with or without cisplatin in carcinosarcoma of the uterus: A Gynecologic Oncology Group study. Gynecol Oncol 2000;79:147–53.
83. Sutton G, Blessing JA, Malfetano JH. Ifosfamide and doxorubicin in the treatment of advanced leiomyosarcomas of the uterus: a Gynecologic Oncology Group study. Gynecol Oncol 1996;62:226–9.
84. Leyvraz S, Bacchi M, Lissoni A, et al High response rate with the combination of high-dose ifosfamide and doxorubicin for the treatment of advanced gynecologic sarcomas. J Clin Oncol 1998; 17:354a.
85. Hensley ML, Maki R, Venkatraman E, et al. Gemcitabine and docetaxel in patients with unresectable leiomyosarcoma: results of a phase II trial. J Clin Oncol 2002;20:2824–31.
86. Omura GA, Blessing JA, Major F, et al. A randomized clinical trial of adjuvant Adriamycin in uterine sarcomas: a Gynecologic Oncology Group study. J Clin Oncol 1985;3:1240–5.
87. Sutton G, Kauderer J, Carson LF, et al. Adjuvant ifosfamide and cisplatin in patients with completely resected stage I or II carcinosarcomas (mixed mesodermal tumors) of the uterus: a Gynecologic Oncology Group study. Gynecol Oncol 2005;96:630–4.

Section 31

THE BREAST

107

Neoplasms of the Breast

Gabriel N. Hortobagyi, MD, FACP
Laura Esserman, MD
Thomas A. Buchholz, MD

Female breast cancer is a major medical problem with significant public health and societal ramifications. Despite major advances that have been made in the past 35 years in understanding the biologic and clinical nature of the disease, and notwithstanding dramatic changes in its treatment, the problem persists and has become more complex.[1] The National Cancer Institute estimates that there are currently more than 2 million breast cancer survivors in the United States.[2] The lifetime risk for women of being diagnosed with breast cancer is currently between 1 in 7 and 1 in 8 (Table 107-1).[2] The risk is even higher for women with certain risk factors, such as a strong family history or known *BRCA1* or *BRCA2* mutations. However, these statistics portray only one aspect of the problem. As new information accumulates, new paradigms of management compete for acceptance with existing ones. It is axiomatic that good scientific data provides the bedrock for good clinical management. Information obtained from molecular, biologic, and pathologic investigations and from clinical trials provides the major focus of this chapter.

Table 107-1 Lifetime Probability of Developing Breast Cancer, Females, All Races

Age	Cumulative Probability
By age 25	1 in 11,571
By age 30	1 in 2,082
By age 35	1 in 589
By age 40	1 in 228
By age 45	1 in 103
By age 50	1 in 54
By age 55	1 in 32
By age 60	1 in 22
By age 65	1 in 16
By age 70	1 in 13
By age 75	1 in 11
By age 80	1 in 9
By age 85	1 in 8

Feuer EJ, Wun LM. DEVCAN: Probability of developing or dying of cancer software, Version 4.2. National Cancer Institute, 2002.

EPIDEMIOLOGY

Breast cancer is the most common malignancy in North American women and for women throughout the industrialized world. In the United States, breast cancer accounts for 32% of all cancers in women.[3] The American Cancer Society estimates that during 2005, 211,240 women will be diagnosed as having breast cancer.[3] The incidence rate of breast cancer has increased steadily over the past 40 years, by about 4% per year in the 1980s (Table 107-2). Incidence rates in women leveled off in the 1990s to about 110 cases per 100,000, however, and for the last 9 years for which complete statistics are available, there has been a modest but continued decrease in incidence.[2]

Some experts believe that the earlier gradual increase in incidence can be explained by the more frequent and systematic use of screening mammography and the lead-time bias associated with earlier diagnosis. Another significant cause of the increasing incidence of breast cancer is that the average age of the population is increasing, and more women are moving into the ages where breast cancer is most common. The incidence of breast cancer has also increased worldwide. In 1985, it was estimated that more than 500,000 new cases would be diagnosed, with about half of the cases occurring in the Western, industrialized countries and the other half occurring in developing countries. By 1990, it was estimated that close to 900,000 new cases of breast cancer would be diagnosed, and during 2002, more than 1,100,000 women developed breast cancer. Incidence rates vary substantially around the world. The incidence rates reported range 4 and 6 per 100,000 (Mozambique and Gambia, respectively) to 28.61 per 100,000 women (Japan) and contrast with incidence rates higher than 110 new cases per year per 100,000 women from the United States and Northern Europe.[4,5] Some of these differences have been attributed to diet, whereas others might be related to behavioral modification associated to the changing roles of women in modern industrialized societies (earlier onset of menses, delayed parity, use of oral contraceptives and hormone replacement therapy, later onset of menopause, longer life-expectancy, and increased consumption of alcohol).[6,7]

The mortality rate of breast cancer in the United States remained essentially stable from the

Table 107-2 Rates by Race or Ethnicity, United States, 1996–2000

	All Races	White	African-American	Hispanic-Latino	American Indian/Asian/Pacific Islander	Alaskan Native
Incidence rates (per 100,000)[2,3]	135.0	140.8	121.7	89.8	58.0	97.2
Mortality rates (per 100,000)[2,3]	27.7	27.2	35.9	17.9	14.9	12.5

1950s to 1989. According to the most recent data, however, mortality rates declined significantly between 1990 and 1999, with the largest decreases in younger women—both white and African American.[2] These decreases are probably the result of earlier detection and improved treatment. The American Cancer Society estimated that in 2005, 40,870 deaths related to breast cancer would be reported, 40,410 of them in women. That figure represents 15% of all cancer-related deaths in American women.[3] National statistics suggest that there has been a decrease in the mortality rate of breast cancer in women of all ages over the past decade, being most prominent in white women under the age of 50 years and least notable in African American women older than 50 years. Similar decreases in breast cancer–related mortality obtained from population-based figures were recently released from British Columbia (Canada), Austria, Germany, Sweden, and the United Kingdom. However, these favorable trends are not universal and have not been evident in other countries.[8–9] Breast cancer is the second leading cause of cancer-related deaths in women in the United States (after lung cancer), but it is the leading cause of cancer-related deaths in women between the ages of 20 and 59.[3] The relative 5-year survival rates increased from 63 to 89% for white women between 1960 and 2000 and from 46 to 75% for black women during the same period.[3]

Sixty-three percent of new breast cancer cases in the United States are diagnosed while in the localized (node-negative) stage; another 29% are diagnosed in a regional stage, and 6% have metastasized to distant sites at the time of initial diagnosis (stage was unknown for the remaining 2%).[3] The percentage of patients with localized breast cancer is even higher among women who follow a systematic screening strategy; among these patients, between 20 and 30% of breast cancer cases are diagnosed in a noninvasive stage, and of those with invasive breast cancer, up to 79% have negative axillary lymph nodes.[10] In contrast, at least 50% of breast cancer cases in Latin America and other parts of the developing world are reported in stage III or IV at the time of diagnosis.[11,12] This is a substantial public health challenge for these countries, and, despite lower incidence rates, it results in higher mortality rates than those observed in Western Europe and the United States.[13] The mortality-to-incidence ratios ranged from 0.19 in North America to 0.46 in Southeast Asia to a high of 0.73 in Middle Africa. In 2000 it was estimated that 471,000 deaths were attributed to breast cancer around the world.[12]

RISK FACTORS

The incidence of breast cancer varies substantially according to the presence or absence of certain well-established risk factors (Table 107-3).[6,14,15] Among these factors, the two most prominent are gender and age.

Gender The age-adjusted breast cancer incidence rate is approximately 100 times higher in women than in men in the United States, a ratio that is fairly consistent around the world, although some reports suggest that the incidence of male breast cancer might be several fold higher in some African countries.[2,4] A number of risk factors have been identified in women. Because of the small number of male breast cancers, risk factors for male breast cancer are much less well established.

Table 107-3 Risk Factors Associated with the Development of Breast Cancer

Major increase
Mutations in *BRCA1*, *BRCA2*, Li-Fraumeni syndrome
Increasing age
Western culture
Family history of breast or ovarian cancer in first-degree relatives
Benign breast disease with atypical hyperplasia
Exposure to ionizing radiation
Prior diagnosis of breast cancer
Moderate increase
Early menarche
Late menopause
Nulliparity or delayed first full-term pregnancy (above age 30)
High socioeconomic status
Alcohol intake
Height
Obesity (postmenopausal women only)
Unfavorable mammographic parenchymal pattern
Diagnosis of soft-tissue sarcoma in son or daughter
Prior diagnosis of uterine, ovarian, or colon cancer
Benign breast disease with hyperplasia but without atypia
Oral contraceptives (for longer than 10 years)
Postmenopausal estrogen replacement therapy
Questionable increase
Interrupted first pregnancy
Psychosomatic factors
High-fat diet
Complex fibroadenoma
Exposure to low-frequency electromagnetic fields
Decrease
Full-term pregnancy before age 20
Multiple pregnancies
Ovariectomy before age 45
Regular exercise, especially during adolescence and early adulthood
Breast feeding
No effect
Breast size
Fibrocystic disease without proliferative changes
Smoking
Organochlorine exposure

Age It is evident that the incidence of breast cancer increases dramatically with age, ranging from fewer than 10 cases per 100,000 women between the ages of 20 and 30 to more than 200 cases per 100,000 women over the age of 60.[2] The probabilities of developing invasive breast cancer are 0.48, 4.18, 7.49 and 13.39 percent for women age 39 or younger, 40 to 59, 60 to 79 and lifetime, respectively.[3] However, the correlation of age and increase in incidence is not linear. The slope of the correlation curve is steepest in younger women; it decreases dramatically during and shortly after the menopause, to resume a steeper correlation several years after menopause. The median age at diagnosis of breast cancer in the United States is 64 years. In other parts of the world, where life expectancy is shorter, the median age at which breast cancer develops is 10 to 15 years younger. Age-related mortality rates parallel this pattern.

Socioeconomic Class Breast cancer is found more frequently in women of higher economic class and educational status.[14] This finding is probably related to lifestyle factors such as diet, age at first childbirth, exogenous hormonal use, and alcohol consumption. However, mortality is higher in women of underprivileged groups, suggesting that access to care and compliance with treatment remain important obstacles for optimal diagnosis and treatment.

Ethnicity There have been multiple reports to suggest that there are important differences in breast cancer incidence and mortality rates among various minority groups in the United States (see Table 107-2).[3] The incidence rates of female breast cancer for 1996 to 2000 were 119.9 per 100,000 among African Americans, 89.6 per 100,000 among Hispanic Americans, 54.2 per 100,000 for American Indians/Alaskan Natives, 96.8 per 100,000 for Asians/Pacific Islanders, and 135.2 per 100,000 for white women.[2] These represent increases compared to the previous 5-year period.[2,3] In contrast, the estimated mortality rates for 1992 to 1999 for the same ethnic groups were 35.4, 17.3, 13.6, 12.6, and 26.4, respectively. Although breast cancer was diagnosed in a localized stage in 64% of white women, it was diagnosed in that stage in only 53% of African Americans.[3] Studies have suggested that Jewish women, especially those with a family history of breast cancer in a first-degree relative, have a risk of breast cancer almost four times that of women in other ethnic groups. In fact, it was recently shown that a single *BRCA1* mutation can be found in as many as 1% of the Ashkenazi Jewish population.[16] Studies of migrant populations have shown that when low-risk groups (eg, Chinese or other Far-Eastern groups) move to high-risk regions (Hawaii or mainland United States), their incidence of breast cancer increases rapidly, approaching the rates of the host population within one or two generations.[17]

Family History/Genetics Approximately one-third of women with breast cancer have one or more first-degree relatives with breast cancer.[18] About 4 to 9% are considered to have hereditary breast cancer.[19] Individuals with a first-degree relative with a history of breast cancer have a substantially increased risk of developing breast cancer themselves compared to women without such a family history (Table 107-4).[14] The identification and cloning of *BRCA1* and *BRCA2,* two genes associated with familial breast (and ovarian) cancer, have highlighted the importance of taking a careful family history during the initial evaluation of breast cancer risk factors. Linkage analysis

Table 107-4 Risk Model and Associated Relative Risks*

Risk Factor (Code No.)		Associated Relative Risk	No. Cases (n = 2,852)	No. Controls (n = 3,146)
Age at menarche (yr)				
≥14 (0)		1.000	790	926
12–13 (1)		1.099	1,554	1,735
< 12 (2)		1.207	508	485
No. previous breast biopsies				
Age < 50 yr				
0 (0)		1.000	635	794
1 (1)		1.698	113	93
≥2 (2)		2.882	66	24
Age ≥ 50 yr				
0 (0)		1.000	1,551	1,817
1 (1)		1.273	312	300
≥ 2 (2)		1.620	175	118
Age at first live birth (yr)	No. relatives with breast cancer			
< 20 (0)	0 (0)	1.000	167	285
	1 (1)	2.607	44	40
	≥ 2 (2)	6.798	8	0
20–24 (1)	0 (0)	1.244	708	1,042
	1 (1)	2.681	208	123
	≥ 2 (2)	5.775	25	5
25–29 or nulliparous (2)	0 (0)	1.548	986	1,106
	1 (1)	2.756	247	178
	≥2 (2)	4.907	46	20
≥ 30 (3)	0 (0)	1.927	307	291
	1 (1)	2.834	87	50
	≥ 2 (2)	4.169	19	6

*Relative risk compared to an individual of the same age without any risk factors is estimated by locating the person's associated relative risk for AGEMEN, NBIOPS, and the combination AGEFLB and NUMREL and multiplying these three numbers together.

From Gail MH, et al.[57]

localized *BRCA1* to chromosome 17q21, and loss of heterozygosity studies suggested that this gene acts as a tumor suppressor gene. Its physiological function is related to DNA repair. *BRCA2* was localized to chromosome 13q12. *BRCA2* mutations are associated with early-onset breast and ovarian cancer and male breast cancer, as well as prostate and pancreatic cancer.[16,20,21] The prevalence of *BRCA1* mutations in high-risk families ranges from less than 20% to more than 80% in different countries. The prevalence is higher in families with ovarian cancer or both ovarian and breast cancer. In population-based series of patients who had breast cancer diagnosed before age 35 years, *BRCA1* mutations were detected in 6.2%.[22,23] The great majority of *BRCA1* mutations are found in individuals with moderate- to high-risk families. For those individuals with *BRCA1* or *BRCA2* mutations, the lifetime risk of developing breast cancer ranges from 40 to 85%. The characteristics of *BRCA1*-related breast cancers include earlier age at onset, lower diploidy rate, higher proliferative rate, higher mitotic counts, higher proportion of estrogen receptor–negative and progesterone receptor–negative tumors, and more lymphocytic infiltration than sporadic cancers.[23] *BRCA2*-associated cancers had lower mitotic counts, higher score for tubule formation, and greater proportion of continuous pushing margins than sporadic tumors.[23] Despite the association with adverse prognostic characteristics, *BRCA1*-associated breast cancers have prognoses similar to or better than sporadic tumors of similar stage.[23,24]

Characteristic *BRCA1* (185delAG, 5382insC) and *BRCA2* (6174delT) mutations have been identified in Ashkenazi Jews; the combined frequency of these genes in the general population exceeds 2%.[16,25] Similar "founder" mutations have been identified in Belgium, Denmark, Finland, France, Holland, Hungary, Iceland, Norway, and Russia, among other ethnic communities.[26] Familial breast cancer, however, accounts for less than 10% of all breast cancers, and *BRCA1*- and *BRCA2*-related familial breast cancers appear to be responsible for only half to two-thirds of these cases. Other genetic abnormalities and less common familial cancer syndromes (Li-Fraumeni and others) are responsible for an additional small number of breast cancers. The cloning of *BRCA1* and *BRCA2* and the presumed appearance of additional molecular genetic markers of risk have brought the issue of genetic screening and counseling to the forefront. Both negative and positive test results are associated with a variety of emotional, legal, economic, and work-related issues. Ongoing clinical trials are in the process of determining who the optimal subjects for screening are, how screening and counseling should be performed, and what approaches are needed to prevent unexpected risks and adverse consequences of genetic testing.

Endocrine and Reproductive Risk Factors Numerous studies suggest a strong link between the female hormone estrogen and the development of breast cancer. In experimental systems, estrogen is required for optimal development of mammary carcinomas. Breast cancer is almost exclusively a disease of women and is rare in males. Ovarian ablation reduces dramatically the risk of mammary cancers in women and in experimental animals. Clinical reports suggest that the younger the age when ovarian ablation is performed, the greater the protective effect. Epidemiologic studies have demonstrated repeatedly that the absence of full-term pregnancies is a risk factor for breast cancer.[15] Early onset of menarche, late onset of menopause, and a greater number of years with ovulatory cycles have all been associated with an increased risk of breast cancer. Thus, women who start menses before the age of 12 have twice the incidence of breast cancer as do those who undergo menarche after age 12.[15] This is probably related to longer exposure of the breast parenchyma to physiologic levels of estrogens. External influences that delay the onset of menses, such as poor nutrition or strenuous physical activity, might, therefore, reduce the incidence of breast cancer.[27] Some epidemiologic studies have suggested that delayed menopause is also associated with an increased incidence of breast cancer. Menopause occurring after age 54 increases risk of breast cancer twofold, compared to the risk of women who have their menopause before age 45. Women who have their first full-term pregnancy before age 18 have an incidence of breast cancer that is one-third that of women who have their first pregnancy after age 35. This has led to speculation that the initial mutagenic event usually occurs before age 18, probably during the rapid growth of the breast at puberty, and that the hormonal milieu of pregnancy diminishes the oncogenicity of the mutated cells. In fact, women who have their first child after age 30 have a higher risk of breast cancer than nulliparous women. The possible mechanism for this apparent enhancement in risk might be the stimulatory effect of pregnancy (and its altered hormonal environment) on an otherwise involuting epithelium. Additional factors include the number of pregnancies and lactation. Most epidemiologic studies have suggested that long periods of lactation reduce breast cancer risk, but that the effect of short periods of lactation that are typical of women in most developed nations is likely to be small. In a recent meta-analysis, each birth decreased the relative risk of breast cancer by 7%, and each year of breastfeeding decreased the relative risk by an additional 4.3%.[28]

Insulin-like growth factor type 1 (IGF-1) is a mitogenic peptide that enhances the proliferation of breast epithelial cells and is thought to have a role in breast cancer.[29] A recent case-control study within the prospective Nurses' Health Study cohort showed a positive relation between circulating IGF-1 concentration and risk of breast cancer among premenopausal women. This correlation was absent in the postmenopausal group. Additional studies to determine the potential clinical utility of this observation are needed.

Exogenous Hormones The relationship of exogenous hormone replacement or oral contraceptives to risk of breast cancer has been under intense scrutiny for the past several decades.[30,31] The composition of oral contraceptives has changed considerably over the years; the type and dose of estrogens, the presence or absence of a progestin, duration of administration, and age at onset all vary from study to study. Until recently, published studies have presented inconsistent and often contradictory conclusions. Both topics have been the subject of meta-analysis. In a large meta-analysis, the Collaborative Group on Hormonal Factors in Breast Cancer found that current or recent use of hormone replacement therapy was associated with a modest increase in risk of breast cancer.[30] The RR was 1.35 (ie, a 35% increase) for women who had used hormone replacement therapy for 5 years or longer. On an annualized basis, this increase is comparable in magnitude with the effect on breast cancer of delaying menopause.

Five or more years after cessation of hormone replacement therapy, there was no significant excess in breast cancer risk. Definitive results were recently provided by the Women's Health Initiative randomized controlled trial. In this study, 16,608 postmenopausal women were randomly assigned to conjugated estrogen plus medroxyprogesterone acetate or placebo.[31] After a 5.2-year mean follow-up, there was a 29% increase in coronary heart disease, a 26% increase in breast cancer, a 41% increase in stroke and a 13% increase in pulmonary embolism associated with hormone replacement therapy. Simultaneously, there was a 47% reduction in colorectal cancer and a 34% reduction in hip fractures among women on hormonal replacement. No protective effects were found for memory loss or other measures of intellectual function. The Million Women Study and the HERS II study reached similar conclusions.[32,33] The increase in the RR of breast cancer was greater for women of lower rather than women of higher weight or body mass index.[30] Combined estrogen-progestin treatments conferred a significantly higher risk than estrogen alone. Cancers diagnosed in women who had received hormone replacement therapy tended to be less advanced clinically than those diagnosed in women who had never received hormone replacement therapy. Some have suggested that the increased risk is predominantly for lobular but not ductal carcinomas. The increase in risk of breast cancer is substantially less than that for endometrial cancer associated with estrogen replacement therapy. The United States Preventive Services Task Force concluded that the harmful effects of estrogen and progestin are likely to exceed the chronic disease prevention effects in most women. Although short-term use of hormone replacement therapy might be beneficial for control of vasomotor symptoms related to menopause, long-term use is not indicated.

Recent, detailed analyses of the many epidemiologic studies correlating oral contraceptive use with risk of breast cancer have reached somewhat similar conclusions.[34] Current or recent users of oral contraceptives have a small increase in the RR of having breast cancer (RR for current users = 1.24), but this excess risk disappears 10 years after stopping use. Women who began using oral contraceptives before age 20 had higher RRs of having breast cancer diagnosed. As was stated in relation to hormone replacement therapy, the cancers diagnosed in association with oral contraceptive use tended to be less advanced clinically than the cancers diagnosed in those who have never used oral contraceptives.[34]

Abortion Several epidemiologic studies suggested that a history of abortion correlated with a higher incidence of breast cancer. Additional studies have not provided confirmation of these findings, however, and at the moment there is insufficient evidence to support an association of abortion with breast cancer risk.

Physical Activity Regular physical activity, especially during adolescence, has been associated with significant reductions in the risk of early onset of breast cancer in some studies.[27] Strenuous exercise has profound effects on menstrual activity during adolescence. Exercise delays menarche and produces amenorrhea in ballet dancers and females participating in college athletic programs. Participation in even moderate levels of physical activity can significantly reduce the frequency of ovulatory cycles.[35] Any factor that reduces the frequency of ovulation, and therefore the cumulative exposure to ovarian hormones, may reduce a woman's lifetime risk of developing breast cancer. On the basis of this information, one might hypothesize that regular physical exercise during adolescence and early adulthood would be beneficial, even if its effect on reducing breast cancer risk remains unproven.

Environmental Factors, Obesity, and Diet The incidence of breast cancer varies markedly throughout the world.[13] There is a six- to ten-fold difference in incidence between the United States and Western Europe (highest incidence) and most middle-African countries (lowest incidence), with Asian, Latin American, and Eastern and Southern European countries reporting an intermediate incidence.[13] The incidence rates in some of the low-risk regions have been increasing over the past several decades. Furthermore, epidemiologic studies have indicated that immigrant groups from low- to high-risk regions evidence increasing incidence rates that approach those of the higher risk host region.[17,35] These marked differences in incidence of breast cancer and the rapid changes in risk observed in migrant populations suggest that environmental factors might influence the risk of developing breast cancer; in fact, environmental factors might be more important than the influence of genetic factors, perhaps with the notable exception of the familial breast cancer syndromes. Variations in weight, height, and reproductive factors represent confounding variables in these studies. In addition, most confounding risk factors point to dietary differences between high-and low-risk regions.[36] Many studies have attempted to establish a correlation between dietary intake of animal proteins, total calories, animal fat, fiber, micronutrients, and risk of breast cancer.[6,36,37] Virtually all these studies were retrospective in nature. Whereas some earlier studies suggested that increased caloric and saturated fat intake may be correlated with increased risk of breast cancer, more recent and definitive studies have failed to confirm this hypothesis. Ongoing laboratory and epidemiologic studies are attempting to assess the influence of dietary fiber intake on breast cancer risk.[38] Studies in animal models point to the potential role of dietary fat in breast carcinogenesis. Even in preclinical experiments, there is ongoing controversy about the relative role of total caloric intake and saturated fat in mammary carcinogenesis.[39]

On the basis of these conflicting experimental and clinical data, one might conclude that the association between diet and risk of breast cancer is weak, at best, and possibly nonexistent. Nevertheless, substantial epidemiologic literature is the basis of the hypothesis that a high caloric intake, especially a high intake of saturated fats, might be linked to increased breast cancer risk. Dietary interventions have been tested in preclinical animal experiments with mixed results. In some models and animal species used, decreased caloric intake and a low-fat diet have been associated with a decreased risk of breast cancer or no change in the incidence of mammary carcinoma. Despite the lack of agreement on the impact of diet on the risk of breast cancer, there are currently several ongoing trials in which dietary interventions are being evaluated for breast cancer prevention.

Dietary interventions (mostly low-fat diets that limit daily caloric intake from fat to less than 15 to 20%) have proven feasible in preliminary or pilot studies.[40,41] The lessons learned from these studies are being applied in large, controlled, multicenter cancer prevention trials.[41] The Women's Health Initiative is a randomized, placebo-controlled, multicenter trial involving postmenopausal women aged 50 to 79 years. Three different interventions were built into this study, one of which was designed to reduce fat intake to 20% of all caloric intake while increasing the intake of fruits and vegetables. Whether this modest reduction in dietary fat intake can result in a tangible reduction in breast cancer risk or not, the reduction in dietary fat may have salutary effects on the prevention or control of cardiovascular disease, osteoarthritis, endometrial cancer, diabetes, and other chronic illnesses. Because obesity in post-menopausal women is a risk factor that is associated with a greater risk of breast cancer, weight reduction should be encouraged in middle-aged and older adults, even in the absence of demonstrated clear-cut benefits in terms of reduction of breast cancer incidence because other health benefits may be associated with this intervention. This study completed patient accrual and results are eagerly awaited. Additional studies should clarify the role of diet in the etiology of breast cancer. Finally, there is some evidence that women with a high intake (as measured by excretion) of phytoestrogens, particularly the isoflavonic phytoestrogen equol and the lignan enterolactone, have a lower breast cancer risk.

The relation of body weight to breast cancer is complex.[42–44] An inverse association between relative weight and breast cancer risk has been found among premenopausal women in most case-control and prospective studies. Obesity may reduce breast cancer risk slightly in premenopausal women through its association with anovulatory menstrual cycles. In many case-control studies, body mass index has been positively associated with postmenopausal breast cancer.[43] However, prospective studies have generally suggested only a weak, if any, positive association.[42,43] Postmenopausal women who are obese have higher estrogen levels resulting from greater conversion of adrenal androgens to estrogens in adipose tissue, and they have lower levels of sex hormone–binding globulin, resulting in more free estrogen.[44] Dietary fat reduction has been shown to reduce body weight and plasma estradiol concentration in postmenopausal women.[44] This provides additional evidence in support of interventional studies to reduce chances of developing breast cancer. Other studies suggest that total body size, rather than weight-to-height ratio, and increased central-to-peripheral body fat distribution may be more important than degree of adiposity.[42] In summary, the role of specific dietary factors in breast cancer causation is not completely resolved. Results from prospective studies do not support the concept that fat intake in middle life has a major relation to breast cancer risk. However, weight gain in middle life contributes substantially to breast cancer risk. Alcohol is the best-established dietary risk factor, probably by increasing endogenous estrogen levels. Hypotheses relating diet during youth to risk decades later will be difficult to test. Nevertheless, available evidence is strong that breast cancer risk can be reduced by avoiding weight gain during adult years, and by limiting alcohol consumption.

Alcohol Consumption Epidemiologic studies have consistently found that women who drink alcohol are at increased risk of developing breast cancer.[45,46] In multivariate analyses controlled for age, race, body mass, and smoking, the RR ranged from 1.5, for one to two drinks per day, to 3.3, for six or more drinks per day. There were no significant differences in this association depending on the type of alcoholic beverage. Early exposure to alcohol may be a key risk factor. Alcohol consumption in pre-menopausal women has been associated with increased total estrogen levels and bioavailable estrogens. The association of alcohol consumption and postmenopausal obesity with subsequent breast cancer risk might be mediated, at least in part, through alteration of plasma estrogen levels. Recent epidemiologic data suggested that the excess risk of breast cancer associated with alcohol consumption may be reduced by adequate folate intake.[47]

Viral Particles For several decades there have been suggestions that breast cancer might be associated with oncogenic viruses. Such reports were strengthened by the demonstration that mouse mammary tumor virus (MMTV) caused mammary carcinomas in mice. Recent reports have shown that sequences highly homologous to segments of MMYV are present in human malignant breast tumors.[48] This finding is present in 30 to 40% of breast cancers in Western Europe and the United States, whereas in the Far East it is found in about 10% of breast cancers. Such sequences have not been found in normal breast tissue. Whether these viral particles are causally related to human breast cancer remains to be established.

Radiation Exposure Exposure to ionizing radiation is a known risk factor for breast cancer. Atomic bomb survivors and patients treated with irradiation for postpartum mastitis, acne, hirsutism, or arthritic conditions all have an increased incidence of breast cancer, even after low or moderate radiation doses. Repeated fluoroscopic chest radiography, as used for monitoring the treatment of tuberculosis in the past, is also associated with increased risk of breast cancer. However, the risk of developing breast cancer as a result of common diagnostic radiologic procedures is minimal, and radiology technologists do not have an increased incidence of breast cancer. The incidence of breast cancer is also increased in patients who received radiotherapy with the mantle technique for Hodgkin's disease.[49] The adolescent and young adult breast appear most susceptible to the carcinogenic effects of ionizing radiation, but irradiation during infancy and childhood also increases breast cancer risk. The latency period between radiation exposure and the development of breast cancer is long (median 30 years). Recent evidence suggests that therapeutic radiation administered to treat primary breast cancer increases modestly (about 30%) the risk of developing a contralateral breast cancer more than 5 years after treatment.[50]

Environmental Factors Cigarette smoking does not appear to increase the overall risk of developing breast cancer, but a recent study showed that there was a significant increase in the risk if young women begin smoking within 5 years of menarche. Although there is substantial interest in evaluating the influence of other occupational and environmental exposures on the risk of breast cancer, no definitive correlation has been found.

Benign Breast Disease Benign breast disease includes a broad array of different, unrelated pathologic entities. However, a number of studies suggest that the presence (or history) of benign breast disease is associated with an increase in breast cancer risk.[51] Other studies have found that women who have had a previous breast biopsy for benign disease are also at increased risk. This association is limited to a large extent, however, to biopsy-proven lesions with histologic demonstration of atypia or proliferative lesions (atypical ductal or lobular hyperplasia) (Table 107-5).[52] When compared with women who had never had a breast biopsy, women with benign breast disease without hyperplasia had an odds ratio of breast cancer of 1.5; women with hyperplasia without atypia had an odds ratio of 1.8, and women with hyperplasia and atypia had an odds ratio of 2.6 to 4.3.[52,53] Although there has been ongoing controversy regarding the definitions used to diagnose these various pathologic entities, there has been growing consensus among pathologists to adopt the classification proposed by Page and colleagues.[51] In this system, the joint occurrence of family history of breast cancer and atypical hyperplasia had a strong synergistic effect on breast cancer risk. Women with papillomas with atypical hyperplasia and those with fibroadenoma also have increased risk of breast cancer. Most other forms of benign breast disease appear to be unrelated to an increased breast cancer risk. Therefore, the majority of women with lumpy breasts, and most of those with benign breast disease, does not have a significantly increased risk of breast cancer. Cytogenetic and molecular genetic studies have suggested that some alterations found in breast cancer are first detected earlier in the biological continuum between normal breast epithelium and frank carcinoma.[54] Although some abnormalities have been detected more often than others, no characteristic molecular abnormalities for various benign breast syndromes have been determined.

Table 107-5 Relative Risk* of Invasive Breast Carcinoma Based on Histologic Examination of Breast Tissue without Carcinoma

No increased risk (no proliferative disease)
Adenosis
Apocrine change
Duct ectasia
Mild epithelial hyperplasia of usual type
Slightly increased risk (1.5–2 times) (proliferative disease without atypia)
Hyperplasia of usual type, moderate or florid
Papilloma (probably)
Sclerosing adenosis
Moderately increased risk (4–5 times) (atypical hyperplasia or borderline lesion)
Atypical ductal hyperplasia
Atypical lobular hyperplasia
High risk (8–10 times) (carcinoma in situ)†
Lobular carcinoma in situ—both breasts
Ductal carcinoma in situ (noncomedo)—unilateral, local

*Women in each category are compared with women matched for age who have had no breast biopsies for the risk of invasive breast cancer during the ensuing 10 to 20 years. These risks are not lifetime risks.

†Only smaller examples of noncomedo ductal carcinoma have consistently been assessed as risk indicators after biopsy only.

From Dupont WD and Page DL.[51]

Mammographic Parenchymal Pattern In 1976, Wolfe proposed that mammographic parenchymal patterns are predictive of breast cancer risk.[55] The P2 pattern, defined as prominent ducts occupying 25% or more of the breast volume, and the DY pattern, characterized by irregular, sheet-like radiographic densities, pose the highest risk. Subsequent studies have been inconsistent in confirming this observation, perhaps because of a lack of standardization and poor reproducibility in accurately classifying mammograms. Nevertheless, the cumulative data suggest that the P2 and DY patterns are moderate risk factors for breast cancer.

Other Risk Factors Several other factors that influence the risk of breast cancer have been reported. Patients with a previous history of ovarian, uterine, or bowel cancer have a higher breast cancer risk. Mothers of children with soft-tissue sarcoma have been reported to have a two- to threefold increased risk of breast cancer. Caffeine consumption does not increase breast cancer risk, and its ability to exacerbate the symptoms of benign breast disease remains unproven. Recent studies suggesting that various psychosomatic factors increase breast cancer risk lack confirmation, as does the recent report suggesting that exposure to extremely low-frequency electromagnetic fields causes excess mortality from breast cancer.

Breast Cancer Risk Assessment Models A number of statistical models can be used to estimate a woman's risk of breast cancer. Some models predict the risk of developing breast cancer framing both short-term and lifetime risk. The models are highly dependent on the age of the person; thus, a very low short-term risk for a young woman may be accompanied by a high lifetime risk. The Gail Risk Assessment model[57,58] and the Claus model[59,60] are the most frequently used models to predict a woman's risk of breast cancer.[61] Other models, such as BRCA-PRO,[62,63] Frank,[64] and Couch[65] predict the risk or probability of carrying a genetic mutation. These models should be used to guide decisions to perform genetic testing for the presence of cancer causing mutations in BRCA1 or BRCA2. They do not identify the risk of developing cancer; rather, prediction will depend on the results of the test looking for inherited predisposition for breast cancer. The interpretation of the results of genetic testing results depends on the knowledge of whether the proband (person with a cancer) is the one being tested, and whether or not there is a known cancer causing mutation in the family.

Gail Model The Gail Risk Assessment Model is the most commonly used statistical model for estimating the risk of developing breast cancer in women undergoing annual screening. Gail and colleagues used data from 284,780 predominantly white women in 28 participating centers of the Breast Cancer Detection Demonstration Project to develop the model. This is an unconditional logistic regression model based on the ratio of risk in a woman with specified risk factors compared with the risk in a woman with no risk factors. The risk factors used in this model include age, age at menarche, age at first live birth, number of first-degree relatives with breast cancer (mother, sisters, or daughters only), number of breast biopsies, and breast pathology exhibiting atypical hyperplasia (see Table 107-5).[66]

The Gail model is applicable to the largest number of women. A score of 1.67 (which is the average 5-year Gail score for a 60 year-old woman) was used as the minimum risk criterion to join the NSABP P-01 prevention trial in the United States. When the trial was stopped early, because women on tamoxifen were shown to have a benefit, the NCI promoted the use of the Gail Risk model to help clinicians assess the risk for breast cancer in their office. It is now fairly widely and easily used, with many forms of access (NCI Web site, handheld and computer applications)[66] and often used for clinical decision making for individual patients. The Gail model is good at predicting the risk for a population, but a cutoff of 1.67 does not show great discriminatory power.[67,68] Ozanne and colleagues have developed improved methods for incorporating Gail Risk by comparing a woman's Gail Risk in context with other women. In particular, showing women if they are in the highest quartile or decile of risk is much more discriminatory, and much more helpful in identifying truly high risk women.[68,69] Another limitation of the model is the treatment of family history. Neither paternal family history of breast cancer nor age at onset in affected relatives is accounted for in the model, both of which are significant in predicting hereditary breast cancer risk. The model is currently being revised to improve the prediction of risk in the African American population.

The Claus model estimates the probability that a woman will develop breast cancer based on her family history of cancer. This includes the number of first and second-degree relatives with breast cancer and the age of cancer onset. This model was developed from the Cancer and Steroid Hormone (CASH) population-based, case-control study involving 4,730 patients with histologically documented breast cancer and 4,688 matched controls.

The statistical calculation of this model is based on the premise that breast cancer risk is transmitted as an autosomal dominant trait, and uses the genetic relationships between the affected relatives and the woman in question to predict risk. Claus and colleagues have published risk tables for clinical use. Risks can be calculated as lifetime probabilities of developing cancer, or as an estimated risk for a woman to develop cancer over 10-year intervals. A handheld application is also available for clinical use. The main limitation of this model is that it relies only on family history to predict risk and does not include personal risk factors.

Hereditary Models Models such as BRCA-PRO,[62,63] Frank,[64] and Couch,[65] are designed to predict who is a *BRCA1* or *BRCA2* gene mutation carrier. These models assist in predicting the chance of carrying a *BRCA1* or *BRCA2* mutation based on an autosomal dominant pattern of inheritance and the incidence of mutations within high-risk populations, but they do not predict the risk of developing a cancer, specifically. They are based on both the maternal and paternal cancer history, and include age and number of first-degree relatives with breast cancer. Most women do not fall into this risk category.

The hereditary models are used clinically for women with a positive family history of breast cancer and are discriminatory and well calibrated for predicting the presence of a *BRCA* mutation. However, the use of these models is restricted to a small subset of the population who are likely to have one of these mutations. It is predicted that at most, 5 to 10% of diagnosed breast cancers are in women with either the *BRCA1* or *BRCA2* mutation. BRCAPRO performs as well in predicting mutations in families of African American descent as it does for Caucasian families. However, it is suspected that approximately 20% of breast cancers are due to unidentified hereditary factors. The remaining 70% are thought to be sporadic or non-hereditary cancers.[70] These tests are helpful in deciding whether to test for the BRCA mutations, but they are not helpful in predicting the likelihood of developing breast cancer and cannot be applied to women without a family history of the disease.

Biomarkers The models described above predict risk based on family risk and internal hormonal exposure. They do not incorporate biological markers that can be assessed and measured over time. Mutations in BRCA 1 and 2 certainly predict lifetime risk, and risk at earlier age, but are not accurate predictors of short-term risk. It is essential to identify biologic markers that can serve as quantifiable markers of risk. The availability of such a marker would dramatically change the field of breast cancer prevention, and enable smaller clinical studies to proceed based on changes in surrogate markers. In this manner, only the most promising interventions would need to be tested using cancer development as the primary endpoint, thus substantially shortening the cycle time and cost for prevention studies. A number of candidate biomarkers are emerging that have the potential to both stratify risk and predict the benefit of intervention. The optimal application of biomarkers in the prevention setting is to have markers that both predict an increased short-term risk and benefit from a targeted intervention.[69] The biomarkers that are potentially changeable and that have consistently been shown to be associated with greater risk for breast cancer include atypia,[71] and breast density. Atypia has been shown to be associated with a three- to fivefold increase in risk whether detected by histology or cytology. Atypia has also been shown to predict a greater benefit from the use of tamoxifen, with a risk reduction of up to 89% in the NSABP P-1 study.[72] It has been shown that women whose breasts appear mammographically dense in greater than 50% of total breast tissue area have a three- to fivefold increased risk of breast cancer compared to women who have less than 25% mammographically dense breasts.[73] This relationship has recently been shown to be even stronger in women with a family history of breast cancer.[74] There are a number of investigators who are conducting biomarker studies to determine if these markers are reliable surrogate markers that change in response to interventions.[75,76]

BREAST CANCER BIOLOGY

Regulation of Breast Cancer Growth

The adult female breast is composed of epithelial lactiferous ducts terminating in secretory alveoli embedded in a fibrous tissue framework and fat. Normal breast growth and development are regulated by the complex interaction of many hormones and growth factors, some of which are secreted by the mammary cells themselves and may have autocrine functions. Estradiol regulates the expression of several genes corresponding to peptides and proteins involved in mammary cell growth control mechanisms. Binding to specific receptors triggers effects of these growth factors and hormones. Polypeptide hormone receptors are typically located on the cell membrane, whereas receptors of the steroid hormone family are found mostly in the nuclear compartment of the cell. However, steroid hormone receptors can also be found localized to the cell membrane. The interaction of growth factors, cytokines, and hormones with specific membrane receptors triggers a cascade of intracellular biochemical signals, resulting in the activation and repression of various subsets of genes. Several of these hormones have been shown to play an active role in breast epithelial cell growth and development and in lactation. Because these hormones and their receptors regulate normal breast tissue, it is not surprising that malignant cells arising from breast tissue might also express receptors for many of these hormones and might retain some degree of hormonal dependence. Numerous studies using cultured cells, as well as human breast cancer tissue, have demonstrated the presence of receptors for most of these hormones in human breast cancer cells. Genetic aberrations in growth factor signaling pathways, for the most part acquired, are inextricably linked to developmental abnormalities and to a variety of chronic diseases, including cancer. Malignant cells arise as a result of a stepwise progression of genetic events that include the unregulated expression of growth factors or components of their signaling pathways.

Growth regulation of breast cancer cells by hormones and growth factors is shown schematically in Figure 107-1. The biological role of estrogens is mediated through high-affinity binding to ER by molecules belonging to a family of ligand-inducible nuclear receptors that have steroid and thyroid hormones and vitamins as known ligands.[78]

Recent studies suggest that breast cancer cells under estrogen control can synthesize and secrete their own growth factors that could autostimulate breast cancer cells or adjacent stromal tissues through autocrine or paracrine mechanisms. Aromatase is abundantly expressed in many breast cancers, providing the malignant cell with the ability to synthesize its own major growth factor. Stromal tissues may also secrete IGF-1 and IGF-2 that can stimulate breast cancer cells. Potential autocrine/paracrine growth factors identified include EGF, TGF-α, IGF-2, platelet-derived growth factor, and fibroblast growth factor. EGF, TGF-α, IGF-1, and IGF-2 have been found to be expressed and secreted by cultured breast cancer cells and by human breast cancer tissue specimens. They are potential mitogens for the epithelial (malignant) component of the tumor. Platelet-derived growth factor and fibroblast growth factor are secreted by breast cancer cells and may be responsible for the proliferation of the mesenchymal stromal component evident in many breast cancers.

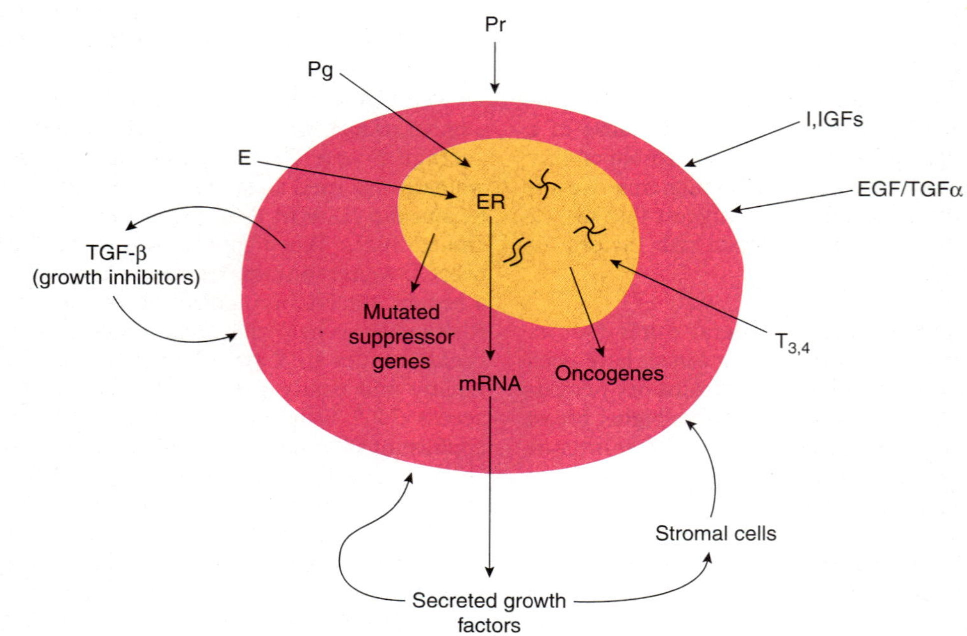

Figure 107-1 Growth regulation of breast cancer by hormones and growth factors. E = Estrogen; Pg = progesterone; Pr = prolactin; I = insulin; IGFs = insulin-like growth factors; EGF = epidermal growth factors; TGF-α = transforming growth factor alpha; T3,4 = thyroid hormones; TGF-β = transforming growth factor beta.

Human breast cancer cells also secrete several peptides that may have autocrine inhibitory activity. TGF-β is a family of growth factors that inhibit the proliferation of epithelial tissues and stimulate the proliferation of stromal tissues.[54] Studies suggest that ER-negative breast cancer cells are more sensitive to TGF-β than are cells expressing ER. The malignant potential of breast cancer is likely to depend, in part, on the balance between growth stimulators and growth inhibitors produced by the tumors. The epithelial and/or stromal cells within the tumor also secrete proteases, such as the cathepsins, stromelysins, gelatinases, or urokinase plasminogen activator, which may participate in tumor invasiveness and metastatic potential.

In ER-positive breast cancer cells, expression and secretion of certain autocrine growth factors, such as TGF-α and IGF-2, are stimulated by estrogen and inhibited by antiestrogens. In ER-negative breast cancer cells, secretion of these factors is not estrogen regulated. Investigators have hypothesized that changes in the expression of these secreted factors may mediate to some extent the growth effects of estrogens and antiestrogens. Estrogens and antiestrogens have a variety of other effects on breast cancer cells. Estrogen stimulates RNA, DNA, and protein synthesis and the activity of key regulatory enzymes. Antiestrogens have the opposite effects in most tissues. Estrogens ultimately regulate movement of the cells through the cell cycle and mitosis. Cell kinetic studies suggest that antiestrogens, such as tamoxifen, slow the transit of cells through the cell cycle by causing a block in the G_1 phase.

Disturbance of normal growth control mechanisms within a cell can result in uncontrolled cell division and the development of cancer. Such cellular transformation occurs through the activation of oncogenes, loss or mutation of tumor suppressor genes, or both. The normal counterparts of oncogenes, termed proto-oncogenes, function as growth regulators in normal cells. Alterations of proto-oncogenes are associated with the initiation, promotion, and/or maintenance of tumors in animals and humans. The products of oncogenes are frequently growth factors, growth factor receptors, molecular switching or transcription factors. Oncogenes often found overexpressed in human breast cancer tissue include members of the *myc* and *ras* family *(c-myc, Ha-ras-1), int-2,* which is involved in mouse (and, presumably, human) mammary gland carcinogenesis; the members of the EGF receptor (EGFR, *erbB)* family, including *erbB-2* (also known as *HER2* or *neu), HER3, and HER4.* Overexpression and mutation of growth factor receptors often lead to constitutive activation of these receptors (ie, signaling in the absence of their cognate ligands). Growth-promoting signals may be continuously transmitted into the cells, resulting in activation of multiple intracellular signal transduction pathways and unregulated cell growth. Genes normally involved in cell cycle control, especially members of the cyclin D family, may also function as oncogenes. Over-expression of these oncogenes may contribute to the initiation and maintenance of the malignant phenotype. Tissue-specific expression of *myc, ras,* and *HER2* in mammary glands of transgenic mice has been shown to result in an increased incidence of both benign and malignant breast pathology. Altered expression of these otherwise normal genes can have profound effects on growth homeostasis of breast epithelium. Recent studies have shown that blockade of these growth factor receptors or pathways has therapeutic implications.[79] These studies have shown that, both in preclinical models and in human breast cancer, monoclonal antibodies to *HER2* have dramatic antitumor effects. Furthermore, these antibodies have synergistic interactions with cytotoxic agents, such as the anthracyclines, the platinum analogs, vinorelbine and the taxanes. The EGFR, when overexpressed, confers an adverse prognosis to patients with EGFR-overexpressing tumors. However, EGFR does not seem to be a critical driver of malignant behavior in breast cancer, and monoclonal antibodies against this target have had only marginal success in clinical trials. Quantification of the expression of these oncogenes in human breast cancer specimens has been shown to provide valuable information on tumor aggressiveness, prognosis, and sensitivity to therapy.[80] *Bcl2* is another gene frequently overexpressed in breast cancer; its overexpression is associated with unfavorable prognosis, resistance to apoptosis and decreased responsiveness to cytotoxic therapy. Signaling molecules downstream from the cell surface receptors are often activated or otherwise altered in malignant cells. Thus, the PI3 kinase pathway, and the MAP kinase pathway are frequently activated in breast cancer, even in the absence of EGFR or HER2 overexpression.

Tumor suppressor genes also play a role in breast carcinogenesis. Loss of the normal "suppressor" function of these genes through mutations or deletion may cause cancer. Alterations in known suppressor genes, such as the retinoblastoma gene *(RB1)* and the human *TP53* gene, have been identified in human breast cancer cells, as well as in other solid tumors. Mutations in the *TP53* gene have been found in families with the Li-Fraumeni syndrome, who have a markedly increased incidence of breast cancer and other neoplasms. In addition, up to 50% of breast cancers have been shown to have mutations in the *TP53* gene. The two mutated genes associated with familial breast cancer, *BRCA1* and *BRCA2,* are also considered tumor suppressor genes. The normal function of the protein products of these genes is to control cell proliferation (*RB1* and *TP53*) or to facilitate/mediate DNA repair (*TP53, BRCA1, BRCA2*). Mutations lead to mutated proteins and thus to dysregulated transit of cells through the cell cycle. Recognition that mutational inactivation of suppressor genes is associated with breast cancer could lead to early recognition of high-risk families, as well as to new treatment strategies to reverse the malignant phenotype by introducing normal gene copies through gene therapy or by treatment with the normal suppressor protein itself. Such strategies are under active investigation, both in the laboratory and in early clinical trials.

Estrogen and Progesterone Receptors

Estrogen receptors are members of the nuclear hormone–receptor superfamily and have several functional domains. There are two subtypes, with each subtype having several isoforms and splice variants. The estrogen receptor α (alpha) gene has been mapped to the long arm of chromosome 6 (6q24-q27), whereas the estrogen receptor β (beta) gene is located on band q22-24 of chromosome 14. Certain estrogen-induced proteins, such as the progesterone receptor (PR), are important for specific metabolic processes in the cell. There are at least three PR subtypes and their tissue distribution and function are under active investigation. Other estrogen-induced proteins regulate events leading to cell proliferation. When receptors are bound to antiestrogens, such as tamoxifen, transcription of growth-promoting genes is blocked, although other genes might be activated by tamoxifen.

Assays for ER alpha and PR A are helpful in selecting the patients most likely to benefit from endocrine therapy, and they provide prognostic information on recurrence and survival, since their expression is related to the degree of tumor differentiation. The role of ER beta and the other subtypes of PR in selecting responders to endocrine therapy is less well understood.

Both ER and PR in their classical form are nuclear proteins that can be measured in intact cells or tumor extracts by several assay techniques. Earlier detection techniques by ligand-binding assays have been replaced by immunohistochemical (IHC) or immunocytochemical assays. The availability of monoclonal antibodies that recognize human ER or PR circumvents many of the shortcomings from earlier biochemical assays. In addition, IHC can be performed on small tissue or cytologic specimens; is not affected by endogenous hormone levels, and displays the cellular heterogeneity of receptor expression; most importantly, it can be used on fresh or archival (paraffin-embedded) tissues. The results of IHC assays correlate well with quantitative enzyme-linked immunoassay techniques and those of the older biochemical assays. More important, the results of IHC correlate well with response to hormonal therapy and prognosis. The remaining disadvantage of IHC is that it is only semiquantitative; the scoring of slides is subjective and requires a trained histopathologist. Nevertheless, because of the simplicity and reproducibility of the assay, IHC is considered the assay of choice for ER and PR today. Nuclear localization of ER leads to its genomic effects. Upon binding its ligand, the ER-ligand complex binds to the estrogen responsive element and initiates transcription of estrogen-driven genes. In its cell membrane localization, ER mediates the non-genomic effects of ligand binding, mostly through crosstalk with peptide growth factor receptors (EGFR, HER2). Upon development of antiestrogen resistance, there is marked increase in the non-genomic effects of ER.

ERs are detected (or expressed) in 60 to 80% of breast cancer samples, depending on the assay used and the clinical characteristics of the tumor and patient. The ER concentration varies widely from tumor to tumor (from 0 to more than 1,000 fmol/mg protein, or 0 to 100% of cells, depending on the method used). Higher ER levels are seen in postmenopausal patients. ER assays performed on primary tumors are more frequently positive than are assays done on metastatic lesions, especially those obtained from visceral metastases. This probably reflects the greater propensity for ER-negative tumor cells to metastasize to visceral organs. ER positivity also correlates with histologic demonstration of differentiation (ie, low nuclear grade), with diploid DNA content, and with low proliferative indices (low SPF or Ki-67 expression). ER expression is inversely correlated with HER2 and EGFR expression These associations may explain in part the prognostic significance of ER status.

An important application of the ER assay is the selection of appropriate patients for endocrine therapy. Approximately 50 to 60% of patients with ER-positive tumors benefit from endocrine therapy. This percentage includes patients who achieve a major objective remission (partial or complete) and those who derive long-term (> 6 months) stability of the disease with endocrine therapy; both groups have equivalent survival expectations. The ER status predicts equally well for all modalities of endocrine therapy. Patients with no detectable ER or PR in their tumors do not benefit from endocrine therapy; however, patients with very low but detectable ER and/or PR respond, albeit infrequently, to endocrine therapy. This may explain why some patients with "ER-negative" tumors have been reported to benefit from adjuvant tamoxifen therapy. Until recently, arbitrary cutoff values were used to differentiate between ER-positive and ER-negative tumors. These values were usually around 10 to 20 fmol/mg protein for ligand-binding assays, or >10% positive cells/hpf in IHC assays. More recently, it has been recognized that virtually any ER expression indicates some probability of benefit from endocrine therapy. For this reason, many laboratories have adopted a semiquantitative method that takes into consideration the percent positive cells as well as the intensity of staining as the basis for determining ER-positivity. Quantitative ER assay and the simultaneous determination of PR expression increase the predictive accuracy of these assays. Tumors with high ER concentration (> 100 fmol/mg protein or strong, homogeneous staining) or those positive for both ER and PR have the highest probability of response and clinical benefit from hormonal therapy. Some recent reports suggest that anastrozole is particularly superior to tamoxifen in patients with ER-positive but PR-negative tumors; however, this has not been broadly confirmed. PR information is not as widely available as ER information in clinical trials, so the relevance of ER-status on treatment selection is more clearly established than that of PR status. Tumor ER and PR status can change over time or with intervening therapy; thus, repeat biopsies of accessible tissue may be helpful in selecting sequential therapies. However, ER status on the primary tumor still predicts reasonably well for endocrine response at the time of relapse. There is a strong trend for higher response rate to chemotherapy in ER-negative tumors, so hormone receptor status might be helpful in predicting response to chemotherapy. It is not known why 40 to 50% of ER-positive tumors fail to respond to hormonal therapy despite the presence of receptor. Clearly, an assay that would identify truly hormone-sensitive tumors would be more clinically useful. Variant and/or mutated ERs have been identified in breast cancer tissue. Some of these altered receptors are constitutively active (activate transcription in the absence of estrogen), some are inactive, and some have dominant negative activity. The biologic importance of these variants and their role, if any, in hormone-resistant states remains to be clarified.

BREAST CANCER PREVENTION STRATEGIES

All women are at risk for developing breast cancer. If a woman lives to the age of 80, she has a 1 in 8 chance of developing breast cancer. This does not tell us what type of breast cancer will develop and whether it will be lethal, only that there is a risk of developing some type of breast cancer. Most women are interested in their risk over the next 5 to 10 years, not just their lifetime risk. The timing of risk is important for thinking about surveillance and treatment of high-risk women. Women have about a 12% lifetime risk of getting cancer, but that risk is distributed differently, depending on age, exposures, and genetic composition. The average 25-year old woman has a 1 in 20,000 chance of developing a cancer. That is in contrast, however, to the extreme of someone who is at very high risk based on an inherited mutation in BRCA 1 or 2.

In the setting of a known inherited mutation in BRCA1 or 2, testing a woman family member for the presence of that mutation will update the lifetime probability of developing breast cancer to 40 to 85% if the mutation is found, or to a lifetime risk of 12% if a mutation is not found. More importantly, the risk curve is shifted dramatically to the left, indicating that women with the mutation get cancers at a much earlier age. In fact, most of the risk is between the ages of 30 and 55, which is clearly different from women with average risk. Therefore, a 30-year-old with a known BRCA mutation, who presents with a mass has a much higher likelihood of having a cancer and should be treated accordingly. Interestingly, we now know that mutations in the *BRCA1* gene lead to the development of high-grade, circumscribed tumors (medullary carcinomas). We also know something about the pathways that activate the tumors. The tumors in the setting of a BRCA1 mutation are usually devoid of estrogen and progesterone receptors on the surface and they do not overexpress HER2/neu. Expression profiling has confirmed this observation, demonstrating that the gene expression pattern shows that BRCA1 tumors have the basal cell phenotype, also typically ER-/PR-/HER2/neu -, or "triple negative," and are thought to arise from basal cells within the breast ducts.[82]

Women who develop BRCA2-mutated tumors are more likely to develop ER-positive tumors that are HER2-negative. Mutations in both BRCA1 or 2 result in impaired DNA repair, but the tumors that arise are different. Approximately 15% of breast cancers are considered to be hereditary, but only 5 to 7% can be explained on the basis of inherited mutations in BRCA 1 or 2. Most breast cancers are considered to arise from non-inherited causes, so-called sporadic cancers. Considerable effort is being devoted to improve our ability to find groups at high risk and to develop methods or tools to risk stratify the population. Genetic testing is an example of a tool that has tremendous risk discrimination. In the setting of a family with a known inherited mutation in BRCA1 or 2, an unaffected family member has a 50% chance of carrying that mutation. Clearly, these results would and often do generate very different choices for breast cancer prevention. Women at highest risk often choose prophylactic mastectomy (17–35%). Women more often choose prophylactic oophorectomy (35–50%) because of the increased lifetime risk for developing ovarian cancer (20–40%, depending on the mutation), the ability to remove the ovaries by laparoscopy, the limited ability to effectively screen for that disease, and because of the significant risk reduction in breast cancer risk (see discussion below). However, it is important to remember that a negative genetic test can only be used to assure women that they have the same risk as the average woman if there is a known mutation in the family. Otherwise, a woman from a family where many members have been affected by cancer must continue to be considered high risk.

There are a number of conditions that identify women as "high risk" for developing breast cancer. Table 107-6 shows the risk for progression to invasive cancer for a given diagnosis. The ranges of risk overlap, but the treatment choices are extremely different. As work in the prevention field starts to intersect with the management of cancer, and in particular, in situ cancer, we will begin to merge our ideas of risk and provide a more rational intervention approach for women with a variety of conditions, who now are given very different treatment recommendations. What is the reason for identifying a woman as high risk? One reason is to tailor screening and surveillance strategies, and the other is to offer chemoprevention, prophylactic surgery, or participation in breast cancer prevention trials. Several risk models have been developed and are being used for counseling in the clinic to help women make decisions about breast cancer. Increasingly, scientists and clinicians are thinking about using biomarkers to identify both an increased risk for breast cancer and increased likelihood that a particular drug/intervention will be successful in lowering risk.[69]

Table 107-6 Estimated Yearly Rate for Progression to Invasive Breast Cancer without Treatment

Predisposing Condition	Annual Rate (%)
DCIS	1–3
Atypical hyperplasia	1–4
LCIS	0.5–2
BRCA1 or BRCA2 mutation	1–5
5-year Gail risk of >5	1–2
60-year-old woman with Gail risk ≤2.0	0.3–0.5
CBC invasive cancer	0.5

CBC = contralateral breast cancer; DCIS = ductal carcinoma in situ; LCIS = lobular carcinoma in situ.[92]

Breast Cancer Screening Options for Women at High Risk The standard recommendations for screening are to begin mammographic screening 10 years prior to the onset of cancer in the youngest first- or second-degree relative with breast cancer. However, another option is emerging that should be considered for very high-risk women, magnetic resonance imaging (MRI). The appropriate population for MRI screening includes women with known genetic predisposition, or extremely high risk on the basis of family history, dense breast tissue, and deleterious BRCA1 and mutations. Two large screening studies have now demonstrated that MRI is far more sensitive than mammography in very high risk women.[83,84]

One-third of the mutation carriers with screened cancers had tumors over 2 cm compared to 13 and 19% of the high and moderate risk groups, respectively. The mutation carriers have high-grade tumors with an apparently faster potential for metastatic spread and a higher chance of having nodes involved and perhaps should be screened at different intervals. The high- and moderate-risk groups had far fewer cancers detected (less than a quarter of the rate of the mutation carriers). There did not appear to be a difference in the rate of cancers between the moderate- and high-risk groups, but the biology was not the same. As we go forward, it will be critical to develop tools to improve our ability to predict which cancers women are susceptible to and tailor screening strategies accordingly. For example, BRCA2 carriers may be able to have annual screening, whereas BRCA1 carriers might be better served with more frequent screening. Interestingly, whereas MRI found many more cancers (20 of 45) that were not seen by mammography, there were 8 cancers seen by mammography alone, and one found by clinical exam alone.[85] This suggests that the optimal screening strategy for mutation carriers may be to stagger mammography and MRI at 6-month intervals and an exam should be performed at that time as well.[85]

The Gail model rarely projects a lifetime risk for women beyond 40%, but it is important to look at models for their ability to find higher risk women, rather than a focus on cut-off value. For the purposes of identifying women at sufficiently high risk to justify MRI screening, a reasonable strategy, given the current data, is to evaluate women on the basis of three criteria: age under 50, dense breasts, and at least a threefold higher lifetime risk than the average woman (in the range of 35% or greater).

Risk Reduction Options for Breast Cancer The management of high-risk women is challenging. The degree of underlying risk, patient risk tolerance and preference, and the attendant "price to pay" for each intervention is what should drive these decisions. Although many women are concerned about their risk of developing breast cancer, their options for risk reduction are limited.[86] Current preventative or risk-reducing options include prophylactic surgery, ovarian suppression, chemoprevention with tamoxifen, and lifestyle modifications.

Prophylactic Surgery Evidence suggests that prophylactic mastectomy provides the most breast cancer risk reduction, decreasing a woman's breast cancer risk by greater than 90%.[87,88] Although reconstruction options have improved significantly[89–92] prophylactic mastectomy still comes at high personal cost for most women. Prophylactic oophorectomy for women in their 30s can reduce breast cancer risk by as much as 60%.[93] Early oophorectomy is a particularly good option for women who are at increased risk because of hereditary predisposition (BRCA 1 or 2 mutation carriers) and who face risk of both breast and ovarian cancer, but the decision is dependent on the timing of childbearing.

Prophylactic mastectomy has been shown, in retrospective cohort studies, to dramatically reduce the risk of developing breast cancer.[87,88] This has now been confirmed in a prospective study. Rebeck and colleagues showed that, in a cohort of 483 mutation carriers, 1.9% who had chosen mastectomy developed cancer, versus 98.1% who did not, with a 95% reduction in risk.[93] Prophylactic surgery is estimated to extend life expectancy in women with BRCA1 or 2 mutations in their 30s and 50s by 1.6 and 0.9-years, respectively.[95] Prophylactic oophorectomy alone will also reduce the risk of developing breast cancer, by 60% if the oophorectomy is performed in the patients' 30s, and 50% if it is performed in their 40s. The risk reduction from prophylactic surgery is shown on Figure 107-2 for a woman with high risk on the basis of an inherited mutation in either BRCA1 or 2. The graphic is taken from a prevention tool used for patient education.[68]

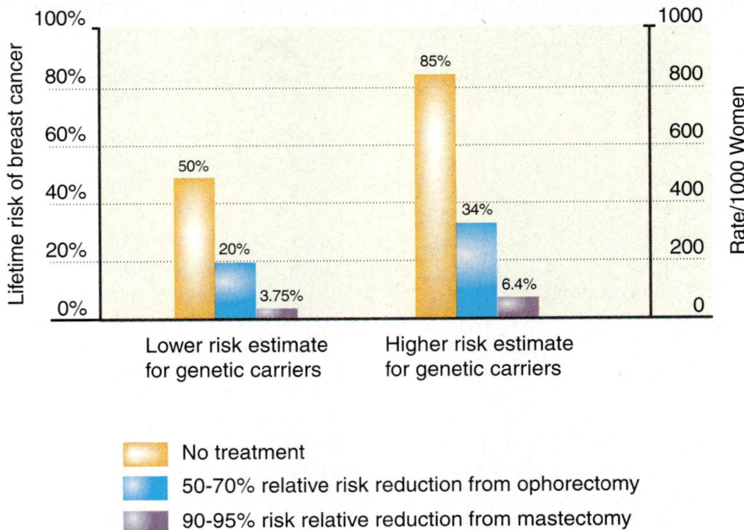

Figure 107-2 Risk reduction from prophylactic surgery for a woman with high risk on the basis of an inherited mutation in either *BRCA1* or *2*.

Lobular Carcinoma In Situ The surgical treatment of lobular carcinoma in situ (LCIS) has changed in recent years as a result of a better understanding of the biology and natural history of this tumor. Treatment strategies for LCIS evolved from considerations relative to its multicentricity, its bilaterality, and its tendency to develop into invasive breast cancer. Formerly, the recommended therapy for LCIS included bilateral total mastectomy, total mastectomy with mirror-image biopsy of the opposite breast, or total mastectomy with elective biopsy of the opposite breast. However, better information about the natural history of LCIS indicates that the majority of patients with the disease do not develop invasive cancer.[96] Furthermore, both breasts are at similar risk for the development of invasive cancer. LCIS is a marker for increased risk for the development of invasive breast cancer of any type in either breast and does not represent a marker of risk in a particular region of breast tissue. The likelihood of developing invasive lobular cancer is much higher (40–50%) relative to the frequency of ductal cancers (10%).[97] Because the risk for developing cancer spans a horizon of 5 to 15 years, and because the in situ lesion does not necessarily predict the geographic location for cancer development, further surgery is not considered the appropriate treatment in a patient with a biopsy-proven LCIS, even if the margins of resection are involved. However, since such patients are at higher risk for developing invasive cancer (a risk estimated to be approximately 10 times the normal), close follow-up with mammography and physical examination is recommended. To date, there is no evidence that breast irradiation is effective in preventing the development of invasive cancer in patients with LCIS.

A more rational approach to the management of LCIS would be an attempt to prevent the development of invasive breast cancer in women with this disease. The National Surgical Adjuvant Breast and Bowel Project (NSABP) breast cancer prevention trial[72] demonstrated that tamoxifen reduced the risk of a woman with diagnosed LCIS progressing to invasive cancer reduced by nearly 50%. Because LCIS is the expression of a phenotype carrying a higher than-normal risk of breast cancer, interventions like tamoxifen represent the promise of ultimate biologic control of these conditions.

Chemoprevention ***Tamoxifen*** An option for women at increased risk is a 5-year course of tamoxifen therapy. The US Food and Drug Administration (FDA) approved this chemoprevention drug for women with a 5-year breast cancer risk equal to or greater than 1.67% as assessed by the Gail risk assessment model. This relatively arbitrary Gail score was chosen as that of an average 60-year-old woman. Tamoxifen data from the NSABP P01 Breast Cancer Prevention Trial (BCPT) demonstrate that the use of tamoxifen, a chemopreventive agent, can decrease a woman's risk of developing breast cancer (Table 107-7). Tamoxifen is currently the only approved agent shown to decrease the incidence of some types of breast cancer, with an average relative risk reduction of 49% in a 4 to 5 year period. Although other tamoxifen prevention studies have not shown as great a reduction in breast cancer, clearly tamoxifen is an agent that is active in reducing the risk of breast cancer. A meta-analysis including the P-1 trial and three other trials utilizing tamoxifen concluded that this agent reduced risk of breast cancer by about 38%, without significantly affecting overall survival yet (Figure 107-3).[98] Women with a known cancer have an elevated risk of developing a contralateral cancer, and tamoxifen in the adjuvant setting confers approximately a 50% reduction in risk of contralateral cancer.

Decisions about the use of tamoxifen can be very difficult for women who are as yet unaffected by breast cancer. The NSABP prevention study demonstrated that of the 13,338 women in the study, only 120 breast cancers were averted. Tamoxifen is associated with both mild and serious side effects. Serious side effects are limited largely to postmenopausal women and include a 1% increase in endometrial cancer (typically low grade) after 5 years and a similar increase in the vascular events (in women over 60). The more

Table 107-7 Rates for Invasive Breast Cancer by Age, 5-Year Predicted Breast Cancer Risk, Number of First-Degree Relatives with Breast Cancer, History of Lobular Carcinoma In Situ (LCIS), or History of Atypical Hyperplasia

Patient Characteristic	Rate per 1,000 Women per 5 Years		Risk Ratio	95% Confidence Interval
	Placebo	Tamoxifen		
Age (yr)				
49	33.5	18.9	0.56	0.4–0.9
50–59	31.4	15.5	0.49	0.3–0.8
≥ 60	36.7	16.6	0.49	0.3–0.7
5-year predicted risk (%)				
≤ 2.00	27.7	10.3	0.37	0.2–0.7
≥ 5.01	66.4	22.6	0.34	0.2–0.6
No. first-degree relatives with breast cancer				
0	32.3	14.9	0.46	0.2–0.8
1	30.0	15.2	0.51	0.4–0.7
2	43.4	23.8	0.55	0.3–1.0
3	68.6	35.1	0.51	0.2–1.6
History of LCIS				
Yes	65.0	28.5	0.44	0.2–1.1
No	32.1	16.5	0.51	0.4–0.7
History of atypical hyperplasia				
Yes	50.6	7.2	0.14	0.0–0.5
No	32.2	18.1	0.56	0.4–0.7

frequent side effects decrease quality of life but the rare side effects can be life threatening.[72] Current estimates suggest that over 10 million women in the United States are eligible for tamoxifen use by FDA guidelines, but it is rarely prescribed by physicians or accepted by women as a preventive option.[99,100] Using more rigorous eligibility criteria for tamoxifen use proposed by Gail and colleagues,[101] it is still estimated that over 2 million women in the United States are eligible for tamoxifen treatment.[101] Approximately 200,000 women are expected to develop breast cancer this year, far less than either of the estimated number of women eligible for tamoxifen use.[3] Thus, better ways of identifying women at high risk are needed (see discussion in LCIS section), The presence of atypia found on surgical biopsy is an example of a biomarker that identifies women at higher risk and greater benefit from tamoxifen, and has been shown to motivate women to choose chemoprevention. However, not all women benefit from tamoxifen, and it does not appear to prevent the development of ER-negative disease, so new agents will be necessary. In order to optimize the use of preventive agents and minimize exposure to side effects, stratification by both risk of breast cancer and benefit from available interventions is necessary.

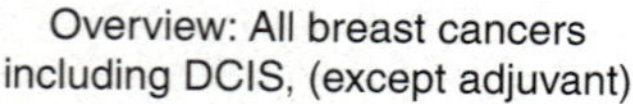

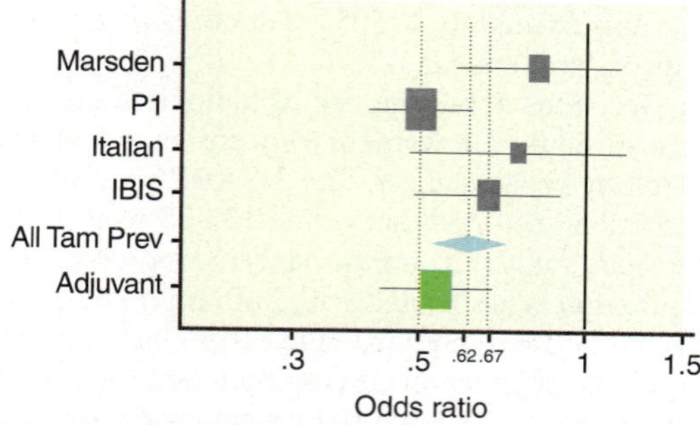

Figure 107-3 Reduction in the incidence of breast cancer by tamoxifen in randomized clinical trials.[98]

Chemoprevention Agents under Investigation Raloxifene, which is a selective estrogen receptor modifier, similar to tamoxifen, has been shown to significantly reduce the risk of estrogen receptor-positive breast cancer in women at risk for osteoporosis, yet it does not appear to increase the risk of developing endometrial cancer.[102] It is currently being tested in a large prevention trial by the NSABP (STAR Trial, NSABP P-2) where women at high risk (Gail Risk above 1.67) are randomized to tamoxifen vs raloxifene. Over the past 10 years, selective aromatase inhibitors were shown to be more effective and better tolerated than megestrol acetate and tamoxifen in treating metastatic and primary breast cancer. A significant reduction in second primary breast cancers was observed in randomized adjuvant trials when selective aromatase inhibitors were compared to tamoxifen. It is estimated that compared to no endocrine treatment, aromatase inhibitors might reduce the risk of second primary breast cancers by up to 75%. Anastrozole is currently under assessment as a chemopreventive agent in three randomized trials: in two, it is being compared to tamoxifen (IBIS II and B-35 DCIS study); in the third, to placebo (IBIS II chemoprevention trial).

Much excitement was generated over the COX-2 inhibitors; however, after several of these agents were pulled from the market because of an associated increased risk in fatal and non-fatal cardiac events, all of the COX-2 inhibitors have come under investigation and most trials have been stopped. This underscores the importance of finding health-promoting or health-neutral interventions for prevention, given the need to expose large populations to the interventions in order to reduce the incidence of cancer. This suggests we should more closely investigate known health promoting drugs such as statins that have been reported to reduce breast cancer risk. It also makes a compelling case for identifying higher risk populations, such as patients with DCIS. We may soon be able to classify pre-malignant and high-risk lesions better by molecular means. Given that high-risk lesions are not an emergency, but rather a marker of predisposition to progress to invasive disease, time can be used to learn more about these lesions. It is possible that the peri-operative period, or a period of neoadjuvant treatment, will help us to learn more about the response characteristics of an individual tumor and lead to better ways of preventing breast cancer.

Lifestyle Changes Lifestyle changes such as increased exercise, decreased consumption of alcohol and animal fat, and refraining from or stopping hormone replacement therapy are thought to have moderate risk reduction potential.[86,103,104] The Nurses' Health Study I and II have demonstrated that lifestyle modifications, especially maintenance of optimal weight after menopause and limiting animal fat intake, can decrease breast cancer risk by 30 to 45%.[105,106] Women thought to be at higher risk for breast cancer should avoid prolonged hormone replacement therapy (HRT) exposure, and no woman should take it unless there is a specific reason or need. Women who drink excessively should take B vitamins, which have shown to be protective in the setting of alcohol.[47]

PATHOLOGY

Recent biologic and clinical advances have made the role of the pathologist in establishing the diagnosis of a breast lesion more, rather than less, important (Figure 107-4). Today, greater expertise is required of the pathologist to establish the diagnosis of cancer from fine-needle aspiration and core biopsy specimens, and to determine the nature of the increasing number of borderline and precancerous lesions. Distinguishing microinvasive from noninvasive lesions, and understanding atypical hyperplasias, all usually diagnosed after discovery by mammography, are new challenges. In addition, pathologic discriminants involving immunohistochemistry are playing a larger role in determining patient prognosis. Finally, the pathologist also provides information that can contribute to a better understanding of the biology of the disease.[107]

Histologic Types Pathologic classifications of mammary carcinoma are frequently confusing to the individual who is not a specialist in breast disease (Table 107-8). If it is appreciated that morphologic studies are based on anatomic or structural units present in an organ, and that in the female breast these units consist of large, medium, and small ducts from which a variety of tumor types arise, a better understanding of breast tumor pathology may ensue. (Only during pregnancy are acinar units present.)

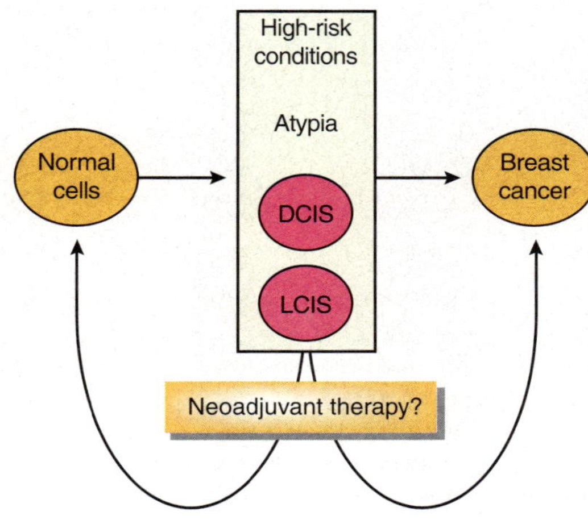

Figure 107-4 Molecular classification of premalignant and high-risk lesions for chemopreventive interventions.

Tumors arising from ductal epithelium may be found only within the lumen of the ducts of origin; that is, the carcinomas are intraductal and do not penetrate the basement membrane or invade surrounding stroma. Most frequently, such tumors arise from large ducts and may present as several types. If they grow into the ducts with a papillary configuration, they are recognized as papillary carcinomas (Figure 107-5). Such lesions are rare, accounting for about 1% of breast cancers. Histologically, pleomorphic duct epithelial cells with disturbed polarity can be demonstrated, as can their "heaping up" into papillae. Difficulty may be encountered in differentiating a papillary carcinoma from a benign atypical papilloma.

Papillary carcinomas rarely invade the surrounding stroma. A survival rate approaching 100% may be anticipated upon complete excision of such tumors. When these tumors do invade surrounding tissue, they grow rather slowly and attain considerable bulk. Skin and fascial attachments are unusual, and axillary node involvement is a late feature. Clinically, noninvasive tumors are found to be movable, circumscribed lesions that have a soft consistency not unlike that of fibroadenomas.

The noninvasive variety of ductal carcinoma, referred to as intraductal carcinoma or ductal carcinoma in situ (DCIS), is a proliferation of a subgroup of epithelial cells confined to the mammary ducts without light microscopic evidence of invasion through the basement membrane into the stroma. The histologic diagnosis of DCIS poses certain problems. It is often difficult to distinguish between benign but highly atypical hyperplasia and DCIS, and it is sometimes difficult to identify small foci of stromal invasion. Occasionally, it is difficult to distinguish between DCIS and lobular carcinoma in situ (LCIS), since DCIS may extend into breast lobules and LCIS may involve extralobular ducts. Some lesions may be intermediate between the two. A variety of histologic patterns of DCIS has been recognized. The most frequently encountered are comedo, cribriform, solid, papillary, and micropapillary (Figure 107-6). The different histologic patterns have been associated with differences in biologic behavior. The proliferative rate has been found to vary according to the histologic characteristics of DCIS. A high proliferative rate has been observed with comedo-DCIS, and a low proliferative rate with cribriform, papillary, and solid DCIS. A type of carcinoma known as comedocarcinoma is characterized by ducts that are dilated and filled with carcinoma cells. These are necrotic and can be expressed as semisolid necrotic plugs. Such cancers are not usually regarded as a separate cell type, but rather represent a descriptive variant of intraductal carcinoma. Patients whose DCIS exhibits comedo features have been shown to have increased rates of local recurrence and may progress more rapidly to invasive breast cancer compared to other types (Figure 107-7). Human EGF-receptor 2 (HER2/neu) protein overexpression has been observed in solid and comedo types of DCIS but not in papillary or cribriform types. Assays for estrogen and progesterone receptors (ER and PR) are an integral part of assessing DCIS lesions and are necessary to select optimal therapeutic interventions. Attempts to gain consensus on pathological classification for DCIS include the EORTC system, the Van Nuys system, and the Philadelphia consensus conference, and have all produced different systems with some overlapping features.

Lobular carcinoma arises from the small end ducts of the breast. The noninvasive variety—the so-called lobular carcinoma in situ—is characterized by small cells of low nuclear grade that fill and expand lobules without penetration of the basement membrane (Figure 107-8). When this lesion extends beyond the boundary of the lobule or terminal duct from which it arises, it is known as inva-

Table 107-8 Incidence of Histologic Types of Invasive Breast Cancers (1,000 Cases from NSABP B-04)[8]

Histologic Type	No.	Percent
Pure tumor groups	526	52.6
Infiltrating duct NOS*		
Medullary	62	6.2
Lobular invasive	49	4.9
Mucinous	24	2.4
Tubular	12	1.2
Adenocystic	4	0.4
Papillary	3	0.3
Carcinosarcoma	1	0.1
Paget's disease	23	2.3
With intraductal carcinoma	2	0.2
Infiltrating duct NOS*	16	1.6
+ Tubular	4	0.4
+ Mucinous	1	0.1
Combinations with infiltrating duct NOS*	280	28.0
Infiltrating duct NOS*		
+ Tubular	165	16.5
+ Lobular invasive	33	3.3
+ Mucinous	16	1.6
+ Lobular invasive + tubular	16	1.6
+ Papillary	12	1.2
+ Adenocystic	10	1.0
+ Tubular + adenocystic	8	0.8
+ Tubular + papillary	8	0.8
+ Mucinous + papillary	4	0.4
+ Adenocystic + mucinous	2	0.2
+ Lobular invasive + adenocystic	1	0.1
+ Lobular invasive + mucinous	1	0.1
+ Lobular invasive + papillary	1	0.1
+ Tubular + mucinous	1	0.1
+ Adenocystic + papillary	1	0.1
+ Lobular invasive + tubular + adenocystic + mucinous	1 16	0.1 1.6
Other combinations of tumor types exclusive of NOS*		
Tubular + papillary	5	0.5
Lobular invasive + tubular	4	0.4
Tubular + mucinous	2	0.2
Lobular invasive + mucinous	1	0.1
Tubular + adenocystic	1	0.1
Adenocystic + mucinous	1	0.1
Mucinous + papillary	1	0.1
Lobular invasive + tubular + adenocystic + papillary	1	0.1
Total	1,000	100.0

* NOS = not otherwise specified

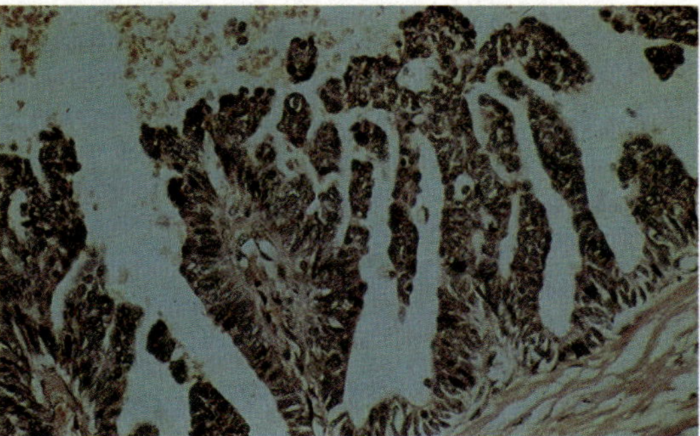

Figure 107-5 Papillary carcinoma of the breast. This uncommon tumor, less than 1%, rarely infiltrates and has a favorable prognosis.

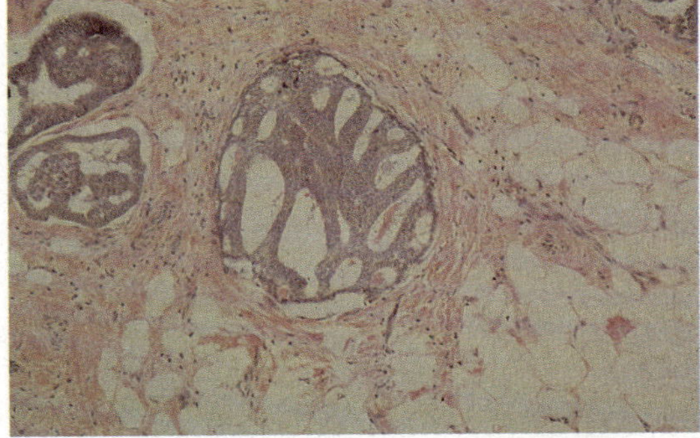

Figure 107-6 Ductal carcinoma in situ (DCIS), cribriform type. Duct spaces are completely involved by a proliferation of ductal cells with relatively uniform nuclei, arranged in back to back (cribriform) glands. The glands are fairly uniform in size and shape and exhibit rigid inner borders (so-called cookie-cutter appearance). (Courtesy Dr. Ira Bleiweiss, Mount Sinai School of Medicine.)

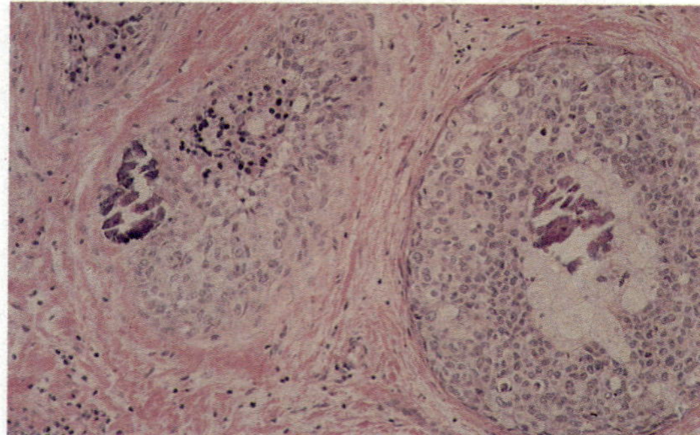

Figure 107-7 Ductal carcinoma in situ (DCIS), comedo type. Two duct spaces contain tumor cells with high nuclear grade, focal necrosis, and calcifications. The combination of high-grade nuclei and central necrosis is diagnostic of comedocarcinoma. (Courtesy Dr. Ira Bleiweiss, Mount Sinai School of Medicine.)

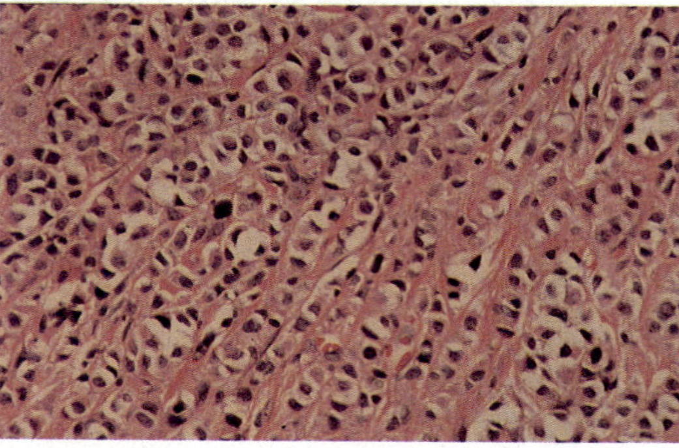

Figure 107-9 Infiltrating lobular carcinoma. Tumor cells with relatively uniform nuclei invade in a single file or linear pattern (so-called Indian file). (Courtesy Dr. Ira Bleiweiss, Mount Sinai School of Medicine.)

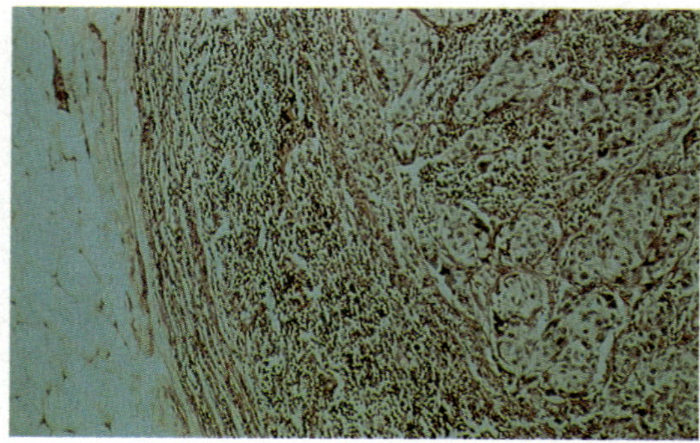

Figure 107-11 Medullary carcinoma of the breast accounts for about 5 to 7% of breast cancers. Despite its relatively poor differentiation, this tumor has a better prognosis than does infiltrating ductal carcinoma.

sive lobular carcinoma. Often the small cells interdigitate between collagen bundles in a single line, so-called "Indian file." At other times, lobular carcinoma may be nearly indistinguishable from the conventional infiltrating ductal carcinoma (Figure 107-9). It has been emphasized that noninvasive mammary carcinomas make up almost 22% of all neoplastic lesions of the female breast and that LCIS accounts for about 60% of these, or 12% of all tumors. Whereas DCIS often accompanies invasive ductal carcinoma, and may well be its usual precursor, LCIS may be followed by invasive ductal or invasive lobular carcinomas in either breast. LCIS thus is more a systemic marker than a local precursor. With the increased use of mammography, a much higher proportion of noninvasive cancers is being detected. Although DCIS and LCIS are both called CIS, they are considered and treated somewhat differently.

Infiltrating duct carcinomas in which no special type of histologic structure is recognized are designated "not otherwise specified" (NOS) and are the most common duct tumors, accounting for almost 80% of breast cancers (Figure 107-10). They are characterized clinically by their stony hardness to palpation. When they are transected, a gritty resistance is encountered, and the tumor retracts below the cut surface. Yellowish, chalky streaks that represent necrotic foci are observed. Histologically, varying degrees of fibrotic response are present. They frequently metastasize to axillary lymph nodes, and their prognosis is the poorest of the various tumor types. More than half (52.6%) of breast cancers are pure infiltrating duct lesions (NOS).

Several other types of invasive carcinomas arise from large ducts, and each has its own distinct histopathologic picture. Medullary carcinoma, composing 3 to 6% of all mammary carcinomas, often attains large dimensions (Figure 107-11). This tumor is formed by cells of relatively high nuclear grade, and usually exhibits an extensive infiltration of the tumor by small lymphocytes. Medullary carcinomas have a relatively well-circumscribed border, sometimes described as a "pushing" border, in contrast to the NOS tumors in which small nests of cells tend to infiltrate the adjacent stroma more extensively. A study of medullary cancer using 336 typical and 273 atypical medullary breast cancers from 6,404 patients enrolled in various stage I and stage II National Surgical Adjuvant Breast Project (NSABP) trials indicated that the survival of patients with typical medullary cancers was better than that for patients with NOS invasive ductal carcinomas. Survival was comparable for those with atypical medullary and NOS types.[108]

Tubular carcinoma is an invasive carcinoma in which tubule formation is highly prominent. This tumor represents 1 to 2% of breast cancers and has a low nuclear grade with some cell polarity (Figure 107-12). Its prognosis is favorable, and, when combined with small size, it is a highly curable tumor. Mucinous or colloid carcinoma, which composes about 1 to 2% of all mammary carcinomas, is characterized on microscopy by its nests and strands of epithelial cells floating in a mucinous matrix. It usually grows slowly and can reach bulky proportions. When the tumor is predominantly mucinous, the prognosis tends to be good. (Figure 107-13).

Two entities represent special manifestations of mammary carcinoma. Paget disease of the breast occurs in 1 to 4% of all patients with breast cancer. Clinically, the patient presents with a relatively long history of eczematoid changes in the nipple, with itching, burning, oozing, and/or bleeding. The nipple changes are associated with an underlying carcinoma in the breast that can be palpated in about two-thirds of the patients. The subjacent tumor may be either intraductal or of the invasive duct type. Prognosis is related to the invasiveness and histologic type of the associated tumor. Histologically, the nipple epithelium contains nests of carcinoma cells.

Inflammatory breast cancer, or "dermal lymphatic carcinomatosis" of the breast, is characterized clinically by skin redness, warmth, edema (peau d'orange), a visible erysipeloid margin, induration of the underlying breast, and a rapid evolution, usually less than 3 months from first sign to diagnosis. These features must be present at the time of primary diagnosis. Biopsies of the erythematous areas and adjacent normal-appearing skin often but not always reveal poorly differ-

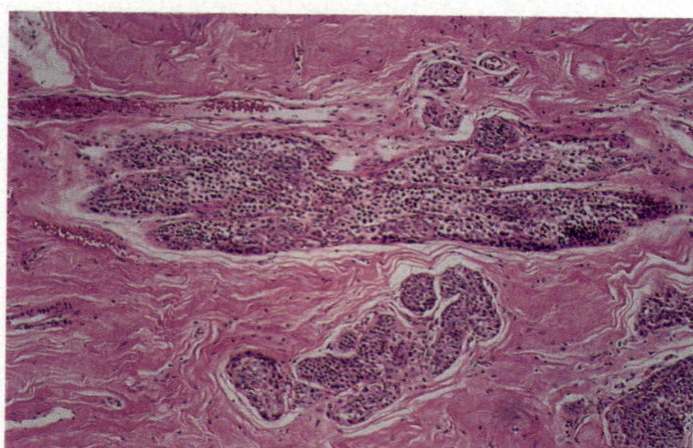

Figure 107-8 Lobular carcinoma in situ (LCIS). Terminal ducts and acini are completely filled and dilated by a uniform small cell proliferation. (Courtesy Dr. Ira Bleiweiss, Mount Sinai School of Medicine.)

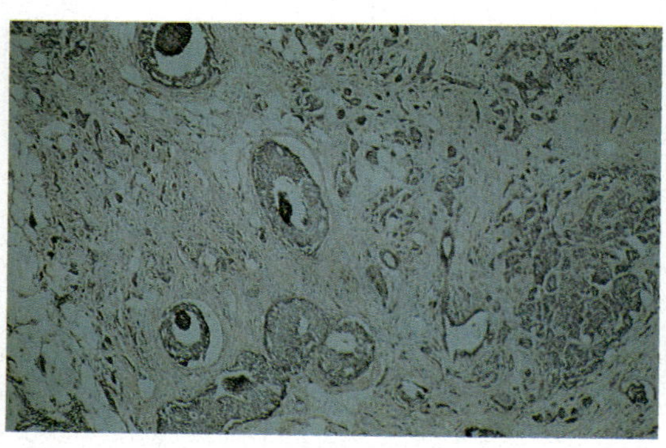

Figure 107-10 Infiltrating ductal carcinoma of the breast, not otherwise specified (NOS). Nearly 80% of breast cancers exhibit this histology, about one-third of the time with additional types of differentiation.

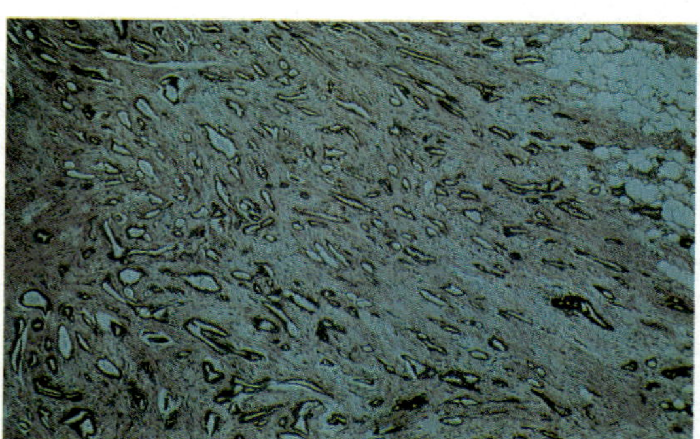

Figure 107-12 Tubular carcinoma of the breast. This tumor is rare in its pure form, less than 1%, but has a better prognosis than infiltrating duct carcinoma not otherwise specified (NOS). Partial tubular differentiation is seen in 20% of infiltrating duct carcinomas NOS.

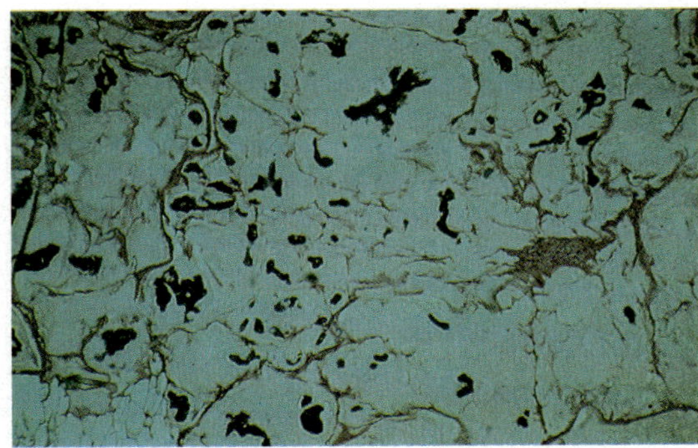

Figure 107-13 Mucinous or colloid carcinoma of the breast. This tumor is uncommon (about 2%) but has a rather favorable prognosis.

Table 107-9 5-Year Breast Cancer-Specific Mortality Rates According to Tumor Size and Axillary Lymph Node Involvement*

	5-Year Breast Cancer Specific Mortality Rate (%)		
Tumor Size in cm	0 Positive Nodes	1 to 3 Positive Nodes	More Than 3 Positive Nodes
< 0.5	0.8	4.7	41.0
0.5–0.9	1.7	6.0	45.8
1.0–1.9	4.2	13.4	32.8
2.0–2.9	7.7	16.6	36.6
3.0–3.9	13.8	21.0	43.1
4.0–4.9	15.4	30.2	47.4
> 5.0	17.8	27.0	54.5

*Information derived from SEER data. No. positive axillary lymph nodes.

entiated cancer cells filling and obstructing the subdermal lymphatics. Inflammatory cells are rarely present. Patients typically have signs of advanced cancer, including palpable axillary nodes, supraclavicular nodes, and/or distant metastases. Inflammatory breast cancer represents about 1% of breast cancers in the United States and Western Europe, although its incidence appears higher in North Africa and the Middle East.

Several other histologic types of mammary carcinomas have been described but are rarely (< 1%) encountered. Adenocystic carcinoma, carcinosarcomas, pure squamous cell carcinoma, metaplastic carcinomas (carcinoma with osseous or cartilaginous stroma), basal cell carcinomas, and so-called lipid-rich carcinomas have been observed. Because of their rarity, clinical correlates are practically nonexistent.

TUMOR CHARACTERISTICS

Tumor Size In addition to being a determinant for optimal local therapy, tumor size has prognostic significance in the determination of additional therapy (Table 107-9). As the size of the tumor increases, the risk of recurrence or metastasis also increases, for both lymph node-negative and node-positive tumors. Because the risk of treatment failure is already high for patients with node-positive breast cancer, increasing tumor size adds relatively little prognostic value. However, tumor size is often the main prognostic indicator in node-negative breast cancer. This variable is particularly important in the decision to use or not to use adjuvant systemic therapy in patients with node-negative breast cancer. Tumor size refers only to the invasive component and should be determined in all three dimensions by the pathologist. Approximately 25 to 30% of patients with negative lymph nodes and a primary tumor less than 2 cm in diameter will experience a recurrence within 20 years of follow-up.[109] Patients with tumors 1 cm or less in diameter have an excellent prognosis, with fewer than 15% recurring at 10 years in the absence of effective adjuvant therapy. The largest database demonstrating the relationship among tumor size, lymph node status, and breast cancer survival comes from the Surveillance, Epidemiology, and End Results (SEER) program (see Table 107-9).[110] Less than 2% of patients with tumors under 1 cm and negative nodes died of breast cancer within 5 years. Considering the excellent prognosis for this group of patients with very small tumors, as well as the expense and toxicity of treatment, routine use of chemotherapy is not indicated. The combination of poor nuclear grade and lymphatic vessel invasion identifies a small subset (approximately 10%) of patients with T1a, b N0 M0 breast cancer with a significant risk of relapse, in the 30 to 40% range, that warrants systemic adjuvant therapy.[108,111]

Axillary Lymph Node Involvement Involvement of the ipsilateral axillary lymph nodes is still the most reliable and reproducible prognostic indicator for primary breast cancer (see Table 107-9).[112,113] In general, 50 to 70% of patients with positive lymph nodes have a relapse, whereas only 15 to 45% of patients with all lymph nodes negative for metastatic disease have a relapse after locoregional treatments only. The risk of tumor recurrence in a patient with primary breast cancer is a continuum related to the number of positive axillary lymph nodes.[113] With each additional positive lymph node found, the risk of recurrence and metastasis increases by a few percentage points. Thus, patients with 4 to 10 positive lymph nodes have a greater risk than those with 1 to 3 positive nodes, and those with 10 or more positive nodes have a greater than 80% probability of recurrence and metastasis. Because nodal status cannot be accurately assessed by clinical means, an axillary lymph node dissection, including levels I and II, is considered the standard of care. Clinical studies have demonstrated that lymph node negativity is reliable only if at least 6, but preferably, 10 axillary lymph nodes are removed and examined. Both macro- and micrometastasis within the lymph nodes have similar prognostic significance.[114] In recent years, primary breast cancer has been diagnosed in earlier and mostly localized stages. A classic axillary lymph node dissection has no therapeutic benefit for patients with node-negative axillae and is associated with considerable short- and long-term morbidity. An alternative (diagnostic) staging procedure for these patients is the sentinel lymph node biopsy.[115] This procedure limits considerably the extent of the surgical procedure in the axilla and, for the great majority of patients with negative axillary lymph nodes, precludes the need for a formal axillary dissection while providing similar (and in some cases superior) diagnostic and prognostic information. The identification of a single (or just a few) sentinel node also permits the pathologist to perform a more detailed assessment to detect micrometastases by combining light microscopy, IHC, and even more sensitive molecular techniques. The prognostic significance of identifying isolated metastatic cells in histologically negative lymph nodes by more sensitive techniques is still undetermined. Sentinel node biopsy and assessment are under extensive evaluation by large cooperative research groups, including the NSABP and the American College of Surgeons Oncology Group. The technique is making substantial inroads in the practice of breast surgery. Preliminary reports of randomized trials comparing axillary dissection with sentinel lymph node biopsy have demonstrated that the latter is associated with significantly reduced morbidity. Because of these results, sentinel lymph node biopsy has replaced classic axillary dissection for early, localized breast cancer in a substantial percentage of patients with clinically negative axillae.

Although axillary lymph node status is still the most powerful prognostic indicator, 15 to 45% of patients whose lymph nodes do not contain metastases still experience a recurrence and die. Conversely, about 15% of patients with >10 positive lymph nodes treated only with surgery and radiotherapy survive without recurrence or metastases. Because of this limitation, other prognostic markers have been developed to improve prognostic accuracy, particularly in the group of patients with node-negative tumors (Table 107-10).

Histologic Type Several histologic variables have been reported to have prognostic significance. Most invasive breast cancers are ductal not otherwise specified (NOS).[107] The prognoses of ductal and lobular carcinomas are similar enough to prompt the same treatment modalities. However, there are several cancers that are less common, but have more favorable prognoses. These include pure tubular carcinoma, mucinous or colloid carcinoma, papillary carcinoma, and all noninvasive breast cancers. These cancers have substantially better prognoses, especially when found in a node-negative stage.[116,117] The more favorable prognosis of these histologic types often justifies omission

Table 107-10 Effect of Lymph Node Involvement on Recurrence and Survival

	Status				
	Relapse Rate %			Survival %	
Axillary Node	18 Mo	5 Yr	10 Yr	5 Yr	10 Yr
N–	5	18	24	78	65
N+	33	65	76	47	25
N+ (1–3)	13	50	65	62	38
N+ (≥ 4)	52	79	86	32	13
All patients	17	40	50	64	46

From Fisher and Slack.[22]

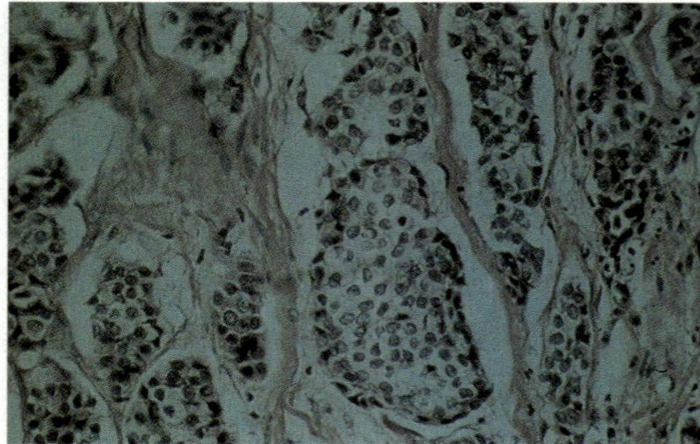

Figure 107-14 Lymphatic invasion by breast cancer. The vessel walls are thin and lined with endothelial cells.

of adjuvant systemic treatment, especially for small tumors (< 3 cm). Because most of these special types have small dimensions when diagnosed and are node-negative, regional treatment is usually all that is required. When stringently defined, medullary carcinoma, when associated with negative axillary lymph nodes, is also considered by some but not all experts to have a better prognosis.[108,117,118] The magnitude of this difference, in terms of 10-year survival, was reported to be 17%. However, atypical medullary carcinomas (those that do not fulfill the necessary histological criteria) or mixed medullary and ductal carcinomas have prognoses similar to those for the common varieties of ductal and lobular breast cancers.

Histologic Grade or Differentiation Tumor grade has been shown to be an important prognostic indicator. In general, tumors expressing features that indicate a high degree of tumor differentiation have the most favorable prognosis. Multiple studies have shown that higher grade is associated with higher rates of recurrence and metastases and poorer survival. These correlations are independent of tumor size and lymph node involvement. High tumor grade is also associated with hormone receptor negativity and increased response to cytotoxic therapy. Conversely, low grade is associated with hormonal sensitivity and lower response to chemotherapy.

The clear definition of various histologic differentiation grades led to the recognition that those grades had reproducible prognostic significance.[119] Trained, experienced breast pathologists can recognize poorly differentiated, moderately well-differentiated, and differentiated tumors without much difficulty; the assessment of the histologic grade for those tumors is quite reproducible. Furthermore, although there is some variation among different pathologists, the concordance rate is quite acceptable. Recent reports based on the SEER tumor registry provided strong evidence supporting the prognostic value of histologic grade determined by "average" pathologists. Something similar can be said for nuclear grade, although some find that histologic grade is a more reliable prognostic indicator because it includes cellular and tissue-related criteria. Nuclear grade can be determined in cytologic specimens. Well-differentiated histologic types, such as tubular, papillary, or colloid (mucinous), have a lower incidence of axillary nodal metastases and a lower risk of distant recurrence than the more common infiltrating ductal carcinomas NOS.[111,117,120] It should be emphasized that pure noninvasive ductal (DCIS) or lobular carcinomas (LCIS) have very low risk for axillary lymph node involvement and virtually no risk for distant metastases. Recent results from clinical trials suggest that the addition of tamoxifen to optimal locoregional therapy reduces the risk of local recurrence and the incidence of second primary breast cancer after non-invasive cancers. Less than 20% of patients with negative nodes having well to moderately well-differentiated (grade 1 or 2) tumors experience a recurrence in 5 years, compared to more than 30% for those with poorly differentiated tumors.[121] Smaller tumors are more often well differentiated, whereas larger tumors are predominantly poorly differentiated. Tumor differentiation is also associated with other prognostic indicators such as ER expression, PR expression, ploidy, and S-phase fraction (SPF).

The grading system most frequently used is the Elston-Ellis modification of the Scarf-Bloom-Richardson system.[122] In this system, invasive ductal breast cancers are categorized into three histologic grades, depending on their degree of tubular and/or gland formation, cellular pleomorphism, and number of mitoses per high-power microscopic field. Within each of these categories, a score of 1 to 3 is assigned, with 1 representing the most favorable findings (for example, prominent gland formation, little cellular pleomorphism, low mitotic rate) and 3 indicating the least favorable. The scores for each of these categories are added together. Grade I carcinoma (well differentiated or low grade) is defined as having a total of 3 to 5 points, grade II (moderately differentiated or intermediate grade) is defined as 6 to 7 points, and grade III (poorly differentiated or high grade) is defined as 8 to 9 points.

OTHER HISTOLOGIC VARIABLES Tumor Necrosis Tumor necrosis of varying degrees was encountered in 60% of 1,539 patients with invasive breast cancer in NSABP protocol B-04. Necrosis, particularly when observed to be of marked degree, was positively correlated with increased rates of treatment failure. Although necrosis was observed to be significantly associated with a number of clinical and histopathologic features purportedly related to an ominous prognosis in this disease, it was not correlated with pathologic nodal status, and multivariate analysis revealed it to influence treatment failure independently of tumor size in lesions less than 5 cm in their greatest diameter. Extrapolation of the data fails to reveal any consistent information that might relate tumor necrosis to tumor growth per se in accounting for such a role.

Circumscription Mammary carcinomas generally assume either a circumscribed structure, or a more infiltrative irregular or stellate configuration. A better prognosis has been ascribed to the former tumor type.

Lymphatic and Blood Vessel Invasion Lymphatic and blood vessel invasion has been associated with poor prognosis in numerous clinical reports. One-third of NSABP patients exhibited extension into lymphatics within the dominant mass, and another 23% were considered questionable (Figure 107-14). Such a finding was associated with other unfavorable characteristics. Blood vessel invasion was observed in only 5% of patients and was associated with the finding of four or more positive axillary nodes, lymphatic invasion, and certain other unfavorable findings (Figure 107-15). In other studies, blood vessel invasion has been reported in 5 to 50%. In one report from Memorial Sloan-Kettering Cancer Center 14% of patients with T1 N0 tumors and in 22% of T1 N1 breast cancer evidenced blood vessel invasion.

Multicentricity Many breast cancers are multicentric in origin. Although several studies have addressed this issue, the number of multicentric, independent cancers that might have been present is difficult to ascertain since no clear indi-

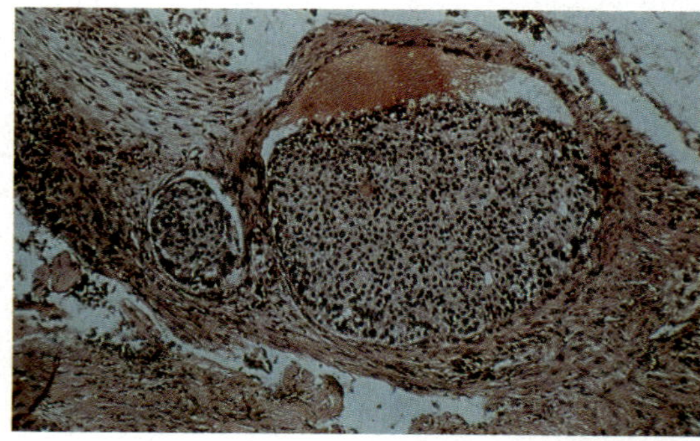

Figure 107-15 Blood vessel invasion by breast cancer. The vessel wall structure is recognizable, together with erythrocytes in the vessel.

cation of actual site or pathologic type of lesion encountered was presented in the reports of study findings. In an examination of 904 NSABP cases, excluding those instances in which the lesion was beneath the nipple or in the tail of the breast, data were collected from only those quadrants in which the primary lesion was not encountered. This method eliminated the difficulty in distinguishing a new focus of carcinoma in the quadrant of the primary from an integral part of the primary lesion. Either invasive or noninvasive cancers regarded as independent were found in 13.4% of the 904 patients. The frequency of invasive and noninvasive multicentric cancers was 4.1% and 9.3%, respectively. The types of noninvasive cancers encountered were intraductal (66.7%), LCIS (22.6%), and a combination of both (10.7%). Increased utilization of magnetic resonance imaging (MRI) of the breast for pre-operative assessment of extent of disease has indicated that multicentricity is much more common than previously determined by mammography. However, the clinical significance of such an observation remains uncertain because of the finding that lumpectomy with or without breast irradiation is as effective as mastectomy in terms of curability. One of the major deterrents to accepting such a limited resection was the realization that such an excision may ignore clinically and pathologically undetected cancers at sites within the breast remote from the dominant mass. Results from the randomized trials of breast conservation indicate that tumors that recur in the ipsilateral breast following lumpectomy are, in the vast majority of instances, found at the site of the initial operation rather than elsewhere in the breast.

Despite the significant incidence of multifocal lesions in both breasts in a woman with a primary breast cancer, two or more clinically overt primary cancers in the primary breast are uncommon. Similarly, synchronous bilateral tumors are uncommon, and the incidence of a second asynchronous primary tumor in the uninvolved or opposite breast (about 4 to 6% in 10 years) fails to approach the incidence predicted by the number of occult lesions detected by random biopsy, autopsy or MRI. It has been noted, for example, that the incidence of clinically latent intraductal carcinomas in the breasts of women over the age of 70 who died of causes other than mammary carcinoma is 19 times greater than the reported incidence of clinical breast cancer.[123] Such findings strongly suggest that not all cancers progress to overt clinical lesions and that they may even undergo regression. These conclusions are similar to and gain support from evidence about adrenal neuroblastomas in children, from thyroid carcinomas, and from carcinomas of the prostate, which are found more frequently pathologically in randomly examined material than clinically in comparable populations.

Nonepithelial Neoplasms of The Breast

A variety of non-epithelial neoplasms of the breast have been described. Fibrosarcomas, leiomyosarcomas, rhabdomyosarcomas, and angiosarcomas are all infrequent.[107] Non-Hodgkin's lymphomas can have their initial onset in the breast and can also occur as a focus of generalized disease. These usually have a B-cell phenotype. Some cases resemble carcinoma on routine histology; immunohistochemistry is often helpful in resolving this question. Only a few cases of Hodgkin's disease and leukemia have been reported with initial manifestation in the breast.

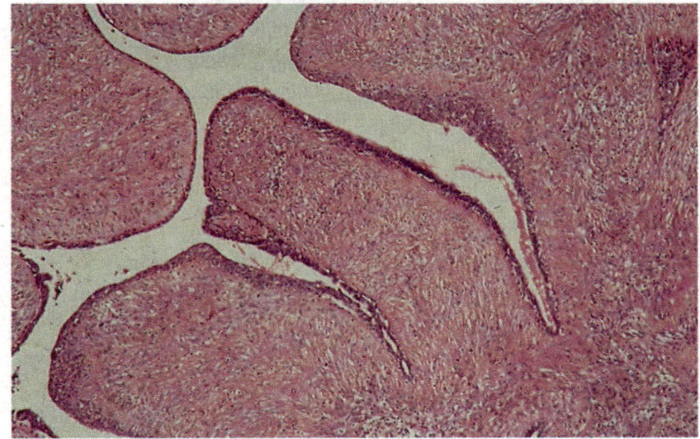

Figure 107-16 Phyllodes tumor (cystosarcoma phyllodes). Leaf-like projections, lined by benign epithelium, contain a hypercellular stroma.

Phyllodes tumor (cystosarcoma phyllodes) is a biphasic neoplasm that is partially epithelial and partially mesenchymal (Figure107-16). Phyllodes tumors may achieve a great size and, not infrequently, demonstrate some invasion of adjacent breast tissue. They are best managed by local excision with a rim of normal breast tissue. Phyllodes tumor has been known to metastasize and to kill. Phyllodes tumors are classified as benign, borderline or indeterminate, or malignant. High mitotic rate, cellular atypia, stromal overgrowth, infiltrative margins, hemorrhage and necrosis are considered features of malignancy. Although it is difficult to determine from clinical or histologic appearance which tumors behave malignantly and will metastasize, malignant histology and stromal overgrowth are predictive of metastasis.[124]

In a report of NSABP findings from 950 women with node-negative invasive breast cancer enrolled in NSABP study B-06, 22 pathologic and four clinical features were evaluated for their prognostic significance.[125] Their assessment in a Cox regression model demonstrated that only nuclear grade, histologic tumor type, and race were prognostically important. Eighty-six percent of patients having tumors of good nuclear grade treated with loco-regional therapy survived for 8 years as opposed to 64% in whom the nuclear grade was scored as poor. Patients with either mucinous, tubular, or papillary cancers fared significantly better than did those with NOS or atypical medullary tumors. Survival for patients with typical medullary, NOS combinations, or lobular invasive cancers was intermediate. Blacks had a worse survival rate than did whites. The NSABP experience suggests that as a predictor of survival in node-negative patients, nuclear grade is as good as, if not better than, information derived from other markers, such as *HER2* gene expression, cathepsin activity, S-phase fraction (SPF), ploidy, tumor size, or estrogen receptors (ER).

In another report, discriminants for treatment failure by the tenth year in 614 patients treated by radical mastectomy were provided.[120] Nodal metastasis was the most significant prognostic discriminant for disease-free survival in the tenth year. Histologic grade and tumor size were significant discriminants in patients with four or more positive nodes, but no additional factors were found to be significant discriminants in patients with one to three positive nodes.

NATURAL HISTORY AND PROGNOSTIC MARKERS

The natural history and prognosis for primary breast cancer vary considerably from patient to patient (see Table 107-10). Some patients present with very indolent disease and either are cured by local therapy or survive for many years even after developing metastases. A small percentage of patients survive more than 10 years without any treatment.[126] In other patients, the disease follows an aggressive, rapidly progressive course that is refractory to treatment.

The heterogeneity in the clinical course of breast cancer is mirrored by great variability in measured doubling time and other cell kinetic parameters. In general, human breast cancer has a low growth fraction (proportion of cells in the active cell cycle) compared with many other tumors, with estimated values ranging from 5 to 30%, depending on the method used. The S-phase fraction (SPF) is an indicator of the rate of cell turnover, or growth rate. In rapidly growing tumors, such as testicular cancer or high-grade lymphomas, it may exceed 50%.

Estimated tumor volume doubling times for primary human breast tumors are also prolonged. In one retrospective study, 147 tumors observed to grow on serial mammograms were evaluated.[127] Doubling times ranged from 44 to more than 1,800 days, with a mean of 212 days. It is not possible to determine the growth rate of breast cancers in their preclinical (microscopic) stage, but if one assumes that a cancer begins with a single cell and grows with a constant doubling time of 200 days, a tumor would need about 20 years of growth to reach 1 to 2 cm in diameter. A tumor with a faster doubling time of 100 days would still require 10 years to become clinically detectable, and a remarkably fast-growing tumor (doubling time of 20 days) could possibly have originated just 2 years earlier. Similarly, a 2 mm tumor with an average doubling time would require about 4 years of growth to reach a size of 1 cm. These growth calculations assume logarithmic growth, whereas Gompertzian growth models indicate that growth rates are not constant throughout the life history of the tumor and that preclinical latency may not be very long. Metastatic lesions may have a slightly faster average rate of growth than primary tumors. These observations may explain the relatively poorer prognosis recorded in several studies for very young women (< 35 years old) with breast cancer. These women may have a higher proportion of faster growing, more aggressive tumors, since indolent, slowly growing tumors would not have had time to become clinically evident by that age. These data also suggest that since most tumors have had a prolonged preclinical life of at least several years, delays in diagnosis of only a few months from the first symptoms of primary breast cancer are unlikely to have a major impact on the presence or absence of metastases or ultimate patient survival. It has been estimated that only 5% of patients would be adversely affected by delays longer than 3 months. Even if primary tumors were diagnosed and treated a full year earlier, only a 30% reduction in the percentage of patients with metastases would result.[128] These estimates are compatible with the documented benefits of mammography screening programs, which detect microscopic, nonpalpable early breast cancers in many patients. The heterogeneity of the natural history of breast cancer complicates patient management. Obviously, patients with virulent, fast-growing tumors might be treated aggressively because of their poor prognosis, whereas other patients with indolent tumors might be spared the morbidity and cost of excessive interventions when their disease is unlikely to compromise survival. A major focus of research in recent years has been the identification of tumor or host factors that would accurately predict patient outcome. The ideal prognostic marker would be one that, if expressed by the tumor, signified early metastases and short survival. Tumors not expressing the marker would be associated with an indolent course, the absence of metastases, and prolonged survival in nearly all patients. Although the ideal prognostic factor does not yet exist, a number of variables have been identified that can help to identify patients according to their relative risk for recurrence (Table 107-11). These factors attempt to measure and quantify the degree of tumor differentiation, tumor aggressiveness or metastatic potential, rate of growth or sensitivity/resistance to planned treatment. Some of the markers shown on Table 107-11 are old and well established; others are new and must be considered investigational until definitive evidence supports their clinical utility.

After surgery has been completed and the surgical specimens have been examined and evaluated by the pathologist, a number of important prognostic indicators are used to determine whether additional therapy is necessary and potentially useful. Indicators that have been demonstrated to have reproducible prognostic value are defined in Table 107-11.

Age and Menopausal Status Both patient characteristics have been extensively evaluated. When other, more important tumor characteristics are considered, age and menopausal status are not important prognostic indicators. A large study with long follow-up indicated that women 45 to 49 years of age had the best prognosis and that the very young (those under age 35 years) or elderly patients had the worst breast cancer specific survival.[129,130]

Table 107-11 Prognostic Factors in Breast Cancer

Predictors of tumor invasiveness or metastatic potential
TNM stage
Axillary lymph node status
Histologic subtype
Angiogenesis markers
Markers of cell proliferation
Oncogene and growth factor receptor expression
Protease expression
Predictors of organ-specific metastases
PTHrP expression
Vimentin expression
Bone marrow micrometastases
L-myc polymorphism
Predictors of tumor growth rate
Tumor differentiation
Estrogen and progesterone receptor expression
HER2/neu, *EGFR*, mutant *TP53*, *Cyclin-D*
Proliferation markers (mitotic index, thymidine labeling index, S-phase fraction, Ki-67, PCNA)
Predictors of efficacy of systemic therapy
Hormone receptor expression (ER and PR)
Growth factor receptor (*EGFR*, *HER2*) expression
TP53 mutation
BCL-2 expression
pgp expression

*Information derived from SEER data.
No. positive axillary lymph nodes.

Angiogenesis Markers In recent years, it has become evident that angiogenesis plays a substantial role in the growth and spread of malignant tumors.[131] Consequently, markers of angiogenic activity have received increasing attention. Counting the number of tumor capillaries immunohistochemically after staining for factor VIII has been shown to have major prognostic value. Tumors with fewer capillaries have a lower metastatic potential and better prognosis.[132] Variations in methodology have led to conflicting results, although the weight of the evidence favors the strong prognostic value of angiogenesis. Markers of angiogenesis have also become putative therapeutic targets.

Markers of Proliferative Capacity Measurement of the proliferation rates of malignant tissues has strong prognostic value for several types of cancer, including breast cancer. Several techniques are used to evaluate the proliferative capacity of the malignant cell, including mitotic indices, thymidine-labeling indices (TLIs) and SPF, and the measurement of proteins expressed preferentially during active phases of the cell cycle. The mitotic index is determined by counting mitotic figures using light microscopy on a tumor specimen stained with hematoxylin and eosin. It is a technique well within the capabilities of any surgical pathology laboratory, and it has been validated by both univariate and multivariate analyses. A commonly used method of evaluating proliferation capacity in the United States is the determination of SPF by flow cytometry.[129] This technique can be performed on fresh or frozen tissues and on archival paraffin-embedded material. It also provides information about DNA ploidy. For both TLI and SPF, a low value indicates a more slowly proliferating tumor and is associated with a slower rate of recurrence regardless of axillary nodal status. A high SPF is strongly correlated with other adverse prognostic factors, such as high histologic and cytologic grades, aneuploidy, and a negative steroid receptor status. Multivariate analyses indicate that SPF is one of the most important prognostic factors in primary breast cancer.

Many proteins play a role in the control of the cell cycle or are expressed at higher levels during certain phases of the cell cycle. Ki-67, MIB1, and proliferating cell nuclear antigen (PCNA) are additional markers for the proliferation rate of malignant tumors.[129,133,134] Of these, Ki-67 has been more extensively studied, and it correlates strongly with the results of SPF determination and, therefore, long-term prognosis. The usefulness of PCNA requires additional evaluation. Other proteins, including mitosin, Ki-S1, and the various cyclins, are currently under evaluation. Cyclin E has been shown to be exceptionally accurate as a prognostic indicator.[134]

Steroid Hormone Receptors Both the ER and the PR have been studied extensively in patients with primary breast cancer.[135] Both clearly have prognostic value, although their ability to discriminate between low- and high-risk patients is quite limited. Patients with ER-positive tumor tend to have a more indolent course and to metastasize preferentially to soft tissue and bone; conversely, those with ER-negative tumors relapse earlier, and metastases to liver, lung, and central nervous system are more likely. ER-positive tumors are more often well differentiated and are associated with other favorable prognostic characteristics. Although patients with ER-positive tumors tend to have better short-term disease-free and overall survival rates than do patients with ER-negative tumors, the differences between the two groups tend to diminish or even disappear with time.[136]

PR appeared in some studies to be a more valuable prognostic indicator than the ER. The best use of steroid hormone receptors is not in the determination of prognosis but in the prediction of response to systemic endocrine therapy and, therefore, the selection of optimal adjuvant systemic treatments. Multiple recent reports have emphasized the strong predictive value of estrogen receptor negativity for response to chemotherapy, especially in the neoadjuvant setting.

Molecular Genetic Alterations Malignant tumors develop as a consequence of multiple critical gene abnormalities secondary to oncogene activation, loss of function of tumor suppressor genes, or alterations of other genes critical for cell control mechanisms. Two members of the type I growth factor receptor family, the EGFR (or HER1) and *HER2/neu*, are frequently amplified and/or overexpressed in breast cancer.[129,137] Overexpression of the proteins encoded by these genes is associated with a more aggressive clinical course, including a higher risk of developing metastases and more rapid growth and tumor progression. HER2 is overexpressed in 20 to 30% of breast cancers and overexpression is almost always the result of gene amplification. Overexpression is inversely correlated with ER expression and associated with poorly differentiated tumors with high growth rate. Survival is shorter for patients with HER2–overexpressing tumors than for patients with normal HER2 expression. Several recent reports suggest, however, that patients with HER2–overexpressing breast cancer derive greater benefit from anthracycline-containing adjuvant chemotherapy than from other regimens, particularly at higher dose.[138]

Whereas some studies suggest that HER2 overexpression is a marker of tamoxifen resistance, other analyses have provided conflicting results. Recent reports suggest that aromatase inhibitors might be more effective than tamoxifen in ER-positive, HER2-positive tumors. For this reason, many experts prefer to use an aromatase inhibitor to tamoxifen for the management of postmenopausal patients with ER-positive, HER2-positive breast cancer. The most important clinical application of HER2 testing is to identify candidates for HER2–directed therapy with trastuzumab (Herceptin).[79,139] Recent reports have suggested that fluorescence in situ hybridization (FISH) is the most definitive testing method to predict response to trastuzumab.[80] The prognostic value of EGFR overexpression is less well established, and there is no FDA–approved diagnostic test or therapeutic intervention that targets this receptor.

TP53 is frequently mutated in breast cancers.[140] Although some studies have found that *TP53* mutation is associated with poor prognosis and others have found correlations with response or resistance to cytotoxic or endocrine agents, no compelling evidence has emerged yet from large, multivariate analysis to support the routine testing for *TP53* gene mutation or abnormal protein expression as either prognostic or predictive factor. Evidence is even less compelling to support testing for *myc, ATM, RB,* or others. The prognostic value of gene mutations for *BRCA1* or *BRCA2* remains to be established.

Bone Marrow Involvement Several investigators have presented data to suggest that the presence of microscopic involvement of the bone marrow, detectable by sensitive IHC analyses, is a major determinant of prognosis.[141] In fact, some have suggested that this finding is superior to axillary lymph node involvement in its prognostic capability.[142] Although these data are increasingly interesting, this marker of prognosis has not been generally accepted or adopted in clinical practice. There is also ongoing work with detection of circulating cancer cells and its correlation with prognosis or response to systemic therapy. Technological advances allow the reproducible detection and quantification of epithelial cells distinct from other nucleated cells in blood. A recent report of a prospective trial indicated that the presence of 5 or more circulating tumor cells/7.5 mL blood at baseline was an adverse prognostic indicator.[143] Furthermore, persistence of 5 or more cells after one month of systemic therapy was associated with a very high probability of short-term progressive disease.

Several other histologic factors, including lymphatic invasion, vascular invasion, tumor necrosis, and mononuclear cell infiltration, have been associated with better or worse prognoses in at least one report. Although extensive clinical experience supports the prognostic value of each of these factors, they have not survived the test of independence in multivariate analysis, nor have they been sufficiently evaluated to date.

Investigational Markers Many biochemical, molecular, genetic, and immunologic markers have been under investigation for the past several years. All of them have been suggested by one or more reports to have prognostic significance. However, evaluation of these markers falls short of determining whether they are independent prognostic factors or valuable additions to other proven, commonly used prognostic indicators. Among the promising investigational markers are heat shock proteins, *nm23,* cathepsin D, urokinase plasminogen activators (Upa), urokinase plasminogen activator receptors (Upar), plasminogen activator inhibitors (PAI-1, PAI-2), *Bcl-2, BAX,* laminin receptors, and apoptotic rate. Tumor levels of Upa and PAI-1, or the ratio of these two markers has been shown, in a prospective multicenter trial designed to validate their prognostic value, to be independently associated with prognosis. Furthermore, the European Organization for Research and Treatment of Cancer-Receptor and Biomarker Group also validated these markers in a prospective trial. A standardized ELISA assay exists. However, because of the need for a fresh, larger tumor sample this assay has not gained wide acceptance.

Some markers can be shown to be relevant as predictors of response to chemotherapy or hormone therapy, whereas others may serve to identify tumors using particular targets of biologic intervention *(HER2/neu,* EGFR). Many genes commonly associated with cancer participate in the regulation of cell proliferation and apoptosis. In a recent report, levels of total cyclin E and low-molecular-weight cyclin E in tumor tissue, as measured by Western blot assay, correlated strongly with survival in patients with breast cancer.[136] Alterations in these genes may be important in determining the chemosensitivity of cancer cells. For instance, cells that express high levels of cyclin D1 mRNA and protein have increased resistance to phase-specific agents like methotrexate but not to doxorubicin or paclitaxel.[133] Mutations or deletions of p53 might be associated with resistance to various DNA-damaging drugs.

Over the years, there have been numerous attempts to reach a consensus on what prognostic factors are of recognized clinical utility. However, with the exception of the basic histopathologic factors, steroid hormone receptors, markers of proliferation, and HER2 expression, the majority of proposed factors fall short of general acceptance as useful clinical tools.

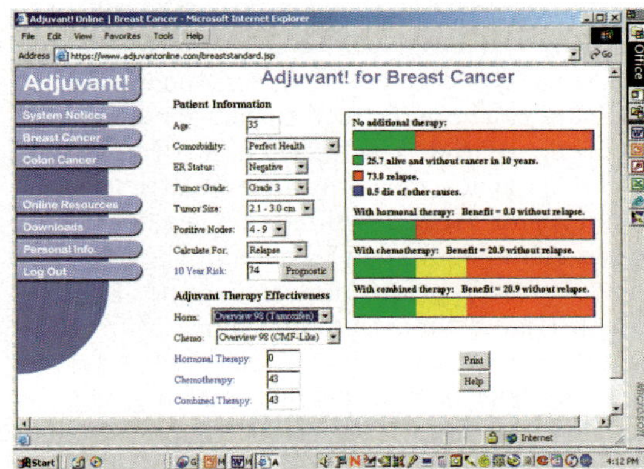

Figure 107-17 On-line prognostic software that predicts 10-year probability of recurrence and mortality, as well as the probability of benefit from various systemic adjuvant treatment options based on individual patient and tumor characteristics.

Prognostic Indices There is no standardized method of integrating prognostic information, and attempts to develop prognostic indices have had limited efficacy. The University of Nottingham index is based on tumor grade, axillary lymph node involvement, and hormone receptor status.[144] It has been validated prospectively and confirmed by an independent center, but it still has limited usefulness in the determination of individual prognosis. The single most useful prognostic index is the Adjuvantonline! Program. (Figure 107-17). This software includes patient age, comorbid conditions, tumor size, grade, number of positive axillary nodes, and estrogen receptor status. With this information, it calculates the 10-year probability of relapse and death for an individual patient.[145] Using this estimated risk level, the program also calculates the absolute benefit the patient would derive from adjuvant tamoxifen, aromatase inhibitors, and various chemotherapy regimens. Investigators from British Columbia recently validated the program, with observed results well within 2% of those predicted. A recent update of the program now includes the possibility to include other, ad hoc prognostic factors.

An emerging area of investigation of prognosis and prediction of sensitivity or resistance to therapy is genomics. CDNA arrays, including 20,000 to 30,000 genes are being used to develop gene expression profiles and correlate them with treatment outcome.[146] Although this is an evolving technology, early results suggest great promise in understanding better the biology of cancers, determining prognosis and predicting drug sensitivity.[147] Gene expression profiling using cDNA arrays or oligonucleotide arrays requires at this time the availability of fresh or fresh-frozen tissue. An alternate approach to develop multigene predictors of prognosis or response to therapy was recently presented.[148] This method, based on RT PCR, can be performed on paraffin-embedded archival material. The assay, as presented, consists of 21 genes, including genes related to estrogen receptor, HER2, proliferation genes and proteases identified from the literature. The results of the assay are expressed as a Recurrence Score, a quantitative estimate of recurrence at 5 years. Updated analyses indicated that the assay had been validated on multiple independent groups of patients, and that the Recurrence Score was also a good predictor of therapeutic benefit from tamoxifen and adjuvant chemotherapy.

Clinical use of Prognostic Factors The major objective of prognostic factors is to calculate the individual risk of recurrence and disease-related mortality for patients with primary breast cancer treated with curative intent. It is considered that patients with a risk of relapse lower than 10% would have only marginal benefit from adjuvant chemotherapy. However, calculations of the benefits of tamoxifen or an aromatase inhibitor administered for 5 years to patients with ER-positive breast cancer and the demonstration that the combination of hormonal therapy and chemotherapy has additive effects on reduction of risk of relapse and mortality have prompted a reassessment of these recommendations. Most patients with invasive primary breast cancer larger than 1 cm should be encouraged to receive adjuvant systemic therapy; some with tumors smaller than 1 cm should also be advised to consider adjuvant therapy, because randomized trials have not identified any subgroups that failed to derive benefit from these interventions. The use of prognostic factors, under these circumstances, serves more to place the benefit:risk ratio for individual patients in the context of their own prognosis. The acceptable benefit:risk ratio varies substantially from person to person; therefore, after a best attempt to calculate individual risk of relapse and mortality, treatment options and the probability of benefit from each should be presented in the light of toxicity and cost to facilitate informed treatment decisions.

DIAGNOSIS AND SCREENING

Historically, the primary presenting symptom of breast cancer was a palpable mass, often first detected by the patient. Today, the increasing use of mammography, especially in screening programs, results in many cancers being found at a preclinical stage. A simple discussion of the signs and symptoms of breast cancer without consideration of these preclinical manifestations would be incomplete. To some extent, this means greater complexity in selecting for biopsy patients who are suspected of having carcinoma. The clinical and mammographic signs and symptoms are best understood against the background knowledge of the anatomy and biology of breast cancer—how it grows and extends locally.

Patient History The patient's history should include standard epidemiologic and reproductive information to assess the relative risk factors. Information about lumps, pain, or any changes in the breast should be obtained and correlated with physical findings. Although pain is probably the most frequent breast complaint that brings a patient to a physician's office, it is uncommonly the presenting factor in cancer. Breast cancer, especially in its early stages, is usually painless. Most breast pain is related to hormone stimulation and swelling of breast tissue (although these symptoms may draw attention to a mass that proves to be cancer). Careful questioning of the patient usually reveals that the pain is cyclic, beginning any time between ovulation and the onset of menstruation, and that commonly it is most intense a few days before menstruation. Pain usually disappears by the first or second day of the menstrual period, only to return again at the next cycle. Cyclic pain is present at a mild level in more than 50% of women of childbearing age. Less frequently, the pain can reach intense proportions. Some patients report that, during the worst days, it is too painful even to take a shower.

The most effective treatment is explanation and reassurance, although some patients who are extremely symptomatic and incapacitated by the pain may require treatments with hormones or hormone-blocking drugs. There are occasional reports that caffeine limitation or low-fat diets help, but relief seems to be individual, and these reports are not supported by persuasive clinical trials.

A patient who reports a lump or any other physical change in her breast needs careful attention. The history should describe any change in the character or size of the lump and whether or not it has been tender. Pain should be described with respect to its timing in the menstrual cycle. Lumpy changes associated with a fibrocystic process may wax and wane, but it is distinctly unusual for a carcinoma to do anything but increase in size. If there is confusion, the patient should be reexamined after the menstrual period.

Other descriptive changes, such as skin thickening or discoloration, the presence of axillary masses, or nipple discharge, should be elicited. Nipple discharge may be serous, watery, or milk-like. It may be clear or have a yellow or greenish hue, or it may be sero-sanguineous or frankly bloody. Although the latter may indicate a neoplasm, this is most commonly an intraductal papilloma, which is benign. It is possible, but rare, for such a discharge to signal an intraductal papillary carcinoma; all bloody discharges require further investigation.

Clear or serous discharge, especially if it involves more than one major duct opening on a nipple, is likely to be benign. Non-bloody discharge that is not spontaneous but requires manual compression to elicit is also likely to be benign. In an apocrine system such as the breast, there is always some cell desquamation and liquefaction and, therefore, some fluid present in the duct system. If this is not well absorbed, it can make its way through the collecting ducts to the nipple and present as a discharge. Similarly, if the duct is blocked by fibrosis or inspissated material, the pressure of secretion can cause dilation and cyst formation. Cytologic examination of the discharge has poor accuracy and is not very useful.

Physical Examination The patient should be examined, first in a sitting, then in a supine position. When the patient is sitting erect, more useful information is obtained visually than by palpation. When the arms are raised and stretched upward, the contour of the skin is pulled tight, allowing for easier detection of contour abnormalities in the upper half of the breast. This position also emphasizes dimpling, especially in the lower half of the breast. Because much of the breast tissue coalesces in the sitting position, it is very difficult when palpating to appreciate true masses and often easy to be confused by confluent tissue. The axilla is palpated by relaxing and adducting the patient's arm, but this is best done with the patient in the sitting position.

With the patient supine and the arm raised so that the hand is behind the head and the elbow lies flat on the pillow, the breast tissue can be spread across the chest wall, allowing for proper palpation. The patient should be slightly turned to the contralateral side to aid this process. It is important to proceed in a pattern, but whether it be performed by quadrants or strips is up to the examiner. Skin changes, such as dimpling, peau d'orange (edema), erythema, or areas of fixation and ulceration, suggest advanced cancer that has invaded the skin or the immediate subcutaneous tissue. Skin retraction is often more easily detected when the patient is sitting and the arms are raised or when the patient is leaning forward. Retraction or asymmetry of the nipple is another worrisome sign unless the patient reports that this has been present all her life. A subtle reddish thickening of the nipple and areola or flaking of the superficial epithelium may suggest Paget's disease.

The examination is concluded with a search for axillary, infraclavicular, and supraclavicular nodes and palpation of the liver to detect enlargement. Although palpably enlarged axillary nodes raise the probability of metastases, careful studies have shown that clinical judgment is highly inaccurate. In a study conducted by the NSABP, a group of cancer patients were judged by their clinicians to have normal axillary nodes, but 38% showed histologic evidence of metastatic tumor when the specimens were examined pathologically.[107] Conversely, in 25% of such cases, nodes that appeared enlarged and were judged to contain cancer were found to be normal.

The most difficult clinical decision is differentiating between a pathologic mass and a physiologic density associated with fibroglandular (or fibrocystic) changes. Many women have the latter condition, which is characterized by a rubbery density without clear margins. A true lump has definite margins. Whether these are smooth, as in a gross cyst or fibroadenoma, or somewhat irregular, as in carcinoma, they delineate a discrete mass that requires further investigation. Invasive ductal carcinomas are usually hard, and dominant in the breast, in contrast to multiple firm masses that may exist in benign breast disease. Lobular carcinomas are not usually so hard and thus are more difficult to recognize.

It is important to measure the size of a tumor with a caliper so that subsequent examinations can more accurately establish any change in size. Mobile lesions are usually considered benign, but this is another area of clinical uncertainty. Advanced cancers may be fixed, but early palpable lesions will certainly be mobile with respect to skin or fascia and muscle of the chest wall. There is, however, a subtle difference in mobility (better called "movability") characteristic of cysts or fibroadenomas, which have capsules and move much more easily within the surrounding breast tissue. Carcinoma, on the other hand, which has no capsule and is surrounded by an infiltrating desmoplastic process, tends to move with the neighboring breast tissue rather than within it, because the process "locks" it into the stroma and surrounding glandular tissues, even when it is not fixed to surrounding structures, such as skin or muscle. Even the most experienced examiner can sometimes fail to distinguish correctly between benign and malignant lesions.

Mammography An ideal screening test should be cheap, easy to administer, and highly sensitive and specific.[149] The current method of screening and diagnosis, mammography, which modestly fits this criteria, is the best tool we currently have and is recommended by most advisory groups including the US Preventive Services Task Force, the American Cancer Society and the National Cancer Institute. In 2000 and 2001, Gotzsche and Olsen performed a meta-analysis of 7 randomized mammography trials,[150] and further analyzed them in a Cochrane review and concluded that there was no reliable evidence that screening mammography reduces breast cancer mortality, and that screening with mammography is unjustified.[151] Another summit on mammography was conducted and the resolution to this crisis in confidence over mammography was to continue to recommend screening on the basis that there is a 20 to 30% reduction in the relative mortality from breast cancer, which translates into a 4 to 6% absolute difference in mortality from screening. Mammography, although the best screening tool we have, is flawed. The prevalence of cancers is 1 to 7 per 1,000 women screened, depending on age. Mammographic screening generates many additional procedures (false negatives), identifies many early lesions, some of which might never come to clinical attention, is expensive, and interpretation varies significantly. Part of the problem is that we do not have a way to identify women for whom mammography is most effective. Mammography is more effective when the prevalence of disease is higher in the population (eg, in older women, or women known to be at higher risk), and performs optimally in the setting of relatively fatty breast tissue. Mammography is much more cost effective for women aged 50 to 70 than it is for women aged 40 to 50,[152] and the aggregate cost of mammography is high, in the range of 6 to 10 billion dollars (US) in the United States alone. Mammograms are most accurate when interpreted by experienced, high-volume readers who review their own data and get feedback on their performance[152]; however, there is a shortage of well-trained breast imagers. Another consequence of mammography is that we have dramatically increased our capacity to identify stage 0 or in situ cancers, which has led to an increase in the use of mastectomy. For all of these reasons, the Institute of Medicine recently made recommendations of how to improve the current practice of screening and detection by a number of interventions, and particularly encouraged a change from opportunistic (encounter-based screening) to population-based organized screening such as is found in some European countries.

MRI is increasingly being used in the management of breast cancer. MRI has the advantages of providing a three-dimensional view of the breast, performing with high sensitivity in dense breast tissue and using non-ionizing radiation. MRI has important disadvantages as well, including its high cost, variability in performance, and moderate specificity that in combination with high sensitivity often leads to unnecessary work-up.[153]

MRI is not appropriate as a general screening tool. It is at least 10 times as expensive as mammography, which would drive the cost of screening in the United States into the 100 billion dollar (US) range. The role of MRI in screening should be limited to screening very high-risk women with dense breast tissue (eg, women with deleterious mutations in *BRCA1* or *BRCA2*). MRI should be reserved for those situations where there is a high prior probability of identifying a cancer and where other, less expensive, robust screening tools (eg, mammography) are known to be less sensitive,[151] such as *BRCA1* or *2* mutation carriers who have an 85% lifetime risk of developing breast cancer, largely between the ages of 30 and 50. Although the average 35-year-old would have a 1/10,000 chance of having a cancer, a mutation carrier would have a risk in the range of 1 to 5/100, and MRI would be much more sensitive in this population than mammography. Women with a very high 5-year Gail risk and very dense breast tissue may also fall into this category.

The true measure of a screening test is not whether it finds more cancers, but whether finding the cancers decreases mortality and morbidity from breast cancer. No study has yet shown that cancers found by MRI decrease mortality from breast cancer. However, two large studies have shown that screening using MRI is much more sensitive in high risk women, with remarkably similar results.[83,84] If tumor size and lymph node involvement is used as a surrogate for outcome, MRI does improve the stage at which tumors are identified in women in the highest risk cohort. In the Netherlands study, the cancers found in the 1,909 women screened with mammography and MRI were compared to two appropriate control groups of mutation carriers and high-risk patients, none of whom had access to MRI screening. In the highest risk group (40–85% estimated life time risk), 63% of mutation carriers with screened cancers had negative nodes in the screening study compared to 47% negative in the controls. In the moderate risk group (15–30% estimated lifetime risk), only 12% had lymph node involvement and 87% had negative nodes (compared to 52–56% positive nodes and 44–48% negative nodes in the control groups). Therefore, MRI appears to be able to find cancers at an earlier stage. However, the rate of detection of cancer was 26.5, 5.4, and 7.8 per 1,000 women years for the mutation carriers, high-risk, and moderate-risk respectively. This should be compared to the detection rate of 5 to 7/1,000 women where mammography is most cost-effective, in women aged 50 to 70 years. This comparison suggests that MRI should be reserved for the highest risk women, and those for whom we would expect mammography would be limited on the basis of young age and high breast density.

Screening comes at a price, both financial and psychological. In the Netherlands study of 1,909 women screened for 10 years, 1,200 extra procedures were performed. In the process of finding the 45 cancers, MRI led to twice as many unneeded extra procedures (420) compared to mammography (207), and three times as many unnecessary biopsies, 24 versus 7 for MRI and mammography, respectively. Mammography is much less sensitive than MRI in this setting, but the false positive rate is double with MRI.[153] MRI should be applied very judiciously as a screening tool and with rigorous criteria, so that we do not misapply resources and inadvertently cause women anguish over false positives which are both more likely and more difficult to follow and resolve, because MRI-directed biopsy tools are not readily available. It is common to recommend 3- or 6-month follow-up studies after an abnormal imaging test. However, MR exams cost $1.000 to 2,000 (US), so it is inappropriate to order these tests unless there truly is a situation where the likelihood of finding an abnormality is much higher than in the general population, and where mammography would be unlikely to be effective. The two key messages are that we need to find ways of stratifying risk to appropriately tailor the use of technology, and MRI screening should be undertaken only in facilities that have the capability of investigating MRI abnormalities, both with ultrasound and MRI-guided biopsy if necessary. The Blue Cross/Blue Shield technology assessment concluded in 2003 that MRI screening was justified in women who carry an inherited predisposition to breast cancer. The Netherlands and Canadian studies[83,84] only strengthened this conclusion. The moderate- and high-risk women probably gain less overall because the risk is not as great, suggesting that MR must become more specific and follow-up of abnormalities easier before we implement widespread screening of intermediate risk women.

Not all MR exams are alike. There is a great deal of variability in technique, sequences, interpretation, and capability for follow-up and biopsy. Although the use of breast MR has proliferated rapidly, standards have not. Clinicians ordering breast MRIs need to know that technique, time of menses (the midcycle is optimal), and that the skill in interpretation impact results. Interpreting images performed in different institutions is also a challenge because of the relative inability to transfer and view images electronically where they are easiest to interpret. Each of these areas is under active investigation, and further research and technological improvements will substantially improve our ability to appropriately integrate MRI into breast cancer management.

MRI has also been used after a diagnostic test reveals an abnormality. The most definitive study on the performance characteristics of MRI for the evaluation of mammographic abnormalities and palpable masses is the multi-institutional International Breast MRI Consortium (IBMC) study. Eight hundred forty-one patients were evaluated using MRI across 14 institutions. All patients received high resolution scans and 500 women with enhancing lesions were returned for a dynamic scan within 48 hours. High sensitivity and moderate specificity were confirmed in this study. It was also found that the high-resolution technique had the same performance characteristics as dynamic scans. High-resolution scans give greater anatomic detail and do not require specialized computer software to perform kinetic analysis. This is important because high-resolution scans are also easier for clinicians to interpret, and thus high resolution scanning is likely to be included in all MRI exams.

Perhaps the most important role for MRI is the staging of known cancer in the breast and monitoring the response to therapy.[152] MRI reveals that tumors form distinct patterns in the breast, and different types of tumors, such as lobular and inflammatory cancers, are more commonly associated with distinct patterns.

Initial imaging characteristics identify women likely to have a particularly poor response, such as diffuse tumors with large volumes.[154] A multicenter trial sponsored by ACRIN, CALGB, and SPORE is underway to validate the role of MRI in predicting and monitoring response to therapy, and to correlate molecular and protein markers to imaging phenotypes.

Biopsy When a woman presents with a diagnostic abnormality, a decision to intervene should be made in context of the likelihood of the lesion being invasive cancer or in situ cancer, as well as the age, underlying health condition, and life expectancy of the patient. A decision about which type of biopsy to perform is made by thinking about the need for future procedures. The goal should be to minimize the total number of procedures (including definitive cancer surgery), to minimize discomfort and scarring, minimize diagnostic wait time and anxiety, and enable the optimal timing of procedures.

There are a number of options available for the diagnosis of masses and mammographic abnormalities.[153] For palpable lesions, the options include fine needle aspiration (FNA), core biopsy, or excisional biopsy. Minimally invasive techniques, core biopsy and FNA, are quite accurate in experienced hands and when the "triple assessment" is used. Triple assessment is the consideration of the imaging, clinical, and pathologic findings. If there is significant discordance, further evaluation should be pursued. In general, excisional biopsy is not the optimal diagnostic procedure. Minimally invasive biopsy techniques can be performed immediately in the office, and facilitate a rapid diagnosis and discussion of options, and full evaluation of the extent of disease in the breast prior to definitive surgery. FNA or core biopsies can also be used to confirm the suspicion of multicentric disease and thereby avoid multiple trips to the operating room, and in general, allow the optimal sequencing of interventions.

The type of biopsy performed should depend on the expertise at a given institution. FNA is highly accurate, with sensitivity and specificity of 98 and 99%, respectively, in the hands of experienced operators. FNA both for palpable and mammographic lesions has been used extensively and successfully in Sweden and the UK where it is the standard diagnostic tool. This technique requires practitioners who have training and experience in sampling the lesion (the aspect prone to greatest error), preparing the slides, and interpreting cytology.[155] The advantage is that it can be performed right away and yield results within a day. Both FNA and core biopsy are preferred when there is a high suspicion of invasive cancer and the anticipation that a sentinel lymph node dissection (SLND) will be performed. When an SLND is performed, the type of biopsy performed affects the accuracy of the SLND. Core and FNA, have a lower false negative rate when compared to excisional biopsy when a subsequent sentinel node dissection is performed, 8% compared to 14.3% for incisional biopsy and 15.2% for excisional biopsy. In the setting of a patient with a large obvious tumor, FNA can facilitate the rapid confirmation of a diagnosis and a discussion of options, including neoadjuvant therapy and clinical trials. For patients who opt for surgical management, no further test is needed. For those who opt for neoadjuvant therapy, a core biopsy should be obtained for histology to confirm invasive disease, to save for future studies in the event of complete pathologic response, and potentially for clinical trials. In the event that cytology expertise does not exist in a given institution, a core biopsy can also be rapidly performed in the office setting.

Recall for mammographic abnormalities is common, and the likelihood of cancer being diagnosed from a mammographic biopsy (cancer to biopsy rate or CBR) is highly variable, anywhere from 10 to 40%. A low CBR is not necessary for high sensitivity, and in fact, the most experienced and highly trained mammographers find more cancers and order fewer biopsies for what turns out to be benign.[156] CBR rates decline over time in settings where quality improvement and feedback on performance is the rule. There are several ways to avoid biopsies of non-cancerous tissue. The first is to take the extra time to get old mammograms for comparison. Circumscribed mass lesions that have been stable for over 2 years will be converted to probably benign and not require a biopsy. If an experienced mammographer has not read the films, a second opinion can always be obtained.

In the event that a biopsy is recommended, it is important to make sure that the lesion is not palpable. If it is, and particularly if the lesion is suspicious for cancer, an FNA not only establishes the diagnosis, but confirms that the palpable mass is indeed the cancer, avoiding the need for wire localization at the time of lumpectomy. An attempt to locate nonpalpable suspicious mammographic masses with ultrasound will enable diagnostic and definitive procedures to be ultrasound guided, which is more comfortable for patients. In the event that a mammographic lesion can only be seen on mammogram, then a stereotactic biopsy can be performed, using digital images to locate the lesion and direct the core biopsy. The sensitivity of this procedure is as high as 98% by experienced practioners.[155] A specimen radiograph is obtained to confirm that the target has been obtained (usually calcifications). If there is a risk that all calcifications will be removed, it is then critical to leave a clip to localize the area later.

It is important to perform procedures in the context of their value to the overall management of the patient. If a cancer is not present, an adequate sampling of the calcifications or lesions should be performed. If cancer is present, the minimal amount to establish the diagnosis is sufficient. At this point, the diagnostic procedure is not definitive and wide excision is needed. Some radiologists take over 30 core biopsy samples. This is not necessary, and can create hematomas, distortion of tissue, and difficulty assessing the true extent of the lesion. It is also unpleasant for the patient.

Some mammographic lesions cannot be biopsied using stereotactic techniques either because the lesion is too close to the chest wall, or the breast compresses to less than 3cm in the direction the biopsy needle would be placed. In this case, an excisional biopsy must be performed. A wire is placed by the radiologists to guide the surgery. Ideally, the tip of the wire should be just under or at the level of the calcifications or mass. The surgeon should use the radiologist's estimate for the likelihood of malignancy to determine the extent of disease. For lesions more likely to be cancer, the lesion and a one-cm rim of tissue should be taken. For lesions of low suspicion, a smaller volume of tissue can be taken. To avoid taking unnecessary tissue, an incision should be made near the tip of the wire or the expected location of the abnormality. Starting the excision at the insertion site of the wire only leads to excessive tissue being removed and usually results in a close margin at the end of the wire. Making the incision over the lesion is helpful in locating the biopsy cavity in the event that an additional resection is necessary. All specimens need to be sent to mammography or evaluated using a Faxitron (if one is available in the operating room) to assure the surgeon that the target lesion has been removed. Mammographers routinely recommend a biopsy of any lesion that is a BIRADS (Breast Imaging Reporting and Data System scale) 4 or greater. However, a BIRADS classification of 4 includes lesions that have a risk of as low as 3% or as high as 75% for being malignant. The lesion may be suspicious for either in situ or invasive cancer—no distinction is implied by the categorization of a BIRADS 4. The surgeon should make sure that they understand both the type of lesion suspected as well as a more specific estimate of risk as it may make a difference in how the patient is evaluated. An older woman with several comorbidities and a mammogram with a BIRADS 4, if she has a lesion that is approximately 90% likely to be benign and 10% likely to be DCIS, may not need a biopsy. This is the type of lesion that could be followed on mammography. In general, we recommend that a minimally invasive biopsy be used to establish a diagnosis, but excisional biopsy may be the procedure of choice for a woman who has a confined cluster of linear calcifications that are highly suspicious for high grade DCIS. In this situation, a core biopsy would likely reveal DCIS, and a negative biopsy would be discordant and require wire localization and excision. If the likelihood of associated, invasive cancer is low, a sentinel node dissection or axillary sampling will not be necessary, and therefore, there is little value in starting with a stereotactic biopsy.

Role of Breast Self-Examination In the HIP study, about one-third of breast cancer cases were found using mammography alone; overall, 75% were detectable on clinical examination. Because mammographic techniques have improved since the 1960s, the value of clinical examination and breast self-examination (BSE) seems less clear today. Many studies have shown that women who perform regular BSEs detect breast cancers at an earlier clinical and pathologic stage of the disease.

The Swedish mammography studies did not include either clinical examination or BSE, which raises the question as to whether those results would have been better, had these modalities been included. The Canadian NBSS included instructions in BSE, and the teaching was reinforced at subsequent annual screenings, but it is uncertain whether the practice had any effect since all participants received instruction. Whereas it seems logical to recommend widespread use of BSE as a screening tool that is free and available to everyone, the evidence in support of it is far from solid and remains controversial. Furthermore, BSE can be expected to prompt a significant number of unnecessary biopsies with their attendant anxiety.

On the other hand, most breast masses are still self-discovered by accident, suggesting that systematic BSE could have diagnosed the disease earlier, or smaller.

Prospective randomized studies of BSE from China and Russia have failed to demonstrate a survival benefit.[157] A meta-analysis from Canadian investigators shows no benefit of routinely teaching BSE to women and concludes that the net effect on the population is a harmful one because the potential for unnecessary biopsies and anxiety is not balanced by any gain in mortality reduction.

Differential Diagnosis In performing breast examinations, the first objective is the detection of potential abnormalities. Discovery of an abnormality is followed by further investigation and evaluation to decide whether intervention is necessary. Mammography and ultrasound can provide additional information, and should be used in most cases. Fibroadenomas cannot be easily distinguished from gross cysts clinically, but a needle aspiration solves the problem instantaneously. Ultrasonography can also differentiate cysts from solid lesions and is useful when mammography detects small lesions, probably cysts that cannot be palpated.

The most common breast lumps are caused by a process previously called fibrocystic disease, more recently labeled fibrocystic or fibroglandular changes or benign breast disease. The process is usually symmetric, and most often situated in the upper outer quadrants because that is where most of the glandular tissue is found. Microscopically, there is a combination of fibrosis and ductal swelling, which gives the process its classic "fibrocystic" name. Clinically, this is a rubbery zone, but focal areas can be quite firm or hard. If a gross cyst is present, it tends to be round, circumscribed, and somewhat movable. The process is usually accompanied by pain or tenderness and tends to be cyclic, with relief as the menstrual period begins. It affects 50% of premenopausal women but usually disappears at menopause (see Figure 107-14). Fibroadenomas are also smooth, round, and mobile and occur from adolescence to menopause.

In older women, the inferior ridge of the breast may be compressed in a crescent-shape pattern due to the weight of the overlying breast. This area represents simple fat compression and is benign. Many poorly defined processes require surgical biopsy to distinguish them from malignancy. Among these are sclerosing adenosis, hyperplasia with or without atypia, and mammary duct ectasia. The last is the end result of the fibrocystic process, with ducts filled with liquid and cellular debris accompanied by fibrous changes and lymphocytic infiltration.

Lesions that are less smooth and less mobile with poorly defined margins, particularly if hard, raise the suspicion of carcinoma. The identification of the nature of a mass requires careful integration of all available information, including mammography. The clinician's responsibility is to establish the diagnosis of cancer when it exists but to minimize the number of unnecessary biopsies. A simplistic approach—biopsy of every clinical abnormality—would certainly identify all of the cancers but would be irresponsible, because of the large numbers of unnecessary operations. Similarly, abstaining from biopsy until the signs are absolutely incontrovertible would be dangerous, even though this approach would minimize unnecessary operations. The proper strategy is to apply all of the available information—history, clinical signs, mammographic and ultrasound information, and needle aspiration cytology—and to biopsy all of those lesions where a reasonable doubt as to their benign nature exists.

STAGING AND CLASSIFICATION

The purposes of staging are to (1) plan a therapeutic strategy that is most appropriate for the patient, (2) allow for more intelligent projection of outcome based on the disease status of the patient, and (3) permit comparison of therapeutic results obtained from different sources by different means. The common staging methods in use today are clinical and pathologic, but newer methods involving biologic assessments are appearing. Regardless of the staging method used, it is important to remember that the stage represents the state of disease or biologic potential of an individual patient's tumor. The usefulness of a particular staging method must be judged against its accuracy in performing this task.

The TNM classification devised by the International Union Against Cancer (UICC) and accepted by the American Joint Commission on Cancer Staging is a world standard.[158] The TNM is based on the clinical features of tumor (T), the regional lymph nodes (N), and the presence or absence of distant metastases (M). The tumor is characterized by its size, so that a T1 is a tumor less than 2 cm, a T2 is 2 to 5 cm, and a T3 is over 5 cm. Similarly, N0 represents negative, or normal, regional lymph nodes, and so on (Table 107-12).

Clinical staging systems generally underestimate the extent of disease. The inclusion of pathologic information improves staging accuracy and is the basis for most modern clinical trials. In all cases, it is wise to remember that the goal is to define the biologic activity of the tumor. Cox regression statistical models demonstrate that the presence of nodal metastases is the most important factor. Furthermore, the number of nodes involved can be used to further subset the prognostic groups (see Table 107-9). It is generally acknowledged that nodal metastases that penetrate the capsule and extend into adjacent perinodal tissue carry a worse prognosis.

The NSABP has evaluated the complete dissection of levels I and II axillary nodes and has shown that this provides an extremely high degree of confidence in establishing whether axillary metastases exist. A comparison of protocols employing Halsted radical mastectomy, modified mastectomy, and lumpectomy with axillary dissection shows that, essentially, the same number of lymph nodes is retrieved for examination, despite the different procedures. Even with multiple positive nodes, axillary recurrence is not common with today's limited axillary dissection. Identification, mapping and biopsy of the sentinel node appears to have promise as a more limited

Table 107-12 TNM Stage Definitions

Primary tumor (T)	
TX:	Primary tumor cannot be assessed
T0:	No evidence of primary tumor
Tis:	Carcinoma in situ
Tis (DCIS):	Ductal carcinoma in situ
Tis (LCIS):	Lobular carcinoma in situ
Tis (Paget's):	Paget's disease of the nipple with no tumor.
T1:	Tumor 2.0 cm or less in greatest dimension
T1mic:	Microinvasion 0.1 cm or less in greatest dimension
T1a:	Tumor more than 0.1 but not more than 0.5 cm in greatest dimension
T1b:	Tumor more than 0.5 cm but not more than 1.0 cm in greatest dimension
T1c:	Tumor more than 1.0 cm but not more than 2.0 cm in greatest dimension
T2:	Tumor more than 2.0 cm but not more than 5.0 cm in greatest dimension
T3:	Tumor more than 5.0 cm in greatest dimension
T4:	Tumor of any size with direct extension to (a) chest wall or (b) skin, only as described below.
T4a:	Extension to chest wall, not including pectoralis muscle
T4b:	Edema (including peau d'orange) or ulceration of the skin of the breast or satellite skin nodules confined to the same breast
T4c:	Both T4a and T4b
T4d:	Inflammatory carcinoma.
Regional lymph nodes (N)	
NX:	Regional lymph nodes cannot be assessed (eg, previously removed)
N0:	No regional lymph node metastasis
N1:	Metastasis to movable ipsilateral axillary lymph node(s)
N2:	Metastasis in ipsilateral axillary lymph node(s) fixed or matted, or in clinically apparent ipsilateral internal mammary nodes in the absence of clinically evident axillary lymph node metastasis
N3:	Metastasis in ipsilateral infraclavicular lymph node(s) with or without axillary lymph node involvement, or in clinically apparent ipsilateral internal mammary lymph node(s) and in the presence of clinically evident axillary lymph node metastasis; or metastasis in ipsilateral supraclavicular lymph node(s) with or without axillary or internal mammary lymph node involvement
Pathologic classification (pN)	
pNX:	Regional lymph nodes cannot be assessed (previously removed, or not removed for pathologic study)
pN0:	No regional lymph node metastasis
pN1:	Metastasis in 1 to 3 axillary lymph nodes, and/or in internal mammary nodes with microscopic disease detected by sentinel lymph node dissection but not clinically apparent
pN2:	Metastasis in 4 to 9 axillary lymph nodes, or in clinically apparent internal mammary lymph nodes in the absence of axillary lymph node metastasis
pN3:	Metastasis in 10 or more axillary lymph nodes, or in infraclavicular lymph nodes, or in clinically apparent ipsilateral internal mammary lymph nodes or in the presence of 1 or more positive axillary lymph nodes with clinically negative microscopic metastasis in internal mammary lymph nodes; or in ipsilateral supraclavicular lymph nodes
Distant metastasis (M)	
MX:	Presence of distant metastasis cannot be assessed
M0:	No distant metastasis
M1:	Distant metastasis present
AJCC stage groupings	
Stage 0	Tis, N0, M0
Stage I	T1,N1, M0
Stage IIA	T0, N1, M0
	T1, N0, M0
	T2, N0, M0
Stage IIB	T2, N1, M0
	T3, N0, M0
Stage IIIA	T0, N2, M0
	T1, N2, M0
	T2, N2, M0
	T3, N1, M0
	T3, N2, M0
Stage IIIB	T4, Any N, M0
	Any T, N3, M0
Stage IV	Any T, Any N, M1

procedure with a high degree of prognostic accuracy and markedly decreased morbidity when compared to conventional level I and II axillary dissection.

Tumor size was seen in a regression analysis model to be closely related to axillary lymph node involvement.[116,125] Tumor size is not an important discriminant within axillary node groups, except for patients with more than four involved nodes. Thus, size, which can be a function of either time or growth rate, is less useful than axillary node involvement, which is a more specific indicator of biologic aggressiveness. Furthermore, some patients with large masses may have slow-growing tumors, ignored for years, that have not metastasized. A similar problem exists in classifying patients with small but aggressive tumors found by screening mammography in whom distant metastases already exist. These patients may die rapidly despite the initial favorable local clinical features. A biologic classification would identify these women more accurately than does the TNM system. These concepts will provide further challenge to the TNM system in the future.

BIOLOGIC MARKERS Detection and Staging Modern molecular biologic techniques will probably change the approach to detecting and staging early breast cancer. The advent of mammography resulted in a change in presenting sign from a clinical mass to a subclinical mammographic abnormality. The search is now on for biologic markers that can indicate the presence of early carcinoma or that can be used as prognostic indicators to select patients for adjuvant therapies. These markers are usually substances produced by a cancer cell or by the host.

Nonspecific antigens, such as carcinoembryonic antigen (CEA), and more characteristic antigens, such as MUC1 (measured with monoclonal antibody-based commercial kits CA 15–3 or CA 27–29), were studied. These are more reliably elevated in advanced disease (stage III or stage IV) than in early stages and are more useful in following the course of a patient who has established cancer than in detecting the presence of cancer in a screening program.[159] Levels of these markers do decline with a good response to chemotherapy and are a useful reflection of changing tumor burden; therefore, they help monitor response to therapy.

Ongoing work in this area has concentrated on receptors for estrogen and progesterone, but EGF, HER2, and IGF-1R are among other receptors now being studied. To date, findings are encouraging, but results are not currently applicable to routine clinical practice.

Current practice requires surgical axillary lymph node removal to determine nodal involvement. This information is used for prognosis and for assignment of patients to adjuvant chemotherapy treatments. Attempts to identify lymph node involvement by radioimmunoscintigraphy or PET scanning have, so far, been of limited usefulness because of the inability to image lesions in the microscopic range, but recent experience with removing the "sentinel node" and studying serial sections with IHC has shown a high degree of accuracy.[115,160] It is not known if clinical correlations can be relied upon. NSABP protocol B-32, which has completed patient accrual, attempts to answer the question of whether an axillary dissection adds any therapeutic benefit to patients with negative sentinel lymph node. The American College of Surgeons Oncology Group's protocols Z-10 and Z-11 will further determine whether in patients with clinically negative lymph nodes a positive sentinel node is an indication for an axillary dissection or whether no additional axillary surgery is needed.

Such less invasive methodology or, better still, the advent of biologic indicators of tumor aggressiveness may well supplant surgical lymph node dissection in the future, but this procedure still provides the most reliable prognostic indicator.

PSYCHOSOCIAL ASPECTS OF BREAST CANCER

In recent decades, there has been increasing awareness of the psychosocial needs of cancer patients. These issues arose in breast cancer patients, in particular, because of the many changes that occurred in therapy. Radical breast surgery gave way to breast-conserving surgery at the same time that adjuvant therapies—many of them accompanied by uncomfortable side effects—were introduced. Axillary dissection is being replaced by sentinel lymph node biopsy in clinically node negative patients. In general, lumpectomy patients report fewer feelings of unattractiveness and loss of femininity and less change in body image. When mastectomy is performed, immediate reconstruction results in a decrease in psychological morbidity.

Surgery Multiple surgical interventions and adjuvant chemotherapy are accompanied by an increased fear of recurrence. This fear is probably due to the perception that these additional therapeutic manipulations imply a more worrisome prognosis. Many adjuvant chemotherapy regimens are accompanied by nausea, vomiting, or by hair loss, and it is not surprising that these side effects have an impact on the psychosocial status of patients. Many studies indicate that breast cancer patients suffer from either increased anxiety states or depressive illness, but these analyses suggest that it is the diagnosis rather than the type of treatment that is responsible. Furthermore, the level of psychological distress at the time of initiating adjuvant chemotherapy had no effect on disease-free survival or survival. Lumpectomy patients are not less anxious or depressed but, in general, adapt more favorably to their surgery and exhibit less functional change. There is increasing agreement that counseling services should be provided to help improve the quality of life of breast cancer patients.

SURGICAL BIOLOGY

Over the past three decades, revolutionary changes have occurred in the locoregional management of primary breast cancer. As a result, radical and extended radical mastectomy have been relegated to the archives of surgical history. Total mastectomy and axillary dissection (modified radical mastectomy) can be considered the "radical" surgery of the present era. This change occurred rapidly, spurred by the publication of a series of randomized controlled clinical trials that resolved decades of controversy. In 1979, an NIH-sponsored consensus development conference recommended that total mastectomy with axillary dissection (modified radical mastectomy) should replace the Halsted radical mastectomy as the current treatment standard. In 1990, another NCI consensus meeting concluded that breast preservation is the preferable treatment for women with stages I and II breast cancer because it provides survival figures equivalent to those of total mastectomy and axillary dissection while, at the same time, preserving the breast.[161]

Information from various sources indicates that many patients with breast cancer have disseminated disease by the time a clinical diagnosis is established. This is not surprising since a breast tumor of 1 cm (usually the minimal size capable of being clinically diagnosed and considered to be an early tumor) has already progressed through 30 of the theoretical 40 doublings that result in a tumor of approximately 1 kg, a size that could be lethal to the patient.

Three of four patients with positive axillary nodal involvement and almost nine of ten patients with four or more involved nodes became treatment failures 10 years after radical mastectomy without adjuvant chemotherapy for what were considered to be clinically "curable" breast cancers. These findings emphasize the systemic nature of the disease [162] and indicate the inadequacy of extensive local and regional surgery when used as sole modalities of treatment.

Breast Conserving Treatments When NSABP B-06 was implemented, surgeons had little familiarity with conducting breast-conserving procedures. Workshops and other educational mechanisms were used to apprise participating surgeons of the methodologies mandated by the protocol. Over time, a number of plastic surgery techniques have been introduced to improve cosmesis.

The goal of breast conservation is to remove the tumor and a rim of normal tissue while preserving the contour and shape of the breast. Tumor left at a margin will increase the risk of recurrence. Recht and colleagues, in a study of 533 patients, showed that recurrence risk depends on the amount of tumor left at the margin: grossly positive margins, focally positive margins, close margins were associated with a recurrence risk of 27%, 14%, and 7%. Close margins did not materially change the recurrence risk in this study where all women received radiation therapy. The presence of extensive intraductal carcinoma, once thought to be a contraindication to breast conservation, has now been shown not to be associated with higher risk of local recurrence if all of the DCIS has been excised. After breast conservation, 90% of all in-breast recurrences, in the first decade after diagnosis, are in the same quadrant and genetically identical to the primary breast cancer. Long-term follow-up studies of breast conservation surgery vs mastectomy, however, show that there is an ongoing risk for developing new cancers in the breast after 10 years, but these often occur in other quadrants.

Breast Biopsy **The Two-Stage Procedure and Fine-Needle Aspiration** With the advent of lumpectomy, there was a need to adopt a two-stage approach to biopsy and then to definitive surgery. One difficulty with this approach was the frequent failure to obtain pathologically clear margins, especially if the surgeon's intent was biopsy and not excision. This created the need for a second procedure in a recently operated site with the likelihood of difficulties in orientation. The wide acceptance of preoperative core needle biopsies, either clinically or radiologically directed, has solved this problem. This approach should be considered standard, so that the surgeon has a definite diagnosis before any surgery takes place and can better plan the operation. A detailed algorithm describing an optimal surgical strategy for the management of primary breast cancer has been described and is presented in Figure 107-18.

If an open breast biopsy must be carried out, it should be done as if a lumpectomy were being performed. Attention must be given to ensuring that specimen margins are likely to be free of tumor should a malignancy be encountered. Today, it is inappropriate to perform a biopsy without paying attention to specimen margins. In all circumstances where breast conservation is feasible, the operation carried out to establish the definitive diagnosis of a breast lesion becomes the definitive treatment whether axillary surgery is done at that time or later. Recent experience has shown that most breast cancer operations—biopsy, lumpectomy, axillary dissection, and even mastectomy—can be performed as out-patient procedures with comparable low levels of surgical complications and equal or better personal and social adjustment to the procedure.

Technique and Cosmetic Considerations To achieve the best cosmetic results, the incision should be planned based on the extent of tumor in the breast, the location of the tumor, and the native shape of the breast. Many options now exist for patients who require breast surgery. The extent of tissue that can be resected depends on the breast size. Plastic surgery techniques can be used to improve symmetry, both with and without cosmetic surgery on the contralateral breast. Once breast tissue is removed, undermining the breast tissue at the level of the fascia provides the opportunity to arrange the closure of the breast tissue in a medial to lateral direction, thereby avoiding the displacement of the nipple either superiorly or inferiorly. Mastopexy or reduction can be performed on the contralateral breast to

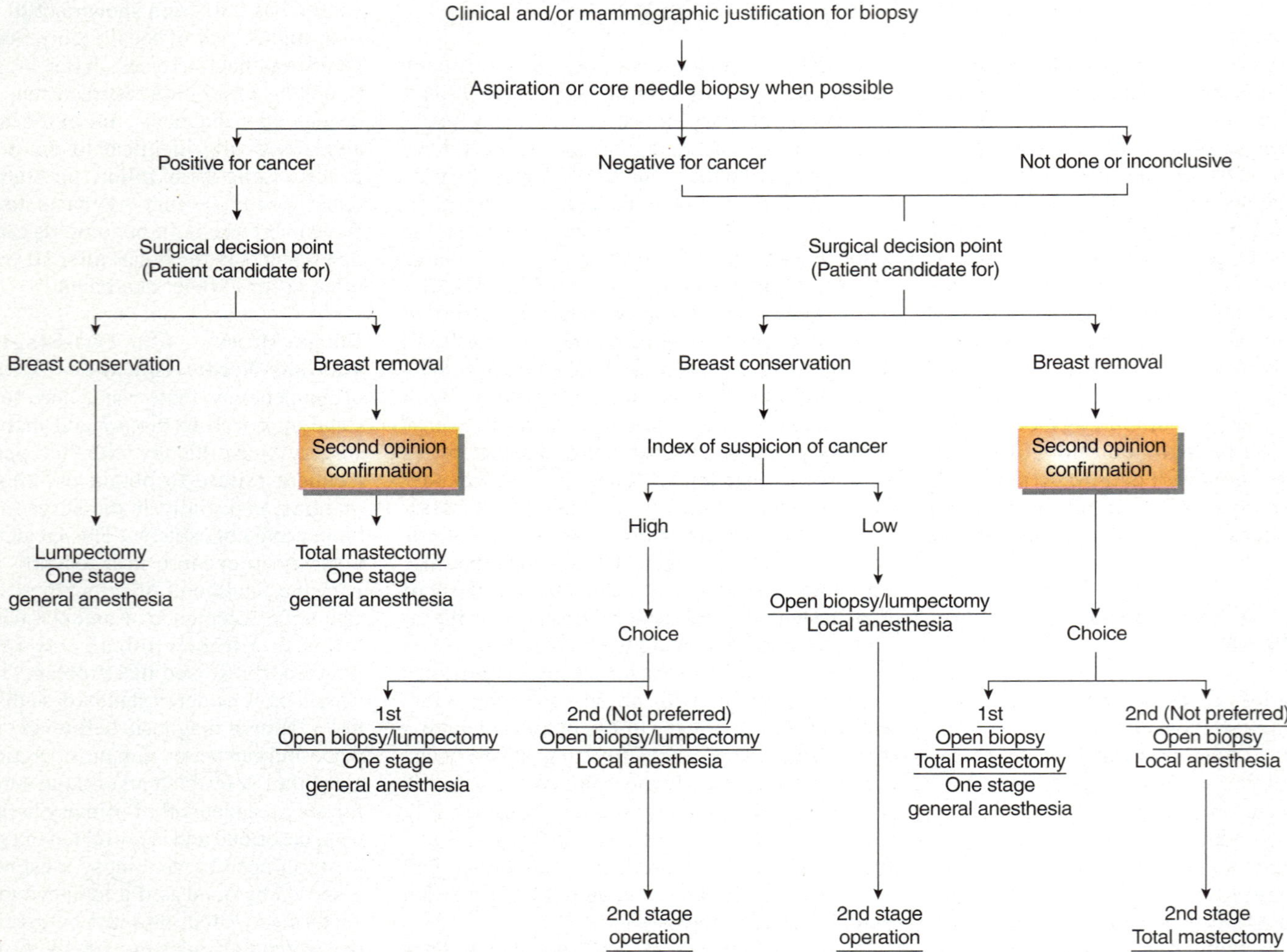

Figure 107-18 Recommended surgical strategy for management of primary breast cancer.

improve symmetry. If there is a significant degree of ptosis in the breast, a partial mastectomy can be accomplished by performing a breast reduction, thereby combining a cosmetic enhancement with the oncologic procedure of removing the breast tissue (Figure 107-19). In a breast reduction procedure, over half of the breast tissue can be removed, thus this technique can be used for larger tumors, or when there is scattered in situ disease in a single quadrant. Figures 107-19, A and B show an example of a patient, with significant discomfort from her large breast size, who had always wanted to undergo breast reduction.

Clear margins were easily obtained by removing over a quadrant of the breast tissue, leaving medial and lateral flaps of at least 1 cm, and achieving a very nice cosmetic result. Pre-operative MRI can be very useful for planning the surgical approach. High-resolution scans should be used to maximize the anatomic detail provided by MRI. When breast surgery is required, it provides an opportunity to change the shape and size of the breast, which, if desired by the patient, may make the surgical resection easier and turn an unpleasant procedure to one that is much more tolerable.

To perform a satisfactory lumpectomy, it is essential that the incision be placed directly over the tumor. The use of a circumareolar incision for removal of a lesion that is not in proximity to the areola not optimal, nor is tunneling through breast tissue to remove a lesion that is not beneath the incision. Tumor-free specimen margins are difficult and often impossible to obtain when such an incision is made. Re-excision of the tumor site to obtain free margins through such an incision is equally difficult. If there is a concern about whether a patient is a candidate for lumpectomy, an MRI prior to operation can be of considerable value if there is a radiologist with expertise interpreting the images. If there is concern that a mastectomy may eventually be necessary, the incision should be made with some thought as to what type of incision would be made if a mastectomy were required. In the instances a lumpectomy cannot be carried out because of the inability to obtain tumor-free margins, the mastectomy incisions can be tailored to accommodate the lumpectomy incision. Preoperative diagnosis with needle biopsy can be of enormous help in planning the incision and should be the standard.

Skin removal is not required for lumpectomy. If a prior biopsy was performed, skin encompassing

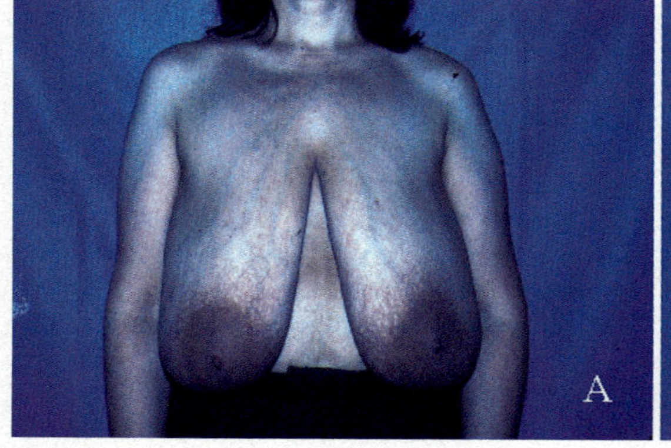

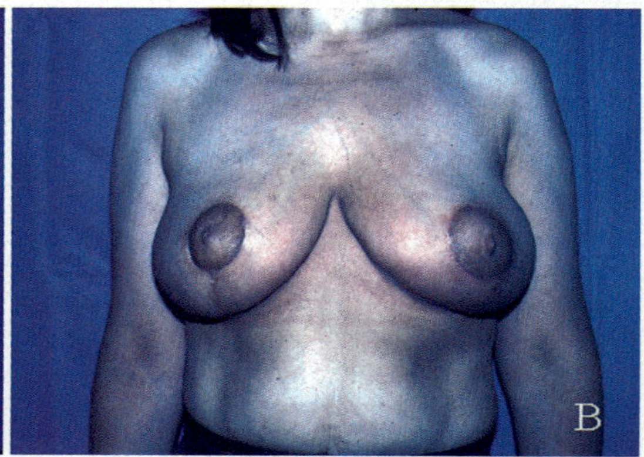

Figure 107-19 Example of a breast reduction technique to accomplish a breast reduction and partial mastectomy in a woman with extremely large, pendulous breasts. **A,** preoperative and **B,** postoperative photographs.

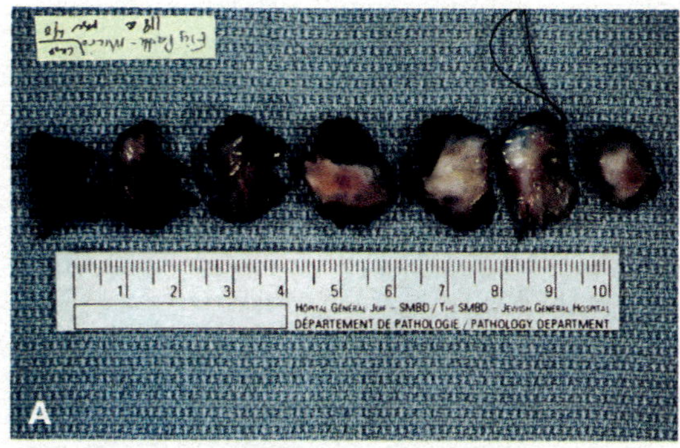

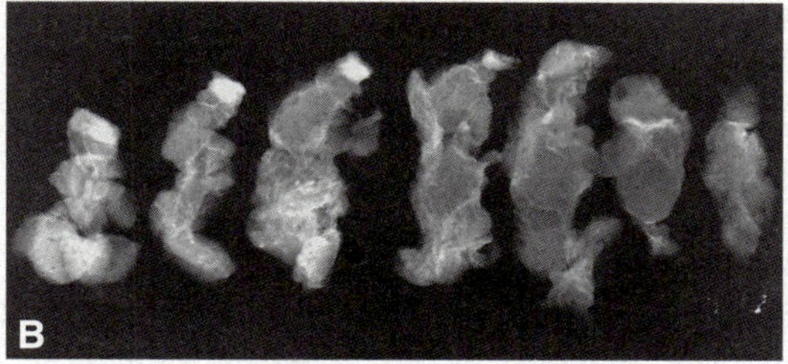

Figure 107-20 **A,** Photo of gross specimen. **B,** Radiograph of gross specimen showing calcifications.

the biopsy scar can be removed when lumpectomy is done but it is not essential. The quality of cosmesis is inversely related to the amount of skin removed. A special point to be emphasized is that skin edges should not be undermined when the excision is being performed; that is, thin skin flaps are not desirable. Undermining of skin can result in an unfavorable cosmetic result, so removal of skin may be the better cosmetic option in some cases.

Tumor Removal and Examination of Specimen Margins The tumor is removed so that it is completely enveloped in normal fat and/or breast tissue. This procedure does not necessitate removal of a predefined amount of normal tissue around the lesion. The aim is to remove the amount adequate to achieve specimen margins grossly free of tumor. Orienting the specimen is especially important. Adopting a standard procedure to orient and ink specimens in your institution will improve communication among pathologists, surgeons, and radiation oncologists. A typical standard is to use a long stitch for the lateral margin and a short stitch for the superior margin, secured to a piece of Telfa posteriorly to improve orientation. This is particularly helpful for those specimens that require specimen radiography, by preserving the shape and improving the chance to identify and further resect a specific margin that may be close to the radiographic lesion (Figure 107-20).

If a prior excisional biopsy was performed and margins were not evaluated, it is obligatory that, at the time of node dissection, a re-resection be performed to ensure tumor-free margins.

The specimen is immediately delivered to the pathologist, or, more ideally, he or she is present in the operating room to receive it and visualize the orientation. The pathologist's role is to confirm or establish the diagnosis of cancer (if a needle biopsy was not done), to aid the surgeon in deciding intraoperatively whether the specimen margins are grossly free of tumor, and to take an aliquot of tumor for any special studies.

The pathologist receives the specimen and carefully orients it by means of the suture tags that the surgeon has placed. After measurement, the uncut specimen is inspected for gross margin involvement. If there is evidence that the tumor has been transected, the surgeon is immediately apprised of the precise location of the margin involvement so that additional tissue can be removed from that area while the pathologist is completing inspection of the specimen. The pathologist then coats the entire surface of the specimen with India ink, blots it dry, and then bisects the tumor and specimen transversely. Some pathologists use multiple colors (eg, for the posterior, anterior superior half, and the anterior inferior half), to improve the ability to pinpoint the location of an involved margin. If tumor is found on gross examination to be close to the resected tissue margin, the pathologist may do a frozen section to determine margin involvement. Additional breast tissue can be removed to obtain a new true margin any time that margin involvement is considered uncertain. A multiplicity of frozen sections should not be carried out to determine whether the margins are tumor free. Margin assessment is better done with permanent sections in a detailed manner.

If the margin is later found to be involved microscopically following re-resection and there is no evidence that gross tumor has been transected, consideration may be given to not removing the breast. In such circumstances, when it is clear that gross tumor has not been transected, it is likely that radiation plus systemic therapy will provide adequate locoregional tumor control and that the majority of patients will remain free of local recurrence. An update on their series of reports on margin control from the Joint Center in Boston demonstrates that recurrence rates are the same for focally positive margins as for true negative ones.[163] Similarly, when a breast tumor recurrence occurs following lumpectomy, it is likely that tumor control will be obtained by repeat lumpectomy if such tumors are small and can be removed with tumor-free specimen margins.

Pathologic criteria used for making a decision about whether the tumor involves specimen margins can vary. Many pathologists have the tendency to infer margin involvement by such subjective designations as tumor "very close" to margin. A review of cases showed that there was residual cancer in only 12% of total mastectomy specimens removed because the margin was close. Thus, it is most appropriate to regard lines of resection as involved only when cancer is transected.

For mammographically detected carcinomas that require radiographic guidance, one or more wires are placed in the breast either to bracket calcifications, or pinpoint the center of the lesion or calcifications. Specimen mammography is required once the lesion is removed to confirm the presence of the lesion as well as the location of the mammographic abnormality relative to the margins. Whenever possible, non-palpable lesions that can be identified using ultrasound should be localized using that technique since these procedures are better tolerated by patients and do not use compression required for mammographic localization. Some surgeons are being trained to use ultrasound so that they can better improve the targeted excision of solid lesions in the operating room. This reduces the need for and time for communication between the operating room and the radiology suite. However, it requires that surgeons be specially trained, very skilled in the technique, and able to determine which lesions they can accurately identify to avoid missing the lesion intraoperatively.

Mastectomy Patients who undergo mastectomy have the option to have reconstruction or not. Cosmetic considerations are important whether a woman chooses reconstruction. It is important to try to leave a flat surface on the chest wall so that wearing a prosthesis is possible and comfortable. Avoiding skin folds in the axillary line can be accomplished through fish tail incisions at the axillary portion of the axilla or contouring the incisions in the axilla using plastic surgery techniques to avoid excess skin.

Immediate reconstruction has been shown to be safe,[164] even in the setting of locally advanced disease (Figure 107-21), when appropriate multimodal therapy is used. Therefore, any woman considering mastectomy should also be told about options for reconstruction both immediate and delayed. Complications after reconstruction are common and should be expected by both the surgeon and the patient. Expectations about outcomes should be appropriately set, and women should be prepared for the possibility of multiple surgical procedures to optimize the reconstructive outcome.

For women who are ambivalent about reconstruction, delayed reconstruction may be optimal. However, cosmetic outcomes are better when reconstruction is performed immediately, and scars can be minimized and tailored to the type of reconstruction that has been chosen. It is difficult to make reconstruction decisions in a matter of days, and women who are deciding should be reassured that an extra week or two to study their options and make good decisions will not affect their survival outcome. They will likely live for decades with the consequence of this decision, so the investment of a

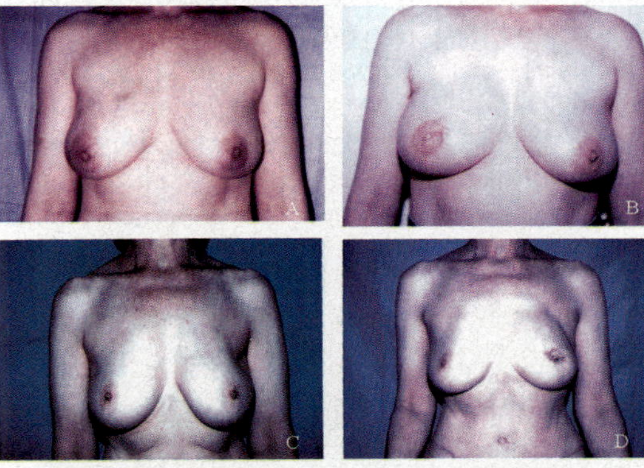

Figure 107-21 Pre- and postoperative photos of a skin sparing mastectomy with immediate reconstruction with TRAM flap, delayed nipple reconstruction in a 37-year-old, **A, B,** and a 65-year-old. Postoperative photos are 12 weeks, **C,** and 8 weeks, **D. D,** shows appearance 5 days after nipple reconstruction.

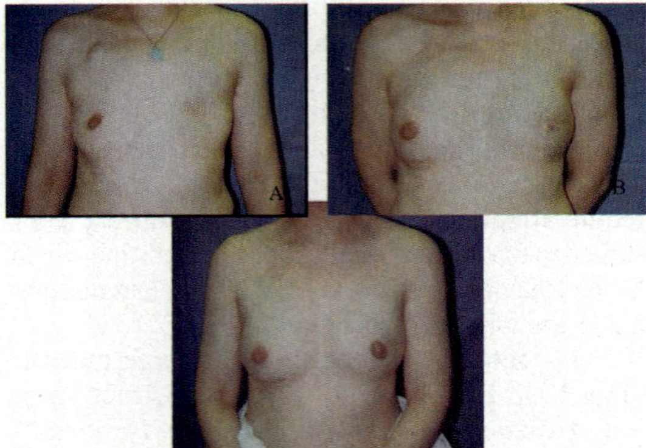

Figure 107-22 Examples of total skin sparing technique combined with various reconstruction techniques. **A,** Placement of immediate implant, using mastopexy incision, and contralateral mastopexy. Mastectomy is on left, photos are 3 weeks post-operative **B,** Bilateral mastectomy with placement of immediate implants in a woman at high risk after recurrence subsequent to lumpectomy for subcentimeter DCIS prior. Pre-operative MRI demonstrated single small focus of lateral recurrence **C,** Mastectomy on right followed by immediate reconstruction using TRAM flap.

few weeks, if necessary, to make sure they are comfortable with their decision is important.

There are two basic types of reconstruction that can be offered. Implant reconstruction or autologous tissue reconstructions. Implants can be placed as expanders or permanent implants. Expanders are the most commonly used form of reconstruction. They are placed under the pectoralis muscle and the pocket is gradually expanded until is it larger than the desired breast size. Then the expander is exchanged for a permanent implant and the breast shape is contoured. The entire process can take 6 to 8 weeks. An alternative technique, used in conjunction with skin sparing mastectomy, is the placement of permanent implants.[165] The majority of implants used for reconstruction are saline; however, silicone implants are again being used. Although silicone implants were pulled off the market because of a concern that they increased the risk for developing autoimmune disease, several large studies have failed to show a definitive connection.[166] There are specific instances where silicone products may be preferred (eg, if a permanent implant is placed immediately, but the ability to expand the implant is desired). Autologous tissue flaps include TRAM, or DIEP flaps or, latissimus dorsi flaps (Figures 107-22, 107-23).

Decisions about type of reconstruction depend largely on patient preference, although treatment considerations can also play an important role. If radiation is anticipated, complications are less if autologous tissue is used. There is controversy about whether TRAM flaps can tolerate radiation, and several published reports suggest that radiation causes significant deleterious effects on the flap. It may be that free flaps, requiring an anastomosis, tolerate radiation as well as pedicle flaps.

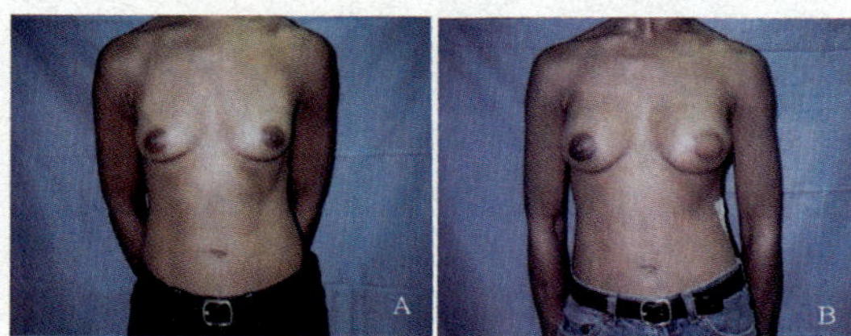

Figure 107-23 **A,** Latissimus dorsi reconstruction with bilateral augmentation in a 39-year-old. Pre- and, **B,** 12-week postoperative photo.

MANAGEMENT OF THE AXILLA

Axillary Dissection Axillary dissection is not used with the intent of enhancing curability since regional lymph nodes are regarded as indicators of distant metastatic disease rather than as instigators of such tumor.

The incision for axillary dissection should be separate from that used for removal of the tumor in the breast. A longitudinal incision placed along the posterolateral margin of the pectoralis major muscle or a transverse incision just below the axillary hairline may be used. An axillary dissection today includes nodes from axillary levels I and II. The anatomic delineation of this dissection is the latissimus dorsi muscle laterally, the axillary vein superiorly, and the medial border of the pectoralis minor muscle medially. Removal of the pectoralis minor muscle is not required. The nerves to the serratus anterior and latissimus dorsi muscles should be identified and preserved. The axillary vein should be visualized and followed under the pectoralis minor muscle to the medial border. These are the minimal limits for the dissection. The average number of nodes removed is about 15. Although the lumpectomy site in the breast is not drained, a suction drain is present in the axilla for several postoperative days.

The management of the axilla has changed significantly since the introduction of sentinel node dissection. This procedure limits considerably the extent of the surgical procedure in the axilla and, for the great majority of patients with negative axillary lymph nodes, precludes the need for a formal axillary dissection while providing similar (and in some cases superior) diagnostic and prognostic information. The identification of a single (or just a few) sentinel node(s) also permits the pathologist to perform a more detailed assessment by assessing multiple level sections of the sentinel node. The detection of micrometastases is significantly increased by combining light microscopy, immunohistochemistry (IHC), and even more sensitive molecular techniques. However, the prognostic significance of identifying isolated metastatic cells in histologically negative lymph nodes by more sensitive techniques is still undetermined; therefore, at this time it is not considered sufficient to constitute stage 2 disease. Any lesion in an axillary node is considered to be N0mic.[158] Sentinel node biopsy and assessment are under extensive evaluation by large cooperative research groups, including the NSABP and the American College of Surgeons Oncology Group (ACOSOG). ACOSOG trial Z-010 required that clinicians not use immunohistochemical analysis in their hospital so that all nodes could be centrally stained and the results blinded in order to assess the prognostic significance of microscopic metastases to the lymph nodes. NSABP B-32 randomized 5,182 women with negative SLN to either SLN biopsy alone or SLN biopsy followed by axillary lymph node dissection (ALND). Women found to have positive SLN also proceeded to full ALND. The strength of the study is that it is the largest randomized trial of SLND and that it is representative of a cross section of surgeons across the country with 232 surgeons participating across 80 centers. Although the longer term outcomes, regional control and survival, are not yet known, the technical results are. The SLN identification rate was 97.2% and improved with surgeon experience, and 26% of patients had a positive sentinel node. In 61.5% of patients with a positive sentinel node, the additional nodes were negative (38.5% had additional positive nodes). The false negative rate (axillary node involvement when the SLN was negative) was 9.7%, which did not change with experience but was significantly affected by the type of biopsy used for diagnosis; the false negative rate went from 8.0%, to 14.3% and 15.2%, for FNA/core, incisional, and excisional biopsy, respectively. The number of SLNs identified also affected SLN false negative rates. Also, the confidence in a negative result is greater if more than 1 SLN is identified, or if the prior probability of having a negative node is high, but may be less for the woman with a higher prior probability of having a positive node.

Sentinel Lymph Node Dissection The use of radiotracer material or visible blue dyes to locate and remove the sentinel node (SLN), (the node that drains the tumor site most directly), is rapidly gaining favor. This technique has been described for melanoma and breast cancer patients and has a high degree of accuracy once the operator has become familiar with the technique. A summary report by Krag and Julian indicates that SN can be successfully removed in a high percentage of cases and that the accuracy of predicting axillary metastases on this basis is very high.[164] Approximately 11% of SN were located outside axillary level one and in 3% they were outside the axilla.

Intraoperative frozen section has not been as accurate in detecting nodal metastases as is specific analysis done later in the laboratory. Imprint cytology has recently been reported to have a very low false-negative rate and may be the preferred method of intraoperative evaluation. In NSABP B-32, cytology was found to indeed have a low false positive rate, 0.4% with a sensitivity of 61.5%. There is value in intraoperative detection of LN metastases because it enables the surgeon to proceed to a full axillary dissection at the time of SLND, thereby avoiding a second procedure. Clinicians should use the technique in their own institution that yields the lowest false positive rate to minimize additional unnecessary surgery.

A mild controversy exists on localization techniques. The two most popular are radioisotope injection and scanning with a hand-held probe, and blue dye injection to provide a visible clue to the sentinel node. Although some authors are strongly in favor of one or the other of these, the majority of reports indicate that the combination of both results in the highest level of successful identification of the sentinel node. There is a small but real risk of anaphylaxis, of just less than 1%, with blue dye, which has been confirmed by many studies. The risk of severe anaphylaxis was shown to be 0.2% in NSABP B-32. Anesthesiologists should be aware of this possibility if blue dye is used.

Need for Axillary Dissection It is frequently asked whether all lumpectomy patients require an axillary dissection. If the need for systemic therapy, as well as the type of systemic therapy, can be determined by patient and tumor characteristics other than the status of the axillary nodes, then the need for axillary node dissection becomes less significant. Furthermore, if all node-negative and node-positive patients were to be given the same systemic adjuvant therapy, as is the case in trials of preoperative chemotherapy, there would seem to be no reason to know the nodal status, except for predicting patient outcome. With the demonstration that adjuvant chemotherapy benefits women with node-negative and node-positive cancers, and that the proportionate reduction in risk of treatment failure is the same for both groups, it seems reasonable to offer adjuvant chemotherapy to all women except those where the proportionate reduction is so low as to be of little real gain. However, the introduction of tailored decision making tools such as Adjuvantonline.com, a well-validated tool for predicting absolute benefit of chemotherapy,[145] or molecular tools which provide a recurrence score,[148] have increased oncologists' ability to refine recommendations for systemic therapy. Certainly, information about the sentinel node becomes very important for the patient who would otherwise choose to forego chemotherapy. In cases where no adjuvant therapy would be given, or the obvious tumors, especially those that are estrogen receptor-negative and have high nuclear grade, where all would be given adjuvant therapy, the value of axillary dissection is not clear. The need for axillary dissection may also be questioned specifically in elderly women, where the status of the axillary nodes does not usually alter the decision about administration of adjuvant therapy. Although it is generally accepted that axillary dissection provides optimal local control on the axilla, a randomized trial comparing total mastectomy with and without axillary dissection suggested that not all patients with positive axillary lymph nodes would develop an axillary recurrence in the absence of an axillary dissection: in fact only about half would. For the present, axillary node surgery is still a standard for women with involved lymph nodes, but with so much uncertainty, the issue remains in flux, and trials of SLND alone with systemic therapy and/or radiation may support a different approach in the future. SN biopsy may be a partial solution.

Local-Regional Treatments for Ductal Carcinoma In Situ Ductal carcinoma in situ (DCIS) is defined by cytologically malignant epithelial cells within the ductal system of the breast that have not invaded through the basement membrane into the breast parenchyma. Figure 107-6 shows a histological example of DCIS. Although once a relatively uncommon condition, the incidence of DCIS has dramatically and consistently increased over the past three decades. It is estimated that over 50,000 new cases of DCIS will be diagnosed in 2005, which makes it the fourth most common cancer in females (behind invasive breast cancers, lung cancer, and colon cancer).[3] Furthermore, over the past 30 years, the incidence of DCIS has increased at a rate 5 times that of invasive breast cancer. The major reason for the significant change in the incidence of DCIS is the increased use of mammographic screening. DCIS was uncommon prior to screening mammography because by the time most malignant breast lesions become palpable they have an invasive component. In contrast, most patients with DCIS diagnosed this year will have asymptomatic, nonpalpable, small lesions detected after a mammogram demonstrates a focal area of pleomorphic calcifications.

DCIS is a premalignant condition, which left untreated has a risk of progressing into an invasive cancer. The genetic and epigenetic events that cause DCIS to develop an invasive phenotype remain unclear and are likely complex. The use of new molecular tools, such as DNA microarray technology, may in the future allow for greater insights into the etiology of disease progression, and help to clarify the risk of subsequent invasive disease in an individual with DCIS. It is clear that DCIS encompasses a spectrum of pathologic disease. High-grade DCIS is defined by frequent cellular mitosis, crowded cellular growth patterns often with comedo necrosis, high rates of genetic mutations, and high proliferative indices. In contrast, well-differentiated DCIS is often very difficult to distinguish from atypical ductal hyperplasia and more frequently grows in a papillary or cribriform pattern. The risk of progressing to an invasive breast cancer and the risk of recurrence after local therapy is in part related to these biological traits.

As DCIS is considered a premalignant condition, the majority of patients currently diagnosed with this disease undergo surgical resection of the disease. Therefore, limited data are available concerning the natural history of untreated DCIS. One of the largest series of untreated DCIS described a group of 28 cases of DCIS followed serially over 30 years.[167] These cases were identified after the initial pathology from an excisional biopsy was subsequently reclassified from a benign condition to low-grade DCIS. All women had small lesions and none had high-grade disease or comedo necrosis. Therefore, it is important to recognize that these patients represent only the most favorable end of the DCIS spectrum. Despite this, over the 30-year period, the majority of patients developed an invasive breast cancer at the site of their DCIS. The risk of developing an invasive breast cancer was nine-fold higher in these patients compared to that of the general population. Furthermore, as many of these patients had an excisional biopsy of their low-grade DCIS, it is possible that some who did not develop invasive ductal carcinoma had been adequately treated by a complete surgical resection.

These data suggest that surgical resection of DCIS is warranted in an effort to reduce the risk of progression to invasive disease. Despite the fact that breast conservation therapy for DCIS has never been formally compared to mastectomy in a randomized trial, breast conservation is currently the standard of care for most patients with DCIS. Mastectomy should be considered when the patient prefers this approach, when there is a strong genetic predisposition to the development of subsequent breast primaries, and when the disease is diffusely present throughout the breast. The reason that breast conservation has become the accepted standard is that it allows for organ preservation, excellent long-term local control rates, and survival rates approaching 100%.

The major ongoing therapeutic questions concerning the treatment of DCIS concern the use of radiation and hormonal therapy. Both of these questions have been the focus of a number of completed phase III clinical trials. Three trials, conducted by the National Surgical Adjuvant Breast and Bowel Project (NSABP B17 trial), the European Organization for Research and Treatment of Cancer (EORTC) and a cooperative effort from the United Kingdom, Australia, and New Zealand (UK/ANZ), have examined the question of radiation benefit by randomizing patients treated with complete excision of DCIS to either whole breast irradiation or observation.[166–170] A summary of the results of these studies is shown in Table 107-13.

As shown in Table 107-13, in aggregate over 3,000 patients were enrolled in these studies. All three trials required the achievement of negative margins as an entry criterion and the majority of patients in the trials had mammographically detected, non-palpable disease. In all three studies, the addition of radiation was found to reduce the rate of ipsilateral breast recurrence. The B-17 trial has the longest follow-up, and after 12 years, the overall rates of ipsilateral breast cancer recurrence were 31.7% for patients treated with surgery only versus 15.7% for those treated with surgery and radiation, $p < .000005$.[168] This 58% proportional reduction of recurrence was roughly of the same magnitude as that seen in the other two trials.[169,170] Furthermore, each trial found that approximately 50% of the recurrences were

Table 107-13 Phase III Randomized Prospective Clinical Trials Investigating the Use of Radiation after Lumpectomy in Patients with Ductal Carcinoma In Situ

Study	No. of Patients	Follow-Up (Yr)	Treatment	Breast Cancer Recurrences		
				Noninvasive	Invasive	Overall
NSABP B-17[168]	818	12	Radiation	8%	7.7%	15.7%
			No radiation	14.6%	16.8%	31.7%
			p	.001	.00001	.000005
EORTC 10853[169]	1,002	4	Radiation	5%	4%	9%
			No radiation	8%	8%	16%
			p	.06	.04	.005
UK/ANZ trial[168]	1,701	5	Radiation	2.3%	2.5%	4.8%
			No radiation	8.4%	5.3%	13.7%

EORTC = European Organization for Research and Treatment of Cancer; NSABP = National Surgical Adjuvant Breast and Bowel Project; UK/ANZ = United Kingdom, Australia, New Zealand.

invasive breast cancer and the risk of developing an invasive breast recurrence within the treated breast was significantly decreased. Each of these trials also confirmed that the risk of breast cancer death in patients with DCIS was very small and not affected by the use of radiation.

Based on the results of these three randomized trials, lumpectomy and whole breast radiation should be considered as the current standard for most patients with DCIS. However, in studies that have evaluated the patterns of care in the United States, it is clear that many patients with DCIS are treated with lumpectomy alone. A recent study using data from the SEER Program found that only 45% of patients treated with lumpectomy for DCIS received radiation in 1992 and this percentage had only increased to 54% by 1999.[171] Furthermore, in a recent survey study of physicians in Australia and New Zealand, only 22% of patients treated with breast conservation surgery for DCIS were referred for a radiation oncology consultation.[172]

The lack of radiation use for women with DCIS is in part attributable to the low risk of dying from breast cancer after treatment with surgery alone. In addition, data from single-institution retrospective studies have suggested that highly selected subsets of patients may have low breast recurrence rates after lumpectomy alone. One of the leading proponents of treating favorable DCIS with lumpectomy alone has been Silverstein and colleagues, who in 1995 developed the Van Nuys Prognostic Index (VNPI) to help define selection criteria for cases with a low recurrence risk.[173] The original VNPI classes were determined from the retrospective analysis of 333 patients treated at two institutions between 1979 and 1995. Patients received 1 to 3 points for three factors: tumor grade and the presence or absence of necrosis (combined into one category), tumor size, and margin status. Over two-thirds of the patients had an intermediate-risk VNPI (cumulative score of 5–7), and, similar to the randomized data, radiation reduced the probability of breast cancer recurrence in this cohort (32% versus 15%; p = .017).[173] Fewer than one-third of their patients had small, low-grade disease with widely negative surgical margins, and the breast cancer recurrence rate was low after breast conservation surgery alone (3% breast cancer recurrence rate among 76 patients treated without radiation). Subsequently, this group has also incorporated patient age into their prognostic index. Similar data were subsequently reported from a population-based cohort study of 1,036 women ≥ 40 years old in the San Francisco area treated with lumpectomy alone for DCIS. This study found overall a relatively high recurrence rate (20% at 5 years), but reported that the subset of patients with mammographically detected low-grade disease treated with surgery that achieved widely negative margins had a low risk of recurrence after surgery alone.[174]

Using an expansion of this original cohort, Silverstein and colleagues reanalyzed their data, focusing on the importance of margin status for patients treated with DCIS. In this analysis,[175] they reported that 93 patients with a margin width of 10 mm or more had an 8-year local recurrence rate of only 3%. The 8-year probability of recurrence was much higher after treatment with lumpectomy without radiation when the margin width was 1 to 10 mm (recurrence rate 20%) and when margins were under 1 mm (58%). Unfortunately, the low recurrence rate noted in the setting of 10 mm margins could not be confirmed in a single-arm prospective trial conducted at the Dana-Farber/Harvard Cancer Center. In this study, 157 patients with grade 1 or 2 DCIS, ≤ 2.5 cm, underwent wide local excision alone with achievement of negative margins of ≥ 1 cm.[176] The trial was closed early because the recurrence rate met pre-defined stopping rules, with an estimated 5-year local recurrence rate of 12.5%. The authors concluded that even in this highly selected group of patients, there was a substantial local recurrence rate.

It is clear that the Van Nuys data are encouraging and very useful for hypothesis generation. However, it is important to recognize that these are single-institution retrospective data, with a relatively small sample size, and they were not reproduced in the prospective Harvard trial. Therefore, based on the completed trials to date, lumpectomy and radiation should be considered as the standard for patients with DCIS treated with breast conservation. There currently is an ongoing Radiation Therapy Oncology Group (RTOG) and Cancer and Leukemia Group B (CALGB) phase III trial being conducted to test the value of radiation in the subpopulation of patients with favorable disease. Only patients with mammographically detected DCIS with nuclear grade 1 to 2 disease who have negative margins of ≥ 3mm are eligible. This study's required sample size is 1,990 patients, and after 6 years, less than one-third of the target population has been entered. The successful completion of this trial is necessary to answer the highly relevant and important question of whether there is a favorable subgroup of patients who may not benefit from radiation because their risk of recurrence after surgery is low.

The second major area of research and controversy regarding the management of DCIS concerns the use of hormonal therapy. After completion of the B-17 trial, the NSABP conducted the B-24 trial, which randomized 1,802 patients treated with lumpectomy and radiation to either receive 5 years of tamoxifen or 5 years of placebo.[177,178] The eligibility of this trial differed from B-17 in that it included patients with positive surgical margins, which ended up being present in 25% of the study population. In addition, the primary endpoint of the study was not ipsilateral breast recurrence but rather the probability of having an ipsilateral recurrence or developing a contralateral breast cancer. Therefore, this trial was designed to investigate the combined therapeutic benefit of tamoxifen against the index DCIS and the chemopreventive benefit of tamoxifen in reducing subsequent independent breast cancers.

The results of the B-24 trial indicated that patients treated with tamoxifen, surgery and radiation had a 5-year rate of non-invasive or invasive breast cancers of 8.2% compared to a 13.4% rate for the patients treated only with surgery and radiation.[177,178] Clearly, a component of this benefit was the chemoprevention effects of tamoxifen. In B-24, the use of tamoxifen resulted in a 41% reduction in the 5-year incidence of contralateral breast cancers. These data are consistent with the reduction in second primary breast cancers seen in the adjuvant tamoxifen trials and the NSABP P-1 trial, which found that tamoxifen decreased breast cancer development in women at increased risk for breast cancer by 49%.[72] In a subsequent retrospective analysis of estrogen receptor (ER) expression from stored tumor material from 628 patients (327 placebo, 301 tamoxifen), it was found that the benefit of tamoxifen was limited to 482 patients (77% of those on study) with ER-positive disease.[179] In this cohort, tamoxifen was associated with a significant reduction in both ipsilateral breast recurrence and the development of contralateral breast cancer. There was no apparent benefit of tamoxifen in those with ER-negative tumors, but the sample size precluded detecting a small benefit.

The UK/ANZ trial provides the most recent information concerning the interaction of radiation and tamoxifen after lumpectomy in patients with DCIS.[170] In this study, tamoxifen use decreased the rate of DCIS recurrence but not invasive recurrence for patients who did not receive radiation. However, in the patients treated with radiation after lumpectomy, tamoxifen provided no benefit in ipsilateral breast events. Unlike the B-24 trial, this study required all patients to have negative surgical margins after lumpectomy and did not include the development of a contralateral breast cancer as an event in their primary outcome measure.

These data suggest that, for patients treated with an adequate lumpectomy that achieves negative surgical margins and subsequently receive radiation, the therapeutic benefits of tamoxifen are likely to be very low. Interestingly, a recent survey found that 56% of United States practitioners routinely recommend tamoxifen for women with DCIS whereas only 22% of European practitioners routinely recommend tamoxifen.[180] Despite the lack of clarity concerning the therapeutic benefits of tamoxifen in DCIS, for patients with ER-positive disease the addition of tamoxifen is likely to have chemopreventive effects and minimize the risks of subsequent new breast cancers. To further evaluate the benefit of hormonal therapy in patients with DCIS, NSABP is currently conducting a phase III trial comparing tamoxifen and anastrozole after lumpectomy and radiation in postmenopausal women.

Local-Regional Treatment of Early Stage Invasive Breast Cancer Over the past two decades, there has been a consistent increase in the percentage of invasive breast cancers diagnosed with T1 or T2 primary disease with no disease present in regional lymphatics. Indeed, by the year 2000, it was estimated that 94% of breast cancers were 5.0 cm or less at the time of diagnosis.[181] Similar to the increase in the diagnosis of DCIS, this shifting of invasive breast cancer toward early stage disease represents the benefits of mammography screening and the increase in breast health education. A number of benefits have resulted from this change. Most important, diagnosing breast cancer at early disease stages has contributed to the decline in the overall breast cancer death rate that has occurred in the United States and the United Kingdom.[4,12] A second major benefit of this trend is that it led to an increasing percentage of breast cancer patients being treated with organ-preserving local-regional therapy, thereby minimizing the impact this disease has on their long-term quality of life.

Similar to screening and education, local-regional therapy of breast cancer has evolved over the past three decades. Breast conservation therapy is now firmly established as an appropriate standard of care for women with early stage breast disease, and therefore should be offered to the majority of patients currently diagnosed with breast cancer.[161] This therapy consists of three important components: removal of the tumor with achievement of negative margins (often called a lumpectomy, tylectomy, or a segmental mastectomy), surgical assessment of axillary lymph nodes with either a sentinel lymph node surgery and/or a level I/II axillary lymph node dissection, and breast irradiation. Most women treated with modern breast conservation approaches achieve excellent outcomes. When combined with systemic therapy, the local recurrence rate after appropriate breast conservation treatments currently is reported to be less than 0.5% per year for women with favorable disease.[182–184] Furthermore, the complication rates of breast conservation therapy are very low and continue to improve with advances in surgical and radiotherapy techniques.

Despite these facts, breast conservation remains underutilized in the United States. In a recent multi-national randomized trial comparing two hormonal therapies for women with early stage disease, the rate of breast conservation in the United States was only 49%.[185] In contrast, the rate of breast conservation in the United Kingdom patients was 58%, and even higher rates were noted in patients from Sweden, Germany or Australia/New Zealand. Previous data had also indicated that the use of breast conservation varies within regions of the United States, with Southern and Midwestern women less likely to be treated with breast conservation compared to women from either the East of West Coast.[186] The reasons for the under-use of breast conservation are likely multifactorial. Unfortunately, some women undergo mastectomy based on a misperception that mastectomy is likely to achieve a superior outcome. Other factors, such as choices celebrity role models make, can influence decisions made by providers and patients. For example, after Nancy Reagan had an early stage breast cancer treated with mastectomy, the rates of breast conservation dropped in the United States. It is critical, therefore, that breast cancer providers understand the data concerning breast conservation so that patients with newly diagnosed disease can be given the option of this treatment if appropriate.

Breast Conservation Therapy versus Mastectomy Breast conservation has been studied as an alternative local-regional treatment to mastectomy for over 30 years. After initial successful results were obtained in single institutions, a number of phase III clinical trials were initiated that directly compared the outcome of patients treated with breast conservation versus those of patients treated with mastectomy.[187–189] One of the more important of these trials was the NSABP B-06 study.[182] This trial began in 1976 and enrolled 1,843 women. Patients with T1 or T2, N0, or N1, M0 breast tumors of 4 cm or less were randomly assigned to one of three treatment groups: (1) modified radical mastectomy, (2) lumpectomy and axillary dissection or (3) lumpectomy, axillary dissection, followed by radiation therapy. This trial demonstrated that lumpectomy and axillary dissection, with or without radiation therapy provides survival equivalent to total mastectomy while preserving the breast.[161]

Contraindications for Breast Conservation Therapy Selected patients with early-stage breast cancer are not suitable for breast conservation therapy because the primary tumor cannot be successfully removed with a lumpectomy. For example, patients presenting with diffuse suspicious calcifications that cannot be resected with a lumpectomy that leaves an acceptable aesthetic result are best treated with a mastectomy. Similarly, patients in whom repeated attempts at breast conservation surgery fail to achieve negative surgical margins are best managed with a mastectomy. A second reason why some patients are not candidates for breast conservation is that they are at high risk for radiation complications. Specific examples of such patients include those previously treated with radiation, women who are pregnant, and patients with certain connective tissue diseases. For women early in the course of their pregnancy, internal radiation scatter from irradiation of the intact breast can reach lethal and teratogenic dose levels.[190] Certain collagen vascular diseases are also associated with significant risks, including breast fibrosis and pain, chest wall necrosis, and brachial plexopathy. Specific disorders associated with radiation injury are systemic scleroderma, polymyositis, dermatomyositis, lupus erythematosus, and mixed-connective tissue disorders. Patients with rheumatoid arthritis do not appear to have elevated rates of late toxicity.[191]

The Role of Radiation after Breast Conservation Surgery for Invasive Disease Breast conservation therapy represented a significant advance in the local-regional treatment of breast cancer. However, one of the downsides of this therapy is that it requires radiation treatments. Although radiation treatments to the breast are relatively well tolerated, with acceptable side effects and low risks of injury to normal tissues, they typically require 6 weeks of daily therapy, resulting in significant inconvenience for patients. Furthermore, the equipment used for modern treatment planning and treatment delivery is expensive and some rural regions of the United States and many other countries do not have the facilities and resources to provide state-of-the-art radiation care. Accordingly, there has always been an interest in determining whether the benefit of radiation after lumpectomy warrants the costs and inconveniences. To investigate this question, over the past 25 years there have been a number of randomized trials designed to directly assess the value of radiation in patients treated with breast conserving surgery.[188,189]

The initial rationale for using radiation after lumpectomy was that when mastectomy specimens were examined in patients who first underwent lumpectomy, the probability of finding residual tumor foci elsewhere in the breast was high. In one of the most important studies, 24% of patients had residual invasive foci, 39% had residual noninvasive foci, and only 37% of breasts were tumor free after lumpectomy.[192] To determine the significance of these data, clinical trials were begun that compared whole breast radiation after lumpectomy versus treatment with lumpectomy alone. The data from such trials have been remarkably consistent, and have clearly indicated that radiation significantly reduces the risk for ipsilateral breast recurrences. Despite the conclusive nature of this evidence, a number of women with early stage

Table 107-14 Radiation after Lumpectomy in Highly Selected Patients with Favorable Invasive Breast Cancer

Study	No. of Patients	Patient Characteristics	Treatment	Follow-Up (Yr)	Breast Recurrence Rates (%)
NSABP B-21[183]	1,009	Tumors ≤ 1 cm	Radiation + tamoxifen	8	3
		Node-negative	Radiation alone		9
			Tamoxifen alone		17
British Columbia[201]	769	Age ≥ 50	Radiation + tamoxifen	5	1
		Node-negative	Tamoxifen alone		8
CALGB[200]	636	Age ≥ 70, clinical stage I, estrogen receptor-positive	Radiation + tamoxifen	5	1
			Tamoxifen alone		4

CALGB = Cancer and Leukemia Group B; NSABP = National Surgical Adjuvant Breast and Bowel Project.

invasive breast cancers are treated with breast-conserving surgery without radiation. Moreover, a study of more than 144,000 cases from the SEER program of the National Cancer Institute found that the percentage of patients with early stage breast cancer who did not receive radiation as a component of their breast conservation therapy increased steadily from approximately 5% in 1983 to over 13% in 1996.[193]

The NSABP B-06 trial was one of the first randomized studies to evaluate the benefit of radiation after lumpectomy. This trial showed that for patients treated with breast conserving surgery, radiation offered a significant clinical benefit. After 20 years, the recurrence rates in the breast were 40% for those treated with lumpectomy alone versus 14% for those treated with lumpectomy plus radiation. The almost two-thirds reduction in the risk of recurrence was very similar to a number of other similarly designed trials.[182]

A number of meta-analyses of the prospective clinical trials that have relatively mature follow-up have been performed. The Early Breast Cancer Trialists' Collaborative Group (EBCTCG), that was able to obtain the individual data sets from each of these trials, conducted the most comprehensive of these. In their analysis of more than 2,200 women, breast radiation reduced the chance of a tumor recurrence within the breast after 20 years from 30.3 to 10.6%.[188] The benefit of radiation was seen both for patients with lymph node–positive disease and for patients with lymph node–negative disease. The most recent presentation of the data from this group has indicated that this reduction in breast recurrence rate was associated with an improvement in overall survival.[194] These data suggest that breast irradiation can eradicate persistent residual local disease left after lumpectomy, which if left untreated can be the source of new metastases and death. A second meta-analyses investigating the outcome of breast conserving surgery with or without radiation also found a survival advantage in the irradiated group.[195]

Although the meta-analyses and large trials such as the NSABP B-06 provide conclusive data that radiation is beneficial for the majority of patients treated with breast-conserving surgery, there remains an interest as to whether subsets of patients may do well with surgery alone. Therefore, some trials have limited eligibility criteria to evaluate only patients with favorable disease characteristics. Investigators from Milan, Italy, conducted a trial to evaluate whether radiation is needed following excision of a small tumor with widely negative margins. In this study, patients with tumors 2.5 cm or less were randomized to undergo quadrantectomy and axillary dissection versus this surgery plus breast radiation. The 10-year results from this trial indicated that radiation reduced the breast recurrence rate from 24 to 6% ($p < .001$).[196]

Patients with stage I disease represent another potentially favorable group. In such patients, data from a Swedish trial indicated that radiation reduced the 5-year breast recurrence rate from 18 to 2% ($p < .0001$).[197] A similar randomized trial from Finland, which was limited to patients with stage I disease who had 1 cm or greater negative margins, also found radiation reduced the breast recurrence rate from 14.1 to 6.2%; $p = .029$.[198]

Data from trials have also indicated that the use of systemic treatment (either chemotherapy or tamoxifen) does not obviate the need for breast radiation. In the NSABP B-06 trial, chemotherapy was used in patients with lymph node–positive disease, and the 20-year breast recurrence rate for these patients was 44% when no radiation was used versus a 9% when radiation was used.[182] A randomized trial from Scotland required systemic treatment for all patients, with approximately 75% of the 589 enrolled patients receiving tamoxifen as the sole systemic treatment.[199] In this trial, the 6-year breast recurrence rates were 6% in the surgery, systemic therapy, and radiation arm versus 25% in the patients randomized to surgery plus systemic therapy without radiation.

Three more recent trials have further refined selection criteria. The results of these three studies are shown in Table 107-14.[182,200,201] In all three of these studies, radiation achieved a statistically significant reduction in breast recurrence rate, although the recurrence rate in some subcategories of patients treated with surgery alone was relatively low. The NSABP B-21 trial enrolled only patients with lymph node–negative breast cancers whose primary tumors measured 1.0 cm or less. All patients underwent lumpectomy and axillary lymph node dissection and were randomized to tamoxifen alone, radiation alone, or tamoxifen and radiation.[183] The British Columbia trial had very similar eligibility criteria and very similar results.[201] Finally, the CALGB/Intergroup study focused on patients over the age of 70 with favorable early stage disease.[200]

In conclusion, nearly all of the clinical studies to date have indicated that breast radiation reduces local recurrences following breast conservation surgery and therefore should be considered a standard component of treatment for all women with early stage invasive disease. The most recent trials that have incorporated both the use of systemic therapy and radiation after lumpectomy indicate the probability of having a breast recurrence after such treatment is very low, less that 0.5% per year.[182,200,201] Thus far, all attempts to define favorable subsets of early-stage breast cancer patients who may not require radiation have been unsuccessful, with the possible exception of women over the age of 70 who have disease that is lymph node-negative and estrogen receptor-positive and who are candidates for tamoxifen. In this cohort, decision as to whether to use radiation or not should be based on the patient's life expectancy.

Factors Affecting Local-Regional Treatment Outcome after Breast Conservation Therapy A number of patient-, tumor-, and treatment-related factors have been found to influence local recurrence rates following breast conservation therapy. The most consistent patient factor demonstrated to influence both local and distant recurrence rates is patient age. Young patient age (most commonly defined as ≤ 40 years old) is associated with an increased risk of distant metastases and lower disease-specific survival[202,203] and an increased risk for ipsilateral breast tumor recurrence following breast conservation therapy.[184,204] Other patient factors, such as African American race/ethnicity have been associated with higher rates of distant metastasis but not clearly been shown to affect ipsilateral breast recurrence rates.[205–207] A number of articles have also indicated that a family history of breast cancer does not predispose to ipsilateral breast recurrence.[208,209] However, breast recurrence rates are likely higher in cases with true familial breast cancer. For example, Haffty and colleagues reported that the breast recurrence rates were 40% or higher for women with BRCA mutations treated with breast conservation therapy.[210] A large percentage of these recurrences occurred many years after treatment and may have been second primary tumors that developed independently from the index cancer. Indeed, the rate of ipsilateral breast recurrence was approximately the same as the rate of development of a contralateral breast cancer.

The status of the surgical margins is one of the most important tumor/pathological factors that affect the rates of local control after breast conservation surgery and radiation. In general, the goal of breast conserving surgery should be to achieve complete tumor resection with 2 mm negative margins, although this definition of negative margins is controversial. In a recent study that evaluated margins according to the density of malignant tissue in addition to distance, margin status highly correlated with breast recurrence risk. This study had the strength of having a central pathology review of 607 cases with mature follow-up and found 12-year recurrence rates of 9% (negative), 6% (near-least), 18% (near-intermediate), 24% (near-greatest), and 30% (positive).[211] Another report suggested that systemic treatment may also influence the prognostic importance of margin status. In this report, the crude local recurrence rate at 8 years was 7% in the 45 patients with focally positive margins treated with systemic therapy versus 18% in the 77 patients with focally positive margins who did not receive systemic therapy.[212] Patients with more extensive margin involvement had unacceptably high local recurrence rates, which were not affected by the use of systemic therapy. A reasonable approach is to recommend re-excision for patients with positive margins and to individualize treatment recommendations for patients with close or focally positive margins, considering breast aesthetics and other factors that also affect recurrence risks.

In addition to complete surgical resection of the primary tumor, there are a number of other treatment-related variables that affect rates of local control. One of these is the use of systemic therapy. In the NSABP B-06 trial, patients with lymph node–positive disease that were treated with radiation and chemotherapy had a 20-year local recurrence rate of 9% compared to a local recurrence rate of 17% in lymph node–negative patients treated with surgery and radiation alone.[182] In NSABP B-21, tamoxifen similarly improved local control rates in patients with lymph node–negative breast cancers measuring less than 1 cm.[183] There was only a 3% crude rate of breast tumor recurrence in women randomized to lumpectomy, radiation, and tamoxifen compared to a 7% rate in women treated with lumpectomy and radiation alone. Data from the University of Texas M. D. Anderson Cancer Center investigating the impact of systemic therapy on local control following breast conservation therapy in patients with lymph node–negative breast cancer further confirmed these data. In that study, 277 patients treated with systemic therapy had improved 5-year (97.5% versus 89.8%) and 10-year (95.6% versus 85.2%) local control rates compared to the 207 patients who received no systemic treatment (p = .004).[185] Finally, in an analysis of NSABP systemic therapy trials, Fisher and colleagues reported a disease-free survival advantage for the use of systemic therapy in tumors less than 1 cm with negative lymph nodes.[213] Most of this benefit was found to be a reduction in ipsilateral breast tumor recurrences.

Another treatment related factor that has been found to affect local control in breast conservation therapy is the use of a tumor bed boost of radiation following whole breast irradiation. The first randomized trial investigating the impact of a 10 Gy boost following 50 Gy of breast irradiation was performed in Lyons, France. The use of a boost led to a small but statistically significant reduction in the rates of local recurrence at 5 years (3.6% versus 4.5%, p = .04).[214] Subsequently, the EORTC completed a much larger trial that randomized over 5,000 patients to 50-Gy delivered to the breast alone or 50 Gy plus a tumor bed boost of 16 Gy. This trial again demonstrated a reduced breast recurrence rate in patients treated with a boost (4.3% versus 7.3% at 5 years; $p < .001$).[215] In a subset analysis, this benefit was most notable in younger women.

New Radiation Treatment Approaches for Early-Stage Breast Cancer As previously noted, some patients treated with breast conservation therapy for an early stage breast cancer do not receive radiation as a component of therapy. In addition, a number of patients who are excellent candidates for breast conservation therapy elect to be treated with mastectomy in order to avoid radiation. A major factor that contributes to both of these scenarios concerns the inconvenience and expense associated with external beam radiation. Conventional external beam radiation treatments for early-stage breast cancer typically require 1 or 2 days of treatment planning followed by 25 to 33 daily treatment visits. The schedule is particularly burdensome for patients who have to travel many hours for access to the nearest radiation facility. In addition, worldwide, there are too few facilities and equipment to offer this type of treatment schedule to all patients with early-stage breast cancer.

For these reasons and others, a number of different strategies are being investigated in order to shorten the radiation treatment schedule. Whelan and colleagues conducted a phase III prospective randomized trial comparing a 3-week fractionation schedule to the conventional 5-week course for women ≥ 50 years old with T1 or T2 N0 disease.[216] After a median follow-up of 4.6 years, there was no difference in local recurrences, survival, or breast aesthetics. This trial has yet to have a major effect on practice patterns in the United States: many feel longer follow-up data are needed concerning late normal tissue risks.

A second strategy for shortening the total treatment time is to minimize the volume of breast tissue being irradiated. The rationale for this strategy is that 80% of patients who undergo lumpectomy for small primary tumors have no residual disease after lumpectomy or disease that is within 2 cm of the index cancer.[192] By limiting the volume of breast irradiated, radiation can potentially be delivered at a higher dose rate, allowing for a 1-week course of treatment. Most of the partial breast irradiation outcome data with follow-up of 5 years have been from studies that investigated interstitial brachytherapy alone as a method to deliver the radiation dose. For this procedure, patients typically have catheters surgically placed to create a volume 2 to 2.5 cm around the tumor bed. Subsequently, high–dose-rate radioactive seeds are temporarily placed within the catheters in two sessions a day for 5 days total.

The placement of the catheters geometrically around the tumor bed to assure 2 cm of coverage can be difficult and requires a skill set that may not be available in every radiation facility. Therefore, other attempts at partial breast radiation have been used. In Milan, Veronesi and colleagues are conducting a phase III clinical trial comparing a single fraction of intraoperative electron beam radiation to a standard course of whole breast irradiation. From an initial phase I/II trial with intraoperative radiation, these authors have reported that there have been minimal complications in the first 100 patients treated.[217] Other commercial vendors have developed intraoperative orthovoltage cones that also can fill the lumpectomy cavity and irradiate the local margin in a single intraoperative fraction.[218] Finally, others have used a similar strategy but deliver therapy through a brachytherapy applicator device, called the Mammosite RTS. The Mammosite utilizes an inflatable balloon within the tumor bed cavity and allows for insertion of a high–dose-rate radioactive source within the center of the balloon.[219]

There are limited data to date concerning the efficacy of partial breast radiation strategies. The most mature data on this subject are single-institution reports of phase II brachytherapy trials. To date, the 5-year outcome data for highly selected patients with favorable disease characteristics using this approach have been excellent.[220] However, others have noted higher rates of clinical fat necrosis and poorer efficacy compared to conventional breast external beam radiation.[221,222] These data suggest that this treatment approach warrants additional study in prospective trials with rigid quality assurance to assure proper volumetric coverage. To date, there are no long-term efficacy data available concerning single-fraction intraoperative radiation therapy with electrons, isotopes, or x-rays.

The concept of partial breast radiation has some additional theoretical downsides. Many devices, such as the Mammosite, treat a volume of only 1 to 1.5 cm around the tumor bed.[223] Therefore, these treatments would be expected to have similar efficacy as a surgical procedure that resected an additional 1 to 1.5 cm of tissue circumferentially around the tumor bed. As noted previously, a randomized trial that compared quadrantectomy versus quadrantectomy and radiation for small primary tumors found a significant disadvantage for quadrantectomy alone (failure rates of 23.5% versus 5.8%, respectively).[196] Although size of margins was not specified in that

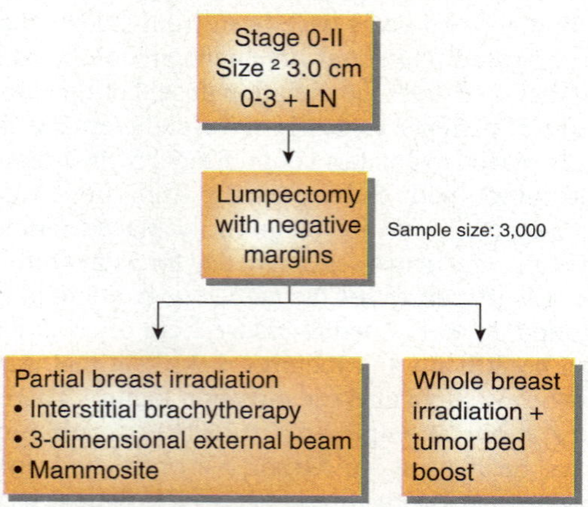

Figure 107-24 Design of the ongoing NSABP/Radiation Therapy Oncology Group phase III trial comparing partial breast irradiation versus whole breast irradiation for patients with stage 0–II breast cancer.

trial, given the ratio of the size of the tumor to the volume of tissue resected, a similar peritumoral volume that is included in some partial breast irradiation strategies was likely excised. For these reasons, breast brachytherapy or limited volume external beam radiation, which has the advantage of treating 2 to 3 cm around the tumor bed, may prove to be a better alternative than the Mammosite for partial breast radiation.

The efficacy and toxicity of partial breast radiation needs to be prospectively compared to fully understand the advantages and shortcomings of this approach. To address this, the NSABP and the Radiation Therapy Oncology Group have jointly sponsored a phase III trial, which is set to open in 2005. The schema of this trial is shown in Figure 107-24.

Management of the Uninvolved Breast Another facet of the uncertainty regarding the proper treatment of clinically curable female breast cancer is the management of the contralateral breast that does not contain a simultaneously clinically recognizable neoplasm. It has been reported that the risk of developing a cancer in the contralateral breast is four to seven times greater than the risk of developing an initial cancer by women in the general population. An NSABP evaluation of 2,734 patients in different protocols revealed that the overall incidence of second contralateral primary carcinomas was 1.9% in 6 years.[224]

Evidence indicates that occult, or subclinical, cancer in the contralateral breast may be much more frequent than previously supposed. These data have been gathered by biopsy of the uninvolved breast at the time of management of the primary breast cancer and by studies utilizing MRI. However, there is a dichotomy between the high incidence of tumor found by random biopsy or MRI and the number of patients who develop overt cancers in the contralateral breast. This strongly suggests that not all cancers progress to overt lesions or that they may undergo regression.

Because of the significant discrepancy in the incidence of positive biopsies and the much smaller number of overt cancers that subsequently appear, a conservative approach using mammography and diligent follow-up examination seems to be more appropriate than random biopsy or prophylactic mastectomy. Studies also indicate a ≈ 50% reduction in the incidence of cancer of the contralateral breast in patients treated with tamoxifen in the adjuvant setting.[188]

Local-Regional Therapy for Locally Advanced Disease ***Breast Conservation after Neoadjuvant Chemotherapy*** Modified radical mastectomy followed by adjuvant chemotherapy and postmastectomy radiation has been the historical standard local-regional therapy for patients with locally or regionally advanced primary tumors. However, over the past three decades the use of neoadjuvant chemotherapy (chemotherapy given prior to surgery) has significantly increased in patients with advanced disease. This strategy was first adopted for patients with unresectable or marginally resectable disease and the initial clinical data from such patients indicated that chemotherapy achieved high rates of tumor response. Subsequently, this approach has also been investigated in patients with large, resectable breast cancers at diagnosis. One reason to investigate the sequencing of chemotherapy prior to surgery was to determine whether breast conservation could be offered to selected patients with larger primary tumors whose residual disease after chemotherapy was amenable to a lumpectomy-type resection. To investigate this, the NSABP and EORTC independently conducted clinical trials that compared neoadjuvant chemotherapy with adjuvant chemotherapy for patients with stage II or III breast cancer (Figure 107-25). Both of these trials found that breast conservation rates were higher in the neoadjuvant chemotherapy arms.[225,226] In the NSABP study, the respective rates of breast conservative surgery were 68% in the neoadjuvant arm and 60% in the adjuvant arm. This increase was directly due to a greater percentage of patients with T3 disease being offered breast conservation after first responding to chemotherapy (22% breast conservation rate versus 8%, respectively).

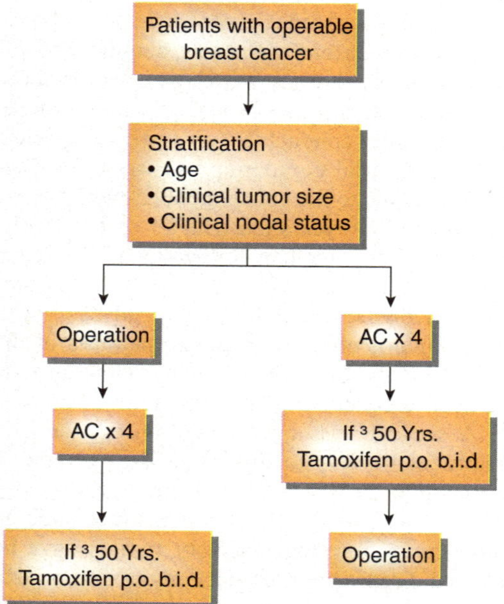

Figure 107-25 NSABP study of B-18 schema.

The goal of breast conservation therapy for patients with advanced disease is to achieve an aesthetically acceptable cosmetic outcome and a low risk of breast recurrence. Accordingly, for patients with large initial primaries, resection must be directed at the post-chemotherapy tumor bed rather than the initial volume of residual disease. However, one concern with resecting only the post-chemotherapy volume of residual disease is that some advanced breast cancers do not shrink concentrically to a solitary nidus in response to neoadjuvant chemotherapy, but rather break up into nests of residual disease over the initially involved volume. In such cases, surgery directed at the primary core may leave a higher burden of microscopic disease around the tumor bed site, which may theoretically be associated with higher rates of breast cancer recurrence.

In the NSABP B-18 trial, the overall rate of breast recurrence did not statistically differ in the patients treated with neoadjuvant chemotherapy compared to those treated with adjuvant chemotherapy (8-year rates of 10% versus 7%, respectively). However, the breast recurrence rate was higher in patients with large primary tumors in whom a response to neoadjuvant chemotherapy permitted a breast conserving surgery. In this subset of patients treated with neoadjuvant chemotherapy, the breast recurrence rate was 16%, which was over twice the rate in the patients with smaller tumors who were treated with breast-conserving surgery first.[225] Other multicenter series have also shown relatively high breast cancer recurrence rates in patients who receive neoadjuvant chemotherapy.[227,228] In general, series that include patients with inflammatory carcinoma and those that use radiation therapy alone (without surgery) in patients who achieve a complete clinical response have also noted higher local recurrence rates.

In contrast to these data, single institution studies with careful selection criteria and a high degree of multidisciplinary coordination have reported excellent rates of local control. Investigators at The University of Texas M. D. Anderson recently published the results of one of the largest studies investigating breast conservation after neoadjuvant chemotherapy.[229] In this study, 340 carefully selected patients who had a favorable response to chemotherapy were treated with breast conserving surgery and radiation. Despite the fact that 72% of patients in the study had clinical stage IIB or III disease, the 5- and 10-year breast cancer recurrence rates were only 5 and 10%, respectively. Four tumor-related factors were associated with breast cancer recurrence and local-regional recurrence: clinical N2 or N3 disease, lymphovascular space invasion, a multifocal pattern of residual disease, and residual disease greater than 2 cm in diameter.[229] Eighty-four percent of patients had either just one of these factors or none of the factors, and in these patients the 10-year breast recurrence rate was only 4%. In contrast, there was a 45% breast cancer recurrence rate in the 4% of patients with 3 of these factors. Interestingly, having a T3 or T4 tumor did not correlate with breast cancer recurrence overall, but those patients with T3 or T4 disease in which the primary tumor broke up and left a multifocal pattern of residual disease had a 20% breast recurrence risk.

In conclusion, the data indicate that breast conservation therapy is an appropriate treatment option for carefully selected patients with advanced primary tumors that have a favorable response to neoadjuvant chemotherapy. When considering breast conservation data in advanced disease, it is also important to recognize that advanced disease status also predicts for local-regional recurrence after postmastectomy radiation and for distant metastases, so that the removal of the breast may not necessarily add to the curability of the patient.

Postmastectomy Radiation There is a strong rationale for combining the beneficial effects of radiation and mastectomy for selected women with breast cancer. For women with locally advanced disease, areas of subclinical disease extending beyond the operative field limit the efficacy of mastectomy. Radiation can often overcome this limitation by treating a larger volume of normal tissue and treating regions such as the supraclavicular fossa, where surgical resections are difficult and can cause significant morbidity. In contrast, the greatest limitation of radiation is its inability to control bulky sites of disease. Fortunately, mastectomy is highly effective in resecting all sites of gross disease for most women with breast cancer.

The initial studies that investigated radiation after mastectomy began in the 1950s and represented some of the first clinical trials in oncology history. It is therefore somewhat surprising that after more than five decades of study there remain significant controversies over the value of postmastectomy radiation and the proper selection criteria for its use. A number of factors have contributed to the continued uncertainties. First, early radiation techniques were found to be associated with life-threatening toxicities that became apparent 10 to 15 years after treatment.[188] Fortunately, technological improvements have lowered the morbidity of postmastectomy radiation, but decades of follow-up were needed to demonstrate this improvement. A second change that has occurred over time has been the addition of chemotherapy as a routine component of care. This change was important because it decreased the competing risk of distant metastases, thereby allowing improvements in local-regional control to have a positive effect on survival.

There have been several meta-analyses conducted to quantify the value and risk of radiation use after mastectomy. The most comprehensive of these has been the work of the EBCTCG. This group was able to obtain the raw data from every randomized prospective trial that has investigated post-mastectomy radiation. These data included over 15,000 women.[188] The 20-year overall survival rates for the postmastectomy radiation and mastectomy alone groups were nearly identical (37.1 to 35.9%, respectively; $p = .06$); however the use of postmastectomy radiation significantly improved survival from breast cancer (20-year rates of 53.4 to 48.6%, $p = .0001$). The reason why breast cancer specific survival did not improve overall survival was that radiation use increased the rate of non–breast cancer deaths ($p = .0003$). These excess deaths were predominantly due to the adverse cardiovascular effects of radiation. There was no increase in deaths due to pulmonary toxicity or treatment-related cancers. The increase in non–breast cancer deaths became significant only after 10-years of follow-up and continued to increase over the subsequent decade.

Most experts consider that the improvement in breast cancer survival noted in these historical trials likely resulted from a reduction in formation of distant metastases that arose from an isolated local-regional recurrence. Indeed, in the meta-analysis of mastectomy studies, radiation reduced the 10-year isolated local-regional recurrence rate for patients with lymph node–positive disease (24 to 9%) and for patients with lymph node–negative disease (9.2 to 2.7%).

It is important to recognize the value and limitations of the EBCTCG and other meta-analyses. The inclusion of data from all available clinical trials provided a number of invaluable insights, such as the potential long-term morbidity associated with radiation. These data led to improvements in radiation techniques that have decreased cardiovascular-related injuries over time, thereby increasing the likelihood that radiation could improve overall survival. However, the outcome data are also of limited clinical value in that many of the early trials were antiquated by today's standards. For example, the early radiation trials had no quality assurance over how radiation was delivered, many had flawed randomization, and many had selection criteria that included patients now known to have very low risk for local-regional recurrence after surgery alone. All of these features likely minimized any real benefit that radiation may have provided and increased radiation associated risks. To attempt to address some of these issues, Van de Steene and colleagues reanalyzed the EBCTCG meta-analysis using only the data from larger trials that began after 1970—trials with a relatively good overall survival rate, and trials that used standard radiation fractionation schedules.[230] By eliminating the poor-quality studies, this meta-analysis showed that postmastectomy radiation improved both breast cancer–specific survival and overall survival. When limiting the analysis to large and more recent clinical trials, the reduction in deaths was 12.4%. Interestingly, this degree of improvement in overall survival is of the same magnitude as that reported by the EBCTCG for the first-generation polychemotherapy trials for patients with lymph-node positive breast cancer.[231]

Modern Postmastectomy Radiation Trials Mature data from three more recent randomized trials investigating postmastectomy radiation were published in 1997. The data from these trials not only provided new insights into the potential benefit of radiation but also further fueled the controversy regarding its use. Importantly, all of these studies used more modern radiation techniques and all patients in these studies received systemic therapy.

The Danish Breast Cancer Cooperative Group (DBCCG) 82b trial is perhaps the most important of these three trials. This study randomized 1,708 premenopausal women with stage II or III breast cancer to mastectomy followed by 9 cycles of CMF chemotherapy or mastectomy, radiation, and 8 cycles of CMF. Radiation therapy consisted of 50 Gy in 25 fractions delivered to the chest wall and draining lymphatics (including the internal mammary lymph nodes) and used electron beams in the regions over the heart to minimize dose to the cardiovascular structures.[232] The majority of patients entered in this trial had 1 to 3 positive lymph nodes. However, most patients in this trial did not undergo a formal level I/II axillary dissection. The median number of axillary lymph nodes resected was only 7, with only 24% of patients having 10 or more lymph nodes removed and 15% having 3 or fewer lymph nodes removed. The most significant finding of this study was that patients randomized to radiation had an improved overall survival rate (10-year rates: 54% vs 45%, respectively; $p < .001$). This survival advantage was likely a consequence of the reduced rate of local-regional recurrence in the patients receiving radiation (9% vs 32%, $p < .001$).

Simultaneously, investigators in Vancouver, British Columbia conducted a smaller trial of similar design. In this trial, 318 premenopausal women with lymph node–positive disease were randomized to receive mastectomy and CMF, or mastectomy, radiation, and CMF.[233] The results were very similar, with radiation use being associated with an improvement in overall survival (10-year rates: 64% vs 54%, respectively; $p = .07$) and local-regional control (10-year rates: 87% vs 75%, respectively; $p = .003$).

Finally, the DBCCG 82c, randomized 1,300 postmenopausal patients to mastectomy and tamoxifen or mastectomy, tamoxifen, and radiation.[234] The stage of disease and extent of axillary surgery were also very similar to the 82b trial. The magnitude of the benefits in overall survival and local control was similar to the two previous studies. The 10-year overall survival rates favored patient randomized to receive radiation (45% vs 36%, respectively; $p = .03$), as did the rates of local-regional control (10-year rates: 92% vs 65%; respectively; $p < .001$).

A number of questions and criticisms have been raised concerning these three studies. Both the extent of axillary surgery and the use of non-anthracycline chemotherapy differed from the standard therapy offered patients in the United States. Despite these relevant criticisms, these studies demonstrated that by reducing postmastectomy local-regional failures, radiation could influence overall survival.

Indications for Postmastectomy Radiation The more recent phase III clinical trials indicate that radiation may well play an important role in the management of selected women treated with mastectomy and chemotherapy. However, because the axillary surgery differed from that commonly used in the United States, these trials are less helpful in defining which subcategories of patients should receive radiation.

There is a general consensus that a modified radical mastectomy achieves excellent rates of local-regional control for women with stage I breast cancer. In addition, there is consensus that patients with stage III disease, (defined by T3 with involved lymph nodes, T4 primaries, or 4 or more involved lymph nodes) should receive postmastectomy radiation.[235] These cohorts of patients have been found to have a 20 to 30% risk of local-regional recurrence after mastectomy, standard axillary dissection, and chemotherapy.

For patients with stage II disease with 1 to 3 positive lymph nodes the use of radiation is controversial. Most of the patients in the Danish and British Columbia trials had 1 to 3 positive lymph nodes, and radiation use in this cohort was associated with a reduction in local-regional recurrence and an improvement in overall survival. However, the rate of local-regional recurrence in the Danish trial was 32% in this cohort, much higher than that reported in United States trials in patients with similar stage breast cancer. The likely reason for this difference is that the axillary sampling procedure used in some patients in the Danish study led to an underestimation of the true number of positive lymph nodes. Correspondingly, many of the patients reported to have 1 to 3 positive lymph nodes would likely have had 4 or more lymph nodes if a more extensive surgical procedure had been performed. Second, the more limited dissection led to a high rate of axillary recurrences in the patients randomized to not receive radiation, which likely would have been avoided with a standard axillary dissection.

A number of recent studies have been conducted to assess the risk of local-regional recurrence in patients with 1 to 3 positive lymph nodes who were treated with a standard modified radical mastectomy and chemotherapy. The data from these studies is shown in Table 107-15 and collectively indicate that the 10-year risk of local-regional recurrence for such patients is approximately 13 to 15%.[232,234,236–238] Within the subgroup of patients with stage II disease with 1 to 3 positive lymph nodes, selected patients have additional features that increase the risk for local-regional recurrence to over 15%. Table 107-16 highlights these additional factors.[236,238–240]

Whether radiation provides a survival benefit for patients with less than a 15% long-term risk of local-regional recurrence is unknown. A randomized trial designed to investigate postmastectomy radiation for patients with stage II breast cancer with 1 to 3 positive lymph nodes did not successfully accrue in the United States and was closed. It is likely that radiation will decrease local-regional recurrence in such patients, but the absolute magnitude of this benefit will be small. Indeed, a study from M. D. Anderson reported that radiation use decreased the rate of local-regional recurrence in this cohort of patients from 13 to 3%.[241]

Table 107-15 Ten-Year Local Regional Recurrence Rates for Patients with 1–3 Positive Lymph Nodes

Study	No. of Patients	Local-Regional Recurrence (%)
Danish 82b[232]	1,708	30
Vancouver[233]	318	33
Danish 82c[234]	1,375	31
Recht et al[235]	2,016	13
Katz et al[236]	1,031	13*
Wallgren et al[238]	5,352	14*
Taghian et al[239]	5,758	13*

*Higher rates were associated with disease features listed in Table 107-16.

Postmastectomy Radiation Therapy after Neoadjuvant Chemotherapy Significantly fewer data are available that address the indications for and efficacy of postmastectomy radiation in patients treated with neoadjuvant chemotherapy. In patients treated with mastectomy first, the decision to administer radiation therapy is predominantly made on the basis of the pathological extent of disease. This is because clinical and radiographic assessment of primary tumor size and number of lymph nodes involved with disease is imprecise. It is clear that neoadjuvant chemotherapy changes the extent of pathological disease in 80 to 90% of cases, and it is apparent that data are needed to determine whether the local-regional recurrence risk after mastectomy is a function of pre-treatment extent of disease, the post-treatment extent of disease or a combination of both. One study attempted to assess whether risk was strictly determined by the post-treatment extent of disease by comparing how the pathological extent of disease correlated with local-regional recurrence after mastectomy for patients treated either with mastectomy followed by chemotherapy or chemotherapy followed by mastectomy.[242] Not surprisingly, this study found that the local-regional recurrence rate associated with a particular pathological extent of disease was higher in patients treated with chemotherapy first than in patients treated with surgery first. These data imply that patients treated with neoadjuvant chemotherapy have a risk of local-regional recurrence that is affected by both the pretreatment clinical stage and the extent of pathologically defined residual disease after chemotherapy. Furthermore, in a separate analysis of the patients treated with neoadjuvant chemotherapy, mastectomy and no radiation, a multivariate analysis of local-regional recurrence predictors found that both pre- and post-treatment factors were independently associated with local-regional recurrence.[243] It is intuitive that the efficacy of radiation in reducing local-regional recurrence would be independent of the sequencing of surgery and chemotherapy. The data appear to indicate this to be so, but to date there is only one published study that has evaluated the efficacy of postmastectomy radiation therapy in patients treated with neoadjuvant chemotherapy. This study compared the outcomes of 579 patients who received neoadjuvant chemotherapy, mastectomy, and radiation therapy with those of 136 patients who were treated with neoadjuvant chemotherapy and mastectomy alone.[244] Although all of these patients were treated on prospective clinical trials, radiation therapy was not a randomized variable in any of them. Therefore, there were significant imbalances in the prognostic factors between the two groups. In general, those treated with radiation therapy had more extensive disease and worse disease characteristics than those treated without radiation. Despite this, the local-regional recurrence rate was significantly lower in the patients treated with postmastectomy radiation therapy than in those treated with neoadjuvant chemotherapy and mastectomy alone (10-year local-regional recurrence rates were 8% and 22%, respectively, $p = .001$). In a multivariate analysis, the hazard ratio for local-regional recurrence associated with not receiving radiation therapy for the endpoint of LRR was 4.7 (95% CI, 2.7–8.1, $p < .0001$). In the subgroup of patients with clinical T4 tumors, clinical stage IIIB/C disease, and in those with 4 or more positive lymph nodes after chemotherapy, the absolute improvement in local-regional recurrence risk was approximately 30 to 40%. The use of radiation in these same subgroups was associated with an approximately 15 to 20% improvement in overall and cause-specific survival. In a multivariate analysis of cause-specific survival for the entire cohort, the hazard ratio for no radiation use was 2.03 (95% CI, 1.41–2.92, $p < .0001$).

Table 107-16 Factors Associated with Higher Local-Regional Recurrence Risk for Patients with 1–3 Positive Lymph Nodes

Author	Factor
Katz et al[236]	Extracapsular extension ≥ 2 mm Tumor size ≥ 4 cm Fewer than 10 lymph nodes recovered > 20% of lymph nodes positive Positive or close margins Pectoralis muscle invasion
Taghian et al[239]	Age under 50 with tumor size over 2 cm
Wallgren et al[238]	Premenopausal: lymphovascular space invasion, G2–3 Postmenopausal: tumor over 2 cm, G3
Cheng et al[240]	Tumor size ≥ 3 cm

That paper also showed that patients with locally advanced clinical disease who had favorable responses to chemotherapy still benefited from the addition of radiation therapy[244] For patients with clinical stage III disease who achieved a pathological complete response, the local-regional recurrence rate for those treated with radiation therapy was 3% versus 33% for those who did not receive radiation therapy ($p = .006$). In addition, for those with clinical stage III disease who after chemotherapy had tumor sizes less than 5 cm and had fewer than 4 positive lymph nodes, local-regional recurrence rates were 9% for those receiving radiation therapy versus 20% for those not receiving radiation therapy.

Whether to use radiation for patients with clinical stage II disease who have positive lymph nodes after chemotherapy remains less clear. A report of 132 patients with clinical stage II disease who did not receive radiation therapy after neoadjuvant chemotherapy and mastectomy indicated that patients with clinical T3N0 disease or 4 or more positive lymph nodes had high rates of local-regional recurrence.[245] The 5-year local recurrence rates in the remaining patients were less than 10%. In the patients with clinical stage II disease who had 1 to 3 positive lymph nodes after neoadjuvant chemotherapy the 5-year rate of local-regional recurrence was 8%. It is important to recognize that this study had a small sample size and that the studied population was prone to selection biases, in that they represented only those patients for whom the treating physicians elected not to use radiation.

On the basis of the available data, it is reasonable to recommend postmastectomy radiation therapy for all patients with clinical stage III disease. It is also reasonable to assume that patients with clinical stage I or II disease who have 4 or more positive lymph nodes after chemotherapy or who have progressive disease leading to a primary tumor size over 5 cm are at high risk for local-regional recurrence and should receive radiation. It is currently not known whether radiation will benefit patients with clinical stage I or II disease who have 1 to 3 positive lymph nodes after neoadjuvant chemotherapy.

Palliative Radiotherapy There is a well-defined role for palliative radiotherapy in the treatment of metastatic breast cancer, which is remarkably responsive to modest doses of radiotherapy.

Painful bony metastases and simple pathologic fractures of non–weight-bearing bones respond well to short courses of radiotherapy, such as 3,000 to 3,500 cGy in 10 to 14 fractions. However, local radiotherapy is no substitute for proper orthopedic fixation in weight-bearing bones.

Radiotherapy is critical for pain relief as well as for the prevention and reversal of neurologic deficits associated with epidural spinal cord compression from metastatic breast cancer. A short course of high-dose corticosteroids and initial large radiation fractions should be used in an attempt to maximize tumor regression as soon as possible. Some authors advocate using radiotherapy without laminectomy in early-stage spinal cord compression and in responsive tumors, such as those in the breast.[246]

Treatment with radiotherapy is the mainstay for multiple intracranial metastases and is preferable to surgical treatment in the presence of widespread, poorly controlled systemic metastases. The generally accepted course of palliative brain irradiation for multiple lesions is 3,000 cGy in 10 to 12 fractions administered in conjunction with high-dose corticosteroids with or without phenytoin (Dilantin). The optimal therapy for a solitary intracranial metastasis in the absence of widespread systemic metastases is less clear. A randomized trial comparing surgical removal plus radiotherapy to radiotherapy alone concluded that patients receiving combined therapy lived longer, had fewer recurrences, and enjoyed a better quality of life.[247] Because 77% of patients in the study had metastatic lung cancer, which is not nearly as responsive to radiotherapy as is breast cancer, the value of surgical resection of brain metastases from breast cancer is certainly not established. It is possible that an external beam radiation boost or a stereotactic radiosurgical boost might be as effective as surgical extirpation.

In patients with less than four brain metastases, none of which measures > 2.5 cm, the addition of stereotactic radiosurgery boosts to these lesions after brain irradiation significantly improves control of intracranial disease.[248] Rapid and dramatic responses to stereotactic radiosurgery have been reported in patients with recurrent brain metastases from a variety of adenocarcinomas.

Details of Radiation Treatment The planning and delivery of radiation treatments for breast cancer is of critical importance. It is clear that radiation treatments can have serious normal tissue consequences and even cause life-threatening radiation injuries. Fortunately, most serious sequelae can be avoided with modern treatment techniques. However, the delivery of radiation and design of the treatment fields is complex and requires modern equipment and attention to detail.

There have been a number of recent advances in the field of radiation oncology that directly benefit breast cancer patients. One of these major advances has been the use of three-dimensional imaging to assist in field design. Computed tomography (CT)-based simulation allows radiation oncologists to design treatment fields on CT images acquired from patients in their treatment positions, thereby permitting better visualization of the targeted regions and the normal tissues that one wishes to avoid, such as the heart. An example of a field design for a stage I left breast cancer treatment after lumpectomy is shown in Figure 107-26. In this image, the tumor bed has been contoured on individual CT slices and reconstructed for the image. The breast is treated with a medial tangentially oriented beam, with a deep edge that enters near the midline and transverses the anterior thorax to exit near the mid axillary line. This field is opposed with a lateral tangent beam to match the fall off of dose as the beam travels through the breast and ultimately provides a homogeneous dose distribution.

Other regions of interest, such as lymph nodes in the axilla, internal mammary chain, or

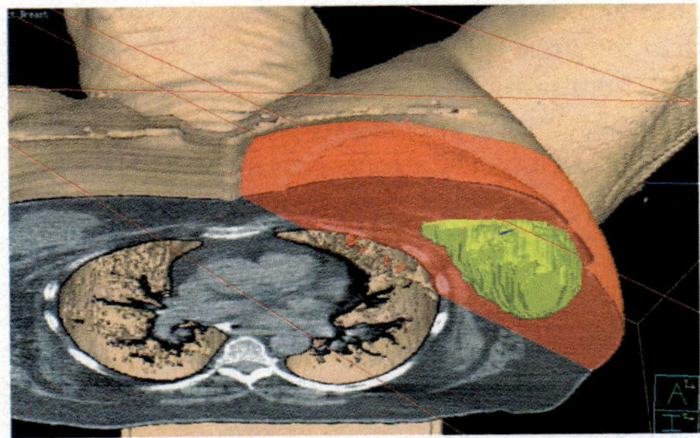

Figure 107-26 Cross-sectional picture of radiation fields used for the treatment of left-sided invasive breast cancer. The red shaded areas represent the volume included within the fields. The solid yellow object represents the tumor bed, which was reconstructed by contouring this region on sequential computed tomography slices. Two opposed treatment fields are used: a medial tangent that obliquely enters the medial breast and exits the lateral breast and an opposed lateral tangent field. The fields are opposed to match the fall-off of radiation dose that occurs as beams travel through tissue.

supraclavicular fossa can likewise be contoured in order to visualize their anatomical location with respect to treatment field borders. Figure 107-27 shows a "beam's eye-view" of a medial tangent beam used to treat the breast (including the tumor bed), the upper internal mammary lymph nodes, and level I and a portion of level II of the axilla.

A second major advance has been the development of three-dimensional dose calculation systems, which more accurately calculate and display the dose on the CT images throughout the three-dimensional treatment volume. Finally, modern treatment tools now also allow the dose to be modulated in three-dimensions. The goal of such modulation is to provide a homogeneous dose distribution, which minimizes the risk of normal tissues receiving more than the prescribed

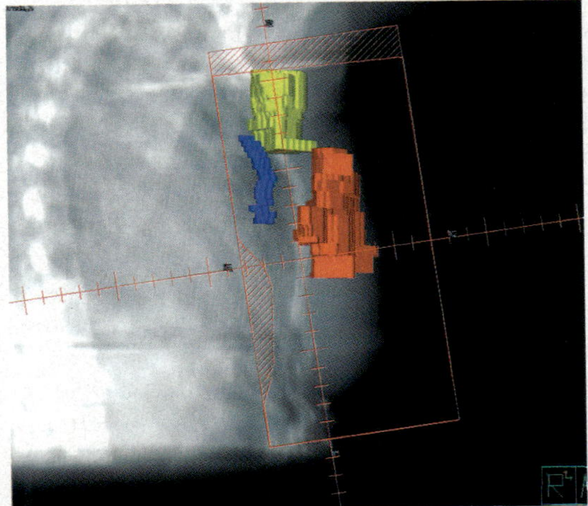

Figure 107-27 A beams' eye-view of a medial tangent radiation treatment field designed to cover the breast, low axilla, and upper internal mammary lymph node chain. The reconstructed contours of a tumor bed (*red*), upper internal mammary lymph node region (*blue*) and the low axilla (*yellow*) are shown.

dose and the risk of targeted areas receiving less than the prescribed dose.

The treatment planning process is the initial critically important step in radiation treatments of breast cancer. Patients are immobilized in a supine position with the ipsilateral arm abducted and externally rotated. They then undergo a CT scan that acquires the image set used for treatment planning. Reference marks are placed on the patient's skin of the breast. The planning process, in which the fields are designed and the dose distribution optimized typically then takes 2 to 3 days and does not require the patient to be present. Following completion of planning, daily treatments begin which typically require 15 minutes each day in the treatment room. The therapy is painless. The most common course of treatment entails 25 to 28 treatments of 180 to 200 cGy per day to the breast or chest wall with or without inclusion of lymphatic regions at risk. This course is typically followed by 5 to 8 supplemental treatments of 180 to 200 cGy per day to the tumor bed region (often called a tumor bed or chest wall boost). In total then, treatments are given 5 days a week for approximately 6 to 6.5 weeks.

Morbidity of Radiation Treatments for Breast Cancer Modern radiation treatments for breast cancer are relatively well tolerated and have low rates for long-term morbidity. Morbidities from radiation are considered as either acute effects or late effects. Acute effects typically occur during or immediately after treatment and for the most part are self-limited. The usual acute effects associated with breast or postmastectomy radiation include treatment-related fatigue and radiation dermatitis. These effects are usually relatively mild for women with early stage disease and patients typically can continue to work and continue their usual daily routines.

Late effects following treatment are also relatively unusual, particularly for patients treated after breast-conserving surgery for early-stage breast cancer or DCIS. For these patients, the most common late effect is a change in breast aesthetics. The cosmetic results after lumpectomy and breast irradiation are influenced by technique, patient body habitus, use of systemic therapy, and the extent of surgery. Approximately 85% of women treated with breast-conserving surgery and radiation consider their aesthetic outcome as good or excellent.[249,250]

The other, more common complication from local-regional therapy is lymphedema. Irradiation of the supraclavicular fossa and axillary apex after a level I-II axillary dissection can double the rate of lymphedema from 8 to 10% (surgery alone) to 15 to 20%. Rates can increase further if level III dissections have been performed and in cases with unresected involved lymph nodes in the infra- or supraclavicular fossa, which necessitate higher radiation dosages to this region. Other patient-related factors that contribute to lymphedema include obesity and subsequent injury or infection of the ipsilateral arm.

Cardiovascular-related morbidity has been the most significant long-term concern associated with breast cancer radiation. It is clear that radiation treatments for breast cancer can cause significant cardiovascular-related deaths if high dose is delivered to underlying cardiovascular structures. Modern radiation treatments for breast cancer are associated with less cardiovascular morbidity and mortality than earlier radiation techniques. In a randomized trial of postmastectomy radiation performed in Stockholm, the investigators noted an increase in cardiovascular death rates when wide treatment fields were used during the early years of the study but noted no increase in cardiovascular mortality after the trials were changed to use electron beam treatments.[251] Similarly, the Danish postmastectomy radiation trials exclusively used an electron beam technique in treating the chest wall to minimize dose to the cardiac structures. After a median follow-up of 117 months, there was no increase in mortality or cardiac-related hospitalizations in the approximately 1,500 patients randomized to receive radiation versus the 1,500 who were randomized to no radiation.[252] Finally, a similar morbidity and mortality analysis was performed in a Canadian study by Vallis and colleagues.[253] The long-term follow-up on 2,128 patients treated with radiation as a component of breast conservative therapy, with a median patient follow-up in excess of 10 years, these authors found that cardiovascular morbidity was not increased in women with left-sided breast cancer compared to those with right breast cancer. Most recently, a report analyzing SEER data found an increase in cardiovascular-related deaths for irradiated breast cancer patients with left-sided tumors versus right-sided tumors during the 1970s. However, this increased risk was not present for patients treated in the 1980s and 1990s.[254]

Other serious late radiation related injuries, such as rib fractures, pulmonary injuries (radiation pneumonitis), brachial plexus injuries, and development of second tumors are rare.

In summary, modern radiation treatments should be considered safe and effective. Treatment techniques and equipment are important to assure that morbidities associated with radiation therapy are minimized.

Sequencing of Local-Regional Breast Cancer Treatment with Systemic Therapies As the beneficial therapeutic effects of surgery, radiation, chemotherapy, and hormonal therapy have become elucidated, important questions concerning the sequencing of therapies have arisen. Most breast cancer patients benefit from multimodality treatment and decisions concerning the sequencing of these treatments are optimally handled in a multidisciplinary fashion, with input from surgeons, medical oncologists, radiation oncologists, pathologists, and diagnostic radiologists.

Sequencing of Surgery and Chemotherapy Definitive surgical therapy has been the historical initial treatment for most patients with breast cancer. However, an increasing percentage of breast cancer patients are treated with chemotherapy prior to definitive surgery. This approach was initially investigated in patients with advanced or inflammatory breast cancer in an attempt to render the disease operable. Subsequently, neoadjuvant chemotherapy was investigated as a strategy to permit breast conservation therapy for patients with large T2 tumors or T3 disease. Even more recently, neoadjuvant chemotherapy has been explored as a treatment option for any woman who is felt to potentially benefit from chemotherapy. These more recent treatment philosophies have permitted the majority of breast cancer patients to be eligible for neoadjuvant chemotherapy.

There are a number of potential advantages and some possible disadvantages for sequencing chemotherapy prior to surgery. Table 107-17 reviews some of these advantages and disadvantages. Neoadjuvant chemotherapy treatment has high anti-tumor activity: numerous studies have indicated that 80 to 90% of breast cancers respond to neoadjuvant chemotherapy, and in 15 to 30% of the cases there is no evidence of residual disease within the surgical specimen at either the primary site or the lymph nodes (termed a pathological complete response [pCR]).[225,226]

From a biologic standpoint, justification for the evaluation of preoperative chemotherapy derives from three hypothetical bases. Laboratory investigations had shown that pulmonary metastases in animals underwent a growth spurt when the primary tumor was amputated, and this could be abro-

Table 107-17 Potential Benefits and Determinants of Using Neoadjuvant Chemotherapy in Breast Cancer

Benefits
- Facilitates the use of mastectomy for patients presenting with inoperable disease or inflammatory breast cancer
- Increases rates of breast conservation surgery for patients presenting with larger primary tumors
- Improves the aesthetic result of a breast conservation surgical procedure if less of the breast is resected after the tumor has responded to chemotherapy
- Allows for identification of resistance to treatment permitting clinicians to stop ineffective chemotherapy regimens and thereby minimize the continued risk of treatment toxicity
- The pathological response of disease to neoadjuvant chemotherapy is prognostic. Therefore, this sequencing strategy has proved to be an invaluable research tool to:
  - Directly compare the effectiveness of two systemic regimens
  - Directly study biological factors that influence chemotherapy sensitivity/resistance
- Identify patients for clinical studies of new agents because of their high risk for recurrence despite receiving the best available standard regimens

Potential determinants
- Information concerning the pathological extent of disease prior to treatment is unknown. Accordingly, the following are less certain:
  - Margin status of a breast conservation surgery
  - The risk of additional lymph node disease when a sentinel lymph node is negative or shows fibrosis and/or treatment-induced changes
  - The indications for postmastectomy radiation

gated with pretreatment with chemotherapy. In addition, early mathematical modeling of growth fractions in cell populations suggested micrometastases might respond differently to preoperative chemotherapy. Finally, the Goldie–Coldman hypothesis suggested that resistance to chemotherapy was a function of time and that early treatment might be better.

During the 1980s, several randomized and nonrandomized studies were conducted to evaluate the worth of preoperative chemotherapy for primary operable breast cancer.[255] Nonrandomized studies were limited to the evaluation of primary tumor response to preoperative chemotherapy and possibly to the correlation of such response to outcome. All of these studies demonstrated that preoperative chemotherapy results in a high rate of primary tumor response. Some authors indicated that a correlation existed between response of the primary tumor to chemotherapy and outcome. In some of these studies, large tumors were reduced in size, allowing breast-conserving surgery.

The most important assessment of preoperative chemotherapy came from randomized trials. The NSABP updated protocol B-18, a randomized trial comparing the preoperative and postoperative administration of four cycles of Adriamycin and cyclophosphamide (AC) in patients with operable breast cancer. The specific aims of this trial were to (1) determine whether preoperative chemotherapy more effectively prolonged disease-free survival and survival than the same chemotherapy given postoperatively; (2) evaluate the response of the primary tumor to preoperative chemotherapy and correlate the response with disease-free survival and survival; and (3) determine whether preoperative chemotherapy, by reducing the size of the primary tumor, allowed more conservative surgery and decreased the frequency of ipsilateral breast tumor recurrence. Patients with palpable operable (T1, T2, T3) breast cancer in whom the diagnosis had been established by fine-needle aspiration cytology were stratified by age, clinical tumor size, and clinical nodal status and randomly assigned to one of two groups. Group I patients underwent a total mastectomy plus axillary dissection, or a lumpectomy plus axillary dissection. They then received four cycles of Adriamycin and cyclophosphamide (60 and 600 mg/m^2 every 21 days × 4). Group II patients received four cycles of Adriamycin and cyclophosphamide as in group I, followed by a total mastectomy or lumpectomy within 4 weeks of the fourth course of chemotherapy. All patients in both groups who were 50 years of age or older received tamoxifen 10 mg twice daily. For patients treated by lumpectomy, breast irradiation was administered after the completion of all chemotherapy.

In the preoperative chemotherapy arm, 36% of patients demonstrated a clinical complete response, and 43% had a clinical partial response, for an overall response rate of 79%. Patients receiving preoperative chemotherapy were more likely to have a lumpectomy than were patients receiving postoperative chemotherapy (68% vs 59%, $p < .01$). Responding patients were significantly more likely to receive a lumpectomy than non-responding patients. Preoperative chemotherapy also resulted in axillary nodal downstaging: 59% versus 42% pathologically negative axillary nodes, for a net axillary nodal downstaging of 34%. There was a highly significant correlation between tumor response to preoperative chemotherapy and pathologic nodal status. Eighty-seven percent of patients with a complete clinical response had pathologically negative nodes, versus 57% with partial response, 50% with stable disease, and 38% with progressive disease. Overall disease-free survival and survival were no different in the preoperative chemotherapy group from the postoperative adjuvant therapy group, however, thus failing to confirm the major hypothesis of this study. The EORTC completed a confirmatory trial of very similar design, with results quite similar to those obtained in NSABP B-18.[226]

One unanswered question arising from this study concerns the need for further therapy following initial treatment. This question was addressed in the Aberdeen trial,[256] the M. D. Anderson Trial 85-01[257] and NSABP protocol B-27.[258] Smith and collaborators reported the results of a multicenter study (the "Aberdeen" trial) in 162 patients with large operable and locally advanced breast cancer. All received four cycles of doxorubicin, cyclophosphamide, vincristine and prednisolone (CVAP); those who responded were randomized to receive four more cycles of CVAP or four cycles of docetaxel (100 mg/m^2). All non-responders received four cycles of docetaxel. The clinical complete remission (CR) and clinical partial remission (PR) rate (94% vs 66%, $p = .001$) and pathologic CR (34% vs 16%, $p = .04$) rates were higher for those who were randomized to receive docetaxel. This improvement in response rates translated into longer relapse-free and overall survival rates. In this small study, treatment was of equal duration in both arms, so the improved outcome could only be attributed to the introduction of docetaxel. The study results confirm that improvements in pathological CR rate are associated with improvement in relapse-free and overall survival.

Thomas and colleagues, from the M. D. Anderson evaluated the use of an alternate, non-cross-resistant adjuvant chemotherapy regimen in women with a poor pathologic response to a preoperative doxorubicin-based regimen.[257] One hundred ninety-three patients with locally advanced breast cancer received three cycles of vincristine, doxorubicin, cyclophosphamide, and prednisone (VACP) every 21 days followed by surgery. Patients with less than 1 cm^3 residual tumor at mastectomy received an additional five cycles of VACP. Those with more than 1 cm^3 residual tumor were randomly assigned to receive an additional five cycles of VACP or five cycles of vinblastine, methotrexate with calcium leucovorin rescue, and fluorouracil (VbMF). Overall clinical response was seen in 83.4% after three cycles of VACP, whereas the pathologic complete response rate was 12.2%. One hundred six patients were randomly assigned to VACP or VbMF. Those receiving VbMF achieved higher relapse-free survival (RFS) and overall survival (OS) than those who received additional VACP, although the differences did not reach statistical significance ($p = .08$). Initial stage of tumor, clinical complete response, and pathologic complete response were all associated with statistically superior survival rates. For patients with a poor response to initial neoadjuvant chemotherapy, treatment with a non-cross-resistant regimen was associated with a trend toward improved RFS and OS compared with those continuing with the doxorubicin regimen.

NSABP B-27 was designed as a three-arm randomized trial where all patients received an initial four courses of preoperative AC therapy. One group received no further adjuvant treatment. A second group received four courses of docetaxel (Taxotere) after surgery, and the third group received four courses of docetaxel before surgery.

Preliminary results indicated that the addition of preoperative docetaxel significantly increased the rate of complete pathological response. In the AC only arms of B-18 and B-27, the clinical complete remission (cCR) rates were 36% and 40%, respectively, in contrast to 65% for the preoperative docetaxel arm in B-27. The pathological CR (pCR) rates were 9% and 9.1% for the two AC arms and 18.9% for the arm with preoperative docetaxel.[258] An update indicated that the administration of preoperative docetaxel following AC was associated with a significant prolongation of relapse-free survival ($p = .03$), although no survival differences had emerged. Since this study confirmed that the rate of pCR predicted relapse-free survival, it also validated the use of pCR as a surrogate marker of long-term benefit from treatment and therefore provided a useful tool for comparing treatment options.

This could provide a useful tool for future chemotherapy regimens. It may be possible to determine the effect of chemotherapy without waiting for long-term results. The response to preoperative chemotherapy becomes a prognostic marker for disease-free survival and survival. Thus, response to preoperative chemotherapy can be used as an intermediate end point in testing new regimens or in testing the additional effect of new drugs administered after well-established regimens, without having to wait for several years until disease-free survival and survival end points can be compared. With the demonstration that preoperative chemotherapy is equivalent to postoperative chemotherapy for disease-free survival and survival, new chemotherapeutic regimens can be tested in this setting without fear of putting patients at a disadvantage. These findings may also help with the evaluation of other prognostic tumor markers in correlating tumor response and outcome.

Even if preoperative chemotherapy does not improve disease-free survival and survival, there are several reasons why it may sometimes be preferred over postoperative chemotherapy. The administration of preoperative chemotherapy results in separating patients into five different groups according to their pathologic and clinical response to chemotherapy: (1) pathologic complete responders, (2) clinical complete responders, (3) clinical partial responders, (4) patients with clinically stable disease, and (5) patients with clinically progressive disease. If these categories continue to predict survival after chemotherapy, we will have a valuable tool for selecting patients for treatment.

The observed reduction in the size of the primary tumor following preoperative chemotherapy, resulting in increased rates of breast-conserving surgery, constitutes an additional advantage. The use of core needle biopsies, which provide histologic diagnosis, is now considered a standard preoperative diagnostic step and will help avoid false-positive diagnoses.

There are some advantages for being able to assess disease response to neoadjuvant chemotherapy. For example, studies have indicated the extent of residual disease after neoadjuvant chemotherapy is prognostic, and therefore more clearly stratifies which patients, such as those who achieve a pCR, have an excellent disease-free survival, and which patients remain at high risk of subsequent systemic relapse despite the chemotherapy treatment.[225,226,259] In addition, the assessment of disease response is of particular value as a research tool, in that it permits the activity of different chemotherapy regimens to be more easily compared. Response data can also provide insights into the biological determinants of chemotherapy response. For example, a study of sequential biopsies taken during the first course of neoadjuvant chemotherapy found that low levels of therapy-induced apoptosis and an increase in bcl-2 expression correlated with a poor response to treatment.[260] A separate study that used microarray technologies, identified and validated a profile of 70 genes that predicted which patients would achieve a pCR to taxane chemotherapy.[261] These types of studies may improve the understanding of chemotherapy resistance and identify new molecular targets for drug development.

Sequencing chemotherapy before surgery increased the percentage of patients treated with breast conservation.[225,226]

Sequencing of Adjuvant Chemotherapy and Radiation Because the majority of breast cancer patients treated in the United States undergo surgery as the initial component of their therapy, the most common treatment-sequencing question concerns the timing of adjuvant chemotherapy and radiation. There has been one relatively small, randomized prospective trial that investigated this question. In this study, patients treated with breast conservation therapy were randomized to radiation followed by 4 cycles of chemotherapy or the same chemotherapy followed by radiation.[262] The initial results of this trial indicated that patients who received chemotherapy prior to radiation had a significantly lower rate of distant metastasis than the group that had radiation immediately following surgery (25% vs 36% at 5 years; $p = .05$).[262] However, with more mature follow-up, there were no differences in local or distant disease control in either arm, or the patterns of first failure. It did appear that patients with close margins did worse with radiation delay, suggesting that such patients may benefit from re-excision.[263] The equivalent first failure pattern noted in this trial was also found in a similar retrospective analysis of patients treated on Southwest Oncology Group trials.[264]

Fewer data are available concerning the sequencing of chemotherapy and radiation for women treated with mastectomy. In the Danish 82b trial, radiation was sequenced very early in the adjuvant course.[232] However, a recent study that examined the timing of radiation delivery in the Cancer and Leukemia Group B 9344 trial, found very low rates of local-regional recurrence after postmastectomy radiation and the rates of local-regional recurrence were lowest in those for whom there was a delay in delivering radiation in order to first treat with taxane chemotherapy.[265]

Until definitive data are obtained in trials, it is reasonable to consider the risks and benefits of any adjuvant sequencing approach according to the particulars of each case. The majority of data suggest that the breast tumor recurrence risk is not increased with radiation delay if negative margins are achieved. Therefore, a reasonable sequencing strategy would be to attempt to achieve negative surgical margins and administer chemotherapy prior to radiation.

Sequencing of Radiation and Hormonal Therapy The final area of clinical controversy surrounding treatment sequencing is whether to administer hormonal therapy concurrently or sequentially with radiation. Historically, sequential treatment was recommended based on preclinical data suggesting that tamoxifen may arrest breast cancer cells in radioresistant cell cycle phases, which theoretically would decrease the efficacy of radiation treatment. However, clinical data suggest that breast recurrence rates are low and independent of tamoxifen-radiation sequencing.[266,267] These data however all come from small retrospective studies.

Another possible drawback of concurrent tamoxifen and radiation use concerns the potential risk of normal tissue injury. Tamoxifen use has been associated with increased levels of circulating TGF-β, which is an important mediator of radiation normal tissue injury. A study of radiation-related lung changes using clinical data from a small prospective randomized trial comparing postmastectomy radiation versus postmastectomy radiation with concurrent tamoxifen reported increased lung fibrosis in the tamoxifen-treated patients.[268] However, no symptom data were reported in this study and the clinical significance of this finding is unknown to date. It is also unclear from these data whether concurrent use would increase lung fibrosis compared to sequential use. Another study recently reported that the concomitant use of tamoxifen and radiation increased the incidence of grade 2 or greater subcutaneous soft tissue fibrosis.[269]

The sequencing question of radiation and tamoxifen will become less clinically relevant as more patients receive aromatase inhibitors as adjuvant therapy. To date there are no data available that have investigated the sequencing of aromatase inhibitors and radiation.

SYSTEMIC THERAPY OF BREAST CANCER

SPECIFIC ENDOCRINE THERAPIES **Suppression of Steroid Hormone Production** This therapeutic objective can be accomplished by the surgical removal of organs that produce and secrete hormones involved in breast cancer growth, radiotherapy-induced ablation, or chemical inhibition of hormone synthesis.

Ovarian Ablation Ovarian ablation is the oldest form of endocrine therapy, first described in 1896. It is ineffective for post-menopausal patients. Ovarian ablation can be performed by surgical removal of the ovaries or by radiotherapy. The latter requires 2 to 3 months for maximal ablation of ovarian function, which is a disadvantage in the treatment of symptomatic patients. Ovarian ablation by radiotherapy is noninvasive, but its effects may not be permanent. Over the short term, ovarian ablation is a safe, well-tolerated procedure. Acute side effects include hot flashes, alterations in mood, and other symptoms of estrogen deprivation. Long-term consequences include accelerated loss of bone mineral density and alterations in the blood lipid profile that indicate an increased risk of coronary artery disease. In the United States, surgical ablation is preferred over radiotherapy-induced ablation. Ovarian ablation has been largely displaced by antiestrogens and LHRH analogs.

Selective Aromatase Inhibitors Aromatase, an enzyme of the cytochrome P-450 superfamily catalyzes the conversion of androgenic precursors to estrogens in peripheral tissues. Aromatase is substantially concentrated in adipose and hepatic tissues and is also found in elevated concentrations in breast cancer.[270] The enzyme has no effect on glucocorticoid, androgen, or mineralocorticoid production. Aromatase inhibitors lower serum and tumor estrogen levels in postmenopausal patients. Therefore, aromatase inhibition is applicable only to postmenopausal (or oophorectomized) women in whom estrogen production is predominantly from peripheral sources. Two types of aromatase inhibitors have been developed: Type 1 aromatase inhibitors (exemestane, formestane) are exclusively steroidal and bind the enzyme covalently and irreversibly; type 2 inhibitors (such as aminoglutethimide, letrozole, anastrozole) reversibly inhibit cytochrome P-450.

Type 1 Aromatase Inhibitors The earliest of the new inhibitors, formestane (or 4-hydroxyandrostenedione), has no estrogenic properties and is rapidly metabolized by the liver. By intramuscular administration, its half-life is 5 to 10 days.

It has an excellent therapeutic index and requires no glucocorticoid replacement. It is commercially available in several European countries.

Exemestane is the most potent and commonly used member of this family.[271] Its potency in inhibiting aromatase is similar to the type 2 inhibitors, and its pharmacokinetic properties make it quite competitive.

Type 2 Aromatase Inhibitors Both anastrozole and letrozole are FDA-approved for treatment of hormone receptor positive breast cancer in postmenopausal women.[271] Both agents inhibit aromatase activity by 96 to 98%, and have excellent antitumor activity and excellent tolerance profile. All three selective AIs are more effective and better tolerated than megestrol acetate and compare favorably with tamoxifen in the metastatic setting. Anastrozole and letrozole are superior to tamoxifen in the adjuvant setting for primary breast cancer. Anastrozole, letrozole, and exemestane have all proven superior to tamoxifen after 2 to 5 years of adjuvant tamoxifen therapy.[271] Fadrozole demonstrated antitumor efficacy similar to that of established AIs or other hormonal agents. It was well tolerated, although nausea, vomiting, anorexia, headache, rash, and other minor adverse effects have been reported. This agent is commercially available in Japan. The major advantage of the selective AIs over their predecessors is a better therapeutic index. Furthermore, anastrozole, exemestane, and letrozole are conveniently administered orally, once daily. There is incomplete cross-resistance between type 1 and type 2 AIs.

Inhibitors of Pituitary Function LHRH analogs (buserelin, goserelin, leuprolide) produce long-lasting inhibition of luteinizing hormone and follicle-stimulating hormone release after a transient initial increase. Their action could also be described as pharmacologic ovarian ablation because they inhibit ovarian estradiol release by about 90%.[272] In addition, some authors have hypothesized that LHRH analogues may have direct effects on breast cancer cells; however, this action remains speculative. LHRH analogs are primarily effective in premenopausal women.

Interference with Hormonal Action The endocrine therapies described in this section act by interfering with the effects of hormones on the end organ (ie, the breast cancer cell).

Selective Estrogen Receptor Modulators (SERMs, or Antiestrogens) Antiestrogens were initially developed in the search for better contraceptives. Although their efficacy as antifertility drugs was limited, they were found to cause regression of breast cancer cells. Tamoxifen is known to bind competitively to the ER, but it also has multiple additional adverse effects on the cancer cell.[273] It can lower the production of IGF-1 and TGF-α; it blocks angiogenesis and induces the production of TGF-β, calmodulin, and protein kinase C. It also has been reported to increase natural killer cell activity. The effects of tamoxifen have been studied mostly in post-menopausal women, although its effects have also been examined in younger patients. The serum estrogen level rises dramatically in some premenopausal patients, but this effect does not mediate tamoxifen resistance. The usual dose of tamoxifen is 20 to 40 mg daily. Higher doses do not appear to be more effective. Tamoxifen and its active metabolites have a prolonged serum half-life (7 days) after reaching steady-state levels.[273] Thus, once-a-day dosing is sufficient, and missing an occasional dose will not alter serum levels dramatically.

Several new SERMs have been extensively tested. Toremifene was approved by the FDA for the management of metastatic, ER-positive breast cancer, based on evidence indicating therapeutic equivalence with tamoxifen.[273] Raloxifene was approved for the prevention of osteoporosis.[274] Limited phase II evaluation suggested modest antitumor efficacy in metastatic breast cancer. Both toremifene and raloxifene appear to lack estrogen agonist activity on the uterus. For this reason, raloxifene is currently being compared with tamoxifen in a large, randomized trial of breast cancer prevention (STAR trial), which completed patient recruitment in early 2004. Other SERMs (idoxifene, droloxifene, LY353381, LY357489, EM-652, and GW5638) are under development.[273] However, to date these agents have not been proven to be more effective or less toxic, than tamoxifen.

Another important group of endocrine agents is the selective estrogen receptor downregulators (SERDs).[273] Fulvestrant (Faslodex) is the first of this family to complete clinical development. This steroidal antiestrogen is a pure estrogen antagonist. Fulvestrant blocks ER transactivation from both the activation function (AF)-1 and AF-2 domains. Fulvestrant also impairs receptor dimerization and induces receptor degradation, resulting in a dramatic reduction of receptor concentration in the cell. Fulvestrant exhibits 100 times greater affinity for the ER than tamoxifen, and it is effective in tamoxifen-resistant cell lines. Furthermore, it is a potent inhibitor of tamoxifen-stimulated breast cancer cells in vivo. Fulvestrant was shown to be equivalent to anastrozole in the treatment of tamoxifen-resistant tumors.

Progestins The development of synthetic progestational agents led to their evaluation for the treatment of breast cancer.[275] The two most commonly used progestational agent for this purpose are megestrol acetate (Megace, 40 mg PO qid), and medroxyprogesterone acetate (Provera, 400 mg/d). Other progestational agents are of historical interest only. Although responses to progestin therapy correlate with ER content, there is no evidence that PR content is a better predictor of response for this group of agents than for other hormonal treatments. Toxicity is clearly dose related. At high doses, substantial weight gain, fluid retention, and other toxicities become prominent. At commonly used doses, the efficacy, and tolerance of progestins appear similar to those of tamoxifen. Based on these studies, progestins were frequently used as first- or second-line therapy for metastatic breast cancer until they were rapidly displaced by selective AIs over the past few years. High-dose progestins stimulate appetite and weight gain and have been used with some success for cancer cachexia. For palliative treatment of patients with advanced cancer, progestins can improve a sense of well being. Low doses of progestins were reported to be effective treatment of vasomotor instability-related symptoms in postmenopausal women.

Androgens Androgen therapy also is an effective approach to the endocrine treatment of breast cancer, but the virilizing effects make it intolerable to many women. Semisynthetic testosterone derivatives, such as fluoxymesterone (10 mg orally bid) and danazol, are better tolerated, with fewer virilizing effects. Nevertheless, with long-term therapy, hirsutism, deepening of the voice, clitoral hypertrophy, male pattern alopecia, and increased libido occur. Like other hormonal agents with intrinsic endocrine effects, androgens also can cause tumor flare. The therapeutic index of the new antiestrogens, AIs, and LHRH analogs is clearly superior to that of androgens. Through their anabolic activity, androgens exhibit an important palliative effect, even in the absence of tumor regression. Increased appetite and weight gain are common. Androgens, like estrogens, can be valuable therapeutic tools when cost is an important consideration, especially when good tolerance can be established in an individual patient.

Estrogens Second to ovarian ablation, estrogens are probably the oldest form of hormonal therapy for breast and other hormone-responsive tumors. It appears paradoxical that both reduction of estrogen levels by ablative therapies and the administration of high doses of estrogen can cause tumor regression. The mechanisms by which high doses of estrogen induce tumor regression are not known, but estrogen therapy is as effective as antiestrogens or progestins for postmenopausal patients. High-dose estrogen therapy was also reported to have therapeutic activity in pre-menopausal women with breast cancer. Diethylstilbestrol 15 mg/day or ethinyl estradiol 1.5 to 3 mg/day are the most common preparations used. The major drawback of estrogen therapy is toxicity. Common side effects include nausea, vomiting, fluid retention, increased risk of thrombotic phenomena, tumor flare, urinary incontinence, and vaginal bleeding. When compared to tamoxifen, estrogens were found to be more toxic and less well tolerated, but also less expensive than tamoxifen or several of the other modern hormonal therapies. For postmenopausal women who have responded to several lines of hormonal therapy (SERMs, SERD, AIs, progestins, and perhaps androgens), estrogen therapy is a viable therapeutic alternative. Starting at a lower dose and escalating to the full therapeutic dose over a 2- to 3-week period lessens gastrointestinal toxicity and improves tolerance.

Corticosteroids The antitumor efficacy of corticosteroids is poorly documented for metastatic breast cancer but is considered to be about 10%. In some trials, no antitumor activity was observed. The long-term administration of glucocorticoids is associated with potentially severe and intolerable side effects. Therefore, glucocorticoids are not recommended as antitumor agents for metastatic breast cancer.

Glucocorticoids have a specific role in the management of well-defined complications of breast cancer, however. High-dose glucocorticoid therapy is administered for short periods to patients with central nervous system metastases and those with spinal cord compression, and some experts also use it during the management of acute hypercalcemia of malignancy. This latter indication has been relegated to the management of bisphosphonate-refractory cases in recent years. Its antiemetic effects are also well known.

Antiandrogens (Flutamide and cyproterone acetate) and antiprogestins (mifepristone, RU 486) have been evaluated in a few clinical trials. Their efficacy against metastatic breast cancer appears limited. At this point, there is no role for these agents in the standard treatment of breast carcinoma.

Side Effects of Hormone Therapy Most types of hormonal therapy can produce hot flashes, mild nausea, fluid retention, and an increase in the incidence of thromboembolic phenomena. Tamoxifen has been associated with an increased risk of endometrial hyperplasia, dysplasia, and carcinoma, as well as the development of ovarian cysts and other benign gynecologic abnormalities. A recent report suggested an increase in the incidence of uterine sarcomas as well. Ocular toxicity has also been attributed to tamoxifen, especially when it is administered at high doses. Progestins are known to cause moderately severe fluid retention, increased appetite, and weight gain, and they can occasionally cause or contribute to glucose intolerance. The newer aromatase inhibitors and LHRH analogs appear to be better tolerated.[271,272] However, diarrhea, nausea, headaches, hot flushes, bone pain, musculoskeletal pain, arthralgias, and alopecia have been reported in association with these agents. Because both types of agent produce estrogen deprivation, symptoms related to estrogen deprivation are relatively common, including hot flashes and vaginal dryness. In addition, loss of bone mineral density and increased rate of osteoporotic fractures have been reported with LHRH analogs and aromatase inhibitors.[271,272]

Cytotoxic Chemotherapy Breast cancer is moderately sensitive to a number of cytotoxic agents. Several classes of agents with different mechanisms of action and only partially overlapping toxic effects have substantial antitumor activity in patients with metastatic breast cancer. The most active drugs include the anthracyclines (doxorubicin, epirubicin, and liposomal formulations of doxorubicin), alkylating agents (cyclophosphamide, melphalan, thiotepa, and platinum salts), the anthraquinones (mitoxantrone), antimetabolites (methotrexate, 5-fluorouracil, capecitabine and gemcitabine), the Vinca alkaloids (vinorelbine, vinblastine, and vincristine) and the taxanes (paclitaxel and docetaxel). Response durations after single-agent therapy are short, in the range of 4 to 6 months and there is no noticeable impact on survival. One of the most important additions in recent years has been capecitabine. This agent is a fluoropyrimidine prodrug, converted to the active compound by thymidine phosphorylase. Many malignant cells produce high concentrations of this enzyme, resulting in preferential activation of the drug at the site of tumor deposits. Some cytotoxic agents, such as the taxanes, induce the production of thymidine phosphorylase, thus further enhancing local drug activation and resulting in a synergistic combination.

Combination Chemotherapy Combination chemotherapy was developed based on the rationale that combining agents with different mechanisms of action and non-overlapping toxicities would increase treatment benefit, prevent or delay the emergence of drug resistance without significantly worsening morbidity or quality of life. (For details of the strategy and tactics of combination chemotherapy see Chapter 38: "Principles of Dose, Schedule, and Combination Chemotherapy.") Combination chemotherapy regimens consisting of cyclophosphamide, methotrexate, 5-fluorouracil (CMF); cyclophosphamide, methotrexate, 5-fluorouracil, vincristine, prednisone (CMFVP); and 5-fluorouracil, doxorubicin (Adriamycin), cyclophosphamide (FAC) produce higher overall response rates, exceeding 50% in most reports, with remission durations that range from 6 to 12 months and survival that approaches 2 years. Randomized trials demonstrated that these combinations were more effective than single agents such as 5-fluorouracil, cyclophosphamide, and melphalan, resulting in higher response rates and longer times to progression.

Since the introduction of the taxanes into the treatment of advanced breast cancer, two competing hypotheses have directed clinical research in chemotherapy for breast cancer. One, the conventional approach based on the Goldie–Coldman hypothesis, called for concurrent administration of two or more cytotoxic agents to prevent or minimize the development of drug resistance and maximize cytoreduction.[276] The other, based on the Norton–Simon hypothesis, proposed the sequential administration of full-dose, single-agent treatments, to maximize dose-intensity and minimize toxicity.[277] In general, sequential single-agent therapy is better tolerated than simultaneous combinations, provided the same doses of all drugs are used. In the metastatic setting, in the absence of life-threatening or symptomatic disease, the sequential use of single agent therapies is a reasonable alternative to simultaneous combinations. However, there is no obvious benefit for using sequential single agents if the active doses can be administered simultaneously.

Side Effects of Cytotoxic Chemotherapy Cytotoxic chemotherapy regimens used for breast cancer treatment have produced considerable side effects. Most cytotoxic agents are myelosuppressive. The most serious toxicity is neutropenia, which can lead to severe infection. The correlation of neutropenia with infection appears when the neutrophil counts fall below 500 cells/μL, and the risk of infection rises greatly when neutrophil count drops below 100 cells/μL or severe neutropenia lasts more than 5 days. Sepsis associated with neutropenia is the most common cause of death during chemotherapy, whether at standard or high doses. The availability of hematopoietic growth factors allows the administration of myelosuppressive agents with minimal myelosuppressive toxicity and rapid recovery, enhancing on-time administration of chemotherapy. Many drugs produce partial or total alopecia. Most produce some degree of nausea and vomiting, and some can produce oral and gastrointestinal mucositis, diarrhea, constipation, and peripheral neuropathy. Modern antiemetics have dramatically reduced the incidence and severity of nausea and vomiting. Many patients receiving chemotherapy report fatigue. Fatigue is often associated with anemia, which can sometimes be prevented or treated with erythropoietin administration. Other important side effects of chemotherapy include ovarian ablation in premenopausal women, which brings with it the short- and long-term consequences of premature menopause and the development of infertility. Premature menopause leads to rapid loss of bone density and the development of osteoporosis.

Long-term side effects include a slight increase in the incidence of myelodysplastic syndromes and acute leukemias. Two types of chemotherapy-related myelodysplastic syndromes have been identified. One, which is related to large cumulative doses of alkylating agents, results in the development of acute hematologic malignancies 5 to 15 years after the initiation of therapy. Since long-term alkylating agent therapy is seldom used, this type of acute leukemia has become less common. A second syndrome, which is attributed to topoisomerase II inhibitors, has been reported to include development of myelomonocytic leukemia (M4M5), mostly within 2 years after the initiation of therapy. This second syndrome has been reported with higher doses of doxorubicin or epirubicin, often in association with an alkylating agent and/or a hematopoietic growth factor. Since anthracycline-containing regimens represent the standard of care for both metastatic and primary breast cancer, this type of leukemia or myelodysplastic syndrome is more commonly seen today.

Targeted Therapies The rapid expansion of our understanding of the biological changes that lead to malignant transformation and the growth-stimulatory and growth-inhibitory factors that influence this process led to the identification of a number of critical steps that can be targeted for therapeutic intervention.[278] Growth factors and their cognate receptors, intracellular signaling pathways, angiogenesis, the metastatic cascade, have all been recognized as potentially useful targets. A very large number of candidate therapeutics that focus on these putative targets is under preclinical and early clinical evaluation. Among these, the type I growth factor receptor (human epidermal growth factor receptor or EGFR) family is in a prominent place. There are four members of this family: *EGFR* or *HER1, HER2, HER3, and HER4. EGFR* is often overexpressed in colorectal, lung and head and neck carcinomas, and less often (10 to 20%) in breast cancer. HER2 is amplified and/or overexpressed in about 20 to 30% of breast cancers. *HER3* and *HER4* are also found overexpressed, but they have been less extensively studied. *HER2* is a normal gene involved in growth regulation. When overexpressed, the cell surface receptors become constitutively activated, producing uninterrupted signaling that stimulates growth, invasion and metastasis.

The cause of overexpression is gene amplification in the great majority of breast cancers. Patients with HER2-overexpressing breast cancers have a higher rate of relapses and relapses tend to occur earlier than in patients with normal HER2 expression. Mortality is also higher in patients with HER2-overexpressing breast cancer. A monoclonal antibody (trastuzumab, Herceptin) that binds to the extracellular domain of the HER2 protein was developed almost 15 years ago. This agent was shown to produce objective regressions in about 11 to 16% of patients with HER2-overexpressing breast cancers with extensive previous exposure to chemotherapy.[279] In previously untreated patients, the activity of the antibody was more pronounced, with response rates exceeding 25%. If candidates for trastuzumab treatment were selected with a fluorescence in situ hybridization assay, the objective response rate in this group increased to 41%. Trastuzumab has increased the response rate to anthracyclines, taxanes, vinorelbine and platinum salts. In combination with paclitaxel or the doxorubicin [Adriamycin]/cyclophosphamide (AC) combination, trastuzumab resulted in significant increases in response rate, time to progression, response duration and survival in a large randomized trial that included over 400 patients with metastatic breast cancer.[280]

Several small molecules with inhibitory effects on the receptor tyrosine kinase have reached clinical development.[281] Dual inhibitors of HER1 and HER2, inhibitors of protein farnesylation, ERK-inhibitors, mTOR inhibitors, angiogenesis inhibitors, protein kinase C-inhibitors, cyclin and cyclin-dependent kinase inhibitors, inhibitors of the proteasome and modulators of apoptosis are also in clinical development. However, none have reached the final clinical evaluation stage. Most seem to have modest single-agent activity to date, and there is much interest in testing two- and three-drug combinations in an attempt to block multiple signaling pathways, or the same pathway in multiple steps. There is also much interest in developing combinations of signaling inhibitors with cytotoxic drugs, hormones or other targeted interventions.

SYSTEMIC ADJUVANT THERAPY

Early Trials One of the most important advances in oncology came out of the acceptance of evidence that most patients with primary breast cancer have disseminated tumor at the time of diagnosis and that increased survival results only from effective systemic therapy used in conjunction with surgical therapy and radiation. This consensus has led to a major change in the concept of the disease and to the implementation of clinical trials to evaluate the efficacy of various systemic treatment regimens as adjuncts to operation.

Ashworth made the earliest observation of tumor cells in the blood in 1869. In 1955, Fisher and Turnbull, and Engell reported the presence of tumor cells in the blood of cancer patients and a surge of interest ensued. Following reports of favorable effects of chemotherapeutic agents on the destruction of disseminated tumor cells in experimental animals, a rationale for embarking on clinical trials of adjuvant therapy was established. Further support for the use of systemic therapy was obtained from early investigations in which it was noted that, although surgical removal of tumors or the use of 6-mercaptopurine failed to "cure" 15-day-old murine mammary tumors, the combination of the two resulted in a 57% cure rate.

As a result of these and other experimental findings, in 1958, under the auspices of the NIH Cancer Chemotherapy National Service Center, the NSABP initiated a trial to determine the efficacy of administering chemotherapy in addition to cancer surgery with curative intent to decrease recurrence and to extend the survival of patients with breast cancer. It was anticipated that such a therapeutic regimen could destroy the tumor cells dislodged into the blood and lymph during surgical manipulation. Participants were treated by either conventional Halsted radical mastectomy and triethylene thiophosphoramide (thiotepa) or by radical mastectomy and placebo. Thiotepa was administered at the time of operation and on each of the first 2 postoperative days. The results reported in 1968 indicated a significant increase in the 5-year survival of premenopausal women who received thiotepa. The difference, which was seen only in patients with four or more positive axillary nodes, persisted after 10 years of follow-up. Thus, it was demonstrated for the first time that the natural history of some breast cancer patients could be altered by systemic therapy.

In the 1960s, new concepts were formulated that led to a second generation of chemotherapy trials. The first of this second generation of clinical trials was conducted jointly by the NSABP and the Eastern Cooperative Oncology Group (ECOG) to evaluate the use of L-phenylalanine mustard (L-Pam) administered orally for 24 months after radical mastectomy to patients with positive nodes. In 1973, a second clinical trial was begun at the Istituto Nazionale Tumori in Milan to evaluate the effectiveness of a three-drug combination, cyclophosphamide, methotrexate, and 5-fluorourocil (CMF) as an adjuvant to mastectomy.

By September 1974, Fisher reported that L-PAM administration could prolong the disease-free interval of patients. Extended follow-up (more than 20 years) has demonstrated not only a significant prolongation of disease-free survival but also a significant benefit in the overall survival of pre-menopausal patients with the use of this single agent.[282] Although a similar trend was initially observed in postmenopausal women, that benefit was not sustained. Women taking L-Pam reported minimal undesirable side effects; mild nausea and vomiting occurred in about one-third of the patients.

In the Italian trial, a significant reduction in treatment failure occurred in all subgroups of patients treated with CMF. About two-thirds of patients experienced some toxicity, indicated by nausea, vomiting, anorexia, alopecia, cystitis, or amenorrhea. The 20-year results from the Milan trial continue to indicate a benefit in premenopausal, but not postmenopausal, women.[283]

Over the next two decades, over 200 controlled clinical trials were initiated to extend the earlier results, define optimal adjuvant systemic therapy, and evaluate a variety of newer treatment regimens. To summarize these results, the NIH organized three consensus development conferences.[161] In addition, the Early Breast Cancer Trialists Collaborative Group (EBCTCG) performed several meta-analyses of all (published and unpublished) prospective randomized trials designed and conducted for operable primary breast cancer.[231,284] Review of the consensus documents and the reports of the EBCTCG's meta-analyses shows the continuous evolution of this field, based on the maturation of clinical trial results and the availability of new data. The information obtained from the individual clinical trials, the consensus process, and the meta-analyses can be summarized as follows:

1. Adjuvant chemotherapy effectively reduces the risk of recurrence and death from breast cancer.
2. Combination chemotherapy is more effective than single-agent chemotherapy.
3. Adjuvant chemotherapy is more effective for women younger than 50 years of age than for older women, but significant benefit is observed in women in all age groups in which chemotherapy has been adequately evaluated.
4. Adjuvant anthracycline-containing regimens are more effective than other combinations lacking an anthracycline. This is particularly true for regimens that use three or more drugs and are given for longer than four cycles.
5. Adjuvant chemotherapy for longer than 6 months with the same regimen is not more effective than chemotherapy for 6 months.
6. The addition of taxanes to adjuvant chemotherapy regimens significantly improves relapse-free and overall survival rates.
7. The administration of chemotherapy with doxorubicin, cyclophosphamide and paclitaxel with hematopoietic growth factor support at two-week intervals instead of the conventional three-week intervals significantly improved relapse-free and overall survival rates.
8. Adjuvant tamoxifen effectively reduces the risk of recurrence and death from breast cancer. This effect is similar for patients in all

prognostic groups, regardless of age, tumor size, or lymph node positivity.

9. Adjuvant tamoxifen is effective only in patients with ER-positive and/or PR-positive breast cancer.
10. The efficacy of adjuvant tamoxifen increases with longer duration of therapy. At this time, data indicate that the optimal duration of adjuvant tamoxifen is 5 years.
11. Adjuvant tamoxifen significantly reduces the incidence of new or contralateral breast cancers.
12. Adjuvant ovarian ablation effectively reduces the risk of recurrence and death from breast cancer.
13. Adjuvant ovarian ablation is effective only for premenopausal women.
14. Adjuvant anastrozole or letrozole is more effective and better tolerated than adjuvant tamoxifen in postmenopausal women.
15. After receiving 5 years of adjuvant tamoxifen, crossover to letrozole for another 5 years significantly improves relapse-free survival and reduces the risk of second primary breast cancer.
16. After receiving 2 to 3 years of adjuvant tamoxifen, cross-over to anastrozole or exemestane for another 2 to 3 years significantly improves relapse-free survival and reduces the risk of second primary breast cancer compared to continuing tamoxifen until completing 5 years of therapy. For patients with positive lymph nodes crossover to exemestane was associated with a significant improvement in survival.
17. The combination of tamoxifen and adjuvant chemotherapy is more effective than chemotherapy alone or tamoxifen alone for patients with hormone receptor-positive tumors.
18. For optimal results, chemotherapy and tamoxifen should not be administered simultaneously. Rather, chemotherapy followed by tamoxifen appears to be appropriate.
19. Patients with steroid hormone receptor negative tumors benefit from chemotherapy to a greater extent than those with receptor positive tumors.

The report of the third EBCTCG meta-analysis included 69 chemotherapy clinical trials (30,000 women), 17 ovarian ablation trials (3,456 women), and 63 tamoxifen trials (42,000 women). A fourth EBCTCG meta-analysis was conducted in the fall of 2000, and the results were recently published as a full manuscript; in addition, the data were presented at the November 2000 NIH Consensus Development Conference.[161,284a] The fourth meta-analysis largely confirmed the conclusions derived from earlier analyses, and solidified the superiority of anthracycline-containing regimens over CMF-type regimens and confirmed that endocrine therapy was useful only for women with estrogen-receptor–positive tumors. The results of adjuvant chemotherapy trials are summarized on Table 107-18. The summary of adjuvant endocrine therapy trials is found on Table 107-19.

Table 107-18 Comparative Efficacy of Adjuvant Chemotherapy Regimens

Therapies	% Reduction in Annual Odds of Recurrence	*p*	Death	*p*
CT vs no CT (CMF vs Nil)	23.5	< .00001	17	< .00001
Doxorubicin vs no doxorubicin	12–30	.006	11–35	.02
Paclitaxel vs no paclitaxel	17–30	.09–.0022	6–18	> .10–.0064
Docetaxel vs no docetaxel	28	.001	30	.008

Adjuvant Therapy for Node-Negative Patients Tumor recurrence and death due to breast cancer affects a significant percentage of the patients with lymph node-negative breast cancer. In one study, treatment failed in approximately 25%, and 15% died during 5 years of follow-up.[284] Unpublished data from other studies indicate that treatment failed in 43% of the patients; 32% had died by 10 years of follow-up. A review of the literature suggests that with longer follow-up, even patients with small (< 1 cm), node-negative tumors have reported recurrence rates ranging up to 20 percent by 10 years, depending on specific tumor characteristics.[285]

Although the 1985 NIH consensus conference counseled against the routine administration of adjuvant systemic therapy in women with histologically negative axillary nodes, the 1990 NIH conference, based on newer data, reversed this advice.[286–288]

Endocrine Therapy **Tamoxifen** Starting more than 20 years ago, several organizations conducted randomized, controlled trials to evaluate the worth of postoperative tamoxifen, 10 to 20 mg twice a day, in node-negative patients with ER-positive tumors.[271,289] A highly significant overall disease-free survival advantage was found for tamoxifen ($p < .0001$). Several trials also reported a significant survival benefit. That benefit was observed in patients 49 years and younger and 50 years and older ($p = .0001$ for both). The tamoxifen-treated patients had fewer locoregional and distant metastases. Of particular interest was the reduction by 58% in ipsilateral breast tumor recurrences in patients treated by lumpectomy and breast irradiation and the reduction by 40% in the number of contralateral breast cancers when tamoxifen was administered. A significant survival advantage was also evident ($p = .02$) Clinical trials testing different durations of tamoxifen concluded that 5 years were superior to shorter durations, while durations exceeding 5 years were not superior to 5 years.

Tamoxifen Toxicity Although hot flashes, vaginal discharge, and irregular menses occurred more often in tamoxifen-treated patients than in those given placebo, the differences were not as pronounced as might have been thought if the placebo control had not been present. Thromboembolic events were more frequent in the tamoxifen-treated than in the placebo-treated group (1.3% vs 0.1%, $p < .001$). Pulmonary embolism occurred in 6 of 1,422 tamoxifen treated patients versus in 1 of 1,439 placebo-treated women ($p = .06$). This excess in thromboembolic complications associated with tamoxifen administration has also been reported in other large controlled trials. Second primary tumors other than endometrial carcinomas occurred equally in the two groups. Liver, gastrointestinal, urinary tract, and non-uterine genital cancers were not increased by tamoxifen treatment.

The relationship of tamoxifen administration to the development of endometrial cancer was investigated retrospectively in several randomized clinical trials. In one of the largest adjuvant tamoxifen trials a 7.5 relative risk for endometrial cancer was reported in the tamoxifen group, compared to placebo. Subsequent trials indicated a more modest increase in risk. In addition, most cases were of good-to-moderate histologic grade and deaths from endometrial cancer occurred in 4 of 23 women. The cumulative hazard rate for endometrial cancer was 6.3 per 1,000 patients. Including all reported endometrial cancers, the annual hazard rate through all follow-up was 0.2 per 1,000 in the placebo-treated group and 0.6 per 1,000 in the randomized, tamoxifen-treated group. Using population-based rates of endometrial cancer from SEER data, the RRs would be 2.2. The 5-year cumulative hazard rate for relapse from breast or endometrial cancer in the randomized tamoxifen group was 38% lower than that in the placebo group.

Additional information about the risk of developing endometrial cancer for patients receiving tamoxifen can be derived from the results of the BCPT.[72] After a median time on study of 47.7 months, 36 invasive endometrial cancers were reported on the tamoxifen arm, compared to 15 on the placebo arm. The RR was

Table 107-19 Comparative Efficacy of Adjuvant Hormonal Therapies

Therapies	% Reduction in Annual Odds of Recurrence	*p*	Death	*p*
Tamoxifen vs no tamoxifen	50	< .00001	33	< .00001
AI vs tamoxifen	19–22	.007	?	?
Tamoxifen × 5 years + AI	43	.00008	?	?
Tamoxifen × 2–3 years + AI	32–64	< .006	?–82	> .05

4 for patients 50 years of age or older, whereas there was no detectable increase in risk for younger women.

Although the risk of endometrial cancer increases after tamoxifen therapy, the net benefit vis-à vis breast cancer greatly outweighs the risk. Endometrial cancers occurring after tamoxifen therapy do not appear to be of a different type or of a worse prognosis than such tumors in patients who have not received tamoxifen.

Aromatase Inhibitors A recent report of the preliminary results of the Arimidex versus Tamoxifen And the Combination (ATAC) trial (*N* = 9,366) showed that, after two and a half years of follow-up, adjuvant anastrozole was significantly superior to tamoxifen in therapeutic efficacy and tolerance.[286] Anastrozole was associated with a 17% relative reduction in risk of recurrences, a figure even greater for patients with ER-positive tumors. There was also a significant reduction in second primary breast cancers compared to the group of patients treated with tamoxifen. Anastrozole was associated with fewer side effects than tamoxifen, although there were more fractures with anastrozole than with tamoxifen. Additional follow up of this large clinical trial will contribute critical information to the choice of adjuvant hormonal therapy. Similar results were recently reported from a randomized trial comparing letrozole to tamoxifen. Other large clinical trials, evaluating the contribution of letrozole or exemestane in the adjuvant setting, are currently in progress.

CHEMOTHERAPY In the early 1980s, three trials probed the use of adjuvant therapy for node-negative women. Investigators at the Instituto Nazionale Tumori activated a prospective randomized trial to assess the efficacy of adjuvant chemotherapy in patients with lymph node–negative and ER-negative primary breast cancer. Women 70 years of age or younger who had completed a modified radical mastectomy or breast-conserving surgery with axillary dissection and had no histological evidence of nodal involvement were randomized to receive either 12 cycles of intravenous cyclophosphamide, methotrexate, and fluorouracil (CMF) or no further treatment. High thymidine-labeling index was reported for two-thirds of the patients, and more than 50% had nuclear grade III tumors. Ninety patients were registered over 5 years in this study. Twelve years after surgery, the relapse-free survival rate for the CMF treated patients was 71%, compared to 43% for those in the control arm (p = .008); overall survival rates were 80 and 50%, respectively (p = .03).

The NSABP trial for node-negative patients (B-13) was initiated in August 1981 and was carried out to assess the worth of sequential treatment with two antimetabolites—methotrexate and fluorouracil (MF) followed by leucovorin (folinic acid)—in node-negative women considered to be at greatest risk for treatment failure, that is, those with ER-negative (less than 10 fmol/mg protein) tumors.[287] Treated patients had significantly increased disease-free survival ($p < .001$) compared with those receiving no chemotherapy (74% vs 59%, average time on study, 114 months). At 8 years, the treatment failure was reduced by 30% in patients aged 49 and younger and by 50% in those 50 years of age and older. Survival benefit in those 50 years old and older was significant (p = .03). Survival for younger patients was marginally better.

In 1981, an Intergroup study was initiated by ECOG for women with no histopathologic evidence of axillary node involvement. In that trial, 536 women who had undergone either a modified radical mastectomy or a total mastectomy with axillary-node dissection were randomized to receive adjuvant chemotherapy or no treatment. Patients were considered at high risk for recurrence because they had either an ER-negative tumor of any size or an ER-positive tumor at least 3 cm in diameter. The chemotherapy consisted of six 4-week cycles of cyclophosphamide, methotrexate, fluorouracil, and prednisone (CMFP).

The 10-year analysis of this trial demonstrated highly significant improvements in disease-free survival (p = .0006) and overall survival (p = .02) for patients who received CMFP.[284] A 37% reduction in risk of recurrence and a 34% reduction in risk of death were observed at 10 years. Treatment benefits were observed regardless of age, menopausal status, or estrogen receptor status. In a subsequent NSABP trial (B-19) 1,095 patients with ER-negative, axillary node–negative primary breast cancer were registered and randomized following appropriate regional therapy.[288] The control arm received six cycles of MF with leucovorin, whereas the investigational arm required six cycles of CMF. After 8 years of study, there was a significant improvement in disease-free survival and overall survival in favor of CMF.[161] The benefits of CMF were greater for women younger than 50 years of age.

A number of other clinical trials demonstrated significant improvement in disease-free survival with perioperative or postoperative adjuvant chemotherapy. The highly significant disease-free and overall survival benefit in the initial trials of adjuvant chemotherapy for patients with node-negative breast cancer was subsequently corroborated and expanded in a meta-analysis of all randomized trials involving node-negative breast cancer.[231] The mature results of these trials pointed out that these patients, previously considered to have an "excellent prognosis," had a 30 to 50% risk of recurrence after locoregional treatment. There is clear evidence that the rate of local and distant recurrence is decreased both by adjuvant combination cytotoxic chemotherapy[231] and by adjuvant tamoxifen.[289] Adjuvant systemic therapy with first-generation regimens reduces the rate of recurrence by approximately one-third, with a broad range. For example, among a group of women with a recurrence rate of 30%, adjuvant therapy would decrease the rate of recurrence to about 20%.

NSABP B-20 compared tamoxifen alone to tamoxifen plus methotrexate-fluorouracil or CMF in a group of 2,306 patients with node-negative, ER-positive breast cancer.[288] After 5 years of follow-up both the disease-free and overall survival were better for patients who received chemotherapy and tamoxifen than for those treated with tamoxifen only (p = .01 and .05, respectively). CMF appeared superior to MF, as also observed in B-19.

The EBCTCG meta-analysis and data from individual randomized trials clearly show that adjuvant chemotherapy, tamoxifen, or ovarian ablation improves survival for patients with node-negative breast cancer.[231,284,289] As is true for node-positive breast cancer, the combination of tamoxifen plus chemotherapy provides incremental benefits, as compared to either treatment alone, for patients with hormone receptor-positive, lymph node-negative breast cancer.[231,288]

Fisher and Redmon reviewed the prognosis of patients with node-negative breast cancer treated in NSABP protocols.[290] In the ER-negative group, the best disease-free survival (77%) was in patients with tumors 1 cm or smaller, and the poorest (55%) was in those with tumors 4.1 cm or larger. In patients with ER-positive tumors, the disease-free survival ranged from 82% in those with the smallest tumors to 55% in those with the largest tumors.[291]

Besides tumor size, other prognostic factors of value in node-negative patients in predicting the risk for recurrence and, consequently, the need for therapy are S-phase fraction (SPF) as determined by flow cytometry, histological or nuclear grade and progesterone receptor. In a multivariate analysis, all but nuclear grade predicted for survival.

In the previously described ECOG/Intergroup trial, patients with primary tumors < 1 cm in largest diameter had a 75% 10-year disease-free survival rate and a 79% overall survival rate. However, other investigators have reported markedly superior survival figures for patients with primary tumors < 1 cm and negative nodes, especially patients with tumors < 0.5 cm, negative nodes, and no other unfavorable prognostic indicators.[292] These observations prompted the analysis of data from five NSABP trials that focused on the prognosis of patients with node-negative tumors < 1 cm in largest diameter and the therapeutic effect of chemotherapy or hormonal therapy. One thousand, two hundred and fifty-nine patients were identified among the population registered in protocols B-06, B-13, B-14, B-19, and B-20.[293] Relapse-free survival rates were available at 8 years for the 1,024 patients with ER-negative tumors: They were 81% for those treated with surgery and 90% for those who received chemotherapy after surgery (p = .06). The 8-year relapse-free survival rates for women with ER-positive tumors treated with surgery alone, surgery plus tamoxifen and surgery, tamoxifen and chemotherapy were 86%, 93%, and 95%, respectively (p = .01 and .07). The authors concluded that even for this highly selected group of patients with favorable prognosis, the relapse rates were higher than previously reported and no subset could be identified that would not benefit from treatment.

The reports of the SEER program and several single-institution reports also highlight the excellent prognosis of patients with special, favorable histologic subgroups: those with pure tubular or mucinous carcinomas. Clearly, there are subgroups of patients with excellent prognosis for whom the benefit from adjuvant chemotherapy (and even tamoxifen) might be so minimal as to be matched or exceeded by the proportion of serious or life-threatening toxicity of the interventions. The challenge is to develop reproducible methods to identify such patients prospectively. One such approach was recently developed utilizing an RT-PCR assay based on 21 genes related to the estrogen receptor, proliferation, HER2 and several stromal proteases.[148] When this assay was performed on paraffin-embedded tissue blocks from patients who participated in several NSABP clinical trials for node-negative breast cancer, the results identified three prognostic subgroups of patients. About 50% of patients fell in the low-risk category with an estimated 10-year relapse rate of 6.8% when treated with adjuvant tamoxifen. This would suggest that about half of the patients with node-negative breast cancer have a low enough risk of recurrence to spare them the rigors of adjuvant chemotherapy. Subsequent extensions of the evaluation of this assay demonstrated that the benefits of tamoxifen were much greater in the low-risk group and those of chemotherapy in the high-risk group. Additional, prospective randomized trials to validate the utility of this assay are in progress or in the planning stage.

Although tamoxifen is successful in reducing local recurrence and distant disease in all categories evaluated, the proportionate reduction remains constant. Therefore, the likelihood of real clinical benefit diminishes as prognosis in general improves. With extremely small and favorable tumors, the use of systemic adjuvant therapies has as much rationale for prevention of new primary cancers as it does for treatment of the index cancer. Until new answers come from ongoing clinical trials, it is probably best in practice to review the available data with each patient concerning whether to use systemic therapy because of their putative "good" prognosis. As indicated earlier, the Adjuvantonline! software is available on the internet at no cost and estimates individual risk of recurrence and mortality as well as probability of benefit from relevant systemic adjuvant interventions.

Should tamoxifen be given to node-negative patients with ER-negative tumors? A recent EBCTCG meta-analysis failed to show a significant disease-free or overall survival benefit for the ER-poor group.[289] NSABP trial B-23 compared six cycles of CMF with four cycles of doxorubicin, cyclophosphamide (AC), with or without tamoxifen in a group of 1,800 patients with node-negative, ER-negative breast cancer. No differences were detected between the two chemotherapy regimens, and tamoxifen had no therapeutic effect in this ER-negative population.[291] The use of tamoxifen is not recommended for women with ER-negative tumors.

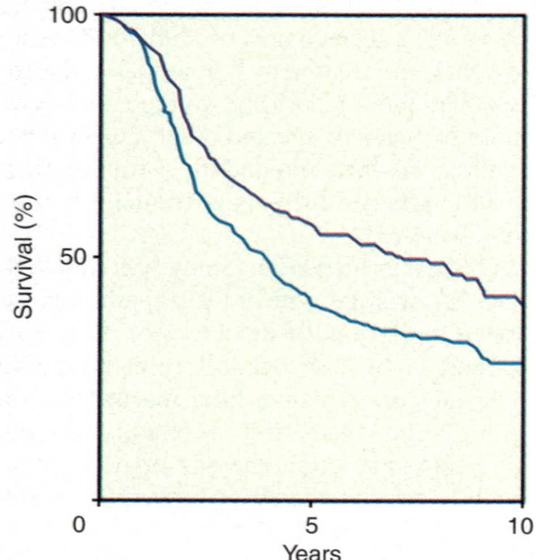

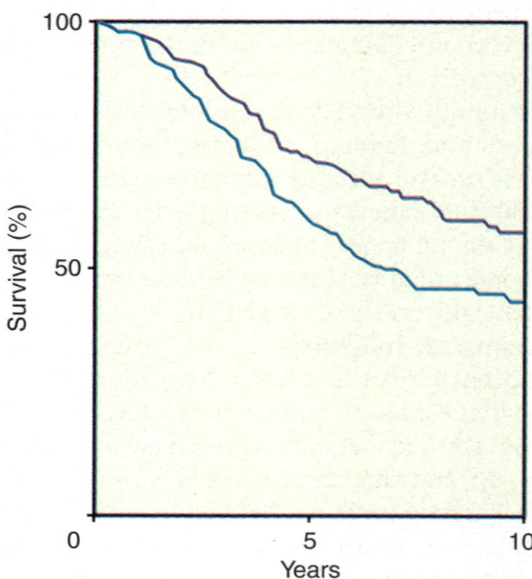

Figure 107-28 Disease-free *(left panel)* and overall survival *(right panel)* of patients with more than three metastatic nodes, who were less than 70 years old. They received four courses of moderately high-dose doxorubicin followed by eight cycles of CMF *(purple line)*, or two courses of CMF alternating with a cycle of doxorubicin four times *(blue line)*. This is the best example so far of a comparison of the Norton-Simon hypothesis and the Goldie-Coldman hypothesis.[296]

ADJUVANT THERAPY FOR NODE-POSITIVE PATIENTS **Chemotherapy** Over the past 30 years, controlled clinical trials provided compelling information in support of the use of adjuvant chemotherapy and adjuvant endocrine therapy for patients with node-positive primary breast cancer. Chemotherapy is considered the treatment of choice for patients with ER-negative breast cancer.[1,231] Although the magnitude of the benefit from chemotherapy is greater for younger women, significant reduction in risk of recurrence and death has been documented for women up to age 69 years. Furthermore, a recent retrospective review of four CALGB trials including women up to age 79 indicated that there was no association between age and disease-free survival.[294] The authors concluded that "age alone should not be a contraindication to the use of optimal chemotherapy regimens in older women who are in good general health."

Whereas CMF therapy was for several years broadly employed as the chemotherapeutic regimen for node-positive breast cancer patients, anthracycline-containing combinations have become more commonly employed. Several prospective randomized trials comparing doxorubicin (or epirubicin)–containing regimens versus non–anthracycline-containing regimens in the adjuvant setting for node-positive and also node-negative breast cancer, and the meta-analysis of all randomized trials has concluded that the anthracycline-containing regimens have superior efficacy.[231] Further analysis of existing randomized trials indicate that those anthracycline-containing regimens that include three or more drugs (FAC, CAF, FEC) have demonstrated superiority over CMF, whereas the doxorubicin (Adriamycin) and cyclophosphamide (AC) combination is equivalent to CMF.[295] Whether these differences in the various regimens are related to the additional drugs or the longer duration of therapy are questions currently being investigated in clinical trials.

HER2/neu overexpression has been associated with increased relapse rates after adjuvant therapy, and apparent relative resistance to certain types of cytotoxic treatment—for instance, the CMF regimen. Several retrospective analyses of prospective clinical trials have suggested that patients with *HER2/neu* overexpressing breast cancer benefit more from treatment with an anthracycline than with the CMF regimen.

NSABP protocol B-15 suggested that AC would be preferable to CMF.[295] Although of shorter duration and in general easier to administer than 6 cycles of CMF, this regimen is not more effective. Unfortunately, its broad acceptance has delayed the introduction of more effective anthracycline-containing regimens (FAC, CAF, FEC) in the management of primary breast cancer. Bonadonna and colleagues compared, in a randomized trial in high-risk patients, sequential administration of Adriamycin at 75 mg/m^2 for four courses followed by IV CMF for eight courses with alternating chemotherapy (two courses of IV CMF followed by one course of Adriamycin), for a total of 12 courses.[296] Results of this study after a median follow-up of 10 years demonstrated a significant improvement in disease-free survival with the sequential regimen versus the alternating regimen. This difference was translated into a significant difference in survival (Figure 107-28). Similar results were reported by other groups with sequential, non-cross-resistant chemotherapy. The Milan trial was an important clinical confirmation for the Norton-Simon hypothesis (as distinct from the Goldie-Coldman hypothesis) and stimulated the design of a later cooperative group trial (C9741).

The clinical evaluation of taxanes (paclitaxel [Taxol] and docetaxel [Taxotere]) in patients with metastatic breast cancer indicated that both agents have marked antitumor activity. Both taxanes retain a high degree of activity in anthracycline-resistant tumors.[297] Based on this information, clinical trials incorporating the taxanes into the adjuvant systemic therapy of high-risk primary breast cancer were initiated. The early results of the first large, multicenter, randomized clinical trial were recently reported.[298] In this study (CALGB 9344), patients with lymph node-positive primary breast cancer were treated with four cycles of doxorubicin at 60, 75, or 90 mg/m^2 plus cyclophosphamide at 600 mg/m^2 every 3 weeks for four cycles and then randomly assigned to no additional chemotherapy or four cycles of single-agent paclitaxel at 175 mg/m^2 every 3 weeks for four cycles. After a median follow-up of 69 months, no differences were seen in the doxorubicin dose escalation, making 60 mg/m^2 the preferred dose. A highly significant difference emerged in patients treated with doxorubicin/cyclophosphamide followed by paclitaxel who had a 17% reduction in odds of recurrence and an 18% reduction in odds of death, translating into a 6% absolute improvement in relapse-free survival and a 6% absolute improvement in overall survival at 7 years. The benefit of adding paclitaxel appeared greater for patients with ER-negative breast cancer than for those with ER-positive tumors. This regimen has been widely adopted in the community.

Several additional randomized trials evaluating the contributions of either paclitaxel or docetaxel to the management of primary breast cancer are maturing. In NSABP protocol B-28, patients with operable breast cancer and positive axillary nodes were randomly assigned to receive four cycles of AC or four cycles of AC followed by four cycles of paclitaxel. More than 3,000 patients were registered. After 5 years of follow-up, a significant difference in relapse-free survival favoring the paclitaxel arm has been reported. No differences in overall survival have been reported yet. Investigators from the University of Texas M. D. Anderson designed a randomized trial to determine the role of paclitaxel in adjuvant therapy. Patients with primary breast cancer received either 8 cycles of 5-fluorouracil, Adriamycin, and cyclophosphamide (FAC) or 4 cycles of paclitaxel followed by 4 cycles of FAC. Five hundred twenty-four patients were registered. After a median follow-up of 60 months, there was a non-significant trend in disease-free survival favoring the paclitaxel-FAC arm ($p = .09$).

The results of the initial analysis of NSABP B-27, in which 2,400 patients with operable breast cancer were randomly assigned to four cycles of AC followed by surgery, or four cycles of AC followed by four cycles of docetaxel and surgery, or four cycles of AC, followed by surgery and four cycles of docetaxel postoperatively, were recently reported. The analysis of this trial indicated that the addition of preoperative docetaxel to preoperative AC increased the overall clinical response from 85 to 91%, the complete clinical remission from 40 to 65% and the pathological complete remission rate from 13.7 to 25.6%.[258] In addition, updated results indicated a significant improvement in relapse-free survival favoring the preoperative docetaxel arm, without an improvement in disease-free or overall survival rates. A multicenter, multinational trial comparing docetaxel (Taxotere), Adriamycin, and cyclophosphamide (TAC) with FAC recruited 1,491 patients with node-positive primary breast cancer.[299] After a median follow-up of 55 months, a highly significant improvement in disease-free survival favoring TAC was reported: 75% versus 68% ($p = .001$). The survival also favored TAC: 87% versus 81% ($p = .008$).

Dose Intensification and Increased Cumulative Dose of Chemotherapy for Patients with Positive Axillary Nodes Among the hypotheses formulated to design more effective adjuvant treatment strategies, the contention that inadequate drug dose administration is a major factor responsible for the failure to achieve a greater therapeutic effect in responsive tumors led to several important clinical trials.

In 1984, Hryniuk and Bush presented arguments for recognizing the importance of dose intensity in the use of chemotherapy for metastatic breast cancer. They defined dose intensity as the amount of drug administered per unit of time, expressing intensity as milligrams per square meter per week using a single-drug regimen. They concluded that the higher the dose intensity, the higher would be the remission rate of patients with advanced breast cancer. Results from several randomized trials were considered to support the Hryniuk thesis. A prospectively randomized trial conducted by Tannock and colleagues to test the relationship between two dose levels of CMF and the remission rate in patients with advanced breast cancer significantly favored the standard rather than the half-dose regimen.

Using the same approaches that they employed for evaluating dose intensity in advanced disease, Hryniuk and his associates correlated the dose intensity of adjuvant chemotherapy with relapse-free survival. Their retrospective review of the literature led them to conclude in 1986 that, as in advanced disease, dose intensity of chemotherapy correlated with relapse-free survival, and that this correlation was independent of the number of positive nodes or menopausal status.

One randomized trial to evaluate the contribution of dose intensity to the results of adjuvant chemotherapy was conducted by the CALGB.[300] In that study, CAF was administered at a high dose for 4 months, at a moderate dose for 6 months, and at a low dose for 4 months. The protocol-specified high dose for CAF was 600 mg/m^2 on day 1 (C), 60 mg/m^2 on day 1 (A), and 600 mg/m^2 on days 1 and 8 (FU) of a 28-day cycle. Moderate and low dose rates were two-thirds and one-half, respectively, of the high dose for all three drugs. The results from the study indicated a significant difference in the 3-year disease-free survival between the high-/moderate-dose group and the low-dose group (high-dose group, 75 ± 2%; moderate-dose group, 70 ± 3%; low-dose group, 64 ± 3%; $p < .00001$).

When colony-stimulating factors became widely available, even higher intensification of cyclophosphamide could be achieved. NSABP developed two consecutive clinical trials to determine the effects of increasing the dose and dose-intensity of cyclophosphamide in the context of the AC combination. B-22 compared standard-dose AC (60 mg/m^2 and 600 mg/m^2, respectively), with 60 and 1200 for two doses and four doses respectively. B-25 adopted the highest dose level achieved in B-22 as the control arm and further increased the dose of cyclophosphamide to 2400 mg/m^2 for two doses or four doses in the other arms. There were more than 2,500 patients randomized in each study, and the average time on study exceeded 4 years; no statistically significant differences were observed for survival or disease-free survival.[301] Toxicity information from B-25 indicated that the maximum acceptable dose of cyclophosphamide given in the outpatient setting had been achieved. Sixteen patients treated on protocol B-25 were diagnosed with myelodysplastic syndrome (MDS) or acute myeloid leukemia (AML). The 4-year cumulative incidence of AML or MDS for patients on protocol B-25 was 0.87%, greater than that observed in previous NSABP studies using standard-dose cyclophosphamide (600 mg/m^2). Thus, the doxorubicin 60 mg/m^2 with cyclophosphamide 600 mg/m^2 regimen proved to be best.

Although dose-intensification has not improved the outcome of adjuvant chemotherapy to date, the application of the Norton-Simon hypothesis in one clinical trial provided improved results. In CALGB 9741, patients with lymph node-positive primary breast cancer were randomly assigned adjuvant chemotherapy with doxorubicin, cyclophosphamide and paclitaxel at standard doses given every 3 weeks, or every 2 weeks with filgrastim support.[302] After a median observation period of 2 years significant prolongation of relapse-free survival and overall survival was observed in the groups treated with the dose-dense or accelerated schedule. These improved results persisted after 5 years of follow-up.

The development of autologous bone marrow (and later, peripheral stem cell) support techniques and the recent availability of hematopoietic growth factors (G-CSF, GMCSF, and erythropoietin) made possible testing of the dose-outcome hypothesis along a much broader range of doses. Following the developmental trials of high-dose chemotherapy in metastatic disease and the early and apparently encouraging results in advanced breast cancer, several centers investigated the contribution of this approach to the management of patients with high-risk primary breast cancer. To evaluate the efficacy of high-dose adjuvant chemotherapy programs including hematopoietic stem cell support, several prospective randomized clinical trials were initiated over the past decade. The early results of several of these trials have now been reported. Although a few of the trials have suggested a modest decrease in recurrences in the high-dose chemotherapy arms, this has not been a universal finding, and morbidity and mortality have been higher in the high-dose arms. To date, no single trial has shown an improvement in survival. A meta-analysis of all randomized trials assessing the value of high-dose chemotherapy is currently in progress. These trials have confirmed that high-dose chemotherapy is a tolerable intervention with substantial morbidity, but a generally acceptable mortality risk. These studies have also shown the power of selection: The short-and intermediate-term outcome for the control groups of all of these adjuvant trials was much better than would have been expected compared to historical experience, based on the rigid criteria of admission to the study. The available evidence does not, however, support the superiority of high-dose chemotherapy for high-risk primary breast cancer.

Targeted Therapy for Patients with HER2-Positive Tumors The monoclonal antibody, trastuzumab, is the only specific therapy for HER2-positive cancers. After demonstration of its efficacy and safety in the management of HER2-positive metastatic breast cancer (vide infra), prospective trials were initiated to determine its contribution to the management of HER2-positive primary breast cancers. Four randomized trials were initiated: in all four trastuzumab was added, either simultaneously or sequentially, to conventional adjuvant chemotherapy and compared to the same chemotherapy without trastuzumab. After follow-ups ranging from one to two and a half years, three trials (NSABP B-31, N9831 and HERA) demonstrated such marked benefit that the trials were stopped and the results reported.[303] Compared to the arms without trastuzumab, trastuzumab-treated patients had about a 50% reduction in risk of recurrence in all three trials. These reductions were very highly significant, and translated into a 3 year absolute reduction in recurrences of 9 to 12% for the two North American trials, and an 8% difference at 2 years for the HERA trial. Despite the short follow-up, significant survival benefits were emerging in the North American trials. While one study suggested that simultaneous administration with chemotherapy was more effective than sequential administration after chemotherapy, definitive assessment of this question will require longer follow-up. There was increased cardiac toxicity associated with the administration of trastuzumab, especially in those treatment arms that called for simultaneous administration of chemotherapy and the antibody. Grade III/IV cardiac toxicity (congestive heart failure) was observed in 0.5 to 4.1% of patients in these trials. The reversibility of these cardiac events is uncertain at this point. However, at this time, the therapeutic benefits appear to exceed by far, the adverse events and for high-risk patients with HER2-positive breast cancer, trastuzumab should be incorporated into adjuvant systemic therapy.

Monitoring Disease Status after Adjuvant Therapy After completion of combined-modality therapy for primary breast cancer, patients are followed at regular intervals to detect recurrent disease, second primary tumors, or complications of therapy. During the first 2 years, patients are seen every 4 months, for the subsequent 3 years every 6 months, and yearly thereafter. A careful history and a complete physical examination are performed at each visit. A yearly mammogram of the remaining breast(s) completes the necessary evaluation for asymptomatic patients. Other tests are performed only if symptoms or physical findings warrant them. No advantage has been demonstrated for performing frequent or extensive imaging studies or tumor markers.[304] Controversy exists on this point, however, because it tacitly assumes that no advantage accrues from the early detection of metastatic disease. The advent of new therapies, such as aromatase inhibitors, monoclonal antibodies, tyrosine kinase inhibitors, and antiangiogenic compounds may change the efficacy of salvage therapy. This, in turn, might make early diagnosis of recurrent or metastatic disease an important step. Even if survival is not prolonged, maintaining an asymptomatic state by effective therapy may be possible and is important for many patients.

Endocrine Therapy **Tamoxifen** As for patients with lymph node negative breast cancer, there is clear evidence that administration of tamoxifen for 5 years is more efficacious than short-term therapy (for example, 2 years or less).[289] Tamoxifen administered for 5 years is equally effective in the management of women (and men) of any age with primary breast cancer with positive ER and/or PR assays. However, there is no evidence that prolonging the administration of tamoxifen for longer than 5 years provides greater benefit than administration for 5 years. There is compelling evidence to limit the use of tamoxifen to patients with ER-and/or PR-positive tumors.[289]

There are conflicting results about whether patients with *HER2/neu* overexpression have associated resistance to hormonal therapy with tamoxifen. Additional prospective clinical trials are needed to clarify this issue. At this time, there is no justification for withholding adjuvant endocrine therapy from patients with ER-positive and *HER2/neu*-positive tumors.

Evidence from the EBCTCG meta-analysis and from large randomized trials showed that tamoxifen combined with chemotherapy provides more effective systemic adjuvant treatment to patients with hormone receptor-positive breast cancer than either tamoxifen alone or chemotherapy alone.[289] Recent reports have indicated, however, that the benefit from chemotherapy is greater for patients with ER-negative breast cancer compared to those with ER-positive tumors. Furthermore, there is emerging information to suggest that patients with strongly ER-positive tumors that are well differentiated derive only marginal benefit from chemotherapy, while the effects of chemotherapy are greater for women with ER-negative or weakly positive tumors.[231] Some investigators have reported an increased risk of thromboembolic complications when tamoxifen and chemotherapy are administered simultaneously. The results of a prospective randomized trial addressing this specific issue were recently reported. SWOG trial 0100 randomized 1,477 patients with hormone receptor–positive breast cancer to receive either tamoxifen alone, concurrent tamoxifen and CAF, or sequential CAF followed by tamoxifen. At a median follow-up of 8.5 years, 8-year disease-free survival (DFS) estimates were 67% for sequential CAF followed by tamoxifen and 62% for concurrent CAF plus tamoxifen (p = .045).[305] The overall survival differences were not significant, although the trend favored the sequential arm. Both FAC plus tamoxifen arms were superior to tamoxifen alone. There were no differences in toxicity between the two combination arms. These results would indicate that the sequential administration of chemotherapy followed by tamoxifen would be the preferred strategy.

Adjuvant Ovarian Ablation Ovarian ablation lowers the odds of recurrence and death to levels that are quantitatively similar to those produced by chemotherapy, a benefit that is restricted to premenopausal women.[306] Ovarian ablation is not commonly employed as adjuvant therapy in the United States, however, largely because adjuvant chemotherapy produces a chemical ovarian ablation in the majority of patients anyway and because there is fear of the long-term effects of the premature menopause caused by ovarian ablation. A direct comparison of ovarian ablation and CMF chemotherapy in premenopausal women with primary breast cancer suggested equivalence of the two interventions. Further analysis indicated that for patients with ER-positive tumors, ovarian ablation was significantly more effective than CMF, whereas for patients with ER-negative breast cancer, CMF produced higher disease-free rates. The combination of chemotherapy and tamoxifen appears to provide superior disease control to patients with hormone receptor–positive breast cancer. However, the data in support of the superiority of the combination of chemotherapy and ovarian ablation for women under the age of 50 years are much less compelling.[306] A nonsignificant trend in some studies suggests that the combination of ovarian ablation and chemotherapy might be superior to chemotherapy alone for premenopausal women with ER-positive tumors. Additional studies to clarify the role of combined hormone therapy and chemotherapy are needed in this population.

The introduction of luteinizing hormone-releasing hormone (LHRH) analogs has also created new treatment opportunities.[272] In metastatic breast cancer, the efficacy of LHRH analogs has been validated: Their efficacy is similar to surgical or radiotherapy-induced ovarian ablation. An international group of investigators recently reported the results of a prospective randomized trial comparing the efficacy and tolerability of goserelin with IV CMF in premenopausal women with node-positive breast cancer.[307] After a median survival of 6 years, 42% of 1,640 women reported an event. In the subgroup with ER-positive tumors, the two treatments were equivalent (p = .94). As expected, in the ER-negative group, CMF was therapeutically superior to goserelin (p = .0006).

Another randomized trial included 2,631 premenopausal patients in a comparison of standard adjuvant therapy, with or without goserelin (ZIPP trial). With follow-up approaching 8 years, a trend favoring the goserelin arm approached statistical significance ($p = .08$). The Cancer Research Campaign conducts a trial comparing tamoxifen to goserelin and to the combination of tamoxifen and goserelin; the International Breast Cancer Study Group (IBCSG VIII) compares goserelin to CMF, and to CMF followed by goserelin; and the North American Intergroup has completed a randomized trial comparing CAF to CAF plus goserelin, and to CAF plus goserelin plus tamoxifen. These studies, and others assessing the contribution of other LHRH analogs alone or in combination with chemotherapy and/or tamoxifen will provide important guidance for the treatment of premenopausal patients with primary breast cancer. There are three important randomized trials assessing the place of LHRH analogs in the management of ER-positive premenopausal breast cancer. Known by their acronyms, the SOFT, TEXT and PERCHE trials will determine whether the combination of an LHRH analog and tamoxifen or an aromatase inhibitor is superior to tamoxifen alone for chemotherapy treated patients (SOFT), whether an LHRH analog and exemestane is superior to the LHRH analog plus tamoxifen, regardless of prior exposure to chemotherapy (TEXT) and whether chemotherapy adds to optimal combination endocrine therapy (PERCHE). These three studies represent a major international effort conducted in Europe, North America and several other regions of the world.

Aromatase Inhibitors Third-generation, selective AIs have potent effects on enzyme activity and reduce estrogen production in postmenopausal women by more than 90%. The updated results of the Arimidex, Tamoxifen, Alone or in Combination (ATAC) trial ($n = 9{,}366$) showed that, after 6 years of follow up, adjuvant anastrozole was significantly superior to tamoxifen in therapeutic efficacy and tolerance in a group of post-menopausal patients with positive or negative nodes.[286] Anastrozole was associated with a 17% relative reduction in risk of recurrences, a figure even greater for patients with ER-positive tumors. There was also a significant reduction in second primary breast cancers compared to the group of patients treated with tamoxifen. No survival differences were reported. Anastrozole was associated with fewer side effects than tamoxifen, although there were more fractures with anastrozole than with tamoxifen. Analysis after a median follow-up of 68 months confirmed the benefit of anastrozole over tamoxifen, with increased separation of the relapse-free survival curves. Additional follow up of this large clinical trial will contribute critical information to the choice of adjuvant hormonal therapy.

The Canadian MA-17 trial randomized postmenopausal patients with ER-positive breast cancer who had completed 5 years of adjuvant tamoxifen to 5 additional years of adjuvant letrozole or placebo.[308] After two and a half years of median follow-up, a 43% reduction in events was observed (HR: 0.57, 0.43–0.75, $p = .00008$). One year later, a significant survival benefit was reported for patients with positive lymph nodes. Another international group of investigators reported the results of a randomized trial of over 4,400 postmenopausal patients with ER-positive breast cancer who had completed 2 to 3 years of adjuvant tamoxifen. At that stage, they were randomly assigned to complete 5 years of tamoxifen or cross over to exemestane for the remainder of the 5 years.[309] After a 42-month median follow-up, there was a 32% reduction in recurrences ($p = .00005$) as well as a significant reduction in contralateral breast cancers, and a trend for a reduction in breast cancer deaths ($p = .08$). A smaller, Italian study of identical design using anastrozole and the combined analysis of an Austrian and a German clinical trial of very similar design provided confirmatory evidence in favor of a crossover to an aromatase inhibitor (anastrozole in these three trials) compared to continued tamoxifen therapy. Thus, evidence is overwhelming that a selective aromatase inhibitor must form part of adjuvant endocrine therapy for postmenopausal women with ER and/or PR-positive breast cancer.[310] Whether starting with an aromatase inhibitor is better than crossing over after some time on adjuvant tamoxifen remains to be established. Similarly, the role of aromatase inhibitors in the management of premenopausal women with hormone-responsive breast cancer is currently under evaluation in the SOFT, TEXT and PERCHE trials. The optimal duration of treatment with aromatase inhibitors is unknown and whether aromatase should be given sequentially or simultaneously with chemotherapy remains to be determined.

MANAGEMENT OF METASTATIC BREAST CANCER

General Consideration Patients with untreated metastatic breast cancer demonstrate considerable heterogeneity in the clinical course of their disease. Some have a rapidly progressing tumor that metastasizes to multiple vital organs and causes death within a few months after detection of the first metastasis. Other patients have an indolent disease course, with slow progression alternating with long periods of stability in metastasis to soft tissues or bone. Some of these patients survive in the absence of active treatment for more than 10 years.[126]

The organ localization of recurrent or metastatic disease and the extent of metastatic breast cancer partially determine the long-term prognosis.[311] The biologic characteristics of the tumor, including its growth rate and relative resistance or sensitivity to available interventions, also contribute to the outcome. Finally, the efficacy of individual treatment modalities determines the success of palliation and the duration of disease control. Most patients with overt distant metastases are presently incurable. However, among those who achieve a complete remission after standard chemotherapy, a few remain progression-free for extended periods of time, occasionally exceeding 20 years.[312] Complete remissions of long duration have also been reported after high-dose chemotherapy programs. The median survival of patients with metastatic breast cancer is 2 to 3 years. It is longer for patients who present with low-volume metastases to skin, lymph nodes, or bone and shorter for patients with multiple organ involvement, especially those with visceral organ (liver, brain, lung) involvement. The survival is longer for patients with ER-positive tumors and for those who achieve a complete remission with chemotherapy (3 to 4 years), compared to patients with hormone receptor-negative tumors or those who fail to respond to systemic treatment.[311]

Diagnostic Evaluation Patients with a previous diagnosis of primary breast cancer who present with findings suspicious for recurrent metastatic disease should be strongly considered for diagnostic biopsy, especially if there has been a long disease-free interval. A biopsy is helpful in excluding benign processes that frequently masquerade as metastases and in ruling out the development of other cancers. Furthermore, the tissue can be assayed for ER, PR, *HER2/neu* and other markers, to assist in treatment decisions. These markers may change from the time primary breast cancer was diagnosed and accurate determination will lead to better choice of therapy.

Metastases from breast cancer are usually multiple and frequently involve more than one organ site. Thus, surgical resection of metastatic lesions is not usually indicated for therapeutic purposes in breast cancer patients. However, it is advisable to remove resectable chest wall recurrences, a solitary brain metastasis in the patient with a long disease-free survival, or when histologic confirmation of a recurrence requires an open biopsy. Occasionally, resection of solitary metastasis to lung, liver or other organs can lead to a long recurrence-free period, especially when combined with systemic therapy.

Diagnostic tests and staging procedures are directed by the organ sites most frequently involved in metastatic breast cancer and by patient signs and symptoms. Documentation of initial metastatic sites is helpful in treatment planning and in later assessment of response to treatment. History and physical examination should focus on the detection of metastases on the chest wall, skin, remaining breast, regional and distant lymph nodes, axial skeleton, lungs, liver, and central nervous system. Laboratory evaluation should include a complete blood count, a platelet count, serum calcium, and liver and renal function studies. A chest radiograph and bone scan are obtained in most patients because these sites are commonly involved with metastatic breast cancer. Suspicious lesions on bone scan need confirmation by radiograph or by other diagnostic tests because of the high false-positive rate. Computed tomography and magnetic resonance imaging are also commonly used for this purpose. In the presence of bone pain unexplained by results of the bone scan, radiographs or MRI of the symptomatic area should be performed. Although bone scans are quite sensitive, they are of limited use in assessing treatment response in the first 2 to 4 months after the start of a new therapy. Increased intensity of uptake in existing lesions or even new lesions can signify either disease progression or disease regression with active bone healing. Bone scan changes must be corroborated by other information. Optimal monitoring of bone lesions during therapy should include symptoms, tumor markers (CA 27–29, CA 15-3, CEA), and radiographs (radiographs, computed tomograms) or MRI of involved areas. Routine brain and liver imaging procedures are expensive and are not indicated in the absence of symptoms, physical findings, or laboratory values suggesting involvement. Patients with ER-positive tumors are especially unlikely to suffer recurrence initially in the brain or liver. Serial blood tumor markers are recommended by some clinicians as an aid for monitoring disease status, especially when no measurable disease exists. The most frequently used markers are CA 153, CA 2729, and carcinoembryonic antigen (CEA). CA 153 and CA 2729 are more sensitive than CEA and are elevated in more than 70% of metastatic breast cancer patients, compared with 55% for CEA. All three markers can be moderately increased in certain benign diseases, especially liver disease, and with other neoplasms, including lung, gastrointestinal, and genitourinary cancers. Levels of all three markers do correlate significantly, although not absolutely, with changing disease status. Increasing levels may signal the need to perform more objective diagnostic tests to confirm worsening of the disease. Decreasing levels may provide greater confidence that a treatment is working. Modifying treatment based solely on changing marker levels, however, is often hazardous and in general should be avoided. For optimal utilization of markers, the clinician must be aware of the normal variations in measurements in the laboratory used (ie, the coefficient of variation) and confirm decreasing or increasing values with additional measurements over time. These markers are of limited value in following patients for recurrence after treatment of primary breast cancer and current guidelines do not recommend them. The average lead-time in the diagnosis of a recurrence is only 4 to 6 months, and there are no data to suggest that early institution of presently available systemic therapy at the time the marker rises affects survival. Positron emission tomography (PET) is an additional diagnostic modality with a number of potential advantages. First, it represents functional, as opposed to anatomical, imaging of tumor deposits. Second, PET scanning (like bone scanning) gives a whole body image and might detect previously unsuspected metastatic lesions. PET scanning might serve to differentiate malignant from benign solitary lesions, and might also be useful in monitoring response to therapy. PET scanning might also serve to advance our understanding of biological correlates and behavior of breast cancer. In combination with computed tomography or magnetic resonance imaging, PET will lead to more precise anatomical localization and functional imaging of suspected metastatic lesions. PET scanning was recently accepted for reimbursement by the federal health care financing authorities, reflecting its increasing importance in the diagnosis, staging, and monitoring of breast cancer.

GENERAL THERAPEUTIC GUIDELINES

Over the past four decades, systemic treatment with endocrine or cytotoxic agents became the fundamental treatment approach of the management of metastatic breast cancer.[1] Treatment decisions can be complicated because of the varied clinical courses among different patients and because many different therapies of apparently similar efficacy are available. Upon diagnosis of metastatic disease, the first task is to assess the extent of metastasis and to determine, based on available clinical information, the likelihood of rapid progression, which could cause vital organ failure or other catastrophic complications. In this sense, patients are often classified into low- and high-risk groups on the basis of clinical information and imaging. Those at low risk include patients who have had a long disease-free interval and have limited metastatic disease, often located in soft tissues or osseous sites. Some patients with limited visceral disease may also qualify. More often than not, low-risk patients are older and postmenopausal, and their tumors are hormone receptor positive. Other than bone pain, symptoms attributed to the disease are minimal. The age of the patient, the presence of comorbid conditions, the organ distribution and extent of metastatic disease, abnormalities in vital organ function, and the likelihood of hormone responsiveness all influence the selection of treatments. Patients with these low-risk characteristics are excellent candidates for hormone therapy as the first intervention for metastatic breast cancer, unless the tumor is clearly receptor negative.[1] Selection of endocrine therapy should be based on a high quality estrogen and progesterone receptor assay, preferably on tumor tissue obtained at the time the decision needs to be made. If such an assay is not available or tumor tissue cannot be obtained for the assay, patient and tumor characteristics are helpful in the determination of whether a tumor is likely to respond to hormonal manipulation. These characteristics include: age, disease-free interval, menopausal status, and location and extent of tumor deposits. Patients with ER-positive metastatic tumors have a 50% or greater probability of clinical benefit from hormone therapy, whereas those with clearly ER-negative tumors have marginal or no probability of response. Those with high ER concentrations have higher probabilities of an objective response than those with lower ER concentration, and patients with both ER and PR expression respond better than those with only one receptor expressed. Recently conducted prospective, randomized clinical trials comparing different hormonal agents as first-line therapy for metastatic breast cancer revealed that overall response rates, using strict definitions of complete and partial remission, ranged from 13 to 40%, even in patients with ER- and PR-positive tumors. Prolonged disease stability (including minor responses) was achieved in an additional 20 to 30% of patients during hormonal therapy. Stable disease for longer than 6 months is associated with survival durations similar to those of patients who achieve a partial or complete response with endocrine therapy. In case of an indolent clinical course, a negative estrogen receptor assay should prompt a repeat assay to make sure a false-negative result does not preclude potentially beneficial endocrine therapy.

Patients who achieve an objective regression or longstanding disease stability after first-line hormone therapy often benefit from second-line and sometimes third- and fourth-line hormonal interventions. The hormonal interventions of choice today include selective AIs such as anastrozole, exemestane, formestane, and letrozole, selective estrogen receptor modulators (tamoxifen, toremifene) and selective estrogen receptor downregulators (fulvestrant). Selective aromatase inhibitors are at least as effective as (and sometimes more effective than) tamoxifen for postmenopausal women and their safety profile is superior to that of tamoxifen. For premenopausal women, tamoxifen remains the endocrine agent of choice. Although oophorectomy is still practiced, it has largely been replaced by antiestrogens (tamoxifen, toremifene) and LHRH analogues (goserelin, leuprolide, buserelin, etc.); the latter provide an effect equivalent to chemical ovarian ablation. Progestins such as megestrol acetate and medroxyprogesterone acetate are also well tolerated when administered at the usual dose and schedule and have replaced estrogens, androgens, and corticosteroids. If an antiestrogen is chosen for first-line therapy, an aromatase inhibitor (for postmenopausal women) or ovarian ablation/suppression (for pre-menopausal women) is chosen for second-line therapy; third-line therapy would include an aromatase inhibitor of a different family (steroidal versus nonsteroidal) an ER downregulator (fulvestrant or Faslodex) or a progestin (megestrol acetate or medroxyprogesterone acetate); androgens or high-dose estrogens are usually chosen for fourth-line interventions or beyond. More commonly, if not used in the adjuvant setting, and aromatase inhibitor will be the first choice; upon progression, tamoxifen or an aromatase inhibitor of a different family (steroidal versus nonsteroidal) would be selected for second line, with an ER-downregulator (fulvestrant or Faslodex) being chosen for third-line treatment. Eventually, most patients with hormone-responsive breast cancer develop resistance to endocrine manipulation and become candidates for cytotoxic chemotherapy.

Ovarian ablation or suppression is also useful for ER-positive tumors in premenopausal women. This effect is permanent, inducing a menopausal state that permits the use of other endocrine therapies, including the selective AIs, for second- and third-line therapy. Although tamoxifen is an effective alternative to surgical ovarian ablation, the two treatments can be used in sequence, since response to one often predicts a high response rate to the other. The LHRH analogs offer another alternative for premenopausal patients by causing a chemical (or medical) castration.[272] Results to date suggest that serum estrogen concentrations are suppressed to postmenopausal levels and that response rates in advanced breast cancer are similar to those obtained after surgical ovarian ablation. Recent randomized trials and a meta-analysis of these trials indicated that the endocrine treatment of choice for premenopausal women with hormone-responsive metastatic breast cancer was a combination of tamoxifen with an LHRH analog.[313] The combination results in higher response rates and longer time to progression and survival than the LHRH agonist alone. One criticism of these trials is that none of them compared the combination to the sequential use of both components.

The time to obtain maximal response with endocrine therapy can be quite prolonged, and treatment should not be abandoned prematurely. Patients should be continued on a therapeutic trial for 6 to 12 weeks in the absence of progressive disease, before other therapies are used. Prolonged stable disease, without objective regression, is one form of clinical benefit associated with endocrine therapy. This effect is particularly acceptable in patients with minimal or no disease-related symptoms. A "tumor flare" with increased bone pain, swelling, or erythema of superficial lesions or hypercalcemia during the first week or two of therapy should not be confused with disease progression. Tumor flare is seen occasionally with endocrine treatments such as high-dose estrogens, tamoxifen, androgens, and progestins, and it frequently reflects hormone-sensitive disease. If tumor flare occurs early, within the first few weeks of starting treatment, endocrine therapy should continue under close observation and appropriate symptomatic support unless life-threatening conditions exist. Management of hypercalcemia with hydration and bisphosphonate therapy and liberal use of analgesics should be applied until the flare resolves.

For patients who initially respond to endocrine therapy, additional responses with second- and third-line endocrine interventions are common. This is especially the case for patients with indolent tumors. These patients should be offered additional endocrine therapies, in the absence of life-threatening disease, before changing to chemotherapy. Some patients derive many months or even years of high-quality life with sequential endocrine therapies. Few patients who fail to benefit from the initial endocrine treatment will respond to second- or third-line hormonal interventions. These patients, those who develop endocrine resistance, and those who manifest life-threatening disease should be offered chemotherapy. Table 107-20 documents the recommended sequence of hormonal treatments. For pre-menopausal women, tamoxifen, toremifene, or ovarian ablation appears to be the treatment of choice. LHRH analogues can substitute for ovarian ablation. The selection between these two modalities depends on patient preference, cost, possibility of follow-up, and predicted compliance with treatment. As indicated above, the concurrent combination of ovarian ablation/suppression and a selective ER modulator was recently proposed as the new standard of care for premenopausal women with hormone receptor–positive metastatic breast cancer. It is certainly a very reasonable choice, although its superiority to the sequential use of ovarian ablation/suppression and SERMs awaits additional evidence from clinical trials.

Table 107-20 Selection of Optimal Hormonal Therapy in the Management of Metastatic Breast Cancer

- Premenopausal patients
  - First-line therapy
    - Antiestrogens (tamoxifen of toremifene) or
      - Ovarian ablation (surgery, radiotherapy) or
      - Luteinizing Hormone-releasing hormone analogues (goserelin, leuprolide)
  - Second-line therapy:
    - If ovarian function persists after first-line therapy:
      - Ovarian ablation (surgery, radiotherapy) or
      - Luteinizing hormone-releasing hormone analogues (goserelin, leuprolide)
    - If ovarian function ceases after first-line therapy:
      - Aromatase inhibitors or Antiestrogens (tamoxifen of toremifene)
  - Third-line therapy
    - Estrogen receptor downregulator (fulvestrant
    - Progestins (megestrol acetate or
      - Medroxyprogesterone acetate)
  - Fourth-line therapy
    - Androgens (fluoxymesterone)
    - Estrogens
- Postmenopausal patients (including premenopausal women with irreversible amenorrhea)
  - First-line therapy
    - Aromatase inhibitors (anastrozole, letrozole or exemestane)
    - Antiestrogens (tamoxifen or toremifene)
  - Second-line therapy
    - Aromatase inhibitors of a different class
      - If antiestrogens were used in first line:
        - aromatase inhibitors
      - Selective estrogen receptor modulators
      - Selective estrogen receptor downregulator
  - Third-line therapy
    - Progestins (megestrol acetate, medroxyprogesterone acetate)
    - Androgens (fluoxymesterone)
    - Estrogens

Whereas some oncologists elect to treat selected patients with solitary lesions with locoregional therapy, the great majority of patients receive systemic therapy from the onset of overt metastatic disease. Certainly, symptomatic patients with widespread disease or aggressive visceral metastases should receive chemotherapy. In addition to bone pain, common symptoms include anorexia, weight loss, and reduced performance status. The disease-free interval for patients with high-risk or aggressive metastatic disease is typically short (less than 2 years), and the tumor is frequently ER negative. Carcinomatous meningitis, extensive liver metastases, lymphangitic lung metastases, or brain metastases usually signify aggressive disease that is unresponsive to endocrine therapy. Patients who have been diagnosed with aggressive disease should be treated with combination chemotherapy, even if the tumor contains ER and PR. Endocrine therapy is less likely to induce remission in this setting, and the more rapid response usually seen with chemotherapy is highly desirable. High-risk patients with receptor-positive tumors can be considered for endocrine therapy at a later date or if they fail to respond to chemotherapy. Patients with brain metastases should also receive regional therapy, usually whole brain irradiation or radiosurgery, which are very effective in palliating symptoms of central nervous system involvement.

Symptomatic Management Pain management, appropriate prevention of chemotherapy-related nausea, appropriate dietary intervention, and psychological support complete the multidisciplinary management of metastatic breast cancer. When used judiciously, all of these interventions contribute to the maintenance or improvement of quality of life while delaying the progression of metastatic breast cancer to the utmost.

Cytotoxic Chemotherapy for Metastatic Breast Cancer Chemotherapy is used in patients with aggressive disease who are not candidates for endocrine therapy and in those with tumors that no longer respond to endocrine therapy. Forty to 50% of previously untreated patients with metastatic breast cancer achieve an objective regression after single-agent anthracycline therapy. Mitoxantrone and the alkylating agents produce partial or complete responses in 30 to 40% of patients, whereas the other drugs are estimated to have a 20 to 30% response rate. Cisplatin was also reported to produce response rates of around 50%, but this information is based on two small studies; the reported response rate with carboplatin was around 30%. Mitomycin is another effective agent, although its use has decreased markedly since the development of the taxanes, vinorelbine, and other new drugs.

Anthracycline-based combinations appear to be more effective than CMF and CMFVP in several randomized trials, producing not only higher overall and complete remission rates but, durations of response (or time to progression).[314] In at least one of the studies, continuous rather than periodic treatment also provided a better quality of life, suggesting that a more substantial antitumor response had a greater influence on quality of life than the negative effects of the regimen-related toxicity. When all published randomized trials addressing the issue of shorter versus longer duration of therapy are pooled in a meta-analysis, there is an important trend for longer duration of survival favoring longer duration of treatment.

Combination chemotherapy regimens commonly used to treat metastatic breast cancer are shown in Table 107-21. The earliest attempts at combining chemotherapeutic agents were reported by Greenspan in 1958. Subsequently, the five-drug combination consisting of cyclophosphamide, methotrexate, 5-fluorouracil, vincristine, and prednisone (CMFVP, or the "Cooper" regimen) initiated the modern era of combined cytotoxic therapy. Multiple modifications in dose, schedule, and the individual drug components were reported over the next 30 years. The most commonly used modification of the original CMFVP regimen is the three-drug (CMF) combination, without vincristine or prednisone. The intravenous combination previously was shown to be inferior to the "classical" CMF.

Doxorubicin-containing combinations are probably the most commonly used regimens today. The 5-fluorouracil, doxorubicin (Adriamycin), cyclophosphamide (FAC) regimen came into use in 1973; shortly thereafter, other doxorubicin-containing combinations were reported. Randomized comparisons between CMF-like and FAC-like regimens have shown a higher response rate and longer time to progression for the anthracycline-containing regimens. Some individual studies and a recent meta-analysis of the contribution of doxorubicin to the "Cooper" regimen also showed a significant prolongation of survival.[315] However, anthracycline-containing regimens produce alopecia, nausea, and vomiting with greater frequency and severity, and cardiomyopathy occurs in a dose-dependent manner. Because the added benefits gained with FAC over CMF are modest, the decision about which regimen to choose should be individualized, based on the stated objectives of treatment, understanding and acceptance of a toxicity profile, and the physician's familiarity with a particular regimen.

Most of these drugs are myelosuppressive, resulting in substantial leucopenia and neutropenia. In addition, they are associated with nausea, vomiting, and, sometimes, mucositis and diarrhea. The anthracyclines produce almost universal (but transient) alopecia, and at high cumulative doses they produce cardiomyopathy. The incidence of cardiomyopathy, nausea, and vomiting decreases markedly when doxorubicin is administered weekly or as a 48- to 96-hour intravenous infusion rather than by bolus. Epirubicin is somewhat less cardiotoxic than doxorubicin; the risk of cardiotoxicity can also be reduced by the co-administration of a cardiac protector, dexrazoxane. Liposome-encapsulated anthracyclines are also considered to have lower cardiac toxicity. The vinca alkaloids and the platinum analogs produce peripheral neuropathy.

Over the past decade several new, moderately effective cytotoxic agents have completed clinical trials and been approved by the FDA for the treatment of breast cancer. These agents include the taxanes, paclitaxel and docetaxel, and the oral fluoropyrimidine analog, capecitabine.[297,316]

The Taxanes Paclitaxel and docetaxel are certainly among the most effective agents for the treatment of breast cancer.[297] Administered as a single agent, paclitaxel has demonstrated activity similar or superior to other first-line chemotherapy regimens. The FDA-approved method to administer paclitaxel is as a 1- to 3-hour infusion every 3 weeks, at the dose of 175 mg/m^2. However, over the past several years evidence has accumulated to show that the weekly administration of paclitaxel, usually at doses ranging between 80 and 90 mg/m^2/week, is more effective and better tolerated than the 3-weekly schedule. The weekly schedule is associated with a different safety profile, with a marked reduction in myelosuppressive and infectious complications, as compared to the 3-weekly schedule of administration. There is no compelling evidence that higher doses or more prolonged durations of administration modify the drug's efficacy in a substantial manner. Paclitaxel and docetaxel are substantially active in previously treated patients with metastatic breast cancer, including a 30 to 50% response rate in patients with anthracycline-resistant breast carcinoma. This degree of activity indicates that these two are the most effective drugs available for anthracycline-refractory breast cancer. Docetaxel and paclitaxel are not completely cross-resistant, and some patients derive clinical benefit from treatment with one taxane after developing resistance to the other. A direct comparison of the two taxanes was recently reported. In a prospective phase III trial 372 patients with metastatic breast cancer were randomly assigned to receive docetaxel 100 mg/m^2 IV every 3 weeks or paclitaxel 175 mg/m^2 IV every 3 weeks. Time to progression favored docetaxel (medians, 5.7 and 3.6 months, $p < .0001$) as did overall survival (15.4 vs 12.7, $p = .03$).[317]

Paclitaxel has been evaluated in combination with various other cytotoxic agents with demonstrated efficacy against breast cancer. In combination with doxorubicin, it produces a higher response rate and duration of response than either paclitaxel alone, doxorubicin alone, or the combination of doxorubicin/cyclophosphamide. However, schedule-dependent pharmacokinetic interactions and increased myelosuppressive and mucosal toxicity were reported by several investigators. Combinations of bolus doxorubicin and 3-hour paclitaxel were initially reported to have very high response rates, approaching 90%, but a 20% rate of congestive heart failure after six to eight cycles of treatment. Separating the administration of the two drugs by 6 to 18 hours reduces the risk of cardiac toxicity substantially. The initial very high response rates have not been replicated; in most trials with this combination, the overall response rate ranges from 50 to 70%. Other successful two-drug paclitaxel combinations included cisplatin, carboplatin, 5-fluorouracil, or vinorelbine.

Table 107-21 Commonly Used Combination Chemotherapy Regimens for Metastatic and High-Risk Primary Breast Cancer

Cytotoxic Agent	Dose (mg/m^2)	Route	Schedule and Days	Frequency
5-Fluorouracil	500	IV	Bolus, days 1 + 8	Every 21 days
Adriamycin (doxorubicin)	50	IV	Bolus, day 1, or 72-hr infusion (days 1–3)	
Cyclophosphamide	500	IV	Bolus day 1	
Cyclophosphamide	100	PO	Days 1–14	Every 28 days
Adriamycin (doxorubicin)	25	IV	Bolus, days 1 + 8	
5-Fluorouracil	500	IV	Bolus, days 1 + 8	
Adriamycin (doxorubicin)	60	IV	Bolus, day 1	Every 21 days
Cyclophosphamide	600	IV	Bolus, day 1	
Doxorubicin	50	IV	Bolus, day 1	Every 21 days
Paclitaxel	220	IV	3-hour infusion, day 2	
Doxorubicin	60	IV	Bolus, day 1	Every 21 days
Paclitaxel	200	IV	3-hour infusion, day 1	
Doxorubicin	60 or 50	IV	Bolus, day 1	
	+ +			
Docetaxel	60 75	IV	1-hour infusion, day 1	Every 21 days
Cyclophosphamide	100	PO	Days 1–14	Every 28 days
Methotrexate	40	IV	Bolus, days 1 + 8	
5-Fluorouracil	600	IV	Bolus, days 1 + 8	
Cyclophosphamide	600	IV	Bolus, day 1	Every 21 days
Methotrexate	40	IV	Bolus, day 1	
5-Fluorouracil	600	IV	Bolus, day 1	
Cyclophosphamide	600	IV	Bolus, day 1	Every 21 days
Novantrone (mitoxantrone)	12	IV	Bolus, day 1	
5-Fluorouracil	600	IV	Bolus, day 1	
Mitomycin	8	IV	Bolus, day 1	Every 42 days
Mitoxantrone	8	IV	Bolus, days 1 + 22	
Methotrexate	35	IV	Bolus, days 1 + 22	
Vinorelbine	25	IV	30-minute IV infusion on days 1 and 8	Every 21 days
Doxorubicin	50	IV	Bolus, day 1	
Docetaxel	100	IV	Over 1 hour, day 1	Every 21 days
Capecitabine	2,000	PO	Daily for 14 days	
Paclitaxel	175	IV	3 hours, day 1	Every 21 days
Gemcitabine	1,250	IV	Bolus, days 1 + 8	

IV = intravenous; PO = oral.

Docetaxel as a single agent produces objective responses in up to 60% of patients with metastatic breast cancer previously unexposed to chemotherapy. The usual method of administering docetaxel is a 1-hour infusion every 3 weeks, at a dose of 75 to 100 mg/m^2. As for paclitaxel, there is great interest in the weekly administration of docetaxel, since this schedule is associated with less myelosuppressive and musculoskeletal toxicity. However, weekly administration is frequently complicated by asthenia, epiphora, nail changes and fluid retention. Docetaxel as a single agent produced a higher response rate and longer time to progression than full-dose doxorubicin, although survival was equivalent for the two drugs. Docetaxel was superior to the combination of vinblastine and mitomycin for all end points considered and superior to the combination of methotrexate/5-fluorouracil in terms of response rate and time to progression. Docetaxel combinations with doxorubicin or epirubicin have also demonstrated substantial efficacy without an apparent increase in cardiac toxicity. A recent preliminary report of a randomized comparison of docetaxel/doxorubicin with cyclophosphamide/doxorubicin in first-line chemotherapy for metastatic breast cancer showed that the former combination was associated with a higher response rate and longer time to progression than the latter.[318] However, no prolongation in overall survival has been reported. Docetaxel is also under evaluation in combination with cisplatin, carboplatin, cyclophosphamide, vinorelbine, 5-fluorouracil, and other agents.

Vinorelbine The Vinca alkaloid vinorelbine has undergone extensive clinical evaluation that showed, in addition to excellent tolerability, objective response rates ranging from 40 to 50% in first-line and 20 to 35% in second-line therapy; however, it has not gained FDA approval for treatment of breast cancer, although it is widely used for the treatment of advanced breast cancer. Vinorelbine is effective in patients with anthracycline-refractory tumors, although, based on indirect comparisons, it would appear to be less effective in this situation than the taxanes. Vinorelbine has been extensively evaluated in combination with anthracyclines, 5-fluorouracil, cisplatin, and the taxanes. The activity of these combinations appears similar to the activity of CMF or even FAC; however, only the vinorelbine/doxorubicin combination has been directly compared to a standard regimen.

Capecitabine Capecitabine is a prodrug that is metabolized to 5-fluorouracil upon absorption from the gastrointestinal tract. Its oral bioavailability is excellent and it is a well-tolerated and effective palliative regimen. Capecitabine retains antitumor activity after prior therapy with an anthracycline-containing regimen and a taxane.[316] Capecitabine is under evaluation in comparative trials against other effective single agents (eg, paclitaxel), in combination therapy and in the adjuvant setting. A recent report showed that the addition of capecitabine to single-agent docetaxel resulted in a significant increase in objective response rate, time to progression and overall survival. Other interventions that mimic the continuous intravenous infusion of 5-fluorouracil (S-1) are also under active development.

Gemcitabine Another new drug with considerable antitumor activity in metastatic breast cancer is gemcitabine. This agent was approved by the FDA for the treatment of metastatic breast cancer in combination with paclitaxel. Gemcitabine produces responses in about 40% of patients with untreated metastatic breast cancer and in 20 to 30% of those with previous exposure to chemotherapy, including anthracycline-refractory tumors. The combination of gemcitabine and doxorubicin was recently reported to have substantial antitumor activity and good tolerance. Triple combinations, including gemcitabine, epirubicin and paclitaxel (Taxol) (GET) have also been reported to have very high response rates and overall, excellent antitumor activity.[319]

Between 50 and 75% of patients with metastatic breast cancer have responses to firstline chemotherapy.[1] In general, patients with a good performance status, normal organ function, and limited extent of disease are more likely to respond than patients with the opposite characteristics. Only 15 to 20% of patients will achieve a complete remission, and most of those patients will develop progressive disease within the subsequent 5 years. About 10% of all complete remissions achieved with anthracycline-containing regimens last more than 10 years.[312]

COMBINED HORMONAL THERAPY AND CHEMOTHERAPY Because hormonal therapy and cytotoxic therapy have different mechanisms of action, and because the two modalities produce different patterns of toxicity, it was hypothesized that their combined use might result in enhanced therapeutic efficacy without increased toxicity. Numerous prospective randomized trials have been conducted using a combination of simultaneous chemotherapy and hormonal therapy. In most cases, the hormonal agent was either ovarian ablation (or LHRH analogues) or tamoxifen, although several trials used progestins or androgens. Some of these trials showed increased response rates, and a few demonstrated a slight prolongation of response duration. However, most individual trials failed to demonstrate an increase in median survival or in long-term survival in patients with metastatic breast cancer. A recent meta-analysis of randomized clinical trials in the setting of metastatic breast cancer suggested, however, a modest but significant prolongation of survival with simultaneous combination of chemotherapy and endocrine therapy.[315] However, this modest advantage must be considered in the context of increased toxicity with combined therapy. Based on these results, the sequential use of hormonal therapy and chemotherapy is considered the optimal way to provide palliative therapy to patients with metastatic breast cancer.

TARGETED THERAPIES FOR METASTATIC BREAST CANCER Trastuzumab, a humanized monoclonal antibody with high binding affinity to the extracellular domain of the HER2 oncoprotein is the only targeted therapy that is in general use today.[79] Trastuzumab was also evaluated in a prospective, randomized trial of first-line chemotherapy for metastatic breast cancer.[280] In this study, patients were offered treatment with doxorubicin and cyclophosphamide if no prior chemotherapy exposure had occurred, or single-agent paclitaxel, if the patient had received prior anthracycline therapy. In addition, patients were randomly assigned to receive trastuzumab by intravenous administration once a week. Four hundred sixty-nine patients were treated. The objective response rates were 32% with chemotherapy alone, and 50% with chemotherapy and trastuzumab ($p < .001$). Time to progression, duration of response, time to treatment failure and overall survival were all significantly improved by the addition of trastuzumab to chemotherapy. The overall survival improvement was particularly gratifying, since over 65% of patients in the control arm of the study received trastuzumab after progressive disease was documented. On the basis of these data, the FDA approved the use of trastuzumab for treatment of patients with HER2-positive metastatic breast cancer. A second randomized trial compared single-agent docetaxel with docetaxel combined with trastuzumab: the combination significantly improved all endpoints. Several other trastuzumab-containing combinations are under clinical evaluation, and the agent is also being explored in adjuvant systemic therapy of high-risk primary breast cancer. Trastuzumab also potentiates chemotherapy with platinum derivatives, vinorelbine and gemcitabine, but not with capecitabine. Based on a randomized trial demonstrating superior survival associated with the addition of carboplatin to paclitaxel and trastuzumab, the triple drug combination is considered by many the initial treatment of choice for patients with HER2-positive metastatic breast cancer. Because the antibody also attaches to heart muscle, heart failure can occur.

A monoclonal antibody with high binding affinity to the vascular endothelial growth factor (VEGF), bevacizumab, was introduced to clinical trials several years ago. As a single agent administered to patients with metastatic breast cancer who had received treatment with conventional therapies, bevacizumab was associated with objective responses in about 10% of patients. Prospective randomized trials to determine its role in the management of metastatic breast cancer were initiated. In one phase III trial, patients with previously treated metastatic breast cancer were offered capecitabine alone or in combination with the anti-VEGF antibody. While objective responses were almost twice as high in the combination arm compared with capecitabine alone, no differences in time to progression or overall survival were detected. In a second phase III trial, patients with metastatic breast cancer who had received no prior treatment were offered paclitaxel alone or in combination with bevacizumab. The preliminary results showed a highly significant improvement in response rate (14 to 28%), as well as a significant prolongation in time to progression (from 6 to 11 months, $p < .001$).[302] An emerging survival trend favoring the bevacizumab arm was also observed. The addition of bevacizumab was associated with hypertension, bleeding, proteinuria, and fatigue in a small number of patients.

SPECIAL ISSUES REGARDING THERAPY

Management of Isolated Local-Regional Recurrence If an isolated chest wall or regional lymph node recurrence is detected, biopsy confirmation and surgical resection are recommended. If not irradiated earlier, radiotherapy to the chest wall and involved regional lymph node-bearing area is indicated. Should the tumor be hormone receptor positive, adjuvant endocrine therapy has been shown to reduce the risk of additional recurrences. Although no controlled trial has been conducted to assess its efficacy, some centers advocate the use of "adjuvant chemotherapy" in these situations to reduce the risk of recurrence and death.

Osseous Metastases Osseous metastases represent the commonest type of metastatic spread in breast cancer: Up to 80% of patients with metastatic breast cancer will develop bone metastases during the clinical course of the illness. Bone metastases are the most frequent source of morbidity and disability related to breast cancer. Radiotherapy to painful sites of bone metastasis or impending fracture sites in weight-bearing bones is commonly used in association with systemic treatments. Bisphosphonates are effective inhibitors of osteoclast activation and, therefore, of bone resorption and the development of osteolytic bone metastases. Treatment with pamidronate, zoledronic acid, or clodronate alone was shown to produce pain relief and radiographic evidence of healing in 20 to 25% of patients with osteolytic bone metastases from breast cancer in several phase II clinical trials. Several large randomized clinical trials demonstrated that the administration of pamidronate disodium combined with chemotherapy or hormone therapy delays the appearance and reduces the severity of bone-related complications of breast cancer. Similar data exist for clodronate, another second-generation bisphosphonate, and more recently, for ibandronate and zoledronic acid.[320] Zoledronic acid, 4 mg IV over 15 minutes every 4 weeks is the preferred bisphosphonate regimen for management of patients with bone metastases. This regimen is more effective and more convenient than pamidronate. Bisphosphonate therapy should start at the first evidence of osteolytic bone metastases and be continued during the clinical course of metastatic breast cancer.

Several bone-seeking radionuclides (^{89}strontium chloride, ^{153}samarium-EDTMP) were shown to target osseous metastases and provide temporary pain relief for patients with systemic bone metastases. Because of protracted myelosuppression associated with these agents, they are often reserved for third-line therapy and beyond.

Pregnancy and Breast Cancer Among women with breast cancer, 1 to 2% are pregnant at the time of diagnosis, their average age being around 35 years.[321] There is no evidence that pregnancy is associated with either the development or the progression of breast cancer, since the patient's prognosis is related to the stage of the disease rather than to the pregnancy itself. The generally worse prognosis for women diagnosed with breast cancer during pregnancy can be attributed to the fact that a diagnosis in such patients is often delayed so that by the time the disease is detected, it has already progressed to an advanced stage. Changes in the breasts during pregnancy that make cancer difficult to detect, as well as the reluctance of physicians to perform mammography in pregnant patients, may account for the delay in diagnosis. With the use of abdominal shields, however, radiation exposure to the fetus is negligible, and adverse effects to the fetus have not been observed with mammography. Therefore, the diagnostic procedures performed in women who present with suspected breast cancer during pregnancy should be the same as those used for non-pregnant women. Similar results can be obtained with non–radiograph-based imaging techniques, such as sonography or magnetic resonance imaging. Treatment is generally similar to that prescribed for non-pregnant breast cancer patients. Although modified radical mastectomy might be considered the treatment of choice in order to avoid the need for postoperative radiation, there is a role for lumpectomy followed by breast irradiation after delivery, particularly in late pregnancy. Avoiding chemotherapy during the first trimester of pregnancy, when organogenesis is taking place, is strongly recommended. In all cases of breast cancer diagnosed during pregnancy, decisions should be based on close interaction between breast surgeon, obstetrician, and medical oncologist, after clear discussions with the patient, to understand and respect her belief and value system, while providing the highest probability of cure (see chapter 63, "Pregnancy and Cancer"). Termination of the pregnancy is rarely warranted, since combined modality therapy can usually be delivered with proper care. If the diagnosis occurs during late pregnancy and the tumor is a low-risk malignancy, the patient can be treated after delivery. In a group of women with a similar stage of breast cancer, there is no significant difference in prognosis between those who are pregnant and those who are not. With regard to subsequent pregnancies for patients who have had breast cancer, several authors have suggested a waiting period of 3 to 5 years, depending on the nodal status of the cancer. Findings from recent studies, however, fail to show a worse prognosis in breast cancer patients who subsequently become pregnant; some have even indicated a better prognosis for such patients compared to breast cancer patients who do not have subsequent pregnancy, but this is best explained by self-selection—patients wait to see if they will be well for a time, so early failures are removed from consideration.

Male Breast Cancer Carcinoma of the breast occurs infrequently in men in the developed countries, the incidence being about 1% of that in women.[2,3] In several African countries, the incidence in hospital registries is 5 to 15% that of female breast cancer. Breast cancer accounts for about 0.1% of all cancers in American men and rarely occurs in males under the age of 40, with the average age at onset about 60 years. Familial associations have been reported. Between 4 and 40% of male breast cancers have recently been reported to have mutations in the *BRCA2* gene.[322] Most are frameshift mutations that result in truncated proteins. Several factors have been implicated in the etiology of the disease, including history of prior radiation, hyperestrogenism, and Klinefelter syndrome. The association between gynecomastia and male breast cancer is less clear.

Histologic tumor characteristics in males are similar to those in females, with two-thirds of patients presenting with intraductal carcinoma. LCIS, however, is not observed in males. ERs have been found in up to 84% of tumors in males who have the disease. The most common presenting symptoms include breast mass, bloody nipple discharge, nipple retraction, axillary mass, and distant or local pain. Breast cancer usually presents in a more advanced stage in men than in women. However, operability rates of from 74 to 95% have been reported. Radical mastectomy has been recommended because of the frequent involvement of the pectoralis major muscle; however, if the muscle is not extensively involved, a modified radical mastectomy can be performed. Postoperative radiation therapy to the chest wall is advocated by some for local control. Patterns of metastasis are similar to those in females. The prognosis for breast cancer in men depends on lymph node status, size of the tumor, and duration of symptoms prior to diagnosis.

The treatment for metastatic breast cancer in men has changed during recent years.[323] Although orchiectomy was once the standard therapy for advanced disease, it has been replaced by tamoxifen as the initial therapy since ER-positive tumors are predominant in males.

As noted earlier, breast cancer is more often hormone receptor—positive in men than in women. This also has been confirmed clinically by the more frequent observation of responses to hormonal therapy in men as compared to women. Tamoxifen is the hormonal treatment of choice for male breast cancer today. More than 50% of unselected patients with metastatic breast cancer respond, as do 70 to 80% of patients with ER-positive tumors.

The experience with other SERMs in male breast cancer is quite limited. Other hormonal agents with demonstrated efficacy against metastatic breast cancer in men are progestins, aminoglutethimide, estrogens, and antiandrogens. Selective aromatase inhibitors have not been formally evaluated in male breast cancer. Case reports suggest stability of metastatic disease but no objective responses to date. Anecdotal reports have shown antitumor activity of androgens and corticosteroids in men with breast cancer. However, these reports are based on only a few patients. Combined hormonal therapy has not been extensively evaluated in males.

In cases of progression after an initial remission with tamoxifen, orchiectomy or gonadotropin-releasing hormone agonist treatment is indicated, with other modalities such as chemotherapy being reserved for further failures. Chemotherapy as the initial therapy for metastatic disease has efficacy similar to that observed in women with breast cancer.

Adjuvant therapy decisions are made on the basis of stage, age, ER/PR, and comorbid conditions. Because no randomized trials have been conducted in male breast cancer, decisions are based largely on extrapolation from female breast cancer.

Inflammatory Breast Cancer At present, the initial treatment of choice for inflammatory carcinoma is chemotherapy followed by surgery and/or radiation therapy for local control in patients who show a response to chemotherapy. However, prolongation of survival has not been shown to be attributable either to surgery or to radiation therapy in this form of the disease.

Inflammatory breast cancer (IBC) is a locally advanced and particularly aggressive form of breast cancer.[324] This disease constitutes 1 to 6% of all newly diagnosed breast cancers (probably closer to 2% in the United States). The diagnosis of IBC is based on a clinical triad of erythema, edema of the skin of the breast (peau d'orange), and ridging, a tactile sensation caused by engorged dermal lymphatics. IBC's evolution is usually rapid, often taking less than 3 months to go from the first detectable abnormality to the establishment of a diagnosis. Because an underlying mass is frequently absent, IBC is often mistakenly treated with antibiotics on the working assumption that the patient has mastitis. The inflammatory process may extend off the breast onto the adjacent chest wall. A core needle biopsy usually provides a definitive diagnosis. Before the advent of systemic adjuvant therapy, the 5-year survival rate for patients with IBC after surgery, radiotherapy, or a combination of the two was reported by multiple investigators to be less than 5%.[255] Median survival seldom reached 1 year, and rapid tumor dissemination to multiple organs was the rule. Since the introduction of primary chemotherapy into the multidisciplinary management for IBC, the prognosis has improved. Most cases of IBC respond dramatically to chemotherapy; in addition, more than 90% of patients with IBC can be rendered free of locoregional disease with a combination of either chemotherapy and surgery or chemotherapy and radiotherapy, and 5-year survival rates now routinely exceed 30% and sometimes 50%. Long-term follow-up of multidisciplinary protocols from several institutions has shown that 25 to 30% of IBC patients survive progression-free for at least 10 and sometimes 15 years. Radiotherapy is a critical component of combined modality therapy for this subset of breast cancer. Although IBC is usually ER-negative, patients with ER-positive IBC should be offered endocrine therapy after completion of chemotherapy and local-regional treatments. Although no randomized trials have been performed involving patients with IBC, those statistics represent such a dramatic departure from the natural history following locoregional therapy only that they provide reasonably compelling evidence of progress.

Despite improvements in both local and systemic control of locally advanced breast cancer and IBC achieved with modern combined-modality treatments, the majority of patients still die of the disease. Therefore, multiple attempts are under way to improve the odds of eradicating micrometastases. Among them, consolidation therapy with paclitaxel, docetaxel, vinorelbine, and several molecularly targeted agents is being tested.

Treatment of the Elderly Few studies have been carried out to clearly define the management of elderly women with breast cancer. Perhaps one of the reasons such efforts have failed relates to difficulty in defining the word "elderly." One may relate this to chronologic age, physiologic age, or life expectancy. Some of the more commonly asked questions relate to whether axillary dissection is necessary in such patients. It is our contention that axillary dissection need be carried out only for (1) determining prognosis, (2) providing information for choosing a particular therapy, or (3) local disease control. In elderly women with clinically negative axillary nodes who will receive systemic therapy, there is little justification for performing an axillary dissection.

Another issue relates to whether endocrine therapy should be given to all elderly patients, regardless of hormone receptor status. At present, the use of aromatase inhibitors or tamoxifen has become standard therapy for the management of women with hormone receptor–positive tumors, regardless of age. Endocrine therapy is not indicated for patients with hormone receptor-negative tumors.

A question frequently asked is whether less than full dose chemotherapy should be given to elderly patients. Unless full-dose chemotherapy can be given, no chemotherapy should be administered. The use of less than full-dose chemotherapy will usually be ineffective, at the cost of unnecessary toxicity. In the CALGB study, however, women who received doxorubicin in a CAF regimen at a dose of 30 mg/m^2 for 4 weeks × 4, did as well as those who received 60 mg/m^2 × 4 or 40 mg/m^2 × 6 if their *HER2/neu* assay was negative. A question also has been raised regarding what chemotherapy is best and how long it should be used. Only recently, has there been interest in devising protocols to evaluate new drugs that may be less toxic in such patients. Vinorelbine (Navelbine) is one such agent; capecitabine (Xeloda) is another commonly used oral agent, whereas others have considered the use of MF as described elsewhere (NSABP B-13). An ongoing trial will compare single-agent oral capecitabine with classical CMF or AC in the adjuvant treatment of patients older than age 65.

PERSPECTIVES

With the rapid rate of change in basic and clinical cancer research, it is sometimes difficult to see things in perspective. Some seemingly new ideas have really been around a long time, and some concepts seem to gain acceptance very slowly. For the first half of the twentieth century, breast cancer thinking was stuck in an anatomic mode leading to radical surgical concepts, and clinical research amounted to little more than counting cases and outcomes in tumor registries. With the advent of chemotherapy and modern endocrine therapy and the realization that breast cancer was more likely to be a systemic disease and that it was a disorder of growth regulation, new ideas quickly took hold.

One avenue of research was to determine the optimal amount of surgery necessary, and determine the indications of and the benefits from radiation therapy. A second was to combine surgery with systemic adjuvant systemic treatments to improve cure rates. When attention then focused on metastasis and issues of drug resistance, there began a happy convergence of basic and clinical researchers into what is now called translational research. From today's perspective, it is easy to see that we have made the transition from anatomic to biologic thinking and have many new and exciting avenues for further progress. In this chapter, we reviewed some of the new biologic approaches with adjuvant systemic therapy, including the recent introduction of trastuzumab into adjuvant therapy. We also reviewed the potential application of preoperative chemotherapy as a drug sensitivity test, and, perhaps most important for the immediate future, in the use of tamoxifen as a chemopreventative agent. In this sense, tamoxifen is presented not as a simple antiestrogen but as a biologic growth factor inhibitor. Another investigative strategy would evaluate other interventions that might interfere with the initiation and/or promotion of breast cancers. Although there are several candidates for evaluation (eg, low-fat diets, other SERMs, COX-2-inhibitors or retinoids), one category that is particularly interesting involves drugs that act as inhibitors of aromatase.

It is clear that systemic therapies have become more effective, and the relative importance of surgery and radiation therapy has shifted. It is easier to obtain local control than it is to control metastases, even the micrometastases at which adjuvant therapies are aimed. Therefore, efforts must be directed at these systemic therapies. New cytotoxic agents, such as capecitabine, gemcitabine, liposomal doxorubicin, vinorelbine have already been tested and show promise. Other efforts to devise progressively better regimens for systemic treatment, both for adjuvant and advanced disease, should certainly persist. The power of endocrine interventions has become manifest as novel agents are moved into the adjuvant setting. Within the past 2 years, the aromatase inhibitors have changed completely our approach to adjuvant endocrine therapy. As our understanding of the crosstalk between the various growth factor pathways, including the estrogen-driven signaling increases, combined therapies will become more effective and better targeted to individual needs.

New therapeutic modalities, such as immunomodulators and vaccines, may one day require evaluation. Targeted immune cells may be used to introduce cytotoxic agents, such as tumor necrosis factor, directly to tumor cells, or to alter tumor cells genetically in order to suppress their growth. Such approaches may be tested alone or in conjunction with chemo- and hormonal therapeutic agents of proven value. Evaluation of methodologies for overcoming drug resistance and for modulating the action of chemotherapeutic agents based on pharmacologic principles should also continue, as should testing of currently available modalities in novel ways.

Efforts at improving our ability for early diagnosis continue. Screening mammography continues to be the centerpiece of approaches to early diagnosis, although magnetic resonance imaging has shown remarkable promise, especially in high-risk groups, such as those with familial syndromes. The exact dimension of the benefits of screening is still controversial, but there is evidence that breast cancer mortality is reduced, at least in women aged 50 to 74. There is marked interest in proteomic approaches to identify markers of risk to select appropriate subjects for mammographic screening or to develop early diagnostic tests based on serology. We must continue to make progress in the areas of breast cancer prevention and of early treatment of systemic metastases as described above. One happy, but still troubling aspect of successful mammographic screening is the continued increase in the proportion of small tumors at diagnosis. Sorting out how much treatment is appropriate in these cases will continue to occupy our attention.

It is likely that any discussion of breast cancer will have as its major component information regarding the mechanisms and feasibility of chemoprevention. The results of the NSABP BCPT, now confirmed by the IBIS study, are of fundamental importance in taking us in new directions. These findings are arguably one of the most important public health advances in breast cancer, mainly because they demonstrate that it is feasible to intervene and reduce breast cancer incidence with a pharmacologic agent, which opens new avenues for research. Ongoing studies in this area (STAR and IBIS II trials) will define the best choice of agents for chemoprevention and identify the role of aromatase inhibitors in primary and secondary prevention. Breast cancer results from DNA damage, and, although it is possible that lifestyle changes can diminish this slightly, it will take intervention with active agents, with their risk of side effects, to control or reverse this fundamental cause.

Last, but probably most important because it brings us to the core of the problem, are all of the new advances in molecular biology and genetics. Along with the discovery of the *BRCA,* genetic mutations are other important insights into how genes work. Among these are p53, the EGFR family, IGF, telomerase, the whole family of targets for SERMS, and mechanisms of angiogenesis and its control. The *BRCA* story has moved from clinical studies and pattern searching to investigations of mechanisms, now known to be in the realm of DNA repair. This also raises interest in the genes involved in sporadic breast cancer. Understanding the *BRCA* mutations and their relationship to causation and progression of breast cancer might expose targets of opportunity for research. Better fundamental understanding of the etiology and pathogenesis of breast cancer should provide new approaches that are likely to have a major impact on therapy, diagnosis, and prevention. As it has for decades, the rate of progress continues to increase. New knowledge continues to offer us new possibilities and new challenges.

REFERENCES

1. Hortobagyi GN. Treatment of breast cancer. N Engl J Med 1998;339:974–84.
2. Ries LAG, Eisner MP, Kosary CL, et al. SEER cancer statistics review, 1973–1999, Bethesda (MD): National Cancer Institute; 2002.
3. Jemal A, Murray T, Ward E, et al. Cancer statistics, 2005. CA Cancer J Clin 2005;55:10–30
4. Parkin DM, Pisani P, Ferlay J. Global cancer statistics. CA Cancer J Clin 1999;49:33–64.
5. Parkin DM, Whelan SL, Ferlay J, et al. Cancer incidence in five continents. Vol. VIII. IARC Scientific Publication No. 155. Lyon (France): IARC; 2002.
6. Colditz GA. Epidemiology of breast cancer. Cancer 1993;71:1480–9.
7. Miller AB. Causes of breast cancer and high-risk groups—incidence and demographics. Radiation risk. In: Harris JR, Hellman S, Henderson IC, Kinne DW, editors. Breast diseases. 2nd ed. Philadelphia: JB Lippincott; 1991. p 119–26.
8. La Vecchia C, Negri E, Levi F, et al. Age, cohort-of-birth, and period-of-death trends in breast cancer mortality in Europe. J Natl Cancer Inst 1997;89:732–4.
9. Hermon C, Beral V. Breast cancer mortality rates are levelling off or beginning to decline in many western countries. Analysis of time trends, age-cohort and age period models of breast cancer mortality in 20 countries. Br J Cancer 1996;73:955–60.
10. Duffy SW, Tabar L, Fagerberg G, et al. Breast screening, prognostic factors and survival—results from the Swedish two county study. Br J Cancer 1991;64:1133–8.
11. Cisneros MT. Situacion epidemiologica del cancer mamario. In: Sanchez Basurto C, editor. Compendio de patologia mamaria. 1st ed. Mexico, DF: Ciencia y Cultura Latinoamerica, SA de CV; 1999. p. 91–4.
12. Globocan 2002. IARC publication. Available at: http://www.depdb.iarc.fr/globocan/GLOBOframe.htm (accessed on February 25, 2005)
13. Mettlin C. Global breast cancer mortality statistics. CA Cancer J Clin 1999;49:138–44.
14. Colditz GA, Willett WC, Hunter DJ, et al. Family history, age, and risk of breast cancer. Prospective data from the Nurses' Health Study. [published erratum appears in JAMA 1993;270:1548] JAMA 1993;270:338–43.
15. Vatten LJ, Kvinnsland S. Pregnancy-related factors and risk of breast cancer in a prospective study of 29,981 Norwegian women. Eur J Cancer 1992;28A:1148–53.
16. Struewing JP, Hartge P, Wacholder S, et al. The risk of cancer associated with specific mutations of *BRCA1* and *BRCA2* among Ashkenazi Jews. N Engl J Med 1997;336:1401–8.
17. Trichopoulos D, Yen S, Brown J, et al. The effect of westernization on urine estrogens, frequency of ovulation, and breast cancer risk. A study of ethnic Chinese women in the Orient and the USA. Cancer 1984;53:187–92.
18. Lynch HT, Lynch JF. Breast cancer genetics in an oncology clinic: 328 consecutive patients. Cancer Genet Cytogenet 1986;22:369–71.
19. Anderson DE, Badzioch MD. Familial breast cancer risks. Effects of prostate and other cancers. Cancer 1993;72:114–9.
20. Couch FJ, Farid LM, Deshano ML, et al. *BRCA2* germline mutations in male breast cancer cases and breast cancer families. Nat Genet 1996;13:123–5.
21. Blackwood MA, Weber BL. *BRCA1* and *BRCA2.* From molecular genetics to clinical medicine. J Clin Oncol 1998;16:1969–77.
22. Malone KE, Daling JR, Thompson JD, et al. *BRCA1* mutations and breast cancer in the general population. Analyses in women before age 35 years and in women before age 45 years with first-degree family history. JAMA 1998;279:922–9.
23. Lakhani SR, Jacquemier J, Sloane JP, et al. Multifactorial analysis of differences between sporadic breast cancers and cancers involving *BRCA1* and *BRCA2* mutations. J Natl Cancer Inst 1998;90:1138–45.
24. Verhoog LC, Brekelmans CT, Seynaeve C, et al. Survival and tumour characteristics of breast-cancer patients with germline mutations of *BRCA1.* Lancet 1998;351:316–21.
25. Neuhausen S, Gilewski T, Norton L, et al. Recurrent *BRCA2* 6174delT mutations in Ashkenazi Jewish women affected by breast cancer. Nat Genet 1996;13:126–8.
26. Thompson D, Easton DF. Breast Cancer Linkage Consortium. Cancer Incidence in BRCA1 mutation carriers. J Nat Cancer Inst 2002;94:1358–65.
27. Bernstein L, Henderson BE, Hanisch R, et al. Physical exercise and reduced risk of breast cancer in young women. J Natl Cancer Inst 1994;86:1403–8.
28. Collaborative group on Hormonal Factors in Breast Cancer. Breast cancer and breastfeeding: collaborative reanalysis of individual data from 47 epidemiological studies in 30 countries, including 50,302 women with breast cancer and 96,973 women without the disease. Lancet 2002;360:187–95.
29. Burroughs KD, Dunn SE, Barrett JC, et al. Insulin-like growth factor-I. A key regulator of human cancer risk? J Natl Cancer Inst 1999;91:579–81.
30. Collaborative Group on Hormonal Factors in Breast Cancer. Breast cancer and hormone replacement therapy. Collaborative reanalysis of data from 51 epidemiological studies of 52,705 women with breast cancer and 108,411 women without breast cancer. Lancet 1997;350:1047–59.
31. Writing Group for the Women's Health Initiative Investigators. Risks and Benefits of Estrogen Plus Progestin in Healthy Postmenopausal Women: Principal Results From the Women's Health Initiative Randomized Controlled Trial. JAMA 2002;288:321–33.
32. Grady D, Herrington D, Bittner V, et al. Cardiovascular disease outcomes during 6.8 years of hormone therapy: Heart and Estrogen/progestin Replacement Study follow-up (HERS II) [comment]. [erratum appears in JAMA 2002 Sep 4;288(9):1064]. JAMA 2002;288:49–57.
33. Beral V. Million Women, Study Collaborators. Breast cancer and hormone-replacement therapy in the Million Women Study. Lancet 2003;362:419–27.
34. Collaborative Group on Hormonal Factors in Breast Cancer. Breast cancer and hormonal contraceptives. Collaborative reanalysis of individual data on 53,297 women with breast cancer and 100,239 women without breast cancer from 54 epidemiological studies. Lancet 1996;347:1713–27.
35. Buell P. Changing incidence of breast cancer in Japanese-American women. J Natl Cancer Inst 1973;51:1479–83.
36. Howe GR, Hirohata T, Hislop TG, et al. Dietary factors and risk of breast cancer. Combined analysis of 12 case-control studies. J Natl Cancer Inst 1990;82:561–9.
37. Ziegler RG, Hoover RN, Nomura AM, et al. Relative weight, weight change, height, and breast cancer risk in Asian-American women. J Nat Cancer Inst 1996;88:650–60.
38. Wu AH, Pike MC, Stram DO. Meta-analysis. Dietary fat intake, serum estrogen levels, and the risk of breast cancer. J Natl Cancer Inst 1999;91:529–34.
39. Albanes D. Caloric intake, body weight, and cancer. A review. Nutr Cancer 1987;9:199–217.
40. Chlebowski RT, Blackburn GL, Buzzard IM, et al. Adherence to a dietary fat intake reduction program in post-

menopausal women receiving therapy for early breast cancer. The Women's Intervention Nutrition Study. J Clin Oncol 1993;11:2072–80.
41. Boyd NF, Greenberg C, Lockwood G, et al. Effects at two years of a low-fat, high carbohydrate diet on radiologic features of the breast. Results from a randomized trial. Canadian Diet and Breast Cancer Prevention Study Group. J Natl Cancer Inst 1997;89:488–96.
42. Ballard–Barbash R, Schatzkin A, Carter CL, et al. Body fat distribution and breast cancer in the Framingham Study. J Natl Cancer Inst 1990;82:286–90.
43. Tretli S. Height and weight in relation to breast cancer morbidity and mortality. A prospective study of 570,000 women in Norway. Int J Cancer 1989;44:23–30.
44. Prentice R, Thompson D, Clifford C, et al. Dietary fat reduction and plasma estradiol concentration in healthy postmenopausal women. The Women's Health Trial Study Group. J Natl Cancer Inst 1990;82:129–34.
45. Schatzkin A, Jones DY, Hoover RN, et al. Alcohol consumption and breast cancer in the epidemiologic follow-up study of the first National Health and Nutrition Examination Survey. N Engl J Med 1987;316:1169–73.
46. Willett WC, Stampfer MJ, Colditz GA, et al. Moderate alcohol consumption and the risk of breast cancer. N Engl J Med 1987;316:1174–80.
47. Zhang S, Hunter DJ, Hankinson SE, et al. A prospective study of folate intake and the risk of breast cancer. JAMA 1999;281:1632–7.
48. Wang Y, Go V, Holland JF, et al. Expression of mouse mammary tumor virus-like env gene sequences in human breast cancer. Clin Cancer Res. 1998;4:2565–8.
49. Goss PE, Sierra S. Current perspectives on radiation-induced breast cancer. J Clin Oncol 1998;16:338–47.
50. Roychoudhuri R, Evans H, Robinson D, Moller H. Radiation-induced malignancies following radiotherapy for breast cancer. Br J Cancer 2004;91:868–72.
51. Dupont WD, Page DL. Risk factors for breast cancer in women with proliferative breast disease. N Engl J Med 1985;312:146–51.
52. Dupont WD, Parl FF, Hartmann WH, et al. Breast cancer risk associated with proliferative breast disease and atypical hyperplasia. Cancer 1993;71:1258–65.
53. McDivitt RW, Stevens JA, Lee NC, et al. Histologic types of benign breast disease and the risk for breast cancer. The Cancer and Steroid Hormone Study Group. Cancer 1992;69:1408–14.
54. Relf M, LeJeune S, Scott PA, et al. Expression of the angiogenic factors vascular endothelial cell growth factor, acidic and basic fibroblast growth factor, tumor growth factor beta-1, platelet-derived endothelial cell growth factor, placenta growth factor, and pleiotrophin in human primary breast cancer and its relation to angiogenesis. Cancer Res 1997;57:963–9.
55. Wolfe JN. Breast patterns as an index of risk for developing breast cancer. AJR Am J Roentgenol 1976; 126:1130–7.
56. Gail MH, Brinton LA, Byar DP, et al. Projecting individualized probabilities of developing breast cancer for white females who are being examined annually. J Nat Cancer Inst 1989;81:1879–86.
57. Gail MH, Brinton LA, Byar DP, et al. Projecting individualized probabilities of developing breast cancer for white females who are being examined annually. J Nat Cancer Inst 1989;81:1879–86.
58. Gail M, Benichou J. Epidemiology and Biostatistics Program of the National Cancer Institute. JNCI. 1994:86;573–607.
59. Claus E, Risch N, Thompson W. Genetic Analysis of breast cancer in cancer and steroid hormone study. Am J of Human Genetics 1991;148:232–42.
60. Claus EB, Risch N, Thompson WD. The calculation of breast cancer risk for women with a first degree family history of ovarian cancer. Breast Cancer Res Treat 1993;128:115–20.
61. Domchek SM, Eisen A, Calzone K, et al.. Application of breast cancer risk prediction models in clinical practice. J Clin Oncol 2003;121593–601.
62. Berry D, ParmigianiA, Sanchez J, Schildkraut J. Probability of carrying a mutation of breast-ovarian cancer gene BRCAI based on family history. JNCI 1997;189:227–38.
63. Pannigiani a, Berry D, Aguilar O. Determining carrier probabilities for breast cancer-susceptibility genes BRCAI and BRCA2. Am J Human Genetics 1998;162:145–58.
64. Frank TS, Manley SA, Olopade 01, et al. Sequence analysis of BRCAI and BRCA2: correlation of mutations with family history and ovarian cancer risk. J Clin Oncol 1998;116:2417–25.
65. Couch FJ, DeShano ML, Blackwood MA, et al. BRCAI mutations in women attending clinics that evaluate the risk of breast cancer. N Engl J Med 2004;336:1409–15.
66. National Cancer Institute: Breast Cancer Risk Assessment Tool. http://bcra.nci.nih.gov/brc [Accessed July 30, 2005.]
67. Rockhill B, Spiegelman D, Byme C, et al. Validation of the Gail et al. model of breast cancer risk prediction and implications for chemoprevention. J Natl Cancer Inst 2001;93:358–66.
68. Ozanne E, Adduci K, Esserman L. Feasibility study of a computerized decision aid for breast cancer prevention. Paper presented at: San Antonio Breast Cancer Symposium 2003; San Antonio, TX.
69. Ozanne E, Esserman L. Evaluation of Breast Cancer Risk Assessment Techniques: A Cost-Effectiveness Analysis. Cancer Epidemiology, Biomarkers, and Prevention 2004;13(12):2043–52.
70. Meijers-Heijboer H, Van Geel B, Van Putten W, et al. Breast Cancer After Prophylactic Bilateral Mastectomy in Women with a BRCAI or BRCA2 Mutation. N Engl J Med 2001;345:159–64.
71. Fabian C, Kimler B, Zalles C, et al. Short-term Breast Cancer Prediction by Random Periareolar Fine-Needle Aspiration Cytology and the Gail Risk Model. J Natl Cancer Inst 2000;92:1217–27.
72. Fisher B, Costantino JP, Wickerham DL, et al. Tamoxifen for prevention of breast cancer: report of the National Surgical Adjuvant Breast and Bowel Project P-I Study [see comments]. J Natl Cancer Inst 1998;90:1371–88.
73. Wolfe IN, Saftlas AF, Salane M. Mammographic parenchymal patterns and quantitative evaluation of marnmographic densities: a case-control study. AJR Am J Roentgenol 1987;1148:1087–92.
74. Boyd NF, Lockwood GA, Martin LJ et al. Mammographic densities and risk of breast cancer among subjects with a family history of this disease. J Natl Cancer Inst 1999;91:1404-8.
75. Ziv E, Tice J, Srnith-Bindman R, et al. Mammographic density and estrogen receptor status of breast cancer. Cancer Epidemiol Biomarkers Prev 2004;1312:2090–5.
76. Fabian CJ, Kimler BF, Simonsen M, et al. Reduction in breast epithelial cell proliferation after six months of letrozole in high risk women on hormone replacement therapy with random periareolar fine needle aspiration evidence of atypia. San Antonio Breast Cancer Symposium, December 8, 2004.
77. Dickson RB, Lipprnan ME. Growth factors in breast cancer. Endocr Rev 1995;16:559–89.
78. Evans RM. The steroid and thyroid hormone receptor superfamily. Science 1988;240:889–95.
79. Baselga J, Tripathy D, Mendelsohn J, et al. Phase II study of weekly intravenous recombinant humanized antipl85 HER2 monoclonal antibody in patients with HER2/neu-overexpressing metastatic breast cancer. J Clin Oncol 1996;14:737–44.
80. Press MF, Jones LA, Godolphin W, et al. HER-2/neu oncogene amplification and expression in breast and ovarian cancers. Prog Clin Biol Res 1990;354:209–21.
81. Gago FE, Tello OM, Diblasi AM, et al. Integration of estrogen and progesterone receptors with pathological and molecular prognostic factors in breast cancer patients. J Steroid Biochem Mol Biol 1998;67:431–7.
82. Sorlie T, Perou C, Tibshirani R, et al. Gene expression patterns of breast carcinomas distinguish tumor subclasses with clinical implications. Proc Natl Acad Sci U S A 2001; 98:10869–74.
83. Wamer E, Plewes DB, Hill KA, et al. Surveillance of BRCAI and BRCA2 mutation camers with magnetic resonance imaging, ultrasound, mammography, and clinical breast examination. JAMA 2004;292:1317–25.
84. Kriege M, Brekelmans CT, Boetes C, et al. Efficacy of MRI and mammography for breast-cancer screening in women with a familial or genetic predisposition. N Engl J Med 2004;351:427–37.
85. Esserman L. Integration of imaging in the management of breast cancer. J Clin Oncol 2005; 23(8):1601–2.
86. Vogel V. Evaluation of risk and preventive approaches to breast cancer. In: Einhorn N, editor. Cancer in Women. Malden (MA): Blackwell Science;1998. p. 58–91.
87. Rebbeck TR, Friebel T, Lynch HT, et al. Bilateral Prophylactic Mastectomy Reduces Breast Cancer Risk in BRCAI and BRCA2 Mutation Carriers: The PROSE Study Group. J Clin Oncol 2004;22(6):1055–62.
88. Hartmann LC, Sellers TA, Schaid DL, et al. Efficacy of bilateral prophylactic mastectomy in BRCAI and BRCA2 gene mutation camers. J Natl Cancer lnst 2001;93:1633–37.
89. Crowe IP Jr, Kim IA, Vetman R, et al Nipple-sparing mastectomy: technique and results of 54 procedures. Arch Surg 2004;139:148–50.
90. Kroll SS, Khoo A, Singletary SE, et al. Local recurrence risk after skin-sparing and conventional mastectomy: a 6-year follow-up. Plast Reconstr Surg 1999;104:421–5.
91. Craigie IE, Allen RJ, DellaCroce FI, Sullivan SK. Autogenous breast reconstruction with the deep inferior epigastric perforator flap. Clin Plast Surg 2003;30:359–69.
92. Foster RD, Esserman U, Anthony IP, et al. Skin-sparing mastectomy and immediate breast reconstruction: a prospective cohort study for the treatment of advanced stages of breast carcinoma. Ann Surg Oncol 2002;9:462–6.
93. Rebbeck TR. Breast Cancer Risk After Bilateral Prophylactic Oophorectomy in BRCA1 Mutation Carriers. JNCI 1999;91:1475–9.
94. Rebbeck TR, Friebel T, Lynch HT, et al.Bilateral prophylactic mastectomy reduces breast cancer risk in BRCA1 and BRCA2 mutation carriers. The PROSE Study Group. J Clin Oncol 2004;22:1055–62.
95. Schrag D, Kuntz K, Garber I, Weeks I. Life Expectancy Gains from Cancer Prevention Strategies for women with Breast Cancer and BRCAI or BRCA 2 Mutations. JAMA 2000;283:617–24.
96. Haagensen CD, Bodian C, Haagensen DE. Lobular neoplasia (lobular carcinoma in situ). In: Haagenson CD, editor. Breast carcinoma. Risk and detection. Philadelphia: WB Saunders; 1981. p. 238.
97. Shelley Hwang E, Nyante SI, et al. Clonality of lobular carcinoma in situ and synchronous invasive lobular carcinoma Cancer 2004;100:2562–72.
98. Cuzick I, Powles T, Veronesi U, et al. Overview of the main outcomes in breast cancer prevention trials. Lancet 2003;361:296–300.
99. Freedman AN, Graubard BI, et al. Estimates of the number of US women who could benefit from tamoxifen for breast cancer chemoprevention. J Natl Cancer lnst 2003;95:526–32.
100. Port ER, Montgomery LL, Heerdt AS, Borgen PI. Patient reluctance toward tamoxifen use for breast cancer primary prevention. Ann Surg Oncol 2001;8:580–5.
101. Gail M, Costantino I, Bryant I, et al. Weighing the risks and benefits oftamoxifen treatment for preventing breast cancer. J Natl Cancer Inst 1999;91:1829–46.
102. Cauley IA, Norton L, Lippman ME, et al. Continued breast cancer risk reduction in postmenopausal women treated with raloxifene: 4-year results from the MORE trial. Multiple outcomes of raloxifene evaluation. Breast Cancer Res Treat 2001;65:125–34.
103. Chlebowski RT, Hendrix SL, Langer RD, et al. Influence of estrogen plus progestin on breast cancer and mammography in healthy postmenopausal women: the Women's Health Initiative Randomized Trial. JAMA 2003;289:3243–53.
104. Key TI, Schatzkin A, Willett WC, et al. Diet, nutrition and the prevention of cancer. Public Health Nutr 2004;7:187–200.
105. Cho E, Spiegelman D, Hunter DJ, et al. Premenopausal fat intake and risk of breast cancer. J Natl Cancer lnst 2003;95:1079–85.
106. Holmes MD, Willett WC. Does diet affect breast cancer risk? Breast Cancer Res 2004;6:170–8.
107. Fisher ER, Gregorio RM, Fisher B, et al. The pathology of invasive breast cancer. A syllabus derived from findings of the National Surgical Adjuvant Breast Project (protocol No.4). Cancer 1975;36:1–85.
108. Fisher ER, Kenny IP, Sass R, et al, and NSABP collaborators. Medullary cancer of breast revisited. Breast Cancer Res Treat 1990;16:215–29.
109. Rosen PP, Groshen S, Kinne DW, et al. Factors influencing prognosis in node-negative breast carcinoma. Analysis of 767 TINOMO/T2NOMO patients with long-term follow-up. J Clin Oncol 1993;11:2090–100.
110. Carter CL, Allen C, Henson DE. Relation of tumor size, lymph node status, and survival in 24,740 breast cancer cases. Cancer 1989;63:181–7.
111. Leitner SP, Swem AS, Weinberger D, et al. Predictors of recurrence for patients with small (one centimeter or less) localized breast cancer (Tla,b No MO). Cancer 1995;76:2266–74.
112. Fisher B, Ravdin RG, Ausman RK, et al. Surgical adjuvant chemotherapy in cancer of the breast. Results of a decade of cooperative investigation. Ann Surg 1968; 168:337–56.
113. Nemoto T, Vana I, Bedwani RN, et al. Management and survival of female breast cancer: results of a national survey by the American College of Surgeons. Cancer 1980;45:2917–24.
114. The International Breast Cancer Study Group. Prognostic importance of occult axillary lymph node rnicrometastases from breast cancers. Lancet 1990;335:1565–8.

115. Giuliano AE, Dale PS, Turner RR, et al. Improved axillary staging of breast cancer with sentinel lymphadenectomy. Ann Surg 1995;222:394–9; discussion 399–400.
116. Fisher ER, Redmond C, Fisher B. Pathologic findings from the National Surgical Adjuvant Breast Project (Protocol No.4). VI. Discriminants for five-year treatment failure. Cancer 1980;46:908–18.
117. Gamel JW, Meyer JS, Feuer E, et al. The impact of stage and histology on the longterm clinical course of 163,808 patients with breast carcinoma. Cancer 1996;77:1459–64.
118. Pedersen L, Holck S, Schiodt T, et al. Medul l ary carcinoma of the breast, prognostic importance of characteristic histopathological features evaluated in a multivariate Cox analysis. Eur J Cancer 1994;30:1792–7.
119. Page DL, Jensen RA, Simpson JF. Routinely available indicators of prognosis in breast cancer. Breast Cancer Res Treat 1998;51:195–208.
120. Fisher ER, Sass R, Fisher B. Pathologic findings from the National Surgical Adjuvant Project for Breast Cancers (Protocol No.4). X. Discriminants for tenth-year treatment failure. Cancer 1984;53:712–23.
121. Rosen PP, Groshen S, Saigo PE, et al. Pathological prognostic factors in stage I (TINOMO) and stage II (TINIMO) breast carcinoma. A study of 644 patients with median follow-up of 18 years. J Clin Oncol 1989;7:1239–51.
122. Elston CW, Ellis IO. Pathologic prognostic factors in breast cancer. I. The value of histologic grade in breast cancer: experience from a large study with long-term follow-up. Histopathol 1991;19:403–10.
123. Kramer WM, Rush BF. Mammary duct proliferation in the elderly. A histopathologic study. Cancer 1973;31:130–7.
124. Chaney AW, Pollack A, McNeese MD, et al. Primary treatment of cystosarcoma phyl1odes of the breast. Cancer 2000;89:1502–11.
125. Fisher ER, Redmond C, Fisher B. Prognostic factors in NSABP studies of women with node-negative breast cancer. Presented at Consensus Development Conference on Treatment of Early-Stage Breast Cancer, Bethesda, Maryland, June 19, 1990. J Natl Cancer Inst Monogr 1992;11:151–8.
126. Bloom HJG, Richardson WW, Halties EJ. Natural history of untreated breast cancer (1805-1933). Comparison of untreated and treated cases according to histological grade of malignancy. Br Med J 1962;213–21.
127. von Fournier D, Weber E, Hoeffken W, et al. Growth rate of 147 mammary carcinomas. Cancer 1980;45:2198-207.
128. Koscielny S, Tubiana M, Le MG, et al. Breast cancer. Relationship between the size of the primary tumour and the probability of metastatic dissemination. Br J Cancer 1984;49:709–15.
129. Ravdin PM. Prognostic factors in breast cancer. ASCO Education Book 1997;Spring:217–27.
130. Adami Ho, Malker B, Holmberg L, et al. The relation between survival and age at diagnosis in breast cancer. N Engl J Med 1986;315:559–63.
131. Thorpe PE. Vascular targeting agents as cancer therapeutics. Clinical Cancer Research 2004;10:415–27s.
132. Weidner N, Semple JP, Welch WR, et al. Tumor angiogenesis and metastasis—correlation in invasive breast carcinoma. N Engl J Med 1991;324:1–8.
133. Steeg PS, Zhou Q. Cyclins and breast cancer. Breast Cancer Res Treat 1998;52:17–28.
134. Keyomarsi K, Tucker SL, Buchholz TA, et al. Cyclin E and Survival in Patients with Breast Cancer. N Engl J Med 2003;347:1566–75.
135. Osborne CK. Steroid hormone receptors in breast cancer management. Breast Cancer Res Treat 1998;51:227–38.
136. Hess KR, Pusztai L, Buzdar AU, Hortobagyi GN. Estrogen receptors and distinct patterns of breast cancer relapse. Breast Cancer Res Treat 2003;78:105–18.
137. Slamon DJ, Clark GM, Wong SG, et al. Human breast cancer. Correlation of relapse and survival with amplification of the HER-2/neu oncogene. Science 1987;235:177–82.
138. Pegrarn MD, Pauletti G, Slamon DJ. HER-2/neu as a predictive marker of response to breast cancer therapy. Breast Cancer Res Treat 1998;52:65–77.
139. Vogel CL, Cobleigh MA, et al. Efficacy and safety of trastuzumab as a single agent in first-line treatment of HER2-overexpressing metastatic breast cancer. Journal of Clinical Oncology 2002;20:719–26.
140. Thor AD, Moore DHI, Edgerton SM, et al. Accumulation of p53 tumor suppressor gene protein: an independent marker of prognosis in breast cancers. J Natl Cancer Inst 1992;84;845.
141. Berger U, Bettelheirn R, Mansi JL, et al. The relationship between micrometastases in the bone marrow, histopathologic features of the primary tumor in breast cancer and prognosis. Am J Clin Pathol 1988;90:1–6.
142. Diel U, Kaufmann M, Costa SD, et al. Micrometastatic breast cancer cells in bone marrow at primary surgery. Prognostic value in comparison with nodal status. J Nat Cancer Inst 1996;88:1652–8.
143. Cristofanilli M, Budd GT, Ellis MJ, et al. Circulating tumor cells, disease progression, and survival in metastatic breast cancer. [see comment]. N Engl J Med 2004;351:781–91.
144. Haybittle JL, Blarney RW, Elston CW, et al. A prognostic index in primary breast cancer. Br J Cancer 1982;45:361–6.
145. Ravdin PM, Siminoff LA, Davis GJ, et al. Computer program to assist in making decisions about adjuvant therapy for women with early breast cancer. J Clin Oncol 2001;19:980–91.
146. van de Vijver MJ, He YD, van't Veer U, et al. A gene-expression signature as a predictor of survival in breast cancer. N Engl J Med 2002;347:1999–2009.
147. Ayers M, Symmans WF, Stec J, et al. Gene expression profiles predict complete pathologic response to neoadjuvant paclitaxel and fluorouracil, doxorubicin, and cyclophosphamide chemotherapy in breast cancer. J Clin Oncol 2004;22:2284–93.
148. Paik S, Shak S, Tang G, et al. A multigene assay to predict recurrence of tamoxifen-treated, node-negative breast cancer. N Engl J Med 2004;351:2817–26
149. Wang L. Mammography and beyond: building better breast cancer screening tests. J Natl Cancer Inst 2003;95:344–6.
150. Gotzsche PC, Olsen O. Is screening for breast cancer with mammography justifiable? Lancet 2000;355:129–34.
151. Esserman L. New Approaches to the Imaging, Biopsy, and Diagnosis of Breast Lesions. Principles and Practice of Oncology 2002.
152. Kerlikowske K, Grady D, Rubin SJ, et al. Efficacy of screening mammography. A meta-analysis. JAMA 1995;273:149–54.
153. Hylton N. Magnetic Resonance Imaging of the Breast: Opportunities to Improve Breast Cancer Management. Journal of Clinical Oncology 2005;23:1678–84.
154. Esserman U, Kaplan E, Partridge S, et al. MRI Imaging Phenotype is Associated With Response to AC Neoadjuvant Chemotherapy in Stage III Breast Cancer. Ann Surg Oncol 2001;8(6):549–59.
155. Ljung B, Drejet A, Chiampi N, et al. Diagnostic accuracy of fine-needle aspiration biopsy is determined by physician training in sampling technique. Cancer 2001;93:263–8.
156. Esserman L, Cowley H, Eberle C, et al. Improving the accuracy of mammography: volume and outcome relationships. J Natl Cancer Inst 2002;94:369–75.
157. Thomas DB, Gao DL, Ray RM, et al. Randomized trial of breast self-examination in Shanghai. Final results. J Natl Cancer Inst 2002;94:1445–57.
158. Greene FL, Balch CM, Page DL, et al, editors. American Joint Committee on Cancer (AJCC) Cancer Staging Manual. 6th ed. New York: Springer-Verlag; 2002.
159. Bast RC Jr, Ravdin P, Hayes, DF, et al. 2000 update of recommendations for the use of tumor markers in breast and colorectal cancer: clinical practice guidelines of the American Society of Clinical Oncology. J Clin Oncol 2001;19:1865–78.
160. Schwartz GF, Giuliano AE, Veronesi U, Consensus Conference Committee. Proceedings of the consensus conference on the role of sentinel lymph node biopsy in carcinoma of the breast, April 19–22, 2001, Philadelphia, PA. Cancer 2002;94:2542–51.
161. NIH consensus conference: treatment of early stage breast cancer. JAMA 1991;265:391–5.
162. Fisher B, Slack N, Katrych D, et al. Ten-year follow-up results of patients with carcinoma of the breast in a cooperative clinical trial evaluating surgical adjuvant chemotherapy. Surg Gynecol Obstet 1975;140:528–34.
163. Schnitt S, Abner A, Gelman R, et al. The relationship between microscopic margins of resection and the risk of local recurrence in patients with breast cancer treated with breast-conserving surgery and radiation therapy. Cancer 1994;74:1746–51.
164. Krag DN, Julian TB. Practice patterns of sentinel node biopsy at five comprehensive cancer centers. Journal of the National Cancer Institute 2003;95:1498–9.
165. Salgarello M, Seccia A, Eugenio F. Immediate breast reconstruction with anatomical permanent expandable implants after skin-sparing mastectomy: aesthetic and technical refinements. Ann Plast Surg 2004;52:358–64.(discussion 365–6)
166. Gabriel SE, O'Fallon WM, Kurland LT, et al. Risk of connective-tissue diseases and other disorders after breast implantation. N Engl J Med 1994;330:1697–702.
167. Page DL, Dupont WD, Rogers LW, et al. Continued local recurrence of carcinoma 15–25 years after a diagnosis of low-grade ductal carcinoma in situ of the breast treated only by biopsy. Cancer 1995;76:1197–1200.
168. Fisher B, Dignam J, Wolmark N, et al. Lumpectomy and radiation therapy for the treatment of intraductal breast cancer: findings from National Surgical Adjuvant Breast and Bowel Project B-17. J Clin Oncol 1998;16:441–52.
169. Julien JP, Bijker N, Fentiman IS, et al. Radiotherapy in breast-conserving treatment for ductal carcinoma in situ: first results of the EORTC randomised phase III trial 10853. Lancet 2000;355:528–33.
170. Houghton J, George WD, Cuzick J, et al. Radiotherapy and tamoxifen in women with completely excised ductal carcinoma in situ of the breast in the UK, Australia, and New Zealand: randomized controlled trial. Lancet 2003;362:95–102.
171. Baxter NN, Virnig BA, Durham SB, et al. Trends in the treatment of ductal carcinoma in situ of the breast. J Natl Cancer Institute 2004;96:443–8.
172. Ottesen GL, Graversen HP, Blichert-Toft M, et al. Carcinoma in situ of the female breast. 10-year follow-up prospective nationwide study. Breast Cancer Res Treat 2000;62:197–210.
173. Silverstein MJ, Lagios MD, Craig PH, et al. A prognostic index for ductal carcinoma in situ of the breast. Cancer 1996;77:2267–74.
174. Kerlikowski K, Molinaro A, Cha I, et al. Characteristics associated with recurrence among women with ductal carcinoma in situ treated by lumpectomy. J Natl Cancer Institute 2003;95:1692–1702.
175. Silverstein MJ, Lagios MD, Groshen S, et al. The influence of margin width on local control of ductal carcinoma in situ of the breast. N Engl J Med 1999;340:1455–61.
176. Wong JS, Gadd MA, Gelman R, et al. Wide excision alone for ductal carcinoma in situ (DCIS) of the breast. Breast Cancer Res Treat 2003;82(Supplement 1):S10 (abst 15).
177. Fisher B, Land S, Mamounas E, et al. Prevention of invasive breast cancer in women with ductal carcinoma in situ: an update of the National Surgical Adjuvant Breast and Bowel Project experience. Semin Oncol 2001;28:400–18.
178. Fisher B, Dignam J, Wolmark N, et al. Tamoxifen in treatment of intraductal breast cancer. National Surgical Adjuvant Breast and Bowel Project B-24 randomised controlled trial. Lancet 1999;353:1993–2000.
179. Allred D, Bryant J, Land S, et al. Estrogen receptor expression as a predictive marker of the effectiveness of tamoxifen in the treatment of DCIS: Findings from NSABP Protocol B-24 [abstract]. Breast Cancer Res Treat 2002;76:Suppl 36.
180. Ceilley E, Jagsi R, Goldberg S, et al. The management of ductal carcinoma in situ in North American and Europe. Results of a survey. Cancer 2004;101:1958–67.
181. Breast Cancer Facts & Figures 2003–2004. Atlanta, GA: American Cancer Society; 2003. p. 1–25.
182. Fisher B, Anderson S, Bryant J, et al. Twenty-year follow-up of a randomized trial comparing total mastectomy, lumpectomy, and lumpectomy plus irradiation for the treatment of invasive breast cancer. N Engl J Med 2002;347:1233–41.
183. Fisher B, Bryant J, Dignam JJ, et al. Tamoxifen, radiation therapy, or both for prevention of ipsilateral breast tumor recurrence after lumpectomy in women with invasive breast cancers of one centimeter or less. J Clin Oncol 2002;20:4141–9.
184. Buchholz TA, Tucker SL, Mathur D, et al. Impact of systemic treatment on local control for lymph-node negative breast cancer patients treated with breast-conservation therapy. J Clin Oncol 2001;19:2240–6.
185. Locker GY, Sainsbury JC Jr. Breast surgery in the 'Arimidex, Tamoxifen alone or in combination' (ATAC) trial. Cancer 2004;101:735–40.
186. Morrow M, White J, Moughan J, et al. Factors predicting the use of breast-conserving therapy in Stage I and II breast carcinoma. J Clin Oncol 2001;19:2254–62.
187. Veronesi U, Cascinelli N, Mariani L, et al. Twenty-year follow-up of a randomized study comparing breast-conserving surgery with radical mastectomy for early breast cancer. N Engl J Med 2002;347:1227–32.
188. Early Breast Cancer Trialists' Collaborative Group. Favourable and unfavourable effects on long-term survival of radiotherapy for early breast cancer: an overview of the randomised trials. Lancet 2000;355:1757–70.
189. Morris AD, Morris RD, Wilson JF, et al. Breast-conserving therapy vs mastectomy in early-stage breast cancer: a meta-analysis of 10-year survival. Cancer J Sci Am 1997;3:6–12.

190. Stovall M, Blackwell CR, Cudiff J, et al. Fetal dose from radiotherapy with photon beams: report of AA PM Radiation Therapy Committee. Med Phys 1995;22:63–82.
191. Morris MM, Powell SN. Irradiation in the setting of collagen vascular disease: acute and late complications. J Clin Oncol 1997;15:2728–35.
192. Holland R, Veling SH, Mravunac M, et al. Histologic multifocality of Tis, T1-2 breast carcinomas. Implications for clinical trials of breast-conserving surgery. Cancer 1985;56:979–90.
193. Nattinger AB, Hoffman RG, Kneusel RT, et al. Relation between appropriateness of primary therapy for early-stage breast carcinoma and increased use of breast-conserving surgery. Lancet 2000;356:1148–53.
194. Peto R. Early Breast Cancer Trialists' Collaborative Group. Meta-analysis on local therapy. 27th San Antonio Breast Cancer Symposium–oral plenary presentation. Dec. 11, 2004, San Antonio, TX; 2004.
195. Vinh-Hung V, Verschraegen C. Breast-conserving surgery with or without radiotherapy: pooled-analysis for risks of ipsilateral breast tumor recurrence and mortality. J Natl Cancer Inst 2004;96:115–21.
196. Veronesi U, Marubini E, Mariani L, et al. Radiotherapy after breast-conserving surgery in small breast carcinoma: long-term results of a randomized trial. Ann Oncol 2001;12:997–1003.
197. Liljegren G, Lindgren A, Bergh J, et al. Risk factors for local recurrence after conservative treatment in stage I breast cancer. Definition of a subgroup not requiring radiotherapy. Ann Oncol 1997;8:235–41.
198. Holli K, Saaristo R, Isola J, et al. Lumpectomy with or without postoperative radiotherapy for breast cancer with favourable prognostic features: results of a randomized study. Br J Cancer 2001;84:164–9.
199. Forrest AP, Stewart HJ, Everington D, et al. Randomised controlled trial of conservation therapy for breast cancer: 6-year analysis of the Scottish trial. Scottish Cancer Trials Breast Group. Lancet 1996;348:708–13.
200. Hughes KS, Schnaper LA, Berry D, et al. Lumpectomy plus tamoxifen with or without irradiation in women 70 years of age or older with early breast cancer. N Engl J Med 2004;351:971–7.
201. Fyles A, McCready DR, Manchul LA, et al. Tamoxifen with or without breast irradiation in women 50 years of age or older with early breast cancer. N Engl J Med 2004;351:963–70.
202. Lee CG, McCormick B, Mazumdar M, et al. Infiltrating breast carcinoma in patients age 30 years and younger. Long-term outcome for life, relapse, and second primary tumors. Int J Radiat Oncol Biol Phys 1992;23:969–75.
203. Nixon AJ, Neuberg D, Hayes DF, et al. Relationship of patient age to pathologic features of the tumor and prognosis for patients with stage I or II breast cancer. J Clin Oncol 1994;12:888–94.
204. Fowble BL, Schultz DJ, Overmoyer B, et al. The influence of young age on outcome in early stage breast cancer. Int J Radiat Oncol Biol Phys 1994;30:23–33.
205. Natarajan N, Nemoto T, Mettlin C, et al. Race-related differences in breast cancer patients. Results of the 1982 national survey of breast cancer by the American College of Surgeons. Cancer 1985;56:1704–9.
206. Eley JW, Hill HA, Chen VW, et al. Racial differences in survival from breast cancer. Results of the National Cancer Institute Black/White Cancer Survival Study. JAMA 1994;272:947–54.
207. Newman LA, Kuerer HM, Hunt KK, et al. Local recurrence and survival among black women with early-stage breast cancer treated with breast-conservation therapy or mastectomy. Ann Surg Oncol 1999;6:241–48.
208. Haas JA, Schulta DJ, Peterson ME, et al. An analysis of age and family history on outcome after breast-conservation treatment. The University of Pennsylvania experience. Cancer J 1998;4:308–15.
209. Vlastos G, Mirza NQ, Meric F, et al. Breast conservation therapy in early-stage breast cancer patients with a positive family history. Ann Surg Oncol 2002;9:912–19.
210. Haffty BG, Harrold E, Kahn AJ, et al. Outcome of conservatively managed early-onset breast cancer by BRCA1/2 status. Lancet 2002;359:1471–7.
211. Vicini FA, Goldstein NS, Pass H, et al. Use of pathologic factors to assist in establishing adequacy of excision before radiotherapy in patients treated with breast-conserving therapy. Int J Radiat Oncol Biol Phys 2004;60:86–94.
212. Park CC, Mitsumori M, Nixon A, et al. Outcome at 8 years after breast-conserving surgery and radiation therapy for invasive breast cancer. Influence of margin status and systemic therapy on local recurrence. J Clin Oncol 2000;18:1668–75.
213. Fisher B, Jeong JH, Dignam J, et al. Findings from recent national surgical adjuvant breast and bowel project adjuvant studies in stage I breast cancer. J Natl Cancer Inst Monogr 2001;:62–6.
214. Romestaing P, Lehingue Y, Carrie C, et al. Role of a 10-Gy boost in the conservative treatment of early breast cancer. J Clin Oncol 1997;15:963–68.
215. Bartelink H, Horiot JC, Poortmans P, et al. Recurrence rates after treatment of breast cancer with standard radiotherapy with or without additional radiation. N Engl J Med 2001;345:1378–87.
216. Whelan TJ, MacKenzie RG, Levine M, et al. A randomized trial comparing two fractionation schedules for breast irradiation postlumpectomy in node-negative breast cancer. Proc Am Soc Clin Oncol 2000;19:2a (abst. 5).
217. Veronesi U, Orecchia R, Luini A, et al. Preliminary report of intraoperative radiotherapy (IORT) in limited-stage breast cancers that are conservatively treated. Eur J Cancer 2001;37:2178–83.
218. Vaidya JS, Baum M, Tobias JS, et al. Targeted intra-operative radiotherapy (Targit). An innovative method of treatment for early breast cancer. Ann Oncol 2001;12:1075–80.
219. Edmundson GK, Vicini FA, Chen PY, et al. Dosimetric characteristics of the MammoSite RTS, a new breast brachytherapy applicator. Int J Radiat Oncol Biol Phys. 2002;52:1132–9.
220. Vicini FA, Kestin L, Chen P, et al. Limited-field radiation therapy in the management of early-stage breast cancer. J Natl Cancer Inst 2003;95:1205–10.
221. King TA, Bolton JS, Kuske RR, et al. Long-term results of wide-field brachytherapy as the sole method of radiation therapy after segmental mastectomy for T(is,1,2) breast cancer. Am J Surg 2000;180:299–304.
222. Wazer DE, Lowther D, Boyle T, et al. Clinically evident fat necrosis in women treated with high-dose-rate brachytherapy alone for early-stage breast cancer. Int J Radiat Oncol Biol Phys 2001;50:107–11.
223. Dickler A, Kirk M, Choo J, et al. Treatment volume and dose optimization of MammoSite breast brachytherapy applicator. Int J Radiat Oncol Biol Phys 2004;59:469–74.
224. Slack NH, Bross IDJ, Nemoto T, Fisher B. Experiences with bilateral primary carcinoma of the breast. Surg Gynecol Obstet 1973;136:433–40.
225. Wolmark N, Wang J, Mamounas E, et al. Preoperative chemotherapy in patients with operable breast cancer: nine-year results from National Surgical Adjuvant Breast and Bowel Project B-18. Journal of the National Cancer Institute Monographs 2001;96–102.
226. van der Hage JA, Cornelis JH, van de Velde CJ, et al. Preoperative chemotherapy in primary operable breast cancer: results from the European Organization for Research and Treatment of Cancer trial 10902. J Clin Oncol 2001;19:4224–37.
227. Mauriac L, MacGrogan G, Avril A, et al. Neoadjuvant chemotherapy for operable breast carcinoma larger than 3 cm: A unicentre randomized trial with a 124-month median follow-up. Ann Oncol 1999;10:47–52.
228. Rouzier R, Extra JM, Carton M, et al. Primary chemotherapy for operable breast cancer: incidence and prognostic significance of ipsilateral breast tumor recurrence after breast-conserving surgery. J Clin Oncol 2001;19:3828–35.
229. Chen AM, Meric-Bernstam F, Hunt KK, et al. Breast-conserving therapy after neoadjuvant chemotherapy: the M. D. Anderson Cancer Center experience. J Clin Oncol 2004;22:2303–12.
230. Van de Steene J, Soete G, Storme G. Adjuvant radiotherapy for breast cancer significantly improves overall survival: the missing link. Radiother Oncol 2000;55:263–72.
231. Early Breast Cancer Trialists' Collaborative Group. Polychemotherapy for early breast cancer. An overview of the randomised trials. Lancet 1998;352:930–42.
232. Overgaard M, Hansen PS, Overgaard J, et al. Postoperative radiotherapy in high-risk premenopausal women with breast cancer who receive adjuvant chemotherapy. N Engl J Med 1997;337:949–55.
233. Ragaz J, Jackson SM, Le N, et al. Adjuvant radiotherapy and chemotherapy in node-positive premenopausal women with breast cancer. N Engl J Med 1997;337:956–62.
234. Overgaard M, Jensen MB, Overgaard J, et al. Randomized trail evaluating postoperative radiotherapy in high risk postmenopausal breast cancer patients given adjuvant tamoxifen: Results from the DBCG 82c trial. Lancet 1999;353:1641–8.
235. Recht A, Edge SB, Solin LJ, et al. Postmastectomy radiotherapy: clinical practice guidelines of the American Society of Clinical Oncology. J Clin Oncol 2001;19:1539–69.
236. Katz A, Strom EA, Buchholz TA, et al. Loco-regional recurrence patterns following mastectomy and doxorubicin-based chemotherapy: implications for postoperative irradiation. J Clin Oncol 2000;18:2817–27.
237. Recht A, Gray R, Davidson NE, et al. Locoregional failure ten years after mastectomy and adjuvant chemotherapy with or without tamoxifen without irradiation: Experience of the Eastern Cooperative Oncology Group. J Clin Oncol 1999;17:1689–1700.
238. Wallgren A, Bonetti M, Gelber RD, et al. Risk factors for locoregional recurrence among breast cancer patients: results from International Breast Cancer Study Group Trials I through VII. J Clin Oncol 2003;21:1205–13.
239. Taghian A, Jeong JH, Mamounas E, et al. Patterns of locoregional failure in patients with operable breast cancer treated by mastectomy and adjuvant chemotherapy with or without tamoxifen and without radiotherapy: results from five National Surgical Adjuvant Breast and Bowel Project randomized clinical trials. J Clin Oncol 2004;22:4247–54.
240. Cheng JCH, Chen CH, Liu MC, et al. Locoregional failure of postmastectomy patients with 1-3 positive lymph nodes without adjuvant radiotherapy. Int J Rad Oncol Biol Phys 2002;52:980–8.
241. Woodward W, Strom EA, Tucker SL, et al. Locoregional recurrence after doxorubicin-based chemotherapy and postmastectomy radiation: Implications for patients with early stage disease and predictors for recurrence after radiation. Int J Rad Oncol Biol Phys 2003;57:336–44.
242. Buchholz TA, Katz A, Strom EA, et al. Pathologic tumor size and lymph node status predict for different rates of locoregional recurrence after mastectomy for breast cancer patients treated with neoadjuvant versus adjuvant chemotherapy. Int J Rad Oncol Biol Phys 2002;53:880–8.
243. Buchholz TA, Tucker SL, Masullo L, et al. Predictors of local-regional recurrence after neoadjuvant chemotherapy and mastectomy without radiation. J Clin Oncol 2002;20:17–23.
244. Huang EH, Tucker SL, Strom EA, et al. Radiation treatment improves local-regional control and cause-specific survival for selected patients with locally advanced breast cancer treated with neoadjuvant chemotherapy and mastectomy. J Clin Oncol 2004;22(23):4691–9.
245. Garg A, Strom EA, McNeese MD, et al. T3 disease at presentation or pathologic involvement of four or more lymph nodes predict for local-regional recurrence in stage II breast cancer treated with neoadjuvant chemotherapy and mastectomy without radiation. Int J Rad Oncol Biol Phys 2004;59:138–45.
246. Gilbert RW, Kim JH, Posner JB. Epidural spinal cord compression from metastatic tumor. Diagnosis and treatment. Ann Neurol 1978;3:40–51.
247. Patchell RA, Tibbs PA, Walsh JW, et al. A randomized trial of surgery in the treatment of single metastases to the brain. N Engl J Med 1990;322:494–500.
248. Loeffler JS, Kooy HM, Wen PY, et al. The treatment of recurrent brain metastases with stereotactic radio-surgery. J Clin Oncol 1990;8:576–582.
249. Taylor ME, Perec CA, Halverson KJ, et al. Factors influencing cosmetic results after conservation therapy for breast cancer. Int J Rad Oncol Biol Phys 1995;31:753–64.
250. Wazer DE, DiPetrillo T, Schmidt-Ullrich R, et al. Factors influencing cosmetic out-come and complication risk after conservative surgery and radiotherapy for early-stage breast carcinoma. J Clin Oncol 1992;10:356–63.
251. Rutqvist LE, Lax I, Fornander T, et al. Cardiovascular mortality in a randomized trial of adjuvant radiation therapy versus surgery alone in primary breast cancer. Int J Rad Oncol Biol Phys 1992;22:887–96.
252. Hojris I, Overgaard M, Christensen JJ, et al. Morbidity and mortality of ischaemic heart disease in high-risk breast-cancer patients after adjuvant postmastectomy systemic treatment with or without radiotherapy: analysis of DBCG 82b and 82c randomised trials. Lancet 1999;354:1425–30.
253. Vallis KA, Pintilie M, Chong N, et al. Assessment of coronary heart disease morbidity and mortality after radiation therapy for early breast cancer. J Clin Oncol 2002;20:1036–42.
254. Giordano SH, Kuo YF, Freeman JL, et al. Decreasing risk of cardiac death after adjuvant radiotherapy for breast cancer. Nat Cancer Inst 2005;97:419–24.
255. Hortobagyi GN, Buzdar AU. Locally advanced breast cancer. A review including the M.D. Anderson experience. In: Rogaz J, Ariel IM, editors. High-risk breast cancer. 1st ed. Berlin: Springer-Verlag; 1991. p. 382–415.
256. Smith IC, Heys SD, Hutcheon AW, et al. Neoadjuvant chemotherapy in breast cancer: significantly enhanced response with docetaxel. J Clin Oncol 2002;20:1456–66.

257. Thomas E, Holmes FA, Smith TL et al. The use of alternate, non-cross-resistant adjuvant chemotherapy on the basis of pathologic response to a neoadjuvant doxorubicin-based regimen in women with operable breast cancer: long-term results from a prospective randomized trial. J Clin Oncol 2004;22:2294–302.
258. Bear HD, Anderson S, Brown A, et al. The effect on tumor response of adding sequential preoperative docetaxel to preoperative doxorubicin and cyclophosphamide: preliminary results from National Surgical Adjuvant Breast and Bowel Project Protocol B-27. J Clin Oncol 2003;21:4165–74.
259. Kuerer HM, Newman LA, Smith TL, et al. Clinical course of breast cancer patients with complete pathologic primary tumor and axillary lymph node response to doxorubicin-based neoadjuvant chemotherapy. J Clin Oncol 1999;17:460–9.
260. Buchholz TA, Davis D, McConkey DJ, et al. Chemotherapy-induced apoptosis and bcl-2 levels correlated with breast cancer response. Cancer J 2003;9:33–41.
261. Ayers M, Symmans WF, Stec J, et al. Gene expression profiles predict complete pathologic response to neoadjuvant paclitaxel and fluorouracil, doxorubicin, and cyclophosphamide chemotherapy in breast cancer. J Clin Oncol 2004;22:2284–93.
262. Recht A, Come SE, Henderson IC, et al. The sequencing of chemotherapy and radiation therapy after conservative surgery for early-stage breast cancer. N Engl J Med 1996;334:1356–61.
263. Bellon JR, Harris JR. Chemotherapy and radiation therapy for breast cancer: what is the optimal sequence? J Clin Oncol 2004;23(1):5–7.
264. Pierce LJ, Lew D, Hutchins L, et al. Patterns of recurrence by sequence of chemotherapy and radiotherapy in early stage breast cancer. Int J Rad Oncol Biol Phys 2003;57:127.
265. Sartor CI, Peterson BL, Woolf S, et al. Effect of addition of adjuvant paclitaxel on radiotherapy delivery and locoregional control of node-positive breast cancer: Cancer and Leukemia Group B 9344. J Clin Oncol 2005;23:30–40.
266. Ahn PH, Vu HT, Lannin D, et al. Sequence of radiotherapy with tamoxifen in conservatively managed breast cancer does not affect local relapse rates. J Clin Oncol 2004;23:17–23.
267. Pierce LJ, Hutchins LF, Green SR, et al. Sequencing of tamoxifen and radiotherapy after breast-conserving surgery in early-stage breast cancer. J Clin Oncol 2004;23:24–29.
268. Bentzen SM, Skoczylas JZ, Overgaard M, et al. Radiotherapy-related lung fibrosis enhanced by tamoxifen. J Natl Cancer Inst 1995;88:918–22.
269. Azria D, Gourgou S, Sozzi WJ, et al. Concomitant use of tamoxifen with radiotherapy enhances subcutaneous breast fibrosis in hypersensitive patients. Br J Cancer 2004;91:1251–60.
270. Silva MC, Rowlands MG, Dowsett M, et al. Intratumoral aromatase as a prognostic factor in human breast carcinoma. Cancer Res 1989;49:2591–2.
271. Smith IE, Dowsett M. Aromatase inhibitors in breast cancer. N Engl J Med 2003;348:2431–42.
272. Robertson JF, Blamey RW. The use of gonadotrophin-releasing hormone (GnRH) agonists in early and advanced breast cancer in pre- and perimenopausal women. European J Cancer 2003;39:861–9.
273. Osborne CK, Zhao H, Fuqua SA. Selective estrogen receptor modulators. Structure, function, and clinical use [review]. J Clin Oncol 2000;18:3172–86.
274. Delmas PD, Bjarnason NH, Mitlak BH, et al. Effects of raloxifene on bone mineral density, serum cholesterol concentrations, and uterine endometrium in post-menopausal women. N Engl J Med 1997;337:1641–7.
275. Buzdar AU, Hortobagyi G. Update on endocrine therapy for breast cancer [review]. Clin Cancer Res 1998;4:527–34.
276. Goldie JH, Coldman AJ. A mathematical model for relating the drug sensitivity of tumors to their spontaneous mutation rate. Cancer Treat Rep 1979;63:1727–33.
277. Norton L, Simon R. Tumor size, sensitivity to therapy and design of treatment schedules. Cancer Treat Rep 1977;61:1307–17.
278. Ross JS, Fletcher JA, Bloom KJ, et al. Targeted therapy in breast cancer: the HER-2/neu gene and protein. Molecular & Cellular Proteomics 2004;3:379–98.
279. Baselga J, Tripathy D, Mendelsohn J, et al. Phase II study of weekly intravenous recombinant humanized antip185HER2 monoclonal antibody in patients with HER2/neu-overexpressing metastatic breast cancer. J Clin Oncol 1996;14:737–44.
280. Slamon DJ, Leyland-Jones B, Shak S, et al. Use of chemotherapy plus a monoclonal antibody against HER2 for metastatic breast cancer that overexpresses HER2. N Engl J Med 2001;344:783–92.
281. Noonberg SB, Benz CC. Tyrosine kinase inhibitors targeted to the epidermal growth factor receptor subfamily–Role as anticancer agents [Review]. Drugs 2000;59:753–67.
282. Fisher B, Redmond C, Poisson R, et al. Eight-year results of a randomized clinical trial comparing total mastectomy and lumpectomy with or without radiation in the treatment of breast cancer. N Engl J Med 1989;320:822–8.
283. Bonadonna G, Valagussa P, Moliterni A, et al. Adjuvant cyclophosphamide, methotrexate, and fluorouracil in node-positive breast cancer. The results of 20 years of follow-up. N Engl J Med 1995;332:901–6.
284. Mansour EG, Gray R, Shatila AH, et al. Survival advantage of adjuvant chemotherapy in high-risk node-negative breast cancer. Ten-year analysis-an intergroup study. J Clin Oncol 1998;16:3486–92.
284a. Early Breast Cancer Trialists' Collaborative Group (EBCTCG). Effects of chemotherapy and hormonal therapy for early breast cancer on recurrence and 15-year survival: an overview of the randomized trials. Lancet 2005;365:1687–1717.
285. Hortobagyi GN. Adjuvant systemic therapy for small, node-negative breast cancer. Decisions based on therapeutic ratio. Breast Dis 2002;12:364–9.
286. Baum M, Buzdar A, Cuzick J, et al. Anastrozole alone or in combination with tamoxifen versus tamoxifen alone for adjuvant treatment of postmenopausal women with early-stage breast cancer: results of the ATAC (Arimidex, Tamoxifen Alone or in Combination) trial efficacy and safety update analyses. Cancer 2003;98:1802-10.
287. Fisher B, Dignam J, Mamounas EP, et al. Sequential methotrexate and fluorouracil for the treatment of node-negative breast cancer patients with estrogen receptor-negative tumors. Eight-year results from National Surgical Adjuvant Breast and Bowel Project (NSABP) B-13 and first report of findings from NSABP B-19 comparing methotrexate and fluorouracil with conventional cyclophosphamide, methotrexate, and fluorouracil. J Clin Oncol 1996;14:1982–92.
288. Fisher B, Dignam J, Wolmark N, et al. Tamoxifen and chemotherapy for lymph node-negative, estrogen receptor-positive breast cancer. J Natl Cancer Inst 1997;89:1673–82.
289. Early Breast Cancer Trialists' Collaborative Group. Tamoxifen for early breast cancer: an overview of the randomised trials. Lancet 1998;351:1451–67.
290. Fisher B, Redmond C. Systemic therapy in node-negative patients. Updated findings from NSABP clinical trials. J Natl Cancer Inst Monogr 1992;11:105–16
291. Fisher B, Anderson S, Tan-Chiu E, et al. Tamoxifen and chemotherapy for axillary node-negative, estrogen receptor-negative breast cancer. Findings from National Surgical Adjuvant Breast and Bowel Project B-23. J Clin Oncol 2001;19:931–42.
292. Carter CL, Allen C, Henson DE. Relation of tumor size, lymph node status, and survival in 24,740 breast cancer cases. Cancer 1989;63:181–7.
293. Fisher B, Dignam J, Tan-Chiu E, et al. Prognosis and treatment of patients with breast tumors of one centimeter or less and negative axillary lymph nodes. J Natl Cancer Inst 2001;93:112–20.
294. Muss HB, Woolf S, Berry D, et al. Adjuvant chemotherapy in older and younger women with lymph node-positive breast cancer. JAMA 2005;293:1073–81.
295. Fisher B, Brown AM, Dimitrov NV, et al. Two months of doxorubicin-cyclophosphamide with and without interval reinduction therapy compared with 6 months of cyclophosphamide, methotrexate, and fluorouracil in positive-node breast cancer patients with tamoxifen non-responsive tumors. Results from the National Surgical Adjuvant Breast and Bowel Project B-15. J Clin Oncol 1990;8:1483.
296. Bonadonna G, Zambetti M, Valagussa P. Sequential or alternating doxorubicin and CMF regimens in breast cancer with more than three positive nodes. Ten-year results. JAMA 1995;273:542–7.
297. Michaud LB, Valero V, Hortobagyi G. Risks and benefits of taxanes in breast and ovarian cancer. Drug Safety 2000;23:401–28.
298. Henderson IC, Berry DA, Demetri GD, et al. Improved outcomes from adding sequential Paclitaxel but not from escalating Doxorubicin dose in an adjuvant chemotherapy regimen for patients with node-positive primary breast cancer. J Clin Oncol 2003;21:976–83.
299. Martin M, Pienkowski T, Mackey J, et al and BCIRG 001 Investigators. TAC improves disease free survival and overall survival over FAC in node positive early breast cancer patients, BCIRG 001: 55 months follow-up [abstract]. Breast Cancer Res Treat 2003; 76 (Suppl 1 [late breaking abstracts]):2..
300. Wood WC, Budman DR, Korzun AH, et al. Dose and dose intensity of adjuvant chemotherapy for stage II, node-positive breast carcinoma [published erratum appears in N Engl J Med 1994;331:139]. N Engl J Med 1994;330:1253–59.
301. Fisher B, Anderson S, DeCillis A, et al. Further evaluation of intensified and increased total dose of cyclophosphamide for the treatment of primary breast cancer. Findings from National Surgical Adjuvant Breast and Bowel Project B-25. J Clin Oncol 1999;17:3374–88.
302. Citron ML, Berry DA, Cirrincione, et al. Randomized trial of dose-dense versus conventionally scheduled and sequential versus concurrent combination chemotherapy as postoperative adjuvant treatment of node-positive primary breast cancer: first report of Intergroup Trial C9741/Cancer and Leukemia Group B Trial 9741. J Clin Oncol 2003;21:1431–9.
303. 2005 ASCO Annual Meeting: Advances in Monoclonal Antibody Therapy for Breast Cancer (Scientific Symposium). Available at: http://www.asco.org/ac/1,1003,_12-002514-00_18-0034-00_19-00934-00_21-001,00.asp
304. American Society of Clinical Oncology. Recommended breast cancer surveillance guidelines. J Clin Oncol 1997;15:2149–56.
305. Albain KS, Green SJ, Ravdin PM, et al. Adjuvant chemohormonal therapy for primary breast cancer should be sequential instead of concurrent. Initial results from Intergroup Trial 0100 (SWOG-8814). Proc Am Soc Clin Oncol 2002;21:36a (abst. 143).
306. Early Breast Cancer Trialists' Collaborative Group. Ovarian ablation in early breast cancer. Overview of the randomised trials. Lancet 1996;348:1189–96.
307. Jonat W, Kaufmann M, Sauerbrei W, et al. Goserelin versus cyclophosphamide, methotrexate, and fluorouracil as adjuvant therapy in premenopausal patients with node-positive breast cancer: The Zoladex Early Breast Cancer Research Association Study.[comment]. J Clin Oncol. 2002;20:4628–35.
308. Goss PE, Ingle JN, Martino S, et al. A randomized trial of letrozole in postmenopausal women after five years of tamoxifen therapy for early-stage breast cancer. New England Journal of Medicine 2003;349:1793–802.
309. Coombes RC, Hall E, Gibson LJ, et al. A randomized trial of exemestane after two to three years of tamoxifen therapy in postmenopausal women with primary breast cancer. N Engl J Med 2004;350:1081–92.
310. Winer EP, Hudis C, Burstein HJ, et al. American Society of Clinical Oncology Technology Assessment on the Use of Aromatase Inhibitors As Adjuvant Therapy for Postmenopausal Women With Hormone Receptor-Positive Breast Cancer: Status Report 2004. J Clin Oncol 2005;23:619–29.
311. Hortobagyi GN, Smith TL, Legha SS, et al. Multivariate analysis of prognostic factors in metastatic breast cancer. J Clin Oncol 1983;1:776–86.
312. Greenberg PA, Hortobagyi GN, Smith TL, et al. Long-term follow-up of patients with complete remission following combination chemotherapy for metastatic breast cancer. J Clin Oncol 1996;14:2197–205.
313. Klijn JG, Blamey RW, Boccardo F, et al. Combined tamoxifen and luteinizing hormone-releasing hormone (LHRH) agonist versus LHRH agonist alone in premenopausal advanced breast cancer. A meta-analysis of four randomized trials. J Clin Oncol 2001;19:343–53.
314. A'Hern RP, Smith IE, Ebbs SR. Chemotherapy and survival in advanced breast cancer. The inclusion of doxorubicin in Cooper type regimens. Br J Cancer 1993;67:801–5.
315. Fossati R, Confalonieri C, Torri V, et al. Cytotoxic and hormonal treatment for metastatic breast cancer. A systematic review of published randomized trials involving 31,510 women [review]. J Clin Oncol 1998;16:3439–60.
316. Blum JL, Jones SE, Buzdar AU, et al. Multicenter phase II study of capecitabine in paclitaxel-refractory metastatic breast cancer. J Clin Oncol 1999;17:485–93.
317. Jones S, Erban J, Overmoyer B, et al. Randomized trial comparing docetaxel and paclitaxel in patients with metastatic breast cancer [abstract]. Breast Cancer Res Treat 2003;82(Suppl 1):S9.
318. Nabholtz JM, Falkson C, Campos D et al. Docetaxel and doxorubicin compared with doxorubicin and cyclophosphamide as first-line chemotherapy for metastatic breast cancer: results of a randomized, multicenter, phase III trial. Journal of Clinical Oncology 2003;21:968–75.

319. Gennari A, Salvadori B, Donati S, et al. Cardiotoxicity of epirubicin/paclitaxel-containing regimens. Role of cardiac risk factors. J Clin Oncol 1999;17:3596–602.
320. Rosen LS, Gordon D, Kaminski M, et al. Long-term efficacy and safety of zoledronic acid compared with pamidronate disodium in the treatment of skeletal complications in patients with advanced multiple myeloma or breast carcinoma: a randomized, double-blind, multicenter, comparative trial. Cancer 2003;98:1735–44.
321. Petrek JA, Theriault RL. Pregnancy-associated breast cancer and subsequent pregnancy in breast cancer survivors. In: Harris JR, Lippman ME, Morrow M, Osborne CK, editors. Diseases of the Breast, 3rd ed. Baltimore: Lippincott Williams & Wilkins; 2004, p. 1035–46.
322. Wooster R, Bignell G, Lancaster J, et al. Identification of the breast cancer susceptibility gene BRCA2. Nature 1995;378:789–92.
323. Giordano SH, Cohen DS, Buzdar AU, et al. Breast carcinoma in men. Cancer. 2004;101:51–7.
324. Jaiyesimi IA, Buzdar AU, Hortobagyi G. Inflammatory breast cancer. A review. J Clin Oncol 1992;10:1014–24.

Section 32

THE SKIN

108

Malignant Melanoma

Donald L. Morton, MD, FACS
Richard Essner, MD, FACS
John M. Kirkwood, MD
Robert C. Wollman, MD

Once an uncommon cancer, cutaneous melanoma is rapidly increasing in incidence throughout the world. Melanoma now accounts for approximately 4% of all cancers diagnosed in the United States.[1] The reasons for this rapidly increasing incidence appear related to changes in sun exposure patterns and perhaps to the reduction in the ozone layer.[2] The prognosis for patients with melanoma is directly related to the depth of invasion of the primary lesion and, in part, to initial treatment. Early-stage melanoma is readily cured by wide surgical excision. However, once melanoma metastasizes, no current treatment reliably affects the course of disease. For this reason, physicians must be cognizant of the classic clinical signs associated with melanoma developing de novo or as part of a nevus (change in color, recent enlargement, nodularity, pruritus, ulceration, or bleeding) and recognize the more subtle clinical characteristics, such as irregular or angular borders or variations in color. These characteristics often signal minimally invasive, early, and curable melanomas.

EPIDEMIOLOGY AND ETIOLOGY

According to the American Cancer Society, 57,700 new cases of melanoma will be diagnosed in the United States in 2005, and there will be approximately 7,700 deaths from the disease.[1] Current projections indicate that 1 in 56 men and 1 in 80 women will develop cutaneous melanoma (lifetime risk).[3] The age-adjusted annual incidence in the United States is approximately 17.2 per 100,000, although some geographic areas have a greater incidence.[3] Australia and New Zealand have the highest melanoma incidence and mortality rate in the world.

Although the etiology of melanoma is not entirely understood, case-control studies have shown that it is largely a disease of individuals with fair complexions. Individuals with red or blond hair and fair skin, who burn easily or have a history of severe sunburn, are at substantially higher risk of developing melanoma than more darkly pigmented, age-matched controls. Individuals with an increased number of nevi or a tendency to develop freckles are also at increased risk for developing melanoma.[4]

Several observations strongly suggest that ultraviolet (UV) light may be a critical factor leading to the development of cutaneous melanoma.[5,6] There is an increasing incidence of melanoma in fair-complected populations and a correlation with increasing distance from the north and south poles. Adults who migrate to sunny climates are at less risk than similar individuals who were born there, suggesting that duration of exposure to UV radiation is important in the development of melanoma. Freckles and nevi induced by solar irradiation are risk factors for the development of melanoma. These epidemiologic observations suggest that sunlight, particularly UV light, has an important role in the induction of cutaneous melanoma and that changes in the pattern of sun exposure have substantially contributed to increases in melanoma incidence during the past several decades. In addition, the depletion of the ozone in the stratosphere and the resulting increased intensity of UV light may be responsible in part for the increasing incidence of cutaneous melanoma. Recent studies have suggested that the ozone layer may have decreased by 3 to 7% since 1969.

Factors other than UV light contribute to the development of melanoma. Melanoma can occur in relatively unexposed areas of skin, such as the palms and soles and even in mucosal sites, albeit at rates considerably lower than for sun-exposed areas. In contrast to squamous and basal cell carcinoma, melanoma risk does not have a direct relationship to cumulative sun exposure. Melanoma is more common among white-collar workers than among individuals whose occupation is largely outdoors. These observations suggest that the relationship between sun exposure and the risk of developing melanoma is related not only to the cumulative level of sun exposure but also to acute, intense, and intermittent exposure. In fact, numerous studies have consistently found that a person's risk of being diagnosed with melanoma is associated with a history of blistering sunburn.[3,6]

The increased incidence of melanoma may be related to two observed patterns. First, younger people appear to have a proportionally greater incidence of melanoma than do people over 65 years old. Second, the incidence of melanoma around the head and face has increased slightly, and there has been a marked increase in the incidence of melanoma on the legs in females and the trunk in males.[7] This trend reflects changes in clothing styles and materials, as well as in recreational habits. Melanoma rarely occurs on the double-covered areas on which brassieres and underpants are worn.

Familial Melanoma UV-mediated induction of melanoma is believed to result from damage to the DNA of melanocytes. This is suggested by the fact that metastatic melanoma cells are usually highly aneuploid, whereas normal melanocytes are diploid. Further evidence for the genetic etiology of melanoma comes from chromosomal alterations involving the short arm of chromosome 1 and both arms of chromosomes 6 and 7 in melanomas and cell lines derived from either primary melanomas or metastases.[8,9] Evidence suggests a 9p21 deletion in familial melanoma, and consistent lesions of 9p have become apparent.[10,11] Common losses also occur on chromosomes 10 and 8p, along with gains in copy number for chromosomes 7, 8, 6p, 19, 20, 17, and 2.[12]

Members of certain families are more susceptible to development of the genetic abnormalities associated with melanoma. Approximately 8 to 12% of all cases of cutaneous melanoma occur in persons with familial predisposition to the development of melanoma.

Like many other heritable malignant and premalignant conditions, familial human melanoma is characterized by an increased risk of developing a primary tumor, a higher incidence of multiple primary tumors, and an earlier age at onset.[13] In individuals with familial melanoma, the locus for cutaneous malignant melanoma–dysplastic nevus resides on the distal portion of the short arm of chromosome 1. Because this region of the human genome is frequently involved in karyotypic abnormalities, chromosomal deletion may represent the second event in a recessive model of tumorigenesis.[8] Two genetic lesions relating to p16, cyclin-dependent kinase 4 (CDK4) and cyclin-dependent kinase inhibitor 2A (CDKN2A), have been identified in familial melanoma; in these patients, the predisposition to melanoma appears to be associated with an increased risk of developing pancreatic cancer and perhaps other cancers.[14,15] The *TP53* tumor suppressor gene, although overexpressed in melanoma, may only be a sign of genetic disruption and not an initiating event.[16] *BRAF* mutations are frequently reported in melanoma and may be related to metastasis.[17] All patients and their families should undergo complete skin surveys as part of their routine medical care.[18]

PRECURSOR LESIONS

Dysplastic Nevus Syndrome (Familial Atypical Mole/Melanoma Syndrome) This familial form of malignant melanoma is distinguished by multiple, large (> 5 mm in diameter) macular moles that have irregular borders and are variable shades of brown, black, and red. Dysplastic nevi have both macular and papular components and may appear anywhere on the body but are most commonly seen on the trunk. The frequent appearance of dysplastic nevi on areas of the body that are normally covered, such as the buttocks, scalp, and breasts, is distinctive of this form of malignant melanoma. Microscopically, these lesions are active junctional or compound nevi with well-described patterns of melanocytic atypia, dermal fibrosis, telangiectasia, and lymphocytic infiltration. The patient with dysplastic nevus syndrome (DNS) may present with 10 to 20 dysplastic nevi.[19]

Histologic confirmation is desirable for initial diagnosis of dysplastic nevi. According to the National Institutes of Health Consensus Conference on Precursors to Malignant Melanoma, these histologic features are superimposed on those of junctional or compound nevus and include melanocytic hyperplasia with elongation of rete ridges; enlarged, hyperchromatic melanocytic nuclei; bridging of aggregated melanocytes at rete ridges; lamellar and concentric dermal fibroplasia; and lymphocytic infiltrates.[20]

Melanoma may arise from dysplastic nevi or from apparently normal skin remote from nevi in patients with DNS. This is one argument against resection of all atypical nevi for melanoma prevention. Melanomas associated with dysplastic nevi are of the superficial spreading type and are often relatively thin. Dysplastic nevi are reportedly contiguous with 20 to 50% of all melanomas. They are considered nonobligate precursors and markers of malignant potential.[21]

The molecular genetic mechanism by which melanoma develops in DNS is not known. DNS was first attributed to an autosomal dominant single gene with incomplete penetrance. Other data suggest that transmission is polygenic from an undetermined number of alleles at separate loci, perhaps influenced by a cytoplasmic component.

Congenital Nevi Congenital melanocytic nevi are collections of nevus cells present in almost 1% of newborn infants.[22] These hamartomas originate in the neural crest. Clinical features of congenital nevi are readily recognizable to the experienced physician. These features include grossly irregular surface, increased pigmentation in varying shades of brown, and hypertrichosis. Although melanoma may arise de novo, it arises in association with congenital nevi at increased frequency, and all congenital nevi should be viewed with suspicion.

Because large congenital nevi are regarded as precursors for human malignant melanoma,[23] they should be followed very closely and excised or a biopsy should be performed if any change is noted. It is not yet clear whether small congenital nevi are precursors to melanoma, but they should be monitored by an experienced dermatologist. The lifetime risk of melanoma in patients with congenital nevi approaches 20%.[20,22]

Melanocytes as Antecedent Lesions Melanocytes arise from the neural crest and migrate to their final destinations in the skin, uveal tract, meninges, and mucosae. Most melanocytes are found at the epidermal-dermal junction of the skin, and the vast majority of melanomas arise from cutaneous sites. However, melanoma has also been reported in the meninges, in the mucosa of the gastrointestinal and respiratory tract, and in the vagina. Clinical and histological observations indicate that melanoma may arise in association with a pre-existing lesion,[24] but most cutaneous melanomas do not appear to originate in previously known or histopathologically documentable nevocellular nevi.

Biologic Growth Phases Most melanomas have two distinctive growth phases: radial and vertical. During the radial phase, neoplastic cells grow in a radial fashion, either above or just below the basal lamina. The radial growth phase is not associated with metastasis. Radial growth may last many years for superficial spreading melanoma and lentigo maligna melanoma but is generally brief or undetected for nodular melanoma. Eventually, the melanoma evolves into the vertical growth phase, the malignant cell population invades the dermis, and cells gain the potential to metastasize.

CLINICAL CHARACTERISTICS

If the diagnosis of melanoma is made early in the course of its natural history, simple wide surgical excision is usually curative. Cutaneous melanoma can occur anywhere on the body but most commonly is found on the lower extremities in women and on the trunk in men. The classic clinical signs of cutaneous melanoma are alterations in a pigmented lesion's color, size, or surface, with nodularity, ulceration, bleeding, and pruritus. However, these manifestations are most often associated with advanced, deeply invasive lesions. More subtle signs, such as irregular borders and variegated color, are more common in early melanomas. About 1% of melanomas lack pigment and are termed amelanotic. Common to all melanomas is change in size, configuration, character, or color. For this reason, pigmented lesions exhibiting any change, particularly in patients with high-risk characteristics, should be biopsied and examined histologically.

Classification The American Joint Committee on Cancer (AJCC) identifies five different forms of extraocular melanoma: lentigo maligna melanoma, superficial spreading melanoma, nodular melanoma, acral-lentiginous melanoma, and mucosal lentiginous melanoma. Between 80 and 85% of melanomas are lentigo maligna melanoma, superficial spreading melanoma, or nodular melanoma. These different forms of melanoma represent distinct pathologic entities that have different clinical and biologic characteristics (Table 108-1).

Superficial Spreading Melanoma Superficial spreading melanoma (SSM) represents approximately 70% of all melanomas. SSM generally arises in a pre-existing lesion and is the lesion most commonly associated with dysplastic nevi or amelanotic melanomas. SSM may have a relatively long natural history. Typically, diagnosis follows an increased rate of change in a precursor lesion. Early in their evolution, SSMs usually appear flat, with irregular borders. Notching of the border is particularly characteristic. The lesions are multiple shades of tan, brown, black, red, and white (Figure 108-1). Amelanotic areas may represent areas of regression. As the lesion grows, it may develop an irregular surface. SSMs tend to occur throughout adulthood, with a peak incidence in the fifth decade of life. Most commonly, they occur on the head, neck, and trunk in males and on the extremities in females.

Table 108-1 Differential Clinical Features of the Common Types of Melanoma

Type of Melanoma	Common Locations	Median Age (Yr)	Sex Predilection	Duration	Identifying Features of Radial Growth Phase*
Lentigo maligna	Sun-exposed surfaces (head and neck most common)	70	None	5–15 yr	Flat. Shades of tan to black Frequent areas of hypopigmentation
Superficial spreading	All body surfaces	56	Males: head, neck, trunk Females: lower legs	1–5 yr	Flat to slightly raised Irregular margins. Shades of brown, black, pink. Areas of hypopigmentation
Nodular	All body surfaces	49	None overall Males: head, neck, trunk	1 mo–2 yr	None
Acral-lentiginous	Volar and subungual areas	59	Slight female predominance	2 mo–10 yr	Tan to dark-brown macule
Mucosal lentiginous	Oral, ocular, and genital mucosa	56	Slight male preponderance but varies from area to area	4–20 yr	Tan to dark-brown macular area

*The invasive tumors in each melanoma subtype vary from low convex to polypoid in shape and from dark blue-black to light tan or even reddish pink (amelanotic) in color. They are usually hairless and may be ulcerated. Reprinted with permission from Cancer Treatment. 3rd ed. Philadelphia: WB Saunders; 1990. p. 102.

Lentigo Maligna Melanoma Lentigo maligna melanoma (LMM), which constitutes approximately 10% of all melanomas, arises from lentigo maligna (melanotic freckle of Hutchinson or precancerous melanosis of Dubreuilh). LMM is found most commonly on sun-exposed skin in elderly individuals (median age 70 years). The lesions are generally large (3–4 cm in diameter) and flat with irregular borders, in variable shades of tan to dark brown (Figure 108-2). Hypopigmented areas in the lesion represent areas of regression. The precursor lesion, lentigo maligna, usually has been present for 5 to 15 years prior to the development of invasive melanoma.

Nodular Malignant Melanoma Nodular malignant melanoma (NM) comprises 10 to 15% of all cutaneous melanomas. NM may develop on any body surface area but most commonly is diagnosed on the trunk of men. NM is thought to be biologically more aggressive than SSM. Clinically, the lesion is dark and most often uniform in color. Histologically, NM is notable for the complete absence of melanocytic abnormalities in the adjacent epidermis (Figure 108-3). Approximately 5% of NMs are amelanotic. Amelanotic NM may have a symmetric appearance but occasionally becomes polypoid or cauliflower in appearance. NM does not have a radial growth phase and is associated with rapid evolution to vertical growth and invasion of the dermis. For this reason, nodular melanomas tend to be thicker, higher risk lesions.

Acral Lentiginous Melanoma Acral lentiginous melanoma (ALM) occurs on the palms, soles, and subungual regions. It represents approximately 3 to 5% of all cutaneous melanomas. ALM constitutes a substantially higher proportion of melanomas in dark-skinned individuals such as African Americans, Asians, and Hispanics. Most ALM lesions are large (3 cm in diameter) with irregular borders and occur in older individuals (median age 59 years). Subungual melanoma most commonly occurs on the great toe or thumb. ALM is often a tan to dark brown macule with an irregular border, but it may be ulcerating or fungating. Although similar in clinical appearance to LMM, ALM is a much more aggressive lesion that quickly evolves to the vertical growth phase.

Mucosal Lentiginous Melanoma Mucosal lentiginous melanoma (MLM) is similar in appearance to ALM. This lesion occurs in a variety of mucosal sites, including the oral cavity, esophagus, anus, vagina, and conjunctiva.

Staging The methods of Clark and colleagues and Breslow have successively dominated the microstaging of primary melanoma.[25,26] Clark's method defines five levels of penetration through the dermis to the subcutaneous fat (Figure 108-4). Level I melanoma lies in the epidermis above an intact basal lamina. When the melanoma has penetrated the basal lamina into the papillary dermis, it is classified as level II. When the melanoma involves the papillary dermis and may extend to the papillary-reticular dermis interface, it is classified as level III; as it extends into the reticular dermis, it becomes level IV; and as it extends into the subcutaneous fat, it becomes level V. The success of Clark's method of microstaging is directly related to the ability to recognize the microscopic anatomy of the skin. Clark's original observation suggested that the deeper the level of penetration, the poorer the prognosis, an observation that has been repeatedly confirmed when primary lesions are microstaged by experienced dermatopathologists.

Breslow's microstaging method, which is simpler and more reproducible than Clark's method, uses an ocular micrometer to measure the vertical thickness of the primary tumor from the granular layer of the epidermis, or the base of an ulcer, to the deepest identifiable contiguous melanoma cell. The technique is a more accurate prognostic parameter than Clark's level of invasion. The thicker the melanoma, the greater the risk for developing metastatic disease.

The first clinical staging system for melanoma was a macrostaging system of three stages: I, localized melanoma; II, regional metastatic melanoma; and III, disseminated melanoma. This original three-stage system offered the advantage of simplicity but failed to account for important prognostic factors derived from microstaging of the primary lesion. It also did not differentiate the

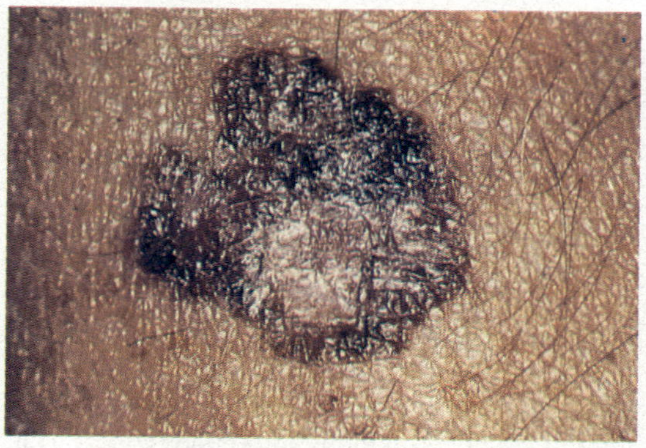

Figure 108-1 Superficial spreading melanoma. Note irregular borders, variations in color, and area of partial regression.

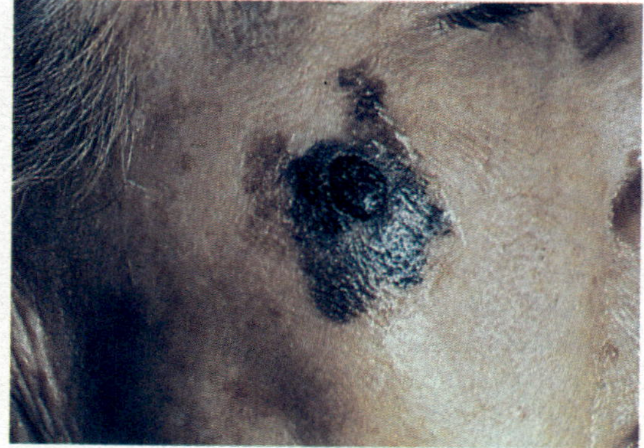

Figure 108-2 Lentigo maligna melanoma with a nodular area of accelerated growth.

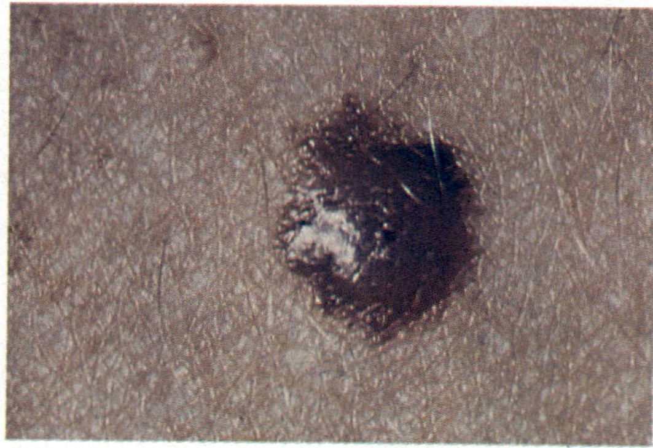

Figure 108-3 Nodular melanoma.

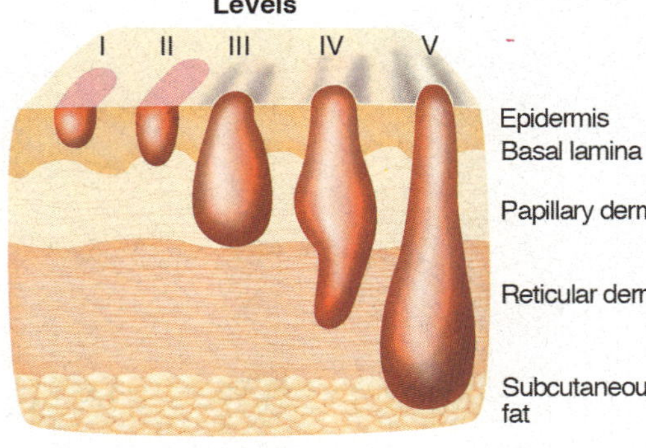

Figure 108-4 Clark's levels of invasion. Redrawn with permission from Eilber FR, Holmes EC, Morton DL. Malignant melanoma. In: Grabb WC, Smith JW, editors. Plastic surgery. A concise guide to clinical practice. Boston: Little Brown; 1968, p. 511.

metastatic risk of the majority of patients with melanoma, because approximately 85% of patients present with clinically localized, stage I melanoma.

The AJCC staging system for melanoma incorporates the histologic characteristics of the primary tumor. This primary tumor–nodes–metastases (pTNM) staging system more accurately assesses the metastatic potential of clinically localized disease and provides a more practical, although more complex, classification for clinicians. In 2001, the AJCC updated its staging system for melanoma based on review of a multicenter-derived database of 17,600 patients.[27] Ulceration was incorporated into the system, and the depth categories were simplified to integer increments of 1, 2, and 4 mm. In addition, nodal disease was classified as microscopic or macroscopic, and distant disease was categorized as soft tissue nonvisceral (M1a); pulmonary (M1b); or other visceral and any distant disease associated with an elevated serum level of lactic dehydrogenase (M1c) (Table 108-2).[28,29]

PROGNOSTIC FEATURES OF CLINICALLY LOCALIZED DISEASE

Melanoma's capricious clinical course makes outcome prediction difficult in patients with clinically localized disease. Variables with prognostic value include the patient's age and gender; the primary tumor's anatomic location, Clark's level, Breslow's thickness, ulceration, and histopathologic type; and the number of regional lymph nodes that contain metastases.[30] Review of a multicenter database of 13,581 patients with localized disease demonstrated that tumor thickness and ulceration were most predictive of survival,[27] and its findings formed the basis of the current AJCC staging system (see Table 108-2).[28] The prognosis for thin, nonulcerated melanomas is excellent (Table 108-3).[29]

Ulceration Ulceration is associated with a biologically more aggressive lesion and a poorer prognosis[31]; 5-year survival rate reportedly drops from 80% for nonulcerated melanomas to 55% for ulcerated melanomas. It is not known why ulcerated primaries have a more aggressive biologic nature. Ulcerated lesions tend to be thicker and have a nodular growth pattern, but the increased thickness does not account for the poorer prognosis. However, the width of surface ulceration has been significantly correlated with survival.

Other Histologic Prognosticators The mitotic rate per square millimeter and the presence of lymphatic or blood vessel invasion are relevant. The histological growth pattern also has prognostic value; LMM may have a more favorable prognosis than SSM or NM. Most of these differences may, however, merely reflect a tendency for NM to be thicker and more invasive, whereas LMM tends to be thinner and exhibit prolonged radial growth.

A faint white halo surrounding a cutaneous melanoma may represent regression of the lesion. Microscopically, partial (> 50%) regression is seen as subtotal loss of the melanocyte nest and replacement with lymphocytes. Although regression is generally associated with thin primaries, these lesions have a less favorable outcome than would be expected on the basis of their thickness alone.[32] The development of new molecular biology techniques may soon allow genetic characteristics to replace histologic features as the most important prognostic indicators.[16,33]

Gender Women with melanoma fare substantially better than men.[34] This survival advantage may be primarily due to the more frequent location of the lesion on the extremities and the less frequent presence of ulceration.

Anatomic Site The anatomic site of the primary lesion is an important prognostic factor. Both male and female patients with melanomas of the extremities have a better survival rate than patients with melanomas of the head and neck; patients with melanomas of the trunk appear to have the worst prognosis.[35,36] Day and colleagues[37] identified a group of patients with thin melanomas, apparently at low risk for developing recurrent disease, who nonetheless had unanticipated higher mortality. These patients had primary lesions on the skin of the upper back, posterior arm, neck, and scalp. The acronym BANS (back, arm, neck, scalp) was introduced to suggest that these particular anatomic sites had prognostic value. The John Wayne Cancer Institute (JWCI) found that patients with primary lesions arising in the BANS region appeared to have a slightly worse outcome than those with lesions in non-BANS regions, particularly in the presence of nodal metastases.[38] Cascinelli and colleagues,[39] however, have questioned the validity of the BANS concept.

Pregnancy Melanoma arising during pregnancy has been associated with a particularly aggressive clinical course and an extremely grave prognosis. However, a study from JWCI found no significant difference in prognostic characteristics or 5-year survival rates between pregnant and nonpregnant females with localized melanoma.[40] Similar results have been reported by others,[41] and a study from the World Health Organization (WHO) found that female melanoma patients presenting during pregnancy had slightly deeper melanomas but not a different prognosis.[42]

PROGNOSTIC FEATURES OF REGIONAL LYMPH NODE METASTASES

Lymph node metastases (AJCC stage III melanoma) may be discovered when a patient presents with palpable lymph nodes or when pathologic examination of nodes removed during selective

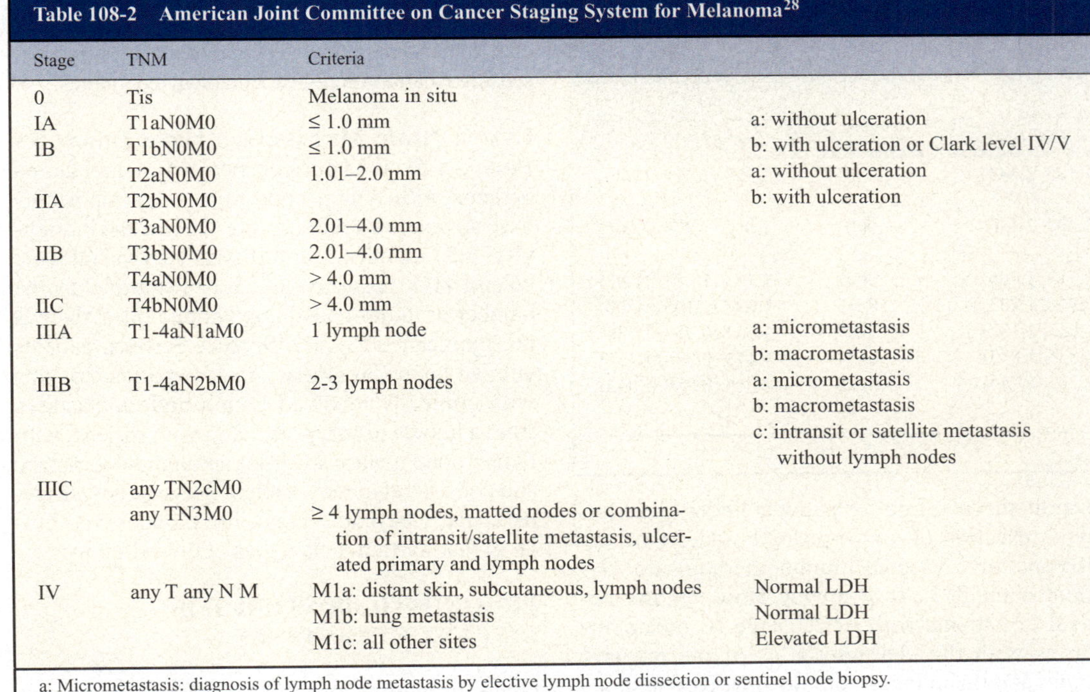

Table 108-2 American Joint Committee on Cancer Staging System for Melanoma[28]

Stage	TNM	Criteria	
0	Tis	Melanoma in situ	
IA	T1aN0M0	≤ 1.0 mm	a: without ulceration
IB	T1bN0M0	≤ 1.0 mm	b: with ulceration or Clark level IV/V
	T2aN0M0	1.01–2.0 mm	a: without ulceration
IIA	T2bN0M0		b: with ulceration
	T3aN0M0	2.01–4.0 mm	
IIB	T3bN0M0	2.01–4.0 mm	
	T4aN0M0	> 4.0 mm	
IIC	T4bN0M0	> 4.0 mm	
IIIA	T1-4aN1aM0	1 lymph node	a: micrometastasis
			b: macrometastasis
IIIB	T1-4aN2bM0	2-3 lymph nodes	a: micrometastasis
			b: macrometastasis
			c: intransit or satellite metastasis without lymph nodes
IIIC	any TN2cM0		
	any TN3M0	≥ 4 lymph nodes, matted nodes or combination of intransit/satellite metastasis, ulcerated primary and lymph nodes	
IV	any T any N M	M1a: distant skin, subcutaneous, lymph nodes	Normal LDH
		M1b: lung metastasis	Normal LDH
		M1c: all other sites	Elevated LDH

a: Micrometastasis: diagnosis of lymph node metastasis by elective lymph node dissection or sentinel node biopsy.
b: Macrometastasis: clinically detected metastases or presence of extracapsular extension of disease.

Table 108-3 Survival According to the New American Joint Committee on Cancer Staging System[29]

Pathologic Stage	TNM	Thickness (mm)	Ulceration	Number of Positive Nodes	5-Year Survival (%)	10-Year Survival (%)
1A	T1a	1	No	0	95	88
1B	T1b	1	Yes or level IV, V	0	91	83
	T2a	1.01–2.0	No	0	89	79
IIA	T2b	1.01–2.0	Yes	0	77	64
	T3a	2.01–4.0	No	0	79	64
IIB	T3b	2.01–4.0	Yes	0	63	51
	T4a	> 4.0	No	0	67	54
IIC	T4b	> 4.0	Yes	0	45	32
IIIA	N1a	Any	No	1	70	63
	N2a	Any	No	2–3	63	57
IIIB	N1a	Any	Yes	1	53	38
	N2a	Any	Yes	2–3	50	36
	N1b	Any	No	1	59	48
	N2b	Any	No	2–3	46	39
IIIC	N1b	Any	Yes	1	29	24
	N2b	Any	Yes	2–3	24	15
	N3	Any	Any	4	27	18
IV	M1a	Any	Any	Any	19	16
	M1b	Any	Any	Any	7	3
	M1c	Any	Any	Any	10	6

Survival is determined from the time of initial presentation of stage I/II, III, or IV melanoma. Patients with recurrent stage III or IV disease have shorter survival from the time of recurrence.

Table 108-4 Long-Term Survival Rates of Patients with Clinical versus Nonclinical Evidence of Regional Node Metastasis*

Source	Nonpalpable/Nonsuspicious Lymph Nodes (%)	Palpable/Suspicious Lymph Nodes (%)	Difference (%)
McNeer and Das Gupta (Surgery 1964;56:512)	52	19	33
Cohen et al (Ann Surg 1977;186:635)	55	38	17
Das Gupta (Ann Surg 1977;186:201)	69	20†	49
Balch et al (Ann Surg 1981;193:77)	48	24	24
Callery et al (Ann Surg 1982;196:69)	48	36	12
Roses et al (Ann Surg 1985;201:103)	44	20	24
Morton et al (Ann Surg 1991;214:491)	59	43	16

*All data are 5-year survival rates except Cohen et al, which are 10-year results.
†Patients with Clark's level III and IV.

Table 108-5 Multivariate Cox Regression Analyses of Prognostic Factors for Survival of Patients with AJCC Stage III Melanoma

Factor	Balch et al[27] *p* Value	Balch et al[27] Risk Ratio (95% CI)	Morton et al[44] *p* Value	Morton et al[44] Risk Ratio (95% CI)
Number of tumor-positive nodes (1 vs 2–3 vs ≥ 4)	< .00001	1.257 (1.185, 1.334)	.0001	1.329 (1.219, 1.449)
Clinical status of nodes/micro- vs macrometastases	< .00001	1.792 (1.497, 2.146)	.0001	1.663 (1.379, 2.006)
Ulceration	< .00001	1.582 (1.313, 1.906)	.0002	1.183 (1.083, 1.293)
Thickness (pT1/2 vs pT3/4)	.1611	1.091 (0.966, 1.233)	.0012	1.287 (1.105, 1.500)
Age	.0003	1.118 (1.053, 1.187)	.1489	1.131 (0.957, 1.336)
Sex	.9407	1.007 (0.836, 1.213)	.0557	1.173 (0.996, 1.381)
Site (extremity vs head/neck vs trunk vs nodal)	.0001	1.461 (1.225, 1.746)	.6108	1.015 (0.959, 1.073)

AJCC = American Joint Committee on Cancer; CI = confidence interval.

elective lymph node dissection or sentinel node biopsy reveals clinically occult tumor deposits. Patients with clinically occult lymph node involvement generally have a better prognosis than those with palpable lymph nodes (Table 108-4); JWCI data indicate a 16% difference in long-term survival.[43] According to Morton and colleagues,[44] the median overall survival and 5-year overall survival rate for patients undergoing surgical resection of tumor-positive nodes (without postoperative vaccine immunotherapy) are 31.9 months and 37%, respectively. However, the survival of patients with AJCC stage III melanoma varies with the characteristics of the primary tumor and the number of tumor-involved regional nodes (see Table 108-3).[29]

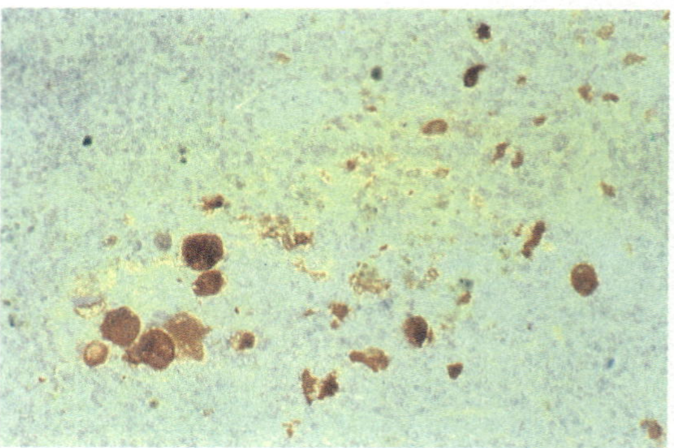

Figure 108-5 Occult melanoma cells in a regional lymph node are detected by immunohistochemical staining using monoclonal antibody to S-100 protein.

Balch and colleagues[27] and Morton and colleagues[44] studied the prognostic significance of age; gender; site, thickness and ulceration of primary; clinical status of regional lymph nodes; and number of histologically positive nodes. By multivariate analysis, the number of tumor-containing lymph nodes, the clinical status of these nodes (palpable versus nonpalpable), and ulceration of the primary were significant in both studies; the number of tumor positive nodes was the strongest predictor of survival (Table 108-5).

Because the number of tumor-positive lymph nodes is the single most important prognostic factor in AJCC stage III melanoma, accurate assessment of these nodes is of paramount importance. Immunohistochemistry permits more detailed microstaging of lymph nodes than conventional histologic techniques using hematoxylin and eosin (H&E) staining, which may underestimate the number of lymph nodes containing tumor. Immunohistochemical assessment of nodal status using antibodies to S-100 protein and other melanoma-associated antigens improves prognostic accuracy and provides a more homogeneous population for trial stratification (Figure 108-5). Molecular assays using reverse transcription polymerase chain reaction (RT-PCR) with specific melanoma-associated markers are even more sensitive than immunohistochemical techniques.[45,46]

Lymph Node Metastases from Unknown Primary Site Fourteen percent of melanoma patients with lymph node metastases reportedly have an unknown primary site.[43] Their median survival is 37 months; 5- and 10-year survival rates are 46 and 41%, respectively.[47] When stratified by the number of tumor-containing lymph nodes, there is no significant survival difference between patients with an unknown primary melanoma and patients with clinically involved lymph node metastases from a known primary site. However, patients with lymph node metastases from an unknown primary site consistently enjoy a slight survival advantage, particularly beyond 5 years. The prognosis is similar to that for thin melanomas of the extremity.

PROGNOSTIC FEATURES OF DISTANT METASTASES

Once melanoma metastasizes to distant sites, median survival is only 4 to 8 months in most

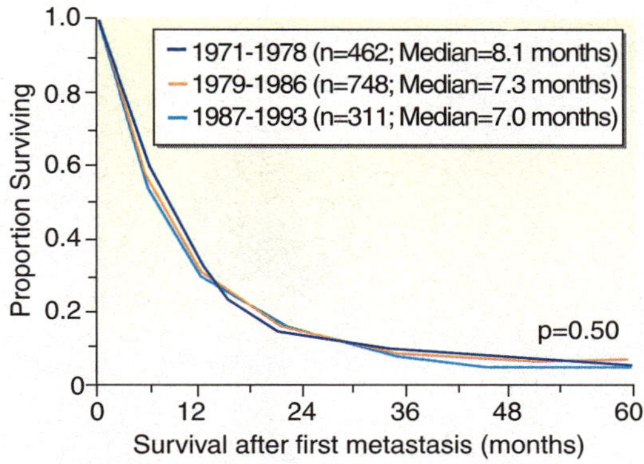

Figure 108-6 John Wayne Cancer Institute melanoma database of American Joint Committee on Cancer stage IV patients (distant metastatic disease) shows the survival of 1,521 patients treated between 1971 and 1993. Reprinted with permission from Barth A et al.[48]

series. A JWCI review of 1,521 melanoma patients with AJCC stage IV disease revealed a median survival of 7.5 months and an estimated 5-year survival rate of 5.5%, with no improvement over the past 22 years (Figure 108-6).[48] Because melanoma has the relatively unusual ability to spread to almost any organ site and does so in a variety of clinical patterns, any symptom in a patient with a history of melanoma must be considered to be potentially secondary to metastatic disease until proven otherwise.

Clinical variables such as age, gender, and primary site and histologic variables such as Clark's level, Breslow's thickness, and ulceration have little bearing on the outcome of distant metastatic disease. The initial site of distant metastasis, the disease-free interval before distant metastases, and stage of disease preceding distant metastases are the three independent clinical variables that predict survival (Table 108-6).[48] AJCC stage IV melanoma patients can be divided into three distinct prognostic groups based on their initial site of metastases: (1) cutaneous, subcutaneous, or nodal metastases (median survival, 12.5 months; estimated 5-year survival rate, 13.5%); (2) lung metastases (median survival, 8.3 months; estimated 5-year survival rate, 3.6%); and (3) gastrointestinal, liver, brain, or bone metastases (median survival, 4.4 months; estimated 5-year survival rate, 2.5%).[29]

The number of metastatic sites is important; median survival is 7 to 12 months for patients with one metastatic site but only 2 to 8 months for patients with multiple metastatic sites.

Disease-Free Interval A multifactorial analysis from the University of Alabama demonstrated significantly improved outcomes among patients whose disease-free interval exceeded 12 months.[49] Review of the JWCI database showed a 5-year survival rate of 6% when the disease-free interval between AJCC stage III and IV disease was at least 18 months, compared to 3% when this interval was shorter (see Table 108-6).[48]

MANAGEMENT OF PRIMARY MELANOMA

Surgical Resection and Biopsy Surgical resection remains the principal curative therapy for melanoma. The first surgical consideration is confirmation of the diagnosis (Figure 108-7). Histologic verification of the diagnosis is essential because surgical recommendations may depend on the microstage of the lesion. There is no evidence that an interval of 1 to 2 weeks between excisional biopsy and wide excision adversely affects outcome. To microstage the lesion accurately, all layers of the skin must be included in the sample. For this reason, shave biopsy or curetting is not recommended. For most lesions less than 2 cm in diameter, where sufficient skin is present to allow a primary closure, an excisional biopsy is appropriate (Figure 108-8). For large lesions or those located where sufficient skin might not be available for primary closure, such as on the face, hands, or feet, incisional biopsy of the most nodular or irregular area is appropriate to establish the diagnosis (Figure 108-9).

Margins of Excision Failure to perform re-excision after biopsy of a primary melanoma is associated with a local recurrence rate as high as 40%. However, although the necessity of re-excision requires little discussion, the margins of excision have been debated. Cochran[50] noted increased numbers of melanocytes in clinically normal skin surrounding many melanomas, supporting the need for a wide margin of excision. Others have claimed that the width of excision may not influence recurrence or survival[51]; Fallowfield and Cook questioned Handley's original recommendation for extensive surgical resection of skin and subcutaneous tissue.[52] It appears that wide local excision as originally described by Handley is not necessary for very thin melanomas; however, increasing level and thickness increase occult permeation of adjacent tissues and probably justify a more extensive resection.

In 1988, the WHO published results of a randomized trial comparing narrow excision (1 cm) and wide surgical excision (3 cm or more) for melanomas less than 2 mm in thickness.[53] Although three patients undergoing narrow excision developed local recurrence, all had melanomas thicker than 1 mm, suggesting that narrow excision for lesions thinner than 1 mm is safe and effective. Studies stratifying patients according to thickness of the primary tumor have demonstrated that the surgical margin has no effect on survival, although a trend toward increasing local recurrence with narrow margins has been observed.[54] A prospective, multiinstitutional randomized intergroup United States trial found that surgical margins could be safely reduced to 2 cm if the primary melanoma was intermediate in thickness (1.0–4.0 mm).[55] Other randomized studies have confirmed that margins of excision do not influence overall survival.[56,57]

Because the time to recurrence is inversely proportional to the thickness of the primary lesion, long-term follow-up (8–10 years) is required to determine the actual local recurrence rate of thin lesions. In sites with sufficient surrounding skin, a wide excision would appear to be the conservative approach, especially for thicker melanomas or those with satellites. There is little cosmetic difference between narrow and wide excision as long as primary closure uses flap rotation and advancement techniques. Skin grafts are rarely necessary except on the scalp and distal to the elbows or knees.

The following surgical guidelines are based on the observation that the risk of local recurrence is directly proportional to the depth of the primary melanoma[58]:

- For Clark's level II melanoma or thin level III lesions that measure less than 1.00 mm in thickness, excise with 1 cm radial margins.
- For Clark's level III melanoma, lesions that are 1.0 to 4.0 mm in thickness, and all Clark's level IV melanomas, excise with 2 cm radial margins.
- For Clark's level V melanoma and all melanomas thicker than 4 mm, excise widely with 2 to 3 cm radial margins around the primary site, including the underlying fascia, because these lesions are more likely to have microsatellites surrounding the primary lesion and involvement of the subdermal lymphatics close to the primary lesion.

Site-Specific Considerations General recommendations regarding the extent of surgical resection are applicable to most areas of the body. However, certain anatomic sites are not amenable to rigid surgical criteria. The appropriate treat-

Table 108-6 Univariate and Multivariate Analyses of Prognostic Factors for Survival of 1,521 Patients with AJCC Stage IV Melanoma

Factor	Univariate	Multivariate* p Value
Gender	.0120	
Age (yr)	.3907	
Site (extremity vs nonextremity)	.3376	
Breslow depth	.0264	
Clark level	.0273	
Year of diagnosis	.1431	
Initial site of metastases	$<$ .0001	$<$ .0001
Number of initial metastatic sites (1 vs 2 vs $\geq$ 3)	.0001	
Preceding AJCC stage (I/II vs III)	.0001	.0001
Disease-free interval ($>$ 18 vs $\leq$ 18 months)	.0004	.0001

AJCC = American Joint Committee on Cancer.
*Data shown only for factors with $p < .10$ by multivariate analysis.
Adapted from Barth A et al.[48]

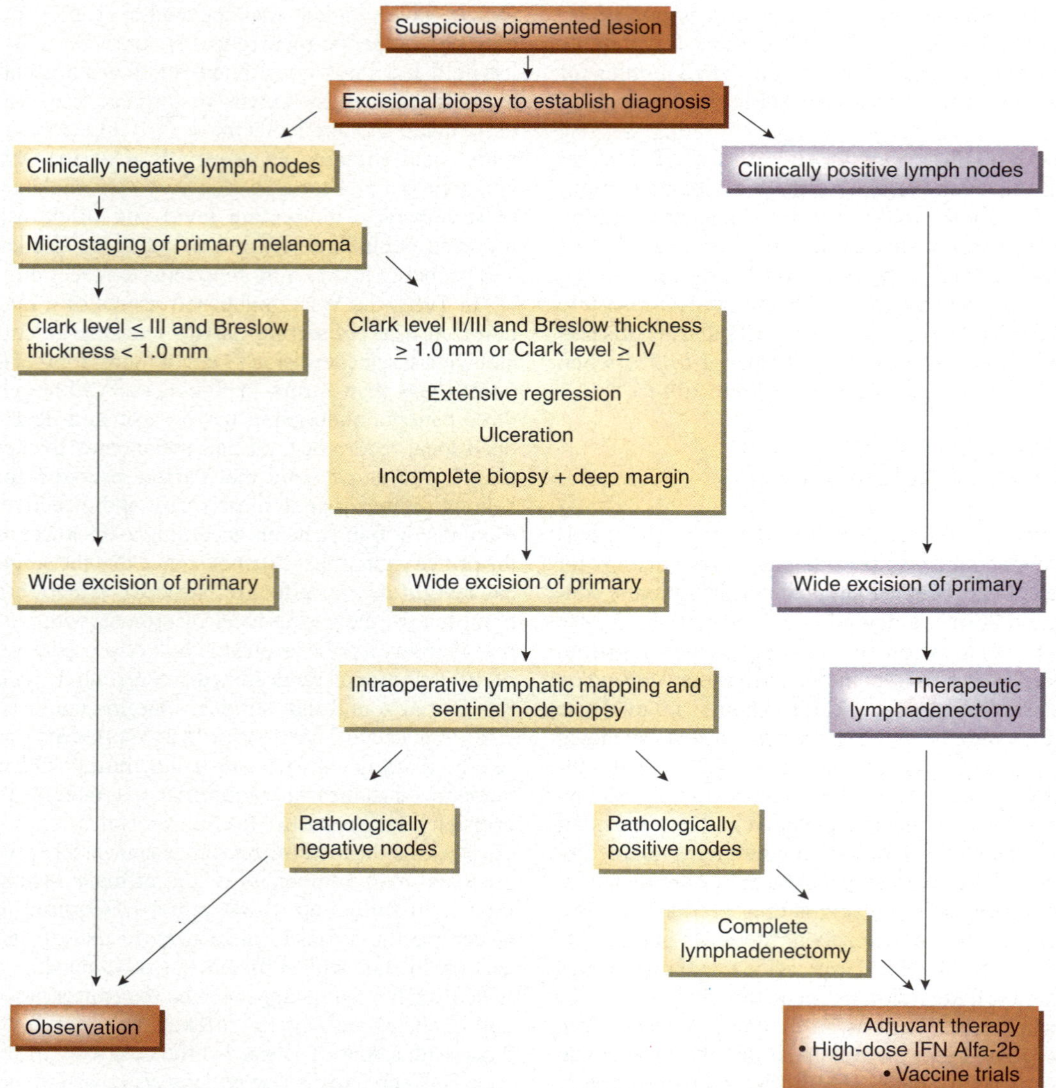

Figure 108-7 Algorithm for the management of primary melanoma. The workup for melanoma comprises chest radiography, complete blood count, and liver function tests for American Joint Committee on Cancer (AJCC) stage I/II disease, plus magnetic resonance imaging of the brain, computed tomography of the chest/abdomen, or positron emission tomography for AJCC stage III disease.

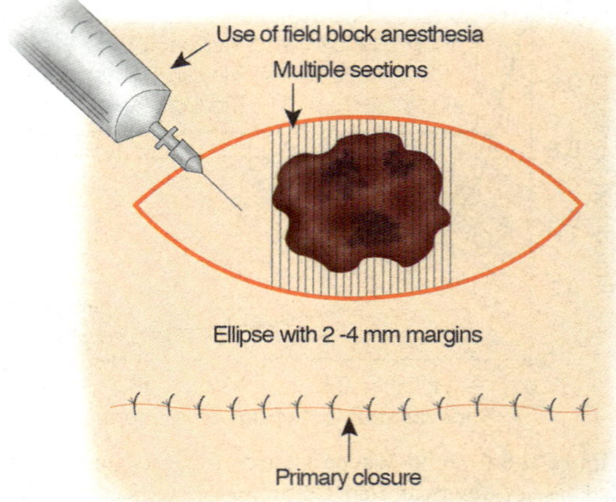

Figure 108-8 Excisional biopsy is preferable because the entire lesion is available for step-section pathologic analysis, providing evidence of the maximum depth of penetration. Redrawn with permission from Sugarbaker EV, Roseman JM, Weingard DN. Malignant melanoma. In: Copeland EM, editor. Surgical oncology. New York: Wiley; 1983.

ment for melanoma in the subungual areas is amputation, usually at the level of the distal interphalangeal joint, although with an extensive lesion, amputation of the whole digit may be necessary. For lesions of the helix of the ear, wedge excision of the lesion with careful plastic reconstruction can achieve excellent cosmetic results without compromising the incidence of local recurrence. Rarely should total amputation of the ear be necessary. Because of the cosmetic defect associated with wide excision on the face, as well as the close proximity of vital structures, lesions on the face generally are excised with margins of 1.0 to 2.5 cm, depending on their location and microstage. Fortunately, the majority of lesions on the face are relatively thin. Moh's micrographic surgery has been used for treating some low-risk melanomas on the face, but there is little support in the literature for use of this technique.

Radiation Therapy In the era of megavoltage radiotherapy, more and more reports have challenged melanoma's purported insensitivity to radiation. Patients with recurrent or metastatic melanoma involving the brain or bones formed the bulk of those initially treated. Numerous reports showed very high rates of response and/or palliation of symptoms (50–70%). Accumulated evidence now shows that the determinants of melanoma's radioresponsiveness are no different from those of other tumors: volume of disease, site of disease, and dose that can be safely administered.[59]

Encouraging reports have suggested a role of radiation after surgical resection in the axillary, vaginal, and head and neck regions. In these sites, where microscopic disease is often present following surgical resection, radiation may enhance local control and/or disease-free survival.[60–62] In fact, it is now clear that some melanomas may be cured solely by radiation. Intermediate-stage choroidal melanomas are usually managed with brachytherapy or with particle irradiation,[63–65] with local control rates of 85 to 97%. On the other hand, radiation is no longer believed to be of benefit in the preoperative treatment of larger choroidal melanomas. The Zimmerman hypothesis, formulated from anecdotal and retrospective studies, held that enucleation leads to increased distant metastases in this rare disease. The Collaborative Ocular Melanoma Study randomized 1,003 patients with choroidal melanomas to surgery versus surgery plus preenucleation radiation therapy (20 Gy in 5 fractions). Patients were accrued from 1986 to 1994 at 43 centers in the United States and Canada. Results at 5 and 8 years have demonstrated no benefit to the preoperative radiation arm.[66,67]

Adjuvant Treatment by Limb Perfusion The role of isolated limb perfusion in the adjuvant treatment of primary cutaneous melanoma of the extremity has generated considerable debate. Single-institution studies have suggested that hyperthermic, isolated limb perfusion with melphalan (L-PAM) substantially reduces the rate of recurrence and improves survival of patients with localized melanoma or regional node metastases when compared to conventional surgical therapy alone.[68,69]

Ghussen and colleagues[70] prospectively randomized patients to wide excision and regional node dissection with or without isolated limb perfusion of melphalan at 42°C. A reportedly significant improvement in disease-free status of patients receiving isolated limb perfusion led to early closure of the study. The findings cannot be

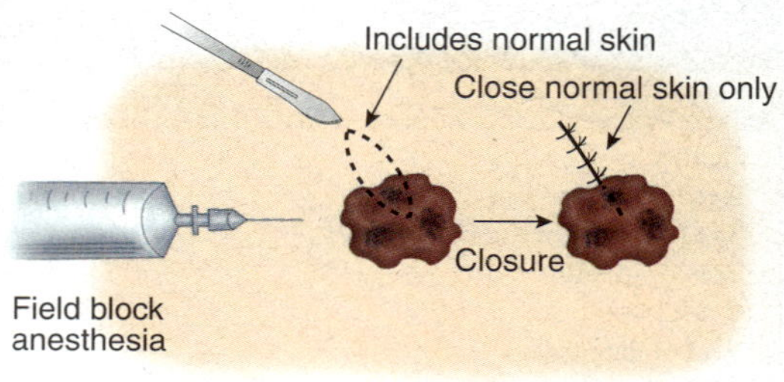

Figure 108-9 Incisional biopsy. Full-thickness excision of a nodular portion of the lesion ensures maximum depth of penetration. This procedure does not worsen the patient's prognosis. Redrawn with permission from Sugarbaker EV, Roseman JM, Weingard DN. Malignant melanoma. In: Copeland EM, editor. Surgical oncology. New York: Wiley; 1983.

accepted, however, because the control-arm relapse rate was substantially worse than the experience at institutions practicing similar management of primary melanoma without isolated limb perfusion. Although benefits from this therapy have been reported for patients with metastatic in-transit recurrence, its adjuvant use after curative surgery has not been substantiated. Randomized multiinstitutional studies of WHO, EORTC, and the North American Perfusion Group have failed to demonstrate the value of this therapy for resected high-risk melanoma.

MANAGEMENT OF REGIONAL LYMPH NODES

Elective versus Therapeutic Lymphadenectomy When melanoma metastasizes, it most commonly spreads initially to the regional lymph nodes. Surgical excision of the involved lymph nodes is currently the only effective treatment for melanoma metastatic to lymph nodes. Lymphadenectomy for individual lymphatic stations has been described in detail.[71] When performed for clinically identifiable disease in the lymph node station, surgical excision is therapeutic; when performed without palpable metastases but because there is sufficient risk of metastases, it is immediate or elective.

There is little argument about the utility of therapeutic lymphadenectomy, because surgical excision is the only effective modality for both local control and potential cure. Long-term survival depends on the number of involved nodes but approaches 25 to 40% at 5 years (see Table 108-4). There has been considerable controversy about elective lymphadenectomy for clinically uninvolved lymph nodes. If melanomas metastasize sequentially to regional lymph nodes and subsequently to distant sites, earlier intervention should improve outcome; this premise is supported by multiple reports that 5- and 10-year survival rates are approximately 25% higher for patients with clinically negative/histopathologically positive lymph nodes versus clinically positive/histopathologically positive nodes (see Table 108-4). However, approximately 80% of patients have tumor-free lymph nodes. In these patients, elective lymphadenectomy introduces a risk for immediate and long-term complications with little or no likely therapeutic benefit. Although the introduction of sentinel node biopsy has deflated the controversy regarding elective lymphadenectomy, the data supporting routine elective lymphadenectomy in primary melanoma remain important.

Prospective and Retrospective Studies of Routine Elective Lymphadenectomy Most large, long-term, retrospective studies from single institutions have demonstrated a small but consistent therapeutic benefit for patients with intermediate-to-thick melanomas treated with immediate lymph node dissection. Nonrandomized prospective studies from the Sydney Melanoma Unit demonstrated improved survival in patients with intermediate to thick lesions (0.76–4.0 mm).[71,72] Similar results have been achieved at the University of Alabama, Duke University, Memorial Sloan–Kettering, JWCI, and in a European trial.[43,73–76]

Four prospective randomized trials have examined whether early dissection of clinically negative lymph nodes offers any therapeutic advantage compared to later dissection of obvious nodal metastases. The WHO Melanoma Group conducted a prospective randomized study of 553 patients with extremity lesions and clinically uninvolved lymph nodes.[77] Two hundred sixty-seven patients underwent wide excision followed by immediate node dissection; 286 underwent wide excision followed by therapeutic node dissection if positive nodes were detected during observation. No statistically significant survival difference was observed. Although no subset of patients appeared to derive a large benefit from immediate node dissection, patients with Clark's level IV, intermediate-thickness lesions had a 10% better 5-year survival rate (20% at 10 years). This survival advantage did not achieve statistical significance, however, because of the small number of patients in this subset of the trial. The results of this trial have been questioned because of the large number of patients for whom lesion thickness was not obtained. In addition, any benefit of immediate lymph node dissection might have been obscured by restriction of melanomas to the extremities, the predominance of females, and the limited number of patients in certain subgroups.

Similar results were reported in a Mayo Clinic study of 171 patients with clinically uninvolved lymph nodes, who were prospectively randomized into three subgroups: no lymphadenectomy, delayed lymphadenectomy, and immediate excision of the regional lymph nodes.[78] No significant difference in total survival or metastasis-free survival was found among the three treatment arms, but most of the primary lesions were low-risk, thin lesions unlikely to recur regardless of therapy. (The study was initiated before the importance of tumor thickness was recognized.)

The randomized prospective study conducted by Balch and colleagues[79] examined elective node dissection in patients who had primaries 1 to 4 mm thick at any cutaneous site. Seven hundred and forty patients were randomized, 379 to elective lymph node dissection and 361 to observation. Because patients were allowed to cross over to the alternative treatment, investigators could examine survival of the "randomized intent" and the "actual treatment" groups. Although there was no survival difference overall, specific subsets of patients appeared to benefit from elective dissection.

Cascinelli and colleagues completed a randomized trial for patients with truncal primaries > 1.5 mm thick.[80] Two hundred fifty-two patients were randomized to one of the two treatments. Overall, these investigators found no difference in survival. This study has been criticized because lymphoscintigraphy was not routine for patients undergoing immediate dissection.

Complications of Lymphadenectomy The most common complications associated with lymph node dissection are those related to the wound itself and may lead to prolongation of hospitalization. However, the severity and type of the complication vary with the site of node dissection. The morbidity associated with axillary and neck dissections generally is minimal. Wound seroma and infection are relatively infrequent in axillary node dissection, whereas significant arm edema occurs in approximately 1% of patients. Similarly, long-term complications associated with neck dissection are infrequent and usually do not involve functional deficits. On the other hand, radical inguinal node dissection may be associated with significant edema, particularly if the iliac and obturator nodes are removed with the superficial inguinal nodes and those of the femoral triangle.[81] In approximately 2 to 10% of patients, this can be a particularly debilitating complication. Regardless of the site of node dissection, the rate of edema formation can usually be minimized by prophylactic measures, such as elevating the extremity while recumbent and wearing elastic compression stockings.

Microstage of Primary Melanoma and Risk of Nodal Metastases Microstaging the primary lesion by Breslow's thickness and Clark's level of invasion can identify patients who have an increased probability of harboring microscopic metastatic disease.[31] Patients with thin melanomas (Clark's level II, Breslow's thickness < 0.76 mm) without evidence of regression rarely have nodal metastases, whereas patients with increasingly thick melanomas (Clark's level III or IV, Breslow's thickness 0.76–4.0 mm) have an increased risk of harboring occult metastatic disease. Microstaging, along with other prognostic variables such as anatomic site, ulceration, and gender, can identify patients at substantial risk for harboring microscopic metastatic disease. These are the patients most likely to benefit from immediate lymph node dissection.

Cutaneous Lymphoscintigraphy Ambiguous lymphatic drainage has been advanced as one argument against immediate lymph node dissection for truncal melanomas. Sappey's line encircles the trunk 2 cm above and below the umbilicus; lesions above this line have been predicted to drain to the axillae and those below to the inguinal nodes. However, certain midline lesions, particularly those of the umbilical area or midline of the back, can drain to all four areas.

Cutaneous lymphoscintigraphy was introduced in the late 1970s by Morton and colleagues to determine the route of lymphatic drainage from a primary melanoma.[82] This procedure is particularly useful for melanomas arising from an axial location on the trunk or the head and neck because these skin sites may drain to one or more lymphatic areas. Morton's group has replaced colloidal gold with technetium (Tc 99m)–labeled dextran and more recently with Tc 99m–labeled human serum albumin or sulfur colloid; Tc 99m is injected into the site of the primary melanoma to identify lymph node stations draining that site.[83] Cutaneous lymphoscintigraphy is used to

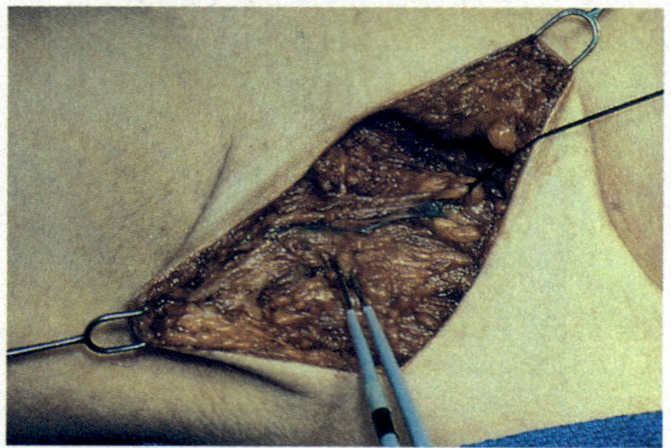

Figure 108-10 Intraoperative lymphatic mapping using a vital blue dye shows the path to the first blue-staining (sentinel) lymph node draining a primary cutaneous melanoma. Excision and histologic examination of this node is used to determine the tumor status of the regional drainage basin.

identify regional lymph node stations at risk for harboring occult microscopic metastatic disease, but it cannot identify nodal metastases.

Intraoperative Lymphatic Mapping and Sentinel Node Biopsy Because of the controversy surrounding immediate lymph node dissection, Morton and colleagues devised a minimally invasive technique to identify occult metastases in the regional lymph nodes of patients with primary cutaneous melanoma.[84] Intraoperative lymphatic mapping is based on the hypothesis that lymph from a primary melanoma drains initially to one or more sentinel lymph nodes, which therefore should be the first nodes at risk for harboring occult metastatic disease.[83,84] Briefly, mapping involves the intradermal injection of a tracer such as vital blue dye and/or radiocolloid. This tracer readily enters the subdermal lymphatics and passes through the lymphatic channels to the regional nodal basin/station draining that particular skin site. This permits identification of the sentinel lymph node(s) (Figure 108-10), which is selectively excised and examined by conventional H&E staining and highly sensitive immunohistochemical techniques. If metastatic melanoma is identified, a complete lymphadenectomy is performed; if not, the procedure is terminated (see Figure 108-7).

Using intraoperative lymphatic mapping and sentinel node biopsy, Morton and colleagues have found that only 20% of patients with clinically localized melanoma have occult regional node metastases.[84] These patients can be treated by standard lymphadenectomy; the other 80% of patients can avoid the complications of radical lymphadenectomy. Many investigators have validated the accuracy of sentinel node biopsy and demonstrated its strength as a lymph node staging procedure.[85,86] Intraoperative lymphatic mapping has been performed using blue dye alone[84] or in combination with a radiopharmaceutical that is tracked by a hand-held gamma probe.[83] The blue dye remains the gold standard for identifying sentinel nodes. The radiopharmaceutical serves as a useful adjunct but is impractical as the sole mapping agent because of its tendency to migrate up the nodal chain beyond the sentinel node.[83]

JWCI investigators have compared the therapeutic value of sentinel node biopsy and standard elective lymph node dissection.[87] The data suggest that these procedures are equal but that sentinel node biopsy is better for staging the regional lymph nodes. With respect to treatment of the primary melanoma, the therapeutic efficacy of sentinel node biopsy is being compared with excision alone as part of a multicenter randomized phase III trial; recently reported interim results of this trial indicate that sentinel node biopsy, followed immediately by complete dissection if the sentinel node contains tumor, clearly prolongs disease-free survival and spares the patient the psychological trauma of anticipating possible nodal recurrence during the traditional "watch and wait" approach.[88] Interim results also show that failure to identify and remove occult sentinel node metastases may allow development of more extensive regional node disease.[89] The diagnostic utility of sentinel node biopsy has already been validated in this multicenter trial.[90]

Adjuvant Therapy The high rate of recurrence (45–70%) in patients with nodal metastases has been the motivation for multiple trials of adjuvant therapy, none of which yielded convincing evidence to justify routine adjuvant therapy outside a clinical trial setting—until the Eastern Cooperative Oncology Group (ECOG) and ECOG-led trials of high-dose interferon (IFN)α-2b. Based on results of these intergroup trials, the United States Food and Drug Administration (FDA) approved IFNα-2b as the first postsurgical adjuvant for AJCC stage IIb and III melanoma. However, the toxicity of high-dose IFN and some inconsistency in the results of randomized trials have generated controversy regarding its international adoption as the standard of care (see below).

Active Specific Immunotherapy: Melanoma Vaccines as Postsurgical Adjuvants Extensive phase II trials have demonstrated that certain patients receiving a polyvalent allogeneic whole-cell vaccine generate immune responses that are correlated with prolonged survival.[91–93] A multicenter, randomized phase III trial of this vaccine (Canvaxin polyvalent specific active immunotherapeutic, CancerVax Corp., Carlsbad, CA) as postsurgical adjuvant therapy for patients with AJCC stage III melanoma has completed accrual. In the meantime, a recent analysis of phase II data using sophisticated statistical methods showed that Canvaxin dramatically and consistently increased overall survival of stage III patients matched with a control group for all known prognostic factors and managed by the same team of surgical and medical oncologists.[44] Survival rates were 49% versus 37% at 5 years and 42% versus 31% at 10 years for 739 vaccine patients versus 739 nonvaccine patients ($p = .0001$).

The Southeastern Cancer Study Group used a viral melanoma oncolysate in an attempt to decrease recurrence of melanoma, but promising results of the phase I/II trial were not validated in a phase III trial.[94] Hersey and colleagues also reported negative results of a phase III trial undertaken after phase II studies demonstrated improved survival with a viral melanoma oncolysate.[95] The Southwestern Oncology Group (SWOG) completed a study of melanoma cell line–derived vaccine (Melacine), which demonstrated no significant overall impact on relapse interval or survival, but subsequent subgroup analysis suggested a benefit for HLA-A2 and HLA-C3 patients; this will be examined in a prospective trial for patients with stage IIA disease.[96,97] The E1694 intergroup trial (see below) of ganglioside GM2 vaccine immunotherapy (GMK, Progenics Inc) for high-risk resected stage IIB and III disease showed statistically significant inferiority of the vaccine compared to high-dose IFNα-2b.[98]

Interferons as Postsurgical Adjuvants

E1684 Pivotal Trial Given the evidence for antitumor activity of maximally tolerated dosages of IFNα-2 in patients with advanced melanoma, ECOG and the North Central Cancer Treatment Group (NCCTG) launched adjuvant trials of IFNα-2a and IFNα-2b in 1983–1984. Patients with lymph node metastases or deep primary lesions (T3 in NCCTG; T4 in ECOG) received a 1-year (ECOG) or 3-month (NCCTG) course of therapy and were compared with patients who underwent observation. ECOG trial E1684 tested IFNα-2b given intravenously at 20 MU/m^2/day, 5 days a week for the first 4 weeks (induction), followed by alternate-day treatment using 10 MU/m^2/day, 3 days a week subcutaneously for the subsequent 11 months (maintenance).[99] These were projected to be the maximally tolerated dosages on the basis of phase I-II trial experience in metastatic melanoma.[100] The NCCTG tested a 3-month regimen of IFNα-2a at maximally tolerated dosages given intramuscularly at 20 MU/m^2/day on an alternate-day schedule, based upon a series of phase II trials at the Mayo Clinic.[101] These two trials reached accrual goals and were closed in 1990. At a median follow-up of 7 years, the ECOG trial showed a statistically significant and clinically meaningful 1-year increase in median disease-free and overall survival for patients treated with IFNα-2b. The NCCTG study failed to demonstrate a survival benefit for a shorter course of high-dose IFNα-2a overall, but showed significant reduction in relapses among patients with higher risk node-positive disease.

United States Intergroup E1690 Trial Intergroup trial E1690 tested the high-dose regimen of E1684 and a lower dosage of 3 MU subcutaneously three times a week for 104 weeks, compared to observation. (The trial was designed before data from E1684 became available.) Findings revealed relapse interval prolongation with high-dose IFN but no survival impact for the high-dose or low-dose regimen.[102] This finding has been a source of confusion in regard to the significance of the survival benefit reported in E1684. However, E1690 did not mandate elective node dissection for patients with deep (> 4 mm Breslow) primary melanomas but no clinically apparent nodal disease; the percentage of patients accrued in this stratification category was more than twice that of E1684 (25% vs 11%). Moreover, because patients assigned to observation developed recurrence in the regional lymph nodes, the FDA's approval of high-dose IFN in 1995 introduced the opportunity for crossover therapy—a possibility that was not anticipated in the design of E1690. An analysis of crossover therapy revealed that all but one of 38 observation patients who had resectable relapses received postrelapse therapy with IFN. This plausible explanation for the discrepancies in survival impact between E1690 and the pivotal E1684 has been validated by the positive results for both relapse-free and overall survival observed in the subsequent E1694 (see below). Postrelapse survival for patients assigned to observation in E1690 was double (at 4.3 years) that observed in the prior E1684 trial (2 years).

United States Intergroup E1694 Trial The E1694 Intergroup Study was the first United States cooperative group trial in which high-dose IFN was adopted as the standard of treatment and used to test the potential benefit of a GM2 vaccine conjugated to the carrier keyhole limpet hemocyanin (GMK vaccine) and administered with the immunomodulator QS21. This trial was based on the results of a single-institution phase III trial showing a trend to improved relapse-free survival for recipients of GM2 with BCG, in comparison to BCG; subset analysis of the benefit for antibody-responders demonstrated significant improvement in relapse-free survival.[103] The E1694 study was unblinded and closed at a median follow-up of 16 months, due to highly significant relapse-free and overall survival benefits of high-dose IFN compared to GMK vaccine. Updates at median follow-up times of 2.1 and 4 years have showed sustained relapse-free and overall survival differences that were significant by both log rank and Cox analyses, using 2-sided or 1-sided tests.[102, 104] The outcome for the GMK vaccine was similar to or better than the outcome for observation in the E1690 and E1684 trials. The vaccine induced an immune response in > 85% of participants, and no data suggest an adverse impact of the vaccine to otherwise explain the outcome of this trial. Given these data, E1694 (the largest United States cooperative group melanoma trial ever conducted) may be a study in which the vaccine appears to have been indistinguishable from observation, although a formal observation arm has been considered untenable since the mature results of E1684 became available.

Results of the E1694 study in conjunction with the pivotal E1684 study are the only prospective, randomized phase III trial data that show significant overall and relapse-free survival prolongation in patients with high-risk melanoma. Hazard ratios for mortality in patients not treated with high-dose IFNα-2b (compared to high-dose IFN normalized to 1.00) in the E1684 and E1694 trials were 1.22 (updated to 12.6 years median follow-up) and 1.32, respectively. Hazard ratios for relapse in patients not treated with high-dose IFN in the E1684 and E1694 studies were 1.38 and 1.33, respectively. These two rigorous, randomized multicenter studies suggest that patients not treated with high-dose IFN have a 22 to 32% increase in the likelihood of death and a 33 to 38% increase in the likelihood of relapse.

An area of controversy in the ECOG and the US Intergroup trials relates to the benefit of high-dose IFN in patients with different stages of disease. In the original results of E1684, this benefit was most evident for node-positive patients (particularly with 1 tumor-involved node; hazard ratio 2.29, p = .001). There was no benefit for the 15 patients with node-negative disease, but this subgroup's uneven distribution of prognostic factors (especially primary tumor ulceration) would not have favored relapse-free survival. The E1690 trial was modestly larger; relapse-free benefit was most significant (hazard ratio 1.92, p = .02) for the subset of patients with 2 or 3 tumor-involved nodes. The E1694 study was twofold larger than either E1684 or E1690; relapse-free benefit was greatest (hazard ratio 2.07, p = .01) for patients without known nodal involvement. The potential benefit of high-dose IFN for any given patient can be determined by using the fractional reduction estimates from E1684 and E1694 (22 to 32% reduction in mortality and 33 to 38% reduction in relapse risk) and the current AJCC prognostic data. A time utility analysis provides a further basis for decisions concerning adjuvant therapy of melanoma.[105]

Current Trials of the US Intergroup If the 4-week induction regimen of intravenous IFN (20 MU/m^2/day), used in all ECOG and subsequent intergroup trials, proves to be as effective as the one-year regimen, the toxicity and cost of high-dose IFN treatment would be substantially reduced. This possibility is under investigation in the E1697 trial, which was initiated by ECOG and has become an intergroup United States trial and an international collaborative trial involving the NCI-Canada, Australia, and the European Organization for Treatment and Research of Cancer (EORTC). El697 has an estimated completion date of 2008 and a target accrual of 1,420 patients with intermediate-risk melanoma (T3-4, N1a).

The possibility that chemobiotherapy with cisplatin, vinblastine, dacarbazine, IFNα-2b and IL-2 given by continuous infusion may have adjuvant benefits superior to those of high-dose IFNα-2b has formed the impetus for a trial led by the Southwest Oncology Group (SWOG 0008). This study will accrue 280 patients with resectable stage IIIB melanoma; its goal is to determine whether 3 cycles of chemobiotherapy administered on an inpatient basis over 3 months is superior to the high-dose IFNα-2b regimen used in the E1684 trial.

Mechanism of High-Dose IFN A prospective laboratory analysis of specimens from patients in the three treatment arms of the E1690 trial demonstrated that high-dose IFN significantly modulated the function and numbers of lymphoid cell subpopulations in the blood.[106] High-dose IFN had significant in vitro effects on tumor cell surface antigen expression, induction of major histocompatibility complex Class II (DR), and inhibition of expression of adhesion molecules (Intercellular Adhesion Molecule–1). None of the variables tested predicted disease-free survival, but the sample size (n = 148) may have been too small to detect changes with potential clinical significance.

Low-Dose IFNα-2 Trials The results of IFNα-2 in several other cancers suggest that protracted periods of treatment may achieve the most beneficial results; however, the maximally tolerated dosages used in ECOG E1684 are not feasible for longer than approximately 1 year. The potential role of chronic or longer-term therapy with low-dose IFNα-2 therefore has been of interest. The Austrian Multicenter Group, French Multicenter Group, UK Clinical Cancer Research Group, and WHO Melanoma Programme reported trials of IFN administered subcutaneously in a dose of 3 MU after resection of intermediate-risk and high-risk melanoma.[107–110] In the WHO trial, a 3-year course of postoperative adjuvant low-dose IFNα-2a was compared to standard observation in 444 patients with lymph node metastases; results showed no impact on disease-free or overall survival.[110] The UK trial also showed no effect on relapse-free and overall survival.[109] The French and Austrian trials demonstrated transient prolongation of relapse-free interval in patients who received low-dose IFN thrice weekly for 1.5 to 2 years. No trial has shown a significant impact of low-dose IFN on overall survival. Its transient impact on relapse-free survival does not compare favorably to the durable relapse-free survival benefit of high-dose IFN at a median follow-up of > 12.6 years in the E1684 trial, or to the survival prolongation observed in E1684 and E1694.[98,111]

Overall Evaluation of High-Dose IFN Pooled and meta-analyses indicate that IFN in low, intermediate and high dosages has a significant and consistent dose-dependent effect on the relapse-free survival of patients with intermediate and high-risk resected melanoma.[104,112] Long-term follow-up data show that the one-year regimen of high-dose IFN used in E1684 controls disease for more than 16 years (patients in the initial trials), or for more than 4 years (patients in all ECOG and US Intergroup trials). By contrast, the lower dose IFN regimens are associated with erosion of relapse-free survival 1 to 2 years after conclusion of treatment.

High-dose IFN clearly is an active agent in melanoma and the only FDA-approved postsurgical adjuvant therapy. The management of its toxicity has been demonstrated in more than 2,000 patients reported in the literature; the percentage of patients completing the 1-year treatment regimen rose from 75% in E1684 to 90% in E1694. The use of high-dose IFN must be considered in relation to its toxicity for each patient, using the best current information and the hazard ratios for relapse and death associated with omission of this therapy.

Chemotherapy Dacarbazine (DTIC) is the only agent approved by the FDA for chemotherapy of disseminated melanoma. However, adjuvant trials with DTIC, either alone or in combination with immunotherapy or other chemotherapeutic agents, have demonstrated no better survival than that associated with surgery alone.[113] Temozolomide (Temodar) was approved for therapy of malignant glioma in 2000; data presented to the FDA and published by Middleton and colleagues.[114] demonstrate a therapeutic efficacy at least equivalent to that of dacarbazine. For this reason, and due to the more favorable pharmacodynamics of this oral agent, which reaches effective levels in the central nervous system (CNS), temozolomide has often been adopted in place of dacarbazine, although its cost is substantially higher.

Radiation Therapy The role of radiation therapy in the adjuvant setting remains controversial. Most reports are small retrospective comparisons of patients treated at a variety of sites, with varying doses and doses per fraction, usually after surgical resections of varying degrees of completeness.[59] Johanson and colleagues reported 54 patients treated with the Princess Margret Hospital's 0-7-21 protocol (8 Gy in three fractions on days 0, 7, and 21).[115] Of these patients, 22 were treated for microscopic residual disease following surgery to 7 different sites. Local control was maintained in 18 of 22 (82%) at 12 to 44 months following irradiation. Creagan and colleagues reported the only randomized prospective study of adjuvant radiation for lymph node–positive melanoma.[116] Fifty-six patients with positive regional lymph nodes following surgical resection (from a variety of sites) were randomized to no further therapy or to irradiation of the involved nodal basin. Radiation was a split-course of 25 Gy in 1.78 Gy fractions followed by a 3- to 4-week break, then a further 25 Gy in 1.78 Gy fractions. Only one field was treated daily. Despite these suboptimal techniques and inadequate numbers of patients, radiation therapy conferred a small advantage in disease-free survival (20 vs 9 months) and median overall survival (33 vs 22 months). These differences did not reach statistical significance.

In what has become an influential study of adjuvant radiation for melanoma, Ang and colleagues treated 174 patients with high-risk cutaneous melanoma of the head and neck.[117] There were three risk groups: (1) clinically node-negative with lesions > 1.5 mm or Clark's level higher than IV ($n = 79$); (2) clinically node-positive ($n = 32$); and (3) nodal relapse but no distant metastases ($n = 63$). Patients underwent surgical resection of the primary tumor in group 1 and surgical resection plus lymph node dissection in groups 2 and 3. Radiation consisted of 6 Gy per fraction twice weekly to a total dose of 30 Gy in 2.5 weeks. Ipsilateral electrons were the most commonly applied modality. Five-year locoregional control and survival rates of 88% and 47%, respectively, greatly exceeded historic control rates. However, more recent JWCI data reported by Shen and colleagues suggest that radiation is of limited benefit except for patients with extracapsular extension and large (> 3 cm) nodal metastases.[118]

The Radiation Therapy Oncology Group (RTOG) initiated a randomized trial of adjuvant radiation for high-risk head and neck melanoma patients, but the trial was closed prematurely due to poor accrual. A subsequent effort to test an adjuvant regimen of hypofractionated radiotherapy plus high-dose IFNα-2b has also been unable to garner adequate accrual, so it is unlikely that any compelling data will emerge to resolve this issue.

Management of Locally Recurrent and In-Transit Melanomas Melanomas recurring within 5 cm of the primary site are referred to as locally recurrent, and melanomas metastasizing between the primary and the regional lymphatic station are referred to as in transit. Locally recurrent melanomas suggest inadequate treatment of the primary lesion, although at least 0.5% will recur regardless of the operative margins.[53] In-transit metastases represent the trapping of melanoma cells in the lymphatics in transit to the regional lymphatic station, although the actual mechanism for this is unknown.

Most patients with locally recurrent melanoma eventually develop systemic metastases, but about 20% are apparently cured by further surgical excision, suggesting that the initial surgical margins were inadequate. In contrast, with only rare exceptions, patients with in-transit metastases develop systemic metastases within 6 to 12 months. The prognosis appears to be related to the number of in-transit lesions and the interval before development of recurrence.[119] The incidence of in-transit lesions is reportedly about 1% of all melanoma cases.[119] Calabro and colleagues from M. D. Anderson Cancer Center reviewed their experience with 1,001 consecutive patients who had nodal metastases.[120] Ten percent subsequently developed in-transit metastases. Lower extremity primaries draining to the groin were associated with an increased risk (19%) of in-transit metastases. The patient's age and gender, the timing of nodal dissection (immediate or delayed), and the number of excised nodes did not affect the incidence of in-transit metastases. Although Calabro's group did not attempt to explain the higher incidence of in-transit metastases associated with primaries on the lower extremities, some investigators suspect that gravity and delayed lymphatic drainage may be responsible.

Because symptoms are rarely associated with in-transit melanoma, it seems reasonable to avoid the toxicities of systemic chemotherapy, which rarely provides long-term complete regression. Rather, these lesions should be treated with aggressive local therapy, which in some patients results in prolonged control, or with active immunotherapy using a whole-cell vaccine.[119,121] Clinicians may use an algorithm for the management of in-transit melanoma (Figure 108-11).

Surgery Surgical excision of in-transit lesions can be considered in patients whose lesions are few in number and slow in development. Because of the eventual development of systemic disease in the majority of these patients, amputation is rarely indicated.

Intralesional Immunotherapy Intralesional immunotherapy with bacille Calmette-Guérin (BCG) has been reported as an alternate means to control the regional manifestations of recurrent inoperable in-transit melanoma (Figure 108-12). BCG incites an inflammatory reaction that may control in-transit metastases in approximately 60% of patients.[122] Another investigational alternative for intralesional treatment of recurrent in-transit melanoma is use of human monoclonal antibodies that recognize melanoma-associated gangliosides GD2 and GM2.[123,124] Intralesional therapy with human monoclonal antibodies directed against these ganglioside antigens has resulted in complete clinical and histologic regression of dermal metastases in approximately 90% of patients whose melanomas contain the target antigen (Figure 108-13).

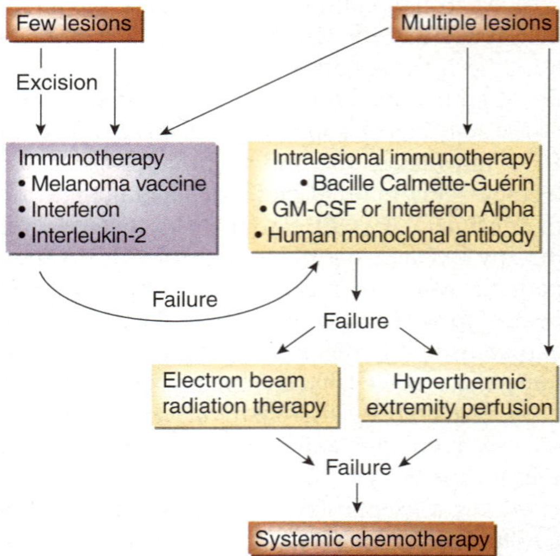

Figure 108-11 Algorithm for management of in-transit melanoma metastases (American Joint Committee on Cancer stage III).

Regional Chemotherapy Chemotherapy administered by arterial infusion or by isolated perfusion of the extremities has been undertaken for more than 40 years for in-transit melanoma recurrence. More recently, hyperthermic isolation/perfusion of melphalan has been used to expose tumor cells to dosages (and physical conditions) that are not systemically feasible.[70] Dramatic results have been achieved by perfusing melphalan at 41.8°C.[125] Other drugs, such as DTIC and cisplatin, may have similar activity, although they have not been as successful as melphalan. Recent studies suggest that biological response modifiers such as tumor necrosis factor and IFNγ may increase the effectiveness of chemotherapy perfusion, but randomized studies thus far have been equivocal.

Systemic Chemotherapy and Biotherapy Local disease rarely undergoes complete regression for prolonged periods, although partial and temporary responses are frequent. Therefore, unless systemic disease becomes manifest, systemic chemotherapy is rarely indicated in the management of in-transit melanoma. The issue is more controversial with biologics like interleukin (IL)-2 and IFNα-2, for which durable complete responses may be possible. These and newer cytokine/growth factor and peptide vaccine combinations are being investigated prospectively in cooperative group trials.

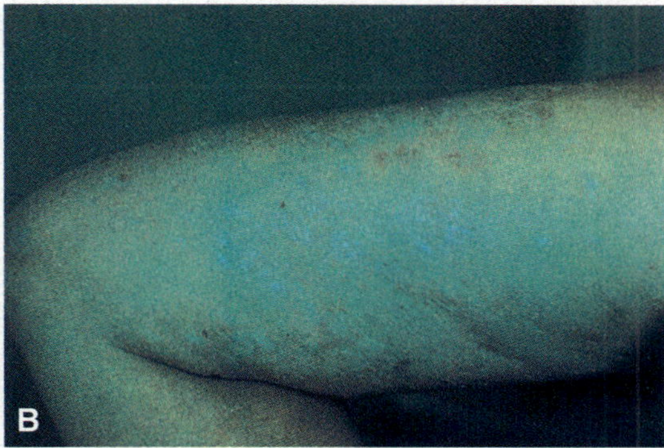

Figure 108-12 **A,** Recurrent melanoma before treatment with intralesional injections of bacille Calmette-Guérin (BCG). **B,** Complete regression 5 years later. Patient remained free of disease at last follow-up 10 years later.

Radiation Therapy Radiation therapy for locally recurrent and in-transit melanoma has been inadequately investigated. Several reports in the literature have shown encouraging response rates. Johanson's report of the Princess Margaret's 0-7-21 protocol (see above) included 23 patients with locally recurrent or in-transit melanoma. Of these, 7 achieved a complete remission, 2 had a complete remission followed by in-field failure, 5 had a partial remission, 3 had disease stabilization, and the remainder (5 patients) had no response. Given the poor survival in these clinical situations, it appears reasonable to consider palliative radiation in those patients who are not candidates for the therapies listed above.

Active Specific Immunotherapy Impressive results in the management of regional skin and soft-tissue metastases (AJCC stage IIIA) have been obtained with active specific immunotherapy using a polyvalent allogeneic whole-cell vaccine (Canvaxin immunotherapeutic).[91,121] During the last 20 years, the median survival associated with local and regional metastatic melanoma has remained constant for patients treated by other modalities, such as intralesional immunotherapy and surgery, with an overall median survival of 28.7 months and a 5-year survival rate of 20%. A study of 54 patients receiving Canvaxin for treatment of in-transit melanoma reported a 17% rate of objective clinical responses (9 of 54 patients), with a 13% rate of complete remission (7 of 54 patients). The median duration of complete remission exceeded 22 months. Median survival was > 53 months for vaccine responders, 42 months for nonresponders, and 53 months overall (Figure 108-14).[121] A subsequent study reported successful vaccine reinduction in patients who developed recurrence after complete resection of AJCC stage III or stage IV melanoma. The median survival time was 37 months for the 94 reinduced patients and 17 months for the 100 other patients (p = .0001). In the reinduction group, there was a significant correlation between reinduced delayed-type hypersensitivity responses to Canvaxin and survival (p = .0178).[126]

MANAGEMENT OF DISTANT METASTASES

At the time of autopsy, the lung, liver, brain, and lymph nodes are the most common sites of metastasis. However, essentially every visceral site, including the heart, adrenal gland, spleen, pancreas, gastrointestinal tract, bone, thyroid, pleura, diaphragm, ovaries, prostate, and genitourinary tract, may be involved. The median survival in this setting is usually only 4 to 6 months. The site of metastasis is an important prognostic variable. Patients with subcutaneous and lymph node metastases (median survival, 11 months) and pulmonary metastases (median survival, 8 to 10 months) have a better prognosis than those with central nervous system and hepatic metastases (median survival, 2–4 months).

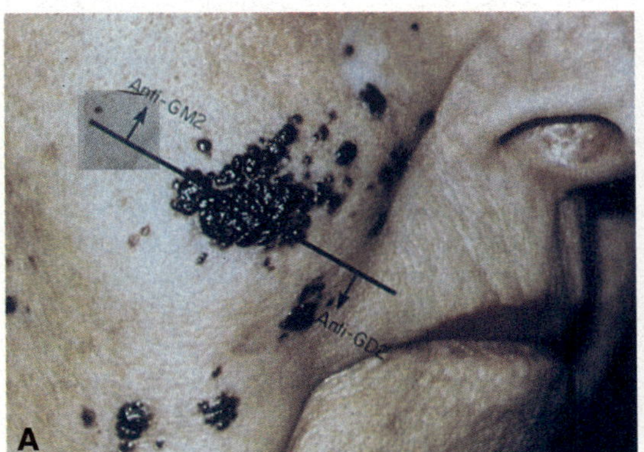

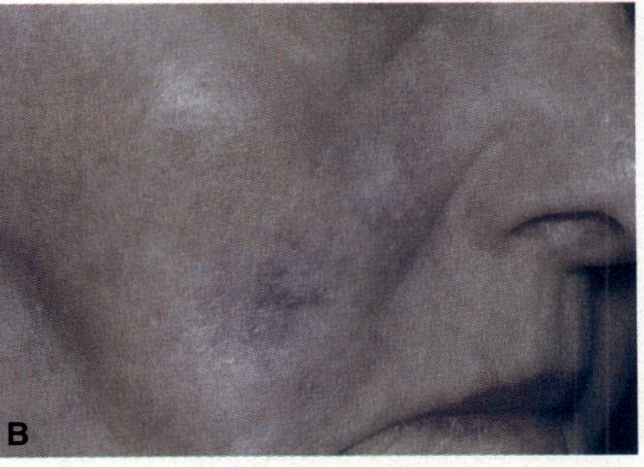

Figure 108-13 **A,** Radioresistant recurrent melanoma before treatment with intralesional injections of human monoclonal antibody to gangliosides GM2 or GD2. **B,** Complete regression of all disease 2.5 years later.

Symptoms associated with disseminated melanoma vary with the site of involvement. In the absence of abnormal physical findings, abnormal serum chemistries or an abnormal chest x-ray, it is unlikely that extensive radiologic evaluations will identify unsuspected metastases. Although some patients have no symptoms, others experience seizures associated with intracranial metastases, gastrointestinal bleeding from small-bowel metastases, and/or pain from masses. Because of this variable presentation, the onset of new and persistent symptoms in individuals previously diagnosed with melanoma should be evaluated by standard radiologic studies, including computed tomography of chest and abdomen and magnetic resonance imaging of the brain. Contrast studies of the small bowel in patients with unexplained anemia or with evidence of blood loss from the gastrointestinal tract often reveal evidence of small-bowel metastases. Positron emission tomography (PET) scanning using fluorine-18 deoxyglucose can evaluate the entire patient with one study, and whole-body PET may prove to be the most accurate and effective staging tool available for patients with malignant melanoma.[127]

Currently, disseminated melanoma is not curable. The clinical course of patients with metastatic melanoma may, however, vary widely. Progression of disease may be extremely rapid, or existing metastases may remain stable for prolonged periods. For these reasons, careful clinical judgment is required for optimal palliation. Modalities available for the treatment of disseminated melanoma include surgical excision, systemic chemotherapy, radiation therapy, immunotherapy with vaccines and biologic response modifiers, and other investigational treatment options. An algorithm for suggested management is given in Figure 108-15.

Surgery Despite the well-recognized tendency of melanoma to disseminate widely, surgical excision of metastases can provide excellent palliation and sometimes long-term survival. The excision of multiple metastases from multiple organ sites does not appear to improve outcome, but complete surgical resection can prolong the survival of patients who have a limited number of lesions in a limited number of organ sites. Some patients with multiple metastases in the same organ, such as the lung, may enjoy long-term survival. A study of 1,574 patients undergoing resection of distant metastases at JWCI revealed a 5-year survival rate of up to 29% for patients with solitary metastases.[128,129] Factors predictive of survival include site and number of metastases, prior stage of disease, and disease-free interval before diagnosis of stage IV melanoma. Surgical excision of sequentially developing metastases can also be beneficial.[130]

Brain Metastases Approximately 50% of patients with disseminated melanoma will develop clinical evidence of brain metastases. Symptoms may be due to mass effect and include headache, double vision, and seizures as well as

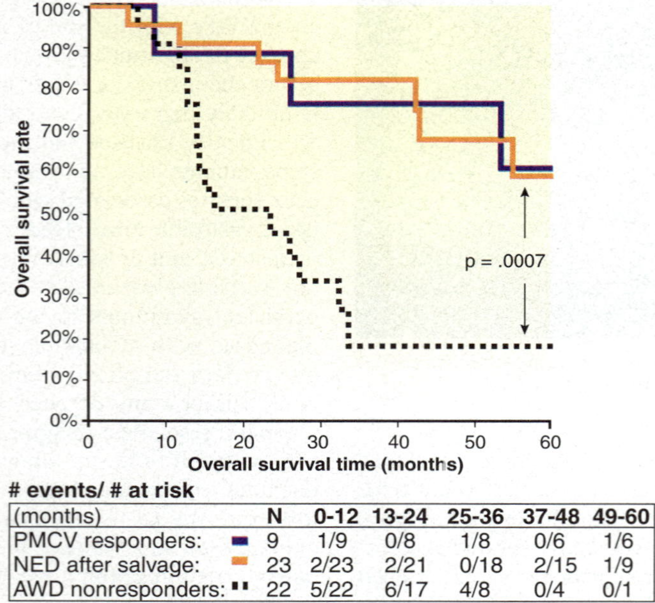

events/ # at risk

(months)	N	0-12	13-24	25-36	37-48	49-60
PMCV responders:	9	1/9	0/8	1/8	0/6	1/6
NED after salvage:	23	2/23	2/21	0/18	2/15	1/9
AWD nonresponders:	22	5/22	6/17	4/8	0/4	0/1

Figure 108-14 Overall survival curves for patients whose in-transit melanoma metastases were treated by a polyvalent melanoma cell vaccine (PMCV) called Canvaxin. (*Solid black line),* PMCV clinical responders (9 patients); (*solid gray line),* PMCV nonresponders rendered clinically free of disease (NED) by salvage therapy (23 patients); (*dashed line),* PMCV nonresponders not rendered NED (22 patients). A partial response was defined as at least a 50% decrease in the products of the greatest tumor dimensions for at least 30 days. Reprinted with permission from Hsueh EC et al.[121]

symptoms associated with the location of the lesion in the brain. Although the symptoms may be improved substantially with the use of steroids, they usually progress in the absence of definitive treatment. Some brain metastases appear to be solitary. Surgical removal of solitary brain metastases may relieve associated symptoms and occasionally results in long-term survival.[131] Postoperative cranial radiotherapy is generally considered of value because other occult lesions may exist. Significant progress in the management of brain metastases with stereotactic radiosurgery using the gamma knife has reduced the need for surgical resection.

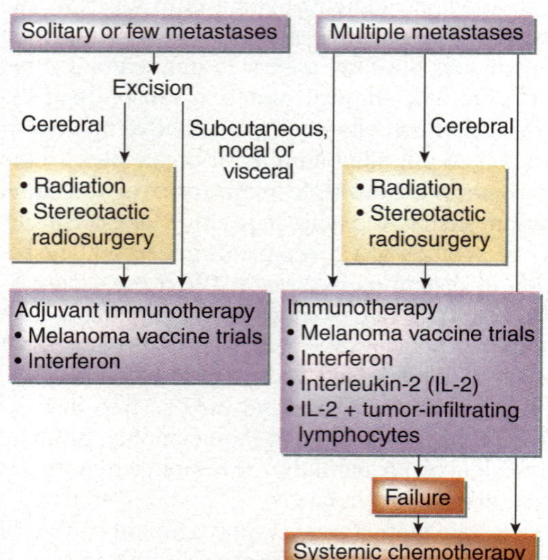

Figure 108-15 Algorithm for the management of melanoma metastatic to distant sites (American Joint Committee on Cancer stage IV).

Subcutaneous and Lymph Node Metastases Metastatic deposits in subcutaneous sites and lymph nodes are frequent in patients with disseminated melanoma and may represent the only manifestation of disease. Surgical excision of these clinically involved sites can be associated with prolonged disease-free periods and a median survival as long as 29 months.[132]

Lung Metastases The lungs represent one of the most frequent sites of metastatic involvement by melanoma. Occasionally, patients present with a solitary pulmonary nodule as the only manifestation of recurrent melanoma. Thoracotomy in this setting can result in substantial (35%) 5-year survival. Isolated pulmonary metastases reportedly account for approximately 5% of disseminated melanomas. These patients may be initially evaluated according to the tumor doubling time and treated with a therapeutic polyvalent cancer vaccine.[133] Patients with a tumor doubling time > 60 days are considered for thoracotomy.[134] Although the best candidates for resection are patients with a solitary pulmonary lesion, no evidence of extrapulmonary intrathoracic metastases, and a tumor doubling time longer than 60 days, patients with multiple metastases and no extrapulmonary intrathoracic disease can still have a 5-year survival rate of 19% and therefore should be considered for resection.

Gastrointestinal Metastases Gastrointestinal metastases from metastatic melanoma may produce highly symptomatic and immediately life-threatening clinical manifestations. Most commonly, gastrointestinal metastases present as the result of occult blood loss or as obstructing lesions at the lead point of an intussuscepting segment of small bowel. Indications for surgery are most frequently associated with acute bowel obstruction from intussuscepting small bowel or chronic gastrointestinal bleeding. Surgical exploration usually reveals multiple sites of involvement. Operative intervention, whether for curative or palliative intent, can be performed with minimal morbidity and mortality. A JWCI study reported a 5-year survival rate of 41% for 46 patients undergoing curative resection of gastrointestinal tract metastases.[135]

IMMUNOTHERAPY The correlation between prognosis and the degree of lymphoid infiltration of a primary tumor suggests that host immunity plays a role in the natural history of melanoma.[136] The prognosis associated with primary melanoma, otherwise defined by the depth of primary invasion and the presence or absence of regional lymph node and distant metastatic disease, may thus be governed by underlying immunologic response. The fact that IFNα-2b, the first active adjuvant medical therapy for patients with resected high-risk melanoma, has major effects on the tumor's major histocompatibility complex (MHC) expression and on the function of T cells, natural killer (NK) cells, and dendritic cells has prompted exploration of newer immunomodulating agents.

The elements of the host response to melanoma may be separated into acute, subacute, and chronic components. The NK system and IFN systems along with the dendritic (antigen-presenting) cell system provide acute/subacute responses, whereas the antigen-specific T-cell and B-cell humoral responses are the more chronic/enduring mechanisms of response, accompanied by the IFN systems. The manner and degree to which host response mechanisms may determine the outcome of melanoma have yet to be determined, but recombinant DNA technology has afforded oncologists the opportunity to test and dissect the therapeutic role of each component.

Active Specific Immunotherapy Based on the observation that antibodies in the sera of melanoma patients recognize surface antigens on melanoma cells, numerous attempts have been made to develop a vaccine to induce active immunity against melanoma to cause the regression of established tumors or, more frequently, to prevent recurrence. The majority of these vaccines are based on whole melanoma cells or extracts obtained from melanoma cells.[136]

In 1992, Morton and colleagues reported a phase II trial of Canvaxin in 75 patients with melanoma metastatic to distant sites (AJCC stage IV).[91] Overall survival significantly ($p < .0001$) increased to a median of 23.1 months, compared to 7.3 months for AJCC stage IV patients in a 20-year historic database. This improvement was evident for all metastatic sites. In addition, the proportion of vaccine patients alive 5 years following appearance of distant metastases was 26%, compared to 6% historically. A more recent analysis of 107 matched pairs of vaccine and nonvaccine patients with resected stage IV melanoma revealed a significant overall survival advantage for postoperative adjuvant treatment with Canvaxin ($p = .0009$): 5-year overall survival was

39% for vaccine patients versus 20% for nonvaccine patients.[128] Morton's group[137] has proposed a management paradigm based on cytoreductive surgery plus adjuvant immunotherapy, and two phase III multicenter trials were initiated to examine postoperative Canvaxin therapy in patients with stage III or stage IV melanoma. However, the phase III clinical trial of Canvaxin in patients with stage IV melanoma was discontinued in 2005 after the data and safety monitoring board responsible for oversight of this clinical trial found that the data were unlikely to provide significant evidence of a survival benefit for treatment with Canvaxin versus placebo.

Interferon Therapy IFNs have served as prototypes of biologic response modifiers. The pleiotropy of the IFNs and other biologic agents represents an alternative to conventional chemotherapy for combating tumor growth; direct, indirect, and composite effects on tumor cell surface markers have been documented. The biologic effects of IFN differ from the chemotherapeutic effects of cytotoxic drugs. Optimal biologic response modification by IFN may not necessarily be obtained at its maximally tolerated dosage, where the maximal antitumor effects of a cytotoxic agent would be anticipated.

IFNα-2 Considerable experience has been gained in the treatment of metastatic melanoma with native IFNα of leukocyte and lymphoblastoid cell origin and with several recombinant subspecies (IFNα-2a [Roferon, Hoffmann–La Roche, Inc], IFNα-2b [Intron, Schering–Plough], IFNα-2c [Boehringer]). A response to IFNα was observed in 8 of 112 subjects treated with the earliest available native IFNα (Le or N1) (Table 108-7). The low dosages (0.5–10 MU daily or alternate-daily) and limited periods of treatment (less than 2 months, generally 4–6 weeks) may have compromised the assessment of antitumor effect. As IFN produced by recombinant DNA became available for clinical trials, the maximally tolerated dosages of IFNα-2a, -b, and - c were defined as 10 to 50 MU administered daily via subcutaneous, intramuscular, or intravenous routes. In phase II studies, 25 of 174 (14.4%) evaluable subjects treated with IFN-2a and 24 of 106 (22.6%) evaluable subjects receiving IFNα-2b had clinical responses to therapy administered by a variety of dosages and routes, in daily or alternate-daily schedules (see Table 108-7).[100,138–141]

Regimens employing intermittent therapy interrupted by one or more weeks of nontreatment have produced inferior response rates.[142,143] The results of treatment with the two subspecies of recombinant IFNα are otherwise comparable, achieving an objective clinical response rate of 17.5% overall. Multiple studies have observed that smaller tumor masses respond more frequently to IFNα than do larger masses, and that the response to IFN follows a time course that may be more characteristic of endocrine hormonal therapy than of chemotherapy: some responses have been observed after protracted periods of treatment. The optimal dosage for therapy, however, has not been rigorously determined, nor have in vitro correlates of response been defined among the multiple mechanisms known to be influenced by IFNα and its subspecies.

Table 108-7 Interferons in Treatment of Metastatic Melanoma

Dose/Schedule	No. of Evaluable Patients	No. of Partial Responses	No. of Complete Responses	Objective Response Rate* (%)
Nonrecombinant interferon-α				
0.5–60 MU/m² daily *or* 15–50 MU/m² three times a week	112	6	2	7 (3–14)
Recombinant interferonα-2a				
3–50 MU/m² three times a week	174	16	9	14 (9–20)
10–100 MU/m² daily	106	15	9	23 (15–31)

*95% confidence interval.

Table 108-8 Clinical Trials in Melanoma: Interferon Gamma Alone and in Combinations

Drug (Dose)	No. of Evaluable Patients	No. of Partial Responses	No. of Complete Responses	Objective Response Rate*(%)
IFNγ (.01–4.5 mg/m²)	69	4	1	7 (2–16)
IFNγ and IFNβ				
IFNγ (2 mg)				
IFNβ (30 MU/m²)	15	0	0	0 (0–22)
IFNγ and IFNα-2a				
IFNγ(.01–.05 mg/m²)				
IFNα-2a (2–10 MU/m²)	20	0	1	5 (0–25)
IFNγ and IFNα-2c				
IFNγ (.05–.2 mg/m²)				
IFNα-2c (2 MU/m²)	15	0	0	0 (0–22)

IFN = interferon.
*95% confidence interval.

IFNγ SWOG has tested the adjuvant activity of IFNγ administered at its putative optimal immunomodulatory dosage to patients with intermediate or deep primary tumor invasion (T2–T4, > 0.76 mm) or positive regional nodes (N1–2). SWOG terminated this study following an interim analysis in early 1990.[144] At the time of study closure, death or relapse was observed among 34 of 58 subjects treated with IFNγ and among 25 of 66 subjects in the control arm; analysis suggested that it would be impossible to demonstrate a 50% improvement in disease-free survival. An ongoing EORTC study of IFNγ versus IFNα or control has been completed in 350 subjects; neither adverse nor beneficial effects were observed (JM Kirkwood, personal communication).

A number of immunologic investigations have been carried out in conjunction with clinical trials of recombinant IFNγ in melanoma (Table 108-8). Two studies are of particular note. One phase I–II trial from the Pittsburgh Melanoma Center evaluated the immunomodulatory effect of IFNγ (Biogen, Inc.) administered in five different dosages (3, 30, 300, 1,000, and 3,000 mg/m² daily) to groups of six patients. Continuous intravenous infusion and 2-hour daily infusions were comparable.[145,146] ECOG assessed immunobiologic correlates in an extended phase II(B) trial (ECOG EST 4687/EST 4987) of IFNγ administered to 98 patients for at least 3 months, three times a week. This study failed to detect antitumor effects of IFNγ at any dose. Although profound immunomodulatory effects were observed, the absence of antitumor activity has halted further single-agent studies of IFNγ for metastatic melanoma.

In the future, the use of cytokines in combined-modality regimens may improve results. IFN and granulocyte-macrophage-colony-stimulating factor (GM-CSF) have been administered in a prospective randomized factorial 2 × 2 design with three peptide vaccines of the lineage category, all related to melanogenesis.[147] Vaccine immune responses were obtained in more than a third of patients with advanced metastatic disease, even when administered in second-line therapy. IFNα-2b and GM-CSF both improved vaccine immune responses measured by ELISPOT assay, and the same three peptide vaccines are now being evaluated in a larger phase III adjuvant trial for resected stage IIIB/IV disease (E4697), which will complete accrual of 800 patients in 2007. In summary, the role of IFNs and cytokines as adjuncts to chemotherapy and biologic therapy of melanoma is being studied intensively (Table 108-9). Encouraging data suggest that IFNs may act through immunological mechanisms, as well as vascular mechanisms that reduce tumor tissue pressure and other physiologic barriers to antitumor therapies and imaging agents.[148]

Interleukin-2 and Adoptive Immunotherapy IL-2 has been intensively explored for therapy of melanoma since this central immunoregulatory cytokine (T cell growth factor) was obtained from lectin-stimulated lymphoid cell lines over a decade ago.

IL-2 and Lymphokine-Activated Killer Cells In 1982, Grimm and colleagues reported that natural IL-2 and recombinant DNA-produced IL-2 could activate large granular lymphocytes to kill a variety of human tumor cells, suggesting that tumor cells might be susceptible to IL-2 with or without lymphokine-activated killer (LAK) cells.[149] Adoptive effector cell transfer was developed pre-

Table 108-9 Clinical Trials in Melanoma: Chemotherapy and Biologic Therapy Combinations

Drug(s)/Dose(s)	No. of Evaluable Patients	No. of Partial Responses	No. of Complete Responses	Objective Response Rate* (%)
rIL-2 and DTIC	86	12	5	20 (12–30)
rIL-2 (2–18 × 10^6 IU/m^2)				
DTIC (850–1000 mg/m^2)				
IFNα-2a and DFMO	16	0	0	0 (0–21)
IFNα-2a (36 × 10^6 U/m^2)				
DFMO (2.25 g/m^2)				
IFNα-2b and cyclophosphamide	17	1	0	6 (0–29)
IFNα-2b (10 × 10^6 IU/m^2)				
Cyclophosphamide (25 mg)				
IFNα-2a and dacarbazine	43	7	6	20 (17–46)
IFNα-2a (3–9 MU/m^2 daily)				
Dacarbazine (200 mg/m^2)				
IFNα-2b and dacarbazine	21	4	0	19 (5–42)
IFNα-2b (10 MU/m^2)				
Dacarbazine (200 mg/m^2 daily)				
IFNβ and chemotherapy	12	0	0	0 (0–27)
IFNβ (30 MU/m^2 daily)				
Dacarbazine (10 mg/m^2)				
Cimetidine (300 mg)				

*95% confidence interval.

clinically and rapidly translated to large-scale clinical studies through recombinant DNA technology.[150,151] Based on experimental studies demonstrating that the greatest antitumor activity is obtained at the maximally tolerated dosages of IL-2 and that IL-2 with LAK cells has greater antitumor effects than IL-2 alone in mice, the Surgery Branch of the National Cancer Institute (NCI) conducted a series of mural and extramural clinical studies of IL-2 with LAK cells.[151,152] In six extramural clinical research centers assembled as the IL-2 Extramural Working Group, high-dose IL-2 with the adoptive transfer of effector cells was intensively pursued to confirm the antitumor activity in melanoma, renal cell carcinoma, and colorectal carcinoma.

With high doses of IL-2 (100,000 U/kg, Cetus [Chiron] Corp.; or 1–6 MU/m^2, Hoffmann–La Roche) administered daily for up to 5 days by intravenous bolus every 8 hours and repeated after 7 to 10 days, partial responses were obtained in 10 of 42 (24%) evaluable melanoma patients.[151,153,154] By comparison, four complete and six partial responses were obtained among 48 subjects treated with IL-2 and LAK (21%). There is no evidence that adoptive transfer of LAK cells has significantly improved the antitumor efficacy of IL-2 as a single agent for therapy of melanoma.[155,156]

A major obstacle for implementation of the high-dose bolus IL-2 regimen of the NCI Surgery Branch has been toxicity related to the induction of a capillary leak syndrome and to the secretion of secondary cytokines by cells of the immune system. Chills, nausea, vomiting, and diarrhea are common and may be associated with hypotension, tachycardia somnolence, disorientation, and coma, as well as respiratory distress, shock, and even death. Despite a significant incidence of side effects, Rosenberg and colleagues reported a treatment-related mortality rate of only 1.5%.[154] West has reported diminished toxicity and comparable antitumor activity from the use of continuous infusions of 18 × 10^6 IU/m^2/d.[157] A study of maximally tolerated doses of IL-2 delivered with LAK cell transfer suggests that the antitumor efficiency of continuous infusion may be less than that of bolus administration for melanoma.[158]

High-dose IL-2 represents an evolving area of research in biologic therapy and forms the basis for the only FDA-approved systemic biologic therapy of disseminated melanoma.

IL-2 and Tumor-Infiltrating Lymphocytes Experimental studies of effector cells derived from tumor-infiltrating lymphocytes (TIL) in mice suggest improved antitumor efficacy and the potential emergence of cytotoxic T cells from these TIL.[159] The first clinical translation of these studies suggested improved antitumor efficacy for melanoma.[160] An inherent problem with the therapeutic use of TIL has been the technical difficulty and low frequency of outgrowth of cells appropriate for adoptive transfer. The possibility of using tumor-specific T cells that are generated from TIL or induced by specific immunization of the host in vivo or in vitro is an evolving area of therapeutic research. To date, it has not been established that TIL add to the benefit of IL-2.

Dendritic Cell Vaccines Tumor cells may escape recognition by a variety of mechanisms. One of the more effective ways to curtail this escape is the use of dendritic cell vaccines. Dendritic cells are the sentinels of the immune system. They take up antigen and process it for secondary lymphoid organs. In recent years, an enormous body of information on dendritic cell biology has allowed development of dendritic cells as vaccines by stimulating cells with peptide antigens, tumor lysates or whole-cell preparations, or RNA or DNA.[161]

Combined-Modality Regimens The use of IL-2 in combined-modality regimens was initiated with IFNα-2 and then applied to IFNγ, TNF, low-dose cyclophosphamide, DTIC, and cisplatin and amifostine (WR2721).[162–165] These combinations have not significantly elevated the response rate to IL-2. The experience to date with IL-2 and IFNα has been the largest; response rates are somewhat above those of IFNα and IL-2 taken individually at 17 to 20%, but there is no evidence of synergism or an additive effect to counterbalance the toxicity of this combination.

CHEMOTHERAPY **Single-Agent Chemotherapy** Systemic medical management has failed to improve significantly the survival of patients with nonresectable melanoma. DTIC, the only agent that has reproducibly caused partial remissions of disease, is the only FDA-approved chemotherapy for melanoma. DTIC has undergone the most extensive clinical trials of any single agent, with an objective response rate of 6 to 28% in reported series of 100 or more patients.[166,167] Although the overall response rate has historically been cited as 20%, more current estimates indicate objective response in no more than 7 to 10% of recipients, with less than a 4% rate of complete responses, primarily in patients with soft-tissue metastases; responses are rare for visceral sites of metastasis.

Temozolomide (Temodar) is an oral, 100% absorbed prodrug for MTIC, the active metabolite derived in the liver from dacarbazine. It is simpler to administer and it penetrates the CNS, which dacarbazine does not. Middleton and colleagues[114] established that temozolomide was not inferior to dacarbazine, although this study failed to demonstrate superiority. A current EORTC study is testing whether a 6-week regimen of daily therapy with temozolomide may achieve results that are superior to dacarbazine.

Combination Chemotherapy In multicenter cooperative group trials, combination chemotherapy regimens have had increased toxicity and until recently have not enhanced response rates significantly (> 20%) over DTIC (Table 108-10). An analysis of three phase III studies of DTIC given alone or in combination with other agents showed that 26 of 580 patients (4.5%) achieved complete remission. Of the 26 remissions, 17 were associated with soft-tissue metastases and 6 (1%) lasted over 30 to 60 months.[168] By contrast, complete remissions were achieved in only 10 of 503 patients (2%) treated with a variety of investigative chemotherapeutic regimens, and only 3 of these survived disease-free for more than 60 months. This experience suggests that durable responses to chemotherapy are indeed rare and, conversely, argues that the benefits observed with DTIC or other biologic and chemotherapeutic agents should not be attributed to spontaneous remission.[169] Although two combinations employing cisplatin have been suggested to show significantly greater activity than DTIC alone, more recent studies indicate that they may be no more effective.[170]

The most recent advance in multiagent chemotherapy for melanoma is triple-agent chemotherapy plus IL-2 and IFNα. Single-institution trials have demonstrated response rates as high as 60%, with short-term complete remission rates of 12 to 15%. The toxicity of sequential and concurrent biochemotherapy regimens limits their use in younger patients with high performance levels, a

Table 108-10 Clinical Trials in Melanoma: Combination Chemotherapy

Drug(s)/Dose(s)	No of. Evaluable Patients	No. of Partial Responses	No. of Complete Responses	Objective Response Rate* (Range)
Cisplatin-based agents + tamoxifen	40	17	4	53% (36–68)
DTIC + CDDP	130	27	6	25% (18–34)
DTIC 200–750 mg/m^2				
CDDP 15–100 mg/m^2				
DTIC + CDDP + Vindesine	155	38	11	32% (24–39)
DTIC 250–450 mg/m^2/d				
CDDP 50–100 mg/m^2/d				
Vindesine 3 mg/m^2/d				
DTIC + CDDP + Vinblastine	157	30	5	22% (16–29)
DTIC 150–800 mg/m^2				
CDDP 20–50 mg/m^2				
Vinblastine 1.6–5 mg/m^2				
DTIC + CDDP + Carmustine	20	1	1	10% (1–25)
DTIC 220 mg/m^2 qod				
CDDP 25 mg/m^2 qod				
Carmustine 150 mg/m^2/6 wk				
Vinblastine + Bleomycin + Cisplatin	20	0	0	0 (0–17)
Vinblastine 6 mg/m^2				
Bleomycin 15 mg/m^2				
Cisplatin 50 mg/m^2				
Vinblastine + Bleomycin + Cisplatin + DTIC + DBD	42	10	1	26% (14–42)
Vinblastine 3–6 mg/m^2				
Bleomycin 15 mg/m^2				
Cisplatin 50 mg/m^2				
DTIC 800 mg/m^2				
DBD 125 mg/m^2				
BCNU + DBD	20	3	1	20% (6–44)
BCNU 180 mg/m^2				
DBD 100 mg/m^2				

*95% confidence interval.

group that traditionally responds to DTIC alone. A large United States Intergroup study led by ECOG did not demonstrate a significant benefit in survival, time to progression, or response rate for the more toxic inpatient biochemotherapy regimen compared to simpler outpatient chemotherapy.[171]

Del Prete and colleagues reported on the combination of DTIC, carmustine (BCNU), cisplatin, and tamoxifen[172]; response rates were about 50% (11/20 objective responses). Phase II and III trials have not corroborated any benefit of tamoxifen in combination chemotherapy for melanoma.[173–175] However, JWCI investigators reported that concurrent biochemotherapy using decrescendo dosing of IL-2, posttreatment G-CSF, and low-dose tamoxifen produced a 57% overall response rate in patients with poor-prognosis metastatic melanoma. This modified regimen was associated with significantly lower toxicity levels than those of standard concurrent biochemotherapy.[176] Several institutions are comparing the efficacy of these newer biochemotherapy regimens with that of DTIC-based combination therapy.[177]

Hormonal Therapy The natural history of malignant melanoma suggests a relationship between estrogen and the onset of malignant activity. Melanoma is infrequently seen before puberty, except in cases of familial melanoma, and the peak incidence of melanoma in females coincides with the late childbearing years and the beginning of menopause. In addition, cases have been reported of spontaneous regression following parturition, as well as periods of widespread dissemination during pregnancy.[178,179] Furthermore, survival rates always favor the female population, especially postmenopausal women.

Estrogen receptors have been reported in benign nevi of melanoma patients and in tumor cells, but not in benign nevi from normal individuals.[180] This supports the theory that malignant melanoma is estrogen dependent and that the binding of estrogen to cell-specific receptors may result in a molecular alteration associated with neoplastic transformation. Other investigators have failed to support these findings.[181] Because estrogen, a steroid hormone, exerts its biologic effect through the mediation of cytoplasmic protein receptors, the presence of an estrogen receptor on the cell surface might be a biologic marker in melanoma patients.

Tamoxifen alone at standard or high doses has little objective antitumor activity in metastatic melanoma. The mechanism of its synergism with chemotherapeutic agents has been a matter of conjecture; the possibility of calcium channel activity and interaction with cisplatin or BCNU has been raised.[170] Cocconi and the Italian Cooperative Multicenter Oncology Group reported the results of a randomized study of DTIC with or without tamoxifen.[182] A significant advantage was demonstrated for DTIC-tamoxifen, and the beneficial impact of tamoxifen seemed to occur chiefly among females.

Radiation Therapy Radiation has been widely used, often with excellent results, in the palliation of symptoms from metastatic melanoma. Metastatic sites where radiation has been of great palliative benefit include the lung, lymph nodes, subcutaneous nodules, bone, brain, spinal cord, and abdomen. Response rates depend on the dose of radiation that can be safely delivered to the involved region, as well as the volume of disease and intrinsic radiosensitivity of the tumor cells. The most appropriate dose per fraction has been the subject of much controversy.[183,184] Certain in vitro features of irradiated melanoma cell lines (a broad shoulder on many radiation cell-survival curves) suggested that a larger-than-standard dose per fraction would be more advantageous in cell kill, but greater late toxicity is associated with larger doses per fraction. An RTOG prospective randomized trial compared 4 fractions of 8 Gy (one fraction per week) to 20 fractions of 2.5 Gy (daily, 5 fractions per week) in patients with measurable melanoma.[185] There was no difference in complete response (24.2 and 23.4%, respectively) or partial response (35.5 and 34.4%, respectively). It was concluded that the most appropriate fractionation should be determined by standard factors (location of lesion, life expectancy, convenience, and efficacy) rather than histology.

Brain Metastases Conventional whole-brain radiation has been used for palliation of symptoms, typically with survival of only 4 to 6 weeks. Patchell and colleagues demonstrated a significant reduction in neurologic sequelae when surgical resection of solitary metastases from a variety of tumor types was followed by whole-brain radiation.[186] More recent studies suggest that stereotactic radiosurgery may provide safe and effective control of disease in patients who are not candidates for resection.[187]

FUTURE HORIZONS

Prevention of melanoma appears possible through education about the etiologic role of sunburn in fair-skinned individuals. Counseling to avoid the sun and to use barrier clothing and sun-blocking agents may influence high-risk behavior patterns. Intensive public health interventions implemented in several regions of Australia and New Zealand, where melanoma incidence rates are the highest in the world, appear to have had a beneficial effect. Intergovernmental action to eliminate the manufacture of chlorofluorohydrocarbons and other measures to preserve the ozone layer are also fundamental to long-range cancer control measures.

Improvements in treatment for malignant melanoma, a cancer that is rapidly increasing in incidence, must be directed to both the early and late stages of the disease. Because thin, early-stage melanomas are highly curable by simple surgical excision, early diagnosis must be the foundation for more effective therapy. The most practical approach is public education and skin screening projects.

There is also an urgent need for improved therapy in the melanoma patient who has metastases. Perhaps the most promising approach to metastases in the regional nodes or distant sites is more aggressive surgery in combination with postsurgical adjuvant therapy. Phase II studies with melanoma vaccines have been promising, and the results of multicenter phase III trials should become available shortly. The last 2 decades have seen no significant progress in extending the survival of patients with distant metastases, despite multiple trials of cytotoxic chemotherapy agents. Some of the newer regimens that use combination chemotherapy plus high-dose IL-2 and IFNα-2 appear to have improved the response rate when compared with DTIC alone, but recent phase III ECOG randomized trials have shown no survival advantage. When combined with biologic response modifiers such as IFN and IL, immunotherapy based upon specific melanoma antigens, whether active or adoptive, probably holds the greatest promise for future progress. Recent reports from NCI's Surgery Branch indicate that lymphodepletion followed by adoptive transfer of autologous tumor-reactive lymphocytes and high-dose IL-2 therapy also holds great promise.[188]

REFERENCES

1. Jemal A, Murray T, Ward E, et al. Cancer statistics 2005. CA A Cancer Clin 2005;55:10–30.
2. Blumthaler M, Ambach W. Indications of increasing solar ultraviolet B radiation flux in Alpine regions. Science 1990;248:206.
3. Ries LAG, Eisner MP, Kosary CL, et al. SEER cancer statistics review, 1973–1999. Bethesda, MD: National Cancer Institute; 2002.
4. MacKie RM, Freudenberger T, Aitchison TC. Personal risk-factor chart for cutaneous melanoma. Lancet 1989;2:487.
5. Fountain JW. Genetic Factors. In: Balch CM, Houghton AN, Sober AJ, Soong S-J, editors. Cutaneous melanoma. St. Louis: Quality Med Pub; 1998. p 475–92.
6. Manson JE, Rexrode KM, Garland FC, et al. The case for a comprehensive national campaign to prevent melanoma and associated mortality. Epidemiology 2000;11:728–34.
7. Gillgren P, Brattstrom G, Frisell J, et al. Body site of cutaneous malignant melanoma—a study on patients with hereditary and multiple sporadic tumors. Melanoma Res 2003;13:279–86.
8. Bale SJ, Dracopoli NC, Tucker MA, et al. Mapping the gene for hereditary cutaneous malignant melanoma-dysplastic nevus to chromosome 1p. N Engl J Med 1989;320:1367.
9. Pedersen MI, Wang N. Chromosomal evolution in the progression and metastasis of human malignant melanoma. A multiple lesion study. Cancer Genet Cytogenet 1989;41:185–201.
10. Cannon–Albright LA, Goldgar DE, Meyer LJ, et al. Assignment of a locus for familial melanoma, MLM, to chromosome 9p13-p22. Science 1992;258:1148.
11. Fountain JW, Karayiorgou M, Ernstoff MS, et al. Homozygous deletions within human chromosome band 9p21 in melanoma. Proc Natl Acad Sci U S A 1992;89:10557.
12. Bastign BC. Molecular genetics of melanocytic neoplasia: practical applications for diagnosis. Pathology 2004;36:458–61.
13. Goldstein AM. Familial melanoma, pancreatic cancer and germline CDKN2A mutations. Hum Mutat 2004;23:630.
14. Tucker MA, Fraser MC, Goldstein AM, et al. A natural history of melanoma and dysplastic nevi. An atlas of lesions in melanoma-prone families. Cancer 2002;94:3192.
15. Ghiorzo P, Ciotti P, Mantelli M, et al. Characterization of ligurian melanoma families and risk of occurrence of other neoplasia. Int J Cancer 1999;83:441.
16. Essner R, Kuo CT, Wen DR, et al. Prognostic implications of p53 overexpression in cutaneous melanoma from sun-exposed and non-exposed sites. Cancer 1998;82:309–16.
17. Shinozaki M, Fujimoto A, Morton DL, Hoon DS. Incidence of BRAF oncogene mutation and clinical relevance for primary cutaneous melanomas. Clin Cancer Res 2004;10:1753–7.
18. Lucchina LC, Barnhill RL, Duke DM, Sober AJ. Familial cutaneous melanoma. Melanoma Res 1995;5:413.
19. Elder DE, Greene MH, Guerry D IV, et al. The dysplastic nevus syndrome. Our definition. Am J Dermatopathol 1982;4:455.
20. Consensus Conference. Precursors to malignant melanoma. JAMA 1984;251:1864.
21. Tucker MA, Halpern A, Holly EA, et al. Clinically recognized dysplastic nevi. A central risk factor for cutaneous melanoma. JAMA 1997;277:1439–44.
22. Rhodes AR, Melski JW. Small congenital nevocellular nevi and risk of cutaneous melanoma. J Pediatr 1982;100:219.
23. Watt AJ, Kotsis SV, Chung KC. Risk of melanoma arising in large congenital melanocytic nevi: a systemic review. Plast Reconstr Surg 2004;113:1968–74.
24. Herlyn M, Clark WH, Rodeck U, Mancianti MC. Biology of tumor progression in human melanocytes. Lab Invest 1987;56:461.
25. Clark WH Jr, From L, Bernardino EA, Mihm MC Jr. The histogenesis and biologic behavior of primary human malignant melanoma of the skin. Cancer Res 1969;29:705.
26. Breslow A. Prognostic factors in the treatment of cutaneous melanoma. J Cutan Pathol 1979;6:208.
27. Balch CM, Soong SJ, Gershenwald JE, et al. Prognostic factors analysis of 17,600 melanoma patients. Validation of the American Joint Committee on Cancer melanoma staging system. J Clin Oncol 2001;19:3622
28. American Joint Committee on Cancer. AJCC Cancer Staging Manual. 6th ed. New York: Springer–Verlag; 2002. p. 209–20.
29. Balch CM, Buzaid AC, Soong SJ, et al. Final version of the American Joint Committee on Cancer staging system for cutaneous melanoma. J Clin Oncol 2001;19:3635.
30. Morton DL, Davtyan DG, Wanek LA, et al. Multivariate analysis of the relationship between survival and the microstage of primary melanoma by Clark level and Breslow thickness. Cancer 1993;71:3737.
31. Balch CM, Soong SJ, Atkins MB, et al. An evidence-based staging system for cutaneous melanoma. CA Cancer J Clin 2004;54:131–49.
32. Shaw HM, McCarthy SW, McCarthy WH, et al. Thin regressing malignant melanoma. Significance of concurrent regional lymph node metastes. Histopathology 1989;15:257.
33. Hoon DSB, Spugnardi M, Kuo C, et al. Profiling epigenetic inactivation of tumor suppressor genes in tumors and plasma from cutaneous melanoma patients. Oncogene 2004;23:4014–22.
34. Shaw HM, McGovern VJ, Milton GW, et al. Histologic features of tumors and the female superiority in survival from malignant melanoma. Cancer 1980;45:1604.
35. Hsueh EC, Lucci A, Qi K, Morton DL. Survival of patients with melanoma of the lower extremity decreases with distance from the trunk. Cancer 1999;85:383–8.
36. Urist MM, Balch CM, Soong S-J, et al. Head and neck melanoma in 534 clinical stage I patients. A prognostic factors analysis and results of surgical treatment. Ann Surg 1984;200:769.
37. Day CL Jr, Mihm MC Jr, Sober AJ, et al. Prognostic factors for melanoma patients with lesions 0.76–1.69 mm in thickness. Ann Surg 1982;195:30.
38. Wong JH, Wanek L, Chang L-JC, et al. The importance of anatomic site in prognosis in patients with cutaneous melanoma. Arch Surg 1991;126:486.
39. Cascinelli N, Vaglini M, Bufalino R, Morabito A. BANS. A cutaneous region with no prognostic significance in patients with melanoma. Cancer 1986;57:441–4.
40. Wong JH, Sterns E, Kopald KH, et al. Prognostic significance of pregnancy in stage I melanoma. Arch Surg 1989;124:1227.
41. Slingluff CL, Reintgen DS, Vollmer RT, Seigler HF. Malignant melanoma arising during pregnancy. A study of 100 patients. Ann Surg 1990;211:552.
42. MacKie RM, Bufalino R, Morabito A, et al. Lack of effect of pregnancy on outcome of melanoma. Lancet 1991;337:653.
43. Morton DL, Wanek LA, Nizze JA, et al. Improved long-term survival after lymphadenectomy of melanoma metastatic to regional nodes. Ann Surg 1991;214:491.
44. Morton DL, Hsueh EC, Essner R, et al. Prolonged survival of patients receiving active immunotherapy with Canvaxin therapeutic polyvalent vaccine after complete resection of melanoma metastatic to regional lymph nodes. Ann Surg 2002;236:438.
45. Shrivers SC, Xang X, Li W, Joseph E, et al. Molecular staging of malignant melanoma. Correlation with clinical outcome. JAMA 1998;280:1410.
46. Morton DL, Hoon DSB, Cochran AJ, et al. Lymphatic mapping and sentinel lymphadenectomy for early-stage melanoma. Therapeutic utility and implications of nodal microanatomy and molecular staging from improving the accuracy of detection of nodal micrometastases. Ann Surg 2003;238:538–50.
47. Wong JH, Cagle LA, Morton DL. Surgical treatment of lymph nodes with metastatic melanoma from an unknown primary site. Arch Surg 1987;122:1380.
48. Barth A, Wanek LA, Morton DL. Prognostic factors in 1,521 melanoma patients with distant metastases. J Am Coll Surg 1995;181:193.
49. Costanzi JJ. DTIC (NSC 45388) studies in the Southwest Oncology Group. Cancer Treat Rep 1976;60:189.
50. Cochran AJ. Studies of the melanocytes of the epidermis adjacent to tumors. J Invest Dermatol 1971;57:38.
51. Goldman LI, Byrd R. Narrow resection margins for patients with low-risk melanoma. Am J Surg 1988;155:242.
52. Fallowfield ME, Cook MG. Re-excisions of scar in primary cutaneous melanoma. A histopathological study. Br J Dermatol 1992;126:47.
53. Veronesi U, Cascinelli N, Adamus J, et al. Thin stage I primary cutaneous malignant melanoma. Comparison of excision with margins of 1 or 3 cm. N Engl J Med 1988;318:1159.
54. Neades GT, Orr DJ, Hughes LE, Horgan K. Safe margins in the excision of primary cutaneous melanoma. Br J Surg 1993;80:731.
55. Balch CM, Urist MM, Karakousis CP, et al. Efficacy of 2-cm surgical margins for intermediate-thickness melanomas (1 to 4 mm). Results of a multi-institutional randomized surgical trial. Ann Surg 1993;218:262.
56. Cohn–Cedermark G, Rutqvist LE, Anderson R, et al. Long-term results of a randomized study by the Swedish Melanoma Study Group on 2cm versus 5cm resection margins for patients with cutaneous melanoma with a tumor thickness of 0.8–2.0mm. Cancer 2000;89:1495.
57. Thomas JM, Newton-Bishop J, A'Hern R, et al. Excision margins in high risk melanoma. N Engl J Med 2004;350:757–66.
58. Morton DL. Current management of malignant melanoma. Ann Surg 1990;212:123.
59. Cooper JS. The evolution of the role of radiotherapy in the management of mucocutaneous melanoma. Hematol Oncol Clin North Am 1998;12:849–62.
60. Strom EA, Ross MI. Adjuvant radiation therapy after axillary lymphadenectomy for metastatic melanoma. Toxicity and local control. Ann Surg Oncol 1995;2:445–9.
61. Ang KK, Peters LJ, Weber RS. Postoperative radiotherapy for cutaneous melanoma of the head and neck region. Int J Radiat Oncol Biol Phys 1994;30:795–8.
62. De Meerleer GO, Vermeersch H, van Eijkeren M, et al. Primary sinonasal mucosal melanoma. Three different therapeutic approaches to inoperable local disease or recurrence and a review of the literature. Melanoma Res 1998;8:449–57.
63. Beitler JJ, McCormick B, Ellsworth RM, et al. Ocular melanoma. Total dose and dose rate effects with cobalt 60 plaque therapy. Radiology 1990;176:275.
64. Munzenrider JE, Gragoudas ES, Seddon JM. Conservative treatment of uveal melanoma. Probability of eye retention after proton treatment. Int J Radiat Oncol Biol Phys 1988;15:553.
65. Courdi A, Caujolle JP, Grange JD. Results of proton therapy of uveal melanomas treated in Nice. Int J Radiat Oncol Biol Phys 1999;45:5–11.
66. Earle JD. Results from the Collaborative Ocular Melanoma Study (COMS) of enucleation versus preoperative radiation therapy in the management of large ocular melanomas. Int J Radiat Oncol Biol Phys 1999;43:1168–9.
67. The Collaborative Ocular Melanoma Study (COMS) randomized trial of pre-enucleation radiation of large choroidal melanoma II: initial mortality findings. COMS report no. 10. Am J Ophthalmol 1998;125:779–96.
68. Janoff KA, Moseson D, Mohlgren J, et al. The treatment of stage I melanoma of the extremities with regional hyperthermic isolation perfusion. Ann Surg 1982;196:316.
69. Krementz ET, Ryanb RF. Chemotherapy of melanoma of the extremities by perfusion. Fourteen years' clinical experience. Ann Surg 1972;182:316.
70. Ghussen F, Kruger I, Groth W, Stutzer H. The role of regional hyperthermic cytostatic perfusion in the treatment of extremity melanoma. Cancer 1988;61:654.
71. Milton GW, Shaw HM, McCarthy WH, et al. Prophylactic lymph node dissection in clinical stage I cutaneous malignant melanoma: results of surgical treatment in 1,319 patients. Br J Surg 1982;69:108.
72. McCarthy WH, Shaw HM, Milton GW. Efficacy of elective node dissection in 2,347 patients with clinical stage I malignant melanoma. Surg Gynecol Obstet 1985;161:575.

73. Balch CM, Soong S–J, Milton GW, et al. A comparison of prognostic factors and surgical results in 1,786 patients with localized (stage I) melanoma treated in Alabama USA, and New South Wales. Aust Ann Surg 1982;196:677.
74. Reintgen DS, Cox EB, McCarthy KS Jr, et al. Efficacy of elective lymph node dissection in patients with intermediate thickness primary melanoma. Ann Surg 1983;198:379.
75. Wanebo HJ, Fortner JG, Woodruff J, et al. Selection of the optimum surgical treatment of stage I melanoma by depth of microinvasion. Ann Surg 1975;182:302.
76. Drepper H, Kohler CD, Bastian B, et al. Benefit of elective lymph node dissection in subgroups of melanoma patients. Cancer 1995;72:741.
77. Veronesi U, Adamus J, Bandiera DC, et al. Inefficacy of immediate node dissection in stage 1 melanoma of the limbs. N Engl J Med. 1977;297:627–30.
78. Sim FH, Taylor WF, Ivins JC, et al. A prospective randomized study of the efficacy of routine elective lymphadenectomy in management of malignant melanoma. Preliminary results. Cancer 1978;41:948.
79. Balch CM, Soong SJ, Bartolucci AA, et al. Efficacy of an elective regional lymph node dissection of 1 to 4 mm thick melanomas for patients 60 years of age and younger. Ann Surg 1996;224:255.
80. Cascinelli N, Morabito A, Santinami M, et al. Immediate or delayed dissection of regional nodes in patients with melanoma of the trunk. A randomised trial. WHO Melanoma Programme. Lancet 1998;351:793.
81. Holmes EC, Moseley HS, Morton DL, et al. A rational approach to the surgical management of melanoma. Ann Surg 1977;185:481.
82. Fee HJ, Robinson DS, Morton DL, et al. The determination of lymph shed by colloidal gold scanning in patients with malignant melanoma. A preliminary study. Surgery 1978;84:626.
83. Bostick P, Essner R, Glass E, et al. Comparison of blue dye and probe-assisted intraoperative lymphatic mapping in melanoma to identify sentinel nodes in 100 lymphatic basins. Arch Surg 1999;134:43.
84. Morton DL, Wen DR, Wong JH, et al. Technical details of intraoperative lymphatic mapping for early stage melanoma. Arch Surg 1992;127:392.
85. Gershenwald JE, Thompson W, Mansfield PF, et al. Multi-institutional melanoma lymphatic mapping experience. The prognostic value of sentinel lymph node status in 612 stage I or II melanoma patients. J Clin Oncol 1999;17:976.
86. Thompson JF, McCarthy WH, Bosch CM, et al. Sentinel lymph node status as an indicator of the presence of melanoma in the regional lymph nodes. Melanoma Res 1995;5:255.
87. Essner R, Conforti A, Kelley MC, et al. Efficacy of lymphatic mapping, sentinel lymphadenectomy, and selective complete lymph node dissection as a therapeutic procedure for early-stage melanoma. Ann Surg Oncol 1999;6:442–9.
88. Morton DL, Thompson JF, Cochran AJ, et al. Interim results of the Multicenter Selective Lymphadenectomy Trial (MSLT-I) in clinical stage I melanoma [abstract 7500]. J Clin Oncol 2005;23(16S):710S.
89. Morton DL, Cochran AJ, Thompson JF, et al. Sentinel node biopsy for early-stage melanoma: accuracy and morbidity in MSLT-I, an international multicenter trial. Ann Surg 2005;242:302.
90. Morton DL, Thompson JF, Essner R, et al. Validation of the accuracy of intraoperative lymphatic mapping and sentinel lymphadenectomy for early-stage melanoma. A multicenter trial. Ann Surg 1999;230:453–65.
91. Morton DL, Foshag LJ, Hoon DSB, et al. Prolongation of survival in metastatic melanoma after active specific immunotherapy with a new polyvalent melanoma vaccine. Ann Surg 1992;216:463.
92. Barth A, Hoon DSB, Foshag LJ, et al. Polyvalent melanoma cell vaccine induces delayed-type hypersensitivity and in vitro cellular immune response. Cancer Res 1994;54:3342.
93. DiFronzo LA, Gupta R, Essner R, et al. Enhanced humoral immune response correlates with improved disease-free and overall survival in American Joint Committee on Cancer stage II melanoma patients receiving adjuvant polyvalent vaccine. J Clin Oncol 2002;20:3242.
94. Wallack MK, Sivanandham M, Balch CM, et al. A phase III randomized, double-blind, multiinstitutional trial of vaccinia melanoma oncolysate-active specific immunotherapy for patients with stage II melanoma. Cancer 1995;75:34.
95. Hersey P, Coates AS, McCarthy WH, et al. Adjuvant immunotherapy of patients with high-risk melanoma using vaccinia viral lysates of melanoma: results of a randomized trial. J Clin Oncol 2002;20:4181.
96. Sondak VK, Lin PY, Tathill RJ, et al. Adjuvant immunotherapy of resected, intermediate-thickness, node-negative melanoma with an allogeneic tumor vaccine. Overall results of a randomized trial of the Southwest Oncology Group. J Clin Oncol 2002;20:2058.
97. Sosman JA, Unger JM, Lin PY, et al. Adjuvant immunotherapy of resected, intermediate-thickness node-negative melanoma with an allogeneic tumor vaccine. Impact of HLA class I antigen expression on outcome. J Clin Oncol 2002;20:2067.
98. Kirkwood JM, Ibrahim JG, Sosman JA, et al. High-dose interferon alfa-2b significantly prolongs relapse-free and overall survival compared with the GM2-KLH/QS-21 vaccine in patients with resected stage IIB-III melanoma: results of intergroup trial E1694/S9512/C509801. Classic Papers and Current Comments. J Clin Oncol 2002;7:565.
99. Kirkwood JM, Strawderman MH, Ernstoff MS, et al. Interferon alfa-2b adjuvant therapy of high-risk resected cutaneous melanoma. The Eastern Cooperative Oncology Group trial EST 1684. J Clin Oncol 1996;14:7.
100. Kirkwood JM, Ernstoff MS, Davis CA, et al. Comparison of intramuscular and intravenous recombinant alfa-2 interferon in melanoma and other cancers. Ann Intern Med 1985;103:32.
101. Creagan ET, Ahmann DL, Frytak S, et al. Recombinant leukocyte A interferon (rIFN-aA) in the treatment of disseminated malignant melanoma. Cancer 1986; 58:2576.
102. Kirkwood JM, Ibrahim JG, Sondak VK, et al. High- and low-dose interferon alfa-2b in high-risk melanoma: first analysis of intergroup trial E1690/S9111/C9190. J Clin Oncol 2000;18:2444–58.
103. Livingston PO, Wong GYC, Adluri S, et al. Improved survival in stage III melanoma patients with GM2 antibodies. A randomized trial of adjuvant vaccination with GM2 ganglioside. J Clin Oncol 1994;12:1036.
104. Kirkwood JM, Manola J, Ibrahim J, et al. A pooled analysis of Eastern Cooperative Oncology Group and intergroup trials of adjuvant high-dose interferon for melanoma. Clin Cancer Res 2004;10:1670–7.
105. Kilbridge KL, Cole BF, Kirkwood JM, et al. Quality-of-life adjusted survival analysis of high-dose adjuvant interferon alfa-2b for high-risk melanoma patients using intergroup clinical trial data. J Clin Oncol 2002;20:1311.
106. Kirkwood JM, Richards T, Zarour HM, et al. Immunomodulatory effects of high-dose and low-dose interferon alpha2b in patients with high-risk resected melanoma: the E2690 laboratory corollary of intergroup adjuvant therapy trial E1690. Cancer 2002;95:1101.
107. Pehamberger H, Soyer P, Steiner A, et al. Adjuvant interferon alfa-2a treatment in resected primary stage II cutaneous melanoma. J Clin Oncol 1998;16:1425.
108. Grob JJ, Dreno B, de la Salmoniere, et al. Randomised trial of interferon alpha-2a as adjuvant therapy in resected primary melanoma thicker than 1.5 mm without clinically detectable node metastases. Lancet 1998;351:1905.
109. Cameron D, Cornbleet M, Mackie RM, et al. Adjuvant interferon alpha 2b in high-risk melanoma: the Scottish Study. Br J Cancer 2001;84:1146.
110. Cascinelli N, Belli F, Mackie RM, et al. Effect of long-term adjuvant therapy with interferon alpha-2a in patients with regional node metastases from cutaneous melanoma. A randomised trial. Lancet 2001;358:866.
111. Cascinelli N, Bufalino R, Morabito A, MacKie R. Results of adjuvant interferon study in WHO melanoma programme. Lancet 1994;343:913.
112. Wheatley K, Ives N, Hancock B, et al. Does adjuvant interferon-alpha for high-risk melanoma provide a worthwhile benefit? A meta-analysis of the randomised trials. Cancer Treat Rev 2003;29:241–52.
113. Veronesi U, Adamus J, Aubert C, et al. A randomized trial of adjuvant chemotherapy and immunotherapy in cutaneous melanoma. N Engl J Med 1982;307:913.
114. Middleton MR, Grob JJ, Aaronson N, et al. Randomized phase III study of temozolomide versus dacarbazine in the treatment of patients with advanced metastatic malignant melanoma. J Clin Oncol 2000;18:158–66.
115. Johanson CR, Harwood AR, Cummings BJ. 0-7-21 Radiotherapy in nodular melanoma. Cancer 1983;51:226.
116. Creagan ET, Cupps RE, Ivins JC, et al. Adjuvant radiation therapy for regional nodal metastases from malignant melanoma. A randomized, prospective study. Cancer 1978;42:2206.
117. Ang KK, Peters LJ, Weber RS, et al. Postoperative radiotherapy for cutaneous melanoma of the head and neck region. Int J Radiat Oncol Biol Phys 1994;30:795.
118. Shen P, Wanek LA, Morton DL. Is adjuvant radiotherapy necessary after positive lymph node dissection in head and neck melanomas? Ann Surg Oncol 2000;7:554.
119. Wong JH, Cagle LA, Kopald KH, et al. Natural history and selective management of in transit melanoma. J Surg Oncol 1990;44:146.
120. Calabro A, Singletary SE, Balch CM. Patterns of relapse in 1001 consecutive patients with melanoma nodal metastases. Arch Surg 1989;124:1051.
121. Hsueh EC, Nathanson L, Foshag LJ, et al. Active specific immunotherapy with polyvalent melanoma cell vaccine in patients with in-transit melanoma metastases. Cancer 1999;85:2160.
122. Morton DL, Hunt KK, Bauer RL, Lee JD. Immunotherapy by active immunization of the host using nonspecific agents. In: DeVita VT Jr, Hellman S, Rosenberg SA, editors. Biologic therapy of cancer. Philadelphia: Lippincott; 1991. p. 627.
123. Irie RF, Matsuki T, Morton DL. Human monoclonal antibody to ganglioside GM2 for melanoma treatment. Lancet 1989;1:786.
124. Irie RF, Morton DL. Regression of cutaneous metastatic melanoma by intralesion injection with human monoclonal antibody to ganglioside GD2. Proc Natl Acad Sci U S A 1986;83:8694.
125. Storm FK, Morton DL. Value of therapeutic hyperthermic limb perfusion in advanced recurrent melanoma of the lower extremity. Am J Surg 1985;150:32.
126. Hsueh EC, Essner R, Foshag LJ, et al. Active immunotherapy by reinduction with a polyvalent allogeneic cell vaccine correlates with improved survival in recurrent metastatic melanoma. Ann Surg Oncol 2002;9:486.
127. Gulec SA, Faries MB, Lee CC, et al. The role of fluorine-18 deoxyglucose positron emission tomography in the management of patients with metastatic melanoma: impact on surgical decision making. Clin Nucl Med 2003;28:961–5.
128. Hsueh EC, Essner R, Foshag LJ, et al. Prolonged survival after complete resection of disseminated melanoma and active immunotherapy with a therapeutic cancer vaccine. J Clin Oncol 2002;20:4549.
129. Essner R, Lee JH, Wanek, LA, et al. Contemporary surgical treatment of advanced-stage melanoma. Arch Surg 2004; 139: 961–6.
130. Ollila DW, Hsueh EC, Stern SL, Morton DL. Metastectomy for recurrent stage IV melanoma. J Surg Oncol 1999;71:209–13.
131. Patchell RA, Tibbs PA, Walsh JW, et al. A randomized trial of surgery in the treatment of single metastases to the brain. N Engl J Med 1990;322:494.
132. Karakousis CP, Velez A, Driscoll BA, Takita H. Metastasectomy in malignant melanoma. Surgery 1994;115:295.
133. Tafra L, Dale PS, Wanek LA, et al. Resection and adjuvant immunotherapy for melanoma metastatic to the lung and thorax. J Thorac Cardiovasc Surg 1995;110:119.
134. Ollila DW, Stern SL, Morton DL. Tumor doubling time. A selection factor for pulmonary resection of metastatic melanoma. J Surg Oncol 1998;69:206.
135. Ollila DW, Essner R, Wanek LA, Morton DL. Surgical resection for melanoma metastatic to the gastrointestinal tract. Arch Surg 1996;131:975.
136. Faries MB, Morton DL. Melanoma: is immunotherapy of benefit? Adv Surg. 2003;37:139–69.
137. Morton DL, Ollila DW, Hsueh EC, et al. Cytoreductive surgery and adjuvant immunotherapy. A new management paradigm for metastatic melanoma. CA Cancer J Clin 1999;49:101.
138. Creagan ET, Ahmann DL, Green SJ, et al. Phase II study of recombinant leukocyte A interferon (rIFN-alfa A) in disseminated malignant melanoma. Cancer 1984;54:2844.
139. Dorval T, Palangie T, Jouve M, et al. Clinical phase II trial of recombinant DNA interferon (interferon alfa 2b) in patients with metastatic malignant melanoma. Cancer 1986;58:215.
140. Legha SS, Papadopoulos NE, Plager C, et al. Clinical evaluation of recombinant interferon alfa-2a (Roferon-A) in metastatic melanoma using two different schedules. J Clin Oncol 1987;5:1240.
141. Sertoli MR, Bernengo MG, Ardizzoni A, et al. Phase II trial of recombinant alfa-2b interferon in the treatment of metastatic skin melanoma. Oncology 1989;46:96.
142. Coates A, Rallings M, Hersey P, Swanson C. Phase II study of recombinant alfa 2-interferon in advanced malignant melanoma. J Interferon Res 1986;6:1.
143. Ron IG, Inbar MJ, Gutman M, et al. Recombinant interferon alfa-2a in combination with dacarbazine in the treatment of metastatic malignant melanoma. Analysis of long-term responding patients. Cancer Immunol Immunother 1993;37:61.

144. Meyskens FL Jr, Kopecky K, Samson M, et al. Recombinant human interferon gamma. Adverse effects in high-risk stage I and II cutaneous malignant melanoma [letter]. J Natl Cancer Inst 1990;82:1071.
145. Trautman T, Kirkwood JM, Ernstoff MS, et al. Phase I-II trial of recombinant interferon gamma (IFN gamma) by 2 or 24 hour infusion in 30 melanoma patients. Proc Am Soc Clin Oncol 1985;4:232.
146. Kirkwood JM, Ernstoff MS, Trautman T, et al. In vivo biological response to recombinant interferon-gamma during a phase I dose-response trial in patients with metastatic melanoma. J Clin Oncol 1990;8:1070.
147. Kirkwood JM, Lee S, Land S, et al. E1696: Final analysis of the clinical and immunological results of a multicenter ECOG phase II trial of multi-epitope peptide vaccination for stage IV melanoma with MART-1 (27-35), gp100 (209-217, 210M), and tyrosinase (368-376, 370D) (MGT)+/IFNα2b and GM-CSF. J Clin Oncol 2004;22:7502.
148. Dvorak E. Experimental design for vaccine preparations against human malignant tumors. Med Hypotheses 1990;20:428.
149. Grimm EA, Mazumder A, Zhang HZ, Rosenberg SA. Lymphokine-activated killer cell phenomenon. Lysis of natural killer-resistant fresh solid tumor cells by interleukin 2-activated autologous human peripheral blood lymphocytes. J Exp Med 1982;155:1823.
150. Mule JJ, Shu S, Schwarz SL, Rosenberg SA. Adoptive immunotherapy of established pulmonary metastases with LAK cells and recombinant interleukin-2. Science 1984;225:1487.
151. Rosenberg SA, Lotze MT, Muul LM, et al. Observations on the systemic administration of autologous lymphokine-activated killer cells and recombinant interleukin-2 in patients with metastatic melanoma. N Engl J Med 1985;313:1485.
152. Papa MZ, Mule JJ, Rosenberg SA. The antitumor efficacy of lymphokine-activated killer cells and recombinant interleukin-2 in vivo. Successful immunotherapy of established pulmonary metastases from weakly- and non-immunogenic murine tumors of three distinct histologic types. Cancer Res 1986;46:4973.
153. Lotze MT, Chang AE, Seipp CA, et al. High dose recombinant interleukin-2 in the treatment of patients with disseminated cancer. Responses, treatment of patients with disseminated findings. JAMA 1986;256:3117.
154. Rosenberg SA, Lotze MT, Yang JC, et al. Experience with the use of high-dose interleukin-2 in the treatment of 652 cancer patients. Ann Surg 1990;210:474.
155. Dutcher JP, Creekmore S, Weiss GR, et al. A phase II study of interleukin-2 and lymphokine-activated killer cells in patients with metastatic malignant melanoma. J Clin Oncol 1989;7:477.
156. Fisher RI, Coltman CA Jr, Doroshow JH, et al. Metastatic renal cancer treated with interleukin-2 and lymphokine-activated killer cells. A phase II clinical trial. Ann Intern Med 1988;108:518.
157. West WH. Continuous infusion recombinant interleukin-2 (rIL-2) in adoptive cellular therapy of renal carcinoma and other malignancies. Cancer Treat Rev 1989;16:83.
158. Dutcher JP, Gaynor ER, Boldt DH, et al. A phase II study of high-dose continuous infusion interleukin-2 with lymphokine-activated killer cells in patients with metastatic melanoma. J Clin Oncol 1991;9:641.
159. Maghazachi AA, Goldfarb RH, Herberman RB. Influence of T cells on the expression of lymphokine-activated killer cell activity and in vivo tissue distribution. J Immunol 1988;141:4039.
160. Rosenberg SA, Packard BS, Aebersold PM, et al. Use of tumor-infiltrating lymphocytes and interleukin-2 in the immunotherapy of patients with metastatic melanoma. A preliminary report. N Engl J Med 1988;319:1676.
161. Nestle FO. Dendritic cell vaccination for cancer therapy. Oncogene 2000;19:6673–9.
162. Mittelman A, Huberman M, Puccio C, et al. A phase I study of recombinant human interleukin-2 and alfa-interferon-2a in patients with renal cell cancer, colorectal cancer, and malignant melanoma. Cancer 1990;66:664.
163. Rosenberg SA, Lotze MT, Yang JC, et al. Combination therapy with interleukin-2 and alfa-interferon for the treatment of patients with advanced cancer. J Clin Oncol 1989;7:1863.
164. Redman BG, Flaherty L, Chou TH, et al. A phase I trial of recombinant interleukin-2 combined with recombinant interferon-gamma in patients with cancer. J Clin Oncol 1990;8:1269.
165. Mitchell MS, Kempf RA, Harel W, et al. Low-dose cyclophosphamide and low-dose interleukin-2 for malignant melanoma. Bull N Y Acad Med 1989;65:1:128.
166. Eggermont AM, Kirkwood JM. Re-evaluating the role of dacarbazine in metastatic melanoma: what have we learned in 30 years? Eur J Cancer 2004; 40:1825–36.
167. Avril MF, Aamdal S, Grob JJ, et al. Fotemustine compared with dacarbazine in patients with disseminated malignant melanoma: a phase III study. J Clin Oncol 2004;22:1118–25.
168. Hill GJ II, Krementz ET, Hill HZ. Dimethyl triazeno imidazole carboxamide and combination therapy for melanoma: IV. Late results after complete response to chemotherapy (Central Oncology Group protocols 7130, 7131, and 7131A). Cancer 1984;53:1299.
169. Ahmann DL, Creagan ET, Hahn RG, et al. Complete responses and long-term survivals after systemic chemotherapy for patients with advanced malignant melanoma. Cancer 1989;63:224.
170. Chapman PB, Einhorn LH, Meyers ML, et al. Phase III multicenter randomized trial of the Dartmouth regimen versus dacarbazine in patients with metastatic melanoma. J Clin Oncol 1999;17:2745–51.
171. Atkins MB, Lee S, Flaherty LE, et al. A prospective randomized phase III trial of concurrent biochemotherapy (BCT) with cisplatin, vinblastine, dacarbazine (CVD), IL-2 and interferon alpha-2b (IFN) versus CVD alone in patients with metastatic melanoma (E3695): An ECOG-coordinated intergroup trial [abstract]. Proc Am Soc Clin Oncol 2003;22:708.
172. Del Prete SA, Maurer LH, O'Donnell J, et al. Combination chemotherapy with cisplatin, carmustine, dacarbazine and tamoxifen in malignant melanoma. Cancer Treat Rep 1984;68:1403.
173. Agarwala SS, Ferri W, Gooding W, Kirkwood JM. A phase III randomized trial of dacarbazine and carboplatin with and without tamoxifen in the treatment of patients with metastatic melanoma. Cancer 1999;85:1979.
174. Falkson CI, Ibrahim J, Kirkwood JM, et al. Phase III trial of dacarbazine versus dacarbazine with interferon alpha-2b versus dacarbazine with tamoxifen versus dacarbazine with interferon alpha-2b and tamoxifen in patients with metastatic malignant melanoma. An Eastern Cooperative Oncology Group study. J Clin Oncol 1998;16:1743.
175. Creagan ET, Suman VJ, Dalton RJ, et al. Phase III clinical trial of the combination of cisplatin, dacarbazine, and carmustine with or without tamoxifen in patients with advanced malignant melanoma. J Clin Oncol 1999;17:1884.
176. O'Day SJ, Gammon G, Boasberg PD, et al. Advantages of concurrent biochemotherapy modified by decrescendo interleukin-2, granulocyte colony-stimulating factor, and tamoxifen for patients with metastatic melanoma. J Clin Oncol 1999;17:2752.
177. Rosenberg SA, Yang JC, Schwartzentraber DJ, et al. Prospective randomized trial of the treatment of patients with metastatic melanoma using chemotherapy with cisplatin, dacarbazine, and tamoxifen alone or in combination with interleukin-2 and interferon alfa-2b. J Clin Oncol 1999;17:968.
178. Allen EP. Malignant melanoma. Spontaneous regression after pregnancy. BMJ 1955;2:1067.
179. Conybeare RC. Malignant melanoma and pregnancy. Report of 3 cases. Obstet Gynecol 1964;24:451.
180. Chaudhuri PK, Walker MJ, Briele HA, et al. Incidence of estrogen receptor in benign nevi and human malignant melanoma. JAMA 1980;244:791.
181. Creagan ET, Ingle JN, Woods JE, et al. Estrogen receptors in patients with malignant melanoma. Cancer 1980;46:1785.
182. Cocconi G, Bella M, Calabresi F, et al. Treatment of metastatic malignant melanoma with dacarbazine plus tamoxifen. N Engl J Med 1992;327:516.
183. Overgaard J. The role of radiotherapy in recurrent and metastatic melanoma. A clinical radiobiological study. Int J Radiat Oncol Biol Phys 1986;12:867.
184. Fenig E, Eidelevich E, Njuguna E, et al. Role of radiation therapy in the management of cutaneous malignant melanoma. Am J Clin Oncol 1999;22:184.
185. Sause WT, Cooper JS, Rush S, et al. Fraction size in external beam radiation therapy in the treatment of melanoma. Int J Radiat Oncol Biol Phys 1991;20:429.
186. Patchell RA, Tibbs PA, Regine WF, et al. Postoperative radiotherapy in the treatment of a single metastasis to the brain. JAMA 1998;280:1485.
187. Lavine SD, Petrovich Z, Cohen–Gadol AA, et al. Gamma knife radiosurgery for metastatic melanoma. An analysis of survival, outcome, and complications. Neurosurgery 1999;44:59.
188. Dudley ME, Wunderlich JR, Yang JC, et al. Adoptive cell transfer therapy following non-myeloablative but lymphodepleting chemotherapy for the treatment of patients with refractory metastatic melanoma. J Clin Oncol 2005;23:2346.

Other Skin Cancers

Victor A. Neel, MD, PhD
Arthur J. Sober, MD

The skin is a heterogeneous organ, consisting of elements of ectodermal, endodermal, and mesodermal origin. Such a diverse group of tissues gives rise to a wide variety of benign and malignant tumors. Many of these tumors are rare and will not be discussed in this chapter. Table 109-1 lists the more common premalignant and malignant tumors, which we discuss in detail. These are tumors relevant to the oncologist because they have the capacity to metastasize and cause serious medical harm. We also touch on several tumor syndromes that may present with unusual benign skin tumors that, if recognized, should prompt the clinician to conduct a detailed search for an internal malignancy. Melanoma, Kaposi sarcoma, the malignant histiocytoses, and the cutaneous lymphomas are discussed elsewhere in this book.

The incidence of keratinocytic skin cancer (KSC), which includes squamous cell carcinoma and basal cell carcinoma, is increasing (Table 109-2). In 1983, approximately 480,000 persons were diagnosed with KSC in the United States.[1] In 2004, over 1 million cases were reported.[2] The ratio of basal cell carcinoma to squamous cell carcinoma among whites in the United States, Australia, and the United Kingdom is about 4:1.[1,3,4] Together, these two tumors account for approximately 90% of all skin cancers.[5] In recent years, the role of the sun in the causation of these common skin tumors has received much attention[6] (see Table 109-2). This aspect of the epidemiology of skin cancers is also discussed in some detail.

ULTRAVIOLET RADIATION IN THE PATHOGENSIS OF SKIN CANCERS

In the past several decades, research on the relationship between the sun and skin cancer has escalated principally because of fear of the consequences of increased ultraviolet B (UVB) radiation on the earth's surface as a result of ozone depletion in the stratosphere. There is now general consensus over the role of sunlight in the etiology of KSC.[7,8] There is also general agreement that the principal action spectrum in sunlight is UVB (280 to 320 nm).[9–12] Chuang and colleagues[13] reported a 45-fold increase in KSC skin cancer in the Japanese population in Kauai, Hawaii, as compared with the Japanese population in Japan. Another study showed the incidence of squamous cell carcinoma, but not basal cell carcinoma, in Maryland watermen (a group of white men who make a living fishing in the Chesapeake Bay), correlated directly with the amount of sun exposure.[14] A population-based study on nearly 12,000 patients also demonstrated the close correlation between chronic cumulative sun exposure and squamous cell carcinoma.[15] Geographically, the incidence of skin cancer in whites increases toward the equator, further supporting the role of sunlight in carcinogenesis.

UVB imprints a unique signature on the deoxyribonucleic acid (DNA) it damages. Cellular attempts to repair this damage can lead to CC->TT mutations or C->T transitions. In the precursors of squamous cell carcinoma (SCC) (known as actinic keratoses), Zeigler and colleagues[16] showed that inactivating mutations of the tumor-suppressor p53 harbor these UV-induced errors. Because p53 is involved in the transcriptional regulation of DNA repair genes, cell-cycle control genes, and the induction of cell death, damage to this important regulator by UV irradiation is one mechanism that allows for the overgrowth of damaged cells.

UVB and UVA (320 to 440 nm) also have direct and indirect effects on the cutaneous immune system, lowering cell-mediated immunity and inducing T-suppressor cell production.[17] Loss of local immunity is thought to be another factor influencing carcinogenesis.

TUMORS ARISING FROM THE EPIDERMIS

Actinic Keratosis **Definition** Actinic keratosis, also known as solar keratosis, is a very common lesion occurring in susceptible persons as a result of prolonged and repeated solar exposures. The action of ultraviolet radiant energy, principally UVB, results in damage to the keratinocytes and produces single or multiple, discrete, dry, rough, adherent scaly lesions. These premalignant lesions may, in time, progress to squamous cell carcinomas.

Epidemiology Actinic keratosis affects predominantly the sun-exposed areas of fair-skinned people. The incidence in elderly whites may approach 100% in some populations.[1,18] The appearance of actinic keratosis may be at a much younger age (under 30 years) if the susceptible individuals have an outdoor occupation, such as farmers, ranchers, and sailors, or have an outdoor

Table 109-1 Common Premalignant and Malignant Neoplasms of the Skin

	Premalignant	Malignant
Epidermis	Keratoacanthoma Actinic keratosis Arsenical keratosis HPV-induced premalignant papules (epidermodysplasia verruciformis, bowenoid papulosis) Mucosal leukoplakia	Basal cell carcinoma Merkel cell carcinoma Squamous cell carcinoma
Dermal		Dermatofibrosarcoma protuberans Malignant fibrous histiocytoma Angiosarcoma
Appendageal	Nevus sebaceous	Sebaceous carcinoma Extramammary Paget disease
Benign cutaneous tumors associated with cancer syndromes Trichilemmomas → Cowden disease (breast/visceral tumors) Sebaceous tumors → Muir–Torre syndrome (GI/GU tumors) Mucosal neuromas → MEN type IIB (thyroid carcinoma/pheochromocytoma)		

GI = gastrointestinal; GU = genitourinary; HPV = human papillomavirus; MEN = multiple endocrine neoplasia.

Table 109-2 Sun-Induced Skin Cancer Statistics (United States 1989)

	Basal and Squamous Cancer	Malignant Melanoma
Magnitude of the problem (yearly)	500,000 new patients	29,000 new patients
Severity of the problem (yearly)	1,600 deaths Disfigurement Disability	6,000 deaths Mortality increasing 3.0% per year

lifestyle in sports or recreation. The lesions are more common in transplant recipients[19,20] and albinos.[21] It is rare in darker-skinned individuals, and almost never affects blacks, East Indians, or other Asians.

Clinical Features The onset of actinic keratosis is insidious as a rule and therefore often passes unnoticed for some time. The characteristic lesion is rough and gritty to palpation, similar to the feel of coarse sandpaper. On close examination, they appear as round-to-oval lesions, often less than 1.0 cm in diameter. They may be flat to nodular, as in the hypertrophic variety of actinic keratosis (Figure 109-1). The lesions are usually skin-colored or yellow-brown, often with a reddish tinge. There may be single or multiple scattered discrete lesions, typically limited to sun-exposed areas. A pigmented variant of actinic keratosis, named spreading pigmented actinic keratosis, is a brown, slowly growing, slightly scaly lesion that tends to appear on the face and may be larger than 1.5 cm in diameter, making it difficult to distinguish from lentigo maligna.[22]

Diagnosis The diagnosis of flat actinic keratosis is usually based on clinical examination alone. In contrast, the hypertrophic variant may sometimes be confused with an early squamous cell carcinoma. Suchniak and colleagues[23] demonstrated histologically the presence of in situ or invasive squamous cell carcinomas in 50% of lesions diagnosed clinically as hypertrophic actinic keratoses.

Treatment The flat actinic keratosis lesions are most easily treated with cryotherapy.[24] Application of liquid nitrogen with either a cotton tipped swab or a spray gun will suffice in the majority of cases. Retreatment may be necessary for the more stubborn lesions. It is not necessary to freeze to the point of blistering. Curettage and electrodesiccation of the lesions are equally effective, but carry a slightly greater risk of scarring and dyspigmentation. The hypertrophic lesions are best evaluated by biopsy to rule out invasive SCC.

Where large areas of skin are involved, applications of 5-fluorouracil preparations twice a day

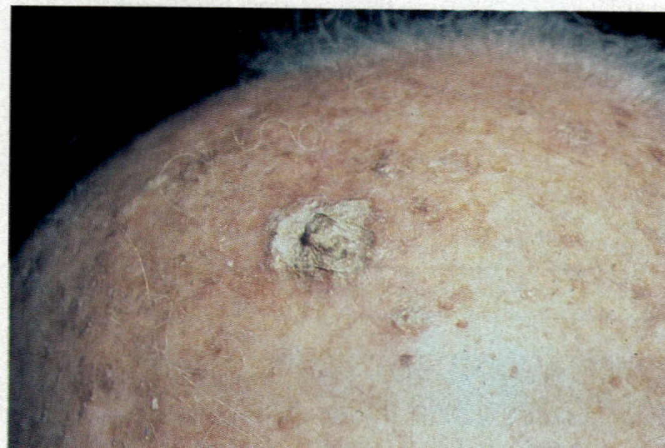

Figure 109-1 Actinic keratosis. Multiple discrete lesions on the scalp. These lesions are "gritty" to palpation. The largest lesion in the center of the picture represents the hypertrophic variant. This must be differentiated from a squamous cell carcinoma in situ.

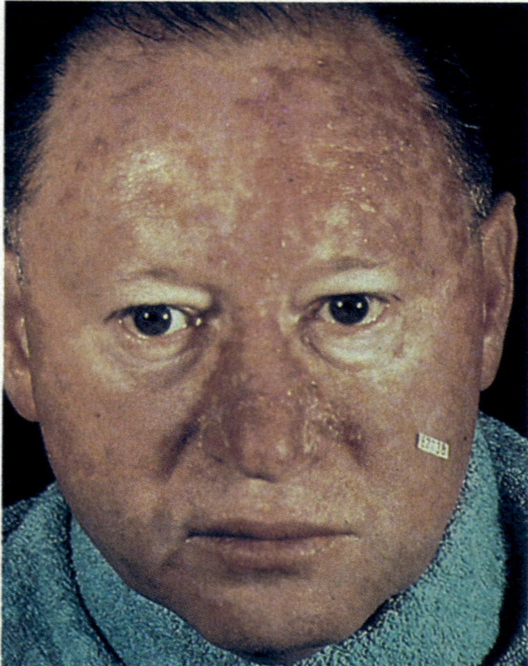

Figure 109-2 Actinic keratosis. Extensive actinic keratosis on the face. Note that the right half has been used as control and the left half of the forehead and the nose were treated with 5% 5-fluorouracil cream for 14 days.

to the affected areas may be used for up to four weeks.[25] This will result in a brisk reaction in the treated areas, ranging from redness, soreness, and weeping, to shallow ulceration and crusting (Figure 109-2). The reaction will gradually subside after discontinuation of the cytotoxic cream. Newer formulations with 0.5% 5-fluorouracil may be equally efficacious and may cause less irritation to the skin.[26] Recently, the nonsteroidal anti-inflammatory diclofenac has been shown to be effective in treating actinic keratoses, the mechanism of action apparently being the inhibition of cyclooxygenase.[27]

Course and Prognosis The lesions of actinic keratosis may rarely disappear spontaneously, but, in general, they persist if not treated. There is an estimated 5 to 20% lifetime risk of transformation into squamous cell carcinoma.[28] Marks and colleagues[29,30] reported that 60% of squamous cell carcinomas arise from preexisting solar keratoses diagnosed within the previous year.

Human Papillomavirus Induced Premalignant Papules Human papillomavirus (HPV) is a double-stranded DNA virus that belongs to the family Papovaviridae. Different HPV types are readily identified by DNA hybridization or PCR reactions. Lesions of the anogenital epithelium, such as bowenoid papulosis and condyloma acuminata, were recently found to be closely linked etiologically to infection with certain types of HPV (HPV 6, 11, 16, 18, and, less commonly, 31, 33, 35, and 45).[31–33] The link of HPV to oncogenicity in nonanogenital epithelium is also well documented in the genetically transmitted disease epidermodysplasia verruciformis (HPV 5, 8 to 10, 12, 14, 15, 17, 19 to 29) and periungual squamous cell carcinomas (HPV 16).[34,35] HPV 5, 8, and 17 genomes have been detected only in carcinomas associated with epidermodysplasia verruciformis. The association of particular HPV types with specific lesions is probably not absolute. Various immunologic abnormalities, such as decreased T-cell mitogenic responses, reduced delayed-type hypersensitivity reaction, and increased natural killer cell activity probably all play a role in carcinogenesis.[36]

Keratoacanthoma **Definition** Keratoacanthoma is a common, rapidly growing but benign tumor that will involute spontaneously, even if untreated. It is believed to originate from the hair follicles.[37–39]

Epidemiology Few studies have been done on the incidence of keratoacanthoma.[40–42] Chuang and colleagues[43] recently reported an incidence rate of 103.6 per 100,000, based on the small population in Kauai, Hawaii. It is most common between the ages of 60 and 65 years[39] and is rare in persons younger than the age of 20 years. In contrast to squamous cell carcinoma and basal cell carcinoma, there is no increase in frequency in old age. It is uncommon in blacks[44] or Japanese, and is approximately two to three times more common in males. The majority of patients have a solitary lesion.

Sun exposure,[41] and exposure to chemical carcinogens such as tar,[39] are thought to be etiologic factors. The possibility of a viral etiology is still being debated.[45–50] The presence of HPV has been demonstrated by DNA hybridization and polymerase chain reaction (PCR) studies.[51,52] The possibility of a genetic defect has also been proposed because these tumors are more common in patients with the Muir–Torre syndrome than in the general population.

Clinical Features Keratoacanthomas characteristically arise on hairy skin. The most common areas are the central parts of the face: the cheeks, nose, ears, lips, eyelids, and forehead. The dorsa of the hands, wrists, and forearms are also common sites.[46] The trunk and scalp are uncommon sites. Typically, the lesion presents as a solitary, rapidly growing, firm, dome-shaped, flesh-colored to slightly pink lesion with a plug of keratin in the central crater (Figure 109-3). The

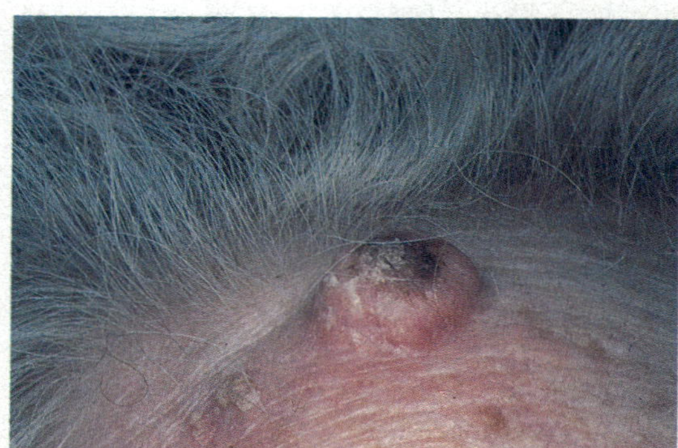

Figure 109-3 Keratoacanthoma. A pink, dome-shaped lesion with a central core of keratin. This rapidly growing lesion is located on the mid-forehead. Courtesy of P.L. McCarthy, MD.

evolving lesion typically grows rapidly for 2 to 4 weeks to a size of up to 2 cm in diameter. The mature lesion involutes spontaneously after a few months, leaving a scar. The complete cycle of growth to spontaneous resolution takes approximately 4 to 6 months.[53] Multiple or recurrent lesions may occur, particularly in cases associated with tar exposure. Multiple lesions associated with defects in cell-mediated immunity and with multiple internal malignant neoplasms and sebaceous adenomas, as part of Muir–Torre syndrome,[54] have been noted. There is no evidence that the solitary type is associated with internal malignancy.[46]

Diagnosis The main differential diagnosis is to distinguish keratoacanthoma from squamous cell carcinoma. The rapid evolution and spontaneous involution, the characteristic dome shape with a central plug of keratin, and the relatively young age of the patient are all clues to the diagnosis. In most cases, a wedge biopsy is essential in order to exclude an invasive squamous cell carcinoma.

Treatment Keratoacanthomas resolve spontaneously as a rule, leaving behind a scar. Surgical excision of the lesion will produce better end results cosmetically as well as provide tissue for histopathologic diagnosis. Radiotherapy[41,55–57] has been used successfully in lesions that cannot be distinguished from squamous cell carcinomas, as well as the so-called giant aggressive keratoacanthomas.[58,59] The dosage used, 4,000 to 6,000 cGy, is the same as the tumoricidal dosage used for squamous cell carcinomas. Topical or intralesional 5-fluorouracil[60,61] and intralesional injections of methotrexate[62] may be effective alternative treatment modalities. Methotrexate, given systemically, is found to be useful in treating multiple, as well as the larger keratoacanthomas.[63,64] Both the solitary[65] and multiple keratoacanthomas[66] have been successfully treated with oral isotretinoin. Intralesional interferon α-2a has also been tried with some success.[67] The lack of histologic confirmation with nonsurgical modalities is a major drawback. A biopsy of the lesion to rule out a squamous cell carcinoma prior to treatment may be prudent.

Course and Prognosis Keratoacanthoma is a benign tumor that carries a very good prognosis. Reports of malignant transformation as well as metastasizing lesions are probably misdiagnosed squamous cell carcinomas.

SQUAMOUS CELL CARCINOMA **Definition** Squamous cell carcinoma is a malignant tumor arising from epidermal or appendageal keratinocytes or from squamous mucosal epithelium. There is often a history of damage by exogenous agents acting as carcinogens, such as sunlight, ionizing radiation, local irritants, or arsenic ingestion. The tumor cells have a tendency toward keratin formation. Bowen disease is an in situ squamous cell carcinoma. Verrucous carcinoma is a variant of low grade squamous cell carcinoma with a clinicopathologically distinct warty appearance. The Buschke–Loewenstein tumor is the subset of verrucous carcinoma found on the genitals.

Epidemiology The incidence of squamous cell carcinoma of the skin varies greatly for different parts of the world and for different races and different people with different life habits and occupations. In 1963, the age-adjusted incidence of squamous cell carcinoma per 100,000 white residents in 8 American cities was 12.1 for males and 6.7 for females.[68] This is in contrast to the rate of 62 per 100,000 among whites in Honolulu County, Hawaii, reported by Quisenbery.[69] In 1983, Scotto and colleagues[1] reported an incidence of 41.4 cases per 100,000, and the incidence of cutaneous squamous cell carcinoma appears to be on the increase. The incidence of all skin cancer in various groups of blacks, including African Americans is only 1 to 2 per 100,000, excluding melanoma,[70] whereas the fraction of newly diagnosed skin cancers in India is only 1.4% of all carcinomas.[71] The incidence of squamous cell carcinoma in Japanese Kauaiians is four times lower than in white Kauaiians.[13] These studies illustrate the marked difference in incidence between light-skinned people and the darker races. Dorn studied the incidence of skin cancer in 10 different areas in the United States and found a much higher frequency in the southern parts of the country than in the north.[72] Eastcott likewise found a much higher incidence of skin cancer in Australia and New Zealand than in England.[73] The latitude gradient is steeper for squamous cell carcinoma than for basal cell carcinoma, suggesting a closer correlation between squamous cell carcinomas and chronic cumulative sun exposure than basal cell carcinoma.[74] Lookingbill and colleagues[21] reported a higher incidence of nonmelanoma skin cancer, particularly that of squamous cell carcinoma, in an albino population in Tanzania, where the prevalence of skin cancer is low among the normally dark-skinned population.

As previously mentioned, mutations in the p53 tumor-suppressor gene have been found in a number of squamous cell carcinomas.[75] Phototherapy patients who had received UVB or psoralen plus ultraviolet A (PUVA) for the treatment of skin diseases, such as psoriasis or mycosis fungoides, are also at increased risk.[76–79] In a study of 368 patients who developed carcinoma of the skin after radiation therapy, one-third of the tumors were squamous cell carcinomas.[80] The incidence of squamous cell carcinoma is known to be much higher in immunosuppressed patients, and these patients should be followed very carefully. Many dermatology departments now have dedicated clinics for immunosuppressed and transplant patients.[81] Depending on the dose of immunosuppressive drugs and previous sun exposure, transplant patients have up to a 65-fold increased risk of developing squamous cell carcinoma.[82] The squamous cell carcinoma to basal cell carcinoma ratio also reverses from 0.25 to 1 in the general population to 1.5–3 to 1 in transplant patients. [83] Tumors in such patients tend to behave more aggressive clinically.[78,84]

Verrucous carcinoma of the skin (epithelioma cuniculatum) is a rare tumor, with more than 100 reported cases.[85] Approximately 80 to 90% of patients are male, with a mean age of 52 to 60 years.[86] The Buschke–Loewenstein tumor is best considered a verrucous carcinoma of the anogenital mucosa. Penile Buschke–Loewenstein tumor is the most common, with an incidence between 5 and 24% of all penile cancers. Vaginal, cervical, perianal, and perirectal Buschke–Loewenstein tumors are less common than penile ones. The etiology of these tumors is linked to HPV, particularly to HPV 6 and 11.[85]

The incidence of Bowen disease has not been extensively investigated. Chute and colleagues[87] reported an incidence of 14 per 100,000 population for Bowen disease in a Rochester, Minnesota, population. In a 5-year prospective study based on the residents of Kauai, Hawaii, Reizner and colleagues[88] reported an incidence of 142 per 100,000 population.

The incidence of squamous cell carcinoma of the oral mucosa also varies significantly for different parts of the world.[89,90] It is high in India, southeast Asia, and Puerto Rico, and is low in Japan, Israel, Norway, and England. The use of betel nut and other spices may be partly responsible for the higher incidence in India and southeast Asia.[91] In the United States, there are approximately 30,000 new cases per year.[92] It is about nine times more common in males. Oral cancer is rare in persons younger than age 35 years. The incidence increases with age until the age of 60 to 64 years, and then declines.[93]

Recently, some squamous cell carcinomas, particularly those in the anogenital and periungual areas, have been linked etiologically to infection with certain types of HPV (HPV 16, 18, and, less commonly, 31, 33, 35, and 45).[34,35,94–96.] These were discussed in more detail under "Human Papillomavirus Induced Premalignant Papules" above.

Clinical Features Squamous cell carcinoma often arises in damaged skin or skin that has been subjected to chronic irritation. Thus, the skin adjacent to the carcinoma may show evidence of solar damage, such as actinic keratosis, wrinkling and dryness, telangiectasia, and irregular pigmentation. Alternatively, there may be features of radiodermatitis from previous radiation therapy,[80,97,98] a sinus tract associated with an underlying osteomyelitis,[99] or scarring from a burn (Marjolin ulcer).[96,100,101] Chronic venous ulcers of the lower extremities are also associated with increased risks of developing squamous cell carcinomas.[102] A chronic ulcer that shows features of proliferation beyond the expected granulation process should raise the suspicion of malignant transformation.

Squamous cell carcinoma usually evolves faster than basal cell carcinoma, but not as rapidly as keratoacanthoma. The earliest lesion, the so-called intraepidermal squamous cell carcinoma or carcinoma in situ, typically appears as a scaly, erythematous plaque on sun-exposed areas. The lesion often has a sharply demarcated but irregular outline (Figure 109-4). Bowen disease is clinically identical to squamous cell carcinoma in

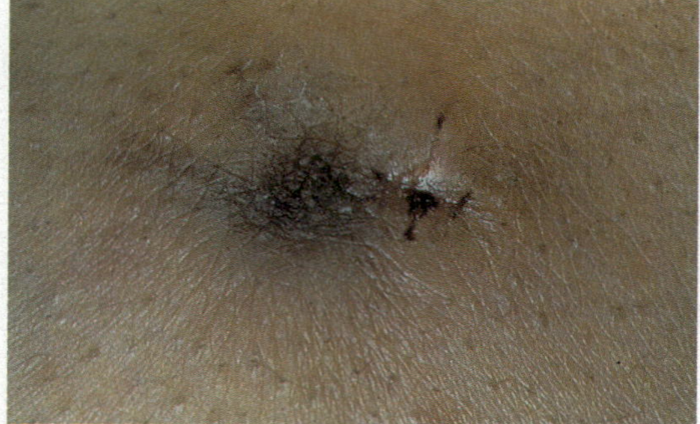

Figure 109-4 Dermatofibrosarcoma protuberans on the back of the neck. Firm papule resembling a dermatofibroma. Courtesy of R.A. Johnson, MD.

situ. Bowen disease on the glans penis is also known as erythroplasia of Queyrat.

Invasive squamous cell carcinoma (Figure 109-5) almost always arises from a preexisting premalignant lesion or from an in situ carcinoma, although de novo squamous cell carcinoma has been reported.[103] The lesion is typically an erythematous, indurated papule, plaque, or nodule. The shape of the lesion may be polygonal, oval, round, or verrucous (Figures 109-6 and 109-7). The tumor tends to increase both in elevation and diameter with time. A hallmark of squamous cell carcinoma is its firmness on palpation. The late lesion is often eroded, crusted, and ulcerated with an indurated margin. The ulcer is often covered with a purulent exudate and bleeds easily (Figure 109-8). Early ulceration is often a marker for anaplastic lesions. Regional lymphadenopathy may be present either as a response to infection of the ulcer or from metastases. In the latter case, they tend to be rubbery and more irregular, and may be fixed to adjacent tissues.

Verrucous carcinoma of the skin is most commonly found on the soles of men.[85] Typically, it presents as a slowly enlarging cauliflower-like mass. It is locally aggressive and may grow to a significant size. The ball of the foot is involved in more than 50% of cases. Other locations include the face, buttocks, oral cavity, trunk, and extremities. The bulk of the tumor is soft and

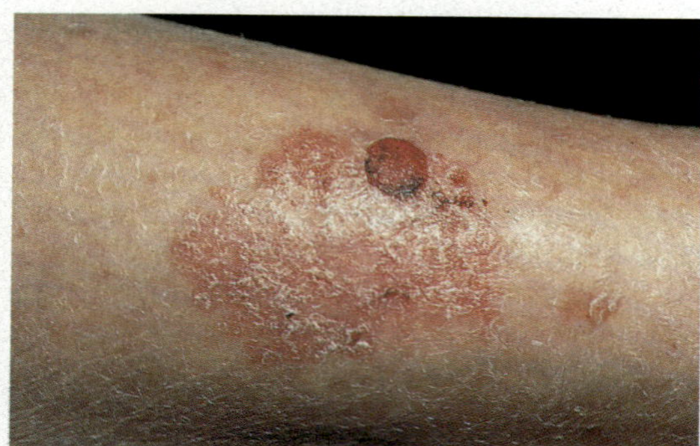

Figure 109-5 Squamous cell carcinoma (SCC) arising in SCC in situ. A nodule of invasive SCC on the lower leg arising within the well-demarcated, erythematous scaly plaque of SCC in situ.

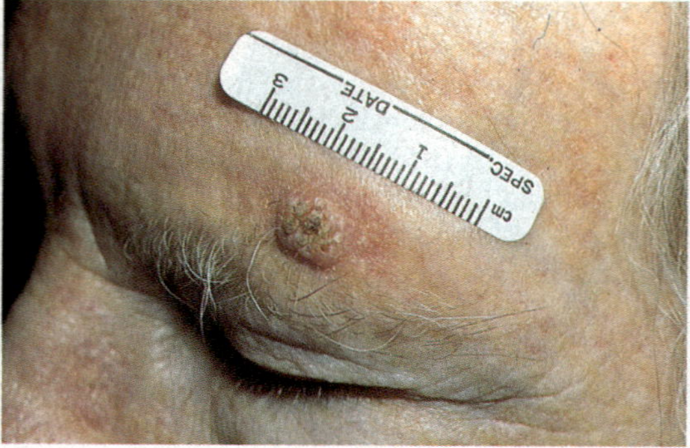

Figure 109-6 Invasive squamous cell carcinoma. Erythematous, hyperkeratotic nodule on the forehead resembling a keratoacanthoma (see Figure 109-3). An incisional or excisional biopsy is necessary to distinguish the two lesions.

"squashy," and may be foul smelling. If left untreated, the tumor will eventually penetrate the underlying soft tissue and bone. However, metastasis is rare.

The Buschke–Loewenstein tumor most commonly affects the penile glans and prepuce of uncircumcised males, presenting as a cauliflower-like, fungating, foul-smelling tumor on the coronal sulcus. In women, it may present on the vagina, cervix, or vulva. The Buschke–Loewenstein tumor has a tendency to infiltrate deeply, causing destruction of underlying tissues.

Squamous cell carcinoma of the oral mucosa may present as an exophytic papillary mass, a discrete ulcer with a raised indurated border, or a firm, slightly raised plaque. The last is characteristic of a deeply infiltrative lesion. There may be hemorrhage, particularly when there is ulceration. An area of leukoplakia may be observed in association with the carcinoma.

Squamous cell carcinoma of the lip may arise from an area of leukoplakia, leukokeratosis, or actinic cheilitis. Approximately 90% of SCCs occur on the lower lip. This tumor is typically much more aggressive than those on glabrous skin and has a high rate of metastasis.

Carcinoma arising in late radiation dermatitis or x-ray keratoses tends to be very anaplastic and

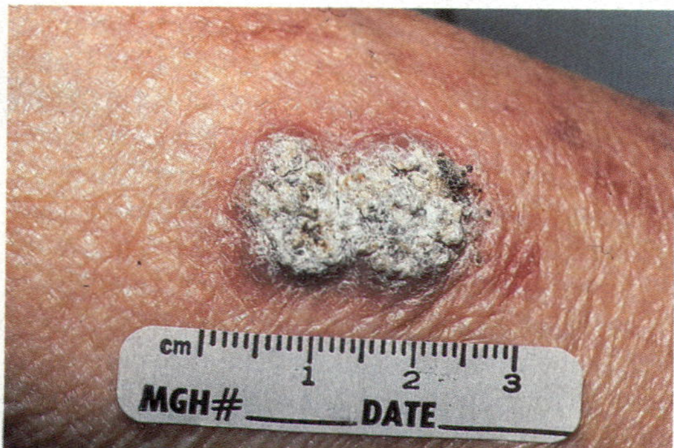

Figure 109-7 Invasive squamous cell carcinoma. A hyperkeratotic, crusty plaque on the forearm. Note the evidence of sun damage in the surrounding skin: wrinkling, bruising, and a lackluster appearance.

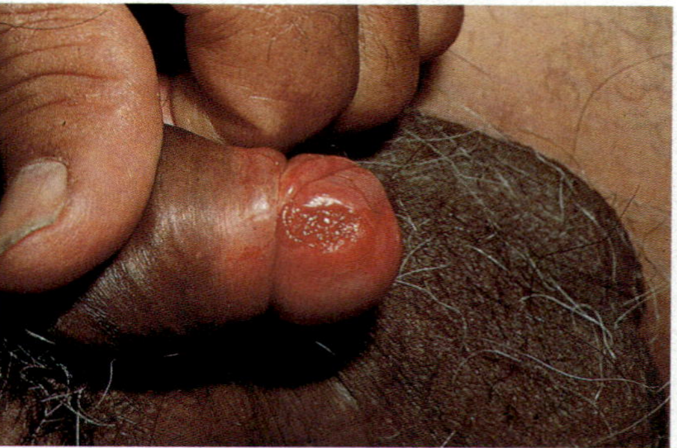

Figure 109-8 Invasive squamous cell carcinoma. An ulcerated lesion on the glans penis with an indurated margin. The ulcer typically bleeds easily.

extremely aggressive. The rate of metastasis is high in such tumors.[104]

Treatment The choice of treatment modality depends on the degree of differentiation of the tumor and the presence or absence of metastasis. The size, shape, location of the tumor, and the predisposing factors should also be considered. In the case of a localized, well-differentiated tumor with no evidence of metastasis, the goal should be complete eradication of the lesion. In the case of a poorly differentiated, recurrent tumor or the presence of lymph node metastases, palliative treatment may be considered, if complete eradication is deemed impossible. The variety of modalities available for consideration include excisional surgery, Mohs surgery, cryosurgery, electrosurgery, and radiation therapy.[5,10,56,105–107] The final result often depends as much on the experience of the surgeon as on the choice of treatment selected. Thus, cooperation among dermatologists, surgeons, and radiotherapists is important.

Excisional Surgery Surgical excision with primary closure or repair with skin graft or flap is the treatment of choice for relatively small lesions with distinct borders. There should be an adequate margin of clearance of 3 to 5 mm to minimize the risk of recurrence. Brodland and Zitelli[108] reported that margins of 4 mm were required to achieve a 95% tumor clearance rate. For invasive or large tumors (> 2 cm), or tumors on high-risk areas such as the scalp, ears, nose, eyelids, or lips, a minimum margin of 6 mm is recommended.

Tumors arising in late radiation dermatitis or x-ray keratosis should also be surgically excised rather than treated with more radiation. Likewise, tumors previously treated with radiation should be excised with the entire radiation scar, if possible, because tumor may exist in multiple foci within the irradiated field.

Large tumors situated near the lip, eyelid, and the anogenital area should be excised in order to preserve the function of the structures and avoid retraction caused by excessive scarring.

Surgery is also preferred for lesions invading bone or cartilage. Treating such lesions with radiation therapy may result in radiation necrosis of the bone or cartilage. Recurrent carcinomas, tumors with indistinct borders, and those arising in scars, ulcers, or sinuses may be treated with surgery to allow histologic examination of the excision margins. Tumors that have metastasized to regional lymph nodes are also best treated with excision surgery and lymph node dissection. Prophylactic lymph node dissection is not recommended because of the relatively low rate of metastasis. The utility of selective lymph node dissection for high-risk tumors is currently being evaluated.

Mohs Surgery Surgery with microscopic control of the excision margins (Mohs micrographic surgery[109]) has become the treatment of choice for extensively invasive and infiltrative tumors or those that are recurrent. This technique allows maximum conservation of "good tissue" while the surgeon can still be reassured of clear margins. This modality of treatment is also associated with a lower local recurrence rate.[82]

Cryosurgery Treatment of squamous cell carcinoma by freezing with liquid nitrogen is best restricted to the most superficial tumors and carcinoma in situ. This modality has the advantage of simplicity with an excellent cure rate when employed in the proper situation.[106,110] Because collagen, cartilage, and bone are less sensitive to injury by freezing than the tumor cells, scarring and damage to underlying bony or cartilaginous structures can be minimized.

Electrosurgery The choice of lesions suitable for treatment by curettage and electrodesiccation is similar to those suitable for cryosurgery. In addition, large superficial tumors on the head and neck, trunk, and upper extremities have been treated with this modality with excellent results.

Radiation Therapy Radiation therapy is often employed for poorly differentiated tumors and for patients who may not be able to tolerate other more invasive treatment modalities. The site of the lesion has to be taken into consideration to minimize the late complications of ionizing radiation. Thus, lesions on the dorsum of the hand and those over bony and cartilaginous structures should not be treated with radiation. Tumors that have a tendency to invade along the planes of embryonic closure, such as those in the nasolabial fold and pre- and postauricular areas, are good candidates for this modality of treatment.[111] Excellent results can also be obtained for small lesions of the nose, lip, eyelid, and canthus. A fractionated dose is usually preferred to a single massive dose for the best cure rate and to minimize the local as well as systemic side effects of radiation.[56] The treatment schedule is determined by the size, depth, and location of the tumor and the particular time-dose-fractionation schedule used. The total dose is typically between 4,000 and 6,000 cGy.

Rapid anaplastic transformation with widespread metastases has been reported in verrucous carcinoma following radiation therapy.[85,86]

Chemotherapy The use of oral isotretinoin in patients with large, recurrent or metastatic squamous cell carcinomas resulted in partial to complete regression of the tumors.[112] Isotretinoin also decreased the incidence of a second primary squamous cell carcinoma, when given as a chemopreventive agent. However, the benefit from such long-term use has to be weighed against the toxicity. In organ transplant recipients, where the risk of developing skin cancer is increased, the use of retinoids may be justified.[113,114] Recently, a new low-dose retinoid regimen has shown promise in suppressing tumor formation in transplant recipients while decreasing the systemic side effects of retinoid.

Course and Prognosis The risk factors correlated with local recurrence and metastatic rates include treatment modality, prior treatment, location, size, depth, histologic differentiation, histologic evidence of perineural involvement, precipitating factors other than ultraviolet light, and host immunosuppression. Squamous cell carcinoma in skin carries an overall metastatic rate of 3 to 6%.[115,116] Those arising from sun-damaged skin typically have a low risk for metastasis,[82,116] whereas those arising from chronic osteomyelitic sinus tracts, irradiated areas, and burn scars have a much higher metastatic rate (31%, 20%, and 18%, respectively). Carcinoma on the lower lip, although mostly sun induced, has a metastatic incidence of about 15%. Tumor arising in areas such as the glans penis (see Figure 109-9), the vulva, and the oral mucosa also have a high rate of metastasis.

Histologically, the best prognostic indicators are level of dermal invasion and vertical tumor thickness.[117] In the study by Immerman and colleagues,[118] all the tumors that recurred were at least 4 mm or more in thickness and involved the deep dermis, whereas all the fatal cases involved tumors more than 1 cm thick, with invasion into the subcutaneous fat or beyond.

With proper treatment, the overall 5-year remission rate is 90%, including squamous cell carcinoma of the lip. Frankel and colleagues[119] recommended followups at least every 3 months for a year after treatment of squamous cell carcinoma, and semiannually thereafter for up to 4 years.

Verrucous carcinoma and the Buschke–Loewenstein tumor rarely metastasizes to regional lymph nodes if left untreated for many years.[114]

BASAL CELL CARCINOMA **Definition** Basal cell carcinoma is a malignant tumor that rarely metastasizes.[120] It is composed of cells that arise from the epidermis and the appendages which resemble the basal layer of the epidermis and is associated with a characteristic stroma.[121] It tends to grow slowly and invade locally over many years, which eventually leads to ulceration, hence the name "rodent ulcer."

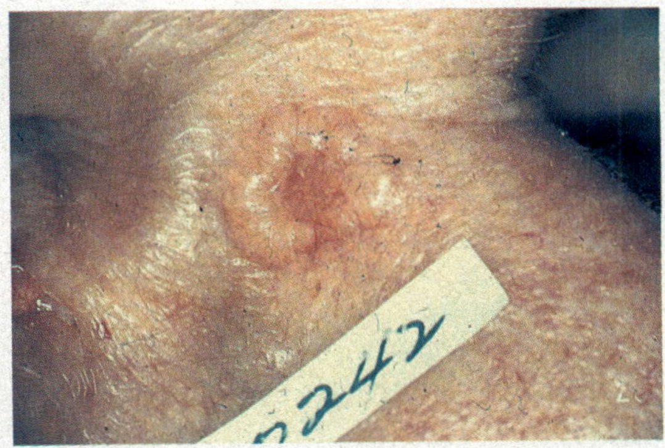

Figure 109-9 Basal cell carcinoma. A pearly nodule with an umbilicated, ulcerated center and telangiectasia.

Epidemiology Basal cell carcinomas account for more than 75% of keratinocytic skin cancers diagnosed in the United States each year.[109,122,123] The incidence of basal cell carcinoma varies from 422 per 100,000 general population in Kauai, Hawaii,[124] to 146 per 100,000 in Rochester, Minnesota.[125] The average annual incidence in the United States is 191 per 100,000 white persons.[126] It is the most common form of skin cancer in whites.[1,12] It is very rare in darkly pigmented people.[127,128] It most frequently occurs in persons older than 40 years of age. The frequency is slightly higher in males. Other risk factors include geographic locations with high solar intensity, exposures to inorganic trivalent arsenic,[129,132] ionizing radiation,[130] and immunosuppression. In a review of 368 patients who developed cancer of the skin after radiotherapy, two-thirds were basal cell carcinomas.[2,38,106] Phototherapy patients receiving UVB or PUVA for treatment of certain dermatoses, such as psoriasis or mycosis fungoides, are also at increased risk.[102] Several recent studies suggest a correlation between basal cell carcinomas and exposures to sunlight in early life and intense intermittent (recreational) sun exposures.[133,134] This is contrary to the previous belief that basal cell carcinomas result from cumulative lifetime sunlight exposures. Genetic studies show that loss-of-function mutations in the tumor-suppressor gene patched, or gain-of-function mutations in the smoothened gene, lead to the formation of sporadic basal cell tumors.[135,136] A genetically inherited form is described in basal cell nevus syndrome.[137,138]

Clinical Features The basal cell carcinoma is characteristically slow growing over months to years. It is usually asymptomatic unless ulceration occurs, and then there is bleeding. It most frequently occurs on sun-exposed areas such as the face and upper trunk, and is rare on the palms and soles.

The early lesions are round-to-oval papules or nodules, often with an umbilicated center that may be ulcerated. The color is pink to red and often has a translucent or pearly quality (Figure 109-9). Basal cell carcinomas (BCCs) are firm to palpation. If left untreated, the lesion enlarges slowly and is destructive to neighboring structures by direct invasion. Longstanding lesions are ulcerated as a rule (Figure 109-10). There are often telangiectasias in the surrounding skin, which also shows other evidence of solar damage, such as actinic keratosis, atrophy, wrinkling, dryness, and irregular pigmentation. Some basal cell carcinomas are pigmented and may exhibit a bluish hue.[141] These may be confused with malignant melanoma (Figure 109-11). The so-called superficial-type basal cell carcinoma usually presents on the trunk as an irregular, atrophic plaque

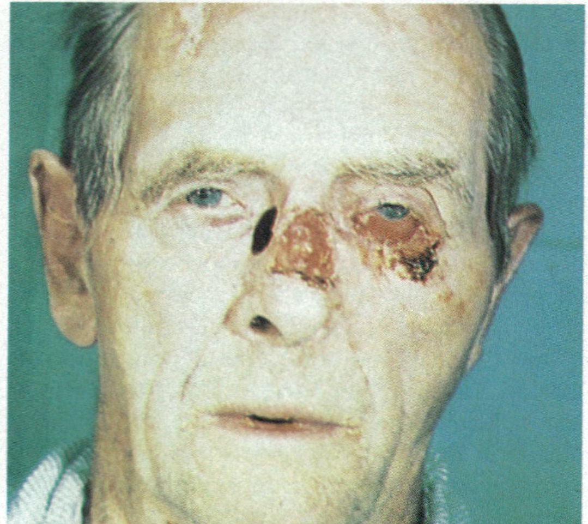

Figure 109-10 Basal cell carcinoma. Note the erosive nature of such a long-standing lesion.

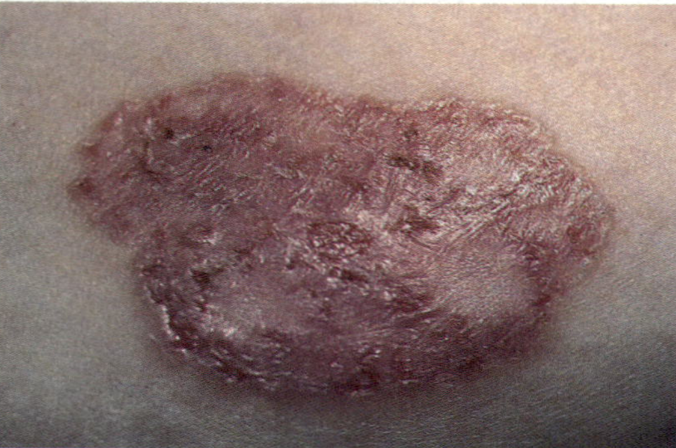

Figure 109-12 Superficial basal cell carcinoma. A large, 5-cm lesion on the abdomen. The pearly, string-like border is the clue to the clinical diagnosis.

with a slightly raised border (Figure 109-12). Flat basal cell carcinomas can be difficult to detect. They are often ivory-white, and may resemble morphea and are therefore called morphea-like basal cell carcinomas.[142,143] This type of lesion usually occurs on the face and has a more aggressive behavior.[144]

Treatment The choice of therapy depends on the type and size of the lesion, the location, the general condition of the patient, the cosmetic considerations, and, not least, the experience and skill of the operator.[145] Morphea-like basal cell carcinomas usually have indistinct borders clinically and may result in underestimation of the extent of the tumor and, consequently, in undertreatment. Lesions situated in the nasolabial crease, around the eye, and behind the ear also tend to undermine deeply and extend far beyond the clinical border (Figure 109-13). Lesions that ulcerate early tend to be more aggressive. A knowledge of the behavior of the different clinical and pathologic types of basal cell carcinoma is essential in determining the choice of therapy. Treatment of basal cell carcinomas should be aimed at a cure in the first instance. Undertreatment will result in recurrence and deep invasion, and there is a 50% recurrence rate for the cases that are treated inadequately.

Surgical Excision Surgical excision of the tumor either with primary closure, a skin graft or local flap produces good cosmetic results and allows the surgical margins to be examined by the pathologist to confirm adequate margins. Tumor present at the lateral excision margins will result in marginal recurrences, which tend to present early and may be reexcised with relative ease. Inadequate deep margins result in recurrences, which tend to present late, together with invasion of deep structures. Surgery is the therapy of choice for lesions with indistinct clinical borders and for the morphea-like lesions.

Mohs Surgery Surgery with microscopic control of the excision margins (Mohs micrographic surgery) is the treatment of choice for the morphea-like lesions and for all extensively invasive or recurrent tumors.[146] This technique allows maximum conservation of "good tissue," while the surgeon can still be reassured of clear margins (see Figure 109-13B).

Radiation Therapy Treatment with ionizing radiation may produce excellent therapeutic and cosmetic results, provided care is taken in patient selection.[147] Radiation therapy is preferred for elderly and fragile patients, particularly those with medium-sized lesions between 1 and 5 cm in diameter. Lesions larger than 5 cm have higher recurrence rates as compared with smaller tumors.[148] Atrophy, necrosis, and scarring may be kept to a minimum when the total dose, typically in the range of 4,000 to 6,000 cGy, is divided into several smaller fractions over several weeks. The choice of a treatment schedule is chosen according to the type, location, size, and depth of the tumor, the total dose of radiation, and the number of fractions that will be given. The appropriate dose schedule may be determined according to the time-dose-fractionation tables.[149,150]

Chemotherapy Topical applications of 5% 5-fluorouracil cream to the tumor twice a day for several weeks is best suited only for small, superficial tumors in the elderly who will not be able to tolerate other more aggressive forms of treatment. The rate of recurrence, however, is considerably higher. Intralesional 5-fluorouracil has also been tried in nodular lesions.[151,152] Imiquimod, a topical immune-response modifier which induces interferon, shows promise in the treatment of superficial basal cell carcinomas, but long-term studies looking at recurrence rates are lacking.[153] Cyclopamine and derivatives of cyclopamine, which specifically block the sonic-hedgehog pathway by inhibiting the smoothened protein, was effective as a topical agent in a very small pilot study and may be shown to have therapeutic value in the future.[154]

Course and Prognosis Basal cell carcinomas are slow growing as a rule. However, if left untreated, they may reach a large size, with consequent extensive tissue destruction. In a comprehensive review of recurrence rates for primary basal cell carcinomas, the results are highly comparable for the various treatment modalities.[146] Most studies reported a 95% or higher cure rate.[7,12,155,156] A lower 5-year recurrence rate has been reported with Mohs surgery than with other commonly used modalities.[146] Metastasis, although rare, may occur, particularly in large and late lesions.[157–159] In such cases, the prognosis is usually poor, with a 1-year survival rate of less than 20%, and a 5-year survival rate of approximately 10%. The 5-year occurrence rate of new basal cell carcinomas developing in patients with a previous basal cell carcinoma may be as high as 45%.[160] No significant benefit was observed in

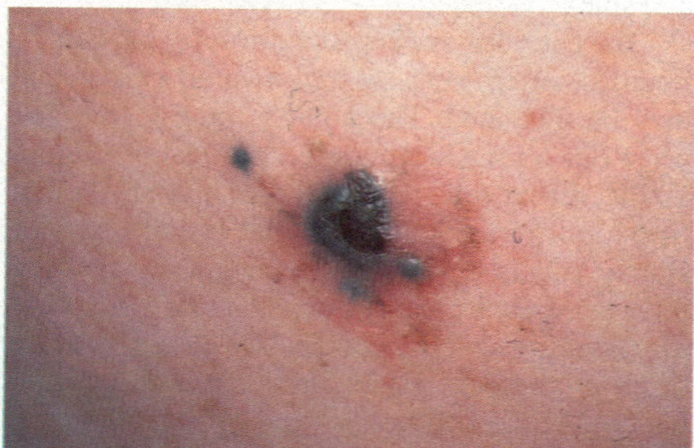

Figure 109-11 Pigmented basal cell carcinoma. A pink, irregular plaque with dark-blue to black pigmentation at the center that mimics a superficial spreading melanoma. The shiny quality is one clue to the diagnosis. Examination with the aid of a dermatoscope may also reveal valuable distinguishing features. A biopsy would yield the definitive diagnosis. Courtesy of P.L. McCarthy, MD.

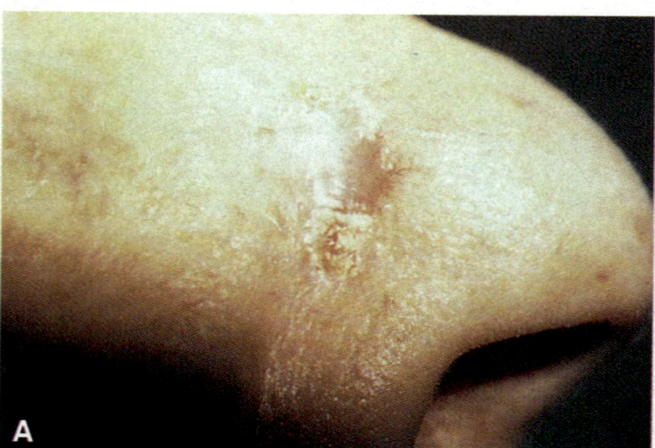

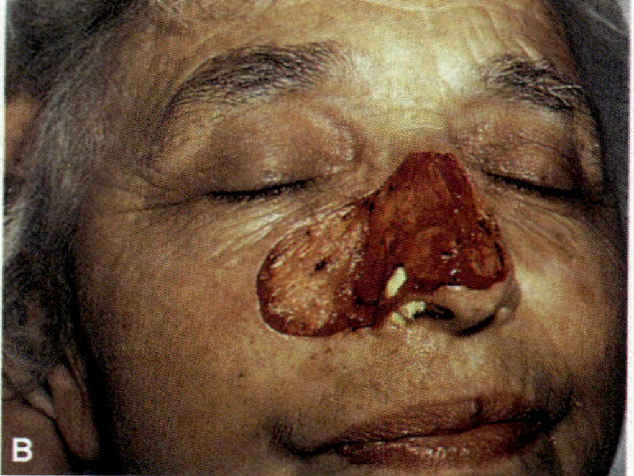

Figure 109-13 **A**, Basal cell carcinoma. The lesion is quite limited clinically. **B**, Same patient after treatment with Mohs surgery, illustrating the cryptic extension far beyond the clinically evident border.

the use of low-dose isotretinoin for the prevention of basal cell carcinomas.[161,162]

Basal Cell Nevus Syndrome (Gorlin Syndrome) **Definition** Basal cell nevus syndrome is an inherited multisystem disorder in which multiple basal cell carcinomas are associated with palmoplantar pits, characteristic facies, and a variety of skeletal, soft-tissue, ocular, neurologic, and endocrine abnormalities.[163,164] The inheritance is autosomal dominant, with variable penetrance.

Epidemiology This disorder is uncommon. The majority of patients are white, although cases have been reported in blacks and Asians. Both sexes are affected equally. The age of onset is early, and some patients may be born with hydrocephalus or blind. A few patients have been found to have chromosome abnormalities. Recently, patched gene mutations were found to be associated with Gorlin syndrome.[165,166]

Clinical Features Although the skin manifestations of basal cell nevus syndrome are characteristic and easily recognizable, the early features are usually extracutaneous. Congenital abnormalities may include absent or undescended testes, hydrocephalus, and blindness from coloboma, cataracts, or glaucoma. The patients have characteristic facies with frontal bossing, broad nasal root, and hypertelorism (ie, excessive interorbital distance) (Figure 109-14).

The most characteristic cutaneous finding is the early onset of multiple basal cell carcinomas on sun-exposed as well as unexposed areas.[167] The number of tumors may vary from a few to hundreds. The distribution is usually bilateral and symmetrical. Areas commonly involved include the face, neck, trunk, and axillae. The scalp is often spared, unless patients have received radiation for medulloblastoma in childhood. Their color varies from flesh-colored to pigmented. The size may vary from 1 mm to more than 1 cm in diameter. The tumors on the eyelids, axillae, and neck tend to be pedunculated and may be confused with skin tags or neurofibromas. The pigmented lesions may be mistaken for melanocytic nevi. Ulceration of the tumors is often a sign for invasion.

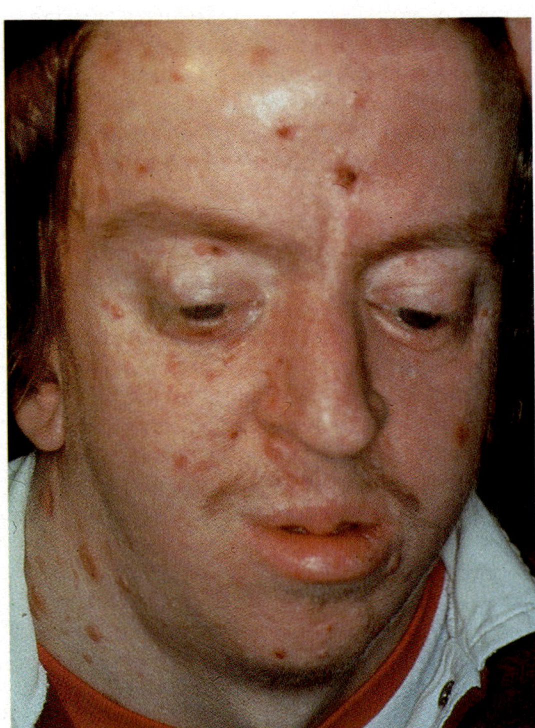

Figure 109-14 Basal cell nevus syndrome. Note the multiple basal cell carcinomas on the face and neck, frontal bossing, broad nasal root, and hypertelorism. Courtesy of R.A. Johnson, MD.

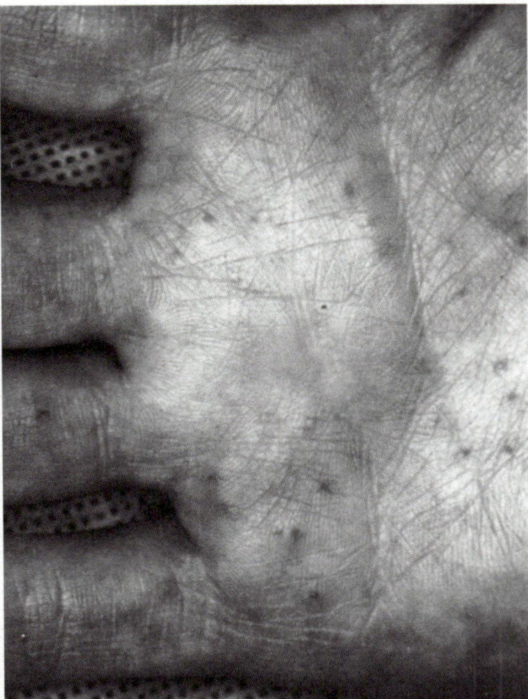

Figure 109-15 Multiple palmar pits in basal cell nevus syndrome.

Approximately 50% of the patients have pin point to several millimeter-sized pits on their palms and soles[168,169] (Figure 109-15). These pits are approximately 1 mm in depth and may number from a few to hundreds. They may concentrate on the lateral surfaces of the palms, soles, and fingers. They are formed as a result of the premature shedding of the horny layer within the epidermis.[168] Other cutaneous lesions include milia, multiple lipomas, fibromas, desmoids, and cysts.

The most common stigma of the syndrome is jaw cysts,[170] which are usually multiple and may be unilateral or bilateral and are odontogenic keratocysts (Figure 109-16). Other osseous abnormalities include defective dentition, bifid or splayed ribs, pectus excavatum, short fourth metacarpals (Albright sign), scoliosis, and kyphosis. Lamellar calcification of the falx is also a useful diagnostic sign.

Ocular abnormalities may include strabismus as well as hypertelorism, dystopia canthorum, and congenital blindness. Mental retardation is uncommon. Other neurologic abnormalities include congenital agenesis of the corpus callosum and medulloblastoma. Treatment of the medulloblastoma with radiotherapy results in marked increase in the number of basal cell carcinomas within the field of irradiation.[171]

Soft tissue abnormalities can include ovarian fibromas, lymphatic mesenteric cysts, ameloblastomas of the oral cavity, teratomas, cystadenomas, and fibrosarcoma of the jaw.

Treatment The therapeutic choices are similar to those for basal cell carcinomas. However, because of the multiple nature of the tumors, maximum preservation of tissue with Mohs surgery may be preferred. The use of oral retinoids as chemopreventive agents is being debated.[172]

Merkel Cell Carcinoma **Definition** The Merkel cell was first described by Merkel in 1875. It is a nondendritic, nonkeratinocytic epithelial clear cell normally found in the epidermis and dermis of mammals and humans. It is believed to be of neuroendocrine origin and functions as a specific slowly adapting sensory touch receptor.

The Merkel cell tumor was first described by Toker in 1972.[173] It is thought to arise from the cutaneous Merkel cell. It is a high-grade malignant tumor, with a high rate of local recurrence and metastasis.

Epidemiology Merkel cell carcinoma is a rare neoplasm. The tumor is most common in the 60- to 80-year-old age group. It is most common in whites. There is no gender predilection. It appears to be more common in the setting of immunodeficiency, particularly HIV infection.

Clinical Features The most common sites of involvement are head and neck (49%), extremities (38%), with the lower extremities more frequently involved than the upper extremities, and trunk (13%), mainly lower back and buttocks.[174] The lesions present as papules or nodules, pink to red to violet, often with overlying telangiectasia. Typically, the tumors are less than 2 cm in size.

Treatment Wide local excision with 2.5 to 3.0 cm margins is the standard treatment modality.[175,176] Alternatively, local excision with margin control by frozen-section histology (Mohs surgery) may be the treatment of choice, if the service is available.[177,178] Lymph node dissection should be done if the nodes are clinically involved, or if there is a single drainage area.[179] Two studies show that selective biopsy of the sentinel lymph nodes is predictive of nodal involvement.[180,181] Radiation may be beneficial for

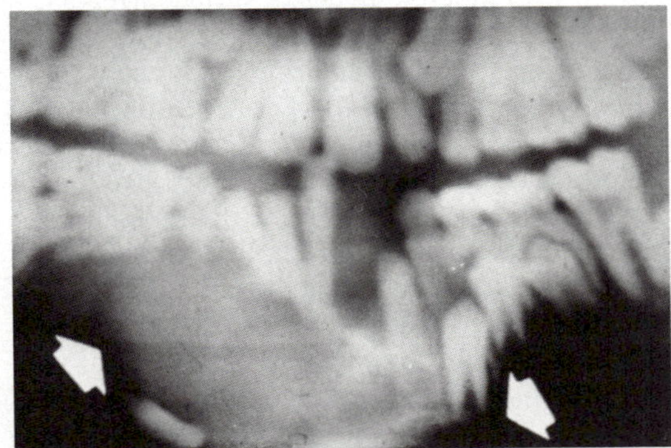

Figure 109-16 Radiograph of a jaw cyst in a patient with basal cell nevus syndrome.

either local recurrences or for local control after node dissection.[182] The dosage used is similar to those used for squamous cell carcinoma (5,000 to 6,000 cGy). Chemotherapy regimens have not been shown to extend life.

Course and Prognosis The rate of local recurrence is approximately 35 to 43%, with the average time to recurrence being 4.3 months. Lymph node metastasis is present in 41% and visceral metastasis in approximately 18% of patients at diagnosis. Sixty percent of patients without local recurrence develop nodal metastasis, whereas 86% of patients with local recurrence also develop nodal metastasis. One-third of patients with positive nodes develop visceral or central nervous system (CNS) metastasis and die of their disease. The overall survival rates are 88% at 1 year, 72% at 2 years, approximately 55% at 3 years, and between 30 and 64% at 5 years.[183] The average time from diagnosis to death is 2.4 years. The factors associated with a poor prognosis are early age at presentation, male sex, lesion location on the head and neck or trunk, and generalized disease.[184] A recent retrospective study of 132 cases showed that cell size, tumor size, and mitotic rate were the most significant clinical and histologic prognosticators.[185]

In view of the high recurrence rate, close follow-up is recommended. Ratner and colleagues[74] recommended monthly visits for the first 6 months, then every 2 to 3 months for the next 2 years, followed by semiannual to annual visits thereafter.

TUMORS ARISING FROM DERMIS

Dermatofibrosarcoma Protuberans Definition Dermatofibrosarcoma protuberans (DFSP) is a locally malignant, slow-growing tumor originating in the dermis. The tumor cells resemble fibroblasts with various degrees of atypia.

Epidemiology This is an uncommon tumor that typically presents during early to mid-adult life. It is reported rarely in children. Males are affected four times as often as females. It may be more common in blacks than in whites.[186] Associations with arsenic exposure, burn or surgical scar, acanthosis nigricans, and rapid growth during pregnancy have been reported.

Clinical Features DFSP is most commonly situated on the trunk and proximal extremities. It typically presents as a solitary, slow-growing nodule with multiple palpable surface irregularities.[187] The early lesion may resemble a dermatofibroma, keloid scar, or squamous cell carcinoma (see Figure 109-4). The lesion is firm to palpation and varies from flesh color to reddish to yellow. The center may be ulcerated. The tumor can achieve an enormous size with multiple satellite nodules, if untreated. The characteristic irregular surface on a firm, plaque-like base may suggest the diagnosis. A biopsy will provide confirmation. The average size at the time of surgery is approximately 5 cm.[188]

Recently, DFSPs were shown to harbor chromosomal translocations that fuse the collagen type I alpha gene with the gene for platelet-derived growth factor B.[189] The presence of this specific t(17;22) translocation permits the diagnosis of DFSP in equivocal cases.

Treatment The treatment of choice is has traditionally been wide surgical excision with subsequent microscopic evaluation of the excision margins. DFSP has a high recurrence rate after conventional surgical excision, with a range of 30 to 50%.[190] Lateral surgical margins of at least 3 cm excised through the deep fascia are the current recommendation for conventional excision. In one large series, this yielded a recurrence rate of approximately 10%.[191] Because of the potential for deforming surgical defects, Mohs surgery, which permits microscopic control of the excision margins, has been advocated. This allows the subclinical margins to be mapped at the time of surgery, and, consequently, the surgical margins more precisely determined. Prophylactic lymph node dissection is not recommended because of the low initial risk of metastasis. Recently, the receptor tyrosine kinase inhibitor imatinib has been used with success in treating multiply recurrent and metastatic cases of DFSP.[192]

Course and Prognosis In a review of 136 cases of DFSP treated with Mohs surgery, a local recurrence rate of 6.6% was determined, although smaller studies have shown fewer recurrences.[193] It is clear that the experience of the Mohs surgeon is critical in preventing tumor recurrence. Historically, late recurrences are frequent, thus long-term follow-up is recommended.

CUTANEOUS ANGIOSARCOMA

Definition Angiosarcoma (AS) is an aggressive malignancy of endothelial cells, arising in the setting of chronic lymphedema, chronic radiation dermatitis or on the face and scalp of the elderly.

Epidemiology Cutaneous AS of the face and scalp is a disease of the elderly, with men affected more often than women. Sun does not appear to be an important factor because the tumor often appears under cover of hair.[194] AS developing in areas of chronic lymphedema (the so-called Stewart–Treves syndrome) is an infrequent complication of mastectomy, axillary node dissection for melanoma, lymphedema secondary to filarial infection and chronic idiopathic lymphedema. Unfortunately, up to 0.5% of women undergoing mastectomy and lymph node dissection develop AS within 1 to 30 years.[195] Radiation-induced AS is a rare iatrogenic complication of radiation that develops in or near the irradiated site. The incubation period may be up to 40 years in some cases.

Clinical Features In all three presentations, the clinical features can be similar. Bruise-like macules, papules, and nodules develop and tend to enlarge quickly. Ulceration can occur in advanced lesions. On the face, facial edema can be the presenting sign. In all cases, the lesions extend beyond the clinical borders.

Treatment Treatment for AS is not promising. One problem facing clinicians is that by the time a diagnosis is made the tumors have spread several centimeters beyond the clinically appreciated borders. AS of the face and scalp is rarely less than 10 cm in diameter at presentation. Wide surgical resection followed by radiotherapy is the mainstay of treatment. In a study of 24 patients with AS of the face and scalp, local control was obtained in 57%. However, of those patients, 47% developed distant metastases.[196] In surgically unresectable tumors, radiation therapy and adjuvant chemotherapy with intralesional recombinant interleukin-2 and interferon-α-2b[197] or liposomal doxorubicin[198] may extend the life of some patients.

Course and Prognosis Survival at 5 years is approximately 12%.[195]

TUMORS ARISING FROM APPENDAGES

Sebaceous Carcinoma Definition Frequently arising on the eyelid, sebaceous carcinoma is a malignant adnexal neoplasm.

Epidemiology Sebaceous carcinoma is the second most frequent malignancy of the eyelid next to basal cell carcinoma.[199]

Clinical Features Misdiagnosis is frequent with sebaceous carcinoma. The tumor usually appears as a painless, flesh-colored papule, or nodule on the upper or lower eyelid where it is easily dismissed as a chalazion or chronic blepharitis. Ulceration is often the feature that stimulates clinical suspicion and biopsy. Focal loss of eyelashes and a yellowish hue are other diagnostic clues. Sebaceous tumors are frequently associated with the Muir–Torre syndrome, as described later in this chapter.

Treatment In a recent evidence-based review on the management of eyelid malignancies, Mohs micrographic surgery and excision with frozen-section control were shown to be superior to other modalities, including radiation therapy.[200]

Course and Prognosis In a study of 18 patients with sebaceous carcinoma treated with the Mohs technique, Spencer and colleagues found an 11% recurrence rate after an average follow-up of 37 months.[201] One patient had metastatic disease (5.6%). This compared favorably to other published rates of recurrence and metastasis, which had been as high as 30 and 22%, respectively.

Extramammary Paget Disease Definition Extramammary Paget disease (EPD) is a neoplasm of apocrine glands that clinically resembles Paget disease of the breast, but occurs in areas rich in apocrine glands, including the perineum and axilla.

Epidemiology More frequent in women and whites, EPD usually strikes after the fifth decade.

Clinical Features EPD is a scaly, sharply marginated plaque, most commonly found in the vulva. Because itching and burning are common symptoms, it is often mistaken for intertrigo or flexural eczema, and the diagnosis is delayed. Progressive enlargement of the plaque in the face of topical steroid or antifungal medications is a diagnostic clue.

Treatment Evaluation to identify the presence of underlying malignancy is crucial. Surgical excision is the treatment of choice for primary EPD. Although conventional surgery can yield a recurrence rate of more than 40%,[202] microscopically controlled excision appears to yield at least as good results while sparing tissue loss.[203,204] High-dose (4,000 cGy) radiotherapy produced local regression in one small study.[205] Ablative carbon dioxide laser treatment is palliative, as recurrence rates are very high.[206,207]

Course and Prognosis When EPD is associated with an adenocarcinoma, the prognosis is poor.[208] However, even primary EPD can eventually ulcerate and become locally invasive and spread to lymph nodes, with depth of invasion > 1 mm being an important prognostic factor.[209] Even after wide excision, local recurrence still approaches 25%.[210]

BENIGN CUTANEOUS TUMORS ASSOCIATED WITH CANCER SYNDROMES

Trichilemmoma (in Cowden Disease) Definition Trichilemmoma is a tumor that exhibits features of outer root sheath differentiation of hair. In Cowden disease, multiple trichilemmomas are associated with multiple hamartomatous neoplasms of ectodermal, mesodermal, and endodermal origin.[211–215]

Epidemiology Cowden disease is a rare autosomal dominant condition with variable expressivity. Less than 100 cases are reported to date. Male patients slightly exceed females among all the cases reported. All reported patients are white, except for one Japanese and two black patients. The age span is between 4 and 75 years, with the median age being 39 years.

Clinical Features In Cowden disease, multiple trichilemmomas are associated with a wide variety of hamartomas and tumors of other organ systems; the most important include fibrocystic disease and carcinoma of the breast, adenoma and follicular adenocarcinoma of the thyroid, gastrointestinal polyps, and lipomas. The trichilemmomas present as small lichenoid, skin-colored to yellow-tan papules with a smooth surface. They are concentrated on the face, especially around the orifices and the ears. Similar papules may appear on the extremities, including palmoplantar surfaces, and the oral cavity, particularly on the gingiva and the tongue (Figures 109-17 and 109-18). The presentation of these papules usually precedes the appearance of breast cancer[211] and, therefore, can serve as a marker of associated cancer.

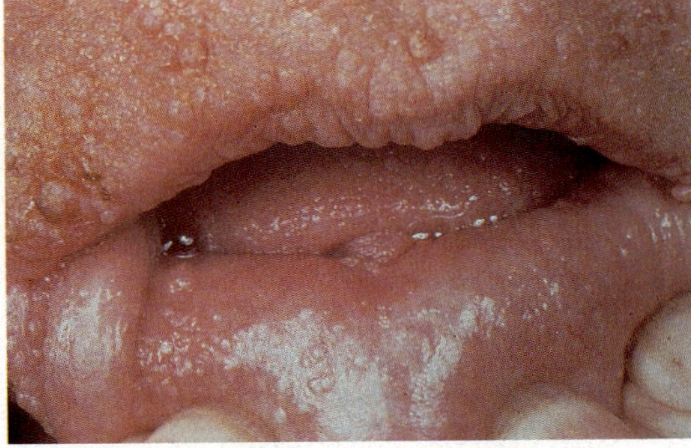

Figure 109-17 Cowden disease. Multiple trichilemmomas on the upper lip. Similar papules are present on the mucosal surface of the lower lip.

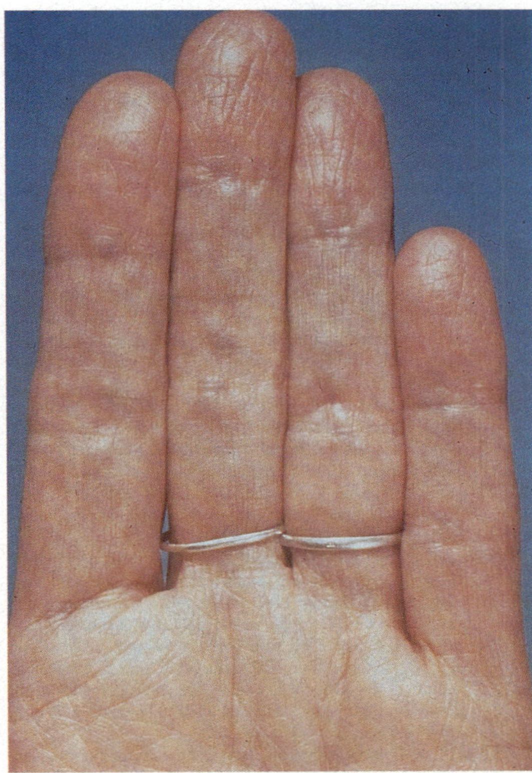

Figure 109-18 Cowden disease. Translucent keratotic papules on the palmar surface. Courtesy of R.A. Johnson, MD.

Genetics Germ line mutations in the protein tyrosine phosphatase PTEN have been linked to multiple families with Cowden disease.[215]

Treatment Therapies are directed toward achieving good cosmetic appearance and treatment of the various associated benign and malignant tumors, as indicated. In view of the high incidence of breast cancer in female patients, which may be as high as 50%, frequent breast examination and mammography are indicated.

Sebaceous Adenoma (in Muir–Torre Syndrome) Definition Sebaceous adenoma is a rare, benign tumor consisting of incompletely differentiated sebaceous lobules within the dermis. In Muir–Torre syndrome, multiple sebaceous adenomas and carcinomas are associated with multiple visceral malignant neoplasms. These sebaceous tumors are rare enough that the presence of a single lesion in an otherwise healthy patient warrants an investigation for internal neoplasms.

Epidemiology Solitary sebaceous adenoma is a rare tumor that occurs in elderly patients of both sexes. The multiple type, associated with Muir–Torre syndrome, is familial, with more than 50% of reported patients having an immediate family member with a history of internal cancer, most frequently of the colon.[216–218]

Clinical Features Sebaceous adenoma typically appears as a firm, flesh-colored to waxy-yellow papule or pedunculated lesion, usually less than 1 cm in size. The surface may be smooth or verrucous. Older lesions may be plaque-like or ulcerated. It is usually located on the face or scalp and is usually slow growing.

In Muir–Torre syndrome, multiple sebaceous tumors, including adenomas and carcinomas, and keratoacanthomas are associated with multiple visceral carcinomas, most commonly carcinoma of the colon and carcinoma of the ampulla of Vater.

Genetics Overlap between Muir–Torre syndrome and kindreds with hereditary nonpolyposis colon cancer allowed the identification of the DNA mismatch repair gene hMSH2 as one of the genes disturbed in Muir–Torre syndrome.[219]

Treatment The treatment of choice is surgical excision. The tumor is also radiosensitive.

Multiple Mucosal Neuromas (Multiple Endocrine Neoplasia 2B, MEN2B) Definition Mucosal neuromas present as small, discrete and coalescing, painless nodules, usually involving the lips, and sometimes studding the margins of the tongue. The association of multiple mucosal neuromas, medullary thyroid carcinoma and pheochromocytoma has been established as a familial syndrome.

Epidemiology Discrete mucosal neuromas are common and often result from direct trauma, as in the typical bite neuroma. More than 150 cases of multiple neuromas associated with endocrine tumors have been described in the literature.[220]

Clinical Features In MEN2B, diffusely enlarged lips are an early feature. Diffuse and symmetric fleshy papules and nodules occur on the tongue by the end of first decade. Any mucosal surface may be involved. Patients often develop a Marfanoid habitus. Most importantly, medullary thyroid carcinoma may develop in early adulthood. These tumors produce calcitonin and can stimulate parathyroid hyperplasia. Pheochromocytomas are frequently present as well.

Genetics In all cases studied to date, mutation in the protooncogene RET, a receptor tyrosine kinase, has been uncovered.[221,222]

Course and Prognosis Medullary thyroid carcinoma is often the cause of death. Routine screening for this tumor with ultrasonography and by measuring serum calcitonin levels is useful, but current recommendations suggest prophylactic thyroidectomy in cases where a RET mutation is documented.[223]

METASTATIC TUMORS TO THE SKIN

Cutaneous metastases of internal cancers are uncommon. In a report of 7,316 nonmelanoma cancer patients by Lookingbill and colleagues,[224] only 1% of patients had cutaneous metastases at the time of diagnosis. In Gates' study of 2,298 patients reported as having died of visceral carcinoma, only 2.7% had evidence of cutaneous metastases.[225] In a more recent retrospective study by Lookingbill and colleagues[226] of 4,020 patients with metastatic carcinomas and melanoma, 10% had cutaneous metastases. In general, the incidence of the various cancers metastatic to the skin correlates well with the incidence of the particular primary tumor.

Hence, the spectrum of metastatic tumors differs slightly between the two sexes.[226–228]

In Lookingbill and colleagues' study,[226] the most common primary sources of metastatic carcinoma to the skin in males were malignant melanoma (32%), lung (12%), large intestine (11%), carcinoma of the oral cavity (9%) and larynx (5.5%), and kidney (5%). In females, breast is by far the most common source (70%), followed by melanoma (12%), and ovary (3%), and large intestine, lung, and oral cavity, each accounting for 1.3 to 2.3% of the cases. In recent years, the incidence of carcinoma of the lung has increased dramatically in females, resulting in a corresponding rise in the incidence of cutaneous metastatic lung carcinoma deposits in females.[229] Other carcinomas that metastasize to the skin include thyroid,[230] pancreas,[231] liver,[232] gallbladder,[233] urinary bladder,[234] endometrium,[235] prostate,[236] and testis.[237] However, these are quite rare.

Typically, metastatic cancer presents as multiple, firm, nonulcerated nodules. When solitary, they may be misdiagnosed as primary skin tumors. Inflammatory skin metastases mimicking cellulitis may occur in 10% of metastases from breast cancer.[226] The most common sites for skin metastases are chest and abdomen, followed by head and neck; metastasis to the extremities is rare. Those metastases situated in the scalp can be associated with alopecia ("alopecia neoplastica"). Dissemination may be via the bloodstream or via the lymphatics. Carcinomas of the breast and of the oral cavity tend to spread through the lymphatics, whereas other carcinomas tend to be hematogenous in their spread. Lymphatic dissemination may explain the observation that skin metastases tend to be close to the site of the primary tumor: chest in lung carcinoma, abdominal wall in gastrointestinal tumors, and lower back in renal cell carcinoma.[228]

The prognosis for patients with cutaneous metastases is generally poor. In Lookingbill and colleagues, the average time from diagnosis of skin metastases to death for the various primary tumors varies from 1 to 34 months.[226] The variability in prognosis may be the result of advances in cancer therapy during the past decades. Some patients with metastatic melanoma to skin as the sole site of metastasis may have prolonged disease-free survival. [238]

REFERENCES

1. Scotto J, Fears TR, Fraumeni JF. Incidence of non-melanoma skin cancer in the United States. Publication No (NIH) 82–2433. Washington, DC: US Dept Health and Human Services; 1983.
2. Jemal A, Murray T, Ward E, et al. Cancer statistics 2005.Ca;Cancer J Clin 2005;55:10–30.
3. Marks R, Staples M, Giles GG. Trends in non-melanocytic skin cancer treated in Australia: the second national survey. Int J Cancer 1993;53:585.
4. Roberts DL. Incidence of non-melanoma skin cancer in West Glamorgan, South Wales. Br J Dermatol 1990;122:399.
5. Albright SD III. Treatment of skin cancer using multiple modalities. J Am Acad Dermatol 1982;7:143.
6. Staehelin J, Blumthaler M, Ambach W, Torhorst J. Skin cancer and the ozone shield. Lancet 1990;2:502.
7. Weinstock MA, Bogaars HA, Ashley M, et al. Non-melanoma skin cancer mortality: a population-based study. Arch Dermatol 1991;127:1194.
8. Weinstock MA. Death from skin cancer among the elderly: epidemiological patterns. Arch Dermatol 1997;133:1207.
9. Bissett DL, Hannon DP, Orr TV. Wavelength dependence of histological, physical, and visible changes in chronically UV-irradiated hairless mouse skin. Photochem Photobiol 1989;50:763.
10. Cole CA, Forbes D, Davoes RE. An action spectrum for UV photocarcinogenesis. Photochem Photobiol 1986;43:275.
11. Freeman R. Actual spectrum for ultraviolet carcinogenesis. NCI Monogr 1978;50:27.
12. Nomura T, Nakajima H, Hongyo T, et al. Induction of cancer, actinic keratosis, and specific p53 mutations by UVB light in human skin maintained in severe combined immunodeficient mice. Cancer Res 1997;57:2081.
13. Chuang T-Y, Reizner GT, Elpern DJ, et al. Non-melanoma skin cancer in Japanese ethnic Hawaiians in Kauai, Hawaii: an incidence report. J Am Acad Dermatol 1995;33:422.
14. Vitasa BC, Taylor HR, Strickland PT, et al. Association of nonmelanoma skin cancer and actinic keratosis with cumulative solar ultraviolet exposure in Maryland watermen. Cancer 1990;65:2811.
15. Franceschi S, Levi F, Randimbison L, La Vecchia C. Site distribution of different types of skin cancers: new aetiological clues. Int J Cancer 1996;67:24.
16. Ziegler A, Jonason AS, Leffell DJ, et al. Sunburn and p53 in the onset of skin cancer. Nature 1994;372:773.
17. Clydesdale GJ, Dandie GW, Muller HK. Ultraviolet light induced injury: immunological and inflammatory effects. Immunol Cell Biol 2001;79:547–68.
18. Gordon D, Silverstone H. The biologic effects of ultraviolet radiation. In: Ubach F, editor. The biologic effects of ultraviolet radiation. Oxford (UK): Pergamon Press; 1969. p. 625.
19. Abel EA. Cutaneous manifestations of immunosuppression in organ transplant recipients. J Am Acad Dermatol 1989;21:167.
20. Marshall V. Premalignant and malignant skin tumors in immunosuppressed patients. Transplantation 1974;17:272.
21. Lookingbill DP, Lookingbill GL, Leppard B. Actinic damage and skin cancer in albinos in northern Tanzania: findings in 164 patients enrolled in an outreach skin care program. J Am Acad Dermatol 1995;32:653.
22. Subrt P, Jorizzo JL, Apisarnthanarax P, et al. Spreading pigmented actinic keratosis. J Am Acad Dermatol 1983;8:63.
23. Suchniak JM, Baer S, Goldberg LH. High rate of malignant transformation in hypertrophic actinic keratoses. J Am Acad Dermatol 1997;37:392.
24. Clark DP, Feinstein RJ, Graham G. Guidelines of care for actinic keratoses. J Am Acad Dermatol 1995;32:95.
25. Goette DK. Topical chemotherapy with 5-fluorouracil. J Am Acad Dermatol 1981;4:633.
26. Gupta AK, Weiss JS, Jorizzo JL. 5-Fluoruracil 0.5% cream for multiple actinic or solar keratoses of the face and anterior scalp. Skin Therapy Lett 2001;6:1–4.
27. Jarvis B, Figgitt DP. Topical 3% diclofenac in 2.5% hyaluronic acid gel: a review of its use in patients with actinic keratoses. Am J Clin Dermatol. 2003;4:203-13
28. Johnson TM, Rowe DE, Nelson BR, Swanson NA. Squamous cell carcinoma of the skin (excluding lip and oral mucosa). J Am Acad Dermatol 1992;26:467.
29. Marks R, Rennie G, Selwood T. The relationship of basal cell carcinoma and squamous cell carcinoma to solar keratoses. Arch Dermatol 1988;124:1039.
30. Marks R, Rennie G, Selwood TS. Malignant transformation of solar keratosis to squamous cell carcinoma. Lancet 1988;1:795.
31. Cobb MW. Human papillomavirus infection. J Am Acad Dermatol 1990;22:547.
32. Gross G, Hagedorn M, Ikenberg H, et al. Bowenoid papulosis. Presence of human papillomavirus (HPV) antigen and HPV-16-related DNA sequences. Arch Dermatol 1985;121:858.
33. Rudlinger R, Grob R, Yu YX, Schnyder UW. Human papillomavirus-35-positive bowenoid papulosis of the anogenital area and concurrent human papillomavirus-35-positive verruca with bowenoid dysplasia of the periungual area. Arch Dermatol 1989;125:655.
34. Moy RL, Eliezri YD, Nuovo GJ, et al. Human papillomavirus type 16 DNA in periungual squamous cell carcinomas. JAMA 1989;261:2669.
35. Eliezri YD, Silverstein SJ, Nuovo GJ. Occurrence of human papillomavirus type 16 DNA in cutaneous squamous and basal cell neoplasms. J Am Acad Dermatol 1990;23:836.
36. Kirchner H. Immunobiology of human papillomavirus infection. Prog Med Virol 1986;33:1.
37. Ghadially FN. The role of hair follicle in origin and evolution of some cutaneous neoplasms in man and experimental animals. Cancer 1961;14:801.
38. Ghadially FN, Barton BW, Kerridge DF. Etiology of keratoacanthoma. Cancer 1963;16:603.
39. Schwartz RA. The keratoacanthoma: a review. J Surg Oncol 1979;12:305.
40. Beare JM. Molluscum sebaceum. Br J Surg 1953;41:167.
41. Belisario JV. Cancer of the skin. London (UK): Butterworths; 1959. p. 80.
42. Reizner GT, Chuang T-Y, Elpern DJ, et al. Basal cell carcinoma and keratoacanthoma in Hawaiians: an incidence report. J Am Acad Dermatol 1993;29:780.
43. Chuang T-Y, Reizner GT, Elpern DJ, et al. Keratoacanthoma in Kauai, Hawaii: the first documented incidence in a defined population. Arch Dermatol 1993;129:317.
44. Binkley GW, Johnson HH. Keratoacanthoma (molluscum sebaceum). Arch Dermatol 1955;71:66.
45. Miyaji T. Skin cancers in Japan: a nationwide 5-year survey 1956–1960. NCI Monogr 1963;10:55.
46. Kingman J, Callen JP. Keratoacanthoma: a clinical study. Arch Dermatol 1984;120:736.
47. Fisher ER, McCoy MM II, Wechsler HL. Analysis of histopathologic and electron microscopic determinants of keratoacanthoma and squamous cell carcinoma. Cancer 1972;29:1387.
48. Ghadially FN. Diagnostic electron microscopy of tumors. London (UK): Butterworths; 1980.
49. Ghadially FN. Ultrastructural pathology of the cell and matrix. London (UK): Butterworths; 1982.
50. Zelickson AS, Lynch FW. Electron microscopy of virus-like particles in keratoacanthoma. J Invest Dermatol 1961;37:79.
51. Magee KL, Rapini RP, Duvic M, Adler-Storthz K. Human papillomavirus associated with keratoacanthoma. Arch Dermatol 1989;125:1587.
52. Hsi ED, Svoboda-Newman SM, Stern RA, et al. Detection of human papilloma virus DNA in keratoacanthomas by polymerase chain reaction. Am J Dermatopathol 1997;19:10.
53. Schwartz RA. Keratoacanthoma. J Am Acad Dermatol 1994;30:1.
54. Muir EG, Bell AJY, Barlow KA. Multiple primary carcinomata of the colon, duodenum, and larynx associated with keratoacanthoma of the face. Br J Surg 1967;54:191.
55. Caccialanza M, Sopelana N. Radiation therapy for keratoacanthomas: results in 55 patients. Int J Radiat Oncol Biol Phys 1983;9:759.
56. Goldschmidt H, Breneman JC, Breneman DL. Ionizing radiation therapy in dermatology. J Am Acad Dermatol 1994;30:157.
57. Shimm DS, Duttenhauer JR, Doucette J. Radiation therapy of keratoacanthoma. Int J Radiat Oncol Biol Phys 1983;9:759.
58. Donahue B, Cooper JS, Rush S. Treatment of aggressive keratoacanthomas by radiotherapy. J Am Acad Dermatol 1990;23:489.
59. Goldschmidt H, Sherwin WK. Radiation therapy of giant aggressive keratoacanthomas. Arch Dermatol 1993; 129:1162.
60. Grupper C. Treatment of keratoacanthomas by local applications of the 5-fluorouracil (5-FU) ointment. Dermatologica 1970;140 Suppl 1:127.
61. Odom RB, Goette DK. Treatment of keratoacanthomas with intralesional fluorouracil. Arch Dermatol 1978;114:1779.
62. Melton JL, Nelson BR, Stough DB, et al. Treatment of keratoacanthomas with intralesional methotrexate. J Am Acad Dermatol 1991;25:1017.
63. Kestel JL, Shelton Blair D. Keratoacanthoma treated with methotrexate [letter]. Arch Dermatol 1973;108:723.
64. Tarnowski WM. Multiple keratoacanthoma. Response of a case to systemic chemotherapy. Arch Dermatol 1966;94:74.
65. Goldberg LH, Rosen T, Becker J, Knauss A. Treatment of solitary keratoacanthomas with oral isotretinoin. J Am Acad Dermatol 1990;23:934.
66. Shaw JC, White CR. Treatment of multiple keratoacanthomas with oral isotretinoin. J Am Acad Dermatol 1986;15:1079.
67. Grob JJ, Suzini F, Richard MA, et al. Large keratoacanthomas treated with intralesional interferon alfa-2a. J Am Acad Dermatol 1993;29:237.
68. Haenszel W. Variations in skin cancer incidence within the United States. NCI Monogr 1963;10:225.
69. Quisenberry WB. Ethnic differences in skin cancer in Hawaii. NCI Monogr 1963;10:141.
70. Oettle AG. Skin cancer in Africa. NCI Monogr 1963;10:197.
71. Mulay DM. Skin cancer in India. NCI Monogr 1963;10:215.

72. Elliott JA, Welton DG. Epithelioma: report on 1742 treated patients. Arch Dermatol Syphilol 1946;53:307.
73. Eastcott DF. Epidemiology of skin cancer in New Zealand. NCI Monogr 1963;10:141.
74. Fears TR, Scotto J, Schneiderman MA. Mathematical models of age and ultraviolet effects on the incidence of skin cancer among whites in the United States. Am J Epidemiol 1977;105:420.
75. Brash DE, Rudolph JA, Simon JA, et al. A role for sunlight in skin cancer: UV-induced p53 mutations in squamous cell carcinoma. Proc Natl Acad Sci USA 1991;88:10124.
76. Roenigk HH, Caro WA. Skin cancer in the PUVA-48 cooperative study. J Am Acad Dermatol 1981;4:319.
77. Chuang T-Y, Heinrich LA, Schultz MD, et al. PUVA and skin cancer: a historical cohort study on 492 patients. J Am Acad Dermatol 1992;26:173.
78. Stern RS, Laird N, Melski J, et al. Cutaneous squamous cell carcinoma in patients treated with PUVA. N Engl J Med 1984;310:1156.
79. Stern RS, Lange R. Nonmelanoma skin cancer occurring in patients treated with PUVA five to ten years after first treatment. J Invest Dermatol 1988;91:120.
80. Martin H, Strong E, Spiro RH. Radiation-induced skin cancer of the head and neck. Cancer 1970;25:61.
81. Christenson LJ, Geusau, A, Ferrandiz F, et al. Specialty clinics for the dermatologic care of solid-organ transplant recipients. Dermatol Surg 2004;30:598-603.
82. Jensen P, Hansen S, Moller B, et al. Skin cancer in kidney and heart transplant recipients and different long-term immunosuppressive therapy regimens. J Am Acad Dermatol 1999;40:177–86.
83. Peter RU, Braun-Falco O, Birioukov A, et al. Chronic cutaneous damage after accidental exposure to ionizing radiation: the Chernobyl experience. J Am Acad Dermatol 1994;30:719.
84. Turner JE, Callen JP. Aggressive behavior of squamous cell carcinoma in a patient with preceding lymphocytic lymphoma. J Am Acad Dermatol 1981;4:446.
85. Schwartz RA. Verrucous carcinoma of the skin and mucosa. J Am Acad Dermatol 1995;32:1.
86. Kao GF, Graham JH, Helwig EB. Carcinoma cuniculatum (verrucous carcinoma of the skin): a clinicopathologic study of 46 cases with ultrastructural observations. Cancer 1982;49:2395.
87. Chute CG, Chuang T-Y, Bergstralh EJ, Su DW-P. The subsequent risk of internal cancer with Bowen's disease: a population-based study. JAMA 1991;266:816.
88. Reizner GT, Chuang T-Y, Elpern DJ, et al. Bowen's disease (squamous cell carcinoma in situ) in Kauai, Hawaii: a population-based incidence report. J Am Acad Dermatol 1994;31:596.
89. Hirayama T. An epidemiological study of oral and pharyngeal cancer in central and South-East Asia. Bull WHO 1966;34:41.
90. Pindborg JJ. Studies in oral cancer epidemiology. J Dent Res 1963;42:348.
91. Muir C, Kirk R. Betel, tobacco and cancer of the mouth. Br J Cancer 1960;14:597.
92. Mashberg A, Samit A. Early diagnosis of asymptomatic oral and oropharyngeal squamous cell cancers. CA Cancer J Clin 1995;45:328.
93. Krolls SO, Hoffman S. Squamous cell carcinoma of the oral soft tissues. A statistical analysis of 14,253 cases by age, sex and race of patients. J Am Dent Assoc 1976;92:571.
94. Grimmel M, de Villiers EM, Neumann C, et al. Characterization of a new human papillomavirus (HPV 41) from disseminated warts and detection of its DNA in some skin carcinomas. Int J Cancer 1988;41:5.
95. Ostrow RS, Shaver MK, Turnquist S, et al. Human papillomavirus-16 in a cutaneous invasive cancer. Arch Dermatol 1989;125:666.
96. Guitart J, Bergfeld WF, Tuthill RJ, et al. Squamous cell carcinoma of the nail bed: a clinicopathological study of 12 cases. Br J Dermatol 1990;123:215.
97. Pousti A. Malignant tumors of the scalp resulting from x-ray treatment of tinea capitis. Br J Plast Surg 1979;32:52.
98. Edwards MJ, Hirsch RM, Broadwater JR, et al. Squamous cell carcinoma arising in previously burned or irradiated skin. Arch Surg 1989;124:115.
99. Johnson LL, Kempson RL. Epidermoid carcinoma in chronic osteomyelitis. Diagnostic problems and management. J Bone Joint Surg Am 1965;47:133.
100. Barr LH, Menard JW. Marjolin's ulcer. The LSU experience. Cancer 1983;52:173.
101. Bartle EJ, Sun JH, Wang X-W, Schneider BK. Cancers arising from burn scars: a literature review and report of twenty-one cases. J Burn Care Rehab 1990;11:46.
102. Baldursson B, Sigurgeirsson B, Lindelof B. Leg ulcers and squamous cell carcinoma: an epidemiological study and a review of the literature. Acta Derm Venereol 1993;73:171.
103. Bendl BJ, Graham JH. New concepts on the origin of squamous cell carcinomas of the skin: solar (senile) keratosis with squamous cell carcinoma—a clinicopathologic and histochemical study. In: Proceedings of the Sixth National Cancer Conference, July 1968. Philadelphia: JB Lippincott; 1970. p. 471.
104. Spoor HJ, Lindo SD, Erlandson RA. Skin cancer comparison of aggressive potentials of sunlight-induced and x-ray–induced tumors. Cutis 1977;20:74.
105. Hruza GJ. Mohs micrographic surgery. Otolaryngol Clin North Am 1990;23:845.
106. Kuflik EG. Cryosurgery updated. J Am Acad Dermatol 1994;31:925.
107. Kwa RE, Campana K, Moy RL. Biology of cutaneous squamous cell carcinoma. J Am Acad Dermatol 1992;26:1.
108. Brodland DG, Zitelli JA. Surgical margins for excision of primary cutaneous squamous cell carcinoma. J Am Acad Dermatol 1992;27:241.
109. Mohs FE, Blanchard L. Microscopically controlled surgery for extramammary Paget's disease. Arch Dermatol 1979;115:706.
110. Graham GF, Detlefs RL, Garrett AB, et al. Guidelines of care for cryosurgery. J Am Acad Dermatol 1994;31:648.
111. Goldschmidt H. Radiotherapy of skin cancer: modern indications and techniques. Cutis 1976;17:253.
112. Lippman SM, Meyskens FL Jr. Treatment of advanced squamous cell carcinomas of the skin with isotretinoin. Ann Intern Med 1987;107:499.
113. Hong WK, Lippman SM, Itri LM, et al. Prevention of second primary tumors with isotretinoin in squamous cell carcinoma of the head and neck. N Engl J Med 1990;323:795.
114. Kelly JW, Sabto J, Gurr FW, Bruce F. Retinoids to prevent skin cancer in organ transplant recipients. Lancet 1991;338:1407.
115. Katz AD, Urbach F, Lilienfeld AM. The frequency and risk of metastases in squamous cell carcinoma of the skin. Cancer 1957;10:1162.
116. Lund HZ. How often does squamous cell carcinoma metastasize? Arch Dermatol 1965;92:635.
117. Friedman HI, Cooper PH, Wanebo HJ. Prognostic and therapeutic use of microstaging of cutaneous squamous cell carcinoma of the trunk and extremities. Cancer 1985;56:1099.
118. Immerman SC, Scanlon EF, Christ M, Knox KL. Recurrent squamous cell carcinoma of the skin. Cancer 1983;51:1537.
119. Frankel DH, Hanusa BH, Zitelli JA. New primary non-melanoma skin cancer in patients with a history of squamous cell carcinoma of the skin: implications and recommendations for follow-up. J Am Acad Dermatol 1992;26:720.
120. Pinkus H. Epithelial and fibroepithelial tumors. Arch Dermatol 1965;91:24.
121. Hashimoto K, Lever WF. Appendage tumors of the skin. Springfield (IL): Charles C Thomas; 1968.
122. Miller SJ. Biology of basal cell carcinoma (part I). J Am Acad Dermatol 1991;24:1.
123. Hoy WE. Nonmelanoma skin carcinoma in Albuquerque, New Mexico: experience of a major health care provider. Cancer 1996;77:2489.
124. Reizner GT, Chuang T-Y, Elpern DJ, et al. Basal cell carcinoma in Kauai, Hawaii: the highest documented incidence in the United States. J Am Acad Dermatol 1993;29:184.
125. Chuang T-Y, Popescu A, Su WPD, Chute CG. Basal cell carcinoma. J Am Acad Dermatol 1990;22:413.
126. Silverberg E, Boring C, Squires T. Cancer statistics 1990. Cancer 1990;40:18.
127. Abreo F, Sanusi ID. Basal cell carcinoma in North American blacks: clinical and histopathologic study of 26 patients. J Am Acad Dermatol 1991;25:1005.
128. Halder RM, Bang KM. Skin cancer in blacks in the United States. Dermatol Clin 1988;6:397.
129. Yeh S. Skin cancer in chronic arsenicism. Hum Pathol 1973;4:469.
130. Mortensen AC, Kjeldsen H. Carcinomas following Grenz ray treatment of benign dermatoses. Acta Derm Venereol (Stockh) 1987;67:523.
131. Peck GL, DiGiovanna JJ, Sarnoff DS, et al. Treatment and prevention of basal cell carcinoma with isotretinoin. J Am Acad Dermatol 1988;19:176.
132. Sommers SC, McManus RG. Multiple arsenical cancers of skin and internal organs. Cancer 1953;6:347.
133. Kricker A, Armstrong BK, English DR. Sun exposure and non-melanocytic skin cancer. Cancer Causes Control 1994;5:367.
134. Kricker A, Armstrong BK, English DR, Heenan PJ. Does intermittent sun exposure cause basal cell carcinoma? A case-control study in Western Australia. Int J Cancer 1995;60:489.
135. Johnson RL, Rothman AL, Xie J, et al. Human homolog of patched, a candidate gene for the basal cell carcinoma syndrome. Science 1996;272:1668–71.
136. Lam CW, Xie J, To KF, et al. A frequent activated smoothened mutation in sporadic basal cell carcinomas. Oncogene 1999;18:833–6.
137. Gorlin RJ. Nevoid basal-cell carcinoma syndrome. Medicine (Baltimore) 1987;66:98.
138. Gorlin RJ, Vickers RA, Kelln E, Williamson JJ. The multiple basal cell nevi syndrome. Cancer 1965;18:89.
139. Unna PG. Die Histopathologie der Hautkrankheiten. Berlin: Hirschwald; 1894.
140. Urbach F, Davies RE, Forbes PD. Ultraviolet radiation and skin cancer in man. In: Montagna W, Dobson RL, editors. Advances in biology of skin. Vol. VII. New York: Pergamon Press; 1966. p. 195.
141. Maloney ME, Jones DB, Sexton FM. Pigmented basal cell carcinoma: investigation of 70 cases. J Am Acad Dermatol 1992;27:74.
142. Howell JB, Caro MR. Morphea-like epithelioma. Arch Dermatol 1957;75:517.
143. Litzow JT, Perry HO, Soderstrom CW. Morpheaform basal cell carcinoma. Am J Surg 1968;116:499.
144. Richman T, Penneys NS. Analysis of morpheaform basal cell carcinoma. J Cutan Pathol 1988;15:359.
145. Miller SJ. Biology of basal cell carcinoma (part II). J Am Acad Dermatol 1991;24:161.
146. Rowe DE, Carroll RJ, Day CL Jr. Long-term recurrence rates in previously untreated (primary) basal cell carcinomas: implications for patient follow-up. J Dermatol Surg Oncol 1989;15:315.
147. Orton CI. The treatment of basal cell carcinoma by radiotherapy. Clin Oncol 1978;4:317.
148. Wilder RB, Kittelson JM, Shimm DS. Basal cell carcinoma treated with radiation therapy. Cancer 1991;68:2134.
149. Ellis F. Dose, time and fractionation: a clinical hypothesis. Clin Radiol 1969;20:1.
150. Weber BM, Simkins GS. A table for the rapid determination of RED and TDF values. Br J Radiol 1975;48:929.
151. Avant WH, Huff RC. Intradermal 5-fluorouracil in the treatment of basal cell cancer of the face. South Med J 1976;69:561.
152. Orenberg EK, Miller BH, Greenway HT, et al. The effect of intralesional 5-fluorouracil therapeutic implant (MPI 5003) for treatment of basal cell carcinoma. J Am Acad Dermatol 1992;27:723.
153. Marks R, Gebauer K, Shumack S, et al. The Australian Multicentre Trial Group. Imiquimod 5% cream in the treatment of superficial basal cell carcinoma: results of a multicenter 6-week dose-response trial. J Am Acad Dermatol 2001;44:807–13.
154. Taipale J, Chen JK, Cooper MK, et al. Effects of oncogenic mutations in Smoothened and Patched can be reversed by cyclopamine. Nature 2000;406:944–5.
155. Silverman MK, Kopf AW, Grin CM, et al. Recurrence rates for treated basal cell carcinomas. Part 2: curettage electrodesiccation. J Dermatol Surg Oncol 1991;17:720.
156. Silverman MK, Kopf AW, Grin CM, et al. Recurrence rates for treated basal cell carcinomas. Part 1: overview. J Dermatol Surg Oncol 1991;17:713.
157. Farmer ER, Helwig EB. Metastatic basal cell carcinoma: a clinicopathologic study of seventeen cases. Cancer 1980;46:748.
158. Lo JS, Snow SN, Reizner GT, et al. Metastatic basal cell carcinoma: report of twelve cases with a review of the literature. J Am Acad Dermatol 1991;24:715.
159. Scanlon EF, Volkmer DD, Oviedo MA, et al. Metastatic basal cell carcinoma. J Surg Oncol 1980;15:171.
160. Marghoob A, Kopf AW, Bart RS, et al. Risk of another basal cell carcinoma developing after treatment of a basal cell carcinoma. J Am Acad Dermatol 1993;28:22.
161. Tangrea JA, Edwards B, Hartman A, et al. Isotretinoin basal cell carcinoma prevention trial. Design, recruitment results and baseline characteristics of the trial participants. The ISO-BCC Study Group. Control Clin Trials 1990;11:433.
162. Tangrea JA, Edwards BK, Taylor PR, et al. Long-term therapy with low-dose isotretinoin for prevention of basal cell carcinoma: a multicenter clinical trial. J Natl Cancer Inst 1992;84:328.
163. Clendenning WE, Block JB, Radde IC. Basal cell nevus syndrome. Arch Dermatol 1964;90:38.
164. Cutler TP, Holden CA, MacDonald DM. Multiple naevoid basal cell carcinoma syndrome (Gorlin's syndrome). Clin Exp Dermatol 1979;4:373.

165. Johnson RL, Rothman AL, Xie J, et al. Human homolog of patched, a candidate gene for the basal cell nevus syndrome. Science 1996;272:1668.
166. Hahn H, Wicking C, Zaphiropoulous PG, et al. Mutations of the human homolog of Drosophila patched in the nevoid basal cell carcinoma syndrome. Cell 1996;85:841.
167. Goldstein AM, Bale SJ, Peck GL, DiGiovanna JJ. Sun exposure and basal cell carcinomas in the nevoid basal cell carcinoma syndrome. J Am Acad Dermatol 1993;29:34.
168. Howell JB, Freeman RG. Structure and significance of the pits with their tumors in the nevoid basal cell carcinoma syndrome. J Am Acad Dermatol 1980;2:224.
169. Howell JB, Mehregan AH. Pursuit of the pits in the nevoid basal cell carcinoma syndrome. Arch Dermatol 1970;102:586.
170. Maddox WD, Winklemann RK, Harrison EG Jr, et al. Nevoid basal cell epithelioma, jaw cysts and skeletal defects. A clinical syndrome. JAMA 1964;188:106.
171. Strong LC. Theories of pathogenesis: mutation and cancer. In: Mulvihill JJ, Miller RW, Fraumeni JF Jr, editors. Genetics of human cancer. New York: Raven Press; 1977. p. 401.
172. Kraemer KH, DiGiovanna JJ, Moshell AN, et al. Prevention of skin cancer in xeroderma pigmentosum with the use of oral isotretinoin. N Engl J Med 1988;318:1633.
173. Toker C. Trabecular carcinoma of the skin. Arch Dermatol 1972;105:107.
174. Ratner D. Nelson BR, Brown MD, Johnson TM. Merkel cell carcinoma. J Am Acad Dermatol Surg Oncol 1986; 29:143.
175. Hitchcock CL, Bland KI, Laney RG III, et al. Neuroendocrine (Merkel cell) carcinoma of the skin: its natural history, diagnosis, and treatment. Ann Surg 1988;207:201.
176. Raaf JH, Urmacher C, Knapper WK, et al. Trabecular (Merkel cell) carcinoma of the skin: treatment of primary, recurrent, and metastatic disease. Cancer 1986;57:178.
177. Roenigk RK, Goltz RW. Merkel cell carcinoma: a problem with microscopically controlled surgery. J Dermatol Surg Oncol 1986;12:332.
178. O'Connor WJ, Roenigk RK, Brodland DG. Merkel cell carcinoma: comparison of Mohs micrographic surgery and wide excision in eighty-six patients. Dermatol Surg 1997;23:929.
179. Zakzouk MD, Ramsay AD, Buchanan G. Merkel cell tumor of the skin. J Laryngol Oncol 1986;100:561.
180. Allen PJ, Zhang ZF, Colt DG. Surgical management of Merkel cell carcinoma. Ann Surg 1999;229:97–105.
181. Messina JL, Reintgen DS, Cruse CW, et al. Selective lymphadenectomy in patients with Merkel cell (cutaneous neuroendocrine) carcinoma. Ann Surg Oncol 1997;4:389–95.
182. Marks ME, Kim RY, Salter MM. Radiotherapy as an adjuvant in the management of Merkel cell carcinoma. Cancer 1990;65:60.
183. Haag ML, Glass LF, Fenske NA. Merkel cell carcinoma. Diagnosis and treatment. Dermatol Surg 1995;21:669.
184. Shaw JHF, Rumball E. Merkel cell tumor: clinical behavior and treatment. Br J Surg 1991;78:138.
185. Skelton HG, Smith KJ, Hitchcock CL, et al. Merkel cell carcinoma: analysis of clinical, histologic, and immunohistologic features of 132 cases with relation to survival. J Am Acad Dermatol 1997;37:734.
186. Garg SK, Subbuswamy SG, Alabi JO, Lawrie JH. Dermatofibrosarcoma protuberans in northern Nigeria: a clinical pathological review of 17 cases. Clin Oncol 1978;4:113.
187. Rademaker B, Angelillo M, Reiman HM, Jackson IT. Dermatofibrosarcoma protuberans: a review of 73 cases. Eur J Plast Surg 1990;13:251.
188. Taylor HB, Helwig EB. Dermatofibrosarcoma protuberans: a study of 115 cases. Cancer 1962;15:717.
189. Wang J, Hisaoka M, Shimajiri S, et al. Detection of COL1A1-PDGFB fusion transcripts in dermatofibrosarcoma protuberans by reverse transcription polymerase chain reaction using archival formalin-fixed, paraffin-embedded tissues. Diagn Mol Pathol 1999;8:113–9.
190. Parker TL, Zitelli JA. Surgical margins for excision of dermatofibrosarcoma protuberans. J Am Acad Dermatol 1995;32:233.
191. McPeak CJ, Cruz T, Nicastri AD. Dermatofibrosarcoma protuberans: an analysis of 86 cases, five with metastasis. Ann Surg 1967;166:803.
192. Maki, RG, Awan RA, Dixon, RH, et al. Differential sensitivity to imatinib of 2 patients with metastatic sarcoma arising from dermatofibrosarcoma protuberans. Int J Cancer 2002;100:623–6.
193. Snow SN, Gordon EM, Larson PO, et al. Dermatofibrosarcoma protuberans: a report on 29 patients treated by Mohs micrographic surgery with long-term follow-up and review of the literature. Cancer 2004; 101:28–38.
194. Holden CA, Spittle MF, Wilson Jones E. Angiosarcoma of the face and scalp, prognosis and treatment. Cancer 1987;59:1046–57.
195. Requena L, Sangueza OP. Cutaneous vascular proliferations. Part III. Malignant neoplasms, other cutaneous neoplasms with significant vascular component, and disorders erroneously considered as vascular neoplasms. J Am Acad Dermatol 1998;38:143–75.
196. Sasaki R, Soejima T, Kishi K, et al. Angiosarcoma treated with radiotherapy: impact of tumor type and size on outcome. Int J Radiat Oncol Biol Phys 2002;52:1032–40.
197. Ulrich L, Krause M, Brachmann A, et al. Successful treatment of angiosarcoma of the scalp by intralesional cytokine therapy and surface irradiation. J Eur Acad Dermatol Venereol 2000;14:412–5.
198. Wollina U, Fuller J, Graefe T, et al. Angiosarcoma of the scalp: treatment with liposomal doxorubicin and radiotherapy. J Cancer Res Clin Oncol 2001;127:396–9.
199. Domingo J, Helwig EB. Malignant neoplasms associated with nevus sebaceus of Jadassohn. J Am Acad Dermatol 1979;1:545.
200. Cook BE Jr, Bartley GB. Treatment options and future prospects for the management of eyelid malignancies: an evidence-based update. Ophthalmology 2001;108: 2088–98; quiz 2099–100, 2121.
201. Spencer JM, Nossa R, Tse DT, Sequeira M. Sebaceous carcinoma of the eyelid treated with Mohs micrographic surgery. J Am Acad Dermatol 2001;44:1004–9.
202. Zollo JD, Zeitouni NC. The Roswell Park Cancer Institute experience with extramammary Paget's disease. Br J Dermatol 2000;142:59–65.
203. Coldiron BM, Goldsmith BA, Robinson JK. Surgical treatment of extramammary Paget's disease. A report of six cases and a reexamination of Mohs micrographic surgery compared with conventional surgical excision. Cancer 1991;67:933–8.
204. O'Connor WJ, Lim KK, Zalla, MJ, et al. Comparison of Mohs micrographic surgery and wide excision for extramammary Paget's disease. Dermatol Surg 2003;29:723–7.
205. Moreno-Arias GA, Conill C, Castells-Mas A, et al. Radiotherapy for genital extramammary Paget's disease in situ. Dermatol Surg 2001;27:587–90.
206. Louis-Syvestre C, Haddad B, Paniel BJ. Paget's disease of the vulva: results of different conservative treatments. Eur J Obstet Gynecol Reprod Biol 2001;99:253–5.
207. Puppala S. Failure of carbon dioxide laser treatment in three patients with penoscrotal extramammary Paget's disease. BJU Int 2001;88:986–7.
208. Yoell JH, Price WG. Paget's disease of the perineal skin with associated adenocarcinoma. Arch Dermatol 1960;82:986–91.
209. Crawford D, Nimmo M, Clement PB, et al. Prognostic factors in Paget's disease of the vulva: a study of 21 cases. Int J Gynecol Pathol 1999;18:351–9.
210. Brownstein MH, Wolf M, Bikowski JB. Cowden's disease. A cutaneous marker of breast cancer. Cancer 1978;41:2393.
211. Salem OS, Steck WD. Cowden's disease (multiple hamartoma and neoplasia syndrome). J Am Acad Dermatol 1983;8:686.
212. Starink TM: Cowden's disease: analysis of fourteen new cases. J Am Acad Dermatol 1984;11:1127.
213. Thyresson HN, Doyle JA. Cowden's disease (multiple hamartoma syndrome). Mayo Clin Proc 1981;56:179.
214. Weary PE, Gorlin RJ, Gentry WC Jr, et al. Multiple hamartoma syndrome (Cowden's disease). Arch Dermatol 1972;106:682.
215. Liaw D, Marsh DJ, Li J, et al. Germline mutations of the PTEN gene in Cowden disease, an inherited breast and thyroid cancer syndrome. Nat Genet 1997;16:64–7.
216. Finan MC, Connolly SM. Sebaceous gland tumors and systemic disease: a clinicopathologic analysis. Medicine (Baltimore) 1984;63:232.
217. Graham R, McKee P, McGibbon D, Heyderman E. Torre–Muir syndrome. An association with isolated sebaceous carcinoma. Cancer 1985;55:2868.
218. Housholder MS, Zeligman I. Sebaceous neoplasms associated with visceral carcinomas. Arch Dermatol 1980; 116:61.
219. Kolodner RD, Hall NR, Lipford J, et al. Structure of the human MSH2 focus and analysis of two Muir–Torre kindreds for msh2 mutations. Genomics 1994;24:516–26.
220. Vasen HF, van der Feltz M, Raue F, et al. The natural course of multiple endocrine neoplasia type IIb. A study of 18 cases. Arch Intern Med 1992;152:1250–2.
221. Elder D, Elenitsas R, Jaworsky C, Johnson B Jr. Lever's histopathology of the skin. 8th ed. Philadelphia: Lippincott-Raven; 1997. p. 998.
222. Santoro M, Carlomagno F, Romano A, et al. Activation of RET as a dominant transforming gene by germline mutations of MEN2A and MEN2B. Science 1995; 267:381–3.
223. Sanso GE, Domene HM, Garcia R, et al. Very early detection of RET proto-oncogene mutation is crucial for preventive thyroidectomy in multiple endocrine neoplasia type 2 children: presence of C-cell malignant disease in asymptomatic carriers. Cancer 2002;94:323–30.
224. Lookingbill DP, Spangler N, Sexton FM. Skin involvement as the presenting sign of internal carcinoma. J Am Acad Dermatol 1990;22:19.
225. Gates O. Cutaneous metastasis of malignant diseases. Am J Cancer 1937;30:718.
226. Lookingbill DP, Spangler N, Helm KF. Cutaneous metastases in patients with metastatic carcinoma: a retrospective study of 4020 patients. J Am Acad Dermatol 1993;29:228.
227. Brownstein MH, Helwig EB. Metastatic tumors of the skin. Cancer 1972;29:1298.
228. Brownstein MH, Helwig EB. Patterns of cutaneous metastases. Arch Dermatol 1972;105:862.
229. Fielding JE. Smoking and women [editorial]. N Engl J Med 1987;317:1343.
230. Ordoiiez NG, Samaan NA. Medullary carcinoma of the thyroid metastatic to the skin. J Cutan Pathol 1987;14:251.
231. Chakraborty AK, Reddy AN, Grosberg SJ, Wapnick S. Pancreatic carcinoma with dissemination to umbilicus and skin. Arch Dermatol 1977;113:838.
232. Bennett AJ, Kalra JK, Cortes EP. Hepatocellular carcinoma. Manifestation as a chest wall metastasis. Arch Dermatol 1982;118:69.
233. Padilla RS, Jarmillo M, Dao A, Chapman W. Cutaneous metastatic adenocarcinoma of gall bladder origin. Arch Dermatol 1982;118:515.
234. Hollander A, Grots IA. Oculocutaneous metastases from carcinoma of the urinary bladder. Arch Dermatol 1968;97:678.
235. Rasbach D, Hendricks A, Stoltzner G. Endometrial adenocarcinoma metastatic to the scalp. Arch Dermatol 1978;114:1708.
236. Peison B. Metastasis of carcinoma of the prostate to the scalp: simulation of a large sebaceous cyst. Arch Dermatol 1971;104:301.
237. Price NM, Kopf AW. Metastases to skin from occult malignant neoplasms. Cutaneous metastases from a teratocarcinoma. Arch Dermatol 1974;109:547.
238. Markowitz, JS, Cosimi LA, Carey RW, et al. Prognosis following initial recurrence of cutaneous melanoma. Arch Surg 1991;126:703–8.

Section 33

BONE AND SOFT TISSUE

110

Bone Tumors

Dempsey Springfield, MD
Gerald Rosen, MD

Primary bone tumors are uncommon. Approximately 2,400 malignant neoplasms of the bones and joints are diagnosed annually in the United States, accounting for 0.18% of all cancer cases. An estimated 1,300 patients die from these cancers each year, representing 0.24% of all deaths from cancer. Osteomyelitis in children, trauma in midlife, and metastatic carcinoma are considerably more common and are often confused for primary skeletal neoplasia. On the other hand, primary bone tumors are not so rare as to be unimportant, and at least some knowledge of them is essential for an oncologist.

Bone tumors can be benign or malignant. The behavior of benign bone tumors can vary considerably from being self-limited and healing spontaneously (eg, unicameral bone cyst, nonossifying fibroma, osteoid osteoma), to inactive but persistent (eg, enchondroma, osteochondroma), to minimally locally aggressive (eg, aneurysmal bone cyst, chondroblastoma, chondromyxofibroma), to locally aggressive (eg, giant cell tumor of bone, osteoblastoma). The treatment of benign bone tumors depends on their growth behavior. Often the behavior of an individual tumor in a specific patient will need to be determined before the proper treatment is chosen. Most primary malignant bone tumors should be surgically resected. Myeloma and lymphoma of bone are exceptions. These two conditions will be mentioned briefly in this chapter but are dealt with in more detail elsewhere in the text. Patients with a primary malignant bone tumor that has a high prevalence of micrometastatic disease at presentation (eg, classic osteosarcoma, Ewing's sarcoma) should be treated with adjuvant chemotherapy. During the past decade, adjuvant chemotherapy has been given both before so-called neoadjuvant chemotherapy and after surgery. Irradiation for bone tumors is routine for myeloma and lymphoma, but otherwise is a secondary treatment option used when an adequate surgical resection would produce unacceptable morbidity or is not technically possible.

Bone tumors arise from the mesenchymal cells normally present in the skeleton. The classification of these tumors is defined by the assumed cell of origin based on the histologic examination. Often it is the matrix of the tumor that indicates the cell type. Therefore, tumors that have a matrix of bone have "osteo" in their name and are believed to have arisen from cells in the osteoblast cell line (eg, osteoid osteoma, osteoblastoma, osteosarcoma). Those with a cartilage matrix have "chondro" in their name and are believed to have arisen from cells in the chondroblast cell line (eg, enchondroma, osteochondroma, chondroblastoma, chondrosarcoma). In addition to these two obvious tumor groupings, there are tumors with a fibrous matrix (eg, nonossifying fibroma, fibrosarcoma, malignant fibrous histiocytoma), a vascular origin (eg, hemangioma, hemangioendothelioma, hemangiopericytoma), and those without a particular matrix (eg, unicameral bone cyst, aneurysmal bone cyst, giant cell tumor of bone, Ewing's sarcoma). Those bone tumors that arise from the marrow elements (eg, Langerhans cell histiocytosis, myeloma, lymphoma) are usually not considered classic primary bone tumors, and their behavior is sufficiently different from primary bone tumors that their clinical distinction is easy. They are included in the differential diagnosis with the more classic primary bone tumors, however, and must be considered in any discussion of them.

This chapter will offer the reader an introductory understanding of the common bone tumors and their current treatments.

STAGING

Malignant The most common staging system used to stage bone tumors is that developed by Enneking (Table 110-1).[1,2] This staging system is based on the histologic grade, anatomic extent, and presence of metastatic disease at presentation. Patients with a metastasis to any site, most commonly lung, are placed in the highest stage III. Those patients who have a so-called skip lesion (a second bone lesion separate from the primary but in the same bone or just across an adjacent joint) should also be considered to have stage III disease. Stage I are those tumors that have less than a 25% frequency of metastasizing, and stage II are those with a higher frequency. The malignant bone tumors that are confined to a single anatomic compartment are subclassified as "A," and those outside a single compartment are subclassified as "B" (Table 110-2). The advantage of this system is that it is simple, but the disadvantage is that most primary malignant bone tumors are stage IIB (Figure 110-1). Although previous versions of the staging system devel-

Table 110-1 Enneking System for Staging of Soft Tissue Sarcoma and Sarcoma of Bone

Stage	Grade	Site	Metastases
IA	G1	T1	M0
IB	G1	T2	M0
IIA	G2	T1	M0
IIB	G2	T2	M0
IIIA	G1–G2	T1–T2	M1
IIIB	G1–G2	T1–T2	M1

Characteristics

Grade (G)
- G1 Low
- G2 High

Site (T)
- T1 Intracompartmental
- T2 Extracompartmental

Metastases (M)
- M0 No regional or distant metastases
- M1 Regional or distant metastases present

From Enneking.[1]

Table 110-2 Surgical Sites

Intracompartmental (T1)	Extracompartmental (T2)
Intraosseous	Soft tissue extension
Intra-articular	Soft tissue extension
Superficial to deep fascia	Deep fascial extension
Paraosseous	Intraosseous or extrafascial
Intrafascial compartments	Extrafascial planes or spaces
Ray of hand or foot	Mid- and hind foot
Posterior calf	Popliteal space
Anterolateral leg	Groin-femoral triangle
Anterior thigh	Intrapelvic
Medial thigh	Mid-hand
Posterior thigh	Antecubital fossa
Buttocks	Axilla
Volar forearm	Periclavicular
Dorsal forearm	Paraspinal
Anterior arm	Head and neck
Posterior arm	
Periscapular	

From Enneking.[1]

oped by the American Joint Committee on Cancer (AJCC) were almost identical to the Enneking system, the most recent version of the AJCC system divides malignancies into stages, IA, IB, IIA, IIB, III, IVA, and IVB based on size, grade, presence of lymph node metastases, and presence of distant metastases.

BIOPSY

Without a biopsy, it is impossible to be absolutely certain of a diagnosis. Not so obviously, sometimes the presentation (clinical and radiographic) of some bone tumors is sufficiently characteristic that a biopsy is not needed. Most nonossifying fibromas, unicameral bone cysts, and enchondromas are diagnosed without histologic confirmation. Most of the other bone tumors can be recognized on the plain radiograph but are biopsied before definite treatment. This is especially true for those lesions that need wide surgical resection and for those that need chemotherapy. When no preresection treatment is needed, the biopsy and definitive surgery may be done during the same anesthetic based on the results of a frozen section diagnosis.

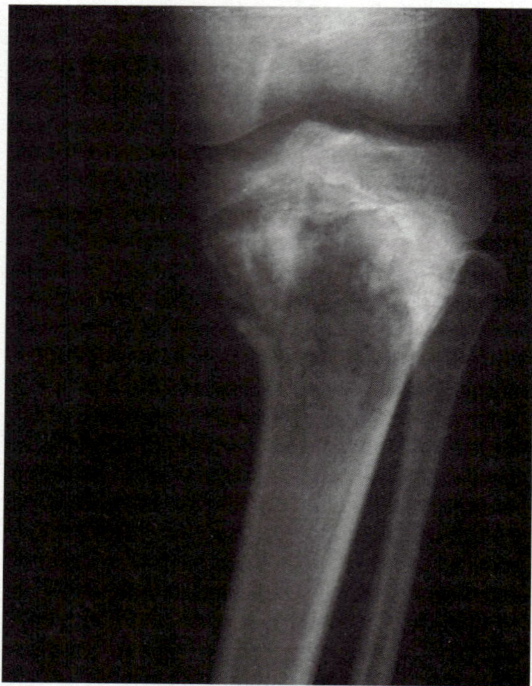

Figure 110-1 Anterior/posterior view of the proximal left tibia. The lesion with bone destruction and bone formation is a high-grade classic osteosarcoma with extension into the soft tissue. This is a typical stage IIB sarcoma.

Planning and doing the biopsy are critical steps that can have impact on the outcome of a patient. Two studies demonstrate the importance of the biopsy and the potential risk.[3,4] In general, mesenchymal tumors have the ability to survive without a direct blood supply and are therefore implantable. When a resection is the required treatment, all tissue exposed during the biopsy must be resected to assure as high local control as possible. This makes the actual biopsy important, especially in an extremity tumor.

There are four types of biopsy: (1) fine-needle aspiration (FNA), (2) needle biopsy, (3) incisional biopsy, and (4) excisional biopsy. Incisional biopsy is the most common type of biopsy and the one against which others are judged. FNA is the easiest for the patient but only obtains individual cells and, therefore, only cytologic details are available. This method is excellent for confirming what is already suspected: Ewing's sarcoma, metastatic carcinoma, infection, and myeloma, but may be insufficient for other bone tumors. Needle biopsy obtains more tissue and the relationships between the cells and matrix is seen. If the tissue is representative and is of sufficient quantity, a diagnosis is usually not that much more difficult to make compared with an open biopsy. The major drawback is that minimal tissue is obtained and often the biopsy must be done with computed tomography (CT) control. Incisional biopsy, if done by the surgeon who will ultimately do the resection, is the least likely to make limb salvage surgery more difficult and risky. It is the most likely to obtain adequate and representative tissue. The major drawback is that anesthesia is needed and it usually must be done in an operating room. An excisional biopsy is intended to be both diagnostic and therapeutic. This is appropriate whenever the morbidity of the excisional biopsy is extremely limited, while at the same time, the biopsy will be adequate surgery.

SURGERY

Not all bone tumors require surgery. Those bone tumors that spontaneously resolve or do not compromise the strength of the bone can be left alone. Fibrous cortical defects, most nonossifying fibromas, many unicameral bone cysts, enchondromas, and osteochondromas are the common bone tumors that do not need to be surgically removed. The vast majority of the remaining bone tumors should be treated by surgical removal.

Unicameral bone cysts and eosinophilic granulomas (isolated Langerhans histiocytosis) are often treated with direct injection of corticosteroids. Various other materials have been used by some for unicameral bone cysts. These injections are usually done under general anesthesia and fluoroscopic control. Rosenthal and colleagues introduced the use of radiofrequency ablation for osteoid osteoma.[5] This treatment has become popular and is used widely.

There are two basic operations used to remove bone tumors. The bone tumor can be removed by curettage or by resection. When curettage is done, the tumor is entered and scraped out from within the tumor. Curettage can be further characterized as being "extended" or "aggressive" when the surgeon extends the breadth of the tissue removal using a power burr to remove surrounding bone. In addition, adjuvants are used by some surgeons to reduce the risk of local recurrence. Phenol has been used for many years, but its role is debatable and there are no controlled studies substantiating its advantage. It is a clinically accepted adjuvant. Freezing the surrounding bone with liquid nitrogen is used by some surgeons. It has been shown to reduce local recurrence of some benign tumors, but is difficult to use and is associated with its own complications. Both these adjuvants are controversial.

Resection of a bone tumor implies that the tumor is removed in toto with surrounding uninvolved bone. The amount of bone depends on the anatomic situation and limitations. Whenever possible, as much surrounding bone as is practical is removed with the tumor. Whenever a bone tumor has penetrated the cortex, the overlying soft tissue is removed with the specimen. Small low-grade lesions in the metaphysis may be safely resected by removing only a portion of the bone. Bone tumors in the diaphysis that require a resection are usually treated with an intercalary resection (Figure 110-2). High-grade tumors that arise in the metaphysis close by or adjuvant to the subchondral bone usually require removal of the adjacent articular surface (Figure 110-3).

TYPES OF RECONSTRUCTION

The main reconstructive options include autogenous bone grafts, structural bone allografts (intercalary or osteoarticular), and metallic endoprosthetics. Allografts and endoprosthetics may be used in conjunction as a composite reconstruction. Autogenous bone grafts may be vascularized

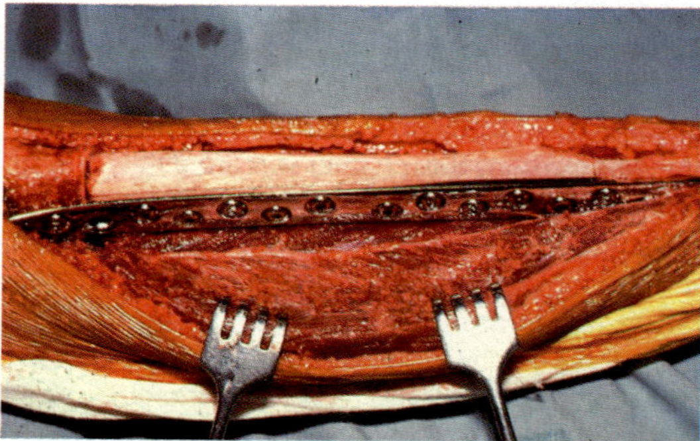

Figure 110-2 Intraoperative photograph of a tibia that has had a resection of its diaphysis with replacement with an intercalary allograft held in place with a bone plate.

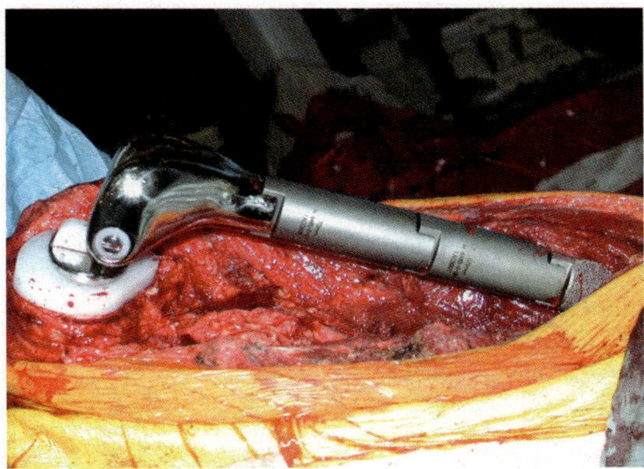

Figure 110-3 Intraoperative photograph of a distal femoral reconstruction with a modular prosthesis reconstruction. The distal femur including the articular surface was resected.

(eg, fibula). All three have inherent advantages and disadvantages. Which technique is employed is a function of the location of the tumor, age of the patient, and types of adjuvant therapies that will be employed (ie, chemotherapy and/or radiation). Large structural allografts and endoprosthetics should generally be reserved for patients older than 8 years. Nonvascularized autografts from the pelvis or other sites may be used in a limited fashion for relatively small defects and work well in children.[6] The advantage is a high incorporation rate, but potential donor site morbidity may occur. Vascularized autografts such as the fibula are attractive because, when successful, the graft incorporates and even may remodel secondary to the forces exerted across it. Again, donor site complications can occur.

Structural allografts have no donor site morbidity. The major drawback to allografts is difficulty incorporating with the host bone (nonunion) and fracture. Their advantage is that they are a biologic solution; if they do heal and do not fracture, they may last the lifetime of the patient. Osteoarticular allografts may be used in the reconstruction of the proximal humerus, distal femur, and proximal tibia, as well as potentially any joint.[6–16] Diaphyseal tumors can be reconstructed with intercalary allografts.[6,13–16] The epiphyseal growth plate may sometimes serve as an adequate tumor barrier allowing preservation of the epiphysis and thus the joint surface. This must be carefully assessed preoperatively with magnetic resonance imaging (MRI). When this is possible, the durability and functional outcome will be superior to cases where the joint proper must be sacrificed.

Metallic endoprosthetics provide an immediate stable reconstruction but suffer from the fact that they eventually fail because of loosening and failure of components. Usually the stem of the prosthesis is cemented in place with PMMA. Prostheses are generally cast from cobalt, chrome, or steel, or machined from titanium (Figure 110-4). Infections are a significant risk with endoprosthetics as well, with rates ranging from 0 to 35%.[17–22]

Durability of endoprostheses is subject to a variety of influences, but the anticipated event-free 5-year survival for proximal femur reconstructions approaches 90%, the distal femur about 60%, and the proximal tibia just over 50%.[23] Prosthetic reconstructions of the proximal humerus tend to be more durable as they are subject to less stress. Failure can result from loosening at the prosthesis-host interface or infection. Improved metallurgy has resulted in a significant reduction in failure of the implants owing to metal fatigue. Articulating, moving components need revision at a rate in direct relation to the cyclical loading of the prosthesis. The more use, the more likely it is that a revision will be necessary. Sometimes failure can be catastrophic, as can be seen with late infections, necessitating a delayed amputation.

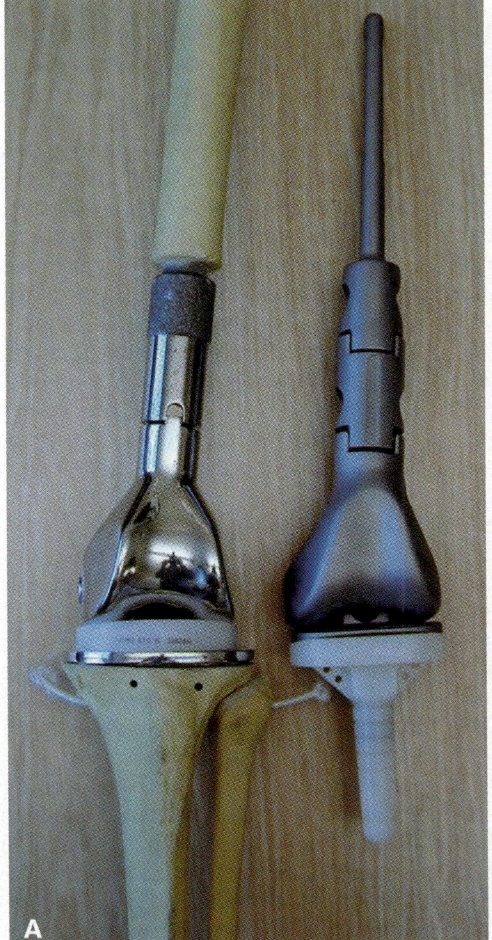

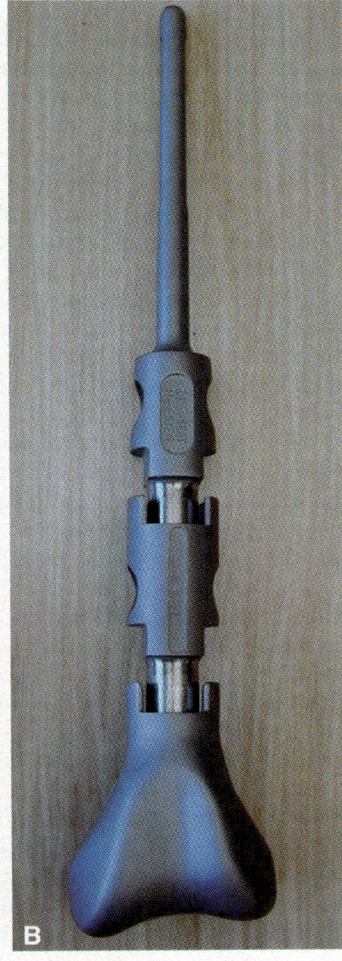

Figure 110-4 Examples of distal femoral endoprostheses. **A,** Nonmodular body on left, modular body on right. **B,** Intercalary bodies may be interchanged to lengthen limb.

Patients with significant growth still to come in the resected bone have the added problem of how the reconstruction can account for this growth. As with any reconstruction in the skeletally immature patient, the construct must be dynamic so as to facilitate skeletal growth. One of the solutions for reconstructions in these patients, usually between 8 and 12 years of age, is the use of a prosthesis that can be lengthened. For such expandable prostheses, the 5-year revision-free survival has been reported as low as 15%.[22] Although some of the expandable mechanisms may be easy to implement, the longevity of prosthetic implants is poor in young children.[20,23–31]

LIMB SALVAGE VERSUS AMPUTATION SURGERY

In general, contemporary limb sparing surgery results in a local recurrence rate of 5 to 10%, which is not statistically significantly different from amputation surgery.[32] Amputation itself does not guarantee absolute local control. Noncontiguous disease ("skip lesions") proximal to the main tumor, if not detected, can result in recurrence within the stump in up to 20% of cases.[32] Historically, this led surgeons to recommend radical resection of the entire bone, which resulted in poor functional and esthetic outcomes and no improvement in overall survival.[32] Currently, with the availability of MRI, the entire involved bone must be imaged to detect any noncontiguous disease. Furthermore, the involvement of neurovascular structures, as meticulously assessed on MRI, may also preclude limb salvage. When carefully screened by experienced orthopedic oncologists, contemporary limb salvage surgery does not appear to impart a survival disadvantage.[33–35]

After induction (neoadjuvant) chemotherapy, a preoperative follow-up assessment of the tumor must be performed. The response to chemotherapy can be assessed by dynamic MRI, although positron emission tomography (PET) and perhaps thallium scanning may also provide useful information.[36–40] In certain cases, an individual who was a questionable candidate for limb salvage may become eligible after induction chemotherapy. Nevertheless, if the margins are precarious at the preoperative staging evaluation, then amputation is necessary.

Complications are far more frequent in limb salvage patients than in those who undergo amputation. However, as techniques evolve, the complication rate is steadily decreasing. Furthermore, patients who present with a pathologic fracture or sustain a fracture during induction chemotherapy may be poor candidates for limb salvage surgery. These are not absolute contraindications, however.[41–43]

The decision to amputate is a complex one and must involve the entire team of health care providers. The age of the patient, location of the tumor, presence or absence of pathologic fracture, and the desires of the patient and family must be considered carefully. Functionally, in the upper extremity, amputation leads to very poor results. Accordingly, aggressive reconstruction with vascular and/or nerve grafting as necessary should be done to save even limited hand and wrist function. If an adequate margin cannot be obtained, however, then amputation is necessary. In the lower extremity, external hemipelvectomy leads to a particularly poor functional result. A hip disarticulation at least permits improved sitting, although prosthetic use remains poor. For tumors above the proximal tibia, limb salvage with one of the above techniques is preferable to amputation and can potentially give equal functional results. Patients undergoing above-knee amputation have increased energy expenditure compared with those undergoing endoprosthetic reconstruction.[44] A knee arthrodesis is intermediate between these two.[45] Tibial diaphyseal lesions often are amenable to limb salvage. However, for malignant tumors about the ankle, a distal, below-knee amputation is generally preferable to limb salvage. In a study evaluating psychosocial adjustment, physical complaints were reported more often in patients undergoing limb salvage, yet amputees tended to have lower self-esteem and experienced more social isolation.[46]

SURGERY FOR METASTATIC DISEASE

The surgical approach to metastatic disease from a bone tumor is a function of the type of sarcoma involved. For osteosarcoma, aggressive surgical resection of all overt metastatic disease is necessary if long-term disease-free survival is to be achieved. Both lung and other bony sites of involvement must be removed.[47–52] To effect cure, metastatic osteosarcoma to other bones must be approached with the same considerations as the primary: to remove the entire diseased site with an uninvolved surgical margin. Most pulmonary lesions can be removed by wedge resection without recurrence and with maximum preservation of lung capacity.[53] Occasionally, more aggressive pulmonary resection is necessary. Bilateral lung involvement can be approached with staged lateral thoracotomies or a single median sternotomy. Although the latter technique allows a single procedure, exposure is limited, as the retrocardiac and left lower lobe are particularly difficult to visualize. Thoracoscopic resection, with or without computerized tomography-assisted localization, is being used more frequently in major centers.[54] However, such techniques may not allow the surgeon to evaluate the entire lung as well as in an open procedure. Furthermore, because of the technical challenges of thoracoscopy, local spread of tumor has been reported.[55] Because Ewing's sarcoma and lymphoma are radiosensitive tumors, radiation is generally used for metastatic foci. In Ewing's sarcoma metastatic lesions must be carefully and individually assessed, as surgery may play a select role in the effort to effect a cure.

CHEMOTHERAPY

Adjuvant chemotherapy for bone tumors will be discussed with the specific tumors. Its use is clearly appropriate for high-grade osteosarcoma, the Ewing's sarcoma family of tumors (ESFT), and malignant fibrous histiocytoma of bone. The treatment of dedifferentiated chondrosarcoma, Paget's-associated and irradiation-associated sarcomas, and angiosarcoma is debatable, but the poor prognosis for these makes chemotherapy trials reasonable. The agents that have had the most use include methotrexate, doxorubicin, cisplatin, ifosfamide, cyclophosphamide, and etoposide. These drugs are used in various combinations. In general, preoperative or neoadjuvant therapy is used in addition to postoperative therapy.

RADIATION THERAPY

Irradiation is the local treatment of choice for myeloma and lymphoma of bone. Its use in the management of ESFT is controversial and debated. This is discussed later. The benefits of irradiation are the treatment of a larger local area than surgery, no operative risk, and no need to replace the normal tissue removed at surgery. The disadvantages are permanent damage to normal tissue, the potential for regrowth of tumor cells not killed by the irradiation, and the risk of a later irradiation-associated tumor. The risk/benefit ratio needs to be weighed before making a decision regarding the use of radiation in the treatment of bone tumors. In general, irradiation is often used for ESFT, myeloma, and lymphoma of bone, but not for the other bone tumors. Postoperative irradiation is used when the surgical margin is close or even positive if additional surgery is either not technically possible or when the additional morbidity is unacceptable to the patient.

SPECIFIC BONE TUMORS

Benign Bone Tumors The World Health Organization has classified the categories of benign bone tumors (Table 110-3).

Table 110-3 World Health Organization Classification of Benign Bone Tumors

Bone-forming tumors
Osteoma
Osteoid osteoma
Osteoblastoma
Cartilage-forming tumors
Chondroma
Osteochondroma
Chondroblastoma
Chondromyxoid fibroma
Giant cell tumor
Benign vascular tumors
Hemangioma
Lymphangioma
Glomus tumor
Other benign connective tissue tumors
Desmoplastic fibroma
Fibrous histiocytoma
Lipoma
Neurilemoma
Neurofibroma
Tumor-like conditions
Solitary bone cyst
Aneurysmal bone cyst
Metaphyseal fibrous defect
Eosinophilic granuloma
Fibrous dysplasia
Osteofibrous dysplasia
Myositis ossificans
Brown tumor of hyperparathyroidism
Intraosseous epidermoid cyst
Giant cell (reparative) granuloma

From Gitelis S, McDonald DJ. General classification and staging. In: Simon MA, Springfield D, editors. Surgery for bone and soft-tissue tumors. Philadelphia: Lippincott-Raven; 1998. p. 120.

Aneurysmal Bone Cyst Aneurysmal bone cyst is a benign bone lesion. It is a radiolucent lesion with expansion or so-called ballooning of the bone (Figure 110-5). It is a lesion seen predominantly in children, rarely before the age of 10 years or after the age of 25 years. The lesion occurs in the metaphyses of long bones, but it can

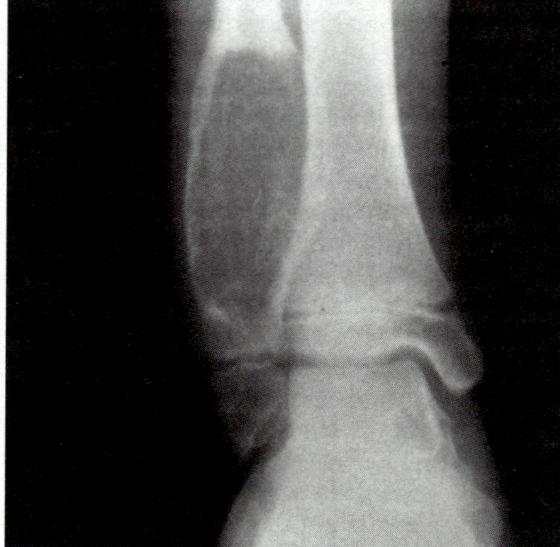

Figure 110-5 An aneurysmal bone cyst arising in the distal fibula of a 14-year-old female. Note the clear and sharply defined margins defining the extent of disease in this lesion. The tumor has thinned and expanded the cortex but has not broken through it. Because of its size and location, this tumor was treated by simple excision of the distal end of the fibula.

also affect the bones of the axial skeleton, including vertebral bodies. When it involves a vertebra it involves the posterior elements and can extend into the body.

Aneurysmal bone cysts may be painless; the patient often presents with swelling of the affected area. Other times the patient complains of an ache in the affected extremity. Rarely, neurologic findings are present when it involves the spine. An occasional patient presents with a pathologic fracture.

Even if the diagnosis is suspected from the clinical presentation and radiographic appearance, a biopsy is necessary to make the diagnosis. Telangiectic osteosarcoma can have the same presentation and must be excluded.

Histologically, aneurysmal bone cysts consist of large vascular channels lined with plump epithelioid cells. Many of the lesions show fibroblastic proliferation that may infiltrate the surrounding bone, and multinucleated giant cells are common (Figure 110-6). These same findings are not uncommon in a variety of benign bone tumors, and some authors say that 50% of aneurysmal bone cysts are secondary lesions. Although this may be literally true, it is not clinically significant, since the vast majority of such secondary aneurysmal bone cysts are not obvious, and the patient presents for the primary lesion.

Aneurysmal bone cysts are active lesions that need surgical treatment. A curettage, usually combined with bone grafting, is an effective treatment. Recurrence is not uncommon, but a repeat curettage most often controls the lesion. Adjuvants such as phenol or freezing (cryosurgery) can be used, but there is no evidence that these are necessary. On very rare occasions a recurrence will behave as an aggressive lesion. It is critical to exclude the possibility that the lesion is a telangiectic osteosarcoma, and if this has been done, a complete resection can be done or local irradiation used.

Radiation therapy is an effective treatment of aneurysmal bone cysts, but should be used with caution. The most significant risk is a secondary radiation-associated sarcoma.[56,57] These are uncommon, and when they occur, do so after 7 or more years. The minimum effective dose of radiotherapy for aneurysmal bone cysts has not been established. Doses varying from 1,100 to 4,000 cGy have been used.[56,58] Although most authors now recommend 1,400 to 2,000 cGy, relapse after 3,850 cGy has been reported.[59]

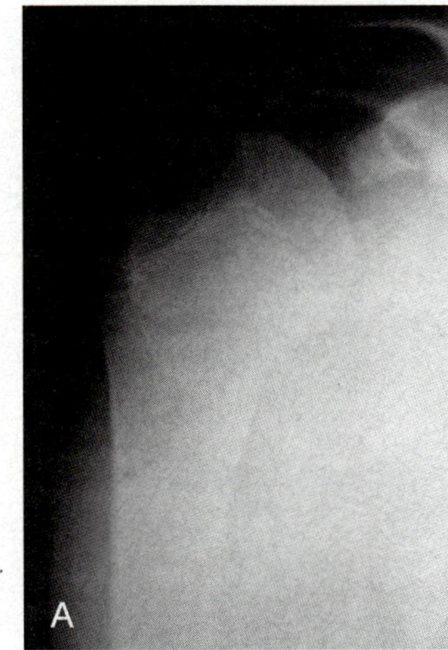

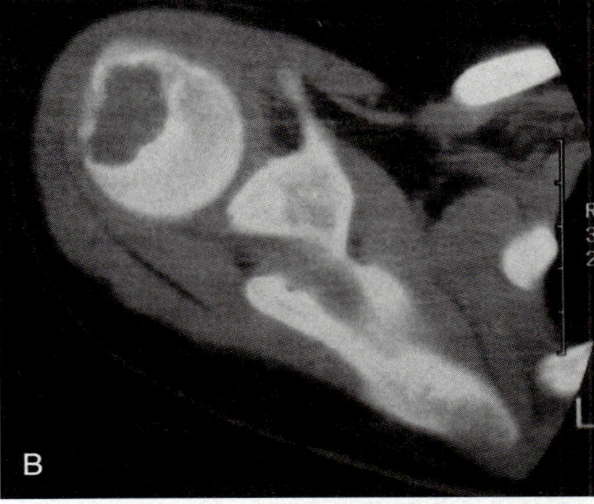

Figure 110-7 **A,** A classic chondroblastoma in a typical location in a 13-year-old girl. The radiograph shows the lesion located in the proximal humeral epiphysis, and the computed tomography scan **(B)** demonstrates the extent and the nature of the benign cartilage tumor.

Chondroblastoma Chondroblastoma is a benign bone tumor. It is an uncommon tumor representing less than 1% of all primary bone tumors. The tumor is more common in males. It occurs most commonly in patients with open growth plates or shortly after they close. Therefore, it is uncommon to see an adult with chondroblastoma. The tumor arises in the secondary ossification center and is most common in the proximal humerus, followed by the epiphyseal centers of the femur and tibia. Patients present with pain and often have loss of motion in the adjacent joint. The lesion can be difficult to see on a radiograph, and it is not uncommon for the symptoms to be thought to be from an intra-articular abnormality.

The radiographic appearance of chondroblastoma is a well-circumscribed small lesion appearing in the epiphysis of a growing adolescent. The lesion is usually well marginated and frequently shows stippled calcification (Figure 110-7). It consists predominantly of chondroblast, which are cuboidal-shaped cells with a prominent nucleus. There is often an amorphous matrix but, rarely, true hyaline cartilage. Fine, lacey calcification is characteristic and is referred as "chicken wire" calcification. Multinucleated giant cells can be quite numerous (Figure 110-8).

Chondroblastoma should are treated with a thorough curettage. Up to a third of chondroblastomas will recur after a curettage, but only rarely will they behave as a locally aggressive neoplasm. Often it is best to approach the lesion through the joint so the epiphysis is not damaged.

Chondromyxoid Fibroma Chondromyxoid fibroma is a rare benign tumor of bone. It is composed of myxoid tissue with scattered foci of chondroid differentiation and fibrous tissue. The tumor can occur in any age group, but is most frequent during the second decade of life. It is slightly more common in females, and although it can occur in all the long bones, short tubular bones of the extremities, and flat bones, it is most common in the tibia.

The patient usually complains of a dull pain. The bone may be tender and a mass is occasionally palpable. The radiographic appearance is

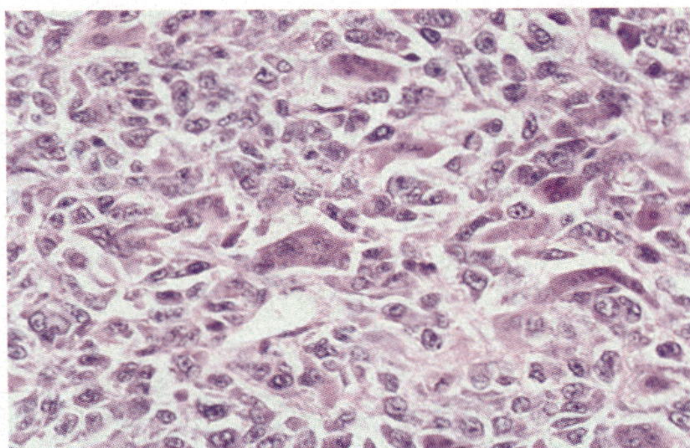

Figure 110-6 Aneurysmal bone cyst. Dilated spaces are separated by variably cellular fibrous septae. The spaces lack either an epithelial or an endothelial lining and instead are bounded by osteoclast-like giant cells, fibroblasts and myofibroblasts.

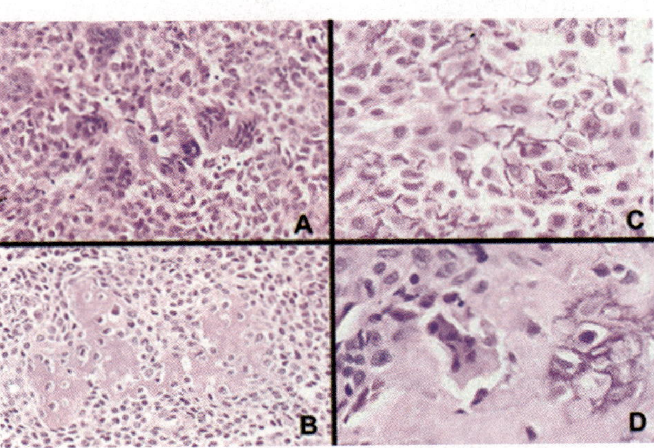

Figure 110-8 Chondroblastoma. **A,** This lesion is characterized by an admixture of mononuclear cells and multinucleated giant cells. **B,** Foci of immature hyaline cartilage. **C,** "Chicken wire" calcification. **D,** Mature hyaline cartilage, often with calcification.

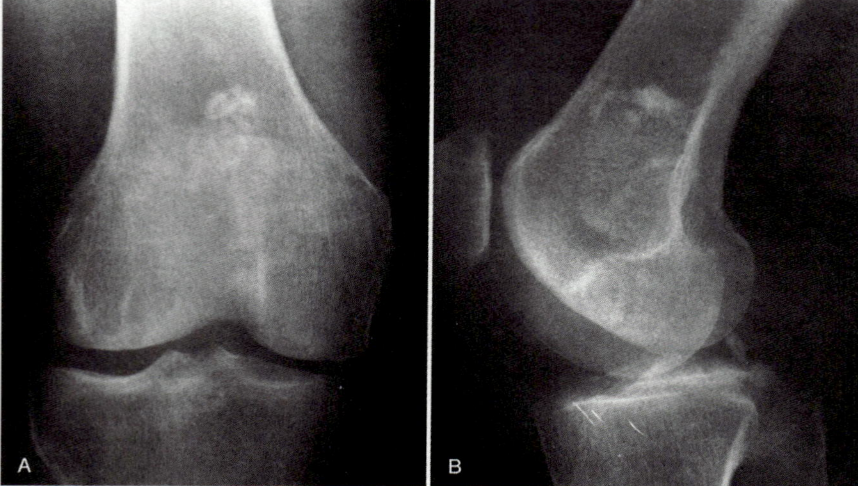

Figure 110-9 **A,** Enchondromas are benign lesions in which the marrow cavity is replaced by often heavily calcified cartilage. **B,** Note that the cortex is intact and the lesion is not actively destroying the bone.

similar to an aneurysmal bone cyst. Chondromyxoid fibroma can be mistaken for a chondrosarcoma by the unsuspecting pathologist.

Whenever possible, chondromyxoid fibroma is best treated with a surgical excision. This can be accomplished with limited morbidity in many cases, as only a portion of the bone needs to be removed and none of the articular cartilage requires removal. When the morbidity of an excision is excessive, a thorough curettage is advised, although the tumor may recur.[60]

Enchondroma Enchondromas are benign cartilaginous lesions within the medullary cavity of the bone. They affect both sexes with equal frequency. They are common in the hands and feet and tend to be diagnosed at these sites earlier than other sites because of either a pathologic fracture or palpable enlargement of the digit. They are diagnosed at other sites most commonly when a radiograph or bone scan is done for an unrelated reason.

Enchondromas probably are residual cartilage from the epiphysis, and are, therefore, located in the metaphysis of long bones. The radiographic appearance depends on when it is found (Figure 110-9). Until the age of about 30 years, enchondromas are radiolucent, but as the patient ages calcification is common. There should be no periosteal reaction or penetration of the cortex.

Enchondromas are composed of nests of hyaline cartilage that have ossified rims around them and often areas of calcification. The normal surrounding marrow spaces are not infiltrated or destroyed by sheets of cartilage, as is seen in chondrosarcomas (Figure 110-10).

The most difficult aspect of enchondroma is differentiating it from low-grade chondrosarcoma. The clinical setting, radiographic appearance, and histologic picture must be combined to accurately differentiate between the two tumors. Enchondroma is rarely associated with pain, while low-grade chondrosarcoma usually causes pain. Enchondroma does not penetrate the cortex or produce periosteal reaction, while chondrosarcoma does both. Enchondroma has inactive cartilage, while low-grade chondrosarcoma is composed of active cartilage cells. The low-power histologic examination of an enchondroma is quite characteristic and is said to be easy to differentiate from a low-grade chondrosarcoma with the criteria developed by Mirra and colleagues.[61] It is not always that easy, and distinguishing between these two tumors is one of the most difficult tasks in musculoskeletal oncology. It is uncommon that a biopsy will allow definitive differentiation of enchondroma from low-grade chondrosarcoma.

If the patient has multiple enchondromas, they are said to have Ollier's disease. They have an increased risk of malignant degeneration compared with patients with a solitary lesion. There is no known inheritance pattern for Ollier's disease. Patients with Ollier's disease and hemangiomas are said to have Maffucci disease. These patients have an almost 100% risk of developing a malignancy, but it is more likely to be a glioma or carcinoma elsewhere than a sarcoma.

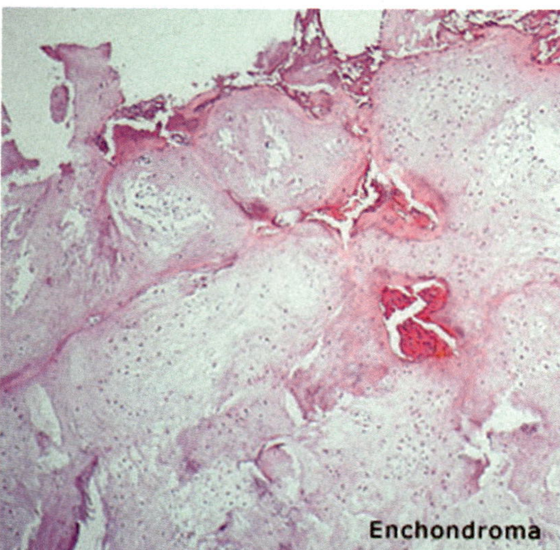

Figure 110-10 Enchondroma. The lobulated pattern that is typical of enchondroma is readily appreciated in this low magnification view. The margins of the lesion appear sharp rather than infiltrative, although the actual relationship to the host bone is difficult to assess in this fragment from a curettage.

Most benign enchondromas do not require surgical treatment. Patients with enchondromatosis may require corrective surgery for both functional and cosmetic deformities produced by the multiple lesions. The major indication for treatment is the possibility of degeneration of the benign enchondroma into a chondrosarcoma, or the differential diagnosis of a large solitary enchondroma to rule out a chondrosarcoma.

Enchondroma is rarely painful, and when the patient has persistent pain from the lesion, it should be removed. The risk of malignant transformation exists, but this is probably extremely rare. As a routine, when the enchondroma is found, it is evaluated with plain radiographs, MRI, and bone scan, and then the patient is followed with periodic radiographs.

When biopsy of an enchondroma is performed to exclude the possibility of chondrosarcoma, it is important to realize that further treatment of a chondrosarcoma may require a radical en bloc resection. The placement of the biopsy incision should, therefore, be done as if it would relate to a possible future radical en bloc resection, should a chondrosarcoma be discovered. In addition, care must be taken to carry out the biopsy in an area where there is suspected malignant degeneration, since malignant degeneration within an enchondroma may take place in only one portion of the tumor. CT and MRI are helpful in guiding the surgeon to the area of suspected rapid growth, which is where the biopsy should be made. When a biopsy is done, if the frozen section is benign, it is best to do a complete curettage. This eliminates the risk of a sampling error and removes the entire lesion.

Eosinophilic Granuloma Eosinophilic granuloma is one of three presentations of what is now called Langerhans cell histiocytoma (LCH). It is a benign bone lesion that can occur in either solitary or multifocal forms.[56,62] Hand-Schüller-Christian disease and Letterer-Siwe disease are two other manifestations of this disorder. The bone lesions are composed of Langerhans cells (a type of histiocyte) mixed with eosinophils, and other types of inflammatory cells. The Langerhans cell is the diagnostic cell. Langerhans cells can be identified on light microscopy, but are best confirmed on electron microscopy. Recent evidence suggests that the lesion is a neoplasm rather than a response to a virus infection, as was previously thought.

Eosinophilic granuloma predominately occurs in childhood and is rarely seen above the age of 30 years. Patients present with mild pain usually without other complaints. Its clinical presentation can be identical to Ewing's sarcoma or osteomyelitis, and these two diagnoses should be in the differential. The multifocal variety tends to occur in younger children and may be progressive, requiring systemic therapy as well as local therapy. The solitary disease is nonprogressive, and the prognosis is excellent for cure.

Eosinophilic granuloma on the plain radiograph is a radiolucent lesion with a so-called punched-out appearance. There can be an acute periosteal reaction. Eosinophilic granuloma can occur in any bone, but the skull is a particularly

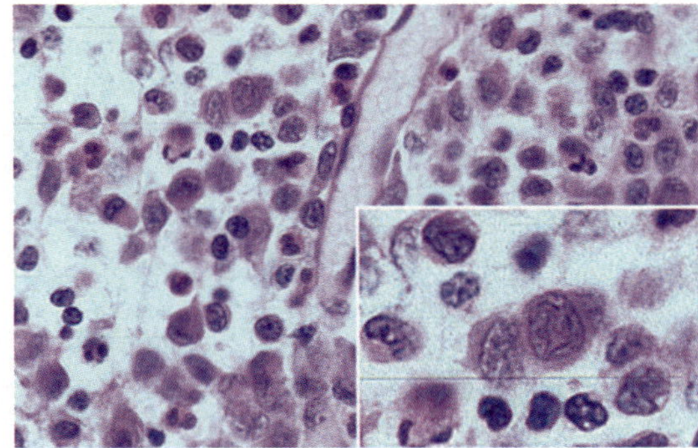

Figure 110-11 Eosinophilic granuloma (Langerhans cell histiocytosis). The lesion is comprised of Langerhans histiocytes and a polymorphous population of inflammatory cells. Langerhans histiocytes are characterized by abundant cytoplasm and large convoluted nuclei (*inset*).

common location. The body of a vertebra is another common location and may lead to a compression fracture. This often leads to an extremely flat vertebra or the so-called vertebra plana.

Biopsy is usually necessary. When the patient does not need stabilization of the bone, a fine-needle aspirate or needle biopsy is usually sufficient.

The Langerhans cells are large cells with a clear cytoplasm. They typically have a large nucleus that is kidney shaped or that has a longitudinal groove. Langerhans cell granules, also known as Birbeck granulaes, are seen on electron microscopy. There may be multinucleated phagocytic giant cells in some areas. The eosinophils present are secondary, and although usually prominent, are not necessary for the diagnosis. (Figure 110-11). Hodgkin's disease has a similar histologic appearance and should be considered in the differential diagnosis.

The world literature on treatment of LCH bone lesions was reviewed in 1980 by Slater and Swarm.[63] The overall local recurrence rate for 545 analyzable sites was 2.8%. Local control following radiotherapy with or without supplemental surgery was reported for 105 of 108 sites and 76 of 80 sites, respectively. Local control following curettage or excision was reported in 90 of 91 and 116 of 118, respectively. Biopsy alone resulted in healing of 13 of 15 lesions. There is no significant difference in the local control rate of bone lesions associated with monostotic LCH compared with polyostotic presentations.[64,65]

Usually the solitary lesions will spontaneously heal or heal after a biopsy, even needle biopsy (Figure 110-12). A curettage is appropriate if an open biopsy is done. Direct injection of corticosteroids will stimulate healing. Irradiation probably has been used too frequently, but can be used for spinal cord compression or recurrent lesions.

Fibrous Dysplasia Fibrous dysplasia is probably a neoplastic condition, but there is debate. It can occur as a single lesion, monostotic fibrous dysplasia, which is more common than the polyostotic variant. When the patient has polyostotic fibrous dysplasia and an endocrine abnormality, they have McCune-Albright syndrome.

Although probably present from late in the first decade or early in the second decade of life, it is usually not found until early adulthood. The patient may present with a pathologic fracture, mild pain with activity, or having had a radiograph for an unrelated reason. The patient may have a pigmented skin lesion called a café-au-lait spot with a highly serrated edge, of the coast of Maine type. This is more common in patients with polyostotic fibrous dysplasia.

Although monostotic fibrous dysplasia can affect any bone in the body, the ribs and the long bones are the most common sites. The radiographic appearance of fibrous dysplasia is characteristic of a benign bone tumor.[66] It usually produces an expansile lesion in the bone that does not break through the bony cortex. The lesion itself appears to be lucent and is frequently described as having a "ground-glass" appearance

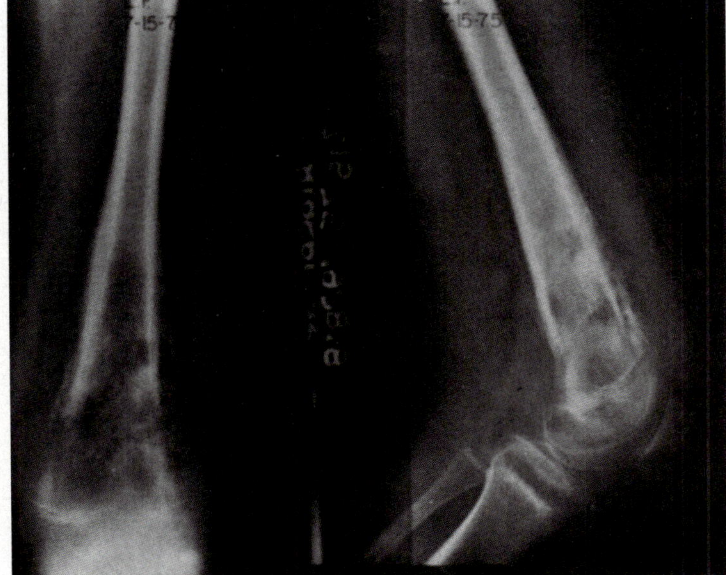

Figure 110-12 A mixed lytic and sclerotic destructive lesion with periosteal elevation and a soft tissue mass. This lesion is characteristic of a malignant lesion on radiographs. However, multiple biopsies were originally thought to represent benign eosinophilic granuloma in this 14-year-old male. After the fifth biopsy this was eventually diagnosed as primary Hodgkin's disease of bone. At the time of staging laparotomy, the patient was noted to have regional lymph node involvement as well as splenic involvement. In the latter areas, the histopathology showed characteristic Reed-Sternberg giant cells that were not present in the primary bone tumor that consisted of mostly a lymphocytic, a histiocytic, and an eosinophilic infiltrate. Initially, a diagnosis of eosinophilic granuloma was entertained; however, on repeat biopsies, an increasing amount of sclerosis or collagen formation was noted, leading to the diagnosis of nodular sclerosing Hodgkin's disease, primary of bone.

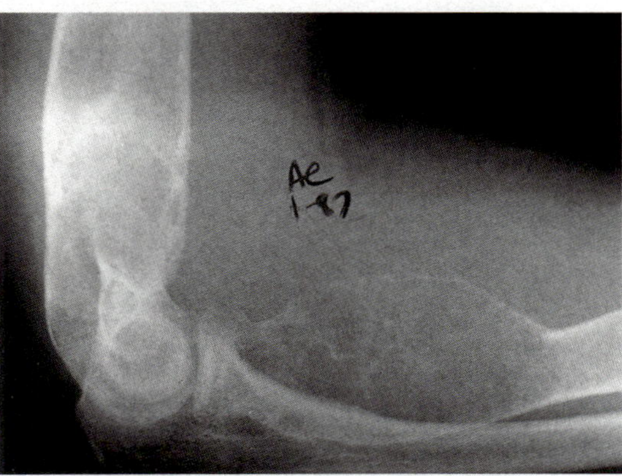

Figure 110-13 Fibrous dysplasia may be monostotic or polyostotic and limited or florid in extent. The proximal radius shows a remarkable degree of expansion with marked thinning of the cortices and a ground-glass appearance to the medullary cavity. The distal humerus shows less marked expansion but similar medullary and cortical abnormalities.

because of bone production within the tumor. When there is not much bone production within the fibrous dysplasia, the lesion may have a "soap-bubble" appearance (Figure 110-13). Often the diagnosis is made based on the clinical presentation and radiographic findings. The lesions usually have a marked uptake on a technetium bone scan.

Microscopic examination reveals that fibrous dysplasia is composed of a benign fibrous stroma and spicules of immature bone. The bone is woven bone and has no organization to its arrangement. Osteofibrous dysplasia is similar microscopically and should be distinguished from fibrous dysplasia. Low-grade osteosarcoma also has a similar appearance.

The treatment of fibrous dysplasia depends on the patient's symptoms and the strength of the bone. When the patient does not have pain and the bones are not significantly weakened, observation is all that is needed. If the patient has pain, curettage and bone grafting are indicated; if the bone is progressively deforming, surgical correction of the deformity is recommended. Sarcoma complicating fibrous dysplasia is a rare but reported event.[67,68]

Giant Cell Tumor The giant cell tumor of bone, sometimes called osteoclastoma, is a benign but aggressive neoplasm representing approximately 5% of all primary bone tumors.[69] The peak incidence of this tumor is in the third decade of life. The tumor is extremely rare in prepubescent adolescents, and the diagnosis of giant cell tumor in this age group should raise suspicion of misdiagnosis. The tumor is slightly more common in females. Giant cell tumors are almost always immediately adjacent to the subchondral bone and usually extend into the metaphysis. The majority are in the distal femur or proximal tibia. Other common sites are the distal radius and distal tibia. Giant cell tumors can occur in the spine and involve the vertebral body when they do.

Most patients present with pain that seems to be coming from the adjacent joint. There may be a palpable mass and the bone is usually tender. The mass may pulsate.

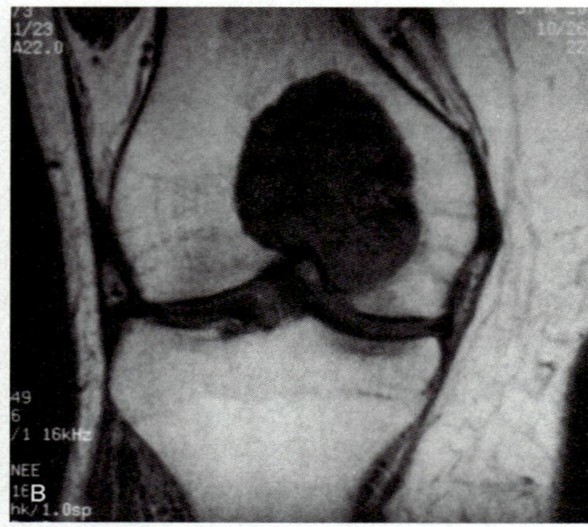

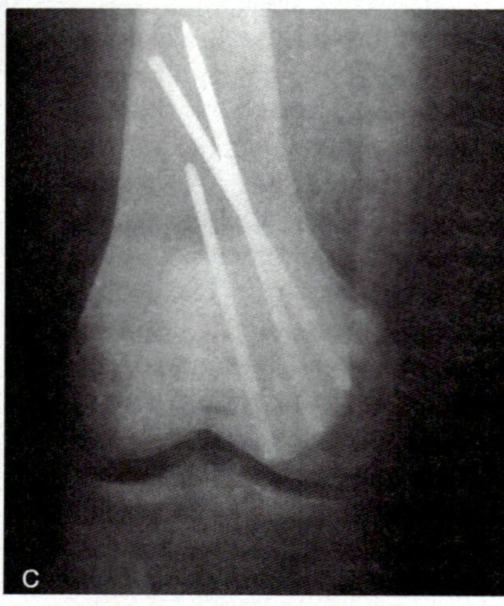

Figure 110-14 **A,** A classic giant cell tumor of the distal femur, purely lytic and thinning the cortex. It is eccentrically located and, as seen on the magnetic resonance image **(B)**, has broken into the joint. **C,** The lesion was curetted, the cavity washed with phenol, and after reconstruction of the breakout area with allograft, the cavity was filled with methyl methacrylate in which were implanted three wires for structural strength.

The radiograph of giant cell tumor is quite typical and includes a well-demarcated lesion that appears to arise in the epiphysis, usually of the distal femur or proximal tibia. There is often destruction of the cortex, although usually there is at least a thin rim of periosteal reactive bone (Figure 110-14). The clinical presentation and plain radiograph are almost diagnostic, although a fibroblastic osteosarcoma could have an identical appearance. A small percent (< 5%) will develop pulmonary lesions of benign giant cell tumor of bone. Therefore, a chest radiograph is done at presentation and repeated until the patient is at least 10 years from their diagnosis.

Histologically, giant cell tumors are composed of a benign spindle-cell stroma with numerous multinucleated giant cells among mononuclear cells that may be round, oval, or spindle-shaped. Characteristically, the nuclei of the benign spindle cells are identical in appearance to the nuclei in the multinucleated giant cells. Mitotic figures are common. Frequently, there is a component of aneurysmal bone cyst associated with the giant cell tumor (Figure 110-15).

The differential diagnosis of a giant cell tumor includes other rare benign conditions, such as reparative granuloma of bone, "brown tumors" associated with hyperparathyroidism, and fibrous dysplasia. Problems in differential diagnosis arise when a giant cell tumor has extended outside the bone or when areas in the tumor show a sparsity of giant cells with a predominance of a spindle-cell stroma. In such instances, it may be difficult to differentiate benign giant cell tumor from the so-called malignant giant cell tumor of bone, which is, in fact, either a telangiectatic osteosarcoma or a malignant fibrous histiocytoma.

Giant cell tumor of bone is treated with curettage. The lesion has a local recurrence rate of up to 40%, and it seems that aggressive curettage can reduce the frequency of local recurrences. Therefore, the most common treatment is thorough curettage with the addition of using a high-speed burr to enlarge the cavity. Often an adjuvant (cryosurgery, laser, or phenol) is used, although none have been shown to be better than curettage alone. The resultant cavity is packed with bone graft (allograft or autograft) or polymethyl methacrylate. Local irradiation can be used for multirecurrent disease or for an aggressive lesion in the spine, but a postirradiation sarcoma is a risk.[70] Total dose determines success of radiotherapy. Virtually all authors now recommend 4,500 to 5,000 cGy. Particular attention must be directed to any soft tissue extension of giant cell tumor during portal design. Bennett recommended 3 to 5 cm margins around the entire lesion.[71]

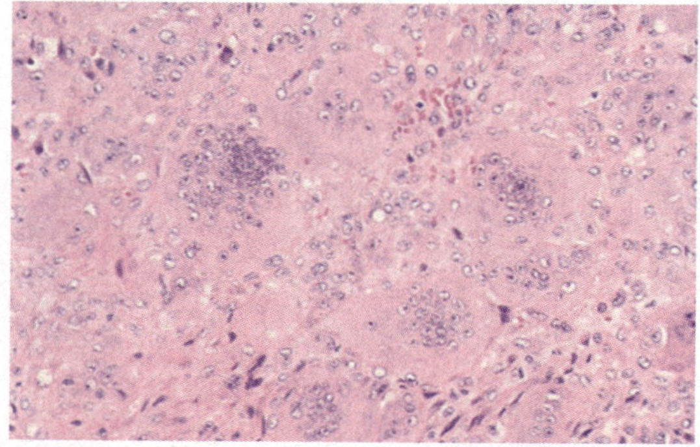

Figure 110-15 Giant cell tumor of bone. Large, multinucleated giant cells with abundant eosinophilic cytoplasm are admixed with spindled mononuclear stromal cells. Note the similarity between the nuclei of the giant cells and stromal cells.

"Benign" giant cell tumors have been noted to metastasize to the lungs. In the case of a solitary pulmonary metastasis, surgical resection of the pulmonary metastasis leads to a cure in most instances. Rarely does a patient develop multiple unresectable pulmonary metastases. This usually occurs in patients who have undergone multiple inadequate surgeries for the primary tumor.

Nonossifying Fibroma and Fibrous Cortical Defects Nonossifying fibroma and fibrous cortical defects are histologically identical. They are common lesions, and it is estimated that 20% of children have one of these two lesions. The vast majority spontaneously heal during the second decade of life. Rarely, a nonossifying fibroma enlarges sufficiently to weaken the bone enough to produce a pathologic fracture. These lesions are most commonly diagnosed based on their clinical presentation and radiographic appearance. Neither lesion causes pain. Nonossifying fibromas are located in the metaphysis of long bones, are eccentric within the medullary canal, and often the cortex is thinned and has not remodeled normally, leaving the metaphysis wider than normal. The endosteal border is marked by a thin rim of reactive bone that is irregular, giving the lesion the appearance of soap bubbles (Figure 110-16). Fibrous cortical defects are small cortical lesions also in the metaphysis of long bones. The lesion is directly under the periosteum with a thin rim of bone separating it from the medullary canal. The lesion is composed of fibrous tissue arranged in a whirling pattern, multinucleated giant cells, and often histiocytes with large amounts of clear cytoplasmic material, so-called foam cells. The risk of malignant degeneration is negligible (Figure 110-17).

Osteoid Osteoma Osteoid osteoma is a benign bone tumor with such a characteristic pain pattern that the diagnosis is usually made based on the pain pattern. The pain is intense, unremitting, usually noticed more at night, and almost always completely relieved with aspirin or a NSAID. The tumor has a peak incidence in the second decade of life. It is uncommon in patients under the age of 10 years and rare in adults over 30 years. The male-to-female ratio is 2.3:1. The most common sites of osteoid osteoma include the femur and tibia, but osteoid osteomas can occur anywhere in the skeleton. Osteoid osteomas of the spine and pelvis can cause considerable pain before they are diagnosed, since routine radiographs of these areas seldom

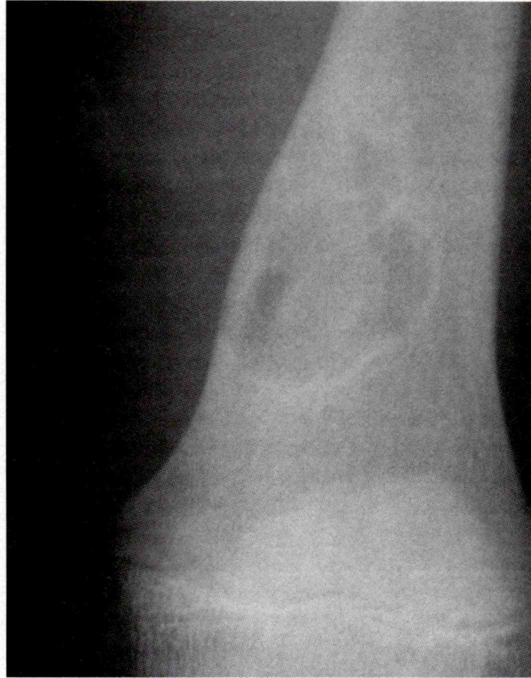

Figure 110-16 Anterior/posterior view of the distal femur. The nonossifying fibroma in the medial aspect of the femoral metaphysis is a typical stage 1 benign tumor. It has a narrow border of transition and easily seen reactive rim. It will heal spontaneously.

demonstrate the diagnostic radiographic findings.[72] Patients with an osteoid osteoma of the spine may have scoliosis.

The radiographic appearance of an osteoid osteoma is often diagnostic: a radiodense lesion with a central radiolucency. It may be on the endosteal surface, within the cortex, or on the periosteal surface (Figure 110-18). This "nidus" is the actual tumor, the density is just reactive bone. Sometimes, there is calcification within the tumor or nidus itself, giving the nidus a very small central density.

On gross inspection, the nidus of the tumor appears to be "cherry red" because of its rich blood supply. The nidus should be less than 2 cm in diameter and usually less than 1. Under

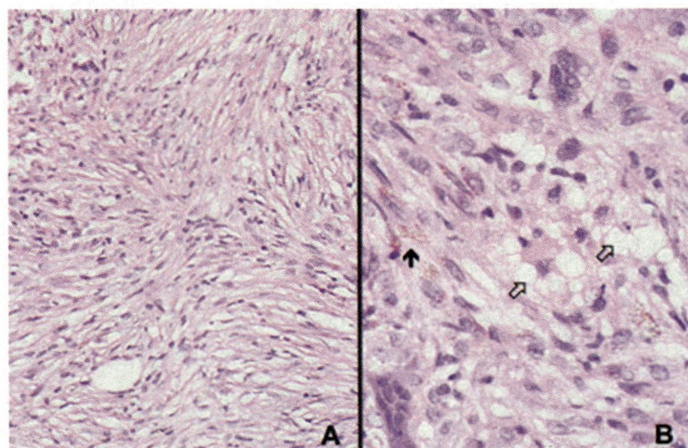

Figure 110-17 Nonossifying fibroma. **A,** The storiform pattern and relatively bland appearance of the spindle cells are evident at low magnification. **B,** In addition to the spindle cells, multinucleated giant cells, foamy histiocytes (*open arrows*), and hemosiderin-laden macrophages (*closed arrow*) are typically present in nonossifying fibroma.

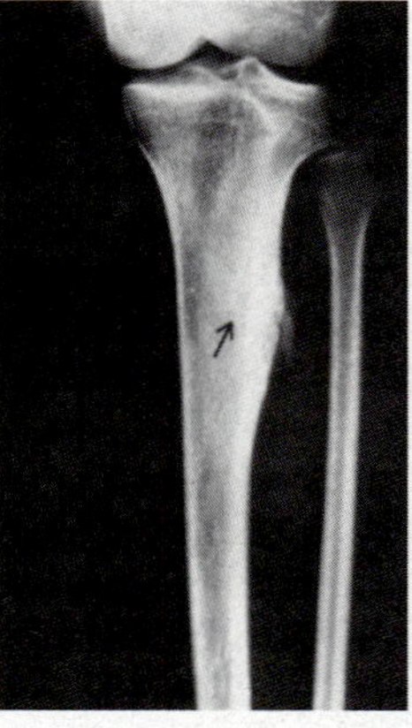

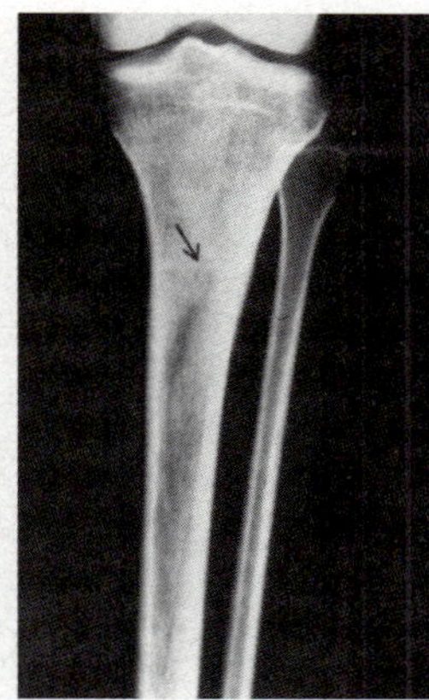

Figure 110-18 Radiograph of an osteoid osteoma in a 17-year-old male. The lesion produces dense cortical sclerosis; however, a characteristic "nidus" can be seen as a central lucent area (*arrow*) diagnostic of an osteoid osteoma.

the microscope, the tumor consists of thin wisps of woven bone lined with osteoblast, with a background rich in vessels (Figures 110-19 and 110-20).

The lesions will spontaneously resolve, but it may take years. The pain is usually so intense that most patients cannot tolerate waiting. Some patients can control their pain with minimal amounts of medication, but most require surgery. The traditional treatment was excision or an open burring, but more recently, percutaneous radiofrequency ablation is most commonly done.[5]

Osteoblastoma Osteoblastoma is a benign bone tumor that has the same histologic appearance as an osteoid osteoma but it is larger than 2 cm in diameter and usually more than 3 to 4 (Figure 110-21).[73] The patient is more commonly a male and usually in the second or third decade of life. Pain is the presenting complaint. Osteoblastoma occurs in the posterior elements of the spine and can produce scoliosis.

Osteoblastomas are usually radiolucent lesions, although some will have sufficiently mineralized bone to be radiodense. They occur in all bones, usually in the metaphysis or posterior elements of the spine[74] (Figure 110-22).

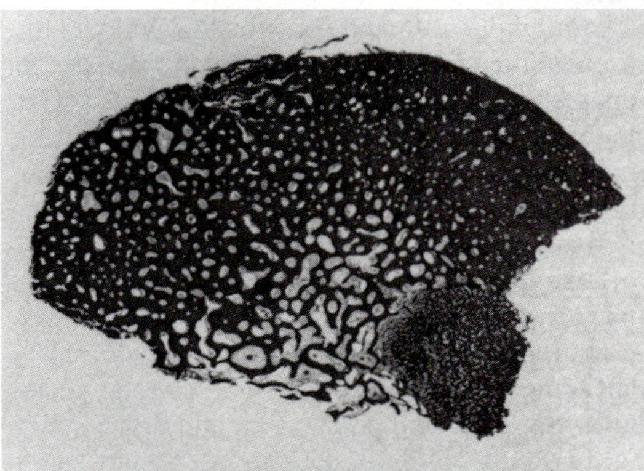

Figure 110-19 The characteristic histologic appearance of a resected osteoid osteoma. The tumor or nidus located in the lower right hand portion of the specimen contains richly anastomosing vascular channels as well as nerve fibers. There is calcification within this lesion. The lesion is surrounded by dense sclerotic reactive bone. (Courtesy of Dr. Joseph Mirra.)

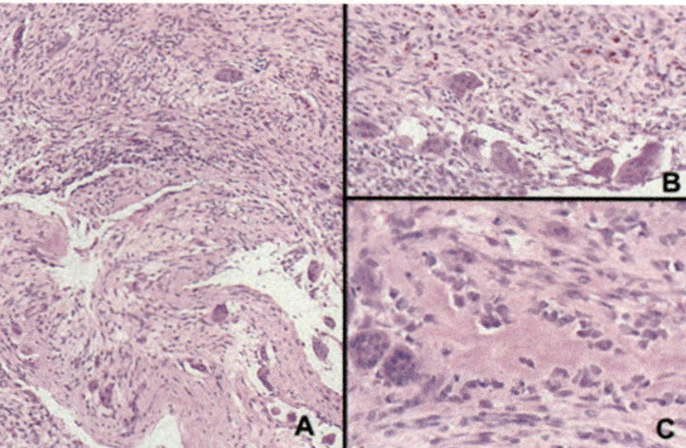

Figure 110-20 Osteoid osteoma. **A,** The more peripheral part of the lesion, seen at the left of the frame, consists of less mature, osteoid-rich trabeculae with prominent osteoblastic rimming and abundant, intervening cellular stroma. The central part of the lesion, seen at the right of the frame, consists of denser, woven bone with less prominent osteoblastic rimming. Osteoclasts present are adjacent to many trabeculae. **B** and **C,** Higher magnification view of osteoid-rich trabecula with osteoblastic rimming.

Surgery is the preferred method of treatment. If an excision can be done with limited morbidity this is best, but often a curettage is done so as to preserve bone. This is usually adequate, but if the lesion recurs, a complete resection is indicated. Irradiation has been used for recurrent lesions in the spine, but is of questionable value.[75–80]

Jackson reviewed the osteoblastoma literature in 1978.[80] Eighteen recurrences were noted in a total population of 181 patients. All recurrences occurred in those patients initially incompletely resected. Seven recurrent patients had been electively irradiated after incomplete tumor removal, while 11 received no adjunctive treatment. Marsh and colleagues also documented progressive osteoblastoma despite postoperative radiotherapy.[79] The natural history of osteoblastoma is unpredictable. Several authors have reported patients free of clinical recurrence years following incomplete curettage alone.[78] Malignant transformation of osteoblastoma to

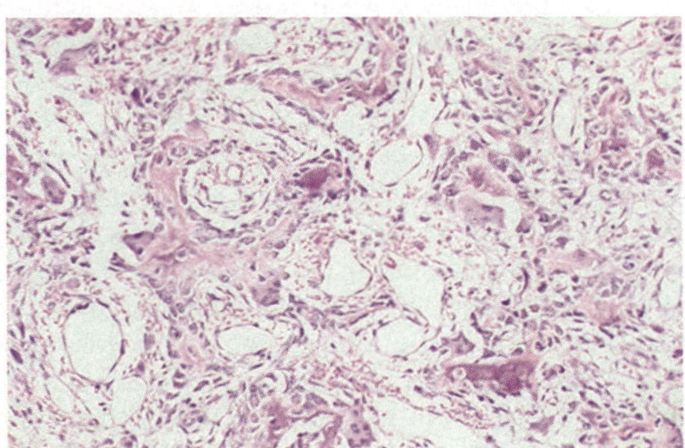

Figure 110-21 Osteoblastoma. The trabeculae have prominent osteoblastic rimming. Dilated capillaries are evident in the intervening fibrovascular stroma.

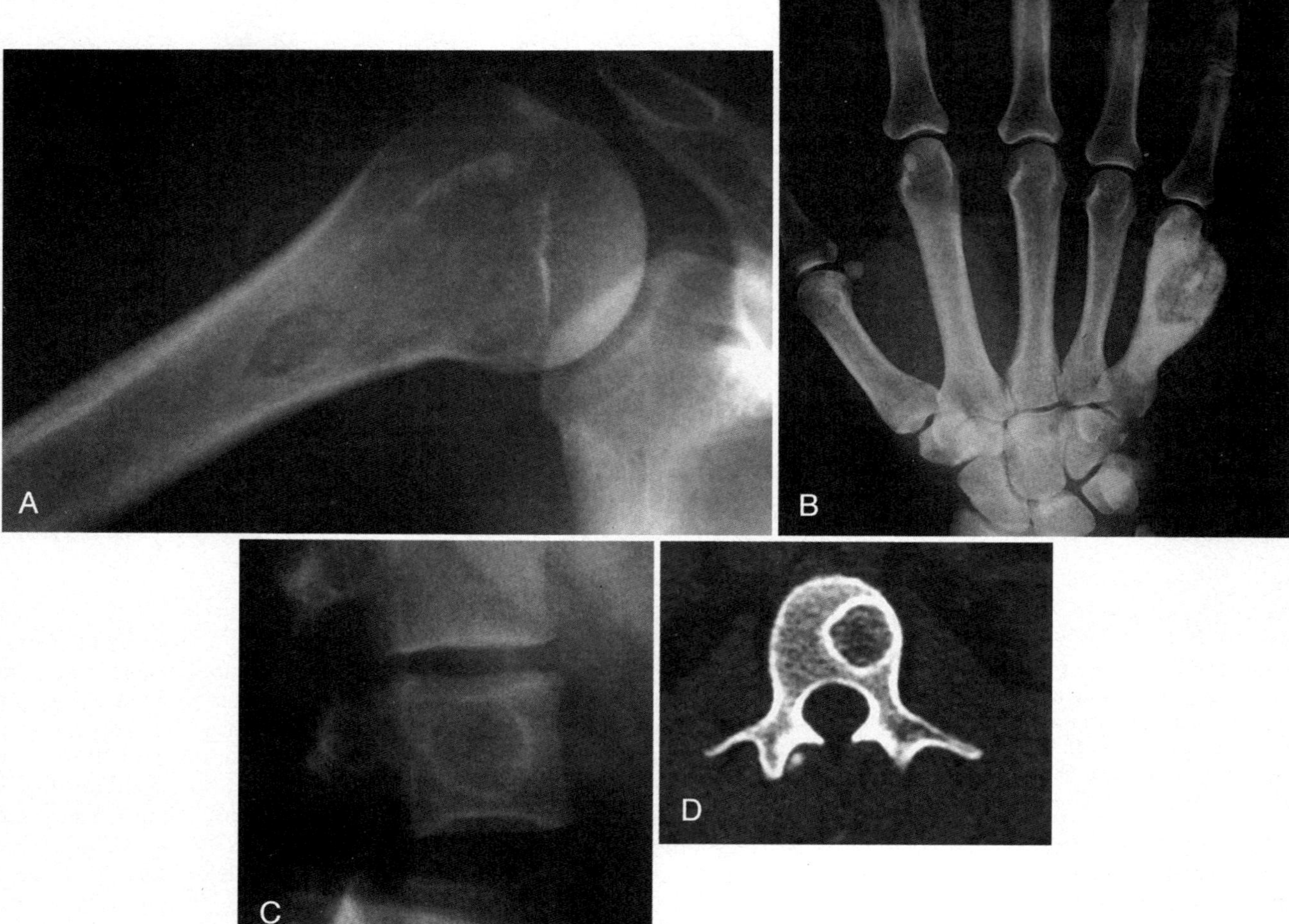

Figure 110-22 Osteoblastoma is a benign lesion of bone. This is an example of a lesion in the 5th metacarpal. The lesions can be radiolucent.

osteosarcoma has also been both with and without prior radiotherapy use.[80]

Osteochondroma Osteochondroma is a benign cartilaginous lesion usually referred to as a benign osteocartilaginous exostosis or simply exostosis. Osteochondromas are developmental defects, probably caused by cartilaginous nests that are left behind at the periphery of the advancing growing epiphyseal plate. There is a hereditary syndrome of multiple osteochondromata (or hereditary multiple cartilaginous exostoses, MHE).

Osteochondromas account for approximately 50% of all benign bone tumors diagnosed and approximately 15% of all primary skeletal lesions. They usually are discovered in growing adolescents when a painless hard mass is noted near the end of a long bone. They occur with equal frequency in males and females. The tumor is more common in the long bones and usually grows in the metaphysis adjacent to the epiphyseal cartilage plate. As the normal bone continues to grow, the osteochondroma appears to be located farther away from the epiphyseal cartilage plate in the metaphysis or metaphysis diaphyseal junction. The majority of osteochondromas occur about the knee, with the femur a slightly more common site than the tibia. Osteochondromas are not uncommon in the humerus and the distal extremities. They can occur in the spine and pelvis, but when they are at these sites they are usually in patients with hereditary multiple exostosis.

In general, biopsy is not necessary, since the radiographic diagnosis of an osteochondroma is usually sufficiently accurate (Figure 110-23). The diagnostic characteristics are that the cortex of the host bone and the cortex of the osteochondroma are in continuity, and the medullary canal of the host bone and medullary canal of the osteochondroma are also in continuity. The lesion has a cartilaginous cap, and some of this will usually have calcifications, giving the lesion an irregular appearance at its top. When patients have MHE, they usually have many characteristic-appearing bones with short broad femoral necks, short forearm bones, and the distal radius or distal tibia is often angulated.

Histologically, the osteochondroma consists of a cap of hyaline cartilage, which is more cellular than articular cartilage and more distorted in appearance, but the cells are small and the nuclei uniformly dark on hematoxylin and eosin staining. In young children, the cap is a site of endochondral ossification leading to the mass of bone that forms the exostosis. As the individual ages, the cartilage becomes considerably thinner and often heavily calcified.

The syndrome of hereditary multiple osteocartilaginous exostoses is one of the most common genetic errors affecting the skeleton. The male-to-female ratio is approximately 3:1. The syndrome is inherited as an autosomal dominant trait. In patients with multiple osteocartilaginous exostoses, follow-up examinations are indicated at frequent intervals during the adolescent years.

Surgical removal is indicated for symptoms related to direct irritation of the overlying tissues, especially nerves and blood vessels. Some lesions become so large that they are cosmetically unattractive. It is best not to resect lesions in the growing child, as recurrence is common. After the patient has reached skeletal maturity, recurrence is much less common. When removing an osteochondroma, it is important not to violate the cartilaginous cap, as this increases the risk of recurrence, even in an adult.

An osteochondroma that enlarges after the patient is 30 years of age is worrisome. A true malignancy from a solitary osteochondroma is exceedingly rare, but lesions with cartilaginous caps that are more than 2 cm thick in an adult patient are usually referred to as a "secondary chondrosarcoma," and excision is advised. Patients with MHE are at greater risk of developing secondary chondrosarcomas than patients with solitary lesions. The incidence is not known but is low.

Unicameral Bone Cysts Unicameral bone cysts, also called simple bone cysts, are common

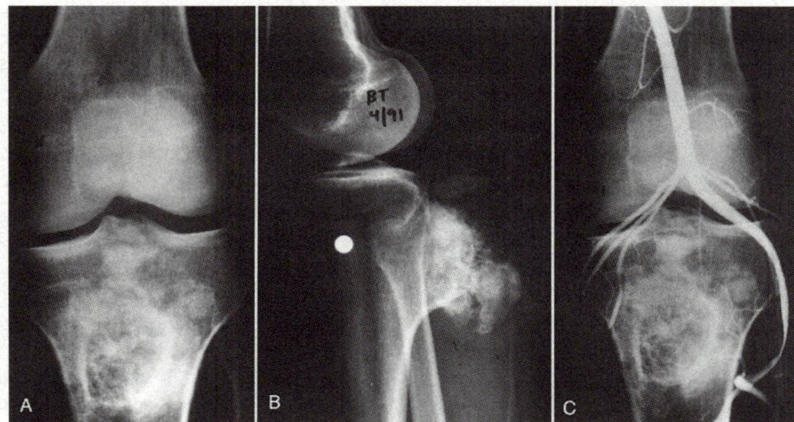

Figure 110-23 **A,** Osteochondroma (osteocartilaginous exostosis) is a benign lesion that may be solitary or multiple and extends from the metaphysis of the long bones into the adjacent soft tissues. **B,** The lesion shares a cortex with the bone. **C,** Such a lesion arising from the proximal tibia compromised the vascular trifurcation, requiring resection.

lesions of childhood.[81] They probably arise during the second half of the first decade of life, and spontaneously heal usually in the middle of the second decade. They may not be true "tumors," but should be considered with the other benign bone tumors because they are often in the differential diagnosis. These lesions, characteristically centrally located, seem to arise from the epiphyseal growth plate. After the patient reaches 10 years of age, the epiphyseal growth plate tends to grow away from the cyst, leaving it in the metaphysis. The lesion is radiolucent and is filled with clear, yellow, synovial-like fluid. Pathologic fractures are a common reason they are discovered. The fracture is usually minimally displaced, is usually treated without surgery, and the fractures heal normally. The only reason to treat the patient with a unicameral bone cyst is to prevent a fracture. The most common treatment is a direct injection of corticosteroids, bone marrow, or a material to stimulate bone formation.

Malignant Bone Tumors Sarcomas of bone are staged using the Enneking Staging System (see Table 110-1) or according to the guidelines of the American Joint Committee (Table 110-4).

Adamantinoma Adamantinoma is a low-grade malignant tumor with a metastatic rate of less than 20%. A mildly painful lesion in the anterior cortex of the tibia in a male between 20 and 40 years of age is the most common presentation. It has been reported in other anatomic locations, but this is unusual. The tumor represents less than 1% of primary bone tumors. The radiographic appearance of the adamantinoma is quite characteristic and usually presents with a mixed lytic and sclerotic lesion eccentrically placed in the tibia (Figure 110-24).

Adamantinoma is composed of a background fibrous stroma, often with a wisp of woven bone that is consistent with osteofibrous dysplasia with foci of epithelioid nests that resemble basal cell carcinoma or carcinoma of the breast scattered throughout the fibrous stroma. An enormous number of histologic variants of adamantinoma have been described: follicular, pigmented, acanthomatous, plexiform, granular cell, stellate, basaloid, ameloblastic fibroma, and adenoameloblastoma.[82] The histologic pattern of these tumors, however, does not reliably predict their clinical course or serve as a guide to therapeutic decision making. Morphologic

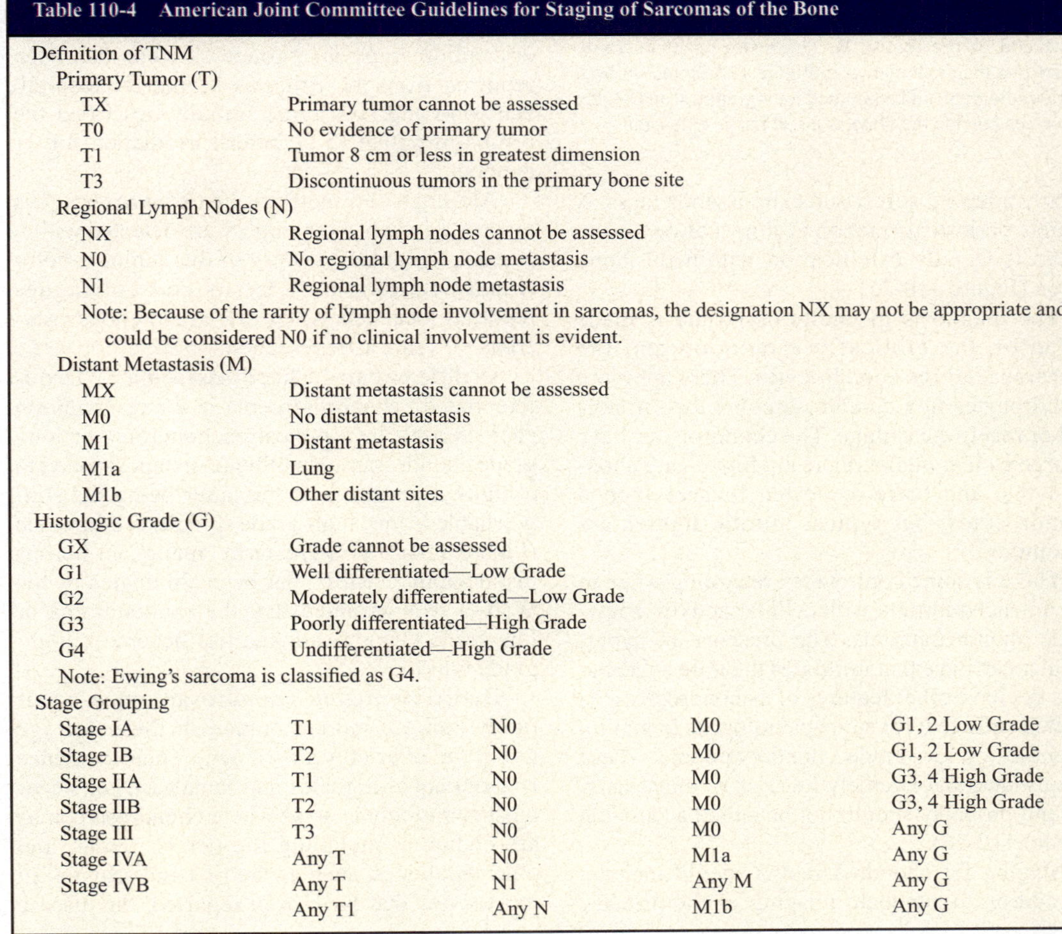

Table 110-4 American Joint Committee Guidelines for Staging of Sarcomas of the Bone

Definition of TNM				
Primary Tumor (T)				
TX	Primary tumor cannot be assessed			
T0	No evidence of primary tumor			
T1	Tumor 8 cm or less in greatest dimension			
T3	Discontinuous tumors in the primary bone site			
Regional Lymph Nodes (N)				
NX	Regional lymph nodes cannot be assessed			
N0	No regional lymph node metastasis			
N1	Regional lymph node metastasis			
Note: Because of the rarity of lymph node involvement in sarcomas, the designation NX may not be appropriate and could be considered N0 if no clinical involvement is evident.				
Distant Metastasis (M)				
MX	Distant metastasis cannot be assessed			
M0	No distant metastasis			
M1	Distant metastasis			
M1a	Lung			
M1b	Other distant sites			
Histologic Grade (G)				
GX	Grade cannot be assessed			
G1	Well differentiated—Low Grade			
G2	Moderately differentiated—Low Grade			
G3	Poorly differentiated—High Grade			
G4	Undifferentiated—High Grade			
Note: Ewing's sarcoma is classified as G4.				
Stage Grouping				
Stage IA	T1	N0	M0	G1, 2 Low Grade
Stage IB	T2	N0	M0	G1, 2 Low Grade
Stage IIA	T1	N0	M0	G3, 4 High Grade
Stage IIB	T2	N0	M0	G3, 4 High Grade
Stage III	T3	N0	M0	Any G
Stage IVA	Any T	N0	M1a	Any G
Stage IVB	Any T	N1	Any M	Any G
	Any T1	Any N	M1b	Any G

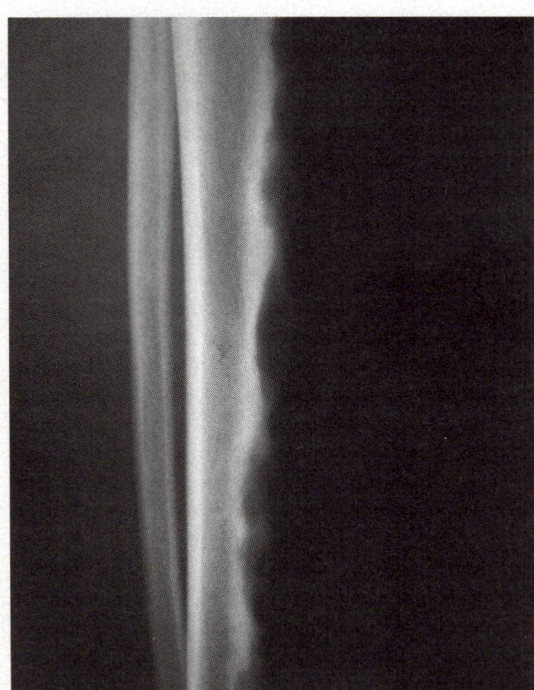

Figure 110-24 Multiple radiolucent lesions in the anterior cortex of the tibia is either osteofibrous dysplasia or adamantinoma. These two bone tumors can have the same radiographic appearance. This patient had an adamantinoma with osteofibrous dysplasia. Other adamantinoma will have extension into the medullary canal and often into the surrounding soft tissues.

subtypes described include unicystic, multicystic, solid, and peripheral.[83] Ameloblastic carcinoma and ameloblastic sarcoma have been described.[82] Ameloblastoma, a tumor of odontogenic origin, is similar but is not related to adamantinoma.

Because adamantinoma metastasizes to the lungs late in the course, staging should include a CT scan of the chest as well as adequate imaging studies of the primary lesional area and careful follow-up for many years. The average interval prior to pulmonary metastatic disease is 8 years.[84]

A wide surgical excision of the lesional area is indicated. The procedure lends itself well to allograft replacement of an intercalary segment. If this procedure does not produce adequate negative soft tissue and bony margins, then amputation may be indicated. Irradiation and chemotherapy are not recommended for adamantinoma unless there are unusual circumstances. Primary radiotherapy should be reserved for inoperable patients or those with unresectable disease. Postoperative radiotherapy may be indicated for those patients with less than optimal surgical clearance of tumor. Patients free of disease for 3 to 20 years have been reported following curettage or partial excision and radiotherapy.[85,86] Local relapse as long as 26 years after incomplete surgery and irradiation implies that prolonged follow-up is also required for patients irradiated adjunctively.[86] When adamantinoma has metastasized, a trial of chemotherapy may be warranted. Because of the rarity of this phenomenon, there are no data on the effects of various chemotherapeutic modalities on metastatic adamantinoma.[87]

Chondrosarcomas Chondrosarcoma is a malignant primary tumor of bone characterized by malignant cartilaginous proliferation. Among malignant bone lesions, chondrosarcoma is second in frequency to osteosarcoma.

Chondrosarcomas represent approximately 20% of all primary bone lesions. They can occur de novo as a primary tumor or as a secondary tumor following malignant degeneration of a benign osteochondroma or a benign enchondroma. The tumor usually occurs in patients > 40 years of age. It occurs with nearly equal frequency in both sexes. Chondrosarcomas can occur in any bone, but there is a preponderance of lesions found in the pelvis and femur. Chondrosarcomas arising in other flat bones, such as the scapula, ribs, and skull, are not uncommon.

Most patients with chondrosarcoma present complaining of a constant mild to moderate pain in the affected extremity. Systemic complaints or findings are rare. On occasion, a mass can be palpable, but not infrequently the physical examination is normal. Lesions in the pelvis can be very large before being detected.

Most chondrosarcomas are suspect by their radiographic appearance before biopsy. They have an ill-defined border, permeate the bone, and usually a have a soft tissue extraosseous mass. A chronic periosteal reaction is almost always seen. There is usually calcification within the bony lesion (Figure 110-25).

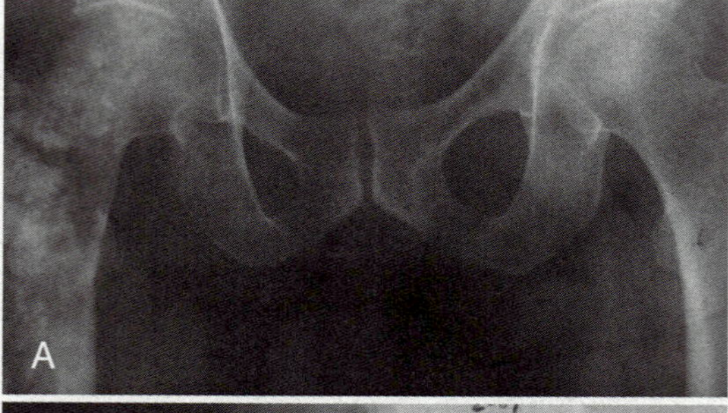

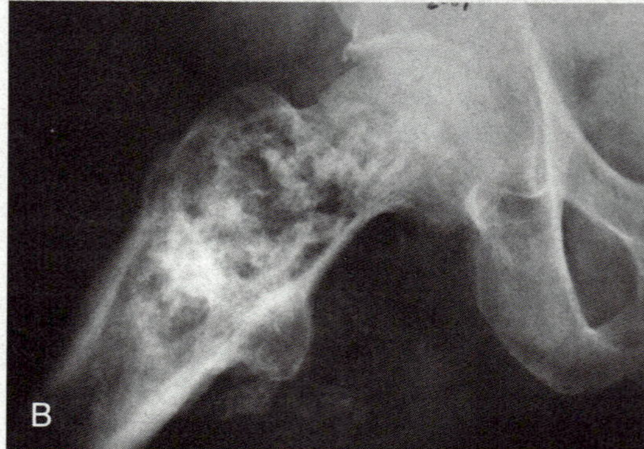

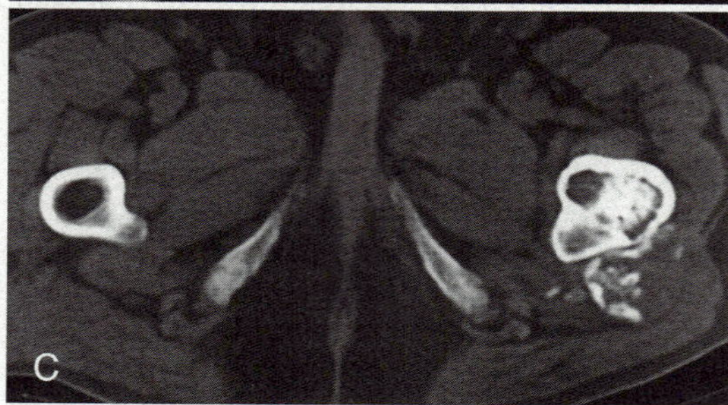

Figure 110-25 **A,** A typical chondrosarcoma of the upper end of the femur. **B,** The lesion is much more destructive than that shown in Figure 110-9, and on both lateral radiograph and computed tomography scan **(C)**, the tumor lies outside the bone as a soft tissue extension.

The diagnosis of chondrosarcoma is made based on the clinical presentation and the appearance of the chondrocytes. There are more chondrocytes in a chondrosarcoma than in normal or reactive cartilage. The chondrocytes have enlarged, clear nuclei, there are binucleate chondrocytes, and there are often bizarre-shaped chondrocytes, but typical mitotic figures are uncommon.

There is some controversy regarding when to call an enchondroma with cellular activity a low-grade chondrosarcoma. The presence of hypercellular cartilage that infiltrates the trabeculae but does not have other features of a chondrosarcoma is often sufficient for some pathologists to make a diagnosis of low-grade chondrosarcoma. These lesions have an extremely low risk of metastasizing and probably should not be called a sarcoma (Figure 110-26).

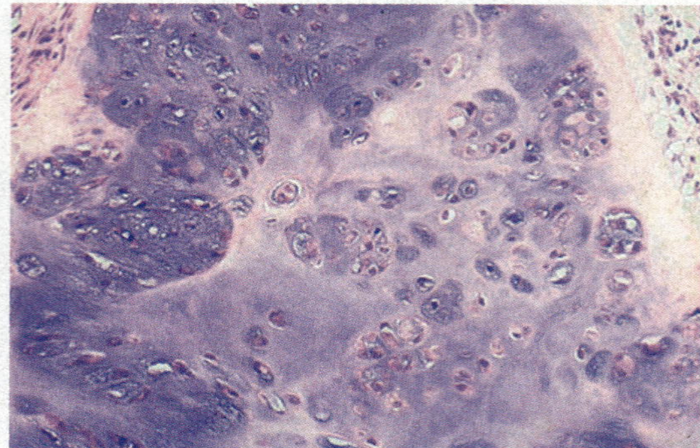

Figure 110-26 Chondrosarcoma. A nodule of hypercellular hyaline cartilage is bounded by fibrovascular tissue (*upper left and right corners*). Even at intermediate magnification, cytologic atypia, and pleomorphism are apparent.

Staging for chondrosarcoma should include, in addition to adequate imaging of the primary lesion (CT scan or MRI), a CT scan of the chest to rule out pulmonary metastases, and a bone scan to rule out the presence of other bony metastases.

Treatment of a chondrosarcoma is wide excision, which sometimes means amputation. Adjuvant chemotherapy or irradiation is not usually advised. There is little evidence that either adds significantly to local control or increases patient survival, but each may be of some benefit when complete resection is not possible or practical. Close analysis of the few well-documented series from the megavoltage era reveal that long-term progression-free survival following radiotherapy is possible for selected patients with chondrosarcoma of bone. The largest experience with modern radiotherapy for chondrosarcoma has been reported from the Princess Margaret Hospital. Harwood and colleagues initially described the results of palliative or radical irradiation for 31 patients.[88]

Although the majority of chondrosarcomas recurring locally after surgery are detected within 5 years, the natural history of this tumor is notoriously capricious.[89] Evans and colleagues reported local relapse of low-grade chondrosarcoma 10 years after resection.[89]

Dedifferentiated Chondrosarcoma "Dedifferentiated" chondrosarcoma is a rare condition characterized by a typical enchondroma or low-grade chondrosarcoma of bone juxtapositioned to a high-grade sarcoma, the latter being indistinguishable from a high-grade spindle-cell sarcoma (Figure 110-27).[90] (The term "malignant fibrous histiocytoma" [MFH] has been eliminated by the WHO.) It is assumed that the enchondroma or low-grade chondrosarcoma has become a high-grade tumor.

Dedifferentiated chondrosarcomas occur rarely and are more common in the older age group (ie, after 60 years of age). Their incidence is about equal in males and females. They occur most commonly in areas where chondrosarcomas are common, including the pelvis, femur, and other flat bones, such as the ribs and scapula. In most series that have been reported, the disease

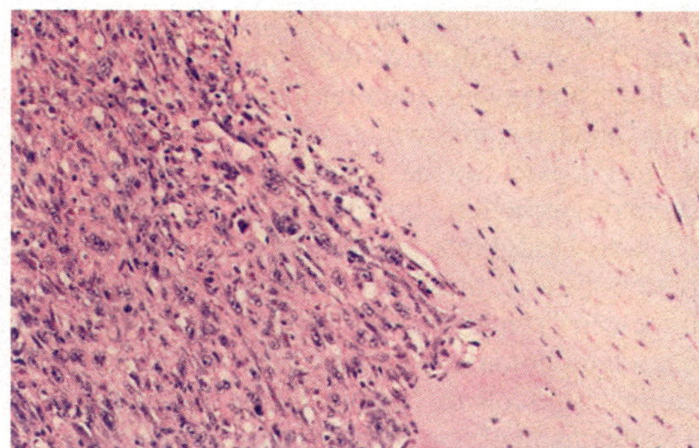

Figure 110-27 Sharp demarcation between the high-grade spindle-cell sarcomatous component (*left*) and the low-grade chondrosarcoma (*right*) is characteristic of dedifferentiated chondrosarcoma.

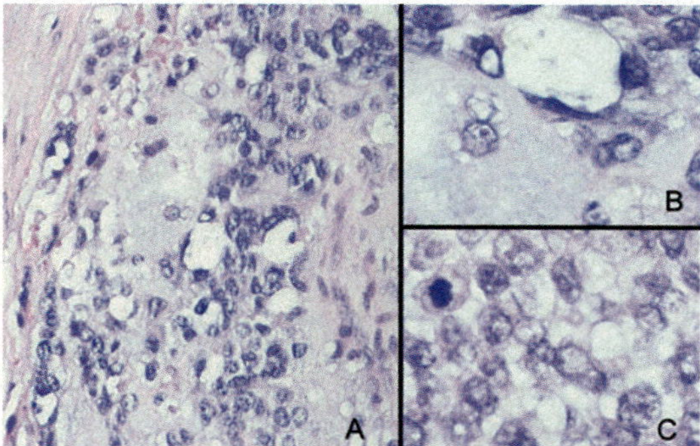

Figure 110-28 Mesenchymal chondrosarcoma. **A,** The tumor is composed of small round cells that are sharply demarcated from the malignant cartilage. **B,** Foci of cartilaginous matrix are often small. **C,** The small round cells have a scant cytoplasm, indistinct cytoplasmic borders, and round or oval nuclei with coarse chromatin and inconspicuous nucleoli.

has an extremely poor prognosis, with the vast majority of patients succumbing to pulmonary metastases early in the course of the disease.

The radiographic appearance of dedifferentiated chondrosarcoma is that of an aggressive lesion, usually adjacent to a more indolent cartilage lesion. A large soft tissue mass may exist.

Surgical resection with a wide margin is recommended. Adjuvant chemotherapy has not been shown to improve survival, but continued trials are in progress because the survival rate is poor (< 10%).[91]

Mesenchymal Chondrosarcoma Mesenchymal chondrosarcoma is an uncommon malignant tumor of bone (that can also occur as a soft tissue primary tumor) that includes islands of neoplastic cartilage among sheets of small, undifferentiated round or spindle-shaped cells.

Mesenchymal chondrosarcoma occurs in the young adult group and is relatively rare below the age of 20 years or above the age of 40 years. It has been shown to affect males and females equally in the few series that have been reported. The most common site is the femur, followed by the flat bones, including the pelvis, ribs, skull, and spine. It is said to have a propensity to occur in the parameningeal areas in the head, neck, and spine.

The radiographic appearance of mesenchymal chondrosarcoma is that of an aggressive bone tumor with an ill-defined border in the medullary canal of the bone, with tumor penetrating the bony cortex, producing a soft tissue mass. The soft tissue mass may contain stippled calcification similar to that seen in classic chondrosarcomas. However, the finding of this characteristic type of malignant lesion in the younger age group and, in particular, in the parameningeal areas, such as the spine or skull, could raise the possibility of mesenchymal chondrosarcoma. The diagnosis is usually arrived at following biopsy of the suspected malignant lesion.

The tumor is composed of sheets of undifferentiated malignant round cells, sometimes quite similar to those seen in a Ewing's sarcoma of bone or small-cell osteosarcoma. Neoplastic cartilage is seen within the tumor (Figure 110-28).

The neoplasm is usually more responsive to radiotherapy and to chemotherapy than the average chondrosarcoma. Mesenchymal chondrosarcoma is an aggressive tumor that should be treated both locally and systemically. Because mesenchymal chondrosarcoma responds to chemotherapy, it needs to be distinguished from classic chondrosarcoma. If tumor shrinkage would make local control easier, preoperative chemotherapy should be used. This frequently results in significant shrinkage of the primary tumor, making it more amenable to radical surgical excision. For those anatomic sites that cannot be totally resected, adjuvant irradiation can also be used to improve local control. This is particularly important in tumors of axial location, such as the spine, skull, scapula, ribs, and pelvis.

The clinical history of mesenchymal chondrosarcoma is one of pain and swelling in the lesional area. The onset of symptoms is usually rapid, since this is a highly malignant tumor. Because of the axial location of many of these tumors, neurologic symptoms may be the first to occur. Early diagnosis of pelvic, sacral, and paraspinal primaries may be possible because of the neurologic pain syndromes produced by these tumors.

Staging for mesenchymal chondrosarcoma includes (in addition to adequate imaging studies of the lesional area) a bone scan to rule out bony metastases, more common with mesenchymal chondrosarcoma than with other chondrosarcomas or osteosarcoma. A CT scan of the lungs to rule out pulmonary metastases is also included in the preoperative staging.

The treatment of mesenchymal chondrosarcoma should be similar to that discussed elsewhere for Ewing's sarcoma. The majority of the malignant stroma of mesenchymal chondrosarcoma consists of small round cells that are usually sensitive to both radiation therapy and chemotherapy with traditional agents, such as doxorubicin, and a high-dose alkylating agent, such as cyclophosphamide or ifosfamide. Radiation therapy is usually given to a dose of between 40 and 45 Gy during the course of preoperative chemotherapy. This usually results in rapid shrinkage of the primary tumor, prevention of early dissemination to bones and lungs, and the tumor's being rendered approachable by wide en bloc excision. Postoperatively, if there is significant tumor necrosis (90%) in the resected specimen, the patient is continued on chemotherapy similar to that used to treat Ewing's sarcoma. Because mesenchymal chondrosarcoma is a pleomorphic tumor, sometimes containing more resistant spindle cells, the finding of residual spindle cells in the resected specimen and < 90% necrosis suggest resistance to the radiation therapy and alkylating agents used preoperatively. Postoperative adjuvant chemotherapy should then be changed to include cisplatin combined with doxorubicin together with high-dose ifosfamide as used in the treatment of osteosarcoma.[91]

Prior to the use of combination multimodality therapy for the treatment of mesenchymal chondrosarcoma, this tumor metastasized in almost 100% of the reported cases. With modern multidisciplinary treatment as described above, the prognosis for mesenchymal chondrosarcoma should be similar to that for Ewing's sarcoma with similar treatment. A caution is that most mesenchymal chondrosarcomas arise in the axial skeleton and are difficult to resect surgically, making the overall prognosis more closely similar to that of axial Ewing's sarcomas, which is worse than for extremity lesions. In addition, the occasional finding of more resistant spindle-cell stroma in the resected specimen indicates that this tumor is somewhat more resistant to combined modality treatment, and the risk of metastases developing late in the course may be somewhat higher than for the more common Ewing's sarcoma that is similarly treated.

Ewing's Sarcoma Please see the discussion of Ewing's sarcoma family of tumors (Chapter 8, "Genomic Alterations and Chromosomal Aberrations in Human Cancer").

Malignant Vascular Tumors The malignant vascular tumors constitute three separate clinical entities.[92] The older literature usually lumped them together under the heading of angiosarcoma of bone. They require separate and distinct treatment, and only the highly malignant round small-cell angiosarcoma of bone is obligatorily treated with systemic chemotherapy.

Hemangiopericytoma Malignant hemangiopericytoma of bone is rare. It is characterized by a low- to intermediate-grade spindle-cell stroma arranged in an irregular pattern consisting of proliferation around blood vessels. Most patients are less than 40 years of age. The tumor has a predilection for the long bones, pelvis, and scapula.

The radiographic appearance of a hemangiopericytoma is nonspecific. It has the radiographic features of a radiolucent aggressive bone lesion. It can occur in the diaphyseal as well as the metaphyseal area of the long bone.

These tumors usually do not respond well to chemotherapy or radiation therapy. Surgery is the primary modality of treatment. Preoperative treatment in the form of embolization may shrink the tumor and make it less vascular, facilitating surgical resection.

Malignant Hemangioendothelioma We prefer to use the term "malignant hemangioendothelioma of bone" for the form of angiosarcoma that is characterized by multifocal occurrence, usually in bones and soft tissue of the affected extremity. This tumor is rare below the age of 50 years. It is more common in the distal extremities and occurs multifocally, usually only in the bones of the involved extremity, perhaps by retrograde venous regional metastases. Involvement of other bones in the skeletal system is uncommon in this multifocal variety of angiosarcoma.

The radiographic appearance is usually that of multiple radiolucent bony lesions. There is increased uptake on the technetium bone scan, as is the case for all aggressive bone tumors.

Malignant hemangioendothelioma of bone is composed of plump endothelial cells that form anastomosing vascular channels. The lining of the vascular channels are the malignant cells themselves, and not normal endothelium. Sometimes, one can see malignant cells being shed into the vascular channels. The stromal cells of the tumor stain positively for factor VIII.

Staging of malignant hemangioendothelioma of the adult should include imaging of the entire affected extremity; MRI is the procedure of choice. CT scans of the chest should also be done to rule out pulmonary metastases, and a technetium bone scan is done.

This tumor is relatively resistant to both combination chemotherapy and irradiation. The treatment of choice is surgical ablation. If radical surgery or amputation (if indicated by the presence of multifocal lesions in the extremity) is performed early, the prognosis is excellent.[93]

Angiosarcoma The authors prefer to reserve this terminology for the rare highly malignant vascular tumors that can usually be recognized histopathologically. Angiosarcoma of bone occurs predominantly in patients under 40 years of age, without predilection for gender. This lesion can affect any bone in the skeletal system, but tends to arise in the axial skeleton, including the flat bones of the pelvis and skull, as well as the ribs and scapula in affected individuals.

The radiographic appearance of angiosarcoma is that of a lytic punched-out lesion in bone. The cortex is destroyed and a soft tissue mass is often present.

Angiosarcomas of bone have malignant spindle cells and epithelioid or small round cells. The latter can mimic a Ewing's sarcoma. Frequently, tumor cells can be seen to be shedding into the small vascular channels individually or in clumps (Figure 110-29). These tumors stain positively for factor VIII, which helps to differentiate them from Ewing's sarcoma.

Angiosarcoma of bone is highly malignant. It is treated in a fashion similar to Ewing's sarcoma of bone, with preoperative chemotherapy, and then a wide resection of the lesional area or local irradiation. Postoperative adjuvant chemotherapy is recommended.

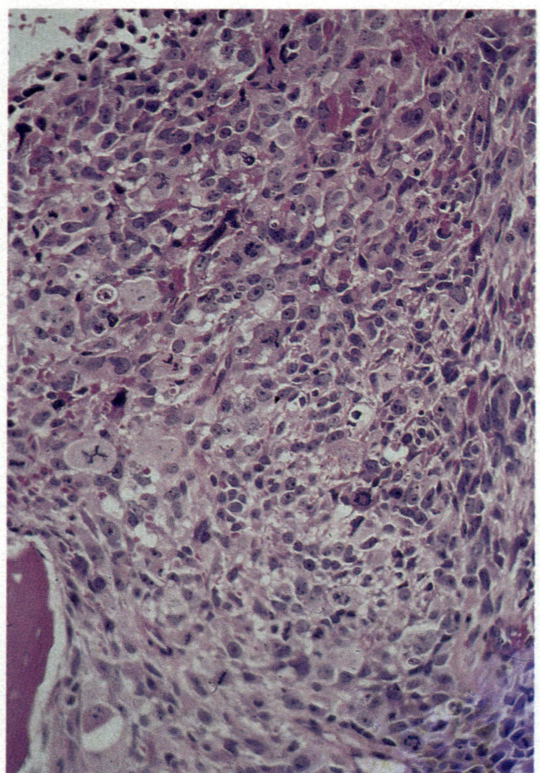

Figure 110-29 Angiosarcoma of bone. The tumor consists of solid sheets of vasoformative polyhedral and spindle-shaped cells (note numerous intracellular erythrocytes and small lumina). The mitotic rate is very high and numerous bizarre mitotic figures are identified (250 ×). (Courtesy of Michael T. Klein, MD, Mount Sinai School of Medicine.)

Lymphoma Lymphoma of bone is most commonly non-Hodgkin's lymphoma. It may present as a solitary site in bone, as multiple sites restricted to bone, or have nonosseous involvement with bone lesions. Patients with involvement of bone usually present complaining of pain. All ages are affected. Patients without nonosseous involvement usually have no systemic complaints and a normal physical examination. The plain radiograph of the involved bone may be normal, but often there is a mixed pattern of destruction and increased density. The bone scan shows increased uptake, and on MRI there is a signal abnormality. PET scans are valuable in searching for other occult foci of tumor.

The diagnostic evaluation of patients with primary lymphoma of bone is similar to that used for patients with lymphomas at other sites. These should include bone scintigraphy; CT of the chest, abdomen, and pelvis; as well as CT scan or MRI of the primary bone involved. PET scanning is recommended. Laboratory evaluation includes a complete blood count, chemistry profile, including the evaluation of lactic dehydrogenase, uric acid, electrolytes, and renal function. Additionally, as for any other patient with lymphoma, a bone marrow aspiration and biopsy from the ilium should be performed to rule out the presence of metastatic disease in the marrow. The Murphy staging system is used for all childhood non-Hodgkin's lymphomas.[94,95] Evaluation of these patients with plain radiographs reveals the presence of single or multiple bone lesions, which can be mostly lytic or sclerotic, and can be located either in the axial skeleton or the long bones.[96,97]

Non-Hodgkin's lymphomas are classified as lymphoblastic, small-cell noncleaved, or diffuse large-cell lymphoma.[95,95] Most patients with primary lymphoma of bone have been reported to have either large-cell or lymphoblastic histology.[96–98] The treatment of non-Hodgkin's lymphoma is based on the stage of disease and histology at the time of initial diagnosis.[94,95] Surgery is not necessary. The prognosis for patients who present with localized disease is excellent and pediatric trials have focused on minimizing therapy while maintaining an excellent outcome.[94,99,100] The duration of therapy and prognosis for patients with advanced-stage disease in the range of 50 to 75%, depends on the histologic diagnosis.[94] The therapy for patients with primary lymphoma of bone has not necessarily followed the same pattern as that for pediatric patients with lymphoma at other sites. The role of radiotherapy has been difficult to assess because most reports of primary lymphoma of bone involve a small number of patients, and the use of radiotherapy has resulted in second malignant neoplasms in a significant proportion of patients.[96–98,101–103] For patients with localized primary lymphoma of bone, a report from 1999 evaluates the use of chemotherapy for 31 patients enrolled on three consecutive Pediatric Oncology Group studies.[104] This study reports the outcome of 11 patients treated between 1983 and 1992 with 8 months of multiagent chemotherapy with or without irradiation, and 20 patients treated since 1992 who received 9 weeks of multiagent chemotherapy without irradiation. The 5-year projected survival and event-free survival were 100% and 95%, respectively, demonstrating that children with primary lymphoma of bone can be treated successfully with chemotherapy regimens of less intensity and duration and without the need for irradiation. The treatment of patients with disseminated primary lymphoma of bone, as with any other type of non-Hodgkin's lymphoma, should be based on histology; however, there are limited data regarding the outcome of these patients.[94–98,101,102]

Malignant Fibrous Histiocytoma and Fibrosarcoma These malignant bone tumors represent similar, and probably identical, entities. The terminology "malignant fibrous histiocytoma" (MFH) has been used more frequently since this malignant primary bone tumor was extensively studied by Huvos in the mid-1970s. Fibrosarcomas and MFHs of bone are composed of a malignant spindle-cell stroma that, in many instances, produces abundant collagen.[104] Multinucleated giant cells are frequently found within this tumor that presumably represent malignant histiocytes in often bizarre forms. These tumors are rare, occur with equal frequency in males and females, and do not occur in any characteristic age group. Many people feel that the MFH of bone represents the response of the tissue to chronic injury, and hence appear with great frequency at the site of radiation, at bone infarcts, in Pagetoid foci, or even as dedifferentiated chondrosarcoma.

The radiographic appearance of an MFH or fibrosarcoma of bone is of an aggressive, lytic lesion. The distribution of skeletal sites of these tumors is similar to that of osteosarcoma, with a majority of lesions occurring in the femur, tibia, and pelvis, although any bone in the skeleton can be affected.

MFH and fibrosarcoma can occur as low-grade as well as high-grade malignant lesions. They may also occur as periosteal lesions similar to parosteal osteosarcoma; indeed, parosteal MFHs are of low-grade malignancy. MFHs tend to have abundant giant cells present as well. The spindle cells of MFH are often arranged in a circular or storiform appearance, whereas those of fibrosarcoma tend to produce a linear or herring-bone pattern of interweaving fascicles of malignant fibroblastic cells, although often they cannot be distinguished from one another.

The main problem in differential diagnosis is from osteosarcoma. Indeed, many of these tumors that occur in the younger age group can be found to produce osteoid. Malignant fibrous tumors that produce small amounts of osteoid in some areas are classified as osteosarcomas by many pathologists; other pathologists may allow osteoid to be produced in small amounts and still classify the tumor as a fibrosarcoma or MFH. The histogenetic name tag given to the tumor is primarily of taxonomic interest; since it is a fully malignant spindle-cell neoplasm of bone, it is treated in a way similar to osteosarcoma and carries with it a similar poor prognosis without adequate treatment.

The clinical history is similar to that for an osteosarcoma: pain and swelling in an area, which usually leads to a radiograph that demonstrates a malignant-appearing bone lesion. Because of the lytic nature of this tumor, patients may sometimes present with a pathologic fracture (Figure 110-30). In this instance, as in any pathologically fractured malignant tumor, the prognosis for performing limb salvage surgery and indeed for ultimate survival appears to be worse.

Staging work-up of this malignant tumor is similar to that for osteosarcoma and includes imaging studies of the lesional area with CT and MRI, a bone scan, and CT scan of the chest.

Treatment is identical to that given for osteosarcoma. Low-grade lesions need only undergo wide surgical resection, but high-grade lesions require preoperative and postoperative chemotherapy. In our experience, MFH of bone has a slightly higher complete response rate to preoperative chemotherapy than does the classic variety of osteosarcoma.[105] Indeed, the prognosis for fully malignant fibrous lesions of bone, as in osteosarcoma, seems to be best predicted from the patient's response to preoperative chemotherapy.

Osseous MFH that is not amenable to neoadjuvant chemotherapy or to surgery may respond to radiotherapy. Campanna and colleagues primarily irradiated 8 patients to doses of 40 to 80 Gy.[106] All four with long bone tumors were locally disease free from 3 to 8 years. Two patients with axial

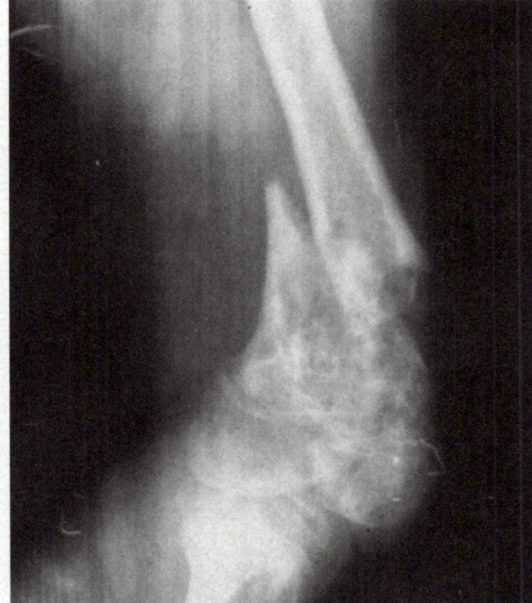

Figure 110-30 Pathologic fracture in a patient with a malignant fibrous histiocytoma of bone. This lesion is usually a lytic lesion, and, therefore, when it occurs in the weight-bearing lower extremities, the presentation with a pathologic fracture is not uncommon.

lesions demonstrated "probable" local relapse at 14 and 23 months. Two others with axial tumors succumbed rapidly to metastatic disease. Dahlin and colleagues also reported significant results of radiotherapy, although details of treatment were not provided.[107] Of those primarily irradiated, 1 patient was palliated for 6 years, 2 were cured, and 1 relapsed locally. One other patient was disease free 18 years after excision and radiotherapy. Spanier and colleagues described a patient receiving radiotherapy for lung metastases and a stump recurrence who was free of tumor in all irradiation sites at necropsy 32 months later.[108] The authors hypothesized that an MFH with an abundance of histiocytes was radiosensitive, while a predominantly fibroblastic tumor was relatively radioresistant. Marked pain reduction after irradiating vertebral MFH has been described.[109] Postoperative radiotherapy may be indicated for MFH with close or inadequate surgical margins.

Campanna and colleagues reported local relapse with wide margins in 17% of resected patients and 21% of amputated patients, compared with 6.5% with a radical margin.[106] Adjuvant chemotherapy did not influence local relapse rates regardless of margin status in their series. Neoadjuvant chemotherapy followed by limb-sparing surgery with adequate margins is also associated with a low risk of local relapse in the absence of routine radiotherapy.[110]

Osteosarcoma There are a variety of osteosarcomas. Classic, high-grade intramedullary osteosarcoma is the tumor most often referred to as just "osteosarcoma." The other types include juxtacortical osteosarcoma (parosteal osteosarcoma and periosteal osteosarcoma), low-grade intramedullary osteosarcoma, multifocal sclerosing osteosarcoma, osteosarcoma of the jaw and skull, osteosarcoma arising from Paget's disease, and postirradiation osteosarcomas.

Classic, high-grade intramedullary osteosarcoma, the most common primary malignant bone tumor, covered in Chapter 124m "Pediatric Bone Tumors," is a Ewing's sarcoma.

Juxtacortical Osteosarcoma Parosteal and periosteal osteosarcoma are usually low- to intermediate-grade osteosarcomas that arise on the surface of bone.[111] They involve the cortex, but rarely penetrate into the intramedullary canal. If there is a high-grade component, they are considered "dedifferentiated."

Parosteal osteosarcoma typically arises in an age group different from the classic osteosarcoma of adolescents (Table 110-5). It is more common in females than males, is most common in the third and fourth decades of life (ages 20–40 years), and typically arises in the posterior aspect of the distal femur, although any bone in the skeleton can be affected (Figure 110-31).

The radiographic appearance is that of an ossified exophytic tumor that is closely applied to the cortex of the bone. The medullary cavity of the bone is invaded infrequently, and although it was thought in the past that this was a poor prognostic sign, recent studies have not supported this view, and the histologic grade of the tumor (usually low grade) is a more significant predictor of outcome and the need for adjuvant therapy. Normally, the histologic appearance of these tumors is quite striking in that they are almost always heavily ossified and show a sparse, or at most, moderately abundant, spindle-cell population, which appears to be making the bone (Figure 110-32).

The differential diagnosis of parosteal osteosarcoma includes osteocartilaginous exostosis and myositis ossificans traumatica or circumscripta. It is important to note that osteocartilaginous exostoses "share a cortex" with the bone, while parosteal osteosarcoma arises from the surface of the bone. Similarly, myositis ossificans can be dis-

Table 110-5 Malignant Cartilage-Producing Tumors

Type	Histologic Grade	Age (Years)	Common Sites
Classic	III–IV	10–20	Femur, tibia, humerus
Parosteal	I–II	20–40	Femur
Periosteal	III	15–25	Tibia, femur
Multifocal	IV	< 15	Multifocal
Jaw tumor	II–III	20–40	Maxilla, mandible
Skull tumor	II–III	20–40	Parietal, occipital, frontal
Paget's sarcoma	III–IV	> 50	Pelvis, long bones
Postirradiation sarcoma	III–IV	> 4 yrs from radiotherapy	Irradiation site(s)

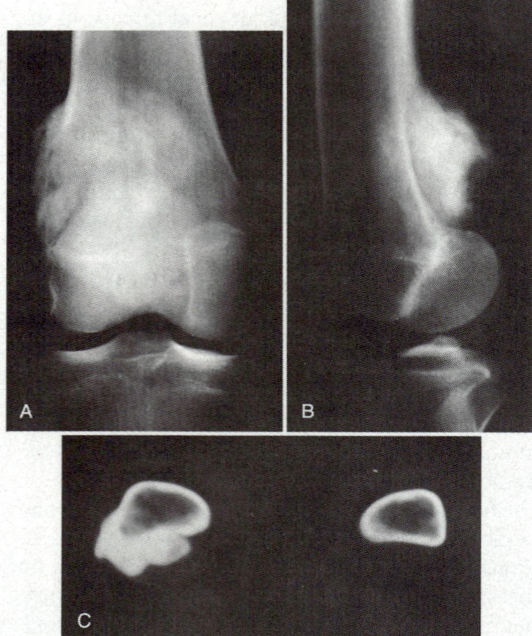

Figure 110-31 The AP and lateral radiographs **(A** and **B)** demonstrate the characteristic presentation of a parosteal osteosarcoma. As can be seen on the computed tomography scan **(C)**, the lesion is located in the popliteal fossa and grows on the surface of the bone extending in irregular fashion posteriorly.

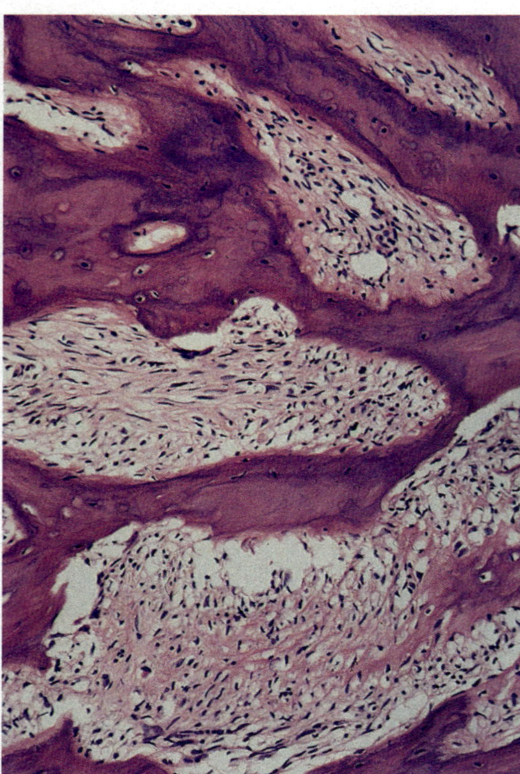

Figure 110-32 Parosteal osteosarcoma. A medium power photograph of the typical low-grade tumor shows rather abundant immature microtrabeculae of tumor bone and an intertrabecular fibrous stroma, which is the actual tumor stroma. The histological changes are rather bland and do not conform to osteosarcoma in its usual grade of pattern (100 ×). (Courtesy of Michael T. Klein, MD, Mount Sinai School of Medicine.)

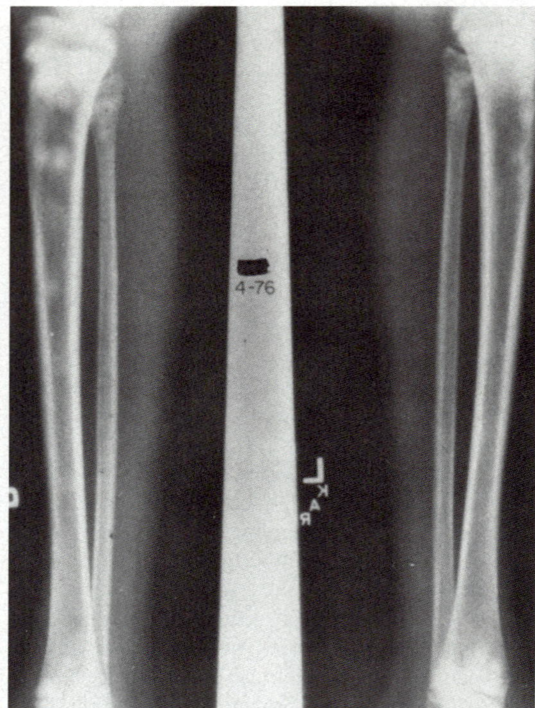

Figure 110-33 Multilocal sclerosing osteogenic sarcoma in a 10-year-old female. This figure demonstrates both the right and left lower extremities. Note the multiple sclerotic lesions appearing in the metaphyseal as well as diaphyseal areas of all four bones. Other bones in the body were similarly involved. This relatively rare variety of osteogenic sarcoma that occurs in young children is uniformly fatal. Although patients may respond initially to systemic chemotherapy, the tumor usually advances in multiple bone sites prior to metastasizing to lungs, eventually killing the patient.

tinguished on imaging studies on the basis of the frequent appearance of a clear space between the lesion and the cortex, rather than being firmly attached, as is noted with parosteal osteosarcoma.

The patient may complain of minimal pain and tenderness over the site and, if the lesion is large, decreased range of motion in the adjacent joint.

The treatment is a wide surgical margin resection. This is usually curative. Late (after 5 years) local recurrences can occur and the patients should be followed for at least 15 years.

Periosteal osteosarcoma is usually of a higher grade than parosteal osteosarcoma, but not as high as classic high-grade osteosarcoma. It often has a significant cartilaginous component. It occurs in a younger age group than the parosteal lesions and slightly more frequently in females. The lesion most often presents as an ossified mass on the anterior aspect of the proximal tibial diaphysis.

Histologically, the tumor may be confused with a fully malignant chondrosarcoma. If the specimen is examined carefully, however, bone is being produced by the malignant spindle cells. Because the periosteal osteosarcoma is more likely to metastasize than the parosteal osteosarcoma, some oncologists prefer to treat this lesion in the same manner as a central osteosarcoma. The likelihood of cure under these conditions is fairly high. If the lesion is small and is easily resectable, this may be sufficient treatment, unless the lesion is histologically of very high grade. Because of the site of the tumor and its proximity to the cortex, the resection should include a segment of bone adjacent to the tumor mass.

Low-Grade Intramedullary Osteosarcoma Low-grade intramedullary osteosarcoma is an unusual tumor seen in young adults. It is often confused, both radiographically and histologically, with fibrous dysplasia. It is treated with a wide surgical resection and adjuvant therapy is not necessary.

Multifocal Sclerosing Osteosarcoma Multifocal sclerosing osteosarcoma is an extremely rare variety of osteosarcoma. It is a fully malignant osteosarcoma that tends to present in one primary site, but on careful examination of the patient, it is evident that there are multiple osteosarcomas throughout most of the skeletal system (Figure 110-33).[112,113]

Multifocal sclerosing osteosarcoma tends to occur in children less than 10 years of age. It represents less than 3% of all primary osteosarcomas. Because of the presentation with multiple bone lesions, it has been postulated that the etiology of this disease could be a blood-borne infectious agent; no proof of this hypothesis has been provided. Because of the rarity of this tumor and its rapid 100% mortality rate, it has been impossible to study the tumor in further detail. The occurrence of this highly malignant form of osteosarcoma might indeed be some "experiment of nature," whose victims could give us some clue to the etiology of osteosarcoma if the disease were more common or the survival of the rare patient who develops this disease more prolonged.

The patient with multifocal sclerosing osteosarcoma usually presents with a primary osteoblastic osteosarcoma that is quite typical on radiographic examination. The clinical history is similar to most other primary osteosarcomas, except for the fact that most patients are young children. Usually, the patient has a biopsy of the suspected osteosarcoma and is referred for a staging work-up. Other multiple lesions are often asymptomatic at that time. The bone scan may not indicate the multifocal nature of this disease, since the disease may attack the growing ends of the bones symmetrically. One can be very suspicious of multifocal osteosarcoma, in the proper clinical setting, if the bone scans show extremely hot metaphyseal ends of all bones. However, younger children tend to have bone scans that show increased uptake in the ends of all bones, since they are growing rapidly. Thus, in this rare entity, the bone scan may be of little use. One should be suspicious of multifocal osteosarcoma in patients who have extremely elevated levels of serum alkaline phosphatase. The finding of multiple sclerotic areas in the lesional area of the primary site might give a clue to the nature of the disease, since the primary tumor sometimes is made up of many discrete round foci of sclerotic lesions that seem to coalesce into one big area. Sometimes the inclusion of other bones in the routine radiograph of the primary lesion will show additional lesions.

In the case of multifocal sclerosing osteosarcoma, a skeletal survey is helpful in defining the entity and demonstrating the multiple lesions (see

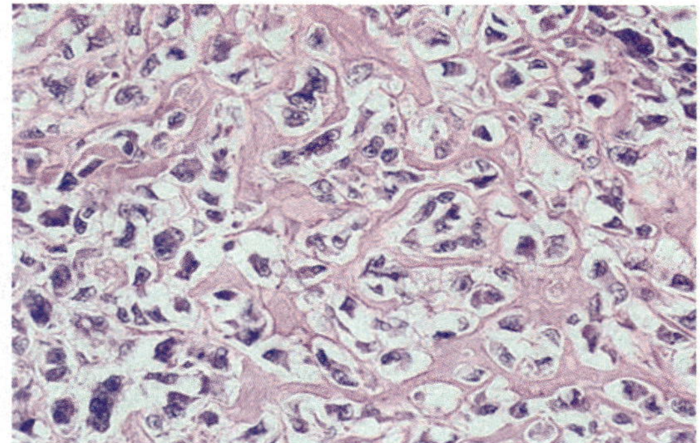

Figure 110-34 Osteosarcoma, conventional. Pleomorphic, obviously malignant cells lie between delicate, interlacing strands of osteoid. Osteoblastic rimming is absent.

Figure 110-33). Because all the bones in the body are involved, surgery is usually futile. Patients can go into remission on aggressive chemotherapy. Sometimes it is necessary to perform surgery on the primary tumor because of uncontrollable pain. Patients should be managed with chemotherapy and pain medication. However, even with the most aggressive chemotherapy, multiple tumors always eventually progress, leading to death, usually within 1 year of diagnosis.

Osteosarcoma of the Jaw and Skull Osteosarcoma of the craniofacial bones represents a clinical syndrome somewhat different from the classic osteosarcoma. Histologically, these tumors are identical to the classic variety of osteosarcoma (Figure 110-34). They tend to occur in an older age group (20–40 years) and, because of their location, are more difficult to resect surgically.

Osteosarcomas of the craniofacial bones are relatively rare and represent less than 10% of all osteosarcomas. The male-to-female ratio is close to one. The most commonly affected bones of the head and neck are the mandible, followed by the maxilla. Osteosarcomas of the other skull bones are extremely rare. The radiographic appearance of osteosarcomas in the head and neck is characteristic of bone-producing osteosarcomas in general. The disease carries a mortality similar to classic osteosarcoma. Because of its location, it tends to be diagnosed earlier, and the tumor can remain localized for a longer period than the classic, fully malignant osteosarcoma of adolescents. Its location precludes very radical surgery, and there is a high incidence of local recurrences following primary surgery. Osteosarcoma of the skull, other than the mandible and maxilla, carries with it an even worse prognosis owing to the difficulty in radically resecting the tumor. Multiple local recurrences often occur prior to the appearance of distant metastases.

The differential diagnoses of a small jaw lesion include various forms of tooth abscess, osteomyelitis of the jaw, and some of the rare benign tumors, such as ossifying fibromas and brown tumors of hyperparathyroidism. In patients older than 50 years, Paget's disease may produce a jaw lesion that mimics early osteosarcoma. In patients with known Paget's disease of the skull, Paget's sarcoma may arise.

Treatment of a fully malignant osteosarcoma occurring in the skull bones is similar to that for classic osteosarcoma. It should include preoperative chemotherapy, which in this setting takes on additional importance because of the limited margins for radical surgical excision. Osteosarcoma of either the mandible or maxilla seems to have a better prognosis than lesions of the skull bones and, indeed, better than the more standard types of classic medullary osteosarcoma. Some believe this is because of the earlier discovery of the lesions, because they are painful and deforming early in the course, but others suggests that these lesions are less malignant and slower to metastasize. In any event, treatment by hemimandibulectomy or segmental resection of the maxilla is successful in eliminating the primary tumor in most cases. Reconstruction of the defect is technically demanding but possible, and most patients achieve a satisfactory result from such surgery. High-dose chemotherapy is advocated for these patients in an effort to prevent metastatic lesions and local recurrence. Lesions of other bones of the skull are frequently considered to have a worse prognosis than those of the mandible and maxilla. This may be associated with the difficulties of gaining a wide margin at surgery and the frequency of local recurrences. In our experience, the only survivors of osteosarcoma of the parietal bone or occipital bones have been patients who have had extremely wide surgical excisions and have escaped local recurrences. These patients have also undergone preoperative and postoperative chemotherapy.[114]

Osteosarcoma Arising in Paget's Disease Osteosarcoma arising in patients with Paget's disease has a very poor prognosis. The lesions are large at the time of their appearance and very destructive, making resective surgery difficult, and pulmonary metastases are often present at the outset. The lesions almost always arise in patients with polyostotic Paget's disease and, in view of the frequency of Paget's disease in the general population (estimated for monostotic or polyostotic disease at 3% of the population over the age of 60 years), are quite rare. The tumors have a predilection for the pelvis, proximal femur, and proximal humerus and are difficult to treat surgically, principally because of the patient's age and the size of the lesion. Amputative surgery is sometimes necessary, especially in the face of a pathologic fracture, which is a frequent occurrence.

The pathology of osteosarcoma arising in Paget's disease is usually that of a fully malignant osteosarcoma.[115,116] Mortality associated with Paget's sarcomas is extremely high because of their location, which often precludes radical removal; the fact that patients with polyostotic Paget's disease sometimes develop multiple synchronous primary osteosarcomas; and the fact that older patients have not, in the past, been treated with aggressive chemotherapy.

The clinical history usually includes increased pain and swelling in the lesional area. Sometimes it is known that the patient has Paget's disease, but frequently radiography reveals a suspected tumor that looks like it is arising in an unsuspected Pagetoid bone. The serum alkaline phosphatase level is almost always elevated in patients with Paget's disease to begin with, and the superimposition of osteosarcoma may serve to elevate the alkaline phosphatase level even more. Because of this, alkaline phosphatase is not valuable as a tumor marker. In addition, in patients with polyostotic Paget's disease, it is sometimes impossible to tell whether the patient has metastatic bone lesions with osteosarcoma or simply polyostotic Paget's disease, with one primary osteosarcoma.

Patients with confirmed osteosarcoma arising in Paget's disease should have a bone scan and radiographic examination of all identified lesions to determine whether changes are due to osteosarcoma or multifocal Paget's disease. A CT scan of the chest should also be done to rule out pulmonary metastases. Osteosarcoma arising in Paget's disease should be treated according to identical principles as those for fully malignant osteosarcoma arising in a younger population. Great care must be taken during the administration of chemotherapy, since many older patients have impaired renal function. Patients who have osteosarcomas arising in Pagetoid lesions appear to have an improved prognosis through the use of preoperative chemotherapy, radical surgical excision of the tumor, and continued postoperative chemotherapy. Tumors of the axial skeleton, including the skull and spine, are sometimes inoperable. In this circumstance, patients should be given chemotherapy and radiation therapy to try to control the primary lesion and delay the appearance of metastatic disease. The patient with osteosarcoma arising in Paget's disease of the ilium depicted in Figure 110-35 was able to undergo preoperative chemotherapy, en bloc resection of the ilium (by internal hemipelvectomy), and postoperative adjuvant chemotherapy successfully. She is surviving, free of disease, more than 3 years after treatment.

Postirradiation Osteosarcomas Osteosarcomas arising in irradiated bones represent fully malignant osteosarcomas. They arise in the irra-

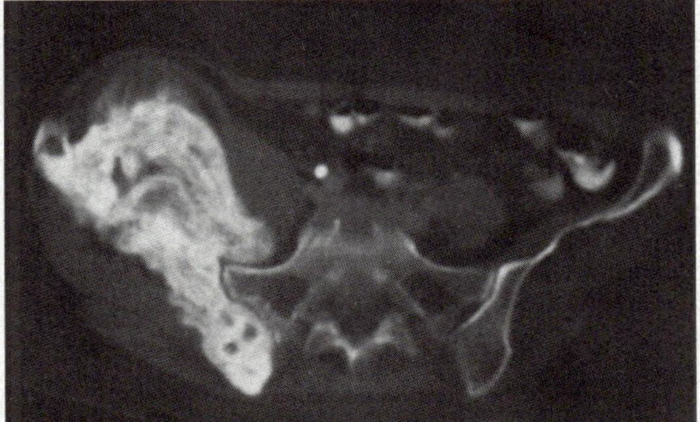

Figure 110-35 Paget's sarcoma occurring in the pelvis of a 60-year-old female. The radiographic appearance of the right ilium is characteristic of advanced pagetoid changes. The benignity of the Paget's disease can be seen by the lack of involvement of the sacroiliac joint space and the confinement of the lesion to the ilium in that area. However, there is a soft tissue mass emanating from the upper part of the iliac crest that is characteristic of malignant degeneration in Paget's disease. This patient responded well to preoperative chemotherapy and is surviving free of disease after limb salvage surgery ("internal hemipelvectomy").

diated area following therapeutic radiation therapy for other diseases. The median time to development of a postirradiation osteosarcoma is 10 years.[117] We have observed postirradiation osteosarcomas as early as 4 years following exposure. Because of the genetic propensity to develop osteogenic sarcoma in patients with familial retinoblastoma owing to reduction to homozygosity of their *Rb* genes, postirradiation sarcomas are more common. The younger the age at the time the patient receives radiation therapy, particularly in infancy, the higher is the incidence of osteosarcoma. In the general population of individuals cured of cancer by radiation therapy, postirradiation sarcomas are rare and develop in less than 5%. Whether or not these patients have some genetic predisposition to developing a second cancer similar to that which has been demonstrated for retinoblastoma is unknown. Evidence suggests that osteosarcomas occur more frequently in patients who receive higher doses of radiation therapy.

The differential diagnosis of postirradiation osteosarcoma is usually that from recurrence of the original irradiated primary tumor. Postirradiation osteosarcomas usually appear on radiographs as osteoblastic or mostly lytic lesions arising in the irradiated site. Some lesions appear to be multifocal osteosarcomas because of separate satellite areas arising within the irradiated site. On histologic examination, in addition to a fully malignant spindle-cell tumor producing osteoid, postirradiation osteosarcomas may also contain areas of radiation osteitis in the non-neoplastic surrounding bone.

The clinical presentation of secondary postirradiation osteosarcoma is one of painful swelling in the irradiated area. After establishing the diagnosis of a postirradiation osteosarcoma by open biopsy, staging is similar to that for other osteosarcomas and should include a bone scan, CT scan, or MRI of the lesional area, and a CT scan of the lungs to rule out the presence of metastases.

Postirradiation sarcomas are treated in a manner similar to other fully malignant osteosarcomas, with preoperative chemotherapy; radical surgical excision of the primary tumor site, when possible; and postoperative adjuvant chemotherapy. The prognosis for postirradiation sarcomas is worse than that for classic osteosarcomas because most are in the axial skeleton following radiotherapy for lymphomas. Osteosarcomas may occur in the sternum, vertebral bodies, shoulder, and bones of the hip. If treatment is to be successful, surgery must be radical.

Radical excision of axial lesions is difficult to perform and almost impossible without the use of preoperative chemotherapy. Preoperative chemotherapy may shrink the primary lesional area and make radical surgery possible. Tumors of the sternum need to be resected en bloc with the adjacent sternoclavicular joints, which otherwise would represent areas destined for local recurrence. The majority of osteosarcomas of the sternum tend to recur in the ribs and to produce malignant pleural effusions. The reconstruction required following radical sternal excision is difficult, but may be achieved by implantation of methylmethacrylate Marlex mesh inserts or transplantation of autograft segments from the iliac wings. We give a protracted course of preoperative chemotherapy and do not perform surgery until good response to preoperative chemotherapy is established. Since chemotherapy in the immediate postoperative period may be precluded by surgical complications, a protracted course of preoperative chemotherapy seems prudent, if the patient is responding well to treatment, prior to subjecting the patient to an attempt at curative surgery.

REFERENCES

1. Enneking WF, Spanier SS, Goodman MA. A system for the surgical staging of musculoskeletal sarcoma. Clin Orthop 1980;153:106.
2. Greene FL, Balch CM, Page DL, et al, editors. American Joint Committee on Cancer (AJCC) Cancer staging manual. 6th ed. New York: Springer-Verlag; 2002. p. 187–92.
3. Mankin HJ, Lange TA, Spanier SS. The hazards of biopsy in patients with malignant primary bone and soft tissue tumors. J Bone Joint Surg Am 1982;64:1121–7.
4. Mankin HJ, Mankin CJ, Simon MA. The hazards of the biopsy, revisited. Members of the Musculoskeletal Tumor Society. J Bone Joint Surg Am 1996;78:656–63.
5. Rosenthal DI, Hornicek FJ, Wolfe MW, et al. Percutaneous radiofrequency coagulation of osteoid osteoma compared with operative treatment. J Bone Joint Surg Am 1998;80:815–21.
6. Alman BA, De Bari A, Krajbich JI. Massive allografts in the treatment of osteosarcoma and Ewing sarcoma in children and adolescents. J Bone Joint Surg Am 1995;77:54–64.
7. Gebhardt MC, Flugstad DI, Springfield DS, Mankin HJ. The use of bone allografts for limb salvage in high-grade extremity osteosarcoma. Clin Orthop 1991;270:181–96.
8. Hornicek FJ Jr, Mnaymneh W, Lackman RD, et al. Limb salvage with osteoarticular allografts after resection of proximal tibia bone tumors. Clin Orthop 1998;352:179–86.
9. Muscolo DL, Ayerza MA, Aponte-Tinao LA. Survivorship and radiographic analysis of knee osteoarticular allografts. Clin Orthop 2000;373:73–9.
10. Clohisy DR, Mankin HJ. Osteoarticular allografts for reconstruction after resection of a musculoskeletal tumor in the proximal end of the tibia. J Bone Joint Surg Am 1994;76:549–54.
11. Gebhardt MC, Roth YF, Mankin HJ. Osteoarticular allografts for reconstruction in the proximal part of the humerus after excision of a musculoskeletal tumor. J Bone Joint Surg Am 1990;72:334–45.
12. Mankin HJ, Gebhardt MC, Jennings LC, et al. Long-term results of allograft replacement in the management of bone tumors. Clin Orthop 1996;324:86–97.
13. Gebhardt MC, Jaffe K, Mankin HJ. Bone allografts for tumors and other reconstructions in children. In: Langlais F, Tomeno E, editors. Limb salvage—major reconstructions in oncologic and nontumoral conditions. Berlin: Springer-Verlag; 1991. p. 561–72.
14. O'Connor MI, Sim FH, Chao EY. Limb salvage for neoplasms of the shoulder girdle. Intermediate reconstructive and functional results. J Bone Joint Surg Am 1996;78:1872–88.
15. Ortiz-Cruz E, Gebhardt MC, Jennings LC, et al. The results of transplantation of intercalary allografts after resection of tumors. A long-term follow-up study. J Bone Joint Surg Am 1997;79:97–106.
16. Weiner SD, Scarborough M, Vander Griend RA. Resection arthrodesis of the knee with an intercalary allograft. J Bone Joint Surg Am 1996;78:185–192.
17. Grimer RJ, Belthur M, Carter SR, et al. Extendible replacements of the proximal tibia for bone tumours. J Bone Joint Surg Br 2000;82:255–60.
18. McDonald DJ, Capanna R, Gherlinzoni F, et al. Influence of chemotherapy on perioperative complications in limb salvage surgery for bone tumors. Cancer 1990;65:1509–16.
19. Wirganowicz PZ, Eckardt JJ, Dorey FJ, et al. Etiology and results of tumor endoprosthesis revision surgery in 64 patients. Clin Orthop 1999;358:64–74.
20. Malawer MM, Chou LB. Prosthetic survival and clinical results with use of large-segment replacements in the treatment of high-grade bone sarcomas. J Bone Joint Surg Am 1995;77:1154–65.
21. Ritschl P, Capanna R, Helwig U, et al. [KMFTR (Kotz Modular Femur Tibia Reconstruction System) modular tumor endoprosthesis system for the lower extremity] Z Orthop Ihre Grenzgeb 1992;130:290–3.
22. Ward WG, Yang R-S, Eckardt JJ. Endoprosthetic bone reconstruction following malignant tumor resection in skeletally immature patients. Orthop Clin North Am 1996;27:493–502.
23. Mnaymneh W, Malinin TI, Makley JT, Dick HM. Massive osteoarticular allografts in the reconstruction of extremities following resection of tumors not requiring chemotherapy and radiation. Clin Orthop 1985;197:76–87.
24. Finn HA, Simon MA. Limb-salvage surgery in the treatment of osteosarcoma in skeletally immature individuals. Clin Orthop 1991;262:108–18.
25. Eckardt JJ, Safran MR, Eilber FR, et al. Expandable endoprosthetic reconstruction of the skeletally immature after malignant bone tumor resection. Clin Orthop 1993;297:188–202.
26. Schiller C, Windhager R, Fellinger EJ, et al. Extendable tumour endoprostheses for the leg in children. J Bone Joint Surg Br 1995;77:608–14.
27. Eckardt JJ, Kabo JM, Kelley CM, et al. Expandable endoprosthesis reconstruction in skeletally immature patients with tumors. Clin Orthop 2000;373:51–61.
28. Schindler OS, Cannon SR, Briggs TW, Blunn GW. Stanmore custom-made extendable distal femoral replacements. Clinical experience in children with primary malignant bone tumours. J Bone Joint Surg Br 1997;79:927–37.
29. Schindler OS, Cannon SR, Briggs TW, et al. Use of extendable total femoral replacements in children with malignant bone tumors. Clin Orthop 1998;357:157–70.
30. Kenan S, Bloom N, Lewis MM. Limb-sparing surgery in skeletally immature patients with osteosarcoma. The use of an expandable prosthesis. Clin Orthop 1991;270:223–30.
31. Lewis MM, Bloom N, Esquieres EM, et al. The expandable prosthesis. An alternative to amputation for children with malignant bone tumors. AORN J 1987;46:457–70.
32. Enneking WF, Kagan A. "Skip" metastases in osteosarcoma. Cancer 1975;36:2192–205.
33. Simon MA. Limb salvage for osteosarcoma. J Bone Joint Surg Am 1988;70:307–10.
34. Lindner NJ, Ramm O, Hillmann A, et al. Limb salvage and outcome of osteosarcoma. The University of Muenster experience. Clin Orthop 1999;358:83–9.
35. Gherlinzoni F, Picci P, Bacci G, Campanacci D. Limb sparing versus amputation in osteosarcoma. Correlation between local control, surgical margins and tumor necrosis: Istituto Rizzoli experience. Ann Oncol 1992;3:S23–7.
36. Schulte M, Brecht-Krauss D, Werner M, et al. Evaluation of neoadjuvant therapy response of osteogenic sarcoma using FDG PET. J Nucl Med 1999;40:1637–43.
37. van der Woude HJ, Bloem JL, Hogendoorn PC. Preoperative evaluation and monitoring chemotherapy in patients with high-grade osteogenic and Ewing's sarcoma: review of current imaging modalities. Skeletal Radiol 1998;27:57–71.
38. Sato O, Kawai A, Ozaki T, et al. Value of thallium-201 scintigraphy in bone and soft tissue tumors. J Orthop Sci 1998;3:297–303.
39. Imbriaco M, Yeh SD, Yeung H, et al. Thallium-201 scintigraphy for the evaluation of tumor response to preoperative chemotherapy in patients with osteosarcoma. Cancer 1997;80:1507–12.
40. Reddick WE, Bhargava R, Taylor JS, et al. Dynamic contrast-enhanced MR imaging evaluation of osteosarcoma response to neoadjuvant chemotherapy. J Magn Reson Imaging 1995;5:689–94.
41. Scully SP, Temple HT, O'Keefe RJ, et al. The surgical treatment of patients with osteosarcoma who sustain a pathologic fracture. Clin Orthop 1996;324:227–32.
42. Scully SP, Ghert MA, Zurakowski D, et al. Pathologic fracture in osteosarcoma: prognostic importance and treatment implications. J Bone Joint Surg Am 2002;84:49–57.
43. Jaffe N, Spears R, Eftekhari F, et al. Pathologic fracture in osteosarcoma. Impact of chemotherapy on primary tumor and survival. Cancer 1987;59:701–9.
44. Otis JC, Lane JM, Kroll MA. Energy cost during gait in osteosarcoma patients after resection and knee replace-

ment and after above-the-knee amputation. J Bone Joint Surg Am 1985;67:606–11.
45. Harris IE, Leff AR, Gitelis S, Simon MA. Function after amputation, arthrodesis, or arthroplasty , for tumors about the knee. J Bone Joint Surg Am 1990;72:1477–85.
46. Postma A, Kingma A, De Ruiter JH, et al. Quality of life in bone tumor patients comparing limb salvage and amputation of the lower extremity. J Surg Oncol 1992;51:47–51.
47. Bacci G, Picci P, Ferrari S, et al. Synchronous multifocal osteosarcoma: results in twelve patients treated with neoadjuvant chemotherapy and simultaneous resection of all involved bones. Ann Oncol 1996;7:864–6.
48. LaQuaglia MP. Osteosarcoma. Specific tumor management and results. Chest Surg Clin N Am 1998;8:77–95.
49. Goorin AM, Delorey MJ, Lack EE, et al. Prognostic significance of complete surgical resection of pulmonary metastases in patients with osteogenic sarcoma: analysis of 32 patients. J Clin Oncol 1984;2:425–31.
50. Saeter G, Hoie J, Stenwig AE, et al. Systemic relapse of patients with osteogenic sarcoma. Prognostic factors for long term survival. Cancer 1995;75:1084–93.
51. Putnam JB Jr, Roth JA, Wesley MN, et al. Survival following aggressive resection of pulmonary metastases from osteogenic sarcoma: analysis of prognostic factors. Ann Thorac Surg 1983;36:516–23.
52. Tabone MD, Kalifa C, Rodary C, et al. Osteosarcoma recurrences in pediatric patients previously treated with intensive chemotherapy. J Clin Oncol 1994;12:2614–20.
53. Telander RL, Pairolero PC, Pritchard DJ, et al. Resection of pulmonary metastatic osteogenic sarcoma in children. Surgery 1978;84:335–41.
54. Kakuda J, Omari B, Renslo R, et al. CT guided needle localization for video-thoracoscopic resection of pulmonary nodules. Eur J Med Res 1997;2:340–2.
55. Aubert A, Chaffanjon P, Peoch M, Brichon PY. Chest wall implantation of a mediastinal liposarcoma after thoracoscopy. Ann Thorac Surg 2000;69:1579–80.
56. Tillman B, Dahlen DC, Lipscomb PR, Stewart FR. Aneurysmal bone cyst. An analysis of 95 cases. Mayo Clin Proc 1968;43:478–95.
57. Saltzman EI, Jun MY. Aneurysmal bone cyst of the mandible: report of a case. J Surg Oncol 1981;17:385–94.
58. Biesecker JL, Marcove RC, Huvos AG, Mike V. Aneurysmal bone cysts. A clinico-pathologic study of 66 cases. Cancer 1970;26:615–25.
59. Parrish FF, Pevey JK. Surgical management of aneurysmal bone cyst of the vertebral column. J Bone Joint Surg Am 1967;49A:1597–604.
60. Arndt CAS, Crist WM. Common musculoskeletal tumors of childhood and adolescence. N Engl J Med 1999;34:342–51.
61. Mirra JM, Gold R, Downs J, Eckardt JJ. A new histologic approach to the differentiation of enchondroma from chondrosarcoma of the bones. A clinico-pathologic analysis of 51 cases. Clin Orthoped 1985;201:214–37.
62. Komp DM. Historical perspectives of Langerhans' cell histiocytosis. Hematol Oncol Clin North Am 1987;1:9–21.
63. Slater JM, Swarm OJ. Eosinophilic granuloma of bone. Med Pediatr Oncol 1980;8:151–64.
64. Greenberger JS, Crocker AC, Vawter G, et al. Results of treatment of 127 patients with systemic histiocytosis (Letterer-Siwe syndrome, Schuller-Christian syndrome and multifocal eosinophilic granuloma). Medicine 1981;60:311–38.
65. Ridley MM, Raney RB, Thawerani H, Meadows AT. Histiocytosis X in children: patterns of disease and results of treatment. Med Pediatr Oncol 1983;11:99–105.
66. Mirra JM. In: Bone tumors: clinical, radiologic and pathologic correlations. Philadelphia, PA: Lea & Febiger; 1989. p 155–73.
67. Yabut SM, Sessons KS, Lewis MM. Malignant transformation of fibrous dysplasia: a case report and review of the literature. Clin Orthoped 1988;228:281–89.
68. Ruggieri P, Sim FH, Bond JR, Unni KK. Malignancies in fibrous dysplasia. Cancer 1994;73:1411–24.
69. Phaler GF, Parry LD. The treatment of giant-cell bone tumors by roentgen irradiation. AJR Am J Roentgenol 1932;28:151–66.
70. Dahlin DC. Giant cell tumor of bone: highlights of 407 cases. AJR Am J Roentgenol 1985;144:955–60.
71. Bennett CJ, Marcus RB, Millian RR, Enneking WF. Radiation therapy for giant cell tumor of bone. Int J Radiat Oncol Biol Phys 1993;26:299–304.
72. Freiberger R, Loitman B, Helpern M, Thompson T. Osteoid osteoma—a report of 80 cases. AJR Am J Roentgenol 1959;82:194–205.
73. Marcove RC, Alpert MA. Pathologic study of benign osteoblastoma. Clin Orthop 1963;30:175–81.
74. Schajowicz F, Lemos C. Osteoid osteoma and osteoblastoma. Closely related entities of osteoblastic derivation. Acta Orthop Scand 1970;41:272–91.
75. Albright F, Buttler AM, Hampton AO, Smith P. Syndrome characterized by osteitis fibrosa disseminata, areas of pigmentation and endocrine dysfunction with precocious puberty in females: report of five cases. N Engl J Med 1937;216:727–46.
76. Jaffee HL. Benign osteoblastoma. Bull Hosp Joint Dis 1956;17:141–51.
77. Mitchell ML, Ackerman LV. Metastatic and pseudomalignant osteoblastoma. A report of two unusual cases. Skeletal Radiol 1986;15:213–8.
78. Campanna R, Ayala A, Bertoni F, et al. Sacral osteoid osteoma and osteoblastoma: a report of 13 cases. Arch Orthoped Trauma Surg 1986;105:205–10.
79. Marsh BW, Bronfiglio M, Brady LP, Enneking WF. Benign osteoblastoma: range of manifestations. J Bone Joint Surg Am 1975;57A:1–9.
80. Jackson RP. Recurrent osteoblastoma. A review. Clin Orthoped Rel Res 1978;131:229–33.
81. Wilkins RM. Unicameral bone cysts. J Am Acad Orthop Surg 2000;8:217–24.
82. Vickers RA, Gorlin RJ. Ameloblastoma: delineation of early histopathologic features of neoplasia. Cancer 1965;26:421–35.
83. Gardner DG, Pecak AM. The treatment of ameloblastoma based on pathologic and anatomic principles. Cancer 1980;46:2514–9.
84. Pantazopolous PE, Nomikos N. Adamantinoma of the maxillary sinus. Ann Otol Rhinol Laryngol 1966;98:1160–8.
85. Shaw HJ, Katsikas DK. Ameloblastoma of the maxilla. A clinical study with four cases. J Laryngol Otol 1973;87:873–84.
86. Sehder MK, Huvos AG, Strong EW, et al. Ameloblastoma of maxilla and mandible. Cancer 1974;33:324–33.
87. Huvos AF, Marcove RC. Adamantinoma of long bones. A clinico-pathological study of 14 cases with vascular origin suggested. J Bone Joint Surg Am 1975;57:148–54.
88. Harwood AR, Krajbich JI, Fornasier VL. Radiotherapy of chondrosarcoma of bone. Cancer 1980;4:2769–77.
89. Evans HL, Ayala AG, Romsdahl MM. Prognostic factors in chondrosarcoma of bone. A clinico-pathologic analysis with emphasis on histologic grading. Cancer 1977;40:818–31.
90. Huvos AG, Rosen G, Dabska M, Marcove RC. Mesenchymal chondrosarcoma. A clinico-pathologic analysis of 35 patients with emphasis on treatment. Cancer 1983;51:1230–7.
91. Rosen G. Spindle cell sarcomas of bone, dedifferentiated, conventional and mesenchymal chondrosarcomas. In: Schein P, editor. Decision making in oncology. Philadelphia: Decker; 1989. p. 170–3.
92. Toretsky JA, Neckers L, Wexler LH. Detection of (11;22)(q24;q12) translocation-bearing cells in peripheral blood progenitor cells of patients with Ewing's sarcoma family of tumors. J Natl Cancer Inst 1995;87:385–6.
93. Fischmeister G, Zoubek A, Jugovic D, et al. Low incidence of molecular evidence for tumour in PBPC harvests from patients with high risk Ewing tumours. Bone Marrow Transplant 1999;24:405–9.
94. Sandlund JT, Downing JR, Crist WM. Non-Hodgkin's lymphoma in childhood. N Engl J Med 1996;334:1238–48.
95. Murphy SB, Fairclough DL, Hutchison RE, Berard CW. Non-Hodgkin's lymphomas of childhood: an analysis of the histology, staging, and response to treatment of 338 cases at a single institution. J Clin Oncol 1989;7:186–93.
96. Wollner N, Lane JM, Marcove RC, et al. Hodgkin's lymphoma in the pediatric age group. Med Pediatr Oncol 1992;20:506–513.
97. Coppes MJ, Patte C, Couanet D, et al. Childhood malignant lymphoma of bone. Med Pediatr Oncol 1991;19:22–7.
98. Furman WL, Fitch S, Hustu HO, et al. Primary lymphoma of bone in children. J Clin Oncol 1989;7:1275–80.
99. Link MP, Donaldson SS, Berard CW, et al. Results of treatment of childhood localized non-Hodgkin's lymphoma with combination chemotherapy with or without radiotherapy. N Engl J Med 1990;322:1169–74.
100. Link MP, Shuster JJ, Donaldson SS, et al. Treatment of children and young adults with early-stage non-Hodgkin's lymphoma. N Engl J Med 1997;337:1259–66.
101. Howat AJ, Thomas H, Waters KD, Campbell PE. Malignant lymphoma of bone in children. Cancer 1987;59:335–9.
102. Loeffler JS, Tarbell NJ, Kozakewich H, et al. Primary lymphoma of bone in children: analysis of treatment results with Adriamycin, prednisone, Oncovin (APO), and local radiation therapy. J Clin Oncol 1986;4:496–501.
103. Jereb B, Wollner N, Kosloff C, Exelby P. The role of local radiation in the treatment of non-Hodgkin lymphoma in children. Med Pediatr Oncol 1981;9:157–66.
104. Suryanarayan K, Shuster JJ, Donaldson SS, et al. Treatment of localized primary non-Hodgkin's lymphoma of bone in children: a Pediatric Oncology Group study. J Clin Oncol 1999;17:456–9.
105. Urban C, Rosen G, Huvos AG, et al. Chemotherapy of malignant fibrous histiocytoma of bone. A report of 5 cases. Cancer 1983;51:795–802.
106. Campanna R, Bertoni F, Bacchini P, et al. Malignant fibrous histiocytoma of bone. The experience at the Rizzoli Institute: report of 90 cases. Cancer 1984;54:177–87.
107. Dahlin DC, Unni KK, Matsuno T. Malignant (fibrous) histiocytoma of bone—fact or fancy? Cancer 1977;39:1508–16.
108. Spanier S, Enneking WF, Enriquez P. Primary malignant fibrous histiocytoma of bone. Cancer 1975;36:2084–98.
109. Feldman F, Lattes R. Primary malignant fibrous histiocytoma (fibrous xanthoma) of bone. Skel Radiol 1977;1:145–60.
110. Bacci G, Avella M, Picci P. Primary chemotherapy and delayed surgery of malignant fibrous histiocytoma of bone in the extremity. Tumor 1990;76:537–42.
111. Ahuja SC, Viljacin AB, Smith J, et al. Juxtacortical (parosteal) osteosarcoma. Histological grading and prognosis. J Bone Joint Surg Am 1977;59:632–47.
112. Rosen G. Preoperative (neoadjuvant) chemotherapy for osteogenic sarcoma. A ten-year experience. Orthopedics 1985;8:658–64.
113. Rosen G, Nirenberg A. Neoadjuvant chemotherapy for osteogenic sarcoma: a five-year follow-up (T-10) and preliminary report of new studies (T-12). In: Wagner DJ, Blijham GH, Smeets JBE, Wils JA, editors. Primary chemotherapy in cancer medicine. New York: Alan R. Liss; 1985. p. 39–52.
114. Huvos AG, Rosen G, Marcove RC. Primary osteosarcoma: pathologic aspects in 20 patients after treatment with chemotherapy, en bloc resection and prosthetic bone replacement. Arch Pathol Lab Med 1977;101:14–8.
115. Stoller RG, Hande KR, Jacobs SA, et al. Use of plasma pharmacokinetics to predict and prevent methotrexate toxicity. N Engl J Med 1977;297:630–4.
116. Rosen G. Preoperative (neoadjuvant) chemotherapy for osteosarcoma. A ten-year experience. Orthopedics 1985;8:659–64.
117. Dickery ID, Rose PS, Fuchs B, et al. Dedifferentiated chondrosarcoma: the role of chemotherapy with updated outcomes. J Bone Joint Surg Am 2004;86:2412–8.

Soft Tissue Sarcomas

Peter W.T. Pisters, MD, FACS
Brian O'Sullivan, MD, FRCPI
Robert G. Maki, MD, PhD

Sarcomas of nonosseous tissues, known traditionally as soft tissue sarcomas (STS), comprise a group of relatively rare malignancies that exhibit tremendous diversity of anatomic site and histopathologic characteristics. These tumors share a common embryologic origin, arising primarily from mesodermal tissues. The notable exceptions are sarcomas of the neural tissues and possibly the Ewing's sarcoma/primitive neuroectodermal tumor (PNET) family of tumors, which are believed to arise from ectodermal tissues. Despite the fact that the somatic nonosseous tissues account for as much as 75% of total body weight, primary neoplasms of these connective tissues are comparatively rare, accounting for 1% of adult malignancies and 15% of pediatric malignancies. About 7,800 new cases of soft tissue sarcoma are diagnosed in the United States each year, with 4,400 deaths annually.[1] Despite their rarity, a thorough understanding of these tumors is important because patients' outcomes might be compromised if initial management is anything less than ideal. Furthermore, biologic insights about sarcomas are providing new strategies for the detection, treatment, and prevention of other, more common malignancies.

This chapter will review current concepts in the diagnosis, staging, and multidisciplinary management of patients with sarcomas of nonosseous tissues. The evolving contributions of molecular biology and basic scientific principles underlying the varied differentiation and clinical behavior of these tumors will also be reviewed. Although histopathologic aspects of sarcomas are increasingly important in categorizing these tumors, the anatomic site of primary disease remains an important variable on which treatment and outcome may depend. Extremity sarcomas account for approximately 50% of all sarcomas and are the focus of the therapy sections of the chapter. Retroperitoneal sarcomas (RPSs), gastrointestinal stromal tumors (GISTs), and dermatofibrosarcoma protuberans (DFSPs) are addressed separately later in the chapter. Sarcomas at other anatomic sites are not discussed because of their rarity. Throughout the chapter, the emphasis is on identifying what is known from definitive data and what requires additional research.

ETIOLOGY

The causes of sarcoma remain obscure in the vast majority of cases. The conceptual frameworks that address the neoplastic transformation of mesenchymal stem cells are in rapid evolution owing to new insights from the molecular analysis of sarcomatous and normal tissues from soft tissue sarcoma patients and family members. Genetics and environmental factors each appear to play a role in the neoplastic transformation of soft tissues into sarcomas.

It has been recognized for more than 30 years that sarcomas can arise in persons with certain genetic predispositions to cancer development. One of the earliest observations of familial cancer development (ie, genetically transmitted predisposition to malignancy) was the development of sarcoma and other tumor types (such as breast cancer) in certain families.[2,3] This autosomal dominant genetic predisposition has now become known as the Li-Fraumeni syndrome, and it has been characterized at the molecular level as a germline mutation of the *TP53* gene, which presumably acts in this context as a faulty tumor suppressor.[4,5]

Other genetic disorders are also associated with an increased risk of developing certain types of sarcoma. The best studied example of this is the predilection of patients with neurofibromatoses to develop malignant peripheral nerve sheath tumors (MPNSTs, also referred to as neurofibrosarcomas or malignant schwannomas).[6] Type 1 neurofibromatosis (von Recklinghausen's disease) is an autosomal dominant disease that can disrupt the function of the *NF1* gene, located on chromosome 17q11.2. The endogenous function of the NF1 gene product, neurofibromin, is incompletely understood, but neurofibromin appears to act as a tumor suppressor via stimulation of guanosine triphosphatase activity. This, in turn, may control *ras* oncogene signaling pathways. Common mutations in *NF1* include truncations, with loss of function leading to uncontrolled signaling through *ras* pathways.[7–9] This may be a fundamental process that facilitates the development of MPNSTs over time in patients with neurofibromatosis. Patients with type 1 neurofibromatosis have up to a 10% cumulative lifetime risk of developing sarcoma (usually MPNST).[10]

Survivors of childhood retinoblastoma have also been noted to have an increased risk of sarcoma development later in life. This provides yet another molecular model of a dysfunctional or deleted tumor suppressor genetic element (in this case, the product of the *Rb* gene on chromosome (13q14).[11–16] The risk of soft tissue sarcoma in retinoblastoma patients and their families is accompanied by the risk of developing several other types of neoplasms, including osteosarcomas, breast cancer, and lung cancer. No reasons have been convincingly posited for the development of one type of malignancy over another in patients with *Rb* mutations, and this remains an important question to be addressed by future research on mechanisms of neoplastic transformation.

Gardner's syndrome represents an important genetic connection between dysfunctional regulation of epithelial and of mesenchymal cells. Gardner's syndrome represents a subset of familial adenomatous polyposis disorders of the bowel (usually the colon); patients with the syndrome also have extracolonic abnormalities such as epidermoid cysts and osteomas. The molecular lesion has been identified as a defect within the *APC* (adenomatous polyposis coli) gene on chromosome 5q21. Patients with Gardner's syndrome are at much increased risk of developing mesenteric and intraperitoneal desmoid tumors. Desmoid tumors are mesenchymal cells proliferating in a pattern of aggressive fibromatosis, characterized by bland cells that—although histologically benign—act in a malignant fashion with uncontrolled proliferation and infiltration of vital structures. It remains poorly understood why some patients with Gardner's syndrome develop desmoid tumors whereas others do not, and the lifetime risk of developing desmoid tumors has been estimated at approximately 10 to 20%, representing a nearly 1,000 times greater risk than that of the general population.

Certain environmental exposures have also been associated with the development of sarcomas. One of the most important is ionizing radiation. Radiation-associated sarcoma is most often a late effect of radiotherapy (RT) given to treat another condition (often a prior malignancy). Sarcomas have been noted as a late effect of (RT) for breast cancer, Hodgkin's disease, non-Hodgkin's lymphomas, and other tumor types.[12] The radiation dose appears to be correlated with the later development of sarcoma, with a very low risk in patients who received less than 10 Gy.[12] However, the molecular mechanisms may be complex, since it has been noted clinically that sarcomas appear at the margins of prior RT fields. This suggests that the mutagenic effect may be maximal at the edges of prior RT where scatter radiation leads to a dose sufficient to induce mutations but insufficient to kill the mutated cells. Traditionally, radiation-associated sarcomas were thought to arise several years following RT, although newer data indicate that a shorter latency period of 2 to

4 years may also be possible.[17–20] MPNSTs, angiosarcomas, and other high-grade unclassifiable histopathologic subtypes comprise the majority of radiation-associated sarcomas. Although they are aggressive, radiation-associated sarcomas may not behave truly differently from other high-grade sarcomas. Clinical outcomes have been reported to be poor in patients with radiation-associated sarcomas, perhaps because of their typically high-grade and because of the inability to use full multimodality treatment (eg, because the patient has already received the maximum tolerable radiation dose or has had extensive prior doxorubicin exposure). Radiation-associated sarcomas should be approached as new primary disease and treated appropriately to optimize the patient's outcomes.

Certain chemical exposures have also been documented to induce sarcomas, and chemical-induced development of sarcomas in animal models has been one of the more widely employed models of studying neoplastic transformation in the laboratory. Hepatic angiosarcomas have been associated with exposure to several classes of chemicals, including polyvinyl chloride, arsenic compounds, and the thorium dioxide colloid Thorotrast (an antiquated contrast agent).[21–29] The possible relationship between exposure and development of sarcoma is less clear for other compounds, including dioxins (such as Agent Orange and other phenoxyacetic acid-based herbicides) and chlorophenols used in wood preservatives.[30]

Chronic irritation of tissues is a controversial potential cause of sarcomas. Certainly, there is an increased sarcoma risk in the lymphedematous arms of women who have undergone radical mastectomy, often with the additional complicating variable of prior RT (the Stewart-Treves syndrome).[31,32] Limited data also suggest that other sources of chronic tissue irritation and inflammation might be associated with the development of sarcoma.[33] Although a history of trauma is not infrequently elicited from patients with soft tissue sarcomas, the impact of such trauma on sarcoma development is in doubt.

Severe and chronic immunosuppression following solid organ transplantation represents yet another risk factor for the development of sarcomas. Sarcomas represent a disproportionate percentage of tumors (10%) in patients following solid organ transplantation, with Kaposi's sarcoma comprising the majority of these.[34]

SCREENING

Given the rarity of sarcomas in the general population, no general screening is indicated beyond routine health care surveillance. However, it is important for physicians to be aware of the predisposing genetic tendencies and environmental exposures that might increase patients' risks of sarcoma development. A complete family history should reveal clues about genetic predispositions, including a family history of polyposis, neurofibromatosis, retinoblastoma, any cancer at a young age in first-degree relatives, or sarcomas. Genetic counseling would be appropriate to discuss issues relating to these predispositions. In patients at increased risk of sarcoma, a more detailed clinical evaluation might be required at a lower threshold of intervention than one might use in general practice. Rapidly growing masses, especially symptomatic ones, in patients with neurofibromatosis should be considered for surgical removal to rule out the potential of sarcomatous transformation of a neurofibroma. Similarly, any superficial or deep abnormalities of skin or soft tissues in patients with a history of prior RT should be evaluated very thoroughly.

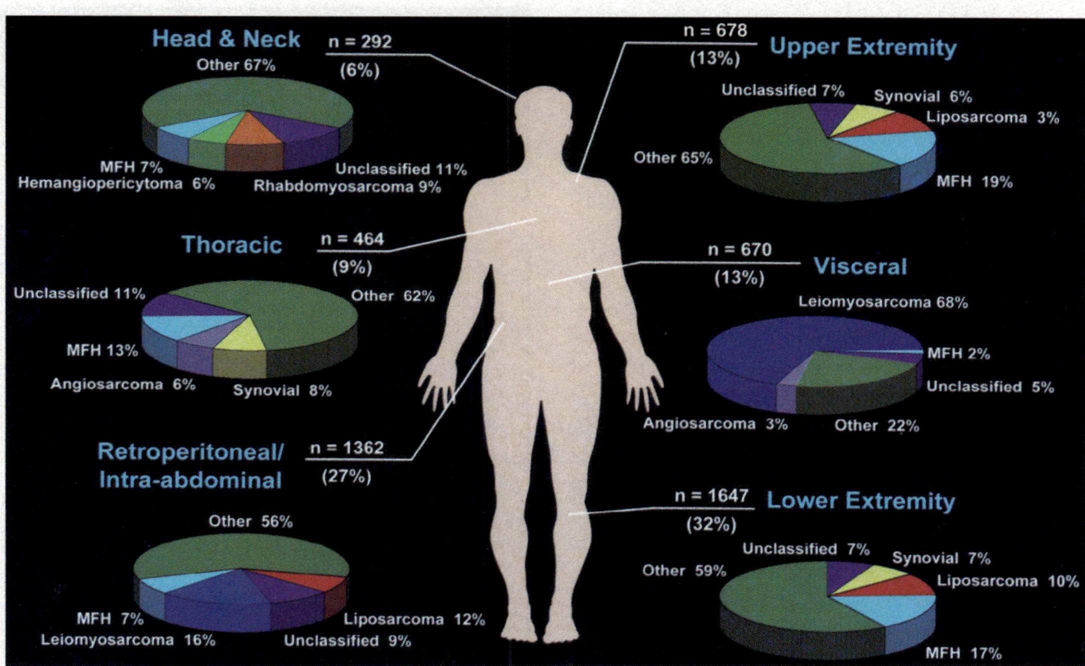

Figure 111-1 Anatomic distribution and site-specific histologic subtypes of 5,113 consecutive soft tissue sarcomas seen at the University of Texas M. D. Anderson Cancer Center Sarcoma Center (MDACC Sarcoma Database, June 1996 to June 2005).

CLINICAL PRESENTATION, CLASSIFICATION, AND DIAGNOSIS

Sites of Origin Sarcomas of nonosseous tissues have been noted to arise at virtually all anatomic sites. The anatomic sites and site-specific histologic subtypes of more than 5,113 sarcomas treated at a single referral institution are outlined in Figure 111-1. Approximately one-third to one-half of all sarcomas of nonosseous tissues occur in the lower extremities, where the most common histopathologic subtypes have traditionally been noted to include liposarcomas as well as the vaguely defined entity "malignant fibrous histiocytoma." With improved pathologic tools to categorize sarcomas (eg, immunohistochemistry and molecular analyses), it is increasingly recognized that sarcomas previously referred to as malignant fibrous histiocytoma are often more accurately categorized as poorly differentiated liposarcomas or leiomyosarcomas, as well as other histologic subtypes.[35] RPSs comprise 15 to 20% of all soft tissue sarcomas, with liposarcoma and leiomyosarcoma being the predominant histologic subtypes. The visceral sarcomas make up an additional 24%, and the head and neck sarcomas approximately 4% of sarcomas.

Clinical Presentation The majority of patients with nonosseous sarcomas present with a painless mass, although pain is noted at presentation in up to a third of cases.[36] Delay in diagnosis of sarcomas is common, with the most common incorrect diagnosis for extremity and trunk lesions being hematoma or "lipoma." Late diagnosis of RPSs is extremely common, since tumors in this area can grow to massive size before causing any symptoms (such as abdominal distention or psoas irritation with back or groin discomfort).

Physical examination should include an assessment of the size and mobility of the mass. Its relationship to the fascia (superficial versus deep) and nearby neurovascular and bony structures should be noted. A site-specific neurovascular examination and assessment of regional lymph nodes should also be performed.

Histopathologic Classification Methods of Classification In broad terms, sarcomas can be classified as neoplasms arising in bone versus those arising from the nonosseous or periosseous soft tissues. Sarcomas of nonosseous tissues can be further grouped into those that arise from the viscera (eg, gastrointestinal or gynecologic organs) and those that originate in nonvisceral soft tissues such as muscle, tendon, adipose tissue, pleura, synovium, and other connective tissues.

The most universally applied classification scheme for soft tissue sarcoma is based on histogenesis, as outlined in the recent World Health Organization classification system for sarcomas.[37,38] This classification system is reproducible between pathologists for the better differentiated tumors. However, as the degree of histologic differentiation declines, the determination of cellular origin becomes increasingly difficult. In particular, despite advanced immunohistochemical techniques[39] and electron microscopy, determining the cellular origin for some spindle cell and round cell soft tissue tumors is difficult to impossible.[39] A discrepancy between the original histologic assessment and that of a subsequent expert review has been noted in as many as 25% of cases of some subgroups of soft tissue sarcomas.[40,41]

Difficulties in establishing the specific cellular origin of soft tissue sarcomas have occasionally been viewed as having limited clinical importance because clinical investigators have not had sufficient data to tie the histologic subtype directly to biologic behavior or to specific therapeutic interventions. Important exceptions to this generalization include epithelioid sarcoma, clear cell sarcoma, angiosarcoma, and embryonal rhabdomyosarcoma, all of which have a greater risk of regional lymph node metastasis.[42,43] In one single-institution study, the overall rate of nodal metastasis at the time of presentation was only 2.7%; however, the rate was much higher for the histologic subtypes angiosarcoma (13.5%), embryonal rhabdomyosarcoma (13.6%), and epithelioid sarcoma (16.7%).[42] Thus, treatment strategies may differ for these histologic subtypes. For the remaining histologic subtypes, biologic behavior appears to be determined more by histologic grade than by histologic subtype.[44] However, as the fundamental biologic and molecular understanding of the mechanisms of malignant transformation in sarcomas increases, in-depth categorization may well prove to have important clinical ramifications. The tools required to categorize or identify sarcomas at the molecular level are now present for certain types, including synovial sarcomas, liposarcomas, GISTs, myofibroblastic sarcomas, Ewing's sarcoma/PNET, and rhabdomyosarcomas (Table 111-1). Future studies will need to take histologic subtype into account in a more sophisticated manner than in the past three decades of research when molecular markers were not available. Recently, there has also been a tendency to significant redefinition within the pathological classification of STS. Thus, malignant fibrous histiocytoma (MFH) has traditionally been regarded as the most common STS in adults, but the true nature and validity of this entity have increasingly been questioned. Available data suggest that most patients with MFH can be subclassified into specific STS types. Specifically, pleomorphic STS showing myogenic differentiation are significantly more aggressive than other subtypes.[28,35] Recent evaluations have shown very profound changes to the classification of previously diagnosed cases with more than 50% of cases undergoing significant modification.[29,45] Of note, Daugaard recently studied a series of cases where the number of MFHs was reduced from 72 to 2, with 22 renamed myxofibrosarcomas and 20 cases (7%) were found not to be sarcomas.[29,45] Contributing reasons are recent advances in immunohistochemistry in addition to changes in nomenclature. The findings are important for several reasons, including the implications they have for retrospective research and potentially also on treatment approaches for some patients.

Table 111-1 Cytogenetic Aberrations in Nonosseous Sarcomas

Histologic Subtype	Cytogenetic Finding	Genes
Myxoid liposarcoma	t(12;16)	TLS/CHOP
Well-differentiated liposarcoma	Rings and giant markers	Amplified 12q13-15
		HMG1-C
		CDK4
		MDM2
Lipoma (minimal atypia)	12q abnormalities	Amplified 12q13-15
Lipoma	12q14-15 abnormalities	
	6p abnormalities	
Synovial sarcoma	t(X;18)	SYT/SSX1 or SSX2
Ewing's family/PNET	t(11;22) and others	EWS/FLI1 (and others)
Rhabdomyosarcoma	t(2;13) or t(1;13)	PAX3 (or 7)/FKHR (alveolar)
Clear cell sarcoma	t(12;22)	EWS/ATF1
Extraskeletal myxoid chondrosarcomas	t(9;22)	EWS/CHN
	t(9;17)	RPB56 / CHN
Dermatofibrosarcoma protuberans	t(17;22)	
Collagen type I alpha1 ring(17;22)	PDGF-B	
Endometrial stromal	t(7;17) sarcoma	
Uterine leiomyosarcoma	t(12;14)	
	7q-	
Desmoplastic small round-cell tumor	t(11;22)	EWS/WT1
Alveolar sarcoma of soft parts	t(X;17)	

PNET = primitive neuroectodermal tumors.

Histologic Grade Biologic aggressiveness can often be predicted based on histologic grade.[44,46] The spectrum of grades varies among specific histologic subtypes (Figure 111-2). In careful comparative multivariate analyses, histo-

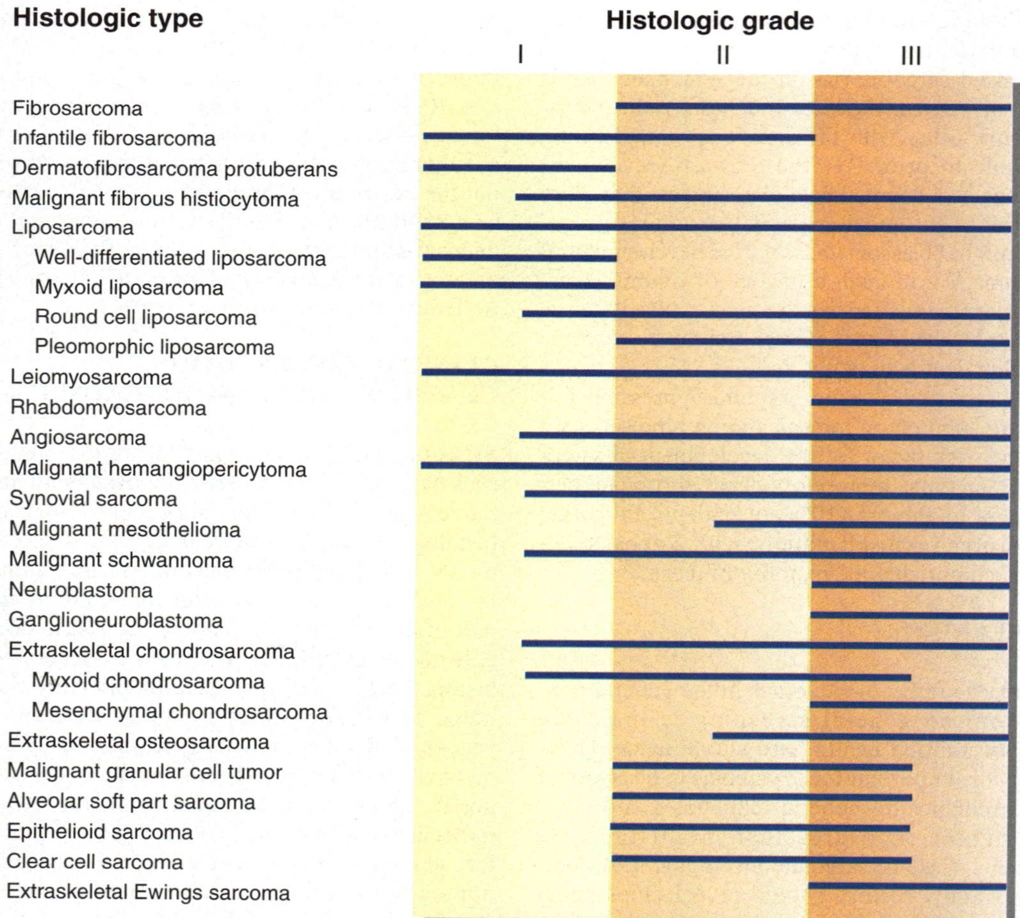

Figure 111-2 Spectrum of grades observed among histologic subtypes of soft tissue sarcoma. (From Enzinger FN and Weiss SW, editors. Soft tissue tumors. 3rd ed. Mosby-Year Book Inc; 1995. With permission.)

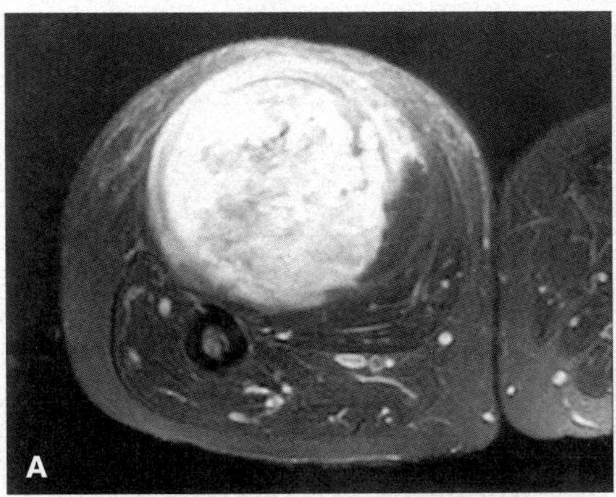

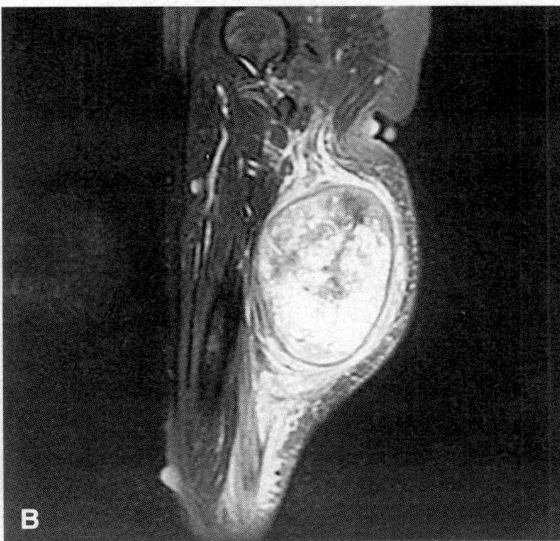

Figure 111-3 A, Weighted T2-fat-saturated magnetic resonance image of a TNM T2b high-grade sarcoma in the posterior thigh compartment of a 55-year-old woman. Note the containment by the superficial fascia overlying the posterior thigh muscles, where there is a "strip" of peritumoral edema. Anteriorly, the lesion can be seen to be separate from the femur, but the edge of the tumor is less clearly defined than its superficial component, presumably because of muscle infiltration. **B,** Sagittal magnetic resonance image of the same patient. The main lesion manifests a well-defined border. However, a clear zone of peritumoral edema is evident tracking proximally toward the head of the femur, seen at the top of the figure. Inferiorly, the edema seems to be even more pronounced as evidenced by the triangular signal enhancement pointing inferiorly. Whether the zone of edema harbors microscopic disease is uncertain, and this uncertainty can complicate accurate treatment planning (see text).

logic grade has been the most important prognostic factor in assessing the risk of distant metastasis and tumor-related death.[44,46] Several grading systems have been proposed, but there is no consensus regarding the specific morphologic criteria that should be employed in the grading of soft tissue sarcomas.

Two of the most commonly employed grading systems are the US National Cancer Institute (NCI) system developed by Costa and colleagues and the system developed by the Federation Nationale des Centres de Lutte Contre le Cancer (FNCLCC) Sarcoma Group.[47,48] The NCI system is based on the tumor's histologic subtype, location, and amount of tumor necrosis, but cellularity, nuclear pleomorphism, and mitosis count are also to be considered in certain situations. The FNCLCC system employs a score generated by the evaluation of three parameters: tumor differentiation, mitotic rate, and amount of tumor necrosis. In a retrospective comparison of these two grading systems, in a population of 410 adult patients with nonmetastatic soft tissue sarcoma, univariate and multivariate analyses suggested that the FNCLCC system has a slightly better ability to predict distant metastasis and tumor-related death.[49] Significant discrepancies in assigned grade were observed in one-third of cases. An increased number of grade 3 tumors, reduced number of grade 2 tumors, and better correlation with overall and metastasis-free survival were observed in favor of the FNCLCC system.[49] Thus, in the absence of other comparative data, the FNCLCC system may be the best presently available grading system.

In discussing grade, it is important to note two well-described characteristics of sarcomas. First, there is often tremendous intratumoral heterogeneity within individual sarcomas. Therefore, diagnoses based on very limited amounts of tumor may be inaccurate (eg, diagnoses based only on fine-needle aspiration biopsy specimens). This is particularly true for such histopathologic subtypes as de-differentiated liposarcomas, where one area of the tumor might have a relatively low-to-intermediate grade appearance and another area within the same tumor might have more evident high-grade components. Any discussion of the clinical relevance of grading must take into account this variability inherent in the diagnostic process, which will add to the clinical variability in outcomes among patients with any given grade of sarcomas.

Second, the grade of tumors may change over time. This process is best described in the evolution of de-differentiated liposarcoma arising in conjunction with well-differentiated liposarcoma in the same patient. Additional examples include the fibrosarcomatous degeneration that can accompany multiple recurrent DFSPs.

Imaging Optimal imaging of the primary tumor is dependent on the anatomic site. For soft tissue masses of the extremities, magnetic resonance imaging (MRI) has been regarded as the imaging modality of choice (Figures 111-3 and 111-4) because MRI enhances the contrast between tumor and muscle and between tumor and adjacent blood vessels and provides multiplanar definition of the lesion.[50,51] However, a study by the Radiation Diagnostic Oncology Group that compared MRI and computed tomography (CT) in patients with malignant bone (n = 183) and soft tissue (n = 133) tumors demonstrated no specific advantage of MRI over CT.[52] On the other hand, although it may be true that the diagnostic evaluation is equally served by both modalities, surgery and RT planning may require additional information provided by the multiplanar capability of MRI and the ability to perform MRI/CT image fusion.[53,54] For pelvic lesions, the multiplanar capability of MRI may provide superior single-modality imaging (see Figure 111-4), whereas in the retroperitoneum and abdomen, CT usually provides satisfactory anatomic definition of the lesion. Occasionally, MRI with gradient sequence imaging can better delineate the relationship of a tumor to midline vascular structures, particularly the inferior vena cava and aorta (Figure 111-5). More invasive studies such as angiography or cavography are almost never required for the evaluation of soft tissue sarcomas.

Cost-effective imaging to exclude the possibility of distant metastatic disease is dependent on the size, grade, and anatomic location of the primary tumor. In general, patients with low- and intermediate-grade tumors or high-grade tumors 5 cm or less in diameter require only a chest radiograph for satisfactory staging of the chest. This directly reflects the comparatively low risk of presentation with pulmonary metastases in these patients.[55] However, patients with high-

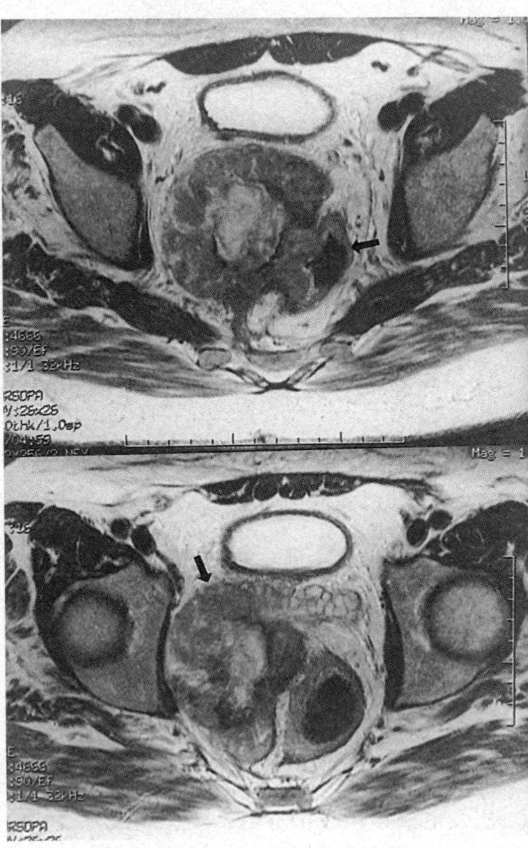

Figure 111-4 A 57-year-old man with T2 pelvic leiomyosarcoma. **Top:** Axial T_2-weighted fast-spin echo magnetic resonance image reveals a heterogeneous mass involving the rectum (*arrow* air in rectal lumen). **Bottom:** Note abutment of mass to right seminal vesicle (*arrow*).

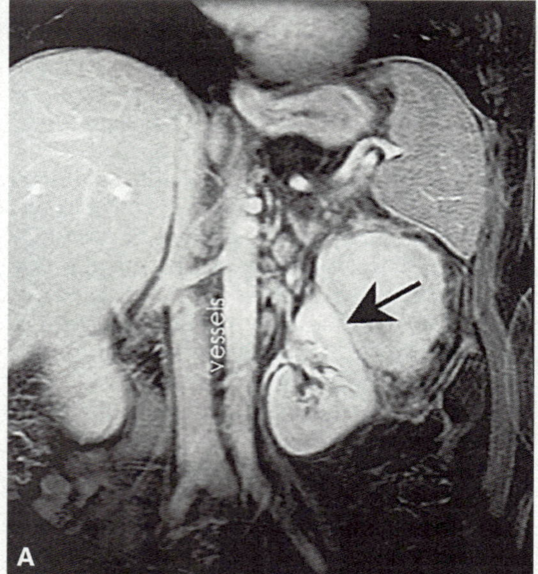

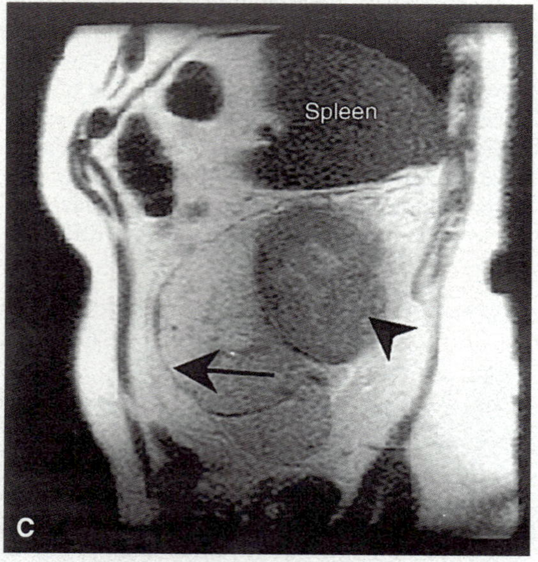

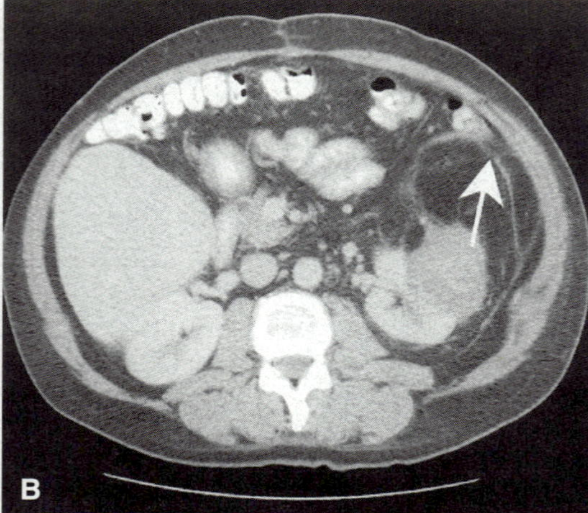

Figure 111-5 **A,** Coronal fat-saturated gadolinium-enhanced magnetic resonance (MR) image showing a solid liposarcoma, 8.3 cm × 6.6 cm, adjacent to and compressing the upper pole of the left kidney. The mass lies below the spleen and is separate from the kidney (see line of demarcation with *arrow*), but is part of a larger fatty tumor. The midline vessels are well visualized. **B,** Computerized tomography (CT) image of the same lesion. The mass can be seen adjacent to the kidney, as before. An additional mass of fatty attenuation with gray areas of edema, inflammation, or increased cellularity can be seen bounded by a rim anteriorly (*arrow*). This mass has the appearance of abnormal fat, which must be considered in treatment planning. Note the displacement of bowel containing contrast. **C,** Sagittal MR image of the same case but without gadolinium. The potential advantage of MR imaging in separating the anterior edge of the retroperitoneal sarcoma (*long arrow*) from the normal fat anteriorly is seen. The more solid component can also be seen (*arrowhead*) inferior to the spleen. In addition, these images can be exported digitally to a three-dimensional radiotherapy treatment planning workstation or CT simulator workstation where the MR images can be fused to the CT planning slices. This can provide more accurate demonstration of tumor in selected cases for contouring the gross tumor volume and clinical target volume than may be possible with CT images alone. This is particularly helpful in situations where CT does not show tumor as well as MR imaging.

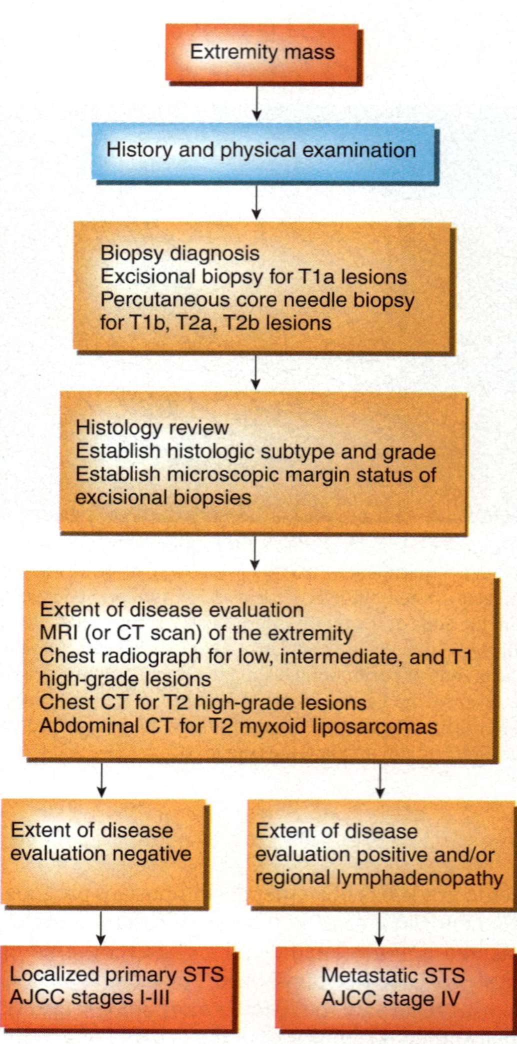

Figure 111-6 Approach for pretreatment evaluation and staging of the patient presenting with a primary extremity soft tissue mass. AJCC, American Joint Committee on Cancer. (From Pisters PWT, Ann Surg Oncol 1998;5:464–72, with permission.)

grade tumors larger than 5 cm (T2) should undergo more thorough staging of the chest by CT owing to the increased risk of presentation with established metastatic disease in this group.[56,57] Patients with RPSs and intra-abdominal visceral sarcomas should undergo imaging of the liver to exclude the possibility of synchronous hepatic metastases; the liver is a more common site of first metastasis from these lesions. CT is usually adequate in these patients to assess the liver, although the increased sensitivity of MRI of the liver may be valuable if any questionable findings are noted on initial CT.

Biopsy Biopsy of the primary tumor is essential for most patients presenting with soft tissue masses. In general, any soft tissue mass in an adult that is enlarging (even if asymptomatic), is larger than 5 cm, or persists beyond 4 to 6 weeks should be biopsied. The preferred biopsy approach is generally the least invasive technique required to allow a definitive histologic diagnosis and assessment of grade. In most centers, core-needle biopsy provides satisfactory tissue for diagnosis and results in substantial cost savings compared with open surgical biopsy.[58–60] However, incisional biopsy may still be required to yield optimal amounts of tissue to assess histopathology over a larger area of tumor volume, given the known heterogeneity of sarcomas, as well as to provide sufficient material for detailed molecular and cytogenetic assays. Direct palpation can be used to guide needle biopsy of most superficial lesions, but less accessible sarcomas often require imaging-guided biopsy for safe percutaneous sampling of the most radiographically suspicious area(s) of the mass. Tumor recurrences within the needle track after percutaneous biopsy are rare but have been reported, leading some physicians to advocate tattooing the biopsy site for subsequent excision.[61] In some centers, fine-needle aspiration may be an acceptable biopsy technique for primary soft tissue masses provided that an experienced sarcoma cytopathologist is available.[62–65] However, because of the frequent difficulty in accurately diagnosing these lesions, even when adequate tissue is available, the major utility of fine-needle aspiration in most centers is in the diagnosis of suspected recurrences of sarcoma.

A practical approach for biopsy and staging of the patient who presents with a primary extremity soft tissue mass is outlined in Figure 111-6. Small superficial lesions on an extremity where the morbidity of excisional biopsy is minimal (ie, remote from joints, tendons, and neurovascular structures that would compromise the surgical margin) are easily biopsied by excisional biopsy with microscopic assessment of surgical margins. T2 lesions, T1 lesions located beneath the investing fascia of the extremity, or superficial T1 lesions situated in proximity to joints, tendons, or neurovascular structures are best biopsied by percutaneous core-needle biopsy.

STAGING AND PROGNOSTIC FACTORS

Staging The relative rarity of soft tissue sarcomas, the anatomic heterogeneity of these lesions, and the presence of more than 50 recognized histologic subtypes of variable grades have made it difficult to establish a functional system that can accurately stage all forms of this disease. The staging system (6th edition) of the American Joint

Table 111-2 American Joint Committee on Cancer Staging System for Soft Tissue Sarcomas						
TX	Primary tumor cannot be assessed					
T0	No evidence of primary tumor					
T1	Tumor 5 cm or less in greatest dimension					
T1a	Superficial tumor					
T1b	Deep tumor					
T2	Tumor more than 5 cm in greatest dimension					
T2a	Superficial tumor					
T2b	Deep tumor					
N1	Regional lymph node metastasis					
G1	Well differentiated					
G2	Moderately differentiated					
G3	Poorly differentiated					
G4	Poorly differentiated or undifferentiated (four-tiered systems only)					
Stage I	T1a, 1b, 2a, 2b	N0	M0	G1-2	G1	Low
Stage II	T1a, 1b, 2a	N0	M0	G3-4	G2-3	High
Stage III	T2b	N0	M0	G3-4	G2-3	High
Stage IV	Any T	N1	M0	Any G	Any G	High or Low
	Any T	N0	M1	Any G	Any G	High or Low

From Freene FL, Page DL, Fleming ID, et al, editors. American Joint Committee on Cancer AJCC cancer staging manual. 6th ed. New York: Springer-Verlag; 2002.
Reprinted with permission from Lippincott-Raven.

Committee on Cancer (AJCC) and the International Union Against Cancer is the most widely employed staging system for soft tissue sarcomas (Table 111-2).[66] All soft tissue sarcoma subtypes are included except DFSPs, a condition considered to have only borderline malignant potential, and lesions of the hollow viscera. The system is designed to optimally stage extremity tumors but is also applicable to torso, head and neck, and retroperitoneal lesions; it should not be used for sarcomas of the gastrointestinal tract.

A major limitation of the present staging system is that it does not take into account the anatomic site of soft tissue sarcomas. Anatomic site, however, has been recognized as an important determinant of outcome.[67,68] Therefore, although site is not a specific component of any present staging system, outcome data should be reported on a site-specific basis.

Conventional Prognostic Factors A thorough understanding of the clinicopathologic factors known to impact outcome is essential in formulating a treatment plan for the patient with soft tissue sarcoma. Several multivariate analyses of prognostic factors for patients with localized sarcoma have been reported.[48,69–83] However, with few exceptions, most studies have analyzed fewer than 300 patients (range, 82–297 patients).[44,46,69,75]

The more recent, larger reports have established the clinical profile of what is now accepted as the high-risk patient with extremity soft tissue sarcoma: the patient with a large (≥ 5 cm), high-grade, deep lesion.[44,46,69] In addition, the previously unappreciated prognostic significance of certain histologic subtypes and the increased risk of adverse outcome associated with a microscopically positive surgical margin or presentation with locally recurrent disease were noted. The type of microscopically positive surgical margins also appears important. Patients with low-grade liposarcomas have a relatively low risk of local recurrence as do those patients in whom the positive margin is planned before surgery to preserve critical structures and RT can sterilize the small amount of residual disease. However, patients with two categories of positive margin are at relatively higher risk of local recurrence. These include patients who underwent "unplanned" excision and still have positive margins on re-excision and those with unanticipated positive margins after primary resection.[84] An "unplanned excision" is defined as an excisional biopsy or resection carried out without adequate preoperative staging or consideration of the need to remove normal tissue around the tumor.

Unlike for other solid tumors, the adverse prognostic factors for local recurrence of a soft tissue sarcoma are different from those that predict distant metastasis and tumor-related death (Table 111-3).[44] In other words, patients with a constellation of adverse prognostic factors for local recurrence are not necessarily at increased risk of distant metastasis or tumor-related death. Therefore, staging systems that are designed to stratify patients for risk of distant metastasis and tumor-related death will not necessarily stratify patients for risk of local recurrence.

Kattan and colleagues from the Memorial Sloan-Kettering Cancer Center (MSKCC) have utilized a database of over 2,000 prospectively followed adult patients with soft tissue sarcoma to predict the probability of sarcoma-specific death by 12 years.[67] The results have been used to construct and internally validate a nomogram to predict sarcoma-specific death (Figure 111-7) This tool is available at <www.nomograms.org> and may be used for patient counseling, follow-up scheduling, and clinical trial eligibility determination.

Potential Molecular Prognostic Factors Specific molecular parameters evaluated for prognostic significance in soft tissue sarcoma have included *TP53, mdm2* mutations, *Ki-67* status, altered expression of the RB gene product in high-grade sarcomas, and the presence of specific molecular subtypes of *SYT-SSX* fusion transcripts in synovial sarcoma or *EWS-FL11* fusion transcripts in Ewing's sarcoma.[16,85–89] Recently, however, conflicting evidence for a relationship to the presence of *SYT-SSX* fusion transcripts in synovial sarcoma has emerged.[90] Histologic grade, but not *SYT-SSX* fusion type, is an important prognostic factor in patients with synovial sarcoma.[90] Complete discussion of the extensive literature on molecular prognostic factors in sarcoma is beyond the scope of this chapter. Readers are referred to recent detailed reviews.[91,92] Data evaluating the prognostic significance of the most widely studied molecular factor, Ki-67, are summarized below.

Table 111-3 Multivariate Analysis of Prognostic Factors in Patients with Extremity Soft Tissue Sarcoma

Endpoint	Adverse Prognostic Factor	Relative Risk
Local recurrence	Fibrosarcoma	2.5
	Local recurrence at presentation	2.0
	Microscopically positive margin	1.8
	Malignant peripheral nerve sheath tumor	1.8
	Age > 50 years	1.6
Distant recurrence	High grade	4.3
	Deep location	2.5
	Size 5.0–9.9 cm	1.9
	Leiomyosarcoma	1.7
	Nonliposarcoma histology	1.6
	Local recurrence at presentation	1.5
	Size ≥ 10.0 cm	1.5
Disease-specific survival	High Grade	4.0
	Deep location	2.8
	Size ≥ 10.0 cm	2.1
	Malignant peripheral nerve sheath tumor	1.9
	Leiomyosarcoma	1.9
	Microscopically positive margin	1.7
	Lower extremity site	1.6
	Local recurrence at presentation	1.5

Adverse prognostic factors identified are independent by Cox regression analysis.
From Pisters PWT et al,[44] with permission from *Journal of Clinical Oncology*.

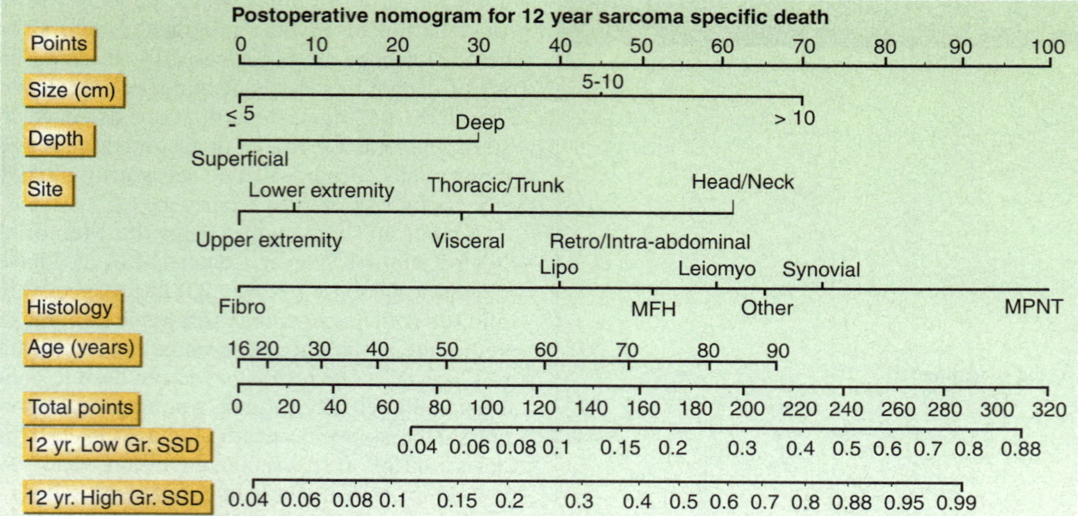

Instructions for physicians: Locate the patient's tumor size on the size axis. Draw a line straight upwards to the points axis to determine how many points towards sarcoma-specific death the patient receives for his tumor size. Repeat this process for the other axes, each time drawing straight upward to the points axis. Sum the points achieved for each predictor and locate this sum on the total points axis. Draw a line straight down to either the low grade or high grade axis to find the patient's probability of dying from sarcoma within 12 years assuming he or she does not die of another cause first.

Instructions for patients: If we had 100 patients exactly like you, we would expect between (predicted percentage from nomogram - 8%) and (predicted percentage + 8%) to die of sarcoma within 12 years if they did not die of another cause first, and death from sarcoma after 12 years is still possible.

Figure 111-7 Postoperative nomogram for 12-year sarcoma-specific deaths, in 2,163 patients treated at Memorial Sloan-Kettering Cancer Center. Fibro = fibrosarcoma; Lipo = liposarcoma; Leiomyo = leiomyosarcoma; MFH = malignant fibrous histiocytoma; MPNT = malignant peripheral-nerve sheath tumor; GR = grade; SSD = sarcoma-specific death. (From Kattan MW et al. J Clin Oncol 2002;20:791–6, with permission.)

Ki-67, an antigen expressed throughout the majority of the cell cycle, is used as a measure of the fraction of cells undergoing division.[93] Preliminary reports of series of heterogeneous sarcomas in adults suggested that the proliferation index as measured by Ki-67 nuclear staining correlated with histologic grade but was not of independent prognostic significance when histologic grade was taken into account.[94,95] However, additional studies in larger numbers of patients have demonstrated that Ki-67 status is an independent prognostic factor.[85,96,97] An initial immunohistochemical analysis of a cohort of 65 soft tissue sarcomas and a subsequent analysis of 132 soft tissue sarcomas by the FNCLCC Sarcoma Group demonstrated the adverse prognostic significance of increased Ki-67 activity.[96,97] More recently, Heslin and colleagues evaluated the potential prognostic significance of Rb, *TP53*, *mdm2*, and *Ki-67* by immunohistochemical techniques in a population of 121 patients with primary, high-grade extremity sarcomas and compared these factors with conventional clinicopathologic prognostic factors (median follow-up, 64 months).[85] Clinicopathologic and molecular factors found to be statistically significant adverse prognostic factors in both univariate and multivariate analyses for the separate end points of distant metastasis and tumor-related death included T2 tumor size, microscopically positive surgical margin, and a Ki-67 score greater than 20 (> 20% nuclear staining). Overexpression of *TP53* or *mdm2* or absence of the Rb gene product did not correlate with an increased risk of distant metastasis or tumor-related death.

Although specific cellular and molecular parameters have been identified as having independent prognostic significance, there is presently no consensus on how these prognostic factors should be used in clinical practice. Until more data are available, molecular prognostic factors proven to be of prognostic significance (eg, *Ki-67*) should be considered for inclusion as stratification criteria in clinical trials.

TREATMENT OF LOCALIZED PRIMARY DISEASE OF THE EXTREMITIES

SURGERY **General Issues** Surgical resection remains the cornerstone of therapy for localized primary soft tissue sarcoma. The discussion that follows focuses on soft tissue sarcomas in the limbs, the most common site of origin, but the principles are equally applicable to sarcomas at other anatomic sites.

Over the past 20 years, there has been a marked decline in the rate of amputation as the primary therapy for extremity soft tissue sarcoma. With the widespread application of multimodality treatment strategies, the vast majority of patients with localized soft tissue sarcoma of the extremities undergo limb-sparing treatment; less than 10% of patients presently undergo amputation.[98,99] In selected patients, limb sparing can be approached with surgery alone.

Amputation Most surgeons consider definite major vascular, bony, or nerve involvement by soft tissue sarcoma as relative indications for amputation. Complex en bloc bone, vascular, and nerve resections with interposition grafting can be undertaken, but the associated morbidity is high. Therefore, for a few patients with critical involvement of major bony or neurovascular structures, amputation remains the only surgical option, but offers the prospect of prompt rehabilitation with excellent local control and survival rates.[100]

Combined-Modality Limb-Sparing Treatment Currently, at least 90% of patients with localized extremity sarcomas can undergo limb-sparing procedures.[98,101] The use of limb-sparing multimodality treatment approaches for extremity sarcoma is based largely on a phase III trial from the NCI, in which patients with extremity sarcomas amenable to limb-sparing surgery were randomly assigned to receive amputation or limb-sparing surgery with postoperative RT.[100,102] Both arms of this trial included postoperative chemotherapy with doxorubicin, cyclophosphamide, and methotrexate. With greater than 9 years of follow-up evaluation, this study established that for patients for whom limb-sparing surgery is an option, limb-sparing surgery combined with postoperative RT and chemotherapy yields disease-related survival rates comparable to those for amputation while simultaneously preserving a functional extremity.[100,102]

Satisfactory local resection involves resection of the primary tumor with a margin of normal tissue around the lesion. Dissection along the tumor pseudocapsule (enucleation) is associated with local recurrence rates ranging between 33 and 63%.[103–105] In contrast, wide local excision with a margin of normal tissue around the lesion is associated with local recurrence rates in the range of 10 to 31%, as noted in the control arms (surgery alone) of randomized trials evaluating postoperative RT and in single-institution reports.[106–108]

In the modern era, a discussion of limb-preserving approaches must be linked to a discussion of the role of adjuvant therapies, most commonly RT. Several randomized controlled trials have addressed issues surrounding the use of adjuvant therapy and collectively have established important milestones in the evolution of the local management of soft tissue sarcomas. With one exception, these trials have focused on extremity lesions and the themes of surgery and adjuvant RT.

Yang and colleagues randomized 91 patients with high-grade extremity lesions following limb-sparing surgery to receive adjuvant chemotherapy alone or concurrent chemotherapy and RT.[107] An additional 50 patients with low-grade tumors were to receive adjuvant RT or no further treatment following limb-sparing surgery. The local control rate for those who received RT was 99% compared with 70% in the no-RT group ($p = .0001$).[107] The results were similar for high- and low-grade tumors (Table 111-4).

Adjuvant RT was also evaluated at MSKCC in a randomized trial of 126 cases treated between 1982 and 1987 (see Table 111-4).[106] Brachytherapy (BRT) was administered postoperatively, via an iridium-192 implant that delivered 42 to 45 Gy over 4 to 6 days. At 5 years, the local control rate for high-grade tumors was 91% with BRT compared with 70% in surgery-alone controls ($p =$

Table 111-4 Phase III Trials of Adjuvant Radiotherapy for Localized Extremity and Trunk Sarcoma Stratified by Grade

Histologic Grade	First Author/Institution	Treatment Group	Radiation Dose, Gy	No. Patients	No. Local Failure (%)	LRFS, %	OS, %
High grade	Pisters/MSKCC(104)	Surgery + BRT	42–45	56	5 (9)	89	27
		Surgery	—	63	19 (30)	66	67
	Yang(105)/NCI	Surgery + XRT	45 + 18 (boost)	47	0 (0)	100	75
		Surgery	—	44	9 (20)	78	74
Low grade	Pisters(104)/MSKCC	Surgery + BRT	42–45	22	8 (36)	73	96
		Surgery	—	23	6 (26)	73	95
	Yang(105)/NCI	Surgery + XRT	45 + 18 (boost)	26	1 (4)	96	NR
		Surgery	—	24	8 (33)	63	NR

BRT = brachytherapy; LRFS = local recurrence-free survival; MSKCC = Memorial Sloan-Kettering Cancer Center; NCI = National Cancer Institute; NR = not reported; OS = overall survival; XRT = external-beam radiotherapy.

.04). Of note, no improvement in local control with BRT was evident for the low-grade tumors (the local control rate was 74% with surgery alone and 64% with BRT). The full explanation for grade-specific differences in local control with BRT remains unresolved, although one suggestion implicates the relatively long cell cycle of low-grade tumors: low-grade tumor cells may not enter the radiosensitive phases of the cell cycle during the relatively short BRT time.[106]

Satisfactory Surgical Margins to Omit Radiotherapy There are no randomized data to define what constitutes a satisfactory gross resection margin for a sarcoma. In general, every effort should be made to achieve a wide margin (2 cm is often an arbitrary choice) around the tumor mass, except in the immediate vicinity of functionally important neurovascular structures, where, in the absence of frank neoplastic involvement, dissection is performed in the immediate perineural or perivascular tissue planes. Technical details of the surgical approach to extremity sarcomas are beyond the scope of this chapter, but are reviewed in Bland and colleagues' *Atlas of Surgical Oncology*.[109] However, the principle remains that adequate clearance of potential tumor-bearing tissues can be achieved if there is sufficient distance between the surgical margin and the edge of any grossly evident tumor (eg, at least 2 cm for the closest margin), or where an intact barrier to tumor spread is excised en bloc with the tumor. In such cases, there is little evidence that RT is required even when potential adverse prognostic factors, such as large high-grade tumors are present. The exception in cases of "unplanned" excision where significant contamination of surrounding tissues may have taken place and the precise extent of the tumor is essentially unknown.

Management of Regional Lymph Nodes Given the low (2–3%) prevalence of lymph node metastasis in adults with sarcomas, there is no role for routine regional lymph node dissection in most patients.[42,43] However, patients with angiosarcoma, embryonal/alveolar rhabdomyosarcoma, and epithelioid sarcoma have an increased incidence of lymph node metastasis and should be carefully examined for lymphadenopathy. These patients may benefit from the inclusion of lymph node regions electively in adjuvant RT fields.

For patients with soft tissue sarcoma, lymph node metastasis has been regarded as a particularly adverse finding conferring similar risk to distant metastasis in the TNM (tumor-nodes-metastasis) stage classification. Nevertheless, therapeutic lymph node dissection results in a 34% actuarial survival rate, and thus the rare patients with regional nodal involvement who have no evidence of extranodal disease should undergo therapeutic lymphadenectomy.[42] In addition, recent information about isolated lymph node metastasis (as opposed to synchronous distant metastasis) indicates that isolated lymph node metastasis, if treated intensively, appear to have a prognosis similar to patients with stage III tumors (ie, those with high-grade, deep lesions and lesions larger than 5 cm). This questions whether the impact of nodal disease should be reconsidered in the future editions of the staging system.[110,111]

Radiotherapy Rationale for Combining Radiotherapy with Surgery The use of RT in combination with surgery for soft tissue sarcomas is supported by two phase III clinical trials (see Table 111-4) and is based on two premises: microscopic nests of tumor cells can be destroyed by RT, and less radical surgery can be performed when surgery and RT are combined.[106,107] Although the traditional belief was that soft tissue sarcomas were resistant to RT, radiosensitivity assays performed on sarcoma cell lines grown in vitro have confirmed that the radiosensitivity of sarcomas is similar to that of other malignancies; this confirmation supports the first premise.[112,113] The second premise stresses the philosophy of preservation of form (including cosmesis where possible) and function as a goal for many patients with extremity, truncal, breast, and head and neck sarcomas.[114–116] Similar principles govern the frequent use of RT for sarcomas at problematic sites, for example, RPSs, high-risk sarcomas of the head and neck with skull base invasion, or spinal canal invasion by paravertebral lesions.

Visceral sarcomas are not ordinarily managed with RT, in part because of the mobile nature of these structures within the pelvic, abdominal, or thoracic compartments. After resection of visceral sarcomas, accurate identification of the field at risk of residual disease is particularly problematic. Contaminated loops of bowel or mesentery may relocate remotely within the abdominal cavity after surgery, and pleural contamination and mediastinal shift may occur following intrathoracic resections. Fixed tumors in the pelvis or tumors attached to internal truncal walls may occasionally be suited to preoperative or postoperative RT. Typically, however, the vast size of the radiation fields needed to cover entire body cavities, coupled with the limited RT doses that can be safely administered to the organs within the cavities, and the overwhelming risk of distant rather than local recurrence, confines adjuvant RT for the investigational setting.

Essential Elements in Treatment Planning of External Beam Radiotherapy Accurate tumor localization is the first essential for RT planning. RT planning primarily uses CT for dosimetric reasons, but MRI can provide complementary information about the tumor extent and can be assimilated in the computer planning workstation through image fusion technology.[53,54] Further essential information is obtained from the pathology and operative reports, and metallic clips placed at the time of surgery may also help define the tumor bed.

It is often helpful to secure the targeted area to minimize set-up variations and eliminate movement during treatment. Simple maneuvers such as comfortable limb positioning or fashioning of customized thermoplastic molds for immobilization will facilitate reliable and consistent treatment set-ups. RT of superficial tissues, including the scar following definitive resection, with appropriate application of tissue-like bolus material should be considered, but with the recognition that fibrosis, atrophy, and telangiectasis may result. Dose uniformity within irregular volumes can be optimized using beam segmentation, compensators, or wedge filters. Whenever possible, the entire limb circumference, whole joints, or pressure areas (eg, elbow or heel) should not be treated with the full RT dose as this may adversely affect limb function and cause distal edema.

It is also prudent to assess baseline function before initiating RT. This is especially important with paired organs, such as eyes or kidneys, if the functional ablation of one organ by RT is expected.

Three-Dimensional Treatment Planning Very complex modulation of the beam is becoming available in many centers with the introduction of intensity-modulated RT (IMRT), but until recently such intensity modulation is reserved for situations in which the target volume is adjacent to critical normal tissues as found at the skull base or within the abdomen.[117–119] This is discussed briefly in the RT sections to follow below. Although there is potential advantage in approaching sarcoma with

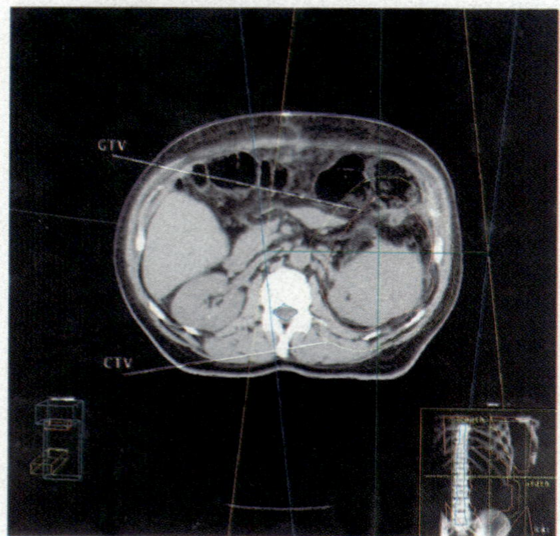

Figure 111-8A The gross tumor volume (GTV) has been contoured on a computed tomography (CT) simulator workstation (red outline). This includes the anterior abnormal fat shown earlier (see Figures 111-5 B and C). This process is performed with many thin CT slices to permit reconstruction of the image later for three-dimensional treatment planning. The clinical target volume (CTV) is outlined in yellow to account for potential microscopic spread beyond the GTV. An additional margin will also be added to account for set-up variation and organ motion. Note the displacement of bowel loops by the tumor mass. The straight lines show the path of the beam for a conventional set-up with opposed anterior and posterior fields.

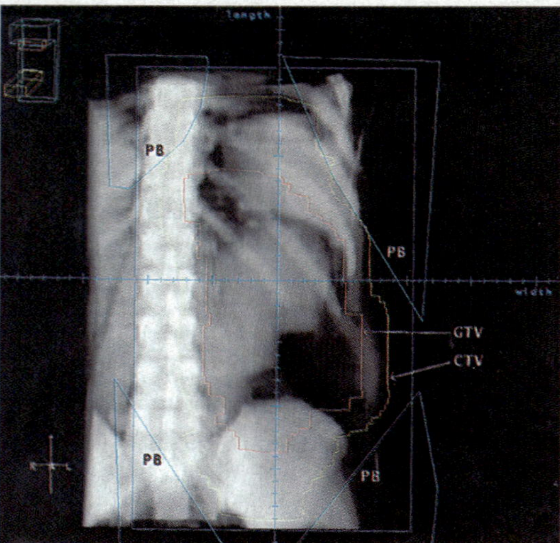

Figure 111-8B The contoured GTV and CTV information displayed in a beam's eye view (BEV) using a digitally reconstructed radiograph created by the CT simulator. Shielding (Pb) can be placed once the path of the beam within the target areas defined is seen on the BEV. One can also discern the opaque tumor partially displacing bowel from target area.

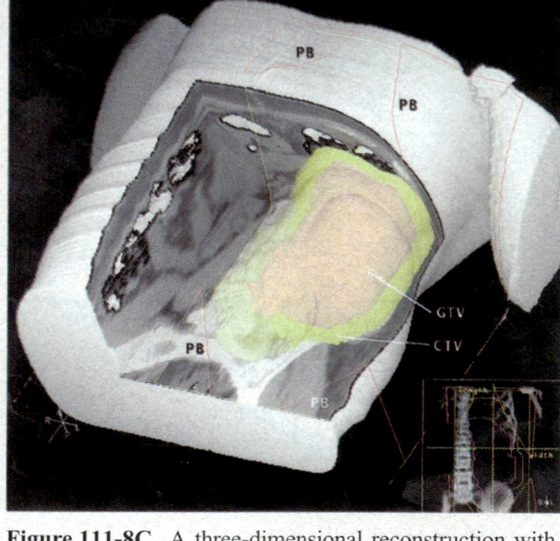

Figure 111-8C A three-dimensional reconstruction with the GTV, CTV, and areas to be shielded (Pb) shown and abdominal wall and anterior structures cut away. Generally, these "cut-away" images are most useful for visualizing the edge of the target volume adjacent to critical anatomy that must be protected and when the spatial relationship cannot be verified precisely with conventional imaging.

more precise targeting, clinical trials are only just commencing to assess the validity and efficacy of these approaches.

Dose-Volume Histograms The treatment of sarcoma often requires large volumes of normal tissue to be irradiated, frequently to high doses. Fortunately, because most sarcomas arise in the limbs, the likelihood of life-threatening sequelae from RT damage to critical organs is low. However, the potential for serious damage to neurologic tissues in the head and neck or intra-abdominal organs including liver and small bowel remains for tumors adjacent to these structures. Because the tolerance of many normal tissues to radiation depends on the irradiated volume, the development of three-dimensional treatment planning has provided tools to quantify the relationships between dose, volume, and normal-tissue complications. Models permit normal-tissue complication probability to be determined for different irradiated volumes of organs or tissues and varying dose levels.[120,121]

These concepts are helpful when treating certain tumors in the retroperitoneum. If right-sided or of great size, an RPS may infiltrate the liver capsule or be "hooded" by the liver, making RT access to an appropriate tissue volume surrounding the tumor extremely difficult. This area may be particularly appropriate for IMRT approaches because of the exquisite conformality that is possible with this approach and permits liver and other normal tissue to be excluded from the irradiated volume.[122,123] Fortunately, although the tolerance of the entire liver to radiation is low, the norma-tissue complication probability model has shown that part of the liver may be safely treated to much higher doses.[124] The "volume effect" can be exploited and cases may be planned more readily and safely using dose-volume histograms.[114] In these instances, if a subsequent liver resection is needed because of tumor infiltration or adherence to the capsule, detailed consultation between the surgical and radiation oncology teams is needed to ensure that an adequate volume of nonirradiated liver is left in situ.

Dose Fractionation Issues Total radiation doses administered postoperatively for sarcoma depend on the tumor grade and involvement of the surgical margin.[107,125,126] Typical total doses are 60 Gy for low-grade and 66 Gy for high-grade tumors, respectively. When RT is given preoperatively, the total dose used in most institutions is approximately 50 Gy in daily fractions administered over 5 weeks.[126,127] However, data regarding radiation dose response are very limited and based on underpowered retrospective studies. Based on current data, higher doses of RT are probably indicated in the postoperative setting (compared with preoperative RT), but the search for an alternative lower dose postoperative schedule seems desirable.

The fraction size used in conventional fractionation schemes varies (usually 1.8 or 2.1 Gy).[126,128] Absence of late effects can be expected with smaller fraction size; this tissue is particularly important when critical structures are irradiated. Several altered fractionation schemes have been described including hyperfractionated, hypofractionated, and accelerated schedules.[129–132] As yet, no apparent benefit from these various strategies is evident compared with conventional RT.

Radiation Target Volume Soft tissue sarcomas generally respect barriers to tumor spread in the axial plane of the extremity, such as bones, interosseous membranes, or major fascial planes. Consequently, extremity soft tissue sarcomas tend to spread longitudinally within the specific muscle groups of the extremity. Therefore, the margins of the RT volume must be wide in the cephalocaudal direction. In the cross-section, there may be much greater security in defining nontarget structures, especially those delimited by an intact barrier to tumor spread. For nonextremity lesions, the preferred direction of spread is also along the direction of the involved musculature, but care must be taken to ensure that the fascial planes are appropriately recognized and encompassed in the radiation target volume.

Earlier, this chapter summarized principles concerning anatomic planes and the preferential pathways for sarcomas to spread within tissues. This information facilitates the design of target areas for RT. The basic elements in RT planning are to first define a gross tumor volume (GTV) and then place a margin around it to encompass tissues at risk of harboring microscopic residual disease (clinical target volume [CTV]) (Figures 111-8 A–C, and Figure 111-9).[133] Generally, RT is phased so that an initial volume (phase I) around the risk zone is treated to doses that are capable of sterilizing microscopic amounts of tumor cells (eg, 50 Gy in 1.8 or 2.0 Gy fractions). It is then customary to have at least one field reduction to permit an augmented dose to a smaller volume surrounding the highest risk zone (phase II). This dose is usually 15 to 16 Gy but can be higher if there is gross residual disease. This postoperative "boost" is generally restricted to patients who received preoperative RT and have margin-positive disease at surgery. This is because the local control rate for margin-negative

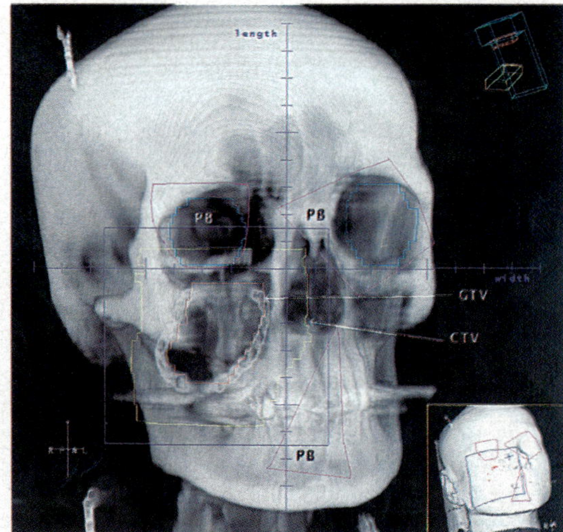

Figure 111-9 A digitally reconstructed radiograph of the head and neck of a young woman with a soft tissue sarcoma of the right cheek. Because of the proximity to the right eye, preoperative radiotherapy has been chosen because of its ability to permit maximal restriction of the clinical target volume (CTV) to the local environment of the tumor. The same process was followed using a computed tomography simulator as described in Figure 111-7. The gross tumor volume (GTV) on the cheek can be seen with the surrounding CTV. Shielding (Pb) is also evident. A hair clip, which the patient was wearing during the CT slice acquisition, is evident in the right parietal area; one can also see her necklace. The smaller insert shows a three-dimensional image of the patient with potential beams applied.

cases is in excess of 90% even when a boost is not provided.[126,134,135] A positive margin is declared when the tumor reaches the inked surface of the specimen, and clear margins can be declared if the tumor does not reach the ink irrespective of how close it is.[126] In the preoperative RT setting, the GTV typically represents the radiologically defined tumor. Some sarcomas have extensive peritumoral edema that extends along fascial planes for some distance beyond the main tumor mass.[136] It is uncertain whether the edema contains viable tumor cells.[137] The inclusion of edema within the GTV can influence the magnitude of the RT field, especially its length. There is no uniform policy or guideline as to whether this area should be considered part of the GTV. Studies to correlate the radiologic imaging appearances of sarcomas with the pathologic findings are needed and would be very relevant in the contemporary era of conformal treatment planning.

When postoperative RT is administered, there is no GTV if one strictly follows the conventions of the International Commission on Radiation Units and Measurements.[133] However, for RT planning, it is still helpful to represent a theoretic GTV as the surgical field comprising all of the tissues handled during the surgical procedure, including undermined skin flaps, drain sites, and scars. A putative zone of potential microscopic residual disease beyond this represents the CTV.

Bone, interosseous membranes, and fascial planes are considered barriers to tumor spread in the axial direction, and, therefore, descriptions of radiation margins employed are principally in the cephalocaudal direction. The RT protocol in the NCI of Canada Clinical Trial performed by the Canadian Sarcoma Group (SR2), which compared preoperative and postoperative RT (see below), required a field margin of 5 cm around the GTV for the initial phase of treatment (50 Gy in 25 fractions).[138] Generally, the GTV included any peritumoral edema seen on MRI, irrespective of tumor grade or size. Subsequently, a reduced volume field was treated to a total combined dose of 66 Gy in all patients who had postoperative RT and in preoperative RT patients with positive resection margins. However, there is variability among centers about what constitutes optimal coverage of tissues at risk of harboring microscopic disease .[128] BRT protocols use margins of only 2 cm around the surgical bed.[106] Despite these differences, the local control rates reported are approximately 90% if low-grade lesions are excluded from the BRT data. This suggests that the zone of microscopic involvement may be less than was previously realized. Recent improvements in surgical technique may lessen the degree of intraoperative tumor dissemination, and irradiation of all surgically handled tissues, scars, and drain sites may be unnecessary. This seems particularly relevant for major centers where surgery is performed by teams with extensive experience in sarcoma management. One must also consider the possibility that case selection factors may explain apparent variations in practice between BRT and external beam RT approaches.

Sequencing of Radiotherapy and Surgery Preoperative RT is delivered to an undisturbed and potentially better oxygenated tumor site, which may be one reason why lower preoperative radiation doses do not appear to compromise local control.[139,140] Nielsen and colleagues repeated RT planning in patients who had undergone preoperative RT and surgery and observed that the field size and number of joints irradiated in preoperative RT were significantly less than if the treatment had been administered postoperatively.[141] This observation was recently validated in a prospective randomized trial and there is evidence that smaller treatment volumes may result in improved limb function.[130,138,142]

Another advantage of preoperative RT is that it promotes collaboration between the surgical and radiation oncologists and facilitates the formulation of a coordinated management plan prior to any treatment. In some circumstances, preoperative RT may provide better tumor control compared to postoperative RT, although this has not yet been substantiated by prospective randomized trial data. A retrospective series from Massachusetts General Hospital suggested that preoperative RT may be more efficacious for larger lesions (> 5 cm).[143] More recently, Pollack and colleagues suggested that preoperative RT is preferable in patients presenting with locally advanced primary disease.[127] Finally, although much of the discussion about preoperative RT is focused on extremity lesions, patients with RPS tolerate preoperative RT substantially better than postoperative RT. This is because the tumor acts as a tissue expander to exclude the bowel from the RT volume (see Figures 111-8 A–C). This is discussed in greater detail later in the section "Retroperitoneal Sarcomas."

Preoperative RT also has certain disadvantages. Definition of the target volume relies almost completely on the imaging characteristics of the tumor, and this may underestimate the true extent of the tumor. In addition, preoperative RT is delivered based on the results of only partially representative biopsy specimens and may interfere with future histopathologic analysis. These two concerns are more academic and theoretical than practical, however. One clinical concern with the preoperative delivery of RT remains the increased risk of serious wound complications following definitive resection (discussed below).

Which approach—preoperative or postoperative RT—is more "correct" is thus controversial.[144] Many competing issues are involved, and the treatment decision algorithm is complex. It is also important to appreciate that conclusions from much of the available data are liable to bias because of the nonrandomized fashion in which treatment was allocated. Often preoperative RT is chosen for patients with more adverse presentations of disease who are therefore in need of more extensive surgery.[140]

The NCI of Canada/Canadian Sarcoma Group SR2 clinical trial represents the only prospective randomized comparison of preoperative versus postoperative RT.[138] The RT parameters for this protocol were briefly addressed earlier. The trial found that wound complications are twice as common with preoperative RT as with postoperative RT (35% vs 17%), although the increased risk is almost exclusively confined to patients with sarcomas of the upper extremity. Of interest, a recent report from the University of Texas M. D. Anderson Cancer Center, using the same criteria for classifying wound complications as were used in the Canadian NCI trial, found almost identical results.[145]

The SR2 trial also found, as anticipated, that larger field sizes are also needed with postoperative RT. In addition, preliminary data concerning RT toxicity rates in the Canadian trial after 2 years differed between the two arms of the study with a tendency to manifest greater fibrosis in the postoperative arm of the study compared to those treated with preoperative radiotherapy.[146] This observation is potentially important because patients with significant fibrosis, joint stiffness, or limb edema, all late treatment responses, had significantly lower limb-function scores at these later time points.[146] Moreover this subsequent analysis also suggested strongly that field size was predictive of greater degrees of fibrosis and joint stiffness and also may be related to edema.[147]

In the initial report of the SR2 trial with 3.3 years median follow-up, an improvement in overall survival (p = .0481) in the preoperative RT arm was noted and partially explained by increased deaths in the postoperative RT unrelated to sarcoma.[138] The local failure rate was identical in the two arms (7%) (Figure 111-10). However, updated results were recently presented and the preliminary

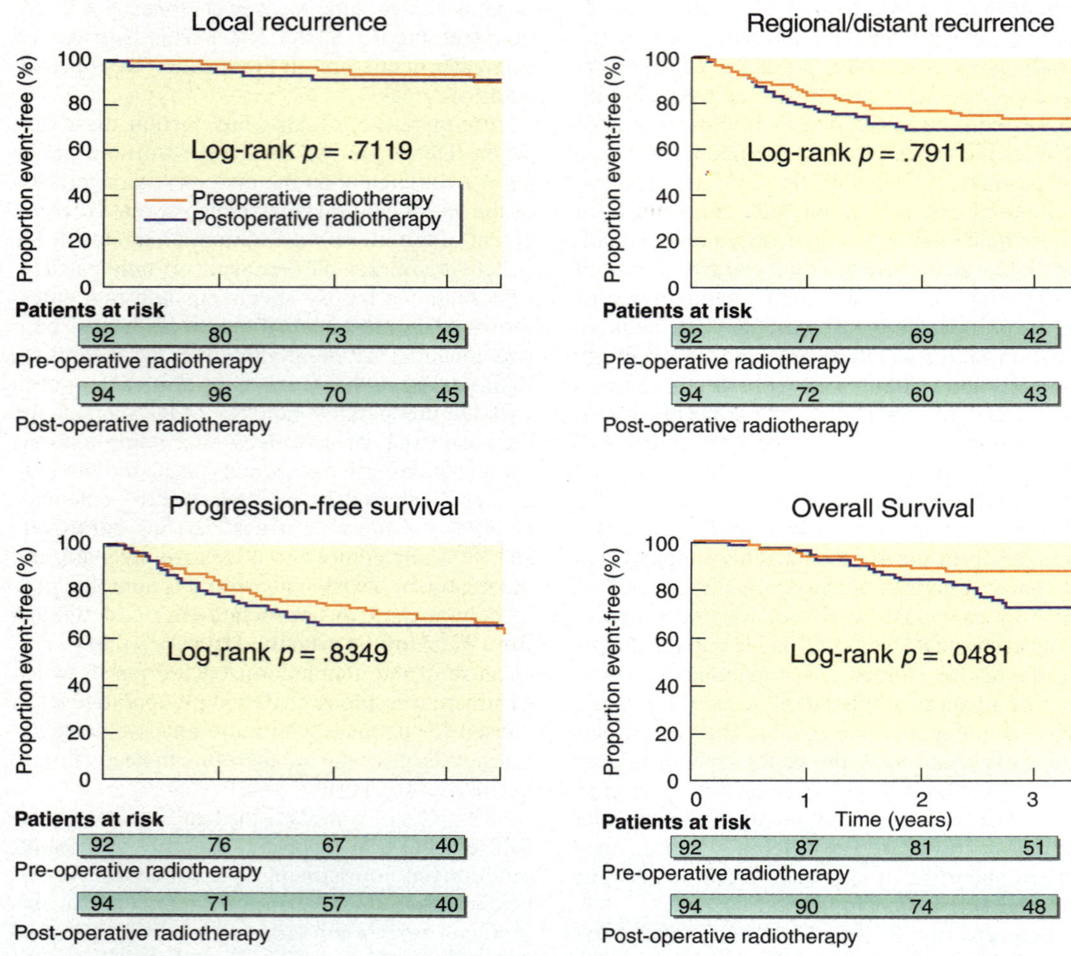

Figure 111-10 Kaplan-Meier plots for probability of local recurrence, metastasis (local and regional recurrence), progression-free survival, and overall survival in the Canadian Sarcoma Group randomized trial of the National Cancer Institute of Canada Clinical Trials Group comparing preoperative and postoperative radiotherapy. Reproduced with permission of The Lancet Ltd. from O'Sullivan B et al.[138]

survival difference has disappeared.[148] The 5-year results for preop vs postop, respectively, were, local control: 93% vs 92%; metastatic relapse-free: 67% vs 69%; recurrence-free survival: 58% vs 59%; overall survival: 73% vs 67% (p = .48); cause-specific survival: 78% vs 73% (p = .64). Cox modeling showed only resection margins as significant for local control. Tumor size and grade were the only significant factors for metastatic-relapse, overall survival, and cause-specific survival. Grade was the only consistent predictor of recurrence-free survival.[148]

For the present, decisions about preoperative versus postoperative RT should be individualized, taking into account tumor location, tumor size, RT field size, comorbidities, and risks. In general, preoperative RT provides some advantages over postoperative RT, but exposes the patient to significantly increased risks of serious postoperative wound complications. A summary of the relative indications that can be used to select patients for preoperative RT is provided in Table 111-5.

Methods of Radiotherapy Delivery No randomized trials directly comparing external beam RT and BRT have been undertaken, but both forms of RT have been compared with surgery alone. BRT has several advantages over external beam, including a shorter overall treatment time (4–6 days vs 5–6.5 weeks) and quicker initiation of RT after surgery while clonogen numbers are at a minimum. Because of its brevity, BRT is also more easily integrated into protocols that include systemic chemotherapy than is external beam RT, with its protracted courses. The irradiated volume is also smaller with BRT, which may confer functional advantages. Furthermore, BRT costs $1,000 US per patient less than external beam.[149] BRT may also have an advantage in situations in which normal-tissue tolerance to RT is compromised.

Table 111-5 Relative Indications for Preoperative RT, Despite Concerns Related to Wound Complications

Treatment Context/Sarcoma Site	Issues of Concern	Comments
Head and neck		
Paranasal sinus	Proximity to optic apparatus (eye, orbit, chiasma)	Major visual functional deficit can be minimized
Skull base	Proximity to spinal cord, brain stem	Other "lesser" morbidities (dental, xerostomia) may also be less due to reduced doses and volumes
Cheek and face		
Split thickness skin graft reconstruction (especially lower limb)	Skin graft breakdown and consequent infection	Many months to years of recreational and/or vocational disability may occur during healing (rare)
Large volume GTV or CTV occupying coelomic cavities		
Retroperitoneum	Proximity to bowel, liver, kidney	Critical organs may be displaced by tumor or not fixed or adherent as is likely in postoperative setting Entire tumor treated prior to possible contamination of cavity
Some small bowel lesions	Proximity to critical anatomy, especially intestine with side wall adherence	Contamination of abdominal cavity renders postoperative RT unsuitable
Thoracic wall/pleura	Proximity to lung or cardiac structures	Lung may be displaced by chest wall or pleural tumor and can be avoided with preoperative RT, or permits GTV to be treated prior to operative contamination
Abdominal trunk walls, pelvic side wall	Proximity to kidney, bowel, liver, ovaries	Avoid CTV encroachment on vulnerable anatomy GTV adjacent to dose limiting critical anatomy
Thoracic inlet/upper chest	Proximity to brachial plexus	Dose limitation of critical anatomy lends itself to preoperative wall low neck RT. Additional volume considerations
Medial thigh (young male)	Proximity to testes	Permanent infertility may be avoided
Central limb tumor	Proximity to other compartments	Permits partial circumferential sparing, which would not be feasible in postoperative setting

CTV = clinical target volume; GTV = gross tumor volume; RT = radiotherapy.
Reproduced with permission from Semin Radiat Oncol 1999;9:335.

One such scenario would be when a postoperative RT boost to the operative bed is desired in patients who received preoperative RT. The use of BRT with surgery in previously irradiated tissues is another situation to achieve limb salvage.[150–153] As noted earlier, no apparent benefit for BRT over surgical excision alone is evident with low-grade lesions, and external beam appears more effective for these tumors (see Table 111-4).[107,143,154]

As noted earlier, an alternative method of delivering RT to a complex shaped target is by means of external beams designed with variable intensity across their profiles, in contrast to the uniform flat profile used in traditional RT. Such variable intensity beams, when shaped according to the needs of the target and in combination with numerous other uniquely characterized beams, all taking account of the dose provided by each other, comprise intensity-modulated RT (IMRT). IMRT is capable of exquisite dose conformation around targets and permits conformal avoidance of structures that would otherwise be damaged by conventional beams, even if delivered by conformal techniques. It may be particularly valuable for tumors of complex shape, such as sarcomas, and has recently been used to treat large intra-abdominal targets such as RPS.[119] Clinical results are awaited from studies of these exciting improvements in RT planning and delivery.

In addition to external beam RT, BRT, and IMRT, several other approaches for RT delivery exist. These include particle beam RT (electrons, protons, pions, or neutrons), intraoperative RT (IORT) using external beam or BRT approaches, and combinations of other techniques (eg, hyperthermia) with RT. IORT has been used most often in the management of RPSs and will be discussed in that section. Some reports also describe IORT for extremity sarcomas.[155,156] Formal clinical trials have not compared the relative merits of these approaches, and their use may be governed as much by the availability of an approach at a given center as by any special advantage that it may confer. In the case of proton beam RT, its ability to achieve accurate targeting provides an advantage when tumors lie in proximity to critical structures.[157,158] In general, however, although reports on the use of many of these approaches exist, the problems of selection bias need to be considered in interpreting these small series in which treatments were not randomly assigned.[159–163]

Chemotherapy Chemotherapy is used widely in the metastatic setting for patients with soft tissue sarcomas. The use of chemotherapy in the adjuvant setting remains controversial. However, if chemotherapy is going to have the same impact as radiation and surgery in the management of sarcomas, effective drugs will have to be identified that help improve the cure rate for patients with primary tumors and unseen microscopic metastatic disease. This section will review the use of chemotherapy in the adjuvant and metastatic settings. A brief discussion of chemotherapy combined with radiation therapy is also included in this section.

Chemotherapy Following Primary Surgical Resection Although local or locoregional recurrence is a problem for a small subset of patients following primary therapy, the major risk to life in sarcoma patients is uncontrolled systemic disease. The availability of systemic therapy with proven, albeit often limited, ability to induce shrinkage of advanced sarcomas has raised the question of whether the early use of systemic treatment might affect microscopic metastatic disease and yield improvements in overall survival and disease-free survival.

Certainly for Ewing's sarcoma/primitive neuroectodermal tumor (PNET), rhabdomyosarcoma, and osteogenic sarcoma, adjuvant or neoadjuvant chemotherapy are an appropriate standard of care.[164–166] However, for more common soft tissue sarcomas such as leiomyosarcoma, liposarcoma, and high-grade undifferentiated pleomorphic sarcoma (formerly known as malignant fibrous histiocytoma, MFH), the benefit for chemotherapy, if there is one, is small.[167] Since adjuvant therapy is utilized by many practitioners for more common diseases where the benefit is a relatively small one, such as stage I breast cancer and stage II colon cancer, this small potential benefit is an issue that needs to be discussed on an individualized basis. Certainly the lack of available effective agents for metastatic sarcoma have impeded progress in this area, but the utility of imatinib in gastrointestinal stromal tumor (GIST) gives hope that new agents will contribute to the ultimate goal of any type of systemic therapy specifically increasing the cure rate for people with new diagnoses.

There have been over a dozen studies of anthracycline-based adjuvant chemotherapy for soft tissue sarcomas that date back nearly as long as the initial development of doxorubicin.[168,169] These will not be reviewed here, since anthracycline/ifosfamide-based therapy constitute a better standard of care in patients offered adjuvant chemotherapy, and only one of the studies completed by 1992 had used ifosfamide. The best summary of anthracycline-containing adjuvant-based chemotherapy for extremity sarcomas to date was the 1997 meta-analysis of 14 studies encompassing sarcomas of all anatomic sites.[170] In this study, 23 potential studies were considered, and 14 ultimately selected, constituting 1,568 patients with soft tissue sarcomas of extremity and nonextremity sites with a median follow-up of 9.4 years. Pathology review was not centralized. The results of the meta-analysis, including the actuarial outcome probabilities and the hazard ratios, are summarized in Figure 111-11 and Table 111-6.

Analyses were stratified by trial, and hazard ratios were calculated for each trial then combined, allowing for an assessment of the risk of death or recurrence in comparison with control patients. Disease-free survival at 10 years was improved with chemotherapy from 45% to a highly statistically significant 55%, as was seen in several of the individual studies that comprised this population. Furthermore, local disease-free survival was also improved at 10 years with chemotherapy, from 75 to 81% ($p = .016$). Most importantly, overall survival also improved from 50 to 54% at 10 years, but was a favorable trend only and not statistically significant ($p = .12$). The largest difference in overall survival was found in a posthoc analysis of the 886 patients examined with extremity sarcomas. Overall survival was shown to improve by 7% in the group receiving chemotherapy ($p = .029$). However, as pointed out in commentary on this meta-analysis,[171] these data have to be interpreted with caution, since (1) this was an unplanned subset analysis, (2) 18% of patients did not have histology available for review, (3) ineligibility rates were high, and (4) ~6% of the patients from the largest contributing study to this meta-analysis did not have sarcoma after a repeat pathology review. Although the meta-analysis cannot replace a well-designed randomized study, it reinforces many of the findings from smaller studies that local and distant recurrence-free survival is definitely improved, but not necessarily overall survival.

Adjuvant and Neoadjuvant Studies Since the 1997 Meta-Analysis Given that the relevance of these older data to more modern practice may be limited, owing to improved imaging, widespread acceptance of limb-sparing surgery, better pathological classification of sarcomas, and the introduction of ifosfamide and supportive care such as offered by hematopoietic growth factors, other groups have re-examined the question of the utility of adjuvant chemotherapy in randomized studies.

In the largest of such studies, the Italian Sarcoma Study Group (ISSG) examined patients with primary or recurrent resected soft tissue sarcoma of the extremity or limb girdle treated or not treated with radiation.[172] One hundred four patients were randomized to receive no chemotherapy or to receive ifosfamide (1,800 mg/m^2/day for 5 consecutive days with mesna) and epirubicin (60 mg/m^2 on 2 consecutive days), with filgrastim support. Interim analysis in 1996 led to early conclusion of the trial because the study had reached its primary endpoint, that of improved disease-free survival. This study was started before the publication of the above-described meta-analysis. It is interesting to speculate that if there had been recognition of the improved disease-free survival (DFS), but not overall survival advantage noted in the meta-analysis, a study with overall survival as a primary endpoint might have been constructed instead. At a median follow-up of 36 months, overall survival in the chemotherapy arm was 72%, compared with 55% for the control arm ($p = .002$). However, with longer-term follow-up, the overall survival difference is now no longer statistically significant on an intention-to-treat analysis.[173] This study was the strongest argument in the literature for the use of adjuvant chemotherapy. Nonetheless, interpretation of the study is made more difficult with the observation of equivalent distant ± local recurrence rates at 4 years. There are also subtle imbalances in the distribution of patients on the control and treatment arms of the study, which are difficult to evaluate given the heterogeneous nature of

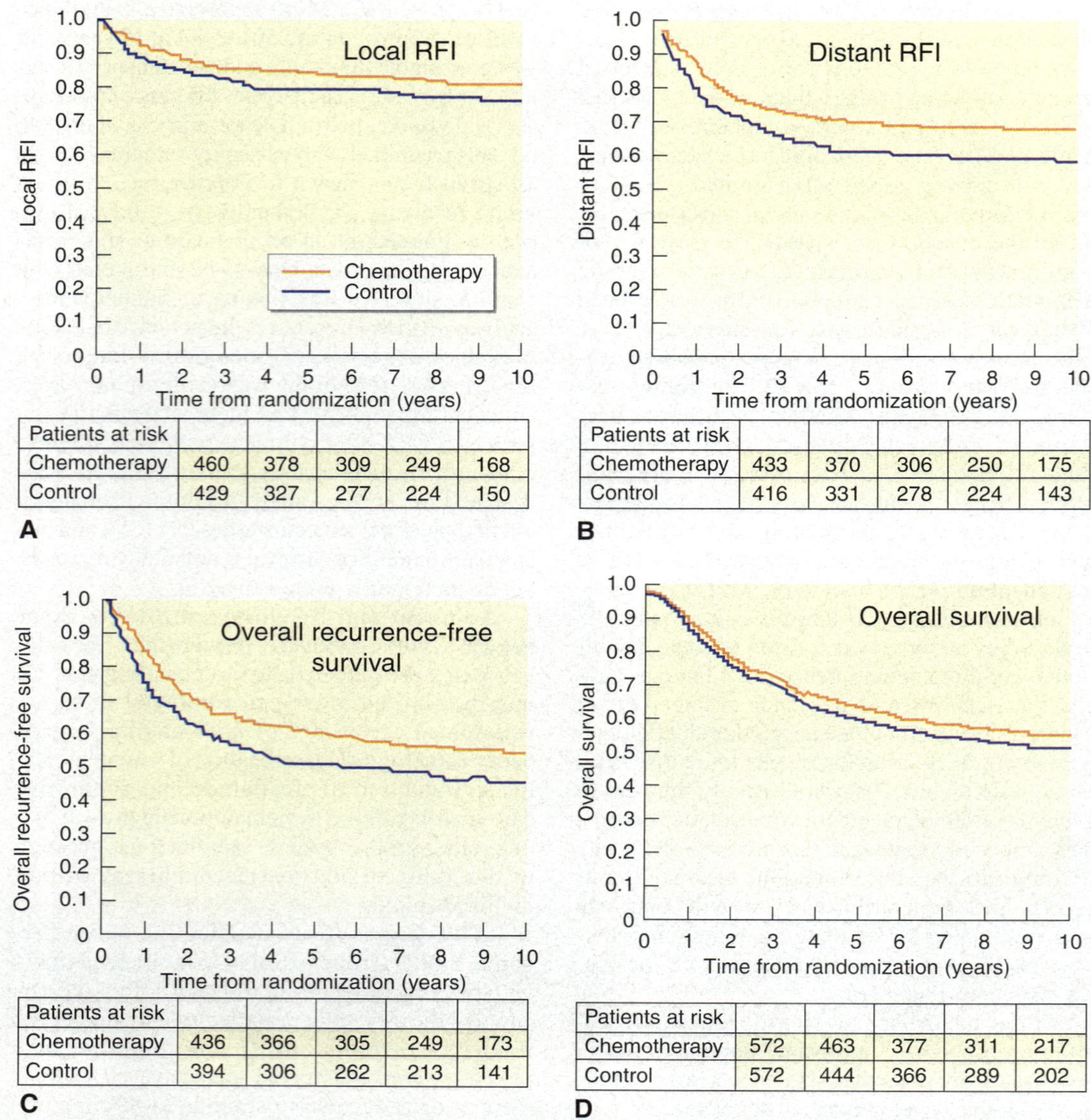

Figure 111-11 Actuarial curves from individual patient data meta-analysis: **A,** local recurrence-free interval (RFI), **B,** distant recurrence-free interval, **C,** overall recurrence-free survival, and **D,** overall survival.[178] (Reproduced with permission of The Lancet Ltd. and The Sarcoma Meta-Analysis Collaboration.)

soft tissue sarcoma histology. We will see over time if there is indeed a new plateau in survival for patients receiving chemotherapy, indicating there is true elimination, not just shrinking, of microscopic metastatic disease.

The data from this well-executed study must also be taken into consideration with other data regarding two smaller studies of adjuvant chemotherapy for extremity sarcomas. To examine the possible benefit of increased dose intensity in an adjuvant setting, an Austrian group studied 59 patients receiving no chemotherapy or doxorubicin 50 mg/m^2/cycle, dacarbazine 800 mg/m^2/cycle, and ifosfamide 6 g/m^2/cycle every 2 weeks with mesna and filgrastim support following surgical resection of the primary sarcoma. Overall survival and relapse-free survival did not differ significantly between the treatment arms at a mean follow-up of 41 months.[174] There were trends to improved recurrence-free survival, but the study was underpowered to detect a small difference in overall survival or disease-free survival. A randomized phase II neoadjuvant study of doxorubicin 50 mg/m^2 and ifosfamide 5 g/m^2 by the EORTC and NCI-Canada also failed to show a survival advantage for the use of chemotherapy (estimated 5-year overall survival 64% for the control arm, 65% for the treatment arm).[175] Neoadjuvant chemotherapy is discussed in greater detail below. Finally, The EORTC have completed accrual in December 2003 to an adjuvant trial (Study 62931) for high-grade soft tissue sarcomas for all sites, utilizing doxorubicin 75 mg/m^2 and ifosfamide 5,000 mg/m^2 with filgrastim. Analysis will not be feasible until there has been sufficient follow-up.

Preoperative (Neoadjuvant) Chemotherapy Preoperative chemotherapy has theoretical advantages over postoperative treatment. First, preoperative chemotherapy provides an in vivo test of chemotherapy sensitivity. Patients whose tumors show objective evidence of response are presumed to be the subset that will benefit most from further postoperative systemic treatment. In contrast, it is assumed that the population of nonresponding patients will derive minimal or no benefit from further chemotherapy and can therefore be spared its toxicity. On the other hand, it is conceivable that the patients whose tumors respond to chemotherapy may not be those who would derive the most from chemotherapy, because these lesions with favorable biology might be those destined to do well irrespective of any systemic treatment. In contrast, those who do not respond may be those with unfavorable disease who could derive the greatest benefit from the discovery of highly effective systemic treatments.

A second potential advantage of preoperative chemotherapy is that it treats occult microscopic metastatic disease as soon as possible after the cancer diagnosis. This may theoretically prevent the development of chemotherapy resistance by isolated clones of metastatic cells or prevent the postoperative growth of microscopic metastases, but given the nature of growth of sarcomas, at most one or two doublings of the tumor would be affected, far fewer than the greater than 35 typically required in the development of a > 1 cm tumor. Chemotherapy-induced cytoreduction may permit a less radical and consequently less morbid surgical resection than would have been required initially. In patients with large soft tissue sarcomas of the extremities, cytoreduction may reduce the morbidity of limb-sparing surgical procedures and possibly even allow patients who might otherwise have required an amputation to undergo limb-sparing surgery.

Investigators from the M. D. Anderson Cancer Center reported long-term results with doxorubicin-based preoperative chemotherapy for AJCC stages IIC and III (formerly AJCC stage IIIB) extremity soft tissue sarcomas.[176] In a series of 76 patients

Table 111-6 Hazard Ratios for Individual Patient Data Meta-Analysis in 1,568 Adults from 14 Trials of Doxorubicin-Based Chemotherapy for Soft Tissue Sarcoma

Hazard Ratio	Outcome	95% Confidence Intervals	*p* Value
Local RFI	0.73	0.56–0.94	.016
Distant RFI	0.70	0.57–0.85	.0003
Overall recurrence-free survival	0.75	0.64–0.87	.0001
Overall survival	0.89	0.76–1.03	.12

RFI = recurrence-free interval.

Data from the Sarcoma Data Base Meta-Analysis Collaboration. Reproduced with permission from Verweij and Seyance, Semin Radiat Oncol 1999;9:352–9 by W.B. Saunders Company.

treated with doxorubicin-based preoperative chemotherapy, radiologic response rates were as follows: complete response, 9%; partial response, 19%; minor response, 13%; stable disease, 30%; and disease progression, 30%. The overall objective major response rate (complete plus partial responses) was 27%. At a median follow-up of 85 months, 5-year actuarial rates of local recurrence-free survival, distant metastasis-free survival, disease-free survival, and overall survival were 83%, 52%, 46%, and 59%, respectively. The event-free outcomes reported from M. D. Anderson are similar to those observed with chemotherapy in the phase III postoperative chemotherapy trials. Furthermore, comparison of responding patients (complete and partial responses) and nonresponding patients did not reveal any significant differences in event-free outcome.

In a prospective study from MSKCC, 29 patients with AJCC (4th edition) stage IIIB soft tissue sarcomas larger than 10 cm were treated with two cycles of a doxorubicin-based regimen prior to local therapy.[177] Subjective changes in the degree of primary tumor firmness and in imaging characteristics of the tumor (intratumoral necrosis and hemorrhage) were observed in many patients but were not quantifiable. Only one patient met the standard criteria for a partial response. Survival results in this population of high-risk patients were similar to those in historic controls treated with postoperative doxorubicin or patients treated with local therapy alone. The reasons for the apparent discrepancy in response rates between the reports from M. D. Anderson and MSKCC remain unclear. Possible explanations include the fact that the population treated at MSKCC appears to be a higher-risk population, with all patients having high-grade lesions larger than 10 cm, as is discussed below in studies examining retrospective data from both institutions. Moreover, the patients treated at MSKCC received a lower doxorubicin dose (60 mg/m^2) for fewer cycles (two). This may be important given the known dose-response relationship with doxorubicin.[178]

Recently, ifosfamide-containing combinations have been used in the preoperative setting. Selected patients treated with aggressive ifosfamide-based regimens have had major responses, and preliminary results suggest that response rates may be higher than in historic controls treated with nonifosfamide-containing regimens.[179] However, as noted above, the randomized phase II neoadjuvant study of doxorubicin and ifosfamide chemotherapy showed no benefit for the treatment arm, although the study was not specifically designed to determine a survival advantage.[175]

Modifying Chemotherapy It has been theorized that the antisarcoma action of adjuvant chemotherapy might be improved by modifying factors related to drug delivery. One such modification is administering chemotherapy regionally rather than systemically. To a great extent, the rationale is based on work in other malignancies that spread predominantly within one segment of the body, such as ovarian cancer, which tends to remain within the peritoneal cavity. Certain sarcomas, such as GISTs and some gastrointestinal leiomyosarcomas, have the tendency to recur repeatedly within the peritoneum, without development of widespread hepatic or lung metastases. For such patients, several investigators have examined intraperitoneal chemotherapy. Limited single-institution data have shown it to be feasible, although the efficacy cannot be rigorously assessed because comparisons have been only with historic controls.[180] Decreases in locoregional recurrence rates have been suggested, but the impact of such treatment on overall survival, if any, may be quite limited since it will not effect the development of hepatic metastases. Accordingly, intraperitoneal chemotherapy remains an investigational modality.

Some investigators have promulgated the use of heated chemotherapy instilled into the peritoneal cavity following resection, based on studies of hyperthermic perfusion for extremity lesions.[181,182] However, no clinical data have been generated to assess objectively the potential contribution of heat in this setting. Others have evaluated whole-body hyperthermia to enhance the efficacy of combination chemotherapy, using methods to increase the temperature of the entire body or a specific region alone to 41°C.[183–185] Despite some limited data regarding clinical responses, this technique remains highly investigational. Given the observed toxicities of hypotension and nephrotoxicity, the clinical outcomes associated with this approach would have to represent significant improvements over conventional treatments in order to be widely accepted.[186] Hyperthermia is not routinely employed in the adjuvant therapy of sarcomas.

Combined Preoperative Chemotherapy and RT With the advances made with combined-modality treatment of other solid tumors, there has been interest in combined-modality preoperative treatment (concurrent or sequential chemotherapy and RT) for patients with localized soft tissue sarcomas. One putative advantage of preoperative chemo-radiation is the potential to shrink selected lesions resectable only by amputation sufficiently that they become amenable to a limb-sparing approach.

Concurrent chemotherapy and radiation has been employed extensively by Eilber and colleagues at UCLA and has been modified and examined by other groups.[187–189] The initial chemo-radiation treatment protocol typically involved intra-arterial doxorubicin with unusually high dose per fraction RT (35 Gy of external beam radiation delivered in 10 daily fractions, which was reduced to 17.5 Gy in 5 daily fractions to minimize local toxicity). Although the intra-arterial route delivers chemotherapy more directly to the tumor, it is more complex, expensive, and prone to complications than intravenous chemotherapy.[190] Indeed, a prospective randomized trial comparing preoperative intra-arterial doxorubicin with intravenous doxorubicin, both followed by 28 Gy of radiation delivered over 8 days and then surgical resection, showed no differences in local recurrence or survival.[191]

The largest study to date directly studying systemic chemotherapy combined with RT examined razoxane as the radiation-sensitizing agent in a randomized study of drug versus no drug in combination with radiation therapy for resectable or unresectable soft tissue sarcomas. Acute skin reactions were enhanced in the razoxane arm, but late toxicity was not greater than in the control arm. Although there are imbalances in the arms of the study, for the 82 of 130 evaluable cases examined with gross disease RT (median dose 56–58 Gy) with razoxane (daily oral doses of 150 mg/m^2 throughout radiotherapy) showed an increased response rate (74% vs 49%), and improved local control rate (64% vs 30%; $p < .05$) compared with external beam radiation alone.[192]

Ifosfamide and cyclophosphamide have been routinely combined with radiation therapy as part of the definitive therapy for Ewing's sarcoma and rhabdomyosarcoma in an attempt to continue systemic therapy at the same time as maximizing local control.[165,166] In general, toxicity does not appear to be greater than that seen for radiation alone. However, skin toxicity from the combination was greater in one study than that seen with radiation alone.[193]

An alternative sequential chemotherapy and radiation strategy in patients with localized, high-grade, large (> 8 cm) extremity soft tissue sarcomas has been examined.[165,166] This treatment protocol involved three courses of doxorubicin, ifosfamide, mesna, and dacarbazine with two 22-Gy courses of radiation (11 fractions each) for a total preoperative radiation dose of 44 Gy. This was followed by surgical resection with careful microscopic assessment of surgical margins. An additional 16-Gy (8 fractions) boost dose was delivered for microscopically positive surgical margins. The outcomes of 48 patients treated with this regimen have been compared with those of matched historic controls and was superior to that of the historical control patients. The 5-year actuarial local control, freedom from distant metastasis, disease-free survival, and overall survival rate were 92% vs 86% ($p = .1155$), 75% vs 44% ($p = .0016$), 70% vs 42% ($p = .0002$), and 87% vs 58% ($p = .0003$) for the MAID and control patient groups, respectively. Febrile neutropenia was a complication in 25% of patients. Wound healing complications were substantial and occurred in 14 (29%) patients receiving the chemotherapy/radiation sequential therapy. One patient who received chemotherapy developed late fatal myelodysplasia. Given the favorable results of this study in comparison to historical controls, the Radiation Therapy Oncology Group is conducting a multi-institutional trial, modifying the chemotherapy in an attempt to address the local toxicity issue.

Although significant toxicity was observed, local control was improved in the prior study, raising the possibility that combined chemotherapy and radiation could be combined safely to decrease local control risk. Pisters and colleagues examined concurrent doxorubicin and irradiation in the neoadjuvant setting in 27 patients with extremity soft tissue sarcomas.[194] Preoperative external beam radiation was administered in 25 fractions of 2 Gy each. Doxorubicin was administered in escalating doses with a bolus followed by 4-day continuous infusion weekly. Radiographic restaging was performed 4 to 7 weeks after chemoradiation. Patients with localized disease underwent surgical resection. The maximum tolerated dose of continuous infusion doxorubicin combined with standard preoperative radiation was 17.5 mg/m^2/wk; 7 of 23 (30%) patients had grade 3 dermatologic toxicity at this dose level. Macroscopically complete resection (R0 or R1) was performed in all 26 patients who underwent surgery. For 22 patients who were treated with doxorubicin at the maximum tolerated dose and subsequent surgery, an encouraging 11 patients (50%) had 90% or greater tumor necrosis, including 2 patients who had complete pathologic responses. This approach is being further studied with other radiation-sensitizing agents, such as gemcitabine.[195] Further studies of combination therapy are also discussed later in the section "Retroperitoneal Sarcomas."

Recent Analyses of Multicenter Data Regarding Adjuvant Therapy for STS It is well recognized that different sarcoma subtypes have different chemotherapy sensitivity patterns. For example, malignant peripheral nerve sheath tumors are typically resistant to doxorubicin, and leiomyosarcomas are typically less sensitive to ifosfamide than other forms of sarcoma. Synovial sarcoma and myxoid/round-cell liposarcoma appear to be more sensitive to chemotherapy in the metastatic setting than other subtypes of sarcoma, and may well be two subtypes that respond to both anthracyclines and ifosfamide.[196] This argues that adjuvant chemotherapy should be examined on a subtype-specific basis. Combined nonrandomized data from UCLA and MSKCC showed that adjuvant chemotherapy may indeed be useful in the setting of synovial sarcomas and myxoid/round-cell liposarcoma, and argued for the use of chemotherapy in the neoadjuvant setting for all types of soft tissue sarcoma, based on MSKCC and Dana-Farber institutional databases.[197–199] Interestingly, data of all patients treated or not treated with chemotherapy from M. D. Anderson and MSKCC indicated in the adjuvant or neoadjuvant setting that there was no statistical difference in overall survival in the group of patients who received chemotherapy versus those who did not.[200] However, these data are inherently biased in that it is likely that younger, healthier patients with larger high-grade tumors were those selected to receive chemotherapy. Even though there was no statistically significant difference between the group of patients who received chemotherapy and those who did not, there were still shifts in the frequency of patients with larger sarcomas with a predominance of liposarcoma toward receiving chemotherapy, perhaps representing the selection bias that allowed a group of patients with an inherently poorer outcome to do as well as those with a better outcome.

In summary, for AJCC stage III soft tissue sarcoma, if there is a benefit to chemotherapy in the adjuvant setting, it appears to be a small one. In such a situation, it is the authors' practice to attempt to compare benefits and risks of systemic therapy and individualize the plan of treatment for a given clinical setting. Younger patients with relatively chemotherapy-sensitive subtypes such as myxoid/round-cell liposarcoma and synovial sarcoma may be those who benefit most among this very heterogeneous patient population. Certainly the finding of 20% or more of soft tissue sarcomas with specific genetic translocations or mutations brings hope that the benefit seen with imatinib and GIST will carry over to the adjuvant setting for a subset of patients with soft tissue sarcomas of the extremities and trunk when adjuvant chemotherapy is combined with one of the new protein kinase-targeted inhibitors.

"Pediatric" Sarcomas and Adjuvant Therapy The standard of care for nearly all sarcomas specific to the pediatric population involves chemotherapy. It is of proven benefit in patients with osteogenic sarcoma, Ewing's sarcoma, and rhabdomyosarcoma. A few brief comments on these chemotherapy-sensitive tumors follow.

Neoadjuvant chemotherapy, established by Rosen and colleagues, is the standard of care for the initial treatment of osteogenic sarcoma.[201] In the era before chemotherapy, cure rates, even in the setting of amputation for primary disease, was only on the order of 15%. With chemotherapy the survival rate is on the order of 70%. Yet the 30% of patients who relapse remain a frustrating problem because the addition of new agents has changed the chance for cure comparatively modestly. The outcome of adjuvant chemotherapy (degree of tumor necrosis after chemotherapy) is directly associated with improved clinical outcome, and provides the opportunity for changing chemotherapy for a poor initial response. The standard of care for adjuvant chemotherapy is a backbone of cisplatin and doxorubicin, with more centers adding ifosfamide in newer regimens. High-dose methotrexate is used in most pediatric patients and is an active drug in metastatic disease. The benefit for multiagent adjuvant therapy was called into question in a 1997 paper in which the combination of doxorubicin and cisplatin alone was shown equivalent to a more complicated and toxic regimen (Rosen T10-like) containing high-dose methotrexate as well.[164] However, the methotrexate component of neoadjuvant therapy has been observed to be an important component of the chemotherapy used for osteosarcoma in some studies.[202]

Through a careful series of international clinical studies, the adjuvant program for rhabdomyosarcoma typically involves an induction course of chemotherapy, followed by combination chemotherapy and radiation, followed by the completion of chemotherapy, which will last approximately 48 weeks in pediatric population. The standard of care is the combination of vincristine, dactinomycin, and cyclophosphamide, since this combination was shown as effective as VAI and VIE and less toxic.[166] The addition of doxorubicin to the vincristine, dactinomycin, and cyclophosphamide regimen did not appear to improve overall survival and is usually omitted in the treatment of rhabdomyosarcoma.[203] The frequent dosing of vincristine is extremely difficult to complete for adults and requires dose adjustment or shorter courses of therapy for adults than for children with this diagnosis. Children with this diagnosis appear to fare better than adults with the same diagnosis stage for stage in most studies.[204]

For patients with Ewing's sarcoma, in distinction from rhabdomyosarcoma, the addition of additional agents (ifosfamide and etoposide) to an existing backbone of vincristine, doxorubicin, and cyclophosphamide chemotherapy improved outcome for localized disease,[165] while data regarding metastatic disease remain unpublished as of January 2005. This five-drug regimen is a good standard of care for patients with a new diagnosis of Ewing's sarcoma. It is often difficult to administer the entire 48 weeks of chemotherapy to adults, abbreviation to the adjuvant therapy program is often necessary. As with rhabdomyosarcoma, children with this diagnosis appear to fare better than adults with the same diagnosis, stage for stage.[205]

TREATMENT OF LOCALLY ADVANCED DISEASE

Hyperthermic Isolated Limb Perfusion Hyperthermic isolated limb perfusion (HILP), an investigational technique in the United States (although recently approved by regulatory agencies in other parts of the world), has received considerable attention in the treatment of locally advanced, unresectable sarcomas of nonosseous tissues. HILP has been evaluated in two settings: (1) attempted limb preservation in cases of locally advanced extremity lesions surgically amenable only to amputation and (2) function extremity preservation for the short survival duration anticipated in cases of locally advanced extremity lesions with synchronous pulmonary metastases (stage IV disease).

A multicenter phase II trial has evaluated a series of 55 patients with radiologically unresectable extremity soft tissue sarcomas using HILP with high-dose tumor necrosis factor-α, interferon-α, and melphalan.[206] A major tumor response was seen in 87% of patients: complete responses in 20 (36%) and partial responses in 28 (51%). Limb salvage was achieved in 84% of patients. Regional toxicity was limited, and systemic toxicity was minimal to moderate. There were no treatment-related deaths. This approach is being further evaluated in ongoing trials in Europe.

Radiation Alone Apart from patients with some very radiosensitive subtypes of sarcomas, most patients who undergo RT as the sole treatment modality for sarcoma have been deemed to have locally advanced unresectable disease. RT alone is a rare treatment choice that should be done only at centers skilled in the management of sarcomas; medically fit patients with grossly

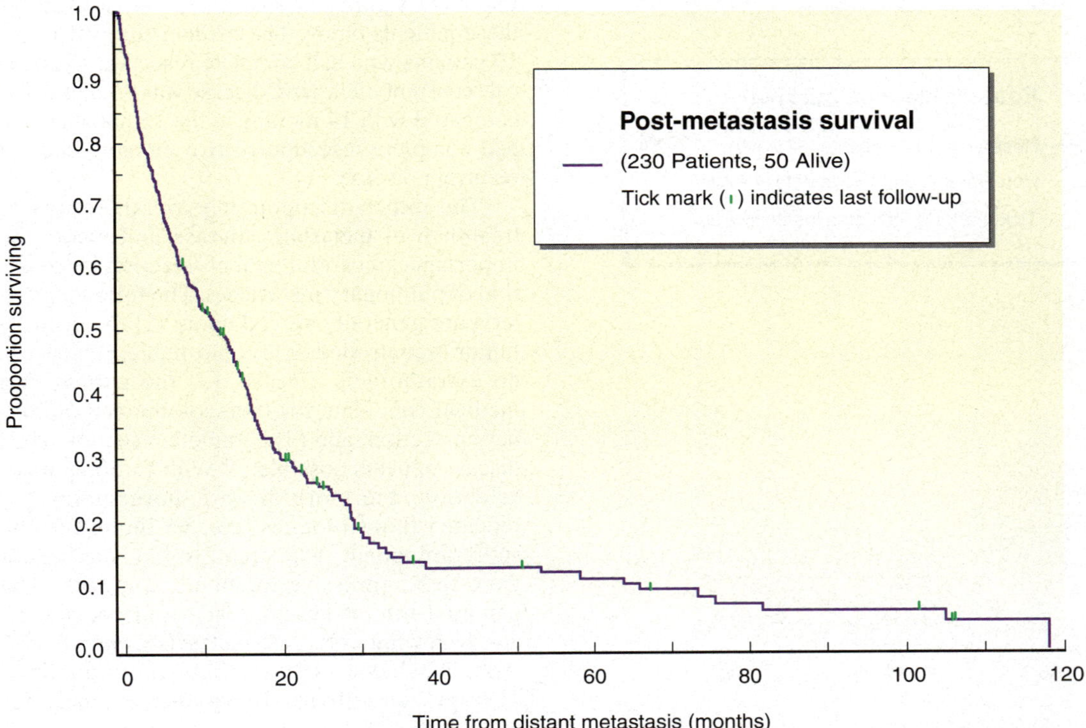

Figure 111-12 Postmetastasis survival (from time of diagnosis of M1 disease) in a cohort of 230 patients with primary soft tissue sarcomas of the extremities. The median postmetastasis survival was 11.6 months. (From Billingsley et al,[208] by permission of *Cancer*.)

"unresectable" but nonmetastatic disease should always be referred to a specialty center for multidisciplinary management, which may combine surgery, RT, and possibly chemotherapy. For example, proximal inguinal or axillary tumors that encircle major vascular structures in the proximal leg or arm may be resected along with the involved vasculature and the vessels reconstructed. Adjuvant RT is also generally used. Rarely, a patient with truly inoperable locally advanced disease may require RT alone, with either photon or particle (proton, neutron, or pion) beams.[157,161,207–209] No formal clinical trials have been performed to compare these strategies with each other, and they are generally administered in an adverse clinical setting. Local control has been reported in 40 to 70% of such cases treated with neutrons; treatment with photons is reported to produce local control in approximately 30% of cases.[161,207]

TREATMENT OF METASTATIC DISEASE

Clinical Problem of Metastases The diagnosis of recurrent or metastatic disease in patients with soft tissue sarcomas is devastating. Patients and physicians are aware that, in general, such a diagnosis significantly worsens the expected outcomes. The role of the multidisciplinary sarcoma team in the management of patients with metastatic sarcoma is to recognize opportunities in which multimodality care might still improve important outcomes such as survival or quality of life. Both surgery and systemic chemotherapy can play an important role in improving these outcomes in selected patients. Overall, it is important to recognize that unresectable metastatic sarcomas of soft tissues are—with rare exceptions—eventually fatal, and that chemotherapy is given with the palliative aim of prolonging life and improving quality of life.

The most common site of metastasis from soft tissue sarcomas of the extremities is the lungs. Indeed, the lungs are the only site of metastasis in approximately 80% of patients with metastases from primary extremity and trunk soft tissue sarcomas.[210,211] Primary visceral and gastrointestinal sarcomas commonly metastasize to the liver as well as the lungs. Extrapulmonary metastases are uncommon forms of first metastasis from extremity sarcomas and usually occur as a late manifestation of widely disseminated disease.[211] The median survival after development of distant metastases is 11.6 months (Figure 111-12).[212] The optimal treatment of patients with metastatic soft tissue sarcoma requires an understanding of the natural history of the disease and individualized selection of treatment options based on patient factors, disease factors, and limitations imposed by prior treatment.

The approach to patients with advanced or metastatic sarcomas is changing over time. We are recognizing that clinical trials must be stratified rationally for data of value to be derived. Studies of "sarcomas" without stratification will soon seem as naïve as studies of "cancer" without further qualification: These mesenchymally derived diseases lumped under the heading of "sarcomas" can be quite different, and studies need to take that into account. To do that and to generate studies of sufficient size and power, large-scale collaborations on a national and international level will be required. Such collaborations are already in place among the nations of Europe (the Soft Tissue and Bone Sarcoma Group of the EORTC), Scandinavian centers, Italian centers, and Canadian centers, and new collaborations are beginning in the United States under the auspices of the American College of Surgeons Oncology Group. With these collaborations, it is hoped that further research will rapidly translate research findings into the novel therapeutics that are so desperately required by patients with sarcomas.

Resection of Metastatic Disease Multiple investigators have reported their experience with pulmonary metastasectomy for metastatic soft tissue sarcoma in adults.[213–222] Three-year survival rates following thoracotomy for pulmonary metastasectomy range from 23 to 54% (Table 111-7).[213–215,222–225] Since the ability to completely resect all metastatic disease is an important determinant of outcome, the reported interinstitution variability in postmetastasectomy survival rates is partially a function of whether survival was reported for all patients who underwent thoracotomy or only for the subset who underwent complete resection.[212,215,224]

It remains difficult to predict which patients with pulmonary metastases will benefit from pulmonary resection. A number of clinical criteria

Table 111-7 Survival Following Complete Resection of Pulmonary Metastases from Soft Tissue Sarcoma in Adults

	No. of Patients					
First Author/Institution	Pulmonary Metastases	Total Metastases	Surgical Treatment	Complete Resection %	Median Survival, Mo.	3-Year Survival %
Creagan[213]/Mayo	112	112	112	64 (57)	18	29
Putnam[223]/NCI	487	93	68	51 (75)	23	32
Jablons[224]/NCI	74	57	57	49 (86)	27	35
Casson[214]/MDACC	68	68	68	58 (85)	25	42
Verazin[231]/Roswell	78	78	78	61 (78)	21	21.5 (5 yr)
Gadd[215]/MSKCC	716	135	78	65 (83)	19	23
van Geel[222]/EORTC	255	255	255	255 (100)	NR	54

Mayo = Mayo Clinic; Roswell = Roswell Park Cancer Institute; NCI = U.S. National Cancer Institute; MDACC = M. D. Anderson Cancer Center; MSKCC = Memorial Sloan-Kettering Cancer Center; EORTC = European Organization Table for Research and Treatment of Cancer.

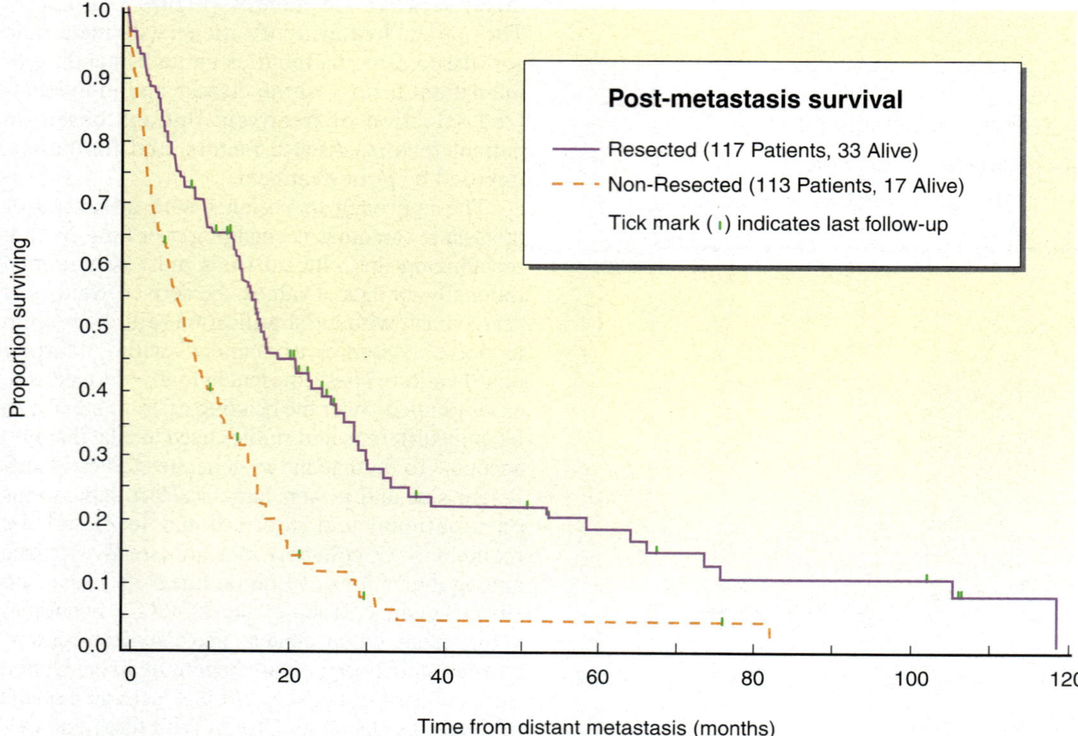

Figure 111-13 Postmetastasis survival stratified by resection of pulmonary metastatic disease. The median survival among patients undergoing complete resection of pulmonary metastatic disease was 20 months. (From Billingsley et al.[212])

have been evaluated by univariate analysis in this regard, including the disease-free interval, number of metastatic nodules, and tumor doubling time.[213,223,225–230] Multivariate analyses from both the NCI and Roswell Park Cancer Institute confirm that a short disease-free interval and incomplete pulmonary resection are adverse prognostic factors for survival for patients with pulmonary metastases.[224,231] A multivariate analysis from M. D. Anderson suggested that, in addition, the presence of more than three metastatic pulmonary nodules on preoperative chest CT is an adverse prognostic sign.[214] Nevertheless, the most important prognostic factor impacting survival appears to be the ability to completely resect all disease.[212,215,224] In the review of postmetastasectomy outcome by Billingsley and colleagues from MSKCC, the median survival among patients who were able to undergo complete resection of metastases was 20 months as compared with 10 months among patients who did not have complete resection (Figure 111-13).[212] In summary, the ability to achieve complete resection and the number of pulmonary nodules present appear to best define the postoperative prognosis for these patients.

Unfortunately, metastasectomy benefits only a small (< 15%) fraction of patients who develop pulmonary metastases. This is best illustrated by data from MSKCC, where a population of 716 patients who presented with primary extremity sarcoma were followed for the subsequent development and treatment of pulmonary metastases (Figure 111-14).[210] Of the initial cohort of 716 patients, 148 patients (21%) developed pulmonary metastases. Isolated pulmonary metastases occurred in 135 (91%) of these 148 patients. Of the 135 patients with pulmonary-only metastases, 78 (58%) were considered to have operable disease, and 65 (83%) of those taken to thoracotomy were able to undergo complete resection of all of their pulmonary metastatic disease. Thus, 44% of all patients with pulmonary metastases were able to undergo complete metastasectomy. The median survival from the time of complete resection was 19 months, and the 3-year survival rate was 23%. All patients who did not undergo thoracotomy died within 3 years. For the entire cohort of 135 patients developing pulmonary-only metastases, the 3-year survival rate was only 11% (see Figure 111-14).

Many investigators believe that repeat thoracotomy to render patients free of disease from pulmonary soft tissue sarcoma metastases is justified in the absence of effective systemic therapy. Several series of repeat pulmonary metastasectomy have been published.[232,233] In a series of 43 patients thus treated at the NCI, 72% of patients could be rendered free of disease at the second thoracotomy, with a median survival duration from the time of second thoracotomy of 25 months.[232] In a report from M. D. Anderson of a series of 39 patients undergoing reoperation for a second pulmonary metastasis after successful initial metastasectomy, factors predicting long-term survival included the presence of a solitary metastasis and the ability to perform a complete resection.[233] The M. D. Anderson study also illustrates the significant survival duration many of these patients enjoy: The median survival in the 19 patients who had complete resection of unifocal recurrent metastatic disease was 65 months as compared with 14 months in the 15 patients who had complete resection of two or more sites of recurrent disease.

The rather disappointing overall results of treatment of metastatic disease underscore the importance of careful patient selection for resection of pulmonary metastases. The following criteria are generally agreed upon: (1) the primary tumor is controlled or is controllable, (2) there is no extrathoracic disease, (3) the patient is a medical candidate for thoracotomy and pulmonary resection, and (4) complete resection of all disease appears possible.[234] With careful patient selection, the morbidity of thoracotomy (or repeated thoracotomies) can be limited to the subset of patients who are most likely to benefit from this aggressive treatment approach. The potential role of systemic adjuvant chemotherapy following complete metastasectomy is discussed below in the section "Individualized Therapy" on individualizing chemotherapy for metastases.

CHEMOTHERAPY FOR METASTATIC DISEASE Natural History of Metastases A good place to begin a discussion of chemotherapy for unresectable metastatic sarcoma is the expected course of the disease. The EORTC has made a major contribution in defining the expected course of unresectable metastatic sarcoma by publishing its large series of more than 2,000 patients with advanced sarcomas of soft tissues to describe prognostic features and the response to anthracycline-based chemotherapy.[235] In this study reviewing more than 20 years of experience, the median overall survival was approximately 1 year for the group as a whole. However, a subset

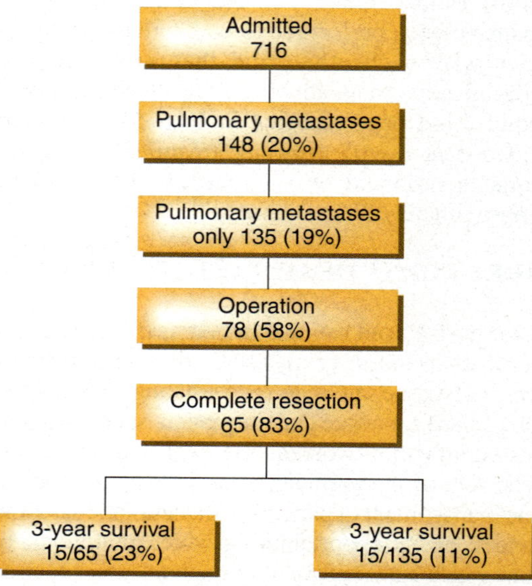

Figure 111-14 Risk and subsequent management of pulmonary metastases in 716 patients with primary or locally recurrent extremity soft tissue sarcoma.[210]

of patients had longer median survival. Such patients were typically those who were younger, had a better performance status, had low-grade sarcoma, had no liver metastases, and had developed metastatic disease following a longer interval from initial diagnosis. Importantly, this study concluded that the variables predicting improved survival were actually different from variables predicting objective response to chemotherapy (the latter variables including such items as high-grade tumor and liposarcoma subtype). Thus, one interpretation that is reasonable is that the most important predictors of survival with metastatic sarcoma are variables dependent on the tumor biology itself, as well as certain patient factors such as age and comorbid disease. These data are critical to understand so that information regarding the impact of new drugs and treatments can be interpreted appropriately, based on a comparison with the correct expectations for the natural or treated history of the disease in past clinical trials.

Individualized Therapy The approach to patients with advanced or metastatic sarcomas is evolving. We increasingly recognize that clinical trials must be stratified rationally for data of value to be derived. Studies of "sarcomas" without stratification will soon seem as naïve as studies of "cancer" without further qualification; each of the greater than 50 mesenchymal cancers lumped under the heading "soft tissue sarcomas" has a distinct biological behavior, and studies need to take that into account. To generate studies of sufficient size and power, large-scale collaborations on a national and international level will be required. Such collaborations are already well established among the nations of Europe (the Soft Tissue and Bone Sarcoma Group of the EORTC), Scandinavian centers, Italian centers, and Canadian centers, and new collaborations are forming in the United States under the auspices of the American College of Surgeons Oncology Group (ACOSOG), Intergroup Committee Against Sarcomas (ICAS), and Sarcoma Alliance for Research through Collaboration (SARC). With these collaborations, it is hoped that further research will rapidly translate research findings into the novel therapeutics that are so desperately required by patients with sarcomas.

Tremendous effort has gone into testing multiple commercially available and experimental agents in soft tissue sarcoma. Nonetheless, with the exception of imatinib in GIST, no new medication has been accepted widely for use in sarcomas since the introduction of ifosfamide. Nonetheless, new data regarding a gemcitabine/docetaxel combination provides a new option for certain subtypes of sarcoma. The data discussed below are a synopsis of many studies, most of which cannot be referenced owing to constraints of space. Special attention to specific subtypes that are sensitive or resistant to particular chemotherapy drugs is noted.

Anthracyclines and Ifosfamide With the caveat that specific sarcomas demonstrate differential sensitivity to different chemotherapy agents, doxorubicin and ifosfamide remain the two most active agents for metastatic sarcoma, with RECIST-defined response rates in the 10 to 20% range for each drug.[236] Depending on the ratio of sensitive versus less sensitive subtypes of soft tissue sarcomas in past studies, the response rate can be significantly higher. For example, synovial sarcoma and myxoid/round-cell liposarcomas are relatively sensitive to ifosfamide (as well as doxorubicin), while GIST, alveolar soft parts sarcoma, and hemangiopericytoma/solitary fibrous tumor are notoriously resistant to both agents. Certain studies have recognized that conventional doxorubicin plus ifosfamide-based chemotherapy is suboptimal for gastrointestinal leiomyosarcomas, and patients with these tumors are excluded from studies of such treatments. However, when this is done, it is impossible to tell whether high rates of response are due to the treatment under study or due to the exclusion of groups of patients who have had lower response rates in other trials.[179]

It is also important to recognize that response rates per se are increasingly being criticized as possibly poor surrogates of clinical benefit. Many sarcomas have densely hyalinized desmoplastic stromal tissues associated with them. Even when chemotherapy successfully induces massive tumor cell kill in vivo, this hyalinized tissue remains unchanged, leading to falsely negative imaging findings of tumor response to chemotherapy. Thus, objective response rates based on imaging may actually underestimate the antitumor efficacy of chemotherapy. Conversely, simply shrinking a tumor and achieving a nondurable response may not be worth the toxicities of aggressive multiagent chemotherapy. Thus, from both standpoints, RECIST-defined responses may not be an ideal indicator of antitumor efficacy in sarcoma management in general, with GIST an excellent case in point.[237] Increasing attention in the field of sarcoma drug development is thus being paid to other important indicators of clinical outcomes, such as progression-free survival duration, percentage survival at a given time point, and overall survival rate.

Some drugs may slow disease progression and prolong survival even if objective response rates are low, although the clinical data to support those claims must be generated with rigor and careful attention to consistency of follow-up. Nonetheless, despite observations that clinical benefit might be underestimated by RECIST, it remains the yardstick by which clinical responses are measured. The measurement of clinical benefit will be an increasingly important question as molecular protein kinase inhibitors such as anti-angiogenic agents become more widely used. It may well be that tumor stasis or "euangiogenesis" is the best possible outcome achieved by some of these newer agents, although it is hoped in and of itself normalization of blood vessels within tumors may allow for reactivation of apoptotic mechanisms within the cell that are suppressed by hypoxia through the action of HIF-alpha.[238] It will be difficult to prove the activity of such agents in comparison with historical control groups because of selection bias issues, and careful statistical designs will be necessary to help identify which newer agents are useful or not.

Notably, taxanes or gemcitabine alone (in the typical 30-minute bolus infusion) were largely inactive.[239,240] However, with gemcitabine given as a controlled rate infusion of 10 mg/m^2/min in combination with docetaxel, activity increased to 40 to 50% in a group of patients with leiomyosarcoma as a dominant histology.[241,242] These data both point out the importance of examining different schedules of drugs as well as the differential sensitivity of different subtypes of sarcomas to different chemotherapy agents.

Dose-Response Relationships The sensitivity of sarcomas to chemotherapy was first convincingly demonstrated with doxorubicin in the early 1970s.[178] Subsequent studies of doxorubicin in sarcomas have widely been viewed as supporting a dose-response relationship, with doses of 50 mg/m^2/cycle or less producing far less antitumor activity than doses of 60 mg/m^2/cycle or higher. Although a dose-response relationship may exist, it is important to recognize that other variables may affect antitumor efficacy, such as histopathologic subtype of sarcoma, as noted above. Nonetheless, since a dose threshold for optimal activity has been documented with doxorubicin in another chemotherapy-sensitive solid tumor, specifically breast cancer, it seems reasonable to conclude that doxorubicin is best used at doses above 60 mg/m^2/cycle. Also analogous to breast cancer, improved response rates above the conventional 60 to 75 mg/m^2/cycle dose range are difficult to demonstrate.

A wide variety of dose- and schedule-ranging studies have been performed with ifosfamide. It is clear that antitumor response is improved by higher doses of ifosfamide.[179] This point has been made most convincingly by the responses to high-dose ifosfamide (> 10,000 mg/m^2/cycle) in patients who had previously failed to respond to the same drug at lower doses (ie, < 6,000 mg/m^2/cycle). However, given the potential toxicities of this drug at high doses, high dose ifosfamide is best reserved for a small subset of patients with disease that is expected to be highly chemotherapy sensitive to achieve meaningful responses (eg, prior to planned surgical extirpation of metastases).

Single-Agent versus Combination Chemotherapy A continuing controversy is whether the optimal approach to patients with advanced sarcomas is combination chemotherapy regimens or sequential single agents. One of the best prospective randomized trials of combination chemotherapy for advanced disease came from a US intergroup study in which ifosfamide was or was not given to previously untreated patients with metastatic or advanced soft tissue sarcomas receiving doxorubicin plus dacarbazine. This study demonstrated no survival advantage for the group receiving ifosfamide in combination with doxorubicin plus dacarbazine, although this group had a statistically significant increase in objective response rate.[243] The role of combination chemotherapy is further called into question for broad use given the statistically significant increase in toxicities when ifosfamide was added. Thus, despite the increased anticancer activity as evidenced by the small but significant improvement in response rates, no survival benefit was obtained by adding a third drug. These data are widely interpreted as supporting aggressive combination chemotherapy for patients with bulky locally advanced disease who may be candidates for limb-sparing surgery after preoperative chemotherapy. However, for patients with widespread advanced disease, such combination chemotherapy may be appropriate only if a rapid induction of response is required to control acute symptoms such as tumor-related pain or obstruction. It is hoped the advent of less toxic kinase-directed therapy will decrease the overall toxicity burden for many patients receiving palliative treatment.

Strategies to Improve the Therapeutic Index of Chemotherapy ***Epirubicin versus Doxorubicin*** Advances in pharmacology and other supportive care have yielded significant changes in the delivery of active chemotherapy for sarcoma patients. The impact of these advances may not yet have been recognized in widespread practice. One of the first such strategies was modifying the chemical structure of the most potent agent, doxorubicin, into another anthracycline, epirubicin. Epirubicin has diminished cardiac toxicity on a milligram-for-milligram basis compared with doxorubicin, allowing the delivery of higher doses. Notably, the efficacy differences between these agents appears small, and it may be that equally myelotoxic doses of epirubicin are no better than an equally myelotoxic dose of doxorubicin. In fact, doxorubicin may have a more favorable therapeutic index than high-dose epirubicin.[244] Larger studies stratified by histology are required before any definitive conclusions could be made concerning the relative worth of these two potent anthracyclines.

Dose Intensification Using Stem Cells An obvious strategy to increase response rates has been to increase dose intensity, adding stem cell support, as examined in hematological malignancies, breast adenocarcinoma, and other malignancies. This was initially attempted solely with provision of autologous bone marrow support and in the past decade has been significantly facilitated by the availability of hematopoietic cytokines to improve hematologic tolerance to myelosuppressive chemotherapy. It is clear that peripheral blood progenitor cells can be mobilized and harvested following standard chemotherapy for sarcoma supported by granulocyte colony-stimulating factor.[245] However, even in chemotherapy-sensitive diseases such as Ewing's sarcoma, dose intensification with autologous stem cell support does not appear to be beneficial for improving survival, although contamination of stem cells with tumors cells may be a contributing factor to its lack of efficacy. The use of high-dose chemotherapy with stem cell and cytokine support remains investigational for sarcomas.

Encapsulated Anthracyclines Another strategy to increase the therapeutic index of anthracyclines is to encapsulate the drug within a liposomal vehicle. At least three liposomal preparations of anthracyclines have been tested, and all have shown some efficacy against sarcomas. Notably, the most widely used agent has decreased cardiac risk in comparison to older preparations of larger liposomes containing doxorubicin. Pegylated liposomal doxorubicin (Doxil/Caelyx) is a small liposome with polyethylene glycol anchored within the lipid bilayer, acting as a hydrophilic coating to preserve the circulating half-life of the liposome and prevent degradation within the reticuloendothelial system. This preparation, given at a dose rate less than that of unencapsulated doxorubicin, is better tolerated than doxorubicin, with substantially less myelotoxicity, cardiac toxicity, and alopecia at the cost of hand-foot syndrome and idiosyncratic reactions to the first dose of therapy. In one randomized phase II study, pegylated liposomal doxorubicin was as effective as doxorubicin.[246] A less toxic anthracycline preparation has yielded a way to extend systemic therapy to patients with poorer performance status and in principle is a novel way of treating very slowly growing connective tissue lesions such as myxoid liposarcomas or desmoid tumors.

New Agents Sarcomas represent a fertile ground for the field of drug development. Doxorubicin was first recognized as an effective agent against sarcomas and subsequently was developed into one of the most widely used anticancer agents ever discovered. A few of the new agents and their utility in sarcoma are noted below, in particular trabectedin (ET-743), which shows specific activity against liposarcomas and leiomyosarcomas. The next edition of this chapter will no doubt contain much more information on small molecule inhibitors kinase and other small molecule inhibitors, many of which are just beginning to be tested now.

Trabectidin (ET-743, Ecteinascidin) Trabectedin (Yondelis) is a marine-derived drug from the marine tunicate *Ecteinascidia turbinata*. It covalently binds to the minor groove of the DNA and blocks the cell cycle in late S and G2, and affects the transcription in part by prevention of binding of transcription factor NF-Y, thus decreasing expression of a variety of genes, including multidrug resistance genes.[247] After initial promising results in phase I studies, multiple phase II trials were performed examining GIST (in which it was inactive), osteogenic sarcoma, and untreated and previously treated metastatic soft tissue sarcoma patients.[248–252]

In the first study of previously treated sarcoma patients, ET-743 was administered at a dose of 1.5 mg/m^2 over 24 hours by ambulatory infusion pump every 3 weeks.[252] Fifty-two patients were assessable for response. Tumor histology included leiomyosarcoma (26 nonuterine, 15 uterine), liposarcoma (n = 11), GIST (n = 7), synovial sarcoma (n = 6), malignant fibrous histiocytoma (n = 6), fibrosarcoma (n = 7), and other sarcomas (n = 22). Patients received a median of three cycles of ET-743. Two partial responses and four minor responses were observed, as well as 9 patients with stable disease as best response. Median progression-free survival was 1.9 months. Twenty-four percent of patients were progression-free at 6 months. Thirty percent of patients were alive at 2 years, with an overall median survival of 12.8 months. Two patients died of treatment-related causes, but both were attributed to protocol eligibility violations. Toxicity included reversible grade 3 to 4 elevations in AST or ALT in half of patients, and 61% of patients had grade 3 to 4 neutropenia, with six episodes of febrile neutropenia.

A confirmatory phase II study of ET-743 was performed in pretreated patients, excluding GIST patients.[251] Patients again received ET-743 as a 24-hour IV continuous intravenous at 1.5 mg/m^2 every 3 weeks. Tumor histology included leiomyosarcoma (n = 13), liposarcoma (n = 10), synovial sarcoma (n = 6), malignant schwannoma (n = 2), and other (n = 5). Overall response rate was 8% (95% confidence interval, 2–23%), with one complete response and two partial responses. The most significant finding was that responses lasted up to 20 months. Including 2 patients with minor responses, the "clinical benefit rate" was 14%. The most common significant toxicities were again grade 3 to 4 neutropenia and grade 3 to 4 transaminitis. One-year estimates for time to progression and overall survival rates were 9% and 53%, respectively. Similar response rates are seen in previously untreated patients. A phase II/III study of ET-743 in patients with metastatic leiomyosarcoma and liposarcoma comparing a weekly schedule of ET-473 with the 24-hour infusion schedule noted above is open and should complete accrual in 2005.

9-Nitrocamptothecin A phase II study of topoisomerase I inhibitor 9-nitrocamptothecin (9-NC) was recently completed, examining patients with gastrointestinal (GI) leiomyosarcomas and other soft tissue sarcomas.[253] 9-NC was given by mouth at 1.5 mg/m^2 daily, 5 days every week. A total of 56 patients were enrolled on this study. Only 1 of 17 patients with GI leiomyosarcoma responded, so that arm of the study was closed; of 39 patients with other sarcomas 3 partial responses were observed, lasting 4, 6, and 13 months. Four patients required hospitalization for nausea, vomiting, and dehydration; other toxicities included anorexia, diarrhea, fatigue, and neutropenia. Its relative lack of activity was consistent with a phase II study of irinotecan in sarcomas (several of which were GIST and therefore resistant to chemotherapy). It should be noted that topoisomerase I agents are active in rhabdomyosarcoma and Ewing's sarcoma/PNET.

Bortezomib Bortezomib (PS-341, Velcade), a therapy targeting the proteasome of the cell, is active against myeloma as well as previously difficult to treat malignancies such as mantle-cell lymphoma. It is believed disruption of the many physiological processes dependent upon proteasome function is the reason for activity of bortezomib in these malignancies, such as regulation

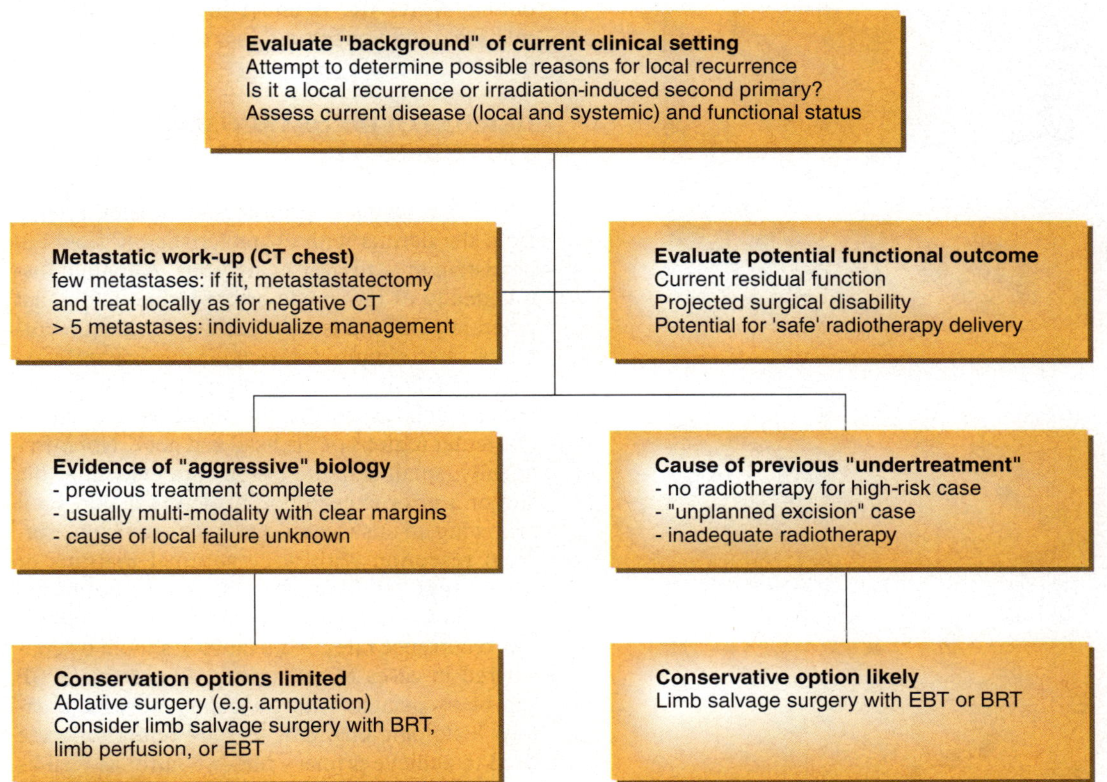

Figure 111-15 Schema for approaching the patient with local recurrence of soft tissue sarcoma. The schema is oriented toward extremity lesions but is equally applicable to other anatomic sites (eg, head and neck and retroperitoneum). BRT = brachytherapy; EBT = external beam radiotherapy. (Reproduced with permission from Catton CN, et al. Semin Radiat Oncol 1999;9:378–88.)

of cell-cycle proteins, TP53, and NF kappa B signaling pathways. A two-arm phase II study was performed examining sarcomas with histologies more commonly seen in adults or in children. Bortezomib was given as a 1.5 mg/m^2 intravenous push twice weekly, 2 weeks on, 1 week off. Only one response (leiomyosarcoma) was seen in 21 evaluable patients and the study was closed.[254] Side effects were significant, and included myalgias, persistent neuropathy, abdominal pain, and fatigue. The authors concluded if bortezomib were to be studied further, it should be in combination with other chemotherapy agents.

MANAGEMENT OF LOCAL RECURRENCE

If an isolated local recurrence is identified, the treatment goals are the same as for patients with primary tumors, namely, optimal local control while maintaining as much function and cosmesis as possible.[152] Early identification of local relapse may improve the chance of successful salvage therapy, and, like newly diagnosed patients, these patients are probably best managed in specialized multidisciplinary sarcoma centers. An approach to the evaluation and management of locally recurrent soft tissue sarcoma is summarized in Figure 111-15. The initial evaluation must include a full review of previous therapy because this will have a bearing on the therapeutic options available. Therefore, all prior surgery and pathology reports should be examined, as should reports on previous chemotherapy and previous RT, especially volume treated, dose, and energy of radiation.

Staging should be performed in the same way as for new cases. The areas adjacent to the original lesion and potentially contaminated by previous surgical interventions should be scrutinized carefully. Both these areas and tissues adjacent to the recurrent tumor, containing potential tumor extensions, should be considered at risk and candidates for resection and/or inclusion in radiation fields.

Several distinct groupings are evident under the rubric of "locally recurrent" disease: (1) cases in which prior treatment did not include RT, (2) cases treated with RT in the past, (3) cases in which distant metastases are also present, and (4) cases in which it is difficult to distinguish between recurrence and secondary tumors induced by RT. Although the therapeutic options available are more limited in recurrent disease and the challenge posed by these cases that much more formidable, a proportion of these patients can be cured. Clinical experience is needed to determine which therapeutic options are appropriate in a given case of recurrent disease.

GASTROINTESTINAL STROMAL TUMORS

No discussion of sarcomas would be complete without noting the remarkable advances made with one particular sarcoma subtype, GIST, which has changed the way people think about sarcomas. With the recognition of c-*kit* as a good marker for GIST to distinguish it from other sarcomas and the recognition of c-*kit* or PDGFR activating mutations that are likely responsible for the constitutive activation of c-*kit*,[255] clinical studies followed rapidly, and have been done in parallel to studies investigating the biology of GIST. Of note, Ewing's sarcomas can mark positive for c-*kit* but kit is not mutated in these tumors and Ewing's sarcomas do not respond to imatinib.

After the recognition of in vivo efficacy of imatinib against a GIST cell line, treatment of metastatic disease has rapidly advanced from treating a single patient (Figure 111-16) to phase I, II, and III studies for patients with metastatic disease.[256–260] The results have been remarkably consistent. Imatinib is at least 10-fold more active than any agent ever examined for treatment of GIST (formerly called GI leiomyosarcoma). The response rate to imatinib is approximately 60%, with 20% with stable disease, and 20% with overt progression on therapy. US phase III data indicate that 400 mg and 800 mg yield equivalent time-to-progression curves, but the European/Australian phase III study indicates that time to progression is improved with the higher dose (800 mg daily) arm.[259] Remarkably, patients' c-*kit* genotype determined their response rate (Figure 111-17).[261] Patients with exon-11 mutation (just inside the cell membrane) had an 80 to 90% response rate, while patients with exon-9 mutation had a response rate only one-third to one-half as high. Patients with no mutation in c-*kit* had a much lower response rate, but still higher than that observed for other chemotherapy drugs. For the time being, regardless of mutation status, imatinib is the standard of care for metastatic GIST. A dosage of 400 mg daily is a reasonable starting point for most patients, with increase toward 800 mg if there is evidence of progression of disease. Therapy should not be interrupted if apparent new hypodense lesions appear in the liver; these likely represent occult metastatic disease.[262]

The median time to progression for patients with metastatic GIST on imatinib is approximately 2 years. Patients with progression on a lower dose of imatinib can respond again with dose increases. The phase I study of imatinib indicated that the maximum tolerated dosage is 800 mg daily (400 mg by mouth bid). Patients with progression of disease have had unusual patterns of progression.[262] In some cases, tumor regrowth in an apparently necrotic tumor is observed, and in others only one metastatic deposit is seen to progress instead of the multiplicity of lesions seen in many patients with advanced GIST. As a result, it is possible to palliate some patients with carefully planned operations to remove problematic single sites of metastatic disease. The benefit of routine debulking of metastatic disease after imatinib is unclear, but is undertaken for some patients with the concern of later progression of metastatic disease, since the complete response rate to imatinib is less than 5%.

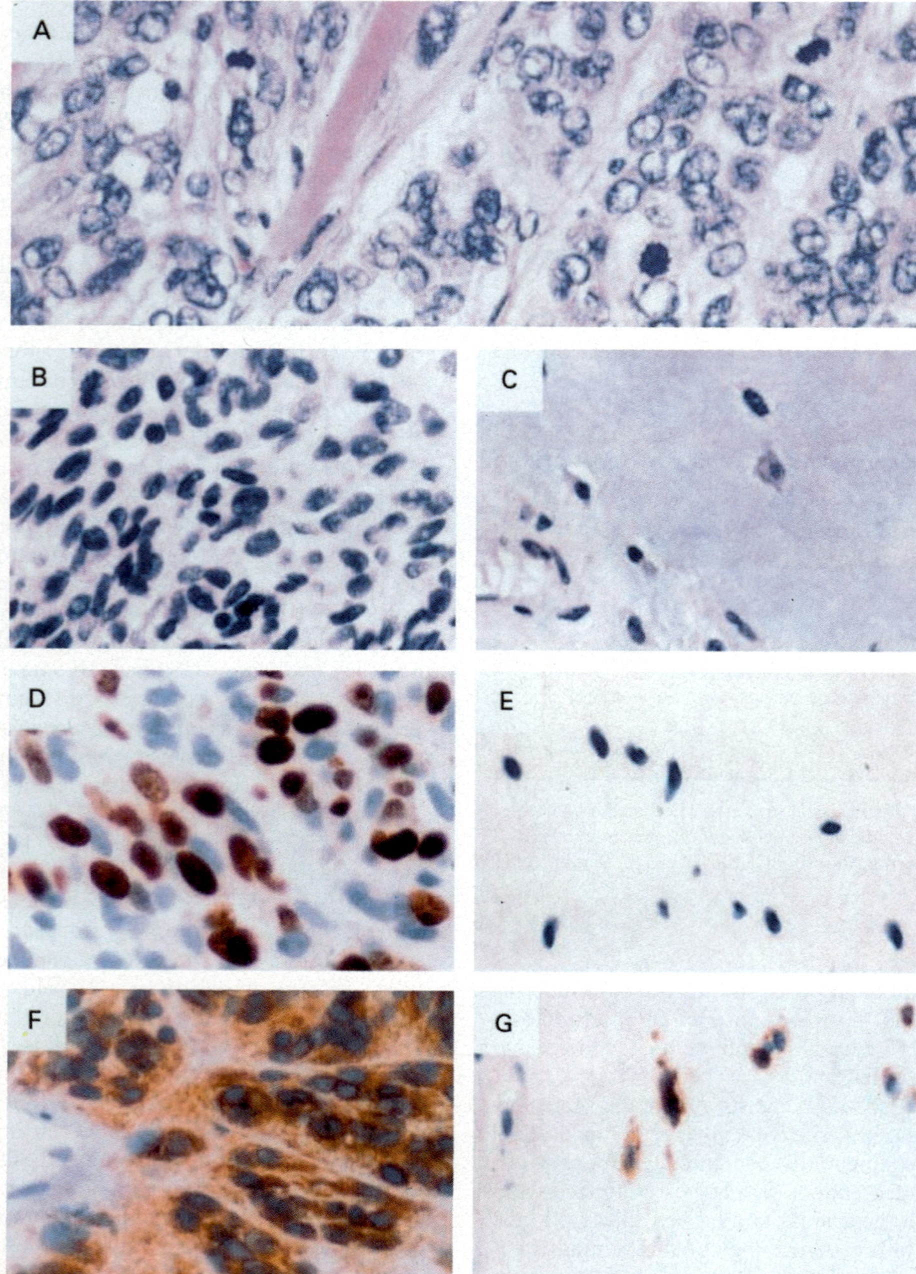

Figure 111-16 Histologic appearance a primary gastrointestinal stromal tumor in hematoxylin and eosin (**A**, **B**, and **C**) and immunostaining for Ki-67 (**D** and **E**) and CD117 (**F** and **G**). In 1996, frequent mitotic figures were present (**A**, ×400). In 2000, a pretreatment biopsy specimen from a cellular liver metastasis (**B**, ×200) had a high frequency of Ki-67–positive nuclei (**D**, ×200) and staining for CD117 (**F**, ×200). After 3 weeks of imatinib treatment, histologic examination of the liver metastasis showed myxoid degeneration and a few pyknotic cells (**C**, ×200), no staining for Ki-67 (**E**, ×200), and only a few scattered CD117-positive cells (**G**, ×200). (From Joensuu H et al,[256] with permission.)

In the era of imatinib resistance, new agents are coming to the fore. The addition of mTOR inhibitor RAD001 was examined in imatinib-resistant patients, since RAD001, like rapamycin, blocks a step downstream from the c-kit molecule and could again inhibit an important pathway keeping the GIST cell alive. Early data are not particularly encouraging, but the study was in its early stages.[263] Better results to date have been observed with c-kit (and flt3 and VEGF receptor) inhibitor SU11248. SU11248 can only be taken intermittently owing to cumulative toxicity, typically mucositis, toxic epidermal necrolysis (deep-seated blister-like rash of the palms and soles), inanition, and thus presently is being investigated in a 4-week-on, 2-week-off daily schedule starting at 50 mg daily. Although the RECIST response rate is only ~10% in the imatinib refractory setting from early phase I/II data, a significant proportion of patients (~50%) are able to remain without progression of disease for more than 6 months, and often have some decrease in size of tumor lesions.[264] PET scan will often indicate inactivation of the tumor, but CT scan responses have been slow to develop in comparison to those seen with imatinib. A similar compound, AMG706, is under investigation in the imatinib refractor setting, as are other newer "targeted therapies."

DERMATOFIBROSARCOMA PROTUBERANS

DFSP is a nodular "protruberant" lesion arising from the dermis with characteristically slow but persistent growth over many years. Although histologically of low grade or borderline malignant potential, DFSP has a propensity for local recurrence after simple excision. Typical manifestations of DFSP are a red to purple lesion on the upper trunk, especially the shoulder and supraclavicular regions of the head and neck. Not infrequently, small satellite lesions are evident at the site of a prior excision or bordering a skin graft following an unsuccessful previous excision. Surgical resection with wide surgical margins or more conservative surgery (facilitating cosmesis) with adjuvant external beam RT results in extremely low recurrence rates. Adjuvant RT should be considered in cases of recurrence. Recurrent DFSP can be associated with secondary fibrosarcomatous histologic changes, thereby reinforcing the need to achieve primary tumor control as well as to optimize cosmesis. In rare instances, metastasis may result in association with fibrosarcomatous transformation.

Imunohistochemical staining for the CD34 antigen is a hallmark of DFSP. In addition, chromosomal translocation and gene fusion products (see Table 111-1) result in the expression of a COL1A1-PDGF-B fusion protein that is processed to mature PDGF-B, resulting in autocrine or paracrine interaction with the PDGF-B receptor on the cell surface of DFSP. Of importance, imatinib inhibits the PDGF tyrosine kinase receptor in the same way that it inhibits the BCR-ABL tyrosine kinase receptor of chronic myeloid leukemia and the c-*Kit* tyrosine kinase receptor of GISTs. Recent clinical data have shown substantial responses to imatinib in patients with metastatic DFSP.[265,266] This suggests the opportunity for targeted molecular therapies, particularly for metastatic or locally advanced DFSP.

RETROPERITONEAL SARCOMAS

RPSs comprise about 15% of soft tissue sarcomas. They present late and are located in regions where the administration of both surgery and RT is often compromised (eg, adjacent to the small bowel and liver). Consequently, the local control rates achieved with combined-modality treatment of extremity soft tissue sarcomas are not seen in RPS. In a series of 102 RPS patients treated at Princess Margaret Hospital, complete excision was achieved in only 45, gross disease remained in 29, and only a biopsy was possible in 28.[267] The overall locoregional relapse-free rates were 28% and 9% at 5 and 10 years, respectively. RT did not improve survival but appeared to significantly lengthen the time to locoregional relapse, especially with higher doses. Complete tumor

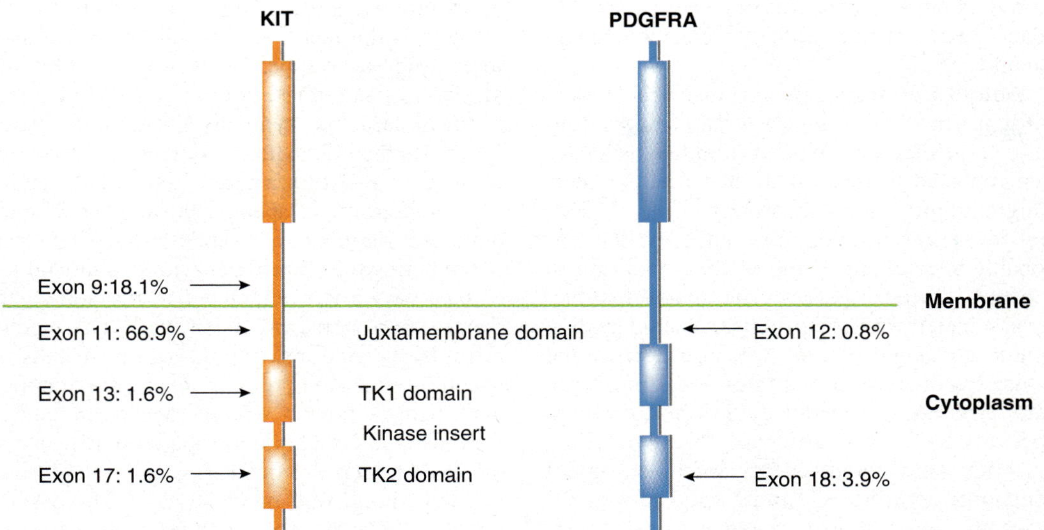

Figure 111-17 Mutation status of gastrointestinal stromal tumors and location on the c-kit or PDGFRA protein. From Heinrich et al.[261]

resection was the only significant prognostic variable for survival and locoregional and distant failure. These results are similar to those reported from MSKCC.[268] Patients with RPS should be evaluated in a multidisciplinary clinic prior to treatment so that patients can benefit from the expertise and investigational approaches available in such centers.

Pre- and Postoperative Radiotherapy Approaches A variety of adjuvant RT approaches have been used for RPS. One approach, evaluated in a prospective randomized trial, used an IORT boost (20 Gy) to the tumor bed followed by postoperative external beam (35–40 Gy); this approach was compared with conventional postoperative RT (50–55 Gy). In this study of 35 patients, the incidence of locoregional recurrence was lower in the experimental treatment arm, but no improvement in survival was demonstrated.[269] IORT was associated with a high rate of peripheral neuropathy when large, sometimes overlapping, RT portals were used to cover the sacral plexus region. However, gastrointestinal complications were more common in the control group, in whom higher doses were delivered to the bowel.

Other researchers have investigated strategies employing preoperative RT. Gieschen and colleagues from the Massachusetts General Hospital reported on 37 patients who underwent preoperative RT, resection, and then, when feasible, electron beam IORT.[270] The grossly complete resection rate was 83%, and the 5-year actuarial overall survival, disease-free survival, local control, and freedom from distant disease rates were 50%, 38%, 59%, and 54%, respectively. Earlier reports from the same group described a 70% complete resection rate and 81% 4-year local control rate.[271] The more recent report also indicates that complete resection and IORT improved overall survival and local control rates (74% and 83%, respectively) compared with no IORT (30% and 61%, respectively). However, the study was not randomized, and potentially more favorable and accessible lesions may have been chosen for IORT. More recently, Petersen and colleagues at the Mayo Clinic found improved local control, at least of primary tumors, using a similar treatment approach.[272]

Another recent report (this from the University of Toronto Sarcoma Group) described an unusually favorable outcome, especially for primary lesions, in a single-arm prospective trial of preoperative RT (median dose of 45 Gy in 25 fractions) plus postoperative BRT in selected cases.[273] Of interest, acute toxicity resulting from preoperative RT was differentiated prospectively from the effects of other treatments. Although the median radiation volume exceeded 7L, preoperative external beam RT was associated with extremely low gastrointestinal toxicity scores. Furthermore, no patient was hospitalized for acute toxicity, and there were no treatment interruptions or cessations of treatment because of acute toxicity. The remarkably low toxicity of the preoperative RT with enormous volumes has been attributed to the displacement of bowel outside the target volume. In contrast, the selective use of postoperative BRT was associated with toxicity, and there was little evidence that BRT contributed to the enhanced tumor outcome reported.[273]

The Mayo Clinic, Massachusetts General Hospital, and University of Toronto series using preoperative RT describe improved outcomes compared with the majority of other reports, especially for primary (as opposed to recurrent) RPS. Furthermore, much of the toxicity in the former two studies was attributed to the IORT rather than the preoperative external beam RT. Here again, however, we would caution against overinterpretation of results that could be explained by surgical technique at major referral centers or by case selection. Similarly, it remains unclear what contribution was provided by the BRT or IORT, which should probably remain protocol-based or be reserved for nonstandard use in selected cases.

The results of these three reports add credence to the advantages posited for preoperative RT in RPS: (1) the tumor bulk often displaces small bowel from the high-dose RT region, resulting in a safer and less toxic treatment; (2) bowel is unlikely to be fixed by surgical adhesions as when RT is given postoperatively, enabling safe delivery of a higher dose to the true area at risk; (3) optimum knowledge of the gross tumor location is possible, permitting better radiation targeting; (4) the tumor is contained by an intact peritoneal covering, providing a physical barrier to immediate tumor dissemination; (5) the risk of intraperitoneal tumor dissemination at the time of surgery may be reduced by the biologic impact of preoperative RT, and (6) using traditional principles of sarcoma RT, the radiation dose believed to be biologically effective is lower in the preoperative setting. Although RT planning for RPS can be complex, the use of conformal techniques or intensity modulation usually permits the RT dosage to be administered safely to the critical organ preoperatively. It is imperative that members of both the surgical and radiation oncology teams be present in the operating room when a significant amount of liver has been irradiated preoperatively to evaluate the planned residual liver volume. We cannot overemphasize that detailed evaluation of dosimetry and treatment planning films is needed to be certain that a sufficient volume of unirradiated liver is left unresected at the time of surgery.[114]

The only standard that exists at present for RPS treatment is that complete surgery should be performed wherever possible. The adjuvant RT approaches described above should be considered experimental and be the subject of further assessment. Recently, it was also suggested that a more scientifically sound approach to study design should be undertaken in RPS, particularly exploring the role of external beam RT through a randomized controlled trial.[274] An intergroup phase III trial of preoperative radiation plus surgery versus surgery alone is currently in the planning stages.

Chemoradiation Approaches Although chemotherapy alone has not been associated with obvious improvements in outcome of RPS, chemoradiation, as in other solid tumors, is a subject of interest as a treatment strategy for RPS. This is especially relevant in high-grade RPSs, which have a more adverse prognosis than the more common low-grade lesions.

Pilot studies using preoperative idoxuridine and doxorubicin plus external beam radiation have been reported, often in patients with extremely large tumors, with acceptable toxicity and with achievement of local control in patients in whom a negative-margin resection was possible.[190,275,276] These reports demonstrate that chemoradiation approaches are feasible. Additional phase II studies will be necessary to clarify response rates and toxicity profiles and determine whether chemoradiation should be tested in phase III trials. The Radiation Therapy Oncology Group is conducting a multicenter phase II trial (RTOG S0124) of preoperative doxorubicin and ifosfamide followed by preoperative RT and then by surgical resection with an intra- or postoperative radiation boost in patients with intermediate- and high-grade RPS. The study is anticipated to yield further information on feasibility and toxicities of combined modality treatment delivered in a multi-institutional setting.

ADDITIONAL ISSUES IN SOFT TISSUE SARCOMA MANAGEMENT

Functional Outcome and Morbidity of Treatment The functional result of extremity sarcoma management has become an important component of outcome assessment. Assessing the functional result is difficult, as it requires methods that are valid and reproducible. Many centers have yet to become experienced in the development and use of these methods, and much of the literature contains significant heterogeneity in patient samples.

Thus far, the variables associated with poorer functional outcome include large tumor size, higher doses and larger volumes of radiation, nerve sacrifice, postoperative fracture, and wound-healing complications.[142,277–279] To evaluate and compare functional outcome, it is imperative that functional data be reported consistently. Three disease-specific scoring scales have been reported as useful in assessing functional outcome.[280] This area has been discussed in detail by Davis, who observed that "function" has many meanings in the literature.[280] The concepts of impairment, disability, and handicap following extremity soft tissue sarcoma are likely misunderstood and certainly not used consistently. Davis noted that impairment is a disorder of structure or function whereas disability is a restriction or lack of ability to perform an activity. Handicap results from impairment and disability and prevents or restricts an individual from performing in a role that is normal for the individual. For sarcoma patients, impairments can be manifested as soft tissue fibrosis, loss of motion at a joint, and decreased muscle strength; disability can be manifested as limited mobility and difficulty performing routine self-care and activities of daily living; and handicap can be evident in limitation in family roles, social functioning, and the capacity for employment.

Impairments are the most frequently reported deficits following limb-preserving therapy for extremity soft tissue sarcoma, and up to 50% of patients appear to experience significant impairments.[280] Disability occurs less frequently, although reports are contradictory. It seems likely that many sarcoma patients learn to accommodate their impairments. Handicap has received little attention in the literature. However, the limited data suggest that up to 50% of patients may experience changes in their employment and vocation status after treatment of extremity soft tissue sarcomas.[280]

The future challenge in treating sarcomas is to define the therapeutic ratio for the patient with sarcoma of the extremity. Specifically, the aim of the multidisciplinary team will be to minimize the amount of treatment while maintaining or improving current standards of disease control to reduce treatment morbidity and enhance patient outcome.[280]

Wound Complications Considerable variability in reporting wound-healing complications exists in the literature. Wound complications have been reported in up to 40% of patients undergoing extremity sarcoma surgery.[129,281–283] Differences in the definition of wound complications probably account for some of the variability in reporting. The retrospective data suggest that factors associated with compromised wound healing include advanced patient age, poor nutritional status, lower extremity tumor location, large tumor size, and preoperative adjuvant treatment, especially RT.[284–287] Particularly high complication rates were noted recently with a protocol using preoperative RT and hyperthermia.[163] Although many authors have reported an association of wound complications with preoperative RT, reports of high rates of surgical complications without RT or chemotherapy also exist.[288] Most likely, these relate to the risk of major wound complications associated with extensive tumor resection, particularly in the lower extremities. The use of vascularized tissue transfers to replace resected tissues and optimize wound closure may decrease the risks of major wound complications and allow for more extensive limb-sparing surgical approaches.[284,289,290] As noted earlier, the SR2 trial results have confirmed the adverse effect of preoperative RT on wound healing in a prospective manner, but did not resolve the contribution of tissue transfer for wound reconstruction as its use was determined on an individual basis at the surgeon's discretion.[138]

Molecularly and Pathobiologically Based Sarcoma Management Management of sarcomas is increasingly being driven by the specific nature of the disease entity, most importantly the pathophysiologic subtype. The work of Pasteur and Koch was fundamental for the recognition and definition of pathogenic microbes; similarly, many laboratories today are identifying molecular and cellular lesions that will redefine the field of sarcoma research. An example of this work is in the recognition of the Ewing's sarcoma/PNET family of tumors as extraosseous soft tissue sarcomas rather than sarcomas of bone. These tumors should be treated with curative intent using an aggressive multimodality approach that begins with multiagent chemotherapy. If primary surgery has removed measurable disease, adjuvant chemotherapy is definitely indicated, with consideration of adjuvant RT if surgical margins were suboptimal. By adopting similar strategies for PNETs and Askin's tumors as for conventional Ewing's sarcomas, outcomes have improved.[205,291] The molecular similarities between tumors of this family have led to the current convention of considering them morphologic and clinicopathologic variants of the same underlying molecular disease process.[89,292]

Molecular diagnostics are also becoming very relevant in synovial sarcomas. Synovial sarcomas have been identified in most series as a very chemotherapy responsive subset of sarcomas.[179,196] Of note is the fact that clinically relevant histologic differences appear to exist even within this subclass of sarcomas, with poorly differentiated synovial sarcomas typically having a far worse prognosis than do synovial sarcomas that exhibit a more well-differentiated histologic profile. Most important, the specific chromosomal breakpoint and rearrangement appear to be important in predicting the clinical behavior of synovial sarcomas, with a rearrangement in the *SSX1* gene conveying a worse prognosis.[87,293] The mechanisms by which translocations transform cells via the chimeric fusion proteins are an area of important scientific inquiry with therapeutic potential.

Finally, the multiple histopathologic subtypes of liposarcomas are becoming increasingly well researched and well understood.[294] Myxoid and round-cell liposarcomas exhibit a characteristic chromosomal rearrangement T(12;16) (q13;p11). These liposarcomas tend to be quite sensitive to doxorubicin-based chemotherapy. Well-differentiated liposarcomas exhibit ring and giant marker chromosomes on cytogenetic analysis, and these karyotypic abnormalities carry through even in de-differentiated liposarcomas, which arise from well-differentiated liposarcomas. Targeting the PPAR-γ nuclear receptor is a particularly promising therapeutic strategy to force the differentiation of sarcoma cells and to decrease the proliferative thrust.[295] Initial proof-of-concept data have been published in a clinical trial using this strategy, and larger randomized trials are planned to assess the clinical worth of this approach.[296]

SUMMARY

It is clear that soft tissue sarcoma management has come a long way in a short time. In less than three decades, the standard of care has shifted toward coordinated multimodality care in specialty centers, with increased rates of function-sparing surgery and better outcomes for patients. Judicious use of aggressive multimodality approaches shows promise to decrease relapse rates and improve survival rates. New scientific approaches are furthering the fundamental understanding of these unusual diseases and providing novel approaches for diagnostic techniques, which will banish the vagaries and lack of consistency that have plagued this field of clinical investigation. Already new therapeutic initiatives are attacking the basic mechanisms of sarcomatous transformation of cells in some subtypes of soft tissue sarcoma, and it is hoped that these initiatives will improve outcomes for patients with less morbidity than current treatments entail. Large collaborative studies will further this work tremendously.

REFERENCES

1. Landis SH, Murray T, Bolden S, Wingo PA. Cancer statistics, 1999. CA: Cancer J Clin 1999;49:8–31.
2. Li FP, Fraumeni JF Jr. Soft-tissue sarcomas, breast cancer, and other neoplasms. A familial syndrome? Ann Intern Med 1969;71:747–52.
3. Li FP. Keynote lecture. The familial syndrome of sarcomas and other neoplasms. Princess Takamatsu Symp 1987;18:243–9.

4. Malkin D, Li FP, Strong LC, et al. Germline p53 mutations in a familial syndrome of breast cancer, sarcomas, and other neoplasms. Science 1990;250:1233–8.
5. Varley JM, Evans DG, Birch JM. Li-Fraumeni syndrome—a molecular and clinical review. Br J Cancer 1997;76:1–14.
6. Sorensen SA, Mulvihill JJ, Nielsen A. Long-term follow-up of von Recklinghausen neurofibromatosis. Survival and malignant neoplasms. N Engl J Med 1986;314:1010–5.
7. Barker D, Wright E, Nguyen K, et al. Gene for von Recklinghausen neurofibromatosis is in the pericentromeric region of chromosome 17. Science 1987;236:1100–2.
8. Fountain JW, Wallace MR, Bruce MA, et al. Physical mapping of a translocation breakpoint in neurofibromatosis. Science 1989;244:1085–7.
9. Menon AG, Anderson KM, Riccardi VM, et al. Chromosome 17p deletions and p53 gene mutations associated with the formation of malignant neurofibrosarcomas in von Recklinghausen neurofibromatosis. Proc Natl Acad Sci U S A 1990;87:5435–9.
10. Pollack IF, Mulvihill JJ. Neurofibromatosis 1 and 2. Brain Pathol 1997;7:823–36.
11. Cavenee WK, Hansen MF, Nordenskjold M, et al. Genetic origin of mutations predisposing to retinoblastoma. Science 1985;228:501–3.
12. Tucker MA, DAngio GJ, Boice JD Jr, et al. Bone sarcomas linked to radiotherapy and chemotherapy in children. N Engl J Med 1987;317:588–93.
13. Hansen MF, Koufos A, Gallie BL, et al. Osteosarcoma and retinoblastoma: a shared chromosomal mechanism revealing recessive predisposition. Proc Natl Acad Sci U S A 1985;82:6216–20.
14. Draper GJ, Sanders BM, Kingston JE. Second primary neoplasms in patients with retinoblastoma. Br J Cancer 1986;53:661–71.
15. Lee EY, To H, Shew JY, et al. Inactivation of the retinoblastoma susceptibility gene in human breast cancers. Science 1988;241:218–21.
16. Cance WG, Brennan MF, Dudas ME, et al. Altered expression of the retinoblastoma gene product in human sarcomas. N Engl J Med 1990;323:1457–62.
17. Cahan WG, Woodward HQ, Higinbotham NL, et al. Sarcoma arising in irradiated bone: report of eleven cases. 1948. Cancer 1998;82:8–34.
18. Arlen M, Higinbotham NL, Huvos AG, et al. Radiation-induced sarcoma of bone. Cancer 1971;28:1087–99.
19. Feigen M. Should cancer survivors fear radiation-induced sarcomas? Sarcoma 1997;1:5–15.
20. Davidson TI, Westbury G, Harmer CL. Radiation-induced soft-tissue sarcoma. Br J Surg 1986;73:308–9.
21. Popper H, Thomas LB, Telles NC, et al. Development of hepatic angiosarcoma in man induced by vinyl chloride, thorotrast, and arsenic. Comparison with cases of unknown etiology. Am J Pathol 1978;92:349–69.
22. Creech JL Jr, Johnson MN. Angiosarcoma of liver in the manufacture of polyvinyl chloride. J Occup Med 1974;16:150–1.
23. Creech JL Jr, Makk L. Liver disease among polyvinyl chloride production workers. Ann N Y Acad Sci 1975;246:88–94.
24. Lloyd JW. Angiosarcoma of the liver in vinyl chloride/polyvinyl chloride workers. J Occup Med 1975;17:333–4.
25. Roth F. Arsen-Lieber Tumoren (Hemangioendothelioma). Krebsforschung 1957;61:468–70.
26. Roth F. The sequelae of chronic arsenic poisoning in Moselle vintners. German Med Mo 1957;2:172–5.
27. MacMahon HE, Murphy AS, Bates MI. Endothelial cell sarcoma of liver following Thorotrast injections. Am J Pathol 1947;23:585–7.
28. DaSilva-Horta J. Late lesions in man caused by colloidal thorium dioxide (Thorotrast). Arch Pathol 1956;62:403–7.
29. DaSilva-Horta J, Abbatt JD, DaMotta LC. Malignancy and other effects following the administration of Thorotrast. Lancet 1965;2:201–4.
30. Kang H, Enzinger FM, Breslin P, et al. Soft tissue sarcoma and military service in Vietnam: a case- control study. J Natl Cancer Inst 1987;79:693–9.
31. Stewart FW, Treves N. Lymphangiosarcoma in post mastectomy lymphedema: a report of six cases of elephantiasis chirurgica. Cancer 1948;1:64–81.
32. Woodward AH, Ivins JC, Soule EH. Lymphangiosarcoma arising in chronic lymphedematous extremities. Cancer 1972;30:562–72.
33. Brand KG. Foreign body induced sarcomas. In: Becker FF, editor. Cancer. New York: Plenum; 1975. p. 485–511.
34. Penn I. Sarcomas in organ allograft recipients. Transplantation 1995;60:1485–91.
35. Fletcher CD, Gustafson P, Rydholm A, et al. Clinicopathologic re-evaluation of 100 malignant fibrous histiocytomas: prognostic relevance of subclassification. J Clin Oncol 2001;19:3045–50.
36. Lawrence WJ, Donegan WL, Natarajan N, et al. Adult soft tissue sarcomas. A pattern of care survey of the American College of Surgeons. Ann Surg 1987;205:349–59.
37. Weiss SW, Sobin LH. Histologic typing of soft tissue tumors. In: Weiss SW, editor. Soft tissue sarcomas. Berlin: Springer-Verlag; 1994. p. 7–14.
38. Association of Directors of Anatomic and Surgical Pathology. Perspectives in pathology: recommendations for the reporting of soft tissue sarcomas. Hum Pathol 1999;30:3–7.
39. Fletcher CDM. The use of immunohistochemistry in the diagnosis of soft tissue tumours. Histopathology 1986;10:771–3.
40. Presant CA, Russell WO, Alexander RW, Fu YS. Soft-tissue and bone sarcoma histopathology peer review: the frequency of disagreement in diagnosis and the need for second pathology opinions. The Southeastern Cancer Study Group experience. J Clin Oncol 1986;4:1658–61.
41. Shiraki MJ, Enterline HT, Brooks JJ, et al. Pathologic analysis of advanced adult soft tissue sarcomas, bone sarcomas, and mesotheliomas. The Eastern Cooperative Oncology Group (ECOG) experience. Cancer 64:484–90.
42. Fong Y, Coit DG, Woodruff JM, Brennan MF. Lymph node metastasis from soft tissue sarcoma in adults. Analysis of data from a prospective database of 1772 sarcoma patients. Ann Surg 1993;217:72–7.
43. Weingrad DN, Rosenberg SA. Early lymphatic spread of osteogenic and soft-tissue sarcomas. Surgery 1978;84:231–40.
44. Pisters PWT, Leung DHY, Woodruff JM, et al. Analysis of prognostic factors in 1041 patients with localized soft tissue sarcomas of the extremities. J Clin Oncol 1996;14:1679–89.
45. Daugaard S. Current soft-tissue sarcoma classifications. Eur J Cancer 2004;40:543–8.
46. Coindre JM, Terrier P, Bui NB, et al. Prognostic factors in adult patients with locally controlled soft tissue sarcoma. A study of 546 patients from the French Federation of Cancer Centers Sarcoma Group. J Clin Oncol 1996;14:869–77.
47. Costa J, Wesley RA, Glatstein EJ, Rosenberg SA. The grading of soft tissue sarcomas. Results of a clinicohistopathologic correlation in a series of 163 cases. Cancer 1984;53:530–41.
48. Trojani M, Contesso G, Coindre JM, et al. Soft-tissue sarcomas of adults: study of pathological prognostic variables and definition of a histopathological grading system. Int J Cancer 1984;33:37–42.
49. Guillou L, Coindre JM, Bonichon F, et al. Comparative study of the National Cancer Institute and French Federation of Cancer Centers Sarcoma Group grading systems in a population of 410 adult patients with soft tissue sarcoma. J Clin Oncol 1997;15:350–62.
50. Chang AE, Matory YL, Dwyer AJ, et al. Magnetic resonance imaging versus computed tomography in the evaluation of soft tissue tumors of the extremities. Ann Surg 1987;205:340–8.
51. Hanna SL, Fletcher BD. MR imaging of malignant soft-tissue tumors. Magn Reson Imaging Clin N Am 1995;3:629–50.
52. Panicek DM, Gatsonis C, Rosenthal DI, et al. CT and MR imaging in the local staging of primary malignant musculoskeletal neoplasms: report of the Radiology Diagnostic Oncology Group. Radiology 1997;202:237–46.
53. Austin-Seymour M, Chen GT, Rosenman J, et al. Tumor and target delineation: current research and future challenges. Int J Radiat Oncol Biol Phys 1995;33:1041–52.
54. Kessler ML, Pitluck S, Petti P, Castro JR. Integration of multimodality imaging data for radiotherapy treatment planning. Int J Radiat Oncol Biol Phys 1991;21:1653–67.
55. Fleming JB, Holtz D, Cantor SB, et al. The utility and cost-effectiveness of computerized tomography (CT) to screen for pulmonary metastases in patients presenting with T1 extremity soft tissue sarcomas (STS). Proc Am Soc Clin Oncol 1998;17:1989.
56. Porter GA, Cantor SB, Ahmad SA, et al. Cost-effectiveness of staging computed tomography of the chest in patients with T2 soft tissue sarcomas. Cancer 2002;94:197–204.
57. Fleming JB, Cantor SB, Varma DG, et al. Utility of chest computed tomography for staging in patients with T1 extremity soft tissue sarcomas. Cancer 2001;92:863–8.
58. Heslin MJ, Lewis JJ, Woodruff JM, Brennan MF. Core needle biopsy for diagnosis of extremity soft tissue sarcoma. Ann Surg Oncol 1997;4:425–31.
59. Ball AB, Fisher C, Pittam M, et al. Diagnosis of soft tissue tumours by Tru-Cut biopsy. Br J Surg 1990;77:756–8.
60. Skrzynski MC, Biermann JS, Montag AG, Simon MA. Diagnostic accuracy and charge-savings of outpatient core needle biopsy compared with open biopsy of musculoskeletal tumors. J Bone Joint Surg Am 1996;78:644–9.
61. Schwartz HS, Spengler DM. Needle tract recurrences after closed biopsy for sarcoma: three cases and review of the literature. Ann Surg Oncol 1997;4:228–36.
62. Akerman M. Fine-needle aspiration cytology of soft tissue sarcoma: benefits and limitations. Sarcoma; 1998;2:155–61.
63. Akerman M, Idvall I, Rydholm A. Cytodiagnosis of soft tissue tumors and tumor-like conditions by means of fine needle aspiration biopsy. Arch Orthop Trauma Surg 1980;96:61–7.
64. Kissin MW, Fisher C, Webb AJ, Westbury G. Value of fine needle aspiration cytology in the diagnosis of soft tissue tumours: a preliminary study on the excised specimen. Br J Surg 1987;74:479–80.
65. Layfield LJ, Anders KH, Glasgow BJ, Mirra JM. Fine-needle aspiration of primary soft-tissue lesions. Arch Pathol Lab Med 1986;110:420–4.
66. Soft tissue sarcoma. In: Greene F, Page D, Fleming ID, et al, editors. American joint committee on cancer (AJCC) staging manual. New York: Springer-Verlag; 2006. p. 193–200.
67. Kattan MW, Leung DH, Brennan MF. Postoperative nomogram for 12-year sarcoma-specific death. J Clin Oncol 2002;20:791–6.
68. Stojadinovic A, Yeh A, Brennan MF. Completely resected recurrent soft tissue sarcoma: primary anatomic site governs outcomes. J Am Coll Surg 2002;194:436–47.
69. Gaynor JJ, Tan CC, Casper ES, et al. Refinement of clinicopathologic staging for localized soft tissue sarcoma of the extremity: a study of 423 adults. J Clin Oncol 1992;10:1317–29.
70. Markhede G, Angervall L, Stener B. A multivariate analysis of the prognosis after surgical treatment of malignant soft-tissue tumors. Cancer 1982;49:1721–33.
71. Sears HF, Hopson R, Inouye W, et al. Analysis of staging and management of patients with sarcoma: a ten-year experience. Ann Surg 1980;191:488–93.
72. Rydholm A, Berg NO, Gullberg B, et al. Prognosis for soft-tissue sarcoma in the locomotor system. A retrospective population-based follow-up study of 237 patients. Acta Pathol Microbiol Immunol Scand [A] 1984;92:375–86.
73. Heise HW, Myers MH, Russell WO, et al. Recurrence-free survival time for surgically treated soft tissue sarcoma patients. Multivariate analysis of five prognostic factors. Cancer 1986;57:172–7.
74. Rooser B, Attewell R, Berg NO, Rydholm A. Survival in soft tissue sarcoma. Prognostic variables identified by multivariate analysis. Acta Orthop Scand 1987;58:516–22.
75. Collin CF, Godbold J, Hajdu SI, Brennan MF. Localized extremity soft tissue sarcoma: an analysis of factors affecting survival. J Clin Oncol 1987;5:601–12.
76. Tsujimoto M, Aozasa K, Ueda T, et al. Multivariate analysis for histologic prognostic factors in soft tissue sarcomas. Cancer 1998;62:994–8.
77. Ueda T, Aozasa K, Tsujimoto M, et al. Multivariate analysis for clinical prognostic factors in 163 patients. Cancer 1988;62:1444–50.
78. Rooser B, Attewell R, Berg NO, Rydholm A. Prognostication in soft tissue sarcoma. A model with four risk factors. Cancer 1988;61:817–23.
79. Mandard AM, Petiot JF, Marnay J, et al. Prognostic factors in soft tissue sarcomas. A multivariate analysis of 109 cases. Cancer 1989;63:1437–51.
80. Bell RS, O'Sullivan B, Liu FF, et al. The surgical margin in soft-tissue sarcoma. J Bone Joint Surg Am 1989;71:370–5.
81. Emrich LJ, Ruka W, Driscoll DL, Karakousis CP. The effect of local recurrence on survival time in adult high-grade soft tissue sarcomas. J Clin Epidemiol 1989;42:105–10.
82. Stotter AT, A'Hern RP, Fisher C, et al. The influence of local recurrence of extremity soft tissue sarcoma on metastasis and survival. Cancer 1990;65:1119–29.
83. Alvegard TA, Berg NO, Baldetorp B, et al. Cellular DNA content and prognosis of high-grade soft tissue sarcoma: the Scandinavian Sarcoma Group experience. J Clin Oncol 1990;8:538–47.
84. Gerrand CH, Wunder JS, Kandel RA, et al. Classification of positive margins after resection of soft-tissue sarcoma of the limb predicts the risk of local recurrence. J Bone Joint Surg Br 2001;83:1149–55.
85. Heslin MJ, Cordon-Cardo C, Lewis JJ, et al. Ki-67 detected by MIB-1 predicts distant metastasis and tumor mortality in primary, high grade extremity soft tissue sarcoma. Cancer 1998;83:490–7.
86. Karpeh MS, Brennan MF, Cance WG, et al. Altered patterns of retinoblastoma gene product expression in adult soft-tissue sarcomas. Br J Cancer 1995;72:986–91.

87. Kawai A, Woodruff JM, Healey JH, et al. SYT-SSX gene fusion as a determinant of morphology and prognosis in synovial sarcoma. N Engl J Med 1998;338:153–60.
88. Zoubek A, Dockhorn-Dworniczak B, Delattre O, et al. Does expression of different EWS chimeric transcripts define clinically distinct risk groups of Ewing tumor patients? J Clin Oncol 1996;14:1245–51.
89. de Alava E, Kawai A, Healey JH, et al. EWS-FLII fusion transcript structure is an independent determinant of prognosis in Ewing's sarcoma. J Clin Oncol 1998;16:1248–55.
90. Guillou L, Benhattar J, Bonichon F, et al. Histologic grade, but not SYT-SSX fusion type, is an important prognostic factor in patients with synovial sarcoma: a multicenter, retrospective analysis. J Clin Oncol 2004;22:4040–50.
91. Pisters PW, Pollock RE. Staging and prognostic factors in soft tissue sarcoma. Semin Radiat Oncol 1999;9:307–14.
92. Pisters PWT, Brennan MF. Sarcomas of soft tissue. In: Abeloff M, Armitage J, Lichter A, Niederhuber J, editors. Clinical oncology. New York: Churchill Livingstone; 2000. p. 2273–313.
93. Gerdes J. Ki-67 and other proliferation markers useful for immunohistological diagnostic and prognostic evaluations in human malignancies. Semin Cancer Biol 1:199–206.
94. Drobnjak M, Latres E, Pollack D, et al. Prognostic implications of p53 nuclear overexpression and high proliferation index of Ki-67 in adult soft-tissue sarcomas. J Natl Cancer Inst 1994;86:549–54.
95. Yang P, Hirose T, Hasegawa T, et al. Prognostic implication of the p53 protein and Ki-67 antigen immunohistochemistry in malignant fibrous histiocytoma. Cancer 1995;76:618–25.
96. Levine EA, Holzmayer T, Bacus S, et al. Evaluation of newer prognostic markers for adult soft tissue sarcomas. J Clin Oncol 1997;15:3249–57.
97. Rudolph P, Kellner U, Chassevent A, et al. Prognostic relevance of a novel proliferation marker, ki-s11, for soft-tissue sarcoma. a multivariate study. Am J Pathol 1997;150:1997–2007.
98. Williard WC, Collin CF, Casper ES, et al. The changing role of amputation for soft tissue sarcoma of the extremity in adults. Surg Gynecol Obstet 1992;175:389–96.
99. Williard WC, Hajdu SI, Casper ES, Brennan MF. Comparison of amputation with limb-sparing operations for adult soft tissue sarcoma of the extremity. Ann Surg 1992;215:269–75.
100. Yang JC, Rosenberg SA. Surgery for adult patients with soft tissue sarcomas. Semin Oncol 1989;16:289–96.
101. Brennan MF, Casper ES, Harrison LB, et al. The role of multimodality therapy in soft-tissue sarcoma. Ann Surg 1991;214:328–37.
102. Rosenberg SA, Tepper JE, Glatstein EJ, et al. The treatment of soft-tissue sarcomas of the extremities: prospective randomized evaluations of (1) limb-sparing surgery plus radiation therapy compared with amputation and (2) the role of adjuvant chemotherapy. Ann Surg 1982;196:305–15.
103. Bowden L, Booher RJ. The principles and techniques of resection of soft parts for sarcomas. Surgery 1958;44:963–77.
104. Cantin J, McNeer GP, Chu FC, Booher RJ. The problem of local recurrence after treatment of soft tissue sarcoma. Ann Surg 1968;168:47–53.
105. Gerner RE, Moore GE, Pickren JW. Soft tissue sarcomas. Ann Surg 1975;181:803–8.
106. Pisters PW, Harrison LB, Leung DH, et al. Long-term results of a prospective randomized trial of adjuvant brachytherapy in soft tissue sarcoma. J Clin Oncol 1996;14:859–68.
107. Yang JC, Chang AE, Baker AR, et al. A randomized prospective study of the benefit of adjuvant radiation therapy in the treatment of soft tissue sarcomas of the extremity. J Clin Oncol 1998;16:197–203.
108. Karakousis CP, Proimakis C, Walsh DL. Primary soft tissue sarcoma of the extremities in adults. Br J Surg 1995;82:1208–12.
109. Karakousis CP. Surgery for soft tissue sarcomas. In: Bland KI, Karakousis CP, Copeland EM, editors. Atlas of surgical oncology. Philadelphia: WB Saunders; 1995. p. 283–400.
110. Behranwala KA, A'Hern R, Omar AM, Thomas JM. Prognosis of lymph node metastasis in soft tissue sarcoma. Ann Surg Oncol 2004;11:714–9.
111. Riad S, Griffin AM, Liberman B, et al. Lymph node metastasis in soft tissue sarcoma in an extremity. Clin Orthop Relat Res 2004;426:129–34.
112. Ruka W, Taghian A, Gioioso D, et al. Comparison between the in vitro intrinsic radiation sensitivity of human soft tissue sarcoma and breast cancer cell lines. J Surg Oncol 1996;61:290–4.
113. Weichselbaum RR, Beckett MA, Simon MA, et al. In vitro radiobiological parameters of human sarcoma cell lines. Int J Radiat Oncol Biol Phys 1988;15:937–42.
114. O'Sullivan B, Wylie J, Catton C, et al. The local management of soft tissue sarcoma. Semin Radiat Oncol 1999;9:328–48.
115. Le Vay J, O'Sullivan B, Catton C, et al. An assessment of prognostic factors in soft-tissue sarcoma of the head and neck. Arch Otolaryngol Head Neck Surg 1994;120:981–6.
116. McGowan TS, Cummings BJ, O'Sullivan B, et al. An analysis of 78 breast sarcoma patients without distant metastases at presentation. Int J Radiat Oncol Biol Phys 2000;46:383–90.
117. Fraass BA, Kessler ML, McShan DL, et al. Optimization and clinical use of multisegment intensity-modulated radiation therapy for high-dose conformal therapy. Semin Radiat Oncol 1999;9:60–77.
118. Boyer AL, Yu CX. Intensity-modulated radiation therapy with dynamic multileaf collimators. Semin Radiat Oncol 1999;9:48–59.
119. Hong L, Alektiar K, Chui C, et al. IMRT of large fields: whole-abdomen irradiation. Int J Radiat Oncol Biol Phys 2002;54:278–89.
120. Burman C, Kutcher GJ, Emami B, Goitein M. Fitting of normal tissue tolerance data to an analytic function. Int J Radiat Oncol Biol Phys 1991;21:123–35.
121. Kutcher GJ, Burman C, Brewster L, et al. Histogram reduction method for calculating complication probabilities for three-dimensional treatment planning evaluations. Int J Radiat Oncol Biol Phys 1991;21:137–146.
122. O'Sullivan B, Ward I, Haycocks T, Sharpe M. Techniques to modulate radiotherapy toxicity and outcome in soft tissue sarcoma. Curr Treat Options Oncol 2003;4:453–64.
123. Ward I, Haycocks T, Sharpe M, et al. Volume-based radiotherapy targeting in soft tissue sarcoma. In: Verweij J, Pinedo R, editors. Targeted treatment of soft tissue sarcoma. Norwell: Kluwer Academic Publishers; 2004. p. 17–42.
124. Lawrence TS, Ten Haken RK, Kessler ML, et al. The use of 3-D dose volume analysis to predict radiation hepatitis. Int J Radiat Oncol Biol Phys 1992;23:781–8.
125. Suit H, Spiro I. Preoperative radiation therapy for patients with sarcoma of the soft tissues. Cancer Treat Res 1993;67:99–105.
126. Wilson AN, Davis A, Bell RS, et al. Local control of soft tissue sarcoma of the extremity: the experience of a multidisciplinary sarcoma group with definitive surgery and radiotherapy. Eur J Cancer 1994;30A:746–751.
127. Pollack A, Zagars GK, Goswitz MS, et al. Preoperative vs. postoperative radiotherapy in the treatment of soft tissue sarcomas: a matter of presentation. Int J Radiat Oncol Biol Phys 1998;42:563–72.
128. Suit HD, Spiro I. Role of radiation in the management of adult patients with sarcoma of soft tissue. Semin Surg Oncol 1994;10:347–56.
129. Brant TA, Parsons JT, Marcus RB Jr, et al. Preoperative irradiation for soft tissue sarcomas of the trunk and extremities in adults. Int J Radiat Oncol Biol Phys 1990;19:899–906.
130. Robinson MH, Spruce L, Eeles R, et al. Limb function following conservation treatment of adult soft tissue sarcoma. Eur J Cancer 1991;27:1567–74.
131. Ashby MA, Ago CT, Harmer CL. Hypofractionated radiotherapy for sarcomas. Int J Radiat Oncol Biol Phys 1986;12:13–7.
132. Le Pechoux C, Le Deley MC, Delaloge S, et al. Postoperative radiotherapy in the management of adult soft tissue sarcoma of the extremities: results with two different total dose, fractionation, and overall treatment time schedules. Int J Radiat Oncol Biol Phys 1999;44:879–86.
133. International Commission on Radiation Units and Measurements. Prescribing, recording, and reporting photon beam therapy. 1993;50:1–72.
134. Sadoski C, Suit HD, Rosenberg AE, et al. Preoperative radiation, surgical margins, and local control of extremity sarcomas of soft tissues. J Surg Oncol 1993;52:223–230.
135. Tanabe KK, Pollock RE, Ellis LM, et al. Influence of surgical margins on outcome in patients with preoperatively irradiated extremity soft tissue sarcomas. Cancer 1994;73:1652–9.
136. Panicek DM, Schwartz LH. Soft tissue edema around musculoskeletal sarcomas at magnetic resonance imaging. Sarcoma 1997;1:189–91.
137. Manaster BJ. Musculoskeletal oncologic imaging. Int J Radiat Oncol Biol Phys 1991;21:1643–51.
138. O'Sullivan B, Davis AM, Turcotte R, et al. Preoperative versus postoperative radiotherapy in soft-tissue sarcoma of the limbs: a randomized trial. Lancet 2002;359:2235–41.
139. Tyldesley S, Fryer K, Minchinton A, Durand R. Effects of debulking surgery on radiosensitivity, oxygen tension and kinetics in a mouse tumour model. Clin Invest Med 1997;20 Suppl 4:S83.
140. Suit HD, Mankin HJ, Wood W, Proppe KH. Preoperative, intraoperative, and postoperative radiation in the treatment of primary soft tissue sarcoma. Cancer 1985;55:2659–67.
141. Nielsen OS, Cummings B, O'Sullivan B, et al. Preoperative and postoperative irradiation of soft tissue sarcomas: effect of radiation field size. Int J Radiat Oncol Biol Phys 1991;21:1595–9.
142. Stinson SF, Delaney TF, Greenberg J, et al. Acute and long-term effects on limb function of combined modality limb sparing therapy for extremity soft tissue sarcoma. Int J Radiat Oncol Biol Phys 1991;21:1493–9.
143. Suit HD, Mankin HJ, Wood WC, et al. Treatment of the patient with stage M0 soft tissue sarcoma. J Clin Oncol 1988;6:854–62.
144. Robinson MH, Keus RB, Shasha D, Harrison LB. Is preoperative radiotherapy superior to postoperative radiotherapy in the treatment of soft tissue sarcoma? Eur J Cancer 1998;34:1309–16.
145. Wayne JD, Langstein H, Pollack A, et al. Preoperative radiotherapy for extremity soft tissue sarcoma (STS): site-specific wound complication rates and the impact of reconstructive surgery. Proc Am Soc Clin Oncol 2000;19:558a.
146. Davis AM, O'Sullivan B, Turcotte R, et al. Late radiation morbidity following randomization to preoperative versus postoperative radiotherapy in extremity soft tissue sarcoma. Radiother Oncol 2005;75:48–53.
147. O'Sullivan B, Davis A. A randomized phase III trial of preoperative compared to postoperative radiotherapy in extremity soft tissue sarcoma. Proc ASTRO 2001;51:151.
148. O'Sullivan B, Davis A, Turcotte R, et al. Five-year results of a randomized phase III trial of pre-operative vs post-operative radiotherapy in extremity soft tissue sarcoma. Proc Am Soc Clin Oncol 2004;23:815.
149. Janjan NA, Yasko AW, Reece GP, et al. Comparison of charges related to radiotherapy for soft tissue sarcomas treated by preoperative external beam irradiation versus interstitial implantation. Ann Surg Oncol 1994;1:415–22.
150. Catton CN, Davis A, Bell RS, et al. Soft tissue sarcoma of the extremity. Limb salvage after failure of combined conservative therapy. Radiother Oncol 1996;41:209–14.
151. Catton C, Swallow C, O'Sullivan B. A pilot study of external beam radiotherapy and pulsed dose rate brachytherapy for resectable retroperitoneal sarcomas [abstract]. Radiother Oncol 1998;47 Suppl 1:S30.
152. Catton CN, Swallow CJ, O'Sullivan B. Approaches to local salvage of soft tissue sarcoma after primary site failure. Semin Radiat Oncol 1999;9:378–88.
153. Pearlstone D, Janjan NA, Feig BW, et al. Re-resection with brachytherapy for locally recurrent soft tissue sarcoma arising in a previously radiated field. Cancer J Sci Am 1999;5:26–33.
154. Pisters PWT, Harrison LB, Woodruff JM, et al. A prospective randomized trial of adjuvant brachytherapy in the management of low grade soft tissue sarcomas of the extremity and superficial trunk. J Clin Oncol 1994;12:1150–5.
155. Dubois JB, Debrigode C, Hay M, et al. Intra-operative radiotherapy in soft tissue sarcomas. Radiother Oncol 1995;34:160–3.
156. Haddock MG, Petersen IA, Pritchard D, Gunderson LL. IORT in the management of extremity and limb girdle soft tissue sarcomas. Front Radiat Ther Oncol 1997;31:151–2.
157. Isacsson U, Hagberg H, Johansson KA, et al. Potential advantages of protons over conventional radiation beams for paraspinal tumours. Radiother Oncol 1997;45:63–70.
158. Suit H. The Gray Lecture 2001: coming technical advances in radiation oncology. Int J Radiat Oncol Biol Phys 2002;53:798–809.
159. Prott FJ, Micke O, Haverkamp U, et al. Treatment results of fast neutron irradiation in soft tissue sarcomas. Strahlenther Onkol 1999;175 Suppl 2:76–78.
160. Schonekaes KG, Prott FJ, Micke O, et al. Radiotherapy on adult patients with soft tissue sarcoma with fast neutrons or photons. Anticancer Res 1999;19:2355–9.
161. Pickering DG, Stewart JS, Rampling R, et al. Fast neutron therapy for soft tissue sarcoma. Int J Radiat Oncol Biol Phys 1987;13:1489–95.
162. Brizel DM, Scully SP, Harrelson JM, et al. Radiation therapy and hyperthermia improve the oxygenation of human soft tissue sarcomas. Cancer Res 1996;56:5347–50.

163. Prosnitz LR, Maguire P, Anderson JM, et al. The treatment of high-grade soft tissue sarcomas with preoperative thermoradiotherapy. Int J Radiat Oncol Biol Phys 1999;45:941–9.
164. Souhami RL, Craft AW, Van der Eijken JW, et al. Randomised trial of two regimens of chemotherapy in operable osteosarcoma: a study of the European Osteosarcoma Intergroup. Lancet 1997;350:911–7.
165. Grier HE, Krailo MD, Tarbell NJ, et al. Addition of ifosfamide and etoposide to standard chemotherapy for Ewing's sarcoma and primitive neuroectodermal tumor of bone. N Engl J Med 2003;348:694–701.
166. Crist WM, Anderson JR, Meza JL, et al. Intergroup rhabdomyosarcoma study-IV: results for patients with nonmetastatic disease. J Clin Oncol 2001;19:3091–102.
167. Bramwell VH. Adjuvant chemotherapy for adult soft tissue sarcoma: is there a standard of care? J Clin Oncol 2001;19:1235–7.
168. Wang JJ, Cortes E, Sinks LF, Holland JF. Therapeutic effect and toxicity of Adriamycin in patients with neoplastic disease. Cancer 1971;28:837–43.
169. Benjamin RS, Wiernik PH, Bachur NR. Adriamycin chemotherapy—efficacy, safety, and pharmacologic basis of an intermittent single high-dosage schedule. Cancer 1974;33:19–27.
170. Sarcoma Meta-analysis Collaboration. Adjuvant chemotherapy for localised resectable soft-tissue sarcoma of adults: meta-analysis of individual data. Lancet 1997;350:1647–54.
171. Verweij J, Seynaeve C. The reason for confining the use of adjuvant chemotherapy in soft tissue sarcoma to the investigational setting. Semin Radiat Oncol 1999;9:352–9.
172. Frustaci S, Gherlinzoni F, De Paoli A, et al. Adjuvant chemotherapy for adult soft tissue sarcomas of the extremities and girdles: results of the Italian randomized cooperative trial. J Clin Oncol 2001;19:1238–47.
173. Frustaci S, De Paoli A, Bidoli E, et al. Ifosfamide in the adjuvant therapy of soft tissue sarcomas. Oncology 2003;65 Suppl 2:80–4.
174. Brodowicz T, Schwameis E, Widder J, et al. Intensified adjuvant IFADIC chemotherapy for adult soft tissue sarcoma: a prospective randomized feasibility trial. Sarcoma 2000;4:151–60.
175. Gortzak E, Azzarelli A, Buesa J, et al. A randomized phase II study on neo-adjuvant chemotherapy for 'high-risk' adult soft-tissue sarcoma. Eur J Cancer 2001;37:1096–103.
176. Pisters PWT, Patel SR, Varma DGK, et al. Preoperative chemotherapy for stage IIIB extremity soft tissue sarcoma: long-term results from a single institution. J Clin Oncol 1997;15:3481–7.
177. Casper ES, Gaynor JJ, Harrison LB, et al. Preoperative and postoperative adjuvant combination chemotherapy for adults with high grade soft tissue sarcoma. Cancer 1994;73:1644–51.
178. O'Bryan RM, Baker LH, Gottlieb JE, et al. Dose response evaluation of Adriamycin in human neoplasia. Cancer 1997;39:1940–8.
179. Patel SR, Vadhan-Raj S, Papadopoulos NJ, et al. High-dose ifosfamide in bone and soft tissue sarcomas: results of phase II and pilot studies—dose-response and schedule dependence. J Clin Oncol 1997;15:2378–84.
180. Eilber FC, Rosen G, Forscher C, et al. Surgical resection and intraperitoneal chemotherapy for recurrent abdominal sarcomas. Ann Surg Oncol 1999;6:645–50.
181. Stehlin JS Jr, Giovanella BC, Gutierrez AE, et al. 15 years' experience with hyperthermic perfusion for treatment of soft tissue sarcoma and malignant melanoma of the extremities. Front Radiat Ther Oncol 1984;18:177–82.
182. Issels RD, Bosse D, Abdel-Rahman S, et al. Preoperative systemic etoposide/ifosfamide/doxorubicin chemotherapy combined with regional hyperthermia in high-risk sarcoma: a pilot study. Cancer Chemother Pharmacol 1993;31 Suppl 2:S233–7.
183. Wiedemann GJ, d'Oleire F, Knop E, et al. Ifosfamide and carboplatin combined with 41.8 degrees C whole-body hyperthermia in patients with refractory sarcoma and malignant teratoma. Cancer Res 1994;54:5346–50.
184. Wiedemann GJ, Robins HI, Gutsche S, et al. Ifosfamide, carboplatin and etoposide (ICE) combined with 41.8C whole body hyperthermia in patients with refractory sarcoma. Eur J Cancer 1996;32A:888–92.
185. Wiedemann GJ, Robins HI, Katschinski DM, et al. Systemic hyperthermia and ICE chemotherapy for sarcoma patients: rationale and clinical status. Anticancer Res 1997;17:2899–902.
186. Brauer LP, Prieshof B, Wiedemann GJ, et al. Whole-body hyperthermia combined with ifosfamide and carboplatin causes hypotension and nephrotoxicity. J Cancer Res Clin Oncol 1998;124:549–54.
187. Eilber FR, Giuliano AE, Huth JH, et al. Neoadjuvant chemotherapy, radiation, and limited surgery for high grade soft tissue sarcoma of the extremity. In: Ryan JR, Baker LO, editors. Recent concepts in sarcoma treatment. Dordrecht, The Netherlands: Kluwer Academic Publishers; 1988. p. 115–22.
188. Wanebo HJ, Temple WJ, Popp MB, et al. Preoperative regional therapy for extremity sarcoma. A tricenter update. Cancer 1995;75:2299–306.
189. Levine EA, Trippon M, DasGupta TK. Preoperative multimodality treatment for soft tissue sarcomas. Cancer 71:3685–9.
190. Eilber FR, Eckardt J, Rosen G, et al. Preoperative therapy for soft tissue sarcoma. Hematol Oncol Clin North Am 1995;9:817–23.
191. Eilber FR, Giuliano AE, Huth JF, et al. Intravenous (IV) vs. intraarterial (IA) Adriamycin, 2800 Gy radiation and surgical excision for extremity soft tissue sarcomas: a randomized prospective trial. Proc Am Soc Clin Oncol 1990;9:309.
192. Rhomberg W, Hassenstein EO, Gefeller D. Radiotherapy vs. radiotherapy and razoxane in the treatment of soft tissue sarcomas: final results of a randomized study. Int J Radiat Oncol Biol Phys 1996;36:1077–84.
193. Cormier JN, Patel SR, Herzog CE, et al. Concurrent ifosfamide-based chemotherapy and irradiation. Cancer 2001;92:1550–5.
194. Pisters PW, Ballo MT, Fenstermacher MJ, et al. Phase I trial of preoperative concurrent doxorubicin and radiation therapy, surgical resection, and intraoperative electron-beam radiation therapy for patients with localized retroperitoneal sarcoma. J Clin Oncol 2003;21:3092–7.
195. Pisters PW, Ballo MT, Bekele N, et al. Phase I trial using toxicity severity weights for dose finding of gemcitabine combined with radiation therapy and subsequent surgery for patients with extremity and trunk soft tissue sarcomas [abstract 9008]. ASCO Meeting 2004.
196. Rosen G, Forscher C, Lowenbraun S, et al. Synovial Sarcoma. Uniform response of metastases to high dose ifosfamide. Cancer 1994;73:2506–11.
197. Eilber FC, Eilber FR, Eckardt JJ, et al. Impact of ifosfamide-based chemotherapy on survival in patients with primary extremity synovial sarcoma [abstract 9017]. ASCO Meeting 2004.
198. Eilber FC, Eilber FR, Eckardt J, et al. The impact of chemotherapy on the survival of patients with high-grade primary extremity liposarcoma. Ann Surg 2004;240:686–95.
199. Grobmyer SR, Maki RG, Demetri GD, et al. Neo-adjuvant chemotherapy for primary high-grade extremity soft tissue sarcoma. Ann Oncol 2004;15:1667–72.
200. Cormier JN, Huang X, Xing Y, et al. Cohort analysis of patients with localized, high-risk, extremity soft tissue sarcoma treated at two cancer centers: chemotherapy-associated outcomes. J Clin Oncol 2004;22:4567–74.
201. Marina N, Gebhardt M, Teot L, Gorlick R. Biology and therapeutic advances for pediatric osteosarcoma. Oncologist 2004;9:422–41.
202. Bacci G, Picci P, Ferrari S, et al. Primary chemotherapy and delayed surgery for nonmetastatic osteosarcoma of the extremities. Results in 164 patients preoperatively treated with high doses of methotrexate followed by cisplatin and doxorubicin. Cancer 1993;72:3227–38.
203. Crist W, Gehan EA, Ragab AH, et al. The Third Intergroup Rhabdomyosarcoma Study. J Clin Oncol 1995;13:610–30.
204. Esnaola NF, Rubin BP, Baldini EH, et al. Response to chemotherapy and predictors of survival in adult rhabdomyosarcoma. Ann Surg 2001;234:215–23.
205. Baldini EH, Demetri GD, Fletcher CD, et al. Adults with Ewing's sarcoma/primitive neuroectodermal tumor: adverse effect of older age and primary extraosseous disease on outcome. Ann Surg 1999;230:79–86.
206. Eggermont AMM, Shraffordt Koops H, Lienard D, et al. Isolated limb perfusion with high-dose tumor necrosis factor-α in combination with interferon-v and melphalan for nonresectable extremity soft tissue sarcomas: a multicenter trial. J Clin Oncol 1996;14:2653–65.
207. Tepper JE, Suit HD. Radiation therapy alone for sarcoma of soft tissue. Cancer 1983;56:475–9.
208. Slater JD, McNeese MD, Peters LJ. Radiation therapy for unresectable soft tissue sarcomas. Int J Radiat Oncol Biol Phys 1986;12:1729–34.
209. Greiner RH, Blattmann HJ, Thum P, et al. Dynamic pion irradiation of unresectable soft tissue sarcomas. Int J Radiat Oncol Biol Phys 1989;17:1077–83.
210. Brennan MF. The surgeon as a leader in cancer care: lessons learned from the study of soft tissue sarcoma. J Am Coll Surg 1996;182:520–9.
211. Potter DA, Glenn J, Kinsella TJ, et al. Patterns of recurrence in patients with high-grade soft-tissue sarcomas. J Clin Oncol 1985;3:353–66.
212. Billingsley KG, Lewis JJ, Leung DHY, et al. Multifactorial analysis of the survival of patients with distant metastasis arising from primary extremity sarcoma. Cancer 1999;85:389–95.
213. Creagan ET, Fleming TR, Edmonson JH, Pairolero PC. Pulmonary resection for metastatic nonosteogenic sarcoma. Cancer 1979;44:1908–12.
214. Casson AG, Putnam JB Jr, Natarajan G, et al. Five-year survival after pulmonary metastasectomy for adult soft tissue sarcoma. Cancer 1992;69:662–8.
215. Gadd MA, Casper ES, Woodruff JM, et al. Development and treatment of pulmonary metastases in adult patients with extremity soft-tissue sarcoma. Ann Surg 1993;218:705–12.
216. Huth JF, Holmes EC, Vernon SE, et al. Pulmonary resection for metastatic sarcoma. Am J Surg 1980;140:9–16.
217. McCormack PM, Martini N. The changing role of surgery for pulmonary metastases. Ann Thorac Surg 1979;28:139–45.
218. Morrow CE, Vassilopoulos PP, Grage TB. Surgical resection for metastatic neoplasms of the lung: experience at the University of Minnesota Hospitals. Cancer 1980;45:2981–5.
219. Mountain CF, McMurtrey MJ, Hermes KE. Surgery for pulmonary metastasis: a 20-year experience. Ann Thorac Surg 1984;38:323–30.
220. Pastorino U, Valente M, Gasparini M, et al. Lung resection for metastatic sarcomas: total survival from primary treatment. J Surg Oncol 1989;4:275–80.
221. Rizzoni WE, Pass HI, Wesley MN, et al. Resection of recurrent pulmonary metastases in patients with soft-tissue sarcomas. Arch Surg 1986;121:1248–52.
222. van Geel AN, Pastorino U, Jauch KW, et al. Surgical treatment of lung metastases: the European Organization for Research and Treatment of Cancer—Soft Tissue and Bone Sarcoma Group study of 255 patients. Cancer 1996;77:675–82.
223. Putnam JB Jr, Roth JA, Wesley MN, et al. Analysis of prognostic factors in patients undergoing resection of pulmonary metastases from soft tissue sarcomas. J Thorac Cardiovasc Surg 1984;87:260–8.
224. Jablons D, Steinberg SM, Roth JA, et al. Metastasectomy for soft tissue sarcoma. Further evidence for efficacy and prognostic indicators. J Thorac Cardiovasc Surg 1989;97:695–705.
225. Roth JA, Putnam JB Jr, Wesley MN, Rosenberg SA. Differing determinants of prognosis following resection of pulmonary metastases from osteogenic and soft tissue sarcoma patients. Cancer 1985;55:1361–6.
226. Takita H, Edgerton F, Karakousis CP, et al. Surgical management of metastases to the lung. Surg Gynecol Obstet 1981;152:191–4.
227. Putnam JB Jr, Roth JA, Wesley MN, et al. Survival following aggressive resection of pulmonary metastases from osteogenic sarcoma: analysis of prognostic factors. Ann Thorac Surg 1983;36:516–23.
228. Regnard JF, Cerrina J, Silbert D. Curative surgical treatment of pulmonary metastases. 3rd European Conference on Clinical Oncology. Stolkholm, Sweden: 1985. p. 58.
229. Ramming KP. Surgery for pulmonary metastases. Surg Clin North Am 1980;60:815–24.
230. Joseph WL, Morton DL, Adkins PC. Prognostic significance of tumor doubling time in evaluating operability in pulmonary metastatic disease. J Thorac Cardiovasc Surg 1971;61:23–32.
231. Verazin GT, Warneke JA, Driscoll DL, et al. Resection of lung metastases from soft-tissue sarcomas. A multivariate analysis. Arch Surg 1992;127:1407–11.
232. Pogrebniak HW, Roth JA, Steinberg SM, et al. Reoperative pulmonary resection in patients with metastatic soft tissue sarcoma. Ann Thorac Surg 1991;52:197–203.
233. Casson AG, Putnam JB Jr, Natarajan G, et al. Efficacy of pulmonary metastasectomy for recurrent soft tissue sarcoma. J Surg Oncol 1991;47:1–4.
234. McCormack PM. Surgical resection of pulmonary metastases. Semin Surg Oncol 1990;6:297–302.
235. van Glabbeke M, van Oosterom AT, Oosterhuis JW, et al. Prognostic factors for the outcome of chemotherapy in advanced soft tissue sarcoma: an analysis of 2,185 patients treated with anthracycline-containing first-line

regimens—a European Organization for Research and Treatment of Cancer Soft Tissue and Bone Sarcoma Group Study. J Clin Oncol 1999;17:150–7.
236. Verweij J, Lee SM, Ruka W, et al. Randomized phase II study of docetaxel versus doxorubicin in first- and second-line chemotherapy for locally advanced or metastatic soft tissue sarcomas in adults: a study of the European organization for research and treatment of cancer soft tissue and bone sarcoma group. J Clin Oncol 2000;18:2081–6.
237. Choi H, Charnsangavej C, de Castro FS, et al. CT evaluation of the response of gastrointestinal stromal tumors after imatinib mesylate treatment: a quantitative analysis correlated with FDG PET findings. AJR Am J Roentgenol 2004;183:1619–28.
238. Jain RK. Normalizing tumor vasculature with anti-angiogenic therapy: a new paradigm for combination therapy. Nat Med 2001;7:987–9.
239. Okuno S, Ryan LM, Edmonson JH, et al. Phase II trial of gemcitabine in patients with advanced sarcomas (E1797): a trial of the Eastern Cooperative Oncology Group. Cancer 2003;97:1969–73.
240. Patel SR, Jenkins J, Papadopoulos N, et al. Preliminary results of a two-arm phase 2 trial of gemcitabine in patients with gastrointestinal leiomyosarcomas and other soft-tissue sarcomas (STS). Proc Am Soc Clin Oncol 1999;18:2091a.
241. Hensley ML, Maki R, Venkatraman E, et al. Gemcitabine and docetaxel in patients with unresectable leiomyosarcoma: results of a phase II trial. J Clin Oncol 2002;20:2824–31.
242. Leu KM, Ostruszka LJ, Shewach D, et al. Laboratory and clinical evidence of synergistic cytotoxicity of sequential treatment with gemcitabine followed by docetaxel in the treatment of sarcoma. J Clin Oncol 2004;22:1706–12.
243. Antman KH, Crowley J, Balcerzak SP, et al. An intergroup phase III randomized study of doxorubicin and dacarbazine with or without ifosfamide and mesna in advanced soft tissue and bone sarcomas. J Clin Oncol 1993;11:1276–85.
244. Nielsen OS, Dombernowsky P, Mouridsen H, et al. High-dose epirubicin is not an alternative to standard-dose doxorubicin in the treatment of advanced soft tissue sarcomas. A study of the EORTC soft tissue and bone sarcoma group. Br J Cancer 1998;78:1634–9.
245. Schwella N, Rick O, Meyer O, et al. Mobilization of peripheral blood progenitor cells by disease-specific chemotherapy in patients with soft tissue sarcoma. Bone Marrow Transplant 1998;21:863–8.
246. Judson I, Radford JA, Harris M, et al. Randomised phase II trial of pegylated liposomal doxorubicin (DOXIL/CAELYX) versus doxorubicin in the treatment of advanced or metastatic soft tissue sarcoma: a study by the EORTC Soft Tissue and Bone Sarcoma Group. Eur J Cancer 2001;37:870–7.
247. Scotto KW. ET-743: more than an innovative mechanism of action. Anticancer Drugs 2002;13 Suppl 1:S3–6.
248. Ryan D, Supko JG, Eder JP, et al. A phase I and pharmacokinetic trial of Ecteinascidin-743 (ET-743) administered as a 72 hour continuous infusion [abstract 725]. Proc Am Soc Clin Oncol 1999.
249. Blay JY, Le Cesne A, Verweij J, et al. A phase II study of ET-743/trabectedin (Yondelis) for patients with advanced gastrointestinal stromal tumours. Eur J Cancer 2004;40:1327–31.
250. Laverdiere C, Kolb EA, Supko JG, et al. Phase II study of ecteinascidin 743 in heavily pretreated patients with recurrent osteosarcoma. Cancer 2003;98:832–40.
251. Garcia-Carbonero R, Supko JG, Manola J, et al. Phase II and pharmacokinetic study of ecteinascidin 743 in patients with progressive sarcomas of soft tissues refractory to chemotherapy. J Clin Oncol 2004;22:1480–90.
252. Yovine A, Riofrio M, Blay JY, et al. Phase II study of ecteinascidin-743 in advanced pretreated soft tissue sarcoma patients. J Clin Oncol 2004;22:890–9.
253. Patel SR, Beach J, Papadopoulos N, et al. Results of a 2-arm phase II study of 9-nitrocamptothecin in patients with advanced soft-tissue sarcomas. Cancer 2003;97:2848–52.
254. Maki RG, Kraft AS, Scheu K, et al. A multicenter phase II study of bortezomib in recurrent or metastatic sarcomas. Cancer 2005;103:1431–8.
255. Tuveson DA, Willis NA, Jacks T, et al. STI571 inactivation of the gastrointestinal stromal tumor c-KIT oncoprotein: biological and clinical implications. Oncogene 2001;20:5054–8.
256. Joensuu H, Roberts PJ, Sarlomo-Rikala M, et al. Effect of the tyrosine kinase inhibitor STI571 in a patient with a metastatic gastrointestinal stromal tumor. N Engl J Med 2001;344:1052–6.
257. van Oosterom AT, Judson IR, Verweij J, et al. Update of phase I study of imatinib (STI571) in advanced soft tissue sarcomas and gastrointestinal stromal tumors: a report of the EORTC Soft Tissue and Bone Sarcoma Group. Eur J Cancer 2002;38 Suppl 5:S83–7.
258. Demetri GD, von Mehren M, Blanke CD, et al. Efficacy and safety of imatinib mesylate in advanced gastrointestinal stromal tumors. N Engl J Med 2002;347:472–80.
259. Verweij J, Casali PG, Zalcberg J, et al. Progression-free survival in gastrointestinal stromal tumours with high-dose imatinib: randomised trial. Lancet 2004;364:1127–34.
260. Rankin C, von Mehren M, Blanke CD, et al. Dose effect of imatinib (IM) in patients (pts) with metastatic GIST—Phase III Sarcoma Group Study S0033. J Clin Oncol 2004;22:14S.
261. Heinrich MC, Corless CL, Demetri GD, et al. Kinase mutations and imatinib response in patients with metastatic gastrointestinal stromal tumor. J Clin Oncol 2003;21:4342–9.
262. Demetri GD, Benjamin RS, Blanke CD. NCCN task force report: optimal management of patients with gastrointestinal stromal tumor (GIST)-expansion and update of NCCN clinical practice guidelines. JNCCN 2004;2:S1–26.
263. Van Oosterom A, Dumez H, Desai J. Combination signal transduction inhibition: a phase I/II trial of the oral mTOR-inhibitor everolimus (E, RAD001) and imatinib mesylate (IM) in patients (pts) with gastrointestinal stromal tumor (GIST) refractory to IM. J Clin Oncol 2004;22:3002.
264. Demetri GD, Desai J, Fletcher JA, et al. SU11248, a multi-targeted tyrosine kinase inhibitor, can overcome imatinib (IM) resistance caused by diverse genomic mechanisms in patients (pts) with metastatic gastrointestinal stromal tumor (GIST) [abstract 3001]. ASCO Meeting 2004.
265. Awan R, Dixon R, Antonescu CR, Maki RG. Patients with metastatic sarcoma arising from dermatofibrosarcoma protruberans (DFSP) may respond to imatinib (STI571, Gleevec) [abstract 1637]. Proc Am Soc Clin Oncol 2002;21:411a.
266. Rubin BP, Schuetze SM, Eary JF, et al. Molecular targeting of platelet-derived growth factor B by imatinib mesylate in a patient with metastatic dermatofibrosarcoma protuberans. J Clin Oncol 2002;20:3586–91.
267. Catton CN, O'Sullivan B, Kotwall C, et al. Outcome and prognosis in retroperitoneal soft tissue sarcoma. Int J Radiat Oncol Biol Phys 1994;29:1005–10.
268. Heslin MJ, Lewis JJ, Nadler E, et al. Prognostic factors associated with long-term survival for retroperitoneal sarcoma: implications for management. J Clin Oncol 1997;15:2832–9.
269. Sindelar WF, Kinsella TJ, Chen PW, et al. Intraoperative radiotherapy in retroperitoneal sarcomas. Final results of a prospective, randomized, clinical trial. Arch Surg 1993;128:402–10.
270. Gieschen HL, Spiro IJ, Suit HD, et al. Long-term results of intraoperative electron beam radiotherapy for primary and recurrent retroperitoneal soft tissue sarcoma. Int J Radiat Oncol Biol Phys 2001;50:127–31.
271. Willett CG, Suit HD, Tepper JE, et al. Intraoperative electron beam radiation therapy for retroperitoneal soft tissue sarcoma. Cancer 1991;68:278–83.
272. Petersen IA, Haddock MG, Donahue JH, et al. Use of intraoperative electron beam radiotherapy in the management of retroperitoneal soft tissue sarcomas. Int J Radiat Oncol Biol Phys 2002;52:469–75.
273. Jones JJ, Catton CN, O'Sullivan B, et al. Initial results of a trial of preoperative external-beam radiation therapy and postoperative brachytherapy for retroperitoneal sarcoma. Ann Surg Oncol 2002;9:346–54.
274. Brennan MF. Retroperitoneal sarcoma: time for a national trial? Ann Surg Oncol 2002;9:324–5.
275. Robertson JM, Sondak VK, Weiss SA, et al. Preoperative radiation therapy and iododeoxyuridine for large retroperitoneal sarcomas. Int J Radiat Oncol Biol Phys 1995;31:87–92.
276. Pisters PWT, Patel SR, Pollock RE, et al. Phase I trial of preoperative doxorubicin-based concurrent chemoradiation and electron-beam intraoperative radiation therapy (IORT) for resectable retroperitoneal sarcomas [abstract]. Cancer J Sci Am 1998;4:103.
277. Pitcher ME, Thomas JM. Functional compartmental resection for soft tissue sarcomas. Eur J Surg Oncol 1994;20:441–5.
278. Karasek K, Constine LS, Rosier R. Sarcoma therapy: functional outcome and relationship to treatment parameters. Int J Radiat Oncol Biol Phys 1992;24:651–6.
279. Bell RS, O'Sullivan B, Davis A, et al. Functional outcome in patients treated with surgery and irradiation for soft tissue tumours. J Surg Oncol 1991;48:224–31.
280. Davis AM. Functional outcome in extremity soft tissue sarcoma. Semin Radiat Oncol 1999;9:360–8.
281. Skibber JM, Lotze MT, Seipp CA, et al. Limb-sparing surgery for soft tissue sarcomas: wound related morbidity in patients undergoing wide local excision. Surgery 1987;102:447–52.
282. Ormsby MV, Hilaris BS, Nori D, Brennan MF. Wound complications of adjuvant radiation therapy in patients with soft tissue sarcomas. Ann Surg 1989;210:93–9.
283. Arbeit JM, Hilaris BS, Brennan MF. Wound complications in the multimodality treatment of extremity and superficial truncal sarcomas. J Clin Oncol 1987;5:480–8.
284. Peat BG, Bell RS, Davis A, et al. Wound-healing complications after soft-tissue sarcoma surgery. Plast Reconstr Surg 1994;93:980–7.
285. Chmell MJ, Schwartz HS. Analysis of variables affecting wound healing after musculoskeletal sarcoma resections. J Surg Oncol 1996;61:185–9.
286. Bujko K, Suit HD, Springfield DS, Convery K. Wound healing after preoperative radiation for sarcoma of soft tissues. Surg Gynecol Obstet 1993;176:124–34.
287. Cheng EY, Dusenbery KE, Winters MR, Thompson RC. Soft tissue sarcomas: preoperative versus postoperative radiotherapy. J Surg Oncol 1996;61:90–9.
288. Saddegh MK, Bauer HC. Wound complication in surgery of soft tissue sarcoma. Analysis of 103 consecutive patients managed without adjuvant therapy. Clin Orthop 1993;247–53.
289. Bell RS, Mahoney J, O'Sullivan B, et al. Wound healing complications in soft tissue sarcoma management: comparison of three treatment protocols. J Surg Oncol 1991;46:190–7.
290. Barwick WJ, Goldberg JA, Scully SP, Harrelson JM. Vascularized tissue transfer for closure of irradiated wounds after soft tissue sarcoma resection. Ann Surg 1992;216:591–5.
291. Amatruda JF, Tran K, Mantel M, et al. Diagnosis in oncology. Askin tumor. J Clin Oncol 1998;16:1997–8.
292. Turc-Carel C, Aurias A, Mugneret F, et al. Chromosomes in Ewing's sarcoma. An evaluation of 85 cases of remarkable consistency of t(11; 22)(q24; q12). Cancer Genet Cytogenet 1988;32:229–38.
293. Nilsson G, Skytting B, Xie Y, et al. The SYT-SSX1 variant of synovial sarcoma is associated with a high rate of tumor cell proliferation and poor clinical outcome. Cancer Res 1999;59:3180–4.
294. Rubin BP, Fletcher CD. The cytogenetics of lipomatous tumours. Histopathology 1997;30:507–11.
295. Tontonoz P, Singer S, Forman BM, et al. Terminal differentiation of human liposarcoma cells induced by ligands for peroxisome proliferator-activated receptor gamma and the retinoid X receptor. Proc Natl Acad Sci U S A 1997;94:237–41.
296. Demetri GD, Fletcher CD, Mueller E, et al. Induction of solid tumor differentiation by the peroxisome proliferator-activated receptor-gamma ligand troglitazone in patients with liposarcoma. Proc Natl Acad Sci U S A 1999;96:3951–6.

Section 34

HEMATOPOIETIC SYSTEM

112

The Myelodysplastic Syndrome

Lewis R. Silverman, MD

The existence of a hematopoietic disorder characterized by anemia and dyspoiesis preceding the onset of acute myelocytic leukemia has been recognized since the early part of the twentieth century. Initially designated as preleukemia, the syndrome was ill defined and could only be established with certainty retrospectively. Moreover, the terminology itself conveyed an unwarranted confidence in predicting the outcome that often belied the facts. The more accurately descriptive and appropriate designation as a myelodysplastic syndrome (MDS) was adopted in 1976 by the French-American-British[1] (FAB) Study Group.[2] The FAB classification permitted the prospective identification of patients within this heterogeneous clonal disorder.

MDS, derived from a multipotent hematopoietic stem cell, is characterized clinically by a hyperproliferative bone marrow, reflective of ineffective hematopoiesis, and is accompanied by one or more peripheral blood cytopenias. Bone marrow failure results, leading to death from bleeding and infection in the majority, while transformation to acute leukemia occurs in up to 40% of patients. The evolution of the disease proceeds in accordance with the multistep pathogenesis theory of carcinogenesis and can thus serve as an important model in furthering our understanding of the processes involved in neoplastic transformation.

This constellation of findings raises the question of whether MDS represents a frank neoplastic state or is merely a preneoplastic condition in transition. The syndrome appears to represent a spectrum, where the initial lesion in the genome, though clinically undetectable, subsequently evolves, with the acquisition of additional lesions, to a state of frank neoplasia.

The designation of this disorder as the myelodysplastic syndrome, rather than preleukemia, permits its distinction from other abnormalities that are known to be associated with the development of acute leukemia. These latter include the classic myeloproliferative syndromes (polycythemia vera, chronic myelocytic leukemia, agnogenic myeloid metaplasia, essential thrombocythemia), aplastic anemia, paroxysmal nocturnal hemoglobinuria (PNH), as well as Fanconi, Bloom, and Down syndromes. These particular "preleukemic states," which can lead to leukemia, are beyond the scope of this chapter.

MDS can be further divided into primary and secondary syndromes. The former arise de novo and are of indeterminate etiology, while the latter are induced by identifiable environmental, occupational, or iatrogenic causes.

Estimates of the incidence of MDS range from 1 case per 100,000 per year to a frequency equal to that of AML, or approximately 14,000 new cases per year in the United States. One recent population-based study demonstrated an incidence almost twice that of AML.[3,4] However, there are no registries that track the disease. The consensus is that the incidence is increasing owing to a number of factors, including greater awareness, greater diagnostic precision, and the aging of the population. The advent of new therapeutic approaches, leading to new hope for improving the outcome of MDS, has stimulated recognition.

HISTORY

Luzzatto first described a case of chronic anemia associated with bone marrow erythroid hyperplasia, which he designated as "pseudo-aplastic anemia."[5] It was not until Rhoads' and Bomford's description of this entity, however, that the designation of the disease as refractory anemia became generally accepted.[6,7]

In the early 1950s, it became apparent that some patients with refractory anemia could develop leukemia, which led to the term preleukemia, coined by Hamilton-Peterson and Block and colleagues.[8,9] In 1956, a special subclass of patients with refractory anemia and ringed sideroblasts, a proportion of whom developed leukemia, was described.[10] Subsequent reports led Dameshek to speculate that sideroblastic anemia might represent an early form of erythroleukemia.[11,12] In patients with sideroblastic anemia, Dacie described one population of hypochromic normocytic cells and another of normochromic macrocytic cells in the blood, suggesting the possibility of a clonal origin for this disorder. Although the clinical features of preleukemia lacked specificity, certain identifiable features could make the diagnosis easier.[13,14] These included frequent cytopenias in the peripheral blood, with morphologic evidence of dyshematopoiesis, associated with a hyperproliferative bone marrow, without clear findings of acute leukemia.

The plethora of terminology applied to the disorder, however, made it difficult to determine whether investigators were describing patients with the same disease. The designation as "preleukemia" often seemed erroneous, since many patients succumbed as a result of bone marrow failure without developing leukemia. In 1976, the FAB established diagnostic criteria for MDS that would permit prospective diagnosis.[2,15]

CLASSIFICATION

Based on bone marrow cellularity, the syndrome was divided into three groups: acquired sideroblastic anemia, refractory anemia with excess blasts, and chronic myelomonocytic leukemia. In 1982, the FAB group updated and expanded their classification to include five categories of MDS based on morphologic characteristics and the percentage of blasts in the bone marrow and peripheral blood.[16] These included (1) refractory anemia (RA), (2) refractory anemia with ringed sideroblasts (RARS), (3) refractory anemia with excess blasts (> 5% to < 20% blasts) (RAEB), (4) chronic myelomonocytic leukemia (CMML), and (5) refractory anemia with excess blasts "in transformation" (20% to < 30% blasts) (RAEB-T). Concerns that the classification might result in an underdiagnosis of M6 myeloid leukemia (erythroleukemia) led to further revision and refinement in 1985.[17] Accordingly, a two-step differential of the bone marrow is required to appropriately determine the FAB subgroup. Patients are initially segregated based on the percentage of erythroid precursors in the bone marrow. For those with 50% erythroid precursors or greater, the percentage of blast cells is calculated based on the number of nonerythroid cells in the marrow. These patients have either M6 leukemia or MDS, dependent on whether there are more or less than 30% blasts, respectively. In those cases where erythroid precursors constitute less than 50% of all the marrow cells, the percentage of blasts is calculated on the basis of all the nucleated cells. The diagnosis is acute myelocytic leukemia, M1 to M5 (≥ 30% blasts) or MDS (< 30% blasts) determined by the percentage of blasts in the marrow.

Some debate focuses on the category of chronic myelomonocytic leukemia and whether this truly represents a subgroup of MDS or should more appropriately be considered a subgroup of the myeloproliferative disorders (MPD). Some patients with CMMoL have features of both MDS and MPD, and thus an overlap syndrome with characteristics of both.[18,19] The biologic behavior appears related most closely to the percentage of blasts in the bone marrow.

The utility of the FAB classification has been validated.[20–22] Several studies have demonstrated differences among the five different categories in both survival and rates of transformation to leukemia, thus confirming its predictive value.[21,23,24] The biologic heterogeneity within each subtype has led to a search for more useful prognostic indicators, however. This led to a number of scoring systems including the Bournemouth, Sanz, Dusseldorf, and Lille scoring systems, which incorporate additional variables and permit further subcategorization of patients within each FAB subgroup based on prognosis.[3,24–26] None of these classifications has proven superior. The International Prognostic Scoring System (IPSS) has been advanced based on the percentage of bone marrow blasts, cytogenetics, and degree of cytopenias.[27] The IPSS has predictive value for both survival and risk of transformation to acute leukemia and classifies patients into four subgroups according to risk: low, intermediate-1, intermediate-2, and high risk (Table 112-1). This system has been validated and has become the standard classification (Table 112-2). If cytogenetic data are not available, however, the predictive power of the model diminishes significantly.

In 1999, another classification system was published by a working group of the World Health Organization (WHO), relying more closely on the FAB system's conventional morphologic criteria, but also considering cytogenetic markers[28] (Table 112-3). Data from 1,600 patients with primary MDS were evaluated, expanding the FAB system by two categories for a total of seven, all having a high degree of correlation with prognosis. CMML with WBC > 13 × 10^9/L was eliminated from the WHO categories and included with myeloproliferative disorders, while those with WBC < 13 × 10^9/L are still classified as MDS/MPD. Refractory anemia (RA) was split into pure refractory anemia (PRA) and refractory cytopenia with multilineage dysplasia (RCMD). Some conditions previously classified as refractory anemia with ringed sideroblasts (RARS) were placed in the pure sideroblastic anemia[29] group, while those with additional dysplastic features were put into the RCMD category, along with refractory anemias without ringed sideroblasts. RAEB was divided into RAEB I and RAEB II, based on medullary and peripheral blast counts. RAEB in transformation (RAEB-T) was included under AML. Additionally, 5q- was separated out as a distinct entity, although its relatively benign nature prevails only if the proportion of medullary blasts is below 5%.

Table 112-2 IPSS Score

Prognostic Variable	Score Value 0	0.5	1.0	1.5	2.0
Bone Marrow Blasts (%)	< 5	5–10	—	11–20	21–29
Karyotype	good	interm	poor		
Cytopenias	0/1	2/3			

Scores:	Cytogenetics:
Low: 0	Good: Normal
Intermediate-1: 0.5–1.0	-y
Intermediate-2: 1.5–2.0	del (5q)
High: > 2.5	del (20q)
	Poor: Chromosome 7 abnormalities
	Complex ≥ 3 abnormalities
	Intermediate: Other

Modified after Greenberg et al.[27]

Table 112-1 International Prognostic Scoring System (IPSS) Classification of MDS According to Prognostic Risk Subgroups

International Prognostic Scoring System (IPSS)	Risk of Transformation to Acute Myeloid Leukemia (in 25% of Patients) (Years)	Median Survival (Years)
Low	9.4	5.7
Intermediate-1	3.3	3.5
Intermediate-2	2.1	1.2
High	0.2	0.4

Modified after Greenberg et al.[27]

Table 112-3 World Health Organization (WHO)

Refractory anemia (RA)
- with ringed sideroblasts
- without ringed sideroblasts

Refractory cytopenia with multilineage dysplasia (RCMD)
- with ringed sideroblasts
- without ringed sideroblasts

Refractory anemia with excess blasts
- RAEB - I (6–10% blasts)
- RAEB - II (11–9% blasts)

5q-syndrome
CMML (MDS/MPD)
Myelodysplastic syndrome, unclassifiable

Modified after Harris et al.[28]

ETIOLOGY

Although the etiologic agent cannot be identified in the majority of patients with MDS, in some, exposure to ionizing radiation, chemicals, drugs, or other environmental agents can be implicated.

Radiation exposure has been clearly linked to the development of stem cell abnormalities.[30] Dogs that survive the transient hematopoietic failure following exposure to continuous total-body gamma irradiation often develop a preleukemic syndrome.[31] In addition, the leukemias that developed in survivors of atomic bomb explosions were often preceded by a preleukemic state.[32] Atomic bomb survivors continue to exhibit an increased incidence of genetic instability manifest as structural and numerical chromosomal abnormalities long after the initial exposure, which may contribute to the development of MDS and AML.[33] Furthermore, long-term population studies demonstrate an increased incidence of MDS and AML among patients exposed to thorium dioxide.[34]

Chemical injury to the marrow is a well-established phenomenon, and an increased risk of leukemogenesis has been noted among workers exposed to petrochemicals, benzene, and rubber.[35,36] The link between leukemia and exposure to benzene is the most strongly established.[37] Many of the initial cases of benzene-induced leukemia were associated with a preleukemic syndrome.[38] Exposure of human cell lines to hydroquinone, a benzene metabolite, is associated with the development of abnormalities of chromosomes 5, 7, and 8 and may be responsible, in part, for the DNA damage associated with the chemical exposure.[39] Farrow and colleagues have demonstrated, in an age and sex matched case-control study of occupational and environmental factors, that exposure to diesel oil fumes ($p < .01$), diesel oil liquids ($p < .01$), or ammonia ($p < .05$) was associated with the development of MDS.[40] A careful history of exposure to environmental and occupational hazards should be an integral part of the work-up of all patients with myelodysplastic syndromes. Additional environmental factors may include hair dye use and cigarette smoking.[41] Further studies will be required to better define the risk. Enzymatic pathways such as glutathione S-transferase (GST) play an important metabolic role in the detoxification of certain mutagens and carcinogens. Genetic differences among individuals to the effects of environmental toxins may contribute to the development of MDS. In one study, patients with MDS had a higher incidence of the GST theta 1 null genotype compared with a population-based control group.[42] This translated to a 4.3-fold higher risk of developing MDS, thus raising the possibility that inability to detoxify certain environmental or endogenous toxins may contribute to the development of MDS. Additional studies have found conflicting results, which may reflect different study populations.[43–45] Larger population-based prospective studies will be required.

Therapy-related myelodysplasia and leukemia following treatment with radiation and/or chemotherapy has been recognized, since this was initially observed in patients treated for Hodgkin's disease.[46] A hematologic disorder characterized by trilineage dysplasia, cytopenias, and panmyelosis following chemotherapy constitutes the least ambiguous cause of MDS.[47–49] Since the initial reports following treatment of Hodgkin's disease, therapy-induced MDS has been reported following treatment of cancers of the breast, lung, ovary, gastrointestinal tract, non-Hodgkin's lymphomas, seminoma, multiple myeloma, polycythemia vera, chronic lymphocytic leukemia, as well as nonmalignant conditions. The leukemogenic potential is greatest for alkylating agents, nitrosoureas, and procarbazine.[49] The risk associated with exposure to these particular agents is further substantiated by the increased frequency of abnormalities involving chromosomes 5 and 7 in comparison with the much lower frequency of abnormalities involving these chromosomes in patients treated with anthracyclines or antimetabolites.[49] Leukemogenicity appears to be a function of both dose and time of exposure, as observed in patients with ovarian cancer treated with melphalan or chlorambucil.[49] The use of etoposide in combination with cisplatin or other alkylating agents in patients treated for germ cell tumors is associated with an increased risk of MDS or AML.[50] The relationship of the cumulative dose of etoposide to development of MDS or therapy-related AML remains to be determined.[51,52] Abnormalities involving deletions of a portion of the short arm of chromosome 17 (17p) associated with either mutations or overexpression of the *TP53* oncogene have also been described related to prior chemotherapy.[53] This has been identified in both patients with lymphoid neoplasms treated with alkylating agents as well as in those with myeloproliferative disorders treated with either hydroxyurea or p.[32] Recently, treatment related MDS has been reported in association with both fludarabine and cladribine.[54]

Whether or not the increase in leukemogenic potential derives as a direct result of exposure to radiation and/or chemotherapy, or more simply reflects a natural predisposition related to the underlying disease, has long been debated. The risk of developing MDS and/or metachronous leukemia has been reported to be increased in association with certain cancers, such as multiple myeloma, lymphoma, carcinoma of the lung, and CLL.[55,56] However, the difference in the rates of developing leukemia after various treatments for polycythemia vera or Hodgkin's disease point to treatment as the most critical etiologic factor. In patients with polycythemia vera, the risk of developing leukemia is significantly elevated in those treated with chlorambucil, compared with those treated with phlebotomy alone.[57] Similarly, patients with Hodgkin's disease treated with ABVD (doxorubicin, bleomycin, vinblastine, and dacarbazine) have a much lower incidence of therapy-related leukemia than those treated with the MOPP (nitrogen mustard, vincristine, procarbazine, and prednisone) regimen.[58] The recognition of this potential risk has led to efforts to develop equally potent, but less leukemogenic, therapies, particularly in diseases with the potential for long-term survival. In a registry review of patients with chronic neutropenia treated with filgrastim, 9% of those patients with congenital neutropenia developed MDS and/or leukemia compared with none of the patients with cyclical or idiopathic neutropenia.[59] The relationship of the use of filgrastim and the development of MDS in these patients is uncertain.

High-dose chemotherapy with stem cell support is being applied as a curative approach in a number of malignancies, non-Hodgkin's lymphoma among them. As noted above, an increased risk of developing MDS or metachronous leukemia in association with lymphoma has been suggested.[55,56] Although therapy-induced MDS in patients with non-Hodgkin's lymphoma treated with standard doses of chemotherapy has been identified, MDS has now been recognized as a late complication of treatment with high-dose chemotherapy regimens.[51,60,61] The reported actuarial risk ranges from 6.4% up to 18% at 6 years.[62–64] The role that the pretransplant chemotherapy and the high-dose regimen contribute to the emergence of the MDS clone are the subject of prospective studies.[65] Strategies currently under study that use high-dose myeloablative treatments earlier in the course of this disease in patients with poor prognosis make the identification of the magnitude of this problem an increasingly important issue.[51,66,67] Studies that track the emergence of abnormal hematopoietic clones poststem cell infusion may provide further insight into the pathogenesis of MDS following high-dose treatments.

PATHOBIOLOGY

Clonal Origin Since originally suggested by Dacie, a substantial body of evidence has accumulated that points to a clonal origin for myelodysplastic syndromes. The identification of nonrandom chromosomal abnormalities detectable in 30 to 70% of patients with MDS confirmed the likelihood that these were clonal disorders.[68–73] Evidence that these disorders originate from pluripotent stem cells was suggested by reports of patients developing biphenotypic and lymphoid leukemias following MDS.[74–77]

Analysis of the patterns of inactivation of an X-linked polymorphic enzyme such as glucose-6-phosphate dehydrogenase (G6PD) has proven to be a useful tool in the analysis of the clonal origin of tumors.[78] Raskind and colleagues have demonstrated that 21 of 24 B lymphoblastoid lines transformed by Epstein-Barr virus expressed a single light chain immunoglobulin and contained only one of the isoenzymes. In contrast, the T cells expressed both the A and B G6PD isoenzymes.[79] The frequency with which the lymphoid lineage is involved as part of the abnormal clone in MDS is quite variable, as demonstrated in a number of studies.[80–84]

Subsequent studies using more refined and sensitive molecular techniques have also suggested that cells of lymphocytic origin belong to the abnormal clone, with B lymphocytes being involved more regularly than T cells.[80,81,83] Other studies have found evidence that only cells committed to the myeloid lineage are involved in the clone, but that lymphocytes are of polyclonal origin.[80–84] Fluorescent in situ hybridization (FISH) or polymerase chain reaction analysis of loss of heterozygosity has confirmed the involvement of an early stem cell that can give rise to CD34+ cells as well as those of erythroid, megakaryocytic, and myelomonocytic lineage, but not lymphocytes.[85] Subsequently, in a study using combined techniques of immunophenotyping and FISH, B-lymphocytes were found to be involved in patients with the 5q- syndrome.[86] Molecular and flow cytometric analysis of T-cell clonality has also suggested involvement of T cells in the MDS clone, at least at the functional level.[87] The reason for the discrepant findings is unclear, but may reflect the heterogeneity of the disease and interpatient variability. This is further suggested in one study where the bone marrow from 2 of 5 patients with MDS manifests evidence of residual polyclonal hematopoiesis.[88] Thus, the diverse heterogeneity of disease biology at the clinical level may simply reflect the degree of heterogeneity of the disease at the cellular level.

In Vitro Progenitor Growth Characteristics A variety of abnormalities in the growth of hematopoietic progenitors has been detected in colony assays in vitro of both bone marrow and peripheral blood from patients with all categories of MDS.[89–93] In a series of studies, 74% of 170 patients had abnormal bone marrow myeloid progenitor growth (CFU-GM). The pattern of colony growth can be classified as either a leukemic or nonleukemic pattern.[90–92] The former are characterized by increased formation of micro- and macroclusters, defective maturation of the colonies formed with the persistence of blasts, or decreased or absent colony formation (< 2 colonies/10^5 bone marrow cells plated). A leukemic type growth pattern is more commonly associated with shortened survival and an increased risk of transformation to acute leukemia than a nonleukemic pattern.[91,92] In patients serially studied, progressive increases in the cluster/colony ratio or progressive decrements in the growth of CFU-GM were seen prior to or concurrent with the transformation to leukemia. A positive correlation between abnormal colony growth and the presence of an abnormal karyotype has been identified and is associated with an increased risk of leukemic transformation. Reports have also indicated decreased to absent growth for other progenitors, including those of erythroid (CFU-E, BFU-E),[80,94,95] mixed lineage (CFU-GEMM),[96–98] and megakaryocytic (CFU-Mk)[99,100] precursors. No consistent pattern of colony growth in association with FAB subtypes has been demonstrated, but some studies have indicated the appearance of increasing growth abnormalities in relation to increasing numbers of bone marrow blasts.[100] Chronic myelomonocytic leukemia is often distinguished by increased CFU-GM growth, even in the absence of exogenous growth factor supplementation.[97]

Production of endogenous regulatory factors influencing the growth of myeloid, erythroid, and megakaryocytic precursors is diminished.[98,99,101] Bone marrow conditioned medium from patients with MDS had both decreased CFU-GEMM$_{CSA}$ and burst promoting activity (BPA) compared with conditioned medium from normal marrow. Both of these activities were completely neutralized by anti–IL-3 antibodies, suggesting that MDS conditioning did not produce IL-3.[98] In addition, accessory cells, including macrophages and NK cells, appear to be capable of directly or indirectly inhibiting bone marrow CFU-GM through the production of soluble factors.[94,102] T cells, although abnormal in number and in their response to mitogens, appear to produce normal levels of growth factors.[103] Partial restoration of colony growth can be accomplished through the addition of exogenous growth factors or other agents to the culture.[95] The addition of rhGM-CSF can result in an increase in CFU-GM, but has little effect on the growth of CFU-GEMM, BFU-E, or CFU-Mk.[93,96] Colony growth of CFU-E and BFU-E in some subgroups of MDS improved with the addition of rhEpo (recombinant human erythropoietin) or kit ligand.[104] Addition of rhG-CSF in vitro partially restored the abnormal function of neutrophils derived from patients with MDS.[105]

Studies of cytokine production by the bone marrow stroma have produced variable results. Stromal cell production of a variety of cytokines, including GM-CSF, IL-6, IL-1β, TNF-α, and IL-8, has been reported to be impaired in some patients with MDS and can be restored, at least in part, by in vitro or in vivo administration of hematopoietic growth factors.[106,107] However, the level of G-CSF, IL-1β, IL-6, IL-8, or stem cell factor messenger ribonucleic acid (mRNA) in a small series has been reported to be normal or increased.[108] Serum cytokine levels have for the most part been found to be normal or increased except for stem cell factor, which in one series was decreased.[109–112]

Bone Marrow Microenvironment Histologic examination of bone marrow trephine biopsies by Tricot and colleagues have pointed to abnormalities of the microenvironment.[113] They noted the presence of clusters of immature precursor cells in the central intertrabecular region of the marrow, rather than along the endosteal surfaces. They cited this as evidence of abnormal localization of immature precursors (ALIP).[113] ALIP was detected even before bone marrow smears revealed an excess of blasts. In a series of 40 patients, the presence of ALIP correlated significantly with shortened survival and was associated with an increased risk of transformation to AML. These findings were independent of the FAB subtype and were detected even in patients with refractory anemia. However, care must be applied to differentiate true ALIP from pseudo-ALIP. In the latter case, the clusters of cells are either of erythroid or megakaryocytic origin and do not convey the same prognostic information compared with the former, where the immature cells are of myeloid origin. The determination of the immature precursor phenotype by immunohistochemical methods may be helpful in distinguishing pseudo- and true ALIP, and thus permit identification of specific subgroups with a poor prognosis,[114] ALIP is not, however, specific to patients with MDS and, therefore, not helpful as a diagnostic tool.[114]

Investigations to define the potential role the bone marrow stroma may play in MDS have been limited and have yielded conflicting data to date. Some studies, however, have suggested that abnormalities of the stroma contribute to the pathophysiology of MDS. In vitro stromal cells either fail to reach confluent growth or their growth is absent in the majority of patients. Furthermore, stromal cell support of normal hematopoiesis in long-term bone marrow cultures can be impaired.[115–118] Cytokine production of LIF and TNF-α by MDS stroma is also impaired. In vivo labeling techniques have demonstrated that the ineffective hematopoiesis in MDS is accompanied by a high cell turnover with an increase in apoptosis of both hematopoietic progenitors and stromal cells. In vitro analyses indicate that the areas of apoptosis are associated with high levels of TNF-α and low levels of GM-CSF.[118–120] Characterization of cellular subsets of bone marrow stroma indicates that fibroblasts and macrophages from some patients with MDS are functionally abnormal, with increased production of TNF-α and IL-6 and an increased apoptotic index.[121]

Signal Transduction Whether the primary pathophysiologic defect(s) resulting in disordered maturation and function are intrinsic to hematopoietic progenitor cells or derive from their interaction with accessory cells and other microenvironmental factors or a combination thereof is uncertain. Hematopoietic cell defects may relate not only to quantitative abnormalities of progenitors, but also reflect abnormalities in signal transduction in response to cytokines or other regulatory molecules that trigger proliferation and differentiation pathways. Hematopoietic cells from MDS patients display impaired responses to a number of cytokines and are unable to respond to external signals owing either to abnormalities in number or function of cytokine receptors or to dysfunctional postbinding signal transduction.[101]

Hematopoietic progenitors have impaired responses to cytokine stimulation with decreased CFU-GM, CFU-GEMM, and BFU-E colony number me.[95,103,122,123] Purified blast cells from MDS patients proliferate but do not mature in response to G- and GM-CSF. Purified populations of CD 34+ cells from MDS patients also demonstrate impaired responses to G-CSF.[124] Receptor abnormalities in MDS are not commonly observed,[125–128] although in some patients their number is either diminished or their structure aberrant.[129] In a small series of patients with congenital neutropenia, analysis of the G-CSF receptor demonstrated a common deletion in 3 nucleotides in the juxtamembrane domain of the G-CSFR. This was associated with an increase in proliferative response to G-CSF but not GM-CSF or IL-3 in cells expressing the mutated G-CSFR. Treatment of these cells with G-CSF was associated with increased and prolonged expression of STAT-3.[130] Further studies will be necessary to determine the role of this mutation in the pathogenesis of the transformation to AML. Progenitor differentiation to erythropoietin is blocked and cells undergo apoptosis in patients with a truncated erythropoietin receptor.[129] On the other hand, defects in signal transduction appear to play a larger role in the aberrant response of hematopoietic progenitors to regulatory molecules.[131,132] This pertains both to the cytokine signal transduction pathways and factors which regulate apoptosis.[131,133] Patients with MDS have defective activation of STAT5 in response to erythropoietin but not IL-3 suggesting a defect in the erythropoietin signaling pathway. Despite the relative impairment, increasing concentrations of cytokines can partially correct the defects.[134,135] Epigenetic changes resulting in transcriptional silencing is another potential mechanism affecting cytokine signaling. Recent evidence demonstrates aberrant hypermethylation of the SOCS-1 gene in 31% of MDS patients associated with increased activity of the JAK/STAT pathway.[136] Hypermethylation which occurs in other genes such as p15 maybe explained in part by the over-expression of DNA methyltransferase 1 and 3A that has been identified in bone marrow of MDS patients.[137]

The majority of patients with MDS have hypercellular bone marrows with evident proliferation of various cellular lineage components. One interpretation of this finding is a compensa-

Table 112-4 Cytogenetics in MDS

	No. with Abnormal Karyotype (%)*						Frequency (%)						
No. of Patients	No. of Abnormal (%)	RA	RARS	RAEB	RAEB-T	CMML	5q-	-5	7q-	-7	20q-	8+	Reference
167	64(38)	13(29)	8(21)	30(43)	6(50)	5(45)	17	7	0	4	8	20	132
244	125(51)	NR	NR	NR	NR	NR	17	9	2	22	8	21	66
77	55(71)	26(63)	4(57)	17(89)	8(73)	2(29)	27	8	0	9	0	13	133
120	50(42)	10(36)	2(14)	25(56)	9(19)	4(29)	11	0	3	3	1	9	134
31	17(55)	NR	NR	12(55)	NR	5(50)	0	5	0	6	0	1	137
49	19(39)	4(29)	1(13)	8(89)	4(80)	2(20)	4	1	2	2	4	5	21
56	44(79)	11(86)	4(31)	21(95)	4(100)	3(100)	5	1	9	9	6	6	67
744	374(50.2)	64(11)	19(3)	113(19)	31(5)	21(4)	81(22)	31(8)	16(4)	55(15)	27(7)	75(20)	

NR = not reported.

*Percent of all patients with FAB subtype specified.

tory response in the marrow to feedback signals secondary to the peripheral blood cytopenias. Yet, the response does not translate into effective hematopoiesis; a role for increased apoptosis has been suggested.[133,138–140] A deficiency in cytokines or relative resistance to their effects could explain this phenomenon of ineffective hematopoiesis. In several recent studies, bone marrow cells from MDS patients have demonstrated increased expression of Fas and Fas-ligand. In marrow cultures, strategies that block TNF mediated signals, such as the use of anti–TNF-α antibody, significantly increased the numbers of hematopoietic colonies compared with untreated cells.[139] Additional studies have implicated a dysregulated Fas pathway and TNF-α as contributing to ineffective hematopoiesis.[138,140,141] Increased apoptosis may be related to mitochondrial encoded cytochrome c-oxidase I gene mutations.[142] Spontaneous release of mitochondrial cytochrome c results in activation of caspase -9 with activation of the apoptotic pathway in patients with low risk MDS. G-CSF can suppress the spontaneous cytochrome c release and reduce apoptosis, particularly in patients with RARS.[143]

Increased apoptosis was identified in both mature cells and immature CD34+ cells by assays for annexin V, measurements of mitochondrial membrane potential and caspase 3 activity from cell lysates in patients with MDS, and compared with patients with de novo AML. These results demonstrated that the patients with MDS had increased apoptosis in all FAB subcategories, which was distinctive compared with patients with AML and was equally applicable to the RAEB-T alone group.[144]

The role of cytokine signaling with apoptosis is less well delineated, but may contribute.[131,145] Progenitors with impaired signal transduction, thus constituting a refractory target cell, could undergo accelerated apoptosis analogous to withdrawal of obligate survival factors. Alternatively, the apoptotic pathway itself may be dysregulated with direct activation of the fas pathway.[145] As MDS evolves to AML, the acceleration of apoptosis declines and AML is characterized by increasing progenitor survival.[146]

Patients may also have myelofibrosis as a component of MDS and another manifestation of the MDS-MPD overlap syndrome. Recent reports suggest that in these patients the increased fibrosis may be secondary to increased production of TGF-β by bone marrow blasts, resulting in fibroblast proliferation.[147]

Cytogenetics Chromosome analysis contributed to the initial determination that MDS is a clonal disorder. In an analysis of studies on a total of 898 patients, 49% were identified as having an abnormal karyotype.[22,27,72,73,148–150] With recent improvements in both banding and high resolution synchronization techniques, 79% of patients in one study had abnormal karyotypes.[73] The chromosomal abnormalities are similar to those seen in patients with AML and involve complete or partial deletions, most frequently involving chromosomes 5(-5,5q-), 7(-7,7q-), and 8(8+) (Table 112-4). Certain karyotypic abnormalities that are associated with core binding factor rearrangements, such as t(15;17) in acute promyelocytic leukemia (M3), t(8;21) in acute myelocytic leukemia (M2), and inv 16 in acute myelocytic leukemia (M4), have only rarely been identified in MDS.[80,151–153] Moreover, patients with these AML subtypes have good prognoses with potential for cure. Thus, they should be viewed as having AML and should be managed accordingly. Furthermore, abnormalities involving partial deletions of the long arm of chromosome 20 (20q-), seen frequently in MDS, particularly RARS, polycythemia vera, and myeloproliferative syndromes, are usually not seen in patients with de novo AML.[22] Abnormalities are identified most frequently in patients with RAEB and RAEB-T compared with those with RA and RARS.[150,154] Although specific chromosomal abnormalities have been identified, unlike AML, no specific abnormality has been associated with any specific FAB category.[22,73,150] Newer techniques using FISH have identified additional chromosomal abnormalities in patients beyond those with banding alone and are complementary to standard techniques.[155]

Many studies have demonstrated that the presence of karyotypic abnormalities is an independent prognostic variable.[22,27,73,150] Several studies have demonstrated that patients with abnormalities present in 100% of the mitoses (AA) examined, or a mix of normal and abnormal mitoses (AN) have poorer survival than patients with normal karyotypes (NN).[22,72,73,154,156] Furthermore, more complex abnormalities are associated with shortened survival compared with either single clonal abnormalities or a normal karyotype.[27,73,149,150,154] Certain specific clonal subtypes have varying prognostic significance for both survival and the risk of leukemic transformation. Monosomy 7 or 5 and 7q- are associated with shortened survival, while deletions of the long arms of chromosome 20 (20q-) and 5(5q- syndrome) and deletion of y[157] as the sole abnormality are associated with prolonged survival.[27,73,149,154,156] In the IPSS, cytogenetic findings are an independent prognostic variable classifying patients according to 3 subgroups: good, intermediate, and poor risk.[27]

Genetic instability as demonstrated by clonal evolution occurs in a substantial percentage of patients. From 20 to 35% have been found to undergo clonal evolution during the course of the disease, independent of karyotypic status at the outset.[72] The significance of clonal evolution with respect to leukemic transformation and survival is contradictory at the outset.[72,150,156,158] In some studies, clonal evolution was associated with a poor prognosis without an increased risk of leukemic transformation.[156] In contrast, Glenn and colleagues have demonstrated karyotypic changes in clinically stable patients.[158] One study of 31 patients evolving to AML from MDS suggests that additional abnormalities involving chromosomes 1, 7, 8, 11, and 17 may contribute to the transformation process.[159] Subclonal evolution suggests genomic instability. Microsatellite instability involving defects in the DNA mismatch repair system has been identified in some MDS patients, particularly those with therapy-related disease.[160]

One particular abnormality involving a deletion of part of the long arm of chromosome 5 (5q-) deserves special note. As originally described, the 5q- syndrome is associated with a refractory macrocytic anemia, a normal or increased platelet count, giant thrombocytes, dyserythropoiesis, hypolobulated megakaryocytes, female predominance, prolonged survival, and a low rate of leukemic transformation.[73,154,161,162] It is important to differentiate the 5q- syndrome from instances where this deletion is found in combination with other chromosomal abnormalities or in association with FAB subtypes other than refractory anemia. It is clear that those patients with the 5q- abnormality, without the characteristic clinical and morphologic features, have a more aggressive clinical course associated with short survival.

Patients with myelodysplastic syndromes secondary to exposure to mutagenic or carcinogenic agents have similar findings in terms of the types and significance of the chromosomal abnormalities.[68,163,164] Patients treated with epidophyllotoxins (etoposide) can develop specific translocations involving the breakpoint at 11q23.[50,165] This leads to transcription of a fusion protein involving the mixed lineage leukemia (*MLL*) gene.[166,167]

Oncogenes Alterations in the control and expression of proto-oncogenes in the cellular genome, leading to abnormalities of cellular proliferation and differentiation, are thought to contribute to the molecular basis of neoplastic transformation.[168] Point mutations of the *ras* family of oncogenes have been identified in association with a number of human tumors, including lung, pancreatic, colorectal, and hematopoietic neoplasms.[151–153,169] Activated *ras* genes with specific point mutations involving codons 12, 13, and 61 have been identified in 20 to 30% of patients with AML and 9 to 48% of patients with myelodysplastic syndromes. These findings have suggested that activation of *ras* genes may either contribute to the development of MDS or, once established, to the process of transformation to AML.[153,170–173]

Table 112-5 *ras* **Oncogene Activation and Mutation in Relation to Leukemic Transformation in Myelodysplastic Syndromes**

Oncogene	No. with Activated or Mutated Gene/Tot. No. Pts. Studied	Pts. Transformed to AML (*ras* (+)/*ras* (–)	Reference
N-*ras*	1/15	–	147
N-*ras*	3/8	3/0	149, 154
Ki-*ras*	2/4	2/0	153
N-*ras*	5/61	2/3	159
ras	0/4	0/4	157
Ki-*ras* or N-*ras*	3/34	0/4	155
N-*ras* or Kiras or Ha-*ras*	20/50	8/4	156
N-*ras*	5/21	1/–	160
N-*ras* or Ki-*ras*	11/27	8/3	158
N-*ras*	6/35	4/8	150
N-*ras*	19/193	13/38	151
N-*ras*	21/50	6/2	161
ras	36/75	14/6	152
ras	5/51	4/17	162
Total	137/628	65/89	

Mutations of all three *ras* genes have been demonstrated in 75 of 628 (12%) patients with MDS (Table 112-5).[153,170,174–179] N-*ras* was most commonly affected, followed by Ki-*ras*, with H-*ras* involved in only a few cases. CMML was the FAB subtype most frequently associated with a *ras* mutation. The abnormality was found in 40% of cases.[180] The association may, however, be a function of the monocytosis, since other FAB subcategories with *ras* mutations were often associated with increased monocyte counts.[179]

In the initial reports, the presence of a mutant *ras* gene was associated with transformation of MDS to AML.[170,174] Overall, 47% (65 of 137) of patients with a *ras* mutation transformed to AML, compared with only 14% (89 of 628) of those without a mutation.[153,159,170–182] A significantly shortened survival of patients with MDS who transformed to AML has been associated with the presence of a *ras* mutation in most but not all.[73,172,183] It is unclear whether the presence of a *ras* mutation is an independent prognostic variable.

The *ras* mutation may confer a selective growth advantage to cells and appears to occur after initiation of leukemogenesis.[175,177,181] These mutations can appear in either the early or late stages of MDS (Figure 112-1). In the early stages, the mutation is present in all bone marrow and peripheral blood cells and involves a totipotent stem cell.[177,179] In other cases, it appears later in the disease and tends to be associated with an evolving and expanding clone of cells.[156,171,175] Its appearance in association with evolving karyotypic changes indicates an underlying genetic instability and suggests that *ras* mutations are not the last step in the transformation pathophysiology.[173] It is also unclear whether *ras* mutations contribute to the transformation from MDS to AML, or merely represent a genetic epiphenomenon in the emergence of a new clone.

Additional insight into a potential role for *ras* mutations. CD34+ progenitors modified to express a mutated N-*ras* were found to have defective differentiation in response to erythropoietin. This was manifest as reduced proliferation, increased doubling time, and decreased number of cells in S/G2M, leading to a failure to express the differentiation program in the late erythroblast stage. These cells also tended to undergo accelerated apoptosis, suggesting that expression of the mutated N-*ras* may be responsible for, at least in part, the pathophysiology underlying MDS.[184] A recent report suggests that activating mutations of FLT3 with internal tandem duplication of fms-like tyrosine kinase 3 at the tyrosine kinase domain may contribute to the transforming events of MDS to AML and interact with *ras* mutations.

Deletion of all or part of chromosome 5 in a substantial number of patients with either de novo or secondary MDS has led to the hypothesis of a tumor suppressor gene located within a short segment of the long arm in the so-called critical region at 5q21-5q34.[185] This region has been the focus of intensive study, and candidate genes either deleted or dysregulated have been identified, narrowing the region of interest.[186] The interferon regulatory factor-1 (IRF-1) is a DNA binding regulatory factor that regulates, in part, expression of interferon and interferon-inducible genes by binding to promoter regions. It functions as an activator, has antiproliferative and antioncogene activity, and can reverse a transformed phenotype.[187] The *IRF-1* gene has been mapped to the 5q31 region.[188] A loss of one or both IRF-1 alleles in patients with MDS[189] or AML with a del 5q has been described.[188,190,191] In vitro studies have suggested that loss of the *IRF-1* gene is associated either with a transformed phenotype and/or chemo- and radiation-induced apoptosis. Although these data suggest a potential role for the *IRF-1* gene, studies have not confirmed these observations.

Point mutations in the *TP53* tumor suppressor gene have been reported in 8% of MDS cases.[192,193] In one series, patients with secondary MDS (sMDS) or therapy-related AML (tAML) were found to have a higher than expected prevalence of *TP53* mutations in leukemic, but not germline tissues. Accumulation of *TP53* abnormalities in patients with sequential follow-up was identified in patients as they transform to AML.[194] Microsatellite instability was identified and was consistent with a mutator phenotype, suggesting that these patients were at higher risk of developing therapy-related MDS/AML.[157] Recently, patients have been described with a 17p- syndrome characterized by dysgranulopoiesis with pseudo–Pelger-Huet hypolobulation and small vacuoles in neutrophils. In one series, 15 of 16 patients with this deletion had an associated deletion of *TP53*, suggesting a potential role for loss of a tumor suppressor gene as a contributing factor to the morphologic, cytogenetic, and molecular phenotype of this syndrome.[195] The expression of several other genes, including *EVI-1*, c-*mpl*, *PDGF*, *MLL*, and the *CSF-1* receptor have recently been described to be dysregulated in some patients with MDS.[167,190,196,197] The *EVI-1* gene, located on chromosome 3, has been shown to play a role in both myeloid and erythroid differentiation. Dysregulation of gene expression is associated with blocks in myeloid and erythroid maturation.[198,199]

Clinical and Laboratory Features The clinical and laboratory picture in patients with MDS is dominated by and derives from the defect involving a multipotent hematopoietic stem cell. Although the disease has occasionally been described in children and adolescents, it is primarily encountered in

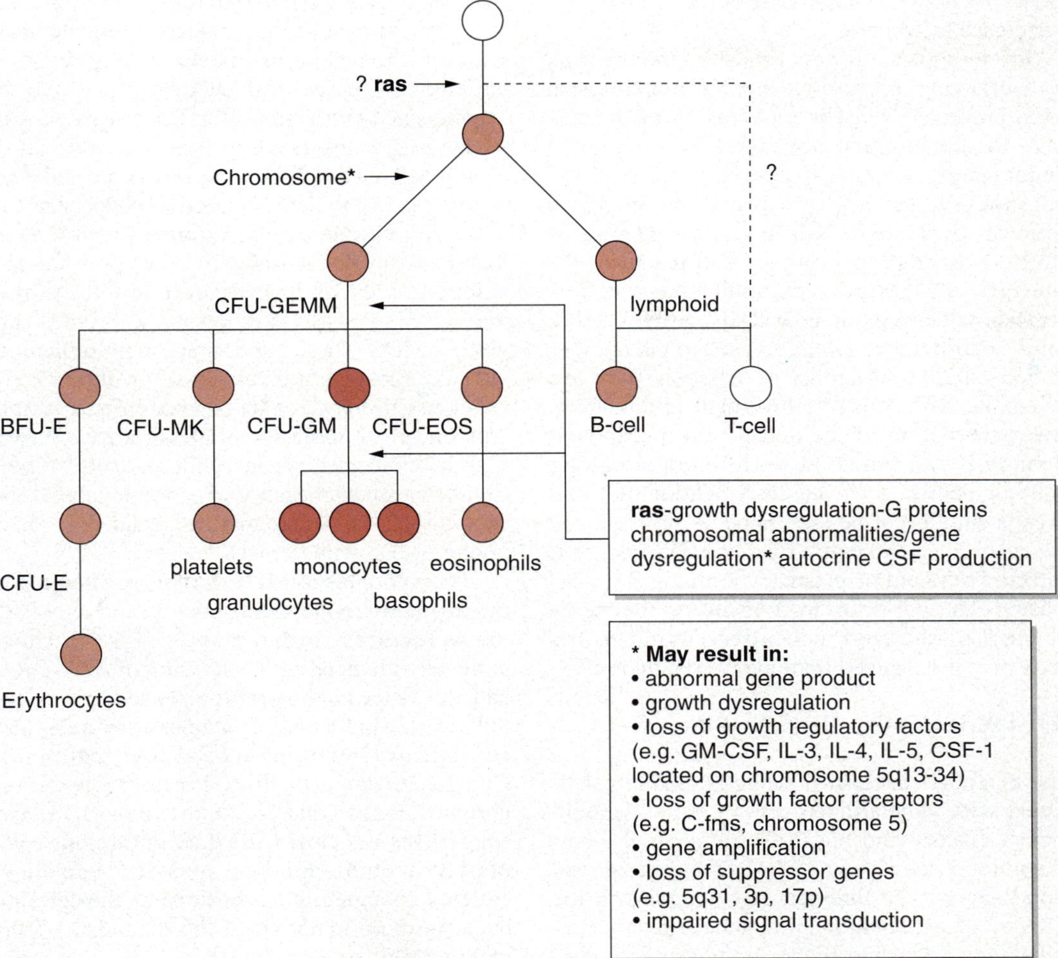

Figure 112-1 Multiple steps involved in the pathogenesis of MDS affecting a pluripotent hematopoietic stem cell (*white circle*). Chromosomal abnormalities and *ras* mutations may occur as early or late events in the pathogenesis of the disease. In younger patients, disease appears to originate in a stem cell committed along a more restricted lineage pathway (dark ●) and is similar to the stem cell origin in some patients with de novo AML. In most patients with MDS the disease originates from a multi-potent stem cell affecting progeny involving multiple hematopoietic lineages (● ●). *May result in abnormal gene product; growth dysregulation; loss of growth regulatory factors (e.g., GM-CSF, IL-3, IL-4, IL-5, CSF-1 located on chromosome 5q13-34); loss of growth factor receptors (e.g., *cfms*, chromosome 5); gene amplification; loss of suppressor genes (e.g., 5q31, 3p, 17p); impaired signal transduction. IL = interleukin; CSF = colony-stimulating factor.

adults in their sixth decade or older.[200] In most reports, the median age is over 65, and there appears to be a male predominance. The clinical presentation is nonspecific. The symptoms relate primarily to the cytopenias, with those attributable to anemia being most common. These include fatigue, weakness, pallor, dyspnea, angina pectoris, and cardiac failure. Other signs and symptoms encountered less frequently include easy bruising, ecchymosis, epistaxis, gingival bleeding, petechiae, and bacterial infections, particularly respiratory and dermal. Physical findings are nonspecific. Hepatic and/or splenic enlargement is reported in 10 to 40% of patients and is most commonly found in CMML. Lymphadenopathy and skin infiltration are uncommon,[21,23,24,26,201,202] although the appearance of leukemia cutis in patients with MDS may herald a transformation to leukemia by weeks or months. Its identification may suggest the development of a more aggressive clinical course, and in one study appeared to be associated with a poor prognosis.[203] Nontherapy-related MDS has been reported in association with other neoplasms, including lymphoproliferative and plasma cell disorders as well as carcinomas.[23]

The characteristic hematologic findings include peripheral blood cytopenias associated with dysmyelopoietic morphology and functional abnormalities involving one or more of the cell lines and are detailed in Table 112-6. The bone marrow is hypercellular in the majority and features the dysmyelopoietic morphology of part of all of the progenitors. Abnormalities involving erythrocyte enzymes, surface antigens, hemoglobin production, and iron metabolism have been described. Some of the changes in enzyme activity, such as pyruvate kinase, may affect red cell survival.[204,205] Impaired activity of A and H transferase and galactosyltransferase has resulted in changes in blood types.[206,207] Hemoglobin production is affected with increased fetal hemoglobin, aberrant globin chain synthesis, and disordered ferrokinetics.[208,209]

The myeloid series often reveals leukopenia with immature forms and increased numbers of large unstained cells (LUC). Neutropenia is more

Table 112-6 Morphologic and Functional Cellular Abnormalities in Myelodysplastic Syndromes

Erythrocytes
Morphology
anisocytosis
poikilocytosis
oval macrocytes
microcytes
basophilic stippling
Howell-Jolly bodies
circulating nucleated red cells
megaloblastoid maturation
multinucleated precursors
nuclear budding
karryohexis
defective hemoglobinization
ringed sideroblasts
increased stainable iron
Enzymes
increased hexokinase
decreased pyruvate kinase
decreased 2,3 diphosphoglycerate mutase
decreased phosphofructokinase
increased adenosine deaminase
increased pyruvate kinase
Decreases or loss of blood group antigens
Increased fetal hemoglobin
Aberrant globin chain synthesis
Disordered ferrokinetics
Leukocytes
Morphology
pseudo–Pelger-Huet cells
abnormal chromatin clumping
abnormal nuclear bridging
monocytosis
defective granule formation (hypogranulation)
megaloblastoid maturation
Auer rods
Increased LAP
Decreased myeloperoxidase
Increased muramidase (CMML)
Loss of granule membrane glycoproteins
Inappropriate surface antigens
Lineage infidelity
Decreased adhesion
Defective chemotaxis
Deficient phagocytosis
Impaired bacteriocidal activity
Megakaryocytes
Morphology
micromegakaryocytes
hypolobulated nuclei
large mononuclear forms
circulating megakaryocyte fragments
giant thrombocytes
Defective platelet aggregation
Deficiency in thromboxane A_2
Bernard-Soulier-like defect
Immune Deficiencies
Decreased T-cell IL-2 receptors
Decreased IL-2 production
Decreased NK activity
Decreased NK response to gamma interferon
Decreased response to mitogens
Decreased T_4 cells
Immunoglobulin abnormalities
Autoantibodies
Autoimmune phenomenon
Impaired self-recognition

commonly found in patients with RAEB and RAEB-T than RA and RARS.[23] Leukocytosis most often accompanies CMML, and by definition, requires an absolute monocytosis ($> 1 \times 10^9$/L) for diagnosis. Monocytosis may, however, also be present in the other MDS subtypes.[23] Cytoplasmic abnormalities result in cells with hypo- or defective granule formation, Auer rods, or abnormal azurophilic granules. Histocytochemical studies reveal cells with increased or decreased levels of leukocyte alkaline phosphatase,[210] decreased myeloperoxidase staining, and loss of granule membrane glycoproteins.[205,211] Surface antigen analysis has shown loss of lineage-specific antigens, with persistent or increased expression of inappropriate antigens and lineage infidelity.[212–215] In some instances, the abnormal persistence of antigens or an increased proportion of cells expressing those antigens was associated with an increased risk of leukemic transformation and shortened survival. Abnormal expression of an activated surface phenotype on monocytes has been demonstrated in patients within all FAB subtypes, while expression of activated surface antigens on granulocytes was almost exclusively seen in patients with excess blasts.[216] Impaired granulocyte function includes impaired respiratory burst, deficit in chemotaxis and superoxide release, as well as a defect in neutrophil stimulation signaling.[216,217] Nuclear and functional abnormalities are outlined in Table 112-6.[102,218]

Megakaryocytes can be decreased and their morphology is often bizarre (see Table 112-6). Patients with RAEB and RAEB-T more commonly have thrombocytopenia, decreased megakaryocytes, and greater degrees of dysmegakaryopoiesis.[23] Megakaryocyte fragments and giant thrombocytes may circulate in the peripheral blood. Hemorrhagic symptoms in these patients may be due not only to thrombocytopenia, but to functionally defective platelets as well. Dysfunction can result from defective platelet aggregation, deficiencies in thromboxane A2 activity, or the development of a Bernard–Soulier-type platelet defect. This latter defect has developed from a deficiency in the membrane glycoprotein GP 1b-IX complex.[219,220]

A small percentage of patients present with hypoplastic bone marrows and cytopenias that morphologically may be difficult to distinguish from aplastic anemia.[221] Cytogenetic analysis with or without interphase FISH may be helpful in establishing a diagnosis.

The relationship of MDS to abnormalities of the immune system is of particular interest given the broad range of abnormalities described. There is a decrease in the number of T-cell interleukin-2 (IL-2) receptors, as well as IL-2 production. The latter is due, in part, to a failure of immunoregulatory B cells.[222] NK cell activity and responsiveness to α-interferon is decreased, as is α-interferon production, while total numbers of NK cells are variable.[94,222] There are decreases in the number of T cells, responsiveness to mitogenic stimulation, the total number of cells, and the T4/T8 ratio.[212,223,224] The latter is due predominantly to a decrease in T4 cells.

Immunoglobulin abnormalities manifest as autoantibodies or a positive direct Coombs' test is often present.[223,225] The relationship of the disease to the immune abnormalities is poorly understood. A general dysregulation of the immune system appears prevalent in many patients. Consistent with this is the finding of altered antibody repertoires of self-reactive IgM and IgG in MDS patients, indicating a disturbance in self-recognition mechanisms.[226] Whether some abnormalities relate, in part, to the number of red cell transfusions, or whether they are reversible with effective treatment is unknown. Given the nature of the defect in a multipotent stem cell with potential to differentiate along multiple pathways,[227] the dysregulation of T and B cells should not be surprising. A report of 20 patients with nontherapy-related MDS and concurrent lymphoid or plasmacytic malignant neoplasms contributes further evidence to the multipotency of the stem cell affected and to the derivative generalized immune dysregulation.[223]

ESTABLISHING A DIAGNOSIS

The diagnosis in most patients is readily established with standardized testing, which should include history and physical examination, complete blood count, and review of the peripheral blood smear. The findings of cytopenias in the absence of explanation from biochemical, vitamin deficiency, hemorrhage, toxin/drug, or infectious etiology should lead to a bone marrow aspirate and biopsy. Routine cytogenetic evaluation should be included as well. The diagnosis of MDS is based primarily on morphologic criteria demonstrating dysmorphic features in the peripheral blood and bone marrow precursors (see Table 112-6). Although some of the classification systems include cytogenetic information (IPSS and WHO), they are based primarily on bone marrow and peripheral blood morphology. Analysis of the marrow population using flow cytometric analysis has become standard for the diagnosis and subtyping in patients with acute leukemia. It is more routinely being applied to establish a diagnosis of MDS as well. Abnormal populations and skewed antigen expression can be identified.[228–234] However, comparative studies of bone marrow morphology and flow cytometry results have not been conducted, and thus one cannot be certain if used alone whether flow cytometry results can reliably establish a diagnosis and classification of MDS. Accurate classification according to FAB, IPSS, or WHO criteria must be based, at least in part, on bone marrow morphology. Thus, flow cytometry should be viewed as a complementary examination but not sufficient to establish the diagnosis and classification.

DIAGNOSTIC DILEMMAS

Some patients with MDS present with features also suggestive of a myeloproliferative disorder (MPD), representing an "overlap syndrome."[235,236] In these patients, cytopenias may present simultaneously with elevated white or platelet counts. In some patients, an increased leucocyte count may be accompanied by monocytosis. Under current classification systems, some of these patients will be clearly defined as MPD, while others are still categorized as MDS, depending on the upper limit of WBC permitted in the classification system. Others may have myelofibrosis with or without marked splenomegaly and peripheral blood cytopenias,[236–239] yet also have dysplastic features suggesting MDS. These patients are more difficult to classify. Those with myelofibrosis with markedly enlarged spleens and a leucoerythroblastic peripheral smear are more likely classic myelofibrosis with myeloid metaplasia, while patients without significant splenomegaly and/or the peripheral leucoerythroblastic picture may be considered to have primary MDS with fibrosis.

The hypoplastic MDS variant is often indistinguishable from aplastic anemia and may have many features in common.[232,240–243] Those patients with increased expression of *HLA-DR15* and the PNH phenotype (decreased expression of CD59), whether MDS or aplastic anemia, may respond to immunomodulatory treatments. Cytogenetic abnormalities, if present, involving chromosomes frequently abnormal in MDS, may suggest the diagnosis of MDS, but do not completely exclude aplastic anemia.[242] In these patients, therapeutic options maybe the determinants in the orientation of the diagnosis absent other criteria.

Finally, there are patients who present with severe pancytopenia and bone marrow findings that are nondiagnostic (ie, minimal, if any, dysmorphic changes; no increase in myeloblasts) and without any cytogenetic abnormalities. Some of these patients may have MDS, and only with continued observation and testing will a diagnosis be unequivocally established. Others may have been exposed to a bone marrow insult (toxin, infectious agent, etc), which may never be identified, but which may permit eventual complete or partial marrow recovery, which takes months or years. In these latter individuals, in the absence of clear diagnostic evidence, patience, continued observation, and supportive care maybe the best approach pending a declarative diagnosis. One other consideration for these patients would be an immune-mediated injury to hematopoietic stem cells. The differential in these patients would include large granular lymphocytic leukemia (LGL), where T-cell receptor and immunoglobulin gene rearrangement studies may be informative.[244]

Pathogenesis and Relation to Leukemic Transformation Initiation and promotion of an abnormality affecting a multipotent stem cell may be related to a variety of factors, including chemical insult, radiation, or infection, leading to modification of gene expression. Since most patients with MDS are in the sixth, seventh, or eighth decades, cell senescence may also play a role. Once established, the clonal lesion follows the multistep process of oncogenesis and results in the transformation to acute leukemia in up to 40% of patients. It is likely that multiple events occur and lead to evolution of the disease and ultimate emergence of a dominant clone of cells.[227] Based on the knowledge of a number of abnormalities that do occur, one may speculate on the possible interrelationship of these events that contribute to the pathogenesis. Mutations of the *ras* oncogene, either as an early or late event in the development of the disease, may be one of the steps in this process.[175,177,179] One model of *ras* mutation results in impaired growth and differentiation along with impaired response to erythropoietin and increased apoptosis, similar to the in vivo phenotype.[184] Such mutations may serve to confer a growth advantage to the mutated cells, resulting in their progressive expansion.[170] As a late event, the selective growth advantage may be sufficient to trigger a leukemic transformation. However, when alteration of the *ras* gene occurs as an early event, it may be insufficient to trigger further progression and may require the concerted action of other factors such as those accompanying chromosomal abnormalities and the attendant gene dysregulation that occurs.

The impaired response of hematopoietic progenitors suggests an underlying abnormality of signal transduction. Mutations of cytokine receptors can result in a signal that is muted or overexpressed. Mutations have been identified of the FLT3 and G-CSF receptor in association with transformation to AML in patients with MDS.[245] Most studies, however, have not identified abnormalities of cytokine receptors, suggesting a defect further downstream from the ligand-receptor interaction. The increase in apoptosis in the bone marrow with apparent dysregulation of TNF-α and TGF-β further suggest cytokine dysregulation. Hematopoietic progenitors with impaired cellular response to cytokine signals could behave as though deprived of obligate survival factors, and thus undergo accelerated apoptosis as a consequence. This would be the predominant phenotype until further genetic or growth regulatory changes occurred that would trigger a proliferative advantage and transformation to AML. In patients with severe congenital neutropenia, evolution to a myelodysplastic syndrome or acute leukemia is usually accompanied by acquired mutations in the *G-CSF* receptor.[246] Point mutations of the *G-CSF* receptor gene cause truncation of the C-terminal cytoplasmic region of the receptor. Cells with this defect fail to undergo terminal maturation to granulocytes in response *G-CSF*.[247] In a mouse model, the equivalent *G-CSF* receptor mutation leads to expansion of the *G-CSF* receptor responsive progenitor population.[248] Treatment with G-CSF leads to neutrophilia, accompanied by increased activation of transcription factors and prolonged external cell surface expression owing to defective internalizaiton. Further genetic mutations in the face of clonal expansion can contribute to leukemogenesis.

Karyotypic abnormalities have been described in up to 79% of patients with MDS[73] and appear to be a later-occurring phenomenon. This is suggested by the identification of karyotypic abnormalities in cells belonging to already established clones derived from a multipotent stem cell[81,220] and by their greater frequency in patients with increased bone marrow blasts.[150,154] The association in some studies of complex karyotypic abnormalities with an increased risk of leukemic transformation[22,27,150] further suggests that these anomalies confer a growth advantage to a clone, as well as reflecting underlying genetic instability. This instability, manifest by clonal evolution with the subsequent acquisition of additional chromosomal abnormalities, has also been associated with disease progression, either to a more malignant subtype or frank AML.[25,27] Finally, most of the karyotypic abnormalities involve complete or partial deletions of chromosomes and suggest that gene loss may play a role in the pathogenesis.[164,185,249,250] The critical region on the long arm of chromosome 5, in the interstitial region q13-q34, contains genes encoding for a number of important proteins, including GM-CSF, IL-3, IL-4, IL-5, CSF-1, and the oncogene c-*fms*, which codes for the CSF-1 receptor.[249–251] Changes in the critical region may result in the production of an abnormal gene product or a point mutation. Deletion or loss of chromosomal material may result in a cell hemizygous for a mutant allele, which can be expressed, or loss of a tumor suppressor gene. Several chromosomal regions that are commonly deleted in patients with MDS have been identified, including del 1q, del 5q, del 17p, and del 3p, and may contain tumor suppressor genes whose loss may contribute to the transformation process.[252,253]

Dysregulation of the cell cycle may occur and contribute to the leukemic transformation. The cyclin-dependent kinase inhibitor (CDKI) gene $p15I^{NK4B}$ undergoes aberrant methylation of the CpG islands in up to 50% of patients with MDS studied in one series. Those patients with high-risk MDS had the highest frequency of hypermethylation, compared with those with lower-risk MDS. In addition, hypermethylation became more prominent as disease progressed.[254] The *EVI-1* gene, with a role in the regulation of erythroid and myeloid maturation, is another involved gene. In patients with translocation t(3;21), a novel chimeric transcription factor, AML1/EVI-1 is formed that appears to block granulocytic differentiation, and thus may play a role in the transformation process.[255] Additionally, unknown factors, including the influence of growth factors on cells, probably participate in leukemogenesis. Additional mutations involving other genes such as the *EVI-1* gene, resulting in impaired cell maturation, or of the *MLL* gene, leading to altered fusion proteins, may be part of the pathogenic process.[167,199] Other candidate tumor suppressor genes may be harbored on chromosomes 1q, 3p, or 17p.

Treatment For many years, the management of patients with MDS has been a frustrating and daunting task, compounded by the age of the patients, their debility secondary to bone marrow failure, comorbidities, and a lack of effective treatments. The mainstay of therapy has been primarily supportive care, consisting of transfusions and antibiotics in an effort to alleviate symptoms, but without impact on the disease outcome. Therapeutic efforts are complicated by the heterogeneity of the disease, which determines individual prognosis. Additional complicating features, including the general lack of randomized trials and the lack of uniform response criteria, made the interpretation of therapeutic results more difficult. The last decade has witnessed an expanded interest in the treatment of MDS, with the identification of new potentially useful therapeutic strategies.

Differentiation-Inducing and Novel-Acting Agents There has been great interest in the potential of differentiation therapy as an antitumor modality since Charlotte Friend and her colleagues first demonstrated that dimethylsulfoxide (DMSO) could induce differentiation of murine erythroleukemic cells in vitro, thus altering their malignant phenotype.[256] The concept, although readily documented in vitro, is more difficult to demonstrate in the clinical setting. A number of agents that have effectively induced differentiation in vitro have been tested in MDS without significant success (eg, *cis*- and *trans*-retinoic acid, vitamin D3, butyrate, hexamethylene bisacetamide [HMBA]).

The hypomethylating agent azacitidine (AzaC) has produced significant benefit (Table 112-7).[257,258] The promoter region of genes that are not expressed are often associated with hypermethylated CpG islands. Aberrant acquired changes in methylation, or epigenetic events, resulting in gene silencing can have important effects on genes regulating the cell-cycle and differentiation programs. A series of experiments by Christman, Acs, and colleagues led to the development of a biochemical model that provided an explanation for the action of azacitidine as an inducer of differentiation through its effects on DNA methylation.[259,260] AzaC, once incorporated into DNA, covalently binds to DNA methyltransferase, the enzyme in mammalian cells responsible for methylation of newly synthesized DNA. This binding results in hypomethylated DNA distal to the binding point and leads to transcription of previously methylated quiescent genes. In patients with β-thalassemia,[261] treatment with AzaC resulted in an increase in fetal hemoglobin production, which was associated with hypomethylation in the region of the gamma globin chain gene. Based on this model, a trial testing the efficacy of AzaC in MDS was undertaken by the Cancer and Leukemia Group B (CALGB).[262] AzaC was administered at 75 $mg/m^2/d$ continuous IV infusion for 7 days repeated in 28-day cycles. Of 43 evaluable patients, 21 (49%) achieved a response. In a second study in the CALGB, AzaC was administered at the same dose and schedule in an ambulatory regimen with comparable efficacy and toxicity profiles.[263] This led to the conduct of a phase III trial of AzaC

Table 112-7 Randomized Controlled Trials in Patients with MDS Drug vs Supportive Care +/– Placebo

Agent	Response to Treatment	Quality of Life	Frequency of Transformation to AML	Time to Progression	Time to AML or Death	Survival at 24 Months	Reference
Cis-retinoic acid	NSSD	–	–	–	–	NSSD	199, 252
Low-Dose Cytarabine	Cytarabine	–	NSSD	NSSD	NSSD	NSSD	239
G-CSF	G-CSF	–	NSSD	NSSD	SC*	SC*	260
GM-CSF	GM-CSF	–	NSSD	–	–	NSSD	255
Azacitidine	Azacitidine†	Azacitidine††	Azacitidine†	Azacitidine‡	Azacotodome§	Azacotodome#	240, 241
Decitabine	Decitabine	Decitabine	NSSD	NSSD	NSSD	NR	SABA

NSSD = no statistically significant difference between agent tested and placebo or supportive care (SC); – = endpoint not assessed in trial; NR = not reported.
SC* = Differences are for patients with RAEB. For those with RAEB-T, there was NSSD between G-CSF and SC.
†$p < .001$
‡$p < .0001$
§$p = .004$
#$p = .03$
††fatigue ($p = .001$); physical functioning ($p = .002$); dyspnea ($p = .0014$); mental health index ($p = .0077$).

compared with supportive care (SC) in the CALGB. In a crossover design, patients with progression could crossover to treatment after a minimum of 4 months in the SC group. Responses occurred in 60% on the AzaC arm (7% CR, 16% PR, 37% improved) compared with 5% (improved) in SC ($p < .0001$). The median time to leukemic transformation or death was significantly delayed for those on AzaC (21 mos vs 13 mos for SC [$p = .007$]) (Figure 112-2). Probability of transformation to AML as the first event was lower on AzaC (15%) than SC[189] ($p = .001$). The quality of life (QOL) of patients on the AzaC arm was significantly superior, according to several test methods, to that experienced by individuals in the control group. On crossover to azacitidine treatment, the same individuals were evaluated for quality of life according to the same serial interviews. Striking improvement in their QOL ensued. Patients on the AzaC arm experienced significantly greater improvement over time in fatigue (EORTC, $p = .001$), physical functioning (EORTC, $p = .002$), dyspnea (EORTC, $p = .0014$), psychosocial distress (MHI, $p = .015$), and positive affect (MHI, $p = .0077$) than patients in the supportive care group. Significant differences persisted after controlling for RBC transfusions. Prior to crossover, the QOL of patients on supportive care was stable or worsening. After crossover to AzaC, significant improvements occurred in fatigue (EORTC, $p = .0001$), physical functioning (EORTC, $p = .004$), dyspnea (EORTC, $p = .0002$), and general well being (MHI, $p = .016$).[45,46] Detailed analyses make unlikely placebo or hawthorne effects as explanations for improvements in QOL by azacitidine. Median survival for AzaC and SC (analyzed by intent to treat regardless of crossover) was 20 and 14 months, respectively ($p = .1$). The probability of survival at 24 months was 41% for AzaC compared with 25% for SC ($p = .03$), respectively. In order to eliminate the confounding effect caused by including the 49 crossover patients in the survival analysis, a landmark analysis was done in which the survival of three subgroups of patients were compared from a 6-month landmark date. These subgroups were[189] supportive care patients who never crossed over or who crossed over only after 6 months,[257] supportive care patients who crossed over before 6 months, and[189] patients who were initially randomized to azacitidine. The 36 patients who died before the landmark date were excluded. The additional median survival (after the 6-month landmark date) for these three groups was 11, 14, and 18 months, respectively. The AzaC group was significantly different from the supportive care subgroup who crossed over late or never ($p = .03$). Supportive care patients who crossed over early (subgroup 2) had a longer median survival than the patients who crossed over late or never (subgroup 1), though this did not reach statistical significance ($p = .11$). Results demonstrate that patients treated with AzaC had significantly higher response rates, improved QOL, delayed time to progression, improved survival at 24 months, delayed time to leukemic transformation or death, and significantly reduced risk of transformation to AML compared with supportive care.[257,258] Thus AzaC is the only agent other than allogeneic bone marrow transplantation to alter the natural history of MDS. Furthermore, AzaC is not age restricted, as is marrow transplantation.

AzaC likely acts via a number of mechanisms. It can be a cytotoxic agent, but in vitro data indicate that it also functions as a biologic response modifier, affecting cytokine signal transduction pathways.[262,264] Another hypomethylating agent, decitabine, (2-deoxy-5-azacitidine) has also been evaluated in a smaller number of patients.[265,266] Although response criteria are different, decitabine, like azacitidine, produces responses. However, there appear to be differences between the two agents, and the impact of decitabine on patient out-

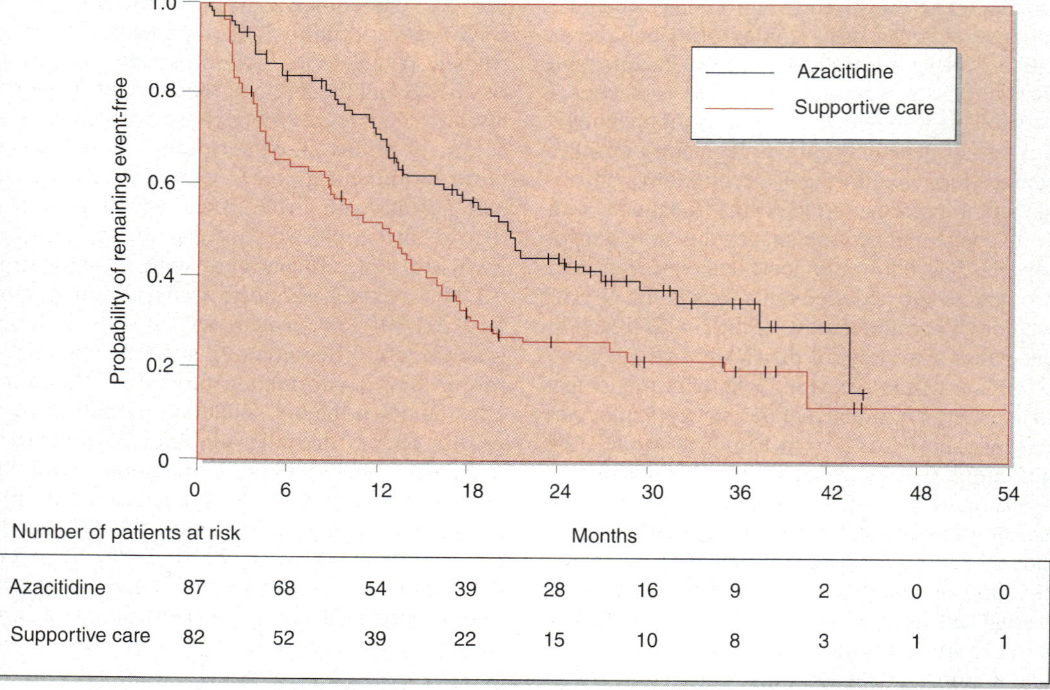

Figure 112-2 Time to transformation or death in patients treated with azacitidine compared to supportive care. Measured from time of study entry to first event, either transformation to AML or death, and estimated according to the method of Kaplan–Meier. Median time 21 vs 13 months, respectively ($p = .007$).[288]

come remains to be determined with more extensive testing. Partial results from a recently completed phase III randomized trial of decitabine versus supportive care were described. Responses occurred in 30% of patients treated with decitabine compared with 7% on supportive care. There was no difference between the two groups in the time to AML or death, or overall survival was not reported.

Cytosine arabinoside has been extensively tested. In an extensive review of the literature, low-dose cytosine arabinoside was found to produce 16% CR in 170 patients reported.[267] Median duration of CR was 10.5 months, but achievement of a response appeared to have little effect on overall survival. In a randomized trial conducted by ECOG and SWOG, patients with MDS were treated with either low-dose cytarabine or supportive care. Patients in supportive care who progressed could cross over and receive treatment with cytarabine. There was no significant difference between the cytarabine and supportive care groups with respect to overall survival, time to progression, or frequency of transformation to AML (see Table 112-7).[268]

Retinoic acid and related compounds, highly effective inducers of differentiation in vitro,[269] have been disappointing in their lack of efficacy in several clinical trials. In trials including some 235 patients reported in the literature, the overall response rate to *cis*-retinoic acid is 20%, and only one patient achieved a CR.[214,270–272] Two randomized controlled trials have not demonstrated a difference in survival compared with control except in one small patient subgroup.[214,272] In that subgroup there were patients with nonsideroblastic MDS and < 5% blasts in the bone marrow. They had a significantly prolonged survival when compared with untreated controls. The survival of the control group was unusually short in comparison with what would normally be observed, however, and may well explain the reason for this isolated finding. All-*trans*-retinoic acid has been studied in 52 patients with only four responses and does not appear to have significant activity.[273]

The observations regarding the potential role of TNF in the pathophysiology of MDS (described above in the section "Signal Transduction") have led to therapeutic strategies targeting TNF in small pilot studies. Etanercept, an anti-TNF fusion protein, has been tested in some small trials with erythroid response in one trial of 30% and a lower response in the other.[274,275] Thalidomide has been tested based on potential anti-TNF activity, but also because of effects on VEGF. Results have identified indicated responses predominantly in the erythroid lineage ranging from 10 to 19%.[276,277] Tolerance to treatment has been difficult in some patients because of somnolence and neuropathy, forcing withdrawal of patients from treatment. This has led to trials of lenalidomide, an analogue with no sedative or neuropathic side effects and more potent in vitro anti-TNF and anti-VEGF effects. In a phase II trial of 43 patients, 49% had a major erythroid response.[278] Patients with low- and intermediate-1–risk disease had a response rate of 60% compared with 20% of patients with intermediate- or high-risk disease. Nine of 12 patients with a del 5q had a complete cytogenetic response. List, 2005 #1349 Preliminary analysis of a large phase II study in patients with low- or intermediate-1–risk disease and del 5q abnormality demonstrates a major erythroid response in 66% of patients, compared with 27% in patients without the del 5q cytogenetic abnormality.[278]

Other agents with antiangiogenesis activity have been tested, including SU-5416. Although improvement in marrow function and blast count was identified in some patients, further trials are not being pursued with this particular agent.[279] The suggestion for a role for *ras* mutations has led to trials using farnesyl transferase inhibitors (FTI). In one trial, R115777 produced responses in some patients with AML and MDS, with responses in the 16 to 30% range. Further studies with this and other signal agents are ongoing.[280,281]

Hormones Although used as a nonspecific stimulant of erythropoiesis in aplastic anemia with some benefit, androgens have not proven to be useful in MDS. Initial observations suggesting that treatment with androgens accelerated the disease and were associated with an increased rate of leukemic transformation were not confirmed in subsequent studies, nor was any efficacy identified.[282,283]

Glucocorticoid therapy yielded an overall response rate of only 9%, and 24% of nonresponding patients experienced significant deleterious side effects.[284]

Danazol has been reported to produce improvements in the thrombocytopenia and anemia in patients with MDS. The effects appear to be mediated, in part, through inhibition of Fc receptor expression on monocytes, which alter the clearance of immunoglobulin-coated platelets and red cells from circulation, rather than a direct stimulatory effect on hematopoiesis. Danazol may be helpful in those patients where immune-mediated cell destruction contributes to the deficit.[285]

Chemotherapy Chemotherapeutic agents, alone and in combination, have been used to treat patients with MDS. These agents have been employed in a variety of regimens ranging from attenuated low-dose schedules[92] to the more conventional antileukemic myelotoxic-type strategies. These have been employed to treat patients at all stages of disease. Antileukemic-type treatments have not substantially altered the outcome of the disease for most patients and have been associated with significant toxicity in many.

The pharmacologic interaction between fludarabine and cytosine arabinoside increases intracellular ara-CTP and has been exploited in a regimen with activity in patients with relapsed AML. Subsequently, the combination with (FLAG) or without (FA) G-CSF has been tested in patients with MDS and de novo AML.[286] The two regimens yielded comparable complete response rates of 60% and 55%, respectively, with the response rate generally higher in the subgroups of MDS with excess blasts. Overall, 27% of patients (MDS and AML) died during induction. The median projected survival was 29 weeks for FA and 39 weeks for FLAG. These differences were not statistically significant. In patients with deletion of chromosome 5 or 7, FLAG produced a response rate of 64% versus 36% for FA. The differences were attributed by the authors to factors other than an effect of treatment, however. Use of G-CSF was associated with a more rapid recovery of neutrophil count, but this did not translate into decreased rates of infection or infection-related mortality.[286] Overall, there were no differences in treatment outcome for patients with MDS compared with AML.

In a successor study, 215 patients (153 AML and 62 RAEB/RAEB-T) were treated with fludarabine (F), cytarabine (A), and idarubicin (I) with or without either G-CSF or all-*trans*-retinoic acid (ATRA) (FAI; FAI + G-CSF; FAI + ATRA; FAI + G-CSF +ATRA).[287] The response was 51%, and the median survival was 28 weeks. Addition of G-CSF ± ATRA to FAI did not affect overall outcome.

In general, results from earlier studies indicated that responses to treatment of patients with either MDS or AML following MDS are less favorable than treatment of de novo AML.[288–290] Age appears to influence the rate and duration of response, with younger patients achieving CR more frequently[291] and remaining in remission longer compared with older patients. Achievement of a CR is associated with improved survival in comparison with nonresponding patients,[288,290] but the duration of the response is substantially shorter in comparison with patients with de novo AML who achieve response. Treatment prior to the transformation to AML,[289] and patients with shorter intervals between the diagnosis of MDS and leukemic transformation,[290] are associated with higher response rates. Aggressive antileukemic-type treatment is associated with high rates of morbidity and mortality, however, with up to 30% of the patients dying from drug-related complications.

The topoisomerase I inhibitor topotecan has demonstrated activity in early phase II trials. As a single agent, topotecan produced a CR rate of 32% in patients with MDS, including a high proportion of patients with CMMoL.[292] The treatment-related mortality rate was 20%, with a median survival of 45 weeks and 38% alive at 12 months. Combination of topotecan and cytarabine yielded a higher response rate, but[293] overall survival was the same as with topotecan as a single agent. In fact, these survival data appear little better than the results for patients treated with FA, FLAG, FAI, FAI + G-CSF, FAI +ATRA, or FAI +ATRA + G-CSF. Thus, although response rates appear better than historical experience, this antileukemic strategic approach does not appear to translate to an effect on overall survival in changing the natural history of the disease.

Bone Marrow Transplantation Results of allogeneic and syngeneic bone marrow transplantation from a series of reports containing small numbers of MDS patients have suggested that 35 to 40% can achieve durable long-term disease-free remissions when treated with this modality.[294,295] This has been substantiated with the results from two larger single-institution series.[296,297] In a large series, 251 patients treated between 1981 and 1996 were evaluated.[294] Appelbaum and colleagues reported an estimated (Kaplan-Meier) 5-year disease-free survival (DFS) of 40%. Younger age, shorter duration of disease, female gender, and de novo MDS were predictors of better DFS. Patients under the age of 20 years had a 60% disease-free survival rate, compared with 40% and 20% for those 20 to 50 years old or over the age of 50, respectively. Patients with low-risk MDS had a 55% DFS at 6 years compared with only 30% for those with high-risk. This difference correlated with a higher rate of relapse among those with more advanced disease. Among patients with low and intermediate-1 risk according to the IPSS score, there were almost no relapses. The 5-year DFS for those in the low and intermediate-1 groups was 60%, 36% for those in intermediate-2, and 28% for those in the high-risk group. Patients undergoing matched unrelated donor (MUD) marrow transplants fare less well. In an analysis of results from the National Marrow Donor Program, patients receiving MUD transplants during the first 4 years of registry data (1986–1990) had a disappointing disease-free survival of only 18% at 2 years and an overall survival at 2 years of 24%.[298] In one study, patients with primary MDS demonstrated a survival advantage over those with secondary MDS (56% vs 27%).[299]

The exact role and timing of bone marrow transplantation remains to be determined, as does the optimal conditioning regimen. A recent analysis suggests for patients with low-risk disease, watchful waiting until evidence of disease progression increases life expectancy compared with immediate transplantation. While for patients with high-risk disease, transplantation shortly after diagnosis was associated with better life expectancy.[300] For patients 40 years or younger with a compatible related donor, however, transplantation should be favored, since no other therapy thus far is curative. Fewer patients over the age of 40 have been transplanted, but limited data for those with related donors suggest that up to 30% may survive disease free.[299] Transplantation for those without a related donor is a more difficult choice in view of the data noted above. Given the age of most patients with MDS and the availability of donors, transplantation in the foreseeable future is likely to be of limited value, benefiting only about 5% of all patients with MDS.

Because of the age of the MDS patients and the potential toxicity of the fully ablative transplantation regimens, interest has developed in reduced-intensity conditioning hematopoietic stem cell transplantation as an alternative. These treatment strategies use conditioning regimens, often fludarabine-based, which are better tolerated and which are not intended to be fully ablative, but permit chimerism to be established with either sibling or VUD-matched donors. Recent reports demonstrate that this strategy can be used in patients over the age of 60 years with mortality rates ranging from 0 to 21%. Chimerism was established in 83% of patients. Duration of remission and relapse are dependant on the IPSS classification, similar to fully ablative transplantation.[301] Thus, this is a feasible approach that can be extended to older patients, but further studies will be necessary to determine its potential role in therapy.

The use of high-dose chemotherapy with either bone marrow or peripheral blood stem cell (PBSC) infusion has been used in a limited fashion. The European Group reported on 79 patients treated with intensive chemotherapy and autologous bone marrow transplantation in first CR. Fifty-five of the 79 in whom the duration of first CR was known were matched with 110 patients with de novo AML. The 2-year survival for all 79 patients was 39%, and the disease-free survival at 2 years was 28% for the 55 patients with MDS/sAML versus 51% for patients with de novo AML. Relapse rates were 69% for MDS/sAML and 40% for de novo AML ($p = .007$).[210] Use of PBSC infusion is more problematic given that adequate collection from patients with MDS is obtained in only half the patients.[302]

Growth Factors The hematopoietic growth factors are regulatory glycoproteins that control the proliferation and differentiation of bone marrow stem cells.[303] Several studies have defined the effects of GM-CSF in MDS. In a controlled study, patients were randomized to observation or treatment with rhGM-CSF.[304,305] Those treated had significant increases in neutrophils, eosinophils, monocytes, and lymphocytes, while the frequency of infections was decreased in comparison with those observed in the absence of this cytokine. There were no differences in platelet count, hemoglobin, or transfusion requirements between the two groups. The risk of leukemic transformation appeared greatest for those patients with > 15% blasts in the bone marrow and may be a critical level with respect to leukemic transformation.[306]

Maintenance therapy, administering GM-CSF on a chronic basis, has met with mixed results, with some reports of benefit or even continued improvement in the granulocyte count, while other reports have shown a progressive deterioration in counts despite continued treatment.[307,308]

Filgrastim (G-CSF) has also been evaluated. In a randomized controlled trial, 102 patients with RAEB or RAEB-T were treated with either G-CSF or supportive care.[309] No differences in frequency or time to progression to AML were seen between the two groups. There was no difference in survival for those with RAEB-T. However, among patients with RAEB, those in the treatment group had a significantly shortened survival compared with patients in the control group, resulting in early termination of the study.

Interleukin-3 (IL-3), another member of the family of hematopoietic growth factors, differs from G-CSF and GM-CSF insofar as its stimulatory effects work on earlier hematopoietic stem cells, which have a multipotential capacity for differentiation. Clinically IL-3 appears similar to G- and GM-CSF in its effects on myeloid cells, has little impact on other lineages, and is significantly more toxic.[310,311]

Human recombinant erythropoietin has also been studied in patients with MDS, with red cell responses being demonstrated in 20 to 25% of the patients tested.[312,313] Responses were confined to the erythroid lineage. A meta-analysis suggests that efficacy declines as bone marrow failure progresses.[314] Those who have lower serum erythropoietin levels and less transfusion need are more likely to respond. The observation that in vitro erythropoiesis improved in patients treated with in vivo G-CSF led to two trials of erythropoietin and G-CSF in combination. The response rate ranged from 35 to 40% and appears to enhance the activity of erythropoietin. Serum erythropoietin levels in these trials, as in others, are of predictive value with few responses in patients with levels above 500 U/L. In one other report, the response-enhancing effect of G-CSF was not substantiated.[315] In a series of 191 patients treated with the combination, the overall response was 39%. Low-risk disease was associated with a higher response, and patients achieving a CR had a longer duration of response.[316] An algorithm based on transfusion need and serum erythropoietin levels maybe a useful guide for patient selection.[317]

For patients with a variant of MDS characterized by severe hypoplasia and pancytopenia, which may resemble severe aplastic anemia (hypoplastic MDS), administration of antithymocyte globulin produced responses in 11 of 25 patients treated (9 of 14 RA; 2 of 6 RAEB).[318] Responses were characterized predominantly by loss of transfusion requirement and 3 of 25 had normalization of their counts. There were no changes in the dysplastic features or in bone marrow cellularity. In the completed study, 61 patients were treated, with 21 (34%) responding. Transfusion requirement was eliminated in 76% of responding patients or 25% overall.[319] The effect may be mediated, in part, through an immunosuppressive effect alleviating a T-cell suppression of hematopoietic progenitors.[320] Patients who are younger, have more cytopenias, shorter duration of red cell transfusion dependence, and the presence of HLA-DRB1-15, appear more likely to respond.

Clinical Management The management of patients with MDS presents a series of difficult choices (Figure 112-3). For patients with RA or RARS, low- or intermediate-1–risk groups, who have better prognoses and in whom the disease is manifest predominantly as asymptomatic anemia, observation and supportive care should be the mainstay. For those who require red cell transfusions, a trial of erythropoietin with or without appears reasonable. Those patients with a karyotypic abnormality (other than the 5q- syndrome, del 20q, or del y) have a less favorable prognosis. Such patients warrant closer follow-up and are candidates for investigational studies, particularly if they manifest an increasing number of blasts in

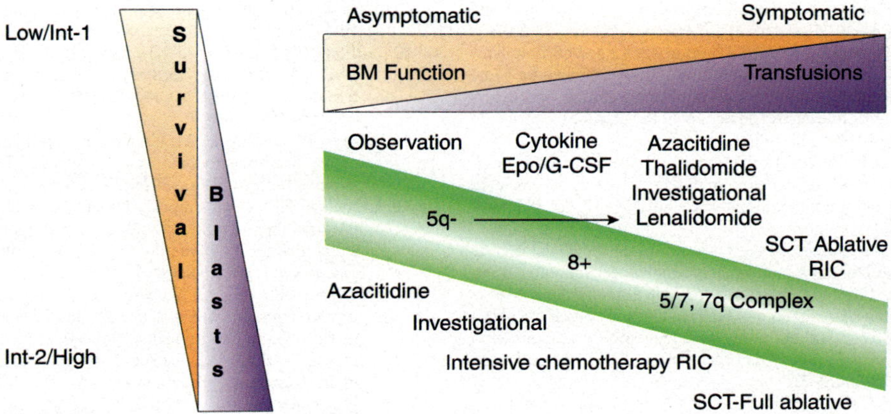

Figure 112-3 Treatment algorithm for patients with the myelodysplastic syndrome.

the bone marrow or develop significant neutropenia or thrombocytopenia. Patients with low-risk disease who fail therapy with erythropoietin with or without G-CSF for anemia or who have severe cytopenias in other lineages can be considered for treatment with azacitidine, which has demonstrated efficacy in low risk disease with amelioration of symptoms. Lenalidomide will likely be of benefit in the future for patients with -5q abnormalities. For patients 40 years or younger who have a compatible donor, allogeneic bone marrow transplantation should be considered, since it is the only therapy that has so far achieved cures. For patients between 41 and 60 years old, the risks associated with bone marrow transplantation appear to be increased, though fewer MDS patients have been treated in this age category. Patients over 60 years may still be considered for bone marrow transplantation, although data are limited, efficacy is low, and complication rates high.

Patients with RAEB or RAEB-T or intermediate-2– or high-risk disease have a poorer prognosis and are candidates for treatment. Those with RAEB I (5–10% blasts) without other poor prognostic features (ie, abnormal karyotype, absence of severe thrombocytopenia) could be closely observed to determine the relative stability of the disease. Those with evidence of progression are candidates for immediate intervention. For patients 40 years or younger who have a compatible donor, allogeneic bone marrow transplantation should be considered, since it is the only therapy that has so far achieved cures.

Patients with RAEB and RAEB-T can benefit from treatment with azacitidine. Azacitidine has demonstrated significant benefit compared with supportive care, induces remission, decreases transfusion requirements, extends survival and improves the quality of life, and likely extends survival.[257,258] This therapy may now represent the standard of care.[321] Alternatively, they can be treated as part of an investigational program. Stem cell transplantation is a consideration for those patients as a potential curative strategy and should be considered early in the evaluation process after the diagnosis is established, if a donor is available, and dependent on the patient's age. However, the rate of relapse is high, and many centers will consider these patients as candidates. Strategies aimed at inducing a remission prior to transplantation may be useful.

For patients who have transformed to leukemia, aggressive antileukemic chemotherapy can be undertaken. The CR rate ranges between 30 and 60%, but is associated with a high rate of treatment-related morbidity and mortality. Most patients relapse. Patients with hypoplastic MDS, particularly if younger, may benefit from antithymocyte globulin with or without cyclosporin.

FUTURE DIRECTIONS

Progress in the prevention and therapy of MDS depends on a better understanding of the basic biochemical and molecular defects that contribute to the development of this syndrome. Well-designed clinical trials using clearly defined biologic end points are critical. Survival is the ultimate goal, but too global a composite to serve as the sole working criterion. Quality of life assessments have gained favor as useful tools in the measure of the effects of treatment. These assessments should be included routinely in phase II and III studies and help as a critical measure of a palliative treatment. Finally, cost analysis is another useful gauge of treatment efficacy. Pharmacoeconomic studies should also be included in future phase III studies.

In a disease characterized by the development of a progressive uncoupling of cellular maturation and proliferation, differentiation induction is an attractive therapy. This has proven to be a highly provocative approach in the treatment of acute promyelocytic leukemia with *trans*-retinoic acid. Azacitidine, which may act in part as a biologic response modifier with effects on signal transduction, may be advantageously combined with other agents. Drugs which interfere with or block abnormal signal transduction (eg, farnesyl transferase inhibitors) may have benefit. Tumor vaccines and the use of allogeneic T cells will be explored in the coming years.

REFERENCES

1. Stiegler G, Sperr W, Lorber C, et al. Red cell antibodies in frequently transfused patients with myelodysplastic syndrome. Ann Hematol 2001;80:330–3.
2. Bennett JM, Catovsky D, Daniel MT, et al. Proposals for the classification of the acute leukaemias. French-American-British (FAB) Co-operative Group. Br J Haematol 1976;33:451–8.
3. Aul C, Gattermann N, Heyll A, et al. Primary myelodysplastic syndromes: analysis of prognostic factors in 235 patients and proposals for an improved scoring system. Leukemia 1992;6:52–9.
4. Groupe Francais de Morphologie Hematologique. French registry of acute leukemia and myelodysplastic syndromes. Age distribution and hemogram analysis of the 4496 cases recorded during 1982–1983 and classified according to FAB criteria. Cancer 1987;60:1385–94.
5. Luzzatto AM. Sull anemia grave megaloblastica sensa reporto ematologica correspondents (anemia pseudo-aplastica). Riv Ven 1907;47:193.
6. Rhoads CP, Barker WH. Refractory anemia: analysis of 100 cases. JAMA 1938;110:794–6.
7. Bomford PR, Rhoads CP. Refractory anaemia. I. Clinical and pathological aspects. Q J Med 1941;10:175.
8. Hamilton-Peterson JL. Preleukemic anaemia. Acta Haematol 1949;2:309.
9. Block M, Jacobson LO, Bethard WF. Preleukemic acute human leukemia. JAMA 1953;152:1018–28.
10. Bjorkman SE. Chronic refractory anaemia with sideroblastic bone marrow. A study of four cases. Blood 1956;11:250–9.
11. Dacie JV, Smith MD, White JC, Mollin DL. Refractory normoblastic anaemia: a clinical and haematological study of 7 cases. Br J Haematol 1959;2:56–82.
12. Dameshek W, Baldini M. The Di Guglielmo syndrome. Blood 1958;13:192–4.
13. Dreyfus B, Rochant H, Sultan C, et al. Les anemies refactaires avec exces de myeloblasties dans la moelle. Etude de onze observations. Nouv Presse Med 1970;78:359.
14. Linman J, Bagby GC. The preleukemic syndrome: clinical and laboratory features, natural course and management. Blood Cells 1976;2:11–31.
15. Gralnick HR, Galton DAG, Catovsky D, et al. Classification of acute leukemia. Ann Intern Med 1977;87:740–53.
16. Bennett JM, Catovsky D, Daniel MT, et al. The French-American-British Cooperative Group. Proposals for the classification of the myelodysplastic syndromes. Br J Haematol 1982;51:189–99.
17. Bennett JM, Catovsky D, Daniel M-T, et al. Proposed revised criteria for the classification of acute myeloid leukemia. A report of the French-American-British Cooperative Group. Ann Intern Med 1985;103:620–5.
18. Neuwirtová R, Mociková K, Jelinek J, et al. [Mixed myelodysplastic and myeloproliferative syndromes]. Cas Lek Cesk 1997;136:724–9.
19. Neuwirtová R, Mociková K, Musilova J, et al. Mixed myelodysplastic and myeloproliferative syndromes. Leuk Res 1996;20:717–26.
20. Economopoulos T, Stathakis N, Foudoulakis A, et al. Myelodysplastic syndromes: analysis of 131 cases according to the FAB classification. Eur J Haematol 1987;38:338–44.
21. Foucar K, Langdon RM 2nd, Armitage JO, et al. Myelodysplastic syndromes. A clinical and pathologic analysis of 109 cases. Cancer 1985;56:553–61.
22. Jacobs RH, Cornbleet MA, Vardiman JW, et al. Prognostic implications of morphology and karyotype in primary myelodysplastic syndromes. Blood 1986;67:1765–72.
23. Vallespi T, Torrabadella M, Julia A, et al. Myelodysplastic syndromes: a study of 101 cases according to the FAB classification. Br J Haematol 1985;61:83–92.
24. Varela BL, Chuang C, Woll JE, Bennett JM. Modifications in the classification of primary myelodysplastic syndromes: the addition of a scoring system. Hematol Oncol 1985;3:55–65.
25. Garcia S, Sanz MA, Amigo V, et al. Prognostic factors in chronic myelodysplastic syndromes: a multivariate analysis in 107 cases. Am J Hematol 1988;27:163–8.
26. Mufti GJ, Stevens JR, Oscier DG, et al. Myelodysplastic syndromes: a scoring system with prognostic significance. Br J Haematol 1985;59:425–32.
27. Greenberg P, Cox C, LeBeau MM, et al. International scoring system for evaluating prognosis in myelodysplastic syndromes [comments] [published erratum appears in Blood 1998;91:1100]. Blood 1997;89:2079–88.
28. Harris N, Jaffe E, Diehold J, et al. World Health Organization classification of neoplastic diseases of the hemato-

poietic and lymphoid tissues: report of the Clinical Advisory Committee Meeting—Airlie House, Virginia, November 1997. J Clin Oncol 1999;17:3835–49.
29. Tsiara S, Economou G, Panteli A, et al. Coexistence of myelodysplastic syndrome and multiple myeloma. J Exp Clin Cancer Res 1999;18:565–6.
30. Mossman KL. Ionizing radiation and cancer. Cancer Invest 1984;2:301–10.
31. Tolle DV, Fritz TE, Norris WP. Radiation induced erythroleukemia in the beagle dog. Am J Pathol 1977;87:499–510.
32. Kamada N, Uchins H. Preleukemic states in atomic bomb survivors. Blood Cells 1976;2:57–65.
33. Nakanishi M, Tanaka K, Shintani T, et al. Chromosomal instability in acute myelocytic leukemia and myelodysplastic syndrome patients among atomic bomb survivors. J Radiat Res (Tokyo) 1999;40:159–67.
34. Visfeldt J, Andersson M. Pathoanatomical aspects of malignant haematological disorders among Danish patients exposed to thorium dioxide. Apmis 1995;103:29–36.
35. Rigolin GM, Cuneo A, Roberti MG, et al. Exposure to myelotoxic agents and myelodysplasia: case-control study and correlation with clinicobiological findings. Br J Haematol 1998;103:189–97.
36. Thomas TL, Waxweiler RJ, Moure-Eraso R, et al. Mortality patterns among workers in three Texas oil refineries. J Occup Med 1982;24:135–41.
37. Cronkite E. Chemical leukemogenesis. Benzene as a model. Semin Hematol 1987;24:2–11.
38. Yin SN, Hayes RB, Linet MS, et al. A cohort study of cancer among benzene-exposed workers in China: overall results [comments]. Am J Ind Med 1996;29:227–35.
39. Stillman WS, Varella-Garcia M, Gruntmeir JJ, Irons RD. The benzene metabolite, hydroquinone, induces dose-dependent hypoploidy in a human cell line. Leukemia 1997;11:1540–5.
40. Farrow A, Jacobs A, West RR. Myelodysplasia, chemical exposure, and other environmental factors. Leukemia 1989;3:33–5.
41. Nagata C, Shimizu H, Hirashima K, et al. Hair dye use and occupational exposure to organic solvents as risk factors for myelodysplastic syndrome. Leuk Res 1999;23:57–62.
42. Chen H, Sandler D, Taylor J, et al. Increased risk for myelodysplastic syndromes in individuals with glutathione transferase theta 1 (GSTT1) gene defect. Lancet 1996;347:295–7.
43. Naoe T, Takeyama K, Yokozawa T, et al. Analysis of genetic polymorphism in NQO1, GST-M1, GST-T1, and CYP3A4 in 469 Japanese patients with therapy-related leukemia/ myelodysplastic syndrome and de novo acute myeloid leukemia. Clin Cancer Res 2000;6:4091–5.
44. Tsabouri SE, Georgiou I, Alamanos I, Bourantas KL. Increased prevalence of GSTM(1) null genotype in patients with myelodysplastic syndrome: a case-control study. Acta Haematol 2000;104:169–73.
45. Woo MH, Shuster JJ, Chen C, et al. Glutathione S-transferase genotypes in children who develop treatment-related acute myeloid malignancies. Leukemia 2000;14:232–7.
46. Arseneau JC, Sponzo RW, Levin DL, et al. Nonlymphomatous malignant tumors complicating Hodgkin's disease. N Engl J Med 1972;287:1119–22.
47. Coltman CA Jr, Dixon DO. Second malignancies complicating Hodgkin's disease: a Southwest Oncology Group 10-year followup. Cancer Treat Rep 1982;66:1023–33.
48. Grunwald HW, Rosner F. Acute myeloid leukemia following treatment of Hodgkin's disease. Cancer 1982;50:676–83.
49. Kantarjian HM, Keating MJ. Therapy-related leukemia and myelodysplastic syndrome. Semin Oncol 1987;14:435–43.
50. Pedersen-Bjergaard J, Daugaard G, Hansen SW, et al. Increased risk of myelodysplasia and leukaemia after etoposide, cisplatin, and bleomycin for germ-cell tumours. Lancet 1991;338:359–63.
51. Kollmannsberger C, Hartmann JT, Kanz L, Bokemeyer C. Risk of secondary myeloid leukemia and myelodysplastic syndrome following standard-dose chemotherapy or high-dose chemotherapy with stem cell support in patients with potentially curable malignancies. J Cancer Res Clin Oncol 1998;124:207–14.
52. Smith A, Watson N, Sharma P. Frequency of trisomy 15 and loss of the Y chromosome in adult leukemia. Cancer Genet Cytogenet 1999;114:108–11.
53. Merlat A, Lai JL, Sterkers Y, et al. Therapy-related myelodysplastic syndrome and acute myeloid leukemia with 17p deletion. A report on 25 cases. Leukemia 1999;13:250–7.
54. Van Den Neste E, Louviaux I, Michaux JL, et al. Myelodysplastic syndrome with monosomy 5 and/or 7 following therapy with 2-chloro-2'-deoxyadenosine. Br J Haematol 1999;105:268–70.
55. Greenberg BR, Miller C, Cardiff RD, et al. Concurrent development of preleukaemic, lymphoproliferative and plasma cell disorders. Brit J Haematol 1983;53:125–33.
56. Lai R, Arber DA, Brynes RK, et al. Untreated chronic lymphocytic leukemia concurrent with or followed by acute myelogenous leukemia or myelodysplastic syndrome. A report of five cases and review of the literature. Am J Clin Pathol 1999;111:373–8.
57. Berk PD, Goldberg JD, Silverstein MN, et al. Increased incidence of acute leukemia in polycythemia vera associated with chlorambucil therapy. N Engl J Med 1981;304:441–7.
58. Valagussa P, Santoro A, Fossati-Bellani F, et al. Second acute leukemia and other malignancies following treatment for Hodgkin's disease. J Clin Oncol 1986;4:830–7.
59. Freedman MH, Bonilla MA, Fier C, et al. Myelodysplasia syndrome and acute myeloid leukemia in patients with congenital neutropenia receiving G-CSF therapy. Blood 2000;96:429–36.
60. Fisher RI, Gaynor ER, Dahlberg S, et al. Comparison of a standard regimen (CHOP) with three intensive chemotherapy regimens for advanced Non-Hodgkin's lymphoma. N Engl J Med 1993;328:1002–6.
61. Sobecks RM, Le Beau MM, Anastasi J, Williams SF. Myelodysplasia and acute leukemia following high-dose chemotherapy and autologous bone marrow or peripheral blood stem cell transplantation. Bone Marrow Transplant 1999;23:1161–5.
62. Miller J, Arthur DC, Litz CE, et al. Myelodysplastic syndrome after autologous bone marrow transplantation: an additional late complication of curative cancer therapy. Blood 1994;12:3780–6.
63. Stone RM. Myelodysplastic syndrome after autologous transplantation for lymphoma: the price of progress? Blood 1994;83:3437–40.
64. Stone RM, Neuberg D, Soiffer R, et al. Myelodysplastic syndrome as a late complication following autologous bone marrow transplantation for non-Hodgkin's lymphoma. J Clin Oncol 1994;12:2535–42.
65. Traweek ST, Slovak ML, Nademanee AP, et al. Myelodysplasia and acute myeloid leukemia occurring after autologous bone marrow transplantation for lymphoma. Leuk Lymphoma 1996;20:365–72.
66. Bearman SI, Overmoyer BA, Bolwell BJ, et al. High-dose chemotherapy with autologous peripheral blood progenitor cell support for primary breast cancer in patients with 4-9 involved axillary lymph nodes. Bone Marrow Transplant 1997;20:931–7.
67. Dillman RO, Barth NM, Nayak SK, et al. High-dose chemotherapy with autologous stem cell rescue in breast cancer. Breast Cancer Res Treat 1996;37:277–89.
68. Auclerc G, Jacquillat C, Auclerc MF, et al. Post-therapeutic acute leukemia. Cancer 1979;44:2017–25.
69. Fialkow PJ, Singer JW, Raskind WH, et al. Clonal development, stem-cell differentiation, and clinical remissions in acute nonlymphocytic leukemia. N Engl J Med 1987;317:468–73.
70. Foucar K, McKenna RW, Bloomfield CD, et al. Therapy-related leukemia. A panmyelosis. Cancer 1979;43:1285–96.
71. Hogge DE, Shannon KM, Kalousek DK, et al. Juvenile monosomy 7 syndrome: evidence that the disease originates in a pluripotent hemopoietic stem cell. Leuk Res 1987;11:705–9.
72. Second International Workshop on Chromosomes in Leukemia. Chromosomes in preleukemia. Cancer Genet Cytogenet 1980;2:108.
73. Yunis JJ, Rydell RE, Oken MM, et al. Refined chromosome analysis as an independent prognostic indicator in de novo myelodysplastic syndromes. Blood 1986;67:1721–30.
74. Barton JC, Conrad ME, Parmley RT. Acute lymphoblastic leukemia in idiopathic refractory sideroblastic anemia. Evidence for a common lymphoid and myeloid progenitor cell. Am J Hematol 1980;9:109–15.
75. Hehlmann R, Zonnchen B, Thiel E, Walther B. Idiopathic refractory sideroachrestic anemia (IRSA) progressing to acute mixed lymphoblastic-myelomonoblastic leukemia. Blut 1983;46:11–21.
76. Nagler A, Brenner B, Tatarsky I. Secondary refractory anemia with excess of blasts in transformation terminating as acute lymphoblastic leukemia. Acta Haemat 1986;76:164–5.
77. San Miguel JF, Gonzales M, Del Canizo MC, Lopez-Borrasca A. Myelodysplastic syndrome evolving to a mixed-lymphoid leukaemia. Hematol Oncol 1986;4:175–6.
78. Wainscoat JS, Fey MF. Assessment of clonality in human tumors: a review. Cancer Res. 1990;50:1355–60.
79. Raskind WH, Tirumali N, Jacobson R, et al. Evidence for a multistep pathogenesis of a myelodysplastic syndrome. Blood 1984;63:1318–23.
80. Gilliland DG, Blanchard KL, Levy J, et al. Clonality in myeloproliferative disorders: analysis by means of the polymerase chain reaction. Proc Natl Acad Sci U S A 1991;88:6848–52.
81. Janssen JWG, Buschle M, Layton M, et al. Clonal analysis of myelodysplastic syndromes: evidence of multipotent stem cell origin. Blood 1989;73:248–54.
82. Kibbelaar RE, van Kamp H, Dreef EJ, et al. Combined immunophenotyping and DNA in situ hybridization to study lineage involvement in patients with myelodysplastic syndromes. Blood 1992;79:1823–8.
83. Tefferi A, Thibodeau SN, Solberg LA Jr. Clonal studies in the myelodysplastic syndrome using X-linked restriction fragment length polymorphisms. Blood 1990;75:1770–3.
84. van Kamp H, Fibbe WE, Jansen RPM, et al. Clonal involvement of granulocytes and monocytes, but not of T and B lymphocytes and natural killer cells in patients with myelodysplasia: analysis by X-linked restriction fragment length polymorphisms and polymerase chain reaction of the phosphoglycerate kinase gene. Blood 1992;80:1774–80.
85. Kroef MJPL, Fibbe WE, Mout R, et al. Myeloid but not lymphoid cells carry the 5q deletion: polymerase chain reaction analysis of loss of heterozygosity using mini-repeat sequences on highly purified cell fractions. Blood 1993;81:1849–54.
86. Jaju RJ, Jones M, Boultwood J, et al. Combined immunophenotyping and FISH identifies the involvement of B-cells in 5q- syndrome. Genes Chromosomes Cancer 2000;29:276–80.
87. Melenhorst JJ, Eniafe R, Follmann D, et al. Molecular and flow cytometric characterization of the CD4 and CD8 T-cell repertoire in patients with myelodysplastic syndrome. Br J Haematol 2002;119:97–105.
88. Asano H, Ohashi H, Ichihara M, et al. Evidence for nonclonal hematopoietic progenitor cell populations in bone marrow of patients with myelodysplastic syndromes. Blood 1994;84:588–94.
89. Gebbia V, Miserendino V, Miceti S, et al. Analysis of human dysplastic haematopoiesis in long-term bone marrow culture. Blut 1989;59:442–8.
90. Greenberg PL, Mara B. The preleukemic syndrome—correlation of in vitro parameters of granulopoiesis with clinical features. Am J Med 1979;66:951–8.
91. Milner GR, Testa NG, Geary CG, et al. Bone marrow culture in refractory cytopenia and "smouldering leukaemia." Br J Haematol 1977;35:251–61.
92. Spitzer G, Verman DS, Dicke KA, et al. Subgroups of oligoleukemia as identified by in vitro agar culture. Leuk Res 1979;3:29–39.
93. Tennant GB, Jacobs A. Effect of 5637-conditioned medium on peripheral blood granulocyte-macrophage progenitors in normal subjects and patients with the myelodysplastic syndrome. Leukemia Res 1989;13:385–9.
94. Kerndrup G, Hokland P. Natural killer cell-mediated inhibition of bone marrow colony formation (CFU-GM) in refractory anaemia (preleukaemia): evidence for patient-specific cell populations. Scand J Haematol 1988;69:457–62.
95. Mayani H, Baines P, Bowen DT, Jacobs A. In vitro growth of myeloid and erythroid progenitor cells from myelodysplastic patients in response to recombinant human granulocyte-macrophage colony-stimulating factor. Leukemia 1989;3:29–32.
96. Carlo-Stella C, Cazzola M, Bergamaschi G, et al. Growth of human hematopoietic colonies from patients with myelodysplastic syndromes in response to recombinant human granulocyte-macrophage colony-stimulating factor. Leukemia 1989;3:363–6.
97. Geissler K, Hinterberger W, Bettelheim P, et al. Colony growth characteristics in chronic myelomonocytic leukemia. Leuk Res 1988;12:373–7.
98. Merchav S, Nagler A, Fleischer-Kurtz G, Tatarsky I. Regulatory abnormalities in the marrow of patients with myelodysplastic syndromes. Br J Haematol 1989;73:158–64.
99. Geissler D, Zwierzina H, Pechlaner C, et al. Abnormal megakaryopoiesis in patients with myelodysplastic syndromes: analysis of cellular and humoral defects. Br J Haematol 1989;73:29–35.
100. Juvonen E, Partanen S, Knuutila S, Ruutu T. Colony formation by megakaryocyte progenitors in myelodysplastic syndromes. Eur J Haematol 1989;42:389–95.

101. Baines P, Masters GS, Lush C, Jacobs A. Enrichment of haemopoietic progenitor cells from the marrow of patients with myelodysplasia. Br J Haematol 1988;68:159–64.
102. Ohmori M, Ohmori S, Ueda Y, et al. Myelodysplastic syndrome (MDS)–associated inhibitory activity on haemopoietic progenitor cells. Br J Haematol 1990;74:179–84.
103. Merchav S, Nagler A, Sahar E, Tatarsky I. Production of human pluripotent progenitor cell colony stimulating activity (CFU-GEMMCSA) in patients with myelodysplastic syndromes. Leuk Res 1987;11:273–9.
104. Backx B, Broeders L, Löwenberg B. Kit ligand improves in vitro erythropoiesis in myelodysplastic syndrome. Blood 1992;80:1213–7.
105. Yuo A, Kitagawa S, Okabe T, et al. Recombinant human granulocyte colony-stimulating factor repairs the abnormalities of neutrophils in patients with myelodysplastic syndromes and chronic myelogenous leukemia. Blood 1987;70:404–12.
106. Maurer AB, Ganser A, Buhl R, et al. Restoration of impaired cytokine secretion from monocytes of patients with myelodysplastic syndromes after in vivo treatment with GM-CSF or IL-3. Leukemia 1993;7:1728–33.
107. Visani G, Zauli G, Tosi P, et al. Impairment of GM-CSF production in myelodysplastic syndromes. Brit J Haematol 1993;843:227–31.
108. Hirayama Y, Kohgo Y, Matsunaga T, et al. Cytokine mRNA expression of bone marrow stromal cells from patients with aplastic anaemia and myelodysplastic syndrome. Br J Haematol 1993;85:676–83.
109. Bowen D, Yancik S, Bennett L, et al. Serum stem cell factor concentration in patients with myelodysplastic syndromes. Br J Haematol 1993;85:63–6.
110. Verhoeif G, De Schouwer P, Ceuppens J, et al. Measurement of serum cytokine levels in patients with myelodysplastic syndromes. Leukemia 1992;6:1268–72.
111. Yoshida Y, Anzai N, Kawabata H, et al. Serial changes in endogenous erythropoietin levels in patients with myelodysplastic syndromes and aplastic anemia undergoing erythropoietin treatment. Ann Hematol 1993;66:175–80.
112. Zwierzina H, Schöllenberger S, Herold M, et al. Endogenous serum levels and surface receptor expression of GM-CSF and IL-3 in patients with myelodysplastic syndromes. Leuk Res 1992;16:1181–6.
113. Tricot G, De Wolf-Peeters C, Hendrickx B, Verwilghen RL. Bone marrow histology in myelodysplastic syndromes: histological findings in myelodysplastic syndromes and comparison with bone marrow smears. Br J Haematol 1984;57:423–30.
114. Mangi MH, Salisbury JR, Mufti GJ. Abnormal localization of immature precursors (ALIP) in the bone marrow of myelodysplastic syndromes: current state of knowledge and future directions. Leuk Res 1991;15:627–39.
115. Aizawa S, Nakano M, Iwase O, et al. Bone marrow stroma from refractory anemia of myelodysplastic syndrome is defective in its ability to support normal CD34-positive cell proliferation and differentiation in vitro. Leuk Res 1999;23:239–46.
116. Coutinho L, Will A, Radford J, et al. Effects of recombinant human granulocyte colony-stimulating factor (CSF), human granulocyte macrophage-CSF, and gibbon interleukin-3 on hematopoiesis in human long-term bone marrow culture. Blood 1990;75:2118–29.
117. Silverman L, Zinzar S, Holland J. Biological consequences of stromal abnormalities in the myelodysplastic syndrome: its influence on the hematopoietic dysregulation. Leuk Res 1997;21:20.
118. Zinzar S, Silverman LR, Holland JF. Stromal defects in the myelodysplastic syndrome (MDS) contribute to the hematopoietic abnormalities. Proc Am Assoc Cancer Res 1997;38:146.
119. Raza A, Mundle S, Iftikhar A, et al. Simultaneous assessment of cell kinetics and programmmed cell death in bone marrow biopsies of myelodysplastics reveals extensive apoptosis as the probable basis for ineffective hematopoiesis. Am J Hematol 1995;48:143–54.
120. Shetty V, Mundle S, Alvi S, et al. Role of the microenvironment and macrophages in understanding the dynamics of myelodysplastic syndrome (MDS). Blood 1994;84 Suppl:314a.
121. Flores-Figueroa E, Gutierrez-Espindola G, Montesinos JJ, et al. In vitro characterization of hematopoietic microenvironment cells from patients with myelodysplastic syndrome. Leuk Res 2002;26:677–86.
122. Mecucci C, Van den Berghe H, Louwagie A. A t(9;11)(q11;p15) translocation in a myelodysplastic syndrome with erythroleukemic trait. Cancer Genet Cytogenet 1986;23:281–2.
123. Merchav S, Wagemaker G, Souza LM, Tatarsky I. Impaired response of myelodysplastic marrow progenitors to stimulation with recombinant haematopoietic growth factors. Leukemia 1991;5:340–6.
124. Sawada K, Sato N, Tarumi T, et al. Proliferation and differentiation of myelodysplastic CD34+ cells in serum-free medium: response to individual colony-stimulating factors. Br J Haematol 1993;83:349–58.
125. Backx B, Broeders L, Hoefsloot LH, et al. Erythropoiesis in myelodysplastic syndrome: expression of receptors for erythropoietin and kit ligand. Leukemia 1996;10:466–72.
126. Mittelman M, Gardyn J, Carmel M, et al. Analysis of the erythropoietin receptor gene in patients with myeloproliferative and myelodysplastic syndromes. Leuk Res 1996;20:459–66.
127. Ohsaka A, Saionji K, Igari J, et al. Altered surface expression of effector cell molecules on neutrophils in myelodysplastic syndromes. Br J Haematol 1997;98:108–13.
128. Shibata S, Asano Y, Yokoyama T, et al. Analysis of the granulocyte colony-stimulating factor receptor gene structure using PCR-SSCP in myeloid leukemia and myelodysplastic syndrome. Eur J Haematol 1998;60:197–201.
129. Shimizu R, Komatsu N, Miura Y. Dominant negative effect of a truncated erythropoietin receptor (EPOR-T) on erythropoietin-induced erythroid differentiation: possible involvement of EPOR-T in ineffective erythropoiesis of myelodysplastic syndrome. Exp Hematol 1999;27:229–33.
130. Awaya N, Uchida H, Miyakawa Y, et al. Novel variant isoform of G-CSF receptor involved in induction of proliferation of FDCP-2 cells: relevance to the pathogenesis of myelodysplastic syndrome. J Cell Physiol 2002;191:327–35.
131. Hoefsloot L, van Amelsvoort M, Broeders L, et al. Erythropoietin-induced activation of STAT5 is impaired in the myelodysplastic syndrome. Blood 1997;89:1690–700.
132. Ohtsuki F, Yamamoto M, Nakagawa T, et al. Granulocyte-macrophage colony-stimulating factor abrogates transforming growth factor-beta 1-mediated cell cycle arrest by up-regulating cyclin D2/Cdk6. Br J Haematol 1997;98:520–7.
133. Fontenay-Roupie M, Bouscary D, Guesnu M, et al. Ineffective erythropoiesis in myelodysplastic syndromes: correlation with Fas expression but not with lack of erythropoietin receptor signal transduction. Br J Haematol 1999.106:464–73.
134. Brada SJ, de Wolf JT, Hendriks DW, et al. CD34+/CD36– cells from myelodysplasia patients have a limited capacity to proliferate but can differentiate in response to Epo and MGF stimulation [comments]. Leukemia 1998;12:882–6.
135. Truran L, Baines P, Hoy T, Burnett AK. GCSF augments post-progenitor proliferation in serum-free cultures of myelodysplastic marrow while ATRA enhances maturation. Leuk Res 1998;22:241–8.
136. Brakensiek K, Langer F, Schlegelberger B, et al. Hypermethylation of the suppressor of cytokine signalling-1 (SOCS-1) in myelodysplastic syndrome. Br J Haematol 2005;130:209–17.
137. Langer F, Dingemann J, Kreipe H, Lehmann U. Up-regulation of DNA methyltransferases DNMT1, 3A, and 3B in myelodysplastic syndrome. Leuk Res 2005;29:325–9.
138. Dar S, Mundle S, Andric T, et al. Biological characteristics of myelodysplastic syndrome patients who demonstrated high versus no intramedullary apoptosis. Eur J Haematol 1999;62:90–4.
139. Gersuk GM, Beckham C, Loken MR, et al. A role for tumour necrosis factor-alpha, Fas and Fas-Ligand in marrow failure associated with myelodysplastic syndrome. Br J Haematol 1998;103:176–88.
140. Greenberg PL. Apoptosis and its role in the myelodysplastic syndromes: implications for disease natural history and treatment. Leuk Res 1998;22:1123–36.
141. Raza A, Mundle S, Shetty V, et al. Novel insights into the biology of myelodysplastic syndromes: excessive apoptosis and the role of cytokines. Int J Hematol 1996;63:265–78.
142. Reddy PL, Shetty VT, Dutt D, et al. Increased incidence of mitochondrial cytochrome c-oxidase gene mutations in patients with myelodysplastic syndromes. Br J Haematol 2002;116:564–75.
143. Tehranchi R, Fadeel B, Forsblom AM, et al. Granulocyte colony-stimulating factor inhibits spontaneous cytochrome c release and mitochondria-dependent apoptosis of myelodysplastic syndrome hematopoietic progenitors. Blood 2003;101:1080–6.
144. Albitar M, Manshouri T, Shen Y, et al. Myelodysplastic syndrome is not merely "preleukemia." Blood 2002;100:791–8.
145. Fontenay-Roupie M, Bouscary D, Guesnu M, et al. Ineffective erythropoiesis in myelodysplastic syndromes: correlation with fas expression but not with lack of erythropoietin receptor signal transduction. Br J Haematol 1999;106:464–73.
146. Parker JE, Fishlock KL, Mijovic A, et al. 'Low-risk' myelodysplastic syndrome is associated with excessive apoptosis and an increased ratio of pro- versus anti-apoptotic bcl-2–related proteins. Br J Haematol 1998;103:1075–82.
147. Akiyama T, Matsunaga T, Terui T, et al. Involvement of transforming growth factor-beta and thrombopoietin in the pathogenesis of myelodysplastic syndrome with myelofibrosis. Leukemia, 2005;19:1558–66.
148. Knapp RH, Dewald GW, Pierre RV. Cytogenetic studies in 174 consecutive patients with preleukemic or myelodysplastic syndromes. Mayo Clin Proc 1985;60:507–16.
149. Musilova J, Michalova K. Chromosome study of 85 patients with myelodysplastic syndrome. Cancer Genet Cytogenet 1988;33:39–50.
150. Suciu S, Kuse R, Weh HJ, Hossfeld DK. Results of chromosome studies and their relation to morphology, course, and prognosis in 120 patients with de novo myelodysplastic syndrome. Cancer Genet Cytogenet 1990;44:15–26.
151. Almoguera C, Shibata D, Forrester K, et al. Most human carcinomas of the exocrine pancreas contain mutant c-K-ras genes. Cell 1988;53:549–54.
152. Bos JL. Ras oncogenes in human cancer: a review. Cancer Res 1989;49:4682–9.
153. Janssen JWG, Steenvoorden ACM, Lyons J, et al. RAS gene mutations in acute and chronic myelocytic leukemias, chronic myeloproliferative disorders, and myelodysplastic syndromes. Proc Natl Acad Sci U S A 1987;84:9228–32.
154. Pierre RV, Catovsky D, Mufti GJ, et al. Clinical-cytogenetic correlations in myelodysplasia (preleukemia). Cancer Genet Cytogenet 1989;40:149–61.
155. Cuneo A, Bigoni R, Cavazzini F, et al. Incidence and significance of cryptic chromosome aberrations detected by fluorescence in situ hybridization in acute myeloid leukemia with normal karyotype. Leukemia 2002;16:1745–51.
156. Horiike S, Taniwaki M, Misawa S, Abe T. Chromosome abnormalities and karyotypic evolution in 83 patients with myelodysplastic syndrome and predictive value for prognosis. Cancer 1988;62:1129–38.
157. Ben-Yehuda D, Krichevsky S, Caspi O, et al. Microsatellite instability and p53 mutations in therapy-related leukemia suggest mutator phenotype. Blood 1996;88:4296–303.
158. Glenn LD, Sanger WG, Kessinger A, Vaughan WP. Failure of karyotypic instability to predict clinical progression in patients with dysmyelopoietic syndromes. Hematol Pathol 1988;2:239–48.
159. de Souza Fernandez T, Menezes de Souza J, Macedo Silva ML, et al. Correlation of N-ras point mutations with specific chromosomal abnormalities in primary myelodysplastic syndrome. Leuk Res 1998;22:125–34.
160. Sheikhha MH, Tobal K, Liu Yin JA. High level of microsatellite instability but not hypermethylation of mismatch repair genes in therapy-related and secondary acute myeloid leukaemia and myelodysplastic syndrome. Br J Haematol 2002;117:359–65.
161. Teerenhovi L. Specificity of haematological indicators for "5q-syndrome" in patients with myelodysplastic syndromes. Eur J Haematol 1987;39:326–30.
162. Mathew P, Tefferi A, Dewald GW, et al. The 5q-syndrome: a single-institution study of 43 consecutive patients. Blood 1993;75:1040–5.
163. Pedersen-Bjergaard J, Philip P. Chromosome characteristics of therapy-related acute non-lymphocytic leukemia and preleukemia: possible implications for pathogenesis of the disease. Leuk Res 1987;11:315–8.
164. Le Beau MM, Albain KS, Larson RA, et al. Clinical and cytogenetic correlations in 63 patients with therapy-related myelodysplastic syndromes and acute nonlymphocytic leukemia: further evidence for characteristic abnormalities of chromosomes no. 5 and 7. J Clin Oncol 1986;4:325–45.
165. Smith MA, Rubinstein L, Anderson JR, et al. Secondary leukemia or myelodysplastic syndrome after treatment with epipodophyllotoxins. J Clin Oncol 1999;17:569–77.
166. Felix CA. Secondary leukemias induced by topoisomerase-targeted drugs. Biochim Biophys Acta 1998;1400:233–55.

167. Super HJ, McCabe NR, Thirman MJ, et al. Rearrangements of the MLL gene in therapy-related acute myeloid leukemia in patients previously treated with agents targeting DNA-topoisomerase II. Blood 1993;82:3705–11.
168. Land H, Parada LF, Weinberg RA. Cellular oncogenes and multistep carcinogenesis. Science 1983;222:771–8.
169. Vogelstein B, Fearon ER, Hamilton SR, et al. Genetic alterations during colorectal tumor development. N Engl J Med 1988;319:525–32.
170. Hirai H, Kobayashi Y, Mano H, et al. A point mutation at codon 13 of the N-ras oncogene in myelodysplastic syndrome. Nature 1987;327:430–2.
171. Horiike S, Misawa S, Nakai H, et al. N-*ras* mutation and karyotypic evolution are closely associated with leukemic transformation in myelodysplastic syndrome. Leukemia 1994;8:1331–6.
172. Paquette RL, Landaw EM, Pierre RV, et al. N-*ras* mutations are associated with poor prognosis and increased risk of leukemia in myelodysplastic syndrome. Blood 1993;82:590–9.
173. Padua RA, Guinn BA, Al-Sabah AI, et al. RAS, FMS and p53 mutations and poor clinical outcome in myelodysplasias: a 10-year follow-up. Leukemia 1998;12:887–92.
174. Liu E, Hjelle B, Morgan R, et al. Mutations of the Kirsten-ras proto-oncogene in human preleukaemia. Nature 1987;330:186–8.
175. Hirai H, Okada M, Mizoguchi H, et al. Relationship between an activated N-ras oncogene and chromosomal abnormality during leukemic progression from myelodysplastic syndrome. Blood 1988;71:256–8.
176. Lyons J, Janssen JWG, Bartram C, et al. Mutation of Ki-ras and N-ras oncogenes in myelodysplastic syndromes. Blood 1988;71:1707–12.
177. Padua RA, Carter G, Hughes D, et al. RAS mutations in myelodysplasia detected by amplification, oligonucleotide hybridization, and transformation. Leukemia 1988;2:503–10.
178. Pedersen-Bjergaard J, Janssen JWG, Lyons J, et al. Point mutation of the ras protooncogenes and chromosome aberrations in acute nonlymphocytic leukemia and preleukemia related to therapy with alkylating agents. Cancer Res 1988;48:1812–7.
179. Yunis JJ, Boot AJM, Mayer MG, Bos JL. Mechanisms of ras mutation in myelodysplastic syndrome. Oncogene 1989;4:609–14.
180. Bartram CR. Mutation in ras genes in myelocytic leukemias and myelodysplastic syndromes. Blood Cells 1988;14:533–8.
181. Bar-Eli M, Ahuja H, Gonzalez-Cadavid N, et al. Analysis of N-RAS exon-1 mutations in myelodysplastic syndromes by polymerase chain reaction and direct sequencing. Blood 1989;73:281–3.
182. Constantinidou M, Chalevelakis G, Economopoulos T, et al. Codon 12 ras mutations in patients with myelodysplastic syndrome: incidence and prognostic value. Ann Hematol 1997;74:11–4.
183. Neubauer A, Dodge RK, George SL, et al. Prognostic importance of mutations in the ras proto-oncogenes in de novo acute myeloid leukemia. Blood 1994;83:1603–11.
184. Darley RL, Hoy TG, Baines P, et al. Mutant N-RAS induces erythroid lineage dysplasia in human CD34+ cells. J Exp Med 1997;185:1337–47.
185. Le Beau MM, Lemons RS, Espinosa R 3rd, et al. Interleukin-4 and interleukin-5 map to human chromosome 5 in a region encoding growth factors and receptors and are deleted in myeloid leukemias with a del(5q). Blood 1989;73:647–50.
186. Boultwood J, Fidler C, Strickson AJ, et al. Narrowing and genomic annotation of the commonly deleted region of the 5q- syndrome. Blood 2002;99:4638–41.
187. Harada H, Kitagawa M, Tanaka N, et al. Anti-oncogenic and oncogenic potentials of interferon regulatory factors-1 and -2. Science 1993;259:971–4.
188. Willman CL, Sever CE, Pallavicini MG, et al. Deletion of *IRF-1*, mapping to chromosome 5q31.1, in human leukemia and preleukemic myelodysplasia. Science 1993;259:968–71.
189. Tennant GB, Jacobs A. Effect of 5637-conditioned medium on peripheral blood granulocyte-macrophage progenitors in normal subjects and patients with the myelodysplastic syndrome. Leukemia Res 1989;13:385–9.
190. Boultwood J, Rack K, Kelly S, et al. Loss of both *CSF1R* (*FMS*) alleles in patients with myelodysplasia and a chromosome 5 deletion. Proc Natl Acad Sci U S A 1991;88:6176–80.
191. Kroef MJ, Bolk MW, Willemze R, Landegent JE. Absence of loss of heterozygosity of the IRF1 gene in some patients with a 5q31 deletion. Blood 1994;83:2382.
192. Jonveaux P, Fenaux P, Quiquandon I, et al. Mutations in the p53 gene in myelodysplastic syndromes. Oncogene 1991;6:2243–7.
193. Preudhomme C, Lubin R, Lepelley P, et al. Detection of serum anti p53 antibodies and their correlation with p53 mutations in myelodysplastic syndromes and acute myeloid leukemia. Leukemia 1994;8:1589–91.
194. Kurotaki H, Tsushima Y, Nagai K, Yagihashi S. Apoptosis, bcl-2 expression and p53 accumulation in myelodysplastic syndrome, myelodysplastic-syndrome-derived acute myelogenous leukemia and de novo acute myelogenous leukemia. Acta Haematol 2000;102:115–23.
195. Soenen V, Preudhomme C, Roumier C, et al. 17p Deletion in acute myeloid leukemia and myelodysplastic syndrome. Analysis of breakpoints and deleted segments by fluorescence in situ. Blood 1998;91:1008–15.
196. Vigon I, Dreyfus F, Melle J, et al. Expression of the c-*mpl* proto-oncogene in human hematologic malignancies. Blood 1993;82:877–83.
197. Golub TR, Barker GF, Lovett M, Gilliland DG. Fusion of PDGF receptor β to a novel *ets*-like gene, *tel*, in chronic myelomonocytic leukemia with t(5;12) chromosomal translocation. Cell 1994;77:307–16.
198. Kreider BL, Orkin SH, Ihle JN. Loss of erythropoietin responsiveness in erythroid progenitors due to expression of the Evi-1 myeloid-transforming gene. Proc Natl Acad Sci U S A 1993;90:6454–8.
199. Morishita K, Parganas E, Matsugi T, Ihle JN. Expression of the *Evi-1* zinc finger gene in 32Dc13 myeloid cells blocks granulocytic differentiation in response to granulocyte colony-stimulating factor. Mol Cell Biol 1992;12:183–9.
200. Creutzig U, Cantu-Rajnoldi A, Ritter J, et al. Myelodysplastic syndromes in childhood. Am J Pediatr Hematol Oncol 1987;9:324–30.
201. Tricot G, Vlietinck R, Boogaerts MA, et al. Prognostic factors in the myelodysplastic syndromes: importance of initial data on peripheral blood counts, bone marrow cytology, trephine biopsy and chromosomal analysis. Br J Haematol 1985;60:19–27.
202. Yunis JJ, Lobell M, Arnesen MA, et al. Refined chromosome study helps define prognostic subgroups in most patients with primary myelodysplastic syndrome and acute myelogenous leukemia. Br J Haematol 1988;68:189–94.
203. Paydas S, Zorludemir S. Leukaemia cutis and leukaemic vasculitis. Br J Dermatol 2000;143:773–9.
204. Tani K, Fujii H, Takahashi K, et al. Erythrocyte enzyme activities in myelodysplastic syndromes: elevated pyruvate kinase activity. Am J Hematol 1989;30:97–103.
205. Breton-Gorius J, Houssay D, Vilde JL, Dreyfus B. Partial myeloperoxidase deficiency in a case of preleukaemia. II. Defects of degranulation and abnormal bactericidal activity of blood neutrophils. Br J Haematol 1975;30:279–88.
206. Dreyfus B, Sultan C, Rochant H, et al. Anomalies of blood group antigens and erythrocyte enzymes in two types of chronic refractory anaemia. Br J Haematol 1969;16:303–12.
207. Yoshida A, Kumazaki T, Dave V, et al. Suppressed expression of blood group B antigen and blood group galactosyltransferase in a preleukemic subject. Blood 1985;66:990–2.
208. Uchida T, Kokubun K, Abe R, et al. Ferrokinetic evaluation of erythropoiesis in patients with myelodysplastic syndromes. Acta Haematol 1988;79:81–3.
209. Peters RE, May A, Jacobs A. Increased alpha:non-alpha globin chain synthesis ratios in myelodysplastic syndromes and myeloid leukaemia. J Clin Pathol 1986;39:1233–5.
210. De Witte T, Van Biezen A, Hermans J, et al. Autologous bone marrow transplantation for patients with myelodysplastic syndrome (MDS) or acute myeloid leukemia following MDS. Chronic and acute leukemia working parties of the European Group for Blood and Marrow Transplantation. Blood 1997;90:3853–7.
211. Elghetany M, MacCallum J, Nelson D, et al. Abnormal granulocytes in myelodysplastic syndromes: a morphologic, cytochemical and immunocytochemical study of 71 patients. Blood 1990;76 Suppl:267a.
212. Hokland P, Kerndrup G, Griffin JD, Ellegaard J. Analysis of leukocyte differentiation antigens in blood and bone marrow from preleukemia (refractory anemia) patients using monoclonal antibodies. Blood 1986;67:898–902.
213. Baumann MA, Keller RH, McFadden PW, et al. Myeloid cell surface phenotype in myelodysplasia: evidence for abnormal persistence of an early myeloid differentiation antigen. Am J Hematol 1986;22:251–7.
214. Clark RE, Ismail SAD, Jacobs A, et al. A randomized trial of 13-cis retinoic acid with or without cytosine arabinoside in patients with the myelodysplastic syndrome. Br J Haematol 1987;66:77–83.
215. Silverman LR, Yagi MJ, Holland JF, Bekesi JG. Lineage infidelity with coexpression of myeloid and lymphoid markers and IL-2 receptor are common in myelodysplastic syndromes. Proc Am Assoc Cancer Res 1992;33:152.
216. Felzman T, Gisslinger H, Krieger O, et al. Immunophenotypic characterization of myelomonocytic cells in patients with myelodysplastic syndrome. Br J Haematol 1993;84:428–35.
217. Lowe GM, Dang Y, Watson F, et al. Identification of a subgroup of myelodysplastic patients with a neutrophil stimulation-signalling defect. Br J Haematol 1994;86:761–6.
218. Felman P, Bryon PA, Gentilhomme O, et al. The syndrome of abnormal chromatin clumping in leukocytes: a myelodysplastic disorder with proliferative features? Br J Haematol 1988;70:49–54.
219. Russell NH, Keenan JP, Bellingham AJ. Thrombocytopathy in preleukaemia: association with a defect of thromboxane A2 activity. Br J Haematol 1979;41:417–25.
220. Raman KS, Van Slyck EJ, Riddle J, et al. Platelet function and structure in myeloproliferative disease, myelodysplastic syndrome, and secondary thrombocytosis. Am J Clin Pathol 1989;91:647–55.
221. Tuzuner N, Cox C, Rowe J, et al. Hypocellular myelodysplastic syndromes: new proposals. Br J Haematol 1995;91:612–7.
222. Sorskaar D, Forre O, Albrechtsen D, Stavem P. Decreased natural killer cell activity versus normal natural killer cell markers in mononuclear cells from patients with smouldering leukemia. Scand J Haematol 1986;37:154–61.
223. Mufti GJ, Figes A, Hamblin TJ, et al. Immunological abnormalities in myelodysplastic syndromes. Br J Haematol 1986;63:143–7.
224. Merchav S, Nagler A, Silvian I, et al. Immunoglobulin synthesis in myelodysplastic syndromes: normal B-cell and immunoregulatory T-cell functions. Clin Immunol Immunopathol 1987;42:195–201.
225. Economopoulos T, Economidou J, Giannopoulos G, et al. Immune abnormalities in myelodysplastic syndromes. J Clin Pathol 1985;38:908–11.
226. Stahl D, Egerer G, Goldschmidt H, et al. Altered self-reactive antibody repertoires are a general feature of patients with myelodysplastic syndrome. J Autoimmun 2001;16:77–86.
227. Prchal JT, Throckmorton DW, Carroll AJ, et al. A common progenitor for human myeloid and lymphoid cells. Science 1978;274:590–1.
228. Ogata K, Nakamura K, Yokose N, et al. Clinical significance of phenotypic features of blasts in patients with myelodysplastic syndrome. Blood 2002;100:3887–96.
229. Chang CC, Cleveland RP. Decreased CD10-positive mature granulocytes in bone marrow from patients with myelodysplastic syndrome. Arch Pathol Lab Med 2000;124:1152–6.
230. Eighetany MT. Diagnostic utility of flow cytometric immunophenotyping in myelodysplastic syndrome. Blood 2002;99:391–2.
231. Ito S, Ishida Y, Murai K, Kuriya S. Flow cytometric analysis of aberrant antigen expression of blasts using CD45 blast gating for minimal residual disease in acute leukemia and high-risk myelodysplastic syndrome. Leuk Res 2001;25:205–11.
232. Kasahara S, Hara T, Itoh H, et al. Hypoplastic myelodysplastic syndromes can be distinguished from acquired aplastic anaemia by bone marrow stem cell expression of the tumour necrosis factor receptor. Br J Haematol 2002;118:181–8.
233. Miller DT, Stelzer GT. Contributions of flow cytometry to the analysis of the myelodysplastic syndrome. Clin Lab Med 2001;21:811–28.
234. Stetler-Stevenson M, Arthur DC, Jabbour N, et al. Diagnostic utility of flow cytometric immunophenotyping in myelodysplastic syndrome. Blood 2001;98:979–87.
235. Bain BJ. The relationship between the myelodysplastic syndromes and the myeloproliferative disorders. Leuk Lymphoma 1999;34:443–9.
236. Gupta R, Abdalla SH, Bain BJ. Thrombocytosis with sideroblastic erythropoiesis: a mixed myeloproliferative myelodysplastic syndrome. Leuk Lymphoma 1999;34:615–9.
237. Lambertenghi-Deliliers G, Annaloro C, Pozzoli E, et al. Cytogenetic and myelodysplastic alterations after autologous hemopoietic stem cell transplantation. Leuk Res 1999;23:291–7.
238. Lambertenghi-Deliliers G, Orazi A, Luksch R, et al. Myelodysplastic syndrome with increased marrow fibrosis: a

distinct clinico-pathological entity. Br J Haematol 1991;78:161–6.
239. Sashida G, Tauchi T, Ando K, et al. Translocation (5;18) in a patient with myelodysplastic syndrome: refractory anemia with excess blasts in transformation. Cancer Genet Cytogenet 2000;121:230–1.
240. Maciejewski JP, Follmann D, Nakamura R, et al. Increased frequency of HLA-DR2 in patients with paroxysmal nocturnal hemoglobinuria and the PNH/aplastic anemia syndrome. Blood 2001;98:3513–9.
241. Maciejewski JP, Risitano A, Kook H, et al. Immune pathophysiology of aplastic anemia. Int J Hematol 2002;76 Suppl 1:207–14.
242. Maciejewski JP, Selleri C. Evolution of clonal cytogenetic abnormalities in aplastic anemia. Leuk Lymphoma 2004;45:433–40.
243. Paquette RL. Diagnosis and management of aplastic anemia and myelodysplastic syndrome. Oncology (Huntingt) 2002;16:153–61.
244. Saunthararajah Y, Molldrem JL, Rivera M, et al. Coincident myelodysplastic syndrome and T-cell large granular lymphocytic disease: clinical and pathophysiological features. Br J Haematol 2001;112:195–200.
245. Horiike S, Yokota S, Nakao M, et al. Tandem duplications of the FLT3 receptor gene are associated with leukemic transformation of myelodysplasia. Leukemia 1997;11:1442–6.
246. Touw IP, Dong F. Severe congenital neutropenia terminating in acute myeloid leukemia: disease progression associated with mutations in the granulocyte-colony stimulating factor receptor gene. Leuk Res 1996;20:629–31.
247. Dong F, Brynes RK, Tidow N, et al. Mutations in the gene for the granulocyte colony-stimulating-factor receptor in patients with acute myeloid leukemia preceded by severe congenital neutropenia [comments]. N Engl J Med 1995;333:487–93.
248. Hermans MH, Antonissen C, Ward AC, et al. Sustained receptor activation and hyperproliferation in response to granulocyte colony-stimulating factor (G-CSF) in mice with a severe congenital neutropenia/acute myeloid leukemia-derived mutation in the G- CSF receptor gene. J Exp Med 1999;189:683–92.
249. Le Beau MM, Epstein ND, O'Brien SJ, et al. The interleukin 3 gene is located on human chromosome 5 and is deleted in myeloid leukemias with a deletion of 5q. Proc Natl Acad Sci U S A 1987;88:5913–7.
250. Huebner K, Isobe M, Croce CM, et al. The human gene encoding GM-CSF is 5q21-q32, the chromosome region deleted in the 5q- anomaly. Science 1985;230:1282–5.
251. Gordon M, Riley GP, Watt SM, Greaves MF. Compartmentalization of a hematopoietic growth factor (GM-CSF) by glycosaminoglycans in the bone marrow microenvironment. Nature 1987;326:403–5.
252. Sankar M, Tanaka K, Kumaravel TS, et al. Identification of a commonly deleted region at 17p13.3 in leukemia and lymphoma associated with 17p abnormality. Leukemia 1998;12:510–6.
253. Najfeld V, Scalise A, Silverman L. Three regions on chromosome 1 identified to be involved in pathogenesis of myelodysplasia. Leuk Res 1999;23:S9.
254. Uchida T, Kinoshita T, Nagai H, et al. Hypermethylation of the p15INK4B gene in myelodysplastic syndromes. Blood 1997;90:1403–9.
255. Tanaka T, Mitani K, Kurokawa M, et al. Dual functions of the AML1/Evi-1 chimeric protein in the mechanism of leukemogenesis in t(3;21) leukemias. Mol Cell Biol 1995;15:2383–92.
256. Friend C, Scher W, Holland J, Sato T. Hemoglobin synthesis in murine virus-induced leukemic cells in vitro: stimulation of erythroid differentiation by dimethyl sulfoxide. Proc Nat Acad Sci U S A 1971;68:378–82.
257. Kornblith AB, Herndon JE 2nd, Silverman LR, et al. Impact of azacytidine on the quality of life of patients with myelodysplastic syndrome treated in a randomized phase III trial: a Cancer and Leukemia Group B study. J Clin Oncol 2002;20:2441–52.
258. Silverman LR, Demakos EP, Peterson BL, et al. Randomized controlled trial of azacitidine in patients with the myelodysplastic syndrome: a study of the cancer and leukemia group B. J Clin Oncol 2002;20:2429–40.
259. Christman J, Mendelsohn N, Herzog D, Schneiderman N. Effect of 5-azacytidine on differentiation and DNA methylation in human promyelocytic leukemia cells (HL-60). Cancer Res 1983;43:763–9.
260. Creusot F, Acs G, Christman J. Inhibition of DNA methyltransferase and induction of Friend erythroleukemia cell differentiation by 5-azacytidine and 5-aza-2'deoxycytidine. J Biol Chem 1982;257:2041–8.
261. Ley T, DeSimone J, Anagrou N, et al. 5-Azacytidine selectively increases, gamma-globin synthesis in a patient with B+ thalassemia. N Engl J Med 1982;307:1469–75.
262. Silverman LR, Holland JF, Weinberg RS, et al. Effects of treatment with 5-azacytidine on the in vivo and in vitro hematopoiesis in patients with myelodysplastic syndromes. Leukemia 1993;7 suppl:21–9.
263. Silverman L, Holland JF, Demakos E, et al. Azacitidine in myelodysplastic syndromes: CALGB studies 8421 and 8921 [abstract 12]. Ann Hematol 1994;68.
264. Silverman L, Zinzar S, Holland J. Azacitidine acts as biologic response modifier on hematopoietic cell response to cytokines [abstract]. Proc Am Assoc Cancer Res 1998;39:405.
265. Wijermans PW, Krulder JW, Huijgens PC, Neve P. Continuous infusion of low-dose 5-Aza-2'-deoxycytidine in elderly patients with high-risk myelodysplastic syndrome. Leukemia 1997;11 Suppl 1:S19–23.
266. Wijermans P, Lubbert M, Verhoef G, et al. Low-dose 5-aza-2'-deoxycytidine, a DNA hypomethylating agent, for the treatment of high-risk myelodysplastic syndrome: a multicenter phase II study in elderly patients. J Clin Oncol 2000;18:956–62.
267. Cheson BD, Jasperse DM, Simon R, Friedman MA. A critical appraisal of low-dose cytosine arabinoside in patients with acute non-lymphocytic leukemia and myelodysplastic syndromes. J Clin Oncol 1986;4:1857–64.
268. Miller KB, Kyungmann K, Morrison FS, et al. The evaluation of low-dose cytarabine in the treatment of myelodysplastic syndromes: a phase III intergroup study. Ann Hematol 1992;65:162–8.
269. Breitman TR, Selonick SE, Collins SJ. Induction of differentiation of the human promyelocytic leukemia cell line (HL-60) by retinoic acid. Proc Natl Acad Sci U S A 1980;77:2936–40.
270. Clark RE, Lush CJ, Jacobs A, Smith SA. Effect of 13-cis-retinoic acid on survival of patients with myelodysplastic syndrome. Lancet 1987;4:763–5.
271. Greenberg BR, Durie BGM, Barnett TC, Meyskens FL Jr. Phase I-II study of 13-cis-retinoic acid in myelodysplastic syndrome. Cancer Treat Rep 1985;69:1369–74.
272. Koeffler HP, Heitjan D, Mertelsmann R, et al. Randomized study of 13-cis retinoic acid v placebo in the myelodysplastic disorders. Blood 1988;71:703–8.
273. Kurzrock R, Estey E, Talpaz M. All-trans retinoic acid: tolerance and biologic effects in myelodysplastic syndrome. J Clin Oncol 1993;11:1489–95.
274. Deeg HJ, Gotlib J, Beckham C, et al. Soluble TNF receptor fusion protein (etanercept) for the treatment of myelodysplastic syndrome: a pilot study. Leukemia 2002;16:162–4.
275. Maciejewski JP, Ristiano AM, Sloand EM, et al. A pilot study of the recombinant soluble human tumour necrosis factor receptor (p75)-Fc fusion protein in patients with myelodysplastic syndrome. Br J Haematol 2002;117:119–26.
276. Raza A, Meyer P, Dutt D, et al. Thalidomide produces transfusion independence in long-standing refractory anemias of patients with myelodysplastic syndromes. Blood 2001;98:958–65.
277. Strupp C, Germing U, Aivado M, et al. Thalidomide for the treatment of patients with myelodysplastic syndromes. Leukemia 2002;16:1–6.
278. List A, Kurtin S, Roe DJ, et al. Efficacy of lenalidomide in myelodysplastic syndromes. N Engl J Med 2005;352:549–57.
279. Giles FJ, Cooper MA, Silverman LR, et al. Phase II study of SU5416, a small molecule vascular endothelial growth factor (VEGF) tyrosine kinase receptor inhibitor, in patients with refractory myeloproliferative diseases. Cancer 2003;97:1920–8.
280. Karp JE, Lancet JE, Kaufmann SH, et al. Clinical and biologic activity of the farnesyltransferase inhibitor R115777 in adults with refractory and relapsed acute leukemias: a phase 1 clinical-laboratory correlative trial. Blood 2001;97:3361–9.
281. Kurzrock R, Albitar M, Cortes JE, et al. Phase II study of R115777, a farnesyl transferase inhibitor, in myelodysplastic syndrome. J Clin Oncol 2004;22:1287–92.
282. Najean Y, Pecking A. Refractory anaemia with excess of myeloblasts in the bone marrow: A clinical trial of androgens in 90 patients. Brit J Haematol 1977;37:25–33.
283. Najean Y, Pecking A. Refractory anemia with excess of blast cells: prognostic factors and effect of treatment with androgens or cytosine arabinoside—results of a prospective trial in 58 patients. Cancer 1979;44:1976–82.
284. Bagby GC, Gabourel JD, Linman JW. Glucocorticoid therapy in the preleukemic syndrome. Ann Int Med 1980;92:55–8.
285. Cines DB, Cassileth PA, Kiss JE. Danazol therapy in myelodysplasia. Ann Intern Med 1985;103:58–60.
286. Estey E, Thall P, Andreeff M, et al. Use of granulocyte colony-stimulating factor before, during, and after fludarabine plus cytarabine induction therapy of newly diagnosed acute myelogenous leukemia or myelodysplastic syndromes: comparison with fludarabine plus cytarabine without granulocyte colony-stimulating factor [comments]. J Clin Oncol 1994;12:671–8.
287. Estey EH, Thall PF, Pierce S, et al. Randomized phase II study of fludarabine + cytosine arabinoside + idarubicin +/– all-trans retinoic acid +/– granulocyte colony-stimulating factor in poor prognosis newly diagnosed acute myeloid leukemia and myelodysplastic syndrome. Blood 1999;93:2478–84.
288. Fenaux P, Lai JL, Jouet JP, et al. Aggressive chemotherapy in adult primary myelodysplastic syndromes. A report on 29 cases. Blut 1988;57:297–302.
289. Larson RA, Wernli M, Le Beau MM, et al. Short remission durations in therapy-related leukemia despite cytogenetic complete responses to high-dose cytarabine. Blood 1988;72:1333–9.
290. Martiat P, Ferrant A, Michaux JL, Sokal G. Intensive chemotherapy for acute non-lymphoblastic leukemia after primary myelodysplastic syndrome. Hematol Oncol 1988;6:299–305.
291. Tricot G, Boogaerts MA. The role of aggressive chemotherapy in the treatment of the myelodysplastic syndromes. Br J Haematol 1986;63:477–83.
292. Beran M, Estey E, O'Brien SM, et al. Results of topotecan single-agent therapy in patients with myelodysplastic syndromes and chronic myelomonocytic leukemia. Leuk Lymphoma 1998;31:521–31.
293. Beran M, Giles F, Cortes J, et al. Comparison of the cyclophosphamide, ara-C, topotecan regimen to ara-C plus topotecan or idarubicin as initial therapy for patients with adverse abnormal karyotype acute myeloid leukemia. Blood 1999;94 Suppl:226b.
294. Appelbaum FR, Anderson J. Allogeneic bone marrow transplantation for myelodysplastic syndrome: outcomes analysis according to IPSS score. Leukemia 1998;12 Suppl 1:S25–9.
295. Bunin NJ, Casper JT, Chitambar C, et al. Partially matched bone marrow transplantation in patients with myelodysplastic syndromes. J Clin Oncol 1988;6:1851–5.
296. Appelbaum FR, Barrall J, Storb R, et al. Bone marrow transplantation for patients with myelodysplasia. Ann Int Med 1990;112:590–7.
297. O'Donnell MR, Nademanee AP, Snyder DS, et al. Bone marrow transplantation for myelodysplastic and myeloproliferative syndromes. J Clin Oncol 1987;5:1822–6.
298. Kernan NA, Bartsch G, Ash RC, et al. Analysis of 462 transplantations from unrelated donors facilitated by the National Marrow Donor Program. N Engl J Med 1993;328:593–602.
299. Longmore G, Guinan EC, Weinstein HJ, et al. Bone marrow transplantation for myelodysplasia and secondary acute nonlymphoblastic leukemia. J Clin Oncol 1990;8:1707–14.
300. Cutler CS, Lee SJ, Greenberg P, et al. A decision analysis of allogeneic bone marrow transplantation for the myelodysplastic syndromes: delayed transplantation for low-risk myelodysplasia is associated with improved outcome. Blood 2004;104:579–85.
301. Ho AY, Pagliuca A, Kenyon M, et al. Reduced-intensity allogeneic hematopoietic stem cell transplantation for myelodysplastic syndrome and acute myeloid leukemia with multilineage dysplasia using fludarabine, busulphan, and alemtuzumab (FBC) conditioning. Blood 2004;104:1616–23.
302. Oosterveld M, Suciu S, Rodts P, et al. Peripheral blood stem cell mobilization after chemotherapy in patients with high risk myelodysplastic syndrome. An ongoing prospective European multicenter study supported by Biomed II. Leuk Res 1999;23:S84.
303. Metcalf D. The granulocyte-macrophage colony-stimulating factors. Science 1985;229:16–22.
304. Schuster MW, Larson RA, Thompson JA, et al. Granulocyte-macrophage colony-stimulating factor (GM-CSF) for myelodysplastic syndrome (MDS): results of a multicenter randomized controlled trial [abstract]. Blood 1990;76:318a.
305. Vadhan-Raj S, Keating M, LeMaistre A, et al. Effects of recombinant human granulocyte-macrophage colony-stimulating factor in patients with myelodysplastic syndromes. N Engl J Med 1987;317:1545–52.
306. Hoelzer D, Ganser A, Vokers B, et al. In vitro and in vivo action of recombinant human GM-CSF (rhGM-CSF) in

patients with myelodysplastic syndromes. Blood Cells 1988;14:551–9.

307. Rose C, Wattel E, Bastion Y, et al. Treatment with very low-dose GM-CSF in myelodysplastic syndromes with neutropenia. A report on 28 cases. Leukemia 1994;8:1458–62.

308. Negrin RS, Haeuber DH, Nagler A, et al. Maintenance treatment of patients with myelodysplastic syndromes using recombinant human granulocyte colony-stimulating factor. Blood 1990;76:36–43.

309. Greenberg P, Taylor K, Larson R, et al. Phase III randomized multicenter trial of G-CSF vs. observation for myelodysplastic syndromes (MDS) [abstract]. Blood 1993;82 Suppl 1:196a.

310. Ganser A, Seipelt G, Lindermann A, et al. Effects of recombinant human interleukin-3 in patients with myelodysplastic syndromes. Blood 1990;76:455–62.

311. Kurzrock R, Talpaz M, Estrov Z, et al. Phase I study of recombinant human Interleukin-3 in patients with bone marrow failure. J Clin Oncol 1991;9:1241–50.

312. Verhoef GEG, Zachee P, Ferrant A, et al. Recombinant human erythropoietin for the treatment of anemia in the myelodysplastic syndromes: a clinical and erythrokinetic assessment. Ann Hematol 1992;64:16–21.

313. Kurzrock R, Talpaz M, Estey E, et al. Erythropoietin treatment in patients with myelodysplastic syndrome and anemia. Leukemia 1991;5:985–90.

314. Hellstrom-Lindberg E. Efficacy of erythropoietin in the myelodysplastic syndrome: a meta-analysis of 205 patients from 17 studies. Br J Haematol 1995;89:67–71.

315. Musto P, Falcone A, Carotenuto M, et al. Granulocyte colony -stimulating factor and erythropoietin for anemia of myelodysplastic syndromes: a real improvement with respect to erythropoietin alone? Blood 1994;1687–8.

316. Jadersten M, Montgomery SM, Dybedal I, et al. Long-term outcome of treatment of anemia in MDS with erythropoietin and G-CSF. Blood 2005;106:803–11.

317. Hellstrom-Lindberg E, Gulbrandsen N, Lindberg G, et al. A validated decision model for treating the anaemia of myelodysplastic syndromes with erythropoietin + granulocyte colony-stimulating factor: significant effects on quality of life. Br J Haematol 2003;120:1037–46.

318. Molldrem JJ, Caples M, Mavroudis D, et al. Antithymocyte globulin for patients with myelodysplastic syndrome. Br J Haematol 1997;99:699–705.

319. Molldrem JJ, Leifer E, Bahceci E, et al. Antithymocyte globulin for treatment of the bone marrow failure associated with myelodysplastic syndromes. Ann Intern Med 2002;137:156–63.

320. Molldrem JJ, Jiang YZ, Stetler-Stevenson M, et al. Haematological response of patients with myelodysplastic syndrome to antithymocyte globulin is associated with a loss of lymphocyte-mediated inhibition of CFU-GM and alterations in T-cell receptor Vbeta profiles. Br J Haematol 1998;102:1314–22.

321. Kantarjian HM. Treatment of myelodysplastic syndrome: questions raised by the azacitidine experience. J Clin Oncol 2002;20:2415–6.

113

Acute Myeloid Leukemia in Adults

Mast Cell Leukemia and Other Mast Cell Neoplasms

Charles A. Schiffer, MD
Richard M. Stone, MD

Acute myeloid leukemia (AML) is the most common variant of acute leukemia occurring in adults, comprising approximately 80% of cases of acute leukemia diagnosed in individuals greater than 20 years of age. Striking advances in transfusion medicine and the treatment of infections, the development of potent antiemetics, as well as improved chemotherapeutic approaches, have eradicated the therapeutic nihilism that characterized many editorials and reports as late as the 1970s. Currently, more than 80% of young adults and 60% of all patients can achieve complete remission (CR) defined as a morphologically normal bone marrow with normal neutrophil and platelet counts.[1] Varying with patient age and other biologic factors, from 10 to 70% of these complete responders can be expected to achieve long-term survival with the likelihood that most of these individuals are cured of their disease (Figure 113-1).

AML affects adults of all ages but is especially common in older adults. The median age of patients with de novo AML entered on recent cooperative group studies is approximately 55 years, and the median age at diagnosis is probably 65 to 70 years.[2] AML can present either as a de novo leukemia without an apparent antecedent illness or as an evolution from obvious marrow disorders such as myelodysplasia, aplastic anemia, and Fanconi anemia, or after the administration of therapy for other types of cancers or nonmalignant disorders. An acute leukemic phase morphologically indistinguishable from AML uniformly terminates chronic myelogenous leukemia (CML) and, less often, other myeloproliferative disorders. De novo AML in young adults is believed usually to derive from stem cells that are more committed to myeloid lineage than the more primitive stem cells that give rise to secondary AML or AML in older patients.[3]

The proper care of patients with AML is a multidisciplinary effort, benefiting from a team

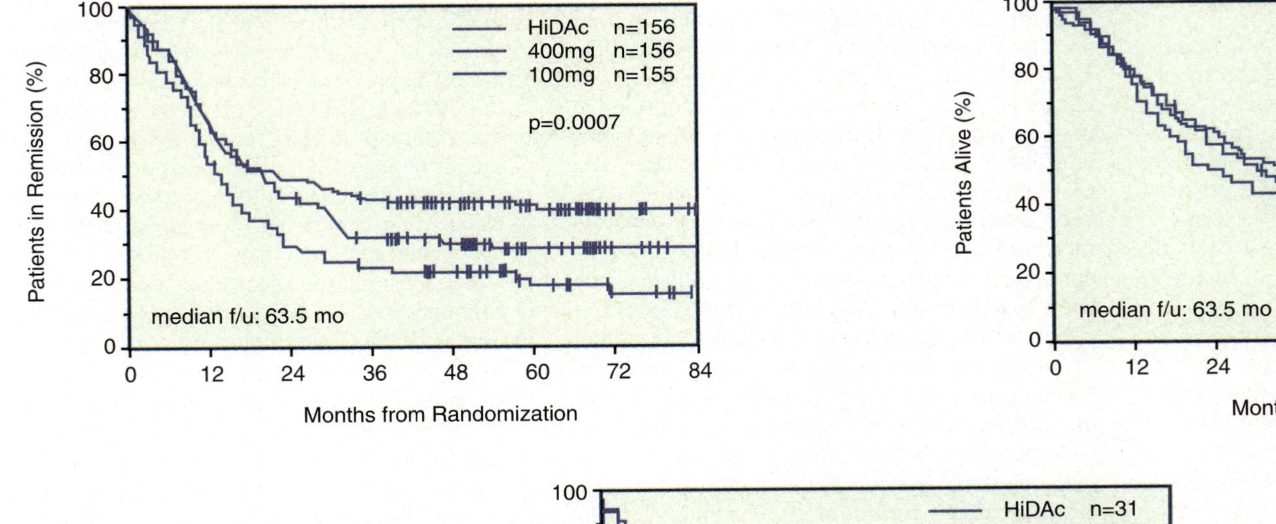

Figure 113-1 Data from the Cancer and Leukemia Group B demonstrating the effect of different ara-C doses and schedules in patients of different ages with acute myeloid leukemia in remission.[2] *Top left*, Complete remission (CR) duration in patients < 60 years old; *Top right*, survival of CR patients < 60 years old; *bottom*, CR duration of patients ≥ 60 year old. These overall long term results are representative of outcomes in trials from leukemia treatment groups around the world.

approach. Expertise in transfusion medicine, infectious disease, placement and care of indwelling catheters, nutrition, and antineoplastic drug pharmacology are required as well as the availability of sophisticated diagnostic laboratory facilities and psychosocial counseling for both patients and their families. These disciplines are described elsewhere in this text, but their critical importance in the care of the leukemia patient cannot be overestimated.

PATHOGENESIS AND ETIOLOGY

The pathophysiology of AML can be explained by the acquisition of genetic changes in bone marrow stem cells that both promote self-renewal and impair normal hematopoietic differentiation, resulting in an accumulation of immature cells. The genetic changes may involve mutations that lead to activation of growth-promoting protooncogenes, inactivation of tumor suppressor genes, or alterations in transcription factors.[4,5] For example, mutations in codons 12, 13, or 61 of the N-*ras* gene that encodes a 21 kDa guanosine nucleotide binding protein involved in signal transduction have been noted in up to 30% of those with AML.[6] Mutations of the flt-3 growth factor receptor are also common,[7,8] suggesting its role in promoting autologous proliferation. Mutations of the tumor suppressor genes *Rb*[9] and *TP53*[10] have been observed and appear to confer a worse prognosis.

The greatest insight regarding AML pathogenesis has been provided by the identification of genes at cytogenetic breakpoints involved in balanced translocations. The fusion proteins generated by the translocation generally result in disruption of transcription factors believed to be critical in myeloid differentiation.[5,11] Many of these chromosomal abnormalities, for example, t(8;21), t(15;17), and inv (16), are associated with specific AML subtypes and carry prognostic importance. Recent murine experiments indicate that transfection of genes that primarily alter cell differentiation, such as *AML1/ETO*, are necessary but not sufficient to produce frank AML.[12] A recent hypothesis, supported by further murine experiments, proposes that additional mutations in genes that provide an increased proliferative signal, such as flt-3, are needed to result in AML.[13] The mechanisms that account for poor prognosis when loss of all or parts of chromosomes occur, remain to be elucidated.

Although more acquired genetic lesions that lead to leukemia are being rapidly defined, DNA damage from a known cause accounts for only a small fraction of patients with AML. Leukemias clearly occur with increased frequency after nuclear bomb[14] or therapeutic[15] radiation exposure, after certain types of chemotherapy, and with heavy and continuous occupational exposures to benzene.[16] It is now recognized that there are two types of chemotherapy-related leukemias: (1) the classic alkylating agent-induced type,[17] in which the leukemia is preceded by a myelodysplastic prodrome and is characterized by clonal abnormalities, often with loss of chromosome 5 and/or 7 and (2) an epipodophyllotoxin topoisomerase II inhibitor associated type with a shorter (median 2- vs 5-year) incubation period that is usually associated with myelomonocytic or monocytic differentiation and abnormalities at the 11q23 region.[18]

There have been a number of large, survey-type epidemiologic studies that have attempted to link a variety of environmental exposures to leukemia incidence. Many of these studies contain relatively small sample sizes and identify modest, if any, increases in risk ratio. Older and retrospective studies may be suspect in that the pathologic diagnoses were not usually reviewed and classified using contemporary criteria, and, therefore, the distinctions between myeloid, lymphoid, and perhaps even acute versus chronic leukemia may not be accurate. Furthermore, as in many epidemiologic studies, it is difficult to quantify the degree of exposure to various environmental insults. There may be a small increased risk associated with cigarette smoking,[19] whereas exposure to electromagnetic radiation[20] seems an unlikely cause of AML. However, occupational exposures, particularly to benzene[16] or petrochemicals,[21] have been implicated in the development of AML.

Nor are the acute leukemias a familial or inherited disorder. Except for the increased incidence of acute leukemia occurring during the first 6 months after diagnosis in the identical twin of an affected child,[22,23] the occurrence of multiple cases of acute leukemia in a given family is extremely rare. Indeed, it is quite important to reassure family members about this because this is often an unasked question when leukemia is first diagnosed in a relative. A few families have been described in which leukemia incidence is increased.[24–27] In some of these families, different types of leukemias and other cancers have been found. In other, potentially more informative families, such as a large family in which seven cases of erythroleukemia or myelodysplasia developed in three successive generations,[26] the morphologic or clinical characteristics of the leukemia have been similar, suggesting a common, heritable genetic mutation. Most of these cases antedated current molecular biologic techniques, and the available cytogenetic data do not suggest a common chromosomal abnormality or linkage to specific human leukocyte antigen (HLA) types. Recently, however, a family has been described in which three patients with AML had identical inherited mutations in *CEBPA*,[27] a gene involved in granulocytic differentiation, while another large kindred with a familial platelet disorder with a predisposition toward AML had been shown to be associated with mutations in the gene encoding CBF alpha (formerly AML1).[28] Lastly, there seems to be a predisposition toward evolution to AML in individuals with inherited polymorphisms in the receptor for granulocyte colony stimulating factor.[29] It is likely that other such associations will be identified as gene array technology is applied to other familial aggregates and that some of these mutations will be detected in "sporadic" cases as well.

MORPHOLOGIC CLASSIFICATION AND CLINICAL AND LABORATORY CORRELATES

The diagnosis of AML depends on the examination of well-prepared specimens of peripheral blood and bone marrow. Both bone marrow aspirates and biopsies should be evaluated. Although the biopsy is usually not helpful in identifying individual cells, it provides the best assessment of cellularity, can occasionally identify aggregates of leukemic cells not seen on aspirate, and is necessary to evaluate marrow fibrosis. In 1976, a group of morphologists from France, the United States, and Great Britain suggested a classification system designed to quantify and standardize definitions of the sometimes clinically and biologically distinct subtypes of AML and acute lymphoblastic leukemia (ALL).[30] This French, American, and British (FAB) classification has been serially modified, most recently in a World Health Organization (WHO)-sponsored undertaking, in an effort to improve concordance among different observers and incorporate new findings from immunologic and cytogenetic studies.[31,32]

According to the widely used WHO classification system,[32] the diagnosis of AML requires that myeloblasts constitute 20% or more of bone marrow cells or circulating white blood cells, generally evaluated on Wright or Wright-Giemsa stained smears. The previous FAB classification required > 30% blasts to distinguish AML from myelodysplasia. Although it is as yet unclear whether this change is biologically well founded or has significant clinical impact, this difference should be kept in mind when comparing older AML trials with more recent studies that may use different eligibility criteria. Neoplastic promyelocytes, monoblasts or promonocytes, and megakaryoblasts are included in this percentage, and their presence defines the various morphologic subtypes described below. An assortment of histochemical stains is used to aid in subclassification and to distinguish AML from ALL. Monoclonal antibodies directed against antigen groups (termed cluster designations [CD]) considered to be restricted to cells committed to myeloid differentiation are also helpful in making this diagnostic distinction. Antibodies against CD11b, CD13, CD14, and CD33 are used most commonly. These antigens are found on normal hematopoietic elements, are not leukemia-specific or unique to different AML FAB subtypes, and generally, do not correlate with prognosis,[33] with the possible exception of CD34. CD34 is detected on undifferentiated hematopoietic progenitors and can be found on the blasts of patients with either AML or ALL. There is a suggestion that patients with AML whose blasts strongly express CD34 have an inferior outcome because of chemotherapy-resistant leukemia,[34,35] particularly in patients with less morphologically differentiated leukemias in which other myeloid-associated antigens are less strongly expressed.

The FAB and WHO nomenclature classify the subtypes of AML according to the normal marrow elements that the blasts most closely resemble. This does not mean, however, that the leukemic event exclusively involves the cell lineage that is most prominently represented morphologically. Until recently, the involvement of other hematopoietic lineages could be inferred only by the presence of prominent morphologic abnormalities in these other cell lines. Thus, in patients with myelodysplasia or erythroleukemia, there is usually morphologic evidence of trilineage dysplasia with the inference that the initial cell that was malignantly transformed was a hematopoietic precursor with capability of multilineage maturation. The ability to pinpoint the lineages involved in an individual patient's leukemia has been enhanced by cytogenetic studies and in situ hybridization techniques using specific molecular probes capable of detecting abnormalities in morphologically identifiable cells, as well as in vitro studies of colonies of different lineages. For example, Fialkow and colleagues,[36] studying female patients with X chromosome-linked polymorphisms of glucose-6-phosphate dehydrogenase, were able to demonstrate involvement of myeloid but not erythroid or megakaryocytic progenitors in some patients with AML. In contrast, using specific chromosomal probes, others demonstrated multiple lineage involvement in patients with erythroleukemia and myelodysplasia.[37,38] There are relatively few studies of this type, and it is unknown how many lineages are affected in most patients with AML. In particular, patients with more differentiated types of AML such as acute progranulocytic leukemia (APL) or monocytic leukemia have not been systematically evaluated, although in a few patients with APL there is a suggestion that the mutation is restricted to the myeloid series.

Representative examples of different subtypes of AML are shown in Figures 113-2 to 113-11. The immunologic, cytogenetic, and (where they exist) clinical correlates of these morphologic subtypes are reviewed (Table 113-1).

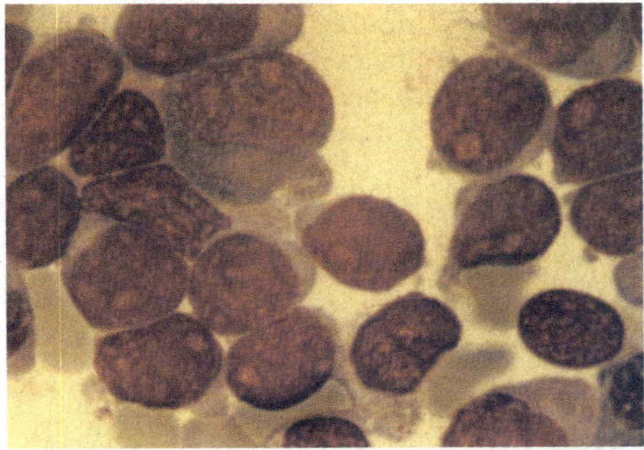

Figure 113-2 FAB M0. Marrow blasts from patients with this undifferentiated type of acute myelogenous leukemia can have variable amounts of agranular cytoplasm. Cells are peroxidase- and Sudan black-negative and can be confused with FAB M7 or FAB L2. Myeloid commitment of these blasts can be confirmed by immunophenotyping with antibodies against myeloid antigens and/or demonstration of ultrastructural peroxidase-positive granules using transmission electron microscopy.

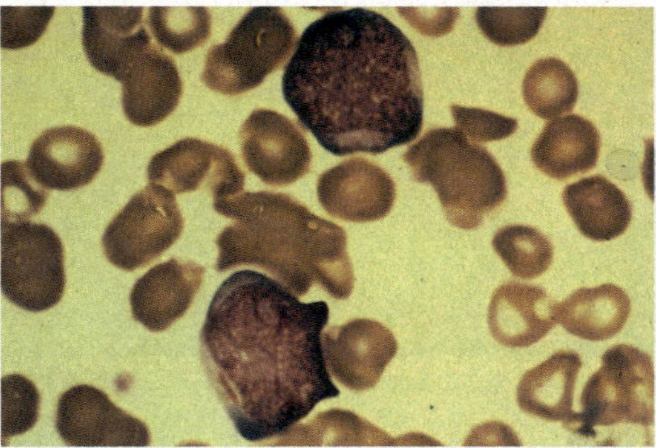

Figure 113-3 One of the blasts from this patient with M1 acute myeloid leukemia contains a prominent Auer rod.

Peripheral Blood Most patients with AML present with anemia (median hemoglobin 8 g%), thrombocytopenia (median platelet count 40,000–50,000/μL), and leukocytosis (median white blood cell count 10,000–20,000/μL). The red blood cell morphology is usually relatively normal. Large, sometimes hypogranular, platelets can be seen and functional defects can contribute to hemorrhagic manifestations. Most patients are neutropenic, and morphologic abnormalities (nuclear hyperlobulation, hypogranulation, Pelger-Huet anomaly) are often noted in the remaining neutrophils. Careful examination will detect blasts in most patients, although it can be difficult to distinguish among leukemia subtypes (or occasionally even to be confident of the diagnosis of acute leukemia) in patients with a low number of circulating blasts. In occasional patients, marked leukopenia at presentation (so-called aleukemic leukemia) may obscure the diagnosis until a marrow examination is performed.

M0 (Minimally Differentiated AML) In most patients, it is relatively simple to distinguish between AML and ALL on morphologic grounds. In general, the blasts from patients with AML are larger, with more abundant cytoplasm and more prominent, often multiple, nucleoli. The definitive diagnosis depends, however, on the presence of Auer rods, which are linear bundles of myeloid-containing granules, or demonstration of at least 3% granulated precursors in AML,[30] usually visible on Wright stain and confirmed by staining with either myeloperoxidase or Sudan black B. It can occasionally be difficult to distinguish between positivity in blasts versus staining in residual maturing myeloid elements in patients with ALL; careful correlation with the Wright stain is mandatory.

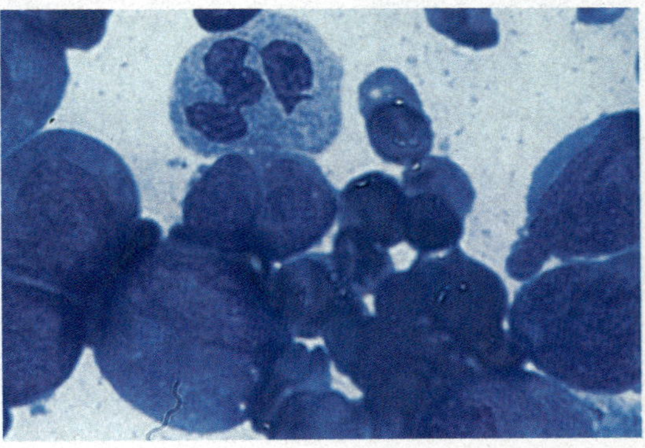

Figure 113-4 M2. Leukemia is characterized by evidence of continued myeloid differentiation with myelocytes and more mature myeloid elements present.

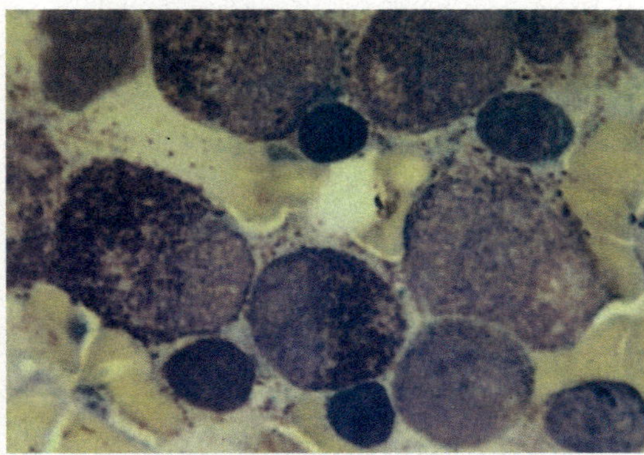

Figure 113-5 FAB M3. Progranulocytic leukemic cells usually have round nuclei with heavily granulated cytoplasm. Extracellular granules are often noted, and blasts with multiple Auer rods (not shown) are common. This leukemia has typical 15;17 translocation and a characteristic clinical picture of disseminated intravascular coagulation.

As shown in Figure 113-2, some patients have blasts that resemble myeloid blasts but are negative at the light microscopic level when examined with myeloperoxidase, Sudan black B, or other histochemical stains. The myeloid nature of these leukemias can be detected, however, by immunologic means or by election microscopy of peroxidase-stained preparations. Electron micrographs reveal ultrastructural peroxidase-positive granules, whereas immunologic phenotyping demonstrates reactivity with antibodies directed against myeloid antigens and nonreactivity with antibodies that characterize lymphoid differentiation.[39,40] The cells are often reactive with antibodies directed against CD34. Terminal deoxynucleotidyl transferase (TdT) is generally absent but can sometimes be detected in a minority of blasts.

Approximately 7% of patients with untreated AML have minimally differentiated AML (so-called M0 AML), which is relatively treatment resistant.[40–42] This undifferentiated leukemia can easily be confused with ALL, and it is, therefore, critically important to obtain immunophenotyp-

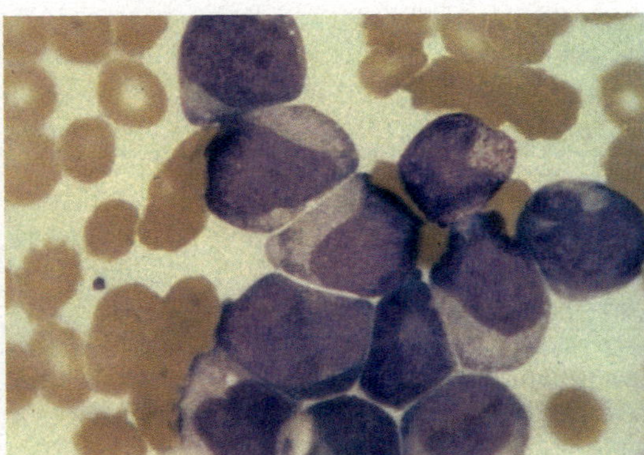

Figure 113-6 M4. Myelomonocytic leukemia has blasts with both myeloid and monocytoid appearance.

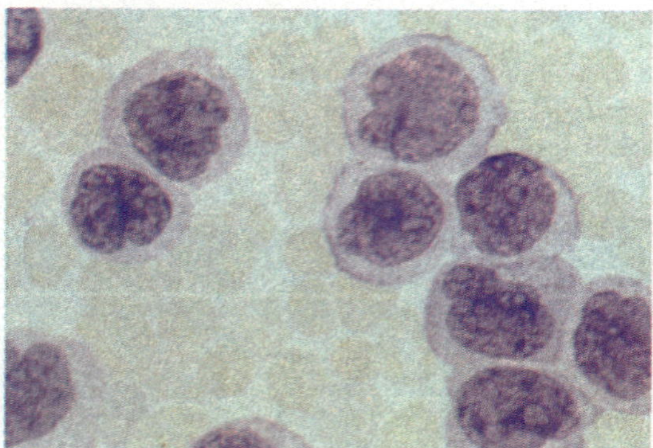

Figure 113-7 FAB M5. Monocytic leukemia. Prominent nuclei filled with nucleoli in some cells, light granulation, and large amounts of lightly basophilic cytoplasm give these cells the appearance of promonocytes.

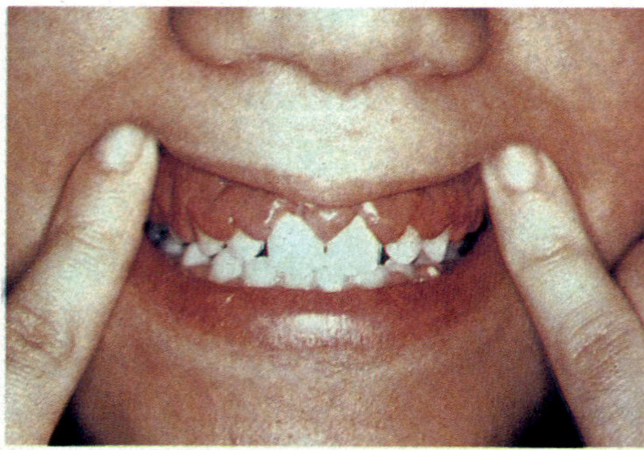

Figure 113-8 M5. Gingival hypertrophy due to infiltration by leukemic cells in acute monocytic leukemia.

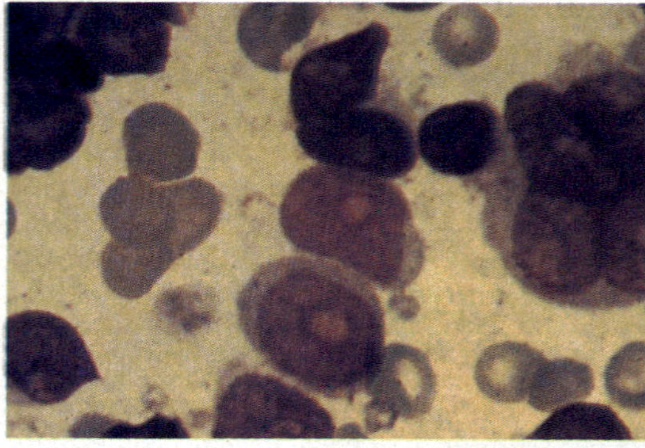

Figure 113-10 FAB M7. Megakaryocytic leukemia. Blasts in this category are often morphologically undifferentiated. The presence of multinucleated cells, dysplastic micromegakaryocytes, and cytoplasmic budding can be helpful diagnostic clues. The diagnosis is confirmed by immunophenotyping or ultrastructural studies.

ing of blasts from patients with morphologically undifferentiated leukemias. Other than resistance to chemotherapy, this M0 variant does not appear to be associated with specific clinical findings. Many M0 patients have complex karyotypic abnormalities.[41] No distinctive cytogenetic pattern has been noted, with the possible exception of trisomy 13, which has been reported to occur in some patients with morphologically less differentiated leukemias.[43]

M1 (Myeloid Leukemia without Maturation) The blasts from patients with FAB M1 have round nuclei with moderate amounts of sometimes lightly granulated cytoplasm, which can contain Auer rods (see Figure 113-3). In contrast to FAB M2, there is little evidence of myeloid maturation, with < 10% of cells beyond the level of the promyelocyte. There is no particular age, gender, clinical feature, or characteristic cytogenetic abnormality associated with this morphologic variant.

M2 (Myeloid Leukemia with Maturation) In contrast to FAB M1, there is obvious continued maturation in the myeloid series with the presence of promyelocytes, myelocytes, and often more mature myeloid elements. Granulation is generally more obvious, Auer rods are often prominent, and there is virtually never any difficulty in distinguishing this variant from ALL (see Figure 113-4). Approximately 20 to 25% of patients with FAB M2 AML have a characteristic translocation between chromosomes 8 and 21 [t(8;21)(q22;22)]; this translocation is seen almost exclusively in patients with FAB M2 and Auer rods. Such patients have a lower median age (approximately 30 years), a very high initial complete response rate (> 85% in most series), a lower relapse rate, and improved long-term disease-free survival, particularly when treated with high-dose cytarabine-based consolidation therapy.[44] The incidence of extramedullary granulocytic sarcomas, often in unusual sites, may be increased in patients with t(8;21) M2 AML whose blasts express the adhesion molecule CD56 on their surface.[45] These can present as discrete tumor masses, sometimes in paraspinous locations, confer a poor prognosis, and are distinct from the gingival and cutaneous involvement found in monocytic leukemia.

The t(8;21) involves what has been termed the *AML1* gene on chromosome 21 and the *ETO* gene on chromosome 8. The *AML1* gene has homology to the Drosophila runt gene and encodes the alpha chain of the heterodimeric transcriptional apparatus, core binding factor (CBF).[46] Normal CBF function is critical for mammalian hematopoietic development. The AML1-ETO protein recruits nuclear corepressor molecules including histone deacetylase, which prevents transcription of genes required for myeloid differentiation.[47,48] The AML1-ETO fusion product can be detected by reverse transcriptase polymerase chain reaction (RT-PCR), which is used for both diagnostic testing and monitoring for minimal residual disease. Of note is that the AML1-ETO has been detectable in the peripheral blood cells of some patients in long-term complete remission (CR) after treatment, suggesting that molecular detection by highly sensitive RT-PCR may not necessarily presage relapse.[49]

M3 (Acute Progranulocytic Leukemia) APL is one of the most distinctive subtypes of AML with regard to morphologic, clinical, cytogenetic features and response to differentiating agent therapies, such as all-*trans*-retinoic acid (ATRA).[50,51] In most patients, the morphologic diagnosis is straightforward, with the marrow being replaced by blasts that resemble unusually heavily granulated progranulocytes. The nuclei are round, with obvious nucleoli, and the cytoplasm is filled with multiple, large, and often coalesced, azurophilic granules (see Figure 113-5). Auer rods are usually seen, and multiple Auer rods (so-called faggot cells) are frequently noted. In a minority of patients, the blasts are hypogranular and granules sometimes can only be seen with electron microscopy.[52] This hypogranular variant often has cells with bilobed or lobulated nuclei, which can sometimes be confused with monocytic variants of AML. In contrast to the typical leukopenic presentation of APL, patients with the hypogranular variant tend to have a high white count. In both types of APL, staining with Sudan black B or myeloperoxidase is strongly positive. Class II HLA antigens (HLA DR), which are found on all hematopoietic precursors, are usually not detected on the surface of the malignant progranulocyte. The explanation for and biologic implications of this finding are not known. In contrast, CD33 is consistently strongly expressed.

Patients with APL tend to be somewhat younger, with a median age of 30 to 40 years, although APL is seen in patients of all ages. APL accounts for approximately 10% of AML and may be more prevalent in Latinos[53] and in obese people.[54] APL is almost uni-

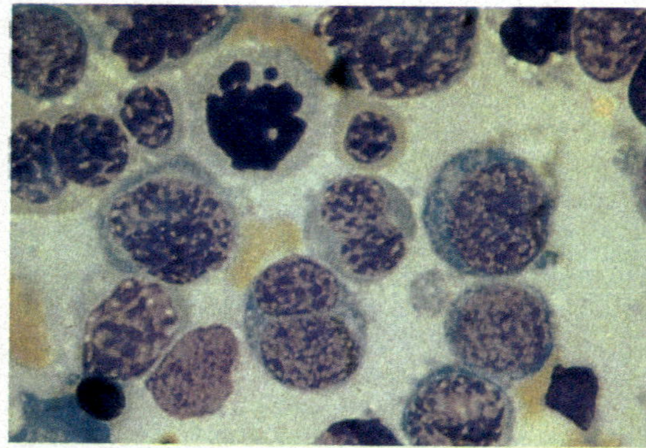

Figure 113-9 M6. Erythroleukemia is characterized by the presence of bizarre megaloblastic and often multinucleated erythroid precursors. Karyorrhexis is seen in some cells. The somewhat arbitrary distinction between FAB M6 and myelodysplastic syndrome with excess blasts in transformation is made by quantification of the fraction of myeloid blasts.

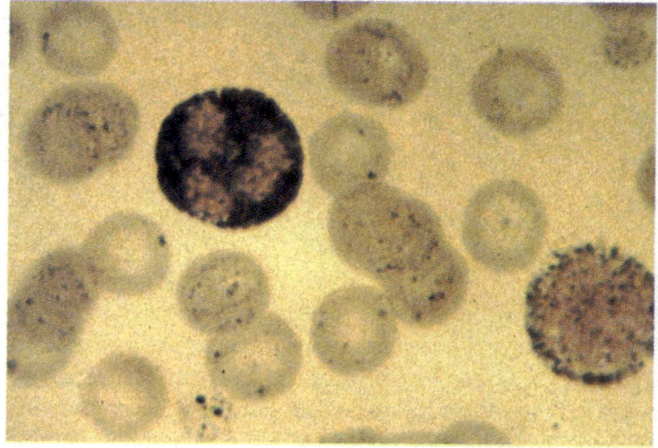

Figure 113-11 Typical granular staining with Sudan black B of a blast and a neutrophil from a patient with FAB M1 acute myeloid leukemia.

Table 113-1 Recurring Karyotypic Abnormalities in AML

Cytogenetic Abnormality	FAB Morphology	Affected Genes	Median Age	Approximate Incidence in De Novo AML	Prognostic Effects	Comments
t (8;21)	M2	*AML1/ETO*	30 yrs	5–7%	Favorable	Auer rods usually present
t (15;17)	M3	*PML-RARa*	40	5–8%	Favorable-high cure rate with ATRA-based therapy	DIC
t(11;17)	Similar to M3	*PLZF/ RARa*	?	< 1%	Poor response to ATRA-based therapy	
abn 16q22	M4 with eosinophilia	*CBFA/MYH11*	35–40	5%	Favorable	High reinduction rate post relapse
abn11q23	M5	*MLL* + many partners	> 50	3%	Poor except t(9;11)	Hyperleukocytosis, extra medullary disease
+8	Varied		> 60	5–10%	Poor	
del 5, del 7, 5q-, 7q-, or combinations	Varied; common in FAB M6		> 60	15–20%	Poor	Common in patients with secondary AML, prior MDS
Inv 3	Abnormal megakaryocytes	Ribophorin/*EVI1*	?	< 1%	Poor	Increased platelet count; other abnormalities common(del 5, del 7)
+13	Varied; sometimes undifferentiated		Probably > 60	~1–2%	Poor	Higher frequency of hybrid features
t(6;9) (p2;q34)	M2/M4 with basophilia	*DEK/CAN*	?	< 1%	Poor	Prominent basophilia
t(9;22)	Usually M1	*BCR/ABL*	Probably > 50	~ 1%	Poor	Splenomegaly
t(1;22)	Often M7	*MOZ/CBP*	Infants	< 1%	Poor	Organomegaly
t(8;16)	M4,5		?	< 1%	Poor	Erythrophagocytosis

AML = acute myelogenous leukemia; ATRA = all-*trans*-retinoic acid; DIC = disseminated intravascular coagulation; FAB = French, American, and British; MDS = myelodysplastic syndrome.

formly characterized by hypofibrinogenemia, variable depletion of other coagulation factors, elevated levels of fibrin degradation products, and accelerated consumption of endogenous and transfused platelets. The granules contain potent procoagulants, and disseminated intravascular coagulation (DIC) is generally accelerated following lysis of blasts by chemotherapy, often with increased bleeding. In some patients, there is evidence that accelerated fibrinolysis may be the primary event triggering the coagulopathy. APL is associated with the highest frequency of hemorrhagic morbidity and mortality, the latter usually related to intracranial hemorrhage. During chemotherapeutic treatment with accelerated cell lysis, these patients need aggressive platelet transfusion support and can require platelet transfusions 2 to 3 times per day during the first few days of treatment. Except for patients with very severe hypofibrinogenemia who may require supplementation with cryoprecipitate, most patients do not require infusion of clotting factors other than the plasma accompanying the platelet transfusion. Aggressive blood product support is probably as effective as heparin, once frequently used to interrupt the clotting cascade during drug therapy.[55] The heparin versus transfusion versus antifibrinolytic[56,57] therapy debate has been largely silenced in recent years, because treatment with ATRA ameliorates DIC within hours of its administration.

Almost all patients with APL have a characteristic translocation involving chromosomes 15 and 17 [t(15;17)(q22;q12)],[58] which may be associated with additional cytogenetic abnormalities, such as trisomy 8.[59] RT-PCR can be used to detect the fusion transcript, is useful for assessing for minimal residual disease,[60] and permits the proper classification of the occasional patient with clinically and morphologically typical APL but with an apparently normal karyotype. The breakpoint on chromosome 17 is in an intron of the retinoic acid receptor alpha gene. A gene that has been termed *PML*, also with DNA-binding capability, is translocated from chromosome 15, resulting in the formation of a fusion protein that functions in a dominant fashion to block transcription of genes controlled by RAR-α, probably by recruiting nuclear corepressor activity. It is likely that retinoic acid treatment relieves the corepression activity, allowing transcription of genes involved in differentiation.[61–63] There is also interest in the use of histone deacetylase inhibitors in patients with APL as another means of enhancing gene expression.[64]

A group of patients with a leukemia similar in morphology to APL but with a t(11;17)(q23;q21) have been described. Although RAR-α is rearranged, these patients fail to respond to ATRA. A novel zinc finger gene termed *PZLF* from chromosome 11 is translocated to the RAR-α, rather than the *PML* gene from chromosome 15, creating a fusion protein that does not allow the ATRA-mediated release of transcriptional corepression activity.[65]

Historically, the initial remission rate in patients with APL treated with chemotherapy was quite high. Initial drug resistance is very unusual, and most failures of therapy are related to hemorrhagic or infectious deaths. APL is uniquely sensitive to anthracycline therapy, and CR rates in excess of 80% can be seen with anthracycline therapy alone.[50,51] In contrast to other types of AML, remission can be attained with chemotherapy in APL without producing bone marrow aplasia.[66,67] Posttreatment bone marrows frequently remain cellular with abnormal progranulocytes, with follow-up marrows demonstrating disappearance of these cells and return of normal hematopoiesis without additional chemotherapy. DIC does not reappear despite the apparent persistence of abnormal cells. Undoubtedly, this unique feature of APL is in some way related to the equally unique sensitivity of APL to agents that have a differentiating and noncytotoxic mechanism of action (see the section "Differentiating Agents and the Therapy of Acute Progranulocytic Leukemia" later in this chapter).

M4 (Myelomonocytic Leukemia) Myelomonocytic leukemia is characterized morphologically by a mixture of myeloid and monocytic elements and represents about 15 to 20% of newly diagnosed patients with AML. According to the FAB criteria, greater than 20% of the leukemic cells must be monocytic in morphology to distinguish this variant from FAB M1 and particularly from FAB M2.[30] The monocytic elements often resemble partially differentiated monocytes with lightly granulated, grayish cytoplasm and folded nuclei, which are frequently seen in the peripheral blood (see Figure 113-6). Monocytic derivation can be confirmed by staining with nonspecific esterases such as α-naphthyl acetate or α-naphthyl butyrate.

There is no distinct clinical picture associated with this variant, perhaps because this classification encompasses a wide spectrum of patients owing to the generous morphologic criteria for inclusion. The median age tends to be somewhat higher, and there may be an increased incidence of hyperleukocytosis and extramedullary leukemic involvement, as can be seen with monocytic leukemia (see below). There is no particular cytogenetic clustering, and it is impossible to reliably predict short- or long-term outcome in patients with M4.

M4Eo (Myelomonocytic Leukemia with Eosinophilia) Approximately 5% of patients with de novo AML have typical morphologic features of myelomonocytic leukemia with the presence of variable numbers of dysplastic eosinophils at various stages of maturation. The distinctive eosinophils usually represent only 5 to 10% of the cells of the marrow.[68,69] These cells generally contain large basophilic granules in addition to typical eosinophilic granules. Occasional patients with M2 morphology with eosinophilia have also been described.

M4Eo tends to occur in patients of younger age (median age 35–40 years) and is associated with an excellent prognosis. CR rates are high (generally > 85%), and failure due to initial drug resistance is unusual. In some series, this variant represents the subtype with the most favorable long-term prognosis. In addition to long initial CRs, second remissions, which are often quite sustained, are generally easier to accomplish in patients with FAB M4Eo.[70,71] Older series suggested that there may be a high rate of central nervous system (CNS) relapse in patients with bone marrow eosinophilia. With more intensive regimens using higher doses of cytosine arabinoside (ara-C), CNS relapse in AML is now an unusual occurrence, and patients with FAB M4Eo do not require prophylactic CNS therapy.

Essentially all patients with FAB M4Eo have a cytogenetic abnormality involving chromosome 16 at band q22. In most patients, the cytogenetic changes involve a pericentric inversion (inv16), although translocations between the two chromosomes 16 with homologous deletions at 16q22 have also been noted.[68,69] This can be a very subtle cytogenetic finding, and cytogeneticists should be prompted to look for these changes by the characteristic morphologic changes. This breakpoint involves a fusion between the CBF-β chain and the gene encoding the smooth muscle myosin heavy chain. The fusion protein thus generated may recruit nuclear corepressor activity (in the form of histone deacetylase), which prevents transcription of genes required for myeloid differentiation in a fashion analogous to the CBF-α ETO fusion in t(8;21) M2 AML.[72] Although it is clear that patients with inv16 leukemia respond very well to intensive chemotherapy (> 60–70% 3 yr DFS rate in those receiving high-dose ara-C[73,74]), the reason for this is uncertain. One group has suggested that the gene coding for the multidrug resistance protein (MRP) is mutated as a consequence of this translocation hypothesizing that the enhanced chemosensitivity may be related to a decrease in the normal amounts of this resistance factor.[75]

M5 (Monocytic Leukemia) Two variants of monocytic leukemia have been described; in both, > 80% of the blasts are of monocytic derivation. Less common is so-called M5a, in which the monocytic blasts have round nuclei and small amounts of sometimes deeply basophilic cytoplasm without evidence of morphologic differentiation. In monocytic leukemia with differentiation (M5b), at least 20% of the blasts resemble promonocytes with folded nuclei and abundant, lightly granulated cytoplasm, generally without Auer rods. The nuclear folding can often be quite marked with rarification of the nuclear chromatin (see Figure 113-7). Phagocytosis of other hematopoietic elements by these cells is frequently noted in bone marrow preparations. These monocytic elements stain prominently with nonspecific esterase that is inhibited by fluoride.

Although seen in patients of all ages, monocytic leukemias are somewhat more common in older adults. Patients with FAB M5 have higher blast counts at diagnosis, and problems with hyperleukocytosis are most common in this morphologic variant (see the section "Complications" later in this chapter).[76] In addition, the incidence of extramedullary leukemia is highest in M5, particularly those with evidence of morphologic differentiation.[77] For example, it is common for patients to present to the dentist with gingival hypertrophy, an example of which is seen in Figure 113-8. Skin infiltration is common both at diagnosis and relapse and frequently represents the initial site of recurrence, sometimes while the bone marrow is still morphologically normal. Other less common areas of extramedullary involvement include the gastrointestinal tract, conjunctivae, and the CNS. It is likely that extramedullary infiltration is related to active migration of the leukemic promonocytes to these sites. These partially differentiated cells are capable of migration to skin windows in vivo as well as phagocytosis of microorganisms and adherence to nylon fibers in vitro.[78]

Serum levels of lysozyme are elevated in most patients with AML, but are generally much higher in patients with monocytic leukemia.[79] Lysozyme can affect renal tubular function, and severe, symptomatic hypokalemia can occur in patients with FAB M4 and M5 leukemia. This problem generally resolves with cytoreduction, but can also be additive to the hypokalemic side effects of antibiotics and amphotericin B, vomiting, and diarrhea.

In addition to the initial problems presented by complications of hyperleukocytosis, patients with monocytic leukemia tend to have lower complete response rates related to drug-resistant disease. Although older studies indicated that CR durations tended to be shorter with consequent very low rates of long-term disease-free survival, a recent analysis of a large number of patients treated by the Eastern Cooperative Oncology Groups (ECOG) suggested similar outcomes to other subtypes of AML when other risk factors are accounted for. [80] A variety of cytogenetic abnormalities can be detected, although the most common findings involve abnormalities of chromosome 11 at band q23. This break point, at what has been termed the *MLL* gene, can be involved in leukemias of myeloid or lymphoid origin as well as in leukemias associated with therapy with epipodophyllotoxins and other drugs directed at topoisomerase II.[18,81] The *MLL* gene, also called *All-1* or *HRX*, may partner with at least 16 different genes in balanced translocation.[5] *MLL* is homologous to a gene important in Drosophila development and includes DNA binding elements.[82,83] The t(9;11) is a relatively common translocation involving the *MLL* gene, which may actually confer a better prognosis than formerly thought, with higher initial CR rates.[84,85] There is an association between M5b with extensive erythrophagocytosis and the t(8;16)(p11;p13), a translocation involving the CBP class of transcation factors that are positive regulators of myeloid differentiation.[86,87]

M6 (Erythroleukemia) Erythroleukemia, often termed de Guglielmo syndrome in earlier literature, is the variant of AML in which morphologic abnormalities of erythropoiesis are most prominent. Cases of pure erythroleukemia, in which the predominant malignant cell is clearly identified as a pronormoblast, are extraordinarily rare. Rather, this is a disease of the myeloid stem cell with marked dysplastic changes in all three hematopoietic lines. Along with the increase in myeloid-appearing blasts, there is persistence of morphologic abnormalities in the erythroid series with profound megablastosis, multinuclearity, karyorrhexis, increased numbers of mitoses, and staining with periodic acid-Schiff (PAS), often in a block pattern (see Figure 113-9). Increased iron stores are usually seen, often with ringed sideroblasts. These changes are morphologically identical to those seen in patients with myelodysplasia, and many observers feel that most cases of erythroleukemia are biologically similar, if not identical, to patients with refractory anemia with excess blasts. This contention is supported by the very poor response to therapy in both groups, the tendency for the disease to occur in patients of older age, and the presence of similar cytogenetic abnormalities (complex karyotypic abnormalities, loss of part or all of chromosomes 5 and/or 7 and marker chromosomes).[88] Nonetheless, in order to provide some consistency in terms of protocol entry and reports of clinical trials, the FAB and WHO groups, somewhat arbitrarily distinguished among M6, myelodysplasia (RAEB), and other FAB subtypes with significant numbers of erythroblasts by quantification of the number of erythroblasts and myeloblasts. M6 is defined by the presence of > 30% blasts among nonerythroid cells when > 50% of the marrow nucleated elements are erythroid. Antibodies against glycophorin A are lineage-specific for erythroblasts, but immunologic phenotyping is rarely needed to identify these morphologic subtypes.

Except for the more advanced age and higher frequency of primary resistance to therapy, there are no distinct clinical or diagnostic karyotypic features associated with FAB M6. In occasional patients, transfusion of red blood cells can result in a marked decrease, if not elimination, of the marrow erythroid elements, suggesting the continued response to normal feedback mechanisms.

FAB M7 (Megakaryocytic Leukemia) Morphologic abnormalities of megakaryocytopoiesis, usually characterized by the presence of mono- or binucleated micromegakaryocytes, are common in many variants of AML and can be particularly prominent in patients with M6 or myelodysplasia. A minority of these patients have thrombocytosis and abnormalities of chromosome 3 [inv(3)(q21;q26)]. This cytogenetic abnormality is often found in association with other chromosomal deletions, with a variety of primary FAB morphologies (M1, M2, M4).[89]

These patients have a poor response to initial treatment and low overall survival. Thrombocytosis is not a unique feature of the inv(3) karyotype but can also be present in other patients with AML at the time of diagnosis.[90] The gene at the chromosome 3q21 break point is associated with the activation of EVI1 transcription factor.[91]

The diagnosis of FAB M7 is reserved for those patients in whom the predominant leukemic cell is of megakaryocytic lineage.[92] In some patients, there is obvious evidence of megakaryocytic dysplasia or multinucleated cells that strongly points toward principal involvement of the megakaryocyte (see Figure 113-10). In others, however, the leukemia is very undifferentiated morphologically, with variable amounts of generally agranular cytoplasm and can sometimes be confused with FAB M1 or even ALL. Sudan black B (see Figure 113-11), myeloperoxidase, and α-naphthyl butyrate stains are negative, whereas PAS and acid phosphatase may be positive, usually in a diffuse, speckled pattern. Histochemical staining is nondiagnostic, however, and the definitive diagnosis depends on either the detection of platelet-specific peroxidase by ultrastructural techniques or, more commonly, by the demonstration of a variety of platelet antigens (usually glycoprotein IIb/IIIa [CD41] or von Willebrand's factor) on the surface of the blasts.[93] At times, the diagnosis can be quite difficult to confirm, particularly because there is increased marrow reticulin in most patients, rendering the marrow fibrotic and inaspirable. Careful evaluation of peripheral blood blasts is necessary in such patients. It is likely that most patients with what has been termed acute myelosclerosis actually have acute megakaryocytic leukemia. Acute megakaryocytic leukemia should not be confused with the late stages of agnogenic myeloid metaplasia, and, indeed, prominent splenomegaly is not a clinical feature of FAB M7.

Although an uncommon variant of AML, most series suggest that this subtype is associated with a very poor prognosis. Prolonged aplasia is common following induction chemotherapy, and, because of the marrow fibrosis, it is often difficult to follow the results of therapy with repeated marrow aspirations. There have been relatively few cytogenetic evaluations of this variant, and except for the inv(3) and a few cases of t(1;22) (p13;q13) found in infants,[94] no consistent abnormality has been identified to date.

Hybrid Leukemias Morphologists have long been perplexed by cases that defy easy categorization or seem to have features of both lymphoid and myeloid histology. A variety of terms have been used to describe such cases including hybrid leukemia, mixed lineage leukemia, biclonal leukemia, lineage infidelity or promiscuity, and biphenotypic leukemia. With the advent of new immunologic and molecular technology, it was hoped that most such leukemias could be assigned to a specific lineage. Paradoxically, the serial application of biochemical, immunologic, and molecular biologic techniques has demonstrated that sharing of myeloid and lymphoid characteristics may be a relatively common feature of both myeloid and lymphoid leukemia. In most such patients, individual cells coexpress myeloid and lymphoid features rather than the simultaneous occurrence of two apparently separate leukemias.

The mechanism of expression of TdT or other lymphoid markers in those with typical myeloperoxidase-positive AML is unclear. Although up to 25% of AML patients may express TdT, there are conflicting data about whether such a feature confers an adverse prognosis.[95,96] In adults with AML treated on Cancer and Leukemia Group B (CALGB) clinical trials, lymphoid antigen expression had no effect on outcome.[97] T-cell antigen expression or T-cell gene rearrangement in children with AML may or may not correlate with a higher level of resistance to regimens designed for AML patients.[98] The significance of a T-cell receptor rearrangement, a finding not uncommon in the AML patient, is even less clear. In fact, CD7 expression is not uncommon in t(8;21) AML, which clearly responds well to chemotherapy.[99,100] Although the phenotypic features of the leukemic blasts are generally constant throughout the patient's course (eg, at diagnosis and relapse), examples of lineage switch, usually AML followed by ALL, have been noted.[101,102]

For patients whose blasts are myeloperoxidase and/or nonspecific esterase positive and express mainly myeloid antigens, but who also display TdT positivity or express one lymphoid antigen, an AML regimen is appropriate. For those ALL patients whose blasts express one or two myeloid antigens, treatment with an ALL protocol is indicated. For the very occasional patient who truly has equal myeloid and lymphoid features, an obvious initial approach would be to combine AML and ALL regimens, but there are few data concerning the outcome of this strategy.

PRESENTING SIGNS AND SYMPTOMS

Patients with AML generally present with symptoms related to complications of pancytopenia including combinations of weakness, easy fatigability, infections of variable severity or hemorrhagic findings such as gingival bleeding, ecchymoses, epistaxis, or menorrhagia (Table 113-2). Occasional patients present because of prominent extramedullary sites of leukemia usually related to either cutaneous or gingival infiltration by leukemia cells. Bone pain is infrequent in adults with AML, although some individuals describe sternal discomfort or tenderness, occasionally with aching in the long bones, particularly of the lower extremities. It is generally difficult to date the onset of AML precisely, at least in part because individuals have different symptomatic thresholds for choosing to seek medical attention. It is likely that most patients have had more subtle evidence of leukemia for weeks, to perhaps months, before diagnosis. This can sometimes make the distinction between de novo leukemia and leukemia associated with prior hematologic disorders arbitrary.

Table 113-2 Initial Diagnostic Evaluation

History and physical examination—In addition to an overall comprehensive evaluation, emphasis should be placed on the following:
Duration of symptoms
Menstrual history
Prior pregnancies, transfusions, history of transfusion reactions
Drug allergies (antibiotics)
Sites of infection: rectum, vagina, oropharynx, gingiva, skin
Signs of hemorrhage
Signs of extramedullary leukemia—skin, gingiva
Dentition status
Bone marrow aspirate and biopsy
Morphologic classification
Cytochemistry
Immunophenotyping
Cytogenetics
Terminal deoxynucleotidyl transferase
Blood chemistries
Blood urea nitrogen, creatinine, electrolytes, uric acid
Transaminases, alkaline phosphatase, bilirubin, lactate dehydrogenase, calcium, phosphorus
Coagulation studies
Prothrombin time, activated partial thromboplastin time, fibrinogen, fibrin split products
Chest radiograph, electrocardiogram, left ventricular ejection fraction if clinically indicated
HLA typing (patient and family); lymphocytotoxic (anti-HLA) antibody screen
Herpes simplex and cytomegalovirus serology
Lumbar puncture (only if symptomatic)

HLA = human leukocyte antigen.

The findings on physical examination are variable and generally nonspecific. If fever is present, it is almost always related to infection, and an infectious site must be vigorously sought and treated empirically with broad-spectrum antibiotics. A small minority of patients have fever related solely to the underlying leukemia, which abates with appropriate chemotherapy; there is a suggestion that this may be more common in patients with promyelocytic leukemia.[66] Examination of the skin can reveal pallor, infiltrative lesions suggestive of leukemic involvement, cutaneous sites of infection, which may be either primary or embolic, or, most commonly, petechiae or ecchymoses related to thrombocytopenia and/or coagulopathy. Examination of the fundus reveals hemorrhages and/or exudates in the majority of patients (see the section "Ophthalmic Complications" later in this chapter). The conjunctivae may be pale, according to the magnitude of the anemia. Careful examination of the oropharynx and teeth is important because of the occasional occurrence of leukemic involvement and the value of applying effective dental prophylaxis with antibiotic coverage, if time permits, prior to chemotherapy. Palpable adenopathy is uncommon in patients with AML, and significant lymph node enlargement is rare. Similarly, hepatomegaly and splenomegaly are uncommon and, if found, may suggest the possibility of ALL or chronic myeloid leukemia in blast crisis. None of these findings is diagnostic of acute leukemia, and the final diagnosis and categorization depends on appropriate evaluation of peripheral blood and bone marrow.

Because of the rigorous nature of the chemotherapy required for the successful treatment of AML, particular attention should be paid to other medical problems that could complicate the patient's management. A history of congestive heart failure or other heart disease may preclude therapy with anthracyclines and mandates careful monitoring of the large amounts of intravenous fluids that accompany the initial chemotherapy, antibiotics, blood and platelet transfusions, hydration for nephrotoxic antimicrobial agents, and parenteral nutrition during the 3 to 4 weeks of chemotherapy-induced pancytopenia. Prior transfusion for other disorders or multiple previous pregnancies may presage difficulties with platelet transfusions or herald the occurrence of transfusion reactions after red blood cell or platelet administration. Careful appraisal for possible drug allergies is critical, since virtually every patient will require antibiotic therapy. A history of prior herpes simplex infections (or the presence of an elevated antibody titer) provides justification for prophylactic administration of acyclovir.[103] In premenopausal women, menses should be suppressed with a GN_r H agonist or estrogens and/or progestational compounds until thrombocytopenia is resolved.

After the diagnosis is established, the physician and staff must present the goals of therapy and the side effects of treatment to the patient and family. For almost all patients, this discussion can rightfully emphasize the potential benefits of treatment with regard to both the short- and long-term outcome. It is frequently appropriate and necessary to repeat this discussion and counsel later during the patient's course. Sometimes, intensive treatment with the intent to achieve CR may be less advisable because of advanced patient age, debility, or prior myelodysplasia. Particularly with de novo leukemia, this represents the exception, and the administration of chemotherapy with the intent to achieve CR affords the greatest potential for even short-term benefit for most patients.

THERAPY

The therapy of AML has traditionally been divided into stages: induction, postremission therapy of varying intensity and duration, and postrelapse therapy. In newly diagnosed patients with AML, the goal of induction therapy is to achieve CR, which then permits the administration of subsequent therapy that, in most treatment protocols, is designed to maximize the probability of disease-free survival and cure. Currently, CR is defined primarily on morphologic grounds and includes the development of a morphologically normal bone marrow containing less than 5% blast elements, absence of any signs of extramedullary leukemia, and return of normal neutrophil (> 1,500/μL) and platelet (> 150,000/μL) counts.[1] Even if the bone marrow contains < 5% blasts, patients are not considered to be in remission if distinctive morphologic signs of leukemia, such as Auer rods, are noted. Low hemoglobin levels and the presence of symptoms unrelated to leukemia no longer exclude CR since they are often treatment-related and slow to normalize.

It has been assumed that CR is accomplished because the cytotoxic chemotherapy markedly decreases the number of cells in the leukemic clone, thereby allowing repopulation of the bone marrow by residual, normal progenitors whose proliferation had been suppressed. This explanation is supported by observations that cytogenetic abnormalities present in the original leukemia cells are either not detectable or constitute a small minority of metaphases during remission. However, in some fraction of patients, intensive chemotherapy eliminates the block in differentiation such that the apparently normal cells seen in the bone marrow and peripheral blood during a CR are actually progeny of the leukemic clone.[104–106] Studies of female patients in CR using X chromosome-linked polymorphisms (glucose-6-phosphate dehydrogenase isoenzymes or restriction fragment-length polymorphisms) have suggested that as many as 20% of adult patients in CR have monoclonally derived hematopoiesis with the same genotype as the leukemic clone. The frequency of this "clonal CR," its possible association with particular subtypes of AML or remission duration, the mechanism by which this important biologic phenomenon occurs, and a number of important technical issues need to be defined further.[107]

INDUCTION THERAPY: GENERAL PRINCIPLES

Induction therapy is designed to produce rapid clearing of leukemic cells from the peripheral blood with subsequent marrow aplasia. Perhaps the only exception to this principle occurs in patients with acute progranulocytic leukemia (FAB M3), in whom remission can be achieved despite the persistence 2 to 3 weeks later of what appear morphologically to be viable leukemia cells.[66,67] Approximately 1 week after standard induction therapy is completed (generally 2 weeks after the initiation of treatment), bone marrow aspirates and biopsies are done to evaluate the magnitude of cytoreduction. If the marrow is profoundly hypoplastic, the marrow is repeated at approximately weekly intervals to assess whether there is return of normal hematopoiesis, leukemia cells, or a mixture of both. If the marrow is not hypoplastic and only leukemia cells are noted on the day 14 marrow, then a second course of therapy is generally administered, although if high-dose cytarabine was used as induction chemotherapy, it is not repeated if leukemia is persistent.

At times, particularly if the marrow is hypocellular, it can be difficult to distinguish between residual leukemia cells and normal undifferentiated hematopoietic progenitors. In this instance, it is advisable to delay a few days and perform another marrow aspirate. If there is no evidence of further maturation, then a second course of treatment is indicated. The presence of erythroid precursors, juvenile megakaryocytes, or increases in the peripheral blood platelet or neutrophil counts serve as clues that normal regeneration is occurring and that a second course of treatment should be delayed. With standard regimens, approximately 30% of patients with AML require two courses of treatment to enter remission. Despite these guidelines, there remains considerable variability and imprecision as to when a second course of therapy is indicated. Some clinicians have advocated performing bone marrow aspirates and biopsies on the day after chemotherapy is completed because of a suggestion that evidence of residual leukemia at this time may be a signal of inadequate cytoreduction and a decreased probability of CR.[108,109] Although it has been suggested that further therapy be administered immediately to such patients, there is no evidence that this approach increases the rate of CR or improves survival; bone marrows that have been so recently exposed to intensive chemotherapy are also often difficult to interpret.

Most papers report results as complete response or no response. It is helpful, however, in investigations of prognostic factors or assessment of the cytotoxic activity of different regimens to more rigorously classify the causes of failure to achieve remission. One such classification divides nonresponders into those with apparent chemotherapy-resistant leukemia, those who die with aplastic bone marrows in whom the response to chemotherapy cannot be determined, and those in whom either early death or failure to obtain adequate bone marrow studies prior to death preclude determination of whether persistent leukemia was present. Patients with drug-resistant leukemia include those patients who survive treatment and those who die but have morphologic evidence of leukemia in the bone marrow or blood antemortem or at autopsy. This categorization is relatively simple to perform in most patients and can be helpful in distinguishing between failure due to drug resistance and failure related to inadequacies of supportive care.

The overall rate of CR in large cooperative group studies is approximately 65%. Patient age and cytogenetics are the most critical clinical variables. Comparisons among studies can be difficult because of imbalances in age and other prognostic factors. In addition, many reports do not stipulate whether patients with secondary leukemias or prior myelodysplasia were included in the trial. Exclusion of such patients, who represent approximately 5 to 10% of adult AML patients overall, and a higher fraction of older patients, can produce apparently improved results. It is preferable to present results in these patients and in patients with de novo leukemia separately. The criteria for CR are generally reached a median of 30 to 35 days after treatment has begun, although patients develop adequate levels of circulating neutrophils (> 500/μL) and no longer require platelet transfusion (at counts of approximately 10–20,000/μL), at least 7 to 10 days earlier.

Although there have been gradual improvements in the CR rates worldwide during the past 10 to 15 years, much of this can be attributed to better supportive care and not to changes in therapy. With the exception of the use of ATRA for patients with APL (see below), relatively few changes in therapy have been made since the introduction of combined therapy with daunorubicin and ara-C, the so-called 7 and 3 regimen.[110] This two-drug combination was derived from observations of single agent activity with either compound. Daunorubicin is generally administered by intravenous push at dosages of 45 to 60 mg/m^2/d for 3 days; ara-C is administered at dosages of 100 to 200 mg/m^2/d by continuous infusion for 7 days (Table 113-3). A series of randomized studies[110–116] by the Cancer and Leukemia Group B (CALGB) demonstrated that (1) results were superior using the 7 and 3 regimen compared with 5 days of ara-C and two doses of daunorubicin; (2) the addition of oral 6-thioguanine (DAT regimen) to the 7 and 3 program did not increase CR rate; (3) continuous infusions of ara-C produced slightly better outcome than twice-daily short intravenous infusions of ara-C when combined with daunorubicin; (4) results were not improved when 10 days of ara-C by continuous infusion were administered compared with 7 days; (5) substitution of doxorubicin for daunorubicin produced almost identical CR rates, although mucosal toxicity was greater with doxorubicin; and (6) there was no overall benefit from doubling the dosage of ara-C from 100 mg/m^2 to 200 mg/m^2/d.

Table 113-3 Representative Regimens for Acute Myeloid Leukemia

	Dose	Route	Days
Induction			
Cytarabine	100–200 mg/m^2	Continuous IV infusion	1–7
+			
Daunorubicin	45–60 mg/m^2	IV	1–3
or			
Idarubicin	12 mg/m^2	IV	1–3
or			
Mitoxantrone	12 mg/m^2	IV	1–3
Postremission			
Cytarabine	3 g/m^2 q12h (over 3 hours)	IV (6 doses)	1, 3, 5
or			
Cytarabine	1.5–2 g/m^2 q12h (over 1 hour)	IV (8 doses)	1–4 (12 doses)
or			
Cytarabine	100 mg/m^2	Continuous IV infusion	1–5

See text for details about number of courses and patient selection for different regimens.

Other attempts to improve the 7 and 3 induction regimen have also been relatively disappointing. Alternative anthracyclines or other agents such as mitoxantrone, rubidazone, aclacinomycin, amsacrine, mitoxantrone, and idarubicin have been used in several trials.[117–121] None of these studies demonstrated a survival or disease-free survival advantage with these different agents, perhaps because most are relatively similar in structure and mechanism of action and, hence, become susceptible to the same mechanisms of resistance. The largest reported experience has been with idarubicin, where three initial trials demonstrated that induction results are at least equivalent to results achieved with daunorubicin and ara-C.[118,120,121] More recent randomized trials have not shown an advantage for idarubicin compared with daunorubicin, particularly in older patients.[122,123] In addition, the duration of myelosuppression was greater in the idarubicin cohorts, calling into question the equitoxicity of the arms. Therefore, the substitution of these compounds has not had a major impact on the long-term disease-free survival rate of patients with AML.

Another trial from Australia added etoposide (VP-16) to the 7 and 3 regimen.[124] The CR rate was similar in older patients when compared with daunorubicin and ara-C alone and possibly slightly increased with a modest prolongation of CR duration in younger patients receiving the etoposide. This was a relatively small study and requires confirmation, since the overall disease-free survival in the group receiving the etoposide during both remission induction and postremission therapy was similar to other larger studies using daunorubicin and ara-C alone. Large phase I studies from the CALGB in which etoposide was added to 7 and 3 had outcomes similar to the past experience with the two drugs alone.[125]

Because high-dose ara-C (HIDAC) is a beneficial postremission therapy (see below), several groups have tested the concept of using this approach during induction in younger patients. Studies have compared standard 7 and 3 to daunorubicin plus intermediate- or high-dose ara-C (2–3 g/m^2 for 8–12 doses).[126–128] These studies failed to show an improved CR rate for the recipients of HIDAC, although an Australian study documented a more prolonged duration of CR (but no change in overall survival) in the patients randomized to HIDAC. The addition of HIDAC to standard daunorubicin/ara-C during induction has also been studied. Although a small trial demonstrated an 87% remission rate in patients under 60 years old,[129] a cooperative group trial[130] failed to confirm those positive results. In addition, a recent randomized trial demonstrated similar results if HIDAC was used either as part of induction or only as postremission therapy.[131] Topotecan-based regimens are now being evaluated[132]; unfortunately, there are few convincing data to suggest that presently known drugs or alternative induction regimens have made a significant difference in either the CR or cure rates.

The reasons for treatment failure vary according to patient age. With improved supportive care, it is uncommon for patients less than 50 years of age to die from complications of treatment and most of the approximately 25% induction failure rate is a consequence of drug-resistant leukemia. In contrast, the CR rate in patients > 60 years of age is approximately 50%, with failures divided equally between drug-resistant leukemia and deaths occurring during marrow aplasia as a consequence of reduced end organ tolerance.

CR can be achieved in approximately 20 to 30% of patients whose leukemia followed treatment of another cancer. Responses may be better in patients who do not have an extended pancytopenic or myelodysplastic period prior to developing frank leukemia. Although responses tend to be short in such patients, intensive induction should be offered, particularly to younger patients in whom subsequent stem cell transplantation may be an option.[133,134] Some younger patients with apparent secondary leukemia have been found to have cytogenetic findings associated with good prognosis de novo AML, such as t(8;21) or t(15;17), and may have a more favorable clinical course than expected.[135,136] These patients should be treated in the same fashion as those with de novo disease.

Whether and how to treat patients with well-documented prior myelodysplastic syndrome (MDS) and leukemia evolving from RAEB can be problematic. CR rates are lower, sustained responses are unusual, prolonged periods of aplasia are common, and these patients are usually older and less able to tolerate pancytopenic complications. Although data from the University of Texas M. D. Anderson Cancer Center suggest that the absolute number of marrow blasts (eg, whether a patient has RAEB, RAEB-T [now categorized as AML] or frank AML) is not of itself of prognostic significance,[137] the presence of major cytogenetic abnormalities and a truly prolonged history of MDS have a profoundly negative prognostic significance. If a histocompatible donor is readily available, initial therapy with allogeneic stem cell transplantation should be considered for selected younger patients with prior MDS.[138,139] There has been some interest in using very low-dose ara-C (10–20 mg/m^2/d) in older patients to decrease acute side effects. Although responses can be seen with low-dose ara-C, many weeks of therapy can be required with consequent pancytopenic complications equivalent to those seen with higher-dose treatment.[140] In addition, the CR rate is lower, and although median survivals may be similar using the two different dosage approaches, the prospect for long-term survival is greater when the intent of treatment is to achieve CR.

Postremission Therapy Morphologic assessments of CR are subjective and relatively insensitive. It is estimated that as many as 10^9 leukemia cells may still be present in patients in apparent CR. Rare patients can remain in CR for 1 to 2 years without further treatment, but it is generally accepted that some form of therapy after CR is required to achieve long-term disease-free survival. In a trial conducted by the German Cooperative Leukemia Group, a subset of 37 patients did not receive postremission therapy for a variety of protocol and medical reasons; all of these individuals relapsed.[141] The Eastern Cooperative Oncology Groups (ECOG) reported a randomized study in which patients achieving CR were randomized to either no therapy, lower-dose maintenance therapy, or an intensive postremission program.[142] All of the patients in the no-treatment arm relapsed rapidly, with a median CR duration of 4 months, resulting in early termination of this arm of the trial. Similar results were noted in a smaller randomized study reported by Embury and colleagues.[143] Although timed sequential therapy, in which patients receive additional chemotherapy during the early postinduction recovery phase, has been associated with prolonged remissions in the absence of postremission chemotherapy,[144] this treatment regimen is more analogous to consolidation therapy. It remains standard practice to administer chemotherapy after remission is achieved with conventional regimens.

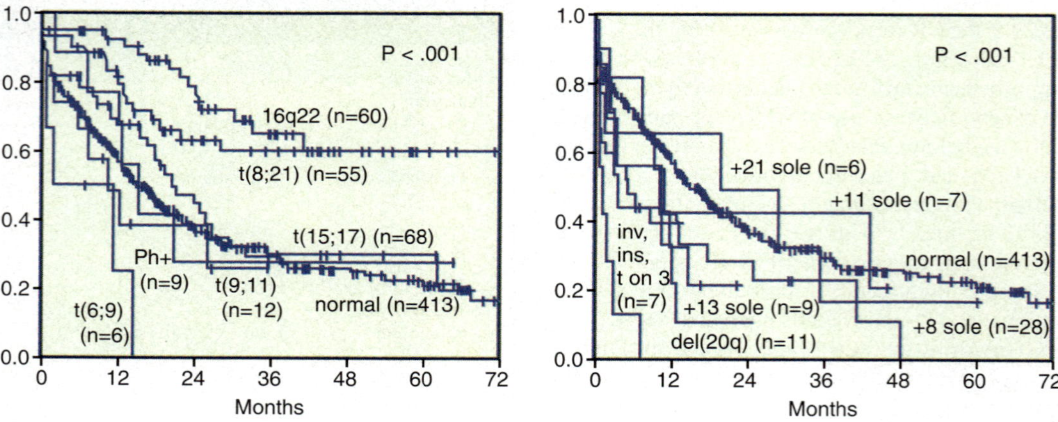

Figure 113-12 Overall survival according to cytogenetic findings in patients with de novo acute myeloid leukemia treated with intensive induction and postremission chemotherapy on CALGB studies.

Chemotherapeutic Approaches Considerable uncertainty and controversy remain about which postremission approach is preferable. These different approaches can be generally categorized according to the intensity of the therapy administered. The terms "consolidation" and "intensification" have been used to describe therapies that are of equal and greater intensity than the regimens used in initial induction therapy. These phrases are used rather loosely, however, and readers are advised to assess carefully the stipulated doses as well as the doses actually delivered, and the periods of aplasia experienced by the recipients. The term "maintenance" has generally referred to lower-dose outpatient therapy administered on an intermittent basis for months to years, patterned on the model successfully used in childhood ALL. Again, however, the ability to deliver such regimens as scheduled varies considerably.

A variety of agents have been used for postremission therapy, including the agents successfully administered in initial induction, with a particular recent focus on high-dose ara-C (HIDAC) as consolidation, as well as different classes of compounds, some of which have proven activity in AML, and others of which may have had only limited activity. Since a variety of prognostic factors significantly affect ultimate outcome, independent of the type of therapy administered, good results in small nonrandomized studies may reflect inadvertent patient selection and must ultimately be confirmed by multi-institutional applicability.

Overall, in adults, it can be expected that the administration of some sort of postremission therapy will result in a median CR duration of 12 to 18 months with approximately 20 to 25% of complete responders remaining as long-term disease-free survivors (Figure 113-12). A large review of CALGB patients who achieved CR demonstrated a relatively constant relapse rate of 4.7% per month during the first 6 months following CR.[145] The failure rate decreased in subsequent 6-month intervals (3.5% per month in months 7–12 and 2.4% per month in months 13–18), with a flattening of the curves after 3+ years of CR. In general, patients relapsing earlier have leukemia that is more drug-resistant than those who relapse late. Older randomized trials of postremission therapy conducted by the CALGB failed to demonstrate long-term benefits from[111–114] (1) an alternate month compared with a monthly schedule of maintenance therapy; (2) 3 years of relatively low-dose maintenance therapy compared with 8 months of a similar program (indeed, there was a modest survival advantage for patients randomized to stop therapy after 8 months); (3) doubling of the dose of ara-C from 100 to 200 mg/m^2 during maintenance therapy; and (4) addition of nonspecific immunotherapy in the form of methanol-extractable residue of Bacille Calinette Grain (MER) to maintenance therapy.

A previous ECOG study demonstrated no benefit from the addition of 2 years of maintenance therapy following two courses of postremission treatment with DAT (daunorubicin, ara-C, thioguanine).[146] Earlier studies from Germany reported by Buchner and colleagues[141] suggested a modest prolongation of CR duration, although with a questionable effect on long-term survival, when long-term maintenance therapy was administered after a single course of postremission DAT. There was less effect of maintenance in a later study when more intensive postremission consolidation was used before the maintenance.[147]

Two important randomized trials have shown that HIDAC in the postremission setting is better than lower doses of the drug. In an ECOG study, patients randomized to receive one course of very intensive postremission consolidation with a HIDAC-type regimen had a longer median duration of remission than patients receiving 2 years of lower-dose maintenance therapy.[148] The CALGB randomized 596 AML patients in CR to receive four courses of ara-C administered at three different dose levels (100 mg/m^2 by continuous IV infusion [CIV] for 5 days, 400 mg/m^2 CIV for 5 days, 3 g/m^2 IV for 3 hours q12h on days 1, 3, and 5 [total 6 doses/course]). There was no benefit from the higher-dose arms in patients > 60 years of age (see Figure 113-1, *bottom*) with a median duration of CR of approximately 13 months and with only 10 to 12% long-term disease-free survival.[2] In addition, there was a substantial incidence of CNS neurotoxicity in the older patients, manifested primarily as cerebellar dysfunction. In contrast, patients younger than 60 years of age benefited substantially from the HIDAC regimen in terms of both relapse-free and overall survival (see Figure 113-1, *top*). The long-term results in patients < 40 years of age were similar to those reported with autologous or allogeneic bone marrow transplant (BMT).

These studies strongly support the use of HIDAC-based consolidation programs in younger patients with AML. It is not known how many courses of such therapy are needed, the optimal dose and schedule of HIDAC, and whether the addition of other active agents will improve on these results. In a recent randomized study, the use of other potentially noncross-resistant regimens substituted for HIDAC was not superior to 3 cycles of HIDAC.[149] The CALGB data suggest that the benefit from HIDAC was most pronounced in patients with favorable cytogenetic findings [t(8;21); and inv (16)] with much less effect in patients with unfavorable karyotypes typically associated with drug resistance.[73,150] When medically feasible, most clinicians attempt to administer at least two to three courses of reasonably intensive HIDAC-based therapy postremission regimens. Programs that use HIDAC in the range of 2 to 3 g/m^2 for 8 to 12 doses are often only able to administer one to two courses of such treatment (see Table 113-3).

The decision about the type of postremission therapy must take into consideration the patient's medical condition and the possible persistence of infection (particularly with fungal organisms) acquired during induction, as well as the ability to provide adequate platelet transfusion therapy, in an attempt to balance the risk of intensive postremission approaches with the potential benefit. Depending on the intensity of the consolidation program, a 5% mortality rate in CR is to be expected and must be carefully explained to the patient.

Between 5 and 15% of patients achieving CR do not receive intensive postremission programs because of concerns about the patient's ability to tolerate and survive this therapy. Such patients should receive some sort of lower-dose treatment if possible, and we frequently use ara-C (100–200 mg/m^2/d by CIV for 5 days or sometimes on a bid, subcutaneous schedule), with or without 1 to 2 doses of an anthracycline for 2 to 4 courses, depending on patient tolerance. It is difficult to recommend a particular postremission approach in older patients not participating in clinical trials. Intensive chemotherapy has not proved beneficial compared with standard doses[151,152]; some form of therapy is required, however, to yield any chance at long-term disease-free survival. Since there is no proven role for HIDAC-based treatment in the older adult in remission, we generally use lower-dose regimens as described above, except in the occasional older patient with t(8; 21) or inv (16) in whom HIDAC is preferred if medically feasible. In view of the lack of proven benefit and the expense and morbidity associated with long-term maintenance therapy, prolonged treatment cannot be recommended.

Stem Cell Transplantation Stem cell transplantation (SCT) represents the other major therapeutic option for postremission therapy. Syngeneic SCT, using identical twins as donors,[153] and allogeneic SCT, using HLA-identical siblings,[154] were first evaluated in patients with advanced, refractory AML. After demonstrating an approximately 10% rate of long-term disease-free survival in this refractory group of patients and a 40 to 50% disease-free survival in patients in first remission receiving syngeneic transplants, studies of allogeneic transplantation in first remission AML were begun.[155] Early small series were promising, demonstrating a low rate of relapse with most of the mortality related to complications of acute and chronic graft-versus-host disease (GVHD). Following these initial results, the suggestion was made that all suitable patients with available donors should be considered for allogeneic transplant. Contentious debate ensued, although the recent completion of several large prospective trials comparing allogeneic or autologous SCT to chemotherapy in the postremission setting has provided relatively consistent data and conclusions.[156–159]

At least in part because of difficulties in identifying suitable donors for many patients as well as the complications of GVHD, considerable attention has also been focused on the use of autologous SCT. Cryopreserved autologous bone marrow can rapidly reconstitute recipients of ablative regimens, although marrow recovery may be delayed compared with allogeneic BMT.[160] Recent experience using cytokine-mobilized peripheral blood stem cells (PBSC) indicates that the duration of neutropenia and particularly thrombocytopenia is shortened compared with the use of bone marrow.[161] Because of the absence of GVHD, the autologous procedure is much better tolerated and can be readily applied to patients up to 65 years of age and perhaps older. The major disadvantages include the absence of a graft-versus-leukemia effect, as well as concern that viable leukemic progenitors will be administered with the autologous stem cells. A number of purging techniques have been used including monoclonal antibodies directed against myeloid blasts, as well as incubation with high concentrations of cytotoxic agents[160] that rather remarkably spare hematopoietic progenitors, although delayed marrow reconstitution is not uncommon.[162] It is unknown whether these in vitro manipulations are necessary, and randomized trials have not been reported. More recently, when unpurged autologous BMT was harvested after high-dose consolidation therapy, retrospective comparisons did not suggest an increased rate of relapse. A number of centers and groups have reported relapse-free survival rates in excess of 40% following autologous SCT in first CR[163–165] Historically, syngeneic transplant experience in this situation demonstrated relapse rates of approximately 50%, which is probably the best that can be expected with the autologous approach. Other evidence of the potential of this approach derive from reports of apparent cure rates of 20% in patients transplanted in second and third remissions of AML.[160]

The controversy about whether a patient in first remission should receive chemotherapy, an autologous SCT, or allogeneic SCT resulted in four prospective trials comparing results in first remission patients "genetically assigned" to allogeneic BMT (usually only in those 45 years old or less) or randomized to autologous BMT versus chemotherapy.[156–159] In the first of these trials, conducted in Europe,[156] 422 patients < 45 years of age (median 33 years) were either allocated to allogeneic BMT if an HLA-identical sibling was available or randomized to autologous BMT or a second course of consolidation chemotherapy with intermediate-dose ara-C and m-amsacrine. Disease-free survival was similar in patients undergoing allogeneic BMT (55% projected at 4 years) and autologous BMT (48%) and superior to the chemotherapy group (30%). Overall survival was similar, however, because many patients relapsing after chemotherapy could be successfully re-induced and then undergo BMT in second CR. Many patients did not undergo treatment as randomized, and no information was provided about responses to the three treatments in different cytogenetic risk groups.

Another similarly designed trial performed in France failed to show a benefit for either type of BMT compared with patients receiving intensive postremission chemotherapy.[157] The Medical Research Council (MRC) 10 trial conducted in Great Britain[158] appeared to show that autologous BMT was beneficial. All patients not assigned to allogeneic BMT received three cycles of post-CR chemotherapy and were then randomized to non-purged autologous BMT or observation. The addition of the autologous transplant prolonged CR duration but there was no significant difference in overall survival between the two groups. Allogeneic BMT was not significantly better than autologous BMT; no modality was clearly better than another in different cytogenetic risk groups. The MRC trials were recently updated with intent to treat analysis of results in patients with and without matched sibling donors. Again there was no apparent survival benefit compared with chemotherapy for patients who had available donors in whom a transplant could have been performed, and no advantage when patients with donors who were and were not transplanted were compared. Exploratory analysis suggested a survival benefit for patients with "intermediate" risk characteristics, although this group of patients is so heterogeneous that it is difficult to begin to apply this finding to recommendations for individual patients.[166]

The most recently published trial conducted by the North American Intergroup[159] found that chemotherapy was at least as good as autologous or allogeneic BMT in leading to cure, based on the intent to treat analysis. As in all the other studies, many patients assigned to autologous BMT did not receive this therapy for a variety of reasons. Randomized trials evaluating allogeneic or autologous PBSC have not been reported.

No firm conclusion can be drawn based on the available evidence. However, some general points can be made concerning the role of allogeneic BMT in the management of patients with AML in first CR:

1. The applicability of the technique is limited by patient age. Mortality from GVHD increases from decade to decade, and many centers do not perform allogeneic transplantation in patients older than 60 years, thereby excluding most patients with AML. Improvements in supportive care and the increased use of "mini-allogeneic" transplants using nonmyeloablative conditioning regimens may allow increased use of transplantation to older individuals. Ongoing studies suggest that the nonmyeloablative approach is clearly feasible in selected older patients.[167] Early side effects are markedly decreased by the nonablative approach, although it appears that the severity and duration of chronic GVHD is increased and further follow-up is needed to assess the ultimate rate of overall survival.
2. Less than one-third of potential recipients have suitable HLA-matched family donors. Although alternatives include the use of matched unrelated donors or partially mismatched family donors, GVHD is increased with both approaches, and administrative delays in identifying suitable donors remain problematic despite the availability of millions of HLA-typed donors throughout the world.[168,169] This is particularly true for patients from minority ethnic groups with less common HLA types and also indicates that there is considerable selection in reports of unrelated donor transplants, since some higher

risk patients relapse while awaiting for a donor to be identified. Umbilical cord blood may offer an alternative source of stem cells for those without matched siblings or unrelated donors. The incidence of graft- versus-host disease is much lower following cord blood transplants with better tolerance of mismatched transplants. Engraftment can be delayed, however, and dosage considerations represent an issue for many adult recipients.[170,171]

3. Although allogeneic SCT can cure some patients with chemotherapy-resistant disease, there remains an appreciable relapse rate and at least some of the factors predictive of drug resistance and relapse after chemotherapy also apply to SCT recipients.[172,173]
4. The antileukemic effect following BMT correlates with the occurrence and severity of GVHD, presumably as a result of a graft-versus-leukemia effect. Attempts to attenuate GVHD with a variety of immunosuppressive approaches are associated with a decrease in GVHD, but also an increase in the relapse rate.[174] Selective T-cell depletion approaches and other immunologic manipulations of the graft are being evaluated in an attempt to make allogeneic SCT safer without an increased relapse risk.[175,176]
5. Although important advances in supportive care directed against cytomegalovirus have been made, the consequences of the immunosuppression and direct organ sequelae of GVHD still represent formidable barriers.
6. As many as 10 to 20% of surviving patients may have significant symptoms and impairment of performance status because of chronic GVHD. There is also a small increase in the frequency of secondary tumors in long-term survivors.[177]

It is hoped that additional ongoing studies, perhaps requiring meta-analysis of results, will clarify many of these issues, particularly with regard to optimal treatments for different risk subgroups of patients. Contradictory results in different cytogenetic subgroups were noted in the randomized trials.[157,178] It would appear, however, that all approaches are in need of considerable improvement. Although the causes of failure are different (high rate of relapse with chemotherapy, lower rate of relapse but high mortality owing to GVHD for BMT), historic results suggest that the outcomes may be similar with the inevitable conclusion that improved cytoreductive approaches are needed in both arenas.

THERAPY OF RELAPSED AND REFRACTORY AML

There are a number of agents available that have clear-cut activity when used alone or in combination in patients with relapsed or refractory AML, including amsacrine, mitoxantrone, diaziquone, idarubicin, fludarabine, 2-chlorodeoxyadenosine, etoposide, homoharringtonine, topotecan, carboplatin, and most recently, clofarabine, cloretazine, and troxacitabine.[179–188] There is considerable heterogeneity among relapsed patients, and a number of factors in addition to the specific drugs used influence the outcome of treatment.[70,189–191] Some consistent trends are evident: (1) Response rates are uniformly low in patients with primarily refractory leukemia, in those with short initial CR durations, or in those who relapsed while receiving postremission chemotherapy; (2) secondary leukemias, leukemias that evolved from a prior hematologic disorder, and patients with poor-risk cytogenetics are particularly resistant to further therapy; and (3) patients in second and subsequent relapse have a poorer prognosis than patients in first relapse, and the durations of subsequent remissions tend to decrease progressively.

Table 113-4 Treatment of AML in Relapse

Duration of First CR	Frequency of Second CR (%)
> 2 years	61
1.5–2 years	53
1–1.5 years	30
7–12 months	19
1–6 months	10
Total	29 (155 of 531 patients)

Patients received a variety of different reinduction regimens.
AML = acute myeloid leukemia; CR, complete response.
Adapted from Rees JKH et al.[191]

Results from the MRC in Britain, which prospectively followed all patients entered on an induction AML trial, are supportive of these conclusions[191] (Table 113-4). In another study, patients whose initial remission was greater than 18 months had a re-induction rate of 64% (37 of 58) compared with a 29% CR rate in 278 patients with shorter initial remissions. Furthermore, the duration of second CR was longer in the former group (8 months vs 3 months). Patient age and cytogenetic findings are also important prognostic factors, emphasizing the enormous influence of patient selection on the results of reported phase II trials. In the absence of comparative trials, differing results may very well be the consequence of patient selection rather than the superiority of a particular regimen.[190,192]

The type and timing of therapy for relapsed patients should be individualized. Patients with other medical problems who have had poor responses to initial therapy have a small likelihood of sustained benefit from re-induction therapy and, indeed, may have life shortened by intensive therapy. Some such patients can be supported for many months, with maintenance of a reasonable quality of life, with a more conservative approach using red blood cell and platelet transfusions and oral hydroxyurea to control elevated white blood cell counts or symptoms such as bone pain. However, there is no potential for long-term benefit. Conversely, younger patients with longer initial responses may derive prolonged benefit from intensive re-induction therapy.

Recurrence of leukemia is often detected when the patient is asymptomatic, blood counts are normal, and there is modest marrow infiltration by blasts. Although it is logical to begin re-induction therapy at the earliest sign of relapse, when tumor burden is presumably the lowest, there are no data to demonstrate the validity of this approach except possibly as preparation for subsequent SCT.[193] The drawback to early treatment is that re-induction therapy is often unsuccessful and may result in excessive early morbidity and premature patient death. Our general policy is to observe such patients until there has been a pattern of deterioration in blood counts, but to initiate therapy while adequate numbers of circulating granulocytes and platelets are still present, prior to the development of symptoms or infection. An important exception is patients who are candidates for allogeneic transplantation (see below). Other patients have relapse diagnosed when bone marrows are done because of falls in blood counts. Such patients usually require re-induction therapy more immediately. In occasional patients, relapse develops in an explosive fashion with high circulating blast counts, fever, and infection. It is likely that the outcome in this group of patients is poorer.

There are essentially no comparative trials providing guidance about choice of agents to be used. The initial decision is generally between reuse of drugs that have previously been effective in a given patient, compared with the use of new drugs, some of which may be investigational. If a patient has relapsed while receiving chemotherapy, it makes little sense to use these same agents for re-induction. The oft-quoted exception to this guideline is the use of HIDAC (2–3 g/m^2 q12h for 8–12 doses), even in patients who had recently received more conventional doses of this agent. Although CR can be achieved in this setting, the duration of CR appears to be short, and it is not clear that the HIDAC approach is of long-term value in such patients.

In contrast, in patients who have longer first remissions, there is logic to reusing initial treatment. Many centers have arbitrarily felt that patients relapsing more than a year after completion of therapy should again receive the standard treatment. Although the CR rate in such patients is probably in excess of 50% when the original drugs are reused, it is not clear whether the same results could have been achieved in this favorable group using other tactics, including new investigational agents.

Gemtuzumab ozogamycin is an anti-CD33 monoclonal antibody that serves as a delivery agent for calicheamicin, a toxin linked to the antibody. It was recently approved for use in older patients with AML in first relapse whose first CR was greater than 3 months in duration.[194] Although it is clearly an active agent with few acute side effects, it produces prolonged myelosuppression (particularly thrombocytopenia) and may be associated with an increased incidence of hepatic veno-occlusive disease, particularly in patients who go on to receive allogeneic transplantation. CR rates have also been lower than initially reported when its use was expanded to other patient populations; further studies are required to assess its long-term role in AML therapeutics.[195]

There is no proven benefit of postremission chemotherapy in patients achieving second or third remissions. The obvious downside is that one is potentially depriving patients of time when they would be asymptomatic and out of hospital by the administration of therapy of variable toxicity but no proven long-term efficacy. At the moment, most re-induction studies do not specify that patients in second or later remission receive either maintenance or consolidation therapy.

It is unclear whether SCT should be offered at the time of initial relapse or whether patients should be re-induced and transplanted when a second remission is achieved. Unfortunately, most patients do not achieve second remission, and some develop medical problems during re-induction therapy that preclude subsequent transplantation. Enthusiasm for transplantation in relapse derives from reports from Seattle indicating that the results of allogeneic transplantation in early relapse were equivalent to or better than those achieved in patients transplanted in second or subsequent remission.[193] It is often a practical problem to identify patients during early relapse and to be able to refer such patients for transplantation rapidly. Nonetheless, it would probably be best to consider allogeneic transplantation for patients in early relapse if a suitable donor is available and the patient is under the age of 55 to 60 years. Similarly, allogeneic BMT can produce long-term survival in some patients with primary refractory leukemia, and it is advisable for HLA-type patients and their families at diagnosis to allow for this possibility. It is more difficult to use nonrelated donors for these purposes because of delays caused by tissue typing, identification of donors, and marrow procurement. Currently, most transplant centers recommend that patients in more florid relapse receive induction chemotherapy first because of poor results with SCT as primary therapy in such patients.

Patients who achieve second remission probably have a greater chance of long-term survival if transplanted in second remission. Data using both allogeneic and autologous approaches are promising in this regard, although it should be kept in mind that all such reports include highly selected patient populations, most of whom have had second remissions lasting a few months prior to transplantation. These patients have thereby identified themselves as having more chemotherapy-sensitive disease. Some centers now obtain and cryopreserve bone marrow from patients in first CR for use in either early relapse or as consolidation in second CR. This is an expensive, administratively cumbersome approach, although it merits study in investigational settings, particularly in high-risk patients, prior to its more widespread application. Lastly, selected patients who relapse following BMT can derive benefit from lymphocyte infusions from their donor or a second BMT and, in general, can receive and tolerate further chemotherapy.[196]

OTHER SUPPORTIVE CARE AND THERAPEUTIC APPROACHES

Hematopoietic Growth Factors Because myelosuppression-associated mortality is so high, particularly in older adults with AML, the development of hematopoietic growth factors (HGFs) held promise to ameliorate such side effects. Granulocyte-macrophage colony-stimulating factor (GM-CSF), granulocyte colony-stimulating factor (G-CSF), and interleukin (IL)-3 have been evaluated as well as the thrombopoietic factors, megakaryocyte growth and development factor (MGDF), and IL-11. The use of these agents in AML lagged behind that in solid tumors because of the concern that pharmacologic doses would lead to blast proliferation and a poor clinical outcome. Although fears regarding this clinical problem have proven unfounded, the HGFs have not lived up to their promise for other reasons.

Multiple randomized studies have been completed in which older patients received an HGF or placebo following the completion of initial induction therapy with the goal of improving CR rate by reducing infectious complications as a consequence of shortened durations of severe myelosuppression [197–205] All trials noted a decrease on the order of 2 to 5 days in the number of days of neutropenia < 500/μL, sometimes in association with a smaller 1- to 2-day reduction in the duration of hospitalization, but with the exception of a smaller trial reported by the ECOG, there was no significant difference in the incidence of severe infection, deaths from infections, CR rate, or survival.[197] One randomized trial using G-CSF after induction therapy for older patients with AML showed an improved CR rate for the G-CSF recipients.[202] Somewhat unexpectedly, the infectious mortality was similar in the two groups of patients, and the reason for the increased CR rate is unclear. There was no difference in overall survival.

In aggregate, it would appear that the benefits of growth factors administered after the completion of induction therapy are modest at best. In contrast, G-CSF following intensive consolidation therapy has appreciably shortened the duration of neutropenia, albeit without improvement in CR duration or survival.[204,206] Because of the potential for eliminating the need for hospitalization, the use of HGF can be recommended following consolidation therapy. Smaller studies with pegylated thrombopoietin failed to demonstrate reduced needs for platelet transfusions during the induction treatment of AML.[207,208]

Although in vitro evidence suggests that HGFs can increase the cytotoxic effects of ara-C, at least in part by increasing the fraction of cells in S-phase,[209,210] clinical results with the priming strategy have been disappointing. An early study from the M. D. Anderson group suggested that GM-CSF administered before and during chemotherapy produced lower response rates and survival than seen in a historical control group treated with chemotherapy alone.[211] Subsequent studies that randomized patients to receive GM-CSF/G-CSF or not before, during, and/or after induction chemotherapy[212–214] also failed to show an advantage for patients primed with growth factor. Some of these studies used HIDAC, whereas others evaluated more conventional continuous-infusion schedules.

Immune Modulation A critical component of the therapeutic benefit associated with allogeneic SCT is related to the graft-versus-leukemia effect. Although this is a complex, multifactorial set of events, further studies may enable the rational application of lymphokines to stimulate the appropriate cells in patients treated with chemotherapy alone. Circulating natural killer (NK) cells that can be cytotoxic to leukemia cell lines, and autologous leukemia cells in vitro, can be detected after both autologous and allogeneic transplantation, but not after chemotherapy.[215] The numbers of these killer cells can be expanded by the post-transplant administration of IL-2.[216] IL-2 itself has some antileukemic effect in patients with AML in relapse.[217,218] Pilot trials have documented the feasibility of administering IL-2 in the postchemotherapy setting; randomized trials are underway. Vaccine-based approaches using dendritic cell fusions to present leukemia-associated agents, or transducing AML cells to express proteins capable of stimulation of immune response, are under development.[219,220]

Circumvention of Drug Resistance The sum of complex and interacting mechanisms determine whether sufficient cytoreduction occurs in a given patient. The pharmacokinetics of antineoplastic agents vary widely among patients receiving the same calculated dose of drug, resulting in marked differences in drug exposure. Cell-cycle kinetics also differ widely, potentially modulating the effectiveness of agents such as ara-C that are largely S-phase–specific.[221] Similarly, there are potential differences in drug transport across leukemia cell membranes and variations among patients, and among individual leukemia cells within a given patient, in the cellular pharmacology of different antineoplastic agents. The ability of individual leukemia cells to repair sublethal damage is a critical variable as well. It is also likely that ultimately drug resistance is conferred by properties of a small fraction of leukemia cells, presumably that fraction capable of efficient self-renewal.[222] Investigations of these phenomena have been hampered by difficulties in reliably and repeatedly cloning leukemic cells from individual patients to allow serial studies to be performed. In addition, a potential sampling bias exists in that the in vitro results are a reflection only of the characteristics of cells obtained at a single point in time that can grow in an artificial environment.

Despite these problems, there have been many important studies done in the area of leukemia drug resistance. Changes in ara-C dose and schedule as well as modifiers of nucleotide metabolism or the cell cycle such as thymidine, L-asparaginase, and fludarabine[223–225] have been evaluated as a means of increasing the amount and rate of incorporation of ara-C into DNA, which appears to be the ultimate lethal event. Except for the apparent beneficial effects of very high-dose ara-C, these maneuvers have not resulted in unequivocal improvement in the therapeutic index.

The multidrug resistance (MDR) phenotype is associated in most cases with increased amounts of a membrane glycoprotein (p-170), which serves as a pump accelerating the efflux of a wide variety of agents, including the anthracycline antibiotics, vincristine, taxanes, and mitoxantrone.[226] Screens of human tumors, including acute leukemia, suggest that the levels of p-170, as can be assessed by immunoperoxidase studies of individual cells, Western blots of cell preparations, and indirectly by mRNA levels and gene expression, are increased in patients refractory to chemotherapy.[227,228] The MDR phenotype is most common in patients with relapsed or refractory disease, older patients, and those with other adverse prognostic factors.[229–231]

Exposure to a variety of compounds in vitro, including calcium channel blockers verapamil, quinine, and cyclosporine A, can reverse the effect of the p-170.[231] Cardiotoxicity occurs at the doses of verapamil required to produce this effect. Cyclosporine can reverse the MDR phenotype in vitro at drug levels that are likely to be clinically acceptable in terms of toxicity. A randomized trial of the addition of cyclosporin A to an ara-C plus continuous-infusion daunorubicin regimen for patients with relapsed AML suggested an overall survival benefit for adults in the experimental arm.[232] PSC–833 is a more potent nonimmunosuppressive cyclosporine analogue, which has been evaluated in randomized trials as an adjunct to standard therapy. Unfortunately, no improvement in CR rates was seen, with some trials demonstrating increased toxicity in the PSC-833 recipients.[233–235] Because of their effects on normal tissues such as the liver and kidney, these modulators also affect the pharmacokinetics of antineoplastic agents, such that the dosage of anthracyclines or etoposide usually have to be attenuated if given with an MDR modulator.[236] Trials with other MDR inhibitors that have minimal effect on drug disposition are in progress.

P-glycoprotein is unlikely to represent the only mechanism of drug resistance in patients with AML. Preliminary evidence suggests overexpression of the multidrug resistant protein (MRP) and breast cancer resistance protein (BCRP) in cells from some patients with AML, particularly in samples from patients in relapse.[237,238] Thus, intervention to circumvent resistance might best be applied during initial treatment prior to the enrichment of subpopulations resistant by other mechanisms and additional trials with these and other MDR modulators, some of which have less effects on chemotherapy drug metabolism, are in progress.

Differentiating Agents and the Therapy of Acute Progranulocytic Leukemia In theory, if leukemic progenitors could be forced to undergo terminal differentiation in vivo, then the leukemic clone could lose the capacity for self-renewal and be eliminated, with fewer side effects than occur with intensive cytotoxic chemotherapy. With the exception of the HL-60 cell line and blasts obtained from patients with APL, it has been difficult to reproducibly induce fresh leukemia cells to differentiate in vitro.

Limited clinical trials evaluating "differentiating" therapies, including vitamin D and low-dose ara-C, have produced disappointing results except for individual patients with APL who derived transient benefit from treatment with *cis*-retinoic acid.[239] The differentiation paradigm was verified, however, by dramatic responses in patients with APL reported from China with all-*trans*-retinoic acid (ATRA) administered orally for 30 to 90 days.[240] CRs were seen in > 80% of both relapsed and previously untreated individuals. Marrow aplasia did not occur, and serial bone marrows demonstrated what appeared to be maturation of the abnormal, hypergranulated promyelocytes.[241,242] Disseminated intravascular coagulation resolved promptly, with a profound reduction in the requirement for platelet transfusions following ATRA treatment. Although the hemorrhagic complications are decreased, approximately 20 to 30% of patients treated with ATRA alone develop significant side effects that can include fever, rapidly evolving pulmonary insufficiency, pericarditis, and pleurisy. This syndrome can occur independently of the leukocytosis frequently observed with ATRA therapy and can be fatal. Optimal management includes the prompt administration of corticosteroids at the first signs of the "ATRA" syndrome.[243,244] Resistance to ATRA eventually develops in patients treated in relapse, and virtually all patients treated with ATRA alone relapse. Possible pharmacokinetic mechanisms include induction of more rapid metabolism of the ATRA and induction of cytoplasmic retinoic acid binding protein in normal tissues that bind the ATRA, thereby decreasing the exposure of residual APL cells to the drug.[245]

A randomized study conducted in Europe first demonstrated the superiority of ATRA (with the addition of chemotherapy as needed) to chemotherapy alone in newly diagnosed patients with APL, both in terms of response to induction therapy and disease-free survival.[246] A large North American trial compared initial ATRA therapy versus chemotherapy as well as ATRA versus observation in the late postremission period.[247] Patients who never received ATRA did very poorly compared with patients receiving ATRA during induction or maintenance. Subsequent studies have demonstrated that optimal results are achieved when ATRA and anthracycline-based chemotherapy are administered concurrently during induction.[248,249] Approximately 70% of patients are cured with ATRA and anthracycline induction followed by anthracycline-based consolidation therapy. Results are less satisfying in older patients and in those presenting with white blood cell count > 10,000/μL. There is some controversy as to whether the addition of ara-C in induction and consolidation improves upon these results with a suggestion that ara-C may add benefit only in the patients in higher risk groups.[250] There appears to be a role for intermittent administration of ATRA as maintenance therapy and possibly further benefit from oral maintenance treatment with methotrexate and 6-mercaptopurine.

An exciting new development in APL has been the demonstration, again in China, that arsenic trioxide administered intravenously, produces a high rate of CR and major tumor burden reduction (four to five orders of magnitude based on PCR testing) even in patients with advanced, multiply relapsed disease.[251,252] Trials are underway evaluating arsenic trioxide as part of the induction and postremission treatment of APL. Although the precise mechanism of action and its relative specificity for APL remain to be elucidated, arsenic trioxide serves to accelerate apoptotic cell death in APL. Recently, tetra-arsenic tetra-sulfide has been shown to be very active in both newly diagnosed and relapsed APL patients with the great advantage of oral administration.[253]

These exciting findings and those related to our understanding of the molecular mechanisms accounting for the block in differentiation in APL and the t(8;21) and inv (16) leukemias have rekindled interest in treatment with other potential differentiating agents. Although the effect of ATRA may be largely limited to APL, presumably related to the unique mutation in the nuclear retinoic acid receptor characteristic of this disorder, other specific small molecules (eg, histone deacetylase inhibitors,[48] which also have a role in APL, and hypomethylating agents such as 5-azacytidine and decitabine) may eventually prove to be useful in other AML subtypes.

MINIMAL RESIDUAL DISEASE

Techniques of varying sensitivity can detect residual leukemia cells in patients in morphologic CR, including (in approximate descending order of sensitivity) conventional cytogenetics,[254] Southern blotting for known gene rearrangements, fluorescent in situ hybridization (FISH), multiparameter flow cytometry, and RT-PCR.[255–257] Technical problems abound, including the requirement for a known and already cloned abnormality when applying molecular techniques, and the potential for changes in antigen expression over time when using immunologic monitoring. There are few large prospective studies available. Although preliminary data tend to be compatible with the logical premise that persistence of detectable disease presages eventual relapse, false-positive (see comments on t(8;21) above)[49] and false-negative rates may be appreciable and could result in incorrect decisions about further treatment. Serial monitoring is cumbersome, and it is hoped that future studies will determine specific time points after completion of therapy when detection of MRD is prognostically significant. This appears to be true of persistence of the t(15;17) in APL after ATRA therapy.[257] The key clinical question is whether intervention with further therapy or allogeneic SCT will be of value if applied earlier, prior to gross relapse. There are no data addressing this issue. Because of the presence of residual disease, autologous collection and high-dose therapy may be predicted to be of less value in this circumstance. Indeed, patients with APL who are in morphologic and cytogenetic CR but are positive for PML/ RAR-α by pcr have a high rate of relapse after autologous transplantation.[258]

Prognostic Factors A number of clinical and laboratory factors have been described that help predict the likelihood of attaining CR and disease-free survival. In general, prognostic factors provide only relative guidelines to be used when discussing the probabilities of treatment outcome with individual patients. Conversely, they are of critical importance in focusing clinical and laboratory research efforts directed toward improving outcome. Most clinical factors are associated with decreased response to initial chemotherapy because they result in poor tolerance of the complications of prolonged pancytopenia. Advanced age (and particularly age > 70 years), renal insufficiency, congestive heart failure, concurrent infection, decreased serum albumin, and history of alloimmunization to blood products are examples.[259] Many can be summed in the assessment of the patient's performance status at the time of presentation.

As supportive care improves, some of these issues become less critical, and the intrinsic biologic characteristics of the patient's leukemia become the dominant factors. Because the major cause of treatment failure tends to be associated with drug resistance, these biologic predictive factors usually are associated with both decreased complete response rates as well as shorter durations of remission. A number of large multivariable analyses have consistently demonstrated that patients with hyperleukocytosis and/or M5 morphology, increases in serum lactate dehydrogenase, prior history of myelodysplasia or other hematologic disorder, and M6 or M7 and probably M0 morphology are associated with poor initial response rates. More advanced age and particularly age > 60 years is associated with decreased CR rates and shorter CR duration because of an increased rate of primarily resistant leukemia as well as difficulties with supportive care. In contrast to patients with ALL, immunologic phenotyping using currently available reagents does not appear to identify distinct biologic or prognostic groups.

Studies have suggested that overexpression of *bcl-2*, with a presumed inhibitory effect on apoptosis,[260] underexpression of *Rb*, a tumor suppressor gene,[9] overexpression of proangiogenic genes, and overexpression of BAALC (Brain and Acute Leukemia Cytoplasmic protein)[261] may be negative prognostic factors. Mutations in the transcription factor CCAAT entamer binding protein encoded by the *CEBPα* gene at 19q13 confers a favorable prognosis in the 7 to 10% of patients with this abnormality,[262] as may nucleophosmin gene mutations.[263] Gene expression array studies[264] will undoubtedly identify other prognostically important mutations or gene expression patterns, presenting the challenge of developing appropriately selected therapies and new agents aimed at these specific changes.

Major attention has focused on the prognostic impact of the nonrandom cytogenetic abnormalities detectable in AML blasts. Clonal abnormalities can be identified in 60 to 75% of patients.[73,265–269] It is reasonable to assume that genetic abnormalities are present in all patients since morphologic evaluation of chromosomal changes represents a relatively crude technique compared with molecular approaches. In addition to the examples cited above, mutations of the *FLT-3* gene, resulting in internal tandem repeats in the transmembrane domain of the flt-3 receptor, are detected by PCR in approximately 30% of patients with "normal" karyotypes, and seem to confer an inferior outcome.[7,8] Activating mutations in this transmembrane tyrosine kinase may be either an in frame base pair repeat (internal tandem duplication) in the region encoding the juxtamembrane part of the molecule, or a point mutation in the C-terminal activation loop. As described earlier, certain recurring abnormalities have a very tight relationship with both morphology and treatment outcome (see Table 113-1). In almost all studies, cytogenetic findings are an independent variable predicting outcome, and in some studies, they represent the major prognostic factor other than patient age. These findings have produced considerable interest in the possibility of specific therapy directed according to different risk groups. Although it is tempting to apply the knowledge of karyotypes to therapeutic decisions, a number of important and unanswered questions remain.

In order for cytogenetic findings or detection of specific mutations to represent more than a simple addition to the descriptive list of clinical factors, dissection of the mechanisms by which these changes are associated with drug sensitivity or resistance are required. With the extraordinary pace of development of molecular, proteomic, and immunologic techniques in the past few years, it is this aspect of the impact of cytogenetics that is most exciting. Although it may be naïve to assume that single DNA abnormalities are at the root of the biologically complex leukemic process, pharmacologic or molecular therapies, such as rationally designed small molecules or antisense fragments, might eventually become available for targeted therapeutic attacks against the products of particular genetic abnormalities. The specific inhibitory effect of imatinib mesylate against bcr/abl serves as the model for this approach and small molecule inhibitors of *FLT-3* are beginning clinical trial.

COMPLICATIONS

Hyperleukocytosis Leukemic blasts are considerably less deformable than mature myeloid cells[270] and are "stickier" than lymphoblasts because of expression of cell surface adhesion molecules. With increasing blast counts, usually at levels greater than 100,000/μL in the myeloid leukemias, blood flow in the microcirculation can be impeded by plugs of these more rigid cells. Local hypoxemia may be exacerbated by the high metabolic activity of the dividing blasts, with endothelial damage and hemorrhage. The situation can be worsened by red blood cell transfusions that rapidly increase whole-blood viscosity in the presence of hyperleukocytosis, thereby further compromising local blood flow. Red blood cell transfusions should, therefore, be administered very slowly or, if possible, withheld until the blast count is reduced. Coagulation abnormalities, including disseminated intravascular coagulation, further increase the risk of local hemorrhage. Liberal use of platelet transfusions is recommended, particularly since the platelet count is frequently overestimated because of the presence of fragments of blasts on blood smears, which can be mistakenly counted as platelets by automated blood cell counters.

Although pathologic evidence of leukostasis can be found in most organs in patients with extremely high blast cell counts, clinical symptomatology is usually related to CNS and pulmonary involvement.[76,271,272] Occasionally, dyspnea with worsening hypoxemia can occur following therapy and lysis of trapped leukemic cells. Spurious elevation of serum potassium occurs because of release from white blood cells during clotting, and it is sometimes necessary to measure potassium levels on heparinized plasma. Similarly, pO_2 can appear falsely decreased because of the enhanced metabolic activity of the white blood cells, even when the specimen is appropriately placed on ice during transport to the laboratory. Pulse oximetry provides an accurate assessment of O_2 saturation in such circumstances. Hyperleukocytosis is more common in patients with myelomonocytic or monocytic leukemia, and it is possible that the clinical manifestations are exacerbated by the migration of leukemic promonocytes into tissue where further proliferation occurs.[78]

The initial mortality rate for patients with AML and symptomatic hyperleukocytosis is high.[76,272] If patients survive the initial period, they tend to have somewhat lower remission rates and shorter CR durations. Symptomatic hyperleukocytosis in AML (and rarely in ALL) constitutes a medical emergency, and efforts should be made to lower the white blood cell count rapidly. In most patients, rapid cytoreduction can be achieved by chemotherapy, with either standard induction agents or with high doses of hydroxyurea (3 g/m^2/d). Some centers also advocate low-dose cranial irradiation, including the retina, in order to prevent further proliferation of leukemic cells in CNS sites where drug delivery may theoretically be compromised. This treatment is well tolerated, although there are no comparative studies to determine whether the results are superior to chemotherapy alone.

In some patients, it is impossible to initiate chemotherapy immediately because of renal insufficiency, metabolic problems, delays in initiating allopurinol therapy so as to prevent hyperuricemia, or similar considerations. In such patients, emergency leukapheresis has been used to lower or stabilize the white count.[273,274] Although intensive leukapheresis, with procedure times often lasting many hours, can produce improvement of pulmonary and CNS symptomatology, there are theoretic and practical limitations to its benefits. It is difficult, for example, for leukapheresis to affect already established vascular plugs, particularly if vascular invasion has taken place. In such cases, chemotherapy is the primary modality, although theoretically, leukapheresis could decrease further accumulation of leukocytes at these sites. Furthermore, it is precisely the patient in whom leukostasis is most likely to occur, that is, the patient with high and rapidly rising blasts counts, in whom the technical limitations of leukapheresis are apparent, in that it is often difficult, even with highly efficient cell separators, to reduce the rising count. In such patients with a high proliferative thrust, cycle-specific chemotherapeutic agents are more likely to be most immediately effective. Leukapheresis is also of modest benefit to patients who develop pulmonary problems during cytotoxic treatment, since in some such patients the symptoms are related at least in part to a local inflammatory response following leukocyte lysis.

CENTRAL NERVOUS SYSTEM LEUKEMIA

Involvement of the CNS is considerably less common in patients with AML than in both adults and children with ALL. Most clinicians have the impression that the incidence has decreased even further in recent years, perhaps related to the use of higher doses of ara-C, which can penetrate into the CNS. The incidence of CNS leukemia has been less than 5% in large AML clinical trials in recent years. Therefore, diagnostic lumbar punctures are not routinely indicated in the absence of CNS symptoms, and chemotherapeutic approaches do not include CNS prophylaxis. The most common symptoms are consequences of increased intracranial pressure and usually consist of a constant headache, sometimes associated with lethargy or other mental changes. Cranial nerve signs (most commonly cranial nerves III or VI) and, occasionally, peripheral nerve manifestations are secondary to nerve root involvement and can be accompanied by headaches or occur alone.[275]

The diagnosis is usually easily confirmed by examination of cytocentrifuge preparations of cerebrospinal fluid (CSF) after lumbar puncture. Cell counts can vary from as few as 5/μL to > 1,000. Most patients have moderate elevations in CSF protein with a moderate decrease in glucose. After the administration of intrathecal therapy, cytocentrifuge preparations can demonstrate reactive ependymal cells that, particularly if the leukocyte count is low, can be difficult to distinguish from leukemia cells. Treatment consists of the administration of intrathecal chemotherapy, with the addition of cranial radiation (usually 2,400 cGy), to patients who do not respond fully to chemotherapy or in whom cranial nerve involvement is present.[275] Either methotrexate (12 mg/dose) or ara-C (50 mg/dose) can be used as initial therapy, with a crossover to the other agents in the event of refractoriness or relapse. A typical schedule includes treatment 2 to 3 times a week until the CSF has cleared, generally occurring after a few injections. Treatment is then given at weekly intervals for two more doses to be followed by monthly administration, for a total of a year. An Ommaya reservoir to permit intraventricular drug administration is frequently needed either because of difficulties in performing repeated lumbar punctures or because of concern that in some individuals, the CSF flow does not deliver sufficient amounts of the drug from the lumbar space to the entire CNS. Successful therapy with systemically administered agents that penetrate the CNS, such as diaziquone (AZQ), high-dose methotrexate, or high-dose ara-C, have also been reported.[276] Slow-release ("depo") preparations of ara-C may be an alternative. Unfortunately, the relapse rate is high, either in association with bone marrow relapse or independently, even after initial successful therapy.

It has been suggested that the incidence of CNS leukemia is higher in patients with FAB M4 E0 morphology and possibly in patients with monocytic leukemia and high circulating blast counts.[277] This may no longer be the case using more contemporary treatment regimens, and prophylactic therapy is not indicated in such individuals. Recent studies have suggested that CNS relapse occurs frequently in patients with APL and some clinicians administer CNS prophylaxis when second CR is achieved.

Ophthalmic Complications Essentially every ocular structure can be involved in the leukemias, sometimes dominating the clinical picture in the prechemotherapy era.[278] Leukemia cells can infiltrate the conjunctiva and lacrimal glands, producing obvious masses that may require treatment with radiation therapy. Involvement of the choroid and retina is most common, however. A prospective study of 53 newly diagnosed adults with AML documented retinal or optic nerve (3 patients) abnormalities in 64% of patients.[279] Hemorrhage and cotton-wool spots (a consequence of nerve fiber ischemia) were most frequent, and the occurrence of these findings was unrelated to patient age, FAB type, white blood cell count, or hematocrit. Initial platelet counts were lower in patients with retinopathy. Ten patients had decreased visual acuity, including five with macular hemorrhages. It was felt that many of the cotton-wool spots were either a consequence of or exacerbated by ischemia due to anemia. Definite leukemic infiltrate of the retina could not be confirmed. All patients received aggressive chemotherapy and platelet transfusion support; no patient received cranial or ocular irradiation. All ocular findings resolved in patients achieving CR, and there was no residual visual deficit in any patient. Infectious ocular problems were not noted and seem to be uncommon, perhaps because the prompt empiric use of antibacterial and antifungal antibiotics has decreased the possibility of hematogenous spread of infections to the eye.

Pregnancy AML is occasionally diagnosed during pregnancy, either because of clinical manifestations or as an incidental finding during blood count checks. If detected during the first trimester, termination of pregnancy followed by treatment of the leukemia is advisable. The management of patients diagnosed later in pregnancy, such as late in the second trimester or during the third trimester, is more problematic. If the leukemia is relatively indolent, it is sometimes possible to manage patients conservatively with leukapheresis and/or transfusion with induction of labor and delivery of the fetus as soon as possible.[280] There have also been many reports of patients treated with chemotherapy later in their pregnancy.[281,282] The majority of these women have not aborted, and there have been no reports of leukemia occurring in the children, or an increased incidence of abnormalities in the infants.

Metabolic Abnormalities Patients receiving therapy for AML can experience a wide range of metabolic problems as a consequence of vomiting, diarrhea, impaired nutrition, or renal dysfunction, usually because of side effects from antibiotics, particularly amphotericin B. Some metabolic disorders are related to the leukemic process itself. Hyperuricemia, occasionally accompanied by urate nephropathy with renal insufficiency, is the most frequent metabolic accompaniment of AML. All patients should receive allopurinol, 300 mg/d or more, as soon as the diagnosis of acute leukemia is established, so that chemotherapy can be administered as soon as is medically appropriate. In most patients, urate nephropathy can be avoided or ameliorated with vigorous hydration and urinary alkalization with systemic or oral administration of sodium bicarbonate. Allopurinol can usually be discontinued within a day or two after chemotherapy is completed. In occasional patients with markedly elevated levels of uric acid, the use of recombinant urate oxidase, which can rapidly lower levels within a few hours, may be advisable.[283] A single dose is almost always sufficient with the decision about subsequent doses dependent on serial monitoring of uric acid.[284]

Tumor lysis syndrome occurs more frequently in patients with ALL, although some AML patients experience hyperphosphatemia, hypocalcemia, hyperkalemia, and renal insufficiency as a consequence of massive leukemic cell death. The inciting cause seems to be release of large amounts of phosphate from lysed blasts, which coprecipitates with calcium in the kidneys, leading to hypocalcemia and sometimes to oliguric renal failure. Hyperuricemia further contributes to this problem, which is usually self-limited and responds to judicious hydration.

Despite markedly hypercellular marrows, hypercalcemia is extremely unusual in patients with AML. Severe, occasionally symptomatic, hypokalemia is not infrequent, particularly in patients with monocytic leukemias. The mechanism appears to be renal potassium loss because of tubular damage induced by the high levels of lysozyme often noted in these patients.[79] Aggressive replacement with parenteral potassium is required; the syndrome usually abates after cytoreduction by chemotherapy. Lastly, rare patients have been described in whom lactic acidosis has been a constant metabolic accompaniment of the leukemia both at the time of presentation and relapse.[285] The mechanism is unclear, although anaerobic metabolism by the leukemia cells at sites of leukostasis has been postulated.

SUMMARY

Largely because of improvements in supportive care and the anticipatory management of complications of the treatment and underlying disease, the overall outlook for adults with AML has improved throughout the world in the past 10 to 15 years. It is equally clear, however, that results have leveled off and that new approaches are needed to increase the fraction of patients cured. Dramatic advances in molecular genetics offer promise both because of increased understanding of leukemia biology and the production of small molecules, monoclonal antibodies, cytokines, and HGF with potential clinical utility. Further clarification of mechanisms of drug resistance with the possibility of enhancement of the effectiveness of currently available drugs is also an exciting and achievable prospect. These strategies, as well as clinical trials designed to assess the appropriate use of SCT and newer chemotherapeutic drugs, provide the hope that therapy for AML will be both more successful and less empiric in the future.

MAST CELL LEUKEMIA AND OTHER MAST CELL NEOPLASMS

Neoplastic mast cell disorders have recently been apportioned into 6 categories by the World Health Organization (WHO).[286] These disorders may be reactive or neoplastic, and they range from benign syndromes with cutaneous involvement to malignant variants with mast cell infiltration of multiple organs, including the bone marrow.

Mast Cell Hyperplasia Mast cell hyperplasia frequently occurs in tissues involved in immediate or delayed-type hypersensitivity reactions, such as in the nasal mucosa during allergic rhinitis. Increased numbers of mast cells in the bone marrow have been noted in association with a wide range of malignant disorders, including lymphoproliferative disorders,[287] hairy cell leukemia,[288] and myeloid neoplasms.[289,290] The mast cells in such patients appear to be reactive rather than derived from the malignant clone. Urticaria pigmentosa is by far the most common manifestation of neoplastic mast cell proliferation.[291] The typical eruption of urticaria pigmentosa consists of multiple discrete hyperpigmented nodulopapular lesions and portends a benign clinical course. Cutaneous symptoms may include the classic urticarial wheals that result from mast cell degranulation in response to mechanical insult (Darier's sign), pruritus, or episodic flushing. A blurred distinction exists between cutaneous mastocytosis (CM)[292] and systemic mast cell disease (SMCD), an indolent disorder in which mast cells may also be found in extracutaneous sites. The serum tryptase level is higher in SMCD than in CM.[293] Systemic mastocytosis may present with a variety of constitutional and/or gastrointestinal symptoms, each of which can be attributed to excessive elaboration of mast cell mediators. Such symptoms, which may also present to a lesser degree in patients with urticaria pigmentosa, include rhinitis, asthma, nausea, vomiting, diarrhea, syncope, chest pain, bone pain, and rectal discomfort.[294] The bony skeleton, the gastrointestinal tract and the spleen can also be sites of mast cell infiltration.

Malignant Mastocytosis Malignant mastocytosis is an aggressive disease characterized by a much less favorable clinical course.[294] Unlike (indolent) systemic mastocytosis, in which an affected patient has a normal life expectancy, survival beyond 1 to 2 years after diagnosis of malignant mastocytosis is uncommon. The bone marrow is always involved, eosinophilia and cytopenias are common, and adenopathy and/or organomegaly are frequently noted.[295] In the early 1990s, it was recognized that mast cells from patients with systemic mastocytosis are capable of growing independently from C-KIT ligand, the critical mast cell growth factor.[296] Cell lines and patient samples demonstrated that the basis for this growth independence was constitutive activation of C-KIT.[297,298] This activation of proliferation is often associated with a mutation at codon 816 in the kinase domain, but juxtamembrane region mutations have also been described. The *ASP-816 VAL* mutation has been detected in both B cells and monocytes from patients, suggesting that systemic mastocytosis is a clonal disorder evolving from an early hematopoietic stem cell.[299] In contrast, blasts from patients with mast cell leukemia do not have this mutation, suggesting an alternative derivation of the leukemia.[300] Unfortunately, the typical *ASP-816 VAL* mutation is insensitive to the C-KIT inhibitor imatinib mesylate.[301]

Mast Cell Leukemia Mast cell leukemia represents a rare and aggressive subtype of malignant mastocytosis characterized by the presence of large numbers of atypical mast cells in the peripheral blood.[302–304] Patients with mast cell leukemia have a median survival of less than 6 months, in contrast to those with the nonleukemic type of malignant mastocytosis, who tend to survive for a longer time. The majority of reported cases of mast cell leukemia arise in patients with preexisting malignant mast cell disease. Criteria required for the diagnosis of mast cell leukemia, outlined in a study by Travis and colleagues,[303] who reviewed the nine cases reported between 1954 and 1986, are (1) the percentage of mast cells in the peripheral white blood cell differential must be 10% or greater; (2) the leukemic mast cells should display features of morphologic atypia; and (3) cytochemical properties of the leukemic cells must be typical of mast cell derivation (presence of metachromatic granules staining with chloroacetate esterase, but not with peroxidase).

Although bone marrow infiltration with atypical mast cells is always present in mast cell leukemia, hematologic findings at the time of diagnosis can vary widely. A mild to moderate degree of anemia is always present; initial leukocyte counts have ranged from normal to 66,300/μL.[303] The percentage of atypical mast cells (hypogranulated metachromatically staining cells with fragmentation, cytoplasmic tails, and multiple nuclei) may be relatively low (but greater than 10%), but almost always increases substantially with time. Karyotypic studies in several patients with mast cell leukemia have been normal, although the lack of dividing cells for metaphase analysis frequently precluded cytogenetic evaluation. Bone marrow cells from patients with systemic mastocytosis often display cytogenetic abnormalities, such as trisomy 8, monosomy 7/7q-, 20q-, typical of those with myeloproliferative disorders.[302,304]

Treatment Treatment of mast cell neoplasms is based on the disease subtype and clinical manifestations. Patients with cutaneous mastocytosis usually require no treatment. Systemic mast cell disease, however, has protean clinical manifestations. For example, those with hematological abnormalities may require supportive care, which could include transfusions or even the empiric use of hematopoietic growth factors. Avoidance of mast cell stimulants such as anesthesia. alcohol, aspirin, and morphine may diminish flushing, pruritus, and diarrhea, symptoms that may be histamine-related.[305–307] H1 and H2 antihistamines or disodium chromoglycolate may offer palliative benefit. Cladribine has activity in systemic mastocytosis.[308] Radiation therapy may control localized disease without causing histamine release.[309] Although an activating mutation of c-*kit* (usually an ASP to VAL substitution in codon 816) often accounts for the cellular proliferation of systemic mastocytosis, this mutated enzyme is insensitive to the c-kit inhibitor imatinib.[298,301] However, preclinical data suggest that the multitargeted kinase inhibitor, PKC412, may be inhibitory for this particular activation mutation.[310] Therapy for those with malignant mastocytosis or frank mast cell leukemia (activating mutations of c-*kit* are not believed to occur in this entity) is not at all standardized, although induction therapy with an anthracycline in combination with cytarabine could be followed by consolidation with high-dose ara-C. Allogeneic hematopoietic stem cell transplantation could be considered in the appropriate patient.

REFERENCES

1. Cheson BD, Bennett JM, Kopecky KJ, et al. Revised recommendations of the International Working Group for Diagnosis, Standardization of Response Criteria, Treatment Outcomes, and Reporting Standards for Therapeutic Trials in Acute Myeloid Leukemia. J Clin Oncology 2003;21:4642–49.
2. Mayer RJ, Davis RB, Schiffer CA, et al. Intensive postremission chemotherapy in adults with acute myeloid leukemia. N Engl J Med 1944;331:896–903.
3. Head DR. Revised classification of acute myeloid leukemia. Leukemia 1996;10:1826–31.
4. Scandura JM, Boccuni P, Cammenga J, et al. Transcription factor fusions in acute leukemia: variations on a theme. Oncogene 2002;21:3422–44.
5. Kelly L, Clark J, Gilliland DG. Comprehensive genotypic analysis of leukemia: clinical and therapeutic implications. Curr Opin Oncol 2002;14:10–8.
6. Toksoz D, Farr CJ, Marshall CJ. Ras genes and acute myeloid leukemia. Br J Haematol 1989;71:1.
7. Thiede C, Steudel C, Mohr B, et al. Analysis of FLT3-activating mutations in 979 patients with acute myelogenous leu-

kemia: association with FAB subtypes and identification of subgroups with poor prognosis. Blood 2002;99:4326–35.

8. Schnittger S, Schoch C, Dugas M, et al. Analysis of FLT3 length mutations in 1003 patients with acute myeloid leukemia: correlation to cytogenetics, FAB subtype, and prognosis in the AMLCG study and usefulness as a marker for the detection of minimal residual disease. Blood 2002;100:59–66.
9. Kornblau SM, Andreeff M, Hu S-X, et al. Low and maximally phosphorylated levels of the retinoblastoma protein confer poor prognosis in newly diagnosed acute myelogenous leukemia: a prospective study. Clin Cancer Res 1998;4:1955–63.
10. Sugimoto K, Hirano N, Toyoshima H, et al. Mutations of the p53 gene in myelodysplastic syndrome (MDS) and MDS-derived leukemia. Blood 1993;81:3022–6.
11. Look AT. Oncogenic transcription factors in the human acute leukemias. Science 1997;278:1059–64.
12. Downing J. The core-binding factor leukemias: lessons learned from murine models. Curr Opin Genet Dev 2003;1:48–54.
13. Kelly LM, Gilliland DG. Genetics of myeloid leukemias. Annual Rev Genomics Hum Genet 2002;3:179–98.
14. Bizzozero OJ, Johnson KG, Ciocco A, et al. Radiation-related leukemia in Hiroshima and Nagasaki, 1946–1964. I. Distribution, incidence and appearance time. N Engl J Med 1966;274:1095–101.
15. Darby SC, Doll R, Gill SK, Smith PG. Long-term mortality after a single treatment course with x-rays in patients treated for ankylosing spondylitis. Cancer 1987;55:179–90.
16. Austin A, Delzell E, Cole P. Benzene and leukemia: a review of the literature and a risk assessment. Am J Epidemiol 1988;127:419–39.
17. Andrieu J-M, Ifrah N, Payen C, et al. Increased risk of secondary acute nonlymphocytic leukemia after extended-field radiation therapy combined with MOPP chemotherapy for Hodgkin's disease. J Clin Oncol 1990;8:1148–54.
18. Pui C-H, Ribeiro RC, Hancock ML, et al. Acute myeloid leukemia in children treated with epipodophyllotoxins for acute lymphoblastic leukemia. N Engl J Med 1991;325:1682–7.
19. Sandler DP, Shore DL, Anderson JR, et al. Cigarette smoking and risk of acute leukemia: associations with morphology and cytogenetics. J Natl Cancer Inst 1993;85:1994–2003.
20. Ahilbom A. A review of the epidemiologic literature on magnetic fields and cancer. Scand J Work Environ Health 1988;14:337–43.
21. Won O, Raabe GK. Critical review of cancer epidemiology in petroleum industry employees, with a quantitative meta-analysis by cancer site. Am J Ind Med 1989;15:283–310.
22. Chaganti RSK, Miller DR, Meyers PA, German J. Cytogenetic evidence of the intrauterine origin of acute leukemia in monozygotic twins. N Engl J Med 1979;300:1032–4.
23. Clarkson BD, Boyse EA. Possible explanation of the high concordance for acute leukemia in monozygous twins. Lancet 1971;1:699–701.
24. Davidson RJL, Walker W, Watt JL, Page BM. Familial erythroleukemia: a cytogenetic and haematological study. Scand J Haematol 1978;20:351–9.
25. Gunz FW, Gunz JP, Vincent PC, et al. Thirteen cases of leukemia in a family. J Natl Cancer Inst 1978;60:1243–50.
26. Lee EJ, Schiffer CA, Misawa S, et al. Clinical and cytogenetic features of familial erythroleukemia. Br J Haematol 1987;65:313–20.
27. Smith ML, Cavenagh JD, Lister TA, Fitxgibbon J. Mutation of CEBPA in familial acute myeloid leukemia. N Engl J Med 2005;351:2403–7.
28. Song WJ, Sullivan MG, Legare RD, et al. Haploinsufficiency of CBFA2 causes familial thrombocytopenia with propensity to develop acute myelogenous leukaemia. Nat Genet 1999;23:166–75.
29. Wolfler A, Erkeland SJ, Bodner C, et al. A functional single-nucleotide polymorphism of the G-CSF receptor gene predisposes individuals to high-risk myelodysplastic syndrome. Blood 2005;105:3731–6.
30. Bennett JM, Catovsky D, Daniel MT, et al. Proposals for the classification of the acute leukaemias. Br J Haematol 1976;33:451–8.
31. Bennett JM, Catovsky D, Daniel MT, et al. Proposed revised criteria for the classification of acute myeloid leukemia. Ann Intern Med 1985;103:620–5.
32. Vardiman JW, Harris NL, Brunning RD. The WHO classification of myeloid neoplasms. Blood 2002;100:2292–302.
33. Bradstock K, Matthews J, Benson E, et al. Prognostic value of immunophenotyping in acute myeloid leukemia. Australian Leukaemia Study Group. Blood 1994;84:1220–5.
34. Campos L, Guyotat D, Archimbaud E, et al. Surface marker expression in adult acute myeloid leukemia: correlations with initial characteristics, morphology and response to therapy. Br J Haematol 1989;72:161–6.
35. Raspadori D, Lauria F, Vetura MA, et al. Incidence and prognostic relevance of CD34 expression in acute myeloblastic leukemia: analysis of 141 cases. Leukemia Res 1997;21:603–7.
36. Fialkow PJ, Singer JW, Adamson JW, et al. Acute nonlymphocytic leukemia: heterogeneity of stem cell origin. Blood 1981;57:1068–73.
37. Kibbelaar RE, van Kamp H, Dreef EJ, et al. Combined immunophenotyping and DNA in situ hybridization to study lineage involvement in patients with myelodysplastic syndromes. Blood 1992;79:1823–8.
38. Keinanen M, Griffin JD, Bloomfield CD, et al. Clonal chromosomal abnormalities showing multiple-cell-lineage involvement in acute myeloid leukemia. N Engl J Med 1988;318:1153–8.
39. Bennett JM, Catovsky D, Daniel M-T, et al. Proposal for the recognition of minimally differentiated acute myeloid leukaemia (AML-M0). Br J Haematol 1991;78:325–9.
40. Lee EJ, Pollak A, Leavitt RD, et al. Minimally differentiated acute non-lymphocytic leukemia: a distinct entity. Blood 1987;71:1400–6.
41. Cuneo A, Ferrant A, Michaux JL, et al. Cytogenetic profile of minimally differentiated (FAB M0) acute myeloid leukemia: correlation with clinicobiologic findings. Blood 1995;85:3688.
42. Stasi R, Del Poeta G, Venditti A, et al. Analysis of treatment in patients with minimally differentiated acute myeloid leukemia (AML-M0). Blood 1994;83:1619.
43. Dohner H, Arthur DC, Ball ED, et al. Trisomy 13—a new recurring chromosome abnormality in acute leukemia. Blood 1990;76:1614–21.
44. Mrozek K, Prior TW, Edwards C, et al. Comparison of cytogenetic and molecular genetic detection of t (8;21) and inv (16) in a prospective series of adults with de novo acute myeloid leukemia: a Cancer and Leukemia Group B Study. J Clin Oncol 2001;19:2482–92.
45. Tallman MS, Hakimian D, Shaw JM, et al. Granulocytic sarcoma is associated with the 8;21 translocation in acute myeloid leukemia. J Clin Oncol 1993;11:690–7.
46. Downing JR, Head DR, Curcio-Brint AM, et al. An AML1/ETO fusion transcript is consistently detected by RNA-based polymerase chain reaction in acute myelogenous leukemia containing the (8;21)(q22;q22) translocation. Blood 1993;81:2860–5.
47. Okuda T, van Deursen J, Hiebert SW, et al. AML1, the target of multiple chromosomal translocations in human leukemia, is essential for normal fetal liver hematopoiesis. Cell 1996;84:321–30.
48. Gelmetti V, Zhang J, Fanelli M, et al. Aberrant recruitment of the nuclear receptor corepressor-histone deacetylase complex by the acute myeloid leukemia partner ETO. Mol Cell Biol 1998;18:7185–91.
49. Nucifora G, Larson RA, Rowley JD. Persistence of the 8;21 translocation in patients with acute myeloid leukemia type M2 in long-term remission. Blood 1993;82:712–5.
50. Fenaux P, Chomienne C, Degos L. All-trans retinoic acid and chemotherapy in the treatment of acute promyelocytic leukemia. Semin Hematol 2001;38:13–25.
51. Tallman MS, Nabhan C, Feusner JH. Acute promyelocytic Leukemia: evolving therapeutic strategies. Blood 2002;99:759–67.
52. Golomb HM, Rowley JD, Vardiman JW, et al. Microgranular acute promyelocytic leukemia: a distinct clinical, ultrastructural, and cytogenetic entity. Blood 1980;55:253–9.
53. Douer D, Preston-Martin S, Chang E, et al. High frequency of acute promyelocytic leukemia among Latinos with acute myeloid leukemia. Blood 1996;87:308–13.
54. Estey E, Thall P, Kantarjian H, et al. Association between increased body mass index and a diagnosis of acute promyelocytic leukemia in patients with acute myeloid leukemia. Leukemia 1997;11:1661–4.
55. Goldberg MA, Ginsburg D, Mayer RJ, et al. Is heparin administration necessary during induction chemotherapy for patients with acute promyelocytic leukemia? Blood 1987;69:187–91.
56. Avvisati G, Wouterten Cate J, Buller HR, Mandelli F. Tranexamic acid for control of hemorrhage in acute promyelocytic leukemia. Lancet 1989;2:122–4.
57. Sanz MA, Tallman MS, Lo-Coco F. Tricks of the trade for the appropriate management of newly diagnosed acute promyelocytic leukemia. Blood 2005;105:3019–25.
58. Larson RA, Kondo K, Vardiman JW, et al. Evidence of a 15;17 translocation in every patient with acute promyelocytic leukemia. Am J Med 1984;76:827–41.
59. Slack JL, Arthur DC, Lawrence D, et al. Secondary cytogenetic changes in acute promyelocytic leukemia-prognostic importance in patients treated with chemotherapy alone and association with the intron 3 breakpoint of the PML gene: a Cancer and Leukemia Group B study. J Clin Oncol 1997;15:1786–95.
60. de The H, Lavau C, Marchio A, et al. The PML-RARα fusion mRNA generated by the t(15;17) translocation in acute promyelocytic leukemia encodes a functionally altered RAR. Cell 1991;66:675.
61. Diverio D, Rossi V, Avvisati G, et al. Early detection of relapse by prospective reverse transcriptase-polymerase chain reaction analysis of the PML/RAR alpha fusion gene in patients with acute promyelocytic leukemia enrolled in the GIMEMA-AIEOP multicenter "AIDA" trial. Blood 1998;92:784–9.
62. Grignani F, De Matteis S, Nervi C, et al. Fusion proteins of the retinoic acid receptor-alpha recruit histone deacetylase in promyelocytic leukemia. Nature 1998;391:815–8.
63. Melnick A, Licht JD. Deconstructing a disease: RARα, its fusion partners, and their roles in the pathogenesis of acute promyelocytic leukemia. Blood 1999;93:3167–215.
64. He LZ, Tolentino T, Grayson P, et al. Histone deacetylase inhibitors induce remission in transgenic models of therapy-resistant acute promyelocytic leukemia. J Clin Invest. 2001;108:1321–30.
65. He LZ, Guidez F, Tribioli C, et al. Distinct interactions of PML-RARalpha and PLZF-RAR alpha with co-repressors determine differential responses to RA in APL. Nat Genet 1998;18:126–35.
66. Daly PA, Schiffer CA, Wiernik PH. Acute promyelocytic leukemia: clinical management of 15 patients. Am J Hematol 1980;8:347–59.
67. Kantarjian HM, Keating MJ, McCredie KB, et al. A characteristic pattern of leukemic cell differentiation without cytoreduction during remission induction in acute promyelocytic leukemia. J Clin Oncol 1985;3:793–8.
68. Arthur DC, Bloomfield CD. Partial deletion of the long arm of chromosome 16 and bone marrow eosinophilia in acute nonlymphocytic leukemia: a new association. Blood 1983;61:994–8.
69. Hogge DE, Misawa S, Parsa NZ, et al. Abnormalities of chromosome 16 in association with acute myelomonocytic leukemia and dysplastic bone marrow eosinophils. J Clin Oncol 1984;2:550–7.
70. Kantarjian HM, Keating MJ, Walters RS, et al. The characteristics and outcome of patients with late relapse acute myelogenous leukemia. J Clin Oncol 1988;6:232–8.
71. Schlenk RF, Benner A, Krauter J, Buchner T, et al. Individual patient data-based meta-analysis of patients aged 16 to 60 years with core binding factor acute myeloid leukemia: a survey of the German Acute Myeloid Leukemia Intergroup. J Clin Oncol 2004;22:3741–50.
72. Marcucci G, Caligiuri MA, Dohner H, et al. Quantification of CBFbeta/MYH11 fusion transcript by real time RTPCR in patients with INV (16) acute myeloid leukemia. Leukemia 2001;15:1072–80.
73. Bloomfield CD, Lawrence D, Byrd JC, et al. Frequency of prolonged remission duration after high dose cytarabine intensification in acute myeloid leukemia varies by cytogenetic subtype. Cancer Res 1998;58:4173–9.
74. Byrd JC, Ruppert AS, Mrozek K, et al. Repetitive cycles of high-dose cytarabine benefit patients with acute myeloid leukemia and inv (16)(p13q22) or t(16;16)(p13;q22): results from CALGB 8461. J Clin Oncol 2004;22:1087–94.
75. Kuss BJ, Deeley RG, Cole SPC, et al. Deletion of the gene for the multidrug resistance associated protein (MRP) is associated with good prognosis in acute myeloid leukemia with the inversion of chromosome 16. Lancet 1994;343:1531–4.
76. Dutcher JP, Schiffer CA, Wiernik PH. Hyperleukocytosis in adult acute nonlymphocytic leukemia: impact on remission rate and duration, and survival. J Clin Oncol 1987;5:1364–72.
77. Scott CS, Strak AN, Limbert JH, et al. Diagnostic and prognostic factors in acute monocytic leukemia: an analysis of 51 cases. Br J Haematol 1988;69:247–52.
78. Schiffer CA, Wiernik PH. Functional evaluation of circulating leukemic cells in acute non-lymphocytic leukemia. Leuk Res 1977;1:271.
79. Sexton C, Buss D, Powell B, et al. Usefulness and limitations of serum and urine lysozyme levels in the classification of acute myeloid leukemia: an analysis of 208 cases. Leuk Res 1996;20:467–72.

80. Tallman MS, Kim HT, Paietta E, et al. Acute monocytic leukemia (French-American-British classification M5) does not have a worse prognosis than other subtypes of acute myeloid leukemia: a report from the Eastern Cooperative Oncology Group. J Clin Oncol 2004;22:1276–86.
81. Rubnitz JE, Behm FG, Pui CH, et al. Genetic studies of childhood acute lymphoblastic leukemia with emphasis on p16, MLL, and ETV6 gene abnormalities: results of St. Jude Total Therapy Study XII. Leukemia 1997;11:1201–6.
82. Rubnitz JE, Behm F, Downing JR. 11q23 rearrangements in acute leukemia. Leukemia 1996;10:74–82.
83. Hunger SP, Cleary ML. What significance should be attributed to the detection of MLL fusion transcripts? Blood 1998;92:709–11.
84. Mrozek K, Heinonen K, Lawrence D, et al. Adult patients with de novo acute myeloid leukemia and t(9;11)(p22;q23) have a superior outcome to patients with other translocations involving band 11q23: a Cancer and Leukemia Group B study. Blood 1997;90:4532–8.
85. Rubnitz JE, Raimondi SC, Tong X, et al. Favorable impact of the t(9;11) in childhood acute myeloid leukemia. J Clin Oncol 2002;20:2302–9.
86. Heim S, Avanzi GC, Billstrom R, et al. A new specific chromosomal rearrangement t(8;16) (p11,p13) in acute monocytic leukemia. Br J Haematol 1987;66:323–6.
87. Giles RH, Dauwerse JG, Higgins C, et al. Detection of CBP rearrangements in acute myelogenous leukemia with t(8;16). Leukemia 1997;11:2087–96.
88. Olopade OI, Thangavelu M, Larson RA, et al. Clinical, morphologic, and cytogenetic characteristics of 26 patients with acute erythroblastic leukemia. Blood 1992;80:2873–82.
89. Bitter MA, Neilly ME, Le Beau MM, et al. Rearrangements of chromosome 3 involving bands 3q21 and 3q26 are associated with normal or elevated platelet counts in acute nonlymphocytic leukemia. Blood 1985;66:1362–70.
90. Lee EJ, Schiffer CA, Tomiyasu T, Testa JR. Clinical and cytogenetic correlations of abnormal megakaryocytopoiesis in patients with acute leukemia and chronic myelogenous leukemia in blast crisis. Leukemia 1990;4:350–3.
91. Suzukawa K, Parganas E, Gajjar A, et al. Identification of a breakpoint cluster region 3' of the ribophorin I gene at 3q21 associated with the transcriptional activation of the EV11 gene in acute myelogenous leukemias with inv(3)(q21q26). Blood 1994;84:2681–8.
92. Bennett JM, Catovsky D, Daniel MT, et al. Criteria for the diagnosis of acute leukemia of megakaryocyte lineage (M7). Ann Intern Med 1985;103:460–2.
93. San Miguel FJ, Gonzalez M, Canizo MO, et al. Leukemias with megakaryoblastic involvement: clinical, hematologic, and immunologic characteristics. Blood 1988;72:402–7.
94. Carroll A, Civin C, Schneider N, et al. The t(1;22)(p13;q13) is nonrandom and restricted to infants with acute megakaryoblastic leukemia: a Pediatric Oncology Group study. Blood 1991;78:748–52.
95. Schachner J, Kantarjian H, Dalton W, et al. Cytogenetic association and prognostic significance of bone marrow blast cell terminal transferase in patients with acute myeloblastic leukemia. Leukemia 1988;2:667–71.
96. Parreira A, Pombo de Oliveira MS, Matutes E, et al. Terminal deoxynucleotidyl transferase positive acute myeloid leukaemia: an association with immature myeloblastic leukaemia. Br J Haematol 1988;69:219–24.
97. Ball ED, Davis R, Griffin JD, et al. Prognostic value of lymphocyte surface markers in acute myeloid leukemia (AML): a Cancer and Leukemia Group B (CALGB) Study. Blood 1991;77:2242–50.
98. Creutzig U, Harbott J, Sperling C, et al. Clinical significance of surface antigen expression in children with acute myeloid leukemia: results of study AML-BFM-87. Blood 1995;86:3097–108.
99. Saxena A, Sheridan DP, Card RT, et al. Biologic and clinical significance CD7 expression in acute myeloid leukemia. Am J Hematol 1998;58:278–84.
100. Kita K, Miwa H, Nakase K, et al. Clinical importance of CD7 expression in acute myelocytic leukemia. Blood 1993;81:2399–405.
101. Pui CH, Dahl GV, Melvin S, et al. Acute leukaemia with mixed lymphoid and myeloid phenotype. Br J Haematol 1984;56:121–30.
102. Stass SA, Mirro J. Lineage heterogeneity in acute leukemia: acute mixed lineage leukemia and lineage switch. Clin Hematol 1986;15:811–27.
103. Saral R, Arminder RF, Burns WH, et al. Acyclovir prophylaxis against herpes simplex virus infection in patients with leukemia: a randomized, double-blind, placebo-controlled study. Ann Intern Med 1983;99:773–6.
104. Fearon ER, Burke PJ, Schiffer CA, et al. Evidence for differentiation of leukemia cells to polymorphonuclear leukocytes in patients with acute non-lymphocytic leukemia. N Engl J Med 1986;315:15–24.
105. Hittelman W, Agbor P, Petkovic I, et al. Detection of leukemic clone maturation in vivo by premature chromosome condensation. Blood 1988;72:1950–60.
106. Jacobson RJ, Temple MJ, Singer JW, et al. A clonal complete remission in a patient with acute nonlymphocytic leukemia originating in multipotent stem cell. N Engl J Med 1984;310:1513–7.
107. Gale RE, Wheadon H, Goldstone AH, et al. Frequency of clonal remission in acute myeloid leukaemia. Lancet 1993;341:138–42.
108. Browman G, Preisler H, Raza A, et al. Use of the day 6 bone marrow to alter remission induction therapy in patients with acute myeloid leukaemia: a leukemia intergroup study. Br J Haematol 1989;71:493–7.
109. Cassileth PA, Gerson SL, Bonner H, et al. Identification of early relapsing patients with adult acute nonlymphocytic leukemia by bone marrow biopsy after initial induction chemotherapy. J Clin Oncol 1984;2:107–11.
110. Yates JW, Wallace J Jr, Ellison RR, Holland JF. Cytosine arabinoside (MSC A63878) and daunorubicin (NSC A83142) in acute non-lymphocytic leukemia. Cancer Chemother Rep 1973;57:485–8.
111. Rai KR, Holland JF, Glidewell OJ, et al. Treatment of acute myelocytic leukemia: a study by Cancer and Leukemia Group B. Blood 1981;58:1203–12.
112. Preisler H, Bjornsson S, Henderson ES, et al. Remission induction in acute nonlymphocytic leukemia: comparison of a seven-day infusion of cytosine arabinoside in combination with Adriamycin. Med Pediatr Oncol 1979;7:269–75.
113. Dillman RO, Davis RB, Green MR, et al. Comparative study of two remission induction regimens of ara-c for acute myelocytic leukemia (AML). Blood 1991;78:2520–6.
114. Wiernik PH, Glidewell OJ, Hoagland C, et al. A comparative trial of daunorubicin, cytosine, arabinoside, and thioguanine, and a combination of the three agents for the treatment of acute myelocytic leukemia. Med Pediatr Oncol 1979;6:261–77.
115. Preisler HD, Anderson K, Rai K, et al. The frequency of long-term remission in patients with acute myelogenous leukemia treated with conventional maintenance chemotherapy: a study of 760 patients with a minimal follow-up time of 6 years. Cancer and Acute Leukemia Group B. Br J Haematol 1989;71:189–94.
116. Yates J, Glidewell O, Wiernik P, et al. Cytosine arabinoside with daunorubicin or Adriamycin for therapy for acute myelocytic leukemia: a CALGB study. Blood 1982;60:454–62.
117. Arlin Z, Case DC Jr, Moore J, et al. Randomized multicenter trial of cytosine arabinoside with mitoxantrone or daunorubicin in previously untreated adult patients with acute nonlymphocytic leukemia (ANLL). Lederle Cooperative Group. Leukemia 1990;4:177–83.
118. Berman E, Heller G, Santorsa J, et al. Results of a randomized trial comparing idarubicin and cytosine arabinoside with daunorubicin and cytosine arabinoside in adult patients with newly diagnosed acute nonlymphocytic leukemia. Blood 1991;77:1666–74.
119. Keating MJ, Gehan EA, Smith TL, et al. A strategy for evaluation of new treatments in untreated patients: application to a clinical trial of AMSA for acute leukemia. J Clin Oncol 1987;5:710–21.
120. Vogler WR, Velez-Garcia E, Weiner RS, et al. A phase-three trial comparing idarubicin and daunorubicin in combination with cytarabine in acute myelogenous leukemia. A Southeaster Cancer Group Study. J Clin Oncol 1992;10:1103–11.
121. Wiernik PH, Banks PL, Case DC, et al. Cytarabine plus idarubicin or daunorubicin as induction and consolidation therapy for previously untreated adult patients with acute myeloid leukemia. Blood 1992;79:313–9.
122. Rowe JM, Neuberg D, Friedenberg W, Bennett JM. A phase III study of three induction regimens and of priming with GM-CSF in older adults with acute myeloid leukemia: a trial by the Eastern Cooperative Oncology Group. Blood 2004;103:479–85.
123. AML Collaborative Group. A systematic collaborative overview of randomized trials comparing idarubicin with daunorubicin (or other anthracyclines) as induction therapy for acute myeloid leukaemia. Br J Haematol 1998;103:100–9.
124. Bishop JF, Lowenthal RM, Josua DE, et al. A randomized trial of cytosine arabinoside, daunorubicin and VP- 16 (73 VS 737) as initial induction in adults with acute nonlymphocytic leukemia. Blood 1990;75:27–32.
125. Kolitz JE, George SL, Dodge RK, Hurd DD. Dose escalation studies of cytarabine, daunorubicin, and etoposide with and without multidrug resistance modulation with PSC-833 in untreated adults with acute myeloid leukemia younger than 60 years: final induction results of Cancer and Leukemia Group B Study 9621. J Clin Oncol 2004;22:4290–301.
126. Weick JK, Kopecky KJ, Appelbaum FR, et al. A randomized investigation of high-dose versus standard-dose cytosine arabinoside with daunorubicin in patients with previously untreated acute myeloid leukemia: a South-west Oncology Group Study. Blood 1996;88:2841–51.
127. Bishop JF, Matthews JP, Young GA, et al. Randomized study of high-dose cytarabine in induction in acute myeloid leukemia. Blood 1996;87:1710–7.
128. Schiller G, Gajewski J, Nimer S, et al. A randomized study of intermediate versus conventional-dose cytarabine as intensive induction for acute myelogenous leukemia. Br J Haematol 1992;81:170–7.
129. Mitus AJ, Miller KB, Schenkein DP, et al. Improved survival for patients with acute myelogenous leukemia. J Clin Oncol 1995;13:560–9.
130. Petersdorf S, Rankin C, Terebelo H, et al. A phase II study of standard dose daunomycin and cytosine arabinoside (ara-C) with high dose ara-C induction therapy followed by sequential high dose ara-C consolidation for adults with previously untreated acute myelogenous leukemia: a Southwest Oncology Group study (SWOG 9500). Proc Am Soc Clin Oncol 1998;17:55a.
131. Bradstock KF, Matthews JP, Lowenthal RM, Baxter H, et al. A randomized trial of high-versus conventional-dose cytarabine in consolidation chemotherapy for adult de novo acute myeloid leukemia in first remission after induction therapy containing high-dose cytarabine. Blood 2005;105:481–8.
132. Beran M, Kantarijian H. Topotecan in the treatment of hematologic malignancies. Semin Hematol 1998;35(3 Suppl 4):26–31.
133. Larson RA, Wernli M, Le Beau M, et al. Short remission duration in the therapy-related leukemia despite cytogenetic complete responses to high dose cytarabine. Blood 1988;72:1333–9.
134. Preisler HD, Raza A, Barcos M, et al. High-dose cytosine arabinoside as the initial treatment of poor-risk patients with acute nonlymphocytic leukemia: a Leukemia Intergroup study. J Clin Oncol 1987;5:75–82.
135. Kantarjian HM, Keating MJ, Walters RS, et al. The association of specific favorable cytogenetic abnormalities with secondary leukemia. Cancer 1986;58:924–7.
136. Fenaux P, Detoumignies L. Therapy-related acute promyelocytic leukemia. Br J Haematol 1995;87:445–6.
137. Estey E, Thall P, Beran M, et al. Effect of diagnosis (refractory anemia with excess blasts, refractory anemia with excess blasts in transformation, or acute myeloid leukemia (AML) on the outcome of AML-type chemotherapy. Blood 1997;90:2969–77.
138. Anderson JE, Appelbaum FR, Fisher LD, et al. Allogenic bone marrow transplantation for 93 patients with myelodysplastic syndrome. Blood 1993;82:677.
139. DeWitte T, Zwaan F, Hermans J, et al. Allogeneic bone marrow transplantation for secondary leukaemia and myelodysplastic syndrome: a survey by the Leukemia Working Party of the European Bone Marrow Trans-plant Group (EBMTG). Br J Haematol 1990;74:151–5.
140. Tilly H, Castaigne S, Bordessoule D, et al. Low-dose cytarabine versus intensive chemotherapy in the treatment of acute nonlymphocytic leukemia in the elderly. J Clin Oncol 1990;7:272–9.
141. Buchner TH, Urbanitz D, Hiddemann W, et al. Intensified induction and consolidation with or without maintenance chemotherapy for acute myeloid leukemia (AML): two multicenter studies of the German AML cooperative group. J Clin Oncol 1985;3:1583–9.
142. Cassileth PA, Harrington DP, Hines JD, et al. Maintenance chemotherapy prolongs remission duration in adult acute nonlymphocytic leukemia. J Clin Oncol 1998;6:583–7.
143. Embury SH, Elias L, Heller PH, et al. Remission maintenance therapy in acute myelogenous leukemia. West J Med 1977;126:267–72.
144. Archimbaud E, Thomas X, Leblond V, et al. Timed sequential chemotherapy for previously treated patients with acute myeloid leukemia: long-term follow-up of the etoposide, mitoxantrone, and cytarabine-86 trial. J Clin Oncol 1995;13:11–8.
145. Schiffer CA, Dodge R, Larson RA. Long term followup of CALGB studies in acute myeloid leukemia. Cancer 1997;80:2210.

146. Cassileth PA, Begg CB, Bennett JM, et al. A randomized study of the efficacy of consolidation therapy in adult acute nonlymphocytic leukemia. Blood 1984;63:843–7.
147. Buchner T, Hiddemann W, Wormann B, et al. Double induction strategy for acute myeloid leukemia: the effect of high-dose cytarabine with mitoxantrone instead of standard-dose cytarabine with daunorubicin and 6-thioguanine: a randomized trial by the German AML Cooperative Group. Blood 1999;93:4116–24.
148. Cassileth PA, Lynch E, Hines JD, et al. Varying intensity of postremission therapy in acute myeloid leukemia. Blood 1992;79:1924–30.
149. Moore JO, George SL, Dodge RK, et al. Sequential multiagent chemotherapy is not superior to high-dose cytarabine alone as postremission intensification therapy for acute myeloid leukemia in adults under 60 years of age: Cancer and Leukemia Group B study 9222. Blood 2005;105:3420–7.
150. Byrd JC, Mrozek K, Dodge RK, et al. Pretreatment cytogenetic abnormalities are predictive of induction success, cumulative incidence of relapse, and overall survival in adult patients with de novo acute myeloid leukemia: results from Cancer and Leukemia Group B (CALGB 8461). Blood 2002;100:4325–36.
151. Stone RM, Berg DT, George SL, et al. Post remission therapy in older patients with de novo acute myeloid leukemia: a randomized trial of comparing mitoxantrone/intermediate dose cytarabine with standard dose cytarabine (CALGB 8923). Blood 2001;98:548–53.
152. Lowenberg B, Suciu S, Archimbaud E, et al. Mitoxantrone versus daunorubicin in induction-consolidation chemotherapy-remission, and an assessment of prognostic factors in acute myeloid leukemia in the elderly: final report of the Leukemia Cooperative Group of the European Organization for the Research and Treatment of Cancer and the Dutch-Belgian Hemato-oncology Cooperative HOVON Group randomized phase III study AML-9. J Clin Oncol 1998;16:872–81.
153. Fefer A, Cheever MA, Thomas ED, et al. Bone marrow transplantation for refractory acute leukemia in 34 patients with identical twins. Blood 1981;57:421–30.
154. Clift RA, Buckner CD, Thomas ED, et al. The treatment of acute nonlymphoblastic leukemia by allogeneic marrow transplantation. Bone Marrow Transplant 1987;2:243–58.
155. Thomas ED, Buckner CD, Clift RA, et al. Marrow transplantation for acute non-lymphoblastic leukemia in first remission. N Engl J Med 1979;301:597–9.
156. Zittoun RA, Mandelli F, Willemze R, et al. Autologous or allogeneic bone marrow transplantation compared with intensive chemotherapy in acute myelogenous leukemia. European Organization for Research and Treatment of Cancer (EORTC) and the Gruppo Italiano Malattie Ematologiche Maligne Dell'Adulto (GIMEMA). Leukemia Cooperative Groups. N Engl J Med 1995;332:217–23.
157. Harousseau JL, Cahn JY, Pignon B, et al. Comparison of autologous bone marrow transplantation and intensive chemotherapy as postremission therapy in adult acute myeloid leukemia. The Groupe Ouest Leucemies Aigues Myeloblastiques (GOELAM). Blood 1997;90:2978–86.
158. Burnett A, Goldstone AH, Stevens RM, et al. Randomized comparison of addition of autologous bone-marrow transplantation to intensive chemotherapy of acute myeloid leukemia in first remission: results of MRC AML 10 trial. UK Medical Research Council Adult and Children's Leukaemia Working Parties. Lancet 1998;351:700–8.
159. Cassileth PA, Harrington DP, Appelbaum FR, et al. Chemotherapy compared with autologous or allogeneic bone marrow transplantation in the management of acute myeloid leukemia in first remission. N Engl J Med 1998;339:1649–56.
160. Yeager AM, Kaizer H, Santos GW, et al. Autologous bone marrow transplantation in patients with acute nonlymphocytic leukemia, using ex vivo marrow treatment with 4-hydroperoxycyclophosphamide. N Engl J Med 1986;315:141–7.
161. Weissinger F, Sandmaier BM, Maloney DG, et al. Decreased transfusion requirements for patients receiving nonmyeloablative compared with conventional peripheral blood stem cell transplants from HLA-identical siblings. Blood 2001;98:3584–8.
162. Gorin NC, Aegerter P, Auvert B, et al. Autologous bone marrow transplantation for acute myelocytic leukemia in first remission: a European survey of the role of marrow purging. Blood 1990;75:1606–14.
163. Linker CA, Ries CA, Damon LE, et al. Autologous bone marrow transplantation for acute myeloid leukemia using busulfan plus etoposide as a preparative regimen. Blood 1993;81:311–8.
164. Gorin NC. Autologous stem cell transplantation in acute myelocytic leukemia. Blood 1998;92:1073–90.
165. Hermans J, Suciu S, Stijnen TH, et al. Treatment of acute myelogenous leukemia. An EBMT EORTC retrospective analysis of chemotherapy versus allogeneic or autologous bone marrow transplantation. Eur J Cancer Clin Oncol 1989;25:545–50.
166. Burnett AK, Wheatley K, Goldstone AH, Stevens RF, Hann IM, et al. The value of allogeneic bone marrow transplant in patients with acute myeloid leukaemia at differing risk of relapse: results of the UK MRC AML 10 trial. Br J Haematol. 2002;118:385–400.
167. Giralt S, Estey E, Albiters, et al. Engraftment of allogeneic hematopoietic progenitor cells with purine analog-containing chemotherapy: harnessing graft-versus-leukemia with myeloablative therapy. Blood 1997;89:4531–6.
168. Aversa F, Tabilio A, Velardi A, et al. Treatment of high-risk acute leukemia with T-cell-depleted stem cells from related donors with one fully mismatched HLA haplotype. N Engl J Med 1998;339:1186–93.
169. Henslee-Downey PJ, Abhyankar SH, Parrish RS, et al. Use of partially mismatched related donors extends access to allogeneic marrow transplant. Blood 1997;89:3864–72.
170. Rocha V, Labopin M, Sanz G, et al. Transplants of umbilical-cord blood or bone marrow from unrelated donors in adults with acute leukemia. N Engl J Med 2004;351:2276–85.
171. Laughlin, MJ, Eapen M, Rubenstien P, et al. Outcomes after transplantation of cord blood or bone marrow from unrelated donors in adults with leukemia. N Engl J Med 2004;351:2265–75.
172. Bostrom B, Brunning RD, McGlave P, et al. Bone marrow transplantation for acute nonlymphocytic leukemia in first remission: analysis of prognostic factors. Blood 1985;65:1191–6.
173. Tallman MS, Kopecky KJ, Amos D, et al. Analysis of prognostic factors for the outcome of marrow transplantation or further chemotherapy for patients with acute nonlymphocytic leukemia in first remission. J Clin Oncol 1989;7:326–37.
174. Sullivan KM, Weiden PL, Storb R, et al. Influence of acute and chronic graft-versus-host disease on relapse and survival after bone marrow transplantation from HLA-identical siblings as treatment of acute and chronic leukemia. Blood 1989;73:1720–8.
175. Soiffer RJ, Fairlough D, Robertson M, et al. CD6-depleted allogeneic bone marrow transplantation for acute leukemia in first complete remission. Blood 1997;89:3039–47.
176. Papadopoulos EB, Carabasi MH, Castro-Malaspina H, et al. T-cell depleted allogeneic bone marrow transplantation as postremission therapy for acute myelogenous leukemia: Freedom from relapse in the absence of graft versus-host disease. Blood 1998;91:1083–90.
177. Witherspoon RP, Fisher LD, Schoch G, et al. Secondary cancers after bone marrow transplantation for leukemia or aplastic anemia. N Engl J Med 1989;321:784–9.
178. Slovak ML, Kopecky KJ, Cassileth PA, et al. Karyotypic analysis predicts outcome of pre-remission and post-remission therapy in adult acute myeloid leukemia: a SWOG/ECOG Intergroup study. Blood 2000;96:4075–83.
179. Brown RA, Herzig RH, Wolff SN, et al. High-dose etoposide and cyclophosphamide without bone marrow transplantation for resistant hematologic malignancy. Blood 1990;76:473–9.
180. Hiddemann W, Kreutzmann H, Straif K, et al. High-dose cytosine arabinoside and mitoxantrone: a highly effective regimen in refractory acute myeloid leukemia. Blood 1987;69:744–9.
181. Ho AD, Lipp T, Ehninger G, et al. Combination of mitoxantrone and etoposide in refractory acute myelogenous leukemia: an active and well-tolerated regimen. J Clin Oncol 1988;6:213–7.
182. Vahdat L, Wong ET, Wile MJ, et al. Therapeutic and neurotoxic effects of 2-chlorodeoyadenosine in adults with acute myeloid leukemia. Blood 1994;84:3429–34.
183. Ghandi V, Estey E, Keating MJ, et al. Fludarabine potentiates metabolism of cytarabine in patients with acute myelogenous leukemia during therapy. J Clin Oncol 1993;11:116–24.
184. Lee EJ, Egorin MJ, Van Echo DA, et al. A phase I and pharmacokinetic trial of carboplatin in refractory adult leukemia. J Natl Cancer Inst 1988;80:131–5.
185. Lee EJ, Van Echo DA, Egorin MJ, et al. Diaziquone given as a continuous infusion is an active agent for relapsed adult acute non-lymphocytic leukemia. Blood 1986;67:182–7.
186. Warrell RP Jr, Coonley CJ, Gee TS. Homoharringtonine: an effective new drug for remission induction in refractory nonlymphoblastic leukemia. J Clin Oncol 1985;3:617–21.
187. Faderl S, Gandhi V, O'Brien S, et al. Results of a phase 1-2 study of clofarabine in combination with cytarabine (ara-C) in relapsed and refractory acute leukemias. Blood 2005;105:940–7.
188. Giles FJ, Kantarjian HM, Cortes JE, G, et al. Adaptive randomized study of idarubicin and cytarabine versus troxacitabine and cytarabine versus troxacitabine and idarubicin in untreated patients 50 years or older with adverse karyotype acute myeloid leukemia. J Clin Oncol 2003;21:1722–7.
189. Hiddemann W, Martin WR, Sauerland CM, et al. Definition of refractoriness against conventional chemotherapy in acute myeloid leukemia: a proposal based on the results of retreatment by thioguanine, cytosine arabinoside and daunorubicin (TAD 9) in 150 patients with relapse after standardized first line therapy. Leukemia 1990;4:184–8.
190. Schiffer CA, Lee EJ. Approaches to the therapy of relapsed acute myeloid leukemia. Oncology 1989;3:23.
191. Rees JKH, Swirsky D, Gray RG, Hayhoe FGJ. Principal results of the Medical Research Councils 8th acute myeloid leukaemia trial. Lancet 1986;2:1236–41.
192. Breems DA, Van Putten WL, Huijgens PC, et al. Prognostic index for adult patients with acute myeloid leukemia in first relapse. J Clin Oncol 2005;23:1969–78.
193. Clift RA, Buckner CD, Appelbaum FR, et al. Allogeneic marrow transplantation during untreated first relapse of acute myeloid leukemia. J Clin Oncol 1992;10:1723–9.
194. Sievers EL, Larson RA, Stadtmauer EA, et al. Efficacy and safety of gemtuzumab ozogamicin in patients with CD33-positive acute myeloid leukemia in first relapse. J Clin Oncol 2001;19:3244–54.
195. Estey EH, Thall PF, Giles FJ, et al. Gemtuzumab ozogamicin with or without interleukin 11 in patients 65 years of age or older with untreated acute myeloid leukemia and high-risk myelodysplastic syndrome: comparison with idarubicin plus continuous-infusion, high-dose cytosine arabinoside. Blood 2002;99:4343–9.
196. Kumar L. Leukemia: management of relapse after allogeneic bone marrow transplantation. J Clin Oncol 1994;12:1710–7.
197. Rowe J, Andersen J, Mazza JJ, et al. A randomized placebo-controlled phase II study of granulocyte-macrophage colony-stimulating factor in adult patients (> 55 to 70 years of age) with acute myelogenous leukemia: a study of the Eastern Cooperative Oncology Group (E1490). Blood 1995;86:457–62.
198. Stone RM, Berg DT, George SL, et al. Granulocyte-macrophage colony-stimulating factor after initial chemotherapy for elderly patients with primary acute myelogenous leukemia. N Engl J Med 1995;332:1671–7.
199. Lowenberg B, Suciu S, Archimbaud OG, et al. Use of recombinant granulocyte-macrophage colony-stimulating factor during and after remission induction chemotherapy in patients 61 years and older with acute myeloid leukemia (AML): final report of AML-11, a phase III randomized study of the Leukemia Cooperative Group of European Organization and Treatment of Cancer (EORTC-LCG) and Dutch Belgian Hematooncology Cooperative Group (HOVON). Blood 1997;90:2952–61.
200. Witz F, Sadoun A, Perrin M-C, et al. A placebo-controlled study of recombinant human granulocyte-macrophage colony-stimulating factor administered during and after induction treatment for de novo acute myelogenous leukemia in elderly patients. Blood 1998;91:2722–30.
201. Godwin JE, Kopecky KJ, Head DR, et al. A double-blind placebo-controlled trial of granulocyte colony-stimulating factor in elderly patients with previously untreated acute myeloid leukemia: a Southwest Oncology Group (9031). Blood 1998;91:3607–15.
202. Dombret H, Chastang C, Fenaux P, et al. A controlled study of recombinant human granulocyte-stimulating factor in elderly patients after treatment for acute myelogenous leukemia. N Engl J Med 1995;332:1678–83.
203. Harousseau JL, Witz B, Lioure B, et al. Granulocyte colony-stimulating factor after intensive consolidation chemotherapy in acute myeloid leukemia: results of a randomized trial of the Groupe Ouest-Est Leucemies Aigues Myeloblastiques. J Clin Oncol 2000;18:780–7.
204. Heil G, Hoelzer D, Sanz MA, et al. A randomized, double-blind, placebo-controlled, phase II study of filgrastim in remission induction and consolidation therapy for adults with de novo acute myeloid leukemia. Blood 1997;90:4710–8.
205. Ohno R, Tomonaga M, Kobayashi T, et al. Effect of granulocyte colony-stimulating factor after intensive induction

therapy in relapsed or refractory acute leukemia. N Engl J Med 1990;323:871–7.

206. Moore JO, Dodge RK, Amrein PC, et al. Granulocyte-colony stimulating factor (Filgrastim) accelerates granulocyte recovery after intensive post-remission chemotherapy for acute myeloid leukemia with aziridinyl benzoquinone and mitoxantrone: Cancer and Leukemia Group B Study 9022. Blood 1997;89:780–8.
207. Schiffer CA, Miller K, Larson RA, et al. A double blind, placebo controlled trial evaluating pegylated recombinant human megakaryocyte growth and development factor (MGDF) as an adjunct to induction and consolidation therapy in patients with acute myeloid leukemia (AML). Blood 2000;95:2530–5.
208. Archimbaud E, Ottmann OG, Yin JA, et al. A randomized double-blind, placebo-controlled study with pegylated recombinant human megakaryocyte growth and development factor (PEG-rHuMGDF) as an adjunct to chemotherapy for adults with de novo acute myeloid leukemia. Blood 1999;94:3694–701.
209. Bhalla K, Tang C, Ibrado AM, et al. Granulocyte macrophage colony-stimulating factor/interleukin-3 fusion protein (pIXY 321) enhances high-dose ara-C-induced programmed cell death or apoptosis in human myeloid leukemia cells. Blood 1992;80:2883–90.
210. Cannistra SA, Groshek P, Griffin JD. Granulocyte-macrophage colony-stimulating factor enhances the cytotoxic effects of cytosine arabinoside in acute myeloblastic leukemia and in the myeloid blast crisis phase of chronic myeloid leukemia. Leukemia 1989;3:328–34.
211. Estey EH, Dixon D, Kantarjian HM, et al. Treatment of poor-prognosis, newly diagnosed acute myeloid leukemia with ara-C and recombinant human granulocyte-macrophage colony-stimulating factor. Blood 1990;75:1766–9.
212. Peterson BA, George SL, Bhalla K, et al. A phase II trial with and without GM-CSF administered before and during high dose cytarabine in patients with relapsed refractory acute myelogenous leukemia. Proc Am Soc Clin Oncol 1996;15:504a.
213. Löwenberg B, van Putten, W, Theobald M, et al. Effect of priming with granulocyte colony stimulating factor on the outcome of chemotherapy for acute myeloid leukemia. N Engl J Med 2003;349:743–52.
214. Amadori S, Suciu S, Jehn U, et al. Use of glycosylated recombinant human G-CSF (lenograstim) during and/or after induction chemotherapy in patients 61 years of age and older with acute myeloid leukemia: final results of AML-13, a randomized phase-3 study. Blood 2005;106:27–34.
215. Reittie JE, Gottlieb D, Heslop HE, et al. Endogenously generated activated killer cells circulate after autologous and allogeneic marrow transplantation but not after chemotherapy. Blood 1989;73:1351–8.
216. Soiffer RJ, Murray C, Gonin R, Ritz J. Effect of low-dose interleukin-2 on disease relapse after T-cell-depleted allogeneic bone marrow transplantation. Blood 1994;84:964–71.
217. Foa R. Does interleukin-2 have a role in the management of acute leukemia? J Clin Oncol 1993;11:1817–25.
218. Meloni G, Foa R, Vignetti M, et al. Interleukin-2 may induce prolonged remissions in advanced acute myelogenous leukemia. Blood 1994;84:2158–63.
219. Cignetti A, Bryant E, Allione B, et al. CD34(+) acute myeloid and lymphoid leukemic blasts can be induced to differentiate to dendritic cells. Blood 1999;94:2048–55.
220. Lu S, Wieder E, Komanduri K, et al. Vaccines in leukemia. .Adv Pharmacol 2004;51:255–70.
221. Raza A, Maheshwari Y, Preisler HD. Differences in cell cycle characteristic among patients with acute nonlymphocytic leukemia. Blood 1987;69:1647–53.
222. Schiffer CA. Hematopoietic growth factors and the future of therapeutic research on acute myeloid leukemia. N Engl J Med 2003;349:727–29.
223. Kufe DW, Spriggs DR. Biochemical and cellular pharmacology of cytosine arabinoside. Semin Oncol 1985;12:34–48.
224. Plunkett W, Liliemark JO, Adams TM, et al. Saturation of 1-(3-D-arabinofuranosylcytosine 5'-triphosphate accumulation in leukemia cells during high-dose 1-P-D-arabinofuranosylcytosine therapy. Cancer Res 1987;47:3005–11.
225. Estey E, Thall P, Andreef M, et al. Use of granulocyte colony-stimulating factor before, during, and after fludarabine plus cytarabine induction therapy of newly diagnosed acute myelogenous leukemia or myelodysplasia syndromes: comparison with fludarabine plus cytarabine without granulocyte colony-stimulating factor. J Clin Oncol 1994;12:671–8.
226. Moscow JA, Cowan KH. Multidrug resistance. J Natl Cancer Inst 1988;80:14–20.
227. Holmes J, Jacobs A, Carter G, et al. Multidrug resistance in haemopoietic cell lines, myelodysplastic syndromes and acute myeloblastic leukaemia. Br J Haematol 1989;72:40–4.
228. Ma DDF, Davey RA, Harman DH, et al. Detection of a multidrug resistant phenotype in acute nonlymphoblastic leukemia. Lancet 1987;1:135–7.
229. Ito Y, Tanimoto M, Kumazawa T, et al. Increased p-glycoprotein expression and multidrug-resistant gene (mdr1) amplification are infrequently found in fresh leukemia cells. Cancer 1989;63:1534–8.
230. Leith CP, Kopecky KJ, Godwin J, et al. Acute myeloid leukemia in the elderly: assessment of multidrug resistance (MDR) and cytogenetics distinguishes biologic subgroups with remarkably distinct responses to standard chemotherapy. A Southwest Oncology Group study. Blood 1997;89:3323.
231. Ross DD, Wooten PJ, Tong Y, et al. Synergistic reversal of multidrug resistance phenotype in acute myeloid leukemia cells by cyclosporine A and Cremophor EL. Blood 1994;83:1337–47.
232. List AF, Kopecky KJ, Willman CL, et al. Benefit of cyclosporine modulation of drug resistance in patients with poor-risk acute myeloid leukemia: a Southwest Oncology Group study. Blood 2001;98:3212–20.
233. Lee EJ, George ST, Caligiuri M, et al. Parallel phase I studies of daunorubicin given with cytosine arabinoside and etoposide with or without the multidrug resistance modulator PSC-833 in previously untreated patients 60 years of age with acute myeloid leukemia: results of Cancer and Leukemia Group B study 9420. J Clin Oncol 1999;17:2831–39.
234. Baer MR, Schiffer CA, George SL, et al. Phase III study of the multidrug resistance modulator PSC-833 in previously untreated patients 60 years of age and older with acute myeloid leukemia: Cancer and Leukemia Group B study 9720. Blood 2002;100:1224–32.
235. Advani R, Saba HI, Tallman M, et al. Treatment of refractory and relapsed acute myelogenous with combination chemotherapy plus the multidrug modulator PSC-833 (Valdospar). Blood 1999;93:787–95.
236. Lum BL, Kaubisch S, Yahanda AM, et al. Alteration of etoposide pharmacokinetics and pharmacodynamics by cyclosporine in a phase I trial to modulate multidrug resistance. J Clin Oncol 1992;10:1635–42.
237. Schneider E, Cowan KH, Bader H, et al. Increased expression of the multidrug resistance-associated protein gene in relapsed acute leukemia. Blood 1995;85:186–93.
238. Schuurhuis GJ, Broxterman HJ, Ossenkoppele GJ, et al. Functional multidrug resistance phenotype associated with combined overexpression of Pgp/MDR1 and MRP together with 1-β-D-arabinofuranosylcytosine sensitivity may predict clinical response in acute myeloid leukemia. Clin Cancer Res 1995;1:81–3.
239. Fontana JA, Rogers JS II, Durham JP. The role of 13 cis-retinoic acid in the remission induction of a patient with acute promyelocytic leukemia. Cancer 1986;57:209–17.
240. Huang ME, Ye YC, Chen SR, et al. Use of all-trans retinoic acid in the treatment of acute promyelocytic leukemia. Blood 1988;72:567–72.
241. Castaigne S, Chomienne C, Daniel MT, et al. All-trans retinoic acid as a differentiation therapy for acute promyelocytic leukemia. I. Clinical results. Blood 1990;76:1704–9.
242. Warrell RP, Frankel SR, Miller WH, et al. Differentiation therapy of acute promyelocytic leukemia with tretinoin (all-trans retinoic acid). N Engl J Med 1991;324:1385–93.
243. Tallman MS, Anderson JW, Schiffer CA, et al. Clinical Description of 44 patients with acute promyelocytic leukemia who developed the retinoic acid syndrome. Blood 2000;95:90–5.
244. De Botton S, Dombret H, Sanz M, et al. Incidence, clinical features, and outcomes of all trans-retinoic acid syndrome in 413 cases of newly diagnosed acute promyelocytic leukemia. The Europe APL Group. Blood 1998;92:2712–8.
245. Warrell RP Jr. Retinoid resistance in acute promyelocytic leukemia: new mechanisms, strategies and implications. Blood 1993;82:1949–53.
246. Fenaux P, Le Deley MC, Castaigne S, et al., the European APL 91 Group. Effect of all trans retinoic acid in newly diagnosed acute promyelocytic leukemia. Results in a multicenter randomized trial. Blood 1993;82:3241–9.
247. Tallman MS, Andersen JW, Schiffer CA, et al. All-transretinoic acid in acute promyelocytic leukemia. N Engl J Med 1997;337:1021–8.
248. Fenaux P, Chastang C, Chevret S, et al. A randomized comparison of all trans retinoic acid (ATRA) followed by chemotherapy and ATRA plus chemotherapy and role of maintenance therapy in newly diagnosed acute promyelocytic leukemia. Blood 1999;94:1192–200.
249. Mandelli F, Diverio D, Avvisati G, et al. Molecular remission in PML/RAR alpha-positive acute promyelocytic leukemia by combined all-trans retinoic acid and idarubicin (AIDA) therapy. Gruppo Italiana-Malattie Ematologiche Maligne dell'Adulto and Associazione Italiana di Ematologia de Oncologia Pediatrica Cooperative Groups. Blood 1997;90:1014–21.
250. Sanz MA, Lo Coco F, Martin G, et al. Definition of relapse risk and role of nonanthracycline drugs for consolidation in patients with acute promyelocytic leukemia: a joint study of the PETHEMA and GIMEMA cooperative groups. Blood 2000;96:1247–53.
251. Niu C, Yan H, Yu T, et al. Studies on treatment of acute promyelocytic leukemia with arsenic trioxide: remission induction, follow-up, and molecular monitoring in 11 newly diagnosed and 47 relapsed acute promyelocytic leukemia patients. Blood 1999;94:3315–24.
252. Soignet SL, Franke SR, Douer D, et al. United States Multicenter study of arsenic trioxide in relapsed acute promyelocytic leukemia. J Clin Oncol 2001;19:3852–60.
253. Dao-Pei Lu, Jing-Ying Qiu, Bin Jiang, et al. Tetra-arsenic tetra-sulfide for the treatment of acute promyelocytic leukemia: a pilot report. Blood 2002;99:3136–43.
254. Marcucci G, Mrozek K, Ruppert AS, Archer KJ, et al. Abnormal cytogenetics at date of morphologic complete remission predicts short overall and disease-free survival, and higher relapse rate in adult acute myeloid leukemia: results from cancer and leukemia group B study 8461. J Clin Oncol 2004;22:2410–8.
255. Campana D, Pui C-H. Detection of minimal residual disease in acute leukemia: methodologic advances and clinical significance. Blood 1995;85:1416–34.
256. San Miguel JF, Vidriales MB, Lopez-Berges C, et al. Early immunophenotypical evaluation of minimal residual disease in acute myeloid leukemia identifies different patient risk groups and may contribute to post induction treatment stratification. Blood 2001;98:1746–51.
257. Diverio D, Rossi V, Avvisati G, et al. Early detection of relapse by prospective reverse transcriptase-polymerase chain reaction analysis of the PML/RAR alpha fusion gene in patients with acute promyelocytic leukemia enrolled in the GIMEMA-AIEOP multicenter "AIDA" trial. GIEMEMA-AIEOP Multicenter "AIDA" Trial. Blood 1998;92:784–9.
258. Meloni G, Diverio D, Vignetti M, et al. Autologous bone marrow transplantation for acute promyelocytic leukemia in second remission: Prognostic relevance of pretransplant minimal residual disease assessment by reverse-transcription polymerase chain reaction of the PML/RAR alpha fusion gene. Blood 1997;90:1321–5.
259. Estey E, Smith TL, Keating MJ, et al. Prediction of survival during induction therapy in patients with newly diagnosed acute myeloblastic leukemia. Leukemia 1989;3:257–63.
260. Campos L, Rouault J-P, Sabido O, et al. High expression of bcl-2 protein in acute myeloid leukemia cells is associated with poor response to chemotherapy. Blood 1993;81:3091–6.
261. Baldus CD, Tanner SM, Ruppert AS, et al. BAALC expression predicts clinical outcome of de novo acute myeloid leukemia patients with normal cytogenetics: a Cancer and Leukemia Group B Study. Blood 2003;102:1613–8.
262. Frohling S, Schlenk RF, Stolze I, et al. CEBPA mutations in younger adults with acute myeloid leukemia and normal cytogenetics: prognostic relevance and analysis of cooperating mutations. J Clin Oncol 2004;22:624–33.
263. Falini B, Mecucci C, Tiacci E, et al. Cytoplasmic nucleophosmin in acute myelogenous leucemia with a normal karyotype. N Engl J Med 2005;352:254–66.
264. Valk PJ, Verhaak RG, Beijen MA, et al. Prognostically useful gene-expression profiles in acute myeloid leukemia. N Engl J Med 2004;350:1617–28.
265. Samuels BL, Larson RA, Le Beau MM, et al. Specific chromosomal abnormalities in acute nonlymphocytic leukemia correlate with drug susceptibility in vivo. Leukemia 1988;2:79–83.
266. Keating MJ, Smith TL, Kantarjian H, et al. Cytogenetic pattern in acute myelogenous leukemia: a major reproducible determinant of outcome. Leukemia 1988;2:403–12.
267. Schiffer CA, Lee EJ, Tomiyasu T, et al. Prognostic impact of cytogenetic abnormalities in patients with de novo acute non-lymphoblastic leukemia. Blood 1989;73:263.
268. Grimwade D, Walker H, Harrison G, et al. The predictive value of hierarchical cytogenetic classification in older adults with acute myeloid leukemia (AML): analysis of 1065 patients entered into the United Kingdom Medical Research Council AML11 trial. Blood 2001;98:1312–20.

269. Byrd JC, Mrozek K, Dodge RK, Carroll AJ. Pretreatment cytogenetic abnormalities are predictive of induction success, cumulative incidence of relapse and overall survival in adult patients with de novo acute myeloid leukemia: results from CALGB 8461. Blood 2002;100:4325–36.
270. Lichtman MA, Weed RI. Peripheral cytoplasmic characteristics of leukocytes in monocytic leukemia: relationship to clinical manifestations. Blood 1972;40:52–61.
271. Lester TJ, Johnson JW, Cuttner J. Pulmonary leukostasis as the single worst prognostic factor in patients with acute myelocytic leukemia and hyperleukocytosis. Am J Med 1985;79:43–8.
272. Vaughan WP, Kimball AW, Karp JE, et al. Factors affecting survival of patients with acute myelocytic leukemia presenting with high WBC counts. Cancer Treat Rep 1981;65:1007–13.
273. Bunin NJ, Kunkel K, Callihan TR. Cytoreductive procedures in the early management in cases of leukemia and hyperleukocytosis in children. Med Pediatr Oncol 1987;15:232–5.
274. Cuttner J, Holland JF, Norton L, et al. Therapeutic leukapheresis for hyperleukocytosis in acute myelocytic leukemia. Med Pediatr Oncol 1983;11:76–8.
275. Bleyer WA, Poplack DG. Prophylaxis and treatment of leukemia in the central nervous system and other sanctuaries. Semin Oncol 1985;12:131–48.
276. Frick J, Ritch PS, Hansen RM, Anderson T. Successful treatment of meningeal leukemia using systemic high-dose cytosine arabinoside. J Clin Oncol 1984;2:365–8.
277. Cassileth PA, Sylvester LS, Bennett JM, Begg CB. High peripheral blast count in adult acute myelogenous leukemia is a primary risk factor for CNS leukemia. J Clin Oncol 1988;6:495–8.
278. Rosenthal AR. Ocular manifestations of leukemia. A review. Ophthalmology 1983;90:899–905.
279. Karesh JW, Goldman EJ, Reck K, et al. A prospective ophthalmic evaluation of patients with acute myeloid leukemia: correlation of ocular and hematologic findings. J Clin Oncol 1989;7:1528–32.
280. Meyer RJ, Cuttner J, Truog P, et al. Therapeutic leukopheresis of acute myelomonocytic leukemia in pregnancy. Med Pediatr Oncol 1978;4:77–83.
281. Bartsch HH, Meyer D, Teichmann AT, Speer CHP. Treatment of promyelocytic leukemia during pregnancy: a case report and review of the literature. Blut 1988;57:51–4.
282. Pizzuto J, Aviles A, Noriega L, et al. Treatment of acute leukemia during pregnancy: presentation of nine cases. Cancer Treat Rep 1980;64:679–83.
283. Pui CH, Jeha S, Irwin D, et al. Recombinant urate oxidase (rasburicase) in the prevention and treatment of malignancy-associated hyperuricemia in pediatric and adult patients: results of a compassionate-use trial. Leukemia 2001;15:1505–9.
284. Liu CY, Sims-McCallum RP, Schiffer CA. A single dose of rasburicase is sufficient for the treatment of hyperuricemia in patients receiving chemotherapy. Leuk Res 2005;29:463–5.
285. Wainer RA, Wiernik PH, Thompson WL. Metabolic and therapeutic studies of a patient with acute leukemia and severe lactic acidosis of prolonged duration. Am J Med 1973;55:255–60.
286. Valent P, Horny HP, Escribano L, et al. Diagnostic criteria and classification of mastocytosis: a consensus proposal. Leuk Res 2001;25:603–25.
287. Yoo D, Lessin LS, Jensen WN. Bone marrow mast cells in lymphoproliferative disorders. Ann Intern Med 1978 88:753–7.
288. Macon WR, Kinney MC, Glick AD, Collins RD. Marrow mast cell hyperplasia in hairy cell leukemia. Mod Pathol 1993;6:695–8.
289. Yoo D, Lessin LS. Bone marrow mast cell content in preleukemic syndromes. Am J Med 1982;73:539–42.
290. Fukuda T, Kakihara T, Kamishima T, et al. Leukemic cell membrane from acute myelogenous leukemias with massive mast cell infiltration has a mast cell differentiation activity under culture containing interleukin-3. Leuk Res 1994;18:749–59.
291. Topar G, Staudacher C, Geisen F, et al. Urticaria pigmentosa: a clinical, hematopathologic, and serologic study of 30 adults. Am J Clin Pathol 1998;109:279–85.
292. Wolff K, Komar M, Petzelbauer P. Clinical and histopathological aspects of cutaneous mastocytosis. Leuk Res 2001;25:519–28.
293. Schwartz LB. Clinical utility of tryptase levels in systemic mastocytosis and associated hematologic disorders. Leuk Res 2001;25:553–62.
294. Parker RI, Metcalfe DD. Basophils, mast cells, and systemic mastocytosis. In: Hoffman R, Benz ES, Shatil SJ, editors. Hematology: basic principles and practice. Philadelphia (PA): Churchill Livingstone; 2000:830–46
295. Horny H-P, Ruck MT, Kaiserling E. Spleen findings in generalized mastocytosis. A clinicopathologic study. Cancer 1992;70:459–68.
296. Durand B, Migliaccio G, Yee NS, et al. Long-term generation of human mast cells in serum-free cultures of CD34 cord blood cells stimulated with stem cell factor and interleukin-3. Blood 1994;84:3667–74.
297. Furitsu T, Tsujimura T, Tono T, et al. Identification of mutations in the coding sequence of the proto-oncogene c-*kit* in a human mast cell leukemia cell line causing ligand independent activation of c-*kit* product. J Clin Invest 1993;92:1736–44.
298. Longley BJ Jr, Metcalfe DD, Tharp M, et al. Activating and dominant inactivating c-KIT catalytic domain mutations in distinct clinical forms of human mastocytosis. Proc Natl Acad Sci U S A 1999;96:1609–14.
299. Yavuz AS, Lipsky PE, Yavuz S, et al. Evidence for the involvement of a hematopoietic progenitor cell in systemic mastocytosis from single-cell analysis of mutations in the c-*kit* gene. Blood 2002;100:661–5.
300. Sperr WR, Walchshofar S, Horny HP, et al. Systemic mastocytosis associated with acute myeloid leukaemia: report of two cases and detection of the c-kit mutation Asp-816 to Val. Br J Haematol 1998;103:740–9.
301. Ma Y, Zeng S, Metcalfe DD, et al. The c-*kit* mutation causing human mastocytosis is resistant to STI571 and other KIT kinase inhibitors; kinases with enzymatic site mutations show different inhibitor sensitivity profiles than wild-type kinases and those with regulatory-type mutations. Blood 2002;99:1741–4.
302. Bain BJ. Systemic mastocytosis and other mast cell neoplasms. Br J Haematol 1999;106:9–17.
303. Travis WD, Li CY, Hoagland HC, et al. Mast cell leukemia: report of a case and review of the literature. Mayo Clin Proc 1986;61:957–66.
304. Dalton R, Chan L, Bitten E, Eridani S. Mast cell leukemia: evidence for bone marrow origin of the pathological clone. Br J Haematol 1986;64:397–406.
305. Valent P, Akin C, Sperr WR, et al. Mastocytosis: pathology, genetics, and current options for therapy. Leuk Lymphoma 2005;46:35–48.
306. Kluin-Nelemans HC, Jansen JH, Breukelman H, et al. Response to interferon alpha-2b in a patient with systemic mastocytosis. N Engl J Med 1992;326:639–40.
307. Frieri M, Alling DW, Metcalfe DD. Comparison of the therapeutic efficacy of cromolyn sodium with that of combined chlorpheniramine and cimetidine in systemic mastocytosis. Am J Med 1985;78:9–14.
308. Tefferi A, Li CY, Butterfield JH, Hoagland JC. Treatment of systemic mast cell disease with cladribine. N Engl J Med 2001;344:307–9.
309. Johnstone PA, Mican JM, Metcalfe DD, DeLaney TF. Radiotherapy of refractory bone pain due to systemic mast cell disease. Am J Clin Oncol 1994;17:328–30.
310. Gotlib J, Berube C, Growney JD, et al. Activity of the tyrosine kinase inhibitor PKC412 in a patient with mast cell leukemia with the D816V KIT mutation. Blood 2005;106:2865–70.

Chronic Myeloid Leukemia

Jorge Cortes, MD
Richard T. Silver, MD
Hagop Kantarjian, MD

Chronic myeloid leukemia (CML) is a clonal myeloproliferative disorder of a pluripotent stem cell[1] with a specific cytogenetic abnormality, the Philadelphia (Ph) chromosome, involving myeloid, erythroid, megakaryocytic, B, and sometimes T, lymphoid cells,[2] but not marrow fibroblasts. Clonality has been demonstrated by cytogenetic,[3] molecular,[4] and glucose-6-phosphate dehydrogenase studies.[5] CML is as one of a group of myeloproliferative disorders clinically resembling polycythemia vera, agnogenic myeloid metaplasia, and essential thrombocythemia, but is distinguished from these diseases by specific chromosome and molecular markers to be discussed later.

Advances in cell biology and molecular genetics, and a plethora of biochemical, cytogenetic, and molecular data have yielded much new information regarding CML. Advances in marrow transplantation and, more recently, the efficacy of imatinib mesylate have radically changed the prognosis of CML. In this chapter we review the hematologic and clinical aspects of CML, discuss the pertinent advances in our understanding of its biology, review treatment programs, and discuss the new strategies and controversies involving the role of stem cell transplant and imatinib. In addition, two new drugs of major importance currently in early clinical trials, dasatinib and AMN107, will also be mentioned.

INCIDENCE AND EPIDEMIOLOGY

The annual incidence of CML is estimated at approximately 10 cases per million. It accounts for approximately 15% of all patients with leukemia.[6,7] Although it occurs relatively infrequently, its importance relates to the cytogenetic and molecular understanding of the disease and to the existence of effective therapy that offers potential for cure. The normal incidence of CML in the United States is 5,000 to 7,000 cases. The prevalence, with older therapies, based on a median survival of 3 to 5 years was 15,000 to 30,000 cases. With imatinib, the annual mortality has been reduced from 15 to 20% to 2%, and the estimated median survival may become 20 years. Thus, the prevalence of CML in the United States in the next decade may exceed 100,000 to 140,000 cases. CML will then change from a rare cancer to a relatively common one.

ETIOLOGY

In the great majority of patients, a causative factor cannot be identified. Ionizing radiation is leukemogenic. The most common type of leukemia following radiation is acute myeloid leukemia, but CML has also been observed in studies following the atom bomb explosions in Japan in 1945[8] and in earlier studies in radiologists and in patients with ankylosing spondylitis treated with radiation therapy.[8,9]

CLINICAL AND HEMATOLOGIC CHARACTERISTICS

The median age of onset of CML is 55 to 65 years, and the incidence increases with age. There is slight male preponderance (ratio 1.3:1). CML typically follows a bi- or triphasic course with a chronic phase, followed by an intermediate or accelerated phase, and finally a blastic phase. Approximately 90% of patients are diagnosed in the chronic phase, which is frequently asymptomatic.[10] When symptoms are present they usually develop insidiously and may be due to splenomegaly (pain, abdominal fullness). Less commonly, patients may present with symptoms of gout, anorexia, weight loss, unexplained fevers, or signs of platelet dysfunction (eg, petechiae, ecchymoses, or hemorrhage), or anemia (eg, fatigue). Leukocytosis is common, with white cell counts frequently higher than 100×10^9/L and occasionally leading to retinal hemorrhage and signs of hyperviscosity (priapism, cerebrovascular accidents, tinnitus, confusion, stupor). Historically, the median survival for patients in the chronic phase has been 3 to 5 years, with an estimated annual risk of transformation to the blastic phase of 5 to 10% in the first 2 years, and 15 to 20% subsequently. Accelerated-phase CML is characterized by increasing maturation arrest heralding transformation to the blastic phase. Different criteria have been used to define the accelerated phase. One common classification defines accelerated phase as the presence of any of the following features: 15% or more blasts, 30% or more blasts plus promyelocytes, 20% or more basophils, platelets lower than 100×10^9/L unrelated to therapy, or cytogenetic clonal evolution.[11] Other criteria have been proposed but some of these classifications, such as the WHO proposal,[12] have not been clinically validated. Median survival for patients in accelerated phase is 1 to 2 years,[13] but the criteria used and the therapy implemented (eg, with imatinib) may affect the expected survival. Symptoms associated with the accelerated phase may include fever, night sweats, or weight loss, or bleeding associated with thrombocytopenia. Occasionally, blood and bone marrow changes that augur transformation to the accelerated phase occur even in patients who are asymptomatic and identified only during routine follow-up. The blastic phase, the last stage of CML, is defined by the presence of at least 30% of blasts in the peripheral blood or the bone marrow, or the presence of extramedullary disease.[14] The WHO classification has proposed this to be changed to ≥ 20% blasts, but this proposal may not be justified.[15] The blastic phase of CML is associated with constitutional symptoms (night sweats, weight loss, fever, bone pain), anemia, an increased risk of infections, and/or bleeding. The blastic phase is of two general types, myeloid and lymphoid, but biphenotypic or mixed lineage lymphoblastic-myeloblastic blastic phase can be observed.[13,16] Lymphoid blastic phase occurs in 20 to 30% of patients, myeloid in 50%, and undifferentiated in 25%.[10,16] Median survival in blastic-phase CML is 3 to 6 months. Patients with lymphoid blast phase have a better prognosis, with a response rate of 60%, to acute lymphoblastic leukemia (ALL)-like therapy, and a median survival of 9 to 12 months.

Laboratory features in the chronic phase include leukocytosis with a left shift including all stages of differentiation, but the myelocyte predominates (Figure 114-1). Basophils and eosinophils are prominent. Thrombocytosis is common but thrombotic phenomena are unusual. A slight degree of anemia is common. A striking biochemical abnormality in CML, still unexplained in the reduction of the leukocyte alkaline phosphatase (LAP) activity, both in intensity and in the number of neu-

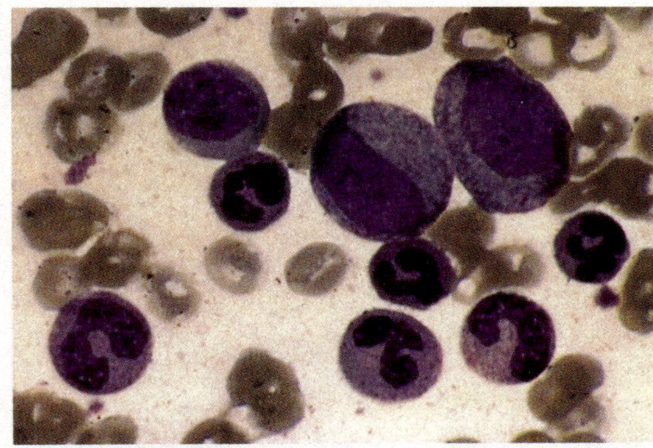

Figure 114-1 Chronic myeloid leukemia. Leukocytosis with myelocytes, metamyelocytes, band cells, and polymorphonuclear leukocytes are characteristic of the peripheral blood in the chronic phase of this disease.

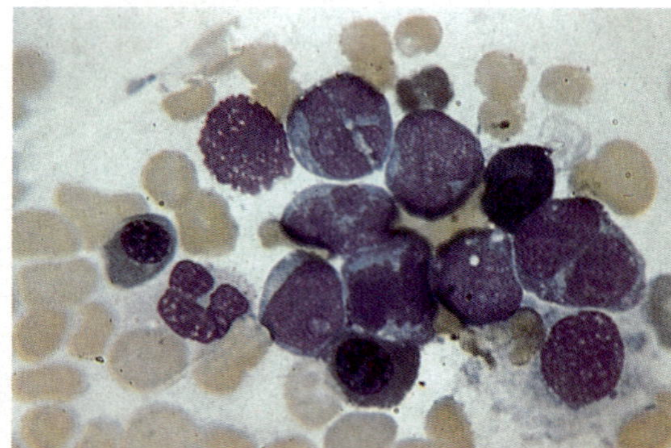

Figure 114-2 Chronic myeloid leukemia, myeloid blast crisis. The marrow aspiration shows predominance of blast forms, which have a myeloid appearance.

trophil band forms that stain positively for the enzyme. Phagocytic function remains essentially normal.[17] Low values may also be seen in agnogenic myeloid metaplasia, but a high value virtually excludes CML. The LAP score may increase in CML in the presence of infection, clinical remission, or with the onset of the blastic phase.

Mature granulocytes synthesize and release into the serum an α-globulin B12-binding protein, transcobalamin 1. The increase in the size of the white blood cell pool is reflected by marked elevation of serum B12 and unsaturated B12 binding capacity. An increase in circulating basophil levels, histamine production, or both, often occur during blastic transformation, but their significance is unknown.[18]

The bone marrow is hypercellular and devoid of fat.[19] During the chronic phase, all stages of differentiation are present, but the myelocyte predominates, whereas myeloblasts and promyelocytes usually account for less than 10% of the marrow cells (Figures 114-2 and 114-3). Early in the disease, megakaryocytes may be increased. Cells morphologically indistinguishable from true Gaucher cells can be seen in 10% of cases.[20] As in other myeloproliferative disorders, biopsy sections may show an increased number of reticulin fibers. As the disease evolves, varying degrees of fibrosis occur.[21] Evidence suggests that the marrow fibrosis may be a secondary phenomenon resulting from an abnormal interaction between the proliferative clone of megakaryocytes and elements regulating marrow fibrosis and collagen, including at least platelet-derived growth factor, transforming growth factor-β, basic fibroblastic growth factor, and other cytokines.

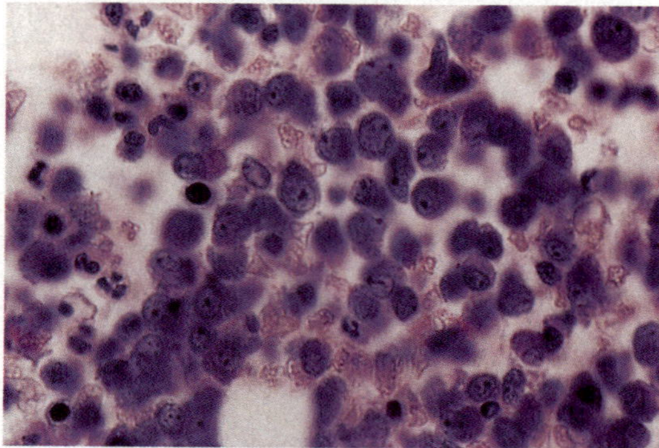

Figure 114-3 Chronic myeloid leukemia, blast phase. This bone marrow biopsy shows "blasts" with prominent nucleoli comprising about 75% of the marrow cells.

In the blastic phase of CML there is an increased number of "blasts," and the cells are morphologically similar to those seen in the acute leukemias. Lymphoid blast cells contain terminal deoxynucleotidyl transferase (TdT), an enzyme that catalyzes the polymerization of deoxynucleoside triphosphates.[22] TdT is found mainly in poorly differentiated normal and malignant lymphoid cells of T-cell and B-cell origin and is lost as these lymphocytes differentiate and mature. The cells in most lymphoid blast phases are of B-cell origin, because the lymphoblasts express CD10, CD19, and CD22 or other B-cell markers. T-cell blast phase occurs in a small proportion of patients.[22] The myeloid blast phase may mimic acute myeloid leukemia since the myeloblasts stain with myeloperoxidase and express myeloid markers, including CD13, CD33, and CD117.

Rarely, patients may present in lymphoid or myeloid blast phase without a recognized antecedent chronic phase. The differentiation between this presentation and Ph-positive acute lymphoblastic or acute myeloid leukemias may be impossible. Megakaryoblastic[23] and erythroblastic[24] transformations and blastic phases marked by basophilia and high blood histamine levels have also been reported.

The basic mechanism by which the chronic phase transforms into the blastic phase is not understood. Cytogenetic abnormalities, in addition to the Ph-chromosome, often develop prior to, or at the time of, transformation, but they may not necessarily be causally related to blastic transformation. Other molecular events, such as alterations of the *TP53* and *p16* genes may be associated with disease transformation.[25] Recently, it has been suggested that granulocyte-macrophage progenitors may be the candidate stem cells in blast phase CML; activation of β-catenin may enhance the self-renewal activity and leukemic potential of these cells.[26]

About 5 to 10% of "typical" CML cases lack the Ph chromosome and its molecular abnormality and have less characteristic clinical and hematologic features, including lower initial white cell and platelet counts and muramidasuria.[27] These Ph-negative cases (called "atypical CML" in the WHO classification) have a median survival of approximately 20 months, for which there is no specific therapy. This type of leukemia is not further discussed in this chapter.

PROGNOSTIC CLASSIFICATION

Prognosis in CML is variable. Risk classifications have been proposed to stratify patients and assist in treatment decisions. The Sokal model is most frequently used.[28] It defines three risk groups, low-risk (about 40–50%), intermediate risk (about 30%), and high risk (about 20%), with median survivals of 4.5, 3.5, and 2.5 years, respectively.[28] Other classifications have been proposed that may be simpler (the "synthesis staging system"),[29] more applicable to patients treated with rIFNα (the Harford score),[30] or specifically oriented for transplant patients (the Gratwohl score).[31] Common poor prognostic factors in CML include older age, splenomegaly, increased blasts or basophils, thrombocytosis, clonal evolution, and fibrosis. With imatinib therapy, the significance of several of these factors has been reduced or eliminated (older age, fibrosis, and 9q abnormality).[32–35]

PATHOPHYSIOLOGY

The characteristic abnormality in CML is an increase in the myeloid component.[36] The total granulocyte pool is from 10 to 150 times normal. This appears to be related to a shift in the number of self-renewal cells toward differentiating cells. It has been suggested that the primary biologic defect in CML is not unregulated proliferation of leukemic stem cells, but rather, discordant maturation, wherein a slight delay in cell maturation within the myeloid compartment results in increased myeloid mass.[37] In contrast to the normal state, in which the primitive progenitors have a large proliferative potential and produce the majority of cells, in CML, early progenitors have reduced proliferative capacity as the leukemic population expands. This occurs because an increased number of divisions take place in the more mature proliferative compartments (late blast, promyelocyte, and myelocyte), which are not under regulatory control, and because the more mature cells have an increased life span. Leukocyte labeling techniques indicate that mature granulocytes equilibrate with the large total granulocyte pool and have a prolonged circulation.[36] In addition, there is a decrease in apoptosis of myeloid cells that contributes to the expansion of this compartment. Defective adherence of immature CML cells to marrow stromal cells in vitro[38] suggests that early release into the circulation in vivo may also play a role in producing an increased white blood cell mass. Attempts have been made to correlate growth abnormalities with variations in hematopoietic factors, such as increased levels of or sensitivity to granulocyte-macrophage colony-stimulating factor (GM-CSF) or decreased levels of sensitivity to inhibitors of myelopoiesis, such as acid lactoferrin or prostaglandin E.[39] The expression and subsequent loss of class II major histocompatibility determinants may also play a role.[39] Whether these events are primary or secondary remains to be determined.[40]

CYTOGENETICS

The cytogenetic hallmark of CML is the Ph chromosome.[41,42] This results from a reciprocal translocation of cytogenetic material following a break on chromosome 9 at band q34.1 that transposes the 3' segment of the *ABL* gene to the 5' segment of the *BCR* gene on chromosome 22 at band q11.21.[42] The cytogenetic nomenclature is t(9;22)(q34.1;q11.21). The chromosomal abnor-

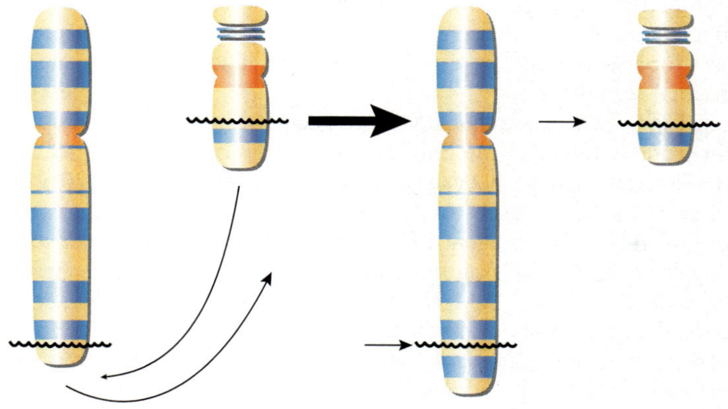

Figure 114-4 Schematic of 9.22 chromosome translocation.

mality creates the chimeric *BCR-ABL* gene (Figure 114-4).

The Ph chromosome is found in approximately 95% of patients with CML. It is also observed in 5% of children and 15 to 30% of adults with acute lymphoid leukemia and in 2% of patients with newly diagnosed acute myeloid leukemia.[43] Some patients were initially described as having translocations involving chromosome 22 and chromosomes other than 9, but it is now believed that 9 is involved in all cases.[44–46] Other patients have complex translocations involving three or more chromosomes that may result in a "masked" Ph.[47,48] Although initially thought to confer poor prognosis,[49] recent data have shown these patients have a similar prognosis compared with patients with the classic Ph chromosome.[50] There is no difference in survival in patients with standard compared with variant translocations. Approximately 5% of patients with the phenotype of typical CML lack the Ph chromosome but demonstrate the *BCR-ABL* rearrangement.[51] The clinical and hematologic characteristics as well as the response to treatment and the course of the disease of CML patients who are Ph negative but express the BCR-ABL rearrangement is the same as that of Ph-positive patients. Thus, the demonstration of the chimeric gene is the sine qua non for the diagnosis of CML.

Progression of CML is frequently accompanied by additional cytogenetic abnormalities.[52,53] The most common abnormalities include a second Ph chromosome, isochromosome 17, trisomy 8, trisomy 19, and 20q-, although any chromosome may be affected. In lymphoid blastic phase, hypodiploidy is common. The molecular counterpart of these cytogenetic abnormalities is not always known. Mutations or deletions of tumor-suppressor genes such as *p16* and *TP53*, may contribute to the more immature phenotype.[54] Hypermethylation of promoter genes such as *ABL*, *BCR*, *p15*, and *cadherin-13* may also contribute to transformation.[55–58]

After successful treatment (eg, with rIFNα or imatinib), chromosomal abnormalities may be found in the Ph-negative cells. The most frequently observed abnormalities are trisomy 8, monosomy 7 or 5, and deletion 20q.[59–61] These occur in as many as 15% of patients treated with imatinib. They usually represent a small percentage of the cells and may regress spontaneously (70% of cases). The clinical significance of this phenomenon is unclear. Rare instances of "secondary" acute leukemias or myelodysplastic syndromes have been reported.[61] This phenomenon (ie, chromosomal abnormalities in Ph-negative cells) differs from clonal evolution where the same cell expresses both the Ph chromosome and additional chromosomal abnormalities.

MOLECULAR BIOLOGY OF CML

The reciprocal translocation of parts of chromosomes 9 and 22 results in a fusion or chimeric gene that codes for a Bcr-Abl oncoprotein with altered tyrosine kinase activity.[62,63]

Although the breakpoints on both chromosomes 9 and 22 are usually restricted to quite specific regions, some heterogeneity exists. On chromosome 9, breakage occurs in a region 200 kb or more in length, resulting in most of the c-*abl* gene being translocated.[62] Depending on the precise location of the breakpoint, c-*abl* exons 1a and 1b may be translocated to the Ph chromosome. However, post-transcriptional splicing of the transcript results in the exclusion of the coding sequence from these two exons from the *bcr-abl* messenger ribonucleic acid (mRNA). Variability in the chromosome 9 break points has no clinical or prognostic consequence.

Depending on the site of the breakpoint in the *BCR* gene, the fusion protein can vary in size from 185 (190) kilodaltons (kDa) to 230 kDa. Each fusion gene encodes the same portion of the *ABL* gene but differs in the length of *bcr* sequence. Transcription of the fusion *BCR-ABL* gene results in a chimeric bcr/abl mRNA that is translated into fusion proteins of varying sizes ranging from p190$^{bcr\text{-}abl}$, *p210*$^{bcr\text{-}abl}$, and p230$^{bcr\text{-}abl}$ according to the break point of the *BCR* gene (Figure 114-5). These cytoplasmic proteins have unregulated constitutive tyrosine kinase activity and activate a number of intracellular signaling pathways that affect cell proliferation, differentiation, and apoptosis rendering the cell independent of cytokine regulation.[64,65] Among the recognized target proteins are STAT, RAS, RAF, JUN kinase, MYC, AKT, and other signal transducers.[64,65] *bcr-abl* may also be involved in cellular adhesion defects because CML cells adhere poorly to marrow stroma.[38,66]

Most patients with typical chronic phase CML express the 210-kDa bcr-abl protein. Two types of *bcr-abl* mRNAs occur as a result of bcr breakpoint heterogeneity. These are known as the b2a2 or b3a2 fusion.[64,65] The clinical features, response to treatment, and prognosis are similar for both groups. Patients with Ph-positive acute lymphocytic leukemia may express either a 210-kDa (30–50%) or a 190-kDa *bcr-abl* protein (50–70%). The latter is also referred to as a 185/190 kDa; in this case, the ribonucleic acid (RNA) is 7.0 kDa. Although frequently thought to be specific for Ph-positive ALL, rare patients with CML in chronic phase may express the 190 kDa protein and may have a worse prognosis than those with typical p210.[67] The larger 230-kDa bcr-abl fusion protein has been reported in a subset of patients with chronic neutrophilic leukemia who have a more benign course and a slower progression to blast phase disease.[68] That fusion proteins of different sizes can be correlated with different clinical outcomes suggests that the 190-kDa bcr-abl protein has more tyrosine kinase activity than the 230-kDa bcr-abl protein, thus affecting the clinical manifestations of the illness.[69] Although many of the molecular abnormalities of CML have been elucidated, the functions of *bcr* and *abl*

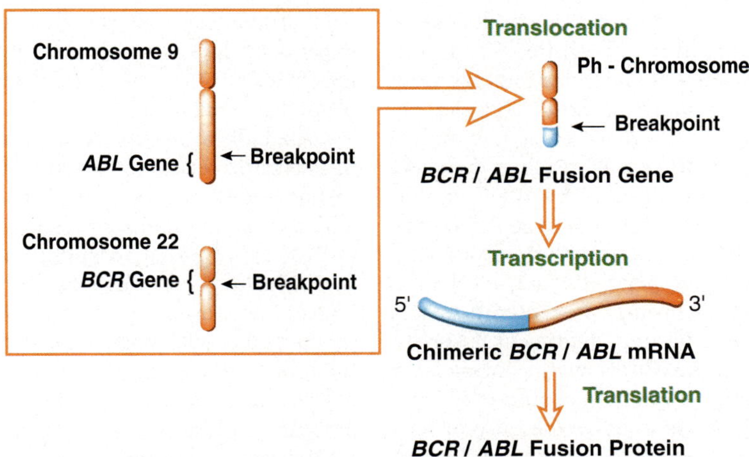

Figure 114-5 Summary of the cytogenetic and molecular effects of the Ph chromosome.

in both normal cells and in CML are still not completely understood.

The molecular test, reverse transcriptase-polymerase chain reaction (RT-PCR), may detect the *bcr-abl* transcript in 10^5 nonleukemic cells.[70] Interestingly, using a more sensitive RT-PCR (sensitivity approximately 10^{-8}) the *bcr-abl* chimerism has been identified in as many as 25 to 30% of normal adults.[71,72] This suggests the presence of bcr-abl positive cells in a sizable number of individuals who never develop CML, indicating that clonal disease requires a critical number of cells and/or a second oncogenic event. Abundant experimental evidence suggests that the *bcr-abl* event is causally related to the clinical development of CML. The relation of c-*abl* to murine leukemia has been mentioned. When murine hemopoietic stem cells are transfected with a retrovirus encoding $p210^{bcr\text{-}abl}$ and transplanted into irradiated syngeneic mice, they develop several hematologic malignancies including a syndrome resembling human chronic myeloid leukemia.[73] The importance of p190 in the pathogenesis of leukemia has also been demonstrated. The progeny of mice made transgenic for a $p190^{bcr\text{-}abl}$ DNA construct were either moribund or died of acute leukemia (myeloid or lymphoid) 10 to 58 days after birth.[63] A causal relationship between the Ph chromosome and human leukemia fortifies the concept that elimination of the Ph chromosome improves the prognosis of patients with CML.

TREATMENT

The most important recent advance in the treatment of CML has been the introduction of imatinib mesylate in patients with CML. Because hydroxyurea, busulfan, recombinant interferon, and marrow transplantation are still relevant to treatment in CML, these modalities are reviewed first.

Hydroxyurea and Busulfan For many years, hydroxyurea (HU) and busulfan (BUS) were the main drugs used to treat patients with CML. However, only recently was HU's superiority established in a randomized clinical comparative trial.[74] The median survival was significantly less with BUS as compared with HU (45 vs 58 months, respectively), as was the 5-year survival (32% vs 44%).[74]

HU is S-phase and cell-cycle specific, and functions as an antimetabolite. It is still useful in temporarily controlling the white blood cell (WBC) and/or platelet count or for patients who have no other treatment options. HU can be started at a dosage of 15 to 50 mg/kg/day orally, depending on the WBC, and increasing, if necessary, or decreasing the dose as the WBC and/or platelet count falls. The drug should be discontinued when the WBC falls to less than 15,000/μL. A rapid decrease in the platelet count in relation to the WBC requires prompt dose modification. On the other hand, additional treatment is sometimes required after the white count is normalized if the platelet count remains substantially elevated. A handy guide is to halve the dose of HU as the WBC is halved. Maintenance treatment may range from 500 to 2,500 mg daily with appropriate dose adjustment up or down. HU side effects include stomatitis, nausea and vomiting, a maculopapular rash, nephrotic syndrome, and pretibial skin ulcers.

BUS is now less frequently used. For patients who cannot tolerate imatinib mesylate, HU, or interferon and who are not candidates for transplantation, BUS can be used. A standard initial daily dose of the alkylating agent BUS is 4 to 6 mg/m^2 body surface (0.06–0.1 mg/kg) orally, with a maximum dose of 8 mg. Like HU, and using the same guide, the dose of BUS is gradually reduced as the WBC falls. Bone marrow hypoplasia in patients receiving BUS is usually dose related but may be idiosyncratic. Exfoliative cytologic studies of the cervix, sputum, and, less often, urine, may reveal dysplastic changes, suggesting that a neoplasm might exist. Should that occur, it may be necessary to discontinue BUS or to undertake other studies to determine whether such cytologic changes represent true neoplasms. Other common toxic effects of BUS include amenorrhea, increased skin pigmentation, a wasting syndrome with features of Addison's disease, cataracts, "busulfan lung," and endocardial fibrosis.

Although both HU and BUS usually cause excellent clinical and hematologic remissions in the great majority of CML patients, the fundamental abnormality, the Ph chromosome, remains in all patients during the otherwise favorable hematologic response. Thus, remission after chemotherapy with either drug in CML reflects quantitative, not qualitative, changes. Refractoriness to either drug is uncommon in the chronic phase of CML, and its occurrence usually signifies impending terminal or blast phase disease.

Interferon Because interferons have a wide range of biologic activities, including antiviral, antiproliferative, immunomodulatory, antiangiogenic, and oncogene regulatory properties,[75] they were evaluated in CML. There is now general agreement that rIFNα-2a or rIFNα-2b, alone or combined with ara-C (and possibly other chemotherapeutic agents) can induce durable suppression of the Ph-positive clone and prolong life of patients with CML. Other interferons have also been evaluated. Although recombinant IFNγ (rIFNγ) shares many of the functional properties of rIFNα, significant differences exist. Based on published clinical experience, however, it is unlikely that rIFNγ will contribute to improved therapeutic response and it is not discussed here.[76,77]

The bulk of the evidence for the effectiveness of interferon relates to the use of rIFNα in at least 30 uncontrolled observational studies.[78] Complete and partial hematologic remission rates after rIFNα are reported in approximately 70% and 10% of patients, respectively. More important than hematologic response after rIFNα, however, is the production of cytogenetic remission, which, unfortunately, occurs significantly less often. Most investigators define cytogenetic response using the percentage of Ph-positive metaphases reported on the most favorable karyotype.[79] Complete cytogenetic response is defined as 0% Ph-positive metaphases, partial cytogenetic response as 5 to 34% Ph-positive, and minor response as 35 to 95%. A major response is defined as the sum of complete plus partial cytogenetic responses. Although response rates differ from center to center, overall, a major response is seen in approximately 20% of patients, of which 8% are complete and 12% are partial responses. The reasons for the difference in response rates have been reviewed in detail.[78] Briefly, they are related to differences in case mix, age, stage of disease, elapsed time from diagnosis to treatment, and prognostic factors that differ among the various centers. In most cases, cytogenetic response occurs more frequently in patients who have low/normal platelet counts, a low percentage of blasts, and a nonpalpable spleen (ie, those defined as "good risk" or who have a favorable or low-risk Sokal or Hasford score).

The achievement of a cytogenetic remission is important because it is accompanied by a superior survival compared with those patients who have an intermediate response or none at all (Figure 114-6).[79] In most, but not all, studies in which a survival advantage is shown, maximally tolerated doses of rIFNα have been given leading to leukocyte counts of 2,000 to 4,000 μL. Usually this dosage is 5 million units (MU) per m^2/day. Of considerable importance, except for one study[80] employing only interferon that did not show survival advantage, all others have employed HU and/or ara-C during induction and during some phase of the maintenance program.

Patients who achieve a complete cytogenetic remission with rIFNα, but have high levels of minimal residual disease measured by quantitative PCR, have a high probability of relapse, whereas 80% of those with low transcript levels (ie, BCR-ABL/ABL $< 0.045\%$) have remained in remission after 3 years.[81] Approximately 30% of patients who achieve a complete cytogenetic remission have undetectable disease by PCR (ie, complete molecular remission); none of these patients has relapsed after a median follow-up of 10 years and may be cured.[82] However, even of those with residual disease by PCR, 40 to 60% have remained in cytogenetic remission after 10 years. This has been called an operational[82] or "biologic cure."[83] Although these data emphasize the importance of achieving a molecular remission with rIFNα, some patients may nevertheless live with low levels of minimal residual disease without clinical evidence of CML. This has been attributed to immune mechanisms induced by rIFNα, which do not occur with imatinib. Cytotoxic T-lymphocytes specific for PR1, a peptide derived from proteinase 3, which is overexpressed in CML, are found in patients in complete remission after rIFNα therapy (or bone marrow transplantation) but not after chemotherapy.[84] These lymphocytes may be responsible for the elimination or control of residual leukemic cells.

The issue of whether interferon improves survival as compared with conventional therapy was established first by the Italian Study Group on Chronic Myeloid Leukemia.[85] Patients, stratified according to risk factors, were randomized to

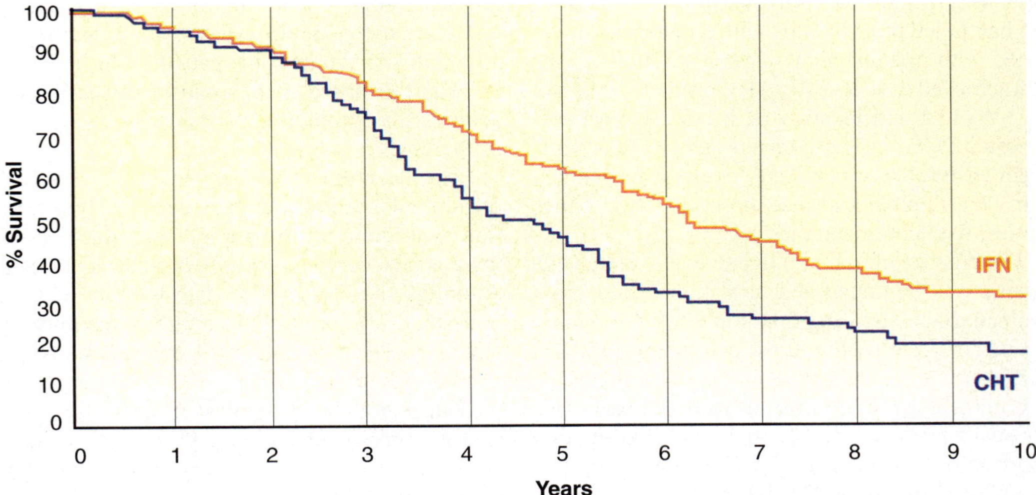

Figure 114-6 Long-term survival of patients with chronic myeloid leukemia treated with interferon-α or conventional chemotherapy. Data of the Italian Cooperative Study Group on Chronic Myeloid Leukemia.[86]

receive rIFNα or hydroxyurea (HU). Patients in the interferon arm were also allowed to receive supplemental HU. After a median follow-up of 68 months, the frequency of hematologic (clinical) remission was the same in both arms. In the interferon arm, however, a complete cytogenetic response was seen in 8% of the complete responders and a major response in 11% of responders. This compared with 0% and 1%, respectively, for the HU-treated group. The time to progression from the chronic phase of leukemia to an accelerated or blastic phase was 72 months in the interferon group compared with 45 months in the HU arm ($p < .001$). Overall, median survival was 72 months in the rIFNα + HU arm compared with 52 months in the HU-only arm. Major cytogenetic responses could be correlated with improved survival.[86] Other randomized trials have confirmed the superiority of interferon over HU in low-risk patients.[87]

A number of single-arm studies employing differing doses and schedules of rIFNα and ara-C indicate that the combination is also effective.[78,83,88,89] In one recent study using a different schedule of rIFNα and ara-C, landmark analysis showed a survival advantage for cytogenetic responses.[90] Two prospective randomized studies confirmed an improved cytogenetic response rate with the combination compared with rIFNα alone,[89,91] but although one (the "French") study showed improved survival for patients treated with the combination,[89] the other (the "Italian") did not.[91]

The side effects of rIFNα are not trivial. They include fever, chills, malaise, fatigue, headache, anorexia, joint pain, vomiting, low backache, myalgia, various types of neuropathy, changes in mood and concentration, abnormalities of liver enzymes, retinal vein thrombosis, leukopenia, and thrombocytopenia. Long-term therapy can be associated with autoimmune effects, including immune-mediated thrombocytopenia, hypothyroidism, and hemolytic anemia. Varying degrees of impotence may occur in approximately 25% of men. Interferon is contraindicated in patients with a psychiatric history of depression or suicidal tendencies.[92]

Bone Marrow Transplantation From 1980 until 2000, allogeneic stem cell transplantation (SCT) was the centerpiece of the management of CML. An overall discussion of SCT and the management of its complications are beyond the scope of this chapter (see Chapter 116, "Chronic Lymphocytic Leukemia"). Important aspects of its use and results in CML and its integration with other treatment options are discussed here.

Allogeneic SCT may be curative in a significant number of eligible patients who receive a transplant from an HLA-identical sibling. Because of the requirements for age, adequate organ function and performance status, availability of donor, and other factors, only a fraction of patients (10–30%) are eligible, particularly because the median age of patients with CML is 65 years (SEER data), and because only one-third of patients have an HLA-matched sibling. The number of potential donors may be increased by using matched unrelated donors,[93] but the cure rate and graft-versus-host disease (GVHD) rate are worse. These may be improved by careful molecular typing, especially HLA-A, -B, and -DRB1,[93] but this also reduces the probability of finding an adequate donor for most patients.

The expected results with modern SCT techniques are illustrated by a recent series from Seattle.[94] This study used busulfan plus cyclophosphamide as the conditioning regimen for 131 patients in early chronic phase (median age of 43 years; range 14 to 66 years). At 3 years, the projected nonrelapse mortality rate was 14%, and 78% were projected to be alive and free of disease. However, 60% had extensive chronic graft-versus-host disease (GVHD) 1 year after transplantation; 11% of patients had minimal residual disease documented by PCR, suggesting immune surveillance could prevent relapse.[94] This would be similar to the "biologic cure" described with rIFNα.

Cure with allogeneic SCT usually refers to the 5- to 6-year EFS rate. Few series have analyzed the very long-term results of SCT and the magnitude of complications, relapse, or death beyond this period. The availability of imatinib therapy has now accentuated the need for a more critical evaluation of risk versus benefit of allogeneic SCT. In the long-term Intermediate Bone Marrow Treatment Registry (IBMTR) studies, the 5-year EFS was 60% for sibling SCT in chronic phase, and the 20-year EFS was 40 to 45%, only partly owing to relapse. Thus, the expected annual mortality (beyond year 5) of a patient after allogeneic SCT may not be the same as normal individuals, perhaps because of subtle but serious effects of SCT or GVHD on organ functions. In an attempt to reduce the risk of GVHD, grafts can be depleted of T-lymphocytes. Although generally effective in reducing the risk of this complication, the risk of graft failure and relapse may increase.[95] Factors such as the method used for T-cell depletion, the ABO blood type match of the donor, and the number of HLA mismatches affect the outcome after T-cell depleted transplants.[96] In addition, allogeneic SCT affects quality of life because of the development of infertility, cataracts, hip necrosis, chronic lung disease, immune disorders, GVHD complications, second cancers, and others. Thus, the role of allogeneic SCT as frontline therapy, even in younger patients, must be reevaluated critically.

Patients transplanted in more advanced stages of CML (accelerated or blastic phase) have significantly worse outcomes, with 5-year survival probabilities of 40% accelerated phase and 10% blastic phase. Patients in blastic phase transplanted after induction of a second chronic phase may have long-term outcomes similar to accelerated phase.[97,98]

Patients who do not have a sibling donor may undergo a matched unrelated donor (MUD) transplantation. This procedure is associated with higher rates of early mortality and graft-versus-host disease. The long-term disease-free survival rate after MUD transplant for patients younger than 30 years of age transplanted within 1 year from diagnosis is 61% compared with 68% for matched siblings.[99] Patients age 30 to 40 years have long-term disease-free survival rates of 57% and 67%, respectively.[99] The results with MUD are improving with the use of molecularly matched donors.

Nonmyeloablative transplants have been used for older patients or those with health considerations that prevent them from receiving a SCT. Early results based on small series (frequently including mostly young patients) report disease-free survival rates as high as 85% at 70 months.[100] There is, however, a higher rate of residual CML after nonablative SCT. Results from larger series followed for longer are required to properly evaluate this technique. The use of alternative donors such as cord blood or haploidentical donors remains investigational.

In deciding on the best treatment strategy for patients eligible for SCT, several considerations must be entertained. One is the ideal timing of SCT. Early results from the IBMTR suggested that SCT performed after 12 months from diagnosis had inferior outcome. Recent studies showed that transplant performed within the first 24 to 36 months have similar outcomes to those performed within the first 12 months.[101] Thus, decisions regarding SCT can be evaluated at early time points in patients who are treated with imatinib but who nevertheless remain transplant candidates. With this approach, a trial with imatinib may be appropriate for most patients.

Another important consideration is the possible effect that prior therapy may have on stem cell transplant results. Most studies have indicated that prior therapy with rIFNα did not adversely affect SCT outcome.[102–104] Recent studies also suggest that prior imatinib therapy has no adverse impact on SCT outcome.[105,106]

Patients who relapse after transplant can frequently be re-induced into remission with donor lymphocyte infusion (DLI).[107–109] In patients who relapse in the chronic phase, a complete remission is achievable in 70%, and may be higher if treated at the time of molecular relapse (compared with cytogenetic or hematologic relapse). The response rate is 20% for those who relapse in accelerated phase and < 10% for patients in blastic phase. Toxicity includes myelosuppression in 20 to 30%, GVHD in 40% as the major toxicity, and a mortality of 10 to 20%. Imatinib has become an alternative for patients who relapse after transplant. A complete hematologic remission can be achieved in most patients treated in chronic phase after relapse from transplant, with complete cytogenetic remission in over 40%.[110–112] Complete hematologic remission occurs in 80 to 40% of those treated in accelerated or blast phase, respectively. The risks of myelosuppression and GVHD are lower with imatinib, but recurrence of GVHD has been reported in 11% of patients.[110] However, the long-term benefits compared with DLI are not known, and thus, DLI remains the treatment of choice.

Imatinib Mesylate The deregulated or constitutively active tyrosine kinase of the bcr-abl chimeric fusion protein is the causative molecular abnormality in CML. Thus, the *bcr-abl* tyrosine kinase is an ideal molecular target. Imatinib mesylate (Gleevec, Glivec, STI-571) is a potent and selective tyrosine kinase inhibitor.[113,114] In addition to *abl* and *abl*-related kinases (eg, *bcr-abl*), it can inhibit the kinase activity of c-kit, PDGF receptor, and probably a few others. By preventing the phosphorylation of the tyrosine residue, effectors that influence cell death, cell signaling, adhesion, and other vital cellular functions cannot be activated, thus disrupting the phenotypic pathway to CML.

Imatinib has become the standard therapy for CML. It was first used in CML after failure or intolerance to rIFNα. Using 400 mg daily, a CHR was achieved in 96% of patients and a complete cytogenetic response in 55%. The estimated 4-year survival rate for the total population was 82%.[115,116] Patients who achieved a major cytogenetic response after 3 months of therapy had an overall survival of 94% and progression-free survival of 78%.[116] With continued therapy, some patients achieved major and complete molecular responses. Among 261 patients in chronic phase who had failed prior therapy with rIFNα who were treated with imatinib in a single-institution study, 31% achieved a BCR-ABL/ABL ratio of < 0.05%, and 15% had undetectable BCR-ABL transcripts by nested PCR.[117] These results suggest that with longer term follow-up, favorable responses to imatinib were durable and that the results over time improve with continued therapy.[117]

The efficacy of imatinib in previously untreated patients was demonstrated in a multicenter randomized trial comparing imatinib to the combination of rIFNα plus low-dose cytarabine (ara-C) (IRIS trial).[118] This study showed significantly higher rates of hematologic and cytogenetic response, improved tolerance, and prolonged progression-free survival with imatinib compared with the combination of rIFNα and ara-C.[118] The improved toxicity profile of imatinib translated into an improved quality of life with imatinib.[119] After 42 months of follow-up, the rate of major cytogenetic response with imatinib was 91%, and complete cytogenetic response 84% (durable for 92%).[120] At 42 months, the estimated rate of freedom from progression to accelerated or blastic phase was 94% and the overall survival 91%. The initial analysis of the IRIS trial did not demonstrate a survival advantage for patients treated with imatinib initially compared with those treated initially with rIFNα and ara-C. This was due to early crossover from rIFNα to imatinib in more than 85% of patients initially randomized to rIFNα.

The standard starting dosage of imatinib in chronic phase is 400 mg daily. The selection of this dosage after the dose-finding phase I study was based on the observation that few responses were observed at lower doses, but no dose-limiting toxicity was identified at dosages up to 1,000 mg daily.[121] Thus, current recommendations are to avoid treating patients with less than 300 mg daily.

Higher dosages of imatinib (600–800 mg daily) may result in improved response rates that may be achieved sooner. Among patients in chronic phase who had failed prior rIFNα therapy, imatinib 800 mg daily resulted in a complete cytogenetic response in 90% of patients, and 50% achieved a complete molecular response.[122] Several single arm, uncontrolled studies in previously untreated patients in early chronic phase have shown higher rates of complete cytogenetic responses (90% or more), major molecular responses (70%), and complete molecular responses (25–40%) with higher doses of imatinib.[123–125] The use of higher doses is associated with increased incidence of myelosuppression, mostly in the first 3 months of therapy. Whether the improved initial results will translate into improved survival remains to be determined in controlled, randomized studies that are currently ongoing.

The response to imatinib at early time points is indicative of the longer-term outcome and should be used for treatment decisions. Among patients receiving imatinib as first-line therapy, patients who are not in CHR after 3 months or who are still 100% Ph positive after 6 months of therapy have ≤ 10% probability of achieving a complete cytogenetic response by 2 years. After 12 months of therapy, only patients who are < 35% Ph positive have a reasonable probability of achieving a complete response with continuation of therapy.[126]

The duration for which imatinib should be prescribed is unknown. The current recommendation is to continue treatment indefinitely unless there is unacceptable toxicity or treatment failure. Although the literature to date is limited, it suggests that discontinuing imatinib in patients who have achieved a complete response is followed by a rapid loss of that response.[127–129]

Management of Adverse Events In general, imatinib is well tolerated. The most common adverse event is myelosuppression. In early chronic phase, grade 3 or higher neutropenia (ie, neutrophils $< 1 \times 10^9$/L) occurs in up to 20% of patients, thrombocytopenia in 10%, and severe anemia in 5%.[115,118,122,124,130] The current recommendation is to interrupt therapy in patients who develop grade 3 or higher neutropenia or thrombocytopenia and not to immediately lower the dose. Upon recovery, treatment is restarted with the same dose if recovery takes less than 2 weeks or with a reduced dose if it takes longer than this time.[131] The use of hematopoietic growth factors (G-CSF for neutropenia, erythropoietin for anemia) has been reported to be safe and effective in patients with recurrent or persistent cytopenias.[132–138] Myelosuppression is frequently seen during the first 2 to 3 months of therapy as the leukemic granulocytes die and are replaced by normal ones. A brief treatment interruption is frequently sufficient to allow recovery, and most patients will not require dose reductions.

Nonhematologic adverse events are relatively common but usually mild and dose related with imatinib. Grade 3 or higher adverse events are rare; only 2 to 3% of patients require permanent discontinuation of therapy because of toxicity. Suggestions for the management of the most common adverse events are presented in Table 114-1. Early intervention is important to avoid more significant problems, unnecessary treatment interruptions, and dose reductions. Administration of other drugs metabolized through the P-450 cytochrome system in the liver should be done with caution as there is the risk of drug interactions.

Monitoring of Patients during Treatment For many years, hematologic response was the goal of therapy with agents such as hydroxyurea and busulfan since the Philadelphia chromosome was not affected. Reduction and even elimination of the Philadelphia chromosome after treatment with rIFNα resulted in cytogenetic responses that translated into a survival advantage.[82,139] Cytogenetic response became the new goal of therapy. In the imatinib era, since most patients achieve complete cytogenetic response, the goal of therapy is now shifting toward achieving a molecular response that will likely translate into further improvement in survival.

Table 114-1 Suggested Management of the Most Common Adverse Events Associated with Imatinib

Adverse Events	Management
Nausea/vomiting	Take with food, fluids Antiemetics
Diarrhea	Loperamide Diphenoxylate atropine
Peripheral edema	Diuretics
Periorbital edema	Steroid-containing cream
Skin rash	Avoid sun exposure Topical steroids Systemic steroids (Early intervention important)
Muscle cramps	Tonic water or quinine Electrolyte replacement as needed Calcium gluconate
Arthralgia, bone pain	Nonsteroidal anti-inflamatory agents
Elevated transaminases (uncommon)	Hold therapy and monitor closely Dose reduction upon resolution
Myelosuppression	
Anemia	Treatment interruption/dose reduction usually not indicated Consider erythropoietin or darbepoetin*
Neutropenia	Hold therapy if grade ≥ 3 (ie, ANC < 1 × 10^9/L)
Consider filgrastim* if recurrent/persistent, or sepsis.	
Thrombocytopenia	Hold therapy if grade ≥ 3 (ie, platelets < 50 × 10^9/L) Consider IL-11* 10 mcg/kg 3–7 days/week

*The use of erythropoietin, darbepoietin, filgrastim and interleukin-11 (IL-11) in this setting is not standard and should be considered investigational.

The significance of molecular monitoring in CML was first documented with SCT. Quantitative PCR (QPCR) has become an important tool to determine the risk of relapse. Patients who have BCR-ABL detectable by polymerase chain reaction (PCR) 6 months after transplant have a significantly higher probability of relapse, and those with the highest level of transcripts had the highest risk.[140,141] Molecular monitoring with quantitative PCR is now routine after SCT, and early intervention (eg, donor lymphocyte infusion, imatinib) is frequently indicated based on increasing levels of BCR-ABL transcripts. It should also be considered a routine test for all patients treated with imatinib or other new drugs.

Despite the shorter follow-up of imatinib studies, it has become evident that molecular responses are important end points. The IRIS trial demonstrated a significantly improved molecular response with imatinib compared with rIFNα at each time point from the achievement of complete cytogenetic response.[142] After a median follow-up of 18 months, 35 to 40% of patients treated with imatinib had a 3-log reduction of BCR-ABL transcripts, and 4 to 10% had undetectable BCR-ABL. These responses had been rare with rIFNα. Among patients who achieved a complete cytogenetic response with imatinib, those with ≥ 3-log reduction in BCR-ABL transcripts at 12 months from the start of therapy had a significantly better probability of progression-free survival at 42 months compared with those who had < 3-log reduction (98% vs 90%, p <.001).[142] In another study of patients in chronic phase who had achieved a complete cytogenetic response after imatinib therapy, those who achieved levels of BCR-ABL/ABL ratio of < 0.05% (ie, major molecular response) had a longer remission duration than those who did not reach these levels.[143]

Adequate molecular responses after the first 1 to 3 months of therapy may improve remission duration and may lower the risk of developing imatinib-resistant mutations. Some studies have suggested that the achievement of a major molecular response at any time is likewise associated with prolonged progression-free survival. Thus, the objective of therapy in the imatinib era should be to achieve a major molecular response that increases the probability of long-term durable responses.

A recommended algorithm for monitoring patients includes a cytogenetic analysis and quantitative PCR (real-time PCR) for all patients at the time of diagnosis. During the first months of therapy, it is appropriate to monitor the patients every 3 months with peripheral blood FISH (see below) until CR, then with quantitative PCR every 3 months and a cytogenetic analysis every 6 months. This last test, although inconvenient, is the only one that gives reliable information regarding the presence of other chromosomal abnormalities. The presence of additional chromosomal abnormalities may reduce the probability of response to imatinib and overall survival.[53,144,145] Also, as many as 15% of patients who respond to imatinib may develop chromosomal abnormalities in the Ph-negative metaphases.[53,60,61] The long-term implications of these abnormalities are still uncertain and most subsequently disappear. Rare patients may develop a myelodysplastic syndrome, or acute leukemia. After cytogenetic CR, quantitative PCR should be performed at least every 6 to 12 months and a routine cytogenetic analysis every 12 months.

Peripheral blood fluorescence in situ hybridization (FISH) can be used to monitor the cytogenetic response between marrow analyses.[146,147] FISH has expanded the sensitivity of the standard karyotype because it can survey many more cells. In addition, it permits the detection of submicroscopic abnormalities that may occur at low frequency. This technique is also important because in situations when the marrow is packed with cells, making aspiration difficult, or when it is hypoplastic following chemotherapy, it is often impossible to obtain adequate marrow specimens for cytogenetic studies to quantify the disease status. FISH can be done in peripheral blood. Variations of the standard FISH test include interphase FISH (i-FISH), hypermetaphase FISH (h-FISH), and the most recently reported dual-color, dual-fusion translocation FISH (D-FISH), which permits analysis of both peripheral blood and marrow specimens.[146] D-FISH uses different colored *bcr* and *abl* DNA probes to detect a single *bcr-abl* fusion signal on the Ph chromosome spanning the common break points of t(9;22)(q34;q11). By using D-FISH, the number of false-positives and false-negatives is minimized. Studies of D-FISH indicate that the percentage of Ph cells in the peripheral blood over the course of therapy is a good predictor of corresponding changes in marrow.[148]

FISH has some disadvantages: (1) even with the newest probes there is a small percentage of false positivity with FISH;[147] (2) routine FISH does not provide information on every chromosome; and (3) although it surveys more cells for the Ph chromosome than a cytogenetic analysis, it is not as sensitive as PCR. A 100% negative FISH test corresponds to only approximately a 2-log reduction in transcript levels, whereas with PCR the limit of detection extends to approximately 4.5 logs. A 3-log reduction of QPCR is approximately equivalent to an absolute QPCR value of 0.05 to 0.1%.

Imatinib Resistance A subset of patients treated with imatinib will develop resistance. Among those treated in chronic phase, the rate of resistance is less than 4% per year, and 2% for those that achieve a complete cytogenetic response. Several mechanisms of resistance have been identified. The most common mechanisms reported are mutations in the abl tyrosine kinase sequence (50–90%) and Bcr-Abl overexpression or amplification (5–10%). Bcr-Abl independent mechanisms such as expression of the MDR phenotype and overexpression of Src-related kinases have been reported less frequently.[149] More than 50 different mutations have been reported. They can involve any of the important domains in the bcr-abl structure, including the P-loop (the area where ATP binds), the activation loop, and the catalytic domain, as well as the amino acids where imatinib makes contact with *bcr-abl*. Currently, detection of mutations requires sequencing the gene to find changes in base pairs. This technique is cumbersome and has low sensitivity. It has been suggested that quantitative PCR could be used as a primary screen to identify patients who have Bcr-Abl kinase domain mutations. In one study, a rise in BCR-ABL of more than twofold was found in 34 of 35 patients with a mutation.[150] Different mutations have considerable variability with respect to resistance to imatinib. Some mutations are inhibited by slightly higher concentrations of imatinib than required to inhibit the wild-type form, whereas others are completely insensitive to imatinib. Patients with mutations in the P-loop domain may have a particularly poor prognosis, with a median survival of 4 to 5 months.[151] Other studies suggest that the prognosis depends on multiple factors other than the specific location of the mutation.

Other drugs are being developed to overcome imatinib resistance. Among them, a second generation of tyrosine kinase inhibitors has been synthesized and is being evaluated in patients resistant to imatinib based on knowledge of the mechanisms of resistance to imatinib (including mutations and expression of other kinases). These drugs are more potent than imatinib and able to inhibit *bcr-abl* even when mutated.[152,153] The first is a selective tyrosine kinase inhibitor called AMN107. It is 10- to 30-fold more potent than imatinib in vitro and active against 32 of 33 mutants against which it has been tested.[152,154] In a phase I study among patients who have failed prior therapy with imatinib, hematologic responses have been observed in 17%, 52%, and 78% of patients in chronic, accelerated, and blastic phases, respectively. The corresponding figures for cytogenetic responses were 41%, 41%, and 14%, respectively.[155]

Another new tyrosine kinase inhibitor is dasatinib (BMS-354825). This is a dual abl- and src-kinase inhibitor, that is ≥ 300-fold more potent than imatinib against wild-type bcr-abl. It is active against 14 of 15 mutants against which it has been tested.[153] In contrast to imatinib, it can bind both the active and the inactive configurations of bcr-abl.[152,153,156] In a phase I study of patients in chronic, accelerated, or blast phases who had failed prior imatinib therapy, hematologic responses were reported in 84%, 80%, and 69%, respectively, and cytogenetic responses in 52%, 40%, and 56%, respectively.[157,158]

TREATMENT RECOMMENDATIONS

The treatment algorithm in CML has changed in the last 5 years. The results with imatinib to date have been excellent, and most responses have been durable, although the treatment follow-up period has been relatively short. With cytogenetic complete responses of 70 to 90%, major molecular responses of 40 to 70%, and annual mortality of 1 to 2%, the estimated median survival may become 10 to 15 years,[159,160] and a significant proportion of patients may have long-term EFS. Thus, it is currently the treatment of choice for most patients. Allogeneic SCT is curative in a significant proportion of eligible patients. Limiting factors include availability of a donor and age of the patient. The major drawbacks are the risk of early mortality and morbidity. Early mortality is usually lowest among the younger patients, particularly those younger than age 20 to 30 years, but these patients need to deal with chronic morbidities and worsened quality of life. Most studies with stem cell transplant emphasize the results of the first few years, but late relapses, higher-than-average mortality, and complications should also be taken into consideration. Extensive chronic graft-versus-host disease can be seen in as many as 60% of patients treated,[94] and late relapses can occur more than 10 years after transplant.[161] All of these issues need to be evaluated when considering allogeneic SCT in view of the positive maturing imatinib experience. When alternative transplant approaches (eg, unrelated donor or cord blood) are considered, the increased risks and lack of long-term data should be recognized. At this time, with current knowledge, it is reasonable to offer all patients with newly diagnosed chronic phase CML initial therapy with imatinib, and consider allogeneic SCT only for those with suboptimal response (eg, no CHR after 3 months, 100% Ph positive after 6 months, or ≥ 35% Ph positive after 12 months of imatinib therapy) or resistance to imatinib.

The decision for young patients who have a fully matched sibling is more controversial. Results with transplant are best among those younger than age 25 to 35 years, and SCT may be given consideration after careful assessment of the risk:benefit ratio compared with imatinib as an alternative. Even at this age, there is known morbidity and mortality, and long-term sequelae must be considered. If the decision is made to start imatinib therapy, it is important to monitor the patient closely for cytogenetic and molecular response. Changing therapy should be considered for patients who have suboptimal response, defined above. More alternatives are now available. Increasing the dosage of imatinib to 800 mg daily is the first choice for patients receiving standard dose imatinib. The option of allogeneic SCT, if appropriate, should be considered for patients already on a higher dose of imatinib. The new tyrosine kinase inhibitors that are effective in patients who fail therapy with imatinib have recently entered clinical trials and should be considered in patients who fail imatinib and who are appropriate for this alternative approach. All the options must be discussed frankly and openly by the physician with the patient in a dialog referred to as "shared decision making." It allows for full informed consent and patient input in the decision process.[78]

Some scenarios are controversial with insufficient information to make strong recommendations. Patients who achieve a complete cytogenetic remission but who have less than a 3-log reduction in transcript levels have a worse prognosis than those who have at least a 3-log reduction.[162] However, the 3-year progression-free survival remains 92%, and a change of therapy to a high-risk approach (eg, allogeneic SCT) is not justified. Patients who show an increase in transcript levels after reaching a nadir also pose a therapeutic dilemma. It has been suggested that a twofold increase may herald the appearance of mutations,[163] but these data have not been confirmed. The short survival of patients with P-loop mutations has not been confirmed. Patients with T315I mutations have a universally poor prognosis and should be referred for allogeneic SCT. At this time, radical treatment changes cannot be recommended based on molecular monitoring alone, particularly when the risks involved with the alternative therapies are high. The same can be said about the appearance of chromosomal abnormalities in Ph-negative metaphases that occur in approximately 15% of patients. The few instances in which such patients have been diagnosed with myelodysplastic syndromes have been based on inadequate criteria. Indeed in many instances these abnormalities may spontaneously disappear. Thus, in the absence of clear data suggesting that these changes affect the long-term outcome of patients, they deserve only careful monitoring.

MANAGEMENT OF CML IN 2006

How, then, should patients be treated in the imatinib era? We believe that patients who are under the age of 25 to 30 years, in good health (other than CML!), with a matched allogeneic donor could receive transplantation because transplant medicine has advanced to the point where the risk:benefit ratio might be in favor of long-term remissions with transplantation. Imatinib is a valid alternative, however, after a thorough discussion of the risks and benefits of both options with the patient. Those patients over 30 years and those who do not have a matched sibling should receive imatinib mesylate until there is evidence of cytogenetic and/or hematologic failure. Matched unrelated transplants may then be considered or the new tyrosine kinase inhibitors may be offered. Despite its limitations, imatinib mesylate remains a model for designer cancer chemotherapy. On this logical molecular approach rest our hopes for the immediate future.

REFERENCES

1. Abramson S, Miller RG, Phillips RA. The identification in adult bone marrow of pluripotent and restricted stem cells of the myeloid and lymphoid systems. J Exp Med 1977;145:1567–79.
2. Schuh AC, Sutherland DR, Horsfall W, et al. Chronic myeloid leukemia arising in a progenitor common to T cells and myeloid cells. Leukemia 1990;4:631–6.
3. Rowley JD. Recurring genetic aberrations in cancer cells: chromosomes as potential targets for nuclear medicine imaging. J Nucl Med 1995;36:22S–4S.
4. Canaani E, Gale RP, Steiner-Saltz D, et al. Altered transcription of an oncogene in chronic myeloid leukaemia. Lancet 1984;1:593–5.
5. Fialkow PJ, Martin PJ, Najfeld V, et al. Evidence for a multistep pathogenesis of chronic myelogenous leukemia. Blood 1981;58:158–63.
6. Cutler SJ, Axtell L, Heise H. Ten thousand cases of leukemia: 1940–62. J Natl Cancer Inst 1967;39:993–1026.
7. Ries LAG, Eisner MP, Kosary CL, et al. SEER cancer statistics review, 1975–2002. Vol. 2004. Bethesda (MD): National Cancer Institute 2004. Available at: http://seer.cancer.gov/csr/1975_2002/ (accessed August 15, 2005). (Based on November 2004 SEER data submission, posted to the SEER Web site 2005.)
8. Bizzozero OJ Jr, Johnson KG, Ciocco A, et al. Radiation-related leukemia in Hiroshima and Nagasaki 1946–1964. II. Ann Intern Med 1967;66:522–30.
9. Corso A, Lazzarino M, Morra E, et al. Chronic myelogenous leukemia and exposure to ionizing radiation—a retrospective study of 443 patients. Ann Hematol 1995;70:79–82.
10. Cortes JE, Talpaz M, Kantarjian H. Chronic myelogenous leukemia: a review. Am J Med 1996;100:555–70.
11. Kantarjian HM, Dixon D, Keating MJ, et al. Characteristics of accelerated disease in chronic myelogenous leukemia. Cancer 1988;61:1441–6.
12. Vardiman JW, Harris NL, Brunning RD. The World Health Organization (WHO) classification of the myeloid neoplasms. Blood 2002;100:2292–302.

13. Cortes J, Kantarjian H. Advanced-phase chronic myeloid leukemia. Semin Hematol 2003;40:79–86.
14. Karanas A, Silver RT. Characteristics of the terminal phase of chronic granulocytic leukemia. Blood 1968;32:445–59.
15. Cortes J, O'Brien S, Garcia-Manero G, et al. Is the proposed World Health Organization (WHO) classification for chronic myeloid leukemia (CML) of clinical value in the imatinib era? [abstract 1014]. Blood 2004;104.
16. Kantarjian HM, Keating MJ, Talpaz M, et al. Chronic myelogenous leukemia in blast crisis. Analysis of 242 patients. Am J Med 1987;83:445–54.
17. Cramer E, Auclair C, Hakim J, et al. Metabolic activity of phagocytosing granulocytes in chronic granulocytic leukemia: ultrastructural observation of a degranulation defect. Blood 1977;50:93–106.
18. Denburg JA, Wilson WE, Bienenstock J. Basophil production in myeloproliferative disorders: increases during acute blastic transformation of chronic myeloid leukemia. Blood 1982;60:113–20.
19. Silver RT. Morphology of the blood and marrow in clinical practice. New York: Grune & Stratton; 1970.
20. Dosik H, Rosner F, Sawitsky A. Acquired lipidosis: Gaucher-like cells and "blue cells" in chronic granulocytic leukemia. Semin Hematol 1972;9:309–16.
21. Castro-Malaspina H, Moore MA. Pathophysiological mechanisms operating in the development of myelofibrosis: role of megakaryocytes. Nouv Rev Fr Hematol 1982;24:221–6.
22. Derderian PM, Kantarjian HM, Talpaz M, et al. Chronic myelogenous leukemia in the lymphoid blastic phase: characteristics, treatment response, and prognosis. Am J Med 1993;94:69–74.
23. Bain B, Catovsky D, O'Brien M, et al. Megakaryoblastic transformation of chronic granulocytic leukaemia. An electron microscopy and cytochemical study. J Clin Pathol 1977;30:235–42.
24. Rosenthal S, Canellos GP, Gralnick HP. Erythroblastic transformation of chronic granulocytic leukemia. Am J Med 1977;63:116–24.
25. Ahuja H, Bar-Eli M, Arlin Z, et al. The spectrum of molecular alterations in the evolution of chronic myelocytic leukemia. J Clin Invest 1991;87:2042–7.
26. Jamieson CH, Ailles LE, Dylla SJ, et al. Granulocyte-macrophage progenitors as candidate leukemic stem cells in blast-crisis CML. N Engl J Med 2004;351:657–67.
27. Perillie PE, Finch SC. Muramidase studies in Philadelphia—chromosome-positive and chromosome-negative chronic granulocytic leukemia. N Engl J Med 1970;283:456–9.
28. Sokal JE, Cox EB, Baccarani M, et al. Prognostic discrimination in "good-risk" chronic granulocytic leukemia. Blood 1984;63:789–99.
29. Kantarjian HM, Keating MJ, Smith TL, et al. Proposal for a simple synthesis prognostic staging system in chronic myelogenous leukemia. Am J Med 1990;88:1–8.
30. Hasford J, Pfirrmann M, Hehlmann R, et al. A new prognostic score for survival of patients with chronic myeloid leukemia treated with interferon alfa. Writing Committee for the Collaborative CML Prognostic Factors Project Group. J Natl Cancer Inst 1998;90:850–8.
31. Gratwohl A, Hermans J, Niederwieser D, et al. Bone marrow transplantation for chronic myeloid leukemia: long-term results. Chronic Leukemia Working Party of the European Group for Bone Marrow Transplantation. Bone Marrow Transplant 1993;12:509–16.
32. Kantarjian HM, Bueso-Ramos CE, Talpaz M, et al. The degree of bone marrow fibrosis in chronic myelogenous leukemia is not a prognostic factor with imatinib mesylate therapy. Leuk Lymphoma 2005;46:993–7.
33. Cortes J, Talpaz M, O'Brien S, et al. Effects of age on prognosis with imatinib mesylate therapy for patients with Philadelphia chromosome-positive chronic myelogenous leukemia. Cancer 2003;98:1105–13.
34. Huntly BJ, Guilhot F, Reid AG, et al. Imatinib improves but may not fully reverse the poor prognosis of patients with CML with derivative chromosome 9 deletions. Blood 2003;102:2205–12.
35. Quintas-Cardama A, Kantarjian H, Talpaz M, et al. Imatinib mesylate therapy may overcome the poor prognostic significance of deletions of derivative chromosome 9 in patients with chronic myelogenous leukemia. Blood 2005;105:2281–6.
36. Galbraith PR, Abu-Zahra HT. Granulopoiesis in chronic granulocytic leukaemia. Br J Haematol 1972;22:135–43.
37. Strife A, Clarkson B. Biology of chronic myelogenous leukemia: is discordant maturation the primary defect? Semin Hematol 1988;25:1–19.
38. Gordon MY, Dowding CR, Riley GP, et al. Altered adhesive interactions with marrow stroma of haematopoietic progenitor cells in chronic myeloid leukaemia. Nature 1987;328:342–4.
39. Pelus LM, Saletan S, Silver RT, Moore MA. Expression of Ia-antigens on normal and chronic myeloid leukemic human granulocyte-macrophage colony-forming cells (CFU-GM) is associated with the regulation of cell proliferation by prostaglandin E. Blood 1982;59:284–92.
40. Gale RP. Chronic myelogenous leukaemia: a model for human cancers. Baillieres Clin Haematol 1987;1:869–886.
41. Nowell PC, Hungerford DA. A minute chromosome in human chronic granulocytic leukemia. Science 1960;132:1497–501.
42. Rowley JD. A new consistent chromosomal abnormality in chronic myelogenous leukaemia identified by quinacrine fluorescence and Giemsa staining [letter]. Nature 1973;243:290–3.
43. Kurzrock R, Gutterman JU, Talpaz M. The molecular genetics of Philadelphia chromosome-positive leukemias. N Engl J Med 1988;319:990–8.
44. Sessarego M, Pasquali F, Bianchi Scarra GL, Ajmar F. Masked Philadelphia chromosome caused by translocation (9;11;22). Cancer Genet Cytogenet 1983;8:319–23.
45. Botti AC, Silver RT, Macera MJ, et al. A new translocation involving chromosomes 8 and 9 in a Philadelphia-negative chronic myelogenous leukemia. Cancer Genet Cytogenet 1988;35:51–4.
46. Chemitiganti S, Verma RS, Silver RT, et al. Unusual translocations involving chromosomes 12;22 and 9;12 in a case of chronic myelogenous leukemia. Cancer Genet Cytogenet 1985;14:61–5.
47. Huret JL. Complex translocations, simple variant translocations and Ph-negative cases in chronic myelogenous leukaemia. Hum Genet 1990;85:565–8.
48. De Braekeleer M. Variant Philadelphia translocations in chronic myeloid leukemia. Cytogenet Cell Genet 1987;44:215–22.
49. Albano F, Specchia G, Pannunzio A, et al. Variant t(9;22) translocation may identify a subgroup of chronic myeloid leukemia patients with poor prognosis [abstract 1354]. Blood 2001;98:321a.
50. El-Zimaity MMT, Kantarjian H, Talpaz M, et al. Results of imatinib mesylate therapy in chronic myelogenous leukaemia with variant Philadelphia chromosome. Br J Haematol 2004;125:187–95.
51. Shtalrid M, Talpaz M, Blick M, et al. Philadelphia-negative chronic myelogenous leukemia with breakpoint cluster region rearrangement: molecular analysis, clinical characteristics, and response to therapy. J Clin Oncol 1988;6:1569–75.
52. Sokal JE, Gomez GA, Baccarani M, et al. Prognostic significance of additional cytogenetic abnormalities at diagnosis of Philadelphia chromosome-positive chronic granulocytic leukemia. Blood 1988;72:294–8.
53. Cortes J, O'Dwyer ME. Clonal evolution in chronic myelogenous leukemia. Hematol Oncol Clin North Am 2004;18:671–84, x.
54. Ahuja H, Bar-Eli M, Advani SH, et al. Alterations in the p53 gene and the clonal evolution of the blast crisis of chronic myelocytic leukemia. Proc Natl Acad Sci U S A 1989;86:6783–7.
55. Issa JP, Kantarjian H, Mohan A, et al. Methylation of c-abl promoter: a prognostic factor in chronic myelogenous leukemia? [abstract 866]. Blood 1997;90:196a.
56. Nguyen TT, Mohrbacher AF, Tsai YC, et al. Quantitative measure of c-abl and p15 methylation in chronic myelogenous leukemia: biological implications. Blood 2000;95:2990–2.
57. Ge XQ, Tanaka K, Mansyur A, et al. Possible prediction of myeloid and lymphoid crises in chronic myelocytic leukemia at onset by determining the methylation status of the major breakpoint cluster region. Cancer Genet Cytogenet 2001;126:102–10.
58. Roman-Gomez J, Castillejo JA, Jimenez A, et al. Cadherin-13, a mediator of calcium-dependent cell-cell adhesion, is silenced by methylation in chronic myeloid leukemia and correlates with pretreatment risk profile and cytogenetic response to interferon alfa. J Clin Oncol 2003;21:1472–9.
59. Fayad L, Kantarjian H, O'Brien S, et al. Emergence of new clonal abnormalities following interferon-alpha induced complete cytogenetic response in patients with chronic myeloid leukemia: report of three cases. Leukemia 1997;11:767–71.
60. Medina J, Kantarjian H, Talpaz M, et al. Chromosomal abnormalities in Philadelphia chromosome-negative metaphases appearing during imatinib mesylate therapy in patients with Philadelphia chromosome-positive chronic myelogenous leukemia in chronic phase. Cancer 2003;98:1905–11.
61. Bumm T, Muller C, Al-Ali HK, et al. Emergence of clonal cytogenetic abnormalities in Ph- cells in some CML patients in cytogenetic remission to imatinib but restoration of polyclonal hematopoiesis in the majority. Blood 2003;101:1941–9.
62. Bernards A, Rubin CM, Westbrook CA, et al. The first intron in the human c-abl gene is at least 200 kilobases long and is a target for translocations in chronic myelogenous leukemia. Mol Cell Biol 1987;7:3231–6.
63. Heisterkamp N, Jenster G, ten Hoeve J, et al. Acute leukaemia in bcr/abl transgenic mice. Nature 1990;344:251–3.
64. Faderl S, Talpaz M, Estrov Z, et al. The biology of chronic myeloid leukemia. N Engl J Med 1999;341:164–72.
65. Sawyers CL. Chronic myeloid leukemia. N Engl J Med 1999;340:1330–40.
66. Bhatia R, Wayner EA, McGlave PB, Verfaillie CM. Interferon-alpha restores normal adhesion of chronic myelogenous leukemia hematopoietic progenitors to bone marrow stroma by correcting impaired beta 1 integrin receptor function [comments]. J Clin Invest 1994;94:384–91.
67. Ravandi F, Cortes J, Albitar M, et al. Chronic myelogenous leukaemia with p185(BCR/ABL) expression: characteristics and clinical significance. Br J Haematol 1999;107:581–6.
68. Pane F, Mostarda I, Selleri C, et al. BCR/ABL mRNA and the P210(BCR/ABL) protein are downmodulated by interferon-alpha in chronic myeloid leukemia patients. Blood 1999;94:2200–7.
69. Lugo TG, Pendergast AM, Muller AJ, Witte ON. Tyrosine kinase activity and transformation potency of bcr-abl oncogene products. Science 1990;247:1079–82.
70. Hochhaus A, Weisser A, La Rosee P, et al. Detection and quantification of residual disease in chronic myelogenous leukemia. Leukemia 2000;14:998–1005.
71. Biernaux C, Loos M, Sels A, et al. Detection of major bcr-abl gene expression at a very low level in blood cells of some healthy individuals. Blood 1995;86:3118–22.
72. Bose S, Deininger M, Gora-Tybor J, et al. The presence of typical and atypical BCR-ABL fusion genes in leukocytes of normal individuals: biologic significance and implications for the assessment of minimal residual disease. Blood 1998;92:3362–7.
73. Daley GQ, Van Etten RA, Baltimore D. Induction of chronic myelogenous leukemia in mice by the P210bcr/abl gene of the Philadelphia chromosome. Science 1990;247:824–30.
74. Hehlmann R, Heimpel H, Hasford J, et al. Randomized comparison of busulfan and hydroxyurea in chronic myelogenous leukemia: prolongation of survival by hydroxyurea. The German CML Study Group. Blood 1993;82:398–407.
75. Gutterman JU. Cytokine therapeutics: lessons from interferon alpha. Proc Natl Acad Sci U S A 1994;91:1198–205.
76. Kurzrock R, Talpaz M, Kantarjian H, et al. Therapy of chronic myelogenous leukemia with recombinant interferon-gamma. Blood 1987;70:943–7.
77. Silver RT, Benn P, Verma RS, et al. Recombinant gamma-interferon has activity in chronic myeloid leukemia. Am J Clin Oncol 1990;13:49–54.
78. Silver RT, Woolf SH, Hehlmann R, et al. An evidence-based analysis of the effect of busulfan, hydroxyurea, interferon, and allogeneic bone marrow transplantation in treating the chronic phase of chronic myeloid leukemia: developed for the American Society of Hematology [comments]. Blood 1999;94:1517–36.
79. Kantarjian HM, Deisseroth A, Kurzrock R, et al. Chronic myelogenous leukemia: a concise update. Blood 1993;82:691–703.
80. Ozer H, George SL, Schiffer CA, et al. Prolonged subcutaneous administration of recombinant alpha 2b interferon in patients with previously untreated Philadelphia chromosome-positive chronic-phase chronic myelogenous leukemia: effect on remission duration and survival: Cancer and Leukemia Group B study 8583. Blood 1993;82:2975–84.
81. Hochhaus A, Reiter A, Saussele S, et al. Molecular heterogeneity in complete cytogenetic responders after interferon-alpha therapy for chronic myelogenous leukemia: low levels of minimal residual disease are associated with continuing remission. German CML Study Group and the UK MRC CML Study Group. Blood 2000;95:62–6.
82. Kantarjian HM, O'Brien S, Cortes JE, et al. Complete cytogenetic and molecular responses to interferon-alpha-based therapy for chronic myelogenous leukemia are associated with excellent long-term prognosis. Cancer 2003;97:1033–41.

83. Silver RT, Szatrowski TP, Peterson B, et al. Combined alfa-interferon (rIFNα-2B) and low dose cytosine arabinoside (Ara-C) for Ph+ chronic phase chronic myeloid leukemia (CML). Blood 1996;88 Suppl 1:638a.
84. Molldrem JJ, Lee PP, Wang C, et al. Evidence that specific T lymphocytes may participate in the elimination of chronic myelogenous leukemia. Nat Med 2000;6:1018–23.
85. The Italian Cooperative Study Group on Chronic Myeloid Leukemia. Interferon alfa-2a as compared with conventional chemotherapy for the treatment of chronic myeloid leukemia. N Engl J Med 1994;330:820–5.
86. The Italian Cooperative Study Group on Chronic Myeloid Leukemia. Long-term follow-up of the Italian trial of interferon-alpha versus conventional chemotherapy in chronic myeloid leukemia. Blood 1998;92:1541–8.
87. Hehlmann R, Heimpel H, Hasford J, et al. Randomized comparison of interferon-alpha with busulfan and hydroxyurea in chronic myelogenous leukemia. The German CML Study Group. Blood 1994;84:4064–77.
88. Kantarjian HM, O'Brien S, Smith TL, et al. Treatment of Philadelphia chromosome-positive early chronic phase chronic myelogenous leukemia with daily doses of interferon alpha and low-dose cytarabine. J Clin Oncol 1999;17:284–92.
89. Guilhot F, Chastang C, Michallet M, et al. Interferon alfa-2b combined with cytarabine versus interferon alone in chronic myelogenous leukemia. French Chronic Myeloid Leukemia Study Group [comments]. N Engl J Med 1997;337:223–9.
90. Silver RT, Peterson BL, Szatrowski TP, et al. Treatment of the chronic phase of chronic myeloid leukemia with an intermittent schedule of recombinant interferon alfa-2b and cytarabine: results from CALGB study 9013. Leuk Lymphoma 2003;44:39–48.
91. Baccarani M, Rosti G, de Vivo A, et al. A randomized study of interferon-alpha versus interferon-alpha and low-dose arabinosyl cytosine in chronic myeloid leukemia. Blood 2002;99:1527–35.
92. Hensley ML, Peterson B, Silver RT, et al. Risk factors for severe neuropsychiatric toxicity in patients receiving interferon alfa-2b and low-dose cytarabine for chronic myelogenous leukemia: analysis of Cancer and Leukemia Group B 9013. J Clin Oncol 2000;18:1301–8.
93. Hansen JA, Gooley TA, Martin PJ, et al. Bone marrow transplants from unrelated donors for patients with chronic myeloid leukemia [comments]. N Engl J Med 1998;338:962–8.
94. Radich JP, Gooley T, Bensinger W, et al. HLA-matched related hematopoietic cell transplantation for chronic-phase CML using a targeted busulfan and cyclophosphamide preparative regimen. Blood 2003;102:31–5.
95. Ash RC, Horowitz MM, Gale RP, et al. Bone marrow transplantation from related donors other than HLA-identical siblings: effect of T cell depletion. Bone Marrow Transplant 1991;7:443–52.
96. Keever-Taylor CA, Bredeson C, Loberiza FR, et al. Analysis of risk factors for the development of GVHD after T cell-depleted allogeneic BMT: effect of HLA disparity, ABO incompatibility, and method of T-cell depletion. Biol Blood Marrow Transplant 2001;7:620–30.
97. Horowitz MM, Rowlings PA, Passweg JR. Allogeneic bone marrow transplantation for CML: a report from the International Bone Marrow Transplant Registry. Bone Marrow Transplant 1996;17 Suppl 3:S5–6.
98. Clift RA, Storb R. Marrow transplantation for CML: the Seattle experience. Bone Marrow Transplant 1996;17 Suppl 3:S1–3.
99. Weisdorf DJ, Anasetti C, Antin JH, et al. Allogeneic bone marrow transplantation for chronic myelogenous leukemia: comparative analysis of unrelated versus matched sibling donor transplantation. Blood 2002;99:1971–7.
100. Or R, Shapira MY, Resnick I, et al. Nonmyeloablative allogeneic stem cell transplantation for the treatment of chronic myeloid leukemia in first chronic phase. Blood 2003;101:441–5.
101. Clift RA, Buckner CD, Thomas ED, et al. Marrow transplantation for patients in accelerated phase of chronic myeloid leukemia. Blood 1994;84:4368–73.
102. Giralt SA, Kantarjian HM, Talpaz M, et al. Effect of prior interferon alfa therapy on the outcome of allogeneic bone marrow transplantation for chronic myelogenous leukemia. J Clin Oncol 1993;11:1055–61.
103. Hehlmann R, Hochhaus A, Kolb HJ, et al. Interferon-alpha before allogeneic bone marrow transplantation in chronic myelogenous leukemia does not affect outcome adversely, provided it is discontinued at least 90 days before the procedure. Blood 1999;94:3668–77.
104. Lee SJ, Klein JP, Anasetti C, et al. The effect of pretransplant interferon therapy on the outcome of unrelated donor hematopoietic stem cell transplantation for patients with chronic myelogenous leukemia in first chronic phase. Blood 2001;98:3205–11.
105. Holowiecki J, Kruzel T, Wojnar J, et al. Allogeneic stem cell transplantation from unrelated and related donors is effective in CML Ph+ and ALL Ph+ patients pretreated with imatinib [abstract 5473]. Blood 2003;102:436b.
106. Prejzner W, Zaucha JM, Szatkowski D, et al. Imatinib therapy prior to myeloablative allogeneic stem cell transplantation does not increase acute transplant related toxicity [abstract 3389]. Blood 2003;102:911a.
107. Kolb HJ, Mittermuller J, Clemm C, et al. Donor leukocyte transfusions for treatment of recurrent chronic myelogenous leukemia in marrow transplant patients. Blood 1990;76:2462–5.
108. Giralt S, Hester J, Huh Y, et al. CD8-depleted donor lymphocyte infusion as treatment for relapsed chronic myelogenous leukemia after allogeneic bone marrow transplantation. Blood 1995;86:4337–43.
109. Slavin S. Immunotherapy of cancer with alloreactive lymphocytes. Lancet Oncol 2001;2:491–8.
110. Olavarria E, Craddock C, Dazzi F, et al. Imatinib mesylate (STI571) in the treatment of relapse of chronic myeloid leukemia after allogeneic stem cell transplantation. Blood 2002;99:3861–2.
111. Kantarjian HM, O'Brien S, Cortes JE, et al. Imatinib mesylate therapy for relapse after allogeneic stem cell transplantation for chronic myelogenous leukemia. Blood 2002;100:1590–5.
112. DeAngelo DJ, Hochberg EP, Alyea EP, et al. Extended follow-up of patients treated with imatinib mesylate (Gleevec) for chronic myelogenous leukemia relapse after allogeneic transplantation: durable cytogenetic remission and conversion to complete donor chimerism without graft-versus-host disease. Clin Cancer Res 2004;10:5065–71.
113. Druker BJ, Tamura S, Buchdunger E, et al. Effects of a selective inhibitor of the Abl tyrosine kinase on the growth of Bcr-Abl positive cells. Nat Med 1996;2:561–6.
114. Beran M, Cao X, Estrov Z, et al. Selective inhibition of cell proliferation and BCR-ABL phosphorylation in acute lymphoblastic leukemia cells expressing Mr 190,000 BCR-ABL protein by a tyrosine kinase inhibitor (CGP-57148). Clin Cancer Res 1998;4:1661–72.
115. Kantarjian H, Sawyers C, Hochhaus A, et al. Hematologic and cytogenetic responses to imatinib mesylate in chronic myelogenous leukemia. N Engl J Med 2002;346:645–52.
116. Silver RT, Talpaz M, Sawyers C, et al. Four years of follow-up of 1027 patients with late chronic phase (L-CP), accelerated phase (AP), or blast crisis (BC) chronic myeloid leukemia (CML) treated with imatinib in three large phase II trials [abstract 23]. Blood 2004;104:287a.
117. Kantarjian HM, Cortes JE, O'Brien S, et al. Long-term survival benefit and improved complete cytogenetic and molecular response rates with imatinib mesylate in Philadelphia chromosome-positive chronic-phase chronic myeloid leukemia after failure of interferon-{alpha}. Blood 2004;104:1979–88.
118. O'Brien SG, Guilhot F, Larson RA, et al. Imatinib compared with interferon and low-dose cytarabine for newly diagnosed chronic-phase chronic myeloid leukemia. N Engl J Med 2003;348:994–1004.
119. Hahn EA, Glendenning GA, Sorensen MV, et al. Quality of life in patients with newly diagnosed chronic phase chronic myeloid leukemia on imatinib versus interferon alfa plus low-dose cytarabine: results from the IRIS Study. J Clin Oncol 2003;21:2138–46.
120. Guilhot F, on behalf of IRIS study group. Sustained durability of responses plus high rates of cytogenetic responses result in long-term benefit for newly diagnosed chronic-phase chronic myeloid leukemia (CML-CP) treated with imatinib (IM) therapy: update from the IRIS study [abstract 21]. Blood 2004;104.
121. Druker BJ, Talpaz M, Resta DJ, et al. Efficacy and safety of a specific inhibitor of the BCR-ABL tyrosine kinase in chronic myeloid leukemia. N Engl J Med 2001;344:1031–7.
122. Cortes J, Giles F, O'Brien S, et al. Result of high-dose imatinib mesylate in patients with Philadelphia chromosome—positive chronic myeloid leukemia after failure of interferon-{alpha}. Blood 2003;102:83–6.
123. Cortes J, Giles F, Salvado A, et al. High-dose imatinib in patients with previously untreated chronic myeloid leukemia in early chronic phase: preliminary results of a multicenter community based trial [abstract 6518]. J Clin Oncol 2005;23:564s.
124. Kantarjian H, Talpaz M, O'Brien S, et al. High-dose imatinib mesylate therapy in newly diagnosed Philadelphia chromosome-positive chronic phase chronic myeloid leukemia. Blood 2004;103:2873–8.
125. Hughes T, Branford S, Matthews J, et al. Trial of higher dose imatinib with selective intensification in newly diagnosed CML patients in the chronic phase [abstract 95]. Blood 2003;102:31a.
126. Druker BJ, Gathmann I, Bolton AE, Larson RA. Probability and impact of obtaining a cytogenetic response to imatinib as initial therapy for chronic myeloid leukemia (CML) in chronic phase [abstract 634]. Blood 2003;102:182a.
127. Cortes J, O'Brien S, Kantarjian H. Discontinuation of imatinib therapy after achieving a molecular response. Blood 2004;104:2204–5.
128. Mauro MJ, Druker BJ, Maziarz RT. Divergent clinical outcome in two CML patients who discontinued imatinib therapy after achieving a molecular remission. Leukemia Res 2004;28:71–3.
129. Ghanima W, Kahrs J, Dahl TG 3rd, Tjonnfjord GE. Sustained cytogenetic response after discontinuation of imatinib mesylate in a patient with chronic myeloid leukaemia. Eur J Haematol 2004;72:441–3.
130. Sneed TB, Kantarjian HM, Talpaz M, et al. The significance of myelosuppression during therapy with imatinib mesylate in patients with chronic myelogenous leukemia in chronic phase. Cancer 2004;100:116–21.
131. Deininger MW, O'Brien SG, Ford JM, Druker BJ. Practical management of patients with chronic myeloid leukemia receiving imatinib. J Clin Oncol 2003;21:1637–47.
132. Quintas-Cardama A, Kantarjian H, O'Brien S, et al. Granulocyte-colony-stimulating factor (filgrastim) may overcome imatinib-induced neutropenia in patients with chronic-phase chronic myelogenous leukemia. Cancer 2004;100:2592–7.
133. Mauro MJ, Kurilik G, Balleisen S, et al. Myeloid growth factors for neutropenia during imatinib mesylate (STI571) therapy for CML: preliminary evidence of safety and efficacy. Blood 2001;98:139a.
134. Marin D, Marktel S, Foot N, et al. G-CSF reverses cytopenia and may increase cytogenetic responses in patients with CML treated with imatinib mesylate [abstract 3091]. Blood 2002;100:782a.
135. Ault P, Kantarjian H, Welch MA, et al. Interleukin 11 may improve thrombocytopenia associated with imatinib mesylate therapy in chronic Myelogenous leukemia. Leuk Res 2004;28:613–8.
136. Cortes J, O'Brien S, Quintas A, et al. Erythropoietin is effective in improving the anemia induced by imatinib mesylate therapy in patients with chronic myeloid leukemia in chronic phase. Cancer 2004;100:2396–402.
137. Mauro MJ, Blasdel C, O'Dwyer ME, et al. Erythropoietin for anemia during imatinib mesylate (STI571) therapy for CML: preliminary evidence of safety and efficacy [abstract 106]. Proc Am Soc Clin Oncol 2002;21:27a.
138. Ault P, Kantarjian H, O'Brien S, et al. Use of darbepoetin alfa for the treatment of anemia occurring during imatinib therapy for CML: preliminary evidence of safety and efficacy [abstract 2467]. Proc Am Soc Clin Oncol 2003;22:613.
139. Talpaz M, Kantarjian H, Kurzrock R, et al. Interferon-alpha produces sustained cytogenetic responses in chronic myelogenous leukemia. Philadelphia chromosome-positive patients. Ann Int Med 1991;114:532–8.
140. Radich JP, Gehly G, Gooley T, et al. Polymerase chain reaction detection of the BCR-ABL fusion transcript after allogeneic marrow transplantation for chronic myeloid leukemia: results and implications in 346 patients. Blood 1995;85:2632–8.
141. Radich JP, Gooley T, Bryant E, et al. The significance of bcr-abl molecular detection in chronic myeloid leukemia patients "late," 18 months or more after transplantation. Blood 2001;98:1701–7.
142. Hughes TP, Kaeda J, Branford S, et al. Molecular responses to Imatinib (STI571) or Interferon + Ara-C as initial therapy for CML; Results of the IRIS study [abstract 345]. Blood 2002;100:93a.
143. Cortes J, O'Brien S, Talpaz M, et al. Clinical significance of molecular response in chronic myeloid leukemia after imatinib (Gleevec) therapy: low levels of residual disease predict for response duration [abstract 1513]. Blood 2003;102:416a.
144. O'Dwyer ME, Mauro MJ, Blasdel C, et al. Clonal evolution and lack of cytogenetic response are adverse prognostic factors for hematologic relapse of chronic phase CML patients treated with imatinib mesylate. Blood 2004;103:451–5.

145. Cortes JE, Talpaz M, Giles F, et al. Prognostic significance of cytogenetic clonal evolution in patients with chronic myelogenous leukemia on imatinib mesylate therapy. Blood 2003;101:3794–800.

146. Buno I, Wyatt WA, Zinsmeister AR, et al. A special fluorescent in situ hybridization technique to study peripheral blood and assess the effectiveness of interferon therapy in chronic myeloid leukemia. Blood 1998;92:2315–21.

147. Dewald GW, Wyatt WA, Juneau AL, et al. Highly sensitive fluorescence in situ hybridization method to detect double BCR/ABL fusion and monitor response to therapy in chronic myeloid leukemia. Blood 1998;91:3357–65.

148. Lesser ML, Dewald GW, Sison CP, Silver RT. Correlation of three methods of measuring cytogenetic response in chronic myelocytic leukemia. Cancer Genet Cytogenet 2002;137:79–84.

149. Donato NJ, Wu JY, Stapley J, et al. Imatinib mesylate resistance through BCR-ABL independence in chronic myelogenous leukemia. Cancer Res 2004;64:672–7.

150. Branford S, Rudzki Z, Parkinson I, et al. Real-time quantitative PCR analysis can be used as a primary screen to identify patients with CML treated with imatinib who have BCR-ABL kinase domain mutations. Blood 2004;104:2926–32.

151. Branford S, Rudzki Z, Walsh S, et al. Detection of BCR-ABL mutations in patients with CML treated with imatinib is virtually always accompanied by clinical resistance, and mutations in the ATP phosphate-binding loop (P-loop) are associated with a poor prognosis. Blood 2003;102:276–83.

152. O'Hare T, Walters DK, Stoffregen EP, et al. In vitro activity of Bcr-Abl inhibitors AMN107 and BMS-354825 against clinically relevant imatinib-resistant Abl kinase domain mutants. Cancer Res 2005;65:4500–5.

153. Shah NP, Tran C, Lee FY, et al. Overriding imatinib resistance with a novel ABL kinase inhibitor. Science 2004;305:399–401.

154. Weisberg E, Manley PW, Breitenstein W, et al. Characterization of AMN107, a selective inhibitor of native and mutant Bcr-Abl. Cancer Cell 2005;7:129–41.

155. Kantarjian H, Ottmann OG, Cortes J, et al. AMN107, a novel aminopyrimidine inhibitor of Bcr-Abl, has significant activity in imatinib-resistant bcr-abl positive chronic myeloid leukemia [abstract 3014]. J Clin Oncol 2005;23:195s.

156. Burgess MR, Skaggs BJ, Shah NP, et al. Comparative analysis of two clinically active BCR-ABL kinase inhibitors reveals the role of conformation-specific binding in resistance. Proc Natl Acad Sci U S A 2005:102:3395–400.

157. Talpaz M, Kantarjian H, Paquette R, et al. A phase I study of BMS-354825 in patients with imatinib-resistant and intolerant chronic phase chronic myeloid leukemia (CML): results from CA180002 [abstract 6519]. J Clin Oncol 2005;23:564s.

158. Sawyers C, Shah NP, Kantarjian H, et al. A phase I study of BMS-354825 in patients with imatinib-resistant and intolerant accelerated and blast phase chronic myeloid leukemia (CML): results from CA180002 [abstract 6520]. J Clin Oncol 2005;23:565.

159. Anstrom KJ, Reed SD, Allen AS, et al. Long-term survival estimates for imatinib versus interferon-alpha plus low-dose cytarabine for patients with newly diagnosed chronic-phase chronic myeloid leukemia. Cancer 2004;101:2584–92.

160. Hasford J, Pfirrmann M, Hochhaus A. How long will chronic myeloid leukemia patients treated with imatinib mesylate live? 2005;19:497–9.

161. Kiss TL, Abdolell M, Jamal N, et al. Long-term medical outcomes and quality-of-life assessment of patients with chronic myeloid leukemia followed at least 10 years after allogeneic bone marrow transplantation. J Clin Oncol 2002;20:2334–43.

162. Hughes TP, Kaeda J, Branford S, et al. Frequency of major molecular responses to imatinib or interferon alfa plus cytarabine in newly diagnosed chronic myeloid leukemia. N Engl J Med 2003;349:1423–32.

163. Branford S, Rudzki Z, Parkinson I, et al. Real-time quantitative PCR analysis can be used as a primary screen to identify imatinib-treated patients with CML who have BCR-ABL kinase domain mutations. Blood 2004;104:2926–32.

Adult Acute Lymphoblastic Leukemia

Stefan Faderl, MD
Hagop M. Kantarjian, MD

Acute lymphoblastic leukemia (ALL) is a heterogeneous group of lymphoid disorders that result from a monoclonal proliferation and expansion of immature lymphoid cells in the marrow, blood, and other organs. Progress in the understanding of the biology of ALL has translated into changes in the pathologic classification of the disease, emergence of new therapies, and institution of risk-adapted therapies. Advances in ALL therapy over recent decades have led to long-term survival rates of better than 80% in children. Although adaptation of successful pediatric ALL treatment strategies into the therapeutic algorithms of adult ALL has resulted in complete response (CR) rates similar to those achieved in children, still only about 30% to 40% of adults achieve long-term disease-free survival (DFS). With further molecular dissection of ALL subtypes, with development of new and targeted drugs, and with the increasing elucidation of biologic and pharmacogenomic differences between childhood and adult ALL, there is hope that the prognosis in adult ALL may continue to improve.

EPIDEMIOLOGY AND CAUSATIVE FACTORS

ALL is the most common childhood acute leukemia and constitutes about 25% of all childhood cancers. In contrast, ALL represents only 20% of adult leukemias, which themselves constitute about 3% of adult malignancies. In most registry studies, the median age of ALL patients is between 25 and 35 years, with 25% of patients being older than 15 years. Although ALL is on average diagnosed with an incidence of 1 to 1.5 per 100,000 population, that incidence shows a bimodal distribution. An early peak is seen at around 4 to 5 years, when the incidence may be as high as 4 to 5 per 100,000 population. That peak is followed by a second, gradual increase at around age 50, when the incidence reaches up to 2 per 100,000 population. ALL is relatively rare during later childhood, adolescence, and young adulthood.[1]

ALL is more frequent among Caucasians than among African Americans.[2] Although little difference is seen in incidence rates among children of either sex, ALL in patients older than 20 years is consistently more predominant in males (1.3:1).[3] Geographic variations in the frequency of ALL have been described, with higher rates occurring in Australia, New Zealand (non-Maori population), and Spain, and among Latin Americans. In contrast, low rates have been demonstrated in Israel and India. Some of the differences are possibly related to socioeconomic factors, because higher frequencies of ALL have also been reported in industrialized countries and urban environments.[4]

In most cases, the cause of ALL remains unknown.[5,6] Exposure to ionizing radiation (atomic bomb explosion, other nuclear exposures such as the Chernobyl accident, therapeutic radiotherapy, in utero exposure) is the only known nongenetic causative factor associated with ALL.[4,7] Although contact with various chemicals (gasoline, diesel and motor exhausts, smoking, hair dyes), exposure to electromagnetic fields, parental occupation, medication use during pregnancy, and dietary habits have been associated with a higher incidence of ALL in some cases, knowledge with regard to most of these associations remains scant and contradictory. A role for genetic factors is suggested by several observations: (1) ALL occurring in a monozygotic twin will develop with a likelihood of 20% to 25% in the second twin within 1 year;[8] (2) an up to fourfold higher risk of leukemia is seen among dizygotic twins as compared with the general population;[9,10] (3) patients with trisomy 21 (Down syndrome) have a 20-fold higher risk of developing ALL;[11,12] and (4) a higher risk of developing ALL has also been observed in patients with Klinefelter's syndrome and inherited diseases with excessive chromosomal fragility, such as Fanconi anemia, Bloom's syndrome, and ataxia–telangiectasia.[13–15] Recent studies have uncovered a protective effect of a polymorphism in the *MTHFR* (methylenetetrahydrofolate reductase) gene in infant and adult ALL, pointing toward genetic susceptibility genes as part of ALL causation.[16,17]

Exposure to infectious agents is increasingly discussed in the context of ALL leukemogenesis.[18,19] Causative associations have been described between the human T-lymphotropic virus 1 and adult T-cell leukemia/lymphoma (ATLL)[20,21] and between the Epstein–Barr virus (EBV) and Burkitt's lymphoma, mature B-cell ALL, and other lymphoproliferative disorders related to the human immunodeficiency virus (HIV).[22,23] Further associations have been suggested with varicella and influenza viruses.[24,25] Greaves[26] and Kinlen[27] have postulated that the incidence peak in childhood ALL is related to a low incidence of infections during childhood in nonimmune populations who are later exposed to common infections. In that context, the observation that ALL is more frequent in patients of higher socioeconomic status may relate to a different spectrum of infectious agents and timing of exposure.[28] The viral causation of lymphoblastic leukemias in mice, cats, cattle, and some primates feeds speculation that a human virus or viruses may exist.

CLINICAL PRESENTATION AND LABORATORY ABNORMALITIES

The clinical signs and symptoms of ALL usually occur suddenly and derive from expansion of the leukemic cell in the marrow and from involvement of the peripheral blood and extramedullary sites such as lymph nodes, liver, spleen, and the central nervous system (CNS). Common symptoms include fatigue, lack of energy, constitutional effects (fevers, night sweats, weight loss), easy bruising or obvious bleeding, dyspnea, dizziness, and infections. Extremity and joint pain may be the only presenting symptoms, leading to a misdiagnosis of arthritis. Diffuse osteopenia or lytic bone lesions are rare.

CNS involvement is rare at diagnosis. If present, cranial nerve deficiencies (especially cranial nerves VI, III, IV, and VII) can lead to double vision, abnormal ocular movements, facial dysesthesias, and facial droop.[29] Nausea and vomiting, headaches, or papilledema may point towards meningeal infiltration and raised intracranial pressure. Chin numbness attributable to mental nerve involvement may be subtle and can easily be missed unless solicited. CNS involvement at presentation is more common in mature B-cell ALL (Burkitt's leukemia) than in other ALL subtypes.

T-lineage ALL presenting with a mediastinal mass can result in stridor and wheezing, pericardial effusions, and superior vena cava syndrome.[30–32] Testicular involvement is rare in adults and occurs with a low frequency predominantly in infant and adolescent boys. It typically presents as an indolent unilateral mass—although bilateral involvement is commonly found on biopsies. Except in mature B-cell ALL, which may cause bleeding or rupture, involvement of the gastrointestinal tract is infrequent.

Physical examination is notable for pallor and ecchymoses or petechiae. Lymphadenopathy and hepatosplenomegaly are noted in 20% of patients These conditions are more frequent with T- and mature B-cell ALL and are rarely symptomatic. Physical examination findings are rarely specific for ALL; they can be elicited in other forms of leukemia as well.

Table 115-1 Features of Adult Acute Lymphoblastic Leukemia (ALL) at Presentation at a Tertiary Care Referral Center (*n* = 403)

Characteristic	Patients (%)
Age (years)	
< 30	30
30–60	47
> 60	23
ECOG performance status > 2	5
Clinical features	
Splenomegaly (> 5 cm BCM)	5
Hepatomegaly (> 5 cm BCM)	3
Lymphadenopathy	30
Mediastinal mass	7
CNS leukemia	7
Laboratory features	
WBC (×10⁹/L)	
< 5	38
5–30	37
> 30	25
Platelets < 100 ×10⁹/L	72
Hemoglobin < 10 g/dL	70
LDH > 2 × ULN	49
Serum creatinine > 1.2 mg/dL	55
Serum bilirubin > 1.2 mg/dL	13
Immunophenotype	
B-lineage	93
T-lineage	7
Cytogenetic profile	
Diploid	26
Philadelphia translocation	17
Hyperdiploid	4
Hypodiploid	4
Other	49
Risk profile	
Standard	23
High	76

BCM = below costal margin; CNS = central nervous system; ECOG = Eastern Cooperative Oncology Group; LDH = lactate dehydrogenase; ULN = upper limit of normal; WBC = white blood cells.

Tumor lysis syndrome is common in patients with mature B-cell ALL, but it can also occur in any other subtype with hyperleukocytosis. It is characterized by hyperuricemia, hyperphosphatemia, hypocalcemia, and hypo- or hyperkalemia. Disseminated intravascular coagulation (DIC) is a frequent laboratory finding, but it rarely manifests as clinical DIC and does not require therapeutic intervention except in the setting of severe hypofibrinogenemia or significant prolongation of other coagulation parameters such as prothrombin time or partial thromboplastin time.[33] The occasional presentation of hypercalcemia and lytic bone lesions suggests a diagnosis of ATLL. Table 115-1 summarizes the clinical and laboratory characteristics of patients with adult ALL presenting to a tertiary referral center.

CLASSIFICATION OF ALL

The classification of ALL is undergoing rapid changes. Although a morphology assessment of ALL blasts remains essential in an ALL work-up, that assessment provides only an unrefined reflection of the biologic heterogeneity of the disease.

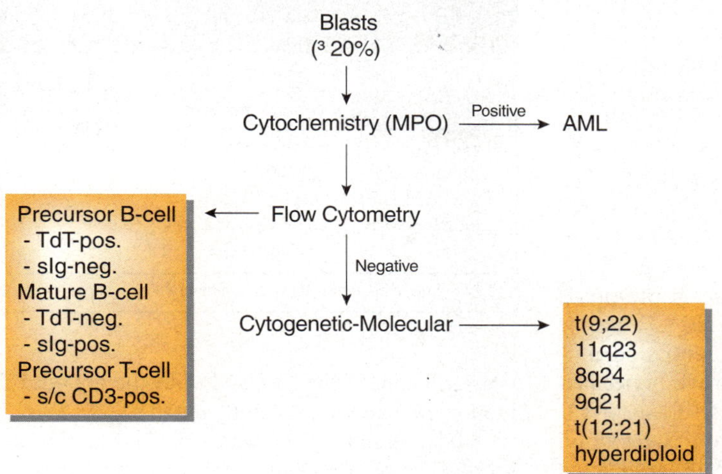

Figure 115-1 Diagnostic scheme for acute lymphoblastic leukemia (ALL).

Identification of distinct immunophenotypes and of cytogenetic–molecular abnormalities has contributed to a more complex view of leukemic blasts and thus has enabled a more accurate assessment of prognosis (Figure 115-1). Current efforts are focused on genomic profiling, which is leading to a new definition of ALL subtypes and to the identification of subgroups of patients with varying treatment outcomes and prognoses. Current diagnostic tools only partially discriminate these subgroups.

Morphology and Cytochemistry ALL blasts are heterogeneous in size and shape.[34] The French–American–British (FAB) Cooperative Group has outlined differences in blast morphology based on cell size, amount of cytoplasm, prominence of nucleoli, degree of cytoplasmic basophilia, and vacuolation.[35]

L1 blasts are smaller and have a high nucleus:cytoplasm ratio and inconspicuous nucleoli. The cytoplasm is sparse and variably basophilic. L2 blasts are larger and more pleomorphic; they have moderately abundant cytoplasm, a lower nucleus:cytoplasm ratio, and more prominent nucleoli.[36] The morphologic distinction between L1 and L2 blasts has lost its prognostic significance with current treatment modalities.

L3 blasts are more homogeneous: they are medium in size and have dispersed chromatin, prominent nucleoli, typically deep blue cytoplasmic basophilia, and sharply demarcated vacuoles. L3 morphology is associated with mature B-cell ALL or Burkitt's lymphoma, although L1 or L2 morphology has been described in some cases ("Burkitt-like").[37,38] Mature B-cell ALL is characterized by a high rate of cell turnover, which is reflected morphologically by the so-called starry sky appearance in marrow biopsy specimens.

No cytochemical stain is diagnostic for ALL. ALL blasts are negative for myeloperoxidase (MPO), and acute myelogenous leukemia (AML) is diagnosed if > 3% of the blasts stain positive for MPO. Low-level MPO positivity (3 to 5%) has been demonstrated in rare cases that otherwise lack expression of myeloid markers by flow cytometry.[39–41] Reactivity patterns of Sudan Black B stains closely resemble those of MPO, but lack of specificity and the ease with which MPO stains can be applied has limited the use of Sudan Black B.[42]

Although terminal deoxynucleotidyl transferase (TdT) is not uniquely specific for ALL, it is a useful marker for distinguishing between reactive and malignant lymphocytosis, especially in cases with predominantly L1 morphology. TdT is usually positive in > 40% of ALL blasts. L3 ALL is typically TdT-negative.[43–46]

About 10% of ALL blasts are strongly positive ("block positivity") for periodic acid–Schiff (PAS), but PAS reactivity (usually diffuse) also occurs in some cases of AML, such as erythroblastic leukemia. Acid phosphatase and α-naphthyl-acetate-esterase reaction are found in almost 80% of T-lineage ALL blasts, exhibiting a strong reaction in the Golgi region of the cytoplasm in contrast to non-T-cell ALL blasts.

The FAB classification lacks integration of immunophenotype and cytogenetic–molecular abnormalities.[47] Recognizing the significance of biologic parameters in the prognosis of ALL, the World Health Organization recently proposed new guidelines for the diagnosis of neoplastic diseases of hematopoietic and lymphoid tissues or lymphomas.[48,49] In addition to establishing a blast count ≥ 20% as sufficient for a diagnosis of ALL, it abandoned the FAB classification into L1, L2, and L3 morphologies as no longer relevant. Instead, it emphasized the importance of immunophenotyping in the diagnostic work-up.

Immunophenotyping Because of ease of application, accuracy in diagnosis, and quantifiability of results, flow cytometry has become the preferred method for lineage assignment and analysis of maturation in ALL.[50,51] Flow cytometry is highly efficient, in that a distinct lineage determination for ALL blasts is possible in more than 98% of the leukemic blasts. Although ALL can be divided into several immunophenotypically recognizable categories, the only distinction of clinical importance is that between precursor B-cell, mature B-cell, and T-cell ALL (Table 115-2).[52]

As a group, precursor B ALL blasts are positive for TdT, for d-related human leukocyte antigens (HLA-DR), and almost always for the B-cell differentiation antigens CD19 and CD79a. With the help of additional markers, precursor B ALL can further be subdivided, based on the stage of maturation of the blasts, into (1) pre-pre-B ALL ("pro-B-ALL"), (2) common ALL, and (3) pre-B ALL.

In the earliest identifiable stage of pre-pre-B ALL, blasts are positive for CD19, CD79a, or CD22, but for no other B-cell differentiation antigens. CD19-positive, CD10-negative, cytoplasmic immunoglobulin-negative B-lineage ALL with myeloid marker coexpression is common among infants with ALL, is typically associated with translocation t(4;11) and *MLL* (mixed-lineage leukemia) gene rearrangements, and has a poor prognosis.[50]

Common ALL ("cALL," "early pre-B ALL") represents an intermediate stage in blast development and is the most common immunophenotype in adults and children. It is characterized by expression of CD10 (common ALL antigen [CALLA]). Common ALL is a frequent immunophenotype with Philadelphia chromosome (Ph)–positive ALL, possibly accounting for the worse prognosis of adult as compared with childhood CD10-positive ALL.

In the more mature stages of pre-B ALL, blasts express cytoplasmic immunoglobulins. The blasts are more differentiated than in early pre-B ALL, and relatively more cases have the t(1;19) translocation.[53] Transitional pre-B ALL is rare (about 1%) and expresses cytoplasmic and surface μ heavy chains, but no surface light chains.[54,55]

In mature B-cell ALL (Burkitt's leukemia), blasts express surface immunoglobulins (sIgs, usually immunoglobulin M [IgM]), are clonal for κ or λ light chains, and lack expression of TdT. About 50% are CD10-positive, which may be associated with a better prognosis. Expression of CD20, which also has therapeutic implications, is almost ubiquitous in mature B-cell ALL.

As with B-lineage ALL, T ALL can be further stratified into subtypes based on various stages of intrathymic differentiation.[56,57] T ALL expresses various levels of CD1a, CD2, CD3, CD4, CD5, CD7, and CD8. CD4 and CD8 are either double-positive or double-negative. CD7 is the most sensitive T-cell marker, but it lacks specificity, because cases of AML or natural killer cell leukemia are sometimes CD7-positive as well.[58]

Surface expression of CD3 (sCD3) is the most lineage-specific marker for T-cell differentiation and is typically positive in mature T ALL. Mature T ALL may be positive for both sCD3 and cytoplasmic CD3 (cCD3), CD2, and either CD4 or CD8, but not both. Earlier stages of differentiation (precursor T ALL) do not express sCD3, but are still positive for cCD3.[59–61] CD3- and CD7-positive T ALL may suggest poor prognosis. Although not lineage-specific, CD52 is expressed in about 30 to 50% of cases with T ALL and may have therapeutic significance when treated with the anti-CD52 monoclonal antibody alemtuzumab.

Table 115-2 Immunophenotypic Classification of Acute Lymphoblastic Leukemia (ALL)[52]

B Lineage		T Lineage	
CD19/CD79a/CD22		CD3 (surface [s]/cytoplasmic [c])	
Pro-B ALL	No further differentiation markers	Precursor-T ALL	CD1a, CD2, CD5, CD7, CD8, cCD3
Common ALL	CD10	Mature-T ALL	Any of the above, plus sCD3
Pre-B ALL	cIgM (±CD10)		
Mature-B ALL	c or sIgκ or λ TdT-negative		

IgM = immunoglobulin M; Igκ = immunoglobulin kappa; Igλ = immunoglobulin lambda; TdT = terminal deoxynucleotidyl transferase.

Coexpression of markers from more than one lineage can be demonstrated in 15 to 50% of adult ALL and in 5 to 35% of childhood ALL.[60,62] Myeloid markers that are frequently coexpressed include CD13 and CD33, CD14, CD15, and CDw65.[63,64] No association exists between myeloid marker expression and the FAB group or karyotype, except in mature B ALL, in which a higher incidence with translocations t(9;22) and t(4;11) and no marker expression are seen.[62]

Although earlier studies had shown a worse outcome in patients whose ALL blasts coexpressed myeloid markers, more recent studies failed to show any prognostic significance.[64–77] A scoring system has been developed in which lineage-specific markers are weighed according to their discriminatory value (myeloid versus lymphoid), but its practical clinical value is limited.[78–81]

Cytogenetic–Molecular Markers Recurrent cytogenetic–molecular abnormalities are common in adult ALL (Table 115-3).[82–85] They provide insights into the underlying molecular events of the leukemic blasts, including the role of fusion transcripts from translocations, tumor suppressor genes from deletions, or the control of cell-cycle regulatory genes. Karyotype analysis, fluorescence in situ hybridization (FISH), Southern blotting of genomic deoxyribonucleic acid (DNA), and reverse transcriptase polymerase chain reaction (RT-PCR) assays can identify molecular abnormalities that characterize subsets of ALL with distinct responses to therapy and distinct prognoses.[86–88] Significant differences exist in the frequency with which good- and poor-prognosis karyotypes occur in childhood and adult ALL. These differences partly explain the differences in outcome between those patient populations. More recently, oligonucleotide or complementary DNA microarray technology has been introduced as an alternative and extension to conventional karyotyping and FISH to identify previously unrecognized molecular ALL subtypes.[89]

Translocation t(9;22) A reciprocal translocation between the long arms of chromosomes 9 and 22, t(9;22)(q34;q11) (Philadelphia chromosome [Ph]), is the most common recurring abnormality in adult ALL, being diagnosed with a frequency of 15 to 30%.[90] This translocation is rare in children with ALL (2 to 5%). Ph is the

Table 115-3 Cytogenetic and Molecular Abnormalities in Acute Lymphoblastic Leukemia (ALL)

		Frequency (%)	
Cytogenetics	Gene Involved	Adults	Children
t(1;14)(p32;q11)	*TAL1*	10–15	5–10
del(5q)	?	< 2	< 2
t(5;14)(q35;q32)	*TLX3*	1	2–3
del(6q), t(6;12)	?	5	< 5
del(7p)	?	5–10	< 5
+ 8	—	10–12	2
t(8;14), t(8;22), t(2;8)	c-*myc*	5	2–5
t(9;22)(q34;q11)	*BCR-ABL1*	15–25	2–6
del(9p21–22)	*CDKN2A, CDKN2B*	6–30	20
t(7;9)(q34;q32)	*TAL2*	< 1	< 1
t(10;14)(q24;q11)	*TLX1*	5–10	< 5
del(11q22–23)	*ATM*	25–30[a]	15[a]
t(4;11), t(9;11), t(11;19), t(3;11)	*MLL*	5–10	< 5
t(12;21)(p12;q22)	*ETV6-RUNX1*	< 1[b]	20–25[b]
del(13)(q14)	*miR15/miR16*	< 5	< 5
t(1;14)(p32;q11)	*TCR-α*	20–25[c]	20–25[c]
t(1;19), t(17;19)	*TCF3-PBX1, TCF3-HLF*	< 5	4–5
Hyperdiploidy	—	2–15	10–26
Hypodiploidy	—	5–10	5–10

[a]As determined by loss of heterozygosity.
[b]As determined by polymerase chain reaction.
[c]In T-ALL, overall incidence is < 10%.

result of a fusion of the *BCR* (breakpoint cluster region) gene on chromosome 22q11 with the *ABL1* (Abelson murine leukemia viral oncogene homolog 1) gene on 9q34. The chimeric *BCR-ABL1* gene is translated into hybrid Bcr-Abl1 oncoproteins of varying size and molecular weight depending on the exact location of the transposed *ABL1* exons within *BCR*[91]: (1) $p190^{BCR\text{-}ABL1}$ (molecular weight 190 kDa), if the breakpoint in *BCR* occurs at the minor breakpoint cluster region (m-*BCR*); (2) $p210^{BCR\text{-}ABL1}$ for transpositions into the major breakpoint cluster region (M-*BCR*); and (3) the longest version, $p230^{BCR\text{-}ABL1}$ if the *BCR-ABL1* fusion is located downstream at the μ-*BCR*. The $p210^{BCR\text{-}ABL1}$ version can be detected in up to 95% of patients with chronic myeloid leukemia, and the $p190^{BCR\text{-}ABL1}$ is detected in 60 to 80% of patients with Ph-positive ALL.

All *BCR-ABL1* proteins are characterized by deregulated and abnormally increased tyrosine kinase activity, leading to the involvement of downstream signaling pathways such as Ras/Raf, Jak/Stat, phosphoinositide-3 kinase, CrkL and Akt, adhesion kinases, and others. Patients with t(9;22) are usually older and frequently have higher white blood cell (WBC) and blast counts at diagnosis than do patients with normal karyotypes.[92] Ph-positive ALL usually exhibits a pre-B-cell immunophenotype and positivity for CD10 and myeloid markers (CD13 and CD33). Although remission rates using current dose-intensive treatment regimens are similar to those in patients with non-Ph-positive ALL, remission durations are notably shorter and long-term DFS is exceedingly rare.[93] Better results have been reported with stem-cell transplant (SCT) and possibly with combinations of anti-ALL chemotherapy regimens plus imatinib mesylate, a tyrosine kinase inhibitor of *BCR-ABL1* activity (see "Maintenance Therapy" later in this chapter).

Aneuploidy Ploidy is a recognized prognostic factor in ALL. Hyperdiploidy denotes a gain of additional chromosomes, so that the modal number of chromosomes exceeds 46; hypodiploidy describes karyotypes with modal numbers less than 46. The incidence of hypodiploidy is about 5% irrespective of age.[94] Distinct subgroups of hypodiploidy have been described. The poorest outcome is associated with near-haploid chromosome sets or multiplications thereof, such as those seen in patients whose blasts harbor near-triploid karyotypes.[95,96] In contrast, hyperdiploidy is usually associated with a precursor B-cell phenotype, low-risk disease features, and a favorable prognosis.

The incidence of hyperdiploidy, especially high hyperdiploidy (> 51 chromosomes), is distinctly higher in children (25% versus < 5%), is associated with favorable prognosis, and is considered to be one of the explanations for the better outcome in children than in adults.[97,98] Blasts with hyperdiploid karyotypes have been shown to accumulate more methotrexate and methotrexate polyglutamate, and to be more sensitive to chemotherapy agents, including mercaptopurine, thioguanine, cytarabine, and L-asparaginase.[87,99,100]

Translocation t(12;21) Translocation t(12;21) involves *ETV6* (Ets variant gene 6), a transcription regulating gene of the Ets family of transcription factors, on 12p11 and *RUNX1 (acute myeloid leukemia 1)* on 21q22, resulting in an *ETV6-RUNX1* fusion gene.[101–103] This cryptic translocation will be missed in most cases when conventional banding techniques alone are used. Using PCR, the translocation can be identified in up to 30% of children with ALL, making *ETV6-RUNX1* the most frequent recurring cytogenetic–molecular abnormality in pediatric pre-B ALL.[104]

ETV6-RUNX1-positive ALL has been associated with a favorable prognosis in children; however, one study suggested that the favorable outcome resulted from the exclusion of patients with other poor-risk cytogenetic abnormalities and from the younger age of the patients as compared with patients having normal karyotypes. Translocation t(12;21) may be associated with late relapses.[105,106]

In contrast to the situation in children, the translocation is rare in adults (1 to 3%), in whom its prognostic significance remains undetermined. ALL blasts carrying the *ETV6-RUNX1* fusion have recently been shown to be significantly more sensitive to doxorubicin and etoposide. That observation further emphasizes the importance of identifying molecular abnormalities, because these abnormalities may define biological characteristics of blasts that may then be exploited therapeutically.[107]

Abnormalities of Chromosome 9p21 Abnormalities of 9p21 occur in up to 15% of patients with ALL.[108,109] These patients represent a prognostically heterogeneous group. They typically present with unfavorable clinical characteristics. The ALL blasts are predominantly of T-cell lineage. Prognosis in the patients is generally unfavorable and is characterized by higher rates of relapse and shorter survival. These prognostic associations are usually stronger in childhood ALL and less well defined in adult ALL.[110–113] Band q21 of chromosome 9 harbors the genes for cyclin-dependent kinase inhibitors (CDKNs) $p16^{CDKN2A}/p14^{CDKN2A}$ and $p15^{CDKN2B}$. Using FISH or PCR, heterozygous or homozygous deletions (or both) of $p16^{CDKN2A}$ have been described in up to 80% of children with T ALL and in 20% of those with pre-B ALL. Hypermethylation of promoter regions of these genes is another mode of inactivation that is being investigated.[114]

***MLL* Rearrangements (11q23)** The common denominator of 11q23 abnormalities is involvement of the mixed lineage leukemia gene *MLL* (previously *ALL-1*, *HRX*, or *HTRX1*). More than 20 chromosomal loci are known to participate in reciprocal rearrangements with 11q23, including 4q21, 9p22, 19p13, and 1p32.[115,116]

The most common translocation involving 11q23 is t(4;11)(q21;23). It is specifically associated with ALL in infants (accounting for up to 85% of cases) and is found in 3 to 8% of adults.[117] Adults with this translocation tend to be older and to have higher WBC counts and organomegaly; sanctuary sites such as the CNS are involved more frequently. The immunophenotype is pre-pre-B ALL, and the blasts are positive for TdT, HLA-DR, and CD19 and variably negative for CD10. Myeloid antigen coexpression is common.[82] The prognosis in adults with 11q23 rearrangements remains poor, and allogeneic SCT in first remission is currently the treatment of choice.[83,84,118,119]

Transcription Factor 3 Gene Rearrangements (19p13) The two known translocations with transcription factor 3 (*TCF3*) rearrangements on chromosome 19p13 are t(1;19)(q23;p13) and t(17;19)(q21;p13). Translocation t(1;19) is strongly associated with pre-B ALL phenotype expressing cytoplasmic immunoglobulin. Its overall frequency in childhood ALL is about 5%, but it can be as high as 25% in pre-B-cell ALL. The frequency in adults is lower.

The translocation juxtaposes the *TCF3* gene on chromosome 19 with the homeobox-containing gene *PBX1* (pre-B-cell leukemia transcription factor 1) to generate the *TCF3-PBX1* fusion gene. The fusion gene functions as a potent transcriptional activator and transforms in vitro a variety of cell types including fibroblasts, myeloid progenitors, and lymphoblasts. Patients with ALL and *TCF3-PBX1* rearrangements have a worse prognosis with standard or less aggressive therapy, but do better with more aggressive approaches.[83,84,120–122]

Translocation t(17;19) is a rare variant. It is more frequent in pre-pre-B ALL, fusing *TCF3* with the leucine zipper transcription factor gene *HLF* (hepatic leukemia factor) on chromosome 17.[123]

8q24 Rearrangements The c-*myc* oncogene is located on 8q24 and is involved in several translocations that rearrange one of the three immunoglobulin chain loci in mature B ALL:

- With a frequency of 80%, t(8;14)(q24;q32) is the most common translocation of 8q24: c-*myc* is juxtaposed to the immunoglobulin heavy chain (IgH) gene locus on 14q32.
- The t(8;22)(q24;q11) translocation occurs in about 15% of B ALL patients and involves the Igλ gene locus on 22q11.
- Of the three translocations involving the Igκ gene locus on 2p12, t(2;8)(p12;q24) is the least frequent.

Translocations of c-*myc* into the T-cell receptor α/δ gene on 14q11 have been described and lead to the same effect of increasing transcription of c-*myc*.[124,125]

T-Cell Receptor Gene Rearrangements T-Cell receptor (*TR*) gene rearrangements are the most common cytogenetic abnormalities in T ALL. Genes for T-cell receptors are located on chromosomes 14q11 (*TRAV23DV6* [alpha variable 23/delta variable 6]), 7q15 (TCR-γ gene λ), and 7q32-36 (TCR-β gene δ). Although no specific cytogenetic abnormality can be linked to a specific clinical subtype of T ALL, a number of distinct chromosomal translocations have been identified. The phenotypic effects of *TR* gene rearrangements are similar to those that have been described with c-*myc* rearrangements in 8q24-containing translocations.[100]

Gene Expression Microarrays Studies of gene-expression profiles are advancing the molecular classification of cancer. DNA microarray technology has rapidly become one of the most-used techniques in the diagnosis and monitoring of a variety of hematologic malignancies.[89] Oligonucleotide microarray technology made it possible to simultaneously quantify the expression of thousands of individual genes, and thus to establish a gene-expression profile for well-defined subgroups of patients. Gene-expression profiling can not only identify genotypic and phenotypic subsets of ALL, it can also provide information to identify genetic alterations that underlie the pathogenesis of individual leukemia subtypes, detect gene-expression clusters that characterize patients with distinct responses to therapy (and thus also provide prognostic information), and establish gene-expression clusters that distinguish blasts in relapse from those unexposed to previous therapy. Application of gene-expression profiling may therefore identify new therapies targeting specific molecular abnormalities and establish leukemia-specific molecular markers that can be monitored as measures for residual disease.[126–128]

In one of the largest studies, which included samples from 360 children with ALL, researchers could identify six known clinical subtypes of ALL that corresponded to known cytogenetic subtypes: t(12;21) (*ETV6-RUNX1*), t(1;19) (*TCF3-PBX1*), t(9;22) (*BCR-ABL1*), 11q23 rearrangements (*MLL*), hyperdiploidy, and T-cell ALL.[129] In addition, a seventh subtype was identified that did not fit any of the described cytogenetic categories and whose clinical relevance remains to be determined.

Gene-expression profiling has succeeded in grouping T-cell ALL according to pathobiologic pathways.[86,130] These pathways identified subsets of patients with distinct molecular signatures and gene clusters, which had cellular counterparts and prognostic significance. Patients identified by a *TLX1* (T-cell leukemia, homeobox 1) or *MLL-MLLT1* (trithorax homolog, Drosophila; translocated to 1) cluster had a survival in excess of 90%; patients identified by the *TAL1* (T-cell acute lymphocytic leukemia 1) cluster had a significantly worse outcome.

The prognostic significance of a particular gene cluster is, however, determined not only by its presence or absence, but also by the treatment administered. Based on gene-expression profiling in adults and children with ALL, distinct subsets of patients have been identified with varying responses to therapy and survival.

However intriguing the results and possibilities of gene-expression profiling have been, numerous technical issues related to the reproducibility, statistical significance, and practical application of such an approach need to be resolved before gene-expression profiling can be recommended for clinical decision-making. In addition, the field of proteomics continues to evolve, and questions remain regarding the significance of gene-expression versus protein-expression profiles.[131]

Epigenetic Alterations in ALL Aberrant methylation of promoter-associated CpG (cytosine–phosphate–guanine) islands and the resultant silencing of tumor-related genes because of hypermethylation has emerged as a distinct molecular pathway in the process of cellular malignant transformation. Aberrant promoter hypermethylation of genes may be at least as common a mechanism for disruption of tumor-suppressor genes as are gene mutations and deletions.[132] The phenomenon is particularly prevalent in ALL both at presentation and at relapse, where methylation of genes can be demonstrated in up to 80% of patients.[133,134]

Analysis of the methylation status of multiple genes in ALL has identified subsets of patients with a "hypermethylator" phenotype that has prognostic significance. Genes frequently involved include *p73* and the cyclin-dependent kinase inhibitors *p15* and *p57*^{CDKN1C}, all of which play a crucial role in cell-cycle regulatory pathways. Although methylation of a single gene such as *p57*^{CDKN1C} does not affect outcome in ALL patients, methylation of at least two genes involved in cell-cycle regulatory pathways has been associated with unfavorable DFS and overall survival.[135–137] These observations have therapeutic consequences, because patients with a defined methylator phenotype may benefit from treatment with hypomethylating agents such as 5-aza-2'-deoxycytidine. Understanding defined genetic and epigenetic changes in adult ALL may lead to risk-adapted therapies that target dominant molecular mechanisms.

THERAPY OF ALL

The goal of ALL therapy is rapid restoration of normal hematopoiesis, prevention of the emergence of resistant subclones, prophylaxis of sanctuary sites such as the CNS, and elimination of minimal residual disease (MRD) through post-remission consolidation strategies. Therapeutic strategies in adult ALL have been patterned after pediatric regimens and typically include multiple drugs in a regimen-specific sequence of dose- and time-intensity. Although various chemotherapy regimens with variations in treatment sequence and choice of agents are applied in adult ALL, all regimens have in common the basic building blocks of an intensive multichemotherapy regimen: (1) induction; (2) consolidation and intensification; and (3) maintenance.[65,66,138–152]

CNS treatment is an essential part of any therapeutic regimen in ALL and is usually delivered during the induction and consolidation phases. Ongoing issues related to adult ALL therapy include (1) the optimal induction strategy; (2) the value of intensified consolidation; (3) the role of duration of maintenance therapy; (4) the optimal approach to CNS prophylaxis; (5) identification of pretreatment prognostic factors, and design of risk-adapted therapy models; (6) the role of SCT; and (7) optimal supportive care measures accompanying leukemia-specific therapy.

Prognostic Factors and Models in ALL ALL is a heterogeneous disease of many subtypes that vary with regard to pathobiology, clinical features, and prognostic characteristics. Identification and validation of these characteristics in prognostic models allows patients to be assigned to therapies of appropriate intensity, with avoidance of unnecessary toxicities where possible. Because remission rates with current regimens are high, prognostic models should ideally achieve most of their impact in predicting progression-free and overall survival. Some of the traditional clinical, laboratory, and biologic variables once thought to be useful predictors of prognosis now have little value, because the treatment for patients with ALL has improved over the last two decades.[153–156]

Outcome in T-lineage ALL and mature B-cell ALL used to be poor, with low CR rates and only a few patients achieving long-term DFS. Recent treatment regimens using cyclophosphamide and cytarabine in T-lineage ALL and short-term dose-intense treatment regimens in mature B-cell ALL increased CR rates to 90% and DFS rates to above 50%.

Persistently valuable prognostic features include age, WBC count at presentation, time to response to therapy, and (with some limitations) immunophenotype.[65,66,157] Cytogenetic–molecular abnormalities are increasingly recognized as powerful predictors of outcome.[82,158,159] Involvement of *BCR-ABL1*, *TCF3*, and *MLL* gene rearrangements are associated with poor prognosis following conventional chemotherapy programs, suggesting SCT in first remission as an appropriate treatment decision. Based on such information, several prognostic models have been developed and are in use in adult ALL (Table 115-4). According to these models, about 75% of adults with ALL are considered "poor risk," with an expected DFS of 25%; the remaining patients are "standard risk," with a projected DFS of better than 50%.

Additional prognostic factors have recently been identified.[161–163]

Sequential monitoring of MRD has become a powerful indicator of treatment outcome, especially in the prediction of relapse after patients have achieved CR. However, large prospective studies for further validation are still lacking (see "MRD in Adult ALL" later in this chapter).

Time to blast clearance in response to steroids, when assessed within 1 to 2 weeks, was found to be of prognostic value in adults as well as in children.[164–166]

Expression of drug resistance markers such as the *ABCB1* (adenosinetriphosphate-binding cassette, subfamily B, member 1) gene was associated with resistance to therapy and with higher relapse probability.[167]

Sensitivity to chemotherapy is determined by molecular events within the leukemic blasts. Cells from patients with hyperdiploid ALL have higher accumulations of methotrexate and its active polyglutamate metabolites. *ETV6-RUNX1*-harboring blasts are exquisitely sensitive to L-asparaginase. Pharmacogenetic information about genes that encode drug-metabolizing enzymes, transporters, or drug targets is increasingly being used in assessing the efficacy and toxicity of chemotherapy regimens.[19,168]

Table 115-4 Adverse Prognostic Factors in Acute Lymphoblastic Leukemia (ALL)

Characteristic	MDACC[65,149,160]	GMALL[139,161] B-Lineage	GMALL[139,161] T-Lineage	CALGB[66,141]	MSKCC[154]
Age (years)	—	> 50	—	> 60	> 60
WBC ($\times 10^9$/L)	> 5	> 30	> 100	> 30	> 20
Time to CR	> 1 course	> 4 weeks	> 4 weeks	—	> 5 weeks
FAB	—	—	—	L3	—
Immunophenotype	B	Pro-B	Pre-T	(B)	Null, B
Karyotype	Ph	Ph, 11q23	—	Ph, 11q23	Ph
CNS disease	Present	—	—	—	—

CALGB = Cancer and Leukemia Group B; CNS = central nervous system; CR = complete remission; FAB = French–American–British Cooperative Group; GMALL = German ALL Study Group; MDACC = M. D. Anderson Cancer Center; MSKCC = Memorial Sloan–Kettering Cancer Center; Ph = Philadelphia chromosome–positive ALL; WBC = white blood cells.

CHEMOTHERAPY Induction Therapy The backbone of induction therapy consists of a combination of vincristine and corticosteroids plus an anthracycline. Vincristine and prednisone alone achieved CR rates of 40 to 65%, but responses were short-lived, with median remission durations of 3 to 7 months. Addition of anthracyclines to the vincristine–prednisone combination increased the CR rates to between 70 and 85%, with median remission durations of about 18 months and with an induction mortality of less than 10%.[149,169] No difference in outcome has been established based on the use of different anthracyclines. Whether higher doses of anthracyclines improve outcome remains under investigation.[147,151,170] Todeschini and colleagues used daunorubicin at total doses of 270 mg/m^2 during induction and high-dose cytarabine during consolidation.[147] The CR rate was 93%, the induction mortality was 8%, and the 6-year event-free survival was 55% in 60 patients with adult ALL. A larger Italian cooperative study is ongoing to confirm those results.

Additional drugs have been incorporated into ALL induction regimens. How L-asparaginase, cyclophosphamide, cytarabine, etoposide, teniposide, m-amsacrine, or other agents influence short- and long-term prognosis remains unclear. This uncertainty exists in part because of the inherent difficulty in ascribing outcome effects of complex treatment regimens to specific single components, and also because it is difficult to demonstrate further improvement in CR rates with the addition of these drugs. Intensification of induction may positively influence remission duration and survival; however, the effect may be related to specific immunophenotypes. Use of cytarabine and cyclophosphamide has increased response rates and DFS in T-lineage ALL, and use of fractionated doses of cyclophosphamide and high doses of methotrexate has improved outcome in mature B-cell ALL.[153,171–174] L-Asparaginase is used less frequently in adults than in children with ALL, mainly because of higher toxicity rates. However, lack of L-asparaginase during induction does not appear to affect remission rates in adults.[175] Pegylated asparaginase, which has a better pharmacologic and more favorable toxicity profile, is currently being investigated in several clinical trials.[176]

Various steroid derivatives have been used. Compared with prednisone, dexamethasone has shown better in vitro antileukemic activity and higher levels of the drug in the cerebrospinal fluid. Dexamethasone was associated with improved outcome in pediatric ALL.[177,178]

Use of hematopoietic growth factors is increasingly being accepted during induction.[179] The rationale includes shortening of the duration of myelosuppression and therefore fewer associated infectious complications. In addition, rapid recovery of marrow function following chemotherapy permits timely administration of dose-intense treatment regimens.

Three randomized trials have demonstrated an advantage with the use of granulocyte colony–stimulating factor (G-CSF).[180–182] In a double-blind, randomized trial by the Cancer and Leukemia Group B (CALGB), 198 adults with ALL were randomized to receive supportive care either with (n = 102) or without G-CSF (n = 96).[180] G-CSF treatment resulted in faster neutrophil recovery to more than 1×10^9/L (16 versus 22 days, p < .001), faster platelet recovery (16 versus 19 days, p = .003), shorter duration of hospital stays (p = .02), higher CR rates (87% versus 71%, p = .01), and less mortality (5% versus 11%, p = .04). G-CSF therapy reduced induction mortality from 25% to 10% (p = .24) in patients older than 60 years. However, G-CSF during induction and consolidation has not been shown to prolong remission duration or overall survival. Because no adverse events have been associated with G-CSF, administration of G-CSF during induction is suggested.[183]

Further measures for supportive care during remission induction consist of prophylactic antibiotics, including antibacterials (eg, levofloxacin, ciprofloxacin, or trimethoprim–sulfamethoxazole), antifungals (eg, fluconazole, itraconazole, or voriconazole), and antivirals (eg, acyclovir).[184] Tumor lysis and DIC should be anticipated in patients with significant leukocytosis and should be treated appropriately. Organ involvement and dysfunction may respond to high-dose steroids (eg, hyperbilirubinemia related to ALL).

Consolidation Therapy In several studies, post-remission intensified consolidation improved outcome, particularly in patients with high-risk disease. Although inclusion of intensified consolidation programs is generally accepted as beneficial, no consensus exists about the optimal type or duration of consolidation. Consolidation programs typically consist of a repetition of the induction sequence or rotational programs that include additional agents, which may benefit particular ALL subtypes. Because the number, schedule, and combination of cytostatic drugs vary considerably between studies, assessing the value of the individual components of various programs remains difficult.

The hyper-CVAD regimen alternates hyperfractionated cyclophosphamide, vincristine, doxorubicin (Adriamycin), and dexamethasone with high doses of cytarabine and methotrexate.[65,160] Compared with the earlier and less intense VAD (vincristine, doxorubicin, dexamethasone) program, hyper-CVAD has shown a superior CR rate (91% versus 75%, p < .01) and survival (p < .01).

In CALGB study 8811, patients underwent early and late intensification courses with eight drugs after a five-drug induction regimen.[66] Maintenance therapy was given until 2 years after diagnosis. The median remission duration was 29 months, and the median survival was 36 months, considerably better than the outcomes observed with earlier, less intense trials.

In a UK study (Medical Research Council [MRC] study UKALL XA), patients were randomized to either early intensification at 5 weeks, late intensification at 20 weeks, both, or neither.[140,146] Early intensification prevented relapses, but DFS at 5 years was increased only slightly.

In an Italian study (Gruppo Italiano Malattie Ematologiche dell' Adulto study ALL 0288), patients were randomized to early post-CR intensification or to maintenance therapy.[138] Of 388 patients, 201 received maintenance alone, and 187 received consolidation followed by maintenance. Intensification of post-CR treatment did not influence the continuous CR rate. At 8 years, 36% of patients on consolidation–maintenance and 37% of patients on maintenance alone remained in CR. Furthermore, only 35% of the patients who were randomized to the intensified consolidation completed their treatment within the expected time frame, raising doubts about the feasibility of prolonged intensified consolidation in adults because of toxicities and compliance problems.

A German multicenter trial (German Multicenter Study Group for Adult ALL 05/93) increased the intensity of consolidation therapy according to ALL subtype: high-dose methotrexate in standard-risk B-lineage ALL, cyclophosphamide and cytarabine in T-lineage ALL, high-dose methotrexate and high-dose cytarabine in high-risk B-lineage ALL.[161] The CR rate was 87% in standard-risk patients, with a median remission duration of 57 months and a 5-year survival probability of 55%. In high-risk patients, intensified induction–consolidation did not improve CR rate or DFS, except in the case of pre-pre-B ALL, in which a continuous CR rate of 41% was achieved versus 19% in other high-risk patients.

In summary, current data suggest that intensification by the addition of high-dose cytarabine, methotrexate, or etoposide may benefit higher risk patients during consolidation as compared with less intense consolidation schedules or maintenance only. SCT should be considered in first remission for high-risk patients, as discussed in "Stem-Cell Transplant" later in this chapter.

Maintenance Therapy The rationale for maintenance is based on the view that monthly administration of prolonged therapy is able to suppress residual leukemic cells with slow proliferation kinetics that might otherwise give rise to relapse. Maintenance treatment consists of a combination of 6-mercaptopurine, methotrexate, and monthly pulses of vincristine and prednisone; it typically extends over 2 to 3 years. Extension of maintenance therapy for more than 3 years has not demonstrated any additional benefits. Omission of maintenance therapy altogether has been associated with significantly shorter DFS rates.[185–187] Use of intensification cycles during maintenance remains investigational without proven benefit.

Maintenance therapy is not usually given in mature B-cell ALL, because these patients typically relapse within the first year of remission and late relapses are rare.[153] In T-cell ALL, the benefit of maintenance chemotherapy has also been questioned; however, recent studies from Japan indicated that shorter maintenance may be associated with higher relapse rates. Innovative approaches to maintenance are being investigated in other well-defined subsets such as Ph-positive ALL, in which the availability of imatinib and other newer tyrosine kinase inhibitors has offered new options.

Stem-Cell Transplant **Allogeneic SCT** Studies of marrow transplant in adult ALL have demonstrated improved outcomes with survival rates of about 50% (range: 20 to 81%) when performed in first complete remission.[188–197] Several studies have compared the outcome of allogeneic SCT with that of autologous SCT or of chemotherapy in patients with ALL in first complete remission. Unbiased comparisons between treatments remain difficult for several reasons. Most patients lack a matched sibling and cannot be allocated to allogeneic SCT in the first place. Furthermore, significant heterogeneity exists in transplant preparative regimens, sources of stem cells (peripheral blood, marrow), and risk profiles of patients (standard risk versus high risk).[197]

Horowitz and colleagues analyzed data from the International Bone Marrow Transplant Registry (IBMTR) and compared outcomes in 484 patients treated with intensive post-remission chemotherapy to outcomes in 251 patients undergoing allogeneic SCT.[198] After adjustments for differences in disease characteristics and time-to-treatment, 5-year survival rates were similar: 38% and 44% respectively. A longer-term follow-up confirmed those results. At 9 years, DFS rates were 32% for chemotherapy and 34% for allogeneic SCT.[196] The causes of treatment failure were different: actuarial relapse probabilities at 9 years were 66% for chemotherapy and 30% for transplant ($p < .001$); treatment-related mortality was 5% and 53% ($p < .0001$) respectively.[164] Outcome was similar in standard-risk and high-risk patients.

In a French multicenter trial (LALA 87), patients with a matched sibling donor were allocated to receive allogeneic SCT if they were in complete remission and younger than 40 years of age ($n = 116$), or they were randomized to receive either chemotherapy ($n = 96$) or autologous SCT ($n = 95$) if they were older or had no sibling donor available.[194] The 5-year survival rates between the two main study arms were not significantly different (48% versus 35%, $p = .08$). However, for patients with high-risk ALL (Ph-positive ALL, undifferentiated ALL, age > 35 years, leukocyte count > 30×10^9/L, time to complete remission > 4 weeks), allogeneic SCT resulted in a better 5-year overall survival (44% versus 20%, $p = .03$) and 5-year DFS (39% versus 14%, $p = .01$) than with chemotherapy or autologous transplant.

In an update of the LALA 87 study, an intent-to-treat analysis of 572 patients showed that overall survival was 46% in the allogeneic SCT arm as compared with 31% in the chemotherapy arm ($p = .04$).[150] In the high-risk group, overall survival rates at 10 years were 44% in the allogeneic SCT arm and 11% in the control arm ($p = .009$); in the standard-risk groups, the corresponding numbers were 49% and 39% ($p = .6$). These results support the role of allogeneic SCT in the first complete remission in patients with high-risk ALL.

The LALA 94 study tried to evaluate the benefits of a risk-adapted post-remission strategy and the role of allogeneic SCT in ALL.[152] A total of 922 patients were divided by risk group (standard-risk, high-risk, Ph-positive, CNS-positive). All patients received a standard 4-week induction and were then assigned to receive either more- or less-intensive post-remission chemotherapy (standard-risk group) or to undergo allogeneic SCT (all other risk groups) if an HLA-identical sibling was available. Alternatively, patients in the defined risk groups were offered either autologous SCT or, in the absence of Ph or CNS disease, randomization to autologous SCT or to chemotherapy. The study was able to demonstrate an improvement of DFS in high-risk ALL patients who underwent allogeneic SCT in first complete remission. On the other hand, autologous transplant did not confer a significant benefit over chemotherapy.

The Groupe Ouest-Est des Leucémies Aiguës et Maladies du Sang (GOELAMS) evaluated the impact of allogeneic SCT for high-risk patients in first complete remission as compared with delayed autologous SCT for patients without matched donors and for those older than 50 years.[199] Allogeneic SCT was performed after two consolidation courses. An intent-to-treat analysis for patients younger than 50 years showed that 6-year overall survival was significantly improved with allogeneic SCT as compared with autologous SCT (75% versus 40%, $p = .0027$).

In a German study, 264 patients with ALL at various disease stages (first complete remission, relapse, primary refractory) received either matched related or unrelated allogeneic SCT.[200] More favorable DFS at 5 years was demonstrated for patients transplanted in first remission rather than later, for B-lineage rather than T-cell ALL, and for Ph-positive ALL.

In the international ALL trial (MRC UKALL XII/Eastern Cooperative Oncology Group E2993), all patients in complete remission after induction therapy were assigned to allogeneic SCT if they had a histocompatible donor ($n = 170$); the others were randomized to standard consolidation and maintenance for another 2.5 years or to autologous SCT ($n = 426$).[201] The 5-year event-free survival (EFS) was 54% for the allogeneic group and 34% for the randomized group ($p = .04$). Among standard-risk patients, the 5-year EFS was 66% for the allogeneic SCT group and 45% for the randomized group ($p = .06$). Among high-risk patients (defined mainly by the presence of Ph), the rates were 44% and 26% respectively ($p = .3$). In contrast to the results in most other studies, the data suggested that allogeneic SCT was beneficial for patients in first complete remission regardless of risk group. A final analysis of the trial is pending.

In summary, given the lack of reliable pre-transplant identification and stratification of prognostic indicators, the role of allogeneic SCT in ALL remains difficult to define. Available data support its early use, at least for patients with high-risk disease; its role in standard-risk patients is not quite so clear.[202] The effect on outcome of combinations of novel therapies (eg, imatinib) with chemotherapy versus SCT needs to be elucidated further and may affect current recommendations for SCT. The roles of newer transplant modalities such as unrelated-donor transplant or reduced-intensity SCT ("mini-SCT") in ALL have yet to be defined.[203–205]

Autologous SCT Several studies did not demonstrate an improvement in outcome of autologous SCT over allogeneic SCT.[194,195,201,206] Although autologous SCT is better tolerated and has lower complication and mortality rates, the absence of the graft-versus-leukemia (GVL) effect and the potential presence of leukemia cell contamination have impaired the effectiveness of autologous SCT.

Adding subsequent maintenance or immunomodulatory therapy to increase the efficacy of autologous SCT has been studied, but does not appear to provide further benefit. In a study by Powles and colleagues, 77 patients received an autologous SCT in first remission, followed by post-transplant maintenance chemotherapy with methotrexate, 6-mercaptopurine, vincristine, and prednisone.[207] The cumulative incidence of relapse at 10 years was 42%. The 10-year probabilities of DFS and overall survival were 50% and 53% respectively. In the GOELAMS study, patients who did not qualify for allogeneic SCT received an autologous transplant and were randomized to interferon-α maintenance. Although the number of patients randomized to interferon-α was small, that maintenance had no effect on relapse or survival.[199]

Autologous SCT may play a role in patients without options for allogeneic transplant who are otherwise noncompliant or unwilling to commit to long-term therapy. Otherwise, autologous SCT currently shows no advantage over chemotherapy.

Additional Aspects of Therapy **CNS Prophylaxis** The value of CNS prophylaxis in reducing the incidence of CNS disease has been clearly established.[208] Although only 5 to 10% of adults with ALL present with CNS leukemia at diagnosis, the incidence of CNS involvement may be as high as 50 to 75% at one year in the absence of prophylaxis. CNS disease may precede overt marrow and peripheral blood relapse.[29,209]

Risk factors for CNS involvement include younger age, T-lineage and mature B-cell ALL immunophenotypes, high WBC count, elevated serum lactate dehydrogenase (LDH), and a high proliferative index (S+G2M > 14%) of the leukemia blasts.[210,211] In a multivariate analysis of potential risk factors, mature B-cell phenotype, high LDH, and high proliferative index emerged as independent factors for CNS disease. In the absence of any risk factor, the probability of CNS involvement was 4%. It was 13% when a high proliferative index only was present, 29% with an elevated LDH only, and 56% if both LDH and proliferative index were high. Assessing the risk of CNS involvement may guide the intensity of CNS prophylaxis applied.[212]

Effective means of CNS prophylaxis include intrathecal chemotherapy (methotrexate, cytarabine, steroids), high-dose systemic chemotherapy (methotrexate, cytarabine, L-asparaginase), and craniospinal irradiation (XRT).[213,214] Combined triple-modality intrathecal therapy is highly effective, but carries a high risk of treatment-related morbidity. Studies in childhood ALL have demonstrated that intrathecal therapy and craniospinal XRT are equivalent even in patients with high risk for CNS disease,[215–217] so that the role of cranial XRT has become controversial, especially in adults. XRT can result in neurologic adverse events including seizures, dementia, and intellectual dysfunction, as well as in other complications such as growth retardation in children.

CNS prophylaxis based on high-dose systemic therapy alone is not sufficient. During the hyper-CVAD regimen, CNS prophylaxis (in addition to systemic high-dose chemotherapy) consisted of 4 intrathecal treatments in the low-risk category (based on normal LDH and low proliferative index), 8 intrathecal treatments with high-risk disease, and 16 intrathecal treatments for mature B-cell ALL or Burkitt's disease.[160] Patients with cranial nerve root involvement may benefit from selective irradiation to the base of the skull.

CNS prophylaxis should start early and extend through the induction and intensified consolidation phases. Delayed CNS prophylaxis has been associated with an increased incidence of CNS disease. The diagnosis of CNS leukemia requires 5 WBCs/μL of cerebrospinal fluid, with the presence of lymphoblasts in a cytocentrifuged sample. The significance of cerebrospinal fluid blasts with WBC counts lower than 5/μL has been disputed, although the presence of blasts with a low WBC cerebrospinal fluid count has been associated with worse risk group. Reliance on cerebrospinal fluid cytology alone may lead to false negative results: in patients with cranial nerve involvement only, no cerebrospinal fluid blasts may be detectable.[215–217]

Pharmacogenetics and Mechanisms of Drug Resistance Different clinical outcomes can be attributed to differences in sensitivity of ALL types to chemotherapy based on cytogenetic–molecular characteristics that determine, among other things, drug disposition and clearance.[100,218] Karyotypes associated with increased sensitivity to therapy include

- Hyperdiploidy: These patients are highly sensitive to antimetabolite-type chemotherapy. On a molecular level, many of these patients harbor additional copies of a gene coding for cellular methotrexate transporters. Also, higher-than-average concentrations of intracellular methotrexate polyglutamates have been demonstrated in vitro after treatment with methotrexate in leukemic blasts from these patients.[219]
- Translocation t(12;21): Patients whose cells harbor an *ETV6-RUNX1* fusion are more sensitive to asparaginase.[220]
- Translocation t(4;11): ALL with *MLL* rearrangements have increased sensitivity to cytarabine, possibly by overexpression of cellular cytarabine receptors.[221]

Phenotypes resistant to standard doses of methotrexate include T-lineage ALL, in which high doses of methotrexate have been associated with better outcome, and ALL associated with translocation t(1;19), which has been associated with resistance to standard antimetabolite-based therapy, but which has a better prognosis using intensified chemotherapy.

In recent years, considerations of drug metabolism and pharmacogenomics have started to play a larger role in the assessment of sensitivity to chemotherapy. Significant interpatient variabilities in the steady-state levels of a number of antineoplastic agents have been observed and may be responsible for variability in outcome.[218] Information from pharmacogenomics (genes encoding drug-metabolizing enzymes, transporters, and drug targets) may influence the efficacy and toxicity of chemotherapy. Polymorphisms in the expression of various genes have been associated with differences in drug absorption, distribution, and metabolism.

Thymidylate synthase (TS) is an important target of methotrexate. Homozygosity for a triple-tandem repeat polymorphism of the thymidylate synthase gene has been associated with increased levels of the enzyme and with inferior outcome in children with ALL.[222]

Polymorphisms of the *MTHFR* gene have been correlated with a higher incidence of adverse events, but also with greater sensitivity of leukemic blasts to methotrexate.[223,224] Evans and colleagues demonstrated a threefold variability in serum concentrations of methotrexate and that patients with low methotrexate concentrations had significantly shorter CR durations. Methotrexate clearance was an independent prognostic factor for remission duration.[225]

Polymorphisms affecting the thiopurine *S*-methyltransferase gene may likewise lead to increased sensitivity to 6-mercaptopurine, and thus to a higher risk of acute hematopoietic adverse events, but also to a more favorable leukemia-free survival because of the higher sensitivity.[226,227]

Because most of these studies have been conducted in children with ALL, it is unknown how these pharmacokinetic variables contribute to outcome in adult ALL. Interest is growing in designing programs that monitor pharmacogenetic properties so as to individualize therapy dose and schedule accordingly.

MRD in Adult ALL MRD describes the presence of disease below the threshold of detection by conventional methods (light microscopy and cytochemical staining). Various methodologies are available to detect and monitor MRD, including FISH, multicolor flow cytometry, and PCR assays, especially real-time quantitative (RQ) PCR.

Multicolor flow cytometry and PCR techniques take advantage of either fusion transcripts resulting from chromosome abnormalities (eg, *BCR-ABL1*, *MLL-AFF1*, *ETV6-RUNX1*) or patient-specific junctional regions of rearranged immunoglobulin and T-cell receptor genes.[228–233]

Measurement of MRD in ALL has become increasingly important as a prognostic factor for assessing the risk of relapse after patients have achieved a clinical remission.[234] The extent to which MRD needs to be controlled or eliminated to prevent leukemic relapse remains uncertain, although several studies have demonstrated a relationship between the ability to control MRD and long-term DFS.[235–243]

Several questions remain:

- What are the most appropriate time points for measurement of MRD?
  - Most patients demonstrate residual disease in clinical remission immediately following the induction sequence; the percentage of MRD-positive patients decreases during consolidation and maintenance. Persistence of MRD early in the treatment sequence typically lacks the clinical significance of detection of residual disease in later stages of therapy.
- Is there a definable threshold of residual disease by quantitative assays that would predict high relapse probability?
  - A number of clinical trials are trying to answer this question, but a reproducible threshold has not been defined in large prospective studies of MRD in adults.

- Is it necessary to revise response criteria and to introduce the concept of a "molecular relapse"?
    - This concept would make sense if treatment at the time of a molecular relapse favorably influenced the outcome of patients. It should also be emphasized that molecular relapse does not always predict clinical relapse; intensification of therapy under these circumstances may not be appropriate.
- Can quantification of MRD over time lead to a new risk classification that affects the choice of consolidation and maintenance strategies?
    - Most of our current knowledge about MRD and its kinetics derive from studies in childhood ALL, and differences between adult and childhood ALL in the pattern and dynamics of clearance of MRD have been described. Foroni and colleagues used PCR to analyze marrow samples from 33 adults and 21 children for immunoglobulin heavy-chain gene rearrangements at specific time points after diagnosis.[236] Among patients who remained in CR, a decrease in the MRD positivity occurred during the first 12 months. The proportion of positive tests decreased faster in children than in adults, suggesting more rapid resolution of MRD, particularly in the first 6 months of CR.
    - More recently, bisulfite PCR assays for detection of methylation patterns have been developed to detect MRD.[244] In a small subset of patients, aberrant DNA methylation predicted disease progression. Studies comparing methylation patterns at initial presentation and at relapse showed these patterns to be stable in 70% in adult ALL, providing the basis for future methylation assays in the detection and monitoring of MRD.[133]
    - As these techniques evolve, and as their prognostic relevance is confirmed, risk-oriented strategies based on tissue methylation patterns may represent an alternative to the markers mentioned earlier and may facilitate risk-adapted therapy.

Disease Subtype–Specific Treatment Approaches **Ph-Positive ALL** The outcome of patients with Ph-positive ALL receiving conventional chemotherapy remains poor, with long-term DFS rates of less than 10%.[245] SCT is therefore currently recommended for all patients with Ph-positive ALL who achieve CR.

In a study by the International ALL Trial group, 167 patients with Ph-positive ALL received either a matched related ($n = 49$), a matched unrelated ($n = 23$), or an autologous SCT ($n = 7$), or continued with chemotherapy alone ($n = 77$).[246] Although the treatment-related mortality was higher with SCT (37% for matched sibling transplant, 43% for matched unrelated donor transplant, 14% for autologous transplant, 8% with chemotherapy), the risk of relapse at 5 years was lower with allogeneic SCT (29%) as compared with the autologous SCT and chemotherapy groups combined (81%). Likewise, the 5-year survival probability was 43% with allogeneic SCT and 19% with autologous SCT or chemotherapy.

Imatinib mesylate (STI571, Gleevec), a small molecule of the group of 2-phenylaminopyrimidines, is a potent and selective inhibitor of the *BCR-ABL1* tyrosine kinase and has become the cornerstone of therapy in chronic myeloid leukemia. Activity of imatinib has also been demonstrated in Ph-positive ALL.[247] Thomas and colleagues combined imatinib with hyper-CVAD for newly diagnosed patients with Ph-positive ALL.[248,249] Hyper-CVAD was alternated with high-dose methotrexate and cytarabine for a total of 8 cycles. Imatinib was given at 400 mg daily for 14 days with each treatment cycle. Maintenance with imatinib at an oral dose of 600 mg daily followed. Of 26 patients, 25 (96%) achieved CR with a median time to response of 21 days. At a median follow-up time of 2 years, 13 patients could proceed to allogeneic SCT, 2 relapsed, and 5 died in CR (2 cases being related to transplant complications). Complete molecular responses (RT-PCR for *BCR-ABL1*) were achieved in 50% of the patients. Outcome appears to be superior to hyper-CVAD alone: 2-year DFS rates were 87% and 28% respectively.

In a study of 56 patients with relapsed and refractory Ph-positive ALL, imatinib was given once daily at a dose of either 400 or 600 mg.[250] The CR rate was 29%, and responses were sustained for at least 4 weeks in 6% of the patients. Median time to progression and overall survival were 2.2 months and 4.9 months respectively.

Although these results document biologic activity of imatinib in relapsed Ph-positive ALL, development of resistance and subsequent disease progression were rapid. Imatinib appears to be more effective when given concurrently with and subsequent to induction and consolidation than when it is alternated with chemotherapy. Under the former conditions, CR rates exceeding 90% and molecular responses of about 50% have been confirmed in other studies.[251,252] The role of novel inhibitors of *ABL1* or v-*src* sarcoma viral oncogene homolog (AMN107, BMS-354825), or both, in ALL is being evaluated.

Burkitt's ALL Outcome for mature B-cell ALL has improved substantially with use of short-term dose-intensive treatment programs. Complete remission rates now exceed 80%, with 2-year DFS rates of 60 to 80%. Relapses are rare after the first year in remission. Intensive early prophylactic intrathecal therapy (with or without cranial irradiation), in addition to intensive systemic administration of methotrexate and cytarabine, significantly reduced the CNS relapse rate.[253,254]

The hyper-CVAD program is a dose-intensive multi-agent chemotherapy program modeled after the Total Therapy B designed by Murphy and colleagues for childhood mature B-cell ALL. The program uses fractionated cyclophosphamide, vincristine, doxorubicin, and dexamethasone alternating with high doses of methotrexate and cytarabine every 3 weeks. CNS prophylaxis consists of 16 intrathecal treatments with methotrexate and cytarabine. Twenty-six patients of median age 58 years were treated. The overall CR rate was 81%.[255] Long-term DFS was 83% for patients under the age of 60 years, but only 16% for those 60 years or older. The addition of the anti-CD20 monoclonal antibody rituximab to hyper-CVAD has improved the survival rate overall and in older patients.

Cortes and colleagues described their experience with hyper-CVAD for newly diagnosed patients with HIV-related mature B-cell ALL.[256] Hyper-CVAD included the anti-CD20 monoclonal antibody rituximab, and all patients continued therapy with highly active antiretroviral treatment (HAART). The CR rate in 13 patients was 92%; nearly 50% of the patients were alive more than 2 years after diagnosis. Outcome was better in the group receiving HAART early in the course of therapy.

SALVAGE THERAPY

Outcome of salvage therapy in adult ALL is poor. Response rates are low (20 to 40%), and response durations short. Salvage therapies are usually modeled after leads from frontline therapy and include: (1) combinations of vincristine, steroids, and anthracyclines; (2) asparaginase and methotrexate combinations; (3) high-dose cytarabine; and (4) allogeneic and autologous SCT.[257] Direct comparisons of various regimens are difficult because of differences in patient characteristics, prior drug exposure and sensitivity, number of salvage attempts, variations in dose and schedule of agents, and the use of SCT as consolidation in some patients.

New agents continue to be assessed in clinical trials (Table 115-5). Rituximab, a chimeric monoclonal antibody against the cell surface protein CD20, has been combined with chemotherapy and has improved outcome in non-Hodgkin's lymphoma and subsets of patients with ALL.[258] Alemtuzumab, a humanized monoclonal antibody against CD52, is active in chronic lymphocytic leukemia and T-cell prolymphocytic leukemia. Its role in CD52-positive ALL and in combination with chemotherapy in aggressive T-lymphocytic malignancies is being explored.[259,260] The role of imatinib and second-generation kinase inhibitors in patients with Ph-positive ALL was mentioned earlier. Other agents of interest include liposomally encapsulated compounds with altered pharmacokinetic properties (eg, liposomal vincristine and liposomal cytarabine), pegylated asparaginase, and nucleoside analogues including nelarabine (compound 506U78), a guanine nucleoside analogue for T-cell ALL, and clofarabine.[261–263] Clofarabine is a second-generation purine nucleoside analogue with activity in acute leukemias (myeloid and lymphoblastic).[264–266] In phase II trials of clofarabine in relapsed or refractory pediatric leukemias, about 30% of patients with ALL responded including 12% CR, 8% CRp

Table 115-5 New Agents in Acute Lymphoblastic Leukemia (ALL)

- Liposomal and pegylated formulations
  - Liposomal vincristine
  - Pegylated asparaginase
  - Liposomal cytarabine (DepoCyt)
- Nucleoside analogs
  - Clofarabine
  - Nelarabine (compound 506U78)
- Purine nucleoside phosphorylase (PNP) inhibitors
  - BCX-1777
- Oligonucleotides
  - Bcl-2 antisense
- Proteasome inhibitors
  - Bortezomib (PS-341)
- Tyrosine kinase inhibitors
  - Imatinib mesylate
  - AMN107
  - BMS-352438
  - SU5416
- Farnesyltransferase inhibitors
  - Tipifarnib (R115777)
  - Lonafarnib (SCH66336)
- Monoclonal antibodies
  - Rituximab (anti-CD20)
  - Alemtuzumab (anti-CD52)
  - Anti-CD7 + ricin
  - Anti-CD19 + ricin/genistein

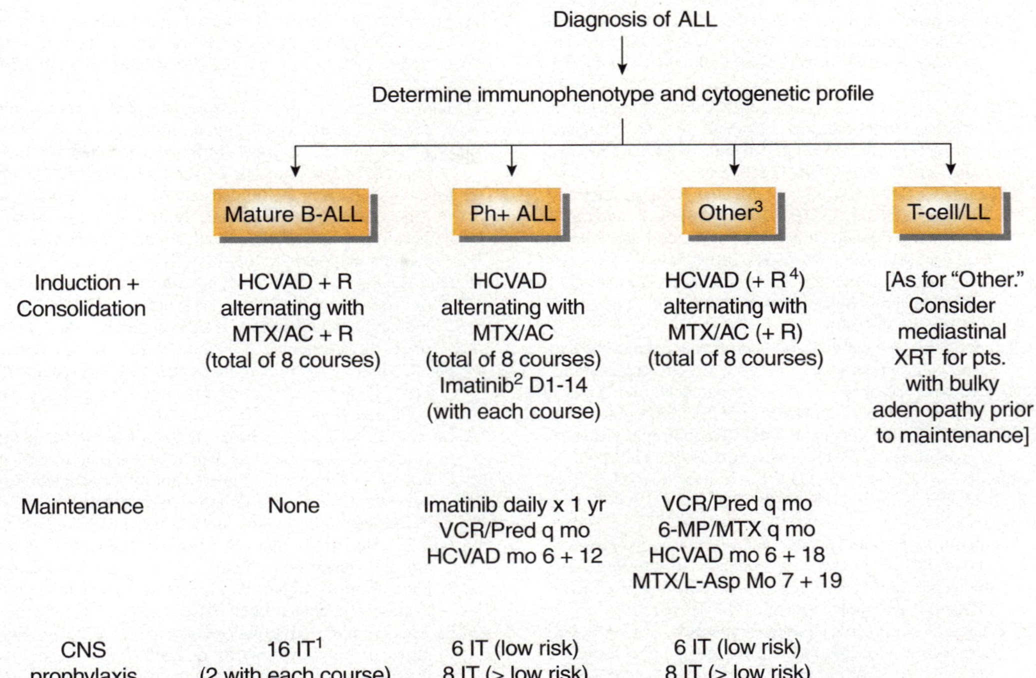

Figure 115-2 The therapeutic approach to acute lymphoblastic leukemia (ALL) at The University of Texas M. D. Anderson Cancer Center. Risk profile is assessed based on lactate dehydrogenase (LDH), proliferative index (% S+G2M), and immunophenotype.[2] Imatinib during induction is administered at 400 mg orally daily during days 1 to 14 concurrently with the chemotherapy. The dose of imatinib is 600 mg orally daily during maintenance.[3] For most patients, "other" refers to pre-B or common ALL antigen–positive immunophenotypes.[4] Rituximab is added if the leukemic blasts express ≥ 20% CD20 by flow cytometry. Two infusions of rituximab are administered with each of the initial 4 courses of chemotherapy. Common to all programs is the use of prophylactic antibiotics, induction therapy in a protective environment (laminar air flow rooms) for patients ≥ 60 years of age, and use of granulocyte colony–stimulating factor (G-CSF) during induction and intensified consolidation. 6-MP = 6-mercaptopurine; AC = cytarabine; HCVAD = hyperfractionated cyclophosphamide, vincristine, Adriamycin, dexamethasone; L-Asp = L-asparaginase;[1] MTX = methotrexate; Pred = prednisone; R = rituximab; VCR = vincristine; IT = intrathecal.

(CR without platelet recovery), and 10% partial responses.[267] Based on the response rate in pediatric relapsed ALL, clofarabine was approved by the US Food and Drug Administration for that indication in December of 2004.

SCT is superior to chemotherapy for ALL patients beyond their first remission.[268–270] Of the 30 to 40% of patients who achieve a second CR and become eligible for SCT, fewer than half have enough time before relapse to undergo SCT. Considering a DFS rate of about 25%, only a fraction of the total population at risk thus benefits from transplant. Identifying unrelated donors in a timely fashion remains challenging.

SUMMARY

Progress in understanding the biology and pathogenesis of adult ALL has helped to improve outcome and prognosis. More-intensive regimens with growth factor support are being evaluated with encouraging results. Consolidation-intensification has improved outcome in pediatric ALL and in some subsets of adult ALL. Prolonged maintenance therapy is beneficial except for mature B-cell ALL and Ph-positive ALL. For some ALL subsets, specific therapies are indicated (Figure 115-2). Patients with mature B-cell ALL respond best to short-term dose-intensive therapies. Patients with Ph-positive ALL have improved outcome when treated with a combination of chemotherapy and imatinib. Outcome in T-cell ALL has been improved with the addition of cyclophosphamide and cytarabine. Allogeneic SCT is beneficial in first remission for patients with high-risk ALL (eg, Ph-positive ALL) and for all adults beyond first remission. Autologous SCT has no advantage over maintenance chemotherapy, but may be useful in patients unwilling to undergo long-term therapy. CNS prophylaxis remains a cornerstone of ALL therapy, and can be performed safely and effectively with a combination of intrathecal and high-dose systemic chemotherapy, obviating the need for radiation therapy.

As with other leukemias, the key to further improving prognosis in adult ALL lies in appreciating and recognizing the heterogeneity of ALL, which should be understood as many and not just as one or a handful of disease states. Increasing appreciation of the biologic characteristics of ALL subsets will lead to more elaborate risk-oriented treatment programs. Treatment regimens in ALL have historically been complex and will continue to be so. Although development of new drugs and agents remains vital to success in adult ALL, a better understanding of the pharmacokinetics of existing drugs, and development of old drugs in new formulations (liposomal or pegylated) continue to be important.

REFERENCES

1. Jemal A, Tiwari RC, Murray T, et al. Cancer statistics. CA Cancer J Clin 2004;54:8–29.
2. Parkin DM, Kramarova E, Draper GJ, et al., editors. International incidence of childhood cancer. Vol 2. [IARC Scientific Publication No. 144] Lyon: International Agency for Research on Cancer; 1998.
3. Groves FD, Linet MS, Devesa SS. Epidemiology of leukemia: overview of patterns of occurrence. In: Henderson ES, Lister TA, Greaves MF, editors. Leukemia. 6th ed. Philadelphia: WB Saunders Company; 1996. p. 145–59.
4. Ries LAG, Smith MA, Gurney JG, et al., editors. Cancer incidence and survival among children and adolescents: United States SEER Program 1975–1995. Bethesda (MD): National Cancer Institute; 1999.
5. Bunin GR. Nongenetic causes of childhood cancers: evidence from international variation, time trends, and risk factor studies. Toxicol Appl Pharmacol 2004;199:91–103.
6. Lightfood TJ, Roman E. Causes of childhood leukaemia and lymphoma. Toxicol Appl Pharmacol 2004;199:104–17.
7. Stewart A, Webb J, Hewitt D. A survey of childhood malignancies. Br Med J 1958;1:1495–508.
8. Pombo De Oliveira MS, Awad El Seed FE, Foroni L, et al. Lymphoblastic leukaemia in Siamese twins: evidence for identity. Lancet 1986;2:969–70.
9. Schmitt TA, Degos L. Leucémies familiales. Bull Cancer 1978;65:83–8.
10. Li FP. Epidemiology of cancer in childhood. In: Nathan DG, Oski FA, editors. Hematology of infancy and childhood. 4th ed. Philadelphia: WB Saunders Company; 1993. p. 1102.
11. Mertens AC, Wen W, Davies SM, et al. Congenital abnormalities in children with acute leukemia: a report from the Children's Cancer Group. J Pediatr 1998;133:617–23.
12. Chessells JM, Harrison G, Richards SM, et al. Down's syndrome and acute lymphoblastic leukaemia: clinical features and response to treatment. Arch Dis Child 2001;85:321–5.
13. Toledano SR, Lange BJ. Ataxia–telangiectasia and acute lymphoblastic leukemia. Cancer 1980;45:1675–8.
14. Shaw MP, Eden OB, Grace E, Ellis PM. Acute lymphoblastic leukemia and Klinefelter's syndrome. Pediatr Hematol Oncol 1992;9:81–5.

15. Janik-Moszant A, Bubala H, Stojewska M, Sonta-Jakimczyk D. Acute lymphoblastic leukemia in children with Fanconi anemia [Polish]. Wiad Lek 1998;51(Suppl 4):285–8.
16. Skibola CF, Smith MT, Kane E, et al. Polymorphisms in the methylenetetrahydrofolate reductase gene are associated with susceptibility to acute leukemia in adults. Proc Natl Acad Sci U S A 1999;96:12810–5.
17. Wiemels JL, Smith RN, Taylor GM, et al. Methylenetetrahydrofolate reductase (*MTHFR*) polymorphisms and risk of molecularly defined subtypes of childhood acute leukemia. Proc Natl Acad Sci U S A 2001;98:4004–9.
18. Greaves MF, Alexander FE. An infectious etiology for common acute lymphoblastic leukemia in childhood? Leukemia 1993;7:349–60.
19. Timonen TT. A hypothesis concerning deficiency of sunlight, cold temperature, and influenza epidemics associated with the onset of acute lymphoblastic leukemia in northern Finland. Ann Hematol 1999;78:408–14.
20. Sarma PS, Graber J. Human T-cell lymphotropic viruses in human diseases. J Natl Cancer Inst 1990;82:1100–6.
21. Mahieux R, Gessain A. HTLV-1 and associated adult T-cell leukemia/lymphoma. Rev Clin Exp Hematol 2003;7:336–61.
22. Lombardi L, Newcomb EW, Dalla-Favera R. Pathogenesis of Burkitt's lymphoma: expression of an activated c-*myc* oncogene causes the tumorigenic conversion of EBV-infected B lymphoblasts. Cell 1987;49:161–70.
23. Lehtinen M, Koskela P, Ogmundsdottir HM, et al. Maternal herpesvirus infections and risk of acute lymphoblastic leukemia in the offspring. Am J Epidemiol 2003;158:207–13.
24. Fredrick J, Alberman ED. Reported influenza in pregnancy and subsequent cancer in the child. Br Med J 1972;2:485–8.
25. Vianna NJ, Polan AK. Childhood lymphatic leukemia: prenatal seasonality and possible association with congenital varicella. Am J Epidemiol 1976;103:321–32.
26. Greaves MF. Aetiology of acute leukaemia. Lancet 1997;349:344–9.
27. Kinlen LJ. Epidemiological evidence for an infective basis in childhood leukaemia. Br J Cancer 1995;71:1–5.
28. Hrusak O, Trka J, Zuna J, et al. Acute lymphoblastic leukemia incidence during socioeconomic transition: selective increase in children from 1 to 4 years. Leukemia 2002;16:720–5.
29. Cortes J. Central nervous system involvement in adult acute lymphocytic leukemia. Hematol Oncol Clin North Am 2001;15:145–62.
30. Ye CC, Echeverri C, Anderson JE, et al. T-cell blast crisis of chronic myelogenous leukemia manifesting as a large mediastinal tumor. Hum Pathol 2002;33:770–3.
31. Attarbaschi A, Mann G, Dworzak M, et al. Mediastinal mass in childhood T-cell acute lymphoblastic leukemia: significance and therapy response. Med Pediatr Oncol 2002;39:558–65.
32. Picozzi VJ Jr, Coleman CN. Lymphoblastic lymphoma. Semin Oncol 1990;17:96–103.
33. Porcu P, Cripe LD, Ng EW, et al. Hyperleukocytic leukemias and leukostasis: a review of pathophysiology, clinical presentation and management. Leuk Lymphoma 2000;39:1–18.
34. Lai R, Hirsch-Ginsberg CF, Bueso-Ramos C. Pathologic diagnosis of acute lymphoblastic leukemia. Hematol Oncol Clin North Am 2000;14:1209–35.
35. Bennett JM, Catovsky D, Daniel MT, et al. Proposals for the classification of acute leukemia. French–American–British Cooperative Group. Br J Haematol 1976;33:451–8.
36. Bennett JM, Catovsky D, Daniel MT, et al. The morphologic classification of acute lymphoblastic leukemia: concordance among observers and clinical correlations. Br J Haematol 1981;47:553–61.
37. Evans AM, Gordon LI. Burkitt's and Burkitt-like lymphoma. Curr Treat Options Oncol 2002;3:291–305.
38. Faber J, Kantarjian H, Roberts MW, et al. Terminal deoxynucleotidyl transferase–negative acute lymphoblastic leukemia. Arch Pathol Lab Med 2000;124:92–7.
39. Ferrari S, Mariano MT, Tagliafico E, et al. Myeloperoxidase gene expression in blast cells with a lymphoid phenotype in cases of acute lymphoblastic leukemia. Blood 1988;72:873–6.
40. Serrano J, Roman J, Sanchez J, Torres A. Myeloperoxidase gene expression in acute lymphoblastic leukemia. Br J Haematol 1997;97:841–3.
41. Wright S, Chucrallah A, Chong YY, et al. Acute lymphoblastic leukemia with myeloperoxidase activity. Am J Hematol 1996;51:147–51.
42. Ho FC, Chan GT, Todd D. Non-specificity of Sudan Black B in the diagnosis of acute myeloid leukemia. Br J Haematol 1993;53:171–2.
43. McCaffrey R, Harrison TA, Parkman P, Baltimore D. Terminal deoxynucleotidyl transferase activity in human leukemic cells and in normal thymocytes. N Engl J Med 1975;292:775–80.
44. Janossy G, Hoffbrand AV, Greaves MF, et al. Terminal transferase enzyme assay and immunological membrane markers in the diagnosis of leukemia: a multiparameter analysis of 300 cases. Br J Haematol 1980;44:221–34.
45. Meenan B, Heavey C, Lichtenstein A, et al. Terminal transferase expression in the differential diagnosis of acute leukemias. Eastern Cooperative Oncology Group. Leuk Lymphoma 1996;22:265–9.
46. Huh YO, Smith TL, Collins P, et al. Terminal deoxynucleotidyl transferase expression in acute myelogenous leukemia and myelodysplasia as determined by flow cytometry. Leuk Lymphoma 2000;37:319–31.
47. Foa R, Vitale A. Towards an integrated classification of adult acute lymphoblastic leukemia. Rev Clin Exp Hematol 2002;6:181–99.
48. Harris NL, Jaffe ES, Diebold J, et al. World Health Organization classification of neoplastic diseases of the hematopoietic and lymphoid tissues: report of the Clinical Advisory Committee Meeting—Airlie House, Virginia, November 1997. J Clin Oncol 1999;17:3835–49.
49. Jaffe ES, Harris NL, Stein H, Vardiman JW, editors. Pathology and genetics of tumours of haematopoietic and lymphoid tissues. Vol 3 of World Health Organization classification of tumours. Lyon: IARC Press. p. 111–87.
50. Paredes-Aguilera R, Romero-Guzman L, Lopez-Santiago N, et al. Flow cytometric analysis of cell-surface and intracellular antigens in the diagnosis of acute leukemia. Am J Hematol 2001;68:69–74.
51. Huh YO, Ibrahim S. Immunophenotypes in adult acute lymphoblastic leukemia. Role of flow cytometry in diagnosis and monitoring of disease. Hematol Oncol Clin North Am 2000;14:1251–65.
52. Bene MC, Castoldi G, Knapp W, et al. Proposals for the immunological classification of acute leukemias. European Group for the Immunological Characterization of Leukemias (EGIL). Leukemia 1995;9:1783–6.
53. Thalhammer-Scherrer R, Mitterbauer G, Simonitsch I, et al. The immunophenotype of 325 adult acute leukemias: relationship to morphologic and molecular classification and proposal for a minimal screening program highly predictive for lineage discrimination. Am J Clin Pathol 2002;117:380–9.
54. Janossy G, Bollum FJ, Bradstock KF, Ashley J. Cellular phenotypes of normal and leukemic hemopoietic cells determined by analysis with selected antibody combinations. Blood 1980;56:430–41.
55. Greaves MF. Differentiation-linked leukemogenesis in lymphocytes. Science 1986;234:697–704.
56. Terstappen LW, Huang S, Picker LJ. Flow cytometric assessment of human T-cell differentiation in thymus and bone marrow. Blood 1992;79:666–77.
57. Onciu M, Lai R, Vega F, et al. Precursor T-cell acute lymphoblastic leukemia in adults: age-related immunophenotypic, cytogenetic, and molecular subsets. Am J Clin Pathol 2002;117:252–8.
58. Wormann B, Safford M, Konemann S, et al. Detection of aberrant antigen expression in acute myeloid leukemia by multiparameter flow cytometry. Recent Results Cancer Res 1993;131:185–96.
59. Rothe G, Schmitz G. Consensus protocol for the flow cytometric immunophenotyping of hematopoietic malignancies. Working Group on Flow Cytometry and Image Analysis. Leukemia 1996;14:877–95.
60. Ludwig WD, Raghavachar A, Thiel E. Immunophenotypic classification of acute lymphoblastic leukaemia. Baillieres Clin Haematol 1994;7:235–62.
61. Gore SD, Kastan MG, Civin CI. Normal human bone marrow precursors that express terminal deoxynucleotidyl transferase include T-cell precursors and possible lymphoid stem cells. Blood 1991;77:1681–90.
62. Borowitz MJ. Immunologic markers in childhood acute lymphoblastic leukemia. Hematol Oncol Clin North Am 1990;4:743–65.
63. Lim LC, Heng KK, Vellupillai M, et al. Molecular and phenotypic spectrum of de novo Philadelphia positive acute leukemia. Int J Mol Med 1999;4:665–7.
64. Czuczman MS, Dodge RK, Stewart CC, et al. Value of immunophenotype in intensively treated adult acute lymphoblastic leukemia. Cancer and Leukemia Group B study 8364. Blood 1999;93:3931–9.
65. Kantarjian HM, O'Brien S, Smith TL, et al. Results of treatment with hyper-CVAD, a dose-intense regimen, in adult acute lymphocytic leukemia. J Clin Oncol 2000;18:547–61.
66. Larson RA, Dodge RK, Burns CP, et al. A five-drug remission induction regimen with intensive consolidation for adults with acute lymphoblastic leukemia: Cancer and Leukemia Group B study 8811. Blood 1995;85:2025–37.
67. Khalidi HS, Chang KL, Medeiros LJ, et al. Acute lymphoblastic leukemia. Survey of immunophenotype, French–American–British classification, frequency of myeloid antigen expression, and karyotype abnormalities in 210 pediatric and adult cases. Am J Clin Pathol 1999;111:467–76.
68. Pui CH, Rubnitz JE, Hancock ML, et al. Reappraisal of the clinical and biologic significance of myeloid-associated antigen expression in childhood acute lymphoblastic leukemia. J Clin Oncol 1998;16:3768–73.
69. Den Boer ML, Kapaun P, Pieters R, et al. Myeloid antigen co-expression in childhood acute lymphoblastic leukaemia: relationship with in vitro drug resistance. Br J Haematol 1999;105:876–82.
70. Bene MD, Bernier M, Casasnovas RO, et al. The reliability and specificity of c-*kit* for the diagnosis of acute myeloid leukemias and undifferentiated leukemias. Blood 1998;92:596–9.
71. EGIL (European Group for the Immunological Classification of Leukemias). The value of c-*kit* in the diagnosis of biphenotypic acute leukemia. Leukemia 1998;12:2038.
72. Nakase K, Kenkichi K, Shiku H, et al. Myeloid antigen, CD13, CD14, and/or CD33 expression is restricted to certain lymphoid neoplasms. Am J Clin Pathol 1996;105:761–8.
73. Guyotat D, Campos L, Shi ZH, et al. Myeloid surface antigen expression in adult acute lymphoblastic leukemia. Leukemia 1990;4:664–6.
74. Wells SJ, Bray RA, Stempora LI, Farhi DC. CD117/CD34 expression in leukemic blasts. Am J Clin Pathol 1996;106:192–5.
75. Putti MC, Rondelli R, Cocito MG, et al. Expression of myeloid markers lacks prognostic impact in children treated for acute lymphoblastic leukemia: Italian experience in AIEOP-ALL 88–91 studies. Blood 1998;92:795–801.
76. Uckun FM, Sather HN, Gaynon PS, et al. Clinical features and treatment outcome of children with myeloid antigen positive acute lymphoblastic leukemia: a report from the Children's Cancer Group. Blood 1997;90:28–35.
77. Preti HA, Huh YO, O'Brien SM, et al. Myeloid markers in adult acute lymphoblastic leukemia. Correlations with patient and disease characteristics and with prognosis. Cancer 1995;76:1564–70.
78. Matutes E, Morilla R, Farahat N, et al. Definition of acute biphenotypic leukemia. Haematologica 1997;82:64–6.
79. Greaves MF, Chan LC, Furley AJW, et al. Lineage promiscuity in hematopoietic differentiation and leukemia. Blood 1986;67:1–11.
80. Ferrara F, Del Vecchio L. Clinical relevance of acute mixed-lineage leukemias. Leuk Lymphoma 1993;12:11–9.
81. Cascavilla N, Musto P, Melillo L, et al. Is the scoring system an effective clinico-biological tool in myeloid antigen positive adult acute lymphoblastic leukemia? Results of a long-term study. Hematol J 2002;3:251–8.
82. Faderl S, Kantarjian HM, Talpaz M, Estrov Z. Clinical significance of cytogenetic abnormalities in adult acute lymphoblastic leukemia. Blood 1998;91:3995–4019.
83. Cytogenetic abnormalities in adult acute lymphoblastic leukemia: correlations with the hematologic findings and outcome. A collaborative study of the Groupe Francais de Cytogenetique Hematologique [published erratum appears in Blood 1996;88:2818]. Blood 1996;87:3135–42.
84. Wetzler M, Dodge RK, Mrozek K, et al. Prospective karyotype analysis in adult acute lymphoblastic leukemia: the Cancer and Leukemia Group B experience. Blood 1999;93:383–93.
85. Secker-Walker LM, Prentice HG, Durrant J, et al. Cytogenetics adds independent prognostic information in adults with acute lymphoblastic leukemia on MRC trial UKALL XA. Br J Haematol 1997;96:601–10.
86. Chiaretti S, Li X, Gentleman R, et al. Gene expression profile of adult T-cell acute lymphocytic leukemia identifies distinct subsets of patients with different response to therapy and survival. Blood 2004;103:2771–8.
87. Moorman AV, Richards SM, Martineau M, et al. Outcome heterogeneity in childhood high-hyperdiploid acute lymphoblastic leukemia. Blood 2003;102:2756–62.
88. Faderl S, Jeha S, Kantarjian HM. The biology and therapy of adult acute lymphoblastic leukemia. Cancer 2003;98:1337–54.
89. Ebert BL, Golub TR. Genomic approaches to hematologic malignancies. Blood 2004;104:923–32.

90. Faderl S, Talpaz M, Estrov Z, et al. The biology of chronic myeloid leukemia. N Engl J Med 1999;341:164–72.
91. Melo JV, Deininger MW. Biology of chronic myelogenous leukemia—signaling pathways of initiation and transformation. Hematol Oncol Clin North Am 2004;18:545–68.
92. Preti HA, O'Brien S, Giralt S, et al. Philadelphia chromosome–positive adult acute lymphocytic leukemia: characteristics, treatment results, and prognosis in 41 patients. Am J Med 1994;97:60–5.
93. Faderl S, Kantarjian HM, Thomas DA, et al. Outcome of Philadelphia chromosome–positive adult acute lymphoblastic leukemia. Leuk Lymphoma 2000;36:263–73.
94. Raimondi SC, Zhou Y, Matthew S, et al. Reassessment of the prognostic significance of hypodiploidy in pediatric patients with acute lymphoblastic leukemia. Cancer 2003;98:2715–22.
95. Harrison CJ, Moorman AV, Broadfield ZJ, et al. Three distinct subgroups of hypodiploidy in acute lymphoblastic leukaemia. Br J Haematol 2004;125:552–9.
96. Charrin C, Thomas X, French M, et al. A report from the LALA-94 and LALA-SA groups on hypodiploidy with 30 to 39 chromosomes and near-triploidy: 2 possible expressions of a sole entity conferring poor prognosis in adult acute lymphoblastic leukemia (ALL). Blood 2004;104:2444–51.
97. Pui CH, Evans WE. Acute lymphoblastic leukemia. N Engl J Med 1998;339:605–15.
98. Faderl S, Albitar M. Insights into the biologic and molecular abnormalities in adult acute lymphocytic leukemia. Hematol Oncol Clin North Am 2000;14:1267–88.
99. Panzer-Grümayer ER, Fasching K, Panzer S, et al. Nondisjunction of chromosomes leading to hyperdiploid childhood B-cell precursor acute lymphoblastic leukemia is an early event during leukemogenesis. Blood 2002;100:347–9.
100. Pui CH, Relling MV, Downing JR. Acute lymphoblastic leukemia. N Engl J Med 2004;350:1535–48.
101. Zelent A, Greaves M, Enver T. Role of the *TEL-AML1* fusion gene in the molecular pathogenesis of childhood acute lymphoblastic leukemia. Oncogene 2004;23:4275–83.
102. Tiensiwakul P. Cloning and sequencing of *ETV6/RUNX1* (*TEL/AML1*) variant acute lymphoblastic leukemia. Cancer Genet Cytogenet 2004;149:85–8.
103. Tsuzuki S, Seto M, Greaves M, Enver T. Modeling first-hit functions of the t(12;21) *TEL-AML1* translocation in mice. Proc Natl Acad Sci U S A 2004;101:8443–8.
104. Codrington R, O'Connor HE, Jalali GR, et al. Analysis of *ETV6/AML1* abnormalities in acute lymphoblastic leukemia: incidence, alternative spliced forms and minimal residual disease value. Br J Haematol 2000;111:1071–9.
105. Harbott J, Viehmann S, Borkhardt A, et al. Incidence of *TEL/AML1* fusion gene analyzed consecutively in children with acute lymphoblastic leukemia in relapse. Blood 1997;90:4933–7.
106. Seeger K, Adams HP, Buchwald D, et al. *TEL-AML1* fusion transcript in relapsed childhood acute lymphoblastic leukemia. The Berlin–Frankfurt–Munster Study Group. Blood 1998;91:1716–22.
107. Cave H, Cacheux V, Raynaud S, et al. *ETV6* is the target of chromosome 12p deletions in t(12;21) childhood acute lymphocytic leukemia. Leukemia 1997;11:1459–64.
108. Quesnel B, Preudhomme C, Fenaux P. $p16^{INK4A}$ gene and hematological malignancies. Leuk Lymphoma 1996;22:11–24.
109. Zhou M, Gu L, Yeager AM, et al. Incidence and clinical significance of $CDKN2/MTS1/p16^{INK4A}$ and $MTS2/p15^{INK4B}$ gene deletions in childhood acute lymphoblastic leukemia. Pediatr Hematol Oncol 1997;14:141–50.
110. Rubnitz JE, Behm FG, Pui CH, et al. Genetic studies of childhood acute lymphoblastic leukemia with emphasis on *p16*, *MLL*, and *ETV6* gene abnormalities: results of St Jude Total Therapy Study XII. Leukemia 1997;11:1201–6.
111. Heerema NA, Sather HN, Sensel MG, et al. Association of chromosome arm 9p abnormalities with adverse risk in childhood acute lymphoblastic leukemia: a report from the Children's Cancer Group. Blood 1999;94:1537–44.
112. Secker-Walker LM, Prentice HG, Durrant J, et al. On behalf of the MRC Adult Leukaemia Working Party: cytogenetics adds independent prognostic information in adults with acute lymphoblastic leukaemia on MRC trial UKALL XA. Br J Haematol 1997;96:601–10.
113. Faderl S, Kantarjian HM, Manshouri T, et al. The prognostic significance of $p16^{INK4A}/p14^{ARF}$ and $p15^{INK4B}$ deletions in adult acute lymphoblastic leukemia. Clin Cancer Res 1999;5:1855–61.
114. Graf Einsiedel H, Taube T, Hartmann R, et al. Deletion analysis of $p16^{INKA}$ and $p15^{INKB}$ in relapsed childhood acute lymphoblastic leukemia. Blood 2002;99:4629–31.
115. Rubnitz JE, Behm FG, Downing JR. 11q23 rearrangements in acute leukemia. Leukemia 1996;10:74–82.
116. Harrison CJ, Cuneo A, Clark R, et al. Ten novel 11q23 chromosomal partner sites. European 11q23 Workshop participants. Leukemia 1998;12:811–22.
117. Heerema NA, Arthur DC, Sather H, et al. Cytogenetic features of infants less than 12 months of age at diagnosis of acute lymphoblastic leukemia: impact of the 11q23 breakpoint on outcome: a report of the Children's Cancer Group. Blood 1994;83:2274–84.
118. Secker-Walker LM, on behalf of the European 11q23 Workshop Participants. General Report on the European Union Concerted Action Workshop on 11q23, London, UK, May 1997. Leukemia 1998;12:776–8.
119. Bloomfield CD, Archer KJ, Mrózek K, et al. 11q23 balanced chromosome aberrations in treatment-related myelodysplastic syndrome and acute leukemia: report from an international workshop. Genes Chromosomes Cancer 2002;33:362–78.
120. Foa R, Vitale A, Mancini M, et al. *E2A-PBX1* fusion in adult acute lymphoblastic leukaemia: biological and clinical features. Br J Haematol 2003;120:484–7.
121. Uckun FM, Sensel MG, Sather HN, et al. Clinical significance of translocation t(1;19) in childhood acute lymphoblastic leukemia in the context of contemporary therapies: a report from the Children's Cancer Group. J Clin Oncol 1998;16:527–35.
122. Khalidi HS, O'Donnell MR, Slovak ML, Arber DA. Adult precursor–B acute lymphoblastic leukemia with translocations involving chromosome band 19p13 is associated with poor prognosis. Cancer Genet Cytogenet 1999;109:58–65.
123. Look AT. *E2A-HLF* chimeric transcription factors in pro–B cell acute lymphoblastic leukemia. Curr Top Microbiol Immunol 1997;220:45–53.
124. Hecht JL, Aster JC. Molecular biology of Burkitt's lymphoma. J Clin Oncol 2000;18:3707–21.
125. Rabbitts TH. Chromosomal translocations in human cancer. Nature 1994;372:143–9.
126. Ross ME, Zhou X, Song G, et al. Classification of pediatric acute lymphoblastic leukemia by gene expression profiling. Blood 2003;102:2951–9.
127. Fine BM, Stanulla M, Schrappe M, et al. Gene expression patterns associated with recurrent chromosomal translocations in acute lymphoblastic leukemia. Blood 2004;103:1043–9.
128. Holleman A, Cheok MH, den Boer ML, et al. Gene-expression patterns in drug-resistant acute lymphoblastic leukemia cells and response to treatment. N Engl J Med 2004;351:533–42.
129. Yeoh EJ, Ross ME, Shurtleff SA, et al. Classification, subtype discovery, and prediction of outcome in pediatric acute lymphoblastic leukemia by gene expression profiling. Cancer Cell 2002;1:133–43.
130. Ferrando A, Neuberg D, Staunton J, et al. Gene expression signatures define novel oncogenic pathways in T cell acute lymphoblastic leukemia. Cancer Cell 2002;1:75–87.
131. Hanash SM, Madoz-Gurpide J, Misek DE. Identification of novel targets for cancer therapy using expression proteomics. Leukemia 2002;16:478–85.
132. Santini V, Kantarjian HM, Issa JP. Changes in DNA methylation in neoplasia: pathophysiology and therapeutic implications. Ann Intern Med 2001;134:573–86.
133. Garcia-Maneroa G, Bueso-Ramos C, Daniel J, et al. DNA methylation patterns at relapse in adult acute lymphoblastic leukemia. Clin Cancer Res 2002;8:1897–903.
134. Garcia-Manero G, Daniel J, Smith TL, et al. DNA methylation of multiple promoter-associated CpG islands in adult acute lymphoblastic leukemia. Clin Cancer Res 2002;8:2217–24.
135. Roman-Gomez J, Castillejo JA, Jimenez A, et al. 5' CpG island hypermethylation is associated with transcriptional silencing of the $p21^{CIP1/WAF1/SDI1}$ gene and confers poor prognosis in acute lymphoblastic leukemia. Blood 2002;99:2291–6.
136. Shen L, Toyota M, Kondo Y, et al. Aberrant DNA methylation of $p57^{KIP2}$ identifies a cell-cycle regulatory pathway with prognostic impact in adult acute lymphoblastic leukemia. Blood 2003;103:4131–6.
137. Roman-Gomez J, Jimenez-Velasco A, Castijello JA, et al. Promoter hypermethylation of cancer-related genes: a strong independent prognostic factor in acute lymphoblastic leukemia. Blood 2004;104:2492–8.
138. Annino L, Vegna ML, Camera A, et al. Treatment of adult acute lymphoblastic leukemia (ALL): long-term follow-up of the GIMEMA ALL 0288 randomized study. Blood 2002;99:863–71.
139. Gökbuget N, Hoelzer D, Arnold R, et al. Treatment of adult ALL according to protocols of the German Multicenter Study Group for Adult ALL (GMALL). Hematol Oncol Clin North Am 2000;14:1307–25.
140. Durrant IJ, Richards SM, Prentice HG, et al. The Medical Research Council trials in adult acute lymphocytic leukemia. Hematol Oncol Clin North Am 2000;14:1327–52.
141. Larson RA. Recent clinical trials in acute lymphocytic leukemia by the Cancer and Leukemia Group B. Hematol Oncol Clin North Am 2000;14:1367–79.
142. Schaison G, Sommelet D, Bancillon A, et al. Treatment of acute lymphoblastic leukemia French protocol Fralle 83-87. Leukemia 1992;6(Suppl 2):148–52.
143. Hussein KK, Dahlberg S, Head D, et al. Treatment of acute lymphoblastic leukemia in adults with intensive induction, consolidation, and maintenance chemotherapy. Blood 1989;73:57–63.
144. GIMEMA Cooperative Group. GIMEMA ALL 0183: a multicentric study on adult acute lymphoblastic leukaemia in Italy. Br J Haematol 1989;71:377–86.
145. Linker C, Damon L, Ries C, Navarro W. Intensified and shortened cyclical chemotherapy for adult acute lymphoblastic leukemia. J Clin Oncol 2002;20:2464–71.
146. Durrant IJ, Prentice HG, Richards SM. Intensification of treatment for adults with acute lymphoblastic leukaemia: results of U.K. Medical Research Council randomized trial UKALL XA. Br J Haematol 1997;99:84–92.
147. Todeschini G, Tecchio C, Meneghini V, et al. Estimated 6-year event-free survival of 55% in 60 consecutive adult acute lymphoblastic leukemia patients treated with an intensive phase II protocol based on high induction dose of daunorubicin. Leukemia 1998;12:144–9.
148. Stryckmans P, Debusscher L. Chemotherapy of adult acute lymphoblastic leukaemia. Baillieres Clin Haematol 1991;4:115–30.
149. Kantarjian HM, O'Brien S, Smith T, et al. Acute lymphocytic leukaemia in the elderly: characteristics and outcome with the vincristine–Adriamycin–dexamethasone (VAD) regimen. Br J Haematol 1994;88:94–100.
150. Thiebault A, Vernant JP, Degos L, et al. Adult acute lymphocytic leukemia study testing chemotherapy and autologous and allogeneic transplantation. A follow-up report of the French protocol LALA 87. Hematol Oncol Clin North Am 2000;14:1353–66.
151. Takeuchi J, Kyo T, Naito K, et al. Induction therapy by frequent administration of doxorubicin with four other drugs, followed by intensive consolidation and maintenance therapy for adult acute lymphoblastic leukemia: the JALSG-ALL93 study. Leukemia 2002;16:1259–66.
152. Thomas X, Boiron JM, Huguet F, et al. Outcome of treatment in adults with acute lymphoblastic leukemia: analysis of the LALA-94 trial. J Clin Oncol 2004;22:4075–86.
153. Hoelzer D, Ludwig WD, Eckhard E, et al. Improved outcome in adult B-cell acute lymphoblastic leukemia. Blood 1996;87:495–508.
154. Gaynor J, Chapman D, Little C, et al. A cause-specific hazard rate analysis of prognostic factors among 199 adults with acute lymphoblastic leukemia: the Memorial Hospital experience since 1969. J Clin Oncol 1988;6:1014–30.
155. Kantarjian HM, Walters RS, Keating MJ, et al. Results of the vincristine, doxorubicin, and dexamethasone regimen in adults with standard- and high-risk acute lymphocytic leukemia. J Clin Oncol 1990;8:994–1004.
156. Hoelzer D, Thiel H, Löffler H, et al. Prognostic factors in a multicenter study for treatment of acute lymphoblastic leukemia in adults. Blood 1988;71:123–31.
157. Boucheix C, David B, Sebban C, et al. Immunophenotype of adult acute lymphoblastic leukemia, clinical parameters, and outcome: an analysis of a prospective trial including 562 tested patients (LALA87). Blood 1994;84:1603–12.
158. Westbrook CA. Molecular subsets and prognostic factors in acute lymphoblastic leukemia. Leukemia 1997;11(Suppl 4):S8–10.
159. Cimino G, Elia L, Mancini M, et al. Clinico-biologic features and treatment outcome of adult pro-B-ALL patients enrolled in the GIMEMA 0496 study: absence of the *ALL/AF4* and of the *BCR/ABL* fusion genes correlates with a significantly better clinical outcome. Blood 2003;102:2014–20.
160. Kantarjian H, Thomas D, O'Brien S, et al. Long-term follow-up results of hyperfractionated cyclophosphamide, vincristine, doxorubicin, and dexamethasone (hyper-CVAD), a dose-intensive regimen, in adult acute lymphocytic leukemia. Cancer 2004;101:2788–801.

161. Gökbuget N, Raff R, Brügge-Mann M, et al. Risk/MRD adapted GMALL trials in adult ALL. Ann Hematol 2004;83(Suppl 1):S129–31.
162. Mortuza FY, Papioannou M, Moreira IM, et al. Minimal residual disease tests provide an independent predictor of clinical outcome in adult acute lymphoblastic leukemia. J Clin Oncol 2002;20:1094–104.
163. Faderl S, Thall PF, Kantarjian HM, Estrov Z. Time to platelet recovery predicts outcome of patients with de novo acute lymphoblastic leukaemia who have achieved a complete remission. Br J Haematol 2002;117:869–74.
164. Miller DR, Coccia PF, Bleyer WA, et al. Early response to induction therapy as a predictor of disease-free survival and late recurrence of childhood acute lymphoblastic leukemia: a report from the Children's Cancer Study Group. J Clin Oncol 1989;7:1807–15.
165. Sandlund JT, Harrison PL, Rivera G, et al. Persistence of lymphoblasts in bone marrow on day 15 and days 22 to 25 of remission induction predicts a dismal outcome in children with acute lymphoblastic leukemia. Blood 2002;100:43–7.
166. Coustan-Smith E, Sancho J, Behm FG, et al. Prognostic importance of measuring early clearance of leukemic cells by flow cytometry in childhood acute lymphoblastic leukemia. Blood 2002;100:52–8.
167. Casale F, D'Angelo V, Addeo R, et al. *P*-Glycoprotein 170 expression and function as an adverse independent prognostic factor in childhood acute lymphoblastic leukemia. Oncol Rep 2004;12:1201–7.
168. Aplenc R, Lange B. Pharmacogenetic determinants of outcome in acute lymphoblastic leukaemia. Br J Haematol 2004;125:421–34.
169. Kantarjian HM, Walters RS, Keating MJ, et al. Experience with vincristine, doxorubicin, and dexamethasone (VAD) chemotherapy in adults with refractory acute lymphocytic leukemia. Cancer 1989;64:16–22.
170. Todeschini G. High-dose anthracycline induction in adult acute lymphocytic leukemia. Hematol Oncol Clin North Am 2001;15:9–20.
171. Kantarjian HM. Adult acute lymphoblastic leukemia. Future research directions. Hematol Oncol Clin North Am 2001;15:207–11.
172. Bassan R, Pogliani E, Lerede T, et al. Fractionated cyclophosphamide added to the IVAP regimen (idarubicin–vincristine–L-asparaginase–prednisone) could lower the risk of primary lymphoblastic leukemia: first results from a phase II clinical study. Haematologica 1999;84:1088–93.
173. Larson RA. Recent clinical trials in acute lymphoblastic leukemia by the Cancer and Leukemia Group B. Hematol Oncol Clin North Am 2000;14:1367–79.
174. Hallbook H, Simonsson B, Ahlgren T, et al. High-dose cytarabine in upfront therapy for adult patients with acute lymphoblastic leukaemia. Br J Haematol 2002;118:748–54.
175. Larson RA, Fretzin MH, Dodge RK, Schiffer CA. Hypersensitivity reactions to L-asparaginase do not impact on the remission duration of adults with acute lymphoblastic leukemia. Leukemia 1998;12:660–5.
176. Graham ML. Pegaspargase: a review of clinical studies. Adv Drug Deliv Rev 2003;55:1293–302.
177. Bostrom BC, Sensel MR, Sather HN, et al. Dexamethasone versus prednisone and daily oral versus weekly intravenous mercaptopurine for patients with standard-risk acute lymphoblastic leukemia: a report from the Children's Cancer Group. Blood 2003;101:3809–17.
178. Lopez-Hernandez MA, Alvarado M, De Diogo J, et al. A randomized trial of dexamethasone before remission induction in de novo childhood acute lymphoblastic leukemia. Haematologica 2004;89:365–6.
179. Weiser MA, O'Brien S, Thomas DA, et al. Comparison of two different schedules of granulocyte-colony-stimulating factor during treatment for acute lymphocytic leukemia with a hyper-CVAD (cyclophosphamide, doxorubicin, vincristine, and dexamethasone) regimen. Cancer 2002;94:285–91.
180. Ottmann OG, Hoelzer D, Gracien E, et al. Concomitant granulocyte colony-stimulating factor and induction chemoradiotherapy in adult acute lymphoblastic leukemia: a randomized phase III trial. Blood 1995;86:444–50.
181. Geissler K, Koller E, Hubmann E, et al. Granulocyte colony-stimulating factor as an adjunct to induction chemotherapy for adult acute lymphoblastic leukemia—a randomized phase-III study. Blood 1997;90:590–6.
182. Larson RA, Dodge RK, Linker CA, et al. A randomized controlled trial of filgrastim during remission induction and consolidation chemotherapy for adults with acute lymphoblastic leukemia: CALGB study 9111. Blood 1998;92:1556–64.
183. Bassan R, Lerede T, Di Bona E, et al. Granulocyte colony-stimulating factor (G-CSF, filgrastim) after or during an intensive remission induction therapy for adult acute lymphoblastic leukaemia: effects, role of patient pretreatment characteristics, and costs. Leuk Lymphoma 1997;26:153–61.
184. Hughes WT, Armstrong D, Bodey GP, et al. 2002 Guidelines for the use of antimicrobial agents in neutropenic patients with cancer. Clin Infect Dis 2002;34:730–51.
185. Cuttner J, Mick R, Budman DR, et al. Phase III trial of brief intensive treatment of adult acute lymphocytic leukemia comparing daunorubicin and mitoxantrone: a CALGB study. Leukemia 1991;5:425–31.
186. Childhood ALL Collaborative Group. Duration and intensity of maintenance chemotherapy in acute lymphoblastic leukaemia: overview of 42 trials involving 12 000 randomized children. Lancet 1996;347:1783–8.
187. Dekker AW, van't Veer MB, Sizoo W, et al. Intensive postremission chemotherapy without maintenance therapy in adults with acute lymphoblastic leukemia. Dutch Hemato-Oncology Research Group. J Clin Oncol 1997;15:476–82.
188. Wingard JR, Piantadosi S, Santos WG, et al. Allogeneic bone marrow transplantation for patients with high-risk acute lymphoblastic leukemia. J Clin Oncol 1990;8:820–30.
189. Blaise D, Gaspard MH, Stoppa AM, et al. Allogeneic or autologous bone marrow transplantation for acute lymphoblastic leukemia in first complete remission. Bone Marrow Transplant 1990;5:7–12.
190. Chao N, Formen S, Schmidt G, et al. Allogeneic bone marrow transplantation for high-risk acute lymphoblastic leukemia during first complete remission. Blood 1991;78:1923–7.
191. Doney K, Fisher LD, Appelbaum FR, et al. Treatment of adult acute lymphoblastic leukemia with allogeneic bone marrow transplantation. Multivariate analysis of factors affecting acute graft-versus-host disease, relapse, and relapse-free survival. Bone Marrow Transplant 1991;7:453–9.
192. Sutton L, Kuentz M, Cordonnier C, et al. Allogeneic bone marrow transplantation for adult acute lymphoblastic leukemia in first complete remission: factors predictive of transplant-related mortality and influence of total body irradiation. Bone Marrow Transplant 1993;12:583–9.
193. DeWitte T, Awwad B, Boezeman J, et al. Role of allogeneic bone marrow transplantation in adolescent or adult patients with acute lymphoblastic leukemia or lymphoblastic lymphoma in first remission. Bone Marrow Transplant 1994;14:767–74.
194. Sebban C, Lepage E, Vernant JP, et al. Allogeneic bone marrow transplantation in adult acute lymphoblastic leukemia in first complete remission: a comparative study. French Group of Therapy of Adult Acute Lymphoblastic Leukemia. J Clin Oncol 1994;12:2580–7.
195. Vey N, Blaise D, Stoppa AM, et al. Bone marrow transplantation in 63 adult patients with acute lymphoblastic leukemia in first complete remission. Bone Marrow Transplant 1994;14:383–8.
196. Zhang MJ, Hoelzer D, Horowitz MM, et al. Long-term follow-up of adults with acute lymphoblastic leukemia in first remission treated with chemotherapy or bone marrow transplantation. The Acute Lymphoblastic Leukemia Working Committee. Ann Intern Med 1995;123:428–31.
197. Martin TG, Gajewski JL. Allogeneic stem cell transplantation for acute lymphocytic leukemia in adults. Hematol Oncol Clin North Am 2001;15:97–120.
198. Horowitz M, Messere D, Hoelzer D, et al. Chemotherapy compared with bone marrow transplantation for adults with acute lymphoblastic leukemia in first remission. Ann Intern Med 1991;115:13–8.
199. Hunault M, Harousseau JL, Delain M, et al. Better outcome of adult acute lymphoblastic leukemia after early genoidentical allogeneic bone marrow transplantation (BMT) than after late high-dose therapy and autologous BMT: a GOELAMS trial. Blood 2004;104:3028–37.
200. Kiehl MG, Kraut L, Schwerdtfeger R, et al. Outcome of allogeneic hematopoietic stem-cell transplantation in adult patients with acute lymphoblastic leukemia: no difference in related compared with unrelated transplant in first complete remission. J Clin Oncol 2004;22:2816–25.
201. Rowe J, Richards S, Burnett A, et al. Favorable results of allogeneic bone marrow transplantation (BMT) for adults with Philadelphia (Ph)-chromosome-negative acute lymphoblastic leukemia (ALL) in first complete remission (CR): results from the International ALL Trial (MRC UKALL XII/ECOG E2993) [abstract]. Blood 2001;98:481a.
202. Chauncey TR. Transplantation for adult ALL—typing and timing. Blood 2004;104:2998–9.
203. Sierra J, Radich J, Hansen JA, et al. Marrow transplant from unrelated donors for treatment of Philadelphia chromosome–positive acute lymphoblastic leukemia. Blood 1997;90:1410–4.
204. Marks DI, Bird JM, Cornish JM, et al. Unrelated donor bone marrow transplantation for children and adolescents with Philadelphia-positive acute lymphoblastic leukemia. J Clin Oncol 1998;16:931–6.
205. Bunin N, Carston M, Wall D, et al. Unrelated marrow transplantation for children with acute lymphoblastic leukemia in second remission. Blood 2002;99:3153–7.
206. Attal M, Blaise D, Marit G, et al. Consolidation treatment of adult acute lymphoblastic leukemia: a prospective, randomized trial comparing allogeneic versus autologous bone marrow transplantation and testing the impact of recombinant interleukin-2 after autologous bone marrow transplantation. Blood 1995;86:1619–28.
207. Powles R, Sirohi B, Treleaven J, et al. The role of posttransplantation maintenance chemotherapy in improving the outcome of autotransplantation in adult acute lymphoblastic leukemia. Blood 2002;100:1641–7.
208. Omura GA, Moffitt S, Vogler WR, Salter MM. Combination chemotherapy of adult acute lymphoblastic leukemia with randomized central nervous system prophylaxis. Blood 1980;55:199–204.
209. Surapeneni UR, Cortes JE, Thomas DA, et al. Central nervous system relapse in adults with acute lymphoblastic leukemia. Cancer 2002;94:773–9.
210. Stewart DJ, Keating MJ, McCredie KB, et al. Natural history of central nervous system acute leukemia in adults. Cancer 1981;47:184–96.
211. Kantarjian HM, Walters RS, Smith TL, et al. Identification of risk groups for development of central nervous system leukemia in adults with acute lymphocytic leukemia. Blood 1988;72:1784–9.
212. Cortes J, O'Brien SM, Pierce S, et al. The value of high-dose systemic chemotherapy and intrathecal therapy for central nervous system prophylaxis in different risk groups of adult acute lymphoblastic leukemia. Blood 1995;86:2091–7.
213. Pinkel D, Woo S. Prevention and treatment of meningeal leukemia in children. Blood 1994;84:355–66.
214. Cortes J, Kantarjian HM. Acute lymphoblastic leukemia. A comprehensive review with emphasis on biology and therapy. Cancer 1995;76:2393–417.
215. Mastrangelo R, Poplack D, Bleyer A, et al. Report and recommendations of the Rome workshop concerning poor-prognosis acute lymphoblastic leukemia in children: biologic bases for staging, stratification, and treatment. Med Pediatr Oncol 1986;14:191–4.
216. Mahmoud HH, Rivera GK, Hancock ML, et al. Low leukocyte counts with blast cells in cerebrospinal fluid of children with newly diagnosed acute lymphoblastic leukemia. N Engl J Med 1993;329:314–9.
217. Gilchrist GS, Tubergen DG, Sather HN, et al. Low numbers of CSF blasts at diagnosis do not predict for the development of CNS leukemia in children with intermediate-risk acute lymphoblastic leukemia: a Children's Cancer Group report. J Clin Oncol 1994;12:2594–600.
218. Pui CH, Relling MV, Evans WE. Role of pharmacogenomics and pharmacodynamics in the treatment of acute lymphoblastic leukaemia. Best Pract Res Clin Haematol 2002;15:741–56.
219. Belkow VM, Krynetski EY, Schuetz JD, et al. Reduced folate carrier expression in acute lymphoblastic leukemia: a mechanism for ploidy but not lineage differences in methotrexate accumulation. Blood 1999;93:1643–50.
220. Ramakers–van Woerden NL, Pieters R, Loonen AH, et al. *TEL-AML1* gene fusion is related to in vitro drug sensitivity for L-asparaginase in childhood acute lymphoblastic leukemia. Blood 2000;96:1094–9.
221. Stam RW, den Boer ML, Meijerink JP, et al. Differential mRNA expression of ara-C-metabolizing enzymes explains ara-C sensitivity in *MLL* gene–rearranged infant acute lymphoblastic leukemia. Blood 2003;101:1270–6.
222. Krajinovic M, Costea I, Chiasson S. Polymorphism of the thymidylate synthase gene and outcome of acute lymphoblastic leukaemia. Lancet 2002;359:1033–4.
223. Ulrich CM, Yasui Y, Storb R, et al. Pharmacogenetics of methotrexate: toxicity among marrow transplantation patients varies with the methylenetetrahydrofolate reductase C677T polymorphism. Blood 2001;98:231–4.
224. Taub JW, Matherly LH, Ravindranath Y, et al. Polymorphisms in methylenetetrahydrofolate reductase and

apoptosis (and resultant longevity of leukemic cells), together with a concurrent proliferation process of leukemic cells. That understanding might also lead to renewed attempts to use antimetabolite chemotherapy in CLL. The "higher" than previously considered proliferative rate of leukemic lymphocytes would also explain why telomeres, which cap the ends of chromosomes, but which shorten with each cell division, are smaller in CLL leukemic lymphocytes than in normal lymphocytes.[75,76]

CLINICAL ASPECTS

Diagnosis **Absolute Lymphocytosis in Blood** CLL is suspected whenever absolute lymphocytosis occurs in the peripheral blood of an adult. Blood lymphocytosis may also occur with viral or other infections (eg, infectious mononucleosis, pertussis, toxoplasmosis) and with neoplastic conditions other than CLL (eg, leukemic phase of lymphomas, hairy cell leukemia, prolymphocytic leukemia [PLL], and large granular cell leukemia).

Until recently, what was meant by "blood lymphocytosis" was not clear. Past publications placed the threshold at 15×10^9/L, but that threshold is widely recognized as being too high. Every hematologist knows that 2.5×10^9/L is the upper limit of normal for the lymphocyte count in blood. Previous investigators had, perhaps, set the threshold high to avoid making an erroneous diagnosis of CLL when a mild degree of blood lymphocytosis (between 2.5 and 15.0×10^9/L) could, in all likelihood, arise from causes other than CLL.

The ready availability of technology to study the phenotypic markers of lymphocytes now makes it possible to distinguish malignant lymphoma and other lymphoproliferative diseases from CLL. Two study groups therefore recommended that the threshold blood lymphocyte count be set at 10×10^9/L, or even 5×10^9/L. The International Workshop on CLL (IWCLL) addressed the generic issue of minimum diagnostic requirements for CLL (which can be applied universally and not restricted only to criteria of protocol entry eligibility) and recommended a blood lymphocyte threshold of 10×10^9/L.[77] The National Cancer Institute–sponsored Working Group (NCIWG) on CLL addressed the issue of diagnosis of CLL solely to define criteria of eligibility to enter prospective protocol studies.[78,79] For those purposes, the NCIWG required studies of lymphocyte phenotype in all patients, with the phenotype having to conform to the pattern detailed in "Minimum Diagnostic Requirements" later in this subsection. If the blood lymphocyte phenotype is clearly that of typical B-CLL, the NCIWG stated that CLL can be diagnosed if the blood lymphocyte count is greater than 5×10^9/L. Therefore, all research protocols in CLL in the United States, especially the ones sponsored by the NCI, recommend a threshold greater than 5×10^9/L of monoclonal phenotypic B cells for the diagnosis of CLL. On the other hand, for worldwide clinical applications of minimum diagnostic criteria (particularly in countries in which lymphocyte phenotyping is not readily available), the IWCLL recommended that a threshold of more than 10×10^9/L be considered appropriate.

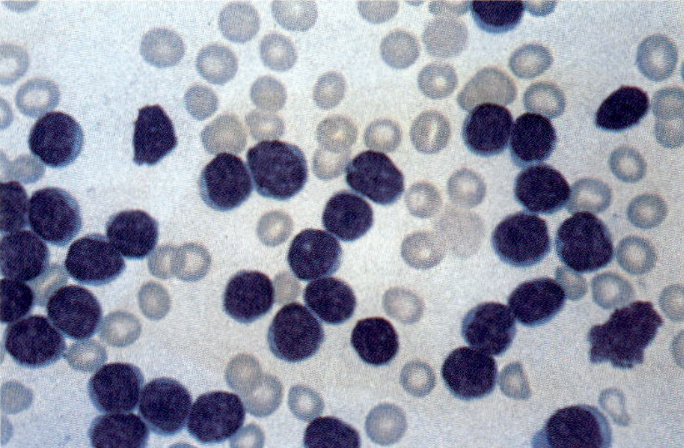

Figure 116-2 Chronic lymphocytic leukemia morphology in peripheral blood smear. Leukocyte count: 100×10^9/L. Most of the lymphocytes are mature-appearing. One smudge cell is present. Platelets are absent in this thrombocytopenic patient (Wright–Giemsa stain; ×100 original magnification).

But these recommendations leave unresolved whether the occasional patient who is discovered to have a normal or relatively low absolute lymphocyte count (between 1.5 and 5.0×10^9/L, for example) but also to have evidence (by flow cytometry) of the presence of monoclonal B cells with features characteristic of CLL should be considered to have the disease and not CLUS.[35,36]

Lymphocyte Morphology Lymphocytes must have the morphologic appearance of normal, mature cells. These are typically uniform populations of small lymphocytes (median volume: 211.5 fL).[80] The nucleus virtually fills the cell, leaving only a thin rim of visible cytoplasm. The nuclear chromatin is clumped, and a nucleolus is usually not discernible (Figures 116-2 and 116-3). A small proportion of cells may be larger lymphocytes with a large, somewhat notched nucleus, lacy-appearing nuclear chromatin, and a clearly visible nucleolus. These prolymphocytes may account for a minority of the overall population of lymphocytes in B-CLL. Most of the other conditions associated with blood lymphocytosis such as hairy cell leukemia, PLL (Figure 116-4), and large granular lymphocytic leukemia have their own characteristic morphologic features, which are distinct from those seen in CLL.

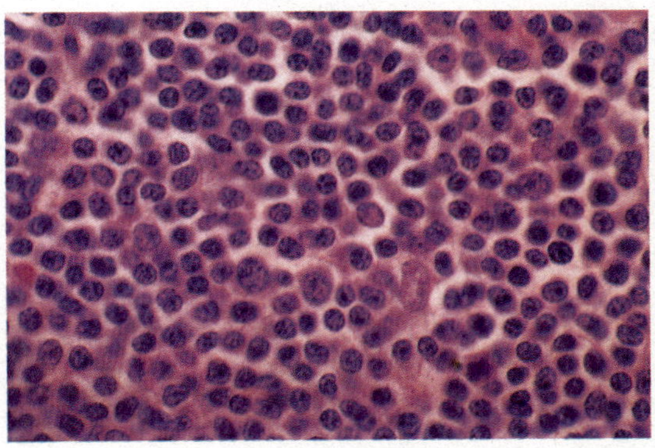

Figure 116-3 Chronic lymphocytic leukemia (CLL). Marrow biopsy with diffuse infiltration by CLL cells (hematoxylin and eosin stain; ×600 original magnification).

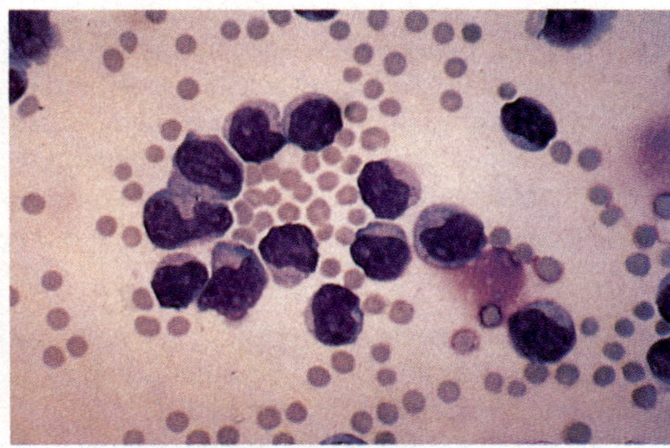

Figure 116-4 Prolymphocytic leukemia. Peripheral blood smear shows cells with prominent nucleoli and abundant cytoplasm (Wright–Giemsa stain; ×1,000 original magnification).

Blood Lymphocytosis Sustained Over Time The requirement that the blood lymphocytosis must be sustained to diagnose CLL was introduced to exclude conditions in which blood lymphocyte counts return to normal after a few weeks (eg, infectious mononucleosis, pertussis, and toxoplasmosis). However, it has not been possible to reach consensus on how often or over how long a period of time blood counts should be repeated to document "sustained" lymphocytosis. Some physicians recommend monthly blood counts for 3 to 6 months; others perform counts weekly for 4 to 6 weeks. This imprecise diagnostic criterion for CLL can be eliminated altogether if bone marrow lymphocytosis is included as one of the minimum requirements.

Only in CLL and similar lymphoid malignancies is lymphocytosis in the blood accompanied by bone marrow lymphocytosis. In small lymphocytic lymphoma (SLL), a disease virtually identical to CLL, but diagnosed by lymph node biopsy, bone marrow lymphocytosis may or may not be present. In infectious mononucleosis and pertussis, bone marrow lymphocytosis does not occur. However, bone marrow lymphocytosis is always present in all cases of CLL at diagnosis. Thus, even though blood lymphocytosis is recognized to be persistent and not transient in CLL, empiric and arguable recommendations for requiring sustained lymphocytosis for a certain period of time can be obviated by requiring that a bone marrow examination be performed to document lymphocytosis.

The characteristic findings of a bone marrow aspirate smear at the time of initial diagnosis of CLL include either hypercellularity or normocellularity (ie, not hypocellularity), with lymphocytes accounting for more than 30% of all nucleated cells (see Figure 116-3). A bone marrow biopsy examination is not required for establishing the diagnosis of CLL, but as discussed in "Criteria Predictive of Course of Disease in the Low- and Intermediate-Risk Groups" later in this chapter,[78,79] it has considerable prognostic value.

Minimum Diagnostic Requirements Minimum requirements for the diagnosis of CLL include an absolute lymphocyte count in the peripheral blood of more than 10×10^9/L, with a preponderant population of morphologically mature-appearing lymphocytes (see Figure 116-2).

In addition, hypercellular or normocellular bone marrow with lymphocytes accounting for more than 30% of all nucleated cells is required. In cases with an absolute lymphocyte count between 5×10^9/L and 10×10^9/L, lymphocyte phenotyping is required and must reveal a majority of the population expressing the following pattern of monoclonal B-cell markers:

- Extremely low levels of surface membrane immunoglobulin (SmIg) and either kappa or lambda light chains (but not both)
- One or more B-cell–associated antigens as demonstrated by CD19, CD20, CD21, and CD24 monoclonal antibodies
- T-cell–associated antigen as demonstrated by CD5 positivity and CD23 positivity

The presence of the T-cell antigen CD5 is a distinguishing property of B cells in B-CLL; CD23 positivity distinguishes CLL from another CD5+ lymphoid malignancy, MCL.

Differential Diagnosis Tables 116-2 and 116-3 list other lymphoproliferative disorders and their respective characteristic lymphocyte phenotypes. The pertinent clinical features distinguishing CLL from these other disorders are highlighted in the next few subsections.

Leukemic Phase of Non-Hodgkin's Lymphomas Sometimes CLL cannot be easily distinguished from the leukemic phase of lymphomas because of overlapping clinical features. In contrast to the phenotypic features of CLL, however, the amount of SmIg is abundant in lymphoma, and the lymphocytes are usually CD5–.

Hairy Cell Leukemia When hairy cell leukemia[81] is associated with an elevated lymphocyte count in the peripheral blood, the distinction from CLL is possible because of the typical morphologic features of hairy cells with cytoplasmic projections. A bone marrow biopsy will show diffuse infiltration by hairy cells in a characteristic loose fashion, with a well-defined rim of cytoplasm, leaving a clear zone around the cells (see Figure 116-2). Cytochemically, a moderately strong acid phosphatase reaction, not inhibited by tartaric acid, will be seen. Characteristically, the hairy cell phenotype consists of CD11c+, CD25+, and CD103+.

Prolymphocytic Leukemia The main feature distinguishing PLL[81,82] from CLL is the morphology of blood lymphocytes: large cells with somewhat immature-appearing nuclear chromatin, a prominent vesicular nucleolus, and abundant cytoplasm (see Figure 116-4). Other characteristics include a very large spleen and hyperlymphocytosis (usually more than 100×10^9/L). Phenotypically, prolymphocytes are B cells that are CD19+, CD20+, CD22+, and CD79b+, and yet are distinct from CLL lymphocytes, having normal amounts of SmIg, and most often being CD5–.

T Cell Chronic Lymphocytic Leukemia Lymphocytes in T cell chronic lymphocytic leukemia (T-CLL)[81,83] are large cells with slightly eccentrically placed nuclei and moderately abundant cytoplasm with fine azurophilic granules. These cells are also described as large granular lymphocytes. They express a mature postthymic phenotype: CD31+, CD42+, CD81+, and CD21+.

Sézary Cells In the leukemic manifestation of cutaneous T-cell lymphoma, the lymphocytes have a cerebriform nucleus (Sézary cells), which are usually CD41+ and CD82+.

Adult T-Cell Leukemia/Lymphoma Adult T-cell leukemia/lymphoma[81] is a viral neoplasm totally different from all other lymphoproliferative disorders. It has a unique incidence in certain parts of the world (Japan and countries of the Caribbean) and in immigrants from those regions. In this disease, the cells have a characteristic cloverleaf nucleus, and patients are rarely asymptomatic at presentation.

CLINICAL PRESENTATION

Like most other human neoplasms, CLL can produce a wide range of symptoms and physical and laboratory abnormalities at the time of its initial discovery in an individual patient.

Symptoms It is not unusual for a patient to feel entirely healthy, with no symptoms whatsoever, when a routine blood count reveals an absolute lymphocytosis requiring additional follow-up investigations that establish a diagnosis of CLL. At the other end of the spectrum is the patient who presents with many or all of the typical "B" symptoms of lymphoma (ie, marked weakness, profuse night sweats, unintended weight loss, and fever without infection). Each of these extremes accounts for approximately 20% of cases at presentation. The remaining 60% have varying symptomatology, with milder constitutional symptoms. Most patients consult a physician because they have noted painless swelling of lymph nodes, often in the cervical area (but also at times in other lymph node–bearing sites), that spontaneously waxes and wanes but does not altogether disappear. Occasionally, the presenting features relate to CLL as an acquired immunodeficiency disorder manifested by infection from opportunistic organisms or herpes zoster virus, or by exaggerated reactions to bee stings or insect bites, or by autoimmune complications such as hemolytic anemia or thrombocytopenia.

Physical Findings at Initial Diagnosis

Lymph Nodes The most consistent abnormal finding on physical examination is lymphadenopathy. Lymph node enlargement may be generalized or localized, and the size of the enlarged nodes may be as small as a few millimeters in diameter or as large as an orange. When cervical nodes are extremely enlarged, they may be easily discernible by simple inspection and may give the patient a "jowly" appearance.

Characteristically, enlarged nodes in CLL are firm, rounded, discrete, nontender, and freely mobile upon palpation. Exceptions to these generalizations are encountered, particularly when the nodes have grown rapidly. Occasionally, several enlarged nodes in the same anatomic site (cervical triangle, axilla, or femoral–inguinal areas) may become confluent with each other, forming large spherical lymphoid masses. New lymph nodes may appear, sometimes in places other than the usual lymph node-bearing sites, such as over the sacrum or the thorax.

Spleen Next to lymph nodes, the spleen is the lymphoid organ most frequently enlarged. It may be palpably enlarged in 30% to 40% of cases. The extent of enlargement varies from an organ barely palpable upon deep inspiration to one so large as to occupy the entire left side of the abdomen and pelvis, to cross the midline, and to encroach upon the right side of the abdomen. As is the case with enlarged lymph nodes, an enlarged spleen in CLL is usually painless. Upon palpation it is nontender, with a sharp edge and a smooth, firm surface. Painful or infarcted splenic enlargement is an unusual presenting feature for CLL.

Liver Enlargement of the liver may be noted at the time of initial diagnosis of CLL in approximately 20% of cases. The liver in CLL generally is not greatly enlarged, ranging from 2 to 6 cm below the right costal margin, with a span of dullness on percussion of 10 to 16 cm. Upon palpation, the liver is usually nontender and firm, with a smooth surface.

Other Tissues In addition to palpably enlarged peripheral lymph nodes, liver, and spleen, virtually any other lymphoid tissue in the body—for example, Waldeyer's ring or the tonsils—may be enlarged at diagnosis. In addition, infiltration with CLL cells may occur in any organ. At the time of diagnosis, skin lesions are the most obvious, but are seen in fewer than 5% of cases. In contrast to lymphoma, gastrointestinal mucosal involvement is rarely seen in CLL. Similarly, meningeal leukemia is unusual in CLL at the time of initial presentation.

Abnormal Radiologic Findings No radiologic examinations are absolutely required as part of evaluation at the time of initial diagnosis of CLL. A chest film is usually ordered and is helpful in detecting hilar and mediastinal adenopathy. If a patient is entered into a therapeutic research protocol, computed tomography imaging of the abdomen and pelvis (and of the chest, if the chest film revealed mediastinal adenopathy) is recommended as a baseline study. The images obtained provide an objective measure of the size of spleen and liver and of the retroperitoneal nodes for comparison with subsequent reexaminations to determine the level of clinical response to protocol-based therapy.

Laboratory Abnormalities **Lymphocytosis** The most noteworthy abnormalities among laboratory findings in CLL are lymphocytosis in the blood and bone marrow. A few additional features related to lymphocytosis are considered here.

Although the absolute blood lymphocyte threshold for diagnosing CLL was placed at more than 10×10^9/L, most patients present with considerably higher counts, usually in excess of 15 × 10^9/L, and occasionally as high as 200 × 10^9/L. Upon examination of a peripheral blood smear, mature-appearing small lymphocytes may be preponderant in the population of leukocytes, ranging from 50% to as much as 99% or 100%. Lymphocytes that appear flattened or smudged in the process of being spread on the glass slide may also be seen. Such "smudge" cells, perhaps reflecting some fragility or vulnerability to distortion upon mechanical manipulation, are considered characteristic of CLL (see Figure 116-2). When blood leukocyte counts are in excess of 200 × 10^9/L, the increased number of cellular elements may result in abnormally high whole-blood viscosity.

In addition to an increased ratio of mature-appearing lymphocytes in the smears of aspirated morrows, three patterns of infiltration by lymphocytes are recognized in trephine biopsy specimens of the bone marrow (see Figure 116-3): nodular, interstitial, and diffuse. Sometimes a given biopsy sample may show a mixture of nodular and interstitial or of nodular and diffuse patterns. It has been observed that patients with diffuse infiltration tend to have advanced disease and relatively worse outlook. For prognostic purposes, nodular and interstitial patterns, which are associated with less-advanced disease and better prognosis, may be grouped together and termed "nondiffuse."[84–86]

Other Abnormalities Anemia and thrombocytopenia may be observed at the time of initial diagnosis, but usually they are of relatively mild degree. Low hemoglobin and platelet levels (below 110 g/L and 100 × 10^9/L respectively) are observed at diagnosis in approximately 20% of CLL patients and herald an overall poor prognosis. A direct antiglobulin (Coombs) test may be positive in approximately 25% of cases, but overt autoimmune hemolytic anemia occurs less frequently. In the absence of a reliable test to demonstrate antiplatelet antibodies, autoimmune thrombocytopenia is most often diagnosed on the basis of the presence of adequate numbers of megakaryocytes in the bone marrow with an abnormally low platelet count in the blood. Agranulocytosis or neutropenia may be encountered. Hypogammaglobulinemia may be present at the time of initial diagnosis, but in most cases it is observed only later in the course of the disease. All three immunoglobulin classes (IgG, IgA, and IgM) are usually decreased, but in some patients, only one or two classes may be low. Significant hypogammaglobulinemia and neutropenia result in increased vulnerability of CLL patients to major bacterial infections.

Blood lymphocyte phenotype characteristics were detailed earlier in this chapter. It should be noted, however, that the normal T:B ratio (2:1) is altered. Instead, a large proportion of cells are B lymphocytes.

No abnormalities in blood chemistry are characteristic of CLL, but elevated levels of serum lactate dehydrogenase, uric acid, hepatic enzymes (alanine aminotransferase [ALT] or aspartate aminotransferase [AST]), and (rarely) calcium may be observed.

NATURAL HISTORY AND TERMINAL EVENTS

It is a generally held belief that CLL is an indolent disease with a prolonged chronic course and that the eventual cause of death may be unrelated to CLL; however, this observation is true for fewer than 30% of all CLL cases. The natural history is heterogeneous in most patients. Some patients die rapidly, within 2 to 3 years of diagnosis, from complications or causes directly related to CLL. Many patients live for 5 to 10 years with an initial course that is relatively benign, but that is almost always followed by a terminal phase lasting 1 to 2 years, during which considerable morbidity ensues both from the disease itself and from complications of therapy. During the initial asymptomatic phase, the patients are able to maintain their usual lifestyle, but during the terminal phase, performance status is poor, with recurring need for hospitalization. The most frequent causes of death are severe systemic infection (especially pneumonia and septicemia), bleeding, and inanition with cachexia.

In approximately 3% of CLL patients, a diffuse large-cell immunoblastic lymphoma supervenes terminally[87] (Richter transformation; Figure 116-5). Richter's syndrome is associated with a rapidly progressive course, refractoriness to all currently known chemotherapy, and death within 6 months.[87] The diagnosis of Richter's syndrome requires histopathologic examination of a lymph node.

In an equally small minority of patients, the terminal event is a morphologic transformation of blood lymphocytes from the typical small, mature-appearing cell to somewhat larger cells with distinct nucleoli and a somewhat less-dense chromatin in the nucleus. This event is called "prolymphocytoid transformation," and it is associated with refractoriness to the usual chemotherapeutic agents.[81]

Acute leukemia is observed only extremely rarely as a terminal event in CLL. When it does occur, it is myeloid in origin (myelocytic, myelomonocytic, or acute erythroleukemia). Prior therapy with alkylating agents has not been clearly implicated in the causation of terminal acute leukemia because a few cases have been observed in patients who did not previously receive such therapy for CLL.

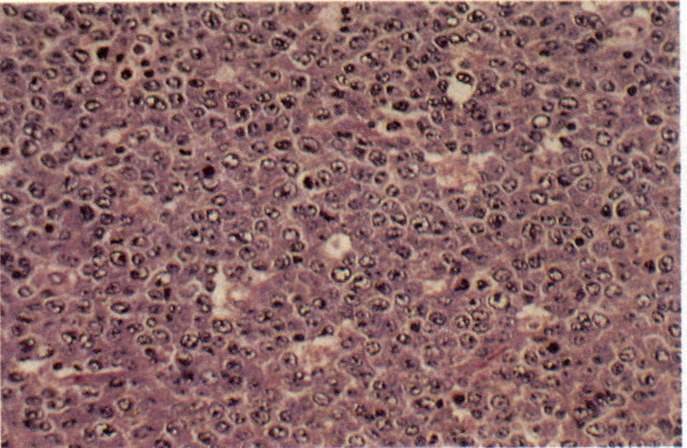

Figure 116-5 Chronic lymphocytic leukemia, Richter's syndrome. Section of lymph node with immunoblastic proliferation consisting of large cells with prominent nucleoli (hematoxylin and eosin stain; ×600 original magnification).

No widely accepted effective therapy is known for terminal transformations in CLL, but anecdotal reports of success with CHOP (cyclophosphamide, hydroxydaunomycin [doxorubicin], Oncovin [vincristine], and prednisone) chemotherapy in Richter syndrome, and fludarabine or deoxycoformycin in prolymphocytoid transformation have been published. Acute leukemia developing in patients known to have had CLL is treated with any of the acute leukemia therapy regimens, but almost invariably with poor outcome.

Patients with CLL are considered to be at a somewhat higher risk of developing another cancer, usually of lung or gastrointestinal tract, than is the general population. Skin cancers occur with considerably greater frequency among CLL patients than among the general population, but those cancers do not result in higher mortality.

CLINICAL STAGING AND OTHER PROGNOSTIC FEATURES

The natural history of CLL can be extremely variable, with survival times from initial diagnosis that range from 2 to 20 years. Until the mid-1970s, no reliable clinically applicable criteria were available to physicians to enable them to prospectively separate patients with a poor outlook for survival from those with an excellent prognosis. Understandably, this difficulty forced physicians to make decisions almost exclusively on an empiric basis about the need for (and timing of) therapeutic interventions in their CLL patients.

With the objective of finding prognostic criteria, Boggs and colleagues published an analysis of the clinical features of a large series of patients with CLL who were continuously followed in their clinic.[11] Their observations indicated that patients with short survival (< 5 years) had evidence of more disease (eg, larger lymphoid masses, more abnormalities in blood counts) at the time of initial diagnosis of CLL than did the patients whose survival time was longer than 5 years. Soon thereafter, Galton[13] and Dameshek[14] almost simultaneously presented their respective ideas, which are remarkably similar and which have since become the classic tenets for understanding the pathophysiology of CLL. These investigators observed that, in CLL, functionally inert lymphocytes progressively accumulate and that the rate and extent of increase of these nonfunctional lymphocytes influence the overall activity of the disease and the outlook for survival of patients. These observations were subsequently confirmed in a study performed by Hansen,[12] in which case histories of a large series of CLL patients followed and treated at a single institution were reported with meticulous precision.

Those reports, published between 1966 and 1973, constituted the basis on which Rai and colleagues[15] developed a system for staging CLL that could prospectively distinguish patients according to their overall outlook for survival. This method of staging was recognized as a simple yet accurate predictor of survival; consequently, it rapidly gained wide acceptance by clinicians. With the advent of reliable criteria for stratification according to survival outlook, the Cancer and Leukemia Group B (CALGB) was able to initiate clinical trials in patients at various stages of CLL to test various therapeutic strategies.[88–91] During the ensuing years, several additional systems of clinical staging were proposed by investigators around the world, each having certain merits. A few of these staging systems are summarized below, but only two—the Rai system[15] and the Binet system[16]—are in wide use in both clinical practice and research.

Table 116-4 Distribution of Cases in Various Series According to Rai Staging

			Stage (% of Cases)				
Reference	Cases (*n*)	Series (Years)	0	I	II	III	IV
Rai et al (1975)	125	18	23	31	17	11	14
Geisler and Hansen (1981)	102	20	36	19	17	8	31
Baccarini et al (1982)	188	26.5	26.5	21	9	17	9
Skinnider (1982)	745	19	21	31	16	13	31
MRC CLL-1* (1989)	660	28	18	29	10	15	31

*The hemoglobin level for stage III in Medical Research Council of Great Britain Chronic Lymphocytic Leukemia Trial I was less than 110 g/L. Reproduced with permission from Catovsky D and Foa R.[81]

Staging System of Rai and Colleagues The Rai system is based on the concept that, in CLL, a gradual and progressive increase in the body burden of leukemic lymphocytes occurs, resulting in sequential clinical manifestations of the disease. Those manifestations start in the blood and bone marrow; then affect the lymph nodes, spleen, and liver; and eventually compromise bone marrow function to a significant degree. The earliest stage is the one in which no stigmata of disease are seen other than the minimum diagnostic requirements for CLL (ie, lymphocytosis in blood and marrow [stage 0]), as detailed in Table 116-4.

At the time of initial diagnosis of CLL, approximately 20% to 25% of patients are in the earliest clinical stage (stage 0), approximately 25% are in the advanced stages (stages III and IV), and the remaining 50% are in stage I or II. Table 116-4 shows the exact stage distributions from various series, revealing a consistent pattern.

The median survival times from the time of diagnosis in the series of patients studied by Rai and coworkers were 150 months for stage 0, 101 months for stage I, 71 months for stage II, 19 months for stage III, and 19 months for stage IV.[15] Although Rai and colleagues noted in their 1975 paper that only three (and not five) distinct actuarial survival patterns emerged from the data (stage 0, stages I and II combined, and stages III and IV combined), they recommended that the five-stage system be maintained to investigate prospectively whether biologic and clinical differences would emerge between stages I and II and between stages III and IV. However, in the 1980s, it became apparent that it was impractical to stratify patients in five categories for prospective randomized trials of CLL therapy. In 1987, therefore, the staging system was modified to consist of three groups: low (Rai stage 0), intermediate (Rai stages I and II combined), and high (Rai stages III and IV combined) risk categories.[92] Figure 116-6 depicts the actuarial survival curves according to clinical stage at the time of diagnosis.

The modified Rai staging system was used for stratification of patients according to their risk category in a large Intergroup comparative study in the front-line therapy of CLL conducted in the 1990s.[90,91]

Method of Binet and Colleagues Binet's method classifies all patients with anemia (defined as hemoglobin below 100 g/L) or thrombocytopenia (platelets less than 100 × 10⁹/L), or both, as stage C.[16] All of the remaining (non-C) patients are divided into two groups, depending on the presence of fewer than three (stage A) or three or more (stage B) sites of palpable enlargement of lymphoid organs. This staging takes into consideration five sites: cervical, axillary, and inguinal lymph nodes (whether unilateral or bilateral, each area is counted as one), and the spleen and liver. This system has been found to be of great value in dividing patients into three types of survival curves, with A, B, and C corresponding, respectively, to the Rai low-, intermediate-, and high-risk groups.

IWCLL Staging Recommendation The IWCLL recommended that, in practice, an integrated system using both methods should be used.[77] According to this recommendation, each Binet stage is to be further identified by the appropriate Rai stage (eg, A-0, A-I, A-II, B-I, B-II, C-III, C-IV). However, this integrated system has not been widely accepted, and most clinicians today use either the Rai or the Binet method for patient management and therapeutic investigation.

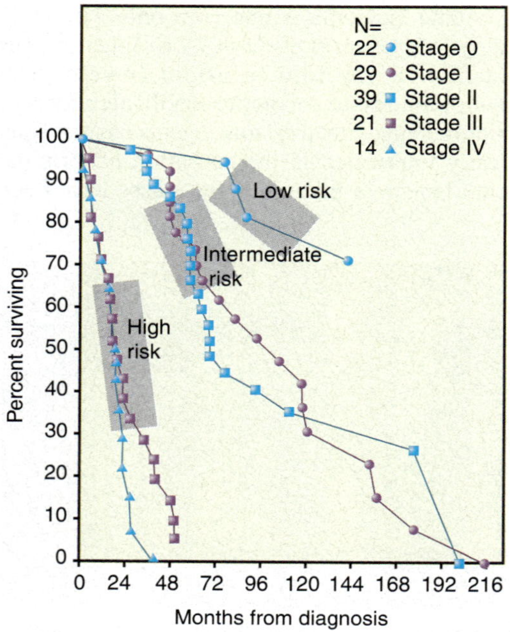

Figure 116-6 Five stages of chronic lymphocytic leukemia modified into a three-stage system: low risk, intermediate risk, and high risk. Adapted with permission from Rai KR et al[15] and from Rai KR.[92]

Method of Jaksic and Vitale Jaksic and Vitale's method is called "total tumor mass score" and is based on blood lymphocyte count and the size of the largest palpably enlarged lymph node and of the spleen.[94] This staging method has found limited acceptance.

Criteria Predictive of Course of Disease in the Low- and Intermediate-Risk Groups Virtually all patients in the high-risk group (stages III and IV) have a relatively rapid clinical course and die within approximately 4 years; however, in the other risk groups, the course of disease is not uniform. Patients in the low- and intermediate-risk groups (stage 0 and stages I and II respectively) may have a benign clinical course in which the disease remains indolent for several years and a long overall survival measurable in years or even decades. Alternatively, the course may be progressive and associated with a short overall survival time. The need to prospectively predict the clinical course of CLL in these risk groups is, therefore, obvious and even crucial; however, neither Rai nor Binet, nor any other currently available method of staging, is of value for this purpose.

Several prognostic factors have been tested and found to be of limited usefulness in predicting the course of disease in non-advanced stages of CLL.[93] These prognostic factors include extent of blood lymphocytosis; morphologic features of blood lymphocytes (ie, the relative proportion of prolymphocytes); presence of normal or abnormal chromosomal karyotype; phenotypic profile of B lymphocytes; age, sex, and levels of serum immunoglobulins; molecular genetics markers; β-2-microglobulin; and adhesion molecules.[95]

In the low-risk group, several investigators have discovered certain clinical criteria that may identify patients whose disease will remain indolent or smoldering, as distinct from those whose disease will progress to higher-risk groups. Spanish workers observed that a relatively low absolute lymphocyte count in blood (below 30 × 10⁹/L), a long projected or actual time of doubling of blood lymphocyte count in low-risk group patients not receiving cytotoxic therapy, a hemoglobin level above 12 g/dL, and a bone marrow biopsy showing a non-diffuse (interstitial or nodular) pattern of lymphoid infiltration are associated with smoldering CLL and survival statistics similar to those of an age- and sex-matched Spanish population.[93,96] French workers found that stage A patients with hemoglobin in excess of 12 g/dL and blood lymphocytosis below 30×10^9/L had a survival time equal to that of the age- and sex-matched French population.[97]

Criteria for defining smoldering CLL notwithstanding, the matter of accurately predicting the clinical course of CLL in all non-advanced stages of the disease (ie, stages 0, I, and II) remains unresolved. In that context, the mutational status of Ig genes on CLL lymphocytes seems promising. Observations suggest that IgV gene mutations correlate with significantly longer survival and a relatively more benign disease course than are seen when such mutations are lacking.[53,71] However, given that testing for gene mutations is not routinely done in hospitals, perhaps CD38 expression, a readily available test, holds the promise of being useful.

Mutated IgV genes were strongly correlated with low expression of CD38 on CLL lymphocytes.[53–55,57,72,73] These findings were especially strong prognostic indicators for patients in the intermediate-risk category. Whether future studies in other laboratories confirm these findings of a correlation between high CD38 expression and unmutated IgV genes will, therefore, be of great interest.

In addition to the prognostic distinction that CD38 expression or lack thereof can provide, cytogenetic abnormalities discovered by applying FISH (and not the conventional banding) techniques can be of immense clinical value in the management of an individual CLL case. The observations of Dohner and colleagues[67] revealed that patients with 13q deletion as the sole abnormality had a median survival duration of 133 months, patients with normal karyotype had 111 months, those with trisomy 12 had 114 months, those with 11q deletion had 79 months, and those with 17p deletion had 32 months.

Table 116-5 Recently Identified Molecular and Cytogenetic Markers of Prognosis in Chronic Lymphocytic Leukemia (CLL)

	Markers of		
	Good Prognosis	Worse Prognosis	Refs.
IgV_H mutation status	Mutated	Unmutated	53,71
ZAP70 on CLL B Lymphocytes	Negative	Positive	39,99–102
CD38 on CLL B lymphocytes	Negative	Positive	53,72,73
FISH cytogenetics	Sole abnormality is 13q del	11q del, 17p del	3,67

***ZAP70* Expression of B-CLL Cells as a Prognostic Marker** Zap-70, an intracellular protein crucial in activation signals delivered to T lymphocytes and natural killer cells under normal circumstances in humans is rarely present in normal B-cells.[98] However, *ZAP70* gene expression in leukemic B-lymphocytes has been observed in CLL patients with unmutated IgV_H genes.[39] This association of *ZAP70* with unmutated IGV_H genes has been confirmed by other investigators.[99] Testing for mutations is laborious and is not usually performed in clinical laboratories. But because *ZAP70* testing can be more readily performed by flow cytometry, such testing is finding favor as a surrogate for testing for mutation status in CLL patients.[99] However, the methodology and reproducibility of testing for *ZAP70* have yet to be standardized, and therefore clinical application will have to wait.[1] We are hopeful that the necessary standardization will be accomplished in the near future. Recent studies have demonstrated that *ZAP70* positivity on CLL lymphocytes is a predictor of disease progression and inferior clinical outcome.[100–102] Table 116-5 summarizes these newly identified prognostic markers.

TREATMENT

In most malignant diseases, early treatment of the malignant process is optimal. The first decision to be made in CLL is whether the patient requires therapy at the time of initial diagnosis. This approach recognizes the extreme heterogeneity of the disease and lack of evidence that early treatment affects long-term survival.

Epidemiology studies, such as those in Olmsted County, Minnesota, illustrate that more patients are now being diagnosed while asymptomatic because of routine examinations or routine testing for other illnesses.[23] These patients remain stable for many years without evidence of developing clinical features of disease progression. Four-parameter flow cytometry analysis in a general hospital outpatient population demonstrated the presence of CLUS in 3.5% of individuals over 40 years of age.[36] The frequency was twice as high for men as for women, increased with age, and was significantly more frequent in relatives of CLL patients.[35,36] These "smoldering" CLL[93] patients have minimal organomegaly, a normal hemoglobin and platelet count, and a survival rate that is the same as an age- and sex-matched population. They could indeed be considered to have CLUS (similar to MGUS in relation to multiple myeloma).

The lack of evidence that CLL can be cured with currently available modalities[96] has resulted in a conservative "watch and wait" approach to the management of CLL. However, the development of new regimens with significant activity in CLL—namely, purine analogs, monoclonal antibodies, and application of autologous and allogeneic hematopoietic stem cells transplantation—has led to consideration of curative attempts in younger patients.

Indications for Treatment The NCIWG has recommended that treatment be initiated for CLL patients with anemia and thrombocytopenia (Rai stage III or IV; Binet stage C) and for patients with disease-related symptoms such as fatigue, night sweats, weight loss, and fever related to CLL.[79] Transient localized lymphadenopathy can occur in response to localized infections and is not an indication for treatment. AIHA or thrombocytopenia (or both) that is poorly responsive to corticosteroid therapy, massive splenomegaly, lymphadenopathy, or a blood lymphocyte doubling time of less than 6 months are indications for treatment. Marked hypogammaglobulinemia per se is not necessarily an indication for initiation of systemic therapy for CLL. These NCIWG guidelines are recommended for patients being entered on clinical research protocols; they also serve as useful guides for treatment in clinical practice.[79]

The recognition of a prognostic significance for CD38, *ZAP70*, IgV_H mutation status, FISH genetic abnormalities, *TP53* mutations and thymidine kinase has led to consideration of earlier intervention in early-stage, low tumor-burden, asymptomatic patients. A report by the IWCLL has urged caution for this approach in clinical practice.[103] Well-designed clinical trials are being initiated, however.

Goals of Therapy Traditionally, treatment of CLL continued until symptoms resolved or clinically troubling lymphadenopathy and splenomegaly were controlled. Complete remission was not an objective of treatment. The idea that most CLL patients die of comorbid conditions has been disproved. In patients with progressive disease, CLL is the major cause of shortening of survival.

In recent years, the availability of regimens with higher complete remission rates in CLL has led both the NCIWG and the IWCLL to develop criteria to define complete remission.[77,79] A complete remission requires the absence of symptoms attributable to CLL, normal findings on physical examination, a lymphocyte count below 4×10^9/L, neutrophils at 1.5×10^9/L or higher, platelets at 100×10^9/L or higher, hemoglobin level of 110 g/L or higher, and a bone marrow lymphocyte differential count below 30%. A partial response was defined as a reduction in previously enlarged nodes, spleen, and liver by 50% or more, with a neutrophil count of 1.5×10^9/L or higher, a platelet count of 100×10^9/L or higher, and a hemoglobin level of 110 g/L or higher (or a 50% or better improvement over pre-therapy deficits in hemoglobin and platelet counts). The IWCLL panel defined partial response by a shift in clinical stage (from stage C to B or from B to A).[77] These responses must persist for a minimum period of 2 months. Initially, both the NCIWG and the IWCLL allowed persistent nodules or lymphoid infiltrates on bone marrow biopsy in patients achieving a complete remission by all other criteria. However, these patients are now classified as nodular partial response because of clear evidence that the duration of nodular partial response is significantly shorter than that of complete response.[104] Flow cytometry studies demonstrated that, in most patients with complete response or nodular partial response, clonal cells co-expressing CD5 and CD19 with an abnormal kappa/lambda light-chain ratio nonetheless persist.[105] Normalization of serum immunoglobulin levels is not a requirement for complete response.

The efforts of the NCIWG and IWCLL in standardizing criteria for clinical research protocols and for evaluating response have allowed results of different trials to be compared and have greatly enhanced the quality of clinical research in CLL.

Chemotherapy For 50 years, the backbone of chemotherapy in CLL was the use of alkylating agents such as chlorambucil or cyclophosphamide, with or without the addition of corticosteroids. Despite evidence that chlorambucil is associated with a lower response rate and shorter response duration than that achieved with purine analogues, chlorambucil is still widely used in older patients because it is well tolerated and inexpensive.

Chlorambucil, 4-[bis(2-chloroethyl)amino]-benzenebutanoic acid, is a bi-functional alkylating agent. It is rapidly and completely absorbed from the gastrointestinal tract.[106] Metabolism is predominantly hepatic. The major metabolite of chlorambucil is phenylacetic acid mustard, which is still pharmacologically active against CLL. Peak plasma concentration of chlorambucil occurs within 1 hour after oral administration; metabolites peak within 2 to 4 hours. Chlorambucil is extensively bound to plasma and tissue proteins. Excretion of chlorambucil and metabolites is predominantly in the urine.

Great variability in the dose and schedule of chlorambucil has been observed. Two commonly used schedules are a daily dose of 0.08 mg/kg (4 to 8 mg total dose per day) or a pulsed intermittent dose of 0.8 mg/kg (40 to 80 mg in a single day) given every 3 to 4 weeks.[107,108] The intermittent schedule was an attempt to prevent myelosuppression, which is the main toxicity. A CALGB study revealed that chlorambucil is equally effective when given daily or on an intermittent basis.[88]

Chlorambucil is usually administered for a period of several weeks until maximum clinical response is reached. Maintenance therapy is uncommon, and recurrence of disease is followed by resumption of therapy. A substantial fraction of patients achieve second and third responses. Chlorambucil is more likely than cyclophosphamide to cause thrombocytopenia.

Cyclophosphamide is 90% absorbed from the gastrointestinal tract. The major active metabolite, 4-hydroxycyclophosphamide (4HC), is formed in the liver and has a terminal half-life of 1.5 to 6 hours.[109] Results from using cyclophosphamide approximate those from using chlorambucil.

Corticosteroids Prednisone has been administered to CLL patients as a single agent, usually in an initial dose of 20 to 60 mg, with dose reductions occurring in a graduated fashion.[110,111] One-third of patients so treated had shrinkage of lymph nodes or spleen. Often, in the first 1 to 2 months, an increase in the lymphocyte count was followed by a subsequent decline, caused by a shift of lymphocytes from lymph nodes and bone marrow into the blood. Anemia and thrombocytopenia improved in approximately two-thirds of patients. Usually, 3 to 6 months of treatment were required. The major side effects were those of chronic corticosteroid therapy and infections.

At the present time, the major indication for prednisone appears to be management of antibody-mediated (autoimmune) anemia and thrombocytopenia. High-dose methylprednisolone has been shown to be effective in shrinking large lymph node masses.[112]

Combination Regimens A study of daily high-dose chlorambucil (15 mg/day) until complete remission or toxicity was compared to 6 doses of chlorambucil 75 mg once weekly, combined with prednisone.[112] A significantly higher response rate was noted for the chlorambucil arm versus the combination regimen. The cumulative dose in the chlorambucil-alone arm was five to six times that in the combination arm, with substantial marrow toxicity. A survival advantage was noted for the chlorambucil-alone arm. The CVP (cyclophosphamide, vincristine, and prednisone) and CHOP regimens have not shown superiority over chlorambucil.[113–115]

French Cooperative Group on CLL In two French Cooperative Group on CLL (FCGCLL) clinical trials involving patients with Binet stage A CLL, immediate treatment with chlorambucil (first trial) or with chlorambucil plus prednisone (second trial) was compared with delay of treatment until progression was noted.[97] The delayed treatment groups each had a slightly superior survival with fewer second malignancies. In Binet stage B patients, the FCGCLL compared chlorambucil with cyclophosphamide, vincristine (Oncovin), and prednisone (COP); similar survival and rate of disease progression were observed between the two groups.[115] In Binet stage C patients,[116] the COP regimen was compared to a mini-CHOP regimen (doxorubicin 25 mg/m^2 on day 1 added to COP). The overall survival was significantly superior for the CHOP group. In both studies, cyclophosphamide was given daily by mouth for 5 days. Those results have been the subject of criticism, because the COP arm survival (2 years) was shorter than when the same regimen was studied by Eastern Cooperative Oncology Group in the United States (4 years).[113]

Purine Analogs Purine analogs have shown major clinical activity in slow-growing lymphoid malignancies. Fludarabine monophosphate (Fludara), 2-chlorodeoxyadenosine (2-CdA), and pentostatin (2'-deoxycoformycin, DCF) are highly active in CLL.

In phase II trials of Fludara, response rates of 40% to 60% were noted in previously treated patients, with 15% achieving complete remission. Higher response rates were seen in earlier-stage disease.[117,118] Addition of prednisone did not improve the response rate.[119] The addition of corticosteroids was associated with an increased incidence of *Pneumocystis carinii* and *Listeria* infections.[119] The major side effects associated with Fludara were myelosuppression and episodes of fever and infection. Subsequent studies have evaluated Fludara with and without prednisone in previously untreated patients, with complete remission rates of 25% to 30% and an overall response rate of 80% being achieved.[119]

The drug 2-CdA, which is extremely potent in hairy cell leukemia, has been studied in CLL with an overall response rate of 30% to 70% in advanced-stage disease.[120–122] Studies in previously untreated patients demonstrated response rates of 56% to 85%, with complete response rates varying between 10% and 47%.[122] Both Fludara and 2-CdA are 50% to 60% bioavailable by mouth and are effective clinically when administered by the oral route.

The response rates for DCF are lower than the rates for Fludara and 2-CdA.[123,124]

The purine analogs have emerged as the major treatment class for CLL. The major causes for concern in using purine analogs are infections and myelosuppression.[125,126] With fludarabine therapy, CD4 and CD8 T-cell counts in CLL patients fell to approximately 200/µL for prolonged periods. Nevertheless, patients in remission off therapy have a very low incidence of infections: approximately 1 febrile episode or infection for every 2.5 patient–years at risk. Serious infections such as pneumonia occurred at a frequency of 1 for every 16 patient–years at risk. Herpes zoster appears to occur more frequently in patients treated with purine analogs: approximately 15% to 20% of patients experienced an outbreak at some time during their course.

Comparative Studies A large Intergroup trial in previously untreated CLL patients in North America showed significantly higher rates of overall response and complete response and longer durations of response and progression-free survival in patients randomized to Fludara than in patients who received CLB. However, there was no significant difference in overall survival between the two arms.[90] A third arm of the study, combining fludarabine and chlorambucil, was discontinued because of an excessive incidence of infections. Major infections and herpes virus infections occurred more often on the Fludara arm than on CLB arm. Advanced stage and low serum levels of immunoglobulin were associated with an increased incidence of infections. More therapy-related leukemias were noted in the Fludara arm than in the chlorambucil arm.[126]

In a multinational clinical trial in Europe, fludarabine was compared with cyclophosphamide, doxorubicin (Adriamycin), and prednisone (CAP) in a randomized fashion.[127] In untreated patients, the response rate was 70% for Fludara versus 58% for CAP; in previously treated patients, it was 45% versus 26% respectively. No survival difference was observed, although time to progression was significantly longer for the Fludara-treated patients.

French investigators have evaluated Fludara versus CAP versus French CHOP.[128] A higher response rate was found with Fludara (71%) and with CHOP (72%) than with CAP (58%). Complete responses were more frequent with Fludara. No difference in survival was noted. The incidences of infections and autoimmune hemolytic anemia were similar in the three groups.

A comparative German CLL Study Group (GCLLSG) study of intravenous fludarabine versus oral chlorambucil in patients older than 65 years demonstrated significantly higher rates of complete response and overall response, and improved quality of life measurements for the purine analog.[129]

A randomized comparative trial of 2-CdA or chlorambucil plus prednisone demonstrated a significantly higher complete response rate for the 2-CdA arm (47% versus 12%), and significantly longer remission duration, but no difference in survival.[122]

New Regimens Recently, based on the ability of fludarabine to inhibit DNA repair,[130] combinations of Fludara and cyclophosphamide have come under investigation. This combination has been reported to have high response rates and acceptable tolerance in both previously treated and untreated patients.[131,132] In the initial study, patients with Fludara-refractory disease had a response rate of 41% to Fludara with cyclophosphamide.[131] Preliminary comparative studies of the combination versus fludarabine alone have demonstrated higher rates of complete response and overall response, and longer progression-free survival for the combination in previously untreated patients.[133,134] Combinations of 2-CdA and cyclophosphamide (Cytoxan) and pentostatin and cyclophosphamide are also effective.[135,136]

A new combination of fludarabine, cyclophosphamide, and mitoxantrone has been developed as a salvage and frontline regimen in CLL.[137,138] High rates of complete response and overall response were demonstrated in previously treated patients, with many responders showing no minimal residual disease (MRD)by flow cytometry and polymerase chain reaction (PCR) for the IgV_H sequence.[137,138]

Monoclonal Antibodies Monoclonal antibodies have been evaluated in CLL because of potential target antigens on the surface of CLL cells. Recent studies have evaluated the role of rituximab against CD20 and that of alemtuzumab (Campath-1H) against CD52.

Rituximab[139] is more active in follicular than in diffuse SLL or CLL; in the latter relapsed or refractory diseases, the response rate is only 12% to 15%.[140] Dose-intensive regimens demonstrated a dose–response relationship; high doses of rituximab in CLL gave higher response rates than did conventional doses.[141,142]

Alemtuzumab has been evaluated in a number of studies. The pivotal clinical trial, in Fludara-refractory patients, demonstrated a response rate of 33%.[143] Alemtuzumab is more effective in clearing disease in blood, bone marrow, and spleen than in bulky lymph nodes. There is an inverse relationship between the size of lymph nodes and probability of response. This phenomenon is not noted with rituximab, which is less effective in clearing bone marrow. These data provide the rationale for recent studies of alemtuzumab plus rituximab, which have response rates of 50% or more in patients with relapsed and refractory CLL.[144]

Alemtuzumab can also be given subcutaneously. In frontline therapy, an overall response rate of 87% was seen, together with 19% complete remissions among 38 evaluable patients. Local reactions can be dose-limiting in some patients, but are usually manageable after the first 1 to 2 weeks.[145] A GCLLSG study demonstrated that subcutaneous alemtuzumab in fludarabine-refractory patients (many of whom showed 17p deletion on FISH analysis) had a similar response rate to the intravenous regimen.[146]

All patients receiving alemtuzumab require prophylaxis against *P. carinii* pneumonia and DNA viruses. Reactivation of cytomegalovirus (CMV) occurs in 15% to 25% of patients. This reactivation is documented by rising CMV antigenemia or by development of PCR positivity for CMV. CMV disease manifested by pneumonitis, hepatitis, or other organ infiltration is much less common. The response to intravenous ganciclovir or foscarnet is usually prompt. Prophylaxis against CMV with valgancyclovir appears to be effective in initial studies.

An emerging area of interest and concern in treatment of CLL with monoclonal antibodies is the detection of soluble CD20 and CD52 in plasma.[147,148] High levels correlate with adverse prognostic factors and may militate against response by forming immune complexes, with rapid clearing of the antibody. A small clinical trial has been conducted with the radioimmunotherapy agent ^{90}Y–ibritumomab tiuxetan (Zevalin).[149]

Table 116-6 Frontline Therapy (Chemoimmunotherapy) for Chronic Lymphocytic Leukemia

Reference	Regimen	Pts.	%CR	%OR	Resp. Duration Med. (Months)
Rai et al[90]	FLU	170	20	63	251
	CLB	181	4	37	14
FCSG[127]	FLU	52	23	71	NR
	CAP	48	17	60	7
Leporrier et al[128]	FLU	336	40	71	32
	CHOP	351	30	71	30
	CAP	237	15	58	27
Robak[122]	CDA+PRED	126	47	87	21
	CLB+PRED	103	12	45	18
O'Brien et al[131]	FC	34	35	88	NR
Robak et al[135]	CDA+C	62	30	88	NR
Flynn et al[133]	FC	141	22	70	41
	F	137	6	50	18
Kay et al[136]	PCR	33	33	94	NR
Byrd et al[91]	FLU	53	47	90	NR
	FLU+RIT	51	28	72	
Keating et al[153]	FLU+CYT+RIT	224	70	95	NR
O'Brien et al[155]	FLU+Alem	36	42	92	NR
Kay et al[154]	FLU+RIT	20	20	85	NR

Alem = alemtuzumab; CAP = cyclophosphamide, doxorubicin, prednisone; CDA = chlorodeoxyadenosine; CHOP = cyclophosphamide, hydroxydaunomycin (doxorubicin), Oncovin (vincristine), prednisone; CLB = chlorambucil; CR = complete response; CYT = cyclophosphamide; F = fludarabine; FC = fludarabine, cyclophosphamide; FLU = fludarabine; NR = not reported; OR = overall response; PCR = pentostatin, cyclophosphamide, rituximab; PRED = prednisone; Pts. = patients; RIT = rituximab.

Chemoimmunotherapy Rituximab sensitizes cells in lymphoid cell lines to a variety of chemotherapeutic agents, including fludarabine and cyclophosphamide.[150] It also downregulates *BCL2*, perhaps by inhibiting interleukin 10.[151] Fludarabine downregulates CD55 and CD59 on CLL cells.[152] The reduction in these antigens is considered to enhance cytotoxicity mediated by complement lysis with rituximab or alemtuzumab therapy.

Three chemoimmunotherapy programs using rituximab have been developed (Table 116-6).[91,153,154] In a CALGB study, fludarabine was combined with either simultaneous or sequential rituximab, followed by consolidation rituximab in both arms.[91] The complete remission rate was higher with the simultaneous protocol (47% vs. 33%), with no additional toxicity apart from neutropenia. No increase in infections was noted. A combination of fludarabine, cyclophosphamide, and rituximab for previously untreated patients had a complete response rate of 70%, and 30% to 40% of patients achieved PCR negativity for the IgV_H gene.[153] Time to treatment failure was significantly longer than in earlier studies. Pentostatin, cyclophosphamide, and rituximab was very active and safe in a small group of patients.[154] Alemtuzumab was combined with fludarabine in a small group of patients.[157] A high response rate occurred in previously treated patients, with a 25% complete response rate. Comparison of two consecutive CALGB studies suggest a higher complete response rate and longer progression-free survival when patients treated with a combination of fludarabine and rituximab are compared with patients treated using fludarabine alone.[157]

SALVAGE THERAPY AND NEW AGENTS

Fewer data are available for salvage therapy in CLL, but discovery of the activity of fludarabine, 2-CdA, and DCF has enlivened this area of research (Table 116-7). Combinations of these regimens with alkylating agents, anthracyclines, or mitoxantrone have been developed.[156–167] In one comparative study, fludarabine had a higher response rate than did CAP.[127]

Single-agent purine analogs have response rates of approximately 50% in relapsed and refractory CLL (10% to 15% complete response). Increasingly, combinations of purine analogs with DNA-active agents such as cyclophosphamide, doxorubicin, or mitoxantrone are being explored, with the achievement of high overall response rates. Comparison of such studies is difficult because of the diversity of patients entered in the protocols. The addition of rituximab or alemtuzumab (or both) appears to increase response rates in salvage regimens.[156,166–168]

And yet more new agents are being investigated in CLL.[169] Depsipeptide (a histone deacetylase inhibitor), flavopiridol (a cyclin-dependent kinase inhibitor),[170] nelarabine (a guanosine analog),[171] and new antibodies such as Hu1D10 and epratuzumab are all under investigation. Flavopiridol and nelarabine have been demonstrated to have significant clinical activity.[169,170]

Table 116-7 Salvage Therapy for Relapsed Refractory Chronic Lymphocytic Leukemia

Regimen	Reference	Patients	%CR	%OR
FLU	Keating et al[118]	68	13	57
FLU	FCSG[127]	48	13	35
CAP	FCSG[127]	48	6	21
FLU+Doxo	Robertson et al[158]	30	3	55
FLU+Mitox	Tsimberidou et al[159]	53	8	55
FLU+Cyclo	O'Brien et al[131]	94	10	70
FLU+Cyclo+Mitox	O'Brien et al[161]	60	50	78
2-CdA	Robak et al[160]	184	13	48
2-CdA+Cyclo	Bosch et al[162]	13	8	62
2-CdA+Cyclo	Van Den Neste et al[163]	29	15	45
DCF+Cyclo	Montillo et al[164]	23	17	74
2-CdA+Ritux	Wierda et al[166]	26	15	68
FLU+Cyclo+Ritux	Weiss et al[165]	177	25	73
FLU+Alem	Elter et al[156]	34	29	85
FLU+Cyclo+Ritux+Alem	Wierda et al[167]	21	14	52

2-CdA = 2-chlorodeoxyadenosine; Alem = alemtuzumab; CAP = cyclophosphamide, doxorubicin, prednisone; CR = complete response; Cyclo = cyclophosphamide; DCF = 2'-deoxycoformycin; Doxo = doxorubicin; FLU = fludarabine; Mitox = mitroxitrone; OR = overall response; Ritux = rituximab.

Immunotherapy The success of cellular therapy in nonablative (minimal) stem cell transplantation (see "Stem Cell Transplantation," next) encouraged exploration of other approaches to immunotherapy. The administration of expanded autologous T cells resulted in a reduction in nodes and spleen in one-third of patients.[172] Autologous CLL cells have been transfused to induce expression of CD154 (CD40 ligand). Such infusions can induce CLL-specific T-cell responses and have been associated with clinical improvement.[173] Likewise, cells expressing both CD40L and interleukin 2 have been studied.[174] Use of agents such as interferon-β, tumor necrosis factor receptor binding agents, interleukin 2, and interleukin 4 has been disappointing.[175–177]

Stem Cell Transplantation Autologous stem cell transplantation (SCT) has been conducted in several series.[178,179] The technique is safe and shows a lower relapse rate in patients transplanted at first response as an intensification procedure, as compared with patients transplanted in the presence of active disease as a salvage regimen. Analysis of patients receiving autologous and allogeneic transplantation suggests a continuing relapse rate in patients receiving autologous transplantation. A number of patients who received allogeneic transplantation are in continuing remission.[180] Patients who become MRD-negative have much longer remission durations.[180]

Allogeneic SCT has not been widely performed in CLL because of the relatively advanced age of most patients. And because complete responses were rare with traditional therapy, collection of autologous stem cells was not an option. More recently, with younger patients being diagnosed, allogeneic SCT is being more seriously considered as an option for patients below the age of 55 years. Patients treated with purine analogs before SCT may have a lower incidence of graft-versus-host disease and a better outcome. Allogeneic transplantation patients have a significantly longer survival if the transplantation procedure occurs while their disease is chemosensitive rather than after their CLL becomes refractory.[181,182]

An interesting new development in the area of allogeneic transplantation in CLL is the development of reduced-intensity transplantation. This procedure is nonmyeloablative and relies on the graft-versus-leukemia effect for efficacy. These transplantations can be performed in patients older than 70 years of age.[182,183] Preliminary results demonstrate that engraftment occurs in almost all patients and that patients with sensitive disease who are transplanted have a better outcome than do patients with resistant disease.

The extent of and response to prior treatments are important prognostic factors for minimal stem cell transplantation.[182] Addition of rituximab to the preoperative immunosuppression regimen may reduce the incidence of graft-versus-host disease and speed engraftment. In the largest study, 18 patients were treated with nonablative conditioning regimens of fludarabine and cyclophosphamide, with or without rituximab.[183] At 1 year, survival and progression-free survival were comparable to that in patients who had received high-dose conventional transplantation. PCR negativity can be achieved with nonablative transplantation—a result that is attributed to the graft-versus-leukemia effect. Future studies will establish the place of this transplantation modality in the context of CLL. Although current studies are investigational, attempts at intensive programs with allogeneic or autologous stem cell support may be an important component of future curative strategies.

Minimal Residual Disease With the advent of higher complete response rates by NCIWG criteria, attention has been directed to developing sensitive methods of detecting residual clonal CLL cells that co-express CD5 and CD19. Four-parameter flow cytometry[184] and a return of IgV_H gene rearrangement to a germline configuration by PCR are two such methodologic approaches.[146,185]

Chemotherapy regimens, monoclonal antibody combination therapy, and alemtuzumab treatment have each demonstrated that MRD-negative patients have an outcome superior to those who are MRD-positive. The fludarabine, cyclophosphamide, and mitoxantrone regimen achieved MRD negativity in 10 of 37 patients (27%), with a marked improvement in survival. Eradication of MRD using alemtuzumab is increasingly being tested in CLL patients in complete or partial remission, but with residual disease by clinical or immunophenotypic findings. PCR negativity for IgV_H in the marrow can be achieved in approximately 40% of patients entered in the clinical trials.[155,185–188] Most patients have reduction in blood and marrow involvement, but nodal disease is more difficult to eradicate.[186] The approach is not without risk, however; opportunistic infections occur in 20% to 60% of patients.[186] Patients who become PCR-negative have a longer time to progression of the CLL.[155,184–189] Maintenance therapy with alemtuzumab has been shown to be associated with long survival in a small group of patients.[190]

Monoclonal antibodies such as rituximab and alemtuzumab are likely to have their maximum benefit in patients with MRD.

Radiation Therapy The major indication for radiation therapy in CLL is large, bulky lymphoid masses causing compression symptomatology, especially if patients are unresponsive to chemotherapy. Splenic irradiation has been performed in patients with painful splenic enlargement or cytopenias thought to be related to hypersplenism. CLL lymphocytes are sensitive to radiation, and shrinkage of lymphoid masses is usual after treatment.[191] Splenic radiation does not usually give long-term control; if the patient is in a satisfactory clinical state, splenectomy is the preferred option.

Leukapheresis Therapy Intensive leukapheresis has been attempted as a method of control of CLL. In one study, 2.9×10^{11} cells could be removed on an alternate-day basis.[192] More than 50% of patients had significant elevations of hemoglobin and platelet counts that coincided with a decrease in lymphocyte counts and size of spleen and lymph nodes. Disease control was maintained for a year.

Apheresis is seldom necessary for leukocytosis per se, because leukostasis rarely causes symptoms such as shortness of breath associated with pulmonary infiltrates or neurologic symptoms unless the white cell count is extremely high ($> 400 \times 10^9$/L). Sustained decreases in white cell count are uncommon, and concurrent administration of effective chemotherapy is necessary.

Splenectomy A number of patients with advanced CLL develop splenomegaly and pancytopenia. This syndrome often responds to effective chemotherapy. A number of studies have suggested hematologic and survival benefits from splenectomy in patients with CLL. Suggested benefits include removal of the major site of disease, control of hypersplenism, and improvement in immune-mediated cytopenias.

In a series of 55 patients, perioperative mortality (9%) was more common in patients with poor performance status. Improvements in platelet count, neutrophil count, and hemoglobin occurred in 81%, 59%, and 33% of patients respectively. The mortality of splenectomy (formerly 20%) has decreased in modern times, especially with laparoscopic procedures.[193] Among Rai stage IV patients, a trend toward improved survival was noted using a case-control method of analysis. Splenectomy is the recommended treatment for patients with massive splenomegaly and cytopenia not responsive to other modalities.

CLINICAL MANAGEMENT OF PATIENTS

A diagnosis of leukemia is a major emotional challenge to patients. Many doctors tell patients that they have CLL but need not be concerned, and that the recommended approach is no treatment. Careful explanation of this approach should be based on the natural history of the disorder, emphasizing that some patients never need treatment and that early treatment has not been shown to be beneficial. Patients need to be reassured that effective treatments are available when treatment becomes necessary because of progressive disease or symptoms. Explanation of newer prognostic factors will reinforce the no-treatment decision. In addition, knowledge that survival in many early-stage (smoldering) CLL patients is the same as in the age- and sex-matched general population is comforting to patients. Development of a close relationship with patients, particularly those in the early phases of disease, and careful responses to questions raised are important in providing psychological and emotional support to the patient and family. The rapidly increasing range of options for therapy, particularly for younger patients, provides a basis for optimism when treatment becomes necessary.

Infections The major complications that occur during the management of CLL are episodes of infection and development of bone marrow and immune system failure with progressive tumor burden.

The immune deficiencies of CLL—hypogammaglobulinemia, impaired T-cell function, and impaired opsonization—have led to the fallacious concept that patients with CLL are immunologic cripples.[194,195] Patients who receive high doses of intravenous gamma globulin experience a reduction in the frequency of infections, mainly moderate ones, and the infections that do occur can then be easily controlled with outpatient antibiotics.[196] The cost of this strategy is substantial.

Rather than treat a low IgG laboratory value, a reasonable clinical recommendation is to treat with prophylactic gamma globulin only those patients with a history of repeated infections, particularly major ones such as pneumonia or septicemia. The usual dose is 200 to 400 mg/kg by intravenous infusion given at 3- to 4-week intervals. If no change is noted in the frequency of infections, the treatment should be discontinued. If a substantial decrease in the incidence of infections is seen, treatment at gradually extended intervals might be considered.

The approach to management of the most common sinobronchial infections is to use broad-spectrum conventional antibiotics such as penicillins, cephalosporins, quinolones, or sulfamethoxazole–trimethoprim. Most patients respond to such treatment, but some develop chronic sinusitis, which may require referral to an ear, nose, and throat specialist. CLL infiltrates of the sinonasal mucosa are common.

Most infections occur late in the disease, after therapy has been initiated, when progressive CLL with neutropenia and possible worsening of immune function occur. During this phase, herpes zoster and herpes simplex infections in particular may occur, and early institution of treatment with antivirals is effective in dealing with these problems. Herpes zoster is usually dermatomal and rarely becomes disseminated.

Following the use of the purine analogs, steroids, and alemtuzumab, opportunistic infections with organisms such as *P. carinii* are a concern. Although some clinicians routinely give sulfamethoxazole–trimethoprim or aerosolized pentamidine prophylaxis, no clinical trial has substantiated the efficacy of this approach. While the incidence of opportunistic infections is low, vigilant observation and early initiation of treatment appears reasonable. Routine prophylaxis may be more cost-effective than expensive diagnostic testing, however. Structured clinical trials to address the efficacy of prophylaxis against bacterial and viral infections should be encouraged.

Despite the immunosuppression that occurs in CLL, mycobacterial infections are uncommon. They should be considered, however, in any patient who develops persistent fever or unexplained pulmonary infiltrates. In patients receiving prophylaxis, early investigation by bronchoalveolar lavage of unexplained or unresponsive pulmonary infiltrates is recommended to identify opportunistic pathogens such as CMV, herpes simplex virus, *P. carinii,* or mycobacteria. The use of growth factors such as granulocyte colony–stimulating factor (G-CSF) or granulocyte macrophage colony–stimulating factor (GM-CSF) in patients with CLL who have neutropenia should follow established guidelines for management of infections in such patients. The addition of G-CSF to Fludara in advanced-stage, previously treated patients reduced the incidence of neutropenia and pneumonia as compared with the incidence in a historical population.[197] An initial trial of antibiotics is usually sufficient, but poor response to antibiotics with persistent neutropenia should lead to the use of G-CSF or GM-CSF. Because alemtuzumab is also intensely immunosuppressive, especially of the T-cell system, similar guidelines for prophylaxis against *P. carinii* have been developed, and antiviral agents are routinely prescribed.

Anemia The anemia of CLL is multifaceted. A number of patients develop anemia without clear evidence of development of progressive disease in other areas, suggesting an inhibitory effect of the leukemia on red-cell production such as occurs in other malignant diseases. In other situations, extensive marrow infiltration is likely to be a cause. AIHA, usually associated with a positive Coombs test, hyperbilirubinemia, reticulocytosis, low haptoglobin, and elevation of serum lactic dehydrogenase is not uncommon. Shortened red-cell survival (as is common in other cancers) may be a factor—and may be accentuated in patients with major splenomegaly. Other patients (usually Coombs-negative) develop pure red-cell aplasia with disappearance of red-cell precursors from the bone marrow.

Management of AIHA should follow established patterns, with the initial use of corticosteroids to try to achieve disease remission. If this tactic fails, splenectomy is usually associated with a satisfactory response. The response of pure red-cell aplasia to cyclosporine is gratifying.[198] Renal function needs to be closely monitored in patients with refractory AIHA or thrombocytopenia (which may also respond to cyclosporine therapy). The effect of cyclosporine may be to diminish the activity of suppressor T cells, which can inhibit marrow erythropoiesis.

Transfusion of packed red cells is usually indicated when patients are clinically symptomatic or have a hemoglobin level below 9 g/dL. The risks of transfusion in patients with CLL are similar to the risks seen in other patients. Leukocyte-trapping filters are useful for patients who are having repeated episodes of fever.

A randomized comparative trial demonstrated that recombinant human erythropoietin therapy in patients with Coombs-negative anemia resulted in an increase in hemoglobin level in a substantial number of patients.[199] As compared with only 1 in 6 patients in the placebo group, half of the erythropoietin-treated group experienced a hematocrit increase of 6%. Treatment was well tolerated and was associated with significant improvement in energy level and a sense of psychological and physical well-being. The dose administered was 150 U/kg subcutaneously three times per week. Response was usually seen within the first 6 to 8 weeks of therapy. More recently, single weekly doses of erythropoietin were demonstrated to be as effective as three-times-per-week dosing. A new form of erythropoietin, darbepoetin (Aranesp) has been demonstrated to be effective in CLL.[200]

Thrombocytopenia Patients can develop thrombocytopenia by mechanisms similar to those for anemia, with suppression of production in the presence of modest or extensive tumor burden or antibody-mediated mechanisms. In addition, dilutional effects associated with splenomegaly are not uncommon. The thrombocytopenia that occurs initially is usually modest. Severe thrombocytopenia (< 50,000/μL) usually occurs only late in the disease process and signals poor prognosis.

Response to treatment of CLL is usually associated with improvement in thrombocytopenia. However, if patients fail to respond to alkylating agent or purine analog treatment with a reduction in tumor burden, thrombocytopenia is often aggravated. Splenectomy is a clinically useful procedure in patients with or without clinical splenic enlargement.[193] Improvement in platelet count occurs in most patients, and for patients with severe thrombocytopenia, platelet transfusion frequency is usually reduced. It has been suggested that splenectomy improves prognosis in Rai stage III and IV disease.[193] Corticosteroids, danazol, high-dose intravenous gamma globulin, and rituximab have all been used judiciously, with variable results, in patients with thrombocytopenia. Cyclosporine is often useful in cases with megakaryocytic hypoplasia.[198]

CLL VARIANTS

The major variants of CLL seen in practice are PLL, which may be of the B- or T-cell type, and splenic lymphoma with circulating villous lymphocytes (SLVL) or marginal zone leukemia (MZL). In addition, patients with MCL can present in a leukemic phase; the differential diagnosis from CLL is sometimes difficult. MCL patients usually have a chromosomal translocation, t(11;14), with additional changes and an increase in cyclin D1 levels, which are characteristic. MCL patients also usually present with massive splenomegaly.[172]

The response to treatment and the prognosis in PLL and MCL are much less satisfactory than in CLL, with only transient responses to alkylating agent regimens, CHOP, or purine analogs. Intensive regimens such as hyper-CVAD (fractionated cyclophosphamide, vincristine, Adriamycin, dexamethasone) followed by transplant are useful in MCL.[201] Bortezomib, a proteasome inhibitor is a promising new agent in MCL.[202] Complete and partial responses have been noted.

The management of SLVL often involves splenectomy, with most patients responding satisfactorily.[203] Purine analogs and rituximab are both active in SLVL and MZL. Rituximab appears to have resulted in a major improvement in prognosis.

Occasionally, patients with follicular lymphoma in a leukemic phase are misdiagnosed as CLL. However, when the correct diagnosis is subsequently made, this disease should be treated as any low-grade lymphoma.

Large granular lymphocytosis characterized by monoclonal proliferation of a T-suppressor cell subset, immunophenotypically characterized as CD3+, CD8+, CD56+, and CD57+, often does not need treatment for substantial periods of time.[204] Antitumor treatment is usually not indicated; the use of G-CSF or GM-CSF for neutropenia is usually satisfactory. Alkylating agents, purine analogs, and cyclosporine all show some activity.

The management of true T-cell CLL (T-CLL) is less satisfactory than that of B-cell CLL.[205] Although purine analogs are highly effective in reducing the number of normal T cells, they are less effective in the management of T-CLL. The drug 2-CdA appears to be more effective than Fludara.[205] Campath-1H is associated with a high response rate in T-CLL/PLL. Two separate studies have demonstrated that alemtuzumab achieves the highest complete remission rates in patients with T-cell CLL/PLL.[206,207] A number of patients have had remissions even if extensively previously treated with other regimens, including pentostatin.

RECOMMENDED APPROACH TO THERAPY

It was noted earlier in this chapter that immediate treatment can be recommended for patients with advanced-stage disease or a large tumor burden, and for patients with symptoms related to their disease or to repeated infections.[79] Otherwise, a period of observation is recommended. During observation, it can be determined whether the patient is developing progressive disease or a rapid doubling time. If the doubling time for the patient's lymphocyte count is less than 12 months, survival is significantly shorter than if the patient shows a longer doubling time. Treatment can be recommended on that basis. In younger patients who are being considered for potentially curative therapy, including autologous or allogeneic SCT, earlier treatment might be considered.

Mature data now show that purine analogs have a higher response rate than do alkylating agent regimens. Initial therapy with purine-based combination regimens is reasonable and is becoming more common. However, the long-term follow-up of comparative trials is necessary before this recommendation can be considered proven.

The goals and duration of therapy for CLL are poorly defined. However, if patients are responding to and tolerating therapy, it appears reasonable to continue until complete remission is obtained or until continued improvement in disease is no longer noted or toxicity supervenes. There is no clear evidence that maintenance or consistent therapy in CLL is of benefit, and the optimal duration of treatment with purine analogs has not yet been established. Many patients receiving these treatments as initial therapy will achieve complete remission after two to three courses. Whether continued treatment after complete remission is of clinical benefit is not known. Most experience has been obtained with the use of purine analogs given for six courses. The promisingly high complete remission rates with chemoimmunotherapy regimens,[91,153] the success of treatment of MRD with alemtuzumab and autologous bone marrow transplantation, and the promising results from nonablative allogeneic transplantation suggest that CLL should begin to be considered a potentially curable disease.

REFERENCES

1. Chioriazzi N, Rai KR, Ferrarini M. Mechanism of disease: chronic lymphocytic leukemia. N Engl J Med 2005;352:804–15.
2. Virchow R. Weisses Blut. Froriep's Notizen 1845;36:148.
3. Bennett JH. Case of hypertrophy of the spleen and liver, in which death took place from suppuration of the blood. Edinburgh Med Surg J 1845;64:413.
4. Bennett JH. Leucocythaemia or white cell blood. Edinburgh: Sutherland and Knox; 1852.
5. Virchow R. Die Leukamie. In: Virchow R, editor. Gesammelte Abhandlungen zur wissenschaftlichen Medizin. Frankfurt: Meidinger; 1856. p. 190.
6. Gowers WR. Splenic leucocythaemia. In: Reynolds JR, editor. System of medicine. Vol. 5. New York: Macmillan; 1879. p. 216.
7. Kundrat H. Uber Lympho-Sarkomatosis. Wien Klin Wochenschr 1893;6:211.
8. Turk W. Ein System der Lymphomatosen. Wien Klin Wochenschr 1903;16:1073.
9. Ehrlich P. Farbenanalytische Untersuchungen zur Histologie und Klinik des Blutes. Berlin: Hirschwald; 1891.
10. Minot GR, Isaacs R. Lymphatic leukemia: age, incidence, duration, and benefit derived from irradiation. Boston Med Surg J 1924;191:1.
11. Boggs DR, Sofferman SA, Wintrobe MM, Cartwright GE. Factors influencing the duration of survival of patients with chronic lymphocytic leukemia. Am J Med 1966;40:243–54.
12. Hansen MM. Chronic lymphocytic leukaemia clinical studies based on 189 cases followed for a long time. Scand J Haematol Suppl 1973;18:3–286.
13. Galton DAG. The pathogenesis of chronic lymphocytic leukemia. Can Med Assoc J 1966;94:1005–10.
14. Dameshek W. Chronic lymphocytic leukemia: an accumulative disease of immunologically incompetent lymphocytes. Blood 1967;29:566–84.
15. Rai KR, Sawitsky A, Cronkite EP, et al. Clinical staging of chronic lymphocytic leukemia. Blood 1975;46:219–34.
16. Binet JL, Auquier A, Dighiero G, et al. A new prognostic classification of chronic lymphocytic leukemia derived from a multivariate survival analysis. Cancer 1981;48:198–206.
17. Schroeder HW Jr, Dighiero G. The pathogenesis of CLL: analysis of the antibody repertoire. Immunol Today 1994;15: 288–94.
18. Chiorazzi N, Ferrarini M. B-cell chronic lymphocytic leukemia: lessons learned from studies of the B-cell antigen receptor. Annu Rev Immunol 2003;21:841–94.
19. Stevenson FK, Caligaris-Cappio F. Chronic lymphocytic leukemia: revelations from the B-cell receptor. Blood 2004;103:4389–95.
20. Jemal A, Murray T, Ward E, et al. Cancer statistics, 2005. CA Cancer J Clin 2005;55:10–30.

21. Hernandez JA, Land KJ, McKenna RW. Leukemias, myeloma, and other lymphoreticular neoplasms. Cancer 1995;75:381–94.
22. Ries LAG, Eisner MP, Kosary CL, et al., editors. SEER Cancer Statistics Review, 1973–1999. Bethesda (MD): National Cancer Institute; 2002.
23. Call TG, Phyliky RL, Noel P, et al. Incidence of chronic lymphocytic leukemia in Olmstead County, Minnesota, 1935 through 1989 with emphasis on changes in initial stage at diagnosis. Mayo Clin Proc 1994;69:323–8.
24. Fleming AF. The epidemiology of lymphomas and leukemias in Africa: an overview. Leuk Res 1985;9:735–40.
25. Yang C, Zhang X. Incidence survey of leukemia in China. Chin Med Sci J 1991;6:65–70.
26. Haenszel W, Kurihara M. Studies of Japanese migrants. I. Mortality from cancer and other diseases among Japanese in the United States. J Natl Cancer Inst 1968;40:43–68.
27. Yanagihara ET, Blaisdell RK, Hayashi T, Lukes RJ. Malignant lymphoma in Hawaii-Japanese: a retrospective morphologic survey. Hematol Oncol 1989;7:219–32.
28. Arp EW, Wolf PH, Chckoway H. Lymphocytic leukemia and exposure to benzene and other solvents in the rubber industry. J Occup Med 1983;25:598–620.
29. Blair A, White D. Leukemia cell types and agricultural practices in Nebraska. Arch Environ Health 1985;40:211–4.
30. Institute of Medicine of the National Academies, Board of Health Promotion and Disease Prevention (HPDP). Committee to review the health effects in Vietnam veterans of exposure to herbicides (4th biennial update). Veterans and Agent Orange, Update 2002. Washington (DC): National Academy Press; 2003. p. 1–299.
31. Waterhouse D, Carman WJ, Schottenfeld D, et al. Cancer incidence in the rural community of Tecumseh, Michigan: a pattern of increased lymphopoietic neoplasms. Cancer 1996;77:763–70.
32. Preston DL, Kusumi S, Tomonoga M, et al. Cancer incidence in atomic bomb survivors. Part II. Leukemia lymphoma and multiple myeloma. Radiat Res 1994;137(Suppl 2):568–97.
33. Yuille MR, Matutes E, Marossy A, et al. Familial chronic lymphocytic leukemia: a survey and review of published studies. Br J Haematol 2000;109:794–9.
34. Capalbo S, Trerotoli P, Ciancio A, et al. Increased risk of lymphoproliferative disorders in relatives of patients with B-cell chronic lymphocytic leukemia: relevance of the degree of familial linkage. Eur J Haematol 2000;65:114–7.
35. Rawstron AC, Yuile MR, Fuller J, et al. Inherited predisposition to CLL is detectable as subclinical monoclonal B-lymphocyte expansion. Blood 2002;100:2289–91.
36. Rawstron AC, Green MJ, Kuzmick A, et al. Monoclonal B-lymphocytes with characteristics of "indolent" chronic lymphocytic leukemias are present in 3.5% of adults with normal blood counts. Blood 2002;100:635–9.
37. Kyle RA, Therneu TM, Rajkumar SV, et al. A long-term study of prognosis in monoclonal gammopathy of undetermined significance. N Engl J Med 2002;346:564–9.
38. Brok-Simoni F, Rechavi G, Katzir N, Ben-Bassat I. Chronic lymphocytic leukemia in twin sisters, monozygous but not identical. Lancet 1987;1:329–30.
39. Chen L, Widhopf G, Huynh L, et al. Expression of ZAP-70 is associated with increased B-cell receptor signaling in chronic lymphocytic leukemia. Blood 2002;100:4609–14.
40. Geisler CH, Larsen JK, Hansen NE, et al. Prognostic importance of flow cytometric immunophenotyping of 540 consecutive patients with B-cell lymphocytic leukemia. Blood 1991;78:1795–802.
41. Ruzickova S, Pruss A, Odendahl M, et al. Chronic lymphocytic leukemia preceded by cold agglutinin disease: intraclonal immunoglobulin light chain diversity in VH4-34 expressing single leukemic B cells. Blood 2002;100:3419–22.
42. Caligaris-Cappio F. New insights into the biology of B-chronic lymphocytic leukemia. Hematology (Am Soc Hematol Educ Program) 1999;:249–54.
43. Caligaris-Cappio F. B-chronic lymphocytic leukemia: a malignancy of anti-self B cells. Blood 1996;87:2615–20.
44. Fais F, Ghiotto F, Hashimoto S, et al. Chronic lymphocytic leukemia B cells express restricted sets of mutated and unmutated antigen receptors. J Clin Invest 1998;102:1515–25.
45. Pangalis GA, Angelopoulou MK, Vassilakopoulos TP, et al. B-chronic lymphocytic leukemia, small lymphocytic lymphoma, and lymphoplasmacytic lymphoma including Waldenström's macroglobulinemia: a clinical and morphologic and biologic spectrum of similar disorders. Semin Hematol 1999;36:104–14.
46. Catovsky D. Immunophenotypic analysis of chronic lymphoid leukemias. Rev Clin Exp Hematol 1997;1:3–14.
47. Kilo MN, Dorfman DM. The utility of flow cytometric immunophenotypic analysis in the distinction of small lymphocytic lymphomas/chronic lymphocytic leukemia from mantle cell lymphoma. Am J Clin Pathol 1996;105:541–7.
48. Zomas AP, Matutes E, Morilla R, et al. Expression of the immunoglobulin-associated protein B29 in B-cell disorders with the monoclonal antibody SN8 (*CD79B*). Leukaemia 1996;10:1966–70.
49. Hamblin TJ, Oscier DH. Chronic lymphocytic leukaemia: the nature of the leukaemic cell. Blood Rev 1997;11:119–28.
50. Zupo S, Isnardi L, Magna M, et al. CD38 expression distinguishes two groups of B-cell chronic lymphocytic leukemias with different responses to anti-IgM antibodies and propensity to apoptosis. Blood 1996;88:1365–74.
51. Summerhill RJ, Jackson DG, Galione A. Human CD38 catalyses the production of cyclic ADP ribose. FEBS Lett 1993;335:231–3.
52. Zupo S, Rugari E, Dono M, et al. CD38 signaling by agonistic monoclonal antibody prevents apoptosis of human germinal center B cells. Eur J Immunol 1994;24:1218–22.
53. Damle RN, Wasil T, Fais F, et al. Immunoglobulin V gene mutation status and CD38 expression as novel prognostic indicators in chronic lymphocytic leukemia. Blood 1999;94:1840–7.
54. Matrai Z, Lin K, Dennis M, et al. CD38 expression and IgV_H gene mutation in B-cell chronic lymphocytic leukemia. Blood 2001;997:1902–3.
55. Ibrahim S, Keating M, Do KA, et al. CD38 coexpression as an important prognostic factor in B-cell chronic lymphocytic leukemia. Blood 2001;98:181–6.
56. Durig J, Maschar M, Schmucker U, et al. CD38 expression is an important prognostic marker in chronic lymphocytic leukemia. Leukemia 2002;16:30–5.
57. Hamblin TJ, Orchard JA, Ibbotson RE, et al. CD38 expression and immunoglobulin variable region mutations are independent prognostic variables in chronic lymphocytic leukemia, but CD38 expression may vary during the course of the disease. Blood 2002;99:1023–9.
58. Chevalier P, Penther D, Avet-Loiseau H, et al. CD38 expression and secondary 17p deletion are important prognostic factors in chronic lymphocytic leukaemia. Br J Haematol 2002;116:142–50.
59. D'Arena G, Nunziata G, Coppola G, et al. CD38 expression does not change in B-cell chronic lymphocytic leukemia. Blood 2002;100:3052–60.
60. Beaume A, Brizard A, Dreyfus B, et al. High incidence of serum monoclonal Igs detected by a sensitive immunoblotting technique in B-cell lymphocytic leukemia. Blood 1994;84:1216–9.
61. Caligaris-Cappio F, Hamblin TJ. B-cell chronic lymphocytic leukemia: a bird of a different feather. J Clin Oncol 1999;17:399–408.
62. Bartik MM, Walker D, Kay NE. Impairments in immune cell function in B cell chronic lymphocytic leukemia. Semin Oncol 1998;25:27–33.
63. Diehl LF, Ketchum LH. Autoimmune disease and chronic lymphocytic leukemia: autoimmune hemolytic anemia, pure red cell aplasia, and autoimmune thrombocytopenia. Semin Oncol 1998;24:80–97.
64. DiRaimondo F, Giustolisi R, Cacciola E, et al. Autoimmune hemolytic anemia in chronic lymphocytic leukemia patients treated with fludarabine. Leuk Lymphoma 1993;11:63–8.
65. Myint H, Copplestone JA, Orchard J, et al. Fludarabine-related autoimmune haemolytic anaemia in patients with chronic lymphocytic leukaemia. Br J Haematol 1995;91:341–40.
66. Mauro FR, Foa R, Cerreti R, et al. Autoimmune hemolytic anemia in chronic lymphocytic leukemia: clinical, therapeutic, and prognostic features. Blood 2000;95:2786–92.
67. Dohner H, Stilgenbauer S, Benner A, et al. Genomic aberrations and survival in chronic lymphocytic leukemia. N Engl J Med 2000;343:1910–6.
68. Bullrich F, Negrini M, Croce CM. Molecular genetics of chronic lymphocytic leukemia. Hematology (Am Soc Hematol Educ Program) 1999;:255–8.
69. Hanada J, Delia D, Aiello A, et al. *Bcl-2* gene hypomethylation and high-level expression in B-cell chronic lymphocytic leukemia. Blood 1993;82:1820–8.
70. Hall PA, Lane DP. Tumour suppressors: a developing role for *p53*? Curr Biol 1997;7:144–7.
71. Hamblin TJ, Davis Z, Gardiner A, et al. Unmutated IgV_H genes are associated with a more aggressive form of chronic lymphocytic leukemia. Blood 1999;94:1848–54.
72. Lin K, Sherrington PD, Dennis M, et al. Relationship between *p53* dysfunction CD38 expression and IgV_H mutation in chronic lymphocytic leukemia. Blood 2002;100:1404–9.
73. Krober A, Seiler T, Benner A, et al. V_H mutation status, CD38 expression level, genomic aberrations, and survival in chronic lymphocytic leukemia. Blood 2002;100:1410–6.
74. Messmer B, Messmer D, Allen SI, et al. In vivo measurements document the dynamic cellular kinetics of chronic lymphocytic leukemia B cells. J Clin Invest 2005;115:755–64.
75. Damle RN, Batliwalla FM, Ghiotto F, et al. Telomere length and telomerase activity delineate distinctive replicative features of the B-CLL subgroups defined by immunoglobulin V gene mutations. Blood 2004;103:375–82.
76. Hultdin M, Rosenquist R, Thunberg U, et al. Association between telomere length and VCH gene mutation status in CLL: clinical and biological implications. Br J Cancer 2003;88:593–8.
77. International Workshop on Chronic Lymphocytic Leukemia. Chronic lymphocytic leukemia: recommendations for diagnosis, staging, and response criteria. Ann Intern Med 1989;110:236–8.
78. Cheson BD, Bennett JM, Rai KR, et al. Guidelines for clinical protocols for chronic lymphocytic leukemia (CLL). Recommendations of the NCI-Sponsored Working Group. Am J Hematol 1988;29:152–63.
79. Cheson BC, Bennett JM, Grever M, et al. National Cancer Institute–sponsored Working Group guidelines for chronic lymphocytic leukemia: revised guidelines for diagnosis and treatment. Blood 1996;87:4990–7.
80. Melo JV, Catovsky D, Galton DAG. The relationship between chronic lymphocytic leukaemia and prolymphocytic leukaemia. II. Patterns of evolution of "prolymphocytoid" transformation. Br J Haematol 1986;64:77–86.
81. Catovsky D, Foa R. The lymphoid leukaemias. London: Butterworths; 1990.
82. Stone RM. Prolymphocytic leukemia. Hematol Oncol Clin North Am 1990;4:457–71.
83. Berliner NT. Gamma lymphocytosis and T cell chronic leukemias. Hematol Oncol Clin North Am 1990;4:473–87.
84. Lipshutz MD, Mir R, Rai KR, Sawitsky A. Bone marrow biopsy and clinical staging in chronic lymphocytic leukemia. Cancer 1980;46:1422–7.
85. Pangalis GA, Boussiotis VA, Kittas C. B-chronic lymphocytic leukemia. Disease progression in 150 untreated stage A and B patients as predicted by bone marrow pattern. Nouv Rev Fr Hematol 1988;30:373–5.
86. Rozman C, Montserrat E, Rodriquez-Fernandez JM, et al. Bone marrow histologic pattern, the best single prognostic parameter in chronic lymphocytic leukemia: a multivariate survival analysis of 329 cases. Blood 1984;64:642–8.
87. Giles FJ, O'Brien SM, Keating MJ. Chronic lymphocytic leukemia in (Richter's) transformation. Semin Oncol 1998;25:117–25.
88. Sawitsky A, Rai KR, Glidewell O, et al. Comparison of daily versus intermittent chlorambucil and prednisone therapy in the treatment of patients with chronic lymphocytic leukemia. Blood 1977;50:1049–59.
89. Shustik C, Mick R, Silver R, et al. Treatment of early chronic lymphocytic leukemia: intermittent chlorambucil versus observation. Hematol Oncol 1988;6:7–12.
90. Rai KR, Peterson BL, Appelbaum FR, et al. Fludarabine compared with chlorambucil as primary therapy for chronic lymphocytic leukemia. N Engl J Med 2000;343:1750–7.
91. Byrd JC, Peterson BL, Morrison VA, et al. Randomized phase 2 study of fludarabine with concurrent versus sequential treatment with rituximab in symptomatic, untreated patients with B-cell chronic lymphocytic leukemia: results from Cancer and Leukemia Group B 9712 (CALGB 9712). Blood 2003;101:6–14.
92. Rai KR. A critical analysis of staging in CLL. In: Gale RP, Rai KR, editors. Chronic lymphocytic leukemia: recent progress and future direction: 1987 UCLA symposia on molecular and cellular biology. New series. Vol. 59. New York: Liss; 1987. p. 253–64.
93. Montserrat E, Vinolas N, Reverter JC, Rozman C. Chronic lymphocytic leukemia in early stage "smoldering" and "active" forms. In: Cheson BD, editor. Chronic lymphocytic leukemia: scientific advances and clinical developments. New York: Marcel Dekker; 1993. p. 281.
94. Jaksic B, Vitale B. Total tumour mass score (TTM): a new parameter in chronic lymphocytic leukaemia. Br J Haematol 1981;49:405–13.
95. Zwiebel JA, Cheson BD. Chronic lymphocytic leukemia: staging and prognostic factors. Semin Oncol 1998;25:42–59.
96. Montserrat E, Rozman C. Chronic lymphocytic leukaemia: prognostic factors and natural history. Bailliere Clin Haematol 1993;6:849–66.

97. Dighiero G, Maloun K, Desablens B, et al. Chlorambucil in indolent chronic lymphocytic leukemia. N Engl J Med 1998;338:1506–14.
98. Chan AC, Iwashima M, Turck CW, Weiss A. Zap-70 a 70 kD protein–tyrosine kinase that associates with the TCR zeta chain. Cell 1992;71:649–62.
99. Crespo M, Bosch F, Villamor V, et al. *ZAP-70* expression as a surrogate for immunoglobulin-variable-region mutations in chronic lymphocytic leukemia. N Engl J Med 2003;348:1764–75.
100. Rassetni LZ, Huynh L, Toy TZ, et al. *ZAP-70* compared with immunoglobulin heavy-chain gene mutation status as a predictor of disease progression in CLL. N Engl J Med 2004;351:893–901.
101. Orchard JA, Ibbotson RE, Davis Z, et al. *ZAP-70* expression and prognosis in chronic lymphocytic leukaemia. Lancet 2004;363:105–11.
102. Wiestner A, Rosenwal A, Barry TS, et al. *ZAP-70* expression identifies a CLL subtype with unmutated immunoglobulin genes, inferior clinical outcome and distinct gene expression profile. Blood 2003;101:4944–51.
103. Binet JL, Caligaris-Cappio F, Catovsky D, et al. Perspectives on the use of new diagnostic tools in the treatment of chronic lymphocytic leukaemia. Blood 2005. [In press]
104. Keating MJ, O'Brien S, Robertson L, et al. Chronic lymphocytic leukemia—correlation of response and survival. Leuk Lymphoma 1993;11:167–75.
105. Robertson LE, Hu YO, Butler JJ, et al. Response assessment in chronic lymphocytic leukemia after fludarabine plus prednisone: clinical, pathologic, immunophenotypic, and molecular analysis. Blood 1992;80:29–36.
106. Alberts DS, Chang SY, Chen HSG, et al. Pharmacokinetics and metabolism of chlorambucil in man: a preliminary report. Cancer Treat Rep 1979;6(Suppl):9–17.
107. Ezdinli EZ, Stutzman L. Chlorambucil therapy for lymphomas and chronic lymphocytic leukemia. JAMA 1965;191:444–50.
108. Knospe WH, Loeb V Jr, Huguley CM Jr. Bi-weekly chlorambucil treatment of chronic lymphocytic leukemia. Cancer 1974;33:555–62.
109. Colvin M. A review of the pharmacology and clinical use of cyclophosphamide. In: Pinedo HM, editor. Clinical pharmacology of antineoplastic drugs. Amsterdam: Elsevier–North Holland; 1978. p. 245.
110. Ezdinli EZ, Stutzman L, Aungst CW, Firat D. Corticosteroid therapy for lymphomas and chronic lymphocytic leukemia. Cancer 1969;23:900–9.
111. Galton DAG, Wiltshaw E, Szur L, Dacie JV. The use of chlorambucil and steroids in the treatment of chronic lymphocytic leukemia. Br J Haematol 1961;7:73–98.
112. Jaksic B, Brugiatelli M. High dose continuous chlorambucil vs intermittent chlorambucil plus prednisone for treatment of B-CLL—IGCI CLL-01 trial. Nouv Rev Fr Hematol 1988;30:437–42.
113. Raphael B, Andersen JW, Silber R, et al. Comparison of chlorambucil and prednisone versus cyclophosphamide, vincristine, and prednisone as initial treatment for chronic lymphocytic leukemia: long-term follow-up of an Eastern Cooperative Oncology Group randomized clinical trial. J Clin Oncol 1991;9:770–6.
114. Jaksic B, Brugiatelli M, Krc I, et al. Comparison of high-dose chlorambucil versus Binet's modified CHOP regimen in B-cell chronic lymphocytic leukemia in advanced phase: results of an international multicentric randomized trial. Cancer 1997;79:2107–14
115. French Cooperative Group on Chronic Lymphocytic Leukemia. A randomized clinical trial of chlorambucil versus COP in stage B chronic lymphocytic leukemia. Blood 1990;75:1422–5.
116. French Cooperative Group on Chronic Lymphocytic Leukaemia. Long-term results of the CHOP regimen in stage C chronic lymphocytic leukaemia. Br J Haematol 1989;73:334–40.
117. Grever MR, Kopecky KJ, Coltman CA, et al. Fludarabine monophosphate: a potentially useful agent in chronic lymphocytic leukemia. Nouv Rev Fr Hematol 1988;30:457–9.
118. Keating MJ, Kantarjian H, Talpaz M, et al. Fludarabine: a new agent with major activity against chronic lymphocytic leukemia. Blood 1989;74:19–25.
119. O'Brien S, Kantarjian H, Beran M, et al. Results of fludarabine and prednisone therapy in 264 patients with chronic lymphocytic leukemia with multivariate analysis derived prognostic model for response to treatment. Blood 1993;82:1695–700.
120. Saven A, Carrera CJ, Carson DA, et al. 2-Chlorodeoxyadenosine treatment of refractory chronic lymphocytic leukemia. Leuk Lymphoma 1991;5(Suppl):133–8.
121. Juliusson G, Liliemark J. High complete remission rate from 2-chloro-2'-deoxyadenosine in previously treated patients with B cell chronic lymphocytic leukemia. J Clin Oncol 1993;11:679–89.
122. Robak T. Cladribine in the treatment of chronic lymphocytic leukemia. Leuk Lymphoma 2001;40:551–64.
123. Dillman RO, Mick R, McIntyre OR. Pentostatin in chronic lymphocytic leukemia: a phase II trial of Cancer and Leukemia Group B. J Clin Oncol 1989;7:433–8.
124. Ho AD, Thaler J, Stryckmans P, et al. Pentostatin in refractory chronic lymphocytic leukemia: a phase II trial of the European Organization for Research and Treatment of Cancer. J Natl Cancer Inst 1990;82:1416–20.
125. Wijermans PW, Gerrits WBJ, Haak HL. Severe immunodeficiency in patients treated with fludarabine monophosphate. Eur J Haematol 1993;50:292–6.
126. Morrison VA, Rai KR, Peterson BL, et al. Therapy-related myeloid leukemias are observed in patients with chronic lymphocytic leukemia after treatment with fludarabine and chlorambucil: results of an Intergroup study, Cancer and Leukemia Group B 9011. J Clin Oncol 2002;20:3878–84.
127. Johnson S, Smith AG, Loffler H, et al. Multicentre prospective randomised trial of fludarabine versus cyclophosphamide, doxorubicin, and prednisone (CAP) for the treatment of advanced-stage chronic lymphocytic leukaemia. The French Cooperative Group on CLL. Lancet 1996;347:1432–8.
128. Leporrier S, Chevret B, Cazin B, et al. Randomized comparison of fludarabine, CAP and CHOP in 938 previously untreated stage B and C chronic lymphocytic leukemia patients. Blood 2001;98:2319–25.
129. Eichhorst BF, Busch R, Stauch M, et al. Fludarabine (F) induces higher response rates in first line therapy of older patients (pts) with advanced chronic lymphocytic leukemia (CLL) than chlorambucil: interim analysis of a phase III study of the German CLL Study Group (GCLLSG) [abstract]. Blood 2003;102:109a.
130. Yamauchi T, Nowak BJ, Keating MJ, et al. DNA repair initiated in chronic lymphocytic leukemia lymphocytes by 4-hydroperoxycyclophosphamide is inhibited by fludarabine and clofarabine. Clin Cancer Res 2001;7:3580–9.
131. O'Brien SM, Kantarjian HM, Cortes J, et al. Results of the fludarabine and cyclophosphamide combination regimen in chronic lymphocytic leukemia. J Clin Oncol 2001;19:1414–20.
132. Flinn IW, Byrd JC, Morrison C, et al. Fludarabine cyclophosphamide with filgrastim support in patients with previously untreated indolent lymphoid malignancies. Blood 2000;96:71–5.
133. Flinn IW, Kumm E, Grever MR, et al. Fludarabine and cyclophosphamide produces a higher complete response rate and more durable remissions than fludarabine in patients with previously untreated CLL: Intergroup Trial E2997 [abstract]. Blood 2004;104:139a.
134. Eichhorst BF, Busch R, Hopfinger G, et al. Fludarabine plus cyclophosphamide (FC) induces higher remission rates and longer progression free survival (PFS) than fludarabine (F) alone in first line therapy of advanced chronic lymphocytic leukemia (CLL): results of a phase III study (CLL4 protocol) of the German CLL Study Group (GCLLSG) [abstract]. Blood 2003;102:72a.
135. Robak T, Blonski JZ, Kasznicki M, et al. Cladribine combined with cyclophosphamide is highly effective in the treatment of chronic lymphocytic leukemia. Hematol J 2002;3:244–50.
136. Weiss MA, Maslak PG, Jurcic JG, et al. Pentostatin and cyclophosphamide: an effective new regimen in previously treated patients with chronic lymphocytic leukemia. J Clin Oncol 2003;21:1278–84.
137. Bosch F, Ferrer A, Lopez-Guillermo A, et al. Fludarabine, cyclophosphamide and mitoxantrone in the treatment of resistant or relapsed chronic lymphocytic leukemia. Br J Haematol 2002;119:976–84.
138. Bosch F, Ferrer A, Villamor M, et al. Combination chemotherapy with fludarabine, cyclophosphamide and mitoxantrone (FCM) induces a high response rate in previously untreated CLL [abstract]. Ann Oncol 2005;16(Suppl 5):v43.
139. McLaughlin P, Grillo-Lopez A, Link BK, et al. Rituximab chimeric anti-CD20 monoclonal antibody therapy for relapsed indolent lymphoma: half of patients respond to a four-dose program. J Clin Oncol 1998;16:2825–33.
140. Huhn D, von Schilling C, Wilhelm M, et al. Rituximab therapy of patients with B-cell chronic lymphocytic leukemia. Blood 2001;98:1326–31.
141. O'Brien SM, Kantarjian H, Thomas DA, et al. Rituximab dose escalation trial in chronic lymphocytic leukemia. J Clin Oncol 2001;19:2165–70.
142. Byrd JD, Murphy T, Howard RS, et al. Rituximab using a thrice weekly dosing schedule in B-cell chronic lymphocytic leukemia and small lymphocytic lymphoma demonstrates clinical activity and acceptable toxicity. J Clin Oncol 2001;19:2153–64.
143. Keating MJ, Flinn I, Jain V, et al. Therapeutic role of alemtuzumab (Campath-1H) in patients who have failed fludarabine: results of a large international study. Blood 2002;99:3554–61.
144. Faderl S, Thomas DA, O'Brien S, et al. Combined use of alemtuzumab plus rituximab in patients with relapsed and refractory lymphoid malignancies [abstract]. Blood 2002;100(11 Pt 2):206b.
145. Lundin J, Kimby E, Bjorkholm M, et al. Phase II trial of subcutaneous anti-CD52 monoclonal antibody alemtuzumab (Campath-1H) as first-line treatment for patients with B-cell chronic lymphocytic leukemia (BCLL). Blood 2002;100:768–73.
146. Stilgenbauer S, Krober A, Winkler D, et al. Efficacy of subcutaneous alemtuzumab (Campath-1H) in genetic high-risk, fludarabine-refractory CLL: CLL^{2}H study of the German CLL Study Group (GCLLSG) [abstract]. Ann Oncol 2005;16:v43.
147. Manshouri T, Do KA, Wang X, et al. Circulating CD20 is detectable in the plasma of patient with chronic lymphocytic leukemia and is of prognostic significance. Blood 2003;101:2507–13.
148. Manshouri T, Giles F, O'Brien S, et al. Soluble CD52 is detectable in the plasma of patients with chronic lymphocytic leukemia [abstract]. Blood 2001;98(11 Pt 2):149a.
149. O'Brien SM, Wierda W, Geisler D, et al. Yttrium-90 ibritumomab tiuxetan for minimal residual disease in CLL [abstract]. Proc Am Soc Clin Oncol 2003;22:579.
150 Demidem A, Lam T, Alas S, et al. Chimeric anti-CD20 (IDEC-C2B8) monoclonal antibody sensitized a B cell lymphoma cell line to cell killing by cytotoxic drugs. Cancer Biother Radiopharm 1997;12:177–86.
151. Alas S, Emmanouilides C, Bonavide B. Inhibition of interleukin 10 by Rituxan results in down-regulation of *BCL-2* and sensitization of B-cell non-Hodgkin's lymphoma to apoptosis. Clin Cancer Res 2001;7:709–23.
152. Golay J, Lazzari M, Facchinetti V, et al. CD20 levels determine the in vitro susceptibility to rituximab and complement of B cell chronic lymphocytic leukemia: further regulation by CD55 and CD59. Blood 2001;98:3383–9.
153. Keating MJ, O'Brien S, Albitar M, et al. Early results of a chemoimmunotherapy regimen of fludarabine, cyclophosphamide, and rituximab as initial therapy for chronic lymphocytic leukemia. J Clin Oncol 2005;23:4079–88.
154. Kay NE, Geyer SM, Lin T, et al. Combination chemotherapy with pentostatin, cyclophosphamide and rituximab induces high rate of remissions including complete responses and achievement of minimal residual disease in previously untreated B-chronic lymphocytic leukemia [abstract]. Blood 2004;104(11 Pt 1):100a.
155. O'Brien SM, Kantarjian HM, Thomas DA, et al. Alemtuzumab as treatment for residual disease after chemotherapy in patients with chronic lymphocytic leukemia. Cancer 2003;98:2657–63.
156. Elter T, Bochmann P, Schulz H, et al. FluCam—a new, 4-weekly combination of fludarabine and alemtuzumab for patients with relapsed chronic lymphocytic leukemia [abstract]. Blood 2004;104(11 Pt 1):690a.
157. Byrd JC, Rai K, Peterson BL, et al. Addition of rituximab to fludarabine may prolong progression-free survival and overall survival in patients with previously untreated chronic lymphocytic leukemia: an updated retrospective comparative analysis of CALGB 9712 and CALGB 9011. Blood 2005;105:49–53.
158. Robertson LE, O'Brien S, Kantarjian H, et al. Fludarabine plus doxorubicin in previously treated chronic lymphocytic leukemia. Leukemia 1995;9:943–5.
159. Tsimberidou AM, Keating MJ, Giles FJ, et al. Fludarabine and mitoxantrone for patients with chronic lymphocytic leukemia. Cancer 2004;100:2583–91.
160. Robak T, Blonski JZ, Kasznicki M, et al. Cladribine with or without prednisone in the treatment of previously treated and untreated B-cell chronic lymphocytic leukaemia—updated results of the multicentre study of 378 patients. Br J Haematol 2000;108:357–68.
161. O'Brien SM, Kantarjian HM, Cortes J, et al. Results of the fludarabine and cyclophosphamide combination regimen in chronic lymphocytic leukemia. J Clin Oncol 2001;19:1414–20.
162. Bosch F, Ferrer A, Lopez-Guillermo A, et al. Fludarabine, cyclophosphamide and mitoxantrone in the treatment of resistant or relapsed chronic lymphocytic leukemia. Br J Haematol 2002;119:976–84.

163. Van Den Neste E, Louviaux I, Michaux JL, et al. Phase I/II study of 2-chloro-2'-deoxyadenosine with cyclophosphamide in patients with pretreated B cell chronic lymphocytic leukemia and indolent non-Hodgkin's lymphoma. Leukemia 2000;14:1136–42.
164. Montillo M, Tedeschi A, O'Brien S, et al. Phase II study of cladribine and cyclophosphamide in patients with chronic lymphocytic leukemia and prolymphocytic leukemia. Cancer 2003;97:114–20.
165. Weiss MA, Maslak PG, Jurcic JG, et al. Pentostatin and cyclophosphamide: an effective new regimen in previously treated patients with chronic lymphocytic leukemia. J Clin Oncol 2003;21:1278–84.
166. Wierda W, O'Brien S, Wen S, et al. Chemoimmunotherapy with fludarabine, cyclophosphamide, and rituximab for relapsed and refractory chronic lymphocytic leukemia. J Clin Oncol 2005;23:4070–8.
167. Wierda W, Faderl S, O'Brien S, et al. Combined cyclophosphamide, fludarabine, alemtuzumab, and rituximab (CFAR) is active for relapsed and refractory patients with CLL [abstract]. Blood 2004;104(11 Pt 1):101a.
168. Robak T, Smolewski P, Urbanska-Rys H, et al. Rituximab followed by cladribine in the treatment of heavily pretreated patients with indolent lymphoid malignancies. Leuk Lymphoma 2004;45:937–44.
169. Byrd JC, Waselenko JK, Keating M, et al. Novel therapies for chronic lymphocytic leukemia in the 21st century. Semin Oncol 2000;27:587–97.
170. Byrd JC, Lin TS, Dalton JT, et al. Flavopiridol administered as a pharmacologically-derived schedule demonstrates marked clinical activity in refractory, genetically high risk, chronic lymphocytic leukemia (CLL) [abstract]. Blood 2004;104:101a.
171. Gandhi V, Plunkett W, Rodriguez CO, et al. Compound GW506U78 in refractory hematologic malignancies—relationship between cellular pharmacokinetics and clinical response. J Clin Oncol 1998;16:3607–15.
172. Castro JE, Wierda WG, Kipps TJ, et al. A phase I/II trial of Xcellerated T cells in patients with chronic lymphocytic leukemia [abstract]. Blood 2004;104(11 Pt 1):687a.
173. Wierda WG, Cantwell MJ, Woods SJ, et al. CD40-ligand (CD154) gene therapy for chronic lymphocytic leukemia. Blood 2000;96:2917–24.
174. Biagi E, Popat U, Raphael R, et al. Immunotherapy of chronic lymphocytic leukemia using CD40L and IL-2 expressing autologous tumor cells [abstract]. Blood 2004;104(11 Pt 1):220a.
175. Rozman C, Montserrat E, Vinolas N, et al. Recombinant β2-interferon in the treatment of B chronic lymphocytic leukemia in early stages. Blood 1988;71:1295–8.
176. Ziegler-Heitbrock HW, Schlag R, Flieger D, Thiel E.. Favorable response of early stage B CLL patients to treatment with IFN-β2. Blood 1989;73:1426–30.
177. Lundin J, Kimby E, Bergmann L, et al. Interleukin 4 therapy for patients with chronic lymphocytic leukaemia: a phase I/II study. Br J Haematol 2001;112:155–60.
178. Provan D, Bartlett-Pandite L, Zwicky C, et al. Eradication of polymerase chain reaction–detectable chronic lymphocytic leukemia cells is associated with improved outcome after bone marrow transplantation. Blood 1996;88:2228–35.
179. Khouri I, Keating M, Champlin R, et al. Hematopoietic stem cell transplantation for chronic lymphocytic leukemia. Curr Opin Hematol 1998;5:454–9.
180. Esteve J, Villamor N, Colomer D, et al. Stem cell transplantation for chronic lymphocytic leukemia: different outcome after autologous and allogeneic transplantation and correlation with minimal residual disease status. Leukemia 2001;15:445–51.
181. Dreger P, Brand R, Hansz J, et al. Treatment-related mortality and graft-versus-leukemia activity after allogeneic stem cell transplantation for chronic lymphocytic leukemia using intensity-reduced conditioning. Leukemia 2003;17:841–8.
182. Khouri KF, Keating M, Korbling M, et al. Transplant-lite: induction of graft-versus-malignancy using fludarabine-based nonablative chemotherapy and allogeneic blood progenitor-cell transplantation as treatment for lymphoid malignancies. J Clin Oncol 1998;16:2817–24.
183. Khouri IF, Lee MS, Saliba RM, et al. Nonablative allogeneic stem cell transplantation for chronic lymphocytic leukemia: impact of rituximab on immunomodulation and survival. Exp Hematol 2004;32:28–35.
184. Rawstron AC, Kennedy B, Evans PA, et al. Quantitation of minimal disease levels in chronic lymphocytic leukemia using a sensitive flow cytometric assay improves the prediction of outcome and can be used to optimize therapy. Blood 2001;98:29–35.
185. Rai KR, Byrd JC, Peterson BI, et al. A phase II trial of fludarabine followed by alemtuzumab (Campath-1H) in previously untreated chronic lymphocytic leukemia (CLL) patients with active disease: Cancer and Leukemia Group B (CALGB) study 19901 [abstract]. Blood 2002;100(11 Pt 1):205a.
186. Montillo M, Cafro AM, Tedeschi A, et al. Safety and efficacy of subcutaneous Campath-1H for treating residual disease in patients with chronic lymphocytic leukemia responding to fludarabine. Haematologica 2002;87:695–700.
187. Wendtner CM, Ritgen M, Schweighofer CD, et al. Consolidation with alemtuzumab in patients with chronic lymphocytic leukemia (CLL) in first remission—experience on safety and efficacy within a randomized multicenter phase III trial of the German CLL Study Group (GCLLSG) [abstract]. Blood 2003;102(11 Pt 1):676a.
188. Rai KR, Byrd JC, Peterson B, et al. Subcutaneous alemtuzumab following fludarabine for previously untreated patients with chronic lymphocytic leukemia (CLL): CALGB study 19901 [abstract]. Blood 2003;102(11 Pt 1):676a.
189. Moreton P, Kennedy B, Lucas G, et al. Eradication of minimal residual disease in B-cell chronic lymphocytic leukemia after alemtuzumab therapy is associated with prolonged survival. J Clin Oncol 2005;23:2971–9.
190. Thieblemont C, Bouafia F, Hornez E, et al. Maintenance therapy with a monthly injection of alemtuzumab prolongs response duration in patients with refractory B-cell chronic lymphocytic leukemia/small lymphocytic lymphoma (B-CLL/SLL). Leuk Lymphoma 2004;45:711–4.
191. Byhardt RW, Brace KC, Wiernik PK. The role of splenic irradiation in chronic lymphocytic leukemia. Cancer 1975;35:1621–5.
192. Cooper IA, Ding JC, Adams PB, et al. Intensive leukapheresis in the management of cytopenias in patients with chronic lymphocytic leukemia (CLL) and lymphocytic lymphoma. Am J Hematol 1979;6:387–98.
193. Seymour JF, Cusack J, Lerner S, et al. A case-control study of the role of splenectomy in chronic lymphocytic leukemia. J Clin Oncol 1997;15:52–60.
194. Rozman C, Montserrat E, Vinolas N. Serum immunoglobulins in B-chronic lymphocytic leukemia. Natural history and prognostic significance. Cancer 1988;61:279–83.
195. Kay NE, Johnson JD, Stanek R, et al. T-cell subpopulations in chronic lymphocytic leukemia: abnormalities in distribution and in in vitro receptor maturation. Blood 1979;54:540–4.
196. Cooperative Group for the Study of Immunoglobulin in Chronic Lymphocytic Leukemia. Intravenous immunoglobulin for the prevention of infection in chronic lymphocytic leukemia. N Engl J Med 1988;319:902–7.
197. O'Brien S, Kantarjian H, Beran M, et al. Fludarabine and granulocyte colony-stimulating factor (G-CSF) in patients with chronic lymphocytic leukemia. Leukemia 1997;11:1631–5.
198. Cortes J, O'Brien S, Loscertales J, et al. Cyclosporin A for the treatment of cytopenia associated with chronic lymphocytic leukemia. Cancer 2001;92:2016–22.
199. Rose E, Rai K, Revicki D, et al. Clinical and health status assessments in anemic chronic lymphocytic leukemia (CLL) patients treated with epoetin alfa (EPO) [abstract]. Blood 1994;84(Suppl 1):2091.
200. Hedenus M, Hansen S, Taylor K, et al. Randomized, dose-finding study of darbepoetin alfa in anaemic patients with lymphoproliferative malignancies. Br J Haematol 2002;119:79–86.
201. Barista I, Romaguera JE, Cabanillas F. Mantle-cell lymphoma. Lancet Oncol 2001;2:141–8.
202. Goy A, Younes A, McLaughlin P, et al. Phase II study of proteasome inhibitor bortezomib in relapsed or refractory B-cell non-Hodgkin's lymphoma. J Clin Oncol 2005;23:667–75.
203. Mulligan SP, Matutes E, Dearden C, et al. Splenic lymphoma with villous lymphocytes: natural history and response to therapy in 50 cases. Br J Haematol 1991;78:206–9.
204. Tefferi A, Li CY, Witzig TE, et al. Chronic natural killer cell lymphocytosis: a descriptive clinical study. Blood 1994;84:2721–5.
205. Matutes E, Catovsky D. Mature T-cell leukemias and leukemia/lymphoma syndromes. Review of our experience in 175 cases. Leuk Lymphoma 1991;4:81–91.
206. Dearden CE, Matutes E, Cazin B, et al. High remission rate in T-cell prolymphocytic leukemia with Campath-1H. Blood 2001;98:1721–6.
207. Keating MJ, Cazin B, Coutre S, et al. Campath-1H treatment of T-cell prolymphocytic leukemia in patients for whom at least one prior chemotherapy regimen has failed. J Clin Oncol 2002;20:205–13.

Hodgkin Disease

Peter M. Mauch, MD
Lawrence Weiss, MD
James O. Armitage, MD

HISTORY

The life and accomplishments of Thomas Hodgkin have been detailed in an excellent biography of this distinguished physician and scientist.[1] Briefly, in his historic paper entitled "On Some Morbid Appearances of the Exorbant Glands and Spleen," presented to the Medical Chirurgical Society in London on January 10, 1832, Thomas Hodgkin described the clinical history and postmortem findings of the massive enlargement of lymph nodes and spleens of patients studied at Guy's Hospital in London.[2] Hodgkin recognized that these patients had suffered from a disease that started in the lymph nodes located along the major vessels in the neck, chest, or abdomen.

Hodgkin began his work at Guy's Hospital in London, in 1825, after graduating from Edinburgh Medical School in Scotland. At Guy's, he assembled and catalogued anatomic specimens relevant to specific diseases that led to his discovery in 1832. Although Hodgkin is best known for his study of malignancy and the abnormalities of the spleen and lymph nodes, he also contributed to the study of heart disease, promoted the use of the microscope, and advocated reforms in medical education and public health. Despite these achievements, Hodgkin was passed over for a teaching position and left Guy's Hospital in 1837, ending his academic career.[1] For the remainder of his life, he devoted himself to the plight of the native populations of colonial countries and their treatment by Western civilization.

It was not until 1865, a year before his death, that Hodgkin was credited with his discovery. This occurred as a result of the work of two physicians at Guy's Hospital. Dr. Richard Bright, an expert on kidney disease, had written a paper on abdominal tumors in 1838.[3] This included the history and postmortem findings of Hodgkin's cases 1 and 2, specifically citing his original discovery. Independently, in 1856, Sir Samuel Wilks, a Guy's Hospital pathologist, described 10 postmortem cases that had "a peculiar enlargement of the lymphatic glands frequently associated with disease of the spleen." Unknown to him, his report included Hodgkin's original cases 1, 2, 3, and 4, which had been preserved in the Gordon Museum at Guy's Hospital. Before completing his work, Wilks came across Bright's reference to Hodgkin's original cases, and he credited Hodgkin with the initial discovery. By 1865, Dr. Wilks had collected 15 cases that were published in a second paper entitled "Cases of the Enlargement of the Lymphatic Glands and Spleen (or Hodgkin's Disease) with Remarks."[4]

Wilks was one of the first physicians to use the microscope to study Hodgkin disease. Although he and other physicians noted the characteristic giant cells present in the lymph nodes and spleens of patients with Hodgkin disease, Dr. W.S. Greenfield, in 1878, was the first to contribute drawings of them from a low microscopic magnification of a lymph node specimen.[5] Providing more detailed descriptions of these cells, Dr. Carl Sternberg, in 1898, and Dr. Dorothy Reed, in 1902, are credited with the first definitive microscopic descriptions of Hodgkin disease.[6,7]

Both Sternberg and Reed, along with many other physicians, believed that Hodgkin disease was caused by an associated infection rather than by a separate malignant process of the lymph nodes. Eight of Sternberg's 13 cases of Hodgkin disease had coexistent tuberculosis, and he believed Hodgkin disease to be a variant of tuberculosis. In contrast, Reed believed that Hodgkin disease was an independent illness with which tuberculosis might sometimes be associated. Still, Reed considered Hodgkin disease to be an inflammatory illness rather than a malignancy. Other physicians believed that Hodgkin disease was a cancer of the lymph nodes. Clinical and pathologic studies, available in the early twentieth century, helped to confirm the view that Hodgkin disease was a malignant neoplasm.[8]

Radiation Therapy The early treatment of Hodgkin disease with crude x-rays in 1901 soon followed the discovery of radiographs by Roentgen, radioactivity by Becquerel, and radium by the Curies at the end of the nineteenth century. Prior to this time, serum and other biologic preparations, arsenic, iodine, and surgery, were all ineffective in the treatment of Hodgkin disease. Thus, the first reports of x-ray radiograph treatments that would dramatically shrink enlarged lymph nodes produced great excitement and premature predictions for the curability of Hodgkin disease.[9,10]

During the first two decades of the twentieth century, physicians used two methods to treat Hodgkin disease with radiation. Small doses of radiation were administered to the entire trunk at weekly intervals for many weeks, or a single massive dose was given just to the tumor. Neither strategy controlled Hodgkin disease and both caused significant side effects.[8] Both techniques shrank enlarged nodes, but recurrence and spread to previously uninvolved nodes invariably followed. After several courses of radiation therapy (RT), Hodgkin disease became more resistant to treatment, and all patients died from it. These multiple recurrences were not attributed to poor radiation therapy techniques, but were viewed as inherent to the disease itself. By 1920, most physicians stopped using radiation as a means of curing Hodgkin disease. For the next 40 years, treatment was mainly palliative, used to shrink large nodes that were painful or interfered with movement, eating, or breathing.

The development of modern radiation therapy techniques for the treatment of Hodgkin disease began in the 1920s with the work of Gilbert, a Swiss radiotherapist. One of the first physicians to point out certain clinical patterns in the behavior of Hodgkin disease, Gilbert attempted to adapt his radiation therapy techniques to these patterns. He began to advocate treatment of apparently uninvolved adjacent lymph node chains that might contain suspected microscopic disease, as well as of the evident sites of lymph node involvement.[11]

Peters used a similar technique to treat patients at the Ontario Institute of Radiotherapy in the late 1930s and early 1940s. In her historic paper, published in the *American Journal of Roentgenology* in 1950, Peters provided evidence that patients with limited Hodgkin disease could be cured with high-dose radiation therapy that treated involved nodal disease and adjacent nodal sites.[12] She reported 5- and 10-year survival rates of 88% and 79%, respectively, for patients with stage I Hodgkin disease, rates that were notably high for a disease in which virtually no one survived 10 years. Despite these results, the concept that early stage Hodgkin disease might be curable with radiation therapy was slow to be accepted. Prior to the 1960s most patients with limited Hodgkin disease were not treated at all, or only with small doses of radiation.

No one deserves greater credit than Henry Kaplan for the development of successful modern treatment for Hodgkin disease. His accomplishments are many. He pioneered work on the development of the linear accelerator, defined radiation field sizes and doses for a curative approach for early Hodgkin disease, refined and improved diagnostic staging techniques, developed models for translating laboratory findings into clinical practice, and promoted early randomized clinical trials in the United States.[13–14]

The development of the linear accelerator that allowed for the use of higher doses and larger radiation fields, the proposal of new classification systems for histologic subtyping[15] and staging, the pioneering of methods for more precise radiographic and surgical staging (bipedal lymphangiography and staging laparotomy), and the development of an effective multiagent chemotherapy regimen,[16] all contributed to the development of curative treatment for early stage Hodgkin disease. From these advances, the philosophy and practice of managing early stage Hodgkin disease changed dramatically by the late 1960s. Early stage patients who 10 years earlier would not have been treated now received extensive staging and radiation therapy with wide fields and high doses, resulting in the cure of a high proportion of patients.

Chemotherapy The history of the development of cytotoxic agents dates to the early part of the twentieth century.[17] By the early 1960s, a number of individual chemotherapeutic agents were known to produce regression of lymph nodes and symptomatic improvement of patients with Hodgkin disease. These agents included the alkylating agent anthracycline, vinblastine, vincristine, and nitrogen mustard. The treatment of Hodgkin disease with multiple chemotherapeutic agents was developed from sequential studies defining curative treatment for acute lymphoblastic leukemia in children.[18] These studies were designed to find combinations of agents, each of which had similar antitumor activity but different normal tissue effects, so that full doses could be given with more than one agent without significantly increasing toxicity.[19] In 1963, a pilot study was initiated to test the feasibility of using a combination of chemotherapeutic agents, cyclophosphamide, vincristine, methotrexate, and prednisone, followed by radiation therapy for the treatment of Hodgkin disease.[20]

The first reports of the use of multiple drug combinations for acute leukemia and Hodgkin disease demonstrated high complete remission rates, rapid tumor regression, and durability with short-term follow-up. By the early 1970s, data were available on nearly 200 patients with stages III and IV Hodgkin disease treated with MOPP (Mustargen [mechlorethamine], Oncovin [vincristine], procarbazine, and prednisone) chemotherapy, a regimen that substituted nitrogen mustard for cyclophosphamide and procarbazine for methotrexate in the original regimen reported by Moxley and colleagues.[16] Nearly 50% of patients who achieved a complete remission remained in remission more than 2 years after treatment. Recurrences were seen primarily in sites of initial nodal involvement.

Meanwhile, other investigators began to design and test new chemotherapeutic regimens to be delivered first in MOPP-resistant patients and then to substitute or complement the four drugs used in the MOPP regimen. The ABVD (Adriamycin [doxorubicin], bleomycin, vinblastine, and dacarbazine) program developed by Gianni Bonadonna in Milan, Italy, was the first and most effective.[21] Over the past 25 years, this regimen has gradually replaced the MOPP regimen as the most commonly used chemotherapeutic regimen for all stages of Hodgkin disease. In head-to-head trials, it has been found to be superior to MOPP in both early stage and advanced-stage disease.[22] Although the regimen carries some risk of cardiac and pulmonary toxicity, it is not associated with leukemogenesis or sterility, the two major complications associated with MOPP.

EPIDEMIOLOGY AND ETIOLOGY

There are approximately 7,600 new cases of Hodgkin disease diagnosed each year in the United States. The incidence has been stable over the last two decades. Slightly more men than women develop this malignancy. In economically developed countries, there is an age-related bimodal incidence for Hodgkin disease. The first peak occurs in the third decade of life, with a second rise in incidence occurring after the age of 50 years.[23]

The incidence of Hodgkin disease by age differs by histologic subtype. Mixed cellularity disease is more common in patients 40 to 45 years of age or older; the nodular sclerosis sub-type occurs more frequently in patients between 15 and 45 years of age.[24] Lymphocyte-predominant histology is more frequently seen in persons younger than age 16 years and in persons 40 to 45 years of age or older, and has a high male to female predominance (4:1), as compared to the other subtypes. The epidemiologic significance of the age- and gender-related differences remains unknown.

Several different theories have been proposed for the epidemiology and etiology of Hodgkin disease. Historically, *Mycobacterium tuberculosis* was first suspected to be the etiologic organism for Hodgkin disease because of the high coexistence of tuberculosis.[6,25] Later, it was appreciated that Hodgkin disease was associated with deficits in the immune system, making the presence of associated infections more likely.[26] Several reports in the 1970s suggested that Hodgkin disease might be contagious because of reports of clustering of the disease. The studies, by Vianna and Poln, noted clustering among high school students exposed to Hodgkin disease.[27] However, population-based studies, using cancer registries in Connecticut and California, convincingly made the argument that the reported clusters occurred by chance alone. A study that repeated the methodology of Vianna and Poln in a different location failed to confirm their findings.[28]

A number of studies have suggested that, under certain circumstances, there is a genetic predisposition for Hodgkin disease. There is an increased incidence in Jews and among first-degree relatives. Siblings appear to have a two- to five-fold increased risk; in siblings of the same sex, there is as much as a nine-fold increased risk.[29,30]An even higher risk has been reported in monozygotic twins of Hodgkin disease cases.[29] There is an increased risk among parent–child pairs but not among spouses, again suggesting a genetic rather than an infectious etiology. In addition, Hodgkin disease has been linked with certain human leukocyte antigens (HLAs).[30]

There is increasing evidence to suggest a viral etiology for Hodgkin disease. In economically developed countries, there is an association between Hodgkin disease in younger patients and increased maternal education, decreased numbers of siblings and playmates, early birth order, and single-family dwellings in childhood.[31,32] This association between Hodgkin disease and childhood factors that decrease exposure to infectious agents at an early age has led to the proposal that Hodgkin disease appears to mimic a viral illness that has an age-related host response to infection (such as seen with polio and infectious mononucleosis). Under this circumstance, a viral infection that would be mild in young children but more persistent and severe in young adults, perhaps with prolonged immunogenic stimulation, would trigger development of Hodgkin disease.[31,32] Supporting this theory is the infrequent occurrence of Hodgkin disease in children younger than 10 years old in economically developed countries.

Epstein–Barr virus (EBV) is a leading candidate as the causative agent for Hodgkin disease.[33,34] EBV is the causative agent in African Burkitt lymphoma, and EBV-associated lymphomas are documented in patients with immunodeficiency disorders and following organ transplantation. There is a two- to three-fold excess in the incidence of Hodgkin disease among patients with a prior history of mononucleosis, a disease caused by EBV. In addition, there appears to be an altered antibody pattern to EBV in patients prior to clinically presenting with Hodgkin disease with elevated titers against the viral capsid antigen and against the EBV nuclear antigen (EBNA).[34] This suggests that these patients may have had more severe initial EBV infections or more frequent viral replication associated with the development of Hodgkin disease.

Recent cellular and molecular biology data have provided additional support for the association of EBV and classic forms of Hodgkin disease (For reviews, see Mueller and colleagues[35] and Ambinder and Weiss[36]). Through the use of sensitive molecular probes, 30 to 50% of Hodgkin' disease specimens have been found to contain EBV genome fragments in the diagnostic Reed–Sternberg cells.[37] EBV genome status appears to be stable over time when studied in initial biopsies and at relapse. EBV genome-positive Reed–Sternberg cells express the so-called type II latency profile, with expression of latent membrane protein (LMP)-1, LMP-2a, EBNA-1, and Epstein–Barr encoded ribonucleic acid (EBER). LMP-1 is critical in transformation and acts as an oncogene in transfection studies, whereas EBNA-

1 is essential for the replication of the episomal viral genome.

Despite these compelling data, direct evidence for EBV as a causative agent for development of Hodgkin disease remains to be determined. The lack of an animal model and the difficulties in studying the malignant cells in Hodgkin disease continues to frustrate investigators. Additional epidemiologic, serologic, and molecular data are needed to determine the precise role of EBV in Hodgkin disease.

There is less support for other proposed causes of Hodgkin disease. Although there are scattered reports of the association of Hodgkin disease with environmental exposure to toxic agents, the data have not been confirmed in case-control studies. It has been suggested that Hodgkin disease might be caused by an altered immune response. Although there are theories that this might occur based on biologic data, there is no clinical evidence that Hodgkin disease is an illness of chronic immune suppression. In contrast to other malignancies, Hodgkin disease is rarely seen as a second malignancy and does not appear to be increased in patients with illness- or treatment-related chronic immunosuppression.

PATHOLOGY

Histopathology Hodgkin disease is unique among lymphomas for its histologic diversity. Involved lymph nodes contain varying degrees of normal reactive and inflammatory cells, fibrosis, and a scattering of the characteristic malignant cells of Hodgkin disease, the Reed–Sternberg cells, and their mononuclear variants. The typical Reed–Sternberg cell has abundant cytoplasm and two or three nuclei, each with a single prominent nucleolus. The large size and unusual appearance of the Reed–Sternberg cell sets it apart from the adjacent smaller background cells. The mononuclear variants have nuclear and cytoplasmic features of Reed–Sternberg cells, but only have a single nucleus, and by themselves are not pathognomonic of Hodgkin disease. Although the diagnosis of Hodgkin disease should rarely be made in the absence of Reed–Sternberg cells, the presence of these cells is not sufficient alone to make the diagnosis. Reed–Sternberg-like cells have been found in infectious mononucleosis, non-Hodgkin lymphomas, and in nonlymphoid malignancies, including carcinomas and sarcomas. Thus, criteria for the diagnosis of Hodgkin disease include both the presence of the Reed–Sternberg cell and the characteristic background of normal lymphocytes, plasma cells, and eosinophils.

In the early twentieth century, physicians began to describe different cellular patterns of Hodgkin disease and to suggest microscopic classifications. But it was not until 1944 that the division of Hodgkin disease, as proposed by Jackson and Parker, into the three subcategories of paragranuloma, granuloma, and sarcoma gained wide acceptance.[38] This classification was not challenged for 20 years, despite its limited clinical utility, perhaps because of the lack of effective treatment. The Jackson–Parker classification identified 10% of patients with the most favorable and 10% with the least favorable prognoses as paragranuloma and sarcoma, respectively; the remaining 80% of patients had the granuloma subtype. An alternative classification, devised by Lukes and Butler, was proposed for international adoption at a conference entitled "Obstacles to the Control of Hodgkin's Disease" held in Rye, New York, in September 1965. Their proposal contained six histologic subtypes. Later, this was simplified to four subtypes. The classification appeared to correlate well with clinical stage and aggressiveness of disease[15] and, as a result, rapidly replaced the Jackson and Parker classification. Most of the Rye classification has been included as part of the newer Revised European–American Lymphoma (REAL) and World Health Organization (WHO) classifications. The REAL classification proposed modest changes in the histopathologic classification of Hodgkin disease.[39,40] These changes mainly reflect the distinct entity of nodular lymphocyte predominant Hodgkin disease (NLPHD) and the new classification of lymphocyte-rich classic Hodgkin disease. The new system includes (1) classic Hodgkin disease: nodular sclerosis, mixed cellularity, lymphocyte depletion, and lymphocyte-rich classic Hodgkin disease (predominance of lymphocytes but Reed–Sternberg cell morphology and immunophenotype of classic Hodgkin disease); (2) NLPHD; and (3) Hodgkin disease unclassifiable.

Although the subtypes proposed in the Rye classification initially correlated with aggressiveness of disease, with modern treatment, subtyping of Hodgkin disease has become less important in guiding clinical management, prognosis, and therapy. Nevertheless, the histologic subtypes of Hodgkin disease are associated with different sites of presentation, distinct natural histories, and variable prognoses. These differences are most evident in the nodular lymphocyte predominance subtype.

Classic Hodgkin Disease For a more detailed review, see Weiss and colleagues.[41]) Mixed cellularity Hodgkin disease (MCHD) has an inflammatory background abundant in normal cells as well as frequent malignant Reed–Sternberg cells and their mononuclear variants with 5 to 15 malignant cells per high-power field (Figures 117-1 and 117-2). Lymphocytes, plasma cells, eosinophils, and histiocytes are frequent. Patients with mixed cellularity histology are older, are more likely to have symptoms of fever, sweats, or weight loss, and often have abdominal involvement or advanced disease. Approximately 25% of patients with Hodgkin disease in the United States present with MCHD. The subtype is more commonly seen in underdeveloped countries. Because of the background cellular pattern, mixed cellularity Hodgkin disease can be confused with peripheral T-cell lymphoma. Immune markers may help to distinguish the two entities.

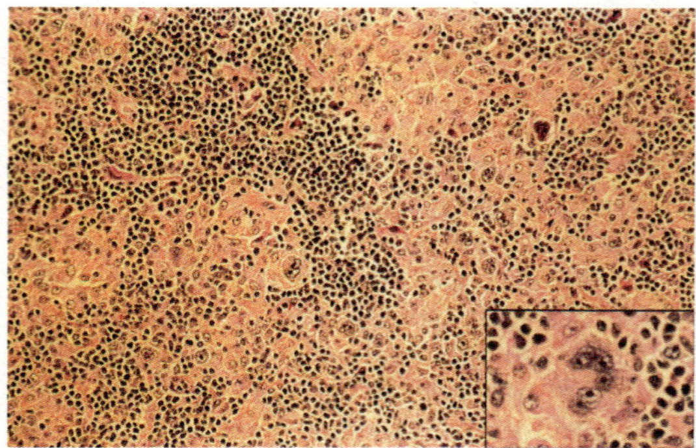

Figure 117-1 Hodgkin disease, mixed cellularity type. Reed–Sternberg cells in histiocyte-rich cellular background. *Insert:* multinucleated Reed–Sternberg cell at higher magnification.

The diagnosis of lymphocyte-depleted Hodgkin disease is rarely made today and accounts for less than 1% of Hodgkin disease in economically advanced countries. Generally, patients with lymphocyte-depleted Hodgkin disease present with advanced disease. With advances in immunohistochemistry, some patients with a prior diagnosis of lymphocyte-depleted Hodgkin disease would now be classified as having non-Hodgkin lymphoma. In lymphocyte-depleted Hodgkin disease, Reed–Sternberg cells and "pleomorphic" variant cells are more frequently seen in comparison to normal lymphocytes. Most cases have only sparse numbers of normal lymphocytes.

Nodular sclerosis Hodgkin disease is morphologically and clinically distinct from the other subtypes. Two histologic features differentiate this form of Hodgkin disease from all others: (1) a proliferation of collagenous bands divide the lymph node into circumscribed nodules and (2) these nodules contain a variant of the Reed–Sternberg cell called the lacunar cell. In formalin-fixed tissue, this cell's abundant pale cytoplasm often retracts and gives the appearance of a cell in space (Figures 117-3, 117-4, and 117-5).

Nodular sclerosis is the only subtype of Hodgkin disease as common in women as in men. It occurs in adolescents and young adults and is

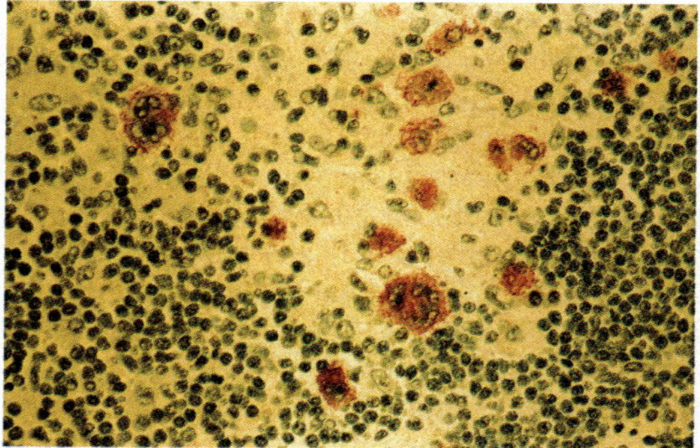

Figure 117-2 Immunostain for Epstein–Barr virus–latent membrane protein in Hodgkin disease, mixed cellularity type (same biopsy as Figure 117-1).

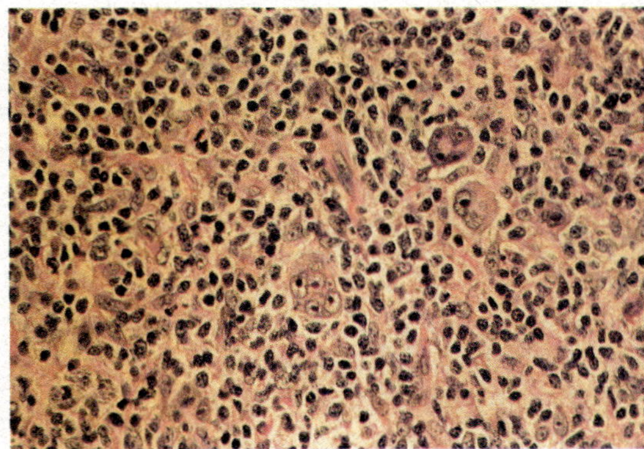

Figure 117-3 Reed–Sternberg cells and variants in Hodgkin disease of the nodular sclerosis type. Large multinucleated or multilobated cells and a few mononuclear cells with macronucleoli stand apart from cellular background elements.

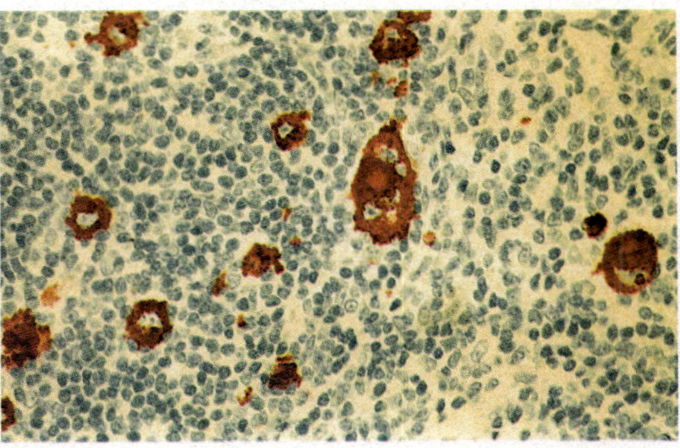

Figure 117-5 Immunostain for CD15 in Hodgkin disease, nodular sclerosis type. Neoplastic Reed–Sternberg cells and mononuclear Hodgkin cells show positive immunoreactivity.

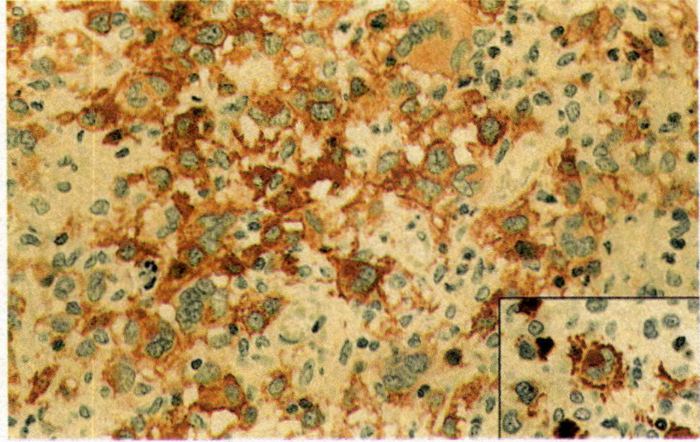

Figure 117-7 Hodgkin disease, nodular sclerosis, British National Lymphoma Investigation grade 2 (same biopsy as Figure 117-7). Neoplastic large cells show diffusely positive immunoreactivity for CD30, positive immunoreactivity for CD15 *(insert)* and variable immunoreactivity for CD20 (not shown).

unusual in patients older than age 50 years. It has a striking propensity to involve lower cervical, supraclavicular, and mediastinal lymph nodes and has an orderly pattern of spread.[24] It makes up 60 to 70% of Hodgkin disease in economically developed countries, but is less commonly seen in underdeveloped countries. Patients with this histology, particularly those with localized disease, have a good prognosis.

The British National Lymphoma Investigation subclassified nodular sclerosis (NS) Hodgkin disease into two subtypes—NS I and NS II—based on the number of Reed–Sternberg cells and variants, the degree of atypia, and the quality and quantity of fibrosis (Figures 117-6 and 117-7).[42] In the British National Lymphoma Investigation study, patients with NS I histology had a better prognosis than patients with NS II histology.[42] The adverse prognosis of NS II histology has been supported by some studies, but not by others.

Lymphocyte-rich classic Hodgkin disease, nodular or diffuse, is a new classification proposed by the REAL classification in 1994. Several recent reports have described the histopathologic and clinical characteristics of nodular lymphocyte predominant Hodgkin disease and lymphocyte-rich classic Hodgkin disease.[43,44] Lymphocyte-rich classic Hodgkin disease may resemble either mixed cellularity, nodular sclerosis, or nodular lymphocyte predominance Hodgkin disease and may be nodular or diffuse. Many cases resemble vaguely nodular appearance on low magnification. Reed–Sternberg cells are relatively rare and the background is dominated by small mature lymphocytes (Figures 117-8 and 117-9). Eosinophils and neutrophils are usually restricted to blood vessels. Some cases of lymphocyte-rich classic Hodgkin disease may show a distinctly nodular appearance that may closely mimic nodular lymphocyte predominance Hodgkin disease. The nodules of lymphocyte-rich classic Hodgkin disease often contain small reactive germinal centers, with Hodgkin and Reed–Sternberg cells present in and near the mantle zones, a pattern that has been called follicular Hodgkin disease.

The immunophenotype of the neoplastic cells in lymphocyte-rich classic Hodgkin disease is identical to that of classic Hodgkin disease, that is, CD15+ and CD30+, whereas that of nodular lymphocyte predominance Hodgkin disease are CD20+ and lack CD15 and CD30. There are, however, differences in the background cells, as many cases of lymphocyte-rich classic Hodgkin disease present with a B-cell–rich infiltrate, in contrast to the marked T-cell predominance usually found in other types of classic Hodgkin disease. This immunohistochemical staining pattern of lymphocytes and follicular dendritic cells of lymphocyte-rich classic Hodgkin disease is similar to that of nodular lymphocyte predominant Hodgkin disease: the nodules are composed predominantly of B cells with nodular meshworks of follicular dendritic cells.

In nodular lymphocyte predominant Hodgkin disease, the lymph node architecture is usually effaced, although a remnant of normal nodal architecture may remain. Nodular lymphocyte predominant Hodgkin disease contains an abundance of benign-appearing cells. True diagnostic Reed–Sternberg cells are not seen, but variant lymphocytic and histiocytic (L and H) cells are typical (Figures 117-10 and 117-11). These cells often have multilobated nuclei and have been called popcorn cells because of their resemblance to a popped kernel of corn. Fibrosis is not usually seen. In the nodular subtype of lymphocyte predominant Hodgkin disease, the L and H or "popcorn" variants of Reed–Sternberg cells occur in background of polyclonal B lymphocytes (see Figure 117-11).[45,46] L and H cells are usually positive for the B-cell CD20, but negative for CD15 and negative or weakly positive for CD30 (Figures 117-12 and 117-13).[46,47] EBV is rarely detected in the nodular LP subtype.[48]

Progressive transformation of germinal centers is associated with NLPHD. The architecture of nodes undergoing progressive transformation of germinal centers is altered by large nodules that contain dispersed follicular center cells in clusters.

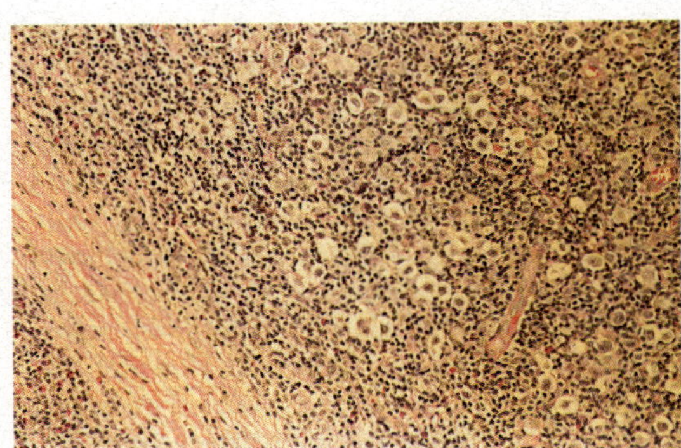

Figure 117-4 Hodgkin disease, nodular sclerosis. A fibrous band is present in the left lower part of the field. Neoplastic lacunar cells having abundant, clear cytoplasm stand out against the lymphocytic background.

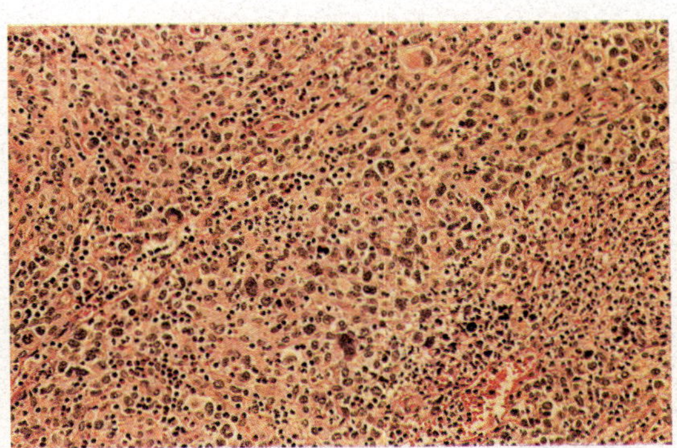

Figure 117-6 Hodgkin disease, nodular sclerosis, British National Lymphoma Investigation grade 2. Sheets of neoplastic large cells (*middle of field*), some with Reed–Sternberg cell morphology, border on a focal area of necrosis (*lower right of field*).

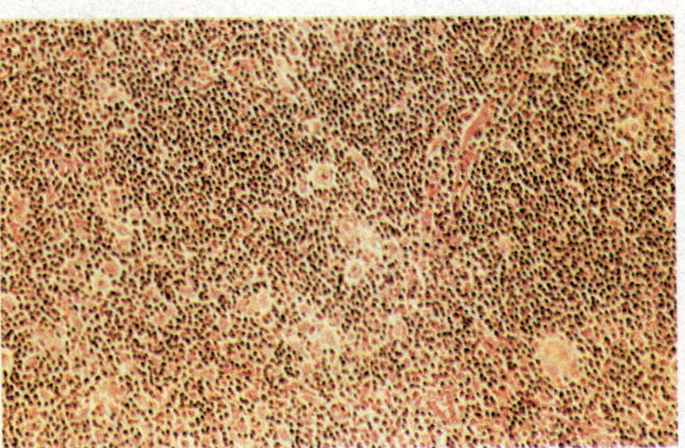

Figure 117-8 Lymphocyte-rich classic Hodgkin disease. Reed–Sternberg cells and mononuclear Hodgkin's cells are relatively rare within the background proliferation of small lymphocytes and histiocytes.

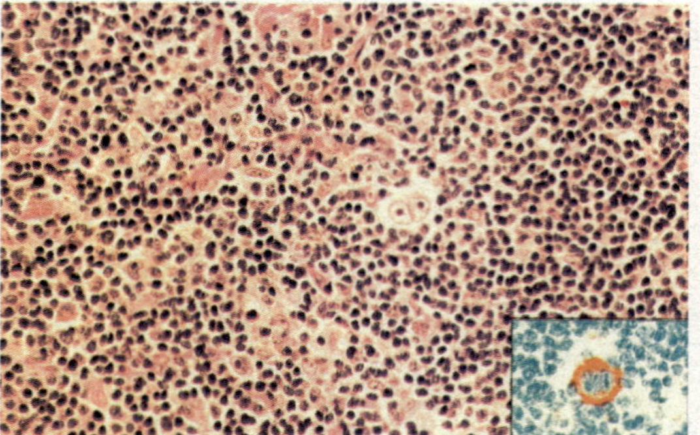

Figure 117-9 Lymphocyte-rich classic Hodgkin disease. Binucleated Reed–Sternberg cell in center of field. In same biopsy, Reed–Sternberg cells immunostained positively for CD15 *(insert)*.

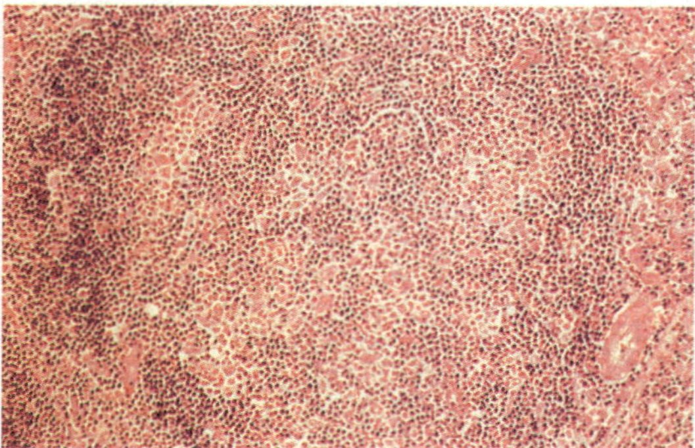

Figure 117-11 Lymphocyte predominant Hodgkin disease. The vaguely nodular histologic pattern is apparent.

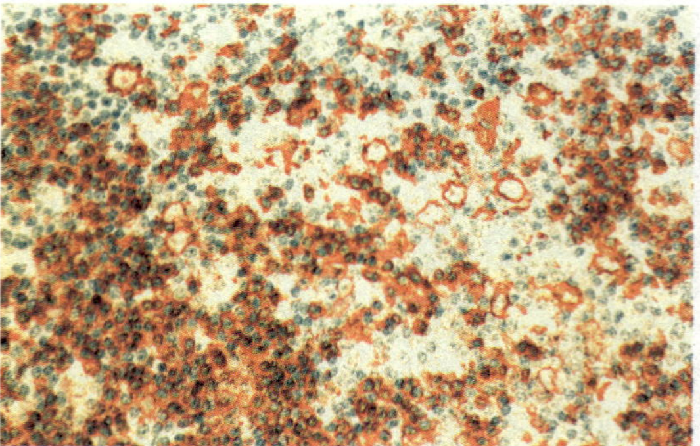

Figure 117-13 Lymphocyte predominant Hodgkin disease (same biopsy as Figures 117-11 and 117-12). Immunostain for CD20 demonstrates positive staining of L and H cells as well as a high percentage of lymphocytes within a nodule.

Reed–Sternberg cells and L and H variants are absent. Progressive transformation of germinal centers also can be seen in association with nodular lymphocyte predominant Hodgkin disease in the same lymph node specimen or follow it in other sites.[47] It is important to distinguish nodular lymphocyte predominant Hodgkin disease from progressive transformation of germinal centers, which is a benign disorder.[47]

Nodular lymphocyte predominant Hodgkin disease makes up 5 to 10% of Hodgkin disease in the United States. It often presents with a long natural history and has the longest time to recurrence of any of the subtypes of Hodgkin disease. Death from this subtype of Hodgkin disease is rare. Nodular lymphocyte predominant Hodgkin disease has distinct patterns of presentation when compared to the other subtypes.

It is often localized to a single peripheral nodal region (high cervical, submandibular, epitrochlear, or inguinal or femoral nodes) and infrequently involves (8%) mediastinal or abdominal nodes. Nodular lymphocyte predominant Hodgkin disease is distinctive, clinically and histologically, from other subtypes of Hodgkin disease; it should be reported separately in clinical studies.

Sometimes Hodgkin disease morphologically resembles certain large-cell non-Hodgkin lymphomas, including anaplastic large-cell lymphoma, T-cell lymphoma, and large-cell lymphoma with sclerosis. Immunohistochemical markers can aid in distinguishing between these entities; however, in some cases, such differentiation remains difficult. Recent molecular profiling studies have shown a close relationship between primary mediastinal large B-cell lymphoma and classic Hodgkin disease, and there may be a true "gray-zone" neoplasm that combines features of both neoplasms.[49]

NATURE OF THE REED–STERNBERG CELL

Surface Antigens The origin of the neoplastic cell in classical Hodgkin disease has been controversial for many years.[50] Theories have included derivation from B lymphocytic, macrophage-reticulum cell, follicular center dendritic cell, or histiocytic lineages. However, more recent evidence indicates a lymphocyte origin for the Reed–Sternberg cells. Reed–Sternberg cells of classical Hodgkin disease may express antigens found on resting or activated lymphocytes, most often B-cell (CD20, PAX5, CD79a) or, more rarely, T-cell surface (CD3, CD4, CD8, T-cell receptor 0 chain) antigens, although Reed–Sternberg cells express neither phenotype in many cases. The L and H cells of nodular lymphocyte predominant Hodgkin disease consistently express B-cell antigens, indicating derivation from B cells. Both CD30 and CD15 antigens are on the surface of most Reed–Sternberg cells and can be detected in paraffin-embedded sections. Nearly all cases of classical Hodgkin disease are CD30+ and approximately 80% of cases are CD15+, whereas CD45 (leukocyte common antigen) is usually negative. In contrast, the Reed–Sternberg cells in nodular lymphocyte predominant Hodgkin disease are CD15–, CD30– or only weakly positive, and CD45+ (leukocyte common antigen).[48]

Molecular Biology Microdissection studies performed on single Hodgkin cells obtained from cases of classical Hodgkin disease have clearly demonstrated clonal immunoglobulin gene rearrangements in the vast majority of cases, confirming the clonality of the cells and moreover definitely establishing a B-cell lineage, despite the aberrant absence of immunoglobulin gene expression.[51,52] In addition, these studies have shown that the Hodgkin cells possess somatically mutated *V* genes, implying a germinal center or post-germinal center origin. However, the pattern of mutations suggests that many of them are nonfunctional. Normal germinal center B cells that develop such "crippling" mutations are usually eliminated within the germinal center through apoptosis; thus, there is some mechanism in Hodgkin cells that renders them resistant to the usual apoptotic mechanism. Unsuccessful germinal center cells usually undergo apoptosis via the FAS/CD95 pathway, a process that is inhibited by *c-FLIP*, a gene that is constitutively expressed by Hodgkin cells.[53] Several hypotheses have been generated to explain this phenomenon, including activation of the NF-κB pathway, general lineage promiscuity, and Epstein-Barr infection. Evidence favoring the NF-κB pathway includes the observation of constitutive expression of NF-κB in Hodgkin disease-derived cell lines, the finding that suppression of NF-κB impairs tumor growth in severe combined immunodeficient mice and growth of cell lines,[54] and an epidemiology study showing that regular aspirin use is associated with a reduced risk of developing Hodgkin disease, presumably through inhibition of NF-κB transcription.[55] Rare cases of classical Hodgkin disease studied by singe-cell techniques show clonal rearrangements of the T-cell receptor genes.

Microdissection studies have shown that L and H cells of lymphocyte predominance Hodgkin disease also undergo clonal immunoglobulin gene rearrangements, again definitively establishing

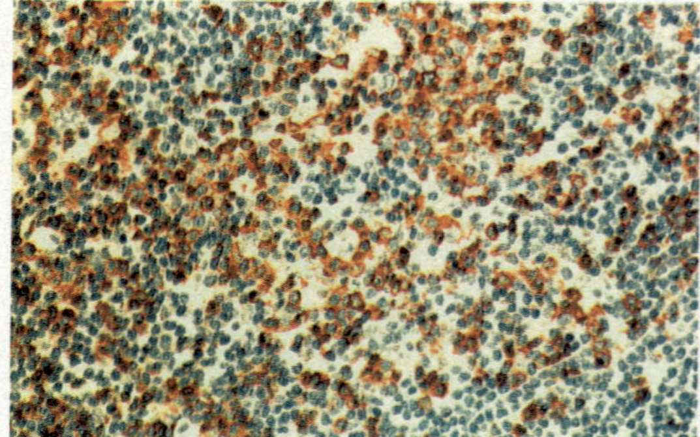

Figure 117-10 Lymphocyte predominant Hodgkin disease (same biopsy as Figures 117-11, 117-12, and 117-13). Immunostain for CD57 reveals a marked increase in immunoreactive cells showing localization around non-immunoreactive L and H cells within a nodule. The CD3 immunostain showed a similar distribution of immunoreactive cells.

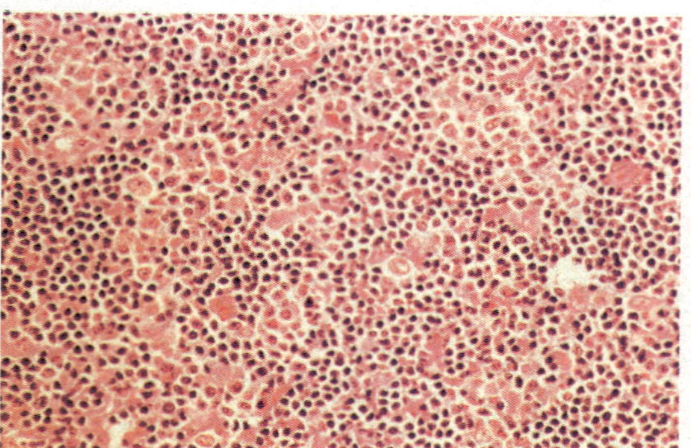

Figure 117-12 Lymphocyte predominant Hodgkin disease at higher magnification (same biopsy as Figure 117-11). Within the background of lymphocytes and histiocytes are scattered large lobated cells having a fine chromatin pattern, relatively small nucleoli, and sparse cytoplasm w so-called L and H cells.

clonality of the process and providing confirmation of a B-cell lineage.[51] In addition to demonstrating somatically mutated *V* genes, intraclonal sequence diversity can also be detected, providing strong evidence that lymphocyte predominance Hodgkin disease is a germinal center lymphoma. In contrast to classical Hodgkin disease, the mutations are compatible with functional antigen receptors.

Cytogenetics Cytogenetic abnormalities are common in Reed–Sternberg cells; however, no consistent pattern has been described.[56,57] The t(14:18) translocation, common in follicular, small cleaved cell B-cell lymphomas, is unusual in Hodgkin disease (less than 2% of cases studied). Comparative genomic hybridization studies demonstrate recurrent gains on chromosomal arms 2p (the site of *NFκBREL* and *BCL11a*), 9p (the site of *JAK2*), and 12q (the site of *MDM2*), and amplifications on chromosomal bands 4p16, 4q23-q24, and 9p23-p24. Recently, recurrent imbalances have been demonstrated in a majority of cases of classic Hodgkin disease using genome-wide GeneScan technology.[58]

Cytokine Secretion It has been hypothesized that cytokines are responsible for the marked inflammatory component, fibrosis, and the diverse histologic patterns of Hodgkin disease, as well as clinical symptoms such as fever, weight loss, and night sweats.[59–61] Many cases of Hodgkin disease are associated with upregulation of tumor necrosis factor receptor (TNFR) and ligand family members, Th2 and to a lesser extent Th1 cytokines, and a variety of chemokines. Necrosis factor receptor (NFR) members may lead to constitutive activation of nuclear factor-kappaB (NFκB), an important factor in proliferation and survival of B lymphocytes. Preferential expression of Th2 cytokines and chemokines may explain the frequent presence of eosinophils and fibroblasts, as well as local suppression of the cellular immune response. EBV may contribute to the production of cytokines, for example, via LMP-1–induced activation of NFκB and stimulation of interleukin (IL)-10, a potent inhibitor of cellular immunity. In some cases, specific cytokines may be associated with specific histologic features. For example, transforming growth factor (TGF)-ai1, a known stimulus for fibroblast proliferation and collagen formation, is associated with the formation of nodular sclerosis Hodgkin disease,[62] and TARC, a lymphocyte-directed CC chemokine secreted by Hodgkin cells, may be responsible for the infiltration by CD4+ T cells.[63] Other cytokines, such as IL-13 may play a role in autocrine stimulation of Hodgkin cells.[64]

IMMUNOLOGIC ABNORMALITIES IN PATIENTS

Hodgkin disease is characterized by functional deficits in cellular immunity and in T-cell–mediated immune responses that exist prior to treatment. These deficits persist in cured patients and include impairment of delayed cutaneous hypersensitivity, depressed proliferative responses to T-cell mitogen stimulation, enhanced immunoglobulin production, and decreased natural killer cell cytotoxicity.[63–65] These abnormalities suggest an immunosuppression secondary to chronic over-stimulation by cytokines. In patients with active Hodgkin disease, these findings are consistent with increased cytokine secretion by Reed–Sternberg cells. However, it has been difficult to explain the persistence of these abnormalities in patients after Hodgkin disease.

Hodgkin disease is characterized by the presence of Hodgkin and Reed–Sternberg cells surrounded by predominantly CD4+ T-lymphocytes. These cells express a variety of activation markers but are incapable of mounting an effective immune response against tumor cells.[65] There appear to be three potential causes of immune suppression after treatment for Hodgkin disease: residual effects from radiation therapy and chemotherapy, immunocompromise from splenectomy after staging laparotomy, and persistence of abnormalities present at diagnosis biologically related to Hodgkin disease.

Treatment-induced immunosuppression returns to normal at varying times after Hodgkin disease but appears to have its greatest effect over the first few years after treatment.[66] One of the clinical consequences of this immunosuppression is the development of herpes zoster. There is an excess of herpes zoster infections during the first year after initiation of treatment for Hodgkin disease. More than 75% of Hodgkin disease-associated herpes zoster cases occur within the first year. Few cases occur after the third year (only 6% of all cases).[67] In addition, the risk of zoster appears highest in patients receiving intensive radiation therapy and alkylating agent chemotherapy (50 to 57%).[67] In contrast, the risk of zoster is only 14 to 23% for patients receiving radiation therapy or chemotherapy alone. The incidence of zoster appears less with the ABVD regimen than with the more immunosuppressive MOPP chemotherapy.

Unlike the deficits in delayed hypersensitivity, most patients with Hodgkin disease at diagnosis appear to have relatively normal B-cell numbers and function.[66] However, B-cell function is adversely affected by treatment with chemotherapy or combined chemotherapy and radiation therapy, and the ensuing consequences may be greater after prior splenectomy.

To counteract the risks of bacterial sepsis, patients in the past were vaccinated prior to staging laparotomy and splenectomy. Antibody response to the 14-valent (and 23-valent) pneumococcus vaccine, combined with *Haemophilus influenzae* type B and meningococcus type C, is normal in patients with untreated Hodgkin disease and similar to that of healthy controls, asplenic controls, and patients treated with radiation therapy alone.

Rarely do patients with Hodgkin disease undergo splenectomy as part of treatment in current practice. However, patients who have had a splenectomy or splenic irradiation in the past as part of management for Hodgkin disease should be revaccinated every 6 years.[68] Even with improvements in vaccines, neither immunization nor antibiotic prophylaxis can be guaranteed to prevent the development of sepsis from encapsulated microorganisms in patients with Hodgkin disease whose staging included splenectomy or who have been heavily treated with combined modality therapy (CMT). Both physicians and patients should remain alert to this risk.

STAGING

Natural History and Patterns of Spread The Swiss radiotherapist Gilbert is credited with first reporting that Hodgkin disease spread by contiguity from one lymph node chain to adjacent regions.[11] Peters, and later Kaplan and others, extended Gilbert's work by employing the use of prophylactic radiation therapy to lymph nodes adjacent to those involved with disease.[69,70] The development of new radiographic studies and the routine use of staging laparotomy improved understanding of the presentation, distribution, and evolution of Hodgkin disease.[71,72] Although there is strong evidence that Hodgkin disease begins in a single group of lymph nodes and then spreads to contiguous lymph nodes, eventually the malignant cells become more aggressive, may invade blood vessels, and spread to organs by hematogenous dissemination.

One study of more than 700 patients evaluated continuous nodal involvement from a combination of clinical and laparotomy staging.[24] Evidence for contiguous spread was most convincing for patients with classic Hodgkin disease. The mediastinum, left side of the neck, and right side of the neck were each involved in more than 60% of patients. These sites were four or more times as common as other nodal sites above or below the diaphragm, suggesting that most cases of classical Hodgkin disease begin in the chest or neck. Significant associations were found between the mediastinum and the right or left neck, the neck and the ipsilateral axilla, the mediastinum and the hilum, and the spleen and abdominal nodal involvement. There was a negative association between the right and left neck if the mediastinum was not involved, suggesting that spread from one neck to the other occurred through the mediastinum.

Most patients with classical Hodgkin disease have a central pattern of lymph node involvement (cervical, mediastinal, paraaortic). In contrast, certain nodal chains (mesenteric, hypogastric, pre-sacral, epitrochlear, popliteal) are seldom involved. The spleen is involved more frequently with adenopathy below the diaphragm, systemic symptoms, and in patients with mixed cellularity histology variants. Involvement of the liver in an untreated patient is rare and almost always occurs with splenic involvement. Infiltration of the bone marrow is usually focal and almost invariably associated with extensive disease and systemic symptoms. The same observation applies to bony involvement, which is a rare event early in the course of the disease. In the great majority of patients, the initial pattern of spread occurs nonrandomly and predictably via lymphatic channels to contiguous lymph node chains. This important observation, first made more than 50 years ago, formed the basis for prophylactic irradiation of adjacent lymph node bearing regions in patients with apparently localized Hodgkin disease treated with radiation therapy alone in the 1970s, 1980s and early 1990s.

Patterns of Relapse A relapse is a new manifestation of disease documented after complete tumor remission. In more than 80% of patients, initial relapses occur within the first 5 years of treatment for Hodgkin disease. The median time to relapse is stage and treatment dependent; recurrences occur earlier in patients with large mediastinal adenopathy than in patients without bulky disease.[73] Late relapses, for example, those occurring beyond the first 5 years, are uncommon and range from 5 to 15% of all recurrences.[74] Relapses among patients treated with radiation therapy generally occur outside the radiation field, whereas relapses among patients treated with chemotherapy occur at previous sites of involvement. True recurrence, that is, relapse within a treated field, is a rare finding when a tumoricidal dose of radiation therapy of greater than 30 Gy is applied. Clinical trials are now testing whether 20 Gy is a sufficient dose to control Hodgkin disease in favorable prognosis patients when administered after ABVD.

Marginal recurrence or relapse appearing at or immediately adjacent to the margin of the irradiated field is more frequent and related to treatment and extent of disease. The risk of a marginal recurrence is partially related to the radiation technique used and to the response to chemotherapy and number of cycles of chemotherapy delivered. Trials are being developed in Europe to test the concept of treating the initially involved nodes as opposed to the initial involved nodal regions.

The sites of initial recurrence after chemotherapy alone correlate with the sites of largest disease prior to therapy[75]; however, recurrences occur even with chemotherapy alone in patients with less-bulky disease. To date, there are no reliable estimates for the risk of nodal recurrence after chemotherapy alone by number of sites or size of disease in patients with less-bulky disease. As standard practice, adjuvant radiation therapy is usually recommended in patients with localized disease after treatment with chemotherapy to reduce the risk of recurrence. In patients who have a favorable prognosis, this has allowed a reduction of the number of cycles of chemotherapy needed. However, a number of trials are exploring the use of chemotherapy alone in this setting, and there are proposals to test the use of negative PET scanning after chemotherapy as a means to forgo adjuvant radiation therapy.

Staging Classification The advent of new imaging modalities and the frequent use of combined modality treatment have made staging procedures simpler and less invasive in recent years. The latest international staging classification was proposed in 1989, during a meeting held in Cotswolds, England.[76] The Cotswolds classification (Table 117-1) is a modification of the Ann Arbor classification using information from staging and treatment obtained in the 1970s and 1980s.

Table 117-1 The Cotswolds Staging Classification for Hodgkin Disease

Stage I	Involvement of a single lymph node region or lymphoid structure (eg, spleen, thymus, Waldeyer ring) or involvement of a single extralymphatic site (IE)
Stage II	Involvement of two or more lymph node regions on the same side of the diaphragm (hilar nodes, when involved on both sides, constitute stage II disease); localized contiguous involvement of only one extranodal organ or site and lymph node region(s) on the same side of the diaphragm (IIE). The number of anatomic regions involved should be indicated by a subscript (eg, II3)
Stage III	Involvement of lymph node regions on both sides of the diaphragm (III), which may also be accompanied by involvement of the spleen (IIIS) or by localized contiguous involvement of only one extranodal organ site (IIIE) or both (III SE)
III1	With or without involvement of splenic, hilar, celiac, or portal nodes
III2	With involvement of paraaortic, iliac, and mesenteric nodes
Stage IV	Diffuse or disseminated involvement of one or more extranodal organs or tissues, with or without associated lymph node involvement
Designations applicable to any disease stage	
A:	No symptoms
B:	Fever (temperature, > 38°C [100.4°F]), drenching night sweats, unexplained loss of > 10% of body weight within the preceding 6 months
X:	Bulky disease (a widening of the mediastinum by more than one-third of the presence of a nodal mass with a maximal dimension greater than 10 cm)
E:	Involvement of a single extranodal site that is contiguous or proximal to the known nodal site
CS:	Clinical stage
PS:	Pathologic stage (as determined by laparotomy)

Adapted from Lister T et al.[76]

Some of the recommended modifications include adding criteria for clinical involvement of the spleen and liver to include evidence of focal defects with two separate imaging techniques and eliminating the findings of abnormal liver function as evidence of liver involvement. The suffix "X" was added to designate bulky disease (greater than 10 cm maximum dimension). A new category of response to therapy, that is, unconfirmed/uncertain complete remission, was introduced to accommodate the difficulty evaluating persistent radiologic abnormalities of uncertain significance following primary therapy. A category of localized extranodal disease (eg, lung, pleura, chest wall, bone) contiguous to involved nodes was added and classified in the appropriate lymph node system stage followed by the subscript E. Patients with localized extranodal disease have a more favorable prognosis than patients with disseminated involvement (stage IV).

Table 117-2 lists recommended staging procedures. An adequate surgical biopsy is required for histopathologic examination. When the diagnosis of Hodgkin disease is made from biopsy of an extranodal site, a concomitant node biopsy confirmation of diagnosis is desirable unless the diagnosis is considered unequivocal.

Radiographic Staging Above the Diaphragm The radiologic assessment of patients with newly diagnosed Hodgkin disease is summarized below. More than 60% of patients have radiographic evidence of intrathoracic involvement. Although frontal and lateral chest radiographs are routinely ordered and represent an easy means for subsequent surveillance, computed (axial) tomography (CT) scanning should be performed on all patients as it provides a much more accurate assessment of the extent and distribution of thoracic disease. CT scanning is especially apt at detecting pulmonary disease, pleural or pericardial involvement, apical cardiac nodal enlargement, and extension into the chest wall, and in defining the extent of involved axillary lymph nodes (Figure 117-14). Such information has considerable potential to alter clinical management. Identification of the extent of thoracic disease will help to define the extent of combination chemotherapy and the dose, extent, and need for radiation therapy.

Massive mediastinal adenopathy (large mediastinal adenopathy) has been variously defined as the ratio greater than one-third between the largest transverse diameter of the mediastinal mass over the transverse diameter of the thorax at the diaphragm on a standing posterior-anterior chest radiograph (Figure 117-15),[77] as greater than 35% of the thoracic diameter at T5-T6, or as measuring

Table 117-2 Recommended Staging

Adequate surgical biopsy reviewed by an experienced hemopathologist
Detailed history with attention to the presence or absence of systemic symptoms
Careful physical examination, emphasizing node chains, size of liver and spleen, and Waldeyer ring inspection
Routine laboratory tests: complete blood count, erythrocyte sedimentation rate, and liver function tests
Chest radiograph (posteroanterior and lateral) with measurement of mass/thoracic ratio
Chest, abdominal, and pelvic computed tomography scans
Radioisotopic evaluation with gallium 67 or positron emission tomography
Core-needle biopsy of bone marrow from the posterior iliac crest in patients with stages IIB to IV disease
Needle or surgical biopsy of any suspicious extranodal (eg, hepatic, osseous, pulmonary, cutaneous) lesion(s)
Cytologic examination of any effusion
Staging laparotomy in rare circumstances in early stage Hodgkin disease where the use of limited radiation therapy alone depends on pathologic staging

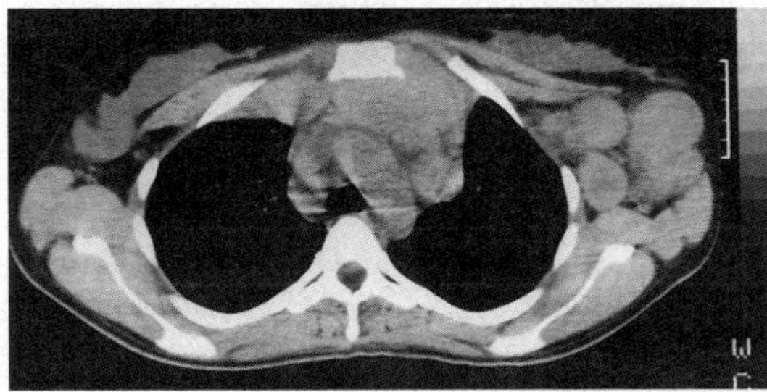

Figure 117-14 Thoracic computed tomography image from a patient with nodular sclerosis Hodgkin disease. Note the very large involvement of the left axillary nodes, involvement of the right pleura, and the anterior mediastinal disease.

greater than 5 or 10 cm in width. Patients with large mediastinal adenopathy have an increased risk of relapsing in nodal and extranodal sites above the diaphragm following radiation therapy alone; this risk is reduced with the use of combined radiation therapy and chemotherapy.[73] These patients make up 20 to 25% of clinical stage I-II patients, generally present with involvement of multiple supradiaphragmatic nodal chains, and may have extension of tumor into the lung, pericardium, or chest wall. Systemic symptoms are frequently present.

Baseline nuclear medicine imaging studies are also routinely recommended both in the initial staging and follow-up of Hodgkin disease patients. Most centers are now replacing gallium 67 scintigraphy with fluorine-18-fluorodeoxyglucose positron emission tomographic (FDG-PET) scanning, that has been shown to be the more sensitive test.[78–80]

Negative follow-up gallium 67 or FDG-PET scanning supports the supposition that there is no active disease after the completion of treatment even in the presence of a residual abnormality on the CT scan. However, these studies are a relative and not absolute indicator of the presence and absence of disease. In the absence of adjuvant-involved field-radiation therapy, recurrences may occur in the initially involved site after chemotherapy alone despite negative gallium or FDG-PET scanning postchemotherapy. At present there is no information supporting the use of these studies to guide whether to use adjuvant involved field radiation in patients with early stage disease.

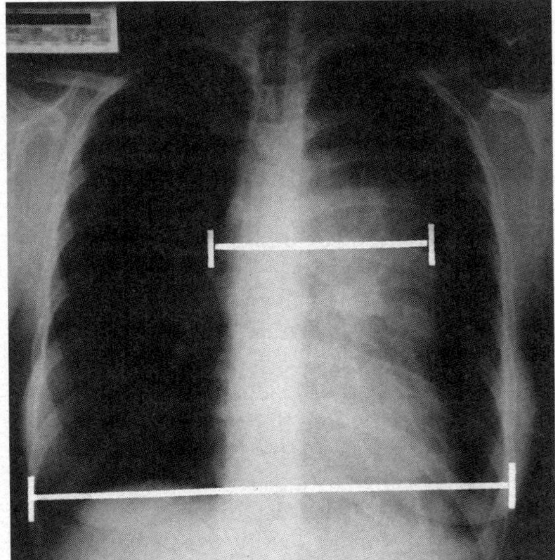

Figure 117-15 Standing posteroanterior chest radiograph of a patient with Hodgkin disease. Measurements of mediastinal mass ratio are made by dividing the width of the mediastinal mass at its widest diameter by the diameter of the thorax (inside rib to inside rib) at the diaphragm. A ratio of greater than 1:3 is classified as bulky mediastinal disease.

Radiographic Staging Below the Diaphragm CT scanning, lymphangiography, FDG-PET, and gallium scanning all have limitations in the radiologic evaluation of the abdominal nodes. No single study is reliable for detecting Hodgkin disease in normal-size nodes, and all studies have a 20 to 35% false-negative rate as a consequence of the inability to detect occult Hodgkin disease in the spleen.[71,72] Comparisons of bipedal lymphangiography and CT scanning suggest that lymphangiography has a small statistical advantage over CT scanning because it provides useful information on lymph node architecture. In contrast, CT scanning can better evaluate adenopathy in the celiac axis, splenic hilus, porta hepatis, and mesentery, relying almost exclusively on increases in the size of the nodes. CT scanning can also demonstrate foci of Hodgkin disease in the liver and spleen. During the past few years, bipedal lymphangiography has given way to CT scanning as the examination of choice. In part, this is because lymphangiography is difficult to perform and interpret and very few departments currently have the expertise to perform the exam. FDG-PET and gallium (with single photon emission computed tomography [SPECT]) scanning are complementary studies to CT scanning. With the infrequent use of staging laparotomy and splenectomy in the staging of Hodgkin disease, the risk of over-staging based on a single radiographic test of abdominal involvement (false positive) has greater potential consequences. Therefore, we strongly recommend that two separate studies (ie, CT scanning and gallium/ FDG-PET scanning) be used to assess abdominal involvement, and that positive findings on both tests be used to confirm radiographically the presence of Hodgkin disease in the abdomen.

Staging Laparotomy Staging laparotomy was extensively used when radiation therapy was the preferred treatment for early stage Hodgkin disease and when it was mandatory to define the extent of abdominal disease to help determine the extent of chemotherapy in early stage Hodgkin disease. However, with many groups using prognostic factors to determine management of Hodgkin disease and with the common use of safer and more effective chemotherapy regimens as part of the treatment in early stage Hodgkin disease, laparotomy has disappeared as a routine staging procedure. Its use should be reserved for rare circumstances in early stage Hodgkin disease for which the use of limited radiation therapy alone depends on pathologic staging.

TREATMENT OF STAGE I-II HODGKIN DISEASE

Randomized Clinical Trials: Meta-Analysis of Trials from the 1970s Significant advances in the treatment of early stage Hodgkin disease have been derived from information obtained from clinical trials. In the 1970s and 1980s, many of the randomized trials evaluated field size in patients treated with radiation therapy alone. A separate set of trials evaluated the role of chemotherapy in stage I-II Hodgkin disease. Specht and colleagues published a meta-analysis of 23 randomized trials involving 3,888 patients with early stage Hodgkin disease treated in the 1970s and 1980s.[81] Early stage Hodgkin disease was defined as patients with clinical or laparotomy stage I-II disease; in some cases, patients with stage III disease were included. Patients with B symptoms and patients with extensive thoracic Hodgkin disease were also included. Specht and colleagues divided the randomized trials into two groups: eight trials compared more extensive radiation therapy to less extensive radiation therapy and 13 trials compared multiagent chemotherapy and radiation therapy alone to radiation therapy alone. Individual patient data including age, stage, date of entry, treatment allocation, date of recurrence, and date and cause of death or date last seen were collected for each patient randomized.

Eight trials evaluated treatment with larger versus smaller radiation field sizes.[81] Larger fields generally included subtotal nodal irradiation (mantle and upper abdomen) or total nodal irradiation; smaller fields included involved fields and regional fields. Although approximately half of the trials showed a significant advantage in disease-free survival with larger field compared to smaller field irradiation, survival differences were not seen in any of the individual eight studies. The combined risk of failure by treatment, in the eight trials at 10 years, was 43.4% for patients treated with less-extensive radiation therapy alone, as compared to 31.3% for those treated with more-extensive radiation therapy alone ($p < .00001$). Ten-year actuarial survival rates were 77% for both groups ($p > .1$). The lack of a survival difference suggests that salvage chemotherapy for relapse after initial radiation therapy alone is effective enough to minimize the impact of the increase in relapse. In addition, the small increased mortality from recurrent Hodgkin disease in patients receiving smaller field irradiation appeared to be balanced by an increased mortality from treatment-related causes in patients receiving more extensive radiation therapy.

Thirteen trials evaluated treatment with multiagent chemotherapy and radiation therapy compared to radiation therapy alone.[81] Most patients received alkylating agent chemotherapy (usually MOPP or an equivalent regimen) for six monthly cycles. Approximately half of the individual trials showed a significant advantage in disease-free survival with combined chemotherapy and radiation therapy, as compared to radiation therapy alone; survival differences were not seen in any of the individual 13 studies. The risk of relapse by treatment for the 13 trials at 10 years was 32.7% for patients treated with radiation therapy alone and 15.8% for those treated with chemotherapy and radiation therapy ($p < .00001$). The 10-year actuarial survival rates were 76.5% for patients treated with radiation therapy alone and 79.4% for those treated with chemotherapy and radiation therapy ($p > .1$).

Long-Term Outcome of Treatment for Early Stage Hodgkin Disease Much of the long-term follow-up data for early stage Hodgkin disease is derived from laparotomy staged patients treated with radiation therapy alone in the 1970s and 1980s. Large, single institutional studies demonstrate approximately an 80% actuarial 10- to 20-year freedom from relapse and less than a 10% mortality from Hodgkin disease following mantle and para-aortic irradiation for PS IA-IIA patients.

The treatment of early stage Hodgkin disease in these studies was so successful that at 15 to 20 years posttreatment, the overall mortality rate from causes other than Hodgkin disease has exceeded that seen from Hodgkin disease.[82–84] Thus, it is in the second and third decades after Hodgkin disease that improved survival of early stage patients might be seen with modern era reduced-treatment regimens.

There are a number of published reports that detail causes of mortality after Hodgkin disease.[82,84–86] Deaths from Hodgkin disease occur most frequently in the first 5 to 10 years; causes of death other than Hodgkin disease are most common after 5 to 10 years. In one recent study, the absolute excess risk of mortality by 5-year interval ranged from 87 to 158 per 10,000 person-years.[82] Thus, on average, these patients had approximately a 1% excess risk of mortality per year over the first 25 to 30 years after Hodgkin disease (Table 117-3).[82] Much of this data is from laparotomy-staged patients treated with wide-field radiation therapy with or without MOPP or MOPP-like regimens. Current clinical trials are based on the data that suggest that reduction of field size and dose of radiation and the use of modified nonalkylating agent regimens results in a reduction of this late mortality incidence.

The three most common causes of death after treatment for Hodgkin disease (Hodgkin disease, secondary malignancy, cardiac disease) are discussed below. Patients who develop recurrent Hodgkin disease after radiation therapy alone are as likely to be cured with combination chemotherapy as if the chemotherapy were used as part of initial treatment. The 10-year actuarial survival rate of patients initially treated with radiation therapy alone after relapse and treatment with multiagent chemotherapy is 57 to 89%.[87,88]

Table 117-3 Excess Mortality after Hodgkin Disease

Time after Hodgkin Disease (Years)	Absolute Excess Risk per 10,000 Person Years
0–5	117
5–10	89
10–15	87
15–20	100
≥ 20	158

Adapted from Ng A et al.[82]

Survival rates are significantly worse for patients who relapse after chemotherapy alone or combined radiation therapy and chemotherapy; most of the data is from patients who initially had advanced Hodgkin disease. Treatment with similar or alternative chemotherapy regimens after relapse from chemotherapy alone yields 5-to 10-year survival rates of only 20 to 32%,[89,90] suggesting cross-resistance among different chemotherapy regimens. Because of the poor overall prognosis of patients who relapse after standard chemotherapy, many centers recommend high-dose chemotherapy and autologous bone marrow rescue at first relapse for patients initially treated with chemotherapy or combined chemotherapy and radiation therapy. Although the results of high-dose therapy are promising, many patients with recurrent disease are not eligible for this approach because of poor tumor response, or occasionally comorbid disease, or advanced age. Patients who undergo transplant, and who are subsequently cured of Hodgkin disease, face significant long-term treatment-related morbidity and mortality risks. One study reports a low rate of survival in patients with early stage disease who relapsed after treatment with chemotherapy alone (9-year actuarial 56% survival rate)[91]; these results await further study. Until more data are available, current information suggests that when chemotherapy is used as definitive treatment for early stage Hodgkin disease, treatment should be designed to minimize relapse. This is probably best achieved with the combined use of both chemotherapy and radiation therapy.

Many years after chemotherapy and/or radiation therapy, patients with Hodgkin disease have an increased risk of developing acute nonlymphoblastic leukemia, non-Hodgkin lymphoma, and second solid tumors.[92–95] This increased risk may be multifactorial, resulting both from the immune dysregulation associated with Hodgkin disease and/or its treatment and the carcinogenic effects of radiation therapy and chemotherapy. Certain cytotoxic agents, especially those contained in the MOPP and ChlVPP (chlorambucil, vinblastine, procarbazine, and prednisone) regimens, are associated with a marked increase in acute nonlymphoblastic leukemia after Hodgkin disease.[96,97] The total incidence of acute leukemia, usually occurring within 10 years of treatment, ranges from 2 to 6%[96,98] The routine use of ABVD has dramatically reduced the risk of leukemogenesis, but there remains concern for secondary leukemia with alternating or hybrid regimens. Regimens that contain significant amounts of alkylating agents known to cause leukemia should not be used in treating favorable prognosis CS I-II patients.

Nearly all cases of non-Hodgkin lymphoma occurring after Hodgkin disease are of intermediate or high-grade histology. The histologies represented are similar to lymphomas seen in patients with immunodeficiency diseases or under chronic immunosuppression for organ transplantation or autoimmune disorders. These lymphomas have a cumulative risk of 1.2 to 2.1% at 15 years.[98,99] The risk is probably not treatment related.

The absolute excess risk of developing a solid tumor is greater than that of developing leukemia or non-Hodgkin lymphoma after Hodgkin disease. Solid tumors constitute 55 to 75% of the second malignancies in long-term studies.[92–94,97,99] The relative risk of solid tumors continues to be elevated more than 20 years after Hodgkin disease.[92] Risk factors for developing a solid tumor after treatment for Hodgkin disease include initial treatment with radiation therapy (solid tumors), treatment with chemotherapy (lung cancer), age at treatment (female patients younger than 35 years of age at treatment and increased breast cancer risk), and environmental factors (ie, smoking and lung cancer).[100] Volume and dose of radiation therapy and type of chemotherapy may all be independent risk factors for the development of second tumors. Additional data are needed to determine the extent to which current treatment reduction strategies will result in a lower second tumor mortality. However, reduction in the radiation field size will almost certainly result in a lower second tumor risk, as many of the radiation-induced tumors occur within or on the edge of the treatment field. Reduction of radiation field size is being studied in stage I-II trials that use combined radiation therapy and chemotherapy years after mantle irradiation. Techniques to combine chemotherapy and radiation limited to involved fields should reduce this risk. In addition, prevention and surveillance strategies are becoming increasingly important in the routine follow-up of long-term survivors of Hodgkin disease and a number of efforts are ongoing to help define these strategies.[101]

Complications related to cardiac irradiation (arrhythmias, myocardial infarction and coronary artery disease, pericarditis, myocarditis, pericardial effusion, and tamponade) have been carefully documented after radiation therapy to the mediastinum. In many of the earlier studies, these complications are related to treatment techniques that resulted in a high radiation dose to the anterior mediastinum and heart (lower energy machinery, anterior weighted fields, doses per fraction of greater than 200 cGy, treatment with one field per day). Current practice, which restricts the dose to the whole heart, blocks the subcarinal region part way into treatment, delivers treatments equally from front and back, and permits lower radiation dose and volume by the use of preradiation chemotherapy, has yielded more satisfactory results. However, even with these advances in treatment, patients will continue to be at some increased for cardiac disease years after Hodgkin disease. Three recent studies detail cardiac risks in long-term survivors of Hodgkin disease and provide recommendations for surveillance.[102–104] Data are now emerging that indicate that patients who received mediastinal irradiation, and have other classic cardiac risk factors, are at significantly increased risk for cardiac disease compared to patients without risk factors.[105] This may allow development of surveillance and prevention strategies for these patients.

Other complications that have factored into the development of clinical trials include pulmonary toxicity and loss of fertility. Radiation pneumonitis typically occurs 1 to 6 months after completion of thoracic irradiation. Symptomatic radiation pneumonitis is characterized by a mild, nonproductive cough, low-grade fever, and dyspnea on exertion and occurs in approximately 5% of patients. Infection and recurrent Hodgkin disease must also be considered in the diagnosis. Radiographically, pneumonitis is characterized by the formation of infiltrates confined to the original radiation fields. Infection, rather than pneumonitis, is more likely if the infiltrates extend into areas of the lung initially protected from radiation by lung shielding. Severe pneumonitis may require treatment with steroids. If the symptoms do not respond to steroid treatment, the presence of a superimposed infection, such as *Pneumocystis carinii,* should be considered. Patients who develop pneumonitis usually do not have long-term pulmonary dysfunction after the acute effects subside.

After bleomycin-containing regimens, a reticulomicronodular pattern located generally at the lower lung zones occurs in 10 to 15% of patients when the cumulative dose of bleomycin exceeds 200 mg/m^2. For lower cumulative doses, such as used in the delivery of four to six cycles of ABVD, early pulmonary toxicity occurs 5% or less of the time, and radiologic findings are reversible with the help of corticosteroids. If left undetected, particularly when bleomycin-containing chemotherapy is administered after prior pulmonary irradiation, the initial findings often evolve into a coarse striking reticulation. In turn, this can evolve into restrictive lung fibrosis.

Gonadal dysfunction is an important iatrogenic toxicity that considerably affects the quality of life in patients after Hodgkin disease. MOPP or MOPP-like combinations induce azoospermia in 90 to 100% of men. Only 10 to 20% of patients eventually show recovery of spermatogenesis, even after long periods. Following MOPP alternated with ABVD, where the cumulative doses of MOPP are 50% of those in full-course MOPP, the incidence of permanent azoospermia is still nearly 50%. Approximately 50% of women become amenorrheic after six courses of MOPP, and premature ovarian failure appears to depend on age (older than age 30 years, 75 to 85%; younger than age 30 years, approximately 20%). In contrast, it has been reported that the administration of ABVD chemotherapy produces only transient germ cell toxicity in men and no drug-induced amenorrhea.[106] Thus, to circumvent chemotherapy-induced sterility, the use of nonalkylating agent regimens is recommended. An alternative for men undergoing MOPP or MOPP–ABVD involves sperm storage prior to chemotherapy. However, approximately one-third of male patients with Hodgkin disease have low sperm count or sperm motility before starting cytotoxic treatment; this may affect the success of the procedure.

PROGNOSTIC FACTORS FOR STAGE I-II HODGKIN DISEASE

Prognostic factors such as age, size of nodal involvement, and presence of systemic symptoms help to determine initial treatment strategies. Patients with stage I-II Hodgkin disease with favorable prognostic factors are candidates for modified chemotherapy and involved field irradiation, or in some cases for chemotherapy alone or radiation therapy alone. Patients with unfavorable prognostic factors should receive chemotherapy and radiation therapy as initial treatment. Although many of the adverse prognostic factors have lost significance as more intensive combined radiation therapy and chemotherapy regimens have been used, these factors continue to be very important in the design of clinical trials that evaluate reduction of radiation therapy and chemotherapy for early stage Hodgkin disease.

Prognostic Factors for Freedom from Treatment Failure and Survival in Stage I-II Patients Prognostic factors have been identified for stage I-II Hodgkin disease that predict for a higher risk of relapse or a lower rate of survival. Many factors predict for recurrence after treatment with radiation therapy alone; fewer predict for relapse after chemotherapy and radiation therapy. Only older age at diagnosis has been consistently reported as a significant adverse factor for survival, both after radiation therapy alone and after combined radiation therapy and chemotherapy.[107,108]

A number of studies have identified prognostic factors for laparotomy-staged (PS)/clinically staged (CS) I-II patients presenting an analysis of significance adjusted for other factors.[109–111] All studies report large mediastinal adenopathy or large tumor burden as a major factor predicting an increased risk of relapse. Patients with a large tumor burden also had a lower survival rate in the Danish study.[109]

Most reports also have identified B symptoms as an important factor for recurrence and survival.

A large retrospective study combining data from PS IB-IIB patients treated at Stanford University Medical School and Harvard Medical School suggested that patients with night sweats without other B symptoms treated with radiation therapy alone had a prognosis similar to that of patients with PS IA-IIA disease. However, the presence of fevers, weight loss, large mediastinal adenopathy, and age 40 years or older all independently predicted for an increased risk of relapse, and survival was impaired in patients who had both fevers and weight loss.[112] Other studies evaluating clinically staged patients have also identified B symptoms as risk factors for relapse.

Two other factors, large number of regions involved and elevated erythrocyte sedimentation rate (ESR), have been identified as adverse factors for freedom from treatment failure in clinically staged patients.[110,111] Many factors, including B symptoms (similar to ESR), male sex, number of sites of involvement, and, to a lesser extent, age, also predict for an increased risk of occult abdominal involvement in CS I-II patients. This may, in part, explain why some of these factors are identified for clinically staged, but not for laparotomy-staged, patients. In current clinical trials, B symptoms are often combined with an elevated ESR in defining an unfavorable prognosis.

Older patients appear to have a lower survival rate, but if treated as younger patients, do not have a higher recurrence rate.[107] Older patients appear to be less-successfully treated at relapse[87,113] and they have a greater absolute excess risk of mortality from causes other than Hodgkin disease, such as second tumors and cardiac disease. Thus, their reduced survival is both disease and treatment related. This argues for treatment strategies that minimize both the risk of recurrence and the risk of long-term complications in this group of patients. Age older than 50 years is used as the criterion for unfavorable prognosis in current trials.

Prognostic Factors Determine Treatment in Clinical Trials Cooperative groups identify favorable and unfavorable prognostic groups for different clinical trials. These prognostic factors predict for likelihood of occult disease in the abdomen and for the effectiveness of treatment in maintaining a high level of freedom from recurrence. Prognostic factors for the current European Organization for the Research and Treatment of Cancer (EORTC) and the German Hodgkin Study Group (GHSG) are listed below. Favorable prognostic factors are listed in Table 117-4 and unfavorable prognostic factors are listed in Table 117-5. For the EORTC and GHSG, favorable prognosis means the absence of each of the factors listed in Table 117-4. Approximately 55% of patients with CS I-II Hodgkin disease will fall into the favorable prognosis group. For the EORTC and GHSG, unfavorable prognosis means the presence of any of the factors listed in Table 117-5. Approximately 35% of patients with CS I-II Hodgkin disease will have either B symptoms or large mediastinal adenopathy, and approximately 10% will have four or more sites involved without B symptoms or large mediastinal disease. The International Prognostic Factor Project analyzed additional prognostic factors in patients with advanced-stage Hodgkin disease to determine poor prognostic groups of patients who might need more aggressive initial treatment (Table 117-6).[114] This international prognostic index is especially valuable for patients with advanced Hodgkin disease.

Reduction of Staging or Treatment: Ongoing and Recently Completed Trials for Favorable Prognosis CS I-II Hodgkin Disease Increasing concern for the long-term consequences of treatment has prompted many investigators to reexamine the aggressive approaches developed for the staging and treatment of early stage Hodgkin disease in the 1970s and 1980s. Many of the ongoing and recently completed studies were developed in an attempt to reduce the long-term complications of treatment without increasing mortality from Hodgkin disease. These include studies that (1) evaluate combined radiation therapy and chemotherapy and attempt to identify the optimal chemotherapy regimen, identify the optimum number of cycles of chemotherapy, or determine the optimal radiation volume and dose when combined with chemotherapy; (2) evaluate combination chemotherapy alone; and (3) define circumstances for radiation

Table 117-4 Favorable Prognosis Stage I-II Hodgkin Disease

EORTC	GHSG
No large mediastinal adenopathy, ESR < 50 without B symptoms, ESR < 30 with B symptoms, age ≤ 50, 1–3 lymph node sites involved	No large mediastinal adenopathy, ESR < 50 without B symptoms, ESR < 30 with B symptoms, no E disease, and 1–2 lymph node sites involved

EORTC = European Organization for the Research and Treatment of Cancer; GHSG =German Hodgkin's Study Group. See review.[107]

Table 117-5 Unfavorable Prognosis Stage I-II Hodgkin Disease

EORTC	GHSG
Any one of the following: Large mediastinal adenopathy, ESR ≥ 50 without B symptoms, ESR ≥ 30 with B symptoms, age > 50, or ≥ 4 lymph node sites involved	Large mediastinal adenopathy, ESR ≥ 50 without B symptoms, ESR ≥ 30 with B symptoms, E disease, or ≥ 3 lymph node sites involved

EORTC = European Organization for the Research and Treatment of Cancer; GHSG = German Hodgkin's Study Group. See review.[108]

Table 117-6 Final Cox Regression Model, International Prognostic Factor Project

Factor	Log Hazard Ratio	Relative Risk
Serum albumin < 4 g/dL	0.40 ± 0.10	1.49
Hemoglobin < 10.5 g/dL	0.30 ± 0.11	1.35
Male sex	0.30 ± 0.09	1.35
Stage IV disease	0.23 ± 0.09	1.26
Age ≥ 45 years	0.33 ± 0.10	1.39
White cell count (WCC) ≥ 15,000/mm^3	0.34 ± 0.11	1.41
Lymphocyte count < 600/ mm^3 or < 8% of WCC	0.31 ± 0.10	1.38

therapy alone and define radiation dose and field size in this setting. Most of the studies discussed in the following sections have relatively short follow-up or are ongoing and would not be expected to demonstrate survival differences. High relapse rates and significant acute toxicity are the main criteria for adverse outcome.

Combination Radiation Therapy and Chemotherapy: Randomized Clinical Trials Using Modified Chemotherapy and Radiation Therapy Randomized trials of combined modality therapy are based on the premise that this approach results in a very high freedom from recurrence in early stage Hodgkin disease, and that the efficacy of combined chemotherapy and radiation can be maintained even when using modified and less toxic regimens. Listed in Table 117-7 are selected trials using modified chemotherapy regimens and radiation therapy. The regimens are combined with involved field radiation therapy. In the Southwest Oncology Cancer Group (SWOG)/Cancer and Leukemia Group B (CALGB) trial and the German Hodgkin Study Group (GHSG) HD7 trial, subtotal nodal and splenic irradiation was used in the combined chemotherapy and radiation therapy arm because of concerns for limited doses of chemotherapy to control abdominal disease. More recent trials have restricted the radiation fields to the involved regions. The newer short-course VAPEC-B (vincristine, doxorubicin [Adriamycin], prednisolone, etoposide [VP-16], cyclophosphamide, and bleomycin) and Stanford V (mechlorethamine, doxorubicin, vinblastine, prednisone, vincristine, bleomycin, and etoposide [VP-16]) trials only use radiation therapy above the diaphragm. Analysis of patterns and frequency of failure will eventually provide better guidelines for such modified regimens to control occult Hodgkin disease not appreciated on physical examination or radiographic evaluation either in adjacent nodes or below the diaphragm.

SWOG/CALGB Study of Three Cycles of Adjuvant Doxorubicin and Vinblastine Plus Subtotal Nodal and Splenic Irradiation versus Subtotal Nodal and Splenic Irradiation Alone in CS IA-IA Hodgkin Disease Patients The trial met stopping rules at the second interim analysis after 348 of the initially planned 420 patients had been enrolled, with the radiation alone group having significantly more recurrences than the combined chemotherapy and radiation group (see Table 117-7). No overall survival differences were seen. There was significantly higher-grade 3-4 hematologic toxicity in the patients receiving both radiation therapy and chemotherapy.[115] Subsequent trials have been designed not to use extended field irradiation when combined with chemotherapy.

The German Hodgkin Study Group HD7 Trial (1994 to 1998) The GHSG HD7 study randomized patients to subtotal nodal and splenic irradiation alone or to two courses of ABVD and the radiation therapy regimen. In the 617 patients available for analysis, there is a significantly improved freedom from treatment failure in the radiation therapy and chemotherapy arm (91%) versus radiation therapy alone (75%, $p < .0001$). No survival differences are seen.

European Organization for the Research and Treatment of Cancer H7F Trial (1988 to 1993) This trial compared EBVP (epirubicin, bleomycin, vinblastine, and prednisone) II and

Table 117-7 Randomized Clinical Trials in Favorable Prognosis Stage I-II Hodgkin Disease: Trials to Identify the Optimum Chemotherapy Combination

Trial	Eligibility	Treatment Regimens	Number of Patients	Outcome
EORTC H7F[116,117]	CS IA-IIB without: age >50, ESR ≥ 50 mm/h in A; ≥ 30 mm/h in B, 4 or more sites of disease, large mediastinal disease (? 0.35 m/t ratio), CS IA, NS/LP, < 40, ESR < 50 mm/h	A. EBVP X 6 + IFRT (36 Gy) B. STLI (S)	168 165	Relapse-free survival (6 year): A = 92%; B = 81%; p = .004 Survival (6 year): A = 98%; B = 96%; p = .156
SWOG 9133/ CALGB 9391[115]	CS IA-IIA without: age < 16, large mediastinal disease	A. doxorubicin and vinblastine for 3 cycles and STLI (S) (36–40 Gy) B. STLI (S) (36–40 Gy)|	348	Failure-free survival (3-year) A= 94%; B=81%, p < .001 Overall survival (3-year) No difference
Stanford V for favorable prognosis	CS I-II without B symptoms for favorable age < 16 and > 60, large mediastinal disease, 2 extranodal sites initial involvement)	Stanford V for 8 weeks and modified FRT	86 (open)	Freedom from progression (3-year) 96% Overall survival (3-year) 98%

CS = clinical stage; EBVP = epirubicin, bleomycin, vinblastine, and prednisone; EORTC = European Organization for the Research and Treatment of Cancer; ESR = erythrocyte sedimentation rate; IF = involved field; LP = lymphocyte predominance histology; NS = nodular sclerosis histology; RT = radiation therapy; Stanford V regimen = mechlorethamine, doxorubicin, vinblastine, prednisone, vincristine, bleomycin, VP- 16; STLI (S) = subtotal nodal irradiation (splenic irradiation).

Table 117-8 Randomized Clinical Trials in Favorable Prognosis Stage I-II Hodgkin Disease: Trials to Identify the Optimal Number of Chemotherapy Cycles

Trial	Eligibility	Treatment Regimens	Number of Patients	Outcome
GHSG HD7	CS IA-IIB without large mediastinal mass, massive splenic disease, localized extranodal disease, ESR ≥ 50 mm/h in A, ≥ 30 mm/h in B, ≥ 3 involved areas	A. RT alone (STLI-spleen) (30 GY) + IFRT (40 Gy) B. ABVD × 2 + RT (RT regimen as in A)	571	FFTF (2-year) A = 84%; B = 96%; $p < .05$ Survival (2-year) A = 98%; B = 98%; p = NS
GHSG HD10[119]	CS IA-IIB without large mediastinal mass, massive splenic disease, localized extranodal disease, ESR ≥ 50 mm/h in A, ≥ 30 mm/h in B, ≥ 3 involved areas	A. ABVD × 2 + IFRT (30 Gy) B. ABVD × 2 + IFRT (20 Gy) C. ABVD × 4 + IFRT (30 Gy) D. ABVD × 4 + IFRT (20 Gy)	1131	FFTF (28 mo) = 97% OS (28 mo) = 99%
EORTC/GELA[121] H8F	CS IA-IIB without age: 50, ESR 50 mm/h in A, 30 mm/h in B, 4 or more sites of disease large mediastinal disease	A. MOPP/ABV × 3 + IFRT (36 Gy) B. STLI (S)	543	FFS (4-year) A = 99%; B = 77%; p < .01 (180) Survival (4-year) A = 99%; B = 96%; p = NS

ABVD = doxorubicin, vinblastine, bleomycin, dacarbazine; CS = clinical stage; EORTC = European Organization for the Research and Treatment of Cancer; ESR = erythrocyte sedimentation rate; FFS = failure-free survival; FFTF = freedom from treatment failure; GELA = French Adult Lymphoma Group; GHSG = German Hodgkin Study Group; IF = involved field; MOPP = mechlorethamine, vincristine, procarbazine, prednisone; NS = no significant difference; RT = radiation therapy; STLI (S) = subtotal nodal irradiation (splenic irradiation).

involved field irradiation (n = 168) to mantle and para-aortic–splenic irradiation (n = 165) for favorable prognosis CS IA-IIA patients. The European Organization for the Research and Treatment of Cancer (EORTC) EBVP II regimen (one dose per cycle) was proposed as a potentially less toxic but similarly effective regimen when compared to ABVD. In the H7F trial, six cycles of EBVP were combined with involved-field radiation and randomly compared with subtotal nodal and splenic irradiation. At 6 years, the relapse-free survival rate was significantly higher for patients on the combined chemotherapy and radiation therapy arm than for those on the radiation therapy alone arm (92% vs 81%, respectively, p = .004). The 6-year survival rate was excellent in both treatment arms (98% vs 96%, respectively, p = .156).[116,117] In contrast, in the H7U trial for patients with unfavorable disease, EBVP and involved-field radiation therapy was inferior to MOPP/ABV (Adriamycin [doxorubicin], bleomycin, and vinblastine) and involved-field radiation therapy, suggesting that defining prognostic factors is crucial in selecting patients for modified chemotherapy and radiation therapy regimens.

BNLI trial (1996–2001) This trial compared VAPEC-B chemotherapy for 4 weeks and involved field irradiation to mantle irradiation alone. With a median follow-up time of 51 months, the five-year relapse-free survival was 87% for the chemotherapy and involved field irradiation versus 70% for mantle irradiation alone (p = .002). the five year survival rates were 98% and 92% respectively (p = .036).[118]

Modified Stanford V for Early Stage Favorable Prognosis Hodgkin Disease The relatively short but intensive Stanford V chemotherapy regimen, given for 12 weeks to patients with poor prognosis stage I-II disease,[119] was modified for favorable prognosis CS IA-IIA patients to 8 weeks of the Stanford V regimen and modified involved field irradiation to sites of initial involvement. The chemotherapy regimen includes mechlorethamine (6 mg/m^2 on weeks 1 and 5), doxorubicin (25 mg/m^2 on weeks 1, 3, 5, and 7), vinblastine (6 mg/m^2 on weeks 1, 3, 5, and 7), prednisone (40 mg/m^2 on days 1 to 36, then taper off), vincristine (1.4 mg/m^2 on weeks 2, 4, 6, and 8), bleomycin (5 U/m^2 on weeks 2, 4, 6, and 8), and VP-16 (60 mg/m^2 on days 15 and 16 and days 43 and 44). Preliminary data in 86 patients reports a 3-year freedom from progression of 96% and overall survival of 98%.

The German Hodgkin Study Group HD10 Trial (1998–2002) This study randomized 1,131 patients to four treatment arms: two cycles of ABVD followed by 30 Gy involved field radiation therapy; two cycles of ABVD followed by 20 Gy involved field radiation therapy; four cycles of ABVD followed by 30 Gy involved field radiation therapy; and four cycles of ABVD followed by 20 Gy involved field radiation therapy. The questions being asked in this trial are how many cycles of ABVD are needed to control occult Hodgkin disease in the abdomen and in apparently uninvolved sites adjacent to known Hodgkin disease and what dose of radiation is needed to control Hodgkin disease when combined with limited chemotherapy? This trial should give physicians further guidelines for reduction of treatment in early stage favorable prognosis Hodgkin disease. At a median follow-up of 28 months, the 2-year freedom from treatment failure was 96.6% and the 2-year overall survival was 98.5%, with no significant differences between the 4 arms.[120]

EORTC/Groupe d'Etude des Lymphomes de l'Adulte (GELA) H8F Trial (1993 to 1998) This trial compared three cycles of MOPP/ABV hybrid and involved field irradiation to mantle and para-aortic–splenic irradiation for favorable prognosis CS IA-IIA patients. Completed in 1998, this trial shows a significant advantage in failure-free survival with three cycles of MOPP/ABV and involved field radiation (99% at 4 years) as compared to subtotal nodal and splenic irradiation alone (80% p = .001). No survival differences were seen.[121] Although very effective, the trial used a hybrid regimen, which conferred some risk of sterility and leukemogenesis in the favorable-prognosis Hodgkin disease patients. Because of this concern, ABVD and EBVP without MOPP are being proposed for subsequent trials.

The GHSG 13 trial is a newly-opened 4-arm study comparing 2 cycles of ABVD, AVD, ABV and AV, all followed by 30 Gy of involved-field irradiation in CS I-II patients without risk factors. The results of this trial will shed light on the feasibility of further reducing the chemotherapy in patients with early-stage, favorable prognosis disease.

Randomized Clinical Trials Identifying the Appropriate Radiation Volume and Dose When Combined with Chemotherapy Two trials in favorable prognosis early stage Hodgkin disease evaluate radiation dose to involved sites after chemotherapy. The GHSG HD10 trial (Table 117-8) evaluates the number of cycles of chemotherapy and radiation dose. Patients are randomized to two or four cycles of ABVD. Patients in complete remission will be randomized to either 20 Gy or 30 Gy involved field radiation. Four groups of patients were randomized: ABVD × 2 and 20 Gy, ABVD × 2 and 30 Gy, ABVD × 4 and 20 Gy, and ABVD × 4 and 30 Gy. The EORTC H9F trial is evaluating 36 Gy, 20 Gy, or no radiation to involved sites in patients who have achieved a complete remission after six cycles of EBVP II.

Chemotherapy Alone **Randomized Clinical Trials of Chemotherapy Alone versus Radiation Therapy Alone** Two randomized trials in PS I-II patients evaluating MOPP chemotherapy alone versus subtotal lymph node irradiation alone have been published. The National Cancer Institute (NCI) study was initially designed to include patients with both favorable and unfavorable prognosis early stage Hodgkin disease. However, the most favorable patients with PS IA Hodgkin disease in peripheral sites were not included in the trial and were treated with radiation therapy alone, and patients with an unfavorable prognosis (B symptoms, large mediastinal adenopathy, and limited stage III disease) were included in the trial so that many of the patients did not have favorable prognosis early stage disease.[122] Patients were randomized to 6 months of MOPP chemotherapy alone or subtotal nodal irradiation alone. After researchers recognized that patients with massive mediastinal involvement and PS IIIA disease were not optimal candidates for the radiation therapy alone arm, the eligibility criteria were changed while the study was

Table 117-9 Randomized Clinical Trials in Favorable Prognosis Stage I-II Hodgkin Disease: Trials of Chemotherapy Alone versus Radiation Therapy Alone

Trial	Eligibility	Treatment Regimens	Number of Patients	Outcome
Italian Prospective Randomized Trial[91]	PS IA-IIA	A. STLI	45	FFP (8-year): A = 76%; B = 64%; $p > .05$
		B. MOPP × 6	44	Survival (8-year): A = 93%; B = 56%; $p < .001$
NCI242[122]	PS IA-IIB without large mediastinal disease	PS IA peripheral nodes STLI	30	30/30 FFFR; 28/30 alive
		PS IA (central), IB, IIA, IIB		
		A. STLI	41	FFP (10-year) A = 67%; B = 82%; $p = .27$
		B. MOPP × 6	41	Survival (10-year) A = 85%; B = 90%; $p = .68$
NCIC CTG HD6	CS IA-IIA without MC or LD histology, age ≥ 40, ESR ≥ 50 mm/h, 4 or more sites of involvement	A. STLI (S) or inverted Y RT B. ABVD × 4–6		PFS (4.2 yr) RT ± CT = 93% CT alone = 87% ($p = .006$)

ABVD = doxorubicin, vinblastine, bleomycin, dacarbazine; CS = clinical stage; ESR = erythrocyte sedimentation rate; FFFR = freedom from first relapse; FFP = freedom from progression; LD = lymphocyte depletion; MC = mixed cellularity; MOPP = mechlorethamine, vincristine, procarbazine, prednisone; NCI = National Cancer Institute; NCIC = National Cancer Institute of Canada; PS = laparotomy staged; RT = radiation therapy; STLI (S) = subtotal nodal irradiation (splenic irradiation).

ongoing. Table 117-9 shows the data for the IA (central sites), IB, IIA, and IIB patients without large mediastinal involvement. No difference in disease-free or overall survival is seen at 10 years.

The Italian prospective randomized study randomized patients with PS IA-IIA Hodgkin disease to receive either 6 months of MOPP alone or subtotal nodal irradiation alone.[91] There were no differences in freedom from progression (see Table 117-9). However, the survival rate was significantly higher in patients treated with radiation therapy alone (93%) than in those treated with chemotherapy alone (56%). The difference in survival was attributed to the inability to salvage patients relapsing after MOPP chemotherapy. These results are similar to the poor results of salvage ABVD in patients who relapsed after MOPP for advanced Hodgkin disease (see earlier discussion in this chapter).

Both the NCI and the Italian studies demonstrated greater acute toxicities in patients who received MOPP chemotherapy. In the Longo study, more than 50% of patients treated with MOPP had at least one hospital admission for fever and neutropenia. Both trials demonstrate freedom from treatment failure rates of only 64 to 82% with MOPP alone. More modern trials are being conducted in clinically staged patients using ABVD or similar regimens without alkylating agent chemotherapy. These are discussed in the following paragraphs.

The National Cancer Institute of Canada (NCIC) and Eastern Cooperative Oncology Group CTG HD6 Study is a modification of the NCI and Italian studies with the randomization of clinically staged patients and the use of ABVD as the chemotherapy regimen. Patients with non-bulky CS I-II disease were stratified into low risk (LP/NS, age < 40, ESR < 50 and < 3 sites of disease) and high risk groups.[123] Low risk patients were randomized to extended-field irradiation versus 4 to 6 cycles of ABVD, and high risk patients were randomized to 2 cycles of ABVD followed by radiation therapy versus 4 to 6 cycles of ABVD. At a median follow-up of 4.2 years, patients treated with chemotherapy alone had a significantly inferior 5-year progression-free survival of 87% versus 93% in patients treated with either extended-field irradiation or combined modality therapy ($p = .006$). There were no significant differences in overall survival. The trial has not reported separately the results among favorable prognosis versus unfavorable prognosis patients. A problem with this trial is the long time to completion of the patient accrual so that the "standard arm" of extended-field irradiation, which had been shown to be inferior to combined modality therapy in several randomized trials even among favorable patients, is currently no longer viewed as standard treatment.

Randomized Clinical Trials of Chemotherapy Alone versus Combined Modality Therapy The ongoing EORTC three-armed trial (H9F) for favorable prognosis CS I-II patients compares six cycles of the EBVP II regimen alone to the same regimen with different doses of involved field irradiation. Patients who achieve a complete remission after the chemotherapy are randomized to 36 Gy involved field irradiation versus 20 Gy involved field irradiation versus no radiation therapy (Table 117-10). This trial is designed to evaluate the role of involved field irradiation in favorable prognosis early stage Hodgkin disease and to evaluate potential differences in the dose of radiation delivered. At the most recent interim analysis, the chemotherapy alone arm was closed due to a higher than expected number of relapses that met stopping rules.[124] A potential criticism of this study is whether inadequate chemotherapy was employed. However, this study was restricted to selected patients with favorable features, and the EBVP II regimen was chosen since its efficacy in combination with involved-field radiation therapy had been proven in the earlier EORTC H7F trial.

The Children's Cancer Group (CCG) randomized 501 patients who received a complete response to chemotherapy to involved field radiation or no further treatment. All stages were included. The chemotherapy alone arm in this trial has been stopped. The interim analysis showed increased recurrences in the no radiation arm that met the stopping rules.[125] At 3 years, based on treatment received, the event-free survival was 93% with involved field radiation and 85% without radiation ($p = .024$).

The Memorial Sloan-Kettering Cancer Center trial randomized CS I-IIIA patients who achieved a complete remission after six cycles of ABVD to

Table 117-10 Randomized Clinical Trials in Favorable Prognosis Stage I-II Hodgkin Disease: Trials of Chemotherapy Alone versus Combined Modality Therapy

Trial	Eligibility	Treatment Regimens	Number of Patients	Outcome
EORTC[123] H9F	CS IA-IIB without age ≥ 50, ESR 50 mm/h in A, ≥ 30 mm/h in B, 4 or more sites of disease, large mediastinal disease (? 0.35 m/t ratio)	A. EBVP II × 6 + IFRT (36 Gy) B. EBVP II × 6 + IFRT (20 Gy) C. EBVP II × 6 alone (closed because of stopping rules).	Open	Open
CCG 5942[125]	All stages	Patients stratified by stage into one of three treatment regimens. Patients in complete remission randomized to A. IFRT or B. no rx	501	EFS A = 93%; B = 85%; $p = .024$
MSKCC[126]	CS/PS IA-IIB, IIIA without large mediastinal disease, peripheral or retroperitoneal nodes >10 cm	A. ABVD ×6 B. ABVD × 6 + Mantle or inverted Y RT (36 Gy); STLI/TLI for stage IIIA		Closed, poor accrual

ABVD = doxorubicin, vinblastine, bleomycin, dacarbazine; CS = clinical stage; EBVP = epirubicin, bleomycin, vinblastine, prednisone; ESR = erythrocyte sedimentation rate; EORTC = European Organization for the Research and Treatment of Cancer; IFRT = involved field radiation therapy; MSKCC = Memorial Sloan-Kettering Cancer Center; PS = laparotomy staged; RT = radiation therapy; STLI/TLI = subtotal nodal/ total nodal irradiation.

either mantle irradiation (35 Gy) or no further treatment. Patients with large mediastinal adenopathy and nodes greater than 10 cm were not eligible; however, CS IIB and CS IIA patients were included, thus, this trial was not restricted to early stage favorable prognosis Hodgkin disease. After 152 patients were accrued at 10 years, the trial was closed due to slow accrual. No significant differences in freedom from progression (86% versus 81%) and overall survival (97% versus 90%) were found at a median follow-up of 60 months. The trial, however, was underpowered to determine if the two treatment approaches are truly equivalent, but preliminary analysis predicts no greater than an 18% point difference in recurrence-free survival favoring the radiation arm.[126]

Pavlovsky and colleagues from the Grupo Argentino de Tratamiento de la Leucemia Aguda (GATLA) randomized 277 patients with CS I-II Hodgkin disease to receive 6 monthly cycles of cyclophosphamide, vinblastine, procarbazine and prednisone (CVPP) followed by involved-field radiation therapy to 30 Gy, versus 6 cycles of CVPP alone.[127] At 84 months, the disease-free survival (DFS) of the combined modality therapy arm was significantly higher than that of the chemotherapy alone arm (71% versus 62%, $p = .01$). On subgroup analysis, the difference between the 2 arms was highly significant among patients with unfavorable features (age > 45, > 2 sites or bulky disease), with DFS of 75% in the combined modality therapy arm versus 34% in the chemotherapy alone arm ($p = .001$). Among favorable patients, the difference in DFS was not significant (77% versus 70%).

Laskar and colleagues reported results of a randomized trial from Tata Memorial Hospital with 6 cycles of ABVD. Complete responders were randomized to involved-field radiation therapy or no further treatment.[128] Patients of all stages were included; 55% had CS I-II disease. Significant differences in 6-year event-free survival (88% versus 76%, $p = .01$) and overall survival (100% versus 89%, $p = .002$) were observed, favoring the combined modality therapy arm. The trial contained a high proportion of pediatric patients. Seventy-one percent of cases were of mixed cellularity histology, reflecting the high proportion of Epstein Barr virus–related cases in developing countries.

RADIATION THERAPY ALONE TRIALS

Risk of Occult Abdominal Involvement in Patients with Clinical Stage I or II Hodgkin Disease Historically, the probability of occult abdominal involvement was factored into treatment approaches for patients with CS I-II Hodgkin disease, however, these probabilities are less important in patients receiving combined radiation therapy and chemotherapy. However for patients with limited disease, a low risk of upstaging may allow the use of limited radiation alone without a staging laparotomy. Twenty percent to 30% of CS IA-IIA and 35% of CS IB-IIB patients with Hodgkin disease have occult splenic or upper abdominal nodal involvement not detected by radiographic staging.[71,72] Studies of the results of staging laparotomy demonstrate that selected prognostic factors can predict for a lower risk of occult abdominal involvement in some CS I-II patients. Selected sub-groups, making up approximately 10 to 15% of all CS I-II patients, including CS IA females, CS IA males with disease limited to the high neck, CS IA patients with interfollicular histology, and CS IA patients with lymphocyte-predominant histology, appear to be at lowest risk for occult abdominal involvement (4 to 6%). CS IIA females age 26 years or younger with three regions or less involved and CS IA males with mediastinal involvement also have been identified in one study as having a low-risk incidence.[71] These patients are candidates for radiation therapy alone (limited to above the diaphragm) in selected circumstances. However, with trials showing the efficacy of safer and shorter course chemotherapy, combined radiation therapy and chemotherapy should still remain the standard treatment for these patients.

Dose–Response Data Only one prospective randomized study has been completed.[129] The multicenter trial by the GHSG evaluated the tumoricidal doses for subclinical involvement by Hodgkin disease. A total of 376 laparotomy staged favorable prognosis IA–IIB Hodgkin disease patients were enrolled. Only patients without adverse risk factors were included in the trial. Patients were randomized to receive either 40 Gy extended field radiation therapy or 30 Gy extended field radiation therapy followed by an additional 10 Gy to involved lymph node regions. The 5-year freedom-from-treatment-failure results favored the 30 Gy extended field plus 10 Gy arm over the 40 Gy extended field arm (81% vs 70%, respectively, $p = .026$). The 5-year survival results also favored the 30 Gy extended field arm (98% vs 93%, respectively, $p = .067$), suggesting that 30 Gy is sufficient for treating subclinical involvement of Hodgkin disease with radiation therapy alone. Several other retrospective and modeling studies have also suggested that 30 Gy may be sufficient for patients treated with radiation therapy alone without bulky disease.[130,131]

Trials with Radiation Therapy Alone Evaluating Radiation Field Size The Princess Margaret Hospital has reported results of treating CS I-II Hodgkin disease with radiation therapy alone. In a report of 250 patients, the 8-year actuarial freedom from relapse rate was 71.6%, with a median follow-up time of 6.3 years.[132] Patients with CS I-II Hodgkin disease with favorable prognostic features (age < 50 years, ESR < 40 mm/h, and lymphocyte predominant/nodular sclerosis histology) treated with mantle and para-aortic–splenic irradiation had only a 12.7% actuarial risk of relapse at 8 years. This treatment approach was used as the control arm in the favorable prognosis EORTC and GHSG trials in the 1990s.

Mantle Irradiation Alone in CS IA-IIA Patients The advantages of mantle irradiation alone for early stage Hodgkin disease include the short treatment time and elimination of the long-term risks of radiation to the upper abdomen. Results from prospective and retrospective studies of mantle irradiation alone for unselected CS I-II patients have been disappointing. The EORTC H1 trial, one of the first studies to evaluate the role of chemotherapy in early stage Hodgkin disease, randomized clinically staged I-II patients to receive mantle irradiation alone or combined with vinblastine chemotherapy. All CS I-II patients were enrolled. Fewer recurrences were seen in patients who received both mantle irradiation and vinblastine chemotherapy. However, relapse rates were high in both groups (freedom from recurrence was only 38% in the mantle alone group, the 15-year survival rate was only 58%), suggesting that mantle irradiation alone was not adequate treatment for unselected patients with CS I-II Hodgkin disease.[133] Similarly, the Toronto series reported that a 10-year rate of freedom from recurrence was only 54%.[134] These high recurrence rates in unselected patients are not surprising, as more than 20% of CS I-II patients have occult abdominal involvement, and absence of treatment (with radiation therapy or chemotherapy) to cover potential abdominal disease therefore results in higher recurrence rates than achieved with more extensive treatment. When mantle irradiation was restricted to clinically staged, asymptomatic patients with a single lymph node region involved (CS IA), better results have been seen with 10- to 15-year freedom-from-recurrence rates of 58 to 81%.[134–136]

Mantle Irradiation Alone in PS IA-IIA Patients To determine the role of prophylactic abdominal irradiation in early stage Hodgkin disease, the EORTC H-5 trial (1977 to 1982) compared the use of mantle and para-aortic–splenic pedicle irradiation to mantle irradiation alone in laparotomy-negative patients with favorable early stage Hodgkin disease.[133,137] This study included only patients with nodular sclerosis or lymphocyte predominant histology, age 40 years or younger, PS I or PS II with mediastinal adenopathy, and an ESR less than 70 mm/h. With 15-year follow-up, no differences were seen between the two treatment arms, either for cumulative treatment failure probability ($p = .62$) or overall survival ($p = .69$). These excellent results with mantle irradiation alone in laparotomy-staged patients have been corroborated in other retrospective studies.[136,138,139] In the single-arm Harvard University Medical School trial for laparotomy-staged IA-IIA Hodgkin disease patients, the freedom from treatment failure at 5-years was 92% for stage IA and 78% for stage IIA disease.[139]

Mantle Irradiation Alone in Patients with a Low Risk of Abdominal Involvement The EORTC defined a subgroup of CS I-II patients (women younger than 40 years of age with CS IA nodular sclerosis Hodgkin disease or nodular lymphocyte predominant Hodgkin disease and an

ESR < 50 mm/h) that were treated with mantle irradiation alone without staging laparotomy in the EORTC H7VF (VF, very favorable) and H8VF trials. In the H7VF trial, 40 patients were treated according to this concept and complete remission was reached in 95%. However, 23% of patients relapsed, yielding a 6-year event-free survival rate of 66%, a relapse-free survival rate of 73%, and overall and cause-specific survival rates of 96%.[140] The relapse rates were thought to be unacceptably high in this selected subgroup of stage IA patients, and these patients are now managed according to the EORTC strategy for the favorable subgroup.

In summary, in most trials the freedom from treatment failure rate with mantle irradiation alone in clinically staged patients is inferior to results with more extensive radiation therapy or combined radiation therapy and chemotherapy. In contrast, following a negative laparotomy, early stage patients have a very good outcome after mantle irradiation alone. In an era when staging laparotomies are rarely performed, most patients should be treated with combined radiation therapy and chemotherapy.

Regional Radiation Alone for Nodular Lymphocyte Predominant Hodgkin Disease The preferred treatment for NLPHD is regional radiation alone. This subtype of Hodgkin disease has the lowest disease-related mortality[44,141] of all the subtypes, and studies suggest that ABVD may not be as effective as in classic Hodgkin disease.[141] In an attempt to reduce the risk of treatment-related second cancers, we and others have suggested treatment with radiation therapy alone with limited fields, usually defined as the involved nodal and adjacent prophylactic nodal regions.[141] For patients with disease above the diaphragm, it may be feasible to avoid treating the mediastinal nodes as the mediastinum is rarely involved.

Recommendations and Future Directions Standard care currently provides a number of treatment options for patients with early stage favorable prognosis Hodgkin disease (see the NCCN guidelines on Hodgkin disease). These options include combination chemotherapy and radiation therapy, often with a modified number of cycles of chemotherapy and some modification of radiation field sizes and doses (preferred option); the use of mantle irradiation alone for selected patients after a negative laparotomy; mantle–para-aortic and splenic irradiation without laparotomy; and chemotherapy alone. Reasonable modification of chemotherapy off-study includes giving ABVD for 3–4 cycles. Reasonable modifications of radiation therapy off-study include involved fields to 30 Gy after a complete remission or an uncertain complete remission. Alternatively, patients can be treated to an involved field to 30 Gy in the involved region (involved field by definition) followed by a cone down to the residual disease to 36 Gy.

Current clinical trials are evaluating the use of alternative chemotherapy combinations, shortened courses of chemotherapy, chemotherapy with smaller radiation fields or lower radiation doses, and chemotherapy without radiation therapy. Fortunately, death from Hodgkin disease in favorable prognosis early stage patients is unusual and mortality from causes other than Hodgkin disease occurs many years later; however, this means that survival is not a useful parameter to evaluate results in early stage Hodgkin disease. Current trials must be judged by freedom-from first-recurrence rates, acute morbidity, and by quality of life and cost-effectiveness. Trial objectives to obtain the highest freedom from first recurrence may not provide the optimum treatment once long-term (10- to 20-year) data are available; thus every effort must be taken to reanalyze trials as data become more mature. New methods in decision analysis should also help in the design of trials and in the analysis of retrospective data.

Despite the increasing availability of guidelines for the treatment of Hodgkin disease, there must remain room for individualization of treatment. With different treatment options, some of which may result in a higher recurrence risk at the gain of less toxic initial treatment (without any difference in long-term survival), patient preferences must be assessed. In addition, treatment should be individualized when a particular treatment approach might result in a higher risk of serious late complications, even when these complications may not influence overall survival (ie, treatment of young female patients with large radiation fields and the risk of late breast cancer; heavy smoking history and risk of lung cancer).

Unfavorable Prognosis CS I-II Hodgkin Disease A number of clinical trials comparing radiation therapy alone to combined modality therapy for unfavorable prognosis stage I–II Hodgkin disease were conducted in the 1970s and 1980s. The high recurrence rates with radiation therapy alone led to the development of strategies in current trials that use various combinations of both combination chemotherapy and radiation therapy. To illustrate, the large EORTC (H5U) trial randomized patients with unfavorable prognostic factors to total nodal irradiation versus MOPP chemotherapy (six cycles) and mantle irradiation. There were differences in treatment failure (35% vs 16%, $p < .001$) favoring the combined chemotherapy and radiation therapy arm, but no overall survival differences (69% in both groups at 15 years).[137]

Trials to Identify the Best Combination of Chemotherapy and Radiation Therapy The evolution of studies to identify the best chemotherapy combination for unfavorable early stage Hodgkin disease paralleled trials to identify the optimal chemotherapy for advanced Hodgkin disease. Early trials evaluated MOPP versus MOPP-like combinations; later trials compared these combinations with ABVD, and, finally, the most recent trials compare new intense chemotherapy combinations with ABVD. Table 117-11 shows representative trials.

The first combined modality trial to test MOPP versus ABVD in unfavorable prognosis patients was the Milan study conducted between 1974 and 1982. Split-course treatment was employed, with three cycles of chemotherapy preceding and following subtotal nodal irradiation. There was no significant difference in 5-year freedom from progression, however, the number of patients enrolled was too small to definitively rule out a difference in outcome.[142] The EORTC H6U trial (1982–1988) also used split-course chemotherapy and radiation therapy and compared MOPP and ABVD.[137] Three hundred sixteen patients were randomized. The 10-year survival was equivalent in both arms, but the freedom-from-treatment-failure rate was significantly higher with ABVD than with MOPP.

A large randomized trial was designed to test whether four cycles of combination chemotherapy and radiation therapy is sufficient treatment compared to six cycles of chemotherapy and radiation therapy. The EORTC H8U study randomized patients to combined modality therapy with four or six cycles of MOPP/ABV, and between involved field and extended field irradiation (Table 117-12). At 4 years there are no differences in failure-free survival or overall survival between the three arms of the trial with 4 cycles of ABVD and involved field irradiation having the same outcome as the two arms with more extensive treatment.[143]

The Grupo Argentino de Tratamiento de la Leucemia Aguda (GATLA) trial and the EORTC H7U trial (see Table 117-11) studied modified nonalkylating regimens versus standard alkylating agent regimens in unfavorable prognosis early stage patients. All patients received combined radiation therapy and chemotherapy. In both trials, the arms using modified chemotherapy were associated with significantly higher recurrence rates. In the GATLA trial, the event-free survival was 66% for doxorubicin, vincristine, prednisone, and etoposide and involved field radiation therapy versus 85% ($p = .009$) for CVPP (cyclophosphamide, etoposide, procarbazine, and prednisone) and involved field radiation therapy.[144] In the EORTC trial, the event-free survival was 68% for EBVP II and involved field radiation therapy versus 90% ($p = .0001$) for MOPP/ABV and involved field radiation therapy.[145] The recurrence rate in this trial was high enough to result in early closure of the trial. These trials illustrate the importance of careful assessment of prognostic factors prior to treatment for early-stage Hodgkin disease. Minimal combined chemotherapy and radiation therapy approaches may not be ideal for patients with unfavorable prognosis CS I-II disease.

Based mainly on trials in advanced Hodgkin disease, ABVD has become the standard regimen used in patients with CS I-II disease. A number of current trials compare combined modality therapy using ABVD with more intense, novel regimens. Both the EORTC H9U and GHSG HD11 studies of combined modality therapy are comparing four cycles of ABVD with four cycles of BEACOPP-baseline (bleomycin, etoposide, Adriamycin [doxorubicin], cyclophosphamide, vincristine, procarbazine, and prednisone). The

Table 117-11 Randomized Clinical Trials in Unfavorable Prognosis Stage I-II Hodgkin Disease: Trials to Identify the Optimal Chemotherapy Combination

Trial	Eligibility	Treatment Regimens	Number of Patients	Outcome
EORTC H6U 1982–1988[137]	CS I-II with large mediastinal mass or ESR ≥ 50 mm/h in A; ≥ 30 mm/h in B or ≥ 3 involved areas	CT ×3 + Mantle + CT ×3 A. MOPP B: ABVD	165 151	FFTF (10-year) A = 68%; B = 90%; $p < .0001$ Survival (10-year) A = 87%; B = 87%; $p = .52$
GATLA 1986–1992[144]	Score of age, B symptoms, stage, number of sites, and bulky disease	A: CVPP × 3 + IFRT (30 Gy) + CVPP × 3 B: AOPE × 3 + IFRT (30 Gy) + AOPE × 3	92 84	EFS (5-year) A = 85%; B = 66%; $p = .009$ Survival (5 year) A = 95%; B = 87%; $p = .16$
EORTC H7U [145] 1988–1992	CS IA-IIA with age > 50 years or ESR ≥ 50 mm/h in A; ≥ 30 mm/h in B or large mediastinal mass (≥\0.33 m/t)	A: EBVP II × 6 + IFRT (36Gy) B: MOPP/ABV × 6 + IFRT	160 156	EFS (6-year) A = 68%; B = 90%; $p < .0001$ Survival (6-year) A = 82%; B = 89%; $p = .18$
EORTC H9U[146]	Same as H7U	A: ABVD × 6 + IFRT (30 Gy) B: ABVD × 4 + IFRT C: BEACOPP × 4 + IFRT	Open	Open
GHSG HD11[147] 1998–	CS IA-IB, IIA with ESR—50 mm/h or CS IIB and ESR > 30 mm/h or large mediastinal disease	A: ABVD × 4 + IFRT (30 Gy) B: ABVD × 4 + IFRT (20 Gy) C: BEACOPP × 4 + IFRT (30 Gy) D: BEACOPP × 4 + IFRT (20 Gy)	Open	Open
ECOG 2496 1998–	Large mediastinal disease	A: ABVD × 6 + IFRT (36 Gy) to bulky sites (> 5 cm) B: 12 weeks Stanford V + IFRT to bulky sites	Open	Open

ABVD = Adriamycin (doxorubicin), bleomycin, vinblastine, and dacarbazine; BEACOPP = bleomycin, etoposide, doxorubicin, cyclophosphamide, vincristine, procarbazine, and prednisone; CS = clinical stage; CVPP = cyclophosphamide, etoposide, procarbazine, and prednisone; ECOG = Eastern Cooperative Oncology Group; EFS = event-free survival; EORTC = European Organization for the Research and Treatment of Cancer; ESR = erythrocyte sedimentation rate; FFTF = freedom from treatment failure; GATLA = Grupo Argentina de Tratamiento de Leucemia Aguda; GHSG = German Hodgkin Study Group; IFRT = involved field radiation therapy; MOPP =Mustargen (mechlorethamine), Oncovin (vincristine), procarbazine, and prednisone; Stanford V = mechlorethamine, doxorubicin, vinblastine, prednisone, vincristine, bleomycin, and etoposide.

EORTC H9U trial randomizes patients between four and six cycles of ABVD or 4 cycles of the BEACOPP regimen, all followed by involved field irradiation.[146] The most recent interim analysis showed 4-year event-free survival and overall survival of 90% and 94%, respectively, for the entire group with no comparison provided for the different treatment arms. The GHSG HD 11 trial randomized patients into 4 arms comparing two doses of involved field radiation therapy (20 vs 30 Gy) and 4 cycles of ABVD versus 4 cycles of BEACOPP.[147] A total of 1,363 patients have been entered on to the trial. At 2-years there are no differences in treatment outcome between chemotherapy regimens and between doses of radiation therapy. The 2-year freedom from treatment failure rate is 90%. In the ECOG 2496 trial of combined modality therapy, six cycles of ABVD are being compared to 3 months of Stanford V. In the recently opened GHSG HD 15 trial, patients with CS I-II disease with risk factors are randomized to 4 cycles of ABVD versus 2 cycles of dose-escalated BEACOPP and 2 cycles of ABVD, followed by involved field irradiation to 30 Gy.

Trials to Identify the Appropriate Radiation Therapy Volume Several randomized trials have studied radiation field size when combined with chemotherapy for unfavorable prognosis early stage Hodgkin disease. The French Cooperative Trial reported by Zittoun and colleagues randomized 218 stage I-II unfavorable prognosis patients to six cycles of MOPP sandwiched around involved field (40 Gy) or extended field (40 Gy) irradiation.[148] The 6-year disease-free survival rates were 87% and 93%, respectively ($p = .15$), for the involved field and extended field arms. The Milan study reported by Santoro incorporated only 4 months of chemotherapy (ABVD), followed by involved field (36 Gy) or subtotal nodal irradiation (30 to 36 Gy). One hundred thirty-three patients were treated; 20% had bulky disease.[149] The 5-year freedom-from-progression rates were 96% and 93%, respectively (see Table 117-12). The EORTC/GELA H8U trial, reported above, randomized patients to four cycles of MOPP/ABV plus involved field versus subtotal nodal irradiation. The GHSG HD8 trial, conducted between 1993 and 1998, used two cycles (4 months) of cyclophosphamide, Oncovin (vincristine), procarbazine, and prednisone (COPP)/ABVD followed by either involved field or extended field irradia-

Table 117-12 Randomized Clinical Trials in Unfavorable Prognosis Stage I-II Hodgkin Disease: Trials to Identify the Appropriate Radiation Volume

Trial	Eligibility	Treatment Regimens	Number of Patients	Outcome
French Cooperative Trial 1976–81	CS I- II without age > 45 years, 3 or more regions of disease, bulky disease	A. MOPP × 3 + IFRT (40 Gy) + MOPP × 3 B. MOPP × 3 + EFRT (40 Gy) + MOPP × 3	82 91	DFS (6-year) A = 87%; B = 93%; p = NS Survival (7-year) A = 92%; B = 91%; p = NS
Milan[142]	All CS I-II	A. ABVD × 4 + STLI B. ABVD × 4 + IFRT	65 68	FFP (5-year) 1990–1997 A = 96%; B = 93%; p = NS
EORTC/GELA H8U 1993–98[143]	CS IA-IIB with age > 50 years, ESR ≥ 50 mm/h in A; > 30 mm/h in B, 4 or more sites of disease, large mediastinal disease	A. MOPP/ABV × 6 + IFRT (36 Gy) B. MOPP/ABV × 4 + IFRT (36 Gy) C. MOPP/ABV × 4 + STLI	995	FFS (4-year); p = NS A= 88%; B = 92%; C = 92% Survival (4-year); p = NS A= 90%; B = 94%; C = 93%
GHSG HD8 1993–98	CS IA-IIB with ESR > 50 mm/h in A; ≥ 30 mm/h in B, 3 or more sites of disease, large mediastinal disease	COPP/ABVD × 4 months + IFRT COPP/ABVD × 4 months + EFRT	Not reported	Not reported

ABV = Adriamycin (doxorubicin), bleomycin, and vinblastine; ABVD = Adriamycin (doxorubicin), bleomycin, vinblastine, and dacarbazine; CS = clinical stage; DFS = disease-free survival; EFRT =extended field radiation therapy; EORTC = European Organization for the Research and Treatment of Cancer; ESR = erythrocyte sedimentation rate; FFP = freedom from progression; FFS = failure-free survival; GELA = Groupe d'Etude des Lymphomes de l'Adulte; GHSG = German Hodgkin Study Group; IFRT = involved field radiation therapy; MOPP = Mustargen (mechlorethamine), Oncovin (vincristine), procarbazine, and prednisone; STLI = subtotal nodal irradiation .

tion to 30 Gy (see Table 117-12). Evidence from these randomized trials suggests that radiation fields may be safely limited to involved regions in most combined chemotherapy and radiation therapy programs.

Trials of Chemotherapy Alone versus Combined Modality Therapy Only one prospective trial of chemotherapy alone versus combined modality therapy in unfavorable prognosis stage I-II has been reported. The GATLA randomized 104 patients with unfavorable disease characteristics to six cycles of CVPP alone or six cycles of CVPP sandwiched around involved field irradiation (30 Gy). The 7-year survival rates were 66% and 84%; the freedom-from-relapse rates were 34% and 75% ($p < .001$), both favoring combined modality treatment.[127]

The ongoing NCIC HD6 trial evaluates patients with unfavorable disease characteristics but excludes patients with large mediastinal adenopathy or nodes greater than 10 cm. Patients are randomized to receive combined modality therapy with two cycles of ABVD followed by irradiation (an extended mantle plus splenic irradiation or mantle plus para-aortic and splenic irradiation) or four to six cycles of ABVD alone (depending on the rapidity of response). Data have not been separately reported for these two groups of patients.[123]

Recommendations and Future Directions The outcome of treatment for patients with unfavorable prognosis stage I-II Hodgkin disease has improved dramatically in the past three decades. Mainly, this is a result of the use of combined modality therapy, because historically fewer than 50% of patients in some subgroups remain free in first remission when radiation therapy alone is used as initial treatment. Combined radiation therapy and chemotherapy not only enhances the likelihood of local tumor control, but it also should control occult nodal and extranodal disease in the majority of patients. Current clinical trials are exploring new combinations of radiation therapy and chemotherapy to try to reduce late morbidity and mortality while maintaining a high probability of freedom from first recurrence.

Continued refinement of the definition of "unfavorable prognosis" is needed in current trials. Whenever possible, individual prognostic factors should be separately analyzed. Detailed analysis of completed clinical trials may permit this redefinition, which would permit some patients to be treated with less aggressive management approaches.

TREATMENT OF ADVANCED HODGKIN DISEASE

The management of Hodgkin disease using chemotherapy represents one of the first major accomplishments of medical oncology. Although patients with localized Hodgkin disease could occasionally be cured with the radiotherapeutic techniques available in the mid-twentieth century, advanced Hodgkin disease was uniformly fatal. Even though mechlorethamine was shown to be an active drug in the 1940s, and numerous other active agents were discovered over the next 20 years,[17] it was not until the 1960s that combination chemotherapy was used for patients with Hodgkin disease.[20] By using single agents, fewer than 5% of the patients survived 5 years.[150] In the mid-1960s, investigators at the NCI first treated patients with a four-drug combination chemotherapy regimen using mechlorethamine, vincristine, methotrexate, and prednisone (MOMP).[20] When procarbazine became available, this drug was substituted for methotrexate (MOPP).[16] The initial results with this regimen demonstrated improved complete remissions and prolonged survival, overcoming the concerns that "using up" all active drugs at one time would shorten survival.[151] Since the curability of advanced Hodgkin disease with MOPP became accepted, numerous other chemotherapy regimens have been developed. These have been aimed at improving the effectiveness of therapy and at reducing toxicity. In recent years, combinations of increasing numbers of drugs, combined modality therapy, and high-dose therapy with autologous bone marrow transplantation have all been studied in an attempt to improve cure rates.

Early in the use of chemotherapy to treat malignancies, the model of leukemia, in which maintenance therapy was used, was often applied. However, randomized trials documented the lack of benefit of maintenance chemotherapy in Hodgkin disease.[19] It also became clear that comparatively brief courses of chemotherapy could affect cure in Hodgkin disease. Between 6 and 12 cycles of treatment have frequently been used. One randomized trial demonstrated that eight cycles of ABVD was comparable to 12 cycles of alternating ABVD and MOPP.[21] At present, the most frequently used duration of chemotherapy is six to eight cycles of ABVD—with the goal of treating two cycles after achieving remission. In some cases of Hodgkin disease, residual masses are apparent on CT scans at the completion of therapy. The distinction between persisting lymphoma and residual fibrous tissue can be difficult. Frequently, gallium or PET scans are used to try to resolve this dilemma, with patients showing a positive scan receiving further therapy.

For many years, the most popular chemotherapy regimen used in the treatment of advanced Hodgkin disease was MOPP (Table 117-13). DeVita and colleagues reported 198 patients treated with this regimen.[16] The complete remission rate was 81%. Eventually, 36% of the complete responders relapsed, giving a 52% 10-year disease-free survival rate. The overall survival at 10 years was 50%, reflecting some deaths from treatment-related toxicity. Several subsequent trials using MOPP[21,152,153] have shown disease-free survivals of 36 to 47%.

A number of variations on the MOPP regimen have been reported (see Table 117-1). The most popular have been MVPP (mechlorethamine, vinblastine, procarbazine, and prednisone),[154,155] ChlVPP,[156,157] and BCVPP (carmustine, cyclophosphamide, vinblastine, procarbazine, and prednisone).[153] These regimens have led to disease-free survival rates approximately comparable to MOPP. The ChlVPP regimen has been reported to have less immediate toxicity and frequently has been used for the treatment of older patients.

The first major alternative to the MOPP regimen was reported by Bonadonna and colleagues in 1975.[158] This regimen used ABVD. Whereas MOPP was administered for 14 days and then no treatment for 14 days, ABVD was administered every other week with all of the drugs given intravenously (see Table 117-1). Several randomized trials have compared MOPP and ABVD.[21,142] In no case has MOPP been found to be superior; it was generally found to have an inferior outcome. In addition, ABVD appeared to have less toxicity.[142,159] A study by Cancer and Leukemia Group B showed a failure-free survival of 61% for ABVD and 50% for MOPP.[21] The results of this study have caused ABVD to be, by far, the most frequently used regimen for treating advanced Hodgkin disease in the United States. Bonadonna and colleagues first reported using a combination of MOPP and ABVD to treat patients with Hodgkin disease.[151] The two regimens have been combined in a variety of ways in subsequent trials. Some patients receive alternating cycles of MOPP and ABVD.[151] Other studies combined MOPP and ABVD in a single cycle with the first 7 days of the cycle using the drugs from MOPP, with the drugs in ABVD being given on day 8. In these studies, the dacarbazine was frequently deleted.[160] Some studies found no difference between the two approaches, whereas others identified superiority to using MOPP/ABV in a "hybrid" regimen. A randomized trial comparing the alternating or hybrid regimens to ABVD alone did not show an advantage to the more complex regimen.[160] This has further solidified the place of ABVD as the "standard" regimen for the treatment of advanced Hodgkin disease.

Unfortunately, 30 to 40% of patients with advanced Hodgkin disease treated with ABVD fail to achieve an initial remission or relapse from remission. The proportion of patients with a large number of adverse risk factors that fail ABVD is even higher. These results have led to attempts at identifying improved treatment regimens. The most popular of these have been Stanford V and BEACOPP (Table 117-14).[161,162] The Stan-ford V regimen uses doxorubicin, vinblastine, mechlorethamine, bleomycin, vincristine, etoposide, and prednisone. The drugs are administered weekly for 12 weeks.[119] The regimen is followed by adjuvant radiation therapy to sites of initial bulky disease of 5 cm or greater. One-hundred forty-two patients with stage III or IV or locally extensive mediastinal stage I or II disease who received Stanford V were reported with a median follow-up of 5.4 years. The overall failure-free survival was 89% and the overall survival was 96%.[163] There were no treatment-related deaths. Patients with 0 to 2 adverse risk factors in the International Prognostic System for Hodgkin disease had a failure-free survival of 94%, versus 75% for patients with a score of 3 or higher. No

Table 117-13 Chemotherapy Regimen Used for Hodgkin Disease

Drug	Dose (mg/m²)	Route	Schedule (Days)	Cycle Length (Days)
MOPP				
Mechlorethamine	6	IV	1.8	21
Vincristine	1.4	IV	1.8	
Procarbazine	100	PO	1–14	
Prednisone	40	PO	1–14	
BCVPP				
Carmustine	100	IV	1	28
Cyclophosphamide	600	IV	1	
Vinblastine	5	IV	1	
Procarbazine	50	PO	1	
	100	PO	2–10	
Prednisone	60	PO	1–10	
ChlVPP				
Chlorambucil	6	PO	1–14	28
Vinblastine	6	IV	1.8	
Procarbazine	100	PO	1–14	
Prednisone	40 total	PO	1–14	
COPP				
Cyclophosphamide	650	IV	1.8	28
Vincristine	1.4	IV	1.8	
Procarbazine	100	PO	1–14	
Prednisone	40	PO	1–14	
MVPP				
Nitrogen mustard	6	IV	1.8	42
Vinblastine	6	IV	1.8	
Procarbazine	100	PO	1–14	
Prednisone	40 total	PO	1–14	
LOPP				
Chlorambucil	10 total	PO	1–10	28
Vincristine	1.4	IV	1.8	
Procarbazine	100	PO	1–10	
Prednisone	25	PO	1–14	
CVPP				
Lomustine	75	PO	1	28
Vinblastine	4	IV	1.8	
Procarbazine	100	PO	1–14	
Prednisone	40	PO	1–14	
ABVD				
Adriamycin (doxorubicin)	25	IV	1.15	28
Bleomycin	10	IV	1.15	
Vinblastine	6	IV	1.15	
Dacarbazine	375	IV	1.15	
MOPP/ABVD hybrid				
Mechlorethamine	6	IV	1	28
Oncovin (vincristine)	1.4[a]	IV	1	
Procarbazine	100	PO	1–7	
Prednisone	40	PO	1–7	
Adriamycin (doxorubicin)	25	IV	15	
Bleomycin	10	IV	15	
Vinblastine	6	IV	15	
Dacarbazine	35	IV	15	
MMOPP/ABV hybrid				
Mechlorethamine	6	IV	1	28
Oncovin (vincristine)	1.4[a]	IV	1	
Procarbazine	100	PO	1–7	
Prednisone	40	PO	1–14	
Adriamycin (doxorubicin)	35	IV	8	
Bleomycin	10	IV	8	
Vinblastine	6	IV	8	

[a]No more than 2.0 mg Oncovin total dose to be delivered.

secondary leukemias were observed. In a recent update for these data[164] 86% of patients treated with stage III or IV Hodgkin disease were free from progression at 8 years follow-up and 83% of the patients were free from progression at 12 years follow-up. The 12-year overall survival was 95%. Fertility seems to be preserved with 72 post treatment conceptions. A recent study from the United Kingdom compared the Stanford V regimen to ABVD and found similar anti-Hodgkin disease efficacy with less toxicity using the Stanford V regimen.[165]

Investigators in Germany have developed a dose-intense regimen named BEACOPP (see Table 117-14).[162] BEACOPP has been given at two dose levels, with the higher dose level requiring hematopoietic growth factors and more intensive supportive care. When compared to COPP/ABVD in a randomized trial, the BEACOPP regimen (ie, both the standard dose BEACOPP and the escalated dose BEACOPP) had a superior freedom from treatment failure at 5 years (69% COPP—ABVD, 76% standard dose BEACOPP, and 87% escalated dose BEACOPP). The overall survival at 5 years was 83%, 88%, and 91% respectively favoring the BEACOPP regimens but not significantly so. However, when the two BEACOPP regimens were combined, there was a significant difference in overall survival. A recent update of these data[166] confirmed the superiority of escalated dose BEACOPP in eradicating Hodgkin disease with an 85% 82-month freedom from treatment failure, which was significantly better than COPP-ABVD, or standard dose BEACOPP. However, secondary acute myeloid leukemia/myelodysplasia was more frequent with the escalated dose BEACOPP arm occurring in 11 of 466 patients versus 5 of 469 patients with standard dose BEACOPP and 1 of 260 patients with COPP ABVD.

The place of combined modality therapy in advanced Hodgkin disease is clear in only a few instances. Patients with bulky mediastinal masses certainly benefit from adjuvant radiation therapy. The Stanford V regimen is a combined modality regimen and has initially been shown to have excellent results. The BEACOPP regimen also uses radiation therapy for bulky sites of disease at the completion of chemotherapy. In patients without bulky disease most clinicians would avoid radiation therapy in an attempt to minimize long-term toxicity.

However, the role of radiation therapy in advanced Hodgkin disease remains somewhat controversial. In part, this is because of the potential morbidity from the large fields of radiation that often are required, the increased risk of extranodal recurrences outside of the radiation fields as the stage of disease increases, and the lack of survival differences in randomized studies. Some randomized trials suggest an improvement in freedom from treatment failure with the use of adjuvant (often low-dose) radiation therapy. In the SWOG trial, when the analysis was restricted to patients of all histologic sub-types who received their randomly assigned therapy, the remission duration of those who received consolidation radiation therapy was significantly better than that of the patients who were treated with chemotherapy alone (85% vs 67%; $p < .002$).[167] In addition, significant improvements in freedom from recurrence were seen in patients with nodular sclerosis histology and in patients with bulky disease. Similar results were reported in a meta-analysis of randomized trials where adjuvant radiation therapy resulted in an 11% advantage in freedom from recurrence, but no overall survival differences when compared to the same chemotherapy regimen alone.[168] In contrast, a recently reported EORTC trial showed no significant difference in event-free survival with adjuvant

Table 117-14 New Chemotherapy Regimen for Hodgkin Disease

Drug	Dose (mg/m²)	Route	Schedule (Days)	RT	Cycle Length
BEACOPP				Bulky, residual	21 days
(Escalated BEACOPP)					
Bleomycin	10	IV	8		
Etoposide	100 (200)	IV	1–3		
Adriamycin (doxorubicin)	25 (35)	IV	1		
Cyclophosphamide	650 (1250)	IV	1		
Oncovin (vincristine)	1.4[a]	IV	8		
Procarbazine	100	PO	1–7		
Prednisone	40	PO	1–14		
G-CSF	–(+)	SQ	8+		
Stanford V					
Mechlorethamine	6	IV	Wk 1, 5, 9	Bulky	12 weeks
Adriamycin (doxorubicin)	25	IV	Wk 1, 3, 5, 9, 11		
Vinblastine	6	IV	Wk 1, 3, 5, 9, 11		
Vincristine	1.4[a]	IV	Wk 2, 4, 6, 8, 10, 12		
Bleomycin	5	IV	Wk 2, 4, 6, 8, 10, 12		
Etoposide	60 × 2	IV	Wk, 3, 7, 11		
Prednisone	40	PO	Wk 1–10 q.o.d.		
G-CSF			Dose reduction or delay		

[a]No more than 2.0 mg Oncovin total dose to be delivered.

involved field irradiation in patients who were in complete remission prior to the randomization to radiation or no further treatment. However, the trial suggested a benefit to radiation therapy in patients who did not achieve a complete remission.[169]

Given the above data and guidelines from standard practice, the following are circumstances in which adjuvant radiation therapy should be considered for use in the management of advanced or recurrent Hodgkin disease: in patients with stage III-IV disease who have not achieved a complete remission with chemotherapy; to sites of large bulky disease such as the mediastinum following a complete response to chemotherapy in other sites[170]; when using chemotherapy regimens that have published data with radiation therapy as part of the upfront management such as Stanford[163]; and as part of systemic treatment (standard dose or high-dose chemotherapy) for localized recurrent disease.

The optimal chemotherapy regimen for the treatment of patients with advanced Hodgkin disease remains unknown. All regimens fail to cure some patients and long-term toxicity is a significant concern. The risk of secondary leukemia seems to be a reflection of the dose of alkylating agents in the treatment regimen. Secondary acute leukemia or myelodysplasia is an unusual complication of treatment with ABVD, but occurs more frequently in patients treated with MOPP-like regimens.[171] The risk of secondary solid tumors seems to be primarily related to the use of radiation therapy in the treatment regimen, although alkylating agents are associated with an increased risk of lung cancer, especially in patients who smoke.[100,172] Other toxicities, including heart disease, lung disease, endocrine dysfunction, and infertility, are seen in a subset of patients. However, in patients with poor-risk Hodgkin disease, the cure rate does not seem to be high enough with available treatments to reduce dose intensity, although in good-risk patients with advanced disease this might be a reasonable consideration.

Very-high-dose therapy and autologous bone marrow transplantation have also been tested as part of the primary therapy in patients with very poor-risk Hodgkin disease. One problem in applying this treatment approach has been the difficulty in identifying patients with Hodgkin disease who have a very poor survival with modern therapies. Italian[173] and Spanish[174] investigators have reported encouraging results in pilot studies. The European Group for Bone and Marrow Transplantation compared 56 patients transplanted in complete remission with 168 patients who were matched by risk factors from the GHSG. Freedom from relapse was superior in patients undergoing transplantation, but overall survival did not differ. An international study of 163 patients with poor risk Hodgkin disease who achieved a complete or partial remission with four courses of a doxorubicin containing chemotherapy regimen were randomly assigned to four more courses of standard chemotherapy or autotransplant. At a median follow up of 48 months, the freedom from failure and overall survival rates were not different. At present, the value of bone marrow transplantation in the primary therapy of patients with Hodgkin disease remains unproven.

ELDERLY PATIENTS WITH HODGKIN DISEASE

Elderly patients with Hodgkin disease have not benefited from chemotherapy to the same degree as younger patients. Patients older than 60 years of age with Hodgkin disease had a very poor outlook, with 5-year failure-free survival rates less than 50%, and even poorer results in those patients with high stage, symptomatic disease. A recent study retrospectively comparing patients older than 60 years of age who were treated with ChlVPP with those receiving the hybrid regimen ChlVPP/ABV showed an advantage in 5-year overall survival (87% vs 39%) and 5-year event-free survival (75% vs 31%) for ChlVPP/ABV.[175] It may be that the addition of doxorubicin to the treatment regimen is even more important in elderly patients whose disease has been chemotherapy resistant. A similar regimen (ChlVPP/EVA) in the study of patients of all ages was found to be superior to a weekly chemotherapy regimen in high-risk patients.[176]

Hodgkin Disease in Patients with HIV Infection The association of Hodgkin disease and infection by the human immunodeficiency virus (HIV) was first noted in 1984.[177] Subsequent studies have shown that Hodgkin disease is 5 to 20 times more frequent in patients with HIV infection. Patients with HIV infection who develop Hodgkin disease are more likely to have mixed cellularity rather than the nodular sclerosis subtype. Patients with HIV infection are more likely to present with advanced stage, extra nodal involvement, and B-symptoms. Before the development of highly active antiretroviral therapy (HAART) the treatment outcome was poorer than in patients without HIV infection.

The development of HAART and its use in HIV infected patients being treated for Hodgkin disease has improved the treatment outcome. In a report of 59 patients treated with the Stanford V regimen while simultaneously receiving HAART and hematopoietic growth factor support, 69 patients were able to complete treatment with no dose reduction or treatment delays.[178] The 3-year overall survival was 51%, 3-year disease-free survival 68%, and 3-year freedom from progression 60%. Patients with a higher International Prognostic Score (IPS) had a poorer outcome (ie, 83% freedom from progression with an IPS score of 2 or lower versus 41% with an IPS score of 3 or higher).

Investigators from Germany treated 12 patients with Hodgkin disease and HIV infection utilizing the standard dose BEACOP regimen.[179] Eight of the 12 patients completed the planned 6 courses of BEACOPP. Two patients died of opportunistic infections and one relapsed. The remaining 9 patients were in complete remission at a median of 49 months at the time of the report. Most but not all the patients in this series were receiving antiretroviral therapy.

A combination of HAART and chemotherapy for Hodgkin disease is practical and achieves treatment outcomes almost as good as seen in HIV negative patients. Except for patients who are seriously ill with opportunistic infections, patients with Hodgkin disease who are HIV positive should be treated with standard regimens and most of these patients can be cured of Hodgkin disease.

Salvage Therapy For the purposes of this section, salvage therapy refers to treatment administered to patients with Hodgkin disease who fail to achieve an initial complete remission or relapse after achieving an initial complete remission. Although seemingly straightforward, the diagnosis of treatment failure is not always easy. Patients with bulky mediastinal or retroperitoneal masses regularly have residual, albeit smaller, masses on imaging studies at the completion of successful therapy. In these patients, previously abnormal gallium scans and elevated ESR usually revert to normal, but this may take some time. In many cases, a biopsy will be required to prove persistent lymphoma. Biopsy should always be done in the patient who achieves a complete remission and then develops new adenopathy or imaging abnormalities. A patient with Hodgkin disease can develop non-Hodgkin lymphoma, other malignancy, and tuberculosis or other infections. Failure to establish a firm diagnosis of relapse can be tragic.

Patients who are treated initially with radiation therapy alone and who progress, have an excellent outcome with salvage chemotherapy.[86–87] When compared to patients who are treated with chemotherapy from the outset, those receiving similar chemotherapy regimens for relapse after radiation therapy have an equivalent or superior outlook.[86] The use of radiation therapy to rescue patients who fail chemotherapy is occasionally an effective treatment maneuver. In patients with localized relapse, extended field radiation therapy can achieve durable remissions in 25 to 50% of cases. It must be emphasized that only occasional patients with nonbulky disease confined to a few node-bearing areas and who do not have systemic systems are candidates for this treatment approach.

Unfortunately, 30 to 60% of patients with advanced Hodgkin disease will either fail to achieve a remission with chemotherapy or will relapse after complete remission. These patients, who are primarily refractory and never achieve an initial remission to an effective chemotherapy regimen, have a particularly poor outlook. Early experience with ABVD showed that some patients who failed MOPP could be successfully treated, whereas the converse was less often true.[88] Even so, the durable remission rate in this setting is less than 20%.[180]

New treatment regimens such as Stanford V and BEACOPP seem to cure a high proportion of patients with advanced Hodgkin disease but expose patients to more drugs and/or higher doses than seen with ABVD. It is possible that salvage therapies after these regimens will not be as effective as have been described for patients treated with ABVD or other earlier treatment regimens.

Early autologous bone marrow transplantation in patients who are primarily refractory to an excellent chemotherapy regimen for Hodgkin disease can produce durable remissions in a significant proportion of patients. The North American Autologous Blood and Marrow Transplant Registry reported 103 such patients. The overall in progression-free survival at 5 years was 40%.[181] The European Group for Blood and Marrow Transplantation described 290 patients with primary refractory Hodgkin disease and reported a 5-year failure-free survival of 30%.[182] Investigators from GELA found that patients with at least a partial response to induction chemotherapy had a better 5-year survival (72%) than did patients with no response or progressive disease (30%).[183] Investigators at Stanford University performed a case-control study for primary chemotherapy failures. They found an event-free survival at 4 years of 52% for transplantation, in contrast to 10% for alternate standard chemotherapy regimens.[184] Patients who fail to achieve remission with primary chemotherapy are best treated with autologous bone marrow transplantation, and this probably represents the clearest indication for autologous transplantation in patients with Hodgkin disease.

Patients who achieve an initial complete remission and relapse represent a heterogeneous group of patients. In general, the longer the initial complete remission, the better the outlook with any form of salvage therapy.[89,185] A follow-up analysis of the original MOPP-treated patients from the NCI found that those patients who had an initial remission longer than 12 months achieved second complete remissions 74% of the time, in contrast to only 28% of the time in patients with initial remissions lasting less than 12 months.[89] However, even in patients with long initial remissions, the eventual survival from first relapse was only 24%. Similar results have been reported from Milan,[185] Vancouver,[186] and Paris.[187] In addition to a brief initial remission, other adverse prognostic factors include advanced age, more extensive initial disease, systemic symptoms, and elevated serum lactate acid dehydrogenase level.[187]

A variety of treatment regimens have been used for patients with relapsed Hodgkin disease. In addition to MOPP or ABVD in patients who received the opposite regimen initially, a number of other treatments have been used. Unfortunately, the number of patients achieving extended survival free of Hodgkin disease is quite poor, although patients with no adverse risk characteristics (see above) have been reported to have 5-year failure-free survivals as high as 50%.[89,185]

An encouraging new drug in the treatment of Hodgkin disease is gemcitabine.[188] Gemcitabine has a significant response rate as a single agent in patients with refractory Hodgkin disease and is now being tested in combinations. It is possible that gemcitabine will some day be used earlier in the treatment of patients with Hodgkin disease. Treatment with the monoclonal antibody rituximab produced objective responses in five of 22 patients with nodular sclerosing classical Hodgkin disease and alleviated system symptoms in a larger number of patients.[189,190] The studies suggested that the responses might be related to the depletion of normal B-cells rather than a direct anticancer effect. Biologic therapies using monoclonal antibodies directed against CD30 have shown early activity in relapse patients and are undergoing clinical trials.[191]

In patients with multiple treatment failures, long remissions are rare. In these patients, there is often a point where further intensive chemotherapy regimens are more likely to do harm than good, and a palliative treatment approach should be adopted. Treatment approaches such as low to moderate doses of vinblastine administered weekly[192] and the judicious use of involved field radiotherapy can alleviate symptoms and produce a reasonable quality of life. Asymptomatic patients might be best followed without therapy. Patients with fevers refractory to other treatment approaches can sometimes be effectively palliated with nonsteroidal anti-inflammatory drugs such as naproxen or indomethacin.

Autologous bone marrow transplantation can rescue occasional patients with multiply relapsed Hodgkin disease. Unfortunately, the results in this setting are usually disappointing. Because of the superior results in patients treated early in the course of the disease, most advocates of bone marrow transplantation would prefer to use it as part of the treatment of the initial relapse after an effective initial chemotherapy regimen. In this setting, patients who receive an alternate standard chemotherapy regimen and achieve at least a partial remission then undergo autologous transplantation. The results in this setting have yielded durable remissions in 47 to 85% of patients.[193–195] In a randomized trial conducted in Europe, patients with relapsed, chemosensitive Hodgkin disease had a significantly better failure-free survival with transplantation rather than continuing standard dose chemotherapy.[196] Patients with long initial remissions had a better failure-free survival, but both early and late relapsers had significant improvement in failure-free survival with the transplant. However, there was not a significant improvement in overall survival. It appears that the International Prognostic Score predicts outcome for patients undergoing autologous transplantation, and that patients with four or more adverse risk factors are probably poor candidates.[197]

Allogeneic bone marrow transplantation has been performed in patients with relapsed Hodgkin disease, but the results have been disappointing. Treatment-related mortality rates have varied from 31 to 61%, but there does seem to be a lower relapse rate in patients surviving allogeneic transplantation in comparison to those surviving autologous transplantation.[198] The explanation for the high treatment-related mortality with allogeneic transplantation might relate to patient selection or other, as yet unidentified, factors making these patients more susceptible to treatment toxicity. At the present time, allogeneic bone marrow transplantation should rarely be selected as the primary salvage treatment for patients with Hodgkin disease. However, one report of patients who had failed an autotransplant for relapsed Hodgkin disease and then underwent a full intensity allotransplant using the BEAM regimen followed by early withdrawal of immunosuppression had a surprisingly good outcome.[199] Ten patients, four of whom received unrelated donor hematopoietic stem cells, were treated with no early deaths. Seven of the ten patients remained in continuous complete remission at 12 months follow up although the majority had chronic graft versus host disease. The lower mortality associated with nonmyeloablative allogeneic transplantation seen in some early trials might lead this form of allotransplant to be more widely used.[200]

SUMMARY

Tremendous progress has been made in the last three decades toward the cure of Hodgkin disease. Additional work, however, is needed to further minimize the morbidity and mortality associated with the disease and its treatment. This includes the need to better understand the etiology and pathology of Hodgkin disease, to optimize control rates, especially in patients with unfavorable prognosis or advanced-stage disease, to modify therapeutic approaches to reduce the long-term complications, and to increase the awareness of physicians and patients to the potential late effects of treatment so that patients will receive appropriate follow-up care.

REFERENCES

1. Kass A, Kass E. Perfecting the world: the life and times of Thomas Hodgkin (1798–1866). New York: Harcourt Brace Jovanovich; 1988.
2. Hodgkin's T. On some morbid appearances of the absorbent glands and spleen. Medico-Chirugical Trans 1832;17:68–97.
3. Bright R. Observations on abdominal tumours and intumescence. Guy's Hosp Rep 1838;3:401–60.
4. Wilks S. Cases of enlargement of the lymphatic glands and spleen (or Hodgkin's disease), with remarks. Guy's Hosp Rep 1865;11:56–67.
5. Greenfield WS. Specimens illustrative of the pathology of lymphadenoma and leukocythemia. Virchows Arch Pathol Anat 1878;20:272.
6. Sternberg C. Uber eine eigenartige unter dem Bilde der Pseudoleukamie verlaufende Tuberculose des lymphatischen Apparates. Ztschr Heilk 1898;19:21–90.
7. Reed D. On the pathological changes in Hodgkin's disease, with special reference to its relation to tuberculosis. Johns Hopkins Hosp Rep 1902;10:133–96.
8. Kaplan HS. Hodgkin's disease: unfolding concepts concerning its nature, management and prognosis. Cancer 1980;45:2439–74.
9. Pusey W. Cases of sarcoma and of Hodgkin's disease treated by exposures to x-rays: a preliminary report. JAMA 1902;38:166–9.
10. Senn N. Therapeutical value of röntgen ray in treatment of pseudoleukemia. N Y Med J 1903;77:665–8.
11. Gilbert R. Radiotherapy in Hodgkin's disease (malignant granulomatosis): anatomic and clinical foundations; governing principles: results. Am J Roentgenol Radium Ther Nucl Med 1939;41:198–241.
12. Peters M. A study of survivals in Hodgkin's disease treated radiologically. Am J Roentgenol 1950;63:299–311.
13. Kaplan H. The radical radiotherapy of regionally localized Hodgkin's disease. Radiology 1962;78:553–61.
14. Kaplan HS. Role of intensive radiotherapy in the management of Hodgkin's disease. Cancer 1966;19:356.
15. Lukes R, Craver, L Hall T, et al. Report of the nomenclature committee. Cancer Res 1966;26:1311.
16. DeVita V, Serpick A, Carbone P. Combination chemotherapy in the treatment of advanced Hodgkin's disease. Ann Intern Med 1970;73:881–95.
17. DeVita, VT, Bonadonna, G. The history of the chemotherapy of Hodgkin's Disease. In: Mauch PM, Armitage JO, Diehl V, et al, editors. Hodgkin's disease. Philadelphia: Lippincott Williams & Wilkins; 1999:9–22.
18. Skipper H, Schabel F, Wilcox W. Experimental evaluation of potential anticancer agents. Cancer Chemotherapy Rep 1964;35:1–111.
19. Frei EI, DeVita VJ, Moxley J, et al. Approaches to improving the chemotherapy of Hodgkin's disease. Cancer Res 1966;26:1284.
20. Moxley J, DeVita VJ, Brace K, et al. Intensive chemotherapy and x-irradiation in Hodgkin's disease. Cancer 1967;27:1258.
21. Bonadonna G, Zucali R, Monfardini S, et al. Combination chemotherapy of Hodgkin's disease with Adriamycin, bleomycin, vinblastine, and imidazole carboxamide versus MOPP. Cancer 1975;36:252–9.
22. Canellos GP, Anderson JR, Propert KJ, et al. Chemotherapy of advanced Hodgkin's disease with MOPP, ABVD, or MOPP alternating with ABVD [see comments]. N Engl J Med 1992;327:1478–84.
23. MacMahon B. Epidemiological evidence of the nature of Hodgkin's disease. Cancer 1957;10:1045–54.
24. Mauch PM, Kalish L, Kadin M, et al. Patterns of presentation of Hodgkin's disease. Cancer 1993;71:2062–71.
25. van Rooyan C. Etiology of Hodgkin's disease with special reference to B. tuberculosis avis. Br Med J 1933;1:50–51.
26. Kaplan H. Hodgkin's disease. Harvard University Press, Cambridge; 1980.
27. Vianna J, Poln A. Epidemiological evidence for transmission of Hodgkin's disease. N Engl J Med 1973;289:499–502.
28. Grufferman S, Cole P, Levitan T. Evidence against transmission of Hodgkin's disease in high schools. N Engl J Med, 1979; 300:1006.
29. Mack M, Riethmuller G, Kufer P. A small bispecific antibody construct expressed as a functional single- chain molecule with high tumor cell cytotoxicity. Proc Natl Acad Sci U S A 1995;92:7021–5.
30. Hors J, Dausset J. HLA and susceptibility to Hodgkin's disease. Immunol Rev 1983;70:167.
31. Gutensohn N, Cole P. Childhood social environment and Hodgkin's disease. N Engl J Med 1981;304:135–40.
32. Mueller N. Hodgkin's disease. In: Schnottenfeld D, Fraumeni J, editors. Cancer epidemiology and prevention. New York: Oxford University Press, 1992:
33. Glaser SL, Lin RJ, Stewart SL, et al. Epstein-Barr virus-associated Hodgkin's disease: epidemiologic characteristics in international data. Int J Cancer 1997;70:375–82.
34. Mueller N, Evans A, Harris N, et al. Hodgkin's disease and Epstein-Barr virus, altered antibody pattern before diagnosis. N Engl J Med 1989;320:689.
35. Mueller NE, Grufferman S. Hodgkin's disease. In: Mauch PM, Armitage JO, Diehl V, et al, editors. Hodgkin's disease. Philadelphia: Lippincott Williams & Wilkins,1999: 61–77.
36. Ambinder RF, Weiss LM. Hodgkin's disease. In: Mauch PM, Armitage JO, Diehl V, et al, editors. Hodgkin's disease. Philadelphia: Lippincott Williams & Wilkins, 1999:79–98.
37. Weiss L, Movahed L, Warnke R, et al. Detection of Epstein-Barr viral genomes in Reed-Sternberg cells of Hodgkin's disease. N Engl J Med 1989;320:502–6.
38. Jackson HJ, Parker FJ. Hodgkin's disease. I. General considerations. N Engl J Med 1944;230:1.
39. Harris N, Jaffe E, Stein H, et al. Perspective: A Revised European-American classification of lymphoid neoplasms: a proposal from the Internation Lymphoma Study Group. Blood, 1994;84:1361–92.
40. Jaffe E, Harris N, Stein H, et al. World Health Organization classification of tumors. Pathology and genetics of tumour of haematopoietic and lymphoid tissue. IARC Press, 2001;Lion:
41. Weiss LM, Chan JKC, MacLennan K, et al. Hodgkin's disease. In: Mauch PM, Armitage JO, Diehl V, et al, editors. Hodgkin's disease, Philadelphia: Lippincott Williams & Wilkins, 1999:101–20.
42. MacLennan K, Bennett M, Tu A, et al. Relationship of histopathologic features to survival and relapse in nodular sclerosing Hodgkin's disease. A study of 1659 patients. Cancer, 1989;64:1686–93.
43. Anagnostostopoulos I, Hansmann ML, Frinssila K, et al. European Task Force on Lymphoma project on lymphocyte predominance Hodgkin disease: histologic and immunohistologic analysis of submitted cases reveals 2 types of Hodgkin disease with a nodular growth pattern and abundant lymphocytes. Blood 2000;96:1889–99.
44. Diehl V, Franklin J, Sextro M, Mauch PM. Clinical presentation and treatment of lymphocyte predominance Hodgkin's disease. In: Mauch PM, Armitage JO, Diehl V, et al, editors. Hodgkin's disease. Philadelphia: Lippincott Williams & Wilkins; 1999. p. 563–82.
45. Poppema S, Brinker MG, Visser L. Evidence for a B-cell origin of the proliferating cells. Cancer Treat Res 1989;41:5–27.
46. Pinkus G, Said J. Hodgkin's disease, lymphocyte predominance type, nodular—further evidence of a B cell derivation: L+H variants of Reed–Sternberg cells express L26, a pan B cell marker. Am J Pathol 1988;133:211.
47. Burns B, Colby T, Dorfman R. Differential diagnostic features of nodular L + H Hodgkin's disease, including progressive transformation of germinal centers. Am J Surg Pathol 1984;8:253.
48. Mason D, Banks P, Chan J, et al. Nodular lymphocyte predominance Hodgkin's disease: a distinct clinicopathologic entity. Am J Surg Pathol 1994;18:526–30.
49. Calvo KR, Traverse-Glehen A, Pittaluga S, Jaffe ES. Molecular profiling provides evidence of primary mediastinal large B-cell lymphoma a distinct entity related to classic Hodgkin lymphoma. Implications for mediastinal gray zone lymphomas as an intermediate form of B-cel lymphoma. Adv Anat Pathol 2004;11:227–38.
50. Stein H, Diehl V, Marafioti T, et al. Hodgkin's disease. In: Mauch PM, Armitage JO, Diehl V, et al, editors. Hodgkin's disease. Philadelphia: Lippincott Williams & Wilkins; 1999. p. 121–37.
51. Kuppers R. Molecular biology of Hodgkin's lymphoma. Adv Cancer Res 2002;84:277–312.
52. Thomas RK, Re D, Wolf J, Diehl V. Part I: Hodgkin' lymphoma—molecular biology of Hodgkin and Reed-Sternberg cells. Lancet Oncol 2004;5:11–18.
53. Mathas S, Lietz A, Anagnostopoulos I, et al. c-FLIP mediates resistance of Hodgkin/Reed-Sternberg cells to death receptor-induced apoptosis. J Exp Med 2004;199:1041–52.
54. Hinz M, Lemke P, Anagnostopoulos I, et al. Nuclear fact kappaB-dependent gene expression profiling of Hodgkin's disease tumor cells, pathogenetic significance, and link to constitutive signal transducer and activator of transcription 5a activity. J Exp Med 2002;196:605–17.
55. Chang ET, Zheng T, Weir EG, et al. Aspirin and the risk of Hodgkin's lymphoma in a population-based case-control study. J Natl Cancer Inst. 2004;96:3015–315
56. Sarris AH, Jhanwar SC, Cabanillas F. Cytogenetics of Hodgkin's disease. In: Mauch PM, Armitage JO, Diehl V, et al, editors. Hodgkin's disease. Philadelphia: Lippincott Williams & Wilkins; 1999. p. 195–212.
57. Fonatsch C, Jox A, Streubel B, et al. Cytogenetic findings in Hodgkin's disease cell lines. In: Mauch PM, Armitage JO, Diehl V, et al, editors. Hodgkin's disease. Philadelphia: Lippincott Williams & Wilkins; 1999. p. 213–9.
58. Re D, Starostik P, Massoudi N, et al. Allelic losses on chromosome 6q25 in Hodgkin and Reed Sternberg cells. Cancer Res 2003;63:2606–9.
59. Stein H, Gerdes J, Lemke H, Mason DY. Hodgkin's disease. A neoplasm of activated lymphoid cells of either T-cell or B-cell type. In: Grignani F, Martelli MF, Mason DY, editors. The Serono Symposium. New York: Raven Press; 1985;26:265.
60. Kadin ME, Liebowitz DN. Cytokines and cytokine receptors in Hodgkin's disease. In: Mauch PM, Armitage JO, Diehl V, et al, editors. Hodgkin's disease. Philadelphia: Lippincott Williams & Wilkins; 1999. p. 139–57.
61. Skinnider BFMT. The role of cytokines in classical Hodgkin's lymphoma. Blood 2002;99:4283–97.
62. Kadin M, Butmarc J, Elovic A, Wong D. Eosinophils are the major source of transforming growth factor-B 1in in nodular sclerosing Hodgkin's disease. Am J Pathol 1993;142:11–6.
63. Peh SC, Kim LH, Poppema S. TARC a CC chemokine, is frequently expressed in classic Hodgkin's lymphoma but not in NLP Hodgkin's lymphoma, T-cell-rich B-cell lymphoma, and most cases of anaplastic large cell lymphoma. Am J Surg Pathol 2001;25:925–9.
64. Skinnider, BF, Kapp U, Mak TW. The role of interleukin 13 in classical Hodgkin lymphoma. Leuk Lymphoma 2002;43:1203–10.
65. Poppema S, Potters M. Dysregulated immune response in Hodgkin's disease. In: Mauch PM, Armitage JO, Diehl V, et al, editors. Hodgkin's disease. Philadelphia: Lippincott Williams & Wilkins; 1999. p. 159–68.
66. Fisher R, DeVita V, Bostick F. Persistent immunological abnormalities in long-term survivors of advanced Hodgkin's disease. Ann Intern Med 1990;92:595–9.
67. Cunningham J, Mauch P, Rosenthal DS, Canellos GP: Long-term complications of MOPP chemotherapy in patients with Hodgkin's disease. Cancer Treat Rep 1982;66:1015–22.
68. Molrine D, George S, Tarbell N, et al. Antibody responses to polysaccharide and polysaccharide-conjugate vaccines following treatment for Hodgkin's disease. Ann Intern Med 1995;123:824–8.
69. Kaplan H. The radical radiotherapy of regionally localized Hodgkin's disease. Radiology 1962;78:553–61.
70. Peters MV, Alison RE, Bush RS. Natural history of Hodgkin's disease as related to staging. Cancer 1966;19:308.
71. Leibenhaut M, Hoppe R, Efron B, et al. Prognostic indicators of laparotomy findings in clinical stage I-II supradiaphragmatic Hodgkin's disease. J Clin Oncol 1989;7:81–91.
72. Mauch P, Larson D, Osteen R, et al. Prognostic factors for positive surgical staging in patients with Hodgkin's disease. J Clin Oncol 1990;8:257–65.

73. Hughes-Davis L, Tarbell N, Coleman C, et al. Stage IA-IIB Hodgkin's disease: management and outcome of extensive thoracic involvement. Int J Radiat Oncol Biol Phys 1997;39:361–9.
74. Bodis S, Henry-Amar M, Bosq J, et al. Late relapses in early stage Hodgkin's disease patients enrolled on European Organization for Research and Treatment of Cancer protocols. J Clin Oncol 1993;11:225–32.
75. Young R, Canellos G, Chabner B, et al. Patterns of relapse in advanced Hodgkin's disease treated with combination chemotherapy. Cancer 1978;42:1001–7.
76. Lister T, Crowther D, Sutcliffe S, et al. Report of a committee convened to discuss the evaluation and staging of patients with Hodgkin's disease: Cotswolds meeting. J Clin Oncol 1989;7:1630–6.
77. Mauch P, Goodman R, Hellman S. The significance of mediastinal involvement in early stage Hodgkin's disease. Cancer 1978;42:1039–45
78. Elstrom R, Guan L, Baker G, et al: Utility of FDG-PET scanning in lymphoma by WHO classification. Blood 2003;101:3875–6.
79. Friedberg JW, Fischman A, Neuberg D, et al: FDG-PET is superior to gallium scintigraphy in staging and more sensitive in the follow-up of patients with de novo Hodgkin lymphoma: a blinded comparison. Leuk Lymphoma 2004;45:85–92.
80. Naumann R, Beuthien-Baumann B, Reiss A, et al: Substantial impact of FDG PET imaging on the therapy decision in patients with early-stage Hodgkin's lymphoma. Br J Cancer 2004;90:620-5.
81. Specht L, Gray RG, Clarke MJ, Peto R. Influence of more extensive radiotherapy and adjuvant chemotherapy on long-term outcome of early stage Hodgkin's disease: a meta-analysis of 23 randomized trials involving 3,888 patients. International Hodgkin's Disease Collaborative Group. J Clin Oncol 1998;16:830–43.
82. Ng A, Bernardo M, Weller E, et al. Long-term survival and competing causes of death in patients with early stage Hodgkin's disease treated at age 50 or younger. J Clin Oncol 2002;20:2101.
83. Cosset J, Henry-Amar M, Meerwaldt J. Long-term toxicity of early stages of Hodgkin's disease therapy: The EORTC experience. Ann Oncol 1991;2:77–82.
84. Hancock S, Hoppe R, Horning S, Rosenberg S. Intercurrent death after Hodgkin's disease therapy in radiotherapy and adjuvant MOPP trials. Ann Intern Med 1988;109:183–9.
85. Ng AK, Hoppe RT, Mauch PM. Life expectancy of patients with Hodgkin's disease. In: Mauch PM, Armitage JO, Diehl V, et al, editors. Hodgkin's disease. Philadelphia: Lippincott Williams & Wilkins; 1999. p. 585–605.
86. Hoppe RT. Hodgkin's disease: complications of therapy and excess mortality. Ann Oncol 1997;8:S115–8.
87. Roach M III, Brophy N, Cox R, et al. Prognostic factors for patients relapsing after radiotherapy for early stage Hodgkin's disease. J Clin Oncol 1990;8:623–9.
88. Ng AK, Li S, Neuberg D, et al. Comparison of MOPP versus ABVD as salvage therapy in patients who relapse after radiation therapy alone for Hodgkin's disease. Ann Oncol 2004; 15:270–5.
89. Santoro A, Bonfante V, Bonadonna G. Salvage chemotherapy with ABVD in MOPP-resistant Hodgkin's disease. Ann Intern Med 1982;96:139–43.
90. Longo D, Duffey P, Young R, et al. Conventional-dose salvage combination chemotherapy in patients relapsing with Hodgkin's disease after combination chemotherapy: the low probability for cure. J Clin Oncol 1992;10:210–8.
91. Biti G, Cimino G, Cartoni C, et al. Extended-field radiotherapy is superior to MOPP chemotherapy for the treatment of pathologic stage I-IIA Hodgkin's disease: eight-year update of an Italian prospective randomized study. J Clin Oncol 1992;10:378–82.
92. Ng A, Bernardo M, Weller E, et al. Second malignancy after Hodgkin's disease treated with radiation therapy with or without chemotherapy: long-term risks and risk factors. Blood 2002;100:1989.
93. Swerdlow A, Barber J, Hudson F, et al. Risk of second malignancy after Hodgkin's disease in collaborative British cohort: the relation to age at treatment. J Clin Oncol 2000;18:498–509.
94. van Leeuwen F, Klokman W, Veer M, et al. Long-term risk of second malignancy in survivors of Hodgkin's disease treated during adolescence or young adulthood. J Clin Oncol 2000;18:487–97.
95. Cutuli B, Borel C, Dhermain F, et al. Breast cancer occurred after treatment for Hodgkin's disease: analysis of 133 cases. Radiother Oncol 2001;59:547–555.
96. van Leeuwen F, Chorus A, van den Belt-Dusebout A, et al. Leukemia risk following Hodgkin's disease: relation to cumulative dose of alkylating agents, treatment with teniposide combinations, number and episodes of chemotherapy, and bone marrow damage. J Clin Oncol 1994;12:1063–73.
97. van Leeuwen FE, Swerdlow AJ, Valaguss P, Tucker MA. Hodgkin's disease. In: Mauch PM, Armitage JO, Diehl V, et al, editors. Hodgkin's disease. Philadelphia: Lippincott Williams & Wilkins; 1999. p. 607–32.
98. Tucker M, Coleman C, Cox R, et al. Risk of second cancers after treatment for Hodgkin's disease. N Engl J Med 1988;318:76–81.
99. Swerdlow A, Douglas A, Hudson G, et al. Risk of second primary cancers after Hodgkin's disease by type of treatment: analysis of 2846 patients in The British National Lymphoma Investigation. BMJ 1992;304:1137–48.
100. Swerdlow A, Schoemaker M, Allerton R, et al. Lung cancer after Hodgkin's disease: a nested case-control study of the relation to treatment. J Clin Oncol 2001;19:1610–8.
101. Mauch P. Late Effects after Hodgkin's Disease: recommendations from the Rockefeller Foundation sponsored workshop on reducing mortality and improving quality of life in long-term survivors of Hodgkin's disease (held in Bellagio, Italy, July 9 through July 16th, 2003). Eur J Haematology 2004; 73 (suppl 65):23–24.
102. Adams MJ, Lipsitz SR, Colan SD, et al. Cardiovascular status in long-term survivors of Hodgkin's disease treated with chest radiotherapy. J Clin Oncol 2004, 22:3139–48.
103. Heidenreich PA, Hancock SL, Lee BK, et al: Asymptomatic cardiac disease following mediastinal irradiation. J Am Coll Cardiol 2003;42:743–9.
104. Hull, M.C., et al., Valvular dysfunction and carotid, subclavian, and coronary artery disease in survivors of Hodgkin lymphoma treated with radiation therapy. JAMA 2003;290:2831–7.
105. Strasser JF, Li S, Neuberg D, et al. Late cardiac toxicity after mediastinal radiation therapy for Hodgkin's disease. Int J Radiat Oncol Biol Phys 2004;60 (Suppl 1):S216–7.
106. Viviani S, Ragni G, Santoro A, et al. Testicular dysfunction in Hodgkin's disease before and after treatment. Eur J Cancer 1991;27:1389–92.
107. Mauch PM, Connors JM, Pavlovsky S, Duhmke E. Treatment of favorable prognosis stage I-II Hodgkin's disease. In: Mauch PM, Armitage JO, Diehl V, et al, editors. Hodgkin's disease. Philadelphia: Lippincott Williams & Wilkins; 1999. p. 435–58.
108. Hoppe RT, Cosset JM, Santoro A, Wolf J. Treatment of unfavorable prognosis stage I-II Hodgkin's disease. In: Mauch PM, Armitage JO, Diehl V, et al, editors. Hodgkin's disease. Philadelphia: Lippincott Williams & Wilkins; 1999. p. 459–81.
109. Specht L, Nordentoft A, Cold S, et al. Tumor burden as the most important prognostic factor in early stage Hodgkin's disease. Relations to other prognostic factors and implications for choice of treatment. Cancer 1988; 61:1719–27.
110. Tubiana M, Henry-Amar M, Carde P, et al. Toward comprehensive management tailored to prognostic factors of patients with clinical stages I and II in Hodgkin's disease. The EORTC Lymphoma Group controlled clinical trials: 1964–1987. Blood 1989;73:47–56.
111. Gospodarowicz M, Sutcliffe S, Clark R, et al. Analysis of supradiaphragmatic clinical stage I and II Hodgkin's disease treated with radiation alone. Int J Radiat Oncol Biol Phys 1992;22:859–65.
112. Crnkovich M, Leopold K, Hoppe R, Mauch P. Stage I to IIB Hodgkin's disease: the combined experience at Stanford University and the Joint Center for Radiation Therapy. J Clin Oncol 1987;5:1041–9.
113. Healey E, Tarbell N, Kalish L, et al. Prognostic factors for patients with Hodgkin's disease in first relapse. Cancer 1993;71:2613–20.
114. Hasenclever D, Diehl V: A prognostic score for advanced Hodgkin's disease. International Prognostic Factors Project on Advanced Hodgkin's Disease. N Engl J Med 1998;339:1506–14.
115. Press O, LeBlanc M, Lichter A, et al. Phase III randomized intergroup trial of subtotal lymphoid irradiation versus doxorubicin, vinblastine, and subtotal lymphoid irradiation for stage IA to IIA Hodgkin's disease. J Clin Oncol 2001;19:4238–44.
116. Noordijk E, Carde P, Hagenbeek A, et al. Combination of radiotherapy and chemotherapy is advisable in all patients with clinical stage I-II Hodgkin's disease. Six-year results of the EORTC-GPMC controlled clinical trials "H7-VF," "H7-F," and "H7-U" [abstract]. Int J Radiat Oncol Biol Phys 1997;39:173.
117. Carde P, Noordijk E, Hagenbeek A, et al. Superiority of EBVP chemotherapy in combination with involved field irradiation over subtotal nodal irradiation in favor-able clinical stage I-II Hodgkin's disease: The EORTCGPMC H7F randomized trial. Proc Am Soc Clin Oncol 1997;16:13.
118. Radford JA, Williams MV, Hancock BW, et al: Minimal initial chemotherapy plus involved field radiotherapy (RT) vs mantle field RT for clinical stage IA/IIA supradiaphragmatic Hodgkin's disease (HD). Results of the UK Lymphoma Group LY07 Trial. Eur J Haematol 2004;73:E08a.
119. Bartlett N, Rosenberg S, Hoppe R, et al. Brief chemotherapy, Stanford V, and adjuvant radiotherapy for bulky or advanced-stage Hodgkin's disease: a preliminary report. J Clin Oncol 1995;13:1080–8.
120. Diehl V, Brilliant C, Engert A, et al: Reduction of combined modality treatment intensity in early stage Hodgkin's lymphoma, interim analysis of HD10 trial of GHSG. Eur J Haematol 2004;73:E03a.
121. Hagenbeek, Eghbali H, Ferme C, et al. Three cycles of MOPP/ABV (M/A) hybrid and involved-field irradiation is more effective than subtotal nodal irradiation (STNI) in favorable supradiaphragmatic clinical stages (CS) I-I Hodgkin's disease (HD): preliminary results of the EORTC-GELA H8-F randomized trial in 543 patients. Blood 2000;96:575a.
122. Longo D, Glatstein E, Duffey P, et al. Radiation therapy versus combination chemotherapy in the treatment of early stage Hodgkin's disease: seven-year results of a prospective randomized trial. J Clin Oncol 1991;9:906–17.
123. Meyer R, Gospodarowicz M, Connors J, et al. A randomized phase III comparison of single-modality ABVD with a strategy that includes radiation therapy in patients with early-stage Hodgkin's disease: the HD-6 trial of the National Cancer Institute of Canada Clinical Trials Group (Eastern Cooperative Oncology Group Trial JHD06). Blood 2004;102:A81.
124. Thomas J, Ferme C, Noordijk E, et al: Six cycles of EBVP followed by 36Gy involved-field irradiation vs. no irradiation in favourable supradiaphragmatic clinical stage I-II Hodgkin's Lymphoma: the EORTC-GELA strategy in 771 patients. Eur J Haematol 2004;73:40.
125. Nachman J, Sposto R, Herzog P, et al. Randomized comparison of low-dose involved-field radiotherapy and no radiotherapy for children with Hodgkin's disease who achieve a complete response to chemotherapy. J Clin Oncol 2002;20:3755–7.
126. Straus DJ, Portlock CS, Qin J, et al: Results of a prospective randomized clinical trial of doxorubicin, bleomycin, vinblastine and dacarbazine (ABVD) followed by radiation therapy (RT) vs. ABVD alone for stages I, II and IIIA non bulky Hodgkin's disease. Blood First Edition Paper prepublished online:10.1182, 2004.
127. Pavlovsky S, Maschio M, Santarelli MT, et al: Randomized trial of chemotherapy versus chemotherapy plus radiotherapy for stage I-II Hodgkin's disease. J Natl Cancer Inst 1988;80:1466–73.
128. Laskar S, Gupta T, Vimal S, et al: Consolidation radiation after complete remission in Hodgkin's disease following six cycles of doxorubicin, bleomycin, vinblastine, and dacarbazine chemotherapy: is there a need? J Clin Oncol 2004;22:62–8.
129. Duhmke E, Diehl V, Loeffler M, et al. Randomized trial with early-stage Hodgkin's disease testing 30 Gy vs. 40 Gy extended field radiotherapy alone. Int J Rad Oncol Biol Phys 1996; 36:305–10.
130. Schewe K, Reavis J, Kuṅ L, Cox J. Total dose, fraction size, and tumor volume in the local control of Hodgkin's disease. Int J Radiat Oncol Biol Phys 1988;15:25–8.
131. Vijayakumar S, Myrianthopoulos L. An updated dose-response analysis in Hodgkin's disease. Radiother Oncol 1992;24:1–13.
132. Gospodarowicz MK, Sutcliffe SB, Bergsagel DE, Chua T. Radiation therapy in clinical stage I and II Hodgkin's disease. The Princess Margaret Hospital Lymphoma Group. Eur J Cancer 1992;28A:1841–6.
133. Tubiana M, Henri-Amar M, Hayat M, et al. The EORTC treatment of early stages of Hodgkin's disease: the role of radiotherapy. Int J Radiat Oncol Biol Phys 1984;10:197–210.
134. Sutcliffe SB, Gospodarowicz MK, Bush RS, et al. Role of radiation therapy in localized non-Hodgkin's lymphoma. Radiother Oncol 1985;4:211–23.
135. Wirth A, Byram D, Chao M, et al. Long-term results of mantle irradiation alone in 261 patients with clinical stage I-II supradiaphragmatic Hodgkin's disease. Int J Radiat Oncol Biol Phys 1997;39:174.
136. Carde P, Burgers J, Henry-Amar M, et al. Clinical stages I and II Hodgkin's disease: a specifically tailored therapy according to prognostic factors. J Clin Oncol 1988;6:239–52.

137. Ganesan T, Wrigley P, Murray P, et al. Radiotherapy for stage I Hodgkin's disease: 20 years of experience at St Bartholomew's Hospital. Br J Cancer 1990;62:314–8.
138. Mandelli F, Cimino G, Mauro F, et al. Prognosis and management of patients affected by multi-pre-treated Hodgkin's disease. Haematology 1986;71:205–8.
139. Backstrand K, Ng A, Takvorian R, et al. Results of a prospective trial of mantle irradiation alone for selected patients with early stage Hodgkin's disease. J Clin Oncol 2001;19:736–41.
140. Noordijk E, Carde P, Hagenbeek A, et al. Combination of radiotherapy and chemotherapy is advisable in all patients with clinical stage I-II Hodgkin's disease. Six-year results of the EORTC-GPMC controlled clinical trials "H7-VF," "H7-F." and "H7-U." Int J Radiat Oncol Biol Phys 1997; 39:173.
141. Bodis S, Kraus M, Pinkus G, et al. Low mortality from lymphocyte predominant Hodgkin's disease with long-term follow-up. J Clin Oncol 1997;15:3060–6.
142. Santoro A, Bonadonna G, Valagussa P, et al. Long-term results of combined chemotherapy–radiotherapy approach in Hodgkin's disease: superiority of ABVD plus radiotherapy versus MOPP plus radiotherapy. J Clin Oncol 1987;5:27–37.
143. Ferme C, Eghabali H, Hagenbeek A, et al. MOPP/ABV (M/A) hybrid and irradiation in unfavorable supradiaphragmatic clinical stages (CS) I-II Hodgkin's disease (HD): comparison of three treatment modalities. Preliminary results of the EORTC-GELA H8-U randomized trial in 995 patients. Blood 2000;96:576a.
144. Pavlovsky S, Schvartzman E, Lastiri F, et al. Randomized trial of CVPP for three versus six cycles in favorable-prognosis and CVPP versus AOPE plus radiotherapy in intermediate-prognosis untreated Hodgkin's disease. J Clin Oncol 1997;15:2652–8.
145. Carde P, Noordijk N, Hagenbeek A, et al. Superiority of MOPP/ABV over EBVP in combination with involved field irradiation in unfavorable clinical stage I-II Hodgkin's disease: the EORTC H7U randomized trial. Proc Am Soc Clin Oncol 1993;12:362
146. Thomas J, Ferme C, Noordijk E, et al: Six cycles of ABVD + IF-RT vs. four cycles of ABVD + RT vs. four cycles of BEACOPP + RT in unfavorable supradiaphragmatic clinical stages I-II Hodgkin's lymphoma: the EORTC-GELA H9U randomized clinical trial in 808 patients. Eur J Haematol 2004;73:40–1.
147. Diehl V, Brillant C, Engert A et al, Intensification of chemotherapy and concomitant reduction of radiotherapy dose in intermediate stage Hodgkin's lymphoma: the results of the fourth interim analysis of the HD11 trial of the GHSG. Eur J Haematol 2004;73:40.
148. Zittoun R, Audebert A, Hoerni B, et al. Extended versus involved field irradiation combined with MOPP chemotherapy in early clinical stages of Hodgkin's disease. J Clin Oncol 1985;3:207–14.
149. Santoro A. Annual Conference of ECCO, Hamburg, Germany, [abstract] 1997.
150. Devita VJ, Hubbard S. Hodgkin's disease. N Engl J Med 1993;328:560–5.
151. DeVita VJ, Simon R, Habbard S, et al. Curability of advanced Hodgkin's disease with chemotherapy: long-term follow up of MOPP-treated patients at the National Cancer Institute. Ann Intern Med 1980;92:587–95.
152. Bonadonna G, Valagussa P, Santoro A. Alternating non–cross-resistant combination chemotherapy or MOPP in stage IV Hodgkin's disease. Ann Intern Med 1986;104:739–46.
153. Bakemeier R, Anderson J, Costello W, et al. BCVPP chemotherapy for advanced Hodgkin's disease: evidence for greater duration of complete remission, greater survival and less toxicity than with a MOPP regimen. Ann Intern Med 1984;101:447.
154. Nicholson W, Beard M, Crowther D, et al. Combination chemotherapy in generalized Hodgkin's disease. Br Med J 1970;3:7–10.
155. Sutcliffe S, Wrigley P, Peto J, et al. MVPP chemotherapy regimen for advanced Hodgkin's disease. Br Med J 1978;1:679.
156. McKendrick J, Mead G, Sweetenham J, et al. ChlVPP chemotherapy in advanced Hodgkin's disease. Eur J Cancer Clin Oncol 1989;25:557–61.
157. McElwain T, Toy J, Smith E, et al. A combination of chlorambucil, vinblastine, procarbazine, and prednisolone for treatment of Hodgkin's disease. Br J Cancer 1977;36:276.
158. Bonadonna G, Beretta G, Tancini G, et al. Adriamycin (NSC-123127) studies at the Instituto Nazionale Tumori, Milan. Cancer Chemother Rep 1975;6:231–45.
159. Viviani S, Santoro A, Ragni G, et al. Gonadal toxicity after combination chemotherapy or Hodgkin's disease. Comparative results of MOPP vs ABVD. Eur J Cancer Clin Oncol 1985;21:601–5.
160. Connors JM, Klimo P, Adams G, et al. Treatment of advanced Hodgkin's disease with chemotherapy—comparison of MOPP/ABV hybrid regimen with alternating courses of MOPP and ABVD: a report from the National Cancer Institute of Canada clinical trials group [published erratum appears in J Clin Oncol 1997;15:2762]. J Clin Oncol 1997;15:1638–45.
161. Horning SJ, Rosenberg SA, Hoppe RT. Brief chemotherapy (Stanford V) and adjuvant radiotherapy for bulky or advanced Hodgkin's disease: an update. Ann Oncol 1996;7:105–8.
162. Diehl V, Sieber M, Ruffer U, et al. BEACOPP: an intensified chemotherapy regimen in advanced Hodgkin's disease. The German Hodgkin's Lymphoma Study Group. Ann Oncol 1997;8:143–8.
163. Horning SJ, Bennett JM, Bartlett NL, et al. 12 weeks of chemotherapy (Stanford V) and involved-field radio-therapy (RT) are highly effective for bulky and advanced-stage Hodgkin's disease: a limited institution ECOG pilot study [abstract]. Blood 1996;88:2681.
164. Horning SJ, Hoppe RT, Advani R, et al. Efficacy and late effects of Stanford V chemotherapy and radiotherapy in untreated Hodgkin's disease: mature data in early and advanced stage patients. Blood 2004;104:92a.
165. Johnson P, Hoskin P, Horwich A, et al. Stanford V (SV) regimen versus ABVD for the treatment of advanced Hodgkin lymphoma (HL): results of a UK NCRI/LTO randomized phase II trial. Blood 2004;104:93a.
166. Diehl V, Brillant C, Franklin J, et al. BEACOPP Chemotherapy for advanced Hodgkin's disease: results of further analyses of the HD9- and HD12- trials of the German Hodgkin Study Group (GHSG). Blood 2004;104:91a.
167. Fabian C, Mansfield C, Dahlberg S, et al. Low-dose involved field radiation after chemotherapy in advanced Hodgkin's disease. Ann Intern Med 1994;120:903–12.
168. Loeffler M, Brosteanu O, Hasenclever D, et al. Meta-analysis of chemotherapy versus combined modality treatment trials in Hodgkin's disease. International Database on Hodgkin's Disease Overview Study Group [see comments]. J Clin Oncol 1998;16:818–29.
169. Aleman BM, Raemaekers JM, Tirelli U, et al: Involved-field radiotherapy for advanced Hodgkin's lymphoma. N Engl J Med 2003;348:2396–406.
170. Longo D, Russo A, Duffey P, et al. Treatment of advanced-stage massive mediastinal Hodgkin's disease: the case for combined modality treatment. J Clin Oncol 1991;9:227–35.
171. Valagussa P, Santoro A, Fossati-Bellani F, et al. Second acute leukemia and other malignancies following treatment for Hodgkin's disease. J Clin Oncol 1986;4:830–7.
172. Kaldor J, Day N, Bell J. Lung cancer following Hodgkin's disease: a case control study. Int J Cancer 1992;52:677–81.
173. Carella A, Prencipe E, Pungolino E, et al. Twelve years experience with high-dose therapy and autologous stem cell transplantation for high-risk Hodgkin's disease patients in first remission after MOPP/ABVD chemotherapy. Leuk Lymphoma 1996;21:63–70.
174. Sureda A, Mataix R, Hernandex-Navarro F, et al. Autologous stem cell transplantation for poor prognosis Hodgkin's disease in first complete remission: a retrospective study from the Spanish GEL-TAMO cooperative group. Bone Marrow Transplant 1997;20:283–8.
175. Weekes C, Vose J, Hynch J, et al. Hodgkin's disease in the elderly: improved treatment outcome with a doxorubicin containing regimen. J Clin Oncol 2002;20:1087–93.
176. Radford J, Rohatiner A, Ryder W, et al. Ch1VPP/EVA hybrid versus the weekly VAPEC-B regimen for previously untreated Hodgkin's disease. J Clin Oncol 2002;20:2988–94.
177. Robert NJ, Schneiderman H. Hodgkin's disease and the acquired immunodeficiency syndrome, Annals of Int Med 1984;101:142-3.
178. Spina M, Gabarre J, Rossi G, et al. , U. Stanford V regimen and concomitant HAART in 59 patients with Hodgkin disease and HIV infection. Blood 2002;100:1984–8.
179. Hartmann P, Rehwald U, Salzberger B, et al. BEACOPP therapeutic regimen for patients with Hodgkin's disease and HIV infection. Ann Oncol 2003,14:1562-9.
180. Longo D, DeVita V. The use of combination chemotherapy in the treatment of early stage Hodgkin's disease. In: DeVita V, Hellman S, Rosenberg S, editors. Important advances in oncology. Philadelphia: JB Lippincott; 1992. p. 155–66.
181. Lazarus HM, Rowlings PA, Phillips GL, et al. Autotransplants for Hodgkin's disease never in complete remission [abstract]. Proc Am Soc Clin Oncol 1997;16:89a.
182. Sweetenham JW, Taghipour G, Linch DC, Goldstone AH. Thirty percent of adult patients with primary refractory Hodgkin's disease (HD) are progression free at 5 years after high-dose therapy (HDT) and autologous stem cell transplantation (ASCT): data from 290 patients reported to the EBMT [abstract]. Blood 1996;88 Suppl 1:486a.
183. Ferme C, Mounier N, Divine M, et al. Intensive salvage therapy with high-dose chemotherapy for patients with advanced Hodgkin's disease in relapse or failure after initial chemotherapy: results of the Groupe d'Etudes des Lymphomes de l'Adulte H89 trial. J Clin Oncol 2002;20:467–75.
184. Yuen AR, Rosenberg SA, Hoppe RT, et al. Comparison between conventional salvage therapy and high-dose therapy with autografting for recurrent or refractory Hodgkin's disease. Blood 1997;89:814–22.
185. Bonfante V, Santoro A, Viviani S, et al. Outcome of patients with Hodgkin's disease failing after primary MOPPA-BVD [see comments]. J Clin Oncol 1997;15:528–34.
186. Lohri A, Barnett M, Fairey R, et al. Outcome of treatment of first relapse of Hodgkin's disease after primary chemotherapy: identification of risk factors from the British Columbia experience 1970–1988. Blood 1991;77:2292–8.
187. Brice P, Bastion Y, Divine M, et al. Analysis of prognostic factors after the first relapse of Hodgkin's disease in 187 patients. Cancer 1996;78:1293–9.
188. Baetz T, Belch A, Couban S, et al. Gemcitabine, dexamethasone and cisplatin is an active and non-toxic chemotherapy regimen in relapsed or refractory Hodgkin's disease: a phase II study by the National Cancer Institute of Canada Clinical Trials Group. Ann Oncol 2003;14:1762–7.
189. Chau I, Watkins D, Cunningham D. Gemcitabine and its combinations in the treatment of malignant lymphoma. Clin Lymphoma 2003;3:97–104.
190. Younes A, Romaguera J, Hagemeister F, et al. A pilot study of rituximab in patients with recurrent, classic Hodgkin disease. Cancer 2003;98:310–4.
191. Borchmann P, Schnell R, Fuss I, et al.. Engert, A. Phase 1 trial of the novel bispecific molecule H22xKi-4 in patients with refractory Hodgkin lymphoma. Blood 2002;100:3101–7.
192. Little R, Wittes RE, Longo DL, Wilson WH. Vinblastine for recurrent Hodgkin's disease following autologous bone marrow transplant. J Clin Oncol 1998;16:584–8.
193. Brandwein JM, Callum J, Sutcliffe SB, et al. Evaluation of cytoreductive therapy prior to high dose treatment with autologous bone marrow transplantation in relapsed and refractory Hodgkin's disease. Bone Marrow Transplantation 1990;5:99–103.
194. Bierman PJ, Anderson JR, Freeman MB, et al. High-dose chemotherapy followed by autologous hematopoietic rescue for Hodgkin's disease patients following first relapse after chemotherapy. Ann Oncol 1996;7:151–6.
195. Poen JC, Hoppe RT, Horning SJ. High-dose therapy and autologous bone marrow transplantation for relapsed/refractory Hodgkin's disease: the impact of involved field radiotherapy on patterns of failure and survival [see comments]. Int J Radiat Oncol Biol Phys 1996;36:3–12.
196. Schmitz N, Pfistner B, Sextro M, et al. Aggressive conventional chemotherapy compared with high-dose chemotherapy with autologous haemopoietic stem-cell transplantation for relapsed chemosensitive Hodgkin's disease: a randomised trial. Lancet 2002;359:2065–71.
197. Bierman PJ, Lynch JC, Bociek RG, et al. The International Prognostic Factors Project score for advanced Hodgkin's disease is useful for predicting outcome of autologous hematopoietic stem cell transplantation. Ann Oncol 2002;13:1370–7.
198. Akpek G, Ambinder R, Piantadosi S, et al. Long-term results of blood and marrow transplantation for Hodgkin's lymphoma. J Clin Oncol 2001;19:4314–21.
199. Cooney JP, Stiff PJ, Toor AA, Parthasarathy M. BEAM allogeneic transplantation for patients with Hodgkin's disease who relapse after autologous transplantation is safe and effective. Biology of Blood and Marrow Transplantation 2002;9:177–82.
200. Porter DL, Stadtmauer, EA, Lazarus HM. "GVHD": graft-versus-host disease or graft-versus-Hodgkin's disease? An old acronym with new meaning. Bone Marrow Transplant 2003;31:739–46.

Non-Hodgkin Lymphoma

Arnold S. Freedman, MD

The malignant lymphomas are neoplastic transformations of cells that reside predominantly within lymphoid tissues. Although Hodgkin and non-Hodgkin lymphomas (NHLs) both infiltrate lymphohematopoietic tissues, their biologic and clinical behaviors are distinct. They clearly differ with regard to the neoplastic cells of origin, sites of disease, presence of specific symptoms, and response to treatment. Although both are among the most sensitive malignancies to radiation and cytotoxic therapy, their cure rates markedly differ. Hodgkin lymphomas are cured in nearly 75% of all patients employing both conventional and salvage treatment strategies whereas NHLs are cured in less than 40% of patients.

EPIDEMIOLOGY AND ETIOLOGY

Incidence and Mortality In 2005 there will be 56,390 new cases of NHL in the United States, 4% of all new cancers in males, 4% in females.[1] This is more than seven times the incidence of Hodgkin lymphoma. There is a slight male-to-female predominance and a higher incidence for Caucasians than for African Americans. The incidence rises steadily with age, especially after age 40 years. The malignant lymphomas are among the most common neoplasms of patients between the ages of 20 and 40 years. Moreover, the incidence of NHL nearly doubled between 1970 and 1990, but the rate of increase has slowed since the mid 1990s.

There are striking differences in the age-dependent incidence of NHL by histologic subtype. In children, Burkitt's, lymphoblastic, and diffuse large B-cell lymphoma (DLBCL) are the most common. Histologic subtypes commonly diagnosed in adults, specifically the indolent lymphomas (small lymphocytic and follicular lymphomas [FLs]) are extremely rare in children. With increasing age, the incidence of FLs and other aggressive lymphomas continues to rise. Small lymphocytic and FLs are most commonly diagnosed in patients over age 60.

NHL ranks as the sixth most common cause of cancer-related death in the United States. In 2005, 19,200 deaths from NHL were predicted, in contrast to 1,320 for Hodgkin lymphoma.[1] In the decades between 20 and 39 years, it ranks fourth for males, and for females 80 or greater, it ranks fifth. The 5-year survival rates for NHL is 60% for Caucasians and 51% for African Americans.

Exposures and Diseases Associated with Increased Risk of Developing NHL Infectious agents are involved in the pathogenesis of some NHLs.(Table 118-1) Epstein-Barr virus (EBV) has a strong association with development of Burkitt's lymphoma and human immunodeficiency virus-1 related lymphoma.[2] Between 45 and 70% of human immunodeficiency virus-1 related NHLs are EBV related. Essentially 100% of the primary central nervous system (CNS) lymphomas are EBV related in human immunodeficiency virus-1 infected individuals. The natural killer cell and natural killer-like T-cell lymphomas that involve the upper aerodigestive tract as well as other extranodal sites also are EBV associated.[3] Human T-cell leukemia virus (HTLV)-1 is responsible for adult T-cell leukemia/lymphoma that is endemic to the Caribbean and southern Japan.[4] The gastric marginal zone lymphomas (MZLs) are associated with *Helicobacter pylori* infection.[5] Splenic MZL has been associated with hepatitis C infection.[6] The ocular adnexal MZL linked with *Chlamydia psittaci* infection,[7] and immunoproliferative small intestinal disease (Mediterranean lymphoma, alpha heavy chain disease) associated with *Campylobacter jejuni*.[8] *Borrelia burgdorferi* infection has been associated with extranodal MZLs of the skin.[9] The Kaposi's sarcoma-associated herpes virus, also known as HHV-8 has been isolated from the neoplastic cells in patients with primary effusion lymphomas in human immunodeficiency virus (HIV) -1 infected individuals.[10]

Table 118-1 Exposures and Diseases Associated with Increased Risk of Developing Non-Hodgkin Lymphoma

Infectious agent association (other than human immunodeficiency virus [HIV])
Epstein-Barr virus
Human T-cell leukemia/lymphoma virus
Helicobacter pylori
HHV-8
Hepatitis C
Chlamydia psittaci
Campylobacter jejuni
Borrelia burgdorferi
Drug or chemical exposures
Diphenylhydantoin
Dioxin, phenoxyherbicides
Radiation
Prior chemotherapy
Prior radiation therapy
Inherited immunodeficiency diseases
Klinefelter's syndrome
Chédiak-Higashi syndrome
Ataxia telangiectasia syndrome
Wiskott-Aldrich syndrome
Common variable immunodeficiency syndrome
Acquired immunodeficiency disease
Iatrogenic immunosuppression
Acquired immunodeficiency virus (HIV-1)
Acquired hypogammaglobulinemia
Autoimmune diseases
Sjögren's syndrome
Celiac sprue
Rheumatoid arthritis and systemic lupus erythematosus

An increased risk of NHL has been associated with a number of exposures and/or disease states (see Table 118-1). There is controversial evidence that certain chemical exposures, specifically the herbicide phenoxyacetic acid, increase the risk of NHL.[11] Other potential environmental associations include exposure to arsenic, pesticides, fungicides, chlorophenols, or organic solvents, halomethane, lead, vinyl chloride, or asbestos. Occupational exposures associated with an increased risk include agricultural work, welding and work in the lumber industry.[12] NHL has been observed as a late complication of prior chemotherapy and/or radiation therapy. Specifically, patients with Hodgkin lymphoma treated with radiation therapy and chemotherapy exhibit an increased risk of developing secondary DLBCL.[13]

Diseases of inherited and acquired immunodeficiency as well as autoimmune diseases are associated with an increased incidence of lymphoma. The association between immunosuppression and induction of NHLs is compelling since if the immunosuppression can be reversed, a percentage of these lymphomas regress spontaneously.[14] The incidence of NHL is nearly 100-fold increased for patients undergoing organ transplantation necessitating chronic immunosuppression, and is greatest in the first year post-transplant. About 30% of these arise as a polyclonal B-cell proliferation that evolves into a clonal B-cell malignancy. The NHLs that occur in the context of immunosuppression or immunodeficiency, including human immunodeficiency virus-1 infection, are frequently associated with EBV.[15] Histologically, DLBCLs are most frequently associated with immunosuppression and autoimmune diseases. The rare inherited immunodeficiency diseases like X-linked lymphoproliferative syndrome, Wiskott-Aldrich syndrome, Chédiak-Higashi syndrome, ataxia telangiectasia, and common variable immunodeficiency syndrome are complicated by highly aggressive lymphomas. The incidence of lymphoma in iatrogenic immunosuppression, AIDS, and autoimmune disease (Felty's syndrome, Sjögren's, celiac disease, Crohn's disease, rheumatoid arthritis and systemic lupus) argues strongly for immune dysregulation contributing in the pathogenesis of some lymphomas.

PATHOLOGY, IMMUNOBIOLOGY, AND NATURAL HISTORY OF NHL

The development of lymphoma classification schemas has evolved over the past 30 years. In

Table 118-2 Classification of Non-Hodgkin Lymphoma

Indolent lymphomas
Follicular lymphoma
B-chronic lymphocytic leukemia/small lymphocytic lymphoma
Lymphoplasmacytic lymphoma
Marginal zone lymphoma (nodal, extranodal, splenic)
T/natural killer large cell granular lymphocyte leukemia
T-chronic lymphocytic leukemia/prolymphocytic leukemia
Aggressive lymphomas
Mantle cell lymphoma
Diffuse large B-cell lymphoma
Peripheral T-cell lymphoma (unspecified)
Peripheral T-cell lymphoma (angioimmunoblastic, angiocentric)
T/natural killer cell, hepatosplenic γ/δ, intestinal T cell lymphoma
Anaplastic large cell lymphomas
Highly aggressive lymphomas
Precursor T or B lymphoblastic leukemia/lymphoma.
Burkitt and Burkitt-like lymphoma.
Adult T-cell leukemia/lymphoma (HTLV-1+)

1995, the Society for Hematopathology and the European Association of Hematopathologists jointly developed a classification of hematologic neoplasms for the World Health Organization (WHO). The goals of the WHO project, in part, were to update and revise the WHO classification of the lymphoid neoplasms, using a combination of morphology, immunotyping, genetic features, and clinical syndromes.[16] To provide a context for this classification, the large numbers of entities will be grouped in "indolent," "aggressive," and "highly aggressive" categories (Table 118-2).

Indolent Lymphomas The indolent NHLs are generally associated with reasonably long survival (years) even if left untreated, but they are usually not curable with conventional treatment. Indolent lymphomas represent 35 to 40% of the NHLs diagnosed in western countries. The most common subtypes are FL, small lymphocytic lymphoma, and MZL, comprising 22, 6, and 5% of all NHLs, respectively. In comparison, lymphoplasmacytic lymphoma, mycosis fungoides/Sézary syndrome, and splenic MZLs are rare diseases, comprising 1% or less of all NHLs.

Follicular Lymphomas FLs are the most common type of indolent NHL, and morphologically recapitulate normal germinal centers of secondary lymphoid follicles. (Figure 118-1) The WHO classification includes 3 grades; grade I (0–5 large cells/high power field) (Figure 118-2); grade II (6–15 large cells/high power field); and grade III (>15 large cells/high power field).[16] Although the grading system remains in place, clinically, grade I and II FLs are approached similarly. Similar to normal germinal centers, small numbers of T cells and follicular dendritic cells are present in the malignant follicles; however, tingible body macrophages, which are macrophages that have ingested apoptotic cells, are not observed. Involvement of the peripheral blood with malignant cells is commonly seen, and morphologically these cells have notches and have been referred to as "buttock cells."

Early studies suggested that FL and normal follicular center B cells were related by their expression of cell surface antigens. Virtually all FLs express monoclonal surface immunoglobulin.[17] Virtually all cases express HLA-DR, the B cell antigens CD19, CD20, CD21, CD10, CD79a, but lack CD5. Cytoplasmic bcl-2 protein is over-expressed in essentially all cases of grade I and II, whereas nuclear bcl-6 is expressed by at least some of the neoplastic cells.[18] The most common cytogenetic abnormality in FL is t(14;18) that leads to over-expression of the anti-apoptotic protein bcl-2 in over 85% of cases (Table 118-3) (see Chapter 8, "Human Genomics and Chromosome Rearrangements in Cancer").

FLs account for about 22% of NHLs, with grade I subtype being most common.[19] Although uncommon until the third and fourth decades, the median age at diagnosis is 60 years. This histologic subtype is less common in Asians and blacks. Patients usually present with painless peripheral adenopathy in cervical, axillary, inguinal, and femoral regions. Often lymph node enlargement has been present for long periods, and the nodes have waxed and waned. Hilar and mediastinal nodes are often involved, but large mediastinal masses are rare. Some patients present with asymptomatic large abdominal masses with or without evidence of gastrointestinal and/or renal obstruction. Staging studies usually demonstrates widely disseminated disease with involvement of spleen (40%), liver (50%), and bone marrow (70%). Bone marrow involvement in FL reveals a unique pattern of paratrabecular infiltration. Very few patients present with extranodal extramedullary disease, and only about 20% present with B symptoms or lactate dehydrogenase (LDH) elevation. Central nervous system involvement is uncommon although peripheral nerve compression and epidural tumor masses causing cord compression may develop.

Many cases of primary cutaneous B cell lymphomas have features of FL.[20] These tumors are often bcl-2 negative, and their relationship to nodal FL is not known. They occur on the head and trunk, and tend to remain localized to the skin, where they are amenable to local therapy.

The course of FL is quite variable. Some patients can be observed with waxing and waning disease for five years or more without the need for therapy.[21] Others present with more disseminated disease and rapid growth, and require treatment because massive nodal or organ enlargement leads to pain, lymphatic obstruction, or organ obstruction. Historically, both disease-free and overall survival for these patients has not significantly changed in spite of many different therapeutic approaches. The median survival for patients with stages III and IV disease is between 7 and 10 years. Regardless of the long natural history, it should be stressed that except for a subset of patients with stage I disease, virtually all patients eventually die of this disease.

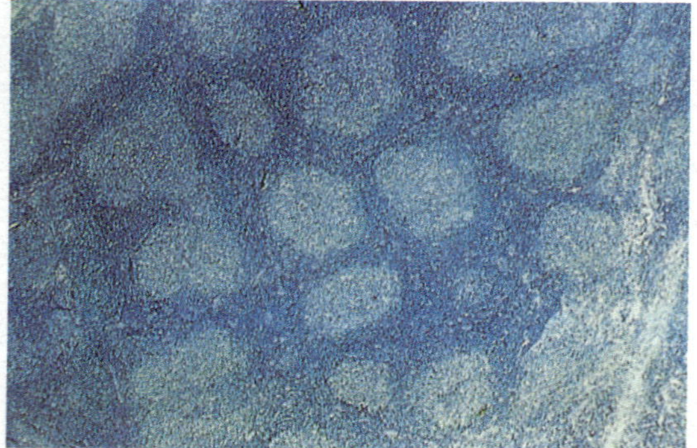

Figure 118-1 Follicular lymphoma grade I (low power).

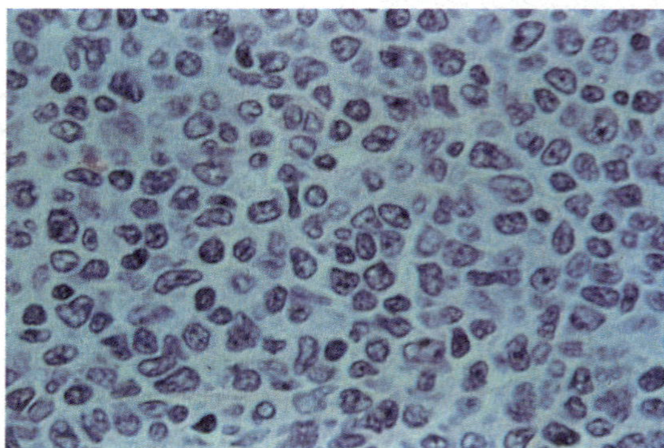

Figure 118-2 Follicular lymphoma grade I (high power).

Histologic transformation to aggressive lymphoma, usually DLBCL, occurs in up to 60% of patients with FL and is characterized by rapid progression of lymphadenopathy, infiltration of extranodal sites, development of B symptoms, elevated LDH, and often a poor prognosis.[22–24] The progression from follicular to DLBCL occurs regardless of whether the FL is treated aggressively or conservatively, and occurs at a rate of 3% per year. Specific genes have been identified as being altered in transformation, including deletions of the cyclin-dependent kinase inhibitors p15 and p16, mutations of p53 and bcl-2, as well as the non-coding regulatory region of the *BCL-6* gene.

FL grade III is synonymous with follicular large cell lymphoma. Although the follicular morphology is preserved, the clinical presentation, and behavior, is very similar to DLBCL.[25,26] In contrast to DLBCL, the relapse rate of FL grade III is higher following combination chemotherapy, but the survival is longer.

Small Lymphocytic Lymphoma Small lymphocytic lymphoma and B-cell chronic lymphocytic leukemia are viewed as the same entity by the WHO classification. Although the major population of cells resembles small normal lymphocytes, larger cells resembling those seen in prolymphocytic leukemia are seen in the nodal tissue in areas known as proliferation centers. (Figure 118-3, and Figures 147-2, 147-3) The small lymphocytic lymphomas are phenotypically nearly identical to B-cell chronic lymphocytic leukemias, by the expression of HLA-DR, B cell antigens CD19, CD20, CD23, weak surface immunoglobulin and CD5. Cytogenetic abnormalities include trisomy 12 present in about 40% of cases, and 13q in 45 to 55%, 11q abnormalities in 17 to 20%, and 17p abnormalities in 7 to 10% of cases.[27]

Recent studies suggest that 30 to 50% of these diseases have non-mutated immunoglobulin vari-

Table 118-3 Consistent Chromosomal Abnormalities Associated with Non-Hodgkin Lymphoma

Histology	Trisomy	Chromosomal Abnormality Translocation/Gene(s)	Deletion
Indolent			
Small lymphocytic lymphoma (B cell)	12	t(11;14)/bcl 1 t(14;19) t(9;14)	—
Follicular lymphoma (B cell)	—	t(14;18)/IgH-bcl 2	6q
Marginal zone lymphoma (B cell)	3	t(14;18), t(11;18) t(1;14), t(11;14)	7q
Aggressive lymphomas			
Mantle cell lymphoma (B cell)	—	t(11;14) bcl-1/IgH	—
Diffuse large cell (B cell)	4, 7, 21, X	t(14;18)/IgH-bcl 2 t(3;22)/bcl 6 t(3;14) t(2;3)	6q,8p,13
Diffuse lymphoma (T cell)	—	t(14;14)(q11;q32)/TCR-tcl 1 inv (14)(q11;q32) t(8;14)(q24;q11) t(10;14)(q24;q11)	iso 7q
Anaplastic large cell lymphoma	—	t(2;5) npm-alk t(1;2)	—
Small noncleaved cell	—	t(8;14)/myc-IgH t(2;8)/Igk-myc t(8;22)/myc-Igl	—

able region genes and correspond to naïve B cells. These cases often express CD38 and the tyrosine kinase ZAP-70, and have a worse prognosis.[27,28] The remaining 50 to 70% of cases have mutated immunoglobulin variable region genes and are derived from germinal center or post-germinal center B cells. These mutated immunoglobulin variable region gene cases are more likely to lack CD38 and ZAP-70, and have a favorable prognosis.

Small lymphocytic lymphomas makes up about 6% of all NHLs.[19] The clinical presentation is similar to FL. Unlike B-cell chronic lymphocytic leukemia, the peripheral blood may be normal or reveal only a mild lymphocytosis (60% have absolute lymphocytosis of < 4,000 per microliter at diagnosis). In contrast, the bone marrow is positive in 70 to 90% of cases. A serum paraprotein is found in about 20% of cases and hypogammaglobulinemia is present in about 40%. Small lymphocytic lymphomas and B-cell chronic lymphocytic leukemia can convert to DLBCL (Richter's syndrome, Figures 118-4 and 118-5).[29]

Lymphoplasmacytic Lymphoma (Immunocytoma) Lymphoplasmacytic lymphoma is an indolent lymphoma composed of diffuse proliferation of small lymphocytes with evidence of maturation to plasma cells.[30] Evidence of immunoglobulin is seen in these cells by special stains or inclusions. These tumors express B cell antigens CD19, CD20, and surface immunoglobulin M isotype, and in general do not express CD5, CD10, or CD23. Up to 50% of the lymphoplasmacytic lymphomas have t(9;14)(p13;q32).[31]

Lymphoplasmacytic lymphoma represents about 1% of all NHLs. Clinically this disease is similar to small lymphocytic lymphomas. The median age is early 60s, and virtually all patients have stage IV disease by virtue of bone marrow involvement. B symptoms and elevated serum LDH are uncommon. Lymph node and splenic involvement are common. A serum M component is commonly seen. As with B-CLL, the paraprotein may have autoantibody or cryoglobulin activity. However, most cases with mixed cryoglobulinemia have been shown to be related to concurrent hepatitis C virus infection.[32] In these cases, treatment with interferon to reduce viral load is associated with regression of the lymphoma. In the WHO clinical study, 5-year overall survival (58%) and failure-free survival (25%) were identical to that of small lymphocytic lymphomas.[33]

Marginal zone lymphomas MZLs are a group of distinct entities including nodal MZL; extranodal MZL also known as the lymphomas of mucosal associated lymphoid tissues; and the splenic MZL.[34,35] In the nodal MZL, the tumor cells cytologically resemble "normal" monocytoid B cells and often involve lymph node sinuses. Phenotypically these tumors express surface immunoglobulin M, B-cell antigens (CD19, CD20). Similar to other indolent lymphomas, MZL can transform into a higher-grade lymphoma. The nodal MZLs constitute 1% of all NHLs.[19] Over 70% of patients present with stage III/IV disease and the majority are asymptomatic. Bone marrow involvement is less common than in most indolent lymphomas, and gastrointestinal involvement unusual. The median survival of these patients is in excess of 12 years.[34]

The extranodal MZL tumor cells express B cells Ags (CD19, CD20) and surface immunoglobulin M. It is hypothesized that these are malignancies of memory B cells. Cytologically, these tumor cells resemble monocytoid B cells. A feature of extranodal MZL is a lymphoepithelial lesion associated with centrocytes. These tumors do not form follicles but the malignant cells surround reactive follicles. When the extranodal MZL spread to lymph nodes, the neoplastic cells involve the marginal zones. The most common cytogenetic abnormality is trisomy 3, occurring in up to 60% of cases (particularly the gastric extranodal MZL) and t(11;18),[36] with t(11;18) occurring in 25 to 40% of cases.[37]

Extranodal MZLs constitute about 5% of all NHLs, and almost 50% of all gastric lymphomas. B symptoms are uncommon and [19] most patients present with stage I or II disease. There is no age predilection for these tumors that most commonly involve the gastrointestinal tract (stomach most commonly), lung, lacrimal and salivary glands, skin, thyroid, and breast. Up to 25% of cases have lymph node or bone marrow involvement.[38] Patients can present with peptic ulcer disease, abdominal pain, and sicca syndrome, or a mass at the site of involvement. These lymphomas can disseminate to other mucosal associated lymphoid tissue sites or bone marrow in about 30% of cases, typically later in the course of the disease. These diseases have high complete remission rates and potentially long survival, as high as 80% at 10 or more years.[38]

The splenic MZLs constitute less than 2% of all NHLs, with a median age of 65, uncommon

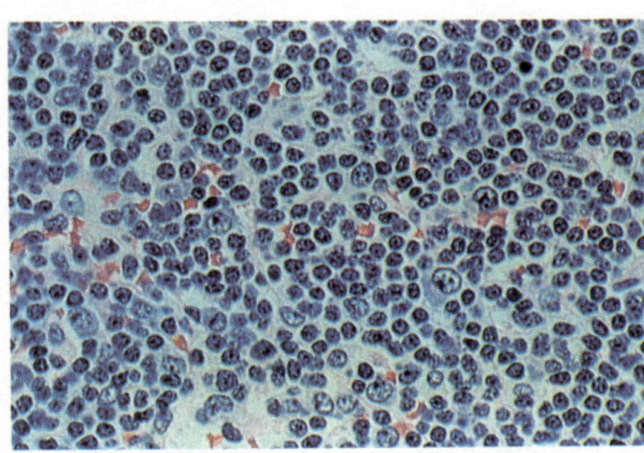

Figure 118-3 Small lymphocytic lymphoma.

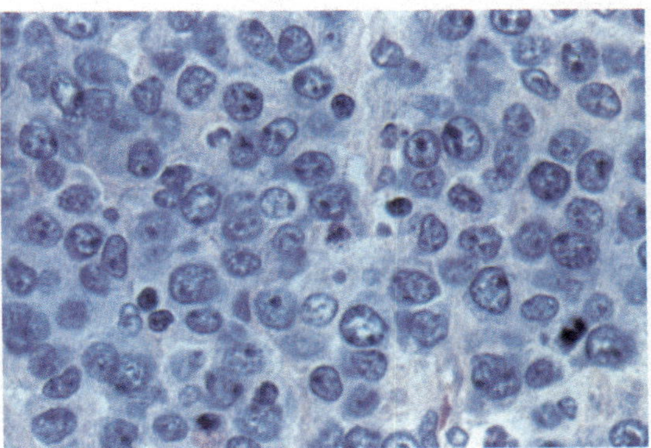

Figure 118-4 Diffuse large B cell lymphoma.

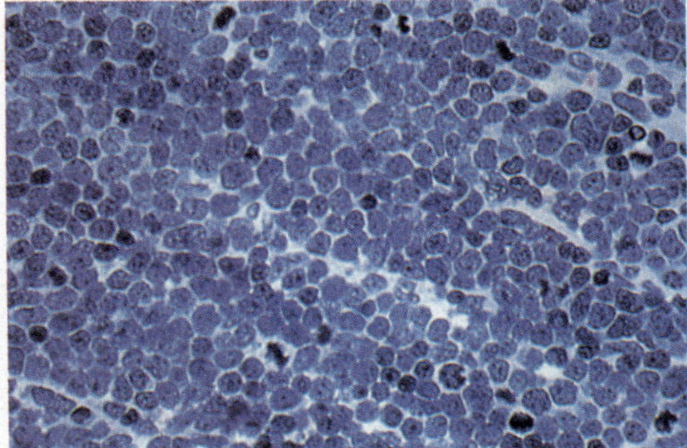

Figure 118-5 T-lymphoblastic lymphoma.

before age 50.[19] In splenic MZL there is expansion of marginal zones in the spleen. Bone marrow and peripheral blood involvement (referred to as splenic lymphoma with villous or non-villous lymphocytes) can also be present. In splenic MZL trisomy 3 is present in 39% of cases. The survival of patients is in excess of 70% at 10 years.[39]

Aggressive Lymphomas **Mantle Cell Lymphoma** Mantle cell lymphoma (MCL) is generally an aggressive disease.[40,41] These tumors are neoplastic counterparts of naive "mantle zone" B cells. Morphologically, MCL can have either diffuse architecture, or a vaguely nodular appearance, occasionally with expansion of the mantle zone of secondary lymphoid follicles. Cytologically, the neoplastic cells are medium sized, with irregular nuclei. Some cases of MCL have a predominance of "blastic" cells with a high mitotic rate. The cells express B cell antigens, surface immunoglobulin M with or without immunoglobulin D, CD5 and CD43, but lack CD10 and CD23, respectively. Over-expression of cyclin D1 protein further distinguishes these tumors from other entities. Approximately 70% of MCLs have t(11;14)(q13;q32) that is rearrangements of *bcl-1* (cyclin D1) gene.

MCL constitutes about 7% of all NHLs. About 75% of patients are males, with median age of 63. Approximately 70% of patients have stage IV disease and B symptoms are observed in approximately one-third of patients. Typical sites of involvement are lymph nodes, spleen, liver, Waldeyer's ring, and bone marrow. Peripheral blood involvement is present in approximately 25% of patients at presentation. MCL can involve any region of the gastrointestinal tract, occasionally presenting as multiple intestinal polyposis. The median survival of patients with MCL is 3 to 4 years, and patients with the blastic variant have a median survival of 18 months.

Diffuse Large B Cell Lymphoma The DLBCLs consist of a diffuse proliferation of large cells that have a high mitotic rate. The cells have a moderate amount of cytoplasm with either cleaved or non-cleaved nuclei often with multiple nucleoli, although there can be great variability in the morphology (see Figure 118-4) Rare cases contain only scattered large cells in a background of small T cells and epithelioid histiocytes, called T cell/histiocyte-rich large B cell lymphoma.[42] Recent studies using gene expression profiling provide evidence that DLBCLs correspond to germinal center B cells or activated B cells.[43,44] The tumor cells generally express B cell antigens (CD19, CD20, CD22), monoclonal surface immunoglobulin M, but occasionally other heavy chain isotypes, with variable expression of CD10 and CD5. Twenty-five to 80% of DLBCLs are reported to express bcl-2 protein, which may be associated with a worse prognosis.[45] Approximately 70% express bcl-6 protein, consistent with a germinal center origin.[46]

Several chromosomal abnormalities have been observed in DLBCL. Bcl 6 is associated with chromosomal rearrangements involving 3q27.[47] Rearrangements of the gene are found in a small proportion of FLs (6–13%) but in 20 to 40% of diffuse aggressive lymphomas.[48] t(14;18) is not specific for FLs and has been observed in approximately 30% of patients with DLBCL. These cases may represent histologic transformations of prior FL.

DLBCL constitutes 31% of all NHLs, and is the most common histologic subtype. Patients who are generally middle aged or older (median age 64 years) present with either nodal enlargement or extranodal disease. These tumors present in a localized (stage I or IE) manner approximately 20% of the time. The disease is confined to one side of the diaphragm (stage I or II) in approximately 30 to 40% of patients. Stage IV disease is seen in approximately 40% of patients. B symptoms are occurring in 30% of patients, and unlike most NHLs, and LDH is elevated in over half the patients. During the course of the disease, the liver, kidneys, and lung may be involved. DLBCL is highly invasive, with local compression of vessels or airways, involvement of peripheral nerves, and destruction of bone. Bone marrow involvement initially is found in only 10 to 20% of patients, and has strong correlation with risk of spread to the central nervous system.[49] Extranodal disease, specifically testicular and paranasal sinus, and elevated LDH are other risks for central nervous system dissemination.

Within the DLBCL is a distinct clinical entity known as primary mediastinal large B-cell lymphoma (7% of all cases of DLBCL).[50] Histologically the cellular infiltrate is heterogeneous, and sclerosis is frequently present. The immunophenotype of these lymphomas includes B-cell antigens (CD19, CD20), but they are often negative for surface and cytoplasmic immunoglobulin. Recent studies suggest that the gene expression profile pattern of primary mediastinal large B-cell lymphoma closely resembles Hodgkin lymphoma Reed-Sternberg cell lines.[51,52]

Primary mediastinal large B-cell lymphomas have a female predominance, with median age of 40. Over 70% of these patients present with stage I/II bulky disease involving the mediastinum, pleural, and pericardial effusions in about one-third of the patients. Superior vena cava syndrome is common in these patients. Similar to DLBCL, an elevated LDH is present in the majority, whereas bone marrow involvement is infrequent. The prognosis of patients with primary mediastinal large B-cell lymphoma is similar to patients with DLBCL.

Rare cases of DLBCL present with a disseminated intravascular proliferation of large lymphoid cells, involving small blood vessels, without an obvious tumor mass.[53] The organs most commonly involved are the central nervous system, kidneys, lungs, and skin, but virtually any site may be involved. Patients present with a variety of symptoms related to organ dysfunction secondary to vascular occlusion. Onset with fever, skin rash, or prominent and rapidly progressive neurologic signs is common. The prognosis of these patients is generally poor.

Peripheral T-cell Lymphomas The category of peripheral T-cell lymphomas (PTCL) includes a number of entities, which constitute 15% of all NHLs in adults. Among these, in decreasing frequency, are the PTCL, not otherwise unspecified; anaplastic large cell lymphoma (ALCL); angioimmunoblastic T-cell lymphoma; the natural killer/T angiocentric lymphomas; and the much rarer entities, panniculitis-like T-cell lymphoma; intestinal T-cell lymphoma; and hepatosplenic γ/δ T-cell lymphoma.[16]

PTCLs can be nodal or entranodal based diseases. The diffuse cellular infiltrates range from a mixture of small and large cells; infiltrates of pleomorphic cells, often with a background of epithelioid histiocytes, plasma cells, eosinophils, and Reed-Sternberg–like cells; or predominantly large cells. In contrast to B-cell lymphomas, the pattern of expression of T-cell surface antigens is very variable. The majority will express CD2, CD3, and CD4, with a subset of tumors expressing CD8. In most cases, one or more "mature" T-cell antigens is lost, such as CD5 or CD7.

Abnormal metaphases are seen in 90% of T-cell lymphomas. The most commonly seen translocations in peripheral T-cell lymphomas are t(7;14), t(11;14), inv(14), and t(14;14).[54] These translocations involve genes for the T-cell receptor (TCR) at 14q11, 7q34-35, and 7p15. Young patients with ALCL have t(2;5) and less commonly t(1;2).[55] ALCL in adults generally lack t(2;5) in the tumor cells but cases with the t(2;5) have a significantly better prognosis than cases lacking the t(2;5). Hepatosplenic γ/δ T-cell lymphomas are associated with isochromosome 7q and trisomy 8.[56]

Histologically, there are uncommon subtypes of PTCL that have unique histologic features. The angioimmunoblastic T-cell lymphoma in addition to a pleomorphic heterogeneous cellular infiltrate, has increased amounts of high endothelial venules present, giving a hypervascular appearance. The subcutaneous panniculitis-like T-cell lymphoma is characterized by subcutaneous nodules with cellular infiltrates in the subcutaneous fat, with generally sparing of the overlying skin.[57] Intestinal T-cell lymphoma, often associated with gluten enteropathy, is characterized by mucosal ulceration or masses in the small bowel. The neoplastic infiltrate consists of anaplastic large cells. Often the adjacent mucosa shows changes seen in celiac disease, with villous atrophy and a lymphocytic infiltrate. These tumor cells are generally CD4–, and express CD103, which is an adhesion receptor on intestinal lymphocytes.[58] Hepatosplenic γ/δ T-cell lymphoma is an extremely rare disease presenting with hepatosplenomegaly, often with marrow involvement and occasionally peripheral blood involvement.[56] The tumor cells infiltrate the red pulp of the spleen and liver sinusoids. The tumor cells are CD2+, CD3+, variably CD8+, but also CD7+ and CD56+. In contrast to most PTCL, which express the α/β T-cell receptor, a unique feature of these tumors is expression of the γ/δ T-cell receptor.

Patients with PTCL have a similar median age as patients with DLBCL. However, 80% of patients with PTCL have stage III/IV disease, and more frequently have B symptoms, hepatosplenomegaly and extranodal disease, such as the skin. PTCL generally have a worse prognosis that DLBCL. Angioimmunoblastic T-cell lymphoma usually affects older adults who present with the acute onset of generalized lymphadenopathy, hepatosplenomegaly, skin rash and B symptoms.[59] Immunologic abnormalities are common and include plasmacytosis, polyclonal hypergammaglobulinemia, and a positive Coombs' test. The median survival is 30 months. Infection is the most common cause of death, followed by the aggressive T-cell lymphoma or development of EBV-positive DLBCL.

Subcutaneous panniculitis-like T-cell lymphoma is also a rare disease that presents with subcutaneous nodules, developing into progressive disseminated disease. Many of these patients have hemophagocytic syndrome either at diagnosis or later on. Hepatosplenic γ/δ T-cell lymphoma is a highly aggressive lymphoma. It typically presents in younger males with hepatosplenomegaly, bone marrow, and peripheral blood involvement. These patients are pancytopenic and have a median survival of 1 to 2 years. The intestinal T-cell lymphomas are rare aggressive diseases that are generally associated with a history of gluten enteropathy. These patients present with intestinal obstruction, perforation, and bleeding. In some patients, there is a brief history of gluten sensitivity or worsening gluten enteropathy. Uncommonly, there is extra-intestinal disease with dissemination to the lungs or skin. These patients have a very poor prognosis, with only occasional patients cured with surgical resection.

The angiocentric natural killer/T-cell lymphomas are characterized by vascular invasion and extensive tissue destruction.[60] EBV is present in the tumor cells in virtually all cases. The tumor cells express the phenotype of natural killer cells CD2, CD56, CD45RO, CD43, but lack surface CD3 and TCR. Occasional cases are reported which express CD4 or CD8. The nasal natural killer/T-cell lymphomas are rare, typically present in males with average age of 60. The vast majority of patients have localized disease with nasal obstruction and a destructive mass. Occasionally the aerodigestive and gastrointestinal tract and testis is involved. B symptoms are uncommon. Over 60% of patients with stage I disease remain in long term remission with treatment, whereas patients with stage II to IV disease have a poor prognosis, with extranodal relapses.

ALCL is a subtype of PTCL, which can have nodal, soft tissue or cutaneous involvement. When involving nodes, ALCL characteristically involves the sinusoids of lymph nodes with bizarre large cells. Neoplastic cells derived from patients with ALCL also generally express the phenotype of mature activated T cells (HLA-DR, CD30, CD25). The ALK protein (anaplastic lymphoma kinase) is detected in 40 to 60% of cases using the ALK1 monoclonal antibody, showing both nuclear and cytoplasmic staining in cases with the t(2;5). ALK positive cases are more common in children and younger adults and have a better prognosis than ALK negative cases.[61]

ALCL constitutes 2% of all NHLs in adults, but is the second most common T-cell lymphoma. The median age of patients with ALCL is 34 with a male predominance. There is a bimodal distribution of this disease, with peaks in childhood/young adults, and late adulthood. In adults, B symptoms, peripheral and retroperitoneal adenopathy are common. Skin is a common site of extranodal disease (about 25% of patients), whereas bone marrow involvement is infrequent. The prognosis of these adult patients with systemic ALCL is similar to patients with DLBCL.[62]

Highly Aggressive Lymphomas Precursor T or B Lymphoblastic Leukemia/Lymphoma There is significant overlap between lymphoblastic lymphoma and acute lymphoblastic leukemia. Cytologically, lymphoblastic lymphoma cells are identical to acute lymphoblastic leukemia cells the majority L1 morphology in the FAB classification. These cells have a high nuclear to cytoplasmic ratio, scant cytoplasm and nuclei with fine chromatin with multiple small nucleoli, and have a high mitotic rate. The nuclei can have folds or convolutions. Typically, nodes involved with lymphoblastic lymphoma are effaced by malignant cells (see Figure 118-5).

The vast majority of lymphoblastic lymphomas are of T-cell lineage. Several investigators have noted that most T-cell lymphoblastic lymphomas correspond to stages of thymocyte differentiation. From a clinical point of view, as well as by cell surface markers, T-cell ALL and T-cell lymphoblastic lymphomas have considerable overlap. Approximately 10 to 15% of lymphoblastic lymphomas have a precursor B cell phenotype.

Although lymphoblastic lymphomas represent a major subgroup of childhood NHLs, they are much more rare in adults (2% of adult NHLs). Patients are usually males in their 20s or 30s who present with lymphadenopathy in cervical, supraclavicular, and axillary regions (50%) or with a mediastinal mass (50–75%). These masses can be associated with superior vena cava syndrome, tracheal obstruction, and pericardial effusions. Less commonly, patients present with extranodal disease (eg, skin, testicular, or bony involvement). More than 80% of patients present with stage III or stage IV disease, and almost 50% have B symptoms, and the majority have elevated LDH. Although the bone marrow is frequently normal at presentation, virtually all patients develop bone marrow infiltration and a subsequent leukemic phase indistinguishable from T-cell acute lymphoblastic leukemia. Patients with bone marrow involvement have a very high incidence of central nervous system infiltration. Prior to aggressive acute leukemia type therapy, this disease was rapidly fatal. B-cell lymphoblastic lymphoma is a very rare variant, affecting patients with a median age of 39.[63] B-cell lymphoblastic lymphomas present without a mediastinal mass but instead involve lymph nodes and extranodal sites. The prognosis for these patients may be better than for adults with T-cell lymphoblastic lymphoma.

Burkitt's and Burkitt-Like Lymphoma Burkitt's lymphoma cells resemble the small noncleaved cells within normal germinal centers of secondary lymphoid follicles. Because of the high mitotic rate, frequent mitotic figures are seen and, analogous to normal germinal centers, tingible body macrophages are seen, giving the classical "starry sky" appearance. Burkitt-like lymphoma cells are more pleomorphic with fewer nucleoli. The pathologic distinction between many cases of Burkitt-like lymphoma and DLBCL remains a challenge. It is generally agreed that the fraction of Ki-67 (proliferating cells) in Burkitt-like lymphoma should be 99%.[16]

Burkitt's lymphoma is a tumor of B lineage derivation by the expression of a variety of B-cell restricted antigens including CD19, CD20, surface immunoglobulin M, HLA-DR, CD10, and nuclear bcl-6 protein.[64] The endemic Burkitt's lymphoma is EBV positive, whereas the vast majority of non-endemic Burkitt's lymphoma is EBV negative. Flow cytometry and gene expression profiling support a germinal center B cell derivation for these lymphomas. The immunophenotype of Burkitt-like lymphomas is similar to Burkitt's lymphomas, although expression of CD10 and CD21 is more variable. Burkitt's lymphoma cells lack bcl-2 protein, whereas Burkitt-like lymphomas are bcl-2 positive.

Burkitt's lymphoma most commonly involves a translocation of chromosome 8q24 in 90% of the cases studied with either chromosome 14, 2, or 22.[65] In contrast, the Burkitt-like lymphomas have c-myc translocations in approximately one-third of cases; dual translocations of bcl-2 and c-myc rearrangements are reported in one-third of cases, and no other abnormality is noted in the remaining one-third of cases.[66]

Burkitt's lymphoma is in general a pediatric tumor that has three major clinical presentations. The endemic (African) form presents as a jaw or facial bone tumor that spreads to extranodal sites including ovary, testis, kidney, breast, and especially to the bone marrow and meninges. The non-endemic form has an abdominal presentation with massive disease, ascites, renal, testis, ovarian involvement, and, like the endemic form, also spreads to the bone marrow and central nervous system. Immunodeficiency-related cases more often involve lymph nodes, and may present as acute leukemia. Burkitt's lymphoma has a male predominance and is typically seen in patients less than 35 years of age. Burkitt-like lymphoma, a rare disease, occurs in patients with a median age of 55, with a male predominance. This is an aggressive disease involving lymph nodes, the nasopharynx, and gastrointestinal tract are involved as well. Occasionally Burkitt-like lymphomas presents as a solitary bone tumor. These tumors have a high propensity to invade the bone marrow and central nervous system.

DIFFERENTIAL DIAGNOSIS AND SITES OF DISEASE AT PRESENTATION

More than two-thirds of patients with NHL present with persistent painless peripheral lym-

Table 118-4 Generalized Lymphadenopathy Potentially Confused with Non-Hodgkin Lymphoma

Infectious
Bacterial (syphilis, brucellosis)
Viral (infectious mononucleosis, cytomegalovirus, human immunodeficiency virus, cat scratch fever)
Mycobacterial (tuberculosis)
Parasitic (toxoplasmosis)
Autoimmune
Systemic lupus erythematosus
Sjögren's syndrome
Hydantoin derivatives
Granulomatosis
Sarcoidosis
Neoplasms
Hodgkin's disease
Chronic lymphocytic leukemia
Small cell carcinoma of the lung
Malignant histiocytosis
Melanoma
Germ cell neoplasms
Other conditions
Reactive lymphoid hyperplasia
Lymphomatoid granulomatosis
Dermatopathic lymphadenopathy
Angioimmunoblastic lymphadenopathy
Giant lymph node hyperplasia (Castleman disease)

phadenopathy. At the time of presentation, differential diagnosis of generalized lymphadenopathy necessitates the exclusion of infectious etiologies including bacteria, viruses (eg, infectious mononucleosis, cytomegalovirus and human immunodeficiency virus), and parasites (toxoplasmosis) (Table 118-4). It is generally agreed that a firm lymph node larger than 1.5 × 1.5 cm that is not associated with a documented infection, and that persists longer than 4 to 6 weeks, and is certainly progressing should be considered for biopsy. However, lymph nodes in several histopathologic subtypes of NHLs frequently wax and wane. In teenagers and young adults, infectious mononucleosis and Hodgkin lymphoma should be placed high in the differential diagnosis. Involvement of Waldeyer's ring, epitrochlear, and mesenteric nodes are more frequently observed in patients with NHL than Hodgkin disease. Unlike patients with Hodgkin lymphoma who frequently present with weight loss, fever, or night sweats, about 40% of all patients with NHL present with systemic complaints. B symptoms are more common in patients with aggressive histologies approaching 50%. Less frequent presenting symptoms include complaints such as fatigue, malaise, and pruritus occurring in less than 20% of patients.

NHLs also present with thoracic, abdominal, and/or extranodal symptoms (Table 118-5). Although much less common than with Hodgkin lymphoma, approximately 20% of patients with NHL present with mediastinal adenopathy. These patients most frequently present with persistent cough, chest discomfort, or without clinical symptoms but have an abnormal chest radiograph. Occasionally, a superior vena cava syndrome accompanies presentation. Differential diagnosis of mediastinal presentation includes infections (eg, histoplasmosis, tuberculosis, infectious mononucleosis), sarcoidosis, Hodgkin lymphoma, as well as other neoplasms. Involvement of retroperitoneal, mesenteric, and pelvic nodes is common in most histologic subtypes of NHL. Unless massive or leading to obstruction, nodal enlargement in these sites usually does not produce symptoms. In contrast, patients with an abdominal mass, massive splenomegaly, or primary gastrointestinal lymphoma present with complaints similar to those caused by other space occupying lesions. These complaints include chronic pain, abdominal fullness, and early satiety—symptoms associated with visceral obstruction, or even acute perforation and gastrointestinal hemorrhage. Rarely, patients present with symptoms of unexplained anemia. Those with aggressive NHLs can present with primary cutaneous lesions, testicular masses, acute spinal cord compression, solitary bone lesions, and rarely lymphomatous meningitis. Symptoms of primary NHL of the central nervous system include headache, lethargy, focal neurologic symptoms, seizures, and paralysis.

When NHL presents in an extranodal site, the differential diagnosis is more difficult. NHL uncommonly presents in the lung as bronchovascular-lymphangitic, nodular, or alveolar patterns of involvement.[67] Between 25 and 50% of patients with NHLs present with hepatic infiltration although relatively few present with large hepatic masses. Of the advanced-stage indolent lymphomas, nearly 75% of patients have microscopic hepatic infiltration at presentation. In contrast, primary hepatic lymphoma is extremely rare and is nearly always aggressive histology. Another extranodal site of presentation occurring in less than 5% of patients is primary lymphoma of bone, presenting as a painful bony site. Most frequently, lytic lesions are observed on standard radiographs. The most common sites of primary lymphoma of bone include femur, pelvis, and vertebrae. Approximately 5% of NHLs present as primary gastrointestinal lymphoma. These patients present with hemorrhage, pain, or obstruction since the stomach is most frequently infiltrated followed by small intestine and colon, respectively. Most gastrointestinal lymphomas are of the diffuse aggressive histologies, specifically DLBCL, MCL and the intestinal T-cell lymphoma. The most common site for extranodal MZLs to involve is the stomach.[68] A subset of MCLs presents as multiple intestinal polyposis involving any sites in the gastrointestinal tract.[69] An uncommon presentation (2–14%) of NHL is renal infiltration, and even less common is localized presentation in the prostate, testis, or ovary. The typical histologic subtypes of these sites are DLBCL or Burkitt's/Burkitt-like lymphomas. Rare sites of primary lymphoma include the orbit, heart, breast, salivary glands, thyroid, and adrenal gland.

Table 118-5 Sites of Disease at Presentation Correlated with Working Formulation

Disease Site	Low Grade	Intermediate Grade	High Grade
Peripheral nodes	Common	Common	Common
Abdominal nodes	Common	Less frequent	Less frequent
Mediastinal nodes	Common	Less frequent	Less frequent
Bone marrow	Common	Less frequent	Common
Liver	Common	Less frequent	Common
Spleen	Common	Less frequent	Less frequent
Extranodal	Uncommon	Common	Common

STAGING AND DISEASE DETECTION

The Ann Arbor staging system developed in 1971 for Hodgkin lymphoma was adapted for staging NHLs.[70] This staging system focuses on the number of tumor sites (nodal and extranodal), location, and the presence or absence of systemic symptoms. Table 118-6 summarizes the essential features of the Ann Arbor system. Because NHLs most frequently disseminate hematogenously, this staging system has proven to be much less useful than for Hodgkin lymphoma.

The concept of staging has less impact in NHL than in Hodgkin lymphoma. Only 10% of patients with FL have localized disease at diagnosis and the majority of patients with aggressive lymphomas have advanced stage disease. There is little therapeutic benefit to distinguishing between stage III and stage IV disease since the treatment options are nearly identical. Multiple studies have demonstrated that prognosis is more dependent on histology and clinical parameters including age, extranodal disease, and performance status. Staging is undertaken in NHLs to identify the small number of patients who can be treated with local therapy or combined modality treatment and to stratify within histologic subtypes in order to determine prognosis and assess the impact of treatment.

Diagnosis and Initial Evaluation Staging must be undertaken in the context of the histology. After the initial biopsy, blood tests should be obtained, including complete blood count, routine chemistries, liver function tests, and serum protein electrophoresis to document the presence of circulating monoclonal paraprotein. The serum beta-2 microglobulin level is useful in patients with indolent lymphomas, for prognostic purposes, as a surrogate measure of disease volume, and for monitoring response to therapy. Serum concentrations of LDH are an important independent predictor of survival in NHL. Waldeyer's ring involvement is associated with intestinal involvement in 20% of cases, and endoscopy should be considered if the patient appears to have localized disease. Chest computed tomography scan has superseded the use of chest radiography. Abdominal/pelvic computed tomography scan is essential for accurate staging to assess

Table 118-6 Ann Arbor Staging System for Non-Hodgkin Lymphoma

Stage I	Involvement of a single lymph node region or of a single extranodal organ or site(IE)
Stage II	Involvement of two or more lymph node regions on the same side of the diaphragm, or localized involvement of an extranodal site or organ (IIE) and one or more lymph node regions on the same side of the diaphragm
Stage III	Involvement of lymph node regions on both sides of the diaphragm, which may also be accompanied by localized involvement of an extranodal organ or site (IIIE) of spleen (IIIS) or both (IIISE)
Stage IV	Diffuse or disseminated involvement of one or more distant extranodal sites.
Fever	> 38°C, night sweats, weight loss > 10% of body weight in the 6 months preceding admission are defined as systemic symptoms and denoted by the suffix B. Other patients are denoted by the suffix A.

lymphadenopathy in retroperitoneal, mesenteric, and retrocrural areas. Unilateral bone marrow biopsies should be performed, since the likelihood of lymphomatous involvement of the marrow is relatively high, especially in most indolent lymphomas, where marrow involvement occurs in most cases. In patients with aggressive lymphomas with marrow involvement, paranasal sinus involvement, paraspinal masses, or if clinically indicated, examination of the cerebral spinal fluid (CSF) by lumbar puncture should be performed.

Radionuclide scans have clinical utility as diagnostic and monitoring studies. Gallium scans are positive in virtually all of the aggressive lymphomas, and in about 50% of indolent lymphomas. Gallium scans, combined with single photon emission computed tomography are very sensitive in detecting tumor infiltration. Gallium scanning is useful in monitoring response to therapy. Positron emission tomography (PET) continues to be evaluated as an imaging tool in lymphoma. Numerous studies indicate that PET using 18F-fluorodeoxyglucose detects actively metabolizing tumor in residual masses following or during chemotherapy. Moreover, persistent abnormal uptake predicts for early relapse and/or reduced survival.[71–73] PET appears to be superior to gallium scanning and was comparable to computed tomography in its capability to detect disease sites in intermediate to high-grade NHL and Hodgkin lymphoma, although the additional findings did not impact on outcome.[74] Magnetic resonance imaging is most valuable for evaluation of the brain and spinal cord.

Immunologic and Molecular Studies Biologic studies including cell surface markers, cytogenetics, and molecular techniques are used in diagnosis, staging, and minimal disease detection. Monoclonal antibodies directed against cell surface antigens expressed on lymphoid cells, and molecular techniques to define immunoglobulin and T-cell receptor gene rearrangements are sensitive tools with which to assess tumor cell infiltration. Immunophenotypic and cytogenetic studies can help to determine histologic subtypes of lymphomas. For those NHLs with known chromosomal translocations, it is possible to identify unique chromosomal breakpoints. For example, detection of the t(14;18) of FLs can be undertaken employing the technique of polymerase chain reaction (PCR).[75] With this approach, one tumor cell in 10^5–10^6 cells can be detected. Studies of minimal disease are providing important insights into whether patients are in molecular remission and whether further therapy is required.

DISEASE PARAMETERS THAT INFLUENCE PROGNOSIS AND ASSESSMENT OF DISEASE RESPONSE

Clinical Prognostic Factors in Aggressive NHL The analysis of a large group (2,031 patients) with diffuse aggressive NHLs treated with an anthracycline containing regimen, led to the establishment of a prognostic model of predicting outcome known as the International Prognostic Index (IPI) (Table 118-7).[76] Of a large number of factors examined for all patients age (≤ 60 vs > 60); serum LDH (≤ normal vs > normal); performance status (0 or 1 vs 2–4); stage (I or II vs. III or IV); and extranodal involvement (≤ site vs >1 site) were independently prognostic for overall survival. These data permitted the identification of four risk groups based on the number of risk factors: low-risk with 0 or 1 factor; low-intermediate with 2 factors; high-intermediate with three factors; and high with four or five factors. The 5-year overall survival rates for patients with scores of 0 to 1, 2, 3, and 4 to 5 were 73, 51, 43, and 26%, respectively. For the patients aged 60 or less, only stage, LDH, and performance status were of prognostic significance. Patients ≤ 60 with 0, 1, 2 or 3 risk factors had five-year survival rates of 83, 69, 46, and 32%, respectively. Survival rates for those > 60 with the same scores were 56, 44, 37, and 21%, respectively.

The IPI has been modified for patients with stage I or II aggressive NHLs [77] with age > 60, LDH, stage II and performance status ≥ 2 being significant factors. When this was applied to patients treated with three courses of cyclophosphamide, Adriamycin, vincristine, and prednisone (CHOP), plus involved region radiation therapy the 10-year overall survival rates for patients with 0, 1 or 2, and 3 or 4 factors were 90, 56, and 40% respectively.[77]

Clinical Prognostic Factors in Indolent NHL A predictive model based on over 4,000 patients with follicular NHL has been developed, known as the FL IPI or FLIPI. This study identified the following prognostic factors: age > 60; stage III/IV, more than 4 nodal sites; elevated serum LDH concentration; and hemoglobin less than 12. The 10-year survival rates for patients with zero to one (low-risk), two (intermediate-risk), or three or more (high-risk) of these adverse factors averaged 71, 51, and 36%, respectively.[78]

In patients under age 60 with indolent NHL, the duration of first remission, partial remission (PR) or complete remission (CR), is related to overall survival. Those patients with CR or PR lasting less than 1 year have median survivals of 2.4 years. In contrast, those patients with CR lasting more than 1 year have a median survival of 5.9 years.[79]

Gene Expression Profiling Gene expression profiling using DNA microarrays has been used to examine DLBCL with one goal of identifying patients with different prognoses.[43,44,80,81] Based on gene expression, DLBCLs have been subclassified into "germinal center" or "activated" B-cell types. Patients with germinal center B-like DLBCL, had significantly better overall survival than those with the activated B-like variant.

Table 118-7 The International Index and Age-Adjusted Index

				RFS of CRs (%)		Survival (%)	
Risk Group	Risk Factors	Distribution of Cases (%)	CR Rate	2-Yr Rate	5-Yr Rate	2-Yr Rate	5-Yr Rate
International index (patients of all ages)							
Low (L)	0.1	35	87	79	70	84	73
Low-intermediate (LI)	2	27	67	66	50	66	51
High-intermediate (HI)	3	22	55	59	49	54	43
High (H)	4.5	16	44	58	40	34	26
Age-adjusted index applied to patients < 60 yr of age							
Low (L)	0	22	92	88	86	90	83
Low-intermediate (LI)	1	32	78	74	66	79	69
High-intermediate (HI)	2	32	57	62	53	59	46
High (H)	3	14	46	61	58	37	32
Age-adjusted index applied to patients > 60 yr of age							
Low (L)	0	18	91	75	46	80	56
Low-intermediate (LI)	1	31	71	64	45	68	44
High-intermediate (HI)	2	35	56	60	41	48	37
High (H)	3	16	36	47	37	31	21

RFS of CRs = relapse free survival of patients who sustained complete remission.

Based on finding from gene expression profiling, immunohistochemistry using tissue microarrays has been used for a limited number of gene products as prognostic markers.[82] Germinal center and non-germinal center B cell derivation can be determined by expression of CD10 and bcl-6, MUM1 and cyclin D2. Using tissue microarrays, 42% of DLBCLs are considered germinal center B cell derivation and 58% are non-germinal center B-cell derivation.

In FL, gene expression profiling has been examined in pretreatment tissue and correlated with survival. This study has shown that genes associated with the non-malignant cell infiltrate segregate patients into subgroups with favorable and unfavorable prognoses. Immune response 1 signature (gene associated with certain T cell and macrophage markers) was favorable, whereas immune response 2 signature (genes highly expressed in macrophages) was unfavorable.[83]

Cell Surface Phenotype With IPI stratification, PTCL patients generally have worse prognoses than DLBCL. More recently, a modification of the IPI was reported for patients with PTCL (not otherwise specified).[84] In this model, 4 prognostic factors were identified: age > 60; PS > 1; LDH greater than normal; and bone marrow involvement. The 10 year overall survival for patients with 0, 1, 2, and 3 or 4 risk factors was 50, 32, 30 and 9%, respectively. Patients with DLBCL whose tumors do not express HLA-DR had a significantly shorter survival duration compared to HLA-DR positive patients. The HLA-DR negative cases had fewer CD8+ T cells infiltrating the tumor tissue. A multivariate analysis, adjusting for prognostic factors of known clinical significance, confirmed the importance of the expression of HLA-DR as a prognostic factor.[85]

Minimal Residual Disease Detection In follicular NHL, following aggressive therapy with high-dose ablative therapy and autologous bone marrow transplantation, those patients whose stem cell product was free of bcl-2 detectable cells, or who consistently lack a bcl-2 translocation in the bone marrow and the peripheral blood in long term follow up, have an increased disease-free survival as compared to patients with PCR detectable disease.[86] It is controversial whether following conventional therapy, the presence in the peripheral blood and marrow of lymphoma cells detected by PCR for t(14;18) in FL patients or t(11;14) in MCL patients correlates with outcome.[87,88]

THERAPEUTIC APPROACHES ACCORDING TO WHO CLASSIFICATION

Indolent Lymphomas **Therapy of Early Stage Indolent Lymphoma** Patients with localized indolent lymphoma should be treated with local radiotherapy with curative intent. The majority of patients with indolent NHL present with advanced disease. Only 10 to 20% of patients have clinical stage I/II disease and less than 10% have pathologic stage I/II. In a study of 177 patients from Stanford, 44% of patients had stage I and 56% had stage II disease.[89] Patients were treated with either involved field, extended field, with a limited number receiving total lymphoid irradiation. Survival rates at 10, 15, and 20 years were 64, 44, and 35%, respectively. The relapse-free survival rates at 10, 15, and 20 years were 44, 40, and 37%, respectively. The freedom from recurrence was significantly better for patients under age 60, and for patients who received radiation to both sides of the diaphragm (although there was no difference in overall survival). This analysis has been extended to outcome after relapse.[90] Most patients (76%) had stage I/II disease at relapse. Actuarial survival rates 5, 10, 15, and 20 years after relapse were 56, 35, 17, and 17%, respectively. The progression-free survival rate for the entire group at 5 years was 44%, and remained at 22% 10, 15, and 20 years following relapse. The development of second solid tumors had been noted in 17% of the patients treated with extensive radiotherapy, whereas the incidence of second solid tumors was 6.8% in patients who received involved- or extended-field radiation. Several studies have employed local radiotherapy with adjuvant chemotherapy, and there appears to be no significant advantage of combined modality over local radiotherapy.[91] A retrospective study by McLaughlin and colleagues reported that the relapse-free survival was 64% versus 37% for patients receiving CHOP chemotherapy plus radiotherapy or radiotherapy alone, respectively.[92] Whether these improved results are because of the more aggressive regimen is unclear, and therefore the benefit of chemotherapy in stage I/II indolent NHL remains uncertain.

The extranodal MZLs often present with localized disease involving the gastrointestinal tract, salivary glands, thyroid, orbit, conjunctiva, breast, and lung.[35,93] Since many cases of gastric MZL appear to be a B-cell clonal expansion in response to *Helicobacter pylori*, treatment has been directed at the chronic gastritis. Therapy with antibiotics (metronidazole, amoxicillin, clarithromycin) and a proton pump inhibitor induce regression of superficial low-grade MZL of the stomach in over 80% of patients. The long-term remission status of these patients remains uncertain. The presence of bcl-10 nuclear expression and/or t(11;18) may be useful to prospectively identify those patients with gastric MZL lymphomas who do not benefit from anti-*Helicobacter pylori* treatment.[94] For patients with localized disease who progress after antibiotic therapy or are *H. pylori* negative, involved field radiotherapy with or without surgical resection has a 10-year disease-free survival of over 90%. For other sites of extranodal MZL, since these diseases tend to remain localized for long periods of time prior to systemic spread, surgery remains a highly effective approach, often with adjuvant involved-field radiotherapy. In a retrospective study of 70 patients with stage IE or IIE MZL, most were treated with involved-field radiation therapy alone.[95] The 5-year disease-free and overall survival for the entire group was 76 and 96%, respectively. Patients with gastric and thyroid disease had 5-year disease-free survival of 93%, whereas disease-free survival for other sites of involvement was 69% ($p = .006$). The response rate for chemotherapy with alkylating agents, fludarabine or rituximab alone for MZL is high.[38,96]

Treatment of Advanced Stage Indolent NHL Asymptomatic patients with low-volume disease can be monitored closely without active therapy. The long natural history of indolent NHLs and the lack of symptoms in some patients at diagnosis have fostered close observation as the initial approach to many of these patients.[21] Moreover, spontaneous remissions of longer than 1 year have been reported in 23% of patients, making treatment unnecessary in this subgroup of patients.[21] In studies from Stanford and the British National Lymphoma Investigation[97] where asymptomatic patients were randomized either to initial therapy or to deferred treatment until the time of symptoms (usually progressive bulky disease), there was no difference in the actuarial survival between the two groups. In the Stanford study the median time until therapy was needed was three years.[98]

The initial treatment of choice for patients with indolent NHL who are not eligible for clinical trials includes either alkylating based regimens (single agent or combinations such as cyclophosphamide, vincristine and prednisone), or purine analogues such as fludarabine. For recurrent disease, outside of clinical trials, patients can often be retreated with alkylating agent regimens, or purine analogues. Rituximab alone is useful for relapsed patients.

Radioimmunotherapy for now should be reserved for patients who are rituximab refractory. Chemotherapy regimens are generally now combined with the anti-CD20 monoclonal antibody rituximab since this increases the response rate and disease-free survival, and this has been the major innovation in treating these diseases in the past 3 decades. The CR rates of previously untreated patients to single alkylating agents range between 30 and 60%. The median duration of response with either single alkylating agents or with combinations such as cyclophosphamide, vincristine, and prednisone (CVP) is only about 2.5 years. In general, only 20 to 25% of patients are disease-free at four years.[99] Following relapse, these diseases continue to be sensitive to single agents and CVP; but the median relapse-free survival progressively decreases with each subsequent relapse.

In an attempt to improve the relapse-free survival and overall survival in patients with indolent NHL, more aggressive combination chemotherapy regimens have been used.[100–103] In general, combination chemotherapy regimens have been observed to give CR rates of 35 to 70%, but the median disease-free survival remains similar to that seen with CVP, in the range of 1.5 to 3 years.

It has been reported that the response of FL grade II (follicular mixed small cleaved and large cell) to aggressive therapy is higher that FL grade I.[104,105] However a prospective randomized trial comparing: cyclophosphamide-prednisone, cyclophosphamide, vincristine, procarbazine and prednisone; and BCNU, cyclophosphamide, vincristine, and prednisone failed to demonstrate significant long term disease-free survival for patients with FL grade II.[106]

Other randomized trials have looked at the impact of combination chemotherapy in patients with advanced FL. CHOP with bleomycin was compared to cyclophosphamide alone in patients with FL. There was no difference in disease-free survival or overall survival for the entire population or the grade I FL patients, but there was a survival advantage for the patients with FL grade II.[107]

Interferon-α is an active agent in relapsed indolent NHL. Several prospective randomized trials have examined the role of interferon when added to combination chemotherapy in advanced stage disease patients.[108–110] These studies have generally reported a significant improvement in progression-free survival, with only two trials that involved maintenance interferon-α having a significant prolongation of survival. A phase III trial compared interferon alfa-2b to observation following induction therapy with aggressive combination chemotherapy for previously untreated patients with indolent NHL, and found no significant difference in progression-free survival or overall survival between the 2 groups.[111]

Purine analogues are active agents in indolent NHL.[112,113] The response rate to fludarabine ranges from 45 to 65% RR, with less than 20% CR. In previously untreated patients the response rate to fludarabine is 65%, with 37% CR.[114] Fludarabine has been used in combination with other drugs including cyclophosphamide[115] as well as mitoxantrone,[116] with encouraging results. A randomized trial compared 8 cycles of either fludarabine or CVP in previously untreated patients with stages III or IV low-grade NHL.[117] Median durations of remission and overall survival at five years were similar in the two treatment arms. A randomized trial compared fludarabine to CVP in previously treated patients with FL. Although the response rates (62 vs 52%) and 2-year overall survival (70 vs 75%) were similar, 2-year progression-free survival was significantly improved with fludarabine (32 vs 14%).[118]

Monoclonal antibody therapies are now an integral part of treatment of indolent NHLs.[119] The "humanized" anti-CD20 monoclonal antibody rituximab has a 50 to 60% response rate, with 6% CR, in patients with previously treated FL.[120] In small lymphocytic lymphoma the response rate is only about 10%. The median duration of responses is about 11 months. The major toxicity of rituximab is largely infusion-related with fevers, rigors, and hypotension, usually associated with the first infusion. A phase II trial studied the safety and efficacy of retreatment with rituximab in patients with relapsed indolent NHL all of whom had previously responded to rituximab.[121] The overall response rate was 40%, with 11% complete remissions and the estimated median time to progression after treatment was 18 months. Phase II trials have employed rituximab as initial therapy in patients with indolent lymphoma with overall response rates of 54 and 73%.[122,123] At a median follow-up of 30 months, median progression-free survival was 34 months in one of the trials. Longer-term follow-up of these studies is necessary before rituximab alone can be recommended as initial therapy.

The addition of rituximab to chemotherapy has created a new paradigm in the treatment of indolent NHLs. CHOP has been given in combination with rituximab, with overall response rates and CR/unconfirmed CR rates of 100 and 87%, respectively.[124] The median time to progression was 83 months. A randomized phase III trial in patients with previously untreated stage III/IV FL compared 8 cycles of CVP or CVP with rituximab.[125] Overall (81 vs 57%) and complete (40 vs 10%) response rates were higher in the CVP plus rituximab treatment arm. At a median follow-up of 18 months, the time to treatment failure was significantly longer in the CVP plus rituximab arm (27 vs 7 months), although no survival advantage for CVP plus rituximab has been noted to date.

Radioimmunoconjugates are Food and Drug Administration (FDA) approved therapies for patients with relapsed follicular NHL. 131-I tositumomab is a murine anti-CD20 mAb conjugated to 131-iodine. The overall response rate in previously treated patients was 65% with 20% CRs.[126] The median duration of remission had not been reached by 47 months. A study in previously untreated patients with FL who received 131I-tositumomab has been reported with the overall response rates and CR rates 95 and 75%, respectively and a 5-year progression-free survival of 59%.[127] The anti-CD20 antibody conjugated to 90-yitrium ibritumomab tiuxetan has an 82% response rate with 26% CR, and median duration of response of greater than 12 months in patients with relapsed disease.[128] In a phase III study of 143 patients with relapsed or refractory low-grade, follicular, or transformed CD20+ NHL, patients were randomized to receive either rituximab or rituximab plus 90-yitrium ibritumomab tiuxetan.[129] The overall response rates to rituximab or the rituximab 90-yitrium ibritumomab tiuxetan combination were 56 and 80%, respectively. The precise role for radioimmunotherapy in indolent lymphoma will need continued investigation.

Histologic Transformation The prognosis for patients following histologic transformation of indolent NHL is generally poor.[22] The median survival of a large series of patients with follicular NHL undergoing histologic conversion was 11 months.[23] In a report from Stanford, the median survival for the entire group of patients was only 22 months, except for patients who achieved a CR with treatment who had an actuarial survival of 75% at five years.[24] As detailed below, a subgroup of patients with a history of indolent NHL who transform to a more aggressive histology may be cured by high-dose therapy and autologous stem cell transplantation (ASCT).[130,131]

Aggressive Lymphomas The aggressive lymphomas within the WHO classification include diffuse large B-cell; MCL; the peripheral T-cell lymphomas (non-specified and the specific subtypes); anaplastic large cell lymphoma, MCL, and FL grade III (follicular large cell). (see Table 118-2).

Therapy of Early Stage Aggressive Lymphoma Less than 20% of patients with diffuse large-cell lymphoma have truly localized disease. The recommended treatment for localized disease outside of clinical trials is abbreviated, combination chemotherapy plus involved field radiotherapy, or full course combination chemotherapy. The benefit of adding radiotherapy to 6 to 8 cycles of chemotherapy is of unclear survival benefit. To address the role of radiotherapy in early stage diffuse aggressive NHL, a randomized trial of patients with localized diffuse aggressive lymphoma compared 8 cycles of CHOP to 3 cycles of CHOP plus involved field radiotherapy.[77] Patients treated with 3 cycles of CHOP plus radiotherapy had a significantly better 5-year progression-free survival and overall survival than patients treated with 8 cycles of CHOP (77 vs 64% for progression-free survival, 82 vs 72% for overall survival). Overall, life-threatening toxicity, and cardiac toxicity were significantly higher in the patients receiving CHOP alone. The benefit of attenuated chemotherapy was largely found in patients over the age of 60. Another randomized trial compared eight courses of CHOP with or without involved field radiotherapy in patients with previously untreated bulky or extranodal stage I or stage II diffuse aggressive NHL. The disease-free survival was greater for CR patients who received radiotherapy (73 vs 56%) although ten year overall survival was similar in the two treatment arms (68 vs 65%).[132] The role of radiation therapy remains uncertain in some patients with stage I or II disease. A recent study provided evidence that in patients aged 60 or less with low-risk disease, an aggressive regimen (ACVBP) was superior to CHOP plus radiation.[133] Similarly, in patients over age 60, the addition of radiation therapy did not improve disease-free or overall survival for patients who received 4 cycles of CHOP alone.[134] The role of rituximab in early-stage disease is presently being investigated.

Therapy of Advanced Stage Aggressive Lymphoma The current recommendation for treatment of advanced stage DLBLC or PTCL if a clinical trial is not available is combination chemotherapy with CHOP plus rituximab or CHOP, respectively. Because the majority of clinical trials used 8 cycles, this is the current recommended number of cycles. Combination chemotherapy for diffuse aggressive NHLs has been a major victory in the treatment of cancer in adults. A number of phase II studies suggested that different combination chemotherapy recipes demonstrated improvement in the treatment of diffuse large cell lymphoma. Because of these studies, the Southwest Oncology Group (SWOG) undertook a phase III study comparing CHOP, m-BACOD, MACOP-B, and ProMACE-CytaBOM.[135] The completed study of 897 eligible patients with intermediate or high-grade NHL found no difference in outcome, at a median follow-up of 31 months for the four regimens. There have been additional randomized trials including comparisons of MACOP-B versus ProMACE-MOPP[136]; escalated versus standard doses of doxorubin in the BACOP regimen.[137]; and CHOP versus m-BACOD,[138] which have clearly demonstrated that more intensive regimens offer no improvement in remission rate, disease-free or overall survival, but increase toxicity.

More aggressive regimens have been examined in phase III studies. A recent randomized trial of the modification of CHOP demonstrated improved results for patients under age 60. The German high-grade NHL study group compared CHOP+ etoposide (CHOPE) to CHOP, given either every 14 or 21 days. The event-free survival at 5 years was improved for the CHOPE regimen.[139] Presently, it is not known if this regimen is superior to standard-dose CHOP with the addition of rituximab. In addition, a number of studies have looked at the role of consolidative high-dose therapy and stem cell support for high-risk patients in first remission (see Stem Cell Transplant section).

For PTCL, similar treatment approaches to DLBCL have been taken for patients with localized and advanced stage disease. When patients are stratified by the IPI, the disease-free survival and overall survival is generally inferior for patients with PTCL than for patients with DLBCL.

Therapy of Aggressive Lymphoma in Older Patients In the analysis that led to the development of the IPI, the outcome for patients over age 60 was significantly different from those aged 60 and less. The reasons for these differences may be related to less-intensive treatment delivered as well as the presence of comorbid diseases.[140] In some studies increased deaths unrelated to lymphoma or its treatment have been reported, whereas in others an increased treatment-related mortality has been reported, often related to poor performance status.[141,142]

Several attempts have been made to modify the chemotherapy for elderly patients.[143] Presently, the standard of care is CHOP plus rituximab. In a randomized trial comparing weekly CHOP with standard dose, the CR rate and PFS were similar, although the OS was better with standard dose CHOP.[144] Substitution of mitoxantrone for Adriamycin has resulted in lower CR rate and 3-year survival.[145,146] The GELA trial in elderly patients (median age 69, range: 60 to 80 years) with previously untreated advanced DLBCL randomized patients to receive either eight cycles of CHOP or CHOP plus rituximab.[147] There was no significant difference in toxicity between the two arms, and the CR rate and overall survival at 3 years for the R-CHOP and CHOP arms were 76 versus 63%, 62 versus 43% (p = .005) and 62 versus 51% (p = .008), respectively. CHOP plus rituximab was also shown to be more effective than CHOP in bcl-2 positive patients.[148] A large United States Intergroup study compared in a similar population, CHOP or CHOP plus rituximab given on a different schedule. Responding patients were randomly assigned to receive either rituximab maintenance therapy or no maintenance. Preliminary results suggest a progression-free survival benefit from the addition of rituximab.[149] However, no overall survival benefit is yet apparent.

FL Grade III (Follicular Large Cell) Follicular large-cell lymphoma is clinically similar to diffuse large cell lymphoma.[25,26] It is generally agreed that all patients should be treated with aggressive combination chemotherapy, with complete remission rates of about 80 and 50%, and overall survival of approximately 70 and 60% for stage I/II and III/IV patients respectively.[25] A study of 100 patients with follicular large-cell lymphoma from a single institution supported this strategy, suggesting prolonged disease-free survival, and an overall favorable prognosis.[26]

Mantle Cell Lymphomas (MCL) The median survival of patients with MCL is 3 to 4 years. The treatment of MCL generally involves alkylating agents to which 30 to 50% of patients will have a CR, with median duration of 1 to 3 years.[40] A randomized trial comparing CVP to CHOP demonstrated no benefit for the addition of doxorubicin in terms of overall survival. Generally, single alkylating agents offer similar results as combination chemotherapy. Newer agents such as fludarabine and rituximab are giving response rates in the range of 30%, with remissions duration similar to alkylating agents.[150–152] CHOP plus rituximab showed a high overall response rate of 96% with CR/CR unconfirmed of 48%. However the median PFS was 16.6 months, which is similar to that seen with CHOP alone.[88] Similarly, the German low-grade lymphoma group has reported that the CR rate is higher with CHOP plus rituximab than CHOP, with no difference in time to treatment failure or OS. The Hyper-CVAD regimen, with escalated doses of cyclophosphamide, high-dose methotrexate and cytarabine has a very high response rate (38% CR).[153] In this report, all patients went on to either autologous or allogeneic stem cell transplantation. The results for previously untreated patients was encouraging with 5-year disease-free survival of 43%, with overall survival of 73%.[154] A report of high-dose sequential therapy in previously untreated patients reported event-free and overall survival at 54 months of 79 and 89%, respectively.[155] The results of high-dose therapy and autologous bone marrow transplantation remain controversial in both previously untreated and relapsed patients with MCL.

Autologous Stem Cell Transplantation for NHL in First Remission Several studies have examined the role of high-dose therapy and autologous stem cell transplantation (ASCT) in first CR/PR for patients with aggressive NHL, and to date no definitive recommendation can be made. ASCT following abbreviated induction therapy generally does not improve outcome when compared to standard induction. The LNH93-3 study included patients younger than 60 years with high-intermediate/high-risk IPI scores who were then randomized to ACVBP plus consolidation or three cycles of dose-escalated cyclophosphamide, epirubicin, vindesine, bleomycin, and prednisone followed by BCNU, etoposide, cytarabine, cyclophosphamide, and ASCT. CR rates were not different between the two treatment arms. The 5-year overall survival and event-free survival rates for ACVBP and ASCT were 60 and 46% (p = .007) and 52% and 39% (p = .01), respectively.[156] In contrast, ASCT after full or very intensive induction may improve outcome for selected patients. Patients with aggressive NHL who obtained a CR with standard therapy were randomly assigned to receive either consolidative sequential therapy (ifosfamide, etoposide, asparaginase, and cytarabine) or high-dose chemotherapy with ASCT. A superior, durable, DFS was observed only in the subgroup of higher-risk patients who underwent ASCT.[157,158] A GOELAMS study of CHOP for 8 cycles versus intensive combination chemotherapy induction followed by consolidation then high-dose BCNU, etoposide, cytarabine, melphalan, and ASCT, found event-free survival at 5 years was 46% versus 63% (p = .037), respectively, but no difference in OS (56 vs 71%). Only patients with high-intermediate IPI, but not low or low-intermediate, had significantly higher event-free and overall survival with high-dose therapy.[159] Development of new strategies, particularly toward resistant cells and minimal residual disease, may make additional impact following high-dose therapy.

HIGH-GRADE LYMPHOMAS Lymphoblastic, Burkitt's and Burkitt-Like Lymphomas Lymphoblastic lymphoma in adults has been treated with some success, although inferior to that seen in children. When treated with regimens initially developed for childhood acute lymphoblastic leukemia, about 40% of adults are reported to survive at 5 years. In a randomized study of autologous stem cell transplantation in first remission there was a trend for improved relapse-free survival, but no improvement in overall survival when compared with conventional therapy.[160] Hyper-CVAD has been studied at MD Anderson Cancer Center, with very high complete response rates.[161]

The Burkitt's and Burkitt-like lymphomas in human immunodeficiency virus-1 negative adults have been similarly treated with regimens designed for the pediatric populations.[162–164] Using an acute lymphoblastic leukemia like regimen, the Cancer and Acute Leukemia Group B has reported results in 75 adults with small non-cleaved cell NHL or the L3 acute lymphoblastic leukemia variant.[165] Complete remission was attained in 80%, with 52% alive and in remission at a median follow-up of 5.1 years. Using the Magrath regimen (CODox-M for low-risk patients, or CODox-M/IVAC for high-risk patients), the event-free survival was 92% at 2 years in 39 adults.[166] A study of 14 patients with median age of 47 reported 64% of patients disease-free at 29 months with a similar intensive regimen.[167]

TREATMENT OF RECURRENT DISEASE Following relapse, at least 50% of patients' disease remains sensitive to conventional treatment, but less than 10% of patients with aggressive NHL experience prolonged disease-free survival with second line treatment regimens, and essentially all patients with indolent disease relapse. Following relapse, the current curative approach for patients with relapsed NHL involves high-dose therapy and stem cell transplantation.

Conventional Salvage Therapy The vast majority of patients with relapsed or refractory NHL have limited benefit from conventional salvage regimens. A number of regimens have been developed for patients with relapsed, aggressive NHL.[168–170] The response rates for these salvage regimens have ranged from 20 to 77% with 20 to 30% CRs reported. The duration of these responses and overall survival of these patients is about 6 months. Although a higher response is seen in indolent NHLs, the response rate of patients with relapsed aggressive NHL to single agent rituximab is 37% (9% CR) and the median duration is 8 months.[152]

Syngeneic and Allogeneic Bone Marrow Transplantation in NHL Only a limited number of patients with NHL have undergone identical twin bone marrow transplantation.[171] In the largest series with 8 patients, 7 achieved CR and four patients were reported to remain in CCR from 12 to 126 months after syngeneic bone marrow transplantation.

Allogeneic stem cell transplantation has received increasing attention for patients with relapsed and refractory NHL.[172–174] Nearly all patients had relapsed disease, many of whom were resistant to conventional dose therapy. The majority of patients treated achieved a CR to high-dose ablative therapy, and the relapse rate was generally less than 20%. However, the treatment associated mortality in these studies ranged from 20% to as high as 50%. The probability of prolonged disease-free survival is between 20 and 40%. In a prospective comparative trial of allogeneic or autologous bone marrow transplantation there was no significant difference in event-free survival between the two sources of stem cells; however the probability of relapse was significantly greater in the autologous patients.[174] In 176 patients with FL, 67% of whom had chemosensitive disease at the time of transplantation, estimates of treatment-related mortality, recurrence rates, and overall survival at five years following allogeneic bone marrow transplantation were 30, 21, and 51%, respectively. During this same period, 597 patients with FL received unpurged autologous transplantation; 82% were chemosensitive at the time of transplant. The estimates of treatment-related mortality, recurrence rates, and overall survival at five years following unpurged autologous bone marrow transplantation were 8, 58, and 55%, respectively.[175] In an effort to reduce the morbidity and mortality associated with GVHD, several groups have employed T-cell depletion for prevention of GVHD.[176] Nonmyeloablative allogeneic transplants are being actively studied in indolent NHLs, with encouraging results to date.[177]

Autologous Stem Cell Transplantation for Relapsed Aggressive NHL The disease sensitivity at the time of ASCT has remained the most significant prognostic variable for predicting treatment outcome.[178] Several large series have shown that patients who undergo ASCT when the disease is resistant to the initial induction therapy have less than 10% probability of disease-free survival. Those relapsed patients whose disease remains sensitive to chemotherapy have a 30 to 60% probability of long-term disease-free survival. In contrast, only 10 to 15% of patients with resistant disease are long term survivors.

ASCT has been compared to conventional salvage therapy for relapsed aggressive NHL in a multicenter trial known as the PARMA trial.[179] Patients with relapsed aggressive NHL (largely DLBCL) received 2 cycles of cisplatin, cytarabine, Solu-Medrol, and if responsive, were randomized to continued chemotherapy for 4 additional cycles or high-dose chemotherapy and autologous bone marrow transplantation. With median follow-up in excess of 5 years, patients randomized to the high-dose arm had superior event-free survival (46 vs 12%) and overall survival (53 vs 32%).

Autologous Stem Cell Transplantation for Relapsed Indolent NHL A number of large phase II studies suggested that a subset of patients with relapsed FL, with chemosensitive disease, who undergo high-dose therapy and ASCT are long-term survivors with disease-free survivals of 40 to 50% at 8 or more years.[180–183] A recent randomized trial compared conventional chemotherapy to autologous stem cell transplantation with purged or unpurged bone marrow, referred to as the European CUP trial.[184] In this study, 89 patients with relapsed or progressive FL received 3 cycles of CHOP. Those patients who achieved a CR or PR, and had less than 20% bone marrow involvement with FL, were randomized to three further cycles of CHOP chemotherapy or to high-dose therapy and autologous stem cell support with immunomagnetic anti-B cell antibody purging or high-dose therapy and autologous stem cell support without purging. At a median follow-up of 69 months, the overall 5-year survival for all registered patients was 50%, but the median survival had not yet been reached for the subset of patients treated with high-dose therapy and autologous stem cell transplantation (either purged or unpurged). Both progression-free and overall survival favored the transplantation arms, but there was no difference between those patients receiving a purged autograft and those receiving an unmanipulated graft.

Patients with histologic conversion from indolent to an aggressive histology generally have a poor prognosis. There have been several reports of ASCT in patients with chemosensitive disease and a good performance status after histologic transformation for FL. In the series from Dana-Farber Cancer Institute, where 21 patients have undergone anti-B cell purged autologous bone marrow transplantation for transformed FL, the estimate of the percentage of patients alive and disease-free at 5 years is 46%, with follow-up from 12 to 120^+ months.[130] When pathology at relapse was available, all patients recurred with DLBCL. Similar results were reported from St. Bartholomew's Hospital and by the European Bone Marrow Transplant Registry.[131,185] Aggressive therapy with ASCT is a reasonable treatment option for selected patients under age 60 who have chemosensitive disease.

New Therapeutic Approaches for NHL

Although strides have been made in the treatment of NHL with conventional, salvage and high-dose ablative therapy, the majority of patients are not cured. Unlike most other cancers, many patients with NHL can achieve a complete remission. This suggests that the major obstacle to cure is subpopulations of resistant neoplastic cells. There are a number of approaches to the treatment of NHL that may potentially overcome resistance, or treat minimal residual disease. Monoclonal antibodies, either unconjugated or conjugated to radionuclides, are effective agents for treating NHLs. Clinical trials with these agents will better define the appropriate sequencing and use of these agents. Further ways to enhance host immunity against the patients' own tumor cells have involved vaccination studies with the immunoglobulin idiotype to induce specific immunotherapy against residual tumor cells. The randomized trials of these tumor vaccines are ongoing and will provide important insights as to whether these are viable adjuncts to treatment. The most significant advance is our understanding of the genetic events and pathways that are aberrant in lymphoma cells as compared to normal cells, and the differences that have been recognized within histologic subtypes of lymphomas. Novel targets may potentially be identified which are more specific to the neoplastic event and less toxic to normal cells. Ongoing and future studies in these areas may provide novel therapies.

REFERENCES

1. Jemal A, Murray T, Ward E, et al. Cancer statistics, 2005. CA Cancer J Clin 2005;55:10–30.
2. Levine A. Acquired immunodeficiency syndrome-related lymphomas. Blood 1992;80:8–16.
3. Borisch B, Hennig I, Laeng R, et al. Association of the subtype 2 of the Epstein-Barr virus with T-cell non-Hodgkin's lymphoma of the mid line granuloma type. Blood 1993;82:828.
4. Robert-Guroff M, Nakao Y, Notake K, et al. Natural antibodies to human retrovirus HTLV in a cluster of Japanese patients with adult T-cell leukemia. Science 1982;215:975.
5. Hussell T, Isaacson PG, Crabtree JE, Spencer J. The response of cells from low-grade B-cell gastric lymphomas of mucosa-associated lymphoid tissue to *Helicobacter pylori*. Lancet 1993;342:571–4.
6. Saadoun D, Suarez F, Lefrere F, et al. Splenic lymphoma with villous lymphocytes, associated with type II cryoglobulinemia and HCV infection: a new entity? Blood 2005;105:74–6.
7. Ferreri AJ, Guidoboni M, Ponzoni M, et al. Evidence for an association between *Chlamydia psittaci* and ocular adnexal lymphomas. J Natl Cancer Inst 2004;96:586–94.
8. Lecuit M, Abachin E, Martin A, et al. Immunoproliferative small intestinal disease associated with *Campylobacter jejuni*. N Engl J Med 2004;350:239–48.
9. Goodlad JR, Davidson MM, Hollowood K, et al. *Borrelia burgdorferi*-associated cutaneous marginal zone lymphoma: a clinicopathological study of two cases illustrating the temporal progression of *B. burgdorferi*-associated B-cell proliferation in the skin. Histopathology 2000;37:501–8.

10. Cesarman E, Chang Y, Moore P, et al. Kaposi's sarcoma-associated herpesvirus-like DNA sequences in AIDS-related body-cavity-based lymphomas. N Engl J Med 1995;332:1186–91.
11. Hardell L, Eriksson M. A case-control study of non-Hodgkin's lymphoma and exposure to pesticides. Cancer 1999;85:1353–60.
12. Persson B, Fredriksson M, Olsen K, et al. Some occupational exposures as risk factors for malignant lymphomas. Cancer 1993;72:1773–8.
13. List A, Greer J, Cousar J, et al. Non-Hodgkin's lymphoma after treatment of Hodgkin's disease: association with Epstein-Barr virus. Ann Intern Med 1986;105:668.
14. Starzl T, Porter K, Iwatsuki S, et al. Reversibility of lymphomas and lymphoproliferative lesions developing under cyclosporin-steroid therapy. Lancet 1984;1:583.
15. Ballerini P, Gaidano G, Gong J, et al. Multiple genetic lesions in acquired immunodeficiency syndrome-related non-Hodgkin's lymphoma. Blood 1993;81:166.
16. Harris NL, Jaffe ES, Diebold J, et al. World Health Organization classification of neoplastic diseases of the hematopoietic and lymphoid tissues: report of the Clinical Advisory Committee meeting-Airlie House, Virginia, November 1997. J Clin Oncol 1999;17:3835–49.
17. Anderson KC, Bates MP, Slaughenhoupt BL, et al. Expression of human B Cell-associated antigens on leukemias and lymphomas: a model of human B cell differentiation. Blood 1984;63:1424–33.
18. Flenghi L, Bigerna B, Fizzotti M, et al. Monoclonal antibodies PG-B6a and PG-B6p recognize, respectively, a highly conserved and a formol-resistant epitope on the human BCL-6 protein amino-terminal region. Am J Pathol 1996;148:1543–55.
19. Armitage J, Weisenburger D. New approach to classifying non-Hodgkin's lymphomas: Clinical features of the major histologic subtypes. J Clin Oncol 1998;16:2780–95.
20. Cerroni L, Arzberger E, Putz B, et al. Primary cutaneous follicle center cell lymphoma with follicular growth pattern. Blood 2000;95:3922–8.
21. Horning SJ, Rosenberg SA. The natural history of initially untreated low-grade non-Hodgkin's lymphoma. N Engl J Med 1984;311:1471–1508.
22. Bastion Y, Sebban C, Berger F, et al. Incidence, predictive factors, and outcome of lymphoma transformation in follicular lymphoma patients. J Clin Oncol 1997;15:1587–94.
23. Johnson P, Rohatiner A, Whelan J, et al. Patterns of survival in patients with recurrent follicular lymphoma: a 20 year study from a single center. J Clin Oncol 1995;13:140–7.
24. Yuen A, Kamel O, Halpern J, Horning S. Long-term survival after histologic transformation of low-grade follicular lymphoma. J Clin Oncol 1995;13:1726–33.
25. Anderson J, Vose J, Bierman P, et al. Clinical features and prognosis of follicular large-cell lymphoma: a report from the Nebraska Lymphoma Study Group. J Clin Oncol 1993;11:218–24.
26. Rodriguez J, McLaughlin P, Hagemeister F, Fayad L. Follicular large cell lymphoma: an aggressive lymphoma that often presents with favorable prognostic features. Blood 1999;93:2202–7.
27. Rassenti LZ, Huynh L, Toy TL, et al. ZAP-70 compared with immunoglobulin heavy-chain gene mutation status as a predictor of disease progression in chronic lymphocytic leukemia. N Engl J Med. 2004;351:893–901.
28. Hamblin TJ, Orchard JA, Gardiner A, et al. Immunoglobulin V genes and CD38 expression in CLL. Blood 2000;95:2455–7.
29. Robertson L, Pugh W, O'Brien S, et al. Richter's syndrome: a report on 39 patients. J Clin Oncol 1993;11:1985–9.
30. Pangalis G, Angelopoulou M, Vassilakopoulos T, et al. B-Chronic lymphocytic leukemia, small lymphocytic lymphoma, and lymphoplasmacytic lymphoma, including Waldenström's macroglobulinemia: a clinical, morphologic, and biologic spectrum of similar disorders. Sem Hematol 1999;36:104–14.
31. Offit K, Parsa N, Jhanwar S, et al. Clusters of chromosome 9 aberrations are associated with clinico-pathologic subsets of non-Hodgkin's lymphoma. Genes Chromosom Cancer 1993;7:1–7.
32. Vallisa D, Bernuzzi P, Arcaini L, et al. Role of Anti-hepatitis C virus (HCV) treatment in HCV-related, low-grade, B-cell, non-Hodgkin's lymphoma: a multicenter Italian experience. J Clin Oncol 2005;23:468–73.
33. A clinical evaluation of the International Lymphoma Study Group classification of non-Hodgkin's lymphoma. The Non-Hodgkin's Lymphoma Classification Project. Blood 1997;89:3909–18.
34. Nathwani B, Drachenberg M, Hernandez A, et al. Nodal monocytoid B-cell lymphoma (nodal marginal zone B-cell lymphoma). Sem Hematol 1999;36:128–38.
35. Isaacson P. Mucosa-associated lymphoid tissue lymphoma. Sem Hematol 1999;36:139–47.
36. Ott G, Katzenberger T, Greiner A, Kalla J. The t(11;18)(q21;q21) chromosome translocation is a frequent and specific aberration in low-grade but not high-grade malignant non-Hodgkin's lymphomas of the mucosa-associated lymphoid tissue (MALT-) type. Cancer Res 1997;57:3944–8.
37. Troussard X, Mauvieux L, Radford-Weiss I, Rack K. Genetic analysis of splenic lymphoma with villous lymphocytes: a Group Francais d'Hematologie Cellulaire (GFHC) study. Br J Haematol 1998;101:712–21.
38. Thieblemont C, Berger F, Dumontet C, et al. Mucosa-associated lymphoid tissue lymphoma is a disseminated disease in one third of 158 patients analyzed. Blood 2000;95:802–6.
39. Catovsky D, Matutes E. Splenic lymphoma with circulating villous lymphocytes/splenic marginal zone lymphoma. Sem Hematol 1999;36:148–54.
40. Fisher R, Dahlberg S, Nathwani B, et al. A clinical analysis of two indolent lymphoma entities: mantle cell lymphoma and marginal zone lymphoma (including mucosal-associated lymphoid tissue and monocytoid B-cell subcatagories): A Southwest Oncology Group study. Blood 1995;85:1075–82.
41. Bertoni F, Zucca E, Cotter FE. Molecular basis of mantle cell lymphoma. Br J Haematol 2004;124:130–40.
42. Boudova L, Torlakovic E, Delabie J, et al. Nodular lymphocyte-predominant Hodgkin lymphoma with nodules resembling T-cell/histiocyte-rich B-cell lymphoma: differential diagnosis between nodular lymphocyte-predominant Hodgkin lymphoma and T-cell/histiocyte-rich B-cell lymphoma. Blood 2003;102:3753–8.
43. Rosenwald A, Wright G, Chan WC, et al. The use of molecular profiling to predict survival after chemotherapy for diffuse large-B-cell lymphoma. N Engl J Med 2002;346:1937–47.
44. Alizadeh A, Eisen M, Davis R, et al. Distinct types of diffuse large B-cell lymphoma identified by gene expression profiling. Nature 2000;403:503–11.
45. Gascoyne RD, Adomat SA, Krajewski S, et al. Prognostic significance of Bcl-2 protein expression and Bcl-2 gene rearrangement in diffuse aggressive non-Hodgkin's lymphoma. Blood 1997;90:244–51.
46. Skinnider BF, Horsman DE, Dupuis B, Gascoyne RD. Bcl-6 and Bcl-2 protein expression in diffuse large B-cell lymphoma and follicular lymphoma: correlation with 3q27 and 18q21 chromosomal abnormalities. Hum Pathol 1999;30:803–8.
47. Kerchaert J, Deweindt C, Tilly H, et al. LAZ3, a novel zinc-finger encoding gene, is disrupted by recurring chromosome 3q27 translocations in human lymphomas. Nat Genet 1993;5:66–70.
48. Bastard C, Deweindt C, Kerckaert J, et al. LAZ3 Rearrangements in non-Hodgkin's lymphoma: correlation with histology, immunophenotype, karyotype, and clinical outcome in 217 patients. Blood 1994;83:2423–7.
49. van Besien K, Ha C, Murphy S, McLaughlin P. Risk factors, treatment, and outcome of central nervous system recurrence in adults with intermediate-grade and immunoblastic lymphoma. Blood 1998;91:1178–84.
50. van Besien K, Kelta M, Bahaguna P. Primary mediastinal B-cell lymphoma: a review of pathology and management. J Clin Oncol 2001;19:1855–64.
51. Rosenwald A, Wright G, Leroy K, et al. Molecular diagnosis of primary mediastinal B cell lymphoma identifies a clinically favorable subgroup of diffuse large B cell lymphoma related to Hodgkin lymphoma. J Exp Med 2003;198:851–62.
52. Savage KJ, Monti S, Kutok JL, et al. The molecular signature of mediastinal large B-cell lymphoma differs from that of other diffuse large B-cell lymphomas and shares features with classical Hodgkin lymphoma. Blood 2003;102:3871–9.
53. DiGiuseppe JA, Nelson WG, Seifter EJ, et al. Intravascular lymphomatosis: a clinicopathologic study of 10 cases and assessment of response to chemotherapy. J Clin Oncol 1994;12:2573–9.
54. Ong ST, Le Beau MM. Chromosomal abnormalities and molecular genetics of non-Hodgkin's lymphoma. Semin Oncol 1998;25:447–60.
55. Kutok JL, Aster JC. Molecular biology of anaplastic lymphoma kinase-positive anaplastic large-cell lymphoma. J Clin Oncol 2002;20:3691–702.
56. Belhadj K, Reyes F, Farcet JP, et al. Hepatosplenic gamma-delta T-cell lymphoma is a rare clinicopathologic entity with poor outcome: report on a series of 21 patients. Blood 2003;102:4261–9.
57. Gonzalez C, Medeiros L, Braziel R, Jaffe E. T-cell lymphoma involving subcutaneous tissue: a clinicopathologic entity commonly associated with hemophagocytic syndrome. Am J Surg Pathol 1991;15:1727–34.
58. Murray A, Cuevas E, Jones D, Wright D. A study of the immunohistochemistry and T-cell clonality of enteropathy associated T-cell lymphoma. Am J Pathol 1995;146:909–13.
59. Dogan A, Attygalle AD, Kyriakou C. Angioimmunoblastic T-cell lymphoma. Br J Haematol 2003;121:681–91.
60. Jaffe E. Classification of natural killer (NK)-cell and NK-like T-cell malignancies. Blood 1996;87:1207–10.
61. Gascoyne RD, Aoun P, Wu D, et al. Prognostic significance of anaplastic lymphoma kinase (ALK) protein expression in adults with anaplastic large cell lymphoma. Blood 1999;93:3913–21.
62. Tilly H, Gaulard P, Lepage E, et al. Primary anaplastic large-cell lymphoma in adults: clinical presentation, immunophenotype, and outcome. Blood 1997;90:3727–34.
63. Soslow R, Baergen R, Warnke R. B-lineage lymphoblastic lymphoma is a clinicopathologic entity distinct from other histologically similar aggressive lymphomas with blastic morphology. Cancer 1999;85:2648–54.
64. Harris N, Jaffe E, Stein H, et al. A revised European-American classification of lymphoid neoplasms: a proposal from the International Lymphoma Study Group. Blood 1994;84:1361–92.
65. Dalla-Favera R, Bregni M, Erikson J, et al. Human c-myc oncogene is located on the region of chromosome 8 that is translocated in Burkitt lymphoma cells. Proc Natl Acad Sci 1982;79:7824.
66. Yano T, van Krieken J, Magrath I, et al. Histogenetic correlations between subcategories of small non-cleaved cell lymphomas. Blood 1992;79:1282–90.
67. Mentzer S, Reilly J, Skarin A, Sugarbaker D. Patterns of lung involvement by malignant lymphoma. Surgery 1993;113:507–14.
68. Isaacson P, Wright D. Malignant lymphoma of mucosal associated lymphoid tissue. A distinct B cell lymphoma. Cancer 1983;52:1410.
69. Mynster T, Hultberg B, Bulow S. Multiple lymphomatous polyposis of the colon and rectum. report of a case and review of the literature. Scand J Gastroenterol 1994;29:545–9.
70. Rosenberg S. Validity of the Ann Arbor Staging Classification for the Non-Hodgkin's Lymphomas. Cancer Treat Rep 1977;61:1023.
71. Naumann R, Vaic A, Beuthien-Baumann B, et al. Prognostic value of positron emission tomography in the evaluation of post-treatment residual mass in patients with Hodgkin's disease and non-Hodgkin's lymphoma. Br J Haematol 2001;115:793–800.
72. Spaepen K, Stroobants S, Dupont P, et al. Prognostic value of positron emission tomography (PET) with fluorine-18 fluorodeoxyglucose ([18F]FDG) after first-line chemotherapy in non- Hodgkin's lymphoma: is [18F]FDG-PET a valid alternative to conventional diagnostic methods? J Clin Oncol 2001;19:414–9.
73. Jerusalem G, Beguin Y, Najjar F, et al. Positron emission tomography (PET) with 18F-fluorodeoxyglucose (18F-FDG) for the staging of low-grade non-Hodgkin's lymphoma (NHL). Ann Oncol 2001;12:825–30.
74. Zijlstra JM, Hoekstra OS, Raijmakers PG, et al. 18FDG positron emission tomography versus 67Ga scintigraphy as prognostic test during chemotherapy for non-Hodgkin's lymphoma. Br J Haematol 2003;123:454–62.
75. Lee M, Chang K, Cabanillas F, Freireich E, et al. Detection of minimal residual cells carrying the t(14;18) by DNA sequence amplification. Science 1987;237:175.
76. International Non-Hodgkin's Lymphoma Prognostic Factors Project: A predictive model for aggressive non-Hodgkin's lymphoma. N Engl J Med 1993;329:987.
77. Miller T, Dahlberg S, Cassady J, Adelstein D. Chemotherapy alone compared with chemotherapy plus radiotherapy for localized intermediate- and high-grade non-Hodgkin's lymphoma. N Engl J Med 1998;339:21–6.
78. Solal-Celigny P, Roy P, Colombat P, et al. Follicular lymphoma international prognostic index. Blood 2004;104:1258–65.
79. Weisdorf D, Andersen J, Glick J, Oken M. Survival after relapse of low-grade non-Hodgkin's lymphoma: implications for marrow transplantation. J Clin Oncol 1992;10:942–7.
80. Shipp MA, Ross KN, Tamayo P, et al. Diffuse large B-cell lymphoma outcome prediction by gene-expression profiling and supervised machine learning. Nat Med 2002;8:68–74.

81. Monti S, Savage KJ, Kutok JL, et al. Molecular profiling of diffuse large B-cell lymphoma identifies robust subtypes including one characterized by host inflammatory response. Blood. 2005;105:1851–61.
82. Hans CP, Weisenburger DD, Greiner TC, et al. Confirmation of the molecular classification of diffuse large B-cell lymphoma by immunohistochemistry using a tissue microarray. Blood 2004;103:275–82.
83. Dave SS, Wright G, Tan B, et al. Prediction of survival in follicular lymphoma based on molecular features of tumor-infiltrating immune cells. N Engl J Med 2004;351:2159–69.
84. Gallamini A, Stelitano C, Calvi R, et al. Peripheral T-cell lymphoma unspecified (PTCL-U): a new prognostic model from a retrospective multicentric clinical study. Blood 2004;103:2474–9.
85. Rimsza LM, Roberts RA, Miller TP, et al. Loss of MHC class II gene and protein expression in diffuse large B-cell lymphoma is related to decreased tumor immunosurveillance and poor patient survival regardless of other prognostic factors: a follow-up study from the Leukemia and Lymphoma Molecular Profiling Project. Blood 2004;103:4251–8.
86. Gribben J, Neuberg D, Freedman A, et al. Detection by polymerase chain reaction of residual cells with the bcl-2 translocation is associated with increased risk of relapse after autologous bone marrow transplantation for B-cell lymphoma. Blood 1993;81:3449–57.
87. Lopez-Guillermo A, Cabanillas F, McLaughlin P, Smith T. The clinical significance of molecular response in indolent follicular lymphomas. Blood 1998;91:2955–60.
88. Howard OM, Gribben JG, Neuberg DS, et al. Rituximab and CHOP induction therapy for newly diagnosed mantle-cell lymphoma: molecular complete responses are not predictive of progression-free survival. J Clin Oncol 2002;20:1288–94.
89. MacManus M, Hoppe R. Is radiotherapy curative for stage I and II low-grade follicular lymphoma? Results of a long-term follow-up study of patients treated at Stanford University. J Clin Oncol 1996;14:1282–90.
90. MacManus MP, Rainer Bowie CA, Hoppe RT. What is the prognosis for patients who relapse after primary radiation therapy for early-stage low-grade follicular lymphoma? Int J Radiat Oncol Biol Phys 1998;42:365–71.
91. Monfardini S, Banfi A, Bonadonna G, et al. Improved five-year survival after combined radiotherapy-chemotherapy for stage I–II non-Hodgkin's lymphoma. Int. J Radiat Oncol Bio Phys 1980;6:125–34.
92. McLaughlin P, Fuller LM, Velasquez WS, et al. Stage I-II follicular lymphoma. Treatment results for 76 patients. Cancer 1986;58:1596–1602.
93. Coiffier B, Thieblemont C, Felman P, et al. Indolent nonfollicular lymphomas: characteristics, treatment, and outcome. Sem Hematol 1999;36:198–208.
94. Starostik P, Patzner J, Greiner A, et al. Gastric marginal zone B-cell lymphomas of MALT type develop along 2 distinct pathogenetic pathways. Blood 2002;99:3–9.
95. Tsang RW, Gospodarowicz MK, Pintilie M, et al. Stage I and II MALT lymphoma: results of treatment with radiotherapy. Int J Radiat Oncol Biol Phys 2001;50:1258–64.
96. Conconi A, Martinelli G, Thieblemont C, et al. Clinical activity of rituximab in extranodal marginal zone B-cell lymphoma of MALT type. Blood 2003;102:2741–5.
97. Ardeshna KM, Smith P, Norton A, et al. Long-term effect of a watch and wait policy versus immediate systemic treatment for asymptomatic advanced-stage non-Hodgkin lymphoma: a randomised controlled trial. Lancet 2003;362:516–22.
98. Hoppe RT, Kushlan P, H.S. K, et al. The treatment of advanced stage favorable histology non-Hodgkin's lymphoma: a preliminary report of a randomized trial comparing single agent chemotherapy, and whole body irradiation. Blood 1981;58:592–8.
99. Gallagher CJ, Gregory WM, Jones AE, et al. Follicular lymphoma: prognostic factors for response and survival. J Clin Oncol 1986;4:1470–80.
100. Ezdinli EZ, Harrington DP, Kucuk O, et al. The effect of intensive intermittent maintenance therapy in advanced low-grade non-Hodgkin's lymphoma. Cancer 1987;60:156–60.
101. Glick JH, Barnes JM, Ezdinli EZ, et al. Nodular mixed lymphoma: results of a randomized trial failing to confirm prolonged disease-free survival with COPP chemotherapy. Blood 1981;58:920–5.
102. Jones SE, Grozea PN, Miller TP, et al. Chemotherapy with cyclophosphamide, doxorubicin, vincristine, and prednisone alone of with levamisole or with levamisole plus BCG for malignant lymphoma: A Southwest Oncology Group study. J Clin Oncol 1985;3:1318–24.
103. Young RC, Johnson RE, Canellos GP, et al. Advanced lymphocytic lymphoma: randomized comparisons of chemotherapy and radiotherapy, alone or in combination. Cancer Treat Rep 1977;61:1153–9.
104. Longo DL, Young RC, Hubard SM, et al. Prolonged initial remission in patients with nodular mixed lymphoma. Ann Intern Med 1984;100:651–6.
105. Cabanillas F, Smith T, Bodey GP, et al. Nodular malignant lymphomas. Factors affecting complete response rate and survival. Cancer 1979;44:1983–9.
106. Ezdinli EZ, Costello WG, Icli F, et al. Nodular mixed lymphocytic-histiocytic lymphoma (NM): response and survival. Eastern Cooperative Oncology Group. Cancer 1980;45:261–7.
107. Peterson BA, Petroni GR, Frizzera G, et al. Prolonged single-agent versus combination chemotherapy in indolent follicular lymphomas: a study of the Cancer and Leukemia Group. Br J Clin Oncol 2003;21:5–15.
108. Smalley R, Andersen J, Hawkins M, et al. Interferon alfa combined with cytotoxic chemotherapy for patients with non-Hodgkin's lymphoma. N Engl J Med 1992;327:1336–41.
109. Hagenbeek A, Carde P, Meerwaldt J, et al. Maintenance of remission with human recombinant interferon alfa-2a in patients with stages III and IV low-grade malignant non-Hodgkin's lymphoma. J Clin Oncol 1998;16:41–7.
110. Solal-Celigny P, Lepage E, Brousse N, et al. Doxorubicin-containing regimen with or without interferon alfa-2b for advanced follicular lymphomas: final analysis of survival and toxicity in the Groupe d'Etude des Lymphomes Folliculaires 86 trial. J Clin Oncol 1998;16:2332–8.
111. Fisher RI, Dana BW, LeBlanc M, et al. Interferon alpha consolidation after intensive chemotherapy does not prolong the progression-free survival of patients with low-grade non- Hodgkin's lymphoma: results of the Southwest Oncology Group randomized phase III study 8809. J Clin Oncol 2000;18:2010–6.
112. Hochster H, Kim K, Green M, et al. Activity of fludarabine in previously treated non-Hodgkin's low-grade lymphoma: results of an Eastern Cooperative Oncology Group Study. J Clin Oncol 1992;10:28–32.
113. Tefferi A, Witzig T, Reid J, et al. Phase I study of combined 2-chlorodeoxyadenosine and chlorambucil in chronic lymphoid leukemia and low-grade lymphoma. J Clin Oncol 1994;12:569–74.
114. Solal-Celigny P, Brice P, Brousse N, et al. Phase II trial of fludarabine monophosphate as first-line treatment in patients with advanced follicular lymphoma: a multicenter study by the Groupe d'Etude des Lymphomes de l'Adulte. J Clin Oncol 1996;14:514–9.
115. Hochster HS, Oken MM, Winter JN, et al. Phase I study of fludarabine plus cyclophosphamide in patients with previously untreated low-grade lymphoma: results and long-term follow-up—a report from the Eastern Cooperative Oncology Group. J Clin Oncol 2000;18:987–94.
116. Velasquez W, Lew D, Miller T, Fisher R. SWOG 95-01: a phase II trial of a combination of fludarabine and mitoxantrone (FN) in untreated advanced low grade lymphoma. An effective, well tolerated therapy [abstract]. Proc ASCO 1999;18:9.
117. Hagenbeek A, Eghbali H, Monfardini S. Fludarabine compared with CVP chemotherapy in newly diagnosed patients with stages III and IV low grade malignant non-Hodgkin's lymphoma. Final analysis of a prospective randomized phase III Intergroup study of 381 patients [abstract]. Blood 2001;98:843.
118. Klasa R, Meyer R, Shustik C, et al. Fludarabine versus CVP in previously treated patients with progressive low grade non-Hodgkin's lymphomas [abstract]. Proc ASCO 1999;18:9.
119. Multani P, Grossbard M. Monoclonal antibody-based therapies for hematologic malignancies. J Clin Oncol 1998;16:3691–710.
120. McLaughlin P, Grillo-Lopez A, Link B, et al. Rituximab chimeric anti-CD20 monoclonal antibody therapy for relapsed indolent lymphoma: half of patients respond to a four-dose treatment program. J Clin Oncol 1998;16:2825–33.
121. Davis TA, Grillo-Lopez AJ, White CA, et al. Rituximab anti-CD20 monoclonal antibody therapy in non-Hodgkin's lymphoma: safety and efficacy of re-treatment. J Clin Oncol 2000;18:3135–43.
122. Hainsworth JD, Burris HA, 3rd, Morrissey LH, et al. Rituximab monoclonal antibody as initial systemic therapy for patients with low-grade non-Hodgkin lymphoma. Blood 2000;95:3052–6.
123. Colombat P, Salles G, Brousse N,. Rituximab (anti-CD20 monoclonal antibody) as single first-line therapy for patients with follicular lymphoma with a low tumor burden: clinical and molecular evaluation. Blood 2001;97:101–6.
124. Czuczman MS, Weaver R, Alkuzweny B, et al. Prolonged clinical and molecular remission in patients with low-grade or follicular non-Hodgkin's lymphoma treated with rituximab plus CHOP chemotherapy: 9-year follow-up. J Clin Oncol 2004;22:4711–6.
125. Marcus R, Imrie K, Belch A, et al. CVP chemotherapy plus rituximab compared with CVP as first-line treatment for advanced follicular lymphoma. Blood 2005;105:1417–23
126. Kaminski MS, Zelenetz AD, Press OW, et al. Pivotal study of iodine I 131 tositumomab for chemotherapy-refractory low-grade or transformed low-grade B-cell non-Hodgkin's lymphomas. J Clin Oncol 2001;19:3918–28.
127. Kaminski MS, Tuck M, Estes J, et al. 131I-tositumomab therapy as initial treatment for follicular lymphoma. N Engl J Med 2005;352:441–9.
128. Witzig TE, White CA, Wiseman GA, et al. Phase I/II trial of IDEC-Y2B8 radioimmunotherapy for treatment of relapsed or refractory CD20(+) B-cell non-Hodgkin's lymphoma. J Clin Oncol 1999;17:3793–803.
129. Witzig T, Leigh B, Gordon L, Smith M. Interim results from a prospective randomized controlled trial comparing Zevalin radioimmunotherapy to rituximab immunotherapy for B-cell non-Hodgkin's lymphoma: resistance to prior chemotherapy versus response rate. Proc Am Soc Clin Oncol 2000;19:29.
130. Friedberg J, Neuberg D, Gribben J, et al. Autologous bone marrow transplantation following histologic transformation of indolent B cell malignancies. Biol Blood Marrow Trans 1999;5:262–8.
131. Williams CD, Harrison CN, Lister TA, et al. High-dose therapy and autologous stem-cell support for chemosensitive transformed low-grade follicular non-Hodgkin's lymphoma: a case-matched study from the European Bone Marrow Transplant Registry. J Clin Oncol 2001;19:727–35.
132. Horning SJ, Weller E, Kim K, et al. Chemotherapy with or without radiotherapy in limited-stage diffuse aggressive non-Hodgkin's lymphoma: Eastern Cooperative Oncology Group Study 1484. J Clin Oncol 2004.
133. Reyes F, Lepage E, Ganem G, et al. Superiority of chemotherapy alone with the ACVBP regimen over treatment with three cycles of CHOP plus radiotherapy in low risk localized aggressive lymphoma [abstract]. Proc ASCO 2003;22:595.
134. Fillet G, Bonnet C, Mounier N, et al. Radiotherapy is unnecessary in elderly patients with localized aggressive non Hodgkin's lymphoma: results of the GELA LNH 93-4 study [abstract]. Blood 2002;100:337.
135. Fisher R, Gaynor E, Dahlberg S, et al. Comparison of a standard regimen (CHOP) with three intensive chemotherapy regimens for advanced non-Hodgkin's lymphoma. N Engl J Med 1993;328:1002.
136. Sertoli M, Santini G, Chisesi T, et al. MACOP-B versus ProMACE-MOPP in the treatment of advanced diffuse non-Hodgkin's lymphoma Cooperative Study Group. J Clin Oncol 1994;12:z1366–74.
137. Meyer R, Quirt I, Skillings J, et al. Escalated as compared with standard doses of doxorubicin in BACOP therapy for patients with non-Hodgkin's lymphoma. N Engl J Med 1993;329:1770–6.
138. Gordon L, Harrington D, Andersen J, et al. Comparison of a second-generation combination chemotherapeutic regimen (m-BACOD) with a standard regimen (CHOP) for advanced diffuse non-Hodgkin's lymphoma. N Engl J Med 1992;327:1342–9.
139. Pfreundschuh M, Trumper L, Kloess M, et al. Two-weekly or 3-weekly CHOP chemotherapy with or without etoposide for the treatment of elderly patients with aggressive lymphomas: results of the NHL-B2 trial of the DSHNHL. Blood 2004;104:634–41.
140. Goss P. Non-Hodgkin's lymphomas in elderly patients. Leuk Lymphoma 1993;10:147–56.
141. Gomez H, Hidalgo M, Casanova L, Colomer R. Risk factors for treatment-related in elderly patients with aggressive non-Hodgkin's lymphoma: results in of a multivariate analysis. J Clin Oncol 1998;16:2065–9.
142. Bastion Y, Blay J, Divine M, Brice P. Elderly patients with aggressive non-Hodgkin's lymphoma: disease presentation, response to treatment, and survival—a Groupe d-Etude des Lymphomas de l'Adulte study on 453 patients older than 69 years. J Clin Oncol 1997;15:2945–53.
143. Zinzani P, Storti S, Zaccaria A, Moretti L. Elderly aggressive-histology non-Hodgkin's lymphoma: first-line VNCOP-B regimen experience on 350 patients. Blood 1999;94:33–8.

144. Meyer R, Browman G, Samosh M, Benger A. Randomized phase II comparison of standard CHOP with weekly CHOP in elderly patients with non-Hodgkin's lymphoma. J Clin Oncol 1995;13:2386–93.
145. Sonneveld P, de Ridder M, van der Lelie H, Neiuwenhuis K. Comparison of doxorubicin and mitoxantrone in the treatment of elderly patients with advanced diffuse non-Hodgkin's lymphoma using CHOP versus CNOP chemotherapy. J Clin Oncol 1995;13:2530–9.
146. Tirelli U, Errante D, Van Glabbeke M, Teodorovic I. CHOP is the standard regimen in patients > or = 70 years of age with intermediate-grade and high-grade non-Hodgkin's lymphoma: results of a randomized study of the European Organization for Research and Treatment of Cancer Lymphoma Cooperative Study Group. J Clin Oncol 1998;16:27–34.
147. Coiffier B, Lepage E, Briere J, et al. CHOP chemotherapy plus rituximab compared with CHOP alone in elderly patients with diffuse large-B-cell lymphoma. N Engl J Med 2002;346:235–42.
148. Mounier N, Briere J, Gisselbrecht C, et al. B. Rituximab plus CHOP (R-CHOP) overcomes bcl-2--associated resistance to chemotherapy in elderly patients with diffuse large B-cell lymphoma (DLBCL). Blood 2003;101:4279–84.
149. Habermann T, Weller E, Morrison V, et al. Phase III trial of rituximab-CHOP (R-CHOP) vs. CHOP with a second randomization to maintenance rituximab or observation in patients 60 years of age and older with diffuse large B-cell lymphoma [abstract]. Blood 2003;102:6.
150. Decaudin D, Bosq J, Tertian G, Nedellec G. Phase II trial of fludarabine monophosphate in patients with mantle-cell lymphomas. J Clin Oncol 1998;16:579–83.
151. Foran J, Rohatiner A, Coiffier B, Barbui T. Multicenter phase II study of fludarabine phosphate for patients with newly diagnosed lymphoplasmacytoid lymphoma, Waldenström's macroglobulinemia, and mantle-cell lymphoma. J Clin Oncol 1999;17:546–53.
152. Coiffier B, Haioun C, Ketterer N, Engert A. Rituximab (anti-CD20 monoclonal antibody) for the treatment of patients with relapsing or refractory aggressive lymphoma: a multicenter phase II study. Blood 1998;92:1927–32.
153. Khouri I, Romaguera J, Kantarjian H, Palmer J. Hyper-CVAD and high-dose methotrexate/cytarabine followed by stem-cell transplantation: an active regimen for aggressive mantle-cell lymphoma. J Clin Oncol 1998;16:3803–9.
154. Khouri IF, Saliba RM, Okoroji GJ, et al. Long-term follow-up of autologous stem cell transplantation in patients with diffuse mantle cell lymphoma in first disease remission: the prognostic value of beta2-microglobulin and the tumor score. Cancer 2003;98:2630–5.
155. Gianni AM, Magni M, Martelli M, et al. Long-term remission in mantle cell lymphoma following high-dose sequential chemotherapy and in vivo rituximab-purged stem cell autografting (R-HDS regimen). Blood 2003;102:749–55.
156. Gisselbrecht C, Lepage E, Molina T, et al. Shortened first-line high-dose chemotherapy for patients with poor- prognosis aggressive lymphoma. J Clin Oncol 2002;20:2472–9.
157. Haioun C, Lepage E, Gisselbrecht C, et al. Benefit of autologous bone marrow transplantation over sequential chemotherapy in poor-risk aggressive non-Hodgkin's lymphoma: updated results of the prospective study LNH87-2. Groupe d'Etude des Lymphomes de l'Adulte. J Clin Oncol 1997;15:1131–7.
158. Haioun C, Lepage E, Gisselbrecht C, et al. Survival benefit of high-dose therapy in poor-risk aggressive non-Hodgkin's lymphoma: final analysis of the prospective LNH87-2 protocol—a groupe d'Etude des lymphomes de l'Adulte study. J Clin Oncol 2000;18:3025–30.
159. Milpied N, Deconinck E, Gaillard F, et al. Initial treatment of aggressive lymphoma with high-dose chemotherapy and autologous stem-cell support. N Engl J Med 2004;350:1287–95.
160. Sweetenham JW, Santini G, Qian W, et al. High-dose therapy and autologous stem-cell transplantation versus conventional-dose consolidation/maintenance therapy as postremission therapy for adult patients with lymphoblastic lymphoma: results of a randomized trial of the European Group for Blood and Marrow Transplantation and the United Kingdom Lymphoma Group. J Clin Oncol 2001;19:2927–36.
161. Kantarjian HM, O'Brien S, Smith TL, et al. Results of treatment with hyper-CVAD, a dose-intensive regimen, in adult acute lymphocytic leukemia. J Clin Oncol 2000;18:547–61.
162. Mashal R, Canellos G. Small non-cleaved cell lymphoma in adults. Am J Hemat 1991;38:40.
163. Schwenn M, Blattner S, Lynch E, Weinstein H. HiC-COM: A 2-month intensive chemotherapy regimen for children with stage III and IV Burkitt's lymphoma and B cell acute lymphoblastic leukemia. J Clin Oncol 1991;9:133.
164. Soussain C, Patte C, Ostronoff M, et al. Small noncleaved cell lymphoma and leukemia in adults. A retrospective study of 65 adults treated with the LMB pediatric protocols. Blood 1995;85:664–74.
165. Lee EJ, Petroni GR, Schiffer CA, et al. Brief-duration high-intensity chemotherapy for patients with small non-cleaved-cell lymphoma or FAB L3 acute lymphocytic leukemia: results of cancer and leukemia group B study 9251. J Clin Oncol 2001;19:4014–22.
166. Magrath I, Adde M, Shad A, et al. Adults and children with small non-cleaved-cell lymphoma have a similar excellent outcome when treated with the same chemotherapy regimen. J Clin Oncol 1996;14:925–34.
167. Lacasce A, Howard O, Lib S, et al. Modified Magrath regimens for adults with Burkitt and Burkitt-like lymphomas: preserved efficacy with decreased toxicity. Leuk Lymphoma 2004;45:761–7.
168. Velasquez WS, Cabanillas F, Salvador P, et al. Effective salvage therapy for lymphoma with cisplatin in combination with high-dose ara-c and dexamethasone (DHAP). Blood 1988;71:117–22.
169. Goss P, Shepherd F, Scott J, et al. Dexamethasone/ifosfamide/cisplatin/etoposide (DICE) as therapy for patients with advanced refractory non-Hodgkin's lymphoma: preliminary report of a phase II study. Ann Oncol 1991;2, Suppl 1:43–6.
170. Velasquez W, McLaughlin P, Tucker S, et al. ESHAP—An effective chemotherapy regimen in refractory and relapsing lymphoma: a 4-year follow-up study. J Clin Oncol 1994;12:1169–76.
171. Applebaum FR, Fefer A, Cheever MA, et al. Treatment of non-Hodgkin's lymphoma with marrow transplantation in identical twins. Blood 1981;58:509–13.
172. van Besien K, Thall P, Korbling M, Pugh W. Allogeneic transplantation for recurrent or refractory non-Hodgkin's lymphoma with poor prognostic features after conditioning with thiotepa, busulfan, and cyclophosphamide: experience in 44 consecutive patients. Biol Blood Marrow Trans 1997;3:150–6.
173. Chopra R, Goldstone A, Pearce R, et al. Autologous versus allogeneic bone marrow transplantation for non-Hodgkin's lymphoma: a case-controlled analysis of the European Bone Marrow Transplant Group Registry data. J Clin Oncol 1992;10:1690–5.
174. Ratanatharathorn V, Uberti J, Karanes C, et al. Prospective comparative trial of autologous versus allogeneic bone marrow transplantation in patients with non-Hodgkin's lymphoma. Blood 1994;84:1050–5.
175. van Besien K, Loberiza FR Jr, Bajorunaite R, et al. Comparison of autologous and allogeneic hematopoietic stem cell transplantation for follicular lymphoma. Blood 2003;102:3521–9.
176. Soiffer R, Freedman A, Neuberg D, et al. CD6+ T-cell depleted allogeneic bone marrow transplantation for non-Hodgkin's lymphoma. Bone Marrow Transplant 1998;21:1177–81.
177. Khouri IF, Saliba RM, Giralt SA, et al. Nonablative allogeneic hematopoietic transplantation as adoptive immunotherapy for indolent lymphoma: low incidence of toxicity, acute graft-versus-host disease, and treatment-related mortality. Blood 2001;98:3595–9.
178. Philip T, Armitage JO, Spitzer G, et al. High-dose therapy and autologous bone marrow transplantation after failure of conventional chemotherapy in adults with intermediate-grade or high-grade non-Hodgkin's lymphoma. N Engl J Med 1987;316:1493–8.
179. Philip T, Guglielmi C, Hagenbeek A, et al. Autologous bone marrow transplantation as compared with salvage chemotherapy in relapses of chemotherapy-sensitive non-Hodgkin's lymphoma. N Engl J Med 1995;333:1540–5.
180. Freedman A, Neuberg D, Mauch P, et al. Long term follow-up of autologous bone marrow transplantation in patients with relapsed follicular lymphoma. Blood 1999;94:3325–33.
181. Apostolidis J, Gupta RK, Grenzelias D, et al. High-dose therapy with autologous bone marrow support as consolidation of remission in follicular lymphoma: long-term clinical and molecular follow-up. J Clin Oncol 2000;18:527–36.
182. Bierman P, Vose J, Anderson J, et al. High-dose therapy with autologous hematopoietic rescue for follicular low-grade non-Hodgkin's lymphoma. J Clin Oncol 1997;15:445–50.
183. Bastion Y, Brice P, Haioun C, et al. Intensive therapy with peripheral blood progenitor cell transplantation in 60 patients with poor-prognosis follicular lymphoma. Blood 1995;86:3257–62.
184. Schouten HC, Qian W, Kvaloy S, et al. High-dose therapy improves progression-free survival and survival in relapsed follicular non-Hodgkin's lymphoma: results from the randomized European CUP trial. J Clin Oncol 2003;21:3918–27.
185. Foran J, Apostolidis J, Papamichael D, et al. High-dose therapy with autologous haematopoietic support in patients with transformed follicular lymphoma: a study of 27 patients from a single centre. Ann Oncol 1998;9:865–9.

Mycosis Fungoides and the Sézary Syndrome

Richard T. Hoppe, MD
Youn H. Kim, MD
Ranjana Advani, MD

Mycosis fungoides (MF) is a cutaneous lymphoma first described by the French dermatologist Alibert in 1806. The mushroom-like appearance of the cutaneous tumor nodules of MF is what gives the disease its name. Mycosis fungoides is included in the spectrum of diseases referred to as cutaneous T-cell lymphomas (CTCL). This group of diseases also includes Sézary syndrome (SS), which is an erythrodermic, leukemic variant of MF.[1]

EPIDEMIOLOGY AND ETIOLOGY

Mycosis fungoides is a rare lymphoma. The estimated annual incidence rate in the US is 0.29 per 100,000, or less than 1,000 new cases annually.[2] It accounts for only 2% of new cases of non-Hodgkin's lymphoma. It commonly affects older adults (median age 55 to 60 years); however, it does not spare younger patients.[3] There is a 2:1 male predominance, without racial predilection.

The etiology of MF is unknown. Some retrospective studies have suggested an etiologic role for environmental chemical exposure. However, a large case-controlled study refutes this hypothesis.[4] A viral etiology was once proposed, based on the isolation of human T-cell leukemia/lymphoma virus 1 (HTLV-1) from the peripheral blood lymphocytes of a patient with a cutaneous lymphoma resembling MF. The clinical characteristics of this entity, HTLV-1–associated T-cell lymphoma, have now been described more precisely[5] and are quite different from those of typical MF. Despite many years of probing patient blood and tissues for HTLV-1, there has not been any conclusive evidence to support an association between the virus and MF.[6]

PATHOLOGY/PATHOGENESIS

The classical histopathology of MF includes abnormal cells infiltrating the epidermis (epidermotropism) as single cells or in clusters (Pautrier's microabscesses) (Figure 119-1). Typically, there is also an upper dermal infiltrate of similar cells, as well as variable proportions of histiocytes, eosinophils, and plasma cells. The neoplastic cells of MF are mononuclear cells. Under oil immersion, the nuclei of these cells have a hyperconvoluted surface. Electron microscopic studies demonstrate marked infolding of the nuclear membrane, which on three-dimensional reconstruction simulates a cerebriform appearance.

Functional studies and monoclonal antibody staining indicate that the majority of cases of MF are associated with the helper T-cell phenotype (CD4+).[7] Immunophenotyping studies demonstrate that the neoplastic cells of MF usually retain the CD4 antigen but lose other mature T-cell antigens, such as Leu-8 or Leu-9 (CD7). This loss of mature T-cell antigens may help in the differential diagnosis of MF from benign dermatoses. Rare cases of MF have been demonstrated to be CD8+ (cytotoxic/suppressor T-cell phenotype).

Analysis of the abnormal cells in MF using the Southern blot and polymerase chain reaction (PCR) methods to assess rearrangements of the T-cell receptor (TCR) have been reported. These studies indicate monoclonal rearrangements of the T-cell receptors in the skin, lymph nodes, and peripheral blood of patients with MF.[7–9] In general, biopsies performed on multiple lesions in a patient at the same time, or different biopsies sequentially performed on lesions in the same patient, demonstrate consistent rearrangements.

The pathology of extracutaneous disease poses special problems. Most commonly, enlarged lymph nodes demonstrate changes of dermatopathic lymphadenitis, including the presence of sinus histiocytosis and an abundance of pigment-laden macrophages. There may also be a variable number of atypical lymphocytes with cerebriform nuclei. The prognostic relevance of the degree of infiltration by these abnormal cells led to the development of a lymph node classification system.[10] In this system, lymph nodes are classified as LN-0 to LN-4 corresponding with involvement ranging from "no atypical lymphocytes" (LN-0) to "complete replacement of nodal architecture by atypical lymphocytes or frankly neoplastic cells" (LN-4). This descriptive system for grading node involvement has prognostic relevance.[11] Detection of abnormal cells in the lymph node is facilitated by the use of Southern blot or PCR analysis. Potential neoplastic involvement with clonal TCR rearrangement may be demonstrated even in lymph nodes that show only dermatopathic changes on routine evaluation.[12]

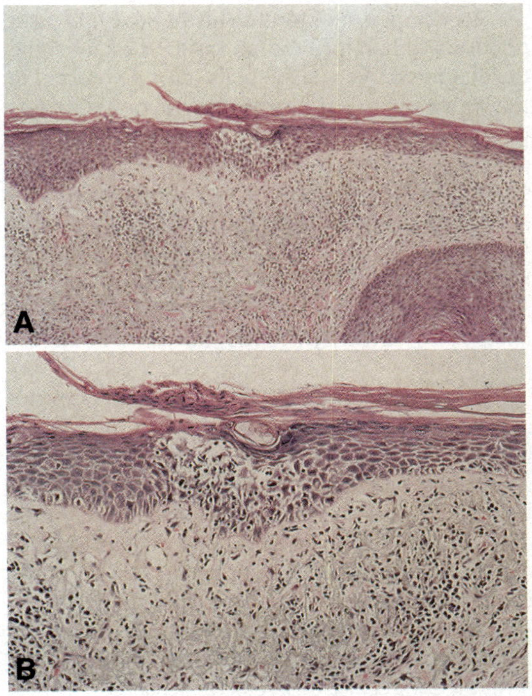

Figure 119-1 **A,** histopathology of mycosis fungoides (MF) showing upper dermal infiltrate and characteristic epidermotropism of atypical lymphocytes (H & E, × 80). **B,** higher magnification of the same field demonstrating cluster of epidermotropic, pleomorphic cells, Pautrier's microabscess, diagnostic of MF (H & E, × 120).

NATURAL HISTORY

Mycosis fungoides often has a long natural history. The disease may present in a premycotic phase with nonspecific, slightly scaling skin lesions that wax and wane for years. Biopsies are generally nondiagnostic during this phase, and patients may respond to topical corticosteroids. Some of these patients will experience an evolution of their disease and develop more typical patches or infiltrated plaques, from which a definitive biopsy may be obtained. The median duration from the onset of skin symptoms to a diagnosis of MF may be 5 years or longer.

The initial presentation of MF may be as patches, plaques, tumors, or generalized erythroderma. A patient may present with more than one morphologic type of skin disease or change from one type to another during the course of disease. The typical patches of MF are slightly scaling and mildly erythematous. Many patients present with involvement in a "bathing trunk" distribution, although lesions may be present on any part of the body. Pruritus is the most common symptom, even in the early phases of the disease and is often the problem that prompts a visit to the dermatologist.

More infiltrated lesions become palpable plaques. These are erythematous, slightly scaling, with well-defined borders. The shape is variable, and the distribution may vary. Infiltrated plaques may eventually develop into ulcerating or fungating tumors (Figure 119-2). Tumors may become

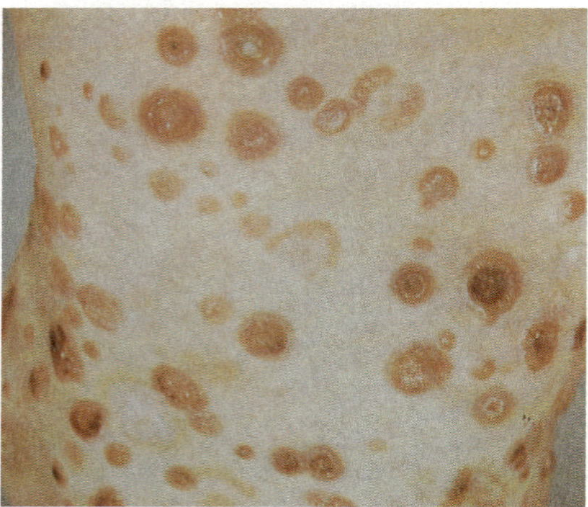

Figure 119-2 The flank of a patient with typical plaques of mycosis fungoides, many of which have evolved into tumors with central ulceration.

infected, and sepsis secondary to infection is often the cause of death in individuals so affected. Generalized dermal thickening from infiltrative disease may cause the classic but rare leonine facies of MF.

Another cutaneous manifestation is generalized erythroderma (Figure 119-3). Plaques or tumors may be superimposed over the erythroderma. These patients suffer from intense pruritus. Patients with erythroderma may also have lymphadenopathy and circulating abnormal cells in the peripheral blood. These cells may have the same microscopic appearance, immunophenotypic, and genotypic characteristics as the cells that infiltrate the epidermis. Patients with this complex of findings have the Sézary syndrome (SS).[13]

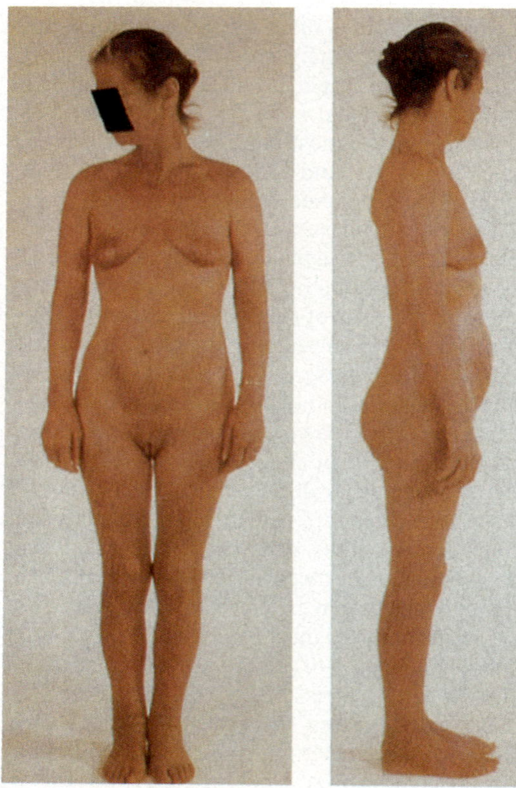

Figure 119-3 Generalized erythroderma (or "l'homme rouge"), often with very atrophic skin, is typical of patients with the Sézary syndrome.

Although MF is usually an indolent disease, and many patients demonstrate only the patch or plaque phase of skin involvement throughout the duration of their disease,[14,15] some will progress to develop cutaneous tumors. The rapidity of this progression is unpredictable. Most patients with MF demonstrate only cutaneous disease throughout the course of their illness. Only 15 to 20% develop clinical problems related to extracutaneous disease. This likelihood is related to the extent of skin involvement. It is exceedingly rare among patients who have only the limited plaque phase of skin involvement, relatively uncommon among those with the generalized plaque phase (8%), and more likely among patients who have developed tumorous involvement of the skin (30%) or generalized erythroderma (25%).[16]

The most commonly identified route of extracutaneous spread is to the regional lymphatics and secondarily to viscera. The organs most commonly involved include the spleen, liver, and lungs, but virtually any organ may be involved at autopsy in patients who have died of the disease.[17]

DIAGNOSIS

A diagnosis of MF or SS may be suspected in patients who present with chronic nonspecific dermatitis or generalized erythroderma. Similar skin lesions can be seen in benign skin conditions, such as psoriasis, parapsoriasis, eczematous dermatitis, photodermatitis, or drug reactions. For patients with tumorous lesions, the differential includes non-MF CTCL or primary cutaneous B-cell lymphoma.

Skin biopsy with routine histology is the most important laboratory tool to assist in establishing the diagnosis. Neoplastic cells must be present in the epidermis (epidermotropism or Pautrier's microabscesses) in order to make a definitive diagnosis of MF (see Figure 119-1). Based on the severity of the epidermal and dermal involvement, the categories "diagnostic of," "consistent with," and "suggestive of" MF have been recommended. Treatment programs specific for MF should be considered only if the biopsy is diagnostic of or consistent with, not merely suggestive of, MF.

Immunophenotyping is used to support the routine histology. Occasionally, when the routine histology is equivocal, the immunophenotyping results may help to confirm or refute the diagnosis. However, results of immunohistochemical studies must be interpreted with caution. There may be discordant expression of antigens between intraepidermal and intradermal T cells in MF and SS.[18] In addition, significant differences of antigen expression in biopsies obtained from different sites from the same patient have been observed.

Evaluation of skin biopsies to detect T-cell receptor (TCR) gene rearrangements, or genotyping, may also be helpful. TCR gene rearrangements can be detected by Southern blot analysis[8] or by methods utilizing PCR amplification.[9] PCR amplification methods for frozen or paraffin tissue analysis are widely available and affordable.[19] Genotyping is becoming an integral diagnostic procedure for patients in whom the routine histology or immunophenotyping is equivocal but whose clinical presentation is strongly suggestive of MF.

Blood and lymph nodes may also be probed for malignant cells. Flow cytometry studies of the peripheral blood may show expansion of the CD4+CD7- population reflective of circulating atypical lymphocytes of Sézary type.[20] PCR methods can be helpful in determination of blood[21] or lymph node involvement.[12]

STAGING AND PROGNOSIS

The intensity of the staging studies performed is dictated by the extent of skin involvement and the results of screening staging procedures. Patients with the limited plaque phase of skin involvement typically will require only a good physical examination, careful mapping of the skin lesions, a complete blood count, Sézary cell detection, screening chemistries, and a chest radiograph. If these are all within normal limits, additional studies need not be performed. Routine imaging studies in patients who have limited disease without peripheral lymphadenopathy is unproductive.[23] Patients with cutaneous tumors, erythroderma, or palpable adenopathy should undergo CT or PET/CT imaging.[24] Any blood or radiographic abnormalities should be evaluated further. Patients who have palpable lymphadenopathy should have a biopsy of the enlarged nodes. Significant bone marrow disease is usually reflected by the presence of readily detectable Sézary cells in the peripheral blood. Therefore, bone marrow biopsy is not routinely used as part of the initial staging.

A Tumor-Node-Metastasis-Blood (TNMB) staging system has proved useful for MF and was introduced at the Workshop on Mycosis Fungoides held at the National Cancer Institute in 1978.[25] Tables 119-1 and 119-2 summarize the staging classification and TNMB categories. The T-classification reflects the extent of skin involvement. The N category indicates the presence of lymph node involvement. Enlarged lymph nodes should be biopsied, since palpable enlargement is often associated only with changes of dermatopathic lymphadenitis. In the M category, suspected disease should also be documented and treatment programs for visceral disease should be considered only if definite proof of disease exists. In the B (blood) category, the presence of a significant proportion of abnormal, cerebriform (Sézary) cells should be noted. However, low levels of Sézary-like cells can be detected in the peripheral blood of patients with benign skin conditions.[13] The current practice by many is to use a criterion of at least 20% of lymphocytes or, an absolute count of at least 1,000/mm^3, or a CD4+:CD8+ ratio greater than 10 to define peripheral blood involvement. Recommendations for a revised stage grouping are currently under consideration by the International Society for Cutaneous Lymphoma.

Table 119-1 Tumor-Node-Metastasis-Blood Classification for Mycosis Fungoides

T (Skin)	
T1	Limited patch/plaque (< 10% of total skin surface)
T2	Generalized patch/plaque (≥ 10% of total skin surface)
T3	Tumors
T4	Generalized erythroderma
N (Nodes)	
N0	Lymph nodes clinically uninvolved
N1	Lymph nodes enlarged, histologically uninvolved (includes "reactive" and "dermatopathic" nodes)
N2	Lymph nodes clinically uninvolved, histologically involved
N3	Lymph nodes enlarged and histologically involved
M (Viscera)	
M0	No visceral involvement
M1	Visceral involvement
B (Blood)	
B0	No circulating atypical (Sézary) cells (< 5% of total lymphocytes)
B1	Circulating atypical (Sézary) cells (≥ 5% of total lymphocytes)

The T-classification and presence of extracutaneous disease are the most important indicators predictive of survival (Figure 119-4).[16,26] Patients with limited patch/plaque (T1, overall stage IA) disease have an excellent prognosis with a long-term life expectancy that is similar to an age-, sex-, and race-matched control population.[14] According to a retrospective study of 122 stage IA patients at Stanford, the median survival was not reached at 33 years. Nearly all patients with stage IA disease who die will die from causes other than MF. Furthermore, only 9% of treated patients at this stage will ever progress to a more advanced stage of disease.

Patients with generalized patch/plaque disease without evidence of extracutaneous involvement (T2, stage IB or stage IIA) have a median survival greater than 11 years.[15] Patients with T2 disease have a greater likelihood of disease progression (24%), and nearly 20% die of causes related to MF.

Patients with cutaneous tumors (T3, stage IIB) or generalized erythroderma (T4, stage III) without extracutaneous disease have median survivals of 3.2 and 4.6 years, respectively. The majority of these patients will die of MF. The long-term outcome in patients with erythroderma (T4) is quite variable and is dependent on patient age at presentation (< 65 years vs > 65 years), overall stage (III vs IV), and peripheral blood involvement (B0 vs B1).[27] The median survival can vary widely depending on the combinations of these independent prognostic factors: three distinct prognostic subgroups were identified, with median survivals of 10.2 years, 3.7 years, and 1.5 years.

Table 119-2 Clinical Staging System for Mycosis Fungoides

Clinical Stages	TNM Classification*		
IA	T1	N0	M0
IB	T2	N0	M0
IIA	T1–2	N1	M0
IIB	T3	N0–1	M0
IIIA	T4	N0	M0
IIIB	T4	N1	M0
IVA	T1–4	N2–3	M0
IVB	T1–4	N0–3	M1

TNM = tumor, node, metastasis.
*The B classification does not alter clinical stage.

Patients with extracutaneous disease at presentation involving either lymph nodes (stage IVA) or viscera (stage IVB) have a median survival of less than 1.5 years.[28] The presence of significant Sézary cells in the peripheral blood (B1) is not factored into the overall clinical stage; however, it usually correlates with more advanced T-stage (usually T4) and the presence of extracutaneous disease.[26]

In a study of patients at the National Cancer Institute, patients with lymph node biopsies showing dermatopathic changes or just a small number of atypical cells (histologic grade LN-1 or LN-2) had a 5-year survival of 80%. Those patients with large clusters of paracortical atypical cells (LN-3) had a 5-year survival of 30%, and those with effaced nodes (LN-4) had a 5-year survival of only 15%.[11] Frank lymph node involvement with MF (N-classification 2 or 3, overall stage IVA) correlates with histologic grade of LN-3 or -4.

Patients with plaque-type or erythrodermic MF may develop cutaneous tumors with large cell histology (large cell transformation); these large cells may often express CD30 (Ki-1). The CD30+ large cell lymphoma arising in these patients shares a common clonal origin with the pre-existing MF and does not represent a new lymphoma.[29] These patients may have more rapid disease progression and require more intensive local or systemic therapy. Thus, transformation of MF to CD30+ large cell lymphoma is associated with a more aggressive clinical course and less favorable outcome.

THERAPY

Nearly all patients with MF will require treatment directed at their skin. Common therapies include topical corticosteroids, psoralen plus ultraviolet A (PUVA), topical chemotherapy, topical retinoids, and irradiation. A minority of patients (10–20%) will also require treatment for systemic disease. There are multiple therapeutic options for MF and SS. Selection of a specific treatment plan is based primarily on the clinical stage of disease (Figure 119-5).

Topical Chemotherapy Topical nitrogen mustard (mechlorethamine, HN2) is a very effective form of management for patients with MF.[30–32] The mechanism of action has not been defined and may not be related simply to its alkylating agent properties. The activity of HN2 may be

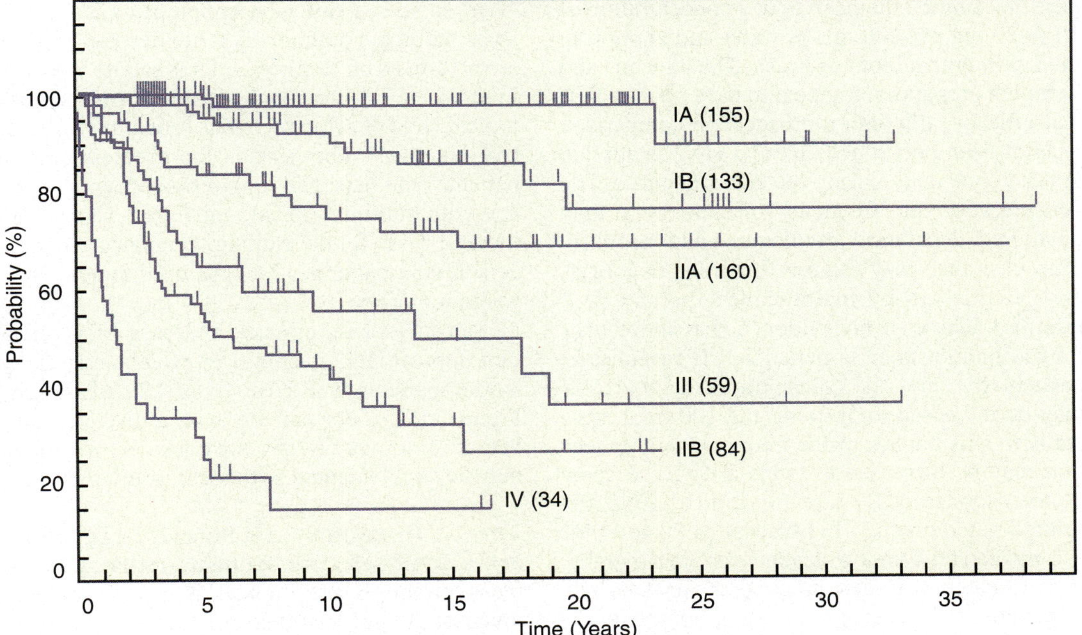

Figure 119-4 Disease-specific survival by initial disease stage for 525 patients with mycosis fungoides treated at Stanford University.

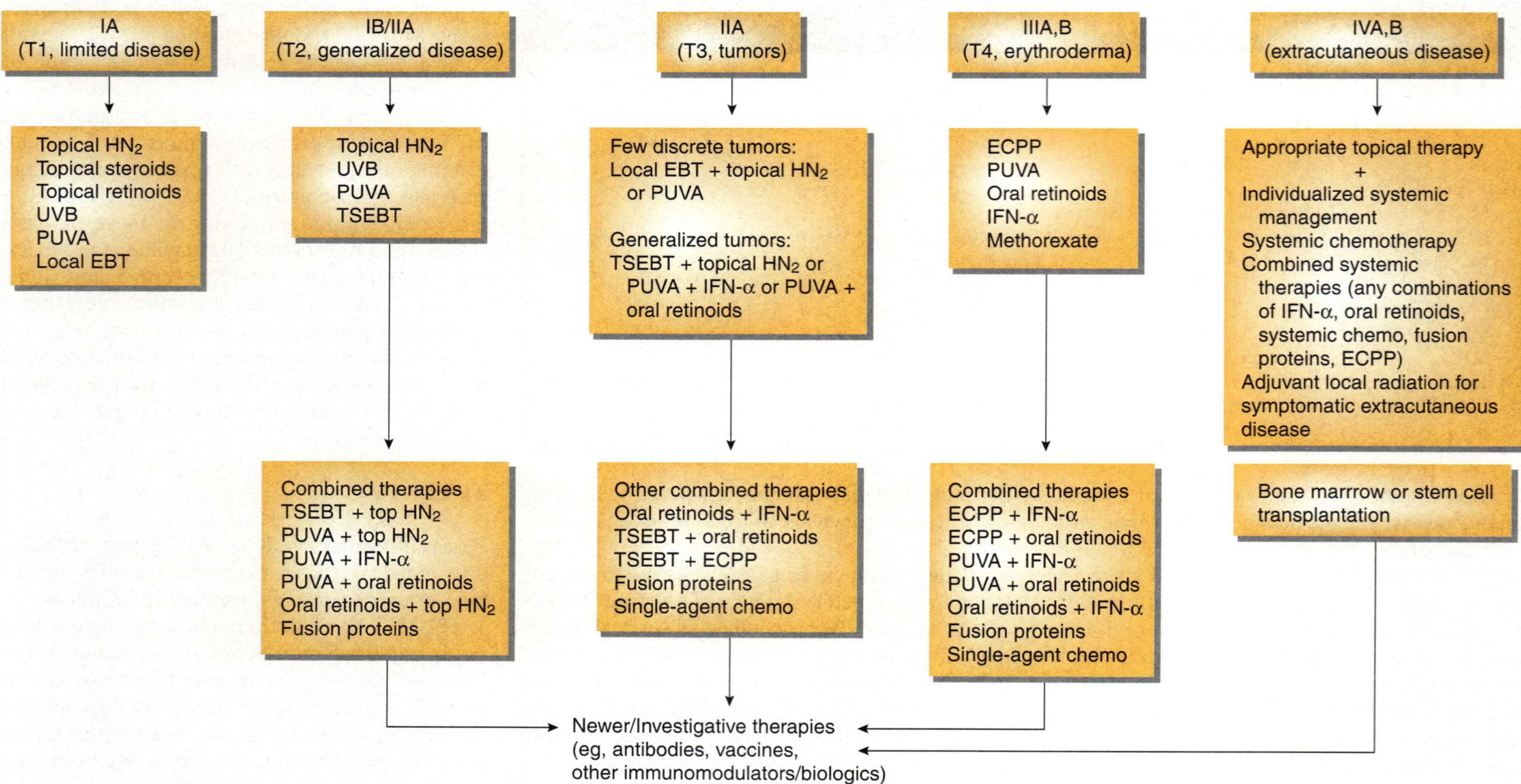

Figure 119-5 Algorithm for the management of patients with clinical suspicion of mycosis fungoides or Sézary syndrome.

mediated by immune mechanisms or by interaction with the epidermal cell–Langerhans cell–T-cell axis.

HN2 may be applied locally, regionally, or to the entire skin. It may be mixed in water or in an ointment base. Nitrogen mustard ointment is prepared by the pharmacist at an initial concentration of 10 to 20 mg of HN2 per 100 grams of Aquaphor. For the aqueous preparation, patients prepare the solution themselves at a concentration of 10 to 20 mg per 100 mL of water and apply it to their skin with a cloth or brush. The aqueous and ointment preparations appear to have similar clinical efficacy, although a prospective comparison has not been performed. Topical HN2 is applied at least once daily during the clearing phase. The concentration and frequency of application may be altered, depending on tolerance and response. Skin clearance may require 6 months or longer, and is followed by maintenance therapy (≥ 2 months). There is no evidence that more prolonged maintenance is beneficial. If response is particularly slow, the concentration of the HN2 may be increased to 30 to 40 mg/100 mL, especially to small areas, or the frequency of application may be increased to twice a day. The complete response (CR) rate for topical HN2 for limited patch/plaque (T1) disease is 70 to 80%. The median time to skin clearance is 6 to 8 months. When treatment is discontinued, more than half of patients will relapse in the skin, but most will respond to a resumption of therapy. The proportion of patients treated with topical HN2 who have a durable complete response (> 10 years) is 20 to 25%.

The primary acute complication of HN2 is a cutaneous hypersensitivity reaction. This may occur in as many as 60% of patients treated with the aqueous preparation but in only about 5% of those treated with the ointment-based preparation. Desensitization may be achieved by a variety of topical or systemic desensitization programs. There is no systemic absorption of topical HN2, so hematologic monitoring is not necessary, there are no effects on fertility, and it is safe to use even in children.[32] Occasionally, patients treated with topical HN2 develop secondary squamoproliferative lesions.[33] This risk is the greatest among patients who have had long-term sequential therapy with multiple topical modalities. There is no increased risk for developing secondary skin cancers among patients who have used topical HN2 as monotherapy.

Because of its efficacy and ease of application, topical HN2 is employed widely, especially among patients who have T1 or T2 disease (see Figure 119-5). For patients with a discrete number of tumorous or refractory lesions, treatment may be supplemented with local irradiation.

Topical Retinoids Bexarotene (Targretin) 1% gel, a RXR-selective synthetic retinoid, is the most commonly used topical retinoid for treating mycosis fungoides. Bexarotene gel is applied with a thin application to the patches or plaques and is most effective and best-tolerated when used twice daily. Due to the irritant effect of the retinoids, it is only feasible to use this agent when there are a discrete number of patches or plaques. It is not intended for generalized application. An early trial reported an overall response rate of 63% with a CR rate of 21%.[34] A phase III trial included 50 patients with refractory or persistent early stage disease (stages IA to IIA).[35] Responses were seen in 62% of patients with stage IA and 50% of patients with stage IB disease. Three patients with stage IIA or IIB disease did not respond. The most common toxicity of bexarotene gel is irritation at the sites of application, which occurs in the majority of patients. Because of the erythema from the irritant reaction, it may be necessary to withhold therapy for a few weeks to assess disease activity.

As a result of these studies, bexarotene gel was approved by the FDA for the topical treatment of cutaneous lesions in patients with stages IA and IB cutaneous T-cell lymphoma who have refractory or persistent disease after other therapies or who have not tolerated other therapies.

Phototherapy Phototherapy includes ultraviolet (UV) radiation in the UVA or UVB wavelengths. The long-wave UVA has the advantage over UVB in its greater depth of penetration into the dermal infiltrates of MF. For early limited diseases, UVB alone[36] or home UV phototherapy (UVA + UVB)[37] may be effective. UVB therapy is initiated as a daily or three times per week regimen with gradual incremental dose delivery. After complete clearance is achieved, the frequency of therapy is gradually reduced during the maintenance period and then discontinued. A CR rate of 83% has been reported using UVB phototherapy in patients with patch-type stage IA disease.[37]

UVA may be used with psoralen, a photosensitizing agent, as psoralen plus UVA or PUVA, referred to as photochemotherapy. In the presence of UVA, psoralen intercalates with DNA, forming monofunctional and bifunctional adducts, which inhibit DNA synthesis. PUVA is clearly the most commonly used form of phototherapy for MF and SS.[38,39] The technique of treatment is for the patient to ingest the psoralen drug (usually 8-methoxypsoralen) followed by controlled exposure to UVA in a specially designed light box, usually commencing 1 to 2 hours later. Only the eyes are shielded routinely. All other body surfaces may be treated; however, selected areas can be shielded to minimize undesired photo damage. Certain "shadowed" areas such as the scalp, perineum, axillae, and other skin fold areas will not receive adequate exposure.

PUVA treatment is initiated thrice weekly until skin clearance is achieved, after which the frequency of treatment is gradually decreased to as infrequently as once every 2 weeks. Maintenance therapy should be discontinued within 1 year in order to minimize the risks of cutaneous carcinogenesis. The usual time to skin clearance is 2 to 6 months and the likelihood of clearance is related to the extent of skin involvement. The complete clearance rate is 50 to 90% in patients with patch or plaque disease. The response is less impressive among patients with erythrodermic or tumor disease. Indications for PUVA treatment include its use as the primary therapy for patients with limited or generalized patch or plaque disease or as a secondary therapy following the failure of other topical modalities (see Figure 119-5). PUVA may also be effective for patients with erythroderma, provided that very low daily exposures are utilized to avoid phototoxicity reactions. In patients with SS, PUVA may be supplemented by systemic therapies; such as interferon alpha[40] or systemic retinoids.[41] The treatment of patients with more advanced cutaneous disease may be facilitated by the addition of localized irradiation to particularly refractory plaques or tumors.

The primary acute complication of PUVA therapy is a phototoxic reaction, with erythroderma and blistering. Patients should shield their skin and eyes for at least 24 hours following psoralen ingestion. The potential long-term complications of PUVA therapy include cataract formation and secondary cutaneous malignancies.[42]

Radiation Therapy Mycosis fungoides is an extremely radiosensitive neoplasm. Individual plaques or tumors of MF may be treated with electron beam radiation therapy (EBT) to total doses of 15 to 25 Gy in 1 to 3 weeks, with a high likelihood of achieving long-term local control.

Techniques have been developed to treat the entire cutaneous surface with electrons (total-skin EBT, or TSEBT).[43] Conventional linear accelerators may be modified to treat patients in the standing position at an extended distance. By having the patient stand in multiple positions, the entire skin surface may be irradiated. The treatment technique employed at Stanford (and adopted at many other centers) uses a six-field technique (anterior, posterior, and four opposed oblique fields). Treatment is administered four times a week, to a total dose of 30 to 36 Gy. Supplementary treatment is required for the soles of the feet, the perineum, and under the breasts. Only the eyes are shielded routinely, but other areas may be shielded during part of the treatment to help control localized cutaneous reactions.

The complications of TSEBT include acute erythema, desquamation, and temporary epilation. Patients also experience temporary loss of their fingernails and toenails, as well as an impaired ability to sweat for up to 12 months. There is an increased risk of secondary squamous and basal cell cancers of the skin, but this is most noticeable in patients who have received protracted therapy with a variety of topical agents, including PUVA and topical HN2.[33]

Several centers have developed expertise in the use of TSEBT.[44,45] Overall response rates are nearly 100%, with complete response rates ranging from 40 to 98%, depending on the extent of skin involvement. As many as 50% of patients with limited plaque disease and 25% of patients with generalized plaque disease may remain free of disease for more than 5 years after completion of a single course of EBT. Although the curative potential of this treatment remains disputed, there is no doubt that it provides an important palliative benefit, especially for patients with extensive disease. Often, when disease recurs, it is in a more limited distribution and may be controlled more readily with localized topical therapies. The use of EBT is often indicated in the primary or secondary management of patients with generalized plaque or tumorous involvement of the skin. After complete skin clearance, adjuvant therapy with topical HN2 may be utilized. Repeat courses of TSEBT may be administered in selected situations.[46]

In patients who have lymph node involvement, traditional megavoltage (4 to 15 MeV) photon irradiation may be helpful in providing important additional palliation. Doses of 30 to 36 Gy in 3 to 4 weeks are often sufficient to achieve local control of lymph node or other extracutaneous disease.[47]

Systemic Chemotherapy Systemic chemotherapy is appropriate for patients with extracutaneous disease and many who present with the Sézary syndrome, however, most chemotherapy regimens result in only temporary palliative responses. Only a minority of patients with MF (10–20%) requires systemic management however it may be an important palliative treatment for patients with Sézary syndrome. Virtually all drugs that are effective as single agents or in combination therapy in the treatment of patients with NHL have been tested in MF/SS.

For single agent chemotherapy, no particular drug is clearly superior and no large, randomized studies comparing agents have been reported. In 526 patients reported in single agent chemotherapy trials, the response rate was 20 to 80% and the median duration of responses ranged from 3 to 22 months.[48] The most data exist for methotrexate, which has activity in many doses and schedules.[49–51] It is not clear that high-dose methotrexate is superior to lower-dose methotrexate therapy. With low dose methotrexate, the overall response rate (ORR) ranges from 33 to 58 %, and the time to treatment failure is 15 to 32 months, depending upon the extent of prior therapy.[52] Another common single agent has been chlorambucil[53] administered daily in 2 mg doses titrating the dose according to hematologic toxicity. Prednisone has been given at 20 mg/day initially with a taper as palliation is achieved. Some newer drugs have shown encouraging single activity in early clinical trials and are summarized in Table 119-3.

The purine analogs are a class of drugs that have demonstrated activity in MF and a variety of other non-Hodgkin's lymphomas. T cells have a high level of adenosine deaminase (ADA), a key enzyme in the purine degradation pathway. The purine analogs pentostatin (deoxycoformycin), fludarabine, and cladribine (2 CDA) are a group of structurally similar agents that were developed to target ADA. They have different interactions with ADA but all result in DNA damage. The

Table 119-3 Results of Chemotherapy Treatment in Mycosis Fungoides

Study	Therapy	Patients	ORR n (%)	CR	Med. Duration of Response (Months)
Single Agent Chemotherapy					
Bunn et al[48]	Single Agent Chemotherapy	528	329 (62)	91 (33)	3–32
Zackheim et al[52]	Low dose methotrexate	69	20 (33)	13 (22)	15
Holmes et al[53]	Chlorambucil + Prednisone	21	11 (57)	3 (14)	Not reported
Tsimberidau et al[55]	Pentostatin	32	13 (54.8)	6 (14)	4.3
Saven et al[56]	2 CDA	15	7 (47)	3 (20)	5
Kuzel et al[57]	2 CDA	21	6 (28)	3 (14)	2–16
Zinzani et al[62]	Gemcitabine	30	21(70)	5 (11)	6–22
Wollina et al[63]	Liposomal doxorubicin	6	5(83)	4/6	Not reported
Combination Chemotherapy					
Bunn et al[48]	Combination	331	(81)	(38)	5–41
Kaye et al[72]	CAVE	52	47 (90)	20 (38)	Not reported
Fierro et al[68]	VICOB-P	25	(80)	(36)	8–7

largest overall experience has been with Pentostatin, although each individual study is small. The response rates vary from 14 to 70%.[54,55] 2-CDA,[56,57] and Fludarabine[58,59] have also been used with a response rate of 20 to 40%. Hematologic toxicity and opportunistic infections are the most common complications associated with this class of drugs. Prophylactic antibiotics against *Pneumocystis carinii* and anti-virals to prevent herpes virus infection are routinely indicated. Combinations of purine analogs with interferon have also been used in small studies and show an increased response rate compared with series using these agents alone.[60]

Gemcitabine (2'2'-difluorodeoxycytidine, Gemzar) a novel nucleoside analog is a deoxycytidine analog with excellent antitumor activity against a number of solid tumors and lymphoproliferative disorders.[61] Gemcitabine must be activated by deoxycytidine kinase and other kinases to its triphosphate form, gemcitabine triphosphate, that can then be incorporated into RNA and DNA. The latter action causes masked chain termination and inhibition of DNA repair and is considered responsible for its antitumor effect. Response rates as high as 70%[62] have been reported, but the complete remission rate is low.

Pegylated liposomes are stable, long-circulating carriers useful for delivering doxorubicin to tumor sites with a lower toxicity than the free drug. In a study of patients who had refractory or relapsed CTCl, pegylated doxorubicin (Doxil) was given as 20 mg/m^2 every month until a CR was achieved or a total dose of 400 mg.[63] An overall response rate of 80% and response duration of 15 months were reported. The most frequent side effects were mild anemia and lymphopenia.

Another new cytotoxic agent is temozolomide that showed encouraging activity in MF in phase I studies[64] and needs prospective further testing. Its mechanism of action is similar to other alkylating agents. It induces DNA damage by cross-linking and resistance has been associated with high levels of the scavenger protein O 6-alkylguanine DNA alkyltransferase in tumor cells. In one series, 22 pts with relapsed stage IB to IVA were treated and there was a 26% overall response rate.[65]

There are no randomized trials comparing combination chemotherapy with single agent regimens. The largest experience is with combinations that include cyclophosphamide, vincristine, and prednisone with or without doxorubicin.[66,67] Complete response rates are generally about 25% (range 11–57%) and response duration 3 to 20 months. Most of the patients treated with combination chemotherapy have advanced disease (IIB to IV), although a few patients with early stage disease (IA–IIA) who had a CR were disease free (with short follow up) at the time of the reports.[48]

An intensive regimen as front line therapy has been reported using VICOB-P (etoposide, idarubicin, cyclophosphamide, vincristine, prednisone, and bleomycin).[68] This intensive regimen was administered weekly for 12 weeks with a response rate of 80% (CR 36%). The median duration of response was 6 to 7 months, similar to that reported for CHOP chemotherapy. No response was seen in patients with Sézary syndrome.

At one time, based on uncontrolled studies, combined modality therapy with combination chemotherapy and total skin irradiation was proposed as a preferred treatment.[69–71] This concept was then tested in a prospective randomized trial at the NCI, which compared an aggressive program of combination chemotherapy (cyclophosphamide, doxorubin, vincristine, and etoposide) and total skin electron beam irradiation with sequential conservative therapies.[72] The objective response rates (90 vs 65%) and CR rates (38 vs 18%) were higher with the combined therapy. However, there was no difference in overall survival and considerably greater toxicity in the combination therapy group.

There are several reports of combining chemotherapy with biological agents such as targeted toxins and immunomodulating agents that appear encouraging and need to be confirmed in large prospective studies.[73]

High Dose Chemotherapy with Hematopoietic Cell Transplant Recent interest has been shown in using high dose chemotherapy followed by peripheral stem cell support (autologous or allogenic) in mycosis fungoides. Given the small number of patients treated thus far, there are no well-defined prognostic factors to identify patients suitable for this therapy. Recent studies are summarized in Table 119-4.

Bigler and associates[74] reported that five of six patients achieved a CR with an autologous transplant. Three of the responses lasted less than 100 days and two patients were disease-free at 1 year. In another study,[75] eight of nine patients achieved a CR of brief duration, 2 months in four of the patients, but three others were disease-free at 11 months. All patients in those two studies ultimately relapsed, suggesting that autologous transplant is not a curative approach.

Auto-transplantation with T-cell depletion has also been reported. In a pilot study,[76] nine patients had their apheresis products treated with immunomagnetic methods for T cell depletion. Eight of nine patients engrafted and seven achieved a CR. Although all patients relapsed, at a median of 7 months, they generally relapsed with less advanced disease that responded to conventional therapy.

The concept of allogenic hematopoietic cell transplantation is provocative, since even in the absence of a CR an allogenic graft versus tumor effect may provide an immune mechanism to control the malignant T-cell process. In a report by Guitart and associates,[77] three patients received an allograft from HLA-matched siblings. Complete and sustained clinical and histologic remissions were achieved in two patients that continued for 4.5+ years, and 15+ months. The third patient was in CR for 9 months followed by a limited cutaneous recurrence.

Molina and associates[78] reported a CR in all six patients transplanted for refractory disease. Five patients remained in CR at a median follow up of 17 months (range 3–65 months). Mild acute and chronic GVHD developed in all patients.

A non-myeloablative approach has also been reported.[79] All three patients achieved a durable CR but there was a high incidence of infection.

Thus, it appears that compared to autologous HSCT, allogenic HSCT may result in durable long-term remissions. With better understanding of the disease biology and with newer molecular characteristics it may be possible to identify patients and develop prognostic factors so that these aggressive approaches can be offered to suitable patients. Larger studies will be required to identify the best conditioning regimen, efficacy, safety, and impact on quality of life.

Extracorporeal Photopheresis Photopheresis (extracorporeal photopheresis [ECPP] or systemic photochemotherapy) is a method of delivering PUVA systemically by using an extracorporeal technique.[80] The patients are first given a photoactivating drug (8-methoxypsoralen, Uvadex), their white blood cells are then collected via leukapheresis and irradiated with UVA, and the irradiated cells are returned to the patient intravenously. The mechanism of action of photopheresis remains unclear. The treatment is believed to induce apoptosis of circulating tumor cells (Sézary cells). The released tumor antigen is then processed by the peripheral dendritic cells leading to the augmentation of systemic antitumor responses.[81] Photopheresis is usually given every 4 weeks, but in patients with severe disease, it can be given as often as every 2 to 3 weeks. Once complete clearance is achieved, the frequency can be gradually reduced and then discontinued.

In erythrodermic (T4) MF and SS, ECPP is considered an initial treatment of choice.[22,82,83] The largest study of erythrodermic patients[84] revealed that the majority experienced some level of response to ECPP, with an overall response rate of 83%. The CR rate was only 21%, but 41% of patients showed at least a 50% improvement in

Table 119-4 Results of High-Dose Therapy and Hematopoietic Cell Transplantation in Mycosis Fungoides

Study	Stage	*n*	# CR	Relapse
Autologous Hematopoietic Cell Transplantation				
Bigler et al[74]	IIB–IV B	5	4	4 pts < 1 y, 1 pt > 1 y
Russel-Jones et al[75]	IIB–IV B	9	8	4 pts < 3 mo, 3 pts > 11 mo
Olavarria et al[76]	IIB–IV B	9	7	All in 1 yr
Allogeneic Hematopoietic Cell Transplantation				
Soligo et al[79]	IV	3	3	16 mo, 12 mo
Guitart et al[77]	IIB–IVA	3	3	10 mo, 26 mo +, 67 mo +

their disease. In another study, a higher proportion of Sézary cells as a percentage of the total white blood cell count correlated with an increased likelihood of a clinical response at 6 months.[85] If the response to ECPP alone is partial or slow, IFN-alpha or systemic bexarotene can be added as a combined modality regimen.[86,87] The efficacy of ECPP in T1, T2, and T3 disease remains unclear.[86]

ECPP has minimal adverse effects. Some patients may experience nausea, mostly due to the ingested psoralen, and some have a transient low-grade fever or slight malaise after treatment. There are no reports of significant organ damage or bone marrow or immune suppression.

Interferon Alpha IFN-alpha is indicated for the palliative management of refractory or advanced disease. It may be used alone, but more often with other topical or systemic therapies. Administration is usually initiated at a low dose of 3 to 5 million units subcutaneously given three times a week. This dose is gradually increased, depending on the clinical response and the severity of adverse effects. Reported overall response rates when used as monotherapy are 53 to 74%, with CR rates of 21 to 35%.[40,88,89] The clinical response and response duration appear to be better with the combined regimen of PUVA and IFN, as compared with either treatment alone, but randomized prospective clinical trials are needed to confirm this impression.[86,90]

Retinoids Systemic retinoid therapy, most commonly bexarotene, has been shown to be beneficial in the management of MF and SS. The initial dose of bexarotene is 100 to 300 mg/m^2/day, which can be adjusted according to clinical response and the severity of adverse effects, especially hyperlipidemia. Systemic retinoids are indicated for palliative therapy for refractory or advanced disease, often in combination with other topical or systemic therapies, including PUVA (Re-PUVA), IFN-α, or total skin electron beam therapy.[41,91–93] The reported response rate is approximately 45%, with a 20% CR rate.[94] When retinoids were used in combination with PUVA (RePUVA), the response rate was similar to that of PUVA alone; however, the responses were obtained with fewer PUVA treatments and with a lower cumulative UVA dose.[41] The duration of remission tended to be prolonged if retinoids were given as maintenance therapy.

The most common complications of systemic bexarotene therapy include photosensitivity, xerosis, myalgia, arthralgia, headaches, and impaired night vision. The well-known teratogenic effects of retinoids must be considered in women of child-bearing age. Because of its potential hepatotoxic and hyperlipidemic effects, liver function and serum lipid levels should be monitored in each patient during treatment. In addition, central hypothyroidism is often induced, so patients are routinely started on levothyroxin immediately before bexarotene and lipid lowering agents are also often required. Most toxicities due to systemic retinoids are reversible after cessation of therapy.

Recombinant Fusion Proteins Recombinant fusion protein therapy, such as the IL-2–diphtheria toxin fusion protein (Ontak, denileukin diftitox), involves the use of growth factor–diphtheria toxin fusion proteins designed specifically to kill defined neoplastic cell populations. Ontak has undergone a multicenter phase III trial in patients with IL-2 receptor (CD25+)-expressing MF.[95] Patients with stage IB to III MF who failed to respond to multiple prior therapies, or stage IVA MF who failed to respond to at least one prior therapy, were included in the phase III trial. The overall response rate was 30%, with CR and PR rates of 10 and 20%, respectively. The main complication related to a "capillary leak" syndrome, which may be ameliorated by pretreatment with corticosteroids. Ontak was approved by the FDA for patients with cutaneous T-cell lymphoma who have persistent or recurrent disease and whose malignant cells express CD25.

Miscellaneous Biologic Agents There have been case reports and anecdotal observations regarding the use of a variety of biologic agents for treating MF, including heat-killed BCG and cord factor,[96] transfer factor,[97] thymidine,[98] acyclovir,[99] cyclosporin,[99] and recombinant interleukin 2.[100] However, none of these has proved to be efficacious over time. In fact, contraindications to the use of cyclosporin have been reported in the literature.[101,102]

Novel Therapies Knowledge of the immunology of MF and its incurability, especially in the advanced stages, has led to the development of a variety of newer therapies. The efficacy of anti–T-cell antibodies has been studied in MF. Early trials using murine monoclonal antibodies were unsuccessful due to the development of human anti–mouse antibodies (HAMA). More recently, a chimeric anti–helper-T-cell (anti-CD4) antibody was used in order to provide more specific treatment against the MF subset of T cells, and to avoid the development of HAMA.[103] In addition, humanized anti-CD3 and anti-CD4 antibodies have been developed and have just entered clinical trials.

The safety and efficacy of alemtuzumab (Campath-1H), a humanized monoclonal antibody directed against CD52, was tested in 22 previously treated patients, most of whom had stage III or IV disease, reduced performance status, and severe pruritus.[94,95] Complete and partial responses were noted in 32 and 23%, respectively, with a median time to treatment failure of 12 months. Serious infections (CMV, generalized herpes simplex, fatal aspergillosis and mycobacterium pneumonia) were noted, especially in patients who had received more than three prior treatment regimens. These patients require antibiotic and antiviral prophylaxis and close observation for the development of infection and cardiac toxicity.

As TLR9 agonists, CpG oligonucleotides (CpG ODNs) are potent immunostimulatory agents being developed for cancer therapy. CPG 7909 is a synthetic 24-mer ODN developed to optimally stimulate the human immune function and is currently undergoing a phase I/II trial in patients with cutaneous T-cell lymphomas.

Histone deacetylase inhibitors (HDAI) are a novel class of agents that can induce tumor cell growth arrest, differentiation, or apoptosis. Suberoylanilide hydroxamic acid (SAHA) is an oral HDAI agent that is currently undergoing a phase IIb multicenter trial in patients with cutaneous T-cell lymphoma.[104,105]

Photodynamic therapy, using nonionizing laser light after topical or systemic application of a photosensitizing agent, such as 5-aminolevulinic acid, has been used for the local treatment of cutaneous lesions in a small number of patients with MF.[106,107] Most of these reports have involved successful treatment of single lesions resistant to treatment with other agents. Toxicity is minimal, and has been limited to local pain, erythema, or blistering.

REFERENCES

1. Kim YH, Hoppe RT. Mycosis fungoides and the Sézary syndrome. Seminars in Oncology 1999; 26:276–89.
2. Weinstock M. Mycosis fungoides in the United States—increasing incidence and descriptive epidemiology. J Clin Oncol 1988; 260:42–60.
3. Crowley JJ, Nikko A, Varghese A, et al. Mycosis fungoides in young patients: clinical characteristics and outcome. Journal of the American Academy of Dermatology 1998;38:696–701.
4. Whittemore A, Holly E, Lee I, et al. Mycosis fungoides in relation to environmental exposures and immune response: a case-control study. J Natl Cancer Inst 1989;81:1560–7.
5. Bunn PA Jr, Schechter GP, Jaffe E, et al. Clinical course of retrovirus-associated adult T-cell lymphoma in the United States. N Engl J Med 1983;309:257–64.
6. Wood G, Savekar A, Schaffer J, et al. Evidence against a role for HTLV-I in the pathogenesis of American cutaneous T-cell lymphoma. J Invest Dermatol 1996;107:301–7.
7. Wood GS, Weiss L, Warnke R, et al. The immunopathology of cutaneous lymphomas: Immunophenotypic and immunogenotypic characteristics. Semin Dermatol 1986;5:334–45.
8. Weiss L, Hu E, Wood GS, et al. Clonal rearrangements of T-cell receptor genes in mycosis fungoides and dermatopathic lymphadenopathy. J Invest Dermatol 1985;85:199–202.
9. Ashton-Key M, Diss TC, Du MQ, et al. The value of the polymerase chain reaction in the diagnosis of cutaneous T-cell infiltrates. Am J Surg Pathol 1997;21:743–7.
10. Clendenning WE, Rappaport H. Report of the Committee on Pathology of Cutaneous T Cell Lymphomas. Cancer Treat Rep 1979;63:719–21.
11. Sausville E, Worsha G, Matthews M, et al. Histologic assessment of lymph nodes in mycosis fungoides/Sézary syndrome (cutaneous T-cell lymphoma): clinical correlations and prognostic import of a new classification system. Am J Clin Pathol 1985;84:610–9.
12. Kern DE, Kidd PG, Moe R, et al. Analysis of T-cell receptor gene rearrangement in lymph nodes of patients with mycosis fungoides. Prognostic implications. Arch Dermatol 1998;134:158–64.
13. Wieselthier JS, Koh HK. Sézary syndrome: diagnosis, prognosis, and critical review of treatment options. J Am Acad Dermatol 1990;22:381–401.
14. Kim YH, Jensen RA, Watanabe GL, et al. Clinical stage IA (limited patch and plaque) mycosis fungoides. A long-term outcome analysis. Archives of Dermatology 1996;132:1309–13.
15. Kim YH, Chow S, Varghese A, et al. Clinical characteristics and long-term outcome of patients with generalized patch and/or plaque (T2) mycosis fungoides. Archives of Dermatology 1999;135:26–32.
16. Kim YH, Liu HL, Mraz-Gernhard S, et al. Longterm outcome of 525 patients with mycosis fungoides and Sézary syndrome at Stanford: Clinical prognostic factors and risks of disease progression and second cancer. Archives of Dermatology 2003;139:857–66.
17. Epstein EH Jr, Levin DL, Croft JD Jr, et al. Mycosis fungoides. Survival, prognostic features, response to therapy,

and autopsy findings. Medicine (Baltimore) 1972;51:61–72.

18. Shiora T, Moriya N, Gotoh C, et al. Differential expression of lymphocyte function-associated antigen 1 (LFA-1) on epidermotropic and non-epidermotropic T-cell clones. J Invest Dermatol 1989;93:804–8.
19. Kohler S, Zehnder JL. Use of the polymerase chain reaction in the evaluation of cutaneous T-cell infiltrates. Dermatol Clin 1999;17:657–66.
20. Harmon C, Witzig T, Katzmann J, et al. Detection of circulating T cells with CD4+CD7-immunophenotype in patients with benign and malignant lymphoproliferative dermatoses. J Am Acad Dermatol 1996;35:404–10.
21. Muche JM, Lukowsky A, Asadullah K, et al. Demonstration of frequent occurrence of clonal T cells in the peripheral blood of patients with primary cutaneous T-cell lymphoma. Blood 1997; 90:1636-42.
23. Kulin PA, Marglin SI, Shuman WP, et al. Diagnostic imaging in the initial staging of mycosis fungoides and Sézary syndrome. Arch Dermatol 1990;126:914–8.
24. Tsai E. Staging accuracy in mycosis fungoides/Sézary syndrome using integrated positron emission tomography and computed tomography. Accepted for publication in Arch Dermatol.
25. Bunn PA, Lambert SI. Report of the Committee on Staging and Classification of Cutaneous T-cell Lymphomas. Cancer Treatment Reports 1979;63:725.
26. Sausville EA, Eddy JL, Makuch RW, et al. Histopathologic staging at initial diagnosis of mycosis fungoides and the Sézary syndrome. Definition of three distinctive prognostic groups. Ann Intern Med 1988;109:372–82.
27. Kim YH, Bishop K, Varghese A, et al. Prognostic factors in erythrodermic mycosis fungoides and the Sézary syndrome [see comments]. Archives of Dermatology 1995;131:1003–8.
28. de Coninck EC, Kim YH, Varghese A, et al. Clinical characteristics and outcome of patients with extracutaneous mycosis fungoides. Journal of Clinical Oncology 2001;19:779–84.
29. Wood GS, Bahler DW, Hoppe RT, et al. Transformation of mycosis fungoides: T-cell receptor beta gene analysis demonstrates a common clonal origin for plaque-type mycosis fungoides and CD30+ large-cell lymphoma. Journal of Investigative Dermatology 1993;101:296–300.
30. Ramsey D, Halperin P, Zeleniuch-Jacquotte A. Topical mechlorethamine therapy for early stage mycosis fungoides. J Am Acad Dermatol 1988;19:684–91.
31. Vonderheid EC, Tan ET, Kantor AF, et al. Long-term efficacy, curative potential, and carcinogenicity of topical mechlorethamine chemotherapy in cutaneous T cell lymphoma. J Am Acad Dermatol 1989;20:416–28.
32. Kim YH, Martinez G, Varghese A, et al. Management with topical nitrogen mustard in mycosis fungoides: update of the Stanford experience. Arch Dermatol 2003;139:165–73.
33. Smoller BR, Marcus R. Risk of secondary cutaneous malignancies in patients with long-standing mycosis fungoides. J Am Acad Dermatol 1994;30:201–4.
34. Breneman D, Duvic M, Kuzel T, et al. Phase 1 and 2 trial of bexarotene gel for skin-directed treatment of patients with cutaneous T-cell lymphoma. Arch Dermatol 2002;138:325–32.
35. Heald P, Mehlmauer M, Martin AG, et al. Topical bexarotene therapy for patients with refractory or persistent early-stage cutaneous T-cell lymphoma: results of the Phase III clinical trial. J Am Acad Dermatol 2003;49:801.
36. Gathers RC, Scherschun L, Malick F, et al. Narrowband UVB phototherapy for early-stage mycosis fungoides. J Am Acad Dermatol 2002;2002:191.
37. Resnik KS, Vonderheid EC. Home UV phototherapy of early mycosis fungoides: long-term follow-up observations in thirty-one patients. J Am Acad Dermatol 1993;29:73–7.
38. Pabsch H, Rutten A, Von Stemm A, et al. Treatment of childhood mycosis fungoides with topical PUVA. J Am Acad Dermatol 2002;47:557.
39. Diederen PV, Van Weelden H, Sanders CJ, et al. Narrowband UVB and psoralen-UVA in the treatment of early stage mycosis fungoides: a retrospective study. J Am Acad Dermatol 2003;48:215.
40. Kuzel TM, Roenigk HH Jr, Samuelson E, et al. Effectiveness of interferon alfa-2a combined with phototherapy for mycosis fungoides and the Sézary syndrome. J Clin Oncol 1995;13:257–63.
41. Thomsen K, Hammar H, Molin L, et al. Retinoids plus PUVA (RePUVA) in mycosis fungoides, plaque stage. A report from the Scandinavian Mycosis Fungoides Group. Acta Dermatol Venereol (Stockh) 1989;69:217–22.
42. Group BP. British Photodermatology Group guidelines for PUVA. Br J Dermatol 1994;130:246–55.
43. Jones GW, Hoppe RT, Glatstein E. Electron beam treatment for cutaneous T-cell lymphoma. Hematology/Oncology Clinics of North America 1995;9:1057–76.
44. Hoppe R. Total skin electron beam therapy in the management of mycosis fungoides. In: Vaeth J, Meyer J, editors. Front Radiat Ther Oncol. The Role of High Energy Electrons in the Treatment of Cancer, Vol. 25. Basel Switzerland: S Karger, 1991. p. 80–89.
45. Jones GW, Tadros A, Hodson DI, et al. Prognosis with newly diagnosed mycosis fungoides after total skin electron radiation of 30 or 35 GY. Int J Radiat Oncol Biol Phys 1994;28:839–45.
46. Becker M, Hoppe RT, Knox SJ. Multiple courses of high-dose total skin electron beam therapy in the management of mycosis fungoides. Int J Radiat Oncol Biol Phys 1995;32:1445–9.
47. Hoppe R. Mycosis fungoides: radiation therapy. Dermatol Ther 2003;16:347–54.
48. Bunn PA Jr, Hoffman SJ, Norris D, et al. Systemic therapy of cutaneous T-cell lymphomas (mycosis fungoides and the Sézary syndrome). Ann Intern Med 1994;121:592–602.
49. McDonald C, Bertino JR. Treatment of mycosis fungoides lymphoma: effectiveness of infusions of methotrexate followed by oral citrovorum factor. Cancer Treat Rep 1978;62:1009–14.
50. Schappell DL, Alper JC, McDonald C. Treatment of advanced mycosis fungoides and Sézary syndrome with continuous infusions of methotrexate followed by fluorouracil and leucovorin rescue. Arch Dermatol 1995;131:307–13.
51. Zackheim HS, Epstein EH Jr. Low-dose methotrexate for the Sézary syndrome. J Am Acad Dermatol 1989;21:757–62.
52. Zackheim HS, Kashani-Sabet M, McMillan AK. Low dose methotrexate to treat mycosis fungoides: a retrospective study in 69 patients. J Am Acad Dermatol 2003;49:873–8.
53. Holmes RC, McGibbon DH, Black MM. Mycosis fungoides: progression towards Sézary syndrome reversed with chlorambucil. Clin Exp Dermatol 1983;8:429–35.
54. Greiner D, Olsen EA, Petroni G. Pentostatin (2'-deoxycoformycin) in the treatment of cutaneous T-cell lymphoma. J Am Acad Dermatol 1997;36:950–5.
55. Tsimberidon AM, Giles F, Duvic M, et al. Phase II study of pentostatin in advanced T-cell lymphoid malignancies: update of an M.D. Anderson Cancer Center series. Cancer 2004;100:342–9.
56. Saven A, Carrera CJ, Carson DA, et al. 2-chlorodeoxyadenosine: an active agent in the treatment of cutaneous T-cell lymphoma. Blood 1992;80:587–92.
57. Kuzel T, Hurria A, Samuelson E, et al. Rose Phase II trial of 2-chlorodeoxyadenosine for the treatment of cutaneous T-cell lymphoma. Blood 1996;87:906–11.
58. Quaglino P, Fierro MT, Rossotto GL, et al. Treatment of advanced mycosis fungoides/Sézary syndrome with fludarabine and potential adjunctive benefit to subsequent extracorporeal photochemotherapy. Br J Dermatol 2004;150:327–36.
59. Von Hoff D, Dahlberg S, Hartsock R, et al. Activity of fludarabine monophosphate in patients with advanced mycosis fungoides: Southwest Oncology Group study. J Natl Cancer Inst 1990;82:1353–5.
60. Foss F, Waldmann TA. Interluekin-2 receptor-directed therapies for cutaneous lymphomas. Oncol Clin North Am 2003;17:1449–58.
61. Fossa A, Santoro A, Hiddemann W, et al. Gemcitabine as a single agent in the treatment of relapsed or refractory aggressive non-Hodgkin's lymphoma. J Clinical Oncology 1999;17:3786–92.
62. Zinzani PL, Baliva G, Magagnoli M, et al. Gemcitabine treatment in pretreated cutaneous T-cell lymphoma: experience in 44 patients. J Clin Oncol 2000;18:2603–6.
63. Wollina U, Graefe T, Karte K. Treatment of relapsing or recalcitrant cutaneous T-cell lymphoma with pegylated liposomal doxorubicin. J Am Acad Dermatol 2000;42(1 Pt 1):40–6.
64. Newlands ES, Blackledge G, Slack JA, et al. Phase I trial of temozolomide (CCRG 81045: M&B 38931:NSC 362856. Br J Cancer 1992;65:287–91.
65. Rosen SG, Guitart J, Martone E, et al. Phase II trial of temozolomide (TMZ) for treatment of mycosis fungoides/Sézary syndrome (MF/SS). Proceedings ASCO 2002;21:286a.
66. Molin L, Thomsen K, Volden G, et al. Combination chemotherapy in the tumour stage of mycosis fungoides with cyclophosphamide, vincristine, vp-16, Adriamycin and prednisone (COP, CHOP, CAVOP): a report from the Scandinavian mycosis fungoides study group. Acta Derm Venereol 1980;60:542–4.
67. Tirelli U, Carbone A, Zagonel V, et al. Staging and treatment with cyclophosphamide, vincristine and prednisone (CVP) in advanced cutaneous T-cell lymphomas. Hematol Oncol 1986;4:83–90.
68. Fierro MT, Doveil GC, Quaglino P, et al. Combination of etoposide, idarubicin, cyclophosphamide, vincristine, prednisone and bleomycin (VICOP-B) in the treatment of advanced cutaneous T-cell lymphoma. Dermatology 1997;194:268–72.
69. Greim ML, Tokars RP, Petras V, et al. Combined therapy for patients with mycosis fungoides. Cancer Treat Rep 1979;63:655–7.
70. Winkler CF, Sausville EA, Ihde DC. Combined modality treatment of cutaneous T cell lymphoma: Results of a 6-year follow up. J Clin Oncol 1986;4:1094–1100.
71. Braverman IM, Yager NB, Chen MG, et al. Combined total body electron beam irradiation and chemotherapy for mycosis fungoides. J Am Acad Dermatol 1987;16:45–60.
72. Kaye FJ, Bunn PA Jr, Steinberg SM, et al. A randomized trial comparing combination electron-beam radiation and chemotherapy with topical therapy in the initial treatment of mycosis fungoides. N Engl J Med 1989;321:1784–90.
73. Duvic M, Apisarnthanarax M, Cohen DS, et al. Analysis of long-term outcomes of combined modality therapy for cutaneous T-cell lymphoma. J Am Acad Dermatol 2003;49:35–49.
74. Bigler RD, Crilley P, Micaily B, et al. Autologous bone marrow transplantation for advanced stage mycosis fungoides. Bone Marrow Transplant 1991;7:133–7.
75. Russell-Jones R, Child F, Olavarria E, et al. Autologous peripheral blood stem cell transplantation in tumor-stage mycosis fungoides: predictors of disease-free survival. Ann N Y Acad Sci 2001;941:147–54.
76. Olavarria E, Child F, Woolford A, et al. T-cell depletion and autologous stem cell transplantation in the management of tumour stage mycosis fungoides with peripheral blood involvement. Br J Haematol 2001;114:624–31.
77. Guitart J, Wickless SC, Oyama Y, et al. Long-term remission after allogeneic hematopoietic stem cell transplantation for refractory cutaneous T-cell lymphoma. Arch Dermatol 2002;138:1359–65.
78. Molina A, Aber D, Collins JL, et al. Clinical, cytogenetic and molecular remission after allogenic hematopoietic stem cell transplantation for refractory Sézary syndrome and tumor stage mycoses fungoides [abstract]. Blood 2001;98(Suppl):409a.
79. Soligo D, Ibatici A, Berti E, et al. Treatment of advanced mycosis fungoides by allogeneic stem-cell transplantation with a nonmyeloablative regimen. Bone Marrow Transplant 2003;31:663–6.
80. Edelson RL, Heald P, Perez M, et al. Photopheresis update. Prog Dermatol 1991;25:1–6.
81. Edelson RL. Cutaneous T-cell lymphoma. the helping hand of dendritic cells. Ann N Y Acad Sci 2001;941.
82. Holloway KB, Flowers FP, Ramos-Caro FA. Therapeutic alternatives in cutaneous T-cell lymphoma. J Am Acad Dermatol 1992;27:367–78.
83. Lim HW, Edelson RL. Photopheresis for the treatment of cutaneous T-cell lymphoma. Hematol Oncol Clin North Am 1995;9:1117–26.
84. Heald P, Rook AH, Perez M, et al. Treatment of erythrodermic cutaneous T-cell lymphoma with extracorporeal photochemotherapy. J Am Acta Dermatol 1992;27:427–33.
85. Evans AV, Wood BP, Scarisbrick JJ, et al. Extracorporeal photopheresis in Sézary syndrome: hematologic parameters as predictors of response. Blood 2001;98:1298.
86. Gottlieb SL, Wolfe JT, Fox FE, et al. Treatment of cutaneous T-cell lymphoma with extracorporeal photopheresis monotherapy and in combination with recombinant interferon alfa: a 10-year experience at a single institution. J Am Acad Dermatol 1996;35:946–57.
87. Suchinal E. Treatment of cutaneous T-cell lymphoma with combined immunomodulatory therapy: a 14-year experience at a single institution. Arch Dermatol 2002;138:1054–60.
88. Chiarion-Sileni V, Bononi A, Fornasa CV, et al. Phase II trial of interferon-alpha-2a plus psoralen with ultraviolet light A in patients with cutaneous T-cell lymphoma. Cancer 2002;95:569.
89. Roenigk HJ, Kuzel TM, Skoutelis A, et al. Photochemotherapy alone or combined with interferon alpha-2a in the treatment of cutaneous T-cell lymphoma. J Invest Dermatol 1990;95(Suppl):198–205.

90. Mostow EN, Neckel SL, Oberhelman L, et al. Complete remissions in psoralen and UV-A (PUVA)-refractory mycosis fungoides-type cutaneous T-cell lymphoma with combined interferon alfa and PUVA. Arch Dermatol 1993;129:747–52.
91. Duvic M, Lemak NA, Redman JR, et al. Combined modality therapy for cutaneous T-cell lymphoma. J Am Acad Dermatol 1996;34:1022–9.
92. Knobler RM, Trautinger F, Radaszkiewicz T, et al. Treatment of cutaneous T cell lymphoma with a combination of low-dose interferon alfa-2b and retinoids. J Am Acad Dermatol 1991;24:247–52.
93. Jones G, McLean J, Rosenthal D, et al. Combined treatment with oral etretinate and electron beam therapy in patients with cutaneous T-cell lymphoma (mycosis fungoides and Sézary syndrome). J Am Acad Dermatol 1992;26:960–7.
94. Duvic M, Martin AG, Kim Y, et al. Phase 2 and 3 clinical trial of oral bexarotene (Targretin capsules) for the treatment of refractory or persistent early-stage cutaneous T-cell lymphoma. Arch Dermatol 2001;137:581–93.
95. Olsen E, Duvic M, Frankel A, et al. Pivotal phase III trial of two dose levels of denileukin diftitox for the treatment of cutaneous T-cell lymphoma. J Clin Oncol 2001;19:376–88.
96. Cohen HA, Bekierkunst A. Treatment of mycosis fungoides with heat-killed BCG and cord factor. Dermatologica 1979; 158:104–16.
97. Zachariae H, Grunnet E, Thestrup-Pedersen K. Transfer factor in mycosis fungoides: A case report on a patient "cured". Arch Dermatovener (Stockholm) 1979;59:375–8.
98. Kufe DW, Wick MM, Moschella S, et al. Effect of high-dose thymidine infusions in patients with mycosis fungoides. Cancer 1981;48:1513–6.
99. Resnick L, Schleider-Kushner N, Horwitz SN, et al. Remission of tumor-stage mycosis fungoides following intravenously administered acyclovir. JAMA 1984;251:1571–3.
100. Nagatani T, Kin S-T, Baba N, et al. A case of cutaneous T cell lymphoma treated with recombinant interleukin 2 (rIL-2). Arch Derm Venereol (Stockh) 1988;68:504–8.
101. Pielop JA, Jones D, Duvic M. Transient CD30+ nodal transformation of cutaneous T-cell lymphoma associated with cyclosporine treatment. Int J Dermatol 2001;40:505–11.
102. Zachkeim HS, Koo J, LeBoit PE, et al. Psoriasiform mycosis fungoides with fatal outcome after treatment with cyclosporine. J Am Acad Dermatol 2002;47:155–7.
103 Knox S, Levy R, Hodgkinson S, et al. Observations on the effect of chimeric-anti-CD4 monoclonal antibody in patients with mycosis fungoides. Blood 1991;77:20–30.
104. Lundin J, Hagberg H, Repp R, et al. Phase 2 study of alemtuzumab (anti-CD52 monoclonal antibody) in patients with advanced mycosis fungoides/Sézary syndrome. Blood 2003;101:4267.
105. Lenihan DJ, Alencar AJ, Yang D, et al. Cardiac toxicity of alemtuzumab in patients with mycosis fungoides/Sézary syndrome. Blood 2004; 104:655.
106. Edstrom DW, Porwit A, Ros AM. Photodynamic therapy with topical 5-aminolevulinic acid for mycosis fungoides: clinical and histological response. Acta Dermato-Venereologica 2001; 81:184.
107. Coors EA, Von Den DP. Topical photodynamic therapy for patients with therapy-resistant lesions of cutaneous T-cell lymphoma. J Am Acad Dermatol 2004;50:363.

Plasma Cell Tumors

Noopur Raje, MD, MB, BS
Teru Hideshima, MD, PhD
Kenneth C. Anderson, MD

MULTIPLE MYELOMA

Multiple myeloma (MM) is a malignant proliferation of plasma cells and plasmacytoid cells in the bone marrow (BM) characterized nearly always by the presence, in the serum and/or urine, of a monoclonal immunoglobulin (Ig) or Ig fragment.[1–4] This disease has probably been recognized since 1845, when the first patient was noted with bone pain and heat soluble "animal matter" in urine.[5,6] The term MM was coined in 1873, reflecting distinct sites of BM involvement. The plasma cell was discovered in 1890 and MM associated with plasmacytosis shortly thereafter, in 1900. The application of electrophoresis in 1939 and immunoelectrophoresis in 1953 allowed for the identification of monotypic Ig characteristic of MM.[7,8]

Diagnostic Criteria Both major and minor criteria for the diagnosis of MM have been defined (Table 120-1).[9] These include the presence of excess monotypic marrow plasma cells, monoclonal Ig in serum and/or urine, decreased normal serum Ig levels, and lytic bone disease. MM must be distinguished from other disorders characterized by monoclonal gammopathies, both malignant and otherwise. These include monoclonal gammopathy of unclear significance (MGUS), macroglobulinemia, non-Hodgkin's lymphoma, primary amyloidosis, idiopathic cold agglutinin disease, essential cryoglobulinemia, and heavy chain disease.

Table 120-1 Durie and Salmon Criteria

Major Criteria
1. Plasmacytomas on tissue biopsy
2. Bone marrow plasmacytosis (>30% plasma cells)
3. Monoclonal immunoglobulin spike on serum electrophoresis immunoglobulin G (IgG) >3.5 g/dL or immunoglobulin A (IgA) >2.0 g/dL; kappa or lambda light chain excretion >1 g/day on 24 hour urine protein electrophoresis

Minor Criteria
1. Bone marrow plasmacytosis (10 to 30% plasma cells)
2. Monoclonal immunoglobulin present but of lesser magnitude than given under major criteria
3. Lytic bone lesions
4. Normal IgM < 50 mg/dL, IgA < 100 mg/dL or IgG < 600 mg/dL

Any of the following sets of criteria will confirm the diagnosis of multiple myeloma:
Any two of the major criteria
Major criterion 1 plus minor criterion 2, 3, or 4
Major criterion 3 plus minor criterion 1 or 3
Minor criterion 1, 2, and 3 or 1, 2 and 4

Monoclonal Gammopathy of Unclear Significance MGUS includes 2% of patients over 50 years old who have less than 3.5 gm/L monoclonal Ig, little or no proteinuria, fewer than 5% monoclonal marrow plasma cells, and no bone lesions, anemia, hypercalcemia, or renal dysfunction.[6] In a large experience of 1,384 patients diagnosed at the Mayo Clinic, 115 patients progressed to MM, IgM lymphoma, primary amyloidosis, macroglobulinemia, chronic lymphocytic leukemia, or plasmacytoma with relative risk of progression of 25.0, 2.4, 8.4, 46.0, 0.9, and 8.5, respectively.[10] The risk of progression of MGUS to MM or related disorders is about 1% per year, and the initial concentration of serum monoclonal protein was a significant predictor of progression at 20 years. Similar results have been published by Cesana and colleagues.[11] Independent prognostic factors influencing MGUS transformation included (1) greater than 5% BM plasmacytosis, (2) Bence Jones proteinuria, (3) decrease in polyclonal serum immunoglobulin, and (4) an elevated erythrocyte sedimentation rate. In some cases, MGUS can be associated with symptomatology requiring therapy. For example, plasma exchange appears to be efficacious in neuropathy associated with IgG or IgA MGUS.[12]

Epidemiology In addition to MGUS, a potential risk factor for the development of MM includes exposure to irradiation or petroleum products. Unlike leukemia, there is no increased risk of MM with benzene exposure.[13] Families with two or more affected individuals have been reported, suggesting a possible genetic predisposition.[14] MM has also been found to occur with somewhat greater frequency (but less than twofold) in farmers, paper producers, furniture manufacturers, and wood workers.

There are two major misconceptions regarding MM. The first is that MM is a rare disease. MM is the second most common hematologic malignancy, accounting for 15,270 new cancer cases in the United States in the year 2004 and approximately 2% of cancer-related deaths.[15] The highest incidence rates have been reported for African Americans and Pacific Islanders; Europeans and North American white people have intermediate rates, while generally low rates have been reported for Asians living in Asia and the United States.[16] Although it has been suggested that the incidence of MM is increasing, data from Olmstead County, Minnesota, demonstrate that the incidence of MM has not changed significantly during the past 46 years.[17] A second misunderstanding is that MM is solely a disease of the elderly. In a large Mayo Clinic series, the mean age was 62 years for men and 61 years for women.[4] Although 98% of MM patients were 40 years of age or older, 35% of men and 41% of women were less than 60 years old. Importantly, 75% of men and 79% of women were younger than age 70. The fact that a significant population of affected individuals is younger than age 70 and therefore can tolerate more aggressive therapeutic approaches influences potential treatment strategies.

Clinical Features The presenting features in 869 cases of MM evaluated from 1960 to 1971 are summarized in Tables 120-2a and b[4] Although there was a slight predominance of men (61%) in this series, other studies suggest that incidence in men and women may be equivalent. Symptoms of bone pain and anemia remain the most common presenting features.

Laboratory Features Laboratory evaluation identifies roentgenographic abnormalities in bone and monoclonal Ig in serum and/or urine in the majority of cases. In most series, 50 to 60% of patients with MM have both serum and urinary monoclonal protein; 20 to 30% of patients have serum without urinary protein; 15 to 20% of patients have monoclonal protein in urine only; and only 1 to 2% of patients do not secrete monoclonal protein in blood and/or urine.[18] IgG or IgA monoclonal proteins are most common, and IgD or IgE are rare. A biclonal process is much more common than previously appreciated, often only documented by immunofixation techniques. Thirty-three percent are IgG and IgA; 24% are IgM and IgG. It appears that patients with biclonal and IgD disease have prognoses similar to those patients with monoclonal disease.[19] Laboratory evaluation of quantitative immunoglobulins can distinguish MGUS from smoldering, indolent, and overt MM (Table 120-3). It provides the basis for staging systems to predict both response and survival. No therapy is an appropriate choice for patients with MGUS, or smoldering and indolent MM, whereas multiple regimens have been employed for therapy of individuals

Table 120-2a Presenting Features of Multiple Myeloma

Percentage of Patients	Presenting Feature
98	More than 40 years old
88	Proteinuria
79	Skeletal roentgenographic abnormalities
68	Bone pain
62	Anemia
61	Male
55	Renal insufficiency
49	Bence Jones proteinuria
30	Hypercalcemia
21	Hepatomegaly
5	Splenomegaly

Source: Kyle RA.[4]

Table 120-2b Presenting Features of Multiple Myeloma

Percentage of Patients	Presenting Feature
83	Monoclonal heavy chain on serum immunoelectrophoresis (IEP)
76	Spike on serum protein electrophoresis (SPEP)
75	Spike on urinary electrophoresis
15	Minor or no abnormalities
9	Hypogammaglobulinemia (SPEP)
8	Monoclonal light chain (IEP)
7	Amyloidosis
0.3	Nonsecretory

Source: Kyle RA.[4]

with overt MM.[20] The natural history of MM is a progressive increase in tumor growth. The M protein doubling time, a measure of the MM growth rate, shortens with each relapse. Eventually, marrow failure develops, with sideroblastic anemia, leukopenia, and thrombocytopenia. The median interval from marrow failure to death is 3 (range 1–9) months.[21] Infection and renal failure account for 52% and 21% of deaths, respectively, in patients with MM.[22]Acute myeloid leukemia develops in a small fraction of patients, but far in excess of the anticipated baseline incidence.[21]

Biology **Cell Surface Phenotype** B-cell–restricted and associated antigens (Ags) have been utilized to delineate stages of normal and malignant B-cell differentiation.[23] Moreover, antigenic profiles are useful not only to identify stages of malignant B-cell differentiation, but also to categorize B-cell tumors. MM cells share cell surface expression of some Ags, for example, CD38 and PCA-1, which are also present on normal plasma cells, suggesting that the normal cellular counterpart of MM is the normal plasma cell. However, a number of other Ags to date have been described on the surface of MM cells, which in some cases react with B cells at stages of differentiation earlier than the plasma cell, but also react with non-B cells.[24–29] Harada and colleagues have shown that normal plasma cells are CD19+CD56–, whereas no MM cells have this phenotype.[30] The core protein of MUC-1 antigen is expressed on MM cells.[31] The expression and function of adhesion molecules on MM cells is described below. This observed heterogeneity in cell surface phenotype has led to controversy as to the cellular origin of MM.

Cellular Origin of MM As is well known, the cells that accumulate in the BM of patients with MM have plasma cell or plasmablast morphology. However, it has been known since the 1970s, based on studies using anti-idiotypic antibodies, that unique idiotypic determinants can identify clones of peripheral blood lymphocytes in patients with macroglobulinemia, MM, MGUS, and chronic lymphocytic leukemia.[32] The presence of idiotypic determinants on cytoplasmic μ-containing pre-B cells in MM BM provided further evidence that the oncogenic event may occur at the pre–B-cell stage. Studies identified B and T cells bearing identical idiotypic determinants, suggesting that target cells for oncogenic transformation could be precursor cells for both B and T cell clones.[33] Aneuploid marrow MM cells can express mRNA for cell surface proteins characteristic of myeloid, erythroid, and platelet lineages, also supporting the view that the malignant clone can extend from an early stage of differentiation.[34] Moreover, monoclonal B lineage cells in peripheral blood of MM patients, which are late-stage B cells (low CD19 and CD20, moderate CALLA and PCA-1, with strong CD45RO antigen expression) are continuously progressing toward the plasma cell stage.[27] However, it remains unclear as to which cell within the malignant clone is "clonogenic" and capable of self-renewal. Some evidence suggests that pre-B and naive B cells migrate from the BM to the lymph node (LN) where antigen recognition, selection, and somatic hypermutation occur. The memory–B-cell compartment is thought to contain the cytoplasmic μ-positive precursor cell of MM, which then undergoes Ig class switching in the LN.[35] Ig variable (*VH*) gene sequence analysis has shown MM tumor cells to be postfollicular, with the mutated homogeneous clonal sequences indicating no continuing exposure to somatic hypermutation mechanism.[36] *VH* gene analysis of IgM MM indicates an origin from a memory cell undergoing isotype switch events.[37] Mutated heterogeneous sequences in MGUS suggest that tumor cells remain under the influence of the mutator.[36] Abnormalities of 14q (the location of IgH) are most common in MM. Since protooncogenes are translocated to this region and overexpressed in B cell malignancies including follicular lymphoma, Burkitt's lymphoma, and chronic lymphocytic leukemia, they may also play a role in the oncogenesis of MM. In addition, translocations involving switch regions indicate that the final oncogenic molecular event in MM occurs late in B-cell ontogeny.[38]

Table 120-3 Classification of Monoclonal Gammopathies

A. Monoclonal gammopathy of unclear significance
  M-component level
  IgG < 3.5 g/dL
  IgA < 2.0 g/dL
  Bence Jones protein < 1.0 g/24 h
  Bone marrow plasma cells < 10%
  No bone lesions
  No symptoms
B. Indolent myeloma (as in A except)
  No bone lesions or only limited bone lesions (< 3 lytic lesions); no compression fractures
  M-component levels
    (a) IgG < 7 gm/dL
    (b) IgA < 5 gm/dL
  No symptoms or associated disease features, ie,
    Performance status > 70%
    Hemoglobin > 10 g/dL
    Serum calcium normal
    Serum creatinine < 2.0 mg/dL
    No infections
C. Smoldering myeloma (as in B except)
  No bone lesions
  Bone marrow plasma cells < 30%

Ig = immunoglobulin.

Role of Adhesion Molecules in MM Adhesion molecules mediate both homotypic adhesion of tumor cells and heterotypic adhesion of tumor cells to either extracellular matrix (ECM) proteins or BM stromal cells (BMSCs) (Figure 120-1).[39] Moreover, they play a critical role in pathogenesis of disease progression. After class switching in the LN, adhesion molecules (eg, CD44, VLA-4, VLA-5, LFA-1, CD56, syndecan-1, and MPC-1) mediate homing of MM cells to the BM.[39–42] Subsequently, binding of MM cells occurs to BMSCs, for example, via VLA-4 to VCAM-1, and to ECM, for example, via syndecan to type I collagen and VLA-4 to fibronectin. Such binding not only localizes tumor cells in the BM microenvironment, but also stimulates interleukin-6 (IL-6) transcription and secretion from BM stromal cells (SCs) with related paracrine growth of MM cells.[43–45] Moreover, triggering via CD40 found on tumor cells induces IL-6 transcription and secretion, with related autocrine MM cell growth.[46] TNF-α upregulates adhesion molecules on MM cells and BMSCs, thereby increasing binding and cell adhesion-mediated (CAM) drug resistance.[47] Syndecan-1 is a multifunctional regulator of tumor cell growth and survival as well as of bone cell differentiation, and elevated serum syndecan-1 correlates with increased tumor cell mass, decreased metalloproteinase-9 activity, and poor prognosis.[48–50] Adhesion also induces matrix metalloproteinase-1, which favors bone resorption and tumor invasion.[51] Syndecan-1 is shed from the surface of most MM cells, induces apoptosis, and can inhibit the growth of MM cells; it also mediates decreased osteoclast and increased osteoblast differentition.[49] As the disease progresses, the development of plasma cell leukemia (PCL) is characterized by decreased expression of certain adhesion molecules (eg, CD56, VLA-5, MPC-1, and syndecan-1), which in turn facilitates tumor cell mobilization. Furthermore, the acquisition of other adhesion molecules on

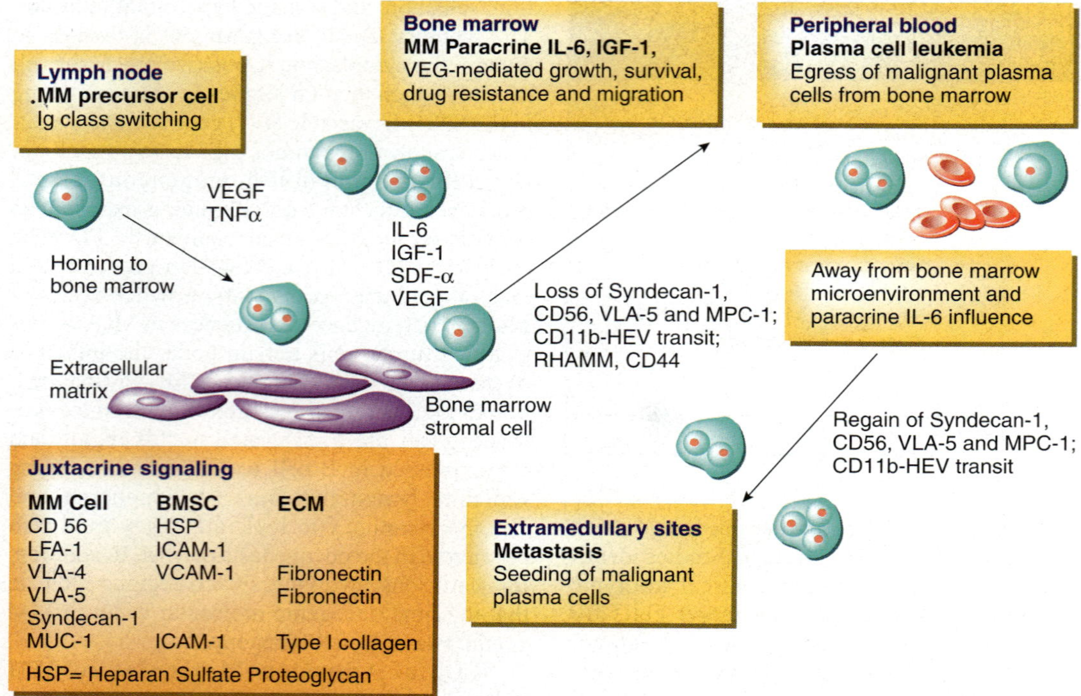

Figure 120-1 Role of adhesion molecules in myeloma pathogenesis.

PCL cells, such as CD11b, CD44, and RHAMM, assists transit through endothelium during egress from the BM. Extramedullary spread of MM cells is facilitated by the reappearance of CD56, VLA-5, MPC-1, and syndecan-1. Since adhesion molecules play a central role in the pathogenesis of MM, therapeutic strategies targeting these molecules have been developed and tested in animal models; for example, anti-ICAM-1 antibodies have been shown to inhibit tumor development in severe combined immunodeficient (SCID) mice.[52] Moreover, a model of MM in SCID mice bearing fetal bone grafts (SCID-hu mice) provides for the first time an in vivo model for the evaluation of homing of human MM cells to human BM ECM proteins and BMSCs, the biologic sequelae of binding, as well as testing of novel treatments based on interruption of this process.[53,54] MM cells resistant to melphalan and doxorubicin typically overexpress VLA-4, and adherence to ECM proteins like fibronectin induces CAM drug resistance, with up-regulation of p27 in tumor cells.[55]As we will discuss below, novel agents, including thalidomide (Thal) and its immunomodulatory derivatives (IMiDs), as well as proteasome inhibitor PS-341 can target both the tumor cell and its BM microenvironment and thereby overcome CAM drug resistance.[47,56–59]

Role of Growth Factors in MM **Interleukin-6** IL-6 was originally described as a factor that promoted differentiation of normal B cells to antibody-producing cells without triggering B-cell proliferation. In contrast, IL-6 is known to be a growth factor both for human MM and mouse plasmacytoma cells.[60] Specifically, multiple reports support an autocrine IL-6–mediated growth mechanism in MM, since some MM cells and derived cell lines both produce and respond to IL-6 in vitro.[61] Moreover, autocrine IL-6–mediated MM cell growth can be induced by triggering tumor cells via their cell surface CD40.[46] Autocrine IL-6 production is associated with a highly malignant phenotype, high proliferative index, and resistance to drug-induced apoptosis.[62] An IL-6–mediated paracrine growth mechanism has also been postulated, based upon these observations: BMSCs are the major source of IL-6 in MM; freshly isolated MM cells cultured without exogenous IL-6 rapidly stop proliferating, and adhesion of MM cells to BMSCs up-regulates IL-6 secretion by BMSCs.[43–45]

IL-6 mediates growth of MM cells via activation of the mitogen-activated protein kinase (MAPK) and phosphatidylinositol-3 kinase/Akt kinase (PI3-K/Akt) signaling cascades, and blockade of these pathways abrogates the proliferative response (Figure 120-2). Moreover, IL-6 is not only a growth factor, but also a survival factor in MM (Figure 120-3).[63,64] Apoptosis of MM cells induced by Fas and gamma irradiation (IR) is associated with activation of various serine/threonine kinases and, in particular, stress-activated protein kinase (SAPK) and p38 kinase.[64] Retinoblastoma (Rb) protein is one of the downstream targets of SAPK, which suggests that Rb is involved in IR-induced apoptosis. In contrast, MM-induced apoptosis is associated with a significant decrease in the activities of MAPK and

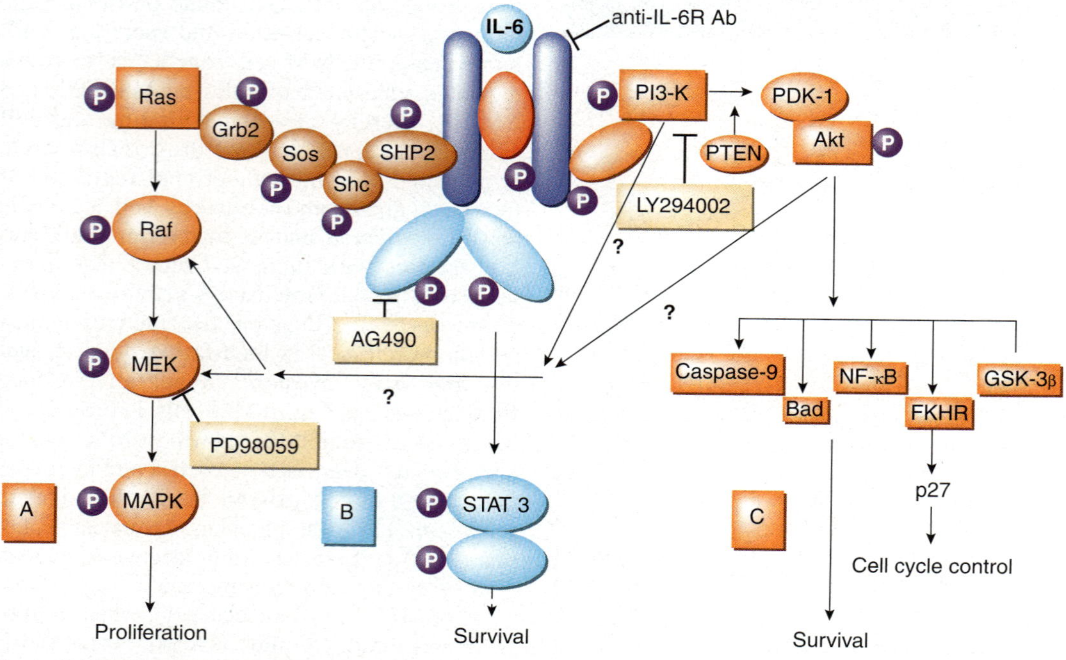

Figure 120-2 Interleukin-6 signaling cascades.

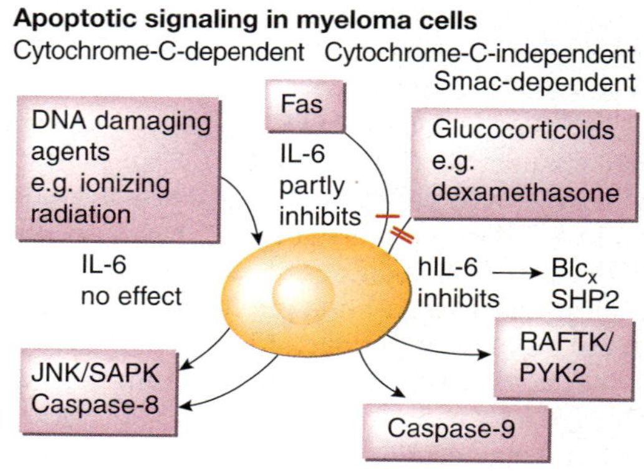

Apoptotic signaling in myeloma cells
Cytochrome-C-dependent Cytochrome-C-independent
Smac-dependent
DNA damaging agents e.g. ionizing radiation
Fas
IL-6 partly inhibits
Glucocorticoids e.g. dexamethasone
IL-6 no effect
hIL-6 inhibits
Blcx SHP2
RAFTK/PYK2
JNK/SAPK Caspase-8
Caspase-9

Figure 120-3 Apoptotic signaling pathways.

p70RSK but is not associated with activation of SAPK and p38 stress kinases.[64,65] Importantly, IL-6 inhibits MM cell apoptosis and associated down-regulation of MAPK, whereas IL-6 does not inhibit either apoptosis or activation of SAPK induced by IR. In addition, IR-induced apoptosis is associated with release of the mitochondrial apoptogenic cytochrome-C (cypt C) into the cytosol, whereas apoptosis induced by MM or anti-Fas has no detectable effect on cyp C release.[66] Therefore, at least two signaling cascades appear to mediate MM cell death.

Recent studies have begun to identify cascades mediating dexamethasone (Dex)-induced MM cell death, as well as resistance to apoptosis conferred by IL-6 (see Figures 120-2 and 120-3). For example, Dex- triggered apoptosis is mediated via activation of related adhesion focal tyrosine kinase (RAFTK).[67] Moreover, Dex-mediated MM apoptosis is not associated with mitochondrial cytochrome c release,[66] but is mediated by second mitochondria activator of caspase (Smac) release from mitochondria[68]; cytosolic Smac disrupts the inhibitor of apoptosis X-linked mammalian inhibitor of apoptosis protein (XIAP)/caspase-9 complex, thereby allowing induction of caspase-9, caspase-3 cleavage, and apoptosis. IL-6 inhibits apoptosis triggered by Dex via PI3-K/Akt signaling[69] and specific activation of src homology 2-domain-containing tyrosine phosphatase 2 (SHP2), thereby blocking activation of RAFTK.[70] Most recently, gene microarrays have been used both to further delineate these cytokine-induced growth and antiapoptotic pathways,[71] and to derive targeted therapeutic strategies to overcome drug resistance based upon interrupting growth or triggering apoptotic signaling cascades.[72] For example, such studies have demonstrated that IL-6 induces the XBP-1 transcription factor,[73] which is implicated in differentiation of normal B cells to plasma cells[74,75] and is markedly up-regulated in freshly isolated MM patient samples.[76] Finally, the constitutive activation of STAT 3 confers resistance to apoptosis in human U266 MM cells.[77] Characterization of these pathways may suggest novel treatment strategies based upon triggering of apoptosis in tumor cells or inhibiting survival signals. For example, it appears that MM cells selected for resistance to Fas-mediated apoptosis are not cross-resistant to cytotoxic drugs, providing evidence for independent mechanisms of caspase activation.[78]

At present, there is also considerable evidence supporting a role for IL-6 in the growth and manifestations of MM in vivo. Elevated IL-6 serum levels in some studies correlate with poor prognosis and higher tumor cell mass.[79,80] Moreover, patients with MGUS or indolent or smoldering MM have serum IL-6 levels similar to those of healthy individuals, in contrast to those with fulminating MM or PCL, who have the highest IL-6 levels. Direct measurement of serum IL-6 levels or of C-reactive protein synthesized in the liver in response to IL-6 may also be a prognostic factor in MM.[80] IL-6 transgenic mice develop histopathologic changes characteristic of MM kidney, IL-6 serves as an osteoclast activating factor in MM bone disease, and anti-IL-6 monoclonal antibody (MoAb) therapy can transiently reverse disease manifestations in patients with MM.[81–83] Several studies suggest potential therapeutic utility of inhibiting IL-6 in MM, antihumanized IL-6R and gp130 antibodies inhibit the growth of IL-6–dependent plasmacytoma cells in vivo, and IL-6 fused to pseudomonas exotoxin or diphtheria toxin effectively and selectively kills MM cell lines.[84–86] IL-6 receptor superantagonists, which bind IL-6 but do not trigger via gp 130, block IL-6–dependent MM cell growth.[87,88] MM has been shown to inhibit IL-6 and IL-6 receptor gene expression, consistent with another possible mechanism for inhibition of tumor cell growth by corticosteroids.[89] Bisphosphonates may also inhibit IL-6 production from MM BMSCs.[90]

Insulin-Like Growth Factor-1 Insulin-like growth factor-1 (IGF-1) is a multifunctional peptide that regulates cell proliferation, differentiation, and apoptosis. In the circulation, IGF-I binds to the main IGF binding protein, IGFBP-3. Several studies on cancer risk including lung,[91] breast,[92] prostate,[93] and colorectal[94] cancer suggest that high concentrations of circulating IGF-I are associated with an increased risk of cancer, and high IGFBP-3 concentrations are associated with a decreased risk.[95] A direct relationship of serum IGF-1 levels and prognosis has not yet been delineated in MM. Standal and colleagues reported that although the mean IGF-1 levels did not differ between myeloma patients and controls, IGF-1 was a strong prognostic indicator with median survival of patients with low levels (< 13 nM) of serum IGF-1 not reached at 80 months.[96]

Recent studies have delineated the biologic sequelae of IGF-1 in MM cells. IGF-1 is mainly produced and secreted by the BMSCs and mediates MM cell growth and survival both in vitro[97–99] and in vivo.[100–102] In contrast to IL-6, IGF-1 activates only ERK and PI3-K/Akt signaling cascades.[98,103] Specifically, IGF-1 stimulates sustained activation of PI3-K/Akt and NF-κB; induces phosphorylation of FKHR (forkhead) transcription factor; up-regulates a series of intracellular antiapoptotic proteins including FLIP, survivin, cIAP-2, A1/Bfl-1, and XIAP; and decreases drug sensitivity of MM cells.[99] IGF-1 also mediates migration via activation of PI3-K/Akt signaling cascade in MM cell lines.[104]

The antiapoptotic effect of IGF-1 has also been studied using an in vitro model system. Specifically, IGF-1 inhibits Dex-induced apoptosis in MM cell lines, without alteration of Bcl-2 or Bcl-X proteins,[105] associated with activation of ERK and PI3-K/Akt signaling pathways.[98,99,106] IGF-1 augments the proliferative and antiapoptotic effects of IL-6.[97,107] It has been demonstrated that IGF-1 increases telomerase activity via PI3-K/Akt activation; conversely, inhibition of PI3-K or NF-κB activity abrogates this effect.[108,109] Most recently, caveolin-1, which is usually absent in blood cells, was noted to be expressed in MM cells and was found to play a crucial role in both IL-6 and IGF-1–mediated signaling cascades.[110] Therapies targeting IGF-1, such as inhibitors of IGF-1 receptor have already have shown preclinical anti-MM activity and will soon undergo clinical evaluation.[102]

Tumor Necrosis Factor-α Tumor necrosis factor-α (TNF-α) has been associated with MM bone disease.[111,112] Although we have shown that TNF-α induces only modest proliferation and activation of MAPK/ERK in MM cells, TNF-α secreted by MM cells up-regulates CD11a, CD54, CD 106, CD 49d, and MUC-1 adhesion molecules on MM cells, as well as CD 54 and CD 106 on BMSCs, thereby increasing binding and triggering-enhanced IL-6 secretion in BMSCs (Figure 120-4).[43,47] Conversely, blockade of NF-κB activation inhibits these sequelae. These studies therefore confirm the central role of TNF-α in the growth and survival of MM cells and its role in the development of cell adhesion-mediated drug resistance (CAM-DR).[113] Novel agents targeting TNFα, including thalidomide (Thal) and the immunomodulatory drugs (IMiDs),[56,59] may act, at least in part, by inhibiting TNFα-mediated sequelae.

Vascular Endothelial Growth Factor Vascular endothelial growth factor (VEGF) is a known angiogenic factor in both solid tumors and hematologic malignancies.[114] In MM, it is produced both by MM cells and BMSCs (Figure 120-5)[59,115,116] and may account, at least in part, for the increased angiogenesis observed in MM patient BM. Increased microvessel density (MVD) in MM patient BM specimens is associated with a poor prognosis,[117–121] and BM MVD at diagnosis is an important prognostic factor for survival of patients who undergo autologous transplantation as front-line therapy. In contrast, BM MVD may not be a good indicator of response to treatment in MM.[122,123] Therefore, the direct evidence linking VEGF level and prognosis in MM patients is not firmly established and the pathophysiological relevance of increased BM angiogenesis in MM therefore remains unclear.

Recent studies show that CD40 activation induces p53-dependent VEGF secretion in human MM cells.[124] Of interest, studies have further shown that some MM cell lines and patient cells express VEGF receptor Flt-1, and that VEGF triggers its phosphorylation.[115,116] Exogenous VEGF triggers ERK activation and proliferation in MM cell lines and patient cells, which can be neutralized by either antibody to VEGF or the VEGF receptor tyrosine kinase inhibitors PTK787[125] and GW654652.[126] Recent studies have looked at the role of VEGF on migration of MM cells'[115,116] development of drug resistance[127,128] via up-regulation of important antiapoptotic proteins, and its effect on immune responses in MM.[129] These direct effects of VEGF on tumor cells, coupled with its induction of cytokines (ie, IL-6) and angiogenesis in the BM milieu, provide the framework for targeting VEGF in treatment strategies. The VEGF receptor tyrosine kinase inhibitor PTK787 is active preclinically and undergoing clinical protocol testing in MM.

Fibroblast Growth Factor Microvessel density of the bone marrow is increased in patients with active MM, parallels disease progression, and

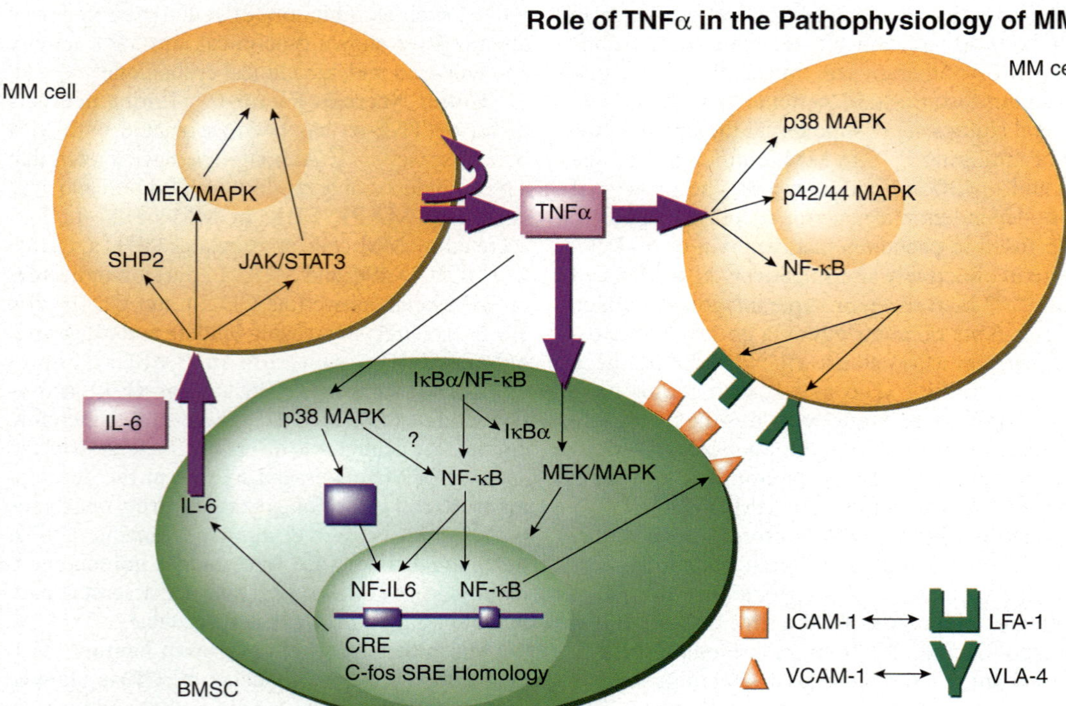

Figure 120-4 Role of tumor necrosis factor-α in myeloma bone marrow microenvironment.

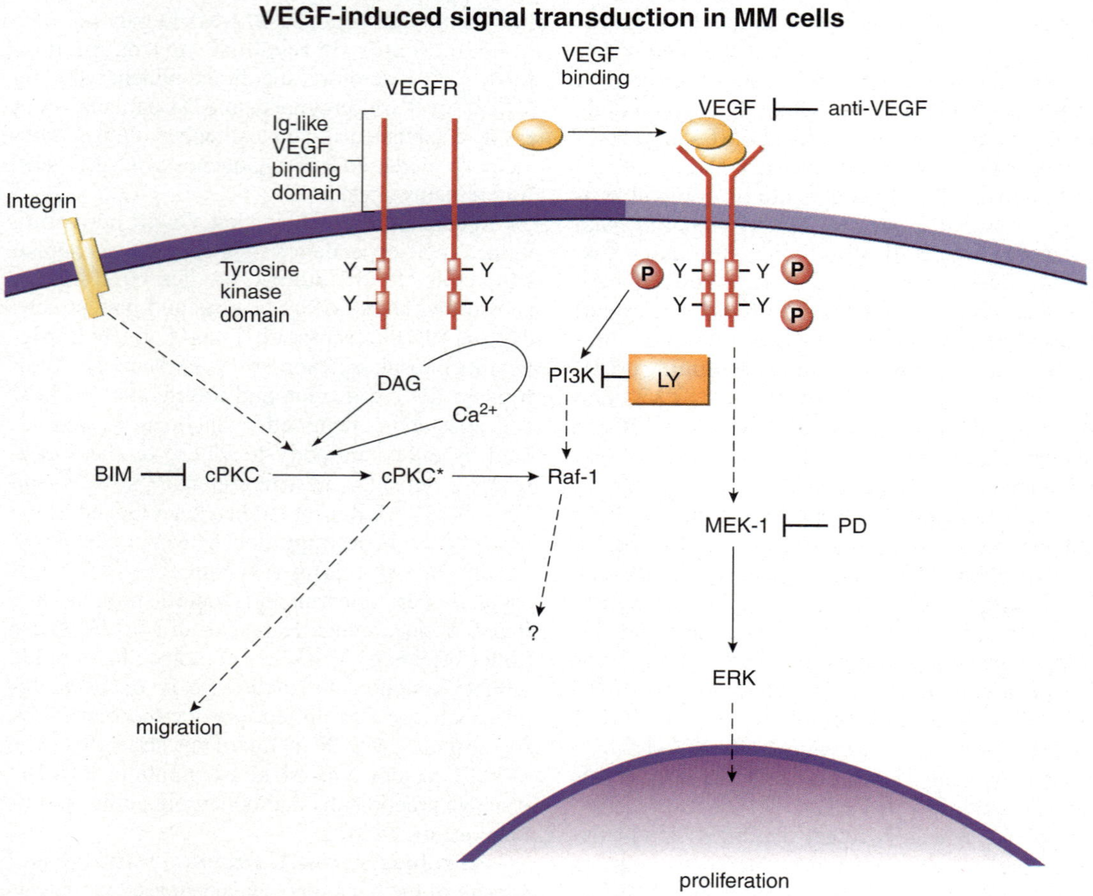

Figure 120-5 Vascular endothelial growth factor signaling cascades.

correlates with poor prognosis[118,130] MM cells express and secrete fibroblast growth factor (bFGF),[117,131] a potent angiogenic cytokine that contributes to the increased angiogenic potential of bone marrow plasma cells in progressive MM. BMSCs from MM patients and control subjects express high-affinity fibroblast growth factor (FGF) receptors R1 through R4. Importantly, stimulation of BMSCs with bFGF induced a time- and dose-dependent increase in IL-6 secretion; conversely, stimulation with IL-6 enhanced bFGF expression and secretion by MM cell lines as well as MM patient cells.[132] This finding suggests paracrine interaction of IL-6 and bFGF between MM and BMSCs, which triggers not only neovascularization, but also MM cell growth and survival in the BM microenvironment.[133] As a surface receptor, FGFR3 may be targeted by monoclonal antibodies, and as a tyrosine kinase, by selective tyrosine kinase inhibitors. Preclinical studies have validated FGFR3 as a therapeutic target in t(4;14) MM[58]; specifically, inhibitors of FGFR3 are being developed, and studies are underway in t(4;14) MM.

Stromal Cell-Derived Factor-1α Chemokines play an important role in lymphocyte trafficking and homing. Stromal cell-derived factor-1α (SDF-1α) is a ligand of CXCR4 and mediates migration of normal hematopoietic stem cells.[134,135] Increased expression of CXCR4 is found on both MM cell lines and patient tumor cells.[136,137] Interestingly, Gazitt and Akay[138] reported that both the levels of SDF-1α and surface expression of CXCR4 significantly decrease on MM cells in four consecutive apheresis collections, compared with premobilization bone marrow specimens. Of note, SDF-1α expression is regulated, at least in part, by TGF-β.[139] SDF-1α promotes proliferation, induces migration, and protects against Dex-induced apoptosis in MM cells.[136] Although SDF-1α plays a role in the pathophysiology of MM, its effects are modest compared with other cytokines.

Wnt Wnt signaling regulates various developmental processes and can lead to malignant formation. Wnts are a family of secreted glycoproteins that bind to frizzled seven-transmembrane span receptors. Intracellularly, the Wnt signaling cascade blocks degradation of β-catenin in proteasomes, thereby leading to accumulation of β-catenin in the cytoplasm. In MM, a canonical Wnt signaling pathway is activated following treatment with Wnt-3a, associated with accumulation of β-catenin. Wnt-3a treatment further led to significant morphological changes in MM cells, accompanied by rearrangement of the actin cytoskeleton.[140] Derksen and colleagues[141] demonstrated that MM cells overexpress β-catenin, including its N-terminally unphosphorylated form, consistent with active β-catenin/T-cell factor-mediated transcription. Further accumulation and nuclear localization of β-catenin, and/or increased cell proliferation, was achieved by stimulation of Wnt signaling with either Wnt-3a, LiCl, or the constitutively active mutant of β-catenin. Interestingly, MM cells in BM-biopsy specimens contained detectable dickkopf 1

(DKK1), a negative regulator of Wnt signaling cascade and a target of the β-catenin/TCF pathway.[142] Moreover, elevated DKK1 levels in BM plasma and peripheral blood from patients with MM correlated with the DKK1 gene-expression patterns and was associated with the presence of focal bone lesions.[143]

Other Growth Factors Transforming growth factor β (TGF-β) is secreted by MM cells and triggers IL-6 secretion in BMSCs, augmenting paracine IL-6–mediated tumor cell growth.[144] TGF-β secreted by MM cells likely also contributes to the immunodeficiency characteristic of MM by down-regulating B cells, T cells, and NK cells without similarly inhibiting the growth of MM cells. Recombinant IL-1 alpha (IL-1α) stimulates MM cells to produce IL-6, which consequently augments proliferation of MM cells.[145] IL-1 beta (IL-1β) mRNA is found within MM cells, and IL-1β mediates bone resorbing activity in MM.[146] These data suggest a possible therapeutic strategy for such antagonists in the treatment of lytic bone disease in MM. Serum levels of IL-1β, as well as IL-6, were found to be chronically elevated in patients with polyneuropathy, organomegaly, endocrinopathy, monoclonal protein, and skin changes (POEMS syndrome), consistent with the view that these cytokines may mediate systemic manifestations of this disease.[147] Recently, it has been suggested that expression of IL-1β by MGUS cells may identify those patients likely to progress to MM.[148] Several reports suggest that the bone-resorbing activity produced by cultured human MM cells can be mostly blocked by neutralizing antibodies to lymphotoxin, suggesting that this factor may be involved in bone disease in vivo.[149] Interleukin-4 inhibits the growth of MM cells in vitro, perhaps by blocking endogenous IL-6 synthesis.[150] However, to date clinical studies are negative. Oncostatin M, leukemia inhibitory factor, and ciliary neurotropic factor induce in vitro DNA synthesis by MM and plasmacytoma cells using the common gp 130 receptor.[151] Granulocyte-macrophage colony-stimulating factor (GMCSF) has been reported to enhance the IL-6 responsiveness of MM cells in vitro and has been utilized to facilitate the development of IL-6–dependent human MM lines.[152] Interleukin-11, a factor that can support the growth of IL-6–dependent cell lines and promote B-cell differentiation, cannot augment DNA synthesis by purified MM cells.[153,154] IL-10 is a proliferation factor, but not a differentiation factor, for human MM cells.[155] Macrophage inflammatory protein-1α is a potential osteoclast stimulatory factor in MM.[156] Autocrine growth mediated by IL-15, and most recently IL-21, has been demonstrated in both MM cell lines and patient cells.[157,158] Long-term engraftment of both MM cell lines and freshly isolated cells from MM BM has been reported in severe combined immunodeficient (SCID) mice and in SCID-hu mice, providing additional models for studying the role of growth factors in the growth of MM in vivo.[53,54,159,160]

Molecular Pathogenesis of MM The malignant plasma cells in MM are localized to the BM in close association with BMSCs. They are long-

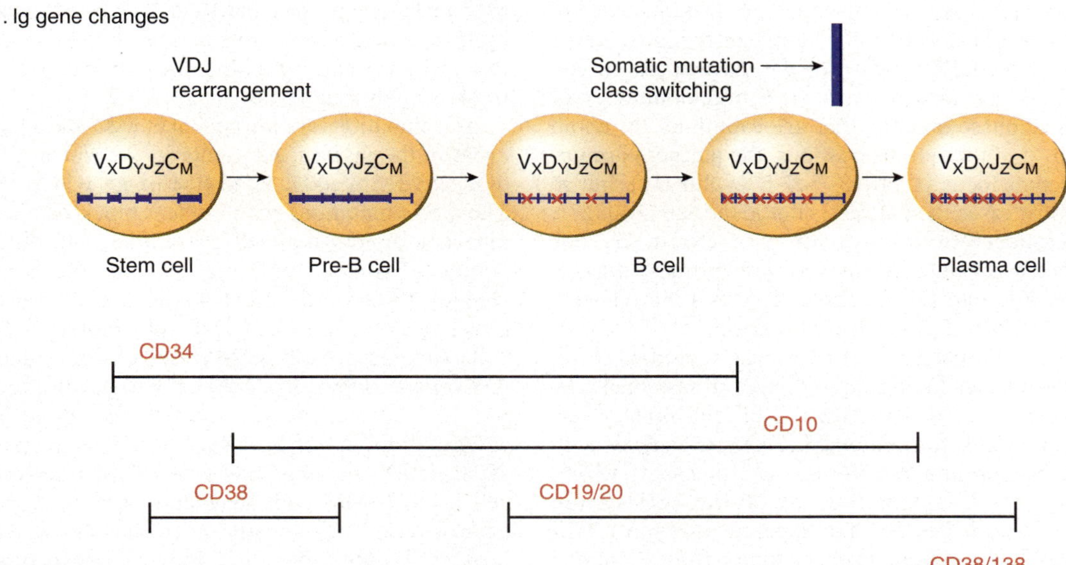

Figure 120-6 Identification of the tumor cell in myeloma.

lived cells with a very low labeling index (LI = 1–2%). The rearranged Ig genes are extensively somatically hypermutated in a manner compatible with antigen selection, with no evidence that the process of hypermutation is continuing (Figure 120-6).[36] However, MM cells have a significantly lower rate of Ig secretion than normal plasma cells. Thus it appears that the critical oncogenic events in MM cells either occur after or do not interfere with most of the normal differentiation process involved in generating a long-lived plasma cell.

By conventional analyses, karyotypic abnormalities are detected in MM at a frequency of 30 to 50% in large studies of MM tumors (Table 120-4).[58,161–163] The frequency and extent of karyotypic abnormalities correlates with the stage, prognosis, and response to therapy. For example, approximately 20% are abnormal in stage I disease, 60% in stage III patients, and > 80% for extramedullary tumor. This analysis is dependent on obtaining reliable metaphase preparations and greatly underrepresents the extent of DNA alterations in these infrequently dividing cell populations. By interphase FISH analysis, two studies report that at least one chromosome is trisomic in 96% or 89% of MM tumor samples, respectively.[164,165] Although conventional karyotypes are not routinely reported for MGUS, it appears that a substantial fraction of MGUS plasma cells are aneuploid as well. By FISH analysis, the incidence of trisomy for at least one chromosome was 43% and 53% in two studies of MGUS cells; in the former, 61% of the cells had an aneuploid DNA content by image analysis.[164,166] The characteristic numerical abnormalities are monosomy 13 and trisomies of chromosomes 3, 5, 7, 9, 11, 15, and 19. Nonrandom structural abnormalities most frequently involve chromosome 1 with no apparent locus specificity; 14q32(IgH) locus occurs in 20 to 40%; 11q13(bcl-1 locus) in about 20%, but mostly translocated to 14q32; 13q14 interstitial deletion in 15%; and 8q24 in about 10%, with about half of these involved in a translocation. Importantly, a recent report documents similar translocations in MGUS and MM, including t(4;14)(p16.3;q32) and t(14;16)(q32;q23), without any obvious clinical or biologic correlation.[167]

The hallmark genetic lesion in many B-lymphocyte tumors involves dysregulation of an oncogene as a consequence of a translocation involving the IgH locus (14q32.3); less frequently, variant translocations involve one of the IgL loci (2p12, kappa or 22q11, lambda) (see Tables 120-4 and 120-5). From conventional karyotypic analyses, translocations involving 14q32 appear to occur in about 20 to 40% of MM

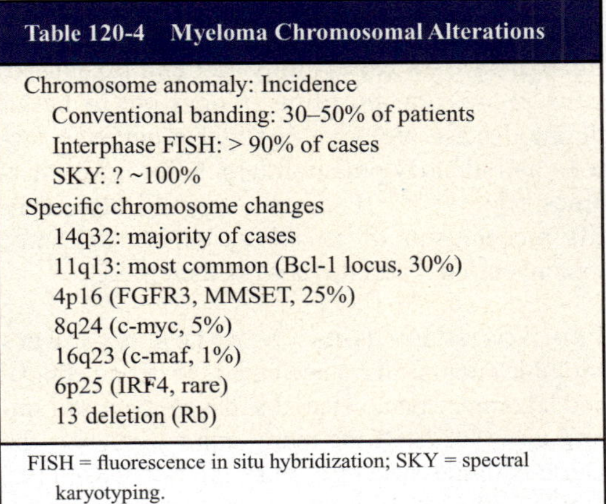

Table 120-4 Myeloma Chromosomal Alterations

Chromosome anomaly: Incidence
- Conventional banding: 30–50% of patients
- Interphase FISH: > 90% of cases
- SKY: ? ~100%

Specific chromosome changes
- 14q32: majority of cases
- 11q13: most common (Bcl-1 locus, 30%)
- 4p16 (FGFR3, MMSET, 25%)
- 8q24 (c-myc, 5%)
- 16q23 (c-maf, 1%)
- 6p25 (IRF4, rare)
- 13 deletion (Rb)

FISH = fluorescence in situ hybridization; SKY = spectral karyotyping.

Table 120-5 Nonimmunoglobulin Sites for Illegitimate Switch Recombination

Chromosome	Gene	Function
11q13	cyclin D_1	Induces growth
4p16	FGFR3, MMSET	Growth factor R
8q24	myc	Growth/apoptosis
16q23	c-maf	Transcription factor
6p25	IRF4	Transcription factor

Source: Kuehl WM. Natl Rev Cancer 2002;3:175.

with an abnormal karyotype.[3,58] The incidence of these translocations is significantly higher in the extramedullary phase of the disease and in cell lines, perhaps because of a higher number of metaphase spreads that are examined. In about 30% of these translocations, the partner chromosomal locus is 11q13 (bcl-1, cyclin D1), but in most cases the partner is not identified (14q32+). Transcriptional activation of cyclin D1 has recently been confirmed in some primary tumors, as has cyclin D3 activation associated with t(6;14)(p21;q32) translocation.[167–169] Other recurrent partner loci have been identified infrequently, including 8q24(c-*myc*) in less than 5%, 18q21(bcl-2), 11q23(MLL-1), and 6p21.1. By combining conventional karyotypic analysis with a comprehensive Southern blot assay, which detects translocations involving IgH switch regions, it has become apparent that most MM cell lines and one primary tumor fully examined have IgH translocations that mainly involve IgH switch regions.[58,170] Recent FISH studies have also shown that IGH gene rearrangements are present in 73% of MM patients.[171] The apparent oncogene dysregulated by the 4;14 translocation is the fibroblast growth factor receptor 3 (*FGFR3*) gene, and it is possible that dysregulated expression of FGFR3, as a result of t(4;14), receives an *FGFR3*-mediated signal from *FGF* produced by stromal cells in the BM microenvironment.[172] The t (4;14) translocation in MM regulates both *FGFR3* and a novel gene, *MMSET,* resulting in IgH/*MMSET* hybrid transcripts.[173] Ectopic expression of *FGFR3* promotes MM cell proliferation and prevents apoptosis, and its oncogenic potential has been tested in a murine model, confirming its capacity to transform hemopoietic cells.[174,175] Finally, there is evidence that elevated expression of c-*myc* and selective expression of one c-*myc* allele may occur frequently in MM, even though structural genetic changes near c-*myc* have been identified in only 10 to 20% of tumors.

Ras mutations occur in about 39% of newly diagnosed MM patients, and the frequency of *ras* mutations increases with disease progression. Mutations of N- and K-*ras* are rarely detected in solitary plasmacytoma and MGUS, but occur more frequently in MM (9–30%) and in the majority of terminal disease or PCL patients (63–70%).[176,177] Activating mutations of the *ras* oncogenes may also result in growth-factor independence and suppression of apoptosis in MM.

Although translocation (14;18) occurs at a low frequency (0–15%) in MM, an overexpression of Bcl-2 is seen in the majority of MM patients and in MM cell lines.[178,179] High levels of Bcl-2 protein are likely to mediate the resistance of MM cells to apoptosis induced by IL-6 deprivation, staurosporine, or other drugs.[180] In a murine MM cell line, Bcl-XL showed a predominant role in preventing apoptosis in response to cycloheximide treatment or IL-6 withdrawal.[181] Similarly, overexpression of Bcl-2 or Bcl-XL could prevent apoptosis induced by IL-6 withdrawal in the B-9 IL-6–dependent cell line.[182] Mcl-1 is overexpressed in MM cells, up-regulated by IL-6, and mediates potent resistance to apoptosis, whereas antisense oligonucleotide to Mcl-1 triggers apoptosis.[183]

p53 mutations are infrequent in MM and a late event in the disease; *p53* mutations occur in 5% of inactive MM and in 20 to 40% of acute PCL.[184] Thus, *p53* mutations may cause a block of plasmablastic apoptosis and differentiation at the final stages of plasma cell maturation. We have recently shown that *p53* status does affect functional sequelae in MM: CD40 activation of MM cells triggers growth of MM cells with mutant *p53* versus apoptosis of MM cells with wild-type *p53*.[124] To date, mutations of the *Rb* gene or abnormalities in *pRb* have been described in up to 70% of MM patients and 80% of MM-derived cell lines.[185] MM cells may show a very strong expression of *pRb*, mostly in its phosphorylated form.[186] Furthermore, IL-6 induces phosphorylation of *pRb*, which in turn releases the suppression of IL-6 transcription mediated by dephosphorylated *pRb* and augments IL-6–mediated MM cell growth. In contrast to its effects on normal B cells, TGF-β does not suppress *pRb* phosphorylation and proliferation of MM cells, and in fact stimulates IL-6 secretion from stromal cells.[144] The p16 INK4A (p16) protein, an inhibitor of cyclin-dependent kinases (CDK) 4 and CDK6, is expressed in MM; its expression correlates with IL-6 responsiveness of more mature (VLA-5+ MPC1+) tumor cells, whereas cyclin D1 is more frequent in immature MM tumors (VLA-5-MPC1–).[187] *P16* gene hypermethylation occurs more frequently in advanced disease (PCL) and in MM cell lines.[188–190] Germline *p16* mutation has recently been implicated in predisposing to MM.[191] Finally, IL-6 down-regulates and IFNγ up-regulates *p21* expression, and this effect correlates with G_1 to S transition in MM cells.[192] *P21* overexpression in MM may induce resistance to apoptosis and slow clinical progression of disease. Induction of *p27* is associated with CAM drug resistance.[55] The overexpression of the MDM2 protein has been reported to enhance cell-cycle progression in MM.[193]

Chromosome 13 deletions are present in over 50% of MM and are associated with poor prognosis.[167,194–196] However, these deletions are also associated with MGUS, and their role in transformation to MM is therefore at present undefined.[167,197,198] With the advent of cDNA microarrays, an expeditious and comprehensive gene expression profiling is possible to better define disease biology, highlight prognostic factors, and identify potential targets for novel therapies.[168,174,199,200] These studies will also identify mechanisms of sensitivity versus resistance to conventional and novel MM therapies.[71,201]

Prognostic Factors **Staging Systems** Multiple attempts have been made to define clinical and laboratory parameters that have prognostic significance.[202–205] Of the many staging systems, the Durie–Salmon system is most commonly utilized (Table 120-6).[203] Tumor cell mass for patients in stage I is low at < 0.6×10^{12} cells/m^2, intermediate for patients with stage II disease at 0.6 to 1.2×10^{12} cells/m^2, and high for patients with stage III disease with > 1.2×10^{12} cells/m^2. In this system, survival duration is 61.2, 54.5, 30.1, and 14.7 months for patients with stage IA, stage IB + IIA + IIB, stage IIIA, and stage IIIB disease, respectively. Gassman and colleagues compared the relative value of seven staging systems in 152 patients with MM.[204] In their analysis, the Cancer and Leukemia Group B (CALGB) and Southeastern Cancer Study Group divided patients into good-risk and poor-risk groups, with significant (albeit small) differences in survival. In the systems of Durie and Salmon, Alexanian Merlini, and Car-bone, some differences in survival were significant while others were not.[203,206–208] The British Medical Research Council staging system was best, with median survival times significantly different in stage A (83 months), stage B (52 months), and stage C (26 months).[209] Stages in this system were defined as follows: Those patients with blood urea nitrogen (BUN) < 8 mmol/L, hemoglobin (Hb) > 10.0 g/L and minimal symptoms as stage A, those with Hb < 7.5 g/L and restricted activity or BUN over 10 mmol/L and restricted activity as stage C, and those patients not in either stage A or C as stage B. Interestingly, none of the staging systems were clearly superior to certain single risk factors, especially the presence of anemia (Hb above or below 8.5 g/L) and renal impairment (creatinine less or more than 177 pmol/L).[204] Bataille and colleagues examined 147 patients with MM using Durie–Salmon, Medical Research Council, and Merlini–Waldenström

Table 120-6 Durie-Salmon Myeloma Staging System Criteria

Stage I
All of the following:
Hemoglobin value > 10 g/L
Serum calcium value normal (< 12 mg/dL)
On roentgenogram, normal bone structure (scale) or solitary bone plasmacytoma only
Low M-component production rates
IgG value < 5 g/dL, IgA value < 3 g/dL
Urine light chain M-component on electrophoresis < 4 g/24 hours
Stage II
Overall data as minimally abnormal as shown for stage I and no single value as abnormal as defined for stage III
Stage III
One or more of the following:
Hemoglobin value < 8.5 g/dL
Serum calcium value > 12 g/dL
Advanced lytic bone lesions (scale 3)
High M-component production rates
IgG value > 7 g/dL, IgA value >> 5 g/dL
Urine light chain M-component on electrophoresis 12 g/24 hours
Subclassification
A = Relatively normal renal function (serum creatinine value < 2.0 mg/dL
B = Abnormal renal function (serum creatinine > 2.0 mg/dL)

Source: Durie BGM, Salmon SE.[203]
Ig = immunoglobulin.

staging criteria as well as serum β2 microglobulin (β2M) and rate of bone resorption.[202] They found serum β2M to be the most powerful indicator of prognosis, with serum albumin the only variable adding to this significantly. These two variables were better than any staging systems. Finally, Cavo and colleagues modified the Durie–Salmon system to include thrombocytopenia, and they demonstrated that platelets above or below 150,000/mm^3 can specifically define intermediate risk groups of Durie–Salmon stages II and III patients.[210] A more recent staging system based on serum albumin and β2M has been proposed and is of prognostic significance.

Single Risk Factors Many additional single parameters have been examined for their value as prognostic features.

Morphology Griepp and colleagues classified 100 cases of MM into mature (28%), intermediate (38%), immature (19%), or plasmablastic (15%) morphology.[211] The median survival of the plasmablastic group in this series was 16 months compared with 35 months for other types. Plasmablastic subtypes had more frequent renal insufficiency and higher plasma cell indices. A study of 453 patients confirmed higher labeling indices, serum IL-6 receptor levels, more *ras* mutations, more aggressive disease, and shortened survival in patients with plasmablast morphology.[212]

Serum β2M Serum β2M represents the light chain of the major histocompatibility complex of the cell membrane. Increased serum β2M results from release by tumors with high growth fraction and cell turnover rates. It is a small protein and is largely excreted in urine; therefore, renal failure can elevate serum β2M. In patients with MM and normal renal function, rising serum β2M predicts for progression. In patients with MM, serum β2M also correlates with clinical stage, as defined by Durie and Salmon, and with response to therapy. For example, Brenning and colleagues related the pretreatment serum β2M levels to creatinine, clinical stage, and survival in 121 patients with MM.[213] Patients in stage III had higher serum β2M levels than patients in stage II or stages I and II. It can be used alone or in combination with other variables for pretreatment stratification.[214] For example, of 612 patients who were similarly treated with combination chemotherapy, 322 patients with serum β2M < 6 mg/L had a significantly longer median survival of 36 months, compared with those 225 patients with serum β2M ≥ 6 mg/L, whose survival was only 23 months ($p < .0001$). Various investigators have chosen different distinct cut off values for serum β2M, but nonetheless serum β2M retains prognostic importance in most studies.

Labeling Index The labeling index (LI), a measure of DNA synthesis by MM cells, predicts for survival. It is usually low (< 1%) at diagnosis, higher at relapse, and lower in MGUS and indolent MM. High plasma cell LI correlates with shorter survival time, independent of tumor cell mass.[205]

Tumor Cell Karyotype Gould and colleagues found that hypodiploidy in patients with Bence Jones proteinuria was associated with resistance to therapy.[162] Investigators at the Mayo Clinic found cytogenetic abnormalities in 18% of patients with newly diagnosed MM, in 63% of patients with aggressive disease, and in 40% of those with PCL.[161] Survival among newly diagnosed patients was shorter in those with abnormalities than for those without abnormalities. Among all patients, survival from the time of chromosomal analysis was shorter for those in whom a chromosomally abnormal clone was found. In proliferating plasma cells, anomalous 1, 11, and 14 chromosomes and t(11;14)(q13:132) abnormalities were most common. Nonrandom chromosomal rearrangements of 14q13.3 and 19p13.3 and preferential deletion of 1p have been reported in patients with MM and PCL.[215] The presence of either partial or complete deletions of chromosome 13q14, deletions of 17p13, or abnormalities involving 11q have an adverse influence.[197,216] By contrast, trisomies of chromosomes 7, 11, and 15, as well as DNA hyperdiploidy, are associated with a favorable outcome.[194] Importantly, the presence of any translocation likewise predicts poor outcome after high-dose therapy and autotransplantation.[217,218] Monosomy 13 has been associated with the transition from MGUS to overt MM.[198] Novel nonrandom translocations can be identified using multicolor spectral karyotyping and double color fluorescent in situ hybridization.[219,220]

Cell Surface Phenotype Cell surface phenotype has been reported to correlate with disease course. Common acute lymphoblastic leukemia Ag-positive (CD10+) MM has been reported to have prognostic significance.[221] Lactic dehydrogenase, although nonspecific, correlates with tumor mass, as in lymphomas.[222] Patients whose MMs produce only λ light chains have a poorer prognosis than those associated with IgG, IgA, or κ light chains only. Moreover, among those with IgG MM, both response rates and median survival are greater in patients with κ than in those with λ MM. Percentages of peripheral blood CD38 and PCA-1 Ag-bearing lymphocytes were reportedly significantly higher at diagnosis of MM as compared to MGUS; furthermore, an additional increase has been observed during relapse, suggesting a correlation between plasma-cell Ag expression and disease activity.[223]

Serum Cytokine/Receptor Levels Serum IL-2 levels were significantly higher in MM patients than in normal controls; moreover, higher serum IL-2 levels were associated with a prolonged actuarial survival.[224] Serum IL-6 levels in some studies appear to correlate both with stage of disease and survival.[79,80] IL-6 stimulates hepatocytes to produce acute phase proteins, such as CRP; CRP, therefore, may reflect the IL-6 level and proliferative status of BM plasma cells. Indeed, CRP levels are significantly lower in patients with MGUS than in those with MM, and survival can be correlated with serum CRP level.[225] High serum soluble IL-6 receptor (sIL-6R) hepatocyte growth factor and syndecan-1 levels, as well as low serum hyaluronate levels, are independent prognostic factors predicting poor outcome.[226–229]

Peripheral Blood Plasma Cells The percentage of circulating plasma cells in peripheral blood and their labeling indices are independent prognostic factors for survival in MM after both conventional and high-dose therapy.[230,231] Plasma cells from primary plasma cell leukemia display singular phenotypic, DNA cell content, and cytogenetic characteristics that lead to a different disease evolution versus MM.[232]

Combinations of Factors Many of these factors are interrelated and, therefore, of limited independent value. Using multivariate analysis, several groups have found that the best combination of variables to predict outcome was serum β2M, reflecting both the tumor burden and the renal function; and the proliferative activity of plasma cells, evaluated by the LI or number of tumor cells in S-phase. Age and performance status also improves the prognostic assessment.[233,234] High levels of sIL-6R or CRP may also be complementary variables. Nevertheless, it is possible that some of the factors that reflect the intrinsic characteristics of the malignant clone may become even more relevant. For example, the presence of K-*ras* mutations is associated with a shorter survival.[235] The presence of circulating plasma cells in the peripheral blood stem harvest of patients about to undergo transplantation has also been associated with poor outcome.[230] Low numbers of circulating CD19+ cells predict for poor outcome.[236] The identification of more accurate prognostic factors is necessary to select patients for whom more aggressive therapy is indicated and for providing accurate assessment of the outcome of treatment approaches.[237] For example, the presence of any translocation predicts poor outcome after high-dose therapy and autotransplantation.[217] Lung resistance-related protein expression predicts for worse outcome after conventional, but not high-dose, therapy, demonstrating that certain prognostic factors may vary with therapeutic strategies.[238]

Complications Complications of MM include bone disease and hypercalcemia, hyperviscosity, recurrent infections, renal failure, and cardiac dysfunction.

Bone Disease and Hypercalcemia As noted earlier, 80% of patients with MM present with bone pain. Bone lesions can be isolated, discrete lytic abnormalities, or diffuse osteopenia. Bone scans and serum alkaline phosphatase are usually not abnormal. Evaluation with roentgenographs is standard; magnetic resonance imaging (MRI) is more sensitive and demonstrates bone healing with bisphosphonate therapy. Active osteoclastic bone resorption is usually evident when > 20% MM cells are present, and lytic bone lesions occur when > 10^{12} cells are present. Bone resorption leads to increased calcium in extracellular fluid. Although patients with normal renal function can increase urine calcium excretion, those with renal failure develop hypercalcemia. Therefore, hypercalcemia is more likely to occur in the setting of Bence Jones proteinuria, MM kidney, chronic infection, or uric acid nephropathy. Overall, hypercalcemia occurs in 20 to 40% of

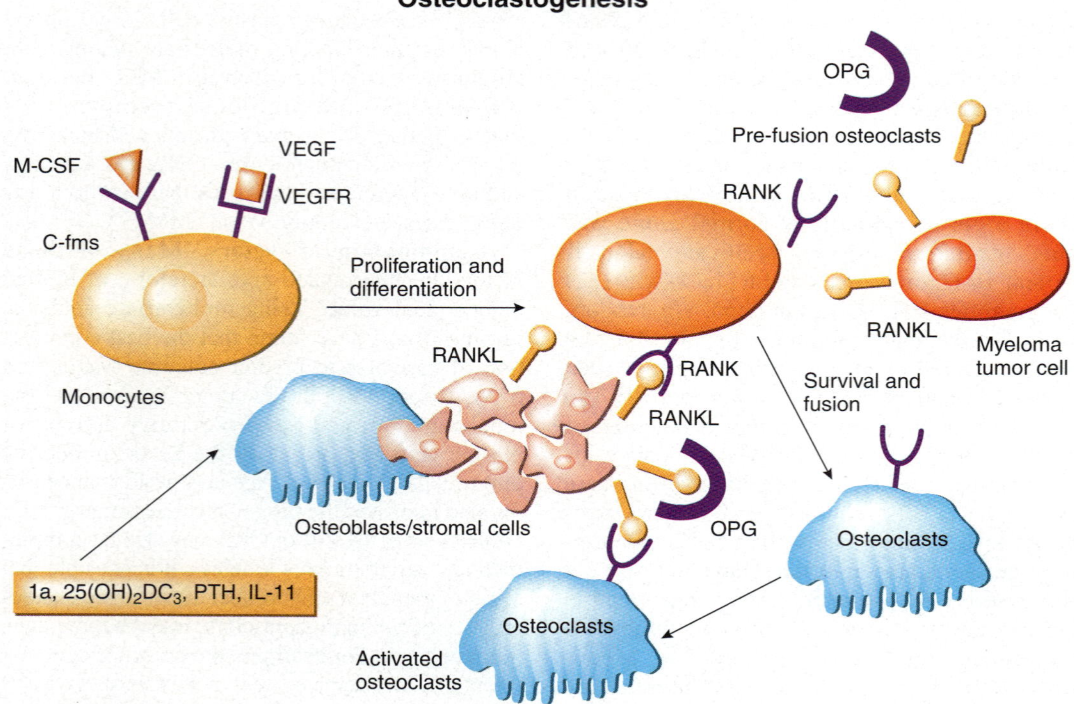

Figure 120-7 Osteoclastogenesis.

patients with MM.[239] Osteosclerosis occurs in < 1% of patients, who may have POEMS syndrome.[240] The differentiation of the POEMS syndrome from so-called osteosclerotic MM with peripheral neuropathy appears to have no clinical value.

Pathogenesis MM cell lines, MM cells, and explants of bone containing MM cells, produce osteoclast-activating factors that are similar biologically and chemically to bone-resorbing activity in normal activated leukocyte culture supernatants (Figure 120-7).[239] These include lymphotoxin (LT), TNF-α, hepatocyte growth factor (HGF), IL-6, IL-1, metalloproteinases (MMP1, MMP2, MMP9), RANKL, and insulin-like growth factor binding protein 4 (IGF-IV).[146,149,241–243] IL-6 can induce TNF-α and IL-1 production in marrow cells and cause bone resorption and hypercalcemia in vivo. Macrophage inflammatory protein Iα (MIP-Iα) has been shown to increase osteoclast stimulatory activity in patients with MM.[156] MIP-Iα mRNA is present in freshly isolated BM from MM patients. More importantly, recombinant hMIP-1α induces OCL formation in human BM cultures.[244] Conversely, blocking MIP-1α in the ARH-77 cell line inhibits tumor growth in an in vivo model of bone disease.[156] The levels of RANKL/osteoprotegerin ligand (OPGL), an OCL activation and differentiation factor, and of osteoprotegerin (OPG), which is a decoy receptor for OPGL, modulate osteoclast formation; furthermore, an imbalance favoring osteoclast activation has been seen in MM patients.[245–247] Although OPG levels are decreased in MM patients with osteolytic lesions, the levels do not correlate with clinical stage or survival. OPG, which neutralizes OPGL, may have therapeutic application in MM bone disease.[243]

An in vivo model of MM bone disease has been developed in which SCID mice injected with ARH-77 tumor cells develop radiologically detectable lytic bone lesions, and their marrow plasma contains a bone-resorbing activity that stimulates osteoclastic bone resorption in bone organ cultures and in human and murine marrow cultures.[248] It appears that a novel cytokine mediates osteoclast activation in this model. Hjorth-Hansen and colleagues have used a different human MM cell line in this model and found similar results.[249] The use of OPG to inhibit osteolytic bone disease has been demonstrated in an in vivo model by Croucher and colleagues.[250] Another antagonist of OPGL is RANK-Fc molecule, a fusion of the Fc portion of immunoglobulin to a soluble form of the RANK receptor. RANK-Fc alone or in combination with bisphosphonates has been evaluated using in vivo models and also blocks bone destruction.[54,251]

Treatment Prior to the advent of effective bisphosphonate therapy, bone healing in MM occurred uncommonly and was delayed in treated patients despite responses to chemotherapy. In this context, a major effort over the last 30 years has been made to either prevent or inhibit further bone resorption in patients with MM. A double-blind study of sodium fluoride treatment in patients with MM offered neither subjective nor objective benefit in this regard.[252] Chloromethylene diphosphonate, an inhibitor of osteoclast activity, decreased urinary excretion of calcium and skeletal pain but has not been widely studied or used.[253] A double-blind randomized trial of clodronate versus placebo in 350 patients revealed that the proportion of patients with progression of osteolytic lesions was twice as high in the placebo group as in the clodronate-treated group.[254] Another randomized trial demonstrated that oral clodronate slowed progressive skeletal disease and associated morbidity but achieved no benefit in survival. Pamidronate has been shown in a prospective randomized trial to reduce skeletal-related events, including pathologic fractures, radiation therapy to bone, and spinal cord compression in patients with Durie–Salmon stage III MM and ≥ 1 lytic bone lesion.[255] This benefit was maintained until 21 months, and it is now recommended that MM patients remain on intravenous bisphosphonates indefinitely to reduce skeletal events and pain, regardless of their response to chemotherapy.[256,257] Interestingly, patients in this study who had failed first-line chemotherapy also had improved survival, suggesting that bisphosphonates may have anti-MM activity.[258] Recent evidence supports the view that bisphosphonates may down-regulate IL-6 production from BMSCs as well as induce apoptosis of both osteoclasts and tumor cells. Pamidronate has been studied in patients with indolent MM. Bone turnover was reduced in treated patients,[90,259] but no significant antitumor activity was noted.[260] More potent bisphosphonates, such as zoledronate, have undergone clinical evaluation and offer the benefit of shorter infusion times than pamidronate.[261–263] On the other hand, ibandronate, a third-generation bisphosphonate, failed to enhance survival or reduce morbidity from bone disease in patients with stage II and III MM.[264] A word of caution should however be exercised with the use bisphosphonate therapy because of reported cases of osteonecrosis of the jaw.[265,266]

The treatment of hypercalcemia consists of treatment of the underlying MM, as well as inhibition of osteoclastic bone resorption with corticosteroids, calcitonin, mithramycin, and/or bisphosphonates. Corticosteroids may impair formation of new osteoclasts; mithramycin is toxic to osteoclasts, but it is also nephrotoxic. Calcitonin and corticosteroids are almost always effective for the short term and useful even in the setting of renal failure. Bisphosphonates bind to the bone surface and inhibit osteoclast activity, and they constitute a mainstay of treatment. Therapeutic recommendations at present, therefore, include initial cytotoxic therapy for MM and cautious forced saline diuresis and bisphosphonate therapy, with the use of calcitonin, prednisone, or mithramycin only for nonresponders to these first-line treatments. In a randomized trial of 287 patients with hypercalcemia of malignancy, zoledronate was found to be superior to pamidronate.[267] A prominent problem exacerbating hypercalcemia relates to patients' becoming immobile because of bone pain or other reasons. Therefore, an important approach is to keep the patient, whenever possible, physically active.

Hyperviscosity Hyperviscosity is characterized clinically by spontaneous bleeding with neurologic and ocular disorders. Hyperviscosity occurred in 4.2% of 238 patients with IgG MM and in 22% of 46 patients with serum IgG M components > 5.0 g/dL.[268] The IgG3 subclass produces hyperviscosity at lower levels than other IgG paraproteins.[269] The severity of the syndrome is not directly related to the serum viscosity. Clinical findings improve with vigorous plasmapheresis, which reduces both MM protein concentration and serum viscosity.

Recurrent Infections Patients with MM had 15 times more infections than a control group of patients with arteriosclerotic heart disease.[270] *Streptococcus pneumoniae* and *Haemophilus* infections usually occur early and typically during response to chemotherapy. Gram-negative infections occur in refractory, advancing disease; in the setting of previous antibiotic therapy; instrumentation; immobilization; colonization with hospital flora; and azotemia. Fatal infections may be hospital-acquired, emphasizing the need to minimize indwelling foreign bodies such as catheters in patients with MM. There is lack of correlation between bacteremia (either gram-negative or -positive) and chemotherapy-induced febrile neutropenia. Fungal, herpes, mycobacterial, and *Pneumocystis* infections are only rarely described in MM patients. Infection is the most common cause of death (20–50% of cases).[22]

The evidence of increased clinical infections in MM has led to attempts at prophylaxis. Although MM patients have normal-fold rises in antibody titers after pneumococcal vaccination, preimmunization titers are markedly diminished.[271] Post-immunization titers are therefore low and considered nonprotective. Nonetheless, because of its low cost and possible benefit to some patients, the use of pneumococcal vaccination has been recommended. In a double-blind randomized trial of gammaglobulin prophylaxis in patients with MM, no benefit of gammaglobulin prophylaxis at reducing infection was noted.[272]At present, gammaglobulin is reserved for those patients with recurrent or life-threatening infections.

The role of prophylactic antibiotics remains controversial and has been evaluated in a prospective randomized clinical trial evaluating whether trimethoprim-sulfamethoxazole (TMP/SMX) given for the first 2 months of chemotherapy would decrease infections during the 3 months from start of chemotherapy.[273,274] Infections occurred in 46% of control and 18% of TMP/SMX treated patients (p = .04) and were less severe in the latter group; however, TMP/SMX was discontinued because of nausea or rash in 25% of patients. A larger, multi-institutional randomized study is therefore needed to better define the role of prophylactic antibiotics in patients with MM.

Renal Failure Renal failure in MM can predict for adverse outcome. One series found that 22% of patients had a serum creatinine > 2 mg/dL at diagnosis; renal function normalized with treatment in 50% of those with creatinine > 2 but < 3.9 mg/dL. In patients with renal dysfunction requiring dialysis, the outcome was quite poor.[275] The causes of renal failure in MM are often multifactorial and include hypercalcemia; MM kidney, with distal and proximal tubules obstructed by large, laminated casts containing albumin, IgG, and κ and λ light chains surrounded by giant cells; hyperuricemia; toxicity from intravenous urography; dehydration; plasma cell infiltration; pyelonephritis; and amyloidosis. The most important predisposing factor is dehydration; aggressive hydration is therefore crucial to avoid irreversible renal dysfunction. Otherwise, treatment is for the underlying disease, along with avoidance of intravenous urography. Combination chemotherapy should be used because of the more rapid response that is observed with melphalan and prednisone. The type and quantity of proteinuria can distinguish MM kidney, with larger amounts of light chains and less albuminuria; light chain deposition disease, characterized by low levels of both light chains and albumin in urine; and amyloidosis, in which large amounts of albuminuria and less light-chain proteinuria occur.[276]

The renal manifestations associated with the production of monoclonal light chains in MM, light-chain deposition disease, and amyloidosis result from the deposition of certain Bence Jones proteins (BJP) as tubular casts, basement-membrane precipitates, or fibrils, respectively.[277–279] For unknown reasons, the severity of the renal manifestations varies greatly from patient to patient. BJP from 40 patients were injected into mice, and 26 (65%) were deposited in mouse kidneys as tubular casts, basement-membrane precipitates, or crystals in a pattern similar to those noted in patients.[279] This experimental model has potential value for the identification and differentiation of nephrotoxic or amyloidogenic light chains. The development of progressive kidney damage and MM kidney has been demonstrated in IL-6 transgenic mice, shedding additional insight into the role of IL-6 in the pathogenesis of MM.[81]

Cardiac Failure The mean and median age of patients with MM is approximately 60 years, and affected patients are also frequently at risk of cardiovascular disease. However, patients can be uniquely susceptible to cardiac ischemia and/or congestive heart failure (CHF) because of myocardial infiltration with amyloid, causing dilated or restricted cardiomyopathy, hyperviscosity syndrome, and/or anemia. MM patients are also susceptible to high output CHF of unclear etiology.[280]

Anemia Anemia in MM can be due to a number of factors, including tumor infiltration of the BM, renal impairment, the myelosuppressive effects of chemotherapy, and a deficient production of erythropoietin (EPO) relative to the degree of anemia. Pilot studies demonstrated efficacy of exogenous EPO administration in MM.[281–283] Osterborg and colleagues have carried out a randomized study of EPO therapy at 10,000 U/d, a titrated dose of EPO starting with 2,000 U/d and escalating stepwise until response, or no EPO for 24 weeks; response was defined as an increase in Hb > 2g/dL and elimination of transfusion need.[284] Sixty percent of EPO-treated groups responded, 72% of those with low EPO levels, and only 20% of those with normal EPO levels. 10,000 units SC three times weekly was the optimal starting dosage, although more recently 40,000 units SC once weekly is a commonly used approach.

Neuropathies A variety of malignant and paraproteinemic disorders can be associated with europathies.[285] In MM, a symmetric, distal sensory or sensorimotor neuropathy is most common and is associated with axonal degeneration, with or without amyloid deposition; there is no specific therapy. In some cases, this is associated with monoclonal antibodies directed against peripheral nerve myelin.[286]

Associated Diseases MM has been described in association with both hematologic disorders and solid tumors. Acute leukemia either is induced by leukemogens, such as radiation and alkylating agents, or is part of the natural history of MM. The mean interval from diagnosis of MM to occurrence of acute leukemia is 60 (17–147) months, consistent with either possibility. The occurrence of acute leukemia in untreated MM patients suggests that it may be part of the natural history of the disease.[287] Furthermore, acute leukemia has been reported in 6 of 125 (4.8%) MM patients treated with alkylating agents, which is significantly higher than the incidence of acute leukemia in ovarian cancer patients treated with irradiation and alkylators.[21] Actuarial risk of leukemia in MM patients treated with melphalan and prednisone or with melphalan, cyclophosphamide, carmustine, and prednisone has been reported to be as high as 17.4% at 50 months from initiation of therapy.[288] Gonzalez and colleagues described 11 of 476 patients with MM who developed myeloid leukemia or sideroblastic anemia.[287] All had received melphalan-prednisone for a median of 3 years and had major cytogenetic abnormalities. This study suggests that leukemia is predominantly treatment related. Finally, in 628 patients with MM, the incidence and diversity of solid tumors were similar to those observed in otherwise healthy persons of the same age.[289]

Treatment Patients undergoing therapy for MM should have clinical and laboratory assessment to assure both safety and efficacy of treatment. Before each course of treatment, a complete blood count, including differential and platelets, should be done. Serum chemistries should be measured at least every 3 months or more often if clinically indicated. Concomitantly, monoclonal protein in the serum and/or urine should be measured by immunoelectrophoresis or, preferably, using more sensitive immunofixation techniques. A skeletal survey should be done annually, with BM examination reserved for diagnosis and time of subsequent change in clinical status, in monoclonal Ig, or in hemogram. It is important to remember that reduction of serum or urine M component as objective evidence of tumor response could reflect increased protein catabolism, decreased protein production, or both. Moreover, non-M protein-secreting MM

Table 120-7 Response Comparison of Southwest Oncology Group (SWOG) and SWOG+ Criteria

Response Criteria	SPEP Reduction (%)	IF (Serum and Urine)	UPEP Reduction (%)	Bone Marrow	Bone Disease	Calcium	Confirmation
CR							
SWOG	75	Not required	90	Not required	Not required	Not required	Yes (3 weeks)
SWOG	100	Negative	100	< 5% PC	Stable	Normal	Yes (6 weeks)
PR							
SWOG	50	Not required	Not required	Not required	Not required	Not required	Yes (3 weeks)
SWOG	50	Not required	90% or < 200 mg	Not required	Normal	Normal	Yes (6 weeks)

Sources: Alexanian R. Cancer 1972;30:382. Blade J, Samson D, Reece D, et al.[292]

CR = complete response; IF = immunofixation; PC = plasma cells; PR = partial response; SPEP = serum protein electrophoresis; UPEP = urine protein electrophoresis.

clones may emerge during treatment, so that even a marked reduction in monoclonal Ig may not correlate with decrease in tumor burden.

Two major definitions of response in MM have been widely utilized, that of the Chronic Leukemia–MM Task Force and that of the Southwest Oncology Group (SWOG).[290,291] The former requires ≥ 50% decrease in monoclonal serum or urine protein, ≥ 50% decrease in cross-sectional areas of plasmacytoma, and some recalcification of bone lesions (without new lesions); whereas the latter requires a 75% or greater reduction in production of MM protein. However, the frequencies of response by either definition are similar in previously untreated patients receiving melphalan and prednisone. Response rates of 32 to 53% were noted by SWOG criteria, and 33 to 56% responses were recorded by Task Force criteria. Need for, and response to, treatment may be a more important determinant of survival than initial tumor stage. For example, a low labeling index may define patients who may not need therapy irrespective of stage; such patients may have a long course prior to need for therapy, a gradual response to treatment, and prolonged survival. Most recently, the Blade criteria to assess response post-transplant were developed for the European Group for Blood and Marrow Transplant (EBMT), the International BM Transplant Registry (IBMTR), and the Autologous Blood and Marrow Transplant Registry (ABMTR).[292] These criteria include a more sensitive and rigorous definition of complete response, including absence of paraprotein assayed by immunofixation, and excludes transient responses (Table 120-7).

Conventional Therapy ***Initial Treatment*** Oral administration of melphalan and prednisone (MP) is a standard form of therapy that produces objective response in up to 50 to 60% of patients.[1,293,294] The dosage of melphalan, because of the variability of absorption, should be modified if necessary so that some reduction in leukocytes and platelets occurs 3 to 4 weeks after the beginning of each cycle. Unless there is disease progression, melphalan and prednisone should be given for at least 1 year until the monoclonal Ig levels in the serum and/or urine have been stable for at least 6 months (plateau state) and then discontinued if the patient has no other evidence of active disease. Typical doses are melphalan at 0.15 mg/kg daily for 7 days (8–10 mg/d) and 20 mg of prednisone three times daily for the same period. Melphalan must be given before meals because food reduces absorption. It is important to remember that the natural course of MM is one of progression, so that alleviation of pain and lack of progressive disease may be beneficial even in the absence of an objective response. In addition, some patients with a low plasma cell proliferative index do not obtain an objective response until the second year. Indeed, in a Canadian study of 457 patients treated with MP, the median survival of those patients who responded, had stable disease, or progressed was 48, 49, and 15 months, respectively.[295] The prognosis is therefore poor in patients who progress despite MP, and second-line chemotherapy is indicated. However, patients who remain stable should not be switched to other therapy, as they appear to do as well as responders. This regimen should, however, be reserved for those patients who are not candidates for stem cell transplantation.[296]

The obvious shortcomings of MP have stimulated investigators to use many combinations of chemotherapeutic agents. A major controversy in treatment of MM is whether MP is as effective as combination chemotherapy (CCT) (Table 120-8).[297] Although some studies have demonstrated that CCT was superior to MP, 10 prospective randomized trials of MP versus a drug combination failed to clearly show that other drug combinations were better than MP.[214,291,298] Improved response rates may not translate into prolonged survival.[299] An earlier SWOG study suggested that combinations of vincristine, melphalan, Cytoxan, and prednisone (VMCP) alternating with vincristine, BCNU, Adriamycin, and prednisone (VBAP) with or without levamisole were superior to vincristine, Cytoxan, and prednisone (VCP) with or without levamisole. However, the results of this trial demonstrated only a 54% response rate and 48-month survival in those receiving VMCP/VBAP without levamisole.[300] Initial CCT with vincristine, doxorubicin, and MM (VAD) produces a high response rate (84%), with 28% of all patients having complete response; however, duration of response was only 18 months.[301] Initial therapy with high-dose steroids achieved response rates approximately 15% less than those seen with VAD and similar to those with MP.[302] Serious complications were less than with VAD, and survival was similar. VAD-like regimens are currently being replaced by use of regimens containing pegylated liposomal doxorubicin.[303,304] This regimen has the obvious advantage of intravenous bolus injection as opposed to continuous infusion circumventing the need for a catheter and comparable efficacy.

Table 120-8 Myeloma Therapies versus Combination Chemotherapy (CCT)

3,814 patients in 18 trials of CCT versus MP
No difference overall: MP superior for good prognosis, inferior for poor prognosis patients.
Source: Gregory WJ. Clin Oncol 1992;10:334
6,333 patients in 27 trials of CCT versus MP
Higher response rates to CCT but equivalent mortality and survival

Source: Myeloma Trialists' Collaborative Group. J Clin Oncol 1998;16:3832.

The inclusion of high doses of corticosteroids increases the frequency of response to chemotherapy and may prolong survival in MM.[305] One of the best-known combinations is the M2 protocol, which includes vincristine, carmustine (BCNU), melphalan, cyclophosphamide, and prednisone (VBMCP). In an Eastern Cooperative Oncology Group (ECOG) study, 220 evaluable patients were randomized to VBMCP and 221 to MP. The objective response was 72% for VBMCP and 51% for MP, but the median survival was not different at 30 versus 28 months, respectively.[306] Elderly, bed-ridden patients had worse survival with VBMCP, but the remaining 85% of patients had a significantly improved survival with the combination of alkylating agents, with the 5-year survival for patients treated with VBMCP at 26% compared with 19% for MP.

In an attempt to determine which patients, if any, do better with more aggressive therapy, Gregory and colleagues examined published reports of 18 randomized controlled trials comparing MP with CCT in the primary treatment of 3,814 patients.[307] The overall results suggested that there was no difference in efficacy between these treatment modalities. Those studies with a high 2-year survival rate showed a survival difference in favor of MP, whereas those with a low rate suggested a difference in favor of CCT. These results imply that, rather than there being no difference between MP and CCT, MP is superior for patients with an intrinsically good prognosis and inferior for those patients with a poor prognosis. A second overview of 6,633 patients from 27 randomized trials of CCT versus MP confirmed higher response rates to CCT but equivalent mortality and survival.[308] In a recent SWOG study, alternate day prednisone at a dose of 50 mg was noted to improve overall survival (OS) and event-free survival (EFS) after induction treatment with a VAD-like induction regimen.[309]

Data from the relapsed refractory setting in MM have prompted the use of alternate strategies including Thal and dexamethasone as initial therapy for MM.[310–312] This is a well tolerated oral regimen with major toxicities being thromboembolic phenomena. Recently, Thal/Dex has been compared with VAP and Dex as initial therapy for patients prior to collection of autologous stem cells and transplantation. Thal/Dex has been compared in a care control analysis where higher response rates were achieved with Thal/Dex compared to VAD. A randomized phase III ECOG trial has also demonstrated higher response rates for Thal/Dex versus Dex. Most recently, Lenalinamide (Revlamid) + Dex has shown superior results compared to Dex alone in the relapsed refractory setting.

Refractory Disease Almost all patients with MM who initially respond to chemotherapy eventually relapse. Patients who progress with initial therapy have a 40% response to high-dose or pulsed corticosteroid therapy.[313] Patients who relapse during therapy or within 6 months of stopping initial treatment have a 75% response rate to VAD chemotherapy.[313–315] Patients who relapse more than 6 months after stopping therapy have a 60 to 70% response rate when initial therapy is reinstituted; if no response is achieved, then VAD or alternate regimens can be used.[293] Tumor cell associated multidrug resistance (MDR) p-glycoprotein (PGP) in aneuploid MM cells correlates with resistance to VAD. Verapamil, tamoxifen, cyclosporine, and PSC 833 have been evaluated as chemosensitizers for reversing multidrug resistance in such MM cells, both in vitro and in clinical trials.[316–318] However, there are multiple mechanisms of drug resistance in MM. Studies have demonstrated that patients who received no prior therapy, cumulative doses of 20 mg of vincristine, 340 mg of doxorubicin, or both vincristine and doxorubicin had 6%, 50%, 83%, and 100% PGP expression, respectively. This suggests that PGP induction is related primarily to therapy.[319] Moreover, PGP is functional in refractory MM; clinical modulation of MDR by cyclosporine (CSA) is mediated through an inhibition of PGP-associated drug efflux, and PGP-expressing plasma cells can be eliminated by combined treatment with VAD and CSA.[318] Unfortunately, even in those patients who respond to salvage therapy, the duration of response is limited. For example, a treatment of refractory MM consisting of etoposide, cisplatin, cytarabine, and MM (EDAP) led to a 40% response in patients resistant to MP, VAD, and high-dose melphalan. However, median survival following EDAP was only 4.5 months.[320] This may be due to alternative potential mechanisms of drug resistance in MM.[318] Topotecan has been shown to have activity in resistant and refractory MM, achieving partial response or better in 16% of patients studied.[321] Of great interest is the observation that cells that are resistant to chemotherapy may also be resistant to Fas-mediated apoptosis, suggesting common downstream effectors.[78]

A major advance in the treatment of resistant MM has been the emergence of Thal as an effective therapy.[122] Despite its potent teratogenicity, the drug is not mutagenic or carcinogenic. The University of Arkansas Cancer Center has evaluated Thal as a sole therapeutic agent for advanced and refractory MM.[122] Prior to receiving Thal, 85% of subjects in this open-label experience underwent at least one cycle of graft-supported high-dose therapy, and 66% had disease relapse/progression after two transplants. The majority of these patients had poor prognostic factors, including IgA subclass and adverse cytogenetic changes. An analysis of the first 83 patients revealed that 32% of patients responded, assessed by SWOG criteria. In a follow-up study, these authors have identified prognostic factors in 169 MM patients with advanced and refractory MM treated with single agent Thal.[322] An overall response rate of 37% was noted; low plasma cell labeling index (PCLI) and normal cytogenetics were associated with higher response rates. The 2-year event-free survival (EFS) and overall survival (OS) were 20% and 48%, respectively; low PCLI, normal cytogenetics, and a β2m < 3 mg/L were good prognostic factors for survival. Based on the impressive results of single agent Thal in refractory relapsed MM and in vitro data suggesting its synergy with Dex, Thal has been coupled with Dex to treat patients with disease refractory to either agent alone; even in this setting, half of patients treated respond.[323] Thal has also been combined with chemotherapy and bisphosphonates in the treatment of refractory MM and is now under evaluation to treat patients earlier in their disease course.[324,325]

Proteosome inhibitors like bortezomib are another significant advance in the therapy of relapsed MM.[57,326] Laboratory-derived studies, coupled with phase I studies of PS-341[327]demonstrating clinical promise in patients with refractory MM, provided the strong rationale for a recently completed multicenter phase II trial of PS-341 in MM (Table 120-9).[326] Two hundred two patients with relapsed and refractory MM were treated on this trial. Of 193 patients who could be evaluated, 92% had been heavily pretreated and the majority of them were refractory to prior therapy. Bortezomib induced a response in 35% of these patients with a median overall survival of 16 months and a median duration of response of 12 months. This therapy was well tolerated with peripheral neuropathy (12%) being the most significant long-term toxicity. Based on this clinical promise, a phase III international randomized trial of PS-341 versus Dex in relapsed MM has demonstrated prolonged TTP in Bortezomib treated patients and the use of Bortezomib in newly diagnosed MM patients is being studied.

Alpha-2B Interferon Therapy The potential mechanisms of action of alpha-2b interferon (IFNα) are both direct and indirect. They include direct cytotoxicity on MM cells, synergism with chemotherapy, a change in the pharmacokinetics of melphalan, inhibition of IL-6, down-regulation of IL-6 receptor on MM cells, down-regulation of activated oncogenes, an increase in NK cells, an increase in tumor cell surface antigens, and/or expansion of specific cytotoxic T cells.[328]

Table 120-9 Conclusions of Phase II Study of Bortezomib
Rate of response to bortezomib: 35%
Median overall survival: 16 months
Median duration of response: 12 months
Manageable toxicity
Reproduced from Richardson PG, et al.[326]

Clinical Studies Several prospective randomized trials have examined the utility of combined IFNα and chemotherapy for induction therapy. The largest was from the Nordic MM Study Group, which utilized MP alone or with IFNα.[329] IFNα prolonged the duration of the plateau phase by 5 to 6 months without a statistically significant increase in median survival. Other trials also found improved response rates and remission duration but no significant prolongation of survival from the addition of IFNα.[330–332] A meta-analysis of 16 randomized trials involving 2,286 patients receiving combined IFNα-chemotherapy for induction treatment yielded higher response rates (CR or PR) in the IFNα arms, but the average gain was only approximately 10%.[330] Similarly, significant but only marginal gains were detected in the IFNα arms in remission duration (median 7 months) and survival (median 5 months).

Mandelli and colleagues were the first to examine the use of IFNα maintenance therapy in a randomized trial in patients who had achieved CR, PR, or stable disease after either MP or VMCP/VBAP.[333] They treated 202 patients with symptomatic MM with 12 monthly courses of either MP or VMCP alternating with VBAP, followed by maintenance IFNα. Although the duration of response and survival was superior with IFNα, subsequent studies had variable results. The remission duration was always longer in the IFNα arm than in patients without maintenance treatment, but the observed differences reached statistical significance in only a few studies and were minimal in others.[305,330,334–336] Substantial increases in survival times were also observed only in some trials.[330,336] Meta-analysis of eight trials of 929 patients receiving maintenance IFNα revealed that both remission duration and survival were significantly longer in the IFNα arm than in the control arm, but median gains were only 6 and 5 months, respectively.[330]

It should be noted that patients may develop flu-like symptoms and anorexia as well as myelosuppression related to IFNα therapy, but only a fraction of patients, primarily the elderly, have required either reduction of the dose or discontinuation of IFNα. A survey of US patients found a 6-month risk/benefit trade off preferred by the majority of interviewed MM patients with regard to IFNα treatment.[337] Quality Adjusted Time Without Symptoms or Toxicity (Q-TWIST) analysis showed that patients treated with maintenance IFNα gained an average of 9.8 months without disease relapse and 5.8 months of overall survival versus the control groups; however, the IFNα group suffered an average of 4.1 months of moderate or worse toxicity.[338] IFNα maintenance treatment, therefore, appears to benefit a subset of patients who have achieved low tumor burden, and its marginal benefit needs to be balanced against side effects in this patient group.

Radiation Therapy Radiation therapy for MM is used for treatment of localized disease, including plasmacytoma or spinal cord compression syndrome, and is frequently used for palliation. Hemibody radiation therapy has been utilized, either as a consolidation following induction combination chemotherapy or as salvage therapy for chemotherapy-resistant MM.[339,340] As is discussed below, total body irradiation (TBI) can be used as a component of ablative therapy prior to hematopoietic stem cell grafting.

High-Dose Therapies The rationale for the administration of alkylating agents (melphalan, cyclophosphamide, busulfan) in a higher than conventional dose with or without TBI, followed by transplantation of syngeneic, allogeneic, and autologous BM or peripheral blood progenitor cells (PBPCs), is as follows: Plasma cell dyscrasias remain uniformly fatal, multiple studies document sensitivity of MM cells to chemotherapy and radiotherapy, and CRs can be obtained with high-dose therapy.

Allogeneic Stem Cell Transplantation An encouraging lead for newer treatment approaches in MM arose from reports of CRs after the administration of alkylating agents in higher-than-conventional doses with or without TBI, followed by syngeneic or allogeneic BM transplantation (BMT).[341,342] Reduction in tumor mass in some cases has been dramatic, with CR rates commonly in the 40% range and a similar number of partial responses (PR). Syngeneic BMT has been done infrequently, but some patients reported from Seattle and in European BM Transplant Group (EBMT) remain progression-free at long intervals post-BMT.[343,344] The EBMT has reported on allografting in MM (Table 120-10).[345–347] Actuarial overall survival (OS) was 32% at 4 years, and 28% at 7 years for the 72 (44%) patients who achieved CR after BMT. However, overall progression-free survival (PFS) was 34% at 6 years, and few patients remain in continuing CR at over 4 years post-allografting. Favorable pre-BMT prognostic factors for both response to and survival after BMT were female gender, IgA MM, low serum β2M, stage I disease at diagnosis, one line of previous treatment, and being in CR prior to BMT. Of major concern is the 40% transplant-related mortality (50% in males) in the EBMT report, which has subsequently been reduced to 20 to 30%.[346,348] In the allografting experience in Seattle, actuarial probabilities of OS and event-free survival for the 36% of patients achieving CR were 0.50 ± 0.21 and 43 ± 0.17, respectively, at 4.5 years. Adverse prognostic factors included transplantation > 1 year from diagnosis, serum β2M > 2.5 mg/dL at transplant, female patients transplanted from male donors, having received > eight cycles of chemotherapy, and Durie–Salmon stage III disease at presentation. Again, toxicity was common, with 35 (44%) patients dying of transplant-related causes within 100 days of BMT.[349] Busulfan/cyclophosphamide ablation achieved 4-year disease-free survival of 26% in a report of 19 patients with MM, but transplant-related mortality (TRM) was 37%.[350] Finally, there were 15 deaths among 36 patients within the first 100 days postallografting in an ongoing multigroup randomized trial in the United States of high-dose versus conventional therapy for MM. Nonetheless, molecular remissions, due in part to a graft versus MM effect, are noted in allogeneic BMT, and the emphasis now is to develop strategies to achieve and maintain high remission rates while avoiding transplant-related morbidity and mortality.

Table 120-10 Representative Studies of Allogeneic Transplantation for Newly Diagnosed Myeloma

	Number of Patients	TRM (%)	CR (%)	OS (Actuarial Months)	EFS (Actuarial Months)
Gahrton et al	162	41	44	28% at 84	45% at 60
Bensinger et al	80	44	36	20% at 54	24% at 54
Alyea et al	61[a]	5	28	40% at 36	20% at 38

Sources: Gahrton G. Br J Haematol 2001;98:934.[349] Bensinger W. Semin Hematol 2001;38:934.[346] Alyea E, Weller E, Schlossman R, et al.[367]
CR = complete response; EFS = event-free survival; OS = overall survival; TRM = transplant-related mortality.
[a]T-cell depleted.

In an attempt to improve the outcome of allografting in MM by avoiding TRM, we carried out T (CD6)-depleted allografting using histocompatible sibling donors in 61 patients with MM whose disease remained sensitive to conventional chemotherapy (see Table 120-10).[351–354] There were 17 (28%) CRs and 34 (57%) PRs, 2 (3%) NR, and only 3 (5%) transplant-related deaths. Forty-seven percent of patients did not develop graft-versus-host disease (GVHD) and 36% had grade I GVHD; only 17% of patients developed ≥ grade II GVHD. Overall survival from time of BMT was a median of 2 years, with approximately 40% of patients surviving beyond 3 years. However, disease-free survival (DFS) after allo-BMT was 1 year, with only 20% of patients disease free at ≥ 4 years post-transplant. The OS and DFS do not significantly differ from our outcome after autografting in MM. Another way to counter transplant-related toxicity is to offer early transplant; the EBMT registry data demonstrate improved survival with low TRM in patients transplanted between 1994 and 1998 because of better patient selection, early trans-plantation, and less pretransplant treatment.[346]

Graft-Versus-MM Effect Molecular remissions are more common after allografting than after autografting, suggesting the ability of an allogeneic graft versus MM effect to mediate sustained remission.[355–358] Data from multiple centers have shown that patients with relapsed hematologic malignancies after allogeneic BMT can achieve marked clinical responses after infusions of lymphocytes collected from the marrow donor (DLI).[359–361] In the setting of relapsed chronic myelogenous leukemia (CML) after allografting, this therapy is most effective in patients with cytogenetic relapse or those in stable phase. However, GVHD occurs in 40 to 60% of patients treated with DLI, contributing to a 13 to 18% treatment-related mortality.[361] Although many investigators have suggested that DLI induces a graft-versus-leukemia (GVL) effect by the induction of GVHD, some patients can obtain a CR in the absence of clinical GVHD, suggesting that the GVL response may be independent of clinical GVHD. Both T-cell number and CD8+ T cells have been implicated in GVHD, and Champlin and colleagues have utilized CD8+ T-cell depletion of donor BM or DLI to avoid GVHD.[362] DLI has been used to treat 3 patients with relapsed MM after allografting, providing the first direct evidence of a GVM effect.[363,364] In these cases, however, GVHD was observed after DLI. Infusion of thymidine kinase gene-transduced DLI, followed by treatment of the recipient with ganciclovir, has been proposed as a potential strategy to treat DLI-associated GVHD.[365]

More recently, we have demonstrated that the GVL effect of DLI can be preserved and GVHD can be abrogated by utilizing CD8-depleted (CD4+) DLI.[366] We have used CD4+ DLI to treat 15 patients with early relapsed CML, 6 patients with advanced CML, 7 patients with MM, and 7 patients with other hematologic malignancies that have recurred after sibling histocompatible CD6-depleted allogeneic BMT. Overall, only 8 of 32 (25%) patients evaluable for toxicity developed acute or chronic GVHD. Treatment-related mortality was low (3%), with one death related to infection in the setting of immunosuppression for GVHD. Complete cytogenetic remissions were noted in 11 of 14 patients with early-phase relapsed CML, including 10 molecular remissions. Five of 7 patients with MM have responded, including three CRs. Overall 6, of 11 patients with CML developed CRs in the absence of clinical GVHD. Given the high response rates, but inevitable relapses, observed in the setting of allografting for MM, we have utilized CD4+ DLI at 6 months post–CD6-depleted BM allografting in order to enhance GVM effect, thereby improving outcome.[345,347,349,353] We have shown that prophylactic DLI induces significant GVM responses after allogeneic BMT but that only 58% of patients were able to receive DLI despite T-cell–depleted BMT.[367] At our institute, the patient outcome after allografting and autografting is equivalent because of the higher toxicity of allografting versus the higher relapse rate postautografting (Table 120-11).[368] Therefore, less toxic transplantation strategies are needed to allow a higher proportion of patients to receive DLI and the benefit from the graft-versus-myeloma effect after transplantation. Our laboratory data demonstrate that patients who receive DLI have a markedly abnormal T-cell repertoire, detected by molecular analysis of T-cell receptor (TCR) *VP* gene rearrangements in peripheral T cells.[369,370] Following infusion of CD4+ DLI, analysis of TCR utilization has identified the expansion of clonal and oligoclonal T-cell populations, which coincides with the elimination of MM cells from marrow and decreases in levels of circulating monoclonal paraprotein. More recently, we have confirmed that prophylactic infusion of

Table 120-11 Dana Farber Cancer Institute Experience

	166 Autografts	6 Allografts	*p*
2 year OS	74%	51%	.006
2 year PFS	48%	28%	.002
4 year OS	41%	39%	
4 year PFS	23%	18%	
4 year non-relapse mortality	13%	24%	.004
Relapse at 4 years	56%	46%	.02
N.B. Need to reduce non-relapse mortality to exploit allografting			

OS = overall survival; PFS = progression free survival.
Reproduced from Alyea EP et al.[368]

CD4+ DLI, besides enhancing reconstitution of donor T cells, helps reconstitute donor hematopoiesis and promotes antitumor immunity.[370] Attempts are also under way to immunize the allogeneic marrow donor to the patient's idiotypic MM protein and thereby transfer specific immunity against MM at the time of allografting.[371] Initial experience demonstrates the transfer of immunity to idiotypic protein, evidenced by the derivation from the patient postallografting of a donor CD4+ T-cell line that proliferates in vitro to the immunizing idiotypic protein. Ongoing studies are defining optimal immunization strategies and may vary in distinct clinical settings. For example, Wimperis and colleagues have shown that preimmunization of both BM donors and BM recipients was required to obtain antigen-specific responses at 3 months post-transplantation in recipients of T-cell–depleted allogeneic sibling marrows.[372]

The use of nonmyeloablative transplantation is an alternative strategy to preserve GVM allogeneic immunity while avoiding the toxicity of allografting (Table 120-12). Melphalan at a dose of 100 mg/m^2 has been used in combination with DLI in high-risk MM patients.[373] Although disease control was achieved in some patients, significant GVHD was noted in this group of patients. Autografting has been performed prior to nonmyeloablative transplant by several investigators, demonstrating the feasibility of this approach to cytoreduce tumor and then enhance anti-MM immunity.[374,375] Although preliminary results are encouraging, follow-up is short, and chronic GVHD may remain a problem.

Autologous Stem Cell Transplantation High-dose chemoradiotherapy followed by transplantation of either autologous BM or PBPCs has also achieved high (40%) CR rates, but the median duration of these responses has, unfortunately, been only 24 to 36 months.[341,376] Patients with sensitive disease and who are less heavily pretreated have the most favorable outcomes. Most important, a national French trial, in which 200 patients with MM who received two courses of VMCP alternating with VBAP were then randomized to receive either conventional chemotherapy (eight additional courses of VMCP/VBAP) or high-dose therapy (melphalan and TBI) followed by autologous BMT, has demonstrated significantly higher response rates, EFS, and OS for those patients treated with high-dose compared with those receiving conventional therapy (Table 120-13).[377] Response rates in the high-dose and conventional arms were 81% versus 57%, respectively. The 5-year probability of EFS and OS was 28% and 52% in recipients of high-dose therapy and only 10% and 12%, respectively, in patients treated with conventional therapy; treatment-related mortality was low and comparable between the two groups. However, the median survival of patients who are less than 65 years of age and respond to initial chemotherapy is 5 years, stressing the importance of randomized trials to assess the relative efficacy of high-dose versus conventional therapy for similar patient groups.[378] Age as a prognostic factor for transplantation has been evaluated in several studies. Moreover, although high-dose therapy is feasible with EFS and OS and outcomes were comparable to those of younger pair mates, increased toxicity is noted in older patients.[379–381] Similarly, excessive toxicity resulted in reduction of melphalan dosage for patients on dialysis.[382] A second randomized trial in MM examined the relative merits of high-dose therapy either early versus late as salvage therapy for relapse after conventional therapy.[383] The overall survival was 64 months in both groups, but the Quality Adjusted Time without Symptoms and Toxicity (Q-TWIST) strongly favored the early-transplant cohort. The IFM has subsequently conducted a randomized trial comparing high-dose melphalan at 200 mg/m^2 versus melphalan at 140 mg/m^2 plus TBI as ablative therapies.[384] Although response rates and EFS were comparable, toxicity and OS was superior in the high-dose melphalan alone arm, suggesting that TBI should not be considered part of the ablation regimen. The Medical Research Council of UK has also completed a randomized trial favoring high-dose therapy.[385] A Scandinavian population-based study demonstrated prolonged survival for patients with MM under 60 years of age treated with intensive therapy compared to historical controls, who received conventional therapy.[386] Although these studies are encouraging and additional randomized trials in the United States, Scandinavia, and Spain are comparing the outcome of conventional therapy versus high-dose therapy and autografting, it is unlikely that patients are cured after a single high dose and stem cell autografting regimen. In all studies to date, the median EFS was prolonged, CR rates were higher in 4 of 5 studies, and OS was improved in 3 of 5 studies.

Improving Outcome of Autografting Attempts to improve the outcome of high-dose therapy followed by autografting include the use of autologous BM or PBPCs either depleted of tumor cells, or processed to select normal hematopoietic progenitor cells by virtue of CD34 expression or multiparameter cell sorting.[353,389–392] Specifically, we have carried out autografting including MoAb-purged BM or PBSCs, or CD34+ PBSCs in 105 patients with MM whose disease remained sensitive to conventional chemotherapy.[353,389,390] Median OS from time of BMT was 4.2 years, with 40% of patients surviving ≥ 5 years. However, median DFS from BMT is only 2.2 years, with < 20% of patients remaining disease free > 4 years post-transplant. More recently, we compared 228 patients undergoing transplantation over a 10-year period, including 166 patients who underwent autografting and 66 patients who received histocompatible T-depleted allografts (see Table 120-11).[368] By 4 years post-transplant, the outcomes were similar, with relapses in the autografting group versus higher toxicity and lower relapse rates in the allograft recipients achieving equivalent long-term outcomes. Therefore, new strategies are needed to treat minimal residual disease after autografting, as relapse remains the major obstacle to progress.

PBPCs are commonly mobilized for collection using filgrastim after chemotherapy, and one study suggests that stem cell factor and filgrastim enhances yield and reduces the number of phereses required.[393] CD34 selection of autologous PBPCs has been used to positively select normal hematopoietic progenitors while depleting MM cells, and can achieve up to 5 log depletion of tumor cells.[391] However, this remains controversial, since CD34+ cells in the blood of MM patients have been reported to express CD19 and IgH mRNA and have patient-specific IgH *VDJ* gene rearrangements.[394] Moreover, after a median follow-up of 28 months,

Table 120-12 Representative Studies of Miniallogeneic Transplantation in Myeloma

Source	Conditioning	Sample Size (*n*)	TRM (%)	Response Rate (%)	Acute GVHD (%)	Chronic GVHD (%)	PFS (%)	OS (%)
Badros et al [373]	Mel or Mel/TBI/Flu	31	10% early, 20% late	CR 61, PR 10	58	32	86 (1 year)	86 (1 year)
Kroger et al[374]	PBSCT + Mel/Flu/ATG	17	18	CR 73, PR 20	63	40	56 (2 year)	74 (2 year)
Maloney et al[375]	PBSCT + TBI/MMF/cyc	31	16	CR 43, PR 31,	45	55	—	81 (1 year)

CR = complete response; GVHD = graft-versus-host disease; OS = overall survival; PFS = progression free survival; PR = partial response; TRM = transplant-related mortality.

Table 120-13 Autologous Transplantation vs Conventional Chemotherapy for Newly Diagnosed Myeloma

Author	Therapy	Patients (*n*)	CR (%)	EFS (Median Months)	OS (Median Months)
Barlogie et al[387]	Conventional *	116	—	22	48
	HDT	123	40	49	62
Lenhoff et al[386]	Conventional*	274	—		46% at 48
	HDT	274	34	27	61% at 48
Attal et al[377]	Conventional	100	5	18	37
	HDT	100	22	27	52% at 60
Fermand et al[383]	Conventional	96	—	18.7	50.4
	HDT	94	—	24.3	55.3
Blade et al[388]	Conventional	83	11	34.3	66.9
	HDT	81	30	42.5	67.4
Child et al[385]	Conventional	200	8.5	19.6	42.3
	HDT	201	44	31.6	54.8

CR = complete response; EFS = event free survival; HDT = hgih dose therapy; OS = overall survival.
* Historical controls.

progression-free survival of 51 patients who underwent high-dose therapy and transplantation of CD34+ PBPCs is only 34 ± 15%, suggesting that the majority of patients, as in other autografting studies, are destined to relapse.[395] A multicenter trial of 193 patients who received either unpurged or CD34+-selected PBPC autografts after ablative chemotherapy with cyclophosphamide and busulfan therapy assessed hematologic engraftment as well as MM burden in the BM and peripheral blood before, at the time of, and after transplantation. Prompt engraftment was noted in both CD34+ and unselected arms. Moreover, in recipients of CD34+ autografts, a median 0.68 and 1.1 log reduction in BM contamination with MM was achieved at 100 and 180 days after grafting, respectively. Peripheral blood MM burden at 100 and 180 days post-transplant was similarly reduced by a median of greater than 1.8 and 1.9 logs, respectively.[396] However, in spite of a median of 3.1 log reduction in MM cells within the CD34+ selected autografts, there was no impact on survival at 2 years.[397,398] A second trial showed that CD34+ selection also had no impact on the outcome of either single or tandem high-dose chemotherapy.[399] Since residual tumor cells are detectable in the graft as well as in the patient after transplant, it would appear that few patients using this approach are likely to be cured.

Several additional strategies have been attempted to improve the outcome of autografting. Barlogie and colleagues[400] are performing multiple high-dose therapies and stem cell transplantation (Table 120-14).[218,395,400,401] Response rates are higher relative to historically matched controls, but the impact on long-term disease-free survival requires further follow-up. A French randomized trial has compared single versus double high-dose therapy and stem cell transplantation.[402] Three hundred and ninety-nine previously untreated patients under the age of 60 years were randomly assigned to receive a single or double transplant. A complete or a very good partial response was achieved by 42% of patients in the single-transplant group and 50% of patients in the double-transplant group ($p = .10$). The probability of surviving event-free for 7 years after the diagnosis was 10% in the single-transplant group and 20% in the double-transplant group ($p = .03$). The estimated overall 7-year survival rate was 21% in the single-transplant group and 42% in the double-transplant group ($p = .01$). Among patients who did not have a very good partial response within 3 months after one transplantation, the probability of surviving 7 years was 11% in the single-transplant group and 43% in the double-transplant group ($p < .001$). When patients who achieved a CR were compared there did not appear to be significant difference in overall survival, suggesting that double transplant may benefit a subset of MM patients who do not achieve a CR with the fist transplant. Four factors were significantly related to survival: base-line serum levels of β2m ($p < .01$), lactate dehydrogenase ($p < .01$), age ($p < .05$), and treatment group ($p < .01$).

Table 120-14 Single vs Double Autologous Transplantation for Newly Diagnosed Myeloma

Author	Therapy	Patients (*n*)	CR (%)	EFS (Median, Month)	OS (Median, Month)
Attal et al	Single	88	42	10% at 84	21% at 84
	Double	92	50	20% at 84	42% at 84
Fermand et al	Single	94	37	No difference	No difference
	Double	99	42		
Cavo et al	Single	81	34	21.5	71% at 48
	Double	97	41	29.5	74% at 48

CR = complete response; EFS = event free survival; OS = overall survival.
Sources: Attal et al. Single versus double autologous stem-cell transplantation for multiple myeloma. N Engl J Med. 2004 Jun17;350(25):2628. Fermand et al. High-dose therapy and autologous peripheral blood stem cell transplantation in multiple myeloma: up-front or rescue treatment? Results of a multicenter sequential randomized clinical trial. Blood. 1998 Nov 1;92(9):3131–6. Cavo et al. Proc VIII Intl Myeloma Wkshp 2001:516:29.

A second trial from France showed no benefit of tandem over single transplant,[403] whereas the Dutch HOVOM, Bologna-96, and GMMG trials all show prolonged event free survival in favor of double autografting. Giralt and colleagues have reported on the use of cyclosporine to induce GVHD postautografting in an attempt to generate associated autologous GVM effect.[404] Finally, it may be possible to stimulate autologous immunity to MM to treat MRD postautografting and thereby improve outcome. Multiple reports suggest that patients may mount an anti-MM immune response.[405] In one study, some MM patients repeatedly immunized with autologous monoclonal Ig demonstrated idiotypic specific T-cell response characterized by γIFN and IL4 secretions, as well as B cells secreting anti-idiotype Ab; however, the induced T-cell response was eliminated during repeated immunization.[406] Hsu and colleagues have vaccinated patients with autologous dendritic cells pulsed ex vivo with tumor-specific idiotypic protein to stimulate host antitumor immunity, and they demonstrated T-cell–mediated anti-idiotype and anti-KLH proliferative responses specific for the immunizing Ig in some patients.[407] Interestingly, anti-idiotypic Abs were not detected, consistent with the view that the idiotype-pulsed DC induced a T helper 1 (TH1) rather than a TH2 response. Further studies are needed to optimize the immunization schedule to achieve long-lasting T-cell immunity against idiotypic determinants on the MM cell and determine its effect on clinical outcome.

FUTURE DIRECTIONS

Evolution of a New Treatment Paradigm for MM Our in vitro and animal model studies have demonstrated the importance of the BM in promoting MM cell growth, survival, drug resistance, and migration in the BM microenvironment and have already derived very promising therapies based on targeting the MM cell in its BM milieu. These studies provide the framework for development of a new treatment paradigm in MM, targeting both the tumor cell and its microenvironment, which is urgently needed since MM remains incurable despite all available therapies.

Identification and Validation of Novel-Targeted MM Therapies In order to overcome resistance to current therapies and improve patient outcome, novel biologically based treatment approaches that target mechanisms whereby MM cells grow and survive in the BM are needed. In our Jerome Lipper MM Center, we are attempting to derive novel therapies to improve patient outcome based on targeting the MM cell as well as its BM microenvironment.[408] To achieve this goal, we have developed systems for studying growth, survival, and drug resistance mechanisms intrinsic to MM cells. Importantly, we have also developed both in vitro systems and in vivo animal models to characterize mechanisms of MM cell homing to BM, as well as factors (MM cell–BMSC interactions, cytokines, angiogenesis) promoting MM cell growth, survival, drug resistance, and migration in the BM microenvironment.[64,66,67,70,115,409–411] These model systems have allowed for the development of several promising biologically based therapies that can target the MM cell in its BM microenvironment and thereby overcome classic drug resistance in vitro, including Thal and its more potent immunomodulatory analogs (IMiDs), the proteasome inhibitor PS-341, and As2O3.[56,57,412]

Once in vitro promise of these novel agents was demonstrated, we have rapidly tested their efficacy in murine models. Thal and the IMiDs, 3-amino-phthalimidoglutaramide, and PS-341 all inhibit human MM cell growth, decrease associated angiogenesis, and prolong host survival in our model where human MM cells and matrigel are injected subcutaneously into SCID mice.[413–415] We have translated our laboratory studies to phase I, II, and III clinical trials to evaluate their clinical utility and toxicity. Most exciting to us, IMiDs and PS-341 have already demonstrated marked clinical anti-MM activity even in patients with refractory relapsed MM, confirming the utility of our preclinical models to identify and validate novel therapeutics.[326,416] Importantly, as in our in vitro gene array studies with conventional Dex and novel (PS-341) therapies, samples obtained from patients treated on these protocols help to identify in vivo targets and mechanisms of novel drug action, on the one hand, versus mechanisms of drug resistance on the other, and also aid in determining whether in vivo targets of these novel therapies correlate with their in vitro anti-MM activities.[76,201] These studies have demonstrated the importance of evaluating the role of the MM cell in its BM microenvironment, both to elucidate MM pathogenesis and to identify targets for novel therapeutics.

Clinical Trials of Agents Targeting MM Cells and Their BM Microenvironment We have begun to translate these studies of Thal/IMiDs, PS-341, and As2O3 from bench to bedside in related clinical trials.[47,56,57,59,115,412,413,417] Specifically, increased angiogenesis in MM BM, coupled with the known antiangiogenesis activity of Thal, provided the rationale for its use to treat refractory MM. There have been remarkable responses even in MM refractory to all other known therapies.[56,122] Importantly, our studies to date demonstrate that Thal and IMiDs not only act to inhibit angiogenesis, but also act directly to induce either apoptosis or G_1 growth arrest in MM cells, even those refractory to conventional therapy; abrogate the adhesion of MM cells to BMSCs and related protection against apoptosis; block the increased secretion of MM growth, survival, and migratory factors (IL-6, VEGF) triggered by binding of MM cells to BMSCs; expand patients' NK cell number and function against human MM cells; and down-regulate protectin expression in MM cells, thereby enhancing their susceptibility to ADCC (Figure 120-8).[56,417,418] Using our SCID model, we have also shown that Thal/IMiDs mediate both anti-MM activity and antiangiogenesis in vivo.[413] Based on this promising preclinical data, we have recently carried out a phase I IMiD CC-5013 (Revlimid) dose escalation (5 mg/d, 10 mg/d, 25 mg/d, and 50 mg/d) study in 27 patients (median age 57, range 40–71) with relapsed and refractory relapsed MM.[416] Patients received a median of 3 (range 2–6) prior regimens, including autologous stem cell transplantation and Thal in 15 and 16 patients, respectively. In 24 evaluable patients, no dose-limiting toxicity (DLT) was observed in patients treated at any dose level within the first 28 days; however, grade 3 myelosuppression developed after day 28 in all 13 patients treated with 50 mg/d CC-5013. In 12 patients, dose reduction to 25 mg/d was well tolerated and therefore considered the maximal tolerated dose (MTD). Importantly, no significant somnolence, constipation, or neuropathy has been seen in any cohort. Best responses of ≥ 25% reduction in paraprotein occurred in 17 of 24 (71%) patients (90% CI: 52–85%), including 11 (46%) patients who had received prior Thal (Table 120-15). Stable disease (< 25% reduction in paraprotein) was observed in an additional 2 (8%) patients. Therefore, 17 of 24 (71%) patients (90% CI: 52%–85%) demonstrated benefit from treatment. Our study therefore provides the basis for the evaluation of CC-5013, either alone or in combination,[419,420] to treat patients with MM at earlier stages of disease. Ongoing studies include CC5013 (Revlimid) as initial therapy, treatment of first relapse, and as maintenance post-high–dose therapy and stem cell transplantation. Phase II studies have confirmed responses and complete responses in relapsed myelema and two phase III randomized trials have confirmed that Revlimid/Dex is superior to Dex in response rates and prolonging time to progression.

Proteasome inhibitors represent a second class of therapeutics targeting the MM cell in its BM microenvironment that have been extensively studied in our laboratory. Previous studies, have demonstrated that IL-6 is a major growth and survival factor for human MM cells, and MM cell adhesion to BMSCs triggers the transcription and secretion of IL-6 in BMSCs via an NF-κB–dependent mechanism. We therefore reasoned that blockade of NF-κB using the proteasome inhibitor PS-341 may mediate anti-MM activity by inhibiting paracrine IL-6 production in BMSCs.[43,58] Our studies demonstrate that PS-341 acts directly on MM cells to induce apoptosis of MM cells resistant to known conventional therapies, overcomes the protective effects of IL-6, and adds to the anti-MM effects of Dex (see Figure 120-8).[57] Importantly, it acts in the BM microenvironment to inhibit the binding of MM cells to BMSCs, the transcription and secretion of IL-6 triggered by MM to BMSC adhesion, and BM angiogenesis. Our recent gene microarray-profiling studies demonstrate that PS-341 induces transcriptional down-regulation of growth/survival signaling pathways, as well as up-regulation of apoptotic cascades, ubiquitin/proteasome pathways, and heat-shock proteins.[201] Our exciting studies, coupled with phase I studies of PS-341,

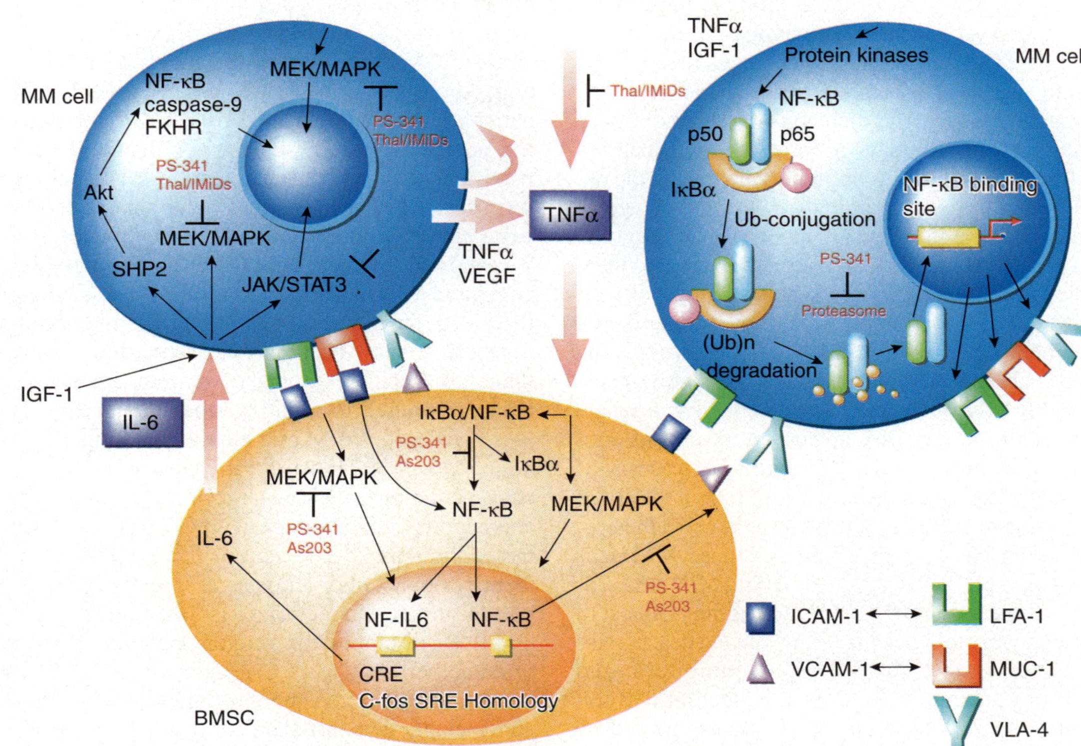

Figure 120-8 Inhibition of signaling pathways by novel therapeutic agents in multiple myeloma.

Table 120-15 Conclusions of Phase I Study of CC-5013 in Multiple Myeloma

Well tolerated with manageable toxicity
No somnolence, constipation, or neuropathy
Significant antitumor activity
More than 25% paraprotein reduction in 63% of patients
Stable disease or better in 79% of patients
Favorable pharmacokinetics
Convenient oral daily dosing

Source: Richardson P et al.[326]

demonstrating clinical promise in patients with refractory MM, provided the strong rationale for a recently completed multicenter phase II trial of PS-341 in MM emanating from our Center.[326] The promising results from our phase II trial were followed by an international phase III randomized study favoring the use of bortezomib in relapsed/refractory MM. Ongoing studies are testing the use of bortezomib in combination with other agents and as upfront in the treatment of MM at diagnosis.

Recent studies in our laboratory have also identified As2O3 as a third agent targeting both the MM cell and interactions with its BM microenvironment (see Figure 120-8). As2O3 at clinically achievable levels induces apoptosis of drug-resistant MM cell lines and patient cells via caspase-9 activation, adds to Dex, and can overcome the anti-apoptotic effects of IL-6.[412] It also decreases MM cell binding to BMSCs, inhibits IL-6 and VEGF secretion in BMSCs induced by MM cell adhesion, and even blocks proliferation of those MM cells adherent to BMSCs. As for Thal/IMiD and PS-341, clinical trials of As2O3 are ongoing. A host of other novel biologics including histone deacetylase inhibitors, heat shock protein inhibitors, and mTOR inhibitors are undergoing preclinical evaluation.[58,420–423] Importantly, our in vitro gene therapy studies with conventional Dex(71) and novel Bortezamib[201] therapies identify novel mechanisms of action and drug resistance, and in vitro data suggest increased cytotoxicity by combining novel agents with conventional treatments.

Immune-Based Strategies Although high response rates can be achieved using high-dose therapy followed by stem cell grafting, patients typically relapse, and few, if any, are cured. Major obstacles to cure are the excessive toxicity noted after allografting in MM, contaminating tumor cells in autografts, and the persistence of minimal residual disease (MRD) after high-dose therapy followed by either allogeneic or autologous stem cell transplantation. In this context, improved strategies to treat MRD after high-dose therapy followed by allogeneic or autologous stem cell grafting are being developed. Most important, multiple approaches for the generation and enhancement of allogeneic and autologous anti-MM immunity in vitro and in animal models are being studied. Based on this research, clinical trials are being designed that couple treatments such as transplant to achieve MRD with novel immune-based therapies, which target MRD post-transplant in an attempt to achieve long-term disease-free survival and potential cure.

Allografting Data from our center and others unequivocally demonstrate that donor lymphocyte infusions (DLI) mediate a GVM effect that can effectively treat relapsed MM postallografting.[366,424] Unfortunately, GVHD is a frequent cause of morbidity and mortality after DLI. However, at our Center, 5 of 7 patients who had relapsed post-CD6–depleted allograft responded (including 3 CRs) to CD4+ T-cell–enriched DLI, in some cases in the absence of GVHD. This raises the possibility that distinct T-cell clones may be mediating GVM versus GVHD. Given the high response rates, but inevitable relapses, observed in the setting of allografting for MM, we are now testing in a clinical protocol whether CD4+ DLI at 6 months post-CD6–depleted allografting may mediate GVM, which will effectively treat MRD and thereby improve outcome.[367] To date, 24 patients have undergone CD6-depleted allografting, and 18 received DLI; 3 are in CR, and 11 have persistent disease post-transplant. GVM responses were seen in 10 of 11 patients with persistent disease, resulting in 6 CRs and 4 PRs; overall, the 2-year EFS for recipients of DLI was improved compared with historical controls. These studies, therefore, suggest that GVM can be adoptively transferred in this fashion. T-cell repertoires, based upon Vβ T-cell receptor gene rearrangement, are being examined to identify those clonal T cells associated with GVM and their target antigens on tumor cells.[369,425] It has already been shown that T cells mediating GVM can target idiotypic antigens, and ongoing studies are presently identifying other target antigens.[370] The goal of these studies is to identify novel tumor antigens as targets for vaccination and to characterize, isolate, and expand GVM T-cell clones for antigen-specific adoptive immunotherapy.

Autografting Although randomized studies convincingly demonstrate a survival advantage for MM patients treated with high-dose therapy and autografting compared with those receiving conventional chemotherapy, this treatment is not curative. Two sites of MRD contribute to the failure of autografting: MRD in the autograft and MRD in the patient postmyeloablative therapy. Monoclonal antibodies have been produced in the laboratory, and these have been used to deplete tumor cells from MM autografts.[353] CD34 selection techniques have also been evaluated to select normal hematopoietic progenitor cells within autografts.[397] However, both of these methods deplete only 2 to 3 logs of tumor cells, and more than 50% of autografts still contained MRD. Based on our laboratory data that MM cells express MUC-1 and adenoviral receptors, we have specifically transduced tumor cells within MM autografts with the thymidine kinase (*tK*) gene using an adenoviral vector with a tumor-selective (MUC-1) promoter, followed by purging tumor cells ex vivo by treatment with ganciclovir.[426] Pilot studies suggest that more than 6 to 7 logs of tumor cells can be purged under conditions that do not adversely affect normal hematopoietic progenitor cells, suggesting one potential method for improved purging prior to autotransplantation.

We are also attempting to generate and expand anti-MM–specific autologous T cells ex vivo for adoptive immunotherapy of MRD in the patient postautotransplant. It is now possible to clone the gene for the patient's specific idiotypic protein, use computer programs to identify gene sequences encoding for peptides predicted to be presented within the groove of Class I HLA of a given patient's HLA type, and expand peptide-specific T cells ex vivo.[427] A similar strategy can be used to expand T cells against peptides within shared antigens that are overexpressed on MM cells, such as the telomerase catalytic subunit (hTERT), MUC-1, or the cytochrome cyp 1B1.[31,428,429] Immunologic responses are also being tested to enhance the immunogenicity of the whole tumor cell. For example, our laboratory studies have shown that autologous T cells do not proliferate in response to the patients' own tumor cells as targets. However, CD40 activation of MM cells up-regulates class I and II HLA, costimulatory, GRP94, and other molecules; and CD40-activated MM cells also trigger a brisk autologous T-cell response.[430] Although T cells can be harvested from MM patients before autografting, expanded ex vivo using CD40-activated autologous MM cells as a stimulus, and given as adoptive immunotherapy to treat MRD post-transplant, this is logistically complex. Therefore, we and others are developing and examining the clinical utility of a variety of MM vaccines. First, based upon our observation that CD40-activated MM cells trigger a brisk autologous T-cell response, we are examining the utility of vaccinations of patients with autologous CD40-activated tumor cells. Second, based on our demonstration of the expression of MUC-1 core protein on freshly isolated MM cells, we are evaluating two vaccines: recombinant vaccinia virus containing the *MUC-1* gene and autologous dendritic cells (DCs) transduced using adenoviral vectors with *MUC-1*.[31] Of interest, we have recently shown that MM cells can be fused to DCs and that the use of the MM DC fusion as an antigen-presenting cell presents the entire MM cell as foreign. In a syngeneic murine MM model, vaccinations with MM cell–DC fusions, but not with either MM cells or DCs alone, demonstrate both protective and therapeutic efficacy.[431] Most important, we have shown that patient MM cells can be fused to autologous DCs, which are readily isolated from either patient BM or peripheral blood, and that autologous MM cell–DC fusions can trigger specific cytolytic autologous T-cell responses in vitro.[432,433] We are translating these findings into clinical trials of MM-DC fusion vaccines to assess in vivo MM-specific T- and B-cell responses, as well as clinical efficacy.

Immunization protocols at other centers have already demonstrated a transient anti-Id T-cell response in 3 of 5 patients by injection of autologous Id. Moreover, 5 of 5 patients injected with autologous Id and GM-CSF had long-lasting MHC class I-restricted Id-specific T-cell responses.[406,434] Massaia and colleagues have also shown generation of T-cell proliferative responses and delayed type hypersensitivity to Id after immunization with Id conjugated to KLH with GM-CSF or IL-2 as immunoadjuvants.[435] Vaccination after autologous peripheral blood stem cell transplantation for MM using idiotype-pulsed dendritic cells can achieve idiotype-specific T-cell responses in a minority of patients.[436] Other strategies currently under evaluation are immunization with idiotypic DNA vaccines as well as dendritic cells pulsed with idiotype.[407,437] *MAGE* antigens and the catalytic subunit of telomerase are expressed by MM and contain peptides that can be effectively presented by HLA class I molecules to generate autologous-specific cytolytic T-cell responses.[428,438] Finally, MM cells can be efficiently transduced with adenoviral vectors, and accessory molecules, for example, CD80 or GM-CSF, are currently being transfected into tumor cells prior to vaccination.[365,439]

Serotherapy A chimeric anti-CD38 antibody has been developed that consists of the Fab portion of the mouse anti-CD38 monoclonal antibody linked by a stable thioether bond to an Fc molecule derived from human IgG1, thereby forming a mouse Fab–human Fc hybrid.[440] In contrast to the parent mouse antibody, the chimeric molecule mediates antibody-dependent cellular cytotoxicity (ADCC) very effectively with human blood mononuclear effector cells and appears effective at low concentration.

Daily intravenous injections of anti-IL-6 monoclonal antibody for 2 months led to a dramatic reduction in the percentage of MM cells in S-phase as well as reduction in serum calcium, serum monoclonal IgG, and CRP levels.[83] This provides further support for the role of IL-6 in MM cell growth in vivo and again suggests that strategies designed to interrupt IL-6-mediated growth may provide new treatments for MM.[87,88,225,441] Several trials of immunotoxin therapy of MM have been attempted. Monoclonal antibody (8A) recognizes a plasma cell-associated antigen and has been conjugated to momordin, a ribosome-inactivating protein similar to the ricin A chain.[442] Specifically, it may be useful for ex vivo purging in autologous marrow grafting in MM. A chimeric toxin composed of IL-6 attached to a portion of Pseudomonas exotoxin devoid of its own recognition domain has also been produced in *Escherichia coli*.[443] This fusion product was cytotoxic to a human MM cell line expressing IL-6 receptors, but it had no effect on IL-6 receptor-negative cells. It therefore may be useful in the selective elimination of MM cells and other cells with high numbers of IL-6 receptors. Anti-CD19 and anti-CD38 monoclonal antibodies have been conjugated to ricin for the in vivo elimination of tumor cells.[444,445] Finally, serotherapy against the plasma cell-specific HM1.24 and other antigens, including CD20 or MUC-1, is also being tested in MM.[31,446,447]

OTHER PLASMA CELL DYSCRASIAS

Plasmacytomas **Clinical Characteristics** Plasmacytomas are collections of monoclonal plasma cells originating either in bone (solitary osseous plasmacytoma, SOP) or in soft tissue (extramedullary plasmacytoma, EMP). They comprise < 10% of plasma cell dyscrasias. MM must be excluded before the diagnosis of either SOP or EMP can be made. Magnetic resonance imaging can be useful to show additional marrow abnormalities consistent with MM.[448] The median age of diagnosis of either SOP or EMP is approximately 50 years, nearly 10 years younger than that for MM.[449–451] Although patients with SOP and EMP can both progress to MM, persons with SOP progress in the majority of cases, in contrast to EMP, where only up to 50% eventually develop MM. The median survival of 86.4 months and 100.8 months for patients with SOP and EMP, respectively, is similar; however, progression-free survival is markedly different, 16% for SOP patients versus 71% for EMP patients. The persistence of stable monoclonal Ig in serum and/or urine after primary treatment of plasmacytoma does not necessitate additional therapy, since it does not influence survival or disease-free survival.[449] In contrast, rising monoclonal Ig levels in a patient with a history of either SOP or EMP should trigger a work-up for either recurrent plasmacytoma or MM. It has been suggested, as is true for MM, that serum β2M has prognostic value in patients with SOP. Specifically, 17 of 19 patients with elevated serum β2M had transformation to MM and shorter survival (31 months) than those with normal serum β2M levels.[452]

Treatment Treatment of SOP and EMP is local therapy, primarily radiotherapy with surgery as needed for structural anatomic support.[449–451] The benefit of chemotherapy, either alone or in combination with radiotherapy and surgery, as primary therapy for SOP or EMP has not been proven. Moreover, the benefit of adjuvant chemotherapy, given to prevent recurrent disease and/or progression to MM, is also undefined. Disappearance of protein after involved-field radiotherapy predicts for long-term disease-free survival and possible cure.[453]

Immunoglobulin M Monoclonal Gammopathy Excess monoclonal IgM in the serum can occur in a variety of diseases. In a Mayo Clinic series of 430 patients in whom a monoclonal IgM protein was identified, 242 (56%) had MGUS, 71 (17%) had Waldenström macroglobulinemia, 28 (7%) had lymphoma, 21 (5%) had chronic lymphocytic leukemia, 6 (1%) had primary amyloidosis, and 62 (14%) had other malignant lymphoproliferative diseases.[454] The duration of time from the recognition of the M protein to the development of a malignant lymphoid disease ranged from 4 to 9 years, suggesting that long-term follow-up of such patients is necessary.

Waldenström Macroblobulinemia The diagnosis of Waldenström macroglobulinemia (WM) requires an IgM serum level of at least 3.0 gm/dL in association with an increase in lymphocytes or plasmacytoid lymphocytes in the marrow.[454–456] WM corresponds most closely to the lymphoplasmacytic lymphoma (LPA) under the World Health Organization (WHO) classification of lymphoid tumors (LPL/immunocytoma of the Revised European–American [REAL] classification of lymphoma). WM accounts for approximately 2% of all hematologic malignancies and is more common in men than in women. Its incidence increases with age, and it is more common among whites than among African Americans.[457,458] Although the etiology of WM is unclear, genetic factors may contribute to the pathogenesis of this disease, since there are reports of families with WM in association with other lymphoproliferative and immunologic disorders.[459] Cytogenetic abnormalities occur in 15 to 90% of cases, but none are specific for WM.[460,461] The WM B-cell clone demonstrates interclonal differentiation from small lymphocytes with large focal deposits of surface immunoglobulins, to lymphoplasmacytic cells and mature plasma cells that contain intracytoplasmic immunoglobulin. This morphologic heterogeneity is reflected by variable expression of phenotypic markers. All WM cells express monoclonal IgM and most cells are CD19, CD20, CD22, and FMC7 positive. High density of CD38 is also detected with variable intensity of the PCA-1 antigen. Predictably, CD45 isoform expression is heterogenous, probably reflecting ongoing monoclonal B-cell differentiation. In approximately 20% of cases, CD5 and CD23 expression are seen, but their coexpression is uncommon.[462] Circulating clonal B cells in WM increase in patients who fail to respond to therapy or who progress.[463] Recent studies suggest that WM originates from a postgerminal center B cell that has undergone somatic mutations and antigenic selection in the lymphoid follicle and has the characteristics of an IgM-bearing memory B cell.[464–466]

The median age of onset of WM is 61 years. Symptoms are characteristically vague and nonspecific, with the most common being weakness, anorexia, and weight loss. Symptoms due to peripheral neuropathy and Raynaud's phenomenon can precede more serious manifestations. Lymphadenopathy, splenomegaly, and/or hepatomegaly are present in 30 to 40% of cases, and at least 20 to 25% lymphoplasmacytoid cells are usually present in the marrow. Visceral involvement of small bowel and peripheral nerves can cause the clinical sequelae of malabsorption and neuropathy, respectively. Hemorrhagic complications are common, attributable to abnormal bleeding times, decreased platelet adhesiveness, or direct interference by the IgM protein with the release of platelet factor 3 and with coagulation factors. An important part of the differential diagnosis is to exclude the less common entity of IgM MM, which is characterized by lytic bone disease and an absence of organomegaly and/or lymphocytic involvement; rarely, WM can itself progress to IgM MM.[467] Amyloidosis occurs rarely in Waldenström macroglobulinemia.[468] Hyperviscosity syndrome, described earlier as a rare complication in MM, occurs more commonly in the setting of excess IgM and is characterized by mucosal bleeding and neurologic, ocular, and cardiovascular abnormalities.[268] Therapy with plasmapheresis is more useful to remove excess IgM than it is in the setting of excess IgG monoclonal proteins and related hyperviscosity in MM.

Plasmapheresis can be considered as only an adjunctive therapy. Treatment regimens utilized are similar to those used to treat low-grade lymphomas and MM, including chlorambucil, cyclophosphamide, melphalan, and corticosteroids, either as single agents or in combinations.[455] Just as for MM, there is no evidence that combined drug regimens are superior to single therapies. The median survival is approximately 50 months, not that dissimilar from the best reported series of patients with MM. In contrast to persons with MM, however, many individuals with WM have indolent disease requiring no therapy for long periods of time, with survivals in excess of 20 years. Pretreatment parameters, including older age, male gender, general symptoms, and cytopenias, define a high-risk population that could perhaps benefit from newer therapeutic approaches.[469,470] Acute leukemia has developed in patients with WM, emphasizing a potential complication of premature and prolonged low-dose therapy with alkylating agents.[471] Nucleoside analogs, including fludarabine and 2-chlorodeoxyadenosine, have been shown to be effective in newly diagnosed as well as in refractory patients with WM and may achieve more rapid cytoreduction than oral chlorambucil.[455,472–474] Prospective randomized trials are needed to assess the effect of nucleoside analogs on survival.[475] In a recent multicenter trial, 92 patients with WM resistant to first-line treatment were treated with fludarabine or combination chemotherapy, including cyclophosphamide, doxorubicin, and prednisone.[476] Although response rates and EFS were significantly higher in patients treated with fludarabine, no survival difference was noted.

Several reports describe responses in patients with WM using recombinant interferon-α or -γ.[477,478] Interestingly, patients who had been treated with prior chemotherapy had an equivalent response rate to those who had not. Future studies are needed to assess its effect as a remission therapy or as part of other strategies.[479] Although high-dose therapy with autologous stem cell support has been shown to be effective in many patients with MM or with low grade lymphoma, relatively few patients with WM have undergone transplant. Nonetheless, preliminary data suggest that high-dose therapy is associated with a high complete response rate and acceptable toxicity, and this approach therefore warrants further investigation, particularly in younger patients with poor prognostic features.[480] Splenectomy has been reported to be effective in chemotherapy-resistant patients with WM and results in a major decrease in monoclonal protein concentration and durable remission.[481,482] Monoclonal antibody therapy with rituximab, a chimeric anti-CD20 monoclonal antibody, produces responses in both treated and untreated patients with low-grade lymphoma. Given that the CD20 antigen is typically present in WM, rituximab has been given to patients and a clinical response was seen in about one-third of previously treated patients in early studies.[483,484] Ongoing studies are looking at combining rituximab with fludarabine in the treatment of WM. Salvage strategies for WM include re-use of first line agents, combination chemotherapy (eg, CHOP, CVP, CAP), thalidimide and bortezomib based therapies.

Heavy-Chain Diseases Since the original description by Franklin and colleagues of a patient with malignant lymphoma whose serum and urine contained large amounts of the Fc fragment of IgG, the clinical and immunochemical scope of gamma-heavy–chain disease (γHCD) has broadened.[485] These diseases are characterized by the presence of a portion of the Ig heavy chain in the serum or urine or both. The median age at diagnosis is similar to that for MM, approximately 60 years.[486] The clinical and laboratory features can be heterogeneous. Most common presenting symptoms are weakness, fatigue, and fever, associated with lymphadenopathy and hepatosplenomegaly. In addition to Ig heavy chain in serum or urine, a lymphoplasmacytic marrow infiltrate is noted in most cases. The clinical course can be fulminant and rapidly progressive; alternatively, the monoclonal heavy chain can persist for years in otherwise asymptomatic patients. Thus, survival is variable, but the median is only 12 months. Treatment options for patients with active disease are similar to those used for lymphoma or MM, whereas patients with indolent disease should be followed expectantly without therapy. Cases of αHCD, μHCD, and δHCD have also been described. HCD is typically associated with non-Hodgkin's lymphoma in the gastrointestinal tract, beginning with plasma cells that produce a heavy chain and aggregate in the intestinal tract and subsequent transformation into a malignant non-Hodgkin's lymphoma of the immunoblastic type, probably arising from the more mature plasma cells.[487] The ideal therapy for heavy-chain disease is not known because of its rarity, but intensive chemotherapy including intravenous cyclophosphamide, doxorubicin, vincristine, and oral prednisone appears to offer some patients long-term remissions.

Amyloidosis Amyloidosis is relatively rare as a clinically significant disease. It has been classified into five categories. These include (1) primary, with or without plasma cell and lymphoid neoplasms; (2) secondary, associated with chronic infections or autoimmune disease; (3) hereditary, associated with familial Mediterranean fever, Portuguese lower limb neuropathy, and others; (4) amyloidosis associated with aging; and (5) amyloidosis of endocrine glands, with medullary thyroid carcinoma and multiple endocrine neoplasia type 2.[468,488] The amyloid found in most cases of amyloidosis can be assigned to one of two types, according to whether the fibrils consist mainly of the variable region of Ig light chains (AL, or primary amyloidosis) or protein A (AA, or secondary amyloidosis). Protein A has a molecular weight of 8,500 daltons and consists of 76 amino acids; it is not related to any known immunoglobulin. In AL, amyloid primarily involves the heart, tongue, gastrointestinal tract, and skin, whereas AA primarily results in fibril deposition in liver, kidney, and spleen. A review of 229 patients with AL documented MM in 47 (21%) patients.[488] Initial presenting symptoms were fatigue and weight loss, with pain more common in those who also had MM. Hepatomegaly and macroglossia were present in up to one-third of patients with AL; renal insufficiency was present in one-half of patients, and proteinuria (defined as albuminuria with immune globulin seen, only in MM) was documented in 82% of patients. Nephrotic syndrome, congestive heart failure, orthostatic hypotension, carpal tunnel syndrome, and peripheral neuropathy were all more common in those without MM (30–70% of patients studied) than in persons with MM (< 20%). Overall median survival was 12 months, 5 months for those with MM in contrast to 13 months for individuals without MM. Although it has been difficult to monitor the distribution and progression of disease, it has been shown that radiolabeled serum amyloid P component, which has specific binding affinity for amyloid fibrils, can be given intravenously and localizes rapidly and specifically in amyloid deposits.[445] This technique may therefore facilitate diagnosis and monitoring of the extent of systemic amyloidosis, including the effects of therapeutic interventions.

Treatment of AL is unsatisfactory. Only 27 of 153 (18%) patients responded to MP, although median survival for responders was prolonged at 89.4 months; only 5% of patients with primary AL survive ≥ 10 years.[468,489] A prospective randomized trial has concluded that MP was superior to colchicine when analyzed from time of entry into the study to time of death or progression of disease.[490] Other retrospective studies suggest that colchicine is superior to placebo for patients with AL.[491] Alkylating agent-based chemotherapy may therefore be beneficial for a subset of patients and result in prolonged survival. One randomized trial of colchicine, MP, or a combination of the three drugs in patients with primary amyloidosis found that therapy with MP results in objective responses and prolonged survival as compared with colchicine.[492] However, therapy with multiple alkylating agents did not achieve either higher response rate or longer survival time than MP.[493] Early reports suggest that dose-intensive melphalan with blood stem cell support can achieve CRs, with improvement in performance status and clinical remission of organ-specific disease.[494] Guidelines have been developed for patient selection to maximize benefit and minimize treatment-related mortality.[495,496] As in MM, a randomized trial is required to assess the true efficacy of high-dose therapy, since those patients eligible for high-dose treatments may also do well with chemotherapy.[497] Attempts to improve outcomes for patients with symptomatic and advanced multisystem disease may require both solid and stem cell transplantation, as well as the use of less intensive conditioning regimens.[495] Novel drugs with promise in the treatment of MM, including Thal, IMiDs, and PS-341, are also being tested in patients with amyloidosis.

REFERENCES

1. Alexanian R, Dimopoulos M. The treatment of multiple myeloma. New Engl J Med 1994;330:484–9.
2. Bataille R, Harousseau J-L. Multiple myeloma. N Engl J Med 1997;336:1657–64.
3. Hallek M, Bergsagel PL, Anderson KC. Multiple myeloma: increasing evidence for a multistep transformation process. Blood 1998;91:3–21.
4. Kyle RA. Multiple myeloma: review of 869 cases. Mayo Clin Proc 1975;50:29–40.
5. Clamp JR. Some aspects of the first recorded case of multiple myeloma. Lancet 1967;2:1354–6.
6. Kyle RA. Multiple myeloma: how did it begin? Mayo Clin Proc 1994;69:680–3.
7. Longsworth LG, Shedlovosky T, MacInnes DA. Electrophoretic patterns of normal and pathological human blood serum and plasma. J Exp Med 1939;70:399–413.
8. Grabar P, Williams CA. Methode permettant l'etude conjuguee des proprietes electrophoretiques et immu-

nochimiques d'un melange de protemes: application au serum sanguin. Biochim Biophys Acta 1953;10:193.
9. Durie BGM. Staging and kinetics of multiple myeloma. Semin Oncol 1986;13:300–9.
10. Kyle RA, Therneau TM, Rajkumar SV, et al. A long-term study of prognosis in monoclonal gammopathy of undetermined significance. N Engl J Med 2002;346:564–9.
11. Cesana C, Klersy C, Barbarano L, et al. Prognostic factors for malignant transformation in monoclonal gammopathy of undetermined significance and smoldering multiple myeloma. J Clin Oncol 2002;20:1625–34.
12. Dyck PJ, Low PA, Windebank AJ, et al. Plasma exchange in polyneuropathy associated with monoclonal gammopathy of undetermined significance. N Engl J Med 1991;325:1482–6.
13. Bergsagel DE, Wong O, Bergsagel PL, et al. Benzene and multiple myeloma: appraisal of the scientific evidence. Blood 1999;94:1174–82.
14. Bourguet CC, Grufferman S, Delzell E, et al. Multiple myeloma and family history of cancer. Cancer 1985;56:2133–9.
15. Jemal A, Tiwari RC, Murray T, et al. Cancer statistics. CA Cancer J Clin 2004;54:8–29.
16. Herrinton LJ, Weiss NS, Olshan AF. Epidemiology of myeloma. In: Malpas JS, Bergsagel DE, Kyle R, Anderson K, editors. Myeloma: biology and management. Oxford: Oxford Medical Publications; 1997. p. 150.
17. Kyle RA, Beard MC, O'Fallon WM, Kurland LT. Incidence of multiple myeloma in Olmsted County, Minnesota: 1978 through 1990, with a review of the trend since 1945. J Clin Oncol 1994;12:1577–83.
18. Pruzanski W, Ogryzlo MA. Abnormal proteinuria in malignant diseases. Adv Clin Chem 1970;13:335–82.
19. Blade J, Lust JA, Kyle RA. Immunoglobulin D multiple myeloma: presenting features, response to therapy, and survival in a series of 53 cases. J Clin Oncol 1994;12:2398–404.
20. Kyle RA. Long-term survival in multiple myeloma. N Engl J Med 1983;308:314–6.
21. Bergsagel DE. Acute leukemia and multiple myeloma: natural history or iatrogenic disease? Drug Ther 1977:8–9.
22. Kapadia SB. Multiple myeloma: a clinicopathologic study of 62 consecutively autopsied cases. Medicine 1980;59:380–92.
23. Anderson KC, Bates MP, Slaughenhoupt B, et al. Expression of human B cell associated antigens on leukemias and lymphomas: a model of human B cell differentiation. Blood 1984;63:1424–33.
24. Anderson KC, Park EK, Bates MP, et al. Antigens on human plasma cells identified by monoclonal antibodies. J Immunol 1983;130:1132–8.
25. Epstein J, Barlogie B, Katzmann J, Alexanian R. Phenotypic heterogeneity in aneuploid multiple myeloma indicates pre-B cell involvement. Blood 1988;71:861–5.
26. Grogan TM, Durie BGM, Lomen C, et al. Delineation of a novel pre-B cell component in plasma cell myeloma: immunochemical, immunophenotypic, genotypic, cytologic, cell culture, and kinetic features. Blood 1987;70:932–42.
27. Jensen GS, Mant MJ, Belch AJ, et al. Selective expression of CD45 isoforms defines CALLA+ monoclonal B lineage cells in peripheral blood from myeloma patients as late stage B cells. Blood 1991;78:711–9.
28. San Miguel JF, Caballero MD, Gonzales M, et al. Immunological phenotype of neoplasms involving the B cell in the last step of differentiation. Br J Haematol 1986;62:75–83.
29. van Camp B, Durie BG, Spier C, et al. Plasma cells in multiple myeloma express natural killer cell-associated antigen: CD56 (NKH-1; Leu-19). Blood 1990;76:377–82.
30. Harada H, Kawano MM, Huang N, et al. Phenotypic difference of normal plasma cells from mature myeloma cells. Blood 1993;81:2658–63.
31. Treon SP, Mollick JA, Urashima M, et al. Muc-1 core protein is expressed on multiple myeloma cells and is induced by dexamethasone. Blood 1999;93:1287–98.
32. Kubagawa H, Vogler LB, Capra JD, et al. Studies on the clonal origin of multiple myeloma. Use of individually specific (idiotypic) antibodies to trace the oncogenic event to its earliest point of expression in B cell differentiation. J Exp Med 1979;150:792–807.
33. Preud'homme JL, Klein M, Labaume S, Seligmann M. Idiotype-bearing and antigen-bearing receptors produced by blood T lymphocytes in a case of human myeloma. Eur J Immunol 1977;7:840–6.
34. Epstein J, Xiao HQ, He XY. Markers of multiple hematopoietic-cell lineages in multiple myeloma. N Engl J Med 1990;322:664–8.
35. Bakkus MHC, Heirman C, van Riet I, et al. Evidence that multiple myeloma Ig heavy chain VDJ genes contain somatic mutations but show no intraclonal variation. Blood 1992;80:2326–35.
36. Vescio RA, Cao J, Hong CH, et al. Myeloma Ig heavy chain V region sequences reveal prior antigenic selection and marked somatic mutation but no intraclonal diversity. J Immunol 1995;155:2487–97.
37. Sahota SS, Garand R, Mahroof R, et al. V_H gene analysis of IgM-secreting myeloma indicates an origin from a memory cell undergoing isotype switch events. Blood 1999;94:1070–6.
38. Bergsagel PL, Chesi M, Nardini E, et al. Promiscuous translocations into immunoglobulin heavy chain switch regions in multiple myeloma. Proc Natl Acad Sci U S A 1996;93(24):13931–6.
39. Teoh G, Anderson KC. Interaction of tumor and host cells with adhesion and extracellular matrix molecules in the development of multiple myeloma. Hematol Oncol Clin North Am 1997;11:27–42.
40. Ahsmann EFM, Lokhorst HM, Dekker HM, et al. Lymphocyte function-associated antigen-1 expression on plasma cells correlates with tumor growth in multiple myeloma. Blood 1992;79:2068–75.
41. Massellis-Smith A, Belch AR, Mant MJ, et al. Hyaluronan-dependent motility of B cells and leukemic plasma cells in blood, but not of bone marrow plasma cells, in multiple myeloma: alternate use of receptor for hyaluronan-mediated motility (RHAMM) and CD44. Blood 1996;87:1891–9.
42. Ridley RC, Xiao H, Hata H, et al. Expression of syndecan regulates human myeloma plasma cell adhesion to type I collagen. Blood 1993;81:767–74.
43. Chauhan D, Uchiyama H, Akbarali Y, et al. Multiple myeloma cell adhesion-induced interleukin-6 expression in bone marrow stromal cells involves activation of NF-κB. Blood 1996;87:1104–12.
44. Lokhorst HM, Lamme T, de Smet M, et al. Primary tumor cells of myeloma patients induce interleukin-6 secretion in long-term marrow cultures. Blood 1994;84:2269–77.
45. Uchiyama H, Barut BA, Mohrbacher AF, et al. Adhesion of human myeloma-derived cell lines to bone marrow stromal cells stimulates IL-6 secretion. Blood 1993;82:3712–20.
46. Urashima M, Chauhan D, Uchiyama H, et al. CD40 ligand triggered interleukin-6 secretion in multiple myeloma. Blood 1995;85:1903–12.
47. Hideshima T, Chauhan D, Schlossman RL, et al. Role of TNF-α in the pathophysiology of human multiple myeloma: therapeutic applications. Oncogene 2001;20:4519–27.
48. Dhodapkar MV, Kelly T, Theus A, et al. Elevated levels of shed syndecan-1 correlate with tumour mass and decreased matrix metalloproteinase-9 activity in the serum of patients with multiple myeloma. Br J Haematol 1997;99:368–71.
49. Dhodapkar MV, Abe E, Theus A, et al. Syndecan-1 is a multifunctional regulator of myeloma pathobiology: control of tumor cell survival, growth, and bone cell differentiation. Blood 1998;91:2679–88.
50. Yang Y, Yaccoby S, Liu W, et al. Soluble syndecan-1 promotes growth of myeloma tumors in vivo. Blood 2002;100:610–7.
51. Barille S, Akhoundi C, Collette M, et al. Metalloproteinases in multiple myeloma: production of metalloproteinase-9 (MMP-9), activation of proMMP-2, and induction of MMP-1 by myeloma cells. Blood 1997;90:1649–55.
52. Huang YW, Richardson JA, Vitetta ES. Anti-CD54 (ICAM-1) has anti-tumor activity in SCID mice with human myeloma cells. Cancer Res 1995;55:610–6.
53. Urashima M, Chen BP, Chen S, et al. The development of a model for the homing of multiple myeloma cells to human bone marrow. Blood 1997;90:754–65.
54. Yaccoby S, Barlogie B, Epstein J. Primary myeloma cells growing in SCID-hu mice: a model for studying the biology and treatment of myeloma and its manifestations. Blood 1998;92:2908–13.
55. Damiano JS, Cress AE, Hazlehurst LA, et al. Cell adhesion mediated drug resistance (CAM-DR): role of integrins and resistance to apoptosis in human myeloma cell lines. Blood 1999;93:1658–67.
56. Hideshima T, Chauhan D, Shima Y, et al. Thalidomide and its analogues overcome drug resistance of human multiple myeloma cells to conventional therapy. Blood 2000;96:2943–50.
57. Hideshima T, Richardson P, Chauhan D, et al. The proteasome inhibitor PS-341inhibits growth, induces apoptosis, and overcomes drug resistance in human multiple myeloma cells. Cancer Res 2001;61:3071–6.
58. Hideshima T, Bergsagel PL, Kuehl WM, Anderson KC. Advances in biology of multiple myeloma: clinical applications. Blood 2004;104:607–18.
59. Gupta D, Treon SP, Shima Y, et al. Adherence of multiple myeloma cells to bone marrow stromal cells upregulates vascular endothelial growth factor secretion: therapeutic applications. Leukemia. 2001;15:1950–61.
60. Klein B, Lu Y, Gaillard JP, et al. Inhibiting IL-6 in human multiple myeloma. Curr Top Microbiol Immunol 1992;182:236–43.
61. Kawano M, Hirano T, Matsuda T, et al. Autocrine generation and requirement of BSF-2/IL-6 for human multiple myelomas. Nature 1988;332:83–5.
62. Frassanito MA, Cusmai A, Iodice G, Dammacco F. Autocrine interleukin-6 production and highly malignant multiple myeloma: relation with resistance to drug-induced apoptosis. Blood 2001;97:483–9.
63. Chauhan D, Kharbanda S, Ogata A, et al. Interleukin-6 inhibits Fas-induced apoptosis and stress-activated protein kinase activation in multiple myeloma cells. Blood 1997;89:227–34.
64. Chauhan D, Pandey P, Ogata A, et al. Dexamethasone induces apoptosis of multiple myeloma cells in a JNK/SAP kinase independent mechanism. Oncogene 1997;15:837–43.
65. Chauhan D, Hideshima T, Treon S, et al. Functional interaction between retinoblastoma protein and stress activated protein kinase in multiple myeloma cells. Cancer Res 1999;59:1192–5.
66. Chauhan D, Pandey P, Ogata A, et al. Cytochrome-c dependent and independent induction of apoptosis in multiple myeloma cells. J Biol Chem 1997;272:29995–7.
67. Chauhan D, Hideshima T, Pandey P, et al. RAFTK/PYK2-dependent and independent apoptosis in multiple myeloma cells. Oncogene 1999;18:6733–40.
68. Epling-Burnette PK, Liu JH, Catlett-Falcone R, et al. Inhibition of STAT3 signaling leads to apoptosis of leukemic large granular lymphocytes and decreased Mcl-1 expression. J Clin Invest 2001;107:351–62.
69. Hideshima T, Nakamura N, Chauhan D, Anderson KC. Biologic sequelae of interleukin-6 induced PI3-K/Akt signaling in multiple myeloma. Oncogene 2001;20:5991–6000.
70. Chauhan D, Pandey P, Hideshima T et al. SHP2 mediates the protective effect of interleukin-6 against dexamethasone-induced apoptosis in multiple myeloma cells. J Biol Chem 2000;275:27845–50.
71. Chauhan D, Auclair D, Robinson EK, et al. Identification of genes regulated by dexamethasone in multiple myeloma cells using oligonucleotide arrays. Oncogene 2002;21:1346–58.
72. Chauhan D, Li G, Sattler M, et al. Superoxide-dependent and -independent mitochondrial signaling during apoptosis in multiple myeloma cells. Oncogene 2003;22:6296–300.
73. Wen XY, Stewart AK, Sooknanan RR, et al. Identification of c-myc promoter-binding protein and X-box binding protein 1 as interleukin-6 target genes in human multiple myeloma cells. Int J Oncol 1999;15:173–8.
74. Reimold AM, Iwakoshi NN, Manis J, et al. Plasma cell differentiation requires the transcription factor XBP-1. Nature 2001;412:300–7.
75. Iwakoshi NN, Lee AH, Vallabhajosyula P, et al. Plasma cell differentiation and the unfolded protein response intersect at the transcription factor XBP-1.Nat Immunol 2003;4:321–9.
76. Chauhan D, Li G, Auclair D, et al. Identification of genes regulated by 2-methoxyestradiol (2ME2) in multiple myeloma cells using oligonucleotide arrays. Blood 2003;101:3606–14.
77. Catlett-Falcone R, Landowski TH, Oshiro MM, et al. Constitutive activation of STAT-3 signaling confers resistance to apoptosis in human U266 myeloma cells. Immunity 1999;10:105–15.
78. Landowski TH, Shain KH, Oshiro MM, et al. Myeloma cells selected for resistance to CD95-mediated apoptosis are not cross-resistant to cytotoxic drugs: evidence for independent mechanisms of caspase activation. Blood 1999;94:265–74.
79. Ludwig H, Nachbaur DM, Fritz E, et al. Interleukin-6 is a prognostic factor in multiple myeloma. Blood 1991;77:2794–5.
80. Bataille R, Jourdan M, Zhang XG, Klein B. Serum levels of interleukin 6, a potent myeloma cell growth factor, as a reflect of disease severity in plasma cell dyscrasias. J Clin Invest 1989;84:2008–11.
81. Fattori E, Della Rocca C, Costa P, et al. Development of progressive kidney damage and myeloma kidney in interleukin-6 transgenic mice. Blood 1994;83:2570–9.
82. Barille S, Collette M, Bataille R, et al. Myeloma cells upregulate IL-6 but downregulate osteocalcin production by osteoblastic cells through cell to cell contact. Blood 1995;86:3151–9.

83. Bataille R, Barlogie B, Yang Z, et al. Biologic effects of anti-interleukin-6 murine monoclonal antibody in advanced multiple myeloma. Blood 1995;86:685–91.
84. Ogata A, Nishimoto N, Shima Y, et al. Inhibitory effect of All-trans retinoic acid on the growth of freshly isolated myeloma cells via interference with interleukin-6 signal transduction. Blood 1994;84:3040–6.
85. Chadwick D, Jamal N, Messner HA, et al. Differential sensitivity of human myeloma cell lines and bone marrow colony forming cells to a recombinant diphtheria toxin-interleukin-6 fusion protein. Br J Haematol 1993;85:25–36.
86. Kreitman R, Siegall CB, Fitzgerald DJP, et al. Interleukin-6 fused to mutant form of pseudomonas exotoxin kills malignant cells form patients with multiple myeloma. Blood 1992;79:1775–80.
87. Ehlers M, de Hon FD, Klasse Bos H, et al. Combining two mutations of human interleukin-6 that affect gp130 activation results in a potent interleukin-6 receptor antagonist on human myeloma cells. J Biol Chem 1995;270:8158–63.
88. Sporeno E, Savino R, Ciapponi L, et al. Human interleukin-6 receptor super antagonists with high potency and wide spectrum on multiple myeloma cells. Blood 1996;87:4510–9.
89. Klein B, Zhang XG, Lu XY, et al. Interleukin-6 in human multiple myeloma. Blood 1995;85:863–72.
90. Savage AD, Belson DJ, Vescio RA, et al. Pamidronate reduces IL-6 production by bone marrow stroma from multiple myeloma patients. Blood 1996;88:105a.
91. Yu H, Spitz MR, Mistry J, et al. Plasma levels of insulin-like growth factor-I and lung cancer risk: a case-control analysis. J Natl Cancer Inst 1999;91:151–6.
92. Hankinson SE, Willett WC, Colditz GA, et al. Circulating concentrations of insulin-like growth factor-I and risk of breast cancer. Lancet 1998;351:1393–6.
93. Chan JM, Stampfer MJ, Giovannucci E, et al. Plasma insulin-like growth factor-I and prostate cancer risk: a prospective study. Science 1998;279:563–6.
94. Ma J, Pollak MN, Giovannucci E, et al. Prospective study of colorectal cancer risk in men and plasma levels of insulin-like growth factor (IGF)-I and IGF-binding protein-3. J Natl Cancer Inst 1999;91:620–5.
95. Yu H, Rohan T. Role of the insulin-like growth factor family in cancer development and progression. J Natl Cancer Inst 2000;92:1472–89.
96. Standal T, Borset M, Lenhoff S, et al. Serum insulin-like growth factor is not elevated in patients with multiple myeloma but is still a prognostic factor. Blood 2002;100:3925–9.
97. Jelinek DF, Witzig TE, Arendt BK. A role for insulin-like growth factor in the regulation of IL-6-responsive human myeloma cell line growth. J Immunol 1997;159:487–96.
98. Ogawa M, Nishiura T, Oritani K, et al. Cytokines prevent dexamethasone-induced apoptosis via the activation of mitogen-activated protein kinase and phosphatidylinositol 3-kinase pathways in a new multiple myeloma cell line. Cancer Res 2000;60:4262–9.
99. Mitsiades CS, Mitsiades N, Poulaki V, et al. Activation of NF-κB and upregulation of intracellular anti-apoptotic proteins via the IGF-1/Akt signaling in human multiple myeloma cells: therapeutic implications. Oncogene 2002;21:5673–83.
100. Vanderkerken K, Asosingh K, Braet F, et al. Insulin-like growth factor-1 acts as a chemoattractant factor for 5T2 multiple myeloma cells. Blood 1999;93:235–41.
101. Ge NL, Rudikoff S. Insulin-like growth factor I is a dual effector of multiple myeloma cell growth. Blood 2000;96:2856–61.
102. Mitsiades CS, Mitsiades NS, McMullan CJ, et al. Inhibition of the insulin-like growth factor receptor-1 tyrosine kinase activity as a therapeutic strategy for multiple myeloma, other hematologic malignancies, and solid tumors. Cancer Cell 2004;5:221–30.
103. Qiang YW, Kopantzev E, Rudikoff S. Insulin-like growth factor-I signaling in multiple myeloma: downstream elements, functional correlates, and pathway cross-talk. Blood 2002;99:4138–46.
104. Tai YT, Podar K, Catley L, et al. Insulin-like growth factor-1 induces adhesion and migration in human multiple myeloma cells via activation of beta1-integrin and phosphatidylinositol 3'-kinase/AKT signaling. Cancer Res 2003;63:5850–8.
105. Xu F, Gardner A, Tu Y, et al. Multiple myeloma cells are protected against dexamethasone-induced apoptosis by insulin-like growth factors. Br J Haematol 1997;97:429–40.
106. Tu Y, Gardner A, Lichtenstein A. The phosphatidylinositol 3-kinase/AKT kinase pathway in multiple myeloma plasma cells: roles in cytokine-dependent survival and proliferative responses. Cancer Res 2000;60:6763–70.
107. Abroun S, Ishikawa H, Tsuyama N, et al. Receptor synergy of interleukin-6 (IL-6) and insulin-like growth factor-I that highly express IL-6 receptor alpha myeloma cells. Blood 2004;103:2291–8.
108. Akiyama M, Hideshima T, Hayashi T, et al. Cytokines modulate telomerase activity in a human multiple myeloma cell line. Cancer Res 2002;62:3876–82.
109. Akiyama M, Hideshima T, Hayashi T, et al. Nuclear factor-kappaB p65 mediates tumor necrosis factor alpha-induced nuclear translocation of telomerase reverse transcriptase protein. Cancer Res 2003;63:18–21.
110. Podar K, Tai YT, Cole CE, et al. Essential role of caveolae in interleukin-6- and insulin-like growth factor I-triggered Akt-1-mediated survival of multiple myeloma cells. J Biol Chem 2003;278:5794–801.
111. Davies FE, Rollinson SJ, Rawstron AC, et al. High-producer haplotypes of tumor necrosis factor alpha and lymphotoxin alpha are associated with an increased risk of myeloma and have an improved progression-free survival after treatment. J Clin Oncol 2000;18:2843–51.
112. Silvestris F, Cafforio P, Calvani N, Dammacco F. Impaired osteoblastogenesis in myeloma bone disease: role of upregulated apoptosis by cytokines and malignant plasma cells. Br J Haematol 2004;126:475–86.
113. Landowski TH, Olashaw NE, Agrawal D, Dalton WS. Cell adhesion-mediated drug resistance (CAM-DR) is associated with activation of NF-kappa B (RelB/p50) in myeloma cells. Oncogene 2003;22:2417–21.
114. Podar K, Anderson KC. The pathophysiological role of VEGF in hematological malignancies: therapeutic implications. Blood 2005;105:1383–95.
115. Podar K, Tai YT, Davies FE, et al. Vascular endothelial growth factor triggers signaling cascades mediating multiple myeloma cell growth and migration. Blood 2001;98:428–35.
116. Podar K, Tai YT, Lin BK, et al. Vascular endothelial growth factor-induced migration of multiple myeloma cells is associated with beta 1 integrin- and phosphatidylinositol 3-kinase-dependent PKC alpha activation. J Biol Chem 2002;277:7875–81.
117. Vacca A, Ribatti D, Presta M, et al. Bone marrow neovascularization, plasma cell angiogenic potential, and matrix metalloproteinase-2 secretion parallel progression of human multiple myeloma. Blood 1999;93:3064–73.
118. Ribatti D, Vacca A, Nico B, et al. Bone marrow angiogenesis and mast cell density increase simultaneously with progression of human multiple myeloma. Br J Cancer 1999;79:451–5.
119. Rajkumar SV, Leong T, Roche PC, et al. Prognostic value of bone marrow angiogenesis in multiple myeloma. Clin Cancer Res 2000;6:3111–6.
120. Kumar S, Fonseca R, Dispenzieri A, et al. Bone marrow angiogenesis in multiple myeloma: effect of therapy. Br J Haematol 2002;119:665–71.
121. Kumar S, Fonseca R, Dispenzieri A, et al. Prognostic value of angiogenesis in solitary bone plasmacytoma. Blood 2003;101:1715–7.
122. Singhal S, Mehta J, Desikan R, et al. Antitumor activity of thalidomide in refractory multiple myeloma. N Engl J Med 1999;341:1565–71.
123. Rajkumar SV, Fonseca R, Witzig TE, et al. Bone marrow angiogenesis in patients achieving complete response after stem cell transplantation for multiple myeloma. Leukemia 1999;13:469–72.
124. Tai YT, Podar K, Gupta D, et al. CD40 activation induces p53-dependent vascular endothelial growth factor secretion in human multiple myeloma cells. Blood 2002;99:1419–27.
125. Lin B, Podar K, Gupta D, et al. The vascular endothelial growth factor receptor tyrosine kinase inhibitor PTK787/ZK222584 inhibits growth and migration of multiple myeloma cells in the bone marrow microenvironment. Cancer Res 2002;62:5019–26.
126. Podar K, Catley LP, Tai YT, et al. GW654652, the pan-inhibitor of VEGF receptors, blocks the growth and migration of multiple myeloma cells in the bone marrow microenvironment. Blood 2004;103:3474–9.
127. Dias S, Shmelkov SV, Lam G, Rafii S. VEGF(165) promotes survival of leukemic cells by Hsp90-mediated induction of Bcl-2 expression and apoptosis inhibition. Blood 2002;99:2532–40.
128. Le Gouill S, Podar K, Amiot M, et al. VEGF induces MCL-1 upregulation and protects multiple myeloma cells against apoptosis. Blood 2004;104:2886–92.
129. Hayashi T, Hideshima T, Akiyama M, et al. Ex vivo induction of multiple myeloma-specific cytotoxic T lymphocytes. Blood 2003;102:1435–42.
130. Vacca A, Ribatti D, Roncali L, et al. Bone marrow angiogenesis and progression in multiple myeloma. Br J Haematol 1994;87:503–8.
131. Otsuki T, Yamada O, Yata K, et al. Expression of fibroblast growth factor and FGF-receptor family genes in human myeloma cells, including lines possessing t(4;14)(q16.3;q32.3) and FGFR3 translocation. Int J Oncol 1999;15:1205–12.
132. Bisping G, Leo R, Wenning D, et al. Paracrine interactions of basic fibroblast growth factor and interleukin-6 in multiple myeloma. Blood 2003;101:2775–83.
133. Chesi M, Brents LA, Ely SA, et al. Activated fibroblast growth factor receptor 3 is an oncogene that contributes to tumor progression in multiple myeloma. Blood 2001;97:729–36.
134. Wang JF, Liu ZY, Groopman JE. The alpha-chemokine receptor CXCR4 is expressed on the megakaryocytic lineage from progenitor to platelets and modulates migration and adhesion. Blood 1998;92:756–64.
135. Wang JF, Park IW, Groopman JE. Stromal cell-derived factor-1alpha stimulates tyrosine phosphorylation of multiple focal adhesion proteins and induces migration of hematopoietic progenitor cells: roles of phosphoinositide-3 kinase and protein kinase C. Blood 2000;95:2505–13.
136. Hideshima T, Chauhan D, Hayashi T, et al. The biological sequelae of stromal cell-derived factor-1alpha in multiple myeloma. Mol Cancer Ther 2002;1:539–44.
137. Moller C, Stromberg T, Juremalm M, et al. Expression and function of chemokine receptors in human multiple myeloma. Leukemia 2003;17:203–10.
138. Gazitt Y, Akay C. Mobilization of myeloma cells involves SDF-1/CXCR4 signaling and downregulation of VLA-4. Stem Cells 2004;22:65–73.
139. Wright N, de Lera TL, Garcia-Moruja C, et al. Transforming growth factor-beta1 down-regulates expression of chemokine stromal cell-derived factor-1: functional consequences in cell migration and adhesion. Blood 2003;102:1978–84.
140. Qiang YW, Endo Y, Rubin JS, Rudikoff S. Wnt signaling in B-cell neoplasia. Oncogene 2003;22:1536–45.
141. Derksen PW, Tjin E, Meijer HP, et al. Illegitimate WNT signaling promotes proliferation of multiple myeloma cells. Proc Natl Acad Sci U S A 2004;101:6122–7.
142. Niida A, Hiroko T, Kasai M, et al. DKK1, a negative regulator of Wnt signaling, is a target of the beta-catenin/TCF pathway. Oncogene 2004;23:8520–6.
143. Tian E, Zhan F, Walker R, et al. The role of the Wnt-signaling antagonist DKK1 in the development of osteolytic lesions in multiple myeloma. N Engl J Med 2003;349:2483–94.
144. Urashima M, Ogata A, Chauhan D, et al. Transforming growth factor β1: differential effects on multiple myeloma versus normal B cells. Blood 1996;87:1928–38.
145. Kawano M, Tanaka H, Ishikawa H, et al. Interleukin-1 accelerates autocrine growth of myeloma cells through interleukin-6 in human myeloma. Blood 1989;73:2145–8.
146. Cozzolino F, Torcia M, Aldinucci D, et al. Production of interleukin-1 by bone marrow myeloma cells. Blood 1989;74:380–7.
147. Gherardi RK, Belec L, Fromont G, et al. Elevated levels of interleukin-1b (IL-1b) and IL-6 in serum and increased production of IL-1b mRNA in lymph nodes of patients with polyneuropathy, organomegaly, endocrinopathy, M protein, and skin changes (POEMS) syndrome. Blood 1994;83:2587–93.
148. Lacy MQ, Donovan DA, Heimbach JH, et al. Comparison of interleukin-1b expression by in situ hybridization in monoclonal gammopathy of undetermined significance and multiple myeloma. Blood 1999;93:300–5.
149. Garrett IR, Durie BG, Nedwin GE, et al. Production of lymphotoxin, a bone-resorbing cytokine, by cultured human myeloma cells. N Engl J Med 1987;317:526–32.
150. Hermann F, Andreff M, Gruss HJ, et al. Interleukin 4 inhibits growth of multiple myeloma by suppressing interleukin 6 expression. Blood 1991;78:2070–8.
151. Chauhan D, Kharbanda S, Ogata A, et al. Oncostatin M induces association of Grb2 with Janus Kinase JAK2 in multiple myeloma cells. J Exp Med 1995;182:1801–6.
152. Zhang XG, Bataille R, Jourdan M, et al. Granulocyte-macrophage colony-stimulating factor synergizes with interleukin-6 in supporting the proliferation of human myeloma cells. Blood 1990;76:2599–605.
153. Anderson KC, Morimoto C, Paul SR, et al. Interleukin-11 promotes accessory cell dependent B cell differentiation in man. Blood 1992;80:2797–804.
154. Paul SD, Barut BA, Cochran MA, Anderson KC. Lack of a role of interleukin-11 in the growth of multiple myeloma. Leukemia Res 1992;16:247–52.

155. Lu ZY, Zhang XG, Rodriguez C, et al. Interleukin-10 is a proliferation factor but not a differentiation factor for human myeloma cells. Blood 1995;85:2521–7.
156. Choi SJ, Cruz JC, Craig F, et al. Macrophage inflammatory protein 1-alpha is a potential osteoclast stimulatory factor in multiple myeloma. Blood 2000;96:671–5.
157. Tinhofer I, Marschitz I, Henn T, et al. Expression of functional interleukin-15 receptor and autocrine production of interleukin-15 as mechanisms of tumor propagation in multiple myeloma. Blood 2000;95:610–8.
158. Brenne AT, Baade Ro T, Waage A, Set al. Interleukin-21 is a growth and survival factor for human myeloma cells. Blood 2002;99:3756–62.
159. Feo-Zuppardi FJ, Taylor CW, Iwato K, et al. Long-term engraftment of fresh human myeloma cells in SCID mice. Blood 1992;80:2843–50.
160. Huang Y-W, Richardson JA, Tong AW, et al. Disseminated growth of a human multiple myeloma cell line in mice with severe combined immunodeficiency disease. Canc Res 1993;53:1392–6.
161. Dewald GW, Kyle RA, Hicks GA, Greipp PR. The clinical significance of cytogenetic studies in 100 patients with multiple myeloma, plasma cell leukemia, or amyloidosis. Blood 1985;66:380–90.
162. Gould J, Alexanian R, Goodacre A, et al. Plasma cell karyotype in multiple myeloma. Blood 1988;71:453–6.
163. Sawyer JR, Waldron JA, Jagannath S, Barlogie B. Cytogenic findings in 200 patients with multiple myeloma. Cancer Genetics Cytogenet 1995;82:41.
164. Drach J, Angerler J, Schuster J, et al. Interphase fluorescence in situ hybridization identifies chromosomal abnormalities in plasma cells from patients with monoclonal gammopathy of undetermined significance. Blood 1995;86:3915–21.
165. Flactif M, Zandecki M, Lai JL. Interphase fluorescence in situ hybridization (FISH) as a powerful tool for the detection of aneuploidy in multiple myeloma. Leukemia 1995;9:2109–14.
166. Zandecki M, Obein V, Bernardi F, et al. Monoclonal gammopathy of undetermined significance: chromosome changes are a common finding within bone marrow plasma cells. Br J Haematol 1995;90:693–6.
167. Fonseca R, Bailey RJ, Ahmann GJ, et al. Genomic abnormalities in monoclonal gammopathy of undetermined significance. Blood 2002;100:1417–24.
168. Zhan F, Hardin J, Kordsmeier B, et al. Global gene expression profiling of multiple myeloma, monoclonal gammopathy of undetermined significance, and normal bone marrow plasma cells. Blood 2002;99:1745–57.
169. Shaughnessy J Jr, Gabrea A, Qi Y, et al. Cyclin D3 at 6p21 is dysregulated by recurrent chromosomal translocations to immunoglobulin loci in multiple myeloma. Blood 2001;98:217–23.
170. Chesi M, Bergsagel PL, Brents LA, et al. Dysregulation of cyclin D1 by translocation into an IgH gamma switch region in two multiple myeloma cell lines. Blood 1996;88:674–81.
171. Avet-Loiseau H, Daviet A, Brigaudeau C, et al. Cytogenetic, interphase, and multicolor fluorescence in situ hybridization analyses in primary plasma cell leukemia: a study of 40 patients at diagnosis, on behalf of the Intergroupe Francophone du Myelome and the Groupe Francais de Cytogenetique Hematologique. Blood 2001;97:822–5.
172. Chesi M, Nardini E, Brents LA, et al. Frequent translocation t(4;14)(p16.3;q32.3) in multiple myeloma: association with increased expression and activating mutations of fibroblast growth factor receptor 3. Nature Genet 1997;16:260–4.
173. Chesi M, Nardini E, Lim RSC, et al. The t(4;14) translocation in myeloma dysregulates both *FGFR3* and a novel gene, *MMSET*, resulting in IgH/MMSET hybrid transcripts. Blood 1998;92:3025–34.
174. Plowright EE, Li Z, Bergsagel PL, et al. Ectopic expression of fibroblast growth factor receptor 3 promotes myeloma cell proliferation and prevents apoptosis. Blood 2000;95:992–8.
175. Li Z, Zhu YX, Plowright EE, et al. The myeloma-associated oncogene fibroblast growth factor receptor 3 is transforming in hematopoietic cells. Blood 2001;97:2413–9.
176. Corradini P, Ladetto M, Voena C, et al. Mutational activation of N- and K- ras oncogenes in plasma cell dyscrasias. Blood 1993;81:2708–13.
177. Neri A, Murphy L, Cro L, et al. RAS oncogene mutation in multiple myeloma. J Exp Med 1989;170:1715–25.
178. Ong F, Nieuwkoop JA, de Groot-Swings GM, et al. Bcl-2 protein expression is not related to short survival in multiple myeloma. Leukemia 1995;9:1282–4.
179. Pettersson M, Jernberg-Wiklund H, Larsson LG, et al. Expression of the bcl-2 gene in human multiple myeloma cell lines and normal plasma cells. Blood 1992;79:495.
180. Tian E, Gazitt Y. The role of p53, bcl-2 and bax network in dexamethasone induced apoptosis in multiple myeloma cell lines. Int J Oncol 1996;8:719.
181. Gauthier ER, Piche L, Lemieux G, Lemieux R. Role of bcl-XL in the control of apoptosis in murine myeloma cells. Cancer Res 1996;56:1451–6.
182. Schwarze MMK, Hawley RG. Prevention of myeloma cell apoptosis by ectopic bcl-2 expression or interleukin-6 mediated up-regulation of bcl-XL. Cancer Res 1995;55:2262–5.
183. Zhang B, Gojo I, Fenton RG. Myeloid cell factor-1 is a critical survival factor for multiple myeloma. Blood 2002;99:1885–93.
184. Portier M, Moles JP, Mazars GR, et al. p53 and RAS gene mutations in multiple myeloma. Oncogene 1992;7:2539–43.
185. Juge-Morineau N, Mellerin MP, Francois S, et al. High incidence of deletions but infrequent inactivation of the retinoblastoma gene in human myeloma cells. Br J Haematol 1995;91:664–7.
186. Urashima M, Ogata A, Chauhan D, et al. Interleukin-6 promotes multiple myeloma cell growth via phosphorylation of retinoblastoma protein. Blood 1996;88:2219–27.
187. Kawano MM, Mahmoud MS, Huang N. Cyclin D1 and p16INK4A are preferentially expressed in immature and mature myeloma cells, respectively. Br J Haematol 1997;99:131–8.
188. Ng MHL, Chung YF, Lo KW, et al. Frequent hypermethylation of *p16* and *p15* genes in multiple myeloma. Blood 1997;89:2500–6.
189. Tasaka T, Berenson J, Vescio R, et al. Analysis of the p16INK4A, p15INK4B and p18INK4C genes in multiple myeloma. Br J Haematol 1997;96:98–102.
190. Urashima M, Teoh G, Ogata A, et al. Characterization of $p16^{INK4A}$ expression in multiple myeloma and plasma cell leukemia. Clin Cancer Res 1997;3:2173–9.
191. Dilworth D, Liu L, Stewart AK, et al. Germline *CDKN2A* mutation implicated in predisposition to multiple myeloma. Blood 2000;95:1869–71.
192. Urashima M, Teoh G, Chauhan D, et al. Interleukin-6 overcomes $p21^{WAF1}$ upregulation and G1 growth arrest induced by dexamethasone and interferon-γ in multiple myeloma cells. Blood 1997;90:279–89.
193. Teoh G, Urashima M, Ogata A, et al. MDM2 protein overexpression promotes proliferation and survival of multiple myeloma cells. Blood 1997;90:1982–92.
194. Tricot G, Barlogie B, Jagannath S, et al. Poor prognosis in multiple myeloma is associated only with partial or complete deletions of chromosome 13 or abnormalities involving 11q and not with other karyotype abnormalities. Blood 1995;86:4250–6.
195. Tricot G, Spencer T, Sawyer J, et al. Predicting long-term (> or = 5 years) event-free survival in multiple myeloma patients following planned tandem autotransplants. Br J Haematol 2002;116:211–7.
196. Facon T, Avet-Loiseau H, Guillerm G, et al. Chromosome 13 abnormalities identified by FISH analysis and serum beta2-microglobulin produce a powerful myeloma staging system for patients receiving high-dose therapy. Blood 2001;97:1566–71.
197. Konigsberg R, Zojer N, Ackermann J, et al. Predictive role of interphase cytogenetics for survival of patients with multiple myeloma. J Clin Oncol 2000;18:804–12.
198. Avet-Loiseau H, Li JY, Morineau N, et al. Monosomy 13 is associated with the transition of monoclonal gammopathy of undetermined significance to multiple myeloma. Intergroupe Francophone du Myelome. Blood 1999;94:2583–9.
199. Schena M, Shalon D, Davis RW, Brown PO. Quantitative monitoring of gene expression patterns with a complementary DNA microarray [see comments]. Science 1995;270:467–70.
200. Davies FE, Dring AM, Li C, et al. Insights into the multistep transformation of MGUS to myeloma using microarray expression analysis. Blood 2003;102:4504–11.
201. Mitsiades N, Mitsiades CS, Poulaki V, et al. Molecular sequelae of proteasome inhibition in human multiple myeloma cells. Proc Natl Acad Sci U S A 2002;99:14374–9.
202. Bataille R, Durie BGM, Grenier J, Sany J. Prognostic factors and staging in multiple myeloma: a reappraisal. J Clin Oncol 1986;4:80–7.
203. Durie BGM, Salmon SE. A clinical staging system for multiple myeloma. Correlation of measured cell mass with presenting clinical features, response to treatment and survival. Cancer 1975;36:842–54.
204. Gassmann W, Pralle H, Haferlach T, et al. Staging systems for multiple myeloma: a comparison. Br J Haematol 1985;59:703–11.
205. Greipp PR. Prognosis in myeloma. Mayo Clin Proc 1994;69:895–902.
206. Alexanian R, Balcerzak S, Bonnet JD, et al. Prognostic factors in multiple myeloma. Cancer 1975;36:1192–201.
207. Merlini G, Waldenström JG, Jayakar SD. A new improved clinical staging system for multiple myeloma based on analysis of 123 patients. Blood 1980;55:1011–9.
208. Carbone PP. A study of the relationship of survival to various clinical manifestations and anomalous protein type in 112 patients. Am J Med 1967;42:937–48.
209. Medical Research Council's Working Party on Leukaemia in Adults. Prognostic features in the third MRC myelomatosis trial. Br J Cancer 1980;42:831–40.
210. Cavo M, Galieni P, Zuffa E, et al. Prognostic variables and clinical staging in multiple myeloma. Blood 1989;74:1774–80.
211. Greipp PR, Raymond NM, Kyle RA, O'Fallon WM. Multiple myeloma: significance of plasmablastic subtype in morphological classification. Blood 1985;65:305–10.
212. Greipp PR, Leong T, Bennett JM, et al. Plasmablastic morphology—an independent prognostic factor with clinical and laboratory correlates: Eastern Cooperative Oncology Group (ECOG) myeloma trial E9486 report by the ECOG Myeloma Laboratory Group. Blood 1998;91:2501–7.
213. Brenning G, Simonsson B, Kallander C, Ahre A. Pretreatment serum beta 2-microglobulin in multiple myeloma. Br J Hematol 1986;62:85–93.
214. Durie BG, Stock-Novack D, Salmon SE, et al. Prognostic value of pretreatment serum beta 2 microglobulin in myeloma: a Southwest Oncology Group Study. Blood 1990;75:823–30.
215. Taniwaki M, Nishida K, Takashima T, et al. Nonrandom chromosomal rearrangements of 14q32.3 and 19p13.3 and preferential deletion of 1p in 21 patients with multiple myeloma and plasma cell leukemia. Blood 1994;84:2283–90.
216. Zojer N, Konigsberg R, Ackermann J, et al. Deletion of 13q14 remains an independent adverse prognostic variable in multiple myeloma despite its frequent detection by interphase fluorescence in situ hybridization. Blood 2000;95:1925–30.
217. Tricot G, Sawyer JR, Jagannath S, et al. Unique role of cytogenetics in the prognosis of patients with myeloma receiving high-dose therapy and autotransplants. J Clin Oncol 1997;15:2659–66.
218. Desikan R, Barlogie B, Sawyer J, et al. Results of high-dose therapy for 1000 patients with multiple myeloma: durable complete remissions and superior survival in the absence of chromosome 13 abnormalities. Blood 2000;95:4008–10.
219. Sawyer JR, Lukacs JL, Munshi N, et al. Identification of new nonrandom translocations in multiple myeloma with multicolor spectral karyotyping. Blood 1998;92:4269–78.
220. Finelli P, Fabris S, Zagano S, et al. Detection of t(4;14)(p16.3;q32) chromosomal translocation in multiple myeloma by double-color fluorescent in situ hybridization. Blood 1999;94:724–32.
221. Durie BGM, Grogan TM. CALLA-positive myeloma: an aggressive subtype with poor survival. Blood 1985;66:229–32.
222. Barlogie B, Smallwood L, Smith T, Alexanian R. High serum levels of lactic dehydrogenase identify a high-grade lymphoma-like myeloma. Ann Intern Med 1989;110:521–5.
223. Omede P, Tarella C, Palumbo A, et al. Multiple myeloma: reduced plasma cell contamination in peripheral blood progenitor cell collections performed after repeated high-dose chemotherapy courses. Br J Haematol 1997;99:685–91.
224. Cimino G, Avvisati G, Amadori S, et al. High serum IL-2 levels are predictive of prolonged survival in multiple myeloma. Br J Haematol 1990;75:373–7.
225. Bataille R, Boccadoro M, Klein B, et al. C-reactive protein and β-2 microglobulin produce a simple and powerful myeloma staging system. Blood 1992;80:733–7.
226. Greipp PR, Gaillard JP, Kalish LA. Independent prognostic value for serum soluble interleukin-6 receptor (sIL-6R) in Eastern Cooperative Oncology Group (ECOG) myeloma trial E9487. Proc Am Soc Clin Oncol 1993;12:404.
227. Seidel C, Borset M, Turesson I, et al. Elevated serum concentrations of hepatocyte growth factor in patients with multiple myeloma. The Nordic Myeloma Study Group. Blood 1998;91:806–12.

228. Seidel C, Sundan A, Hjorth M, et al. Serum syndecan-1: a new independent prognostic marker in multiple myeloma. Blood 2000;95:388–92.
229. Dahl IM, Turesson I, Holmberg E, Lilja K. Serum hyaluronan in patients with multiple myeloma: correlation with survival and Ig concentration. Blood 1999;93:4144–8.
230. Witzig TE, Gertz MA, Lust JA, et al. Peripheral blood monoclonal plasma cells as a predictor of survival in patients with multiple myeloma. Blood 1996;88:1780–7.
231. Rajkumar SV, Fonseca R, Lacy MQ, et al. Plasmablastic morphology is an independent predictor of poor survival after autologous stem-cell transplantation for multiple myeloma. J Clin Oncol 1999;17:1551–7.
232. Garcia-Sanchez R, Orfao A, Gonzalez M, et al. Primary plasma cell leukemia: clinical, immunophenotypic, DNA ploidy, and cytogenetic characteristics. Blood 1999;93:1032–7.
233. Blade J, Kyle RA, Greipp P. Presenting features and prognosis in 72 patients with multiple myeloma who were younger than 40 years. Br J Haematol 1996;93:345–51.
234. San Miguel JF, Caballero MD, Gonzales M, et al. A new staging system for multiple myeloma based on the number of S-phase plasma cells. Blood 1995;85:448–55.
235. Liu P, Leong T, Quam L, et al. Activating mutations of N- and K-ras in multiple myeloma show different clinical associations: analysis of the Eastern Cooperative Oncology Group phase III trial. Blood 1996;88:2699–706.
236. Kay NE, Leong T, Kyle RA, et al. Circulating blood B cells in multiple myeloma; analysis and relationship to circulating clonal cells and clinical parameters in a cohort of patients entered on the Eastern Cooperative Oncology Group phase III E9486 clinical trial. Blood 1997;90:340–5.
237. Kyle RA. Why better prognostic factors for multiple myeloma are needed. Blood 1994;83:1713–6.
238. Raaijmakers HGP, Izquierdo MAI, Lokhorst HM, et al. Lung-resistance-related protein expression is a negative predictive factor for response to conventional low but not to intensified dose alkylating chemotherapy in multiple myeloma. Blood 1998;91:1029–36.
239. Mundy GR, Bertolini DR. Bone destruction and hypercalcemia in plasma cell myeloma. Semin Oncol 1986;13:291–9.
240. Bardwick PA, Zvaifler NJ, Gill GN, et al. Plasma cell dyscrasia with polyneuropathy, organomegaly, endocrinopathy, M protein, and skin changes: the POEMS syndrome. Report on two cases and a review of the literature. Medicine (Baltimore) 1980;59:311–22.
241. Barille S, Bataille R, Rapp MJ, et al. Production of metalloproteinase-7 (matrilysin) by human myeloma cells and its potential involvement in metalloproteinase-2 activation. J Immunol 1999;163:5723–8.
242. Hjertner O, Torgersen ML, Seidel C, et al. Hepatocyte growth factor (HGF) induces interleukin-11 secretion from osteoblasts: a possible role for HGF in myeloma-associated osteolytic bone disease. Blood 1999;94:3883–8.
243. Lacey DL, Timms E, Tan H-L, et al. Osteoprotegerin ligand is a cytokine that regulates osteoclast differentiation and activation. Cell 1998;93:165–76.
244. Han JH, Choi SJ, Kurihara N, et al. Macrophage inflammatory protein-1α is an osteoclastogenic factor in myeloma that is independent of receptor activator of nuclear factor kappaB ligand. Blood 2001;97:3349–53.
245. Giuliani N, Bataille R, Mancini C, et al. Myeloma cells induce imbalance in the osteoprotegerin/osteoprotegerin ligand system in the human bone marrow environment. Blood 2001;98:3527–33.
246. Pearse RN, Sordillo EM, Yaccoby S, et al. Multiple myeloma disrupts the TRANCE/ osteoprotegerin cytokine axis to trigger bone destruction and promote tumor progression. Proc Natl Acad Sci U S A 2001;98:11581–6.
247. Seidel C, Hjertner O, Abildgaard N, et al. Serum osteoprotegerin levels are reduced in patients with multiple myeloma with lytic bone disease. Blood 2001;98:2269–71.
248. Alsina M, Boyce BF, Devlin R, et al. Development of an in vivo model of human multiple myeloma bone disease. Blood 1996;87:1495–501.
249. Hjorth-Hansen H, Borset M, Seidel C, et al. The JJN-3 cell line gives multiple myeloma with bone disease in SCID mice. Blood 1996;88:387a.
250. Croucher PI, Shipman CM, Lippitt J, et al. Osteoprotegerin inhibits the development of osteolytic bone disease in multiple myeloma. Blood 2001;98:3534–40.
251. Oyajobi BO, Anderson DM, Traianedes K, et al. Therapeutic efficacy of a soluble receptor activator of nuclear factor kappaB-IgG Fc fusion protein in suppressing bone resorption and hypercalcemia in a model of humoral hypercalcemia of malignancy. Cancer Res 2001;61:2572–8.
252. Harley JB, Schilling A, Glidewell O. Ineffectiveness of fluoride therapy in multiple myeloma. N Engl J Med 1972;286:1283–8.
253. Siris ES, Sherman WH, Baquiran DC, et al. Effects of dichloromethylene diphosphonate on skeletal mobilization of calcium in multiple myeloma. N Engl J Med 1980;302:310–5.
254. Lahtinen R, Laasko M, Palva I, et al. Randomised, placebo-controlled multicentre trial of clodronate in multiple myeloma. Lancet 1992;340:1049–52.
255. Berenson J, Lichtenstein A, Porter L, et al. Pamidronate disodium reduces the occurrence of skeletal events in patients with advanced multiple myeloma. N Engl J Med 1996;334:488–93.
256. Berenson JR, Lichtenstein A, Porter L, et al. Long-term pamidronate treatment of advanced multiple myeloma patients reduces skeletal events. J Clin Oncol 1998;16:593–602.
257. Bloomfield DJ. Should bisphosphonates be part of the standard therapy of patients with multiple myeloma or bone metastases from other cancers? An evidence-based review. J Clin Oncol 1998;16:1218–25.
258. Dhodapkar MV, Singh J, Mehta J, et al. Anti-myeloma activity of pamidronate in vivo. Br J Haematol 1998;103:530–2.
259. Hyghes DE, Wright KR, Uy HL. Bisphosphonates promote apoptosis in murine osteoclasts in vitro and in vivo. J Bone Miner Res 1995;10:1478–87.
260. Martin A, Garcia-Sanz R, Hernandez J, et al. Pamidronate induces bone formation in patients with smouldering or indolent myeloma, with no significant anti-tumour effect. Br J Haematol 2002;118:239–42.
261. Berenson JR, Lipton A, Rosen LS et al. Phase-1 clinical study of a new bisphosphonate, zoledronate (CGP-42446), in patients with osteolytic bone metastases. Blood 1996;88(Suppl 1):586a.
262. Lipton A, et al. Phase 11 Study of the bisphosphonate, zoledronate in patients with osteolytic lesions [abstract 48]. Second International Conference: Cancer-Induced Bone Diseases; 1999 Mar 27–29; Davos, Switzerland.
263. Lipton A, et al. The effects of the bisphosphonate, zoledronic acid, when administered as a short Intravenous infusion in patients with bone metastases: a phase I study [abstract 848]. American Soceity of Clinical Oncology Annual Meeting; 1997 May 17–20; Denver (CO).
264. Menssen HD, Sakalova A, Fontana A, et al. Effects of long-term intravenous ibandronate therapy on skeletal-related events, survival, and bone resorption markers in patients with advanced multiple myeloma. J Clin Oncol 2002;20:2353–9.
265. Lugassy G, Shaham R, Nemets A, et al. Severe osteomyelitis of the jaw in long-term survivors of multiple myeloma: a new clinical entity. Am J Med 2004;117:440–1.
266. Bagan JV, Murillo J, Jimenez Y, et al. Avascular jaw osteonecrosis in association with cancer chemotherapy: series of 10 cases. J Oral Pathol Med 2005;34:120–3.
267. Major P, Lortholary A, Hon J, et al. Zoledronic acid is superior to pamidronate in the treatment of hypercalcemia of malignancy: a pooled analysis of two randomized, controlled clinical trials. J Clin Oncol 2001;19:558–67.
268. Pruzanski W, Watt JG. Serum viscosity and hyperviscosity syndrome in IgG multiple myeloma. Ann Intern Med 1972;77:853–60.
269. Lindsley H, Teller D, Noonan B, et al. Hyperviscosity syndrome in multiple myeloma. A reversible, concentration-dependent aggregation of the myeloma protein. Am J Med 1973;54:682–8.
270. Twomey JJ. Infections complicating multiple myeloma and chronic lymphocytic leukemia. Arch Intern Med 1973;132:562–5.
271. Jacobsen DR, Zolla-Pazner S. Immunosuppression and infection in multiple myeloma. Semin Oncol 1986;13:282–90.
272. Salmon SE, Samal BA, Hayes DM, et al. Role of gammaglobulin for immunoprophylaxis in multiple myeloma. N Engl J Med 1967;277:1336–40.
273. Gilleece MH, Anderson KC. Multiple myeloma: guarding against infection. Infect Med 2000;17:500–4.
274. Oken MM, Pomeroy C, Weisdorf D, Bennet JM. Prophylactic antibiotics for the prevention of early infection in multiple myeloma. Am J Med 1996;100:624–8.
275. Torra R, Blade J, Cases A, et al. Patient with multiple myeloma requiring long term dialysis: presenting features, response to therapy, and outcome in a series of 20 patients. Br J Haematol 1995;91:854–9.
276. Stone MJ, Frendel EP. The clinical spectrum of light chain myeloma. A study of 35 patients with special reference to the occurrence of amyloidosis. Am J Med 1975;58:601–19.
277. Gallo G, Picken M, Buxbaum J, Frangione B. The spectrum of monoclonal immunoglobulin deposition disease associated with immunocytic dyscrasias. Semin Hematol 1989;26:234–45.
278. Gallo G. Renal complications of B cell dyscrasias. N Engl J Med 1991;324:1889–90.
279. Solomon A, Weiss DT, Kattine AA. Nephrotoxic potential of Bence Jones proteins. N Engl J Med 1991;324:1845–51.
280. McBride W, Jackman JD, Gammon RS, Willerson JT. High output cardiac failure in patients with multiple myeloma. N Engl J Med 1988;319:1651–3.
281. Beguin Y, Yerna M, Loo M, et al. Erythropoiesis in multiple myeloma: defective red cell production due to inappropriate erythropoietin production. Br J Haematol 1992;82:648–53.
282. Cazzola M, Messinger D, Battistel V, et al. Recombinant human erythropoietin in the anemia associated with multiple myeloma or non-Hodgkin's lymphoma: dose finding and identification of predictors of response. Blood 1995;86:4446–53.
283. Ludwig H, Fritz E, Kotzmann H, et al. Erythropoietin treatment of anemia associated with multiple myeloma. N Engl J Med 1990;322:1693–9.
284. Osterborg A, Boogaerts MA, Cimino R, et al. Recombinant human erythropoietin in transfusion-dependent anemic patients with multiple myeloma and non-Hodgkin's lymphoma—a randomized multicenter study. Blood 1996;87:2675–82.
285. Roper AH, Gorson KC. Neuropathies associated with paraproteinemia. N Engl J Med 1998;338:1601–7.
286. Latov N, Sherman WH, Nemni R, et al. Plasma-cell dyscrasia and peripheral neuropathy with a monoclonal antibody to peripheral-nerve myelin. N Engl J Med 1980;303:618–21.
287. Gonzalez F, Trujillo JM, Alexanian R. Acute leukemia in multiple myeloma. Ann Intern Med 1977;86:440–3.
288. Bergsagel DE, Bailey AJ, Langley GR, et al. The chemotherapy of plasma cell myeloma and the incidence of acute leukemia. N Engl J Med 1979;301:743–8.
289. Stegman R, Alexanian R. Solid tumors in multiple myeloma. Ann Intern Med 1979;90:780–2.
290. Chronic Leukemia–Myeloma Task Force, National Cancer Institute. Proposed guidelines for protocol studies II plasma cell myeloma. Cancer Chemother Rep 1973;4:145–58.
291. Salmon SE, Haut A, Bonnet JD, Aet al. Alternating combination chemotherapy and levamisole improves survival in multiple myeloma: a Southwest Oncology Group study. J Clin Oncol 1983;1:453–61.
292. Blade J, Samson D, Reece D, et al. Criteria for evaluating disease response and progression in patients with multiple myeloma treated by high-dose therapy and haemopoietic stem cell transplantation. Myeloma Subcommittee of the EBMT. European Group for Blood and Marrow Transplant. Br J Haematol 1998;102:1115–23.
293. Kyle RA. Newer approaches to the therapy of multiple myeloma. Blood 1990;76:1678–9.
294. Kyle RA, Rajkumar SV. Multiple myeloma. N Engl J Med 2004;351:1860–73.
295. Bergsagel DE. Use a gentle approach for refractory myeloma patients. J Clin Oncol 1988;6:757–8.
296. Boccadoro M, Palumbo A, Bringhen S, et al. Oral melphalan at diagnosis hampers adequate collection of peripheral blood progenitor cells in multiple myeloma. Haematologica 2002;87:846–50.
297. Oken MM. Standard treatment of multiple myeloma. Mayo Clin Proc 1996;69:781–6.
298. Bergsagel DE. Is aggressive chemotherapy more effective in the treatment of plasma cell myeloma? Eur J Cancer Clin Oncol 1989;25:159–61.
299. Blade J, San Miguel JF, Alcala A, et al. Alternating combination VCMP/VBAP chemotherapy versus melphalan/prednisone in the treatment of multiple myeloma: a randomized multicentric study of 487 patients. J Clin Oncol 1993;11:1165–71.
300. Durie BGM, Dixon DO, Carter S, et al. Improved survival duration with combination chemotherapy induction for multiple myeloma: a Southwest Oncology Group study. J Clin Oncol 1986;4:1227–37.
301. Samson D, Gaminara E, Newland A, et al. Infusion of vincristine and doxorubicin with oral dexamethasone as first-line therapy for multiple myeloma. Lancet 1989;ii:882–5.
302. Alexanian R, Dimopoulos MA, Delasalle K, Barlogie B. Primary dexamethasone treatment of multiple myeloma. Blood 1992;80:887–90.

303. Hussein MA, Wood L, Hsi E, et al. A phase II trial of pegylated liposomal doxorubicin, vincristine, and reduced-dose dexamethasone combination therapy in newly diagnosed multiple myeloma patients. Cancer 2002;95:2160–8.
304. Dimopoulos MA, Pouli A, Zervas K, et al. Prospective randomized comparison of vincristine, doxorubicin and dexamethasone (VAD) administered as intravenous bolus injection and VAD with liposomal doxorubicin as first-line treatment in multiple myeloma. Ann Oncol 2003;14:1039–44.
305. Salmon SE, Crowley JJ, Grogan TM, et al. Combination chemotherapy, glucocorticoids, and interferon alpha in the treatment of multiple myeloma: a Southwest Oncology Group study. J Clin Oncol 1994;12:2405–14.
306. Oken MM, Harrington DP, Abramson N, et al. Comparison of melphalan and prednisone with vincristine, carmustine, melphalan, cyclophosphamide, and prednisone in the treatment of multiple myeloma—results of Eastern Cooperative Oncology Group study E2479. Cancer 1997;79:1561–7.
307. Gregory WM, Richards MA, Malpas JS. Combination chemotherapy versus melphalan and prednisolone in the treatment of multiple myeloma: an overview of published trials. J Clin Oncol 1992;10:334–42.
308. Group MTsC. Combination chemotherapy versus melphalan plus prednisone as treatment for multiple myeloma: an overview of 6,633 patients from 27 randomized trials. J Clin Oncol 1998;16:3832–42.
309. Berenson JR, Crowley JJ, Grogan TM, et al. Maintenance therapy with alternate-day prednisone improves survival in multiple myeloma patients. Blood 2002;99:3163–8.
310. Rajkumar SV, Hayman S, Gertz MA, et al. Combination therapy with thalidomide plus dexamethasone for newly diagnosed myeloma. J Clin Oncol 2002;20:4319–23.
311. Weber D, Rankin K, Gavino M, et al. Thalidomide alone or with dexamethasone for previously untreated multiple myeloma. J Clin Oncol 2003;21:16–9.
312. Cavo M, Zamagni E, Tosi P, et al. First-line therapy with thalidomide and dexamethasone in preparation for autologous stem cell transplantation for multiple myeloma. Haematologica 2004;89:826–31.
313. Barlogie B, Smith L, Alexanian R. Effective treatment of advanced multiple myeloma refractory to alkylating agents. N Engl J Med 1984;310:1353–6.
314. Monconduit M, Le Loet X, Bernard JF, Michaux JL. Combination chemotherapy with vincristine, doxurubicin, dexamethasone for refractory or relapsing multiple myeloma. Br J Haematol 1986;63:599–601.
315. Sheehan T, Judge M, Parker AC. The efficacy and toxicity of VAD in the treatment of myeloma and related disorders. Scand J Haematol 1986;37:425–8.
316. Salmon SE, Dalton WS, Grogan TM, et al. Multidrug-resistant myeloma: laboratory and clinical effects of verapamil as a chemosensitizer. Blood 1991;78:44–50.
317. Sonneveld P, Schoester M, de Leeuw K. Clinical modulation of multidrug resistance in multiple myeloma: effects of cyclosporine on resistant tumor cells. J Clin Oncol 1994;12:1584–91.
318. Sonneveld P. Drug resistance in myeloma. VI International Workshop on Multiple Myeloma. Boston; 1997.
319. Grogan TM, Spier CM, Salmon SE, et al. P-glycoprotein expression in human plasma cell myeloma: correlation with prior chemotherapy. Blood 1993;81:490–5.
320. Barlogie B, Valasquez WS, Alexanian R, Cabanillas F. Etoposide, dexamethasone, cytarabine, and cisplatin in vincristine, doxorubicin and dexamethasone-refractory myeloma. J Clin Oncol 1989;7:1514–7.
321. Kraut EH, Crowley JJ, Wade JL, et al. Evaluation of topotecan in resistant relapsing multiple myeloma: a Southwest Oncology Group study. J Clin Oncol 1998;16:589–92.
322. Barlogie B, Desikan R, Eddlemon P, et al. Extended survival in advanced and refractory multiple myeloma after single-agent thalidomide: identification of prognostic factors in a phase 2 study of 169 patients. Blood 2001;98:492–4.
323. Weber DM, Gavino M, Delasalle K, et al. Thalidomide alone or with dexamethasone for multiple myeloma. Blood 1999;94(Suppl 1):604a.
324. Moehler TM, Neben K, Benner A, et al. Salvage therapy for multiple myeloma with thalidomide and CED chemotherapy. Blood 2001;98:3846–8.
325. Garcia-Sanz R, Gonzalez-Porras JR, Hernandez JM, et al. The oral combination of thalidomide, cyclophosphamide and dexamethasone (ThaCyDex) is effective in relapsed/refractory multiple myeloma. Leukemia 2004;18:856–63.
326. Richardson PG, Barlogie B, Berenson J, et al. A phase 2 study of bortezomib in relapsed, refractory myeloma. N Engl J Med 2003;348:2609–17.
327. Orlowski RZ, Stinchcombe TE, Mitchell BS, et al. Phase I trial of the proteasome inhibitor PS-341 in patients with refractory hematologic malignancies. J Clin Oncol 2002;20:4420–7.
328. Portier M, Zhang XG, Caron E, et al. Gamma-interferon in multiple myeloma: inhibition of interleukin 6 dependent myeloma cell growth and downregulation of IL-6 receptor expression in vitro. Blood 1993;81:3076–82.
329. The Nordic Myeloma Study Group. Interferon-alpha 2b added to melphalan-prednisone for initial and maintenance therapy in multiple myeloma. A randomized, controlled trial. Ann Intern Med 1996;124:212–22.
330. Ludwig H, Cohen AM, Polliack A, et al. Interferon-α for induction and maintenance in multiple myeloma: results of two multicenter randomized trials and summary of other studies. Ann Oncol 1995;6:467–76.
331. Montuoro A, De Rosa L, De Blasio A, et al. Alpha-2a-interferon/melphalan/prednisone versus melphalan/prednisone in previously untreated patients with multiple myeloma. Br J Haematol 1990;76:365–8.
332. Osterborg A, Bjorkholm M, Bjoreman M, et al. Natural interferon-α in combination with melphalan/prednisone versus melphalan/prednisone in the treatment of multiple myeloma stages II and III: a randomized study from the Myeloma Group of Central Sweden. Blood 1993;81:1428–34.
333. Mandelli F, Avvisati G, Amadori S, et al. Maintenance treatment with recombinant interferon alpha-2b in patients with multiple myeloma responding to conventional induction chemotherapy. N Engl J Med 1990;322:1430–4.
334. Brockman JA, Scherer DC, McKinsey TA, et al. Coupling of a signal response domain in IκB157} to multiple pathways for NF-κB activation. Mol Cell Biol 1995;15:2809–18.
335. Cunningham D, Powles R, Malpas J, et al. A randomized trial of maintenance therapy with Intron-A following high-dose chemotherapy in multiple myeloma—long-term followup results. Br J Haematol 1998;102:495–502.
336. Westin J, Rodjer S, Turesson I, et al. Interferon α-2b versus no maintenance therapy during the plateau phase in multiple myeloma: a randomized study. Cooperative Study Group. Br J Haematol 1995;89:561–8.
337. Ludwig H, Fritz E, Neuda J, Durie BGM. Patient preferences for interferon-α in multiple myeloma. J Clin Oncol 1997;15:1672–9.
338. Zee B, Cole B, Li T, et al. Quality-adjusted time without symptoms or toxicity analysis of interferon maintenance in multiple myeloma. J Clin Oncol 1998;16:2834–9.
339. MacKenzie MR, Wold H, George C, et al. Consolidation hemibody radiotherapy following induction combination chemotherapy in high-tumor-burden multiple myeloma. J Clin Oncol 1992;10:1769–74.
340. Thomas PJ, Daban A, Bontoux D. Double hemibody irradiation in chemotherapy-resistant multiple myeloma. Can Treat Rep 1984;68:1173–5.
341. Anderson KC. Who benefits from high dose therapy for multiple myeloma? J Clin Oncol 1995;13:1291–6.
342. Kovasics TJ, Delaly A. Intensive treatment strategies in multiple myeloma. Sem Hematol 1997;34:49–60.
343. Bensinger WI, Demirer T, Buckner CD, et al. Syngeneic marrow transplantation in patients with multiple myeloma. Bone Marrow Transplant 1996;18:527–31.
344. Gahrton G, Svensson H, Bjorkstrand B, et al. Syngeneic transplantation in multiple myeloma—a case-matched comparison with autologous and allogeneic transplantation. Bone Marrow Transplantation 1999;7:741–5.
345. Gahrton G, Anderson K, Bensinger W. Allogeneic transplantation in myeloma. In: Berenson J, editor. Totowa (NJ): The Humana Press; 1999.
346. Gahrton G, Svensson H, Cavo M, et al. Progress in allogeneic bone marrow and peripheral blood stem cell transplantation for multiple myeloma: a comparison between transplants performed 1983–93 and 1994–8 at European Group for Blood and Marrow centers. Br J Haematol 2001;113:209–16.
347. Gahrton G, Tura S, Ljungman P, et al. Prognostic factors in allogeneic bone marrow transplantation for multiple myeloma. J Clin Oncol 1995;13:1312–22.
348. Bjorkstrand BB, Ljungman P, Svensson H, et al. Allogeneic bone marrow transplantation versus autologous stem cell transplantation in multiple myeloma: a retrospective case-matched study from the European Group for Blood and Marrow Transplantation. Blood 1996;88:4711–8.
349. Bensinger WI, Buchner CD, Anasetti C, et al. Allogeneic marrow transplantation for multiple myeloma: an analysis of risk factors on outcome. Blood 1996;88:2787–93.
350. Cavo M, Bandini G, Benni M, et al. High dose busulfan and cyclophosphamide are an effective conditioning regimen for allogeneic bone marrow transplantation in chemosensitive multiple myeloma. Bone Marrow Transplantation 1998;22:27–32.
351. Schlossman SF, Alyea E, Orsini E, et al. Immune based strategies to improve hematopoietic stem cell transplantation in multiple myeloma. In: Dicke KA, Keating A, editors. Autologous marrow and blood transplantation. Charlottesville (VA): Carden Jennings Publishing; 1999. p. 207–21.
352. Schlossman SF, Anderson KC. Bone marrow transplantation in multiple myeloma. In: Jones R, editor. Current opinion in oncology. Vol 11. Philadelphia (PA): Lippincott Williams & Wilkins; 1999. p. 102–8.
353. Seiden M, Schlossman R, Andersen J, et al. Monoclonal antibody-purged bone marrow transplantation therapy for multiple myeloma. Leukemia and Lymphoma 1995;17:87–93.
354. Soiffer RJ, Murray C, Mauch P, et al. Prevention of graft-versus-host disease by selective depletion of CD6-positive T lymphocytes from donor bone marrow. J Clin Oncol 1992;10:1191–200.
355. Corradini P, Voena C, Tarella C, et al. Molecular and clinical remissions in multiple myeloma: role of autologous and allogeneic transplantation of hematopoietic cells. J Clin Oncol 1999;17:208–15.
356. Martinelli G, Terragna C, Zamagni E, et al. Molecular remission after allogeneic or autologous transplantation of hematopoietic stem cells for multiple myeloma. J Clin Oncol 2000;18:2273–81.
357. Cavo M, Terragna C, Martinelli G, et al. Molecular monitoring of minimal residual disease in patients in long-term complete remission after allogeneic stem cell transplantation for multiple myeloma. Blood 2000;96:355–7.
358. Willems P, Verhagen O, Segeren C, et al. Consensus strategy to quantitate malignant cells in myeloma patients is validated in a multicenter study. Blood 2000;96:63–70.
359. Antin JH. Graft-versus-leukemia: no longer an epiphenomenon. Blood 1993;82:2273–7.
360. Collins R, Shpilberg O, Drobyski W, et al. Donor leukocyte infusions in 140 patients with relapsed malignancy after allogeneic bone marrow transplantation. J Clin Oncol 1997;15:433–44.
361. Kolb H-J, Schattenberg A, Goldman JM, et al. Graft-versus-leukemia effect of donor lymphocyte transfusions in marrow grafted patients. Blood 1995;86:2041–50.
362. Champlin R, Ho W, Gajewski J, et al. Selective depletion of CD8+ T lymphocytes for prevention of graft-versus-host disease after allogeneic bone marrow transplantation. Blood 1990;76:418–23.
363. Tricot G, Vesole DH, Jagannath S, et al. Graft-versus-myeloma effect: proof of principle. Blood 1996;87:1196–8.
364. Verdonck LF, Lokhorst HM, Dekker AW, et al. Graft-versus-myeloma effect in two cases. Lancet 1996;347:800–1.
365. Munshi NC, Govindarajan R, Drake R, et al. Thymidine kinase (TK) gene-transduced human lymphocytes can be highly purified, remain fully functional and are killed efficiently with ganciclovir. Blood 1997;89:1334–40.
366. Alyea EP, Soiffer RJ, Canning C, et al. Toxicity and efficacy of defined doses of CD4+ donor lymphocytes for treatment of relapse after allogeneic bone marrow transplant. Blood 1998;91:3671–80.
367. Alyea E, Weller E, Schlossman R, et al. T-cell-depleted allogeneic bone marrow transplantation followed by donor lymphocyte infusion in patients with multiple myeloma: induction of graft-versus-myeloma effect. Blood 2001;98:934–9.
368. Alyea E, Weller E, Schlossman R, et al. Outcome after autologous and allogeneic stem cell transplantation for patients with multiple myeloma: impact of graft-versus-myeloma effect. Bone Marrow Transplant 2003;32:1145–51.
369. Orsini E, Alyea EP, Schlossman R, et al. Changes in T cell receptor repertoire associated with graft-versus-tumor effect and graft-versus host disease in patients with relapsed multiple myeloma receiving donor lymphocyte infusions. B Mar Trans 2000;25:623–32.
370. Bellucci R, Alyea EP, Weller E, et al. Immunologic effects of prophylactic donor lymphocyte infusion after allogeneic marrow transplantation for multiple myeloma. Blood 2002;99:4610–7.
371. Kwak LW, Taub DD, Duffey PL, et al. Transfer of myeloma idiotype-specific immunity from an actively immunized marrow donor. Lancet 1995;345:1016–20.
372. Wimperis JZ, Brenner MK, Prentice HG, et al. B cell development and regulation after T cell-depleted marrow transplantation. J Immunol 1987;138:2445–50.

373. Badros A, Barlogie B, Siegel E, et al. Improved outcome of allogeneic transplantation in high-risk multiple myeloma patients after nonmyeloablative conditioning. J Clin Oncol 2002;20:1295–303.
374. Kroger N, Schwerdtfeger R, Kiehl M, et al. Autologous stem cell transplantation followed by a dose-reduced allograft induces high complete remission rate in multiple myeloma. Blood 2002;100:755–60.
375. Maloney D, Sahebi F, Srockerl-Goldstein KE, et al. Combining an allogeneic graft versus myeloma effect with high dose autologous stem cell rescue in the treatment of multiple myeloma. Blood 2001;98:434a.
376. Harousseau J-L, Attal M. The role of autologous hematopoietic stem cell transplantation in multiple myeloma. Sem Hematol 1997;34:61–6.
377. Attal M, Harousseau JL, Stoppa AM, et al. Autologous bone marrow transplantation versus conventional chemotherapy in multiple myeloma: a prospective, randomized trial. N Engl J Med 1996;335:91–7.
378. Blade J, San Miguel JF, Fontanillas M, et al. Survival of multiple myeloma patients who are potential candidates for early high-dose therapy intensification/autotransplantation and who were conventionally treated. J Clin Oncol 1996;14:2167–73.
379. Siegel DS, Desikan KR, Mehta J, et al. Age is not a prognostic variable with autotransplants for multiple myeloma. Blood 1999;93:51–4.
380. Badros A, Barlogie B, Siegel E, et al. Autologous stem cell transplantation in elderly multiple myeloma patients over the age of 70 years. Br J Haematol 2001;114:600–7.
381. Palumbo A, Triolo S, Argentino C, et al. Dose-intensive melphalan with stem cell support (MEL100) is superior to standard treatment in elderly myeloma patients. Blood 1999;94:1248–53.
382. Badros A, Barlogie B, Siegel E, et al. Results of autologous stem cell transplant in multiple myeloma patients with renal failure. Br J Haematol 2001;114:822–9.
383. Fermand J-P, Ravaud P, Chevret S, et al. High-dose therapy and autologous peripheral blood stem cell transplantation in multiple myeloma: up-front or rescue treatment? Results of a multicenter sequential randomized clinical trial. Blood 1998;92:3131–6.
384. Moreau P, Facon T, Attal M, et al. Comparison of 200 mg/m(2) melphalan and 8 Gy total body irradiation plus 140 mg/m(2) melphalan as conditioning regimens for peripheral blood stem cell transplantation in patients with newly diagnosed multiple myeloma: final analysis of the Intergroupe Francophone du Myelome 9502 randomized trial. Blood 2002;99:731–5.
385. Child JA, Morgan GJ, Davies FE, et al. High-dose chemotherapy with hematopoietic stem-cell rescue for multiple myeloma. N Engl J Med 2003;348:1875–83.
386. Lenhoff S, Hjorth M, Holmberg E, et al. Impact on survival of high-dose therapy with autologous stem cell support in patients younger than 60 years with newly diagnosed multiple myeloma: a population-based study. Blood 2000;95:7–11.
387. Barlogie B, Jagannath S, Vesole DH, et al. Superiority of tandem autologous transplantation over standard therapy for previously untreated multiple myeloma. Blood 1997;89:789–93.
388. Blade J, Perales M, Rosinol, L, et al. Thalidomide in multiple myeloma: lack of response of soft-tissue plasmacytomas.Br J Haematol. 2001 May;113(2):422–4.
389. Anderson KC, Barut BA, Ritz J, et al. Monoclonal antibody purged autologous bone marrow transplantation therapy for multiple myeloma. Blood 1991;77:712–20.
390. Anderson KC, Anderson J, Soiffer R, et al. Monoclonal antibody-purged bone marrow transplantation therapy for multiple myeloma. Blood 1993;82:2568–76.
391. Schiller G, Vescio R, Freytes C, et al. Transplantation of CD34 positive peripheral blood progenitor cells following high dose chemotherapy for patients with advanced multiple myeloma. Blood 1995;86:390–7.
392. Gazitt Y, Reading CC, Hoffman R, et al. Purified $CD34^+$ $Lin^- Thy^+$ stem cells do not contain clonal myeloma cells. Blood 1995;86:381–9.
393. Facon T, Harousseau J-L, Maloisel F, et al. Stem cell factor in combination with filgrastim after chemotherapy improves peripheral blood progenitor cell yield and reduces apheresis requirements in multiple myeloma patients: a randomized, controlled trial. Blood 1999;94:1218–25.
394. Szczepek AJ, Bergsagel PL, Axelsson L, et al. $CD34^+$ cells in the blood of patients with multiple myeloma express CD19 and IgH mRNA and have patient-specific igH VDJ gene rearrangements. Blood 1997;89:1824–33.
395. Schiller G, Vescio R, Lee M, et al. Long-term outcome of a phase II study of autologous CD34+ peripheral blood stem cell transplantation as treatment for multiple myeloma. In: Griffin JD, editor. American Society of Hematology Thirty-Eighth Annual Meeting. Orlando (FL): The American Society of Hematology; 1996. p. 483a.
396. Vescio RA, Schiller GJ, Stewart AK, et al. Quantitative assessment of myeloma peripheral blood and bone marrow tumor burden in patients undergoing autologous transplantation. In: Griffin JD, editor. American Society of Hematology Thirty-Eighth Annual Meeting. Orlando (FL): The American Society of Hematology; 1996. p. 641a.
397. Vescio R, Schiller G, Stewart K, et al. Multicenter phase III trial to evaluate CD34+ selected vs. unselected autologous peripheral blood progenitor cell transplantation in multiple myeloma. Blood 1999;93:1858–68.
398. Stewart AK, Vescio R, Schiller G, et al. Purging of autologous peripheral-blood stem cells using CD34 selection does not improve overall or progression-free survival after high-dose chemotherapy for multiple myeloma: results of a multicenter randomized controlled trial. J Clin Oncol 2001;19:3771–9.
399. Lemoli RM, Martinelli G, Zamagni E, et al. Engraftment, clinical, and molecular follow-up of patients with multiple myeloma who were reinfused with highly purified CD34+ cells to support single or tandem high-dose chemotherapy. Blood 2000;95:2234–8.
400. Barlogie B, Jagannath S, Desikan KR, et al. Total therapy with tandem transplants for newly diagnosed multiple myeloma. Blood 1999;93:55–65.
401. Vesole DH, Tricot G, Jagannath S, et al. Autotransplants in multiple myeloma: what have we learned? Blood 1996;88:838–47.
402. Attal M, Harousseau JL, Facon T, et al. Single versus double autologous stem-cell transplantation for multiple myeloma. N Engl J Med 2003;349:2495–502.
403. Fermand JP, Marolleau JP, Alberti C, et al. Single versus tandem high dose therapy supported with autologous stem cell transplantation using unselected of CD 34 enriched ABSC: preliminary results of a two by two designed randomized trial. Blood 2001;98:815a.
404. Giralt S, Weber D, Colome M, et al. Phase I trial of cyclosporine-induced autologous graft-versus-host disease in patients with multiple myeloma undergoing high-dose chemotherapy with autologous stem-cell rescue. J Clin Oncol 1997;15:667–73.
405. Qing Y, Osterborg A. Idiotype-specific T cells in multiple myeloma: targets for an immunotherapeutic intervention? Med Oncol 1996;13:1–7.
406. Bergenbrant B, Yiu Q, Osterborg A, et al. Modulation of antiidiotypic immune response by immunization with the autologous M component protein multiple myeloma patients. Br J Haematol 1996;92:840–6.
407. Hsu FJ, Benike C, Fagnoni F, et al. Vaccination of patients with B-cell lymphoma using autologous antigen-pulsed dendritic cells. Nat Med 1996;2:52–8.
408. Anderson KC. Targeted therapy for multiple myeloma. Semin Hematol 2001;38:286–94.
409. Chauhan D, Hideshima T, Rosen S, et al. Apaf-1/cytochrome c independent and Smac dependent induction of apoptosis in multiple myeloma cells. J Biol Chem 2001;276:24453–6.
410. Ogata A, Chauhan D, Teoh G, et al. Interleukin-6 triggers cell growth via the *ras*-dependent mitogen-activated protein kinase cascade. J Immunol 1997;159:2212–21.
411. Chauhan D, Anderson KC. Apoptosis in multiple myeloma: therapeutic implications. Apoptosis 2001;6:47–55.
412. Hayashi T, Hideshima T, Akiyama M, et al. Arsenic trioxide inhibits growth of human multiple myeloma cells in the bone marrow microenvironment. Mol Cancer Ther 2002;1:851–60.
413. Lentzsch S, LeBlanc R, Podar K, et al. Immunomodulatory analogs of thalidomide inhibit growth of HS Sultan cells and angiogenesis in vivo. Leukemia 2003;17:41–4.
414. Lentzsch S, Rogers MS, LeBlanc R, Birsner AE, et al. S-3-Amino-phthalimido-glutarimide inhibits angiogenesis and growth of B- cell neoplasias in mice. Cancer Res 2002;62:2300–5.
415. LeBlanc R, Catley LP, Hideshima T, et al. Proteasome inhibitor PS-341 inhibits human myeloma cell growth in vivo and prolongs survival in a murine model. Cancer Res 2002;62:4996–5000.
416. Richardson PG, Schlossman RL, Weller E, et al. Immunomodulatory drug CC-5013 overcomes drug resistance and is well tolerated in patients with relapsed multiple myeloma. Blood 2002;100:3063–7.
417. Davies FE, Raje N, Hideshima T, et al. Thalidomide and immunomodulatory derivatives augment natural killer cell cytotoxicity in multiple myeloma. Blood 2001;98:210–6.
418. Treon SP, Mitsiades C, Mitsiades N, et al. Tumor cell expression of CD59 is associated with resistance to CD20 serotherapy in patients with B-cell malignancies. J Immunother 2001;24:263–71.
419. Mitsiades N, Mitsiades CS, Richardson PG, et al. The proteasome inhibitor PS-341 potentiates sensitivity of multiple myeloma cells to conventional chemotherapeutic agents: therapeutic applications. Blood 2003;101:2377–80.
420. Raje N, Kumar S, Hideshima T, et al. Combination of the mTOR inhibitor Rapamycin and RevlimidTM(CC-5013) has synergistic activity in multiple myeloma. Blood 2004;104:4188–93.
421. Mitsiades CS, Mitsiades N, Poulaki V, et al. The HSP90 molecular chaperone as a novel therapeutic target in hematologic malignancies. Blood 2001;98:377a.
422. Mitsiades CS, Mitsiades NS, McMullan CJ, et al. Transcriptional signature of histone deacetylase inhibition in multiple myeloma: biological and clinical implications. Proc Natl Acad Sci U S A 2004;101:540–5.
423. Chauhan D, Li G, Hideshima T, et al. HSP27 inhibits release of mitochondrial protein Smac in multiple myeloma cells and confers Dexamethasone resistance. Blood 2003;102:3379–86.
424. Lokhorst HM, Schattenberg JJ, Cornelissen JJ, et al. Donor lymphocyte infusions are effective in relapsed multiple myeloma after allogeneic bone marrow transplantation. Blood 1997;90:4206–11.
425. Orsini E, Alyea EP, Chillemi A, et al. Conversion to full donor chimerism following donor lymphocyte infusion is associated with disease response in patients with multiple myeloma. Biol Blood Marrow Transplant 2000;6:375–86.
426. Teoh G, Chen L, Urashima M, et al. Adenovirus vector-based purging of multiple myeloma cells. Blood 1998;92:4591–601.
427. Trojan A, Schultze JL, Witzens M, et al. Immunoglobulin framework-derived peptides function as cytotoxic T-cell epitopes commonly expressed in B-cell malignancies. Nat Med 2000;6:667–72.
428. Vonderheide RH, Hahn WC, Schultze JL, Nadler LM. The telomerase catalytic subunit is a widely expressed tumor-associated antigen recognized by cytotoxic T lymphocytes. Immunity 1999;10:673–9.
429. Maecker B, Sherr DH, Shen C, et al. Targeting universal tumor antigens with cytotoxic T cells: potential of CYP1B1 for broadly applicable antigen-specific immunotherapy. Blood 1999;94(Suppl):438a.
430. Schultze JL, Anderson KC, Gilleece MH, et al. A pilot study of combined immunotherapy with autologous adoptive tumor-specific T-cell transfer, vaccination with CD40-activated malignant B cells and interleukin 2. Br J Haematol 2001;113:455–60.
431. Gong J, Koido S, Chen D, et al. Immunization against murine multiple myeloma with fusions of dendritic and plasmacytoma cells is potentiated by interleukin 12. Blood 2002;99:2512–7.
432. Raje N, Gong J, Chauhan D, et al. Bone marrow and peripheral blood dendritic cells from patients with multiple myeloma are phenotypically and functionally normal. Blood 1999;93:1487–95.
433. Raje N, Hideshima T, Davies FE, et al. Tumour cell/dendritic cell fusions as a vaccination strategy for multiple myeloma. Br J Haematol 2004;125:343–52.
434. Osterborg A, Yi Q, Henriksson L, et al. Idiotype immunization combined with granulocyte-macrophage colony-stimulating factor in myeloma patients induced type I, major histocompatibility complex-restricted, CD8 and CD4 specific T cell responses. Blood 1998;91:2459–66.
435. Massaia M, Borrione P, Battaglio S, et al. Idiotype vaccination in human myeloma: generation of tumor-specific immune responses after high -dose chemotherapy. Blood 1999;94:673–83.
436. Reichardt VL, Okada CY, Liso A, et al. Idiotype vaccination using dendritic cells after autologous peripheral blood stem cell transplantation for multiple myeloma-a feasibility study. Blood 1999;93:2411–9.
437. Stevenson FK, Zhu D, King CA, et al. Idiotypic DNA vaccines against B cell lymphoma. Immunol Rev 1995;145:211–28.
438. van Baren N, Brasseur F, Godelaine D, et al. Genes encoding tumor-specific antigens are expressed in human myeloma cells. Blood 1999;94:1156–64.
439. Prince HM, Dessureault S, Gallinger S, et al. Efficient adenoviral mediated transfer of LacZ and B7-1 genes into malignant human plasma cells: relative lymphoid cell resistance. Exp Hematol 1998;26:27–36.
440. Stevenson FK, Bell AJ, Cusack R, et al. Preliminary studies for an immunotherapeutic approach to the treatment of

human myeloma using chimeric anti-CD38 antibody. Blood 1991;77:1071–9.
441. Ogata A, Anderson KC. Therapeutic strategies for inhibition of interleukin-6 mediated multiple myeloma cell growth. Leukemia Res 1996;20:303–7.
442. Dinota A, Barbieri L, Gobbi M, et al. An immunotoxin containing momordin suitable for bone marrow purging in multiple myeloma patients. Br J Cancer 1989;60:315–9.
443. Siegall CB, Chaudhary VK, Fitzgerald DJ, Pastan I. Cytotoxic activity of an interleukin-6 pseudomonas exotoxin fusion protein on human myeloma cells. Proc Natl Acad Sci U S A 1988;85:9738–42.
444. Goldmacher VS, Bourret LA, Levine BA, et al. Anti-CD38-blocked ricin: an immunotoxin for the treatment of multiple myeloma. Blood 1994;84:3017–25.
445. Grossbard M, Fidias P, Kinsella J. Anti-B4 blocked ricin: a phase II trial for 7 day continuous infusion in patients with multiple myeloma. Brit J Hematol 1998;102:509–15.
446. Ozaki S, Kosaka M, Wakatsuki S, et al. Immunotherapy of multiple myeloma with a monoclonal antibody directed against a plasma cell-specific antigen, HM1.24. Blood 1997;90:3179–86.
447. Ozaki S, Kosaka M, Wakahara Y, et al. Humanized anti-HM1.24 antibody mediates myeloma cell cytotoxicity that is enhanced by cytokine stimulation of effector cells. Blood 1999;93:3922–30.
448. Moulopoulos LA, Dimopoulos MA, Weber D, et al. Magnetic resonance imaging in the staging of solitary plasmacytoma of bone. J Clin Oncol 1993;11:1311–5.
449. Frassica DA, Frassica FJ, Schray MF, et al. Solitary plasmacytoma of bone: Mayo Clinic Experience. Int J Radiat Oncol Biol Phys 1989;16:43–8.
450. Knowling MA, Harwood AR, Bergsagel DE. Comparison of extramedullary plasmacytomas with solitary and multiple plasma cell tumors of bone. J Clin Oncol 1983;1:255–62.
451. Wiltshaw E. The natural history of extramedullary plasmacytoma and its relation to solitary myeloma of bone and myelomatosis. Medicine 1976;55:217–38.
452. Aviles A, Huerta J, Zepeda G, Diaz-Maqueo JC. Serum beta 2 microglobulin in solitary plasmacytoma. Blood 1990;76:1663.
453. Dimopoulos MA, Goldstein J, Fuller L, et al. Curability of solitary bone plasmacytoma. J Clin Oncol 1992;10:587–90.
454. Kyle RA, Garton JP. The spectrum of IgM monoclonal gammopathy in 430 cases. Mayo Clin Proc 1987;62:719–31.
455. Dimopoulos MA, Alexanian R. Waldenström's Macroglobulinemia. Blood 1994;83:1452–9.
456. Kyle RA, Anderson KC. A tribute to Jan Waldenström. Blood 1997;89:4245–7.
457. Groves FD, Travis LB, Devesa SS, et al. Waldenström's macroglobulinemia: incidence patterns in the United States, 1988–1994. Cancer 1998;82:1078–81.
458. Herrinton LJ, Weiss NS. Incidence of Waldenström's macroglobulinemia. Blood 1993;82:3148–50.
459. Ogmundsdottir HM, Johannesson GM, Sveinsdottir S, et al. Familial macroglobulinaemia: hyperactive B-cells but normal natural killer function [published erratum appears in Scand J Immunol 1995 Jun;41(6):650]. Scand J Immunol 1994;40:195–200.
460. Calasanz MJ, Cigudosa JC, Odero MD, et al. Cytogenetic analysis of 280 patients with multiple myeloma and related disorders: primary breakpoints and clinical correlations. Genes Chromosomes Cancer 1997;18:84–93.
461. Palka G, Spadano A, Geraci L, et al. Chromosome changes in 19 patients with Waldenström's macroglobulinemia. Cancer Genet Cytogenet 1987;29:261–9.
462. Matutes E, Owusu-Ankomah K, Morilla R, et al. The immunological profile of B-cell disorders and proposal of a scoring system for the diagnosis of CLL. Leukemia 1994;8:1640–5.
463. Smith BR, Robert NJ, Ault KA. In Waldenström's macroglobulinemia the quantity of detectable circulating monoclonal B lymphocytes correlates with clinical course. Blood 1983;61:911–4.
464. Wagner SD, Martinelli V, Luzzatto L. Similar patterns of V kappa gene usage but different degrees of somatic mutation in hairy cell leukemia, prolymphocytic leukemia, Waldenström's macroglobulinemia, and myeloma. Blood 1994;83:3647–53.
465. Aoki H, Takishita M, Kosaka M, Saito S. Frequent somatic mutations in D and/or JH segments of Ig gene in Waldenström's macroglobulinemia and chronic lymphocytic leukemia (CLL) with Richter's syndrome but not in common CLL. Blood 1995;85:1913–9.
466. Klein U, Goossens T, Fischer M, et al. Somatic hypermutation in normal and transformed human B cells. Immunol Rev 1998;162:261–80.
467. Johansson B, Waldenström J, Hasselblom S, Mitelman F. Waldenström's macroglobulinemia with the AML/MDS-associated t(1;3)(p36;q21). Leukemia 1995;9:1136–8.
468. Gertz MA, Kyle RA, Noel P. Primary systemic amyloidosis: a rare complication of immunoglobulin M monoclonal gammopathies and Waldenström's Macroblobulinemia. J Clin Oncol 1993;11:914–20.
469. Facon T, Brouillard M, Duhamel A, et al. Prognostic factors in Waldenström's macroglobulinemia: a report of 167 cases. J Clin Oncol 1993;11:1553–8.
470. Gobbi PG, Bettini R, Montecucco C, et al. Study of prognosis in Waldenström's Macroglobulinemia: a proposal for a simple binary classification with clinical and investigational utility. Blood 1994;83:2939–45.
471. Martelli MF, Falini B, Firenze A, et al. Acute leukemia complicating Waldenström's macroglobulinemia. Haematologica 1981;66:303–10.
472. Dimopoulos MA, Kantarjian H, Estey E, et al. Treatment of Waldenström Macroglobulinemia with 2-chlorodeoxyadenosine. Ann of Intern Med 1993;118:195–8.
473. Foran J, Rohatiner AZS, Coiffier B, et al. Multicenter phase II study of fludarabine phosphate for patients with newly diagnosed lymphoplasmacytoid lymphoma, Waldenström's macroglobulinemia and mantle cell lymphoma. J Clin Oncol 1999;17:546–53.
474. Leblond V, Ben-Othman T, Deconinck E, et al. Activity of fludarabine in previously treated Waldenström's macroglobulinemia: a report of 71 cases. J Clin Oncol 1998;16:2060–4.
475. Dimopoulos MA, Panayiotidis P, Moulopoulos LA, et al. Waldenström's macroglobulinemia: clinical features, complications, and management. J Clin Oncol 2000;18:214–26.
476. Leblond V, Levy V, Maloisel F, et al. Multicenter, randomized comparative trial of fludarabine and the combination of cyclophosphamide-doxorubicin-prednisone in 92 patients with Waldenström macroglobulinemia in first relapse or with primary refractory disease. Blood 2001;98:2640–4.
477. Quesada JR, Alexanian R, Kurzrock R, et al. Recombinant interferon gamma in hairy cell leukemia, multiple myeloma, and Waldenström's macroglobulinemia. Am J Hematol 1988;29:1–4.
478. Rotoli B, De Renzo A, Frigeri F, et al. A phase II trial on alpha-interferon (alpha IFN) effect in patients with monoclonal IgM gammopathy. Leuk Lymphoma 1994;13:463–9.
479. Legouffe E, Rossi JF, Laporte JP, et al. Treatment of Waldenström's macroglobulinemia with very low doses of alpha interferon. Leuk Lymphoma 1995;19:337–42.
480. Desikan R, Dhodapkar M, Siegel D, et al. High-dose therapy with autologous haemopoietic stem cell support for Waldenström's macroglobulinaemia. Br J Haematol 1999;105:993–6.
481. Humphrey JS, Conley CL. Durable complete remission of macroglobulinemia after splenectomy: a report of two cases and review of the literature. Am J Hematol 1995;48:262–6.
482. Takemori N, Hirai K, Onodera R, et al. Durable remission after splenectomy for Waldenström's macroglobulinemia with massive splenomegaly in leukemic phase. Leuk Lymphoma 1997;26:387–93.
483. Byrd JC, White CA, Link B, et al. Rituximab therapy in previously treated Waldenström's macroglobulinemia: preliminary evidence of activity [abstract]. Blood 1998;(suppl 1):106a.
484. Dimopoulos MA, Zervas C, Zomas A, et al. Treatment of Waldenström's macroglobulinemia with rituximab. J Clin Oncol 2002;20:2327–33.
485. Franklin EC, Lowenstein J, Bigelow B, Meltzer M. Heavy chain disease—a new disorder of serum γ-globulins: report of the first case. Am J Med 1964;37:332–50.
486. Kyle RA. The heavy chain diseases. In: Wiernick PH, Canellos GP, Kyle RA, Schiffer CA, editors. Neoplastic diseases of the blood. New York: Churchill Livingston; 1985. p. 593.
487. Guardia J, Rubies-Prat J, Gallart MT, et al. The evolution of alpha heavy chain disease. Am J Med 1976;60:596–602.
488. Kyle RA, Greipp PR. Amyloidosis (AL)—clinical and laboratory features in 229 cases. Mayo Clin Proc 1983;58:665–83.
489. Kyle RA, Gertz MA, Greipp PR, et al. Long-term survival (10 years or more) in 30 patients with primary amyloidosis. Blood 1999;93:1062–6.
490. Kyle RA, Greipp PR, Garton JP, Gertz MA. Primary systemic amyloidosis. Comparison of melphalan/prednisone versus colchicine. Am J Med 1985;79:708–16.
491. Cohen AS, Rubinow A, Anderson JJ, et al. Survival of patients with primary (AL) amyloidosis. Colchicine-treated cases from 1976 to 1983 compared with cases seen in previous years (1961 to 1973). Am J Med 1987;82:1182–90.
492. Kyle RA, Gertz MA, Greipp PR, et al. A trial of three regimens for primary amyloidosis: colchicine alone, melphalan and prednisone, and melphalan, prednisone, and colchicine. N Engl J Med 1997;336:1200–7.
493. Gertz MA, Lacy MQ, Lust JA, et al. Prospective randomized trial of melphalan and prednisone versus vincristine, carmustine, melphalan, cyclophosphamide, and prednisone in the treatment of primary systemic amyloidosis. J Clin Oncol 1999;17:262–7.
494. Comenzo RL, Vosburgh E, Simms RW, et al. Dose-intensive melphalan with blood stem cell support for the treatment of AL amyloidosis: one-year follow-up in five patients. Blood 1996;88:2801–6.
495. Comenzo RL, Vosburgh E, Falk RH, et al. Dose-intensive melphalan with blood stem-cell support for the treatment of AL (amyloid light-chain) amyloidosis: survival and responses in 25 patients. Blood 1998;91:3662–70.
496. Comenzo RL, Gertz MA. Autologous stem cell transplantation for primary systemic amyloidosis. Blood 2002;99:4276–82.
497. Dispenzieri A, Lacy MQ, Kyle RA, et al. Eligibility for hematopoietic stem-cell transplantation for primary systemic amyloidosis is a favorable prognostic factor for survival. J Clin Oncol 2001;19:3350–6.

121

Chronic Myeloproliferative Disorders: Essential Thrombocythemia, Myelofibrosis with Myeloid Metaplasia, and Polycythemia Vera

David P. Steensma, MD
Ayalew Tefferi, MD

The chronic myeloid disorders are a diverse group of malignant bone marrow conditions that originate in a transformed multipotential hematopoietic progenitor cell or pluripotential stem cell.[1] These heterogeneous diseases share an initially indolent biologic behavior and a dangerous propensity to evolve into overt acute leukemia—a tendency that may be encouraged by the well-intentioned use of genotoxic therapeutic agents. Even in the absence of leukemic transformation, the consequences of the cellular excesses or deficiencies characteristic of the myeloid disorders are troublesome for patients and all too frequently fatal.

The major entities in this broad syndromic group include (1) the myelodysplastic syndromes (MDSs; discussed in Chapter XXX); (2) the molecularly defined myeloid disorders, the most prominent of which is chronic myeloid leukemia (CML; discussed in Chapter XXX)—several rarer and more recently described entities (eg, the platelet-derived growth factor receptor–rearranged eosinophilic disorders and *Kit*-mutated systemic mastocytosis) also have a known fundamental molecular etiology; (3) a poorly delineated cluster of atypical myeloid disorders without molecular definition—a group that includes the myeloproliferative or myelodysplastic overlap syndromes, the idiopathic hypereosinophilic syndromes, chronic eosinophilic leukemia, chronic neutrophilic leukemia, chronic basophilic leukemia, and a few defiantly unclassifiable cases; and (4) the classic Philadelphia chromosome–negative chronic myeloproliferative disorders (CMPDs; Figure 121-1), the topic of this chapter.

The last group includes three distinct clinicopathologic entities: essential thrombocythemia (ET), polycythemia vera (PV), and myelofibrosis with myeloid metaplasia (MMM).[2] The first clear descriptions of ET, PV, and MMM were relatively recent; credit for priority is customarily given to Epstein and Goedel (Vienna, 1934) for ET, Vaquez (Paris, 1892) for PV, and Heuck (Heidelberg, 1879) for MMM.[3–5] However, descriptions of plethoric patients extend back to the Hippocratic corpus, and it is quite likely that some of these cases represented PV and were one of the situations in which the Galenic practice of bloodletting was beneficial for patients.[6] Dameshek (Boston, 1951) observed that ET, PV, MMM, and CML share several overlapping clinical and pathologic features, and he classified them together under the diagnostic rubric "CMPD."[7] Clonality has been assumed to be a hallmark of CMPD since monoclonal hematopoiesis was first demonstrated in the late 1960s by Fialkow and colleagues via assays based on the X-chromosome linkage of glucose-6-phosphate dehydrogenase (G6PD).[8]

Since 1960, CML has been defined by the presence of the Philadelphia chromosome, t(9;22)(q34q11).[9] In the 1980s, the aberrant *bcr-abl* translocation—the molecular equivalent of the Philadelphia chromosome—was found to be diag-

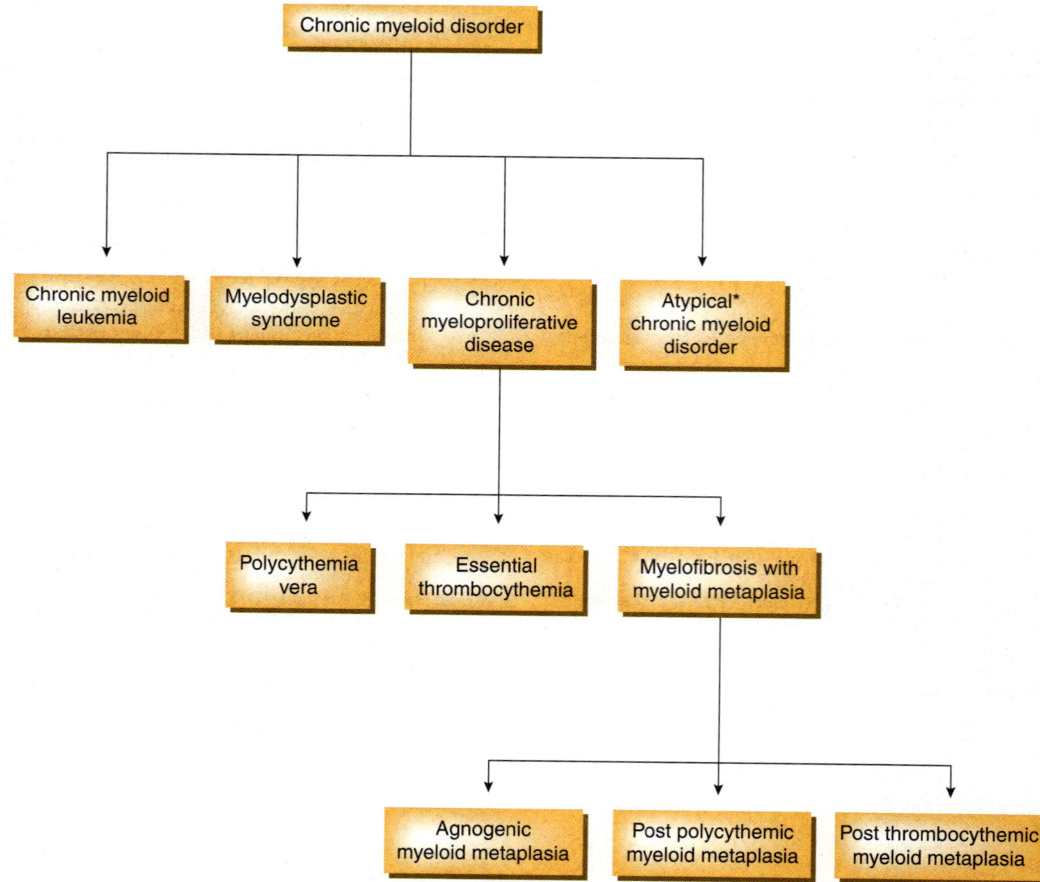

Figure 121-1 A working classification of chronic myeloid disorders. The list of molecularly defined chronic myeloid disorders is expected to grow and will likely make classification challenging, controversial, and subject to continuous revision, especially if most myeloid disorders turn out to be the product of multiple molecular lesions. Chronic myeloid leukemia (CML) is characterized by the presence of the Philadelphia chromosome or its molecular equivalent, the *bcr-abl* translocation; numerous studies have demonstrated that this single mutation is both necessary and sufficient to cause classic CML. The myelodysplastic syndromes are characterized by cytologic dysplasia, which almost always involves the erythroid series and often affects all three myeloid cell lineages. Myelofibrosis with myeloid metaplasia can occur de novo (in which case, it is sometimes referred to as agnogenic myeloid metaplasia) or may be preceded by a polycythemic phase or a thrombocythemic phase. Atypical chronic myeloid disorders include chronic neutrophilic leukemia, chronic basophilic leukemia, hypereosinophilic syndromes and eosinophilic leukemia, mast cell proliferative disorders, and the chronic myeloid processes that display overlapping features of both a myelodysplastic syndrome and a chronic myeloproliferative disorder.

nostic of CML and sufficient to cause the disease in a mouse model.[10] Today, CML is the most well-defined and clearly characterized of Dameshek's original CMPD group. Because of its distinct pathogenesis and treatment, CML is usually considered separately from the other traditional CMPD, which are diseases for which a unifying pathogenetic lesion has yet to be discovered. Because the Philadelphia chromosome–negative CMPDs lack diagnostic markers that are as clear and convincing as that which exists for CML, at present, the non-CML CMPDs remain diagnoses of exclusion. Each of the three classic CMPDs can be diagnosed only after eliminating the presence of a series of look-alike disorders, and even then some uncertainty may remain, especially for cases with atypical features.

The CMPDs lurk under many synonyms in the medical literature. Among other names, ET is also known as essential thrombocytosis, idiopathic thrombocytosis or thrombocythemia, primary thrombocytosis or thrombocythemia, Mortenson syndrome, and Epstein-Goedel syndrome. MMM has been called agnogenic myeloid metaplasia, osteomyelofibrosis, osteomyelosclerosis, idiopathic myelofibrosis, and primary myelofibrosis. PV has been indexed under polycythemia rubra vera (PRV), primary erythrocytosis, Osler-Vaquez disease, myelopathic polycythemia, cryptogenic polycythemia, and true polycythemia. A thorough library archive excavation will uncover even more synonyms, most with extremely limited usage. The terms used in this chapter (ET, MMM, PV) are chosen because they are simple and widely recognized.

ESSENTIAL THROMBOCYTHEMIA

Epidemiology ET is an uncommon disorder; estimates of its age- and gender-adjusted incidence range widely, from 0.2 to 2.5 cases per 100,000 persons per year.[11–13] Among younger people (ages 30–50 years), the disease appears to be more common in women, but this gender imbalance is not as clearly found in other age groups. Case ascertainment bias owing to the symptom of recurrent fetal loss unique to young women may confound such analyses. No clear environmental risk factor has been identified. The incidence of ET (and also of PV and MMM) appears to be increased among Ashkenazi Jews.[14] The median age at diagnosis for all three CMPDs is approximately 60 years. Familial clustering of ET has been described but is exquisitely rare; some familial cases are associated with mutations in the thrombopoietin (*TPO*) gene that result in increased TPO production (a megakaryocyte growth factor) with consequent megakaryocyte hyperstimulation.[15,16] Mutations in TPO and its receptor, c-Mpl, have been sought but not found in the more common nonfamilial cases of ET.[17]

Diagnosis The chief clinical challenge with respect to ET diagnosis is differentiating genuine autonomous thrombocytosis from the myriad causes of "secondary" or "reactive" thrombocytosis (RT). Platelets, like fibrinogen, are an acute-phase reactant; this nonspecific procoagulant response may have evolutionary significance by promoting organism survival in the setting of serious physiologic stress, including wounding. As a consequence, in more than 80% of unselected cases of thrombocytosis, the elevated platelet count is polyclonal and represents a reaction to the presence of a nonmyeloid disorder.[18,19] The thrombocytosis associated with inflammatory, infectious, and malignant conditions is thought to be due to the action of megakaryocyte stimulatory cytokines such as interleukin (IL)-6, whereas the peculiar thrombocytosis seen occasionally in iron-deficient states remains poorly understood and may be mediated by erythropoietin (EPO) cross-stimulation of precursor cells committed to platelet production.[20]

Often the presence of RT is obvious, but, in some instances, the distinction between ET and RT may be difficult because several of the many potential causes of RT can be occult. The degree of thrombocytosis is unfortunately of little diagnostic help. Reactive thrombocytosis can result in platelet counts above 2,000,000/μL.[19] Platelet morphology and platelet functional differences are also not reliable for separating ET from RT, and serum TPO levels are also of little use in distinguishing ET from RT or other non-ET causes of primary thrombocytosis.[21]

The distinction between ET and RT is clinically important because there is an increased risk of thrombosis and bleeding associated with ET, but the risk with RT appears to be much lower.[18] If the presence of RT is not obvious, serum ferritin and C-reactive protein (CRP; a surrogate marker for IL-6 levels) may be diagnostically useful in excluding iron deficiency and inflammation, respectively.[20] Elevated CRP levels suggest RT and should prompt a more thorough search for an obscure source of reactive cytokines. Of course, an elevated CRP does not strictly rule out ET because a patient may potentially have ET and a comorbid inflammatory condition, but this is uncommon.[20] Ferritin levels must also be interpreted with caution: although a low value is consistent with iron deficiency and a high value suggests RT, neither definitively excludes ET.

Surgical hyposplenism is usually obvious from a patient's history, but functional hyposplenism owing to amyloidosis, celiac sprue, or another cause may not be so blatant.[22] Therefore, examination of a blood smear, searching specifically for Howell-Jolly bodies, should be made during the initial evaluation of each patient with chronic thrombocytosis.

Once these steps have been taken and there is no evidence of RT or hyposplenism, ET increases in likelihood. However, another diagnostic hurdle remains: it is important to distinguish ET from other myeloid disorders that may have a very different prognosis and require different therapy. Clonal ET look-alike disorders include some cases of MDS, CML, and the other two non-ET classic CMPDs, PV and MMM, including the potentially confusing "cellular phase" of MMM.

Most cases of MDS have fairly striking erythroid dysplasia and/or morphologic changes in the granulocytic lineage; these features are not consistent with ET. If dysplasia is limited to cells of the megakaryocyte lineage, however, the distinction between MDS and ET may be more difficult because atypical megakaryocytes are often associated with ET. The most difficult distinction between MDS and ET can arise in the setting of the so-called 5q syndrome, which is often associated with thrombocytosis, minimal evidence of dysplasia in the erythroid and granulocytic lineages, a clinically indolent course, and an increased number of small, hypolobated megakaryocytes.[23] In such cases, cytogenetics should be definitive.

Some individuals consider Philadelphia chromosome–positive ET to be a unique diagnostic entity, but most clinicians are not convinced and would consider anyone with a chronic myeloid disorder and *bcr-abl* positivity to have CML, especially because such patients may respond to CML-specific therapy (ie, imatinib).[24,25] If conventional cytogenetic analysis in a suspected ET patient does not reveal a Philadelphia chromosome, it is prudent to obtain peripheral blood or bone marrow fluorescent in situ hybridization (FISH) or RT-PCR (reverse transcriptase polymerase chain reaction) studies at least once to exclude the possibility of karyotypically occult CML.

The distinction between ET and PV may be subtle. Neither an outright elevation of hematocrit nor a substantial increase in hematocrit from a measured baseline value is associated with ET. Unfortunately, other findings that have been reported to be characteristic of PV, including endogenous (ie, spontaneous, autonomous, erythropoietin independent) erythroid colony growth, an inappropriately low serum EPO level, and aberrant expression of the *PRV1* gene on neutrophils, are not specific enough to rule out ET.[26,27] In the past, red cell mass (RCM) measurement was commonly used to distinguish PV from ET in equivocal cases, but it is now widely recognized that hematocrit correlates quite closely with true RCM, so RCM analysis is being ordered less often.[28–30] For some cases that are initially confusing, the distinction between PV or ET may become clearer over time.

Distinguishing ET from MMM is usually not difficult, but there can be exceptions. The heavy marrow fibrosis characteristic of MMM is an atypical finding in ET, although mild (grade 1 or 2) reticulin fibrosis can be found in approximately 15% of ET cases.[31] Massive splenomegaly and a leukoerythroblastic peripheral blood picture are also much more typical of MMM than ET. However, the cellular phase of MMM, characterized by marrow hypercellularity with florid atypical megakaryocytic hyperplasia but not heavy fibrosis, can mimic ET in presentation.[32] Abnormal megakaryocyte clusters on the bone marrow biopsy (Figure 121-2)—megakaryocytes are solitary creatures and do not normally cluster—are typical of ET. Additionally, the overall cellularity is generally not as dense in ET as in cellular phase MMM. However, such distinctions can be diffi-

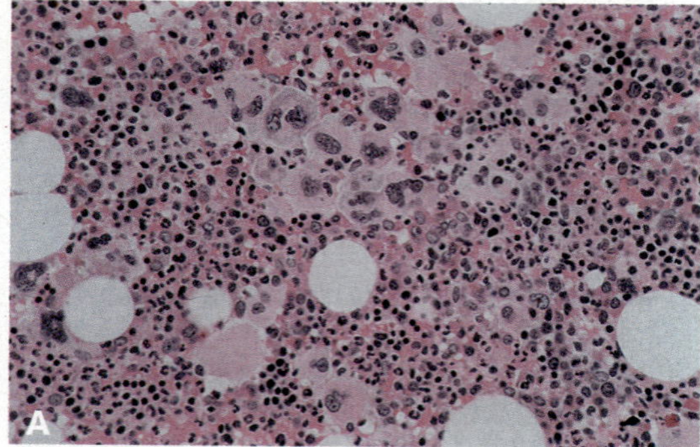

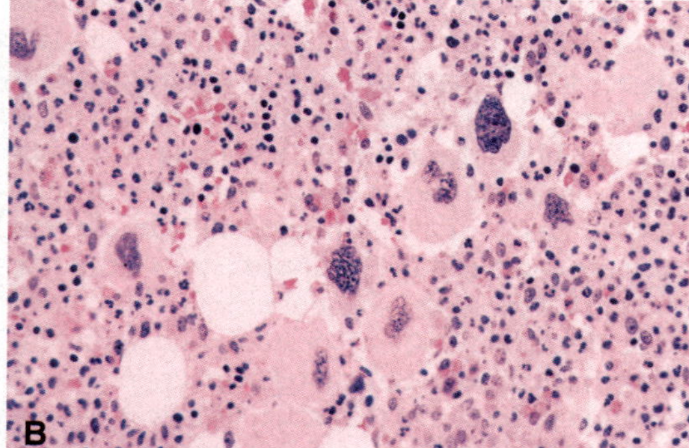

Figure 121-2 **A** and **B,** Bone marrow megakaryocytic clusters in essential thrombocythemia. Reproduced with permission from Tefferi A.[35]

cult, and the opinion of an experienced hematopathologist should be sought. Clonal karyotypic abnormalities are more typical of MMM and other myeloid disorders than they are of ET. Cytogenetic abnormalities are present in fewer than 10% of patients at diagnosis.[25] As with PV and ET, sometimes a distinction between MMM and ET is not possible initially, and an expectant, observant approach is appropriate.[32]

Pathogenesis. As mentioned above, clonal myeloproliferation involving the megakaryocytic lineage and sometimes other myeloid lineages (even in cases in which the white count and hematocrit are normal) is demonstrable in the majority of female patients with ET via X chromosome–linked DNA or gene product analysis.[33,34] Surprisingly, a portion of ET patients has been shown to have polyclonal hematopoiesis, and these patients appear to have less thrombosis risk than those with "monoclonal" ET.[36,37] It is important to keep in mind that clonality is not equal to malignancy. For example, apparently monoclonal X chromosome inactivation patterns can be demonstrated in the hematopoietic cells of some healthy elderly controls.[38] The prevalence of this finding depends in part on what degree of skewed X inactivation (eg, 75% of identical X-chromosomes inactivated vs 90%) is accepted as consistent with monoclonality.

In ET, megakaryocyte proliferation and platelet production are apparently autonomous, and normal regulatory pathways are apparently defective. The mechanism remains obscure in most cases. Megakaryocytes from ET patients are not inhibited by antibodies against key growth and differentiation cytokines, including IL-3, IL-6, granulocyte-monocyte colony-stimulating factor (GM-CSF), and TPO.[39,40] TPO and its receptor, c-Mpl, comprise the major feedback loop controlling megakaryocyte growth and development, but TPO and c-Mpl dynamics in ET and related disorders appear to be complex. TPO levels are often normal or elevated in ET despite the increased megakaryocyte mass but are not reproducibly different among normal marrow and ET or RT cases, whereas c-Mpl expression is often (but not always) markedly down-regulated in ET (Figure 121-3). However, c-Mpl expression is also down-regulated in other CMPDs, so its diagnostic utility for ET is limited.[41,42] The specific cytokines driving megakaryocyte proliferation in ET have not been worked out in detail, but megakaryocyte progenitors from ET patients may display unexplained hypersensitivity to both IL-3 and TPO.[43,44]

Clinical Manifestations ET is often an incidental finding, a consequence of the fact that hemograms are ordered for a great many clinical indications. At least half of patients with ET are asymptomatic at presentation; with appropriate therapy, many can remain asymptomatic throughout the course of their illness and enjoy a normal life expectancy.[45,46] At presentation, microvascular and vasomotor symptoms are found in 25 to 50% of ET patients. Major thrombosis is seen in 11 to 25% of patients at diagnosis and 10 to 22% during follow-up, whereas major hemorrhage is observed in 2 to 5% at diagnosis and 1 to 7% during follow-up.[13,46–48] Bleeding complications can be exacerbated by the use of acetylsalicylic acid (ASA) and nonsteroidal anti-inflammatory drugs (NSAIDs), which have platelet inhibitory effects. In contrast to other CMPDs, in which splenomegaly is very common, less than 25% of ET patients have palpable splenomegaly at the time of initial presentation.[45]

Vasomotor disturbances (eg, headaches, lightheadedness, visual symptoms such as blurring and scotomata, palpitations, chest pain, erythromelalgia, and distal paresthesias) are troublesome but not generally life threatening. The proximate cause of such symptoms remains poorly defined; speculation has focused on abnormal platelet-endothelium interactions in the microvasculature, which can be associated with inflammation and transient thrombotic occlusion.[49] Various platelet products, such as thromboxane A_2, are vasoactive, and some of these probably also play a role in the pathobiology. Erythromelalgia is the most dramatic vasomotor symptom, characterized by erythema, warmth, and pain in distal extremities; this symptom is rare but not entirely specific for ET (Figure 121-4).[50] The presence of vasomotor microvessel disturbances does not clearly predict hemorrhage or thrombosis in large vessels.

There are several potentially life-threatening complications of ET: large-vessel thrombosis (both arterial and venous), hemorrhage, and transformation of the disease into either a fibrotic phase resembling MMM or acute myeloid leukemia (AML).

Arterial thrombosis can lead to cerebrovascular events, cardiovascular ischemia, organ infarction, and digital gangrene. Venous thrombosis in ET occurs both in sites common to other thrombotic diatheses (eg, pulmonary embolism and lower extremity deep venous thrombosis) and in more unusual sites (eg, cerebral sinus thrombosis, retinal vein thrombosis, and hepatic and portal vein thrombosis).[46]

Mucocutaneous bleeding (epistaxis, gingival bleeding, ecchymoses, and petechiae) can be a major nuisance. This is the most common hemorrhagic problem in ET.[51] Because epistaxis and easy bruising are very common in the general public, it can be difficult to assess the contribution

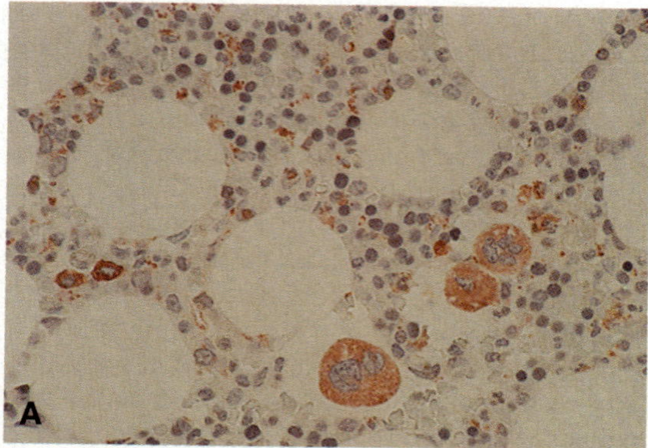

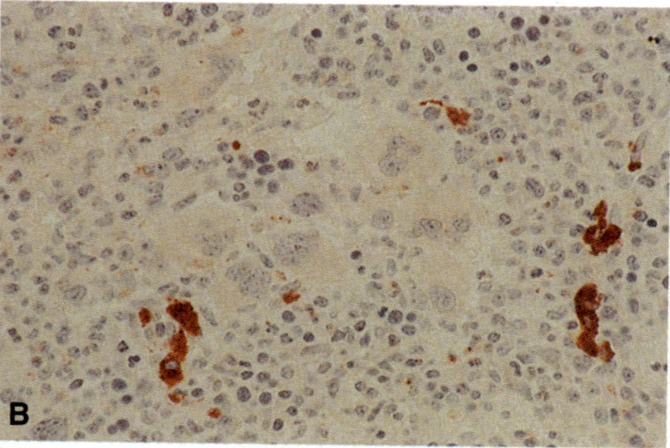

Figure 121-3 **A,** Normal megakaryocyte c-Mpl immunohistochemical staining (*left*) and, **B,** decreased megakaryocyte c-Mpl staining in a myeloproliferative disorder (*right*). Reproduced with permission from Tefferi A.[35]

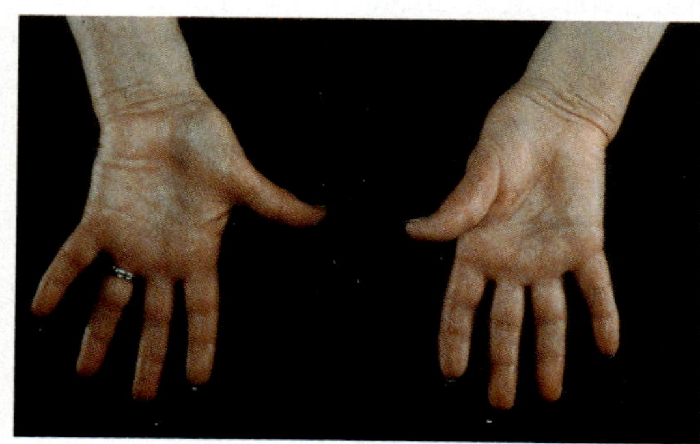

Figure 121-4 Erythromelalgia: dramatic acral erythema associated with pain and warmth and easily relieved by aspirin. Reproduced with permission from Tefferi A.[35]

Table 121-1 Clinical Properties of Platelet-Lowering Agents Used in Chronic Myeloproliferative Disorders

	Drug (Class)				
	Hydroxyurea (Myelosuppressive)	Anagrelide (Platelet Specific)	Interferon-α2a (Myelosuppressive)	Phosphorus 32 (Myelosuppressive)	Pipobroman (Myelosuppressive)
Mechanism of action	Antimetabolite	Unknown	Biologic agent with immunomodulatory actions	Radionucleide	Alkylating agent
Pharmacology	Half-life 5 h, renal excretion	Half-life ≈ 1.5 h, renal excretion	Kidney is main site of metabolism	Half life ≈ 14 d	Insufficient information
Suggested starting dose	500 mg PO bid	0.5 mg PO tid	3 million units SC 3 times per week (peginterferon can be given weekly)	2.3 mCi/m² IV	1 mg/kg/d PO (comes in 25 mg tablets) ≈ 16 d
Onset of action	≈ 3–5 d	≈ 6–10 d	1–3 wk	4–8 wk	
Frequent side effects	Leukopenia, oral ulcers, anemia, hyperpigmentation, nail discoloration, xerodermia	Headache, palpitations, diarrhea, fluid retention, anemia	Flu-like syndrome, fatigue, malaise, anorexia, weight loss, alopecia	Transient mild cytopenia	Nausea, abdominal pain, diarrhea
Infrequent side effects	Leg ulcers, nausea, diarrhea, alopecia, skin atrophy	Arrhythmias, lightheadedness, nausea	Confusion, depression, autoimmune thyroiditis, myalgia, arthritis	Prolonged pancytopenia in elderly patients	Leukopenia, thrombocytopenia, hemolysis
Rare side effects	Fever, cystitis platelet oscillations	Cardiomyopathy	Pruritus, hyperlipidemia, transaminasemia	Leukemogenic	
Absolute contraindications	Pregnancy	Pregnancy		Pregnancy	Pregnancy
Relative contraindications		Cardiomyopathy		Young age	
Cost*	Annual ≈ $1,752 for 500 mg tid dose	Annual ≈ $10,512 for 0.5 mg qid dose	Annual ≈ $7,488 for 3 million units 3 d/wk	Approximately $1,025 for 4 mCi	Not available in USA

bid = twice daily; IV = intravenously; PO = orally; qid = 4 times daily; SC = subcutaneously; tid = 3 times daily.

*Approximate cost to patient for brand name drug purchased from a typical hospital pharmacy (except for phosphorus 32). Prices checked September 2004.

of ET to these symptoms in afflicted patients. If careful control of the platelet count controls the mucocutaneous symptoms, it is reasonable to assume that thrombocytosis was contributory. Serious hemorrhage in ET is most common in the gastrointestinal tract and may be precipitated by ASA or NSAID use.[52] Hemorrhage also occurs in the central nervous system and the retina, but such events are, fortunately, uncommon. Paradoxically, patients with extreme thrombocytosis may be at special risk of bleeding, in part related to the development of an acquired von Willebrand's factor (vWF) deficiency that is thought to be related to platelet adsorption of large multimers of vWF. This phenomenon can be seen with extreme thrombocytosis of any cause.[53]

Fibrotic and leukemic evolution of ET are rare events (< 5% of patients) during the first 10 years after diagnosis.[45,46] High-quality long-term studies evaluating the incidence of these problems in the second and third decades of disease are not yet available.

Prognosis and Therapy When considering therapy for ET, it is important to keep in mind two facts: (1) ET is generally an indolent disorder, with a life expectancy (at least in the first decade of the disease) quite close to that of an age- and gender-matched control population, and (2) no treatment to date has been shown to influence overall survival.[45,54] Therefore, the maxim *primum non nocere* ("first, do no harm") should not be forgotten. Therapy for ET is usually initiated to palliate microvascular symptoms or to prevent thrombotic or hemorrhagic complications.

Vasomotor disturbances in ET can often be relieved with low-dose ASA; 81 mg per day is usually enough. When ASA does not alleviate these symptoms, it is reasonable to add a platelet-lowering agent (Table 121-1), and this is often successful.

There are only a few randomized trials assessing the most appropriate therapy for diminishing the thrombotic risk in patients with ET, so clinical decisions must usually be based on prospective cohort studies and large retrospective analyses. Therapy should be guided by an individualized assessment of thrombotic risk. Two clinical parameters appear to be quite important in making this judgment: a history of thrombosis and age above 60 years.[48,55] Based on the presence or absence of these two risk factors, patients with ET have been grouped into low-risk, high-risk, and indeterminate-risk groups and therapeutic decisions are made accordingly (Tables 121-2 and 121-3).[56] This classification will need to be refined as more data on thrombotic risk become available, but it is useful to guide management at present. It is likely that other factors also significantly affect the intensity of the clotting diathesis in ET patients, such as cigarette smoking, male gender, and the coexistence of plasma hypercoagulability owing to abnormalities such as the factor V Leiden mutation, but these have not yet been subject to multivariate analysis and remain controversial.[57–59] More recently, monoclonal hematopoiesis in ET has also been associated with a higher thrombotic risk than polyclonal hematopoiesis.[36]

Table 121-2 Risk Stratification in Polycythemia Vera and Essential Thrombocythemia

Risk	
Low risk	Age below 60 yr, and No history of thrombosis, and Platelet count below 1.5 million/μL
Indeterminate risk	Age below 60 yr, and No history of thrombosis, and Platelet count above 1.5 million/μL
High risk	Age 60 yr or older or A positive history of thrombosis

The use of ASA (81–325 mg/d) to decrease thrombotic risk in all classes of patients with ET seems reasonable in view of the recently demonstrated antithrombotic benefit in PV,[60] especially if there are other compelling indications for its use (eg, coexisting cardiovascular disease).[61] Data are lacking on the prophylactic utility of other anticoagulants, such as Coumadin and heparin, in high-risk groups. The more common approach for high-risk ET patients is to try to lower the platelet count into the normal range. One important randomized trial demonstrated a 20% absolute risk reduction (24% to 3.6%) in thrombotic events with the use of hydroxyurea (HU) in ET patients in a high-risk group.[62] Other cytoreductive agents have not yet been shown in a randomized fashion to reduce thrombotic events. It is not clear precisely how low the goal platelet count should be in the high-risk group—thrombotic events can happen even with a platelet count in the normal range—but < 400,000/μL seems to be a reasonable target and is supported by retrospective data.[63,64] For low-risk and indeterminate-risk patients, it is not clear that platelet-lowering agents are of any benefit because thrombotic events are much less common in this group.

Table 121-1 summarizes information regarding currently used platelet-lowering agents in CMPD. HU should be the first choice in ET because of the high-quality evidence supporting its use. There has been concern about the leukemogenicity of HU, but in two recent studies of HU-treated patients with ET, no cases of leukemia were reported after 5 to 14 and 2 to 12 years of therapy.[65,66] It is reasonable to substitute anagrelide or pipobroman (where available) for patients intolerant to HU.[67,68] Interferon-α2a (IFN-α) and, more recently, longer-acting pegylated forms of interferon (peginterferon) provide therapeutic alternatives, but interferon's well-known toxicity limits use, especially since many

Table 121-3 Proposed Risk-Adjusted Therapy in Essential Thrombocythemia

Risk Category*	Cytoreductive Therapy	Aspirin Therapy	Childbearing Potential†
Low	No	Yes	ASA
High	Yes	Yes	Interferon-α + ASA
Indeterminate	Sometimes	Yes (unless aVWD)	ASA (unless acquired VWD)

ASA = acetylsalicylic acid (low-dose aspirin); aVWD = acquired von Willebrand's disease.
*See Table 121-2 for algorithm regarding risk category assignment.
†Suggestions for drug therapy in women of childbearing potential are based on anecdotal evidence of safety.

high-risk ET patients are elderly and have a difficult time tolerating the necessary doses.[69–71] IFN-α is the drug of choice for ET patients requiring cytoreduction during pregnancy (see below). Radiophosphorus (^{32}P) and alkylating agents such as chlorambucil may still be useful "backup" regimens for nonpregnant patients but are clearly leukemogenic in PV, so caution is indicated.

Major bleeding (ie, enough blood loss to drop the hemoglobin level or cause bleeding in a critical organ, such as the central nervous system) occurs in less than 10% of ET patients.[45,46] Extreme thrombocytosis (eg, platelet count > 1 million/μL) appears to be a risk factor for bleeding, in part because of the acquired vWF deficiency described above. Therapy designed to lower the platelet count and indirectly raise vWF levels may be indicated in the presence of a substantial reduction in large vWF multimers. In an emergency situation, platelet apheresis is the fastest way to lower the platelet count, but its utility has not been proven conclusively.

Special Considerations **Pregnancy** ET is associated with first trimester spontaneous abortions in at least one-third of patients who become pregnant, and recurrent fetal loss occasionally is the presenting symptom of ET.[72] There does not appear to be a postpartum thrombosis risk.[73] There is no clear association between the increased risk of spontaneous abortion and either the degree of thrombocytosis or the concurrent use of aspirin, nor is there any clear benefit from prophylactic platelet apheresis.[72] High-risk pregnant women with ET (ie, women with previous thrombosis—pregnancy in women over 60 years is, at least at present, quite rare) require cytoreductive therapy just as other high-risk patients do. There is anecdotal evidence of the safety of IFN-α in pregnancy, but no controlled data. HU and pipobroman are considered teratogenic (US Food and Drug Administration [FDA] pregnancy class D), and anagrelide also crosses the placenta and has unknown effects on the developing fetus (FDA pregnancy class C). The teratogenicity of HU, however, does not appear to be severe enough to justify elective abortion in cases of inadvertent early fetal exposure.[74]

MYELOFIBROSIS WITH MYELOID METAPLASIA

Epidemiology Among the three classic CMPDs, ET is the most benign and indolent disorder, whereas MMM is the most aggressive. Fortunately, MMM is a rare scourge; the incidence is only 0.4 to 1.5 cases per 100,000 persons per year, with a median age at diagnosis above 60 years and a slight male predominance.[11,12] MMM has been associated with exposure to ionizing radiation (eg, atomic bomb survivors in Hiroshima), heavy exposure to petroleum derivatives, and thorium dioxide (Thorotrast) contrast medium, but in the vast majority of cases, there is no such exposure history.[75,76]

Pathogenesis As with other CMPDs, myeloid-derived cells in MMM have been shown to be monoclonal by analysis of X-linked genes and gene products.[77] In contrast, the marrow fibroblasts in MMM are polyclonal.[77,78] The florid bone marrow stromal reaction that is so characteristic of MMM includes fibroblast hyperproliferation, a dramatic increase in extracellular matrix proteins such as collagen (mostly type I and type III), increased blood vessel formation (angiogenesis), and increased bone synthesis and osteoblast activity (osteosclerosis).[79,80] Such marrow microenvironmental changes are mediated by a cytokine storm elaborated by the clonal myeloid cells. Indeed, increased cellular and extracellular levels of multiple cytokines with fibrogenic, angiogenic, and/or osteogenic potential have been detected in MMM, lending support to this hypothesis.[81]

There are several murine models in which marrow fibrosis and/or extramedullary hematopoiesis have been observed. Mice forced to overexpress TPO develop marrow fibrosis and osteosclerosis, which may be due to hypersecretion of osteoprotegerin, an osteoclast-inhibiting factor.[82,83] Mice that underexpress the transcription factor GATA-1, which is important in the development and differentiation of hematopoietic cells, suffer impaired megakaryocyte differentiation and diminished platelet production and eventually develop extramedullary hematopoiesis and marrow fibrosis.[84] However, it is not clear to what extent these germline mouse mutants are faithful models of the neoplastic disorder in humans, in whom any mutations would be expected to be restricted to hematopoietic cells. Mutations or expression changes in TPO or its receptor (c-Mpl) or GATA-1 have not been found in human MMM, and mutations in FOG-1 (Friend of GATA-1), the major GATA-1 cofactor, are also generally absent.[85]

The molecular lesions underlying MMM have not been worked out. Recurrent karyotypic abnormalities seen in the disease include del(13q), del(20q), trisomy 8, trisomy 9, del(12p), and abnormalities of chromosomes 1 and 7, all of which are found in other chronic myeloid disorders and have no specificity for MMM.[86] About half of patients with MMM have a cytogenetic abnormality at diagnosis, but there is no predominant lesion and no individual cytogenetic abnormality affects more than 15 to 20% of patients. The relevant genes corresponding to the common karyotypic lesions are uncertain. Occasional mutations of the *ras* gene family or the *TP53* gene have been observed and are associated with progression to leukemia.[87] A global genomic approach will likely be necessary to sort out the aberrant transcriptional signals that lead to the MMM phenotype. Given the clinical heterogeneity of MMM cases, great complexity can be expected. Only initial results from a small MMM transcript microarray study have been reported to date.[88]

Diagnosis Like ET, MMM is a diagnosis of exclusion. Several consensus diagnostic criteria have been proposed; there is no agreement about their validity. Characteristic features of MMM include a hypercellular marrow with heavy fibrosis; extramedullary hematopoiesis, which is most often manifest as splenomegaly; anemia; and a so-called myelophthisic peripheral blood picture (*myelophthisis* is Greek for "marrow wasting"; the typical blood findings are described below).[81] Marrow fibrosis and a myelophthisic blood picture alone are not diagnostic of MMM because myelofibrosis is associated with a diverse litany of conditions, including metastatic cancer, other hematologic disorders, and rheumatologic and granulomatous diseases (Table 121-4).

Table 121-4 Causes of Bone Marrow Fibrosis

Myeloid Disorders	Nonhematologic Disorders	Other Hematologic Disorders
Myelofibrosis with myeloid metaplasia	Metastatic cancer	Hairy cell leukemia
Chronic myeloid leukemia	Connective tissue disorders (eg, lupus and systemic sclerosis)	Multiple myeloma
Essential thrombocythemia	Infections (eg, granulomatous disease, tuberculosis, kala-azar)	Lymphoproliferative disorders
Atypical chronic myeloid disorders	Vitamin D deficiency (rickets)	Gray platelet syndrome
Hypereosinophilic syndromes	Renal osteodystrophy	
Polycythemia vera	Paget's disease	
Myelodysplastic syndrome with fibrosis	Hyperparathyroidism	
Malignant histiocytosis		
Systemic mastocytosis		
Acute myelofibrosis		
Acute megakaryoblastic leukemia (AML-M7)		
Other acute myeloid leukemias		

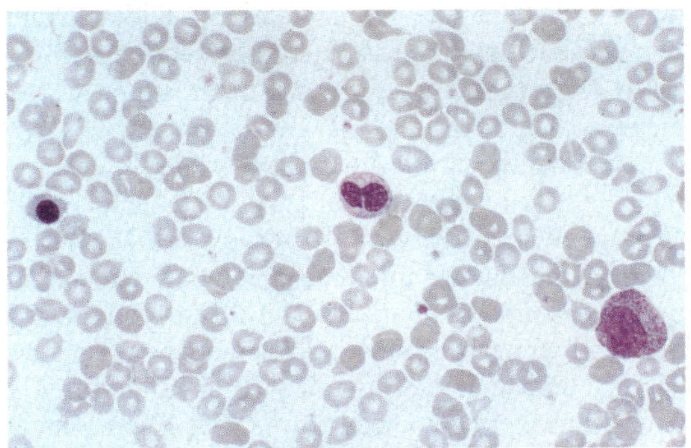

Figure 121-5 Typical peripheral blood findings in myelofibrosis with myeloid metaplasia: erythrocyte poikilocytosis, dacryocytes, a nucleated red blood cell, and an immature myeloid precursor cell (myelocyte).

The presence of marrow fibrosis markedly alters normal control of egress of blood cells from the marrow and also results in morphologic abnormalities. The consequent myelophthisic peripheral blood findings include marked anisocytosis, poikilocytosis, teardrop-shaped red cells (dacryocytes), and left-shifted granulocytopoiesis (Figure 121-5). Basophilia is also common but is not specific for MMM and can be observed in other CMPDs, especially CML. The mechanism is unclear. Even extramedullary hematopoiesis is not completely specific for MMM because it can be observed in other conditions in which the bone marrow is replaced (eg, metastatic cancer) or marrow hematopoiesis is inadequate (eg, β-thalassemia).[89,90]

Because of hypercellularity and fibrosis, the bone marrow in MMM is often difficult to aspirate, resulting in a dry tap. However, an aspirate can sometimes still be obtained. The consequent clear glimpse at cellular morphology may help rule out MDS with fibrosis and might be worth the effort. The more reliably obtainable core marrow biopsy usually shows heavy collagen fibrosis, osteosclerosis, intrasinusoidal hematopoiesis, and atypical megakaryocyte hyperplasia (Figure 121-6). Marrow fibrosis can be difficult to assess on standard hematoxylin-eosin stains and may be better estimated by the use of special stains, such as that for reticulin (a silver impregnation technique that stains a glycoprotein elaborated by stromal cells) or the trichrome stain for collagen. In some cases of MMM, the degree of bone marrow fibrosis may initially be minimal. This finding is often called the cellular phase of MMM (discussed further above) and can be diagnostically challenging. Fibrosis grading schemes have been developed but are of relatively limited clinical utility.[91]

Although ET and PV can also be associated with marrow fibrosis, this is relatively uncommon, and the fibrosis in these conditions usually is not heavy. As discussed above, the diagnostic distinction between ET and MMM may at times be difficult because features such as thrombocytosis, a hypercellular marrow with some fibrosis, and splenomegaly can be seen in both conditions. Extensive megakaryocyte clustering and the presence of vasomotor symptoms favor ET, whereas heavy fibrosis, massive splenomegaly, and anemia favor MMM. MMM is not associated with an elevated RCM, so a high hematocrit is consistent with PV and not MMM. "Spent-phase" fibrotic PV behaves identically to primary MMM, so a struggle to retrospectively diagnose PV is not necessary because management will not be affected.

Circulating myeloid progenitor cell numbers are more dramatically elevated in MMM than in other chronic myeloid conditions. $CD34^+$ cells can be quantified as a surrogate marker of this phenomenon, which may have diagnostic utility in ambiguous cases.[92,93] Although the $CD34^+$ phenotype is considered a marker for very early myeloid progenitor status, it is not clear that the $CD34^+$ circulating cells in MMM actually represent true hematopoietic stem cells. These cells are easy to collect in large numbers at leukapheresis, but their ability to reconstitute hematopoiesis is not hearty, which has important implications for stem cell transplantation.

The bone marrow morphologic features of MMM may sometimes be difficult to distinguish from those of MDS with fibrosis (MDS-F) and so-called "acute myelofibrosis." The latter entity has substantial overlap with megakaryocytic acute leukemia (AML-M7).[91] Megakaryocytes alone often appear dysplastic in routine cases of MMM, but significant dysplasia in other cell lines favors a diagnosis of MDS-F.[91] Acute myelofibrosis (also known as malignant myelosclerosis or acute myelosclerosis) is suggested when constitutional symptoms are prominent, development of the illness is rapid (ie, over the course of a few weeks), and the spleen is not palpable. Special stains for megakaryoblasts (eg, CD61 or vWF) may reveal the presence of an otherwise unrecognized cell population. Sometimes, despite the best efforts of clinicians and pathologists, the diagnosis is simply not clear and patients must be treated expectantly.

Cytogenetic studies should be performed on the marrow to exclude atypical forms of CML that can have substantial bone marrow fibrosis. If cytogenetic studies cannot be performed (eg, a dry tap), FISH or RT-PCR testing for *bcr-abl* translocation is necessary and may be reasonable to obtain on an initial evaluation even if cytogenetic findings are normal, to rule out a cryptic translocation.

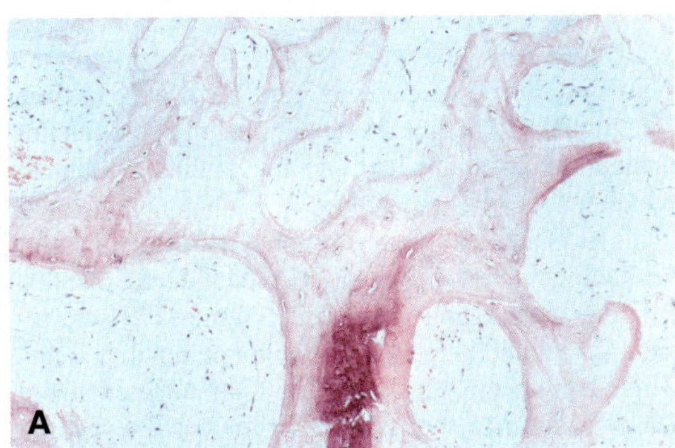

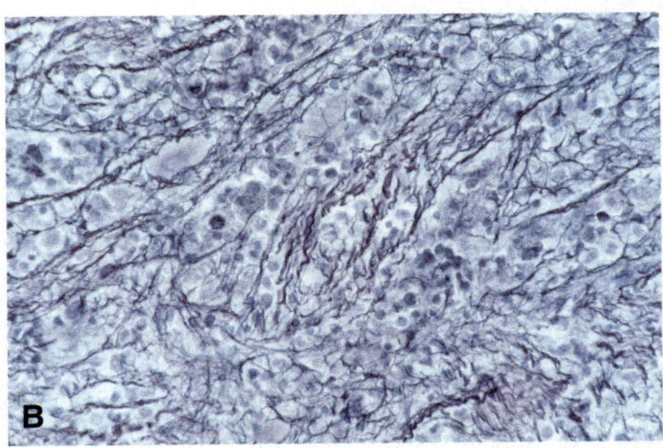

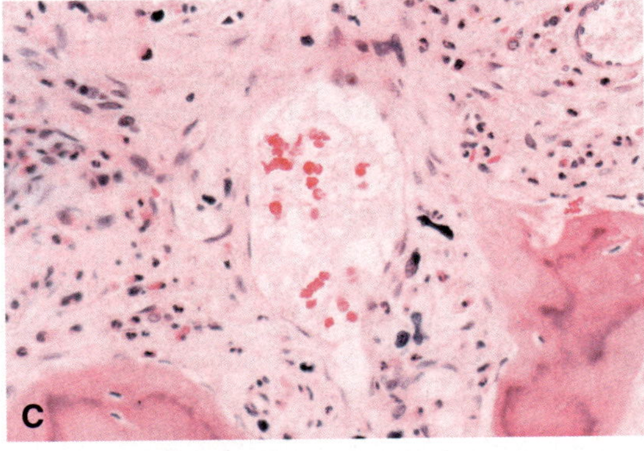

Figure 121-6 Bone marrow biopsy findings in myelofibrosis with myeloid metaplasia, demonstrating osteosclerosis and reduced hematopoietic progenitors (**A**), reticulin fibrosis (**B**), and intrasinusoidal hematopoiesis (**C**). Reproduced with permission from Tefferi A.[81]

Clinical Manifestations About 25% of patients with MMM are asymptomatic at diagnosis. Most patients have anemia and at least some degree of splenomegaly at presentation. The anemia of MMM is multifactorial. Contributing problems include replacement of normal hematopoietic tissue with fibrosis, ineffective hematopoiesis in the remaining myeloid tissue, and hypersplenism. Hemolysis also occurs in a minority of patients, and a paroxysmal nocturnal hemoglobinuria phenotype may be seen. Splenomegaly in MMM may be massive, and the spleen is usually very firm (Figure 121-7). Spleen and liver enlargement in MMM is secondary to extramedullary hematopoiesis and may be associated with hypercatabolic symptoms (profound fatigue, weight loss, night sweats, low-grade fever), peripheral edema (from venous compression), diarrhea (possibly related to splanchnic vascular congestion), early satiety (from gastric compression), and, occasionally, portal hypertension (from portal hyperemia). It was formerly believed that splenic hematopoiesis in MMM was due to a homeostatic "recall" of normal fetal hematopoiesis in the setting of advanced marrow failure.

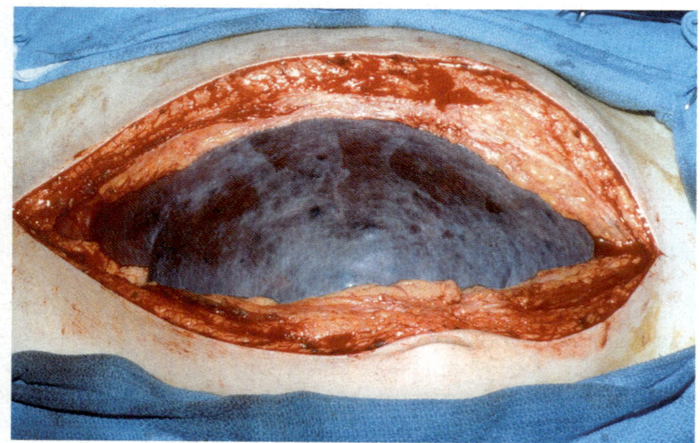

Figure 121-7 Splenomegaly in myelofibrosis with myeloid metaplasia is a result of extramedullary hematopoiesis and can be massive. Reproduced with permission from Tefferi A.[81]

However, evidence now suggests that the extremely high numbers of neoplastic circulating progenitor cells in MMM find a receptive microenvironment in the spleen. In patients with MMM who have karyotypic abnormalities and undergo splenectomy, the spleen karyotype corresponds to marrow karyotype.[94]

Splenomegaly in MMM may be complicated by infarction, an event heralded by moderate to severe pain that may be referred to the left shoulder and often requires opiate analgesics to control.[95] Computed tomography in such cases can be unremarkable or may show wedge-shaped or rounded low-attenuation lesions in the spleen. Spontaneous hepatic infarction may also occur but is uncommon.

Extramedullary hematopoiesis (EMH) occurs in a great diversity of sites throughout the body. Common sites besides the spleen and the liver include the lymph nodes, skin, pleura, peritoneum, lung, and the paraspinal and epidural spaces. The latter may result in spinal cord and/or nerve root compression, which is a medical emergency requiring corticosteroids to reduce edema and immediate radiotherapy.[96] It is fortunate that localized EMH responds promptly to low doses of gamma irradiation (100–150 cGy), which are often administered several times in the case of cord compression; an optimal total dose has not been defined. Irradiation can also be administered to the liver and spleen, but this is perilous and often ineffective, and the duration of success is limited.[97] Such treatment is usually reserved for those patients with symptomatic splenic EMH who are abysmal surgical candidates. Pulmonary hypertension in MMM can be due to chronic thromboembolism but can also result from interstitial EMH in the lung, which may not be seen on conventional radiography and may be detectable only via biopsy. On technetium sulfur colloid scintigraphy, increased uptake in the lung suggests EMH. This dangerous complication can be successfully treated with a single dose of 100 cGy of whole-lung radiotherapy.[98]

In addition to anemia, the majority of MMM patients have leukocytosis, and some have thrombocytosis.[81] Thrombocytopenia is more common (especially in the setting of massive splenomegaly), whereas leukopenia is less frequently seen. Red cell transfusion dependence is widespread, but most patients do not live long enough to develop significant problems from iron overload. Serum levels of lactate dehydrogenase are often elevated, reflecting both ineffective hematopoiesis and injury to the liver by EMH. Hyperuricemia and consequent episodes of gout are not uncommon and reflect ineffective hematopoiesis with high cell turnover. Bone pain is seen and is multifactorial, related to marrow replacement and periostitis. Sweet's syndrome (neutrophilic dermatosis) is associated with MMM, and this lesion must be distinguished from cutaneous EMH because treatment differs.[99]

Death in MMM can come from many directions. Fatal infection and transformation to a resistant myeloid leukemia are common. Overt leukemia occurs in approximately 20% of patients over the first 10 years.[100] Less frequent causes of death include thrombohemorrhagic events and heart failure, often secondary to pulmonary hypertension.

Prognosis The overall median survival for MMM is on the order of 3 to 5 years.[81,100] A number of potential prognostic factors have been identified that may help identify subgroups at lower or higher risk.[101] These include the presence of anemia (hemoglobin < 10 g/dL), hypercatabolic symptoms, hepatomegaly, left-shifted granulocytosis (white blood cell count [WBC] of > 30,000/μL or the presence of circulating blasts), and advanced age (> 60 years).[101,102] A lack of any of these features is associated with a median survival of at least 10 years. Dupriez and colleagues developed a simple and useful prognostic scoring scheme (the Lille Scoring System) for MMM based on the presence or absence of two adverse prognostic factors: a hemoglobin of < 10 g/dL and WBC of either < 4,000 or > 30,000/μL.[102] Using these two criteria, they were able to separate patients into three risk groups: low risk (no factors), intermediate risk (one factor), and high risk (two factors). These three groups lived a median of 93, 26, and 13 months, respectively. Among low-risk patients, those with del(13q) and del(20q) appear to do better than those with trisomy 8 and del(12p). The former group may live longer than 10 years, more than twice the average for the disease.[103] Overall, patients with normal karyotypes at diagnosis live longer than those with abnormal cytogenetics. Spleen size and the degree of marrow fibrosis do not appear to have value for forecasting the course of the illness.

Therapy Conventional therapy for MMM is largely palliative and has not been shown to improve survival. Patients should be considered for clinical trials of new treatments whenever feasible. The use of radiotherapy for localized EMH and pulmonary hypertension is discussed above. Older treatments for anemia include androgen preparations (eg, oral fluoxymesterone 10 mg two times a day or danazol 400 to 600 mg per day), which, given the older age of the typical male MMM patient, should be initiated only after ruling out occult prostate cancer.[104] Corticosteroids may also give transient benefit in this setting (eg, oral prednisone at a starting dose of 30 to 40 mg/d for 1 month and then tapered off over the second month). Unfortunately, responses to androgens and steroids are uncommon; they occur in less than one-third of MMM patients and are usually of brief duration (less than 1 year).

If the endogenous EPO level is less than 200 mIU/mL, a brief trial of EPO therapy is reasonable, although response rates are low, and the most severely anemic patients, who most need the treatment, are the group least likely to respond.[105] The use of at least 60,000 units of erythropoietin weekly during the trial eliminates any concerns over the possibility of failure owing to inadequate dosing. There is anecdotal evidence of a similar rate of response to darbepoeitin.

For control of leukocytosis, thrombocytosis, or splenomegaly associated with MMM, HU is the first choice.[106] An initial dose of 500 mg of HU three times per day typically brings salutary results within 1 to 2 weeks, and the dose can then be adjusted to optimal effect. Anagrelide does not appear to have any unique beneficial effects in MMM.[107]

Thalidomide can improve cytopenias and reduce spleen size in MMM.[108] Reported response rates range between 20 and 62% for anemia, 25 and 80% for thrombocytopenia, and 7 and 30% for splenomegaly.[108,109] In conventional doses similar to those used for multiple myeloma (eg, 200 mg/d and above), thalidomide has been associated with severe myeloproliferative reactions, including accelerated EMH.[110] Lower doses of thalidomide (eg, 50 mg/d) appear to be better tolerated, and responses are often durable.[109,111] There is no clear dose response with respect to the therapeutic effects of thalidomide in MMM, but there is a dose-response effect with respect to the cost of the drug and toxicity. The addition of prednisone to the lower-dose schedule improves tolerance and may enhance the erythropoietic activity of the drug.[109,111]

Patients with MMM often suffer from troubling constitutional symptoms, such as debilitating fatigue, unintentional weight loss, night sweats, and low-grade fevers in the absence of infection. Etanercept, a soluble tumor necrosis factor (TNF) chimeric receptor, has shown efficacy in relieving these symptoms when administered in the usual dose of 25 mg subcutaneously twice weekly, and the drug occasionally also has a beneficial effect on hematopoiesis.[112] Etanercept and other anti-TNF approaches may prove to be useful palliative tools in MMM. Etanercept can be safely combined with thalidomide and prednisone.

Splenectomy can be considered for patients with refractory splenic pain, disabling constitutional symptoms, symptomatic portal hypertension, and/or a need for frequent red cell transfusions. In one series of 223 MMM patients who underwent splenectomy, durable remissions in constitutional symptoms, transfusion-dependent anemia, portal hypertension, and severe thrombocytopenia were achieved in 67%, 23%, 50%, and 0% of patients, respectively.[113] However, even in experienced centers, the perioperative mortality rate of splenectomy in MMM may be as high as 9%, and overall survival may not be affected; the median postsplenectomy survival is about 2 years.[113] An elevated D-dimer, even in the absence of overt disseminated intravascular coagulopathy, may predict a higher surgical risk. Up to 25% of surgical survivors will develop marked hepatomegaly or extreme thrombocytosis.[113] Presplenectomy thrombocytopenia correlates with the risk of postsplenectomy leukemic transformation, for unclear reasons. Extreme postsplenectomy thrombocytosis is significantly associated with perioperative thrombosis. HU can be used perioperatively to prevent a postsplenectomy rise in platelet count. It is customary to administer immunizations for encapsulated organisms prior to splenectomy, but data are lacking on the effectiveness and frequency of high-titer antibody responses in MMM. Patients who have undergone splenectomy should carry a medical alert bracelet or necklace and be treated promptly with antimicrobial agents when they develop signs of infection. In poor surgical candidates with symptomatic splenomegaly, the palliative use of splenic irradiation is reasonable, but success is irregular and of brief duration.[97]

Imatinib mesylate (STI-571, Gleevec) is not effective in MMM and may be associated with spontaneous splenic rupture.[114] It should not be used for this condition.

The use of allogeneic hematopoietic stem cell transplantation (HSCT) in MMM was initially limited because of concerns regarding potential failure of stem cells to engraft in the fibrotic marrow. This concern has not been substantiated. Marrow fibrosis delays post-transplantation platelet recovery by about 3 days and increases platelet transfusion needs slightly but is not clearly associated with graft failure or other unique transplantation-related problems.[115] Interest in allogeneic HSCT in patients with MMM is now growing, but appropriate patient selection and timing remain challenging. Whereas engraftment has not been especially problematic, toxicity continues to be a major issue, even with the newer reduced-intensity "nonmyeloablative" conditioning regimens.[116] In one study of allogeneic HSCT in myelofibrosis, the 5-year survival rate was only 14% for patients older than 44 years, and in another study, the 2-year survival rate was just 41%.[117,118] Rates of chronic graft-versus-host disease of up to 59% have been reported.[119] Younger patients do somewhat better, with post-transplant survival rates of up to 60%, but the decision to proceed to transplantation must be made only after careful deliberation, and the patients chosen should be those with a particularly limited life expectancy.[117,119]

There is also interest in autologous HSCT in MMM, in an attempt to "reset the clock" on the process of marrow fibrosis and EMH by interrupting the ongoing disease process and allowing time for healing. Autologous HSCT approaches presume that the sheer bulk of malignant cells and fibrosis in MMM contribute substantially to ineffective hematopoiesis and disease-related symptoms. (Investigators operating under a similar paradigm are currently examining the role of bone marrow curettage in MMM to alter the marrow microenvironment, with relatively little success thus far.) A recent report of autologous HSCT in 21 patients using a busulfan-based conditioning regimen suggests that the procedure is feasible (a second stem cell infusion was required in 5 of 21 patients owing to delayed engraftment) and may alleviate symptoms, decrease splenomegaly, improve cytopenias, and reduce bone marrow fibrosis.[117,120] The ideal dose of $CD34^+$ cells or marrow mononuclear cells to administer for autologous transplantation in MMM remains uncertain.

POLYCYTHEMIA VERA

Epidemiology The incidence of PV is 0.8 to 2.6 cases per 100,000 persons per year, with most studies giving figures at the upper end of that range, and this incidence appears to be relatively stable over time.[121,122] As is the case with the other CMPDs, the incidence of PV increases with age. The median age at diagnosis is approximately 60 years; the disease can also be seen in young people, and 7% of cases are diagnosed before the age of 40 years.[123,124] There may be a slight male preponderance (on the order of a 1.2:1 male-to-female case ratio), and the disease is more common in Jews, especially Ashkenazi Jews.[14,125] In a few cases, true PV may be familial, but apparently familial erythrocytosis is often proven to be a result of a shared high–oxygen-affinity hemoglobin or a common exposure (eg, a residence at high altitude or cobalt intoxication).[126,127]

Pathogenesis X-linked (G6PD) enzyme analysis first demonstrated the clonal nature of hematopoietic cells in PV in 1976.[128] But three decades later, much about the etiology of the disease remains obscure. Neoangiogenesis is seen in the marrow in PV (as in other CMPDs) but is not a reaction to low marrow oxygen levels, which have been measured and are normal.[129] The erythroid colony-forming progenitor cells (burst forming unit-erythroid [BFU-E] and colony forming unit-erythroid [CFU-E]) in PV are very sensitive to or independent of normal growth and differentiation signals, including EPO, GM-CSF, stem cell factor, and IL-3.[130,131] Although this finding is characteristic of PV, it is not specific and is also observed in ET and MMM. Serum EPO levels in PV patients are generally very low or inappropriately normal in the setting of erythrocytosis, and excessive EPO-independent BFU-E and CFU-E proliferation leads to an increased RCM.[132,133] As is the case with the TPO receptor in ET, some families with recurrent PV have been found to harbor EPO receptor mutations, but structural changes in the EPO receptor have been diligently sought in nonfamilial PV but not found.[134,135] EPO receptor expression patterns may be abnormal in PV (eg, loss of the normal high-affinity EPO receptor), but this finding is not consistent.[136] Cells from patients with PV are consistently observed to be hypersensitive to insulin-like growth factor 1 (IGF-1), which appears to be due to alterations in IGF-1 binding proteins, including increased baseline phosphorylation of the IGF-1 receptor.[137] Decreased activity of the SH2-homology domain containing phosphatase-1 (SHP-1) phosphatase (which associates with the receptors for EPO, stem cell factor, and IL-3 and is a negative regulator of signals generated during ligand binding), constitutive activation of signal transduction and activator of transcription-3 (STAT-3), increased levels of antiapoptotic proteins such as Bcl-X_L, and several other biochemical abnormalities have been reported in subsets of patients; their general pathobiologic relevance is unclear.[138–140]

The genetic basis of PV is uncertain. Karyotypic abnormalities are found in about 10 to 20% of untreated patients.[141,142] The lesions seen are those nonspecific abnormalities typical of chronic myeloid disorders, such as trisomy 8, trisomy 9, del(20q), del(13q), loss of the Y chromosome in men, and abnormalities of chromosomes 5 and 7.[142] Recently, a novel gene with homology to the uPAR/Ly6/CD59/snake toxin receptor superfamily was cloned and found to be overexpressed in PV neutrophils but not in normal neutrophils and was subsequently named *PRV1*.[27,143] The pathophysiologic significance of this gene, if any, continues to be a subject of active investigation.

Clinical Features The signs and symptoms frequently associated with PV are listed in Table 121-5. Many of the clinical features of PV are a direct consequence of the increased RCM and are common to all causes of erythrocytosis, but pruritus and splenomegaly strongly suggest PV. A ruddy, plethoric complexion was a classic finding seen often in the *fin de siècle* world of master clinicians such as Osler and Vaquez, but dramatic skin rubor is less common in the present era of routine hemograms, when erythrocytosis is usually detected much earlier. Increased RCM can lead to blood hyperviscosity, which leads to a plethora of symptoms and signs. Headaches are frequent, but blurry vision, altered hearing,

Table 121-5 Polycythemia Vera–Related Clinical and Laboratory Features

Symptoms and Physical Findings	Frequency, %
Systolic hypertension	72
Splenomegaly	70
Skin plethora ("ruddy cyanosis")	67
Conjunctival plethora	59
Headache	48
Weakness	47
Engorged retinal veins	46
Pruritus	43
Dizziness	43
Palpable liver	40
Sweating	33
Diastolic hypertension	32
Visual disturbances	31
Weight loss	29
Paresthesias	29
Dyspnea	26
Joint symptoms	26
Epigastric distress	24

Adapted from Berlin NI.[144]

mucous membrane bleeding, shortness of breath, and malaise are also observed. Hypertension may be a consequence of increased RCM.

At least two-thirds of PV patients have splenomegaly, so the combination of splenomegaly and erythrocytosis should strongly suggest PV.[144] Thrombosis occurs in about 40% of patients, most commonly arterial thrombosis.[123] Clots occur at a rate of about 3.9% of patients per year.[123] Arterial thromboses are more likely to be fatal than venous thromboses. As in ET, venous thrombosis can occur in unusual sites, such as mesenteric or hepatic vessels. Bleeding, especially gastrointestinal, is seen in PV but less often than thrombosis.[123]

Pruritus is a common and classic PV-associated complaint, may be provoked by warm water ("aquagenic"), and may be related to serotonin release by platelets and elevated histamine levels.[145,146] Erythromelalgia (described above under ET) also troubles patients with PV, as do other vasomotor symptoms; paresthesias and headaches may be in part a result of vasomotor imbalance. Bone pain and neutrophilic dermatosis do occur in PV but are uncommon and much more typical of MMM.

Leukocytosis and thrombocytosis are present in less than half of PV patients. The unsaturated vitamin B_{12}–binding level is high in PV owing to excess transcobalamin I and III released by granulocytes.[147] Measured vitamin B_{12} levels may be elevated in PV, and this can be useful diagnostically.

Diagnosis The major diagnostic difficulty with respect to PV is distinguishing PV from the many other causes of erythrocytosis (Table 121-6) because clonal myeloid disorders other than PV are only very rarely associated with an elevated RCM. To make the diagnosis of PV, erythrocytosis must first be determined to be due to a true increase in RCM (ie, exclusion of relative erythrocytosis that is due to a decrease in plasma volume), and then the genuine elevation in RCM must be shown to be a primary, EPO-independent erythrocytosis (ie, exclusion of secondary EPO-driven erythrocytosis, such as that caused by hypoxia, high–oxygen-affinity hemoglobin, EPO-producing tumors, EPO doping, and cobalt intoxication).

The 1975 Polycythemia Vera Study Group (PSVG) diagnostic criteria[144] were an advancement in their time but are now chiefly of historical interest.[30,148] These criteria included direct measurement of the RCM, which is a cumbersome procedure that is no longer strictly necessary in most cases. The availability of new diagnostic tools and better appreciation of the tight relationship between hematocrit and RCM have undermined the use of RCM measurement in the diagnosis of PV.[27,29,148–151]

The first steps toward determining the cause of erythrocytosis should include taking a careful history to rule out the possibility of dehydration or dramatic fluid volume shifts that might be consistent with relative erythrocytosis. These are usually obvious, and clinicians should not worry about subtle fluid shifts owing to antihypertensive agents or a "stressful lifestyle" causing confusion with true PV. "Gaisbock's syndrome," a chronic mild erythrocytosis purportedly due to a chronically contracted plasma volume, is frequently encountered on medical board examinations but not in the clinic.[29] Oxygen saturation should be measured to exclude hypoxia and a family history taken to ensure that erythrocytosis is not familial (or due to a common environmental exposure).

The next test should be a measurement of the serum EPO level. Serum EPO is generally low in true PV but may be in the normal range, even in untreated cases.[132] The presence of other PV-related features, such as splenomegaly, thrombosis, erythromelalgia, leukocytosis with a left shift, or pruritus, should nudge the clinician toward a tentative diagnosis of PV in polycythemic patients with inappropriately normal serum EPO levels. A high serum EPO level is not consistent with PV and should prompt a careful search for the usual instigators of secondary erythrocytosis with tests such as hemoglobin electrophoresis, measurement of the hemoglobin oxygen dissociation curve (ie, a "P50" determination), cobalt measurement, and appropriate imaging for EPO-producing tumors (eg, cerebellar and liver vascular tumors and renal cell carcinoma).[132,152]

Bone marrow sampling is sometimes helpful in the diagnosis of PV.[32,148] The marrow in PV may show hypercellularity, relative erythroid excess, increased megakaryocyte numbers with some cluster formation, giant megakaryocytes, and decreased iron stores. Karyotypic abnormalities support the diagnosis of a clonal disorder but are not specific for PV. Some fibrosis may be seen in 10 to 15% of patients.[153] The demonstration of markedly decreased megakaryocyte c-Mpl expression supports the histologic diagnosis of PV and may be helpful when there is diagnostic ambiguity.[150,151] Measurement of spontaneous (EPO independent) marrow erythroid colony growth may also be useful for the diagnosis of PV, but limited availability of the test and the need for special

Table 121-6 Classification of Erythrocytosis

- Apparent polycythemia
  - Relative polycythemia owing to major fluid shifts
  - Extreme "high normal" values
- True polycythemia
  - Polycythemia vera
  - Secondary polycythemia
    - Erythropoietin (EPO) mediated
      - Hypoxia driven
        - Central hypoxic process
          - Chronic lung disease
          - Right-to-left cardiopulmonary vascular shunts
          - High-altitude habitat
          - Carbon monoxide poisoning and smoker's polycythemia
          - Hypoventilation syndromes, including sleep apnea
        - Peripheral hypoxic process
          - Localized
      - Renal artery stenosis
        - Diffuse
      - High–oxygen-affinity hemoglobinopathy (congenital; autosomal dominant)
      - 2,3-Diphosphoglycerate mutase deficiency (congenital; autosomal recessive)
      - Hypoxia independent (pathologic EPO production)
        - Malignant tumors
          - Hepatocellular carcinoma
          - Renal cell cancer
          - Cerebellar hemangioblastoma
          - Parathyroid carcinoma
        - Nonmalignant conditions
          - Uterine leiomyomas
          - Renal cysts (polycystic kidney disease)
          - Pheochromocytoma
          - Meningioma
        - Abnormally elevated set point for EPO production (congenital)
        - Chuvash polycythemia (congenital; abnormal oxygen homeostasis)
      - Intentional EPO doping
        - EPO receptor mediated
      - Activating mutation of the erythropoietin receptor
      - Some cases of autosomal dominant congenital polycythemia
        - Drug associated
      - Treatment with androgen preparations
      - Treatment with novel erythropoietic agents such as CERA
        - Unknown mechanisms
      - Most cases of autosomal dominant congenital polycythemia
      - Some forms of autosomal recessive congenital polycythemia
      - Post–renal transplant erythrocytosis

CERA = continuous erythropoiesis receptor activator.

expertise in setting up and interpreting the assay restrict its use.[154,155] Altered expression of *PRV-1* on neutrophils is seen in more than 80% of PV patients but is not specific and is elevated in 21% of ET patients, 42% of MMM, and 18% of those with secondary polycythemia.[27,156] An elevated LAP score correlates highly with elevated *PRV-1* expression and may help clinicians who do not have access to *PRV-1* testing. These assays are complementary to the clinical impression, EPO level, and bone marrow findings and may help support the diagnosis of PV in difficult cases.

Prognosis The median life expectancy for patients diagnosed with PV exceeds 10 years but is worse than a gender- and age-matched control population.[54] Thrombohemorrhagic complications and transformation into AML account for much of the inferior survival.[157] As with ET, older age (> 60 years) appears to be a risk factor for thrombosis.[158] Other clearly prognostic factors in PV beyond old age and a history of thrombosis have not been determined. In about 15 to 20% of cases, PV terminates in a "spent phase," an MMM-like state to which use of ^{32}P might contribute.[159] This transition is usually characterized by worsening anemia and increasing WBC and spleen size.

Treatment As is the case with ET, PV-associated vasomotor symptoms are usually alleviated by low doses of ASA, which inhibit the synthesis of vasoactive thromboxane A_2 by platelets. (The use of ASA for thrombosis prevention in PV is discussed below.) PV-associated pruritus can be treated with selective serotonin reuptake inhibitors, such as paroxetine.[145] Antihistamines, such as hydroxyzine and diphenhydramine, may be effective but are sedating. There are no data about the efficacy of less sedating H1-selective antihistamines, such as loratadine and fexofenadine.

The primary goal of treatment in PV is to prevent disastrous thrombotic events without increasing the risk of other life-threatening problems, such as bleeding, or altering the potential for transformation to a fibrotic marrow or acute leukemia. The main tool used to accomplish this goal is therapeutic phlebotomy. The importance of regular phlebotomy as part of a successful treatment program for PV cannot be overemphasized; marrow-suppressing drugs play only a supplementary role. In the first few decades after the disease's description, before aggressive phlebotomy became *de rigueur*, the median survival for patients with PV was on the order of 2 years, and most deaths were due to thrombotic events.[160,161] Today, most PV-related deaths are still due to thrombosis, but patients treated initially with phlebotomy alone have a median survival of more than 15 years.[123]

Based on studies that have shown an improved cerebral blood flow and normalization of blood viscosity with a hematocrit below 45%, as well as less thrombosis in patients with hematocrits in this range, dropping the hematocrit to below this level and keeping it there should be the goal of phlebotomy-based treatment in PV.[162,163] It has also been widely recommended that females be reduced to a hematocrit of less than 42% because their normal hemoglobin range is lower, but this has not been rigorously tested, and whole blood viscosity should not depend significantly on gender.

Some patients need extremely frequent phlebotomy to keep the hematocrit below goal levels, which is an inconvenience, and phlebotomy can also lead to iron deficiency, which can exacerbate thrombocytosis. In addition, patients treated with phlebotomy alone still suffer from thrombosis. Therefore, there has been a long-standing interest in the addition of other therapies to try to further decrease that risk. Just when these other agents should be added to phlebotomy is controversial. An elevated platelet count does not appear to be a major thrombotic risk factor in PV, and a very elevated platelet count (eg, > 1 million/μL), as in ET, is a risk factor for bleeding in PV.[164] Therefore, young PV patients without a history of thrombosis and with a near-normal platelet count are probably quite safe with phlebotomy alone.

Table 121-7 Suggested Treatment Algorithm for Patients with Polycythemia Vera

Risk Category*	Age < 60 Yr	Age ≥ 60 Yr	Childbearing Age
Low	Phlebotomy + ASA	Not applicable	Phlebotomy + ASA
Indeterminate	Phlebotomy + ASA if no avWD	Not applicable	Phlebotomy + ASA if no avWD
High	Phlebotomy + ASA + HU or IFN-α	Phlebotomy + HU + ASA	Phlebotomy + ASA + IFN-α

ASA = acetylsalicylic acid (low-dose aspirin; if no contraindications), HU = hydroxyurea, IFN-α = interferon-α2a; avWD = acquired von Willebrand's disease.

*See Table 121-2 for a risk stratification algorithm.

In view of a recent large randomized placebo-controlled study that showed a large reduction in thrombotic events (but not an overall survival improvement) with low-dose aspirin (100 mg/d, a dose not available in the United States), all patients with PV who do not have a contraindication should receive aspirin.[60] In this trial, the combined end point of nonfatal myocardial infarction, nonfatal stroke, or death from cardiovascular causes and the risk of the combined end point of nonfatal myocardial infarction, nonfatal stroke, pulmonary embolism, major venous thrombosis, or death from cardiovascular causes were both reduced (relative risk 0.41 and 0.40 compared with placebo, respectively). The risk of bleeding at this dose was elevated slightly above those treated with placebo (relative risk 1.6).[60] In an early PVSG randomized study, an aggressive regimen using high doses of aspirin (900 mg/d) in combination with dipyridamole increased the risk of bleeding in PV, particularly gastrointestinal bleeding, but had little effect on thrombosis.[165] The bleeding risk in that study was highest in those with very elevated platelet counts, perhaps owing to acquired vWF deficiency.[164]

There has been interest in myelosuppressive agents in PV for several decades, and opinion about the optimal regimen continues to evolve. In a landmark three-arm randomized study that originated in the 1960s, two specific agents, oral chlorambucil and intravenous ^{32}P, were each found to decrease the risk of thrombosis when added to phlebotomy.[157] However, overall survival was inferior with either of the additional treatments because of an increased incidence of acute leukemia compared with phlebotomy alone. The incidence of acute leukemia over 13 to 19 years was 1.5, 9.6, and 13.2% for phlebotomy, ^{32}P, and chlorambucil, respectively, and the corresponding median survival was 12.6, 9.1, and 10.9 years, respectively.[157] Several cases of lymphoma were seen in patients treated with chlorambucil, and the incidence of gastrointestinal and skin cancer was also increased. Another alkylating agent, busulfan, improves overall survival above that achievable with ^{32}P but is also leukemogenic.[166]

Other agents have the potential to decrease thrombosis without the same degree of leukemia risk as ^{32}P or alkylators. One of these agents is HU, which decreases thrombotic risk when used as a supplement to phlebotomy but appears to be less leukemogenic than chlorambucil and ^{32}P. In one PVSG study, HU was associated with a lower risk of thrombosis in the first 2 years after diagnosis (6.6% vs 14%) when compared with a historical cohort of patients treated with phlebotomy alone, and only 5.9% of patients had transformed to acute leukemia after a median follow-up of 8.6 years.[167] Because the true leukemogenic risk of HU is unknown, it is used most often as a supplement to phlebotomy for groups at especially high risk of thrombosis, such as the elderly and those with prior thrombosis (Table 121-7). Occasionally, oscillatory thrombopoiesis may develop in PV patients treated with HU, and this can make dose adjustment very difficult.[168] Alternatives to HU include pipobroman, which is not available in the United States but may be associated with a slight reduction in the risk of progression of PV to the "spent phase."[169]

IFN-α2a has salutary effects in PV and is the drug of choice for PV patients who wish to become pregnant because of anecdotal reports of successful maternal and fetal outcomes. This drug controls erythrocytosis in approximately 80% of the patients who can tolerate the necessary dose, which ranges from 4.5 to 27 million units per week (the usual starting dose is 3 million units subcutaneously three times a week), and IFN-α2a has a beneficial effect on thrombocytosis.[69,170,171] IFN can also reduce spleen size and frequently gives relief from intractable pruritus. However, at least 20% of patients discontinue therapy because of drug side effects, including fatigue, malaise, fevers, psychological effects, myalgias, and arthralgias.[171] IFN-α2a is also more expensive than HU. In addition to women of childbearing potential, it is reasonable to choose IFN-α2a for high-risk patients who need a supplement to phlebotomy where the potential benefit of relief from refractory pruritus is desired or for patients who are particularly concerned about the potential leukemogenicity of HU.

Anagrelide lowers platelet production and at higher doses can also inhibit platelet aggregation.[172] The mechanism of action may include interference of the drug with megakaryocyte maturation.[173,174] More than 80% of previously treated and untreated patients with thrombocytosis experience a reduction in platelet count with anagrelide.[67] Anagrelide also results in modest red cell suppression via an unclear mechanism. The toxicity and other relevant properties of anagrelide and other myelosuppressive agents are outlined in Table 121-1.[175] The optimal role of anagrelide in PV is currently undefined, and we rarely use it.

Bone marrow transplantation has been successfully performed in PV but is generally reserved for patients who have transformed to a "spent phase" or for those rare, young, treatment-refractory patients with multiple thrombohemorrhagic complications. The optimal timing and conditioning regimen remain undefined.

REFERENCES

1. Tefferi A. Chronic myeloid disorders: classification and treatment overview. Semin Hematol 2001;38:1–4.
2. Tefferi A. The Philadelphia chromosome negative chronic myeloproliferative diseases. Mayo Clin Proc 1998;73:1177–84.
3. Epstein E, Goedel A. Hämorrhagische Thrombocythämie bei vascularer Schrumpfmilz. Virchows Arch Pathol Anat Physiol Klin Med 1934;292:233–48.
4. Vaquez H. Sur une forme speciale de cyanose s'accompanant d'hyperglobulie excessive et persistante. C R Soc Biol (Paris) 1892;4:384.
5. Heuck G. Zwei Falle von Leukamie mit eigenthumlichem Blut- resp. Knochenmarksbefund. Arch Pathol Anat Physiol Virchows 1879;78:475–96.
6. Wasserman LR. Polycythemia Vera Study Group: a historical perspective. Semin Hematol 1986;23:183–7.
7. Dameshek W. Some speculations on the myeloproliferative syndromes. Blood 1951;6:372–5.
8. Fialkow PJ, Gartler SM, Yoshida A. Clonal origin of chronic myelocytic leukemia in man. Proc Natl Acad Sci U S A 1967;58:1468–71.
9. Nowell PC, Hungerford DA. A minute chromosome in human chronic granulocytic leukemia. J Natl Cancer Inst 1960;25:85.
10. Daley GQ, Van Etten RA, Baltimore D. Induction of chronic myelogenous leukemia in mice by the P210bcr/abl gene of the Philadelphia chromosome. Science 1990;247:824–30.
11. Mesa RA, Silverstein MN, Jacobsen SJ, et al. Population-based incidence and survival figures in essential thrombocythemia and agnogenic myeloid metaplasia: an Olmsted County study, 1976-1995. Am J Hematol 1999;61:10–5.
12. Kutti J, Ridell B. Epidemiology of the myeloproliferative disorders: essential thrombocythaemia, polycythaemia vera and idiopathic myelofibrosis. Pathol Biol (Paris) 2001;49:164–6.
13. Jensen MK, de Nully Brown P, Nielsen OJ, Hasselbalch HC. Incidence, clinical features and outcome of essential thrombocythaemia in a well defined geographical area. Eur J Haematol 2000;65:132–9.
14. Chaiter Y, Brenner B, Aghai E, Tatarsky I. High incidence of myeloproliferative disorders in Ashkenazi Jews in northern Israel. Leuk Lymphoma 1992;7:251–5.
15. Kondo T, Okabe M, Sanada M, et al. Familial essential thrombocythemia associated with one-base deletion in the 5′-untranslated region of the thrombopoietin gene. Blood 1998;92:1091–6.
16. Wiestner A, Schlemper RJ, Vandermaas APC, Skoda RC. An activating splice donor mutation in the thrombopoietin gene causes hereditary thrombocythaemia. Nat Genet 1998;18:49–52.
17. Harrison CN, Gale RE, Wiestner AC, et al. The activating splice mutation in intron 3 of the thrombopoietin gene is not found in patients with non-familial essential thrombocythaemia. Br J Haematol 1998;102:1341–3.
18. Griesshammer M, Bangerter M, Sauer T, et al. Aetiology and clinical significance of thrombocytosis: analysis of 732 patients with an elevated platelet count. J Intern Med 1999;245:295–300.
19. Buss DH, Cashell AW, O'Connor ML, et al. Occurrence, etiology, and clinical significance of extreme thrombocytosis: a study of 280 cases. Am J Med 1994;96:247–53.
20. Tefferi A, Ho TC, Ahmann GJ, et al. Plasma interleukin-6 and C-reactive protein levels in reactive versus clonal thrombocytosis. Am J Med 1994;97:374–8.
21. Wang JC, Chen C, Novetsky AD, et al. Blood thrombopoietin levels in clonal thrombocytosis and reactive thrombocytosis. Am J Med 1998;104:451–5.
22. Doll DC, List AF, Yarbro JW. Functional hyposplenism. South Med J 1987;80:999–1006.
23. Koike T, Uesugi Y, Toba K, et al. 5q-Syndrome presenting as essential thrombocythemia: myelodysplastic syndrome or chronic myeloproliferative disorders? Leukemia 1995;9:517–8.
24. Kwong YL, Chiu EK, Liang RH, et al. Essential thrombocythemia with BCR/ABL rearrangement. Cancer Genet Cytogenet 1996;89:74–6.
25. Steensma DP, Tefferi A. Cytogenetic and molecular genetic aspects of essential thrombocythemia. Acta Haematol 2002;108:55–65.
26. Dobo I, Pineau D, Zandecki M, et al. Endogenous erythroid and megakaryocytic colony formation in serum-free, cytokine-free collagen gels. J Hematother Stem Cell Res 1999;8:601–7.
27. Tefferi A, Lasho TL, Wolanskyj AP, Mesa RA. Neutrophil PRV-1 expression across the chronic myeloproliferative disorders and in secondary or spurious polycythemia. Blood 2004;103:3547–8.
28. Murphy S. Diagnostic criteria and prognosis in polycythemia vera and essential thrombocythemia. Semin Hematol 1999;36:9–13.
29. Fairbanks VF, Klee GG, Wiseman GA, et al. Measurement of blood volume and red cell mass—re-examination of Cr-51 and I-125 methods. Blood Cells Mol Dis 1996;22:169–86.
30. Tefferi A. Diagnosing polycythemia vera: a paradigm shift. Mayo Clin Proc 1999;74:159–62.
31. Thiele J, Kvasnicka HM, Diehl V, et al. Clinicopathological diagnosis and differential criteria of thrombocythemias in various myeloproliferative disorders by histopathology, histochemistry and immunostaining from bone marrow biopsies. Leuk Lymphoma 1999;33:207–18.
32. Dickstein JI, Vardiman JW. Hematopathologic findings in the myeloproliferative disorders. Semin Oncol 1995;22:355–73.
33. Elkassar N, Hetet G, Briere J, Grandchamp B. Clonality analysis of hematopoiesis in essential thrombocythemia—advantages of studying T lymphocytes and platelets. Blood 1997;89:128–34.
34. Fialkow PJ, Faguet GB, Jacobson RJ, et al. Evidence that essential thrombocythemia is a clonal disorder with origin in a multipotent stem cell. Blood 1981;58:916–9.
35. Tefferi A. Thrombocytosis. In: Michelson A, editor. Platelets. London: Academic Press; 2003. p. 667–80.
36. Harrison CN, Gale RE, Machin SJ, Linch DC. A large proportion of patients with a diagnosis of essential thrombocythemia do not have a clonal disorder and may be at lower risk of thrombotic complications. Blood 1999;93:417–24.
37. Chiusolo P, La Barbera EO, Laurenti L, et al. Clonal hemopoiesis and risk of thrombosis in young female patients with essential thrombocythemia. Exp Hematol 2001;29:670–6.
38. Champion KM, Gilbert JG, Asimakopoulos FA, et al. Clonal haemopoiesis in normal elderly women: implications for the myeloproliferative disorders and myelodysplastic syndromes. Br J Haematol 1997;97:920–6.
39. Li Y, Hetet G, Maurer AM, et al. Spontaneous megakaryocyte colony formation in myeloproliferative disorders is not neutralizable by antibodies against IL3, IL6 and GM-CSF. Br J Haematol 1994;87:471–6.
40. Taksin AL, Couedic JPL, Dusanter-Fourt I, et al. Autonomous megakaryocyte growth in essential thrombocythemia and idiopathic myelofibrosis is not related to a c-Mpl mutation or to an autocrine stimulation by Mpl-L. Blood 1999;93:125–39.
41. Horikawa Y, Matsumura I, Hashimoto K, et al. Markedly reduced expression of platelet c-Mpl receptor in essential thrombocythemia. Blood 1997;90:4031–8.
42. Yoon SY, Li CY, Tefferi A. Megakaryocyte c-Mpl expression in chronic myeloproliferative disorders and the myelodysplastic syndrome: immunoperoxidase staining patterns and clinical correlates. Eur J Haematol 2000;65:170–4.
43. Kobayashi S, Teramura M, Hoshino S, et al. Circulating megakaryocyte progenitors in myeloproliferative disorders are hypersensitive to interleukin-3. Br J Haematol 1993;83:539–44.
44. Axelrad AA, Eskinazi D, Correa PN, Amato D. Hypersensitivity of circulating progenitor cells to megakaryocyte growth and development factor (PEG-rHu MGDF) in essential thrombocythemia. Blood 2000;96:3310–21.
45. Tefferi A, Fonseca R, Pereira DL, Hoagland HC. A long-term retrospective study of young women with essential thrombocythemia. Mayo Clin Proc 2001;76:22-8.
46. Fenaux P, Simon M, Caulier MT, et al. Clinical course of essential thrombocythemia in 147 cases. Cancer 1990;66:549–56.
47. Besses C, Cervantes F, Pereira A, et al. Major vascular complications in essential thrombocythemia: a study of the predictive factors in a series of 148 patients. Leukemia 1999;13:150–4.
48. Cortelazzo S, Viero P, Finazzi G, et al. Incidence and risk factors for thrombotic complications in a historical cohort of 100 patients with essential thrombocythemia. J Clin Oncol 1990;8:556–62.
49. Michiels JJ, Abels J, Steketee J, et al. Erythromelalgia caused by platelet-mediated arteriolar inflammation and thrombosis in thrombocythemia. Ann Intern Med 1985;102:466–71.
50. van Genderen PJ, Michiels JJ. Erythromelalgia: a pathognomonic microvascular thrombotic complication in essential thrombocythemia and polycythemia vera. Semin Thromb Hemost 1997;23:357–63.
51. Randi ML, Stocco F, Rossi C, et al. Thrombosis and hemorrhage in thrombocytosis: evaluation of a large cohort of patients (357 cases). J Med 1991;22:213–23.
52. Colombi M, Radaelli F, Zocchi L, Maiolo AT. Thrombotic and hemorrhagic complications in essential thrombocythemia. A retrospective study of 103 patients. Cancer 1991;67:2926–30.
53. Budde U, van Genderen PJ. Acquired von Willebrand disease in patients with high platelet counts. Semin Thromb Hemost 1997;23:425–31.
54. Rozman C, Giralt M, Feliu E, et al. Life expectancy of patients with chronic nonleukemic myeloproliferative disorders. Cancer 1991;67:2658–63.
55. Ruggeri M, Finazzi G, Tosetto A, et al. No treatment for low-risk thrombocythaemia: results from a prospective study. Br J Haematol 1998;103:772–7.
56. Tefferi A, Murphy S. Current opinion in essential thrombocythemia: pathogenesis, diagnosis, and management. Blood Rev 2001;15:121–31.
57. Watson KV, Key N. Vascular complications of essential thrombocythaemia: a link to cardiovascular risk factors. Br J Haematol 1993;83:198–203.
58. Jantunen R, Juvonen E, Ikkala E, et al. The predictive value of vascular risk factors and gender for the development of thrombotic complications in essential thrombocythemia. Ann Hematol 2001;80:74–8.
59. Bucalossi A, Marotta G, Bigazzi C, et al. Reduction of antithrombin III, protein C, and protein S levels and activated protein C resistance in polycythemia vera and essential thrombocythemia patients with thrombosis. Am J Hematol 1996;52:14–20.
60. Landolfi R, Marchioli R, Kutti J, et al. Efficacy and safety of low-dose aspirin in polycythemia vera. N Engl J Med 2004;350:114–24.
61. van Genderen PJ, Mulder PG, Waleboer M, et al. Prevention and treatment of thrombotic complications in essential thrombocythaemia: efficacy and safety of aspirin. Br J Haematol 1997;97:179–84.
62. Cortelazzo S, Finazzi G, Ruggeri M, et al. Hydroxyurea for patients with essential thrombocythemia and a high risk of thrombosis. N Engl J Med 1995;332:1132–6.
63. Storen EC, Tefferi A. Long-term use of anagrelide in young patients with essential thrombocythemia. Blood 2001;97:863–6.
64. Regev A, Stark P, Blickstein D, Lahav M. Thrombotic complications in essential thrombocythemia with relatively low platelet counts. Am J Hematol 1997;56:168–72.
65. Randi ML, Fabris F, Girolami A. Second malignancies in patients with essential thrombocythaemia. Br J Haematol 2002;116:923–4.
66. Finazzi G, Ruggeri M, Rodeghiero F, Barbui T. Efficacy and safety of long-term use of hydroxyurea in young patients with essential thrombocythemia and a high risk of thrombosis. Blood 2003;101:3749.
67. Anagrelide, a therapy for thrombocythemic states: experience in 577 patients. Anagrelide Study Group. Am J Med 1992;92:69–76.
68. Mazzucconi MG, Francesconi M, Chistolini A, et al. Pipobroman therapy of essential thrombocythemia. Scand J Haematol 1986;37:306–9.
69. Elliott MA, Tefferi A. Interferon-alpha therapy in polycythemia vera and essential thrombocythemia. Semin Thromb Hemost 1997;23:463.
70. Alvarado Y, Cortes J, Verstovsek S, et al. Pilot study of pegylated interferon-alpha 2b in patients with essential thrombocythemia. Cancer Chemother Pharmacol 2003;51:81–6.

71. Tsimberidou AM, Giles FJ. Essential thrombocythemia (ET): moving from palliation to cure. Hematology 2002;7:315–23.
72. Wright CA, Tefferi A. A single institutional experience with 43 pregnancies in essential thrombocythemia. Eur J Haematol 2001;66:152–9.
73. Michiels JJ. Essential thrombocythaemia is not associated with postpartum thrombosis or an increased risk of venous thromboembolism. Thrombocythemia Vera Study Group and European Working Group on Myeloproliferative Disorders. Eur J Haematol 1998;60:138–9.
74. Diav-Citrin O. Hydroxyurea use during pregnancy: a case report in sickle cell disease and review of the literature. Am J Hematol 1999;60:148–50.
75. Anderson RE, Hioshino T, Yammamoto T. Myelofibrosis with myeloid metaplasia in survivors of the atomic bomb in Hiroshima. Ann Intern Med 1964;60:1–18.
76. Tondel M, Persson B, Carstensen J. Myelofibrosis and benzene exposure. Occup Med (Lond) 1995;45:51–2.
77. Jacobson RJ, Salo A, Fialkow PJ. Agnogenic myeloid metaplasia: a clonal proliferation of hematopoietic stem cells with secondary myelofibrosis. Blood 1978;51:189–94.
78. Wang JC, Lang HD, Lichter S, et al. Cytogenetic studies of bone marrow fibroblasts cultured from patients with myelofibrosis and myeloid metaplasia. Br J Haematol 1992;80:184–8.
79. McCarthy DM. Fibrosis of the bone marrow: content and causes. Br J Haematol 1985;59:1–7.
80. Mesa RA, Hanson CA, Yoon SY, et al. Clinical relevance of increased angiogenesis in essential thrombocythemia: a clinicopathologic study of 164 patients [abstract]. Blood 2000;96:743a.
81. Tefferi A. Myelofibrosis with myeloid metaplasia. N Engl J Med 2000;342:1255–65.
82. Chagraoui H, Tulliez M, Smayra T, et al. Stimulation of osteoprotegerin production is responsible for osteosclerosis in mice overexpressing TPO. Blood 2003;101:2983–9.
83. Yan XQ, Lacey D, Hill D, et al. A model of myelofibrosis and osteosclerosis in mice induced by overexpressing thrombopoietin (mpl ligand): reversal of disease by bone marrow transplantation. Blood 1996;88:402–9.
84. Vannucchi AM, Bianchi L, Cellai C, et al. Development of myelofibrosis in mice genetically impaired for GATA-1 expression (GATA-1(low) mice). Blood 2002;100:1123–32.
85. Fisher C, Steensma D, Janmohamed R, et al. Absence of mutations in the key megakaryocyte transcriptional regulator FOG-1 in patients with idiopathic myelofibrosis. Br J Haematol 2004;126:750–2.
86. Tefferi A, Mesa RA, Schroeder G, et al. Cytogenetic findings and their clinical relevance in myelofibrosis with myeloid metaplasia. Br J Haematol 2001;113:1–10.
87. Gaidano G, Guerrasio A, Serra A, et al. Mutations in the P53 and RAS family genes are associated with tumor progression of BCR/ABL negative chronic myeloproliferative disorders. Leukemia 1993;7:946–53.
88. Jones LC, Tefferi A, Wachsman W, et al. Detection of aberrant signaling pathways in CD34+ cells from patients with myelofibrosis with myeloid metaplasia using oligonucleotide microarrays. Blood 2001;98:626a.
89. O'Keane JC, Wolf BC, Neiman RS. The pathogenesis of splenic extramedullary hematopoiesis in metastatic carcinoma. Cancer 1989;63:1539–43.
90. Newton KL, McNeeley SG Jr, Novick M. Extramedullary hematopoiesis presenting as a pelvic mass in a patient with beta-thalassemia intermedia. JAMA 1983;250:2178–9.
91. Steensma DP, Hanson CA, Letendre L, Tefferi A. Myelodysplasia with fibrosis: a distinct entity? Leuk Res 2001;25:829–38.
92. Tefferi A, Diehn FE, Baek J, et al. Clinical and bone marrow histologic correlates of peripheral blood CD34 count in myelofibrosis with myeloid metaplasia. Blood 2001;98:627a.
93. Barosi G, Viarengo G, Pecci A, et al. Diagnostic and clinical relevance of the number of circulating CD34(+) cells in myelofibrosis with myeloid metaplasia. Blood 2001;98:3249–55.
94. Mesa RA, Li CY, Schroeder G, Tefferi A. Clinical correlates of splenic histopathology and splenic karyotype in myelofibrosis with myeloid metaplasia. Blood 2001;97:3665–7.
95. Jaroch MT, Broughan TA, Hermann RE. The natural history of splenic infarction. Surgery 1986;100:743–50.
96. Price F, Bell H. Spinal cord compression due to extramedullary hematopoiesis. Successful treatment in a patient with long-standing myelofibrosis. JAMA 1985;253:2876–7.
97. Elliott MA, Tefferi A. Splenic irradiation in myelofibrosis with myeloid metaplasia: a review. Blood Rev 1999;13:163–70.
98. Steensma DP, Hook CC, Stafford SL, Tefferi A. Low-dose, single-fraction, whole-lung radiotherapy for pulmonary hypertension associated with myelofibrosis with myeloid metaplasia. Br J Haematol 2002;118:813–6.
99. Loewy G, Mathew A, Distenfeld A. Skin manifestation of agnogenic myeloid metaplasia. Am J Hematol 1994;45:167–70.
100. Cervantes F, Barosi G, Demory JL, et al. Myelofibrosis with myeloid metaplasia in young individuals: disease characteristics, prognostic factors and identification of risk groups. Br J Haematol 1998;102:684–90.
101. Barosi G. Myelofibrosis with myeloid metaplasia: diagnostic definition and prognostic classification for clinical studies and treatment guidelines. J Clin Oncol 1999;17:2954–70.
102. Dupriez B, Morel P, Demory JL, et al. Prognostic factors in agnogenic myeloid metaplasia: a report on 195 cases with a new scoring system. Blood 1996;88:1013–8.
103. Tefferi A, Mesa RA, Schroeder G, et al. Cytogenetic findings and their clinical relevance in myelofibrosis with myeloid metaplasia. Br J Haematol 2001;113:763–71.
104. Levy V, Bourgarit A, Delmer A, et al. Treatment of agnogenic myeloid metaplasia with danazol: a report of four cases. Am J Hematol 1996;53:239–41.
105. Rodriguez JN, Martino ML, Dieguez JC, Prados D. rHuEpo for the treatment of anemia in myelofibrosis with myeloid metaplasia. Experience in 6 patients and meta-analytical approach. Haematologica 1998;83:616–21.
106. Lofvenberg E, Wahlin A. Management of polycythaemia vera, essential thrombocythaemia and myelofibrosis with hydroxyurea. Eur J Haematol 1988;41:375–81.
107. Yoon SY, Li CY, Mesa RA, Tefferi A. Bone marrow effects of anagrelide therapy in patients with myelofibrosis with myeloid metaplasia. Br J Haematol 1999;106:682–8.
108. Marchetti M, Barosi G, Balestri F, et al. Low-dose thalidomide ameliorates cytopenias and splenomegaly in myelofibrosis with myeloid metaplasia: a phase II trial. J Clin Oncol 2004;22:424–31.
109. Mesa RA, Steensma DP, Pardanani A, et al. A phase 2 trial of combination low-dose thalidomide and prednisone for the treatment of myelofibrosis with myeloid metaplasia. Blood 2003;101:2534–41.
110. Tefferi A, Elliot MA. Serious myeloproliferative reactions associated with the use of thalidomide in myelofibrosis with myeloid metaplasia. Blood 2000;96:4007.
111. Mesa RA, Elliott MA, Schroeder G, Tefferi A. Durable responses to thalidomide-based drug therapy for myelofibrosis with myeloid metaplasia. Mayo Clin Proc 2004;79:883–9.
112. Steensma DP, Mesa RA, Li CY, et al. Etanercept, a soluble tumor necrosis factor receptor, palliates constitutional symptoms in patients with myelofibrosis with myeloid metaplasia: results of a pilot study. Blood 2002;99:2252–4.
113. Tefferi A, Mesa RA, Nagorney DM, et al. Splenectomy in myelofibrosis with myeloid metaplasia: a single-institution experience with 223 patients. Blood 2000;95:2226–33.
114. Elliott MA, Mesa RA, Tefferi A. Adverse events after imatinib mesylate therapy. N Engl J Med 2002;346:712–3.
115. Soll E, Massumoto C, Clift RA, et al. Relevance of marrow fibrosis in bone marrow transplantation: a retrospective analysis of engraftment. Blood 1995;86:4667–73.
116. Devine SM, Hoffman R, Verma A, et al. Allogeneic blood cell transplantation following reduced-intensity conditioning is effective therapy for older patients with myelofibrosis with myeloid metaplasia. Blood 2002;99:2255–8.
117. Guardiola P, Anderson JE, Gluckman E. Myelofibrosis with myeloid metaplasia. N Engl J Med 2000;343:659; discussion 659–60.
118. Daly A, Song K, Nevill T, et al. Stem cell transplantation for myelofibrosis: a report from two Canadian centers. Bone Marrow Transplant 2003;32:35–40.
119. Deeg HJ, Gooley TA, Flowers ME, et al. Allogeneic hematopoietic stem cell transplantation for myelofibrosis. Blood 2003;102:3912–8.
120. Anderson JE, Tefferi A, Craig F, et al. Myeloablation and autologous peripheral blood stem cell rescue result in hematologic and clinical responses in patients with myeloid metaplasia with myelofibrosis. Blood 2001;98:586–93.
121. Ania BJ, Suman VJ, Sobell JL, et al. Trends in the incidence of polycythemia vera among Olmsted County, Minnesota residents, 1935-1989. Am J Hematol 1994;47:89–93.
122. Najean Y, Rain JD, Billotey C. Epidemiological data in polycythaemia vera: a study of 842 cases. Hematol Cell Ther 1998;40:159–65.
123. Polycythemia vera: the natural history of 1213 patients followed for 20 years. Gruppo Italiano Studio Policitemia. Ann Intern Med 1995;123:656–64.
124. Najean Y, Mugnier P, Dresch C, Rain JD. Polycythaemia vera in young people: an analysis of 58 cases diagnosed before 40 years. Br J Haematol 1987;67:285–91.
125. Modan B, Kallner H, Zemer D, Yoran C. A note on the increased risk of polycythemia vera in Jews. Blood 1971;37:172–6.
126. Brubaker LH, Wasserman LR, Goldberg JD, et al. Increased prevalence of polycythemia vera in parents of patients on Polycythemia Vera Study Group protocols. Am J Hematol 1984;16:367–73.
127. Jefferson JA, Escudero E, Hurtado ME, et al. Excessive erythrocytosis, chronic mountain sickness, and serum cobalt levels. Lancet 2002;359:407–8.
128. Adamson JW, Fialkow PJ, Murphy S, et al. Polycythemia vera: stem-cell and probable clonal origin of the disease. N Engl J Med 1976;295:913–6.
129. Lundberg LG, Lerner R, Sundelin P, et al. Bone marrow in polycythemia vera, chronic myelocytic leukemia, and myelofibrosis has an increased vascularity. Am J Pathol 2000;157:15–9.
130. Casadevall N, Vainchenker W, Lacombe C, et al. Erythroid progenitors in polycythemia vera: demonstration of their hypersensitivity to erythropoietin using serum free cultures. Blood 1982;59:447–51.
131. Dai CH, Krantz SB, Dessypris EN, et al. Polycythemia vera. II. Hypersensitivity of bone marrow erythroid, granulocyte-macrophage, and megakaryocyte progenitor cells to interleukin-3 and granulocyte-macrophage colony-stimulating factor. Blood 1992;80:891–9.
132. Cotes PM, Dore CJ, Yin JA, et al. Determination of serum immunoreactive erythropoietin in the investigation of erythrocytosis. N Engl J Med 1986;315:283–7.
133. Messinezy M, Westwood NB, El-Hemaidi I, et al. Serum erythropoietin values in erythrocytoses and in primary thrombocythaemia. Br J Haematol 2002;117:47–53.
134. Kralovics R, Indrak K, Stopka T, et al. Two new EPO receptor mutations—truncated EPO receptors are most frequently associated with primary familial and congenital polycythemias. Blood 1997;90:2057–61.
135. Hess G, Rose P, Gamm H, et al. Molecular analysis of the erythropoietin receptor system in patients with polycythaemia vera. Br J Haematol 1994;88:794–802.
136. Means RT Jr, Krantz SB, Sawyer ST, Gilbert HS. Erythropoietin receptors in polycythemia vera. J Clin Invest 1989;84:1340–4.
137. Mirza AM, Ezzat S, Axelrad AA. Insulin-like growth factor binding protein-1 is elevated in patients with polycythemia vera and stimulates erythroid burst formation in vitro. Blood 1997;89:1862–9.
138. Wickrema A, Chen F, Namin F, et al. Defective expression of the SHP-1 phosphatase in polycythemia vera. Exp Hematol 1999;27:1124–32.
139. Roder S, Steimle C, Meinhardt G, Pahl HL. STAT3 is constitutively active in some patients with polycythemia rubra vera. Exp Hematol 2001;29:694–702.
140. Silva M, Richard C, Benito A, et al. Expression of Bcl-x in erythroid precursors from patients with polycythemia vera. N Engl J Med 1998;338:564–71.
141. Diez-Martin JL, Graham DL, Petitt RM, Dewald GW. Chromosome studies in 104 patients with polycythemia vera. Mayo Clin Proc 1991;66:287–99.
142. Rege-Cambrin G, Mecucci C, Tricot G, et al. A chromosomal profile of polycythemia vera. Cancer Genet Cytogenet 1987;25:233–45.
143. Temerinac S, Klippel S, Strunck E, et al. Cloning of PRV-1, a novel member of the uPAR receptor superfamily, which is overexpressed in polycythemia rubra vera. Blood 2000;95:2569–76.
144. Berlin NI. Diagnosis and classification of the polycythemias. Semin Hematol 1975;12:339–51.
145. Tefferi A, Fonseca R. Selective serotonin reuptake inhibitors are effective in the treatment of polycythemia vera-associated pruritus. Blood 2002;99:2627.
146. Gilbert HS, Warner RR, Wasserman LR. A study of histamine in myeloproliferative disease. Blood 1966;28:795–806.
147. Rachmilewitz B, Manny N, Rachmilewitz M. The transcobalamins in polycythaemia vera. Scand J Haematol 1977;19:453–62.
148. Michiels JJ, Juvonen E. Proposal for revised diagnostic criteria of essential thrombocythemia and polycythemia vera by the Thrombocythemia Vera Study Group. Semin Thromb Hemost 1997;23:339–47.
149. Fairbanks VF, Tefferi A. Normal ranges for packed cell vol-

ume and hemoglobin concentration in adults: relevance to apparent polycythemia. Eur J Haematol 2000;65:285–96.
150. Moliterno AR, Hankins WD, Spivak JL. Impaired expression of the thrombopoietin receptor by platelets from patients with polycythemia vera. N Engl J Med 1998;338:572–80.
151. Tefferi A, Yoon SY, Li CY. Immunohistochemical staining for megakaryocyte c-Mpl may complement morphologic distinction between polycythemia vera and secondary erythrocytosis. Blood 2000;96:771–2.
152. Najean Y, Schlageter MH, Toubert ME, Podgorniak MP. Radioimmunoassay of immunoreactive erythropoietin as a clinical tool for the classification of polycythemias. Nouv Rev Fr Hematol 1990;32:237.
153. Ellis JT, Peterson P, Geller SA, Rappaport H. Studies of the bone marrow in polycythemia vera and the evolution of myelofibrosis and second hematologic malignancies. Semin Hematol 1986;23:144–55.
154. Zanjani ED, Lutton JD, Hoffman R, Wasserman LR. Erythroid colony formation by polycythemia vera bone marrow in vitro. Dependence on erythropoietin. J Clin Invest 1977;59:841–8.
155. Shih LY, Lee CT. Identification of masked polycythemia vera from patients with idiopathic marked thrombocytosis by endogenous erythroid colony assay. Blood 1994;83:744–8.
156. Bock O, Serinsoz E, Neusch M, et al. The polycythaemia rubra vera-1 gene is constitutively expressed by bone marrow cells and does not discriminate polycythaemia vera from reactive and other chronic myeloproliferative disorders. Br J Haematol 2003;123:472–4.
157. Berk PD, Wasserman LR, Fruchtman SM, Goldberg JD. Treatment of polycythemia vera: a summary of clinical trials conducted by the Polycythemia Vera Study Group. In: Wasserman LR, editor. Polycythemia vera and the myeloproliferative disorders. London: W. B. Saunders; 1995. p. 166–94.
158. Orlandi E, Castelli G, Brusamolino E, et al. Hemorrhagic and thrombotic complications in polycythemia vera. A clinical study. Haematologica 1989;74:45–9.
159. Silverstein MN. The evolution into and the treatment of late stage polycythemia vera. Semin Hematol 1976;13:79–84.
160. Rosenthal N. Course of polycythemia. Arch Intern Med 1938;62:903–17.
161. Lawrence JH. The nature and treatment of polycythemia. Medicine 1953;33:323–88.
162. Thomas DJ, du Boulay GH, Marshall J, et al. Cerebral blood-flow in polycythaemia. Lancet 1977;2:161–3.
163. Wade JPH. Transport of oxygen to the brain in patients with elevated hematocrit values before and after venesection. Brain 1983;106:513–23.
164. Mohri H. Acquired von Willebrand disease in patients with polycythemia rubra vera. Am J Hematol 1987;26:135–46.
165. Tartaglia AP, Goldberg JD, Berk PD, Wasserman LR. Adverse effects of antiaggregating platelet therapy in the treatment of polycythemia vera. Semin Hematol 1986;23:172–6.
166. Treatment of polycythaemia vera by radiophosphorus or busulphan: a randomized trial. "Leukemia and Hematosarcoma" Cooperative Group, European Organization for Research on Treatment of Cancer (E.O.R.T.C.). Br J Cancer 1981;44:75–80.
167. Fruchtman SM, Mack K, Kaplan ME, et al. From efficacy to safety—a Polycythemia Vera Study Group report on hydroxyurea in patients with polycythemia vera. Semin Hematol 1997;34:17–23.
168. Steensma DP, Harrison CN, Tefferi A. Hydroxyurea-associated platelet count oscillations in polycythemia vera: a report of four new cases and a review. Leuk Lymphoma 2001;42:1243–53.
169. Najean Y, Rain JD. Treatment of polycythemia vera—the use of hydroxyurea and pipobroman in 292 patients under the age of 65 years. Blood 1997;90:3370–7.
170. Silver RT. Interferon alfa—effects of long-term treatment for polycythemia vera. Semin Hematol 1997;34:40–50.
171. Lengfelder E, Berger U, Hehlmann R. Interferon alpha in the treatment of polycythemia vera. Ann Hematol 2000;79:103–9.
172. Silverstein MN, Petitt RM, Solberg LA Jr, et al. Anagrelide: a new drug for treating thrombocytosis. N Engl J Med 1988;318:1292–4.
173. Mazur EM, Rosmarin AG, Sohl PA, et al. Analysis of the mechanism of anagrelide-induced thrombocytopenia in humans. Blood 1992;79:1931–7.
174. Solberg LA, Tefferi A, Oles KJ, et al. The effects of anagrelide on human megakaryocytopoiesis. Br J Haematol 1997;99:174–80.
175. Spencer CM, Brogden RN. Anagrelide. A review of its pharmacodynamic and pharmacokinetic properties, and therapeutic potential in the treatment of thrombocythaemia. Drugs 1994;47:809–22.

Section 35

NEOPLASMS IN AIDS

122

Neoplasms in Acquired Immunodeficiency Syndrome

David T. Scadden, MD

Immunodeficiency of multiple etiologies is associated with an increased risk of malignancy, particularly lymphoma. The risk is variable, dependent on the severity and extent of the immunologic abnormality. In the setting of the acquired immunodeficiency syndrome (AIDS) secondary to human immunodeficiency virus type 1 (HIV-1) infection, the range of tumor types is more extensive. Yet, the tumors are generally associated with oncogenic viruses and may be considered secondary, opportunistic neoplasms. Etiologic factors contributing to them include poor control of oncogenic viruses, altered cytokine regulation owing to HIV effects on immune cells and tissue stimulation from other AIDS-associated events. The interplay of immunity, infection and oncogenesis is central to AIDS-related malignancies.[1]

The spectrum of the tumor types seen in the context of immunodeficiency extends beyond that of lymphoma, but is quite limited. There appears to be little interaction between the conditions that predispose to the emergence of epithelial malignancies seen in the general population and immunodeficiency. Rather, immunodeficiency tumors represent a narrow subset of neoplasms, some of which are seen with only very low incidence in the general population. For example, primary central nervous system (PCNS) lymphoma and Kaposi's sarcoma are extremely rare entities in all but the immunodeficient population, where they compose a large proportion of tumors. In addition, the incidence of specific tumor types does vary according to the immunodeficient state. Non-Hodgkin's lymphoma is a common theme among all the immunodeficiencies, yet in AIDS, there is a broader spectrum of histologic subtypes than are seen in any other immunodeficiency. Kaposi's sarcoma is increased in subgroups of patients with HIV-related and pharmacologically induced immunodeficiency. Cutaneous tumors are common in many immunodeficient states, but the increase in squamous cell tumors of the skin is higher in the postsolid-organ-transplantation population than in those with HIV-related immunodeficiency. In the latter, papillomavirus-related squamous cell neoplasia of the anogenital region predominates (Table 122-1).

Shared among the tumors related to immunodeficient states is the frequent association with an infectious pathogen. The presence of Epstein–Barr virus (EBV) in immunodeficiency-related lymphomas is well known and likely a result of the direct stimulation that virus provides to B-cell proliferation. In the absence of effective immunologic targeting of cells expressing EBV latency gene products, the overgrowth of cells may proceed unchecked, with the subsequent emergence of a transformed cell. This model for the direct ability of viruses to induce cell proliferation is a paradigm that may be applied to papillomavirus-related tumors as well. However, the model is less easily applied to the Kaposi's sarcoma-associated herpesvirus (KSHV)-related tumors. The tumors associated with KSHV are more varied and are of less clear pathophysiologic relationship to viral gene products—issues that are discussed in greater depth in sections that follow. In general, the tumors that do emerge in immunodeficiency are those in which a secondary pathogen can be implicated (Table 122-2). In that sense, the concept of inadequate immunologic control provides a unifying mechanism, and the tumors may be considered as opportunistic malignancies, much the way in which specific infections are considered opportunistic infections. Indeed, the opportunistic malignancies of the immunocompromised patient represent the overlap between infectious diseases and oncology and provide unique insight into the intersection of immune function and tumor development.

Table 122-1 Tumor Types with Increased Incidence in HIV Disease

Definite
Kaposi's sarcoma
Non-Hodgkin's lymphoma
Squamous cell neoplasia
Hodgkin's disease
Leiomyosarcoma (in children)
Plasmacytoma
Possible
Seminoma

Table 122-2 Secondary Virus Infections Associated with AIDS-Related Malignancies

Virus	Tumor
EBV	NHL (PCNS; some systemic ARL; oropharyngeal T cell)
	HD
	Leiomyosarcoma (children)
KSHV	KS
	NHL (PEL)
HPV	Squamous cell neoplasia

ARL = AIDS-related lymphoma; EBV = Epstein–Barr virus; HD = Hodgkin's disease; HPV = human papillomavirus; KS = Kaposi's sarcoma; KSHV = Kaposi's sarcoma herpesvirus; NHL = non-Hodgkin's lymphoma; PCNS = primary central nervous system; PEL = primary effusion lymphoma.

EPIDEMIOLOGY

The spectrum of tumors in the context of HIV-1 infection varies on the basis of risk group and is substantially affected by the use of potent or highly active antiretroviral therapy (HAART).

Pre-HAART The use of HAART is largely restricted to the developed world and did not become available until 1996, with the introduction of the protease-inhibitor class of anti-HIV medications. Widespread use of protease inhibitors rapidly occurred in the United States, Western Europe, and Australia, altering the death rate and complication rate of HIV disease. The spectrum of opportunistic diseases also changed,[2] with an impact on malignant disease, discussed below in the section "Post-HAART." Given the lack of access to HAART in much of the developing world, the unclear durability of HAART efficacy, and the number of patients unable to take or having failed HAART, the profile of AIDS-related malignancies in the pre-HAART era is still of considerable importance.

One of the first manifestations of the AIDS epidemic was the cluster of cases of a rare malignancy among homosexual men in United States coastal cities. That tumor, Kaposi's sarcoma (KS), was identified as an AIDS-defining illness with the first attempt at classifying the immunodeficiency syndrome by the Centers for Disease Control and Prevention (CDC).[3] The prevalence of KS was documented as approximately 20% early in the AIDS epidemic, but clearly was noted to be highest among patients whose risk factor for HIV transmission was men having sex with men.[4] KS prevalence was substantially lower in the groups infected by blood products or through parenteral drug use.[5] Subsequent behavioral studies indicated that specific types of sexual practice, including promiscuity and oral–fecal contact,[6] had the highest risk and substantiated the impression that KS might be a manifestation of a secondary, transmissible pathogen. Indeed, it was strong epidemiologic data that galvanized efforts to identify a pathogen and that led to the molecular cloning of KSHV.[7]

The second most common malignancy, which was recognized in 1984 to be increased among young homosexual men, was non-Hodgkin's lymphoma. This disease was added to the list of AIDS-defining complications in the first revision of the CDC criteria for AIDS. It was noted that the lymphomas that occurred in this population were generally of high-grade histology and followed extremely aggressive clinical courses. Unlike KS, this complication was much more broadly based in the risk groups for HIV infection. All groups had a high relative risk, estimated to be approximately 60-fold above that of the general population.[6,8–10] Subsets of infected individuals have been noted to have somewhat greater or lesser risk, such as the hemophiliac population, in which at least one study has noted an increased risk.[6,10] Similarly, it has been noted that risk among intravenous drug users or those from the Caribbean basin may be lower, but concern about confounding issues of care and surveillance complicate that analysis. However, the potential for important cofactors of lymphomagenesis within these subsets remains, and attention to this possibility may yield important information about the process of lymphocyte transformation.

The third most common oncologic complication of HIV disease is anogenital squamous cell neoplasms. These are invariably associated with human papillomavirus (HPV) infection of oncogenic serotype.[11,12] The impact of antiretroviral therapy on these neoplasms is at present unclear, but with the improved survival of patients with HIV disease, it is considered likely that HPV-related neoplasms will become increasingly problematic.

Post-HAART The introduction of HAART has resulted in profound and dramatic changes in the nature of HIV disease. The inexorable decline in immune function and its attendant ravaging secondary infections and tumors in many cases is stopped and indeed reversed when combination therapy with protease inhibitors is introduced. The improvement in those patients with advanced disease has led to widespread use of the agents, including among those individuals who have recently acquired HIV-1 infection. The result has been a precipitous decline in the rate of death from AIDS in populations with access to the medications. Although death and debility from AIDS has decreased dramatically, there has not been a similar decline in new cases of HIV infection. Therefore, the total population with HIV infection in the West is rising, and those infected are living longer; globally, the epidemic goes unabated. Some changes in the epidemiology of malignancies in HIV infection have been immediately evident since HAART was introduced, but the impact of longer periods of more modest immune dysfunction or even of the antiretroviral drugs themselves remains to be fully defined.

An observation immediately evident in the clinical care of patients with advanced HIV disease was the regression of KS following successful HIV suppression on HAART. The impact on new cases of KS was also rapidly noticeable, and epidemiologic data have substantiated the magnitude of those clinically apparent effects. Multiple studies from sites in the United States, Europe, and Australia indicate the widespread decline in KS, with estimates of decline in incidence as high as 80-fold.[13–15]

As with KS, changes in the incidence of primary central nervous system (CNS) lymphoma are dramatic. Although this complication of far-advanced HIV disease was much less common than KS, and its decline was therefore less well documented, the impact in clinical terms has been comparable in magnitude. Cases are rarely seen except among those who have failed or not been receiving antiretroviral therapy. This is a complication of severe immune suppression that, like the post-transplantation setting, is virtually uniformly associated with EBV detectable in tumor tissue. In general, the EBV latency genes expressed in these tumors are type III or those of lymphoproliferative disease (*EBNA1-6*, *LMP1*, and *LMP2*).[16,17] These and other features distinguish PCNS lymphoma from other AIDS-related lymphomas and may be the basis for clear differences in the impact of HAART.

The incidence of systemic AIDS-related lymphomas appears to be more modestly affected by the introduction of HAART and is approximately two- to threefold reduced.[18] One large study involved a cohort of 8,500 HIV-positive individuals across much of Europe.[19] The incidence of all subtypes of lymphoma in this observational study was significantly reduced after the use of combination antiretroviral therapy was commonplace (March 1999), as compared with those followed prior to the introduction of potent antiretroviral therapy (September 1995). Similarly, an international multicohort study found a reduction of approximately threefold following the introduction of HAART.[20] Of note, this series assessed subtypes of lymphomas and observed the greatest difference in immunoblastic and PCNS lymphoma. Burkitt's lymphoma and Hodgkin's disease appear to be largely unaffected.[20,21] The changes evident within only some lymphoma subsets does highlight biologic differences between these tumor types and suggests differential immune participation in tumor development.

KAPOSI'S SARCOMA

It was the announcement of clustered cases of KS in Los Angeles that made headlines and first brought the AIDS epidemic to public awareness in 1982. Previously, KS was regarded as a tumor that generally had an indolent course in elderly men of Mediterranean extraction, but which could be problematic in the context of immunosuppressive medication for organ transplantation. It was this latter association that helped focus attention on an immune alteration spreading among subcommunities in urban centers. Recognized as a common entity among homosexual men infected with HIV-1, but not among groups with other risk factors for HIV infection (such as blood product exposure),[5,21] it was long suspected as being related to a second cofactor.[22] A number of potential culprits were examined; none proved tenable until the identification of KSHV, also termed *human herpesvirus-8* (HHV-8). This virus was first recognized through the use of a genetic comparison of tissues from individuals with and without KS. A deoxyribonucleic acid (DNA) fragment was consistently noted that had partial homology with other members of the gamma-herpesvirus family.[7] This subset of the herpesviruses includes several viruses with oncogenic potential, such as EBV, associated with a number of tumors and *herpesvirus saimiri*, associated with the ability to transform T cells. Because of the company KSHV kept and the high frequency of detectable signature DNA sequences in KS lesions, this virus rapidly and justifiably became the focus of investigation for a pathophysiologic basis of KS.

Viral Epidemiology KSHV is a 165-kilobase (kb) double-stranded DNA virus[22] with features strongly supporting its causative role in clinical KS. There are data indicating that KSHV infection precedes tumor formation,[22,23] that populations with high seroprevalence for KSHV are also those with a high incidence of KS,[21] and that the virus infects cell types within tumors.[22]

The definition of prior exposure to KSHV depends on documentation of antibodies specifically reactive against the virus. There have been a number of assays that have been tested with variable results. Current data indicate seropositivity estimated at 3.5% in North America, up to 25% in the peoples of the Mediterranean basin, and up to 89% in sub-Saharan African populations.[24–26]

The much-suspected role of sexual transmission has been convincingly demonstrated in a longitudinal study of men in San Francisco followed over a 10-year period. Among exclusively heterosexual men, no KSHV seropositivity was detected; however, among homosexual or bisexual men, the incidence of seroconversion was linearly related to the number of male sexual-intercourse contacts.[27] Men who had more than 250 sexual partners in the preceding 2 years had a seropositivity rate of 65%. Yet, sexual transmission is not the exclusive basis of virus spread. KSHV can be identified in saliva, and it is thought that oral transmission can occur based on an association with "deep kissing" among homosexual men.[28] The higher incidence of KSHV seropositivity among family members in areas of endemic KS, and given that children are often infected in sub-Saharan Africa, nonsexual means of transmission occur, but the specific basis is still to be fully defined.

Clinical Manifestations KS characteristically appears as pigmented macular-papular lesions on mucocutaneous surfaces (Figures 122-1 and 122-2). It is typically violaceous or erythematous in hue and may be associated with an ecchymotic halo. Typically, the lesions are multifocal and do not have a predictable order or pace of progression. Lesions may present as solitary nodules or plaques, but may also occur in clusters or simultaneously in multiple well-segregated sites. Although classic or endemic KS often favors the lower extremities, the pattern of involvement is much less predictable in the setting of HIV infection. Virtually any mucocutaneous site may be involved. On the face, the ears and nose are often affected, resulting in profound disfigurement. In addition to the disabling cosmetic effects of KS, lesions do occasionally become thick, uncomfortable plaques and can ulcerate with possible superinfection. Lesions are not generally destructive, however. The integument or mucous membrane overlying a lesion is most often intact, and deep invasion into muscle or bone generally does not occur.

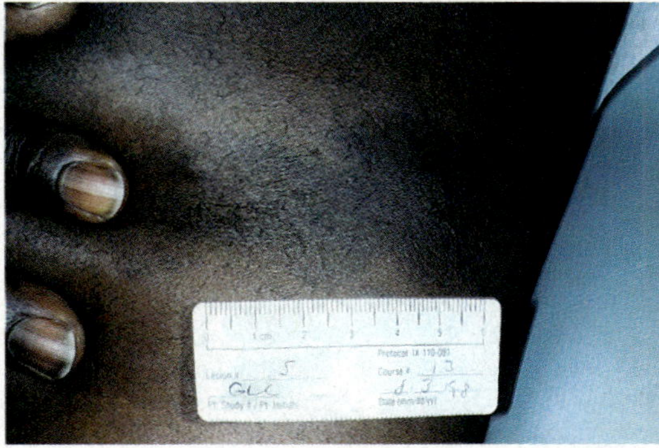

Figure 122-2 Kaposi's sarcoma in an African American male with HIV-1 infection. Skin tone can make the lesions less readily distinguishable from other cutaneous processes and quite distinct from the appearance in lighter-skinned individuals.

Edema often accompanies KS either locally or at a dependent site distal to KS lesions (Figure 122-3). The edema can be marked, with profound compromise of extremity mobility or occasionally with periorbital, peripubic, or genital edema. Two mechanisms are thought to contribute to the development of edema. One is the involvement of lymphatic vessels or lymph nodes with KS, thereby causing a mechanical obstruction to lymphatic flow. The other is the elaboration of permeability factors by KS lesions. The vessels that compose a KS lesion are themselves leaky with extravasation of plasma proteins and cells into surrounding soft tissue. In addition, the vascular endothelial growth factor (VEGF) produced by KS lesions can alter the integrity of surrounding otherwise-normal vessels, increasing their permeability, and thus, their contribution of fluid to interstitial fluid. The increased demand on lymphatic drainage and the compromised egress of lymph results in thickened skin locally and frank edema distally.

Involvement of organs other than lymph nodes occurs frequently. The most common site is the gastrointestinal (GI) tract, where mucosal-based lesions are commonly observed in the course of endoscopic procedures. The physiologic significance of these lesions is often minimal, however. Most patients will be unaware of GI involvement, and serendipitous observation of a mucosal KS lesion should not trigger a reflex to undertake aggressive therapy. However, there are some individuals for whom GI KS can be a symptomatic and even life-threatening complication. Massive bleeding has been observed, as has intussusception.

Pulmonary involvement may take several forms. Pleural-surface studding with KS lesions can result in pleural effusions, which are often bloody, but which do not have a characteristic set of diagnostic findings or cytologic abnormalities. Bronchial mucosa may be involved and, like GI mucosal surfaces, may be incidentally noted during bronchoscopic examination. The lesions are generally not destructive, but depending on location, they may be responsible for bronchial irritation, coughing, and hemoptysis. Involvement of the parenchyma of the lung occurs and is arguably the most serious complication of KS, because it is associated with life-threatening respiratory compromise and a high mortality rate if unsatisfactorily treated.[29] Radiographically, involvement often takes the appearance of peribronchiolar cuffing on computed tomography (CT). Pathologically, this infiltration may extend into fine interstitial tissue and affect airspace function. This results in either a patchy or diffuse reticulonodular appearance on x-rays. The diagnosis of KS involvement of the lung is often difficult to firmly establish short of parenchymal thoracoscopic or open biopsy. Bronchoscopy is useful in assessing alternative infectious explanations for clinical findings and may identify mucosal lesions. However, mucosal lesions do not necessarily coincide with parenchymal infiltration, and transbronchial biopsy is often unrevealing. Nuclear medicine scans have some usefulness, with a negative gallium scan and a positive thallium scan reportedly having a high specificity for pulmonary KS.[30,31] In some circumstances, the use of a therapeutic trial may also be helpful in establishing a presumptive diagnosis. If thorough microbiologic evaluation has been unrevealing, the chemotherapeutic agents discussed below have been well tolerated and associated with high rates of response, such that their use in select patients may be justified as a test for chemotherapy responsiveness of a parenchymal infiltrate. Such a strategy is generally reserved for those patients in whom (1) there is a diagnosis of KS already established from involvement of other sites, (2) there are no symptoms suggesting infec-

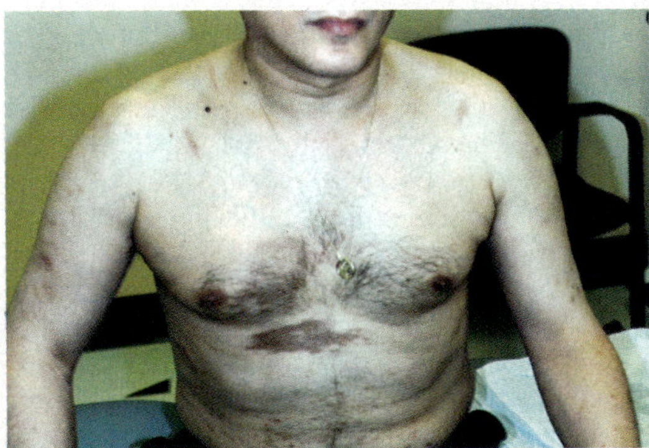

Figure 122-1 Cutaneous Kaposi's sarcoma in a white patient with advanced HIV disease. The violaceous plaques on the chest are of characteristic appearance. These lesions have entirely resolved on paclitaxel chemotherapy and antiretroviral medication.

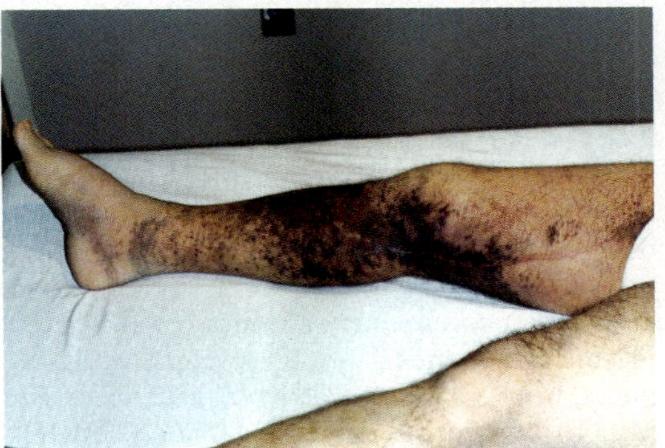

Figure 122-3 Lower extremity involvement by Kaposi's sarcoma can result in marked edema and limited mobility. This patient had pedal edema that had limited response to chemotherapy despite marked improvement in the circumferential Kaposi's sarcoma.

tion, or (3) aggressive assessment for infection is negative and there are no other contraindications to cytotoxic chemotherapy.

In addition to lung, GI tract, and lymph nodes, special sites of concern are areas of the upper airway. Involvement of the mucosa of the mouth, sinuses, pharynx, and larynx can result in distortion of soft tissues such that airway compromise or alteration of food ingestion can occur. These are lesions that generally respond rapidly to therapy and do not invade deeper structures. Therapeutic approaches are discussed below in the section "Treatment."

Given the common occurrence of involvement beyond the readily apparent skin or oral mucous membranes, extensive staging evaluations are often considered. Although the bulk of tumor does have some influence on prognosis, other characteristics of overall status of the patient's immune and general health dictate prognosis to a greater extent[32] (Table 122-3). The staging performed then is often based on clinical presentation, with radiographic studies limited to a chest x-ray unless symptoms dictate otherwise. If localizing symptoms do suggest organ involvement, then more extensive radiographic and procedural interventions are appropriate, but they cannot be recommended routinely. Criteria for staging do include assessment of the underlying HIV infection, and all patients should have a careful history regarding medications, other complications of HIV infections, and documentation of the CD4 count in the blood.

Establishing the diagnosis of KS generally depends on simple punch biopsy of the skin or a snip biopsy of mucosal surfaces. The CDC criteria for an AIDS-defining diagnosis of KS do not require histologic confirmation if assessment is by an experienced clinician. However, biopsy is recommended, given the differential diagnosis for nonblanching lesions resembling KS,[32] such as bacillary angiomatosis (usually caused by *Bartonella* infection, with increased frequency in advanced HIV-infection patients); hematoma; purpura; sarcoid plaques; lichen planus; pyogenic granuloma;[33] mycosis fungoides; secondary syphilis; pityriasis rosea; drug-related erythema multiforme; prurigo nodularis; nevi; vascular lesions of the phakomatoses; epithelioid hemangioendothelioma; angiosarcoma; melanoma; and basal cell carcinoma.

Table 122-3 Staging Classification for AIDS-Related Kaposi Sarcoma

	Good Risk[a]	Poor Risk (1)[b]
Tumor (T)	Small tumor burden with limited involvement of one or more Lymph nodes Skin Other[c]	Large tumor burden Oral Gastrointestinal Pulmonary Other visceral with involvement of tumor associated edema or ulceration
Immune system (I)	CD4$^+$ cells > 200 mm^3	CD4$^+$cells < 200 mm^3
Systematic illness (S)	No opportunistic infection (including thrush), or B symptoms[d]	History of opportunistic infection or thrush B symptoms[d] Other HIV-related illness (eg, NHL or other malignancy, neurologic disease, wasting syndrome)

HIV = human immunodeficiency virus; NHL = non-Hodgkin's lymphoma.

[a]All the parameters listed.

[b]Any of the parameters listed.

[c]Limited oral disease is confined to the palate and is not nodular.

[d]B symptoms are unexplained fever, night sweats, weight loss of more than 10% of body weight, or diarrhea persisting for more than 2 weeks. Modified from Krown SE, Metroka C, Wernz JC. Kaposi's sarcoma in the acquired immunodeficiency syndrome; a proposal for uniform evaluation, response, and staging criteria. J Clin Oncol 1989;7:1201–7.

Pathology and Pathogenesis The histologic appearance of KS belies its unclear association with the term sarcoma. No monomorphic array of mesenchymally derived cells is seen. Rather, the lesions are composed of endothelial cells lining ectatic vascular spaces surrounded by spindle cells of variable extent admixed with mononuclear immune cells and extravasated red blood cells. It is the red blood cells that provide the pigment to KS lesions and their breakdown that leads to the ecchymotic halo seen in actively growing lesions. The hemosiderin deposited locally yields a pigmented lesion that may remain even after effective therapy reverses the proliferative spindle and endothelial cell components. Cutaneous lesions are generally within the dermis. Deep invasion to muscle is generally not seen.

The origins of the endothelial and spindle cell components remain controversial. Recent reports indicate that the endothelial cells of KS lesions express the VEGF-C receptor characteristic of lymphatic endothelium[34] and do not have detectable nitric oxide synthase, generally present in vascular endothelium.[35] The finding that the spindle cell expresses the mannose-binding receptor and CD68 suggests that the origin may be a macrophage-like cell type, perhaps emanating from the sinuses of secondary lymphoid organs and circulating in the blood before ultimately assuming its role in a KS lesion.[36]

The difficulty in defining the cell of origin emanates from its complex histology and the limitations of the available in vitro or in vivo models. In vitro culture has been established for some cell types, and outgrowth of cell lines has been documented, although the relationship to the primary disease process is unclear. In vivo transplantation of KS tissue into immunodeficient mice has resulted in tumors, but these are of murine origin. The potential for cytokine elaboration driving lesion development was hypothesized, and studies have extensively characterized cytokine production by KS lesions.[37–40] The cytokines, particularly VEGF and basic fibroblast growth factor (bFGF), may play a role in the paracrine or autocrine sustenance of KS. Antibodies to bFGF block the proliferation of KS cells and prevent them from entering the S-phase of the cell cycle, even in the presence of exogenous growth factors like the interleukin (IL)-6–IL-6R complex, IL-10, tumor necrosis factor (TNF)-α, and oncostatin M.[41] But exogenous growth factors do not completely explain the phenotype and growth potential of KS cells, which overexpress the antiapoptotic *bcl-2* gene independently of any factors contained in conditioned medium from these cells.[42]

HHV-8 appears necessary for the induction of KS and is found in KS lesions regardless of whether the underlying context is HIV disease, organ transplantation, or endemic KS. However, the specific mechanism by which the virus participates in the oncogenic process is unclear and does not readily fit into paradigms established by other virus-related neoplastic disease. The latent genes implicated in EBV-induced transformation do not have homologs in KSHV. The genes of *Herpesvirus saimiri* (HVS), which are known to transform cells, have homology only in the genome of a KSHV gene, *K1*, that is capable of transforming an immortalized cell line.[43] However, this gene is not expressed in the latent phase of the KSHV life cycle. Similarly, a chemokine receptor-like KSHV gene product, ORF 74, is constitutively activated and is capable of transforming cells when transduced as a single gene, but it is also a lytic-phase gene.[44] Two other gene products, K9 (a homolog of the interferon regulatory factor family) and K12 (with no clear gene family homology), are capable of transforming cell lines when transduced but are not expressed in latent phase.[45–48] The lack of clear association with the latent phase would argue that these gene products are not transforming in *cis*, but whether they may transform in *trans* cannot be excluded. A number of other mechanisms, including those that may be capable of acting at a distance, have been raised as possibilities for KSHV. These include the chemokine-related gene products, vMIP-I (K6) and vMIP-II (K4), or the IL-6 homolog, K2. Each is capable of interacting with cognate receptors on target cells, either acting as agonists (K2 and K6) or antagonists (K4).[49,50] Finally, there are KSHV gene products that have antiapoptotic effects and that may enhance tumorigenicity. ORF 16 encodes a *bcl-2*–related gene product,[51] and ORF 71 (K131) encodes a functional member of the Fas-associated death domain-like IL-10–converting enzyme-inhibitory protein (FLIP) family of antiapoptotic genes.[52]

The vFLIP of KSHV protects cells from Fas-mediated cell death and can enhance tumor progression of cell lines transplanted in vivo. Thus, KSHV encodes a range of gene products with potential for altering the growth, death, and immunologic characteristics of infected cells. Which of these will be shown to play a dominant role in oncogenesis is not clear, but investigation into the process will no doubt lead to new insights into viral-induced tumors and will potentially open new avenues for therapeutic attack.

The prevalence of KS in populations that are HIV-infected, have undergone solid organ transplantation, are elderly and of Mediterranean extraction, or live in economically disadvantaged parts of tropical Africa suggests that expression of a KS disease phenotype requires a degree of immunosuppression. The advent of HAART for HIV infection treatment offers dramatic support to a central role for immune suppression: Complete remissions of cutaneous[53] and pulmonary KS are well recognized in the context of increases in CD4 count and declines in HIV load induced by HAART.[54]

Retrospective analysis of the incidence of KS among HIV-infected patients receiving antiherpesvirus medications has suggested a direct role of replicating KSHV in the pathologic process. In several studies, there was a decline in KS in the context of patients treated with ganciclovir[55–57] or foscarnet.[58] In one such treatment program, it was shown that those patients who received systemic ganciclovir had a lower incidence of KS compared with those in whom the drug was delivered by intraocular implant.[55] Therefore, suppression of replicating virus appears to lower the risk of KS. Although transformation is generally associated with the latent phase of herpesvirus infection, control of the lytic phase (the only time at which the antiherpesvirus medications have known activity) may limit the potential for transformation.

Control of virus by immunologic means also appears to be highly relevant to the risk of developing KS. It has long been known that there is an increased risk of KS in the context of multiple types of immunologic deficiency. The recent definition of epitopes of the virus that are recognized by cytotoxic T lymphocytes will allow for further definition of this important point and potentially lead to vaccine strategies. Although HIV-induced immunodeficiency is only one type of immune abnormality that may predispose to KS, the relative risk among the population co-infected with HIV and KSHV is strikingly high, which suggests the potential for interaction between the two viruses in the development of tumor. The tat gene product of the HIV-1 genome is of particular interest and affects KSHV replication itself,[59] as well as alters cytokine (IL-6)[60] or cytokine receptor expression in target cells, and leads to a proangiogenic effect.[61] Additive effects of HIV-1 and KSHV may thereby particularly increase the potential for development of KS.

Treatment Treatment of KS should be guided by the impact of the tumor on the patient.[62] The adage that KS is "a tumor that people die with rather than from" was generally applied to the endemic KS seen in the elderly. However, variability in the course of HIV-infected patients with KS and the lack of clear association of tumor control with mortality suggests that aggressive therapy may not always be an appropriate response to the diagnosis of KS. This is particularly true among patients with advanced HIV disease or untreated HIV disease. In that setting, the toxicity of cytotoxic therapy may be daunting, and the potential therapeutic effect of anti-HIV medications is considerable. Suppressing HIV replication is associated with a rise in CD4 count, with attendant improvement in immunologic function, and also reduction in whatever the direct contribution of HIV to the pathophysiology of KS might be. The net result is a high frequency of clinical improvement among patients with established KS and, at times, complete eradication, simply by the introduction of antiretroviral therapy. Therefore, for patients in whom the impact of KS is not threatening, a therapeutic trial of antiretroviral therapy alone is appropriate first-line therapy (Figure 122-4). In patients in whom a more aggressive "up-front" approach is warranted, attention to optimizing anti-HIV therapy is also a crucial parameter in the overall management of their oncologic care. Anti-HIV therapy is regarded as an important component of KS treatment of all patients with AIDS-associated KS. However, it should be recognized that not all patients will experience an improvement in their KS with anti-HIV medications, and that the improvement is generally slow, often noted only after 4 to 8 weeks of therapy. For those patients who have not had an improvement in KS by 12 weeks after initiation of anti-HIV therapy, it is unlikely that their disease will be controlled by that intervention alone.

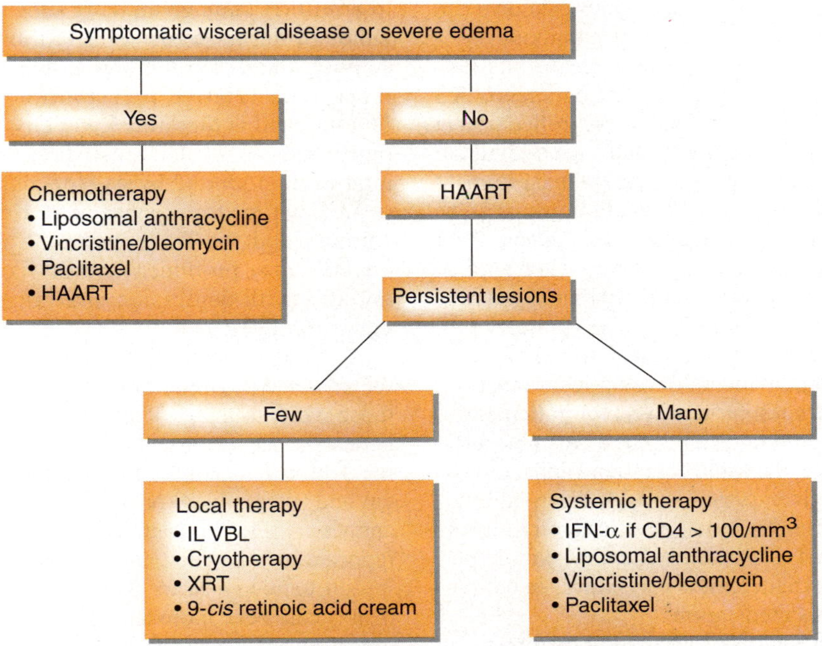

Figure 122-4 Treatment schema for patients with Kaposi's sarcoma. HAART = highly active antiretroviral therapy; IFN-α = interferon-α; IL = interleukin; VBL = vinblastine; XRT = radiation therapy.

In contrast to antiretroviral drugs, antiherpesvirus medications have a less-clear role in the management of KS. Although the studies mentioned above do indicate an impact of certain anticytomegalovirus drugs on KS, the overall impact is modest and does not offset the considerable toxicity and cost of these therapies. Antiherpesvirus agents currently available, therefore, cannot be recommended as anti-KS therapy at this time.

Local Antitumor Chemotherapy Therapies directed at KS tumors can be divided into either local or systemic therapies. The selection of a local therapy may be influenced by certain factors, such as the extent and location of the lesions (eg, small, singular lesions on the trunk or on an extremity) and the rapidity of clinical change (eg, indolent development of new lesions over months rather than weeks). The standard options for local therapy are liquid nitrogen, intralesional injection of vinblastine, and radiation.

Photosensitizing agents are currently being tested, and intralesional interferon-α has been reported to be active, but the former is still investigational, and the latter may more appropriately be considered systemic therapy.

For patients who have a small number of lesions and who are unresponsive to anti-HIV medications or who require more rapid improvement than the anti-HIV medications may offer, intralesional injection of vinblastine is a reasonable first-line approach. In particular, palatal or buccal mucosa lesions respond promptly to intralesional vinblastine,[7] although rarely is such therapy durable for more than a few months, and the discomfort of injection may be considerable. In general, practitioners use vinblastine at 0.1 to 0.4 mg/mL, injecting approximately 0.1 to 0.2 mL into a 1 cm^2 lesion; it may be admixed 1:1 with Xylocaine to reduce local discomfort. Local reaction is generally modest, but skin breakdown can occur, and regrowth of lesions is common.

Topical 9-*cis*-retinoic acid cream has also been approved for treatment of cutaneous KS based on a randomized placebo-controlled trial in 82 patients, which demonstrated a sixfold higher response rate in the retinoic acid-treated group, as compared with the placebo-treated group.[63] The difficulty with this medication is its potential for inducing an irritating local reaction when applied to normal skin. Consequently, patients must be counseled to be fastidious in their application of the cream exclusively to affected skin. Even with such care, some patients develop local reactions that may be troubling; however, for patients who tolerate the compound, it may be a desirable alternative. Of note, the same compound appears to be active when given systemically. In open-label trials, tumor response was noted in approximately 37% of patients.[64,65] Headache, dry skin, hyperlipidemia, and pancreatitis may, however, complicate use of this medication.

Radiation Therapy Radiation therapy using either orthovoltage or electron beam may be useful for some patients.[66] The response rate is high, as shown by a French study of 643 patients with AIDS-associated KS in whom a complete response rate of 92% was noted when 20 Gy was delivered over 2 weeks, followed 2 weeks later by 10 Gy over 1 week.[67] For patients with a limited number of lesions or with large plaque-like lesions, this may be an effective approach.[68] Modifications in dose schedule may reduce the complexity for patients, as in the experience from one center that used a single 8 Gy dose, observing a 77% response.[69] Tolerance of therapy is generally good; however, caution must be used when targeting mucous membranes. The sensitivity of patients with AIDS to mucositis from radiation therapy appears to be heightened, and severe, debilitating complications can occur.

Systemic Antitumor Chemotherapy Type I interferons have long been used for the treatment of KS, with theoretic appeal because of their antiviral, antiproliferative, antiangiogenic, and proimmunologic activities.[70] Whether interferons affect KSHV replication has not been well defined at this time, but interferon-α can decrease HIV-1 replication and may thereby alter the production of HIV tat. Interferons also alter cytokine profiles that may participate in KS development. For example, circulating levels of soluble TNF receptor and IL-1-receptor antagonist are increased,[71,72] and bFGF production by tumor cell lines are decreased.[73,74] Thus, interferons may be considered a pathophysiologically based therapy for KS, yet their use is affected by a number of considerations. As a single agent, interferon-α has antitumor effect but generally requires doses (> 9 mU/d or 3 times weekly) that are difficult to tolerate. When used in combination with zidovudine (azidothymidine [AZT]), lower doses of interferon may be used. Interferon-α-2 induces remission of KS in a dose-dependent fashion when given in combination with AZT, with 31% of 54 patients responding to 8 million units given daily subcutaneously,[70] although doses as low as 2 million units have activity. Interferon therapy is most effective in those with relative preservation of immune function and is therefore generally reserved for those with ≥ 100 CD4 cells/mm^3. The use of interferon is limited by its slow onset of action (a median time to response of 10 weeks in some studies) and the frequency of troubling side effects. Most prominent are flu-like symptoms initially, with depression and fatigue common after prolonged use.

Cytotoxic chemotherapy for KS is appropriate for advanced symptomatic KS, particularly for those patients with edema, extensive mucocutaneous disease, and pulmonary or symptomatic GI involvement. Combination therapies of bleomycin and vincristine[75] or doxorubicin, bleomycin, and vincristine[76] are active, with tumor responses reported over a wide range (57–88%).[77] The definition of response to chemotherapy in KS has historically been more ambiguous than with most other tumors because of the limitations of the bidimensional measurement in KS. KS can undergo complete regression of identifiable tumor on histology, yet the region of hyperpigmentation may not change in size. What does change is the nodularity of the lesion, the color characteristics (from a violaceous or salmon color to a gray-brown hemosiderin stain), and when present initially, associated edema. Thus, responses in the older literature are difficult to assess, while more recent studies have benefited by the introduction of standard response criteria initially defined within the AIDS Clinical Trials Group (ACTG) and, more recently, refined by a joint effort of the AIDS Malignancy Consortium, the National Cancer Institute, and the US Food and Drug Administration (FDA).

Combination cytotoxic therapy with doxorubicin, bleomycin, and vincristine has served as a standard for comparison with newer treatment regimens. Although combined doxorubicin, bleomycin, and vincristine has a substantial response rate, side effects are common, most prominently nausea, alopecia, fatigue, peripheral neuropathy, acral cyanosis, and Raynaud's phenomenon.[78] These toxicities can be quite debilitating in a patient population on numerous other medications and often dealing with numerous other medical problems. The impetus for an active but more easily tolerated treatment program has therefore been particularly acute in KS. The liposomal encapsulated chemotherapy agents have provided that option and have a number of characteristics that are appealing for use in KS. The leaky vasculature composing KS lesions predisposes to deposition of the drug, and lesion concentrations of drug have been shown to be almost an order of magnitude higher than in noninvolved tissue.[79] Furthermore, the side-effect profiles of these agents are more favorable. Two phase III studies, with roughly 250 HIV-related KS patients each, found a 25% response rate to this triple therapy or to bleomycin plus vincristine; this finding compared with 46% and 58% for liposomal doxorubicin in the two studies, respectively.[80,81] In contrast, a large randomized study comparing the doxorubicin bleomycin-vincristine combination with liposomal daunorubicin found the liposomal drug to have less toxicity, but the tumor response rate was equivalent and not as high as that found for liposomal doxorubicin.[82] Whether liposomal doxorubicin is truly superior to liposomal daunorubicin is unclear and is the subject of an ongoing clinical trial. These liposomal agents are different in their liposomal as well as their anthracycline composition and have different kinetic profiles. The longer half-life of liposomal doxorubicin may account for its differential activity and association with the hand-and-foot syndrome, not seen with the currently formulated liposomal daunorubicin. Many practitioners use these agents interchangeably for first-line therapy for patients with advanced, symptomatic KS, although current FDA approval for liposomal doxorubicin is only for use in refractory or relapsed KS.

The taxane tubulin stabilizer paclitaxel has emerged as a highly active, well-tolerated agent for KS. In a phase I trial involving 28 patients, a major response was observed in 71%,[83] including those previously treated with anthracyclines. This treatment appears to have both profound activity and highly durable responses. Tumor breakthrough is relatively rare, and patients can tolerate low-dose paclitaxel (100 mg/m^2 every 2 weeks) extremely well. In a phase II study, the response rate was 59%, with a longer duration of response than had been seen with any other therapy.[84] Some patients have received this therapy for over 2 years at our center and have maintained excellent tumor control. As with other agents, the antitumor effect is rapidly lost if the drug is stopped, unless intervening improvement in immunologic function has occurred and can contribute to tumor control.

The highly vascular nature of KS lesions and their ready accessibility to study have made KS a candidate disease for assessment of antiangiogenesis agents. A number of clinical trials involving a range of different agents have occurred or are under way. The agent thalidomide has a number of properties, including inhibiting angiogenesis, and has been assessed in early phase studies in patients with KS. A phase II trial of 13 patients demonstrated a partial response in 4 patients, and the drug was generally well tolerated over a 52-week period.[85] Fumagillin (TNP-470) was well tolerated in a study of 38 patients, but had poor activity.[86] The membrane metalloproteinase inhibitor col-3 and inhibitors of VEGF-signaling pathways have been shown to have antiangiogenic activity in animal models and continue to be tested in KS. Col-3 has demonstrated reasonable tolerability and tumor reactivity and is being further studied.[87] It is envisioned that these agents may play a role for patients with relatively early stage disease to prevent progression or to maintain a remission induced by a cytotoxic agent.

The viral process underlying KS and the relationship of the disease to immune function also suggests that immunologic approaches may ultimately have therapeutic value. KSHV can alter both macrophage and cytotoxic T lymphocyte (CTL) function. Macrophage inhibitory chemokines are encoded by the virus and produced in KSHV-infected cells. The cells also produce an OX-2 homologue termed K-14. OX-2 receptors are present on monocyte/macrophages and stimulation dampens the ability of macrophages to be activated by other stimuli. K14 is capable of reducing activated macrophage production of inflammatory cytokines, possibly restricting host response to KSHV.[88] In addition, KSHV encodes genes that alter the ability of infected cells to be targeted by CTLs. The K3 and K5 viral gene products limit CTL engagement of MHC class I molecules, and K5 also inhibits interaction with the coreceptor (B7) complex necessary for CTL activation.[89] However, a number of reports have defined epitopes within KSHV gene products that are recognized by cytotoxic T lymphocytes.[90,91] Definition of whether reactivity to certain epitopes associates with protection from disease and whether immune inhibitory pathways can be altered will pave the way for the development of vaccine or adoptive cell therapies of the future.

NON-HODGKIN'S LYMPHOMA

Lymphoproliferation occurs in the context of immunodeficiency of many different types. It is a common complication of individuals born with congenital abnormalities of T-cell function, of individuals receiving immunosuppressive medications for organ transplantation, and of individuals with HIV infection. The common theme among these is the role of EBV going unchecked in its ability to induce B-cell proliferation. However, the minority of AIDS-related lymphomas resemble the lymphoproliferative disease of the congenital or post-transplantation setting. AIDS-related lymphoma is a complex set of tumors with challenging clinical scenarios. It has been and remains the most lethal complication of HIV infection, demanding new approaches and new understanding of the pathophysiology underlying it.[2]

Epidemiology The association of non-Hodgkin's lymphoma (NHL) with HIV infection was evident within the first half-decade of the AIDS epidemic, when an unusual number of lymphomas among young men became evident in cancer registries in California. The first revision of the definition of AIDS by the US Centers for Disease Control and Prevention, in 1987, included NHL, and it has remained an important and devastating manifestation of HIV-induced immunosuppression. Unlike KS, in which select subsets of HIV-infected individuals have a unique risk, NHL is more uniformly distributed among risk groups for HIV, with little variation. What variation is present may be attributable partly to issues of care.

The risk of NHL among HIV-infected individuals is in part determined by the level of immunosuppression, with higher risk noted among those with low CD4 cell counts. However, specific subsets of lymphoma have a stronger association with severe immunosuppression than others. The occurrence of PCNS lymphoma is restricted to those with very advanced immunodeficiency, as is the primary effusion lymphoma (PEL) subset of systemic lymphomas. These manifestations of profound immune dysfunction appear to have decreased in incidence since the advent of HAART. Among the non-PEL systemic lymphomas, the immunoblastic histologic subset appears to occur more commonly in those with more profound immunosuppression, whereas the small noncleaved-cell Burkitt's tumors are often seen in a group with more preserved immune function.[92] The median CD4 counts in most treatment reports of systemic lymphoma are in the range of 50 to 189 cells/mm^3, with the small-cell group having a median CD4 count of 193. In contrast, reports of patients with PCNS lymphomas demonstrate a profound CD4 count depression (30 cells/mm^3 in one study).[93] Thus, NHL may occur across a broad range of contexts in HIV disease, including those with virtually no other manifestations of immunosuppression. Possible underlying, unrecognized HIV infection should be considered in any person presenting with a highly aggressive lymphoma. The recent cohort studies of patients on HAART do not indicate the length of time because infection or the nadir CD4 cell count are themselves predictive of AIDS-related lymphoma (ARL) risk. Rather, the severity of persistent immunosuppression is important, with a relative hazard of approximately 1.4 for each 50% decline in CD4 count. Reassuringly, as the CD4 count responds to HAART, the risk of lymphoma reduces, but there is a lag time of approximately 1 year, somewhat longer than for many other opportunistic diseases.[19] Interestingly, the reduction in risk appears to proceed with longer time on HAART in parallel and likely reflecting the gradual repair in immune function seen over long periods of time on HAART. Immune function is accompanied by HIV RNA as a predictor of ARL risk.[19] In the EuroSIDA study, each log of HIV ribonucleic acid (RNA) was associated with a relative hazard of 1.51. Therefore, controlling HIV is a critical determinant of ARL, presumably because of the immunologic alterations it engenders, though other pathophysiologic mechanisms may also participate.

Pathology and Pathogenesis The development of lymphoma among HIV-infected patients is virtually always associated with transformation of a B cell, a cell type that HIV itself is unable to infect. Thus, HIV does not play a direct role in the development of most ARL; rather, it provides the background immunosuppression either for transforming viruses or for proliferative triggers for B cells to go unabated. The rare exception to this is a small subset of tumors of T-cell origin.

T-cell malignancies in HIV infection are uncommon, but include a spectrum of clinicopathologic entities.[94–102] In one subset, the HIV genome has been identified either in the T cells or in tumor-associated macrophages. Definition of the HIV chromosomal integration site revealed a preferential localization to a region upstream of the c-*fes* proto-oncogene, a finding that suggests a direct role for HIV in tumor pathogenesis.[103]

Although HIV may not be present in any but the rare T-cell malignancy, other viruses often are present. Most particularly, EBV is common in a subset of systemic lymphomas and virtually all primary CNS lymphomas. The biology by which this gamma-herpesvirus exerts its effects is being unraveled through molecular analyses and perhaps is most clearly defined for the PCNS lymphomas and post-transplantation lymphoproliferative diseases. In that context, specific expression of latent virus genes is characteristic of a so-called type III pattern. These genes include the *LMP1*, *LMP2*, and *EBNA1* through *EBNA6*. The *LMP1* gene has been extensively studied as a potentially direct mediator of B-cell proliferation and has been shown to interact with the tumor necrosis factor receptor (TNFR)-signaling pathway.[104,105] It was recently shown that this gene is expressed in primary tumor tissue from patients with post-transplantation lymphoproliferative disease (PTLD) and ARL and is associated with activation of NFκB.[106]

LMP1 is a six-transmembrane-spanning molecule with a cytoplasmic carboxy terminus capable of interacting with the TNFR II-associated factors (TRAFs) that mediate downstream transcription factor activation.[105,107–110]

Aggregation of the cytoplasmic domains of LMP1 mimic activated TNFR II, thereby providing a stimulus resembling constitutively activated receptor.[111] The activated pathways are similar to those of the TNFR family member CD30, involving the transcriptional regulators NFκB and c-jun.[111,112] Potential downstream targets of these regulators are the proproliferative cytokines, IL-6 and IL-10.

A number of mutations within the carboxy terminus of LMP1 have been noted, and there are some data to support the possibility that these are associated with ARL- or HIV-related Hodgkin's disease.[110,113–115] However, other studies have indicated that the frequency of such mutations is no greater among those with lymphoproliferative disease than it is among patients in an unaffected control group.[113] The concept that molecular evolution of persistent EBV infection may lead to alteration in the malignant potential of select latently infected B cells is an appealing hypothesis that remains speculative at this time.

The proportion of tumors associated with EBV has been variably reported, ranging from 33 to 67%.[116–118] This finding leaves a large fraction of systemic ARLs without a clear association with an oncogenic virus; among these, a small proportion is linked to KSHV. The clinicopathologic entity, PEL, is typically seen in those patients with profound immunosuppression and presents as fluid without tumor mass in the involved body cavity.[119,120] The tumor cells generally do not express B-, T-, or even hematopoietic-cell surface markers (they are

CD45, CD3, and CD19 negative). Molecular analysis of the cells demonstrates that they have undergone immunoglobulin gene rearrangement consistent with an origin in the B-cell lineage. All such tumors identified to date include the KSHV genome, and some have evidence of EBV co-infection.[121,122]

The ability of KSHV to infect B cells in vitro has been shown, whereas the impact of that infection has been difficult to discern in vitro. No clear association of virus infection with altered B-cell growth kinetics, such as is observed with EBV, has been noted with KSHV. However, the close clinical and pathologic relationship of KSHV to PEL is compelling evidence for a direct relationship between KSHV and B-cell oncogenesis mediated by mechanisms not yet understood.

Among the possible contributions of viruses to malignant transformation is alteration in the immunologic reactivity to neoplastic cells. Mechanisms include the ability of EBV EBNA1 to alter antigen-processing pathways and thereby potentially mask EBV-infected cells from cytotoxic T lymphocyte (CTL) reactivity.[123–125] Although the specific details of the mechanism remain to be elucidated, it appears that KSHV exerts a similar effect on infected transformed cells. In addition, viral gene products may be elaborated by infected cells and may impact immune effector cells. For example, EBV encodes a viral IL-10 homolog (BRCF-1) with biologic activity mimicking that of endogenous IL-10.[126–128] Cell lines and tumors from AIDS patients and animal models of ARL indicate that IL-10 is produced,[126,128–131] and that it potentially exerts an inhibitory influence on the T-helper-cell (TH1) response. IL-10 potently suppresses interferon-γ and IL-2 production by effector cells of the TH1 response and is a B-cell mitogen.[127]

Other cytokines potentially participating in altered reactivity to malignant cells include IL-6, which, in addition to serving as a proliferative stimulus to B cells, may act to alter cell sensitivity to immune killing. Specifically, IL-6 has been shown to reduce the ability of EBV-positive cells to be lysed by antigen-specific CTL from HIV-1–positive individuals.[132] IL-6 levels have been noted to be elevated in the serum of patients with AIDS and may be associated with the development of NHL.[133] The CD40 and CD40 ligand (CD40L) interaction has also been hypothesized to participate in the development of HIV-related lymphomas. Activation of this TNFR family pathway alters the proliferation, differentiation, and survival of B cells that serve as a key mechanism of interaction of the B- and T-cell–mediated immune mechanisms. The infection of microvascular endothelial cells from the bone marrow and CNS has been shown to result in altered CD40 signaling that up-regulates adhesive interactions with B cells and possibly explains the potential for extranodal lymphoma in HIV-infected individuals.[134]

Chemokine pathways may also contribute to the unique susceptibility of HIV-infected patients for lymphomagenesis. Patients with a genetic variant in the CXC chemokine, stroma-derived growth factor-1 (SDF-1), have an excess risk of developing the Burkitt's lymphoma subtype of ARL.[135] This chemokine is a known B-cell mitogen and by exerting chemokinetic effects, may contribute to a proliferative stimulus for patients with the genetic variant. The presence of this variant has been suggested to possibly provide a method of identifying those patients with increased risk of lymphoma, although the potential for this risk factor remains speculative at this time.

Genetic mutations in the tumor cells have been well characterized and are related to the specific histologic subtype. Large cell lymphomas exhibit a *Bcl-6* rearrangement in approximately 33% of cases, a c-*myc* rearrangement in 40%, and a *TP53* mutation in 25%.[134] In contrast, the small-cell lymphomas seen in AIDS have c-*myc* rearrangements but not *Bcl-6*, and rarely have *TP53* mutations.[136–140] The presence of EBV is variably associated with either the c-*myc* or *Bcl-6* rearrangements in the small- and large-cell lymphomas, respectively.[137–140] The finding that rearranged c-*myc* gene juxtaposes with the immunoglobulin gene heavy chain switch region[139,141–144] suggests that the malignant event is occurring proximate to the time of immunoglobulin class switching. This relatively late event in B-cell ontogeny is indicative of transformation in a relatively mature germinal center B cell.

The tumor types seen can be broadly categorized as large cell, immunoblastic, and small cell. Among the small noncleaved cell tumors are the subtypes called Burkitt's lymphoma and Burkitt's-like lymphoma. The Burkitt's-like lymphoma subtype more closely resembles the large-cell clinical phenotype. Characteristics that distinguish Burkitt's-like lymphoma from Burkitt's lymphoma include a higher frequency of EBV, CD39, CD70, and CD11a. Although Burkitt's lymphoma is often found in a patient population with higher CD4 counts, the Burkitt's-like lymphoma patients have been noted to have lower counts similar to the large-cell subsets.[145,146]

Clinical Setting Lymphoma in the context of HIV infection may be broken down into two major groups: those with PCNS lymphoma presenting with parenchymal brain disease alone or those with systemic lymphoma who may or may not also have CNS involvement. Among the patients with systemic lymphoma, there is a rare subset of individuals presenting without a mass lesion, but rather with PEL, as noted above. All of these groups represent B-cell neoplasms of high grade with a very aggressive pace of disease. In addition, there is a recently appreciated subset of systemic lymphomas that are plasmablastic in histology.

PCNS lymphoma is generally a manifestation of far advanced immunosuppression. Mean CD4 counts are < 30 cells/mm^3, there is commonly a previous history of an AIDS-defining complication, and the EBV genome is invariably present in the tumor.[93] Histologically, these tumors have an immunoblastic appearance and express a type III pattern of EBV latent gene products.[147] The clinical approach to these patients is detailed in a later section.

Systemic lymphomas may occur in a much earlier stage of HIV disease, although there remains an association of incidence with more advanced immunosuppression. This situation is particularly true of PEL, which is an end-stage complication of HIV-induced immunosuppression and which has been observed in other types of immunosuppression, including that associated with organ transplantation.[148] The common sites of involvement with this tumor are the peritoneum, the pleural space, and the pericardium.[149] Involvement of the bone marrow has been observed with progressive disease, and at least one report documents the development of a mass lesion with immunochemical characteristics of PEL.[150] The approach to this patient population is a staging process similar to any systemic NHL, including the evaluation of the CNS. Whether a distinct approach to therapy should be undertaken is unclear at this point, as standard treatment regimens generally have had unfavorable outcomes.

Systemic ARL, which is not PEL, is quite distinct from lymphoma outside the context of HIV. Involvement of extranodal sites is the rule rather than exception, occurring in up to 95% of patients, and is frequently the site of diagnostic biopsy.[138,151–153,154–167] Lymphoma restricted to extranodal sites may be seen in up to 56% of patients.[167] Particular sites of involvement are favored by specific histologic types. Among those patients with small noncleaved histology, bone marrow and meningeal disease occurs in approximately one-quarter, while large-cell tumors favor the GI tract and brain parenchyma. A summary of the sites of involvement reported in three series is presented in Table 122-4, and indicates the frequency of involvement of the most common sites: bone marrow, CNS, GI tract, and the liver.

Clinical Manifestations AIDS-related lymphomas are generally extremely aggressive, high-grade lymphomas of B-cell origin. However, lymphoproliferative disease in AIDS may include a number of entities, including infrequent T-cell malignancies. Large granular lymphocyte disease, large-cell or anaplastic T-cell lymphoma, Sézary

Table 122-4 Sites of Extranodal Involvement for AIDS High-Grade B-Cell Lymphomas

Author	No. of Patients	% Extranodal	% CNS	% GI	% Marrow	% Liver
Ziegler et al.	90	98	42[a]	17	33	9
Kaplan et al.	84	76	17	4	31	26
Knowles et al.	89	74	21	28	21	16

CNS = central nervous system; GI = gastrointestinal.
[a]Meningeal and primary CNS involvement.

syndrome, and angiocentric T-cell proliferation have been reported.[94–100,102,168] Pathologic and pathogenetic variability in these rare tumors is broad. Some have integrated HIV-1, as previously noted,[100,103] some have integrated human T-cell leukemia/lymphoma virus-1 (HTLV-1),[101] and some have integrated EBV in a subset with oropharyngeal T-cell lymphoma.

Multicentric Castleman disease (MCD) or angiofollicular lymph node hyperplasia has been reported in patients with advanced HIV disease.[169] MCD is a disease that is uniformly associated with KSHV in the HIV-infected patient and is often a rapidly progressive, lethal illness. Presenting findings are fever, splenomegaly, and anemia in virtually all patients. Lymphadenopathy occurs in ~ 90% and marked weight loss in 70%; pancytopenia is seen in 35%.[169] Some have hypothesized that this syndrome represents an acute or subacute KSHV infection syndrome.[170] Acute KSHV infection can also be accompanied by bone marrow failure resembling aplastic anemia.[171]

Both the hyalin-vascular and plasma cell subtypes of Castleman disease have been reported in AIDS, but the multicentric plasma cell histology type is far more common. KSHV is found in the involved nodes, and there is a high prevalence of co-incident or subsequent Kaposi's sarcoma.[119,169,172,173]

Plasma cell disorders are increased in the setting of HIV infection and are also fairly heterogeneous. Plasmablastic lymphomas of the oral cavity[174] with frequent absence of typical lymphoid markers, such as CD45 (leukocyte common antigen) or CD20, have been noted. This is a relatively uncommon subset of AIDS-related lymphomas and is now recognized to not be restricted to the oral cavity. Histopathology has indicated that these tumors mark as plasma cells with MUM1, CD138, and CD38 and are generally EBV+ with a lower frequency of KSHV in the tumor.[175,176] Extramedullary plasmacytomas and overt multiple myeloma with paraprotein specific for HIV antigens have been reported.[177,178] The clinical course of these disorders is highly variable, and the clinical approach should be based on standard guidelines for these diseases outside the context of HIV infection. Some cases of plasmablastic lymphoma have responded to antiretroviral therapy alone; however, such an approach must be very cautiously considered as many of these tumors are also highly aggressive.

Clinical Approach Evaluation of patients with ARL follows staging procedures for other types of NHL, with several caveats specific to the HIV-infected population. First, the frequent involvement of the CNS mandates a more thorough assessment of the CNS, including an imaging study of the brain and sampling of the cerebrospinal fluid (CSF). Second, the potential for co-incident opportunistic infection must be kept in mind when evaluating a patient with "B symptoms." Microbiologic evaluation is particularly important for that population with CD4 counts < 200 cells/mm^3 in whom the risk of opportunistic disease is increased and is a necessity for those with < 50 cells/mm^3. Depending on the clinical scenario, particular concern should be paid to the possible presence of active *Pneumocystis carinii*, *Cytomegalovirus*, *Toxoplasma gondii*, *Mycobacterium avium* complex, *Mycobacterium tuberculosis*, and *Cryptococcus*. Third, assessment of the status of the HIV disease is critical in defining the therapeutic approach. CD4 cells should be measured as well as plasma HIV RNA, and a detailed history of previous antiretroviral therapy and opportunistic disease should be obtained. Those patients for whom NHL represents a manifestation of end-stage, treatment-refractory HIV disease should be regarded with palliative intent. In contrast, the patient with viral suppression on HAART may have an open-ended prognosis from HIV-1 infection, and the emphasis should be on curing the lymphoma—a concept not realistically considered in the pre-HAART era, but of substantial importance since the availability of HAART in 1996. Experience with long-term ARL survivors now free of any clinical evidence of HIV disease emphasizes the importance of that perspective. Selecting a regimen appropriate for the patient involves weighing where the patient may lie in the continuum of HIV disease.

Prognostic Factors Prognosis in patients with ARL has generally been poor, but with the advent of HAART, the improved prognosis from HIV-1 itself, as well as the improved tolerance of chemotherapy, are expected to substantially alter long-term results. Factors that have been indicative of higher risk have been variably reported, based on the specific clinical trial. The largest experience, with 192 patients and comparing the moderate-dose m-BACOD (methotrexate, bleomycin, Adriamycin, cyclophosphamide, Oncovin, and dexamethasone) regimen with the modified or low-dose (Table 122-5) m-BACOD regimen, identified a CD4 count of < 100 cells/mm^3, age > 35 years, intravenous drug use, and stages III/IV disease as independent prognostic indicators.[179] Overall survival in the setting of one or none of these factors was 46 weeks; of two factors, 44 weeks; and of three or four factors, 18 weeks.

The International Prognostic Index (IPI)[180] has been applied to patients with ARL and was predictive in at least one study of 46 patients.[181] A more recent multicenter, randomized trial also found that IPI was an important predictor of outcome among 100 patients in the United States[182] Other studies have also identified an increase in lactate acid dehydrogenase (LDH)[183] or age > 40 years as factors independent of CD4 cell counts. Prior AIDS-defining illness, Karnofsky performance status, and the presence of extranodal disease have also been reported to be predictive of risk. Kaplan and colleagues also noted that the presence of polyclonality was a favorable indicator, particularly in the absence of EBV in the tumor and a CD4 count of > 300 cells/mm^2.[184] Postgerminal center markers (BCL-6 and CD10 negative, MUM1/IRF4, or CD138 positive) have been associated with a shorter disease-free survival.[185] Remarkably, only a single study has shown the small noncleaved-cell histology to be of prognostic importance, and histologically guided therapies have generally not been applied to this population. However, the use of regimens tailored for Burkitt's tumor histology is likely to be developed in the future.

Treatment **Low-Dose Therapy** Early in the AIDS epidemic, the aggressive nature of the lymphomas observed was met with an aggressive clinical approach to therapy. The result was severe toxicity and frequent treatment-related death. As prophylactic therapy for opportunistic infections has improved, and with the advent of growth factors, the tolerability of chemotherapy has also improved. However, given the overall poor prognosis of patients with HIV-1 infection and the frequent necessity of concurrent treatment of other opportunistic illnesses, there was an effort to identify a low-intensity antitumor regimen. This effort resulted in the modified m-BACOD regimen,[156] which was tested in a randomized phase III trial comparing it directly with the full-dose regimen.[186] The modified m-BACOD was essentially half dose (see Table 122-5), and the full-dose regimen was given with concurrent granulocyte-macrophage colony-stimulating factor (GM-CSF). Surprisingly, the results revealed no statistically meaningful differences in the incidence of complete remission (50% vs 46%), relapse after complete remission (19% vs 23%), time to progression (22 weeks vs 28 weeks), overall median survival (31 weeks vs 34 weeks), death from AIDS (20 patients vs 12 patients), and death from lymphoma (24 patients vs 36 patients). The major difference between the two arms of the trial was that grade 4 neutropenia occurred with greater frequency in patients receiving the standard-dose regimen, despite the fact that all such patients received GM-CSF as a part of their treatment program. The utility of this regimen has been called into question, however, with the better tolerability of full-dose regimens in the era of HAART and the demonstration in the non-HIV–infected population that a regimen of cyclophosphamide, hydroxydauno, half dose Bleomycin, Adriamycin, Oncovin, and prednisone (CHOP) to be at least as effective as M-BACOD, but with fewer side effects in a randomized phase III trial.[187] For those patients in whom advanced HIV disease precludes use of full-dose chemotherapy, a modified m-BACOD or CHOP regimen may be appropriate. However, use of the modified regimens in patients with retroviral control cannot be advocated without further definition of equivalent control of the lymphoma.

Standard-Dose Therapies For patients with control of HIV-1, the options are those of standard chemotherapy regimens such as CHOP (see Table 122-5), in which response rates slightly lower than that of the uninfected population have been observed.

European investigators have evaluated more chemotherapy-intensive regimens for patients with AIDS lymphoma. The French-Italian Cooperative Group tested the LNH84 regimen in 140

Table 122-5 Commonly Used Therapy Regimens for AIDS-Related Lymphoma

Therapy Regimen	Standard-Dose Therapy	Low-Dose Therapy
m-BACOD		
Methotrexate (IV)	200 mg/m^2, day 15	200 mg/m^2, day 15
Bleomycin (IV)	4 U/m^2, day 1	4 U/m^2, day 1
Doxorubicin (IV)	45 mg/m^2, day 1	25 mg/m^2, day 1
Cyclophosphamide (IV)	600 mg/m^2, day 1	300 mg/m^2, day 1
Vincristine (IV)	1.4 mg/m^2, day 1	1.4 mg/m^2, day 1
Dexamethasone (po)	6 mg/m^2, days 1–5	3 mg/m^2, days 1–5
GM-CSF (SC)	5 g/kg, days 4–13	5 μg/kg, days 4–13, prn
Pneumocystic prophylaxis	Trimethoprim-sulfamethoxazole, dapsone, or inhaled pentamidine	
	Standard	**Modified**
CHOP		
Cyclophosphamide	750 mg/m^2, IVPB, day 1	375 mg/m^2, day 1
Doxorubicin	50 mg/m^2, IVPB day 1	25 mg/m^2, day 1
Vincristine	1.4 mg/m^2 (not to exceed 2 mg), IVPB, day 1	1.4 mg/m^2 (max 2 mg), day 1
Prednisone (each cycle q 21–28 d)	100 mg, po, days 1–5	50–100 mg po, days 1–5
CDE		
Cyclophosphamide	187.5 mg/m^2, CI, days 1–4	
Doxorubicin	12.5 mg/m^2, CI, days 1–4	
Etoposide	60 mg/m^2, CI, days 1–4	
ACVB dose-intensive chemotherapy		
Induction		
Adriamycin	75 mg/m^2, day 1	
Cyclophosphamide	1,200 mg/m^2, day 1	
Vindesine	2 mg/m^2, days 1, 5	
Bleomycin	10 mg, days 1, 5	
Prednisolone	60 mg/m^2, days 1–5	
Consolidation		
Methotrexate (IV)	3 g/m^2, days 1,5	
Folinic acid rescue (po)	25 mg × 4, days 1–3, 15–17	
Ifosfamide (IV)	1.5 g/m^2, days 29,33	
VP-16 (IV)	300 mg/m^2, days 29,33	
L-Asparaginase (IM)	50,000 U/m^2, days 57, 64	
Ara-C (SC)	50 mg/m^2 q12 h × 8, days 78, 92	
CNS prophylaxis		
Methotrexate (IT)	12 mg, days 1, 15, 29	
CNS treatment		
Methotrexate (IT)	12 mg 2 × week, for 5 weeks	
RT	24,000 cGy	
EPOCH regimen		
Etoposide	50/m^2, CI, days 1–4	50/m^2, CI, days 1–4
Vincristine	0.4 mg/m^2, CI, days 1–4	0.4 mg/m^2, CI, days 1–4
Doxorubicin	10 mg/m^2, CI, days 1–4	10 mg/m^2, CI, days 1–4
Prednisone	60 mg/m^2, po, days 1–5	60 mg/m^2, po, days 1–5
Cyclophosphamide	375 mg/m^2, IV, day 5	187 mg/m^2, IV, days

ACVB = Adriamycin (doxorubicin), cyclophosphamide, vindesine, bleomycin, prednisolone; CDE = cyclophosphamide, doxorubicin, etoposide; CHOP = cyclophosphamide, hydroxydaunomycin, Oncovin, prednisone; CNS = central nervous system; GM-CSF = granulocyte macrophage colony-stimulating factor; IM = intramuscularly; IV = intravenously; po = per os (orally); prn = pro re nata (according as circumstances may require); RT = radiation therapy; SC = subcutaneously.

patients and observed a complete remission rate of 65%, with a relapse rate of 24%.[188] A follow-up study of patients with CD4 count > 100 cells/mm^3, no prior AIDS-defining illnesses, and good performance status has been conducted comparing CHOP chemotherapy with ACVB (doxorubicin 75 mg/m^2 on day 1, cyclophosphamide 1.2 mg/m^2 on day 1, vindesine 2 mg/m^2 on day 1, bleomycin 10 mg on days 1 to 5, prednisolone 60 mg on days 1 to 5) with granulocyte colony-stimulating factor (G-CSF) support. Preliminary results indicate that hematologic toxicity was more severe in the ACVB arm, but that a higher response rate was seen.[189] Further analysis of this data is required before firm conclusions can be drawn. However, the potential for dose-intensive regimens for those in this patient population with good prognostic factors is suggested and needs to be further explored.

Continuous-infusion regimens have also been tested for patients as first-line therapy. The CDE regimen (cyclophosphamide 800 mg/m^2, doxorubicin 50 mg/m^2, etoposide 240 mg/m^2, all per day for 4 days), to which dideoxy inosine (ddI) was added, resulted in a complete response rate of 58% with a median response duration exceeding 18 months in a phase II trial.[190] A trial employing the infusional EPOCH (etoposide, vincristine, doxorubicin, cyclophosphamide, oral prednisone) regimen has been very encouraging.[182] Complete remission was achieved in 74% of patients, and at 53 months median follow-up, disease-free and overall survival were 92% and 60%, respectively. This study is now being tested in a cooperative group setting with and without the addition of anti-CD20 antibody therapy.

Standard Cytotoxic Chemotherapy plus Antiretroviral Therapy The idea of combining antiretroviral and antitumor therapy has advocates who suggest that the ability of the immune system to participate in combating the malignancy will be maximized by suppressing HIV-1 replication. This view is balanced by the opinion of those who regard the viral infection as a secondary priority in the setting of life-threatening tumor growth and believe that adding the potential risks of drug-drug interaction does not justify combining these two groups of agents. This dichotomous opinion is reflected in two recent clinical trials. One study involved the use of a set triple drug, protease inhibitor-containing regimen in combination with CHOP chemotherapy and assessed clinical outcomes and pharmacologic parameters. The other involved a trial of continuous-infusion chemotherapy (adjusted EPOCH), in which antiretroviral therapy was held and viral and immune outcomes were measured in addition to tumor responses.

The trial of CHOP plus indinavir, d4T, and 3TC was conducted by the United States National Cancer Institute-supported AIDS Malignancy Consortium and involved a cohort of patients receiving low-dose CHOP and a subsequent cohort receiving full-dose CHOP plus the same antiretroviral regimen. This study indicated that the combination did not result in unexpected severe or more-frequent toxicities. Pharmacologic analysis tested the possibility both of antineoplastic drugs affecting protease inhibitor levels and of antiviral therapies altering cytotoxic drug metabolism. No alterations in levels of indinavir or doxorubicin were noted, although a reduction in cyclophosphamide clearance of approximately 50% was observed.[191]

The United States National Cancer Institute conducted a trial of infusional chemotherapy in which all antiretroviral therapies were held during cancer treatment.[182] The results indicate that holding antiviral therapy results in a rise in HIV RNA during cancer chemotherapy that reverts to entry levels when antivirals are resumed. Whether either maintaining or holding antiretroviral drugs affects long-term outcomes is not known, but the short-term consequences of holding such therapy appear to be acceptable, and combining select antivirals and antitumor therapy appears not to be associated with unacceptable adverse events.

High-Dose Therapy or Combined-Modality Therapy Efforts to improve the currently poor outcome for patients with ARL have included the addition of immunotoxins to enhance tumor killing. Although this combination was reasonably well tolerated, activity of the immunotoxin was limited, and the outcomes were not sufficiently different from concurrent chemotherapy-alone trials to merit further pursuit. With the availability of the humanized anti-CD20 antibody (rituximab) and its apparent activity even for high-grade B-cell malignancies, the concept of combined immunoglobulin and standard cytotoxic chemotherapy is being reconsidered. A multicenter randomized phase III trial testing CHOP versus CHOP plus rituximab, however, demonstrated that in the setting of AIDS, patients did not have any improvement in overall outcome with the addition of rituximab. (Kaplan LD et al Blood 2005).[192] There was a trend toward improved response (58% vs 47%) with rituximab, but any benefit was offset by an increase in infectious death, particularly among patients with CD4 < 50 cells/mm^3. The use of rituximab in this setting must be carefully considered, therefore, and prophylactic antibiotics may be warranted in highly immune-compromised individuals.

Bone marrow transplantation in patients with HIV disease has been reported; however, most reports for allogeneic transplant antedate protease inhibitor combination therapy regimens. In 1989, an allogeneic bone marrow transplantation in a patient with ARL was reported by Holland and colleagues.[193] Cyclophosphamide (50 mg/kg/d on days 9 through 5 preceding transplant) and total-body irradiation(300 cGy/d on days 4 through 1 preceding transplant) were given, followed by allogeneic bone marrow transplantation and intermediate-dose AZT (1.33 mg/kg IV q4h). Bone marrow engraftment occurred by day 17, and complete chimerism was documented by PCR analysis. (The patient died 47 days after transplantation because of relapsed tumor; HIV could not be detected by PCR analysis in autopsy tissue.) In a population of 12 patients in Marseilles who were HIV-seropositive at some point during care for their autologous or allogeneic bone marrow transplantation, 2 were known to be seropositive at the time of transplantation, and no untoward problems with myeloablation or engraftment were reported.[194]

A single HIV-positive patient treated with allogeneic transplantation for aplastic anemia (cyclophosphamide and total-body irradiation were used in unspecified doses) was reported to experience cryptosporidiosis and cerebral toxoplasmosis post-transplantation with normal engraftment.[195] Other reports have similarly noted engraftment, but have noted progressive underlying neoplasia or HIV disease, when allogenic transplantation has been attempted.[196–201]

In the era since the availability of HAART, there have been several more encouraging reports using autologous transplantation. High-dose therapy with autologous stem cell rescue of 20 patients at a single center resulted in a durable remission in 85% of patients.[202] Independent studies from other sites have less impressive disease-free survival statistics (65%, 50%, and 28% respectively), but all studies noted excellent engraftment and safety outcomes.[202–205] Minimally myeloablative allogeneic transplantation has not yet been tested in this patient group and can only be recommended in the context of clinical trials, because the unique mixture of immune-based tumors, active virus infection, and graft-versus-host disease demand intensive evaluation. With these adoptive stem cell transplant approaches, genetic modification of the transferred cells to render the cell insensitive to HIV infection is being tested. Trials performed to date have been disappointing,[206,207] but methods of stem cell gene transfer are still in evolution and it is too early to determine the real potential of this approach.

CNS Prophylaxis The role of CNS prophylaxis has been much debated. Although early studies indicated a very high incidence of CNS involvement or relapse (8 of 12 patients in one study[158]), the usefulness of routine CNS prophylaxis has never been rigorously studied in this patient population. Approach to this issue is very center-dependent, and some centers treat all patients with 4 weekly doses of intrathecal ara-C or methotrexate. The practice at many centers has been to reserve this treatment for patients who have small noncleaved-cell histology or bone marrow, testicular, or Waldeyer's ring involvement. However, data from Cingolani and colleagues suggest that other features may be associated with risk of CNS relapse. In particular, the presence of EBV in the primary tumor and extranodal involvement were highly associated with eventual CNS involvement ($p = .003$ and $p = .006$, respectively).[208] Whether CNS prophylaxis can be restricted to such patients is not clear and it would be prudent to add these features to those that raise particular concern and should prompt serious consideration of prophylactic therapy.

Supportive Care All patients should be considered for prophylaxis for opportunistic infections. Reduction in CD4 count by approximately half can be expected during chemotherapy, and *Pneumocystis carinii* prophylaxis is generally initiated even if entry CD4 counts exceed 200 cells/mm^3. The therapies standardly used in advanced HIV disease are applied to this population.

Growth factor use is often required, given the noted increased sensitivity to myelotoxic injury in patients with HIV disease. A single randomized trial of CHOP versus CHOP plus GM-CSF found a significant difference in the incidence of fever and neutropenia and days of hospitalization in the cohort receiving prophylactic growth factor.[163] This trial antedated the use of protease inhibitors, which has generally improved patients' tolerance of chemotherapy. Therefore, many practitioners use guidelines similar to those for other patients receiving chemotherapy when deciding about growth factor use.[209]

The use of growth factors in the HIV-1–infected population has been of some concern because of the potential for growth factor stimulation of HIV-1 replication.[210,211] This issue has been raised particularly for GM-CSF, in which direct activation of the HIV-1 transcriptional control regions has been documented in vitro. Data regarding the increase in viral load in vivo, however, have been conflicting. Some studies have demonstrated a rise in markers of viral load (HIV p24 at the time of these studies),[163,212] and others show either no increase or a transient increase.[213–215] The trial involving GM-CSF and CHOP observed an increase in HIV-1 p24 that was noted in the early cycles but that by the end of the trial was not different compared with controls. The data with G-CSF use are similarly conflicting. G-CSF does not have effects on inflammatory cytokine release or notable induction of HIV-1 in vitro seen with GM-CSF, but has been shown to induce increases in HIV RNA in half the patients receiving it at doses sufficient for stem cell mobilization.[216] These increases were transient and returned to baseline following cessation of the growth factor. The long-term consequences of growth factor use and its relationship to control of virus replication by antiretroviral drugs are not presently known. Concerns regarding long-term consequences generally do not discourage use of growth factors in the context of patients with otherwise strong indications for their benefit.[209]

Treatment of Multicentric Castleman Disease There is no accepted standard for treating AIDS-related MCD. Small series or anecdotal studies have been reported for successful use of single-agent, low-dose etoposide, thalidomide, interferon-α, retinoids, anti-IL6 antibody, and combination chemotherapy.[217,218] Rituxan (anti-CD20 antibody) has become increasingly more commonly used for several reasons. First, the B cell is clearly a target of KSHV and is involved in the pathologic process of MCD. Second, early reports of this rare tumor type indicate antitumor activity of Rituxan even among patients who have failed more aggressive cytotoxic chemotherapies.[219–222] Complete remissions have been reported with Rituxan associated with an early decrease in viral DNA in peripheral blood and a decline in C-reactive protein and IL-6.[223,224] There are, however, some reports of KS worsening with Rituxan therapy of MCD, so caution must be used.[223]

The association of MCD with KSHV infection has led some to use antiviral medications with varying success. The data regarding this therapy are still very preliminary, and the agents are generally active only in the lytic phase of the viral life cycle, a phase of unclear significance for pathophysiology. Therefore, antiherpesvirus medication can be endorsed only as an experimental approach at this time. Whether anti-HIV medication can play a role in treating MCD similarly remains unknown, though there are reports of this also affecting MCD clinical course.

In caring for patients with MCD, attention must be paid to the high incidence of these patients ultimately developing full blown lymphoma. Either plasmablastic lymphoma[225] or primary effusion lymphoma (PEL) may occur in these patients and are extremely difficult to treat.[226]

Primary CNS Lymphoma A brain mass in the context of HIV infection can be caused by a number of infectious and neoplastic processes, and thereby poses a substantial diagnostic challenge. Most commonly seen in AIDS patients are *Toxoplasma gondii* abscess, PCNS lymphoma, mycobacterial or bacterial abscess, and progressive multifocal leukoencephalopathy (PML). Criteria for distinguishing between these entities remain imperfect without tissue sampling, but for those patients in whom biopsy is not possible or is refused, certain parameters can raise or lower the likelihood of a lymphoma diagnosis, and the use of PCR analysis has greatly improved the reliability of a diagnosis without histologic confirmation.

In general, PCNS lymphoma, PML, and toxoplasmosis are complications of far advanced immunosuppression with CD4 counts of < 50 cells/mm^3. This patient population is often on trimethoprim-sulfamethoxazole prophylaxis for *Pneumocystis*, which provides excellent protection against *Toxoplasma*. For those patients in whom a *Toxoplasma* antibody titer is negative and who have been on such prophylaxis, the likelihood of a lymphoma diagnosis in the setting of a CNS mass lesion has been documented to be 74%.[227] Additional information can be gained from PCR analysis for the EBV genome in CSF samples. Detection of EBV in the CSF has been reported to have specificity for lymphoma approximating unity.[227,228] Sensitivity may be only 80% and there are rare cases of EBV+ CSF where no lymphoma is diagnosed, but this test has become extremely useful in assessing the patient who is unable or unwilling to undergo a definitive histologically defining procedure.

Radiographic features more suggestive of lymphoma include central location, lack of multifocality, and size > 2 cm.[157,229] In addition, a lesion that crosses the midline is highly likely to be a neoplastic process. Single-photon emission computed tomography (SPECT) or positron emission tomography (PET) can also help distinguish lymphoma from abscess. The combination of one of these imaging techniques with a positive DNA PCR for EBV is now often considered sufficient evidence for initiation of therapy. If these tests do not clearly delineate the process and a biopsy is not feasible, empiric anti-*Toxoplasma* therapy may be used as a diagnostic as well as therapeutic tool. Initiation of sulfadiazine or clindamycin with pyrimethamine generally halts the progression by 5 days and results in clinical or radiographic improvement by 14 days.[230,231] For those in whom these milestones are not met, the likelihood of toxoplasmosis is low.

Therapy for PCNS lymphoma remains very limited and with poor outcome. Radiation therapy has been the mainstay of care, with response rates ranging from 60 to 79%, but durable remissions are uncommon.[157,232–234] There are some encouraging reports, however, that the control of HIV replication with antiretroviral therapy associated with a subsequent increase in CD4+ cells may provide therapeutic benefit above that of radiation therapy alone.

Alternative antitumor approaches such as high-dose methotrexate have limited experience in this population, but reports of small trials have been encouraging.[235] Combining cytotoxic chemotherapy and radiation therapy has been tested, with disappointing effect on the tumors and unacceptable toxicity. Although the EBV genome is associated with PCNS lymphoma, it is generally noted to be in latent phase, and therefore unlikely to be sensitive to lytic-phase-specific antiviral agents. Nonetheless, limited experience with the use of ganciclovir in combination with zidovudine and IL-2 has suggested antitumor activity.[236] The ultimate use of these agents or other EBV-directed genetic[237] or chemical[238] manipulations awaits careful assessment in clinical trial. The relationship of the disease to poor immunologic function does provide rationale, however, for emphasizing optimization of anti-HIV therapy as a component of antitumor therapy. The overall poor outcome for these patients also strongly argues for the encouragement of patients to participate in clinical protocols testing novel approaches.

The use of steroids in this patient population has engendered concern because of the potential worsening of immunosuppression. There is an absence of data regarding this point, but the opportunity to reduce edema and mass effect should not be avoided out of concern for immunosuppression. Rather, the tapering of steroids should be as rapid as is tolerated, and vigilance regarding the development of concurrent infection should be maintained. In the era preceding HAART, death was as commonly caused by secondary events as by tumor.[239] For those patients who present with PCNS lymphoma who have not been receiving HAART, initiating antiretroviral therapy should be considered a priority, as anecdotal reports have emerged of long-term survivors among the group gaining control of HIV-1.[240]

HODGKIN'S DISEASE

Although not an AIDS-defining tumor, Hodgkin's disease (HD) is increased in frequency in HIV disease and in the number of unique characteristics distinguishing it from HD outside the context of AIDS.

Epidemiology The risk of Hodgkin's disease in patients infected with HIV-1 is estimated to be 2.5- to 8.5-fold above that of the uninfected population.[241–242] Several analyses of cancer registries have confirmed this increase, including a linkage analysis of cancers and AIDS surveillance data collected by registries in several regions of the United States.[9] A 7.6-fold increased risk of HD was observed in patients with AIDS. In Australia and Italy, similar types of analyses have indicated up to an 18.3-fold increase in the risk of HD. The risk of HD appears to be uniformly increased across the risk groups for HIV infection, independent of age or gender.[243] Despite the increase in relative risk in the HIV-infected population, the overall magnitude of the problem is still relatively small compared with that of NHL.

Pathology and Pathogenesis HD in the context of HIV infection has pathologic features that distinguish it from the seronegative population. In particular, there is a much higher frequency of the mixed-cellularity subtype, with a corresponding reduction in the relative proportion of patients with nodular sclerosis histology.[192] The overall frequency of mixed-cellularity or lymphocyte-depleted histology was found to be two-thirds of the cases in the HIV-1–positive context compared with only 29% in uninfected patients.[244]

In addition, the presence of EBV in Hodgkin's disease tissue is markedly increased in HIV-infected individuals. Estimates ranged from 80 to 100% in contrast to the HIV-negative population.[245–247] Of note, expression of the EBV *LMP1*, but not *EBNA2*, latency genes is in a type 2 pattern.[247] Thus, the EBV genome is identified with high frequency in HIV-infected HD and is considered likely to play an etiologic role.

In addition to the presence of EBV, there are other molecular characteristics of HD unique to the HIV-infected population. Although the transcription factor Bcl-6, expressed in germinal-center B cells, is present on Reed–Sternberg cells from both HIV-1-infected and uninfected individuals, syndecan-1 (a proteoglycan associated with the post-terminal center) is restricted to the HIV-1–positive population.[248,249] Therefore, the postgerminal-center B cell may be the cell of origin in HIV-1–related HD, as opposed to the germinal-center cell of origin presumed to be the source of Reed–Sternberg cells in the uninfected population.

Clinical Features HD in patients with HIV is typically of advanced stage and associated with B symptoms.[250] Stage III or IV disease has been documented in 91% of patients with HIV-associated HD at the time of diagnosis, as compared with 46% in individuals without HIV.[111] Like ARL, the location of HD in the setting of HIV-1 infection is often extranodal, involving the bone marrow in up to 50% of patients.[251,252] Other sites include the tongue, rectum, skin, and lung,[250] and extranodal disease may be the site of presentation. Staging strategies should be the same as those in HD patients outside the context of HIV-1, with particular attention to possible microbiologic explanations for B symptoms.

Treatment The clinical treatment approach to patients with HD in the setting of HIV infection is similar to that in other contexts, and radiation therapy, chemotherapy, or combined radiation and chemotherapy should be applied as appropriate for stage, similar to guidelines for treatment outside the setting of HIV infection. The underlying level of immunosuppression and overall performance status of the patient must be considered before embarking on these therapies, and in general, prophylaxis for *Pneumocystis carinii* is provided. Treatment complications, including myelosuppression and opportunistic infections, may be expected to be more severe among patients with advanced AIDS. However, cure of HD is a realistic aim in the setting of HIV infection, and antitumor therapy dose attenuation should be contemplated only in patients with advanced AIDS or who have demonstrated intolerance to the standard-dose regimens.

SQUAMOUS CELL NEOPLASIA

The issue of human papillomavirus-related disease is an increasing concern in the HIV epidemic for several reasons, including (1) the increasing frequency of women infected by HIV, (2) the rampant progression of HIV disease in parts of the world where there is already a high incidence of cervical cancer and limited screening for cervical disease, and (3) the extension in overall survival of HIV-infected individuals. The nature of the abnormalities is fairly broad in scope and includes anogenital, conjunctival, oropharyngeal, and cutaneous neoplasia.

Epidemiology The increased frequency of squamous cell neoplasia in HIV-infected individuals has been documented in a number of studies. The single AIDS-defining disease among the HPV-related tumors is that of invasive cervical carcinoma, though there is controversy as to whether this malignancy is increased in frequency in the setting of HIV infection. However, it is very clear that intraepithelial neoplasia of both the uterine cervix and the anus is increased. Homosexual HIV-infected men have a particularly high incidence of squamous cell abnormalities and a markedly increased risk of anal cancer.[253] Whether the incidence of invasive cancer is greater in the HIV-infected as compared with the HIV-seronegative homosexual male cohort also remains controversial. Indirect evidence that immune suppression augments this cancer risk comes from an analysis of AIDS and cancer registries. In a study by Frisch and colleagues, the incidence of in situ and invasive cancers was significantly higher in the 5 years following an AIDS-defining illness than in the 5 years preceding it.[254] Among women, cervical, vulvar/vaginal, and anal cancers were increased, while among men, anal, penile, tonsillar, and conjunctival cancers were increased.

Pathology and Pathogenesis The association of specific subtypes of HPV with a potential for epidermal cell transformation has been long established, and the frequency of HPV-16, -18, and -19, is reported to be increased in HIV-infected individuals.[255] The frequency of multiple subtypes of HPV has also been assessed and found to be markedly increased in the HIV-infected population (73% of HIV-1–infected homosexual men, as compared with 23% of uninfected homosexual men).[255,256] The incidence of high-grade intraepithelial neoplasia of the anus has been estimated to be as high as 48% among HIV-1–positive homosexual men over a 4-year interval and was associated with the presence of multiple HPV subtypes, persistent anal infection, and high-level infection with oncogenic HPV subtypes.[257] Screening for intraepithelial neoplasia among HIV-1–infected homosexual men has demonstrated a prevalence of high-grade anal intraepithelial neoplasia (or carcinoma in situ) of 36% compared with 7% of HIV-1–negative homosexual men.[258] Most often, these lesions on the anus and uterine cervix are not solitary sites but rather represent one of multiple areas of dysplasia and are therefore difficult to satisfactorily treat,[259] particularly on the anus. Patients with a history of high-grade intraepithelial neoplasia may often have recurrence following attempts at excision, cryotherapy, or topical treatment because of the ubiquitous nature of the HPV infection locally and the tendency of that virus to continue to have effects on local tissue.

A critical issue in evaluating the magnitude of this problem is the risk of progression of intraepithelial neoplasia to frank invasive cancer. This issue remains ill defined and highly controversial. If the risk is estimated at 1% or above, cost-benefit analyses have indicated that ongoing screening is justified.[260] The lack of large increases in the frequency of invasive anogenital cancer among HIV risk groups suggests that the risk is relatively small. However, the potential for frank invasion is not zero, and therefore, vigilance among patients with HIV disease is warranted.

The risk of some opportunistic neoplasms is clearly diminished in the context of aggressive therapy for HIV and suppression of HIV replication. There have been conflicting reports of whether HPV-related tumors are among those responsive to improved anti-HIV therapy. Some reports have indicated that some individuals may experience improvement in HPV-related neoplasia[261]; however, the bulk of data suggests that antiretroviral therapy has little impact on the incidence of dysplasia or invasive anal cancer.[262,263] At present, the complete suppression of HIV should not be regarded as fail-safe defense against the development of HPV-related tumors.

Clinical Presentation HPV disease may present anywhere along the continuum of condyloma acuminatum to invasive anal cancer. Patients who have anal dysplasia may or may not have symptoms associated with it. Common practice among patients with a history of high-grade anal dysplasia is to perform an anoscopic examination and possible biopsy, even if the diagnostic lesion is on the anal verge, to assess for possible invasive disease out of the external examination field. Some centers are initiating anal Papanicolaou (Pap) evaluation for HIV-infected individuals, but this approach is highly controversial.

For women with HIV infection, the standard practices and recommendations for cervical screening are to be followed, with increased vigilance for those with severe immunosuppression. For HIV-infected women with CD4 counts of < 200 cells/mm^3, the recommendation is for Pap smears to be performed semiannually.

Treatment Treatment guidelines for dysplasia and carcinoma of the uterine cervix are well defined and should be followed in the setting of HIV infection. Management of anal disease is less clear.

For patients with invasive carcinoma of the anus, treatment guidelines recommending a combination of chemotherapy and radiation therapy should be followed; this treatment has been reasonably well tolerated in the HIV-infected population.[264,265] There is a distinct increased sensitivity to mucosal injury with radiation in HIV disease, and, therefore, close interaction of the medical and radiation oncologist is essential. If patients have very advanced HIV disease failing antiretrovirals, a conservative approach to management of the malignancy may be warranted, but this requires case-by-case assessment.

The ambiguity of risk of invasion if high-grade intraepithelial neoplasia or carcinoma in situ is diagnosed has led to considerable variability in treatment practices for these patients. Our practice has been to surgically remove any lesions identifiable to the eye, but not to attempt wide excisions. For those patients with recurrent anal warts or with tissue discoloration seen with HPV disease, imiquimod cream has been useful and is generally well tolerated. For lesions within the anal canal, satisfactory topical therapy is not available, and vigilant monitoring is the general approach.

Lesions on other sites are generally approached with similar principles. For invasive disease, resect and use standard guidelines for care. For noninvasive disease, excise overt lesions locally and attempt topical therapies such as imiquimod or 5-fluorouracil.

REFERENCES

1. Palella FJ Jr, Delaney KM, Moorman AC, et al. Declining morbidity and mortality among patients with advanced human immunodeficiency virus infection. HIV Outpatient Study Investigators [comments]. N Engl J Med 1998;338:853–60.
2. Chaisson RE, Gallant JE, Keruly JC, Moore RD. Impact of opportunistic disease on survival in patients with HIV infection. AIDS 1998;12:29–33.
3. Centers for Disease Control and Prevention. Update: acquired immunodeficiency syndrome(AIDS)—United States. MMWR Morb Mortal Wkly Rep 1983;32:465–7.
4. Centers for Disease Control and Prevention. First 500,000 AIDS cases–United States. MMWR Morb Mortal Wkly Rep 1995;44:849–53.
5. Biggar RJ, Rabkin CS. The epidemiology of AIDS–related neoplasms. Hematol Oncol Clin North Am 1996;10:997–1010.
6. Beral V, Peterman T, Berkelman R, Jaffe H. AIDS-associated non-Hodgkin lymphoma [comments]. Lancet 1991;337:805–9.
7. Chang Y, Cesarman E, Pessin MS, et al. Identification of herpesvirus-like DNA sequences in AIDS-associated Kaposi's sarcoma [comments]. Science 1994;266:1865–9.
8. Beral V, Bull D, Darby S, et al. Risk of Kaposi's sarcoma and sexual practices associated with faecal contact in homosexual or bisexual men with AIDS [comments]. Lancet 1992;339:632–5.
9. Goedert JJ, Cote TR, Virgo P, et al. Spectrum of AIDS-associated malignant disorders [comments]. Lancet 1998;351:1833–9.
10. Rabkin CS, Hilgartner MW, Hedberg KW, et al. Incidence of lymphomas and other cancers in HIV-infected and HIV-uninfected patients with hemophilia. JAMA 1992;267:1090–4.
11. Frizzera G, Rosai J, Dehner LP, et al. Lymphoreticular disorders in primary immunodeficiencies: new findings based on an up-to-date histologic classification of 35 cases. Cancer 1980;46:692–9.
12. Zulman J, Jaffe R, Talal N. Evidence that the malignant lymphoma of Sjögren's syndrome is a monoclonal B-cell neoplasm. N Engl J Med 1978;299:1215–20.
13. Jacobson LP, Yamashita TE, Detels R, et al. Impact of potent antiretroviral therapy on the incidence of Kaposi's sarcoma and non-Hodgkin's lymphomas among HIV-1-infected individuals. Multicenter AIDS Cohort Study. J Acquir Immune Defic Syndr 1999;21 Suppl 1:S34–41.

14. Rabkin CS, Testa MA, Huang J, Von Roenn JH. Kaposi's sarcoma and non-Hodgkin's lymphoma incidence trends in AIDS Clinical Trial Group study participants. J Acquir Immune Defic Syndr 1999;21 Suppl 1:S31–3.

15. Buchbinder SP, Holmberg SD, Scheer S, et al. Combination antiretroviral therapy and incidence of AIDS-related malignancies. J Acquir Immune Defic Syndr 1999;21 Suppl 1:S23–6.

16. Young L, Alfieri C, Hennessy K, et al. Expression of Epstein-Barr virus transformation-associated genes in tissues of patients with EBV lymphoproliferative disease. N Engl J Med 1989;321:1080–5.

17. Kieff E, Liebowitz D. Epstein-Barr virus and its replication. In: Fields B, Knipe D, editors. Virology. Philadelphia: Lippincott-Raven; 1990. p. 1889.

18. Grulich AE. AIDS-associated non-Hodgkin's lymphoma in the era of highly active antiretroviral therapy. J Acquir Immune Defic Syndr 1999;21 Suppl 1:S27–30.

19. Kirk O, Pedersen C, Cozzi-Lepri A, et al. Non-Hodgkin lymphoma in HIV-infected patients in the era of highly active antiretroviral therapy. Blood 2001;98:3406–12.

20. International Collaboration on HIV and Cancer. Highly active antiretroviral therapy and incidence of cancer in human immunodeficiency virus-infected adults. J Natl Cancer Inst 2000;92:1823–30.

21. Kedes DH, Operskalski E, Busch M, et al. The seroepidemiology of human herpesvirus 8 (Kaposi's sarcoma- associated herpesvirus): distribution of infection in KS risk groups and evidence for sexual transmission [comments] [published erratum appears in Nat Med 1996;2:1041]. Nat Med 1996;2:918–24.

22. Russo JJ, Bohenzky RA, Chien MC, et al. Nucleotide sequence of the Kaposi sarcoma-associated herpesvirus (HHV8). Proc Natl Acad Sci U S A 1996;93:14862–7.

23. Ganem D. KSHV and Kaposi's sarcoma: the end of the beginning? Cell 1997;91:157–60.

24. Pellett PE, Wright DJ, Engels EA, et al. Multicenter comparison of serologic assays and estimation of human herpesvirus 8 seroprevalence among US blood donors. Transfusion 2003;43:1260–8.

25. Mbulaiteye SM, Pfeiffer RM, Whitby D, et al. Human herpesvirus 8 infection within families in rural Tanzania. J Infect Dis 2003;187:1780–5.

26. Cattani P, Cerimele F, Porta D, et al. Age-specific seroprevalence of Human Herpesvirus 8 in Mediterranean regions. Clin Microbiol Infect 2003;9:274–9.

27. Martin JN, Ganem DE, Osmond DH, et al. Sexual transmission and the natural history of human herpesvirus 8 infection. N Engl J Med 1998;338:948–54.

28. Pauk J, Huang ML, Brodie SJ, et al. Mucosal shedding of human herpesvirus 8 in men. N Engl J Med 2000;343:1369–77.

29. Gill PS, Akil B, Colletti P, et al. Pulmonary Kaposi's sarcoma: clinical findings and results of therapy. Am J Med 1989;87:57–61.

30. Lee VW, Fuller JD, O'Brien MJ, et al. Pulmonary Kaposi sarcoma in patients with AIDS: scintigraphic diagnosis with sequential thallium and gallium scanning. Radiology 1991;180:409–12.

31. Abdel-Dayem HM, Bag R, DiFabrizio L, et al. Evaluation of sequential thallium and gallium scans of the chest in AIDS patients. J Nucl Med 1996;37:1662–7.

32. Krown SE, Testa MA, Huang J. AIDS-related Kaposi's sarcoma: prospective validation of the AIDS Clinical Trials Group staging classification. AIDS Clinical Trials Group Oncology Committee. J Clin Oncol 1997;15:3085–92.

33. Wyatt ME, Finlayson CJ, Moore-Gillon V. Kaposi's sarcoma masquerading as pyogenic granuloma of the nasal mucosa. J Laryngol Otol 1998;112:280–2.

34. Jussila L, Valtola R, Partanen TA, et al. Lymphatic endothelium and Kaposi's sarcoma spindle cells detected by antibodies against the vascular endothelial growth factor receptor-3. Cancer Res 1998;58:1599–604.

35. Weninger W, Rendl M, Pammer J, et al. Nitric oxide synthases in Kaposi's sarcoma are expressed predominantly by vessels and tissue macrophages. Lab Invest 1998;78:949–55.

36. Uccini S, Sirianni MC, Vincenzi L, et al. Kaposi's sarcoma cells express the macrophage-associated antigen mannose receptor and develop in peripheral blood cultures of KS patients. Am J Pathol 1997;150:929–38.

37. Miles SA. Pathogenesis of AIDS-related Kaposi's sarcoma. Evidence of a viral etiology. Hematol Oncol Clin North Am 1996;10:1011–21.

38. Miles SA, Martinez-Maza O, Rezai A, et al. Oncostatin M as a potent mitogen for AIDS-Kaposi's sarcoma-derived cells. Science 1992;255:1432–4.

39. Miles SA, Rezai AR, Salazar-Gonzalez JF, et al. AIDS Kaposi sarcoma-derived cells produce and respond to interleukin 6. Proc Natl Acad Sci U S A 1990;87:4068–72.

40. Ensoli B, Gendelman R, Markham P, et al. Synergy between basic fibroblast growth factor and HIV-1 Tat protein in induction of Kaposi's sarcoma. Nature 1994;371:674–80.

41. Murakami-Mori K, Mori S, Nakamura S. Endogenous basic fibroblast growth factor is essential for cyclin E- CDK2 activity in multiple external cytokine-induced proliferation of AIDS-associated Kaposi's sarcoma cells: dual control of AIDS-associated Kaposi's sarcoma cell growth and cyclin E-CDK2 activity by endogenous and external signals. J Immunol 1998;161:1694–704.

42. Simonart T, Degraef C, Noel JC, et al. Overexpression of Bcl-2 in Kaposi's sarcoma-derived cells. J Invest Dermatol 1998;111:349–53.

43. Lee H, Veazey R, Williams K, et al. Deregulation of cell growth by the K1 gene of Kaposi's sarcoma-associated herpesvirus. Nat Med 1998;4:435–40.

44. Bais C, Santomasso B, Coso O, et al. G-protein-coupled receptor of Kaposi's sarcoma-associated herpesvirus is a viral oncogene and angiogenesis activator [comments] [published erratum appears in Nature 1998;392:210]. Nature 1998;391:86–9.

45. Li M, Lee H, Guo J, et al. Kaposi's sarcoma-associated herpesvirus viral interferon regulatory factor. J Virol 1998;72:5433–40.

46. Zimring JC, Goodbourn S, Offermann MK. Human herpesvirus 8 encodes an interferon regulatory factor (IRF) homolog that represses IRF-1-mediated transcription. J Virol 1998;72:701–7.

47. Gao SJ, Boshoff C, Jayachandra S, et al. KSHV ORF K9 (vIRF) is an oncogene which inhibits the interferon signaling pathway. Oncogene 1997;15:1979–85.

48. Muralidhar S, Pumfery AM, Hassani M, et al. Identification of kaposin (open reading frame K12) as a human herpesvirus 8 (Kaposi's sarcoma-associated herpesvirus) transforming gene [published erratum appears in J Virol 1999;73:2568]. J Virol 1998;72:4980–8.

49. Dairaghi DJ, Fan RA, McMaster BE, et al. HHV8-encoded vMIP-I selectively engages chemokine receptor CCR8. Agonist and antagonist profiles of viral chemokines. J Biol Chem 1999;274:21569–74.

50. Endres MJ, Garlisi CG, Xiao H, et al. The Kaposi's sarcoma-related herpesvirus (KSHV)-encoded chemokine vMIP-I is a specific agonist for the CC chemokine receptor (CCR)8. J Exp Med 1999;189:1993–8.

51. Cheng EH, Nicholas J, Bellows DS, et al. A Bcl-2 homolog encoded by Kaposi sarcoma-associated virus, human herpesvirus 8, inhibits apoptosis but does not heterodimerize with Bax or Bak. Proc Natl Acad Sci U S A 1997;94:690–4.

52. Djerbi M, Screpanti V, Catrina AI, et al. The inhibitor of death receptor signaling, FLICE-inhibitory protein defines a new class of tumor progression factors [In Process Citation]. J Exp Med 1999;190:1025–32.

53. Murphy M, Armstrong D, Sepkowitz KA, et al. Regression of AIDS-related Kaposi's sarcoma following treatment with an HIV-1 protease inhibitor [letter]. AIDS 1997;11:261–2.

54. Aboulafia D. Regression of AIDS-related pulmonary Kaposi's sarcoma after highly active antiretroviral therapy. Mayo Clin Proc 1998;73:439–43.

55. Martin DF, Kuppermann BD, Wolitz RA, et al. Oral ganciclovir for patients with cytomegalovirus retinitis treated with a ganciclovir implant. Roche Ganciclovir Study Group [comments]. N Engl J Med 1999;340:1063–70.

56. Mocroft A, Youle M, Gazzard B, et al. Anti-herpesvirus treatment and risk of Kaposi's sarcoma in HIV infection. Royal Free/Chelsea and Westminster Hospitals Collaborative Group. AIDS 1996;10:1101–5.

57. Glesby MJ, Hoover DR, Weng S, et al. Use of antiherpes drugs and the risk of Kaposi's sarcoma: data from the Multicenter AIDS Cohort Study. J Infect Dis 1996;173:1477–80.

58. Robles R, Lugo D, Gee L, Jacobson MA. Effect of antiviral drugs used to treat cytomegalovirus end-organ disease on subsequent course of previously diagnosed Kaposi's sarcoma in patients with AIDS. J Acquir Immune Defic Syndr Hum Retrovirol 1999;20:34–8.

59. Harrington W Jr, Sieczkowski L, Sosa C, et al. Activation of HHV-8 by HIV-1 tat [letter]. Lancet 1997;349:774–5.

60. Ambrosino C, Ruocco MR, Chen X, et al. HIV-1 Tat induces the expression of the interleukin-6 (IL6) gene by binding to the IL6 leader RNA and by interacting with CAAT enhancer- binding protein beta (NF-IL6) transcription factors. J Biol Chem 1997;272:14883–92.

61. Albini A, Soldi R, Giunciuglio D, et al. The angiogenesis induced by HIV-1 tat protein is mediated by the Flk- 1/KDR receptor on vascular endothelial cells. Nat Med 1996;2:1371–5.

62. Von Roenn JH, Krown SE. Management of AIDS-associated Kaposi's sarcoma: a multidisciplinary perspective. Oncology (Huntingt) 1998;12:1–24.

63. Bodsworth N. Topical 9-cis-retinoic acid (Panretin) gel as treatment of cutaneous AIDS-related Kaposi's sarcoma: interim results of an international, placebo-controlled trial (ALRT 1057-503) [abstract 22277]. International Panretin KS Study Group. Int Conf AIDS 1998;12:317.

64. Friedman-Kien A, Conant A. Phase 2 study (protocol L1057-28) of PANRETIN capsules (LGD1057, ALRT1057) for the AIDS-related Kaposi's sarcoma [abstract 22278]. The North American Panretin Gel KS Study Group. Int Conf AIDS 1998;12:318.

65. Miles S, Dezube B, Lee J, et al. Anti-tumor activity of oral 9-cis-retinoic acid in AIDS-related Kaposi's sarcoma: AIDS malignancy consortium study 002 [abstract 22276]. Int Conf AIDS 1998;12:317.

66. Swift PS. The role of radiation therapy in the management of HIV-related Kaposi's sarcoma. Hematol Oncol Clin North Am 1996;10:1069–80.

67. Belembaogo E, Kirova Y, Frikha H, et al. Radiotherapy of epidemic Kaposi's sarcoma: the experience of the Henri-Mondor Hospital (643 patients). Cancer Radiother 1998;2:49–52.

68. Kroll M, Shandera W. AIDS-associated Kaposi's sarcoma. Hosp Pract 1998;33:85–102.

69. Harrison M, Harrington KJ, Tomlinson DR, Stewart JS. Response and cosmetic outcome of two fractionation regimens for AIDS-related Kaposi's sarcoma. Radiother Oncol 1998;46:23–8.

70. Shepherd FA, Beaulieu R, Gelmon K, et al. Prospective randomized trial of two dose levels of interferon alfa with zidovudine for the treatment of Kaposi's sarcoma associated with human immunodeficiency virus infection: a Canadian HIV Clinical Trials Network study. J Clin Oncol 1998;16:1736–42.

71. Tilg H, Mier JW, Vogel W, et al. Induction of circulating IL-1 receptor antagonist by IFN treatment. J Immunol 1993;150:4687–92.

72. Tilg H, Vogel W, Dinarello CA. Interferon-alpha induces circulating tumor necrosis factor receptor p55 in humans. Blood 1995;85:433–5.

73. Fidler I, Singh R, Gutman M, et al. Interferons alpha and beta down regulate the expression of basic fibroblast growth factor (bFGF) in human carcinomas [abstract]. Proc Am Assoc Cancer Res 1994;35:47.

74. Dinney CP, Bielenberg DR, Perrotte P, et al. Inhibition of basic fibroblast growth factor expression, angiogenesis, and growth of human bladder carcinoma in mice by systemic interferon-alpha administration. Cancer Res 1998;58:808–14.

75. Gompels MM, Hill A, Jenkins P, et al. Kaposi's sarcoma in HIV infection treated with vincristine and bleomycin [published erratum appears in AIDS 1992;6:following 1410] [comments]. AIDS 1992;6:1175–80.

76. Gill PS, Rarick MU, Espina B, et al. Advanced acquired immune deficiency syndrome-related Kaposi's sarcoma. Results of pilot studies using combination chemotherapy. Cancer 1990;65:1074–8.

77. Lee FC, Mitsuyasu RT. Chemotherapy of AIDS-related Kaposi's sarcoma. Hematol Oncol Clin North Am 1996;10:1051–68.

78. Reiser M, Bruns C, Hartmann P, et al. Raynaud's phenomenon and acral necrosis after chemotherapy for AIDS-related Kaposi's sarcoma. Eur J Clin Microbiol Infect Dis 1998;17:58–60.

79. Northfelt DW, Martin FJ, Working P, et al. Doxorubicin encapsulated in liposomes containing surface-bound polyethylene glycol: pharmacokinetics, tumor localization, and safety in patients with AIDS-related Kaposi's sarcoma. J Clin Pharmacol 1996;36:55–63.

80. Northfelt DW, Dezube BJ, Thommes JA, et al. Pegylated-liposomal doxorubicin versus doxorubicin, bleomycin, and vincristine in the treatment of AIDS-related Kaposi's sarcoma: results of a randomized phase III clinical trial. J Clin Oncol 1998;16:2445–51.

81. Stewart S, Jablonowski H, Goebel FD, et al. Randomized comparative trial of pegylated liposomal doxorubicin versus bleomycin and vincristine in the treatment of AIDS-related Kaposi's sarcoma. International Pegylated Liposomal Doxorubicin Study Group. J Clin Oncol 1998;16:683–91.

82. Gill PS, Wernz J, Scadden DT. Randomized phase III trial of liposomal daunorubicin versus doxorubicin, bleomycin, and vincristine in AIDS-related Kaposi's sarcoma. J Clin Oncol 1996;14:2353–64.
83. Welles L, Saville MW, Lietzau J, et al. Phase II trial with dose titration of paclitaxel for the therapy of human immunodeficiency virus-associated Kaposi's sarcoma. J Clin Oncol 1998;16:1112–21.
84. Gill P, Tulpule A, Espina B, et al. Paclitaxel is safe and effective in the treatment of advanced AIDS-related Kaposi's sarcoma. J Clin Oncol 1999;17:1876–83.
85. Yarchoan R, Little R, Wyvill K, et al. A phase II study of oral thalidomide in patients with AIDS-related KS [abstract 22280]. Int Conf AIDS 1998;12:318.
86. Dezube BJ, Von Roenn JH, Holden-Wiltse J, et al. Fumagillin analog in the treatment of Kaposi's sarcoma: a phase I AIDS Clinical Trial Group study. AIDS Clinical Trial Group No. 215 Team. J Clin Oncol 1998;16:1444–9.
87. Cianfrocca M, Cooley TP, Lee JY, et al. Matrix metalloproteinase inhibitor COL-3 in the treatment of AIDS-related Kaposi's sarcoma: a phase I AIDS malignancy consortium study. J Clin Oncol 2002;20:153–9.
88. Foster-Cuevas M, Wright GJ, Puklavec MJ, et al. Human herpesvirus 8 K14 protein mimics CD200 in down-regulating macrophage activation through CD200 receptor. J Virol 2004;78:7667–76.
89. Ishido S, Wang C, Lee BS, et al. Downregulation of major histocompatibility complex class I molecules by Kaposi's sarcoma-associated herpesvirus K3 and K5 proteins. J Virol 2000;74:5300–9.
90. Brander C, O'Connor P, Suscovich T, et al. Definition of an optimal Cytotoxic T lymphocyte epitope in the latently expressed Kaposi's sarcoma-associated herpesvirus kaposin protein. J Infect Dis 2001;184:119–26.
91. Osman M, Kubo T, Gill J, et al. Identification of human herpesvirus 8-specific cytotoxic T-cell responses. J Virol 1999;73:6136–40.
92. Carbone A, Gloghini A, Gaidano G, et al. AIDS-related Burkitt's lymphoma. Morphologic and immunophenotypic study of biopsy specimens. Am J Clin Pathol 1995;103:561–7.
93. Levine AM, Sullivan-Halley J, Pike MC, et al. Human immunodeficiency virus-related lymphoma. Prognostic factors predictive of survival [comments]. Cancer 1991;68:2466–72.
94. Presant CA, Gala K, Wiseman C, et al. Human immunodeficiency virus-associated T-cell lymphoblastic lymphoma in AIDS. Cancer 1987;60:1459–61.
95. Ruff P, Bagg A, Papadopoulos K. Precursor T-cell lymphoma associated with human immunodeficiency virus type 1 (HIV-1) infection. First reported case. Cancer 1989;64:39–42.
96. Tirelli U, Serraino D, Carbone A. Hodgkin disease and HIV [letter; comment]. Ann Intern Med 1993;118:313; discussion 313–4.
97. Shibata D, Brynes RK, Rabinowitz A, et al. Human T-cell lymphotropic virus type I (HTLV-I)-associated adult T-cell leukemia-lymphoma in a patient infected with human immunodeficiency virus type 1 (HIV-1). Ann Intern Med 1989;111:871–5.
98. Sternlieb J, Mintzer D, Kwa D, Gluckman S. Peripheral T-cell lymphoma in a patient with the acquired immunodeficiency syndrome. Am J Med 1988;85:445.
99. Gonzalez-Clemente JM, Ribera JM, Campo E, et al. Ki-1+ anaplastic large-cell lymphoma of T-cell origin in an HIV- infected patient. AIDS 1991;5:751–5.
100. Ciobanu N, Andreeff M, Safai B, et al. Lymphoblastic neoplasia in a homosexual patient with Kaposi's sarcoma. Ann Intern Med 1983;98:151–5.
101. Harper ME, Kaplan MH, Marselle LM, et al. Concomitant infection with HTLV-I and HTLV-III in a patient with T8 lymphoproliferative disease. N Engl J Med 1986;315:1073–8.
102. Gold JE, Ghali V, Gold S, et al. Angiocentric immunoproliferative lesion/T-cell non-Hodgkin's lymphoma and the acquired immune deficiency syndrome: a case report and review of the literature. Cancer 1990;66:2407–13.
103. Shiramizu B, Herndier BG, McGrath MS. Identification of a common clonal human immunodeficiency virus integration site in human immunodeficiency virus-associated lymphomas. Cancer Res 1994;54:2069–72.
104. Wang D, Liebowitz D, Kieff E. An EBV membrane protein expressed in immortalized lymphocytes transforms established rodent cells. Cell 1985;43:831–40.
105. Mosialos G, Birkenbach M, Yalamanchilli R, et al. The Epstein-Barr virus transforming protein LMP1 engages signaling proteins for the tumor necrosis factor receptor family. Cell 1995;80:389–99.
106. Liebowitz D. Epstein-Barr virus and a cellular signaling pathway in lymphomas from immunosuppressed patients [comments]. N Engl J Med 1998;338:1413–21.
107. Gregory CD, Dive C, Henderson S, et al. Activation of Epstein-Barr virus latent genes protects human B cells from death by apoptosis. Nature 1991;349:612–4.
108. Klein G. Viral latency and transformation: the strategy of Epstein-Barr virus. Cell 1989;58:5–8.
109. Burkhardt AL, Bolen JB, Kieff E, Longnecker R. An Epstein-Barr virus transformation-associated membrane protein interacts with src family tyrosine kinases. J Virol 1992;66:5161–7.
110. Knecht H, Raphael M, McQuain C, et al. Deletion variants within the NF-kappa B activation domain of the LMP1 oncogene prevail in acquired immunodeficiency syndrome-related large cell lymphomas and human immunodeficiency virus-negative atypical lymphoproliferations. Blood 1996;87:876–81.
111. Kieff E. Current perspectives on the molecular pathogenesis of virus-induced cancers in human immunodeficiency virus infection and acquired immunodeficiency syndrome. J Natl Cancer Inst Monogr 1998;23:7–14.
112. Huen DS, Henderson SA, Croom-Carter D, Rowe M. The Epstein-Barr virus latent membrane protein-1 (LMP1) mediates activation of NF-kappa B and cell surface phenotype via two effector regions in its carboxy-terminal cytoplasmic domain. Oncogene 1995;10:549–60.
113. Sandvej K, Gratama JW, Munch M, et al. Sequence analysis of the Epstein-Barr virus (EBV) latent membrane protein-1 gene and promoter region: identification of four variants among wild-type EBV isolates. Blood 1997;90:323–30.
114. Dolcetti R, Zancai P, De Re V, et al. Epstein-Barr virus strains with latent membrane protein-1 deletions: prevalence in the Italian population and high association with human immunodeficiency virus-related Hodgkin's disease. Blood 1997;89:1723–31.
115. Ometto L, Menin C, Masiero S, et al. Molecular profile of Epstein-Barr virus in human immunodeficiency virus type 1-related lymphadenopathies and lymphomas. Blood 1997;90:313–22.
116. Levine A, Shibata D, Weiss L. Molecular characteristics of intermediate/high (I/H) grade lymphomas (NHL) arising in HIV-positive vs. HIV-negative PTS: preliminary data from a population (POP) based study in the county of Los Angeles. Blood 1992;80:1028.
117. Hamilton-Dutoit SJ, Pallesen G, Franzmann MB, et al. AIDS-related lymphoma. Histopathology, immunophenotype, and association with Epstein-Barr virus as demonstrated by in situ nucleic acid hybridization. Am J Pathol 1991;138:149–63.
118. Hamilton-Dutoit SJ, Pallesen G, Karkov J, et al. Identification of EBV-DNA in tumour cells of AIDS-related lymphomas by in-situ hybridisation [letter]. Lancet 1989;1:554–62.
119. Cesarman E, Chang Y, Moore PS, et al. Kaposi's sarcoma-associated herpesvirus-like DNA sequences in AIDS-related body-cavity-based lymphomas [comments]. N Engl J Med 1995;332:1186–91.
120. Karcher DS, Alkan S. Human herpesvirus-8-associated body cavity-based lymphoma in human immunodeficiency virus-infected patients: a unique B-cell neoplasm. Hum Pathol 1997;28:801–8.
121. Knowles DM. Etiology and pathogenesis of AIDS-related non-Hodgkin's lymphoma. Hematol Oncol Clin North Am 1996;10:1081–109.
122. Knowles DM. Molecular pathology of acquired immunodeficiency syndrome-related non-Hodgkin's lymphoma. Semin Diagn Pathol 1977;14:67–2.
123. McClain KL, Leach CT, Jenson HB, et al. Association of Epstein-Barr virus with leiomyosarcomas in children with AIDS [comments]. N Engl J Med 1995;332:12–8.
124. Levitskaya J, Coram M, Levitsky V, et al. Inhibition of antigen processing by the internal repeat region of the Epstein-Barr virus nuclear antigen-1. Nature 1995;375:685–8.
125. Levitskaya J, Sharipo A, Leonchiks A, et al. Inhibition of ubiquitin/proteasome-dependent protein degradation by the Gly-Ala repeat domain of the Epstein-Barr virus nuclear antigen 1. Proc Natl Acad Sci U S A 1997;94:12616–21.
126. Moore KW, Vieira P, Fiorentino DF, et al. Homology of cytokine synthesis inhibitory factor (IL-10) to the Epstein-Barr virus gene BCRFI [published erratum appears in Science 1990;250:494]. Science 1990;248:1230–4.
127. Moore KW, O'Garra A, de Waal Malefyt R, et al. Interleukin-10. Annu Rev Immunol 1993;11:165–90.
128. Howard M, O'Garra A. Biological properties of interleukin 10. Immunol Today 1992;13:198–200.
129. Hsu DH, de Waal Malefyt R, Fiorentino DF, et al. Expression of interleukin-10 activity by Epstein-Barr virus protein BCRF1. Science 1990;250:830–2.
130. Masood R, Zhang Y, Bond MW, et al. Interleukin-10 is an autocrine growth factor for acquired immunodeficiency syndrome-related B-cell lymphoma [comments]. Blood 1995;85:3423–30.
131. Benjamin D, Knobloch TJ, Dayton MA. Human B-cell interleukin-10: B-cell lines derived from patients with acquired immunodeficiency syndrome and Burkitt's lymphoma constitutively secrete large quantities of interleukin-10 [comments]. Blood 1992;80:1289–98.
132. Liu M, Matinez-Maza O, Johnson M, et al. IL-6 induces target cell resistance to HIV-specific cytotoxic lysis. J Acquir Immune Defic Syndr Hum Retrovirol 1995;9:321–31.
133. Pluda JM, Venzon DJ, Tosato G, et al. Parameters affecting the development of non-Hodgkin's lymphoma in patients with severe human immunodeficiency virus infection receiving antiretroviral therapy. J Clin Oncol 1993;11:1099–107.
134. Moses AV, Williams SE, Strussenberg JG, et al. HIV-1 induction of CD40 on endothelial cells promotes the outgrowth of AIDS-associated B-cell lymphomas. Nat Med 1997;3:1242–9.
135. Rabkin CS, Yang Q, Goedert JJ, et al. Chemokine and chemokine receptor gene variants and risk of non-Hodgkin's lymphoma in human immunodeficiency virus-1-infected individuals. Blood 1999;93:1838–42.
136. Gaidano G, Lo Coco F, Ye BH, et al. Rearrangements of the BCL-6 gene in acquired immunodeficiency syndrome-associated non-Hodgkin's lymphoma: association with diffuse large-cell subtype. Blood 1994;84:397–402.
137. Shiramizu B, Herndier B, Meeker T, et al. Molecular and immunophenotypic characterization of AIDS-associated, Epstein-Barr virus-negative, polyclonal lymphoma. J Clin Oncol 1992;10:383–9.
138. Levine AM. Acquired immunodeficiency syndrome-related lymphoma. Blood 1992;80:8.
139. Pelicci PG, Knowles DMd, Arlin ZA, et al. Multiple monoclonal B cell expansions and c-myc oncogene rearrangements in acquired immune deficiency syndrome-related lymphoproliferative disorders. Implications for lymphomagenesis. J Exp Med 1986;164:2049–60.
140. Ballerini P, Gaidano G, Gong JZ, et al. Multiple genetic lesions in acquired immunodeficiency syndrome-related non-Hodgkin's lymphoma. Blood 1993;81:166–76.
141. Chaganti RS, Jhanwar SC, Koziner B, et al. Specific translocations characterize Burkitt's-like lymphoma of homosexual men with the acquired immunodeficiency syndrome. Blood 1983;61:1265–8.
142. Petersen JM, Tubbs RR, Savage RA, et al. Small noncleaved B cell Burkitt-like lymphoma with chromosome t(8;14) translocation and Epstein-Barr virus nuclear-associated antigen in a homosexual man with acquired immune deficiency syndrome. Am J Med 1985;78:141–8.
143. Haluska FG, Russo G, Kant J, et al. Molecular resemblance of an AIDS-associated lymphoma and endemic Burkitt lymphomas: implications for their pathogenesis. Proc Natl Acad Sci U S A 1989;86:8907–11.
144. Neri A, Barriga F, Knowles DM, et al. Different regions of the immunoglobulin heavy-chain locus are involved in chromosomal translocations in distinct pathogenetic forms of Burkitt lymphoma. Proc Natl Acad Sci U S A 1988;85:2748–52.
145. Davi F, Delecluse HJ, Guiet P, et al. Burkitt-like lymphomas in AIDS patients: characterization within a series of 103 human immunodeficiency virus-associated non-Hodgkin's lymphomas. Burkitt's Lymphoma Study Group. J Clin Oncol 1998;16:3788–95.
146. Gaidano G, Pastore C, Gloghini A, et al. Genetic heterogeneity of AIDS-related small non-cleaved cell lymphoma. Br J Haematol 1997;98:726–32.
147. Knowles DM. Immunodeficiency-associated lymphoproliferative disorders. Mod Pathol 1999;12:200–17.
148. Jones D, Ballestas ME, Kaye KM, et al. Primary-effusion lymphoma and Kaposi's sarcoma in a cardiac-transplant recipient [comments]. N Engl J Med 1998;339:444–9.
149. Nador RG, Cesarman E, Chadburn A, et al. Primary effusion lymphoma: a distinct clinicopathologic entity associated with the Kaposi's sarcoma-associated herpesvirus. Blood 1996;88:645–56.
150. DePond W, Said J, Tasaka T, et al. Kaposi's sarcoma-associated herpesvirus and human herpesviirus 8 (KSHV/HHV8)-associated lymphoma of the bowel. Am J Surg Pathol 1997;21:719–24.
151. Katler SP, Riggs SA, Cabanillas F. Aggressive non-Hodgkin's lymphoma in immunocompromised homosexual males. Blood 1985;66.

152. Ioachim HL, Dorsett B, Cronin W, et al. Acquired immunodeficiency syndrome-associated lymphomas. Hum Pathol 1991;22:659–73.
153. Ziegler JL, Beckstead JA, Volberding PA. Non-Hodgkin's lymphoma in 90 homosexual men. N Engl J Med 1984;311:565.
154. Lowenthal DA, Straus DJ, Campbell SW. AIDS-related lymphoid neoplasia: the Memorial Hospital experience. Cancer 1988;61:2325.
155. National Cancer Institute sponsored study of classifications of non-Hodgkin's lymphomas: summary and description of a working formulation for clinical usage. The Non-Hodgkin's Lymphoma Pathologic Classification Project. Cancer 1982;49:2112–35.
156. Levine AM, Wernz JC, Kaplan L. Low-dose chemotherapy with central nervous system prophylaxis and zidovudine maintenance in AIDS-related lymphoma. JAMA 1991;266:84–8.
157. Gill PS, Levine AM, Meyer PR, et al. Primary central nervous system lymphoma in homosexual men. Clinical, immunologic, and pathologic features. Am J Med 1985;78:742–8.
158. Gill PS, Levine AM, Krailo M. AIDS-related malignant lymphoma: results of prospective treatment trials. J Clin Oncol 1987;5:1322–8.
159. Knowles DM, Chamulak GA, Subar M. Lymphoid neoplasia associated with the acquired immunodeficiency syndrome (AIDS): the New York University Medical Center experience with 105 patients. Ann Intern Med 1988;108:744–53.
160. Bermudez MA, Grant KM, Rodvien R, Mendes F. Non-Hodgkin's lymphoma in a population with or at risk for acquired immunodeficiency syndrome: indications for intensive chemotherapy. Am J Med 1989;86:71.
161. Kaplan LD, Abrams DI, Feigal E. AIDS-associated non-Hodgkin's lymphoma in San Francisco. JAMA 1989;261:719–24.
162. Kaplan MH, Susin M, Pahwa SG, et al. Neoplastic complications of HTLV-III infection. Lymphomas and solid tumors. Am J Med 1987;82:389–96.
163. Kaplan LD, Kahn JO, Crowe S. Clinical and virologic effects of recombinant human granulocyte-macrophage colony-stimulating factor in patients receiving chemotherapy for human immunodeficiency virus-associated non-Hodgkin's lymphoma: results of a randomized trial. J Clin Oncol 1991;9:929.
164. Remick SC, McSharry JJ, Wolf BC. Novel oral combination chemotherapy in the treatment of intermediate-grade and high-grade AIDS-related non-Hodgkin's lymphoma. J Clin Oncol 1993;11:1691–702.
165. Freter C. Acquired immunodeficiency syndrome associated lymphoma. NCI Monographs 1990;10:45.
166. von Gunten CF, Von Roenn JH. Clinical aspects of human immunodeficiency virus-related lymphoma. Curr Opin Oncol 1992;4:894–9.
167. Raphael M, Gentilhomme O, Tulliez M, et al. Histopathologic features of high-grade non-Hodgkin's lymphomas in acquired immunodeficiency syndrome. The French Study Group of Pathology for Human Immunodeficiency Virus-Associated Tumors. Arch Pathol Lab Med 1991;115:15–20.
168. Karp JE, Broder S. The pathogenesis of AIDS lymphomas: a foundation for addressing the challenges of therapy and prevention. Leuk Lymphoma 1992;8:167–88.
169. Oksenhendler E, Duarte M, Soulier J, et al. Multicentric Castleman's disease in HIV infection: a clinical and pathological study of 20 patients. AIDS 1996;10:61–7.
170. Oksenhendler E, Cazals-Hatem D, Schulz TF, et al. Transient angiolymphoid hyperplasia and Kaposi's sarcoma after primary infection with human herpesvirus 8 in a patient with human immunodeficiency virus infection. N Engl J Med 1998;338:1585–90.
171. Luppi M, Barozzi P, Schulz TF, et al. Bone marrow failure associated with human herpesvirus 8 infection after transplantation. N Engl J Med 2000;343:1378–85.
172. Herndier BG, Shiramizu BT, Jewett NE, et al. Acquired immunodeficiency syndrome-associated T-cell lymphoma: evidence for human immunodeficiency virus type 1-associated T-cell transformation. Blood 1992;79:1768–74.
173. Soulier J, Grollet L, Oksenhendler E, et al. Kaposi's sarcoma-associated herpesvirus-like DNA sequences in multicentric Castleman's disease [comments]. Blood 1995;86:1276–80.
174. Delecluse HJ, Anagnostopoulos I, Dallenbach F, et al. Plasmablastic lymphomas of the oral cavity: a new entity associated with the human immunodeficiency virus infection. Blood 1997;89:1413–20.
175. Vega F, Chang CC, Medeiros LJ, et al. Plasmablastic lymphomas and plasmablastic plasma cell myelomas have nearly identical immunophenotypic profiles. Mod Pathol 2005;18:873.
176. Deloose ST, Smit LA, Pals FT, et al. High incidence of Kaposi sarcoma-associated herpesvirus infection in HIV-related solid immunoblastic/plasmablastic diffuse large B-cell lymphoma. Leukemia 2005;19:851–5.
177. Lowenthal DA, Filippa DA, Richardson ME, et al. Generalized lymphadenopathy with morphologic features of Castleman's disease in an HIV-positive man. Cancer 1987;60:2454–8.
178. Ng VL, Hwang KM, Reyes GR, et al. High titer anti-HIV antibody reactivity associated with a paraprotein spike in a homosexual male with AIDS-related complex. Blood 1988;71:1397–401.
179. Straus DJ, Huang J, Testa MA, et al. Prognostic factors in the treatment of human immunodeficiency virus-associated non-Hodgkin's lymphoma: analysis of AIDS Clinical Trials Group protocol 142—low-dose versus standard-dose m-BACOD plus granulocyte-macrophage colony-stimulating factor. National Institute of Allergy and Infectious Diseases. J Clin Oncol 1998;16:3601–6.
180. Shipp MA, Harrington DP, Klatt MM, et al. Identification of major prognostic subgroups of patients with large- cell lymphoma treated with m-BACOD or M-BACOD. Ann Intern Med 1986;104:757–65.
181. Navarro JT, Ribera JM, Oriol A, et al. International prognostic index is the best prognostic factor for survival in patients with AIDS-related non-Hodgkin's lymphoma treated with CHOP. A multivariate study of 46 patients. Haematologica 1998;83:508–13.
182. Little RF, Pittaluga S, Grant N, et al. Highly effective treatment of acquired immunodeficiency syndrome-related lymphoma with dose-adjusted EPOCH: impact of antiretroviral therapy suspension and tumor biology. Blood 2003;101:4653–9.
183. Vaccher E, Tirelli U, Spina M, et al. Age and serum lactate dehydrogenase level are independent prognostic factors in human immunodeficiency virus-related non-Hodgkin's lymphomas: a single-institute study of 96 patients. J Clin Oncol 1996;14:2217–23.
184. Kaplan LD, Shiramizu B, Herndier B, et al. Influence of molecular characteristics on clinical outcome in human immunodeficiency virus-associated non-Hodgkin's lymphoma: identification of a subgroup with favorable clinical outcome. Blood 1995;85:1727–35.
185. Hoffmann C, Tieman M, Schrader C, et al. AIDS-related B-cell lymphomas (ARL): correlation of prognosis with differentiation profiles assessed by immunophenotyping. Blood 2005.
186. Kaplan LD, Straus DJ, Testa MA, et al. Low-dose compared with standard-dose m-BACOD chemotherapy for non-Hodgkin's lymphoma associated with human immunodeficiency virus infection. N Eng J Med 1997;336:1641–8.
187. Fisher RI, Gaynor ER, Dahlberg S, et al. Comparison of a standard regimen (CHOP) with three intensive chemotherapy regimens for advanced non-Hodgkin's lymphoma [comments]. N Engl J Med 1993;328:1002–6.
188. Levine AM, Tulpule A, Espina B, et al. Low dose methotrexate, bleomycin, doxorubicin, cyclophosphamide, vincristine, and dexamethasone with zalcitabine in patients with acquired immunodeficiency syndrome-related lymphoma. Effect on human immunodeficiency virus and serum interleukin-6 levels over time. Cancer 1996;78:517–26.
189. Gisselbrecht C, Oksenhendler E, Tirelli U. Human immunodeficiency virus-related lymphoma: treatment with intensive combination chemotherapy. Am J Med 1993;95:188–96.
190. Sparano JA, Wiernik PH, Hu X, et al. Pilot trial of infusional cyclophosphamide, doxorubicin, and etoposide plus didanosine and filgrastim in patients with human immunodeficiency virus-associated non-Hodgkin's lymphoma. J Clin Oncol 1996;14:3026–35.
191. Ratner L, Lee J, Tang S, et al. Chemotherapy for human immunodeficiency virus-associated non-Hodgkin's lymphoma in combination with highly active antiretroviral therapy. J Clin Oncol 2001;19:2171–8.
192. Kaplan LD, Lee JY, Ambinder RF, et al. Rituximab does not improve clinical outcome in a randomized phase 3 trial of CHOP with or without rituximab in patients with HIV-associated non-Hodgkins lymphoma. Blood 2005;106:1538–43.
193. Holland HK, Saral R, Rossi JJ, et al. Allogeneic bone marrow transplantation, zidovudine, and human immunodeficiency virus type 1 (HIV-1) infection. Studies in a patient with non-Hodgkin lymphoma. Ann Intern Med 1989;111:973–81.
194. Cooper MH, Maraninchi D, Gastaut JA, et al. HIV infection in autologous and allogeneic bone marrow transplant patients: a retrospective analysis of the Marseille bone marrow transplant population. J Acquir Immune Defic Syndr 1993;6:277–84.
195. Vilmer E, Rhodes-Feuillette A, Rabian C, et al. Clinical and immunological restoration in patients with AIDS after marrow transplantation, using lymphocyte transfusions from the marrow donor. Transplantation 1987;44:25–9.
196. Hassett JM, Zaroulis CG, Greenberg ML, Liegal FP. Bone marrow transplantation in AIDS [letter]. N Engl J Med 1983;309:665.
197. Bowden RA, Coombs RW, Nikora BH, et al. Progression of human immunodeficiency virus type-1 infection after allogeneic marrow transplantation. Am J Med 1990;88:49N–52N.
198. Bardini G, Re MC, Rosti G, Belardinelli AR. HIV infection and bone-marrow transplantation [letter; comment]. Lancet 1991;337:1163–4.
199. Giri N, Vowels MR, Ziegler JB. Failure of allogeneic bone marrow transplantation to benefit HIV infection. J Paediatr Child Health 1992;28:331–3.
200. Torlontano G, DiBartolomeo P, DiGirolamo G, et al. AIDS-related complex treated by antiviral drugs and allogeneic bone marrow transplantation following conditioning protocol with busulphan, cyclophosphamide and cyclosporin. Haematologica 1992;77:287–90.
201. Contu L, LaNasa G, Arras M, et al. Allogeneic bone marrow transplantation combined with multiple anti-HIV-1 treatment in a case of AIDS. Bone Marrow Transplant 1993;12:669–71.
202. Krishnan A, Molina A, Zaia J, et al. Durable remissions with autologous stem cell transplantation for high-risk HIV-associated lymphomas. Blood 2005;105:874–8.
203. Gabarre J, Marcelin AG, Azar N, et al. High-dose therapy plus autologous hematopoietic stem cell transplantation for human immunodeficiency virus (HIV)-related lymphoma: results and impact on HIV disease. Haematologica 2004;89:1100–8.
204. Re A, Cattaneo C, Michieli M, et al. High-dose therapy and autologous peripheral-blood stem-cell transplantation as salvage treatment for HIV-associated lymphoma in patients receiving highly active antiretroviral therapy. J Clin Oncol 2003;21:4423–7.
205. Serrano D, Carrion R, Balsalobre P, et al. HIV-associated lymphoma successfully treated with peripheral blood stem cell transplantation. Exp Hematol 2005;33:487–94.
206. Krishnan A, Molina A, Zaia J, et al. Autologous stem cell transplantation for HIV-associated lymphoma. Blood 2001;98:3857–9.
207. Kohn DB, Bauer G, Rice CR, et al. A clinical trial of retroviral-mediated transfer of a rev-responsive element decoy gene into CD34(+) cells from the bone marrow of human immunodeficiency virus-1-infected children. Blood 1999;94:368–71.
208. Cingolani A, Gastaldi R, Fassone L, et al. Epstein-Barr virus infection is predictive of CNS involvement in systemic AIDS-related non-Hodgkin's lymphomas [In Process Citation]. J Clin Oncol 2000;18:3325–30.
209. Ozer H. American Society of Clinical Oncology guidelines for the use of hematopoietic colony-stimulating factors. Curr Opin Hematol 1996;3:3–10.
210. Koyanagi Y, O'Brien WA, Zhao JQ. Cytokine alter the production of HIV-1 from primary mononuclear phagocytes. Science 1988;241:1673.
211. Wang J, Roderiquez G, Oravecz T, Norcross MA. Cytokine regulation of human immunodeficiency virus type 1 entry and replication in human monocytes/macrophages through modulation of CCR5 expression. J Virol 1998;72:7642–7.
212. Pluda JM, Yarchoan Y, Smith PD. Subcutaneous recombinant granulocyte-macrophage colony-stimulating factor used as a single agent and in alternating regimen with azidothymidine in leukopenia patients with severe human immunodeficiency virus infection. Blood 1990;76:463.
213. Scadden DT, Bering HA, Levine JD. Granulocyte-macrophage colony-stimulating factor mitigates the neutropenia of combined interferon alfa and zidovudine treatment of acquired immunodeficiency syndrome associated Kaposi's sarcoma. J Clin Oncol 1991;9:802.
214. Davey RT, Davey VJ, Metcalf JA. A phase I/II trial of zidovudine, interferon-alpha, and granulocyte-macrophage colony-stimulating factor in the treatment of human immunodeficiency virus type 1 infection. J Infect Dis 1991;164:43.
215. Scadden DT, Pickus O, Hammer SM, et al. Lack of in vivo effect of granulocyte-macrophage colony-stimulating

factor (GM-CSF) on human immunodeficiency virus-type 1 (HIV-1). AIDS Res and Human Retroviruses 1996;12:1151–9.
216. Schooley RT, Mladenovic J, Sevin A, et al. Reduced mobilization of CD34+ stem cells in advanced human immunodeficiency virus type 1 disease. J Infect Dis 2000;181:148–57.
217. Beck JT, Hsu SM, Wijdenes J, et al. Brief report: alleviation of systemic manifestations of Castleman's disease by monoclonal anti-interleukin-6 antibody. N Engl J Med 1994;330:602–5.
218. Pavlidis NA, Briassoulis E, Klouvas G, Bai M. Is interferon-a an active agent in Castleman's disease? Ann Oncol 1992;3:85–6.
219. Corbellino M, Bestetti G, Scalamogna C, et al. Long-term remission of Kaposi sarcoma-associated herpesvirus-related multicentric Castleman disease with anti-CD20 monoclonal antibody therapy. Blood 2001;98:3473–5.
220. Kofteridis DP, Tzagarakis N, Mixaki I, et al. Multicentric Castleman's disease: prolonged remission with anti CD-20 monoclonal antibody in an HIV-infected patient. AIDS 2004;18:585–6.
221. Marrache F, Larroche C, Memain N, et al. Prolonged remission of HIV-associated multicentric Castleman's disease with an anti-CD20 monoclonal antibody as primary therapy. AIDS 2003;17:1409–10.
222. Ide M, Ogawa E, Kasagi K, et al. Successful treatment of multicentric Castleman's disease with bilateral orbital tumour using rituximab. Br J Haematol 2003;121:818–9.
223. Marcelin AG, Aaron L, Mateus C, et al. Rituximab therapy for HIV-associated Castleman disease. Blood 2003;102:2786–8.
224. Newsom-Davis T, Bower M, Wildfire A, et al. Resolution of AIDS-related Castleman's disease with anti-CD20 monoclonal antibodies is associated with declining IL-6 and TNF-alpha levels. Leuk Lymphoma 2004;45:1939–41.
225. Dupin N, Diss TL, Kellam P, et al. HHV-8 is associated with a plasmablastic variant of Castleman disease that is linked to HHV-8-positive plasmablastic lymphoma. Blood 2000;95:1406–12.
226. Oksenhendler E, Boulanger E, Galicier L, et al. High incidence of Kaposi sarcoma-associated herpesvirus-related non-Hodgkin lymphoma in patients with HIV infection and multicentric Castleman disease. Blood 2002;99:2331–6.
227. Antinori A, Ammassari A, De Luca A, et al. Diagnosis of AIDS-related focal brain lesions: a decision-making analysis based on clinical and neuroradiologic characteristics combined with polymerase chain reaction assays in CSF. Neurology 1997;48:687–94.
228. Cingolani A, De Luca A, Larocca LM, et al. Minimally invasive diagnosis of acquired immunodeficiency syndrome-related primary central nervous system lymphoma [comments]. J Natl Cancer Inst 1998;90:364–9.
229. Gill PS, Graham RA, Boswell W, et al. A comparison of imaging, clinical, and pathologic aspects of space-occupying lesions within the brain in patients with acquired immune deficiency syndrome. Am J Physiol Imaging 1986;1:134–41.
230. Antinori A, Cingolani A, De Luca A, et al. Epstein-Barr virus in monitoring the response to therapy of acquired immunodeficiency syndrome-related primary central nervous system lymphoma. Ann Neurol 1999;5:259–61.
231. Luft BJ, Hafner R, Korzun AH, et al. Toxoplasmic encephalitis in patients with the acquired immunodeficiency syndrome. Members of the ACTG 077p/ANRS 009 Study Team. N Engl J Med 1993;329:995–1000.
232. Epstein L, DiCarlo F, Joshi V, et al. Primary lymphoma of the CNS in children with AIDS. Pediatrics 1988;82:355.
233. Baumgartner JE, Rachlin JR, Beckstead JH, et al. Primary central nervous system lymphomas: natural history and response to radiation therapy in 55 patients with acquired immunodeficiency syndrome. J Neurosurg 1990;73:206–11.
234. Hoffmann C, Tabrizian S, Wolf E, et al. Survival of AIDS patients with primary central nervous system lymphoma is dramatically improved by HAART-induced immune recovery. AIDS 2001;15:2119–27.
235. Jacomet C, Girard PM, Lebrette MG, et al. Intravenous methotrexate for primary central nervous system non-Hodgkin's lymphoma in AIDS [comments]. AIDS 1997;11:1725–30.
236. Raez L, Cabral L, Cai JP, et al. Treatment of AIDS-related primary central nervous system lymphoma with zidovudine, ganciclovir, and interleukin 2. AIDS Res Hum Retroviruses 1999;15:713–9.
237. Franken M, Estabrooks A, Cavacini L, et al. Epstein-Barr virus-driven gene therapy for EBV-related lymphomas. Nat Med 1996;2:1379–82.
238. Robertson KD, Hayward SD, Ling PD, et al. Transcriptional activation of the Epstein-Barr virus latency C promoter after 5-azacytidine treatment: evidence that demethylation at a single CpG site is crucial. Mol Cell Biol 1995;15:6150–9.
239. Formenti SC, Gill PS, Lean E, et al. Primary central nervous system lymphoma in AIDS. Results of radiation therapy. Cancer 1989;63:1101–7.
240. McGowan JP, Shah S. Long-term remission of AIDS-related primary central nervous system lymphoma associated with highly active antiretroviral therapy [letter]. AIDS 1998;12:952–4.
241. Hessol NA, Katz MH, Liu JY, et al. Increased incidence of Hodgkin disease in homosexual men with HIV infection [comments]. Ann Intern Med 1992;117:309–11.
242. Serraino D, Pezzotti P, Dorrucci M, et al. Cancer incidence in a cohort of human immunodeficiency virus seroconverters. HIV Italian Seroconversion Study Group [comments]. Cancer 1997;79:1004–8.
243. Franceschi S, Dal Maso L, Arniani S, et al. Risk of cancer other than Kaposi's sarcoma and non-Hodgkin's lymphoma in persons with AIDS in Italy. Cancer and AIDS Registry Linkage Study. Br J Cancer 1998;78:966–70.
244. Tirelli U, Errante D, Dolcetti R, et al. Hodgkin's disease and human immunodeficiency virus infection: clinicopathologic and virologic features of 114 patients from the Italian Cooperative Group on AIDS and Tumors. J Clin Oncol 1995;13:1758–67.
245. Carbone A, Weiss LM, Gloghini A, Ferlito A. Hodgkin's disease: old and recent clinical concepts. Ann Otol Rhinol Laryngol 1996;105:751–8.
246. Carbone A, Dolcetti R, Gloghini A, et al. Immunophenotypic and molecular analyses of acquired immune deficiency syndrome-related and Epstein-Barr virus-associated lymphomas: a comparative study. Hum Pathol 1996;27:133–46.
247. Spina M, Sandri S, Tirelli U. Hodgkin's disease in HIV-infected individuals [In Process Citation]. Curr Opin Oncol 1999;11:522–6.
248. Carbone A, Gloghini A, Larocca LM, et al. Human immunodeficiency virus-associated Hodgkin's disease derives from post-germinal center B cells. Blood 1999;93:2319–26.
249. Carbone A, Gloghini A, Gaidano G, et al. Expression status of BCL-6 and syndecan-1 identifies distinct histogenetic subtypes of Hodgkin's disease. Blood 1998;92:2220–8.
250. Levine AM. Hodgkin's disease in the setting of human immunodeficiency virus infection. J Natl Cancer Inst Monogr 1998;23:37–42.
251. Andrieu JM, Roithmann S, Tourani JM, et al. Hodgkin's disease during HIV1 infection: the French registry experience. French Registry of HIV-associated Tumors. Ann Oncol 1993;4:635–41.
252. Serrano M, Bellas C, Campo E, et al. Hodgkin's disease in patients with antibodies to human immunodeficiency virus. A study of 22 patients. Cancer 1990;65:2248–54.
253. Northfelt DW, Swift PS, Palefsky JM. Anal neoplasia. Pathogenesis, diagnosis, and management. Hematol Oncol Clin North Am 1996;10:1177–87.
254. Frisch M, Biggar R, Goedert J. Human papillomavirus-associated cancers in patient with human immunodeficiency virus infection and acquired immunodeficiency syndrome. J Nat Can Inst 2000;92:1500–10.
255. Sun XW, Kuhn L, Ellerbrock TV, et al. Human papillomavirus infection in women infected with the human immunodeficiency virus [comments]. N Engl J Med 1997;337:1343–9.
256. Palefsky JM, Holly EA, Ralston ML, Jay N. Prevalence and risk factors for human papillomavirus infection of the anal canal in human immunodeficiency virus (HIV)-positive and HIV-negative homosexual men. J Infect Dis 1998;177:361–7.
257. Palefsky JM, Holly EA, Ralston ML, et al. High incidence of anal high-grade squamous intra-epithelial lesions among HIV-positive and HIV-negative homosexual and bisexual men. AIDS 1998;12:495–503.
258. Palefsky JM, Holly EA, Ralston ML, et al. Anal squamous intraepithelial lesions in HIV-positive and HIV-negative homosexual and bisexual men: prevalence and risk factors. J Acquir Immune Defic Syndr Hum Retrovirol 1998;17:320–6.
259. Kuhn L, Sun XW, Wright TC Jr. Human immunodeficiency virus infection and female lower genital tract malignancy. Curr Opin Obstet Gynecol 1999;11:35–9.
260. Goldie SJ, Kuntz KM, Weinstein MC, et al. The clinical effectiveness and cost-effectiveness of screening for anal squamous intraepithelial lesions in homosexual and bisexual HIV-positive men. JAMA 1999;281:1822–9.
261. Heard I, Schmitz V, Costagliola D, et al. Early regression of cervical lesions in HIV-seropositive women receiving highly active antiretroviral therapy [comments]. AIDS 1998;12:1459–64.
262. Palefsky JM. Anal squamous intraepithelial lesions: relation to HIV and human papillomavirus infection. J Acquir Immune Defic Syndr 1999;21 Suppl 1:S42–8.
263. Bower M, Powles T, Newsom-Davis T, et al. HIV-associated anal cancer: has highly active antiretroviral therapy reduced the incidence or improved the outcome? J Acquir Immune Defic Syndr 2004;37:1563–5.
264. Hoffman R, Welton ML, Klencke B, et al. The significance of pretreatment CD4 count on the outcome and treatment tolerance of HIV-positive patients with anal cancer. Int J Radiat Oncol Biol Phys 1999;44:127–31.
265. Peddada AV, Smith DE, Rao AR, et al. Chemotherapy and low-dose radiotherapy in the treatment of HIV-infected patients with carcinoma of the anal canal. Int J Radiat Oncol Biol Phys 1997;37:1101–5.

Section 36

UNKNOWN PRIMARY SITE

123

Neoplasms of Unknown Primary Site

John D. Hainsworth, MD
F. Anthony Greco, MD

Cancer of unknown primary site is a common clinical entity, accounting for 2% of all cancer diagnoses in the Surveillance, Epidemiology, and End Results (SEER) registries.[1] In spite of the frequency of this syndrome, relatively little attention has been given to this group of patients, and systematic study of the entity has lagged behind that of other areas in oncology. Widespread pessimism concerning the therapy and prognosis of these patients has been the major reason for the lack of effort in this area. The patient with carcinoma of unknown primary site is commonly stereotyped as an elderly, debilitated individual with metastases at multiple visceral sites. Early attempts at systemic therapy yielded low response rates and had a negligible effect on survival, thereby strengthening arguments for a nihilistic approach to these patients. The heterogeneity of this group has also made the design of therapeutic studies difficult; it is well recognized that cancers with different biologies from many primary sites are represented.

Several treatable subgroups of patients within this heterogeneous group have been characterized, and initial identification of these patients is imperative for optimal management. Treatable subsets of patients are recognized either on the basis of specific clinical presentations, or by the use of specialized pathologic techniques that aid in tumor characterization. Empiric chemotherapy for patients who do not fit into any of the specific subsets has also improved, and a trial of therapy should be considered for all patients with good performance status.

The typical patient with cancer of unknown primary site develops symptoms at a metastatic site, but routine history, physical examination, chest radiography, and laboratory studies fail to identify the primary site. The initial light microscopic diagnosis usually identifies one of four histologies and should be used as the initial guideline for further evaluation of these patients. These four light-microscopic diagnoses include poorly differentiated neoplasm, adenocarcinoma, squamous cell carcinoma, and poorly differentiated carcinoma. These four groups are discussed separately, because they vary with respect to clinical characteristics, recommended diagnostic evaluation, treatment, and prognosis.

POORLY DIFFERENTIATED NEOPLASMS

The diagnosis of poorly differentiated neoplasm implies the inability of the pathologist to distinguish between carcinoma and other cancers, such as lymphoma, melanoma, and sarcoma. Establishing a more precise diagnosis is essential in this group of patients, because highly treatable cancers are common. The most frequent tumor for which specific, highly effective therapy is available is non-Hodgkin lymphoma; in reported series, 34 to 66% of poorly differentiated neoplasms were found to be lymphomas after further pathologic evaluation.[2–4] A second important, and potentially treatable, group of patients are those with poorly differentiated neuroendocrine carcinoma, accounting for another 10 to 15% of this group. Most of the remaining patients have poorly differentiated carcinoma; other tumors, including melanoma and sarcoma, collectively account for less than 15% of all cases.

The evaluation of the poorly differentiated neoplasm requires specialized pathologic studies. Immunoperoxidase staining, electron microscopy, and chromosomal analysis are techniques of proved value in the differential diagnosis of these tumors. However, it is important to remember that an inadequate biopsy specimen is a common cause of a non-specific light microscopic diagnosis. Fine-needle aspiration (FNA) biopsy provides adequate amounts of tissue for definitive diagnosis of differentiated tumors (eg, squamous carcinoma, adenocarcinoma), but is frequently inadequate for definitive characterization of poorly differentiated cancers.[5] When recognition of a tumor's pattern of growth or the ability to perform special studies is limited by a FNA specimen's small size, a specific diagnosis can often be made simply by obtaining a larger biopsy. Close communication with the surgeon and the pathologist is important if repeat biopsy is performed, because some pathologic studies require special tissue processing. Some neoplasms remain unclassifiable by light microscopy, however, even with an adequate biopsy specimen; in these cases, additional evaluation is essential.

Immunoperoxidase Staining Immunoperoxidase staining is currently the most widely available adjunctive tool for the classification of neoplasms. In contrast to most other pathologic techniques, immunoperoxidase staining can be performed on formalin-fixed, paraffinized tissue, which broadens its applicability. Immunoperoxidase methods use monoclonal or polyclonal antibodies directed at specific cell components or products, which can include enzymes (eg, prostatic acid phosphatase, neuron-specific enolase), intermediate filaments and other normal tissue components (eg, keratin, desmin, vimentin, neurofilaments, common leucocyte antigen), hormones (eg, chorionic gonadotropin), oncofetal antigens (eg, alpha-fetoprotein, carcinoembryonic antigen), and other tumor markers (eg, S-100 protein). Specific diagnoses cannot be made on the basis of immunoperoxidase staining alone, because none of these reagents are directed at tumor-specific antigens. Therefore, results must be interpreted in conjunction with the light microscopic appearance. At times, clinical features can also be used to support a diagnosis. Clinical information (eg, gender, age, location of

Table 123-1 Examples of Immunoperoxidase Staining Patterns Useful in the Differential Diagnosis of Poorly Differentiated Neoplasms

Tumor Type	Cytokeratin	Epithelial Membrane Antigen	Leukocyte Common Antigen	S-100 Protein	Vimentin	Neuron-Specific Enolase	Human Chorionic Gonadotrophin	α-Fetoprotein	Prostate-Specific Antigen	Estrogen/Progesterone Receptor	Desmin	Factor VIII Antigen	Chromogranin/Synaptophysin
Carcinoma	+	+[a]	–	–	–	±[b]	±	±	±	±	–	–	±
Lymphoma	–	±[c]	+	–	–	–	–	–	–	–	–	–	–
Melanoma	–	–	–	+	+	+	–	–	–	–	–	–	–
Sarcoma	–	±[d]	–	–	+	–	–	–	–	–	+[e]	+[f]	–
Neuroendocrine tumor	+	+	–	–	–	+	–	–	–	–	–	–	+
Germ cell tumor	+	+	–	–	–	–	+	±	–	–	–	–	–
Prostate cancer	+	+	–	–	–	–	–	–	+	–	–	–	–
Breast cancer	+	+	–	–	–	–	–	–	–	+	–	–	–

a = adenocarcinoma; b = neuroendocrine carcinoma; c = anaplastic large cell lymphoma (Ki-1 or CD30-positive lymphoma); d = epithelioid sarcoma, synovial sarcoma; e = leiomyosarcoma, rhabdomyosarcoma; f = angiosarcoma.

metastases and symptoms) may help the pathologist narrow the differential diagnosis, thereby reducing the number of special stains required to reach a diagnosis and the expense of testing.

Specific staining patterns associated with several types of neoplasms are summarized in Table 123-1. In the evaluation of poorly differentiated neoplasms, several important questions can usually be answered by immunoperoxidase staining. First, and most important, these stains can be used to make the distinction between lymphoma and carcinoma.[6–8] Second, staining for chromogranin or synaptophysin can suggest a neuroendocrine carcinoma (eg, small-cell lung cancer, carcinoid, islet cell tumor).[9] Third, staining for prostate-specific antigen (PSA) strongly suggests prostate carcinoma in a male patient with metastatic adenocarcinoma.[10] Fourth, certain staining characteristics can suggest amelanotic melanoma (positive staining for S-100 protein, Hmb-45 antigen, and vimentin) or sarcoma (positive staining for desmin, vimentin, or factor VIII antigen).[11,12]

Several potential problems must be recognized when interpreting immunoperoxidase stains. Considerable technical expertise is required to perform these tests accurately and reproducibly, and proper interpretation requires an experienced pathologist. In addition, care must be taken to avoid overinterpretation, because no staining pattern is entirely specific. Certain stains, particularly leukocyte common antigen and PSA, are quite specific; however, false-positive or false-negative staining is more frequent with most of the other stains.

Some data now exist to verify that diagnoses based on immunoperoxidase staining in patients with poorly differentiated neoplasms can be used to plan therapy and predict outcome. Undifferentiated neoplasms that are identified as lymphoma on the basis of positive leukocyte common antigen staining respond well to the combination chemotherapy treatments used for aggressive non-Hodgkin lymphoma.[4] In a group of 35 such patients, treatment with a variety of standard lymphoma regimens resulted in an actuarial disease-free survival of 45% at 30 months. This treatment outcome was similar to that for a group of concurrently treated patients who had aggressive lymphomas with typical histology (ie, diagnosed by light microscopy). On the basis of this evidence, aggressive non-Hodgkin lymphomas can be reliably identified using immunoperoxidase staining, and specific treatment can be administered with confidence to these patients. Limited data exist concerning the treatment of poorly differentiated neoplasms given the diagnoses other than lymphoma on the basis of immunoperoxidase staining (see "Poorly Differentiated Carcinoma of Unknown Primary Site").

Electron Microscopy The identification of specific ultrastructural features by electron microscopy enables a definitive diagnosis in some poorly differentiated neoplasms. Because it is less widely available, requires special tissue fixation at the time of biopsy or rebiopsy, and is relatively expensive, electron microscopy should probably be reserved for the study of neoplasms whose lineage is unclear after routine light microscopy and immunoperoxidase staining. Like immunoperoxidase staining, electron microscopy is extremely reliable in distinguishing lymphoma from carcinoma and is probably superior in the identification of poorly differentiated sarcoma. Other specific structures, such as neurosecretory granules (neuroendocrine tumors) or premelanosomes (melanoma), are also seen in some poorly differentiated neoplasms and allow specific diagnoses to be made. However, undifferentiated tumors often lose specific ultrastructural features in addition to typical histology; therefore, the absence of a particular ultrastructural finding cannot be used to rule out a specific diagnosis.

In some cases, electron microscopy provides evidence for adenocarcinoma or squamous cell carcinoma. Features of adenocarcinoma include inter- and intracellular lumina and surface microvilli. Squamous cell carcinomas are characterized by frequent and prominent desmosomes and prominent bundles of prekeratin filaments in the adjacent cytoplasm. It is impossible, however, to pinpoint the origin of poorly differentiated adenocarcinoma or squamous carcinoma by electron microscopic features. Treatment implications for adenocarcinoma and squamous cell carcinoma diagnosed only by ultrastructural features are currently unclear (see "Adenocarcinoma of Unknown Primary Site").

Chromosomal Analysis The identification of chromosomal abnormalities associated with neoplasms is becoming increasingly important in predicting prognosis. The use of tumor-specific chromosomal abnormalities in diagnosis is still limited, but it is likely that more of these abnormalities will be identified in the future.

Chromosomal and molecular genetic abnormalities have been best studied in hematopoietic and lymphoid neoplasms. Most B-cell and T-cell non-Hodgkin lymphomas are associated with detectable tumor-specific rearrangements of immunoglobulin genes or T-cell antigen-receptor genes.[13] In the unusual case when the diagnosis of lymphoma cannot be definitively established with either immunoperoxidase staining or flow cytometric immunophenotyping, the detection of these specific gene rearrangements provides definitive diagnostic information.

A few chromosomal rearrangements associated with specific solid tumors have been identified. These specific abnormalities include a chromosomal translocation (rcp [11:22] [q 24; q 12]) found in all peripheral neuroepitheliomas and most Ewing's tumors,[14,15] and an isochromosome of the short arm of chromosome 12 (i12p) found in a large percentage of testicular and extragonadal germ cell tumors in men.[16]

The clinical relevance of molecular and cytogenetic studies in identifying treatable neoplasms has been studied in young patients with poorly differentiated carcinoma or adenocarcinoma involving primarily midline structures or having elevated serum levels of human chorionic gonadotropin (hCG) or alpha-fetoprotein.[17] Specific diagnoses were suggested by genetic studies in 17 of 40 patients (42%): germ cell tumor (12); melanoma (2); lymphoma (1); peripheral neuroepithelioma (1); and desmoplastic small cell tumor (1). Patients with the diagnosis of germ cell tumor had 75% overall and 45% complete response rates to cisplatin-based therapy, as compared with 17% and 0% overall and complete response rates in the remaining patients.[17] The diagnosis of germ cell tumor based on typical cytogenetic abnormalities, therefore, accurately identifies patients with highly responsive neoplasms. The recent development of a comparative genomic hybridization technique that can detect extra 12p material using paraffin-embedded tissue specimens may make this procedure more clinically applicable, by avoiding the need to obtain fresh tissue by repeat biopsy.[18] Likewise, fluorescence in situ hybridization (FISH) can be applied to fresh or paraffin-embedded tissue for detecting translations and gain or loss of specific chromosomes.

In the future, it is likely that analysis of multiple genes using microarray techniques will aid in the diagnosis of unknown primary cancers. Patterns of abnormal gene expression specific for several solid tumors have already been identified.[19,20] However, the clinical applicability of these techniques in identifying primary sites in unknown primary cancers has not yet been validated.

ADENOCARCINOMA OF UNKNOWN PRIMARY SITE

Clinical Characteristics Adenocarcinoma is the most frequent light microscopic diagnosis in patients with neoplasms of unknown primary site and accounts for approximately 70% of cases. The incidence of this diagnosis increases with age; most patients have metastatic tumor at more than one site. The clinical presentation is determined by the sites of tumor involvement, which frequently include the liver, lungs, nodes, and bones.

The clinical course is usually dominated by symptoms related to the sites of metastases. During the clinical course, the primary site becomes obvious in only 15 to 20% of patients.[21] Even at autopsy, 20 to 30% of patients have no primary site detected. Unfortunately, large autopsy series in patients evaluated with modern radiologic techniques (eg, computed tomography [CT]) are not available; therefore, the primary sites detected may not accurately represent the current patient population. The most common primary sites identified in historical autopsy series included the pancreas, hepatobiliary tree, and lung, accounting for approximately 40 to 50% of all cases.[22,23] Other gastrointestinal sites were also frequent, and adenocarcinomas from a wide variety of other primary sites were occasionally encountered. Adenocarcinomas of the breast and prostate were identified infrequently in this group of patients, in spite of being common cancer types.[23]

Many patients with adenocarcinoma of unknown primary site have widespread metastases and poor performance status at the time of diagnosis. The outlook for most of these patients is poor, with median survival of 4 to 6 months. However, subsets of patients with a much more favorable outlook are contained within this large group, and optimal initial evaluation enables the identification of these treatable subsets. In addition, empiric chemotherapy incorporating newer agents has produced higher response rates and probably improves the survival of patients with good performance status.

Pathology The light microscopic diagnosis of adenocarcinoma is usually made without difficulty based on the formation of glandular structures by neoplastic cells. Because this histologic feature is shared by most adenocarcinomas, the site of the primary adenocarcinoma cannot usually be ascertained by routine histologic examination. Certain histologic features are typically associated with a particular tumor type ("papillary features" with ovarian and thyroid cancer, "signet ring cells" with gastric cancer); however, even these are not specific enough to be used as definitive evidence of the primary site. Immunoperoxidase stains are also of limited utility in identifying the site of origin of most adenocarcinomas. One exception is the stain for PSA, which is quite specific for prostate cancer and should be included in the evaluation of men with adenocarcinoma of unknown primary site. Positive immunoperoxidase staining for estrogen receptor suggests metastatic breast cancer in women with metastatic adenocarcinoma. Although multiple other "tumor-specific" immunoperoxidase stains, or batteries of stains, have been evaluated, none has demonstrated sufficient specificity to be recommended in identifying a primary site.[24–26]

The diagnosis of poorly differentiated adenocarcinoma should be interpreted with caution, since these patients may be distinctive as to both their tumor biology and their responsiveness to systemic therapy. The diagnosis of poorly differentiated adenocarcinoma is usually made when only minimal glandular formation is seen on histologic examination. However, it is sometimes made for tumors that exhibit positive staining for mucin but have no glandular features on histologic examination. It is clear that adenocarcinoma, poorly differentiated adenocarcinoma, and poorly differentiated carcinoma are diagnoses that represent parts of a spectrum of tumor differentiation rather than specific, sharply demarcated entities. Different pathologists may use slightly different criteria for making each of these three diagnoses. It is, therefore, appropriate to perform additional pathologic evaluation with immunoperoxidase staining on poorly differentiated adenocarcinomas to identify those that might respond to therapies. At present, evaluation and treatment of patients with poorly differentiated adenocarcinoma should follow the guidelines outlined for poorly differentiated carcinoma (see "Poorly Differential Carcinoma of Unknown Primary Site").

The identification of increasing numbers of oncoproteins that define the malignant phenotype and are prognostically important marks an emerging focus in the characterization of tumors. Some of these substances (eg, epidermal growth factor receptor [EGFR], HER-2 receptor) are now targets for novel therapeutic agents. Although information is currently limited in unknown primary cancer, a substantial percentage of these tumors overexpress p53, Bcl-2, Cmyc, Ras, and EGFR.[27,28] Overexpression of HER-2 is less common: in a group of 94 patients with poorly differentiated carcinoma or poorly differentiated adenocarcinoma, only 10 patients (11%) had 2+ or 3+ HER-2 overexpression by using immunoperoxidase methods.[29] The value of these markers in predicting prognosis or determining therapy is currently undefined.

Diagnostic Evaluation The detection of a primary site is unusual in a patient presenting with adenocarcinoma of unknown primary site; initial staging evaluation, therefore, should be performed to evaluate any clinical signs or symptoms and to determine the extent of metastatic disease. Routine initial evaluation should include a thorough history and physical examination (including pelvic examination in women), standard laboratory screening tests (complete blood count, channel biochemistry profile, urinalysis, stool examination for occult blood), and chest radiography. All men should have a serum PSA determination, and women with a clinical presentation compatible with metastatic breast cancer should undergo mammography, because palliative therapy is available for patients with advanced prostate or breast cancer. Computed tomography of the abdomen can identify a primary site in 10 to 35% of patients; in addition, it is frequently useful in identifying additional sites of metastatic disease.[30,31] Positron emission tomography (PET) identifies a primary site in approximately 30% of patients, and is therefore a useful diagnostic procedure.[32,33] Additional signs or symptoms should be evaluated with appropriate radiologic studies. Extensive radiologic evaluation of asymptomatic areas is rarely useful in identifying a primary site and often results in confusing or false-positive information. Endoscopy of the stomach and colon is also of low yield in asymptomatic patients, although small, occult primary sites are occasionally identified. Commonly used tumor markers (carcinoembryonic antigen [CEA], cancer antigen [CA]19-9, CA 15-3, CA 125, hCG, α-fetoprotein) are not useful as diagnostic or prognostic tests; however, they are commonly elevated and may be useful in monitoring response to therapy.[34,35]

Treatment The group of patients with adenocarcinoma of unknown primary site contains several clinically defined subgroups for which specific therapy is available. Patients who do not fit into one of these subgroups should be considered for a trial of empiric chemotherapy.

Women with Peritoneal Carcinomatosis In women, adenocarcinoma causing diffuse peritoneal involvement usually originates in the ovary, although carcinomas arising in the gastrointestinal tract or breast can occasionally produce this syndrome. However, peritoneal carcinomatosis also occurs in women with normal ovaries and no other evident intra-abdominal primary site. This syndrome has occasionally developed in women from families at high risk for ovarian cancer despite prophylactic oophorectomy,[36] and is increased in incidence in women with *BRCA1* mutations.[37] Many of these patients have histologic features typical of ovarian carcinoma, such as papillary configuration or psammoma bodies. Clinical features are typical

Table 123-2 Results of Treatment in Women with Adenocarcinoma Involving the Peritoneal Cavity

Author	Number of Patients	Chemotherapy Regimen(s)	Response Rate	5-Year Survival Rate
Strnad[39]	18	Cisplatin-based	39%	28% (3-year)
Dalrymple[40]	31	Cisplatin-based, chlorambucil	32%	0
Ransom[41]	33	Cisplatin-based	NA	20%
Fromm[42]	44	CP	64%	22%
Bloss[43]	33	PAC, CP	64%	15%
Piver[44]	46	PAC, TP	66%	NA

A = doxorubicin; C = cyclophosphamide; NA = not available; P = cisplatin; T = paclitaxel.

of advanced ovarian cancer, with tumor involvement limited to the peritoneal surfaces and elevated serum levels of CA 125 antigen. When histologic features suggest ovarian carcinoma, this syndrome has been termed "multifocal extraovarian serous carcinoma" or "peritoneal papillary serous carcinoma." Occasionally, men with peritoneal carcinomatosis, papillary adenocarcinoma, and elevated serum CA 125 levels have also been reported.[38]

Patients with this syndrome often respond well to the chemotherapy regimens effective in the treatment of advanced ovarian carcinoma. Several investigators have documented high initial response rates, with long-term remissions in 15 to 20% of patients (Table 123-2).[39–44] Chemotherapy regimens containing cisplatin and cyclophosphamide have been used most frequently in these patients; however, recent reports have documented the activity of platinum/paclitaxel regimens.[45] As in ovarian cancer, most long-term remissions have been observed in patients who had successful surgical cytoreduction prior to receiving chemotherapy.

The peritoneal epithelium is now accepted as a site of origin for some of these carcinomas. The contiguity of the peritoneal and ovarian epithelial surfaces may explain the similar biology and response to treatment observed in these two tumor types. In fact, these tumors are now thought to be similar enough that women with peritoneal papillary serous carcinoma are routinely included in clinical trials for stage III ovarian carcinoma. Optimal management of women with peritoneal carcinomatosis should therefore include initial maximal surgical cytoreduction followed by taxane/platinum chemotherapy.[45,46] Some patients in this group can be expected to have a complete response to therapy, and a minority will have a prolonged disease-free survival.

Women with Axillary Lymph Node Metastases Metastatic breast cancer should be suspected in women who have axillary lymph node involvement with adenocarcinoma. Initial lymph node biopsy should include measurement of estrogen and progesterone receptors; elevated levels provide strong evidence for the diagnosis of breast cancer.[47] Breast MRI scanning can identify a primary site even when mammography is normal, and should be performed.[48,49] PET scanning may also be a useful procedure, but further evaluation is required.[50]

Women who have metastases isolated to axillary lymph nodes after completion of routine staging evaluation are potentially curable and should be managed according to standard guidelines for stage II breast cancer. Primary therapy should include either modified radical mastectomy or axillary lymph node dissection followed by radiation therapy to the breast.[51–53] When mastectomy is performed, an occult breast cancer is identified in 44 to 82% of patients, even when physical examination and mammograms are normal.[52] Primary tumors are usually less than 2 cm in diameter; in occasional patients, only carcinoma in situ is identified in the breast.[54] Axillary dissection alone is not recommended, because primary breast tumors will subsequently become manifest in approximately 50% of patients.[51–53] Selection of adjuvant therapy should also follow standard guidelines for patients with node-positive breast cancer.

Women with metastatic sites in addition to axillary lymph nodes may also have metastatic breast cancer. These women should receive a trial of systemic therapy using the guidelines for the treatment of metastatic breast cancer. Determination of estrogen receptor status is of particular importance in these patients, because those with positive estrogen receptors may derive major palliative benefit from hormonal therapy. Testing for overexpression of the *HER-2* gene using FISH techniques may define a group who will benefit from treatment with trastuzumab.[55]

Men with Skeletal Metastases Metastatic prostate carcinoma should be suspected in men with adenocarcinoma predominantly involving bone, particularly if the metastases are blastic. Elevated serum levels of PSA or tumor staining with PSA provides confirmatory evidence of prostate cancer in this clinical setting, and treatment should follow guidelines for advanced prostate cancer.

Occasionally, patients have been reported with clinical presentations atypical for prostate cancer, in whom the diagnosis was suggested either by elevated serum PSA levels or by tumor staining for PSA.[56,57] In general, these patients presented with metastases to the lung, mediastinal lymph nodes, or upper abdominal lymph nodes, with no concomitant involvement of bone or pelvic lymph nodes. Even in the absence of a demonstrable primary tumor in the prostate, initial treatment should include androgen deprivation therapy, according to treatment guidelines for advanced prostate cancer.

Most men with adenocarcinoma of unknown primary site and bone involvement have lytic lesions and normal serum PSA levels. Such patients are unlikely to respond to androgen deprivation therapy; potential occult primary sites include lung, kidney, colon, and thyroid. A trial of empiric chemotherapy should be considered (see "Empiric Chemotherapy for Adenocarcinoma of Unknown Primary Site").

Adenocarcinoma Presenting as a Single Metastatic Lesion Occasionally, only a single metastatic lesion can be identified after a complete staging evaluation. Such single lesions have been described in a variety of sites, including lymph nodes, brain, lung, adrenal gland, liver, bone, and skin. The possibility of an unusual primary site (eg, primary cutaneous apocrine, eccrine, or sebaceous carcinomas) mimicking a metastatic lesion should be considered, but this possibility can usually be excluded on the basis of clinical or pathologic features.

In most of these patients, other metastatic sites become evident within a relatively short time. However, local treatment sometimes results in long disease-free intervals, and occasional patients have prolonged survival. Prior to initiating local treatment, a PET scan is useful to rule out the presence of other metastatic sites.[58] If no other metastases are detectable, resection of the solitary lesion should be undertaken, if technically feasible. In some instances (eg, after resection of a solitary brain metastasis), local radiation therapy may also be appropriate to maximize the chance of local control.[59] The role of systemic chemotherapy in addition to definitive local therapy is undefined; however, patients with poorly differentiated adenocarcinoma may benefit from platinum-based therapy (see "Poorly Differentiated Carcinoma of Unknown Primary Site").

Empiric Chemotherapy for Adenocarcinoma of Unknown Primary Site Most patients with adenocarcinoma of unknown primary site do not fit into any of the specific clinical subgroups outlined above. Empiric chemotherapy with 5-fluorouracil (5-FU) or doxorubicin-based regimens developed for the treatment of gastrointestinal primary tumors produced relatively low response rates and few complete responses. Various cisplatin-based regimens have also been evaluated, but were more toxic and showed no greater efficacy than other non–cisplatin-containing treatments. Table 123-3 summarizes results with various empiric chemotherapy regimens.[59–84] Results of small phase II studies using similar or identical regimens have been pooled in this summary.

The recent introduction of several novel antineoplastic agents with broad-spectrum clinical activity has changed the standard treatment of several common epithelial cancers.

These drugs include the taxanes, the topoisomerase I inhibitors irinotecan and topotecan, gemcitabine, and vinorelbine. Although none of these agents has been thoroughly evaluated, experience with various taxane-platinum regimens suggests improved response rates and survival when compared retrospectively to earlier regimens. Our initial experience with the combination of paclitaxel, carboplatin, and oral etoposide

Table 123-3 Empiric Chemotherapy for Patients with Adenocarcinoma of Unknown Primary Site: Pooled Results of Phase II Trials Using Traditional Regimens

Regimens	Number of Patients	Median Response Rate, % (Range)	Median Survival Months (Range)	References
Single agents				
5-FU ± leucovorin	190	9 (0–16)	4 (3–5)	21, 59–61
Cisplatin	21	19	5	62
Etoposide (oral)	24	8	5	63
Mitomycin C	40	17	5	64
5-FU or anthracycline-based combinations				
AM	159	28 (7–39)	5 (4–8)	65–68
FAM	99	25 (13–37)	9 (5–11)	69–72
CAV	54	33 (24, 50)	6 (5,8)	73, 74
CAF/CmeF	51	4 (0–8)	4 (3–7)	21, 68, 75
Platinum-based combinations				
CAP + F	70	24 (17, 28)	7 (6, 7)	76, 77
PveB	50	39	5	67
PE	52	21 (19–25)	5 (4–6)	74, 78, 79
PEF	36	22	5	80
PFL	31	32	18	81
PF Epi	36	28	9	82
CaE	33	23	6	83
CaE Epi	62	43	10	89

A = doxorubicin; B = bleomycin; C = cyclophosphamide; Ca = carboplatin; Epi = epirubicin; F = fluorouracil; M = mitomycin C; L = leucovorin; Me = methotrexate; NA = not available; P = cisplatin; V = vincristine; Ve = vinblastine.

gave a 47% response rate and 13-month median survival in a group of 53 patients.[85] Table 123-4 summarizes and updates results with this regimen and other combinations containing newer chemotherapeutic agents. Although response rates vary, median survival with these newer regimens is 9 to 12 months, with 2-year survival in the 20 to 25% range.[85–93,95] The addition of a third drug to a taxane/platinum-based combination does not appear to improve efficacy. Unfortunately, the lack of comparative trials and the marked heterogeneity of this patient population prevents confident determination of the most efficacious regimen.

Experience with second-line empiric chemotherapy is limited. Single-agent gemcitabine (1,000 mg/m^2 weekly 3 of 4 weeks) has modest activity in this setting.[96] The combination of gemcitabine (1,000 mg/m^2 days 1 and 8) and irinotecan (100 mg/m^2 days 1 and 8, repeated every 21 days) also has modest activity. In a group of 31 patients, most of whom had previously received a taxane/platinum combination, a response rate of 15% was observed.[97]

Retrospective analyses by several investigators have identified clinical and pathologic features associated with a favorable response to treatment with empiric chemotherapy. These features include tumor location in lymph nodes or soft tissue, fewer sites of metastatic disease, female sex, and poorly differentiated carcinoma histology.[98–100] Patients with involvement of the liver or bones have relatively poor prognosis.[84]

At present, all patients with good performance status should be considered for a trial of empiric chemotherapy. Although the most effective combination regimen has not been defined by means of randomized trials, the taxane/platinum combinations recently evaluated have produced higher response rates and have probably prolonged median survival. With these regimens, a substantial minority (approximately 20 to 25%) of patients is alive at 2 years, and a small fraction has prolonged disease-free survival. Patients with poor performance status are much less likely to benefit from chemotherapy, and optimal management may include supportive measures only.

SQUAMOUS CARCINOMA OF UNKNOWN PRIMARY SITE

Squamous cell carcinoma at a metastatic site is unusual in the absence of an obvious primary site. Effective treatment is available for patients who fit certain clinical syndromes, and, therefore, appropriate evaluation of these patients is essential.

Squamous Cell Carcinoma Involving Cervical Lymph Nodes The cervical lymph nodes are the most common metastatic site for squamous cell carcinoma of unknown primary origin. Patients are usually middle-aged or elderly, and many have a history of substantial tobacco and alcohol use. Diagnostic evaluation results in identification of the primary site in the large majority of these patients.[101] When the upper or midcervical lymph nodes are involved, a primary tumor in the head and neck region should be suspected. Optimal evaluation includes a thorough examination of the oropharynx, hypopharynx, nasopharynx, larynx, and upper esophagus by direct vision and fibroscopy, with biopsy of any suspicious areas. Computed tomography of the neck is useful in defining the extent of disease and occasionally in identifying a primary site. PET scanning identifies a primary site in 25% of patients even after other procedures are unrevealing, and should be included as a standard diagnostic procedure.[102] When the lower cervical or supraclavicular lymph nodes are involved, a primary lung cancer should be suspected. Fiberoptic bronchoscopy is indicated if chest radiography and head and neck examination are unrevealing.

In selected patients, chromosomal analysis aids in the characterization of squamous carcinoma involving cervical lymph nodes. Genetic alterations in "benign" mucosal biopsies from the upper aerodigestive tract were identical to those found in metastatic tumor involving cervical nodes in 10 of 18 patients (55%) studied.[103] Three of these patients subsequently developed primary head and neck tumors at the site of abnormal genetic findings. Identification of chromosomal abnormalities on surveillance biopsies may therefore aid in treatment planning in this group of patients. Detection of the Epstein–Barr virus genome in tumor tissue from cervical lymph nodes may also aid in diagnosis. Among occult head and neck cancers, the presence of the Epstein-Barr virus genome indicates a nasopharyngeal origin; therefore, its presence in a metastatic cervical node could lead to identification of an unsuspected primary site.[104] This evaluation can be performed on tissue obtained by fine-needle aspiration biopsy and should be considered, particularly in young patients with poorly differentiated squamous histology.

When no primary site is identified, patients should be treated according to guidelines for locally advanced squamous carcinoma of the head and neck. Treatment with definitive local radiation therapy to the pharyngeal axis and bilateral neck, radical neck dissection, or a combination of these local modalities has resulted in long-term disease-free survival for 30 to 60% of these patients.[105–109] Recently, combined modality therapy with concurrent chemotherapy and radiation therapy has improved treatment results in locally advanced head and neck cancer.[110,111]

Table 123-4 Summary of Treatment Results Using Newer Chemotherapeutic Agents

Regimen	Number of Patients	Response Rate	Median Survival (Mo)	2-Year Survival
PC[87]	77	39%	13	20%
DC[88,89]	92	43%	10	24%
PCE[86,90]	71	48%	11	20%
PCG[91]	113	25%	9	23%
GC[92]	40	55%	8	NA
IC[92]	40	38%	6	NA
DG[93]	35	40%	10	7%
PCE/GI[94]	132	30%	9	16%

C = cisplatin or carboplatin; D = docetaxel; E = etoposide; G = gemcitabine; I = irinotecan; P = paclitaxel.

Although limited experience with combined modality therapy in patients with cervical adenopathy, and an occult primary site is available,[112–114] this approach seems reasonable in these patients. As in patients with known primary sites in the head and neck, extensive involvement in neck nodes and poorly differentiated tumor histology are poor prognostic features.[109,115]

Patients with low cervical or supraclavicular lymph nodes are more likely to have a primary lung cancer, and treatment results are inferior in this group of patients. Nevertheless, patients with no detectable disease below the clavicle should be treated with the same approach as are patients with higher cervical nodes, since occasional patients will have long-term disease-free survival.

Squamous Cell Carcinoma Involving Inguinal Lymph Nodes Most patients with squamous cell carcinoma involving inguinal lymph nodes have a detectable primary site in the genital or anorectal area. In women, careful examination of the vulva, vagina, and cervix is important, with biopsy of any suspicious areas. Men should undergo a careful inspection of the penis. Digital examination and anoscopy should be performed in both sexes to exclude lesions in the anorectal area. Identification of a primary site in these patients is important, since potentially curative therapy is available for carcinomas of the vulva, vagina, cervix, and anus even after they spread to regional lymph nodes. For the occasional patient in whom no primary site is identified, definitive local therapy with inguinal lymph node dissection or radiation therapy sometimes results in long-term survival.[116] Because platinum-based chemotherapy administered concurrently with radiation therapy has improved survival of patients with squamous cancer arising in this region (eg, cervix, anus, bladder), the addition of similar chemotherapy should be considered in patients with an unknown primary site.

Squamous Cell Carcinoma Metastatic to Other Sites Metastatic squamous cell carcinoma in areas other than the cervical or inguinal lymph nodes usually represents metastasis from a primary lung cancer. Computed tomography of the chest and fiberoptic bronchoscopy should be undertaken if other clinical features suggest the possibility of lung cancer. Chemotherapy with regimens employed in the treatment of non–small-cell lung cancer may be considered in patients with good performance status.

Patients with the diagnosis of "poorly differentiated squamous cell carcinoma" should be evaluated carefully, particularly if other clinical features are unusual for lung cancer (ie, young patient, nonsmoker, unusual metastatic sites). As with the diagnosis of "poorly differentiated adenocarcinoma," this histologic diagnosis is sometimes based on scant histologic criteria. Additional pathologic evaluation with immunoperoxidase stains or electron microscopy should be considered. When the diagnosis remains unclear, such patients should be considered for a trial of therapy for poorly differentiated carcinoma (see below).

POORLY DIFFERENTIATED CARCINOMA OF UNKNOWN PRIMARY SITE

Patients with poorly differentiated carcinoma account for approximately 20% of patients with carcinoma of unknown primary site; an additional 10% of patients have poorly differentiated adenocarcinoma. Most early empiric chemotherapy trials included these patients along with the more common patients with adenocarcinoma of unknown primary origin, since no clinical differences between these two groups were recognized. It is now clear that some patients with poorly differentiated carcinoma of unknown primary site have extremely responsive neoplasms, and some are curable with combination chemotherapy. Appropriate clinical and pathologic evaluations, therefore, are critical in patients with poorly differentiated carcinoma, so that optimal therapy can be administered.

Pathologic Evaluation Examination of poorly differentiated carcinoma using routine light microscopy alone is inadequate to assess these tumors optimally. No histologic features have been identified that can distinguish chemotherapy-responsive from nonresponsive tumors.[117] Moreover, it is clear that even with careful retrospective reviews of these cases, some responsive tumors of well-defined types (eg, germ cell tumor, lymphoma) cannot be identified.[117]

Patients with the light microscopic diagnosis of poorly differentiated carcinoma thus should undergo additional pathologic studies with immunoperoxidase staining. Electron microscopy should be considered if immunoperoxidase staining results are inconclusive. The information that can be provided by these additional studies was summarized above in the section on poorly differentiated neoplasms. Because the initial diagnosis of poorly differentiated carcinoma is more specific than "poorly differentiated neoplasm," the frequency of identifying unsuspected tumors of other types (particularly lymphoma) is much lower in this group. However, unsuspected diagnoses may still be suggested; in a series of 87 patients with poorly differentiated carcinoma in whom a large battery of immunoperoxidase stains was performed, other diagnoses were suggested in 16 patients (18%).[118]

Diagnostic Evaluation The initial diagnostic evaluation of these patients is similar to that described for patients with adenocarcinoma of unknown primary site. A thorough history, physical examination, routine laboratory testing, and chest radiograph should be obtained in all patients. Computed tomography of the chest and abdomen should be performed in all patients in this group, because of the frequency of mediastinal and retroperitoneal involvement. Serum levels of hCG and α-fetoprotein should be obtained in all patients, because significant elevations of these markers suggest the diagnosis of germ cell tumor. Other serum tumor markers, such as carcinoembryonic antigen, CA 125, CA 19-9, and CA 15-3, are often elevated but are not helpful in predicting response to therapy.

Treatment When specialized pathologic studies identify a treatable neoplasm, therapy should be administered following guidelines established for the specific tumor identified. Examples of treatable tumor types occasionally identified in this group of patients include lymphoma, Ewing tumor, neuroendocrine carcinoma, and a variety of primitive sarcomas.

It is now well recognized that a few patients in this heterogeneous group have extragonadal germ cell tumors that are unrecognizable by standard pathologic criteria. These patients are usually young males with predominant tumor location in the mediastinum or retroperitoneum. Some also have marked elevations of the serum tumor markers hCG or α-fetoprotein. In some of these patients, molecular genetic analysis enables definitive diagnosis by detecting the i(12p) chromosomal abnormality specific for germ cell tumors.[17] Most young males with poorly differentiated carcinoma and clinical features of extragonadal germ cell tumor have excellent responses to chemotherapy, and some are cured with treatment following guidelines for extragonadal germ cell tumors.[99,119,120] Therefore, all patients with poorly differentiated carcinoma or poorly differentiated adenocarcinoma of unknown primary site who also have clinical characteristics suggestive of an extragonadal germ cell tumor should be treated according to the guidelines established for poor-prognosis germ cell tumors.

Treatment of patients with poorly differentiated carcinoma of unknown primary site who do not have characteristics of extragonadal germ cell tumor remains a subject of controversy. In a group of 220 patients prospectively identified and treated between 1978 and 1989, we reported a 62% overall response rate with 26% complete responses.[99] These patients were treated with intensive cisplatin-based combination regimens used in the treatment of advanced testicular cancer (ie, cisplatin, vinblastine, and bleomycin [PVB] or cisplatin, etoposide, and bleomycin [PEB]). A minority of patients (14%) remained tumor free after a minimum follow-up of 8 years.[121] Most of the patients in this group did not have clinical characteristics strongly suggestive of extragonadal germ cell tumor. However, many patients were young (median age, 39 years), and approximately 40% had predominant tumor location in the mediastinum or retroperitoneum. In a multivariate analysis, clinical features predictive of a favorable treatment outcome included tumor location in the retroperitoneum or peripheral lymph nodes, fewer sites of metastases, younger age, and no history of cigarette smoking.

In a retrospective analysis of a large series of patients with unknown primary cancer, Lenzi and colleagues could not identify a subset of patients with poorly differentiated carcinoma and long-term survival following chemotherapy.[122] In this group, patients with clinical features of extragonadal germ cell tumor were excluded. Patients received a wide variety of treatments, and only a minority of patients with poorly differentiated carcinoma received cisplatin-based therapy used in the treatment of germ cell tumors. Although no long-term survivors were identified, several of the same favorable prognostic factors were detected and included tumor location in lymph nodes, fewer metastatic sites, younger age, female sex, and poorly differentiated carcinoma histology (versus poorly differentiated adenocarcinoma). Other investigators have also documented higher response rates in patients with poorly differentiated carcinoma (versus adenocarcinoma) when treated with cisplatin-based chemotherapy.[100,123]

At present, a trial of combination chemotherapy should be considered for most patients with poorly differentiated carcinoma or poorly differentiated adenocarcinoma of unknown primary site. Patients with clinical features of extragonadal germ cell tumor should receive intensive cisplatin-based chemotherapy with a regimen used for the treatment of germ cell tumors. For the remaining patients in this group, cisplatin-based regimens have also yielded relatively high response rates. However, recent experience with carboplatin-containing regimens suggests that this drug is an acceptable substitute for cisplatin.[86–88,90,91,93,94] By reducing the toxicity of therapy, an empiric trial of treatment becomes feasible in a larger percentage of these patients. Taxane-based combination regimens have also yielded high response rates with moderate toxicity and are also a good choice for this group of patients.[86–91]

NEUROENDOCRINE CARCINOMA OF UNKNOWN PRIMARY SITE

A broad spectrum of neuroendocrine neoplasia is now recognized, in part due to improved pathologic methods for making the diagnosis. Most well-described adult neuroendocrine tumors have indolent biologies and typical histologic features (eg, carcinoid tumors, islet cell tumors, paragangliomas, pheochromocytomas). A second group of neuroendocrine tumors, typified by small cell lung cancer, has high-grade tumor biology and a typical "small cell" anaplastic appearance by light microscopy. A third group of neuroendocrine tumors has high-grade biology and no distinctive neuroendocrine features by light microscopy. In this group, the initial diagnosis is usually "poorly differentiated carcinoma" or "poorly differentiated adenocarcinoma"; neuroendocrine features are only recognized when immunoperoxidase staining or electron microscopy is performed. Neuroendocrine tumors of unknown primary site occur in each of these three categories and are considered separately.

Low-Grade Neuroendocrine Carcinoma Metastatic carcinoid or islet cell tumors are occasionally found at metastatic sites without an obvious primary site. In this situation, the metastatic tumor almost always involves the liver. Some patients have clinical syndromes produced by tumor secretion of bioactive substances. Primary sites in the intestine or pancreas are occasionally identified during the clinical course.

Carcinoid or islet cell tumors of unknown primary site usually exhibit an indolent biology, and management should follow guidelines established for metastatic tumors of these types with known primary sites. Depending on the clinical situation, appropriate management may include local therapy (resection of isolated metastasis, radiofrequency ablation, hepatic artery chemoembolization), treatment of associated syndromes with somatostatin analogues, 5-FU–based systemic therapy, or symptomatic management. Platinum-based chemotherapy has not been useful in these patients.

Small-Cell Carcinoma Patients with small cell anaplastic carcinoma at a metastatic site usually have a bronchogenic primary. Computed tomography of the chest and fiberoptic bronchoscopy should be performed, as they often identify the primary site. A large number of extrapulmonary primary sites have also been described (eg, salivary gland, esophagus, bladder, prostate, ovary, cervix), and patients with localizing symptoms should have appropriate diagnostic studies performed.

Most patients in this group have tumors with a high mitotic rate and aggressive biology. Many patients have disseminated cancer at the time of diagnosis. Unlike carcinoid-type neuroendocrine tumors, these tumors are responsive to chemotherapy, and all patients should be considered for a trial of treatment at the time of diagnosis. Although the "optimum" chemotherapy regimen is not defined, combination regimens effective in the treatment of small-cell lung cancer are recommended.

Poorly Differentiated Neuroendocrine Carcinoma In 10 to 15% of poorly differentiated carcinomas, immunoperoxidase staining or electron microscopy identifies neuroendocrine features; these tumors are called "poorly differentiated neuroendocrine tumors" or "primitive neuroectodermal tumors" on this basis.[124] Neuroendocrine features are observed by light microscopic examination in some of these tumors, whereas in others, the light microscopic diagnosis is "poorly differentiated carcinoma." Table 123-5 summarizes the clinical features and treatment results in a group of 51 such patients. Most patients had clinical evidence of a high-grade tumor, and most had metastases in multiple sites. The retroperitoneum, lymph nodes, and mediastinum were frequently involved. None of these patients had carcinoid syndrome or other syndromes associated with low-grade neuroendocrine carcinoma. Thirty-three of 43 evaluable patients responded to chemotherapy, with either a cisplatin-based combination or a combination regimen used in the treatment of small-cell lung cancer. Thirteen patients had complete responses and eight remain continuously disease-free more than 2 years after completion of therapy. Five patients with involvement at only one site received local modalities only (three received surgical excision; two received radiation therapy), and four have had long-term disease-free survival. A few similar patients, some with long-term survival following chemotherapy, have been reported by other investigators and have been classified as "extrapulmonary small-cell carcinoma of unknown primary site."[125,126]

Table 123-5 Clinical Characteristics, Treatment, and Response of 51 Patients with Poorly Differentiated Neuroendocrine Tumors of Unknown Primary Site

Clinical Characteristics	Patients *(n)*
Median age, y (range)	46 (18–81)
Male/female	34/17
Cigarette use (> 10 pack years)	25 (50%)
Dominant tumor site	
Retroperitoneum	13
Peripheral lymph nodes	7
Mediastinum	6
Bone	5
Liver	6
Other	8
Multiple sites without dominant site	6
Treatment	
Cisplatin-based combinations	38
Cyclophosphamide, doxorubicin-based combinations	8
Surgical excision	3
Radiation therapy	2
Response to chemotherapy (*n* = 46)	
Complete response	13 (28%)
Partial response	20 (43%)
No response	10 (22%)
Inevaluable	3 (7%)
Continuously disease-free	8 (16%)

Preliminary results of a recent prospective phase II trial have documented the activity of combination chemotherapy with paclitaxel/carboplatin/etoposide in patients with poorly differentiated or small cell neuroendocrine carcinoma of unknown primary site. Twenty-one of 39 patients (55%) responded to this treatment; 34% had 2-year survival.[127]

The origin of these poorly differentiated neuroendocrine tumors remains unclear, but it is likely that the group is heterogeneous. Some patients may have small-cell lung cancer with an "occult" primary site. However, many of these patients have no smoking history, and the absence of pulmonary involvement makes this diagnosis unlikely in most patients. As previously discussed, the clinical behavior and histologic appearance of these poorly differentiated tumors are also atypical of most of the other recognized adult neuroendocrine tumors, which are well-defined clinical entities with indolent biologies. However, some of these tumors probably are undifferentiated variants of well-recognized neuroendocrine tumors (eg, carcinoid tumor), albeit without a recognizable primary site. In the undifferentiated form, the clinical as well as the pathologic characteristics no longer resemble the characteristics of the more differentiated counterpart. Metastatic anaplastic neuroendocrine carcinomas

Table 123-6 Carcinoma of Unknown Primary Site: Recommended Evaluation and Treatment of Subsets

Histopathology	Clinical Evaluation (in addition to history, physical exam, routine laboratory, chest radiography)	Special Pathologic Studies	Specific Subsets for Therapy	Therapy
Adenocarcinoma (well-differentiated or moderately differentiated)	CT scan of abdomen, chest PET scan Men: serum PSA Women: Mammograms Additional studies to evaluate signs, symptoms	Men: PSA stain Women: ER, PR stain	1)Women, axillary note involvement 2)Women, peritoneal carcinomatosis 3) Men, blastic bone metastases, or high serum PSA or tumor PSA staining 4) Solitary metastatic lesion	Treat as primary breast cancer Treat as stage III ovarian cancer Treat as stage IV prostate cancer Definitive local therapy
Squamous carcinoma	Cervical presentation: Direct laryngoscopy, nasopharyngoscopy, bronchoscopy	—	Cervical adenopathy Inguinal adenopathy	Treat as locally advanced head/neck cancer Inguinal LND + radiation therapy
Poorly differentiated carcinoma	PET scan CT abdomen, chest Serum HCG, AFP Additional studies to evaluate signs, symptoms	Immunoperoxidase staining, electron microscopy, cytogenetic studies	1) Features of EGCT 2) Other patients	Treat as nonseminomatous EGCT Empiric platinum or paclitaxel/platinum regimen
Neuroendocrine carcinoma	CT scan of abdomen, chest Additional studies to evaluate signs, symptoms	Immunoperoxidase staining	1) Low grade 2) Small cell carcinoma or poorly differentiated	Treat as advanced carcinoid tumor Empiric platinum/etoposide or platinum/etoposide/paclitaxel

AFP = α-fetoprotein; CT = computed tomography; EGCT = extragonadal germ cell tumor; ER = estrogen receptor; HCG = human chorionic gonadotropin; LND = lymph node dissection; PR = progesterone receptor; PSA = prostate-specific antigen.

of gastrointestinal origin have also demonstrated sensitivity to cisplatin-based chemotherapy.[128] It is also possible that some of these neoplasms may represent a previously unrecognized type of neuroendocrine tumor.

Although the nature of these tumors remains undefined, the diagnosis of poorly differentiated neuroendocrine carcinoma identifies a highly treatable subgroup. All of these patients should be considered for a trial of therapy with either a platinum- or taxane/platinum-based regimen. Some patients with a single tumor site may be curable with local treatment modalities alone; however, a course of adjuvant chemotherapy should be considered in these patients, if clinically feasible.

SUMMARY AND FUTURE DIRECTIONS

The recognition of treatable subsets within the large heterogeneous population of patients with carcinoma of unknown primary site represents a definite advance in the management and treatment of these patients. Treatable subsets can be defined with appropriate clinical and pathologic evaluation; Table 123-6 provides a summary of the subsets and outlines the recommended evaluation and treatment. It is likely that further improvements in the molecular characterization of tumors will facilitate the identification of additional primary sites in this group of patients, and will enable the identification of additional favorable prognostic features. Molecular profiling of tumors has already resulted in recognition of patterns of genetic abnormalities typical of specific tumor types.[19]

Empiric chemotherapy for patients who do not fit into any defined subset has improved. Treatment with taxane/platinum-based chemotherapy has produced median survival of 9 to 11 months and 2-year survival of 20 to 25%, and should be considered in all patients with adequate performance status. Several other combinations containing newer agents have also shown activity and require further evaluation. Randomized trials to better define a treatment standard are indicated.

During the next few years, many novel targeted agents will be evaluated in the treatment of cancer. At present, characterization of the frequency of expression of various oncoproteins in unknown primary tumors is very limited. However, it seems likely that the novel targeted agents being evaluated in many solid tumors (eg, epidermal growth factor inhibitors, anti-angiogenesis agents, m-Tor inhibitors, raf kinase inhibitors, histone deacetylase inhibitors) will have a role in the treatment of patients with carcinoma of unknown primary site. Improvements in the treatment of these patients will almost certainly parallel improvements in treatment of other relatively resistant epithelial tumors, as new, targeted treatments are successfully incorporated.

REFERENCES

1. Muir C. Cancer of unknown primary site. Cancer 1995;75:353–6.
2. Azar HA, Espinoza CG, Richman AV, et al. "Undifferentiated" large cell malignancies. An ultrastructural and immunocytochemical study. Hum Pathol 1982; 13:323–33.
3. Gatter KC, Alcock C, Heryet A, Mason DY. Clinical importance of analysing malignant tumors of uncertain origin with immunohistochemical techniques. Lancet 1985;2:1302–5.
4. Horning SJ, Carrier EK, Rouse RV, et al. Lymphomas presenting as histologically unclassified neoplasms: characteristics and response to treatment. J Clin Oncol 1989;7:1281–7.
5. Reyes CV, Thompson KS, Jensen JD, Chouelhury AM. Metastasis of unknown origin: the role of fine needle aspiration cytology. Diagn Cytopathol 1998;18:319–22.
6. Battifora H, Trowbridge IS. A monoclonal antibody useful for the differential diagnosis between malignant lymphoma and nonhematopoietic neoplasms. Cancer 1983;51:816–21.
7. Nagle RB, McDaniel RK, Clark VA, Payne CM. The use of antikeratin antibodies in the diagnosis of human neoplasms. Am J Clin Pathol 1983;79:458–66.
8. Warnke RA, Gatter KC, Falini B, et al. Diagnosis of human lymphoma with monoclonal antileukocyte antibodies. N Engl J Med 1983;209:1275–81.
9. O'Connor DT, Burton D, Deftos LJ. Immunoreactive human chromogranin A in diverse polypeptide hormone-producing human tumors and normal endocrine tissues. J Clin Endocrinol Metab 1983;57:1084–6.
10. Allhof EP, Proppe KH, Chapman CM. Evaluation of prostate-specific acid phosphatase and prostate-specific antigen. J Urol 1983;129:316–9.
11. Kahn HJ, Marks A, Thom H, Baumal R. Role of antibody to S-100 protein in diagnostic pathology. Am J Clin Pathol 1983;79:341–7.
12. Osborn M, Weber K. Biology of disease. Tumor diagnosis by intermediate filament type: a novel tool for surgical pathology. Lab Invest 1983;48:372–94.
13. Arnold A, Cossman J, Bakhshi A, et al. Immunoglobulin gene rearrangements as unique clonal markers in human lymphoid neoplasms. N Engl J Med 1983;309:1593–9.
14. Turc-Carel C, Philip I, Berger MP, et al. Chromosomal translocation in Ewing's sarcoma. N Engl J Med 1983;309:497–8.
15. Whang-Peng J, Triche TJ, Knutsen T, et al. Chromosome translocation in peripheral neuroepithelioma. N Engl J Med 1984;311:584–5.
16. Bosl GJ, Ilson DH, Rodriguez E, et al. Clinical relevance of the i(12p) marker chromosome in germ cell tumors. J Natl Cancer Inst 1994;86:349–55.
17. Motzer RJ, Rodriguez E, Reuter VE, et al. Molecular and cytogenetic studies in the diagnosis of patients with midline carcinomas of unknown primary site. J Clin Oncol 1995;13:274–2.
18. Summersgill B, Goker H, Osin P, et al. Establishing germ cell origin of undifferentiated tumors by identifying gain of 12p material using comparative genomic hybridization analysis of paraffin-embedded samples. Diag Mol Pathol 1998;7:260–6.
19. Su AI, Welsh JB, Sapinoso LM, et al: Molecular classification of human carcinomas by use of gene expression signatures. Cancer Res 2001;61:7388-93.
20. Moraleda J, Grove N, Tran Q, et al: Gene expression data analytics with interlaboratory validation for identifying anatomical sites of origin of metastatic carcinomas [abstract]. Proc Am Soc Clin Oncol 2004;23:862 .
21. Shildt RA, Kennedy PS, Chen TT, et al. Management of patients with metastatic adenocarcinoma of unknown origin: a Southwest Oncology Group study. Cancer Treat Rep 1983;67:77–9.
22. Mayordomo JI, Guerra JM, Guijarro C, et al. Neoplasms of unknown primary site. A clinicopathological study of autopsied patients. Tumori 1993;79:321–4.
23. Nystrom JS, Weiner JM, Heffelfinger-Juttner J, et al. Metastatic and histologic presentations in unknown primary cancer. Semin Oncol 1977;4:53–8.
24. Brown RW, Campagna LB, Dunn JK, Cagle PT. Immunohistochemical identification of tumor markers in metastatic adenocarcinoma. A diagnostic adjunct in the determination of primary site. Am J Clin Pathol 1997;107:12–5.

25. Lagendijk JH, Mullink H, VanDiest PJ, et al. Tracing the origin of adenocarcinomas with unknown primary using immunohistochemistry: differential diagnosis between colonic and ovarian carcinomas as primary sites. Hum Pathol 1998;29:491–5.
26. Tot T. Adenocarcinomas metastatic to the liver: the value of cytokeratins 20 and 7 in the search for unknown primary tumors. Cancer 1999;85:171–4.
27. Briasoulis E, Tsakos M, Fountzilas G, et al. Bc12 and p53 protein expression in metastatic carcinoma of unknown primary origin; biological and clinical implications. A Hellenic Cooperative Oncology Group study. Anti-cancer Res 1998;18:1907–14.
28. Pavlidis N, Briasoulis E, Baj M, et al. Overexpression of C-myc, Ras and C-erB-2 oncoproteins in carcinoma of unknown primary origin. Anticancer Res 1995; 15:2563–8.
29. Hainsworth JD, Lennington WJ, Greco FA. Overexpression of Her-2 in patients with poorly differentiated carcinoma or poorly differentiated adenocarcinoma of unknown primary site. J Clin Oncol 2000;18:632–5.
30. Karsell PR, Sheedy PF, O'Connell MJ. Computerized tomography in search of cancer of unknown origin. JAMA 1982;248:340–3.
31. McMillan JH, Levine E, Stephens RH. Computed tomography in the evaluation of metastatic adenocarcinoma from an unknown primary site. Radiology 1982; 143:143–6.
32. Kole AC, Nieweg OE, Pruim J, et al. Detection of unknown occult primary tumors using positron emission tomography. Cancer 1998;82:1160–6.
33. Bohuslavski KH, Klutmann S, Kroger S, et al: FDG PET detection of unknown primary tumors. J Nucl Med 2000;41:816-22.
34. Currow DC, Findlay M, Cox K, Harnett PR. Elevated germ cell markers in carcinoma of unknown primary site do not predict response to platinum-based chemotherapy. Eur J Cancer 1996;32A:2357–9.
35. Pavlidis N, Kalef-Ezra J, Briasoulis E, et al. Evaluation of six tumor markers in patients with carcinoma of unknown primary. Med Pediatr Oncol 1994;22:162–7.
36. Tobacman JK, Greene MH, Tucker MA, et al. Intra-abdominal carcinomatosis after prophylactic oophorectomy in ovarian cancer-prone families. Lancet 1982;2:795–6.
37. Schorge JO, Muto MG, Welch WR, et al. Molecular evidence for multifocal papillary serous carcinoma of the peritoneum in patients with germ-line BRCA1 mutations. J Natl Cancer Inst 1998;90:841–5.
38. Shah IA, Jayram L, Gani OS, et al. Papillary serous carcinoma of the peritoneum in a man: a case report. Cancer 1998;82:860–6.
39. Strnad CM, Grosh WW, Baxter J, et al. Peritoneal carcinomatosis of unknown primary site in women. Ann Intern Med 1989;111:213–7.
40. Dalrymple JC, Bannatyne P, Russell P, et al. Extraovarian peritoneal serous papillary carcinoma. A clinicopathologic study of 31 cases. Cancer 1989;64:110–5.
41. Ransom DT, Patel SR, Kenney GL, et al. Papillary serous carcinoma of the peritoneum: a review of 33 cases treated with cisplatin-based chemotherapy. Cancer 1990;66:1091–4.
42. Fromm GL, Gershenson DM, Silva EG. Papillary serous carcinoma of the peritoneum. Obstet Gynecol 1990;75:75–9.
43. Bloss JD, Liao SY, Buller RE, et al. Extraovarian peritoneal serous papillary carcinoma: a case-control retrospective comparison to papillary adenocarcinoma of the ovary. Gynecol Oncol 1993;50:347–51.
44. Piver MS, Eltabbakh GH, Hempling RE, et al. Two sequential studies for primary peritoneal carcinoma: induction with weekly cisplatin followed by either cisplatin/doxorubicin/cyclophosphamide or paclitaxel/cisplatin. Gynecol Oncol 1997;67:141–6.
45. McGuire WP, Hoskins WJ, Brady MF, et al. Cyclophosphamide and cisplatin compared with paclitaxel and cisplatin in patients with stage III and stage IV ovarian cancer. N Engl J Med 1996;334:1–6.
46. Vasey PA, Jayson GC, Gordon A, et al: Phase III randomized trial of docetaxel-carboplatin versus paclitaxel-carboplatin as first-line chemotherapy for ovarian carcinoma. J Natl Cancer Inst 2004;96:1682-91.
47. Bhatia SK, Saclarides TJ, Witt TR, et al. Hormone receptor studies in axillary metastases from occult breast cancers. Cancer 1987;59:1170–2.
48. Henry-Tillman RS, Harms SE, Westbrook KC, et al: Role of breast magnetic resonance imaging in determining breast as a source of unknown metastatic lymphadenopathy. Am J Surgery 1999;178:496-503.
49. Schorn C, Fischer U, Luftner-Nagel S, et al. MRI of the breast in patients with metastatic disease of unknown primary. Eur Radiol 1999;9:470–3.
50. Block EF, Meyer MA. Positron emission tomography in diagnosis of occult adenocarcinoma of the breast. Am Surg 1998;64:906–8.
51. Ellerbroek N, Holmes F, Singletary E, et al. Treatment of patients with isolated axillary nodal metastases from an occult primary carcinoma consistent with breast origin. Cancer 1990;66:1461–7.
52. Merson M, Andreola S, Galimberti V, et al. Breast carcinoma presenting as axillary metastases without evidence of a primary tumor. Cancer 1992;70:504–11.
53. Foroudi F, Tiver KW. Occult breast carcinoma presenting as axillary metastases. Int J Rad Oncol Biol Phys 2000; 47:143–7.
54. Rosen PP. Axillary lymph node metastases in patients with occult noninvasive breast carcinoma. Cancer 1980;46:1298–306.
55. Slamon DJ, Leyland-Jones B, Shak S, Fuchs H, et al: Use of chemotherapy plus a monoclonal antibody against Her 2 for metastatic breast cancer that overexpresses Her2. N Engl J Med 2001;344:783-92.
56. Gentile PS, Carloss HW, Huant T-Y, et al. Disseminated prostatic carcinoma simulating primary lung cancer. Cancer 1988;62:711–5.
57. Tell DT, Khoury JM, Taylor HG, Veasey SP. Atypical metastasis from prostate cancer: clinical utility of the immunoperoxidase technique for prostate specific antigen. JAMA 1985;253:3574–5.
58. Rades D, Kuhnel G, Wildfang I, et al: Localised disease in cancer of unknown primary (CUP): The value of positron emission tomography (PET) for individual therapeutic management. Ann Oncol 2001;12:1605–9.
59. Nguyen LN, Maor MH, Oswald MJ. Brain metastases as the only manifestation of an undetected primary tumor. Cancer 1998;83:2181–4.
60. Johnson RO, Castro R, Ansfield FJ. Response of primary unknown cancers to treatment with 5-fluorouracil. Cancer Chemother Rep 1964;38:63–4.
61. Moertel CG, Reitemeier RJ, Schutt AJ, Hahn RG. Treatment of the patient with adenocarcinoma of unknown origin. Cancer 1972;30:1469–72.
62. Nole F, Colleoni M, Buzzoni R, Bajetta E. Fluorouracil plus folinic acid in metastatic adenocarcinoma of unknown primary site suggestive of a gastrointestinal primary. Tumori 1993;79:116–8.
63. Wagener DJT, de Mulder PHM, Burghouts JT, et al, for the IKZ/IKO Clinical Research Group. Phase II trial of cisplatin for adenocarcinoma of unknown primary site. Eur J Cancer 1991;27:755–7.
64. Van der Gaast A, Henzen Logmans NC, Planting AS, et al. Phase II study of oral administration of etoposide for patients with well- and moderately differentiated adenocarcinomas of unknown primary site. Ann Oncol 1993;4:789–90.
65. Falkson CI, Cohen GL. Mitomycin C, epirubicin and cisplatin versus mitomycin C alone as therapy for carcinoma of unknown primary origin. Oncology 1998;33:116–21.
66. Eagan RT, Therneau TM, Rubin J, et al. Lack of value for cisplatin added to mitomycin/doxorubicin combination chemotherapy for carcinoma of unknown primary site. Am J Clin Oncol 1987;10:82–5.
67. Kambhus SA, Kelsen D, Niedzwiecki D, Ochoa M Jr. Phase II trial of mitomycin C, vindesine, and Adriamycin and predictive variables in the treatment of patients with adenocarcinoma of unknown primary site [abstract]. Proc Am Assoc Cancer Res 1986;27:185.
68. Milliken ST, Tattersall MH, Woods RL, et al. Metastatic adenocarcinoma of unknown primary site. A randomized study of two combination chemotherapy regimens. Eur J Cancer Clin Oncol 1987;23:1645–8.
69. Woods RL, Fox RM, Tattersall MHN, et al. Metastatic adenocarcinomas of unknown primary: a randomized study of two combination chemotherapy regimens. N Engl J Med 1980;303:87–8.
70. Goldberg RM, Smith FP, Ueno W, et al. Fluorouracil, Adriamycin, mitomycin in the treatment of adenocarcinoma of unknown primary. J Clin Oncol 1986;4:395–9.
71. Sulkes A, Uziely B, Isaacson R, et al. Combination chemotherapy in metastatic tumors of unknown origin. Int J Med Sci 1988;24:604–10.
72. Treat J, Falchuk SC, Tremblay C, et al. Phase II trial of methotrexate-FAM (m-FAM) in adenocarcinoma of unknown primary. Eur J Clin Oncol 1989;25:1053–5.
73. Van der Gaast AVD, Verweij J, Planting ASTH, Stoter G. 5-Fluorouracil, doxorubicin, and mitomycin C (FAM) combination chemotherapy for metastatic adenocarcinoma of unknown primary. Eur J Cancer Clin Oncol 1988;24:765–8.
74. Anderson H, Thatcher N, Rankin E, et al. VAC (vincristine, Adriamycin and cyclophosphamide) chemotherapy for metastatic carcinoma from an unknown primary site. Eur J Cancer Clin Oncol 1983;19:49–52.
75. de Campos ES, Menasce LP, Radford J, et al. Metastatic carcinoma of uncertain primary site: a retrospective review of 57 patients treated with vincristine, doxorubicin, cyclophosphamide (VAC), or VAC alternating with cisplatin and etoposide (VAC/PE). Cancer 1994;73:470–95.
76. Valentine J, Rosenthal S, Arseneau JC. Combination chemotherapy for adenocarcinoma of unknown primary origin. Cancer Clin Trials 1979;2:265–8.
77. Jadega J, Legha S, Burgess M, et al. Combination chemotherapy with 5-FU, Adriamycin, cyclophosphamide, and cisplatin in the treatment of adenocarcinoma of unknown primary and undifferentiated carcinoma [abstract]. Proc Am Soc Clin Oncol 1983;2:926.
78. Pasterz R, Savoraj N, Burgess M. Prognostic factors in metastatic carcinoma of unknown primary. J Clin Oncol 1986;4:1652–7.
79. Gill I, Guaglianone P, Grunberg SM, et al. High-dose intensity of cisplatin and etoposide in adenocarcinoma of unknown primary. Anticancer Res 1991;11:1231–6.
80. Liu JM, Chen YM, Chao U, et al. Continuous-infusion cisplatin and etoposide chemotherapy for cancer of unknown primary site in Taiwan, a region with a high prevalence of endemic viral infections. Jpn J Clin Oncol 1998;28:431–5.
81. Raber MN, Faintuch J, Abbruzzese JL, et al. Continuous-infusion 5-fluorouracil, etoposide and cis-diammine-dichloroplatinum in patients with metastatic carcinoma of unknown primary origin. Ann Oncol 1991;2:519–20.
82. Lenzi R, Abbruzzese J, Amato R, et al. Cisplatin, 5-fluorouracil and folinic acid for the treatment of carcinoma of unknown primary. A Phase II study [abstract]. Proc Am Soc Clin Oncol 1991;10:301.
83. Karapetis CS, Yip D, Virik K, et al. The treatment of carcinoma of unknown primary with epirubicin, cisplatin, and 5-fluorouracil (ECF) [abstract]. Proc Am Soc Clin Oncol 1999;18:642a.
84. Warner E, Goel R, Chang J, et al. A multicentre Phase II study of carboplatin and prolonged oral etoposide in the treatment of cancer of unknown primary site (CUPS). Br J Cancer 1998;77:2376–80.
85. Briasoulis E, Tsavaris N, Fountzilas G, et al. Combination regimen with carboplatin, epirubicin and etoposide in metastatic carcinomas of unknown primary site: a Hellenic Cooperative Oncology Group Phase II study. Oncologia 1998;55:426–30.
86. Hainsworth JD, Erland JB, Kalman LA, et al. Carcinoma of unknown primary site: treatment with one-hour paclitaxel, carboplatin, and extended-schedule etoposide. J Clin Oncol 1997;15:2385–93.
87. Briasoulis E, Kalofonos H, Bafaloukos D, et al. Carboplatin plus paclitaxel in unknown primary carcinoma: a Phase II Hellenic Cooperative Oncology Group study. J Clin Oncol 2000;18:3101–7.
88. Greco FA, Erland JB, Morrissey LH, et al. Carcinoma of unknown primary site: Phase II trials with docetaxel plus cisplatin or carboplatin. Ann Oncol 2000;11:211–5.
89. Mukai H, Watanabe T, Ando M, et al: A safety and efficacy trial of docetaxel and cisplatin in patients with cancer of unknown primary [abstract]. Proc Am Soc Clin Oncol 2003;22:286.
90. Greco FA, Burris HA, Erland JB, et al. Carcinoma of unknown primary site: long-term follow-up after treatment with paclitaxel, carboplatin, and etoposide. Cancer 2000;89:2655–60.
91. Greco FA, Burris HA, Litchy S, et al. Gemcitabine, carboplatin and paclitaxel for patients with carcinoma of unknown primary site: a Minnie Pearl Cancer Research Network study. J Clin Oncol 2002;20:1651–6.
92. Culine S, Lortholary A, Voigt JJ, et al: Cisplatin in combination with either gemcitabine or irinotecan in carcinomas of unknown primary site: Results of a randomized phase II study—trial for the French Study Group in Carcinomas of Unknown Primary (GEFCAPI 01). J Clin Oncol 2003;21:3479–82.
93. Pouessel D, Culine S, Becht C, et al: Gemcitabine and docetaxel as front-line chemotherapy in patients with carcinoma of an unknown primary site. Cancer 2004;100:1257–61.
94. Greco FA, Rodriguez GI, Shaffer DW, et al: Carcinoma of unknown primary site: sequential treatment with paclitaxel/carboplatin/etoposide and gemcitabine/irinotecan: A Minnie Pearl Cancer Research Network phase II trial. Oncologist 2004;9:644–52.

95. Greco FA, Gray J, Burris HA, et al. Taxane-based chemotherapy for patients with carcinoma of unknown primary site. Cancer J 2001;7:203–12.
96. Hainsworth JD, Burris HA, Calvert SW, et al. Gemcitabine in the second-line therapy of patients with carcinoma of unknown primary site: a Phase II trial of the Minnie Pearl Cancer Research Network. Cancer Invest 2001;19:335–9.
97. Doss HH, Hainsworth JD, Spigel DR, et al: Gemcitabine and irinotecan in patients with previously treated carcinoma of unknown primary site: A Minnie Pearl Cancer Research Network phase II trial [abstract]. Proc Am Soc Clin Oncol 2004;23:354.
98. Abbruzzese JL, Abbruzzese MC, Hess KR, et al. Unknown primary carcinoma: natural history and prognostic factors in 657 consecutive patients. J Clin Oncol 1994;12:1272–81.
99. Hainsworth JD, Johnson DH, Greco FA. Cisplatin-based combination chemotherapy in the treatment of poorly differentiated carcinoma and poorly differentiated adenocarcinoma of unknown primary site: results of a 12-year experience. J Clin Oncol 1992;10:912–22.
100. van der Gaast A, Verweij J, Henzen-Logmans SC, et al. Carcinoma of unknown primary; identification of a treatable subset. Ann Oncol 1991;1:119–21.
101. Jones AS, Cook JA, Phillips DE, Roland NR. Squamous carcinoma presenting as an enlarged cervical lymph node. Cancer 1993;72:1756–61.
102. Rusthoven KE, Koshy M, Paulino AC: The role of fluorodeoxyglucose positron emission tomography in cervical lymph node metastases from an unknown primary tumor. Cancer 2004;101:2641-49.
103. Califano J, Westra WH, Koch W, et al. Unknown primary head and neck squamous cell carcinoma: molecular identification of the site of origin. J Natl Cancer Inst 1999;91:599–604.
104. Feinmesser R, Miyazaki I, Cheung R, et al. Diagnosis of nasopharyngeal carcinoma by DNA amplification of tissue obtained by fine-needle aspiration. N Engl J Med 1992;326:17–21.
105. Carlson LS, Fletcher GH, Oswald MJ. Guidelines for the radiotherapeutic techniques for cervical metastases from an unknown primary. Int J Radiat Oncol Biol Phys 1986;12:2101–10.
106. Reddy SP, Marks JE. Metastatic carcinoma in the cervical lymph nodes from an unknown primary site: results of bilateral neck plus mucosal irradiation vs ipsilateral neck irradiation. Int J Radiat Oncol Biol Phys 1997;37:797–802.
107. Spiro RH, DeRose G, Strong EW. Cervical node metastasis of occult origin. Am J Surg 1983;146:441–6.
108. Yang ZY, Hu YH, Yan JH, et al. Lymph node metastases in the neck from an unknown primary. Report on 113 patients. Acta Radiol Oncol 1983;22:17–22.
109. Grau C, Johansen LV, Jakobsen J, et al. Results from a national survey by the Danish Society for Head and Neck Oncology. Radiother Oncol 2000;55:121–9.
110. Brizel DM, Albers ME, Fisher SR, et al. Hyperfractionated irradiation with or without concurrent chemotherapy for locally advanced head and neck cancer. N Engl J Med 1998;338:1798–804.
111. Wendt TG, Grabenbauer GG, Rodel CM, et al. Simultaneous radiochemotherapy versus radiotherapy alone in advanced head and neck cancer: a randomized multi-center study. J Clin Oncol 1998;16:1318–24.
112. de Braud F, Heilbrun LK, Ahmed K, et al. Metastatic squamous cell carcinoma of an unknown primary localized to the neck. Advantages of an aggressive treatment. Cancer 1989;64:510–5.
113. Jeremic B, Zivic L, Jevremovic S. Radiotherapy and cisplatin in metastatic squamous cell carcinoma of an unknown primary tumor localized to the neck. A Phase II study. J Chemother 1992;4:399–402.
114. Smith SM, Argiris A, Stenson K, et al: Combined modality therapy with chemoradiation for squamous cell carcinoma of the head and neck from an occult primary [abstract]. Proc Am Soc Clin Oncol 2002;21:235a.
115. Fernandez JA, Suarez C, Martinez JA, et al. Metastatic squamous cell carcinoma in cervical lymph nodes from an unknown primary tumor: prognostic factors. Clin Otolaryngol 1998;23:158–63.
116. Guarischi A, Keane TJ, Elhakim T. Metastatic inguinal nodes from an unknown primary neoplasm. A review of 56 cases. Cancer 1987;59:572–7.
117. Hainsworth JD, Wright EP, Gray FG Jr, Greco FA. Poorly differentiated carcinoma of unknown primary site: correlation of light microscopic findings with response to cisplatin-based combination chemotherapy. J Clin Oncol 1987;5:1275–80.
118. Hainsworth JD, Wright EP, Johnson DH, et al. Poorly differentiated carcinoma of unknown primary site: clinical usefulness of immunoperoxidase staining. J Clin Oncol 1991;9:1931–8.
119. Fox RM, Woods RL, Tattersall MHN. Undifferentiated carcinoma in young men: the atypical teratoma syndrome. Lancet 1979;1:1316–8.
120. Greco FA, Vaughn WK, Hainsworth JD. Advanced poorly differentiated carcinoma of unknown primary site: recognition of a treatable syndrome. Ann Intern Med 1986;104:547–53.
121. Greco FA, Thomas M, Hainsworth JD. Poorly differentiated carcinoma (PDC) or adenocarcinoma (PDA) of unknown primary site: long-term follow-up after cisplatin-based chemotherapy [abstract]. Proc Am Soc Clin Oncol 1997;16:274a.
122. Lenzi R, Hess KR, Abbruzzese MC, et al. Poorly differentiated carcinoma and poorly differentiated adenocarcinoma of unknown origin: favorable subsets of patients with unknown primary carcinoma? J Clin Oncol 1997;15:2056–62.
123. Pavlidis N, Kosmidis P, Skarlos D, et al. Subsets of tumors responsive to cisplatin or carboplatin combinations in patients with carcinoma of unknown primary site. A Hellenic Cooperative Oncology Group study. Ann Oncol 1992;3:631–4.
124. Hainsworth JD, Johnson DH, Greco FA. Poorly differentiated neuroendocrine carcinoma of unknown primary site: a newly recognized clinicopathologic entity. Ann Intern Med 1988;109:364–72.
125. Kasimis BS, Wuerker RB, Malefatto JP, Moran EM. Prolonged survival of patients with extrapulmonary small cell carcinoma arising in the neck. Med Pediatr Oncol 1983;11:27–30.
126. van der Gaast A, Verweij J, Prins E, Splinter TAW. Chemotherapy as treatment of choice in extrapulmonary undifferentiated small cell carcinomas. Cancer 1990;65:422–4.
127. Miranda FT, Spigel DR, Hainsworth JD, et al. Paclitaxel/carboplatin/etoposide (PCE) therapy for advanced poorly differentiated neuroendocrine carcinoma: A Minnie Pearl Cancer Research Network phase II trial [abstract]. Proc Am Soc Clin Oncol 2005;23:322s
128. Moertel CG, Evols LF, O'Connell MJ, Rubin J. Treatment of neuroendocrine carcinomas with etoposide and cisplatin: evidence of major therapeutic activity in anaplastic variants of these neoplasms. Cancer 1991;68:227–32.

Section 37

PEDIATRIC ONCOLOGY

124

Pediatric Oncology: Principles and Practice

Gregory H. Reaman, MD

Cancer in the pediatric age group, which spans the period from neonate through adolescence, differs considerably from cancer in adults. The differences extend from the diagnostic type, which ultimately influences etiology, biology, and natural history, relative incidence and distribution frequency, clinical presentation and manifestations, and response to therapy and outcome.[1] Epithelial malignancies frequently observed in adults rarely exist in children, and the spectrum of pediatric cancer types varies in distribution frequency by age group.[2,3]

The age-dependent variation in frequency and the relative incidence in children of cancers arising from the embryonic mesenchyme appropriately suggest the extremely close connection between oncogenesis and developmental biology in childhood malignancies. In general, childhood malignancies tend to be associated with shorter latency periods, to grow rapidly, and frequently to be disseminated at the time of presentation. They are generally not amenable to surgical extirpation as primary modality. In addition, because most pediatric cancers do not arise from hollow viscera, wide-scale approaches to screening are generally unavailable.[4]

Although recent experience using detection of increased urinary concentration of catecholamine metabolites to screen infant populations for neuroblastoma detected the disease earlier and with favorable subtypes in some infants, such screening had no impact on the timeliness of therapeutic intervention or ultimate outcome.[5] The value of newborn screening for neuroblastoma could not, therefore, be supported based on cost–benefit considerations in regard to changing the natural history of the disease.[6]

Acute leukemia—more specifically, acute lymphoblastic leukemia—is the most common form of malignancy seen in the pediatric age group. With respect to solid tumors, primary neoplasms of the central nervous system outnumber all other solid tumors in the pediatric age group. In children, most such tumors arise in the posterior fossa and are of primitive neuroectodermal rather than glial origin, a distribution pattern that is distinct from that seen in adults. Figure 124-1 shows the distribution frequency of pediatric cancer types. As the figure shows, not only is the distribution frequency of tumor types different when the entire pediatric population is compared to adults, but an age-specific distribution pattern is also seen, separating the adolescent and young-adult population from the rest of the pediatric age group.[7]

The last several decades of the 20th century have been a period of enormous accomplishment in pediatric clinical cancer research, resulting in the preservation of millions of person-years of life. Since the early 1960s, cancer has moved from being a nearly uniformly fatal disease to being one in which more than 75% of children can be expected to achieve disease-free survival in excess of 5 years and presumably be cured of their disease. Data from the most recent Surveillance Epidemiology and End Results (SEER) publications of the National Cancer Institute (NCI) demonstrate a consistent reduction in the rate of childhood cancer mortality through the year ending 1998.[8] As shown in Figure 124-2, the past 23 years have seen a 50% decline in the death rate from childhood cancer, to approximately 25 per million from 50 per million. A 25% decrease in childhood cancer mortality has been observed since the mid 1990s alone.

The explanation for this significant progress relates to improvements in the treatment of child-

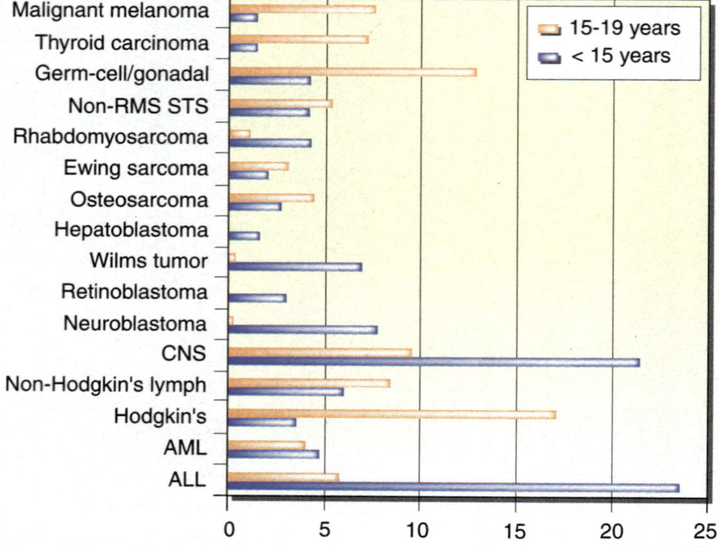

Figure 124-1 Distribution of pediatric cancer diagnoses by age group. ALL = acute lymphoblastic leukemia; AML = acute myelogenous leukemia; CNS = central nervous system; RMS = rhabdomyosarcoma; STS = soft-tissue sarcoma.

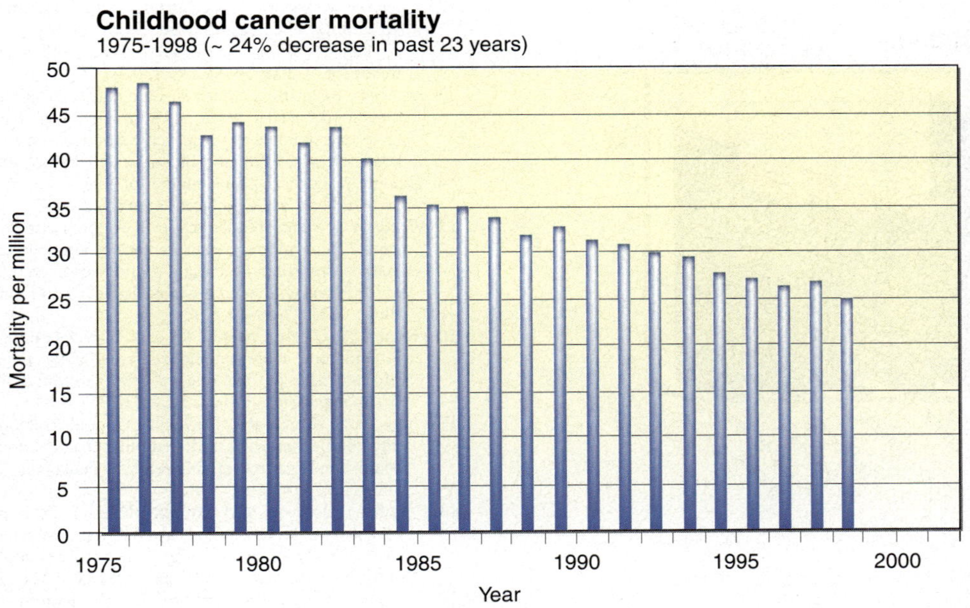

Childhood cancer mortality
1975-1998 (~ 24% decrease in past 23 years)

Mortality per million: 0, 5, 10, 15, 20, 25, 30, 35, 40, 45, 50
Year: 1975, 1980, 1985, 1990, 1995, 2000

Figure 124-2 Childhood cancer mortality. Data from the Surveillance Epidemiology and End Results Program of the National Cancer Institute.

hood cancer that have resulted from hypothesis-driven clinical trials performed, for the most part, by pediatric cancer cooperative groups. Unfortunately, similar improvements in outcome have not been demonstrated for adolescents and young adults.[9] The most graphic evidence validating this contribution of multicenter cooperative group trials to the improvement in outcome for children with cancer is the progressive improvement in survival of children treated for acute lymphoblastic leukemia (Sather HN and Reaman G. Unpublished observations. 2002). Figure 124-3 demonstrates the 10-year survival rate by period of treatment for nearly 25,000 children during consecutive time periods in which clinical trials for pediatric acute lymphoblastic leukemia were conducted. As shown, 10-year survival has increased to more than 80% from 5%. As demonstrated in Figure 124-4, improvements in 5-year survival rates vary by individual cancer type. The smallest improvements are seen in diseases where the previous rate approached 90%—except in Hodgkin's disease.[10]

The success of the pediatric cancer cooperative groups has resulted in protocol-directed therapy as a near-standard of care. Currently, more than 90% of American children younger than age 15 years receive their care in a pediatric cancer treatment center that is a member of the Children's Oncology Group, the single NCI-sponsored pediatric cancer cooperative clinical trials group.[11] Comprehensive, multidisciplinary treatment has been instrumental in improving outcomes. The presence of this multidisciplinary expertise at approved pediatric cancer treatment centers, in accordance with guidelines put forth by the American Academy of Pediatrics and the American Society of Pediatric Hematology/Oncology, guarantees a commitment to comprehensive care throughout all phases of illness and in all treatment settings.[12,13]

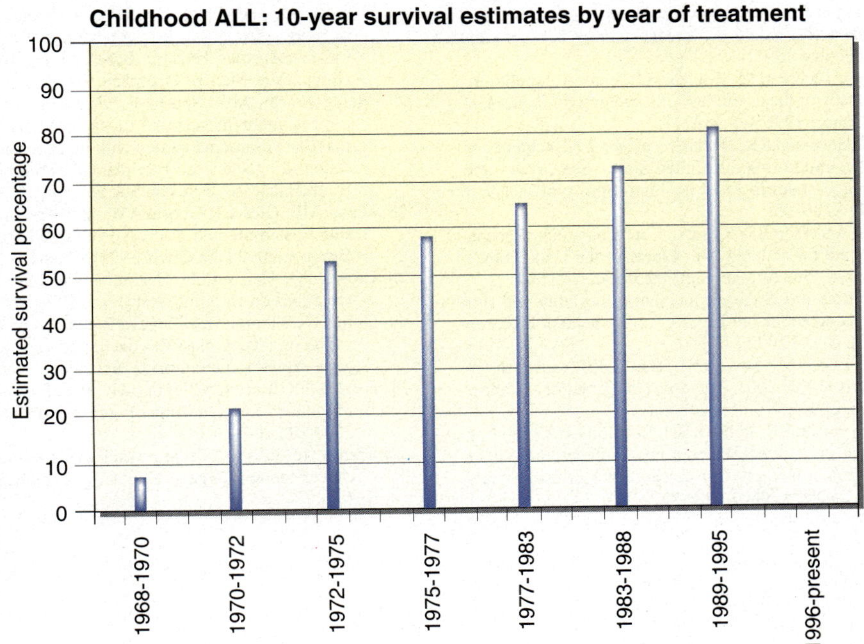

Figure 124-3 Ten-year survival estimates by year of treatment for childhood acute lymphoblastic leukemia.

An important distinguishing feature of pediatric cancer care is the need for long-term follow-up care for possible sequelae of the disease and for anticancer treatment.[14] The emergence of the Children's Oncology Group has resulted in a consolidated, unified North American–based clinical trials consortium, providing an extraordinary opportunity for a focused, coordinated, international agenda to maintain, and hopefully exceed, past progress toward increased survival and cure with increased attention to quality of life and survivorship alike. In addition, this unification provides an unprecedented opportunity for population-based clinical trials and outcomes research in pediatric cancer.

Despite the dramatic improvements in outcome, cancer remains the leading cause of death from disease in children and adolescents, evidence that considerable challenges remain in the effort to cure all children and to mitigate the risk of long-term sequelae of therapy. These challenges relate in part to an incomplete understanding of the mechanisms of intrinsic or acquired resistance of certain tumors to therapy, as well as of the widely variable host differences in distribution, metabolic rate, and clearance of the pharmacologic agents used to treat cancer. These factors appear to be particularly relevant to specific clinical situations in which the risk for treatment failure is increased, ultimately accounting for most of the cancer deaths in the pediatric age group.

The high-risk childhood cancers in which current 5-year survival rates are less than 50% include acute myelogenous leukemia[15]; relapsed acute lymphoblastic leukemia[16,17]; acute lymphoblastic leukemia with specific structural chromosomal abnormalities [t(9;22), t(4,11), and other *MLL* gene rearrangements][18–20]; biologically unfavorable subgroups of neuroblastoma (age > 1 year, chromosome 1p deletions, *myc*-N amplified, TrkC expression increased)[21–23]; supratentorial high-grade and brainstem gliomas[24,25]; and metastatic sarcomas of bone and soft tissue.[26–28] These diseases represent an area for focused, coordinated, basic, translational, and clinical research to elucidate mechanisms of resistance and to explore the potential of novel therapeutic approaches, especially those directed at unique molecular targets. An exploitable consequence of targeted molecular therapy in pediatric cancer is the equally important diminution of non–cell-specific collateral acute and long-term toxicity associated with conventional, cytotoxic anticancer therapy. Because nearly 80% of children with cancer can be expected to be long-term survivors, enhanced efforts to reduce treatment-related toxicities have never been more warranted.

The extensive search for the genetic origin of cancer has resulted in observations of genomic alterations consisting of point mutations, viral

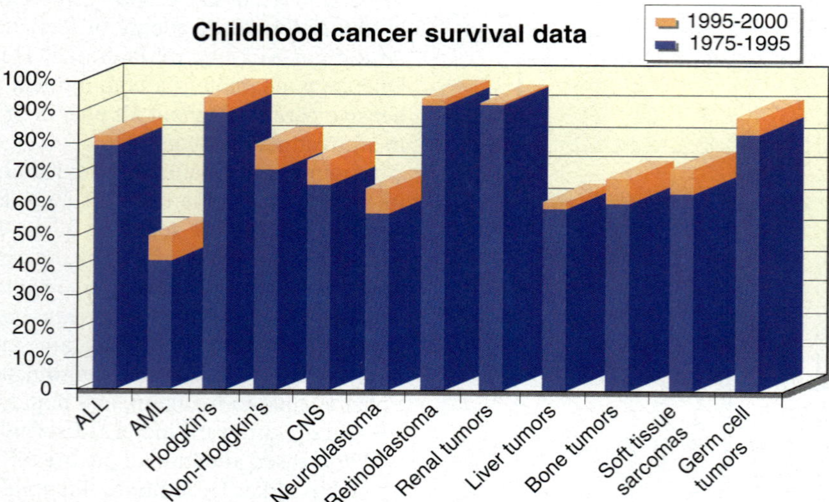

Figure 124-4 Improvement in 5-year survival rate by cancer type.

insertions, amplification, deletions, and rearrangements, each of which may alter the process of normal cell growth and development. The specific gene defect involved dictates the extent of its potential incremental contribution to oncogenesis and the magnitude of its disruption of an orderly and highly regulated growth process.[29–31] Exploiting specific genetic alterations to design novel treatments for pediatric cancer is critical to planned success for achieving or exceeding target childhood cancer survival rates in the next decade.[32] Continued progress is much more likely to come from such exploitation than from further intensification of currently available chemotherapy agents, because the chemotherapy approach has nearly reached its maximum potential as a result of limitations imposed by short-term and long-term cumulative toxicities.

Key to the successful integration of molecularly targeted therapy is increased understanding of the genetic causes of cancer and the impact of gene–environment interactions. Although each child's genome may be inherently unstable, that instability can be influenced significantly by both inheritance and environmental exposure. The necessity of integrating correlative biologic investigations with population-based clinical trials will not only provide extremely useful information identifying potential genetic risk for cancer, but also explain epigenetic differences in outcome in groups of patients treated identically. Given that most children with cancer will be treated at institutions that are members of the Children's Oncology Group, the resulting opportunity to establish a North American cancer registry provides the potential for near population-based clinical trials with integrated investigations of genetic alterations and of single-nucleotide polymorphisms, and for population-based investigation of epidemiologic associations.

Clearly, continued progress in improving the outcome of childhood cancer requires the coordinated integration of correlative biology studies with well-controlled clinical trials and the translation of basic molecular genetics into refinement of risk groups, development of risk-adjusted therapy, and ultimately, therapy directed to specific molecular lesions.

REFERENCES

1. Ries LA, Percy CL, Bunin GR. SEER pediatric monograph. In: Ries L, Smith M, Gurney JG, et al. editors. Cancer incidence and survival among children and adolescents: United States SEER program 1975–1999 [NIH Pub. No. 99-4649]. Bethesda (MD): National Cancer Institute, SEER program; 1999.
2. Gurney JG, Davis S, Severson RK, et al. Trends in cancer incidence among children in the US. Cancer 1996;78:532–41.
3. Adamson P, Law G, Roman E. Assessment of trends in childhood cancer. Lancet 2005;365:753.
4. Bleyer WA. The impact of childhood cancer on the United States and the world. CA Cancer J Clin 1990;40:355–67.
5. Bessho F, Hashizume K, Nakajo T, Kamoshita S. Mass screening in Japan increased the detection of infants with neuroblastoma without a decrease in cases in older children. J Pediatr 1991;119:237–41.
6. Woods WG, Tuchman M, Robison LL, et al. A population-based study of the usefulness of screening for neuroblastoma. Lancet 1996;348:1682–7.
7. Gurney JG Severson RK, Davis S, Robison LL. Incidence of cancer in children in the United States. Sex-, race-, and 1-year age-specific rates by histologic type. Cancer 1995;79:2186–95.
8. Smith MA, Anderson BD, Ries LA. Continuing improvements in outcome for children with cancer in the United States 1979–1998. Proc Am Soc Clin Oncol 2002;21:1551.
9. Bleyer A, Ries L. US cancer incidence, mortality and survival: young adults are lagging further behind. Proc Am Soc Clin Oncol 2002;21:1552.
10. Ries LAG, Eisner MP, Kosary CL, et al. SEER cancer statistics review 1975–2001. Bethesda (MD): National Cancer Institute; 2004
11. Ross JA, Severson RK, Pollock BH, Robison LL. Childhood cancer in the United States: a geographical analysis of cases from the pediatric cooperative clinical trials groups. Cancer 1996;77:201–7.
12. American Academy of Pediatrics Section statement on hematology/oncology. Guidelines for the pediatric cancer center and the role of such centers in diagnosis and treatment. Pediatrics 1997;99:139–41.
13. Arceci R, Reaman G, Cohen A, Lampkin B. Position statement for the need to define pediatric hematology/oncology programs: a model of subspecialty care for chronic childhood diseases. J Pediatr Hematol Oncol 1998;20:98–103.
14. Simone JV, Lyons J. The evolution of cancer care for children and adults. J Clin Oncol 1998;16:2904–5.
15. Woods WG, Neudorf S, Gold S, et al. A comparison of allogeneic bone marrow transplantation, autologous bone marrow transplantation, and aggressive chemotherapy for children with acute myeloid leukemia in remission. Blood 2001;97:56–62.
16. Gaynon PS, Qu RP, Chappell RJ, et al. Survival after relapse in childhood acute lymphoblastic leukemia: impact of site and time of first relapse—the Children's Cancer Group experience. Cancer 1998;82:1387–95.
17. Hongeng S, Krance RA, Bowman LC, et al. Outcomes of transplantation with matched-sibling and unrelated-donor bone marrow in children with leukemia. Lancet 1997;350:767–71.
18. Barrett AJ, Horowitz MM, Pollack BH, et al. Bone marrow transplants from HLA-identical siblings as compared with chemotherapy for children with acute lymphoblastic leukemia in a second remission. N Engl J Med 1994;331:1253–8.
19. Behm FG, Raimondi SC, Frestedt JL, et al. Rearrangement of the *MLL* gene confers a poor prognosis in childhood acute lymphoblastic leukemia, regardless of presenting age. Blood 1996;87:2870–7.
20. Arico M, Valsecchi MG, Camitta B, et al. Outcome of treatment in children with Philadelphia chromosome–positive acute lymphoblastic leukemia. N Engl J Med 2000;342:998–1006.
21. Brodeur GM, Ambros PF. Genetic and biological markers of prognosis in neuroblastoma. In: Brodeur GM, Sawada T, Tsuchida Y, Voute PA, editors. Neuroblastoma. Amsterdam: Elsevier Science; 2000. p. 355–69.
22. Kaneko Y, Cohn SL. Ploidy and cytogenetics of neuroblastoma. In: Brodeur GM, Sawada T, Tsuchida Y, Voute PA, editors. Neuroblastoma. Amsterdam: Elsevier Science; 2000. p. 41–56.
23. Maris JM, Matthay KK. Molecular biology of neuroblastoma. J Clin Oncol 1999;17:2264–79.
24. Mandell LR, Kadota R, Freeman C, et al. There is no role for hyperfractionated radiotherapy in the management of children with newly diagnosed diffuse intrinsic brainstem tumors: results of a Pediatric Oncology Group phase III trial comparing conventional vs. hyperfractionated radiotherapy. Int J Radiat Oncol Biol Phys 1999;43:959–64.
25. Pollack IF, Boyett JM, Finlay JL. Chemotherapy for high-grade gliomas of childhood. Childs Nerv Syst 1999;15: 529–44.
26. Koscielniak E, Klingenbiel TH, Peters L, et al. Do patients with metastatic and recurrent rhabdomyosarcoma benefit from high-dose therapy with hematopoietic rescue? Report of the German/Austrian Pediatric Bone Marrow Transplantation Group. Bone Marrow Transplant 1997;19:227–31.
27. Malogolowkin MH, Sposto R, Grovas L, et al. Lack of improvement in survival of children with metastatic rhabdomyosarcoma treated with intensive chemotherapy followed by stem cell transplant for control of minimal residual disease. Proc Am Soc Clin Oncol 1999;18:555.
28. Harris MB, Gieser P, Goorin AM, et al. Treatment of metastatic osteosarcoma at diagnosis: a Pediatric Oncology Group study. J Clin Oncol 1998;16:3641–8.
29. Brown PO, Hartwell L. Genomics and human disease—variations on variation. Nat Genet 1998;18:91–3.
30. Golub TR, Slonion DK, Tamayo P, et al. Molecular classification of cancer: class discovery and class prediction by gene expression monitoring. Science 1999;286:531–7.
31. Hughes TR, Marton MJ, Jones AR, et al. Functional discovery via a compendium of expression profiles. Cell 2000;102:109–26.
32. Uren A, Toretsky JA. Pediatric malignancies provide unique cancer therapy targets. Curr Opin Pediatr 2005;17:14–19.

124a

Incidence, Origins, and Epidemiology

Leslie L. Robison, PhD

In the United States, it is estimated that nearly 10,000 new cases of cancer will be diagnosed in 2006 in children under the age of 15 years.[1] Although pediatric cancers represent only approximately 2% of all cancers diagnosed in the United States each year, they remain the leading cause of death in children because of disease.[2] It has long been observed that, internationally, there are striking differences in the annual incidence of reported childhood cancers.[3,4] However, a number of possible explanations must be considered when interpreting international data, including potential differences in medical care systems, diagnostic acumen, differences in classification, thoroughness of cancer surveillance and reporting, the size of the population and accuracy of census, and the true occurrence of cancer among the various populations. Although temporal changes in the incidence of childhood cancer have been described and clusters observed, the significance of these patterns of occurrence remains unclear.[4–10]

Summarized below is a brief description of the incidence and epidemiology of the major forms of childhood cancer. Incidence data are provided for the United States and are derived from the National Cancer Institute's Surveillance, Epidemiology and End Results Program (SEER). The SEER pediatric monograph (<http://www-seer.ims.nci.nih.gov>) represents one of the most current and extensive assessments available.[11] Summarized in Table 124a-1 are the age-adjusted and age-specific rates for childhood cancers in the United States between 1975 and 2002.

ACUTE LEUKEMIA

In the United States, leukemias are the most common childhood cancer, representing approximately 31% of all cancer cases occurring in children under the age of 15 years.[11] Acute lymphoblastic leukemia (ALL) represents approximately 75% of all leukemias within this age group, whereas acute myeloid leukemia (AML) accounts for 20%. Childhood ALL is characterized by a sharp peak in the annual incidence occurring between the ages of 2 and 3 years, with a subsequent decrease in the rate occurring by 8 to 10 years of age. Leukemia occurs at a much higher rate in white children than in black children (4.3 vs 2.7 per 100,000), with an approximate threefold higher incidence in whites during the early childhood peak.[5] In the United States, the annual incidence of acute leukemia in children has demonstrated a very modest but consistent increase, which has led to ongoing speculation regarding the significance, if any, of this observed trend.[5,7]

Although childhood leukemias have been the subject of numerous epidemiologic investigations, the etiology of the vast majority of cases remains unknown.[12,13] There are a number of genetic conditions associated with risk, including Down syndrome, neurofibromatosis, Shwachman syndrome, Bloom syndrome, and ataxia telangiectasia. Factors that are generally agreed to infer an increased risk of childhood ALL include male gender, age 2 to 5 years, white race, higher socioeconomic status, in utero radiation exposure, and postnatal exposure to radiation (ie, therapeutic doses, atomic bomb exposure). There are a number of other less well-characterized factors that have been reported to be associated with risk of childhood ALL, such as increased birth weight, maternal history of fetal loss, older maternal age, and selected environmental exposures. Recent investigations have provided evidence against a role for environmental factors such as low-frequency electromagnetic fields (EMF) and indoor radon,[14,15] although pooled analyses have found some evidence of elevated risks for very high EMF exposures, specifically levels above 0.4 microT.[16] Hypotheses have been proposed for a potential etiologic role to postnatal infections, specifically, exposure to common and/or specific infectious agents in susceptible populations.[17,18] Some studies using day-care exposure as a surrogate for postnatal exposures have provided support for this hypothesis,[19,20] although others have not.[21]

With respect to childhood AML, risk factors include Hispanic race and exposure to chemotherapeutic agents (specifically, alkylating agents or DNA topoisomerase-II inhibitors). Genetic conditions including Down syndrome, neurofibromatosis, Shwachman syndrome, Bloom syndrome, familial monosomy, and Fanconi anemia are also associated with an increased risk of myeloid leukemia during childhood.[9,22] Although substantially less research has been conducted to identify environmental risk factors for childhood

Table 124a-1 Age-Adjusted and Age-Specific Annual Incidence Rates per Million Population for Childhood Cancer

	Age at Diagnosis						
Cancer Type (ICCC Group)	0–14	0–19	< 1	1–4	5–9	10–14	15–19
All groups combined	139.5	154.3	223.9	188.3	107.9	118.0	198.4
All leukemia	42.2	37.5	35.7	77.2	35.0	24.2	23.5
Acute lymphoblastic leukemia (ALL)	32.9	27.6	18.1	65.2	28.3	15.8	11.9
Acute nonlymphocytic leukemia	6.3	6.8	11.2	8.0	4.4	6.1	8.1
All other leukemias	2.9	3.1	6.4	4.0	2.3	2.3	3.6
All CNS	29.7	27.0	29.4	35.4	30.4	24.6	19.2
Ependymoma	2.7	2.3	4.4	5.3	1.6	1.5	0.9
Astrocytoma	14.6	13.9	11.3	15.1	15.2	14.4	11.9
PNET	6.6	5.5	8.5	9.1	7.1	3.8	2.2
All other CNS	6.8	5.3	5.2	5.9	6.5	4.8	4.3
Hodgkin's lymphoma	5.9	13.4	0.3	0.5	4.0	12.9	35.8
Non-Hodgkin's lymphoma	5.6	7.2	1.3	4.1	5.6	7.5	12.1
Burkitt's lymphoma	2.3	2.1	0.0	1.9	2.7	2.5	1.6
Neuroblastoma and ganglioneuroblastoma	10.3	7.9	61.9	19.7	3.0	0.8	0.6
Retinoblastoma	4.0	3.0	26.8	8.2	0.5	0.1	0.1
Wilms' tumor	8.3	6.3	20.2	18.8	5.6	0.9	0.3
Hepatoblastoma	1.5	1.2	8.7	3.3	0.3	0.1	0.1
Osteosarcoma	3.5	4.7	0.0	0.5	2.4	7.4	8.3
Ewing's sarcoma	2.4	3.0	0.2	0.7	2.3	4.3	4.8
Soft tissue sarcomas	10.1	11.5	14.6	9.7	8.7	10.9	15.6
Rhabdomyosarcoma and embryonal sarcoma	4.8	4.5	5.7	6.7	4.9	3.0	3.6
All other soft tissue sarcomas	5.3	7.0	8.9	3.0	3.8	8.0	12.1
Germ cell	4.5	9.4	14.8	3.8	1.8	6.0	25.9
Carcinomas	5.4	14.8	3.3	1.1	3.1	11.3	42.7
Adrenocortical carcinoma	0.2	0.2	0.8	0.3	0.2	0.1	0.3
Thyroid carcinoma	1.8	5.3	0.0	0.1	0.9	4.3	15.7
Nasopharyngeal carcinoma	0.3	0.5	0.2	0.1	0.0	0.7	1.4
Malignant melanoma	1.6	4.8	1.3	0.5	1.1	2.9	14.4

Adapted from Ries et al.[11] Surveillance, Epidemiology and End Results program, 1975–2002.

AML, studies have identified an association between maternal alcohol consumption during pregnancy and increased risk of childhood AML, as well as exposures of parents and children to pesticides and specific solvents.[23–25] However, these environmental exposures require confirmation within populations where the exposure assessment is of high quality.

CENTRAL NERVOUS SYSTEM TUMORS

Central nervous system (CNS) malignancies are the second most common malignancy in childhood and the most common form of solid tumor.[11] Approximately 17% of all pediatric cancers arise in the CNS, of which 90% are located within the brain. In contrast to CNS tumors occurring in adults, pediatric CNS tumors have a relatively high rate of occurrence within the cerebellum and brain stem. Histologically, approximately 50% of CNS tumors are astrocytomas, 20% medulloblastoma/primitive neuroectodermal tumor (PNET), 15% other gliomas, and 10% ependymomas. The incidence of CNS tumors is higher in males than in females and higher in whites than in blacks. In contrast to the age-specific pattern for childhood leukemia, CNS tumors do not demonstrate a marked variation in age. The incidence of childhood brain tumors has been reported to be increasing over the past several decades and is thus the topic of considerable speculation.[5] Assessment of the secular trends in CNS tumors suggests that improvements in diagnostic technology may account for some of the observed increases.[26]

Review of the literature reveals that currently there are no known risk factors that account for a substantial proportion of CNS tumors in children.[27–32] Factors known to be associated with an increased risk of CNS tumors include male gender (medulloblastoma/PNET, ependymomas), ionizing radiation (therapeutic doses), and genetic conditions such as neurofibromatosis, tuberous sclerosis, nevoid basal cell syndrome, Turcot's syndrome, and Li-Fraumeni syndrome. Although the Li-Fraumeni syndrome is characterized by presence of germline *TP53* mutations, there is an absence of germline somatic mutations of that gene among sporadic pediatric brain tumors.[33] Exposure to *N*-nitroso compounds, primarily through dietary intake of cured meats, has been actively pursued as an etiologic risk factor in childhood brain tumors, with results suggestive of an increased risk. There has been some interest in the potential role of polyoma viruses (ie, simian virus 40, JC, BK) in the etiology of childhood brain tumors, but further investigation is necessary to elucidate the possible association and mechanisms.[34–38]

LYMPHOMAS

The third most common form of childhood cancer in the United States is the lymphomas, accounting for 15% of all childhood malignancies.[11] The pediatric lymphomas are composed of two prominent forms including Hodgkin's disease and non-Hodgkin's lymphoma (NHL), with annual rates (per million population) in populations under 15 years of age of 5.9 and 7.9, respectively. When considering populations under the age of 20 years, the rate for Hodgkin's disease increases substantially to 13.4 per million. Pediatric Hodgkin's disease is composed of histologically distinct subgroups, including nodular sclerosis (70%), mixed cellularity (16%), lymphocytic predominance (7%), and lymphocytic depletion (< 2%). The frequency of mixed cellularity and nodular sclerosis subtypes are age and gender dependent, with both forms increasing with older age at diagnosis. NHL represents a heterogeneic group of tumors with Burkitt's and Burkitt's-like tumors predominating in children diagnosed between the ages of 5 and 14 years. Moreover, in contrast to Hodgkin's disease, NHL varies less by age. Males and whites have a higher incidence of NHL.

Only limited information is available on the etiology of Hodgkin's disease during childhood.[39] Risk of pediatric Hodgkin's disease is associated with a positive family history of Hodgkin's disease among siblings, and particularly among monozygotic twins. Epstein-Barr virus (EBV) infections have been documented to be associated with Hodgkin's disease (primarily of mixed cellularity subtype), with detection of EBV genomic material in the Reed-Sternberg cells, that varies in frequency internationally.[40–42] Based on epidemiologic observations in young adults with Hodgkin's disease (primarily the nodular sclerosis subtype), there is also speculation of an infectious etiology given the reported associations with socioeconomic status and social contacts. Some evidence supports an interaction between EBV exposure and social contacts.[43] Similarly, there is limited information relating to risk factors for childhood NHL, with only immunodeficiency, either congenital or acquired, and EBV (within "African-type" Burkitt's lymphoma) as established associations.[44]

NEUROBLASTOMA

In the United States, it is estimated that approximately 700 children are diagnosed annually with tumors of the sympathetic nervous system, of which approximately 650 are neuroblastoma.[11] Neuroblastoma, most commonly occurring in the adrenal gland, is predominantly a tumor of infancy, with 16% of children diagnosed within the first month of life and 41% diagnosed within the first 3 months of life. There are no appreciable differences in the occurrence of neuroblastoma according to sex or race.

Research stimulated by Japanese investigators has demonstrated that neuroblastoma can be detected preclinically through urinary screening of catecholamine metabolites (homovanillic acid and vanillylmandelic acid).[45] Results from population-based screening at 3 weeks and 6 months of age have shown that the incidence of neuroblastoma is increased twofold; thus, a large proportion of tumors spontaneously regress and never come to clinical diagnosis.[46]

Little is known about the etiology of neuroblastoma. Clinical and biologic characteristics, such as the very early age at onset, spontaneous regression, amplification of the *myc-n* oncogene, hyperdiploidy, and loss of heterozygosity on 1p, have generated a great deal of interest in the etiology of neuroblastoma.[47] The relatively limited number of epidemiologic studies conducted have provided some suggestions of risk associated with maternal use of medications, hormones, tobacco, and alcohol during the index pregnancy; birth characteristics (eg, increased birth weight); and a variety of parental occupations.[48] Recent research has identified a significant protective effect of maternal vitamin use during pregnancy,[49] increased risk associated with congenital anomalies,[50] day-care and childhood infections,[51] and maternal medication use,[52] but these findings require confirmation before being considered as risk factors for neuroblastoma.

RETINOBLASTOMA

Although retinoblastoma accounts for only 3% of all childhood cancers (approximately 300 cases annually in the United States), it does account for 12% of all malignancies occurring within the first year of life.[11] As seen in neuroblastoma, retinoblastoma is a tumor of infancy, with 63% diagnosed within the first 2 years and 95% within the first 5 years. Bilateral retinoblastoma is associated with younger age at diagnosis. In 42% of affected children less than 1 year old, the disease is bilateral in 21% of those 1 year of age, and only in 9% of those 2 or more years of age. The annual incidence rate of retinoblastoma is similar for males versus females and whites compared with blacks.

Based on the observed age-specific incidence patterns for children with the hereditary and nonhereditary forms of retinoblastoma, the concept of tumor suppressor genes was proposed and validated.[53] Thus, the retinoblastoma gene at 13q23 was identified.[54] Each child of a parent with familial bilateral retinoblastoma has a 50% risk of inheriting the defective retinoblastoma gene; of these, 90% will develop retinoblastoma.[55] The etiology of the nonhereditary form of retinoblastoma (sporadic retinoblastoma) is not known.

WILMS' TUMOR

Approximately 6% of all childhood cancers arise in the kidney (annual incidence rate of 8.3 per million population under age 15 years).[11] In the United States, approximately 91% of the 550 renal tumors diagnosed are Wilms' tumors, with the remaining consisting of rhabdoid tumors and clear cell sarcoma of the kidney. The vast majority of Wilms' tumors occur within the first 5 years of life. Females have a somewhat higher incidence of Wilms' tumors than males, and black children have a higher incidence compared with white children. It is notable that the rate of Wilms' tumor is substantially lower in Asians.

In contrast to many of the less common childhood malignancies, Wilms' tumor has been relatively extensively studied from an epidemiologic perspective.[11,27,56] The only established associations include race and presence of congenital and genetic conditions, including aniridia, genitourinary anomalies, WAGR syndrome (Wilms' tumor, aniridia, genitourinary abnormalities, mental retardation), Beckwith-Wiedemann syndrome, Perlman syndrome, Denys-Drash syndrome, and Simpson-Golabi-Behmenl syndrome.[57] Some studies have reported increased risks associated with paternal occupations, including welders and mechanics. A variety of other risk factors have been observed, but the evidence is limited or inconsistent, including increased birth weight, parental exposure to pesticides, in utero radiation exposure, maternal pregnancy factors such as consumption of coffee and tea, hair dye use, medication use, and occupational exposures.

BONE TUMORS

With an annual incidence rate of 8.6 per million population under the age of 20 years, malignant bone tumors account for approximately 6% of all cancers in children and young adults under the age of 20 years in the United States.[11] The age-specific incidence of bone tumors is characterized by very low rates before the age of 5 years, followed by increasing rates that peak around 13 to 15 years of age. Of the estimated 650 to 700 malignant bone tumors diagnosed each year, approximately 400 are osteosarcomas and 200 are Ewing's sarcoma. The primary site for osteosarcoma is usually in the long bones of the lower extremities (78%), which differs from the most common primary site for Ewing's sarcoma, which is the central axis (45%). For both osteosarcoma and Ewing's sarcoma, the incidence rates are generally comparable for males and females. Incidence rates for osteosarcoma are higher among blacks than whites. In contrast, the incidence of Ewing's sarcoma is approximately six times higher in whites than in blacks.

Known risk factors for bone tumors during childhood and adolescence include exposure to radiation/chemotherapy for the treatment of other childhood malignancies and genetic conditions, including hereditary retinoblastoma and Li-Fraumeni syndrome.[58–61] Because of the peak incidence that coincides with the pubertal growth spurt, several investigations have assessed a potential association with stature and/or growth velocity during pubertal development with limited or inconsistent findings.[62,63]

RHABDOMYOSARCOMA

In the United States, there are approximately 850 to 900 children and young adults diagnosed annually with soft tissue sarcoma, including approximately 350 cases of rhabdomyosarcoma, which represents 50% of soft tissue sarcomas under the age of 15 years and 60% of those under 5 years of age.[11] Approximately 75% of rhabdomyosarcomas are of embryonal histology (annual incidence of 3.0 per million), whereas alveolar histology is less common (annual incidence of 0.7 per million). Blacks have a slightly higher incidence of soft tissue sarcomas, whereas males have a somewhat higher incidence than females.

Assessment of risk factors has, by and large, been confined to children with rhabdomyosarcoma.[27] A higher frequency of congenital anomalies has been reported among rhabdomyosarcoma cases as have genetic conditions including Li-Fraumeni syndrome and neurofibromatosis type 1.[64,65] Limited information suggests a potential association with lower socioeconomic status, in utero x-ray exposure, and parental use of recreational drugs during pregnancy.

REFERENCES

1. American Cancer Society. Cancer facts and figures 2005. Atlanta: American Cancer Society; 2005.
2. Landis SH, Murray T, Bolden S, Wingo PA. Cancer statistics, 1999. CA Cancer J Clin 1999;49:8–31.
3. Parkin DM, Kramarova E, Draper GJ, et al. International incidence of childhood cancer. Vol 2. Lyon, France: IARC Scientific Publication No. 144; 1998.
4. Steliarova-Foucher E, Stiller C, Kaatsch P, et al. Geographical patterns and time trends of cancer incidence and survival among children and adolescents in Europe since the 1970s (the ACCIS project): an epidemiological study. Lancet 2004;364:2097–105.
5. Gurney JG, Davis S, Severson RK, et al. Trends in cancer incidence among children in the U.S. Cancer 1996;78:532–41.
6. McNally RJQ, Kelsey AM, Cairns DP, et al. Temporal increases in the incidence of childhood solid tumors seen in northwest England (1954–1998) are likely to be real. Cancer 2001;92:1967–76.
7. Linet MS, Ries LAG, Smith MA, et al. Cancer surveillance series: recent trends in childhood cancer incidence and mortality in the United States. J Natl Cancer Inst 1999;91:1051–8.
8. Ross JA, Severson RK, Swensen AR, et al. Seasonal variations in the diagnosis of childhood cancer in the United States. Br J Cancer 1999;81:549–53.
9. Alexander FE. Clusters and clustering of childhood cancer: a review. Eur J Epidemiol 1999;15:847–52.
10. Adamson P, Law G, Roman E. Assessment of trends in childhood cancer incidence. Lancet 2005;365:753.
11. Ries LAG, Eisner MP, Kosary CL, et al, editors. SEER cancer statistics review, 1975–2002. National Cancer Institute. Bethesda (MD): National Cancer Institute; based on November 2004 SEER data submission, posted to the SEER Web site 2005. Available at: http://seer.cancer.gov/csr/1975_2002/ (accessed September 3, 2005).
12. Ross JA, Davies SM, Potter JD, et al. Epidemiology of childhood leukemia, with a focus on infants. Epidemiol Rev 1997;7:172–9.
13. Buffler PA, Kwan ML, Reynolds P, Urayama KY. Environmental and genetic risk factors for childhood leukemia: appraising the evidence. Cancer Invest 2005;23:60–75.
14. Linet MS, Hatch EE, Kleinerman RA, et al. Residential exposure to magnetic fields and acute lymphoblastic leukemia in children. N Engl J Med 1997;337:1–7.
15. Lubin JH, Linet MS, Boice JD, et al. Case-control study of childhood acute lymphoblastic leukemia and residential radon exposure. J Natl Cancer Inst 1998;90:294–300.
16. Ahlbom IC, Cardis E, Green A, et al. ICNIRP (International Commission for Non-Ionizing Radiation Protection) Standing Committee on Epidemiology. Review of the epidemiologic literature on EMF and health. Env Health Perspect 2001;6:911–33.
17. Greaves MF. Speculations on the cause of childhood acute lymphoblastic leukemia. Leukemia 1988;2:120–5.
18. Kinlen LJ. Epidemiological evidence for an infective basis for childhood leukaemia. Br J Cancer 1995;71:1–5.
19. Gilham C, Peto J, Simpson J, et al. Day care in infancy and risk of childhood acute lymphoblastic leukemia: findings from UK case-control study. Br Med J 2005;330:1294–9.
20. Ma X, Buffler PA, Selvin S, et al. Daycare attendance and risk of childhood acute lymphoblastic leukaemia. Br J Cancer 2002;86:1419–24.
21. Neglia JP, Linet MS, Shu XO, et al. Patterns of infection and day care utilization and risk of childhood acute lymphoblastic leukaemia. Br J Cancer 2000;82:234–40.
22. Sandler DP, Ross JA. Epidemiology of acute leukemia in children and adults. Semin Oncol 1997:24:3–16.
23. Buckley JD, Robison LL, Swotinsky R, et al. Occupational exposures of parents of children with acute nonlymphocytic leukemia: a report from the Children's Cancer Study Group. Cancer Res 1989;49:4030–7.
24. Shu XO, Gao YT, Brinton LA, et al. A population-based case-control study of childhood leukemia in Shanghai. Cancer 1988;62:635–44.
25. Shu XO, Ross JA, Pendergrass TW, et al. Parental alcohol consumption, cigarette smoking, and risk of infant leukemia: a Children's Cancer Group study. J Natl Cancer Inst 1996;88:24–81.
26. Smith MA, Feidlin B, Ries LAG, Simon R. Trends in reported incidence of primary malignant brain tumors in children in the United States. J Natl Cancer Inst 1998;90:1269–77.
27. Little J. Epidemiology of childhood cancer. Lyon, France: IARC Scientific Publication No. 149; 1999.
28. Davis FG, Preston-Martin S. Epidemiology: incidence and survival. In: Bigner DD, McLennon RE, Bruner JM (editors). Russell & Rubinstein's pathology of tumors of the nervous system. Vol 1. London: Arnold; 1998. p. 5–45.
29. Bondy ML, Wrensch MR. Epidemiology of primary malignant brain tumors. Baillieres Clin Neurol 1996;5:251–70.
30. Kuijten RR, Bunin GR. Risk factors for childhood brain tumors. Cancer Epidemiol Biomarkers Prev 1993;2:277–88.
31. Cordier S, Mandereau L, Preston-Martin S, et al. Parental occupations and childhood brain tumors: results of an international case-control study. Cancer Causes Control 2001;12:865–74.
32. Filippini G, Maisonneuve P, McCredie M, et al. Relation of childhood brain tumors to exposure of parents and children to tobacco smoke: the Search International case-control study. Int J Cancer 2002;100:206–13.
33. Portwine C, Chilton-MacNeill S, Brown C, et al. Absence of germline and somatic p53 alterations in children with sporadic brain tumors. J Neuro Oncol 2001;52:227–35.
34. Stickler HD, Rosenberg PS, Devesa SS, et al. Contamination of poliovirus vaccines with simian virus 40 (1955–1963) and subsequent cancer rates. JAMA 1998;279:292–5.
35. Bergsagel DJ, Finegold MJ, Butel JS, et al. DNA sequences similar to those of simian virus 40 in ependymomas and choroid plexus tumors of childhood. N Engl J Med 1992;326:988–93.
36. Huang H, Reis R, Yonekawa Y, et al. Identification in human brain tumors of DNA sequences specific for SV40 large T antigen. Brain Pathol 1999;9:33–42.
37. Krynska B, Del Valle L, Croul S, et al. Detection of human neurotropic JC virus DNA sequence and expression of the viral oncogenic protein in pediatric medulloblastoma. Proc Natl Acad Sci U S A 1999;96:11519–24.
38. Kim JY, Koralnik IJ, LeFave M, et al. Medulloblastomas and primitive neuroectodermal tumors rarely contain polyomavirus DNA sequences. Neuro-Oncol 2002;4:165–70.
39. Stiller CA. What causes Hodgkin's disease in children? Eur J Cancer 1998;34:523–8.
40. Ambinder R, Browning P, Lorenzana I, et al. Epstein-Barr virus and childhood Hodgkin's disease in Honduras and the United States. Blood 1993;81:462–7.
41. Chang KL, Albujar PF, Chen YY, et al. High prevalence of Epstein-Barr virus in the Reed-Sternberg cells of Hodgkin's disease. Am J Pathol 1993;81:496–501.
42. Weinreb M, Day PJ, Niggli F, et al. The role of Epstein-Barr virus in Hodgkin disease from different geographical areas. Arch Dis Child 1996;74:27–31.
43. Flavell KJ, Biddulph JP, Powell JE, et al. South Asian ethnicity and material deprivation increase the risk of Epstein-Barr virus infection in childhood Hodgkin's disease. Br J Cancer 2001;85:350–6.
44. Robison LL, Ross JA. Epidemiology of leukemias and lymphomas in childhood. Baillieres Clin Pediatr 1995;3:639–58.
45. Parker L, Powell J. Screening for neuroblastoma in infants younger than 1 year of age: review of the first 30 years. Med Pediatr Oncol 1998;31:455–69.
46. Woods WG, Tuchman M, Robison LL, et al. A population-based study of the usefulness of screening for neuroblastoma. Lancet 1996;348:1682–7.
47. Brodeur GM, Castleberry RP. Neuroblastoma. In: Pizzo PA, Poplack DG, editors. Principles and practices of pediatric oncology. 3rd Ed. Philadelphia: Lippincott-Raven; 1997. p. 761–97.

48. Olshan AF, Bunin GR. Epidemiology of neuroblastoma. In: Brodeur GM, Sawada T, Tsuchida Y, Voute PA, editors. Neuroblastoma. Amsterdam: Elsevier Science, BV; 2000. p. 33–9.
49. Olshan AF, Smith JC, Bondy ML, et al. Maternal vitamin use and reduced risk of neuroblastoma. Epidemiology 2002;13:575–80.
50. Menegaux F, Olshan AF, Reitnauer PJ, et al. Positive association between congenital anomalies and risk of neuroblastoma. Pediatr Blood Cancer 2005;45:649–55.
51. Menegaux F, Olshan AF, Neglia JP, et al. Day care, childhood infections, and risk of neuroblastoma. Am J Epidemiol 2004;159:843–51.
52. Cook MN, Olshan AF, Guess HA, et al. Maternal medication use and neuroblastoma in offspring. Am J Epidemiol 2004;159:721–31.
53. Knudson AG. Mutation and cancer: statistical study of retinoblastoma. Proc Natl Acad Sci U S A 1971;68:820–3.
54. Dryja TP, Rapaport JM, Joyce JM, et al. Molecular detection of deletions involving band q14 of chromosome 13 in retinoblastoma. Proc Natl Acad Sci U S A 1986;83:7391–4.
55. Li F. Familial aggregation. In: Schottenfeld D, Fraumeni J, editors. Cancer epidemiology and prevention. New York: Oxford University Press; 1996. p. 546–58.
56. Sharpe CR, Franco EL. Etiology of Wilms' tumor. Epidemiol Rev 1995;17:415–32.
57. Green D, Coppes M, Breslow N, et al. Wilms' tumor. In: Pizzo PA, Poplack DG, editors. Principles and practices of pediatric oncology. 3rd Ed. Philadelphia: Lippincott-Raven; 1997. p. 733–59.
58. Tucker MA, D'Angio GJ, Boice JD, et al. Bone sarcomas linked to radiotherapy and chemotherapy in children. N Engl J Med 1987;317:588–93.
59. Hawkins MM, Wilson LMK, Burton HS, et al. Radiotherapy, alkylating agents, and risk of bone cancer after childhood cancer. J Natl Cancer Inst 1996;88:270–8.
60. Hansen MF, Koufos A, Gallie BL, et al. Osteosarcoma and retinoblastoma: a shared chromosomal mechanism revealing recessive predisposition. Proc Natl Acad Sci U S A 1985;82:6216–20.
61. Li FP, Fraumeni JF, Mulvihill JJ, et al. A cancer family syndrome in twenty-four kindreds. Cancer Res 1988;48:5358–62.
62. Winn DM, Li FP, Robison LL, et al. A case-control study of the etiology of Ewing's sarcoma. Cancer Epidemiol Biomarkers Prev 1992;1:525–32.
63. Buckley JD, Pendergrass TW, Buckley CM, et al. Epidemiology of osteosarcoma and Ewing's sarcoma in childhood: a study of 305 cases by the Children's Cancer Group. Cancer 1998;83:1440–8.
64. Malkin D, Li FP, Strong LC, et al. Germ line p53 mutations in a familial syndrome of breast cancer, sarcomas, and other neoplasms. Science 1990;250:1233–8.
65. Hartley AL, Birch JM, Marsden HB, et al. Neurofibromatosis in children with soft tissue sarcoma. Pediatr Hematol Oncol 1988;5:7–16.

124b

Late Effects of Cancer in Children and Adolescents

Smita Bhatia, MD, MPH

With the use of risk-based therapies, the overall 5-year survival rate of the more than 12,000 children and adolescents diagnosed with cancer each year in the United States is approaching 80%,[1] resulting in a growing population of childhood cancer survivors. In 1997, there were an estimated 270,000 survivors of childhood cancer; more than two-thirds were older than 20 years of age.[2] This translates into about 1 in 810 individuals under the age of 20 being a childhood cancer survivor, and 1 in 640 individuals between the ages 20 and 39 years having successfully survived childhood cancer.

The use of cancer therapy at an early age can produce complications that may not become apparent until years later, hence the term "late effects" for late-occurring or chronic outcomes—either physical or psychological—that persist or develop beyond 5 years from diagnosis of cancer. These complications involve all organ systems. Approximately two out of every three survivors will experience at least one late effect,[3–6] and about one out of four will experience a late effect that is severe or life threatening.[3,5,6] Psychosocial problems in survivors and members of the family may be more prevalent.

Table 124b-1 summarizes the topics that will be reviewed in detail in this chapter. These issues are related to the potential adverse events faced by the survivors and the options for obtaining health care. The relationship between known late effects and therapeutic modalities (surgery, radiation, or chemotherapy) (Table 124b-2) are reviewed. Challenges faced in the clinical management of childhood cancer survivors and the future research opportunities are described in Table 124b-3.

Table 124b-1 Issues Relating to Childhood Cancer Survivorship

- Medical Issues Faced by this Population
  - Cancer survivors are at increased risk of the following adverse outcomes:
    - Early deaths
    - Second neoplasms
    - Organ dysfunction (eg, cardiopulmonary, gonadal, etc)
    - Impaired growth and development
    - Decreased fertility
    - Neurocognitive impairment
    - Difficulties obtaining employment and insurance
    - Overall reduced quality of life
- Delivery of Care to the Survivor Population
  - Models of care delivery:
    - Pediatric oncology-based
    - Adult oncology-based
    - Community medicine-based
  - Guidelines for ongoing screening and management:
    - Screening for potential complications
    - Health protective counseling/interventions
    - Management of identified complications

Research regarding late effects has been ongoing for the last three decades, using populations treated at single institutions or creating multi-institution consortia. With the recognition that large cohorts of survivors would be needed to evaluate the effects of multiple therapies on individuals treated for a variety of neoplasms at different ages, and with funding from the National Cancer Institute, the Childhood Cancer Survivor Study (CCSS) was established.[7] The Web site can be accessed for more details at <www.cancer.umn.edu/ltfu#ccss>.

LATE MORTALITY AMONG CHILDHOOD CANCER SURVIVORS

Overall mortality among childhood cancer survivors has been described to be 10-fold that of the general population.[8,9] The CCSS assessed overall and cause-specific mortality in a retrospective cohort of 20,227 5-year survivors and demonstrated a 10.8-fold excess in overall mortality.[8] Risk of death was statistically significantly higher in females, individuals diagnosed with cancer before the age of 5 years, and those with an initial diagnosis of leukemia or brain tumor. The excess mortality was due to death from primary cancer, second cancer, cardiotoxicity and noncancer death, and existing up to 25 years after the initial cancer diagnosis.

SECOND MALIGNANT NEOPLASMS

Several studies following large cohorts of childhood cancer survivors have reported a three- to six-fold increased risk of a second cancer when compared with the general population, and this risk continues to increase as the cohort ages.[10,11] The magnitude of risk and the type of second malignancy differ with the primary diagnosis, type of therapy received, and presence of genetic conditions. Patients with the following diagnoses are at particularly high risk: Hodgkin's disease, hereditary retinoblastoma, genetic form of Wilms' tumor, von Recklinghausen's neurofibromatosis, xeroderma pigmentosum, Klinefelter's disease, or immunodeficiency, and those who received high doses of radiation therapy or alkylating agents. Several large cohorts have documented clearly that the risk of solid tumors continues to climb with increasing follow-up, while that of secondary leukemia plateaus after 15 years.[12]

Younger age at treatment of the primary cancer has been reported to be associated with an increased risk of second cancers,[10] with the exception of secondary myelodysplasia and acute myeloid leukemia, where older age at treatment of the primary cancer is associated with an increased risk.[13,14] Female sex is associated with an increased risk of second primary cancers, owing primarily to the excess number of secondary breast cancers and, to some extent, to the increased occurrence of thyroid cancer in female survivors.[10] Ionizing radiation can cause most types of cancer, but different organs vary in their susceptibility. The risk is highest when the exposure occurs at a younger age.[10,15] It increases with the total dose of radiation[16–20] and with increasing follow-up after radiation.[21] Examples of radiation-associated tumors include breast and lung cancer, thyroid cancer, brain tumors, and osteosarcoma. The large majority of radiation-associated second cancers develop within the radiation field.[12]

The more commonly reported second primary cancers are breast, bone, and thyroid cancers, therapy-related myelodysplasia, and acute myeloid leukemia. Female survivors who were treated with chest or mantle radiation for a pediatric malignancy face a significantly increased risk of breast cancer. In a recent report, the 30-year cumulative incidence of breast cancer in female survivors following radiation was 17%.[12] The cumulative incidence by age 40 years was 14%, increasing to 20% by 45 years of age. Female patients treated with mantle radiation before the age of 21 years are at a significantly higher risk of developing radiation-related breast cancer, in comparison with those treated in their adult years.[22,23] However, recent studies have not shown a difference in risk between prepubertal and adolescent girls. The risk of breast cancer begins to increase about 8 years after radiation.[12,22,24] The large majority of women are diagnosed at a relatively young age, often before 40 years of age. Since outcome is closely linked to stage at diagnosis, early diagnosis should confer survival advantage.[25,26] Mammography has been shown to detect most radiation-related breast cancers.[25–27] It is too early to determine whether girls treated during the last two decades when lower radiation doses and smaller volumes were used have a lesser risk or a longer latent period for the development of breast cancer.

Lung cancer has been reported after chest radiation, although it is relatively infrequent. The risk is known to increase among smokers, and appears to increase with increasing follow-up of this cohort of survivors.[12,28,29] Smoking has been

Table 124b-2 Commonly Occurring Late Effects after Conventional Therapy for Childhood Cancer

Adverse Outcomes	Therapeutic Exposures	Risk Factors
Growth and Development		
Neurocognitive deficits	Cranial radiation, intravenous cytarabine, intrathecal or intravenous methotrexate	Females, younger age at treatment, increasing dose
Endocrine Dysfunction		
Hypothyroidism	Radiation to the thyroid gland (neck, mantle, etc)	Increasing dose, females, age at treatment
Hypogonadism	Alkylating agents, craniospinal radiation, abdomino-pelvic radiation, gonadal radiation	Males, treatment during peripubertal or postpubertal period in girls, higher cumulative doses of alkylators
Growth hormone deficiency	Cranial radiation	Younger age at treatment, radiation dose > 18 Gy
Subsequent Cancers		
Therapy-related myelodysplasia/ Acute myeloid leukemia	Alkylating agents, topoisomerase II inhibitors	Increasing doses of alkylating agents, older age at therapeutic exposure
Thyroid cancer	Radiation to the thyroid gland (neck, mantle, etc)	Increasing doses, females, younger age at radiation
Skin cancer (basal cell, squamous cell, melanoma)	Radiation therapy	Orthovoltage radiation (prior to 1970) – delivery of greater dose to skin, additional excessive exposure to sun, tanning booths
Secondary CNS tumor	Cranial radiation	Increasing dose, younger age at treatment
Cardiopulmonary Dysfunction		
Cardiomyopathy/Congestive heart failure	Anthracyclines	High cumulative doses (> 550 mg/m^2 in patients > 18 years of age; > 300 mg/m^2 for patients < 18 years of age), females, younger than 5 years at treatment, African-American race
Pulmonary fibrosis/Interstitial pneumonitis	Bleomycin, radiation to chest, carmustine	Younger age at treatment, bleomycin dose > 400 U/m^2
Musculoskeletal disorders		
Osteopenia/Osteoporosis	Corticosteroids, craniospinal radiation, gonadal radiation, total-body irradiation	Associated hypothyroidism, hypogonadism, growth hormone deficiency
Avascular necrosis	Corticosteroids, high-dose radiation to any bone	Dexamethasone, adolescence
Miscellaneous		
Dental abnormalities	Cranial radiation	Younger age at treatment
Cataracts	Cranial radiation, steroids	Higher radiation dose, combination of steroids and radiation, single daily fraction
Chronic hepatitis C and HCV-related sequelae (cirrhosis, hepatic failure, hepatocellular carcinoma)	Transfusions before 1993	Living in hyperendemic area
Obesity	Cranial radiation	Younger age at treatment (< 5 years), females, higher cranial radiation dose

linked with lung cancer occurring as a second primary cancer among survivors of Hodgkin's disease, with the risk increasing with higher doses of radiation received, suggesting a multiplicative positive interaction.[30] Moreover, the increase in risk of lung cancer with increasing radiation dose was much greater among the patients who smoked after the diagnosis of Hodgkin's disease than among those who refrained from smoking ($p = .04$).[30]

Table 124b-3 Childhood Cancer Survivorship: Challenges and Future Directions

- Major Clinical and Research Challenges
  - Continual change in landscape of cancer survivorship research because of introduction of
    - New therapeutic agents or combination of agents
    - Radiation oncology techniques
    - Surgical procedures
    - Supportive care techniques
  - Attrition to follow-up (due to mobility of survivor population, insurance coverage, denial regarding need for medical follow-up)
    - Inaccurate assessment of magnitude of risk (selection bias)
  - Standardized exposure and risk-based follow-up of survivors
    - Education of health care providers regarding the unique needs of survivor population
    - Education of survivors to encourage behavior that would lead to actively seeking health care
- Future Directions
  - Identification of late-occurring adverse outcomes (beyond the first decade after diagnosis)
  - Identification of genetic predisposition to adverse outcomes
  - Identification of role of life-style choices (alcohol, tobacco, diet, exercise) as risk modifiers
  - Development of effective intervention strategies

The risk of thyroid cancer has been described after radiation therapy for several primary cancers, including Hodgkin's disease, ALL, brain tumors, and after total-body irradiation (TBI).[31–37] The long-term risk of developing a thyroid tumor in 4,096 3-year survivors of childhood cancer treated between 1942 and 1985 in France and Britain was reported to rise with increasing dose of radiation: a dose of 0.5 Gy was associated with a 35-fold increased risk of developing a thyroid cancer when compared with the general population, whereas the risk increased to 73-fold when the exposure increased to 3.6 Gy.[34] Radiation therapy at a young age has been identified as a risk factor for the development of secondary thyroid cancers.[33] The risk of thyroid cancer was reported to be 18-fold that of the general population among 1,791 5-year survivors of Hodgkin's disease followed as part of the CCSS cohort.[35] A recent CCSS report noted a linear dose response relationship between thyroid cancer and radiation up to 20 to 29 Gy, but a downturn in the odds ratio from a peak of 9.8-fold at higher doses, especially in children less than 10 years at treatment.[38] Thyroid cancer has also been reported among patients receiving radiation to the craniospinal axis for ALL.[32,37]

The risk of subsequent bone tumors estimated among 9,170 2-year survivors of childhood cancer was reported to be 133-fold that of the general population (95% CI, 98–176), with an estimated 20-year cumulative risk of 2.8 ± 0.7%.[39] Patients who had received radiation therapy had a 2.7-fold risk over other survivors (95% CI, 1–7.7) of developing a bone tumor, and a sharp dose-response gradient reaching a 40-fold risk after doses to the bone of more than 60 Gy. After adjustment for radiation therapy, treatment with alkylating agents was also linked to bone cancer (RR = 4.7, 95% CI, 1.0–22.3), with the risk increasing with cumulative drug exposure.

A report from the population-based National Registry of Childhood Tumours in Britain of a cohort of 13,175 3-year survivors of childhood cancer diagnosed between 1940 and 1983 revealed the cumulative probability of secondary bone cancer to be 0.9% at 20 years, except following hereditary retinoblastoma (7.2%), Ewing's sarcoma (5.4%), and other malignant bone tumors (2.4%).[18] The risk of bone cancer increased substantially with increased cumulative dose of radiation to the bone ($p < .001$, linear trend). At the highest level of exposure, the risk appeared to decline ($p = .07$). The risk of bone cancer increased linearly ($p = .04$, one-tailed test) with increased cumulative dose of alkylating agents.

A cohort study of 4,400 3-year survivors of a first solid cancer during childhood diagnosed in France or United Kingdom between 1942 and 1986 revealed the risk of osteosarcoma to be a linear function of the local dose of radiation.[40] Bilateral retinoblastoma, Ewing's sarcoma, and soft tissue sarcoma were found to be associated with an increased risk of subsequent osteosarcoma.

These three studies therefore demonstrate that the risk of second primary bone tumors among survivors of childhood cancer is not very high, except among certain specific tumor types, and that the risk is associated with radiation therapy and alkylating agents. These studies, therefore, provide a rational basis for targeted surveillance in certain high-risk groups and consideration regarding modification of therapeutic protocols.

Secondary myelodysplasia and acute myeloid leukemia have been associated with certain chemotherapeutic agents, such as alkylating agents[13] and topoisomerase II inhibitors.[41] A dose-dependent relationship is noted with alkylating agents, which typically cause leukemias after latencies of 5 to 10 years. Cytogenetic abnormalities in the alkylating agent associated secondary leukemias characteristically involve chromosomes 5 or 7. Topoisomerase II inhibitor-associated secondary leukemias classically have a shorter latency, no preceding dysplastic phase, and cytogenetic abnormalities involving chromosome 11q23.

Genetic predisposition was first noted to have a substantial impact on the risk of secondary sarcomas among patients with the genetic form of retinoblastoma. This risk is further increased by radiation treatment and increases with the total dose of radiation delivered. Patients with a family history of early-onset cancers have also been shown to be at an increased risk of developing a second cancer. Members of families with Li-Fraumeni syndrome have been reported to be at increased risk of multiple subsequent cancers, with the highest risk observed among survivors of childhood cancer.[42] The subsequent cancers reported in this population were characteristic of Li-Fraumeni syndrome. It therefore appears that germline mutations in tumor suppressor genes, as occurring in Li-Fraumeni syndrome, might interact with therapeutic exposures to result in an increased risk of second cancers.

Several genetic polymorphisms of enzymes capable of metabolic activation or detoxification of anticancer drugs, such as NAD(P)H:quinone oxidoreductase (NQO1), glutathione S-transferase (GST)-M1 and -T1, and CYP3A4, have been examined for their role in the development of therapy-related leukemia or myelodysplasia. These studies indicate that NQO1 polymorphism is significantly associated with the genetic risk of therapy-related acute leukemia and myelodysplasia. In addition, individuals with CYP3A4-W genotype may be at increased risk of treatment-related leukemia, presumably by increasing the production of reactive intermediates that damage DNA.[43–49]

Since subsequent malignancies remain a significant threat to the health of survivors treated for cancer during childhood, vigilant screening is important for those at risk. Risk of secondary acute myeloid leukemia is associated with exposure to topoisomerase II inhibitors (ie, epipodophyllotoxins and anthracyclines) for up to 10 years and with alkylating agents for up to 15 years. Monitoring should include yearly complete blood count (CBC) with differential and platelet count for 10 to 15 years post-therapy, depending on exposure. Most other subsequent malignancies are associated with radiation exposure. Screening recommendations include careful annual physical examination of the skin and soft tissues in the radiation field with radiographic or other cancer screening evaluations as indicated. Specialized recommendations for females who received radiation with potential impact to the breast (ie, mantle, mediastinal, whole lung, spinal at doses of 30 Gy or higher) include monthly self-breast examination beginning at puberty, yearly clinical breast examinations beginning at puberty until age 25 years, and then every 6 month clinical breast examination, with yearly mammograms beginning 8 years after radiation or at age 25 (whichever comes last).

Evaluation of those at risk of early-onset colorectal cancer (ie, radiation doses of 25 Gy or higher to the abdomen, pelvis, or spine) should begin at age 35 years or 15 years following radiation (whichever occurs last) and should include colonoscopy every 10 years, double contrast barium enema every 5 years, or yearly fecal occult blood testing combined with flexible sigmoidoscopy every 5 years.

Patients with chronic hepatitis, most often resulting from blood exposure, are at higher risk of developing hepatocellular carcinoma and should have serum alpha-fetoprotein (AFP) monitoring on an annual basis; patients who develop cirrhosis should also have an annual liver ultrasound.

NEUROCOGNITIVE SEQUELAE

Neurocognitive sequelae of treatment of childhood cancer occur as a consequence of radiation to the whole brain, systemic therapy with high-dose methotrexate or cytarabine, or with intrathecal methotrexate and other agents. Children with a history of brain tumors, ALL, or non-Hodgkin's lymphoma (NHL) are most likely to be affected. Risk factors include increasing radiation dose, young age at the time of treatment, treatment with both cranial radiation and systemic or intrathecal chemotherapy, and female gender.[50] Severe deficits are most frequently noted in children with brain tumors treated with radiation therapy, and in children who were less than 5 years of age at the time of treatment.

Neurocognitive deficits usually become evident within 1 to 2 years following radiation and are progressive in nature. Affected children may experience information-processing deficits resulting in academic difficulties. These children are particularly prone to problems with receptive and expressive language, attention span, and visual and perceptual motor skills. They most often experience academic difficulties in the areas of reading, language, and mathematics. Children in the younger age groups and those treated for brain tumors may experience significant drops in IQ scores, with irradiation- or chemotherapy-induced destruction in normal white matter, partially explaining intellectual and academic achievement deficits.[51] In a series of 120 children with medulloblastoma treated from 1967 to 1987, Hoppe-Hirsch and colleagues reported that by 5 years following therapy, 42% had a full-scale intelligence quotient (FSIQ) of less than 80, and by 10 years after therapy, 75% scored less than 80, including 46% who were below 60.[52] The CCSS reported that 18% of the 18- to 24-year-old brain tumor survivors had not completed high school.[53] Recent studies show that treating medulloblastoma with a lower dose of whole-brain radiation (23.5 Gy) (while maintaining a higher boost to the posterior fossa) is associated with less neurocognitive dysfunction.[54,55] Treatment of ALL patients with cranial radiation at a dose of 24 Gy is also associated with cognitive deficits—with a mean decrease in FSIQ of 10 points.[56] Verbal IQ scores are more likely to be affected than performance IQ, and changes are progressive. Treatment with 18 Gy cranial irradiation is associated with less neuropsychological toxicity than 24 Gy.[57] Survivors treated with 24 Gy are more likely to enter special education or learning disabled programs. Moreover, those treated with 24 Gy or treated before the age of 6 years are less likely to enter college.[58]

Evidence suggests that direct effects on intracranial endothelial cells and brain white matter, as well as immunologic mechanisms, play a role in the pathogenesis of central nervous system damage. A spectrum of clinical syndromes may occur, including radionecrosis, necrotizing leukoencephalopathy, and mineralizing microangiopathy with dystrophic calcification, cerebellar sclerosis, and spinal cord dysfunction.[59] Mulhern and colleagues have shown an association between FSIQ and the volume of white matter loss determined by quantitative neuroimaging.[51,55]

For survivors who have received radiation involving the brain, a baseline brain MRI is recommended and ongoing annual surveillance for new-onset neurologic complications is advisable. Patients who received therapy that may potentially impact neurocognitive function (ie, cranial irradiation, intrathecal methotrexate, intermediate to high-dose methotrexate, and/or cytarabine) should undergo a baseline neuropsychological evaluation, and periodic assessment of their vocational or educational progress should be repeated as clinically indicated.

CARDIOVASCULAR FUNCTION

Chronic cardiotoxicity usually manifests itself as cardiomyopathy, pericarditis, and congestive heart failure. Childhood cancer survivors in the CCSS who were treated with chest or spinal radiation had a more than twofold increased risk of death related to cardiac disease in comparison with the standard U.S. population.[8]

The anthracyclines doxorubicin and daunomycin are well-known causes of cardiomyopathy.[60–62] Anthracyclines have a wide range of clinical activity against pediatric cancers, and about 40 to 50% of childhood cancer survivors have been treated with anthracyclines, making it one of the more common exposures. The incidence of cardiomyopathy is dose-dependent and may exceed 30% among patients who received cumulative doses of anthracyclines in excess of 600 mg/m^2. With a total dose of 500 to 600 mg/m^2, the incidence is 11%, falling to less than 1% for cumulative doses less than 500 mg/m^2.[63] This has formed the basis for considering 500 mg/m^2 as the threshold cumulative dose for cardiotoxicity. However, a lower cumulative dose of anthracyclines may place children at increased risk of cardiac compromise than previously described.[64] Kremer and colleagues have evaluated the cumulative incidence of anthracycline-induced clinical heart failure in a cohort of 607 children who had been treated with a mean cumulative anthracyclines dose of 301 mg/m^2 and were followed for a median of 6.3 years. A cumulative dose of anthracyclines greater than 300 mg/m^2 was associated with an increased risk of clinical heart failure (relative risk 11.8) compared with a cumulative dose lower than 300 mg/m^2. The estimated risk of clinical heart failure increased with time, and approached 5% after 15 years.

Several investigators have described subclinical anthracycline-induced myocardial damage. Steinherz and colleagues found 23% of 201 patients to have echocardiographic abnormalities, a median of 7 years after therapy.[65] The median cumulative dose of doxorubicin received by these patients was 450 mg/m^2 (range: 200–1,275 mg/m^2). Lipshultz and colleagues evaluated survivors of childhood cancer who had received a median doxorubicin dose of 334 mg/m^2 (range: 12–550 mg/m^2). They concluded that doxorubicin causes progressive elevation of afterload or depression of left ventricular contractility in about 75% of the patients. Pathologic specimens in 7 patients showed myocyte hypertrophy. These investigators speculated that doxorubicin administered in childhood results in acute asymptomatic loss of myocytes, which, in turn, results in hypertrophy of the remaining myocytes with inadequate left ventricular mass and secondary heart disease later in life.[66] However, the clinical relevance of subclinical myocardial injury is not clearly established, in part owing to widely varying methods used to define and assess such injury.

These studies and others emphasize that cardiomyopathy can occur many years after completion of therapy (15–20 years) and that the onset may be spontaneous or coincide with exertion or pregnancy. During the third trimester, the cardiac volume increases, increasing the cardiac workload, leading to overt symptomology in women with left ventricular dysfunction.[67,68] Risk factors known to be associated with anthracycline-related cardiac toxicity include mediastinal radiation; uncontrolled hypertension; exposure to other chemotherapeutic agents, especially cyclophosphamide, dactinomycin, mitomycin, dacarbazine, vincristine, bleomycin, and methotrexate; younger age; dyselectrolytemia such as hypokalemia and hypomagnesemia; and female gender.[69]

Chronic cardiac toxicity associated with radiation alone most commonly involves pericardial effusions or constrictive pericarditis, sometimes in association with pancarditis.[70] Although 40 Gy of total-heart radiation dose appears to be the usual threshold, pericarditis has been reported after as little as 15 Gy, even in the absence of radiomimetic chemotherapy. Symptomatic pericarditis, which usually develops 10 to 30 months after radiation, is found in 2 to 10% of patients.[71] Subclinical pericardial and myocardial damage as well as valvular thickening may be common in this population,[72] and symptomatic pericarditis may first appear as late as 45 years after therapy.[73,74]

Coronary artery disease has been reported following radiation to the mediastinum, although the mortality rate was not significantly higher in patients with Hodgkin's disease (HD) who had received mediastinal radiation than in the general population.[75] A Dutch study of HD survivors reported a cumulative risk of ischemic heart disease of 21% at 20 years after radiation.[76] In another study following 415 HD survivors, 10% developed coronary heart disease.[77]

Prevention of anthracycline-related cardiotoxicity has been a major focus of investigation for the past few years. Certain analogs of doxorubicin and daunomycin and liposomal anthracyclines, which appear to have decreased cardiotoxicity, with equivalent antitumor activity, are being explored. The anthracyclines chelate iron, and the anthracycline-iron complex catalyzes the formation of hydroxyl radicals. Agents such as dexrazoxane that are able to remove iron from the anthracyclines have been investigated as cardioprotectants. Clinical trials of dexrazoxane have been conducted in children, with encouraging evidence of short-term cardioprotection,[78,79] although the long-term avoidance of cardiotoxicity with the use of this agent needs to be determined. In a recent prospective, randomized study of pediatric ALL patients, Lipshultz and colleagues have demonstrated that patients treated with doxorubicin at 300 mg/m^2 alone were more likely than those treated with dexrazoxane and doxorubicin to have cardiac injury as reflected by elevated troponin T levels (50% vs 21%, $p < .001$) and extremely elevated troponin T levels (32% vs 10%, $p < .001$), without compromising the antileukemic efficacy of doxorubicin (event-free survival was 83% at 2.5 years for both arms).[80] However, longer follow-up is necessary to determine the influence of dexrazoxane on echocardiographic findings and, hence, the clinical significance of these findings. Lower doses of anthracyclines and reduced port sizes of radiation therapy may also help in decreasing the incidence of carditis. Management of survivors with asymptomatic deterioration of left ventricular function is controversial. Angiotensin converting enzyme (ACE) inhibitors have been known to improve morbidity and mortality in patients with cardiomyopathy. There appear to be theoretic risks with such therapy in the childhood years, since the ACE inhibitors, while lowering the afterload in the short-term, may also limit the cardiac growth potential by inhibiting cardiac growth factors. Thus, the role of ACE inhibitors and beta-blockers in asymptomatic survivors with cardiac dysfunction remains in question.[81,82]

Patients who received anthracycline chemotherapy need ongoing monitoring for late-onset cardiomyopathy, with the frequency of evaluation based on total cumulative dose and age at the time of initial therapy. In addition to monitoring for cardiomyopathy, survivors who received radiation potentially impacting the heart (ie, chest, spine, upper abdomen, or TBI) also need monitoring for potential early-onset atherosclerotic heart disease, valvular disease, and pericardial complications. Specific recommendations for monitoring, based on age and therapeutic exposure, are delineated within the Children's Oncology Group (COG) long-term follow-up guidelines (described below).

PULMONARY FUNCTION

Pulmonary fibrosis and pneumonitis can result from pulmonary radiation. Thus, these problems are seen most often in patients with thoracic malignancies, notably Hodgkin's disease. Asymptomatic radiographic findings or restrictive changes on pulmonary function testing have been reported in more than 30% of such individuals.[83–85] Of 25 HD survivors treated with standard mantle radiation before age 35, 60% had an abnormal chest radiograph at a mean follow-up of 9 years.[86] Of the 19 who had pulmonary function testing, 89% had an abnormality, with 72% having a reduced diffusion capacity. None of the patients were symptomatic. These changes have been detected months to years after radiation therapy, most often in patients who suffered radiation pneumonitis during or shortly after therapy.[87] Clinically apparent pneumonitis with cough, fever, or dyspnea occurs in only 5 to 15% of patients, and is generally limited to those who received more than 30 Gy in standard fractions to more than 50% of the lung.[87] Craniospinal radiation for patients with malignant brain tumors and scatter from abdominal ports contribute to the development of late restrictive lung disease.[88] Obstructive changes have also been reported after conventional radiation therapy. Self-reported pulmonary problems were assessed in 12,390 long-term survivors participating in CCSS.[89] The cumulative incidence of pulmonary fibrosis by 20 years after chest radiation was 3.5%. Chest radiation was associated with chest wall hypoplasia, chronic cough, and exercise-related dyspnea.

Following hematopoietic cell transplantation (HCT), both restrictive and obstructive lung disease, including bronchiolitis obliterans are well described.[90,91] In one series,[90] after 10 Gy TBI in a single fraction, 8% of patients had a forced expiratory volume in 1 second (FEV1)/vital capacity (VC) (a measure of obstructive lung disease) below 50% of normal at 3 years, and 29% had an FEV1/VC below 70% by that time.

On a molecular level, radiation-related pulmonary injuries in older patients are likely mediated by cytokine production, which stimulates septal fibroblasts, increasing collagen production and resulting in pulmonary fibrosis.[92,93] The basis for respiratory damage in young children appears to be different from that in the adult or adolescent. In one study of 12 survivors of Wilms' tumor 7 to 14 years after treatment with bilateral pulmonary radiation for metastatic disease, several patients had dyspnea on exertion and radiographic evidence of interstitial and pleural thickening. Mean total lung volumes and DLCO were reduced to approximately 60% of predicted values after median total doses of approximately 20 Gy. In contrast to older children and adults, in whom, as noted previously, radiation for thoracic malignancy results in pulmonary fibrosis with loss of lung volume alone, these data were thought to be consistent with a proportionate interference with the growth of both the lung and the chest wall. Restrictive lung changes after lower doses of whole-lung radiation (11–14 Gy) have been reported in several other studies of children with various malignancies.[94–96] Some investigators have suggested that children younger than 3 years old at the time of therapy experience more chronic toxicity.[94] Following HCT, children seem to be at less risk of significant late pulmonary dysfunction than adults,[97,98] although both restrictive and obstructive pulmonary changes have been described in children.

The incidence of radiation-induced late pulmonary toxicity has dramatically decreased in the last decade secondary to refined techniques of radiation therapy.[99–101] In a recently published study of patients with stage I and IIA Hodgkin's disease treated with radiation alone (40–45 Gy to involved fields), the late pulmonary effects observed were minimal.[101] Although vital capacity (VC), residual volume (RV), forced expiratory volume in one second (FEV1), DLCO, and total lung capacity (TLC) were significantly decreased at completion of radiation therapy compared with pretreatment studies, all except DLCO returned to near normal within 1 year. The decrease in DLCO remained stable, but the forced expiratory flow rate between 25 and 75% of VC (FEF 25–75) had a significant decline at 3 years post-treatment compared with baseline studies. Use of more modest radiation doses also has contributed to decreased pulmonary toxicity.[102]

In addition to radiation therapy, a growing list of chemotherapeutic agents appears to be responsible for pulmonary disease in long-term survivors. Bleomycin toxicity is the prototype for chemotherapy-related lung injury. Although interstitial pneumonitis and pulmonary fibrosis have been reported in children,[103] clinically apparent bleomycin pneumonopathy is most frequent in older adults.[104] The chronic lung toxicity usually follows persistence or progression of abnormalities developing within 3 months of therapy. Like the acute toxicity, it is dose-dependent above a threshold cumulative dose of 400 units/m^2 and is exacerbated by concurrent or previous radiation therapy.[105] Above 400 units in the absence of other risk factors, 10% of patients experience fibrosis.[105] At lower doses, fibrosis occurs sporadically in less than 5% of patients, with a 1 to 2% mortality rate. In some reports, bleomycin toxicity was anticipated on the basis of DLCO abnormalities.

Alkylating agents also are believed to cause chronic lung injury. As with bleomycin, BCNU and CCNU pulmonary toxicity is dose-related. Cumulative BCNU doses greater than 600 mg/m^2 result in a 50% incidence of symptoms.[106] In a careful clinicopathological review of children with brain tumors, O'Driscoll and colleagues reported restrictive changes with lung fibrosis up to 17 years after treatment, the common feature of which was BCNU at a dose of 100 mg/m^2 every 6 to 8 weeks for as long as two years.[107] Four of the patients still alive at the time of study experienced shortness of breath and coughing, 6 showed a characteristic pattern of upper zone fibrosis on chest radiograph and CT scan, and all had restrictive pulmonary function testing with vital capacities ~50% of normal. Toxicity increases with more intensive dose scheduling.[106] A marked increase in pulmonary fibrosis appears at doses exceeding 1,500 mg/m^2.[106] Pulmonary fibrosis has also been observed in 16 to 40% of transplant recipients treated with cytotoxic conditioning agents including BCNU at doses of 500 to 600 mg/m^2; the incidence of fibrosis declines considerably when doses are limited to less than 300 to 450 mg/m^2.[108,109] Female patients are at a higher risk of this complication than their male counterparts. Case reports and small series suggest that cyclophosphamide can cause delayed-onset pulmonary fibrosis with severe restrictive lung disease in association with marked reduction in the anteroposterior diameter of the chest.[104,110] Melphalan and busulfan are also known to cause pulmonary fibrosis in a dose-related manner. Busulfan toxicity is most predictable in transplantation doses exceeding 500 mg and may be associated with a progressive, potentially fatal restrictive lung disease. Lung injury associated with busulfan is characterized by diffuse interstitial fibrosis and bronchopulmonary dysplasia.

Additional factors contributing to chronic pulmonary toxicity include superimposed infection, underlying pneumonopathy (eg, asthma), cigarette or respiratory toxicity, chronic graft-versus-host disease (GVHD), and the effects of chronic pulmonary involvement by tumor or reaction to tumor.[111] Increased oxygen concentrations associated with general anesthesia or scuba diving also have been found to exacerbate pulmonary fibrosis.[112,113]

Monitoring for pulmonary dysfunction in childhood cancer survivors includes asking about symptoms such as chronic cough (with or without fever) or dyspnea on yearly follow-up. All patients must understand the risks of smoking. The best approach to chronic pulmonary toxicity of anticancer therapy is preventive and includes respecting cumulative dosage restrictions of bleomycin and alkylators, limiting radiation dosage and port sizes, and avoiding primary or secondhand smoke. Pulmonary function tests (including DLCO and spirometry) have been recommended as a baseline on entry into long-term follow-up for patients at risk, in patients with symptoms, or in those who require general anesthesia for any reason. Patients with risk factors for lung disease are discouraged from scuba diving.

GASTROINTESTINAL FUNCTION

Fibrosis and enteritis are the most common pathologic abnormalities of the gastrointestinal tract in long-term survivors of cancer. These can arise as late complications of radiation to any site from the esophagus to the rectum[114–119] and have been associated with adhesions or stricture formation, sometimes with obstruction, ulcers, fistulae, and chronic enterocolitis or incontinence. Their frequency depends on the radiation dosage delivered by external beam or by brachytherapy. The stomach and small intestine appear to be more radiation sensitive than the colon or rectum. Overall, the incidence of fibrosis after 40 to 50 Gy is 5% and as high as 36% after 60 Gy or more. Most complications of intestinal fibrosis arise within 5 years, but strictures have developed as late as 20 years after treatment.[114,117,119,120] Once they occur, radiation-induced gastrointestinal strictures may be progressive or recurrent. The incidence of clinically significant problems is enhanced by radiomimetic chemotherapy[115] or abdominal surgery.[115,120] Abdominal surgery even without radiation can result in late-onset obstruction.[121,122]

Chronic fibrosis of the liver is associated with radiation. The degree of damage increases with the volume irradiated, prior partial hepatectomy, concomitant use of dactinomycin, the presence of large intraabdominal masses compressing the liver or hepatic venous system, and, possibly, younger age.[123,124] There also has been a trend, toward increasing damage (both clinically appreciable and asymptomatic) with increasing doses between 12 and 58 Gy. A dose of 20 to 30 Gy to the entire liver is thought to carry the highest risk of fibrosis and cirrhosis.[125]

Chemotherapy, even in the absence of radiation therapy, may be a cause of chronic hepatopathy. In several early prospective studies of patients given methotrexate for ALL or psoriasis, the incidence of biopsy-proven hepatic fibrosis was as high as 80% after 3 to 5 years of low-dose daily oral methotrexate.[126,127] With intermediate doses of intravenous methotrexate, the incidence of fibrosis has been below 5%.[128] In general, and apparently in contrast to what occurs after radiation therapy, methotrexate-related hepatic fibrosis stabilizes or resolves after discontinuation of the drug. Cirrhosis has been documented in small numbers of survivors of stage 4S neuroblastoma with extensive hepatic tumor treated with a number of nonantimetabolite drugs, limited doses of radiation only (< 10 Gy), or even after resolution of tumor in the absence of any therapy.[129]

Viral hepatitis, most often related to transfusion of blood products prior to 1992, is another cause of chronic liver disease in long-term survivors.[130–132] In one retrospective series of 658 survivors of childhood cancer who had been treated before routine screening of blood products, 117

(17.8%) were seropositive for hepatitis C[131]; 35% of these also were positive for hepatitis B with or without delta virus. Eighty percent of the seropositive patients had been transfused, so that in 20%, other risk factors appeared to have been responsible. Of long-term survivors of HCT for pediatric leukemia diagnosed prior to 1991, as many as 35% are estimated to be seropositive for hepatitis B or C. In one series of 10-year survivors of HCT for hematologic malignancy, hepatitis C was the major risk factor for late development of cirrhosis: of 16 patients with cirrhosis, 15 had disease attributable to hepatitis C.[133] Hepatitis B has largely been eliminated in populations treated after 1972.[134]

Other late effects involving the gastrointestinal tract include postsurgical blind loop syndromes, iron overload (sometimes with secondary cirrhosis), secondary malignancies, and complications of gut or liver GVHD.[135]

The true incidence of hepatic pathology undoubtedly is higher than current numbers suggest because the presence of cirrhosis is seldom reflected by abnormal liver function tests or hepatomegaly, because hypertransaminasemia may be asymptomatic, and because liver biopsies or liver scans are not routinely recommended after therapy. It is therefore difficult to suggest guidelines for long-term follow-up. Patients at risk of gastrointestinal complications should be monitored by history or physical examination for hepatomegaly, icterus, and malabsorption. For patients with acute hepatotoxicity during therapy or patients treated with hepatectomy, methotrexate, or hepatic radiation, the potential consequences of excessive alcohol and other high-risk behaviors are emphasized. In such patients, a post-treatment baseline screen including transaminase and bilirubin levels is advised. Prothrombin time and serum albumin for evaluation of liver synthetic function may be indicated. If persistent, abnormalities should be evaluated further in collaboration with a gastroenterologist. The Centers for Disease Control and Prevention (CDC) recommendations for hepatitis C screening include patients transfused or transplanted before 1992, even when transaminases are normal.[136] Hepatitis A and B testing should be considered in unimmunized patients with abnormal liver function tests. Given the trend toward lower doses of hepatic radiation, shorter courses of oral methotrexate, and the infrequent development of clinically apparent end-stage liver disease with current anticancer regimens, routine liver scans or biopsies are not recommended.

GENITOURINARY ABNORMALITIES

Renal Cisplatin, ifosfamide, and radiation are the agents most commonly implicated in long-term renal damage in children treated for cancer. Cisplatin damages the glomerulus and distal renal tubules, potentially causing diminished glomerular filtration rate (GFR) and electrolyte wasting, most commonly involving magnesium, calcium, potassium, and sodium.[137] Ifosfamide damages the proximal renal tubule, potentially resulting in Fanconi renal syndrome (hypokalemia, hypophosphatemia, glucosuria, proteinuria, renal tubular acidosis, and rickets).[138] Children at particular risk include those who received treatment with more than one nephrotoxic agent and those with concomitant renal damage related to surgery or radiation. Although GFR may improve over time, electrolyte wasting associated with ifosfamide therapy and hypomagnesemia associated with cisplatin therapy appear to persist in some children.[139,140] Yearly surveillance should include monitoring of serum creatinine, blood urea nitrogen and serum chemistries, urinalysis, and measurement of blood pressure. Ongoing management includes electrolyte replacement, treatment of hypertension, and avoidance of further nephrotoxic agents. In children with a history of radiation to the renal artery who develop hypertension, radiologic studies for stenosis of the renal artery should be done and, if present, surgical correction of the stenosis should be undertaken.[141] Patients with a history of nephrectomy need counseling regarding the importance of protecting the remaining single kidney. These patients should be cautioned to avoid potentially nephrotoxic agents (eg, ibuprofen, aminoglycosides), maintain normal weight, obtain early intervention for urinary tract infections, and consult with their physician prior to participating in contact sports.

Bladder Cyclophosphamide and ifosfamide are both capable of inducing hemorrhagic cystitis as a result of accumulation of acrolein in the bladder.[142] Radiation to the pelvis or bladder can result in fibrosis and scarring, with resultant decreased bladder capacity and predisposition to urinary tract infections.[143] Bladder cancer has developed in some patients who received bladder-toxic agents during treatment of childhood cancer.[142] Yearly urinalysis should be done in these patients to evaluate for the presence of microscopic hematuria.

GROWTH

Decreased linear growth is a common problem during therapy in children with cancer. Although catch-up growth may occur, such that the premorbid growth status is regained, in some instances short stature is permanent or even progressive. Severe growth retardation, defined as a standing height below the fifth percentile, has been observed in as many as 30 to 35% of survivors of childhood brain tumors[144–146] and in 10 to 15% of patients treated with some antileukemia regimens.[147–149] Reports indicate the potential for severe growth retardation in patients with tumors involving the head and neck, other than the brain, as well.[147,150–154] As long-term survivors of childhood ALL actually reach adulthood and their final heights can be measured rather than projected, the degree of loss of final height appears to be greater than previously believed.[147,155,156]

Whole-brain irradiation is a major risk factor for short stature,[148,157] especially in doses exceeding 18 Gy.[158] Although severe growth retardation is seen in more than 50% of patients with brain tumors after 30 Gy or more to the hypothalamus or pituitary gland,[144,146] long-term growth retardation after 18 or 24 Gy is less frequent and is generally milder.[159–162] The effects of cranial irradiation also are age-related, with younger children being more susceptible to its growth-inhibiting properties.[147]

The precise mechanism by which cranial irradiation induces short stature is not clear. Biochemical evidence of growth hormone deficiency, including low plasma IGF-1 (somatomedin C) levels and blunted growth hormone responses to different provocative stimuli, have varied, with less than complete correlation with the degree of failure.[163] Early onset of puberty in girls with ALL may contribute to loss of final height. Direct inhibition of vertebral growth by spinal irradiation also contributes to short stature, especially when the entire spinal column is irradiated in doses exceeding 35 Gy.[164] Moreover, a third of children with ALL treated with abdominal irradiation in addition to 18 to 24 Gy of craniospinal irradiation have been reported to have standing heights less than the fifth percentile resulting from irradiation to gonads or thyroid, or from scatter radiation to femoral heads.[149] Mathematic models have allowed the degree of stature loss to be predicted on the basis of radiation dose, radiation port, patient gender, and ideal adult height.[164,165] When lower doses (10–25 Gy) have been given to ports including part or all of the spine, patients have reduced sitting heights.[144,165–167] This problem has been seen particularly in children who are either less than 6 years old or who are undergoing their adolescent growth spurt at the time of radiation therapy. Thoracoabdominal preparative radiation in the setting of hematopoietic cell transplantation (HCT) also has been associated with short stature.[168] Experience with the long-term effects on height of total-body irradiation (TBI) indicate that after 10 Gy given as a single fraction, long-term, severe decreases in growth rates are seen in most children, although fractionation of TBI appears to decrease growth retardation.[169–171] The pathogenesis of short stature in these children includes factors other than radiation, notably GVHD and its therapy. In contrast to the effects of radiation, when chemotherapy is given alone, growth retardation is usually temporary, and patients catch up with their peers. Treatment with growth hormone prior to closure of epiphyses in patients with documented growth hormone deficiency usually results in near normalization of final height, unless the spinal axis has also been irradiated.

Observational studies indicate that obesity as measured by weight or body mass index (BMI) has been reported in small groups of children with ALL and brain tumors treated with conventional therapy or BMT.[155,168,172] This problem has its onset either during therapy or within the first year after discontinuation of therapy and may either progress or stabilize. The majority, but not all patients, have been treated with cranial radiation or TBI, and the contribution of adrenocorticosteroids to the development of obesity is unclear. Other risk factors for the development of obesity include higher radiation dosage (exceeding 20 Gy to the hypothalamus); age less than 4 years at treatment; female gender; associated medical conditions, including hypothyroidism; and familial dyslipidemias.[172] A recent study suggests that doses as low as 15 to 18 Gy are associated with increased body fat when examined by dual x-ray absorptiometry (DEXA).[173] Among the brain tumor survivors, only females treated with high doses of cranial irradiation at a young age have been identified to be at an increased risk of obesity.[174] Obesity developing during adolescence or young adulthood is strongly associated with several common adult health problems, including adult-onset diabetes mellitus, hypertension, dyslipidemias, cardiovascular disease, endometrial cancer, osteoarthritis, and possibly breast and colon cancer. Two small studies suggest that survivors of childhood ALL treated with cranial irradiation may be at an increased risk of cardiovascular risk factors, mediated in part through the radiation-associated obesity.[175,176] The immediate pathogenesis of posttherapy obesity appears to be related to hyperleptinism and is associated with excess insulin secretion. Treatment with octreotide, a somatostatin agonist, results in normalization of insulin secretion, decreased leptin levels, and weight loss.[177] Another study of survivors of posterior fossa tumors who had been treated with radiation reported a reduction in body mass index (BMI) after initiation of growth hormone for short stature.[178]

Monitoring long-term survivors for growth problems relies on the use of standardized curves familiar to the pediatrician and available online at <www.cdc.gov/growthcharts>. Because single values for heights and weights are unreliable for children, frequent serial measurements to establish each child's pattern of growth are recommended. For children whose height crosses percentiles, is less than the third percentile, or whose growth velocity is < 4 to 5 cm/yr, endocrine consultation may be indicated. Because of the foregoing concerns about obesity after the termination of antileukemia therapy, particular attention also needs to be paid to weight during that time, especially during the first year.

Current therapeutic approaches have attempted to prevent growth retardation by using high-dose methotrexate, cytosine arabinoside or both, or intrathecal chemotherapy alone in lieu of radiation for CNS prophylaxis for children with ALL. Similarly, hyperfractionation schedules for radiation therapy and chemotherapy-only regimens are being implemented for treatment of brain tumors and as conditioning regimens in HCT.

THYROID FUNCTION

Hypothyroidism is a common late effect and almost always is due to radiation to the neck for a nonthyroid malignancy. At a mean of 7 years (1.5–16 years) after radiation doses of 15 to 70 Gy, laboratory evidence of primary hypothyroidism (increased serum thyrotropin [TSH] with normal or low thyroxine [T4] levels) has been demonstrated in 30 to 90% of patients with Hodgkin's disease, non-Hodgkin's lymphoma, and primary intracranial or head and neck tumors,[35,144,179–182] and in as many as 50% of children after HCT for hematologic malignancy.[183] Hancock and colleagues reported the risk of hypothyroidism to be 44% at 25 years in 1,787 Hodgkin's disease survivors diagnosed between 1961 and 1989.[181] In the recent CCSS experience of 1,791 Hodgkin's disease survivors, the risk of developing hypothyroidism was increased 17-fold when compared with sibling controls.[35]

The magnitude of risk is dose-dependent. In the CCSS study, among patients treated with radiation doses exceeding 45 Gy, the actuarial risk of hypothyroidism at 20 years was 50%.[35] Adolescents may experience more severe abnormalities with higher thyroid-stimulating hormone levels than those seen in young children.[35,180] Other factors that may contribute to the development of hypothyroidism in survivors of cancer include female sex, hemithyroidectomy, and use of iodide-containing contrast material as in lymphangiography. In some instances, hypothyroidism has been reversible after as long as 3 years, even without replacement therapy.[182] The risk of thyroid nodules has been reported to be 27-fold that of sibling controls, occurring at a mean latency of 14 years after treatment.[35] Female sex and radiation dose exceeding 25 Gy are independent risk factors. About 7% of nodules have been found to be malignant. Secondary hypothyroidism with low thyrotropin and T4 levels appears to be uncommon after radiation to the head or neck.[144,179]

Hyperthyroidism has been described in about 5% of patients after radiation for Hodgkin's disease[35,181,184] or other nonthyroid neoplasms of the neck[185] and after TBI.[170]

Patients at risk of hypothyroidism should be routinely screened with serum thyrotropin and free T4 levels, as well as with a physical examination indefinitely. Evaluation and treatment by an endocrinologist are recommended if any abnormalities are detected. Careful shielding of the thyroid during irradiation, elimination of radiation or the use of lower doses, and avoidance of the concurrent use of radiation and iodide-containing contrast materials should help to decrease the incidence of thyroid abnormalities.

GONADAL FUNCTION

MALES All therapeutic modalities (radiation, surgery, or chemotherapy) cause both germ cell depletion and abnormalities of gonadal endocrine function among male cancer survivors. Radiation to the testes is known to result in germinal loss with decreases in testicular volume and sperm production, and increases in follicle-stimulating hormone (FSH). Effects are dose-dependent, following fractionated exposures of 0.1 to 6 Gy.[186] All males treated with inverted-Y radiation for Hodgkin's disease at a cumulative testicular dose of 1.4 to 3.0 Gy become azoospermic without recovery after 2 to 40 months of follow-up, despite lead shielding of the scrotum.[187] At doses of 4 to 6 Gy, azoospermia may persist for at least 3 to 5 years, and at doses above 6 Gy, usually appears to be irreversible.[188,189] In Seattle, the Bone Marrow Transplantation Team has monitored gonadal function in a large group of male patients who were past puberty at the time of total-body irradiation at a dose of 10 Gy delivered in a single fraction. Azoospermia was universal, although 2 of 41 patients had recovery of sperm production 6 years after HCT.[170]

Radiation therapy may also be toxic to Leydig cells, although at doses higher than those that are toxic to germ cells. Leydig cell damage is dose-dependent and inversely related to age at treatment.[190] Boys treated prepubertally or peripubertally with ≥ 20 Gy for testicular leukemia, in addition to suffering germ cell depletion, are at high risk of delayed sexual maturation associated with decreased testosterone levels, despite increased luteinizing hormone (LH) levels.[191–194] Of 16 boys with hematologic malignancy treated prepubertally with TBI, 11 had delayed onset of puberty.[170] Fractionated doses of less than 12 Gy to the prepubertal testis are compatible with normal pubertal maturation in most patients, although often at the expense of compensated Leydig cell failure (normal testosterone levels with elevated LH levels).[190] Adolescent and young adult male testes are relatively radioresistant, and fractionated doses greater than 30 Gy to the testes may induce Leydig cell failure in only about 50%.[195] Cranial or craniospinal irradiation results in variable testicular dysfunction. Some studies have suggested that this treatment does not harm the testes.[196,197] However, a recent study of young men treated for brain tumors during childhood suggested that secondary hypogonadism with low levels of LH may be seen.[198] Precocious onset of puberty also has been reported in this setting.[199]

Alkylating agents decrease spermatogenesis in long-term survivors of cancer, and the effects are dose-dependent. Gonadal damage following cumulative doses lower than 7.5 mg/m^2 of mechlorethamine or 200 mg/kg of cyclophosphamide as used in HCT has been shown to be reversible in up to 70% of patients after therapy-free intervals of several years.[200,201] Although long-term follow-up of patients who received single-agent cyclophosphamide[202] suggests that prepubertal testicular germ cells may be relatively resistant to chronic toxicity, others have reported that damage to spermatogenesis from alkylating agents in the developing testis may be severe and permanent.[203] Among pubertal or adult males treated for Hodgkin's disease, exposure to more than three cycles of mechlorethamine, vincristine, prednisone, and procarbazine (MOPP) conveys a risk of azoospermia.[204,205] This effect is reversible in only about 20% of cases even 7 years after therapy, a percentage that may increase with fewer MOPP cycles and may decrease with pelvic irradiation.[206] After doxorubicin (Adriamycin), bleomycin, vinblastine, and dacarbazine (ABVD), the incidence of azoospermia appears to be lower (36%) and the incidence of recovery higher (100%) than after MOPP.[207]

Chemotherapy effects are less striking on slowly dividing Leydig cells and may be age-related. Following MOPP in prepubertal boys, normal pubertal progression and normal adult levels of testosterone are the rule; gynecomastia with low testosterone and increased LH have been reported in patients treated during adolescence, and compensated Leydig cell failure (increased LH with low normal testosterone levels or exaggerated FSH and LH responses to LH-releasing hormone) without gynecomastia is common in adults.[201,204,205]

Impotence or retrograde ejaculation are the possible consequences of bilateral retroperitoneal lymph node dissection or partial or complete pelvic exenteration. In patients with primary CNS tumors involving the hypothalamus or pituitary, surgical resection may cause secondary hypogonadism.[208] Hydroceles have been seen in long-term survivors of Hodgkin's disease,[209] Wilms' tumor,[210] and paratesticular rhabdomyosarcoma[118] after surgery or radiation therapy.

The gonadal toxicities are of serious concern to patients and their families. This concern has popularized pretreatment sperm banking. Although many men with Hodgkin's disease, primary testicular cancer, and diverse metastatic cancers have lower-than-expected sperm counts and decreased sperm motility at the time of diagnosis,[211,212] discussion of sperm banking storage with adolescent male patients and their parents is advisable.

Screening for problems of gonadal function with an age-appropriate history with specific attention to problems with libido, impotence, or fertility and examination for gynecomastia, Tanner staging of body hair, and penile and testicular size should be part of the follow-up of all male survivors. Hormonal evaluation, including at least a single measurement of serum LH, FSH, and testosterone levels, has been recommended as a baseline at age 11 years, and in boys whose puberty appears to be delayed. Males at risk of infertility may request semen analysis. When abnormalities in testicular function are detected, close cooperation with an endocrinologist is essential in planning hormonal replacement therapy or in monitoring patients for spontaneous recovery. When no abnormalities are noted on history and physical examination, but sexual maturity has not been completed, these studies should be repeated every 1 to 2 years. Conversely, reminders about contraception should be given in light of the potential for recovery of spermatogenesis and interpatient variations in gonadal toxicity. The value of trying to prevent gonadal dysfunction is obvious. The use of chemotherapeutic regimens such as ABVD that may be less toxic but as effective, as well as refinement of radiation techniques, has been advocated.

Female Gonadal Function Unlike the males, germ cell failure and loss of ovarian endocrine function usually occur concomitantly in females. Following radiation therapy, manifestations are both age- and dose-dependent. In women older than 40 years at the time of treatment, irreversible ovarian failure (amenorrhea, increased LH and FSH levels with or without symptoms of menopause and loss of libido) is an almost universal result of 4 to 7 Gy conventionally fractionated radiation delivered to both ovaries.[213] Prepubertal ovaries are relatively radioresistant, and despite higher doses (12–50 Gy), primary amenorrhea and delayed puberty eventually occurred in 68% of patients treated at a mean age of 6.9 years.[214] In one series, only 23% of prepubertal and adolescent girls in whom at least one ovary was at the edge of the radiation field (and therefore had received a dose of 0.9–10 Gy) had ovarian failure.[215] When secondary amenorrhea results from such modest doses, which are similar to those administered to the ovaries after midline oophoropexy and lead shielding with pelvic radiation in Hodgkin's disease, it appears to be reversible within several months to 4 years in 50 to 60% of patients.[215] In some series, TBI (10 Gy single fraction) has been associated with primary amenorrhea and absent secondary sexual characteristics in most patients treated as young girls and followed for as long as 10 years.[170,183] However, others have reported normal pubertal progression, although with elevated FSH levels following TBI during early childhood.[216,217] As with standard radiation, increasing age at the time of TBI has been found to predict ovarian failure.[218] Premature menopause also has been reported in the setting of HCT.[183] The effect of ovarian scatter from craniospinal radiation is less clear. In one report, girls with medulloblastoma treated with craniospinal radiation alone (30 Gy to the spine) did not experience gonadal toxicity.[196] In contrast, among similarly aged girls with ALL, those receiving craniospinal (18–24 Gy) or craniospinal plus abdominal (12 Gy) radiation experienced incidences of increased FSH and LH of 49% and 93%, respectively, and a large proportion of these children had delayed menses.[219]

Ovarian failure has also been associated with chemotherapy, such as single alkylating agents (cyclophosphamide, busulfan, nitrogen mustard) or as combination therapy (MOPP).[220–222] As with radiation therapy, chemotherapy results in dose- and age-dependent toxicity. Women older than 40 years may develop amenorrhea with as little as one to four cycles of MOPP. In contrast, 30% of women less than 35 years of age require 3 to 12 cycles to become amenorrheic.[222] Young girls treated with conventional doses of single alkylating agents or MOPP generally are capable of normal puberty,[205,221] although they may have biopsy-proven or transient clinical evidence of ovarian failure.[223–225] Moreover, measurement of serum anti-müllerian hormone and inhibin levels, and sonographic measure of ovarian size suggest that subclinical abnormalities of ovarian function may occur despite normal menses and gonadotropin levels.[226]

The diagnostic evaluation of ovarian dysfunction rests on history (primary or secondary amenorrhea, menstrual irregularity, and pregnancies or difficulties becoming pregnant), Tanner staging of breast and genital development, and serum gonadotropin and estradiol levels. In the absence of clinical evidence of puberty (menarche, development of secondary sexual characteristics), baseline studies should be obtained at expected time of onset of puberty in order to assess the need for hormone therapy to induce puberty. However, because young women may progress to early menopause, they should have ongoing follow-up. In an attempt to prevent gonadal failure, some investigators have studied the use of oral contraceptives to suppress ovulation and thus prevent loss of ova.[227] Harvesting and freezing of ova prior to therapy that is likely to cause premature ovarian failure is under investigation.[228] Survivors with concerns regarding fertility are urged to seek consultation with reproductive endocrinologists.

PREGNANCY OUTCOME

Numerous series and case reports have suggested that intensive chemotherapy completed before pregnancy, including myeloablative chemotherapy prior to HCT,[229] is compatible with normal offspring.[230] A recent report from the CCSS of 4,029 pregnancies in 1,915 female 5-year survivors of childhood cancer did not identify excess adverse outcomes for chemotherapeutic agents.[231] A companion study of 2,323 pregnancies in partners of 1,427 male survivors reported 69% live births, 1% stillbirths, 13% miscarriages, and 13% abortions (5% of outcomes were not accounted for).[232] The probability of a pregnancy ending in a live birth was significantly less than that for partners of male sibling controls (RR = 0.8, $p = .007$). Previous studies did not detect any significant malformations, problems with school performance, or excess of minor abnormalities after various intensive combinations commonly used in the treatment of leukemia, Hodgkin's disease, and sarcomas.[231,233] Radiation involving the pelvis is more likely than chemotherapy to result in pregnancy complications. Reports document an increased risk of perinatal death, prematurity, and low birth weight in the offspring of female long-term survivors,[234,235] especially those of Wilms' tumor[232,236] and Hodgkin's disease.[237] Malposition of the fetus, early or threatened labor, birth weight less than 2,500 g, and gestations less than 36 weeks correlated in a dose-related manner with radiation among survivors of Wilms' tumor treated with flank radiation.[238] Studies of offspring of long-term survivors who had been treated during childhood or adolescence with chemotherapy with or without radiation therapy have failed to demonstrate an increased overall risk of childhood cancer in offspring of childhood cancer survivors.[230,239,240] However, survivors with a genetic predisposition to cancer may have children with the same predisposition to malignancy.

Patients who desire to have children after completion of therapy may require care in high-risk obstetrical clinics, especially those who have received abdominal or pelvic irradiation. Because much remains unknown about the problems of children born to survivors of childhood cancer, long-term general follow-up should be emphasized.

AUDITORY COMPLICATIONS

Several potentially ototoxic agents are commonly used in the treatment of children with malignancies, including platinum-based chemotherapy, aminoglycoside antibiotics, loop diuretics, and radiotherapy. These agents are all capable of causing sensorineural hearing loss. Significant risk factors for hearing loss include age less than 4 years at the time of treatment, diagnosis of central nervous system neoplasm, treatment with platinum-based chemotherapy in combination with cranial irradiation, and treatment involving multiple ototoxic agents.[241] Children whose renal function was diminished at the time of treatment, often as a result of treatment with nephrotoxic chemotherapeutic agents, are also at increased risk of ototoxicity.[242] Diagnoses commonly associated with hearing loss include brain and germ cell tumors, neuroblastoma, and osteosarcoma. Very young children who received ototoxic agents during their cancer treatment and whose speech has not yet developed should undergo audiologic evaluations to determine whether they require intervention.

Interventions to assist children experiencing hearing loss as a result of cancer treatment include the use of hearing aids and other assistive devices, along with preferential seating in the front of the classroom. For more severely affected children, placement in special educational environments for the hearing impaired may be required. Affected patients should be counseled to avoid exposure to loud noise, to use ear protection in noisy environments, and to avoid further exposure to ototoxic medications (eg, aminoglycosides, loop diuretics) in order to prevent additional hearing loss. All children with hearing loss related to cancer treatment should receive an evaluation and ongoing follow-up from a pediatric audiologist or otologist.[243]

OCULAR FUNCTION

Children at risk of cataract formation related to cancer treatment include those who received treatment with busulfan or long-term corticosteroids, total-body irradiation (TBI) or radiation to the brain, head, or orbit.[244] Surgical removal of cataracts is indicated when visual impairment interferes with the child's ability to carry out normal activities.[245] Systemic corticosteroid therapy also places children at risk of glaucoma and uveitis. TBI and cranial radiation may result in dry eyes (Sjögren's syndrome) related to decreased lacrimation. Orbital radiation also places children at risk of corneal ulceration, dry eyes, optic nerve damage, retinitis, iritis, glaucoma, blepharitis, and orbital hypoplasia.[245] An ophthalmologist should see children who received radiation therapy to the orbit annually, and those with other risk factors at least once within 5 years of completing therapy. Management of ocular sequelae of cancer therapy should be done collaboratively with an ophthalmologist. Surgical interventions, including cataract extraction and photocoagulation, as well as use of ophthalmic drops and ointments may be indicated,[245] with preservation of the child's sight being the overall goal.

MUSCULOSKELETAL AND RELATED TISSUES

Musculoskeletal problems after childhood cancer involve bony abnormalities, such as scoliosis, atrophy, or hypoplasia; avascular necrosis (AVN); and osteoporosis (bone density ≥ 2.5 SD below mean)/ osteopenia (bone density 1–2.5 SD below mean). Scoliosis is a delayed consequence of radiation therapy to segments of the spinal column. As such, it is seen almost exclusively in patients with solid tumors.[119,167,246] With current techniques including symmetric radiation of the entire spine, sparing large volumes of the adjacent soft tissue, as in the treatment of medulloblastoma[166] or as in total-nodal radiation for Hodgkin's disease, the risk of scoliosis is slight.

Atrophy or hypoplasia has been reported to follow radiation to most other bones, including the long bones of children with soft tissue sarcomas of an extremity and the facial skeleton.[154,247] Doses of radiation exceeding 20 Gy and involvement of epiphyses in the radiation field increase the risk.

Young adult survivors of childhood cancer are at risk of reduced bone density.[248–250] Decreased bone density has been described at diagnosis in children with ALL.[251] Osteopenia in survivors of childhood ALL, as documented by quantitative computed tomographic (CT) scans, also has been related to cranial irradiation.[252] Osteopenia and osteoporosis may progress following steroids or radiation therapy in doses used in children with soft tissue sarcomas or Ewing's sarcoma.[253] Following methotrexate, osteoporosis appears primarily during therapy and resolves once the drug has been discontinued.[254] Both genders are at risk of reduced bone mineral density. Whites may be at greater risk than blacks.[250] Contributing factors include treatment-related gonadal and growth hormone failure, hyperthyroidism, poor calcium intake, and increased body weight.[255,256]

Avascular necrosis is a radiographic diagnosis, which may be asymptomatic until the involved bone is subject to fracture or infection. Although AVN usually develops during therapy, the latency period has been as long at 13 years after treatment. Major risk factors are radiation therapy and systemic corticosteroids. Clinically significant AVN presenting as pain is well described in Hodgkin's disease and non-Hodgkin's lymphoma, and in children with ALL in whom the overall incidence has been about 5%, but in a more significant number of adolescents[257–259] Dexamethasone appears to have more bone toxicity than equivalent doses of prednisone and increased cumulative exposure conveys increased risk.[258] In one retrospective review, almost 15% of adolescents treated with dexamethasone experienced symptomatic AVN.[59] Avascular necrosis most commonly involves the femoral heads, where it may be accompanied by slipped capital femoral epiphysis, but it has been described in virtually all locations and commonly is multifocal.

Dental and maxillofacial abnormalities are a composite of radiation effects on bone and soft tissue. Delayed or arrested tooth development has been reported after 18 Gy or more to the cranium in children with ALL and to the neck or whole mantle for Hodgkin's disease using megavoltage equipment.[260–262] Severe structural tooth abnormalities including malocclusion and caries are almost uniformly seen after 45 to 65 Gy to ports involving the nasopharynx in children treated for soft tissue sarcomas of the head and neck.[263] The effects of radiation, including TBI, on dentition are most severe when this therapy is administered to children younger than 6 years.[171,247] Chemotherapy also appears to contribute to cavity formation and gingivitis, as well as to the development of cosmetically significant grooves, pits, and discoloration.[264]

Detection and diagnosis of musculoskeletal and connective tissue toxicities depend largely on anticipating these issues in vulnerable hosts, taking a careful history, and performing a thorough physical examination. Because of progress with various interventions (including the use of calcium supplementation, calcitonin, bisphosphonates and sex hormone replacement in postmenopausal patients), a baseline DEXA scan has been recommended when survivors reach 18 years of age, with repeat studies as clinically indicated. Regular dental care should be performed twice yearly. Scrupulous oral hygiene, including flossing and fluoride supplementation, may minimize the dental abnormalities.

DELIVERING SURVIVORSHIP CARE

Providing appropriate health care for survivors of cancer is emerging as one of the major challenges in medicine. Childhood cancer survivors, an especially high-risk population, seek and receive care from a wide variety of health care professionals, including oncologists, medical and pediatric specialists, surgeons, primary care physicians, gynecologists, nurses, psychologists, and social workers.[2] The challenge arises from the heterogeneity of this patient population treated with numerous therapeutic modalities in an era of rapidly advancing understanding of late effects. The Institute of Medicine has recognized the need for a systematic plan for lifelong surveillance that incorporates risks based on therapeutic exposures, genetic predisposition, lifestyle behaviors, and comorbid health conditions.[2] Providing comprehensive risk-based care that is readily accessible to survivors is a significant challenge. Although the number of childhood cancer survivors is ever increasing, health care professionals outside academic centers are unlikely to see more than a handful of survivors in their practice, and unless those patients share a similar diagnosis and received similar treatment, there will likely be little similarity in their required follow-up care. Academic settings may allow for establishment of a specialized multidisciplinary follow-up team to care for large numbers of survivors; however, the paucity of such centers and their limited geographic access make such centers an option only for survivors who live nearby or who can afford time and expenses in order to travel to a distant center. Therefore, finding ways to educate local health care providers regarding needed follow-up is a priority. Efforts focusing on educating survivors regarding indicated follow-up may be efficacious, with survivors in turn providing the necessary link in order to direct health care providers to specialized information regarding appropriate long-term follow-up care.

The Children's Oncology Group (COG) has recently released risk-based, exposure-related guidelines (*Long-Term Follow-Up Guidelines for Survivors of Childhood, Adolescent, and Young Adult Cancers*, [Landier, 2004 #741]) specifically designed to direct follow-up care for patients who were diagnosed and treated for pediatric malignancies. These guidelines represent a set of comprehensive screening recommendations that are clinically relevant and can be used to standardize and direct the follow-up care for this group of cancer survivors with specialized health care needs. Implementation of these guidelines is intended to provide ongoing monitoring that facilitates early identification of and intervention for treatment-related complications in order to increase quality of life for these patients. Specially tailored patient education materials, known as "Health Links" accompany the guidelines, offering detailed information on guideline-specific topics in order to enhance health maintenance and promotion among this population of cancer survivors. The entire set of guidelines, with associated Health Links, can be downloaded from <www.survivorshipguidelines.org>.

CANCER SURVIVORSHIP—FUTURE RESEARCH OPPORTUNITIES

Because of its heterogeneity, the growing childhood cancer survivor population provides remarkable opportunities for research relating to the etiopathogenesis of cancer and early detection and prevention of adverse outcomes. Table 124b-3 summarizes the issues related to the future research opportunities that can and should be explored. Therapeutic exposures occurring at known time points, accompanied with close follow-up after the exposure, enables researchers to study testable hypotheses and determine the effects of host- and therapy-related factors in the development of adverse outcomes ranging from carcinogenesis and organ dysfunction to psychosocial consequences. Opportunities also exist to explore gene-environment interactions that may modify individual responses to treatment, as well as susceptibility to develop adverse outcomes, thus providing insights into the identification of high-risk populations. The Children's Oncology Group Late Effects Committee is currently examining the role of gene-environment interactions in the development of key adverse events, such as congestive heart failure, second malignancies, avascular necrosis, myocardial infarction, and stroke, within the setting of a group-wide study entitled "Key Adverse Events after Childhood Cancer – COG ALTE03N1."

Nevertheless, several challenges exist to the conduct of survivorship research. Cancer survivorship research is an evolving issue. With more than 20% of pediatric cancer patients in need of better treatment options, new agents and combinations of agents are being developed.[265] Targeted therapies such as imatinib mesylate and other growth factor inhibitors likely will contribute to increased survivorship. Evaluation of their late effects will need to keep in step with their increased usage. Recent refinements in radiation therapy, such as conformal irradiation, and popularization of surgical techniques, such as laparoscopy, have been intended to minimize late effects. Evidence-based medicine will need to determine whether they will live up to this expectation. Again, the Children's Oncology Group Late Effects Committee has a currently open study comparing the adverse treatment-related sequelae after Hodgkin's disease from two different treatment eras (Title: "Health-related Outcomes after Hodgkin's disease – COG – ALTE04N1"). Advances in supportive care, including transfusions and hematopoietic growth factors, also require ongoing surveillance for identification of late effects. Furthermore, the influence of genetic profiles on susceptibility to late effects, as well as their interaction with lifestyle exposures, such as tobacco, alcohol, and diet, is of growing interest and has not been fully explored. However, the multifactorial etiology of the adverse effects, coupled with the heterogeneous nature of the patient population necessitates large sample sizes within the context of well-characterized cohorts with complete long-term follow-up, and this remains the biggest challenge in conducting sound survivorship research.

REFERENCES

1. Reis LAG, Eisner MP, Kosary CL, et al. SEER cancer statistics review, 1973–1998. Bethesda (MD): National Cancer Institute; 2001.
2. Hewitt M, Weiner SL, Simone JV, editors. Childhood cancer survivorship: improving care and quality of life. Washington, DC: National Academies Press; 2003.
3. Garre ML, Gandus S, Cesana B, et al. Health status of long-term survivors after cancer in childhood. Results of an uniinstitutional study in Italy. Am J Pediatr Hematol Oncol 1994;16:143–52.
4. Oeffinger KC, Eshelman DA, Tomlinson GE, et al. Grading of late effects in young adult survivors of childhood cancer followed in an ambulatory adult setting. Cancer 2000;88:1687–95.
5. Stevens MC, Mahler H, Parkes S. The health status of adult survivors of cancer in childhood. Eur J Cancer 1998;34:694–8.
6. Vonderweid N, Beck D, Caflisch U, et al. Standardized assessment of late effects in long-term survivors of childhood cancer in Switzerland: results of a Swiss Pediatric Oncology Group (SPOG) pilot study. Int J Pediatr Hematol Oncol 1996;3:483–90.
7. Robison LL, Mertens AC, Boice JD Jr, et al. Study design and cohort characteristics of the Childhood Cancer Survivor Study: a multi-institutional collaborative project. Med Pediatr Oncol 2002;38:229–39.
8. Mertens AC, Yasui Y, Neglia JP, et al. Late mortality experience in five-year survivors of childhood and adolescent cancer: the Childhood Cancer Survivor Study. J Clin Oncol 2001;19:3163–72.
9. Moller TR, Garwicz S, Barlow L, et al. Decreasing late mortality among five-year survivors of cancer in childhood and adolescence: a population-based study in the Nordic countries. J Clin Oncol 2001;19:3173–81.
10. Neglia JP, Friedman DL, Yutaka Y, et al. Second malignant neoplasms in five-year survivors of childhood cancer: Childhood Cancer Survivor Study. J Natl Cancer Inst 2001;93:618–29.
11. Olsen JH, Garwicz S, Hertz H, et al. Second malignant neoplasms after cancer in childhood or adolescence. Nordic Society of Paediatric Haematology and Oncology Association of the Nordic Cancer Registries. BMJ 1993;307:1030–6.
12. Bhatia S, Yasui Y, Robison LL, et al. High risk of subsequent neoplasms continues with extended follow-up of childhood Hodgkin's disease: report from the Late Effects Study Group. J Clin Oncol 2003;21:4386–94.
13. Bhatia S, Ramsay NKC, Steinbuch M, et al. Malignant neoplasms following bone marrow transplantation. Blood 1996;87:3633–9.
14. Darrington DL, Vose JM, Anderson JR, et al. Incidence and characterization of secondary myelodysplastic syndrome and acute myelogenous leukemia following high-dose chemoradiotherapy and autologous stem cell transplantation for lymphoid malignancies. J Clin Oncol 1994;12:2527–34.
15. Bhatia S, Robison LL, Oberlin O, et al. Breast cancer and other second neoplasms after childhood Hodgkin's disease. N Engl J Med 1996;334:745–51.
16. Wong FL, Boice JD Jr, Abramson DH, et al. Cancer incidence after retinoblastoma. Radiation dose and sarcoma risk. JAMA 1997;278:1262–7.
17. Zang EA, Wynder EL. Differences in lung cancer risk between men and women: examination of the evidence. J Natl Cancer Inst 1996;88:183–92.
18. Hawkins MM, Wilson LM, Burton HS, et al. Radiotherapy, alkylating agents, and risk of bone cancer after childhood cancer. J Natl Cancer Inst 1996;88:270–8.
19. Breslow NE, Takashima JR, Whitton JA, et al. Second malignant neoplasms following treatment of Wilm's tumor: report from the National Wilms' Tumor Study Group. J Clin Oncol 1995;13:1851–9.
20. Garwicz S, Anderson H, Olsen JH, et al. Second malignant neoplasms after cancer in childhood and adolescence: a population-based case-control study in the 5 Nordic countries. The Nordic Society for Pediatric Hematology and Oncology. The Association of the Nordic Cancer Registries. Int J Cancer 2000;88:672–8.
21. de Vathnaire F, Hawkins M, Campbell S, et al. Second malignant neoplasms after first cancer in childhood: temporal pattern of risk according to type of treatment. Br J Cancer 79:1884–93.
22. Ng AK, Bernardo MV, Weller E, et al. Second malignancy after Hodgkin disease treated with radiation therapy with or without chemotherapy: long-term risks and risk factors. Blood 2002;100:1989–96.
23. Dores GM, Metayer C, Curtis RE, et al. Second malignant neoplasms among long-term survivors of Hodgkin's disease: a population-based evaluation over 25 years. J Clin Oncol 2002;20:3484–94.
24. Metayer C, Lynch C, Clarke EA, et al. Second cancers among long-term survivors of Hodgkin's disease diagnosed in childhood and adolescence. J Clin Oncol 2000;18:2435–43.
25. Diller L, Medeiros Nancarrow C, Shaffer K, et al. Breast cancer screening in women previously treated for Hodgkin's disease: a prospective cohort study. J Clin Oncol 2002;20:2085–91.
26. Wolden SL, Hancock ML, Carlson RW, et al. Management of breast cancer after Hodgkin's disease. J Clin Oncol 2000;18:765–72.
27. Yahalom J, Petrek JA, Biddinger PW, et al. Breast cancer in patients irradiated for Hodgkin's disease: a clinical and pathological analysis of 45 events in 37 patients. J Clin Oncol 1992;10:1674–81.
28. Van Leeuwen FE, Somers R, Taal BG, et al. Increased risk of lung cancer, non-Hodgkin's lymphoma, and leukemia following Hodgkin's disease. J Clin Oncol 1989;7:1046–58.
29. Travis LB, Gospodarowicz M, Curtis RE, et al. Lung cancer following chemotherapy and radiotherapy for Hodgkin's disease. J Natl Cancer Inst 2002;94:182–92.

30. Van Leeuwen FE, Klokman WJ, Stovall M, et al. Roles of radiotherapy and smoking in lung cancer following Hodgkin's disease. J Natl Cancer Inst 1995;87:1530–7.
31. Gurney JG, Davis S, Severson RK, et al. The influence of subsequent neoplasms on incidence trends in childhood cancer. Cancer Epidemiol Biomarkers Prev 1994;3:349–51.
32. Neglia JP, Meadows AT, Robison LL, et al. Second neoplasms after acute lymphoblastic leukemia in childhood. N Engl J Med 1991;325:1330–6.
33. Tucker MA, Jones PH, Boice JDJ, et al. Therapeutic radiation at a young age is linked to secondary thyroid cancer. The Late Effects Study Group. Cancer Res 1991;51:2885–8.
34. De Vathaire F, Hardiman C, Shamsaldin A, et al. Thyroid carcinomas after irradiation for a first cancer during childhood. Arch Intern Med 1999;159:2713–9.
35. Sklar C, Whitton J, Mertens A, et al. Abnormalities of the thyroid in survivors of Hodgkin's disease: data from the Childhood Cancer Survivor Study. J Clin Endocrinol Metab 2000;85:3227–32.
36. Acharya S, Sarafoglou K, LaQuaglia M, et al. Thyroid neoplasms after therapeutic radiation for malignancies during childhood or adolescence. Cancer 2003;97:2397–403.
37. Bhatia S, Sather HN, Pabustan OB, et al. Low incidence of second neoplasms among children diagnosed with acute lymphoblastic leukemia after 1983. Blood 2002;99:4257–64.
38. Sigurdson AJ. Radiation dose and thyroid cancer. 2004. [In review]
39. Tucker MA, D'Angio GL, Boice JD Jr, et al. Bone sarcomas linked to radiotherapy and chemotherapy in children. N Engl J Med 1987;317:588–93.
40. Le Vu B, de Vathaire F, Shamsaldin A, et al. Radiation dose, chemotherapy and risk of osteosarcoma after solid tumours during childhood. Int J Cancer 1998;77:370–7.
41. Smith MA, Rubinstein L, Anderson JR, et al. Secondary leukemia or myelodysplastic syndrome after treatment with epipodophyllotoxins. J Clin Oncol 1999;17:569–7.
42. Hisada M, Garber JE, Fujng CY, et al. Multiple primary cancers in families with Li-Fraumeni syndrome. J Natl Cancer Inst 1998;90:606–11.
43. Naoe T, Takeyama K, Yokozawa T, et al. Analysis of genetic polymorphism in NQO1, GST-M1, GST-T1, and CYP3A4 in 469 Japanese patients with therapy-related leukemia/myelodysplastic syndrome and de novo acute myeloid leukemia. Clin Cancer Res 2000;6:4091–5.
44. Felix CA, Walker AH, Lange BJ, et al. Association of CYP3A4 genotype with treatment-related leukemia. Proc Natl Acad Sci U S A 1998;95:13176–81.
45. Hayes JD, Pulford DJ. The glutathione S-transferase supergene family: regulation of GST and the contribution of the isoenzymes to cancer chemoprotection and drug resistance. Crit Rev Biochem Mol Biol 1995;30:445–600.
46. Smith G, Stanley LA, Sim E, et al. Metabolic polymorphisms and cancer susceptibility. Cancer Surv 1995;25:27–65.
47. Raunio H, Husgafvel-Pursianen K, Anttila S, et al. Diagnosis of polymorphisms in carcinogen-activating and inactivating enzymes and cancer susceptibility. Gene 1995;159:113–21.
48. Wrighton S, Stevens J. The human hepatic cytochromes P450 involved in drug metabolism. Crit Rev Toxicol 1992;22:1–21.
49. Rebbeck TR, Walker AH, Lange BJ, et al. Association of CYP3AQ4 genotype with treatment related leukemia. Proc Natl Acad Sci U S A 1998;95:13176–81.
50. Brown RT, Sawyer MB, Antoniou G, et al. A 3-year follow-up of the intellectual and academic functioning of children receiving central nervous system prophylactic chemotherapy for leukemia. J Dev Behav Pediatr 1996;17:392–8.
51. Mulhern RK, Reddick WE, Palmer SL, et al. Neurocognitive deficits in medulloblastoma survivors and white matter loss. Ann Neurol 1999;46:834–41.
52. Hoppe-Hirsch E, Renier D, Lellouch-Tubiana A, et al. Medulloblastoma in childhood: progressive intellectual deterioration. Childs Nerv Syst 1990;6:60–5.
53. Mitby PA, Robison LL, Whitton JA, et al. Utilization of special education services and educational attainment among long-term survivors of childhood cancer: a report from the Childhood Cancer Survivor Study. Cancer 2003;97:1115–26.
54. Ris MD, Packer RJ, Goldwein J, et al. Intellectual outcome after reduced-dose radiation therapy plus adjuvant chemotherapy for medulloblastoma: a Children's Cancer Group study. J Clin Oncol 2001;19:3470–6.
55. Mulhern RK, Kepner JL, Thomas PR. Neuropsychologic functioning of survivors of childhood medulloblastoma randomized to receive conventional or reduced-dose craniospinal irradiation: a Pediatric Oncology Group Study. J Clin Oncol 1998;16:1723–8.
56. Cousens P, Waters B, Said J, et al. Cognitive effects of cranial irradiation in leukemia: a survey and meta-analysis. J Child Psychol Psychiatry 1988;29:839–52.
57. Waber DP, Tarbell N, Fairclough D, et al. Cognitive sequelae of treatment in childhood acute lymphoblastic leukemia: cranial irradiation requires an accomplice. J Clin Oncol 1995;13:2490–6.
58. Haupt R, Fears TR, Robison LL, et al. Educational attainment in long-term survivors of childhood acute lymphoblastic leukemia: a report from the NIH and the CCG. JAMA 1994;272:1427–32.
59. Packer RJ, Meadows AT, Rorke LB, et al. Long-term sequelae of cancer treatment on the central nervous system in childhood. Med Pediatr Oncol 1987;15:241–53.
60. Reddick WE, White HA, Glass JO, et al. Developmental model relating white matter volume to neurocognitive deficits in pediatric brain tumor survivors. Cancer 2003;97:2512–9.
61. Shan K, Lincoff AM, Young JB. Anthracycline induced cardiotoxicity. Ann Intern Med 1996;125:47–58.
62. Grenier MA, Lipshultz SE. Epidemiology of anthracycline cardiotoxicity in children and adults. Semin Oncol 1998;25:72–85.
63. Bossi G, Lanzarini L, Laudisa ML, et al. Echocardiographic evaluation of patients cured of childhood cancer: a single center study of 117 subjects who received anthracyclines. Med Pediatr Oncol 2001;36:593–600.
64. Kremer LCM, van Dalen EC, Offringa M, et al. Anthracycline-induced clinical heart failure in a cohort of 607 children: long-term follow-up study. J Clin Oncol 2001;19:191–6.
65. Steinherz LJ, Steinherz PG, Tan CTC, et al. Cardiac toxicity 4 to 20 years after completing anthracycline therapy. JAMA 1991;266:1672–7.
66. Lipshultz SE, Colan SD, Gelber RD, et al. Late cardiac effects of doxorubicin therapy for acute lymphoblastic leukemia in childhood. N Engl J Med 1991;324:808–15.
67. Pan PH, Moore CH. Doxorubicin-induced cardiomyopathy during pregnancy: three case reports of anesthetic management for cesarian and vaginal delivery in two kyphoscoliotic patients. Anesthesiology 2002;97:513–5.
68. Hinkle AS, Proukou CB, Deshpande SS, et al. Cardiovascular complications: cardiotoxicity caused by chemotherapy. In: Wallace H, Green DM, editors. Late effects of childhood cancer. New York: Oxford University Press; 2004.
69. Lipshultz SE, Lipshultz SR, Mone SM, et al. Female sex and higher drug dose as risk factors for late cardiotoxic effects of doxorubicin therapy for childhood cancer. N Engl J Med 1995;332:1738–43.
70. Adams MJ, Hardenbergh PH, Constine LS, et al. Radiation-associated cardiovascular disease. Crit Rev Oncol Hematol 2003;45:55–75.
71. Mill WB, Baglan RJ, Kurichetz P, et al. Symptomatic radiation induced pericarditis in Hodgkin's disease. Int J Radiat Oncol Biol Phys 1984;10:2061–5.
72. Perraut DJ, Levy M, Herman JD, et al. Echocardiographic abnormalities following cardiac irradiation. J Clin Oncol 1985;3:546–51.
73. Scott DL, Thomas RD. Late onset constrictive pericarditis after thoracic radiotherapy. Br Med J 1978;1:341–2.
74. Haas JM. Symptomatic constrictive pericarditis developing 45 years after radiation therapy to the mediastinum: a review of radiation pericarditis. Am Heart J 1969;77:89–95.
75. Boivin JF, Hutchinson GB, Lubin JH, et al. Coronary artery disease in patients treated for Hodgkin's disease. 1992;69:1241–7.
76. Reinders JG, Heijman BJ, Olofsen-van Acht MJ, et al. Ischemic heart disease after mantlefield irradiation of Hodgkin's disease in long-term follow-up. Radiother Oncol 1999;51:35–42.
77. Hull MC, Morris CG, Pepine CJ, et al. Valvular dysfunction and carotid, subclavian, and coronary artery disease in survivors of Hodgkin lymphoma treated with radiation therapy. JAMA 2003;290:2831–7.
78. Bu'Lock FA, Gabriel HM, Oakhill A, et al. Cardioprotection by ICRF187 against high dose anthracycline toxicity in children with malignant disease. Br Heart J 1993;70:185–8.
79. Wexler L. Ameliorating anthracycline cardiotoxicity in children with cancer: clinical trials with dexrazoxane. Semin Oncol 1998;25:86–92.
80. Lipshultz SE, Rifai N, Dalton VM, et al. The effect of dexrazoxane on myocardial injury in doxorubicin-treated children with acute lymphoblastic leukemia. N Engl J Med 2004;351:145–53.
81. Lipshultz SE, Lipsitz SR, Sallan SE, et al. Long-term enalapril therapy for left ventricular dysfunction in doxorubicin-treated survivors of childhood cancer. J Clin Oncol 2002;20:4517–22.
82. Silber JH, Cnaan A, Clark BJ, et al. Design and baseline characteristics for the ACE Inhibitor After Anthracycline (AAA) study of cardiac dysfunction in long-term pediatric cancer survivors. Am Heart J 2001;142:577–85.
83. Horning SJ, Adhikari A, Rizk N. Effect of treatment for Hodgkin's disease on pulmonary function: results of a prospective study. J Clin Oncol 1994;12:297–305.
84. Mefferd JM, Donaldson SS, Link MP. Hodgkin's disease: pulmonary, cardiac, and thyroid function following combined modality therapy. Int J Radiat Oncol Biol Phys 1989;16:679–85.
85. Nysom K, Holm K, Hertz H, et al. Risk factors for reduced pulmonary function after malignant lymphoma in childhood. Med Pediatr Oncol 1998;30:240–8.
86. Morgan GW, Freeman AP, McLean RG, et al. Late cardiac, thyroid, and pulmonary sequelae of mantle radiotherapy for Hodgkin's disease. Int J Radiat Oncol Biol Phys 1985;11:1925–31.
87. Wara WM, Phillips TL, Margolis LW, et al. Radiation pneumonitis: a new approach to the derivation of time-dose factors. Cancer 1973;32:547–52.
88. Jakacki RI, Schramm CM, Bernadine R, et al. Restrictive lung disease following treatment for malignant brain tumors: a potential late effect of craniospinal irradiation. J Clin Oncol 1995;13:1478–85.
89. Mertens AC, Yasui Y, Liu Y, et al. Pulmonary complications in survivors of childhood and adolescent cancer. A report from the Childhood Cancer Survivor Study. Cancer 2002;95:2431–41.
90. Springmeyer SC, Flournay N, Sullivan KM, et al. Pulmonary function changes in long-term survivors of allogeneic marrow transplantation. In: Gale RP, editor. Recent advances in bone marrow transplantation. New York: Alan R. Liss; 1983. p. 343.
91. Griese M, Rampf U, Hofmann D, et al. Pulmonary complications after bone marrow transplantation in children: twenty-four years of experience in a single pediatric center. Pediatr Pulmonol 2000;30:393–401.
92. Kikkawa Y, Smith F. Cellular and biochemical aspects of pulmonary surfactant in health and disease. Lab Invest 1993;49:122–39.
93. Rubin P, M. F, Shapiro D. Molecular biology mechanisms in the radiation induction of pulmonary injury syndromes: interrelationship between the alveolar macrophages and septal fibroblast. Int J Radiat Oncol Biol Phys 1992;24:93–101.
94. Miller RW, Fusner JE, Fink RJ, et al. Pulmonary function abnormalities in long-term survivors of childhood cancer. Med Pediatr Oncol 1986;14:202–7.
95. Benoist MR, Lemerle J, R. J, et al. Effects on pulmonary function of whole lung irradiation for Wilms' tumour in children. Thorax 1982;37:175–80.
96. Littman P, Meadows AT, Polgar G, et al. Pulmonary function in survivors of Wilms' tumor: patterns of impairment. Cancer 1976;37:2773–6.
97. Fort JA, Graham-Pole J. Pulmonary complications of bone marrow transplantation. In: Johnson L, Pochedly C, editors. Bone marrow transplantation in children. New York: Raven Press; 1990.
98. Quigley PM, Yeager AM, Loughlin GM. The effects of bone marrow transplantation on pulmonary function in children. Pediatr Pulmonol 1994;18:361–7.
99. Wohl ME, Griscom NT, Traggis DG, et al. Effects of therapeutic irradiation delivered in early childhood upon subsequent lung function. Pediatrics 1975;55:507–16.
100. Hassink EAM, Souren TS, Boersma LJ, et al. Pulmonary morbidity 10-18 years after irradiation for Hodgkin's disease. Eur J Cancer 1993;29A:343–7.
101. Villani F, Viviani S, Bonfante V, et al. Late pulmonary effects in favorable stage I and IIA Hodgkin's Disease treated with radiotherapy alone. Am J Clin Oncol 2000;23:18–21.
102. Salloum E, Tanoue LT, Wackers FJ, et al. Assessment of cardiac and pulmonary function in adult patients with Hodgkin's disease treated with ABVD or MOPP/ABVD plus adjuvant low-dose mediastinal irradiation. Cancer Invest 1999;17:171–80.
103. Eigen H, Wyszomierski D. Bleomycin lung injury in children: pathophysiology and guidelines for management. Am J Pediatr Hematol Oncol 1985;7:71–8.
104. Comis RL. Bleomycin pulmonary toxicity. In: Carter SK, Crooke ST, Umezawa H, editors. Bleomycin: current sta-

tus and new developments. New York:, Academic Press; 1978. p. 279.
105. Samuels ML, Johnson DE, Holoye PY, et al. Large-dose bleomycin therapy and pulmonary toxicity: a possible role of prior radiotherapy. JAMA 1976;235:1117–20.
106. Aronin PA, Mahaley MSJ, Rudnick SA, et al. Prediction of BCNU pulmonary toxicity in patients with malignant gliomas: an assessment of risk factors. N Engl J Med 1980;303:183–8.
107. O'Driscoll BR, Hasleton PS, Taylor PM, et al. Active lung fibrosis up to 17 years after chemotherapy with carmustine (BCNU) in childhood. N Engl J Med 1990;323:378–82.
108. Wheeler C, Antin JH, Churchill WH, et al. Cyclophosphamide, carmustine, and etoposide with autologous bone marrow transplantation in refractory Hodgkin's disease and non-Hodgkin's lymphoma: a dose-finding study. J Clin Oncol 1990;8:648–56.
109. Rubio C, Hill ME, Milan S, et al. Idiopathic pneumonia syndrome after high-dose chemotherapy for relapsed Hodgkin's disease. Br J Cancer 1997;75:1044–8.
110. Bauer KA, Skarin AT, Balikian JP, et al. Pulmonary complications associated with combination chemotherapy programs containing bleomycin. Am J Med 1983;74:557–63.
111. Komp DM. Long-term sequelae of histiocytosis X. Am J Pediatr Hematol Oncol 1981;3:165–8.
112. Goldiner PL, Schweizer O. The hazards of anaesthesia and surgery in bleomycin-treated patients. Semin Oncol 1979;6:121–4.
113. Schwerzmann M, Seiler C. Recreational scuba diving, patent foramen ovale and their associated risks. Swiss Med Wkly 2001;131:365–74.
114. Mahboubi S, Silber RJ. Radiation-induced esophageal strictures in children with cancer. Eur Radiol 1997;7:119–22.
115. Donaldson SS, Jundi S, Ricour C, et al. Radiation enteritis in children: a retrospective review, clinco-pathologic correlation, and dietary management. Cancer 1975;35:1167–78.
116. Ehinger DS, Slavin RE. Chronic radiation enteritis complicating non-Hodgkin's lymphoma. South Med J 1977;70:960–1.
117. Localio SA, Stone A, Friedman M. Surgical aspects of radiation enteritis. Surg Gynecol Obstet 1969;129:302–7.
118. Heyn R, Raney RB, Hayes DM, et al. Late effects of therapy in patients with paratesticular rhabdomyosarcoma. J Clin Oncol 1992;10:614–23.
119. Paulino A, Wen BC, Brown CK, et al. Late effects in children treated with radiation therapy for Wilms tumor. Int J Radiat Oncol Biol Phys 2000;46:1239–46.
120. Roswit B. Complications of radiation therapy: the alimentary tract. Semin Roentgenol 1974;9:115–31.
121. Olver IN, Pearl P, Wiernik PH, et al. Small bowel obstruction as a late complication of the treatment of Hodgkin's disease. Aust N Z J Surg 1990;60:585–8.
122. Ritchey ML, Kelalis P, Breslow N, et al. Small bowel obstruction following nephrectomy for Wilms' tumor. Ann Surg 1993;218:654–9.
123. D'Angio GJ, Farber S, Maddock CL. Potentiation of x-ray effects by actinomycin D. Radiology 1959;73:175–7.
124. Philips TL. Chemical modifications of radiation effect. Cancer 1977;39:987–99.
125. Tefft M, Mitus A, Das L, et al. Irradiation of the liver in children: review of experience in the acute and chronic phases and in the intact normal and partially resected. AJR Am J Roentgenol 1970;108:365–85.
126. Sharp H, Nesbit M, White J, et al. Methotrexate liver toxicity. J Pediatr 1969;74:818–9.
127. Dahl MGC, Gregory MM, Schever PJ. Liver damage due to methotrexate in patients with psoriasis. Br Med J 1971;1:625–30.
128. McIntosh S, Davidson DL, O'Brien RT, et al. Methotrexate hepatotoxicity in children with leukemia. J Pediatr 1977;90:1019–21.
129. Claviez A, Hero B, Schneppenhim R, et al. Hepatopathy in patients with stage 4S neuroblastoma. Klin Pediatr 1996;208:221–8.
130. Strickland DK, Riely CA, Patrick CC, et al. Hepatitis C infection among survivors of childhood cancer. Blood 2000;95:3065–70.
131. Locasciulli A, Testa M, Pontisso P, et al. Prevalence and natural history of hepatitis C infection in patients cured of childhood leukemia. Blood 1997;90:4628–33.
132. Cesaro S, Petris MG, Rosetti R, et al. Chronic hepatitis C virus infection after treatment for pediatric malignancy. Blood 1997;90:1315–20.
133. Strasser SI, Sullivan KM, Myerson D, et al. Cirrhosis of the liver in long-term marrow transplant survivors. Blood 1999;93:3259–66.
134. Dodd RY. The risk of transfusion-transmitted infection. N Engl J Med 1992;327:419–21.
135. Knapp AB, Crawford JM, Rappeport JM, et al. Cirrhosis as a consequence of graft versus host disease. Gastroenterology 1987;392:513–9.
136. Rose VL. CDC issues new recommendations for the prevention and control of hepatitis C virus infection. Am Family Phys 1999;59:1321–3.
137. Raney B, Heyn R, Cassady R, Marks L. Late effects of cancer therapy on the genitourinary tract in children. In Schwartz CL, Hobbie WL, Constine LS, Ruccione KS, editors. Survivors of childhood cancer: assessment and management. St. Louis: Mosby; 1994. p. 245–62.
138. Pratt CB, Meyer WH, Jenkins JJ, et al. Ifosfamide, Fanconi's syndrome and rickets. J Clin Oncol 1991;9:1495–9.
139. Neglia JP, Nesbit ME. Care and treatment of long-term survivors of childhood cancer. Cancer 1993;71:3386–91.
140. Grossi M. Management of long-term complications of pediatric cancer. Pediatr Clin North Am 1998;45:1637–58.
141. Green DM. Effects of treatment for childhood cancer on vital organ systems. Cancer 1993;71:3299–305.
142. Raney B, Heyn R, Cassady R, Marks L. Late effects of cancer therapy on the genitourinary tract in children. In: Schwartz CL, Hobbie WL, Constine LS, Ruccione KS, editors. Survivors of childhood cancer: assessment and management. St. Louis: Mosby; 1994. p. 245–62.
143. Marina N. Long-term survivors of childhood cancer: the medical consequences of cure. Pediatr Clin North Am 1997;44:1021–42.
144. Oberfield SE, Allen JC, Pollack J, et al. Long-term endocrine sequelae after treatment of medulloblastoma: prospective study of growth and thyroid function. J Pediatr 1986;108:219–23.
145. Danoff BF, Cowchock FS, Marquette C, et al. Assessment of the long-term effects of primary radiation therapy for brain tumors in children. Cancer 1982;49:1580–6.
146. Onoyama Y, Mitsuyuki A, Takahashi M, et al. Radiation therapy of brain tumors in children. Radiology 1977;115:687–93.
147. Noorda EM, Somers R, van Leeuwen FE, et al. Dutch Late Effects Study Group. Adult height and age at menarche in childhood cancer survivors. Eur J Cancer 2001;37:605–12.
148. Oliff A, Bode U, Bercu BB, et al. Hypothalamic-pituitary dysfunction following CNS prophylaxis in acute lymphocytic leukemia: correlation with CT scan abnormalities. Med Pediatr Oncol 1979;7:141–51.
149. Robison LL, Nesbit ME, Sather HN, et al. Height of children successfully treated for acute lymphoblastic leukemia: a report from the Late Effects Study Committee of Children's Cancer Study Group. Med Pediatr Oncol 1985;13:14–21.
150. Rappaport R, Brauner R. Growth and endocrine disorders secondary to cranial irradiation. Pediatr Res 1989;25:561–7.
151. Bajorunas DR, Chavimi F, Jereb B, et al. Endocrine sequelae of antineoplastic therapy in childhood and head and neck malignancies. J Clin Endocrinol Metab 1980;50:329–35.
152. Braunstein GD, Kohler PO. Endocrine manifestations of histiocytosis. Am J Pediatr Hematol Oncol 1981;3:67–75.
153. Samaan NA, Vieto R, Schultz PN. Hypothalamic, pituitary and thyroid function after radiotherapy to the head and neck. Int J Radiat Oncol Biol 1982;8:1857–67.
154. Heyn R, Ragab A, Raney RBJ, et al. Late effects of therapy in orbital rhabdomyosarcoma in children: a report from the Intergroup Rhabdomyosarcoma Study. Cancer 1986;57:1738–43.
155. Birkebaek NH, Clausen N. Height and weight pattern up to 20 years after treatment for acute lymphocytic leukaemia. Arch Dis Child 1998;79:161–4.
156. Schriock EA, Schell MJ, Carter M, et al. Longitudinal growth patterns and final height of long term survivors of childhood leukemia. J Clin Oncol 1991;9:400–5.
157. Wells RJ, Foster MB, D'Ercole AJ, et al. The impact of cranial irradiation on the growth of children with acute lymphocytic leukemia. Am J Dis Child 1983;137:37–9.
158. Sklar CA, Mertens AC, Walter A, et al. Final height after treatment for childhood acute lymphoblastic leukemia: comparison of no cranial irradiation with 1800 and 2400 centigrays of cranial irradiation. J Pediatr 1993;123:59–64.
159. Melin AE, Adan L, Leverger G, et al. Growth hormone secretion, puberty and adult short height after cranial irradiation with 18 Gy for leukemia. Eur J Pediatr 1998;157:703–7.
160. Sklar CA. Growth and neuroendocrine dysfunction following therapy for childhood cancer. Pediatr Clin N Am 1997;44:489–503.
161. Shalet SM, Price DA, Beardwell CG, et al. Normal growth despite abnormalities of growth hormone secretion in children treated for acute leukemia. J Pediatr 1979;94:719–22.
162. Hakimi N, Mohammad A, Mayer JW. Growth and growth hormone of children with acute lymphocytic leukemia following central nervous system prophylaxis with and without cranial radiation. Am J Pediatr Hematol Oncol 1980;2:311.
163. Shalet SM, Beardwell CG, Morris-Jones PH, et al. Growth hormone deficiency after treatment of acute leukaemia in children. Arch Dis Child 1976;51:489–93.
164. Silber JH, Littman PS, Meadows AT. Stature loss following skeletal irradiation for childhood cancer. J Clin Oncol 1990;8:304–12.
165. Schell MJ, Ochs JJ, Schriock EA, et al. A method of predicting adult height and obesity in long-term survivors of childhood acute lymphoblastic leukemia. J Clin Oncol 1992;10:128–33.
166. Bloom HJ, Wallace EN, Henk JM. The treatment and prognosis of medulloblastoma in children: a study of 82 verified cases. AJR Am J Roentgenol 1969;105:43–62.
167. Thomas PRM, Griffith KD, Fineberg BB, et al. Late effects of treatment for Wilms' tumor. Int J Radiat Oncol Biol Phys 1983;9:651–7.
168. Cohen A, Duell T, Socie G, et al. Nutritional status and growth after bone marrow transplantation (BMT) during childhood: EBMT Late-Effects Working Party retrospective data. European Group for Blood and Marrow Transplantation. Bone Marrow Transplant 1999;23:1043–7.
169. Cohen A, Roselli A, Bakker B, et al. Final height of patients who underwent bone marrow transplantation for hematological disorders: a study by the Working Party for Late-Effects EBMT. Blood 1999;93:4109–15.
170. Sanders J. Late effects after bone marrow transplantation. In: Schwartz CL, Hobbie WL, Constine LS, Ruccione KS, editors. Survivors of childhood cancer: assessment and management. St. Louis: Mosby; 1994. p. 293.
171. Kolb HJ, Bender-Gotze C. Late complications after allogeneic bone marrow transplantation for leukaemia. Bone Marrow Transplant 1990;6:61–72.
172. Oeffinger KC, Mertens AC, Sklar CA, et al. Obesity in adult survivors of childhood acute lymphoblastic leukemia: a report from the childhood cancer survivor study group. J Clin Oncol 2003;21:1359–65.
173. Nysom K, Holm K, Michaelsen KF, et al. Degree of fatness after treatment for acute lymphoblastic leukemia in childhood. J Clin Endocrinol Metab 1999;84:4591–6.
174. Gurney JG, Ness KK, Stovall M, et al. Final height and body mass index among adult survivors of childhood brain cancer: childhood cancer survivor study. J Clin Endocrinol Metab 2003;88:4731–9.
175. Talvensaari KK, Lanning M, Tapanainen P, et al. Long-term survivors of childhood cancer have an increased risk of manifesting the metabolic syndrome. J Clin Endocrinol Metab 1996;81:3051–5.
176. Oeffinger KC, Buchanan GR, Eshelman DA, et al. Cardiovascular risk factors in young adult survivors of childhood acute lymphoblastic leukemia. J Pediatr Hemotol Oncol 2001;23:424–30.
177. Lustig RH, Rose SR, Burghen GA, et al. Hypothalamic obesity caused by cranial insult in children: altered glucose and insulin dynamics and reversal by a somatostatin agonist. J Pediatr 1999;135:162–8.
178. Hamre M, Smietana S, Sood S, et al. Obesity in survivors of posterior fossa PNETs and ependymomas is related to hormonal insufficiency. Proceedings of the 5th International Conference on Long-term Complications of Treatment of Children and Adolescents for Cancer. Niagara-on-the-Lake (ON); 1998. p. 164
179. Richards GE, Wara WM, Grumbach MM, et al. Delayed onset of hypopituitarism: sequelae of therapeutic irradiation of central nervous system, eye, and middle ear tumors. J Pediatr 1976;89:553–9.
180. Constine LS, Donaldson SS, McDougall IR. Thyroid dysfunction after radiotherapy for children with Hodgkin's disease. Cancer 1984;53:878–83.
181. Hancock SL, Cox RS, McDougall IR. Thyroid diseases after treatment of Hodgkin's disease. N Engl J Med 1991;325:599–605.
182. Devney RB, Sklar CA, Nesbit MEJ, et al. Serial thyroid function measurements in children with Hodgkin's disease. J Pediatr 1984;105:223–7.
183. Liesner RJ, Leiper AD, Hann IM, et al. Late effects of intensive treatment for acute myeloid leukemia and myelodysplasia in childhood. J Clin Oncol 1994;12:916–24.
184. Jackson R, Rosenberg C, Kleinmann R, et al. Ophthalmopathy following neck irradiation for Hodgkin's disease. Cancer Treat Rep 1979;63:1393–5.
185. Wasnich RD, Grumet CF, Payne RO, et al. Grave's ophthalmopathy following external neck irradiation for nonthy-

roidal neoplastic disease. J Clin Endocrinol Metab 1973;37:703–13.
186. Rowley MM, Leach DR, Warner GA, Heller CG. Effect of graded doses of ionizing radiation on the human testes. Radiat Res 1974;59:665–78.
187. Speiser B, Rubin P, Casarett G. Aspermia following lower truncal irradiation in Hodgkin's disease. Cancer 1973;32:692–8.
188. Hahn EW, Feingold BS, Simpson L, Batata M. Recovery from aspermia induced by low dose radiation in seminoma patients. Cancer 1982;50:337–40.
189. Clifton DK, Bremner WJ. The effect of testicular x-irradiation on spermatogenesis in man. J Androl 1983;4:387–92.
190. Sklar C. Reproductive physiology and treatment-related loss of sex hormone production. Med Pediatr Oncol 1999;33:2–8.
191. Shalet SM, Horner A, Ahmed SR, Morris-Jones PH. Leydig cell damage after testicular irradiation for lymphoblastic leukaemia. Med Pediatr Oncol 1985;13:65–8.
192. Blatt J, Sherins RJ, Niebrugge D, et al. Leydig cell function in boys following treatment for testicular relapse of acute lymphoblastic leukemia. J Clin Oncol 1985;3:1227–31.
193. Brauner R, Czernichow P, Cramer P, et al. Leydig-cell function in children after direct testicular irradiation for acute lymphoblastic leukemia. N Engl J Med 1983;309:25–8.
194. Leiper AD, Grant DB, Chessells JM. Gonadal function after testicular radiation for acute lymphoblastic leukaemia. Arch Dis Child 1986;61:53–6.
195. Izard MA. Leydig cell function and radiation: a review of the literature. Radiother Oncol 1995;34:1–8.
196. Ahmed SR, Shalet SM, Campbell RH, Deakin DP. Primary gonadal damage following treatment of brain tumors in childhood. J Pediatr 1983;103:562–5.
197. Blatt J, Poplack DG, Sherins RJ. Testicular function in boys after chemotherapy for acute lymphoblastic leukemia. N Engl J Med 1981;304:1121–4.
198. Schmiegelow M, Lassen S, Poulsen HS, et al. Gonadal status in male survivors following childhood brain tumors. J Clin Endocrinol Metab 2001;86:2446–52.
199. Brauner R, Czernichow P, Rappaport R. Precocious puberty after hypothalamic and pituitary irradiation in young children. N Engl J Med 1984;311:920.
200. Schamberger, Schilsky RL, Sherins RJ. Gonadal dysfunction. In: DeVita VT Jr, Hellman S, Rosenberg SA, editors. Cancer: principles and practice of oncology. Philadelphia: JB Lippincott; 1982. p. 1713.
201. Sherins RJ, DeVita VT. Effect of drug treatment for lymphoma on male reproductive capacity. Ann Intern Med 1973;79:216–20.
202. Sanders JE, Buckner CD, Leonard JM, et al. Late effects on gonadal function of cyclophosphamide, total body irradiation, and marrow transplantation. Transplantation 1983;36:252–5.
203. Kenney LB, Laufer MR, Grant FD, et al. High risk of infertility and long term gonadal damage in males treated with high dose cyclophosphamide for sarcoma during childhood. Cancer 2001;91:613–21.
204. Sherins RJ, Olweny CLM, Ziegler JL. Gynecomastia and gonadal dysfunction in adolescent boys treated with combination chemotherapy for Hodgkin's disease. N Engl J Med 1978;299:12–6.
205. Whitehead E, Shalet SM, Morris-Jones PH, et al. Gonadal function after combination chemotherapy for Hodgkin's disease in childhood. Arch Dis Child 1982;57:287–91.
206. da Cunha MF, Meistrich ML, Fuller LM, et al. Recovery of spermatogenesis after treatment for Hodgkin's disease with limiting dose of MOPP chemotherapy. J Clin Oncol 1984;2:571–7.
207. Santoro A, Bonadonna G, Valagussa P, et al. Long-term results of combined chemotherapy-radiotherapy approach in Hodgkin's disease: superiority of ABVD plus radiotherapy versus MOPP plus radiotherapy. J Clin Oncol 1987;5:27–37.
208. Thomsett MJ, Conte FA, Kaplan SL, Grumbach MM. Endocrine and neurologic outcome in childhood craniopharyngioma: review of effect of treatment on 42 patients. J Pediatr 1980;97:728–35.
209. Duffey P, Campbell EW, Wiernik PH. Hydrocele following treatment for Hodgkin's disease. Cancer 1982;50:305–7.
210. Ginsberg JP, Hobbie WL, Ogle SK, et al. Prevalence of and risk factors for hydrocele in survivors of Wilms' tumor. Pediatr Blood Cancer 2004;42:361–3.
211. Chapman RM, Sutcliffe SB, Malpas JS. Male gonadal dysfunction in Hodgkin's disease: a prospective study. JAMA 1981;245:1323–8.
212. Vigersky RA, Chapman RM, Berenberg J, Glass AR. Testicular dysfunction in untreated Hodgkin's disease. Am J Med 1982;73:482–6.
213. Lushbaugh CC, Casarett GW. The effects of gonadal irradiation in clinical radiation therapy: a review. Cancer 1976;37:1111–25.
214. Stillman RJ, Schinfeld JS, Schiff I, et al. Ovarian failure in long-term survivors of childhood malignancy. Am J Obstet Gynecol 1981;139:62–6.
215. Ortin TTS, Shostak CA, Donaldson SS. Gonadal status and reproductive function following treatment for Hodgkin's disease in childhood: the Stanford experience. Int J Radiat Oncol Biol Phys 1990;19:873–80.
216. Matsumoto M, Shinohara O, Ishiguro H, et al. Ovarian function after bone marrow transplantation performed before menarche. Arch Dis Child 1999;80:452–4.
217. Mayer EI, Dopfer RE, Klingebiel T, et al. Longitudinal gonadal function after bone marrow transplantation for acute lymphoblastic leukemia during childhood. Pediatr Transplantation 1999;3:38–44.
218. Couto-Silva AC, Trivin C, Thibaud E, et al. Factors affecting gonadal function after bone marrow transplantation during childhood. Bone Marrow Transplant 2001;28:67–75.
219. Hamre MR, Robison LL, Nesbit ME, et al. Effects of radiation on ovarian function in long-term survivors of childhood acute lymphoblastic leukemia: a report from the Children's Cancer Study Group. J Clin Oncol 1987;5:1759–65.
220. Rose DP, Davis TE. Ovarian function in patients receiving adjuvant chemotherapy for breast cancer. Lancet 1977;1:1174–6.
221. Siris ES, Leventhal BG, Vaitukaitis JL. Effects of childhood leukemia and chemotherapy on puberty and reproductive function in girls. N Engl J Med 1976;294:1143–6.
222. Chapman RM, Sutcliffe SB, Malpas JS. Cytotoxic-induced ovarian failure in women with Hodgkin's disease. JAMA 1979;242:1877–81.
223. Nicosia SV, Matus-Ridley M, Meadows AT. Gonadal effects of cancer therapy in girls. Cancer 1985;55:2364–72.
224. Himelstein-Braw R, Peters H, Faber M. Influence of irradiation and chemotherapy on the ovaries of children with abdominal tumours. Br J Cancer 1977;36:269–75.
225. Morris-Jones PH, Beardwell CG, Deakin DP. Gonadal function after combination chemotherapy for Hodgkin's disease in childhood. Arch Dis Child 1982;47:287–91.
226. Bath LE, Wallace WH, Shaw MP, et al. Depletion of ovarian reserve in young women after treatment for cancer in childhood: detection by anti-Müllerian hormone, inhibin B and ovarian ultrasound. Hum Reprod 2003;1811:2368–74.
227. Chapman RM, Sutcliffe SB. Protection of ovarian function by oral contraceptives in women receiving chemotherapy for Hodgkin's disease. Blood 1981;58:849–51.
228. Wallace WH, Anderson R, Baird D. Preservation of fertility in young women treated for cancer. Lancet Oncol 2004;5:269–70.
229. Gulati SC, Van Poznak C. Pregnancy after bone marrow transplantation. J Clin Oncol 1998;16:1978–85.
230. Blatt J. Pregnancy outcome in long-term survivors of childhood cancer. Med Pediatr Oncol 1999;33:29–33.
231. Green DM, Whitton J, Stovall M, et al. Pregnancy outcome of female survivors of childhood cancer: a report from the Childhood Cancer Survivor Study. Am J Ob Gyn 2002;187:1070–80.
232. Green DM, Whitton JA, Stovall M, et al. Pregnancy outcome of partners of male survivors of childhood cancer: A report from the Childhood Cancer Survivor Study. J Clin Oncol 2003;21:716–21.
233. Blatt J, Mulvihill JJ, Ziegler JL, et al. Pregnancy outcome following cancer chemotherapy. Am J Med 1980;69:828–32.
234. Green DM, Peabody EM, Nan B, et al. Pregnancy outcome after treatment for Wilms' tumor: a report from the National Wilms' Tumor Study Group. J Clin Oncol 2002;20:2506–13.
235. Olsson H, Brandt L. Sex ratio in offspring of patients with non-Hodgkin's lymphoma. N Engl J Med 1982;306:367–8.
236. Li FP, Gimbrere K, Gelber RD, et al. Outcome of pregnancy in survivors of Wilms' tumor. JAMA 1987;257:216–9.
237. Holmes GE, Holmes FF. Pregnancy outcome of patients treated for Hodgkin's disease. Cancer 1978;41:1317–22.
238. Kalapurakal JA, Peterson S, Peabody EM, et al. Pregnancy outcomes after abdominal irradiation that included or excluded the pelvis in childhood Wilms tumors survivors: a report from the National Wilms Tumor Study. Int J Radiat Oncol Biol Phys 2004;58:1364–8.
239. Mulvihill JJ, Myers MH, Connelly RR, et al. Cancer in offspring of long-term survivors of childhood and adolescent cancer. Lancet 1987;2:813–7.
240. Hawkins MM, Draper GJ, Winter DL. Cancer in the offspring of survivors of childhood leukaemia and non-Hodgkin's lymphomas. Br J Cancer 1995;71:1335–9.
241. Schell MJ, McHaney VA, Green AA, et al. Hearing loss in children and young adults receiving cisplatin with or without prior cranial irradiation. J Clin Oncol 1989;7:754–60.
242. lveskoski I, Saarinen UM, Wiklund T, et al. Ototoxicity in children with malignant brain tumors treated with the "8 in 1" chemotherapy protocol. Med Pediatr Oncol 1996;27:26–31.
243. Landier W. Hearing loss related to ototoxicity in children with cancer. J Pediatr Oncol Nurs 1998;15:195–206.
244. Soysal T, Bavunoglu I, Baslar Z, Aktuglu G. Cataract after prolonged busulfan therapy. Acta Haematol 1993;90:213.
245. Abramson DH, Servodidio CA. Ocular complications due to cancer treatment. In: Schwartz CL, Hobbie WL, Constine LS, Ruccione KS, editors. Survivors of childhood cancer: assessment and management. St. Louis: Mosby; 1994. p. 111–31.
246. Heaston DK, Libshitz HI, Chan RC. Skeletal effects of megavoltage irradiation in survivors of Wilms tumor. AJR Am J Roentgenol 1979;113:389–95.
247. Larson DL, Kroll S, Jaffe N, et al. Long-term effects of radiotherapy in childhood and adolescence. Am J Surg 1990;160:348–51.
248. Aisenberg J, Hsieh K, Kalaitzoglou G, et al. Bone mineral density in young adult survivors of childhood cancer. J Pediatr Hematol Oncol 1998;20:241–5.
249. Arikoski P, Voutilainen R, Kroger H. Bone mineral density in long-term survivors of childhood cancer. J Pediatr Endocrinol Metab 2003;16:343–53.
250. Kaste SC, Jones-Wallace D, Rose SR, et al. Bone mineral decrements in survivors of childhood acute lymphoblastic leukemia: frequency of occurrence and risk factors for their development. Leukemia 2001;15:728–34.
251. van der Suis IM, Keizer-Schrama S, van den Heuvel-Eibrink MM. Bone mineral density in childhood acute lymphoblastic leukemia during and after treatment. Pediatr Blood Cancer 2004;43:182–3.
252. Gilsanz V, Carlson ME, Roe TF, Ortega JA. Osteoporosis after cranial irradiation for acute lymphoblastic leukemia. J Pediatr 1990;117:238–44.
253. Tefft M, Lattin PB, Jereb B, et al. Acute and late effects on normal tissue following combined chemo- and radiotherapy for childhood rhabdomyosarcoma and Ewing's sarcoma. Cancer 1976;37:1201–17.
254. Nesbit M, Krivit W, Heyn R, et al. Acute and chronic effects of methotrexate on hepatic, biliary, and skeletal systems. Cancer 1976;37:1048–54.
255. Aisenberg J, Hsieh K, Kalaitzoglou G, et al. Bone mineral density in young adult adult survivors of childhood cancer. J Ped Hematol Oncol 1998;20:241–5.
256. Henderson RC, Madsen CD, Davis C, Gold SH. Bone density in survivors of childhood malignancies. J Pediat Hematol Oncol 1996;18:367–71.
257. Felix C, Blatt J, Goodman MA, Medina J. Avascular necrosis of bone following combination chemotherapy for acute lymphocytic leukemia. Med Pediatr Oncol 1985;13:269–72.
258. Halton JM, Wu B, Atkinson SA, et al. Comparative skeletal toxicity of dexamethasone and prednisone in childhood acute lymphoblastic leukemia [abstract]. J Pediatr Hematol Oncol 2000;22:369.
259. Mattano LA Jr, Sather HN, Trigg ME, Nachman JB. Osteonecrosis as a complication of treating acute lymphoblastic leukemia in children: a report from the Children's Cancer Group. J Clin Oncol 2000;18:3262–72.
260. Jaffe N, Toth BB, Hoar RE, et al. Dental and maxillofacial abnormalities in long term survivors of childhood cancer: effects of treatment with chemotherapy and radiation to the head and neck. Pediatrics 1984;73:816–23.
261. Sonis AL, Tarbell N, Valachovic RW, et al. Dentofacial development in long term survivors of acute lymphoblastic leukemia. Cancer 1990;66:2645–52.
262. Kaste SC, Hopkins KP, Jones D, et al. Dental abnormalities in children treated for acute lymphoblastic leukemia. Leukemia 1997;11:792–6.
263. Raney RB, Asmar L, Vassilopoulou-Sellin R, et al. Late complications of therapy in 213 children with localized, nonorbital soft-tissue sarcoma of the head and neck: a descriptive report from the Intergroup Rhabdomyosarcoma studies (IRS)-II and -III. Med Pediatr Oncol 1999;33:362–71.
264. Dens F, Boute P, Otten J, et al. Dental caries, gingival health, and oral hygiene of long term survivors of paediatric malignant diseases. Arch Dis Child 1995;72:129–32.
265. Albritton K, Bleyer WA. The management of cancer in the older adolescent. Eur J Cancer 2003;39:2584–99.

124c

Childhood Acute Lymphoblastic Leukemia

Paul S. Gaynon, MD
Anne L. Angiolillo, MD
Janet L. Franklin, MD
Gregory H. Reaman, MD

Acute lymphoblastic leukemia (ALL) is the most common malignancy in children, with a yearly incidence of 31 of 1,000,000 children younger than 15 years of age (Table 124c-1).[1,2] Children may present with signs and symptoms of leukemic proliferation, such as bone pain and/or marrow replacement, anemia, and thrombocytopenia. The peak incidence is between 3 and 6 years of age, with a male predominance, except for infants younger than 1 year of age, where girls predominate.

Diagnosis requires greater than 25% FAB L1 or L2 lymphoblasts in the marrow. About 85% of cases of childhood ALL express membrane markers consistent with B-precursor lineage, and about 15% express T-lineage markers. Flow cytometry excludes FAB M7 acute megakaryoblastic leukemia. Patients with lymphoid appearing, myeloperoxidase negative blasts expressing lymphoid-associated antigens, but co-expressing myeloid-associated membrane antigens are included as ALL. Patients with FAB L3 morphology and/or characteristic translocations are excluded. FAB M0 acute myeloblastic leukemia provides a rare diagnostic challenge. Flow cytometry may provide critical clues.[3] Over time, flow cytometry is increasing in importance, while histochemistry is diminishing.

Contemporary therapies include several components, namely, induction, presymptomatic central nervous system therapy, postinduction intensification, and maintenance, and may cure more than 80% of patients overall. Childhood ALL is unique among malignancies in the proven value of prolonged therapy for 2 to 3 years.[4]

Conventionally, children aged 1 to 9 years with presenting white blood counts (WBC) less than 50,000/μL are designated standard risk (SR). Children aged 1 to 9 years with presenting WBC ≥ 50,000/μL and adolescents age 10 years and older with any WBC are designated higher risk (HR).[5,6] The presence or absence of extramedullary leukemia, clonal cytogenetic or molecular abnormalities, and/or initial response to therapy may modify this initial designation. Patients with T-lineage disease are at greater risk of CNS relapse and/or early marrow relapse and lesser risk of later marrow relapse. T-lineage patients, at any age or WBC, may benefit from therapy employed for "HR" B-precursor patients.[7,8] In terms of morphology, immunophenotype, cytogenetics, molecular findings, initial response to therapy, and clinical outcome, childhood ALL is a heterogeneous disease. Gene expression microarrays have added appreciation of a new dimension of complexity. Differences in gene expression among cases of childhood ALL are said to exceed differences between lung adenocarcinoma or melanoma and bladder carcinoma.[9,10] Deeper understanding of the biology of ALL requires an integration of clinical, cellular, and molecular findings with the physiology and evolution of the malignant cell. Host factors—adherence to therapy, pharmacokinetics, pharmacodynamics, and target sensitivity—add additional layers of complexity. Pharmacogenomics[11] may provide new insights into disease relapse and treatment complications such as avascular necrosis of bone.

Gains in outcome in childhood ALL equal or surpass gains in other areas of childhood cancer. Since 1978, researchers have obtained major advances in childhood ALL. Gains have been realized for both HR and SR and both B-precursor and T-lineage patients[12–22] (Table 124c-2). The gains continue and are similar to the best obtained in other areas of childhood cancer.[23–26]

Strategies such as postinduction intensification, which were successful at one level (eg, delayed intensification or Protocol II) have been successfully employed at higher levels (eg, double delayed intensification or the augmented intensive regimen). Strategies successful in one patient population have been extended to other populations with similar success. Others have achieved similar success with other postinduction intensification strategies.[27–31]

A number of lessons have emerged from this experience. Several of these have already found confirmation:

- Substitution of dexamethasone for prednisone improves outcome for SR and HR patients.
- Initial response to therapy—whether determined by Day 8/15 marrow morphology or by PCR or flow cytometry assessment of minimal residual disease (MRD)—is an important predictor of outcome.
- Postinduction intensification (PII) improves outcome for both higher and standard risk, B-precursor and T-lineage patients.
- Longer and stronger PII "rescues" many HR patients with a poor day 8 response and many SR patients with a poor day 15 response.
- Improved systemic therapy allows elimination of cranial irradiation for most patients.
- Outcomes remain poor after marrow relapse, especially after early marrow relapse (first remission [CR1] < 36 months).

HETEROGENEITY

Many have described the considerable heterogeneity among children with ALL. Despite similar age and WBC, outcomes differ among and within ethnic, cytogenetic/molecular, and Day 8/15 response subsets.[31–35] High hyperdiploidy with trisomy 10 or 18, or triple trisomy 4, 10, and 17 describe overlapping patient subsets with an excellent outcome.[36–39] The occult translocation, t(12;21) also carries a good prognosis, though patients are subject to late relapse.[40,41] Some late relapses have been shown to be "second" leukemia rather than leukemic relapses.[42] Outcomes after such relapses are better than average. Cells with t(12;21) have been found in the cord blood of infants who later developed ALL.[43]

Table 124c-1 Incidence of Childhood Cancer Diagnoses in the United States[1,2,6]

Diagnosis	Number in U.S. per Year, Age < 15 Years	Incidence in U.S. per Million, Age < 15 Years
ALL	2,484	30.9
Brain tumors	2,205	27.6
Neuroblastoma	754	9.7
Non-Hodgkin's lymphoma	666	8.4
Wilms' tumor	638	8.3
Treatment failure in ALL	617	7.7
Hodgkin's disease	511	6.6
AML	454	5.6
Rhabdomyosarcoma	354	4.5
Retinoblastoma	309	3.9

Table 124c-2 Improved Outcome for Children with ALL

Population Trial (Reference)	*n*	Intervention 5-Year EFS	% Change in Rate of Failure
Lower Risk		± V/P pulses	36
CCG-161[16]	631	77% vs 64%	
Average Risk		± DI	41
CCG-105[20]	625	77% vs 61%	
Higher Risk		BFM vs CCG standard	38
CCG-106[17,18]	545	63% vs 40%	
Higher Risk		BFM vs LSA2L2	33
CCG-123[19]	694	67% vs 53%	
Lower Risk		± DI	62
BFM '83	199	82% vs 61%	
Lower Risk		± DI	29
CCG-1881[21]	700	85% vs 79%	
Average Risk		DI × 2 vs DI × 1	30
CCG-1891[22]	802	84% vs 77%	
Higher Risk		augmented vs standard intensification	44
CCG-1882/SER[23]	310	75% vs 55%	
Standard Risk		Dex vs Prednisone	40
CCG-1922[24]	1,060	88% vs 80%	
Higher Risk		stronger intensification	37
CCG-1961/RER[25]	1,293	81% vs 70%	
All risk groups		Dex vs Prednisolone	33
MRC (UK) ALL97[26]	1,693	84% vs 76%	

BFM = Berlin-Frankfurt-Munster Group; CCG = Children's Cancer Study Group; Dex = dexamethasone; DI = delayed intensification (Protocol II); LSA2L2 = "lymphosarcoma-2 leukemia-2" regimen; NY I = "New York I" regimen; RER = rapid early response; SER = slow early (Day 7) responder; V/P = vincristine prednisone pulses.

Excellent outcomes in specific subsets have been ascribed to increased sensitivity to glucocorticosteroids or to asparaginase in in vitro cytotoxicity assays,[44,45] or to increased accumulation of methotrexate polyglutamates.[46,47] Neither the methylthiazol-tetrazolium (MTT) assay nor methotrexate polyglutamate accumulation explains the occasional treatment failure in the generally favorable subsets, however.

Philadelphia chromosome positive ALL t(9;22) and severe hypodiploidy (modal chromosome number < 45) carry an adverse prognosis.[48,49] Poor outcomes are also seen for patients with 11q23 rearrangements, especially infants and older patients with a slow initial response to therapy.[50]

Conventional cytogenetics alone does not reveal the full extent of chromosomal abnormalities. The common translocation t(12;21) is rarely identified without molecular studies.[40] The reverse transcriptase polymerase chain reaction (RT-PCR) may ascertain additional cases with translocations missed by conventional cytogenetics.[51] Molecular studies may identify abnormalities even when 20 normal metaphases are found on conventional cytogenetics.[52]

Just as age, WBC, and immunophenotype fail to define homogeneous patient populations, so do single cytogenetic or molecular findings.[53–56] Leukemia is the end result of a number of genetic and/or epigenetic changes. Occult point mutations may be as important as additions or deletions of entire chromosomes. Underlying host factors may modify the clinical phenotype. With a bit of perspective, the quaint notion that a case might be defined completely by the single, most visually obvious chromosomal abnormality seems naïve.

The heterogeneity of childhood ALL is reflected in emerging gene-expression microarray data. Expression of more than 10,000 genes may be assessed simultaneously with complementary DNA (cDNA) microarrays.[57] Gene expression may be assessed at baseline, either at presentation or after relapse, and changes in gene expression may be assessed in the first hours after treatment. Specific expression patterns characterize immunophenotypic and cytogenetic subtypes. Holleman and colleagues identified 124 genes in B-lineage ALL where altered expression was associated with in vitro resistance, specifically to vincristine (40 genes), prednisolone (33 genes), L-asparaginase (35 genes), or daunomycin (20 genes), and a combined resistance score predictive of relapse in multivariate analyses.[58,59]

Unlike most other malignancies occurring in children and adults, a majority of cases of ALL occur in children and adolescents. Adult ALL is more likely to exhibit FAB L2 morphology,[60] in vitro steroid resistance,[61,62] and the Philadelphia chromosome or *bcr-abl*.[63] Perhaps 30% of adults with ALL have t(9;22) compared with about 3% of children.[64] Adult ALL is less likely to exhibit the favorable trisomy of chromosomes 10[65] or t(12;21).[66] Among adults, T-lineage is a favorable prognostic factor—largely excluding cases with Philadelphia chromosome.[67] Adult patients seem more tolerant of anthracyclines and less tolerant of vincristine and L-asparaginase than children. The value of anthracycline is more obvious in adults[68] than in children[18,69] among patients who also receive asparaginase.

Stock and colleagues compared the outcome of adolescents, age 16 to 21 years, with ALL treated on either Cancer and Leukemia Group B (CALGB) or the Children's Cancer Group (CCG) protocols. One hundred three patients treated on adult protocols achieved a 6-year event-free survival (EFS) of 38%, similar to that obtained for young adults aged 21 to 29 years on CALGB protocols; however, 196 patients treated on pediatric protocols achieved a 6-year EFS of 64%.[70] Findings from the French and Dutch groups are similar.[71–72] Adolescents and young adults achieve better outcomes when treated on pediatric protocols at pediatric centers. However, treatment mortality comprises a larger percentage of adverse events than in younger children.[73]

With better outcomes, avascular necrosis (AVN) of bone has emerged as a significant complication in adolescents and young adults.[74,75] AVN is usually multifocal and affects weight-bearing bone. It may be debilitating and require surgical joint replacement. The recent CCG-1961 study decreased the use of dexamethasone in intensification from 3 weeks to 7 days on, 7 days off, and 7 days on and halved the incidence of AVN to 8% in older patients.[76]

INDUCTION

Induction therapy invariably includes vincristine and a glucocorticoid. Attempts to defer these agents to the second month of therapy and substitute agents active in relapsed patients were unsuccessful.[77] Induction always contains a third agent, usually asparaginase, but sometimes an anthracycline. Induction often includes four agents, namely, vincristine, a glucocorticoid; asparaginase; and an anthracycline, and may include a fifth—usually cyclophosphamide. Addition of daunomycin to a vincristine, prednisone, and asparaginase induction was unhelpful for standard-risk patients[14] or overall.[69] However, four or more agents are usually employed for higher-risk patients.

Based on observations that dexamethasone impeded egress of granulocytes from the circulation less completely than prednisone, the CALGB compared dexamethasone and prednisone in childhood ALL between 1971 and 1977 with the hope that dexamethasone would be less immunosuppressive. They found that dexamethasone resulted in fewer central nervous system (CNS) relapses, but overall EFS was similar for dexamethasone and prednisone.[78]

Balis and colleagues showed that dexamethasone provided higher relative cerebrospinal fluid (CSF) levels than prednisone.[79] The Dutch Group found that in vitro sensitivity to glucocorticoid is an important predictor of outcome[80] and that dexamethasone was 16-fold more potent than prednisolone in vitro.[81] On the other hand, Ito and colleagues suggested that the cytotoxicity of dexamethasone and prednisone were more in keeping with the conventional 1:6 to 7 activity ratio.[82] The Dutch Group changed to dexamethasone with the Dutch ALL VI study with promising results relative to historical controls.[83]

Between 1992 and 1995, CCG conducted a randomized comparison of prednisone and dexamethasone in about 1,000 SR patients receiving a three-drug induction with no anthracycline. Patients received either prednisone 40 mg/m^2 or dexamethasone 6 mg/m^2 in induction and maintenance. All patients received dexamethasone in delayed intensification (DI). At 5-years, the EFS for dexamethasone was 87% versus 81% for prednisone, $p < .01$.[24] About one-half of the benefit was in CNS relapse and one-half in marrow relapse. Dexamethasone provided a 36% reduction in hazard. A previous study had found no benefit for higher-dose prednisone 60 mg/m^2 with daunomycin, cyclophosphamide, and cytosine arabinoside versus prednisone 40 mg/m^2 in SR patients.[14] A subsequent, even larger study by the Medical Research Council of the United Kingdom (MRC) found a similar advantage for dexamethasone in both standard- and higher-risk patients receiving induction anthracycline.[22] A smaller Japanese study obtained similar excellent outcomes with either prednisone and dexamethasone in about 400 patients.[84] Several attempts to employ dexamethasone in an anthracycline-containing induction regimen encountered problems with excessive toxicity.[85,86]

MORPHOLOGICAL RESPONSE AND OUTCOME

Failure to achieve remission, that is, fewer than 5% blasts by day 29 of induction, remains a consistent adverse prognostic factor. On the CCG 1988 to 1995 series trials, 1.6% of children survived induction with an M2 marrow (between 5 and 24% blasts) and 1.0% of children survived induction with an M3 marrow (more than 25% marrow blasts). M2 patients have 5-year EFS of 50%. Of M3 patients, one-third never achieve remission and have a dismal outcome and two-thirds ultimately achieve remission and have a 5-year EFS of 40%.[87] The vast majority of relapses still occur among patients with a good morphologic marrow response at the end of induction.

Day 8 and 15 marrow response continues to identify groups with disparate treatment outcomes[88–92] (Table 124c-3). However, the day 15 response is relatively insensitive and "captures" no more than 12 to 27% of events on three recent CCG studies. Among an SR population with an 85% EFS, if 20% of events are found among the 10% of patients with a poor response on day 15, then the EFS for the better and worse response subsets are about 87% and 70%, respectively. The day 8 response data on four recent CCG studies are fairly consistent and somewhat more sensitive but less specific. The poor response group captures about 60% of events, but is relatively nonspecific with a relative hazard less than 2. In an SR population with an 85% EFS, if 60% of events are found among the 50% of patients with a poor response on day 8, then the EFS for the better and worse response subsets are about 88% and 82%, respectively.

CCG and now the Children's Oncology Group employs early marrow response to allocate therapy. On a past HR trial, Nachman and colleagues showed that many patients with more than 25% marrow blasts on day 8 might be rescued with the augmented regimen.[19] On the 1995 to 1999 SR CCG trial, patients with more than 25% marrow blasts on day 15 were allocated to the augmented intensive regimen. Benefit has now been demonstrated.[93] Rescue has now been extended to all patients who are M3 on day 8 and M2 or M3 on day 15. The Berlin-Frankfurt-Munster (BFM) Group has similarly employed the peripheral blood response after one dose of methotrexate and 1 week of prednisone for treatment allocation.[94] Successful rescue of slow-response patients improves their outcome and abrogates the prognostic significance of delayed early response. Conversely, less morbid therapy may be adequate for rapid response patients. Data in one study suggest that SR patients with a rapid day 8 response obtain a similarly excellent outcome with less extensive postinduction intensification, that is, one delayed intensification (DI) phase. Slower response patients in general, however, benefited from more extensive postinduction intensification, that is, two delayed intensification phases.[16]

Table 124c-3 "Early" Marrow Response

Study/Risk	Percent M2 or M3 (%)	Percent of Total Events in Poor Response Subset (%)	Relative Hazard
CCG-105/AR Day 14 marrow	117/1,320 (9)	12	1.6
CCG-123/HR Day 14 marrow	30/205 (15)	27	2.8
CCG-1881/LR Day 14 marrow	64/711 (9)	18	2.5
CCG-123/HR Day 7 marrow	86/220 (39)	58	2.7
CCG-1891/AR Day 7 marrow	525/1,074 (49)	60	1.7
CCG-1922/SR Day 7 marrow	458/977 (47)	61	1.8

From Gaynon PS et al.[92]

The value of measures of response is limited by the quality of marrow samples and by the ability to identify residual leukemia. A dilute specimen may not be representative of marrow disease. Schultz and colleagues found substantial differences between estimates of marrow blast percentage based on marrow aspirates and biopsies.[95] The burden of leukemia in a single marrow aspirate may not be representative because leukemia may be anatomically heterogeneous.[96]

Precise identification of marrow blasts on day 8 or 15 by light microscopy may be difficult. Thomson and colleagues found 3 of 15 marrows on day 8 had fewer than 5% marrow blasts by microscopy, but more than 25% marrow blasts by flow cytometry.[97]

MINIMAL RESIDUAL DISEASE

Laboratory assays may allow more accurate assessment of early response. Conventional light microscopy has allowed classification of marrow responses in three categories: M1 (< 5% blasts), M2 (5–25% blasts), and M3 (> 25% blasts). Detection of leukemic blasts below the conventional level for remission or 5% may still have clinical significance. Sandlund and colleagues have identified patients with < 1% and 1 to 4% marrow lymphoblasts on day 15 and 22 to 25 by light microscopy and shown divergent outcomes[98] when provided similar therapy. In fact, patients in complete remission by conventional microscopy may harbor up to 10^{10} leukemic blasts.[99]

Residual leukemia at levels too low for detection by conventional microscopy has been termed minimal residual disease (MRD).[99,100] Candidate measures of MRD include multidimensional flow cytometry,[101,102] PCR amplification of immunoglobulin heavy chain (IgH), and/or T-cell receptor (TCR) gene rearrangements,[103–106] and RT-PCR amplification of specific fusion transcripts.[107] These strategies may provide an opportunity to identify rapid and slow responders more precisely and better allocate treatment.

Multiparameter flow cytometry can identify a leukemia-specific or leukemia-associated immunophenotype in a substantial proportion of cases. Two-marker flow cytometry can identify a leukemia specific pattern in 35% of cases.[108] Three-marker flow cytometry can identify a leukemia-specific pattern in 90% of cases,[109] and four-marker flow cytometry in > 95% of cases.[110] Quantification of the percentage of cells bearing the leukemia-specific immunophenotype allows an assessment of disease burden at the level of 1 cell in 10^4.

Coustan-Smith and colleagues have demonstrated prognostic significance for MRD assessed by multidimensional flow cytometry (Table 124c-4); flow cytometry identified a poor response group including about 25% of patients with about 50% of events.[101] Specificity and sensitivity appear better than early marrow response. Dworzak and colleagues analyzed 329 bone marrow samples from 108 children with ALL at four treatment time points. They found that the presence of distinct levels of MRD correlated with high probability of early relapse at each of the time points studied. Day 33 and week 12 were the most predictive of outcome, independent of clinical risk groups.[111] The Children's Oncology Group (COG), successor to the Pediatric Oncology Group (POG) and CCG, now employs day 15 marrow morphology (marrow blasts < 5%) *and* day 29 MRD by flow cytometry (blasts < 10^{-3}) to define a rapid early response.

PCR can be used to identify clonotypic IgH gene or TCR gene rearrangements in a substantial proportion of cases. IgH gene undergoes rear-

Table 124c-4 End Induction Disease Burden

Report Method (Reference)	Positive at End Induction (%)	Events in Positive Subset (%)	Relative Hazard
Coustan-Smith, et al, flow cytometry[101]	30/128 (23)	49	3.1
Goulden, et al, PCR[105]	38/66 (58)	82	3.4
Cave, et al, PCR[106]	63/151 (42)	78	5.7
Van Dongen, et al, PCR[103]	98/169 (58)	95	14.5

PCR = polymerase chain reaction.

rangement in 95% of cases of B-lineage ALL. TCR gene undergoes rearrangement in 95% of cases of T-lineage ALL and greater than 50% of cases of B-lineage ALL. Reaction product may be quantified by dot blot,[112] limit dilution,[113,114] competitive,[115] or real-time assays[116,117] in order to provide an estimate of leukemic burden on the order 10^{-3} to 10^{-4}.

Goulden and colleagues,[105] Cave and colleagues,[106] and van Dongen and colleagues[103] have demonstrated prognostic significance of MRD assessed by PCR (see Table 124c-4). About one-half of patients are found to have a poor response with end-induction leukemic levels between 10^{-3} and 10^{-2} and an increased likelihood of relapse.[100] The poor response group includes about 80% of events. Significance is not restricted to the initial stages of therapy; 5 of the 6 patients who relapsed in the van Dongen study after maintenance had persistently detectable MRD at the end of their maintenance therapy.[103] Specificity and sensitivity again appear better than early marrow response.

MRD may also be employed to assess the efficacy of treatment. Roberts and colleagues found that more recent patients who had received postinduction intensification had disease burden one log less than earlier patients who had not received intensification.[118] Zur Stadt and colleagues treated 73 patients with a three-drug (vincristine, prednisone, and daunomycin) induction and found end-induction MRD at 10^{-2} in 33% and at 10^{-3} in 33%;[119] van Dongen and colleagues employed a four-drug (vincristine, prednisone, daunomycin, and L-asparaginase) induction and found 16% at 10^{-2} and 22% at 10^{-3}.[103] MRD determinations, like assessment of early marrow response, depend on the quality of marrow samples. The number of cells or amount of DNA studied limits sensitivity. Marrow disease may be present in the absence of peripheral blood disease.[100] Sykes and colleagues found levels fourfold higher in marrow trephine material than in aspirate material.[120] The variation was higher at lower levels of disease. As with early marrow response, blasts must be identified. Identified cells may share a clonotypic feature but may be nonleukemogenic. Both detailed immunophenotype and TCR/immunoglobulin gene rearrangements are subject to oligoclonality and drift.[99,121–123] Both may change between diagnosis and relapse. Van Wering and colleagues found changes in immunophenotype between diagnosis and relapse in 29 of 40 cases studied.[124] Beishuizen and colleagues found changes in Ig or TCR gene rearrangements at diagnosis and relapse in 25 of 40 studied cases.[125] Either could lead to an inaccurate assessment of disease burden.

Thorough evaluation may improve the odds, however. In cases with oligoclonal immunoglobulin gene rearrangements, the variability of the DN-J junctional sequences is less than that of the VH-D sequences. When novel Ig or TCR gene rearrangements appear at relapse, one rearrangement, present at initial diagnosis, will usually persist.[100] Definition of the leukemic clone by multiparameter flow cytometry can lessen the impact of immunophenotypic drift.[124] Variability occurs because neither detailed immunophenotype nor immunoglobulin nor TCR gene rearrangements are central to the cell proliferation and malignant process.

The clinical significance of response and MRD, however measured, may be confounded by the underlying heterogeneity of childhood leukemia. The significance of residual E2A PBX1 fusion transcript positive cells may differ from the significance of residual BCR-ABL fusion transcript positive cells.[107] Relapse may arise from a small, resistant subclone, completely hidden at diagnosis among a more sensitive majority population.[126] However, laboratory assessment of end-induction disease burden may offer an opportunity to distinguish more precisely patients for whom current therapies are adequate or even excessive from patients who require innovative treatment strategies and to compare treatment strategies. The best time and technique with which to assess MRD are not yet clear. Better assessment of response may allow more precise treatment allocation.[18]

POSTINDUCTION INTENSIFICATION

In 1976, the BFM Group added Protocol II or delayed intensification (DI) to the intensive induction/consolidation (Protocol I) that they had introduced in 1970.[127] Two subsequent CCG trials for higher-risk patients showed the superiority of this approach—Protocol I and Protocol II—over then current CCG strategies.[17–19,91]

CCG also showed that DI improved EFS for average-risk patients.[18] However, administration of Protocol I provided no additional benefit for Rome/National Cancer Institute (NCI) SR patients who also received DI. Protocol I appeared to benefit eligible patients older than 10 years, all of whom presented with WBC < 50,000/µL. The value of Protocol I has not been tested rigorously for Rome/NCI HR patients.

CCG built on these results and then showed that DI alone also improved outcome for the subset of patients believed at lowest risk of relapse as defined by age, WBC, and early marrow response.[19] However, the impact of DI in the CCG study, 85% versus 79% (see Table 124c-2), was less than in the BFM-83 trial where addition of Protocol II increased EFS from 61 to 82%. Unlike BFM '83,[128] the CCG trial employed no induction anthracycline and no Protocol Ib (cyclophosphamide and cytarabine). On the other hand, CCG employed maintenance intrathecal methotrexate and vincristine/ prednisone pulses.[12] These two interventions may have improved the outcome of the no-DI arm, while adding nothing for patients who also received DI. Interventions that are useful individually may be redundant in combination, in whole or in part. A current international BFM Group (I-BFM) trial is examining the role of vincristine/dexamethasone pulses when patients also receive Protocol II. CCG also showed that two courses of DI were superior to one course of DI for average-risk patients.[18] Four months of intensive therapy were better than 2 months. However, outcomes with dexamethasone in induction and one DI phase were as good as outcomes with prednisone in induction and two DI phases.

The augmented intensive regimen provides longer and stronger postinduction intensification. Patients receive 10 pulses of Capizzi I,[129] namely, sequential vincristine, escalating-dose intravenous methotrexate (with no rescue), and L-asparaginase, two DI phases, and additional vincristine and asparaginase. The duration of intensification is 10 months instead of 4 months. Nachman and colleagues showed that HR patients with a poor marrow response on day 8 of therapy might be "rescued" with longer and stronger postinduction intensification.[19,130] The DFS at 5 years was 75% for augmented versus 55% for standard postinduction intensification. Treatments diverged fully 5 weeks after the day 8 response determination.

Seibel and colleagues recently reported a test of longer and stronger postinduction intensification in higher-risk patients with a rapid day 8 response. Almost 1,300 patients were randomized. Stronger postinduction intensification increased the 5-year EFS from 70 to 81%, although longer postinduction intensification provided no benefit. Ten or 6 months of intensification was no better than 7 or 4 months. B-precursor and T-lineage patients, children, adolescents, and young adults all showed benefit. An intervention shown useful in one patient subset, slow early responders, was shown beneficial in another, rapid early responders. More was not better, however.[8,25,73]

PARENTERAL METHOTREXATE AND RESCUE

Parenteral methotrexate and rescue provide an alternative postinduction intensification approach. Pursuant of earlier studies in CALGB,[131–133] both Pediatric Oncology Group (POG) and St. Jude investigators employ a postinduction intensification "backbone" of intermediate-dose methotrexate with rescue (IDM).[134–137] BFM family regimens include IDM in an "M" phase between Protocol I and Protocol II.[138]

Unambiguous demonstration of the contribution of IDM to postinduction intensification has been lacking, however. St. Jude Study Total X showed an advantage for a complex regimen including IDM relative to a second complex regimen excluding IDM.[134,135] Two CCG trials examined the role of IDM for SR patients and found no advantage for either methotrexate 0.5 g/m^2 [139] or for 33.6 g/m^2 [140] over conventional oral methotrexate. More recently, UKALL XI found no advantage for methotrexate 6 to 8 g/m^2,[141] and FRALLE 93 found no EFS advantage for methotrexate 8 g/m^2 [142] for intermediate-risk patients.

CCG has achieved good outcomes with no IDM and avoided significant neurotoxicity and additional hospital stays. The dexamethasone/oral 6-MP arm of CCG-1922 provided an 87% 5-year EFS for Rome/NCI standard-risk patients with no IDM.[24] Omission of IDM accounts for a 25-day-per-patient advantage in median hospital stay versus a contemporary IDM regimen.[143] IDM was implicated in a 10 to 16% incidence of CNS toxicity in three recent trials.[136,144,145] The ultimate neurocognitive consequences of these studies have not yet been reported. Neurotoxicity may be prevented with less frequent IDM and earlier or more generous rescue. However, earlier and more generous use of leucovorin may diminish any therapeutic benefit.[146]

Much remains to be learned about methotrexate. Although Chessells and colleagues found no advantage for intramuscular over oral methotrexate in maintenance,[147] two randomized trials show an advantage for intravenous versus oral methotrexate.[148,149] Long-term follow-up on a study comparing whole brain irradiation with additional intrathecal methotrexate found the early excess of CNS relapses on the methotrexate arm more than balanced by an eventual excess of marrow relapse on the radiation arm.[150] Additional vincristine, methotrexate, and asparaginase rescues standard-risk patients with a slow day 15 response in the context of double delayed intensification.[91]

PRESYMPTOMATIC CENTRAL NERVOUS SYSTEM THERAPY

Effective presymptomatic central nervous system therapy, pioneered by Pinkel and colleagues at St. Jude Children's Research Hospital, is prerequisite to all subsequent advances in the treatment of childhood ALL.[151,152] Nesbit and colleagues showed that 24 Gy craniospinal irradiation might be replaced with 24 Gy cranial radiation and 6 doses of intrathecal methotrexate,[153] and that 24 Gy cranial irradiation might be safely replaced with 18 Gy.[154] Bleyer and colleagues devised a widely adopted age-based dosage schedule for intrathecal methotrexate.[155]

Elimination of cranial irradiation has been a priority for more than two decades. Cranial irradiation has been linked to second malignancies[156,157] and neurocognitive damage.[158–160] Lesser problems are seen in patients who received no cranial irradiation.[161] However, other elements of therapy may also be neurotoxic. IDM was implicated in a 10 to 16% incidence of CNS toxicity in three recent trials.[111,118,119] Questions have been raised about dexamethasone.[162] The ultimate neurocognitive consequences of these studies have not yet been reported.

Improved systemic therapy has allowed elimination of cranial irradiation for most patients. Freeman and colleagues showed that cranial irradiation might be replaced safely with IDM.[131–133] CCG showed that cranial irradiation might be replaced with maintenance intrathecal methotrexate in the lowest-risk patients by age and WBC.[14] Then CCG showed that cranial irradiation might be replaced with maintenance intrathecal methotrexate in average-risk patients, providing that patients received either intensive induction/consolidation (BFM Protocol I) or DI (BFM Protocol II).[163] Finally, CCG showed that cranial irradiation might be replaced with additional intrathecal methotrexate in higher-risk patients with a rapid initial response to therapy in the context of BFM-based systemic therapy.[150] The Children's Oncology Group now limits cranial irradiation to patients with overt CNS leukemia at diagnosis, patients with T-lineage disease and HR features, and patients with B-precursor disease, higher-risk features, and a slow initial response to therapy, about 25% of patients in all. Contrary to the experience of some,[164] CCG studies found that neither overt nor occult CNS disease at diagnosis adversely impacts on prognosis.[165–167]

Current intrathecal therapy on some United States regimens may be excessive for some subsets of patients in the context of today's effective systemic therapy. Children on COG trials receive more than 20 doses of intrathecal therapy over the course of treatment. Children on BFM trials receive only 11 doses of intrathecal therapy over the first 6 months of treatment and no subsequent maintenance intrathecal treatment.[138]

BONE MARROW TRANSPLANTATION IN FIRST REMISSION

Marrow ablative therapy and stem cell rescue or, more simply, BMT, has been advocated as a compelling strategy for postinduction intensification of children with ALL and very high risk features in first complete remission (CR1). Waiting time bias, selection bias, and variability in the details of prior chemotherapy, in marrow ablative therapy, and in graft-versus-host disease prophylaxis have confounded rigorous evaluation. Outcome after BMT begins with BMT and does not include the experience of patients who never achieved remission or relapsed before a BMT could be performed. Patients with severe organ dysfunction or deep-seated infection may be refused BMT, and thus, never appear in BMT statistics.

The European Bone Marrow Transplant Registry has reported the preliminary results of an international retrospective trial.[168] Three hundred fifteen children were identified with ALL and very high risk features. Two hundred thirty-eight received chemotherapy only, 45 underwent BMT from matched related donors, 20 from matched unrelated donors, and 12 from other donors. The death rate for BMT ran 30%. After correction for time to transplant, the 2-year disease-free survival was 58% for transplant versus 53% for chemotherapy (not significant). A difference may still emerge with longer follow-up.

The Medical Research Council of the United Kingdom addressed the challenge in a prospective trial.[169] Four hundred seventy-three (13%) of 3,676 patients were designated very high risk on the basis of WBC > 100,000/μL, certain cytogenetic abnormalities, and/or a slow response to induction therapy. Four hundred fifty-two achieved remission. Two hundred eighty-six patients underwent tissue typing. Ninety-nine had a matched related donor. Of these, 76 patients received transplants in first remission. In addition, 25 of 187 patients with no matched related donor also underwent transplantation. The median time to transplant was 5 months and the median follow-up at the time of the report was 8 years. By treatment actually received the 10-year unadjusted EFS was similar at 45% for transplant patients versus 39% for chemotherapy patients. In the critical intent to treat analyses, the 10-year EFS was 40% for patients with a matched related donor versus 50% for patients with no matched related donor. Transplant mortality ran 18% versus 3% for chemotherapy. Relapses ran 55% for chemotherapy versus 31% for transplant.

The value of BMT may differ in different patient subsets. Arico and colleagues, summarizing the results from 10 groups worldwide, showed an important advantage for matched sibling donor BMT for children with Philadelphia chromosome-positive ALL. No advantage was shown for matched unrelated donor BMT.[48] Contrary to the poor result with matched unrelated donors in that overview, Marks and colleagues report a more positive experience.[170] No advantage for BMT was found for patients with 11q23 abnormalities in a similar overview.[50]

BMT is not a complete answer to the problem of very high risk ALL. Donor availability is not the primary constraint to the clinical utility of BMT. Although the clinical decision between BMT options and chemotherapy options is critical, any single study compares one BMT approach and one chemotherapy approach. Generalization to all BMT approaches and all chemotherapy approaches is perilous. Efforts should focus on improving chemotherapy and BMT outcomes rather than endless comparisons of the two strategies.

RELAPSE

Despite signal progress to date in the treatment of newly diagnosed ALL, relapsed ALL remains a major problem in pediatric oncology.[1,2] Numerically, more children have ALL and relapse than have new diagnoses of a number of relatively common childhood cancers (see Table 124c-1).

Outcome after relapse depends on the duration of first remission and the site of relapse. Table 124c-5 summarizes the experience of

Table 124c-5 Survival after Relapse on the CCG-100 Series

		n	*n* (%)	6-Year Freedom from 2nd Adverse Event (SD)
Isolated marrow		642		16% ± 2%
	Early		223 (36)	5% ± 2%
	Intermediate		194 (30)	10% ± 4%
	Late		215 (33)	33% ± 4%
Combined marrow		120		29% ± 4%
	Early		34 (28)	9% ± 5%
	Intermediate		26 (22)	11% ± 6%
	Late		60 (50)	48% ± 7%
Isolated CNS		220		37% ± 3%
	Early		102 (46)	24% ± 5%
	Intermediate		84 (38)	44% ± 5%
	Late		34 (17)	59% ± 9%
Isolated Testes		112		64% ± 5%
	Early		22 (20)	48% ± 11%
	Intermediate		24 (21)	44% ± 11%
	Late		66 (59)	76% ± 6%

Early = < 18 months; Intermediate = 19–36 months; Late = > 36 months.
From Gaynon P et al.[171]

patients with relapse who had been diagnosed between 1983 and 1988 and enrolled on the CCG-100 series trials.[171] Seventy percent of relapses involve the bone marrow.

Outcomes are particularly unfavorable for marrow relapse prior to 3 years from diagnosis and for isolated CNS relapse prior to 18 months. Outcomes are somewhat better for testicular relapse and for late marrow relapse. As first reported by the BFM Groups, outcomes are good for late combined marrow and extramedullary relapse and poor for T-cell disease after marrow relapse.[172] British data are similar.[173]

Matched sibling donor BMT has been proposed as the treatment of choice for children with bone marrow relapse. Retrospective studies support this assertion. For patients in second remission (CR2), Barrett and colleagues examined 255 matched pairs from the International Bone Marrow Transplant Registry and found a 5-year disease-free survival (DFS) of 40% for BMT versus 17% for a historical chemotherapy control.[174] Hoogerbrugge and colleagues compared 25 BMT patients with 97 matched controls and found DFS of 44% and 24%.[175] Uderzo and colleagues reported a DFS of 37% for 57 BMT patients and 22% for 230 matched chemotherapy patients.[176] Schroeder and colleagues reported a DFS of 35% for BMT versus 15% for chemotherapy in an analysis of 63 cases and 126 matched controls.[177] Boulad and colleagues reported 62% DFS for 37 BMT patients and 26% for 29 chemotherapy patients.[178] Adjusting for prognostic factors and allowing for waiting time bias, Wheeler and colleagues found 4-year DFS of 43% and 28% for BMT and chemotherapy, respectively (p = .05).[179] Some found a greater advantage for BMT for patients with earlier marrow relapse,[176,177,180] and others did not.[174,175] p-Values may vary with sample size as well as with the exact magnitude of the differences, but a trend seems clear.

Matched sibling donor BMT requires that patients achieve and maintain a remission and possess a matched sibling donor. If 80% of relapsed patients achieve CR2 and 80% of these maintain remission long enough to undergo BMT, then only 64% of patients with matched sibling donors may undergo BMT in CR2. A post–BMT-DFS of 40% corresponds to a postrelapse EFS (starting from relapse) of only 25%.

Most patients lack a matched sibling donor. Alternative stem cell sources such as matched unrelated donor (MUD) marrow or umbilical cord blood, haplo-identical related donors and purged autologous marrow have been proposed.[181,182] Neither Wheeler and colleagues nor Borgmann and colleagues found any advantage for purged autologous marrow BMT over chemotherapy.[179,183]

Interest in MUD BMT remains high. Results for MUD BMT are generally similar to those for matched sibling donor BMT.[184] However, the time from CR2 to transplant may be longer, introducing greater waiting time and a shrinking subset of CR2 patients, some of whom relapse or suffer major complications that preclude BMT while waiting for BMT. Balduzzi and colleagues report a 47% DFS for 15 patients transplanted in CR1 or CR2.[185] Oakhill and colleagues report a 2-year DFS of 53% for 50 patients transplanted in CR2 after T-cell depletion.[186] Davies and colleagues report a 20% 2-year DFS for 19 patients.[187] Whether the results of single centers can be replicated more widely remains to be demonstrated. Adequately controlled trials are lacking.

Retrospective and case-control analyses can compensate for waiting time bias, but selection bias may still confound comparisons. Comparison of BMT experience from the past 20 years to chemotherapy experience from the last several years may be misleading.[188]

Results from prospective trials are somewhat different. Harrison and colleagues studied 206 children in second remission with human leukocyte antigen typing.[189] Sixty-seven had a family donor and 64 underwent BMT. One hundred thirty-nine had no family donor, 40 underwent matched unrelated donor BMT, and 9 underwent autologous BMT. The 5-year EFS was 46% overall, 45% in the donor group and 45% in the no-donor group. Adjustment for time to and site of relapse yielded 45% in the donor group and 37% in the no-donor group. Adjustment for time to relapse, site of relapse, and waiting time yielded 45% in the BMT group and 40% in the chemotherapy group by treatment received. Gaynon and colleagues reported 123 children in second remission after an initial bone marrow relapse within 12 months of the completion of primary therapy.[190] Fifty-one had matched family donors. Forty underwent BMT in second remission and achieved a DFS of 40% from BMT. For the entire matched family donor subset, the 3-year DFS was 29% from the end of induction. Patients with no donors were randomized between chemotherapy and alternative donor BMT. The 3-year DFS was 28% for patients allocated to chemotherapy and 18% for patients allocated to alternative donor BMT. Ten of 35 patients allocated to chemotherapy received alternative donor BMT; 4 died of complications and 3 relapsed after BMT. Only 20 of 37 patients allocated to alternative donor BMT actually underwent BMT in CR2; 14 relapsed prior to any BMT. Retrospective studies with constructed controls may exaggerate any benefit of BMT. BMT is not a complete answer to the problem of marrow relapse any more than for very high risk ALL. Too many patients never achieve CR2. Too many patients who achieve CR2 relapse before a BMT can be performed. Too many patients die of BMT complications or relapse after BMT. Wheeler and colleagues report only 2 survivors among 16 BMTs in CR2 following an on-therapy marrow relapse.[179]

Prompt identification of a stem cell source for every patient who relapses will have minimal impact on outcome after relapse if the post–BMT-DFS is no better than 30%. Post-BMT interventions, such as minimization of graft-versus-host prophylaxis,[191] can have little benefit for the majority of patients who can never get as far as a BMT.

A recent CCG AML trial may point to a more useful strategy.[24] Intensively timed induction presumably led to lower disease burden and better outcome after allogeneic BMT, autologous BMT, or chemotherapy consolidation. Knechtli and colleagues showed that outcome after BMT is related to disease burden prior to BMT in ALL.[192]

Our challenge is the reduction of disease burden. Better asparagine depletion may lead to better response for patients in relapse after prior exposure to native *Escherichia coli* asparaginase. Kurtzberg and colleagues showed that the appearance of anti-asparaginase antibodies was associated with poor response to vincristine, prednisone, and asparaginase therapy in second relapse.[193] Abshire and colleagues found similarly that the appearance of anti-asparaginase antibodies was associated with poor response to vincristine, prednisone, asparaginase, and daunomycin therapy in first relapse.[194] The recent CCG trial also found that induction response was strongly linked to asparagine depletion in first relapse.[195] More effective asparaginase schedules might be employed or noncross-reactive products might be substituted to guarantee asparagine depletion.

Steroid resistance is a hallmark of relapsed ALL[196] and identification of ligands with activity against prednisolone-resistant blasts may make a major contribution to therapy. The MTT response to prednisolone is a reliable predictor of outcome.[80] Klumper and colleagues found that the median 50% lethal concentration (LC50) of prednisolone was 100-fold higher at relapse than at presentation, representing relapse of steroid-resistant patients rather than late emergence of prednisolone resistance.[196] Cortivazol, a pyrazolosteroid, induces apoptosis in several classes of prednisolone-resistant lymphoblasts.[197] Six of 10 multiply relapsed patients achieved complete or partial remission after treatment with single-agent cortivazol.[198]

The combination of monoclonal antibodies and cytotoxic chemotherapy has shown benefit in a number of adult malignancies and may hold promise for childhood ALL. Randomized trials showed benefit for rituximab in lymphoma and CLL,[199] trastuzumab in breast cancer,[200] and bevacizumab in colon cancer[201] and nonsmall cell lung cancer.[202] The combination of epratuzumab, and anti-CD22 monoclonal antibody,[203] and chemotherapy is under study in childhood ALL.

Many chemotherapeutic agents work through p53, including, for example, cyclophosphamide, etoposide, anthracyclines, ara-c, and methotrexate.[204] Utility against blasts with diminished p53 function may be limited. Loss of p53 function is common in ALL with primary resistance[205] or at relapse.[206,207] Vincristine, an antitubulin agent, asparaginase, and glucocorticoids may not require p53 function and may provide more benefit.[201,208] A past CCG trial showed that addition of vincristine, a p53-independent agent, to Capizzi I sequential methotrexate/asparaginase doubled the duration of CR2.[128] Other antitubulin agents are in development.

CONCLUSIONS

Treatment outcome depends on disease, host, and treatment factors. Treatment factors are paramount and may alter the clinical significance of disease and host factors. Disease factors include features apparent at diagnosis, features that may appear in response to therapy, and factors that become apparent only at relapse. Single, isolated cytogenetic or molecular findings no more define outcome than blast morphology or immunophenotype. Host factors refer to differences among patients with regard to drug absorption, metabolism, and sensitivity. Considerable heterogeneity has been described with respect to host pharmacology of thiopurines[209] and vincristine.[210,211] Population variability has been described with respect to sensitivity to glucocorticoids.[212,213] Disease factors at diagnosis will never completely define outcome.

Much has been accomplished but much still remains. We understand little about why our therapy so often succeeds and less about why it sometimes fails. Better treatment allocation through molecular ascertainment of common cytogenetic subsets and more precise assessment of response via laboratory assays can assure that fewer patients are overtreated and fewer patients denied needed therapy. Disease at relapse often retains sensitivity to conventional agents. More effective use of conventional agents up front might prevent emergence of relapse. Introduction of novel agents with activity against resistant blasts provides a strategy to treat relapse or to prevent the emergence of otherwise resistant disease that becomes apparent only at relapse. To date, BMT has not provided an adequate answer to the problem of very high risk disease or relapse. If disease burden can be reduced prior to BMT, however, BMT may be more useful. Better understanding of the biology of early and late marrow and extramedullary relapses may lead to new insights and new treatment strategies. Lessons learned in the treatment of childhood ALL might have value in the treatment of other cancers in other populations.

REFERENCES

1. Gurney JG, Severson RK, Davis S, Robison LL. Incidence of cancer in children in the United States. Sex-, race-, and 1-year age-specific rates by histologic type. Cancer 1995;75:2186–95.
2. Miller RW, Young JL Jr, Novakovic B. Childhood cancer. Cancer 1995;75:395–405.
3. Kaleem Z, Crawford E, Pathan MH, et al. Flow cytometric analysis of acute leukemia. Diagnostic utility and critical analysis of data. Arch Pathol Lab Med 2003;127:42–8.
4. Childhood ALL Cooperative Group. Duration and intensity of maintenance chemotherapy in acute lymphoblastic leukaemia: overview of 42 trials involving 12,000 randomised children. Lancet 1996;347:1783–8.
5. Mastrangelo R, Poplack D, Bleyer A, et al. Report and recommendations of the Rome workshop concerning poor-prognosis acute lymphoblastic leukemia in children: biologic bases for staging, stratification, and treatment. Med Pediatr Oncol 1986;14:191–4.
6. Smith M, Arthur D, Camitta B, et al. Uniform approach to risk classification and treatment assignment for children with acute lymphoblastic leukemia [comments]. J Clin Oncol 1996;14:18–24.
7. Matloub Y, Asselin BL, Stork LC, et al. Outcome of children with T-cell acute lymphoblastic leukemia (T-ALL) and standard risk (SR) features: results of CCG-1952, CCG-1991, and POG 9404 [abstract 680]. Blood 2004;104:195a.
8. Seibel NL, Asselin BL, Nachman JB, et al. Treatment of high risk T-cell acute lymphoblastic leukemia (T-ALL): comparison of recent experience of the Children's Cancer Group (CCG) and Pediatric Oncology Group (POG) [abstract 681]. Blood 2004;104:195a.
9. Yeoh EJ, Ross ME, Williams WK, et al. Classification, subtype discovery, and prediction of outcome in pediatric acute lymphoblastic leukemia by gene expression profiling. Cancer Cell 2002;1:133–43.
10. Fine BM, Stanulla M, Schrappe M, et al. Gene expression patterns associated with recurrent chromosomal translocations in acute lymphoblastic leukemia. Blood 2004;103:1043–9.
11. Evans WE, Relling MV. Moving towards individualized medicine with pharmacogenomics. Nature 2004;429:464–8.
12. Bleyer WA, Sather HN, Nickerson HJ, et al. Monthly pulses of vincristine and prednisone prevent bone marrow and testicular relapse in low-risk childhood acute lymphoblastic leukemia: a report of the CCG-161 study by the Children's Cancer Study Group. J Clin Oncol 1991;9:1012–21.
13. Gaynon PS, Steinherz PG, Bleyer WA, et al. Intensive therapy for children with acute lymphoblastic leukaemia and unfavourable presenting features. Early conclusions of study CCG-106 by the Children's Cancer Study Group. Lancet 1988;2:921–4.
14. Gaynon PS, Steinherz PG, Bleyer WA, et al. Improved therapy for children with acute lymphoblastic leukemia and unfavorable presenting features: a follow-up report of the Children's Cancer Group Study CCG-106. J Clin Oncol 1993;11:2234–42.
15. Steinherz P, Gaynon P, Breneman J, et al. Treatment of acute lymphoblastic leukemia with bulky extramedullary disease and T-cell phenotype or other poor prognostic features: randomized control trial from the Children's Cancer Group. Cancer 1998;82:600–12.
16. Tubergen D, Gilchrist G, O'Brien A, et al. Improved outcome with delayed intensification for children with acute lymphoblastic leukemia and intermediate presenting features. J Clin Oncol 1993;11:527–37.
17. Hutchinson R, Neerhout R, Bertolone S, et al. Should therapy be intensified for patients with good risk ALL? Blood 1996;88:668a.
18. Lange B, Bostrom B, Cherlow JM, et al. Double-delayed intensification improves event free survival for children with intermediate-risk acute lymphoblastic leukemia: a report from the Children's Cancer Group. Blood 2002;99:825–33.
19. Nachman JB, Sather HN, Sensel MG, et al. Augmented post-induction therapy for children with high-risk acute lymphoblastic leukemia and a slow response to initial therapy. N Engl J Med 1998;338:1663–71.
20. Bostrom BC, Sensel MR, Sather HN, et al. Dexamethasone versus prednisone and daily oral versus weekly intravenous 6-mercaptopurine for patients with standard-risk acute lymphoblastic leukemia: a report from the Children's Cancer Group. Blood 2003;101:3809–17.
21. Seibel NL, Steinherz P, Sather H, et al. Early intensification improves outcome in children and adolescents with acute lymphoblastic leukemia (ALL) presenting with unfavorable features who show a rapid early response to induction chemotherapy: a report of CCG-1961 [abstract 787]. Blood 2003;102:224a.
22. Mitchell CD, Richards SM, Kinsey SE, et al. Benefit of dexamethasone compared with prednisolone for childhood acute lymphoblastic leukaemia: results of the UK Medical Research Council ALL97 randomised trial. Br J Haematol 2005;129:734–45.
23. Link M, Goorin A, Miser A, et al. The effect of adjuvant chemotherapy on relapse-free survival in patients with osteosarcoma of the extremity. N Engl J Med 1986;314:1600–6.
24. Woods WG, Kobrinsky N, Buckley JD, et al. Timed-sequential induction therapy improves postremission outcome in acute myeloid leukemia: a report from the Children's Cancer Group. Blood 1996;87:4979–89.
25. Grier HE, Krailo MD, Tarbell NJ, et al. Addition of ifosfamide and etoposide to standard chemotherapy for Ewing's sarcoma and primitive neuroectodermal tumor of bone. N Engl J Med 2003;348:694–701.
26. Matthay KK, Villablanca JG, Seeger RC, et al. Treatment of high-risk neuroblastoma with intensive chemotherapy, radiotherapy, autologous bone marrow transplantation, and 13-cis-retinoic acid. Children's Cancer Group. N Engl J Med 1999;341:1165–73.
27. LeClerc JM, Billett AL, Gelber RD, et al. Treatment of childhood acute lymphoblastic leukemia: results of Dana-Farber ALL Consortium Protocol 87-01. J Clin Oncol 2002;20:237–46.
28. Silverman LB, Gelber RD, Dalton VK, et al. Improved outcome for children with acute lymphoblastic leukemia: results of the Dana-Farber Consortium protocol 91-01. Blood 2001;97:1211–8.
29. Evans WE, Relling MV, Rodman JH, et al. Conventional compared with individualized chemotherapy for childhood acute lymphoblastic leukemia. N Engl J Med 1998;338:499–505.
30. Pui CH, Mahmoud HH, Rivera GK, et al. Early intensification of intrathecal chemotherapy virtually eliminates central nervous system relapse in children with acute lymphoblastic leukemia. Blood 1998;92:411–5.
31. Pui CH, Sandlund JT, Pei D, et al. Improved outcome for children with acute lymphoblastic leukemia: results of Total Therapy Study XIIIB at St. Jude Children's Research Hospital. Blood 2004;104:2690–6.
32. Chessells JM, Swansbury GJ, Reeves B, et al. Cytogenetics and prognosis in childhood lymphoblastic leukaemia: results of MRC UKALL X. Medical Research Council Working Party in Childhood Leukaemia. Br J Haematol 1997;99:93–100.
33. Pui CH. Recent advances in the biology and treatment of childhood acute lymphoblastic leukemia. Curr Opin Hematol 1998;5:292–301.
34. Heerema NA, Sather HN, Sensel MG, et al. Frequency and clinical significance of cytogenetic abnormalities in pediatric T-lineage acute lymphoblastic leukemia: a report from the Children's Cancer Group. J Clin Oncol 1998;16:1270–8.
35. Jackson JF, Boyett J, Pullen J, et al. Favorable prognosis associated with hyperdiploidy in children with acute lymphocytic leukemia correlates with extra chromosome 6. A Pediatric Oncology Group study. Cancer 1990;66:1183–9.

36. Harris MB, Shuster JJ, Carroll A, et al. Trisomy of leukemic cell chromosomes 4 and 10 identifies children with B-progenitor cell acute lymphoblastic leukemia with a very low risk of treatment failure: a Pediatric Oncology Group study. Blood 1992;79:3316–24.
37. Heerema NA, Sather HN, Sensel MG, et al. Prognostic impact of trisomies of chromosomes 10, 17, and 5 among children with acute lymphoblastic leukemia and high hyperdiploidy (> 50 chromosomes). J Clin Oncol 2000;18:1876–87.
38. Suttcliffe MJ, Shuster JJ, Sather HN, et al. High concordance from independent studies by the Children's Cancer Group (CCG) and the Pediatric Oncology Group (COG) associating favorable prognosis with combined trisomies 4, 10, and 17 in children with NCI standard-risk, B-precursor acute lymphoblastic leukemia: a Children's Oncology Group (COG) initiative. Leukemia 2005;19:734–40.
39. Moorman MV, Richards SM, Martineau M, et al. Outcome heterogeneity in childhood high-hyperdiploid acute lymphoblastic leukemia. Blood 2003;102:2756–62.
40. Shurtleff SA, Buijs A, Behm FG, et al. TEL/AML1 fusion resulting from a cryptic t(12;21) is the most common genetic lesion in pediatric ALL and defines a subgroup of patients with an excellent prognosis. Leukemia 1995;9:1985–9.
41. Sawinska M. Ladon D. Mechanism, detection and clinical significance of the reciprocal translocation t(12;21)(p12:q22) in the children suffering from acute lymphoblastic leukemia. Leuk Research 2004;28:35–42.
42. Ford AM, Fasching K, Panzer-Grumayer ER, et al. Origins of "late" relapse in childhood acute lymphoblastic leukemia with TEL-AML1 fusion genes. Blood 2001;98:558–64.
43. Hjalgrim LL, Madsen Mo, Melbye M, et al. Presence of clone-specific markers at birth in children with acute lymphoblastic leukemia. Br J Cancer 2002;87:994–9.
44. Kasper GJ, Smets LA, Pieters R, et al. Favorable prognosis of hyperdiploid common acute lymphoblastic leukemia may be explained by sensitivity to antimetabolites and other drugs: results of an in vitro study. Blood 1995;85:751–6.
45. Stams WA, den Boer ML, Beverloo HB, et al. Sensitivity to L-asparaginase is not associated with expressin levels of asparagine synthetase in t(12;21)+ pediatric ALL. Blood 2003;101:2743–7.
46. Whitehead VM, Vuchich MJ, Lauer SJ, et al. Accumulation of high levels of methotrexate polyglutamates in lymphoblasts from children with hyperdiploid (greater than 50 chromosomes) B-lineage acute lymphoblastic leukemia: a Pediatric Oncology Group study. Blood 1992;80:1316–23.
47. Whitehead VM, Payment C, Cooley L, et al. The association of the TEL-AML1 chromosomal translocation with accumulation of methotrexate polyglutamates in lymphoblasts and with ploidy in childhood B-progenitor cell acute lymphoblastic leukemia: a Pediatric Oncology Group study. Leukemia 2001;15:1081–8.
48. Arico M, Valsecchi MG, Camitta B, et al. Outcome of treatment in children with Philadelphia chromosome-positive acute lymphoblastic leukemia. N Engl J Med 2000;342:998–1006.
49. Harrison CJ, Moorman AV, Broadfield ZJ, et al. Three distinct groups of hypodiploidy in acute lymphoblastic leukemia. Br J Haematol 2004;125;552–9.
50. Pui CH, Gaynon PS, Boyett JM, et al. Outcome of treatment in childhood acute lymphoblastic leukemia with rearrangements of the 11q23 chromosomal region. Lancet 2002;359;1909–15.
51. Gaynon PS, Crotty ML, Sather HN, et al. Expression of BCR-ABL, E2A-PBX1, and MLL-AF4 fusion transcripts in newly diagnosed children with acute lymphoblastic leukemia: a Children's Cancer Group initiative. Leuk Lymphoma 1997;26:57–65.
52. Wu SQ, Weinberg KI, Joo WJ, et al. Preponderant mitotic activity of nonleukemic cells plays an important role in failures to detect abnormal clone in childhood acute lymphoblastic leukemia. J Pediatr Hematol Oncol 2003;25:520–5.
53. Secker-Walker LM, Berger R, Fenaux P, et al. Prognostic significance of the balanced t(1;19) and unbalanced der(19)t(1;19) translocations in acute lymphoblastic leukemia. Leukemia 1992;6:363–9.
54. Ribeiro RC, Broniscer A, Rivera GK, et al. Philadelphia chromosome-positive acute lymphoblastic leukemia in children: durable responses to chemotherapy associated with low initial white blood cell counts. Leukemia 1997;11:1493–6.
55. Schrappe M, Arico M, Harbott J, et al. Philadelphia chromosome-positive (Ph+) childhood acute lymphoblastic leukemia: good initial steroid response allows early prediction of favorable treatment outcome. Blood 1998;92:2730–41.
56. Cazzaniga G, Lanciotti M, Rossi V, et al. Prospective monitoring of BCR/ABL transcript in children with Ph+ acute lymphoblastic leukemia unravels differences in treatment response. Br J Haematol 2002;119:445–53.
57. Golub TR, Slonim DK, Tamayo P, et al. Molecular classification of cancer: class discovery and class prediction by gene expression monitoring. Science 1999;286:531–7.
58. Holleman A, Cheok MH, den Boer ML, et al. Gene-expression patterns in drug-resistant acute lymphoblastic leukemia cells and response to treatment. N Engl J Med 2004;351:533–42.
59. Lughart S, Cheok MH, den Boer ML, et al. Identification of genes associated with chemotherapy cross resistance and treatment response in childhood acute lymphoblastic leukemia. Cancer Cell 2005;7:375–86.
60. Bennett JM, Catovsky D, Daniel MT, et al. The morphological classification of acute lymphoblastic leukaemia: concordance among observers and clinical correlations. Br J Haematol 1981;47:553–61.
61. Maung ZT, Reid MM, Matheson E, et al. Corticosteroid resistance is increased in lymphoblasts from adults compared with children: preliminary results of in vitro drug sensitivity study in adults with acute lymphoblastic leukaemia. Br J Haematol 1995;91:93–100.
62. Styczynski J, Pieters R, Huismans DR, et al. In vitro drug resistance profiles of adult versus childhood acute lymphoblastic leukaemia. Br J Haematol 2000;110:813–8.
63. Westbrook CA, Hooberman AL, Spino C, et al. Clinical significance of the BCR-ABL fusion gene in adult acute lymphoblastic leukemia: a Cancer and Leukemia Group B Study (8762). Blood 1992;80:2983–90.
64. Wetzler M, Dodge RK, Mrozek K, et al. Prospective karyotype analysis in adult acute lymphoblastic leukemia: the Cancer and Leukemia Group B experience. Blood 1999;93:3983–93.
65. Wetzler M. Cytogenetics in adult acute lymphocytic leukemia. Hematol Oncol Clin North Am 2000;14:1237–49.
66. Cayuela JM, Baruchel A, Orange C, et al. TEL-AML1 fusion RNA as a new target to detect minimal residual disease in pediatric B-cell precursor acute lymphoblastic leukemia. Blood 1996;88:302–8.
67. Thomas X, Danaila C, Le QH, et al. Long-term follow-up of patients with newly diagnosed adult acute lymphoblastic leukemia: a single institution experience of 378 consecutive patients over a 21-year period. Leukemia 2001;15:1811–22.
68. Gottlieb A, Weinberg V, Ellison R, et al. Efficacy of daunorubicin in the therapy of adult acute lymphoblastic leukemia: a prospective randomized trial by Cancer and Acute Leukemia Group B. Blood 1984;64:267–274.
69. Eden OB, Lilleyman JS, Richards S, et al. Results of Medical Research Council Childhood Leukaemia Trial UKALL VIII (report to the Medical Research Council on behalf of the Working Party on Leukaemia in Childhood). Br J Haematol 1991;78:187–96.
70. Stock W, Sather H, Dodge R, et al. Outcome of adolescents and young adults with ALL: a comparison of Children's Cancer Group (CCG) and Cancer and Leukemia Group B (CALGB) regimens. Blood 2000;96:467a.
71. Boissel N, Auclerc MF, Lheritier V, et al. Should adolescents with acute lymphoblastic leukemia be treated as old children or young adults? Comparison of the French FRALLE-93 and LALA-94 trials. J Clin Oncol 2003;21:774–80.
72. de Bont JM, van der Holt B, Dekkar AW, et al. [Adolescents with acute lymphatic leukemia achieve significantly better results when treated following Dutch paediatric oncology protocols than with adult protocols]. Ned Tijdschr Geneeskd 2005;149:400–6.
73. Nachman J, Seibel N, Sather H, et al. Outcome for adolescent and young adults 16–21 years of age (AYA) with acute lymphoblastic leukemia (ALL) treated on the Children's Cancer Group (CCG) 1961 study [abstract 683]. Blood 2004;104:196a.
74. Mattano LA Jr, Sather HN, Trigg ME, et al. Osteonecrosis as a complication of treating acute lymphoblastic leukemia in children. A report from the Children's Cancer Group. J Clin Oncol 2000;18:3262–72.
75. Bürger B, Beier R, Zimmermann M, et al. Osteonecrosis: a treatment related toxicity in childhood acute lymphoblastic leukemia (ALL)—experiences from trial ALL-BFM 95. Pediatr Blood Cancer 2005;44:220–5.
76. Mattano LA, Sather HN, La MK, et al. Modified dexamethasone (DXM) reduces the incidence of treatment-related osteonecrosis (ON) in children and adolescents with higher risk acute lymphoblastic leukemia (HR ALL): a report of CCG-1961 [abstract 777]. Blood 2003;102:221a.
77. Ekert H, Waters K, Matthews R, et al. A randomized study of corticosteroid and noncorticosteroid containing therapy in childhood ALL. Cancer Ther Control 1990;1:87–95.
78. Jones B, Freeman AI, Shuster JJ, et al. Lower incidence of meningeal leukemia when prednisone is replaced by dexamethasone in the treatment of acute lymphocytic leukemia. Med Pediatr Oncol 1991;19:269–75.
79. Balis FM, Lester CM, Chrousos GP, et al. Differences in cerebrospinal fluid penetration of corticosteroids: possible relationship to the prevention of meningeal leukemia. J Clin Oncol 1987;5:202–7.
80. Pieters R, Kaspers GJ, Klumper E, Veerman AJ. Clinical relevance of in vitro drug resistance testing in childhood acute lymphoblastic leukemia: the state of the art. Med Pediatr Oncol 1994;22:299–308.
81. Kaspers GJ, Veerman AJ, Popp Snijders C, et al. Comparison of the antileukemic activity in vitro of dexamethasone and prednisolone in childhood acute lymphoblastic leukemia. Med Pediatr Oncol 1996;27:114–21.
82. Ito C, Evans W, Ninch LM, et al. Comparative cytotoxicity of dexamethasone and prednisolone in childhood acute lymphoblastic leukemia. J Clin Oncol 1996;14:2370–6.
83. Veerman AJ, Hahlen K, Kamps WA, et al. Dutch Childhood Leukemia Study Group: early results of Study All VI (1984-1988). Hamatologie und Bluttransfusion 1990;33:473–7.
84. Igarashi S, Tsuchida M, Manabe A, et al. No advantage of dexamethasone over prednisolone for the outcome of standard and intermediate risk childhood acute lymphoblastic leukemia in the Tokyo Children's Cancer Study Group L95-14 protocol [abstract 3270]. Blood 2003;102:879a.
85. Hurwitz CA, Silverman LB, Schorin MA, et al. Substituting dexamethasone for prednisone complicates induction in children with acute lymphoblastic leukemia. Cancer 2000;88:1964–9.
86. Belgaumi AF, Al-Bahrah M, al-Mahr M, et al. Dexamethasone-associated toxicity during induction chemotherapy for childhood acute lymphoblastic leukemia is augmented by concurrent use of daunomycin. Cancer 2003;97:2898–903.
87. Schultz K, Bostrom B, Cairo M, et al. Very high risk (VHR) features in childhood acute lymphoblastic leukemia (ALL) in recent Children's Cancer Group (CCG) therapeutic trials. Med Pediatr Oncol 1999;33:169.
88. Gaynon PS, Bleyer WA, Steinherz PG, et al. Day 7 marrow response and outcome for children with acute lymphoblastic leukemia and unfavorable presenting features. Med Pediatr Oncol 1990;18:273–9.
89. Hutchinson R, Bertolone S, Cooper H, et al. Early marrow response predicts outcome for patients with low risk ALL: results of CCG-1881. Proc Am Soc Clin Oncol 1994;13:319.
90. Lange B, Sather H, Weetman R, et al. Predictive value of early response in intermediate risk acute lymphoblastic leukemia in children, Children's Cancer Group (CCG) 1891. Blood 1995;86:767a.
91. Steinherz PG, Gaynon PS, Breneman JC, et al. Cytoreduction and prognosis in acute lymphoblastic leukemia—the importance of early marrow response: report from the Children's Cancer Group. J Clin Oncol 1996;14:389–98.
92. Gaynon PS, Desai AA, Bostrom BC, et al. Early response to therapy and outcome in childhood acute lymphoblastic leukemia: a review. Cancer 1997;80:1717–26.
93. Stork L, Sather H, Nachman J, et al. Intensive therapy 'rescues' children with standard risk ALL (SR-ALL) and slow early response to induction: CCG-1952 results [abstract 2007]. Blood 2000;96:466a.
94. Riehm H, Reiter A, Schrappe M, et al. Corticosteroid-dependent reduction of leukocyte count in blood as a prognostic factor in acute lymphoblastic leukemia in childhood (therapy study ALL-BFM 83). Klin Padiatr 1987;199:151–60.
95. Schultz K, Massing B, Spinelli J, et al. The importance of the day 7 bone marrow biopsy as a prognostic measure of the outcome in children with acute lymphoblastic leukemia. Med Pediatr Oncol 1997;29:16–22.
96. Martens AC, Schultz FW, Hagenbeek A. Nonhomogeneous distribution of leukemia in the bone marrow during minimal residual disease. Blood 1987;70:1073–8.
97. Thomson B, Green C, Loken M, et al. Minimal residual disease detection during induction therapy in pediatric acute lymphoblastic leukemia with multi-dimensional flow cytometry (MDF). Proc Am Soc Clin Oncol 1998;17:530a.
98. Sandlund J, Harrison P, Rivera G, et al. Persistence of lymphoblasts in bone marrow on day 15 and days 22 to 25 of remission induction predicts a dismal treatment outcome

in children with acute lymphoblastic leukemia. Blood 2002;100:43–7.

99. Campana D, Pui CH. Detection of minimal residual disease in acute leukemia: methodologic advances and clinical significance. Blood 1995;85:1416–34.
100. Foroni L, Harrison C, Hoffbrand A, Potter M. Investigation of minimal residual disease in childhood and adult acute lymphoblastic leukaemia by molecular analysis. Br J Haematol 1999;105:7–24.
101. Coustan-Smith E, Behm FG, Sanchez J, et al. Immunological detection of minimal residual disease in children with acute lymphoblastic leukaemia. Lancet 1998;351:550–4.
102. Farahat N, Morilla A, Owusa-Ankomah K, et al. Detection of minimal residual disease in B-lineage acute lymphoblastic leukaemia by quantitative flow cytometry. Br J Haematol 1998;101:158–64.
103. van Dongen JJ, Seriu T, Panzer-Grumayer ER, et al. Prognostic value of minimal residual disease in acute lymphoblastic leukaemia in childhood. Lancet 1998;352:1731–8.
104. Roberts WM, Estrov Z, Ouspenskaia MV, et al. Measurement of residual leukemia during remission in childhood acute lymphoblastic leukemia [comments]. N Engl J Med 1997;336:317–23.
105. Goulden NJ, Knechtli CJ, Garland RJ, et al. Minimal residual disease analysis for the prediction of relapse in children with standard-risk acute lymphoblastic leukaemia. Br J Haematol 1998;100:235–44.
106. Cave H, van der Werff ten Bosch J, Suciu S, et al. Clinical significance of minimal residual disease in childhood acute lymphoblastic leukemia. European Organization for Research and Treatment of Cancer—Childhood Leukemia Cooperative Group [comments]. N Engl J Med 1998;339:591–8.
107. Hunger SP, Fall MZ, Camitta BM, et al. E2A-PBX1 chimeric transcript status at end of consolidation is not predictive of treatment outcome in childhood acute lymphoblastic leukemias with a t(1;19)(q23;p13): a Pediatric Oncology Group study. Blood 1998;91:1021–8.
108. Campana D, Coustan-Smith E, Janossy G. The detection of minimal residual disease in acute leukemia. Blood 1990;76:163–71.
109. Griesinger F, Piro-Noack M, Kaib N, et al. Leukaemia-associated immunophenotypes (LAIP) are observed in 90% of adult and childhood acute lymphoblastic leukaemia: detection in remission marrow predicts out-come. Br J Haematol 1999;105:241–55.
110. Weir EG, Cowan K, LeBeau P, Borowitz MJ. A limited antibody panel can distinguish B-precursor acute lymphoblastic leukemia from normal B precursors with four color flow cytometry: implications for residual disease detection. Leukemia 1999;13:558–67.
111. Dworzak M, Froeschi G, Printz D, et al. Prognostic significance and modalities of flow cytometric minimal residual disease detection in childhood acute lymphoblastic leukemia. Blood 2002;99:1952–8.
112. Pongers-Willemse MJ, Seriu T, Stolz F, et al. Primers and protocols for standardized detection of minimal residual disease in acute lymphoblastic leukemia using immunoglobulin and T cell receptor gene rearrangements and TAL1 deletions as PCR targets: report of the BIOMED-1 CONCERTED ACTION: investigation of minimal residual disease in acute leukemia. Leukemia 1999;13:110–8.
113. Sykes PJ, Neoh SH, Brisco MJ, et al. Quantitation of targets for PCR by use of limiting dilution. Biotechniques 1992;13:444–9.
114. Ouspenskaia MV, Johnston DA, Roberts WM, et al. Accurate quantitation of residual B-precursor acute lymphoblastic leukemia by limiting dilution and a PCR-based detection system: a description of the method and the principles involved [comments]. Leukemia 1995;9:321–8.
115. Cave H, Guidal C, Rohrlich P, et al. Prospective monitoring and quantization of residual blasts in childhood acute lymphoblastic leukemia by polymerase chain reaction study of delta and gamma T-cell receptor genes. Blood 1994;83:1892–902.
116. Gibson UE, Heid CA, Williams PM. A novel method for real time quantitative RT-PCR. Genome Res 1996;6:995–1001.
117. Heid CA, Stevens J, Livak KJ, Williams PM. Real time quantitative PCR. Genome Res 1996;6:986–94.
118. Roberts W, Johnston D, Ouspenskaia M, et al. Evaluating protocol efficacy by measuring submicroscopic disease reduction during treatment for childhood ALL. Blood 1996;88:74a.
119. zur Stadt U, Harms DO, Schluter S, et al. [Minimal residual disease analysis in acute lymphoblastic leukemia of childhood within the framework of COALL Study: results of an induction therapy without asparaginase]. Klin Padiatr 2000;212:169–73.
120. Sykes P, Brisco M, Hughes E, et al. Minimal residual disease in childhood acute lymphoblastic leukaemia quantified by aspirate and trephine: is the disease multifocal? Br J Haematol 1998;103:60–5.
121. Steward CG, Goulden NJ, Katz F, et al. A polymerase chain reaction study of the stability of Ig heavy-chain and T-cell receptor delta gene rearrangements between presentation and relapse of childhood B-lineage acute lymphoblastic leukemia. Blood 1994;83:1355–62.
122. Steenbergen EJ, Verhagen OJ, Nibbering CP, et al. Clonal evolution of immunoglobulin heavy chain rearrangements in childhood B-precursor acute lymphoblastic leukemia after engraftment in SCID mice. Leukemia 1996;10:1471–8.
123. Szczepanski T, Beishuizen A, Pongers-Willemse MJ, et al. Cross-lineage T cell receptor gene rearrangements occur in more than ninety percent of childhood precursor-B acute lymphoblastic leukemias: alternative PCR targets for detection of minimal residual disease. Leukemia 1999;13:196–205.
124. van Wering ER, Beishuizen A, Roeffen ET, et al. Immunophenotypic changes between diagnosis and relapse in childhood acute lymphoblastic leukemia. Leukemia 1995;9:1523–33.
125. Beishuizen A, Verhoeven M, van Wering E, et al. Analysis of Ig and T-cell receptor genes in 40 childhood acute lymphoblastic leukemias at diagnosis and subsequent relapse: implications for the detection of minimal residual disease by polymerase chain reaction analysis. Blood 1994;83:2238–47.
126. Brisco MJ, Sykes PJ, Dolman G, et al. Early resistance to therapy during induction in childhood acute lymphoblastic leukemia [In Process Citation]. Cancer Res 2000;60:5092–6.
127. Henze G, Langermann HJ, Bramswig J, et al. [The BFM 76/79 acute lymphoblastic leukemia therapy study]. Klin Padiatr 1981;193:145–54.
128. Henze G, Fengler R, Reiter A, et al. Impact of early intensive reinduction therapy on event-free survival in children with low-risk acute lymphoblastic leukemia. Hamatol Blood Transfus 1990;33:483–8.
129. Baum E, Nachman J, Ramsay N, et al. Prolonged second remissions in childhood acute lymphocytic leukemia: a report from the Children's Cancer Study Group. Med Pediatr Oncol 1983;11:1–7.
130. Nachman J, Sather HN, Gaynon PS, et al. Augmented Berlin-Frankfurt-Munster therapy abrogates the adverse prognostic significance of slow early response to induction chemotherapy for children and adolescents with acute lymphoblastic leukemia and unfavorable presenting features: a report from the Children's Cancer Group. J Clin Oncol 1997;15:2222–30.
131. Freeman AI, Weinberg V, Brecher ML, et al. Comparison of intermediate-dose methotrexate with cranial irradiation for the post-induction treatment of acute lymphocytic leukemia in children. N Engl J Med 1983;308:477–84.
132. Brecher ML, Weinberg V, Boyett JM, et al. Intermediate dose methotrexate in childhood acute lymphoblastic leukemia resulting in decreased incidence of testicular relapse. Cancer 1986;58:1024–8.
133. Freeman A, Boyett J, Glicksman A, et al. Intermediate-dose methotrexate versus cranial irradiation in childhood acute lymphoblastic leukemia: a ten-year follow-up. Med Pediatr Oncol 1997;28:98–107.
134. Abromowitch M, Ochs J, Pui CH, et al. High-dose methotrexate improves clinical outcome in children with acute lymphoblastic leukemia: St. Jude Total Therapy Study X. Med Pediatr Oncol 1988;16:297–303.
135. Abromowitch M, Ochs J, Pui CH, et al. Efficacy of high-dose methotrexate in childhood acute lymphocytic leukemia: analysis by contemporary risk classifications. Blood 1988;71:866–9.
136. Land VJ, Shuster JJ, Crist WM, et al. Comparison of two schedules of intermediate-dose methotrexate and cytarabine consolidation therapy for childhood B-precursor cell acute lymphoblastic leukemia: a Pediatric Oncology Group study. J Clin Oncol 1994;12:1939–45.
137. Mahoney DH Jr, Shuster J, Nitschke R, et al. Intermediate-dose intravenous methotrexate with intravenous mercaptopurine is superior to repetitive low-dose oral methotrexate with intravenous mercaptopurine for children with lower-risk B-lineage acute lymphoblastic leukemia: a Pediatric Oncology Group phase III trial [comments]. J Clin Oncol 1998;16:246–54.
138. Schrappe M, Reiter A, Sauter S, et al. [Concept and interim results of the ALL-BFM 90 therapy study in treatment of acute lymphoblastic leukemia in children and adolescents: the significance of initial therapy response in blood and bone marrow]. Klin Padiatr 1994;206:208–21.
139. Lange BJ, Blatt J, Sather HN, Meadows AT. Randomized comparison of moderate-dose methotrexate infusions to oral methotrexate in children with intermediate risk acute lymphoblastic leukemia: a Children's Cancer Group study. Med Pediatr Oncol 1996;27:15–20.
140. Poplack D, Reaman G, Bleyer W, et al. Successful prevention of central nervous system (CNS) leukemia without cranial radiation in children with high risk acute lymphoblastic leukemia (ALL): a preliminary report. Proc Am Soc Clin Oncol 1989;8:213.
141. Hill F, Gibson B, Eden T, Richards S. Comparison of high dose methotrexate with continuing intrathecal methotrexate versus intrathecal methotrexate alone in low white blood count childhood acute lymphoblastic leukemia: preliminary results from the UKALLXI randomised trial. Blood 1998;92 Suppl 1:398a.
142. Leblanc T, Auclerc M-F, Landman-Parker J, et al. Impact of HD-MTX on the outcome of children with intermediate -risk ALL: results from the FRALLE93: a randomized study. Blood 1998;92 Suppl 1:399a.
143. Mahoney DH Jr, Shuster J, Nitschke R, et al. Intermediate-dose intravenous methotrexate with intravenous mercaptopurine is superior to repetitive low-dose oral methotrexate with intravenous mercaptopurine for children with lower-risk B-lineage acute lymphoblastic leukemia: a Pediatric Oncology Group phase III trial. J Clin Oncol 1998;16:246–54.
144. Bell B, Abish S, Shuster J, Camitta B. Neurotoxicity (NT) in children with standard-risk acute lymphoblastic leukemia (ALL) on Pediatric Oncology Group (POG) 9405. Blood 1997;90:559a.
145. Mahoney DH Jr, Shuster JJ, Nitschke R, et al. Acute neurotoxicity in children with B-precursor acute lymphoid leukemia: an association with intermediate-dose intravenous methotrexate and intrathecal triple therapy—a Pediatric Oncology Group study. J Clin Oncol 1998;16:1712–22.
146. Jurgens H, Janka G, Ibrahim M, et al. Prognostic significance of exposure to intermediate dose methotrexate in children with standard risk ALL: the COALL 82/85 experience. Haematol Blood Transfus 1992;34:338–42.
147. Chessells J, Leiper A, Tiedemann K, et al. Oral methotrexate is as effective as intramuscular methotrexate in maintenance therapy of acute lymphoblastic leukaemia. Arch Dis Child 1987;62:172–6.
148. Koizumi S, Fujimoto T, Takeda T, et al. Comparison of intermittent or continuous methotrexate plus 6-mercaptopurine in regimens for standard-risk acute lymphoblastic leukemia in childhood(JCCLSG-S811). The Japanese Children's Cancer and Leukemia Study Group. Cancer 1988;61:1292–300.
149. Winkler K, Beron G, Thone I, et al. [Therapy of Acute Lymphoblastic Leukemia in Childhood. Multicenter Prospective Therapy Study Coall-80]. Onkologie 1983;6:26–32.
150. Nachman J, Sather HN, Cherlow JM, et al. Response of children with high-risk acute lymphoblastic leukemia treated with and without cranial irradiation: a report from the Children's Cancer Group. J Clin Oncol 1998;16:920–30.
151. Hustu HO, Aur RJ, Verzosa MS, et al. Prevention of central nervous system leukemia by irradiation. Cancer 1973;32:585–97.
152. Pinkel D, Woo S. Prevention and treatment of meningeal leukemia in children [review]. Blood 1994;84:355–66.
153. Nesbit ME, Sather H, Robison LL, et al. Sanctuary therapy: a randomized trial of 724 children with previously untreated acute lymphoblastic leukemia: a report from Children's Cancer Study Group. Cancer Res 1982;42:674–80.
154. Nesbit ME, Robison LL, Littman PS, et al. Presymptomatic central nervous system therapy in previously untreated childhood acute lymphoblastic leukaemia: comparison of 1800 rad and 2400 rad. A report for Children's Cancer Study Group. Lancet 1981;8218:461–6.
155. Bleyer WA, Coccia PF, Sather HN, et al. Reduction in central nervous system leukemia with a pharmacokinetically derived intrathecal methotrexate dosage regimen. J Clin Oncol 1983;1:317–25.
156. Neglia JP, Meadows AT, Robison LL, et al. Second neoplasms after acute lymphoblastic leukemia in child-hood. N Engl J Med 1991;325:1330–6.
157. Bhatia S, Sather H, Pabustan OB, et al. Low incidence of second neoplasms among children diagnosed with acute lymphoblastic leukemia after 1983. Blood 2000;99:4257–64.
158. Haupt R, Fears T, Robison L, et al. Educational attainment in long-term survivors of childhood acute lymphoblastic leukemia. JAMA 1994;272:1427–32.

159. Jankovic M, Brouwers P, Valsecchi MG, et al. Association of 1800 cGy cranial irradiation with intellectual function in children with acute lymphoblastic leukaemia. ISPACC. International Study Group on Psychosocial Aspects of Childhood Cancer [comments]. Lancet 1994;344:224–7.
160. Hill JM, Kornblith AB, Jones D, et al. A comparative study of the long term psychosocial functioning of childhood acute lymphoblastic leukemia survivors treated by intrathecal methotrexate with or without cranial radiation. Cancer 1998;82:208–18.
161. Brown RT, Madan-Swain A, Walco GA, et al. Cognitive and academic late effects among children previously treated for acute lymphocytic leukemia receiving chemotherapy as CNS prophylaxis. J Pediatr Psychol 1998;23:333–40.
162. Waber DP, Carpentieri SC, Klar N, et al. Cognitive sequelae in children treated for acute lymphoblastic leukemia with dexamethasone or prednisone. J Pediatr Hematol Oncol 2000;22:193–6.
163. Tubergen DG, Gilchrist GS, O'Brien RT, et al. Prevention of CNS disease in intermediate-risk acute lymphoblastic leukemia: comparison of cranial radiation and intrathecal methotrexate and the importance of systemic therapy: a Children's Cancer Group report. J Clin Oncol 1993;11:520–6.
164. Mahmoud HH, Rivera GK, Hancock ML, et al. Low leukocyte counts with blast cells in cerebrospinal fluid of children with newly diagnosed acute lymphoblastic leukemia. N Engl J Med 1993;329:314–9.
165. Gilchrist GS, Tubergen DG, Sather HN, et al. Low numbers of CSF blasts at diagnosis do not predict for the development of CNS leukemia in children with intermediate-risk acute lymphoblastic leukemia: a Children's Cancer Group report. J Clin Oncol 1994;12:2594–600.
166. Cherlow JM, Sather H, Steinherz P, et al. Craniospinal irradiation for acute lymphoblastic leukemia with central nervous system disease at diagnosis: a report from the Children's Cancer Group [comments]. Int J Radiat Oncol Biol Phys 1996;36:19–27.
167. Gilchrist G, Sather H, Gaynon P, et al. Outcome effect of low cerebrospinal fluid (CSF) leukocyte count with blasts at diagnosis of childhood acute lymphoblastic leukemia (ALL). Proc Am Soc Clin Oncol 1997;16:516a.
168. Uderzo C, Balduzzi A, De Lorenzo P, et al. Prospective study on allogeneic bone marrow transplantation (allo BMT) versus chemotherapy (chemo) for very high-risk (VHR) childhood acute lymphoblastic leukemia in first complete remission. Bone Marrow Transplant 2001;28:S22–4.
169. Wheeler KA, Richards SM, Bailey CC, et al. Bone marrow transplantation versus chemotherapy in the treatment of very high-risk childhood acute lymphoblastic leukemia in first remission: results from medical research council UKALL X and XI [In Process Citation]. Blood 2000;96:2412–8.
170. Marks DI, Bird JM, Cornish JM, et al. Unrelated donor bone marrow transplantation for children and adolescents with Philadelphia-positive acute lymphoblastic leukemia. J Clin Oncol 1998;16:931–6.
171. Gaynon P, Qu R, Chappell R, et al. Survival after relapse in childhood acute lymphoblastic leukemia: impact of site and time to first relapse, the Children's Cancer Group experience. Cancer 1998;82:1387–95.
172. Buhrer C, Hartmann R, Fengler R, et al. Superior prognosis in combined compared to isolated bone marrow relapses in salvage therapy of childhood acute lymphoblastic leukemia. Med Pediatr Oncol 1993;21:470–6.
173. Chessells J. Relapsed lymphoblastic leukemia in children: a continuing challenge. Br J Haematol 1998;102:423–38.
174. Barrett AJ, Horowitz MM, Pollock BH, et al. Bone marrow transplants from HLA-identical siblings as compared with chemotherapy for children with acute lymphoblastic leukemia in a second remission. N Engl J Med 1994;331:1253–8.
175. Hoogerbrugge PM, Gerritsen EJ, vd Does-van den Berg A, et al. Case-control analysis of allogeneic bone marrow transplantation versus maintenance chemotherapy for relapsed ALL in children. Bone Marrow Transplant 1995;15:255–9.
176. Uderzo C, Valsecchi MG, Bacigalupo A, et al. Treatment of childhood acute lymphoblastic leukemia in second remission with allogeneic bone marrow transplantation and chemotherapy: ten-year experience of the Italian Bone Marrow Transplantation Group and the Italian Pediatric Hematology Oncology Association. J Clin Oncol 1995;13:352–8.
177. Schroeder H, Gustafsson G, Saarinen-Pihkala UM, et al. Allogeneic bone marrow transplantation in second remission of childhood acute lymphoblastic leukemia: a population-based case control study from the Nordic countries. Bone Marrow Transplant 1999;23:555–60.
178. Boulad F, Steinherz P, Reyes B, et al. Allogeneic bone marrow transplantation versus chemotherapy for the treatment of childhood acute lymphoblastic leukemia in second remission: a single-institution study. J Clin Oncol 1999;17:197–207.
179. Wheeler K, Richards S, Bailey C, Chessells J. Comparison of bone marrow transplant and chemotherapy for relapsed childhood acute lymphoblastic leukaemia: the MRC UKALL X experience. Br J Haematol 1998;101:94–101.
180. Dopfer R, Henze G, Bender-Gotze C, et al. Allogeneic bone marrow transplantation for childhood acute lymphoblastic leukemia in second remission after intensive primary and relapse therapy according to the BFM- and CoALL-protocols: results of the German Cooperative Study. Blood 1991;78:2780–4.
181. Dini G, Cornish JM, Gadner H, et al. Bone marrow transplant indications for childhood leukemias: achieving a consensus. The EBMT Pediatric Diseases Working Party. Bone Marrow Transplant 1996;18 Suppl 2:4–7.
182. Sanders JE. Bone marrow transplantation for pediatric malignancies [review]. Pediatr Clin North Am 1997;44:1005–20.
183. Borgmann A, Schmid H, Hartmann R, et al. Autologous bone-marrow transplants compared with chemotherapy for children with acute lymphoblastic leukaemia in a second remission: a matched-pair analysis. The Berlin-Frankfurt-Munster Study Group. Lancet 1995;346:873–6.
184. Hongeng S, Krance RA, Bowman LC, et al. Outcomes of transplantation with matched-sibling and unrelated-donor bone marrow in children with leukaemia. Lancet 1997;350:767–71.
185. Balduzzi A, Gooley T, Anasetti C, et al. Unrelated donor marrow transplantation in children. Blood 1995;86:3247–56.
186. Oakhill A, Pamphilon DH, Potter MN, et al. Unrelated donor bone marrow transplantation for children with relapsed acute lymphoblastic leukaemia in second complete remission. Br J Haematol 1996;94:574–8.
187. Davies SM, Wagner JE, Shu XO, et al. Unrelated donor bone marrow transplantation for children with acute leukemia. J Clin Oncol 1997;15:557–65.
188. Lausen BF, Heilmann C, Vindelov L, Jacobsen N. Outcome of acute lymphoblastic leukaemia in Danish children after allogeneic bone marrow transplantation. Superior survival following transplantation with matched unrelated donor grafts. Bone Marrow Transplant 1998;22:325–30.
189. Harrison G, Richards S, Lawson S, et al. Comparison of allogeneic transplant versus chemotherapy for relapsed childhood acute lymphoblastic leukaemia in the MRC UKALL R1 trial. Ann Oncol 2000;11:999–1006.
190. Gaynon P, Harris R, Trigg M, Stram D. Chemotherapy (CT) vs BMT for children (pts) with acute lymphoblastic leukemia (ALL) and early marrow relapse (MR) :CCG-1941. Blood 2000;96:418a.
191. Locatelli F, Zecca M, Rondelli R, et al. Graft versus host disease prophylaxis with low-dose cyclosporine-A reduces the risk of relapse in children with acute leukemia given HLA-identical sibling bone marrow transplantation: results of a randomized study. Blood 2000;95:1572–9.
192. Knechtli CJ, Goulden NJ, Hancock JP, et al. Minimal residual disease status before allogeneic bone marrow transplantation is an important determinant of successful outcome for children and adolescents with acute lymphoblastic leukemia. Blood 1998;92:4072–9.
193. Kurtzberg J, Asselin B, Pollack B, et al. PEG-L-asparaginase (PEGasp) vs native *E. coli* asparaginase (asp) for reinduction of relapsed acute lymphoblastic leukemia (ALL): Pediatric Oncology Group (POG) 8866 phase II trial. Proc Annu Meet Am Soc Clin Oncol 1993;12:A1079.
194. Abshire T, Pollock BH, Billett AL, et al. Weekly polyethylene glycol conjugated L-asparaginase compared with biweekly dosing produces superior induction remission rates in childhood relapsed acute lymphoblastic leukemia: a Pediatric Oncology Group (POG) study. Blood 2000;96:1709–15.
195. Gaynon P, Harris R, Stram D, et al. Asparagine (ASN) depletion and treatment response in childhood acute lymphoblastic leukemia (ALL) after an early marrow relapse; a Children's Cancer Group trial (CCG-1941). Blood 1999;94:628a.
196. Klumper E, Pieters R, Veerman AJ, et al. In vitro cellular drug resistance in children with relapsed/refractory acute lymphoblastic leukemia. Blood 1995;86:3861–8.
197. Juneja HS, Harvey WH, Brasher WK, Thompson EB. Successful in vitro purging of leukemic blasts from marrow by cortivazol, a pyrazolosteroid: a preclinical study for autologous transplantation in acute lymphoblastic leukemia and non-Hodgkin's lymphoma. Leukemia 1995;9:1771–8.
198. Castillo L, Brunetto A, Conchin C, et al. Cortivazol (RU 3625) for children with acute lymphoblastic leukemia in marrow relapse. Med Pediatr Oncol 1999;33:276.
199. Plosker GL, Figgitt DP. Rituximab: a review of its use in non-Hodgkin's lymphoma and chronic lymphocytic leukaemia. Drugs 2003;63:803–43.
200. Marty M. Cognetti F, Maraninchi D, et al. Randomized phase II trial of the efficacy and safety of trastuzumab combined with docetaxel in patients with human epidermal growth factor receptor 2-positive metastatic breast cancer administered as first-line treatment: the M77001 study group. J Clin Oncol 2005;23:4265–74.
201. Kabbinavar FF, Schulz J, McCleod M, et al. Addition of bevacizumab to bolus fluorouracil and leucovorin in first-line metastatic colorectal cancer: results of a randomized phase II trial. J Clin Oncol 2005;23:3697–705.
202. Herbst RS, Sandler AB. Non-small cell lung cancer and antiangiogenic therapy: what can be expected of bevacizumab? Oncologist 2004;9 Suppl 1:19–26.
203. Coleman M, Goldenberg DM, Siegel AB, et al. Epratuzumab: targeting B-cell malignancies through CD22. Clin Cancer Res 2003;9:3991S–4S.
204. Hannun Y. Apoptosis and the dilemma of cancer chemotherapy. Blood 1997;89:1845–53.
205. Marks DI, Kurz BW, Link MP, et al. High incidence of potential p53 inactivation in poor outcome childhood acute lymphoblastic leukemia at diagnosis. Blood 1996;87:1155–61.
206. Kawamura M, Kikuchi A, Kobayashi S, et al. Mutations of the p53 and ras genes in childhood t(1;19)-acute lymphoblastic leukemia. Blood 1995;85:2546–52.
207. Diccianni MB, Yu J, Hsiao M, et al. Clinical significance of p53 mutations in relapsed T-cell acute lymphoblastic leukemia. Blood 1994;84:3105–12.
208. Harris C. Structure and function of the p53 tumor suppressor gene: clues for rationale cancer therapeutic strategies. J Natl Cancer Inst 1996;88:1442–5.
209. Lilleyman JS, Lennard L. Mercaptopurine metabolism and risk of relapse in childhood lymphoblastic leukaemia. Lancet 1994;343:1188–90.
210. Crom WR, de Graaf SS, Synold T, et al. Pharmacokinetics of vincristine in children and adolescents with acute lymphocytic leukemia. J Pediatr 1994;125:642–9.
211. de Graaf S, Bloemhoff H, Vendrig E, Uges D. Vincristine disposition in children with acute lymphoblastic leukemia. Med Pediatr Oncol 1995;24:235–40.
212. Werner S, Bronnegard M. Molecular basis of glucocorticoid-resistant syndromes. Steroids 1996;61:216–21.
213. Huizenga NA, Koper JW, De Lange P, et al. A polymorphism in the glucocorticoid receptor gene may be associated with an increased sensitivity to glucocorticoids in vivo. J Clin Endocrinol Metab 1998;83:144–51.

Acute Myeloid Leukemia in Children

Richard Aplenc, MD, MSCE
Beverly Lange, MD

INTRODUCTION

Leukemia is the most common pediatric malignancy. Acute myeloid leukemia (AML) comprises about 20% of pediatric leukemia, acute lymphoblastic leukemia (ALL) almost 80%, and subacute or chronic myeloid leukemia the remaining 1 to 2%.[1] Compared with ALL, pediatric AML is less responsive to the available drugs, both in vitro[2] and in vivo.[1] Although cure rate in ALL has exceeded 50% for over 25 years, only recently, with marked intensification of both therapy and supportive care, have cure rates approached and exceeded 50% in pediatric AML.[3–5]

Except in the very young and the very old, AML in children and adults (Chapter 12, "The Myelodysplastic Syndrome") are quite similar. However, given the same treatment, children usually have better outcomes than adults with what appears to be biologically the same disease (Table 124d-1).[6] Despite differences in outcome, investigation of etiology and pathogenesis in pediatric AML provides information relevant to adult AML. In parallel, information gained in adult trials may be applied to pediatric patients.

EPIDEMIOLOGY

The incidence of pediatric AML is 5.2 cases per 1,000,000 children under age 15 years or about 500 cases per year in the United States.[1] Males and females are equally affected. The incidence peaks in the first year of life, and then declines until adolescence, when it begins to rise.[1] The incidence rate is higher in Hispanic ethnic groups, and acute promyelocytic leukemia (APL) comprises approximately one-third of pediatric AML in Latin countries, and less than 10% in non-Latin nations.[7,8] The Middle East, India, China, the Maori in New Zealand, and indigenous populations in Hawaii also have higher incidence rates.[9] Geographic differences in AML subtypes and presentation occur. For example, in Turkey, almost 30% of patients present with isolated orbital chloromas.[10]

Table 124d-1 Medical Research Council-Acute Myeloid Leukemia-10: 5-Year Survival by Age

Age (Yr)	DAT	ADE
0–14	60%	53%
15–24	47%	46%
25–34	52%	46%
35–44	33%	33%
45+	26%	34%

DAT = daunomycin, ara-C, 6-thioguanine; ADE = ara-C, daunomycin, etoposide induction.
Hann IM et al.[6]

ETIOLOGY AND PATHOGENESIS

Although 90% of children with AML have no known risk factors, a number of predisposing constitutional disorders have been identified in the remaining 10% (Table 124d-2). Trisomy-21 is associated with a 15- to 20-fold increased risk of acute leukemia, with AML occurring three times more frequently than ALL in the first 3 years of life.[11] Although constitutional trisomy-8 is much less frequent than trisomy-21, children with trisomy-8 also are at increased risk of developing AML.[12] About 1 of 200 children with Down syndrome (DS) or mosaic DS develops AML, with a peak incidence of age 2 years. Some of these children have a documented transient myeloproliferative disorder (TMD) in the neonatal period that usually regresses spontaneously, but in 10 to 30% of cases, it may recrudesce months later as megakaryoblastic or erythro/megakaryoblastic AML (AMKL). Many of these patients typically have an antecedent myelodysplastic syndrome that precedes the AMKL.[13] The pathogenesis of AML in Down syndrome is not understood, but may be related to an unidentified gene or genes predisposing to leukemia on chromosome 21 band q 22. However, acquired mutations of the hematopoietic transcription factor *GATA1* on chromosome 17 are a unique and obligatory feature of AMKL in DS cases: These mutations are present in all cases of TMD and AMKL in DS, are absent in cases of ALL and non-AMKL myeloid leukemia in DS, and are also absent in cases of AMKL or MDS in patients without DS.[14–16] The mutations introduce a stop codon in the N-terminal activation domain, leading to an incomplete *GATA1* with reduced transactivation potential.[15] The relation between *GATA1* mutation and trisomy 21 is as yet unclear.

Patients with neurofibromatosis 1 (NF1) are genetically predisposed to many forms of cancer, including AML and juvenile myelomonocytic leukemia (JMML).[17] NF1 disease is caused by mutations of the *NF1* gene, which is located on the long arm of chromosome 17. Children with this disease have increased risk of AML or JMML. Neurofibromin, the protein product of the *NF1* gene, is a GTPase-activating protein for p21^{ras} Ras.[18] Most hematopoietic growth factors stimulate growth through Ras activation. Ras proteins have a slow intrinsic rate of GTP hydrolysis; neurofibromin accelerates Ras hydrolysis several thousandfold, that is, neurofibromin is a negative regulator of Ras output. Thus *NF1* might function as a tumor suppressor gene by restraining Ras signaling. JMML bone marrows and other tumors from NF1 patients show frequent loss of heterozygosity, a hallmark of

Table 124d-2 Risk Factors for Pediatric Acute Myeloid Leukemia

Risk Factor	Approximate Risk	Reference
Monozygotic infant twin	1:5	9
Constitutional		
Shwachman's syndrome	1:3	128
Fanconi anemia	1:10	129
Kostmann syndrome	1:10	130
Down syndrome	1:100 to 1:200	131
Neurofibromatosis type 1	1:200	132
CBFA2 mutations	Unknown	50
Bloom syndrome	Unknown	131
Trisomy 8	Unknown	12
Carcinogen Exposure		
Benzene	OR > 1.8	57
Ionizing radiation	OR = 2.4 (NS)	58
Maternal drug use	OR = 11	59
Maternal ETOH use	OR = 2.6–3.0	60,62
Maternal smoking	OR = 0.97–2.4	60,61
Maternal topoisomerase inhibitor II intake	OR = 10	68
Radon exposure	Under investigation	1
Chemotherapy Exposure		
Alkylating agents	1:10 to 1:50	51
Topoisomerase II inhibitors	1:8 to 1:80	55

tumor suppressor gene inactivation.[18,19] JMML cells from children with NF1 have elevated levels of Ras-GTP and activation of downstream effector kinase cascades.[20] One of the characteristics of JMML is hyperproliferation in vitro in the presence of granulocyte-monocyte colony-stimulating factor (GMCSF). In NF1 mutant mice, GM-CSF enables establishment and maintenance of the abnormal myelopoiesis.[21]

Children with Noonan's syndrome (NS) are commonly predisposed to transient monocytosis as well as thrombocytopenia, and rarely predisposed to transient myeloproliferative disorders and JMML.[22,23] The pathogenesis of JMML in NS is similar to that in NF1. Linkage analysis mapped about 50% of NS cases to germline missense mutations of exon 3 or 8 of *PTPN11* within the NS locus on chromosome band 12q24. *PTPN11* encodes SHP-2, a nonreceptor tyrosine phosphatase.[24,25] In hematopoietic and nonhematopoietic cells, SHP-2 relays signals from growth factor receptors, at least in part, through the Ras/RAF/ERK cascade.[24–26] Molecular studies implicate hyperactive Ras in the pathogenesis of JMML in patients with NS. JMML cells from patients with NS have mutations in *PTPN11* that encode amino acid substitutions that are relatively uncommon in NS patients without JMML.[27,28] Somatic *PTPN11* mutations with amino acid substitutions distinct from those in NS are found in JMML specimens from about 35% of children with de novo JMML, in 4% of de novo pediatric AML, and uncommonly in adult myelodysplastic syndrome (MDS) and chronic myelomonocytic leukemia.[27–30]

Children with bone marrow failure syndromes are at increased risk of developing AML. Those with Fanconi anemia have a 1 in 10 chance of developing AML, often with monosomy 7 and an antecedent myelodysplastic syndrome.[31,32] Their predisposition to AML is attributed to the function of one of the 12 or more FA genes that collectively function as a DNA damage response pathway.[33] FA cells are hypersensitive to damage induced by DNA cross-linking agents such as diepoxybutane, mitomycin C, and ionizing radiation. Molecular cloning of the genes discloses a multicomponent DNA repair pathway, composed of distinct FA proteins.[32,33] DNA damage activates a complex consisting of Fanconi proteins A, C, G, and F, and it results in monoubiquination of the FANCD2 protein.[34] Modified FANCD2 protein relocalizes in the nucleus where it directly interacts with the breast cancer susceptibility protein BRCA1. In response to ionizing radiation, FANCD2 protein is phosphorylated by the ATM protein kinase.[32] Mutations in the *BRCA2* gene, encoding a DNA repair enzyme, are the underlying abnormality in FA patients previously assigned to complementation groups B and D1.[33–35] Just how these defects in DNA repair lead to bone marrow failure followed by MDS and AML is unknown.

About 1 in 3 children with Shwachman-Bodian-Diamond syndrome (SBDS) develops MDS or AML, frequently with deletions of chromosome 7 or 7q.[36] SBDS is associated with recurring mutations in *SBDS* on chromosomal band 7q11[37] Near *SBDS* is a pseudogene, *SBDSP*, with 97% sequence homology to *SBDS*. Recombination of *SBDS* with *SBDSP* results in gene conversion, an established mechanism of mutagenesis.[37] The pathogenesis of MDS and AML in SBDS is presumably a result of a number of intrinsic abnormalities in the marrow progenitors, but the specific mechanism is unknown.[38] Compared with normal controls, the CD 34+, CD34–/CD38+, and CD34–/CD38– fractions of marrow from SBDS patients with and without MDS showed significantly higher FAS expression and greater apoptosis in vitro.[33–37]

The use of granulocyte-colony stimulating (G-CSF) has prevented children with Kostmann's syndrome (severe congenital neutropenia [SCN]) from dying of infection in the first or second year of life.[39] About 10% of the patients treated with G-CSF develop AML, frequently with monosomy 7. SCN is the result of an intrinsic defect in myeloid progenitors. Myeloid progenitor cells of SCN patients undergo accelerated apoptosis compared with normal controls, and granulocyte-macrophage colony-formation in vitro is impaired,[39,40] while G-CSF production and G-CSF receptor expression on neutrophil precursors are normal.[41–44] Mutations in the neutrophil elastase (*ELA2*) gene are associated with cyclic neutropenia,[45] and mutations in different segments of *ELA2* are detected in a most patients with SCN.[46] Somatically acquired mutations in the G-CSF receptor that truncate the carboxyl terminus and/or *ras* mutations may contribute to the pathogenesis of AML in these patients.[44–46]

Rare familial forms of monosomy 7 have been described.[47] A familial form of AML has been mapped to 16q22, although the gene is not yet defined.[48] In contrast, the very high risk of AML or ALL among monozygotic infant twins with leukemia is not heritable: The leukemic clone in both twins is identical and is due to in utero twin-to-twin transfusion of a premalignant clone that undergoes malignant transformation in each individual sibling.[49]

Haploinsufficiency of the transcription factor CBFA2 on chromosome 21 has been shown to be associated with the autosomal dominant familial platelet disorder, in which affected children and adults are at increased risk of AML.[50] Conceivably, altered expression of CBFA2 may be relevant to the development of megakaryoblastic leukemia in DS.

AML has also been associated with prior chemotherapy. Therapy-related AML occurs in two distinct clinical phenotypes: in adults, the first phenotype occurs 5 to 10 years after administration of alkylating agents, is dose-dependent, and is frequently preceded by myelodysplasia with monosomy 7.[51] The latency in children is shorter, often within 3 years of diagnosis of the primary malignancy.[52] The second phenotype occurs months to several years after exposure to the epipodophyllotoxins teniposide and etoposide[53] and other topoisomerase II inhibitors.[54] This association may be related to the schedule of epipodophyllotoxin administration, rather than to the individual or cumulative dose.[55] Translocations of chromosome 11q23, t(8;21), t(15;17), or inv(16) are present in over half the cases.[53,55,56]

Multiple chemical and physical exposures have been associated with AML. Benzene,[57] ionizing radiation,[58] and chemotherapeutics have the strongest associations. Maternal marijuana,[59] cigarette,[60,61] and ETOH use,[60,62,63] as well as prior maternal fetal loss[64] are more weakly associated with AML. Although several small studies demonstrated an association between electromagnetic fields and AML,[65,66] the largest and best-designed study to date has shown no association.[67] Most recently, infant AML has been associated with maternal intake of topoisomerase II inhibitor-containing foods.[68] In general, these associations are weak and account for only a small proportion of cases of AML.

CLASSIFICATION AND DIAGNOSIS

For nearly 2 decades, the French-American-British (FAB) classification system has been the standard for AML (Chapter 12). This system is based on morphology, histologic staining, and, in the cases of undifferentiated AML (FAB M0) and megakaryoblastic leukemia (FAB M7), immunophenotyping. The diagnosis of AML is made on marrow aspirate and biopsy showing greater than 30% blasts, or with biopsy of an extramedullary mass composed of myeloblasts.[69] The WHO classification is now replacing the FAB.[70] In the WHO system, 20% marrow blasts are sufficient to diagnose AML. Cytogenetics and fluorescent in situ hybridization (FISH) are becoming standard: They provide useful diagnostic and prognostic information. These assays, as well as the polymerase chain reaction (PCR) that uses commercially available molecular probes for translocation breakpoint sequences, are sensitive tools for following minimal residual disease.

Typically, blasts from over 90% of pediatric patients with AML express one or more of the myeloid-associated antigens CD13, CD14, CD33 and myeloperoxidase.[71] T-cell or B-cell lymphoid markers may be present in 30 to 60% of cases.[72] Some correlation between immunophenotype, morphology, and cytogenetic findings has been noted: $CD19^+$ and $CD56^+$ with FAB AML M2/t(8;21), $CD2^+$ and $CD7^+$ with FAB AML M2/t(8;21 negative), and $CD33^+$, $CD34^-$ with FAB AML M3/t(15;17).[71,73] Moreover, individual pediatric AML patients will have conserved clonotypic immunophenotype expression that can serve as a "molecular fingerprint" of the patient's leukemia. Such a fingerprint may be very helpful in disease monitoring.[74,75]

Seventy to 80% of de novo AML blasts have an abnormal karyotype.[76,77] Approximately 40% of cytogenetic abnormalities are miscellaneous clonal abnormalities, while 60% fall into known cytogenetic subgroups.[78] Table 124d-3 lists the major subgroups and their relative contribution to the total of cytogenetic abnormalities. The roles of t(8;21), inv(16), and t(15;17) in leukemia pathogenesis are discussed in Chapters 6, "Oncogenes," and 124a, "Incidence, Origins, and Epidemiology."

Although the diagnosis of AML is usually straightforward, other malignancies may mimic

Table 124d-3 Cytogenetic Abnormalities

Patients	% of Total
Normal	15–31
t(8;21)(q22;q22)	8–17
t(15;17)(q22;q21)	4–10
Inv(16)(p13;q22)	4–12
t(9;11)(p21-22;q23)	0–9
Other 11q23	6–11
t(6;9)(p23;q24)	< 1
t(1;22)(p13;q13)	< 3
(–7) + del(7)(q)	3–5
(–5) + del(5)(q)	< 1.5
Hyperdiploidy	14–21

AML. Most notably, metastatic alveolar rhabdomyosarcoma,[79] undifferentiated leukemia, or FAB L2 ALL may appear morphologically like megakaryoblastic (M7) AML.[80] Neuroblastoma and alveolar rhabdomyosarcoma may also look like monoblastic FAB (M5) AML.[81] A high index of suspicion and histochemical, immunologic, cytogenetic, and molecular genetic studies are essential for the correct diagnosis.

PRESENTATION

The clinical presentation of AML stems from over 10^{12} leukemia cells crowding out normal hematopoietic cells in the marrow and invading extramedullary sites, such as soft tissues, skin (leukemia cutis), gingiva, orbit, and brain. Patients usually present with signs and symptoms of diminished numbers of normal red blood cells, white blood cells, and platelets, as well as the presence of blasts on blood smears. Marrow replacement causes neutropenia that places patients at risk of opportunistic bacterial infections. Thus, patients often have fever or other signs of a focal or systemic infection. Patients may also present with anemia, which gives rise to fatigue, pallor, and, in extreme cases, hemodynamic instability. Thrombocytopenia may cause petechiae, purpura, mucosal bleeding, or rarely, CNS hemorrhage. Thrombocytopenia may be exacerbated by coagulopathy, especially in the M3 and M5 subtypes. Although the mechanism for disseminated intravascular coagulation (DIC) is not known in M5 AML, there is convincing evidence that expression of annexin II, a receptor for fibrinolytic proteins, facilitates plasminogen activation by associating plasminogen and its activator, t-PA, at the APL (M3) leukemic blast cell surface.[82] Patients with peripheral blast counts greater than 200,000/mm^3 are at risk of central nervous system (CNS) stroke owing to hyperviscosity or vessel wall invasion. About 5% of patients with AML have CNS disease at diagnosis, and a smaller percentage present with CNS chloromas.[83] These patients may have headaches, cranial nerve palsies, focal neurological deficits, or rarely, seizures.

THERAPY

Pediatric AML protocols begin with a remission induction regimen. Induction therapy has two goals: first, to reduce the malignant blast bone marrow percentage to less than 5% and/or to eliminate overt extramedullary disease, and second, to restore normal hematopoiesis. Therapy continues with CNS prophylaxis and with either postremission chemotherapy or with marrow or stem cell transplantation.

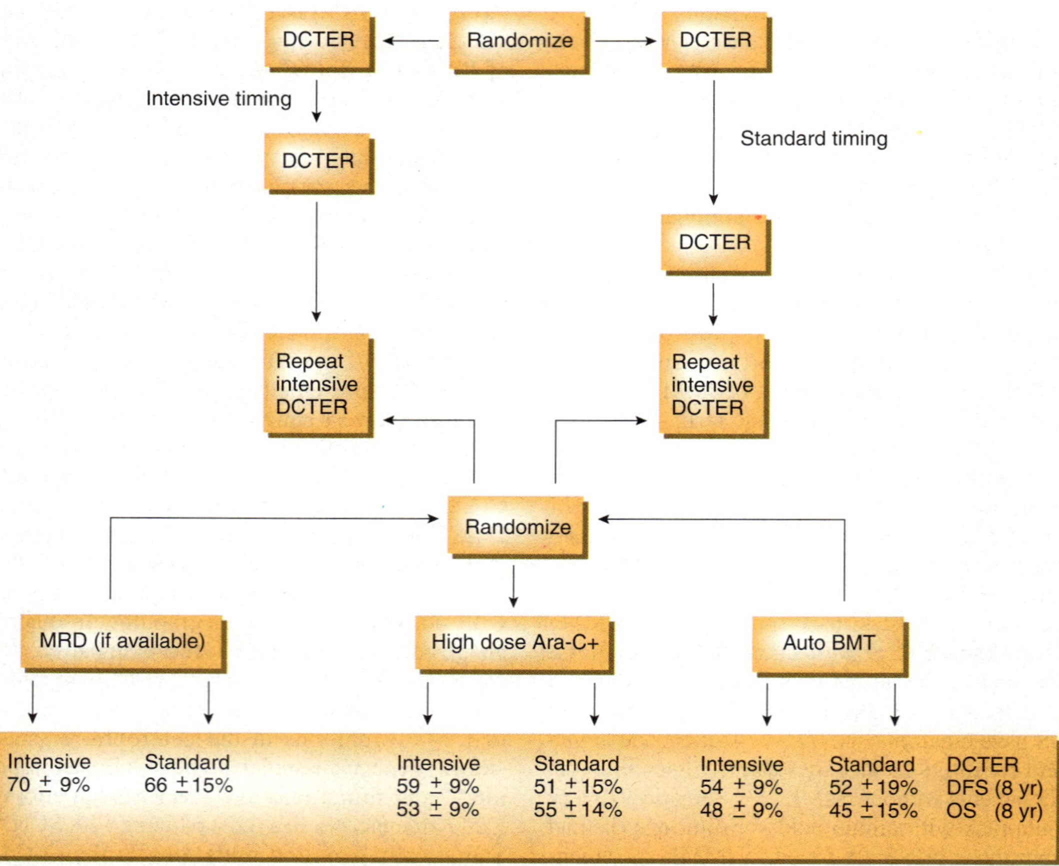

Figure 124d-1 The Children's Cancer Group's (CCG) therapeutic strategies.

Figures 124d-1 to 124d-3 illustrate recent, relatively successful therapeutic strategies of large, published trials of three pediatric cooperative groups, these being the Berlin-Frankfurt-Munster (BFM), the Medical Research Council (MRC),[84] and the Children's Cancer Group (CCG). Common to all are the use of cytarabine (ara-C), anthracyclines +/– etoposide, or 6-thioguanine in induction and consolidation. Traditionally, the BFM group adds a maintenance phase similar to pediatric ALL therapy and central nervous system prophylaxis with cranial irradiation.[3,85,86] The MRC focuses on a 10-day induction, followed by postremission therapy with sequential combinations of high-dose ara-C and alternating anthracyclines.[6] The CCG-2891 intensive timing regimen uses two cycles of sequentially timed five-drug induction and consolidation, followed by timed sequential Capizzi, high-dose ara-C, or marrow transplantation.[5] Five-year survival of pediatric patients with de novo AML in studies of these groups is currently 50% or higher.[3,5,87]

Postremission therapy at a minimum consists of consolidation chemotherapy, which uses agents similar to those in induction and intensification chemotherapy regimens. Most postremission chemotherapy consolidation regimens rely heavily on ara-C in high doses. Although the various pediatric cooperative oncology groups use high-dose ara-C in consolidation and intensification, they differ in the use of bone marrow transplant (BMT) and maintenance therapy.

Considerable debate exists over the appropriate role of matched related bone marrow transplantation (MRD BMT) in postremission therapy. Trials in the United States and France have demonstrated that MRD BMT significantly improves event-free survival (EFS) and overall survival (OS), compared with intensive chemotherapy or autologous bone marrow transplant (AUTO BMT).[5,88,89] Thus, in CCG, in the Pediatric Oncology Group (POG), and in the French Cooperative AML Group (LAME), intensive induction therapy with appropriately matched related donor

ADE
Randomize
TAD
ADE
TAD
MACE
MIDAC
MRD BMT If family donor available
No further therapy
Early Auto BMT
60% OS (3 yr) 72%
48% EFS (3 yr) 68%
ADE: Daunorubicin, cytarabine, 6-thioguanine
TAD: Daunorubicin, cytarabine, etoposide
MACE: Amsacrine, cytarabine, etoposide
MIDAC: Mitoxantrone, cytarabine
Auto BMT: Autologous bone marrow transplant
OS: overall survival
EFS: event-free survival

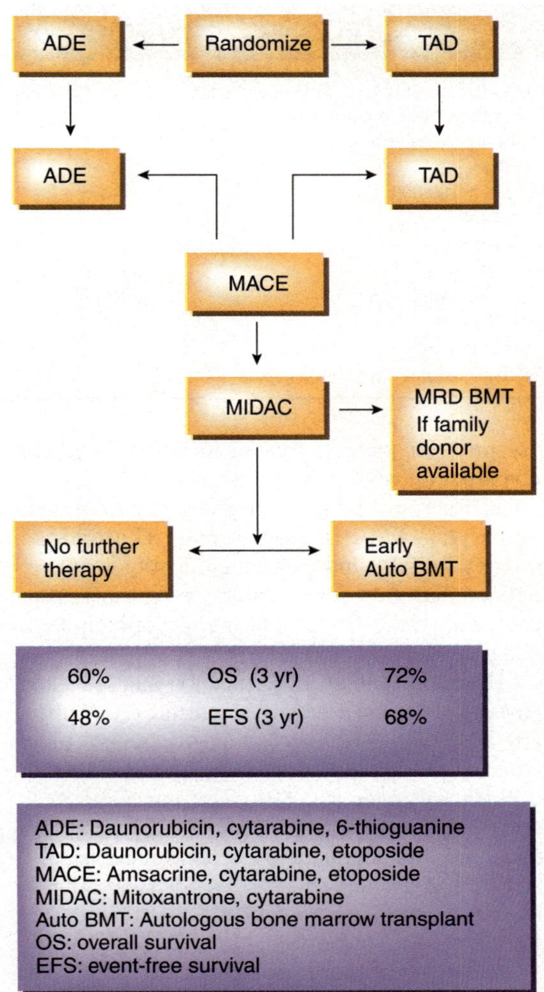

Figure 124d-2 The Medical Research Council's (MRC) therapeutic strategies.

Randomize
ADE
AIE
Risk stratification
Standard risk
High risk
Randomize
Consolidation
HAM
Consolidation
HD Ara-C VP-16
Consolidation
HAM
HD Ara-C VP-16
HD Ara-C VP-16
XRT
Maintenance for 1 year
74 ± 4% 58 ± 5% 57 ± 6% OS (5yr)
65 ± 4% 52 ± 5% 45 ± 5% EFS (5yr)
ADE: Cytarabine, daunorubicin, etoposide
AIE: Cytarabine, idarubicin, etoposide
Consolidation: 6-Thioguanine, prednisolone, vincristine, Adriamycin, cyclophosphamide
HAM: High dose cytarabine and mitoxantrone
HD Ara-C: High dose cytarabine
VP-16: etoposide
XRT: Craniospinal irradiation
Maintenance: 6-Thioguanine, cytarabine
OS: overall survival
EFS: event-free survival

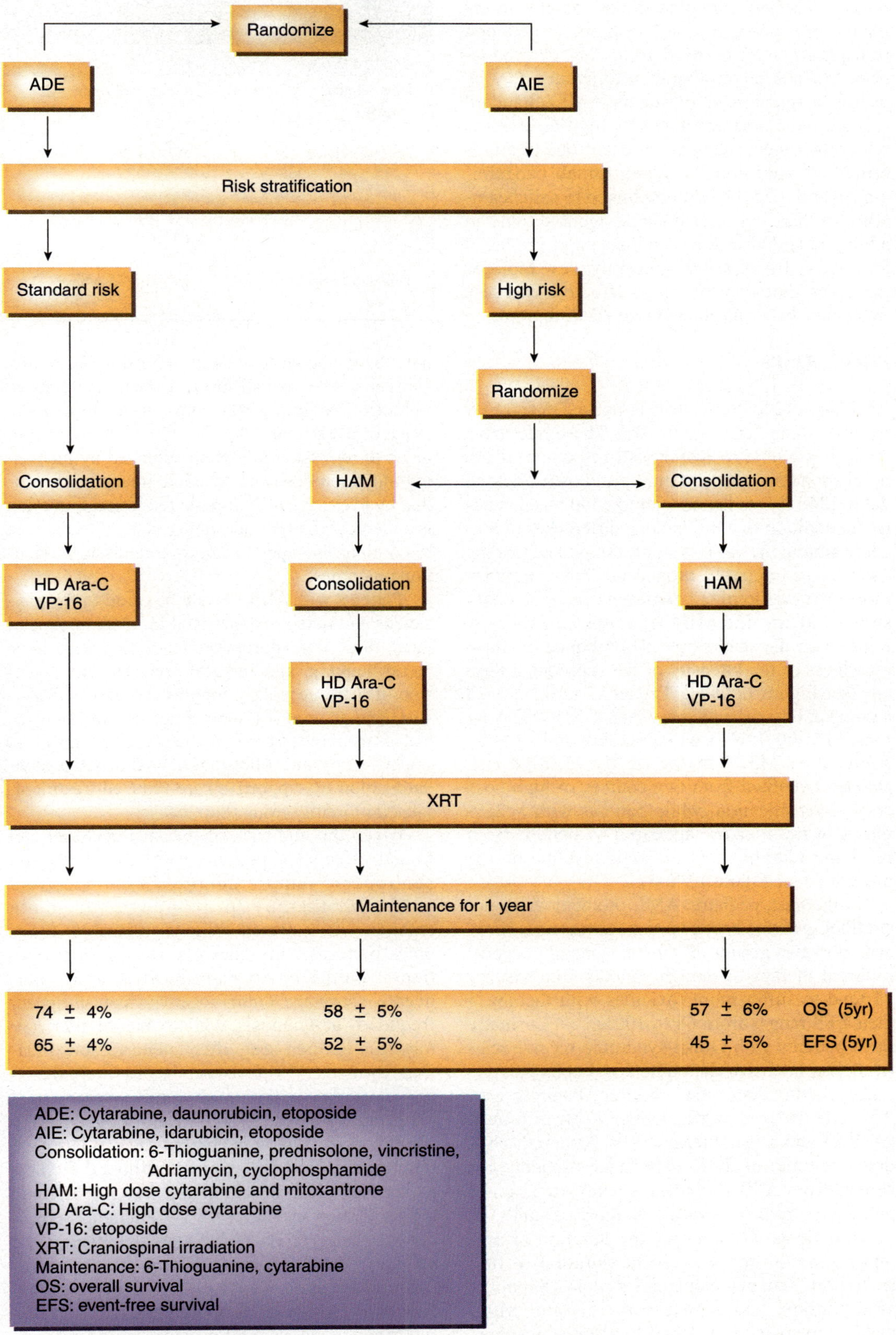

Figure 124d-3 The Berlin-Frankfurt-Munster (BFM) groups therapeutic strategies.

transplantation is now front-line therapy for patients in first remission. However, the MRC AML-10 trial in England[84] and the BFM 93 trial in Germany[3] have not shown a statistically significant advantage to MRD BMT for patients with "standard risk" AML, as defined by each trial. The discordant results of these trials may stem from the different patient populations and treatment protocols of each cooperative group, from statistical limitations of relatively small numbers, and from biases of parents, guardians, and physicians regarding postinduction therapies.[84] Most pediatric groups are no longer recommending transplantation in first remission for patients with AML with the cytogenetic abnormalities t(15;17), t(8;21), and (inv 16).

If MRD BMT is not available or selected, then consolidation and intensification chemotherapy regimens are given. Although the various pediatric cooperative oncology groups use ara-C in consolidation and intensification, they differ in the use of AUTO BMT and maintenance therapy. Although CCG,[5] POG,[88] and LAME[89] have shown no benefit to AUTO BMT, the combined pediatric and adult experience in MRC AML10 demonstrated a significant benefit to AUTO BMT compared with no further therapy after four courses of intensive chemotherapy.[84] The Italian Pediatric Group for Bone Marrow Transplantation favors melphalan with and without TBI in single-arm studies for patients with AML.[90,91] Although the BFM group relies heavily on maintenance therapy,[71,85] CCG and LAME have shown that maintenance therapy may decrease OS.[89,92]

Refractory disease and relapse remain the major causes of treatment failure in AML, and there is general agreement that marrow or stem cell transplant is the treatment of choice. If the tumor burden is low and the donor readily available, there is some success in transplanting without cytoreduction; if there is no matched related donor, matched unrelated donor (MUD) transplant—or in younger, smaller patients, cord blood transplant—may be used following cytoreduction. Various chemotherapeutic agents may be useful in relapsed or refractory AML. Standard salvage chemotherapy includes high-dose ara-C with other agents such as mitoxantrone or amsacrine.[93,94] Additionally, gemtuzumab ozogamicin, an anti–CD-33 antibody linked to calicheamicin, has had impressive single-agent activity in adult and pediatric AML and is being introduced into phase III trials.[95,96] Recently, new biologic therapies that may be more effective and less toxic have been introduced into AML therapy.

Table 124d-4 Prognostic Factors in Pediatric Acute Myeloid Leukemia (AML)

Factor	Favorable	Unfavorable	Variable
Host-related	Down syndrome	Germline DNA repair defect	
		Obesity; malnutrition	
		Older age	
Disease-related	WBC < 20,000	WBC > 100,000	
		FAB M7	
		Treatment-related AML	
	Inv(16)	del(7)/7q-	t(8;21)
	t(15;17)	Complex karyotype	t(9;11)
		FLT3/ITD[1]	
Treatment-related	Day 15: < 5% blasts	Induction failure	
		Relapse within a year of diagnosis	

PROGNOSIS

As Figures 124d-1 to 124d-3 indicate, OS and EFS for AML range from 40 to 70%. These rates have made it possible to distinguish responders from nonresponders and to define prognostic factors. Table 124d-4 lists factors identified in recent studies. In addition to these factors, differences in outcome among the various studies implicate therapy itself as an important prognostic factor. Furthermore, the randomized regimens in CCG-2891 show that the intensity of induction therapy impacts on the success of all subsequent therapy, regardless of the intensity of the subsequent therapy (see Figure 124d-1).[5] The BFM group defined a group of low-risk patients who had M1 with Auer rods, M2 with less than 20,000 blast cells, M4 eo subtype, or M3.[97] In the BFM '93, high-risk patients benefited from two courses of high-dose ara-C intensification, while patients with > 25% blasts in the marrow appeared to benefit from receiving idarubicin as the anthracycline during induction (see Figure 124d-3).[3]

In the past, pediatric AML protocols have not stratified patients based on risk assessment. However, now two groups of patients generally receive different therapy. Although patients with trisomy 21 tend to suffer more toxicities with therapy,[11] their EFS ranges from 68 to 100%.[11,98] Currently most patients with Down syndrome receive relatively less intensive chemotherapy, but fare significantly better than other children. Patients with APL are treated with all-*trans*-retinoic acid (ATRA) and chemotherapy.[99,100] Although children are more likely to experience pseudotumor cerebri from ATRA,[101] their rates of rapid onset pulmonary failure are similar to those of adults.[102]

In patients who relapse, the duration of second remission depends on the duration of first remission: Patients relapsing less than 18 months after therapy had a 10% survival rate, while patients relapsing more than 18 months posttherapy had a 40% survival rate.[103] Although investigators have proposed therapy stratification based on time to relapse,[104] such risk stratification is not presently used in pediatric AML.

COMPLICATIONS

AML protocols are becoming increasingly intensive. Although more intensive induction regimens have been shown to induce more durable remissions and better overall survival, the more intensive induction regimens also have mortality in the range of 6% to over 10%.[11,71,84,88,89] Thus, overall gains in remission induction achieved by increasing induction dose and schedule intensity are limited by toxicity. Since durable remission induction is a prerequisite for cure, future clinical trials need to continue in order to improve remission induction outcomes.

Patients with AML should be cared for by physicians and nurses experienced in AML therapy at institutions with appropriate laboratory, radiology, blood banking, and surgical services. The provision of these necessary support services is expensive, and it requires substantial commitment as well as resources from both the patient's family and society. Riley and colleagues have shown that standardization of supportive care reduced treatment-related mortality from 18 to 9%.[105]

Given the high risk of invasive bacterial and fungal infections, patients who are febrile and neutropenic require empiric broad-spectrum antibiotic therapy until their neutropenia resolves.[106,107] Based on local microbial resistance patterns, appropriate antibiotic combinations would include gram-positive and gram-negative coverage. Gram-negative organisms occur frequently at diagnosis, while α-hemolytic streptococcus is often seen after intensive consolidation regimens.[108] If fever persists for more than 3 to 5 days after initiation of empiric therapy or if recurrent fever occurs, empiric antifungal therapy should begin. Although amphotericin B has been traditionally used for empiric antifungal therapy, newer, equally efficacious and less nephrotoxic agents are now available.[109,110] Although *Pneumocystis carinii* is rare in pediatric AML outside of the setting of BMT, prophylaxis with trimethoprim-sulfamethoxazole (TMP-SMZ) is often given. However, TMP-SMZ is no longer used for bacterial prophylaxis. Penicillin prophylaxis for *Streptococcus viridans* may prevent sepsis syndromes in centers where *S. viridans* remain penicillin-sensitive; however, penicillin resistance is becoming common. HEPA air filtration has been proven to diminish *Aspergillus* infection in marrow transplant patients, and because *Aspergillus* infection is becoming increasingly common in AML patients receiving chemotherapy, HEPA filtration is generally recommended.[111] Such filtration is probably essential for patients treated in hospitals where construction work is being done.

Patients are at risk of coagulopathy from their underlying AML or from sepsis. The optimal therapy for APL-induced coagulopathy is not yet defined, but most investigators prefer supportive care with fresh frozen plasma, cryoprecipitate, and platelets.[112]

Hematopoietic toxicity, infection mucositis and emesis are universal acute side effects of AML therapy. BMT with TBI may cause acute nephritis and an acute pneumonitis that is usually fatal.[113] Both cyclophosphamide and TBI cause infertility,[114,115] and TBI may cause growth retardation, cataracts,[116,117] endocrine dysfunction, pulmonary[118] and cardiac dysfunction.[119,120] Aside from infertility and cataracts, the late effects of BMT and chemotherapy are similar.[121]

Allogeneic donor transplants carry additional risks of graft-versus-host disease (GVHD). Although the risks of veno-occlusive disease and GVHD preclude the use of matched unrelated donor bone marrow transplant (MUD-BMT) in first remission, most salvage regimens for relapsed AML incorporate MUD transplantation if a suitable donor is available.[122] Risk of GVHD MRD BMT is approximately 40% and may reach 80% in the MUD setting.[123] Methotrexate, cyclosporine, tacrolimus (FK506), and steroids are used in various combinations for acute GVHD prophylaxis and management, while cyclosporine, FK506, and steroids are primarily used to treat chronic GVHD. The observation that patients with acute GVHD are less likely to relapse than those without acute GVHD has led to a postulated graft-versus-leukemia (GVL) effect.[124] Unlike acute GVHD, chronic GVHD has no GVL effect. Transplant-related mortality is proportional to the extent of donor recipient mismatch, age, and the extent of pretreatment. Allogenic transplant-related mortality from unrelated or mismatched donors may reach 50%.[122]

CONCLUSION

Although progress has been made in the treatment of pediatric AML by intensifying chemotherapy and improving supportive care, at the rate of 1% gains in survival per year, there is substantial room for improvement.[125] Moreover, the high treatment-associated mortality rates indicate that chemotherapy may have been maximally intensified, and new active agents and strategies are thus needed. These agents and strategies may include histone deacetylase inhibitors, translocation breakpoint targeted therapy, monoclonal antibody therapy targeted to membrane antigens, and differentiation therapy that has worked well with APL.[126] Finally, development of predictive models of relapse risk may allow for individualization of therapy.[127]

REFERENCES

1. Smith M, Gloecker Ries L, Gurney J, Ross J. Leukemia SEER pediatric monograph. National Cancer Institute; 1999.
2. Zwaan CM, Kaspers GJ, Pieters R, et al. Different drug sensitivity profiles of acute myeloid and lymphoblastic leukemia and normal peripheral blood mononuclear cells in children with and without Down syndrome. Blood 2002;99:245–51.
3. Creutzig U, Ritter J, Zimmerman M, et al. Improved treatment results in high-risk pediatric acute myeloid leukemia patients after intensification with high-dose cytarabine and mitoxantrone: results of Study Acute Myeloid Leukemia—Berlin-Frankfurt-Munster 93. J Clin Oncol 2001;19:2705–13.
4. Stevens RF, Hann IM, Wheatley K, Gray RG. Marked improvements in outcome with chemotherapy alone in paediatric acute myeloid leukemia: results of the United Kingdom Medical Research Council's 10th AML trial. MRC Childhood Leukaemia Working Party. Br J Haematol 1998;101:130–40.
5. Woods WG, Neudorf S, Gold S, et al. A comparison of allogeneic bone marrow transplantation, autologous bone marrow transplantation, and aggressive chemotherapy in children with acute myeloid leukemia in remission. Blood 2001;97:56–62.
6. Hann IM, Stevens RF, Goldstone AH, et al. Randomized comparison of DAT versus ADE as induction chemotherapy in children and younger adults with acute myeloid leukemia. Results of the Medical Research Council's 10th AML trial (MRC AML10). Adult and Childhood Leukaemia Working Parties of the Medical Research Council. Blood 1997;89:2311–8.
7. Biondi A, Rovelli A, Cantu-Rajnoldi A, et al. Acute promyelocytic leukemia in children: experience of the Italian Pediatric Hematology and Oncology Group (AIEOP). Leukemia 1994;8:1264–8.
8. Douer D, Preston-Martin S, Chang E, et al. High frequency of acute promyelocytic leukemia among Latinos with acute myeloid leukemia [comments]. Blood 1996;87:308–13.
9. Bhatia S, Neglia JP. Epidemiology of childhood acute myelogenous leukemia [comments]. J Pediatr Hematol Oncol 1995;17:94–100.
10. Turker A, Cadvar A, Yavuz G, et al. Cytogenetic abnormality in Turkish children with acute myeloid leukemia (AML) and orbito-ocular granulocytic sarcoma (chloroma). Blood 1993;82:550a.
11. Lange BJ. The management of malignant disorders of hematopoiesis in children with Down syndrome. Br J Haematol 2000;110:64:1–9.
12. Mili F, Khoury MJ, Flanders WD, Greenberg RS. Risk of childhood cancer for infants with birth defects. I. A record- linkage study, Atlanta, Georgia, 1968–1988. Am J Epidemiol 1993;137:629–38.
13. Lange BJ, Kobrinsky N, Barnard DR, et al. Distinctive demography, biology, and outcome of acute myeloid leukemia and myelodysplastic syndrome in children with Down syndrome: Children's Cancer Group Studies 2861 and 2891. Blood 1998;91:608–15.
14. Hitzler JK, Cheung J, Li Y, et al. GATA1 mutations in transient leukemia and acute megakaryoblastic leukemia of Down syndrome. Blood 2003;101:4301–4.
15. Wechsler J, Greene M, McDevitt MA, et al. Acquired mutations in GATA1 in the megakaryoblastic leukemia of Down syndrome. Nat Genet 2002;32:148–52.
16. Mundschau G, Gurbuxani S, Gamis AS, et al. Mutagenesis of GATA1 in an initiating event in Down syndrome leukemogenesis. Blood 2003;101:4298–300.
17. Stiller CA, Chessells JM, Fitchett M. Neurofibromatosis and childhood leukemia/lymphoma: a population-based UKCCSG study. Br J Cancer 1994;70:969–72.
18. Shannon KM, O'Connell P, Martin GA, et al. Loss of the normal NF1 allele from the bone marrow of children with type 1 neurofibromatosis and malignant myeloid disorders [comments]. N Engl J Med 1994;330:597–601.
19. Side LE, Emanuel PD, Taylor B, et al. Mutations of the NF1 gene in children with juvenile myelomonocytic leukemia without clinical evidence of neurofibromatosis, type 1. Blood 1998;92:267–72.
20. Bos JL. *ras* oncogenes in human cancer: a review. Cancer Res 1989;49:4682–9.
21. Birnbaum RA, O'Marcaigh A, Wardak Z, et al. Nf1 and GM-CSF interact in myeloid leukemogenesis. Mol Cell 2000;5:189–195.
22. Tartaglia M, Kalidas K, Shaw A, et al. PTPN11 mutations in Noonan syndrome: molecular spectrum, genotype- phenotype correlation, and phenotypic heterogeneity. Am J Hum Genet 2002;70:1555–63.
23. Tartaglia M, Mehler EL, Goldberg R, et al. Mutations in PTPN11, encoding the protein tyrosine phosphatase SHP-2, cause Noonan syndrome. Nat Genet 2001;29:465–8.
24. Barford D, Neel BG. Revealing mechanisms for SH2 domain mediated regulation of the protein tyrosine phosphatase SHP-2. Structure 1998;6:249–54.
25. Neel BG, Gu H, Pao L. The 'Shp'ing news: SH2 domain-containing tyrosine phosphatases in cell signaling. Trends Biochem Sci 2003;28:284–93.
26. Feng GS. Shp-2 tyrosine phosphatase: signaling one cell or many. Exp Cell Res 1999;253:47–54.
27. Van Vactor D, O'Reilly AM, Neel BG. Genetic analysis of protein tyrosine phosphatases. Curr Opin Genet Dev 1998;8:112–26.
28. Itho T, Liu R, Yokota T, et al. Definition of the role of tyrosine residues of the common beta subunit regulating multiple signaling pathways of granulocyte-macrophage colony-stimulating factor receptor. Mol Cell Biol 1998;18:742–52.
29. Loh ML, Reynolds MG, Vattikuti S, et al. PTPN11 mutations in pediatric patients with acute myeloid leukemia: results from the Children's Cancer Group. Leukemia 2004;18:1831–4.
30. Loh ML, Martinelli S, Cordeddu V, et al. Acquired PTPN11 mutations occur rarely in adult patients with myelodysplastic syndromes and chronic myelomonocytic leukemia. Leuk Res 2005;29:459–62.
31. Kutler DI, Singh B, Satagopan J, et al. A 20-year perspective on the International Fanconi Anemia Registry (IFAR). Blood 2003;101:1249–56.
32. Alter BP. Fanconi's anemia and malignancies. Am J Hematol 1996;53:99–110.
33. Taniguchi T, Dandrea AD. Molecular pathogenesis of Fanconi anemia. Int J Hematol 2002;75(2):123-8.
34. Garcia-Higuera I, Taniguchi T, Ganesan S, et al. Interaction of the Fanconi anemia proteins and BRCA1 in a common pathway. Mol Cell 2001;7:249–62.
35. Howlett NG, Taniguchi T, Olson S, et al. Biallelic inactivation of BRCA2 in Fanconi anemia. Science 2002;297(5581):606–9.
36. Smith OP, Hann IM, Chessells JM, et al. Haematological abnormalities in Shwachman-Diamond syndrome. Br J Haematol 1996;94:279–84.
37. Boocock GRB, Morrison JA, Popovic M, et al. Mutations in SBDS are associated with Schwachman-Diamond Syndrome. Nature Genetics 2003;33:97–101.
38. Dror Y, Freedman MH. Shwachman-Diamond syndrome marrow cells show abnormally increased apoptosis mediated through the Fas pathway. Blood 2001;97(10):3011–6.
39. Kobayashi M, Yumiba C, Kawaguchi Y, et al. Abnormal responses of myeloid progenitor cells to recombinant human colony-stimulating factors in congenital neutropenia. Blood 1990;75:2143–9.
40. Hestdal K, Welte K, Lie SO, et al. Severe congenital neutropenia: abnormal growth and differentiation of myeloid progenitors to granulocyte colony-stimulating factor (G-CSF) but normal response to G-CSF plus stem cell factor. Blood 1993;82:2991–7.
41. Banerjee A, Shannon KM. Leukemic transformation in patients with severe congenital neutropenia. J Pediatr Hematol Oncol 2001;23:487–95.
42. Bernhardt TM, Burchardt ER, Welte K. Assessment of G-CSF and GM-CSF mRNA expression in peripheral blood mononuclear cells from patients with severe congenital neutropenia and in human myeloid leukemic cell lines. Exp Hematol 1993;21:163–8.
43. Guba SC, Sartor CA, Hutchinson R, et al. Granulocyte colony-stimulating factor (G-CSF) production and G-CSF receptor structure in patients with congenital neutropenia. Blood 1994;83:1486–92.
44. Mempel K, Pietsch T, Menzel T, et al. Increased serum levels of granulocyte colony-stimulating factor in patients with severe congenital neutropenia. Blood 1991;77:1919–22.
45. Horwitz M, Benson KF, Person RE, A et al. Mutations in ELA2, encoding neutrophil elastase, define a 21-day biological clock in cyclic haematopoiesis. Nat Genet 1999;23:433–6.
46. Dale DC, Person RE, Bolyard AA, et al. Mutations in the gene encoding neutrophil elastase in congenital and cyclic neutropenia. Blood 2000;96:2317–22.
47. Shannon KM, Watterson J, Johnson P, et al. Monosomy 7 myeloproliferative disease in children with neurofibromatosis, type 1: epidemiology and molecular analysis. Blood 1992;79:1311–8.
48. Horwitz M, Benson KF, Li FQ, et al. Genetic heterogeneity in familial acute myelogenous leukemia: evidence for a second locus at chromosome 16q21-23.2. Am J Hum Genet 1997;61:873–81.
49. Ford AM, Bennett CA, Price CM, et al. Fetal origins of the TEL-AML1 fusion gene in identical twins with leukemia. Proc Natl Acad Sci U S A 1998;95:4584–8.
50. Song WJ, Sullivan MG, Legare RD, et al. Haploinsufficiency of CBFA2 causes familial thrombocytopenia with propensity to develop acute myelogenous leukaemia [comments]. Nat Genet 1999;23:166–75.
51. Kaldor JM, Day NE, Clarke EA, et al. Leukemia following Hodgkin's disease [comments]. N Engl J Med 1990;322:7–13.
52. Barnard DR, Lange BJ, Alonzo TA, et al. Acute myeloid leukemia and myelodysplastic syndrome in children treated for cancer: comparison with primary presentation. Blood 2002. [In press]
53. Pui CH, Behm FG, Raimondi SC, et al. Secondary acute myeloid leukemia in children treated for acute lymphoid leukemia [comments]. N Engl J Med 1989;321:136–42.
54. Spector LG. Xie Y, Robison LL, et al. Maternal diet and infant leukemia: the DNA topoisomerase II inhibitor hypothesis: a report from the children's oncology group. Cancer Epidemiol Biomarkers Prev 2005;14:651–5.
55. Pui CH, Ribeiro RC, Hancock ML, et al. Acute myeloid leukemia in children treated with epipodophyllotoxins for acute lymphoblastic leukemia. N Engl J Med 1991;325:1682–7.
56. Felix CA, Hosler MR, Winick NJ, et al. ALL-1 gene rearrangements in DNA topoisomerase II inhibitor-related leukemia in children. Blood 1995;85:3250–6.
57. Savitz DA, Andrews KW. Review of epidemiologic evidence on benzene and lymphatic and hematopoietic cancers. Am J Ind Med 1997;31:287–95.
58. Magnani C, Pastore G, Luzzatto L, Terracini B. Parental occupation and other environmental factors in the etiology of leukemias and non-Hodgkin's lymphomas in childhood: a case-control study. Tumori 1990;76:413–9.
59. Robison LL, Buckley JD, Daigle AE, et al. Maternal drug use and risk of childhood nonlymphoblastic leukemia among offspring. An epidemiologic investigation implicating marijuana (a report from the Children's Cancer Study Group). Cancer 1989;63:1904–11.
60. Shu XO, Ross JA, Pendergrass TW, et al. Parental alcohol consumption, cigarette smoking, and risk of infant leukemia: a Children's Cancer Group study. J Natl Cancer Inst 1996;88:24–31.
61. Brondum J, Shu XO, Steinbuch M, et al. Parental cigarette smoking and the risk of acute leukemia in children. Cancer 1999;85:1380–8.
62. van Duijn CM, van Steensel-Moll HA, Coebergh JW, van Zanen GE. Risk factors for childhood acute non-lymphocytic leukemia: an association with maternal alcohol consumption during pregnancy? Cancer Epidemiol Biomarkers Prev 1994;3:457–60.
63. Guengerich FP, Shimada T, Yun CH, et al. Interactions of ingested food, beverage, and tobacco components involving human cytochrome P4501A2, 2A6, 2E1, and 3A4 enzymes. Environ Health Perspect 1994;102 Suppl 9:49–53.
64. Yeazel MW, Buckley JD, Woods WG, Ret al. History of maternal fetal loss and increased risk of childhood acute leukemia at an early age. A report from the Children's Cancer Group. Cancer 1995;75:1718–27.
65. Savitz DA, Calle EE. Leukemia and occupational exposure to electromagnetic fields: review of epidemiologic surveys. J Occup Med 1987;29:47–51.
66. Wertheimer N, Savitz DA, Leeper E. Childhood cancer in relation to indicators of magnetic fields from ground current sources. Bioelectromagnetics 1995;16:86–96.
67. Linet MS, Hatch EE, Kleinerman RA, et al. Residential exposure to magnetic fields and acute lymphoblastic leukemia in children [comments]. N Engl J Med 1997;337:1–7.
68. Ross JA. Maternal diet and infant leukemia: a role for DNA topoisomerase II inhibitors? Int J Cancer Suppl 1998;11:26–8.

69. Cheson BD, Cassileth PA, Head DR, et al. Report of the National Cancer Institute-sponsored workshop on definitions of diagnosis and response in acute myeloid leukemia. J Clin Oncol 1990;8:813–9.
70. Jaffe ES, Harris NL, Stein H, Vardeman JW, editors. World Health Organization classification of tumours. Pathology and genetics of tumours of hematopoietic and lymphoid tissue. Lyon, France: IARC Press; 2001.
71. Creutzig U, Harbott J, Sperling C, et al. Clinical significance of surface antigen expression in children with acute myeloid leukemia: results of study AML-BFM-87. Blood 1995;86:3097–108.
72. Smith FO, Lampkin BC, Versteeg C, et al. Expression of lymphoid-associated cell surface antigens by childhood acute myeloid leukemia cells lacks prognostic significance. Blood 1992;79:2415–22.
73. Barnard DR, Kalousek DK, Wiersma SR, et al. Morphologic, immunologic, and cytogenetic classification of acute myeloid leukemia and myelodysplastic syndrome in childhood: a report from the Children's Cancer Group. Leukemia 1996;10:5–12.
74. Lo Coco F, Diverio D, Pandolfi PP, et al. Molecular evaluation of residual disease as a predictor of relapse in acute promyelocytic leukaemia. Lancet 1992;340:1437–8.
75. Sievers EL, Loken MR. Detection of minimal residual disease in acute myelogenous leukemia. J Pediatr Hematol Oncol 1995;17:123–33.
76. Thirman MJ, Larson RA. Therapy-related myeloid leukemia. Hematol Oncol Clin North Am 1996;10:293–320.
77. Mitelman F, editor. Catalog of chromosome aberrations in cancer. 5th ed. New York: Wiley-Liss; 1994.
78. Look AT. Oncogenic transcription factors in the human acute leukemias. Science 1997;278:1059–64.
79. Douglass EC, Valentine M, Etcubanas E, et al. A specific chromosomal abnormality in rhabdomyosarcoma [published erratum appears in Cytogenet Cell Genet 1988;47:following 232]. Cytogenet Cell Genet 1987;45:148–55.
80. Penchansky L, Taylor SR, Krause JR. Three infants with acute megakaryoblastic leukemia simulating metastatic tumor. Cancer 1989;64:1366–71.
81. Boyd JE, Parmley RT, Langevin AM, Saldivar VA. Neuroblastoma presenting as acute monoblastic leukemia. J Pediatr Hematol Oncol 1996;18:206–12.
82. Menell JS, Cesarman GM, Jacovina AT, et al. Annexin II and bleeding in acute promyelocytic leukemia. N Engl J Med 1999;340:994–1004.
83. Pui CH, Dahl GV, Kalwinsky DK, et al. Central nervous system leukemia in children with acute nonlymphoblastic leukemia. Blood 1985;66:1062–7.
84. Burnett AK, Goldstone AH, Stevens RM, et al. Randomised comparison of addition of autologous bone-marrow transplantation to intensive chemotherapy for acute myeloid leukaemia in first remission: results of MRC AML 10 trial. UK Medical Research Council Adult and Children's Leukaemia Working Parties. Lancet 1998;351:700–8.
85. Creutzig U, Ritter J, Riehm H, et al. Improved treatment results in childhood acute myelogenous leukemia: a report of the German cooperative study AML-BFM-78. Blood 1985;65:298–304.
86. Creutzig U, Ritter J, Zimmermann M, Schellong G. Does cranial irradiation reduce the risk for bone marrow relapse in acute myelogenous leukemia? Unexpected results of the Childhood Acute Myelogenous Leukemia Study BFM-87. J Clin Oncol 1993;11:279–86.
87. Awan A, Malcolm Taylor G, Gokhale DA, et al. Increased frequency of Fanconi anemia group C genetic variants in children with sporadic acute myeloid leukemia [letter]. Blood 1998;91:4813–4.
88. Ravindranath Y, Yeager AM, Chang MN, et al. Autologous bone marrow transplantation versus intensive consolidation chemotherapy for acute myeloid leukemia in childhood. N Engl J Med 1996;334:1428–34.
89. Michel G, Leverger G, Leblanc T, et al. Allogeneic bone marrow transplantation vs aggressive post-remission chemotherapy for children with acute myeloid leukemia in first complete remission. A prospective study from the French Society of Pediatric Hematology and Immunology (SHIP). Bone Marrow Transplant 1996;17:191–6.
90. Cesaro S, Meloni G, Messina C, et al. High-dose melphalan with autologous hematopoietic stem cell transplantation for acute myeloid leukemia: results of a retrospective analysis of the Italian Pediatric Group for Bone Marrow Transplantation. Bone Marrow Transplant 2001;28:131–6.
91. Bonetti F, Zecca M, Pession A, et al. Total-body irradiation and melphalan is a safe and effective conditioning regimen for autologous bone marrow transplantation in children with acute myeloid leukemia in first remission. The Italian Association for Pediatric Hematology and Oncology-Bone Marrow Transplantation Group. J Clin Oncol 1999;17:3729–35.
92. Wells RJ, Woods WG, Lampkin BC, et al. Impact of high-dose cytarabine and asparaginase intensification on childhood acute myeloid leukemia: a report from the Children's Cancer Group. J Clin Oncol 1993;11:538–45.
93. Wells RJ, Woods WG, Buckley JD, et al. Treatment of newly diagnosed children and adolescents with acute myeloid leukemia: a Children's Cancer Group study. J Clin Oncol 1994;12:2367–77.
94. Weitman S, Ochoa S, Sullivan J, et al. Pediatric phase II cancer chemotherapy trials: a Pediatric Oncology Group study. J Pediatr Hematol Oncol 1997;19:187–91.
95. Sievers EL, Larson RA, Stadtmauer EA, et al. Mylotarg Study Group. Efficacy and safety of gemtuzumab ozogamicin in patients with CD33-positive acute myeloid leukemia in first relapse. J Clin Oncol 2001;19:3244–54.
96. Arceci RJ, Sande J, Lange B, et al. Safety and efficacy of gemtuzumab ozogamicin (Mylotarg) in pediatric patients with advanced CD33-positive acute myeloid leukemia. Blood 2005. [In press]
97. Creutzig U, Ritter J, Schellong G. Identification of two risk groups in childhood acute myelogenous leukemia after therapy intensification in study AML-BFM-83 as compared with study AML-BFM-78. AML-BFM Study Group. Blood 1990;75:1932–40.
98. Ravindranath Y, Abella E, Krischer JP, et al. Acute myeloid leukemia (AML) in Down's syndrome is highly responsive to chemotherapy: experience on Pediatric Oncology Group AML Study 8498 [comments]. Blood 1992;80:2210–4.
99. Huang ME, Ye YC, Chen SR, et al. Use of all-trans retinoic acid in the treatment of acute promyelocytic leukemia. Blood 1988;72:567–72.
100. Tallman MS, Anderson JW, Schiffer CA, et al. All-trans-retinoic acid in acute promyelocytic leukemia. N Engl J Med 1997;337:1021–8.
101. Mahmoud HH, Hurwitz CA, Roberts WM, et al. Tretinoin toxicity in children with acute promyelocytic leukaemia [comments]. Lancet 1993;342:1394–5.
102. Frankel SR, Eardley A, Lauwers G, et al. The "retinoic acid syndrome" in acute promyelocytic leukemia [comments]. Ann Intern Med 1992;117:292–6.
103. Stahnke K, Boos J, Bender-Gotze C, et al. Duration of first remission predicts remission rates and long-term survival in children with relapsed acute myelogenous leukemia. Leukemia 1998;12:1534–8.
104. Estey E, Thall P, David C. Design and analysis of trials of salvage therapy in acute myelogenous leukemia. Cancer Chemother Pharmacol 1997;40 Suppl:S9–12.
105. Riley LC, Hann IM, Wheatley K, Stevens RF. Treatment-related deaths during induction and first remission of acute myeloid leukaemia in children treated on the Tenth Medical Research Council acute myeloid leukaemia trial (MRC AML10). The MCR Childhood Leukaemia Working Party. Br J Haematol 1999;106:436–44.
106. Pizzo PA. Fever in immunocompromised patients. N Engl J Med 1999;341:893–900.
107. Chanock SJ, Pizzo PA. Infectious complications of patients undergoing therapy for acute leukemia: current status and future prospects. Semin Oncol 1997;24:132–40.
108. Gamis AS, Howells WB, DeSwarte-Wallace J, et al. Alpha hemolytic streptococcal infection during intensive treatment for acute myeloid leukemia: a report from the Children's Cancer Group Study CCG-2891. J Clin Oncol 2000;18:1845–55.
109. Walsh TJ, Pappas P, Winston DJ, et al. Voriconazole compared with liposomal amphotericin B for empirical antifungal therapy in patients with neutropenia and persistent fever. N Engl J Med 2002;346:225–34.
110. Walsh TJ, Teppler H, Donowitz GR, et al. Caspofungin versus liposomal amphotericin B for empirical antifungal therapy in patients with persistent fever and neutropenia. N Engl J Med 2004;351:1391–402.
111. Sheretz RJ, Belani A, Kramer BS, et al. Impact of air filtration on nosocomial Aspergillus infections. Unique risk of bone marrow transplant recipients. Am J Med 1989;83:709–18.
112. Levi M, Ten Cate H. Disseminated intravascular coagulation. N Engl J Med 1999;341:586–92.
113. Bortin MM, Kay HE, Gale RP, Rimm AA. Factors associated with interstitial pneumonitis after bone-marrow transplantation for acute leukaemia. Lancet 1982;1:437–9.
114. Sanders JE. The impact of marrow transplant preparative regimens on subsequent growth and development. The Seattle Marrow Transplant Team. Semin Hematol 1991;28:244–9.
115. Teinturier C, Hartmann O, Valteau-Couanet D, et al. Ovarian function after autologous bone marrow transplantation in childhood: high-dose busulfan is a major cause of ovarian failure. Bone Marrow Transplant 1998;22:989–94.
116. Cohen A, Rovelli A, Bakker B, et al. Final height of patients who underwent bone marrow transplantation for hematological disorders during childhood: a study by the Working Party for Late Effects-EBMT. Blood 1999;93:4109–15.
117. Leiper AD, Stanhope R, Lau T, et al. The effect of total body irradiation and bone marrow transplantation during childhood and adolescence on growth and endocrine function. Br J Haematol 1987;67:419–26.
118. Beinert T, Dull T, Wolf K, et al. Late pulmonary impairment following allogeneic bone marrow transplantation. Eur J Med Res 1996;1:343–8.
119. Kupari M, Volin L, Suokas A, et al. Cardiac involvement in bone marrow transplantation: serial changes in left ventricular size, mass and performance. J Intern Med 1990;227:259–66.
120. Hogarty AN, Leahey A, Zhao H, et al. Longitudinal evaluation of cardiopulmonary performance during exercise after bone marrow transplantation in children. J Pediatr 2000;136:311–7.
121. Leahey AM, Teunissen H, Friedman DL, et al. Late effects of chemotherapy compared to bone marrow transplantation in the treatment of pediatric acute myeloid leukemia and myelodysplasia. Med Pediatr Oncol 1999;32:163–9.
122. Szydlo R, Goldman JM, Klein JP, et al. Results of allogeneic bone marrow transplants for leukemia using donors other than HLA-identical siblings. J Clin Oncol 1997;15:1767–77.
123. Lange B, Bunin N. Treatment of acute myeloid leukemia in children. In: Lilleyman JS, Hann IM, Blanchette VS, editors. Textbook of pediatric hematology. London, U.K.: 1999. p. 387–402.
124. Weaver CH, Clift RA, Deeg HJ, et al. Effect of graft-versus-host disease prophylaxis on relapse in patients transplanted for acute myeloid leukemia. Bone Marrow Transplant 1994;14:885–93.
125. Lange B. Progress in acute myelogenous leukemia: the one hundred years' war [editorial; comment]. J Pediatr Hematol Oncol 1995;17:91–3.
126. Perentesis JP, Sievers EL. Targeted therapies for high-risk acute myeloid leukemia. Hematol Oncol Clin North Am 2001;16:677–701.
127. Wheatley K, Burnett AK, Goldstone AH, et al. A simple, robust, validated and highly predictive index for the determination of risk-directed therapy in acute myeloid leukaemia derived from the MRC AML 10 trial [In Process Citation]. Br J Haematol 1999;107:69–79.

Central Nervous System Tumors of the Infant and Child

Tobey J. MacDonald, MD
Brian R. Rood, MD

Significant differences in epidemiology, molecular genetics, and biology distinguish central nervous system (CNS) tumors of the infant and child from those arising in adulthood. As a result of these differences, important aspects of clinical presentation, treatment and outcome are uniquely related to childhood CNS tumors.

GENERAL EPIDEMIOLOGY

Malignant CNS tumors are the most common solid tumor of childhood, with 2,200 new cases per year in the United States.[1] This figure would be approximately 28% higher if non-malignant brain tumors were included. The second most common cancer following leukemia, brain tumors comprise 16.6% of all cancers in children less than 20 years of age.[1] Worldwide, approximately 30,000 to 40,000 children develop CNS tumors each year.[2]

Pediatric brain tumors vary considerably in their histological, topographical, and gender distribution throughout childhood and adolescence. Boys are 24% more commonly affected than girls in all age groups, but this increase is accounted for mostly by medulloblastoma, primitive neuroectodermal tumor (PNET), and ependymoma[1] Over 90% of CNS tumors in children are primary brain tumors and only rarely do children experience CNS metastases from extraneural tumors.[1] Survival has improved from 60% in 1975 to 1984 to 65% in 1985 to 1994, and survival is noted to improve with increasing age: 45% in those aged less than 1 year, 59% in those aged 1 to 4 years, 64% in 5- to 9-year-olds, 70% in 10- to 14-year-olds, and 77% in 15- to 19-year-olds.[1] The main histological entities are pilocytic astrocytomas (23.5%), followed by medulloblastomas (16.3%), ependymomas (10.1%), anaplastic astrocytomas and glioblastomas (7.2% each), and craniopharyngiomas (5.6%).[3] In aggregate, astrocytomas are most common, accounting for 52.2% of all pediatric brain tumors.[1] Rarer entities include germ cell tumors, gangliogliomas, and meningiomas (2.5% each), supratentorial PNET and pineal parenchymal tumors (1.9% each), atypical teratoid/rhabdoid tumors (1.3%), choroid plexus tumors (0.9%), and desmoplastic infantile astrocytomas and dysembryoplastic neuroepithelial tumors (0.6% each).[3]

In the United States, CNS tumors are the most common cause of death due to cancer in childhood, accounting for 24%.[1] Although overall mortality decreased from 1973 to 1994, the incremental gain in patient survival over this period lags far behind other childhood cancers. Furthermore, despite the modest improvement in survival, treatment-related morbidity of childhood CNS tumors remains high. Morbidity includes cognitive, memory and learning impairment, neuroendocrine deficiencies, hearing deficits, sterility, and secondary cancers.

The etiology of CNS tumors remains mostly unknown. The known risk factors include (1) gender (medulloblastoma and ependymoma rates are higher in males, although little difference is noted in other CNS cancers), (2) therapeutic doses of ionizing radiation to the head (ie, leukemia or prior brain tumor), and (3) genetic syndromes such as neurofibromatosis, tuberous sclerosis, nevoid basal cell carcinoma syndrome (Gorlin's syndrome), Turcot's syndrome, and Li-Fraumeni syndrome. Suggestive, but not conclusive, risk factors include (1) maternal diet during pregnancy (cured meat consumption, 1.5- to 2-fold increased risk), (2) parent or sibling with brain tumor (3.9-fold increase, presumably due to the inherited genetic risks listed above), and (3) family history of bone cancer, leukemia or lymphoma (possibly due to familial Li-Fraumeni syndrome).[1,4]

TUMOR BIOLOGY

Molecular Pathogenesis With the mapping of the human genome, the molecular pathogenesis of pediatric CNS tumors is becoming more clearly defined and gene expression patterns or "genetic fingerprints" are beginning to emerge that demonstrate the molecular diversity among childhood CNS tumors.

Embryonal Tumors A recent study using microarray profiling revealed that morphologically identical tumors such as medulloblastoma and supratentorial PNET could be separated based solely on their specific patterns of gene expression.[5] Histologic subclassification of medulloblastoma yields three main subtypes of medulloblastoma: classic, nodular/desmoplastic, and large/cell anaplastic (LCA) morphologies. Gene expression profiling is able to distinguish the desmoplastic type of medulloblastoma from classic appearing medulloblastoma, predominantly due to differential expression of the sonic hedgehog (Shh) signaling pathway, and was able to predict clinical outcome.[5] Mutations of the Shh receptor Patched1 (Ptc1), and other members of the Shh pathway that similarly result in constitutive activation of Shh signaling, are associated with medulloblastomas.[6–8] Ptc1 (+/–) heterozygous mice spontaneously develop medulloblastomas, which can be induced to regress with Shh pathway antagonists.[9–11] Inactivation of the Shh target gene Gli1 has also been most recently shown to significantly reduce medulloblastoma formation in this tumor model.[12] As these molecular alterations are becoming increasingly better understood, it is anticipated that novel agents specifically targeting the pathway intermediates will undergo investigation in clinical trials in the very near future.

Approximately 10% of medulloblastomas harbor amplification of the MYC oncogene, which has been associated with the LCA phenotype and poor prognosis.[13] Similarly, expression of the tyrosine kinase receptor ERBB2 has been demonstrated in 40% of medulloblastomas, most frequently LCA type, and has also been shown to be an independent poor prognostic indicator.[14] Small molecule inhibitors of ERBB2 are currently under clinical investigation. Recently, amplification of the OTX2 homeobox gene, whose product can be targeted by retinoids, was identified in LCA medulloblastoma, suggesting that OTX2 is another potentially therapeutically susceptible medulloblastoma oncogene.[15,16]

The most common chromosomal event in medulloblastoma, 17p deletion, occurs in 35–50% of tumors.[17,18] The minimal area of deletion at 17p13.3 encompasses regulatory elements of HIC1, a tumor suppressor gene that is epigenetically inactivated in the majority of medulloblastoma tumors.[18,19] Evidence also exists for a possible connection between alterations in chromosome 17 and the Ptch/Shh genes.[17] Atypical teratoid/rhabdoid tumor (AT/RT) has been misdiagnosed as medulloblastoma or PNET; however, mutation of the hSNF5/INI1 gene is observed in most AT/RT and can now be used as a molecular diagnostic tool for this tumor.[20] Together, these recent discoveries, derived substantially from the rapid technological advancement in the molecular interrogation of tumors, have led to an emerging new view of medulloblastoma and other embryonal tumors.

Glial Tumors Pediatric and adult astrocytomas of the same WHO histologic classification have been shown to have significant differences in the incidence of p53 and PTEN mutations, EGFR amplification or expression, and loss of heterozygosity (LOH) at 17p13.1, 9p21, and 10q23–25.[21–24] Pediatric high grade astrocytomas (HGA) lack amplification of the EGFR gene compared with EGFR amplification in one-third of adult glioblastomas.[22] In another pediatric series, EGFR amplification was not detected in any case; however, PTEN mutations were significantly associated with decreased survival among grade III and grade IV patients.[23] These data indicate that the development of pediatric HGA may follow different pathways from the paradigm of adult glioblastomas. Oligodendroglioma (OG), although rare in children, also appears to be molecularly divergent from OG in adults since alterations in 1p or 19q in one study were much less frequently seen in childhood OG.[25] Ependymoma, a more frequent glial tumor of childhood, has been shown to overexpress the ERBB2 and ERBB4 receptors in 75% of tumors, and similar to medulloblastoma, is associated with more aggressive behavior.[26]

Angiogenesis The regulation of angiogenesis in pediatric CNS tumors remains largely unknown. Two reports have investigated the microvessel density (MVD) and angiogenic profile of childhood PNETs/medulloblastomas (MB). The expression of eight angiogenic factors, (vascular endothelial growth factors [VEGF, VEGF-B, VEGF-C], basic fibroblast growth factor [bFGF], angiopoietins [Ang-1, Ang-2], transforming growth factor [TGF-alpha], and platelet-derived growth factor [PDGF-A]) was examined in 28 primary PNET/MB. The mRNA expression levels of the angiogenic factors were compared with MVD, TrkC mRNA expression, clinical variables and survival outcomes. The results showed that all PNET/MB tested produce a wide range of angiogenic factors, although no clear associations with MVD, gene expression, or outcome were observed.[27,28] A more recent expression profiling study of angiogenesis genes in childhood astrocytomas revealed increased expression of the EGFR/HIF/IGFBP2 pathway in malignant tumors.[24]

INVASION AND METASTASIS

The mechanisms promoting invasion and metastasis in pediatric CNS tumors are relatively undefined. A study compared gene expression profiles of metastatic (M+) versus non-metastatic (M0) medulloblastomas at the time of diagnosis and found the platelet-derived growth factor receptor beta (PDGFR-β) and members of the Ras/MAP kinase pathways significantly upregulated in the M+ tumors. These results suggest that this growth factor-mediated signal pathway may be critical in the control of metastasis of these tumors.[29] In another study, ERBB2 was found to upregulate S100A4 and other prometastatic genes, including several targets of the PDGFR pathway, in medulloblastoma.[30]

In adult gliomas, matrix metalloproteinases (MMPs) appear to play an important role in facilitating invasion by remodeling the extracellular matrix (ECM). One pediatric study examined 24 astrocytomas for MMP immunoreactivity. Positive staining for MMP-3 and -10 was observed in the ECM surrounding over 90% of the tumor cells. However, no immunoreactivity was detected for MMP-2, -9, and -13, the most commonly expressed MMPs in adult astrocytomas.[31]

In another pediatric study, p53, bcl-2, Mib-1, MVD, and correlation with metastasis was examined. None of the parameters studied were associated with metastasis nor any of the biological markers tested.[32]

Identification of cancer initiating stem cells in human brain tumors, including childhood medulloblastoma, has been demonstrated which should provide invaluable insight into the molecular alterations and mechanistic pathways for tumor development.[33] Further characterization of these molecular changes is expected to have a profound impact on the diagnosis, prognosis and future treatment of pediatric CNS tumors. The molecular alterations associated with specific subtypes of childhood CNS tumors are summarized in Table 124e-1.

Table 124e-1 Common Molecular Genetic Associations with Childhood CNS Tumors

Epidermal Growth Factor Receptor (EGFR)
HGA: protein over-expressed (80%), amplification rare[24,84]
TP53
HGA: mutated (34%), < 3 yrs.(12%), > 3 yrs. (40%)[85]
5-yr PFS-low expression (44 %), high expression (17%)[86]
EP: mutations not found[87]
IGCT: mutated (6%), over-expression (75%)[88]
Chromosome 17p
HGA: deletions (75%)[89]
JPA: deletions (10%)[89]
MB: deletions (35–50%), most common MB alteration[17–19,90]
SPNET: deletions not found[87,91]
EP: deletions (50–78%)[87]
Rb
HGA: deletions for p16INK4a and p14ARF (10%)[92]
IGCT: p14ARF mutated (71%); GGCT (90%), NGGCT (55%)[93]
TrkC (neurotrophin-3 receptor)
MB: expression correlates with good outcome[94,95]
ErbB2 oncogene (EGFR/HER family)
MB: expression (40%), correlates with poor outcome[14]
C-Myc oncogene
MB: expression correlates with poor survival[13]
PTCH/Sonic Hedgehog (chromosome 9q22)
MB: mutated (2–10%)[6–12]
Other genetic alterations
MB: del 10q, 11; gains 17q, 7 (60%)[96]
EP: del 6q, 22q, X ; gains 1q, 9[97]
hSNF5/INI1 mutations (del 22q)
ATRT: mutations diagnostic[20]

ATRT = atypical teratoid rhabdoid tumor; CNS = central nervous system; EP = ependymoma; GGCT = germinomatous germ cell tumor; HGA = high-grade astrocytoma; IGCT = intracranial germ cell tumor; JPA = juvenile pilocytic astrocytoma; MB = medulloblastoma; NGGCT = non-germinomatous germ cell tumor; SPNET = supratentorial primitive neuroectodermal tumor.

TREATMENT

Special Considerations in the Treatment of the Infant Approximately 70% of brain tumors in children under 2 years of age are made up of three distinct types: medulloblastoma, ependymoma, and low-grade astrocytoma. Less commonly, infants may be diagnosed with teratomas (mature or immature) or the atypical teratoid/rhabdoid tumor (AT/RT).

Historically, brain tumors in children have been treated by surgical excision and, for those tumors with a propensity toward recurrence with metastasis, craniospinal irradiation. Of special concern with regard to the treatment of CNS tumors in children, especially in the child under the age of 3, is the immaturity of the CNS and its sensitivity to the long-term effects of radiation. Thus, the volume and dose that can be safely given without causing extensive neuro-cognitive and endocrinologic sequelae is limited. In general, CNS tumors are more chemo-responsive in children than in adults. Because of this, attention has been directed toward exploiting the potential therapeutic advantage of chemotherapy and newer biologic agents with the aim of delaying or avoiding radiation therapy.

Non-radiotherapy treatment strategies for childhood CNS tumors can be broadly separated into two categories: methods that increase the amount of drug delivered to the sites of disease and therapeutics that exploit the biological characteristics of the tumor. These novel treatment strategies are summarized in Table 124e-2.

Focal Radiotherapy Techniques Despite recent advances, chemotherapy alone has not produced durable responses in a significant proportion of patients. It continues to be necessary in most cases to use limited field irradiation to prevent local recurrences. 3-D conformal radiotherapy attempts to minimize toxicity by integrating many beams, precisely directing radiotherapy to the tumor site although leaving untargeted areas minimally exposed. The success of this technique depends upon precise localization of the tumor and normal structures by integrating CT or MR imaging with reproducible patient positioning.

Intensity-modulated radiation therapy (IMRT) is a new conformal technique that makes use of 3-D based treatment planning and non-uniform radiation beams. The high-dose treatment volume can then be made to conform to an irregular target. In one study, the incidence of radiation-induced ototoxicity was retrospectively assessed in twenty-six pediatric patients treated for medulloblastoma with either conventional radiotherapy (RT) or IMRT. In the IMRT Group, only 68% of the radiation dose was delivered to the auditory apparatus and only 13% had Grade 3 or 4 hearing loss, compared to 64% of the RT Group.[34]

ASTROCYTIC TUMORS

The incidence of cortical astrocytomas increases with age, having a first peak at age 5 and again at age 13.[1] In children, brain stem and cerebellar astrocytomas are as common as cortical tumors.

Table 124e-2 Novel Treatment Strategies in Childhood CNS Tumors

A. Treatment strategies that increase drug delivery to tumor
High-Dose Systemic Therapy
Thiotepa/Busulfan: relapsed tumors, 26% response rate[98]
Carboplatin/Thiotepa/VP-16: relapsed MB, 3-year EFS (34%)[72]
Newly diagnosed, 3-yr EFS (25%)[99]
Regional Therapy
Intraventricular Mafosfamide: disseminated tumors, CR/PR (68%)[100]
Blood-Brain Barrier Disruption
Bradykinin agonist (RMP-7): in combination with carboplatin[101]
B. Treatment strategies targeting tumor biology
Angiogenesis Inhibitors
SU5416: inhibits VEGF
Cilengitide: integrin antagonist
Thalidomide and thalidomide analogues: mechanism unknown
Radiosensitizers
Topotecan and Taxol
Gd-texaphyrin: porphyrin compound conjugated to gadolinium[102]
Immunotherapy
Interferon and interferon-inducers[103]
Poly-IC double stranded RNA[104]
Differentiation Therapy
ATRA and Fenretinide: retinoic acid and retinoid derivatives
Phenylacetate and phenylbutyrate[105,106]
Gene Therapy
HSV 1-TK gene and ganciclovir: phase I, recurrent supratentorial tumors[107]
Signal Transduction Inhibitors
Gleevec: inhibits bcr/abl, PDGFR, and c-kit[108–111]
Iressa: inhibits EGFR
Lapatinib/Erlotinib: inhibits ERBB family receptors
Farnesyl transferase inhibitors: inhibits Ras and other farnesylated proteins

EFS = event free survival; EGFR = epidermal growth factor receptor; ERBB = avian erythroblastic leukemia viral oncogene homolog; HSV 1-TK = herpes simplex virus type 1-thymidine kinase; PDGFR = platelet-derived growth factor receptor.

Cerebellar Astrocytoma This tumor is found almost exclusively in children, occurring most frequently between ages 4 to 9. Juvenile pilocytic astrocytoma (JPA) is the most common subtype, accounting for 85% of cerebellar astrocytomas.[3] Diffuse astrocytoma is the next most common, whereas malignant astrocytoma is rare in this location.

Children typically present with headache, vomiting, papilledema, and gait disturbance.

CT and MRI reveal either a large solid (20%) or mixed solid and cystic (80%) circumscribed mass that enhances with contrast (Figure 124e-1).[35]

Pilocytic tumors are well circumscribed and characterized by a biphasic pattern with varying proportion of bipolar cells with Rosenthal fibers and loose multipolar cells with microcysts (Figure 124e-2).[36]

Total surgical resection is curative in 95 to 100%.[37,38] JPAs may stabilize for long periods of time or even spontaneously regress; however, the behavior of cerebellar astrocytomas in children with

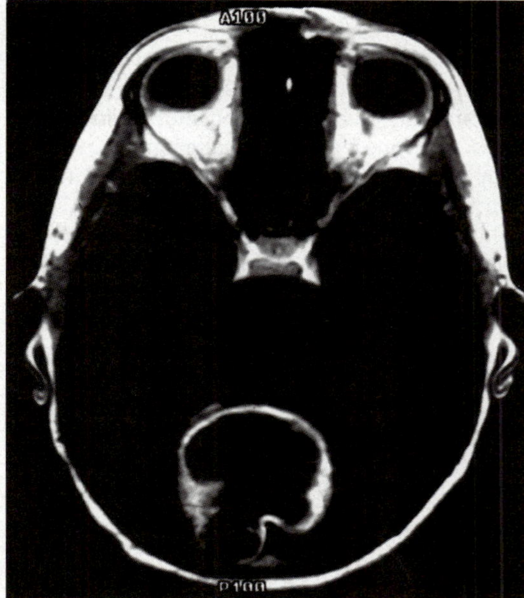

Figure 124e-1 T_1-weighted magnetic resonance image of a juvenile pilocytic astrocytoma with prominent cyst formation.

neurofibromatosis type I (NF-1) may be more aggressive. Those children whose lesions are inoperable due to brain stem involvement may require additional therapy, though residual tumor may remain quiescent for years, and thus irradiation and/or chemotherapy should be reserved for tumors that demonstrate clear growth or symptomatic change.[39] Rare malignant cerebellar astrocytomas have a poor outcome and require aggressive treatment similar to supratentorial high-grade astrocytomas.

Diencephalic Glioma Gliomas of the visual pathway, hypothalamus, and thalamus comprise a relatively common form of childhood astrocytoma. Tumors of the optic chiasm and hypothalamus are usually low-grade, whereas thalamic tumors tend to be more variable. Twenty percent of children with NF-1 will develop visual pathway tumors, predominantly JPA, during childhood.[40]

Visual pathway tumors may cause visual loss, strabismus, proptosis, and/or nystagmus. Hypothalamic tumors usually present with endocrinologic disturbances, including precocious puberty. Thalamic tumors present more commonly with unilateral motor deficits contralateral to the site of the lesion.[40]

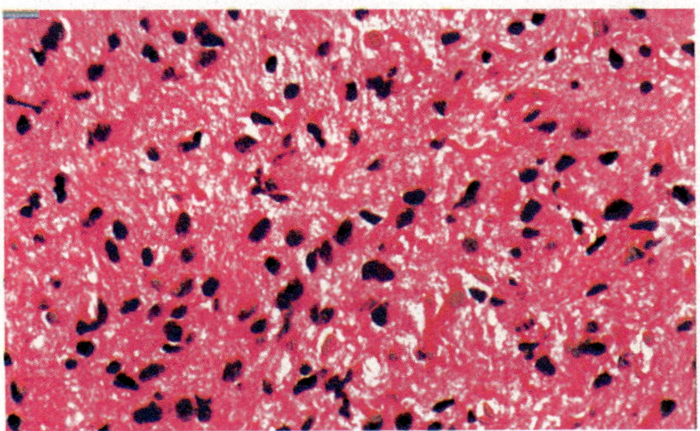

Figure 124e-2 Hematoxylin-eosin stained section (400×) of a juvenile pilocytic astrocytoma demonstrating prominent Rosenthal fibers.

Imaging demonstrates similar characteristics of low-grade and high-grade gliomas that present elsewhere. Optic pathway lesions have limited capacity to spread as they are confined to migrate between optic nerve and chiasm.[40]

Following surgical resection, radiation therapy from 5,000 to 5,500 cGy is generally reserved for older children with progressive or symptomatic diencephalic tumors, especially thalamic gliomas. Therapy with carboplatin and vincristine has demonstrated tumor shrinkage and/or stabilization in over 90% of children less than 5 years of age.[41,42] In children with NF-1, tumor biopsy for histologic confirmation is not necessary owing to the highly characteristic appearance on MRI. In these children, lesions may be detected by routine screening before the onset of symptoms and thus many will not require any treatment. Thalamic high-grade gliomas are treated as malignant cortical gliomas.

Low-Grade Cortical Glioma Most low-grade cortical gliomas in children are JPAs or diffuse fibrillary astrocytoma. Other forms, such as oligodendroglioma, oligoastrocytoma, and mixed glioma are much less common.[1]

Low-grade cortical gliomas most commonly present with headache and seizure.

On CT, diffuse astrocytomas appear as ill-defined, homogeneous masses of low density without contrast enhancement. MRI usually shows a mass that is hypodense on T_1-weighted and hyperintense on T_2-weighted images with little enhancement. Imaging of JPA lesions are similar to the cerebellar counterpart.[43]

Complete surgical resection is curative for most, and even with incomplete excision, long-term progression-free survival is common.[44] If subsequent progression occurs then re-resection is generally undertaken. For patients with progressive disease not amenable to resection, irradiation from 5,000 to 5,500 cGy is warranted. Chemotherapy is reserved for very young children and infants. Overall, 5-year survival is 95%; whereas progression-free survival is 88%. Less favorable results have been seen in patients with non-pilocytic astrocytoma.[45]

High-Grade Cortical Glioma These tumors present most frequently between 5 to 10 years of age.[46]

Patients may present with headaches, motor weakness, personality changes, and seizures; however, seizures are more typical of low-grade cortical lesions.[47]

On CT and MRI, HGA typically appear as irregularly shaped lesions with partial contrast enhancement and peritumoral edema with or without mass effect.[36]

Radical (> 90%) surgical resection is the most powerful predictor of favorable outcome in HGA when followed by irradiation.[48,49] However, only 49% of tumors in the superficial hemisphere and 8% of tumors in the midline or deep cerebrum are amenable to radical resection. Local or wide-field irradiation from 5,000 to 6,000 cGy is the mainstay of therapy. The addition of radiation therapy has improved 5-year survival rates (10–30%) compared to surgery alone (0%).[50] Although initial reports demonstrated a benefit of adjuvant chemotherapy with prednisone, CCNU, and vincristine (pCV) compared to radiotherapy alone (46% vs 18%), a subsequent trial comparing pCV to the "8-in-1" regimen failed to show the same benefit (26%).[51,52] A review of the histology from the original trial with pCV suggested that a significant portion of patients (69/250) actually did not meet the central consensus definition of HGA. To date, no large randomized clinical trial has clearly demonstrated a benefit of chemotherapy. High-dose chemotherapy for HGA has shown effective responses, however, and despite significant associated toxicity, may warrant further investigation.[53]

Brain Stem Glioma Brain stem gliomas (BSG) comprise 10 to 15% of all pediatric CNS tumors and are generally uncommon in the adult population. Peak incidence is between the ages of 5 to 9 years of age, but may occur anytime during childhood.[1]

BSGs most commonly arise in the pons (diffuse intrinsic), in which location they typically resemble adult glioblastomas multiforme (GBM) and have an almost uniformly dismal prognosis. In contrast, those arising from midbrain or medulla are likely to be low-grade lesions that have a more indolent course and better outcome. BSGs commonly present with multiple cranial nerve deficits, especially sixth and seventh nerve palsies, long track signs, and cerebellar deficits.[54]

Diffuse pontine gliomas show CT and MRI characteristics similar to HGA within an enlarged pons (Figure 124e-3). Low-grade BSGs are relatively discrete, often exophytic and contrast enhancing with cyst formation.[36]

Treatment is local irradiation from 5,500 to 6,000 cGy. Over 90% of patients with diffuse intrinsic lesions transiently respond, but ultimately succumb to disease progression within 18 months of diagnosis. Neither hyperfractionated radiotherapy nor chemotherapy has been shown to add benefit.[55] Low-grade lesions are treated with similar irradiation doses, but overall respond less favorably than their counterparts in other locations.[54,56]

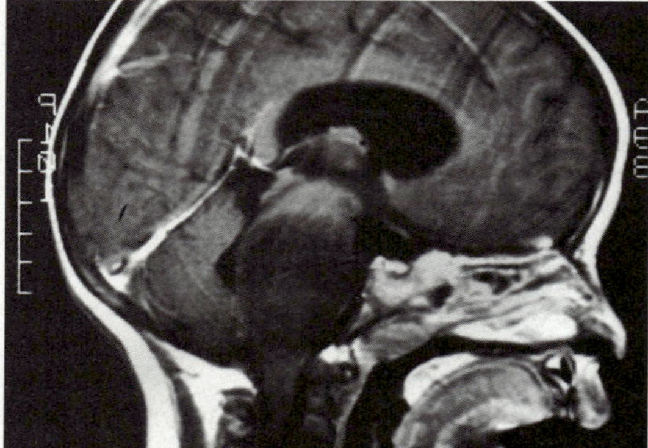

Figure 124e-3 T_1-weighted image of an intrinsic brainstem glioma.

EMBRYONAL TUMORS

Embryonal tumors of the central nervous system comprise a group of tumors that share a histologically similar, undifferentiated morphology, and represent the most common malignant brain tumor group in children (21%). The incidence is constant from infancy to 3 years of age (11.6 to 10.2 per million) and then a steady decline is observed thereafter.[1] This group includes the primitive neuroectodermal tumors (PNET), ependymoblastoma, and atypical teratoid/rhabdoid tumor (AT/RT). PNETs are further subdivided by anatomic location into medulloblastoma (posterior fossa) and supratentorial PNET. Controversy has existed regarding the class division between supratentorial PNET and medulloblastoma but the preponderance of molecular genetic, biologic and clinical evidence validates this division.[5]

PNET/Medulloblastoma Medulloblastoma is the most common malignant CNS tumor of childhood, comprising 40% of all posterior fossa tumors and 20% of all pediatric brain tumors. The peak incidence occurs between 3 to 4 years of age and there is a male predilection of 1.5- to 2-fold.[1] Dissemination at diagnosis is found 11 to 43% of the time and remains one of the most important clinical predictors of outcome.[57,58] Extraneural spread can occur to the bones, bone marrow, lymph nodes, liver, and lung although this is a rare occurrence.

Medulloblastoma typically arises in the midline of the cerebellum, growing into and compressing the fourth ventricle. Therefore, it often presents with the findings associated with increased intracranial pressure such as nausea, vomiting, irritability, lethargy, gait ataxia, and dysmetria.

On CT scan, medulloblastoma appears as a well-defined cerebellar mass. Calcification is present in up to 20% of cases.[59] MRI reveals a homogeneous hypointense T_1 signal and contrast enhancement is similarly homogeneous (Figure 124e-4). Other

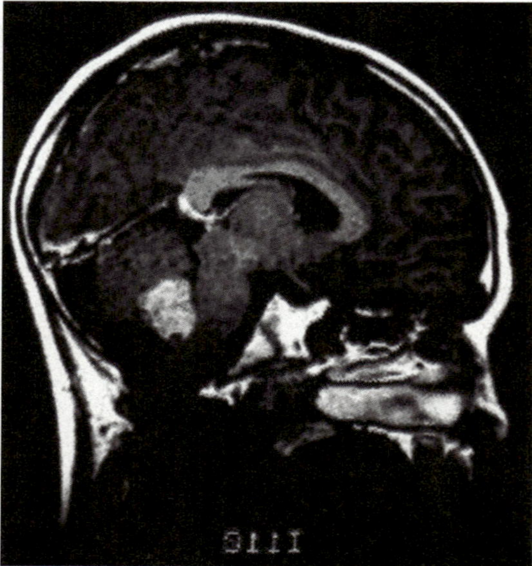

Figure 124e-4 T_1 weighted gadolinium enhanced magnetic resonance image of a medulloblastoma.

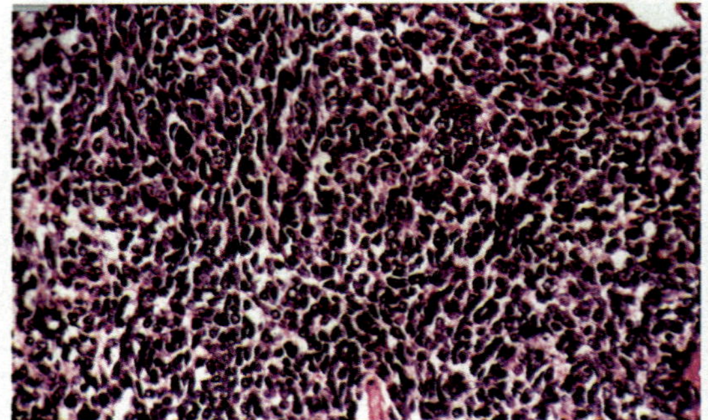

Figure 124e-5 Hematoxylin-eosin stained section (250×) of classic medulloblastoma/primitive neuroectodermal tumor.

characteristic findings of the tumor include cyst formation, necrosis, and hemorrhage.[60]

Medulloblastoma is a tumor characterized on light microscopy by sheets of small round blue cells with dense, hyperchromatic nuclei, and very little cytoplasm (Figure 124e-5).

Treatment groups designated high risk and standard risk are created based upon the criteria of age greater than or less than 3 years, residual tumor greater than or less than 1.5 cm^2, and the presence or absence of metastatic disease on neuroimaging or cerebrospinal fluid (CSF) sampling.[61] Age younger than 3 years is predictive of a poor outcome. This fact is difficult to separate from the finding that younger children more commonly present with metastatic disease,[62] are less likely to be treated with conventional doses of radiotherapy,[63] and are more likely to have subtotal tumor resection.[64] Extent of resection was found to correlate with better survival for patients without metastatic disease in the Children's Cancer Group study 921.[65] Metastatic disease at the time of diagnosis has been repeatedly correlated with poor survival, the exception being M1 disease, defined as CSF cytology positive for medulloblastoma cells.[66,67]

The goal of surgical resection is complete removal of tumor whenever possible while maintaining acceptable postoperative morbidity. Approximately 10% of patients suffer from the cerebellar mutism syndrome postoperatively which consists of pseudobulbar signs and an inability to speak.[68]

Medulloblastoma is a very radiosensitive tumor and radiotherapy has historically been the cornerstone of treatment for this tumor. Given the ability of this tumor to disseminate, especially upon relapse, craniospinal radiotherapy has been necessary to maximize survival.[69] Unfortunately, the neuropsychological and endocrine effects of radiation to the developing neuraxis have exacted a high price for this protection. Chemotherapy has been explored as a means to allow for a reduction in the radiation dose that is administered to the entire neuraxis. Medulloblastoma responds to a range of alkylator and platinum based drugs. A Children's Cancer Group protocol reduced the craniospinal dose from the standard 3,600 cGy to 2,340 cGy with the addition of adjuvant chemotherapy consisting of vincristine, cisplatin, and CCNU. Progression free survival was 86% at 3 years and 79% at 5 years.[70] These rates compare favorably with historical controls. A nationwide trial has been completed using an identical radiation dose scheme and a randomization between the maintenance chemotherapy regimen described above and one substituting cyclophosphamide for CCNU. The outcome of this study is awaited to confirm these promising results for reduced dose craniospinal radiation. For relapsed medulloblastoma, future Children's Oncology Group studies will focus on the utility of high-dose chemotherapy and stem cell rescue followed by retinoids as a differentiating agent. Strategies for high-risk medulloblastoma are still not clear, although the addition of methotrexate to high-dose chemotherapy regimens is under consideration.

Despite this reduction in the dose of craniospinal radiation dose, neurocognitive deficits were still noted in a companion study to the above treatment protocol. Forty-three of the enrolled patients underwent longitudinal intelligence testing. The estimated rate of change from baseline was –4.3 Full Scale Intelligence Quotient points per year, –4.2 Verbal IQ points per year, and –4.0 Nonverbal IQ points per year ($p < .001$ for all three outcomes). Females, children less than 7 years of age, and those with higher baseline IQs were at greatest risk.[71]

In very young children, for whom the long-term neurocognitive sequelae of radiotherapy are unacceptable, chemotherapy has been used in an attempt to delay or obviate the need for radiation. One method for increasing the delivered dose of chemotherapy is to increase the administered dose to a level that would otherwise be toxic to the bone marrow and then infusing autologous stem cells (ASC) to rescue the hematopoietic system. In a study of 23 relapsed medulloblastoma patients who received a high-dose chemotherapy regimen consisting of carboplatin, thiotepa, and etoposide with ASC rescue, a 3-year EFS of 34% and an 3-year overall survival of 46% was achieved.[72] Trials of high-dose chemotherapy with ASC rescue are ongoing as a strategy to delay or obviate the need for radiotherapy in the patient less than 3 years of age with a malignant brain tumor and preliminary results are promising, especially in the patients with completely resected, non-disseminated disease.

Supratentorial PNET This rare malignant primitive tumor is most often found in the cerebrum, suprasellar, or pineal region of children in their first decade of life.[73]

Supratentorial PNET presents with symptomatology dependent upon location. Paresis and seizures can occur when the tumor involves the cortex, symptoms of increased intracranial pressure (ICP) are seen when the flow of CSF is disrupted, and endocrinopathies or visual deficits result from suprasellar tumors. Infants in whom the cranial sutures have not fused can present with a rapidly increasing head circumference.

These tumors are characterized by hemorrhage, calcifications, necrosis, and cyst formation. The former two findings result in increased T_1 signal and the latter two in increased T_2 signal on MR imaging.[74] As with all malignant brain tumors of childhood, imaging of the entire neuraxis and CSF sampling should be performed to define the extent of disease.

Histological findings are basically similar to medulloblastoma and common to all PNETs. The predominant cell type is termed the small round blue cell that is characterized by little differentiation, a deeply basophilic nucleus, and very little cytoplasm. Homer-Wright rosettes, necrosis, hemorrhage, Flexner-Wintersteiner rosettes, and occasional melanotic cells are also found.[36]

The role of complete surgical resection has not been established in this tumor. Given the propensity of supratentorial PNET to invade local structures as well as their large size, complete resection is often not possible with acceptable surgical morbidity.

Doses of 3,600 cGy craniospinal with boost to 5,400 cGy have been used to treat this tumor when neurodevelopmentally appropriate. When used as the only postoperative treatment, results are dismal.

Supratentorial PNET has been shown to be sensitive to various chemotherapeutic agents and responses are seen in up to 50% of patients. Regimens of postoperative chemoradiotherapy for non-pineal supratentorial PNET have produced 5-year survival in approximately one-third of patients with children less than 2 years of age faring more poorly.[64] Although infants presenting with tumor localizing to the pineal region did poorly, older patients with tumor in this location may represent a subset with a better prognosis.[64,75]

Atypical Teratoid/Rhabdoid Tumor Atypical teratoid/rhabdoid tumor is an aggressively malignant, primitive tumor most often arising in children younger than 2 years of age.[36,76] These tumors have only recently been recognized as an entity distinct from PNET due to their histological similarity with two-thirds containing foci morphologically indistinct from PNET.

Approximately half of AT/RTs arise in the infratentorial compartment with a propensity to invade the cerebello-pontine angle.[77] Because of its association with chromosome 22 deletion and INI1-mutation, analysis of these markers in infants with presumed MB/PNET should be considered for all children with brain tumors who are less than 1 year of age.

Signs and symptoms at presentation include those attributed to increased ICP. Focal findings related to cranial nerve involvement, especially the sixth and seventh nerves, are common in tumors invading the cerebello-pontine angle. The ability of these tumors to disseminate along CSF pathways is well known.

Heterogeneous enhancement, cyst formation, and hemorrhage are common findings on CT imaging.[77]

The histological hallmark of AT/RT is the presence of rhabdoid cells. These cells are characterized by a variable size, eccentric nucleus with a prominent nucleolus and a cytoplasmic inclusion that is pink (Figure 124e-6). These rhabdoid foci occur variously in conjunction with a small round cell embryonal or a mesenchymal component.[36] AT/RT are briskly mitotic with an MIB-1/Ki-67 labeling index of up to 80%.[77]

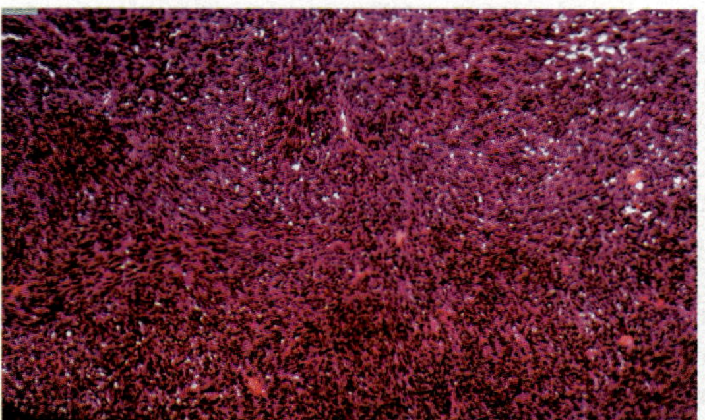

Figure 124e-6 Hematoxylin-eosin stained section (100×) of an atypical teratoid/rhabdoid tumor.

No effective treatment for AT/RT has yet been found. Strategies employed have been those common to the treatment of malignant embryonal tumors in young children, namely surgical resection followed by chemotherapy and radiation where neuro-developmentally appropriate. The role of complete resection is unclear and often complicated by proximity to the cerebello-pontine angle and brainstem. These tumors are often found to be chemosensitive, although they typically recur within 6 months and progress rapidly. The majority of patients die within 1 year of diagnosis and no prognostic factors have been elucidated.

EPENDYMAL TUMORS

As the third most common CNS tumor of childhood, ependymoma makes up 9% of childhood CNS tumors with approximately two-thirds occurring infratentorially. Greater than half of these tumors occur in children less than 5 years of age with a peak during the second year of life (8.6 per million).[1]

Ependymal tumors are usually found adjacent to the normal sites of ependymal cell residence; namely along the surface of the ventricles or in the parenchyma adjacent to the ventricles. Tumor extension occurs along the ventricular and subarachnoid CSF spaces. Based upon the degree of histologic anaplasia, ependymoma is divided into high-grade and low-grade tumors.

Infratentorial tumors often present with signs and symptoms of increased intracranial pressure. They may also present with signs of cerebellar dysfunction and deficits of cranial nerves VI to X. Supratentorial tumors may present with focal findings including visual field defects, focal seizures, or non-specific symptoms of headache, nausea, or vomiting.

Characteristic features of ependymoma that may yield findings upon neuroimaging include frequent calcification, cyst formation, hemorrhage, and necrosis. Gadolinium enhancement is often heterogeneous and patchy. The entire neuraxis should be imaged at the time of diagnosis to evaluate for metastatic disease.

The mainstay of therapy for ependymoma of all grades is surgery with complete resection as the goal. Unfortunately, complete tumor removal is only achieved in 40% and most of these are supratentorial in location.

Postoperative radiotherapy has been practiced since the 1950s and has become standard therapy owing to the substantial improvement in survival that it provides. In a comparison of patients treated with surgery alone or surgery plus radiation therapy, the survival rates were 17 and 40%, respectively.[78] The extent of the field involved has been the subject of some debate. Progression and recurrence is typically local with a less than 10% incidence for distant spread. The relative rarity of distant relapse has called into question the practice of prophylactic craniospinal radiotherapy regardless of site and histology of primary tumor and it is no longer recommended. The exception to this is in tumors with evidence of subarachnoid dissemination. Spinal tumors, which are completely resected, do not necessitate radiotherapy. For infratentorial tumors, the radiation field must be planned to account for the propensity of these tumors to invade the spine to the level of C2 to C4.

The addition of chemotherapy to surgery and radiotherapy for childhood ependymoma has not been proven effective. However, the clinical scenarios in which chemotherapy is achieving greater enthusiasm are in infants less than 3 years of age as a means to delay radiation therapy and as neoadjuvant therapy prior to second look surgery for incompletely resected tumors. In the Pediatric Oncology Group study of postoperative vincristine, cyclophosphamide, cisplatin, and etoposide chemotherapy with deferred irradiation for infants less than 3 with malignant brain tumors, the 2-year progression-free survival for children with ependymoma was 42%, with a 2-year survival of 74%.[64] The single prospective randomized trial (CCG-942) completed in children compared postoperative craniospinal radiation to radiation in combination with chemotherapy consisting of vincristine, CCNU, and prednisone. The 5-year progression-free survival was 45% in patients receiving chemotherapy plus radiation therapy, and 35% in patients receiving radiation therapy alone; the difference was not statistically significant.[79] However, chemotherapy may make residual tumor more amenable to second surgery, which could potentially improve outcome. The current Children's Oncology Group study for ependymomas is investigating this concept. This study is also investigating whether completely resected supratentorial ependymomas without anaplasia require no further intervention to maintain good outcome.

Spinal ependymoma enjoys an overall 5-year survival of greater than 95%. In contrast, ependymoma of childhood has an unfavorable prognosis with a 5-year overall survival of approximately 45% in aggregate and a median time to progression of 18 months. Unfortunately, in many cases, survival carries the high price of focal neurologic, neuroendocrinologic, psychological, and neurocognitive sequelae.

GERM CELL TUMORS

Intracranial germ cell tumors (IGCTs) account for less than 5% of pediatric CNS tumors but are primarily seen in children and adolescence, with 90% occurring in those less than 20 years.[36] Incidence peaks at age 10 to 12 years. They account for nearly 50% of all pineal region tumors of childhood. The incidence is higher in Japan and Asia.[36] More than 80% arise in the midline. IGCTs consist of a variety of histologic entities including germinoma, malignant germ cell (embryonal carcinoma, yolk sac/endodermal sinus tumor, choriocarcinoma), mature and immature teratoma, teratoma with malignant transformation, and mixed germ cell.

Tumors of the pineal region often obstruct the cerebral aqueduct, resulting in hydrocephalus and raised ICP. These lesions are also likely to compress the tectal plate, producing a characteristic upward gaze palsy and loss of convergence known as Parinaud syndrome. Suprasellar tumors typically impinge the optic chiasm and cause visual field deficits and disturb the hypothalamic-pituitary axis resulting in diabetes insipidus, retarded growth, and sometimes-precocious puberty.[80]

On CT and MRI scan IGCTs usually appear as solid midline masses that show prominent contrast enhancement. Teratoma is suggested by midline lesions containing intratumoral cysts with calcifications and fat.[36]

Germinoma is composed of primitive germ cells with large vesicular nuclei and clear cytoplasm. Germinomas may contain synciotrophoblastic giant cells that secrete β-hCG. This marker may be detected in both serum and CSF, but usually at much lower levels than that expressed by malignant IGCTs. Teratomas may be mature, composed of differentiated tissue (ie, bone, fat, and muscle) with low mitotic activity, or immature, composed of undifferentiated tissues. Yolk sac tumors demonstrate primitive epithelial cells in a myxoid matrix resembling embryonic mesoblast and are immunoreactive for AFP, which may be detected as a secreted marker in the serum and/or CSF. Embryonal carcinoma contains large cells with clear cytoplasm that line irregular, gland-like spaces. These malignant tumors show high mitotic activity and immunoreactivity for cytokeratins. Choriocarcinoma is characterized by cytotrophoblastic differentiation and synciotrophoblastic giant cells. Immunohistochemical staining as well as serum and/or CSF are usually highly positive for β-hCG.[36]

The most important predictive feature of IGCT outcome is histologic subtype. Pure germinomas, which have negative serum and CSF markers for AFP and negative to low β-hCG, are sensitive to craniospinal irradiation, and as such, have > 95% survival rate.[80] Current clinical studies are looking at whether the addition of chemotherapy will allow volume and dose reduction of irradiation.[81] Attempts to treat these tumors with chemotherapy alone have shown complete response rates of 78%, but only 60 to 70% OS.[82] Patients with malignant IGCT have a much worse prognosis. The best results have been obtained with platinum-based chemotherapy and full-dose craniospinal RT, although 5-year OS remains 40 to 50%. Pure teratomas are typically unresponsive to chemotherapy or radiotherapy and surgery is the only proven treatment.[83]

REFERENCES

1. Gurney JG SM, Bunin GR. CNS and miscellaneous intracranial and intraspinal neoplasms. In: Ries LAG, SM Gurney JG, editors. Cancer incidence and survival among children and adolescents: United States SEER Program 1975–1995. NIH Pub No 99-4649. Bethesda: National Cancer Institute SEER Program; 1999. p. 51–63.
2. Bleyer WA. Epidemiologic impact of children with brain tumors. Childs Nerv Syst 1999;15:758–63.
3. Rickert CH, Paulus W. Epidemiology of central nervous system tumors in childhood and adolescence based on the new WHO classification. Childs Nerv Syst 2001;17:503–11.
4. Bunin G. What causes childhood brain tumors? Limited knowledge, many clues. Pediatr Neurosurg 2000;32:321–6.
5. Pomeroy SL, Tamayo P, Gaasenbeek M, et al. Prediction of central nervous system embryonal tumour outcome based on gene expression. Nature 2002;415:436–42.
6. Zurawel RH, Allen C, Chiappa S, et al. Analysis of PTCH/SMO/SHH pathway genes in medulloblastoma. Genes Chromosomes Cancer 2000;27:44–51.
7. Hallahan AR, Pritchard JI, Hansen S, et al. The SmoA1 mouse model reveals that notch signaling is critical for the growth and survival of sonic hedgehog-induced medulloblastomas. Cancer Res 2004;64:7794–800.
8. Taylor MD, Liu L, Raffel C, et al. Mutations in SUFU predispose to medulloblastoma. Nat Genet 2002;31:306–10.
9. Wetmore C, Eberhart DE, Curran T. Loss of p53 but not ARF accelerates medulloblastoma in mice heterozygous for patched. Cancer Res 2001;61:513–6.
10. Berman DM, Karhadkar SS, Hallahan AR, et al. Medulloblastoma growth inhibition by hedgehog pathway blockade. Science 2002;297:1559–61.
11. Romer JT, Kimura H, Magdaleno S, et al. Suppression of the Shh pathway using a small molecule inhibitor eliminates medulloblastoma in Ptc1(+/–)p53(–/–) mice. Cancer Cell 2004;6:229–40.
12. Kimura H, Stephen D, Joyner A, Curran T. Gli1 is important for medulloblastoma formation in Ptc1(+/-) mice. Oncogene 2005;
13. Eberhart CG, Kratz J, Wang Y, et al. Histopathological and molecular prognostic markers in medulloblastoma: c-myc, N-myc, TrkC, and anaplasia. J Neuropathol Exp Neurol 2004;63:441–9.
14. Gajjar A, Hernan R, Kocak M, et al. Clinical, histopathologic, and molecular markers of prognosis: toward a new disease risk stratification system for medulloblastoma. J Clin Oncol 2004;22:984–93.
15. Boon K, Eberhart CG, Riggins GJ. Genomic amplification of orthodenticle homologue 2 in medulloblastomas. Cancer Res 2005;65:703–7.
16. Di C, Liao S, Adamson DC, et al. Identification of OTX2 as a medulloblastoma oncogene whose product can be targeted by all-trans retinoic acid. Cancer Res 2005;65:919–24.
17. Zakrzewska M, Rieske P, Debiec-Rychter M, et al. Molecular abnormalities in pediatric embryonal brain tumors--analysis of loss of heterozygosity on chromosomes 1, 5, 9, 10, 11, 16, 17, and 22. Clin Neuropathol 2004;23:209–17.
18. Rood BR, Zhang H, Weitman DM, Cogen PH. Hypermethylation of HIC-1 and 17p allelic loss in medulloblastoma. Cancer Res 2002;62:3794–7.
19. Waha A, Waha A, Koch A, et al. Epigenetic silencing of the HIC-1 gene in human medulloblastomas. J Neuropathol Exp Neurol 2003;62:1192–201.
20. Judkins AR, Mauger J, Ht A, et al. Immunohistochemical analysis of hSNF5/INI1 in pediatric CNS neoplasms. Am J Surg Pathol 2004;28:644–50.
21. Cheng Y, Ng HK, Zhang SF, et al. Genetic alterations in pediatric high-grade astrocytomas. Hum Pathol 1999;30:1284–90.
22. Sung T, Miller DC, Hayes RL, et al. Preferential inactivation of the p53 tumor suppressor pathway and lack of EGFR amplification distinguish de novo high-grade pediatric astrocytomas from de novo adult astrocytomas. Brain Pathol 2000;10:249–59.
23. Raffel C, Frederick L, O'Fallon JR, et al. Analysis of oncogene and tumor suppressor gene alterations in pediatric malignant astrocytomas reveals reduced survival for patients with PTEN mutations. Clin Cancer Res 1999;5:4085–90.
24. Khatua S, Peterson KM, Brown KM, et al. Overexpression of the EGFR/FKBP12/HIF-2alpha pathway identified in

childhood astrocytomas by angiogenesis gene profiling. Cancer Res 2003;63:1865–70.
25. Raghavan R, Balani J, Perry A, et al. Pediatric oligodendrogliomas: a study of molecular alterations on 1p and 19q using fluorescence in situ hybridization. J Neuropathol Exp Neurol 2003;62:530–7.
26. Gilbertson RJ, Bentley L, Hernan R, et al. ERBB receptor signaling promotes ependymoma cell proliferation and represents a potential novel therapeutic target for this disease. Clin Cancer Res 2002;8:3054–64.
27. Huber H, Eggert A, Janss AJ, et al. Angiogenic profile of childhood primitive neuroectodermal brain tumours/medulloblastomas. Eur J Cancer 2001;37:2064–72.
28. Grotzer MA, Wiewrodt R, Janss AJ, et al. High microvessel density in primitive neuroectodermal brain tumors of childhood. Neuropediatrics 2001;32:75–9.
29. MacDonald TJ, Brown KM, LaFleur B, et al. Expression profiling of medulloblastoma: PDGFRA and the RAS/MAPK pathway as therapeutic targets for metastatic disease. Nat Genet 2001;29:143–52.
30. Hernan R, Fasheh R, Calabrese C, et al. ERBB2 up-regulates S100A4 and several other prometastatic genes in medulloblastoma. Cancer Res 2003;63:140–8.
31. Bodey B, Bodey B Jr, Siegel SE, Kaiser HE. Matrix metalloproteinase expression in childhood astrocytomas. Anticancer Res 2000;20:3287–92.
32. Miralbell R, Tolnay M, Bieri S, et al. Pediatric medulloblastoma: prognostic value of p53, bcl-2, Mib-1, and microvessel density. J Neurooncol 1999;45:103–10.
33. Singh SK, Hawkins C, Clarke ID, et al. Identification of human brain tumour initiating cells. Nature 2004;432:396–401.
34. Huang E, Teh BS, Strother DR, et al. Intensity-modulated radiation therapy for pediatric medulloblastoma: early report on the reduction of ototoxicity. Int J Radiat Oncol Biol Phys 2002;52:599–605.
35. Lapras C, Patet JD, Lapras C Jr, Mottolese C. Cerebellar astrocytomas in childhood. Childs Nerv Syst 1986;2:55–9.
36. Kleihues P, Cavenee W. Pathology and Genetics: Tumours of the Central Nervous System. In: Kleihues P, Sobin L, editors. World Health Organization Classification of Tumours. Lyon, France: IARC Press; 2000. p. 314.
37. Pencalet P, Maixner W, Sainte-Rose C, et al. Benign cerebellar astrocytomas in children. J Neurosurg 1999;90:265–73.
38. Undjian S, Marinov M, Georgiev K. Long-term follow-up after surgical treatment of cerebellar astrocytomas in 100 children. Childs Nerv Syst 1989;5:99–101.
39. Kayama T, Tominaga T, Yoshimoto T. Management of pilocytic astrocytoma. Neurosurg Rev 1996;19:217–20.
40. Burger PC, Cohen KJ, Rosenblum MK, Tihan T. Pathology of diencephalic astrocytomas. Pediatr Neurosurg 2000;32:214–9.
41. Gropman AL, Packer RJ, Nicholson HS, et al. Treatment of diencephalic syndrome with chemotherapy: growth, tumor response, and long term control. Cancer 1998;83:166–72.
42. Packer RJ. Chemotherapy: low-grade gliomas of the hypothalamus and thalamus. Pediatr Neurosurg 2000;32:259–63.
43. Finizio FS. CT and MRI aspects of supratentorial hemispheric tumors of childhood and adolescence. Childs Nerv Syst 1995;11:559–67.
44. Pollack IF. The role of surgery in pediatric gliomas. J Neurooncol 1999;42:271–88.
45. Pollack IF, Claassen D, al-Shboul Q, et al. Low-grade gliomas of the cerebral hemispheres in children: an analysis of 71 cases. J Neurosurg 1995;82:536–47.
46. Ciurea AV, Vasilescu G, Nuteanu L, et al. Neurosurgical management of cerebral astrocytomas in children. Ann N Y Acad Sci 1997;824:237–40.
47. Marchese MJ, Chang CH. Malignant astrocytic gliomas in children. Cancer 1990;65:2771–8.
48. Wolff JE, Gnekow AK, Kortmann RD, et al. Preradiation chemotherapy for pediatric patients with high-grade glioma. Cancer 2002;94:264–71.
49. Wisoff JH, Boyett JM, Berger MS, et al. Current neurosurgical management and the impact of the extent of resection in the treatment of malignant gliomas of childhood: a report of the Children's Cancer Group trial no. CCG-945. J Neurosurg 1998;89:52–9.
50. Bloom HJ, Glees J, Bell J, et al. The treatment and long-term prognosis of children with intracranial tumors: a study of 610 cases, 1950-1981. Int J Radiat Oncol Biol Phys 1990;18:723–45.
51. Sposto R, Ertel IJ, Jenkin RD, et al. The effectiveness of chemotherapy for treatment of high grade astrocytoma in children: results of a randomized trial. A report from the Children's Cancer Study Group. J Neurooncol 1989;7:165–77.
52. Finlay JL, Boyett JM, Yates AJ, et al. Randomized phase III trial in childhood high-grade astrocytoma comparing vincristine, lomustine, and prednisone with the eight-drugs- in-1-day regimen. Children's Cancer Group. J Clin Oncol 1995;13:112–23.
53. Coppes MJ, Lau R, Ingram LC, et al. Open-label comparison of the antiemetic efficacy of single intravenous doses of dolasetron mesylate in pediatric cancer patients receiving moderately to highly emetogenic chemotherapy. Med Pediatr Oncol 1999;33:99–105.
54. Farmer JP, Montes JL, Freeman CR, et al. Brainstem Gliomas. A 10-year institutional review. Pediatr Neurosurg 2001;34:206–14.
55. Mandell LR, Kadota R, Freeman C, et al. There is no role for hyperfractionated radiotherapy in the management of children with newly diagnosed diffuse intrinsic brainstem tumors: results of a Pediatric Oncology Group phase III trial comparing conventional vs. hyperfractionated radiotherapy. Int J Radiat Oncol Biol Phys 1999;43:959–64.
56. Rubin G, Michowitz S, Horev G, et al. Pediatric brain stem gliomas: an update. Childs Nerv Syst 1998;14:167–73.
57. Allen JC, Epstein F. Medulloblastoma and other primary malignant neuroectodermal tumors of the CNS. The effect of patients' age and extent of disease on prognosis. J Neurosurg 1982;57:446–51.
58. Deutsch M, Reigel DH. The value of myelography in the management of childhood medulloblastoma. Cancer 1980;45:2194–7.
59. Evans AE, Jenkin RD, Sposto R, et al. The treatment of medulloblastoma. Results of a prospective randomized trial of radiation therapy with and without CCNU, vincristine, and prednisone. J Neurosurg 1990;72:572–82.
60. Vezina LG, Packer RJ. Infratentorial brain tumors of childhood. Neuroimaging Clin N Am 1994;4:423–36.
61. Packer RJ, Cogen P, Vezina G, Rorke LB. Medulloblastoma: clinical and biologic aspects. Neuro-oncol 1999;1:232–50.
62. Deutsch M. Medulloblastoma: staging and treatment outcome. Int J Radiat Oncol Biol Phys 1988;14:1103–7.
63. Saran FH, Driever PH, Thilmann C, et al. Survival of very young children with medulloblastoma (primitive neuroectodermal tumor of the posterior fossa) treated with craniospinal irradiation. Int J Radiat Oncol Biol Phys 1998;42:959–67.
64. Duffner PK, Horowitz ME, Krischer JP, et al. Postoperative chemotherapy and delayed radiation in children less than three years of age with malignant brain tumors. N Engl J Med 1993;328:1725–31.
65. Albright AL, Wisoff JH, Zeltzer PM, et al. Effects of medulloblastoma resections on outcome in children: a report from the Children's Cancer Group. Neurosurgery 1996;38:265–71.
66. Kortmann RD, Kuhl J, Timmermann B, et al. Postoperative neoadjuvant chemotherapy before radiotherapy as compared to immediate radiotherapy followed by maintenance chemotherapy in the treatment of medulloblastoma in childhood: results of the German prospective randomized trial HIT '91. Int J Radiat Oncol Biol Phys 2000;46:269–79.
67. Zeltzer PM, Boyett JM, Finlay JL, et al. Metastasis stage, adjuvant treatment, and residual tumor are prognostic factors for medulloblastoma in children: conclusions from the Children's Cancer Group 921 randomized phase III study. J Clin Oncol 1999;17:832–45.
68. Pollack IF, Polinko P, Albright AL, et al. Mutism and pseudobulbar symptoms after resection of posterior fossa tumors in children: incidence and pathophysiology. Neurosurgery 1995;37:885–93.
69. Bouffet E, Bernard JL, Frappaz D, et al. M4 protocol for cerebellar medulloblastoma: supratentorial radiotherapy may not be avoided. Int J Radiat Oncol Biol Phys 1992;24:79–85.
70. Packer RJ, Goldwein J, Nicholson HS, et al. Treatment of children with medulloblastomas with reduced-dose craniospinal radiation therapy and adjuvant chemotherapy: A Children's Cancer Group Study. J Clin Oncol 1999;17:2127–36.
71. Ris MD, Packer R, Goldwein J, et al. Intellectual outcome after reduced-dose radiation therapy plus adjuvant chemotherapy for medulloblastoma: a Children's Cancer Group study. J Clin Oncol 2001;19:3470–6.
72. Dunkel IJ, Boyett JM, Yates A, et al. High-dose carboplatin, thiotepa, and etoposide with autologous stem-cell rescue for patients with recurrent medulloblastoma. Children's Cancer Group. J Clin Oncol 1998;16:222–8.
73. Yang HJ, Nam DH, Wang KC, et al. Supratentorial primitive neuroectodermal tumor in children: clinical features, treatment outcome and prognostic factors. Childs Nerv Syst 1999;15:377–83.
74. Zimmerman RA, Bilaniuk LT, Rebsamen S. Magnetic resonance imaging of pediatric posterior fossa tumors. Pediatr Neurosurg 1992;18:58–64.
75. Cohen BH, Zeltzer PM, Boyett JM, et al. Prognostic factors and treatment results for supratentorial primitive neuroectodermal tumors in children using radiation and chemotherapy: a Children's Cancer Group randomized trial. J Clin Oncol 1995;13:1687–96.
76. Burger PC, Yu IT, Tihan T, et al. Atypical teratoid/rhabdoid tumor of the central nervous system: a highly malignant tumor of infancy and childhood frequently mistaken for medulloblastoma: a Pediatric Oncology Group study. Am J Surg Pathol 1998;22:1083–92.
77. Rorke LB, Packer RJ, Biegel JA. Central nervous system atypical teratoid/rhabdoid tumors of infancy and childhood: definition of an entity. J Neurosurg 1996;85:56–65.
78. Mork SJ, Loken AC. Ependymoma: a follow-up study of 101 cases. Cancer 1977;40:907–15.
79. Evans AE, Anderson JR, Lefkowitz-Boudreaux IB, Finlay JL. Adjuvant chemotherapy of childhood posterior fossa ependymoma: cranio-spinal irradiation with or without adjuvant CCNU, vincristine, and prednisone: a Children's Cancer Group study. Med Pediatr Oncol 1996;27:8–14.
80. Packer RJ, Cohen BH, Cooney K. Intracranial germ cell tumors. Oncologist 2000;5:312–20.
81. Zissiadis Y, Dutton S, Kieran M, et al. Stereotactic radiotherapy for pediatric intracranial germ cell tumors. Int J Radiat Oncol Biol Phys 2001;51:108–12.
82. Balmaceda C, Heller G, Rosenblum M, et al. Chemotherapy without irradiation—a novel approach for newly diagnosed CNS germ cell tumors: results of an international cooperative trial. The First International Central Nervous System Germ Cell Tumor Study. J Clin Oncol 1996;14:2908–15.
83. Jakacki R. Central Nervous System Germ Cell Tumors. Curr Treat Options Neurol 2002;4:139–145.
84. Bredel M, Pollack IF, Hamilton RL, James CD. Epidermal growth factor receptor expression and gene amplification in high-grade non-brainstem gliomas of childhood. Clin Cancer Res 1999;5:1786–92.
85. Pollack IF, Finkelstein SD, Burnham J, et al. Age and TP53 mutation frequency in childhood malignant gliomas: results in a multi-institutional cohort. Cancer Res 2001;61:7404–7.
86. Pollack IF, Finkelstein SD, Woods J, et al. Expression of p53 and prognosis in children with malignant gliomas. N Engl J Med 2002;346:420–7.
87. von Haken MS, White EC, Daneshvar-Shyesther L, et al. Molecular genetic analysis of chromosome arm 17p and chromosome arm 22q DNA sequences in sporadic pediatric ependymomas. Genes Chromosomes Cancer 1996;17:37–44.
88. Iwato M, Tachibana O, Tohma Y, et al. Molecular analysis for p53 and mdm2 in intracranial germ cell tumors. Acta Neuropathol (Berl) 2000;99:21–5.
89. Willert JR, Daneshvar L, Sheffield VC, Cogen PH. Deletion of chromosome arm 17p DNA sequences in pediatric high-grade and juvenile pilocytic astrocytomas. Genes Chromosomes Cancer 1995;12:165–72.
90. Burnett ME, White EC, Sih S, et al. Chromosome arm 17p deletion analysis reveals molecular genetic heterogeneity in supratentorial and infratentorial primitive neuroectodermal tumors of the central nervous system. Cancer Genet Cytogenet 1997;97:25–31.
91. Fruhwald MC, O'Dorisio MS, Dai Z, et al. Aberrant hypermethylation of the major breakpoint cluster region in 17p11.2 in medulloblastomas but not supratentorial PNETs. Genes Chromosomes Cancer 2001;30:38–47.
92. Newcomb EW, Alonso M, Sung T, Miller DC. Incidence of p14ARF gene deletion in high-grade adult and pediatric astrocytomas. Hum Pathol 2000;31:115–9.
93. Iwato M, Tachibana O, Tohma Y, et al. Alterations of the INK4a/ARF locus in human intracranial germ cell tumors. Cancer Res 2000;60:2113–5.
94. Segal RA, Goumnerova LC, Kwon YK, et al. Expression of the neurotrophin receptor TrkC is linked to a favorable outcome in medulloblastoma. Proc Natl Acad Sci U S A 1994;91:12867–71.
95. Grotzer MA, Janss AJ, Fung K, et al. TrkC expression predicts good clinical outcome in primitive neuroectodermal brain tumors. J Clin Oncol 2000;18:1027–35.

96. Biegel JA. Cytogenetics and molecular genetics of childhood brain tumors. Neuro-oncol 1999;1:139–51.
97. Reardon DA, Entrekin RE, Sublett J, et al. Chromosome arm 6q loss is the most common recurrent autosomal alteration detected in primary pediatric ependymoma. Genes Chromosomes Cancer 1999;24:230–7.
98. Kalifa C, Hartmann O, Demeocq F, et al. High-dose busulfan and thiotepa with autologous bone marrow transplantation in childhood malignant brain tumors: a phase II study. Bone Marrow Transplant 1992;9:227–33.
99. Mason WP, Grovas A, Halpern S, et al. Intensive chemotherapy and bone marrow rescue for young children with newly diagnosed malignant brain tumors. J Clin Oncol 1998;16:210–21.
100. Slavc I, Schuller E, Czech T, et al. Intrathecal mafosfamide therapy for pediatric brain tumors with meningeal dissemination. J Neurooncol 1998;38:213–8.
101. Elliott PJ, Hayward NJ, Huff MR, et al. Unlocking the blood-brain barrier: a role for RMP-7 in brain tumor therapy. Exp Neurol 1996;141:214–24.
102. Young SW, Qing F, Harriman A, et al. Gadolinium(III) texaphyrin: a tumor selective radiation sensitizer that is detectable by MRI. Proc Natl Acad Sci U S A 1996;93:6610–5.
103. Rosenblum MG, Yung WK, Kelleher PJ, et al. Growth inhibitory effects of interferon-beta but not interferon-alpha on human glioma cells: correlation of receptor binding, 2',5'- oligoadenylate synthetase and protein kinase activity. J Interferon Res 1990;10:141–51.
104. Nakamura O, Shitara N, Matsutani M, et al. Phase I–II trials of poly(ICLC) in malignant brain tumor patients. J Interferon Res 1982;2:1–4.
105. Ponzoni M, Bocca P, Chiesa V, et al. Differential effects of N-(4-hydroxyphenyl)retinamide and retinoic acid on neuroblastoma cells: apoptosis versus differentiation. Cancer Res 1995;55:853–61.
106. Samid D, Hudgins WR, Shack S, et al. Phenylacetate and phenylbutyrate as novel, nontoxic differentiation inducers. Adv Exp Med Biol 1997;501–5.
107. Packer RJ, Raffel C, Villablanca JG, et al. Treatment of progressive or recurrent pediatric malignant supratentorial brain tumors with herpes simplex virus thymidine kinase gene vector-producer cells followed by intravenous ganciclovir administration. J Neurosurg 2000;92:249–54.
108. Druker BJ, Tamura S, Buchdunger E, et al. Effects of a selective inhibitor of the Abl tyrosine kinase on the growth of Bcr-Abl positive cells. Nat Med 1996;2:561–6.
109. Kilic T, Alberta JA, Zdunek PR, et al. Intracranial inhibition of platelet-derived growth factor-mediated glioblastoma cell growth by an orally active kinase inhibitor of the 2-phenylaminopyrimidine class. Cancer Res 2000;60:5143–50.
110. Pollack IF, Randall MS, Kristofik MP, et al. Response of low-passage human malignant gliomas in vitro to stimulation and selective inhibition of growth factor-mediated pathways. J Neurosurg 1991;75:284–93.
111. Vassbotn FS, Ostman A, Langeland N, et al. Activated platelet-derived growth factor autocrine pathway drives the transformed phenotype of a human glioblastoma cell line. J Cell Physiol 1994;158:381–9.

Hodgkin Disease

James Nachman, MD

Hodgkin disease (HD) is unique among cancers in that the malignant cell, the Reed–Sternberg (RS) cell, accounts for only a small fraction of the tumor cellularity. HD accounts for approximately 5% of pediatric malignancies in developed countries. The cure rate for pediatric patients with HD is greater than 90%. Standard therapy for pediatric patients with HD includes combination chemotherapy and low-dose involved-field radiotherapy (RT). Clinical research in pediatric HD aims to (1) delineate minimal treatment necessary for cure and (2) eliminate or minimize late sequelae of treatment. Study of the biology of the RS cell in an effort to identify new therapeutic targets is also receiving significant attention.

BIOLOGY

Microdissection techniques that facilitate the harvesting of individual tumor cells have led to significant advances in understanding the biology of HD. RS cells from an individual patient show identical immunoglobulin heavy chain gene rearrangements in 90% of cases, supporting derivation from a single, transformed B cell.[1,2] In cases of lymphocyte predominant HD, tumor cells (so-called L and H cells) express CD20 and J chain, and are negative for CD30 and CD15. L and H cells also express additional B lineage antigens. RS cells (characteristics of classic HD: nodular sclerosis, mixed cellularity, lymphocyte-depleted, and lymphocyte-rich HD) express CD30 and CD15, but lack CD20 and J chain expression. RS cells also express receptors seen on antigen presenting dendritic cells such as restin and fascin.[3]

Rearrangement and somatic hypermutation of immunoglobulin heavy chain genes implies that RS cells derive from germinal center B cells carrying nonproductive immunoglobulin genes.[4] Under normal circumstances, such cells are eliminated through apoptosis. RS cells show high levels of NF1cB, which may prevent apoptosis.[5]

B-cell fate is determined by a dynamic balance between death receptor-ligand interactions and survival proteins that inhibit transduction of these signals to the death machinery (caspases, mitochondria). This balance is regulated by NF1cB. NF1cB dimers are bound in an inactive cytoplasmic complex with inhibitory protein-I1cBs. B-cell stimulation by diverse signals results in activation of I1cB kinase,[6–9] which phosphorylates two critical serine residues of I1cBs, targeting them for ubiquitin mediated proteasomal degradation. Active NF1cB dimers are then released and translocated to the nucleus. In RS cells, CD40–CD40L interactions,[10,11] overexpression of tumor necrosis factor receptor-associated factors (TRAFs),[9] and CD30 expression[7] all facilitate activation of NF1cB.

RS cells are both cytokine-producing and cytokine-responding cells. Many systemic symptoms and pathologic features of HD result from cytokine production by RS cells and neighboring inflammatory cells. Unique histologic features such as fibrosis and tissue eosinophilia may relate to the expression of interleukin (IL)-4, IL-5, eotaxin, and basic fibroblast growth factor.[12] B symptoms at diagnosis have been associated with high levels of IL-6 and immunosuppression with expression of transforming growth factor (TGF)-R.[12]

CLINICAL PRESENTATION AND STAGING

As in adults, most pediatric patients with HD present with upper torso disease (neck, 80%; mediastinum, 60%). Cervical adenopathy may be present for a long period prior to diagnosis. Approximately 25% of patients will have systemic symptoms at diagnosis (B) including fever (otherwise unexplained, > 100.4°F [> 38°C]), weight loss (unintended and > 10% of body weight), and drenching night sweats. Pruritus may occur as well. Because of the frequency of mediastinal involvement, chest radiography is an important initial step in the evaluation of cervical adenopathy.

Diagnosis is usually established by biopsy of a clinically enlarged node. The most common histologic subtype is nodular sclerosis (70%); lymphocyte predominant and mixed cellularity subtypes account for the rest of cases and are more common in children younger than 10 years of age. Nodular sclerosis may be subdivided into two categories based on the relative frequency of RS cells in the biopsy specimen.

Following biopsy, a staging workup is performed that includes a computed tomography (CT) scan of the neck, chest, abdomen, and pelvis, and a gallium and/or positron emission tomography (PET) scan, which may be particularly useful in the assessment of residual radiographic abnormalities often present at the end of the initial chemotherapy.[13] Currently, PET scans have replaced gallium scans as the functional imaging procedure of choice. Bone marrow aspiration and biopsy should be performed in patients with disease on both sides of the diaphragm or with B symptoms. Bone scan is only undertaken if the patient has bone pain.

The Ann Arbor staging system is used for pediatric HD.[14] Stage I patients have involvement of a single lymph node region, whereas stage II patients have involvement of two or more lymph node regions on the same side of the diaphragm (almost always upper torso). Stage III patients have lymphatic disease on both sides of the diaphragm (may include the spleen). Patients with stage IV disease have noncontiguous involvement of an extralymphatic organ such as liver, lung, or bone marrow. A biopsy of liver and/or lung lesions discovered on routine scanning should be performed to confirm stage IV disease. An area of positivity on PET scan without an anatomic correlate is not used to upstage a patient. Lymphatic disease is usually classified as bulky (> 6 cm maximum diameter) or nonbulky. Determination of erythrocyte sedimentation rate may provide important prognostic information. Baseline tests of lung or cardiac function should be performed. Postpubertal males should be encouraged to bank sperm prior to chemotherapy that includes alkylating agents.

TREATMENT

Chemotherapy The skeletal consequences of full-dose radiation therapy are unacceptable in prepubertal patients. Therefore, all pediatric patients with HD receive combination chemotherapy as initial treatment. The majority of patients then received low dose involved field radiation (15–25 Gy). MOPP (nitrogen mustard, [Oncovin], procarbazine, prednisone) was the first chemotherapy regimen that produced cures in patients with HD.[15] However, there was a high incidence of infertility in males, and cases of therapy-related acute myelogenous leukemia (AML) and myelodysplasia were noted. These late effects were related to the use of procarbazine and nitrogen mustard.

Italian investigators developed a nonalkylator combination chemotherapy regimen, ABVD (Adriamycin [doxorubicin], bleomycin, vinblastine, and dacarbazine).[16] Although infertility and therapy-related AML were eliminated, cardiac toxicity (doxorubicin) and pulmonary toxicity (bleomycin) were noted. Hybrid regimens were then developed. The COPP/ABV combination (cyclophosphamide [Cytoxan] replacing nitrogen mustard) was widely used.[17] This regimen produced excellent complete response rates and limited the exposure to doxorubicin, bleomycin, and alkylating agents. This regimen was used in a recently completed Children's Cancer Group Pediatric HD study.

German investigators have replaced procarbazine with etoposide in initial therapy for males with HD.[18] Males receive two initial cycles of OEPA (Oncovin, etoposide, prednisone, doxorubicin

[Adriamycin]), whereas females receive two initial cycles of OPPA (Oncovin, procarbazine, prednisone, doxorubicin [Adriamycin]). Patients then receive either none, two, or four cycles of COPP therapy based on initial extent of disease.

A consortium of United States centers studied VAMP (vincristine, Adriamycin [doxorubicin], methotrexate and prednisone) in conjunction with low dose involved field radiation (15 Gy)[33] 5-year event-free survival (EFS) and S were 93 and 99%, respectively. The same group studied VAMP/COP chemotherapy plus involved field radiation for patients with advanced stage HD: The regimen was abandoned because of an unacceptably high relapse rate.[34] Investigators of the Pediatric Oncology Group developed a hybrid regimen including Adriamycin [doxorubicin], bleomycin, vinblastine, etoposide, prednisone, and cyclophosphamide (ABVE-PC). This regimen is used in the first Children's Oncology Group HD trial.

Radiotherapy Ongoing until recently, almost all pediatric HD patients received low-dose involved-field RT following chemotherapy; doses ranged from 15 to 25 cGy. In a recently completed Children's Cancer Group study, patients who achieved an initial complete response to chemotherapy were randomized to receive either low-dose involved-field RT or no further therapy. Patients achieving a partial response received RT. Five-year EFS and survival were 85 and 96%, respectively.[19] Although there was a significant EFS advantage for patients receiving low-dose involved-field RT, there was no survival advantage.

In the German HD 95 trial, all patients achieving a complete response to initial chemotherapy received no further treatment.[20] Twenty-two percent of patients received no low-dose involved-field RT. Comparing patients receiving RT to those receiving no further therapy, patients with advanced disease who received RT had a significantly better EFS than did those who received chemotherapy alone. However, to date, there is no difference in survival.

In the ongoing Children's Oncology Group HD trial, patients who show a rapid response to 2 cycles of ABVE-PC and a complete response after 4 cycles will be randomized to receive or not receive low dose involved field RT. It may be feasible to use PET scans at end therapy to determine which patients would be eligible for treatment with chemotherapy alone. In the new German HD study, stage I and II patients with a negative PET scan at the end of chemotherapy will receive no radiation.

LATE EFFECTS OF TREATMENT

Assessing late effects of treatment for pediatric HD is a frustrating endeavor. Many of these complications may take 20 years or more to develop, requiring long and careful follow-up. In addition, certain late effects seen with prior treatment strategies such as high-dose radiation therapy (4,400 cGy) and extensive alkylator chemotherapy are unlikely to be seen with more modern treatment regimens. It is hard to determine a best regimen to minimize late effects while maintaining cure rates if the late effects are unknown.

Second Malignant Neoplasms The most devastating complication of therapy for HD is the development of a second malignant neoplasm (SMN). Secondary leukemia, most notably AML, is associated with alkylating agent therapy and with etoposide.[21–25] The rate of secondary leukemia reaches a plateau approximately 10 years after treatment of HD and few cases are noted thereafter. In the ABVE-PC regimen, which will be used in the new Children's Oncology Group trials, etoposide exposure is limited and cumulative alkylating agent dose is lower than in previous regimens.

The risk for developing a second solid tumor peaks after 10 years and there does not appear to be a plateau.[21–25] The most common second solid tumor is carcinoma of the breast; increased risk is related to young age at diagnosis and high RT dose to fields including breast tissue. In some series, the incidence of secondary breast cancer approached 35%.[26] In current pediatric HD trials, limiting field size and tailoring fields leads to fewer female patients receiving RT to breast tissue and those that do receive only lower dose RT (approximately 20 cGy). Only in the next decade will data mature sufficiently to determine whether RT treatment modifications will be successful in reducing the risk for secondary breast cancer.

Cardiac Disease Doxorubicin cardiotoxicity is a potential late effect of therapy for pediatric HD.[27] In most protocols, the dose of doxorubicin is between 200 and 300 mg/m^2. Radiation therapy including the heart may increase the risk for cardiomyopathy. In adults, an increased risk of ischemic heart disease, pericarditis, and valvular heart damage has been reported after standard-dose radiation.[28] No data on risk for ischemic heart disease is available for patients receiving low-dose radiation. Pediatric HD patients treated with doxorubicin should have serial echocardiograms as part of long-term follow-up.

Pulmonary Toxicity Pulmonary toxicity is related to the use of bleomycin as well a pulmonary radiation. Radiation pneumonitis and both restrictive and obstructive changes on pulmonary function testing have been described.[29] In most pediatric HD protocols, cumulative bleomycin dose is less than 100 units/m^2 and few patients receive pulmonary radiation. The risk for long-term pulmonary toxicity in pediatric HD patients is low.

Fertility Issues It is well known that male patients with HD may be azoospermic prior to any therapy. The natural history of pretreatment azoospermia is not clear. HD patients, especially males, are at risk for infertility following treatment with alkylating agents (nitrogen mustard, procarbazine, cyclophosphamide) and risk is directly related to cumulative dose. Most pediatric HD protocols reduce alkylating agent exposure through the use of hybrid regimens such as COPP/ABV or ABVE-PC or eliminate alkylating agents altogether (OEPA, ABVE, VAMP).[30,31] Assessment of fertility following use of such regimens requires longer follow-up.

Hypothyroidism Because the majority of pediatric HD patients present with disease in the neck, radiation fields often include the thyroid gland. Patients who receive neck radiation should have annual thyroid function tests for at least a decade after treatment. Twenty-five to 30% of pediatric HD patients who receive radiation involving the thyroid gland will develop abnormal thyroid function tests, generally, normal thyroxine and an elevated thyroid-stimulating hormone (TSH).[32] If TSH elevation is persistent, patients should receive thyroid hormone replacement.

REFERENCES

1. Mason D, Banks P, Chan J, et al. Nodular lymphocyte predominance Hodgkin's disease: a distinct clinico-pathological entity. Am J Surg Pathol 1994;18:526–30.
2. Harris N, Jaffe E, Stein, et al. A revised European-American classification of lymphoid neoplasms: a proposal from the International Lymphoma Study Group. Blood 1994;84:1361–92.
3. Stein H, Diehl V, Marafioti T, et al. The nature of Reed–Sternberg cells, lymphocytic and histiocytic cells and their molecular biology in Hodgkin's disease. In: Mauch PM, Armitage JO, Diehl V, et al, editors. Hodgkin's disease. Philadelphia: Lippincott Williams & Wilkins; 1999. p. 121–38.
4. Kuppers R, Rajewsky K. The origin of Hodgkin and Reed–Sternberg cells in Hodgkin's disease. Ann Rev Immunol 1998;16:471–94.
5. Bargou R, Leng C, Krappmann D, et al. High-level nuclear NF-κB and Oct-2 is a common feature of cultured Hodgkin/Reed–Sternberg cells. Blood 1996;87:4340–7.
6. Aizawa S, Nakano H, Ishida T, et al. TRAF5 and TRAF2 are involved in CD30-mediated NF-κB activation. J Biol Chem 1997;272:2042–5.
7. Lee S, Kandala G, Liou M, et al. CD30/TNF receptor-associated factor-interaction: NF-κB activation and binding specificity. Proc Natl Acad Sci U S A 1996; 93:9699–703.
8. Duckett C, Thompson C. CD30-dependent degradation of TRAF2: implications for negative regulation of TRAF signaling and the control of cell survival. Genes Dev 1997; 11:2810–21.
9. Ansieau S, Scheffrahn I, Mosialos G, et al. Tumor necrosis factor receptor-associated factor (TRAF)-1, TRAF-2, and TRAF-3 interact in vivo with the CD30 cytoplasmic domain: TRAF-2 mediates CD30-induced nuclear factor kappa B activation. Proc Natl Acad Sci U S A 1996;93:14053–8.
10. Datta S, Brunet A, Greenberg M. Cellular survival: a play in three Akts. Genes Dev 1999;13:2905–27.
11. Kane L, Sharpiro V, Stokoe D, et al. Induction of NF-κB by the Akt/PKB kinase. Curr Biol 1999;9:601–4.
12. Kadin M, Liebowitz D. Cytokines and cytokine receptors in Hodgkin's disease. In: Mauch PM, Armitage JO, Diehl V, et al, editors. Hodgkin's disease. Philadelphia: Lippincott Williams & Wilkins; 1999. p. 139–258.
13. Weiner M, Leventhal B, Canto A, et al. Gallium-67 scans as an adjunct to CT scans for the assessment of a residual mediastinal mass in pediatric patients with Hodgkin's disease: a Pediatric Oncology Group study. Cancer 1991;68:2478–80.
14. Carbone P, Kaplan H, Husshoff K, et al. Report of the committee on Hodgkin's disease staging classification. Cancer Res 1971;31:1860–1.
15. DeVita V, Simon R, Hubbaard S. Curability of advanced Hodgkin's disease with chemotherapy. Long-term follow up of MOPP-treated patients at the National Cancer Institute. Ann Intern Med 1980;92:587–95.
16. Santoro N, Bonadonna G, Bonfante V, et al. Alternative drug combinations in the treatment of advanced Hodgkin's disease. N Engl J Med 1982;306:770–5.

17. Hamilton V, Norris C, Bunin M, et al. Cyclophosphamide based, seven-drug hybrid and low dose involved field radiation for the treatment of childhood and adolescent Hodgkin's Disease. J Pediatr Hematol Oncol 2001;23:84–8.
18. Schellong G. Pediatric Hodgkin's disease: treatment in the late 1990s. Ann Oncol 1998; 9 (Suppl 5):115–9.
19. Nachman J, Sposto R, Herzog P, et al. Randomized comparison of low-dose involved-field radiotherapy and no radio-therapy for children with Hodgkin's disease who achieve a complete response to chemotherapy. J Clin Oncol 2002;20:3765–71.
20. Ruhl U, Albrecht M, Dieckmann, et al. Response-adapted radiotherapy in the treatment of pediatric Hodgkin's disease: an interim report at 5 years of the German GPOH-HD 95 trial. Int J Radiat Oncol Biol Phys 2001;51:1209–18.
21. Woldin S, Lamborn K, Cleary S, et al. Second cancers following pediatric Hodgkin's disease. J Clin Oncol 1998;16:536–44.
22. Beaty O, Hudson M, Greenwald C, et al. Subsequent malignancies in children and adolescents after treatment for Hodgkin's disease. J Clin Oncol 1995;13:103–9.
23. Sankila R, Garwicz S, Olsen J, et al. Risk of subsequent malignant neoplasms among 1,641 Hodgkin's disease patients diagnosed in childhood and adolescence: a population-based cohort study in the five Nordic countries. J Clin Oncol 1996;14:1442–6.
24. Green D, Hyland H, Barlos M, et al. Second malignant neoplasms after treatment for Hodgkin's disease in childhood or adolescence. J Clin Oncol 2000;18:1492–9.
25. Metayer C, Lynch C, Clarke E, et al. Second cancers among long-term survivors of Hodgkin's disease diagnosed in childhood and adolescence. J Clin Oncol 2000;18:2435–43.
26. Bhatia S, Robison L, Oberlin O, et al. Breast cancer and other second neoplasms after childhood Hodgkin's disease. N Engl J Med 1996;334:745–51.
27. Hancock S, Donaldson S, Hoppe R, et al. Cardiac disease following treatment of Hodgkin's disease in children and adolescents. J Clin Oncol 1993;11:1208–15.
28. Constine L, Schwartz R, Savage D, et al. Cardiac function, perfusion, and morbidity in irradiated long-term survivors of Hodgkin's disease. Int J Radiat Oncol Biol Phys 1997;39:897–906.
29. Marina N, Greenwald C, Fairclough D, et al. Serial pulmonary function studies in children treated for newly diagnosed Hodgkin's disease with mantle radiotherapy plus cycles of cyclophosphamine, vincristine, and procarbazine alternating with cycles of doxorubicin, bleomycin, vinblastine, and dacarbazine. Cancer 1995;75:1706–11.
30. Mackie E, Radford M, Shalet S, et al. Gonadal function following chemotherapy for childhood Hodgkin's disease. Med Pediatr Oncol 1996;27:74–8.
31. Gerres L, Bramsudig J, Schlegel W, et al. The effects of etoposide on testicular function in boys treated for Hodgkin's disease. Cancer 1998;83:2217–22.
32. Sklar C, Whitton J, Mertens A, et al. Abnormalities of the thyroid in survivors of Hodgkin's disease: data from the childhood cancer survivor study. J Clin Endocrinol Metab 2000;85:3227–32.
33. Donaldson S, Hudson M, Lamborn K, et al. VAMP and low-dose, involved-field radiation for children and adolescents with favorable, early-stage Hodgkin's disease: results of a prospective clinical trial. J Clin Oncol 2002;20:3081–87.
34. Hudson M, Krasin M, Link M, et al. Risk-adapted, combined-modality therapy with VAMP/COP and response-based, involved-field radiation for unfavorable pediatric Hodgkin's disease. J Clin Oncol 2004;22:4541–50.

Non-Hodgkin Lymphoma in Children

Mitchell S. Cairo, MD
Elizabeth Raetz, MD
Sherrie Perkins, MD, PhD

EPIDEMIOLOGY

Approximately 15% of all childhood cancers diagnosed in the United States are lymphomas. Sixty percent of all childhood lymphomas have been classified as non-Hodgkin lymphoma, representing 3% of all childhood malignancies for children younger than 5 years, and 8 to 9% for children and adolescents 5 to 19 years of age. In the United States, 750 to 800 cases of non-Hodgkin lymphoma are diagnosed annually in children and young adults younger than 20 years of age. There is a two- to threefold increase in frequency of childhood non-Hodgkin lymphoma in males compared with females. The incidence of non-Hodgkin lymphoma in white children is approximately twice that found in African-American children, with approximately 9.2 cases per million versus 4.6 cases per million (white vs black children).[1–3] The incidence of non-Hodgkin lymphoma in children who are less than 15 years of age has been fairly constant over the past two decades, while there has been an overall increase in the incidence in adolescents ages 15 to 19 years.[4] There is also an increased incidence of non-Hodgkin lymphomas, especially B-cell lymphomas, in children with inherited and/or acquired immunodeficiencies. Specific, primary, or inherited immunodeficiencies associated with an increased risk of non-Hodgkin lymphoma include Wiskott-Aldrich syndrome, severe combined immune deficiency, ataxia-telangiectasia, and common variable immune deficiency.[5–10] Patients on immunosuppressive medication, especially those following solid organ transplantation, children with acquired immunodeficiency syndrome (AIDS), and children following allogeneic stem cell transplantation that used certain methods of in vitro allogeneic stem cell T-cell depletion is another large group of children susceptible to an increased risk of developing B-cell lymphomas.[5–8,11,12]

Traditionally, non-Hodgkin lymphoma has been classified into low, intermediate, or high grade and, more recently, by morphologic, immunologic, and molecular and genetic variables. Additional subclassification has divided non-Hodgkin lymphomas according to their spectrum of clinical behavior into two major subgroups: indolent or aggressive. Over the past 30 years, the most common histologic classifications of childhood non-Hodgkin lymphoma have included the morphologic schema developed by Rappaport, the morphologically and immunologically based schema of Lukes and Collins, the Kiel classifications, the prognostic subgrouping of the National Cancer Institute's Working Formulation, the Revised European-American Lymphoma (REAL) classification, and, most recently, the World Health Organization (WHO) classification.[5–8,13–18] With the current understanding of the biologic and pathologic characteristics of non-Hodgkin lymphoma, recent classification systems, such as the REAL[17] or WHO classifications,[18] incorporate morphologic, immunophenotypic, and molecular characteristics to define the type of lymphoma. Non-Hodgkin lymphomas are subtyped on the basis of morphology, B- or T-cell phenotype and/or molecular features into subcategories that are defined by the REAL or WHO classifications.[17,18] The vast majority of childhood non-Hodgkin lymphomas are high-grade tumors with aggressive clinical behavior. In contrast, the majority of adult non-Hodgkin lymphomas are low to intermediate grade indolent tumors.[2,3,5] Unlike adult non-Hodgkin lymphoma that is predominantly B-cell phenotype, pediatric lymphomas are almost equally divided between B- and T-cell neoplasms, and follicular or low-grade lymphomas are distinctly uncommon.[19–21] There are four major subtypes of childhood non-Hodgkin lymphoma: Burkitt's lymphoma (classic and atypical Burkitt's lymphoma), lymphoblastic lymphoma, diffuse large B-cell lymphoma (DLBCL), and anaplastic large-cell lymphoma (ALCL). The distribution of these four main histologic subtypes includes approximately 40% Burkitt's lymphoma, 30% lymphoblastic lymphoma, 20% diffuse large B-cell, and 10% anaplastic large-cell lymphoma (Tables 124g-1 and 124g-2).[22]

CLINICAL PRESENTATION/STAGING

The clinical presentation of childhood non-Hodgkin lymphoma depends primarily on the histologic subtype and the primary site of involvement. Childhood variants are commonly extranodal at the time of presentation compared with nodal involvement at diagnosis in adult non-Hodgkin lymphoma. The most common extranodal sites involved at presentation include head and neck (30%), abdominal disease (30%), and intrathoracic or mediastinal and/or hilar adenopathy (25%).[2,23] Childhood non-Hodgkin lymphoma commonly presents with advanced and/or metastatic disease at the time of diagnosis. Approximately 70% of children who present with non-Hodgkin lymphoma have advanced disease (ie, stage III or IV) and/or have metastatic involvement including bone marrow, central nervous systems (CNS), and/or bone.[2,23] Depending on its geographic origin, Burkitt's lymphomas (classic and atypical subtypes) have a significantly different mode of clinical presentation. Children in equatorial Africa will commonly present with head and neck involvement, including, most specifically, jaw involvement and, less commonly, orbital and paraspinal disease. The sporadic form of Burkitt's lymphoma, which occurs more commonly in North America and Europe, commonly presents with abdominal involvement and much less commonly with head and neck or paraspinal disease. Children with the endemic form commonly present with a painful mass in the jaw and less commonly with abdominal symptomatology or paraspinal disease. Children with the sporadic type will commonly present with abdominal involvement that is manifested by abdominal pain, nausea and vomiting, and signs of acute bowel obstruction. Often the diagnosis of Burkitt's lymphoma in the sporadic form is not recognized until an intraoperative procedure has been performed and is often confused with other forms of acute surgical abdominal disease.[2,5,13] The sporadic forms of Burkitt's lym-

Table 124g-1 Non-Hodgkin Lymphoma in Children

Histology	%	Immunophenotyping	Organs Involved
Burkitt's (BL)	40	B-Cell 100%	Abdomen, head, neck, BM, CNS
Lymphoblastic (LL)	30	T-Cell 90% B-Cell 10%	Mediastinum, lymph nodes, CNS, BM, bone
Diffuse Large B Cell (DLBCL)	20	B-Cell 100%	Mediastinum, abdomen, lymph nodes
Anaplastic Large Cell (ALCL)	10	T-Cell 70% Null 20% B-Cell 10%	Skin, mediastinum, liver, spleen, abdomen

BM = bone marrow; CNS = central nervous system.

Table 124g-2 Morphologic, Immunologic, Molecular, and Cytogenic Findings in Pediatric NHL

	DLBCL	Burkitt's	Lymphoblastic	ALCL
Morphology				
Cell size	Large	Intermediate	Small to intermediate	Variable, small to large, multinucleated
Nuclear chromatin	Clumped, vesicular	Coarse	Fine, blastic	Clumped, vesicular
Nucleoli	Variable, single, prominent, or inconspicuous	Variable, multiple, inconspicuous	Absent	Variable
Cytoplasm	Moderate to abundant	Moderate to scanty with prominent vacuoles	Scanty	Moderate to abundant
Nodal pattern	Diffuse	Diffuse, starry-sky pattern	Diffuse, starry-sky pattern	Sinusoidal or diffuse
Immunophenotype	Mature B cell	Mature B cell	Precursor T cell (80%) Precursor B cell (20%)	T cell, null cell, CD30+
Molecular Genetics	Ig gene rearrangements	Ig gene rearrangements	TCR or Ig gene rearrangements	TCR rearrangements
Cytogenetics	t(8;14) may be seen in 35% of cases. Complex cytogenetics, multiple abnormalities	t(8;14), t(8;22), t(2;8). Additional abnormalities including der(13q), −1q +7q common	T cell: t(7;14), t(1;14), t(14;14), t(8;14), t(11;13), B cell: hyperdiploid, additional 21q material	t(2;5), ALK translocation with chromosome 1, 2, 3, and 17

DLBCL = diffuse large B-cell lymphoma; ALCL = anaplastic large-cell lymphoma; TCR = T-cell receptor; Ig = immunoglobulin.

phoma often are associated with metastatic spread to the bone marrow and/or the CNS. Patients with bone marrow involvement will often present with various forms of cytopenias and have evidence of L3 lymphoblasts within the bone marrow. Children with greater than 25% involvement with L3 lymphoblasts in the bone marrow have been defined as having a form of acute lymphoblastic leukemia (ALL), L3 subtype, often called B-ALL. Children with CNS involvement often present with spinal cord compression, cranial and/or peripheral nerve palsies, and/or seizures and require immediate clinical attention.[2,5,24] Since the rapid doubling time of the Burkitt's lymphoma histologic subtype ranges between 12 hours and a few days, a rapid diagnosis and treatment plan are usually required.

Childhood lymphoblastic lymphoma in North America is commonly manifested by a supradiaphragmatic mass, usually either intrathoracic and/or mediastinal. The clinical presentation often includes various forms of respiratory distress and/or signs and symptoms associated with a superior vena cava syndrome.[2,5,13] Besides involving an intrathoracic mass, lymphoblastic lymphoma in children and adolescents often includes bilateral pleural effusions and hepatosplenomegaly. Although less frequent than Burkitt's lymphoma, childhood lymphoblastic lymphoma may also involve spread to the bone marrow and/or the CNS. Children presenting with more than 25% of lymphoblastic lymphoma cells in the bone marrow are often diagnosed and treated as acute lymphoblastic leukemia (ALL) and treated on ALL treatment protocols.[2,5,13]

There are two common forms of childhood large-cell lymphoma, diffuse large B-cell lymphoma (DLBCL) and anaplastic large-cell lymphoma (ALCL), each with a different clinical presentation. The more common diffuse large B-cell type presents similarly to other forms of B-cell Burkitt's lymphoma. Approximately 75% of children and adolescents with DLBCL have advanced disease, that is, stage III (70%) or, rarely, stage IV (5%).[22] The majority of children and adolescents with advanced DLBCL present with an abdominal primary lesion and, to a lesser extent, a primary lesion in the mediastinum. There is an increased incidence of mediastinal involvement in DLBCL versus Burkitt's lymphoma. DLBCL rarely involves both the CNS and bone marrow (less than 3%).[25]

Anaplastic large-cell lymphomas (ALCL) have a somewhat different clinical presentation, resulting in two categories: systemic and primary cutaneous ALCL.[18] The majority of children and adolescents with ALCL have advanced, stage III/IV disease at diagnosis.[26] In systemic ALCL, 40 to 60% of patients have extranodal disease, most commonly involving the skin, bone, and soft tissue. In contrast, primary cutaneous ALCL is limited to the skin and tends to occur in older patients and is rare in children.[27–30]

Critically important in designing the appropriate treatment plan for each histologic subtype is the staging of childhood non-Hodgkin lymphoma. Diagnostic work-up often involves a variety of laboratory studies, including a complete blood count; serum chemistries, including electrolytes, uric acid, calcium, phosphorus, and lactate dehydrogenase; and diagnostic tests for the human immunodeficiency virus. Additionally, laboratory studies might also include T- and B-cell subsets and T- and B-cell functional studies if a congenital and/or acquired immune deficiency syndrome is being considered. Recommended radiographic imaging studies also include ultrasound, computed tomography and/or magnetic resonance imaging, and nuclear medicine studies including positron emission tomography (PET), gallium, and bone scanning. To accurately stage the patient, diagnostic lumbar puncture and bone marrow aspirate and/or biopsy are also critically important for determining the specific histologic subtype and for accurate staging.[2,5]

Additionally, correct staging is critically important at the time of diagnosis since most children present with advanced disease at diagnosis. Historically, the staging system for childhood non-Hodgkin lymphoma modified the one proposed in Ann Arbor for Hodgkin disease.[5] The St. Jude Children's Research Hospital staging classification, modified from the Ann Arbor system for Hodgkin disease, took into consideration the common presentations of childhood non-Hodgkin lymphoma, including increased extranodal involvement, metastatic spread to the bone marrow and CNS, and noncontinuous spread of disease (Table 124g-3). Limited-stage disease (stage I and II) is defined as one or two masses on one side of the diaphragm, whereas more advanced disease (stages III and IV) has been defined as either metastatic disease including the CNS and/or bone marrow disease or disease on both sides of the diaphragm and extensive intrathoracic and intra-abdominal disease (see Table 124g-3).[31] However, the St. Jude's staging classification is unclear on the definition of extensive primary disease and considers all primary abdominal and thoracic tumors as extensive stage III disease, despite original surgical debulking, which may occur at diagnosis.[31] Subsequently, a new French, American, and British (FAB) staging classification was developed (Table 124g-4) that better defines the staging

Table 124g-3 St. Jude's Staging Classification for Childhood Non-Hodgkin Lymphoma

Stage I
A single tumor (extranodal) or single anatomic area (nodal) with the exclusion of mediastinum or abdomen
Stage II
A single tumor (extranodal) with regional node involvement
Two or more nodal areas on the same side of the diaphragm
Two single (extranodal) tumors with or without regional node on the same side of the diaphragm
A primary gastrointestinal tract tumor with or without mesenteric nodes, grossly and completely excised
Stage III
Two single tumors (extranodal) on opposite sides of the diaphragm
Two or more nodal areas above and below the diaphragm
All of the primary intrathoracic tumors (mediastinal, pleural, thymic)
All extensive primary intra-abdominal disease
All paraspinal or epidural tumors, regardless of the other tumor site(s)
Stage IV
Any of the above with initial CNS and/or bone marrow involvement (< 25% malignant cells)

From Murphy SB. Childhood non-Hodgkin's lymphoma. N Engl J Med 1978;299:1446–8.

Table 124g-4 FAB* Staging System for Childhood Large B-Cell and Burkitt's Lymphoma

Group A
- Completely resected stage I (St. Jude)
- Completely resected abdominal stage II (St. Jude)

Group B
- All patients not eligible for Group A or Group C

Group C
- Any CNS involvement† and/or bone marrow involvement (≥ 25% blasts)

*FAB: French, American, British.
†CNS: Any L3 blast, cranial nerve palsy or compression, intracerebral mass, and/or parameningeal compression.
From Cairo et al., Med Pediatr Oncol 1997;29:320a.

of childhood large B-cell and Burkitt's lymphoma of childhood.[32] This staging classification was applied in the DLBCL and Burkitt's lymphoma international study (LMB-FAB) within the Children's Cancer Group (CCG), the United Kingdom Children's Cancer Study Group (UKCCSG), and the Société Française d'Oncologie Pediatrique (SFOP) study group.[32]

GENERAL PRINCIPLES OF TREATMENT

The primary modality of treatment of all histologic types and stages of childhood non-Hodgkin lymphoma is multiagent chemotherapy. The exact regimen of chemotherapy with or without intrathecal therapy and the intensity and length of treatment are usually dictated by the extent of disease and the histologic subtype. The role of surgery is critically important in the diagnosis and staging process, but recently has had limited importance in the overall treatment of childhood non-Hodgkin lymphoma.[1,2,33] Surgery can be beneficial in a variety of instances, including biopsy for initial diagnosis, exploratory laparotomy in patients with acute abdominal disease, and surgical resection during acute emergencies. There is, however, little role for surgery in tumor debulking or for second-look surgery. Similarly, the role of radiotherapy is also of limited use in the present-day management of childhood non-Hodgkin lymphoma.[1,2,34] Radiotherapy is occasionally required as emergency treatment of acute CNS involvement and/or for superior vena cava obstruction. The prophylactic use, however, of radiation in limited-stage disease and/or active CNS involvement has recently been demonstrated to provide no advantage to current multiagent chemotherapy approaches.[34]

Newly diagnosed childhood non-Hodgkin lymphoma, however, is associated with several acute emergent conditions that require specific forms of immediate treatment. Because of the high tumor burden and short doubling time in several forms of childhood non-Hodgkin lymphoma, especially in Burkitt's lymphoma, children are susceptible to several complications, including uric acid nephropathy and acute tumor lysis syndrome.[1,2,35] In addition to the high risk of acute tumor lysis syndrome, children are susceptible to other emergencies, including superior vena cava syndrome, respiratory distress, acute abdominal emergencies, cardiac tamponade, and/or cranial and peripheral nerve compression and/or palsies.[2] Tumor lysis syndrome (TLS) requires rapid treatment with vigorous alkaline hydration, diuresis, allopurinol therapy, and, recently, the use of recombinant urate oxidase enzyme therapy.[36] A new recombinant form of urate oxidase, rasburicase, has recently been developed and investigated in patients with hematologic malignancies at risk of TLS. In a phase I/II study of rasburicase in children and young adults with hematologic malignancies, rasburicase was demonstrated to be well tolerated at 0.2 mg/kg/d IV × 5 to 7 days, had a mean $T_{1/2}$ of 21.2 ± 12.0 hours, and a median decrease in uric acid (UA) from 9.7 to 1.0 mg/dL ($p < .0001$) by 4 hours after the first dose.[37] In a follow-up compassionate study of 255 patients with hematologic malignancies (82 adults and 173 children), rasburicase significantly ($p < .001$) lowered the median uric acid levels in children during prophylaxis (2.7 vs 0.5 mg/dL) and treatment (9.7 vs 0.4 mg/dL), and in adults (4.0 vs 0.7 and 12.0 vs 0.6 mg/dL, respectively).[38] We recently demonstrated in a randomized prospective trial comparing rasburicase versus allopurinol in children with hematologic malignancies and a high risk of tumor lysis syndrome that rasburicase versus allopurinol significantly lowered mean uric acid $AUC_{0->96}$ (128 ± 70 vs 329 ± 129 mg/dL/h) ($p < .0001$) and 4 hours post-UA by 86% versus 12%, respectively ($p < .0001$).[36] Furthermore, in the hyperuricemic group, the baseline creatinine level decreased from 144 to 102% by 96 hours following rasburicase compared with an increase from 132 to 147% following allopurinol.[36] Current use of rasburicase suggests that only 1 to 3 doses are probably required for prophylaxis and/or treatment of TLS.[35]

Diffuse Large B-Cell Lymphoma (DLBCL)

Treatment and Prognosis of Limited-Stage Childhood and Adolescent Diffuse Large B-Cell Lymphoma (DLBCL) Children and adolescents with limited-disease DLBCL, either St. Jude's stage I and II, CCG limited stage, or FAB group A, have an excellent prognosis with an estimated 5-year event-free survival (EFS) of 90 to 95% (Table 124g-5). Over the past 10 to 15 years, there has been significant progress in reducing the amount of therapy required for limited-stage childhood DLBCL and eliminating the need for radiotherapy. Although surgery plays a major role in the diagnosis and/or complete resection of limited DLBCL, multiagent chemotherapy in large part accounts for the excellent survival recently reported.[34,39–42] The length of treatment of childhood limited-stage DLBCL currently ranges between 6 weeks and 6 months of multiagent chemotherapy. Current chemotherapy regimens that have been successfully used in this clinical setting include COMP (CCG and the Pediatric Oncology Group [POG]) (3–6 months), cyclophosphamide, oncovin, prednisone, adriamycin (COPAD) (× 6 weeks) (FAB), or cyclophosphamide and prednisone (CP) followed by dexamethasone/ifosfamide/Ara-C/VP-16/methotrexate and dexamethasone/cyclophosphamide/ methotrexate/doxorubicin (12 weeks) (BFM) (see Table 124g-5).[34,39–43]

Treatment and Prognosis of Childhood and Adolescent Advanced DLBCL The prognosis of advanced childhood and adolescent DLBCL has improved significantly over the past decade.[39,42,44–47] The chemotherapy combinations that have been used for advanced large B-cell (nonanaplastic) childhood lymphoma include Adriamycin, Prednisone, Oncovin ("APO") + Ara-C/VP-16 (POG), "ORANGE" (CCG), Lymphoma, Mature B (LMB) (FAB), and BFM-NHL (BFM).[39,42,44–47] The recent use, however, of short but intense chemotherapy such as FAB/LMB 96 (FAB), ORANGE (CCG), or BFM NHL90 (BFM) has now resulted in a greater than 90% 3-year survival rate in children with advanced large B-cell (nonanaplastic) lymphoma.[39,42,47,48] The CCG hybrid regimen "ORANGE," which consists of Cyclophosphamide, Adriamycin, Oncovin, Prednisone (CHOP)-based induction, VP-16/ifosfamide intensification, and Dexamethasone, Etoposide, Cytosine, Arabinoside, L-Asparaginase (DECAL) intensification, and a similar maintenance phase with a slight decrease in intensity, results in a 90% overall survival rate in children and adolescents with advanced DLBCL.[46,49] Similarly, Patte and colleagues, using a FAB/LMB-type regimen of Cyclophosphamide, Oncovin, Prednisone (COP) reduction, COPADM intensification, and Cytosine, Arabinoside, Methotrexate (CYM) consolidation in children and adolescents with advanced DLBCL, demonstrated a 90% 5-year EFS (Figure 124g-1).[39,48] Reiter and colleagues, using a BFM approach of CP, ifosfamide, methotrexate, dexa-

Table 124g-5 Treatment and Outcome of Limited-Stage (Localized) Diffuse Large B-Cell Lymphoma (DLBCL) and Burkitt's Lymphoma in Children and Adolescents

	CCG	POG	SFOP	BFM	FAB
	Meadows et al[40]	Link et al[41]	Patte et al[39]	Woessman et al[70]	Gerrard et al[43]
Patients (N)	52	27	52	81	132
Protocol	COMP	COMP	COPAD	CP, DX, IFOS, MTX, ARA-C,VP-16, DX, MTX, CTX, DOX	COPAD
Duration	6 mo	8 mo	1.5 mo	3 mo	6 weeks
5-yr EFS (Est)	95%	88%	99%	100%	99%

CCG = Children's Cancer Group; POG = Pediatric Oncology Group; SFOP = Société Française d'Oncologie Pediatrique; BFM = Berlin-Frankfurt-Munster Group; FAB = French-American-British; EFS = event-free survival; COMP = cyclophosphamide, vincristine, methotrexate, prednisone; COPAD = cyclophosphamide, vincristine, prednisone, doxorubicin; CP = cyclophosphamide, prednisone; DX = dexamethasone; IFOS = ifosfamide; MTX = methotrexate; ARA-C = cytosine arabinoside; VP-16 = etoposide; CTX = cyclophosphamide; DOX = doxorubicin; Est = estimate.

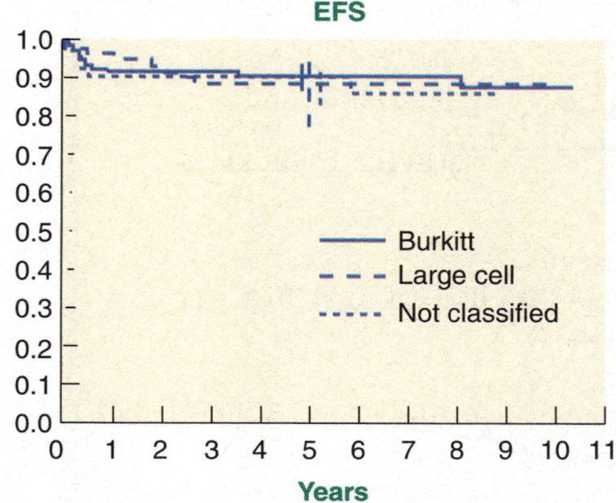

At risk

420 388 381 350 290 240 161 94 41 10 2

63 61 59 50 41 26 16 12 5 1

78 71 66 63 43 31 19 10 8

Figure 124g-1 Event-free survival (EFS) according to histology for cases reviewed by the national panel. From Patte C, Auperin A, Michon J, et al, The Société Française d'Oncologie Pediatrique LMB89 protocol: highly effective multiagent chemotherapy tailored to the tumor burden and initial response in 561 unselected children with B-cell lymphomas and L3 leukemia. Blood 2001;97:3370–9. Copyright American Society of Hematology, used by permission.

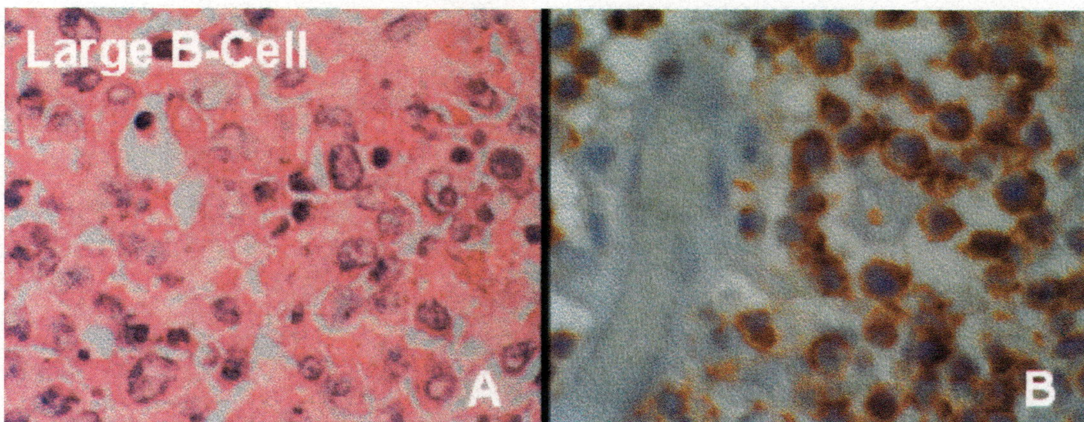

Figure 124g-2 B-LCL. Panel **A** demonstrates the large, noncleaved neoplastic lymphocytes (Hematoxylin and eosin, 400×). Panel **B** demonstrates staining with the B-cell marker, CD20, by immunohistochemistry (400×).

methasone, Ara-C, VP-16, and cytarabine/methotrexate/cyclophosphamide/dexamethasone/doxorubicin, demonstrated a 95% 3-year EFS.[42] All three of the above advanced B-LCL approaches have used a chemotherapy regimen designed to treat Burkitt's (classic and atypical) lymphoma. Laver and colleagues, however, using an approach more designed for large-cell lymphoma (LCL) and not Burkitt's lymphoma (APO + VP-16/Ara-C), demonstrated only a 78% EFS with this approach (Table 124g-6).[45] Patients with advanced DLBCL who still have a somewhat inferior outcome include those with a primary mediastinal DLBCL and patients with bulky tumors (stage III) with elevated LDH levels.[43,48]

Pathology of Childhood DLBCL DLBCLs are characterized by a mature B-cell phenotype and B-cell gene rearrangement. Unlike adults, where follicular architecture is more common, childhood DLBCLs are predominantly diffuse neoplasms occurring in lymph nodes or the mediastinum.[19] A small proportion (< 1% of DLBCL) may be predominantly follicular, with a high proportion occurring in extranodal sites, such as testis.[50] Similar to adult, specific subtypes of DLBCL, such as primary mediastinal large-cell lymphoma[51] or T-cell rich large B-cell lymphoma,[52] have been described in pediatric and adolescent populations. DLBCL may occur in both nodal and extranodal sites, and this is the most common type of non-Hodgkin lymphoma associated with immunodeficiency states.[19]

DLBCLs may display a variety of morphologic appearances, including large noncleaved cells, large cleaved cells, polylobated cells, and immunoblastic cells (exhibiting a single prominent eosinophilic nucleolus) (Figure 124g-2A). Although in earlier classifications these morphologic subtypes were separated out, in the REAL and WHO classifications they are all considered together as DLBCLs.[17,18] The neoplastic cells should have a nucleus that is larger than the size of a tissue histiocyte or twice the size of a small lymphocyte. The cytoplasm may vary from pale to plasmacytoid. There may be a significant accompanying infiltrate of reactive T cells accompanying the malignant cells, which in some cases may obscure the malignant large B cells (see Table 124g-2).[52]

All DLBCL will demonstrate a mature B-cell immunophenotype, including expression of CD20, CD22, and CD79a in paraffin sections,[53] and CD19, CD20, and CD22 by flow cytometry (Figure 124g-2B).[19] Most will demonstrate monoclonal cell surface expression of immunoglobulin light chains but will lack CD10, CD5, or TdT.[17]

Cytogenetic and Molecular Features of Childhood DLBCL There are no characteristic cytogenetic abnormalities associated with DLBCL in children and adolescents. Most cases of DLBCL will demonstrate complex abnormalities, and hyperdiploidy is common, with > 80% of cases demonstrating more than 3 cytogenetic abnormalities. 11q abnormalities as well as of chromosomes appear to be common in pediatric DLBCL.[54] About 30% of adult cases of DLBCL will have a t(14;18)(q32;q21), the translocation seen in follicular center-cell lymphomas involving the *bcl-2* oncogene and associated with bcl-2 protein overexpression that is detectable by immunohistochemistry.[55] However, this translocation is very rare in pediatric DLBCL.[54,56] In light of the paucity of follicular lymphomas in the pediatric populations,[19] it is unclear whether adult and pediatric DLBCL are derived from similar follicular center cells, and identification of the cell(s) of origin for pediatric DLBCL is currently the subject of intense investigation. Translocations associated with the c-*myc* oncogene, such as t(8;14) may also be seen in pediatric DLBCL and appear with a much higher frequency than is seen in adult cases (described in 35% of pediatric cases vs < 10% of adult cases), suggesting a possible relationship with Burkitt's lymphomas.[54,57] The significance of c-*myc* translocation in DLBCL remains uncertain.

Molecular analysis of DLBCL will demonstrate monoclonal immunoglobulin gene rearrangements. Further molecular characterization of DLBCL has been attempted in adult populations by microarray [58] and protein expression studies[59] that have identified expression of the oncogenes such as *bcl-6*[58,60] and c-*myc*[61] as well as identification of a germinal center genetic expression pattern[62,63] as possible prognostic markers in DLBCLs. Unfortunately, similar prognostic molecular studies in childhood DLBCL are not currently available.

Table 124g-6 Treatment and Prognosis of Advanced Diffuse Large B-Cell Lymphoma (DLCBL) in Children and Adolescents

	CCG	POG	SFOP	BFM	CCG
	Cairo et al[47]	Laver et al[45]	Patte et al[39]	Woessmann et al[70]	Cairo et al[46]
Patients (N)	18	33	62	67	212
Protocol	"ORANGE"	"APO"	"LMB"	"BFM"	COMP, D-COMP, ORANGE
Duration	6 mo	12 mo	6 mo	5 mo	6–18 mo
3-yr EFS (Est)	90%	78%	90%	95%	50–90%

CCG = Children's Cancer Group; POG = Pediatric Oncology Group; SFOP = Société Française d'Oncologie Pediatrique; BFM = Berlin-Frankfurt-Munster Group; ORANGE = CHOP (cyclophosphamide, vincristine, Adriamycin, prednisone) + (IFOS + VP-16) + DECAL (dexamethasone, etoposide, cisplatin, high-dose cytarabine, L-asparaginase); APO + = doxorubicin, prednisone, vincristine + VP-16, ARA-C; LMB = lymphoma mature B; COMP = cyclophosphamide, vincristine, methotrexate, prednisone; D-COMP = daunomycin, cyclophosphamide, vincristine, methotrexate, prednisone; EFS = event-free survival; Est = estimate.

Burkitt's Lymphoma in Children and Adolescents

Treatment and Prognosis in Limited-Stage Childhood and Adolescent Burkitt's Lymphoma (BL) Similar to limited-stage DLBCL, children and adolescents with limited stage, either

St. Jude stage I and stage II, CCG limited stage, or FAB group A, with Burkitt's lymphoma have a superb prognosis with an estimated 5-year EFS of 90 to 95% (see Table 124g-5). Similar to limited-stage childhood DLBCL, the requirement for radiotherapy has been eliminated over the past decade as a requirement for treatment in children with limited-stage Burkitt's lymphoma. Surgery is critically important for diagnosis and accurate staging and likely contributes to the success of treatment because of the requirement of complete surgical resection and pinpoint staging for limited-stage patients with Burkitt's lymphoma. With minimal chemotherapy (range 6 weeks to 6 months), the prognosis is excellent, ranging between 90 and 95% 5-year EFS.[34,39–43] There are several multiagent chemotherapy regimens that have been used by a variety of pediatric cooperative groups that have resulted in this excellent outcome, including COPAD (6 weeks) (FAB), Cyclophosphamide, Oncovin, Methotrexate, Prednisone (COMP) (3–6 months) (CCG and POG), or CP followed by dexamethasone/ifosfamide/Ara-C/VP-16/methotrexate and dexamethasone/cyclophosphamide/methotrexate/doxorubicin (BFM) (12 weeks) (see Table 124g-5).[34,39–43] Further investigations will require an elucidation of which multiagent chemotherapy regimen and duration of therapy is required to maintain the high cure rate of limited-stage childhood and adolescent Burkitt's lymphoma.

Treatment and Prognosis of Childhood and Adolescent Advanced Burkitt's Lymphoma The most dramatic advances in the cure of childhood non-Hodgkin lymphoma have been the significant improvement in disease-free and overall survival of advanced Burkitt's lymphoma over the past 20 years. In four consecutive CCG studies from 1977 through 1995, there has been a steady improvement in the 3-year disease-free survival in children and adolescents with advanced Burkitt's lymphoma (Figure 124g-3).[64] In the original CCG-551 study conducted from 1977 through 1983 using COMP or LSA_2L_2, the 3-year disease-free survival for advanced disease was approximately 45% (see Figure 124g-3). In the most recent CCG study, CCG-5911 conducted from 1993 through 1995 and using short but intensive chemotherapy consisting of CHOP, ifosfamide + etoposide and DECAL or LMB-89 type therapy, the 3-year disease-free survival improved significantly to 82% (see Figure 124g-3).[47] Similarly, Patte and colleagues, using an LMB-type regimen of COP reduction, Cyclophosphamide, Oncovin, Prednisone, Adriamycin, Methotrexate (COPADM) intensification, and Cytosine, Arabinoside, VP-16 (CYVE) consolidation in children and adolescents with advanced Burkitt's lymphoma, recently demonstrated a 90% 3-year disease-free survival (see Figure 124g-1) (Table 124g-7).[39] Reiter and colleagues, using a BFM approach (BFM95) (R2 and R3) regimens in children with advanced Burkitt's lymphoma, reported an estimated 4-year EFS of 89% and 74% for bulky disease B-NHL and B-ALL, respectively (see Table 124g-7).[42] Additionally, in building on the original success of Total-B therapy,[65–67] the POG has intensified Total-B therapy with the addition of VP-16 and Ara-C and has recently reported an 83% 3-year disease-free survival in children and adolescents with advanced Burkitt's lymphoma (see Table 124g-7).[68] Most recently, the international FAB/LMB 96 study has demonstrated that with standard FAB therapy, children and adolescents with bone marrow involvement have a ≥ 90% 3-year EFS and patients with CNS involvement have a 71% 3-year EFS with short and intensive chemotherapy.[69]

Children and adolescents with bone marrow and/or CNS involvement have an inferior outcome if they have no response to reduction chemotherapy with COP, or have combined bone marrow and CNS disease.[69] Although elevated lactate dehydrogenase (LDH) is still a poor-risk factor for both stage III BL and DLBCL, LDH has not been shown to be prognostically important in patients with BM and/or CNS disease.[48,69] Furthermore, in the most recent FAB/LMB 96 and BFM NHL 95 studies, both studies have demonstrated that cranial irradiation can be eliminated in patients with CNS positive disease with the substitution of more aggressive high-dose methotrexate and additional intrathecal chemotherapy.[69,70]

Pathology of Burkitt's Lymphoma Burkitt's and Burkitt's-like lymphomas were previously placed together under the category of small noncleaved-cell lymphomas. Whereas Burkitt's lymphoma is a well-defined clinical, morphologic, and cytogenetic entity, Burkitt's-like lymphoma was poorly defined. Because of difficulties among pathologists in diagnostic reproducibility[71] and heterogeneous molecular, cytogenetic, and morphologic features, Burkitt's-like lymphoma is considered only as a provisional diagnostic category in the REAL classification.[17] Burkitt's-like lymphoma is not a recognized specific category in the WHO classification, where it is included under Burkitt's lymphoma as "atypical Burkitt's" lymphoma and shows more morphologic and immunophenotypic diversity than classic Burkitt's lym-

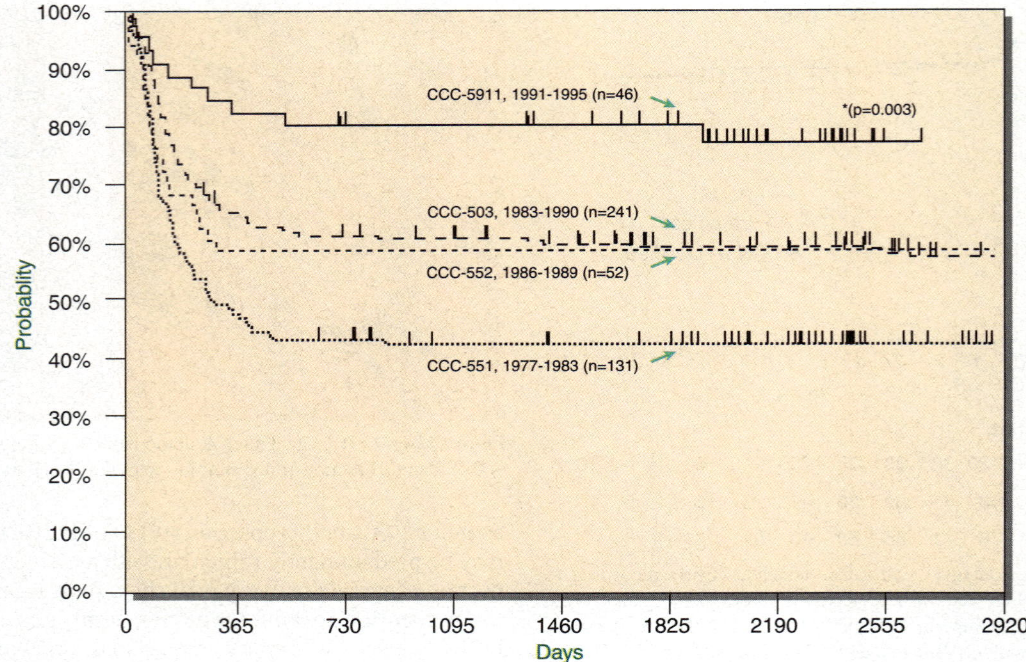

Figure 124g-3 Comparison of event-free survival by Children's Cancer Group (CCG) study among 470 disseminated small noncleaved cell non-Hodgkin lymphoma patients from CCG studies 551, 503, 552, and 5911. *CCG-5911 versus all other studies (CCG-551, -503, and -552), 4-year EFS (80 ± 6% vs 54 ± 2%, $p = .003$).

Table 124g-7 Treatment and Prognosis of Advanced Burkitt's Lymphoma in Children and Adolescents

	CCG	POG	SFOP	BFM	FAB
	Cairo et al[47]	Schwenn et al[68]	Patte et al[39]	Woessmann et al[70]	Cairo et al[69]
Patients (N)	46	327	368	430	50
Protocol	"ORANGE"	"TOTAL B" + ARA-C/VP-16	"LMB" Group B & C	"BFM" R2, R3, R4	FAB/LMB 96
Duration	6 mo	4–5 mo	6 mo	5 mo	5 mo
EFS	Stage IV 82%	Stage IV 83%	BM – 90% CNS – 79%	BM – 89% CNS – 65–70%	BM – 90% CNS – 71%

CCG = Children's Cancer Group; POG = Pediatric Oncology Group; SFOP = Société Française d'Oncologie Pediatrique; BFM = Berlin-Frankfurt-Munster Group; FAB = French-American-British; ORANGE = CHOP (cyclophosphamide, vincristine, Adriamycin, prednisone) + (IFOS + VP-16) + DECAL (dexamethasone, etoposide, cisplatin, high-dose cytarabine, L-asparaginase); Total B = B-Cell Lymphoma Therapy; LMB = lymphoma mature B; FAB/LMB = French-American-British/lymphoma mature B; EFS = event-free survival.

phoma.[18] Burkitt's lymphomas often occur in extranodal sites, including the gut (terminal ileum) and nasopharynx, or in the African endemic form of Burkitt's lymphoma in the bones of the face.[19,72]

The morphologic features of classic Burkitt's lymphoma include a diffuse, homogeneous proliferation of intermediate-sized cells that are larger than a resting lymphocyte but smaller than a centrocyte or large cell (see Table 124g-2). The cells have smooth round to ovoid nuclear contours and usually three to five inconspicuous nucleoli (Figure 124g-4A). The cytoplasm is scanty, is intensely basophilic owing to a high content of polyribosomes, and contains numerous cytoplasmic vacuoles that are filled with lipid that may be demonstrated with neutral fat stains. This distinctive pattern of cytoplasmic vacuoles is best appreciated in cytologic or touch preparations made from the tumor. These cells are analogous to those seen in ALL-L3 leukemias. It should be noted that cytoplasmic vacuoles may be seen in other tumor cells, particularly those that are undergoing early apoptosis and are not specific for Burkitt's lymphoma.[19] This lymphoma has an extremely high mitotic rate (usually in excess of 90%),[17] and a starry-sky pattern of reactive macrophages is present. Atypical Burkitt's lymphomas share many morphologic features with Burkitt's lymphomas, but will have more cellular pleomorphism, variable nuclear irregularities, and variable numbers of nucleoli. Some cases may have slightly more abundant cytoplasm with a central nucleolus, termed Burkitt's lymphoma with plasmacytoid differentiation.[18] The ability to reproducibly distinguish Burkitt's from Burkitt's-like or atypical Burkitt's lymphomas strictly on the basis of morphology has been shown to be highly unreliable, with poor consensus among pathologists.[71] The most common considerations in the differential diagnosis of atypical Burkitt's lymphoma include classic Burkitt's lymphoma or diffuse large-cell lymphoma, and the ability to confidently distinguish between these entities requires optimally fixed and sectioned tissues. Often immunophenotypic analysis or molecular studies may help in the differential if morphologic features are not diagnostic.[18,73]

Immunophenotypic features of both classic Burkitt's and atypical Burkitt's lymphomas are similar. Both are mature B cells (Figure 124g-4B), expressing CD19, CD20, CD22, CD10, and cell surface immunoglobulin (usually IgM) that is light chain restricted.[19,73] Burkitt's lymphomas have a very high mitotic index as evidenced by staining with MIB-1 or Ki-67 proliferation markers, with classic Burkitt's lymphoma showing 99 to 100% more variability in cell surface antigen expression (CD10) and mitotic rate than is seen in the atypical Burkitt's lymphomas.[74] Some studies also suggest that atypical Burkitt's lymphomas have higher immunophenotypic expression of *bcl-6*, similar to DLBCL, than classic Burkitt's lymphomas.[75]

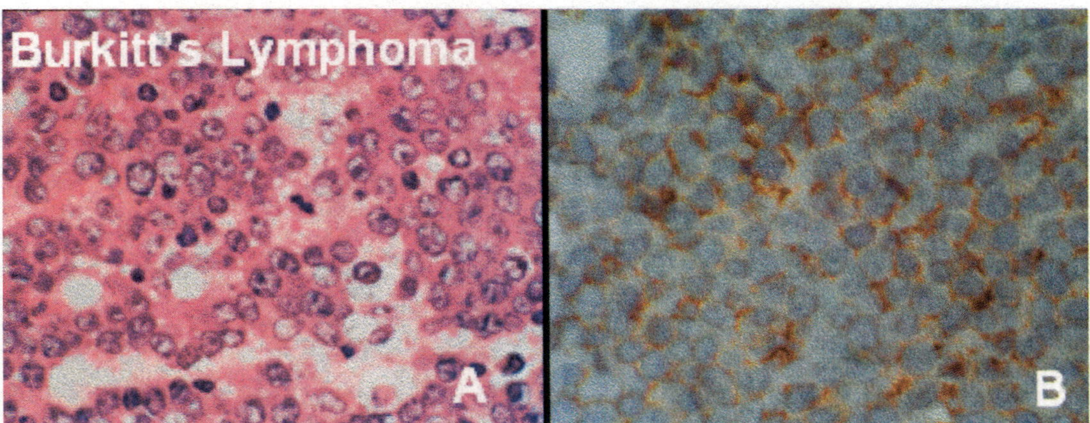

Figure 124g-4 Burkitt's lymphoma. Panel **A** demonstrates the uniform, intermediately sized neoplastic cells. (Hematoxylin and eosin stain, 400×). Panel **B** demonstrates staining with the B-cell marker, CD20, by immunohistochemistry (400×).

Cytogenetic and Molecular Features of Burkitt's Lymphoma Cytogenetic analysis of Burkitt's lymphomas will demonstrate characteristic translocations involving the c-*myc* oncogene locus on chromosome 8, including t(8;14)(q24;q32) in about 80% of cases with the remaining 20% of cases demonstrating a t(2;8)(p11;q24) or t(8;22)(q24;q11). These translocations will juxtapose c-*myc* to immunoglobulin genes (heavy chain, kappa, or lambda light chain loci), leading to inappropriate overexpression of the oncogene.[56,76] By definitions set forth in the WHO classification, atypical Burkitt's lymphomas must also have a c-*myc* translocation. In addition to the c-*myc* translocations that define this disorder, up to 70% of pediatric classic Burkitt's lymphomas have additional cytogenetic abnormalities that include +1q, dup (1q), –6q, +7q and der (13q). Approximately 75% will have one to three cytogenetic abnormalities, but approximately 25% will have more than three abnormalities.[77] The translocations seen in atypical Burkitt's or Burkitt's-like lymphomas are similar and include translocations involving one or more components of the c-*myc* locus[18] and other translocations that are not associated with c-*myc*, similar to those seen in classic Burkitt's lymphoma. The atypical Burkitt's lymphoma cases tend to have a higher incidence (approximately 50% of cases) with more than three cytogenetic abnormalities.[77] The number of cytogenetic abnormalities may correlate with prognosis with der (13q), +7q, and greater than three abnormalities appearing to impact on prognosis.[77,78]

Molecular analysis will demonstrate monoclonal immunoglobulin gene rearrangements with germline T-cell receptor genes in all Burkitt's and atypical Burkitt's lymphomas.[56] Endemic (African) Burkitt's lymphoma consistently demonstrates amplification of the EBV genome, although in sporadic Burkitt's lymphoma EBV is demonstrated in only about 30% of cases. When EBV is present, it is monoclonal, suggesting a possible role in clonal expansion of the neoplastic cells.[79]

Anaplastic Large-Cell Lymphoma (ALCL)

Treatment and Prognosis of Localized Anaplastic Large-Cell Lymphoma The prognosis for patients with anaplastic large-cell lymphoma (ALCL) has improved significantly over the past two decades, although children are susceptible to late relapse.[80] Treatment approaches have varied, with some groups using shortened, intensive B-NHL therapy[80–83] and others using ALL-type treatment based on the T-cell immunophenotypes that are commonly present in these tumors (Table 124g-8).[84–87] As the majority (approximately two-thirds) of children present with advanced-stage disease, optimal therapeutic approaches for localized disease have not been well defined.[26] Children with localized (stage I/stageII resected) ALCL have achieved 100% EFS with 2 months of intensive chemotherapy using the combination of dexamethasone, ifosfamide, methotrexate, cytarabine, etoposide, and prophylactic intrathecal therapy.[80] Five-year EFS rates of 75% have also been reported in a small number of children with localized CD30+ large-cell lymphoma, treated at St. Jude Children's Research Hospital with three courses of CHOP, either with or without continuation treatment with mercaptopurine and methotrexate.[82]

Treatment and Prognosis of Advanced-Stage Anaplastic Large-Cell Lymphoma Systemic chemotherapy has been the mainstay of treatment of advanced disease, with favorable outcomes reported. Long-term disease-free survival rates have ranged from 56 to 76% using a variety of approaches.[45,81–83,88] Some of the most promising results have been reported by the BFM group.[80,83] Children with advanced ALCL treated on NHL-BFM 90 have achieved event-free survival rates of 76% after receiving short courses of intensive B-NHL therapy, stratified according to disease stage, without local radiotherapy. The maximal duration of treatment was 5 months. Features of this regimen that may have contributed to its success were the use of dexamethasone versus prednisone, the incorporation of ifosfamide, and 24-hour methotrexate infusions with delayed leucovorin rescue. Similar outcomes (72% 4-yr EFS) were observed in the Pediatric Oncology Group study using an APO (doxorubicin, prednisone, vincristine)-based regimen in children with advanced-stage ALCL.[89] This study compared a standard APO regimen with one incorporating intermediate-dose methotrexate and high-dose cytarabine.[89] Greater toxicity and

Table 124g-8 Treatment and Outcome of Anaplastic Large-Cell Lymphoma in Children and Adolescents

	BFM	POG	SFOP	UKCCSG	St. Jude	MSKCC
	Seidemann et al[80]	Laver et al[89]	Brugieres et al[81]	Williams et al[183]	Sandlund et al[82]	Mora et al[84]
Patients (N)	89	86	82	72	18	19
Protocol	NHL-BFM 90	POG 9315	HM89-91	NHL 9000 series	CHOP-based	LSA_2L_2, LSA_4
Duration	2–5 mo	12 mo	7–8 mo	6 mo	6–18 mo	14–36 mo
EFS (Est)	76% (5-yr)	72% (4-yr)	66% (3-yr)	59% (5-yr)	57% (5-yr)	56% (5-yr)
OS	NR	88% (4-yr)	83% (3-yr)	65% (5-yr)	84% (5-yr)	84% (5-yr)

BFM = Berlin-Frankfurt-Munster Group; POG = Pediatric Oncology Group; SFOP = Société Française d'Oncologie Pediatrique; UKCCSG = United Kingdom Children's Cancer Study Group; St. Jude = St. Jude Children's Research Hospital; MSKCC = Memorial Sloan Kettering Cancer Center; EFS = event-free survival; Est = estimate; OS = overall survival; NR = not reported.

no improvement in disease-free survival was seen with the inclusion of methotrexate and cytarabine, and the current Children's Oncology Group study has therefore been based on the standard APO backbone with the inclusion of vinblastine.

Several prognostic parameters have been identified in ALCL. With small numbers of patients enrolled on current studies and heterogeneous treatment approaches, however, the findings have been inconsistent. Poor-risk prognostic factors that have been identified include organ involvement (liver, lung, spleen), mediastinal involvement, an elevated LDH, and/or disseminated skin disease.[81,90] In the NHL-BFM 90 experience, only the presence of B symptoms was significantly associated with a poor outcome in multivariate analysis.[80] Other factors that had been previously identified as negative prognostic indicators during the earlier phases of this trial, such as skin involvement, were no longer associated with a risk of treatment failure. Anaplastic lymphoma kinase (ALK) expression was not associated with outcome in this group of patients, in contrast to reports of other groups, where it has been associated with a favorable outcome.[27] This suggests that larger numbers of pediatric patients, treated uniformly, will be needed to accurately identify true prognostic variables.

Treatment of Relapsed Anaplastic Large-Cell Lymphoma Unlike other histologic subtypes of NHL, chemosensitivity at the time of relapse is a hallmark of ALCL and has made salvage strategies for ALCL generally very effective.[80,84,86,88] Relapses in ALCL also tend to occur later than in other histologic subtypes of large-cell lymphoma.[84] The clinical behavior after relapse has been variable with some patients developing rapidly progressive disease, and others having an indolent, waxing and waning course.[83] These differences have made uniform treatment approaches difficult. Of 20 patients who relapsed following treatment with NHL-BFM 90, 9 are in second complete remission after salvage chemotherapy with or without the addition of stem cell transplantation.

In 41 patients treated for consecutive relapses of ALCL following initial treatment on a series of three clinical trials in France over two decades, overall and disease-free survival rates were 69% and 44%, respectively, at 3 years.[91] Fifteen patients underwent myeloablative therapy with autologous or allogeneic stem cell transplantation (SCT) in second remission (CR2). Twenty-one patients received chemotherapy alone, commonly with CVBA (CCNU, vinblastine, bleomycin, cytarabine), or alternatively, with weekly vinblastine alone. Factors associated with a higher risk of treatment failure included earlier relapse and more intensive initial treatment. Three-year disease-free survival did not differ in patients who underwent SCT in CR2 when compared with those treated with chemotherapy alone (45% vs 52% 3-yr disease-free survival). Furthermore, the chemosensitivity of relapsed disease was highlighted by the unexpectedly favorable outcome of 12 children treated with weekly vinblastine alone. Ten of these 12 children achieved a complete remission, and the overall CR2 rate with chemotherapy alone was 85%. Prospective future trials will help to define the optimal treatment strategies for refractory disease. Given the distinctive biologic features of this disease, novel targeted therapies may be beneficial.

The distinctive biologic features of ALCL provide a compelling rationale for the development of novel targeted therapies, such as those that modulate the activity of ALK or its downstream signaling pathways. Examples of agents that are entering clinical trials include anti-CD30 monoclonal antibodies,[92] as well as inhibitors of the PI3/AKT pathway proteins (eg, UCN-01), which are targets of ALK.[93] As the majority of ALCLs also express CD52, anti-CD52 immunotherapy with alemtuzumab (Campath-1H) may also prove to be a beneficial approach.

Pathology of ALCL ALCL is a peripheral T-cell lymphoma characterized by expression of CD30 that includes two broad categories of disease: systemic (S-ALCL) and primary cutaneous ALCL (C-ALCL), with slightly different pathologic features.[18,30] These tumors show a broad morphologic spectrum, but usually contain large, pleomorphic, multinucleated cells or cells with eccentric horseshoe-shaped nuclei and abundant, clear to basophilic cytoplasm with an area of eosinophilia near the nucleus (termed "hallmark cells") (Figure 124g-5A).[94] These cells may resemble Reed-Sternberg cells, although hallmark cells tend to have less conspicuous nucleoli.

There is much morphologic diversity in ALCL, and several morphologic variants have been recognized in the REAL and WHO classifications.[17,18] These include the common variant (more than 75% of ALCLs) composed primarily of hallmark cells, the lymphohistiocytic variant (10% of ALCL) that has a large number of benign histiocytes admixed that may obscure the neoplastic cells, which tend to be smaller and clustered around vessels, and the small-cell variant (10% of ALCL), where small neoplastic cells predominate and only scattered hallmark cells are seen. Other, less well described variants include a sarcomatoid variant, signet-ring variant, neutrophil-rich variant, and giant-cell variant (see Table 124g-2).[28,95] In the lymph nodes, the neoplastic cells tend to infiltrate in a sinusoidal pattern,

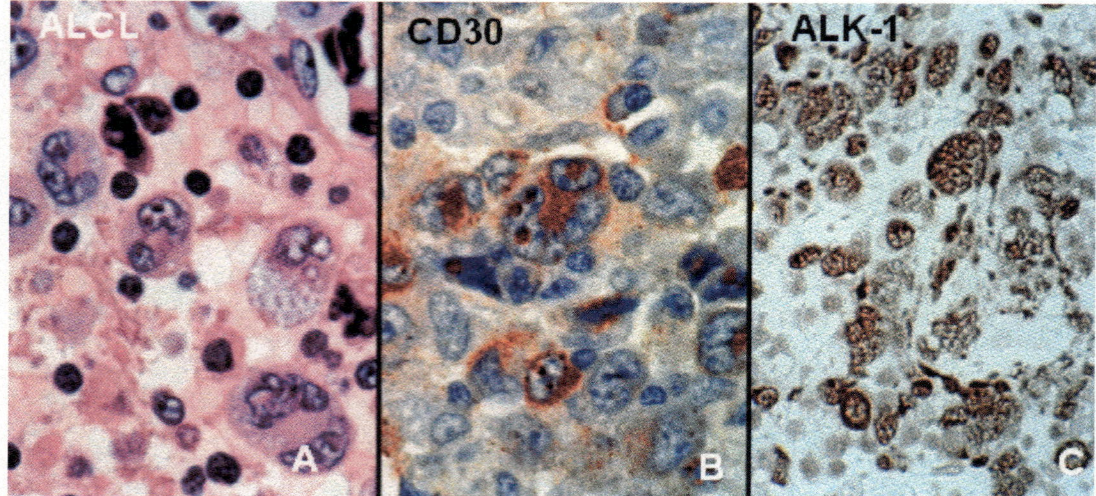

Figure 124g-5 Systemic ALCL. Panel **A** demonstrates the large, multinucleated neoplastic "hallmark cells" (Hematoxylin and eosin stain, 400×). Panel **B** demonstrates staining with the CD30 showing characteristic Golgi and cytoplasmic staining by immunohistochemistry (400×). Panel **C** shows nuclear staining for the NPM-ALK fusion protein using ALK-1 antibodies by immunohistochemistry in a patient known to have a t(2;5) (200×).

mimicking metastatic disease, although diffuse effacement of nodes is also seen. Vascular invasion is often prominent in the lymphohistiocytic and small-cell variants. There is a high propensity of S-ALCL for involvement of extranodal tissues (skin, bone, soft tissues) either as the only sites of disease or, more commonly, in association with nodal disease.[30,95] Rare cases of S-ALCL may present with leukemic blood involvement, a high propensity for CNS involvement, and an extremely poor prognosis.[96]

C-ALCL is separated both clinically and pathologically from S-ALCL.[28] C-ALCL is part of a spectrum of CD30+ T-cell lymphoproliferative disorders that includes the benign entity of lymphomatoid papulosis.[97,98] Because CD30+ cutaneous lymphoproliferative disorders share overlapping pathologic and clinical features, diagnosis requires careful assessment of clinical, histologic, immunophenotypic, and genetic features. C-ALCL is a T-cell lymphoma of large, anaplastic cells that are CD30+ and is limited to the skin at the time of diagnosis by extensive staging. This usually is as a solitary tumor, nodule, or papule that is composed of larger, pleomorphic cells that infiltrate the upper and deep dermis and extend into the subcutaneous tissues. Epidermal invasion is not frequently seen, and background inflammation is usually modest.[98]

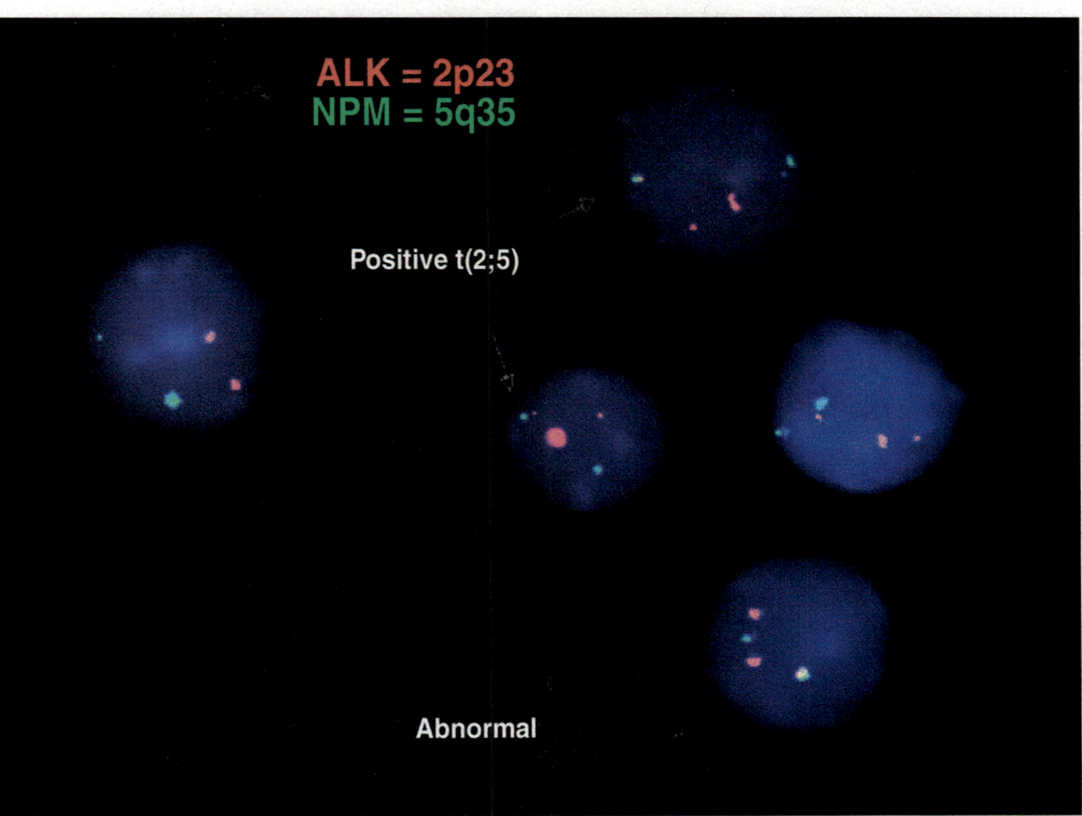

Figure 124g-6 Fluorescent in situ hybridization (FISH) analysis on paraffin tissues from a patient with systemic ALCL demonstrating fusion of the NPM and ALK probe signals, indicative of t(2;5).

Both S-ALCL and C-ALCL will show expression of CD30 by immunohistochemistry (Figure 124g-5B). CD30 is an activation marker that is found in the tumor necrosis factor superfamily.[99] It should be noted that expression of CD30 is not diagnostic of ALCL. CD30 is also an activation marker that may be expressed in B-LCL as well as benign cells. The majority of ALCL have been shown to be of T-cell phenotype by molecular studies, although immunophenotypic analysis may show staining with T-cell markers (CD2, CD3, CD5, CD7, CD45RO, CD43) or may fail to demonstrate staining with either T- or B-cell markers (null cell). Antigen deletion, especially of CD3, CD5, and/or CD7 is common. Most tumors will express CD4. Expression of cytotoxic antigens, such as TIA-1 or granzyme, and epithelial membrane antigen (EMA) is frequently seen. ALK expression detects the fusion protein generated by translocations associated with S-ALCL (see below) is also seen (Figure 124g-5C). ALK staining is very specific for S-ALCL, and is otherwise noted only in brain cells, some rhabdomyosarcomas, and inflammatory myofibroblastic tumors. ALK staining is absent in C-ALCL and, if observed, indicates the likelihood that systemic disease is present.[100]

Cytogenetic and Molecular Features of ALCL Nearly all S-ALCL and C-ALCL will demonstrate T-cell receptor gene rearrangements, even when immunophenotypic analysis fails to demonstrate expression of T-cell antigens.[28] Cytogenetic and molecular analyses often demonstrate a characteristic genetic alteration involving the ALK locus on chromosome 2. Classically, this is manifested as the t(2;5)(p23;q35) translocation that places a nucleolar phosphoprotein gene (*NPM1*) adjacent to the ALK tyrosine kinase gene. Less common translocations include translocation of ALK to partner genes on chromosomes 1, 2, 3, and 17 that also result in up-regulation of ALK expression.[101,102] ALK translocations may be detected by conventional cytogenetics, polymerase chain reaction, or fluorescent in situ hybridization (FISH) using ALK-specific probes (Figure 124g-6). The gene product of these translocations is detected by immunohistochemistry using ALK antibodies. The pattern of ALK staining is usually nuclear with or without cytoplasmic staining for the t(2;5) and is only in the cytoplasm for many of the alternative translocations.[18,28] There are studies correlating specific translocations with either disease presentation or prognosis. There is a high expression of ALK translocations in pediatric S-ALCL, probably in excess of 90% of cases, when a combination of ALK immunostaining, cytogenetics, and FISH is employed.[103]. ALK translocations are absent in C-ALCL and seen with lower frequency in adults.[28,101,102] The presence of an ALK translocation or ALK protein expression appears to be associated with a better prognosis in adults, but this association has not been observed in pediatric patients.[28,104]

Lymphoblastic Lymphoma **Limited-Stage Lymphoblastic Lymphoma** Children with limited-stage lymphoblastic lymphoma, St. Jude's stages I and II, have a favorable prognosis with long-term survival rates of 85 to 90%[2] and reported disease-free survival rates of 63 to 73% (Table124g-9).[40,105,106] The excellent overall survival rates have been attributed to effective salvage strategies for patients who have relapsed after initial shorter courses of therapy. Even in the case of localized disease, systemic multidrug chemotherapy, with central nervous system prophylaxis, is needed to achieve favorable cure rates. Variable responses to treatment have been seen among children with different histologic subtypes of localized NHL. In general, children with localized lymphoblastic lymphoma have achieved better outcomes with ALL-based treatment regimens.[87,106–108]

Over the past 10 to 15 years, the need for local radiotherapy has been eliminated.[34] Although surgery plays a major role in the diagnosis and/or complete resection of limited-stage disease, combination chemotherapy is the cornerstone of treatment. Initially, localized lymphoblastic lymphoma was treated with the same regimens as other localized non-Hodgkin lymphomas within many cooperative groups. Therapeutic approaches varied and have included CHOP with mercaptopurine and methotrexate (POG),[105] LSA_2L_2 (a drug combination therapy developed at Memorial Sloan Kettering Cancer Center) and COMP (CCG).[40,87] and modified LSA_2L_2 with the addition of high-dose methotrexate[106] (see Table 124g-9). Because of the reports of treatment failures after shortened courses of B-NHL chemotherapy,[40,105,106,109] many international cooperative groups have now adopted histology-specific treatment strategies for localized disease that are similar or identical to the treatment approaches used for advanced-stage (III or IV) lymphoblastic lymphoma.[106,108,110]

Table 124g-9 Treatment and Outcome of Limited-Stage (Localized) Lymphoblastic Lymphoma in Children and Adolescents

	CCG	POG	SFOP
	Meadows et al[40]	Link et al[105]	Patte et al[106]
Patients (*n*)	15	50	8
Protocol	COMP vs LSA_2L_2	CHOP, MP, MTX	LMT81
Duration	6–18 mo	9 weeks–8 mo	24 mo
5-yr EFS (Est)	67%	63%	73%

CCG = Children's Cancer Group; POG = Pediatric Oncology Group; SFOP = Société Française d'Oncologie Pediatrique; EFS = event-free survival; COMP = cyclophosphamide, vincristine, methotrexate, prednisone; LSA_2L_2 = cyclophosphamide, vincristine, prednisone, daunomycin, methotrexate, cytarabine, thioguanine, asparaginase, carmustine; CHOP = cyclophosphamide, doxorubicin, vincristine, prednisone; MP = mercaptopurine; MTX = methotrexate; LMT81 = modified LSA_2L_2 with high-dose methotrexate; Est = estimate.

Treatment and Prognosis of Advanced-Stage Lymphoblastic Lymphoma The prognosis for children with advanced lymphoblastic lymphoma improved significantly after the introduction of the 9-drug LSA_2L_2 regimen originally developed by Wollner and colleagues.[111] The selective advantage of this regimen in the treatment of lymphoblastic compared with nonlymphoblastic lymphoma also helped to underscore the importance of histology-specific treatment strategies in childhood NHL. The 5-year event-free survival rates for patients with advanced lymphoblastic lymphoma treated with LSA_2L_2 in comparison with COMP were significantly better (64% vs 34%, $p = .001$).[107] The principal component of treatment of advanced-stage lymphoblastic lymphoma is multiagent chemotherapy. Excellent outcomes have been achieved without the addition of local radiotherapy.[110] Since the introduction of the LSA_2L_2 regimen, treatment approaches for advanced lymphoblastic lymphoma have varied, with many groups adopting ALL-based therapeutic regimens.[110,112–115] Historically, 60 to 80% survival rates have been seen using a variety of multiagent chemotherapy regimens, with treatment durations of 12 to 32 months.[108,113–121] (Table 124g-10). More recently, very favorable results have been observed with the BFM adaptation of ALL therapy. The NHL-BFM-90 regimen, which used high-dose methotrexate, dexamethasone, moderate doses of anthracyclines and cyclophosphamide, as well as prophylactic cranial radiation, with a treatment stratification based on tumor response to induction therapy, resulted in a 90% EFS.[110]

Relapsed Lymphoblastic Lymphoma The prognosis for children who develop recurrent disease is poor, with reported 5-year survival rates of 10% after recurrence of lymphoblastic lymphoma following initial treatment on CCG-551.[107] In an effort to improve outcome for patients with relapsed disease, intensive re-induction chemotherapy followed by hematopoietic stem cell transplantation (HSCT) is often pursued if partial or complete responses are achieved. This approach has led to disease-free survival rates of 23 to 58% in pediatric and adult patients with refractory NHL (including multiple histologic subtypes).[122–125] Although re-induction chemotherapy regimens used in this setting vary, many advocate an approach identical to that used in relapsed ALL. Alternatively, intensive NHL regimens such as DECAL (dexamethasone, etoposide, cisplatin, high-dose cytarabine, and L-asparaginase)[49] or ICE (ifosfamide, carboplatin, etoposide)[126] have been used. The response to salvage chemotherapy is an important predictor of outcome following HSCT, with improved survival seen in those patients with chemosensitive disease.[122,124,127] Few studies have reported the outcome following HSCT for pediatric patients with recurrent or refractory lymphoblastic lymphoma. Outcomes following autologous versus allogeneic stem cell transplantation for recurrent lymphoblastic lymphoma, from the International Bone Marrow Transplant Registry and Autologous Blood and Marrow Transplant Registry, were recently compared. Significantly lower relapse rates were observed following allogeneic SCT; however, higher treatment-related mortality offset any survival benefit.[128] Potential benefits of an allogeneic stem cell source include a graft-versus-lymphoma effect,[127] as well as elimination of the risk of infusing tumor cells, or stem cells damaged by prior therapy. Randomized trials may help to better define optimal therapy in the future.

Given the poor prognoses for the majority of patients with recurrent lymphoblastic lymphoma, biologically targeted and less toxic treatment approaches are needed. One example of an agent of promise for treatment of T-cell hematopoietic disease is compound 506U78. Compound 506U78 (2-amino-9-B-D-arabinofuranosyl-6-methoxy-9H-purine) is a water-soluble prodrug of ara-G (9-B-arabinofuranosylguanine), which is selectively toxic to T-lymphoblasts.[129–131] Cytotoxicity is mediated by the accumulation of ara-G nucleotides, which preferentially occurs in T- versus B-lymphoblasts, and results in inhibition of DNA synthesis. This agent is currently being used in combination with chemotherapy for the treatment of T-ALL (COG study AALL00P2).

Immunotherapeutic approaches also offer potential benefit for lymphoblastic lymphoma owing to the specificity and favorable toxicity profiles of these agents. Alemtuzumab (Campath-1H) is a humanized monoclonal antibody that targets the CD52 molecule that is widely expressed on both B- and T-lineage lymphoid tumors, and favorable responses to Campath-1H have been observed in patients with recurrent T-ALL.[132] Another agent of potential promise is denileukin diftitox ($DAB_{389}IL2$), an interleukin-2 receptor (IL-2R)–targeted diphtheria toxin that causes T-cell death through inhibition of protein synthesis.[133] Favorable responses to this agent have been observed in cutaneous T-cell lymphoma and small numbers of patients with NHL expressing IL-2R and suggest that future treatment initiatives in lymphoblastic lymphoma may be warranted.[134,135] Finally, the high frequency of *NOTCH1* activating mutations in T-cell leukemia[136] provides rationale for the potential future use of NOTCH-pathway inhibitors in precursor T-cell malignancies.

Pathology of Lymphoblastic Lymphoma Lymphoblastic lymphomas are neoplasms of immature or precursor lymphoid cells, analogous to the neoplastic cells of ALL. Often the immature lymphoid neoplasms have both lymphomatous and leukemic components and may demonstrate a spectrum of disease. This spectrum of disease is reflected in the REAL[17] and WHO[18] classifications, where these are termed precursor T (or B) lymphoblastic leukemia/lymphomas. The designation lymphoma is preferred when the primary presentation is as a mass lesion with minimal blood and bone marrow involvement, whereas leukemia is used for primary presentation in the blood and > 25% blasts in the marrow.[17,18] When the primary presentation pattern is not clear, the designation of leukemia/lymphoma is appropriate. Whereas precursor B-cell disease predominates in ALL, most of the lymphomatous presen-

Table 124g-10 Treatment and Outcome of Advanced (Disseminated) Lymphoblastic Lymphoma in Children and Adolescents

	BFM	St. Jude	EORTC-CLCG	DFCI	UKCCSG	CCG
	Reiter et al[108]	Dahl et al[113]	Millot et al[116]	Weinstein et al[118]	Eden et al[120]	Abromowitch et al[121]
Patients (*n*)	101	24	60	21	95	102
Protocol	NHL-BFM-90	Total Therapy-X	EORTC 58881	APO	UKCCSG 8503	CCG 5941
Duration	24 mo	32 mo	24 mo	24 mo	24 mo	12 mo
EFS (Est)	90% (5-yr)	73% (4-yr)	76% (6-yr)	58% (3-yr)	65% (4-yr)	79% (3-yr)

EFS = event-free survival; Est = estimate.

tations are of precursor T-cell derivation (80–90% T-cell vs 10–20% B-cell). Precursor T-cell lymphoblastic lymphomas tend to present as mediastinal or upper torso nodal masses, whereas precursor B-cell lymphoblastic lymphomas are more likely to present in skin, soft tissue, bone, tonsil, and peripheral lymph nodes.[19,137–140]

Morphologic features of lymphoblastic lymphoma include diffuse or partial effacement of lymph nodes. Particularly in T-cell disease, the neoplastic cells may infiltrate in interfollicular zones with sparing of benign, reactive follicles. Owing to rapid proliferation, a starry-sky pattern derived from the presence of tingible body macrophages ingesting apoptotic debris may be present. Cytologically, the neoplastic cells are indistinguishable from those seen in ALL. The cells have an immature, blast-like appearance with fine ("dusty") chromatin, inconspicuous or absent nucleoli, and scanty cytoplasm that ranges from pale to slightly basophilic in color. Cells may have rounded or irregular nuclear contours with infoldings. The cells will demonstrate a high mitotic rate.[17–19,140] Some "large-cell" variants may have more abundant cytoplasm and visible nucleoli as well as significant nuclear pleomorphism, corresponding to the L2 morphologic variant seen in ALL (see Table 124g-2).[115,141]

Most immature B- or T-lymphoid cells will express terminal deoxytidyl transferase (TdT), which may be detected by flow cytometric, immunohistochemical, or cytochemical methods and is a useful marker of lymphoblastic lymphoma.[19] Precursor T-lymphoblastic lymphomas will display a cortical thymocyte immunophenotype, usually reflecting middle to late stages of differentiation. Although antigenic deletion is common, most neoplasms will express some combination of CD1, CD2, CD5, and CD7 along with coexpression of CD4 and/or CD8. Occasionally, both CD4 and CD8 may be absent. Cell surface CD3 and T-cell receptors are usually not expressed, but may be present within the cytoplasm. CD10 is expressed in 15 to 40% of cases, and occasionally natural killer antigens such as CD57 or CD16 may be seen.[19,115] Precursor B-lymphoblastic lymphomas most often display the immunophenotype early pre-B or pre–B-phenotypes (CD19, CD10, and TdT with variable CD20, CD22, HLA-DR, and cytoplasmic immunoglobulin).[19,139]

Cytogenetic and Molecular Features of Lymphoblastic Lymphoma Molecular analysis and cytogenetic findings in the lymphoblastic lymphomas mirror those found in ALL.[56,115,142,143] Precursor T-lymphoblastic lymphomas will display early T-cell gene rearrangements (TCRδ, TCRγ, TCRα, and/or TCRβ) by molecular studies, although some very immature cells may not demonstrate a rearrangement and others may also demonstrate immunoglobulin gene rearrangements (lineage infidelity).[143] Precursor B-lymphoblastic lymphomas will usually show monoclonal immunoglobulin gene rearrangements, and will lack evidence of somatic hypermutation.[144] Cytogenetic abnormalities are common in both B- and T-lymphoblastic lymphomas, with a frequency of 50 to 80%.[115] Although no unique translocation for T-lymphoblastic lymphoma has been identified, chromosomal breakpoints associated with T-cell receptor (TCR) genes or specific oncogenes are most commonly reported. TCRαδ (14q11), TRCβ (7q32-36), and TCRγ (7p15) sites are characteristic sites of chromosomal abnormalities, with the more immature cellular phenotypes favoring the TCRγ or TCRδ loci. Often the TCR enhancer or promoter elements are translocated and juxtaposed to putative transcription factors.[115,143] Specific oncogenes associated with T-lymphoblastic lymphomas include *tcl-1* (14q32) involved in t(7;14)(q35;q32) or t(14;14)(q11;q32), the *tcl-2* oncogene (11p13) involved in t(11;13)(p13;q11), the *tcl-3* oncogene (10q24) seen in t(8;14)(q24;q11), and *tal-1* (1p32) involved in t(1;14)(q32;q11). Approximately 30% of precursor T-cell neoplasms will demonstrate cytogenetic abnormalities involving these specific loci.[56] Cytogenetic abnormalities in B-lymphoblastic lymphoma include hyperdiploidy as well frequent observation of additional material from the 21q locus (near the locus involved in the t(12;21) translocation that gives rise to the *TEL/AML1* fusion gene).[139]

Post-Transplant Lymphoproliferative Disorders (PTLD) Treatment and Prognosis of PTLD in Children and Adolescents The mainstay of treatment of PTLD in children following solid organ transplantation has been a reduction in the intensity of immunosuppressive medications.[145,146] Although this approach has a reasonable success rate in patients with polymorphic histology, less than one-third of children with monomorphic histology respond to simple reduction of immunosuppressive medications.[146] Furthermore, reducing immunosuppressive medications following solid organ transplantation for the treatment of PTLD significantly increases the risk of organ allograft rejection. Successful eradication of childhood PTLD requires controlling EBV-induced B-cell proliferation and transformation and enhancing the development of specific EBV cytotoxic T lymphocytes (EBV-CTL).[147] Antiviral therapy including acyclovir and, recently, ganciclovir, have not been demonstrated to be effective.[148–150]

Immunomodulation with interferon and/or intravenous gamma globulin has been studied in adult patients with PTLD following solid organ transplantation, but has been associated with mixed results.[151,152] The most successful therapy for EBV-associated PTLD following allogeneic stem cell transplantation has been the infusion of donor leukocytes (DLI) from the original donor.[153] Recently, patients with PTLD post solid organ transplantation have also received partially HLA-matched allogeneic EBV-specific CTLs from a frozen bank of CTLs derived from healthy blood donors.[154]

Patients who do not respond to reduction/withdrawal of immunosuppression or develop allograft rejection (refractory PTLD) have had a poor prognosis. Chemotherapy has been used for refractory PTLD because it provides cytotoxic therapy for B-cell lymphoproliferation and immunosuppression to prevent/treat allograft rejection. Because of the concerns of toxicity and the theoretic risk of standard-dose chemotherapy inhibiting EBV T-cell immunity development, Gross and colleagues conducted an institutional pilot study using a low-dose chemotherapy regimen of cyclophosphamide and prednisone (Cy/Pred) for 36 children with refractory PTLD.[155,156] Gross and colleagues demonstrated Cy/Pred to be safe and effective, with a 69% 2-year event-free survival, but the relapse rate was higher than expected (22%), and there was a 10% allograft failure rate.[155,156]

A recently developed chimeric antibody that consists of variable regions from the heavy and light chains of the murine anti-CD20 antibody and human IgG1 and kappa constant regions (rituximab) was demonstrated to induce significant responses with and without chemotherapy in adults with low and intermediate de novo (non-PTLD–associated) B-NHL.[157,158] Most recently, Coiffier and colleagues demonstrated that chemoimmunotherapy (using rituximab and CHOP chemotherapy) compared with chemotherapy alone with CHOP in elderly patients with DLBCL resulted in a significant improvement in disease free survival (DFS) and overall survival (OS).[159] Initial studies using monoimmunotherapy (rituximab) in adult patients with PTLD reported a 65% response rate with an 18% relapse rate and a 16% mortality rate following rituximab alone.[160] However, in a much larger cohort and with longer follow-up in a multicenter open-label phase II trial of rituximab therapy in patients with PTLD, the overall response rate was only 46%, with the remainder of patients either progressing or dying on study.[161] These results suggest that single-agent rituximab therapy is not likely to result in a high percentage of long-term sustained complete remissions.

We (MSC) recently conducted a pilot study combining cyclophosphamide and prednisone (Cy/Pred) with rituximab (CPR).[162] Six children, two with fulminant PTLD, were treated with cyclophosphamide (600 mg/m^2 day 1), prednisone (2 mg/kg/day for 5 days) and rituximab (375 mg/m^2/dose IV weekly for 3 weeks) for two to four courses of therapy. Two patients each had a cardiac, liver, and renal transplant with a median onset of PTLD of 39 (10–144) months post solid organ allograft. The overall response rate was 100% (five complete and one partial response). All five complete responders are currently without disease and the one partial responder with fulminant PTLD eventually developed progressive disease and died.[162] These results have led to the development of a pilot phase II study of CPR in children and adolescents with CD20 positive PTLD who fail reduced immunosuppressive therapy after solid organ transplantation with the Children's Oncology Group (COG ANHL-0221).

Pathology of PTLD There are three major morphologic categories of PTLD: (1) lymphoid hyperplasia, (2) polymorphic PTLD, and (3) lymphomatous or monomorphic PTLD.[163] This classification also recognizes another category that includes other unusual presentations of PTLD such as plasmacytoma, myeloma, Hodgkin disease, and T-cell PTLD.[163,164] The majority of children and adolescents with PTLD express a B-cell immunophenotype such as CD20 or CD79a, although a small percentage (approximately 3–10%) may be of T-cell phenotype.[165–168] Furthermore, 90% of PTLD demonstrate intratumoral EBV by either in situ hybridization to detect EBV early RNA (EBER) or LMP-1 by immunohistochemistry.[163,169] PTLD following solid organ transplantation in children occurs most commonly in the following highest-risk groups: lung, bowel, combined organ solid organ transplantation, use of T-cell, antibody tacrolimus or sirolimus, EBV seronegativity at time of transplant, and age less than 5 years.[170–174] In contrast, the risk of PTLD following allogeneic stem cell transplantation in children occurs in the following poor-risk groups: unrelated adult stem cell donors, mismatched donors, T-cell depletion, and recipients who develop grade II-IV acute graft-versus-host disease.[175] The most prominent immune defect in both groups of children who develop PTLD following either a solid organ graft or allogeneic stem cell graft is delayed T-cell reconstitution or suppression of specific T-cell EBV cytotoxic T-lymphocytes (EBV-CTL).[174,176]

Cytogenetic and Molecular Genetics in PTLD The underlying cytogenetic and molecular genetic subtypes of childhood PTLD have yet to be described. Polymorphic subtypes may be monoclonal, but are more likely to show a polyclonal or oligoclonal pattern, whereas monomorphic PTLDs are more likely to show monoclonal gene rearrangements.[163,164,168] T-cell PTLDs demonstrate clonal T-cell receptor gene rearrangements.[164,177] In adults with monomorphic or lymphomatous PTLD, molecular abnormalities of *TP53*, N-*ras*, and/or c-*myc* have been previously described.[178] Recently, up to 40% of polymorphic PTLDs have been described in adults to have *bcl-6* mutations, which have been associated with refractoriness to therapy.[179] COG ANHL0221, using CPR for childhood PTLD unresponsive to reduced immunosuppression, will also investigate the cytogenetic and genetic aberrations associated with childhood PTLD.

SUMMARY/FUTURE CONSIDERATIONS

The prognosis for children and adolescents with non-Hodgkin lymphoma, both with limited- and advanced-stage disease, has improved significantly over the past two decades. Except for rare subtypes, the chance of being alive and disease free at 5 years for limited- and advanced-stage disease B-NHL is 95% and 80%, respectively. The prognosis for advanced lymphoblastic non-Hodgkin lymphoma in children and adolescents has now increased to over 85% survival. The prognosis, however, for the most advanced childhood and adolescent ALCL is still less than 70% at 7-year follow-up. The improved outlook for childhood non-Hodgkin lymphoma, however, has not come without a certain price. The use of short but intense chemotherapy, especially in B-NHL, has resulted in long hospitalizations and severe hematopoietic and nonhematopoietic toxicity. Furthermore, long-term complications or late effects, such as sterility, cardiomyopathy, and secondary malignancies, still occur following the use of the aggressive multiagent chemotherapy in children and adolescents with advanced non-Hodgkin lymphoma.

The recent improvements in EFS and survival in DLBCL in the elderly age group with the combination of targeted monoclonal antibody therapy (rituximab) and chemotherapy (CHOP) suggests that chemoimmunotherapy may be a future treatment strategy to consider in children and adolescents with B-LCL.[159] The introduction of targeted immunotherapy may not only enhance the prognosis, but also provide a synergistic strategy of using combination chemotherapy and immunotherapy in hopes of decreasing the acute and chronic toxicities associated with current chemotherapy regimens. The COG is currently piloting a new protocol combining rituximab with FAB-type therapy (COMRAP) (cyclophosphamide, vincristine, methotrexate, rituximab, Adriamycin, prednisone) in their new open advanced B-NHL trial (COG ANHL01P1) (personal communication, M. Cairo, MD, Chair).

The COG is also investigating the benefit of adding vinblastine, an active agent in ALCL, in combination with an APO backbone in the treatment of children and adolescents with advanced ALCL (ANHL0131). Additionally, COG is investigating the benefit of a BFM-NHL backbone approach compared with an aggressive pre–B-ALL regimen in children and adolescents with advanced T-cell lymphoblastic lymphoma (A5971).

Recent advances in genomic scale gene expression profiling of adult DLBCL have recently been reported.[58] Staudt and colleagues, using a “Lymphochip” developed at the NCI and containing approximately 3,500 genes expressed in lymphocytes, performed microarray analyses of a large cohort of adults with DLBCL.[58,180,181] They demonstrated the clustering of two distinctive subgroups of DLBCL, an activated B-like and GC (germinal center)-like. The adults with DLBCL with a GC-like profile had a significantly improved survival compared with the activated B-like (65% vs 30%) ($p < .01$).[58] More recently, Staudt and colleagues have demonstrated five different genetic signatures by microarray in adult DLBCL that predict for prognosis.[180,181] Similarly, Dalla Favera and colleagues, using the Affymetrix oligonucleotide microarray approach, have demonstrated a homogeneity of adult chronic lymphocytic leukemia with memory B cells.[182] We are currently performing gene expression profiling of childhood and adolescent B-NHL in the ongoing COG ANHL01P1 study to determine if similar diagnostic and prognostic subgroups can be identified by this molecular genetic approach in childhood B-NHL as had been demonstrated in adults with B-LCL.

Future therapeutic strategies for childhood non-Hodgkin lymphoma will likely incorporate immunophenotyping, cytogenetics, and molecular genetic features. Surface, intracellular and molecular targets will likely be identified that will alter our treatment approach over the next decade. Furthermore, prevention of the development of childhood non-Hodgkin lymphoma and the reduction of acute and long-term complications resulting from the treatment of childhood and adolescent non-Hodgkin lymphoma will be two major strategies to pursue in years to come.

REFERENCES

1. Shad A, Magrath I. Malignant non-Hodgkin lymphomas in children. In: Pizzo PA, Poplack DG, editors. Principles and practice of pediatric oncology. 3rd ed. Philadelphia: Lippincott-Raven Publishers; 1997. p. 545–87.
2. Sandlund JT, Downing JR, Crist WM. Non-Hodgkin lymphoma in childhood. N Engl J Med 1996;334:1238–48.
3. Young JL Jr, Ries LG, Silverberg E, et al. Cancer incidence, survival, and mortality for children younger than age 15 years. Cancer 1986;58:598–602.
4. Percy CL, Smith MA, Linet M, et al. Lymphomas and reticuloendothelial neoplasms. In: Ries LAG, Smith MA, Gurney JG, et al., editors. Cancer incidence and survival among children and adolescents: United States SEER Program 1975–1995. Pub. No. 99-4649. Bethesda (MD): National Cancer Institute, Seer Program; 1999. p. 35–50.
5. Perkins SL, Segal GH, Kjeldsberg CR. Classification of non-Hodgkin lymphomas in children. Semin Diagn Pathol 1995;12:303–13.
6. Purtilo DT, Strobach RS, Okano M, Davis JR. Epstein-Barr virus-associated lymphoproliferative disorders. Lab Invest 1992;67:5–23.
7. Levine AM. Acquired immunodeficiency syndrome-related lymphoma. Blood 1992;80:8–20.
8. Filipovich AH, Mathur A, Kamat D, Shapiro RS. Primary immunodeficiencies: genetic risk factors for lymphoma. Cancer Res 1992;52:5465s–7s.
9. Fisher S, Fisher R. The epidemiology of non-Hodgkin lymphoma. Oncogene 2004;23:6524–34.
10. Hennessy B, Hanrahan E, Daly P. Non-Hodgkin lymphoma: an update. Lancet Oncol 2004;5:341–53.
11. Chiu B, Weisenburger D. An update of the epidemiology of non-Hodgkin lymphoma. Clin Lymphoma 2003;4:161–8.
12. Thirlwell C, Sarker D, Stebbing J, Bower M. Acquired immunodeficiency syndrome-related lymphoma in the era of highly active antiretroviral therapy. Clin Lymphoma 2003:86–92.
13. Rappaport H. Tumors of the hematopoietic system. Atlas of tumor pathology. Washington DC: Armed Forces Institute of Pathology; 1966. p. 10–4.
14. Lukes RJ, Collins RD. Immunologic characterization of human malignant lymphomas. Cancer 1974;34(4 suppl):1488–503.
15. Lennert K, Feller A. Histopathology of non-Hodgkin lymphoma. New York: Springer-Verlag; 1992.
16. The non-Hodgkin Lymphoma Pathologic Classification Project. National Cancer Institute-sponsored study of classification of non-Hodgkin lymphomas: summary and description of a working formulation for clinical usage. Cancer 1982;49:2112–35.
17. Harris N, Jaffe E, Stein H, et al. A revised European-American classification of lymphoid neoplasms: a proposal from the International Lymphoma Study Group. Blood 1994;84:1361–92.
18. Jaffe E, Harris N, Stein H, Vardiman J, editors. World Health Organization classification of tumors. Tumours of haematopoietic and lymphoid tissues. Washington DC: IARC Press; 2000.
19. Perkins SL. Work-up and diagnosis of pediatric non-Hodgkin lymphomas. Pediatr Dev Pathol 2000;3:374–90.
20. Lorsbach R, Shay-Seymore D, Moore J, et al. Clinicopathologic analysis of follicular lymphoma occurring in children. Blood 2002;99:1959–64.
21. Swerdlow S. Pediatric follicular lymphomas, marginal zone lymphomas and marginal zone hyperplasia. Am J Clin Pathol 2004;122:S98–109.

22. Cairo MS. Current advances and future strategies in B-large cell lymphoma in children and adolescents. Proc Am Soc Clin Oncol 2002;21:512–9.
23. Murphy SB, Fairclough DL, Hutchison RE, Berard CW. Non-Hodgkin lymphomas of childhood: an analysis of the histology, staging, and response to treatment of 338 cases at a single institution. J Clin Oncol 1989;7:186–93.
24. Hoover-Regan ML, Sposto R, Morris E, et al. Significant improvement in survival over the past 20 years with short and intense therapy in children with disseminated small non-cleaved cell lymphoma (SNCCL): analysis of 465 Children's Cancer Group (CCG) patients [abstract]. Proc Am Soc Clin Oncol 1998;17:533a.
25. Hoover-Regan M, Meadows AT, Sposto R, et al. Treatment and outcome of pediatric large cell lymphoma over 18 years (n=279): the Children's Cancer Group (CCG) experience [abstract]. Proc Am Soc Clin Oncol 1997;16:517a.
26. Murphy SB. Pediatric lymphomas: recent advances and commentary on Ki-1-positive anaplastic large-cell lymphomas of childhood. Ann Oncol 1994;5:31–3.
27. Falini B, Pileri S, Zinzani PL, et al. ALK+ lymphoma: clinico-pathological findings and outcome. Blood 1999;93:2697–706.
28. Stein H, Foss HD, Durkop H, et al. CD30(+) anaplastic large cell lymphoma: a review of its histopathologic, genetic, and clinical features. Blood 2000;96:3681–95.
29. Kinney MC, Kadin ME. The pathologic and clinical spectrum of anaplastic large cell lymphoma and correlation with ALK gene dysregulation. Am J Clin Pathol 1999;111:S56–67.
30. Jaffe E. Mature T-cell and NK-cell lymphomas in the pediatric age group. Am J Clin Pathol 2004;122 Suppl:S110–21.
31. Murphy SB. Classification, staging and end results of treatment of childhood non-Hodgkin lymphoma: dissimilarities from lymphomas in adults. Semin Oncol 1980;7:332–9.
32. Cairo MS, Gerrard M, Patte C. A new protocol for treatment of mature B-cell lymphoma/leukaemia (BCLL): FAB LMB 96, a SFOP LMB 96/CCG-5961/UKCCSG NHL 9600 international cooperative study [abstract]. Med Pediatr Oncol 1997;29:320a.
33. Magrath I, Lee YJ, Anderson T, et al. Prognostic factors in Burkitt's lymphoma: importance of total tumor burden. Cancer 1980;45:1507–15.
34. Link MP, Donaldson SS, Berard CW, et al. Results of treatment of childhood localized non-Hodgkin lymphoma with combination chemotherapy with or without radiotherapy. N Engl J Med 1990;322:1169–74.
35. Cairo MS, Bishop M. Tumour lysis syndrome: new therapeutic strategies and classification. Br J Haematol 2004;127:3–11.
36. Goldman SC, Holcenberg JS, Finklestein JZ, et al. A randomized comparison between rasburicase and allopurinol in children with lymphoma or leukemia at high risk for tumor lysis. Blood 2001;97:2998–3003.
37. Pui CH, Mahmoud HH, Wiley JM, et al. Recombinant urate oxidase for the prophylaxis or treatment of hyperuricemia in patients with leukemia or lymphoma. J Clin Oncol 2001;19:697–704.
38. Pui CH, Jeha S, Irwin D, Camitta B. Recombinant urate oxidase (rasburicase) in the prevention and treatment of malignancy-associated hyperuricemia in pediatric and adult patients: results of a compassionate-use trial. Leukemia 2001;15:1505–9.
39. Patte C, Auperin A, Michon J, et al. The Societe Francaise d'Oncologie Pediatrique LMB89 protocol: highly effective multiagent chemotherapy tailored to the tumor burden and initial response in 561 unselected children with B-cell lymphomas and L3 leukemia. Blood 2001;97:3370–9.
40. Meadows AT, Sposto R, Jenkin RD, et al. Similar efficacy of 6 and 18 months of therapy with four drugs (COMP) for localized non-Hodgkin lymphoma of children: a report from the Children's Cancer Study Group. J Clin Oncol 1989;7:92–9.
41. Link MP, Shuster JJ, Donaldson SS, et al. Treatment of children with localized non-Hodgkin lymphoma (NHL) with nine weeks of chemotherapy without radiotherapy [abstract]. Med Pediatr Oncol 1993;21:532a.
42. Reiter A, Schrappe M, Tiemann M, et al. Improved treatment results in childhood B-cell neoplasms with tailored intensification of therapy: a report of the Berlin-Frankfurt-Munster Group Trial NHL-BFM 90. Blood 1999;94:3294–306.
43. Gerrard M, Cairo MS, Patte C, et al. Results of the FAB international study in children and adolescents (C+A) with localised B-NHL (large cell [LCL], Burkitt's [BL] and Burkitt's-like [BLL]) [abstract]. Proc Am Soc Clin Oncol 2003;22:3197.
44. Weinstein H, Lack E, Cassady J. APO therapy for malignant lymphoma on large cell "histiocytic" type of childhood: analysis of treatment for 29 patients. Blood 1984;64:422–6.
45. Laver JH, Weinstein HJ, Hutchison RE, et al. Lineage-specific differences in outcome for advanced stage large cell lymphoma in children and adolescents: results of a randomized phase III Pediatric Oncology Group Trial [abstract]. Blood 2001;87:345a.
46. Cairo MS, Sposto R, Hoover-Regan M, et al. Childhood and adolescent large-cell lymphoma (LCL): a review of the Children's Cancer Group experience. Am J Hematol 2003;72:53–63.
47. Cairo MS, Krailo MD, Morse M, et al. Long-term follow-up of short intensive multiagent chemotherapy without high-dose methotrexate ("Orange") in children with advanced non-lymphoblastic non-Hodgkin lymphoma. A Children's Cancer Group report. Leukemia 2002;16:594–600.
48. Patte C, Gerrard M, Auperin A, et al. Results of the randomised international trial FAB LMB 96 for the "intermediate risk" childhood and adolescent B-cell lymphoma: reduced therapy is efficacious [abstract]. Proc Am Soc Clin Oncol 2003;22:796.
49. Kobrinsky NL, Sposto R, Shah NR, et al. Outcomes of treatment of children and adolescents with recurrent non-Hodgkin lymphoma and Hodgkin disease with dexamethasone, etoposide, cisplatin, cytarabine, and l-asparaginase, maintenance chemotherapy, and transplantation: Children's Cancer Group Study CCG-5912. J Clin Oncol 2001;19:2390–6.
50. Finn LS, Viswanatha DS, Belasco JB, et al. Primary follicular lymphoma of the testis in childhood. Cancer 1999;85:1626–35.
51. Lones MA, Perkins SL, Sposto R, et al. Large-cell lymphoma arising in the mediastinum in children and adolescents is associated with an excellent outcome: a Children's Cancer Group report. J Clin Oncol 2000;18:3845–53.
52. Lones MA, Cairo MS, Perkins SL. T-cell-rich large B-cell lymphoma in children and adolescents: a clinicopathologic report of six cases from the Children's Cancer Group Study CCG-5961. Cancer 2000;88:2378–86.
53. Chu PG, Chang KL, Arber DA, Weiss LM. Practical applications of immunohistochemistry in hematolymphoid neoplasms. Ann Diagn Pathol 1999;3:104–33.
54. Heerema N, Poirel H, Swansbury J, et al. Chromosomal abnormalities of pediatric (ped) and adult diffuse large B-cell lymphoma (DLBCL) differ and may reflect potential differences in oncogenesis. An international pediatric mature B-cell non-Hodgkin lymphoma study (FAB/LMB96) [abstract]. Blood 2003;102:3139.
55. Gascoyne RD, Adomat SA, Krajewski S, et al. Prognostic significance of Bcl-2 protein expression and Bcl-2 gene rearrangement in diffuse aggressive non-Hodgkin lymphoma. Blood 1997;90:244–51.
56. Goldsby RE, Carroll WL. The molecular biology of pediatric lymphomas. J Pediatr Hematol Oncol 1998;20:282–96.
57. Le Beau MM, Rowley JD. Chromosomal abnormalities in leukemia and lymphoma: clinical and biological significance. Adv Hum Genet 1986;15:1–54.
58. Alizadeh AA, Eisen MB, Davis RE, et al. Distinct types of diffuse large B-cell lymphoma identified by gene expression profiling. Nature 2000;403:503–11.
59. Falini B, Mason DY. Proteins encoded by genes involved in chromosomal alterations in lymphoma and leukemia: clinical value of their detection by immunocytochemistry. Blood 2002;99:409–26.
60. Lossos IS, Jones CD, Warnke R, et al. Expression of a single gene, BCL-6, strongly predicts survival in patients with diffuse large B-cell lymphoma. Blood 2001;98:945–51.
61. Chang CC, Liu YC, Cleveland RP, Perkins SL. Expression of c-Myc and p53 correlates with clinical outcome in diffuse large B-cell lymphomas. Am J Clin Pathol 2000;113:512–8.
62. Davis RE, Staudt LM. Molecular diagnosis of lymphoid malignancies by gene expression profiling. Curr Opin Hematol 2002;9:333–8.
63. Siebert R, Rosenwald A, Staudt L, Morris S. Molecular features of B-cell lymphoma. Curr Opin Oncol 2001;13:316–24.
64. Cairo MS, Sposto R, Perkins SL, et al. Burkitt's and Burkitt-like lymphoma in children and adolescents: a review of the Children's Cancer Group experience. Br J Haematol 2003;120:660–70.
65. Brecher ML, Schwenn MR, Coppes MJ, et al. Fractionated cyclophosphamide and back to back high dose methotrexate and cytosine arabinoside improves outcome in patients with stage III high grade small non-cleaved cell lymphomas (SNCCL): a randomized trial of the Pediatric Oncology Group. Med Pediatr Oncol 1997;29:526–33.
66. Griffin TC, Bowman WP, Winick NJ, Buchanan GR. Treatment of advanced stage diffuse, small non-cleaved cell lymphoma in childhood: further experience with total therapy B. Med Pediatr Oncol 1994;23:393–9.
67. Bowman WP, Shuster JJ, Cook B, et al. Improved survival for children with B-cell acute lymphoblastic leukemia and stage IV small noncleaved-cell lymphoma: a Pediatric Oncology Group study. J Clin Oncol 1996;14:1252–61.
68. Schwenn MR, Mahmoud HH, Bowman WP, et al. Successful treatment of small noncleaved cell (SNCC) lymphoma and B cell acute lymphoblastic leukemia (B-ALL) with central nervous system (CNS) involvement: a Pediatric Oncology Group (POG) study [abstract]. Proc Am Soc Clin Oncol 2000;19:580a.
69. Cairo MS, Gerrard M, Sposto R, et al. Poor response to initial reduction therapy (COP) and combined bone marrow and CNS disease are poor prognostic factors in children with advanced (BM+CNS) B-NHL treated on the international study FAB/LMB96) [abstract]. Blood 2003;102:492.
70. Woessmann W, Seidemann K, Mann G, et al. The impact of the methotrexate administration schedule and dose in the treatment of children and adolescents with B-cell neoplasms: a report of the BFM Group Study NHL-BFM95. Blood 2005;105:948–58.
71. Lones MA, Auperin A, Raphael M, et al. Mature B-cell lymphoma/leukemia in children and adolescents: intergroup pathologist consensus with the revised European-American Lymphoma Classification. Ann Oncol 2000;11:47–51.
72. Wright D, McKeever P, Carter R. Childhood non-Hodgkin lymphomas in the United Kingdom: findings from the UK Children's Cancer Study Group. J Clin Pathol 1997;50:128–34.
73. Frost M, Newell J, MA L, et al. Comparative immunohistochemical analysis of pediatric Burkitt lymphoma and diffuse large B-cell lymphoma. Am J Clin Pathol 2004;121:384–92.
74. Braziel RM, Arber DA, Slovak ML, et al. The Burkitt-like lymphomas: a Southwest Oncology Group study delineating phenotypic, genotypic, and clinical features. Blood 2001;97:3713–20.
75. Hutchison RE, Finch C, Kepner J, et al. Burkitt lymphoma is immunophenotypically different from Burkitt-like lymphoma in young persons. Ann Oncol 2000;11:35–8.
76. Macpherson N, Lesack D, Klasa R, et al. Small noncleaved, non-Burkitt's (Burkitt-Like) lymphoma: cytogenetics predict outcome and reflect clinical presentation. J Clin Oncol 1999;17:1558–67.
77. Sanger W, Swansbury J, Poirel H, et al. Primary (8q24) and secondary chromosome abnormalities (1q, 6q, 13q, & 17p) are similar in pediatric Burkitt lymphoma/Burkitt leukemia & Burkitt-like lymphoma: a report of the international pediatric B-cell non-Hodgkin lymphoma study (FAB/LMB 96) [abstract]. Blood 2003;102:1355.
78. Lones M, Sanger W, LeBeau M, et al. Chromosomal abnormalities may correlate with prognosis in Burkitt/Burkitt-like lymphomas of children and adolescents: a report from the Children's Cancer Study Group Study CCG-E08. J Pediatr Hematol Oncol 2004;26:169–78.
79. Pagano JS, Huang CH, Levine P. Absence of Epstein-Barr viral DNA in American Burkitt's lymphoma. N Engl J Med 1973;289:1395–9.
80. Seidemann K, Tiemann M, Schrappe M, et al. Short-pulse B-non-Hodgkin lymphoma-type chemotherapy is efficacious treatment for pediatric anaplastic large cell lymphoma: a report of the Berlin-Frankfurt-Munster Group Trial NHL-BFM 90. Blood 2001;97:3699–706.
81. Brugieres L, Deley MC, Pacquement H, et al. CD30(+) anaplastic large-cell lymphoma in children: analysis of 82 patients enrolled in two consecutive studies of the French Society of Pediatric Oncology. Blood 1998;92:3591–8.
82. Sandlund JT, Pui CH, Santana VM, et al. Clinical features and treatment outcome for children with CD30+ large-cell non-Hodgkin lymphoma. J Clin Oncol 1994;12:895–8.
83. Reiter A, Schrappe M, Tiemann M, et al. Successful treatment strategy for Ki-1 anaplastic large-cell lymphoma of childhood: a prospective analysis of 62 patients enrolled in three consecutive Berlin-Frankfurt-Munster group studies. J Clin Oncol 1994;12:899–908.
84. Mora J, Filippa DA, Thaler HT, et al. Large cell non-Hodgkin lymphoma of childhood: analysis of 78 consecutive patients enrolled in 2 consecutive protocols at the

Memorial Sloan-Kettering Cancer Center. Cancer 2000;88:186–97.

85. Massimino M, Gasparini M, Giardini R. Ki-1 (CD30) anaplastic large-cell lymphoma in children. Ann Oncol 1995;6:915–20.
86. Vecchi V, Burnelli R, Pileri S, et al. Anaplastic large cell lymphoma (Ki-1+/CD30+) in childhood. Med Pediatr Oncol 1993;21:402–10.
87. Anderson J, Wilson J, Jenkin D, et al. Childhood non-Hodgkin lymphoma. The results of a randomized therapeutic trial comparing a 4-drug regimen (COMP) with a 10-drug regimen (LSA_2-L_2). N Engl J Med 1983;308:559–65.
88. Sandlund JT, Pui CH, Roberts WM, et al. Clinicopathologic features and treatment outcome of children with large-cell lymphoma and the t(2;5)(p23;q35). Blood 1994;84:2467–71.
89. Laver JH, Kraveka JM, Hutchison RE, et al. Advanced-stage large-cell lymphoma in children and adolescents: results of a randomized trial incorporating intermediate-dose methotrexate and high-dose cytarabine in the maintenance phase of the APO regimen: a Pediatric Oncology Group phase III trial. J Clin Oncol 2005;23:541–7.
90. Massimino M, Spreafico F, Luksch R, Giardini R. Prognostic significance of p80 and visceral involvement in childhood CD30 anaplastic large cell lymphoma (ALCL). Med Pediatr Oncol 2001;37:97–102.
91. Brugieres L, Quartier P, Le Deley MC, et al. Relapses of childhood anaplastic large-cell lymphoma: treatment results in a series of 41 children—a report from the French Society of Pediatric Oncology. Ann Oncol 2000;11:53–8.
92. Borchmann P, Treml JF, Hansen H, et al. The human anti-CD30 antibody 5F11 shows in vitro and in vivo activity against malignant lymphoma. Blood 2003;102:3737–42.
93. Senderowicz AM. Novel direct and indirect cyclin-dependent kinase modulators for the prevention and treatment of human neoplasms. Cancer Chemother Pharmacol 2003;52 Suppl 1:S61–73.
94. Benharroch D, Meguerian-Bedoyan Z, Lamant L, et al. ALK-positive lymphoma: a single disease with a broad spectrum of morphology. Blood 1998;91:2076–84.
95. Jaffe ES. Anaplastic large cell lymphoma: the shifting sands of diagnostic hematopathology. Mod Pathol 2001;14:219–28.
96. Onciu M, Behm FG, Raimondi SC, et al. ALK-positive anaplastic large cell lymphoma with leukemic peripheral blood involvement is a clinicopathologic entity with an unfavorable prognosis. Report of three cases and review of the literature. Am J Clin Pathol 2003;120:617–25.
97. Willemze R, Beljaards RC. Spectrum of primary cutaneous CD30 (Ki-1)-positive lymphoproliferative disorders. A proposal for classification and guidelines for management and treatment. J Am Acad Dermatol 1993;28:973–80.
98. Vergier B, Beylot-Barry M, Pulford K, et al. Statistical evaluation of diagnostic and prognostic features of CD30+ cutaneous lymphoproliferative disorders: a clinicopathologic study of 65 cases. Am J Surg Pathol 1998;22:1192–202.
99. Falini B, Pileri S, Pizzolo G, et al. CD30 (Ki-1) molecule: a new cytokine receptor of the tumor necrosis factor receptor superfamily as a tool for diagnosis and immunotherapy. Blood 1995;85:1–14.
100. DeCoteau JF, Butmarc JR, Kinney MC, Kadin ME. The t(2;5) chromosomal translocation is not a common feature of primary cutaneous CD30+ lymphoproliferative disorders: comparison with anaplastic large-cell lymphoma of nodal origin. Blood 1996;87:3437–41.
101. Drexler HG, Gignac SM, von Wasielewski R, et al. Pathobiology of NPM-ALK and variant fusion genes in anaplastic large cell lymphoma and other lymphomas. Leukemia 2000;14:1533–59.
102. Duyster J, Bai RY, Morris SW. Translocations involving anaplastic lymphoma kinase (ALK). Oncogene 2001;20:5623–37.
103. Liang X, Meech S, Odom L, et al. Assessment of t(2;5)(p23;q35) translocation and variants in pediatric ALK+ anaplastic large cell lymphoma. Am J Clin Pathol 121:496–506.
104. Gascoyne RD, Aoun P, Wu D, et al. Prognostic significance of anaplastic lymphoma kinase (ALK) protein expression in adults with anaplastic large cell lymphoma. Blood 1999;93:3913–21.
105. Link MP, Shuster JJ, Donaldson SS, et al. Treatment of children and young adults with early-stage non-Hodgkin lymphoma. N Engl J Med 1997;337:1259–66.
106. Patte C, Kalifa C, Flamant F, et al. Results of the LMT81 protocol, a modified LSA2L2 protocol with high dose methotrexate, on 84 children with non-B-cell (lymphoblastic) lymphoma. Med Pediatr Oncol 1992;20:105–13.
107. Anderson J, Jenkin R, Wilson J, et al. Long-term follow-up of patients treated with COMP or LSA_2L_2 therapy for childhood non-Hodgkin lymphoma: a report of CCG-551 from the Children's Cancer Group. J Clin Oncol 1993;11:1024–32.
108. Reiter A, Schrappe M, Parwaresch R, et al. Non-Hodgkin lymphomas of childhood and adolescence: results of a treatment stratified for biologic subtypes and stage—a report of the Berlin-Frankfurt-Munster group. J Clin Oncol 1995;13:359–72.
109. Neth O, Seidemann K, Jansen P, et al. Precursor B-cell lymphoblastic lymphoma in childhood and adolescence: clinical features, treatment, and results in trials NHL-BFM 86 and 90. Med Pediatr Oncol 2000;35:20–7.
110. Reiter A, Schrappe M, Ludwig WD, et al. Intensive ALL-type therapy without local radiotherapy provides a 90% event-free survival for children with T-cell lymphoblastic lymphoma: a BFM group report. Blood 2000;95:416–21.
111. Wollner N, Burchenal JH, Lieberman PH, et al. Non-Hodgkin lymphoma in children. A comparative study of two modalities of therapy. Cancer 1976;37:123–34.
112. Asselin B, Shuster JJ, Amylon M, et al. Improved event-free survival (EFS) with high dose methotrexate (HDM) in T-cell lymphoblastic leukemia (T-ALL) and advanced lymphoblastic lymphoma (T-NHL): a Pediatric Oncology Group (POG) study [abstract]. Proc Am Soc Clin Oncol 2001;20:1464.
113. Dahl GV, Rivera G, Pui CH, et al. A novel treatment of childhood lymphoblastic non-Hodgkin lymphoma: early and intermittent use of teniposide plus cytarabine. Blood 1985;66:1110–4.
114. Goldberg JM, Silverman LB, Levy DE, et al. Childhood T-cell acute lymphoblastic leukemia: the Dana-Farber Cancer Institute acute lymphoblastic leukemia consortium experience. J Clin Oncol 2003;21:3616–22.
115. Thomas DA, Kantarjian HM. Lymphoblastic lymphoma. Hematol Oncol Clin North Am 2001;15:51–95.
116. Millot F, Suciu S, Philippe N, et al. Value of high-dose cytarabine during interval therapy of a Berlin-Frankfurt-Munster-based protocol in increased-risk children with acute lymphoblastic leukemia and lymphoblastic lymphoma: results of the European Organization for Research and Treatment of Cancer 58881 randomized phase III trial. J Clin Oncol 2001;19:1935–42.
117. Sullivan MP, Boyett J, Pullen J, et al. Pediatric Oncology Group experience with modified LSA2-L2 therapy in 107 children with non-Hodgkin lymphoma (Burkitt's lymphoma excluded). Cancer 1985;55:323–36.
118. Weinstein HJ, Cassady JR, Levey R. Long-term results of the APO protocol (vincristine, doxorubicin [Adriamycin], and prednisone) for treatment of mediastinal lymphoblastic lymphoma. J Clin Oncol 1983;1:537–41.
119. Hvizdala EV, Berard C, Callihan T, et al. Lymphoblastic lymphoma in children—a randomized trial comparing LSA2-L2 with the A-COP+ therapeutic regimen: a Pediatric Oncology Group Study. J Clin Oncol 1988;6:26–33.
120. Eden OB, Hann I, Imeson J, et al. Treatment of advanced stage T cell lymphoblastic lymphoma: results of the United Kingdom Children's Cancer Study Group (UKCCSG) protocol 8503. Br J Haematol 1992;82:310–6.
121. Abromowitch M, Sposto R, Prkins S, et al. Outcome of Children's Cancer Group (CCG) 5941: a pilot study for the treatment of newly diagnosed pediatric patients with disseminated lymphoblastic lymphoma [abstract]. Proc Am Soc Clin Oncol 2000;19:2295.
122. Bureo E, Ortega JJ, Munoz A, et al. Bone marrow transplantation in 46 pediatric patients with non-Hodgkin lymphoma. Spanish Working Party for Bone Marrow Transplantation in Children. Bone Marrow Transplant 1995;15:353–9.
123. Hartmann O, Pein F, Beaujean F, et al. High-dose polychemotherapy with autologous bone marrow transplantation in children with relapsed lymphomas. J Clin Oncol 1984;2:979–85.
124. Mills W, Chopra R, McMillan A, et al. BEAM chemotherapy and autologous bone marrow transplantation for patients with relapsed or refractory non-Hodgkin lymphoma. J Clin Oncol 1995;13:588–95.
125. Sweetenham JW, Liberti G, Pearce R, et al. High-dose therapy and autologous bone marrow transplantation for adult patients with lymphoblastic lymphoma: results of the European Group for Bone Marrow Transplantation. J Clin Oncol 1994;12:1358–65.
126. Kleiner S, Kirsch A, Schwaner I, et al. High-dose chemotherapy with carboplatin, etoposide and ifosfamide followed by autologous stem cell rescue in patients with relapsed or refractory malignant lymphomas: a phase I/II study. Bone Marrow Transplant 1997;20:953–9.
127. Jones RJ, Ambinder RF, Piantadosi S, Santos GW. Evidence of a graft-versus-lymphoma effect associated with allogeneic bone marrow transplantation. Blood 1991;77:649–53.
128. Levine JE, Harris RE, Loberiza FR Jr, et al. A comparison of allogeneic and autologous bone marrow transplantation for lymphoblastic lymphoma. Blood 2003;101:2476–82.
129. Gandhi V, Plunkett W, Rodriguez CO Jr, et al. Compound GW506U78 in refractory hematologic malignancies: relationship between cellular pharmacokinetics and clinical response. J Clin Oncol 1998;16:3607–15.
130. Rodriguez CO Jr, Stellrecht CM, Gandhi V. Mechanisms for T-cell selective cytotoxicity of arabinosylguanine. Blood 2003;102:1842–8.
131. Shewach DS, Daddona PE, Ashcraft E, Mitchell BS. Metabolism and selective cytotoxicity of 9-beta-D-arabinofuranosylguanine in human lymphoblasts. Cancer Res 1985;45:1008–14.
132. Pawson R, Dyer MJ, Barge R, et al. Treatment of T-cell prolymphocytic leukemia with human CD52 antibody. J Clin Oncol 1997;15:2667–72.
133. Talpur R, Apisarnthanarax N, Ward S, Duvic M. Treatment of refractory peripheral T-cell lymphoma with denileukin diftitox (ONTAK). Leuk Lymphoma 2002;43:121–6.
134. LeMaistre CF, Saleh MN, Kuzel TM, et al. Phase I trial of a ligand fusion-protein (DAB389IL-2) in lymphomas expressing the receptor for interleukin-2. Blood 1998;91:399–405.
135. Olsen E, Duvic M, Frankel A, et al. Pivotal phase III trial of two dose levels of denileukin diftitox for the treatment of cutaneous T-cell lymphoma. J Clin Oncol 2001;19:376–88.
136. Weng AP, Ferrando AA, Lee W, et al. Activating mutations of NOTCH1 in human T cell acute lymphoblastic leukemia. Science 2004;306:269–71.
137. Soslow RA, Baergen RN, Warnke RA. B-lineage lymphoblastic lymphoma is a clinicopathologic entity distinct from other histologically similar aggressive lymphomas with blastic morphology. Cancer 1999;85:2648–54.
138. Lin P, Jones D, Dorfman DM, Medeiros LJ. Precursor B-cell lymphoblastic lymphoma: a predominantly extranodal tumor with low propensity for leukemic involvement. Am J Surg Pathol 2000;24:1480–90.
139. Maitra A, McKenna RW, Weinberg AG, et al. Precursor B-cell lymphoblastic lymphoma. A study of nine cases lacking blood and bone marrow involvement and review of the literature. Am J Clin Pathol 2001;115:868–75.
140. Reddy K, Perkins S. Advances in the diagnostic approach to childhood lymphoblastic malignant neoplasms. Am J Clin Pathol 2004;122:S3–18.
141. Picozzi VJ Jr, Coleman CN. Lymphoblastic lymphoma. Semin Oncol 1990;17:96–103.
142. Raimondi SC. Current status of cytogenetic research in childhood acute lymphoblastic leukemia. Blood 1993;81:2237–51.
143. Pilozzi E, Muller-Hermelink HK, Falini B, et al. Gene rearrangements in T-cell lymphoblastic lymphoma. J Pathol 1999;188:267–70.
144. Hojo H, Sasaki Y, Nakamura N, Abe M. Absence of somatic hypermutation of immunoglobulin heavy chain variable region genes in precursor B-lymphoblastic lymphoma: a study of four cases in childhood and adolescence. Am J Clin Pathol 2001;116:673–82.
145. Starzl TE, Nalesnik MA, Porter KA, et al. Reversibility of lymphomas and lymphoproliferative lesions developing under cyclosporin-steroid therapy. Lancet 1984;1:583–7.
146. Hayashi RJ, Kraus MD, Patel AL, et al. Posttransplant lymphoproliferative disease in children: correlation of histology to clinical behavior. J Pediatr Hematol Oncol 2001;23:14–8.
147. Gross TG. Treatment of Epstein-Barr virus-associated post-transplant lymphoproliferative disorders. J Pediatr Hematol Oncol 2001;23:7–9.
148. Cohen JI. Epstein-Barr virus lymphoproliferative disease associated with acquired immunodeficiency. Medicine (Baltimore) 1991;70:137–60.
149. Katz BZ, Raab-Traub N, Miller G. Latent and replicating forms of Epstein-Barr virus DNA in lymphomas and lymphoproliferative diseases. J Infect Dis 1989;160:589–98.
150. Sixbey JW, Pagano JS. Epstein-Barr virus transformation of human B lymphocytes despite inhibition of viral polymerase. J Virol 1985;53:299–301.
151. Shapiro RS, Chauvenet A, McGuire W, et al. Treatment of B-cell lymphoproliferative disorders with interferon alfa

and intravenous gamma globulin. N Engl J Med 1988;318:1334.

152. Davis CL, Wood BL, Sabath DE, et al. Interferon-alpha treatment of posttransplant lymphoproliferative disorder in recipients of solid organ transplants. Transplantation 1998;66:1770–9.
153. Papadopoulos EB, Ladanyi M, Emanuel D, et al. Infusions of donor leukocytes to treat Epstein-Barr virus-associated lymphoproliferative disorders after allogeneic bone marrow transplantation. N Engl J Med 1994;330:1185–91.
154. Haque T, Wilkie GM, Taylor C, et al. Treatment of Epstein-Barr-virus-positive post-transplantation lymphoproliferative disease with partly HLA-matched allogeneic cytotoxic T cells. Lancet 2002;360:436–42.
155. Gross TG. Low-dose chemotherapy for treatment of children with PT-LPD. In: Oertel SH, Riess HB, editors. Recent results in cancer research, immunosurveillance, immunodeficiencies and lymphoproliferations. Berlin-Heidelberg: Springer-Verlag; 2002.
156. Gross TG, Park J, Bucuvalas J, et al. Low-dose chemotherapy for refractory EBV associated post-transplant lymphoproliferative disease (PTLD) following solid organ transplant (SLT) in children [abstract]. Blood 2002;100:159a.
157. Maloney DG, Grillo-Lopez AJ, Bodkin DJ, et al. IDEC-C2B8: results of a phase I multiple-dose trial in patients with relapsed non-Hodgkin lymphoma. J Clin Oncol 1997;15:3266–74.
158. Czuczman MS, Grillo-Lopez AJ, White CA, et al. Treatment of patients with low-grade B-cell lymphoma with the combination of chimeric anti-CD20 monoclonal antibody and CHOP chemotherapy. J Clin Oncol 1999;17:268–76.
159. Coiffier B, Lepage E, Briere J, et al. CHOP chemotherapy plus rituximab compared with CHOP alone in elderly patients with diffuse large-B-cell lymphoma. N Engl J Med 2002;346:235–42.
160. Milpied N, Vasseur B, Parquet N, et al. Humanized anti-CD20 monoclonal antibody (Rituximab) in post transplant B-lymphoproliferative disorder: a retrospective analysis on 32 patients. Ann Oncol 2000;11:113–6.
161. Choquet S, Herbrecht R, Socie G, et al. Multicenter, open label, phase II trial to evaluate the efficacy and safety of treatment with rituximab in patients suffering from B-cell posttransplantation lymphoproliferative disorders (B-PTLD) (M39037 trial) [abstract]. Ann Oncol 2002;110:137.
162. Orjuela M, Gross TG, Cheung YK, et al. A pilot study of chemoimmunotherapy (cyclophosphamide, prednisone, and rituximab) in patients with post-transplant lymphoproliferative disorder following solid organ transplantation. Clin Cancer Res 2003;9:3945S–52S.
163. Harris NL, Ferry JA, Swerdlow SH. Posttransplant lymphoproliferative disorders: summary of Society for Hematopathology Workshop. Semin Diagn Pathol 1997;14:8–14.
164. Nalesnik MA. The diverse pathology of post-transplant lymphoproliferative disorders: the importance of a standardized approach. Transpl Infect Dis 2001;3:88–96.
165. George T, Jeng M, Berquist N, et al. Epstein-Barr virus-associated peripheral T-cell lymphoma and hemophagocytic syndrome arising after liver transplantation: case report and review of the literature. Pediatr Blood Cancer 2005;44:270–6.
166. Rajakariar R, Bhattacharyya M, Norton A, et al. Post transplant T-cell lymphoma: a case series of four patients from a single unit and review of the literature. Am J Transplant 2004;4:1534–8.
167. Lundell R, Elinitoba-Johnson K, Lim M. T-cell post-transplant lymphoproliferative disorder occurring in a pediatric solid-organ transplant patient. Am J Surg Pathol 2004;28:967–73.
168. Pickhardt PJ, Siegel MJ, Hayashi RJ, Kelly M. Posttransplantation lymphoproliferative disorder in children: clinical, histopathologic, and imaging features. Radiology 2000;217:16–25.
169. Ifthikharuddin JJ, Mieles LA, Rosenblatt JD, et al. CD-20 expression in post-transplant lymphoproliferative disorders: treatment with rituximab. Am J Hematol 2000;65:171–3.
170. Ho M, Jaffe R, Miller G, et al. The frequency of Epstein-Barr virus infection and associated lymphoproliferative syndrome after transplantation and its manifestations in children. Transplantation 1988;45:719–27.
171. Opelz G, Henderson R. Incidence of non-Hodgkin lymphoma in kidney and heart transplant recipients. Lancet 1993;342:1514–6.
172. Morgan G, Superina RA. Lymphoproliferative disease after pediatric liver transplantation. J Pediatr Surg 1994;29:1192–6.
173. Cox KL, Lawrence-Miyasaki LS, Garcia-Kennedy R, et al. An increased incidence of Epstein-Barr virus infection and lymphoproliferative disorder in young children on FK506 after liver transplantation. Transplantation 1995;59:524–9.
174. Haque T, Thomas JA, Parratt R, et al. A prospective study in heart and lung transplant recipients correlating persistent Epstein-Barr virus infection with clinical events. Transplantation 1997;64:1028–34.
175. Curtis RE, Travis LB, Rowlings PA, et al. Risk of lymphoproliferative disorders after bone marrow transplantation: a multi-institutional study. Blood 1999;94:2208–16.
176. Lucas KG, Small TN, Heller G, et al. The development of cellular immunity to Epstein-Barr virus after allogeneic bone marrow transplantation. Blood 1996;87:2594–603.
177. Sivaraman P, Lye WC. Epstein-Barr virus-associated T-cell lymphoma in solid organ transplant recipients. Biomed Pharmacother 2001;55:366–8.
178. Knowles DM, Cesarman E, Chadburn A, et al. Correlative morphologic and molecular genetic analysis demonstrates three distinct categories of posttransplantation lymphoproliferative disorders. Blood 1995;85:552–65.
179. Cesarman E, Chadburn A, Liu YF, et al. BCL-6 gene mutations in posttransplantation lymphoproliferative disorders predict response to therapy and clinical outcome. Blood 1998;92:2294–302.
180. Rosenwald A, Wright G, Chan WC, et al. The use of molecular profiling to predict survival after chemotherapy for diffuse large-B-cell lymphoma. N Engl J Med 2002;346:1937–47.
181. Staudt LM. Molecular diagnosis of the hematologic cancers. N Engl J Med 2003;348:1777–85.
182. Klein U, Tu Y, Stolovitzky GA, et al. Gene expression profiling of B cell chronic lymphocytic leukemia reveals a homogeneous phenotype related to memory B cells. J Exp Med 2001;194:1625–38.
183. Williams DM, Hobson R, Imeson J, et al. Anaplastic large cell lymphoma in childhood: analysis of 72 patients treated on the United Kingdom Children's Cancer Study Group chemotherapy regimens. Br J Haematol 2002;117:812–20.

124h

Less-Frequently Encountered Tumors of Childhood

Carlos Rodriguez-Galindo, MD
Alberto S. Pappo, MD

Individually, carcinomas, germ cell tumors, retinoblastoma, and liver tumors are relatively rare in pediatric patients.[1,2] Collectively, however, these neoplasms account for up to 18% of all cancers seen in young people (ie, those younger than 20 years old; Figures 124h-1A and 124h-1B). Furthermore, the incidence of some of these tumors, such as germ cell malignancies and certain carcinomas, is significantly higher in older patients (ie, those aged between 15 and 19 years; Figure 124h-1B), a population that has been under-represented in prospective NCF cooperative national trials.[3] This chapter describes the principles of diagnosis and therapy for rare pediatric tumors, including hepatoblastoma, germ cell tumors, and retinoblastoma, and discusses the epidemiological aspects of various carcinomas and melanoma.

RETINOBLASTOMA

Retinoblastoma is the most frequent neoplasm of the eye in childhood and represents 3% of all pediatric cancers. The average incidence of retinoblastoma in the United States is 1 in 14,000 to 18,000 live births. Thus, an estimated 200 to 300 children develop retinoblastoma each year.[2]

Retinoblastoma presents in two distinct clinical forms: (1) Bilateral or multifocal, hereditary (40% of cases), characterized by the presence of germline mutations of the *RB1* gene. Multifocal retinoblastoma may be inherited from an affected survivor (25%) or be the result of a new germline mutation (75%). (2) Unilateral or unifocal, usually nonhereditary (60% of cases). Retinoblastoma is discussed in detail in Chapter 74, "Neoplasms of the Eye." Only a few supplementary points will be presented here.

Biology The human retina is far from having completed its maturation at the completion of gestation, and it is not considered to be terminally differentiated until 3 years of age. It is during this period of time, in which primitive photoreceptor cells are stimulated to differentiate into the mature retina, that cells are at high risk of sustaining oncogenic events that result in the development of a neoplasm. Retinoblastoma is among the best understood of human neoplasms and has served as an important model for understanding tumorigenesis.[4] The *RB1* gene, located in chromosome 13q14, was identified and cloned in 1986.[5,6] Its product (pRb) is a 110 kd nuclear phosphoprotein that acts by binding and inhibiting several proteins with growth-stimulatory activity, and it appears to function as a tumor suppressor by inhibiting cell-cycle progression past the G_1-S restriction point. Thus, pRb stands as the major gatekeeper to control this critical point in growth regulation. The lack of pRb or its inactivation removes the pRb constraint on cell-cycle control, with the consequence of deregulated cell proliferation.[7] The *RB1* gene is a large gene, containing 27 exons over about 200 kb of DNA, and mutations ("first hit") have been described in almost every exon. Nonsense and frameshift are the most common germline and somatic mutations, although deletions and duplications are also frequently encountered.[7] There are no mutational hotspots, although new germline mutations have an overwhelming preference for the paternal allele, suggesting that deamination of methylated CpG pairs has an important role in mutagenesis.[8] In both hereditary and nonhereditary retinoblastoma, the second tumorigenic event ("second hit") is chromosomal in nature, often as a result of mitotic recombination errors.[9] This second hit occurs at a much higher frequency than the first hit, and it is more sensitive to environmental factors such as ionizing radiation, thus the increased risk of radiation-induced malignancies in survivors of retinoblastoma. After the "second hit" has taken place, retinoblastoma cells rapidly accumulate additional genetic damage.[10] In fact, it is possible that an additional mutation ("third hit"), probably involving a gene of the apoptotic pathway, is necessary for final retinal tumor formation.[7]

Genetic Counseling Retinoblastoma is a unique neoplasm, in which the hereditary type shows an autosomal dominant inheritance, with almost complete penetration (85–95%).[11] However, some families display an inheritance pattern characterized by reduced penetrance and expressivity. These low-penetrance retinoblastoma mutations either cause a reduction in the amount of normal pRb produced, or result in a partially functional mutant pRb.[12] Also, the *RB1* gene mutation can occur at a late stage of embryogenesis, resulting in a variable expression depending on the tissue, causing mosaicisms in 10 to 15% of family members.[13] Genetic counseling is of utmost importance to determine the heritability of a given case and to estimate the risk in relatives. Because of the size of the *RB1* gene and the lack of mutational hot spots, exhaustive analysis of the *RB1* gene is required for clinical DNA testing.[14] With the refinement in methods of mutational analysis over the last decade, detection rates have increased to greater than 90%.[15–17] In general, however, based on the inheritance pattern and considering the existence of mosaicisms, the following risk estimates can be made[11]:

1. Risk to offspring of survivors of retinoblastoma: The risk of retinoblastoma arising in the offspring of survivors of bilateral (hereditary) disease is 45%, whereas it is 2.5% for the offspring of survivors of unilateral retinoblastoma.
2. Risk to siblings of patients with retinoblastoma: In those cases with positive family history, the siblings of bilaterally affected cases have a risk of 45% of developing retinoblastoma, and the siblings of unilaterally affected cases have a risk of 30%. For those cases without family history, the risk is 2% for siblings of bilateral cases and 1% for siblings of unilateral cases.

Although most patients with bilateral retinoblastoma carry a germline mutation of the *RB1* gene, a small proportion (5–6%) carry a deletion involving the 13q14 locus, which is large enough to be detected by karyotype analysis, either as a deletion or as part of a balanced translocation.[18] In those cases, retinoblastoma is part of a more complex syndrome resulting from the loss of additional genetic material. In addition to developing retinoblastoma, patients with the 13q– syndrome are characterized by typical facial dysmorphic features, subtle skeletal abnormalities, and different degrees of mental retardation and motor impairment.[19–21]

Because their orbital growth is still in progress, children treated for retinoblastoma are at risk of functionally and cosmetically significant bony orbital abnormalities. These sequelae become evident by early adolescence, when orbital growth is largely complete, and results in the "hourglass facial deformity."[22] Both enucleation, which causes orbital contraction, and radiotherapy, which induces arrest of bone growth, adversely affect orbital growth. In children treated for bilateral retinoblastoma, the impact of enucleation in orbital development is not different from that of irradiation. However, final orbital volumes after enucleation correlate with the size of the prosthetic implant.[23]

Patients with germline mutation of the *RB1* gene are at risk of developing second cancers. These patients normally have multifocal, bilateral disease and are thus often treated with radiation therapy, further enhancing the susceptibility of a second cancer. The cumulative incidence of sec-

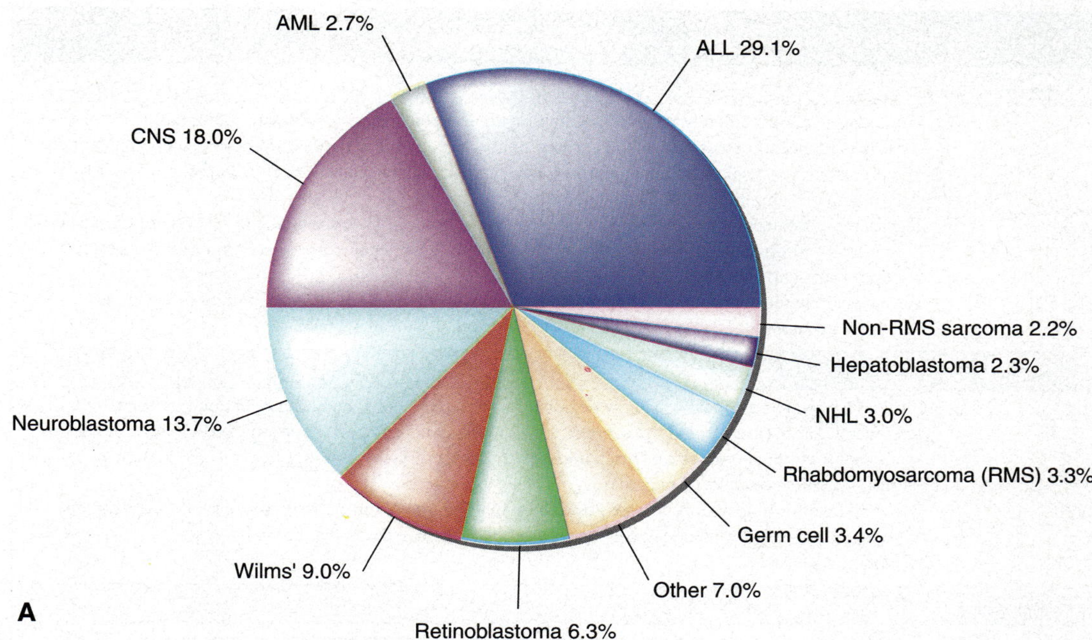

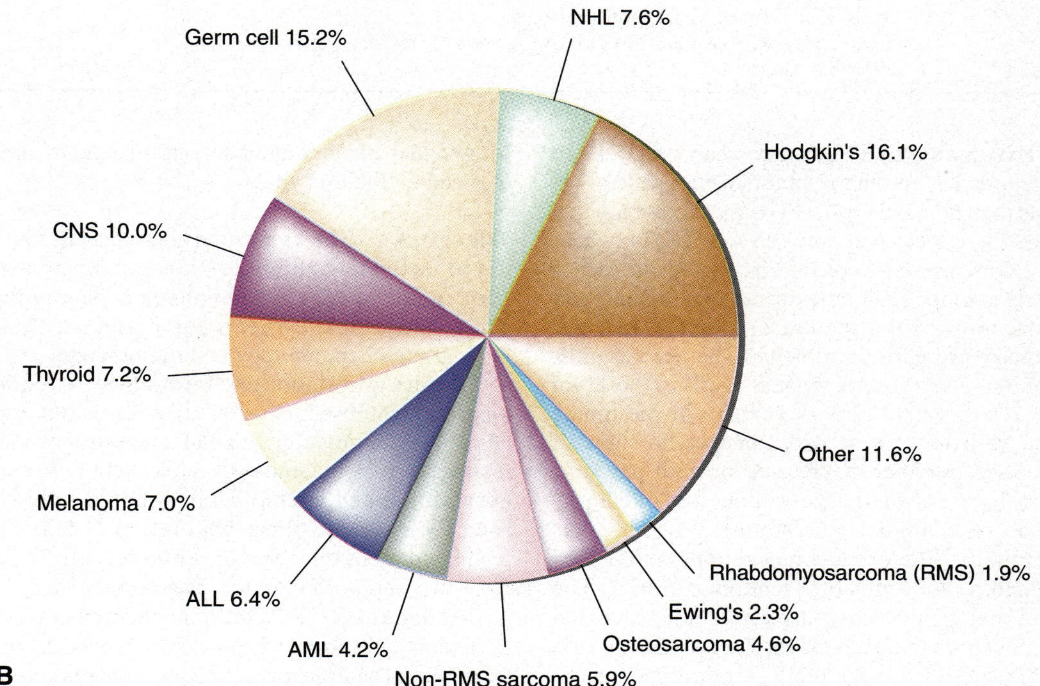

Figure 124h-1 Distribution of cancer types **A,** in children < 5 years of age and **B,** in patients 15–19 years of age (SEER 1986–1995). AML = acute myelogenous leukemia; ALL = acute lymphoblastic leukemia; CNS = central nervous system; NHL = non-Hodgkin's lymphoma.

ond malignancies is 4% at 10 years, 18% at 35 years, and 51% at 50 years.[24–26] The tumors most commonly encountered are soft tissue sarcomas, melanomas, and osteosarcomas. There appears to be an age effect on the sarcoma risk; patients receiving radiation during the first year of life are at higher risk of developing a sarcoma.[27]

GERM CELL TUMORS

Epidemiology Germ cell tumors (GCT) are rare in children, with an incidence of 2.4 cases per million children per year, accounting for less than 3% of all pediatric malignancies.[2] This incidence is, however, underestimated, since most tumor registries are biased in favor of malignant types, excluding most mature teratomas. The age distribution follows a bimodal pattern, with a peak during the first 3 years of life and a second peak in late adolescence. In general, females have a higher overall incidence of GCT, although males are more at risk of malignant GCT.[28] The only two well-established predisposing factors are males with cryptorchidism and patients with gonadal dysgenesias. In children, GCT comprise a variety of distinct entities that differ in their histology, molecular biology, and clinical behavior.

Pathology GCT arise from primitive pluripotential germ cells, and thus represent a very heterogeneous group of tumors that range from benign teratomas to very aggressive neoplasms.[29] Close to half of the tumors present at extragonadal sites.[28] For these tumors, it is hypothesized that aberrant or incomplete migration of primordial cells has taken place. Alternatively, totipotential embryonal cells could have escaped the influence of embryogenic organizers controlling normal differentiation.[29] The biology, histology, and clinical behavior of the different GCT are dependent on the site of origin, the stage of development of the germ cell at the time of neoplastic transformation, and the gender and age of the patient. A germ cell tumor may have many different types of tissue, both benign and malignant, and the most malignant component always dictates the behavior. Therefore, the tumor must be sampled very extensively before the final diagnosis and the treatment plan are made.

Benign GCT:

1. Mature teratomas are usually composed of mature representatives of all three embryogenic germ cell layers. They occur most commonly in ovaries, sacrococcygeal area, and mediastinum, in this order. Sacrococcygeal teratomas occur almost exclusively in neonates, whereas ovarian and mediastinal teratomas occur during the second decade.
2. Gonadoblastomas represent a mixture of immature germ cells and gonadal sex cord cells. They are always located in a dysgenetic gonad in patients with aberrant sexual differentiation. They may be associated with germinomas.

GCT of Indeterminate Behavior:

1. Immature teratomas, in which immature components are identified. The immature component is almost always of neuroepithelial origin, but can also be immature mesenchyma or renal blastema. Immature teratomas usually occur in the ovaries, and rarely in extraovarian sites. They are graded into four different grades according to the degree of maturation. Grades 0 to 2 usually have a benign behavior.[30]
2. Malignant GCT. Malignant childhood GCT differ significantly from their adult counterparts in composition, distribution, and site. For example, more than 40% of malignant GCT in children occur in extragonadal sites.
3. Germinomas are the least aggressive tumors of this group, and they are very chemo- and radiosensitive. They can occur in the ovaries (dysgerminomas), central nervous system (pineal region), or very rarely in the testes (seminomas). They are composed of large cells with clear cytoplasm, arranged in nests separated by bands of fibrous tissue.
4. Yolk sac tumor (YST) or endodermal sinus tumor is the most common malignant germ cell

tumor in prepubertal children, and it is usually the only malignant germ cell component in sacrococcygeal and infantile testicular malignancies.[31] An elevation of alpha-fetoprotein (AFP) is diagnostic of this malignancy.

5. Embryonal carcinoma seldom occurs in children. It is often a major component of a mixed GCT of the testes or the mediastinum in adolescents and much less likely a part of an ovarian tumor. Microscopically, embryonal carcinomas are very similar to YST, but cells are larger, with a major epithelial pattern.
6. Choriocarcinomas are very rare, may be pure in infants, but in older children usually occurs as a component of a mixed GCT. In infants choriocarcinoma usually represents a maternal or placental metastasis, and thus is actually a gestational trophoblastic tumor rather than a germ cell tumor.[32] Both cytotrophoblast and syncytiotrophoblast cells must be present for diagnosis. Elevated serum levels of beta-HCG (B-HCG) are usually diagnostic of this malignancy.
7. Mixed malignant germ cell tumors. In younger children, teratomas usually have YST or germinoma components. In older, usually postpubertal children, more malignant components are seen, usually embryonal carcinoma, YST, germinoma, and choriocarcinoma.

Table 124h-1	Staging of Testicular, Ovarian, and Extragonadal Tumors
Testicular	
I	Limited to testis, completely resected by high inguinal orchiectomy; no clinical, radiographic, or histologic evidence of disease beyond the testis; tumor markers normal after appropriate half-life decline; patients with normal or unknown markers at diagnosis must have negative ipsilateral retroperitoneal lymph node sampling to confirm stage I disease
II	Transscrotal orchiectomy; microscopic disease in scrotum or high in spermatic cord (< 5 cm from proximal end); retroperitoneal lymph node involvement (< 2 cm) and/or increased tumor markers after appropriate half-life decline
III	Tumor-positive retroperitoneal lymph nodes (> 2 cm); no visceral or extra-abdominal involvement
IV	Distant metastases
Ovarian	
I	Limited to ovary, peritoneal washings negative for malignant cells; no clinical, radiologic, or histologic evidence of disease beyond the ovaries; tumor markers negative after appropriate half-life decline
II	Microscopic residual or positive lymph nodes (< 2 cm); peritoneal washings negative for malignant cells; tumor markers positive or negative
III	Gross residual or biopsy only; tumor-positive lymph nodes (> 2 cm); contiguous visceral involvement (omentum, intestine, bladder); peritoneal washings positive for malignant cells
IV	Distant metastases
Extragonadal	
I	Complete resection at any site; coccygectomy included as management for sacrococcygeal site; negative tumor margins
II	Microscopic residual; lymph nodes negative
III	Gross residual or biopsy only; regional lymph nodes positive or negative
IV	Distant metastases

MOLECULAR BIOLOGY Cytogenetic and molecular studies have confirmed that childhood germ cell tumors constitute a group of distinct entities. A distinct chromosomal aberration, i(12p), is often seen in adult GCT.[33] In children, however, the i(12p) is found almost exclusively in gonadal and extragonadal (usually mediastinal) tumors of adolescent males.[34] As in adults, the i(12p) has also been found in hematopoietic malignancies in adolescents with extragonadal GCT.[35] Contrary to their adult counterparts, in children there is a wide array of cytogenetic abnormalities that appear to define biologically distinct subgroups that cluster based on age and sex and site of origin.[36] Gains in chromosomes 1q, 2, 3, 7, 8, 12, and 14 have been described in tumors originating in prepubertal females, whereas tumors in prepubertal males have been found to have gains in chromosomes 1q, 7, and 21, and losses in chromosome 1p.[34] Central nervous system germinomas have a high frequency of sex chromosome abnormalities, usually increased number of copies of chromosome X. Finally, del 1p36 is a common finding in extragonadal and testicular tumors in young children with YST.[37]

CLINICAL PRESENTATION **Gonadal GCT** Ovarian tumors account for approximately 25% of all GCT and usually develop in pubertal and postpubertal girls, who often present with acute or chronic pain and enlarged abdomen. Testicular tumors account for 18 to 20% of all GCT. In infants, they usually present as a painless mass in the scrotum, and distant metastases are rare. In contrast, in older boys and adolescents, testicular tumors tend to disseminate early into the retroperitoneal lymph nodes and lung.[28]

Extragonadal GCT Over half of GCT are extragonadal, and these tumors have worse prognosis than gonadal GCT.[38] The most common site is the sacrococcygeal area (25% of GCT), where tumors are present at birth. Virtually all sacrococcygeal tumors have an external component, and obstruction of the rectum or urinary tract are common presenting problems. The second most common site of extragonadal GCT is the brain (18–20%), where tumors develop in the pineal area. Patients present with nonspecific signs of increased intracranial pressure or with paralysis of conjugate upward gaze without loss of convergence (Parinaud's syndrome). Germinomas account for 60% of these pineal tumors, followed by mature and immature teratomas (30%). The more malignant embryonal carcinoma, YST and choriocarcinoma account for the remaining 10% of brain GCT. Intracranial germinomas have a high tendency for craniospinal dissemination.[39] Less frequently encountered extragonadal GCT are mediastinal and retroperitoneal.

GCT have an infiltrative growth pattern and may disseminate by both lymphogenous and hematogenous routes. Most common sites of hematogenous metastases are lungs and liver. Serologic markers are very useful for diagnosis, monitoring of response, and prediction of recurrence. AFP levels are usually elevated in tumors with YST components. However, normal newborns have elevated levels of AFP, and they remain elevated above adult levels during most of the first year of life. Also, hepatoblastomas and other conditions, such as liver damage, may results in elevation of the serum AFP levels. Finally, the syncytiotrophoblastic component of choriocarcinomas, and some germinomas, secrete B-HCG. Staging of GCT is individualized for gonadal and extragonadal tumors, and is summarized in Table 124h-1.

TREATMENT The successful treatment of GCT has to include a multimodal strategy, where surgery, chemotherapy, and radiotherapy play a role. The histological subentities differ in their response to chemotherapy and radiotherapy.

Mature and Immature Teratomas A complete surgical resection is curative for mature teratomas. For immature gonadal and extragonadal teratomas, the outcome is also excellent with surgery alone, and chemotherapy should only be used for the rare patient who recurs.[40] Surveillance with determination of serum levels of AFP for 3 to 5 years after surgery is recommended.

Malignant GCT Different chemotherapeutic agents and combinations are effective in the treatment of malignant GCT. However, platinum-based regimens are considered to be the standard of therapy.[38,41,42] In the United States, the intergroup POG-CCG studies prospectively explored the PEB regimen (cisplatin 20 $mg/m^2/d \times 5$ days, etoposide 100 $mg/m^2/d \times 5$ days, and bleomycin 15 mg/m^2 day 1).[43,44] For patients with stage II testicular or stages I/II ovarian tumors, the POG9048/CCG8891 trial used surgery and 4 courses of PEB, with a 6-year EFS of 100% in patients with testicular tumors, and 92.9% in patients with ovarian tumors.[43] For patients with gonadal stages III–IV and extragonadal stages I–IV malignant GCT, the POG9049/CCG8882 trial evaluated the use of cisplatin intensification, and patients were randomized to receive standard (cisplatin 20 $mg/m^2/d$) or high-dose (cisplatin 40 $mg/m^2/d$) PEB.[44] Overall, there was a trend toward improved outcome for patients receiving high-dose PEB; the 6-year EFS distributions were

89.6% and 80.5% for patients receiving high-dose and standard-dose cisplatin, respectively. However, the overall survival was not different, and the high-dose arm was significantly more toxic. A subsequent Children's Oncology Group (COG) study explored the use of amifostine to decrease the cisplatin-related toxicity of the high-dose regimen. The preliminary results of this study did not show any advantage of the addition of amifostine, and approximately 70% of the patients developed severe hearing loss.[45]

An alternative to the PEB regimen is the JEB regimen (etoposide 120 mg/m^2/d × 3 days, carboplatin 600 mg/m^2 day 2, and bleomycin 15 mg/m^2 day 3), which appears to have comparable efficacy and less toxicity.[46] However, there have been no randomized studies comparing the efficacy of the PEB and JEB regimens.

Based on these results, a more refined risk-adapted therapy, based on stage and site, is possible. The new classification proposed by the COG stratifies patients into three groups (Table 124h-2).

1. Low risk: Patients with stage I immature teratomas (with or without malignant elements) and gonadal malignant germ cell tumors, which can be cured with surgery alone. Boys with stage I testicular tumors originally treated with surgical resection and observation can usually be salvaged if relapse occurs by using further surgical excision and standard PEB chemotherapy.[43,47] European studies also have reported encouraging salvage rates for stage I ovarian GCT patients originally treated with surgery and observation.[48] Therefore, surgery alone is indicated for stage I gonadal tumors; however, a close follow-up observation to document a normalization of the tumor markers after surgery is mandatory.
2. Intermediate risk: Patients with stage II–IV gonadal, and stage I–II extragonadal tumors have an excellent outcome (survival > 90%) with the standard PEB[44] or JEB[46] regimens. These good results suggest that a reduction in therapy may be possible for this group of patients in the future. The current COG-GCT132 study is investigating a modified, reduced-dose PEB regimen. However, the subgroups of patients older than 15 years of age with metastatic testicular tumors, and patients with metastatic ovarian tumors appear to have worse outcome (survival < 85%), and therefore should be considered to represent a higher risk group and are not candidates for dose reduction.
3. High risk: Patients with stage III/IV extragonadal tumors. For these patients, survival with the standard PEB or JEB regimens is not better than 80%. Although high-dose PEB may provide some advantage, the incidence and severity of long-term toxicities is very significant and cannot be decreased with the use of amifostine.[44,45] Therefore, new strategies are needed. The current COG study (GCT1P1) is exploring the addition of cyclophosphamide to standard PEB.

Table 124h-2 Standard Treatment Approaches for Children with Extracranial Germ Cell Tumors

Histology	Site	Stage	Treatment
Mature teratoma	All sites	I	Surgery + observation
Immature teratoma	All sites	I	Surgery + observation
Malignant germ cell tumor	Testicular	I	Surgery + observation*
		II–IV	Surgery + PEB/JEB
	Ovarian	I	Surgery + observation*
		II–IV	Surgery + PEB/JEB
	Extragonadal	I–II	Surgery + PEB/JEB
		III–IV	Surgery + PEB/JEB New regimens

*Normalization of tumor markers after surgery is required.
B = bleomycin; E = etoposide; J = carboplatin; P = cisplatin.

With the more widespread use of cisplatin-based regimens, the previous prognostic factors such as histology, site, and tumor stage have, in part, lost their prognostic relevance. Patients with metastatic disease can be cured, and the completeness of tumor resection appears to be the new, more relevant prognostic factor. In advanced, infiltrating tumors, the rate of complete resections can be significantly increased by preoperative chemotherapy, and extended, mutilating surgeries can be avoided.

TUMORS OF THE LIVER

Approximately 60% of all liver tumors are malignant,[49] accounting for 1.1% of all childhood cancers. Of the estimated 150 new cases of liver cancer seen in children under the age of 20 years, each year in the United States, hepatoblastoma accounts for two-thirds of these.[1,2]

EPIDEMIOLOGY AND ETIOLOGY

Hepatoblastoma Hepatoblastoma preferentially affects boys and occurs in infants or very young children with a median age of presentation of 16 months.[1,49] The incidence of this disease has steadily increased over the past 30 years, but has been most marked over the past 10 years, and more rapidly among those aged 1 to 4 years of age.[50] Most cases of hepatoblastoma are sporadic; they rarely occur in association with specific predisposition syndromes and commonly arise within the setting of normal hepatic function. Hepatoblastoma is strongly associated with premature birth, particularly among neonates that weigh < 1,000 g, where an excess risk of up to 21-fold has been described.[50–52] A prospective case-controlled trial will be conducted by the Children's Oncology Group to determine the risk factors associated with hepatoblastoma in low birth weight infants. Hepatoblastoma occurs in children from families affected by familial adenomatous polyposis, which is associated with an inherited germline mutation of the adenomatous polyposis coli (*APC*) gene.[53,54] Among the 8% of patients with hepatoblastoma who had a highly suggestive family history of *APC*, all had germline mutations within the *APC* gene, but no definitive "hot spot" could be identified (Gail Tomlinson, personal communication, 2005). Hepatoblastoma is also seen in association with Beckwith–Wiedemann syndrome (BWS), where the relative risk of developing this disease is 2,280 times higher than that for other embryonal tumors.[55] Finally, hepatoblastoma has also been observed in patients with Li–Fraumeni syndrome and trisomy 18.[56,57]

Hepatocellular Carcinoma Hepatocellular carcinoma is rare during the first 20 years of life, but its incidence is substantially higher among those aged 15 to 19 years and is the most common malignant hepatic tumor in adolescents.[1] Patients with hepatocellular carcinoma commonly have a preexisting parenchymal liver disorder. The association of hepatitis B infection with hepatocellular carcinoma in adults is well recognized and has been documented with increasing frequency in children in Southeast Asia and South Africa[2,58–60]; hepatitis C infection may be an emerging risk factor following therapy for childhood cancer and among infected Asian Americans with evidence of cirrhosis.[61–63] The institution of national programs of universal vaccination such as those implemented in Taiwan may sharply decrease the incidence of hepatocellular carcinoma.[64] Other diseases associated with hepatocellular carcinoma include hereditary tyrosinemia type I, glycogen storage disease type I, a1-antitrypsin deficiency, ataxia-telangiectasia, neurofibromatosis type 1, Alagille syndrome, and Fanconi anemia.[65–69]

PATHOLOGY AND MOLECULAR GENETIC ABNORMALITIES

Hepatoblastomas are embryonal neoplasms akin to Wilms' tumors, embryonal rhabdomyosarcomas, and pancreatoblastomas that recapitulate embryonic and fetal hepatocyte development. They are most often unifocal and nonencapsulated, and they can contain epithelial and mesenchymal elements and undifferentiated small cells. The epithelial element can include fetal or embryonal cells; most hepatoblastomas contain both types of cell. Patients with tumors containing only fetal cells, as shown by histology of resected material, appear to have a better prognosis than do those whose tumors contain small undifferentiated cells, the presence of which has been associated with an increased risk of recurrence of the tumor.[70]

Table 124h-3 Staging Systems for Hepatoblastoma

POG/CCG Classification	Outcome after Surgical Resection
Stage 1	Complete gross resection with pathologically negative margins
Stage 2	Total gross resection with microscopic, residual disease at margin of resection
Stage 3	Total gross resection with nodal involvement or tumor spill, or gross intrahepatic disease after incomplete resection or biopsy
Stage 4	Metastatic disease, incomplete resection, or biopsy

CCG = Children's Cancer Group; POG = Pediatric Oncology Group.

Cytogenetic abnormalities of hepatoblastoma cells are seen in half of the cases. Seventy-three percent of cases with an abnormal karyotype have numerical anomalies, most commonly trisomies of chromosomes 2, 8, and 20.[71] In one study, structural abnormalities were seen in 39% of cases of hepatoblastoma, and it most commonly affected the 1q12-21 region (Gail Tomlinson, personal communication, 2005). A chromosomal translocation, t(1;4)(q12;q34), unique to hepatoblastoma cells has also been reported.[72] In sporadic hepatoblastoma, the *APC* gene is only occasionally mutated, although the beta-*catenin* gene is mutated in at least half of these cases.[73–75] The genetic locus for BWS is at chromosome 11p15.5, a region of the genome containing several key genes known to undergo genomic imprinting (ie, silencing of gene expression from one specific parental chromosome).[55] Loss of heterozygosity at chromosome 11p15.5, with a consistent loss of alleles derived from maternal DNA, has been described in hepatoblastoma. In tumor cells that do not demonstrate loss of heterozygosity at chromosome 11p15.5, loss of imprinting with subsequent gene expression from both parental alleles may occur.[76,77]

A specific *TP53* mutation has been reported in association with aflatoxin B exposure in hepatocellular carcinoma, and the presence of *TP53* mutations or serum antibodies against *TP53* has been reported to be associated with a reduced survival probability in these patients.[78,79]

Clinical Presentation and Abnormalities in Laboratory Findings Most liver tumors present as an asymptomatic, palpable mass. Weight loss, loss of appetite, vomiting, and abdominal pain are usually associated with more advanced disease and are more commonly seen in patients with hepatocellular carcinoma. Occasionally, pseudoprecocious puberty is seen in boys at initial examination. Laboratory findings are usually nonspecific and may include normochromic normocytic anemia and thrombocytosis. Jaundice and hyperbilirubinemia are rare. Radiographs and imaging usually demonstrate a right upper quadrant mass; calcifications can be seen in up to 6% of patients. Diagnostic work-up should include CT or MRI of the abdomen, and signs of metastatic disease, most commonly seen in the lungs, should be sought. α-Fetoprotein is the most valuable indicator in the diagnosis and monitoring of hepatic tumors. This normal globulin, which is present during fetal life and whose half-life is 5 to 7 days, is present at elevated concentrations in more than 90% of patients with hepatoblastoma and in a significant number of patients with hepatocellular carcinoma. The rate of decline and maximum concentration of α-fetoprotein have been correlated with clinical outcome.[80] Tumor staging is necessary to determine the prognosis and to plan therapy. The two most commonly used staging systems are depicted in Table 124h-3 and in Figure 124h-2. In North America, the most widely used staging system is based on the extent of tumor and its surgical resectability (see Table 124h-3). The International Society of Pediatric Oncology (SIOP) uses the PRETEXT staging system (see Figure 124h-2). This system is based on preoperative radiological observations of the tumor and divides the liver into four parts or sectors. In Figure 124h-2, the letter A corresponds to PRETEXT group I (three adjacent sectors free of disease), the letter B corresponds to group II (two adjacent sectors free of tumor or one sector in each hemi-liver), the letter C depicts the PRETEXT group III (one sector free of tumor or two sectors in one hemi-liver and one nonadjacent sector in the other hemi-liver), and the letter D depicts PRETEXT group IV (no tumor-free sectors). In addition, extrahepatic growth of tumor (involvement of portal vein, vena cava, distant metastases) is also annotated with the letters P, V, or M.[81] A recent analysis suggests that the PRETEXT staging system is reproducible and more accurate in predicting survival than the COG-based system.[81]

Treatment Surgical resection is required to achieve a cure for patients with liver tumors. Unfortunately, most patients (60%) are not amenable to surgical resection at the time of initial diagnosis. Fortunately, however, most hepatoblastomas that are initially deemed unresectable are highly responsive to various chemotherapeutic regimens that commonly incorporate cisplatin and doxorubicin. The results of the best-known national and international chemotherapeutic trials for the treatment of hepatoblastoma are depicted in Table 124h-4. Adjuvant chemotherapy with a cisplatin-based regimen has proven useful for patients who initially undergo surgical resection, resulting in overall survival rates that exceed 90%.[82–84] Preoperative chemotherapy using agents such as cisplatin, doxorubicin, ifosfamide, vincristine, and 5-FU for patients with unresectable tumors induces tumor responses in over 75% of cases with concomitant survival rates in excess of 65%.[83–86] Patients with complete resections after induction chemotherapy fare significantly better than those who have residual disease.[83] Liver transplantation offers an attractive alternative for patients with unresectable disease with cures rates in excess of 80%.[87]

Patients with hepatocellular carcinoma fare significantly worse than do those with hepatoblastoma. Given their dismal outcome and poor response to therapies used for hepatoblastoma, patients with hepatocellular carcinoma desperately need alternative therapeutic approaches.[88–91] Antiangiogenic therapies may offer an attractive therapeutic alternative for this disease, and trials using these drugs are being actively pursued.[92,93] Chemoembolization has proven effective for the treatment of unresectable tumors after systemic therapy,[94] and liver transplantation offers the possibility of cure in patients with cirrhosis and limited disease.[95] Radiofrequency ablation has successfully been used in selected patients with localized disease with encouraging results.[96] More recently, proton beam radiotherapy has been used to control limited disease in selected patients with

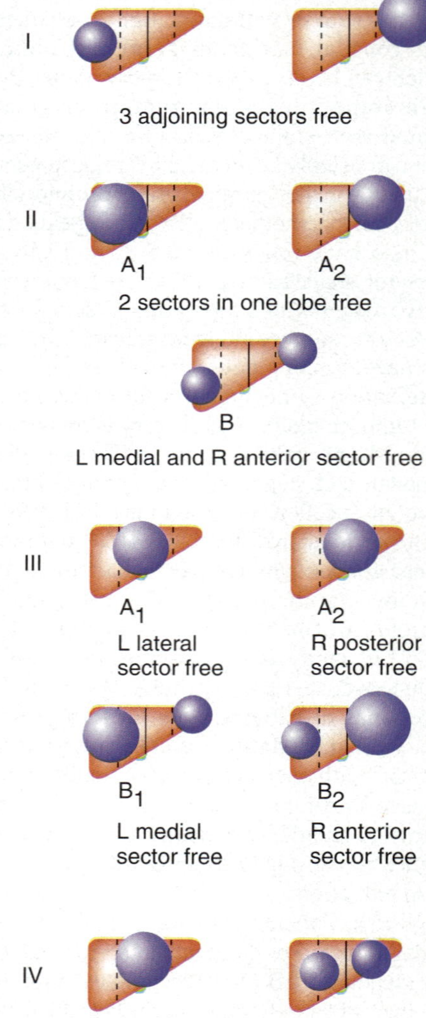

Figure 124h-2 SIOPEL "PRETEXT" system to determine extent of pretreatment required for pediatric liver tumors. This system describes the site and spread of the disease according to pretreatment imaging with ultrasonography, computed tomography, or magnetic resonance imaging.

Table 124h-4 Treatment Results for Pediatric Hepatoblastoma and Hepatocellular Carcinoma

Group	Regimen	No. of Patients	Outcome
Hepatoblastoma			
POG/CCG[83]*	A: CDDP, 100 mg/m^2; V, 1.5 mg/m^2; 5-FU, 600 mg/m^2	173	5-yr survival rate, 69%
	B: CDDP, 100 mg/m^2; dox, 80 mg/m^2		5-yr survival rate, 72%
COG P9645[101]	A: CDDP, 100 mg/m^2; V, 1.5 mg/m^2; 5-FU, 600 mg/m^2	112	1-yr EFS 57%
	B: CBDCA 700mg/m2 day 0 and CDDP 100mg/m2 day 14		1-yr EFS 37%**
SIOPEL 1[102]	CDDP, 80 mg/m^2; dox, 60 mg/m^2	154	5-yr survival rate, 75%
SIOPEL 2[103]	SR PRETEXT I,II,III: CDDP, 80 mg/m^2	67	3-yr survival rate, 91%
	HR PRETEXT IV, M: CDDP, 80 mg/m^2; CBDCA, 500 mg/m^2; dox, 60 mg/m^2	58	3-yr survival rate, 53%
GHB 89[104]	IF, 3.5 g/m^2; CDDP, 100 mg/m^2; dox, 60 mg/m^2	72	64-month survival rate, 75%
GHB 94[84]	IF, 3.5 g/m^2; CDDP, 100 mg/m^2; dox, 60 mg/m^2; ± CBDCA, VP16	69	58-month survival rate, 77%
Hepatocellular carcinoma			
POG/CCG[89]	A: CDDP, 100 mg/m^2; V, 1.5 mg/m^2; 5-FU, 600 mg/m^2	46	Overall 5-yr EFS, 19%
	B: CDDP, 100 mg/m^2; dox, 80 mg/m^2		
SIOPEL 1[90]	CDDP, 80 mg/m^2; dox, 60 mg/m^2	39	5-yr survival rate, 28%

POG = Pediatric Oncology group; CCG = Children's Cancer Group; SIOPEL = International Society of Pediatric Oncology; GHB = Cooperative German Pediatric Liver Tumor Study 89 and 94; S = standard risk (tumor confined to liver, involving 3 sectors at most); H = high risk (tumor involving all 4 sectors, or metastases, or both); CDDP = cisplatin; 5-FU = 5-fluorouracil; V = vincristine; dox = doxorubicin; CBDCA = carboplatin; IF = ifosfamide; VP16 = etoposide.

*Randomized trial. Survival and EFS rates were similar for both regimens. However, patients on regimen A had a higher progression rate and patients on regimen B had a higher incidence of grades 3 and 4 neutropenia, anemia, stomatitis, thrombocytopenia, and adverse cardiac events.

***p* value .013.

cirrhosis and hepatocellular carcinoma.[97] Table 124h-4 outlines the treatment results for pediatric hepatocellular carcinoma.

Carcinomas and Melanoma Carcinomas and melanoma account for approximately 9% of all cases of cancer in children.[1] In the SEER database, the distribution of these malignancies is as follows: thyroid carcinoma, 35%; common melanomas, 31%; adrenocortical carcinomas, 1.3%; nasopharyngeal carcinoma, 4.5%; and other skin carcinomas, 0.5%. Most carcinomas (75%) occur in the 15- to 19-year-old age group. In patients aged 15 to 19 years, thyroid cancer and melanoma account for more than 14% of the malignancies seen in this age group. Melanoma accounts for approximately 1.3% of all cases of cancer among persons younger than 20 years old in the United States, and more girls or young women are affected by melanoma than boys or young men (ratio of female to male patients = 1:6). At initial examination, most patients (89%) have localized disease, the most common site being the trunk, although patients younger than 20 years old are more likely than adults to have disease primarily in the head and neck. Survival rates are similar for patients younger than 20 and older than 20 years of age, and the prognosis appears to be stage dependent.[98] There is a higher incidence of melanoma among those aged between 10 and 19 years in the southern registries, but the incidence of melanoma among patients younger than 10 years old does not vary geographically. In the 15- to 19-year old age group, the incidence of cutaneous melanoma increased at a rate of 2.6% per year between 1975 and 1995. Two recent single institutional trials have documented the feasibility of administering "adult-type therapies" such as adjuvant interferon-alpha 2b to pediatric patients with high-risk localized disease.[99,100] These findings strongly support the need for combined trials with adult cooperative groups to better define the best therapies for pediatric melanoma. The Children's Oncology Group (COG) has recognized such a need, and through its rare tumor committee is developing active liaisons with adult cooperative groups such as ECOG and SWOG to better study these malignancies.

REFERENCES

1. Ries LAG, Smith MA, Gurney JG, et al, editors. Cancer incidence and survival among children and adolescents: United States SEER Program 1975–1995. Bethesda (MD): National Cancer Institute, SEER Program. NIH Pub No 99–4649; 1999.
2. Gurney JG, Severson RK, Davis S, Robison LL. Incidence of cancer in children in the United States. Sex-, race-, and 1-year age-specific rates by histologic type. Cancer 1995;75:2186–95.
3. Bleyer WA. Cancer in older adolescents and young adults: epidemiology, diagnosis, treatment, survival, and importance of clinical trials. Med Pediatr Oncol 2002;38:1–10.
4. Knudson AG, Jr. Mutation and cancer: statistical study of retinoblastoma. Proc Natl Acad Sci U S A 1971;68:820–3.
5. Lee WH, Bookstein R, Hong F, et al. Human retinoblastoma susceptibility gene: cloning, identification, and sequence. Science 1987;235:1394–9.
6. Friend SH, Bernards R, Rogelj S, et al. A human DNA segment with properties of the gene that predisposes to retinoblastoma and osteosarcoma. Nature 1986;323:643–6.
7. Brantley MA Jr, Harbour JW. The molecular biology of retinoblastoma. Ocul Immunol Inflamm 2001;9:1–8.
8. Dryja TP, Mukai S, Petersen R, et al. Parental origin of mutations of the retinoblastoma gene. Nature 1989;339:556–8.
9. Zhu X, Dunn JM, Goddard AD, et al. Mechanisms of loss of heterozygosity in retinoblastoma. Cytogenet Cell Genet 1992;59:248–52.
10. Weinberg RA. Tumor suppressor genes. Science 1991; 254:1138–46.
11. Draper GJ, Sanders BM, Brownbill PA, Hawkins MM. Patterns of risk of hereditary retinoblastoma and applications to genetic counselling. Br J Cancer 1992;66:211–9.
12. Harbour JW. Molecular basis of low-penetrance retinoblastoma. Arch Ophthalmol 2001;119:1699–704.
13. Sippel KC, Fraioli RE, Smith GD, et al. Frequency of somatic and germ-line mosaicism in retinoblastoma: implications for genetic counseling. Am J Hum Genet 1998;62:610–9.
14. Yandell DW, Campbell TA, Dayton SH, et al. Oncogenic point mutations in the human retinoblastoma gene: their application to genetic counseling. N Engl J Med 1989;321:1689–95.
15. Houdayer C, Gauthier-Villars M, Lauge A, et al. Comprehensive screening for constitutional RB1 mutations by DHPLC and QMPSF. Hum Mutat 2004;23:193–202.
16. Blanquet V, Turleau C, Gross-Morand MS, et al. Spectrum of germline mutations in the RB1 gene: a study of 232 patients with hereditary and non hereditary retinoblastoma. Hum Mol Genet 1995;4:383–8.
17. Richter S, Vandezande K, Chen N, et al. Sensitive and efficient detection of RB1 gene mutations enhances care for families with retinoblastoma. Am J Hum Genet 2003;72:253–69.
18. Bunin GR, Emanuel BS, Meadows AT, et al. Frequency of 13q abnormalities among 203 patients with retinoblastoma. J Natl Cancer Inst 1989;81:370–4.
19. Pratt CB, Raimondi SC, Kaste SC, et al. Outcome for patients with constitutional 13q chromosomal abnormalities and retinoblastoma. Pediatr Hematol Oncol 1994;11:541–7.
20. Kaste SC, Pratt CB. Radiographic findings in 13q-syndrome. Pediatr Radiol 1993;23:545–8.
21. Baud O, Cormier-Daire V, Lyonnet S, et al. Dysmorphic phenotype and neurological impairment in 22 retinoblastoma patients with constitutional cytogenetic 13q deletion. Clin Genet 1999;55:478–82.
22. Yue NC, Benson ML. The hourglass facial deformity as a consequence of orbital irradiation for bilateral retinoblastoma. Pediatr Radiol 1996;26:421–3.
23. Kaste SC, Chen G, Fontanesi J, et al. Orbital development in long-term survivors of retinoblastoma. J Clin Oncol 1997;15:1183–9.
24. Wong FL, Boice JD Jr, Abramson DH, et al. Cancer incidence after retinoblastoma. Radiation dose and sarcoma risk. JAMA 1997;278:1262–7.
25. Eng C, Li FP, Abramson DH, et al. Mortality from second tumors among long-term survivors of retinoblastoma. J Natl Cancer Inst 1993;85:1121–8.
26. Mohney BG, Robertson DM, Schomberg PJ, Hodge DO. Second nonocular tumors in survivors of heritable retinoblastoma and prior radiation therapy. Am J Ophthalmol 1998;126:269–77.
27. Abramson DH, Frank CM. Second nonocular tumors in survivors of bilateral retinoblastoma: a possible age effect on radiation-related risk. Ophthalmology 1998;105:573–9; discussion 579–80.
28. Gobel U, Schneider DT, Calaminus G, et al. Germ-cell tumors in childhood and adolescence. GPOH MAKEI and the MAHO study groups. Ann Oncol 2000;11:263–71.
29. Hawkins EP, PE. Germ Cell Tumors. In: Parham D, editor. Pediatric Neoplasia: morphology and biology. Philadelphia: Lippincott-Raven; 1996. p. 297–330.
30. Heifetz SA, Cushing B, Giller R, et al. Immature teratomas in children: pathologic considerations: a report from the combined Pediatric Oncology Group/Children's Cancer Group. Am J Surg Pathol 1998;22:1115–24.
31. Hawkins EP. Pathology of germ cell tumors in children. Crit Rev Oncol Hematol 1990;10:165–79.
32. Belchis DA, Mowry J, Davis JH. Infantile choriocarcinoma. Re-examination of a potentially curable entity. Cancer 1993;72:2028–32.
33. Chaganti RS, Houldsworth J. The cytogenetic theory of the pathogenesis of human adult male germ cell tumors. Review article. Apmis 1998;106:80–3; discussion 83–4.

34. Bussey KJ, Lawce HJ, Olson SB, et al. Chromosome abnormalities of eighty-one pediatric germ cell tumors: sex-, age-, site-, and histopathology-related differences—a Children's Cancer Group study. Genes Chromosomes Cancer 1999;25:134–46.
35. Ladanyi M, Samaniego F, Reuter VE, et al. Cytogenetic and immunohistochemical evidence for the germ cell origin of a subset of acute leukemias associated with mediastinal germ cell tumors. J Natl Cancer Inst 1990;82:221–7.
36. Castleberry RP, Cushing B, Perlman E, et al. Germ Cell Tumors. In: Pizzo PA, Poplack DG, editors. Principles and practice of pediatric oncology. Philadelphia: Lippincott Williams & Wilkins; 2002. p. 1091–113.
37. Perlman EJ, Hu J, Ho D, et al. Genetic analysis of childhood endodermal sinus tumors by comparative genomic hybridization. J Pediatr Hematol Oncol 2000;22:100–5.
38. Baranzelli MC, Kramar A, Bouffet E, et al. Prognostic factors in children with localized malignant nonseminomatous germ cell tumors. J Clin Oncol 1999;17:1212.
39. Packer RJ, Cohen BH, Cooney K. Intracranial germ cell tumors. Oncologist 2000;5:312–20.
40. Marina NM, Cushing B, Giller R, et al. Complete surgical excision is effective treatment for children with immature teratomas with or without malignant elements: a Pediatric Oncology Group/Children's Cancer Group Intergroup Study. J Clin Oncol 1999;17:2137–43.
41. Rescorla F, Billmire D, Stolar C, et al. The effect of cisplatin dose and surgical resection in children with malignant germ cell tumors at the sacrococcygeal region: a pediatric intergroup trial (POG 9049/CCG 8882). J Pediatr Surg 2001;36:12–7.
42. Billmire D, Vinocur C, Rescorla F, et al. Malignant mediastinal germ cell tumors: an intergroup study. J Pediatr Surg 2001;36:18–24.
43. Rogers PC, Olson TA, Cullen JW, et al. Treatment of children and adolescents with stage II testicular and stages I and II ovarian malignant germ cell tumors: a pediatric intergroup study—Pediatric Oncology Group 9048 and Children's Cancer Group 8891. J Clin Oncol 2004;22:3563–9.
44. Cushing B, Giller R, Cullen JW, et al. Randomized comparison of combination chemotherapy with etoposide, bleomycin, and either high-dose or standard-dose cisplatin in children and adolescents with high-risk malignant germ cell tumors: a pediatric intergroup study—Pediatric Oncology Group 9049 and Children's Cancer Group 8882. J Clin Oncol 2004;22:2691–700.
45. Marina N, Malogolowkin M, London WB, et al. Amifostine does not protect against the ototoxicity associated with high-dose cisplatin, etoposide and bleomycin (HD-PEB) in pediatric germ cell tumors (PGCT): a PGCT Intergroup Study. Proc Amer Soc Clin Oncol 2003;22:798.
46. Mann JR, Raafat F, Robinson K, et al. The United Kingdom Children's Cancer Study Group's second germ cell tumor study: carboplatin, etoposide, and bleomycin are effective treatment for children with malignant extracranial germ cell tumors, with acceptable toxicity. J Clin Oncol 2000;18:3809–18.
47. Schlatter M, Rescorla F, Giller R, et al. Excellent outcome in patients with stage I germ cell tumors of the testes: a study of the Children's Cancer Group/Pediatric Oncology Group. J Pediatr Surg 2003; 38:319–24; discussion 319–24.
48. Baranzelli MC, Bouffet E, Quintana E, et al. Non-seminomatous ovarian germ cell tumours in children. Eur J Cancer 2000;36:376–83.
49. Perilongo G, Shafford EA. Liver tumours. Eur J Cancer 1999;35:953–8.
50. Spector LG, Feusner JH, Ross JA. Hepatoblastoma and low birth weight. Pediatr Blood Cancer 2004;43:706.
51. Feusner J, Plaschkes J. Hepatoblastoma and low birth weight: a trend or chance observation? Med Pediatr Oncol 2002;39:508–9.
52. Ikeda H, Matsuyama S, Tanimura M. Association between hepatoblastoma and very low birth weight: a trend or a chance? J Pediatr 1997;130:557–60.
53. Garber JE, Li FP, Kingston JE, et al. Hepatoblastoma and familial adenomatous polyposis. J Natl Cancer Inst 1988;80:1626–8.
54. Giardiello FM, Offerhaus GJ, Krush AJ, et al. Risk of hepatoblastoma in familial adenomatous polyposis. J Pediatr 1991;119:766–8.
55. Debaun MR, Tucker MA. Risk of cancer during the first four years of life in children from the Beckwith-Wiedemann Syndrome Registry. J Pediatr 1998;132:398–400.
56. Sameshima Y, Tsunematsu Y, Watanabe S, et al. Detection of novel germ-line p53 mutations in diverse-cancer-prone families identified by selecting patients with childhood adrenocortical carcinoma. J Natl Cancer Inst 1992;84:703–7.
57. Mamlok V, Nichols M, Lockhart L, Mamlok R. Trisomy 18 and hepatoblastoma. Am J Med Genet 1989;33:125–6.
58. Pontisso P, Morsica G, Ruvoletto MG, et al. Latent hepatitis B virus infection in childhood hepatocellular carcinoma. Analysis by polymerase chain reaction. Cancer 1992;69:2731–5.
59. Crivellaro C, Cadrobbi P, Perilongo G, et al. Chronic type B hepatitis and primary hepatocellular carcinoma in children. Eur J Pediatr 1991;150:685.
60. Pontisso P, Basso G, Perilongo G, et al. Does hepatitis B virus play a role in primary liver cancer in children of Western countries? Cancer Detect Prev 1991;15:363–8.
61. Nguyen MH, Whittemore AS, Garcia RT, et al. Role of ethnicity in risk for hepatocellular carcinoma in patients with chronic hepatitis C and cirrhosis. Clin Gastroenterol Hepatol 2004;2:820–4.
62. Nguyen MH, Keeffe EB. Chronic hepatitis B and hepatitis C in Asian Americans. Rev Gastroenterol Disord 2003;3:125–34.
63. Strickland DK, Jenkins JJ, Hudson MM. Hepatitis C infection and hepatocellular carcinoma after treatment of childhood cancer. J Pediatr Hematol Oncol 2001;23:527–9.
64. Tsai HL, Liu CS, Chin TW, Wei CF. Hepatoblastoma and hepatocellular carcinoma in children. J Chin Med Assoc 2004;67:83–8.
65. Farhi DC, Shikes RH, Murari PJ, Silverberg SG. Hepatocellular carcinoma in young people. Cancer 1983;52:1516–25.
66. Weinberg AG, Mize CE, Worthen HG. The occurrence of hepatoma in the chronic form of hereditary tyrosinemia. J Pediatr 1976;88:434–8.
67. Chiaretti A, Zampino G, Botto L, Polidori G. Alagille syndrome and hepatocarcinoma: a case report. Acta Paediatr 1992;81:937.
68. Krishna KG, Al Saadi A, Yang SS, McCaughey RS. Ataxia-telangiectasia and hepatocellular carcinoma. Am J Med Sci 1979;278:157–60.
69. Lieberman J, Silton RM, Agliozzo CM, McMahon J. Hepatocellular carcinoma and intermediate alpha1-antitrypsin deficiency (MZ phenotype). Am J Clin Pathol 1975;64:304–10.
70. Haas JE, Feusner JH, Finegold MJ. Small cell undifferentiated histology in hepatoblastoma may be unfavorable. Cancer 2001;92:3130–4.
71. Sainati L, Leszl A, Surace C, et al. Fluorescence in situ hybridization improves cytogenetic results in the analysis of hepatoblastoma. Cancer Genet.Cytogenet 2002;134:18–20.
72. Schneider NR, Cooley LD, Finegold MJ, et al. The first recurring chromosome translocation in hepatoblastoma: der(4)t(1;4)(q12;q34). Genes Chromosomes Cancer 1997;19:291–4.
73. Koch A, Denkhaus D, Albrecht S, et al. Childhood hepatoblastomas frequently carry a mutated degradation targeting box of the beta-catenin gene. Cancer Res 1999;59:269–73.
74. Wei Y, Fabre M, Branchereau S, et al. Activation of beta-catenin in epithelial and mesenchymal hepatoblastomas. Oncogene 2000;19:498–504.
75. Oda H, Imai Y, Nakatsuru Y, et al. Somatic mutations of the APC gene in sporadic hepatoblastomas. Cancer Res 1996;56:3320–3.
76. Albrecht S, von Schweinitz D, Waha A, et al. Loss of maternal alleles on chromosome arm 11p in hepatoblastoma. Cancer Res 1994;54:5041–4.
77. Weksberg R, Smith AC, Squire J, Sadowski P. Beckwith-Wiedemann syndrome demonstrates a role for epigenetic control of normal development. Hum Mol Genet 2003;12 Spec No 1:R61–8.
78. Honda K, Sbisa E, Tullo A, et al. p53 mutation is a poor prognostic indicator for survival in patients with hepatocellular carcinoma undergoing surgical tumour ablation. Br J Cancer 1998;77:776–82.
79. Hsu IC, Metcalf RA, Sun T, et al. Mutational hotspot in the p53 gene in human hepatocellular carcinomas. Nature 1991;350:427–8.
80. Van Tornout JM, Buckley JD, Quinn JJ, et al. Timing and magnitude of decline in alpha-fetoprotein levels in treated children with unresectable or metastatic hepatoblastoma are predictors of outcome: a report from the Children's Cancer Group. J Clin Oncol 1997;15:1190–7.
81. Aronson DC, Schnater JM, Staalman CR, et al. Predictive value of the pretreatment extent of disease system in hepatoblastoma: results from the International Society of Pediatric Oncology Liver Tumor Study Group SIOPEL-1 Study. J Clin Oncol 2005;23:1245–52.
82. Evans AE, Land VJ, Newton WA, et al. Combination chemotherapy (vincristine, Adriamycin, cyclophosphamide, and 5-fluorouracil) in the treatment of children with malignant hepatoma. Cancer 1982;50:821–6.
83. Ortega JA, Douglass EC, Feusner JH, et al. Randomized comparison of cisplatin/vincristine/fluorouracil and cisplatin/continuous infusion doxorubicin for treatment of pediatric hepatoblastoma: a report from the Children's Cancer Group and the Pediatric Oncology Group. J Clin Oncol 2000;18:2665–75.
84. Fuchs J, Rydzynski J, von Schweinitz D, et al. Pretreatment prognostic factors and treatment results in children with hepatoblastoma: a report from the German Cooperative Pediatric Liver Tumor Study HB 94. Cancer 2002;95:172–82.
85. Perilongo G, Shafford E, Brugieres L, et al. Cisplatin (CDDP) alone and delayed surgery, an effective treatment for standard risk (SR) hepatoblastoma (HB), the most relevant finding of the SIOPEL2. Proc Amer Soc Clin Oncol 2002;21.
86. Perilongo G, Shafford E, Plaschkes J. SIOPEL trials using preoperative chemotherapy in hepatoblastoma. Lancet Oncol 2000;1:94–100.
87. Otte JB, Pritchard J, Aronson DC, et al. Liver transplantation for hepatoblastoma: results from the International Society of Pediatric Oncology (SIOP) study SIOPEL-1 and review of the world experience. Pediatr Blood Cancer 2004;42:74–83.
88. Nowak AK, Chow PK, Findlay M. Systemic therapy for advanced hepatocellular carcinoma: a review. Eur J Cancer 2004;40:1474–84.
89. Katzenstein HM, Krailo MD, Malogolowkin MH, et al. Hepatocellular carcinoma in children and adolescents: results from the Pediatric Oncology Group and the Children's Cancer Group Intergroup Study. J Clin Oncol 2002;20:2789–97.
90. Czauderna P, Mackinlay G, Perilongo G, et al. Hepatocellular carcinoma in children: results of the first prospective study of the International Society of Pediatric Oncology Group. J Clin Oncol 2002;20:2798–804.
91. Leung TW, Tang AM, Zee B, et al. Factors predicting response and survival in 149 patients with unresectable hepatocellular carcinoma treated by combination cisplatin, interferon-alpha, doxorubicin and 5-fluorouracil chemotherapy. Cancer 2002;94:421–7.
92. Graepler F, Verbeek B, Graeter T, et al. Combined endostatin/sFlt-1 antiangiogenic gene therapy is highly effective in a rat model of HCC. Hepatology 2005;41:879–86.
93. Zhang ZL, Liu ZS, Sun Q. Effects of thalidomide on angiogenesis and tumor growth and metastasis of human hepatocellular carcinoma in nude mice. World J Gastroenterol 2005;11:216–20.
94. Malogolowkin MH, Stanley P, Steele DA, Ortega JA. Feasibility and toxicity of chemoembolization for children with liver tumors. J Clin Oncol 2000;18:1279–84.
95. Steinmuller T, Jonas S, Neuhaus P. Review article: liver transplantation for hepatocellular carcinoma. Aliment Pharmacol Ther 2003;17 Suppl 2:138–44.
96. Harrison LE, Koneru B, Baramipour P, et al. Locoregional recurrences are frequent after radiofrequency ablation for hepatocellular carcinoma. J Am Coll Surg 2003;197:759–64.
97. Kawashima M, Furuse J, Nishio T, et al. Phase II study of radiotherapy employing proton beam for hepatocellular carcinoma. J Clin Oncol 2005;23:1839–46.
98. Hamre MR, Chuba P, Bakhshi S, et al. Cutaneous melanoma in childhood and adolescence. Pediatr Hematol Oncol 2002;19:309–17.
99. Navid F, Furman WL, Fleming M, et al. The feasibility of adjuvant interferon alpha-2b in children with high-risk melanoma. Cancer 2005;103:780–7.
100. Chao MM, Schwartz JL, Wechsler DS, et al. High-risk surgically resected pediatric melanoma and adjuvant interferon therapy. Pediatr Blood Cancer 2005;44:441–448.
101. Malogolowkin MH, Katzenstein H, Krailo M, et al. Intensive versus standard platinum therapy for the treatment of children with hepatoblastoma (HB): a report of the Intergroup Hepatoblastoma Study P9645, American Society of Clinical Oncology, New Orleans (LA). J Clin Oncol 2004;23 Suppl 14:799.
102. Pritchard J, Brown J, Shafford E, et al. Cisplatin, doxorubicin, and delayed surgery for childhood hepatoblastoma: a successful approach--results of the first prospective study of the International Society of Pediatric Oncology. J Clin Oncol 2000;18:3819–28.
103. Perilongo G, Shafford E, Maibach R, et al. Risk-adapted treatment for childhood hepatoblastoma. Final report of the second study of the International Society of Paediatric Oncology–SIOPEL 2. Eur J Cancer 2004;40:411–21.
104. von Schweinitz D, Byrd DJ, Hecker H, et al. Efficiency and toxicity of ifosfamide, cisplatin and doxorubicin in the treatment of childhood hepatoblastoma. Study Committee of the Cooperative Paediatric Liver Tumour Study HB89 of the German Society for Paediatric Oncology and Haematology. Eur J Cancer 1997;33:1243–9.

Renal Tumors of Childhood

Paul E. Grundy, MD
Jeffrey S. Dome, MD
John A. Kalapurakal, MD
Elizabeth J. Perlman, MD
Michael L. Ritchey, MD

Wilms' tumor is the most common primary malignant renal tumor of childhood and a paradigm for multimodal treatment of a pediatric malignant solid tumor. Developments in surgical techniques and postoperative care, recognition of the sensitivity of Wilms' tumor to irradiation, the availability of several active chemotherapeutic agents, and a multidisciplinary approach to clinical research have led to very good outcomes with progressively less therapy for most children.

EPIDEMIOLOGY

During 1975–1995, the annual incidence of Wilms' tumor was 7.6 cases per million children under 15 years of age.[1] During that period, Wilms' tumor represented 6% of childhood cancers in the United States, the total incidence being estimated at 500 cases per year. Relative to Caucasians, the incidence rate for Wilms' tumor is higher in African Americans and lower in East Asians.[2]

Wilms' tumor is slightly less frequent in boys than in girls. The male:female ratio for patients with a unilateral tumor is 0.92:1; for those with bilateral tumors, it is 0.60:1.[3] The tumor presents at an earlier age among males, with the mean age at diagnosis for patients with unilateral tumors being 41.5 months and 32.6 months and, for those with bilateral tumors, 29.5 months and 46.9 months for males and females respectively.[3]

Children with Wilms' tumor may have associated anomalies, including aniridia, hemihypertrophy, cryptorchidism, and hypospadias.[4] The constellation of Wilms' tumor, aniridia, ambiguous genitalia, and mental retardation (WAGR syndrome) occurs in association with an interstitial deletion of the Wilms' tumor 1 (*WT1*) gene on chromosome 11: del(11p13).[5] Children with pseudohermaphroditism or renal disease (glomerulonephritis or nephrotic syndrome), alone or in combination, who develop Wilms' tumor may have the Denys–Drash or Frasier syndrome, which is associated with mutations in the *WT1* gene.[6,7] Hemihypertrophy may occur as an isolated abnormality or as a component of Beckwith–Wiedemann syndrome (BWS), which includes macroglossia, omphalocele, and visceromegaly. About 5 to 10% of children with BWS develop an embryonal tumor, most commonly Wilms' tumor.[8] Interestingly, homozygous mutations of the *BRCA2* gene in patients with Fanconi anemia group D seem clearly related to Wilms tumorigenesis in a rare subset of Wilms patients.[9]

The role of parental environmental exposures in the causation of Wilms' tumor is unknown. No consistent positive findings have emerged from a series of case-control studies.[10–12]

MOLECULAR BIOLOGY AND GENETICS

Wilms' tumor was first thought to represent one of the paradigms for Knudson's "two hit" hypothesis,[13] but it is now clear that several genetic events contribute to Wilms tumorigenesis.[14]

The first evidence that a specific chromosomal locus was associated with Wilms' tumor was the demonstration that patients with WAGR syndrome had a constitutional interstitial deletion encompassing the short am of chromosome 11, region 1, band 13.[5] The underlying tumor-suppressor gene, *WT1,* appears to be a transcription factor, although its in vivo targets have still not been conclusively identified.[15] The normal function of *WT1* is required for normal genitourinary development;[16,17] it is important for differentiation of the renal blastema.[18] Constitutional mutations of single base pairs within the *WT1* gene result in the rare Denys–Drash syndrome.[19] However, mutations of *WT1* have been found in only about 10% or fewer of sporadic Wilms' tumors.[20]

Involvement of the Wnt signaling pathway is suggested by the discovery of activating β-catenin mutations in some Wilms' tumors.[21] Intriguingly, these mutations are restricted to tumors with inactivation of the *WT1* gene.[22]

In association with Beckwith–Wiedemann syndrome, a second Wilms' tumor locus (*WT2*) maps to an imprinted region of chromosome 11 (11p15.5).[23] It now seems apparent that inactivation of the maternally imprinted, expressed untranslated mRNA gene (*H19*), whether by genetic or epigenetic mechanisms, is the critical tumorigenic event.[24,25] However, the expression of a number of other imprinted loci is also altered, because loss of heterozygosity, which exclusively affects the maternal chromosome arm 11p, has the effect of upregulating paternally active genes and silencing maternally active ones. A loss or switch of the imprint for genes in this region has also been frequently observed and results in the same functional aberrations.[26] Recent observations suggest genetic heterogeneity in the causation of BWS, with varying levels of association with risk for tumor formation.[24,27,28]

Familial predisposition to Wilms' tumor is rare: it accounts for only 1 to 2% of all cases.[29] Constitutional mutations of the *WT1* gene have been implicated in only a few Wilms' tumor families, and genetic linkage analysis excluded 11p13 as the predisposing locus in many others.[30,31] Analysis of two families revealed linkage with chromosome arm 17q, and the putative Wilms' tumor gene at that locus has been named familial Wilms' tumor 1 (*FWT1*).[32,33] Interestingly, neither familial nor sporadic Wilms' tumors have undergone loss of heterozygosity (LOH) for this region, as would be expected if *FWT1* were a tumor-suppressor locus.[32] A second locus, *FWT2,* has been mapped to chromosome 19 (19q13.3–q13.4).[34] However, given that some families exhibit evidence against linkage to *WT1*, *FWT1,* and *FWT2,*[33–35] the existence of yet another Wilms' tumor loci must be assumed.

Additional tumor-suppressor or tumor-progressor genes may lie on chromosome arms 16q and 1p, as evidenced by LOH for these regions in subsets of Wilms' tumors.[36] The relevance of these alterations is underscored by the fact that patients classified by tumor-specific loss of 1p and 16q have significantly worse relapse-free and overall survival rates.[37] Recurrent losses of chromosome arm 7p have also been documented,[38] and two candidate tumor-associated genes have been identified.[39,40] Likewise, cloning of a translocation breakpoint involving chromosome arm 5q has led to the identification of another candidate tumor gene, *HACE1* (homologous to E6AP C-terminus [HECT] domain and ankyrin repeat–containing, E3 ubiquitin protein ligase 1).[41]

Mutations of the *TP53* tumor-suppressor gene have also been reported in a few Wilms' tumors.[42] A striking association between *TP53* mutation and the anaplastic histology (86%), as compared with favorable histology (0.8%), suggests that mutation of *TP53* may underlie the anaplastic phenotype.

In summary, Wilms' tumor, like many other cancers, is characterized by alterations in multiple genes, some that regulate cell growth, others differentiation, and yet others the cell's proliferative potential, although it is not clear how many genes are involved in each tumor.

PATHOLOGY

Although most Wilms' tumors are single lesions, 7% are bilateral, and 12% are multifocal within a single kidney. Most are sharply demarcated spherical masses with a "pushing" border relative to the renal parenchyma, resulting in a fibrous pseudocapsule. That feature may help to distinguish Wilms' tumor from other malignant renal tumors, most of which have infiltrative borders. However, cysts are also common. The texture of a Wilms' tumor may vary from soft and friable to firm, depending on the predominant histologic differentiation.

Microscopically, the classic nephroblastoma consists of varying proportions of three cell types: blastemal, stromal, and epithelial. Not all specimens are triphasic, and monophasic patterns often present diagnostic difficulties. Monophasic blastemal Wilms' tumor must be differentiated from other small, round, blue-cell tumors such as primitive neuroepithelial tumor, neuroblastoma, and lymphoma. Monophasic undifferentiated stromal Wilms' tumor may simulate primary sarcomas such as clear cell sarcoma of the kidney (CCSK), congenital mesoblastic nephroma, or synovial sarcoma. Purely tubular and papillary variants may at times be difficult to distinguish from papillary renal cell carcinoma (RCC) and metanephric adenoma.

The absence of anaplastic nuclear changes allows Wilms' tumor to be classified as "favorable histology." Anaplasia, which may be focal or diffuse, is characterized by the presence in cells of markedly enlarged nuclei (diameter more than three times that of nuclei in neighboring cells), and the presence of multipolar or obviously polyploid mitotic figures.[43] Resected tumors with circumscribed, small areas of anaplasia confined to the kidney and surrounded by non-aplastic tissue are defined as focal anaplasia; otherwise, the anaplasia is defined as diffuse. Because anaplasia adversely affects prognosis, meticulous documentation and photographs should be part of the pathology examination.[44]

CCSK must enter the differential diagnosis, although it is not a variant of Wilms' tumor. The name is based on the staining characteristics of the predominant cell type, which commonly demonstrate clear cytoplasm. When unrecognized, the tumor has a propensity for bone metastases, brain metastases, and early death. Although the classic appearance of CCSK is histologically quite distinctive, many tumors show epithelioid, spindle, myxoid, and other variants that can be confused with other renal tumors.[45]

Rhabdoid tumor of the kidney (RTK) is a highly malignant tumor previously not distinguished from Wilms' tumor. The name derives from the prominently acidophilic cytoplasm, which causes the cells to resemble rhabdomyoblasts. However, no ultrastructural or other features of skeletal muscle appear, and the cell of origin is unknown.[46] Patients with rhabdoid tumors of the kidney at times also develop separate primary tumors of the brain variously called atypical teratoid or rhabdoid tumors. Like renal rhabdoid tumors, the brain tumors are now known to show mutations or deletions of the *SMARCB1* gene (SWI/SNF [mating type switching/sucrose nonfermenting]–related, matrix-associated, actin-dependent regulator of chromatin, subfamily B, member 1) on chromosome arm 22q.[47]

RCCs may present in childhood and in fact constitute approximately 6% of pediatric renal tumors.[48] They often show histologic and genetic features that are different from carcinomas of the same kind found in adults.[49] Pediatric papillary RCC represents the counterpart to adult papillary RCC and is thought to be the most common type of pediatric RCC. Translocation RCC, which accounts for approximately 20% of pediatric RCCs, contains translocations involving the *TFE3* (transcription factor binding to IGHM enhancer 3) gene at chromosome X (Xp11.2). The most prevalent fusion partners are the papillary renal cell carcinoma (*PRCC*) gene at chromosome 1 (1q21),[50,51] and the *ASPL* (alveolar soft part sarcoma chromosome region, candidate 1) gene at chromosome 17 (17q25).[52,53] These tumors are composed of cells with voluminous clear cytoplasm, often arranged in papillary or tubular formation. Conventional clear cell carcinoma represents less than 20% of pediatric RCC cases; in contrast to clear cell RCCs in adults, pediatric cases rarely show mutation or LOH of the von Hippel–Lindau tumor suppressor (*VHL*) gene at chromosome 3 (3p25–26).[49] A small number of pediatric RCCs contain t(6;11)(p21.1;q12), which involves a fusion between the transcription factor EB *(TFEB)* and *Alpha* genes.[52,54] Renal medullary carcinoma affects individuals with sickle cell trait and typically presents at an advanced stage with metastatic disease; it is associated with very poor prognosis.[55] Other types of renal cell carcinoma, including collecting duct carcinoma, chromophobe RCC, RCC arising from Wilms' tumor, and oncocytoid RCC arising in survivors of neuroblastoma have been described.[49,56,57] Approximately 30% of pediatric RCCs cannot be classified according to the new WHO criteria.[49]

CLINICAL PRESENTATION

Most children with Wilms' tumor come to medical attention because of abdominal swelling or because an abdominal mass is felt, often first by a family member. Abdominal pain, gross or microscopic hematuria, hypertension, and fever are other frequent findings at diagnosis.

During the physical examination, noting the location and size of the abdominal mass and its movement with respiration is important to help differentiate Wilms' tumor from splenomegaly or neuroblastoma. A varicocele, particularly if persistent when supine, may be associated with the presence of a tumor thrombus in the renal vein or inferior vena cava. Any specific signs of Wilms' tumor–associated syndromes—presence of aniridia, of genitourinary abnormalities such as hypospadias and cryptorchidism, of partial or complete hemihypertrophy, of macroglossia, or of omphalocele—are also important to note.

PREOPERATIVE EVALUATION

The preoperative evaluation should include a complete blood count; tests of coagulation, liver and kidney function, and serum calcium; a urinalysis; and imaging studies. The main purpose of the imaging studies is to assist the physicians, primarily the surgeon, in planning management. The studies are therefore performed to (1) establish the presence of a renal tumor and a normally functioning contralateral kidney, (2) determine the presence of tumor in the contralateral kidney, (3) document the patency of the inferior vena cava, and (4) demonstrate the presence or absence of pulmonary metastases.

The initial study is often an abdominal ultrasound examination. Contrast-enhanced computed tomography (CT) of the abdomen will provide further evaluation of extension of the tumor into adjacent structures such as the liver, spleen, or colon; however, most children identified as having possible invasion of the liver on CT are found at surgical exploration to have hepatic compression rather than hepatic invasion.[58] In addition, CT and sonography may demonstrate small lesions in the opposite kidney; these may be nephrogenic rests or Wilms' tumor.[59] Inclusion in the CT of a supine view of the abdomen following contrast injection is important, because this view is necessary for planning and review of radiation therapy. Magnetic resonance imaging (MRI) of the abdomen may be used in place of CT imaging and may be particularly valuable for assessing nephrogenic rests.[60,61]

The patency of the inferior vena cava may be demonstrated relatively inexpensively using real-time sonography. When tumor is identified within that vessel, the proximal extent of the thrombus must be established before surgery; extension of the thrombus to the right atrium may not be suspected because clinical signs of such extension are few.[62] Sudden death has been reported at laparotomy following dislodgement and mobilization of tumor lying within the draining vessels.[63]

A number of other neoplasms, benign and malignant (most commonly, neuroblastoma or benign renal cysts), can mimic the clinical and radiographic findings of Wilms' tumor. The results of the radiographic studies and real-time sonography provide information sufficient to make a decision for laparotomy in most children.

Chest CT scans should be obtained to determine whether pulmonary metastases are present. CT has been compared with conventional chest radiographic studies in Wilms' tumor patients; CT is more sensitive, but it identifies some lesions that are not metastases, suggesting a need for lung biopsy in some cases.[64]

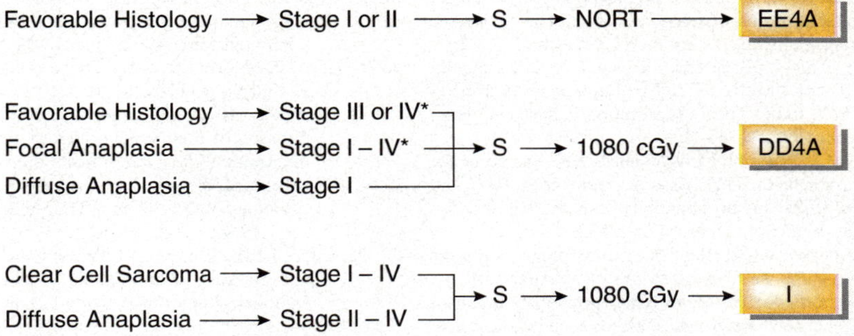

Figure 124i-2 Treatment algorithms by tumor histology and stage for regimens that represent a reasonable standard of care for treatment. IV* = stage IV patients receive abdominal radiation therapy depending on the local stage of the abdominal primary.

although recent case reports have shown transient responses to gemcitabine/cisplatin/paclitaxel and methotrexate/vinblastine/doxorubicin/cisplatin.[98–100] On the upcoming COG trial for high-risk renal tumors, patients with localized RCCs (including those with regional lymph node involvement) will not receive adjuvant therapy after surgical resection. Patients with metastatic or incompletely resected RCCs will be candidates for phase II studies.

Treatment of Recurrent Disease Most recurrences are found within 2 years of diagnosis. The most common sites of recurrence are the lungs and pleura, tumor bed, and liver. Less frequently, recurrences in bone, brain, and distant lymph nodes are seen. Most "recurrences" in the contralateral kidney likely represent second primary tumors rather than true relapses.

Children with relapsed favorable-histology Wilms' tumor have a variable prognosis, depending on the site of relapse, the time from initial diagnosis to relapse, and their previous therapy. Favorable prognostic factors include no prior treatment with doxorubicin, relapse more than 12 months after diagnosis, and intra-abdominal relapse in a patient not previously treated with abdominal irradiation.[101–103]

Children in this more favorable group should be treated aggressively, because they generally have a good response to retrieval therapy. Although surgical excision of pulmonary metastases does not improve outcome,[104] surgical biopsy should be considered to confirm recurrent disease histologically. Treatment regimens for recurrent Wilms' tumor are designed to include chemotherapy agents that were not used during primary therapy and so should include doxorubicin, if not used previously. Several highly effective chemotherapy combinations, including ifosfamide/carboplatin/etoposide (ICE), cyclophosphamide/etoposide, and carboplatin/etoposide are considered first-line treatment for recurrent disease.

For patients with adverse prognostic factors at the time of relapse, management using high-dose chemotherapy with stem-cell rescue has been suggested,[103,105–107] although whether stem-cell transplant is more efficacious or less toxic than conventional chemotherapy (or both) remains unproven. In general, these children should be referred to centers that are conducting research in the treatment of children with recurrent solid tumors.

PROGNOSTIC FACTORS

The distinction between favorable and anaplastic histology Wilms' tumor has been identified as the most important determinant of prognosis.[44] Recent analyses have also confirmed the importance of lymph node involvement. The prognostic significance of previously identified factors, such as age and tumor size, has lessened as treatment efficacy has improved.[108]

The results of NWTS-4 predicted that the 4-year relapse-free and overall survival percentages that can be expected with use of the regimens outlined in Figure 124i-1 are (1) 92% and 98% for stage I favorable-histology Wilms' tumor, (2) 85% and 96% for stage II favorable-histology Wilms' tumor, (3) 90% and 95% for stage III favorable-histology Wilms' tumor, and (4) 80% and 90% for stage IV favorable histology Wilms' tumor.[87,88] Regimens for other histologies are new in NWTS-5; but, using the NWTS-3 and -4 regimens, 4-year relapse-free and overall survival rates were (1) 82.5% and 81.8% for stages II to IV diffuse anaplasia, (2) 70.6% and 74.8% for stages I to IV CCSK, and (3) 23.1% and 25.4% for stages I to IV RTK.[84,109]

Current research is focused on identifying additional prognostic factors that could be used to further stratify therapy according to risk of recurrence. NWTS-5 demonstrated that tumor-specific LOH for chromosome arms 1p and 16q, present in 5% of Wilms' tumors, is associated with a significantly increased risk of relapse and death. In the next COG study, this criterion will be used for treatment stratification to attempt to improve the outcome for this subset of patients.

LONG-TERM FOLLOW-UP

Because Wilms' tumor is usually a curable malignancy, limiting iatrogenic sequelae is essential. Although the damage from the primary treatment, nephrectomy, may be limited to the kidney, additional treatment modalities may cause acute and chronic damage to several organs (heart, lungs, liver, bones, and gonads, for example). Chemotherapy and radiation both can also induce second malignant neoplasms. It is therefore important that children treated for Wilms' tumor be examined regularly by a physician who is familiar with the natural history of the disease and the complications of therapy.

REFERENCES

1. Bernstein L, Linet M, Smith MA, Olshan AF. Renal tumors. In: Ries LAG, Smith MA, Gurney JG, et al., editors. Cancer incidence and survival among children and adolescents: United States Surveillance Epidemiology and End Results (SEER) Program 1975–1995. [NIH Publication No. 99-4649] Bethesda (MD): National Cancer Institute, SEER Program; 1999. p. 79–.
2. Stiller CA, Parkin DM. International variations in the incidence of childhood renal tumors. Br J Cancer 1990;62:1026–30.
3. Breslow N, Olshan A, Beckwith JB, Green DM. Epidemiology of Wilms tumor. Med Pediatr Oncol 1993;21:172–81.
4. Miller RW, Fraumeni JF, Manning MD. Association of Wilms' tumor with aniridia, hemihypertrophy and other congenital anomalies. N Engl J Med 1964;270:922–7.
5. Riccardi VM, Sujansky E, Smith AC, Francke U. Chromosomal imbalance in the aniridia–Wilms' tumor association: 11p interstitial deletion. Pediatrics 1978;61:604–10.
6. Coppes MJ, Huff V, Pelletier J. Denys–Drash syndrome: relating a clinical disorder to genetic alterations in the tumor suppressor gene *WT1*. J Pediatr 1993;123:673–8.
7. Koziell AB, Grundy R, Barratt TM, Scambler P. Evidence for the genetic heterogeneity of nephropathic phenotypes associated with Denys–Drash and Frasier syndromes. Am J Hum Genet 1999;64:1778–80.
8. Beckwith JB. Macroglossia, omphalocele, adrenal cytomegaly, gigantism, and hyperplastic visceromegaly. Birth Defects 1969;188–196.
9. Hirsch B, Shimamura A, Moreau L, et al. Association of biallelic *BRCA2/FANCD1* mutations with spontaneous chromosomal instability and solid tumors of childhood. Blood 2004;103:2554–9.
10. Sanders BM, White GC, Draper GJ. Occupations of fathers of children dying from neoplasm. J Epidemiol Commun Health 1981;35:245–50.
11. Olshan AF, Breslow NE, Daling JR, et al. Wilms' tumor and paternal occupation. Cancer Res 1990;50:3212–7.
12. Olshan AF, Breslow NE, Falletta JM, et al. Risk factors for Wilms tumor. Report from the National Wilms Tumor Study. Cancer 1993;72:938–44.
13. Knudson AG, Strong LC. Mutation and cancer: a model for Wilms' tumor of the kidney. J Natl Cancer Inst 1972;48:313–24.
14. Dome JS, Huff V. Wilms tumor overview. Gene Rev 2003;1–18.
15. Madden SL, Cook DM, Morris JF, et al. Transcriptional repression mediated by the *WT1* Wilms tumor gene product. Science 1991;253:1550–3.
16. van Heyningen V, Bickmore WA, Seawright A, et al. Role for the Wilms tumor gene in genital development? Proc Natl Acad Sci U S A 1990;87:5383–6.
17. Pritchard-Jones K, Fleming S, Davidson D. et al. The candidate Wilms' tumour gene is involved in genitourinary development. Nature 1990;346:194–7.
18. Kreidberg JA, Sariola H, Loring JM, et al. *WT-1* is required for early kidney development. Cell 1993;74:679–91.
19. Pelletier J, Bruening W, Cashtan CE, et al. Germline mutations in the Wilms' tumor suppressor gene are associated with abnormal urogenital development in Denys–Drash syndrome. Cell 1991;67:437–47.
20. Varanasi R, Bardeesy N, Ghahremani M, et al. Fine structure analysis of the *WT1* gene in sporadic Wilms tumor. Proc Natl Acad Sci U S A 1994;91:3554–8.
21. Koesters R, Ridder R, Kopp-Schneider A, et al. Mutational activation of the β-catenin proto-oncogene is a common event in the development of Wilms' tumors. Cancer Res 1999;59:3880–2.
22. Maiti S, Alam R, Amos CI, Huff V. Frequent association of β-catenin and *WT1* mutations in Wilms tumors. Cancer Res 2000;60:6288–92.
23. Koufos A, Grundy P, Morgan K, et al. Familial Wiedemann–Beckwith syndrome and a second Wilms' tumor locus both map to 11p15.5. Am J Hum Genet 1989;44:711–9.
24. DeBaun MR, Niemitz EL, McNeil E, et al. Epigenetic alterations of *H19* and *LIT1* distinguish patients with Beckwith–Wiedemann syndrome with cancer and birth defects. Am J Hum Genet 2002;70:604–11.

25. Bliek J, Maas SM, Ruijter JM, et al. Increased tumour risk for BWS patients correlates with aberrant *H19* and not *KCNQ1OT1* methylation: occurrence of *KCNQ1OT1* hypomethylation in familial cases of BWS. Hum Mol Genet 2001;10:467–76.
26. Steenman MJC, Rainier S, Dobry CJ, et al. Loss of imprinting of *IGF2* is linked to reduced expression and abnormal methylation of *H19* in Wilms tumour. Nat Genet 1994;7:433–9.
27. Smith AC, Squire JA, Thorner P, et al. Association of alveolar rhabdomyosarcoma with the Beckwith–Wiedemann syndrome. Pediatr Dev Pathol 2001;4:550–8.
28. Weksberg R, Nishikawa J, Caluseriu O, et al. Tumor development in the Beckwith–Wiedemann syndrome is associated with a variety of constitutional molecular 11p15 alterations including imprinting defects of *KCNQ1OT1*. Hum Mol Genet 2001;10:2989–3000.
29. Breslow N, Olsen J, Moksness J, et al. Familial Wilms tumors: a descriptive study. Med Pediatr Oncol 1996;27:429–33.
30. Grundy P, Koufos A, Morgan K, et al. Familial predisposition to Wilms' tumour does not map to the short arm of chromosome 11. Nature 1988;336:374–6.
31. Huff V, Compton DA, Chao L, et al. Lack of linkage of familial Wilms' tumour to chromosomal band 11p13. Nature 1988;336:377–8.
32. Rahman N, Arbour L, Tonin P, et al. Evidence for a familial Wilms' tumour gene (*FWT1*) on chromosome 17q12–q21. Nat Genet 1996;13:461–3.
33. Rahman N, Abidi F, Ford D, et al. Confirmation of *FWT1* as a Wilms' tumour susceptibility gene and phenotypic characteristics of Wilms' tumour attributable to *FWT1*. Hum Genet 1998;103:547–56.
34. McDonald JM, Douglass EC, Fisher R, et al. Linkage of familial Wilms' tumor predisposition to chromosome 19 and a two-locus model for the etiology of familial tumors. Cancer Res 1998;58:1387–90.
35. Huff V, Amos CI, Douglass EC, et al. Evidence for genetic heterogeneity in familial Wilms tumor. Cancer Res 1997;57:1859–62.
36. Grundy PE, Telzerow PE, Breslow N, et al. Loss of heterozygosity for chromosomes 16q and 1p in Wilms' tumors predicts an adverse outcome. Cancer Res 1994;54:2331–3.
37. Grundy P, Breslow N, Li S, et al. The relationship between loss of heterozygosity for chromosomes 1p and 16q and prognosis in Wilms tumor. A report from the National Wilms Tumor Study Group. J Clin Oncol 2005. [In press]
38. Wilmore HP, White GFJ, Howell RT, Brown KW. Germline and somatic abnormalities of chromosome 7 in Wilms' tumor. Cancer Genet Cytogenet 1994;77:93–8.
39. Perotti D, De Vecchi G, Testi MA, et al. Germline mutations of the *POU6F2* gene in Wilms tumors with loss of heterozygosity on chromosome 7p14. Hum Mutat 2004;24:400–7.
40. Vernon EG, Malik K, Reynolds P, et al. The parathyroid hormone–responsive *B1* gene is interrupted by a t(1;7)(q42;p15) breakpoint associated with Wilms' tumour. Oncogene 2003;22:1371–80.
41. Anglesio MS, Evdokimova V, Melnyk N, et al. Differential expression of a novel ankyrin containing E3 ubiquitin–protein ligase, *HACE1*, in sporadic Wilms' tumor versus normal kidney. Hum Mol Genet 2004;13:1–14.
42. Bardeesy N, Falkoff D, Petruzzi MJ, et al. Anaplastic Wilms' tumour, a subtype displaying poor prognosis, harbours *p53* gene mutations. Nat Genet 1994;7:91–7.
43. Bonadio JF, Storer B, Norkool P, et al. Anaplastic Wilms tumor: clinical and pathologic studies. J Clin Oncol 1985;3:513–20.
44. Faria P, Beckwith JB, Mishra K, et al. Focal versus diffuse anaplasia in Wilms tumor—new definitions with prognostic significance. Am J Surg Pathol 1996;20:909–20.
45. Argani P, Perlman EJ, Breslow N, et al. Clear cell sarcoma of the kidney (CCSK): a review of 351 cases from the National Wilms Tumor Study Group Pathology Center. Am J Surg Pathol 2000;24:4–18.
46. Weeks DA, Beckwith JB, Mierau GW, Luckey DW. Rhabdoid tumor of kidney: a report of 111 cases from the National Wilms' Tumor Study Pathology Center. Am J Surg Pathol 1989;13:439–58.
47. Biegel JA, Zhou JY, Rorke LB, et al. Germ-line and acquired mutations of *INI1* in atypical teratoid and rhabdoid tumors. Cancer Res 1999;59:74–9.
48. United States, Department of Health and Human Services, National Cancer Institute. SEER Cancer Statistics Review, 1975–2000. Bethesda (MD): National Cancer Institute, Surveillance Epidemiology and End Results Program; 2004.
49. Bruder E, Passera O, Harms D, et al. Morphologic and molecular characterization of renal cell carcinoma in children and young adults. Am J Surg Pathol 2004;28:1117–32.
50. Sidhar SK, Clark J, Gill S. The t(X;1)(p11.2;q21.2) translocation in papillary renal cell carcinoma fuses a novel gene *PRCC* to the *TFE3* transcription factor gene. Hum Mol Genet 1996;5:1333–8.
51. Weterman MA, Wilbrink M, van Geurts KA. Fusion of the transcription factor *TFE3* gene to a novel gene, *PRCC*, in t(X;1)(p11;q21)-positive papillary renal cell carcinomas. Proc Natl Acad Sci U S A 1996;93:15294–8.
52. Argani P, Antonescu CR, Illei PB. Primary renal neoplasms with the *ASPL–TFE3* gene fusion of alveolar soft part sarcoma: a distinctive tumor entity previously included among renal cell carcinomas of children and adolescents. Am J Pathol 2001;159:179–92.
53. Tomlinson GE, Nisen PD, Timmons CF, Schneider NR. Cytogenetics of a renal cell carcinoma in a 17-month-old child. Evidence for Xp11.2 as a recurring breakpoint. Cancer Genet Cytogenet 1991;57:11–7.
54. Kuiper RP, Schepens M, Thijssen J, et al. Upregulation of the transcription factor *TFEB* in t(6;11)(p21;q13)-positive renal cell carcinomas due to promoter substitution. Hum Mol Genet 2003;12:1661–9.
55. Davis CJJ, Mostofi FK, Sesterhenn IA. Renal medullary carcinoma. The seventh sickle cell nephropathy. Am J Surg Pathol 1995;19:1–11.
56. Medeiros LJ, Palmedo G, Krigman HR, et al. Oncocytoid renal cell carcinoma after neuroblastoma: a report of four cases of a distinct clinicopathologic entity. Am J Surg Pathol 1999;23:772–80.
57. Fleitz JM, Wootton-Gorges SL, Wyatt-Ashmead J, et al. Renal cell carcinoma in long-term survivors of advanced stage neuroblastoma in early childhood. Pediatr Radiol 2003;33:540–5.
58. Ng YY, Hall-Graggs MA, Dicks-Mireaux C, Pritchard J. Pre- and post-chemotherapy CT appearances. Clin Radiol 1991;43:255–9.
59. Ritchey ML, Green DM, Thomas P, et al. Accuracy of current imaging modalities in the diagnosis of synchronous bilateral Wilms' tumor: a report from the National Wilms' Tumor Study Group [abstract]. J Urol 1994;151:329A.
60. Gylys-Morin V, Hoffer FA, Kozakewich H, Shamberger RC. Wilms tumor and nephroblastomatosis: imaging characteristics at gadolinium-enhanced MR imaging. Radiology 1993;188:517–21.
61. Rorschneider WK, Weirich A, Rieden K, et al. US, CT, MR imaging characteristics of nephroblastomatosis. Pediatr Radiol 1998;28:435–43.
62. Ritchey ML, Kelalis PP, Haase GM, et al. Preoperative therapy for intracaval and atrial extension of Wilms tumor. Cancer 1993;71:4104–10.
63. Shurin SB, Gauderer MWL, Dahms BB, Contrad WG. Fatal intraoperative pulmonary embolization of Wilms' tumor. J Pediatr 1982;101:559–62.
64. Green DM, Fernbach DJ, Norkool P, et al. The treatment of Wilms tumor patients with pulmonary metastases detected only with computed tomography: a report from the National Wilms Tumor Study. J Clin Oncol 1991;9:1776–81.
65. Feusner JH, Beckwith JB, D'Angio GJ. Clear cell sarcoma of the kidney: accuracy of imaging methods for detecting bone metastases. Report from the National Wilms Tumor Study. Med Pediatr Oncol 1990;18:225–7.
66. Green DM, Breslow NE, Beckwith JB, et al. Treatment of children with clear-cell sarcoma of the kidney: a report from the National Wilms' Tumor Study Group. J Clin Oncol 1994;12:2132–7.
67. Beckwith JB. National Wilms Tumor Study: an update for pathologists. Pediatr Dev Pathol 1998;1:79–84.
68. Shamberger RC, Guthrie KA, Ritchey ML, et al. Surgery-related factors and local recurrence of Wilms tumor in National Wilms Tumor Study 4. Ann Surg 1999;229:292–7.
69. Ehrlich P, Ritchey M, Hamilton T, et al. Quality assessment for Wilms tumor: a report from the National Wilms' Tumor Study 5. J Pediatr Surg 2005;40:208–13.
70. Ritchey ML, Kelalis PP, Breslow N, et al. Surgical complications after nephrectomy for Wilms tumor. Surg Gynecol Obstet 1992;175:507–14.
71. Tournade MF, Com-Nougue C, Voute PA, et al. Results of the Sixth International Society of Pediatric Oncology Wilms' Tumor Trial and Study: a risk-adapted therapeutic approach in Wilms' tumor. J Clin Oncol 1993;11:1014–23.
72. Shamberger RC, Ritchey ML, Haase GM, et al. Intravascular extension of Wilms tumor. Ann Surg 2001;234:116–21.
73. Godzinski J, Tournade MF, DeKraker J. Rarity of surgical complications after postchemotherapy nephrectomy for nephroblastoma. Experience of the International Society of Paediatric Oncology Trial and Study "SIOP-9." Eur J Pediatr Surg 1998;8:83–6.
74. Tournade MF, Com-Nougue C, DeKraker J, et al. Optimal duration of preoperative therapy in unilateral and non-metastatic Wilms' tumor in children older than 6 months: results of the Ninth International Study of Pediatric Oncology Wilms' Tumor Trial and Study. J Clin Oncol 2001;19:488–500.
75. Ritchey ML, Pringle KC, Breslow NE, et al. Management and outcome of inoperable Wilms tumor. A report of National Wilms Tumor Study 3. Ann Surg 1994;220:683–90.
76. Ritchey ML, Green DM, Thomas PRM, et al. Renal failure in Wilms' tumor patients: a report from the National Wilms' Tumor Study Group. Med Pediatr Oncol 1996;26:75–80.
77. Breslow NE, Takashima JR, Ritchey ML, et al. Renal failure in the Denys–Drash and Wilms' tumor–aniridia syndromes. Cancer Res 2000;60:4030–2.
78. Weirich A, Leuschner I, Harms D. Clinical impact of histologic subtypes in localized non-anaplastic nephroblastoma treated according to the trial and study SIOP-9/GPOH. Ann Oncol 2001;12:311–19.
79. D'Angio GJ, Evans AE, Breslow N, et al. The treatment of Wilms' tumor. Cancer 1976;38:633–46.
80. D'Angio GJ, Evans A, Breslow N, et al. The treatment of Wilms' tumor: results of the Second National Wilms' Tumor Study. Cancer 1981;47:2302–11.
81. Thomas PR, Tefft M, Compaan PJ, et al. Results of two radiotherapy randomizations in the third National Wilms' Tumor Study (NWTS-3). Cancer 1991;68:1703–7.
82. Kalapurakal JA, Li SM, Breslow NE, et al. Influence of radiation therapy delay on abdominal tumor recurrence in patients with favorable histology Wilms' tumor treated on NWTS-3 and NWTS-4: a report from the National Wilms' Tumor Study Group. Int J Radiat Oncol Biol Phys 2003;57:495–9.
83. Meisel JA, Guthrie KA, Breslow NE, et al. Significance and management of computed tomography detected pulmonary nodules: a report from the National Wilms Tumor Study Group. Int J Radiat Oncol Biol Phys 1999;44:579–85.
84. Green DM, Beckwith JB, Breslow NE, et al. Treatment of children with stages II to IV anaplastic Wilms' tumor: a report from the National Wilms' Tumor Study Group. J Clin Oncol 1994;12:2126–31.
85. Green DM, Breslow NE, Evans I, et al. The effect of chemotherapy dose intensity on the hematological toxicity of the treatment for Wilms' tumor. A report of the National Wilms Tumor Study. Am J Pediatr Hematol Oncol 1994;16:207–12.
86. Green DM, Breslow NE, Evans I, et al. Relationship between dose schedule and charges for treatment on National Wilms' tumor Study 4. A report from the National Wilms' Tumor Study Group. J Natl Cancer Inst Monographs 1995;19:21–5.
87. Green DM, Breslow NE, Beckwith JB, et al. Comparison between single-dose and divided-dose administration of dactinomycin and doxorubicin for patients with Wilms' tumor: a report from the National Wilms' tumor study group. J Clin Oncol 1998;16:237–45.
88. Green DM, Breslow NE, Beckwith JB, et al. Effect of duration of treatment on treatment outcome and cost of treatment for Wilms' tumor: a report from the National Wilms' Tumor Study Group. J Clin Oncol 1998;16:3744–51.
89. Green DM, Moksness J, Breslow NE, et al. The treatment of children with clear cell sarcoma of the kidney (CCSK). A report from the National Wilms Tumor Study (NWTS) [abstract]. Proc Annu Meet Am Assoc Cancer Res 1994;35:A1428.
90. Miser J, Drailo M, Hammond GD. The combination of ifosfamide (IFOS), etoposide (VP-16) and MESNA (M): a very active regimen in the treatment of recurrent Wilms tumor (WT) [abstract]. Proc Am Soc Clin Oncol 1993;12:417.
91. Kung FH, Pratt CB, Vega RA, et al. Ifosfamide/etoposide combination in the treatment of recurrent malignant solid tumors of childhood. A Pediatric Oncology Group phase II study. Cancer 1993;71:1898–903.
92. Gururangan S, Bowman LC, Parham DM, et al. Primary extracranial rhabdoid tumors: clinicopathologic features and response to ifosfamide. Cancer 1993;71:2653–9.
93. Waldron PE, Rodgers BM, Kelly MD, Womer RB. Successful treatment of a patient with a stage IV rhabdoid tumor

of the kidney: case report and review. J Pediatr Hematol Oncol 1999;21:53–7.

94. Wagner L, Hill DA, Fuller C, et al. Treatment of metastatic rhabdoid tumor of the kidney. J Pediatr Hematol Oncol 2002;24:385–8.
95. Geller JI, Dome JS. Local lymph node involvement does not predict poor outcome in pediatric renal cell carcinoma. Cancer 2004;101:1575–83.
96. Bauer M, Reaman GH, Hank JA, et al. A phase II trial of human recombinant interleukin-2 administered as a 4-day continuous infusion for children with refractory neuroblastoma, non-Hodgkin's lymphoma, sarcoma, renal cell carcinoma, and malignant melanoma. A Children's Cancer Group study. Cancer 1995;75:2959–65.
97. MacArthur CA, Isaacs H Jr, Miller JH, Ozkaynak F. Pediatric renal cell carcinoma: a complete response to recombinant interleukin-2 in a child with metastatic disease at diagnosis. Med Pediatr Oncol 1994;23:365–71.
98. Strouse JJ, Spevak, Mack AK, et al. Significant responses to platinum-based chemotherapy in renal medullary carcinoma. Pediatr Blood Cancer 2005;44:407–11.
99. Pirich LM, Chou P, Walterhouse DO. Prolonged survival of a patient with sickle cell trait and metastatic renal medullary carcinoma. J Pediatr Hematol Oncol 1999;21:67–9.
100. Stahlschmidt J, Cullinane C, Roberts P, Picton SV. Renal medullary carcinoma: prolonged remission with chemotherapy, immunohistochemical characterisation and evidence of *BCR/ABL* rearrangement. Med Pediatr Oncol 1999;33:551–7.
101. Grundy P, Breslow NE, Green DM, et al. Prognostic factors of children with recurrent Wilms tumor: Results from the second and third National Wilms Tumor Study. J Clin Oncol 1989;7:638–47.
102. Dome JS, Liu T, Krasin M, et al. Improved survival for patients with recurrent Wilms tumor: the experience at St. Jude Children's Research Hospital. J Pediatr Hematol Oncol 2002;24:192–8.
103. Pein F, Michon J, Valteau-Couanet D, et al. High-dose melphalan, etoposide, and carboplatin followed by autologous stem-cell rescue in pediatric high-risk recurrent Wilms' tumor: a French Society of Pediatric Oncology Study. J Clin Oncol 1998;16:3295–301.
104. Green DM, Breslow N, Li Y, et al. The role of surgical excision in the management of relapsed Wilms' tumor patients with pulmonary metastases. J Pediatr Surg 1991;26:728–33.
105. Garaventa A, Hartmann O, Bernard JL, et al. Autologous bone marrow transplantation for pediatric Wilms' tumor: the experience of the European Bone Marrow Transplantation Solid Tumor Registry. Med Pediatr Oncol 1994;22:11–4.
106. Kremens B, Gruhn B, Klingebiel T, et al. High-dose chemotherapy with autologous stem cell rescue in children with nephroblastoma. Bone Marrow Transplant 2002;30:893–8.
107. Campbell AD, Cohn SL, Reynolds M, et al. Treatment of relapsed Wilms' tumor with high-dose therapy and autologous hematopoietic stem-cell rescue: the experience at Children's Memorial Hospital. J Clin Oncol 2004;22:2885–90.
108. Breslow N, Sharples K, Beckwith JB, et al. Prognostic factors in nonmetastatic favorable histology Wilms' tumor. Results of the Third National Wilms' Tumor Study. Cancer 1991;68:2345–53.
109. D'Angio GJ, Breslow N, Beckwith B, et al. Treatment of Wilms' tumor. Results of the Third National Wilms' Tumor Study. Cancer 1989;64:349–60.

Neuroblastoma

John M. Maris, MD
Suzanne Shusterman, MD

Neuroblastoma is a common solid malignancy of childhood that remains responsible for significant childhood cancer-related morbidity and mortality. It is an embryonal malignancy of the postganglionic sympathetic nervous system and has remarkably diverse clinical and biological characteristics and behavior. Some tumors undergo spontaneous regression or differentiation to a benign neoplasm, whereas others exhibit an extremely malignant phenotype with regional or disseminated disease that is resistant to intensive therapy. Although neuroblastoma remains responsible for approximately 15% of all childhood cancer deaths, there has been substantial improvement in the overall outcome of children with neuroblastoma in the last 30 years. Recent review of the Surveillance, Epidemiology and End Results (SEER) database showed a significant improvement in overall survival rates from 52.2% in 1974 to 1976 to 68.5% in 1992 to 1998 (<http://seer.cancer.gov>). Our ever-increasing ability to distinguish subsets of patients with different relative risks for recurrent disease based on both clinical and biological features has led to risk-related therapy that is likely responsible for much of the improvement in survival (Figure 124j-1). This chapter reviews the clinical and biologic features of neuroblastoma and relates these characteristics to prognosis as well as to current and future treatment strategies.

EPIDEMIOLOGY

Neuroblastoma accounts for 7.2% of all cancers diagnosed between the ages of 0 to 14 years (<http://seer.cancer.gov>). The prevalence is approximately 1 case per 7,000 live births, and there are about 600 to 650 new cases of neuroblastoma per year in the United States corresponding to an incidence of 10.4 per million per year.[1] The tumor is slightly more common in boys than in girls, with a male:female gender ratio of 1.1:1 in most large studies. There also appears to be a preponderance of cases in whites compared to other races.

Neuroblastoma is almost exclusively a pediatric neoplasm. The incidence rate is 28.5 per million in the 0- to 4-year-old age group, making up 14.7% of all childhood cancers within this age group, but falls to 3.0 per million in the 5- to 9-year-old group and 0.8 per million in the 10- to 14-year-old group. Neuroblastoma is the most common malignancy diagnosed during infancy.[1] Review of 3,666 neuroblastoma patients registered on cooperative group studies at Children's Oncology Group (COG) institutions from 1986 to 2001 showed a median age at diagnosis of 18.8 months.[2] In this cohort, 36% of patients were diagnosed as infants, 89% at less than 5 years of age, and 97% were diagnosed by 10 years of age.

The etiology of neuroblastoma is unknown in most cases, and no causal environmental factor has been isolated. Given the usual young age of diagnosis, associations with prenatal and postnatal environmental exposures have been widely investigated. Despite a large literature showing modestly increased relative risks for neuroblastoma in association with a variety of environmental exposures,[3–5] none of these associations have been seen consistently or confirmed by large studies. Thus, no prenatal or postnatal exposure to drugs, chemicals, viruses, electromagnetic fields, or radiation has been associated strongly or consistently associated with an increased incidence of neuroblastoma.

MOLECULAR PATHOGENESIS

Neuroblastomas are presumed to originate from neural crest-derived cells destined to form the sympathoadrenal lineage of the peripheral nervous system. Considerable progress has been made in the past decade toward understanding human neuroblastoma at a cellular and molecular level. These studies have contributed to better methods of tumor diagnosis and subclassification, and provide useful information for predicting clinical behavior. Most cooperative groups used assays to detect molecular genetic alterations in diagnostic neuroblastoma specimens to help assign patients to risk stratified therapies. In addition to providing insights into mechanisms of malignant transformation and progression, these studies may identify critical genes, proteins, and pathways that may serve as targets for future therapy. In turn, these novel approaches to treatment may prove to be more effective and less toxic than current therapeutic modalities.

Genetic Predisposition Although neuroblastoma usually occurs sporadically, a family history of the disease can be found in 1 to 2% of cases.[6–8] Familial neuroblastoma is inherited in an autosomal dominant Mendelian fashion with incomplete penetrance. Patients from these families differ from those with sporadic disease in that they are often diagnosed at an earlier age (usually infancy) and/or they have multiple primary tumors.[9–11] There is remarkable heterogeneity among patients with familial neuroblastoma. Within individual families, the disease can vary from asymptomatic ganglioneuroma or spontaneously regressing neuroblastoma to rapidly progressive and fatal disease.[6] The clinical heteroge-

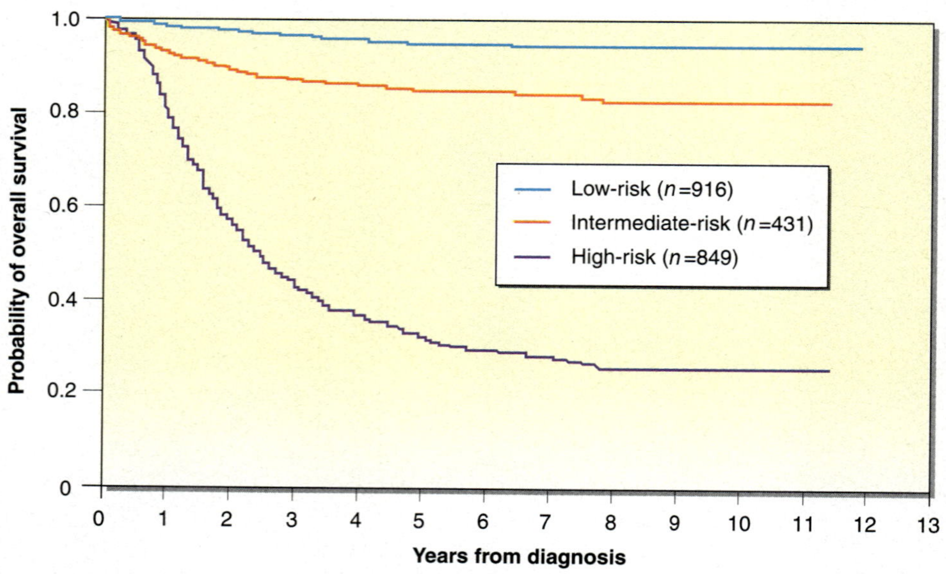

Figure 124j-1 Overall survival stratified by risk group. Comparison of overall survival of 2,196 patients treated at Children's Oncology Group (COG) institutions stratified by risk group. Low-risk, $n = 916$, intermediate-risk, $n = 431$, high risk, $n = 849$. (Courtesy of W.B. London, Children's Oncology Group Statistical Office, Gainesville, Florida.)

neity of familial neuroblastoma may partially explain its rarity, because some tumors remain occult or regress and thus are never detected, whereas others result in death prior to reproductive age. Although a putative hereditary neuroblastoma predisposition locus has been mapped to the short arm of chromosome 16,[12] no causal gene at this location has yet been identified. Recently, mutations in the paired homeobox gene *PHOX2B* (located on chromosome 4) have been found to segregate with neuroblastoma in a few pedigrees.[13,14] Although mutations in this master regulator of noradrenergic nervous system development are implicated in only a small subset of all neuroblastoma cases,[15] these cases may implicate the *PHOX2B* pathway as a likely target for initiating mutations in hereditary and/or sporadic neuroblastoma.

Neuroblastoma may also occur coincident with congenital anomalies, although this is relatively uncommon. Both sporadic and familial neuroblastoma has been reported in patients with Hirschsprung disease, congenital central hypoventilation syndrome (CCHS; Ondine's curse), pheochromocytoma, and/or neurofibromatosis type 1 (NF1) suggesting the existence of a global disorder of neural crest-derived cells (neurocristopathy).[16–21] Interestingly, PHOX2B mutations were first identified in CCHS,[22] but these are typically expansions of a polyalanine tract in the carboxy terminal end of the gene, whereas the neuroblastoma mutations identified to date typically are nonsense mutations or missense alterations in highly conserved regions.[13–15] Neuroblastoma has been postulated to be associated with global neurodevelopmental abnormalities,[23,24] congenital heart disease [25] and Turner's syndrome,[26] and there is also a suggestion of a lower incidence of neuroblastoma among patients with Down syndrome,[27] but these findings have not been independently confirmed and the reason for these possible associations are unclear. Several patients with constitutional chromosomal rearrangements have been described, including patients with constitutional deletions overlapping putative tumor suppressor gene loci at chromosome bands 1p36 and 11q14-23.[24,28,29] These rare patients suggest that predisposition to neuroblastoma may be genetically heterogeneous.

Neurotrophins Neuroblastoma cells can undergo spontaneous or induced differentiation to ganglioneuroblastoma or ganglioneuroma. Thus, malignant transformation of neuroblasts may result in part from a failure to respond to normal differentiation signals. The factors responsible for regulating normal differentiation in the sympathetic nervous system are not completely understood, but they at least in part involve the neurotrophin receptor pathways.[30] Neurotrophins critical to these pathways include nerve growth factor (NGF),[31,32] as well as brain-derived neurotrophin growth factor (BDNF), neurotropin-3 (NT-3), and neurotrophin-4 (NT-4).[33] To date, three high affinity receptor tyrosine kinases for this family of neurotrophins have been identified. The genes TrkA, TrkB, and TrkC encode the primary receptors for NGF, BDNF, and NT-3, respectively.[33] The primary receptor for NT-4 is not known, but it appears to function through TrkB.

The expression pattern of the Trk neurotrophin receptors is correlated with biological and clinical features of neuroblastoma. High TrkA expression has been shown to be associated with younger age (< 1 year), lower stage (stage 1, 2, and 4S), and a favorable outcome.[34–37] In addition, Nakagawara and colleagues have demonstrated that there is an inverse correlation between TrkA expression and *MYCN* amplification and that the combined assessment of *MYCN* copy number and TrkA expression provides additional prognostic information over either variable alone.[34,38] Furthermore, primary neuroblastoma cells with high TrkA expression differentiate in the presence of NGF in vitro, whereas the same cells die in the absence of NGF.[34] Thus, the NGF/TrkA pathway may explain the propensity for some neuroblastomas to differentiate or to regress spontaneously.

The studies of TrkB and TrkC expression in neuroblastomas are more limited. TrkB is expressed in about a third of neuroblastomas.[39] The truncated form of TrkB, lacking the tyrosine kinase domain, is expressed predominantly in more differentiated tumors (ganglioneuroblastomas and ganglioneuromas), whereas the full-length TrkB transcript is expressed in tumors with *MYCN* amplification often in association with its cognate ligand BDNF.[39] Thus, the TrkB/BDNF pathway may serve as an autocrine or paracrine pathway to promote survival in *MYCN*-amplified, and perhaps other, high-risk tumors. In addition, constitutively active BDNF/TrkB signaling seems to confer (or at least be associated with) resistance to conventional chemotherapeutic agents.[40,41] TrkC expression is present in about 25% of neuroblastomas tested, and its pattern of expression resembles that of TrkA,[42,43] and may represent an alternate or additional pathway for neuronal differentiation in these tumors.

DNA Index Flow cytometric analysis of DNA content is a method of measuring total cell DNA content, which correlates well with modal chromosome number. Infants with tumors that have a hyperdiploid DNA content are more likely to have lower stages of disease and to respond to initial therapy; whereas those with a diploid DNA content are more likely have advanced stages of disease and not to respond to therapy.[44,45] Currently, the Children's Oncology Group (COG) uses this biological variable to assign treatment intensity for infants with stages 3, 4, or 4S tumors that do not have *MYCN* amplification. The influence of this variable seems especially important for the 4S subset of patients.[45,46]

MYCN Amplification and Expression Cytogenetic analyses of neuroblastoma frequently show extrachromosomal double minutes or chromosomally integrated homogeneously staining regions, both of which are manifestations of gene amplification. The region amplified is virtually always derived from the distal short arm of chromosome 2, and contains the proto-oncogene *MYCN*.[47] Brodeur, Seeger and colleagues originally demonstrated that *MYCN* amplification occurs in about 20 to 25% of primary neuroblastomas from untreated patients; and amplification is associated with advanced stages of disease, rapid tumor progression and a poor prognosis.[48,49] Amplification is found in 30 to 40% of patients with advanced disease and only 5 to 10% of patients with low stages of disease and stage 4S.[50–53] *MYCN* amplification is almost always present at the time of diagnosis, if it is going to occur,[54] so it appears to be an intrinsic biologic property of a subset of very aggressive tumors. Interestingly, targeted over-expression of a *MYCN* transgene to the murine peripheral neural crest causes neuroblastic tumors with high penetrance and with remarkably similar phenotype as that seen in humans.[55]

In general, there is a correlation between *MYCN* copy number and expression at the mRNA and protein levels.[56] Thus, *MYCN* overexpression in the context of amplification consistently identifies a subset of neuroblastomas with highly malignant behavior. However, it is controversial whether or not overexpression of *MYCN* has prognostic significance in nonamplified tumors.[56,57] Some rare neuroblastoma cell lines express high levels of *MYCN* mRNA or protein without gene amplification.[56–58] This may be due to alterations in normal protein degradative pathways, rather than loss of *MYCN* transcriptional autoregulation.[59,60] A review of 69 advanced stage neuroblastoma cases with non-amplified *MYCN* for the prognostic influence of *MYCN* mRNA copy number showed no detectable influence of this variable on disease outcome.[61] Further studies in a larger cohort of consistently treated patients will be necessary to determine if quantitative assessment of *MycN* expression in tumors lacking *MYCN* amplification provides additional prognostic information.

Unbalanced Gain of 17q Unbalanced gain of distal 17q material is perhaps the most common genetic abnormality detected in primary neuroblastoma tissue specimens. Unbalanced 1;17 translocations occur frequently in primary neuroblastomas and often result in loss of distal 1p with concomitant gain of distal 17q material.[62–64] However, the 17q translocation breakpoints are heterogeneous and often involve other partner chromosomes, most notably 11q.[65] Unbalanced 17q gain is associated with adverse prognostic features and is present in the vast majority of neuroblastomas with *MYCN* amplification.[66–69] Bown and colleagues demonstrated that 54% of 313 neuroblastomas analyzed at diagnosis had unbalanced 17q21-qter gain and that this was associated with an adverse outcome.[70] Thus, 17q21-qter is likely to harbor a gene (or genes) that contributes to neuroblastoma tumorigenesis when present in increased copy number and/or over-expressed.

Chromosomal Deletions Deletions of the short arm of chromosome 1 (1p) are found in

Table 124j-1 International Neuroblastoma Pathology Classification[99]

International Neuroblastoma	Pathology Classification	Original Shimada Classification	Prognostic Group
Neuroblastoma	(Schwannian stroma-poor)[a]	Stroma-poor	
Favorable		Favorable	Favorable
< 1.5 years	Poorly differentiated or differentiating and low or intermediate MKI tumor		
1.5–5 years	Differentiating and low MKI tumor		
Unfavorable		Unfavorable	Unfavorable
< 1.5 years	1) Undifferentiated tumor[b] 2) High MKI tumor		
1.5–5 years	1) Undifferentiated or poorly differentiated tumor 2) Intermediate or high MKI tumor		
≤ 5 yrs	All tumors		
Ganglioneuroblastoma Nodular	(composite Schwannian stroma-rich) (stroma-dominant with stroma poor)	Stroma-rich nodular (unfavorable)	Unfavorable
Ganglioneuroblastoma Intermixed	(Schwannian stroma-rich)	Stroma-rich intermixed (favorable)	Favorable
Ganglioneuroma	(Schwannian stroma-dominant)		
Maturing Mature		Well-differentiated (favorable) Ganglioneuroma	Favorable[c]

MKI: mitosis-karyorrhexis index.
[a]Subtypes of neuroblastoma are described in detail elsewhere.[99]
[b]Rare subtype, especially diagnosed in this age group. Further investigation and analysis is required.
[c]Prognostic grouping for these tumor categories is not related to patient age.
Modified with permission from Shimada H, et al.[99]

approximately 25 to 35% of primary tumors and are highly correlated with the presence of *MYCN* amplification.[71–73] Bader and colleagues showed that addition of an intact human chromosome 1p to a 1p-deleted neuroblastoma cell line induced cellular differentiation and/or death.[74] It therefore appears likely that a neuroblastoma suppressor gene is located on the short arm of chromosome 1, and that this gene is inactivated in at least one-third of primary neuroblastomas. However, the majority of 1p deletions are large and the proximal breakpoints heterogeneous, suggesting that distal 1p may contain more than one suppressor gene critical for malignant transformation or progression.[75–78]

Hemizygous deletions of the long arm of chromosome 11 occur in about 40% of human neuroblastomas.[65,79–81] In addition, constitutional rearrangements of chromosome 11q, including interstitial deletions, have been observed in neuroblastoma patients.[24,82] Thus, 11q also likely harbors a neuroblastoma suppressor gene, but in contrast to 1p deletions, there is a striking inverse relationship of 11q LOH with *MYCN* amplification, despite the fact that this abnormality is correlated with advanced stage disease.[81] In a recent study of almost 1,000 patients registered on COG studies, unbalanced deletions of 11q (11q loss with either retention or gain of 11p material) was independently prognostic for outcome in a multivariate analysis that included all other currently used prognostic markers.[83]

Allelic loss at multiple other chromosomal loci has been reported. Recent evidence suggests that 3p deletions often occur co-incident with 11q deletions and help define the subset of patients with aggressive disease without the oncogenic influence of deregulated MycN [84,85] Array-based genomic studies have recently revealed the true complexity of chromosomal alterations in neuroblastoma, with multiple other areas of recurrent deletions (and gains) scattered throughout the genome.[86–88] However, homozygous deletions are only very rarely identified in this disease,[88,89] thus complicating traditional approaches for identifying the tumor suppressor genes postulated to be targeted by the hemizygous deletions noted above.

PATHOLOGY

Neuroblastomas arise from primitive, pluripotential sympathetic cells derived from the neural crest. The three classic histopathologic patterns of neuroblastoma appear to correlate with the normal differentiation patterns of the sympathetic nervous system and include neuroblastoma, ganglioneuroblastoma, and ganglioneuroma. These subtypes reflect a spectrum of maturation and differentiation that varies from immature small, round blue cells to mature ganglion cells surrounded by Schwannian stroma. The typical neuroblastoma is composed of small, uniform cells that contain dense, hyperchromatic nuclei and scant cytoplasm as well as characteristic neuritic processes or neuropil. The Homer-Wright pseudorosette, consisting of a ring of neuroblasts surrounding eosinophilic neuropil, is a classic finding in neuroblastoma, but is only rarely observed in tumor tissue or bone marrow containing metastatic disease. Immunohistochemistry (eg, immunoperoxidase techniques) can be helpful in distinguishing neuroblastoma from other "small, round blue-cell" tumors of childhood. Neuroblastomas stain with monoclonal antibodies recognizing neurofilament proteins, synaptophysin, cell surface proteins such as GD2 and NCAM, and neuron-specific enolase.

Several prognostic classification systems based on histopathologic features have been proposed.[90–93] Shimada and colleagues have developed a system that classifies tumors as favorable or unfavorable based on age at diagnosis, the presence or absence of Schwannian stroma; the degree of differentiation; and the mitosis-karyorrhexis index (MKI).[93] In a retrospective analysis of 295 Children's Cancer Group (CCG) patients, these histologic patterns were independently predictive of outcome and stage was prognostically less important than histologic grade.[94–96] Joshi and colleagues developed a modification of this classification system based on mitotic ratio and presence or absence of calcification.[97,98] A retrospective analysis of pathologic data collected in the Pediatric Oncology Group (POG) from 211 patients with neuroblastoma showed that the presence of calcification and a low mitotic rate (≤ 10 mitoses/10 high power fields) predicted a favorable outlook, independent of stage or age. The Joshi method provided greater simplicity in determining the histologic features and prognostic categories, but did not demonstrate the same prognostic power as the Shimada system. An International Neuroblastoma Pathology Classification (INPC) that combines the best features of these two systems has been developed (Table 124j-1).[99,100] This classification is based primarily on the Shimada system but incorporates other features that should permit improved concordance among pathologists around the world. Although it is clear that the INPC can add prognostic information, the use of age at diagnosis within the classification system makes its independent prognostic power difficult to evaluate since age alone is also used for patient risk assignment. Work on developing an international consensus for implementing the INPC is ongoing.

CLINICAL PRESENTATION

Signs and Symptoms Because neuroblastomas can arise from any site along the sympathetic nervous system chain, the locations of primary tumors at the time of diagnosis are varied and change with age. Most primary tumors occur within the abdomen (65%). The frequency of adrenal tumors is slightly higher in children (40%) compared to infants (25%), whereas infants have more thoracic

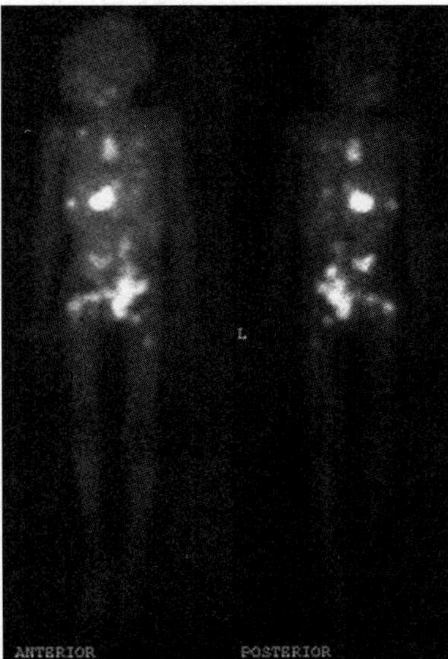

Figure 124j-2 ^{123}I-MIBG scan showing extensive metastatic disease throughout the chest, abdomen, pelvis as well as both appendicular and axial skeleton.

and cervical primary tumors. Infrequently, a primary tumor cannot be found.

Metastatic extension of neuroblastoma occurs in lymphatic and hematogenous patterns (Figure 124j-2). Regional lymph node metastases are noted in one-third of patients with apparently localized tumors. Spread of tumor to lymph nodes outside the cavity of origin is considered to be disseminated disease. However, these children may have a better outlook if there is no other metastatic disease noted.[101] Hematogenous spread occurs most frequently to bone marrow and bone. Liver is also a common site of metastases, especially in International Neuroblastoma Staging System INSS 4S patients (see below), and this often occurs with subcutaneous metastatic deposits. Rarely, metastatic disease may be present in the lung and brain parenchyma at diagnosis, although these sites are more often seen at disease relapse. Metastatic disease is more commonly seen in older children compared to infants.

The signs and symptoms of neuroblastoma at diagnosis vary according to the location of primary disease and the degree of dissemination. Abdominal disease can be asymptomatic or present with complaints of fullness, discomfort, or, rarely, obstruction. Sudden and dramatic enlargement of abdominal tumors with resultant increased abdominal distention and discomfort can result from spontaneous hemorrhage into the tumor. When primary tumors arise from the organ of Zuckerkandl in the pelvis, bladder, and bowel symptoms may occur. Massive involvement of the liver with metastatic disease is particularly frequent in infants (eg, INSS 4S) and may result in respiratory compromise. Patients may also experience renin-mediated hypertension caused by compromise of renal vasculature.[102]

Primary thoracic tumors often are diagnosed incidentally. High thoracic and cervical masses can be associated with Horner syndrome, which consists of unilateral ptosis, miosis, and anhydrosis.[103] Occasionally, large thoracic tumors are associated with mechanical obstruction and resultant superior vena cava syndrome. Paraspinal tumors in the thoracic, abdominal, and pelvic regions may extend into the neural foramina of the vertebral bodies and result in symptoms related to compression of nerve roots and spinal cord. The range of symptomatology can include radicular pain, subacute or acute paraplegia, as well as bladder or bowel dysfunction.

Several classical signs and symptoms are associated with metastatic neuroblastoma. Proptosis and periorbital ecchymoses are frequent and result from tumor infiltration of the bony orbit.[103] Widespread bone and bone marrow disease causes bone pain, which can lead to limping, and irritability in a younger child. In addition, there may be bone marrow replacement and symptoms of bone marrow failure, such as anemia, bleeding, or infection. Subcutaneous tissue involvement is seen almost exclusively in infants with INSS 4S tumors and is characterized by variable numbers of c, bluish nodules.[104] Constitutional symptoms associated with disseminated disease can include failure to thrive and fever; fever observed most often in the presence of extensive bone metastases.

Neuroblastoma in adolescent and adult patients represents a unique diagnostic and therapeutic challenge. Although rare, teenagers and adults with neuroblastoma typically show a much more indolent course, although the distribution of primary sites and pattern of metastases is similar to that seen in children.[105–107] Neuroblastomas from adolescents and adults frequently lack *MYCN* amplification, but are typically poorly sensitive to chemotherapy and treatment failures are common.[105,107]

Paraneoplastic Syndromes Two unique paraneoplastic syndromes may be associated with neuroblastoma. Opsoclonus-myoclonus (OMS) a syndrome of random eye movement, myoclonus and/or cerebellar ataxia, has been observed in 2 to 4% of children diagnosed with neuroblastoma.[108] Although most children with this syndrome have favorable tumor biology and a high survival rate, the majority also appear to have long-term neurologic deficits, including cognitive and motor delays, language deficits, and behavioral abnormalities.[109–111] The syndrome, as well as the sequelae, are thought to be caused by antineural antibodies directed against the tumor that cross-react with neural cells in the cerebellum or elsewhere in the brain.[112,113] Some children have improvement of symptoms following tumor removal or following administration of glucocorticoids or adrenocorticotropic hormone, although the majority have persistent or recurrent symptoms, especially in association with intercurrent illnesses.[110,114,115] A retrospective review of OMS cases within the Pediatric Oncology Group suggests that patients who received chemotherapy as part of their initial tumor management had fewer long-term side effects, implying that immunosuppression at diagnosis may be beneficial,[114] but this was not observed in a similar review done by the Children's Cancer Group.[110] Intravenous immune globulin has also been used in the treatment of opsomyoclonus with varying success. A trial to determine the efficacy of low dose chemotherapy and prednisone at diagnosis has recently been initiated within the COG with a randomization looking at the additive effect of intravenous gamma globulin. When caring for patients with OMS, it is important to anticipate long-term neurologic abnormalities and use early intervention to help minimize these deficits. OMS can occur without associated neuroblastoma, and it is not clear if some of these cases are due to tumors that have spontaneously regressed. All children with OMS should have a complete diagnostic workup for neuroblastoma including ^{123}I-MIBG scintigraphy,[116] but a tumor will only be detected in 50% of cases.

A syndrome of intractable secretory diarrhea, associated with hypokalemia and dehydration is a manifestation of tumor secretion of vasoactive intestinal peptide (VIP).[117,118] Most tumors secreting VIP are mature histologically (ganglioneuroblastomas or ganglioneuroma), and these patients almost always have a favorable outcome.[119] Surgical removal of the tumor usually results in complete resolution of symptoms.

DIAGNOSIS AND EVALUATION

In general, a diagnosis of neuroblastoma is made by histopathologic evaluation of primary tumor material obtained from a patient with a consistent clinical presentation. Immunohistochemistry will confirm that the tissue is of neural origin by staining positive for neuron specific enolase and/or chromogranin, and Schwannian stroma will stain positive with S-100. Select patients may be diagnosed with neuroblastoma based on the presence of "unequivocal" neuroblasts involving the bone marrow as long as the urinary catecholamine metabolites are elevated (see below).

Increased urinary catecholamine metabolites can be detected in > 90% of neuroblastomas if sensitive techniques such as high performance liquid chromatography are used.[120,121] This provides a great advantage in establishing the diagnosis of neuroblastoma, as well as in following disease activity in those patients whose tumors are secretors. The two enzymes primarily responsible for the catabolism of catecholamines are catechol-O-methyl transferase and monamine oxidase. Dihydroxyphenylalanine (DOPA) and dopamine are converted primarily to homovanillic acid (HVA), whereas norepinephrine and epinephrine are converted primarily to vanillylmandelic acid (VMA). Most laboratories involved in neuroblastoma diagnosis measure both urinary HVA and VMA. Symptoms of catecholamine excess such as hypertension, flushing, and sweating are uncommon in neuroblastoma, in contrast to pheochromocytoma, likely because of the relatively low concentrations of active catecholamines in the circulation.

In addition to establishing the diagnosis, primary tumor material is essential for prognostic purposes, as evaluation of tumor-specific variables is an essential component of risk stratification. The only current exception is the large subset of patients older than 1.5 to 2 years of age with metastatic disease. These patients will be classified as high-risk regardless of tumor biology. Consequently, demonstration of unequivocal neuroblasts in the bone marrow in conjunction with elevated urinary HVA or VMA is sufficient for diagnosis.[122,123] This may need to be reevaluated in the future if tumor-specific biological information becomes prognostically relevant as new data become available.

Differential Diagnosis Because of the many potential clinical presentations, neuroblastoma may be confused with a variety of other neoplasms as well as non-neoplastic conditions. Adrenal neuroblastomas detected in the perinatal period may be confused with adrenal hemorrhage.[124] Disseminated neuroblastoma may mimic many inflammatory, infectious, and/or rheumatologic disorders, especially in children older than 5 years of age with a more indolent course. Histologically, neuroblastoma tissue from primary or metastatic sites may be undifferentiated, and therefore confused with other embryonal pediatric cancers such as rhabdomyosarcoma, Ewing's sarcoma, lymphoma, or even leukemia (especially megakaryoblastic leukemia). Fortunately, molecular, biochemical, and immunologic characterization can usually distinguish among these various diagnostic entities.[125,126]

Table 124j-2 International Neuroblastoma Staging System[122,123]

STAGE 1	Localized tumor with complete gross excision, with or without microscopic residual disease; representative ipsilateral lymph nodes negative for tumor microscopically (nodes attached to and removed with the primary tumor may be positive).
STAGE 2A	Localized tumor with incomplete gross excision; representative ipsilateral nonadherent lymph nodes negative for tumor microscopically.
STAGE 2B	Localized tumor with or without complete gross excision, with ipsilateral nonadherent lymph nodes positive for tumor. Enlarged contralateral lymph nodes must be negative microscopically.
STAGE 3	Unresectable unilateral tumor infiltrating across the midline[a], with or without regional lymph node involvement; or localized unilateral tumor with contralateral regional lymph node involvement; or midline tumor with bilateral extension by infiltration (unresectable) or by lymph node involvement.
STAGE 4	Any primary tumor with dissemination to distant lymph nodes, bone, bone marrow, liver, skin and/or other organs (except as defined for stage 4S).
STAGE 4S	Localized primary tumor (as defined for stage 1, 2A, or 2B), with dissemination limited to skin, liver and/or bone marrow[b] (limited to infants younger than 1 year of age).

Note: Multifocal primary tumors (e., bilateral adrenal primary tumors) should be staged according to the greatest extent of disease, as defined above, followed by a subscript "M" (eg, 3_M).

[a]The midline is defined as the vertebral column. Tumors originating on one side and "crossing the midline" must infiltrate to or beyond the opposite side of the vertebral column.

[b]Marrow involvement in Stage 4S should be minimal, ie, less than 10% of total nucleated cells identified as malignant on bone marrow biopsy or on marrow aspirate. More extensive marrow involvement would be considered to be stage 4. The MIBG scan (if done) should be negative in the marrow.

Clinical and Laboratory Evaluation A standard set of recommended tests to define the clinical stage and extent of disease has been established.[122] For evaluation of the primary tumor, computed tomography (CT) provides volumetric data and is typically the modality of choice for evaluation of lesions in the abdomen, pelvis, and posterior mediastinum. Magnetic resonance imaging (MRI) should be used for paraspinal lesions and is essential for evaluation of possible spinal cord compression. Either modality can be used to evaluate primary tumors in the neck.

CT is the method of choice to evaluate solid organ metastases. Although rare at diagnosis, parenchymal brain metastases are seen as a site of disease relapse in high-risk patients and head imaging should be considered in heavily pretreated patients.[127] Evaluation of bone and bone marrow disease is critically important in all patients at diagnosis. In young infants with a low risk of bony metastases (localized tumors with favorable biologic features), plain radiographs may be sufficient to detect cortical bone metastases.[128,129] ^{99m}Tc-diphosphonate scintigraphy (bone scan) is classically used to survey for occult bony metastases in all other patients and is relatively sensitive and somewhat specific. Enhanced sensitivity and specificity for detecting bone metastases, as well as occult soft tissue masses is afforded by metaiodobenzylguanidine (MIBG) scintigraphy (Figure 124j-2). MIBG is an adrenergic neuron blocking agent that is selectively concentrated in more than 90% of neuroblastomas making radiolabeled MIBG scintigraphy a highly specific method for assessment of the primary tumor and metastatic disease.[130,131] MIBG scintigraphy may be performed with either ^{131}I or ^{123}I isotopes, with the latter giving enhanced sensitivity. ^{123}I- or ^{131}I-MIBG scintigraphy should be considered as part of the diagnostic evaluation for patients with high-risk features, especially because response at metastatic sites as judged by MIBG may be of prognostic importance.[132,133] Because up to 10% of patients may have tumors that are not MIBG avid, it is common practice to obtain both MIBG and bone scan at diagnosis. For patients with MIBG avid disease, it may not be necessary to use both modalities to restage patients during or after therapy. The sensitivity and specificity of positron emission tomography with fluorine-18 fluorodeoxyglucose (PET scan) for detection and follow-up of metastatic disease is currently being evaluated and compared to MIBG scintigraphy. It may play a role in disease evaluation in the future.[134,135]

There has been considerable variation in the number of bone marrow aspirates and/or biopsies done in different institutions for the assessment of bone marrow disease. Studies suggest that marrow biopsies add substantially to the detection of marrow involvement by tumor compared to marrow aspirates alone.[136,137] Furthermore, it is clear that obtaining more samples will increase the likelihood of detecting marrow involvement, but the clinical relevance of marrow involvement detected with additional studies is uncertain. To provide uniformity, the international conferees on neuroblastoma staging recommend two marrow aspirates and two biopsies, that is, one aspirate and one biopsy from each of the iliac crests.[122,123] Only a single study positive for tumor is required to document bone marrow involvement, but all four studies are required if the findings are negative.

Immunocytochemical analysis of bone marrow aspirates with monoclonal antibodies directed against neural-specific antigens (eg, GD2, NCAM) increases the sensitivity of detecting marrow involvement to at least 1:100,000 nucleated cells. The clinical significance of not clearing immunocytologically detectable disease has been established in high-risk patients[138] and thus immunocytochemical analysis is used in patients with high-risk disease to follow response to therapy. However, the clinical relevance of finding immunocytologically detectable disease at diagnosis in otherwise low-risk patients is not yet understood and is therefore not recommended as a diagnostic tool. Additional sensitivity, greater than 1:1,000,000 nucleated cells, may be added with reverse transcriptase polymerase chain reaction (PCR) methodologies that target the expression of neuroblastoma-specific messages such as tyrosine hydroxylase, PGP 9.5, or GD2 synthase.[139] The clinical significance of positivity at this level, however, remains to be determined.

Staging Until recently, two major staging systems were used for neuroblastoma, the Evans system used by the CCG and others[104]; and the system used by St. Jude Children's Research Hospital and the POG.[140] However, some of the differences between the staging systems are substantial, particularly as applied to patients with intermediate stages, making comparison of clinical trials and biology studies difficult. For this reason, an International Neuroblastoma Staging System (INSS) has been established based on clinical, radiographic, and surgical evaluation of children with neuroblastoma (Table 124j-2).[122,123] The INSS has gained acceptance worldwide and will be used by all major cooperative groups prospectively.

Definition of Response to Treatment Table 124j-3 lists internationally proposed criteria to determine response to therapy in patients with neuroblastoma.[122] It is important to note that determination of overall response requires assessment of both primary and metastatic sites. The same tests that are used for determining extent of disease should be used to assess response of primary and metastatic sites of disease. Newly diag-

Table 124j-3 Definitions of Response to Treatment[122,123]

Response[a]	Primary[b]	Metastases[b]	Markers[b]
1) CR	No tumor	No tumor (chest, abdomen, liver, bone, bone marrow, nodes, etc)	HVA/VMA normal
2) VGPR	Reduction > 90% but < 100%	No tumor (as above except bone); no new bone lesions, all preexisting lesions improved.	HVA/VMA decreased > 90%
3) PR	Reduction 50–90%	No new lesions; 50–90% reduction in measurable sites; 0–1 bone marrow samples with tumor; bone lesions same as VGPR.	HVA/VMA decreased 50–90%
4) MR	No new lesions; > 50% reduction of any measurable lesion (primary or metastases) with < 50% reduction in any other; < 25% increase in any existing lesion.[c]		
5) NR	No new lesions; < 50% reduction but < 25% increase in any existing lesion.[c]		
6) PD	Any new lesion; increase of any measurable lesion by > 25%; previous negative marrow positive for tumor.		

[a]CR = complete response; VGPR = very good partial response; PR = partial response; MR = mixed response; NR = no response; PD = progressive disease.
[b]Evaluations of primary and metastatic disease as outlined in the text.
[c]Quantitative assessment does not apply to marrow disease.

nosed patients should have response evaluated at the end of induction, at the end of treatment, before and after surgical procedures, before stem cell transplant, and as clinically indicated.

NEUROBLASTOMA SCREENING

Because neuroblastomas frequently produce increased levels of catecholamines whose metabolites are detectable in the urine, mass screening of infants for occult neuroblastoma has been investigated to determine whether early detection improves outcome [141–150] Data from these studies show that when screening infants 6 months of age or younger, the prevalence of neuroblastoma overall is increased by 50 to100%, but the prevalence of neuroblastoma in patients older than 1 year of age is not changed appreciably. In addition, clinical and cytogenetic features of tumors identified as a result of mass screening of infants suggest that the majority of patients have low-stage disease and biologically favorable features.[151–154] This suggests that screening is detecting tumors in a substantial number of patients who likely would never develop symptomatic disease because their tumors would have regressed or matured without therapy.

Several studies in Japan and Europe have screened at later times, between 8 to14 months of age.[148,149,155,156] From these studies it appears that the prevalence of "overdiagnosis" by screening at a later time is less, and there is a greater frequency of patients with unfavorable clinical and biologic features, but there is no decrease in the mortality of these patients. Because of these results, mass screening efforts have essentially stopped throughout the world.

PROGNOSTIC CONSIDERATIONS

There has been substantial progress made in risk stratification for neuroblastoma patients based on the analysis of a panel of clinical and biological variables. Despite the growing number of putative prognostic markers for this disease, the easily measured clinical variables of age at diagnosis and disease stage remain two of the most important predictors for disease outcome. Introduction of any new marker into the algorithm used to assign risk must be done in multivariable comparisons including each of the currently used clinical and biological prognostic markers.

Clinical Variables The most important clinical variables predictive of disease outcome are the age of the patient and stage of disease at diagnosis.[157–160] Traditionally, age has been analyzed as a binary function, with a cut point at the first birthday being used by most groups, and this has proven clinical utility. However, because age is a continuous variable, alternative ages have recently been explored as surrogates for tumor behavior. A recent review of 3,666 patients by London and colleagues reached the conclusion that 18 months of age more clearly discriminated outcome in patients with INSS stage 4 disease and no *MYCN* amplification.[2] It is important to recognize that the children aged 12 to 18 months in the studies cited here were all treated with significant chemotherapeutic dose intensity and many received myeloablative chemotherapy. Whether or not therapy can be safely reduced in this patient population should be explored in a controlled research setting. Although the INSS staging system is in worldwide use,[161,162] controversy exists on the best management of stage 3 tumors with favorable biological characteristics. Most clinicians are reluctant to simply observe, or to recommend aggressive surgery for tumors often entrapped in major vessels and/or nerves. The COG will continue to treat most stage 3 patients with adjuvant chemotherapy, and will likely develop a response-based algorithm to determine the duration of therapy. In addition, there appears to be no major difference in either relapse-free or overall survival between INSS stages 2A and 2B, and this sub-categorization may ultimately be dropped.

Biological Variables Several biological variables (pathology, urine markers, serum markers, and genetic features) appear to have prognostic value in patients with neuroblastoma. Detailed analysis of histology by the classifications of Shimada[93] or Joshi[92] has provided important prognostic information (see Pathology). These systems are now being replaced by a new INPC system that should provide worldwide uniformity in the application of this variable.[99,100] The ratio of easily measurable urinary metabolites of catecholamine metabolism correlate with prognosis. In general, homovanillic/vanillylmandelic acid ratios > 2 are associated with more undifferentiated tumors and a more aggressive clinical course.[163,164] Serum markers reported to be associated with disease outcome when elevated at diagnosis include ferritin, neuron-specific enolase (NSE), the cell membrane ganglioside GD2, and lactate dehydrogenase (LDH).[165–169] Although each of these markers is associated with disease outcome, their independent prognostic value appears to be limited in light of modern molecular genetic prognostic markers. The genetic features of the tumor that have been proposed as prognostic markers include tumor cell DNA index, *MYCN* gene copy number, deletion of 1p, 3p, 11q or 14q, unbalanced gain of 17q, and relative expression of the neurotrophin receptor TrkA.[170] DNA index and *MYCN* amplification status are currently used to assign risk in the COG and by most cooperative groups, and some cooperative groups have begun to integrate 1p and 11q LOH status into treatment stratification systems. Addition of the other genetic markers awaits completion of ongoing clinical correlative studies where these, and other, markers are studied in multivariable analyses with each of the five variables currently used to assign risk (see below).

PRINCIPLES OF INITIAL THERAPY

The treatment modalities traditionally employed in the management of neuroblastoma are surgery, chemotherapy, and radiotherapy. The role of each is determined by the anticipated clinical behavior of the tumor in individual cases considering age, stage, and biological features.

Surgery Surgery plays a pivotal role in the management of neuroblastoma, both for diagnosis and for treatment.[171] The goals of primary surgical procedures, performed prior to any therapy, are to establish the diagnosis, to provide tissue for biological studies, to stage the tumor surgically, and to attempt to excise the tumor if feasible without injury to vital structures. In delayed primary or second-look surgery, the surgeon will determine response to therapy and remove residual disease when possible. For the majority of patients with localized disease, surgery is the only treatment required for cure, even if a complete resection is not obtained. In addition, data from mass screening studies discussed above, show that a subset of neuroblastomas detected early in life are likely to spontaneously regress.[172] The COG has an ongoing observation only study for perinatally detected adrenal tumors to explore the hypothesis that surgery is not required for these tumors that are very likely to show favorable biological features.

The role of complete surgical resection of the primary tumor for patients with metastatic dissemination remains controversial. A retrospective review of 141 cases at Memorial Sloan-Kettering Cancer showed that gross total resection of the primary tumor correlated with improved survival ($p < .01$).[173] Chamberlain and colleagues[174] also saw improved survival at 3 years (40% vs 15%) in patients undergoing complete versus partial surgical resection. However, 2 recent reports analyzing patients treated on single protocols do not show a survival advantage for gross total resection. Adkins and colleagues showed no statistically significant impact of gross total resection on EFS (event-free survival) for patients treated on the CCG high-risk protocol 3891.[175] von Allmen and colleagues reporting on a tandem transplant protocol, also showed that although there were no local treatment failures if greater than 90% resection was achieved, there was no significant difference in EFS or OS (overall survival).[176] Further examination of this area is needed, but it is likely that resectability is a surrogate for tumor biology and that gross total resection should be the goal, but not at the risk for loss of vital structures or significant post-operative morbidity particularly that might lead to a delay in further cytotoxic chemotherapy.

Table 124j-4 Children's Oncology Group Risk Group Classification System

INSS Stage	Age	MYCN Status[a]	INPC[b]	DNA Ploidy	Risk Group
1	0–21years	Any	Any	Any	Low
2A/2B	< 365 days	Any	Any	Any	Low
	> 365 days–21years	Non-Amp	Any	—	Low
	≥ 365 days–21 years	Amp	FH	—	Low
	≥ 365 days–21 years	Amp	UH	—	High
3	< 365 days	Non-Amp	Any	Any	Intermediate
	< 365 days	Amp	Any	Any	High
	≥ 365 days–21 years	Non-Amp	FH	—	Intermediate
	≥ 365 days–21 years	Non-Amp	UH	—	High
	≥ 365 days–21 years	Amp	Any	—	High
4	< 365 days	Non-Amp	Any	Any	Intermediate
	< 365 days	Amp	Any	Any	High
	≥ 365 days – 21 years	Any	Any	—	High
4S	< 365 days	Non-Amp	FH	> 1	Low
	< 365 days	Non-Amp	Any	= 1	Intermediate
	< 365 days	Non-Amp	UH	Any	Intermediate
	< 365 days	Non-Amp	Any	Any	High

[a]MYCN amplification status: Amp = amplified; Non-Amp = not amplified.
[b]International Neuroblastoma Pathology Classification: FH = favorable histology; UH = unfavorable histology.

Radiation Therapy Neuroblastoma is generally considered a radiosensitive tumor, although local control of neuroblastoma on a clinical level has been variable.[177] Accepted tumoricidal doses of ionizing radiation range from 15 to 30 Gy, depending on patient age, tumor volume and tumor location.[178,179] A dose response effect is assumed and supporting evidence was suggested by improved local control rates in high-risk neuroblastoma patients who received total body irradiation (TBI) in addition to conventional external beam radiation compared to those who received external beam radiation only.[180] Historically, radiation has been used in the multimodality management of residual neuroblastoma, bulky unresectable tumors, and disseminated disease. External beam radiation therapy is also an effective modality for emergency management of progressive liver enlargement (INSS 4S patients) and spinal cord impingement causing neurologic compromise, but most investigators now consider radiation second line to chemotherapy in these situations. External beam radiotherapy is also very effective for palliation of painful bony metastases. Lastly, targeted radiotherapy with ^{131}I-MIBG is effective with manageable toxicity only to the hematopoietic compartment, and this novel approach may play a more prominent role in front line management in the future.[181–186]

Chemotherapy Chemotherapy is the predominant modality of management in neuroblastoma patients who have intermediate- or high-risk disease. Single agent phase II trials conducted in patients with recurrent or advanced neuroblastoma have identified a number of effective drugs that form the backbone of current induction chemotherapy regimens.[187–198] In particular, these studies have established the activity of alkylating agents and platinum analogs in this disease. Cyclophosphamide, cisplatin, doxorubicin, and the epidophyllotoxins have yielded CR and PR rates ranging from 34 to 45% in patients with refractory disease, and they have become the cornerstone of most multi-agent regimens. More recently, the camptothecin analogs topotecan and irinotecan have shown activity in the relapse setting.[199–201] The use of topotecan in newly diagnosed high-risk patients is currently being explored within the COG.

The Concept of Risk-Related Therapy A large body of data supports the hypothesis that the clinical behavior of human neuroblastoma may be reliably predicted based upon the analysis of a panel of prognostic variables.[30,170] Thus, most pediatric oncology clinical trials groups currently stratify patients into "risk groups" based upon analysis of well-defined prognostic factors. The COG Risk Stratification System is based on the experience of both the POG and CCG and is outlined in Table 124j-4.[170] This system uses analysis of the clinical factors of patient age at diagnosis and INSS, and the biological factors of tumor histopathology, DNA index and *MYCN* amplification status, to assign patients to one of three distinct risk groups (low, intermediate, and high), with dramatically different overall survival probabilities (see Figure 124j-1). A major goal of ongoing clinical trials is to prospectively validate the existing risk stratification schema as well as integrate newly discovered prognostic markers with independent prognostic impact into future risk assignment algorithms. There is also movement toward creating an international risk group system, similar to the INSS, based on the combined worldwide experience.

Treatment of Low-Risk Disease Treatment of patients with low-risk localized neuroblastoma (INSS 1 and 2) consists of surgical removal of the primary tumor. Unlike other cancers, a complete resection is not necessary in the setting of neuroblastoma that is localized and shows favorable biological features. Patients with INSS 1 tumors (gross total resection) can be expected to have an outstanding probability of relapse-free and overall survival.[202–204] A recent prospective CCG study reported a 93% EFS rate and a 99% OS rate for 141 Evans stage I patients.[205] Surgery alone followed by close observation is also the initial treatment for patients with INSS 2 neuroblastoma with greater than 50% initial tumor resection. The recent prospective CCG study included 233 Evans stage II patients (56% INSS 2) with single copy *MYCN* and showed a 4-year EFS of 81% with surgery alone and a 4-year OS of 98%.[205] INSS 2 patients with < 50% surgical resection at diagnosis are currently treated with 4 cycles of intermediate-risk style chemotherapy (see below), although upcoming cooperative group studies will examine a further reduction in therapy in these patients who have biologically favorable features. Local recurrences in low-risk patients can be managed with second surgeries, and metastatic recurrences are rare but often salvageable with chemotherapy.

Table 124j-5 Induction Chemotherapy Cumulative Dose (mg) and Dose Intensity (mg/M²/week) in Recent United States Clinical Trials for Neuroblastoma Patients with Intermediate- and High-Risk Disease. CCG-3881 Was the Immediate Predecessor to COG-A3961, and CCG-3891 Was the Immediate Predecessor to COG-A3973.

	Duration of Induction (Days)	Doxorubicin	Etoposide	Vincristine	Cyclophosphamide	Cisplatin	Carboplatin	Effective Platinum
CCG-3881	267							
Cumulative Dose (mg)		205	2,495	0.0	8,100	510	0	510
Dose Intensity (mg/M²/d)		0.8	9.3		30.3	1.9	0.0	1.9
COG-A3961	168							
Cumulative Dose (mg)		120	1,800	0.0	5,000	0	2,800	510
Dose Intensity (mg/M²/d)		0.7	10.7		29.8	0.0	0.0	3.0
CCG-3891	154							
Cumulative Dose (mg)		150	1,000	0.0	9,000	300	0	300
Dose Intensity (mg/M²/d)		1.0	6.5		58.4	1.9	0.0	1.9
COG-A3973	126							
Cumulative Dose (mg)		300	1,200	8.0	16,800	400	0	400
Dose Intensity (mg/M²/d)		2.4	9.5		133.3	3.2	0.0	3.2

Management of the rare patient with INSS 1 or 2 tumors with *MYCN* amplification is somewhat controversial. In 1995 Cohn and colleagues reported probability that 5 of 6 patients with *MYCN* amplification and INSS 1 (n = 3) 2A (n = 2) tumors survived without evidence of disease at 7+ to 38+ months following surgery. However, in 2000 Perez and colleagues showed that 4 of 7 INSS 1 (n = 4) and 2b (n = 3) patients with *MYCN* amplification had relapse (3 metastatic) between 2 and 22 months from surgery and 3 of these patients died from disease progression.[205]Further prospective evaluation of these rare patients is needed to determine a consensus treatment strategy.

The majority of patients with INSS 4S disease fall into the low-risk category (hyperdiploid, favorable Shimada, and single copy *MYCN*). Retrospective analyses have shown overall survival rates ranging from 57 to 97% for stage 4S patients taken as a whole.[206–213] Recent prospective analyses have confirmed these observations and show overall survival probabilities of 85% (n = 110) to 92% (n = 80).[214] The indications for intervening and the methods of managing infants with stage 4S neuroblastoma are becoming standardized. A diagnostic biopsy is indicated for evaluation of tumor biological features, but resection of the primary tumor does not appear to influence outcome.[214] Thus, the safest surgical procedure, such as removal of a subcutaneous nodule, should be performed. Patients with favorable biological features should be observed closely for symptomatology from tumor expansion, especially when younger than 2 months of age at diagnosis. If respiratory compromise becomes evident, moderately intensive chemotherapy is indicated, such as that currently recommended for intermediate-risk disease.[46,208,214] Radiation therapy should be reserved for those patients who progress despite chemotherapy. If necessary, a minimal dose of radiation, such as 450 to 600 cGy in three to four fractions, is generally sufficient to halt tumor progression and often induce regression. Lastly, the rare stage 4S patients with unfavorable biological features should be considered for either intermediate-risk (diploidy and/or unfavorable Shimada pathology) or high-risk (*MYCN* amplification) treatment strategies.

Intraspinal tumor extension and cord compression is frequently identified in children who otherwise would be considered low-risk. Many of these patients are quite young and so extensive laminectomies or radiation to the spine can result in significant long-term morbidity. Retrospective analyses show no survival or neurological outcome advantage for surgical decompression over external beam radiation therapy.[215,216] In addition, Hoover and colleagues documented mild to severe spinal deformities in 11 of 15 patients treated initially with laminectomy.[217] The French NBL90 Study prospectively evaluated the role of initial chemotherapy for 42 nonmetastatic neuroblastomas presenting with intraspinal extension.[218] It showed that chemotherapy alone was successful in reducing the tumor volume in 58% of cases and was associated with improved neurologic function in 92%. Thus, chemotherapy appears to be a safe and effective initial modality to manage spinal canal invasion, and it has less long-term morbidity than surgery or radiation therapy.

Treatment of Intermediate-Risk Disease Retrospective comparison of intermediate-risk treatment strategies is difficult because the group of patients currently defined as INSS 3 were treated in a heterogeneous fashion in the past, mainly owing to differences in the staging systems used by the various cooperative groups. Implementation of a standardized staging and risk stratification system should allow for a more-uniform approach to treatment planning for this subset of patients.

Matthay and colleagues reported the CCG experience with Evans stage III disease (92% INSS 3).[159] Of 228 Evans stage III patients prospectively evaluated for risk status by analysis of age, stage, *MYCN* amplification status, Shimada pathology and serum ferritin, 143 met the current criteria for intermediate-risk disease. These patients were treated with moderately dose-intensive chemotherapy including cyclophosphamide, doxorubicin, cisplatin, and etoposide, as well as local radiation for any gross residual disease following delayed surgery. Patients with Evans stage III disease and normal *MYCN*, favorable Shimada and low serum ferritin had a 4-year EFS of 100%. Infants with Evans stage III disease and at least one unfavorable biological feature had 4-year EFS and OS rates of 90 and 93%, respectively.

The role of radiation therapy for advanced locoregional neuroblastoma remains controversial. In a randomized study of children with POG stage C disease (INSS 2B and 3), 46% of 28 patients treated with chemotherapy alone achieved complete response and 32% were free of disease at 2 years.[219] In comparison, 75% of 29 children treated with chemotherapy plus radiation therapy achieved a complete response, and 59% were free of disease at two years. In contrast, de Bernardi and colleagues found no advantage for radiotherapy in a randomized trial (chemotherapy +/- radiotherapy) in 29 nonmetastatic patients with residual tumor or positive lymph nodes (INSS 2 and 3) following initial surgery.[220] Nonrandomized addition of radiation therapy for patients with gross residual disease following second surgery for Evans stage III disease also had no apparent influence on disease outcome.[159] Currently most cooperative groups are withholding radiation therapy for the majority of intermediate-risk patients, except for the patients with disease progression despite surgery and chemotherapy, or patients with unresectable primary tumors with unfavorable biological features at the end of chemotherapy.

Infants with INSS 4 neuroblastomas that do not have amplified *MYCN* typically have a much less aggressive clinical course and respond to moderate intensity chemotherapy, classifying them as intermediate risk. Schmidt and colleagues reviewed the recent CCG experience and reported a 3-year EFS rate of 93% for infants with *MYCN* single-copy neuroblastomas treated with moderately intensive chemotherapy.[221] This is in contrast to the 10% EFS noted for those infants with *MYCN* amplified tumors, many of whom were treated with much more intensive therapy. As discussed above, there may be a subset of patients between 12 and 24 months of age with metastatic disease that have tumor biology more consistent with infant patients. These patients may benefit from reduction in therapy if they can be reliably identified and will likely be studied prospectively in upcoming studies.

In summary, the current approach to intermediate-risk neuroblastoma centers on moderately intensive chemotherapy (Table 124j-5) and avoids radical surgery and external beam radiotherapy in the majority of patients with the goal of a greater than 90% EFS rate and minimal treatment-related morbidity. The current COG intermediate-risk neuroblastoma strategy consists of four or eight cycles of combination chemotherapy including carboplatin, etoposide, cyclophosphamide, and doxorubicin, with duration of therapy based on tumor biology. The next COG intermediate-risk study will attempt to further reduce chemotherapy exposure to this very young group of patients by using initial chemotherapy response to determine duration of therapy. In addition, this will be the first COG study to use 1p and 11q LOH analyses to identify patients not eligible for the planned dose reductions because of the presence of one of these aberrations in the diagnostic tumor specimen.

Treatment of High-Risk Disease Children with metastatic neuroblastoma diagnosed after the first birthday remain one of the greatest challenges to pediatric oncologists. Before the mid-1980s, this group of patients had a dismal prognosis with little hope for cure.[222–227] With the advent of comprehensive treatment approaches that include (1) intensive induction chemotherapy; (2) myeloablative consolidation therapy with stem cell rescue, and (3) targeted therapy for minimal residual disease, overall survival rates have improved (Figure 124j-3). However, the current survival rates remain poor and have come at the expense of significant immediate and long-term morbidity.[228]

The vast majority of neuroblastoma patients classified as high-risk is over 1 year of age with stage 4 disease. The COG also includes any INSS stage 3 patients with amplified *MYCN*, INSS stage 3 patients over 1 year at diagnosis with unfavorable Shimada pathology, INSS stage 2 patients with amplified *MYCN* and unfavorable Shimada pathology, and INSS stage 4S patients with amplified *MYCN*. These latter categories are relatively rare, and some (INSS stage 3 disease with unfavorable Shimada histology) remain controversial. Recent evidence suggesting that patients 12 to 18 months of age with metastatic disease and favorable prognostic features have superior survival probabilities[2] has made many groups reconsider the traditional 1 year cut point for determining if a patient with metastatic neuroblastoma should be classified as intermediate- or high-risk.

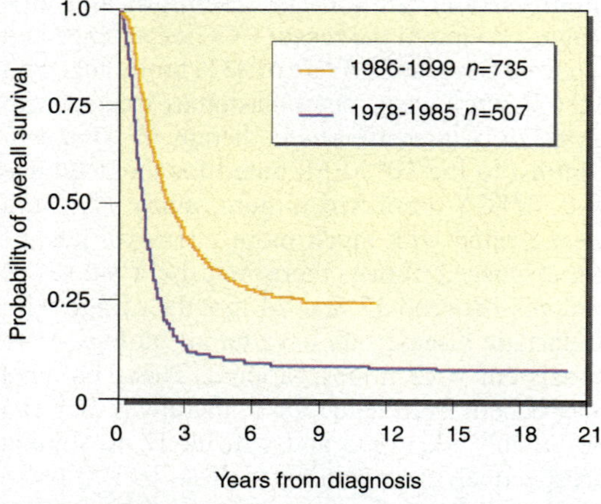

Figure 124j-3 Improving survival for high-risk neuroblastoma patients. Comparison of overall survival of 1,242 consecutive patients with stage 4 neuroblastoma diagnosed at age older than 1 year and treated at a CCG institution from 1978 to 1999. (Courtesy of W.B. London, Children's Oncology Group Statistical Office, Gainesville, Florida.)

Induction Therapy After assuring diagnosis is safely established and sufficient tumor material and other biological samples are submitted for processing, alkylator- and platinum-based chemotherapy is typically administered to induce maximum reduction in tumor bulk at primary and metastatic sites. Neuroblastoma is typically sensitive to initial chemotherapy, even in cases with amplified *MYCN*. Retrospective analyses have shown an association of chemotherapy dose intensity, especially the platinating agents, with response and survival rates[229,230]. Most induction chemotherapy regimens prescribed 5 to 7 dose-intensive cycles of therapy using alternating combinations of agents including cisplatin, etoposide, vincristine, doxorubicin, cyclophosphamide, and perhaps ifosfamide, carboplatin or more recently topotecan. A comparison of the relative chemotherapy dose intensities used on recent United States trials is shown in Table 124j-5. The current COG trial has adopted the Memorial Sloan Kettering Cancer Center approach,[231] although recent experience in a French multicenter study was not able to reproduce the original very high response rates previously reported.[232]

The efficacy of induction chemotherapy regimens is assessed by the response rate, typically determined after a second surgical procedure. Although not definitively proven, there is a substantial body of evidence suggesting that the quality of remission at the end of induction chemotherapy is associated with long-term survival probability.[230,233–237] In a multivariable analysis performed with 549 high-risk neuroblastoma patients registered on the European Bone Marrow Transplantation Solid Tumor Registry, Ladenstein and colleagues showed that persisting cortical bone lesions (p = .004) and bone marrow involvement (p = .03) were the only independent adverse prognostic factors.[235] Thus, patients who achieve a CR or VGPR with induction chemotherapy have a better chance of cure, although some patients with a PR can be converted to CR with high-dose myeloablative therapy.[238] Ever-improving sensitivity of imaging, most importantly nuclear imaging such as ^{123}I-MIBG and PET, makes comparison of current studies with those in the past challenging.

Consolidation Therapy Initial limited success with chemotherapy in the 1980s led investigators to hypothesize that myeloablative chemotherapy could consolidate a remission and eradicate chemotherapy resistant minimal residual disease. Since the first published trial of myeloablative consolidation therapy using high-dose melphalan alone,[239] multiple single arm trials and registry reviews have been reported in the literature.[233,235,240–254] These studies are difficult to compare due to the heterogeneity of induction and consolidation regimens as well as varying strategies for stem cell harvesting and reinfusion. However, the majority of studies reported at least a trend towards improved survival probabilities compared with nonrandomized control groups and historical controls.

Matthay and colleagues completed the first randomized trial of myeloablative consolidation with immunomagnetically purged bone marrow support compared to intensive consolidation chemotherapy.[255] A total of 539 eligible patients were enrolled onto this clinical trial designed with two sequential randomizations (± myeloablative chemotherapy with autologous purged marrow rescue, and ± 13-*cis*-retinoic acid, see below). A total of 379 patients were randomly assigned to autologous marrow rescue (n = 189) or continuation chemotherapy (n = 190). An intent-to-treat analysis showed a significant improvement in 3-year EFS probability for the patients assigned to myeloablative therapy (34 ± 4% versus 22 ± 4%; p = .03; Figure 124j-4A). Importantly, autologous transplantation appeared to have the largest impact on survival for the ultra-high risk subset of patients, such as those with *MYCN* amplified metastatic disease diagnosed after age 2 years. However, follow-up is relatively short, and these data will need further analysis due to the potential for late relapse in the transplant group. Long-term comparisons may be difficult because many of the patients who subsequently had relapse in the non-transplant arm were treated with myeloablative chemotherapy and purged bone marrow rescue.

It has recently become clear that using peripheral blood stem cells provides superior engraftment kinetics compared to conventional bone marrow grafts, and this technique likely abrogates some transplant-related morbidity.[253,256] In addition, because peripheral blood stem cell harvests typically occur after 2 to 4 cycles of induction chemotherapy, and therefore follow an "in vivo purging," pheresis products may be less likely to contain contaminating tumor cells.[253,256] Thus, all current clinical trials for high-risk neuroblastoma patients use autologous peripheral blood stem cells for myeloablative rescue. The current COG clinical trial is testing the hypothesis that rare tumor cells in the peripheral blood stem cell pheresate can contribute to relapse. Patients are randomized to ex vivo purging using a strategy similar to that used for bone marrow in the past,[257–260] versus no stem cell manipulation at all. In order to be eligible for the randomization, the stem cell product must be negative by immunocytochemical methods with a sensitivity of at least 1:100,000.

The potential that two myeloablative consolidations might be better than one is currently being investigated. The main theoretical advantage of a tandem transplant approach involves providing multiple non-cross resistant agents at maximal doses in a relatively rapid sequence. Philip and colleagues demonstrated that this approach, when supported by purged, autologous bone marrow, was associated with significant

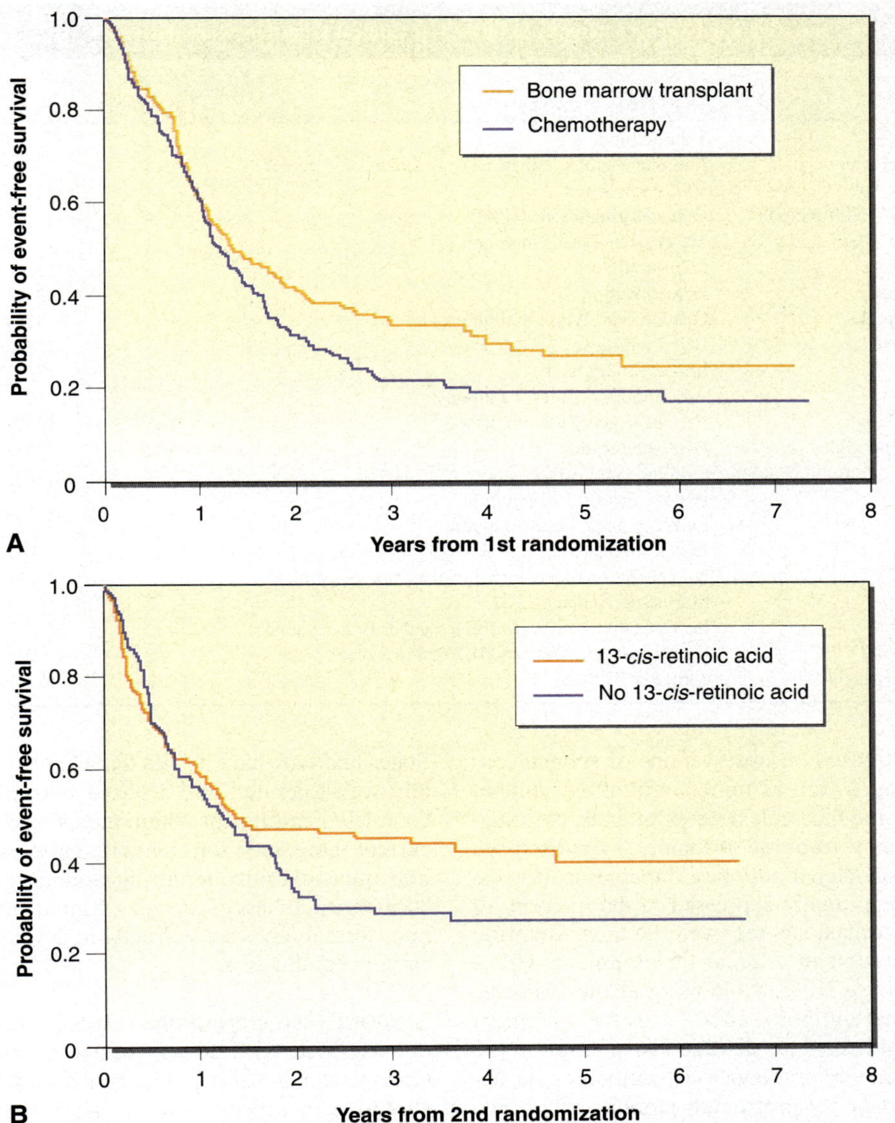

Figure 124j-4 Results of CCG study 3891. Autologous bone marrow transplantation (ABMT) and 13-*cis*-retinoic acid improve event-free survival for high-risk neuroblastoma patients. All patients were treated with identical induction chemotherapy and were first randomized to either purged ABMT or continuation chemotherapy, and then were randomized to receive either 13-*cis*-retinoic acid or no further therapy. **A,** Event-free survival for patients randomized to ABMT ($n = 189$) or intensive but non-myeloablative continuation therapy ($n = 190$) ($p = .03$). **B,** Event-free survival from time of randomization to 13-*cis*-retinoic acid ($n = 130$) to no further therapy ($n = 128$) ($p = .03$). (Redrawn with permission from Matthay KK, Villablanca JG, Seeger RC, et al. Treatment of high risk neuroblastoma with intensive chemotherapy, radiotherapy, autologous bone marrow transplantation, and 13-*cis*-retinoic acid. Children's Cancer Group. N Engl J Med 1999; 341:1165–73.)

transplant related morbidity and mortality, but an encouraging 5-year survival of 32%, in a cohort of 33 very high risk patients with relapsed and/or refractory disease.[261] More recently, Grupp and colleagues showed that a tandem myeloablative consolidation with peripheral blood stem cell support was feasible with rapid myeloid engraftment in a limited institution pilot study of 39 patients.[253] Transplant-related mortality was 8% (3/39) and the 3-year EFS was estimated at 58%. Similarly, Kletzel and colleagues recently documented a 57% 3-year EFS in a cohort of 25 consecutive patients treated with a triple myeloablative consolidation regimen.[254] A randomized trial of single versus tandem myeloablative consolidations will be necessary to determine the true impact of a tandem high-dose myeloablative consolidation strategy.

Minimal Residual Disease Therapy Relapse occurs all to frequently after autologous transplantation, suggesting that chemotherapy resistant malignant stem cells can survive dose intensive therapy. Because the original observations that retinoids and other agents can induce differentiation of neuroblastoma cells in vitro, a biological-based therapy against minimal residual disease has been sought.

Several novel agents specifically targeted to the unique biology of neuroblastoma may be effective for eliminating minimal residual disease. The retinoids are a class of compounds that have been known for two decades to induce cellular differentiation with a concomitant decrease in proliferation of neuroblastoma cells in vitro.[262] The efficacy of 13-*cis*-retinoic acid was recently tested in the CCG randomized trial mentioned above using a factorial design following a randomization to myeloablative or continuation chemotherapy.[255] A total of 130 patients were randomized to receive either six cycles of high dose, pulsed 13-*cis*-retinoic acid or no further therapy. The cohort of patients assigned to receive post-transplant therapy with 13-*cis*-retinoic acid had a significantly improved EFS probability (46 ± 6% versus 29 ≤ 6% from second randomization; $p = .03$; Figure 124j-4B). Other retinoids such as 9-*cis*-retinoic acid, all trans-retinoic acid, and/or fenretinide may also have activity for minimal residual disease in high-risk neuroblastoma patients. Fenretinide is an interesting retinoid that appears to be directly cytotoxic to neuroblastoma cells, even in neuroblastoma cells that are resistant to 13-cis-retinoic acid. Phase I experience with the current oral formulation showed poor bioavailability.[263] Phase II results are pending, and new oral and intravenous formulations are being pursued.

An alternative, or perhaps complementary, strategy that appears promising for application during the minimal residual disease phase of therapy is targeted molecules directed against neuroblastoma-specific cellular antigens. Murine, chimeric, and humanized antibodies specific to the cell surface ganglioside GD2, either alone or with cytokines, have shown activity in preclinical models[264–267] as well as phase I[268–273] and phase II[274,275] clinical trials. The murine monoclonal antibodies 3F8[276] and GD2a,[272] and the human-mouse chimeric monoclonal antibody ch14.18[268] have received the most clinical attention. Measurable responses have been observed in refractory neuroblastoma patients[270,277,278] justifying further examination in phase III clinical trials. Limiting the broad application of this strategy are difficulties with antibody production and the development of neutralizing antibodies, even to the chimeric molecules.[270,277,278] Neuropathic pain is also a significant immediate toxicity and can be dose limiting.[270,277,278] Although a nonrandomized trial of ch14.18 alone did not show obvious profound clinical benefit in a German study,[279] a randomized clinical trial designed to test the efficacy of ch14.18 with IL-2 and GM-CSF versus no antibody/cytokine therapy following myeloablative chemotherapy is ongoing within the COG, and another randomized trial is ongoing in Europe. Additional strategies early in clinical development that may be exploited in this phase of therapy include immunocytokines ("fusion antibodies"), vaccines (both cellular and anti-idiotypic), and engineered T-cells for cellular immunotherapy.

High-risk patients are at the greatest risk of experiencing late effects of treatment including problems with linear growth, cardiac function, renal function and cognition.[280–282] Ototoxicity, secondary to the use of platinum-containing regiments to treat very young children, has been a particular problem in these patients.[283] In addition, the extensive use of alkylating agents and topoisomerase II inhibitors results in a higher prevalence of sterility as well as second malignancies, particularly myelodysplastic syndromes and acute nonlymphoblastic leukemias.[228,284]

NEW APPROACHES TO HIGH-RISK DISEASE

Although there are highly effective salvage options for patients with low- and intermediate-risk disease with local relapses, refractory high-risk disease remains a significant clinical challenge with no known curative approach. Over the past several years an expanding portfolio of novel therapeutic agents with efficacy in the relapsed setting have been developed (Table 124j-6) and several are highlighted in this section.

Table 124j-6 Investigational Agents Currently in Phase I–II Clinical Trials for Neuroblastoma

Agent	Mechanism of Action/Target	Phase of Development	Reference
ABT-751	Tubulin binding	1	(323)
beta-D-glucan	Immune response enhancer/iC3b leukocyte receptor	1	(324)
Bevacizumab	VEGF inhibition		(325)
Buthionine Sulfoximine	Depletes glutathione (GSH)	1	(326)
CEP-701	Trk tyrosine kinase inhibitor	1	(319)
CCI-779	mTor inhibitor	1	(327,328)
Decitabine	Demethylation	1	(320)
Depsipeptide	Histone deacetylase inhibitor	1	(329)
Genasense	BCL2 antisense	1	(330)
IL12	Immune modulator	1	(331,332)
mAb1A7	Anti-anti-GD2 (anti-id antibody)	1	(303)
MS-27-275	Histone deacetylase inhibitor	1	(322)
Pyrazoloacridine	DNA intercalator	1	(333,334)
safingol	Ceramide modulator	1	(306,335)
SAHA	Histone deacetylase inhibitor	1	(321)
ZD1839 (Iressa)	EGFR tyrosine kinase inhibitor	1	(336)
zoledronic acid	Bisphosphonate	1	(337)
^{131}I-MIBG	Norepinephrine receptor/targeted radiotherapeutic	2	(183–186,297)
3F8	Murine-derived anti-GD2	2	(296)
Fenretinide	Increases reactive oxygen species and de novo ceramides	2	(305)
hu14.18-IL2	Humanized anti-GD2 and IL2 fusion protein	2	(299)
Imatinib mesylate	c-kit, PDGFR	2	(338)

Cytotoxic Agents The topoisomerase 1 inhibitors, topotecan and irinotecan, are often used early in the relapse setting because of their proven efficacy and low toxicity profile.[199,200,285,286] Although both have efficacy as single agents, a recent randomized trial showed that topotecan combined with low dose cyclophosphamide was superior to topotecan alone (CR + PR 31% vs 19%).[287] Irinotecan combined with temozolomide has been shown to be tolerable in the phase I setting,[199] and efficacy will soon be tested in a COG phase II study. The most common toxicity related to irinotecan is diarrhea, which can potentially be prevented with the concomitant use of oral antibiotics.[288] The combination of irinotecan and topotecan has been studied in the phase I setting, but unacceptable toxicity has limited further development.[289] A promising novel cytoxic agent is ABT-751, an oral tubulin-binding agent that is not a classic multi-drug resistance pump substrate. Early clinical trials suggest activity against refractory neuroblastoma,[290] and ABT-751 will be studied in an upcoming COG phase II trial.

Targeted Delivery of Radionucleotides Because neuroblastoma is a radiation sensitive, but also systemic tumor, there has been interest in targeting delivery of radioactive molecules that are selectively concentrated in neuroblastoma cells. Approaches have included attachment of radionuclide to MIBG,[183,291,292] somatostatin analogs,[293–295] and anti-GD2 antibodies.[270,274,296] The compound ^{131}I-MIBG is furthest in clinical development. Low-dose ^{131}I-MIBG has been shown to be highly effective for disease palliation,[184] and a phase I dose escalation trial established 12 mCi/kg of ^{131}I-MIBG as the maximum tolerated dose with the only significant toxicity being hematopoeitic.[183] This trial further showed that doses up to 18 mCi/kg are tolerable with stem cell support for the one-third of patients with protracted grade 4 hematopoietic toxicity. A recently completed phase II study showed an objective response rate of approximately 40% in heavily pretreated patients receiving 18 mCi/kg with acceptable toxicity.[185,186] Current clinical investigation is focusing on further dose intensification of MIBG as well as combining ^{131}I-MIBG with myeloablative therapies for high-risk patients with a poor response to initial treatment.[297] Future trials will likely combine ^{131}I-MIBG with potential radiosensitizing agents.

Immunotherapy Immunotherapeutic strategies for treating neuroblastoma were originally postulated based on observations of spontaneous regression, as well as tumor infiltrating lymphocytes in some favorable neuroblastomas, both suggesting a host response to tumor.[298] As discussed above, monoclonal antibody directed against the GD2 antigen, highly expressed in the majority of neuroblastomas, has received the most attention and is furthest in clinical development with a current phase III study looking at the chimeric monoclonal antibody ch14.18 in the treatment of minimal residual disease. To maximize the immunogenicity of monoclonal antibodies, particularly in heavily pretreated patients who have chemotherapy-suppressed function of immune effector cells, immunocytokines or tumor-specific monoclonal antibodies linked with cytokines are in development. A humanized GD2 antibody fused to IL2 (hu14.18-IL2)[299,300] will soon be investigated in a COG phase II trial. Other immunotherapeutic strategies early in development include DNA,[301] cellular[302] and anti-idiotypic vaccination strategies[303] as well as using engineered cytolytic T lymphocytes for cellular immunotherapy.[304]

Retinoids Based on the results from the randomized trial of 13-cis-retinoic acid following myeloablative chemotherapy,[255] most investigators consider this agent standard of care for high-risk neuroblastoma patients who have a complete or very good partial response following myeloablative chemotherapy and stem cell rescue. Current investigation is focused on finding the retinoid compound that gives optimal systemic exposure allowing for maximal anti-tumor effect without excess toxicity.[139] Fenretinide is currently the lead retinoid in development because it has been shown to achieve multi-log cell kill in multiple neuroblastoma cell lines, even those resistant to other retinoic acids, at least in part through ceramide upregulation.[305,306] Phase I studies done in the United States and Italy have shown that the drug is generally well-tolerated and a phase II trial recently completed enrollment within the COG.[263,307] The current fenretinide formulation, however, has low oral bioavailability requiring young children to take large numbers of capsules. Liquid and intravenous formulations are currently in development to circumvent this issue.

Angiogenesis Inhibitors Tumor vascularity is correlated with an aggressive phenotype in neuroblastoma making angiogenesis inhibitors an attractive therapeutic option. High-risk tumors are highly vascular, and the tumor vascular index is strongly correlated with adverse prognostic features including *MYCN* amplification and poor-survival probability.[308] In addition, several pro-angiogenic factors, including VEGF, have been shown to be differentially expressed in primary neuroblastomas in a pattern suggesting promotion of an angiogenic phenotype in high-risk tumors,[309,310] whereas low-risk neuroblastomas are characterized by a rich stromal component that produces angiogenesis inhibitors.[311,312] Preclinical therapeutic studies, however, have shown variable efficacy in neuroblastoma [313–317] that is not always predicted by activity seen in adult and other pediatric tumors, making the translation to the clinic somewhat slow. Strategies focused on neutralization of circulating VEGF are currently in early clinical trials with specific development for neuroblastoma underway. The challenge of providing neovascular inhibition strategies in young children with a developing cardiovascular system need to be considering during preclinical and clinical development.

Other Strategies The MycN protein provides an obvious potential therapeutic target, but it is so massively dysregulated in neuroblastoma cells with amplification that this has been difficult to date. Constitutive activation of the BDNF:TrkB signaling pathway in high-risk neuroblastoma provides another rational target that might be exploited. Evans and colleagues showed that small molecule inhibition of the Trk tyrosine kinases causes significant growth inhibition of neuroblastoma xenografts,[318,319] providing the rationale for an ongoing phase I trial. Another strategy currently being explored is the use of demethylating agents such as decitabine. The rationale for this approach is that methylation of genes critical for apoptosis such as caspase 8 appear to occur frequently in neuroblastomas, particularly in association with *MYCN* amplification.[320] Histone deacetylase inhibitors have demonstrated preclinical activity against neuroblastoma,[321,322] and there are several in clinical trials for patients with refractory solid tumors. With the relatively small number of pediatric patients available for experimental therapeutic trials and the growing number of potential drugs to be tested, it is becoming increasingly important to have firm biological rationale and evidence of efficacy in appropriate preclinical models to help prioritize drug development. Many other strategies, some of which are listed in Table 124j-6, are under development in the laboratory or in early phase clinical trials.

CONCLUSIONS AND FUTURE CONSIDERATIONS

Considerable progress has been made in understanding the genetic basis of clinical heterogeneity observed in neuroblastoma. Patients can now be more reliably categorized as having a low-, intermediate- or high-risk for disease relapse, and this has resulted in more rational treatment choices. Although low-risk patients are currently mostly cured with minimal therapy, high-risk disease remains a significant pediatric problem. It is apparent that although short-term improvements in outcome are likely to come from more effective use of existing treatment modalities, including newer cytotoxic agents and stem cell support, further dose intensification of conventional chemoradiotherapeutics is unlikely to be tolerated in young children. Thus, the challenge for the future is to translate new insights concerning the biology of neuroblastoma into novel treatment approaches that target critical pathways involved in tumor cell survival or maintenance of the malignant state.

REFERENCES

1. Gurney JG, Ross JA, Wall DA, et al. Infant cancer in the US: histology-specific incidence and trends, 1973 to 1992. Journal of Pediatric Hematology and Oncology 1997;19:428–32.
2. London WB, Castleberry RP, Matthay KK, et al. Evidence for an Age Cut-off Greater than 365 days for Neuroblastoma Risk Group Stratification in the Children's Oncology Group (COG). Journal of Clinical Oncology [in press].
3. Kinney H, Faix R, Brazy J. The fetal alcohol syndrome and neuroblastoma. Pediatrics 1980;66:130–2.
4. Kramer S, Ward E, Meadows AT, et al. Medical and drug risk factors associated with neuroblastoma: A case-control study. Journal of the National Cancer Institute 1987;78:797–804.
5. Olshan AF, Smith J, Cook MM, et al. Hormone and fertility drug use and the risk of neuroblastoma: A report from the Children's Cancer Group and the Pediatric Oncology Group. American Journal of Epidemiology 1999;150:930–8.
6. Maris JM, Tonini GP. Genetics of familial neuroblastoma. In: Brodeur GM, Sawada T, Tsuchida Y, Voute PA, editors. Neuroblastoma. Amsterdam: Elsevier Science B.V.; 2000. p. 125–36.
7. Maris JM, Brodeur GM. Genetics. In: Cheung N-KV, Cohn SL, editors. Neuroblastoma. Berlin, Heidelberg, New York: Springer; 2005. p. 21–6.
8. Shojaei-Brosseau T, Chompret A, Abel A, et al. Genetic epidemiology of neuroblastoma: A study of 426 cases at the Institut Gustave-Roussy in France. Pediatric Blood and Cancer 2004;42:99–105.
9. Maris JM, Kyemba SM, Rebbeck TR, et al. Molecular genetic analysis of familial neuroblastoma. Eur J Cancer 1997;33:1923–8.
10. Kushner BH, Gilbert F, Helson L. Familial neuroblastoma. Case reports, literature review, and etiologic considerations. Cancer 1986;57:1887–93.
11. Knudson AG Jr, Strong LC. Mutation and cancer: neuroblastoma and pheochromocytoma. Am J Hum Genet 1972;24:514–32.
12. Maris JM, Weiss MJ, Mosse Y, et al. Evidence for a hereditary neuroblastoma predisposition locus at chromosome 16p12-13. Cancer Res 2002;62(22):6651–8.
13. Trochet D, Bourdeaut F, Janoueix-Lerosey I, et al. Germline Mutations of the Paired-Like Homeobox 2B (PHOX2B) Gene in Neuroblastoma. Am J Hum Genet 2004;74:761–4.
14. Mosse YP, Laudenslager M, Khazi D, et al. Germline PHOX2B Mutation in Hereditary Neuroblastoma. Am J Hum Genet 2004;75:727–30.
15. van Limpt V, Schramm A, van Lakeman A, et al. The Phox2B homeobox gene is mutated in sporadic neuroblastomas. Oncogene 2004;23:9280–8.
16. Bolande RP. The neurocristopathies: A unifying concept of disease arising in neural crest maldevelopment. Human Pathol 1974;5:409–29.
17. Bower RJ, Adkins JC. Ondine's curse and neurocristopathy. Clinical Pediatrics 1980;19:665–8.
18. Knudson AGJ, Meadows AT. Developmental genetics of neuroblastoma. J Natl Cancer Inst 1976;57:675–82.
19. Knudson AG Jr, Amromin GD. Neuroblastoma and ganglioneuroma in a child with multiple neurofibromatosis. Implications for the mutational origin of neuroblastoma. Cancer 1966;19:1032–7.
20. Kushner BH, Hajdu SI, Helson L. Synchronous neuroblastoma and von Recklinghausen's disease: a review of the literature. J Clin Oncol 1985;3:117–20.
21. Maris JM, Chatten J, Meadows AT, et al. Familial neuroblastoma: A three generation pedigree and a further association with Hirschsprung disease. Med Pediatr Oncol 1997;28:1–5.
22. Amiel J, Laudier B, Attie-Bitach T, et al. Polyalanine expansion and frameshift mutations of the paired-like homeobox gene PHOX2B in congenital central hypoventilation syndrome. Nat Genet 2003;33:459–61.
23. Blatt J, Hamilton RL. Neurodevelopmental anomalies in children with neuroblastoma. Cancer 1998;82:1603–8.
24. Mosse Y, Greshock J, King A, et al. Identification and high-resolution mapping of a constitutional 11q deletion in an infant with multifocal neuroblastoma. Lancet Oncol 2003;4:769–71.
25. Bellah R, D'Andrea A, Darillis E, et al. The association of congenital neuroblastoma and congenital heart disease. Is there a common embryologic basis? Pediatr Radiol 1989;19:119–21.
26. Blatt J, Olshan AF, Lee PA, et al. Neuroblastoma and related tumors in Turner's syndrome. J Ped 1997;131:666–70.
27. Satge D, Sasco AJ, Carlsen NL, et al. A lack of neuroblastoma in Down syndrome: a study from 11 European countries. Cancer Res 1998;58:448–52.
28. Satge D, Moore SW, Stiller CA, et al. Abnormal constitutional karyotypes in patients with neuroblastoma: a report of four new cases and review of 47 others in the literature. Cancer Genet Cytogenet 2003;147:89–98.
29. Biegel JA, White PS, Marshall HN, et al. Constitutional 1p36 deletion in a child with neuroblastoma. Am J Hum Genet 1993;52:176–82.
30. Brodeur GM. Neuroblastoma: Biological insights into a clinical enigma. Nat Rev Cancer 2003;3:203–16.
31. Azar C, Scavarda NJ, Reynolds CP, et al. Multiple defects of the nerve growth factor receptor in human neuroblastomas. Cell Growth Differ 1990;1:421–8.
32. Baker DL, Reddy UR, Pleasure D, et al. Analysis of nerve growth factor receptor expression in human neuroblastoma and neuroepithelioma cell lines. Cancer Res 1989;49:4142–6.
33. Brodeur GM, Nakagawara A, Yamashiro DJ, et al. Expression of TrkA, TrkB, and TrkC in human neuroblastomas. J Neuroncol 1996;12:37–41.
34. Nakagawara A, Arima-Nakagawara M, Scavarda NJ, et al. Association between high levels of expression of the TRK gene and favorable outcome in human neuroblastoma. N Engl J Med 1993;328:847–54.
35. Tanaka T, Sugimoto T, Sawada T. Prognostic discrimination among neuroblastomas according to Ha-ras/Trk A gene expression. Cancer 1998;83:1626–33.
36. Suzuki T, Bogenmann E, Shimada H, et al. Lack of high-affinity nerve growth factor receptors in aggressive neuroblastomas. J Natl Cancer Inst 1993;85:377–84.
37. Kogner P, Barbany G, Dominici C, et al. Coexpression of messenger RNA for TRK protooncogene and low affinity nerve growth factor receptor in neuroblastoma with favorable prognosis. Cancer Res 1993;53:2044–50.
38. Nakagawara A, Arima M, Azar CG, et al. Inverse relationship between trk expression and N-myc amplification in human neuroblastomas. Cancer Res 1992;52:1364–8.
39. Nakagawara A, Azar CG, Scavarda NJ, et al. Expression and function of TRK-B and BDNF in human neuroblastomas. Mol Cell Biol 1994;14:759–67.
40. Jaboin J, Kim CJ, Kaplan DR, et al. Brain-derived neurotrophic factor activation of TrkB protects neuroblastoma cells from chemotherapy-induced apoptosis via phosphatidylinositol 3'-kinase pathway. Cancer Res 2002;62:6756–63.
41. Ho R, Eggert A, Hishiki T, et al. Resistance to chemotherapy mediated by TrkB in neuroblastomas. Cancer Res 2002;62:6462–6.
42. Ryden M, Sehgal R, Dominici C, et al. Expression of mRNA for the neurotrophin receptor trkC in neuroblastomas with favourable tumour stage and good prognosis. Br J Cancer 1996;74:773–9.
43. Yamashiro DJ, Nakagawara A, Ikegaki N, et al. Expression of TrkC in favorable human neuroblastomas. Oncogene 1996;12:37–41.
44. Look AT, Hayes FA, Nitschke R, et al. Cellular DNA content as a predictor of response to chemotherapy in infants with unresectable neuroblastoma. N Engl J Med 1984;311:231–5.
45. Look AT, Hayes FA, Shuster JJ, et al. Clinical relevance of tumor cell ploidy and N-myc gene amplification in childhood neuroblastoma. A Pediatric Oncology Group Study. J Clin Oncol 1991;9:581–91.
46. Katzenstein HM, Bowman LC, Brodeur GM, et al. Prognostic significance of age, MYCN oncogene amplification, tumor cell ploidy, and histology in 110 infants with stage D(S) neuroblastoma: the pediatric oncology group experience—a pediatric oncology group study. J Clin Oncol 1998;16:2007–17.
47. Schwab M, Alitalo K, Klempnauer KH, et al. Amplified DNA with limited homology to myc cellular oncogene is shared by human neuroblastoma cell lines and a neuroblastoma tumour. Nature 1983;305:245–8.
48. Brodeur G, Seeger RC, Schwab M, et al. Amplification of N-*myc* in untreated human neuroblastomas correlates with advanced disease stage. Science 1984;224:1121–4.
49. Seeger RC, Brodeur GM, Sather H, et al. Association of multiple copies of the N-myc oncogene with rapid progression of neuroblastomas. N Engl J Med 1985;313:1111–6.
50. Brodeur GM, Ambros PF. Genetic and biological markers of prognosis in neuroblastoma. In: Brodeur GM, Sawada T, Tsuchida Y, Voute PA, editors. Neuroblastoma. Amsterdam, The Netherlands: Elsevier Science, B.V.; 2000. p. 355–69.
51. Brodeur GM, Fong CT. Molecular biology and genetics of human neuroblastoma. Cancer Genet Cytogenet 1989;41:153–74.
52. Brodeur GM. Molecular basis for heterogeneity in human neuroblastomas [abstract]. Eur J Cancer 1995;31:505–10.
53. Brodeur GM, Maris JM, Yamashiro DJ, et al. Biology and genetics of human neuroblastomas. J Ped Hemat Oncol 1997;19:93–101.
54. Brodeur GM, Hayes FA, Green AA, et al. Consistent N-myc copy number in simultaneous or consecutive neuroblastoma samples from sixty individual patients. Cancer Res 1987;47:4248–53.
55. Weiss WA, Aldape K, Mohapatra G, et al. Targeted expression of MYCN causes neuroblastoma in transgenic mice. EMBO J 1997;16:2985–95.

56. Slavc I, Ellenbogen R, Jung WH, et al. Myc gene amplification and expression in primary human neuroblastoma. Cancer Res 1990;50(5):1459–1463.
57. Seeger RC, Wada R, Brodeur GM, et al. Expression Of N-myc by neuroblastomas with one or multiple copies of the oncogene. Prog Clin Biol Res 1988;271:41–9.
58. Wada RK, Seeger RC, Brodeur GM, et al. Human neuroblastoma cell lines that express N-myc without gene amplification. Cancer 1993;723346–54.
59. Sivak LE, Tai KF, Smith RS, et al. Autoregulation of the human N-myc oncogene is disrupted in amplified but not single-copy neuroblastoma cell lines. Oncogene 1997;15:1937–46.
60. Cohn SL, Salwen H, Quasney MW, et al. Prolonged N-Myc protein half-life in a neuroblastoma cell line lacking N-Myc amplification. Oncogene 1990;5:1821–7.
61. Cohn SL, London WB, Huang D, et al. MYCN expression is not prognostic of adverse outcome in advanced-stage neuroblastoma with nonamplified MYCN. J Clin Oncol 2000;18:3604–13.
62. Savelyeva L, Corvi R, Schwab M. Translocation involving 1p and 17q is a recurrent genetic alteration of human neuroblastoma cells. Am J Human Genet 1994;55(2):334–340.
63. Van Roy N, Laureys G, Cheng NC, et al. 1;17 translocations and other chromosome 17 rearrangements in human primary neuroblastoma tumors and cell lines. Genes Chromosomes Cancer 1994;10:103–14.
64. Van Roy N, Laureys G, Van Gele M, et al. Analysis of 1;17 translocation breakpoints in neuroblastoma: implications for mapping of neuroblastoma genes. Eur J Cancer 1997;33:1974–78.
65. Lastowska M, Roberts P, Pearson AD, et al. Promiscuous translocations of chromosome arm 17q in human neuroblastomas. Genes Chromosomes Cancer 1997;19:143–9.
66. Meddeb M, Danglot G, Chudoba I, et al. Additional copies of a 25 Mb chromosomal region originating from 17q23.1-17qter are present in 90% of high-grade neuroblastomas. Genes Chromosomes Cancer 1996;17:156–65.
67. Bown N, Cotterill S, Lastowska M, et al. European multicentre study of 274 neuroblastoma tumours demonstrates that 17q gain is a powerful prognostic indicator. Med Pediatr Oncol 1998;31:190.
68. Lastowska M, Cotterill S, Pearson AD, et al. Gain of chromosome arm 17q predicts unfavourable outcome in neuroblastoma patients. U.K. Children's Cancer Study Group and the U.K. Cancer Cytogenetics Group. Eur J Cancer 1997;33:1627–33.
69. Morowitz M, Shusterman S, Mosse Y, et al. Detection of single-copy chromosome 17q gain in human neuroblastomas using real-time quantitative polymerase chain reaction. Mod Pathol 2003;16:1248–56.
70. Bown N, Cotterill S, Lastowska M, et al. Gain of chromosome arm 17q and adverse outcome in patients with neuroblastoma. N Engl J Med 1999;340:1954–61.
71. Fong CT, Dracopoli NC, White PS, et al. Loss of heterozygosity for the short arm of chromosome 1 in human neuroblastomas: Correlation with N-*myc* amplification. Proceedings of the National Academy of Sciences of the United States of America 1989;86:3753–7.
72. White PS, Maris JM, Beltinger C, et al. A region of consistent deletion in neuroblastoma maps within 1p36.2-.3. Proc Natl Acad Sci U S A 1995;92:5520–4.
73. Maris JM, Weiss MJ, Guo C, et al. Loss of heterozygosity at 1p36 independently predicts for disease progression, but not decreased overall survival probability, in neuroblastoma patients: A Children's Cancer Group Study. J Clin Oncol 2000;18:1888–99.
74. Bader SA, Fasching C, Brodeur GM, et al. Dissociation of suppression of tumorigenicity and differentiation in vitro effected by transfer of single human chromosomes into human neuroblastoma cells. Cell Growth Differ 1991;2:245–55.
75. Martinsson T, Sjoberg RM, Hedborg F, et al. Deletion of chromosome 1p loci and microsatellite instability in neuroblastomas analyzed with short-tandem repeat polymorphisms. Cancer Res 1995;55:5681–6.
76. Schleiermacher G, Peter M, Michon J, et al. Two distinct deleted regions on the short arm of chromosome 1 in neuroblastoma. Genes Chromosomes Cancer 1994;10:275–81.
77. Caron H, Peter M, van Sluis P, et al. Evidence for two tumour suppressor loci on chromosomal bands 1p35-36 involved in neuroblastoma: one probably imprinted, another associated with N-myc amplification. Hum Mol Genet 1995;4:535–9.
78. White PS, Thompson PM, Gotoh T, et al. Definition and characterization of a region of 1p36.3 consistently deleted in neuroblastoma. Oncogene 2005;24:2684–94.
79. Takita J, Hayashi Y, Kohno T, et al. Allelotype of neuroblastoma. Oncogene 1995;11:1829–34.
80. Srivatsan ES, Ying KL, Seeger RC. Deletion of chromosome 11 and of 14q sequences in neuroblastoma. Genes Chromosomes Cancer 1993;7:32–7.
81. Guo C, White PS, Weiss MJ, et al. Allelic deletion at 11q23 is common in *MYCN* single copy neuroblastomas. Oncogene 1999;18:4948–57.
82. Kaneko Y, Cohn SL. Ploidy and cytogenetics of neuroblastoma. In: Brodeur GM, Sawada T, Tsuchida Y, Voute PA, editors. Neuroblastoma. Amsterdam: Elsevier Science B.V.; 2000. p. 41–56.
83. Attiyeh E, Mossé Y, Wang Q, et al. Chromosome 11q deletion is an independent marker for neuroblastoma patient outcome: a Children's Oncology Group Study. J Clin Oncol 2004. [In press]
84. Spitz R, Hero B, Ernestus K, et al. Deletions in chromosome arms 3p and 11q are new prognostic markers in localized and 4s neuroblastoma. Clin Cancer Res 2003;9:52–8.
85. Breen CJ, O'Meara A, McDermott M, et al. Coordinate deletion of chromosome 3p and 11q in neuroblastoma detected by comparative genomic hybridization. Cancer Genet Cytogenet 2000;120:44–49.
86. Beheshti B, Braude I, Marrano P, et al. Chromosomal localization of DNA amplifications in neuroblastoma tumors using cDNA microarray comparative genomic hybridization. Neoplasia 2003;5:53–62.
87. Chen QR, Bilke S, Wei JS, et al. cDNA array-CGH profiling identifies genomic alterations specific to stage and MYCN-amplification in neuroblastoma. BMC Genomics 2004;5:70.
88. Mosse YP, Greshock J, Margolin A, et al. High-resolution detection and mapping of genomic DNA alterations in neuroblastoma. Genes Chromosomes Cancer 2005;43:390–403.
89. Thompson PM, Maris JM, Hogarty MD, et al. Homozygous deletion of CDKN2A (p16INK4a/p14ARF) but not within 1p36 or at other tumor suppressor loci in neuroblastoma. Cancer Res 2001;61:679–86.
90. Hughes M, Marsden HB, Palmer MK. Histologic patterns of neuroblastoma related to prognosis and clinical staging. Cancer 1974;34:1706–11.
91. Hassenbusch S, Kaizer H, White JJ. Prognostic factors in neuroblastic tumors. J Ped Surg 1976;11:287–97.
92. Joshi VV, Cantor AB, Brodeur GM, et al. Correlation between morphologic and other prognostic markers of neuroblastoma. A study of histologic grade, DNA index, N-myc gene copy number, and lactic dehydrogenase in patients in the Pediatric Oncology Group. Cancer 1993;71:3173–81.
93. Shimada H, Chatten J, Newton W Jr, et al. Histopathologic prognostic factors in neuroblastic tumors: definition of subtypes of ganglioneuroblastoma and an age-linked classification of neuroblastomas. J Natl Cancer Inst 1984;73:405–16.
94. Shimada H, Stram DO, Chatten J, et al. Identification of subsets of neuroblastomas by combined histopathologic and N-myc analysis. J Natl Cancer Inst 1995;87:1470–6.
95. Silber JH, Evans AE, Fridman M. Models to predict outcome from childhood neuroblastoma: the role of serum ferritin and tumor histology. Cancer Res 1991;51:1426–33.
96. Evans AE, D'Angio GJ, Propert K, et al. Prognostic factors in neuroblastoma. Cancer 1987;59:1853–9.
97. Joshi VV, Cantor AB, Altshuler G, et al. Recommendations for modification of terminology of neuroblastic tumors and prognostic significance of Shimada classification. A clinicopathologic study of 213 cases from the Pediatric Oncology Group. Cancer 1992;69:2183–96.
98. Joshi VV, Cantor AB, Altshuler G, et al. Age-linked prognostic categorization based on a new histologic grading system of neuroblastomas. A clinicopathologic study of 211 cases from the Pediatric Oncology Group. Cancer 1992;69:2197–211.
99. Shimada H, Ambros IM, Dehner LP, et al. The International Neuroblastoma Pathology Classification (Shimada) System. Cancer 1999;86:364–72.
100. Shimada H, Ambros IM, Dehner LP, et al. Terminology and morphologic criteria of neuroblastic tumors: recommendations by the International Neuroblastoma Pathology Committee. Cancer 1999;86:349–63.
101. Rosen EM, Cassady JR, Frantz CN, et al. Neuroblastoma; The Joint Center for Radiation Therapy/Dana-Farber Cancer Institute/Children's Hospital experience. J Clin Oncol 1984;2:714–32.
102. Weinblatt ME, Heisel MA, Siegel SE. Hypertension in children with neurogenic tumors. Pediatrics 1983;71:947–57.
103. Musarella MA, Chan HS, DeBoer G, et al. Ocular involvement in neuroblastoma: prognostic implications. Ophthalmology 1984;91:936–40.
104. Evans AE, D'Angio GJ, Randolph JA. A proposed staging for children with neuroblastoma: Children's Cancer Study Group A. Cancer 1971;27:374–8.
105. Franks LM, Bollen A, Seeger RC, et al. Neuroblastoma in adults and adolescents: an indolent course with poor survival. Cancer 1997;79:2028–35.
106. Blatt J, Gula MJ, Orlando SJ, et al. Indolent course of advanced neuroblastoma in children older than 6 years at diagnosis. Cancer 1995;76:890–4.
107. Kushner BH, Kramer K, LaQuaglia MP, et al. Neuroblastoma in adolescents and adults: the Memorial Sloan-Kettering experience. Med Pediatr Oncol 2003;41:508–15.
108. Matthay KK, Blaes F, Hero B, et al. Opsoclonus myoclonus syndrome in neuroblastoma a report from a workshop on the dancing eyes syndrome at the advances in neuroblastoma meeting in Genoa, Italy, 2004. Cancer Lett 2005.
109. Hayward K, Jeremy RJ, Jenkins S, et al. Long-term neurobehavioral outcomes in children with neuroblastoma and opsoclonus-myoclonus-ataxia syndrome: relationship to MRI findings and anti-neuronal antibodies. J Pediatr 2001;139:552–9.
110. Rudnick E, Khakoo Y, Antunes NL, et al. Opsoclonus-myoclonus-ataxia syndrome in neuroblastoma: clinical outcome and antineuronal antibodies-a report from the Children's Cancer Group Study. Med Pediatr Oncol 2001;36:612–22.
111. Koh PS, Raffensperger JG, Berry S, et al. Long-term outcome in children with opsoclonus-myoclonus and ataxia and coincident neuroblastoma. J Pediatr 1994;125:712–6.
112. Antunes NL, Khakoo Y, Matthay KK, et al. Antineuronal antibodies in patients with neuroblastoma and paraneoplastic opsoclonus-myoclonus. J Pediatr Hematol Oncol 2000;22:315–20.
113. Connolly AM, Pestronk A, Mehta S, et al. Serum autoantibodies in childhood opsoclonus-myoclonus syndrome: an analysis of antigenic targets in neural tissues [see comments]. J Pediatr 1997;130:878–84.
114. Russo C, Cohn SL, Petruzzi MJ, et al. Long-term neurologic outcome in children with opsoclonus-myoclonus associated with neuroblastoma: a report from the Pediatric Oncology Group. Med Pediatr Oncol 1997;28:284–8.
115. Veneselli E, Conte M, Biancheri R, et al. Effect of steroid and high-dose immunoglobulin therapy on opsoclonus-myoclonus syndrome occurring in neuroblastoma. Med Pediatr Oncol 1998;30:15–7.
116. Swart JF, de Kraker J, van der Lely N. Metaiodobenzylguanidine total-body scintigraphy required for revealing occult neuroblastoma in opsoclonus-myoclonus syndrome. Eur J Pediatr 2002;161:255–8.
117. El Shafie M, Samuel D, Klippel CH, et al. Intractable diarrhea in children with VIP-secreting ganglioneuroblastomas. J Pediatr Surg 1983;18:34–6.
118. Kaplan S, Holbrook C, McDaniel H, et al. Vasoactive intestinal peptide secreting tumors of childhood. Am J Dis Child 1980;134:21–4.
119. Qualman SJ, O'Dorisio MS, Fleshman DJ, et al. Neuroblastoma. Correlation of neuropeptide expression in tumor tissue with other prognostic factors. Cancer 1992;70:2005–12.
120. LaBrosse EH, Com-Nougue C, Zucker JM, et al. Urinary excretion of 3-methoxy-4-hydroxymandelic acid and 3-methoxy-4-hydroxyphenylacetic acid by 288 patients with neuroblastoma and related neural crest tumors. Cancer Res 1980;40:1995–2001.
121. Graham-Pole J, Salmi T, Anton AH, et al. Tumor and urine catecholamines (CATS) in neurogenic tumors. Correlations with other prognostic factors and survival. Cancer 1983;51:834–9.
122. Brodeur GM, Pritchard J, Berthold F, et al. Revisions of the international criteria for neuroblastoma diagnosis, staging, and response to treatment. J Clin Oncol 1993;11:1466–77.
123. Brodeur GM, Seeger RC, Barrett A, et al. International criteria for diagnosis, staging and response to treatment in patients with neuroblastoma. J Clin Oncol 1988;6:1874–81.
124. Black J, Williams DI. Natural history of adrenal haemorrhage in the newborn. Arch Dis Child 1973;48:183–90.
125. Kemshead JT, Goldman A, Fritschy J, et al. Use of panels of monoclonal antibodies in the differential diagnosis of neuroblastoma and lymphoblastic disorders. Lancet 1983;1:12–5.

126. Sugimoto T, Sawada T, Arakawa S, et al. Possible differential diagnosis of neuroblastoma from rhabdomyosarcoma and Ewing's sarcoma by using a panel of monoclonal antibodies. Gann 1985;76:301–7.
127. Matthay KK, Brisse H, Couanet D, et al. Central nervous system metastases in neuroblastoma: radiologic, clinical, and biologic features in 23 patients. Cancer 2003;98:155–65.
128. Heisel MA, Miller JH, Reid BS, et al. Radionuclide bone scan in neuroblastoma. Pediatrics 1983;71:206–9.
129. Kaufman RA, Thrall JH, Keyes JW, et al. False negative bone scans in neuroblastoma metastatic to the ends of long bones. Roentgenology 1978;130:131–5.
130. Geatti O, Shapiro B, Sisson JC, et al. Iodine-131 metaiodobenzylguanidine scintigraphy for the location of neuroblastoma: Preliminary experience in ten cases. J Nucl Med 1985;26:736–42.
131. Voute PA, Hoefnagel CA, Marcuse HR, et al. Detection of neuroblastoma with 131I-meta-iodobenzylguanidine. Prog Clin Biol Res 1985;175:389–98.
132. Katzenstein HM, Cohn SL, Shore RM, et al. Scintigraphic Response by 123I-Metaiodobenzylguanidine Scan Correlates With Event-Free Survival in High-Risk Neuroblastoma. J Clin Oncol 2004;22:3909–15.
133. Matthay KK, Edeline V, Lumbroso J, et al. Correlation of early metastatic response by 123I-metaiodobenzylguanidine scintigraphy with overall response and event-free survival in stage IV neuroblastoma. J Clin Oncol 2003;21:2486–91.
134. Kushner BH, Yeung HW, Larson SM, et al. Extending positron emission tomography scan utility to high-risk neuroblastoma: fluorine-18 fluorodeoxyglucose positron emission tomography as sole imaging modality in follow-up of patients. J Clin Oncol 2001;19:3397–405.
135. Scanga DR, Martin WH, Delbeke D. Value of FDG PET imaging in the management of patients with thyroid, neuroendocrine, and neural crest tumors. Clin Nucl Med 2004;29:86–90.
136. Franklin IM, Pritchard J. Detection of bone marrow invasion by neuroblastoma is improved by sampling at two sites with both aspirates and trephine biopsies. J Clin Pathol 1983;36:1215–8.
137. Bostrom B, Nesbit ME, Brunning RD. The value of bone marrow trephine biopsy in the diagnosis of metastatic neuroblastoma. American Journal of Pediatric Hematology and Oncology 1985;7:303–5.
138. Seeger RC, Reynolds CP, Gallego R, et al. Quantitative tumor cell content of bone marrow and blood as a predictor of outcome in stage IV neuroblastoma: a Children's Cancer Group Study. J Clin Oncol 2000;18(24):4067–76.
139. Reynolds CP. Detection and treatment of minimal residual disease in high-risk neuroblastoma. Pediatr Transplant 2004;8 Suppl 5:56–66.
140. Hayes FA, Green AA, Hustu HO, et al. Surgicopathologic staging of neuroblastoma: Prognostic significance of regional lymph node metastases. J Pediatr 1983;102:59–62.
141. Sawada T, Kidowaki T, Sakamoto I, et al. Neuroblastoma. Mass screening for early detection and its prognosis. Cancer 1984;53:2731–5.
142. Kaneko Y, Kanda N, Maseki N, et al. Current urinary mass screening for catecholamine metabolites at 6 months of age may be detecting only a small portion of high-risk neuroblastomas: A chromosome and N-myc amplification study. J Clin Oncol 1990;8:2005–13.
143. Bessho F, Hashizume K, Nakajo T, et al. Mass screening in Japan increased the detection of infants with neuroblastoma without a decrease in cases in older children. J Pediatr 1991;119:237–41.
144. Woods WG, Tuchman M, Robison LL, et al. A population-based study of the usefulness of screening for neuroblastoma. Lancet 1996;348:1682–7.
145. Woods WG, Tuchman M, Robison LL, et al. Screening for neuroblastoma is ineffective in reducing the incidence of unfavourable advanced stage disease in older children. Eur J Cancer 1997;33:2106–12.
146. Bergeron C, Tafese T, Kerbl R, et al. European Experience with screening for neuroblastoma before the age of 12 months. Med Pediatr Oncol 1998;31:442–9.
147. Parker L, Powell J. Screening for neuroblastoma in infants younger than 1 year of age: Review of the first 30 years. Med Pediatr Oncol 1998;31:455–69.
148. Schilling FH, Spix C, Berthold FE, R., et al. German neuroblastoma mass screening study at 12 months of age: statistical aspects and preliminary results. Med Pediatr Oncol 1998;31:435–41.
149. Erttmann R, Tafese T, Berthold F, et al. 10 years' neuroblastoma screening in Europe: preliminary results of a clinical and biological review from the Study Group for Evaluation of Neuroblastoma Screening in Europe (SENSE). Eur J Cancer 1998;34:1391–7.
150. Woods WG, Gao RN, Shuster JJ, et al. Screening of infants and mortality due to neuroblastoma. N Engl J Med 2002;346:1041–6.
151. Sawada T, Matsumura T, Kawakatsu H, et al. Long-term effects of mass screening for neuroblastoma in infancy. American Journal of Pediatric Hematology/Oncology 1991;13:3–7.
152. Nakagawara A, Zaizen Y, Ikeda K, et al. Different genomic and metabolic patterns between mass screening-positive and mass screening-negative later-presenting neuroblastomas. Cancer 1991;68:2037–44.
153. Hayashi Y, Hanada R, Yamamoto K. Biology of neuroblastomas in Japan found by screening. American Journal of Pediatric Hematology/Oncology 1992;14:342–7.
154. Brodeur GM, Ambros PF, Favrot MC. Biological aspects of neuroblastoma screening. Med Pediatr Oncol 1998;31:394–400.
155. Nishi M, Miyake H, Takeda T, et al. Mass screening for neuroblastoma targeting children age 14 months in Sapporo City: A preliminary report. Cancer 1998;82:1973–7.
156. Schilling FH, Spix C, Berthold F, et al. Neuroblastoma screening at one year of age. N Engl J Med 2002;346:1047–53.
157. Jereb B, Bretsky SS, Vogel R, et al. Age and prognosis in neuroblastoma. Review of 112 patients younger than 2 years. Am J Pediatr Hematol Oncol 1984;6:233–243.
158. Cheung NK, Heller G, Kushner BH, et al. Stage IV neuroblastoma more than 1 year of age at diagnosis: Major response to chemotherapy and survival durations correlated strongly with dose intensity. Prog Clin Biol Res 1991;366:567–73.
159. Matthay KK, Perez C, Seeger RC, et al. Successful treatment of stage III neuroblastoma based on prospective biologic staging: a Children's Cancer Group study. J Clin Oncol 1998;16:1256–64.
160. West DC, Shamberger RC, Macklis RM, et al. Stage III neuroblastoma over 1 year of age at diagnosis: improved survival with intensive multimodality therapy including multiple alkylating agents. J Clin Oncol 1993;11:84–90.
161. Ikeda H, Iehara T, Tsuchida Y, et al. Experience with International Neuroblastoma Staging System and Pathology Classification. Br J Cancer 2002;86:1110–6.
162. Castel V, Garcia-Miguel P, Canete A, et al. Prospective evaluation of the International Neuroblastoma Staging System (INSS) and the International Neuroblastoma Response Criteria (INRC) in a multicentre setting. Eur J Cancer 1999;35:606–11.
163. Laug WE, Siegel SE, Shaw KN, et al. Initial urinary catecholamine metabolite concentrations and prognosis in neuroblastoma. Pediatrics 1978;62:77–83.
164. Nishi M, Miyake H, Takeda T, et al. The relationship between homovanillic/vanillylmandelic acid ratios and prognosis in neuroblastoma. Oncol Rep 1998;5:631–3.
165. Hann HW, Evans AE, Siegel SE, et al. Prognostic importance of serum ferritin in patients with Stages III and IV neuroblastoma: the Children's Cancer Study Group experience. Cancer Res 1985;45:2843–8.
166. Zeltzer PM, Marangos PJ, Evans AE, et al. Serum neuron-specific enolase in children with neuroblastoma. Relationship to stage and disease course. Cancer 1986;57:1230–4.
167. Shuster JJ, McWilliams NB, Castleberry R, et al. Serum lactate dehydrogenase in childhood neuroblastoma. A Pediatric Oncology Group recursive partitioning study. American J Clin Oncol 1992;15:295–303.
168. Ladisch S, Wu ZL. Detection of a tumour-associated ganglioside in plasma of patients with neuroblastoma. Lancet 1985;1:136–8.
169. Schulz G, Cheresh DA, Varki NM, et al. Detection of ganglioside GD2 in tumor tissues and sera of neuroblastoma patients. Cancer Res 1984;44:5914–20.
170. Maris JM. The biologic basis for neuroblastoma heterogeneity and risk stratification. Curr Opin Pediatr 2005;17:7–13.
171. Smith EI, Castleberry RP. Neuroblastoma. In: Wells SA, Jr., editor. Current problems in pediatric surgery. St. Louis: C. V. Mosby; 1990. p. 577–620.
172. Nishihira H, Toyoda Y, Tanaka Y, et al. Natural course of neuroblastoma detected by mass screening: s 5-year prospective study at a single institution. J Clin Oncol 2000;18(:3012–7.
173. La Quaglia MP, Kushner BH, Su W, et al. The impact of gross total resection on local control and survival in high-risk neuroblastoma. J Pediatr Surg 2004;39:412–7; discussion 412–7.
174. Chamberlain RS, Quinones R, Dinndorf P, et al. Complete surgical resection combined with aggressive adjuvant chemotherapy and bone marrow transplantation prolongs survival in children with advanced neuroblastoma. Ann Surg Oncol 1995;2:93–100.
175. Adkins ES, Sawin R, Gerbing RB, et al. Efficacy of complete resection for high-risk neuroblastoma: a Children's Cancer Group study. J Pediatr Surg 2004;39:931–6.
176. von Allmen D, Grupp S, Diller L, et al. Aggressive surgical therapy and radiotherapy for patients with high-risk neuroblastoma treated with rapid sequence tandem transplant. J Pediatr Surg 2005;40:936–41; discussion 941.
177. Halperin E. Neuroblastoma. In: Halperin E, Kun L, Constine L, Tarbell N, editors. Pediatric radiation oncology. New York: Raven Press; 1989. p. 134.
178. Jacobson GM, Sause WT, O'Brien RT. Dose response analysis of pediatric neuroblastoma to megavoltage radiation. Am J Clin Oncol 1984;7:693–7.
179. Halperin EC, Cox EB. Radiation therapy in the management of neuroblastoma. The Duke University Medical Center Experience 1967–1984. Int J Radiat Oncol Biol Phys 1986;12:1829.
180. Haas-Kogan DA, Swift PS, Selch M, et al. Impact of radiotherapy for high-risk neuroblastoma: a Children's Cancer Group study. Int J Radiat Oncol Biol Phys 2003;56(1):28–39.
181. Hoefnagel CA, De Kraker J, Valdes Olmos RA, et al. [^{131}I]MIBG as a first line treatment in advanced neuroblastoma. Q J Nucl Med 1995;39(4 Suppl 1):61–4.
182. Mastrangelo R, Tornesello A, Riccardi R, et al. A new approach in the treatment of stage IV neuroblastoma using a combination of [^{131}I]meta-iodobenzylguanidine (MIBG) and cisplatin. Eur J Cancer 1995;31A(4):606–11.
183. Matthay KK, DeSantes K, Hasegawa B, et al. Phase I dose escalation of ^{131}I-metaiodobenzylguanidine with autologous bone marrow support in refractory neuroblastoma. J Clin Oncol 1998;16:229–36.
184. Kang TI, Brophy P, Hickeson M, et al. Targeted radiotherapy with submyeloablative doses of 131I-MIBG is effective for disease palliation in highly refractory neuroblastoma. J Pediatr Hematol Oncol 2003;25:769–73.
185. DuBois SG, Messina J, Maris JM, et al. Hematologic toxicity of high-dose iodine-131-metaiodobenzylguanidine therapy for advanced neuroblastoma. J Clin Oncol 2004;22:2452–60.
186. Howard JP, Maris JM, Kersun LS, et al. Tumor response and toxicity with multiple infusions of high dose (131)I-MIBG for refractory neuroblastoma. Pediatr Blood Cancer 2005;44:232–9.
187. Carli M, Green AA, Hayes FA, et al. Therapeutic efficacy of single drugs for childhood neuroblastoma: A review. In: Raybaud C, Clement R, Lebreuil G, et al, editors. Pediatric oncology. Amsterdam,: Excerpta Medica; 1982. p. 141–50.
188. Starling KA, Sutow WW, Donaldson MH, et al. Drug Trials in neuroblastoma: cyclophosphamide (NSC-26271) alone; vincristine (NSC-67574) plus cyclophosphamide; 6-mercaptopurine (NSC-755) plus 6-methylmercaptopurine riboside (NSC-40774); and cytosine arabinoside (NSC-63878) alone. Cancer Chemotherapy Reports 1974;58:683–8.
189. Thurman WG, Fernbach DJ, Sullivan MP, et al. Cyclophosphamide therapy in childhood neuroblastoma. N Engl J Med 1964;270:1336–40.
190. Kontras SB, Newton WA. Cyclophosphamide (Cytoxan) therapy of childhood neuroblastoma: preliminary report. Cancer Chemotherapy Reports 1961;12:39–50.
191. Green AA, Hayes FA, Pratt CB, et al. Phase II evaluation of cisplatin in children with neuroblastoma and other malignant solid tumors. In: Prestyko AW, Crooke ST, Carter SK, editors. Cisplatin: current status and new developments. New York: Academic Press; 1980. p. 477–84.
192. Evans AE, Baehner RL, Chard RL, et al. Comparison of Daunorubicin (NSC-83142) with Adriamycin (NSC-123127 in the treatment of late-stage childhood solid tumors. Cancer Chemotherapy Reports 1974;58:671–6.
193. Pratt CB, Shanks EC. Doxorubicin in treatment of malignant solid tumors in children. American Journal of Diseases in Childhood 1974;127:534–7.
194. Bleyer WA, Krivit W, Chard RL, et al. Phase II study of VM-26 in acute leukemia, neuroblastoma, and other refractory childhood malignancies; a report from the Children's Cancer Study Group. Cancer Treatment Reports 1979;63:977–81.
195. Rivera G, Green A, Hayes A, et al. Epipodophyllotoxin VM-26 in the treatment of childhood neuroblastoma. Cancer Treatment Reports 1977;61:1243–8.
196. Windmiller J, Berry DH, Haddy TB, et al. Vincristine sulfate in the treatment of neuroblastoma in children. American Journal of Diseases in Childhood 1966;3:75–8.

197. Sullivan MP, Nora AH, Kulapongs P, et al. Evaluation of vincristine sulfate and cyclophosphamide chemotherapy for metastatic neuroblastoma. Pediatrics 1969;44:685–94.
198. Sutow WV, Fernbach DJ, Thurman WG, et al. Daunomycin (NSC-82151) in the treatment of metastatic neuroblastoma. Cancer Chemotherapy Reports 1970;54:283–9.
199. Wagner LM, Crews KR, Iacono LC, et al. Phase I trial of temozolomide and protracted irinotecan in pediatric patients with refractory solid tumors. Clin Cancer Res 2004;10:840–8.
200. Vassal G, Doz F, Frappaz D, et al. A phase I study of irinotecan as a 3-week schedule in children with refractory or recurrent solid tumors. J Clin Oncol 2003;21:3844–52.
201. Saylors RL, 3rd, Stine KC, Sullivan J, et al. Cyclophosphamide plus topotecan in children with recurrent or refractory solid tumors: a Pediatric Oncology Group phase II study. J Clin Oncol 2001;19:3463–9.
202. Matthay KK, Sather HN, Seeger RC, et al. Excellent outcome of stage II neuroblastoma is independent of residual disease and radiation therapy. J Clin Oncol 1989;7:236–44.
203. Kushner BH, Cheung NK, LaQuaglia MP, et al. International neuroblastoma staging system stage 1 neuroblastoma: a prospective study and literature review. J Clin Oncol 1996;14:2174–80.
204. Evans AE, Silber JH, Shpilsky A, et al. Successful management of low-stage neuroblastoma without adjuvant therapies: a comparison of two decades, 1972 through 1981 and 1982 through 1992, in a single institution. J Clin Oncol 1996;14:2504–10.
205. Perez CA, Matthay KK, Atkinson JB, et al. Biologic variables in the outcome of stages I and II neuroblastoma treated with surgery as primary therapy: a children's cancer group study. J Clin Oncol 2000;18:18–26.
206. Evans AE, Chatten J, D'Angio GJ, et al. A review of 17 IV-S neuroblastoma patients at the children's hospital of Philadelphia. Cancer 1980;45:833–839.
207. Evans AE, Baum E, Chard R. Do infants with stage IV-S neuroblastoma need treatment? Archives of Diseases in Childhood 1981;56:271–274.
208. McWilliams NB. Stage IV-S neuroblastoma: treatment controversy revisited. Med Pediatr Oncol 1986;14:41–4.
209. Mancini AF, Rosito P, Vitelli A, et al. IV-S neuroblastoma: a cooperative study of 30 children. Med Pediatr Oncol 1984;12:155–61.
210. Suarez A, Hartmann O, Vassal G, et al. Treatment of stage IV-S neuroblastoma: a study of 34 cases treated between 1982 and 1987. Med Pediatr Oncol 1991;19:473–7.
211. Martinez DA, King DR, Ginn-Pease ME, et al. Resection of the primary tumor is appropriate for children with stage IV-S neuroblastoma: An analysis of 37 patients. J Pediatr Surg 1992;27:1016–20.
212. Strother D, Shuster JJ, McWilliams N, et al. Results of pediatric oncology group protocol 8104 for infants with stages D and DS neuroblastoma. Journal of Pediatric Hematology and Oncology 1995;17(3):254–259.
213. Hsu LL, Evans AE, D'Angio GJ. Hepatomegaly in neuroblastoma stage 4s: criteria for treatment of the vulnerable neonate. Med Pediatr Oncol 1996;27:521–8.
214. Nickerson HJ, Matthay KK, Seeger RC, et al. Favorable biology and outcome of stage IV-S neuroblastoma with supportive care or minimal therapy: a Children's Cancer Group study. J Clin Oncol 2000;18:477–86.
215. De Bernardi B, Pianca C, Pistamiglio P, et al. Neuroblastoma with symptomatic spinal cord compression at diagnosis: treatment and results with 76 cases. J Clin Oncol 2001;19:183–90.
216. Katzenstein HM, Kent PM, London WB, et al. Treatment and outcome of 83 children with intraspinal neuroblastoma: the Pediatric Oncology Group experience. J Clin Oncol 2001;19:1047–55.
217. Hoover M, Bowman LC, Crawford SE, et al. Long-term outcome of patients with intraspinal neuroblastoma. Med Pediatr Oncol 1999;32:353–9.
218. Plantaz D, Rubie H, Michon J, et al. The treatment of neuroblastoma with intraspinal extension with chemotherapy followed by surgical removal of residual disease. A prospective study of 42 patients—results of the NBL 90 Study of the French Society of Pediatric Oncology. Cancer 1996;78:311–9.
219. Castleberry RP, Kun L, Shuster JJ, et al. Radiotherapy improves the outlook for children older than one year with POG stage C neuroblastoma. J Clin Oncol 1991;9:789–95.
220. de Bernardi B, Rogers D, Carli M, et al. Localized neuroblastoma. Surgical and pathologic staging. Cancer 1987;60:1066–72.
221. Schmidt ML, Lukens JN, Seeger RC, et al. Biologic factors determine prognosis in infants with stage IV neuroblastoma: A prospective Children's Cancer Group study. J Clin Oncol 2000;18:1260–8.
222. Bernard JL, Philip T, Zucker JM, et al. Sequential cisplatin/VM26 and vincristine/cyclophosphamide/doxorubicin in metastatic neuroblastoma; an effective alternating non-cross resistant regimen? J Clin Oncol 1987;5:1952–9.
223. Jaffe N. Neuroblastoma: review of the literature and an examination of factors contributing to its enigmatic character. Cancer Treatment Reviews 1976;3:61–82.
224. Finklestein JZ, Klemperer MR, Evans A, et al. Multiagent chemotherapy for children with metastatic neuroblastoma; a Report from Children's Cancer Study Group. Med Pediatr Oncol 1979;6:179–188.
225. Berthold F, Treuner J, Brandeis WE, et al. Neuroblastoma study NBL-79 of the German Society for Pediatric Oncology; report after 2 years. 1982;194:262–9.
226. Nitschke R, Cangir A, Crist W, et al. Intensive chemotherapy for metastatic neuroblastoma: A Southwest Oncology Group study. Med Pediatr Oncol 1980;8:281–8.
227. Bernard JL, Hartmann O, Zucker JM, et al. Alternating induction chemotherapy with cyclophosphamide - Adriamycin - vincristine (CAD) and high dose cisplatin - etoposide (CVP) for children with metastatic neuroblastoma (NB) over 1 year of age. Preliminary results of the French Cooperative NB87 Protocol [abstract]. Med Pediatr Oncol 1990;18:385.
228. Meadows AT, Tsunematsu Y. Late effects of treatment for neuroblastoma. In: Brodeur GM, Sawada T, Tsuchida Y, Voute PA, editors. Neuroblastoma. Amsterdam: Elsevier Science B.V.; 2000. p. 561–70.
229. Helson L, Helson C, Peterson RF, et al. A rationale for the treatment of metastatic neuroblastoma. J Natl Cancer Inst 1976;57:727–9.
230. Cheung NV, Heller G. Chemotherapy dose intensity correlates strongly with response, median survival, and median progression-free survival in metastatic neuroblastoma [see comments]. J Clin Oncol 1991;9:1050–8.
231. Kushner BH, LaQuaglia MP, Bonilla MA, et al. Highly effective induction therapy for stage 4 neuroblastoma in children over 1 year of age. J Clin Oncol 1994;12:2607–13.
232. Valteau-Couanet D, Michon J, Boneu A, et al. Results of induction chemotherapy in children older than 1 year with a stage 4 neuroblastoma treated with the NB 97 French Society of Pediatric Oncology (SFOP) protocol. J Clin Oncol 2005;23:532–40.
233. Philip T, Zucker JM, Bernard JL, et al. Improved survival at 2 and 5 years in the LMCE1 unselected group of 72 children with stage IV neuroblastoma older than 1 year of age at diagnosis: is cure possible in a small subgroup? J Clin Oncol 1991;9:1037–44.
234. Saarinen UM, Wikstrom S, Makipernaa A, et al. In vivo purging of bone marrow in children with poor-risk neuroblastoma for marrow collection and autologous bone marrow transplantation. J Clin Oncol 1996;14:2791–802.
235. Ladenstein R, Philip T, Lasset C, et al. Multivariate analysis of risk factors in stage 4 neuroblastoma patients over the age of one year treated with megatherapy and stem-cell transplantation: a report from the European Bone Marrow Transplantation Solid Tumor Registry. J Clin Oncol 1998;16:953–65.
236. Hartmann O, Berthold F. Treatment of advanced neuroblastoma: the European experience. In: Brodeur GM, Sawada T, Tsuchida Y, Voute PA, editors. Neuroblastoma. Amsterdam: Elsevier Science B.V.; 2000. p. 437–52.
237. Hartmann O, Valteau-Couanet D, Vassal G, et al. Prognostic factors in metastatic neuroblastoma in patients over 1 year of age treated with high-dose chemotherapy and stem cell transplantation: a multivariate analysis in 218 patients treated in a single institution. Bone Marrow Transplant 1999;23:789–95.
238. Matthay KK, Castleberry RP. Treatment of advanced neuroblastoma: the U.S. experience. In: Brodeur GM, Sawada T, Tsuchida Y, Voute PA, editors. Neuroblastoma. Amsterdam: Elsevier Science B.V.; 2000. p. 417–36.
239. Pritchard J, McElwain TJ, Graham-Pole J. High dose melphalan with autologous marrow for treatment of advanced neuroblastoma. Br J Cancer 1982;45:86–94.
240. August CS, Serota FT, Koch PA, et al. Treatment of advanced neuroblastoma with supralethal chemotherapy, radiation and allogeneic or autologous marrow reconstitution. J Clin Oncol 1984;2:609–616.
241. Hartmann O, Kalifa C, Benhamou E, et al. Treatment of advanced neuroblastoma with high-dose melphalan and autologous bone marrow transplantation. Cancer Chemotherapy and Pharmacology 1986;16:165–9.
242. Dini G, Lanino E, Garaventa A, et al. Myeloablative therapy and unpurged autologous bone marrow transplantation for poor-prognosis neuroblastoma: report of 34 cases. J Clin Oncol 1991;9:962–9.
243. Philip T, Ladenstein R, Zucker JM, et al. Double megatherapy and autologous bone marrow transplantation for advanced neuroblastoma: the LMCE2 study. Br J Cancer 1993;67:119–27.
244. Ladenstein R, Lasset C, Hartmann O, et al. Comparison of auto versus allografting as consolidation of primary treatments in advanced neuroblastoma over one year of age at diagnosis. Report from the European Group for Bone Marrow Transplantation. Bone Marrow Transplantation 1994;14:37–46.
245. Matthay KK, Seeger RC, Reynolds CP, et al. Allogeneic versus autologous purged bone marrow transplantation for neuroblastoma: a report from the Children's Cancer Group. J Clin Oncol 1994;12:2382–9.
246. Evans AE, August CS, Kamani N, et al. Bone marrow transplantation for high risk neuroblastoma at the Children's Hospital of Philadelphia: an update. Med Pediatr Oncol 1994;23:323–7.
247. Ohnuma N, Takahashi H, Kaneko M, et al. Treatment combined with bone marrow transplantation for advanced neuroblastoma: an analysis of patients who were pretreated intensively with the protocol of the Study Group of Japan. Med Pediatr Oncol 1995;24:181–7.
248. Shuster JJ. The role of autologous bone marrow transplantation in advanced neuroblastoma. J Clin Oncol 1996;14:2413–4.
249. Stram DO, Matthay KK, O'Leary M, et al. Consolidation chemoradiotherapy and autologous bone marrow transplantation versus continued chemotherapy for metastatic neuroblastoma: a report of two concurrent Children's Cancer Group studies. J Clin Oncol 1996;14:2417–26.
250. Garaventa A, Rondelli R, Lanino E, et al. Myeloablative therapy and bone marrow rescue in advanced neuroblastoma. Report from the Italian Bone Marrow Transplant Registry. Italian Association of Pediatric Hematology-Oncology, BMT Group. Bone Marrow Transplant 1996;18:125–30.
251. Cohn SL, Moss TJ, Hoover M, et al. Treatment of poor-risk neuroblastoma patients with high-dose chemotherapy and autologous peripheral stem cell rescue. Bone Marrow Transplant 1997;20:543–51.
252. Kletzel M, Abella EM, Sandler ES, et al. Thiotepa and cyclophosphamide with stem cell rescue for consolidation therapy for children with high-risk neuroblastoma: a phase I/II study of the Pediatric Blood and Marrow Transplant Consortium. Journal of Pediatric Hematology-Oncology 1998;20:49–54.
253. Grupp SA, Stern JW, Bunin N, et al. Tandem high-dose therapy in rapid sequence for children with high-risk neuroblastoma. J Clin Oncol 2000;18:2567–75.
254. Kletzel M, Katzenstein HM, Haut PR, et al. Treatment of high-risk neuroblastoma with triple-tandem high-dose therapy and stem-cell rescue: results of the Chicago Pilot II Study. J Clin Oncol 2002;20:2284–92.
255. Matthay KK, Villablanca JG, Seeger RC, et al. Treatment of high-risk neuroblastoma with intensive chemotherapy, radiotherapy, autologous bone marrow transplantation, and 13-cis-retinoic acid. Children's Cancer Group. N Engl J Med 1999;341:1165–73.
256. Kletzel M, Longino R, Rademaker AW, et al. Peripheral blood stem cell transplantation in young children: experience with harvesting, mobilization and engraftment. Pediatric Transplantation 1998;2:191–6.
257. Reynolds CP, Seeger RC, Vo DD, et al. Model system for removing neuroblastoma cells from bone marrow using monoclonal antibodies and magnetic immunobeads. Cancer Res 1986;46:5882–6.
258. Berthold F, Schumacher R, Schneider A, et al. Removal of neuroblastoma cells from bone marrow by a direct monoclonal antibody rosetting technique. Bone Marrow Transplant 1989;4:273–8.
259. Gee A, Moss T, Mansour V, et al. Large-scale immunomagnetic separation system for the removal of tumor cells from bone marrow. Prog Clin Biol Res 1992;377:181–7.
260. Canals C, Punti C, Picon M, et al. Immunomagnetic purging in autologous bone marrow transplantation: experience in fourteen patients. Prog Clin Biol Res 1992;377:289–96.
261. Philip T, Zucker JM, Bernard JL, et al. Bone marrow transplantation in an unselected group of 65 patients with stage IV neuroblastoma. In: Dicke KA, Spitzer G, Jagannath S, editors. Autologous bone marrow transplantation III. Houston: Univ. of Texas; 1987. p. 407.

262. Sidell N. Retinoic acid-induced growth inhibition and morphologic differentiation of human neuroblastoma cells in vitro. J Natl Cancer Inst 1982;68:589–96.
263. Garaventa A, Luksch R, Lo Piccolo MS, et al. Phase I trial and pharmacokinetics of fenretinide in children with neuroblastoma. Clin Cancer Res 2003;9:2032–9.
264. Cheung NK, Landmeier B, Neely J, et al. Complete tumor ablation with iodine 131-radiolabeled disialoganglioside GD2-specific monoclonal antibody against human neuroblastoma xenografted in nude mice. J Natl Cancer Inst 1986;77:739–45.
265. Lode HN, Moehler T, Xiang R, et al. Synergy between an antiangiogenic integrin alphav antagonist and an antibody-cytokine fusion protein eradicates spontaneous tumor metastases. Proceedings of the National Academy of Sciences of the United States of America 1999;96:1591–6.
266. Kushner BH, Cheung NK. GM-CSF enhances 3F8 monoclonal antibody-dependent cellular cytotoxicity against human melanoma and neuroblastoma. Blood 1989;73(7):1936–41.
267. Barker E, Mueller BM, Handgretinger R, et al. Effect of a chimeric anti-ganglioside GD2 antibody on cell-mediated lysis of human neuroblastoma cells. Cancer Res 1991;51:144–9.
268. Uttenreuther-Fischer MM, Huang CS, Reisfeld RA, et al. Pharmacokinetics of anti-ganglioside GD2 mAb 14G2a in a phase I trial in pediatric cancer patients. Cancer Immunology & Immunotherapy 1995;41:29–36.
269. Uttenreuther-Fischer MM, Huang CS, Yu AL. Pharmacokinetics of human-mouse chimeric anti-GD2 mAb ch14.18 in a phase I trial in neuroblastoma patients. Cancer Immunology & Immunotherapy 1995;41:331–8.
270. Yu AL, Uttenreuther-Fischer MM, Huang CS, et al. Phase I trial of a human-mouse chimeric anti-disialoganglioside monoclonal antibody ch14.18 in patients with refractory neuroblastoma and osteosarcoma. J Clin Oncol 1998;16:2169–80.
271. Frost JD, Hank JA, Reaman GH, et al. A phase I/IB trial of murine monoclonal anti-GD2 antibody 14.G2a plus interleukin-2 in children with refractory neuroblastoma: a report of the Children's Cancer Group. Cancer 1997;80:317–33.
272. Handgretinger R, Baader P, Dopfer R, et al. A phase I study of neuroblastoma with the anti-ganglioside GD2 antibody 14.G2a. Cancer Immunol Immunother 1992;35:199–204.
273. Cheung NK, Lazarus H, Miraldi FD, et al. Ganglioside GD2 specific monoclonal antibody 3F8: a phase I study in patients with neuroblastoma and malignant melanoma [see comments]. J Clin Oncol 1987;5:1430–40.
274. Cheung NK, Kushner BH, Yeh SDJ, et al. 3F8 monoclonal antibody treatment of patients with stage 4 neuroblastoma: a phase II study. Int J Oncol 1998;12:1299–306.
275. Yu AL, Batova A, Alvarada C, et al. Usefulness of a chemeric anti-GD2 (ch 14.18) and GM-CSF for refractory neuroblastoma: a POG Phase II study. Proceedings of the American Society of Clinical Oncology 1997;16:513a.
276. Cheung NK, Von Hoff DD, Strandjord SE, et al. Detection of neuroblastoma cells in bone marrow using GD2 specific monoclonal antibodies. J Clin Oncol 1986;4:363–9.
277. Murray JL, Cunningham JE, Brewer H, et al. Phase I trial of murine monoclonal antibody 14G2a administered by prolonged intravenous infusion in patients with neuroectodermal tumors. J Clin Oncol 1994;12:184–93.
278. Cheung NK, Kushner BH, Cheung IY, et al. Anti-G(D2) antibody treatment of minimal residual stage 4 neuroblastoma diagnosed at more than 1 year of age. J Clin Oncol 1998;16:3053–60.
279. Simon T, Hero B, Faldum A, et al. Consolidation treatment with chimeric anti-GD2-antibody ch14.18 in children older than 1 year with metastatic neuroblastoma. J Clin Oncol 2004;22:3549–57.
280. Hank JA, Surfus J, Gan J, et al. Treatment of neuroblastoma patients with antiganglioside GD2 antibody plus interleukin-2 induces antibody-dependent cellular cytotoxicity against neuroblastoma detected in vitro. Journal of Immunotherapy 1994;15:29–37.
281. Yoshida H, Tanabe M, Miyauchi M, et al. Induced immunity by expression of interleukin-2 or GM-CSF gene in murine neuroblastoma cells can generate antitumor response to established tumors. Cancer Gene Therapy 1999;6(5):395–401.
282. Bowman LC, Grossmann M, Rill D, et al. Interleukin-2 gene-modified allogeneic tumor cells for treatment of relapsed neuroblastoma. Human Gene Therapy 1998;9:1303–11.
283. Parsons SK, Neault MW, Lehmann LE, et al. Severe ototoxicity following carboplatin-containing conditioning regimen for autologous marrow transplantation for neuroblastoma. Bone Marrow Transplant 1998;22:669–74.
284. Kushner BH, Cheung NK, Kramer K, et al. Neuroblastoma and treatment-related myelodysplasia/leukemia: the Memorial Sloan-Kettering experience and a literature review. J Clin Oncol 1998;16:3880–9.
285. Saylors RL, 3rd, Stine KC, Sullivan J, et al. Cyclophosphamide plus topotecan in children with recurrent or refractory solid tumors: a Pediatric Oncology Group phase II study. J Clin Oncol 2001;19:3463–9.
286. Langler A, Christaras A, Abshagen K, et al. Topotecan in the treatment of refractory neuroblastoma and other malignant tumors in childhood—a phase-II-study. Klin Padiatr 2002;214:153–6.
287. Frantz CN, London WB, Diller L, et al. Recurrent neuroblastoma: Randomized treatment with topotecan + cyclophosphamide (T+C) vs. topotecan alone(T). A POG/CCG Intergroup Study. Journal of Clinical Oncology, 2004 ASCO Annual Meeting Proceedings 2004;22(14S):8512.
288. Alimonti A, Satta F, Pavese I, et al. Prevention of irinotecan plus 5-fluorouracil/leucovorin-induced diarrhoea by oral administration of neomycin plus bacitracin in first-line treatment of advanced colorectal cancer. Ann Oncol 2003;14:805–6.
289. Rodriguez-Galindo C, Crews KR, Stewart CF, et al. Phase I study of the combination of topotecan and irinotecan in children with refractory solid tumors. Cancer Chemother Pharmacol 2005:1–10.
290. Cho SY, Adamson PC, Hagey AE, et al. Phase I trial and pharmacokinetic (PK) study of ABT-751, an orally bioavailable tubulin binding agent, in pediatric patients with refractory solid tumors. Proc Annu Meet Am Soc Clin Oncol 2004;22(Suppl 14):2080.
291. Tepmongkol S, Heyman S. ^{131}I MIBG therapy in neuroblastoma: mechanisms, rationale, and current status. Med Pediatr Oncol 1999;32:427–31; discussion 432.
292. Garaventa A, Bellagamba O, Lo Piccolo MS, et al. ^{131}I-metaiodobenzylguanidine (^{131}I-MIBG) therapy for residual neuroblastoma: a mono-institutional experience with 43 patients. Br J Cancer 1999;81:1378–84.
293. Wiseman GA, Kvols LK. Therapy of neuroendocrine tumors with radiolabeled MIBG and somatostatin analogues. Semin Nucl Med 1995;25:272–8.
294. O'Dorisio MS, Hauger M, Cecalupo AJ. Somatostatin receptors in neuroblastoma: diagnostic and therapeutic implications. Semin Oncol 1994;21(5 Suppl 13):33–7.
295. Borgstrom P, Hassan M, Wassberg E, et al. The somatostatin analogue octreotide inhibits neuroblastoma growth in vivo. Pediatr Res 1999;46:328–32.
296. Kushner BH, Kramer K, Cheung NK. Phase II trial of the anti-GD2 monoclonal antibody 3F8 and granulocyte-macrophage colony-stimulating factor for neuroblastoma. J Clin Oncol 2001;19:4189–94.
297. Yanik GA, Levine JE, Matthay KK, et al. Pilot study of iodine-131-metaiodobenzylguanidine in combination with myeloablative chemotherapy and autologous stem-cell support for the treatment of neuroblastoma. J Clin Oncol 2002;20:2142–9.
298. Cooper R, Khakoo Y, Matthay KK, et al. Opsoclonus-myoclonus-ataxia syndrome in neuroblastoma: histopathologic features-a report from the Children's Cancer Group. Med Pediatr Oncol 2001;36:623–9.
299. Neal ZC, Yang JC, Rakhmilevich AL, et al. Enhanced activity of hu14.18-IL2 immunocytokine against murine NXS2 neuroblastoma when combined with interleukin 2 therapy. Clin Cancer Res 2004;10:4839–47.
300. King DM, Albertini MR, Schalch H, et al. Phase I clinical trial of the immunocytokine EMD 273063 in melanoma patients. J Clin Oncol 2004;22:4463–73.
301. Bolesta E, Kowalczyk A, Wierzbicki A, et al. DNA vaccine expressing the mimotope of GD2 ganglioside induces protective GD2 cross-reactive antibody responses. Cancer Res 2005;65:3410–8.
302. Rousseau RF, Haight AE, Hirschmann-Jax C, et al. Local and systemic effects of an allogeneic tumor cell vaccine combining transgenic human lymphotactin with interleukin-2 in patients with advanced or refractory neuroblastoma. Blood 2003;101:1718–26.
303. Yu A, Batova A, Strother D, et al. Promising results of a pilot trial of a GD2 directed anti-idiotypic antibody as a vaccine for high risk neuroblastoma. In: Advances in neuroblastoma research; 2004; Genoa, Italy; 2004. p. 75.
304. Gonzalez S, Naranjo A, Serrano LM, et al. Genetic engineering of cytolytic T lymphocytes for adoptive T-cell therapy of neuroblastoma. J Gene Med 2004;6:704–11.
305. Maurer BJ, Melton L, Billups C, et al. Synergistic cytotoxicity in solid tumor cell lines between N-(4-hydroxyphenyl)retinamide and modulators of ceramide metabolism. J Natl Cancer Inst 2000;92:1897–909.
306. Maurer BJ, Metelitsa LS, Seeger RC, et al. Increase of ceramide and induction of mixed apoptosis/necrosis by N-(4-hydroxyphenyl)- retinamide in neuroblastoma cell lines [see comments]. J Natl Cancer Inst 1999;91:1138–46.
307. Reynolds CP, Matthay KK, Villablanca JG, et al. Retinoid therapy of high-risk neuroblastoma. Cancer Lett 2003;197:185–92.
308. Meitar D, Crawford SE, Rademaker AW, et al. Tumor angiogenesis correlates with metastatic disease, N-Myc amplification, and poor outcome in human neuroblastoma. J Clin Oncol 1996;14:405–14.
309. Eggert A, Ikegaki N, Kwiatkowski J, et al. High-level expression of angiogenic factors is associated with advanced tumor stage in human neuroblastomas. Clin Cancer Res 2000;6:1900–8.
310. Fotsis T, Breit S, Lutz W, et al. Down-regulation of endothelial cell growth inhibitors by enhanced MYCN oncogene expression in human neuroblastoma cells. Eur J Biochem 1999;263:757–64.
311. Huang D, Rutkowski JL, Brodeur GM, et al. Schwann cell-conditioned medium inhibits angiogenesis. Cancer Res 2000;60:5966–71.
312. Chlenski A, Liu S, Crawford SE, et al. SPARC is a key Schwannian-derived inhibitor controlling neuroblastoma tumor angiogenesis. Cancer Res 2002;62:7357–63.
313. Shusterman S, Grupp SA, Barr R, et al. The angiogenesis inhibitor TNP-470 effectively inhibits human neuroblastoma xenograft growth, especially in the setting of subclinical disease. Clin Cancer Res 2001;7:977–84.
314. Shusterman S, Barr R, McMahon G, et al. Targeted inhibition of the VEGF, PDGF, and bFGF signaling pathways can potentiate the antiangiogenic effect of low-dose chemotherapy in human neuroblastoma xenografts. [Submitted]
315. Morowitz MJ, Barr R, Wang Q, et al. Methionine aminopeptidase 2 inhibition is an effective treatment strategy for neuroblastoma in preclinical models. Clin Cancer Res 2005;11:2680–5.
316. Katzenstein HM, Rademaker AW, Senger C, et al. Effectiveness of the angiogenesis inhibitor TNP-470 in reducing the growth of human neuroblastoma in nude mice inversely correlates with tumor burden. Clin Cancer Res 1999;5:4273–8.
317. Erdreich-Epstein A, Shimada H, Groshen S, et al. Integrins alpha(v)beta3 and alpha(v)beta5 are expressed by endothelium of high-risk neuroblastoma and their inhibition is associated with increased endogenous ceramide. Cancer Res 2000;60:712–21.
318. Evans AE, Kisselbach KD, Liu X, et al. Effect of CEP-751 (KT-6587) on neuroblastoma xenografts expressing TrkB. Med Pediatr Oncol 2001;36:181–4.
319. Evans AE, Kisselbach KD, Yamashiro DJ, et al. The antitumor activity of CEP-751 (KT-6587) on human neuroblastoma and medulloblastoma xenografts. Clin Cancer Res 1999;5:3594–3602.
320. Teitz T, Wei T, Valentine MB, et al. Caspase 8 is deleted or silenced preferentially in childhood neuroblastomas with amplification of MYCN. Nat Med 2000;6:529–35.
321. Coffey DC, Kutko MC, Glick RD, et al. The histone deacetylase inhibitor, CBHA, inhibits growth of human neuroblastoma xenografts in vivo, alone and synergistically with all-trans retinoic acid. Cancer Res 2001;61:3591–4.
322. Jaboin J, Wild J, Hamidi H, et al. MS-27-275, an inhibitor of histone deacetylase, has marked in vitro and in vivo antitumor activity against pediatric solid tumors. Cancer Res 2002;62:6108–15.
323. Segreti JA, Polakowski JS, Koch KA, et al. Tumor selective antivascular effects of the novel antimitotic compound ABT-751: an in vivo rat regional hemodynamic study. Cancer Chemother Pharmacol 2004.
324. Cheung NK, Modak S. Oral (1-->3),(1-->4)-beta-D-glucan synergizes with antiganglioside GD2 monoclonal antibody 3F8 in the therapy of neuroblastoma. Clin Cancer Res 2002;8:1217–23.
325. Yang JC, Haworth L, Sherry RM, et al. A randomized trial of bevacizumab, an anti-vascular endothelial growth factor antibody, for metastatic renal cancer. N Engl J Med 2003;349:427–34.
326. Anderson CP, Reynolds CP. Synergistic cytotoxicity of buthionine sulfoximine (BSO) and intensive melphalan (L-PAM) for neuroblastoma cell lines established at relapse after myeloablative therapy. Bone Marrow Transplant 2002;30:135–40.

327. Galanis E, Buckner JC, Maurer MJ, et al. Phase II Trial of TEM sirolimus (CCI-779) in Recurrent Glioblastoma Multiforme: North Central Cancer Treatment Group. J Clin Oncol 2005.
328. Chan S, Scheulen ME, Johnston S, et al. Phase II study of TEM sirolimus (CCI-779), a novel inhibitor of mTOR, in heavily pretreated patients with locally advanced or metastatic breast cancer. J Clin Oncol 2005.
329. Marks PA, Richon VM, Breslow R, et al. Histone deacetylase inhibitors as new cancer drugs. Curr Opin Oncol 2001;13:477–83.
330. Banerjee D. Genasense (Genta Inc). Curr Opin Investig Drugs 2001;2(4):574-80.
331. Siapati KE, Barker S, Kinnon C, et al. Improved antitumour immunity in murine neuroblastoma using a combination of IL-2 and IL-12. Br J Cancer 2003;88:1641–8.
332. Lode HN, Xiang R, Duncan SR, et al. Tumor-targeted IL-2 amplifies T cell-mediated immune response induced by gene therapy with single-chain IL-12. Proc Natl Acad Sci U S A.. 1999;96:8591–6.
333. Berg SL, Blaney SM, Sullivan J, et al. Phase II trial of pyrazoloacridine in children with solid tumors: a Pediatric Oncology Group phase II study. J Pediatr Hematol Oncol 2000;22:506–9.
334. Keshelava N, Tsao-Wei D, Reynolds CP. Pyrazoloacridine is active in multidrug-resistant neuroblastoma cell lines with nonfunctional p53. Clin Cancer Res 2003;9:3492–502.
335. Reynolds CP, Maurer BJ, Kolesnick RN. Ceramide synthesis and metabolism as a target for cancer therapy. Cancer Lett 2004;206:169–80.
336. Ho R, Minturn JE, Hishiki T, et al. Proliferation of human neuroblastomas mediated by the epidermal growth factor receptor. Cancer Res 2005. [In press]
337. Sohara Y, Shimada H, Scadeng M, et al. Lytic bone lesions in human neuroblastoma xenograft involve osteoclast recruitment and are inhibited by bisphosphonate. Cancer Res 2003;63:3026–31.
338. Beppu K, Jaboine J, Merchant MS, et al. Effect of imatinib mesylate on neuroblastoma tumorigenesis and vascular endothelial growth factor expression. J Natl Cancer Inst 2004;96:46–55.

Soft Tissue Sarcomas of Childhood

William H. Meyer, MD

The soft tissue sarcomas are a heterogeneous group of connective tissue neoplasms that arise in soft tissues throughout the body. These tumors represent 7.4% of cancer cases in children and adolescents ages 0 to 20 years.[1] Traditionally, pediatric oncologists have arbitrarily divided these tumors into two major groups: rhabdomyosarcoma (RMS), uniformly high-grade tumors; and the remaining group that contains many biologically and clinically heterogeneous tumors, together referred to as nonrhabdomyosarcoma soft tissue sarcomas (NRSTS). Surveillance, Epidemiology, and End Results (SEER) data estimate that 850 to 900 new cases of soft tissue sarcomas are diagnosed in children each year in the United States. Rhabdomyosarcoma is the most common soft tissue sarcoma in children ages 0 to 14 years, with an annual incidence of 4.6 cases per million children, representing nearly 50% of soft tissue sarcomas in this age range (Figure 124k-1). The nonrhabdomyosarcoma soft tissue sarcomas include fibrosarcoma, synovial sarcoma, leiomyosarcoma, liposarcoma, and others; each histology is rare in children and adolescents.

RHABDOMYOSARCOMA

Rhabdomyosarcoma is one of the "small round, blue cell tumors" of childhood. It is the third most common extracranial solid tumor occurring in children. Almost two-thirds of RMS cases develop in children under the age of 10 years.[1–5] Since the inception of the pediatric cooperative group process, over 4,000 patients with rhabdomyosarcoma have been enrolled in therapeutic trials in North America, conducted by the Intergroup Rhabdomyosarcoma Study Group (IRSG) and the Children's Oncology Group (COG). These multidisciplinary studies led to successive improvements in outcome for children with RMS. The proportion of patients alive at 5 years after start of therapy has increased: 55% on IRS-I,[2] 63% on IRS-II,[3] 69% on IRS-III, and 73% on IRS-IV protocols.[4,6]

Rhabdomyosarcoma can occur in almost any soft tissue site in the body. The most common primary sites are genitourinary (29%), parameningeal (24%), extremity (15%), retroperitoneal (13%), orbit (8%), other head and neck (7%), and miscellaneous other sites (4%).[7] Most often RMS presents as a mass, however, the presenting signs and symptoms often correspond with the site of primary tumor. Genitourinary tumors may present with hematuria, difficulty voiding or urinary obstruction, and/or a scrotal or vaginal mass, occasionally associated with vaginal bleeding. Parameningeal tumors may present with cranial nerve dysfunction, signs suggestive of sinusitis, ear discharge, headaches, and facial pain. Proptosis or periorbital swelling are common manifestations of orbital tumors. Extremity tumors and those occurring at other sites most often present as a rapidly enlarging, firm mass lesion.

There are no clear predisposing risk factors for the development of RMS in most cases. Although rhabdomyosarcoma has been reported in association with neurofibromatosis type 1,[8,9] Beckwith-Wiedemann syndrome,[10,11] Li-Fraumeni syndrome,[12,13] cardio-facio-cutaneous syndrome,[14] Costello syndrome,[15] Noonan's syndrome,[16,17] a variety of congenital anomalies,[18] and parental use of cocaine and marijuana,[19] the vast majority of cases appear to be sporadic.

Accurate and specific diagnosis of rhabdomyosarcoma is critical for appropriate treatment assignment and analysis of outcome data. Rhabdomyosarcoma must be distinguished from the other small round, blue cell tumors, including neuroblastoma, Ewing's tumor, and lymphoma. The hallmark for diagnosis of RMS is the demonstration of malignant skeletal muscle differentiation. On light microscopy, occasionally cross striations in tumor cells characteristic of skeletal muscle or plump rhabdomyoblasts are noted. Often immunohistochemical staining (eg, myogenin, MyoD, muscle specific actin, myoglobin, and/or desmin) is required for accurate diagnosis.[20] Tumors are classified using the modified International Classification of Rhabdomyosarcoma.[21,22] This system identifies a favorable histologic group comprising the embryonal histology tumors, including the spindle cell and botryoid variants, and an unfavorable group comprising tumors with alveolar histology and undifferentiated sarcoma.

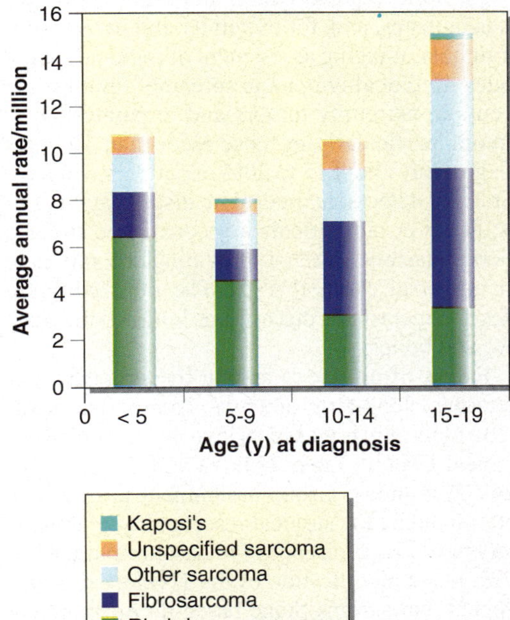

Figure 124k-1 Soft tissue sarcoma age-specific incidence rates by International Classification of Childhood Cancer subcategory, all races, both sexes, SEER, 1975–95.

Embryonal RMS (ERMS) is most common, comprising over half of all RMS cases. ERMS tends to occur in younger children; these tumors typically occur in the orbit, head and neck, and genitourinary system. Histologically, ERMS is characterized by primitive spindle cells, often with more myxoid areas. The botryoid variant often arises in mucosa-lined hollow organs (nasopharynx, vagina, and bladder), presenting as a grape-like protruding mass and characterized histologically by a subepithelial condensation of tumor cells ("cambium layer") (Figure 124k-2). Analysis of histologic subtypes of RMS may have additional prognostic significance.[23] For example, spindle cell RMS histology, accounting for 3% of all RMS, is associated with a superior prognosis (95% 5-yr survival).[21] The prognosis of conventional embryonal RMS is intermediate; this group may include tumors with either favorable or unfavorable features. Although a grading system often used for other soft tissue sarcomas

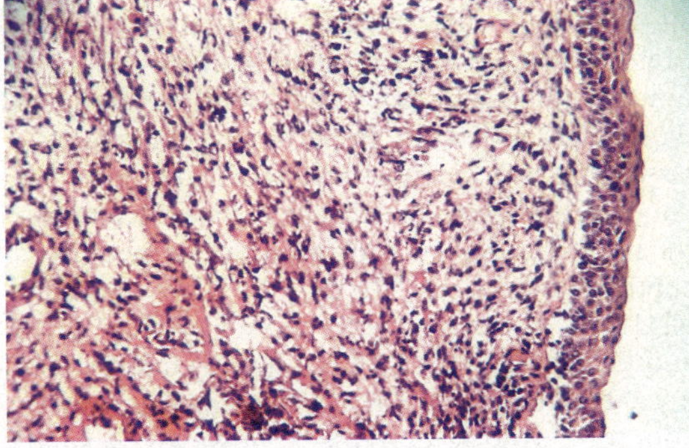

Figure 124k-2 High-power photomicrograph of embryonal rhabdomyosarcoma, botryoid variant, with primitive spindle-shaped cells and the characteristic "cambium" layer of ovoid cells in the submucosal zone.

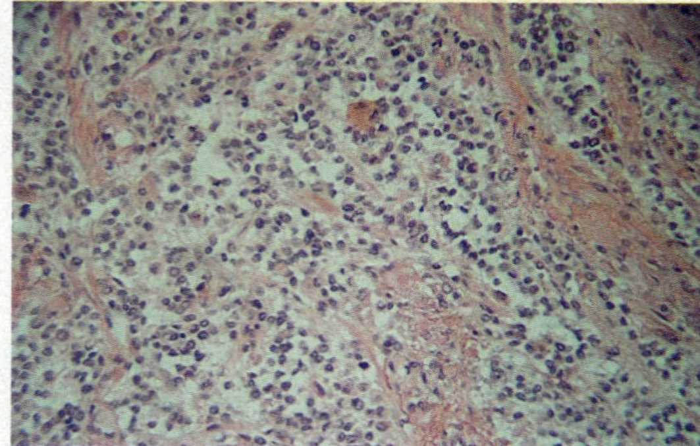

Figure 124k-3 High-power photomicrograph of alveolar rhabdomyosarcoma, with fibrovascular septae, loss of cellular cohesion, and occasional giant cells.

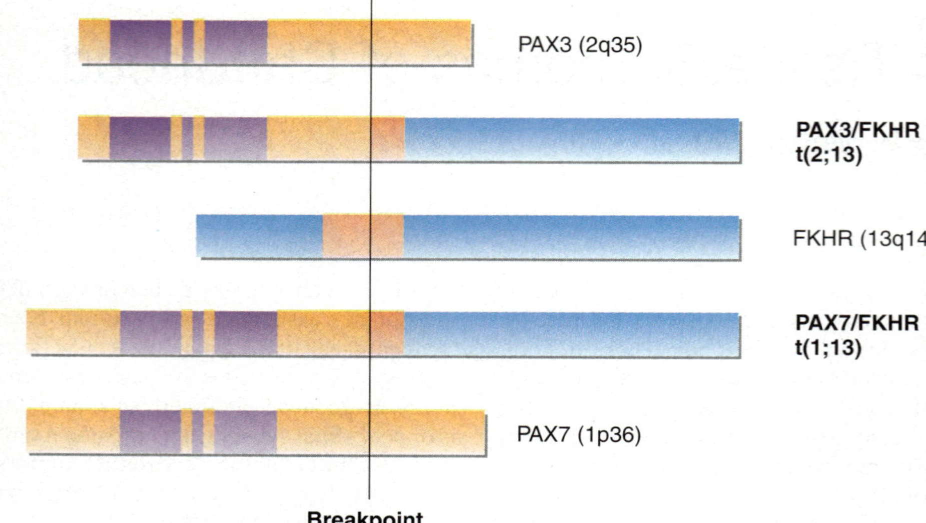

Figure 124k-4 Gene fusions in alveolar rhabdomyosarcoma. *PAX3/FKHR* [t(2;13)] is created by fusion of *PAX3*, localized to 2q25, and *FKHR*, localized to 13q14; *PAX7/FKHR* [t(1;13)] is created by fusion of *PAX7*, localized to 1q36, and *FKHR*, localized to 13q14.

has not been routinely used for RMS, grading of ERMS by degree of maturation, proliferation, and apoptosis may serve, in lieu of known biologic markers, to further subdivide this intermediate prognostic category of RMS into better defined prognostic subgroups. Embryonal RMS with diffuse anaplasia (2% of all RMS) has a poor prognosis (45% 5-year survival).[21] The fate of RMS with focal anaplasia (2% of RMS) is less clear. ERMS is characterized by loss of heterozygosity on the short arm of chromosome 11 (11p15.5), suggesting inactivation of a tumor-suppressor gene.[24,25] This is the region of the *IGF-2* gene that is overexpressed in rhabdomyosarcoma.[26]

Alveolar histology tumors comprise about 25% of RMS. This histology is more common in tumors arising in adolescents and in extremity primary tumors. Histologically, ARMS is composed of ill-defined round or oval cell tumor aggregates, often with loss of cellular cohesion, forming "alveolar" spaces surrounded by a framework of fibrous septae (Figure 124k-3). A solid variant of ARMS with cellular nests separated by fibrovascular septae is less common. Numerous studies have demonstrated that fusions of *PAX3* or *PAX7* and the *FKHR* (*FOXO1a*) gene that are generated by t(2;13) and t(1;13) chromosomal translocations are specific and consistent features of the alveolar subtype of RMS (Figure 124k-4).[27,28] The fusion transcripts expressed from these gene fusions can be detected by highly sensitive PCR-based and FISH assays.[29,30] In conjunction with standard histopathologic analysis, this molecular testing facilitates accurate identification and subclassification of RMS tumors and subsequent assignment to risk-based therapeutic protocols. In particular, this molecular testing provides valuable confirmation of the "higher risk" alveolar subtype in cases where histopathologic evidence of an alveolar pattern is subtle or equivocal. The *PAX3-FKHR* fusion of t(2;13) is associated with classic cystic ARMS and giant cells; *PAX7-FKHR* t(1;13) tumors may have a more subtle ARMS histology and lower apoptotic/mitotic activity.[31] However, a small population of ARMS tumors, determined by histologic criteria, are translocation negative.[32] Many RMSs of both histiotypes have increased expression of *MYCN*, which may be correlated with patient outcome.[33] The ability to screen the entire genome using gene expression profiles clearly demonstrates differences in gene expression between ERMS and ARMS.[34,35]

Open biopsy is usually required to obtain sufficient tissue for accurate diagnosis and also provides invaluable tissue for molecular characterization and other investigations. Complete clinical and radiologic evaluation should be done prior to consideration of primary tumor resection. The primary tumor should be assessed by either MRI or CT imaging to determine location, size, invasiveness, and anatomic boundaries that will determine the necessary local therapy. Appropriate metastatic evaluation includes CT scanning of lungs, bone scan, bilateral bone marrow aspirates/biopsies, and, for extremity and paratesticular tumors, imaging assessment of regional lymph nodes. Regional lymphatic spread of tumor often occurs in extremity tumors and in paratesticular tumors, particularly in those older than 10 years of age. Only about 15 to 20% of patients will have clinically detectable metastatic disease at diagnosis; however, all patients are considered to have micrometastatic disease, providing the rationale for universal chemotherapy. The most common sites for metastatic disease are lungs, bone marrow, and bones.

Extent of disease is among the strongest predictors for long-term outcome. Appropriate treatment planning is based primarily on the IRSG Clinical Group (Table 124k-1) and Stage (Table 124k-2). Clinical Group assignment primarily is determined by the surgical resectability of the primary tumor and presence of metastatic disease.[2] In 1991, a site modification of the TNM system was adopted that assigns Stage based on pretreatment assessment of tumor site, size, and regional and systemic tumor spread.[36,37] Patients with completely excised tumors (Group I), tumors arising in favorable sites (Stage 1), and those without regional node involvement (N_0) consistently have the most favorable outcomes, while patients with alveolar histology tumors and metastatic disease have significantly poorer outcomes. The recent generation of Children's Oncology Group protocols for rhabdomyosarcoma assigned patients to one of three risk groups. For the present series of COG studies started in 2004 and 2005, a similar risk stratification is used. All children with metastatic disease are enrolled on the high-risk trial (Table 124k-3). Multidisciplinary evaluation, including assessment by the surgical subspecialist and radiation oncologist, is critical for appropriate treatment planning.

Complete surgical excision of tumor is correlated with better outcome and, for embryonal tumors, obviates the need for local irradiation. However, rhabdomyosarcoma arises in many sites that do not permit primary surgical excision without significant morbidity or loss of function. Fewer than 20% of patients have tumors that are completely excised with negative tumor margins (Clinical Group I). Data from IRS II and III demonstrate a benefit for pretreatment reexcision of primary tumors occurring in the trunk and extremities to assure adequate resection margins[38]; such reexcision of the tumor bed is recommended for these sites when necessary. Better methods are needed to assess adequacy of tumor margins and are proposed for future studies. In some studies, delayed resection after a period of chemotherapy for selected tumors has minimized surgical morbidity and decreased doses of radiotherapy required. About one-half of patients over the age of 10 years with paratesticular RMS[39–41] and a similar proportion of patients with extremity and trunk primaries (regardless of age) have regional node involvement.[42,43] For these two groups, regional lymph node sampling is required. Regional node involvement in extremity RMS is associated with significantly poorer EFS ($p < .001$).[42,43] The recent ability to assess sentinel node involvement[44,45] potentially provides a refined method for risk assessment in RMS.

Table 124k-1 IRS Clinical Grouping for Rhabdomyosarcoma

IRS Clinical Grouping	Classification
Group I:	Localized disease, completely resected (Regional nodes not involved—lymph node biopsy or dissection is highly advised except for head and neck lesions) (a) Confined to muscle or organ of origin (b) Contiguous involvement—infiltration outside the muscle or organ of origin, as through fascial planes. NOTATION: This includes both gross inspection and microscopic confirmation of complete resection. Any nodes that may be inadvertently taken with the specimen must be negative. If the latter should be involved microscopically, then the patient is placed in the Group IIb or IIc (see below).
Group II:	Total gross resection with evidence of regional spread (a) Grossly resected tumor with microscopic residual disease (Surgeon believes that he has removed all of the tumor, but the pathologist finds tumor at the margin of resection and additional resection to achieve clean margin is not feasible). No evidence of gross residual tumor. No evidence of regional node involvement. Once radiotherapy and/or chemotherapy have been started, reexploration and removal of the area of microscopic residual does not change the patient's group. (b) Regional disease with involved nodes, completely resected with no microscopic residual. NOTATION: Complete resection with microscopic confirmation of no residual disease makes this different from Groups IIa and IIc. Additionally, in contrast to Group IIa, regional nodes (which are completely resected, however) are involved, but the most distal node is histologically negative. (c) Regional disease with involved nodes, grossly resected, but with evidence of microscopic residual and/or histologic involvement of the most distal regional node (from the primary site) in the dissection. NOTATION: The presence of microscopic residual disease makes this group different from IIb, and nodal involvement makes this group different from Group IIa.
Group III:	Incomplete resection with gross residual disease (a) After biopsy only (b) After gross or major resection of the primary (> 50%)
Group IV:	Distant metastatic disease present at onset (Lung, liver, bones, bone marrow, brain, and distant muscle and nodes) NOTATION: The above excludes *regional* nodes and adjacent organ infiltration, which places the patient in a more favorable grouping (as noted above under Group II). The presence of positive cytology in CSF, pleural or abdominal fluids as well as implants on pleural or peritoneal surfaces are regarded as indications for placing the patient in Group IV.

Table 124k-2 IRS Modified TNM Pretreatment Staging Classification

Stage	Sites	T	Size	N	M
1	Favorable	T_1 or T_2	a or b	N_0 or N_1 or N_2	M_0
2	Unfavorable	T_1 or T_2	a	N_0 or N_x	M_0
3	Unfavorable	T_1 or T_2	a	N_1	M_0
			b	N_0 or N_1 or N_x	M_0
4	All	T_1 or T_2	a or b	N_0 or N_1	M_1

Favorable sites = orbit, head and neck (excluding parameningeal) genitourinary (excluding bladder/prostate tumor, biliary tract; Unfavorable sites = bladder/prostate, extremity, cranial parameningeal, and other (includes trunk, retroperitoneum, but excludes biliary); T_1 – confined to anatomic site of origin, T_2 – extension and/or fixation to surrounding tissue; Size, a = ≤ 5 cm in diameter, b = > 5 cm in diameter; Regional nodes N_0 = regional nodes not clinically involved, N_1 = regional nodes clinically involved by neoplasm, N_x = clinical status of regional nodes unknown (especially sites that preclude lymph node evaluation); Metastasis M_0 = no distant metastasis, M_1 = metastasis present. Pretreatment size is determined by external measurement using MRI or CT depending on the anatomic location. For less accessible primary sites, CT will be employed as a means of lymph node assessment as well. Metastatic sites will require some form of imaging (but not histologic confirmation, except for bone marrow examination) confirmation.

Table 124k-3 Estimated Outcome for Rhabdomyosarcoma—COG Risk Groups*

Risk Group	Histology/Group/Stage	Proportion of Patients	Predicted 5-Yr FFS	Predicted Overall Survival
Low	Embryonal histology Group I, II Group III, Stage 1	33%	88%	95%
Intermediate	Embryonal histology Group III, Stage 2, 3 (unfavorable sites) Alveolar histology Groups I-III	48%	70%	75%
High	Group IV (regardless of histology)	19%	25%	27%

*Patients entered on IRS-IV or topotecan window study between 1/1/1992 and 6/30/1996.

Multiagent chemotherapy is indicated for all patients with rhabdomyosarcoma. Combination therapy including vincristine, dactinomycin, and cyclophosphamide (VAC) continues to be the mainstay of effective, curative therapy. Several other antineoplastic agents are active against RMS, but to date have not improved outcome. The overall 5-year survival for the most favorable subset of patients with low-risk RMS is 95% when treated with vincristine and dactinomycin chemotherapy administered for 48 weeks. European studies suggest that excellent outcomes may be achieved with shorter therapy in this group of patients.[46] In 2004, COG began a new low-risk study, testing whether further substantial decreases in length of therapy will maintain excellent outcomes. For the less favorable low-risk patients, three-drug therapy is necessary to achieve similar excellent outcome. Patients at intermediate risk of treatment failure also require three-drug chemotherapy. Based on activity of ifosfamide[47] and ifosfamide/etoposide in trials by IRSG and others and in phase II trials of relapsed patients,[48,49] the IRS-IV study prospectively randomized patients with intermediate-risk RMS to VAC or to vincristine, dactinomycin, ifosfamide (VAI), or to vincristine, ifosfamide, etoposide (VIE). The 3-year failure-free survivals were 75%, 77%, and 77%, respectively, indicating no advantage for ifosfamide-containing regimens.[6] Recently, the topoisomerase I poisons demonstrated clinical activity, as predicted from human tumor xenograft models of RMS.[50–52] Both topotecan alone and topotecan/cyclophosphamide caused tumor regression in about one-half of patients enrolled on phase II window trials;[53,54] the two-drug combination also is active in patients with recurrent RMS.[55] The present cooperative group study is comparing VAC alone to VAC plus vincristine, topotecan, and cyclophosphamide in a prospective, randomized trial for patients with intermediate-risk rhabdomyosarcoma. This study should reach its accrual goal in 2005; a successor study will test VAC against VAC plus irinotecan, vincristine.

The highest-risk population comprises patients who have macrometastatic disease at diagnosis. Fewer than one-third of these children will survive,[4] although some lower-risk subsets have been identified.[56,57] The IRSG has used the phase II window strategy[58,59] to assess the activity of several new agent combinations, prioritizing for clinical evaluation those agents with high levels of activity in the preclinical human rhabdomyosarcoma xenograft model. Using this strategy, several single agents and two-drug combinations have shown substantial clinical activity, including vincristine/melphalan, ifosfamide/etoposide,[60] ifosfamide/doxorubicin,[61] topotecan[53] and topotecan/cyclophosphamide.[54] The most recently completed study tested the combination of irinotecan/vincristine, based on the preclinical[51] and clinical activity for prolonged exposures to irinotecan,[62–64] the activity of single-agent vincristine, and the predicted synergism of this combination.[65] In the absence of a promising new candidate agent for phase II window testing, the next study will test a dose compression strategy of known effective agents, including alternating cycles of vincristine, doxorubicin, cyclophosphamide and ifosfamide, etoposide, on a backbone similar to the prior study.

For patients with embryonal RMS and microscopic or gross residual disease after surgical excision (Clinical Groups II-IV) and for all patients with alveolar RMS, radiation therapy plays a critical role for successful local tumor control. The dose of radiotherapy required varies dependent on tumor site, Group, and response to chemotherapy, with total doses ranging from 36 to 50.4 Gy. Higher doses are indicated for patients with gross residual disease after initial surgery and chemotherapy. The IRS-IV study was the first prospective evaluation of radiation therapy technique in children, comparing once-daily conventional fractionation with a twice-daily hyperfractionation schedule.[66] No benefit was found for the hyperfractionation schedule. For patients with tumors that erode the skull base or extend into the intracranial space or cause spinal cord compression, immediate initiation of radiotherapy is indicated.[67,68] In recent studies, radiotherapy was delayed for most other patients until either week 3 or 12 of therapy. Patients with tumors arising in the vagina may have local control delayed even longer so that late effects of therapy may be minimized.[69,70] The local failure rate continues to be unacceptably high, however.[71] The next COG intermediate-risk trial will therefore evaluate the early introduction of irradiation for all patients. To minimize the late effects of radiotherapy and decrease toxicity to surrounding normal tissues, new innovative techniques may be indicated in selected patients, including brachytherapy, three dimensional conformal treatment planning,[72] and intensity-modulated radiation therapy.

Most children and adolescents with favorable and intermediate-risk rhabdomyosarcoma can be cured with presently available multidisciplinary therapeutic approaches. Strategies in these groups to minimize the late effects of therapy are warranted. For the lower-risk patients, efforts are underway to decrease treatment length and minimize exposure to alkylating agents, thus decreasing the risk of infertility and second malignancies. Newer radiotherapy guidelines and treatment techniques are aimed at decreasing late toxicities,[73] including neuroendocrine dysfunction, bladder dysfunction,[74] soft tissue and skeletal growth effects,[75] and development of secondary sarcomas.

Of the children who relapse, a small subset is potentially curable who had Group I embryonal histology tumors at diagnosis and recurrent tumor only at the primary site. Over 80% with tumor recurrence have a dismal outcome, however.[76] In these very poor risk patients, new and innovative approaches to therapy must be attempted. Combinations of irinotecan and vincristine, shown to be synergistic in the xenograft model, and tirapazamine, an agent particularly active in a hypoxic milieu,[77,78] are now being evaluated in the ongoing cooperative group relapse study. In addition, other potential modalities and targets for therapeutic interventions that are being evaluated in early clinical trials or preclinical models include vaccines generated against small peptide fragments spanning the *PAX3-FKHR* fusion,[79] epidermal growth factor receptor tyrosine kinase inhibitors,[80,81] tumor necrosis factor alpha-related apoptosis-inducing ligand (TRAIL),[82,83] modified oncolytic herpes simplex virus,[84,85] CpG oligo peptides,[86] and rapamycin analogues.[87–89]

NONRHABDOMYOSARCOMA SOFT TISSUE SARCOMAS

Based on SEER data, NRSTS comprise approximately 4% of childhood malignancies and affect about 500 patients under the age of 20 years in the United States each year.[1] NRSTS include many histologically and biologically distinct entities, including fibrosarcoma, malignant peripheral nerve sheath tumors, synovial sarcoma, leiomyosarcoma, liposarcoma, and others. All are rare in children and often are more diagnostically challenging than rhabdomyosarcoma. Most NRSTS developing in children and adolescents are biologically similar to adult soft tissue sarcomas. The common primary tumors sites include extremities, trunk, abdomen, and pelvis. Most often the presenting symptom is a growing, sometimes painful mass. Adequate initial assessment is important and should include complete tumor imaging using MRI or CT and evaluation for metastatic lesions. Although therapeutic recommendations for older children and adolescents with NRSTS are often similar to those for adults with these tumors, differences between children and adults in risks for acute and late complications of treatment often require modifications in those treatment recommendations.

Only three prospective multi-institutional clinical trials for pediatric NRSTS have been conducted,[90–92] with fewer than 200 patient enrollments. Therefore, definitive data are lacking to determine (1) which children with resected NRSTS require adjuvant therapy, (2) the appropriate dose and field of radiotherapy needed to achieve adequate local/regional control in resected and unresected NRSTS, (3) the optimal type and duration of chemotherapy for patients at high risk of developing metastatic disease, (4) the most effective approach for patients with unresectable NRSTS, and (5) what the acute and late side effects of treatment are for childhood NRSTS.

The childhood NRSTS are graded histologically as low-, intermediate-, or high-grade tumors, using a modification of the AJCC tumor grading system that recognizes the unique features of some soft tissue sarcomas in young children.[93] Histologic grading is highly predictive of outcome. Low-grade tumors tend to be smaller, less invasive and more easily excised. High-grade tumors are often larger, invasive, more difficult to remove surgically, and more often present with established metastases.[94–96] Other unfavorable prognostic features include intra-abdominal primary site, positive microscopic margin after initial surgery, initially unresectable tumor, and older age.[94,96]

Although these prognostic factors are similar to those found in studies of adults with soft tissue sarcomas,[97,98] childhood NRSTS differ from adult soft tissue sarcomas in several important ways. Although liposarcoma and malignant fibrous histiocytoma are the most common soft tissue sarcomas in adults,[97,98] synovial sarcoma and malignant peripheral nerve sheath tumor predominate in pediatric populations.[94,95] Certain unique histologies (eg, infantile fibrosarcoma [IFS]) occur only in the pediatric age group,[99] requiring adjustments of standard tumor grading systems. IFS characteristically has a novel cryptic translocation between the *TEL* gene on chromosome 12p12 and the *TRK C* on chromosome 15.[100–102] Surgical excision is the treatment of choice for IFS, but may result in significant long-term morbidity.[103] Radiation therapy is typically reserved for palliation. The outcome with chemotherapy is much more favorable than for adults with fibrosarcoma.[104–106] Infantile hemangiopericytoma is another rare infantile soft tissue sarcoma (STS) that behaves in a clinically similar fashion, with infants appearing to have a more favorable outcome than older children.[107,108]

Surgical excision is the mainstay of treatment of children with soft tissue sarcomas. For small and low-grade lesions, complete excision is the only required treatment. For incompletely excised tumors, local irradiation is usually indicated. Ongoing debate surrounds many aspects of therapy, including the role and timing of chemotherapy for high-grade NRSTS.[109–111] The sole pediatric study addressing this showed no benefit for adjuvant chemotherapy,[90] and other studies suggest that some adults with soft tissue sarcomas may also be managed safely without adjuvant therapy.[112,113] For those who are candidates for radiotherapy, the optimal dose and timing of this treatment modality have not been clearly defined.[114,115] Finally, a recent retrospective review suggests better responses when chemotherapy/radiotherapy precedes surgery in adults with extremity sarcomas.[116] For those patients who require chemotherapy, including those with established metastatic disease, the most active agents are ifosfamide and doxorubicin; fewer than half the children receiving this therapy respond, however.[117] Such patients may be considered for phase II trials. Several histiotype-specific protocols are now being conducted for adults with soft tissues sarcomas; some of these trials may become available for selected children and adolescents through an intergroup coalition.

FUTURE RESEARCH

Further refinements of risk-group assignment are needed to better identify patient subsets at lower risk of disease recurrence and potentially to identify new targets for therapeutic intervention for patients with higher-risk soft tissue sarcomas. This may be accomplished by analyzing clinical, pathologic, and new molecular and gene expression profile features that will better characterize these tumors. For patients with rhabdomyosarcoma identified to be at the lowest risk of treatment failure, the goal is to maintain excellent cure rates while decreasing treatment intensity. For patients at highest risk of tumor recurrence and ultimate treatment failure, new therapeutic interventions that ultimately will improve cure rates need to be identified. The NRSTS are much more heterogeneous, and appropriate therapeutic interventions are more controversial. Research efforts should be directed at enabling risk-directed therapeutic interventions for children and adolescents with soft tissue sarcomas that are based on leads from preclinical models adult sarcoma results and on the identification of potential molecular targets for therapeutic intervention.

REFERENCES

1. Ries LAG, Smith MA, Gurney JG, et al. Cancer incidence and survival among children and adolescents: United States SEER Program 1975–1995. [NIH Pub No. 99-4649]. Bethesda (MD). National Cancer Institute SEER Program; 1999.
2. Maurer HM, Beltangady M, Gehan EA, et al. The Intergroup Rhabdomyosarcoma Study-I. A final report. Cancer 1988;61:209–20.
3. Maurer HM, Gehan EA, Beltangady M, et al. The Intergroup Rhabdomyosarcoma Study-II. Cancer 1993;71:1904–22.
4. Crist W, Gehan EA, Ragab AH, et al. The Third Intergroup Rhabdomyosarcoma Study. J Clin Oncol 1995;13:610–30.
5. Arndt CAS, Crist WM. Common musculoskeletal tumors of childhood and adolescence. N Engl J Med 1999;341:342–52.
6. Crist WM, Anderson JR, Meza JL, et al. Intergroup Rhabdomyosarcoma Study-IV: results for patients with nonmetastatic disease. J Clin Oncol 2001;19:3091–102.
7. Pappo AS, Shapiro DN, Crist WM, Maurer HM. Biology and therapy of pediatric rhabdomyosarcoma. J Clin Oncol 1995;13:2123–39.
8. Yang P, Grufferman S, Khoury MJ, et al. Association of childhood rhabdomyosarcoma with neurofibromatosis type I and birth defects. Genet Epidemiol 1995;12:467–74.
9. Sung L, Anderson JR, Arndt C, et al. Neurofibromatosis in children with rhabdomyosarcoma: a report from the Intergroup Rhabdomyosarcoma study IV. J Pediatr 2004;144:666–8.
10. Smith AC, Squire JA, Thorner P, et al. Association of alveolar rhabdomyosarcoma with the Beckwith-Wiedemann syndrome. Pediatr Dev Pathol 2001;4:550–8.
11. Cohen PR, Kurzrock R. Miscellaneous genodermatoses: Beckwith-Wiedemann syndrome, Birt-Hogg-Dube syndrome, familial atypical multiple mole melanoma syndrome, hereditary tylosis, incontinentia pigmenti, and supernumerary nipples. Dermatol Clin 1995;13:211–29.
12. Malkin D, Li FP, Strong LC, et al. Germ line p53 mutations in a familial syndrome of breast cancer, sarcomas, and other neoplasms. Science 1990;250:1233–8.
13. Heyn R, Haeberlen V, Newton WA, et al. Second malignant neoplasms in children treated for rhabdomyosarcoma. Intergroup Rhabdomyosarcoma Study Committee. J Clin Oncol 1993;11:262–70.
14. Bisogno G, Murgia A, Mammi I, et al. Rhabdomyosarcoma in a patient with cardio-facio-cutaneous syndrome. J Pediatr Hematol Oncol 1999;21:424–7.
15. Gripp KW, Scott CIJ, Nicholson L, et al. Five additional Costello syndrome patients with rhabdomyosarcoma: proposal for a tumor screening protocol. Am J Med Genet 2002;108:80–7.
16. Jung A, Bechthold S, Pfluger T, et al. Orbital rhabdomyosarcoma in Noonan syndrome. J Pediatr Hematol Oncol 2003;25:330–2.
17. Agras PI, Baskin E, Sakallioglu AE, et al. Neurofibromatosis--Noonan's syndrome with associated rhabdomyosarcoma of the urinary bladder in an infant: case report. J Child Neurol 2003;18:68–72.
18. Ruymann FB, Maddux HR, Ragab A, et al. Congenital anomalies associated with rhabdomyosarcoma: an autopsy study of 115 cases. A report from the Intergroup Rhabdomyosarcoma Study Committee (representing the Children's Cancer Study Group, the Pediatric Oncology Group, the United Kingdom Children's Cancer Study Group, and the Pediatric Intergroup Statistical Center). Med Pediatr Oncol 1988;16:33–9.
19. Grufferman S, Schwartz AG, Ruymann FB, Maurer HM. Parents' use of cocaine and marijuana and increased risk of rhabdomyosarcoma in their children. Cancer Causes Control 1993;4:217–24.
20. Sebire NJ, Malone M. Myogenin and MyoD1 expression in paediatric rhabdomyosarcomas. J Clin Pathol 2003;56:412–6.
21. Qualman SJ, Coffin CM, Newton WA, et al. Intergroup Rhabdomyosarcoma Study: update for pathologists. Pediatr Dev Pathol 1998;1:550–61.
22. Qualman SJ, Bowen J, Parham DM, et al. Protocol for the examination of specimens from patients (children and young adults) with rhabdomyosarcoma. Arch Pathol Lab Med 2003;127:1290–7.
23. Newton WAJ, Gehan EA, Webber BL, et al. Classification of rhabdomyosarcomas and related sarcomas. Pathologic aspects and proposal for a new classification—an Intergroup Rhabdomyosarcoma Study. Cancer 1995;76:1073–85.
24. Scrable HJ, Witte DP, Lampkin BC, Cavenee WK. Chromosomal localization of the human rhabdomyosarcoma locus by mitotic recombination mapping. Nature 1987;329:645–7.
25. Loh WEJ, Scrable HJ, Livanos E, et al. Human chromosome 11 contains two different growth suppressor genes for embryonal rhabdomyosarcoma. Proc Natl Acad Sci U S A 1992;89:1755–9.
26. El-Badry OM, Minniti C, Kohn EC, et al. Insulin-like growth factor II acts as an autocrine growth and motility factor in human rhabdomyosarcoma tumors. Cell Growth Differ 1990;1:325–31.
27. Barr FG, Galili N, Holick J, et al. Rearrangement of the PAX3 paired box gene in the paediatric solid tumour alveolar rhabdomyosarcoma. Nat Genet 1993;3:113–7.
28. Bois PR, Grosveld GC. FKHR (FOXO1a) is required for myotube fusion of primary mouse myoblasts. EMBO J 2003;22:1147–57.
29. Barr FG, Chatten J, D'Cruz CM, et al. Molecular assays for chromosomal translocations in the diagnosis of pediatric soft tissue sarcomas. JAMA 1995;273:553–7.
30. Biegel JA, Nycum LM, Valentine V, et al. Detection of the t(2;13)(q35;q14) and PAX3-FKHR fusion in alveolar rhabdomyosarcoma by fluorescence in situ hybridization. Genes Chromosom Cancer 1995;12:186–92.
31. Collins MH, Zhao H, Womer RB, Barr FG. Proliferative and apoptotic differences between alveolar rhabdomyosarcoma subtypes: a comparative study of tumors containing PAX3-FKHR or PAX7-FKHR gene fusions. Med Pediatr Oncol 2001;37:83–9.
32. Barr FG, Qualman SJ, Macris MH, et al. Genetic heterogeneity in the alveolar rhabdomyosarcoma subset without typical gene fusions. Cancer Res 2002;62:4704–10.
33. Williamson D, Lu YJ, Gordon T, et al. Relationship between MYCN copy number and expression in rhabdomyosarcomas and correlation with adverse prognosis in the alveolar subtype. J Clin Oncol 2005;23:880–8.
34. Wachtel M, Dettling M, Koscielniak E, et al. Gene expression signatures identify rhabdomyosarcoma subtypes and detect a novel t(2;2)(q35;p23) translocation fusing PAX3 to NCOA1. Cancer Res 2004;64:5539–45.
35. Schaaf GJ, Ruijter JM, van Ruissen F, et al. Full transcriptome analysis of rhabdomyosarcoma, normal and fetal skeletal muscle: statistical comparison of multiple SAGE libraries. FASEB J 2005;19:404–6.
36. Lawrence WJ, Gehan EA, Hays DM, et al. Prognostic significance of staging factors of the UICC staging system in childhood rhabdomyosarcoma: a report from the Intergroup Rhabdomyosarcoma Study (IRS-II). J Clin Oncol 1987;5:46–54.
37. Lawrence WJ, Anderson JR, Gehan EA, Maurer H. Pretreatment TNM staging of childhood rhabdomyosarcoma: a report of the Intergroup Rhabdomyosarcoma Study Group. Children's Cancer Study Group. Pediatric Oncology Group. Cancer 1997;80:1165–70.
38. Hays DM, Lawrence WJ, Wharam M, et al. Primary reexcision for patients with 'microscopic residual' tumor following initial excision of sarcomas of trunk and extremity sites. J Pediatr Surg 1989;24:5–10.
39. Raney RBJ, Tefft M, Lawrence WJ, et al. Paratesticular sarcoma in childhood and adolescence. A report from the Intergroup Rhabdomyosarcoma Studies I and II, 1973–1983. Cancer 1987;60:2337–43.
40. Wiener ES, Anderson JR, Ojimba JI, et al. Controversies in the management of paratesticular rhabdomyosarcoma: is staging retroperitoneal lymph node dissection necessary for adolescents with resected paratesticular rhabdomyosarcoma? Semin Pediatr Surg 2001;10:146–52.
41. Stewart RJ, Martelli H, Oberlin O, et al. Treatment of children with nonmetastatic paratesticular rhabdomyosarcoma: results of the Malignant Mesenchymal Tumors studies (MMT 84 and MMT 89) of the International Society of Pediatric Oncology. J Clin Oncol 2003;21:793–8.
42. Lawrence WJ, Hays DM, Heyn R, et al. Lymphatic metastases with childhood rhabdomyosarcoma. A report from the Intergroup Rhabdomyosarcoma Study. Cancer 1987;60:910–5.
43. Andrassy RJ, Corpron CA, Hays D, et al. Extremity sarcomas: an analysis of prognostic factors from the Intergroup Rhabdomyosarcoma Study III. J Pediatr Surg 1996;31:191–6.
44. Paganelli G, De Cicco C, Chinol M. Sentinel node localization by lymphoscintigraphy: a reliable technique with widespread applications. Recent Results Cancer Res 2000;157:121–9.
45. McMulkin HM, Yanchar NL, Fernandez CV, Giacomantonio C. Sentinel lymph node mapping and biopsy: a potentially valuable tool in the management of childhood extremity rhabdomyosarcoma. Pediatr Surg Int 2003;19:453–6.
46. Koscielniak E, Harms D, Henze G, et al. Results of treatment for soft tissue sarcoma in childhood and adolescence: a final report of the German Cooperative Soft Tissue Sarcoma Study CWS-86. J Clin Oncol 1999;17:3706–19.
47. Pappo AS, Etcubanas E, Santana VM, et al. A phase II trial of ifosfamide in previously untreated children and adolescents with unresectable rhabdomyosarcoma. Cancer 1993;71:2119–25.
48. Miser JS, Kinsella TJ, Triche TJ, et al. Ifosfamide with mesna uroprotection and etoposide: an effective regimen in the treatment of recurrent sarcomas and other tumors of children and young adults. J Clin Oncol 1987;5:1191–8.
49. Kung FH, Pratt CB, Vega RA, et al. Ifosfamide/etoposide combination in the treatment of recurrent malignant solid tumors of childhood. A Pediatric Oncology Group Phase II study. Cancer 1993;71:1898–903.
50. Houghton PJ, Cheshire PJ, Myers L, et al. Evaluation of 9-dimethylaminomethyl-10-hydroxycamptothecin against xenografts derived from adult and childhood solid tumors. Cancer Chemother Pharmacol 1992;31:229–39.
51. Houghton PJ, Cheshire PJ, Hallman JC, et al. Therapeutic efficacy of the topoisomerase I inhibitor 7-ethyl-10- (4-[1-piperidino]-1-piperidino)-carbonyloxy-camptothecin against human tumor xenografts: lack of cross-resistance in vivo in tumors with acquired resistance to the topoisomerase I inhibitor 9- dimethylaminomethyl-10-hydroxycamptothecin. Cancer Res 1993;53:2823–9.
52. Vassal G, Pondarre C, Boland I, et al. Preclinical development of camptothecin derivatives and clinical trials in pediatric oncology. Biochimie 1998;80:271–80.
53. Pappo AS, Lyden E, Breneman J, et al. Up-front window trial of topotecan in previously untreated children and adolescents with metastatic rhabdomyosarcoma: an intergroup rhabdomyosarcoma study. J Clin Oncol 2001;19:213–9.
54. Walterhouse DO, Lyden ER, Breitfeld PP, et al. Efficacy of topotecan and cyclophosphamide given as a phase II window in children with newly diagnosed metastatic rhabdomyosarcoma: a report from the Soft Tissue Sarcoma Committee of the Children's Oncology Group. J Clin Oncol 2004;22:1398–403.
55. Saylors RL 3rd, Stine KC, Sullivan J, et al. Cyclophosphamide plus topotecan in children with recurrent or refractory solid tumors: a Pediatric Oncology Group phase II study. J Clin Oncol 2001;19:3463–9.
56. Carli M, Colombatti R, Oberlin O, et al. European intergroup studies (MMT4-89 and MMT4-91) on childhood metastatic rhabdomyosarcoma: final results and analysis of prognostic factors. J Clin Oncol 2004;22:4735–42.
57. Breneman JC, Lyden E, Pappo AS, et al. Prognostic factors and clinical outcomes in children and adolescents with metastatic rhabdomyosarcoma—a report from the Intergroup Rhabdomyosarcoma Study IV. J Clin Oncol 2003;21:78–84.
58. Horowitz ME, Etcubanas E, Christensen ML, et al. Phase II testing of melphalan in children with newly diagnosed rhabdomyosarcoma: a model for anticancer drug development. J Clin Oncol 1988;6:308–14.

59. Meyer WH, Houghton PJ, Horowitz ME, et al. Use of investigational drugs as initial therapy for childhood solid tumors. Hamatol Bluttransfus 1989;32:141–8.
60. Breitfeld PP, Lyden E, Beverly RR, et al. Ifosfamide and etoposide are superior to vincristine and melphalan for pediatric metastatic rhabdomyosarcoma when administered with irradiation and combination chemotherapy: a report from the Intergroup Rhabdomyosarcoma Study Group. Am J Pediatr Hematol Oncol 2001;23:225–33.
61. Sandler ES, Lyden E, Ruymann F, et al. Efficacy of ifosfamide and doxorubicin given as a phase II "window" in children with newly diagnosed metastatic rhabdomyosarcoma: a report from the Intergroup Rhabdomyosarcoma Study Group. Med Pediatr Oncol 2001;37:442–8.
62. Furman WL, Stewart CF, Poquette CA, et al. Direct translation of a protracted irinotecan schedule from a xenograft model to a phase I trial in children. J Clin Oncol 1999;17:1815–24.
63. Cosetti M, Wexler LH, Calleja E, et al. Irinotecan for pediatric solid tumors: the Memorial Sloan-Kettering experience. J Pediatr Hematol Oncol 2002;24:101–5.
64. Pappo AS, Lyden E, Breitfeld PP, et al. Irinotecan (CPT-11) is active against pediatric rhabdomyosarcoma(RMS): a phase II window trial from the Soft Tissue Sarcoma Committee (STS) of the Children's Oncology Group (COG). Proc Annu Meet Am Soc Clin Oncol 2002;21:393a.
65. Thompson J, George EO, Poquette CA, et al. Synergy of topotecan in combination with vincristine for treatment of pediatric solid tumor xenografts. Clin Cancer Res 1999;5:3617–31.
66. Donaldson SS, Meza J, Breneman JC, et al. Results from the IRS-IV randomized trial of hyperfractionated radiotherapy in children with rhabdomyosarcoma—a report from the IRSG. Int J Radiat Oncol Biol Phys 2001;51:718–28.
67. Raney RBJ, Tefft M, Newton WA, et al. Improved prognosis with intensive treatment of children with cranial soft tissue sarcomas arising in nonorbital parameningeal sites. A report from the Intergroup Rhabdomyosarcoma Study. Cancer 1987;59:147–55.
68. Raney RB, Meza J, Anderson JR, et al. Treatment of children and adolescents with localized parameningeal sarcoma: experience of the Intergroup Rhabdomyosarcoma Study Group protocols IRS-II through -IV, 1978–1997. Med Pediatr Oncol 2002;38:22–32.
69. Andrassy RJ, Wiener ES, Raney RB, et al. Progress in the surgical management of vaginal rhabdomyosarcoma: a 25-year review from the Intergroup Rhabdomyosarcoma Study Group. J Pediatr Surg 1999;34:731–4.
70. Arndt CA, Donaldson SS, Anderson JR, et al. What constitutes optimal therapy for patients with rhabdomyosarcoma of the female genital tract? Cancer 2001;91:2454–68.
71. Wharam MD, Meza J, Anderson J, et al. Failure pattern and factors predictive of local failure in rhabdomyosarcoma: a report of group III patients on the third Intergroup Rhabdomyosarcoma Study. J Clin Oncol 2004;22:1902–8.
72. Wolden SL, La TH, LaQuaglia MP, et al. Long-term results of three-dimensional conformal radiation therapy for patients with rhabdomyosarcoma. Cancer 2003;97:179–85.
73. Punyko JA, Mertens AC, Gurney JG, et al. Long-term medical effects of childhood and adolescent rhabdomyosarcoma: a report from the childhood cancer survivor study. Cancer 2005;103:1475–83.
74. Arndt C, Rodeberg D, Breitfeld PP, et al. Does bladder preservation (as a surgical principle) lead to retaining bladder function in bladder/prostate rhabdomyosarcoma? Results from intergroup rhabdomyosarcoma study iv. J Urol 2004;171:2396–403.
75. Estilo CL, Huryn JM, Kraus DH, et al. Effects of therapy on dentofacial development in long-term survivors of head and neck rhabdomyosarcoma: the memorial Sloan-Kettering cancer center experience. J Pediatr Hematol Oncol 2003;25:215–22.
76. Pappo AS, Anderson JR, Crist WM, et al. Survival after relapse in children and adolescents with rhabdomyosarcoma: a report from the Intergroup Rhabdomyosarcoma Study Group. J Clin Oncol 1999;17:3487–93.
77. Brown JM. The hypoxic cell: a target for selective cancer therapy—eighteenth Bruce F. Cain Memorial Award lecture. Cancer Res 1999;59:5863–70.
78. Siim BG, Menke DR, Dorie MJ, Brown JM. Tirapazamine-induced cytotoxicity and DNA damage in transplanted tumors: relationship to tumor hypoxia. Cancer Res 1997;57:2922–8.
79. Dagher R, Long LM, Read EJ, et al. Pilot trial of tumor-specific peptide vaccination and continuous infusion interleukin-2 in patients with recurrent Ewing sarcoma and alveolar rhabdomyosarcoma: an inter-institute NIH study. Med Pediatr Oncol 2002;38:158–64.
80. Miller VA, Johnson DH, Krug LM, et al. Pilot trial of the epidermal growth factor receptor tyrosine kinase inhibitor gefitinib plus carboplatin and paclitaxel in patients with stage IIIB or IV non-small-cell lung cancer. J Clin Oncol 2003;21:2094–100.
81. Stewart CF, Leggas M, Schuetz JD, et al. Gefitinib enhances the antitumor activity and oral bioavailability of irinotecan in mice. Cancer Res 2004;64:7491–9.
82. Petak I, Douglas L, Tillman DM, et al. Pediatric rhabdomyosarcoma cell lines are resistant to Fas-induced apoptosis and highly sensitive to TRAIL-induced apoptosis. Clin Cancer Res 2000;6:4119–27.
83. Petak I, Vernes R, Szucs KS, et al. A caspase-8-independent component in TRAIL/Apo-2L-induced cell death in human rhabdomyosarcoma cells. Cell Death Differ 2003;10:729–39.
84. Bharatan NS, Currier MA, Cripe TP. Differential susceptibility of pediatric sarcoma cells to oncolysis by conditionally replication-competent herpes simplex viruses. J Pediatr Hematol Oncol 2002;24:447–53.
85. Currier MA, Adams LC, Mahller YY, Cripe TP. Widespread intratumoral virus distribution with fractionated injection enables local control of large human rhabdomyosarcoma xenografts by oncolytic herpes simplex viruses. Cancer Gene Ther 2005;12:407–16.
86. Weigel BJ, Rodeberg DA, Krieg AM, Blazar BR. CpG oligodeoxynucleotides potentiate the antitumor effects of chemotherapy or tumor resection in an orthotopic murine model of rhabdomyosarcoma. Clin Cancer Res 2003;9:3105–14.
87. Dilling MB, Dias P, Shapiro DN, et al. Rapamycin selectively inhibits the growth of childhood rhabdomyosarcoma cells through inhibition of signaling via the type I insulin-like growth factor receptor. Cancer Res 1994;54:903–7.
88. Hosoi H, Dilling MB, Shikata T, et al. Rapamycin causes poorly reversible inhibition of mTOR and induces p53-independent apoptosis in human rhabdomyosarcoma cells. Cancer Res 1999;59:886–94.
89. Gallicchio MA, van Sinderen M, Bach LA. Insulin-like growth factor binding protein-6 and CCI-779, an ester analogue of rapamycin, additively inhibit rhabdomyosarcoma growth. Horm Metab Res 2003;35:822–7.
90. Pratt CB, Pappo AS, Gieser P, et al. Role of adjuvant chemotherapy in the treatment of surgically resected pediatric nonrhabdomyosarcomatous soft tissue sarcomas: a Pediatric Oncology Group Study. J Clin Oncol 1999;17:1219–26.
91. Pratt CB, Maurer HM, Gieser P, et al. Treatment of unresectable or metastatic pediatric soft tissue sarcomas with surgery, irradiation, and chemotherapy: a Pediatric Oncology Group study. Med Pediatr Oncol 1998;30:201–9.
92. Pappo AS, Devidas M, Jenkins J, et al. Vincristine (V), ifosfamide (I), doxorubicin (D), and G-CSF (G) for pediatric unresected metastatic non-rhabdomyosarcomatous soft tissue sarcomas (NRSTS): a Pediatric Oncology Group (POG) Study. Proc Annu Meet Am Soc Clin Oncol 2001;20:378a.
93. Parham DM, Webber BL, Jenkins JJ, et al. Nonrhabdomyosarcomatous soft tissue sarcomas of childhood: formulation of a simplified system for grading. Mod Pathol 1995;8:705–10.
94. Spunt SL, Poquette CA, Hurt YS, et al. Prognostic factors for children and adolescents with surgically resected nonrhabdomyosarcoma soft tissue sarcoma: an analysis of 121 patients treated at St Jude Children's Research Hospital. J Clin Oncol 1999;17:3697–705.
95. Marcus KC, Grier HE, Shamberger RC, et al. Childhood soft tissue sarcoma: a 20-year experience. J Pediatr 1997;131:603–7.
96. Spunt SL, Hill DA, Motosue AM, et al. Clinical features and outcome of initially unresected nonmetastatic pediatric nonrhabdomyosarcoma soft tissue sarcoma. J Clin Oncol 2002;20:3225–35.
97. Pisters PW, Leung DH, Woodruff J, et al. Analysis of prognostic factors in 1,041 patients with localized soft tissue sarcomas of the extremities. J Clin Oncol 1996;14:1679–89.
98. Coindre JM, Terrier P, Bui NB, et al. Prognostic factors in adult patients with locally controlled soft tissue sarcoma. A study of 546 patients from the French Federation of Cancer Centers Sarcoma Group. J Clin Oncol 1996;14:869–77.
99. Coffin CM, Dehner LP. Soft tissue tumors in first year of life: a report of 190 cases. Pediatr Pathol 1990;10:509–26.
100. Knezevich SR, McFadden DE, Tao W, et al. A novel ETV6-NTRK3 gene fusion in congenital fibrosarcoma. Nat Genet 1998;18:184–7.
101. Rubin BP, Chen CJ, Morgan TW, et al. Congenital mesoblastic nephroma t(12;15) is associated with ETV6-NTRK3 gene fusion: cytogenetic and molecular relationship to congenital (infantile) fibrosarcoma. Am J Pathol 1998;153:1451–8.
102. Knezevich SR, Garnett MJ, Pysher TJ, et al. ETV6-NTRK3 gene fusions and trisomy 11 establish a histogenetic link between mesoblastic nephroma and congenital fibrosarcoma. Cancer Res 1998;58:5046–8.
103. Cofer BR, Vescio PJ, Wiener ES. Infantile fibrosarcoma: complete excision is the appropriate treatment. Ann Surg Oncol 1996;3:159–61.
104. Grier HE, Perez-Atayde AR, Weinstein HJ. Chemotherapy for inoperable infantile fibrosarcoma. Cancer 1985;56:1507–10.
105. Ninane J, Rombouts JJ, Cornu G. Chemotherapy for infantile fibrosarcoma. Med Pediatr Oncol 1991;19:209.
106. Kynaston JA, Malcolm AJ, Craft AW, et al. Chemotherapy in the management of infantile fibrosarcoma. Med Pediatr Oncol 1993;21:488–93.
107. Rodriguez-Galindo C, Ramsey K, Jenkins JJ, et al. Hemangiopericytoma in children and infants. Cancer 2000;88:198–204.
108. Dennis TR, Spallone PA, Kurlinski JP, Stock AD. Molecular cytogenetic study of a hemangiopericytoma in a newborn. Cancer Genet Cytogenet 2000;121:146–9.
109. Sarcoma Meta-Analysis Collaboration. Adjuvant chemotherapy for localised resectable soft-tissue sarcoma of adults: meta-analysis of individual data. Lancet 1997;350:1647–54.
110. Frustaci S, Gherlinzoni F, De Paoli A, et al. Adjuvant chemotherapy for adult soft tissue sarcomas of the extremities and girdles: results of the Italian randomized cooperative trial. J Clin Oncol 2001;19:1238–47.
111. Bramwell VH. Adjuvant chemotherapy for adult soft tissue sarcoma: is there a standard of care? J Clin Oncol 2001;19:1235–7.
112. Baldini EH, Goldberg J, Jenner C, et al. Long-term outcomes after function-sparing surgery without radiotherapy for soft tissue sarcoma of the extremities and trunk. J Clin Oncol 1999;17:3252–9.
113. Rydholm A, Gustafson P, Rooser B, et al. Limb-sparing surgery without radiotherapy based on anatomic location of soft tissue sarcoma. J Clin Oncol 1991;9:1757–65.
114. Cheng EY, Dusenbery KE, Winters MR, Thompson RC. Soft tissue sarcomas: preoperative versus postoperative radiotherapy. J Surg Oncol 1996;61:90–9.
115. Wolfson AH, Benedetto PW, Mnaymneh W, et al. Does a radiation dose-response relation exist concerning survival of patients who have soft-tissue sarcomas of the extremities? Radiation dose-response relation for soft-tissue sarcomas. Am J Clin Oncol 1998;21:270–4.
116. Eilber FC, Rosen G, Eckardt J, et al. Treatment-induced pathologic necrosis: a predictor of local recurrence and survival in patients receiving neoadjuvant therapy for high-grade extremity soft tissue sarcomas. J Clin Oncol 2001;19:3203–9.
117. Walter AW, Shearer PD, Pappo AS, et al. A pilot study of vincristine, ifosfamide, and doxorubicin in the treatment of pediatric non-rhabdomyosarcoma soft tissue sarcomas. Med Pediatr Oncol 1998;30:210–6.

Unique Pathologic Features of Childhood Cancer

Kadria Sayed, MD
David M. Parham, MD

Although childhood neoplasia is rare everywhere in the world, it nevertheless constitutes the second leading cause of death in the pediatric population, following accidents.[1] Generally, one classifies cancer by individual organs, each with its own frequency and demographic pattern. However, childhood cancers are histologically diverse and it is more appropriate to classify them based on histologic type rather than organ of origin.[2] This way of classification helps to understand their etiology, progression of disease, and response to therapy. An assortment of unique features distinguishes pediatric tumors from adult ones. These features include their ability to recapitulate different stages of embryogenesis, their differing morphologic appearances, the unique pathobiologic processes that affect their tumorigenesis and prognosis, their association with congenital anomalies, the frequent occurrence of primitive undifferentiated neoplasms, and the infrequent association of childhood neoplasms with precursor lesions. In this chapter, the features of childhood cancers that differ as a group from adult malignancies are discussed and the implications of these characteristics on diagnosis, treatment, and prognosis are noted.

RESEMBLANCE TO EMBRYONAL TISSUE

A large percentage of malignant neoplasms in children are dysontogenetic tumors whose morphologic and biologic features resemble or recapitulate those of developing organs and tissues.[3] Approximately 30% of childhood cancers fall into this category. Table 124I-1 lists the major types of embryonic tumors in childhood and their occurrence relative to other childhood cancers.

Table 124I-1 Occurrence of Major Embryonic Childhood Tumors

Type	Frequency of Occurrence (%)
Neuroblastoma	8
Wilms' and other renal tumors	6.5
Medulloblastoma	4
Rhabdomyosarcoma	4
Retinoblastoma	3
Ewing sarcoma	2
Hepatoblastoma	1
Pancreatoblastoma	<1
Sialoblastoma	<1
Pleuropulmonary blastoma	<1

Neuroblastoma constitutes the fourth most common malignant tumor and the most common extracranial solid tumor in children. It represents approximately 7 to 10% of childhood malignancies. Neuroblastic tumors develop from neuronal crest cells that normally migrate to form the adrenal medulla, sympathetic ganglia, and other autonomic organs. Similar to normal neuroblasts, neuroblastomas variably differentiate along gangliocytic and Schwannian lineages.[4] Thus the term "neuroblastic tumor" encompasses non-paragangliomatous tumors of the sympathetic nervous system that possess a wide array of differentiation patterns recapitulating normal ganglionic development. For the purposes of pathologic classification, lesions are separated into neuroblastoma, ganglioneuroblastoma, and ganglioneuroma (Figures 124I-1 and 124I-2). Neuroblastomas arise most commonly in young children, and three-fourths of affected patients are less than 4 years of age.[5] Although more mature tumors, for instance, ganglioneuromas, may become manifest during childhood, many are clinically silent until adolescence or adult life and may represent maturation of a clinically silent neuroblastoma.[6] Conversely, true neuroblastomas are extremely rare in adults.[7]

Embryonal tumors of the central nervous system (CNS) constitute approximately 20% of the childhood tumors and are the second in frequency among CNS tumors in children.[8] They encompass a group of undifferentiated tumors and are referred to as primitive neuroectodermal tumors of the CNS. Medulloblastomas make up 85% of this group of tumors, most commonly occur in the first 2 years of life and are located in the cerebellar vermis. Histologically, they are composed of densely packed undifferentiated cells with occasional Homer Wright pseudorosettes. These tumors can display neuronal and/or glial differentiation. Other less common embryonal tumors include other supra-tentorial tumors (ie, pineoblastomas, central neuroblastoma, and ganglioneuroblastoma), ependymoblastoma, and medulloepithelioma. The histogenesis of CNS embryonal tumors is unclear. One theory suggests an origin from common pluripotent precursor cells. During tumorigenesis, these cells recapitulate ontogenetic development to varying degrees up to end-stage differentiation.[9]

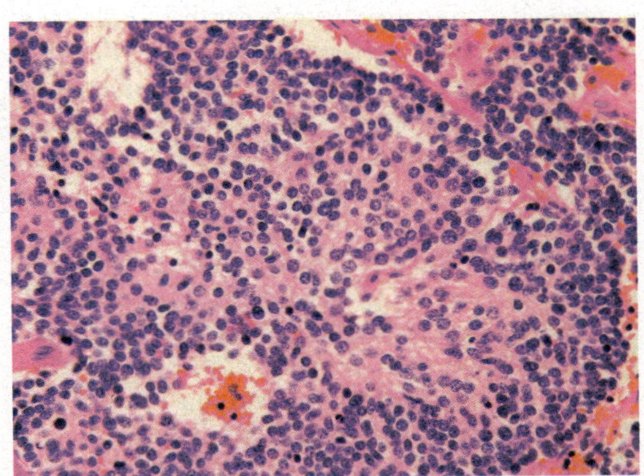

Figure 124I-1 Neuroblastoma showing sheets of undifferentiated neuroblastic cells and immature neurofibrillary stroma.

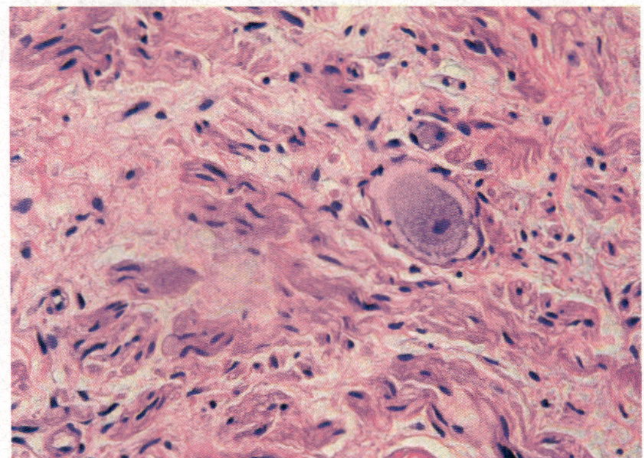

Figure 124I-2 Ganglioneuroma: mature ganglion cells and Schwann cell–rich stroma.

Renal neoplasms constitute an important childhood tumor category and are sixth in frequency among pediatric cancers. Wilms' tumor, or nephroblastoma, is by far the most common of these lesions. The histologic features of Wilms' tumor closely recapitulate those of the developing kidney, which arises as the protruding ureteric bud abuts the mesodermal blastema.[10] Microscopically, both the developing kidney and Wilms' tumor are composed of three basic elements: blastema, stroma, and epithelium (Figure 124I-3). The mixture of these maturing components gives Wilms' tumors a heterogeneous histologic appearance that often bears a startling resemblance to normal embryonic kidney. Blastemal elements comprise undifferentiated small blue cells that are analogous to the metanephric blastema. Blastema-predominant Wilms' tumors tend to present as higher-stage lesions and therefore have a propensity for aggressive behavior,[11] although this factor was not significant in a multivariate analysis. However, tumors with persistent blastemal predominance after preoperative chemotherapy are now considered to be high risk by the International Society for Paediatric Oncology (SIOP).[12] Conversely, epithelial predominant

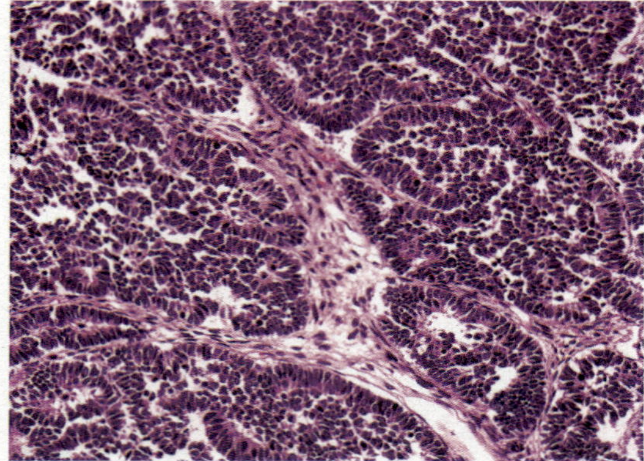

Figure 124I-3 Wilms' tumor with mixed blastemal, epithelial, and mesenchymal component.

Wilms' tumors tended to be lower stage and have a better prognosis in older series.[13] Heterologous mesenchymal tissues, most commonly muscle, bone, adipose tissue, and cartilage, can be seen in Wilms' tumors. This differentiation presumably represents mesodermal elements that have escaped nephrogenic induction. The term "teratoid" Wilms' tumor signifies a subset of tumors in which these mesenchymal elements predominate.[14] Wilms' tumors usually arise in infants and young children, as predicted by the embryonic content of these lesions. Rare examples may arise in adults.[15]

Rhabdomyosarcoma follows neuroblastoma in order of frequency among childhood cancers. Rhabdomyosarcomas comprise the most common malignant soft tissue sarcomas of children and constitute approximately 70% of pediatric mesenchymal malignancies.[16] Rhabdomyosarcomas are composed of cells with features of fetal skeletal muscle at 10 to 12 weeks gestation. Because rhabdomyosarcomas commonly occur in areas devoid of skeletal muscles, such as the prostate or nasopharynx, they may arise in mesenchymal stem cells that have myogenic potential, rather than from true skeletal myocytes.

Several morphologically distinct subtypes comprise rhabdomyosarcomas; these include embryonal, botryoid, alveolar, and pleomorphic tumors. Although each subtype possesses a distinct morphologic appearance, the essential ingredient for the diagnosis of these tumors is the rhabdomyoblast (Figure 124I-4), an embryonic cell whose features closely recapitulate the stages of prenatal myogenesis. Embryonal rhabdomyosarcomas contain a mixture of loose myxoid and dense spindle cell areas, similar to primitive skeletal muscle arising from embryonic mesenchyme (Figure 124I-5). Terminally differentiated rhabdomyoblasts contain cross-striations and resemble myofibers. Maturation, or terminal differentiation, of rhabdomyoblasts occurs following combination chemotherapy and radiation.[17] On the other hand, some rhabdomyosarcomas possess a latent capacity for myogenesis that is evident only with immunohistochemical stains.[18]

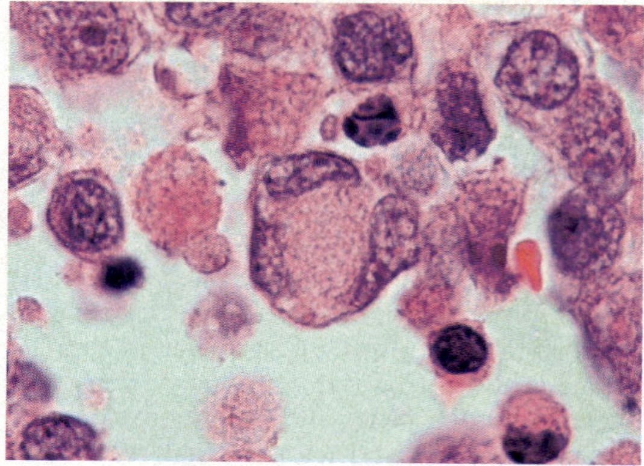

Figure 124I-4 Alveolar rhabdomyosarcoma: giant rhabdomyoblast and small, immature, discohesive blue cells.

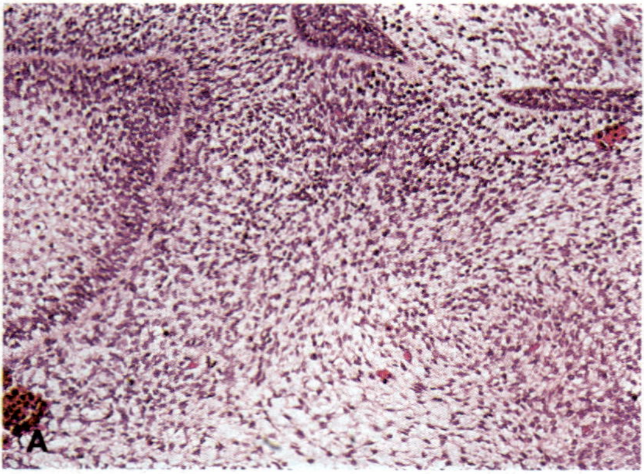

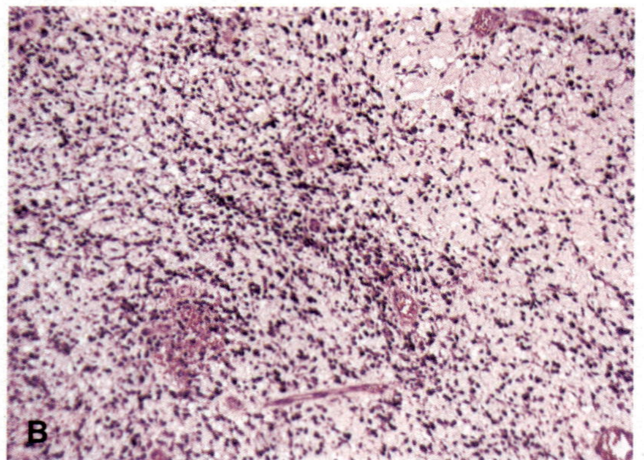

Figure 124I-5 **A,** Embryonic muscle at 12 weeks' gestation. **B,** Embryonal rhabdomyosarcoma.

Retinoblastoma, a rare intraocular childhood cancer, derives from primitive photoreceptor cells that express photoreceptor cell-associated proteins.[19] The average age at retinoblastoma discovery is 24 months. Histologically, retinoblastomas are composed of immature neuroblasts that focally may differentiate into well-formed rosettes (Flexner-Wintersteiner rosettes), which are considered an attempt of the tumor to form photoreceptor cells. Further differentiation is manifested by the formation of fleurettes, a further recapitulation of retinal epithelium.

Hepatoblastoma is another classic embryonic neoplasm. Similar to the preceding embryonic tumors, the peak incidence of hepatoblastoma is in early childhood, with 80 to 90% presenting before 5 years of age.[20] Hepatoblastoma mimics the developing fetal or embryonal liver and, like Wilms' tumor, exhibits a large range of histopathologic patterns that include mesenchymal and epithelial elements (Figure 124I-6). The epithelial component can display a range of differentiation including small primitive "anaplastic" cells, poorly differentiated "embryonal" cells, well-differentiated "fetal" hepatocytes, and large atypical hepatocytes. The mesenchymal component is usually represented by osteoid-appearing matrix and, less commonly, cartilage and skeletal muscle. In 80 to 90% of cases, there is a dramatic increase in serum alpha-fetoprotein because of its secretion by the tumor cells in a manner similar to fetal hepatocytes; patients with elevated levels have a better outcome than those with normal ones.[21]

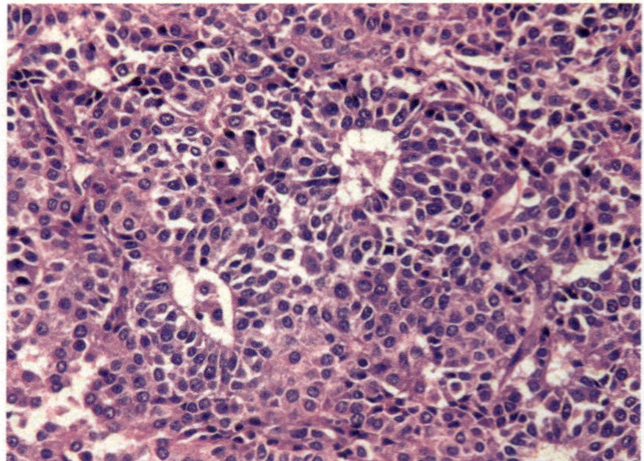

Figure 124I-6 Hepatoblastoma resembling embryonal liver.

Pancreatoblastoma is an extremely rare childhood tumor and again tends to present in young children.[22] It also recapitulates normal organogenesis, in this case by acinar differentiation, squamoid cell nests, and occasional endocrine cells. A mesenchymal component of cartilage and bone may also be present. Eosinophilic acinar cells contain zymogen granules demonstrated by electron microscopy.[23] Other rare embryonic neoplasms of childhood that recapitulate developing organs are sialoblastoma, a distinctive infantile tumor of salivary gland, and pleuropulmonary blastoma of lung, a primitive tumor of the thorax. Sialoblastomas are composed of nests of primitive epidermoid cells embedded in a fibrous stroma, architecturally similar to the embryonic salivary gland.[24] Pleuropulmonary blastomas are composed of blastemal and mesenchymal elements that resemble embryonic lung at the pseudoglandular stage of development.[25]

DISTINCT MORPHOLOGIC FEATURES

Some pediatric cancers have unique morphologic features that are not shared with adult malignancies and should be classified based on histology rather than by the site of the tumor. Table 124I-2 lists some examples of this phenomenon. Pediatric renal neoplasms often exhibit special distinguishing histolo-

Table 124I-2 Examples of Pediatric Neoplasms with Unique Morphologic Appearances
Clear cell sarcoma of the kidney
Malignant rhabdoid tumor
Congenital mesoblastic nephroma
Melanotic neuroectodermal tumor
Fibrolamellar carcinoma of the liver
Inclusion body fibromatosis

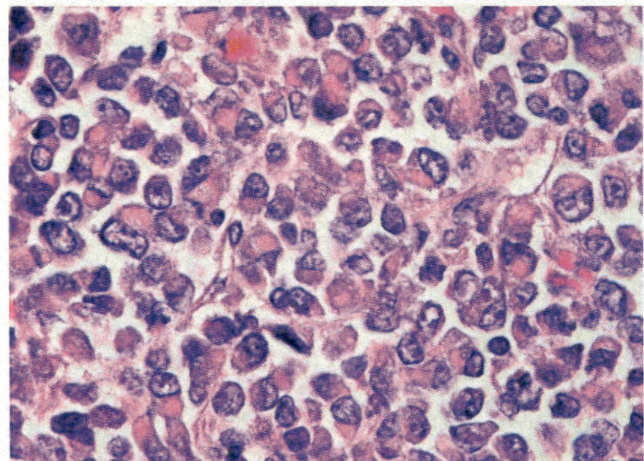

Figure 124I-7 Malignant rhabdoid tumor composed of cells with eccentric nuclei, prominent nucleoli, and hyaline cytoplasmic inclusions.

gies. Examples include clear cell sarcoma, rhabdoid tumor (Figure 124I-7), and mesoblastic nephroma. Beckwith and Palmer originally recognized the unique features of clear cell sarcomas and rhabdoid tumors and characterized them as special forms of Wilms' tumor.[26] In their retrospective analysis of National Wilms' Tumor Study cases treated with uniform therapy, they realized that certain recurring histologic features differed from those of typical Wilms' tumors and were associated with poor outcome independent of stage. These features do not recapitulate embryonic nephrogenesis, as do Wilms' tumors, but instead have an identity based purely on their unique morphology. Mesoblastic nephroma, also known as congenital mesoblastic nephroma, was also initially thought to represent a histologic variant of non-nephrogenic Wilms' tumor.[27] Subsequently, it has been classified as a benign fetal tumor with unique clinical or prognostic features, totally different from Wilms' tumor.[28]

A pertinent non-renal pediatric neoplasm with a unique histology is fibrolamellar carcinoma, a distinctive morphologic variant of hepatocellular carcinoma. It occurs predominantly in adolescents without underlying cirrhosis, fibrosis, viral infection, or metabolic abnormality and has a favorable outcome.[29] Fibrolamellar carcinoma is distinguished from adult hepatocellular carcinoma by its distinctive pattern of large acidophilic cells embedded in a fibrous stroma, and it is noted for its differing clinical behavior and hypothesized relationship to nodular hyperplasia (Figure 124I-8).

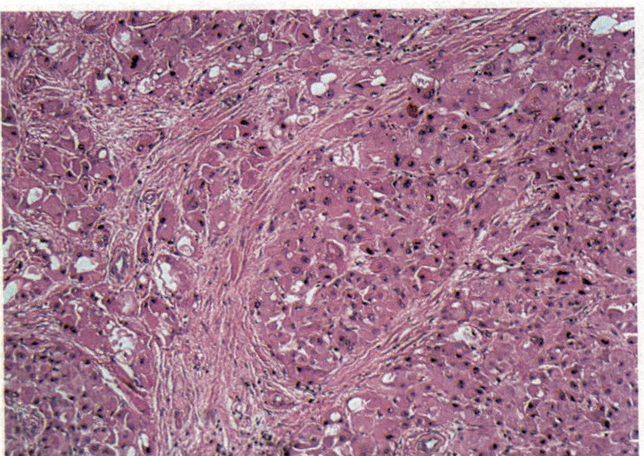

Figure 124I-8 Fibrolamellar variant of hepatocellular carcinoma with large polygonal hepatocytes and bands of fibrosis.

Another morphologically distinctive tumor is melanotic neuroectodermal tumor. It usually occurs in infants and very young children and behaves in a relatively benign fashion in spite of its alarming histology.[30] Melanotic neuroectodermal tumors contain a mixture of primitive neuroectodermal cells and neuroepithelial cells with melanin production and exhibit a unique immunohistochemical profile with positivity for epithelial, mesenchymal, neural, and melanocytic markers.[30] In adults, these features might lead to a diagnosis of malignant melanoma, but in children they connote a much more benign prognosis.[31]

Another distinctive pediatric lesion, inclusion body fibromatosis (also known as digital or infantile fibromatosis), occurs almost exclusively in the fingers and toes of infants and young children.[32] In addition to these distinctive clinical features, the lesions contain characteristic distinct perinuclear inclusions present in some of the constituent fibroblastic cells, which extend from the overlying epidermis into the subcutaneous tissue.[33] As with the other lesions noted above, rare examples occur in adults, but the rarity of these occurrences makes them worthy of case reports.[34]

The tumors in the preceding section highlight the uniqueness of some pediatric tumors by virtue of their distinct morphology and clinical history. This histologically distinct category has a potpourri of biologic bases. Some lesions have a distinctive fusion protein created by a unique translocation, such as the t(12;15) seen in cellular forms of mesoblastic nephroma.[35] Still others, much as rhabdoid tumor, exhibit deletions in key developmental genes. Others, such as the melanotic neuroectodermal tumor, have no biologically distinguishing features discovered to date.

FREQUENT OCCURRENCE OF UNDIFFERENTIATED TUMORS

Undifferentiated tumors occur frequently in childhood, and as a group, account for a more prominent proportion of neoplasms than in adults. The term "small round cell tumor" has been applied to these entities when they form sheets of malignant cells with high nuclear-cytoplasmic ratio and no differentiation. Table 124I-3 lists the most commonly encountered small round cell tumors of childhood. Blast cell leukemias comprise the great majority of childhood hematologic malignancies and in conceptual parallel, small round cell tumors constitute approximately 20% of childhood malignant solid tumors. Clinical behavior, prognostic implication, and therapeutic approach can be significantly different among small round cell tumors requiring precise diagnosis. Because of the primitive nature of the cells, multiple diagnostic approaches, supported by the clinical impression, are often required. In addition to routine histology, ancillary studies may include immunohistochemistry, electron microscopy, cytogenetics, and molecular genetics.

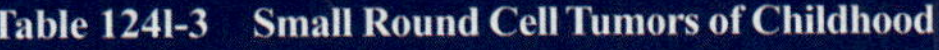

Table 124I-3 Small Round Cell Tumors of Childhood

Neuroblastoma
Ewing's sarcoma/peripheral primitive neuroectodermal tumor
Rhabdomyosarcoma
Non-Hodgkin's lymphoma
Desmoplastic small round cell tumor
Osteosarcoma, small cell type
Blastemal Wilms' tumor
Small cell variants of malignant peripheral nerve sheath tumor
Synovial sarcoma
Undifferentiated sarcoma
Extramedullary leukemia

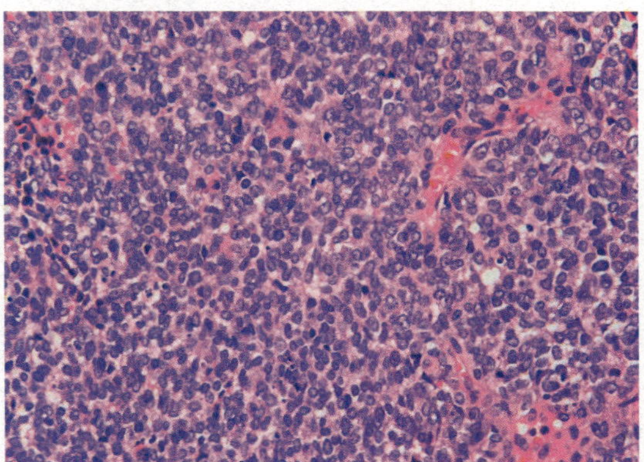

Figure 124I-9 Ewing sarcoma: undifferentiated small round cell tumor.

The Ewing sarcoma family of tumors (ie, peripheral primitive neuroectodermal tumor [PNET], Askin tumor, and Ewing sarcoma) is a prominent subset of undifferentiated malignant childhood neoplasms (Figure 124I-9). Their content ranges from small, uniform round cells growing in no specific pattern to larger cells focally arranged in Homer Wright pseudorosettes. These tumors comprise perhaps the archetypal "small round blue cell tumor" of childhood and until recently were diagnosed primarily by means of clinical setting and pathologic exclusion. All members of this tumor family usually possess an identical chromosomal translocation, the t(11;22)(q24;q12), and express a relatively unique surface marker termed CD99. The biologic evidence thus indicates that these lesions comprise a single entity with a morphologic spectrum of differentiation, with PNET representing the most differentiated form and Ewing sarcoma the most primitive.

Despite great advances in molecular biology and ancillary techniques, the most important component of small cell tumor diagnosis remains the routine microscopic examination. One must recognize architectural patterns, including fibrosis, a myxoid background, pseudoalveolar spaces, tumor rosettes and pseudorosettes, and vascular proliferation. Also important are unique cytologic features such as the size and shape of nuclei, cytoplasmic features, mitotic and karyorrhectic bodies, and most important, the presence of focally differentiated cells such as rhabdomyoblasts.

Immunohistochemical studies have been a major tool in discriminating small round cell tumors.[36] Certain tumors express specific markers in a combination that may help in diagnosis. Interpretation of immunohistochemical studies requires critical assessment to ensure diagnostic accuracy. Interpretation difficulties may be encountered due to staining and fixation artifacts, immunologic cross-reactivity between certain tumors, loss of staining in poorly differentiated forms, and aberrant expression of antibodies in others.

The advent of immunohistochemistry has decreased reliance on ultrastructural examination by electron microscopy (EM). Undifferentiated pediatric neoplasms, however, still may require electron microscopic examination to resolve diagnostic uncertainty. EM can be particularly important in cases with unusual immunologic reactivity on immunostaining, and some authors claim that EM yields better accuracy than immunohistochemistry.[37,38]

MOLECULAR ABERRATIONS IN CERTAIN PEDIATRIC TUMORS

Many childhood cancers are associated with genetic aberrations or genetic diseases. Some childhood tumors have persistent chromosomal translocations that involve a single somatic cell at the early stage of tumorigenesis. Fusion genes biologically tend to characterize a group of primitive small round cell tumors of childhood (Table 124I-4). These genes arise by chromosomal fusion resulting from either translocation or inversion, and they constitute a group of unique genetic sequences not found in non-neoplastic cells. In most cases, these fusions affect the cell cycle and result in unrestrained growth impulses leading to tumorigenesis.[39] They occur frequently in both solid and hematologic malignancies that contain primitive cells. Genetic fusions are by no means unique to pediatric tumors but they tend to be more consistent than those seen in adult neoplasms. Moreover, they have important indications for our understanding of the biology of childhood small cell tumors, as well as implications for diagnosis and treatment.[40]

The use of molecular markers as diagnostic and prognostic tools has been increased dramatically.[41] Examples include *EWSR1/FLI1* fusion and t(11;22)(q24;q12) in Ewing sarcoma/primitive neuroectodermal tumor, the *PAX3/FOXOIA* fusion and t(2;13)(q35;q14) in alveolar rhabdomyosarcoma, and the *SSX/SYT* fusion and t(X;18)(p11.2;q11.2) in synovial sarcoma. Cytogenetic technique was initially the most commonly used technique in detecting these abnormalities. Currently, the use of reverse transcriptase-polymerase chain reaction (RT-PCR) and in situ hybridization has made investigation of these molecular abnormalities more readily accessible and they are becoming a standard component of our diagnostic armamentarium.

Other pediatric tumors are associated with point mutations, genome deletions, and other forms of genetic damage. These tumors can be a part of genetic disorder or can occur sporadically. Table 124I-5 lists some genes involved in inherited cancer syndromes.[42] The following tumors are examples of the different types of molecular aberrations seen in pediatric tumors.

Genetically, rhabdomyosarcomas are associated with two important molecular events that differ among the subtypes of embryonal and alveolar tumors. Loss of heterozygosity characterizes the former group, whereas *PAX3/FOXOIA* fusion gene formation characterizes the latter.[43] Loss of heterozygosity of chromosome 11p15, the locus associated with Beckwith–Wiedemann syndrome, characterizes not only many embryonal rhabdomyosarcomas but also other embryonal neoplasms such as hepatoblastoma, Wilms' tumor and pancreatoblastoma.[44] A closely related genetic phenomenon, parental imprinting, also appears to affect this group of neoplasms causing failure of transcription without mutations in the genetic code.[45] A combination of inherited mutations in cancer genes from one parent and imprinting from the other essentially results in total absence of gene function. Loss of imprinting can have the opposite effect of increased genetic dosing.[46] The reciprocal translocation t(2;13)(q35;q14) is specific for alveolar rhabdomyosarcoma,[41,43,45] where the t(2;13) fusion joins the *PAX3* gene sequence with *FOXOIA* gene.[47,48] Variant chromosomal aberrations, all involving chromosome 13, have also been reported in this tumor[49–52]; primarily these involve PAX7, located on chromosome 1.[41,43,45]

The large majority of Ewing sarcoma/peripheral neuroectodermal tumors exhibit t(11;22)(q24;q12), whereas other tumors show other molecular aberrations. This translocation results in a unique fusion gene uniting the *FLI1* gene on chromosome 11 and the *EWSR1* gene on chromosome 22. In a minority of cases, other *ETS* family genes, such as *ERG*, form the *EWSR1* fusions seen in these tumors.[53]

Inherited cases of retinoblastoma are a classic example of tumors associated with constitutional mutation of a tumor suppressor gene, are commonly bilateral, and may be associated with pineoblastomas and other midline intracranial tumors (trilateral retinoblastoma).[54] The survivors of these tumors have a significant increase in the incidence of other nonocular tumors, most commonly soft tissue sarcomas, particularly following radiation therapy. Investigation into the genetics of this particular group of tumors paved the way for discoveries of tumor-suppressor genes, which encode proteins important to maintenance of the cell cycle.[55] Inherited mutations and deletions of these "anti-oncogenes" are an important factor in the development of many types of childhood cancers, particularly the "embryonic" neoplasms. The combination of mutations and genetic imprinting aberrations is a potent mechanism for childhood tumorigenesis. These comprise two-step combinations that lead to childhood cancer as elegantly stated by Knudson and Strong in a classic hypothesis.[56] In distinction, typical adult cancers have a multi-step combination of genetic events that lead to tumorigenesis.[57]

Neuroblastomas, biologically, can be divided into three major groups.[58] Chromosomal multiplication and hyperdiploidy characterize one group associated with a good clinical prognosis. Hyperdiploid adult tumors, on the other hand, typically have a worse prognosis.[59,60] In neuroblastomas, gene amplification affecting *MYC-N* characterizes a group of highly aggressive neoplasms with a poor prognosis. *MYC* gene amplification, however,

Table 124I-4 Representative Genetic Fusions in Small Round Cell Tumors of Childhood

Tumor	Fusion
Ewing's sarcoma/PNET	*EWSR1/FLI1, EWSR1/ERG*
Alveolar rhabdomyosarcoma	*PAX3/FOXO1A, PAX7/FOXO1A*
Synovial sarcoma	*SSX1/SYT, SSX2/SYT*
Desmoplastic small cell tumor	*EWSR1/WT1*
Burkitt's lymphoma	*MYC/IGH, MYC/IGKC, MYCC/IGL*
Lymphoblastic lymphoma	*LOMI/TCRB*
Acute lymphoblastic leukemia	*PBX1/TCF3, MLLT2/MLL, ABL1/BCR, LOMI/TCRB, MYC/IGH*
Acute myeloblastic leukemia (AML M2)	*CBFA2TI/RUNX1*
Acute promyelocytic leukemia (AML M3)	*PML/RARA*
Acute myelomonocytic leukemia (AML M4)	*MYH11/CBFB*
Acute monoblastic leukemia (AML M5)	*MLLT3/MLL*

PNET = primitive neuroectodermal tumor.

Table 124I-5 Some of the Genes Involved in Inherited Cancer Syndrome

Gene	Classification	Tumors	Cancer Syndrome
TP53	Tumor suppressor	Osteosarcoma, rhabdomyosarcoma, leukemia, breast carcinoma, brain tumors, adrenocortical carcinoma	Li–Fraumeni syndrome
RB1	Tumor suppressor	Retinoblastoma, osteosarcoma, pineal tumors	Familial retinoblastoma
WT1	Tumor suppressor	Wilms' tumor	WAGR syndrome, Denys–Drash syndrome
NF1	Tumor suppressor	Neurofibroma, malignant peripheral nerve sheath tumor, leukemia	Neurofibromatosis type 1
NF2	Tumor suppressor	Acoustic neuroma, meningioma, schwannoma, ependymoma	Neurofibromatosis type 2
VHL	Tumor suppressor	Renal cell carcinoma, vascular tumors, pheochromocytoma	von Hippel–Lindau syndrome
RET	Oncogene	Medullary carcinoma of the thyroid, parathyroid carcinoma, pheochromocytoma	Multiple endocrine neoplasia type 2

Table 124I-6 Some Syndromes and Congenital Malformations Associated with Childhood Tumors

Congenital Malformation	Tumor
Beckwith–Wiedemann syndrome	Wilms' tumor, adrenocortical adenoma and carcinoma, hepatoblastoma, pancreatoblastoma
Central nervous system defects	Central nervous system tumors
Immunodeficiency disorders	Lymphoma
Genitourinary system anomalies and Perlman syndrome	Nephroblastomatosis, Wilms' tumor
Hirschsprung disease	Neuroblastoma
Tuberous sclerosis	Cardiac rhabdomyoma, angiomyolipoma, astrocytoma

Table 124I-7 Examples of Chromosomal Abnormalities Associated with Childhood Tumors

Chromosomal Defect	Childhood Tumor
del 11p13	Wilms' tumor
del 13q14	Retinoblastoma
del 1p32p36, double minute	Neuroblastoma
Trisomy 18	Wilms' tumor
Trisomy 21 (Down syndrome)	Myelodysplastic syndrome and leukemia
Gonadal dysgenesis	Gonadoblastoma, germinoma
Klinefelter's syndrome	Teratoma

is seen also in some relatively common adult cancers and so does not necessarily distinguish them from pediatric neoplasms.[61] Similar to neuroblastoma, hyperdiploid forms of acute lymphoblastic leukemia (ALL) tend to have a good prognosis.[62]

Wilms' tumors are associated with at least two major biologic events: deletion of a tumor-suppressor gene, *WT1*, associated with the Wilm's tumor, aniridia, genitourinary abnormalities or gonadoblastoma, and mental retardation (WAGR) syndrome, or allele-specific alterations at a gene associated with Beckwith–Wiedemann syndrome, an overgrowth syndrome associated with a variety of congenital malformations.[63,64] Loss of heterozygosity of a tumor suppressor gene at 16q appears to be a later event that enhances the malignant potential of these tumors.[65]

Chromosomal translocations in childhood leukemia involve a diverse set of genes whose fusions are associated with tumors of specific cell lineages. This includes the 11q23 translocations of infantile ALL and AML, the *TEL/AML1, E2A/PBX1*, and *BCR/ABL* fusions of B-cell precursor ALL, the *SIL/SCL* fusion of T-cell precursor ALL, and the *AML1/ETO* fusion of AML. These translocations appear to be the result of errors in DNA breakage and repair mechanisms that may be active in prenatal hematopoiesis. Gene fusions of various types may occur often during embryogenesis and fetal development, but a strict set of requirements must be met for them to be functional in tumorigenesis. Thus, childhood leukemia is a relatively rare event (although still the most common childhood neoplasm). Screening data from RT-PCR analysis of blood smears indicates however, that the fusions detailed above occur relatively frequently and can be found in up to 100% of normal neonatal blood spots. Thus, secondary events must be necessary for the activation of the stem cells containing these aberrations. This supposition conforms to the "two-hit" hypothesis of Knudson and Strong mentioned above.[66]

Similar data regarding pediatric solid tumors are lacking, but a conditional model of the *PAX3/FKHR* fusion gene also indicates that secondary events are necessary for tumorigenesis. Targeted fusion gene activation in differentiated muscle produces alveolar rhabdomyosarcoma-like tumors at a relatively low frequency unless the antioncogenes *Trp53* or *Ink4a/ARF* are secondarily disrupted.[67]

Another factor likely to play a role in production of childhood lymphomas is the initial exposure of infants to antigenic stimulation. Recombination of the immunoglobulin genes, a normal mechanism in this process, likely leads to fusions with proto-oncogenes during the process of DNA breakage and repair. These fusions in turn are associated with B-cell lymphomas and leukemias. Epidemiologic evidence suggests that abnormal exposure of the nascent immune system to childhood infections increases the likelihood of this occurrence.[66,68] T-cell receptor fusions and their associated leukemia/lymphomas may arise through a similar mechanism.

ASSOCIATION WITH CONGENITAL MALFORMATION

Children with congenital malformations are at increased risk of developing cancer.[69] The association with congenital malformations occurs relatively frequently in childhood neoplasms and further distinguishes them from adult tumors.[70] This frequent occurrence suggests that childhood neoplasia is more akin to teratogenesis or dysontogenesis as a process than it is to adult cancer formation. Table 124I-6 lists some examples of this phenomenon.

Patients with chromosomal abnormalities also have increased risk of developing tumors. A classic example is Down syndrome and its association with myelodysplastic syndrome and leukemia. In addition, patients with gonadal dysgenesis are at risk of developing gonadoblastoma and germinoma. Table 124I-7 lists examples of chromosomal abnormalities associated with childhood tumors.

Several hereditary syndromes characterized by DNA repair defects are associated with increased risk for malignancies. Examples include xeroderma pigmentosum (skin tumors), ataxia telangiectasia (lymphoma), Fanconi anemia (leukemia), and Bloom syndrome (leukemia).

INFREQUENT ASSOCIATION OF CHILDHOOD NEOPLASMS WITH PRECURSOR LESIONS

As a general rule, the origin of frank adult neoplasia proceeds from progressive somatic genetic dysfunction that affects incipient precursor lesions. Cervical neoplasia forms the paradigm for this model of cancer evolution, and today we recognize similar processes in many other adult cancers. Examples include the adenomatous polyp to cancer sequence of colonic neoplasia and the intraductal to infiltrative pattern of breast tumors. In general, recognizable precursors are missing in the bulk of pediatric tumors. Genetic evidence, however, indicates that stem cells with latent tumorigenic properties may be present in unaffected children.[66]

Some childhood tumors, usually embryonic tumors, arise from a malformative, immature organ field that persists after birth or after the expected organ development period. These immature embryonal tissues may evolve into malignant tumors and therefore are designated precursor lesions. They fundamentally differ from precursor lesions of adults by their close resemblance to embryonic tissues. Adult lesions, on the other hand, are recognized by cytologic and architectural atypia.

The most famous and well-documented examples of pediatric precursor lesions are nephrogenic rests and neuroblastoma in situ. About one-third of Wilms' tumors are associated with precursor embryonal lesions, termed "nephrogenic rests," present in the adjacent kidney.[71] Their presence has also been demonstrated in 1% of neonatal autopsies. These nephrogenic rests are composed of immature blastemal tissue that resembles embryonic kidney. Multiple or diffuse forms have been called nephroblastomatosis. Beckwith classified the nephrogenic rests as hyperplastic and neoplastic based on their configuration and spatial relationship to the adjacent kidney.[71] These lesions contain DNA sequence abnormalities also recognized in full-blown Wilms' tumors.[72]

Neuroblastoma in situ, although rare, is another well-known example of these precursor lesions.[73] Beckwith and Perrin described neuroblastoma in situ as small lesions incidentally found at autopsy in the adrenal medulla of neonates and infants who died from other causes.[74] The next most common sites include abdominal sympathetic ganglia, followed by the sympathetic ganglia of the thorax, neck, and pelvis. Beckwith and Perrin predicted that most of the neuroblastomas in situ regress during early infancy and only rarely become full-fledged neuroblastoma. With the onset of pre-natal screening by means of ultrasonography, neonatal neuroblastomas have been detected with much greater frequency.[75] Because of the usual regression of these lesions, the best clinical management has become an issue. The biologic and clinical characteristics of these lesions indicate that mass screening is unnecessary and that genetic progression into full-blown cancer typically occurs with lesions arising after birth.[76,77]

SUMMARY

This brief review only superficially touches on a full comparison between tumors that arise in adults and those presenting during childhood. Pediatric neoplasms differ in a number of fundamental ways that separate them as a class from adult cancers. These features include their histologic and biologic characteristics, frequent resemblance to embryonal tissues and composition of undifferentiated cells, consistent molecular aberrations, association with congenital malformation, and relative paucity of morphologically recognizable precursor lesions. Proper diagnosis and management of childhood cancers require recognition of these unique features and are thus best accomplished by pathologists and clinicians familiar with them. Thankfully, survival rates for childhood cancer have markedly improved during the past several decades, and proper clinical management has been key to this success. Liberal use of pediatric specialists is therefore advisable when generalists are confronted with the many pathologic and clinical issues that arise when dealing with this group of diseases.

REFERENCES

1. Jemal A, Tiwari RC, Murray T, et al. Cancer statistics, 2004. CA Cancer J Clin 2004;54:8–29.
2. Steliarova-Foucher E, Stiller C, et al. International classification of childhood cancer, third edition. Cancer 2005;103:1457–67.
3. Willis RA. The Borderland of embryology and pathology. 2 ed. London: Butterworths; 1962.
4. Parham DM. Neuroectodermal and neuroendocrine tumors principally seen in children. Am J Clin Pathol 2001;115(Suppl):113–28.
5. Shimada H, Umehara S, Monobe Y, et al. International neuroblastoma pathology classification for prognostic evaluation of patients with peripheral neuroblastic tumors: a report from the Children's Cancer Group. Cancer 2001;92:2451–61.
6. Shimada H, Ambros IM, Dehner LP, et al. The International Neuroblastoma Pathology Classification (the Shimada system). Cancer 1999;86:364–72.
7. Moody AM, Norman AR, Tait D. Paediatric tumours in the adult population—the experience of the Royal Marsden Hospital 1974–1990. Med Pediatr Oncol 1996;26:153–9.
8. Koeller KK, Rushing EJ. From the archives of the AFIP: medulloblastoma: a comprehensive review with radiologic-pathologic correlation. Radiographics 2003;23:1613–37.
9. Rorke LB, Trojanowski JQ, Lee VM, et al. Primitive neuroectodermal tumors of the central nervous system. Brain Pathol 1997;7:765–84.
10. Mierau GW, Beckwith JB, Weeks DA. Ultrastructure and histogenesis of the renal tumors of childhood: an overview. Ultrastruct Pathol 1987;11:313–33.
11. Webber BL, Parham DM, Drake LG, Wilimas JA. Renal tumors in childhood. Pathol Annu 1992;27:191–232.
12. Vujanic GM, Sandstedt B, Harms D, et al. Revised International Society of Paediatric Oncology (SIOP) working classification of renal tumors of childhood. Med Pediatr Oncol 2002;38:79–82.
13. Beckwith JB, Zuppan CE, Browning NG, et al. Histological analysis of aggressiveness and responsiveness in Wilms' tumor. [Review] [20 refs]. Med Pediatr Oncol 1996;27:422–8.
14. Park CM, Kim WS, Cheon JE, et al. Teratoid Wilms tumor in childhood: CT and ultrasonographic appearances. Abdom Imaging 2003;28:440–3.
15. Terenziani M, Spreafico F, Collini P, et al. Adult Wilms' tumor: A monoinstitutional experience and a review of the literature. Cancer 2004;101:289–93.
16. Crist WM, Anderson JR, Meza JL, et al. Intergroup rhabdomyosarcoma study-IV: results for patients with nonmetastatic disease. J Clin Oncol 2001;19:3091–102.
17. Coffin CM, Rulon J, Smith L, et al. Pathologic features of rhabdomyosarcoma before and after treatment: a clinicopathologic and immunohistochemical analysis. Mod Pathol 1997;10:1175–87.
18. Wijnaendts LCD, van der Linden JC, van Unnik AJM, et al. Histologic classification of childhood rhabdomyosarcomas: relationship with clinical parameters and prognosis. Hum Pathol 1994;25:900–7.
19. Dyer MA, Bremner R. The search for the retinoblastoma cell of origin. Nat Rev Cancer 2005;5:91–101.
20. Emre S, McKenna GJ. Liver tumors in children. Pediatr Transplant 2004;8:632–8.
21. Fuchs J, Rydzynski J, Von SD, et al. Pretreatment prognostic factors and treatment results in children with hepatoblastoma: a report from the German Cooperative Pediatric Liver Tumor Study HB 94. Cancer 2002;95:172–82.
22. Shorter NA, Glick RD, Klimstra DS, et al. Malignant pancreatic tumors in childhood and adolescence: The Memorial Sloan-Kettering experience, 1967 to present. J Pediatr Surg 2002;37:887–92.
23. Cooper JE, Lake BD. Use of enzyme histochemistry in the diagnosis of pancreatoblastoma. Histopathology 1989;15:407–14.
24. Garrido A, Humphrey G, Squire RS, Nishikawa H. Sialoblastoma. Br J Plast Surg 2000;53:697–9.
25. Hill DA. USCAP Specialty Conference: case 1-type I pleuropulmonary blastoma. Pediatr Dev Pathol 2005;8:77–84.
26. Beckwith JB, Palmer NF. Histopathology and prognosis of Wilms tumors: results from the First National Wilms' Tumor Study. Cancer 1978;41:1937–48.
27. Bolande RP, Brough AJ, Izant RJ Jr. Congenital mesoblastic nephroma of infancy. A report of eight cases and the relationship to Wilms' tumor. Pediatrics 1967;40:272–8.
28. Glick RD, Hicks MJ, Nuchtern JG, et al. Renal tumors in infants less than 6 months of age. J Pediatr Surg 2004;39:522–5.
29. El-Serag HB, Davila JA. Is fibrolamellar carcinoma different from hepatocellular carcinoma? A US population-based study. Hepatology 2004;39:798–803.
30. Barrett AW, Morgan M, Ramsay AD, et al. A clinicopathologic and immunohistochemical analysis of melanotic neuroectodermal tumor of infancy. Oral Surg Oral Med Oral Pathol Oral Radiol Endod 2002;93:688–98.
31. Banerjee SS, Menasce LP, Eyden BP, Brain AN. Malignant melanoma showing ganglioneuroblastic differentiation: report of a unique case. Am J Surg Pathol 1999;23:582–8.
32. Sungur N, Kilinc H, Ozdemir R, et al. Infantile digital fibromatosis: an unusual localization. J Pediatr Surg 2001;36:1587–9.
33. Yun K. Infantile digital fibromatosis. Immunohistochemical and ultrastructural observations of cytoplasmic inclusions. Cancer 1988;61:500–7.
34. Viale G, Doglioni C, Iuzzolino P, et al. Infantile digital fibromatosis-like tumour (inclusion body fibromatosis) of adulthood: report of two cases with ultrastructural and immunocytochemical findings. Histopathology 1988;12:415–24.
35. Knezevich SR, Garnett MJ, Pysher TJ, et al. ETV6-NTRK3 gene fusions and trisomy 11 establish a histogenetic link between mesoblastic nephroma and congenital fibrosarcoma. Cancer Res 1998;58:5046–8.
36. Devoe K, Weidner N. Immunohistochemistry of small round-cell tumors. Semin Diagn Pathol 2000;17:216–24.
37. Mierau GW, Berry PJ, Orsini EN. Small round cell neoplasms: can electron microscopy and immunohistochemical studies accurately classify them. Ultrastruct Pathol 1985;9:99–111.
38. Mierau GW, Berry PJ, Malott RL, Weeks DA. Appraisal of the comparative utility of immunohistochemistry and electron microscopy in the diagnosis of childhood round cell tumors. Ultrastruct Pathol 1996;20:507–17.
39. Barr FG. The malevolence of matchmaking [news; comment]. Nat Genet 1996;12:113–4.
40. Tomescu O, Barr FG. Chromosomal translocations in sarcomas: prospects for therapy. Trends Mol Med 2001;7:554–9.
41. Bennicelli JL, Barr FG. Chromosomal translocations and sarcomas. Curr Opin Oncol 2002;14:412–9.
42. Ganjavi H, Malkin D. Genetics of childhood cancer. Clin Orthop 2002;401:75–87.
43. Xia SJ, Pressey JG, Barr FG. Molecular pathogenesis of rhabdomyosarcoma. Cancer Biol Ther 2002;1:97–104.
44. Koufos A, Hansen MF, Copeland NG, et al. Loss of heterozygosity in three embryonal tumours suggests a common pathogenetic mechanism. Nature 1985;316:330–4.
45. Anderson J, Gordon A, Pritchard-Jones K, Shipley J. Genes, chromosomes, and rhabdomyosarcoma. Genes Chromosomes Cancer 1999;26:275–85.
46. Ravenel JD, Broman KW, Perlman EJ, et al. Loss of imprinting of insulin-like growth factor-II (IGF2) gene in distinguishing specific biologic subtypes of Wilms tumor. JNCI 2001;93:1698–703.
47. Barr FG. Fusions involving paired box and fork head family transcription factors in the pediatric cancer alveolar rhabdomyosarcoma. Curr Top Microbiol Immunol 1997;220:113–29.
48. Sorensen PH, Lynch JC, Qualman SJ, et al. PAX3-FKHR and PAX7-FKHR gene fusions are prognostic indicators in alveolar rhabdomyosarcoma: a report from the Children's Oncology Group. J Clin Oncol 2002;20:2672–9.
49. Dal Cin P, Brock P, Sayed Aly M, et al. A variant (2;13) translocation in rhabdomyosarcoma. Cancer Genet Cytogenet 1991;55:191–5.
50. Douglass EC, Rowe ST, Valentine M, et al. Variant translocations of chromosome 13 in alveolar rhabdomyosarcoma. Genes Chromosom Cancer 1991;3:480–2.
51. Harrison CJ, Johnson PRE, Yin JAL, Bhavnani M. Alveolar rhabdomyosarcoma with del(13q14). Cancer Genet Cytogenet 1991;55:257–9.
52. Voullaire LE, Petrovic V, Sheffield LJ, Campbell P. Two forms of ring 13 in a child with rhabdomyosarcoma. Am J Med Genet 1991;39:285–7.
53. De Alava E, Gerald WL. Molecular biology of the Ewing's sarcoma/primitive neuroectodermal tumor family [review]. J Clin Oncol 2000;18:204–13.
54. Brodeur GM. Genetics of embryonal tumours of childhood: retinoblastoma, Wilms' tumour and neuroblastoma. Cancer Surv 1995;25:67–99.
55. Knudson AG. Antioncogenes and human cancer. Proc Natl Acad Sci U S A 1993;90:10914–21.
56. Knudson AG, Jr., Strong LC. Mutation and cancer: a model for Wilms' tumor of the kidney. J Natl Cancer Inst 1972;48:313–24.
57. Weinberg RA. Tumor suppressor genes. Science 1991;254:1138–46.
58. Brodeur GM. Neuroblastoma: biological insights into a clinical enigma. Nat Rev Cancer 2003;3:203–16.
59. Maris JM, Matthay KK. Molecular biology of neuroblastoma. J Clin Oncol 1999;17:2264–79.
60. Herman CJ. Cytometric DNA analysis in the management of cancer. Clinical and laboratory considerations. Cancer 1992;69(6 Suppl):1553–6.
61. Makela TP, Saksela K, Alitalo K. Amplification and rearrangement of L-myc in human small-cell lung cancer. Mutat Res 1992;276:307–15.
62. Behm FG. Malignancies of the bone marrow. In: Parham DM, editor. Pediatric neoplasia: morphology and biology. Philadelphia: Lippincott-Raven; 1996. p. 449–504.
63. Grundy P, Coppes MJ, Haber D. Molecular genetics of Wilms tumor. Hematol Oncol Clin North Am 1995;9:1201–15.
64. Jones KP, Grundy PE, Coppes MJ. Recent advances in the genetics of childhood renal cancers: a report of the 3rd International Conference on the Molecular and Clinical Genetics of Childhood Renal Tumors, together with the Mitchell Ross symposium on anaplastic and other high risk embryonal tumors of childhood, 8–10th April 1999, Wistar Institute, Philadelphia, PA. Med Pediatr Oncol 2000;35:126–30.
65. Safford SD, Goyeau D, Freemerman AJ, et al. Fine mapping of Wilms' tumors with 16q loss of heterozygosity localizes the putative tumor suppressor gene to a region of 6.7 megabases. Ann Surg Oncol 2003;10:136–43.
66. Greaves MF, Wiemels J. Origins of chromosome translocations in childhood leukaemia. Nat Rev Cancer 2003;3:639–49.
67. Keller C, Arenkiel BR, Coffin CM, et al. Alveolar rhabdomyosarcomas in conditional Pax3:Fkhr mice: cooperativity of Ink4a/ARF and Trp53 loss of function. Genes Dev 2004;18:2614–26.
68. Goldsby RE, Carroll WL. The molecular biology of pediatric lymphomas. J Pediatr Hematol Oncol 1998;20:282–96.
69. Altmann AE, Halliday JL, Giles GG. Associations between congenital malformations and childhood cancer. A register-based case-control study. Br J Cancer 1998;78:1244–9.
70. Agha MM, Williams JI, Marrett L, et al. Congenital abnormalities and childhood cancer. Cancer 2005;103:1939–48.
71. Beckwith JB, Kiviat NB, Bonadio JF. Nephrogenic rests, nephroblastomatosis, and the pathogenesis of Wilms' tumor. Pediatr Pathol 1990;10:1–36.
72. Hennigar RA, O'Shea PA, Grattan-Smith JD. Clinicopathologic features of nephrogenic rests and nephroblastomatosis. Adv Anat Pathol 2001;8:276–89.
73. Ikeda Y, Lister J, Bouton JM, Buyukpamukcu M. Congenital neuroblastoma, neuroblastoma in situ, and the normal fetal development of the adrenal. J Pediatr Surg 1981;16(4 Suppl 1):636–44.
74. Beckwith JB, Perrin EV. In situ neuroblastoma: a contribution to the natural history of the neural crest tumors. Am J Pathol 1963;43:1089–104.
75. Bessho F. Effects of mass screening on age-specific incidence of neuroblastoma. Int J Cancer 1996;67:520–2.
76. Craft AW, Parker L. Screening for neuroblastoma: 20 years and still no answer [abstract]. Eur J Cancer 1996;32:1540–3.
77. Brodeur GM, Look AT, Shimada H, et al. Biological aspects of neuroblastomas identified by mass screening in Quebec. Med Pediatr Oncol 2001;36:157–9.

124m

Pediatric Bone Tumors

Richard G. Gorlick, MD, FAAP
Mark L. Bernstein, MD, FRCP(C)
Jeffrey A. Toretsky, MD
R. Lor Randall, MD, FACS
Mark C. Gebhardt, MD
Lisa A. Teot, MD
Suzzane Wolden, MD
Neyssa Marina, MD

INTRODUCTION

This chapter will focus on malignant primary bone tumors occurring in pediatric patients and young adults. Malignant primary bone tumors that occur in both younger and older patients have important differences in pathophysiology, presentation, and treatment, and these differences will be highlighted. In pediatric patients, as in adults, metastatic bone lesions are more common than primary bone tumors, but the predominant histologies among pediatric patients include neuroblastoma, lymphoma, and rhabdomyosarcoma.[1–3] Although primary bone tumors are rare, they are the sixth most common malignant neoplasm in children and the third most frequent neoplasm in adolescents and young adults.[4] Malignant bone tumors occur in the United States at an annual rate of approximately 8.7 cases per million children and adolescents younger than 20 years. Only half the bone tumors in childhood are malignant, and of these, osteosarcoma is the most frequent, accounting for approximately 35% of all primary sarcomas of bone. Ewing's sarcoma, the second most frequent primary bone cancer, is more common than osteosarcoma in children younger than 10 years.

OSTEOSARCOMA

Osteosarcoma, the most common primary malignant bone tumor, is composed of spindle cells producing osteoid. It is a highly aggressive neoplasm for which dramatic progress has been made in treatment and outcome during the past several decades. Osteosarcoma is primarily a disease of adolescents and young adults, although it can also occur in older patients.[1]

Presentation The most common clinical presentation is pain with or without an associated soft tissue mass in the involved region of bone. Among young patients, the most common location is the metaphysis of a long bone. Approximately half of all osteosarcomas originate around the knee joint. Involvement of the axial skeleton, most commonly the pelvis, occurs in less than 10% of cases in the pediatric age group.[5]

Similar to other sarcomas in young patients (typically high grade), osteosarcoma metastasizes very early in its evolution. Approximately, 20% of patients present with radiographically detectable metastases, most frequently to the lung. However, virtually all patients have subclinical, microscopic metastasis.[6] Much less frequently, metastases at initial diagnosis occur in other bones, soft tissues, or lymph nodes. When osteosarcoma is widely metastatic, more frequently at recurrence than at the time of initial diagnosis, it can spread to the central nervous system or gastrointestinal tract. Death from osteosarcoma is almost always the result of progressive pulmonary metastasis with respiratory failure, pulmonary hemorrhage, pneumothorax, or superior vena cava obstruction. Other lesions, although extremely painful, are usually not life threatening.[6]

The diagnosis of osteosarcoma is typically suspected by the radiographic appearance of the affected lesion. Osteosarcoma can present as a lytic, sclerotic, or a mixed lytic-sclerotic lesion. As with other malignant tumors of bone, plain films reveal permeative destruction with poorly defined zones of transition with surrounding normal bone and lack of endosteal response. Ossification in the soft tissue in a radial or "sunburst" pattern is classic for osteosarcoma, but is not a sensitive or specific feature. Periosteal new bone formation with lifting of the cortex leads to the appearance of a Codman's triangle. The extent of osteosarcoma in both bone and soft tissue is best appreciated with cross-sectional imaging techniques such as computed tomography or magnetic resonance imaging. The differential diagnosis includes infection and other tumors, including aneurysmal bone cyst, Ewing's sarcoma, and chondrosarcoma. Features such as the eccentric location of the tumor in the metaphyseal portion of the bone and the skeletal location help to distinguish osteosarcoma and Ewing's sarcoma, the second most frequent tumor in this age group. Bony metastases from other primary tumors are less frequent in the young than in adult patients, but must also be considered in the differential.[5]

The diagnosis of osteosarcoma is dependent on a biopsy for histologic examination providing a pathological diagnosis. Osteosarcoma is a pleomorphic, spindle cell tumor that forms an extracellular matrix consisting mostly of osteoid. Rarely, the diagnosis cannot be made on a biopsy because the sample is not representative. When the tumor is removed by definitive surgical resection, it may become possible to confirm the diagnosis.[5]

Patients with osteosarcoma should undergo a staging work-up to determine the extent of disease at presentation (local and distant). Diagnostic studies indicated as part of the evaluation include a radionuclide bone scan, with methylene diphosphonate labeled with technetium-99m, computed tomography of the chest and/or chest radiograph, and magnetic resonance imaging of the primary tumor. The bone scan helps define the extent of the primary tumor as well as a safe margin for surgical planning. Radionuclide bone scanning is also useful in the detection of "skip lesions" within the same bone, as well as distant bone metastases. Routine posteroanterior and lateral radiographs of the chest allow detection of metastases in the majority of cases. CT of the chest is more sensitive in detecting pulmonary metastases and has become the imaging procedure of choice. However, there are false positive results, particularly with smaller lesions.[7] If a reasonable doubt exists that a lesion on CT scan represents metastatic disease, biopsy for confirmation may be indicated.

Successful treatment of osteosarcoma requires the use of systemic chemotherapy. Since many of the agents have acute and long-term toxicity, baseline evaluation prior to initiation of chemotherapy is important. All patients need baseline evaluation of renal function, usually with a creatinine clearance or glomerular filtration rate determination.

Additional studies include baseline cardiac evaluation with either an echocardiogram or a radionuclide scan of cardiac function, a baseline audiogram, as well as sperm banking. Although newer techniques for maintaining fertility in young women are being developed, their indications are not completely established, and, therefore, recommendations cannot be made at the moment.

The most widely used staging system for osteosarcoma is the system developed by Enneking and colleagues based on a retrospective review of cases of primary malignant tumors of bone treated by primary surgical resection.[8] This system categorizes localized malignant bone tumors by grade (low grade, stage I or high grade, stage II) and by local anatomic extent (intracompartmental, A or extracompartmental, B). The compartmental status is determined by whether or not the tumor extends through the cortex. Patients with distant metastases are classified as stage III. There are very few high-grade intramedullary lesions (ie, stage IIA), because most high-grade osteosarcomas break through the cortex early in their natural history. In younger age groups, the vast majority of osteosarcomas are high-grade lesions, hence, virtually all patients are stage IIB or III, distinguished by the presence or absence of detectable metastatic disease.[8]

Epidemiology Osteosarcoma has a bimodal age distribution, with the first peak in the second decade of life during the adolescent growth spurt, and the second among older adults. Osteosarcoma is a rare tumor of children and young adults with an estimated frequency of 4.8 per million.[9] It is estimated that approximately 400 children and adolescents < 20 years are diagnosed each year in the United States. It is extremely rare before the age of 5 years, and the modal age is 16 years for girls and 18 years for boys. Boys are affected more frequently in most series, and the incidence in black children is slightly higher than in whites.[1,5] In older patients, osteosarcoma arises in abnormal bones, such as those affected by long standing Paget's disease.

Pathogenesis There is limited knowledge about the etiology of osteosarcoma. The peak age coincides with a period of rapid bone growth in young people, suggesting a correlation between rapid bone growth and the evolution of osteosarcoma. Other evidence supporting this relationship includes the higher incidence of osteosarcoma in large dog breeds as compared with small breeds, and the earlier peak age in girls as compared with boys, corresponding to the earlier age of their growth spurt. At the same time, it must be recognized that osteosarcoma arises in many patients both well before and long after the adolescent growth spurt. Radiation exposure is a well-documented etiologic factor, but since the interval between irradiation and appearance of osteosarcoma is typically long, this is not relevant to most pediatric patients.[1,5] The incidence of osteosarcoma is dramatically increased among survivors of retinoblastoma. The majority of second malignancies in these patients are sarcomas, and almost 50% of these are osteosarcomas. In the hereditary form of this disorder, germline mutations of the retinoblastoma gene are common. This is the likely basis for the increased frequency of secondary cancers in this population, since the rate in survivors of unilateral sporadic retinoblastoma is much less.[10] Germline mutations in the *TP53* gene can lead to a high risk of developing malignancies, including osteosarcoma, which has been described as the Li-Fraumeni syndrome.[11] Numerous oncogenes are altered in osteosarcoma tumor cells, and although it is clear that alterations in tumor suppressor genes and oncogenes are necessary to produce osteosarcomas, it is not clear which of these events occurs first and why or how it occurs.

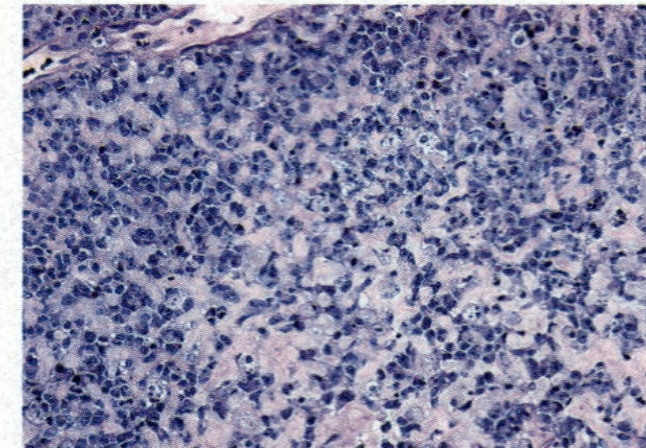

Figure 124m-1 Osteoblastic osteosarcoma.

Histology As defined by the World Health Organization (WHO), osteosarcoma is a malignant tumor in which the neoplastic cells produce osteoid.[12] Because these tumors arise from mesenchymal cells capable of differentiating toward bone, cartilage, or fibrous tissue, osteosarcomas can have osteoblastic, chondroblastic, and fibroblastic components and vary greatly in histologic appearance and extent of osteoid production. Most osteosarcomas, including those in children and adolescents, are of the osteoblastic subtype. Osteoblastic osteosarcoma is composed of cytologically malignant osteoblastic cells, spindle cells, and multinucleated tumor giant cells with interspersed osteoid (Figure 124m-1). The current WHO classification recognizes two additional subtypes of conventional osteosarcoma: chondroblastic (Figure 124m-2) and fibroblastic (Figure 124m-3), based on the predominant pattern of differentiation.[12] The value of subclassification is unclear because it is highly dependent on sampling and no difference in clinical behavior or outcome based solely on subtype has been discerned. Telangiectatic osteosarcoma[12] is a rare subtype, which appears as a purely lytic lesion on plain radiographs and, thus, may be confused with aneurysmal bone cyst or giant cell tumor. Telangiectatic osteosarcomas are grossly cystic and microscopically have dilated blood-filled spaces separated by fibrous septae containing tumor cells and scant osteoid. With current chemotherapy regimens, the prognosis is similar to conventional osteosarcoma. Small-cell osteosarcoma[12] is a rare subtype, notable for its histologic similarity to Ewing's sarcoma. Immunohistochemical or molecular studies may be required to make the distinction. Other subtypes of osteosarcoma, such as parosteal, periosteal, and low-grade central, are uncommon in pediatric patients and therefore will not be discussed. An unusual presentation of osteosarcoma is multifocal osteosarcoma,[13] a rare entity in which multiple synchronous skeletal tumors are present at diagnosis, with each lesion resembling the primary tumor radiographically, suggesting a multicentric origin. It is unclear whether such sarcomas arise at multiple sites or if one of the lesions is the true primary that has metastasized rapidly to other skeletal sites in the absence of lung metastases. This presentation is associated with a very poor prognosis.

Chemotherapy Almost all newly diagnosed patients with osteosarcoma have at least micrometastatic disease as evidenced by the fact that if treated by surgical resection, 80% will relapse in the lung within 2 years.[6] These findings suggested the need for systemic chemotherapy, which has now become the standard of care.[14] Despite the effectiveness of chemotherapy against the presence of microscopic disease, it cannot control clinically detectable disease. Tumors detected by conventional techniques, both at the primary and metastatic sites, require local control. Osteosarcoma is resistant to radiation therapy, and, therefore, local control usually

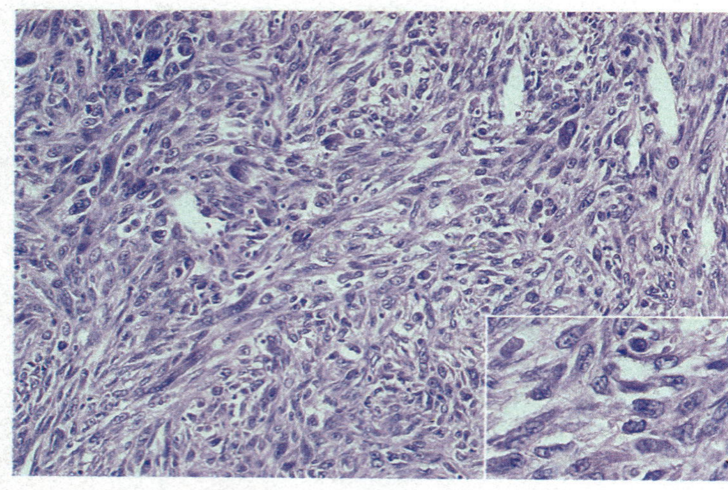

Figure 124m-2 Chondroblastic osteosarcoma.

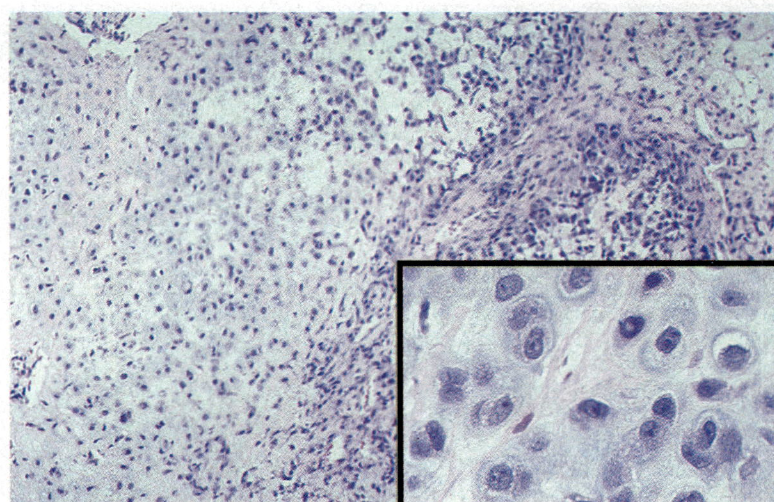

Figure 124m-3 Fibroblastic osteosarcoma.

consists of surgical resection. Advances made in surgical techniques have significantly improved the clinical practice and options available for patients.

Prior to the early 1970s, therapy for osteosarcoma consisted mostly of surgical interventions. Despite the use of radical surgery, the outcome was poor, with 2-year survival rates of approximately 15%, since 85 to 90% of patients who presented with apparently localized disease developed recurrences mostly to the lung.[6] In the 1970s, several investigators reported that chemotherapy had activity against relapsed or metastatic osteosarcoma. The agents reported to be effective included doxorubicin, cisplatin, and high-dose methotrexate with leucovorin rescue.[15–17] When these agents were administered to patients with relapsed or metastatic disease, tumor responses were observed. It was recognized that in the absence of any clinically detectable or bulk disease, chemotherapy may be even more effective and may result in long-term disease-free survival. With this rationale, several investigators embarked on trials of adjuvant chemotherapy for osteosarcoma. In the 1970s and early 1980s, all of these trials were single arm, nonrandomized treatments employing adjuvant chemotherapy, comparing results against historical controls.[18,19] Every reported trial of adjuvant chemotherapy reported a disease-free survival superior to the historical rate of 20%.

However, not all investigators were convinced that chemotherapy was appropriate for all patients with osteosarcoma because the use of historical comparisons can be flawed. Other changes in the management of osteosarcoma had also occurred during that period, such as the routine use of computed tomography to assess for pulmonary metastases. As trials of chemotherapy were limited to those without clinically detectable metastases, the improved outcome might be the result of selection of a cohort of patients with a better outcome. Earlier diagnosis or improved surgical technique could also have contributed to the reported improved outcome.[20]

In the early 1980s, investigators at the Mayo Clinic carried out the first randomized trial of adjuvant chemotherapy for osteosarcoma. All patients had surgical resection of the primary tumor and had no evidence of clinically detectable metastatic disease. Patients were randomly assigned to observation or to adjuvant chemotherapy. Results of this study revealed no difference between the two groups with a disease-free survival of 40%.[21] This was interpreted as a change in the natural history of the disease.[20,22]

To clarify the value of adjuvant chemotherapy, the Multi-Institution Osteosarcoma Study (MIOS) was initiated. Patients were eligible for study entry after amputation or tumor resection if they did not have clinically detectable metastatic disease. The intent of the study was to randomize patients between observation and adjuvant multiagent chemotherapy. Many of the patients enrolled on the study were not randomized; however, most were being treated with chemotherapy. The randomized patients and the larger nonrandomized group had identical results. Patients who did not receive chemotherapy after surgical resection had a 2-year probability of disease-free survival of 11% compared with 66% for those who received chemotherapy.[14] This study unequivocally demonstrated that the natural history of osteosarcoma had not changed, and adjuvant chemotherapy was clearly beneficial.

In the same era, Rosen, who had much earlier reported excellent results with the combination of doxorubicin and methotrexate, introduced the concept of chemotherapy prior to surgical resection, referred to as preoperative or induction chemotherapy.[23] The concept of induction chemotherapy arose from the need for time to make the custom endoprosthesis required for limb salvage procedures, creating an interval during which chemotherapy could be administered. In addition, theoretic advantages of induction chemotherapy included early treatment of micrometastatic disease and facilitation of the eventual surgical procedure, because of tumor shrinkage and decreased vascularity. It also provided the ability to examine the histologic response of the tumor to induction chemotherapy as a way to evaluate the effectiveness of therapy. A strong correlation between the degree of necrosis and the probability of subsequent disease-free survival was observed,[24] which has subsequently been confirmed in multiple clinical trials. A theoretic concern with this approach was that delay in tumor removal could lead to the emergence of chemotherapy resistance. A prospective trial by the Pediatric Oncology Group addressed this concern, however, by randomizing patients to immediate definitive surgery or induction chemotherapy followed by resection. The total dose of chemotherapy was identical in both arms. There was no advantage to immediate surgery.[25] Since preoperative therapy provides facilitation of limb salvage and the ability to assess chemotherapeutic response, induction chemotherapy for osteosarcoma has become the standard of care.

Soon after the identification of the prognostic value of the degree of necrosis following induction chemotherapy, it was suggested that chemotherapy be modified for the patients with less necrosis (currently referred to as either standard or poor responders) variably defined as $< 90\%$ or $< 98\%$ tumor necrosis, in order to increase their probability of disease-free survival.[24] Despite an early report of benefit, changed and intensified regimens have not improved outcome for poor responders.[26,27] The standard treatment of patients with nonmetastatic osteosarcoma, although variable, includes the use of cisplatin and doxorubicin with the addition of high-dose methotrexate in North American countries, and the addition of ifosfamide in Cooperative Osteosarcoma Studies (COSS) (Table 124m-1). The survival of patients with osteosarcoma appears to have reached a plateau. To see differences from new therapeutic regimens, randomized trials involving large numbers of patients will be needed. European and North American investigators have thus agreed to collaborate in future trials (EURAMOS).

Based on the promising activity of ifosfamide, with or without etoposide in patients with metastatic osteosarcoma,[28] and the encouraging results from a nonrandomized Italian study suggesting that addition of this drug pair improves the outcome for patients with a poor histologic response,[29] EURAMOS investigators have agreed to evaluate the addition of this drug pair to the standard postoperative therapy for patients with a poor histologic response. Because of toxicity in patients with a good histologic response, EURAMOS investigators have agreed to ask a different question in these patients. Scandinavian investigators have reported encouraging results in osteosarcoma with the use of interferon following surgical resection. The development of a long-acting interferon with fewer side effects has prompted interest in evaluating this agent. Patients with a good histologic response will be randomized to the administration of interferon following standard three-drug therapy.

METASTATIC DISEASE

The standard management for patients with metastatic disease at the time of initial diagnosis follows the same general principles as those who present

Table 124m-1 Osteosarcoma Treatment Regimens

Regimens of Chemotherapy	Drug	Dose	Reference
COG	HDMTX	12 g/m^2 × 12 (LCV 10 mg q 6 h) (wk 3, 4; 8, 9*; 15, 16; 20, 21; 25, 26; 30, 31)	Meyers P: J Clin Oncol 23(9):2004, 2005
	CDDP/DOX	120 mg/m^2 & 75 mg/m^2 × 4 (wk 0, 5, 12, 17)	
	DOX	75 mg/m^2 × 2 (wk 22, 27)	
COSS	HDMTX	12 g/m^2 × 12–14 (wk 3, 4; 13, 14; 18, 19; 22, 23, 27, 28; 31, 32; 36,37)	Fuchs N: Ann Oncol 9:893, 1998
	DOX	90 mg/m^2 × 4–5 (wk 1, 11, 20, 29)	
	Ifos/CDDP	3 g/m^2 × 2 d/120 mg/m^2 × 5, (wk 5, 8, 15, 24, 33)	
EOI	CDDP/DOXO	100 mg/m^2 & 25 mg/m^2/dx3 × 5 (wk 1, 4, 7**, 12, 15, 18)	

HDMTX: high-dose methotrexate.
LCV: leucovorin rescue 10 mg every 6 hours administered until MTX level is < 0.1 μM
CDDP/DOXO: cisplatin/doxorubicin-only administered once the absolute neutrophil count > 500 and platelet count > 75,000.
Ifos/CDDP: ifosfamide/cisplatin-only administered once the absolute neutrophil count > 500 and platelet count > 75,000.
Filgrastin may be used.
*Surgery usually performed at week 10.
**Surgery usually performed at week 9.
Editor's Note: HDMTX in adults is usually limited to 8 g/m^2. Alkalinization and hydration are important to avoid precipitation in renal tubules. Leukovorin rescue 25 mg q h 6 until MTX level is < 0.1 μM.

with localized disease.[30] Patients undergo surgery to remove all evidence of bulk disease. Several chemotherapy and surgical timing approaches have been reported for the treatment of these patients. Survival has clearly been enhanced by aggressive treatment designed with a curative intent.

In general, radical surgery is the best option for local control, and patients unable to undergo complete resection have a poor outcome. Therapeutic alternatives for patients who are unable or refuse to have surgery are limited, and although a recent report suggests a small number of patients can be cured without radical surgery,[31] the standard of care involves the use of multiagent therapy and radical surgery. Recent data also suggest that the administration of radiotherapy may be useful in patients treated with multiagent therapy who are unable to undergo complete resection or who have microscopic residual following attempted resection.[32]

Prognosis The outcome of osteosarcoma patients depends on several factors. The most consistent prognostic factor at diagnosis is the presence of clinically detectable metastases, which confers an unfavorable prognosis. Among patients presenting with localized disease, few factors are sufficiently predictive to allow stratification of therapy or more precise determination of a patient's likelihood of survival. The site of the primary tumor has some prognostic significance, with axial lesions prognostically inferior to tumors of the appendicular skeleton. Both serum lactate dehydrogenase and alkaline phosphatase correlate with outcome; higher levels of either enzyme predict an inferior prognosis. These factors most likely influence outcome by reflecting the size of the tumor or its resectability.[1] The histologic response to induction chemotherapy is a consistent prognostic factor but cannot be assessed at the time of diagnosis. In patients with metastatic disease at diagnosis, the number of pulmonary nodules as well as whether they are unilateral or bilateral is also of prognostic significance.

With currently available regimens, approximately 60 to 70% of patients with nonmetastatic osteosarcoma of the extremity will survive without evidence of recurrence. In most large reported studies, only 10 to 20% of patients who present with clinically detectable metastatic disease are continuously disease-free.[30] In some series, 5-year survival of patients presenting with metastatic disease has been reported to be as high as 50%, but these reports typically included patients with isolated pulmonary nodules that were not histologically confirmed.[33]

EWING'S SARCOMA

James Ewing first described Ewing's sarcoma (ES) in 1921, based on his observation of a radiosensitive bone tumor.[34] In the early 1980s, ES and peripheral primitive neuroectodermal tumor (PPNET) were both found to contain the same reciprocal translocation between chromosomes 11 and 22, t(11;22)(q24;q12).[35,36] Later that decade, similar patterns of oncogene expression (c-*myc*, N-*myc*, c-*myb*, and c-*mil/raf-1*) were seen among these tumors.[37] The combination of the shared translocation, cellular physiology, and clinical response has led to categorizing these tumors into the Ewing's Sarcoma Family of Tumors (ESFT). The ESFT includes ES, peripheral primitive neuroectodermal tumor, neuroepithelioma, atypical ES, and Askin's tumor (an ESFT of the chest wall).

Presentation ESFT patients usually present with pain and a palpable mass. Frequent primary sites include the pelvis (25%), femur (16%), ribs (12%), and spine (8%) (Figure 124m-4). Lesions in long bones can present with a pathologic fracture; while back pain may indicate a vertebral, paraspinal, retroperitoneal, or deep pelvic tumor. Neuropathic pain can be a sign of nerve compression, warranting comprehensive neurologic examination. Occasionally, the presence of vertebral lesions with an associated extradural mass can lead to progressive paraparesis and the rapid onset of paraplegia, with sphincter dysfunction. Primary lesions of the ribs may expand sufficiently to cause lung compression and a mediastinal shift. Systemic symptoms of fever and weight loss can also occur and often indicate the presence of metastatic disease.

Approximately 25% of patients present with metastatic disease. Of these, 37% (or 9% of all patients) have metastases confined to the lung or pleura. Infrequently, patients with lung metastases can present with asymmetric breath sounds, pleural signs, or rales. The remaining patients have bone and/or bone marrow metastases, either alone or in addition to pulmonary/pleural disease. Rarely, patients with bone marrow metastases have extensive infiltration and present with petechiae or purpura from thrombocytopenia. The presence of a pelvic tumor, a high LDH, fever, an interval between onset of symptoms and diagnosis > 3 months, and age older than 12 years are risk factors for clinically evident metastatic disease. There are no pathognomonic or suggestive blood studies to diagnose ESFT. The presence of an elevated serum LDH level can suggest malignancy; while the presence of anemia, neutropenia, or thrombocytopenia may suggest bone marrow infiltration, but none of these are specific for ESFT.

Differential Diagnosis ESFT should be included in the differential diagnosis of any bone or soft tissue mass in patients from age 2 years through the fourth decade of life. The differential diagnosis of a bone lesion should include both primary and secondary tumors. Primary lesions include osteomyelitis, osteogenic sarcoma, reticulum cell sarcoma, eosinophilic granuloma, and lymphoma.

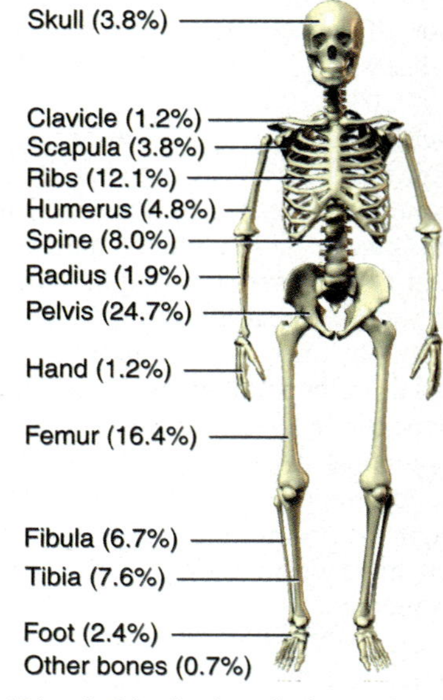

Figure 124m-4 Distribution of primary sites.

Metastatic deposits may result from neuroblastoma, rhabdomyosarcoma, or lymphoma. The differential diagnoses of soft tissue lesions include rhabdomyosarcoma, neuroblastoma, nonrhabdomyosarcomatous soft-tissue sarcoma, and lymphoma.

Radiographic Appearance Patients who present with a palpable bone lesion or those reporting persistent bone pain should undergo evaluation with plain radiographs. Although there are no pathognomonic lesions diagnostic of ESFT, the radiologic findings of a lamellar (onion skin) lesion on plain film is highly suggestive. ESFT cells do not produce bone, but do stimulate normal osteoblasts to produce sheets of new cortical bone. Additional radiographic findings include bone sclerosis, elevation of periosteum with periosteal reaction (Codman's triangle), and radial streaks of bone beyond the cortical walls. If a patient presents with a large pelvic mass and pulmonary metastases, ESFT is likely. MRI of the region can help to identify the extent of disease and is generally more precise than CT scan, which can, however, help delineate bone involvement. Tumors that are adjacent to critical neurologic structures require immediate MRI scanning and consideration of emergency therapy to prevent neurologic deterioration. Metastatic radiographic evaluation includes chest CT scan and radioisotope bone scan. The role of positron emission tomography (PET) scan remains to be defined. Bone marrow aspiration and biopsy are required to exclude malignant infiltration. The definitive diagnosis for ESFT requires a biopsy.

Epidemiology Based on the Surveillance, Epidemiology and End Results (SEER) data, the incidence of ESFT in persons < 20 years is 2.9 per million per year.[9] The incidence of ESFT in females is 2.6 per million and in males is 3.3 per million. The incidence of ESFT peaks in the latter half of the second decade of life. The age distribution for ESFT shows that 27% occur in the first decade, 64% in the second decade, and 9% in the third decade. An enigma in ESFT is its racial distribution. The incidence in whites is at least ninefold higher than in blacks. This is in contrast to osteogenic sarcoma, which has a relatively equal race distribution.[9] African countries report similar osteosarcoma incidence rates, with a paucity of ESFT.

Pathophysiology The cause of ESFT is unknown. Cases are thought to be sporadic, but family members of ESFT patients have an increased incidence of neuroectodermal and stomach malignancies.[38] Growth parameters such as height and weight have not been linked to the development of ESFT.[39] ESFT rarely occurs as a second neoplasm, although the exact incidence is unknown.

ESFT are thought to derive from cells of neuroectodermal origin, possibly postganglionic cholinergic neurons, although the exact cell of origin has yet to be identified. The translocation t(11;22)(q24;q12), or another related translocation, occurs in greater than 95% of ESFT. Some argue that such a translocation is pathognomonic and is both necessary and sufficient for a diagnosis of ESFT. The classic t(11;22)(q24;q12) translocation joins the Ewing's sarcoma (*EWS*) gene located on chromosome 22 to an *ets*-family gene, *FLI1* (Friend Leukemia Insertion), located on chromosome 11.[40]

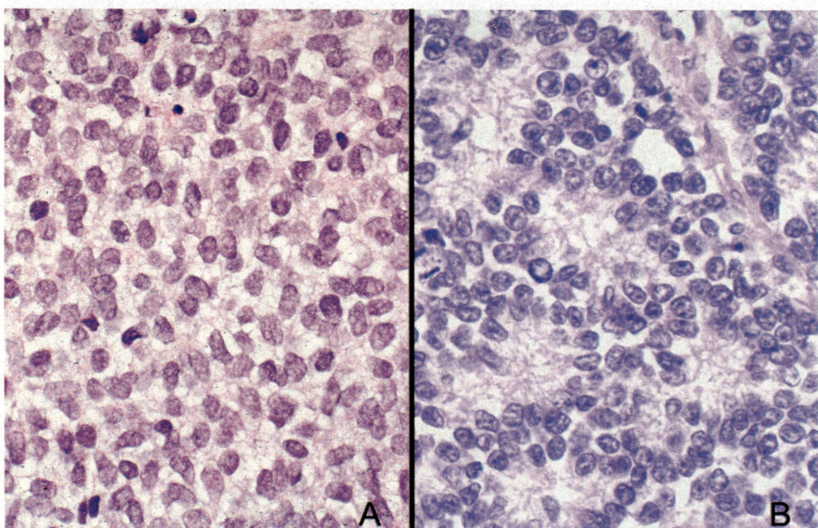

Figure 124m-5 Ewing's sarcoma family of tumors. **A,** Undifferentiated Ewing's sarcoma. **B,** Peripheral primitive neuroectodermal tumor with pseudorosette formation.

The EWS/FLI1 fusion transcript encodes a 68-kDa protein with two primary domains. The EWS domain is a potent transcriptional activator, while the FLI1 domain contains a highly conserved *ets* DNA binding domain. The EWS/FLI1 fusion protein thus acts as an aberrant transcription factor and transforms mouse fibroblasts. To effect this transformation, both the EWS and FLI1 functional domains must be intact.[41] In addition, the IGF-I receptor (IGF-IR) is required for EWS/FLI1 to transform fibroblasts.[42] Thus, the EWS/FLI1 fusion protein is implicated in the pathogenesis of ESFT. When the expression level of EWS/FLI1 is reduced by antisense RNA or antisense oligonucleotides, ESFT cell lines die and tumors in nude mice regress.[43–45] These studies have established the critical nature of the EWS/FLI1 to ESFT cells and the role of EWS/FLI1 as a therapeutic target. Effective strategies for reducing the activity of EWS/FLI1 in ESFT patients through novel delivery systems of small interfering (si) RNA are in development.[46,47] Early investigations of EWS/FLI1-induced transformation of mouse fibroblasts demonstrated that not all fibroblasts could be equally transformed. The fibroblasts that were transformable were immortalized and were found to lack some component of the G1 checkpoint, most often $p16^{INK4a}$.[48] Over half of all ESFT from patients have been shown to lack some component of the G1 checkpoint, either *p16*, *p15*, *p14*, *TP53*, or *p21*.[49] The role of the loss of these checkpoint genes on patient survival is discussed in the section on prognosis.

Histologic Findings When ESFT is suspected clinically, consultation with a pediatric oncologist and an orthopedic oncologist should occur *prior* to biopsy. Likewise, the pathologist should be alerted to ensure appropriate handling and triaging of the tissue. Biopsies should be performed with consideration of eventual local therapy. Inappropriate biopsy or resection often results in increased morbidity or mortality. A small piece of tumor should be snap frozen in liquid nitrogen to allow for molecular studies, including reverse transcriptase-polymerase chain reaction (RT-PCR). Whereas diagnosis can often be made on routine and immunohistochemical stains, there is increasing emphasis on identification of the t(11;22) or a related translocation by cytogenetics, RT-PCR, or fluorescent in situ hybridization (FISH) to confirm the diagnosis and exclude other entities.

ESFT is one of the small round blue cell tumors and spans a spectrum from undifferentiated (Ewing's sarcoma) to differentiated (peripheral primitive neuroectodermal tumor) (Figure 124m-5). Pseudorosette formation is seen with increasing differentiation. The immunohistochemical hallmark of ESFT is diffuse membranous staining for CD99 (MIC2),[50] which is present in greater than 90% of ESFT. Undifferentiated tumors are negative for other markers except vimentin and Fli-1, whereas more differentiated tumors variably express additional markers, including neuron specific enolase, S-100, neurofilaments, CD57, and synaptophysin. Muscle and lymphoid markers are negative. A Kiel modified classification proceeds from the least to the most differentiated: ES (0–2 markers), atypical ES (3–5 markers), and PPNET (requires rosettes or 4–5 markers).[51] The current WHO classification does not distinguish between these entities[12] because many statistically mature patient cohorts do not identify a prognostic advantage to classification based on differentiation or diagnosis of ES versus PPNET.[51–53]

Molecular Diagnosis Identifying an ESFT-specific translocation is pathognomonic for the diagnosis. This includes chromosomal break points t(11;22), t(21;22), and t(7;22). These break points are often seen with standard cytogenetic karyotyping. Standard cytogenetics and FISH can also reveal additional karyotypic abnormalities,

Table 124m-2 Ewing's Sarcoma Treatment Regimens

Regimens of Chemotherapy	Drug	Dose	Reference
COG: alternating cycles of VDC & IE (cumulative ifosfamide 72 g/m^2)	VDC	V-1.5 mg/m^2, D-75 mg/m^2, C-1.2 g/m^2, (wk 0, 6, 12, 18, 24, 30, 36, 42, 48)	Grier: N Engl J Med 348:694, 2003
	IE	I-1.8 $g/m^2/d \times 5$ E-100 $mg/m^2/d \times 5$, (wk 3, 9, 15, 21, 27, 33, 39, 45)	
EURO-Ewing	VIDE × 6	V-1.5 mg/m^2 I-3 $g/m^2/d \times 3$ D-20 $mg/m^2/d \times 3$ E-150 $mg/m^2/d \times 3$, (wk 0, 3, 6, 9, 12, 15)	Schuck: Int J Radiat Oncol Biol Phys 55:168, 2003
	VAI or VAC × 7	V-1.5 mg/m^2 A-0.75 mg/m^2 I-3 $g/m^2/d \times 2$ C-1.5 g/m^2, (wk 18, 21, 24, 27, 30, 33, 36, 39)	

Chemotherapy administered at 3 week intervals once absolute neutrophil count > 500 and platelet count > 75,000. Filgrastin may be used.
VDC: vincristine, doxorubicin, cyclophosphamide* doxorubicin eliminated after a total dose of 375 mg/m^2 (wk 30, 36, 42, 48 VC only administered). Maximum vincristine dose in adults = 2 mg.
IE: ifosfamide, etoposide.
VIDE: vincristine, ifosfamide, doxorubicin, etoposide-administered at 3 week intervals once absolute neutrophil count > 1,000; platelet count > 80,000.
VAI: vincristine, actinomycin, ifosfamide administered at 3 week intervals once absolute neutrophil count > 1,000; platelet count > 80,000.
VAC: vincristine, actinomycin, cyclophosphamide administered at 3 week intervals once absolute neutrophil count > 1,000; platelet count > 80,000.

including trisomies 8 and 12, and chromosomes 1 and 16 abnormalities.[54] Some of the t(21;22) translocations remain cryptic by standard cytogenetic techniques and require RT-PCR or FISH. Ideally, every small round blue cell tumor should be evaluated by a multiplex RT-PCR assay that will identify any of the known translocations and identify translocations of histologically similar small round blue cell tumors such as rhabdomyosarcoma.

Chemotherapy Before the use of chemotherapy, studies for patients with ESFT reported a 5-year survival of approximately 10%.[55] The first chemotherapeutic agents with efficacy in ESFT were cyclophosphamide (C), actinomycin-D (A), and vincristine (V). Patients with ESFT started receiving these agents individually in the early 1960s and in combination by the late 1960s. The most consistent prognostic factor is the presence of metastatic disease at diagnosis. Alkylating agents (cyclophosphamide, ifosfamide, melphalan, and busulfan) and doxorubicin are the most active single agents in ESFT, while the combination of ifosfamide plus etoposide showed significant activity in a classic phase II setting.[56] Platinum derivatives have not shown significant efficacy in ESFT.[55]

Localized Disease The successful management of patients with ESFT requires the use of both local and systemic therapy. In 1973, the first Intergroup Ewing's Sarcoma Study (IESS-1) evaluated the efficacy of VAC compared with VAC plus lung radiation or VAC plus doxorubicin (D). This study showed that for patients with localized disease, VAC alone provided 24%, VAC plus lung RT 44%, and VAC plus D 60% 5-year disease-free survival (DFS).[57] Besides the dramatic improvement in overall survival, IESS-1 identified patients with large primary tumors, particularly pelvic, as having a shorter survival. The addition of ifosfamide and etoposide to the three-drug VDC regimen produced further improvement in outcome.[58] The most recently published trials for localized ESFT are summarized in Table 124m-2. Most recently, the IESS compared a 30-week dose-intensive regimen of alkylators with the previous 48-week regimen and showed no difference between therapeutic arms.[59] The successor study, the current Children's Oncology Group (COG) study, is examining the role of dose-intensive therapy administered every 2 weeks with filgrastin support compared with the conventional every-3-week therapy for patients with initially localized disease. The current European study, Euro-E.W.I.N.G. 99, randomly assigns patients with initially localized, small (< 200 mL) primary tumors to ifosfamide or cyclophosphamide in combination with vincristine and actinomycin following standard induction therapy with vincristine-ifosfamide-doxorubicin-etoposide.

Metastatic Disease ESFT patients with disease metastatic at initial diagnosis have been identified as having a poor outcome since early multiagent trials.[60] The most recent multicenter trials with greater than 40 patients are summarized in Table 124m-3. Patients with multiple sites of metastases have the lowest survival rates. Patients with metastases confined to the lungs may represent a group of patients with better prognosis than patients with bone or bone marrow metastases. For example, in the European Intergroup Ewing's Sarcoma Study (EICESS 92) study, patients with pulmonary only metastases had a 40% 4-year disease-free survival when treated with whole-lung irradiation in addition to multiagent chemotherapy.[61]

Early chemotherapy regimens included low-dose regimens, such as oral cyclophosphamide 150 mg/m^2 for 7 days followed by intravenous doxorubicin 35 mg/m^2 on day 8, alternating with vincristine (1.5 mg/m^2), dactinomycin (1.5 mg/m^2), and bischloroethylnitrosourea (BCNU) 50 mg/m^2.[62] To improve survival, high-dose regimens consisting of VDC induction followed by total-body irradiation/melphalan 180 mg/m^2 or thiotepa 900 mg/m^2/carboplatin 1,500 mg/m^2 have been used.[63] These studies assured the feasibility of high-dose regimens requiring stem cell support, but also demonstrated significant toxicity. They were driven by the hypothesis that the dose response to alkylator therapy for ESFT cells is very steep and that, therefore, increasing the dose intensity of these agents would increase the tumor cell kill and improve patient survival. This is particularly true for melphalan and busulfan, where therapeutic dosing requires stem cell support. However, despite dose intensification to megadose therapy followed by stem cell rescue, survival has not significantly improved.[63] It is equally unclear whether the addition of ifosfamide/etoposide to standard dose VACD results in an improvement in outcome in the setting of initially metastatic disease.[64]

More recently, poor prognosis patients were treated with melphalan, busulfan, and thiotepa with or without total-marrow irradiation in a pilot study using a tandem autologous stem cell rescue. This study, which included patients with recurrent disease (who historically have had dismal survival chances), showed encouraging results, with a 36% 2-year disease-free survival.[65]

One possible mechanism for disease recurrence in the patients who have undergone autologous transplant could be the presence of tumor in the stem cell preparation.[66] The actual incidence of ESFT tumor cells in pheresed stem cell preparations is likely dependent on many factors including chemotherapy prior to harvest, method of stem cell mobilization, and, possibly, stem cell handling. Some studies report a low incidence of tumor contamination. A quantitative method to estimate tumor cell contamination in stem cell preparations has the potential to clarify the role of contaminating tumor cells in recurrent disease as well as for use in tumor cell purging strategies.[67]

As suggested in earlier studies, the role of megatherapy with stem cell support for ESFT is

Table 124m-3 Outcome for Patients with Metastatic ESFT Treated with Conventional Therapy

First Author (Ref)	Institution/ Group	Type of Study	Patients (No.)	Therapy	F/U Time	EFS	OS
Miser[64]	IESS	multi	121	VAC(1.2 g/m^2)D vs VAC(1.2 g/m^2)D/I(9 g/m^2)E	4 yr	19%	38%
Miser[64]	IESS	multi	60	VAC(2.2 g/m^2)D/I(14 g/m^2)E	2 yr	26%	35%
Craft[89]	UKCCSG	multi	42	IVAD	5 yr	23%	
Paulussen[61]	EICESS	multi	171	IVAD ± E (36 patients received megatherapy)	4 yr	27%	

A = actinomycin; C = cyclophosphamide; D = doxorubicin, EICESS = European Intergroup Cooperative Ewing Sarcoma Study; E = etoposide; I = ifosfamide; IESS = Intergroup Ewing Sarcoma Study; V = vincristine; UKCCSG = United Kingdom Children's Cancer Study Group.

best evaluated in the context of controlled clinical trials. The ongoing Euro-E.W.I.N.G. study randomizes patients with large primary tumors or tumors with a poor histologic response to induction chemotherapy to standard chemotherapy versus megatherapy using busulfan and melphalan. COG is participating in the part of that therapeutic question that assigns patients with isolated pulmonary metastases at initial diagnosis to standard chemotherapy and pulmonary irradiation compared with megatherapy using busulfan and melphalan followed by stem cell re-infusion.

Toxicity Toxicity is an important consideration in the therapy of ESFT, because the doses of effective agents are administered at the maximum tolerated dose. Good multidisciplinary (nutrition, psychological, occupational, and physical therapy) supportive care is therefore essential to patient management. Most patients develop severe neutropenia after alkylating agent and doxorubicin treatment, but despite G-CSF support, cytopenias, particularly neutropenia, sometimes complicated by fever, infection, and mucositis develop. In addition, cumulative cardiotoxicity from doxorubicin may complicate therapy. In one small randomized study, patients who received the cardioprotectant dexrazoxane (ICRF-187) tolerated higher doses of doxorubicin with less cardiotoxicity but no effect on disease outcome.[68] High doses of alkylating agents, in particular ifosfamide, can result in Fanconi syndrome (renal electrolyte wasting), and at the extreme, may result in hypophosphatemic rickets.

Second Malignancy Patients treated for ESFT are at risk of the development of second malignancy. The majority of second malignancies are acute myeloid leukemia, myelodysplastic syndrome, and sarcomas in the radiation field. The overall likelihood of developing a second malignancy is approximately 2%, with most leukemias occurring within 3 years from diagnosis.[69–71] Radiation dosage is important to the rate of development of secondary cancers, with the vast majority of induced tumors being osteosarcomas.[70,72] As a result of these studies, recommendations for radiation usage and dosage are being modified. Patients who have received radiation therapy should be evaluated for the development of secondary sarcomas in the radiation field because the development of these cancers continues to increase more than 15 years after treatment. Since the risk of osteosarcoma has been shown to rise after as little as 10 Gy, evaluation should not be limited to the irradiated bone.

LOCAL CONTROL

ESFT, unlike osteosarcoma, is quite radioresponsive, and radiotherapy is considered a standard option for definitive local control. Radiotherapy can be used as an alternative to disfiguring surgery such as amputation. In large prospective studies, patients who receive radiotherapy for local control have a similar disease-free and overall survival to those patients treated with surgery.[73] Although some retrospective reports have shown an advantage to surgery, these results are extremely influenced by selection bias because patients with large tumors of the axial skeleton or metastatic disease are typically referred for radiotherapy, while patients with the better prognosis extremity tumors are managed surgically.[74]

The standard dose for definitive treatment of ESFT is 55.8 Gy in standard once daily fractions of 1.8 Gy. Although single institution results using hyperfractionation are excellent, an advantage to altered fractionation has not been proven in a randomized trial. The target volume for treatment consists of the initial tumor extent plus a 2 cm margin in all directions. In the 1980s, the Pediatric Oncology Group studied involved field (tumor plus 2 cm margin) versus whole bone radiotherapy and found no difference in event-free survival.[75] Initial tumor volume may be a significant prognostic factor for patients treated with definitive radiation therapy.[76]

If surgery is performed and adequate (≥ 10 mm of bone or 5 mm of soft tissue) surgical margins are obtained, postoperative radiotherapy is not indicated.[76] Postoperative radiotherapy should be administered when surgical margins are close or positive. The postoperative target consists of the pretreatment tumor extent plus a 2 cm margin with a dose of 45 to 50.4 Gy. Radiotherapy is also indicated to sites of Ewing's sarcoma metastases, including the lungs. The dose for treatment of the lungs is 15 Gy in 1.5 Gy fractions. With modern radiotherapy doses (< 60 Gy), the risk of radiation-induced second cancers is less than 5% and should be weighed against other factors when deciding between surgery and radiotherapy for local control.[70]

Prognosis ESFT survival is highly dependent on the initial presentation and, therefore, potentially the biologic properties of the disease. Overall survival in patients with ESFT is 60%. For patients with localized disease it approaches 70%, while patients with metastatic disease have less than a 25% likelihood of long-term survival. The presence of metastatic disease at initial presentation is the most significant adverse prognostic factor despite aggressive chemotherapy.[52] Other prognostic factors that have been evaluated include age at diagnosis, sex, serum LDH levels, size and location of tumor, and neural differentiation. In general, larger tumors (often axial) had a poorer prognosis and correlated with other poor prognostic factors. Aggressive multiagent chemotherapy as well as effective local management has somewhat reduced the prognostic importance of size. Most studies show a trend to improved survival in patients who are less than 10 or 15 years.[58]

Molecular markers as prognostic indicators in patients with ESFT are under study. Several of these include translocation break-point regions, other chromosomal abnormalities, cell-cycle/checkpoint genes and p-glycoprotein expression. The t(11;22) in any individual patient fuses one of many observed combinations of exons together from EWS and FLI1 to form the fusion message. The most common combination is the EWS exon 7 fused to FLI1 exon 6 (type 1 translocation), which occurs in approximately 50 to 64% of ESFT. Retrospective analyses have shown that patients with localized tumors and the 7/6 fusion have a 70% 4-year survival, while patients with the other variants had a 20% 4-year survival.[77]

In addition to the well-described t(11;22) and related translocations, additional chromosomal abnormalities have been described including trisomy 8 and chromosome 1p and 1q rearrangements. Loss of chromosome segment 1p36 has been associated with poor prognosis in patients with localized disease.[78] Additional abnormalities including +8 and +12 may portend a better prognosis.[78]

Cell-cycle and checkpoint genes have been evaluated as prognostic markers in ESFT. Although particular checkpoint genes have been found mutated or deleted in small numbers of tumors; as a group, these abnormalities are found in over 50% of ESFT. In patients with ESFT, 80% of $p16^{INK4a}$ mutations or deletions were found in patients with metastatic disease.[49] Other studies confirmed that patients with $p16^{INK4a}$ abnormalities had a poor prognosis.

TP53 mutations are often identified by overexpression (or delayed catabolism) of *TP53* measured by increased immunoreactivity in tissues. Increased *TP53* occurs in approximately 10% of ESFT samples.[49] In retrospective studies the presence of *TP53* has been shown to identify patients with a poor prognosis.

Research Studies and Future Directions In order to improve survival and reduce morbidity, novel combinations of established chemotherapeutic agents and molecular targeted therapies are being tested in ESFT. Since EWS-FLI1 is a specific molecular target, future therapies are likely to focus on inactivating EWS-FLI1 function, although no drugs are currently available.[79] In patients with recurrent disease, a classic phase II trial of cyclophosphamide (250 mg/m^2)/topotecan (0.75 mg/m^2) administered daily for 5 days induced complete or partial responses in 6 of 17 patients and stable disease in another 6.[80] In an upfront window study of patients with ESFT metastatic at initial diagnosis, topotecan/cyclophosphamide showed a 56% partial response rate.[81]

Imatinib (Gleevac, STI-571), a small molecule tyrosine kinase inhibitor is active against platelet-derived growth factor receptor (PDGF-R) and c-kit, the receptor for stem cell factor (SCF), both of which are expressed on ESFT cells. Inhibition of the PDGF-R in ESFT cell lines causes both reduced cell growth and motility.[82] The concentration required to inhibit Ewing cell growth, however, was above that achievable with standard dosage imatinib.[83,84] A phase II study using imatinib showed minimal activity in patients with recurrent disease. However, it is possible that imatinib may sensitize cells to doxorubicin-induced apoptosis, a possibility that will first be investigated in the laboratory.

The tumor necrosis factor-related apoptosis-inducing ligand (TRAIL) can activate tumor necrosis factor-modulated apoptotic pathways in ESFT. TRAIL-activated apoptosis occurs through caspase-8 in ESFT, and most ESFT cell lines express caspase-8. TRAIL may represent a biologic approach to inducing apoptotic cell death in ESFT.[85–87]

The insulin-like growth factor type I receptor is critical for transformation and growth of ESFT.[42,88] New small molecule inhibitors of IGF-IR, either alone or in combination with established chemotherapeutic agents deserve study.

Other bone tumors are discussed in Chapter 110, "Bone Tumors."

REFERENCES

1. Link MP, Eilber F. Osteosarcoma. In: Pizzo PA, Poplack DG, editors. Principles and practice of pediatric oncology. 3rd ed. Philadelphia: Lippincott-Raven; 1997. p. 889–920.
2. Rosen G, Forscher CA, Mankin HJ. Neoplasms of bone and soft tissue: bone tumors. In: Holland JF, Frei E, editors. Cancer medicine. 5th ed. Hamilton (ON): BC Decker; 2000. p. 1870–902.
3. Meyers PA, Gorlick R. Osteosarcoma. Pediatr Clin North Am 1997;44:973–89. Available at: http://www.ncbi.nlm.nih.gov/entrez/query.fcgi?cmd=Retrieve&db=PubMed&dopt=Citation&list_uids=9286295 (accessed August 16, 2005).
4. Dahlin DC, Unni KK. Osteosarcoma. In: Dahlin DC, Unni KK, editors. Bone tumors. General aspects and data on 8542 cases. Springfield (IL): Charles C. Thomas; 1986. p. 269–307.
5. Dorfman HD, Czerniak B. Bone cancers. Cancer 1995;75(1 Suppl):203–10. Available at: http://www.ncbi.nlm.nih.gov/entrez/query.fcgi?cmd=Retrieve&db=PubMed&dopt=Citation&list_uids=8000997 (accessed August 16, 2005).
6. Dahlin DC, Coventry MB. Osteogenic sarcoma. A study of six hundred cases. J Bone Joint Surg Am 1967;49:101–10.
7. Johnson H Jr, Fantone J, Flye MW. Histological evaluation of the nodules resected in the treatment of pulmonary metastatic disease. J Surg Oncol 1982;21:1–4. Available at: http://www.ncbi.nlm.nih.gov/entrez/query.fcgi?cmd=Retrieve&db=PubMed&dopt=Citation&list_uids=6955574 (accessed August 16, 2005).
8. Enneking WF, Spanier SS, Goodman MA. Current concepts review. The surgical staging of musculoskeletal sarcoma. J Bone Joint Surg Am 1980;62:1027–30. Available at: http://www.ncbi.nlm.nih.gov/entrez/query.fcgi?cmd=Retrieve&db=PubMed&dopt=Citation&list_uids=7000786 (accessed August 16, 2005).
9. Gurney JG, Swensen AR, Bulterys M. Malignant bone tumors. In: Ries LAG, Smith MA, Gurney JG, et al., editors. Cancer incidence and survival among children and adolescents: United States SEER program 1975–1995. Bethesda (MD): National Cancer Institute, SEER Program; 1999. p. 99–110.
10. Abramson DH, Ellsworth RM, Kitchin FD, Tung G. Second nonocular tumors in retinoblastoma survivors. Are they radiation-induced? Ophthalmology 1984;91:1351–5. Available at: http://www.ncbi.nlm.nih.gov/entrez/query.fcgi?cmd=Retrieve&db=PubMed&dopt=Citation&list_uids=6595610 (accessed August 16, 2005).
11. Friend SH, Bernards R, Rogelj S, et al. A human DNA segment with properties of the gene that predisposes to retinoblastoma and osteosarcoma. Nature 1986;323:643–6. Available at: http://www.ncbi.nlm.nih.gov/entrez/query.fcgi?cmd=Retrieve&db=PubMed&dopt=Citation&list_uids=2877398 (accessed August 16, 2005).
12. Fletcher CDM, Unni K, editors. World Health Organization classification of tumours: pathology and genetics of tumours of soft tissue and bone. Lyons: IARC Press; 2002.
13. Parham DM, Pratt CB, Parvey LS, et al. Childhood multifocal osteosarcoma. Clinicopathologic and radiologic correlates. Cancer 1985;55:2653–8.
14. Link MP, Goorin AM, Miser AW, et al. The effect of adjuvant chemotherapy on relapse-free survival in patients with osteosarcoma of the extremity. N Engl J Med 1986;314:1600–6. Available at http://www.ncbi.nlm.nih.gov/entrez/query.fcgi?cmd=Retrieve&db=PubMed&dopt=Citation&list_uids=3520317 (accessed August 17, 2005).
15. Cores EP, Holland JF, Wang JJ, Sinks LF. Doxorubicin in disseminated osteosarcoma. JAMA 1972;221:1132–8. Available at: http://www.ncbi.nlm.nih.gov/entrez/query.fcgi?cmd=Retrieve&db=PubMed&dopt=Citation&list_uids=4512088 (accessed August 17, 2005).
16. Jaffe N, Frei E, Traggis D, Bishop Y. Adjuvant methotrexate and citrovorum-factor treatment of osteogenic sarcoma. N Engl J Med 1974;291:994–7. Available at: http://www.ncbi.nlm.nih.gov/entrez/query.fcgi?cmd=Retrieve&db=PubMed&list_uids=4606174&dopt=Citation (accessed August 17, 2005).
17. Ochs JJ, Freeman AI, Douglass HO, et al. cis-Dichlorodiammineplatinum (II) in advanced osteogenic sarcoma. Cancer Treat Rep 1978;62:239–45. Available at: http://www.ncbi.nlm.nih.gov/entrez/query.fcgi?cmd=Retrieve&db=PubMed&list_uids=346212&dopt=Abstract (accessed August 17, 2005).
18. Pratt CB, Rivera G, Shanks E, et al. Combination chemotherapy for osteosarcoma. Cancer Treat Rep 1978;62:251–7. Available at: http://www.ncbi.nlm.nih.gov/entrez/query.fcgi?cmd=Retrieve&db=PubMed&dopt=Citation&list_uids=346214 (accessed August 17, 2005).
19. Goorin AM, Frei E 3rd, Abelson HT. Adjuvant chemotherapy for osteosarcoma: a decade of experience. Surg Clin North Am 1981;61:1379–89. Available at: http://www.ncbi.nlm.nih.gov/entrez/query.fcgi?cmd=Retrieve&db=PubMed&dopt=Citation&list_uids=6976007 (accessed August 17, 2005).
20. Lange B, Levine AS. Is it ethical not to conduct a prospectively controlled trial of adjuvant chemotherapy in osteosarcoma? Cancer Treat Rep 1982;66:1699–704. Available at: http://www.ncbi.nlm.nih.gov/entrez/query.fcgi?cmd=Retrieve&db=PubMed&dopt=Citation&list_uids=6749284 (accessed August 17, 2005).
21. Edmonson JH, Green SJ, Ivins JC, et al. A controlled pilot study of high-dose methotrexate as postsurgical adjuvant treatment for primary osteosarcoma. J Clin Oncol 1984;2:152–6. Available at: http://www.ncbi.nlm.nih.gov/entrez/query.fcgi?cmd=Retrieve&db=PubMed&dopt=Citation&list_uids=6366150 (accessed August 17, 2005).
22. Carter SK. Adjuvant chemotherapy in osteogenic sarcoma: the triumph that isn't? J Clin Oncol 1984;2:147–8. Available at: http://www.ncbi.nlm.nih.gov/entrez/query.fcgi?cmd=Retrieve&db=PubMed&dopt=Citation&list_uids=6583329 (accessed August 17, 2005).
23. Rosen G, Marcove RC, Caparros B, et al. Primary osteogenic sarcoma: the rationale for preoperative chemotherapy and delayed surgery. Cancer 1979;43:2163–77.
24. Rosen G, Caparros B, Huvos AG, et al. Preoperative chemotherapy for osteogenic sarcoma: selection of postoperative adjuvant chemotherapy based on the response of the primary tumor to preoperative chemotherapy. Cancer 1982;49:1221–30. Available at: http://www.ncbi.nlm.nih.gov/entrez/query.fcgi?cmd=Retrieve&db=PubMed&dopt=Citation&list_uids=6174200 (accessed August 17, 2005).
25. Goorin AM, Schwartzentruber DJ, Devidas M, et al. Presurgical chemotherapy compared with immediate surgery and adjuvant chemotherapy for nonmetastatic osteosarcoma: Pediatric Oncology Group Study POG-8651. J Clin Oncol 2003;21:1574–80. Available at: http://www.ncbi.nlm.nih.gov/entrez/query.fcgi?cmd=Retrieve&db=PubMed&dopt=Citation&list_uids=12697883 (accessed August 17, 2005).
26. Meyers PA, Heller G, Healey J, et al. Chemotherapy for nonmetastatic osteogenic sarcoma: the Memorial Sloan-Kettering experience [comments]. J Clin Oncol 1992;10:5–15.
27. Meyers PA, Gorlick R, Heller G, et al. Intensification of preoperative chemotherapy for osteogenic sarcoma: results of the Memorial Sloan-Kettering (T12) protocol. J Clin Oncol 1998;16:2452–8. Available at: http://www.ncbi.nlm.nih.gov/entrez/query.fcgi?cmd=Retrieve&db=PubMed&dopt=Citation&list_uids=9667263 (accessed August 17, 2005).
28. Goorin AM, Harris MB, Bernstein M, et al. Phase II/III trial of etoposide and high-dose ifosfamide in newly diagnosed metastatic osteosarcoma: a pediatric oncology group trial. J Clin Oncol 2002;20:426–33. Available at: http://www.ncbi.nlm.nih.gov/entrez/query.fcgi?cmd=Retrieve&db=PubMed&dopt=Citation&list_uids=11786570 (accessed August 17, 2005).
29. Bacci G, Picci P, Ferrari S, et al. Primary chemotherapy and delayed surgery for nonmetastatic osteosarcoma of the extremities. Results in 164 patients preoperatively treated with high doses of methotrexate followed by cisplatin and doxorubicin. Cancer 1993;72:3227–38. Available at: http://www.ncbi.nlm.nih.gov/entrez/query.fcgi?cmd=Retrieve&db=PubMed&dopt=Citation&list_uids=8242546 (accessed August 17, 2005).
30. Meyers PA, Heller G, Healey JH, et al. Osteogenic sarcoma with clinically detectable metastasis at initial presentation. J Clin Oncol 1993;11:449–53. Available at: http://www.ncbi.nlm.nih.gov/entrez/query.fcgi?cmd=Retrieve&db=PubMed&dopt=Citation&list_uids=8445419 (accessed August 17, 2005).
31. Jaffe N, Carrasco H, Raymond K, et al. Can cure in patients with osteosarcoma be achieved exclusively with chemotherapy and abrogation of surgery? Cancer 2002;95:2202–10. Available at: http://www.ncbi.nlm.nih.gov/entrez/query.fcgi?cmd=Retrieve&db=PubMed&dopt=Citation&list_uids=12412175 (accessed August 17, 2005).
32. Ozaki T, Flege S, Kevric M, et al. Osteosarcoma of the pelvis: experience of the Cooperative Osteosarcoma Study Group. J Clin Oncol 2003;21:334–41. Available at: http://www.ncbi.nlm.nih.gov/entrez/query.fcgi?cmd=Retrieve&db=PubMed&dopt=Citation&list_uids=12525527 (accessed August 17, 2005).
33. Harris MB, Gieser P, Goorin AM, et al. Treatment of metastatic osteosarcoma at diagnosis: a Pediatric Oncology Group Study. J Clin Oncol 1998;16:3641–8.
34. Ewing J. Diffuse endothelioma of bone. Proc N Y Pathol Soc 1921;21:17–24.
35. Turc-Carel C, Aurias A, Mugneret F, et al. Chromosomes in Ewing's sarcoma. I. An evaluation of 85 cases of remarkable consistency of t(11;22)(q24;q12). Cancer Genet Cytogenet 1988;32:229–38.
36. Whang PJ, Triche TJ, Knutsen T, et al. Chromosome translocation in peripheral neuroepithelioma. N Engl J Med 1984;311:584–5.
37. McKeon C, Thiele CJ, Ross RA, et al. Indistinguishable patterns of protooncogene expression in two distinct but closely related tumors: Ewing's sarcoma and neuroepithelioma. Cancer Res 1988;48:4307–11. Available at: http://www.ncbi.nlm.nih.gov/entrez/query.fcgi?cmd=Retrieve&db=PubMed&dopt=Citation&list_uids=3390826 (accessed August 17, 2005).
38. Novakovic B, Goldstein AM, Wexler LH, Tucker MA. Increased risk of neuroectodermal tumors and stomach cancer in relatives of patients with Ewing's sarcoma family of tumors [comments]. J Natl Cancer Inst 1994;86:1702–6.
39. Buckley JD, Pendergrass TW, Buckley CM, et al. Epidemiology of osteosarcoma and Ewing's sarcoma in childhood: a study of 305 cases by the Children's Cancer Group. Cancer 1998;83:1440–8.
40. Delattre O, Zucman J, Plougastel B, et al. Gene fusion with an ETS DNA-binding domain caused by chromosome translocation in human tumours. Nature 1992;359:162–5. Available at: http://www.ncbi.nlm.nih.gov/entrez/query.fcgi?cmd=Retrieve&db=PubMed&dopt=Citation&list_uids=1522903 (accessed August 17, 2005).
41. May WA, Lessnick SL, Braun BS, et al. The Ewing's sarcoma EWS/FLI-1 fusion gene encodes a more potent transcriptional activator and is a more powerful transforming gene than FLI-1. Mol Cell Biol 1993;13:7393–8. Available at: http://www.ncbi.nlm.nih.gov/entrez/query.fcgi?cmd=Retrieve&db=PubMed&dopt=Citation&list_uids=8246959 (accessed August 17, 2005).
42. Toretsky JA, Kalebic T, Blakesley V, et al. The insulin-like growth factor-I receptor is required for EWS/FLI-1 transformation of fibroblasts. J Biol Chem 1997;272:30822–7. Available at: http://www.ncbi.nlm.nih.gov/entrez/query.fcgi?cmd=Retrieve&db=PubMed&dopt=Citation&list_uids=9388225 (accessed August 17, 2005).
43. Toretsky JA, Connell Y, Neckers L, Bhat NK. Inhibition of EWS-FLI-1 fusion protein with antisense oligodeoxynucleotides. J Neurooncol 1997;31:9–16. Available at: http://www.ncbi.nlm.nih.gov/entrez/query.fcgi?cmd=Retrieve&db=PubMed&dopt=Citation&list_uids=9049825 (accessed August 17, 2005).
44. Ouchida M, Ohno T, Fujimura Y, et al. Loss of tumorigenicity of Ewing's sarcoma cells expressing antisense RNA to EWS-fusion transcripts. Oncogene 1995;11:1049–54. Available at: http://www.ncbi.nlm.nih.gov/entrez/query.fcgi?cmd=Retrieve&db=PubMed&dopt=Citation&list_uids=7566963 (accessed August 17, 2005).
45. Tanaka K, Iwakuma T, Harimaya K, et al. EWS-Fli1 antisense oligodeoxynucleotide inhibits proliferation of human Ewing's sarcoma and primitive neuroectodermal tumor cells. J Clin Invest 1997;99:239–47. Available at: http://www.ncbi.nlm.nih.gov/entrez/query.fcgi?cmd=Retrieve&db=PubMed&dopt=Citation&list_uids=9005992 (accessed August 17, 2005).

46. Chansky HA, Barahmand-Pour F, Mei Q, et al. Targeting of EWS/FLI-1 by RNA interference attenuates the tumor phenotype of Ewing's sarcoma cells in vitro. J Orthop Res 2004;22:910–7. Available at: http://www.ncbi.nlm.nih.gov/entrez/query.fcgi?cmd=Retrieve&db=PubMed&dopt=Citation&list_uids=15183454 (accessed August 17, 2005).
47. Dohjima T, Sook Lee N, Li H, et al. Small interfering RNAs expressed from a Pol III promoter suppress the EWS/Fli-1 transcript in an Ewing sarcoma cell line. Mol Ther 2003;7:811–6. Available at: http://www.ncbi.nlm.nih.gov/entrez/query.fcgi?cmd=Retrieve&db=PubMed&dopt=Citation&list_uids=12788655 (accessed August 17, 2005).
48. Deneen B, Denny CT. Loss of p16 pathways stabilizes EWS/FLI1 expression and complements EWS/FLI1 mediated transformation. Oncogene 2001;20:6731–41. Available at: http://www.ncbi.nlm.nih.gov/entrez/query.fcgi?cmd=Retrieve&db=PubMed&dopt=Citation&list_uids=11709708 (accessed August 17, 2005).
49. Kovar H, Jug G, Aryee DN, et al. Among genes involved in the RB dependent cell cycle regulatory cascade, the p16 tumor suppressor gene is frequently lost in the Ewing family of tumors. Oncogene 1997;15:2225–32. Available at: http://www.ncbi.nlm.nih.gov/entrez/query.fcgi?cmd=Retrieve&db=PubMed&dopt=Citation&list_uids=9393981 (accessed August 17, 2005).
50. Kovar H, Dworzak M, Strehl S, et al. Overexpression of the pseudoautosomal gene MIC2 in Ewing's sarcoma and peripheral primitive neuroectodermal tumor. Oncogene 1990;5:1067–70. Available at: http://www.ncbi.nlm.nih.gov/entrez/query.fcgi?cmd=Retrieve&db=PubMed&dopt=Citation&list_uids=1695726 (accessed August 17, 2005).
51. Parham DM, Hijazi Y, Steinberg SM, et al. Neuroectodermal differentiation in Ewing's sarcoma family of tumors does not predict tumor behavior. Hum Pathol 1999;30:911–8.
52. Cotterill SJ, Ahrens S, Paulussen M, et al. Prognostic factors in Ewing's tumor of bone: analysis of 975 patients from the European Intergroup Cooperative Ewing's Sarcoma Study Group. J Clin Oncol 2000;18:3108–14. Available at: http://www.jco.org/cgi/content/full/18/17/3108 and http://www.jco.org/cgi/content/abstract/18/17/3108 (accessed August 17, 2005).
53. Terrier P, Henry-Amar M, Triche TJ, et al. Is neuro-ectodermal differentiation of Ewing's sarcoma of bone associated with an unfavourable prognosis? Eur J Cancer 1995;31A:307–14. Available at: http://www.ncbi.nlm.nih.gov/entrez/query.fcgi?cmd=Retrieve&db=PubMed&dopt=Citation&list_uids=7786593 (accessed August 17, 2005).
54. Hattinger CM, Rumpler S, Ambros IM, et al. Demonstration of the translocation der(16)t(1;16)(q12;q11.2) in interphase nuclei of Ewing tumors. Genes Chromosomes Cancer 1996;17:141–50. Available at: http://www.ncbi.nlm.nih.gov/entrez/query.fcgi?cmd=Retrieve&db=PubMed&dopt=Citation&list_uids=8946192 (accessed August 17, 2005).
55. Horowitz ME, Malawer MM, Woo SJ, Hicks MJ. Ewing's Sarcoma family of tumors: Ewing's sarcoma of bone and soft tissue and the peripheral primitive neuroectodermal tumors. In: Pizzo PA, Poplack DG, editors. Principles and practice of pediatric oncology. 3rd ed. Philadelphia: Lippincott-Raven; 1997. p. 831–63.
56. Miser JS, Kinsella TJ, Triche TJ, et al. Ifosfamide with mesna uroprotection and etoposide: an effective regimen in the treatment of recurrent sarcomas and other tumors of children and young adults. J Clin Oncol 1987;5:1191–8. Available at: http://www.ncbi.nlm.nih.gov/entrez/query.fcgi?cmd=Retrieve&db=PubMed&dopt=Citation&list_uids=3114435 (accessed August 17, 2005).
57. Nesbit ME Jr, Gehan EA, Burgert EO Jr, et al. Multimodal therapy for the management of primary, nonmetastatic Ewing's sarcoma of bone: a long-term follow-up of the First Intergroup study. J Clin Oncol 1990;8:1664–74.
58. Grier HE, Krailo MD, Tarbell NJ, et al. Addition of ifosfamide and etoposide to standard chemotherapy for Ewing's sarcoma and primitive neuroectodermal tumor of bone. N Engl J Med 2003;348:694–701. Available at: http://www.ncbi.nlm.nih.gov/entrez/query.fcgi?cmd=Retrieve&db=PubMed&dopt=Citation&list_uids=12594313 (accessed August 17, 2005).
59. Granowetter L, Womer R, Devidas M. Comparison of dose intensified and standard dose chemotherapy for the treatment of non-metastatic Ewing's sarcoma and primitive neuroectodermal tumor of bone and soft tissue: a Pediatric Oncology Group-Children's Cancer Group phase III trial [abstract]. Med Pediatr Oncol 2001;37:A-038.
60. Cangir A, Vietti TJ, Gehan EA, et al. Ewing's sarcoma metastatic at diagnosis. Results and comparisons of two intergroup Ewing's sarcoma studies. Cancer 1990;66:887–93.
61. Paulussen M, Ahrens S, Burdach S, et al. Primary metastatic (stage IV) Ewing tumor: survival analysis of 171 patients from the EICESS studies. European Intergroup Cooperative Ewing Sarcoma Studies. Ann Oncol 1998;9:275–81. Available at: http://www.ncbi.nlm.nih.gov/entrez/query.fcgi?cmd=Retrieve&db=PubMed&dopt=Citation&list_uids=9602261 (accessed August 17, 2005).
62. Hayes FA, Thompson EI, Hustu HO, et al. The response of Ewing's sarcoma to sequential cyclophosphamide and Adriamycin induction therapy. J Clin Oncol 1983;1:45–51.
63. Kushner BH, Meyers PA. How effective is dose-intensive/myeloablative therapy against Ewing's sarcoma/primitive neuroectodermal tumor metastatic to bone or bone marrow? The Memorial Sloan-Kettering experience and a literature review. J Clin Oncol 2001;19:870–80. Available at: http://www.jco.org/cgi/content/full/19/3/870, http://www.jco.org/cgi/content/abstract/19/3/870, and http://www.ncbi.nlm.nih.gov/entrez/query.fcgi?cmd=Retrieve&db=PubMed&dopt=Citation&list_uids=11157041 (accessed August 17, 2005).
64. Miser JS, Krailo MD, Tarbell NJ, et al. Treatment of metastatic Ewing's sarcoma or primitive neuroectodermal tumor of bone: evaluation of combination ifosfamide and etoposide—a Children's Cancer Group and Pediatric Oncology Group study. J Clin Oncol 2004;22:2873–6. Available at: http://www.ncbi.nlm.nih.gov/entrez/query.fcgi?cmd=Retrieve&db=PubMed&dopt=Citation&list_uids=15254055 (accessed August 17, 2005).
65. Hawkins D, Barnett T, Bensinger W, et al. Busulfan, melphalan, and thiotepa with or without total marrow irradiation with hematopoietic stem cell rescue for poor-risk Ewing- Sarcoma-Family tumors. Med Pediatr Oncol 2000;34:328–37.
66. Toretsky JA, Neckers L, Wexler LH. Detection of (11;22)(q24;q12) translocation-bearing cells in peripheral blood progenitor cells of patients with Ewing's sarcoma family of tumors. J Natl Cancer Inst 1995;87:385–6. Available at: http://www.ncbi.nlm.nih.gov/entrez/query.fcgi?cmd=Retrieve&db=PubMed&dopt=Citation&list_uids=7853420 (accessed August 17, 2005).
67. Merino ME, Navid F, Christensen BL, et al. Immunomagnetic purging of Ewing's sarcoma from blood and bone marrow: quantitation by real-time polymerase chain reaction. J Clin Oncol 2001;19:3649–59. Available at: http://www.ncbi.nlm.nih.gov/entrez/query.fcgi?cmd=Retrieve&db=PubMed&dopt=Citation&list_uids=11504746 (accessed August 17, 2005).
68. Wexler LH, Andrich MP, Venzon D, et al. Randomized trial of the cardioprotective agent ICRF-187 in pediatric sarcoma patients treated with doxorubicin. J Clin Oncol 1996;14:362–72.
69. Dunst J, Ahrens S, Paulussen M, et al. Second malignancies after treatment for Ewing's sarcoma: a report of the CESS-studies. Int J Radiat Oncol Biol Phys 1998;42:379–84.
70. Kuttesch JF Jr, Wexler LH, Marcus RB, et al. Second malignancies after Ewing's sarcoma: radiation dose-dependency of secondary sarcomas. J Clin Oncol 1996;14:2818–25.
71. Miser J, Krailo M, Smith M, et al. Secondary leukemia (SL) or myelodysplastic syndrome (MDS) following therapy for Ewing's sarcoma (ES) [abstract]. Proc Am Soc Clin Oncol 1997;16:518a.
72. Le Vu B, de Vathaire F, Shamsaldin A, et al. Radiation dose, chemotherapy and risk of osteosarcoma after solid tumours during childhood. Int J Cancer 1998;77:370–7.
73. Dunst J, Jurgens H, Sauer R, et al. Radiation therapy in Ewing's sarcoma: an update of the CESS 86 trial. Int J Radiat Oncol Biol Phys 1995;32:919–30. Available at: http://www.ncbi.nlm.nih.gov/entrez/query.fcgi?cmd=Retrieve&db=PubMed&dopt=Citation&list_uids=7607966 (accessed August 17, 2005).
74. Schuck A, Hofmann J, Rube C, et al. Radiotherapy in Ewing's sarcoma and PNET of the chest wall: results of the trials CESS 81, CESS 86 and EICESS 92. Int J Radiat Oncol Biol Phys 1998;42:1001–6. Available at: http://www.ncbi.nlm.nih.gov/entrez/query.fcgi?cmd=Retrieve&db=PubMed&dopt=Citation&list_uids=9869222 (accessed August 17, 2005).
75. Donaldson SS, Torrey M, Link MP, Glicksman A, Gilula L, Laurie F, et al. A multidisciplinary study investigating radiotherapy in Ewing's sarcoma: end results of POG #8346. Pediatric Oncology Group. Int J Radiat Oncol Biol Phys 1998;42(1):125–-35. Available at: http://www.ncbi.nlm.nih.gov/entrez/query.fcgi?cmd=Retrieve&db=PubMed&dopt=Citation&list_uids=9747829 (accessed August 17, 2005).
76. Oberlin O, Deley MC, Bui BN, et al. Prognostic factors in localized Ewing's tumours and peripheral neuroectodermal tumours: the third study of the French Society of Paediatric Oncology (EW88 study). Br J Cancer 2001;85(11):1646–-54. Available at: http://www.ncbi.nlm.nih.gov/entrez/query.fcgi?cmd=Retrieve&db=PubMed&dopt=Citation&list_uids=11742482
77. Zoubek A, Dockhorn-Dworniczak B, Delattre O, et al. Does expression of different EWS chimeric transcripts define clinically distinct risk groups of Ewing tumor patients? J Clin Oncol 1996;14:1245–51. Available at: http://www.ncbi.nlm.nih.gov/entrez/query.fcgi?cmd=Retrieve&db=PubMed&dopt=Citation&list_uids=8648380 (accessed August 17, 2005).
78. Hattinger CM, Rumpler S, Strehl S, et al. Prognostic impact of deletions at 1p36 and numerical aberrations in Ewing tumors. Genes Chromosomes Cancer 1999;24:243–54. Available at: http://www.ncbi.nlm.nih.gov/entrez/query.fcgi?cmd=Retrieve&db=PubMed&dopt=Citation&list_uids=10451705 (accessed August 17, 2005).
79. Uren A, Toretsky JA. Pediatric malignancies provide unique cancer therapy targets. Curr Opin Pediatr 2005;17:14–9. Available at: http://www.ncbi.nlm.nih.gov/entrez/query.fcgi?cmd=Retrieve&db=PubMed&dopt=Citation&list_uids=15659957 (accessed August 17, 2005).
80. Saylors RL 3rd, Stine KC, Sullivan J, et al. Cyclophosphamide plus topotecan in children with recurrent or refractory solid tumors: a Pediatric Oncology Group phase II study. J Clin Oncol 2001;19:3463–9. Available at: http://www.ncbi.nlm.nih.gov/entrez/query.fcgi?cmd=Retrieve&db=PubMed&dopt=Citation&list_uids=11481351 (accessed August 17, 2005).
81. Bernstein M, Goorin A, Devidas M, et al. Topotecan and topotecan, cyclophosphamide window therapy in patients with Ewing sarcoma metastatic at diagnosis: an intergroup Pediatric Oncology Group study. SIOP 2001;37:0–51.
82. Uren A, Merchant MS, Sun CJ, et al. Beta-platelet-derived growth factor receptor mediates motility and growth of Ewing's sarcoma cells. Oncogene 2003;22:2334–42. Available at: http://www.ncbi.nlm.nih.gov/entrez/query.fcgi?cmd=Retrieve&db=PubMed&dopt=Citation&list_uids=12700668 (accessed August 17, 2005).
83. Merchant MS, Woo CW, Mackall CL, Thiele CJ. Potential use of imatinib in Ewing's Sarcoma: evidence for in vitro and in vivo activity. J Natl Cancer Inst 2002;94:1673–9. Available at: http://www.ncbi.nlm.nih.gov/entrez/query.fcgi?cmd=Retrieve&db=PubMed&dopt=Citation&list_uids=12441322 (accessed August 17, 2005).
84. Scotlandi K, Manara MC, Strammiello R, et al. C-kit receptor expression in Ewing's sarcoma: lack of prognostic value but therapeutic targeting opportunities in appropriate conditions. J Clin Oncol 2003;21:1952–60. Available at: http://www.ncbi.nlm.nih.gov/entrez/query.fcgi?cmd=Retrieve&db=PubMed&dopt=Citation&list_uids=12743148 (accessed August 17, 2005).
85. Mitsiades N, Poulaki V, Mitsiades C, Tsokos M. Ewing's sarcoma family tumors are sensitive to tumor necrosis factor-related apoptosis-inducing ligand and express death receptor 4 and death receptor 5. Cancer Res 2001;61:2704–12. Available at: http://www.ncbi.nlm.nih.gov/entrez/query.fcgi?cmd=Retrieve&db=PubMed&dopt=Citation&list_uids=11289151 (accessed August 17, 2005).
86. Takita J, Yang HW, Bessho F, et al. Absent or reduced expression of the caspase 8 gene occurs frequently in neuroblastoma, but not commonly in Ewing sarcoma or rhabdomyosarcoma. Med Pediatr Oncol 2000;35:541–3. Available at: http://www.ncbi.nlm.nih.gov/entrez/query.fcgi?cmd=Retrieve&db=PubMed&dopt=Citation&list_uids=11107112 (accessed August 17, 2005).
87. Van Valen F, Fulda S, Truckenbrod B, et al. Apoptotic responsiveness of the Ewing's sarcoma family of tumours to tumour necrosis factor-related apoptosis-inducing ligand (TRAIL). Int J Cancer 2000;88:252–9. Available at: http://www.ncbi.nlm.nih.gov/entrez/query.fcgi?cmd=Retrieve&db=PubMed&dopt=Citation&list_uids=11004677 (accessed August 17, 2005).
88. Scotlandi K, Benini S, Nanni P, et al. Blockage of insulin-like growth factor-I receptor inhibits the growth of Ewing's sarcoma in athymic mice. Cancer Res 1998;58:4127–31. (accessed August 17, 2005).
89. Craft AW, Cotterill SJ, Bullimore JA, Pearson D. Long-term results from the first UKCCSG Ewing's Tumour Study (ET-1). United Kingdom Children's Cancer Study Group (UKCCSG) and the Medical Research Council Bone Sarcoma Working Party. Eur J Cancer. 1997 Jun;33(7):1061–9.

Section 38

COMPLICATIONS OF CANCER AND THEIR TREATMENT

125

Cancer in Young Adults and Older Adolescents

W. Archie Bleyer, MD
Karen Albritton, MD

During the past half-century, since the advent of modern oncology, children (younger than 15 years of age) with cancer have been a singular focus of treatment and research. The advances among patients in this age group have been among the most dramatic in the history of medicine, and the cooperative infrastructure that has supported this success has been among the most organized in the history of science. In 1971, the National Cancer Act led to another highly organized effort, which has significantly improved the outcome of adults with cancer, in whom the median age is in the sixties. Meanwhile, substantially less attention has been given to the next oldest age group of cancer patients. Yet, cancer develops in nearly three times more people in the 15- to 29-year-old age group than in those younger than 15 years of age, and the incidence of cancer has increased more rapidly in this older age group than in the younger population. In addition, the relative improvement in the survival rate in young adults has not kept pace with that achieved in younger patients.

The reasons for this lack of progress certainly include issues specific to this age group: some inherent in the disease or the patient (differences in biology or intolerance of therapy), some inherent in the system (treatment by physicians less familiar with the disease, delay in recognition of malignancy, lack of available clinical trials, or failure to enroll patients in available trials), and some influenced by the psychosocial milieu of the patient (unwillingness to participate in clinical trials, delays in seeking medical attention with symptoms of cancer, poor compliance with treatment). A further consideration is that the physical, emotional, and social challenges posed by cancer in adolescence and early adult life are often unique and especially difficult for patients, families, and health care providers alike.

In contradistinction to younger and older patients with cancer, until recently, adolescents and young adults with cancer have had no national program to address their special problems. This review describes these issues relevant and specific to adolescents and young adults with cancer and their caregivers. The ultimate goal is to heighten awareness of a relatively neglected group of patients who, during the next half-century, deserve better.

DEFINITION OF OLDER ADOLESCENT AND YOUNG ADULT

For the purposes of this review, the older adolescent–young adult age range is considered to be 15 to 29 years of age. Most of the published analyses that have been performed on this age group were performed on subgroups in this age range, such as 15 to 19, 20 to 29, and 16 to 21 years of age. When known, the age range is specified in this review.

EPIDEMIOLOGY

Incidence Data from the National Cancer Institute's (NCI) Surveillance, Epidemiology, and End Results (SEER) Program indicate that in the United States each year, nearly 24,000 persons between 15 and 30 years of age are diagnosed with invasive cancer (Table 125-1). This age group has a cancer incidence that is 2.6 times that of children less than 15 years of age (see Table 125-1).[1] Specifically, the average annual rate per million Americans during the period 1993 to 2000 was 409 among 15- to 29-year-olds and 151 among 0- to 15-year-olds (see Table 125-1).

Table 125-1 Incidence of Invasive Cancer, SEER Program, 1975–2000*

	Age at Diagnosis, Yr								
	<5	5–9	10–14	15–19	20–24	25–29	30–34	35–39	40–44
US population, 2000 census	19,175,798	20,549,505	20,528,072	20,219,890	18,964,001	19,381,336	20,510,388	22,706,664	22,441,863
Average annual increase in invasive cancer, %, 1975–1999, SEER Program	1.0	0.4	0.9	0.7	1.0	1.9	1.6	1.1	0.4
Estimated incidence of invasive cancer, 2000, per million	216.6	112.59	128.5	216.3	365.3	662.0	983.0	1,462.0	2,156.0
Estimated number of persons diagnosed with invasive cancer, 2000, US	4,153	2,314	2,638	4,374	6,928	12,830	20,162	33,197	48,385

SEER = Surveillance, Epidemiology, and End Results.
*SEER Program data adapted from Ries LAG et al[1] and population data from the US Census Bureau.

Among 15- to 29-year-old females, the incidence of cancer was 3.0 times greater, and among males, it was 2.4 times greater than in the younger females and males, respectively.

The most common cancers among 15- to 19-year-olds in the United States are Hodgkin's lymphoma (16%), germ cell tumors (15%), central nervous system tumors (10%), non-Hodgkin's lymphoma (NHL) (8%), thyroid cancer (7%), malignant melanoma (7%), and acute lymphoblastic leukemia (ALL) (6%) (Figure 125-1, upper panel). In 20- to 29-year-olds, the most frequent malignancies are lymphomas (including Hodgkin's disease) (18%), germ cell tumors (primarily testicular and ovarian carcinoma) (17%), malignant melanoma (12%), thyroid carcinoma (10%), and sarcomas (primarily soft tissue) (10%) (see Figure 125-1, lower panel). From the distribution, it is obvious that adolescents and young adults rarely develop the cancers that predominate in older adults, such as carcinomas of the aerodigestive and genitourinary tracts.[2,3] Similarly, most of the common "developmental" malignancies in children younger than 5 years of age are virtually absent in 15- to 19-year-olds, including the embryonal malignancies of Wilms' tumor, neuroblastoma, medulloblastoma, ependymoma, hepatoblastoma, and retinoblastoma.

One example of how young adults fall in a gap between pediatric and adult oncology becomes apparent when one attempts to analyze cancer incidence in this age group; one must chose between two classification systems. The one for children, the World Health Organization or International Classification of Childhood Cancer (ICCC) classification, is based on histology.[4] The International Classification of Diseases (ICD) system, used for adults, is based primarily on organ site. For the cancers of older adolescents and young adults, the childhood cancer system has proved to be more applicable.[5–7] This is illustrated in Figure 125-2, which shows that between two-thirds and three-fourths of 15- to 19-year-old patients have a pediatric type of cancer (upper panel) and about half of the types in 20- to 29-year-olds are pediatric in nature (lower panel). Although uncommon, many of the cancers of older patients or younger children do occur in adolescents.[8–16] Adolescents may also develop two cancers simultaneously.[17] Thus, neither histology nor topography provides a completely accurate basis on which to classify the cancers of adolescents and young adults.

Some authors advocate using the childhood cancer classification scheme, with minor modifications, for analyzing cancer incidence in older adolescent age groups.[5–7] One recommendation is to enumerate colorectal, salivary, and lung carcinomas separately from "other carcinomas" within the group of "carcinoma and other epithelial tumors."[5] Breast cancer also should probably be dealt with in this way.[8,9] A separate nosologic system for patients 15 to 29 years of age may be the best solution because of the uniqueness of the distribution of cancers in this age group.

Osteosarcoma, Ewing's sarcoma, gonadal germ cell tumors, and Hodgkin's lymphoma have a peak in incidence during adolescence and young adulthood. The two bone sarcomas peak between 15 and 19 years of age and the gonadal tumors and Hodgkin's lymphoma peak between 20 and 29 years of age (Figure 125-3). The types of soft tissue sarcoma that occur in 15-to 19-year-olds are also distinct from those seen in younger patients. Specifically, rhabdomyosarcoma predominates among the sarcomas of childhood, accounting for more than 60% of the soft tissue sarcomas among

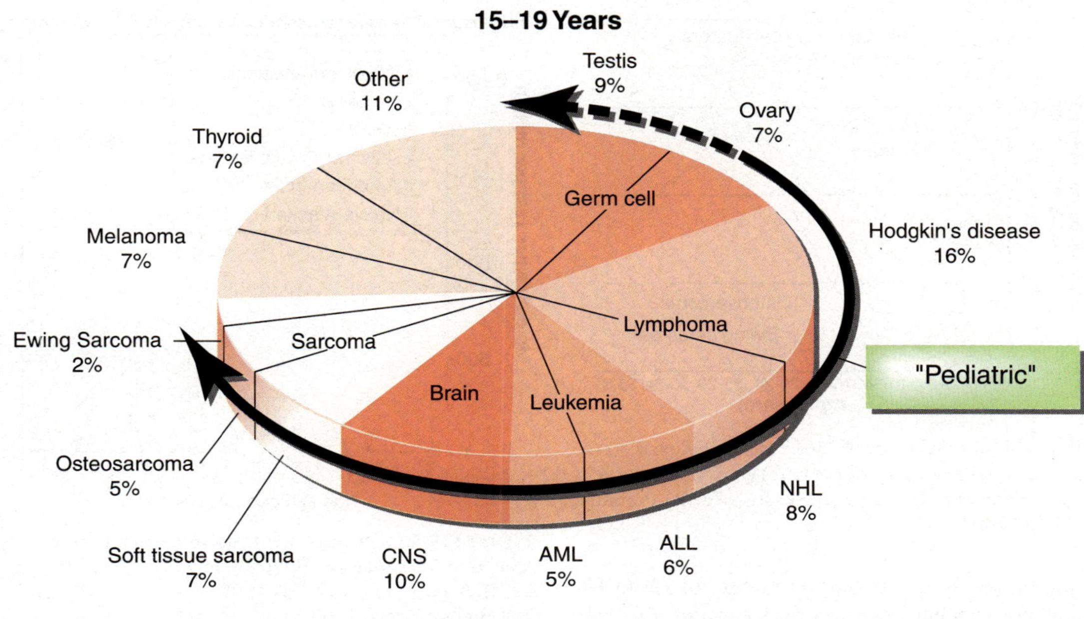

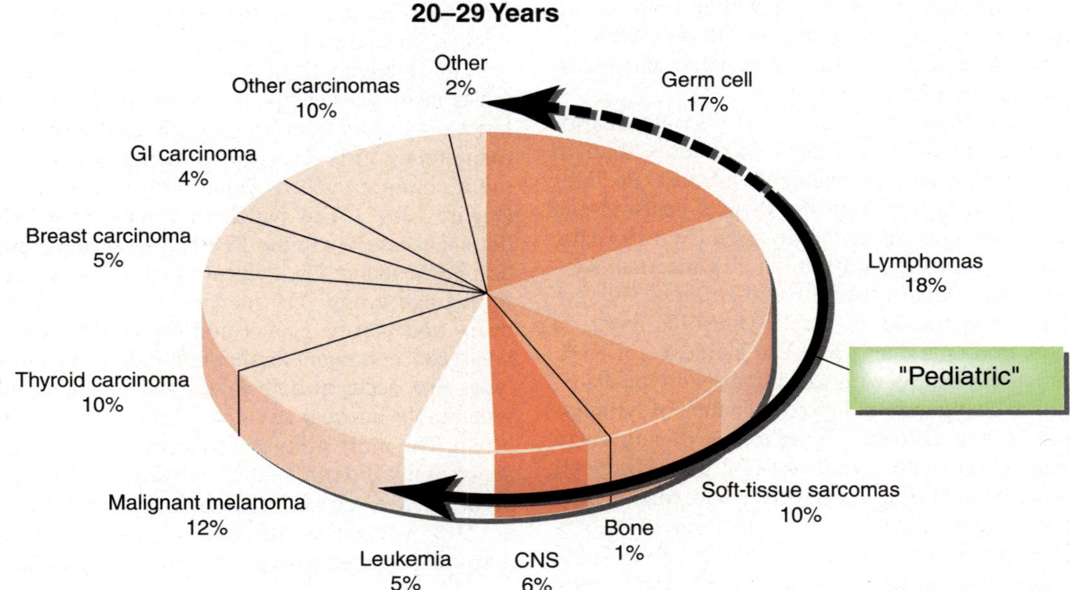

Figure 125-2 Common malignancies diagnosed at ages 15 to 19 years (*upper panel*) and 20 to 29 years (*lower panel*). Data from the Surveillance, Epidemiology, and End Results (SEER) Program, 1986 to 1995.[1] The *arrow* circumscribes those cancers that are common in children.

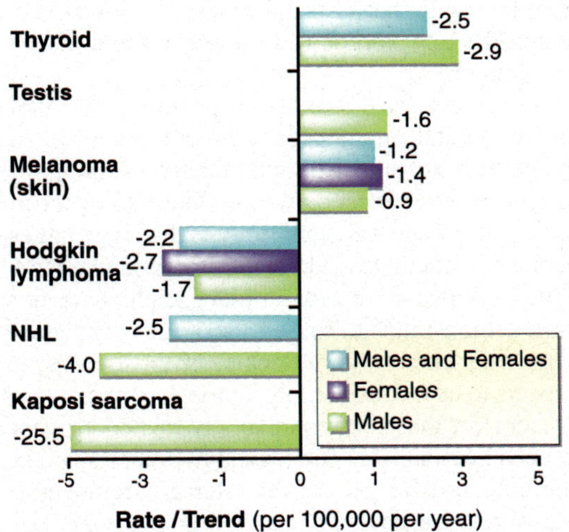

Figure 125-1 Cancer incidence trends, Surveillance, Epidemiology, and End Results (SEER) Program, 1992 to 2001, ages 20 to 29 years at diagnosis. NHL = non-Hodgkin's lymphoma.

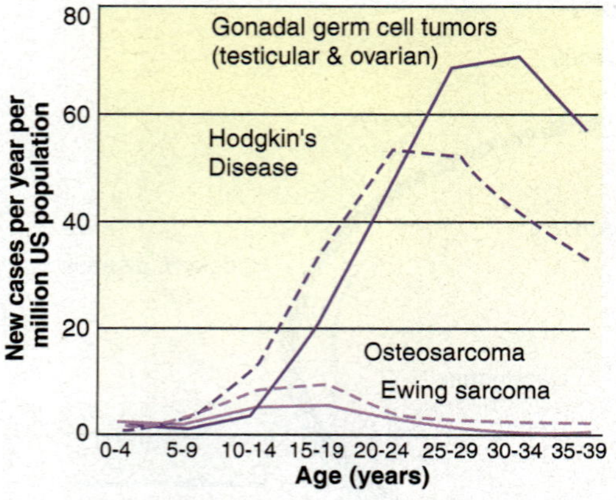

Figure 125-3 Incidence of four cancers that peak in the adolescent–young adult age range. Data from the Surveillance, Epidemiology, and End Results (SEER) Program, 1986 to 1995.[1]

children younger than 5 years of age. In 15- to 19-year-olds, rhabdomyosarcoma accounts for only 25% of soft tissue sarcomas. Nonrhabdomyosarcoma soft tissue sarcomas, including synovial sarcoma,[10] liposarcoma, malignant fibrous histiocytoma, and malignant peripheral nerve sheath tumors, account for most of the rest.

Leukemias and lymphomas also are distributed differently in older adolescents than in young children. The incidence of ALL declines steadily with age from the 0- to 5-year-old age group and upward, so that by ages 15 to 19 years, ALL accounts for only 6% of all cancers in adolescents, in contrast to 30% in children younger than 15 years. In 15- to 19-year-olds, NHL is more common than ALL. The incidence of NHL increases steadily with age, but the subtype distribution changes from a predominance of lymphoblastic and Burkitt's lymphomas during early childhood to a predominance of diffuse large-cell lymphoma during adolescence and early adulthood. Acute myelogenous leukemia (AML) is nearly as common as ALL in 15- to 19-year-olds and is more common than ALL in 20- to 29-year-olds. The incidence of chronic myelogenous leukemia (CML) increases steadily with age from birth on but is not as common as either ALL or AML from 15 to 29 years of age. Juvenile myelomonocytic leukemia is uncommon in all four 5-year age groups before age 20 years, but this is especially true in 15- to 19-year-olds.

Ethnic and racial differences in incidence become apparent by 15 years of age, such that the 15- to 29-year age group clearly demonstrates a higher incidence of cancer among the non-Hispanic white population and a lower incidence among native Americans and Alaskans (Figure 125-4). African Americans, Hispanics and Latinos, and Asian Americans have intermediate incidence rates (see Figure 125-4). The incidence of Ewing's sarcoma and of melanoma is strikingly higher in whites, a difference that occurs at all age levels affected by these malignancies. ALL, testicular carcinoma, and thyroid cancer also are substantively more common in whites than in African Americans. Among the common cancers in this age group, only soft tissue sarco-

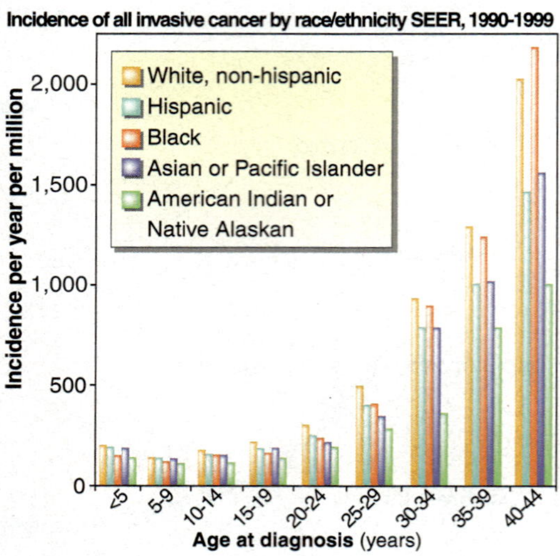

Figure 125-4 Incidence of invasive cancer by race or ethnicity, Surveillance, Epidemiology, and End Results (SEER) Program, 1990 to 1999, ages 0 to 44 years. Adapted from Ries LAG et al.[1]

mas, considered as a group, are more common in African Americans than in whites.[3]

The relative risk of cancer in females versus males increases steadily as a function of age from birth to 44 years from being nearly 20% less common among girls than boys to being nearly 70% more common among females by age 44 years (Figure 125-5). The switch from male to female dominance occurs in the 15- to 29-year age group despite the increasing incidence in testicular cancer in this age group. The increase in cancer of the ovary and uterine cervix and the emergence of breast cancer account for the shift. Individual tumor types that occur in both males and females have remarkably unequal sex distributions in this age group. The most striking difference is in the incidence of thyroid carcinoma, with females 10 times more likely to develop this disease. Females also are 50% more likely than males to develop melanoma and approximately 15% more likely to have

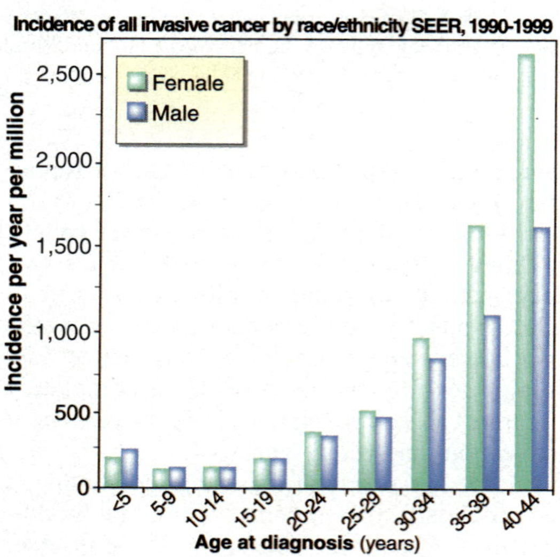

Figure 125-5 Incidence of invasive cancer by gender, Surveillance, Epidemiology, and End Results (SEER) Program, 1990 to 1999, ages 0 to 44 years. Adapted from Ries LAG et al.[1]

Hodgkin's lymphoma.[3] Alternatively, young males are more than twice as likely to develop ALL, twice as likely to be diagnosed with NHL or Ewing's sarcoma, 50% more likely to sustain osteosarcoma, and 20 to 30% more likely to have a brain tumor.[3]

Several cancers important in this age group have marked international variations in incidence rates.[18] The rates of melanoma among members of this age group are 3 to 50 times higher in Australia, where the incidence of melanoma is the highest in the world among both adults and children.[5,18] In Asia and India, Hodgkin's lymphoma is far less frequent than in the rest of the world. Testicular cancer has a similarly low incidence in these countries and in blacks in the United States. Thyroid cancer is more prominent in Canada, whites in the United States, Hong Kong, and Israel and is uncommon in Costa Rica, Puerto Rico, blacks in the United States, Japan, India, and the Netherlands. These variations in incidence provide fertile ground for research into etiology.

ETIOLOGY

As in younger patients, little is known about the causes of cancer in adolescents and young adults. Whereas cancers in infants and young children are likely to be strongly influenced by congenital and prenatal factors and cancers in the elderly population are most strongly linked to environmental causes, the pathogenesis of cancer in young adults and older adolescents may be a combination of both, or the mechanisms may be entirely different. Very few cancers in this age group have been attributed directly to single environmental or inherited factors. An exception is clear cell adenocarcinoma of the vagina or cervix in adolescent females, with most cases caused by diethylstilbestrol taken prenatally by their mothers in an attempt to prevent spontaneous abortion.[19] Radiation-induced cancers may occur in adolescents and young adults after exposure during early childhood. In fact, many of the adolescent and young adult cancers that have been linked to an identifiable cause are second malignant neoplasms in patients who were treated with chemotherapy and/or radiotherapy for a previous cancer.

Given that the duration of exposure to potential environmental carcinogens is directly proportional to age, it is not surprising that tobacco-, sunlight-, or diet-related cancers are more likely to occur in older adolescents and young adults than in younger persons. Nonetheless, these environmental agents known to be carcinogens in older adults have not been demonstrated to cause cancer with any significant frequency in adolescents. In most cases, it appears to take considerably longer than one or two decades for these environmentally related cancers to become manifest. The logical hypothesis is that adolescents who get cancer after a carcinogenic exposure must have a predisposing genotype. For example, melanoma is more common among Australian adolescents than among those elsewhere in the world, as described above. This suggests that solar exposure may be able to induce skin cancer before the end of the second decade of life, at least in that part of the world.

Besides intense sun exposure, exposure to other environmental carcinogens (including tobacco), recreational drugs, alcohol, and sexually transmitted diseases begins or intensifies during this age period. Cancer control efforts to reduce teenage exposure to these carcinogens are unlikely to affect the rates of cancers in adolescents but should decrease the rates in older adults.

Skin cancer, lymphoma, sarcoma, and thyroid and hepatic cancers may also occur at higher frequency during this period of life in persons with inherited conditions (Chapter 13, "Genetic Predisposition to Cancer"). In the aggregate, however, these cancers account for only a small proportion of the cancers that occur during adolescence and early adulthood.

DIAGNOSIS

Signs and Symptoms With few exceptions, the signs and symptoms of cancer in young adults and older adolescents are similar to those of the same cancer in younger and older patients. Nonetheless, knowing the most common sites of disease in the age group helps in directing the evaluation of the symptoms and in formulating the most appropriate differential diagnosis. The examiner who is not aware of the prominence of sarcomas, thyroid and testicular cancer, and melanoma in this age group may overlook these possibilities when taking the history and performing the physical examination.

Because of psychological and social factors in adolescents and young adults, patients in this age range may be at higher risk of a delay in diagnosis, a factor that may impact their cancer survival. In a study of the interval between symptom onset and diagnosis in 2,665 children participating in Pediatric Oncology Group therapeutic protocols between 1982 and 1988, Pollock and colleagues found by multivariate analysis that for all solid tumors except Hodgkin's lymphoma, as age increased, lag time increased.[20]

The reasons for delay in seeking medical care and obtaining a diagnosis are multiple:

1. Adolescents and young adults have a strong sense of invincibility. Out of denial, they may delay seeing a physician for symptoms. Even when seen, they may give poor historical information, especially to a physician untrained to "read between the lines" of an adolescent's history. Some of the most advanced disease presentations occur in adolescents. We have had older adolescents with extraordinarily large masses of the breast, testes, abdomen, pelvis, and extremity that they had harbored for months because they were too embarrassed to bring the problem to anyone's attention.
2. Too many young adults are not receiving routine medical care. Young adults and older adolescents have the lowest rate of primary care use of any age group in the United States.[21] Regardless of health insurance status, adolescents and young adults are more likely than younger children to lack a usual source of care. Without a primary physician who knows the patient's baseline heath status, the symptoms of cancer can be missed.
3. Physicians may be poorly trained or unwilling to care for adolescents.
4. Adolescents and young adults are not "supposed to" have cancer. Clinical suspicion is low, and symptoms are often attributed to physical exertion, fatigue, and stress.
5. Young adults are the most underinsured age group, falling in the gap between parental coverage and programs designed to provide universal health insurance to children (Medicaid and Children's Health Insurance Programs) and the coverage supplied by a full-time secure job.[22,23]

Data from The University of Texas M. D. Anderson Cancer Center indicate that among 15- to 29-year-olds with newly diagnosed, previously untreated cancer, the lag time to diagnosis was correlated with the quality of health insurance. Those with public or no health insurance had statistically longer lag times in five of the six cancers evaluated.[24,25] In multivariate analysis, only the type of cancer and quality of health insurance were significantly correlated with lag time. Gender, age subgroup, race or ethnicity, religion, marital status, rural versus urban residence, and median household income and population density of the zip code of residence were not correlated.

Given the lack of routine care, empowering young adults and older adolescents for self-care and detection is important. Certainly, self-examination of the skin and, in females, of the breasts should be encouraged. However, at this age, it may be most difficult to teach the importance of early detection of cancer because at no other time in life is the sense of invincibility more pervasive. Adolescents should be taught especially to examine themselves for cancers that increase in incidence during this time period. This is particularly true for testicular self-examination, a subject that is obviously difficult to bring up and teach at this age.[26] On the other hand, there is little evidence that testicular self-examination screening is effective. The American Cancer Society encourages self-examination of the skin and breasts and increasing the awareness of testicular cancer in young men, but routine testicular self-examination is not recommended by the organization. Teaching testicular cancer awareness to high school and college students may not be as difficult as it may seem. A preliminary assessment of teaching testicular self-examination showed that anxiety was no greater in students who were exposed to presentations on testicular cancer and testicular self-examination than in those who did not receive this training.[27] Additionally, efforts should be made to educate teenagers about the treatment and cure rates of cancer in children and young adults to dispel the fatalistic perception that arises from knowing older individuals (grandparents and others) who have died from cancer.

Radiologic and Pathologic Diagnosis Compared with the diagnosis of cancer in children, the diagnosis of cancer in adolescents and young adults is facilitated by the older patient's ability to describe and localize the symptoms and signs caused by the malignancy and the greater ease with which biopsies can be obtained. Knowing the most common sites and histology of malignancies in the age group assists in evaluating symptoms and in selecting the most appropriate imaging and biopsy procedures. Noninvasive imaging without the need for sedation, endoscopy, and minimally invasive surgery are all available for patients in this age group. Although these are used more often in adolescents and young adults than in children because they are easier to obtain, it is possible that they are underused in this group, in comparison with older patients, because of a lack of insurance and other economic constraints, difficulty taking time off from work, transportation limitations, and a lack of understanding on the part of professional staff as to what diagnostic and staging procedures are appropriate.

TREATMENT

As is true at any age, treatment depends on the type and stage of the tumor. In general, however, the therapeutic management of cancers in adolescents and young adults differs from that in adults because of physiologic, psychological, and social differences. Although there is a dearth of publications that address these issues, several provide advice on how to manage the cancers that occur in this age group.[28–38]

Choice of Treatment Setting and Specialist A central, complex issue is the appropriate specialist to manage the treatment of the young adult and adolescent—a pediatric oncologist or an adult oncologist (medical, radiation, surgical or gynecologic oncologist). Leonard and colleagues surmised that, at least in the United Kingdom, adult oncologists are "untutored in arranging ancillary medical, psychological, and educational supports that are so important to people who are facing dangerous diseases and taxing treatment at a vulnerable time in their lives" and "unpracticed in managing rare sarcomas," and pediatric oncologists "have little to no experience in epithelial tumours or some of the other tumours common in late adolescence."[39] The (admittedly biased) American Academy of Pediatrics issued a consensus statement, in 1997, in which it indicated that referral to a board-eligible or board-certified pediatric hematologist-oncologist and to pediatric subspecialty consultants was the standard of care for all pediatric and adolescent cancer patients.[40] A wider consensus panel that included adult oncologists, the American Federation of Clinical Oncologic Societies, also concluded that "payors must provide ready access to pediatric oncologists, recognizing that childhood cancers are biologically distinct" and that the "likelihood of successful outcome in children is enhanced when treatment is provided by pediatric cancer specialists."[41] However, neither of these statements defines an age cutoff for the recommendation.

Currently, the choice of specialist is made haphazardly and probably depends on the decision of the referring physician. Younger children primarily obtain care from pediatricians who refer to pediatric centers and specialists. Young adult and older adolescent patients are seen by a breadth of specialists for their presenting symptoms of cancer. These include internists, family physicians, gynecologists, emergency room physicians, dermatologists, gastroenterologists, neurologists, and other specialists. These physicians may have very different referral patterns.[42] And when a referral of a young adult or adolescent patient is made to an oncologist subspecialist, the latter may be a medical, radiation, surgical, or gynecologic oncologist or other oncologic specialist.

The switch from predominantly pediatric specialist management to adult management occurs not at age 21 years or even at age 18 years, as might be expected, but around age 15 years. A cancer registry review in Utah, a state that has only one pediatric oncology treatment facility, showed that only 36% of oncology patients aged 15 to 19 years were ever seen at the pediatric hospital.[43] A study of the National Cancer Data Base found that for nearly 20,000 cases of cancer in adolescents aged 15 to 19 years, only 34% were treated at centers that had NCI pediatric cooperative group affiliation.[44] Research is only now being done to ascertain the reasons for this practice pattern.

The answer to which specialist is most appropriate certainly varies from case to case. Patients at any age who have a "pediatric" tumor, such as rhabdomyosarcoma, Ewing's sarcoma, and osteosarcoma, will probably benefit from the expertise of a pediatric oncologist, at least in the form of consultation. Children younger than age 18 years and their parents may benefit from the social and supportive culture of a pediatric hospital regardless of the diagnosis. Individuals between the ages of 16 and 24 years may have varying levels of maturity and independence, and the choice of physician and setting for their care should be individually determined. Pediatric oncologists may be less adept at a nonpaternalistic relationship with the patient (and potentially his or her spouse) and less inclined to consider issues such as sexuality, body image, fertility, and the like. Adult oncologists are more accustomed to dose delays and adjustments and may be less willing to be aggressive with dosing that can be tolerated by the younger patient.

In the end, the decision should be based in large part on which setting will provide the patient with the best outcome. If these are equivalent, "social" or "supportive" factors should weigh into the decision. Few comparative outcome data are available. Stock and colleagues compared patients between the ages of 16 and 21 years who were registered on either a pediatric (Children's Cancer Group [CCG]) or an adult (Cancer and Leukemia Group B [CALGB]) treatment protocol between 1988 and 1998. The remarkably significant results were a 6-year event-free survival of 64% for those treated in the CCG study and 38% for those treated in the CALGB study.[45] At M. D. Anderson, the results of treatment for AML in adults improved substantively after treatment derived from pediatric trials was introduced into the institution's trials.[46] The analysis of data from the National Cancer Data Base revealed that adolescents (ages 15–19 years) with NHL, leukemia, liver cancer, and bone tumors have a survival advantage if treated at an NCI pediatric group institution.[44]

The British, although hindered by the limited size of their patient population (only 600 cancer cases per year between the ages of 13 and 20 years), have pioneered the solution of treating young adult and adolescent patients at a unique "adolescent oncology unit."[29] This provides the adolescent with age-specific nursing care, recreation therapy, and peer companionship. Perhaps it is appropriate to have as a goal centers and oncologists devoted solely to the care of this group of patients.

Surgery In general, surgery is performed more readily and anesthesia is easier to administer in larger patients. Another advantage is that young adults are generally healthier than older patients. The main disadvantage in fully grown patients relative to children is that the older patients generally have fewer compensatory mechanisms to overcome deficits and disabilities resulting from the surgical resection of large tumors. Decisions to use sedation and anesthesia commonly employed in younger children (eg, topical anesthetic for venipunctures) should be individualized to the adolescent or young adult patient but should not be dismissed as unnecessary just because of the patient's "maturity."

Radiation Therapy Compared with children, adolescents and young adults are less vulnerable to the adverse effects of ionizing radiation. This is particularly true for the central nervous system, the cardiovascular system, connective tissue, and the musculoskeletal system, each of which may be irradiated to higher doses and/or larger volumes with less long-term morbidity than in younger patients. By analogy, older adolescents who are still maturing may be more vulnerable to radiation toxicities than older persons at those sites and tissues that are still undergoing development, such as the breast and gonads. Breast cancer, for example, is more likely in women who received radiation for Hodgkin's lymphoma if the radiation was administered between the onset of puberty and the age of 30 years.[47] Remarkably little is actually known about the differential normal tissue effects of radiotherapy in patients between 15 and 30 years of age.

Chemotherapy The acute and chronic toxicities of chemotherapeutic agents are generally similar in children, adolescents, and young adults. Exceptions are that older patients in this age range may experience a greater degree of anticipatory vomiting, have a somewhat less rapid recovery from myeloablative agents, and have fewer stem cells in the peripheral blood available for autologous rescue. Adolescents and young adults certainly can tolerate more intensive chemotherapeutic regimens than older adults because of better organ (especially renal) function. This should encourage those treating patients in this age group to push the limits of dose intensification. At M. D. Anderson, the more rigorous pediatric regimen for ALL was adopted successfully years ago. Subsequently, the center also integrated the more intensive AML regimen used by pediatric oncologists into the adult therapy program for AML. In London, Verrill and colleagues found the use of pediatric regimens for the treatment of young adults (ages 16–48 years) with Ewing's sarcoma "rational and feasible," without excessive dose delays or modifications.[48]

Adherence to therapeutic regimens, particularly oral chemotherapy, is also much more problematic in teenagers and young adults than in younger and older patients.[49–52]

Psychosocial and Supportive Care The greatest difference in the management of adolescents and young adult patients is in the supportive care, particularly psychosocial care, that they require. These patients have special needs that are not only unique to their age group but are also broader in scope and more intense than those at any other time in life.

Young adult and older adolescent patients are on the cusp of autonomy, starting to gain success at independent decision making, when the diagnosis of cancer renders them "out of control" and often throws them back to a dependent role with parents and authority figures (by circumstance and/or by choice). Sometimes the patient has become distanced from his or her nuclear family but has not yet developed a network of adult support relationships. Young adults or adolescent patients usually have many new roles that they are just trying to master when the cancer diagnosis hits: high school student, college student, recent graduate, newlywed, new employee, or new parent. How can they succeed when, in addition to all of these stresses, cancer intervenes? How can they plan and begin their future when they suddenly realize that they may not have one? What will happen if they cannot graduate, keep their friends, finish their education, get a good job, marry, have children, or be whatever they aspire to be?

Because of the complex issues of dependence, decision making during cancer therapy is different for the patient, family, and physician of an adolescent or young adult than for either the younger patient (which is more paternalistic) or the older adult (more patient centered). The young adult patient may wish to make his or her own decisions, but his or her understanding of the illness may be incomplete or flawed.[53]

Honing social and interpersonal skills is an important developmental milestone during adolescence. Cancer treatment for these patients must accommodate this important developmental process. We discharged a patient from the intensive care unit to allow her to attend her senior prom and readmitted her when the party was over. Yet boundaries must be set, so that treatment effectiveness is not compromised to keep a "social calendar." Certainly, cancer therapy causes practical problems in social arenas. Adolescent and young adult patients, who are developmentally dependent on peer group approval, often feel isolated from peers by their experience; the cancer patient's issues are illness and death, whereas their peers are consumed by lipstick and homework. All adolescents agonize over their personal appearance and hate to be singled out or to appear different. In adolescents with cancer, having to be isolated from peers and society by having a disease that makes them different and having to be treated separately are often devastating. In addition, many of the adverse effects of therapy can be overwhelming to an adolescent's or young adult's self-image, which is often tenuous under the best of circumstances. Weight gain, alopecia, acne, stunted growth, and mutilating surgery to the face and extremities are examples of adverse consequences that can be devastating to an adolescent's self-image. In particular, hair loss is cited over and over as a huge blow to the adolescent or young adult (especially the female) with cancer.

Other challenges include the time away from school, work, and community that therapy requires and the financial hardships that occur at an age when economic independence from family is an objective. There may be guilt if not attending to these responsibilities or stress and fatigue if trying to keep up a semblance of normal activity.

This is a period when sexuality, intimacy, and reproduction are central. In our culture, a young adult is supposed to attract a mate and reproduce. But the young adult with cancer may feel or look unattractive, may be uninterested in or unable to have sex, and may be infertile. A feeling of impotence can pervade.

Most patients are in a relationship or hope to be in one. However, the relationship will be tested by the strain of the cancer diagnosis and its therapy. Patients may wonder whether the partner stays in the relationship out of guilt or sympathy. Some significant others may feel ignored by medical staff because they are not formally a "family member." After treatment, commitment to the relationship in the face of fear of relapse or infertility can be difficult for both parties. Those contemplating having children often worry about passing on a genetic predisposition to cancer.

A wide range of financial situations is seen in the young adult population. Some patients are still happily dependent on their parents. If at a university, they usually (but not always) have health insurance. Some are just striking out on their own but, without a long-standing job or savings, may have to return to dependence on parents or get public assistance. Others are trying to begin a career, but long work absences threaten their job security or growth. As stated above, this age range is the most uninsured. As a result, many young adult patients incur high medical bills at a time in life when they may be least able to afford them.

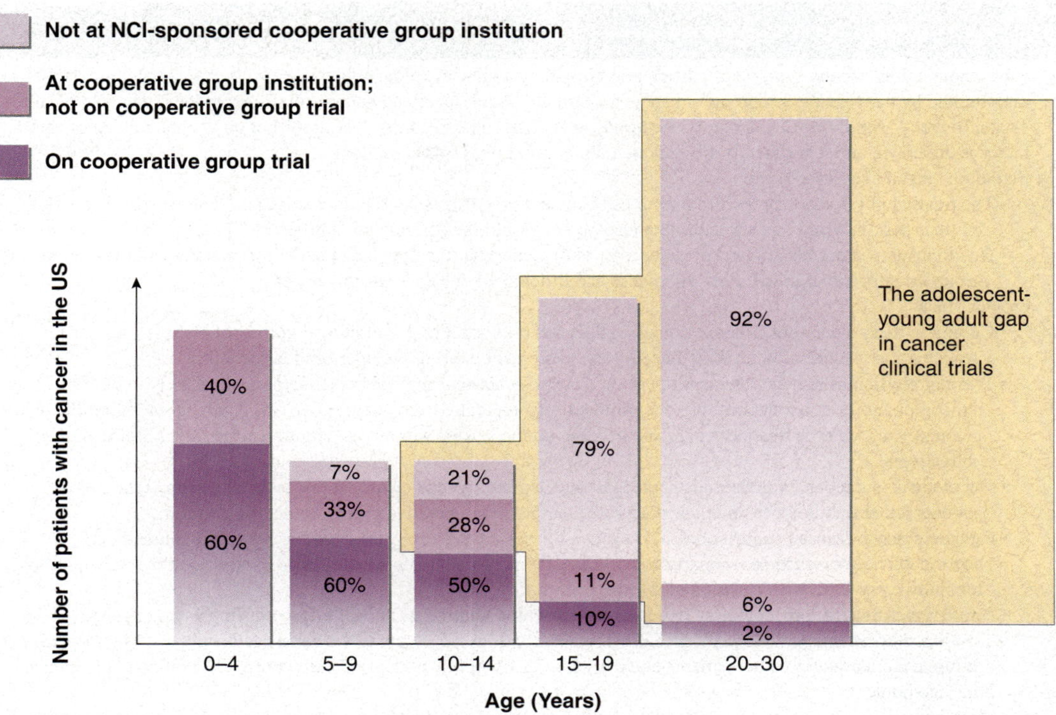

Figure 125-6 The "adolescent and young adult gap" in cancer clinical trials.

Future insurability is certainly a stressful issue for all of these patients.

Medical professionals caring for adolescents and young adults may be used to the psychosocial problems more common in either younger children or older adults. Extra effort, including patient and family support groups specifically geared to this age bracket, should be made to uncover and address these needs, to increase compliance, reduce stress, and improve the quality of life during cancer therapy. Established theories of developmental behavior should be used to systematically improve our care of these patients. As Eiser states, "only by seeing adolescents with cancer as adolescents will we ultimately be acceptable as sources of support."[54] Only by seeing young adults with cancer as young adults will we ultimately be able to optimize their care.

Lack of Participation in Clinical Trials

More than 90% of children with cancer who are younger than 15 years of age are managed at institutions that participate in NCI-sponsored clinical trials, and 55 to 65% of these young patients are entered into clinical trials. In contrast, only 20 to 35% of 15- to 19-year-olds with cancer are seen at such institutions, and only approximately 10% are entered into a clinical trial (Figure 125-6).[52,53] Among 20- to 29-year-olds, the participation rate is even lower, with fewer than 10% being seen at member institutions of the cooperative groups, either pediatric or adult, and only approximately 1% of 20- to 29-year-olds entering clinical trials of the pediatric or adult cooperative groups. Among older patients, the trial participation rate is higher, putatively between 3 and 5%. The high proportion of older adolescent and young patients who are not entered into clinical trials is referred to as the "adolescent and young adult gap." This gap has been observed throughout the United States and spares no geographic region or ethnic group.[55]

The reasons for the gap are to a large extent unknown and are undoubtedly multifactorial. Table 125-2 summarizes the reasons that were identified at an NCI-sponsored workshop on the topic. A factor that does not explain the discrepancy is the participation of minority adolescent patients in clinical trials. Although minority patients are known to be underrepresented in visits to physician offices,[21] they have equal or higher rates of entry into clinical trials. The participation rate of older adolescent patients is lower than the rates of younger patients of corresponding ethnicity and socioeconomic status.

The dramatically lower clinical trial participation rate by young adults helps explain the lower than expected improvement in their outcome, relative to younger and older patients, as summarized in the next section. Studies of younger children have certainly shown a survival advantage to children enrolled in clinical trials for ALL,[56] NHL,[57] Wilms' tumor,[58] and medulloblastoma.[59] Similar analyses of data for adolescents are sparse. In the United States and Canada, a comparison of 16- to 21-year-olds with ALL or AML showed that the outcome was superior in patients with either cancer treated in CCG trials than in those not entered.[60] In France, Holland, and North America, older adolescents with ALL treated with pediatric clinical trials have fared considerably better than those treated in adult leukemia treatment trials.[61–63] In Germany, older adolescents with Ewing's sarcoma who were treated at pediatric cancer centers had a better outcome than those treated at other centers.[64] In Italy, young adults with rhabdomyosarcoma fared better if they were treated according to pediatric

Table 125-2 Barriers to Participation in Clinical Trials

Possible explanations for the low rate of participation of young adults and older adolescents with cancer on clinical trials, as compiled by the NCI Workshop on Enhancing Accrual of Adolescent and Young Adult Cancer Patients on Clinical Trials, Bleyer A, Smith M, Coordinators, Bethesda, Maryland, June 17, 1999. The contribution and magnitude of each factor is unknown, and other factors are undoubtedly missing from this compilation.

Economic, insurance-based factors

- The treating physician may be reluctant to use clinical trials because of the time, cost, and effort involved, not only on their part (and that of their team) but also on the part of the patient and family.
- Health insurance organizations may deter referral of adolescents and young adults to a cancer center or cooperative group or entry into clinical trials. Attendees had little direct evidence for this factor.

Provider bias

- Coping with an older adolescent or young adult is difficult. Adding the additional burden of clinical trial participation is more difficult to achieve for the adolescent than for younger or older patients.
- Treating physicians may be reluctant to use clinical trials because they perceive the patient as likely to be noncompliant (or nonadherent) with the protocol requirements. The patient is perceived to have enough difficulty in complying with the treatment plan and keeping up their lives, without the additional burden of protocol obligations.
- Oncologists (surgeons, radiotherapists, medical oncologists, gynecologists) in private practice may retain these patients rather than refer them to a tertiary-care facility or cooperative group member institution.
- Providers may be biased against clinical trials in adolescents and young adults. Reasons may include the historically better results in comparison to older and younger patients, and the need to explain and obtain consent for study entry from both patient and family.
- Family practitioners, gynecologists, and internists may not regard multimodal therapy as important in young adults or older adolescents as in younger or older patients. Reasons may include the better results obtained in this age group in comparison to older patients and a higher rate of single-modality therapy normally applied to patients in this age range.
- Providers may be unaware of opportunities for clinical trials participation for adolescents and young adults with cancer.

Patient/family preferences

- Patients and/or parents are more inclined to refuse referral to a cooperative group member institution or to be entered into a clinical trial.
- Patients and/or parents may be unaware of opportunities for clinical trials participation for adolescents and young adults with cancer.

Provider age policies

- The age policies of hospitals may prevent patient access to clinical trials that are under way at the institution. Children's hospitals may have upper age limits that deny the older patient or deny the treating physician who does not have clinical privileges. The reverse may be true for younger patients accessing clinical trials primarily intended for adult patients.
- The clinical trial itself may have age limits that prohibit entry of an otherwise eligible patient.

Cooperative group limitations

- Pediatric cooperative group and adult cooperative group clinical trials may not allow adolescents and young adults because of restrictive eligibility criteria.
- A clinical trial may not be available.
- Adult cooperative groups may lack treatment protocols for the youngest patients.
- Vice versa, pediatric cooperative groups may lack treatment protocols for older patients.
- Clinical trials for the types of cancer that predominate among adolescents and young adults may not be a priority of the cooperative group enterprise.

standards of therapy than if treated ad hoc or on an adult sarcoma regimen.[65]

On the other hand, a population-based study of 15- to 29-year-olds with acute leukemia in England and Wales showed no difference between patients treated in national clinical trials and those not entered or between those managed at teaching hospitals as opposed to nonteaching hospitals.[66] This observation appears to be exceptional, however, in that subsequent national AML trials in the United Kingdom have shown some of the best results reported to date.[67]

SURVIVAL

In the United States, cancer and suicide are the leading causes of nonaccidental death among adolescents and young adults. Among 20- to 29-year-olds, cancer causes more deaths than heart disease, human immunodeficiency virus (HIV) infection, diabetes mellitus, chronic liver disease (including cirrhosis), cerebrovascular disease, and congenital anomalies (Table 125-3).[68] In females, deaths caused by cancer occur at more than twice the frequency of the second leading cause of death caused by disease (see Table 125-3).

Absolute Survival Figure 125-7 shows the 5-year relative survival rates for all invasive cancer as a function of age at and era of diagnosis. Children with cancer currently enjoy a 5-year survival rate that is estimated to exceed 80%. Among those diagnosed between 15 and 30 years of age, however, the 5-year survival rate is not as good, despite the prominence in this age group of cancers that carry a good prognosis, such as testicular cancer, thyroid cancer, Hodgkin's lymphoma, and melanoma. Moreover, the relative degree of survival improvement during the past quarter-century has been less among 15- to 29-year-olds than in either younger or older patients (see Figure 125-7). In 25- to 34-year-old Americans, there has been no demonstrable improvement in survival from invasive cancer once it is diagnosed.

A recent report on 38,144 young adults with sarcoma diagnosed during 1975–1998 and followed by the SEER Program may help explain the relative lack of progress.[69] In this study, the average annual percent change in 5-year survival as a function of patient age was compared with national sarcoma treatment trial data obtained on 3,242 patients entered into NCI-sponsored trials during 1997–2002. For bone and soft tissue sarcomas except Kaposi's sarcoma, the least survival improvement occurred between the ages of 15 and 45 years. For Kaposi's sarcoma, the pattern was reversed, with the greatest survival increase occurring in 30 to 44-year-olds. The lowest participation rate in NCI-sponsored sarcoma treatment trials occurred in 20- to 44-year-olds. For Kaposi's sarcoma patients, the highest accrual rate occurred in 35- to 44-year-olds. The age-dependent survival improvement and clinical trial accrual patterns were directly correlated (soft tissue sarcomas, $p < .005$; bone sarcomas, $p < .05$; Kaposi's sarcoma, $p = .06$) regardless of whether the accrual profile demonstrated a decline or a peak (Kaposi's sarcoma) during early adulthood. Thus, the lack of survival prolongation in 15- to 44-year-old Americans with non–Kaposi's sarcomas may be a result of their relative lack of participation in clinical trials. If so, reversing the shortfall in survival among young adults with sarcomas, as was accomplished in Kaposi's sarcoma patients, should benefit from increased clinical trial availability, access, and participation.

Table 125-3 Top 8 Causes of Death owing to Disease, Ages 20 to 39 Years, United States, 2002

	Male and Female	Deaths		Males	Deaths		Females	Deaths
1	Suicide	10,684	1	Suicide	8,771	1	Cancer	5,403
2	Cancer	10,029	2	Heart diseases	5,590	2	Heart diseases	2,640
3	Heart diseases	8,230	3	Cancer	4,626	3	Suicide	1,913
4	HIV disease	4,597	4	HIV disease	3,206	4	HIV disease	1,391
5	Diabetes mellitus	1534	5	Diabetes mellitus	905	5	Cerebrovascular disease	740
6	Chronic liver disease	1327	6	Chronic liver disease	852	6	Diabetes mellitus	629
7	Cerebrovascular disease	1482	7	Cerebrovascular disease	742	7	Chronic liver disease	475
8	Congenital anomalies	983	8	Congenital anomalies	552	8	Congenital anomalies	431

HIV = human immunodeficiency virus.

*Accidents and homicides excluded; adapted from Jemal A et al.[68]

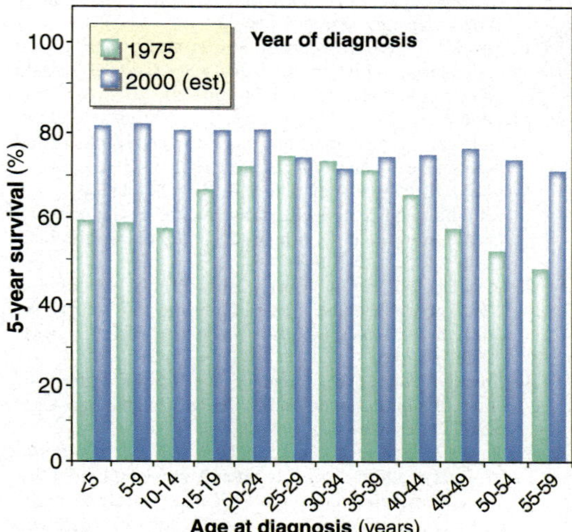

Figure 125-7 Five-year survival, all invasive cancers, 2000 versus 1975, Surveillance, Epidemiology, and End Results (SEER) Program, ages 0 to 59 years. Adapted from Ries LAG et al.[1]

Quality of Survival The quality of survival, both during and after therapy, is a critical issue in adolescents and young adults. Quality of life is poor during the months and years when most adolescents and young adults with cancer are treated, and the acute and delayed toxicities of cancer therapy are undeniably among the worst associated with the treatment of any chronic disease. The acute toxicities of nausea, vomiting, mucositis, alopecia, weight gain (or excessive loss), acne, bleeding, and infection are generally harder for adolescents to cope with than for either younger or older persons. Delayed complications may be of low concern to patients in this age group during treatment, but after therapy has been completed, these complications can be frightening and real. Cardiomyopathies, growth disturbances, and neuropsychological side effects are examples of adverse late effects that are hard to describe in a meaningful way before initiating therapy to an adolescent or young adult. A particularly tragic example of unanticipated late effect is the development of a second malignancy in a patient cured of the original disease.

Many adolescent and young adult cancer survivors cite fertility as a primary concern that impacts the quality of their life. Most do not recall an adequate discussion of the risks of infertility or methods to decrease the risks with their physician at the initiation of therapy. The risk of infertility is very hard to predict for an individual. The effect on fertility of direct radiation to the gonads is relatively easy to predict: permanent ovarian damage occurs between 5 and 20 Gy, with higher doses required in younger females, and testicular damage occurs between 22 and 30 Gy. Cranial radiation impairs gonadal hormone synthesis and can result in decreased production of luteinizing and follicle-stimulating hormones. Alkylating chemotherapeutic agents carry a high risk of infertility, but the exact dose required or the rates associated with combination agents are unavailable. Table 125-4 lists available methods to preserve fertility prior to the initiation of cancer therapy.

Table 125-4 Strategies for Maintaining Fertility in Young Adult Cancer Patients Treated with Chemotherapy

1. Modification of chemotherapy regimen
2. Relocation of gonads outside radiation field
3. Medical suppression of ovulation
4. Sperm banking
5. Oocyte cryopreservation
6. Testicular wedge or aspiration

The quality of life issues that arise during and after cancer therapy have been the focus of studies in children and older adults but have not received the same attention or study in adolescents and young adults. A few studies have found certain trends that should be tested in future studies. A higher risk-taking behavior has been noted among survivors of Hodgkin's lymphoma occurring during childhood and adolescence,[70] an observation that does not appear to be limited to this disease. On the other hand, evidence also suggests that adolescent and young adult cancer survivors show better attendance and performance at school and work.[71] Persistent anxiety over relapse, death, or late effects is likely to be higher in adolescents who were cognitively aware of the severity of their illness than in those treated in early childhood (Damocles syndrome).[72] The paucity of quality of life data in this age group is another manifestation of the general neglect of these patients.

SUMMARY

There are nearly three times as many cases of cancer in individuals 15 to 29 years of age as in those ages 0 to 15 years. Yet the former has its own organized cooperative oncology group, whereas the latter does not. Adolescent and young adult oncology patients should be viewed as a distinct age group that—like pediatric, adult, and geriatric patients—has unique medical and psychosocial needs. This mindset will help bring the problem into focus and will help those caring for adolescents or young adults to find solutions. A specific discipline for this special population is just beginning to evolve.[73] Meanwhile, resources should be devoted to educating the public, health professionals, insurers, and legislators about the special needs of these patients. The overriding issues to be addressed are the lagging improvements in survival and the special psychosocial needs of this age group.

During the last 25 years, the incidence of cancer in this age range has increased more and the reduction in cancer mortality has been lower than in younger or older patients. A major reason for this gap in outcome may be the poor participation by older adolescents and young adults with cancer in clinical trials: in the United States, only approximately 1% of 15- to 29-year-olds with cancer are entered into clinical trials, in contrast to more than 50% of younger patients. And as is intuitively obvious (we have all been through this phase of life), adolescents and young adults with cancer also face unique psychosocial challenges in the arenas of self-image, independence and dependence, finances, and relationships.

To address this problem, the NCI and the NCI-sponsored pediatric and adult cooperative groups launched a national initiative to improve the accrual of adolescents and young adults with cancer into clinical trials. In North America and Australia, the Children's Oncology Group has taken a leadership role in this effort. In conjunction with the NCI and NCI-sponsored adult cooperative groups, four initiatives were identified as priorities for development: (1) improving access to care through understanding barriers to participation; (2) developing a cancer resource network that provides information about clinical trials to patients, families, providers, and the public; (3) enhancing adolescent treatment adherence (compliance with protocol-prescribed therapy); and (4) increasing adolescent accrual and adult participation in sarcoma trials specifically designed for patients in this age group. However, reasons other than poor clinical trial participation, such as undescribed differences in biology, delays in diagnosis, poor compliance or intolerance of therapy, and treatment by physicians less familiar with the disease, may contribute to this outcome disparity as well and need to be studied.

Surviving adolescence and young adulthood is difficult enough even when all is well and health is not limiting. Cancer makes this phase of life extraordinarily more challenging and demanding. The medical community caring for these patients should pay special attention to the unique transitions faced by adolescents and young adults with cancer at the times of diagnosis, informed consent, initiation of therapy, school and employment reentrance, completion of therapy, post-treatment follow-up, and switching from pediatric to adult care.[74,75] Ideally, specialized adolescent and young adult cancer units should be developed in the anticipation that the centralization of care and the availability of age-targeted clinical trials will lead to improved treatment, survival, and quality of life.

Thus, cancer during adolescence and early adult life is an underestimated challenge that merits specific resources, solutions, and a national focus. Future research should elucidate why the outcomes have lagged behind and identify the efforts, including better clinical trial accrual, that will remedy the disparity. Lastly, more scholarly and focused attention on the unique psychosocial needs of this population will improve the quality of their cancer care and the quality of their survival.

REFERENCES

1. Ries LAG, Eisner MP, Kosary CL, et al, editors. SEER cancer statistics review, 1975-2001. Bethesda (MD): National Cancer Institute. Available at: http://seer.cancer.gov/csr/1975_2001/, 2004 (accessed March 15, 2005).
2. Canadian cancer statistics 2002, as reported by Reuters Medical News May, 2002.
3. Smith MA, Gurney JG, Ries LA. Cancer in adolescents 15–19 years old. In: Ries LAG, Smith MA, Gurney JG, et al, editors. Cancer incidence and survival among children and adolescents: United States SEER Program 1975–1997. Bethesda (MD): National Cancer Institute, SEER Program; 1999. NIH Publication No.: 99–4649.

4. Kramarova E, Stiller CA. The International Classification of Childhood Cancer. Int J Cancer 1996;68:759–65.
5. Fritschi L, Coates M, McCredie M. Incidence of cancer among New South Wales. adolescents: which classification scheme describes adolescent cancers better? Int J Cancer 1995;60:355–60.
6. Hoff J, Schymura MJ, McCrea Curren MG. Trends in the incidence of childhood and adolescent cancer in Connecticut, 1935–1979. Med Pediatr Oncol 1988;16:78–87.
7. Martos MC, Winther JF, Olsen JH. Cancer among teenagers in Denmark, 1943–1979. Int J Cancer 1993;55:57–62.
8. Ashikari H, Jun MY, Farrow JH, et al. Breast carcinoma in children and adolescents. Clin Bull 1977;7:55–62.
9. Corpron CA, Black CT, Singletary SE, et al. Breast cancer in adolescent females. J Pediatr Surg 1995;30:322–4.
10. Okcu M, Munsell M, Treuner J, et al. J Clin Oncol 2003;21:1602–11.
11. Franks LM, Bollen A, Seeger RC, et al. Neuroblastoma in adults and adolescents: an indolent course with poor survival. Cancer 1997;79:2028–35.
12. Raney RB, Sinclair L, Uri A, et al. Malignant ovarian tumors in children and adolescents. Cancer 1987;59:1214–20.
13. McNall RY, Nowicki PD, Miller B, et al. Adenocarcinoma of the cervix and vagina in pediatric patients. Pediatr Blood Cancer 2004;43:289–94.
14. Indolfi P, Terenziani M, Casale F, et al. Renal cell carcinoma in children: a clinicopathologic study. J Clin Oncol 2003;21:530–5.
15. French C, Kutok JL, Faquin WC, et al. Midline carcinoma of children and young adults with NUT rearrangement. J Clin Oncol 2004;22:4135–9.
16. Hamre MR, Chuba P, Bakhshi S, et al. Cutaneous melanoma in childhood and adolescence. Pediatr Hemat Oncol 2002;19:309–17.
17. Pianovski MAD, Filno LDL. A teenager with simultaneous Hodgkin disease and thyroid carcinoma. Med Pediatr Oncol 2003;40:91–2.
18. Parkin DM, Whelan SL, Ferlay J, et al, editors. Cancer incidence in five continents. Vol VII, no. 143. Lyon: IARC Scientific Publications; 1997.
19. Melnick S, Cole P, Anderson D, et al. Rates and risks of diethylstilbestrol-related clear cell adenocarcinoma of the vagina and cervix: an update. N Engl J Med 1987;316:514–9.
20. Pollock BH, Krischer JP, Vietti TJ. Interval between symptom onset and diagnosis of pediatric solid tumors. J Pediatr 1991;119:725–32.
21. Ziv, A, Boulet JR. Slap GB. Utilization of physician offices by adolescents in the United States. Pediatrics 1999;104:35–42.
22. US Congress Office of Technology. Adolescent health. Vol I: summary and policy options. Washington (DC): US Congress Office of Technology; 1991.
23. McCormick MC, Kass B, Elixhauser A, et al. Annual review of child health care access and utilization: annual report on access to and utilization of health care for children and youth in the United States—1999. Pediatrics 2000;105 Suppl:219–30.
24. Bleyer A, Ulrich C, Martin S, et al. Status of health insurance predicts time from symptom onset to cancer diagnosis in young adults. Proc Am Soc Clin Oncol 2005;23:547.
25. Martin S, Ulrich C, Munsell M, et al. Time to cancer diagnosis in young Americans depends on type of cancer and health insurance status. Value in Health 2005;8:344.
26. Friman PC, Finney JW, Glasscock SG, et al. Testicular self-examination: validation of a training strategy for early cancer detection. J Appl Behav Anal 1986;19:87–92.
27. Wiest MD, Finney JD. Training in early cancer detection and anxiety in adolescent males: a preliminary report. Dev Behav Pediatr 1996;17:98–9.
28. Albritton K, Bleyer A. The management of cancer in the older adolescent. Eur J Cancer 2003;39:2548–99.
29. Lewis IJ. Cancer in adolescence. Br Med Bull 1996;52:887–97.
30. Reaman G, Bonfiglio J, Krailo M, et al. Cancer in adolescents and young adults. Cancer 1993;71 Suppl 10:3206–9.
31. Selby P, Bailey C, editors. Cancer and the adolescent. London: BMJ Publishing Group; 1996. p. 276–83.
32. Yarcheski A, Scoloveno MA, Mahon NE. Social support and well-being in adolescents: the mediating role of hopefulness. Nurs Res 1994;43:288–92.
33. Manne S, Miller D. Social support, social conflict and adjustment among adolescents with cancer. J Pediatr Psychol 1998;23:121–30.
34. Nichols ML. Social support and coping in young adolescents with cancer. Pediatr Nurs 1995;21:235–40.
35. Novakovic B, Fears TR, Wexler LH, et al. Experience of cancer in children and adolescents. Cancer Nurs 1996;19:54–9.
36. Pelcovitz D, Libov BG, Mandel F, et al. Post-traumatic stress disorder and family functioning in adolescent cancer. J Trauma Stress 1998;11:205–21.
37. Blum RW, Garell D, Hodgman CH, et al. Transition from child-centered to adult health care systems for adolescents with chronic conditions: a position paper of the Society for Adolescent Medicine. J Adolesc Health 1993;14:570–6.
38. Rait DS, Ostroff J, Smith K, et al. Lives in a balance: perceived family functioning and the psychosocial adjustment of adolescent cancer survivors. Fam Process 1992;4:383–97.
39. Leonard RCG, Gregor A, Coleman RE, et al. Strategy needed for adolescent patients with cancer. BMJ 1995;311:387.
40. American Academy of Pediatrics, Section on Hematology/Oncology. Guidelines for the pediatric cancer center and role of such centers in diagnosis and treatment. Pediatrics 1997;99:139–41.
41. American Federation of Clinical Oncologic Societies. Consensus statement on access to quality cancer care. J Pediatr Hematol Oncol 1998;20:279–81.
42. Goldman S, Stafford C, Lenarsky C, et al. Older adolescents vary greatly from children in their route of referral to the pediatric oncologist and national trials [abstract]. Proc Am Soc Clin Oncol 2000;19:1766.
43. Albritton K, Wiggins C. Adolescents with cancer are not referred to Utah's pediatric center [abstract]. Proc Am Soc Clin Oncol 2001;20:990.
44. Rauck AM, Fremgen AM, Menck HR, et al. Adolescent cancers in the United States: a National Cancer Data Base (NCDB) report. J Pediatr Hematol Oncol 1999;21:310.
45. Stock W, Sather H, Dodge RK, et al. Outcome of adolescents and young adults with ALL: a comparison of Children's Cancer Group (CCG) and Cancer and Leukemia Group B (CALGB) regimens. Blood 2000;96:467a.
46. Kantarjian HM, O'Brien S, Smith TL, et al. Results of treatment with hyper-CVAD, a dose-intensive regimen, in adult acute lymphocytic leukemia. J Clin Oncol 2000;18:547–61.
47. Clemons M, Loijens L, Goss P. Breast cancer risk following irradiation for Hodgkin's disease. Cancer Treat Rev 2000;26:291–302.
48. Verrill MW, Judson IR, Fisher C, et al. The use of paediatric chemotherapy protocols at full dose is both a rational and feasible treatment strategy in adults with Ewing's family tumours. Ann Oncol 1997;8:1099–105.
49. Festa RS, Tamaroff MH, Chasalow F, et al. Therapeutic adherence to oral medication regimens by adolescents with cancer. I. Laboratory assessment. J Pediatr 1992;120:807–11.
50. Tamaroff MH, Festa RS, Adesman AR, et al. Therapeutic adherence to oral medication regimens by adolescents with cancer. II. Clinical and psychologic correlates. J Pediatr 1992;120:813–7.
51. Tebbi CK. Treatment compliance in childhood and adolescence. Cancer 1993;71 Suppl 10:3441–9.
52. Kyngas HA, Kroll T, Duffy ME. Compliance in adolescents with chronic diseases: a review. J Adolesc Med 2000;26:379–88.
53. Everhart C. Overcoming childhood cancer misconceptions among long-term survivors. J Pediatr Oncol Nurs 1991;8:46–8.
54. Eiser C. The impact of treatment: adolescent view. In: Selby P, Bailey C, editors. Cancer and the adolescent. London: BMJ Publishing Group; 1996.
55. Bleyer WA, Tejeda H, Murphy SM, et al. National cancer clinical trials: children have equal access; adolescents do not. J Adolesc Health 1997;21:366–73.
56. Meadows AT, Kramer S, Hopson R, et al. Survival in childhood acute lymphocytic leukemia. Effect of protocol and place of treatment. Cancer Invest 1983;1:49–55.
57. Wagner HP, Dingeldein-Bettler I, Berchthold W, et al. Childhood NHL in Switzerland: incidence and survival in 120 study and 42 non-study patients. Med Pediatr Oncol 1995;24:281–6.
58. Lennox EL, Stiller CA, Morris-Jones PH, Wilson-Kinnier LM. Nephroblastoma: treatment during 1970–3 and the effect on survival of inclusion in the first MRC trial. BMJ 1979;2:567–9.
59. Duffner K, Cohen ME, Flannery JT. Referral patterns of childhood brain tumors in the state of Connecticut. Cancer 1982;50:1636–40.
60. Nachman J, Sather HN, Buckley JD, et al. Young adults 16–21 years of age at diagnosis entered onto Children's Cancer Group acute lymphoblastic leukemia and acute myeloblastic leukemia protocols. Results of treatment. Cancer 1993;71 Suppl 10:3377–85.
61. Stock W, Sather H, Dodge RK, et al. Outcome of adolescents and young adults with ALL: a comparison of Children's Cancer Group and Cancer and Leukemia Group B regimens. Blood 2000;96:467a.
62. de Bont JM, van der Holt B, Dekker AW, et al. Significant difference in outcome for adolescents with acute lymphoblastic leukemia treated on pediatric versus adult ALL protocols in the Netherlands. Leukemia 2004;18:2032–53.
63. Boissel N, Auclerc MF, Lheritier V, et al. Should adolescents with acute lymphoblastic leukemia be treated as old children or young adults? Comparison of the French FRALLE-93 and LALA-94 trials. J Clin Oncol 2003;21:774–80.
64. Paulussen S, Ahrens S, Juergens HF. Cure rates in Ewing tumor patients aged over 15 years are better in pediatric oncology units. Results of GPOH CESS/EICESS studies. Proc Am Soc Clin Oncol 2003;22:816.
65. Ferrari A, Dileo P, Casanova M, et al. Rhabdomyosarcoma in adults. A retrospective analysis of 171 patients treated at a single institution. Cancer 2003;98:571–80.
66. Stiller CA, Benjamin S, Cartwright RA, et al. Patterns of care and survival for adolescents and young adults with acute leukemia—a population-based study. Br J Cancer 1999;79:658–65.
67. Webb DK, Harrison G, Stevens RF, et al. Relationships between age at diagnosis, clinical features, and outcome of therapy in children treated in the Medical Research Council AML 10 and 12 trials for acute myeloid leukemia. Blood 2000;98:1714–20.
68. Jemal A, Murray T, Ward E, et al. Cancer statistics, 2005. CA Cancer J Clin 2005;55:10–30.
69. Bleyer A, Montello M, Budd T, Saxman S. National survival trends of young adults with sarcoma: lack of progress is associated with lack of clinical trial participation. Cancer [In press]
70. Wasserman AL, Thompson EI, Wilmas JA, et al. The psychological status of survivors of childhood/adolescent Hodgkin's disease. Am J Dis Child 1987;141:626–31.
71. Hays DM, Landsverk J, Sallan SE, et al. Educational, occupational, and insurance status of childhood cancer survivors in their fourth and fifth decades of life. J Clin Oncol 1992;10:1397–406.
72. Koocher GP, O'Malley JE. The Damocles syndrome. Psychosocial consequences of surviving childhood cancer. New York: McGraw-Hill; 1981.
73. Barr RD. On cancer control and the adolescent. Med Pediatr Oncol 1999;32:404–10.
74. MacLean WE, Foley GV, Ruccione H, et al. Transitions in the care of adolescent and young adult survivors of childhood cancer. Cancer 1996;78:1340–5.
75. Glasson JE. A descriptive and exploratory pilot study into school re-entrance for adolescents who have received treatment for cancer. J Adv Nurs 1995;22:753–8.

Cancer Anorexia and Cachexia

Takao Ohnuma, MD, PhD

INTRODUCTION

The term cachexia is derived from the Greek words κακοζ (cacos) and ηξισ (hexis), meaning "bad" "condition."

Cachexia may be defined as reduced carcass weight. Cachexia is a complex syndrome presenting anorexia; early satiety; wasting of muscle and adipose tissues; weight loss; fatigue; anemia; hyperlipidemia; systemic inflammatory responses, including elevated proinflammatory cytokines; and a hypercatabolic state. Cachexia is induced not only by cancer, but also by AIDS and other chronic infections, for example, tuberculosis, rheumatoid arthritis, chronic heart failure, chronic kidney disease, and chronic obstructive pulmonary disease.

Cachexia is different from simple starvation or anorexia nervosa. In cancer, cachexia anorexia develops at an early phase of disease, body mass index is predictive of mortality, hypoalbuminemia occurs early, hypocholesterolemia is often observed, and total lymphocyte counts are low.[1] There is extensive loss of skeletal muscle mass and adipose tissue.[2,3] This contrasts with simple starvation, in which fat replaces glucose as the preferred fuel to spare lean body mass. Cancer cachexia results from altered metabolism rather than just an energy deficit, and it cannot be reversed by simple feeding.[4,5] We will focus on cachexia commonly seen in patients with upper gastrointestinal and lung cancers, as well as with advanced cancer.

INCIDENCE

Anorexia and early satiety are common symptoms in patients with cancer. Anorexia has been reported in 43 to 53%, and early satiety in 13 to 62% of patients with cancer.[6,7] As many as 45% of all hospitalized cancer patients had lost more than 10% of their initial body weight, and 25% had lost more than 20%. Weight loss often tended to be underestimated because a significant number of patients had edema. The frequency of weight loss ranged from 31% in favorable histology non-Hodgkin's lymphoma to 87% in patients with measurable gastric carcinoma. Gastric and pancreatic cancer patients had lost the greatest amount of weight. Small-cell and nonsmall-cell lung cancer patients had a high frequency of weight loss, probably secondary to systemic effects. Weight loss and survival are correlated with systemic inflammatory response as measured by the magnitude of the C-reactive protein concentrations.[8,9] In a longitudinal study, 20 patients with unresectable pancreatic cancer underwent nutritional analysis monthly until death.[10] They had lost a median of 14.2% of their preillness body weight at the time of diagnosis. Weight loss progressed to a median of 24.5% by the time of the last assessment. There was a significant reduction in lean body mass from a median of 43.4 kg/m^2 at initial study to 40.1 at the time of last assessment, and a reduction of fat mass from 12.5 kg/m^2 to 9.6. Albumin and hemoglobin levels also correlated with survival in patients with small-cell lung cancer.[11] In a series of 400 autopsies, cachexia was blamed for 22% of cancer deaths and was implicated as an ancillary contributor in many other patients.[12]

Pretreatment weight loss and malnutrition in cancer patients often lead to poor tolerance of surgery, chemotherapy, and radiotherapy. Preoperative nutritional parameters are predictive of operative complications.[13] Good performance status correlated positively with tolerance to chemotherapy and radiotherapy, response rates to chemotherapy, as well as survival in patients with lung and colorectal cancer.[14,15]

ETIOLOGY

The causes of cancer-related cachexia are multifold and can be grouped into three interrelated categories: anorexia and early satiety, mechanical obstruction of the alimentary tract, and metabolic derangement.

Anorexia and Early Satiety Anorexia may be defined as the loss of desire to eat or the lack of hunger. Anorexia may result from early satiety, nausea, or a change in taste. Early satiety is the desire to eat associated with an inability to eat adequately.[6]

Anorexia in cancer patients can be divided into disease-related, treatment-related, and that caused by emotional distress.

Abnormalities of taste sensation and olfaction for food aromas have been demonstrated in cancer patients.[16,17] These patients displayed an elevated threshold for sweet compared with healthy subjects, which correlated with a loss of taste sensation. Patients experiencing early satiety found the odors of pork, ham, and coffee less pleasant than those without early satiety.

Many factors have been postulated as causes of anorexia. These include increases in serum lactate, known to be produced abundantly by tumor; appearance of ketosis during fasting; hypercalcemia, a common paraneoplastic syndrome; toxohormone-L, a lipolytic factor purified from ascitic fluid of patients with hepatoma; bombesin, a neuropeptide produced by small-cell lung cancer; satietins, proteins isolated from human plasma; glucagon or glucagon-like peptides; increases in serotonin levels in serum and the central nervous system (CNS) in cancer patients; certain cytokines; and possibly dysfunction of neuropeptidergic circuits in the brain.[18–27] These findings suggest that the causes of tumor-induced anorexia are multifactorial. Among these factors, serotonin, cytokines, and prostaglandins, as well as neuropepidergic circuit dysfunction are worthy of additional comments.

Serotonin Abnormal utilization by tumor cells of tryptophan, the precursor of serotonin, with resultant excess levels of free tryptophan in plasma has been reported in cancer patients.[28] Increases in blood tryptophan levels result in excess tryptophan levels in the cerebrospinal fluid, which appears to lead to increased serotonin synthesis/secretion in the ventromedial hypothalamic (VMH) serotonergic system. A close relationship between elevated plasma-free tryptophan and anorexia with reduced food intake was observed in patients with cancer.[25] As described below, studies of cytokines and neuropeptide circuits have led to identification of CNS serotonin as a major mediator of cancer anorexia.[29]

Cytokines and Prostaglandins Cytokines, such as tumor necrosis factor-α (TNF-α) and interleukin (IL)-1 released by the tumor or the host immune system have been shown to be mediators of anorexia. Although TNF-α induces IL-1, both TNF-α and IL-1 appear to be operative in mediating their anorectic effect through the brain as well as directly on the gastrointestinal tract, for example, decrease in gastric emptying.[30,31] Peripherally infused IL-1 increased brain tryptophan and serotonin concentrations, whereas intracerebrally infused IL-1 increased neural firing rate and serotonin release in the VMH, suggesting that IL-1 production during tumor growth facilitated tryptophane conversion in the brain. Although interferon-γ (IFN-γ) infusion produced anorexia in patients with renal cell cancer, the appearance of anorexia in mice associated with tumor growth was similar whether mice were IFN-γ knockout or intact, suggesting that endogenous IFN-γ plays little role in producing anorexia in the tumor-bearing host.[32,33] Interleukin-6 (IL-6) appears to have no direct anorectic effect.[34,35]

An opposing view was recently presented. Thus, immunohistochemical image analyses of the time course of cytokines in the CNS of tumor-bearing mice did not find that up-regulation of brain cytokines could explain cancer anorexia.[36] Further studies indicated that transcription of prostaglandin-E receptors in liver, fat, and skeletal muscle tissue may be a control mechanism for host metabolic alterations during tumor progression.[37] Overall, prostaglandin-E and prostaglandin-I receptor expression in the CNS did not seem to have significant control of appetite regulation in a mouse model, however, despite prostanoid-related anorexia.

Animal studies showed development of tolerance to injections of TNF-α and IL-1.[38] IL-1 infusion was not anorexigenic in food-deprived rats.[39] Serum levels of circulating TNF-α, IL-1, IL-6, and IFN-γ did not correlate with anorexia or weight loss in cancer patients.[40] These studies imply that anorexigenic actions of these cytokines are processed by intermediate mediator molecules, such as melanocortins.[41] Cytokines not only produce anorectic effects, but also exert direct catabolic activity on muscle and adipose tissues. This will be discussed in separate sections later.

Dysregulation of Neuropeptidergic Circuits Both insulin, secreted from the exocrine pancreas, and leptin, produced primarily by adipocytes, circulate at levels proportional to body fat content and enter the CNS in proportion to their plasma levels. As weight increases, insulin secretion is increased both at the basal state and in response to meals to compensate for insulin resistance. Increased insulin secretion as obesity progresses promotes insulin delivery to the brain, where it helps to limit further weight gain. Insulin also promotes both fat storage and leptin synthesis by fat cells. Leptin has a more important role than insulin in the CNS control of energy homeostasis. Thus, leptin deficiency causes severe obesity with hyperphagia that persists despite high insulin levels. In contrast, obesity is not induced by insulin deficiency.[42]

Several studies have dealt with the role of leptin in cancer-induced anorexia. In cachectic tumor-bearing animals, lower circulating levels of leptin together with decreased adipose tissue mRNA content for leptin have been described.[43] Similarly, serum leptin levels were also reduced in patients with both advanced lung cancer and colon cancer, suggesting that cancer anorexia and cachexia are not solely due to the dysregulation of leptin production.[44,45]

Ghrelin, secreted predominantly from the stomach, is the natural ligand for the growth hormone secretagogue receptor in the pituitary gland. It has profound orexigenic, adipogenic, and somatotrophic properties, thereby increasing food intake and body weight.[46] The brain-gut axis is the effector of anabolism, regulating feeding, metabolism, and growth via vagal efferents mediating ghrelin signaling.

Recent work has shown that endogenous levels of the biologically active (octanoylated) form of ghrelin and of IL-6 were increased in patients with cancer-induced cachexia when compared with individuals with stable body weight with or without cancer.[47,48] Active ghrelin and IL-6 levels correlated positively and albumin correlated negatively with weight loss over the preceding 6 months. IL-6 but not ghrelin levels were associated with the degree of anorexia. The increase in active ghrelin levels was considered to be a compensatory response to weight loss.[48,49] Lack of correlation between appetite and ghrelin levels was explained by the concept that cachexia may be a state of ghrelin resistance.[47] Changes in the active:total ghrelin ratio suggest that a mechanism other than increased secretion must be responsible for the increase in active ghrelin levels.

Both insulin and leptin interact with several distinct hypothalamic neuropeptide-containing pathways.[50] Neuropeptides implicated in the control of energy homeostasis are divided into orexigenic (anabolic) and anorexigenic (catabolic) signaling molecules (Table 126-1). Peripheral leptin enters into the CNS where leptin receptors exist in the hypothalamus. Leptin interacts with numerous hypothalamic neuropeptidergic effector molecules, which are downstream of the leptin signal. Leptin suppresses hypothalamic orexigenic neuropeptides, which include neuropeptide Y (NPY), agouti-related protein (AgRP), melanin-concentrating hormone (MCH), and orexin. Contrarily, leptin stimulates anorexigenic neuropeptides including α-melanocytes-stimulating hormone (α-MSH), cocaine and amphetamine-related transcript (CART), and corticotropin-releasing hormone (CRH). The arcuate nucleus transduces leptin signals from the periphery. The leptin receptor is coexpressed with NPY and AgRP in the arcuate nucleus neurons, and is also expressed in pro-opiomelanocortin/CART neurons. NPY/AgRP neurons are inhibited by leptin and activated by a decrease in leptin levels. NPY stimulates food intake and decreases energy expenditure, primarily from a reduction in thermogenesis in brown adipose tissue and by facilitating fat deposition in white adipose tissue, partly through increased insulin activity. Recently, both insulin and leptin were shown to activate the hypothalamic phosphoinositol-3-kinase pathway.[51] From these apparently contradictory observations, possible mechanisms of insulin and leptin resistance were inferred.[52]

Table 126-1 Orexigenic (Anabolic) and Anorexigenic (Catabolic) Neuropeptides

Orexigenic molecules
Neuropeptide Y (NPY)
Agouti-related protein (AGRP)
Melanin-concentrating hormone (MCH)
Hypocretin 1 and 2 (Orexin A and B)
Galanin
Norepinephrine
Opioids
Anorexigenic molecules
Melanocyte-stimulating hormone (MSH)
Corticotropin-releasing hormone (CRH)
Thyrotropin-releasing hormone (TRH)
Cocaine- and amphetamine-regulated transcript (CART)
Urocortin
Glucagon-like peptide 1 (GLP-1)
Oxytocin
Neurotensin
Serotonin

Adapted from Schwartz MW et al.[42]

Dysregulation of this neuropeptidergic circuit controlling food intake and energy expenditure, and thus energy homeostasis, may play a role in the development of the cancer anorexia-cachexia syndrome.[27] Thus, rats bearing methylcholanthrene-induced sarcomas exhibited refractory feeding response to intrahypothalamic injection of NPY compared with controls.[53] Reduced affinity of hypothalamic NPY receptors as well as refractory adenylate cyclase in response to NPY suggested that the postsynaptic NPY-signaling systems were altered in the hypothalamus of tumor-bearing rats.[54,55]

Cytokines produce a more potent effect on feeding and metabolism when injected directly into the CNS rather than peripherally. A central mechanism of action in the production of cachexia has been postulated for many cytokines, including interleukin-1, interleukin-6, interleukin-8, TNF-α, interferon-α and other chemokines/intercrines.[50,56]

TNF-α acts peripherally to increase leptin mRNA and centrally upon neural activity of glucose-sensitive neurons within the ventromedial nucleus and the lateral hypothalamic area. Episodic TNF administration has been reported to induce anorexia, but does not appear to be able to induce cachexia. It appears that tolerance to cytokine develops and food intake and body weight return to normal.[57]

IL-1β blocked hypothalamic NPY mRNA levels and decreased NPY-induced feeding, whereas it stimulated CRH in parallel with suppression of food intake.[57,58] Conversely, at different doses, NPY blocked and reversed IL-1β–induced anorexia.[59] IL-1–induced anorexia is mainly due to development of early satiety, and such early satiety has long been linked to enhanced serotonergic activity.[60] In addition, TNF-α and IFN-γ were also shown to stimulate CRH expression and/or release.[61] Cytokines may play an important role in long-term inhibition of feeding by mimicking the hypothalamic effect of excessive negative feedback signaling from leptin by persistent stimulation of anorexigenic neuropeptides such as CRH or by inhibition of the NPY orexigenic network (Figure 126-1).[27]

It is of note that there are reports that describe an opposite view. Thus, NPY mRNA levels are not always increased in anorectic tumor-bearing rats when compared with pair-fed or control animals.[62] Although synthesis and secretion of leptin appear to be stimulated by cytokines such as IL-1, circulating leptin levels are not elevated in cachectic cancer patients.[63,64]

In summary, a number of factors have been proposed as putative mediators of cancer anorexia, including hormones (eg, leptin), neuropeptides (eg, NPY), cytokines (eg, IL-1, TNF), and neurotransmitters (eg, serotonin and dopamine). Rather than representing separate and distinct pathogenic entities, it appears that close interrela-

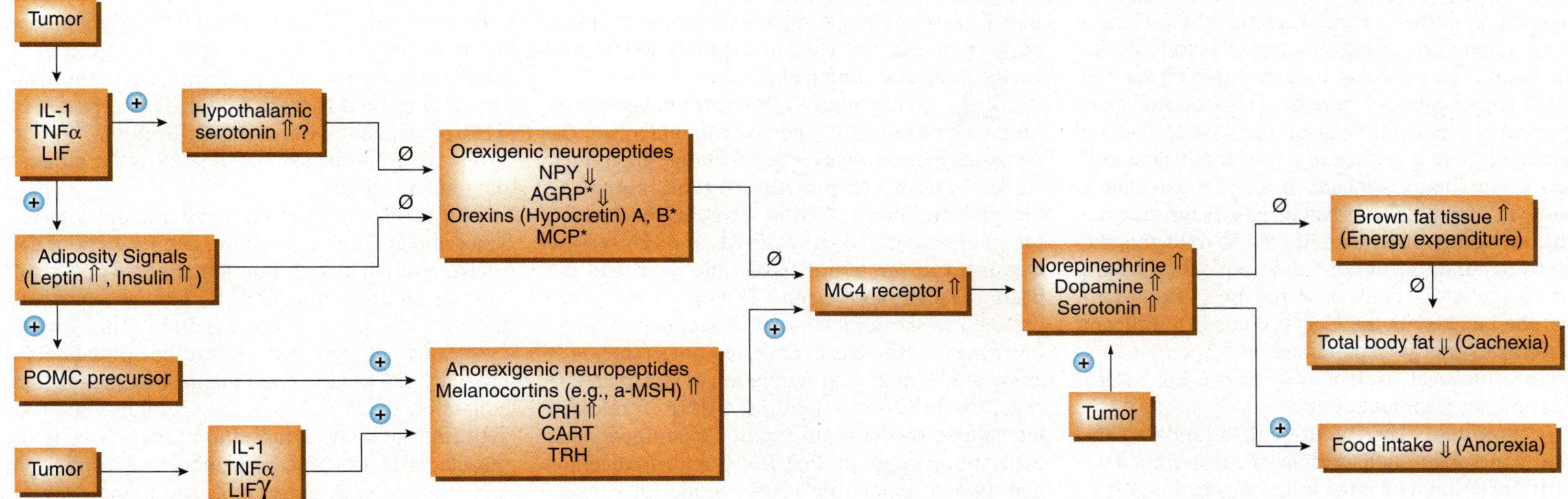

Figure 126-1 A simplified provisional model for the central nervous system circuitry of food intake and energy balance in cancer, anorexia, and cachexia. AGRP = agouti-related protein; CART = cocaine- and amphetamine-regulated transcript; CRH = corticotropin-releasing hormone; IFN-γ = interferon-γ; IL-1 = interleukin-1; LIF = leukemia inhibitory factor; MC4 = melanocortin receptor 4; MCP = melanine concentrating hormone; NPY = neuropeptide Y; POMC = pro-opiomelanocortin; TNF-α = tumor necrosis factor-α; TRH = thyrotropin-releasing hormone; *compensatory signal when NPY is not present; ⇑ increases in expression, release. or amount; ⇓ decreases in expression, release, or amount; →⊕, positive signaling: activation, increased synthesis or secretion; →Ø, negative signaling: inhibition, decreased synthesis or secretion.

tionships exist among these factors. Indeed, many studies suggest that different anorexia-related factors converge on a common final pathway as a major target, that is, hypothalamic monoaminergic neurotransmission and serotonergic activity.[65,66] In patients with cancer, it is likely that cytokines and anorexia are related, but compelling evidence is lacking because the biological effects of cytokines may be released episodically and many of their effects are mediated by paracrine and autocrine mechanisms. Circulating concentrations of cytokines may not reliably reflect their role in determining specific biological responses, including cachexia.[42,50,67]

Emotional Distress Anorexia may occur with emotional distress, for example, at the time cancer is diagnosed, prior to major treatment decisions, and upon discovering that cancer is advancing. Anorexia from emotional distress is usually transient, however, and the impact of this type of anorexia on cancer cachexia in patients (and in rodents and other species) is insufficient to explain it. One cause of weight loss can be a psychotic depression, which may be unrecognized because many of the symptoms and effects are attributed directly to the cancer. The use of antidepressants for a true psychotic depression established by psychiatric consultation can have a profound positive effect on appetite.

Anorexia vs Cachexia Anorexia should not be equated with cachexia. In cachectic cancer patients the measured food intake fails to correspond with the degree of malnutrition.[68] Loss of both muscle and adipose tissue precedes the decrease in food intake.[69] Some patients present initially with significant weight loss as their first and only symptom in the face of dietary intake that ordinarily would be normal.[70]

Alimentary Tract Dysfunction Abnormalities in perception of taste and smell have been described in cancer patients. Tumors of the mouth, oropharynx, esophagus, stomach, pancreas, liver, and peritoneum may compromise oral intake from mechanical interference with anatomical structures. Intestinal obstruction is a common complication of cancer. Malabsorption secondary to pancreatic insufficiency owing to pancreas carcinoma or secondary to the infiltration of the intestine or mesentery by lymphoma has been described.[71,72]

Direct encroachment of a tumor on the gastrointestinal tract; atrophic changes in the mucosa and muscles of the stomach; a reduction in the duration or activity of digestive enzymes, which may lead to delayed gastric emptying; and slowing of peristalsis are all pathogenic mechanisms that may contribute to early satiety.[6,7] Early satiety is common in patients with decreased upper gastrointestinal motility.[73]

Major surgery for cancer, particularly on the gastrointestinal tract, may produce abnormalities in taste and difficulties in swallowing, digestion, or absorption that may contribute indirectly to anorexia. Chemotherapy commonly induces abnormal perception of taste, mucositis, and nausea and vomiting. Radiotherapy to the head and neck can induce stomatitis, xerostomia, and alterations in taste and smell. Radiotherapy to the abdomen can induce anorexia, nausea, vomiting, diarrhea, and malabsorption.

Biochemical and Metabolic Derangement The situation of cancer cachexia is similar to that seen with AIDS or sepsis: Weight loss can result from complex metabolic events. Several biochemical and metabolic derangements are considered to be causally related to the pathogenesis of cancer cachexia.

Increased Glucose Utilization and Futile Substrate Cycles High rates of glucose utilization with production of lactic acid are characteristic features of the neoplastic cell. In mice bearing transplantable colon tumors, glucose utilization by the tumors was second only to that by the brain.[74] Hexokinase, which catalyzes the first step of the glycolytic pathway and which is often highly overexpressed in tumor cells, is a major player in this process. Binding of tumor hexokinase to the outer mitochondrial membrane provides the enzyme with preferential access to mitochondrially generated ATP and increases the activity and stability of the enzyme.[75] The end product of the hexokinase reaction, glucose-6-phosphate, serves not only as a source of ATP via glycolysis, but is also a key intermediate in the metabolic processes essential for cell growth and proliferation. Alteration of an isozyme appears closely linked to this process. Thus, the promoter activity of the type II isoform of hexokinase, the dominant form expressed in AS-30 hepatoma cells, was found to be resistant to normal hormonal control.[76] Recently, the distal region of the promoter was found to display consensus motifs for hypoxia-inducible factor-1 (HIF-1). Subjecting transfected hepatoma cells to hypoxic conditions activated the type II hexokinase promoter almost sevenfold in the presence of glucose.[77] The tumor cell was able to maintain glycolysis regardless of the metabolic state of surrounding normal cells.

Lactic acid produced via glucose metabolism may be utilized by other tissues for energy purposes or may be transported to the liver for resynthesis to glucose. The cyclic metabolic pathway, in which glucose is converted to lactic acid by glycolysis in tumor tissue and then reconverted to glucose in the liver, is referred to as the Cori cycle. Conversion of glucose to lactate in cancer cells yields two ATPs, whereas lactate to glucose conversion in the liver requires six ATPs. Thus, a systemic energy-losing or futile substrate cycle, involving this interplay of tumor glycolysis and host gluconeogenesis may be an important cause of cancer cachexia.[78] Assuming that all lactate produced is recycled to glucose, the cancer cell acts as an energy parasite. It may be calculated, however, that if 85% of lactate passes through the gluconeogenic pathway and 15% is oxidized, the host's handling of tumor-produced lactate would be energetically neutral. It has been suggested that the increase in the Cori cycle is insignificant in terms of energy expenditure and that increased glucose turnover itself is responsible for weight loss and development of cachexia.[79]

Cytokines TNF-α, IL-1, IL-6 (and its subfamily members such as ciliary neurotrophic factor [CNTF] and leukemia inhibitory factor [LIF]) and IFN-γ produced by host immune cells and/or tumor cells have all been implicated as mediators of cancer cachexia.[80–83] These cytokines are characterized by the induction of anorexia, weight loss, an acute-phase protein response, protein and fat breakdown, rises in levels of cortisol and glucagon and falls in insulin level, insulin resistance, anemia, fever, and elevated energy expenditure in animals. Direct interaction with leptin, neuropeptides, and serotonin as mechanisms of induction of cancer anorexia has been described above.

TNF-α TNF-α was simultaneously discovered as cachectin because it caused systemic suppression of lipoprotein lipase and development of hypertriglyceridemia, a state frequently seen in cachectic animals.[84] One mechanism by which TNF-α induces a net catabolic state in the host is by mediating increased catabolism at the level of specific tissues, such as muscle and fat.[85] TNF-α increases activities of both phosphofructokinase and fructose bisphosphate phosphatase in myocytes in culture, producing an increased substrate cycling between fructose-6-phosphate and fructose-1,6-bisphosphate. Each of the fructose-6-phosphate/fructose-1,6-bisphosphate cycles loses one ATP. TNF also increased ubiquitin gene expression in isolated rat muscle. Total cellular ubiquitin-conjugated muscle protein in C2C12 myotubules was increased, and protease activities of the 20S proteasome and the lysosomal-proteolytic enzymes cathepsins B and B + L were reduced.[85]

Elevation of serum TNF-α and/or TNF-α–receptor levels has been associated with the clinical status of patients with B-cell chronic lymphocytic leukemia and with endometrial carcinoma and other solid tumors.[86,87] Administration of TNF-α in humans induced anorexia, negative nitrogen balance, and increases in serum triglycerides and in very-low-density lipoprotein.[88,89] In contrast, TNF-α was rarely detected in patients with clinical cancer cachexia, and administration of recombinant TNF-α did not produce demonstrable cachexia.[90] Patients with type I hyperlipidemia caused by an inherited deficiency in lipoprotein-lipase have normal fat stores and are not cachectic. These observations suggest neither TNF-α nor suppression of lipoprotein-lipase alone can explain loss of adipose tissue and cachexia in cancer patients.

IL-1 Using methylcholanthrene-induced tumors in rats, various specific components of the cytokine-induced anorectic reactions, including: IL-1β system components (ligand, signaling receptor, receptor accessory proteins, and receptor antagonist); TNF-α; TGF-β1; and IFN-γ were examined in the tumor tissue, the liver, and the brain. IL-1β, TNF-α and IFN-γ mRNA were detected in the tumor tissue of anorectic tumor-bearing rats, whereas in brain regions, anorexia is associated with the up-regulation of IL-1β and its receptor mRNA. All other mRNA remained unchanged in the brain regions examined. This observation suggests that IL-1β and its receptor may play a major role in this model of cancer-associated anorexia.[91]

The genotype for a diallelic polymorphism of the *IL-1β* gene was examined in patients with pancreatic cancer.[92] The possession of a genotype resulting in increased IL-1β production was associated with shortened survival and increased serum C-reactive protein (CRP) level. This may reflect the role of IL-1β in inducing an acute-phase protein response and cachexia in cancer.

IL-6 Involvement of IL-6 in the development of cancer cachexia has been suggested from a number of animal models. Prevention of muscle atrophy in tumor-bearing mice by anti–IL-6 receptor antibody appears to be mediated by modulation of lysosomal and ATP-ubiquitin–dependent proteolytic pathways.[93] In vivo, however, IL-6 administration produced no changes in ubiquitin gene expression and no effect on body weight or food intake, despite being associated with increased acute-phase protein production.[35]

The influence of IL-1 on cachexia appears to be mediated through IL-6, and IL-6 seems to act in concert with other cytokines in a final common pathway of cachexia.[94,95]

In patients with lung cancer, increased IL-6 levels were correlated with extensive disease, impaired performance status, enhanced acute phase response, weight loss, and malnutrition.[96,97]

The exact role of IL-1 and IL-6 in the development of cancer cachexia in humans remains speculative, however. Serum IL-6 concentrations were significantly elevated in tumor-bearing animals, but only minimally in patients with cancer.[98] IL-1 and IL-6 serum levels were not always measurable.[99] Administration of IL-6 failed to produce cachexia. Transgenic mice constitutively expressing IL-6 did not develop cachexia.[100,101] It has been suggested that IL-6 is necessary but not sufficient for the induction of cachexia, and that additional factor(s) besides IL-1β control production of IL-6 and other cachexigenic factors.[91]

The superfamily of IL-6 includes LIF and CNTF. LIF will be discussed in the section "Tumor By-Products." The role of CNTF in cancer anorexia/cachexia in humans has not been established.

IFN-γ IFN-γ may have a bearing on the development of cancer cachexia. Interferons and TNFs were shown to have similar catabolic effects on NIH 3T3 cells in vitro.[102] Monoclonal antibody against IFN-γ given prior to injection of Lewis lung tumor cells prevented cachexia from developing.[103] IFN-γ was found to be increased in 51% of patients with multiple myeloma.[104] The levels of IFN-γ had no correlation with clinical parameters, however.

As to the link between inflammatory cytokines and energy expenditure, involvement of the transcriptional coactivator, peroxisome proliferator-activated receptor (PPAR) gamma coactivator-1 (PGC-1), has been suggested. Thus, many cytokines activate PGC-1 through phosphorylation by p38 kinase, resulting in stabilization and activation of PGC-1 protein. Cytokine-induced activation of PGC-1 in cultured muscle cells or muscle tissue in vivo caused increased respiration and expression of genes linked to mitochondrial uncoupling and energy expenditure. These data illustrated a direct thermogenic action of cytokines through PGC-1.[105]

Recently, the actual muscle gene product was identified as the target for down-regulation during the wasting state. In myogenic cell cultures, treatment with a combination of TNF-α and IFN-γ resulted in selective and progressive depletion of myosin heavy chain, whereas none of other core myofibrillar proteins, troponin T, tropomyosin α and β, actin, and actinin were affected.[106] Treatment with TNF-α alone or IFN-γ alone had negligible effect on the myosin heavy chain depletion. Depletion of myosin heavy chain of cultured myotubes with TNF-α and IFN-γ resulted in a decrease in MyoD, the nuclear transcription factor. These results imply that TNF-α and IFN-γ selectively trigger a reduction in the expression of the myosin heavy chain through a MyoD-mediated block in gene transcription. The implantation of cells expressing both TNF-α and IFN-γ into muscles of mice led to a similar, specific reduction in the synthesis of the myosin heavy chain relative to that of other myofibrillar proteins such as actin and tropomyosin. Interestingly, transplantation of C-26 adenocarcinoma, which is known to produce IL-6 rather than TNF-α and IFN-γ resulted in down-regulation of myosin heavy chain, but from a different mechanism, via ubiquitin-dependent proteasome-mediated protein degradation. These observations highlight the importance of myosin heavy chain as a target of cachexia, which occurs through different pathways.

Tumor By-Products Various pharmacologically active tumor by-products have been reported as causal factors of cachexia.

Lipolytic Factors Three different lipolytic factors have been characterized or purified. First, a lipolytic factor termed toxohormone-L was found in pleural effusions of patients with malignant lymphoma as well as in ascites from patients with ovarian carcinoma and hepatoma.[20] It is an acidic protein with a molecular weight of 65 to 75 kDa. *Toxohormone-L* elicited fatty acid release in rat adipose tissue in vitro, and injections into rat resulted in suppression of food and water intake. Toxohormone-L and related substances were considered responsible for the cancer cachexia syndrome in nude mice bearing human cancer cell lines.[107]

Second, *leukemia inhibitory factor* (*LIF*) was originally isolated from conditioned medium of Krebs II ascites tumor cells. This factor has a differentiation-inducing activity on myeloid leukemia cell lines. In an independent work, the identical material was purified from conditioned medium of human melanoma cell line SEKI. The substance was found to be an effective lipoprotein-lipase inhibitor.[108] Comparisons among nude mice bearing various human melanoma cell lines revealed that the degree of LIF mRNA expression correlated with the development of cachexia.[108] LIF caused smaller increases in lipolysis and catabolic effects than those of TNF.[109,110]

Third, British workers purified and characterized what they termed *lipid-mobilizing factor* (LMF), which was derived from MAC16 murine adenocarcinoma and from urine of cancer patients with cachexia.[111,112] LMF, an acidic peptide, lacked triglyceride lipase activity and was different from natural lipolytic hormones, which were all basic. LMF isolated from the murine tumor and that from the patients' urine both had an apparent *M*w of 43 kDa and was homologous with the plasma protein Zn-α2-glycoprotein (ZAG).[111] Both caused direct lipolysis in isolated murine adipocytes and caused selective loss of adipose tissue in exbreeder male mice.[112] Both caused stimulation of adenylate cyclase in murine adipocyte plasma membranes in a GTP-dependent process and release of glycerol from isolated adipocytes. Adenylate cyclase stimulation and, thus, oxygen consumption in brown adipose tissue (BAT) by LMF is mediated by a β3-adrenergic receptor.[113,114] Brown adipocytes express abundant amounts of β3-adrenergic receptors. An increase in oxygen uptake by interscapular brown adipose tissue suggested that LMF exerted its effect by increases in energy expenditure.[112] This increase may be related to changes in expression of uncoupling proteins (UCP), because mice bearing MAC16 tumor showed higher UCP-1 mRNA levels in BAT than controls.[115] Three types os UCPs are known. UCP-1 is present only in BAT, UCP-2 is expressed ubiquitously, and UCP-3 is expressed abundantly and specifically in skeletal muscle in humans and also in BAT of rodents. LMP increased expression of UCP-1, -2, and -3 in brown adipose tissue and UCP-2 in liver and skeletal muscle.[116] UCPs function as a mitochondrial protein carrier that stimulate heat production by dissipating the proton gradient generated during respiration across the inner mitochondrial membrane, thereby uncoupling respiration from ATP synthesis. In rodents, UCP-2 and UCP-3 mRNAs were elevated in skeletal muscle during tumor growth; TNF was able to mimic this increase in the gene expression.[117]

Recent studies showed that ZAG is produced not only by certain tumors, but also by BAT and white adipose tissue.[118] Glucocorticoids were shown to stimulate ZAG gene expression, suggesting that increased cortisol levels seen in cachectic cancer patients may lead to an increased lipolysis through ZAG overexpression.

In cancer patients with weight loss, LMF/ZAG levels found in serum and urine were much higher than those in noncancer control patients with comparable weight loss and were proportional to the degree of weight loss.[119] Patients who responded to therapy showed a decrease in the plasma levels of LMF/ZAG, which correlated with the levels of response.[120]

Proteolysis-Inducing Factor Serum from cachectic mice bearing MAC16 adenocarcinoma as well as urine and plasma from cancer patients with weight loss contained factors that induced proteolysis in skeletal muscles.[2,121–123] These factors are termed proteolysis-inducing factor (PIF). The PIFs derived from murine and human sources are identical: Both are characterized as a sulfated glycoprotein with a molecular weight of 24 kDa, with a unique amino acid sequence. A murine monoclonal antibody can attenuate weight loss induced by human PIF in mice. PIF was readily detected in the urine of cachectic cancer patients, whereas it was absent in the urine of normal subjects and of patients with weight loss owing to trauma or sepsis.

Body composition analysis of mice with weight loss from PIF showed specific depletion of the nonfat carcass mass. Weight loss was associated with loss of skeletal muscles, but there was no effect on the heart and there was an increase in liver weight.[123] Protein degradation induced by PIF appears to be mediated through the ubiquitin-proteasome pathway specifically in skeletal muscle.[124] Increased muscle proteasome activity was correlated with disease severity in gastric cancer patients.[125] Effects of PIF on increased expression of proteasome subunits and the ubiquitin conjugating enzyme E2(14k) were also demonstrated in vitro. The action of PIF on the protein degradation was mediated by the phospholipase A2 catalyzed release of arachidonic acid from membrane phospholipid and its conversion to the lipoxygenase product 15-hydroxyeicosatetraenoic acid.[124]

Production of PIF appears to be associated specifically with cancer cachexia, and it was not found in the urine of patients undergoing major surgery or in those with burns, multiple injuries, sepsis, or sleeping sickness, even though the rate of weight loss exceeded that found in cancer patients.[126] Patients with cancer of the pancreas, lung, colon, breast, rectum, liver, and ovary, in whom the rate of weight loss was greater than or equal to 1 kg/month showed evidence of PIF excretion in the urine.[122] Eighty percent of patients with pancreas cancer excreted PIF in the urine.[126]

It is of note that in humans, muscle protein degradation may not necessarily be mediated though the ubiquitin-proteasine pathway. Thus, mRNA levels of lysosomal protease cathepsin B were shown to be much higher in early stages of lung cancer patients with weight loss. In the early stages of the disease lysosomal proteases appear to play a significant role in muscle wasting.[127]

Hormonal Aberration Hormonal aberration may be a contributory factor to cancer cachexia. In a unique endocrine animal tumor model estrogen was incriminated as the cause of cancer cachexia.[128] Abnormally low levels of testosterone or hypogonadism have been described in male patients with advanced cancer; these findings correlated with weight loss and adverse outcome.[129,130] Plasma cortisol values and arterial glucagon levels in patients with malignant tumors were significantly increased, however, compared with patients with benign surgical disorders.[131,132] This finding is in accord with the hypothesis that glucocorticoids are involved in the increased protein catabolism of skeletal muscles and other organs in cachectic cancer patients.

Prostaglandin Elevation In animal systems, marked weight loss and wasting of muscle and adipose tissue after tumor transplantation were associated with the presence of circulating TNF-α and high levels of prostaglandin-E2.[133] Indomethacin reduced weight loss and increased survival of mice with transplantable tumors receiving chemotherapy.[134] Ibuprofen, a cyclo-oxygenase inhibitor, abrogated IL-1–induced anorexia in rats.[135] Close interaction of host- and tumor-derived cytokines and prostaglandins in the CNS were suggested from animal models.[135] These observations indicated that prostaglandin-E2 contributes to cancer anorexia and cachexia. Recent studies using an animal model showed that prostaglandin-E and prostaglandin-I receptor levels in the CNS had little role in cancer anorexia/cachexia. Rather, expressions of overall prostaglandin-E receptors in the liver, fat, and skeletal muscles appeared to be directly contributory to metabolic alterations in cancer cachexia.[136]

Tumor Parasitism Selective parasitism of the host by the tumor in the form of a successful competition for substrates with limited availability may be a cause of cachexia. Animal studies demonstrated that translocation of nitrogen from host to tumor constitutes nearly the total nitrogen depression of the host.[137] Tumors are effective nitrogen traps independent of protein intake, despite the wasting of normal host tissue.[138] Since cachexia can appear in patients with very small tumors, however, and the total tumor mass in the majority of cancer patients at death rarely exceeds 0.5 kg, it is unlikely that a simple competition of available nitrogen between tumor and host is responsible for the development of cachexia, especially in early-stage cancer.

Dysfunction of Neuropeptidergic Circuit Dysfunction of neuropeptidergic circuits as the mechanism of the cancer anorexia-cachexia syndrome has been discussed in the section on anorexia above.

Metabolic Derangement Produced by Treatment Postoperative weight loss results from increased energy expenditure owing to the stress response and a decreased dietary intake.[139] Pancreatic resection can result in pancreatic exocrine and endocrine insufficiency, creating major nutritional problems such as steatorrhea and hyperglycemia. In addition, major hepatic resections cause metabolic abnormalities in the immediate postoperative period. Extensive resection of the small bowel can lead to malabsorption of many nutrients.

A majority of chemotherapeutic agents are toxic, producing a variety of metabolic effects. L-asparaginase and IL-12 exemplify this: Profound weight loss and/or hypoalbuminemia are among the common manifestations in patients treated with these compounds.[140–142]

LABORATORY MANIFESTATIONS OF CANCER CACHEXIA

Energy Expenditure In cancer patients, resting energy expenditure and metabolic rates are often elevated and the increases are regarded as a contributing factor to weight loss.[143] An elevation of 12% in the metabolic rate was estimated to account for the loss of body weight of 1 to 2 kg per month.[144] In other studies, minimal or no elevation in metabolic rates were observed in many cancer patients. Measurements of resting energy expenditure in cancer patients showed that only one-third of them were hypermetabolic, one-half were hypometabolic, and the rest normometabolic.[145,146] Following curative resection, resting energy expenditure normalized or remained normal, but after palliative resection, resting energy expenditure remained hypermetabolic or significantly increased toward hypermetabolism. There are substantial metabolic differences depending on the anatomic site and histologic type of cancer. Thus, patients with lung cancer showed an increase in resting energy expenditure compared with healthy controls, whereas patients with gastrointestinal cancer had no elevation in resting energy expenditure.[147] Increases in resting energy expenditures were more pronounced in patients with an acute-phase response.[148] Patients with lower gastrointestinal tract cancer were metabolically similar to normal volunteers, while patients with upper gastrointestinal cancer had elevated rates of lipolysis, glucose turnover, and an increased reliance on glucose as an energy substrate.[149,150] Patients with advanced head and neck cancer, as well as those with sarcoma, were also metabolically abnormal, having accelerated rates of glucose turnover, glucose recycling, and a loss of the protein-sparing response to starvation.[151,152]

Carbohydrate Metabolism Abnormalities of carbohydrate metabolism in tumor-bearing animals may include abnormal glucose tolerance, elevated blood lactate, and changes in glucose turnover, pool size, and half-life. In cancer patients with progressive weight loss, enhanced glucose utilization with increases in both complete oxidation and the Cori cycle, and "diabetic glucose" tolerance have been described.[153,154] Glucose uptake and lactate release by human colon carcinomas have been found to exceed the peripheral tissue exchange rate by 30-fold and 43-fold, respectively.[155] A positive correlation was found between tumor bulk and rate of plasma glucose appearance, plasma glucose clearance, the percent of tissue glucose uptake recycled to lactate, and oxygen consumption.[156] In these patients insulin:glucose ratios were increased, decreased, or unchanged, but the insulin:glucagon ratio was always decreased.[157] Hyperglucagonemia may be an important hormonal alteration in the tumor-bearing host. Increases in glucagon levels caused anorexia, enhanced tumor protein synthesis, and stimulated tumor growth.[158] Inhibition of glucagon secretion and reversal of insulin:glucose ratios were associated with increased carcass weight, increased muscle weight, increased liver cellular protein, and decreased tumor protein content compared with untreated tumor-bearing controls.[159]

In patients with advanced cancer, hypoglycemia is also occasionally found.[160] The explanation for hypoglycemia in islet cell tumors is the production of ectopic insulin or proinsulin. In patients with large hepatic carcinomas, hypoglycemia occurs because of poor hepatic glycogen reserves and liver failure. Possible pathogenesis of hypoglycemia in large abdominal sarcomas and adrenocortical and gastrointestinal carcinomas include excessive consumption of glucose by the neoplasms; elaboration of tryptophan derivatives, which inhibit hepatic gluconeogenesis; and production of insulin or insulin-like growth factor I and II.[161–164]

Fat Metabolism Lipid metabolism in animal systems is altered by cancer, including loss of body fat early in tumor growth, induction of hyperlipidemia, changes in a variety of serum lipid and lipoprotein fractions, suppression of the postprandial rise in fatty acid synthesis in the liver, and reduction in the rate of excretion of $^{14}CO_2$ after intraperitoneal injections of ^{14}C-tripalmitin.[165–167]

Likewise, human cancer cachexia involves an impairment of both lipid and cholesterol metabolism, including reduced adipose tissue mass and increased plasma levels of free fatty acids and triglycerides.[168,169] High-density lipoprotein levels are decreased and very-low-density lipoprotein levels are elevated.[170] In cancer hosts, the activity of lipoprotein lipase, the enzyme responsible for the movement of fatty acids from blood into adipocytes, is decreased and the decrement correlated with the loss of body fat.[171,172] As the result of a decline in the activity of lipoprotein lipase in the adipose tissue, hyperlipidemia ensues, which is a common characteristic in cancer patients.[173] Decreases in lipoprotein lipase are mediated by TNF-α and IL-1, the latter via IL-6.[173] LMF/ZAG causes stimulation of adenylate cyclase in a GTP-dependent process and induces direct lipolysis in adipocytes.[112] Plasma total lipoprotein lipase activity in cancer patients with varying degrees of weight loss was decreased by 35% compared with that of normal volunteers.[174] In addition, cancer patients were found to have higher rates of fat oxidation compared with control subjects with equal weight loss.[145,175] The increased fat oxidation has been explained by tumor production of LMF.[176] The magnitude of the increase in fat oxidation suggests that this occurs in the host rather than in tumor tissue, contributing to fat loss in cancer patients. The inability of glucose loading to suppress fatty acid oxidation in cachectic patients suggests that there is a disturbance in normal homeostatic mechanisms involving the integration of glucose.[74]

Patients with ovarian and endometrial tumors were found to have lower concentrations of linoleic acid in subcutaneous adipose tissue than cancer-free controls, suggesting mobilization of structural lipid to supply the tumor.[177] Linoleic acid is also a stimulator of tumor growth.[178] Lipolysis of host fat, hyperlipidemia and resynthesis of the fatty acid within a tumor cell may represent another futile cycle contributing to cancer cachexia.

In a study of autopsy samples, BAT comprised 80% of periadrenal tissue in cachectic cancer patients compared with 13% in age-matched controls dead of other causes.[179] The most unique feature of brown adipocytes is their expression of UCP-1, a 32-kDa protein of the inner mitochondrial membrane, which functions to uncouple mitochondrial respiration, that is, the failure to make high-energy phosphate bonds. The physiologic consequence of uncoupling protein activity is unrestrained oxidation of fuels with the sole by-product being the generation of heat, leading to increased energy expenditure. BAT also plays an important role in regulating total-body fat stores.[113]

In the loss of adipose tissue in cancer cachexia, increased lipolysis, rather than decreased synthesis, appears to play the most important role.

Protein Metabolism Protein-calorie undernutrition is universally prevalent in patients with advanced cancer.[180] Whole-body protein turnover is increased in most patients with advanced cancer compared with starved normal individuals and weight-losing noncancer patients.[181] The energy cost of this increased protein turnover has been estimated to be 100 Kcal/d.[187] Loss of skeletal-muscle protein, a hallmark of cancer cachexia, occurs through increased rate of skeletal muscle protein breakdown, whereas there is only secondary or no reduction in the rate of muscle protein synthesis.[182–184]

Three major proteolytic pathways responsible for the catabolism of protein in skeletal muscle are known: (1) the cytosolic calcium-activated pathway, which is responsible mainly for tissue injury, necrosis and autolysis; (2) the lysosomal system, which is involved mainly in the proteolysis of extracellular proteins and cell surface receptors; and (3) the ATP-ubiquitin–dependent proteolytic system, which is involved in breakdown of myofibrillar proteins in starvation, sepsis, metabolic acidosis, and cancer cachexia.[2,185]

Protein degradation in cachectic cancer patients is mediated primarily through the ubiquitin-proteasome proteolytic pathway. In cancer cachexia, cytokines such as TNF-α and tumor-derived glycoprotein, PIF, induces proteolysis in skeletal muscle by increasing expression of proteasome subunits and the ubiquitin carrier protein, E2(14k).[2,186,187] In this system, ubiquitin is bound covalently to the protein substrate, which acts as a signal for degradation by the multisubunit proteasome. Since this process requires ATP, this may be another process contributing to the elevated energy expenditure observed in cancer cachexia.[188] Induction of proteasome expression by glucocorticoids during sepsis appears to be a direct result of the down-regulation of the activity of nuclear factor kappa B (NF-κB), while PIF acts through 15-hydroxyeicosatetraenoic acid as an intracellular transducer.[2,186,187] The mechanism behind overexpression of the ubiquitin gene under these conditions may be related to β2-adrenoreceptor overactivity.[189]

E3 ubiquitin ligases control polyubiquitination, a rate-limiting step in the ubiquitin-proteasome system. E3α-II, a novel "N-end rule" ubiquitin ligase is highly enriched in skeletal muscle, and its expression is regulated by proinflammatory cytokines. In two different animal models of cancer cachexia, E3α-II was significantly induced at the onset and during the progression of muscle wasting. The E3α-II activation in skeletal muscle was accompanied by a sharp increase in protein ubiquitination, which could be blocked by arginine methylester, an E3α-selective inhibitor. Treatment of myotubes with TNF-α or IL-6 elicited marked increases in E3α-II but not E3α-I expression and ubiquitin conjugation activity in parallel. E3α-II transfection markedly accelerated ubiquitin conjugation to endogenous cellular proteins in muscle cultures. These findings show that E3α-II plays an important role in muscle protein catabolism during cancer cachexia. E3α-II may be a potential therapeutic target for muscle wasting.[190]

Although ubiquitin-proteasome–dependent proteolysis is the predominant mechanism of muscle protein loss, there is evidence that several other regulatory mechanisms may also be important in producing muscle cachexia induced by sepsis, severe injury, and cancer.[191] Participation of the putrescine/spermine pathway in muscle tissue in tumor-bearing animals has been suggested.[192] In experimental cancer-associated cachexia, TNF-induced apoptosis has been observed.[193]

There is an imbalance between the amino acid composition of skeletal muscle and acute-phase proteins.[194] In fasting state, the synthetic rate of fibrinogen, a positive acute-phase protein, is higher in cancer patients than in healthy controls. In cancer patients in the fed state, fibrinogen synthetic rate rose by a median of 38%, whereas in controls there was no significant change.[195] These findings demonstrate significant up-regulation by feeding of acute-phase protein synthesis in cachectic cancer patients. This may provide a mechanism whereby a proportion of supplied nutrients is diverted from normal anabolism in cancer cachexia.

Recently, longitudinal body composition measurements of 311 patients with a variety of cancers who were treated with an anti-inflammatory agent, indomethacin, and erythropoietin (if Hg < 12.5 gm/dL) were reported.[196] There was a significant loss of body fat, preferentially from trunk, but lean tissue was maintained or even increased slightly. Lean tissue loss occurred in arm tissues. Maintenance of lean tissue in trunk and loss in the arm may reflect differences in skeletal muscle versus visceral protein. Percent decreases in body weight and serum albumin were correlated with increases in ESR and C-reactive protein, serum insulin, and lowered daily caloric intake. Serum albumin, whole-body fat, and caloric intake were significant predictors of survival, whereas lean tissue lacked predictive significance.

Specific protein abnormalities in cancer patients also include anemia, which may be due to acute or chronic blood loss, marrow involvement by tumor cells, marrow suppressive effects of chemotherapy or radiation therapy, "anemia of chronic disease," or due to production of inflammatory cytokines; hypoalbuminemia, probably secondary to decreases in albumin synthesis by inflammatory cytokines in the liver; acute phase protein response, a reprioritization of liver protein synthesis often seen in trauma, inflammation, and infection; and hepatic catalase depression, as a remote effect of cancer. Recently, a suggestion was made that toxohormone, a hepatic catalase-depressing agent in patients with cancer, is derived from proteolytic digestion of fibrin and fibronectin by tumor cells.[197]

Neuroendocrine System A variety of hormonal abnormalities has been reported in cancer patients. These abnormalities include increases in plasma cortisol, increase in urinary excretion of cortisol and its metabolites and catecholamines, decreases in testosterone levels or hypogonadism, and diabetic glucose tolerance secondary to insulin resistance and/or to increased rate of insulin clearance.[129,130,198,199] The elevated basal metabolic rate observed in cancer patients has been associated with an increase in heart rate and may be due to an elevated adrenergic state.[143]

Water and Electrolytes Hyponatremia is common in patients with advanced cancer. The cause of hyponatremia may include ectopic secretion of antidiuretic hormone (ADH) or an ADH-like substance by the tumor; cardiac, renal, or adrenal cortical insufficiency; and excessive loss of sodium from gastrointestinal fistulae, diarrhea, salt-losing nephropathy, and diuretic use. Cyclophosphamide and vinca alkaloids are also known to produce hyponatremia either as a direct neurotoxic effect on the central nervous system with release of ADH from its site of formation and storage or as direct renal tubular toxicity. Hyponatremia occurs quite frequently in patients with intracranial tumors. This may result from excessive use of dextrose-water solutions, inadequate salt intake in obtunded patients under improper dietary supervision, and, rarely, from excessive ADH release. The search for a specific cause of hyponatremia in cancer patients is not always successful.

A subclinical or overt increase in total-body water may occur in patients with cancer. Malnutrition, hypoalbuminemia, "nonspecific" adrenal response, and mechanical obstruction of venous or lymphatic return may play a role. Fluid overload may also be produced by zealous hydration as a part of treatment. New sodium-free water may arise from excessive loading by mouth or vein, oxidation of fat, and catabolism of cellular tissue.

ASSESSMENT OF CANCER CACHEXIA IN HUMANS

Because of the strong relationship between nutritional status and various clinical outcomes, including quality of life, survival and the ability to tolerate treatment, it is important to assess patients at nutritional risk and to provide early interventions and potentially to improve the untoward outcomes.

Nutritional Screening Various screening questionnaires have been developed to identify patients who are at the greatest risk of developing nutritional problems. Examples are Patient-Generated Subjective Global Assessment (PG-SGA),[200] Nestle Mini Nutritional Assessment (MNA),[201] and Malnutrition Screening Tool (MST).[202] Usefulness of PG-SGA has been validated in populations with cancer, MNA in geriatric populations, and MST in patients on radiotherapy. There are other methods of assessment of nutritional status, such as the Malnutrition Universal Screening Tool and the Nutrition Risk Assessment Tool. Attempts to validate the former in a population with cancer showed that it was unsuitable for use because of low sensitivity and specificity.[203]

Nutritional Assessment Nutritional assessment is different from nutritional screening. When high-risk patients are identified by nutritional screening, systemic assessment and a clearly outlined plan for intervention should ensue. This is commonly done by a registered dietician or nutrition professional. It incorporates medical history, a detailed dietary history, physical examination, anthropometric measurements, and laboratory data. Nutritional assessment includes an assessment of body compartments and an analysis of the structure and function of organ systems and their effect on metabolism. Nutritional intervention requires multidisciplinary approach to care. There is a recent review article available, which details nutritional screening, assessment, medical nutritional treatment, and nutritional care plan.[204] Results of such nutritional counseling and intervention are discussed in the next sections "Treatment of Cachexia" and "Supportive Care."

TREATMENT OF CACHEXIA

The definitive treatment of cancer cachexia is removal of the causative tumor. Short of achieving this goal, various measures have been undertaken with limited success.

Supportive Care Patients with anorexia from decreased physical activity, concomitant infection, and toxicities to the alimentary tract from chemotherapy and radiotherapy are managed symptomatically for maintenance of nutritional status and quality of life. Such management includes the use of mouthwash for stomatitis, frequent small-volume feedings, antiemetics, antibiotics, transfusions of blood components, and/or oral and parenteral nutritional supplement. Consideration of the patient's food preferences and service of food in a dining room atmosphere may also be important to stimulate appetite. When a patient is unable to consume a regular diet to obtain adequate nutrition, food supplements, both homemade and commercially available, are an effective means of providing additional calories, protein, fat, vitamins, and minerals, although overall consumption may not increase much. In specific instances, such as the malabsorption syndrome secondary to pancreas carcinoma, exogenous pancreas extract improves fat and protein absorption.[71]

The effect of frequent nutritional counseling on oral food intake, body weight, response rate, survival, and quality of life was examined in patients with cancer undergoing chemotherapy.[205,206] In a randomized study, the counseling increased daily energy and protein intake as well as triceps skinfold measurements. Response rates and overall survival did not differ from control patients who received no intervention, however.[205] In randomized studies of colorectal cancer and head and neck cancer patients undergoing radiotherapy, both dietary counseling and nutritional supplements positively influenced outcomes, including less weight loss, less nutritional deterioration, and maintenance of quality of life (QoL).[207,208] In another randomized study by the Rural Physician Cancer Prevention Project, the intervention group demonstrated significant improvement in dietary fat and fiber behaviors and intentions to change fat and fiber intake. Whether or not cancer prevention was achieved or longevity in the study population was improved was not reported. This study, however, provided an effective model for achieving public health-level dietary health behavior changes among a rural, minority, and low-literacy/low-education population.[209]

Pharmacologic Management Various agents have been administered in attempts to retard or halt progressive cachexia in cancer patients. In addition, a number of agents are currently being studied in animals. These agents are arranged in Table 126-2 based on their major mechanism of action. It is of note that each of these agents exerts a variety of other pharmacologic activities.

Table 126-2 Pharmacologic Treatment of Cancer Cachexia in Humans

	Reported Activities	Were Favorable Effects Seen in Randomized Studies?	References
Corticosteroids			
Prednisolone	Euphoriant activity	Yes?; ↑appetite, ↑BW, ↑sense of well being, but effects were transient	7, 210–213
Methylprednisolone	↓prostaglandin metabolism		
Dexamethasone	↓IL-1.	No improvements in OS	
Progestational agents			
Megestrol acetate	↑appetite, ↓IL–1α, , ↓IL–β, ↓TNF-α, ↑NPY,↑BW	Yes; ↑appetite, ↑body weight	216, 218–222
Medroxyprogesterone acetate	↑appetite, ↓serotonin ↓IL-1β, IL-6, TNF-α	Yes; ↑appetite but no BW gain	224–226
Anabolic steroids			
Nandrolone decanoate	↑BW in noncancer patients	Yes?; ↓BW loss but response to chemotherapy and survivals were same as controls	227–230
Fluoxymesterone		No; less appetite enhancement and unfavorable toxicity profile as compared with megestrol acetate or dexamethasone	213
Cannabinoids (dronabinol)	antiemetic, ↑appetite	No; megestrol + dronabinol not better than megestrol alone	232
Hormones	↑muscle weight, ↑muscle protein		
Growth hormone/insulin	Whole body and skeletal protein net balance was higher than control.	ND	326
	No data on BW or QoL.	ND	
GHRP-2	↑fat and bone mass, ↑food intake	ND	238
IGF-1	↑amino acid uptake, ↑protein synthesis,↓lipolysis, ↓host muscle protein loss.	ND	
rhGH/ rhIGF-1		ND; (no significant anabolic effect in HIV pts)	243
Prokinetic agents			
Metoclopramide	↑appetite, ↓dyspeptic symptoms	No; unable to improve appetite or weight loss	247
Cisapride			
Inhibitor of phosphoenolpyruvate carboxykinase			
Hydrazine sulfate	Interruption of gluconeogenesis ↑appetite, ↑BW, ↑PS, ↑muscle strength, ↓pain	No; no improvements in appetite, weight, QOL, or OS	249–251
Inhibitors of prostaglandin synthesis and COX-2			
Indomethacin, ibuprofen	↓fever, ↓C-reactive protein	ND	
Celecoxib	↓BW loss	ND	
Ibuprofen/megestrol		Yes; ↑BW, ↑QoL	263
Indomethacin/erythropoietin		Yes; prevented anemia, exercise capacity preserved, ↑BW, but no ↑ in OS	264, 265
Methylxanthine analogues			
Pentoxifylline, lisofylline	Anti-inflammatory properties, ↓TNF-α, ↑appetite, ↑sense of well being, ↑BW in patients with normal TNF-α	No; no improvements in appetite or BW. Rate of infection or mortality rates unchanged from controls	269, 270
NF-κB inhibitors			
Curcumin	↓protein degradation in myotubes,	ND	
Resveratrol	↓PIF-induced increases in ubiquitin-proteasome pathway		
	↓BW loss and protein degradation in cachexia animal model (Resveratrol)		
2-Adrenoceptor agonist			
Clenbuterol	↓muscle protein wasting in animals and noncancer patients	ND	

(Continued)

Table 126-2 Pharmacologic Treatment of Cancer Cachexia in Humans *(Continued)*

	Reported Activities	Were Favorable Effects Seen in Randomized Studies?	References
Thalidomide	Immunomodulatory activity and antiangiogenic properties	Yes; ↓BW loss and ↑arm muscle mass	284
Nucleosides and nucleoids			
Adenosine triphosphate	Extracellular ATP is involved in regulation of a variety of biologic processes including muscle contraction and liver glucose metabolism, ↓BW loss ↓QoL deterioration	Yes; prevented anorexia, loss of fat mass, arm muscle area, body cell mass, and BW loss	285, 286
5'-dFUrd	↓PIF	ND	
Cytokines and anticytokines			
Anti-TNF Ab	↓skeletal muscle loss, ↓BW loss	ND; (not effective in patients with severe sepsis)	295
Anti-IL-1 Ab			
Anti-IL-1R Ab			
Etanercept, Infliximab		ND; (not effective in patients with chronic heart failure)	296
Suramin	↓binding of IL-6 to cell receptor	ND	
Anti-IL-6 Ab	↓cancer cachexia in mice	ND	
IL-12	↓serum	ND	
Eicosapentaenoic acid	↓prostaglandin synthesis, ↓PMF, ↓IL-6, ↑BW, ↑lean body mass	Yes; EPA/Vit E: ↑T4/T8 ratio, ↑OS in both nourished and malnourished patients	315
		No; no advantage over placebo or regular nutritional supplement or megestrol	316–318
TPN		No; TPN does not augment chemotherapy or radiotherapy effects, does not prolong OS	322–326
Amino acids			
Branched-chain amino acids	↓protein catabolism ↑protein synthesis, ↑appetite	Yes; supplement of branched chain amino acids to TPN improved nitrogen balance, ↑albumin and protein synthesis	329, 330
		No; not better than balanced amino acid solution alone	331
Glutamine		No; (effective in transplant patients)	336
Orexigenic and anorexigenic mediators:			
Insulin	↑food intake, ↓muscle wasting Major side effect is hypoglycemia	ND	
Ghrelin	↑food intake	ND	
Melatonin	Immunologic modulation, antioxidative and anti-inflammatory activities, ↓circulating TNF	Yes; in combination with IL-2, ↑PS, reduced weight loss, ? ↑OS. With chemotherapy no survival advantage but ↓toxicities and ↓BW loss	345, 346
Melatonin/EPA		Yes; BW stabilization only	347
Serotonin antagonist			
Cyproheptadine	↑BW	Yes; ↓nausea and ↑appetite (mild), but no BW gain	348

Ab = antibody; BW = body weight; GHRP = growth hormone releasing peptide; IGF = insulin-like growth factor; IL = interleukin; ND = has not been done; NPY = neuropeptide Y; OS = overall survival; PMF = proteolysis-mobilizing factor; PS = performance status; QoL = quality of life; TNF = tumor necrosis factor; TPN = total parenteral nutrition.

Corticosteroids A number of uncontrolled studies have suggested that corticosteroids can alleviate such symptoms as anorexia, asthenia, and pain in patients with cancer. The mechanism of action may include a euphoriant activity, anti-inflammatory action through the inhibition of TNF release, and suppression of IL-1β activity, as well as inhibition of prostaglandin metabolism. Significant improvements in appetite and a sense of well-being have been reported in randomized trials with *prednisolone*, *methylprednisolone*, or *dexamethasone*.[8,210–212] Unfortunately, the improvements were not long lasting, and upon completion of the studies, all nutritional parameters returned to their baseline. There were no differences in mortality rate or in survival.

In a randomized comparison of dexamethasone and megestrol acetate, both drugs caused a similar degree of appetite enhancement and similar changes in nonfluid weight status, but dexamethasone was found to be less favorable.[213] Dexamethasone had more corticosteroid-type toxicity and a higher rate of drug discontinuation because of toxicity and/or patient refusal than megestrol acetate.

Although corticosteroids have been postulated to be responsible for muscle wasting and cancer cachexia, studies involving treatment with RU38486, a glucocorticoid receptor antagonist, of experimental animals bearing cachexia-producing tumors suggested that glucocorticoids are not involved in skeletal muscle wasting associated with cancer cachexia, and receptor blockade did not abrogate tumor-induced cachexia.[214,215]

Megestrol Acetate and Medroxyprogesterone Acetate *Megestrol acetate*, a progestational agent, is frequently used in the treatment of patients with metastatic breast cancer. It is generally well tolerated, except that it may cause undesirable weight gain. Subsequently, it was shown that megestrol acetate produced weight gain in a variety of cachectic cancer patients. Significant reduction in serum levels of IL-1α and β, IL-2, IL-6, and TNF-α were observed in cancer patients treated with megestrol acetate, which may bear on the mechanism of improved appetite and body weight gain.[216] It has also been postulated that the effect is, at least in part, mediated by neuropeptide Y, a potent central appetite stimulant.[217]

In a review of 15 randomized clinical trials including more than 2,000 patients, there was a statistically significant advantage for high-dose progestins in regard to improved appetite and gain of body weight.[218] Treatment morbidity was low because of the brief period of the treatment in most of the studies. A meta-analysis of 26 studies confirmed the usefulness of megestrol acetate in gaining appetite and body weight of cancer patients with anorexia-cachexia syndrome.[219]

Weight gain produced by megestrol acetate was found to be mainly from increased body fat stores rather than accretion of lean tissue.[220,221] It has been argued that the gain of adipose tissue as opposed to lean tissue during treatment with megestrol acetate, although suboptimal, should not be considered inherently negative because depletion of body fat is generally an undesirable outcome of cancer.

The addition of megestrol acetate to chemotherapy for patients with melanoma resulted in a high objective response and prolonged median survival compared with historical controls with chemotherapy alone.[222] Megestrol acetate is contraindicated in pediatric cachectic patients, since a significant proportion of such patients developed adrenal insufficiency.[223]

Medroxyprogesterone acetate is a more widely used synthetic progestogen. Medroxyprogesterone reduced production of cytokines and serotonin that are involved in anorexia/cachexia in cancer patients.[224] Two placebo-controlled randomized studies have been reported in which increased appetite was described.[225,226] In one study, significant increases in rapid turnover proteins such as serum thyroid-binding prealbumin and retinol-binding protein were reported.[225] In spite of increased appetite, no weight gain was produced in either study.

Anabolic Steroids Anabolic androgenic steroids have been used by athletes to promote muscle growth and strength. In MCG sarcoma-bearing mice with progressive cachexia, administration of *nandrolone propionate* resulted in significant weight gain.[227] The weight gain was, however, mainly attributed to water retention, and food intake and survival were not affected. Randomized clinical trials were carried out to test whether supplements of *nandrolone decanoate* influenced the outcome of chemotherapy in patients with nonsmall-cell lung cancer.[228,229] Although the treated group experienced less weight loss, response to chemotherapy and survival were comparable. In a three arm phase III randomized clinical trial comparing a progestational agent, a corticosteroid, and an anabolic corticosteroid for the treatment of cancer anorexia/cachexia, the *fluoxymesterone* group showed significantly less appetite enhancement and did not have as favorable a toxicity profile compared with megestrol acetate or dexamethasone.[213]

Cannabinoids (Dronabinol) While using *dronabinol* (delta 9-tetrahydocannabinol, THC) as an antiemetic it was found that the agent enhanced the appetite in healthy individuals and in cancer patients. To study this phenomenon further, an open dose-ranging study was carried out in patients with cancer.[230,231] All patients reported improvement in appetite. Higher dosages, 5.0 mg or 7.5 mg/day, were more effective than the low dosage of 2.5 mg/day. Patients in all groups continued to lose weight, although the rate of weight loss decreased with therapy. It is of note that these effects were observed at doses lower than those producing antiemetic effects and without overt psychotropic symptoms.

Recently, a randomized study was carried out to determine whether dronabinol administered alone or with megestrol acetate was more, less, or equal in efficacy to single-agent megestrol acetate for palliating cancer-associated anorexia.[232] Megestrol acetate provided superior anorexia palliation among advanced cancer patients compared with dronabinol alone. Combination of megestrol and dronabinol did not appear to have conferred additional benefit.

Growth Hormone, Somatostatin, and Growth Hormone Releasing Peptide-2 Anabolic properties of growth hormone have been examined in animals. Administration of growth hormone to tumor-bearing rats resulted in increased muscle weight and muscle protein content and preserved host-body composition.[233] Growth hormone did not stimulate tumor growth.[234] The effect of a combination of insulin, growth hormone, and somatostatin on tumor growth, metastasis, and host metabolism was evaluated in rats bearing MAC33 mammary tumor.[235] The triple therapy supported host anabolism, increased hamstring muscle weight and protein content, and inhibited tumor growth kinetics. The advantage of the inclusion of somatostatin in the treatment relied on the fact that insulin treatment alone led to limited success in treating cancer cachexia due to insulin-induced hypoglycemia and subsequent glucagon secretion. Somatostatin alone is known to have antitumor activity, however, and the contribution of each component to the observed changes was not clear.

The effect of recombinant human growth hormone and insulin administration on protein kinetics was examined in 28 cancer patients.[236] Whole-body protein net balance was higher in patients treated with both growth hormone and insulin than in insulin only or growth hormone only controls. Skeletal muscle protein net balance in the growth hormone/insulin group was higher than no-treatment controls. Recombinant human growth hormone and insulin reduced whole-body and skeletal muscle protein loss in cancer patients. Simultaneous use of these agents during nutritional therapy may benefit the cancer patient.[236]

Daily subcutaneous injections of a more stable synthetic ghrelin receptor agonist GHRP-2 (*growth hormone releasing peptide-2*) in mice produced dose-dependent increases in food intake and body weight.[237] Pre- and post-treatment analysis of body composition indicated increased fat and bone masses but not lean mass. GHRP-2–induced positive energy balance leading to fat gain occurred in the absence of involvement of hypothalamic NPY neurons. Indeed, GHRP-2 administration to healthy volunteers resulted in increased food intake.[238] Ghrelin receptor agonists may offer a treatment option for syndromes like anorexia nervosa, cancer cachexia, or AIDS wasting.

Insulin-Like Growth Factor-1 *Insulin-like growth factor-1* (IGF-1), also known as somatomedin-C, mediates many of the anabolic properties of growth hormone including stimulation of amino acid uptake and protein synthesis.[239] Other studies have shown its important role in muscle cell proliferation and differentiation,[240] as well as inhibition of lipolysis.[239] Continuous subcutaneous IGF-1 administration in rat bearing methylchanthrene-induced sarcoma resulted in host preservation of lean tissue and attenuation of host muscle protein depletion.[241] Interestingly, the treatment did not stimulate tumor growth.

Ten subjects with AIDS-associated cachexia received either low- or high-dose IV recombinant IGF-1 daily for 10 days.[242] Cumulative nitrogen retention was positive for both dosage groups, but a significant increase in daily nitrogen retention occurred only in the low-dose group. The anabolic response was transient, however. Repeated administration of IGF-1 decreased IGF-binding protein-3 levels, producing lower intrainfusion levels of IGF-1 and limiting its therapeutic efficacy. The basal metabolic rate increased with high-dose IGF-1 and may have contributed to the lack of anabolic effect. The authors concluded that partial growth hormone resistance occurred in AIDS-associated cachexia.

A randomized placebo-controlled 12-week trial of a combination of recombinant human growth hormone (rhGH, Nutropin) and rhIGF-1 was carried out in 142 subjects with HIV wasting.[243] At 3 weeks, the treatment group had a significantly larger weight increase, but this difference was not observed at any later time point. Similarly, fat-free mass, calculated from skinfold measurements, increased transiently in the treatment group at 6 weeks. No significant differences in isokinetic muscle strength or endurance testing or in quality of life were observed between the groups. Authors concluded that the combination of rhIGF-I and low-dose rhGH had no significant anabolic effect in HIV wasting.[243] IGF-I has not been tested in patients with cancer cachexia.

Metoclopramide and Cisapride In advanced cancer patients with delayed gastric emptying or gastroparesis, oral administration of a prokinetic agent, *metoclopramide*, 10 mg orally 4 times daily before meals and at bedtime, was shown to be effective in stimulating appetite and relieving other dyspeptic symptoms associated with anorexia.[244,245] A controlled release preparation appears to be more effective than immediate release drug because of its control of nausea associated with advanced cancer, even without demonstrated abnormalities of the gastrointestinal (GI) tract.[246] Patients with head and neck cancer undergoing radiotherapy were randomized to 3 groups, megestrol acetate, cisapride, and placebo. Megestrol significantly prevented body weight loss and deterioration of appetite, whereas cisapride lacked these clinical benefits.[247]

Hydrazine Sulfate *Hydrazine sulfate*, an inhibitor of the enzyme phosphoenolpyruvate carboxykinase, has been shown to interrupt gluconeogenesis in animals.[248] Based on a theory that increased gluconeogenesis and enhanced Cori cycle activity were the central mechanism of tumor-induced cachexia, clinical studies of hydrazine sulfate attempted to prevent or reverse cancer-related cachexia and weight loss. Three multicenter group studies were carried out in patients with nonsmall-cell lung cancer or colorectal cancer.[249–251] All three studies failed to show beneficial results in appetite, body weight, quality of life, or survival from hydrazine sulfate.

Indomethacin, Ibuprofen, and Celecoxib It has been proposed that cell growth may be controlled by the interconversion of different types of prostagladins.[252–254] Animal studies of the prostaglandin biosynthesis inhibitors' ability to reverse cancer cachexia are not universally positive. In one study, *indomethacin*, *ibuprofen*, or aspirin inhibited growth of Walker 256 carcinoma in rats.[255] All drug-treated rats partially recovered body weight and food intake compared with a saline-treated group. In another study using the same tumor system, however, indomethacin and ibuprofen retarded tumor growth and lowered body temperature compared with controls, but these agents had no effect on food intake or body weight of tumor-bearing animals.[256] *Celecoxib*, a COX-2 inhibitor, was reported to rapidly reverse weight loss in two murine models, colon 26, which induced high levels of circulating IL-6 and human head and neck tumor 1483 HNSCC xenograft.[257]

In clinical trials, indomethacin reduced fever and granulocytosis and was claimed to have improved the well-being of cancer patients.[258,259] In cachectic cancer patients, indomethacin or ibuprofen was reported to decrease resting energy expenditure and C-reactive protein values to produce body weight gain and to improve survival.[260–262] In a randomized study in patients with advanced gastrointestinal cancer with more than 5% weight loss, megestrol acetate alone resulted in weight loss and deterioration of quality of life, whereas the combination of megestrol/ibuprofen appeared to reverse weight loss and appeared to improve quality of life.[263] Impact of erythropoietin was studied in a randomized fashion in unselected weight-losing cancer patients who were treated with indomethacin. The combination resulted in an improvement of hematocrit together with increased serum albumin levels, decreases in C-reactive protein, improved body weight, and greater exercise capacity compared with indomethacin-alone controls.[264,265] Study and control patients did not differ in survival, however. Well-designed randomized clinical studies are needed to assess therapeutic values of prostaglandin inhibitors alone and in combination with other anticachectic agents in patients with cancer cachexia.

Pentoxifylline and Lisofylline These agents are methylxanthine analogues shown to have anti-inflammatory properties. They have been shown to have profound stimulatory effects on vascular endothelial production of noninflammatory prostaglandins-I2 and –E2, while inhibiting TNF-α synthesis by blocking gene transcription.[266] *Pentoxifylline* was originally used for the treatment of various types of vascular insufficiency because of its hemorheological property. Pentoxifylline prevented muscle atrophy and suppressed increased protein breakdown in tumor-bearing rats by inhibiting the activation of a nonlysosomal, Ca(2+)-independent ubiquitin-proteasome proteolytic pathway.[267] Pentoxifylline suppressed the enhanced expression of ubiquitin, the 14-kDa ubiquitin conjugating enzyme E2, and the C2 20S proteasome subunit in muscle from cancer-bearing rats.

Prophylactic oral administration of pentoxifylline in allograft recipients together with chemotherapy and radiotherapy resulted in significant reduction in the incidence and severity of treatment-related complications: mucositis, hepatic veno-occlusive disease, renal insufficiency, and the incidence of graft-versus-host disease.[268] In an initial study in cancer patients, pentoxifylline suppressed TNF-α mRNA levels, increased the sense of well-being, improved appetite, and improved the ability to perform activities of daily living. Patients with normal TNF levels also had a weight gain. In a randomized controlled trial in patients with solid tumors, however, pentoxifylline failed to provide improvement in appetite or body weight compared with a placebo group.[269] Likewise, for patients with acute myelocytic leukemia or myelodysplastic syndrome once in complete remission with idarubicin/ara-C chemotherapy, lisofylline provided no favorable effects in terms of rates of infection, overall mortality rates, or outcome.[270] Lisofylline did not alter the toxicities of high-dose IL-2, and thus did not impact the overall dose intensity in the treatment of advanced renal cancer and malignant melanoma.[271]

Proteasome Inhibitors and NF-κB Inhibitors As detailed previously, ubiquitin-proteasome pathway plays an important role in muscle protein catabolism during cancer cachexia and may be a potential therapeutic target for muscle wasting.[190] *Arginine methylester* and alanine methylester, ubiquitin ligase E3α-selective inhibitors, have not been examined in cachectic cancer patients.

Activation of nuclear factor-κB (NF-κB) leads to the induction of proteasome expression and protein degradation by PIF. The cell permeable NF-κB inhibitor SN50 attenuated the expression of 20S proteasome α-subunits, two subunits of the 19S regulator MSS1 and p42, and the ubiquitin-conjugating enzyme E2(14k). It also decreased myosin expression in murine myotubes. The potential for inhibitors of NF-κB activation, *curcumin* and *resveratrol*, to act as inhibitors of muscle protein degradation in cancer cachexia was evaluated both in vitro and in vivo. Both agents completely attenuated total protein degradation in murine myotubes at all concentrations of PIF, and attenuated the PIF-induced increase in expression of the ubiquitin-proteasome proteolytic pathway. Curcumin was ineffective in preventing weight loss and muscle protein degradation in the animal tumor model, however, whereas resveratrol significantly attenuated weight loss and protein degradation in skeletal muscle and produced a significant reduction in NF-κB DNA-binding activity.[272,273] The inactivity of curcumin was probably due to a low bioavailability. These results suggest that agents that inhibit nuclear translocation of NF-κB may prove useful for the treatment of muscle wasting in cancer cachexia.[273]

Clenbuterol *Clenbuterol* is a β2-adrenoceptor agonist. It prevented muscle protein wasting in tumor-bearing animals and increased muscle mass and function in healthy animals.[274–276] There was no change in food intake or tumor growth. Combinations of naproxen, clenbuterol, insulin, and EPA supplement ameliorated cancer cachexia and reduced tumor growth in Walker 256 tumor-bearing rats.[277,278] In patients after knee surgery, clenbuterol was able to improve muscle strength in a randomized trial.[279] Its effects on muscle preservation appeared to occur without the need for exercise. Clenbuterol has not yet been studied in patients with cancer cachexia.

Thalidomide *Thalidomide*, a drug associated with over 10,000 cases of severe malformation in newborn children, was revived recently because of its ability to suppress TNF production in monocytes in vitro and to normalize elevated TNF levels in animals. The drug also possesses antiangiogenic properties. Thalidomide inhibited TNF-α production in patients with leprosy, tuberculosis, AIDS, and cancer.[280,281] In a preliminary study, 72 cancer patients with anorexia and weight loss were given thalidomide 100 mg a day.[282] By day 10, 50 to 70% of 37 evaluable patients reported improvements in anorexia, nausea, fatigue, and sense of well-being. In another study, 11 patients with nonobstructing and inoperable esophageal cancer were established on an isocaloric diet for 2 weeks, followed by 2 weeks on thalidomide at 200 mg daily.[283] Ten patients completed the study protocol. The average caloric intake remained the same throughout the study period in all patients. Nine of 10 patients lost weight on diet alone. The mean weight gain on thalidomide in the following 2 weeks was 1.29 kg. A similar trend was shown in the lean body mass. Eight of 9 patients initially lost lean body mass on diet alone. The mean gain in lean body mass on thalidomide in the following 2 weeks was 1.75 kg. Thalidomide treatment appeared to reverse the loss of weight and lean body mass over the 2-week trial period.[283] In a randomized placebo-controlled trial, 50 patients with advanced pancreatic cancer who had lost at least 10% of their body weight received thalidomide 200 mg daily or placebo for 24 weeks.[284] At 4 weeks, patients who received thalidomide had gained on average 0.37 kg in weight and 1.0 cm^3 in arm muscle mass compared with a loss of 2.21 kg and 4.46 cm^3, respectively, in the placebo group. At 8 weeks, patients in the thalidomide group had lost 0.06 kg in weight and 0.5 cm^3 in arm muscle mass compared with a loss of 3.62 kg and 8.4 cm^3, respectively, in the placebo group. Improvement in physical functioning correlated positively with weight gain. Thalidomide was well tolerated and appeared effective at attenuating loss of weight and lean body mass in patients with cachexia due to advanced pancreatic cancer. Beneficial effects of thalidomide have not been compared with other anticachexia agents such as megestrol acetate.

Adenosine Triphosphate Patients with nonsmall-cell lung cancer, stage IIIB or IV, were randomized to receive either 10 intravenous, 30-hour ATP infusions every 2 to 4 weeks, or no ATP.[285,286] No change in body composition over the 28-week follow-up period was found in the ATP group, whereas the control group lost 0.6 kg of fat mass, 0.5 kg of fat-free mass, 1.8% of arm muscle area, and 0.6% of body cell mass/kg body weight per 4 weeks. Appetite also remained stable in the ATP group, but decreased significantly in the control group, 568 KJ/d in energy intake. These effects were ascribed to maintenance of energy intake by exogenous ATP.

These reports contrast with a strategy of ATP suppression as a means of cancer therapy. ATP suppression in tumor tissue by means of direct intra-arterial delivery of 3-bromopyruvate, a potent inhibitor of cell ATP production, to the site of the primary tumor, or a combination of 6-methylmercaptopurine riboside, a purine de novo synthesis inhibitor, and 6-aminonicotinamide, an inhibitor of glycolysis, which were given concomitant with a pyrimidine synthesis inhibitor was reported to show marked therapeutic enhancement.[287–289]

5'-Deoxy-5-fluorouridine The fluorinated pyrimidine nucleoside, 5'-deoxy-5-fluorouridine (5'-dFUrd), was shown to effectively attenuate the progress of cachexia in mice bearing the murine adenocarcinomas MAC16 or colon 26, as well as in the human uterine cervical carcinoma xenograft, Yumoto. The anticachexia effect of 5'-dFUrd was shown to be independent of its antitumor activity and appears to be, at least in part, related to its inhibition of proteolysis-inducing factor (PIF), thought to be responsible for the development of cachexia in the murine MAC16 model.[290,291] 5'-dFUrd has not yet been evaluated as an anticachectic agent in humans.

Proinflammatory-Cytokine Inhibitors, Proinflammatory-Cytokine Antibodies, and Anti-Inflammatory Cytokines In addition to pentoxifylline and thalidomide, a number of cytokine inhibitors and antibodies have been developed.

Anti–TNF-α antibody, *anti–IL-1 antibody*, and *anti–IL-1 receptor antibody* were reported to have attenuated the cachexia produced by either chronic TNF-α administration or implantation of a tumor in experimental animals.[292,293] Administration of TNF-α antibody to tumor-bearing rats decreased protein degradation rates in skeletal muscle, heart, and liver as compared with controls; the antibody was unable to prevent a reduction in body weight, however.[294] Decreases in protein degradation in skeletal muscle by TNF-α antibody appear to be due to inhibition of tumor-induced increases in muscle ubiquitin gene expression.[294] Anti-TNF antibodies have not been evaluated in patients with cancer cachexia. Randomized clinical trials using anti-TNF treatment failed to increase survival or reverse the protein catabolism associated with severe sepsis or septic shock compared with those who received standard supportive care and antimicrobial therapy.[295] Similarly, clinical trials involving anti-TNF strategies such as *etanercept* (a dimeric fusion protein consisting of the extracellular ligand-binding portion of the human 75 kilodalton tumor necrosis factor receptor [TNFR] linked to the Fc portion of human IgG1) or *infliximab* (monoclonal antibody against TNF-α) in patients with chronic heart failure showed no improvements in clinical outcome as compared with placebo controls.[296]

Suramin, an antitrypanosomal polyanion, prevented the binding of IL-6 to its cell surface receptor subunits in vitro and inhibited colon-26–mediated cancer cachexia in mice.[297] Treatment of mice bearing AB 22 mesothelioma with *anti–IL-6 antibody* curtailed the clinical symptoms, as did treatment with recombinant human (rhu) IFN-α.[298] Neither anti–IL-6 antibody nor rhuIFN-α had a direct growth-inhibitory effect on the tumor cell line in vitro; however, in vivo rhuIFN-α attenuated both IL-6 mRNA expression in the tumors and serum IL-6 levels, ameliorated the depression of lymphocyte activities, and enhanced the number of tumour-infiltrating lymphocytes and macrophages. A combination therapy of rhuIFN-α and anti–IL-6 antibody may be beneficial in the palliative treatment of patients with malignant mesothelioma.[298]

The administration of an anti–IL-6 antibody in patients seropositive for human immunodeficiency virus-1 and suffering from an immunoblastic or a polymorphic large-cell lymphoma resulted in partial remission or stabilization of the disease.[299] The neutralizing effect of the anti–IL-6 antibody as measured by C-reactive protein levels in the serum was accompanied by abrogation of B clinical symptoms, including fever and cachexia. Paradoxically, administration of purified human rIL-6 alone or in combination with subtherapeutic doses of TNF was effective against syngeneic tumors in mice and rat.[99]

Production of anti-inflammatory cytokine IL-12 and type 2 immune responses is markedly decreased in cachectic patients with colorectal and gastric cancer.[300] Administration of *IL-12* was reported to reduce serum levels of IL-6 in mice bearing colon 26 carcinoma and prevented development of cachexia.[301] The IL-12 activity was T-cell–dependent and the anticachexia effect resulted from at least 2 mechanisms: the down-regulation of IL-6 and the up-regulation of IFN-α. Similarly, a gene transfer of IL-10, another IL-6 inhibitor, prevented cachexia in an animal model.[302] *IL-15* treatment partly inhibited skeletal muscle wasting in AH-130–bearing rats by decreasing protein degradative rates to values even lower than those observed in nontumor-bearing animals.[303] These alterations in protein breakdown rates were associated with an inhibition of the ATP-ubiquitin–dependent proteolytic pathway. Administration of IL-15 to rats bearing ascites hepatoma resulted in a significant reduction of muscle wasting and reversal of the increased DNA fragmentation observed in skeletal muscle.[304] IL-15 decreased apoptosis apparently by affecting TNF-α signaling. Administration of IL-15 decreased the inducible nitric oxide synthase protein levels by 73%, suggesting that nitric oxide formation and muscle apoptosis during tumor growth could be related. IL-12, IL-10, and IL-15 have not been evaluated as anticachectic agents in humans.

Eicosapentaenoic Acid ω-3 Polyunsaturated fatty acids are an essential component of the diet and are involved in the synthesis of eicosanoids (prostaglandins, leukotrienes, and thromboxanes) and in membrane, receptors and enzyme functions. Eicosapentaenoic acid (EPA), an ω-3 polyunsaturated fatty acid found in oily fish, such as sardines, salmon, and mackerel, has been shown to possess antitumor as well as anticachexia activities in animal cachexia models.[305,306] EPA-induced inhibition of weight loss was accompanied by increases in total-body fat and muscle mass. EPA administration resulted in suppression of well-characterized mediators of cancer-associated wasting, including IL-6, and an attenuation of protein degradation by the ubiquitin-proteasome proteolytic pathway mediated by PIF in cachectic mice.[307,308] PIF in skeletal muscle releases arachidonic acid, which is rapidly metabolized to prostaglandins E2 and F2α as well as 5-, 12-, and 15-hydroxyeicosatetraenoic acids (HETEs). Of all the metabolites, only 15-HETE produces a significant increase in protein degradation. EPA induced inhibition of arachidonic acid release and subsequent decreases in 15-HETE, which serves as a second messenger, abrogate the enhancer effect on the promoter region of the proteasome C3 subunit gene.[309] EPA also decreased glucose utilization of skeletal muscle and inhibited lipolysis in adipocytes by preventing prostaglandin synthesis and by a rising cyclic AMP in response to the LMF and by inhibiting nuclear translocation of the transcription factor NF-κB, by preventing degradation of the inhibitor protein I-κB in the cytosol.[310–312]

Early clinical trials were encouraging. Patients with pancreas cancer treated with supplements of fish oil capsules (EPA and docosahexaenoic acid) showed body weight gain accompanied by significant reduction in acute-phase protein production and by stabilization of resting energy expenditure.[313] Although nutritional supplement alone did not attenuate the development of weight loss in cachectic cancer patients, nutritional supplement enriched with EPA produced significant weight gain along with an improvement in appetite and performance status.[314] Significant rises of lean body mass noted in body composition analysis was noteworthy among various therapeutic interventions reported. A randomized controlled study was carried out to investigate the effects of dietary EPA plus vitamin E on the immune systems and survival of well-nourished and of malnourished cancer patients.[315] EPA had a considerable immunomodulating effect by increasing the ratio of T-helper cells to T-suppressor cells in the subgroup of malnourished patients. EPA doubled the survival of patients compared with the placebo arm.

More recent randomized clinical studies cast a serious doubt as to any unique benefit of EPA, however. In a first trial, 60 patients with advanced cancer and loss of both weight and appetite were randomized to fish oil capsules or placebo.[316] No significant differences in symptomatic or nutritional parameters were found. The majority of the patients were not able to swallow more than 10 fish oil capsules per day. They concluded that fish oil did not significantly influence appetite, tiredness, nausea, well-being, caloric intake, nutritional status, or function after 2 weeks of treatment compared with placebo. In an international multicenter randomized double-blind trial, 200 patients with weight-losing inoperable pancreas cancer were randomized to receive EPA (2.2 gm/day) plus nutritional supplement or the nutritional supplement alone.[317] Enrichment with EPA did not provide a therapeutic advantage over nutritional supplement alone. Both treatment groups equally benefited in arresting weight loss. There were no differences in body mass index, lean body mass, QoL, or survival. In a third trial, 221 patients with cancer-associated wasting were randomized to either EPA supplement alone, megestrol acetate alone, or EPA plus megestrol acetate.[318] Weight gain of ≥ 10% was seen in a higher percentage of patients with megestrol acetate than EPA. Overall weight gain, functional assessment of anorexia/cachexia therapy (FAACT), and QoL were essentially identical among the three groups. Thus, available data do not support the value of EPA in the treatment of cancer cachexia in humans.

Enteral and Parenteral Nutrition Cancer cachexia is different from simple starvation in that nutritional support, either enteral or parenteral, has only limited value. For the correction of cancer-related malnutrition, therefore, enteral and parenteral administration of nutrient solutions must be used discreetly. In patients with oropharyngeal dysfunction from head and neck neoplasm or esophageal obstruction, blenderized food and liquid supplement can often achieve an adequate level of nutritional repletion. When necessary, percutaneous gastrostomy or jejunostomy offer bypass feeding. For patients who cannot tolerate the use of the gastrointestinal tract because of nausea, vomiting, obstruction, malabsorption, or absence, it may be necessary to begin total parenteral nutrition (TPN, "hyperalimentation").

The needs of nutritional support in cancer patients during tumor progression and the role of TPN in cancer surgery, chemotherapy, and radiotherapy should be considered at several different levels. Benefits of TPN in patients who underwent cancer surgery included improved wound healing, a decreased rate of infection, fewer major complications, and a decrease in postoperative mortality. In other studies, however, no advantage of TPN was found; one report described an increase in the rate of major postoperative complications.[319] TPN in cancer patients with obstructions of the gastrointestinal tract, gastrointestinal fistulae, evisceration, and intra-abdominal infection appears justified during and after surgery.[320] Although strong data are lacking, when enteral nutrition cannot be encouraged or applied, TPN is considered beneficial in patients who have not been eating for at least 10 days or in those who have lost more than 10% of their usual body weight.[321]

No significant benefit of TPN was demonstrated, however, in patients undergoing chemotherapy and/or radiotherapy in terms of treatment tolerance, response to chemotherapy or radiotherapy, or in survival.[322,323] Furthermore, other authors have reported that TPN is detrimental. Controversies related to TPN in the treatment of cancer cachexia have been reviewed.[324–326]

Recently, in a randomized trial of more than 300 patients with malignant neoplasms who experienced progressive cachexia, indomethacin and Epogen, or indomethacin and Epogen plus oral or parenteral nutritional support were compared.[327] The patients in the latter group had significant improvements in food intake, energy balance, and overall survival. Authors suggested palliation of patients with cancer can be fortified using treatments that attenuate systemic inflammation, prevent anemia, and improve energy balance via the provision of nutritional support. It is unclear, however, whether improved survival was due to combined effects of two drugs plus nutritional intervention or nutritional intervention alone. This question is important because in this study, a large percentage (92.1%) of patients with gastrointestinal cancer was accrued, suggesting that many patients might have had nausea and vomiting, GI obstruction, ascites, diarrhea, or other GI-specific causes of weight loss rather than simply cancer cachexia. Confirmatory studies are needed, specifically accruing patients with non-GI malignancies.

Because of limited nutritional reserves, children with cancer suffer more often from malnutrition than adults with neoplasms. Therefore, combined chemotherapy/radiotherapy protocols for children with neuroblastoma and Wilms' tumor often incorporate parenteral and enteral nutritional support. Recently, enteral nutritional support has become more popular than TPN, mainly for economic reasons. An algorithm for nutritional support has been developed that requires a compelling rationale for choosing parenteral over enteral support in children with a functional GI tract.[328] Such a plan resulted in increased choice of enteral nutritional support.

Branched-Chain Amino Acids Branched-chain amino acids (leucine, isoleucine, and valine) are utilized by skeletal muscle but not by the liver. They have been shown to be uniquely effective in regulating nitrogen balance in muscle by reducing protein catabolism and increasing protein synthesis in both injured and tumor-bearing animals. Randomized studies have shown improved nitrogen retention, improved protein utilization, and increased protein and albumin synthesis in patients who received parenteral nutritional support with a high content of branched-chain amino acids.[329,330] In contrast, in another randomized study, the effects of a balanced amino acid solution with or without supplementation of α-ketoisocaproate or a branched-chain amino acid solution were compared in patients with gastrointestinal cancer who underwent surgery.[331] The balanced amino acid solution itself with an adequate energy supply had an optimal nitrogen-sparing effect. Branched-chain amino acids or α-ketoisocaproate did not improve nitrogen balance or reduce protein degradation.

Interestingly, the tryptophan (precursor of serotonin) uptake into the brain is competitive with that of branched-chain amino acids.[332] A trial to reduce tryptophan uptake by increasing plasma levels of branched-chain amino acids resulted in a decrease in the severity of anorexia in cancer patients.[333]

Glutamine Tumor cells are major glutamine consumers, both for protein synthesis and for oxidation.[334] A glutamine-enriched solution has been used to compensate for the uptake of the amino acid by the tumor to enhance host immune response against tumor growth.[335] In patients undergoing bone marrow transplantation for hematological malignancies, glutamine supplementation was found to be beneficial, improving nitrogen balance and diminishing the incidence of clinical infection.[336]

Orexigenic and Anorexigenic Mediators

Insulin Some of the metabolic alternations associated with cancer cachexia include glucose intolerance, increased gluconeogenesis, and Cori cycle activation. These metabolic changes are accompanied by insulin resistance. These observations led to the study of exogenous insulin administration. Animal studies show that insulin administration has improved the degree of food intake, muscle wasting, and host preservation of nitrogen, fat, and potassium.[337,338] Indeed, daily subcutaneous insulin administration resulted in a marked weight gain in AIDS patients.[339] Insulin administration has not been evaluated in the treatment of cancer cachexia.

Ghrelin Ghrelin, an orexigenic mediator has recently been reported to have a key role in increasing appetite and food intake. The circulating levels of ghrelin have been reported to be increased in patients with chronic heart failure and muscle wasting and in patients with cancer cachexia.

Anticachexic effects of ghrelin have been demonstrated in nude mice bearing human melanoma cells.[340] Ghrelin has not been tested in patients with cancer cachexia.

Melatonin Melatonin is an indole amine primarily secreted from the pineal gland during the hours of darkness. The functions of melatonin are obscure, but it has been claimed to modulate sleep, cardiac rhythms, sexual behavior, the reproductive system, immunologic functions, as well as antioxidative and anti-inflammatory activities. Melatonin decreased the level of circulating TNF in patients with advanced cancer, prevented body weight loss and reduced chemotherapy-induced malaise and asthenia as well as thrombocytopenia.[341–344]

Based on observations that melatonin amplified IL-2–induced antitumor effects in animals, a randomized study was carried out in patients with metastatic solid tumors comparing a combination of low-dose IL-2 plus melatonin with best supportive care.[345] In the treated group, the percentage of patients with improved performance status as well as overall survival were significantly higher than the controls. Another randomized study of chemotherapy with cisplatin and etoposide plus/minus melatonin was carried out in patients with advanced nonsmall-cell lung cancer with poor clinical status.[346] There was no significantly different survival between groups, but the melatonin group had less frequent myelosuppression, neuropathy, and cachexia. In a recent Swedish trial, the effect of fish oil, melatonin, or their combination were investigated in 24 patients with advanced gastrointestinal cancer. Fish oil, melatonin, or their combination did not induce major biochemical changes indicative of a strong anti-cachectic effect. Nonetheless, the interventions used may have produced a weight-stabilizing effect.[347] Additional clinical studies appear indicated to define the role of melatonin in the treatment of cancer cachexia.

Cyproheptadine As has been discussed earlier, anorexia may be mediated by an increased serotonergic activity in the brain. Cyproheptadine is a serotonin antagonist with antihistaminic properties, usually used for the treatment of allergies. In several clinical situations the agent produced appetite stimulation and weight gain. A randomized trial in patients with advanced malignant neoplasms showed that cyproheptadine produced a decrease in nausea and mild enhancement in appetite. The agent did not abate progressive weight loss in these patients, however.[348] Additional studies are needed with the use of other antiserotogenic drugs.

EPILOGUE

In patients with cancer, cachexia may appear even when the total tumor is the size of "pinheads."[349] In the majority of cancer patients the tumor mass seldom exceeds 500 g at autopsy.[69] Cachexia is a function of the type of tumor and its stage and location. Since cancer itself represents multiple diseases, cachexia can be an end result of multiple causes and of multifactorial etiology. Studies of the mechanisms of cachexia have focused on an early effect of the tumor on a host with a small tumor burden. In such a situation, elaboration of pharmacologically active mediator(s), either from tumor or from the host, is more likely the cause of cachexia than simple competition for available nitrogen and other nutrients between tumor and host. In contrast, metabolic abnormalities in cachectic patients with advanced cancer appear to be far different from the metabolic changes that occur in patients with minimal disease. Complex and often confusing features of the pathophysiology of cachexia stem from this difference. Clearly, major mediator(s) of cachexia are different for different cancer types and different disease stages. Identification of specific cachexia-producing mediator(s) for individual patients may lead to the development of treatments specific for each patient.

Cachexia contributes to a poor quality of life, and every effort should be made to reverse or halt the advancement of cachexia, even if such measures have little survival advantage. For patients with anorexia, dietary counseling may include a discussion of the concept of food choices and preparation, alternative nutritional supplements, as well as an assessment of additional issues, such as swallowing dysfunction. If cachectic cancer patients who present with intestinal obstruction are judged to be potentially curable (eg, untreated ovarian cancer) parenteral nutritional support should be started without delay. In advanced cancer patients with cachexia, generous administration of megestrol acetate and other appetite stimulants is often a part of good clinical management.

Although traditional TPN does not prevent progressive cachexia in humans, various modifications of TPN have been reported to improve nitrogen retention and to prevent weight loss. Eicosapentaenoic acid has emerged as a potent anticachexia agent, but recent randomized studies are not encouraging. Perhaps, combinations of so-called anticachexia agents may have a value. Clinical extrapolation of these studies with robust experimental design is needed to determine their usefulness.

REFERENCES

1. Thomas DR. Distinguishing starvation from cachexia. Clin Geriatr Med 2002;18:883–91.
2. Tisdale MJ. Tumor-host interactions. J Cell Biochem 2004;93:871–7.
3. Giordano A, Calvani M, Petillo O, et al. Skeletal muscle metabolism in physiology and in cancer disease. J Cell Biochem 2003;90:170–86.
4. Nixon DW, Lawson DH, Kutner M, et al. Hyperalimentation of the cancer patient with protein-calorie undernutrition. Cancer Res 1981;41:2038–45.
5. Brennan MF. Uncomplicated starvation versus cancer cachexia. Cancer Res 1977;37:2359–64.
6. Armes PJ, Plant HJ, Allbright A, et al. A study to investigate the incidence of early satiety in patients with advanced cancer. Br J Cancer 1992;65:481–4.
7. Willox JC, Corr J, Shaw J, et al. Prednisolone as an appetite stimulant in patients with cancer. Br Med J 1984;288:27.
8. Scott HR, McMillan DC, Forrest LM, et al. The systemic inflammatory response, weight loss, performance status and survival in patients with inoperable non-small cell lung cancer. Br J Cancer 2002;87:264–7.
9. Maltoni M, Amadori D. Prognosis in advanced cancer. Hematol Oncol Clin North Am 2002;16:715–29.
10. Wigmore SJ, Plester CE, Richardson RA, Fearon KC. Changes in nutritional status associated with unresectable pancreatic cancer. Br J Cancer 1997;75:106–9.
11. Cohen MH, Makuch R, Johnston-Early A, et al. Laboratory parameters as an alternative to performance status in prognostic stratification of patients with small cell lung cancer. Cancer Treat Rep l981;65:187–95.
12. Warren S. The immediate cause of death in cancer. Am J Med Sci l932;184:610–5.
13. Mullen JL, Gertner MH, Buzby GP, et al. Implications of malnutrition in the surgical patient. Arch Surg 1979;114:121–5.
14. Evans WK, Nixon DW, Daly JM, et al. A randomized study of oral nutritional support versus ad lib nutritional intake during chemotherapy for advanced colorectal and non-small-cell lung cancer. J Clin Oncol 1987;5:113–24.
15. Osterlind K, Hansen HH, Dombernowsky P, et al. Determinants of complete remission induction and maintenance in chemotherapy with or without irradiation of small cell lung cancer. Cancer Res 1987;47:2733–6.
16. DeWys WD, Walters K. Abnormalities of taste sensation in cancer patients. Cancer 1975;36:1888–96.
17. Nielsen SS, Theologides A, Vickers ZM. Influence of food odors on food aversion and preference in patients with cancer. Am J Clin Nutr 1980; 33:2253–61.
18. Baile CA, Zinn WM, Mayer J. Effects of lactate and other metabolites on food intake of monkeys. Am J Physiol 1970;219:1606–13.
19. Bajorunas DR. Clinical manifestations of cancer-related hypercalcemia. Semin Oncol 1990;17 (2 Suppl 5):16–25.
20. Masuno H, Yoshimura M, Ogawa N, Okuda H. Isolation of lipolytic factor (toxohormone-L) from ascites fluid of patients with hepatoma and its effects on feeding behavior. Eur J Cancer Clin Oncol 1984;20:1177–85.
21. Moody TW, Pert CB, Gazdar AF, et al. High levels of intracellular bombesin characterize human small cell lung cancer. Science 1981;214:1246–8.
22. Knoll J. Endogenous anorectic agent-satietins. Annu Rev Pharmacol Toxicol 1988;28:247–68.
23. Hamilton J, Cabanac M, Lafrance L, Nagy J. Ingestive response shows absence of taste aversion after bovine satietin in rats. Physiol Behav 1995;57:125–8.
24. Jensen PB, Blume N, Mikkelsen, JD, et al. Transplantable rat glucagonomas cause acute onset of severe anorexia and adiposia despite highly elevated NPY mRNA levels in the hypothalamic arcuate nucleus. J Clin Invest 1998;101:503–10.
25. Cangiano C, Testa U, Muscaritoli M, et al. Cytokines, tryptophan and anorexia in cancer patients before and after surgical tumor ablation. Anticancer Res 1994;14:1451–5.
26. Cubeddu LX, Hoffmann IS, Fuenmayor NT, Finn AL. Efficacy of ondansetron (GR 38032F) and the role of serotonin in cisplatin-induced nausea and vomiting. N Engl J Med l990;322:810–6.
27. Inui A. Cancer anorexia-cachexia syndrome: are neuropeptides the key? Cancer Res 1999;59:4495–501.
28. Krause R, Humphrey C, von Meyenfeldt M, et al. A central mechanism for anorexia in cancer: a hypothesis. Cancer Treat Res 1981;65 Suppl 5:15–21.
29. Laviano A, Meguid MM, Yang ZJ, et al. Cracking the riddle of cancer anorexia. Nutrition 1996;12:706–10.
30. Bodnar RJ, Pasternak GW, Mann PE, et al. Mediation of anorexia by human recombinant tumor necrosis factor through a peripheral action in the rat. Cancer Res 1989;49:6280–4.
31. Plata-Salaman CR, Oomura Y, Kai Y. Tumor necrosis factor and interleukin-1 beta: suppression of food intake by direct action in the central nervous system. Brain Res 1988;448:106–14
32. Phase II study of recombinant human interferon gamma (S-6810) on renal cell carcinoma. Summary of two collaborative studies. Recombinant Human Interferon Gamma (S-6810) Research Group on Renal Cell Carcinoma. Cancer 1987;60:929–33.
33. Cahlin C, Korner A, Axelsson H, et al. Experimental cancer cachexia: the role of host-derived cytokines interleukin (IL)-6, IL-12, interferon-gamma, and tumor necrosis factor alpha evaluated in gene knockout, tumor-bearing mice on C57 Bl background and eicosanoid-dependent cachexia. Cancer Res 2000;60:5488–93.
34. Llovera M, Carbo N, Lopez-Soriano J, et al. Different cytokines modulate ubiquitin gene expression in rat skeletal muscle. Cancer Lett 1998;133:83–7.
35. Espat NJ, Auffenberg T, Rosenberg JJ, et al. Ciliary neurotrophic factor is catabolic and shares with IL-6 the capacity to induce an acute phase response. Am J Physiol 1996;271(1 Pt 2):R185–90.
36. Wang W, Lonnroth C, Svanberg E, et al. Cytokine and cyclooxygenase-2 protein in brain areas of tumor-bearing mice with prostanoid-related anorexia. Cancer Res 2001;61:4707–15.
37. Wang W, Andersson M, Lonnroth C, et al. Prostaglandin E and prostacyclin receptor expression in tumor and host tissues from MCG 101-bearing mice: a model with prostanoid-related cachexia. Int J Cancer 2005;115:582–90
38. Otterness IG, Seymour PA, Golden HW, et al. The effects of continuous administration of murine interleukin-1α in the rat. Physiol Behav 1988;43:797–804.
39. Mrosovsky N, Molony LA, Conn CA, et al. Anorexic effects of interleukin 1 in the rat. Am J Physiol 1989;257:R1315–21.
40. Maltoni M, Fabbri L, Nanni O, et al. Serum levels of tumour necrosis factor alpha and other cytokines do not correlate with weight loss and anorexia in cancer patients. Support Care Cancer 1997;5:130–5.
41. Wisse BE, Schwartz MW, Cummings DE. Melanocortin signaling and anorexia in chronic disease states. Ann N Y Acad Sci 2003;994:275–81.
42. Schwartz MW, Woods SC, Porte D Jr, et al. Central nervous system control of food intake. Nature 2000;404:661–71.
43. Lopez-Soriano J, Carbo N, Tessitore L, et al. Leptin and tumor growth in rats. Int J Cancer 1999;81:726–9.
44. Aleman MR, Santolaria F, Batista N, et al. Leptin role in advanced lung cancer. A mediator of the acute phase response or a marker of the status of nutrition? Cytokine 2002;19:21–6.
45. Arpaci F, Yilmaz MI, Ozet A, et al. Low serum leptin level in colon cancer patients without significant weight loss. Tumori 2002;88:147–9.
46. Wu JT, Kral JG. Ghrelin: integrative neuroendocrine peptide in health and disease. Ann Surg 2004;239:464–74.
47. Garcia JM, Garcia-Touza M, Hijazi RA, et al. Active ghrelin levels and active/total ghrelin ratio in cancer-induced cachexia. J Clin Endocrinol Metab 2005;90:2920–6.
48. Shimizu Y, Nagaya N, Isobe T, et al. Increased plasma ghrelin level in lung cancer cachexia. Clin Cancer Res 2003;9:774–8.
49. Inui A, Meguid MM. Ghrelin and cachexia. Diabetes Obes Metab 2002;4:431.
50. Ramos EJ, Suzuki S, Marks D, et al. Cancer anorexia-cachexia syndrome: cytokines and neuropeptides. Curr Opin Clin Nutr Metab Care 2004;7:427–34.
51. Niswender KD, Morton GJ, Stearns WH, et al. Intracellular signalling. Key enzyme in leptin-induced anorexia. Nature 2001;413:794–5.
52. Niswender KD, Schwartz MW. Insulin and leptin revisited: adiposity signals with overlapping physiological and

intracellular signaling capabilities. Front Neuroendocrinol 2003;24:1–1047.
53. Chance WT, Bakasubramaniam A, Thompson H, et al. Assessment of feeding response of tumor-bearing rats to hypothalamic injection and infusion of neuropeptide Y. Peptides 1996;17:797–801.
54. Chance WT, Bakasubramaniam A, Fischer JE. Neuropeptide Y and the development of cancer anorexia. Ann Surg 1995;221:579–89.
55. Chance WT, Bakasubramaniam A, Borchers M, Fischer JE. Refractory hypothalamumic adenylate cyclase in anorectic tumor-bearing rats. Brain Res 1995;691:180–4.
56. Sarraf P, Frederich RC, Turner EM, et al. Multiple cytokines and acute inflammation raise mouse leptin levels: potential role in inflammatory anorexia. J Exp Med 1997;185:171–5.
57. Argiles JM, Moore-Carrasco R, Busquets S, et al. Catabolic mediators as targets for cancer cachexia. Drug Discov Today 2003;8:838–44.
58. Gayle D, Ilyin SE, Plata-Salaman CR. Central nervous system IL-1 beta system and neuropeptide Y mRNAs during IL-1 beta-induced anorexia in rats. Brain Res Bull 1997;44:311–7.
59. Hellerstein MK, Meydani SN, Maydani M, et al. Interleukin-induced anorexia in the rat. J Clin Invest 1989;84:228–35.
60. Sato T, Laviano A, Meguid MM, et al. Involvement of plasma leptin, insulin and free tryptophan in cytokine-induced anorexia. Clin Nutr 2003;22:139–46.
61. Sonti G, Ilyin SE, Plata-Salaman CR. Neuropeptide Y blocks and reverses interleukin-1 beta-induced anorexia in rats. Peptides 1996;17:517–20.
62. Rossi-Fanelli F, Laviano A. Role of brain tryptophan and serotonin in secondary anorexia. Adv Exp Med Biol 2003;527:225–32.
63. Plata-Slaman CR. Immunoregulators in the nervous system. Neurosci Biobehav Rev 1991;15:185–215.
64. Chance WT, Sheriff S, Moore J, et al. Reciprocal changes in hypothalamic receptor binding and circulating leptin in anorectic tumor-bearing rats. Brain Res 1998;803:27–33.
65. Simons JP, Schols AM, Campdfield LA, et al. Plasma concentration of total leptin and human lung cancer-associated cachexia. Clin Sci Colch 1997;93:273–7.
66. Wallace AM, Satter N, McMillan DC. Effect of weight loss and the inflammatory response on leptin concentrations in gastrointestinal cancer patients. Clin Cancer Res 1998;4:2977–9.
67. Laviano A, Russo M, Freda F, Rossi-Fanelli F. Neurochemical mechanisms for cancer anorexia. Nutrition 2002;18:100–5.
68. Costa G, Lane WW, Vincent RG, et al. Weight loss and cachexia in lung cancer. Nutr Cancer 1980;2:98–104.
69. Costa G. Cachexia, the metabolic component of neoplastic disease. Cancer Res 1977;37:2327–35.
70. Vlachopapadopoulou E, Tracey KJ, Capella M, et al. Increased energy expenditure in a patient with diencephalic syndrome. J Pediatr l993;122:922–4.
71. Perez MM, Newcomer AD, Moertel CG, et al. Assessment of weight loss, food intake, fat metabolism, malabsorption, and treatment of pancreatic insufficiency in pancreatic cancer. Cancer 1983;52:346–52.
72. Ramot B. Malabsorption due to lymphomatous diseases. Ann Rev Med 1971;22:19–24.
73. Nelson KA, Walsh TD, Sheehan FG, et al. Assessment of upper gastrointestinal motility in the cancer-associated dyspepsia syndrome (CSDS). J Palliat Care 1993;9:27–31.
74. Mulligan HD, Tisdale MJ. Metabolic substrate utilization by tumour and host tissue in cancer cachexia. Biochem J 1991;277:321–6.
75. Pedersen PL, Mathupala S, Rempel A, et al. Mitochondrial bound type II hexokinase: a key player in the growth and survival of many cancers and an ideal prospect for therapeutic intervention. Biochim Biophys Acta 2002;1555:14–20.
76. Mathupala SP, Rempel A, Pedersen PL. Glucose metabolism in cancer cells: isolation, sequence, and activity of the promotor for type II hexokinase. J Biol Chem 1995;270:16918–25.
77. Mathupala SP, Rempel A, Pedersen PL. Glucose catabolism in cancer cells: identification and characterization of a marked activation response of the type II hexokinase gene to hypoxic conditions. J Biol Chem 2001;276:43407–12.
78. Gold J. Cancer cachexia and gluconeogenesis. Ann N Y Acad Sci 1974;230:103–10.
79. Lundholm K, Edstrom S, Karlberg I, et al. Glucose turnover, gluconeogenesis from glycerol and estimation of net glucose cycling in cancer patients. Cancer 1982;50:1142–50.
80. Ramos EJ, Suzuki S, Marks D, et al. Cancer anorexia-cachexia syndrome: cytokines and neuropeptides. Curr Opin Clin Nutr Metab Care 2004;7:427–34.
81. Tisdale MJ. Pathogenesis of cancer cachexia. J Support Oncol 2003;1:159–68.
82. Deans C, Wigmore SJ. Systemic inflammation, cachexia and prognosis in patients with cancer. Curr Opin Clin Nutr Metab Care 2005;8:265–9.
83. Henderson JT, Mullen BJM, Roder JC. Physiological effects of CNTF-induced wasting. Cytokins 1996;8:784–93.
84. Beutler B, Greenwald D, Hulmes JD, et al. Identity of tumour necrosis factor and the macrophage-secreted factor cachectin. Nature (Lond) 1985;316:552–4.
85. Tisdale MJ. Loss of skeletal muscle in cancer: biochemical mechanisms. Front Biosci 2001;6:D164–74.
86. Adami F, Guarini A, Pini M, et al. Serum levels of tumor necrosis factor-α in patients with B-cell chronic lymphocytic leukemia. Eur J Cancer 1994;30A:1259–63.
87. Aderka D, Englemann H, Hornik V, et al. Increased serum levels of soluble receptors for tumor necrosis factor in cancer patients. Cancer Res 1991;15:5602–7.
88. Sherman ML, Spriggs DR, Arthur KA, et al. Recombinant human tumor necrosis factor administered as a five-day continuous infusion in cancer patients: phase I toxicity and effects on lipid metabolism. J Clin Oncol 1988;6:344–50.
89. Starnes HF Jr, Warren RS, Jeevanandam M, et al. Tumor necrosis factor and the acute metabolic response to tissue injury in man. J Clin Invest 1988; 82:1321–5.
90. Socher SH, Martinez D, Craig JB, et al. Tumor necrosis factor not detectable in patients with clinical cancer cachexia. J Natl Cancer Inst 1988;80:595–8.
91. Turrin NP, Ilyin SE, Gayle DA, et al. Interleukin-1beta system in anorectic catabolic tumor-bearing rats. Curr Opin Clin Nutr Metab Care 2004;7:419–26.
92. Barber MD, Powell JJ, Lynch SF, et al. A polymorphism of the interleukin-1 beta gene influences survival in pancreatic cancer. Br J Cancer 2000;83:1443–7.
93. Fujita J, Tsujinaka T, Yano M, et al. Anti-interkeukin-6 receptor antibody prevents muscle atrophy in colon-25 adenocarcinoma-bearing mice with modulation of lysosomal and ATP-ubiquitin-dependent proteolytic pathways. Int J Cancer 1996;68:637–43.
94. Oldenburg HS, Rogy MA, Lazarus DD, et al. Cachexia and the acute phase protein response in inflammation are regulated by Interleukin-6. Eur J Immunol l993;23:1889–94.
95. Strassmann G, Masui Y, Chizzonite R, Fong M. Mechanism of experimental cancer cachexia. Local involvement of IL-1 in colon 26 tumor. J Immunol l993;150:2341–5.
96. Scott HR, McMillan DC, Crilly A, et al. The relationship between weight loss and interleukin 6 in non-small-cell lung cancer. Br J Cancer 1996;73:1560–2.
97. Martin F, Santolaria F, Batista N, et al. Cytokine levels (IL-6 and IFN-gamma), acute phase response and nutritional status as prognostic factors in lung cancer. Cytokine 1999;11:80–6.
98. Jablons DM, McIntosh JK, Mule JJ, et al. Induction of interferon β2/interleukin-6 (IL-6) by cytokine administration and detection of circulating interleukin-6 in the tumor-bearing state. Ann N Y Acad Sci 1989;557:157–60.
99. McNamara MJ, Alexander HR, Norton JA. Cytokines in their role in the pathophysiology of cancer cachexia. J Parenter Enteral Nutr 1992;16 Suppl 6:50S–5S.
100. Mule JJ, McIntosh JK, Jablons DM, Rosenberg SA. Antitumor activity of recombinant interleukin-6 in mice. J Exp Med 1990;171:629–36.
101. Suematsu S, Matsuda T, Aozasa K, et al. IgG1 plasmacytosis in interleukin-6 transgenic mice. Proc Natl Acad Sci U S A 1989;86:7547–51.
102. Patton JS, Shepard HM, Wilking H, et al. Interferon and tumor necrosis factors have similar catabolic effects on 3T3 L1 cells. Proc Natl Acad Sci U S A 1986;83:8313–7.
103. Matthys P, Heremans H, Opdenakker G, Billiau A. Anti-interferon-γ antibody treatment, growth of Lewis lung tumours in mice and tumour-associated cachexia. Eur J Cancer 1991;27:182–7.
104. Pisa P, Stenke L, Bernell P, et al. Tumor necrosis factor-α and interferon-γ in serum of multiple myeloma patients. Anticancer Res 1990;10:817–20.
105. Puigserver P, Rhee J, Lin J, et al. Cytokine stimulation of energy expenditure through p38 MAP kinase activation of PPARgamma coactivator-1. Mol Cell 2001;8:971–82.
106. Acharyya S, Ladner KJ, Nelsen LL, et al. Cancer cachexia is regulated by selective targeting of skeletal muscle gene products. J Clin Invest 2004;114:370–8.
107. Kajimura N, Iseki H, Tanaka R, et al. Toxohormones are responsible for cancer cachexia syndrome in nude mice bearing human cancer cell lines. Cancer Chemother Pharmacol 1996;38 Suppl:S48–52.
108. Mori M, Yamaguchi K, Honda S, et al. Cancer cachexia syndrome developed in nude mice bearing melanoma cells producing leukemia-inhibitory factor. Cancer Res l991;51:6656–9.
109. Marshall MK, Doerrler W, Feingold KR, Grunfeld C. Leukemia inhibitory factor induces changes in lipid metabolism in cultured adipocytes. Endocrinology 1994;135:141–7.
110. Berg M, Fraker DL, Alexander HR. Characterization of differentiation factor/leukemia inhibitory factor effect on lipoprotein lipase activity and mRNA in 3T3-L1 adipocytes. Cytokine 1994;6:425–32.
111. Todorov PT, McDevitt TM, Meyer DJ, et al. Purification and characterization of a tumor lipid-mobilizing factor. Cancer Res 1998;58:2353–8.
112. Hirai K, Hussey HJ, Barber MD, et al. Biological evaluation of a lipid-mobilizing factor isolated from the urine of cancer patients. Cancer Res 1998;58:2359–65.
113. Lowell BB, Flier JS. Brown adipose tissue, beta 3-adrenergic receptors, and obesity. Annu Rev Med 1997;48:307–16.
114. Hyltander A, Daneryd P, Sandstrom R, et al. Beta-adrenoceptor activity and resting energy metabolism in weight losing cancer patients. Eur J Cancer 2000;36:330–4.
115. Bing C, Brown M, King P, et al. Increased gene expression of brown fat uncoupling protein (UCP)1 and skeletal muscle UCP2 and UCP3 in MAC16-induced cancer cachexia. Cancer Res 2000;60:2405–10.
116. Bing C, Russell ST, Beckett EE, et al. Expression of uncoupling proteins-1, -2 and -3 mRNA is induced by an adenocarcinoma-derived lipid-mobilizing factor. Br J Cancer 2002;86:612–8.
117. Busquets S, Sanchis D, Alvarez B, et al. In the rat, tumor necrosis factor alpha administration results in an increase in both UCP2 and UCP3 mRNAs in skeletal muscle: a possible mechanism for cytokine-induced thermogenesis? FEBS Lett 1998;440:348–50.
118. Bing C, Bao Y, Jenkins J, et al. Zinc-alpha2-glycoprotein, a lipid mobilizing factor, is expressed in adipocytes and is up-regulated in mice with cancer cachexia. Proc Natl Acad Sci U S A 2004;101:2500–5.
119. Groundwater P, Beck SA, Barton C, et al. Alterations of serum and urinary lipolytic activity with weight loss in cachectic cancer patients. Br J Cancer 1990;62:816–21.
120. Beck SA, Groundwater P, Barton C, Tisdale MJ. Alteration in serum lipolytic activity in cancer patients with response to therapy. Br J Cancer 1990;62:822–5.
121. Belizario JE, Katz M, Chenker E, Raw I. Bioactivity of skeletal muscle proteolysis-inducing factors in the plasma proteins from cancer patients with weight loss. Br J Cancer l991;63:705–10.
122. Todorov PT, McDevitt TM, Cariuk P, et al. Induction of muscle protein degradation and weight loss by a tumor product. Cancer Res 1996;56:1256–61.
123. Cariuk P, Lorite MJ, Todorov PT, et al. Induction of cachexia in mice by a product isolated from the urine of cachectic cancer patients. Br J Cancer 1997;76:606–13.
124. Lorite MJ, Thompson MG, Drake JL, et al. Mechanism of muscle protein degradation induced by a cancer cachectic factor. Br J Cancer 1998;78:850–6.
125. Bossola M, Muscaritoli M, Costelli P, et al. Increased muscle proteasome activity correlates with disease severity in gastric cancer patients. Ann Surg 2003;237:384–9.
126. Wigmore SJ, Todorov PT, Barber MD, et al. Characteristics of patients with pancreatic cancer expressing a novel cancer cachectic factor. Br J Surg 2000;87:53–8.
127. Jagoe RT, Redfern CP, Roberts RG, et al. Skeletal muscle mRNA levels for cathepsin B, but not components of the ubiquitin-proteasome pathway, are increased in patients with lung cancer referred for thoracotomy. Clin Sci (Lond) 2002;102:353–61.
128. Mordes JP, Longcope C, Flatt JP, et al. The rat LTW (m) Leydig cell tumor: cancer cachexia due to estrogen. Endocrinology 1984;115:167–73.
129. Greenway B, Iqbal MJ, Johnson PJ, Williams R. Low serum testosterone concentrations in patients with carcinoma of the pancreas. Br Med J (Clin Res Ed) 1983;286:93–5.
130. Heber D, Tchekmedyian NS. Pathophysiology of cancer: hormonal and metabolic abnormalities. Oncology 1992;49 Suppl 2:28–31.
131. Schaur RJ, Fellier H, Gleispach, et al. Tumor host relations. I. Increased plasma cortisol in tumor-bearing humans compared with patients with benign surgical diseases. J Cancer Res Clin Oncol 1997;93:281–5.
132. Knapp ML, al-Sheibani S, Riches PG, et al. Hormonal factors associated with weight loss in patients with advanced breast cancer. Ann Clin Biochem 1991;28:480–6.

133. Tessitore L, Costelli P, Baccino FM. Humoral mediation for cachexia in tumour-bearing rats. Br J Cancer 1993;67:15–23.
134. Bennett A, Berstock DA, Carroll MA. Increased survival of cancer- bearing mice with inhibitors of prostaglandin synthesis, alone or with chemotherapy. Br J Cancer 1982;45:762–8.
135. Noriki S, Imamura Y, Ikeda T, et al. Multi-organ damage (MOD) induced by cancer cachexia and its pathogenesis. Basic Appl Histochem 1989;33:337–46.
136. Wang W, Andersson M, Lõnnroth C, et al. Prostaglandin E and prostacyclin receptor expression in tumor and host tissues from MCG 101-bearing mice: a model with prostanoid-related cachexia. Int J Cancer 2005;115,582–90.
137. Radcliffe JD, Morrison SD. Histidine deficiency, food intake and growth in normal and Walker 256 carcinoma-bearing rats. Nutr Cancer 1981;3:40–5.
138. Torosian MH, Nguyen HQ. Tumors—effective nitrogen traps independent of protein intake. J Surg Res 1989;47:456–9.
139. Ulander K, Jeppsson B, Grahn G. Postoperative energy intake in patients after colorectal cancer surgery. Scand J Caring Sci 1998;12:131–8.
140. Ohnuma T, Holland JF. Nutritional consequences of cancer chemotherapy and immunotherapy. Cancer Res 1977;37:2395–406.
141. Ohnuma T, Holland JF, Freeman A, Sinks LF. Biological and pharmacological studies with asparaginase in man. Cancer Res 1970;30:2297–305.
142. Atkins MB, Robertson MJ, Gordon M, et al. Phase I evaluation of intravenous recombinant human interleukin 12 in patients with advanced malignancies. Clin Cancer Res 1997;3:409–17.
143. Hyltander A, Drott C, Körner U, et al. Elevated energy expenditure in cancer patients with solid tumours. Eur J Cancer 1991;27:9–15.
144. Lindmark L, Bennegard K, Eden E, et al. Resting energy expenditure in malnourished patients with and without cancer. Gastroenterology 1984;87:402–8.
145. Knox LS, Crosby LO, Feurer ID, et al. Energy expenditure in malnourished cancer patients. Ann Surg 1983;197:152–62.
146. Luketich JD, Mullen JL, Feurer ID, et al. Ablation of abnormal energy expenditure by curative tumor resection. Arch Surg 1990;125:337–41.
147. Fredix EW, Soeters PB, Wouters EF, et al. Effect of different tumor types on resting energy expenditure. Cancer Res 1991;51:6138–41.
148. Falconer JS, Fearon KC, Plester CE, et al. Cytokines, the acute phase response, and resting energy expenditure in cachectic patients with pancreatic cancer. Ann Surg 1994;219:325–31.
149. Shaw JH, Wolfe RR. Fatty acid and glycerol kinetics in septic patients and in patients with gastrointestinal cancer. The response to glucose infusion and parenteral feeding. Ann Surg 1987;205:368–76.
150. Shaw JH, Wolfe RR. Glucose and urea kinetics in patients with early and advanced gastrointestinal cancer: the response to glucose infusion, parenteral feeding, and surgical resection. Surgery 1987;101:181–91.
151. Shaw JH, Humberstone DA, Holdaway C. Weight loss in patients with head and neck cancer: malnutrition or tumour effect? Aust N Z J Surg 1988;58:505–9.
152. Shaw JH, Humberstone DM, Wolfe RR. Energy and protein metabolism in sarcoma patients. Ann Surg 1988;207:283–9.
153. Holroyde CP, Skutches CL, Boden G, et al. Glucose metabolism in cachectic patients with colorectal cancer. Cancer Res 1984;44:5910–3.
154. Moldawer LL, Rogy MA, Lowry SF. The role of cytokines in cancer cachexia. J Parenter Enteral Nutr l992;16:43S–9S.
155. Holm E, Hagmuller E, Staedt U, et al. Substrate balance across colonic carcinoma in humans. Cancer Res 1995;55:1373–8.
156. Koea JB, Shaw JF. The effect of tumor bulk on the metabolic response to cancer. Ann Surg 1992;215:282–8.
157. Rofe AM, Bourgeois CS, Coyle P, et al. Altered insulin response to glucose in weight-losing cancer patients. Anticancer Res 1994;14:647–50.
158. Hartl WH, Demmelmair H, Jauch KW, et al. Effect of glucagon on protein synthesis in human rectal cancer in situ. Ann Surg 1998;227:390–7.
159. Bartlett DL, Charland SL, Torosian MH. Reversal of tumor-associated hyperglucagonemia as treatment for cancer cachexia. Surgery 1995;118:87–97.
160. Marks LJ, Steinke J, Podolsky S, Egdahl RH. Hypoglycemia associated with neoplasia. Ann N Y Acad Sci 1974;230:147–60.
161. Pourmotabbed G, Kitabchi AE. Hypoglycemia. Obstet Gynecol Clin North Am 2001;28:383–400.
162. Rose MG, Tallini G, Pollak J, Murren J. Malignant hypoglycemia associated with a large mesenchymal tumor: case report and review of the literature. Cancer J Sci Am 1999;5:48–51.
163. Silverstein MN, Wakim KG, Bahn RC, Decker RH. Role of tryptophan metabolites in the hypoglycemia associated with neoplasia. Cancer 1966;19:127–33.
164. Zapf J, Futo E, Peter M, Froesch ER. Can 'big' insulin-like growth factor II in serum of tumor patients account for the development of extrapancreatic tumor hypoglycemia? J Clin Invest 1992;90:2574–84.
165. Costa G, Lyles K, Ullrich L. Effects of human and experimental cancer on the conversion of 14C tripalmitin to 14C02. Cancer 1976;38:1259–65.
166. Emery PW, Carpenter TT, Obeid OA. Alterations in post-prandial glycogen and lipid synthesis in cachectic tumor-bearing rats. Nutr Cancer 1993;20:231–40.
167. Ogilvie GK, Ford RB, Vail DM, et al. Alterations in lipoprotein profiles in dogs with lymphoma. J Vet Intern Med 1994;8:62–6.
168. Klein S, Wolfe RR. Whole-body lipolysis and triglyceride-fatty acid cycling in cachectic patients with esophageal cancer. J Clin Invest 1990;86:1403–8.
169. Kern KA, Norton JA. Cancer cachexia. JPEN J Parenter Enteral Nutr 1988;12:286–98.
170. Dessi S, Batetta B, Pulisci D, et al. Total and HDL cholesterol in human hematologic neoplasms. Int J Hematol 1991;54:483–6.
171. Nomura K, Noguchi Y, Yoshikawa T, Kondo J. Plasma interleukin-6 is not a mediator of changes in lipoprotein lipase activity in cancer patients. Hepatogastroenterology 1997;44:1519–26.
172. Carbo N, Costelli P, Tessitore L, et al. Anti-tumour necrosis factor-alpha treatment interferes with changes in lipid metabolism in a tumour cachexia model. Clin Sci (Lond) 1994;87:349–55.
173. Grunfeld C, Adi S, Soued M, et al. Search for mediators of the lipogenic effects of tumor necrosis factor: potential role for interleukin 6. Cancer Res 1990;50:4233–8.
174. Vlassara H, Spiegel RJ, San Doval D, Cerami A. Reduced plasma lipoprotein lipase activity in patients with malignancy-associated weight loss. Horm Metab Res 1986;18:698–703.
175. Barber MD, McMillan DC, Preston T, et al. Metabolic response to feeding in weight-losing pancreatic cancer patients and its modulation by a fish-oil-enriched nutritional supplement. Clin Sci (Lond) 2000;98:389–99.
176. Russell ST, Tisdale MJ. Effect of a tumour-derived lipid-mobilising factor on glucose and lipid metabolism in vivo. Br J Cancer 2002;87:580–4.
177. Yam D, Ben-Hur H, Fink A, et al. Insulin and glucose status, tissue and plasma lipids in patients with tumours of the ovary or endometrium: possible dietary implications. Br J Cancer 1994;70:1186–7.
178. Hussey HJ, Tisdale, MJ. Effects of polyunsaturated fatty acids on the growth of murine colon adenocarcinomas in vitro and in vivo. Br J Cancer 1994;70:6–10.
179. Shellock FG, Riedinger MS, Fishbein MC. Brown adipose tissue in cancer patients: possible cause of cancer-induced cachexia. J Cancer Res Clin Oncol 1986;111:82–5.
180. Nixon DW, Heymsfield SB, Cohen AE, et al. Protein calorie undernutrition in hospitalized cancer patients. Am J Med 1980;68:683–90.
181. Fearon KC, Hansell DT, Preston T, et al. Influence of whole body protein turnover rate on resting energy expenditure in patients with cancer. Cancer Res 1988;48:2590–5.
182. Dworzak F, Ferrari P, Gavazzi C, et al. Effects of cachexia due to cancer on whole body and skeletal muscle protein turnover. Cancer 1998;82:42–8.
183. Baracos VE. Regulation of skeletal-muscle-protein turnover in cancer-associated cachexia. Nutrition 2000;16:1015–8.
184. Argiles JM, Moore-Carrasco R, Fuster G, et al. Cancer cachexia: the molecular mechanisms. Int J Biochem Cell Biol 2003;35:405–9.
185. Lecker SH, Solomon V, Mitch WE, Goldberg AL. Muscle protein breakdown and the critical role of the ubiquitin-proteasome pathway in normal and disease states. J Nutr 1999;129(1S Suppl):227S–37S.
186. Williams A, Sun X, Fischer JE, Hasselgren PO. The expression of genes in the ubiquitin-proteasome proteolytic pathway is increased in skeletal muscle from patients with cancer. Surgery 1999;126:744–9.
187. Lazarus DD, Destree AT, Mazzola LM, et al. A new model of cancer cachexia: contribution of the ubiquitin-proteasome pathway. Am J Physiol 1999;277(2 Pt 1):E332–41.
188. Tisdale MJ. Biochemical mechanisms of cellular catabolism. Curr Opin Clin Nutr Metab Care 2002;5:401–5.
189. Costelli P, Garcia-Martinez C, Llovera M, et al. Muscle protein waste in tumor-bearing rats is effectively antagonized by a beta 2-adrenergic agonist (clenbuterol). Role of the ATP-ubiquitin-dependent proteolytic pathway. J Clin Invest 1995;95:2367–72.
190. Kwak KS, Zhou X, Solomon V, et al. Regulation of protein catabolism by muscle-specific and cytokine-inducible ubiquitin ligase E3alpha-II during cancer cachexia. Cancer Res 2004;64:8193–8.
191. Hasselgren PO, Fischer JE. Muscle cachexia: current concepts of intracellular mechanisms and molecular regulation. Ann Surg 2001;233:9–17.
192. Ushmorov A, Hack V, Droge W. Differential reconstitution of mitochondrial respiratory chain activity and plasma redox state by cysteine and ornithine in a model of cancer cachexia. Cancer Res 1999;59:3527–34.
193. Carbo N, Busquets S, van Royen M, et al. TNF-alpha is involved in activating DNA fragmentation in skeletal muscle. Br J Cancer 2002;86:1012–6.
194. Reeds PJ, Fjeld CR, Jahoor F. Do the differences between the amino acid compositions of acute-phase and muscle proteins have a bearing on nitrogen loss in traumatic states? J Nutr 1994;124:906–10.
195. Barber MD, Fearon KC, McMillan DC, et al. Liver export protein synthetic rates are increased by oral meal feeding in weight-losing cancer patients. Am J Physiol Endocrinol Metab 2000;279:E707–14.
196. Fouladiun M, Korner U, Bosaeus I, et al. Body composition and time course changes in regional distribution of fat and lean tissue in unselected cancer patients on palliative care—correlations with food intake, metabolism, exercise capacity, and hormones. Cancer 2005;103:2189–98.
197. Rubin H. Cancer cachexia: its correlations and causes. Proc Natl Acad Sci U S A 2003;100:5384–9.
198. Byerley LO, Heber D, Bergman RN, et al. Insulin action and metabolism in patients with head and neck cancer. Cancer l991;67:2900–6.
199. Drott C, Svaninger G, Lundholm K. Increased urinary excretion of cortisol and catecholamines in malnourished cancer patients. Ann Surg 1988;208:645–50.
200. Ottery FD. Definition of standardized nutritional assessment and interventional pathways in oncology. Nutrition 1996;12(1 Suppl):S15–9.
201. Guigoz Y, Vellas B, Garry PJ. Assessing the nutritional status of the elderly: the Mini Nutritional Assessment as part of the geriatric evaluation. Nutr Rev 1996;54(1 Pt 2):S59–65.
202. Ferguson M, Capra S, Bauer J, Banks M. Development of a valid and reliable malnutrition screening tool for adult acute hospital patients. Nutrition 1999;15:458–64.
203. Bauer J, Capra S. Comparison of a malnutrition screening tool with subjective global assessment in hospitalised patients with cancer—sensitivity and specificity. Asia Pac J Clin Nutr 2003;12:257–6.
204. Huhmann MB, Cunningham RS. Importance of nutritional screening in treatment of cancer-related weight loss. Lancet Oncol 2005;6:334–43.
205. Ovesen L, Allingstrup L, Hannibal J, et al. Effect of dietary counseling on food intake, body weight, response rate, survival and quality of life in cancer patients undergoing chemotherapy: a prospective randomized study. J Clin Oncol 1993;11:2043–9.
206. Bauer JD, Capra S. Nutrition intervention improves outcomes in patients with cancer cachexia receiving chemotherapy—a pilot study. Support Care Cancer 2005;13:270–4.
207. Ravasco P, Monteiro-Grillo I, Vidal PM, Camilo ME. Dietary counseling improves patient outcomes: a prospective, randomized, controlled trial in colorectal cancer patients undergoing radiotherapy. J Clin Oncol 2005;23:1431–8.
208. Isenring EA, Capra S, and Bauer JD. Nutrition intervention is beneficial in oncology outpatients receiving radiotherapy to the gastrointestinal or head and neck area, Br J Cancer 2004;91:447–52.
209. Fries E, Edinboro P, McClish D, et al. Randomized trial of a low-intensity dietary intervention in rural residents: the Rural Physician Cancer Prevention Project. Am J Prev Med 2005;28:162–8.
210. Bruera E, Roca E, Cedaro L, et al. Action of oral methylprednisolone in terminal cancer patients: a prospective randomized double-blind study. Cancer Treat Rep l985;69:751–4.
211. Popiela T, Lucchi R, Giongo F. Methylprednisolone as palliative therapy for female terminal cancer patients. The Methylprednisolone Female Preterminal Cancer Study Group. Eur J Cancer Clin Oncol l989;25:1823–9.
212. Della Cuna GR, Pellegrini A, Piazzi M. Effect of methylprednisolone sodium succinate on quality of life in preterminal cancer patients: a placebo-controlled multicenter study. Eur J Cancer Clin Oncol 1989;25:1817–21.

213. Loprinzi CL, Kugler JW, Sloan JA, et al. Randomized comparison of megestrol acetate versus dexamethasone versus fluoxymesterone for the treatment of cancer anorexia/cachexia. J Clin Oncol 1999;17:3299–306.
214. Llovera M, Garcia-Martinez C, Costelli P, et al. Muscle hypercatabolism during cancer cachexia is not reversed by the glucocorticoid receptor antagonist RU38486. Cancer Lett 1996;99:7–14.
215. Rivadeneira DE, Naama HA, McCarter MD, et al. Glucocorticoid blockade does not abrogate tumor-induced cachexia. Nutr Cancer 1999;35:202–6.
216. Mantovani G, Maccio A, Bianchi A, et al. Megestrol acetate in neoplastic anorexia/cachexia: clinical evaluation and comparison with cytokine levels in patients with head and neck carcinoma treated with neoadjuvant chemotherapy. Int J Clin Lab Res 1995;25:135–41.
217. McCarthy HD, Crowder RE, Dryden S, Williams G. Megestrol acetate stimulates food and water intake in the rat: effects on regional hypothalamic neuropeptide Y concentrations. Eur J Pharmacol 1994;265:99–102.
218. Pascual Lopez A, Roque i Figuls M, Urrutia Cuchi G, et al. Systematic review of megestrol acetate in the treatment of anorexia-cachexia syndrome. J Pain Symptom Manage 2004;27:360–9.
219. Maltoni M, Nanni O, Scarpi E, et al. High-dose progestins for the treatment of cancer anorexia-cachexia syndrome: a systematic review of randomized clinical trials. Ann Oncol 2001;12:289–300.
220. Loprinzi CL, Schaid DJ, Dose AM, et al. Body-composition changes in patients who gain weight while receiving megestrol acetate. J Clin Oncol 1993;11:152–4.
221. McMillan DC, Simpson JM, Preston T, et al. Effect of megestrol acetate on weight loss, body composition and blood serum of gastrointestinal cancer patients. Clin Nutr 1994;13:85–9.
222. Nathanson L, Meelu MA, Losada R. Chemohormone therapy of metastatic melanoma with megestrol acetate plus dacarbazine, carmustine, and cisplatin. Cancer 1994;73:98–102.
223. Orme LM, Bond JD, Humphrey MS, et al. Megestrol acetate in pediatric oncology patients may lead to severe, symptomatic adrenal suppression. Cancer 2003;98:397–405.
224. Mantovani G, Maccio A, Esu S, et al. Medroxyprogesterone acetate reduces the in vitro production of cytokines and serotonin involved in anorexia/cachexia and emesis by peripheral blood mononuclear cells of cancer patients. Eur J Cancer 1997;33:602–7.
225. Downer S, Joel S, Allbright A, et al. A double blind placebo controlled trial of medroxyprogesterone acetate (MPA) in cancer cachexia. Br J Cancer 1993;67:1102–5.
226. Simons JP, Aaronson NK, Vanateenkiste JF, et al. Effects of medroxyprogesterone acetate on appetite, weight and quality of life in advanced-stage non-hormone-sensitive cancer: a placebo-controlled multicenter study. J Clin Oncol 1996;14:1077–84.
227. Lyden E, Cvetkovska E, Westin T, et al. Effects of nandrolone propionate on experimental tumor growth and cancer cachexia. Metabolism 1995;44:445–51.
228. Spiers AS, DeVita SF, Allar MJ, et al. Beneficial effects of an anabolic steroid during cytotoxic chemotherapy for metastatic cancer. J Med 1981;12:433–45.
229. Chlebowski RT, Herrold J, Ali I, et al. Influence of nandrolone decanoate in weight loss in advanced non-small cell lung cancer. Cancer 1986;58:183–6.
230. Plasse TP, Gorter RW, Krasnow SH, et al. Recent clinical experience with dronabinol. Pharmacol Bioch Behav 1991;40:695–700.
231. Nelson K, Walsh D, Deeter P, Sheehan F. A phase II study of delta-9-tetrahydrocannabinol for appetite stimulation in cancer-associated anorexia. J Palliat Care 1994;10:14–8.
232. Jatoi A, Windschitl HE, Loprinzi CL, et al. Dronabinol versus megestrol acetate versus combination therapy for cancer-associated anorexia: a North Central Cancer Treatment Group study. J Clin Oncol 2002;20:567–73.
233. Wolf RF, Ng B, Weksler B, et al. Effect of growth hormone on tumor and host in an animal model. Ann Surg Oncol 1994;1:314–20.
234. Fiebig HH, Dengler W, Hendriks HR. No evidence of tumor growth stimulation in human tumors in vitro following treatment with recombinant human growth hormone. Anticancer Drugs 2000;11:659–64.
235. Bartlett DL, Charland S, Torosian MH. Growth hormone, insulin, and somatostatin therapy of cancer cachexia. Cancer 1994;73:1499–504.
236. Wolf RF, Pearlstone DB, Newman E, et al. Growth hormone and insulin reverse net whole body and skeletal muscle protein catabolism in cancer patients. Ann Surg 1992;216:280–8.
237. Tschop M, Statnick MA, Suter TM, Heiman ML. GH-releasing peptide-2 increases fat mass in mice lacking NPY: indication for a crucial mediating role of hypothalamic agouti-related protein. Endocrinology 2002;143:558–68.
238. Laferrere B, Abraham C, Russell CD, Bowers CY. Growth hormone releasing peptide-2 (GHRP-2), like ghrelin, increases food intake in healthy men. J Clin Endocrinol Metab 2005;90:611–4.
239. Froesch ER, Schmid C, Schwander J, Zapf J. Actions of insulin-like growth factors. Annu Rev Physiol 1985;47:443–67.
240. Florini JR. Hormonal control of muscle growth. Muscle Nerve 1987;10:577–98.
241. Ng EH, Rock CS, Lazarus DD, et al. Insulin-like growth factor I preserves host lean tissue mass in cancer cachexia. Am J Physiol 1992;262(3 Pt 2):R426–31.
242. Lieberman SA, Butterfield GE, Harrison D, Hoffman AR. Anabolic effects of recombinant insulin-like growth factor-I in cachectic patients with the acquired immunodeficiency syndrome. J Clin Endocrinol Metab 1994;78:404–10.
243. Lee PD, Pivarnik JM, Bukar JG, et al. A randomized, placebo-controlled trial of combined insulin-like growth factor I and low dose growth hormone therapy for wasting associated with human immunodeficiency virus infection. J Clin Endocrinol Metab 1996;81:2968–75.
244. Nelson KA, Walsh TD. Metoclopramide in anorexia caused by cancer-associated dyspepsia syndrome (CADS). J Palliat Care 1993;9:14–8.
245. Shivshanker K, Bennett RW Jr, Haynie TP. Tumor-associated gastroparesis: correction with metoclopramide. Am J Surg 1983;145:221–5.
246. Bruera ED, MacEachern J, Spachynski KA, et al. Comparison of the efficacy, safety, and pharmacokinetics of controlled release and immediate release metoclopramide for the management of chronic nausea in patients with advanced cancer. Cancer 1994;74:3204–11.
247. Chen HC, Leung SW, Wang CJ, et al. Effect of megestrol acetate and propulside on nutritional improvement in patients with head and neck cancers undergoing radiotherapy. Radother Oncol 1997;43:75–9.
248. Ray PD, Hanson RL, Lardy HA. Inhibition by hydrazine of glyconeogenesis in the rat. J Biol Chem 1970;245:690–6.
249. Kosty MP, Fleischman SB, Herndon JE 2nd, et al. Cisplatin, vinblastine and hydrazine sulfate in advanced, non-small-cell lung cancer: a randomized placebo-controlled, double-blind phase III study of the Cancer and Leukemia Group B. J Clin Oncol 1994;12:1113–20.
250. Loprinzi CL, Goldberg RM, Su JQ, et al. Placebo-controlled trial of hydrazine sulfate in patients with newly diagnosed non-small-cell lung cancer. J Clin Oncol 1994;12:1126–9.
251. Loprinzi CL, Kuross SA, O'Fallon JR, et al. Randomized placebo-controlled evaluation of hydrazine sulfate in patients with advanced colorectal cancer. J Clin Oncol 1994;12:1121–5.
252. Kikawa Y, Narumiya S, Fukushima M, et al. 9-Deoxy-delta 9, delta 12-13,14-dihydroprostaglandin D2, a metabolite of prostaglandin D2 formed in human plasma. Proc Natl Acad Sci U S A 1984;81:1317–21.
253. Fischer SM, Furstenberger G, Marks F, Slaga TJ. Events associated with mouse skin tumor promotion with respect to arachidonic acid metabolism: a comparison between SENCAR and NMRI mice. Cancer Res 1987;47:3174–9.
254. Bennett A, Houghton J, Leaper DJ, Stamford IF. Cancer growth, response to treatment and survival time in mice: beneficial effect of the prostaglandin synthesis inhibitor flurbiprofen. Prostaglandins 1979;17:179–91.
255. Homem-de-Bittencourt Junior PI, Pontieri V, Curi R, Lopes OU. Effects of aspirin-like drugs on Walker 256 tumor growth and cachexia in rats. Braz J Med Biol Res 1989;22:1039–42.
256. McCarthy DO, Daun JM. The effects of cyclooxygenase inhibitors on tumor-induced anorexia in rats. Cancer 1993;71:486–92.
257. Davis TW, Zweifel BS, O'Neal JM, et al. Inhibition of cyclooxygenase-2 by celecoxib reverses tumor-induced wasting. J Pharmacol Exp Ther 2004;308:929–34.
258. Bredt AB, Girey GJ. Antipyretic effects of indomethacin in liver metastasis of solid tumors. Cancer 1982;50:1430–3.
259. Romeu J, Chadha N, Fukilman O, et al. Indomethacin therapy in symptomatic hepatic neoplasms. Am J Gastroent 1982;77:655–9.
260. Preston T, Fearon KC, McMillan DC, et al. Effect of ibuprofen on the acute phase response and protein metabolism in patients with cancer and weight loss. Br J Surg 1995;82:229–34.
261. Wigmore SJ, Falconer JS, Plester CE, et al. Ibuprofen reduces energy expenditure and acute-phase protein production compared with placebo in pancreatic cancer patients. Br J Cancer 1995;72:185–8.
262. Lundholm K, Gelin J, Hyltander A, et al. Anti-inflammatory treatment may prolong survival in undernourished patients with metastatic solid tumors. Cancer Res 1994;54:5602–6.
263. McMillan DC, Wigmore SJ, Fearon KC, et al. A prospective randomized study of megestrol acetate and ibuprofen in gastrointestinal cancer patients with weight loss. Br J Cancer 1999;79:495–500.
264. Daneryd P. Epoetin alfa for protection of metabolic and exercise capacity in cancer patients. Semin Oncol 2002;29(3 Suppl 8):69–74.
265. Daneryd P, Svanberg E, Korner U, et al. Protection of metabolic and exercise capacity in unselected weight-losing cancer patients following treatment with recombinant erythropoietin: a randomized prospective study. Cancer Res 1998;58:5374–9.
266. Han J, Thompson P, Beutler B. Dexamethasone and pentoxifylline inhibit endotoxin-induced cachectin/tumor necrosis factor synthesis at separate points in the signaling pathway. J Exp Med 1990;172:391–4.
267. Combaret L, Ralliere C, Taillandier D, et al. Manipulation of the ubiquitin-proteasome pathway in cachexia: pentoxifylline suppresses the activation of 20S and 26S proteasomes in muscles from tumor-bearing rats. Mol Biol Rep 1999;26:95–101.
268. Bianco JA, Appelbaum FR, Nemunaitis J, et al. Phase I-II trial of pentoxifylline for prevention of transplant-related toxicities following bone marrow transplantation. Blood 1991;78:1205–11.
269. Goldberg RM, Loprinzi CL, Mailliard JA, et al. Pentoxifylline for treatment of cancer anorexia and cachexia? A randomized, double-blind, placebo-controlled trial. J Clin Oncol 1995;13:2856–9.
270. Estey EH, Thall PF, Reed P, et al. Treatment of newly diagnosed AML, RAEB-t or RAEB with lisofylline or placebo in addition to chemotherapy. Leukemia 1999;13:850–4.
271. Margolin K, Atkins M, Sparano J, et al. Prospective randomized trial of lisofylline for the prevention of toxicities of high-dose interleukin 2 therapy in advanced renal cancer and malignant melanoma. Clin Cancer Res 1997;3:565–72.
272. Busquets S, Carbo N, Almendro V, et al. Curcumin, a natural product present in turmeric, decreases tumor growth but does not behave as an anticachectic compound in a rat model. Cancer Lett 2001;167:33–8.
273. Wyke SM, Russell ST, Tisdale MJ. Induction of proteasome expression in skeletal muscle is attenuated by inhibitors of NF-kappaB activation. Br J Cancer 2004;91:1742–50.
274. Carbo N, Lopez-Soriano J, Tarrago T, et al. Comparative effects of beta 2-adrenergic agonists on muscle waste associated with tumour growth. Cancer Lett 1997;115:113–8.
275. Chance WT, Cao LQ, Zhang FS, et al. Clenbuterol treatment increases muscle mass and protein content of tumor-bearing rats maintained on total parenteral nutrition. J Parenter Enteral Nutr 1991;15:530–5.
276. Costelli P, Garcia-Martinez C, Llovera M, et al. Muscle protein waste in tumor-bearing rats is effectively antagonized by a β2-adrenergic agonist (clenbuterol). Role of the ATP-ubiquitin-dependent proteolytic pathway. J Clin Invest 1995;95:2367–72.
277. Piffar PM, Fernandez R, Tchaikovski O, et al. Naproxen, clenbuterol and insulin administration ameliorates cancer cachexia and reduce tumor growth in Walker 256 tumor-bearing rats. Cancer Lett 2003;201:139–48.
278. Pinto JA Jr, Folador A, Bonato SJ, et al. Fish oil supplementation in F1 generation associated with naproxen, clenbuterol, and insulin administration reduce tumor growth and cachexia in Walker 256 tumor-bearing rats. J Nutr Biochem 2004;15:358–65.
279. Maltin CA, Delday MI, Watson JS, et al. Clenbuterol, a beta-adrenoceptor agonist, increases relative muscle strength in orthopaedic patients. Clin Sci 1993;84:651–4.
280. Kaplan G. Cytokine regulation of disease progression in leprosy and tuberculosis. Immunobiol 1994;191:564–8.
281. Tramontana JM, Utaipat U, Molloy A, et al. Thalidomide treatment reduces tumor necrosis factor alpha production and enhances weight gain in patients with pulmonary tuberculosis. Mol Med 1995;1:384–97.
282. Bruera E, Neumann CM, Pituskin E, et al. Thalidomide in patients with cachexia due to terminal cancer: preliminary report. Ann Oncol 1999;10:857–9.
283. Khan ZH, Simpson EJ, Cole AT, et al. Oesophageal cancer and cachexia: the effect of short-term treatment with thalidomide on weight loss and lean body mass. Aliment Pharmacol Ther 2003;17:677–82.

284. Gordon JN, Trebble TM, Ellis RD, et al. Thalidomide in the treatment of cancer cachexia: a randomised placebo controlled trial. Gut 2005;54:540–5.
285. Agteresch HJ, Dagnelie PC, van der Gaast A, et al. Randomized clinical trial of adenosine 5′-triphosphate in patients with advanced non-small-cell lung cancer. J Natl Cancer Inst 2000;92:321–8.
286. Agteresch HJ, Rietveld T, Kerkhofs LG, et al. Beneficial effects of adenosine triphosphate on nutritional status in advanced lung cancer patients: a randomized clinical trial. J Clin Oncol 2002;20:371–8.
287. Martin DS, Bertino JR, Koutcher JA. ATP depletion + pyrimidine depletion can markedly enhance cancer therapy: fresh insight for a new approach. Cancer Res 2000;60:6776–83.
288. Martin DS, Spriggs D, Koutcher JA. A concomitant ATP-depleting strategy markedly enhances anticancer agent activity. Apoptosis 2001;6:125–31.
289. Geschwind JF, Ko YH, Torbenson MS, et al. Novel therapy for liver cancer: direct intraarterial injection of a potent inhibitor of ATP production. Cancer Res 2002;62:3909–13.
290. Eda H, Tanaka Y, Ishitsuka H. 5'-Deoxy-5-fluorouridine improves cachexia by a mechanism independent of its antiproliferative action in colon 26 adenocarcinoma-bearing mice. Cancer Chemother Pharmacol 1991;29:1–6.
291. Hussey HJ, Todorov PT, Field WN, et al. Effect of a fluorinated pyrimidine on cachexia and tumour growth in murine cachexia models: relationship with a proteolysis inducing factor. Br J Cancer 2000;83:56–62.
292. Sherry BA, Gelin J, Fong Y, et al. Anticachectin/tumor necrosis factor-α antibodies attenuate development of cachexia in tumor models. FASEB J 1989;3:1956–62.
293. Costelli P, Carbo N, Tessitore L, et al. Tumor necrosis factor-alpha mediates changes in tissue protein turnover in a rat cancer cachexia model. J Clin Invest 1993;92:2783–9.
294. Llovera M, Carbo N, Garcia-Martinez C, et al. Anti-TNF treatment reverts increased muscle ubiquitin gene expression in tumour-bearing rats. Biochem Biophys Res Commun 1996;221:653–5.
295. Reinhart K, Wiegand-Lohnert C, Grimminger F, et al. Assessment of the safety and efficacy of the monoclonal anti-tumor necrosis factor antibody-fragment, MAK 195F, in patients with sepsis and septic shock: a multicenter, randomized, placebo-controlled, dose-ranging study. Crit Care Med 1996;24:733–42.
296. Anker SD, Coats AJ. How to recover from renaissance? The significance of the results of recover, renaissance, renewal and attach. Int J Cardiol 2002;86:123–30.
297. Strassmann G, Fong M, Freter CE, et al. Suramin interferes with interleukin-6 receptor binding in vitro and inhibits colon-26-mediated experimental cancer cachexia in vivo. J Clin Invest 1993;92:2152–9.
298. Bielefeldt-Ohmann H, Marzo AL, Himbeck RP, et al. Interleukin-6 involvement in mesothelioma pathobiology: inhibition by interferon alpha immunotherapy. Cancer Immunol Immunother 1995;40:241–50.
299. Emilie D, Wijdenes J, Gisselbrecht C, et al. Administration of an anti-interleukin-6 monoclonal antibody to patients with acquired immunodeficiency syndrome and lymphoma: effect on lymphoma growth and on B clinical symptoms. Blood 1994;84:2472–9.
300. Shibata M, Nezu T, Kanou H, et al. Decreased production of interleukin-12 and type 2 immune responses are marked in cachectic patients with colorectal and gastric cancer. J Clin Gastroenterol 2002;34:416–20.
301. Mori K, Fujimoto-Ouchi K, Ishikawa T, et al. Murine interleukin-12 prevents the development of cancer cachexia in a murine model. Int J Cancer 1996;67:849–55.
302. Fujiki F, Mukaida N, Hirose K, et al. Prevention of adenocarcinoma colon 26-induced cachexia by interleukin 10 gene transfer. Cancer Res 1997;57:94–9.
303. Carbo N, Lopez-Soriano J, Costelli P, et al. Interleukin-15 antagonizes muscle protein waste in tumour-bearing rats. Br J Cancer 2000;83:526–31.
304. Figueras M, Busquets S, Carbo N, et al. Interleukin-15 is able to suppress the increased DNA fragmentation associated with muscle wasting in tumour-bearing rats. FEBS Lett 2004;569:201–6.
305. Tisdale MJ, Dhesi JK. Inhibition of weight loss by omega-3 fatty acids in an experimental cachexia model. Cancer Res 1990;50:5022–6.
306. Dagnelie PC, Bell JD, Williams SC, et al. Effect of fish oil on cancer cachexia and host liver metabolism in rats with prostate tumors. Lipids 1994;29:195–203.
307. Wigmore SJ, Fearon KC, Maingay JP, Ross JA. Down-regulation of the acute-phase response in patients with pancreas cancer cachexia receiving oral eicosapentaenoic acid is mediated via suppression of interleukin-6. Clin Sci (Colch) 1997;92:215–21.
308. Whitehouse AS, Smith HJ, Drake JL, Tisdale MJ. Mechanism of attenuation of skeletal muscle protein catabolism in cancer cachexia by eicosapentaenoic acid. Cancer Res 2001;61:3604–9.
309. Belda-Iniesta C, de Castro Carpeno J, Fresno Vara JA, et al. Eicosapentaenoic acid as a targeted therapy for cancer cachexia. J Clin Oncol 2003;21:4657–8.
310. Tisdale MJ, Beck SA. Inhibition of tumor-induced lipolysis in vitro and cachexia and tumour growth in vivo by eicosapentaenoic acid. Biochem Pharmacol 1991;41:103–7.
311. Hussey HJ, Tisdale MJ. Effect of a cachectic factor on carbohydrate metabolism and attenuation by eicosapentaenoic acid. Br J Cancer 1999;80:1231–5.
312. Smith HJ, Lorite MJ. Tisdale MJ. Effect of a cancer cachectic factor on protein synthesis/degradation in murine C2C12 myoblasts. Modulation by eicosapentaenoic acid. Cancer Res 1999;59:5507–13.
313. Wigmore SJ, Ross JA, Flaconer JS, et al. The effect of polyunsaturated fatty acids on the progress of cachexia in patients with pancreatic cancer. Nutrition 1996;12:527–30.
314. Barber MD, Ross JA, Voss AC, et al. The effect of an oral nutritional supplement enriched with fish oil on weight loss in patients with pancreatic cancer. Br J Cancer 1999;81:80–6.
315. Gogos CA, Ginopoulos P, Salsa B, et al. Dietary omega-3 polyunsaturated fatty acids plus vitamin E restore immunodeficiency and prolong survival for severely ill patients with generalized malignancy: a randomized control trial. Cancer 1998;82:395–402.
316. Bruera E, Strasser F, Palmer JL, et al. Effect of fish oil on appetite and other symptoms in patients with advanced cancer and anorexia/cachexia: a double-blind, placebo-controlled study. J Clin Oncol 2003;21:129–34.
317. Fearon KC, von Meyenfeldt MF, Moses AGW, et al. Effect of a protein and energy dense n-3 fatty acid enriched oral supplement on loss of weight and lean tissue in cancer cachexia: a randomised double blind trial. Gut 2003;52:1479–86.
318. Jatoi A, Rowland K, Loprinzi CL, et al. An eicosapentaenoic acid supplement versus megestrol acetate versus both for patients with cancer-associated wasting: a North Central Cancer Treatment Group and National Cancer Institute of Canada collaborative effort. J Clin Oncol 2004;22:2469–76.
319. Detsky AS, Baker JP, O'Rourke K, Goel V. Perioperative parenteral nutrition: a meta-analysis. Ann Intern Med 1987;107:195–203.
320. Jensen S. Clinical effects of enteral and parenteral nutrition preceding cancer surgery. Med Oncol Tumor Pharmacother 1985;2:225–9.
321. American College of Physicians. Parenteral nutrition in patients receiving cancer chemotherapy. Ann Intern Med 1989;110:734–6.
322. Donaldson, SS. Nutritional support as an adjunct to radiation therapy. J Parenter Enteral Nutr 1984;8:302–10.
323. McGeer AJ, Detsky AS, O'Rourke K. Parenteral nutrition in cancer patients undergoing chemotherapy: a meta-analysis. Nutrition l990;6:233–40.
324. Barber MD, Fearon KC, Delmore G, Loprinzi CL. Should cancer patients with incurable disease receive parenteral or enteral nutritional support? Eur J Cancer 1998;34:279–85.
325. Copeland EM 3rd. Historical perspective on nutritional support of cancer patients. CA Cancer J Clin 1998;48:67–8.
326. Iestra JA, Fibbe WE, Zwinderman AH, et al. Parenteral nutrition following intensive cytotoxic therapy: an exploratory study on the need for parenteral nutrition after various treatment approaches for hematological malignancies. Bone Marrow Transplant 1999;23:933–9.
327. Lundholm K, Daneryd P, Bosaeus I, et al. Palliative nutritional intervention in addition to cyclooxygenase and erythropoietin treatment for patients with malignant disease: effects on survival, metabolism, and function. Cancer 2004;100:1967–77.
328. Bowman LC, William R, Sanders M, et al. Algorithm for nutritional support: evidence of the Metabolic and Infusion Support Service of Saint Jude Children's Research Hospital. Int J Cancer 1998;11(Suppl 1):76–80.
329. Hunter DC, Weintraub M, Blackburn GL, Bistrian BR. Branched chain amino acids as the protein component of parenteral nutrition in cancer cachexia. Br J Surg 1989;76:149–53.
330. Okada A, Mori S, Totsuka M, et al. Branched-chain amino acids metabolic support in surgical patients: a randomized, controlled trial in patients with subtotal or total gastrectomy in 16 Japanese institutions. J Parenter Enteral Nutr 1988;12:332–7.
331. Sandstedt S, Jorfeldt L, Larsson J. Randomized, controlled study evaluating effects of branched chain amino acids and alpha-ketoisocaproate on protein metabolism after surgery. Br J Surg 1992;79:217–20.
332. Fernstrom JD. Dietary effects on brain serotonin synthesis: relationship to appetite regulation. Am J Clin Nutr 1985;42(5 Suppl):1072–82.
333. Cangiano C, Laviano A, Meguid MM, et al. Effects of administration of oral branched-chain amino acids on anorexia and caloric intake in cancer patients. J Natl Cancer Inst 1996;88:550–2.
334. Rivera S, Azcon-Bieto J, Lopez-Soriano FJ, et al. Amino acid metabolism in tumour-bearing mice. Biochem J 1988;249:443–9.
335. Souba WW. Glutamine and cancer. Ann Surg 1993;218:715–28.
336. Ziegler TR, Young LS, Benfell K, et al. Clinical and metabolic efficacy of glutamine-supplemented parenteral nutrition after bone marrow transplantation. A randomized, double-blind, controlled study. Ann Intern Med 1992;116:821–8.
337. Moley JF, Morrison SD, Norton JA. Preoperative insulin reverses cachexia and decreases mortality in tumor-bearing rats. J Surg Res 1987;43:21–8.
338. Tessitore L, Costelli P, Baccino FM. Pharmacological interference with tissue hypercatabolism in tumour-bearing rats. Biochem J 1994;299(Pt 1):71–8.
339. Kabadi UM, Reust CS, Kabadi MU. Weight gain, improvement in metabolic profile, and CD4 count with insulin administration in an AIDS patient. AIDS Patient Care STDS 2000;14:575–9.
340. Hanada T, Toshinai K, Kajimura N, et al. Anti-cachectic effect of ghrelin in nude mice bearing human melanoma cells. Biochem Biophys Res Commun 2003;301:275–9.
341. Lissoni P, Barni S, Tancini G. Role of the pineal gland in the control of macrophage functions and its possible implementation in cancer: a study of interactions between tumor necrosis factor-alpha and the pineal hormone melatonin. J Biol Regul Homeost Agents 1994;8:126–9.
342. Lissoni P, Tancini G, Barni S, et al. Treatment of cancer chemotherapy-induced toxicity with the pineal hormone melatonin. Supportive Care Cancer 1997;5:126–9.
343. Lissoni P, Tancini G, Paolorossi F, et al. Chemoneuroendocrine therapy of metastatic breast cancer with persistent thrombocytopenia with weekly low dose epirubicin plus melatonin: a phase II study. J Pineal Res 1999; 26:169–73.
344. Lissoni P, Paolorossi F, Tancini G, et al. Is there a role for melatonin in the treatment of neoplastic cachexia? Eur J Cancer 1996;32A:1340–3.
345. Lissoni P, Barni S, Fossati V, et al. A randomized study of neuroimmunotherapy with low-dose subcutaneous interleuken-2 plus melatonin compared to supportive care alone in patients with untreated metastatic solid tumour. Supportive Care Cancer 1995;3:194–7.
346. Lissoni P, Paolorossi F, Ardizzoia A, et al. A randomized study of chemotherapy with cisplatin plus etoposide versus chemoendocrine therapy with cisplatin, etoposide and the pineal hormone melatonin as a first-line treatment of advanced non-small cell lung cancer patients in a poor clinical state. J Pineal Res 1997;23:15–9.
347. Persson C, Glimelius B, Ronnelid J, Nygren P. Impact of fish oil and melatonin on cachexia in patients with advanced gastrointestinal cancer: a randomized pilot study. Nutrition 2005;21:170–8.
348. Kardinal CG, Loprinzi CL, Schaid DJ, et al. A controlled trial of cyproheptadine in cancer patients with anorexia and/or cachexia. Cancer 1990;65:2657–62.
349. Nathanson L, Hall TC. A spectrum of tumors that produce paraneoplastic syndromes. Lung tumor: how they produce their syndromes. Ann N Y Acad Sci 1974;230:367–7.

Antiemetic Therapy

David S. Ettinger, MD
Tara L. Lin, MD

Chemotherapy-induced nausea and vomiting (CINV) remains a significant problem for many cancer patients despite recent advances in pharmacologic therapy.[1] It may have a dramatic impact on a patient's quality of life, in addition to physical consequences, including dehydration, nutritional compromise, and metabolic disturbances.[2] Despite the publication of guidelines for preventive antiemetic therapy, some patients continue to receive suboptimal prophylaxis against CINV. Nausea and vomiting occurring after chemotherapy may be more difficult to manage than if the symptoms had been prevented with appropriate pharmacologic intervention. In addition, patients may develop a psychological component to their nausea and vomiting as a result of inadequate management in the past. We discuss the pathophysiology of CINV, the emetogenic potential of common chemotherapeutics, classes of antiemetic therapy, and guidelines for prevention and acute management of CINV.

Historically, approximately 70 to 80% of all cancer patients receiving chemotherapy experienced emesis,[3] and, fortunately, there have been dramatic improvements since the introduction of effective antiemetic therapy.[1] Studies over the last 20 years have attempted to quantify the impact of chemotherapy side effects on cancer patients. Repeatedly, nausea and vomiting are mentioned as "major physical side effects"[4] and "most troublesome."[5] Although there have been recent advances in pharmacologic prevention of CINV, a 1997 study by de Boer-Dennert and colleagues revealed that nausea and vomiting ranked as the first and third most distressing side effects of chemotherapy, despite a decrease in the overall incidence and severity with the introduction of 5-hydroxytryptamine 3 (5-HT_3) antagonists.[6] Grunberg and colleagues surveyed patients, medical oncologists, and oncology nurses in 2001 to 2002 to assess the frequency and provider perception of CINV.[1] Although improvements in the prevention of acute nausea and vomiting were seen (acute nausea in approximately 35% and acute emesis in 13%), delayed symptoms were seen more frequently (50 to 60% with nausea and 30 to 50% with emesis, depending on the chemotherapy used). Strikingly, more than 75% of physicians and nurses underestimated the occurrence of delayed nausea and vomiting. Progress in relieving the symptoms of CINV will only come with greater awareness of the problem and more aggressive use of current medications.

PATHOPHYSIOLOGY OF NAUSEA AND VOMITING

Vomiting is controlled by the central nervous system via a complex pathway of varied afferent inputs and neurotransmitters (Figure 127-1). In the 1950s, studies by Borison and Wang identified two areas of the brainstem involved in nausea and vomiting: the chemoreceptor trigger zone (CTZ) and the emetic center.[7] The CTZ is located in the area postrema in the floor of the fourth ventricle. Because it lies outside the blood-brain barrier, the CTZ is susceptible to emetogenic stimuli from the bloodstream, such as chemotherapeutic drugs or, more likely, their metabolites.[8] Muscarinic, dopamine D_2, serotonin (5-HT_3), neurokinin 1 (NK-1) and histamine H_1 receptors have been identified in the CTZ. Impulses from the CTZ are then transmitted to the emetic center. In addition to those from the CTZ to the emetic center, afferent pathways from the gastrointestinal tract and pharynx via the vagus and splanchnic nerves are coordinated in the emetic center.[9] Inputs from the cerebral cortex may also be involved, especially in anticipatory emesis.

The emetic center receives afferent impulses and coordinates the efferent activities of the salivation center, abdominal muscles, respiratory center, and autonomic nerves that result in vomiting. The emetic center, composed of these indistinct receptor and effector nuclei, is located in the nucleus tractus solitarius of the brainstem.[8]

The most critical neuroreceptors involved in these afferent and efferent pathways are serotonin, dopamine, and substance P. Others include acetylcholine, corticosteroid, histamine, cannabinoid, opiate, and NK-1 receptors.[10] Three receptors with clinical relevance, as demonstrated by the clinical benefit of blockade, are dopamine, serotonin (5-HT_3), and substance P. The most significant advance in antiemetic therapy came in the early 1990s when the 5-HT_3 receptor antagonists became available.[6] Substance P, which binds to the NK-1 receptor, is an emerging target in antiemetic therapy,[11] and one approved NK-1 receptor antagonist, aprepitant, has shown clinical utility.[12–14]

It is unknown how and where along these pathways chemotherapy and its metabolites have their emetic effects. Metabolites may stimulate the CTZ directly. Serotonin and other neurotransmitters may be released from intestinal cells damaged by chemotherapy. Sensory neurons release substance P, and numerous NK-1 receptors have been identified in both the CTZ and the nucleus tractus solitarius.

Despite increasing knowledge of the central nervous system and pathways involved in control of vomiting, no single common pathway has been discovered, and it is unlikely that any single agent will be able to provide complete antiemetic protection from chemotherapy.

TYPES OF EMESIS

Three distinct types of chemotherapy-induced emesis have been identified: acute, delayed, and anticipatory. Acute emesis is defined as nausea and vomiting within 24 hours of chemotherapy. It has its onset within 1 to 2 hours of chemotherapy and peaks in the first 4 to 6 hours without adequate prophylaxis. Delayed emesis refers to symptoms that start more than 24 hours after chemotherapy. It typically peaks at 48 to 72 hours and may last for 6 to 7 days. Although delayed emesis may be less frequent and severe than acute emesis, it is less well controlled than acute emesis. Cisplatin is most frequently associated with delayed emesis, and it is also seen with carboplatin, cyclophosphamide, and anthracyclines.

Anticipatory emesis is seen in patients who have previously experienced significant nausea and vomiting following chemotherapy. In these patients, symptoms develop as a conditioned response and before the chemotherapy is administered. It may be triggered by sights and activities associated with the chemotherapy (eg, driving to the treatment center). As control of CINV has improved, the incidence of anticipatory emesis has declined.[15]

In addition to chemotherapy-induced emesis, other potential causes of nausea and vomiting in cancer patients include partial or complete bowel obstruction, brain metastases, uremia, electrolyte disturbances (ie, hyperglycemia, hypercalcemia, hyponatremia), and gastroparesis. Other medications commonly prescribed in cancer patients, such as opiates, may cause emesis as well.

EMETOGENIC CHEMOTHERAPY

The severity and frequency of CINV are affected by variables of both the patient and the chemotherapy. Patient-related factors predicting a higher incidence of CINV include a history of chemotherapy, a history of CINV, female sex, younger age, a history of motion sickness, and no or a minimal history of alcohol use. Chemotherapy-related factors include the route and rate of administration and drug dosage. The most predictive factor is the specific chemotherapy agent used.[16]

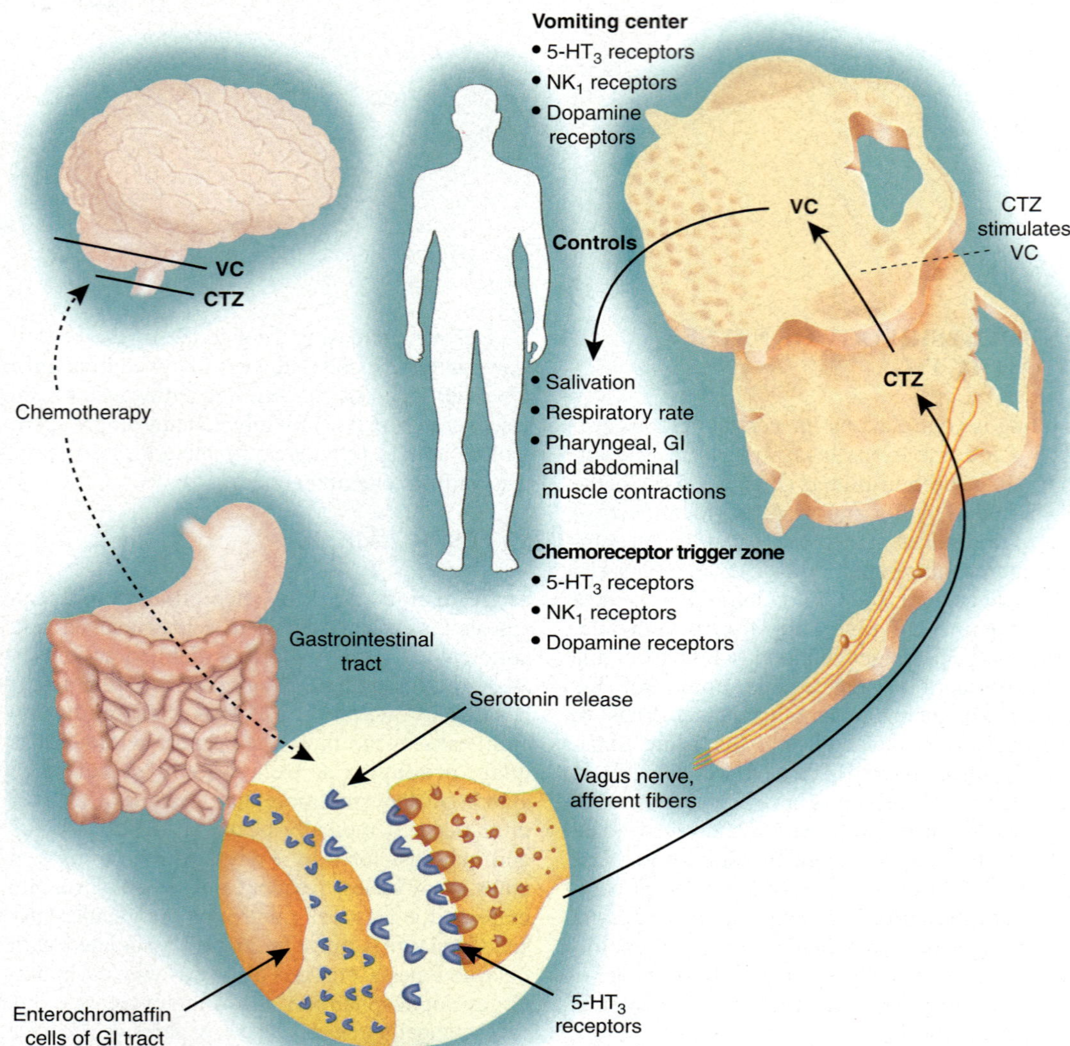

Figure 127-1 Two sites in the brainstem—the vomiting center and the chemoreceptor trigger zone—are important to emesis control. The vomiting center consists of an intertwined neural network in the nucleus tractus solitarius that controls patterns of motor activity. The chemoreceptor trigger zone, located in the area postrema, is the entry point for emetogenic stimuli. Enterochromaffin cells in the gastrointestinal tract respond to chemotherapy by releasing serotonin. Serotonin binds to 5-hydroxytryptamine 3 (5-HT_3) receptors, which are located not only in the gastrointestinal tract but also on vagal afferent neurons and in the nucleus tractus solitarius and area postrema. The activated 5-HT_3 receptors signal the chemoreceptor trigger zone via pathways that may include the afferent fibers of the vagus nerve. Serotonin may also bind with 5-HT_3 receptors in the brainstem. Other neurotransmitters, including dopamine and substance P, also influence the chemoreceptor trigger zone. Afferent impulses from the chemoreceptor trigger zone stimulate the vomiting center, which initiates emesis. Grunberg SM, Hesketh PJ. Control of chemotherapy-induced emesis. N Engl J Med 1993;329:1790–6. Reproduced with permission of MGI Pharma.

There is no universally accepted classification system of chemotherapy agents by emetogenic potential (Table 127-1). The most widely accepted, devised by Hesketh and colleagues, divides chemotherapy into five levels of emetogenicity based on the percentage of patients who experience nausea and vomiting following each without any antiemetic prophylaxis. Level 1 drugs result in emesis in less than 10% without antiemetic therapy; level 2, 10 to 30%; level 3, 30 to 60%; level 4, 60 to 90%; and level 5, more than 90% of patients experiencing emesis without prophylaxis.[17] A recently proposed modification would classify chemotherapy into four risk categories: high risk (level 5, more than 90%), moderate risk (levels 3 and 4, 30–90%), low risk (level 2, 10–30%), and minimal risk (level 1, less than 10%).[18]

These classification systems were developed with a focus on acute emesis. It is clear from recent data that the frequency and severity of delayed symptoms are often underestimated and remain a significant problem for many patients.[1] Adequate antiemetic prophylaxis is required for the duration of days that symptoms are anticipated.

CLASSES OF ANTIEMETICS

Our knowledge of the known neurotransmitters involved in the central nervous system pathways that regulate the vomiting response has provided targets for antiemetic therapy (Table 127-2). In return, successful clinical application of these agents has confirmed the importance of these neurotransmitters and receptors in the vomiting pathway. Neuroreceptors involved in the control of emesis include muscarinic (M_1), dopamine (D_2), histamine (H_1), 5-HT_3 (receptor site for serotonin), and NK-1 (receptor site for substance P).[19,20] The most effective and most commonly used classes of agents are the 5-HT_3 receptor antagonists, the dopamine antagonists, and corticosteroids. An emerging class of agents, the NK-1 receptor antagonists, further expands the repertoire of antiemetic agents.

5-HT_3 Receptor Antagonists Since the early 1990s, four 5-HT_3 receptor antagonists have been approved in the United States: ondansetron, granisetron, dolasetron, and, most recently, palonosetron. These agents revolutionized the antiemetic prophylaxis of highly and moderately emetogenic chemotherapy. Studies of 5-HT_3 receptor antagonists used alone demonstrated superior efficacy compared with high-dose metoclopramide alone[21] and equivalence to the combination of high-dose metoclopramide and dexamethasone, the previous standard of care for these patients.[22] However, the combination of 5-HT_3 receptor antagonist and dexamethasone was the most effective combination tested.[23] Significantly, the 5-HT_3 receptor antagonists were well tolerated, with few adverse effects.

Before 2003, there were three 5-HT_3 receptor antagonists approved by the US Food and Drug Administration (FDA): ondansetron, granisetron, and dolasetron. Numerous subsequent clinical trials demonstrated the clinical equivalence of these three agents, despite differences seen in preclinical models.[24–29] A single dose prechemotherapy was shown to be as effective as repeat dosing.[30–32] In addition, there was no significant difference whether the agent was given orally or intravenously.[33,34]

In July 2003, a new 5-HT_3 receptor antagonist, palonosetron, was approved by the FDA for antiemetic prophylaxis. Palonosetron may have advantages over the other serotonin antagonists because of its higher binding affinity to the 5-HT_3 receptor and its longer half-life. Two phase III randomized clinical trials demonstrated the superiority of palonosetron compared with ondansetron and dolasetron, particularly in preventing delayed nausea and vomiting. In the first, 592 patients were randomized to receive palonosetron at either 0.25 or 0.75 mg or dolasetron at 100 mg 30 minutes prior to moderately emetogenic chemotherapy. Less than 5% of patients received concomitant corticosteroids. A statistically significant difference was observed between the palonosetron 0.25 mg and dolasetron arms in complete response (CR, defined as absence of emesis and no rescue medication in the first 24 hours). CR rates were 63% in the palonosetron 0.25 mg arm versus 52.9% in the dolasetron arm (p = .049) and 57% for the palonosetron 0.75 mg arm (p = .412). For complete control (defined as no emesis, no need for rescue medication, and no symptoms other than mild nausea) of delayed nausea and vomiting (24–120 hours), palonosetron 0.25 and 0.75 mg demonstrated statistically significant improvements compared with dolasetron 100 mg (48.1% for palonosetron 0.25 mg compared with 36.1% for dolasetron, p = .027; 51.9% for palonosetron 0.75 mg, p = .016). There was no difference among the groups in observed adverse effects, including headache, constipation, and fatigue.[35]

Table 127-1 Emetogenic Potential of Single Chemotherapy Agents

Level	Agent
High risk, level 5 (> 90% predicted frequency of emesis without prophylaxis)	Carmustine > 250 mg/m^2 Cisplatin ≥ 50 mg/m^2 Cyclophosphamide > 1,500 mg/m^2 Dacarbazine Mechlorethamine Streptozocin
Moderate risk, level 4 (60–90% predicted frequency of emesis without prophylaxis)	Amifostine > 500 mg/m^2 Busulfan > 4 mg/d Carboplatin Cisplatin < 50 mg/m^2 Cyclophosphamide > 750 mg/m^2 and ≤ 1,500 mg/m^2 Cytarabine > 1 g/m^2 Dactinomycin Doxorubicin > 60 mg/m^2 Epirubicin > 90 mg/m^2 Melphalan > 50 mg/m^2 Methotrexate > 1,000 mg/m^2 Procarbazine (oral dosing)
Moderate risk, level 3 (30–60% predicted frequency of emesis without prophylaxis)	Amifostine > 300 mg/m^2 and ≤ 500 mg/m^2 Arsenic trioxide Cyclophosphamide ≤ 750 mg/m^2 Cyclophosphamide (oral dosing) Doxorubicin 20 mg/m^2 and < 60 mg/m^2 Epirubicin ≤ 90 mg/m^2 Ifosfamide Interleukin-2 > 12–15 million units/m^2 Irinotecan Lomustine Methotrexate 250–1,000 mg/m^2 Mitoxantrone < 15 mg/m^2 Oxaliplatin > 75 mg/m^2
Low risk, level 2 (10–30% predicted frequency of emesis without prophylaxis)	Amifostine ≤ 300 mg/m^2 Bexarotene Cytarabine 100–200 mg/m^2 Capecitabine Docetaxel Doxorubicin (liposomal formulation) Etoposide 5-Fluorouracil < 1,000 mg/m^2 Gemcitabine Methotrexate > 50 mg/m^2 and < 250 mg/m^2 Mitomycin Paclitaxel Temozolomide Topotecan
Minimal risk, level 1 (< 10% predicted frequency of emesis without prophylaxis)	Alemtuzumab Asparaginase Alpha Interferon Bleomycin Bortezomib Chlorambucil (oral dosing) Cladribine Dexrazoxane Denileukin diftitox Fludarabine Gefitinib Gemtuzumab ozogamicin Hydroxyurea Imatinib mesylate Melphalan (low dose, oral dosing) Methotrexate ≤ 50 mg/m^2 Pentostatin Rituximab Thioguanine (oral dosing) Trastuzumab Valrubicin Vinblastine Vincristine Vinorelbine

In the second study, palonosetron was compared with ondansetron 32 mg. Five hundred seventy patients receiving moderately emetogenic chemotherapy were randomized to one of two doses of palonosetron (0.25 or 0.75 mg) or ondansetron 32 mg on day 1 of chemotherapy. No patients received corticosteroids. CR rates were superior for the palonosetron 0.25 mg arm compared with the ondansetron group in prevention of both acute (81% vs 68.6%, $p = .009$) and delayed (74.1% vs 55.1%, $p < .001$) symptoms. Although palonosetron 0.75 mg demonstrated numeric improvement over ondansetron, the results were not statistically significant. Side effects were similar in all groups and included headache, diarrhea, constipation, and fatigue.[36]

The 5-HT$_3$ antagonists remain the cornerstone of prophylaxis for both highly and moderately emetogenic chemotherapy. Initial data show the superiority of palonosetron over the others, particularly in the prevention of delayed symptoms. Further studies are needed to define the differences between palonosetron and the other 5-HT$_3$ antagonists. All of the 5-HT$_3$ antagonists are well tolerated; the most common adverse effect is headache, occurring in 15 to 20% of patients. Less common side effects include constipation and dizziness.

Dopamine Receptor Antagonists Three classes of dopamine receptor antagonists are effective in the prevention and treatment of nausea and vomiting: phenothiazines, butyrophenones, and benzamides. In the 1960s, the phenothiazines were the first drugs proven to have efficacy in the prevention of CINV. Prochlorperazine is the most commonly used in this class and has efficacy in all classes except the most highly emetogenic chemotherapy.[37] Extrapyramidal effects, including dystonia, may be seen. These are treated with diphenhydramine and cessation of the drug. The butyrophenones, including haloperidol, are less frequently used for CINV and have adverse effects similar to those of the phenothiazines. They may be effective in the treatment of breakthrough nausea and vomiting.

Of the benzamides, metoclopramide is the best studied and most widely used in CINV. It blocks central and peripheral D$_2$ receptors at low doses and exhibits weak 5-HT$_3$ inhibition at high doses. In addition, it speeds gastric emptying and increases sphincter tone at the gastroesophageal junction. Prior to the introduction of the 5-HT$_3$ antagonists, a combination of high-dose intravenous metoclopramide and dexamethasone was the most effective antiemetic prophylaxis for highly emetogenic chemotherapy.[38] Because metoclopramide crosses the blood-brain barrier, side effects, including dystonia and tardive dyskinesia, may be seen, particularly at high doses and in elderly patients. Diphenhydramine was commonly given as part of the combination regimen to prevent these adverse effects. This regimen has generally been replaced by a combination containing a 5-HT$_3$ receptor antagonist because of its improved efficacy and safety profile.[21–23] The

Table 127-2 Classes and Recommended Doses of Selected Antiemetics

Agent	Class	Route	Dose
Ondansetron	5-HT_3 receptor antagonist	IV	8–12 mg
		PO	12–24 mg
Granisetron	5-HT_3 receptor antagonist	IV	1 mg or 0.01 mg/kg
		PO	2 mg
Dolasetron	5-HT_3 receptor antagonist	IV	100 mg or 1.8 mg/kg
		PO	100 mg
Palonosetron	5-HT_3 receptor antagonist	IV	0.25 mg
Aprepitant	NK-1 receptor antagonist	PO	125 mg day 1
			80 mg day 2, 3
Dexamethasone	Steroid	IV	8–20 mg
		PO	8–20 mg
Prochlorperazine	Dopamine receptor antagonist	IV	10 mg
		PO	10 mg
		Spansule suppository	15 mg
			25 mg
Metoclopramide	Dopamine receptor antagonist	IV	1–2 mg/kg
		PO	20–40 mg
Haloperidol	Dopamine receptor antagonist	IV	1–3 mg
		PO	1–2 mg
Dronabinol	Cannabinoid	PO	5–10 mg

IV = intravenous; 5-HT_3 = 5-hydroxytryptamine 3; NK = neurokinin; PO = orally.

regimen of metoclopramide, dexamethasone, and diphenhydramine may be useful in patients intolerant of 5-HT_3 receptor antagonists or those who have failed first-line treatment.

Corticosteroids Corticosteroids, most commonly dexamethasone, are effective in preventing nausea and vomiting when used alone or in combination for all emetogenic classes of chemotherapy. For moderately to highly emetogenic chemotherapy, dexamethasone plus a 5-HT_3 receptor antagonist is used. A meta-analysis of 32 randomized clinical trials including 5,613 patients from 1984 to 1998 demonstrated the efficacy of dexamethasone in both moderately and highly emetogenic chemotherapy either alone or in combination with other agents.[39] Later studies revealed the superiority of a combination of 5-HT_3 receptor antagonist and dexamethasone compared with either agent alone in highly emetogenic chemotherapy.[40] The site of action of corticosteroids along the vomiting reflex pathway is unknown. Side effects include insomnia, increased energy, and mood disturbances.

NK-1 Receptor Antagonists NK-1 receptors are found in the nucleus tractus solitarius and the area postrema and are activated by substance P.[11] Inhibitors of the NK-1 receptor have demonstrated antiemetic effects and represent a new target for antiemetic therapy. The first approved medication in this class, aprepitant, has been shown to prevent both acute and delayed emesis resulting from highly emetogenic chemotherapy.[13,14]

Following promising preliminary data, two randomized phase III multicenter trials demonstrated the efficacy of aprepitant for the prevention of both acute and delayed nausea and vomiting. Five hundred twenty-three patients receiving highly emetogenic chemotherapy (cisplatin > 70 mg/m^2) received as emetic prophylaxis either aprepitant in combination with 5-HT_3 receptor antagonists and dexamethasone (aprepitant 125 mg orally [PO], ondansetron 32 mg intravenously [IV], and dexamethasone 12 mg PO on day 1, followed by aprepitant 80 mg PO and dexamethasone 8 mg PO on days 2 to 3 and dexamethasone 8 mg PO on day 4) or a regimen of a 5-HT_3 receptor antagonist and dexamethasone alone (ondansetron 32 mg IV plus dexamethasone 20 mg PO on day 1, followed by dexamethasone 8 mg PO twice daily on days 2 to 4). In the first study, the overall CR (absence of emesis and no need for rescue medication in the first 24 hours) was 62.7% in the aprepitant arm versus 43.3% in the standard therapy arm ($p < .001$). CR rates for the aprepitant arm and the standard therapy arm, respectively, for acute (82.8% vs 68.4%, $p < .001$) and delayed (67.7% compared with 46.8%, $p < .001$) symptoms demonstrated the superiority of the aprepitant arm.[13] The second study, which evaluated the same regimens in 521 patients receiving high-dose cisplatin chemotherapy, confirmed these results. Overall CR rates were 72.7% in the aprepitant group versus 52.3% in the standard arm ($p < .001$). CR rates in both acute and delayed emesis were also superior in the aprepitant arm (89.2% vs 78.1%, respectively, $p < .001$, and 75.4% vs 55.8%, respectively, $p < .001$).[14] These data led to the FDA approval of aprepitant in 2003.

Aprepitant is a substrate for and moderate inducer and moderate inhibitor of the cytochrome P-450 enzyme 3A4 (CYP3A4).[41] Chemotherapy and other drugs are metabolized by this enzyme, and caution must be used when adding aprepitant in these patients. Docetaxel, paclitaxel, etoposide, irinotecan, ifosfamide, imatinib, vinorelbine, vinblastine, and vincristine are metabolized by CYP3A4. Although, in clinical trials, aprepitant was given to patients receiving these agents without any alteration in dose and no observed adverse effect or decreased efficacy, caution is urged. In addition, aprepitant may interact with other, nonchemotherapy agents. It may induce metabolism of warfarin, leading to reduced levels. Aprepitant appears to increase the active levels of oral dexamethasone and methylprednisolone, and reduced dosing of prophylactic dexamethasone is recommended when used in combination with aprepitant. Other drugs with interactions include oral contraceptives, midazolam, ketoconazole, erythromycin, carbamazepine, rifampin, and phenytoin.

Other Classes of Antiemetics Additional classes of antiemetic agents that may be useful in patients include the benzodiazepines, anticholinergics, and cannabinoids. The most commonly used benzodiazepines, lorazepam and alprazolam, although not antiemetics, have their greatest utility in the treatment of anticipatory nausea and reduction in the anxiety associated with chemotherapy when used in addition to the classic antiemetics.[42] The anticholinergic promethazine and, less frequently, transdermal scopolamine may be used for treatment of breakthrough CINV. There are fewer randomized clinical trial data to recommend the use of cannabinoids such as marijuana or its synthetic versions, nabilone and dronabinol,[43] although there is anecdotal evidence to support their use in patients who do not respond to conventional antiemetics.

RECOMMENDATIONS FOR PREVENTION AND TREATMENT OF CHEMOTHERAPY-INDUCED EMESIS

The goal of antiemetic therapy is complete prevention of CINV (Table 127-3). In patients receiving highly and moderately emetogenic chemotherapy, the period of risk for nausea and vomiting lasts at least 4 days following chemotherapy, and protection with antiemetics is needed throughout this period. The choice of antiemetic prophylaxis is driven by the emetogenic potential of the specific chemotherapy agents and patient risk factors.

Table 127-3 Guidelines for Prevention of Acute and Delayed Nausea and Vomiting in Patients Depending on Emetic Risk

Emetic Risk	Acute	Delayed
High (> 90%)	Aprepitant + 5-HT_3 antagonist + dexamethasone	Aprepitant + dexamethasone
Moderate (30–90%)	5-HT_3 antagonist* + dexamethasone	Dexamethasone
Low (10–30%)	Dexamethasone or phenothiazine or metoclopramide	None
Minimal (< 10%)	None	None

5-HT_3 = 5-hydroxytryptamine 3.

*Palonosetron is preferred and is administered on day 1 only.

Highly Emetogenic Chemotherapy Cisplatin and cyclophosphamide are the most frequently used highly emetogenic chemotherapy agents. Nausea and vomiting are virtually ensured without adequate prophylaxis. Prior to the approval of the NK-1 receptor antagonist aprepitant, the previous recommendation was a combination of a 5-HT3 antagonist and dexamethasone. A regimen of a 5-HT3 receptor antagonist, aprepitant (125 mg PO), and dexamethasone (12 mg PO or IV) on day 1 followed by aprepitant (80 mg PO) and dexamethasone (8 mg PO or IV) on days 2 to 4 is recommended in all patients receiving highly emetogenic chemotherapy. All prophylaxis should begin prior to the administration of chemotherapy.

Moderately Emetogenic Chemotherapy A combination of a 5-HT3 receptor antagonist and dexamethasone is recommended in all patients receiving moderately emetogenic chemotherapy. Given recent data and its superior efficacy in preventing delayed symptoms, palonosetron (0.25 mg on day 1 only) is the preferred 5-HT3 receptor antagonist. If others are used, they should be given on day 1 prior to chemotherapy and then repeated daily on days 2 to 4. Dexamethasone is given as 12 mg IV or PO on day 1 and then at a daily dose of 8 mg on days 2 to 4 (either 8 mg daily or 4 mg in divided doses twice daily). In selected patients (those with breakthrough nausea and vomiting despite adequate prophylaxis or those with other patient variables that suggest a higher risk of symptoms), aprepitant (125 mg PO on day 1 followed by 80 mg PO on days 2 to 3) should be considered.

Low-Risk Chemotherapy Options for antiemetic prophylaxis in patients receiving chemotherapy of low emetogenic potential include dexamethasone (12 mg PO or IV) or prochlorperazine (10 mg PO or IV every 4 to 6 hours) or metoclopramide (20 to 40 mg PO every 4 to 6 hours or 1 to 2 mg/kg IV every 3 to 4 hours with diphenhydramine to prevent extrapyramidal symptoms). All prophylaxis should be given prior to the administration of chemotherapy.

Minimally Emetogenic Chemotherapy No routine prophylaxis is recommended. Should nausea and vomiting occur, the use of dexamethasone, prochlorperazine, or metoclopramide is recommended. Prophylactic use of these medications should be considered prior to the next cycle of therapy.

SPECIAL SITUATIONS

Breakthrough Nausea and Vomiting Ideally, the best treatment for breakthrough nausea and vomiting is to prevent it from occurring at all. At times, despite aggressive prophylaxis, symptoms still occur. The best therapy for breakthrough symptoms is the addition of agents from another class of antiemetics. In addition, an alternative route other than oral, such as intravenous or rectal, may need to be used. These medications work best if taken on a schedule rather than on an as-needed basis. When breakthrough nausea and vomiting occur, the prophylactic regimen should be reevaluated and enhanced prior to the next cycle of therapy.

Anticipatory Nausea and Vomiting The key to preventing anticipatory nausea and vomiting is preventing symptoms from occurring with each cycle of chemotherapy. Once the symptoms have developed, agents such as the benzodiazepines may be added to the prophylactic regimen.[42] Other strategies that have been proven useful for some patients include behavioral therapy, systemic desensitization, and hypnosis.[44,45]

Radiation-Induced Nausea and Vomiting Radiation-induced nausea and vomiting (RINV) is seen is nearly all patients receiving total body irradiation prior to bone marrow transplantation and in more than 80% of those receiving radiation to the upper abdomen.[46] Studies have demonstrated the efficacy of prophylactic 5-HT3 receptor antagonists compared with placebo[47] and the superiority of prophylaxis with 5-HT3 receptor antagonists compared with combinations with metoclopramide and prochlorperazine.[48,49] The recommendation is for all patients undergoing either upper abdominal radiation therapy or total body irradiation to receive prophylaxis with an oral 5-HT3 receptor antagonist dosed either twice or three times daily with or without oral dexamethasone.[50]

CONCLUSIONS

Dramatic progress has been made in the prevention and treatment of chemotherapy-induced emesis, especially since the introduction of the 5-HT3 receptor antagonists in the early 1990s and the 2003 introduction of the NK-1 receptor antagonist aprepitant. Recent surveys indicate the need for heightened awareness of the frequency and severity of acute and, especially, delayed nausea and vomiting from chemotherapy. Fortunately, new agents have been added to the antiemetic arsenal to further enhance the efficacy of antiemetic prophylaxis. Appropriate implementation of guidelines for prophylaxis based on the specific chemotherapy agents used will ensure that fewer patients experience these most distressing of side effects.

REFERENCES

1. Grunberg SM, Deuson RR, Mavros P, et al. Incidence of chemotherapy-induced nausea and emesis after modern antiemetics. Cancer 2004;100:2261–8.
2. Mitchell EP. Gastrointestinal toxicity of chemotherapeutic agents. Semin Oncol 1992;19:566–79.
3. Morran C, Smith DC, Anderson DA, McArdle CS. Incidence of nausea and vomiting with cytotoxic chemotherapy: a prospective randomised trial of antiemetics. BMJ 1979;1:1323–4.
4. Coates A, Abraham S, Kaye SB, et al. On the receiving end—patient perception of the side-effects of cancer chemotherapy. Eur J Cancer Clin Oncol 1983;19:203–8.
5. Lindley C, McCune JS, Thomason TE, et al. Perception of chemotherapy side effects: cancer versus noncancer patients. Cancer Pract 1999;7:59–65.
6. de Boer-Dennert M, de Wit R, Schmitz PI, et al. Patient perceptions of the side-effects of chemotherapy: the influence of 5HT3 antagonists. Br J Cancer 1997;76:1055–61.
7. Borison HL, Wang SC. Physiology and pharmacology of vomiting. Pharmacol Rev 1953;5:193–230.
8. Miller AD, Leslie RA. The area postrema and vomiting. Front Neuroendocrinol 1994;15:301–20.
9. Carpenter DO. Neural mechanisms of emesis. Can J Physiol Pharmacol 1990;68:230–6.
10. Dodds LJ. The control of cancer chemotherapy-induced nausea and vomiting. J Clin Hosp Pharm 1985;10:143–66.
11. Saito R, Takano Y, Kamiya HO. Roles of substance P and NK(1) receptor in the brainstem in the development of emesis. J Pharmacol Sci 2003;91:87–94.
12. de Wit R, Herrstedt J, Rapoport B, et al. Addition of the oral NK1 antagonist aprepitant to standard antiemetics provides protection against nausea and vomiting during multiple cycles of cisplatin-based chemotherapy. J Clin Oncol 2003;21:4105–11.
13. Poli-Bigelli S, Rodrigues-Pereira J, Carides AD, et al. Addition of the neurokinin 1 receptor antagonist aprepitant to standard antiemetic therapy improves control of chemotherapy-induced nausea and vomiting: results from a randomized, double-blind, placebo-controlled trial in Latin America. Cancer 2003;97:3090–8.
14. Hesketh PJ, Grunberg SM, Gralla RJ, et al. The oral neurokinin-1 antagonist aprepitant for the prevention of chemotherapy-induced nausea and vomiting: a multinational, randomized, double-blind, placebo-controlled trial in patients receiving high-dose cisplatin—the Aprepitant Protocol 052 Study Group. J Clin Oncol 2003;21:4112–9.
15. Moher D, Arthur AZ, Pater JL. Anticipatory nausea and/or vomiting. Cancer Treat Rev 1984;11:257–64.
16. Pollera CF, Giannarelli D. Prognostic factors influencing cisplatin-induced emesis. definition and validation of a predictive logistic model. Cancer 1989;64:1117–22.
17. Hesketh PJ, Kris MG, Grunberg SM, et al. Proposal for classifying the acute emetogenicity of cancer chemotherapy. J Clin Oncol 1997;15:103–9.
18. Koeller JM, Aapro MS, Gralla RJ, et al. A. Antiemetic guidelines: creating a more practical treatment approach. Support Care Cancer 2002;10:519–22.
19. Mitchelson F. Pharmacological agents affecting emesis. A review (part I). Drugs 1992;43:295–315.
20. Bountra C, Gale JD, Gardner CJ, et al. Towards understanding the aetiology and pathophysiology of the emetic reflex: novel approaches to antiemetic drugs. Oncology 1996;53 Suppl 1:102–9.
21. Chevallier B, Cappelaere P, Splinter T, et al. A double-blind, multicentre comparison of intravenous dolasetron mesilate and metoclopramide in the prevention of nausea and vomiting in cancer patients receiving high-dose cisplatin chemotherapy. Support Care Cancer 1997;5:22–30.
22. Warr D, Wilan A, Venner P, et al. A randomised, double-blind comparison of granisetron with high-dose metoclopramide, dexamethasone and diphenhydramine for cisplatin-induced emesis. An NCI Canada Clinical Trials Group phase III trial. Eur J Cancer 1992;29A:33–6.
23. Heron JF, Goedhals L, Jordaan JP, et al. Oral granisetron alone and in combination with dexamethasone: a double-blind randomized comparison against high-dose metoclopramide plus dexamethasone in prevention of cisplatin-induced emesis. The Granisetron Study Group. Ann Oncol 1994;5:579–4.
24. Bonneterre J, Hecquet B. Granisetron (IV) compared with ondansetron (IV plus oral) in the prevention of nausea and vomiting induced by moderately-emetogenic chemotherapy. A cross-over study. Bull Cancer 1995;82:1038–43.
25. Stewart A, McQuade B, Cronje JD, et al. Ondansetron compared with granisetron in the prophylaxis of cyclophosphamide-induced emesis in out-patients: a multicentre, double-blind, double-dummy, randomised, parallel-group study. Emesis Study Group for Ondansetron and Granisetron in Breast Cancer Patients. Oncology 1995;52:202–10.
26. Martoni A, Angelelli B, Guaraldi M, et al. An open randomised cross-over study on granisetron versus ondansetron in the prevention of acute emesis induced by moderate dose cisplatin-containing regimens. Eur J Cancer 1996;32A:82–5.
27. Hesketh P, Navari R, Grote T, et al. Double-blind, randomized comparison of the antiemetic efficacy of intravenous dolasetron mesylate and intravenous ondansetron in the prevention of acute cisplatin-induced emesis in patients with cancer. Dolasetron Comparative Chemotherapy-

Induced Emesis Prevention Group. J Clin Oncol 1996;14:2242–9.
28. Audhuy B, Cappelaere P, Martin M, et al. A double-blind, randomised comparison of the anti-emetic efficacy of two intravenous doses of dolasetron mesilate and granisetron in patients receiving high dose cisplatin chemotherapy. Eur J Cancer 1996;32A:807–13.
29. Lofters WS, Pater JL, Zee B, et al. Phase III double-blind comparison of dolasetron mesylate and ondansetron and an evaluation of the additive role of dexamethasone in the prevention of acute and delayed nausea and vomiting due to moderately emetogenic chemotherapy. J Clin Oncol 1997;15:2966–73.
30. Seynaeve C, Schuller J, Buser K, et al. Comparison of the anti-emetic efficacy of different doses of ondansetron, given as either a continuous infusion or a single intravenous dose, in acute cisplatin-induced emesis. A multicentre, double-blind, randomised, parallel group study. Ondansetron Study Group. Br J Cancer 1992;66:192–7.
31. Ettinger DS, Eisenberg PD, Fitts D, et al. A double-blind comparison of the efficacy of two dose regimens of oral granisetron in preventing acute emesis in patients receiving moderately emetogenic chemotherapy. Cancer 1996;78:144–51.
32. Harman GS, Omura GA, Ryan K, et al. A randomized, double-blind comparison of single-dose and divided multiple-dose dolasetron for cisplatin-induced emesis. Cancer Chemother Pharmacol 1996;38:323–8.
33. Perez EA, Hesketh P, Sandbach J, et al. Comparison of single-dose oral granisetron versus intravenous ondansetron in the prevention of nausea and vomiting induced by moderately emetogenic chemotherapy: a multicenter, double-blind, randomized parallel study. J Clin Oncol 1998;16:754–60.
34. Gralla RJ, Navari RM, Hesketh PJ, et al. Single-dose oral granisetron has equivalent antiemetic efficacy to intravenous ondansetron for highly emetogenic cisplatin-based chemotherapy. J Clin Oncol 1998;16:1568–73.
35. Eisenberg P, Figueroa-Vadillo J, Zamora R, et al. Improved prevention of moderately emetogenic chemotherapy-induced nausea and vomiting with palonosetron, a pharmacologically novel 5-HT3 receptor antagonist: results of a phase III, single-dose trial versus dolasetron. Cancer 2003;98:2473–82.
36. Gralla R, Lichinitser M, Van Der V, et al. Palonosetron improves prevention of chemotherapy-induced nausea and vomiting following moderately emetogenic chemotherapy: results of a double-blind randomized phase III trial comparing single doses of palonosetron with ondansetron. Ann Oncol 2003;14:1570–7.
37. Moertel CG, Reitemeier RJ, Gage RP. A controlled clinical evaluation of antiemetic drugs. JAMA 1963;186:116–8.
38. Kris MG, Gralla RJ, Tyson LB, et al. Improved control of cisplatin-induced emesis with high-dose metoclopramide and with combinations of metoclopramide, dexamethasone, and diphenhydramine. results of consecutive trials in 255 patients. Cancer 1985;55:527–34.
39. Ioannidis JP, Hesketh PJ, Lau J. Contribution of dexamethasone to control of chemotherapy-induced nausea and vomiting: a meta-analysis of randomized evidence. J Clin Oncol 2000;18:3409–22.
40. Dexamethasone, granisetron, or both for the prevention of nausea and vomiting during chemotherapy for cancer. The Italian Group for Antiemetic Research. N Engl J Med 1995;332:1–5.
41. Shadle CR, Lee Y, Majumdar AK, et al. Evaluation of potential inductive effects of aprepitant on cytochrome P450 3A4 and 2C9 activity. J Clin Pharmacol 2004;44:215–23.
42. Razavi D, Delvaux N, Farvacques C, et al. Prevention of adjustment disorders and anticipatory nausea secondary to adjuvant chemotherapy: a double-blind, placebo-controlled study assessing the usefulness of alprazolam. J Clin Oncol 1993;11:1384–90.
43. Sallan SE, Zinberg NE, Frei E III. Antiemetic effect of delta-9-tetrahydrocannabinol in patients receiving cancer chemotherapy. N Engl J Med 1975;293:795–7.
44. Morrow GR, Morrell C. Behavioral treatment for the anticipatory nausea and vomiting induced by cancer chemotherapy. N Engl J Med 1982;307:1476–80.
45. Redd WH, Andrykowski MA. Behavioral intervention in cancer treatment: controlling aversion reactions to chemotherapy. J Consult Clin Psychol 1982;50:1018–29.
46. Horiot JC. Prophylaxis versus treatment: is there a better way to manage radiotherapy-induced nausea and vomiting? Int J Radiat Oncol Biol Phys 2004;60:1018–25.
47. Franzen L, Nyman J, Hagberg H, et al. A randomised placebo controlled study with ondansetron in patients undergoing fractionated radiotherapy. Ann Oncol 1996;7:587–92.
48. Okamoto S, Takahashi S, Tanosaki R, et al. Granisetron in the prevention of vomiting induced by conditioning for stem cell transplantation: a prospective randomized study. Bone Marrow Transplant 1996;17:679–83.
49. Priestman TJ, Roberts JT, Upadhyaya BK. A prospective randomized double-blind trial comparing ondansetron versus prochlorperazine for the prevention of nausea and vomiting in patients undergoing fractionated radiotherapy. Clin Oncol (R Coll Radiol) 1993;5:358–63.
50. Feyer PC, Maranzano E, Molassiotis A, et al. Radiotherapy-induced nausea and vomiting (RINV): antiemetic guidelines. Support Care Cancer 2004.

128

Neurologic Complications

Lisa M. DeAngelis, MD

Disorders of the central or peripheral nervous system affect approximately 15% of patients with cancer.[1] The disorders usually appear in patients with advanced metastatic disease, often as only one of several organ systems involved by the cancer. However, sometimes the neurologic disorder is the first symptom of cancer; for example, approximately 10% of patients with lung cancer present with symptoms of brain metastasis. Regardless of whether neurologic complications occur early or late in the course of the patient's cancer, they uniquely threaten the patient's quality of life by causing such distressing symptoms as dementia, paralysis, incontinence, and pain; in addition, neurologic dysfunction itself often shortens survival.

Neurologic complications of cancer are increasing in frequency. In part, this represents increased opportunity for metastases to the nervous system to develop because systemic tumors are better controlled for longer periods.[2,3] Part of the increase also results from more vigorous treatment of the primary tumor with modalities that cause toxicity to the nervous system. Because these toxic effects are often delayed (eg, radiation-induced dementia), the longer the patient lives, the more likely the toxicity is to appear.

Early diagnosis and appropriate treatment of the neurologic symptoms significantly lessen the impact of neurologic complications on many patients. Thus, it is important for the physician to recognize these complications early. This requires knowledge of those disorders associated with cancer that are likely to affect the nervous system, and also the symptoms and signs that distinguish one neurologic disorder from another. This chapter systematically approaches the diagnosis and treatment of nervous system complications of systemic cancer.

Neurologic complications of cancer can be either metastatic or nonmetastatic (Table 128-1). Metastatic lesions affect the nervous system by direct invasion (eg, brachial plexus metastasis), by compression (eg, epidural spinal cord compression), or by compromise of vascular supply (eg, sagittal sinus occlusion from skull metastases). Brain metastases are discussed in Chapter 73, "Brain Metastases." Although any tumor can metastasize to the nervous system, certain tumors have a predilection for causing particular central or peripheral nervous system disorders, for example, leukemias and lymphomas frequently metastasize to the leptomeninges, but rarely to the brain. Tumors arising in the pelvis are less likely to metastasize to the brain than lung cancer, but when they do, they have a predilection for involving the cerebellum rather than the cerebral hemispheres.[4] Prostate cancer commonly causes epidural spinal cord and cauda equina compression[5] because of its tendency to metastasize to the vertebral bodies, but leptomeningeal or brain involvement is much less common.[6]

Nonmetastatic neurologic complications are often tumor specific. Metabolic derangements are more likely to occur with tumors that metastasize widely to vital organs, such as liver (colon cancer), or that cause changes in fluid and electrolyte balance, such as hypercalcemia (breast cancer) or inappropriate antidiuretic hormone secretion (small-cell lung cancer). Central nervous system (CNS) infections are more common in patients whose cancer is associated with immune suppression, as in Hodgkin's disease. Vascular complications are more common in hematologic malignancies than in solid tumors.[7] Paraneoplastic syndromes affecting the nervous system are much more frequent with certain tumors, such as small-cell lung cancer and ovarian cancer, than with the more common adenocarcinomas of lung, colon, and breast.[8]

The physician encountering a cancer patient with neurologic symptoms may begin by considering the disorders listed in Table 128-1. From a more practical point of view, it is often easier to identify the site of neurologic dysfunction by its signs and symptoms and to consider first only those neurologic complications likely to affect that particular site. This approach to diagnosis is listed in Table 128-2.

METASTASES

Spinal Metastases Metastatic lesions compressing the spinal cord or cauda equina are, after brain metastases, the most common symptomatic neurologic complication of metastatic cancer.[1,9,10]

Table 128-1 Neurologic Complications of Cancer

Metastases
Intracranial (usually to brain)
Spinal (usually epidural)
Leptomeningeal (usually base of brain and cauda equina)
Cranial nerves (usually from base of skull lesions)
Peripheral nerves (usually brachial or lumbosacral plexus)
Muscle (rare)
Nonmetastatic
Complications of treatment (radiation, chemotherapy)
Vascular disorders (hemorrhage, infarcts)
Metabolic, nutritional disorders
Paraneoplastic syndromes
Infections

Table 128-2 Neurologic Complications in Cancer Patients by Site

Site	Usual Causes	Typical Symptoms and Signs
Brain	Metastasis Leptomeningeal metastasis Metabolic/toxic encephalopathy Infection (meningitis, brain abscess) Radiation encephalopathy Cerebral hemorrhage or infarction Paraneoplastic (limbic encephalopathy)	Headache Confusion Hemiparesis Seizures Ataxia
Spinal cord and cauda equina	Epidural metastasis Leptomeningeal metastasis Intramedullary metastasis Epidural abscess or hematoma Radiation myelopathy Myelopathy following intrathecal chemotherapy Paraneoplastic myelopathy	Back pain Paraparesis Sensory level Incontinence
Cranial and peripheral nerves	Extrinsic compression by tumor or other mass (eg, hematoma) Direct infiltration by tumor Drug toxicity Varicella-zoster infection Radiation plexopathy Paraneoplastic neuropathy	Focal pain Sensory loss Motor weakness Decreased reflexes in nerve distribution (focal lesion) or distally in hands and feet (polyneuropathy)
Neuromuscular junction	Drugs (aminoglycoside antibiotics) Paraneoplastic disorders (Eaton-Lambert myasthenic syndrome, myasthenia gravis)	Diffuse weakness without sensory loss Respiratory insufficiency
Muscle	Metastasis Steroid myopathy Cachectic myopathy Paraneoplastic polymyositis or dermatomyositis	Proximal weakness Weakness without sensory loss

The spinal cord ends at the L-1 or L-2 vertebral body but compression of the cauda equina below that level is usually also considered spinal cord compression (SCC) because the diagnosis and treatment are identical.[1] SCC causes pain and, if untreated, paralysis and incontinence. Patients who become paraplegic as a result of cancer usually die within a matter of months. On the other hand, clinical studies indicate that early diagnosis (while the patient is still ambulatory) and prompt treatment maintain a patient's independent ambulation, and usually result in longer survival.[1,11,12]

Approximately 5% of patients dying of cancer have evidence of SCC at autopsy, suggesting 18,000 to 20,000 new cases of SCC annually in the United States.[13] Approximately 10% of new patients referred to a large cancer center have metastases to the spinal column.[14] Breast,[15,16] lung, prostate,[17] and lymphoma[18] are the most common primary cancers causing SCC (Table 128-3). SCC usually occurs in the late stages of metastatic cancer, but in up to 20% of patients being treated for neoplastic SCC, cancer was unsuspected prior to the neurologic symptoms. Lymphoma, kidney, and lung primaries each account for approximately 20% of such cases.

Vertebral metastases are common in patients with metastatic cancer. The cancer usually spreads hematogenously to the vertebral column, via either the arterial system or Batson venous plexus.[19] SCC then results when the vertebral body metastasis extends into the spinal canal or paraspinal tumor invades the epidural space through a neural foramen (Figure 128-1). Lymphomas and neuroblastomas often invade the spinal canal through neural foramina without destruction of bone. Epidural lesions may also result when tumors in the colon, kidney, prostate, or head and neck area grow directly into vertebral structures. Less common causes of spinal cord dysfunction result from metastases to a vertebral pedicle, lamina, or arch, or hematogenous metastasis to the epidural space, or to the spinal cord itself. When a metastasis causes the vertebral body to collapse, bone, tumor, and ligament may extend into the spinal canal to compress the spinal cord.

The thoracic spine is the most common location of SCC, followed by the lumbosacral and cervical spine in a ratio of about 4:2:1. Colon cancer preferentially involves the lumbosacral spine. Two or more contiguous vertebral bodies are involved by metastatic disease in approximately 25% of patients with SCC, but, unlike infection, the intervertebral disc space is preserved.[20] As many as 32% of patients have other sites of SCC in addition to the clinically suspected location,[21] emphasizing the importance of imaging the entire length of the spinal canal when evaluating a patient for suspected epidural disease. Multiple sites of vertebral metastases predict a poor prognosis.

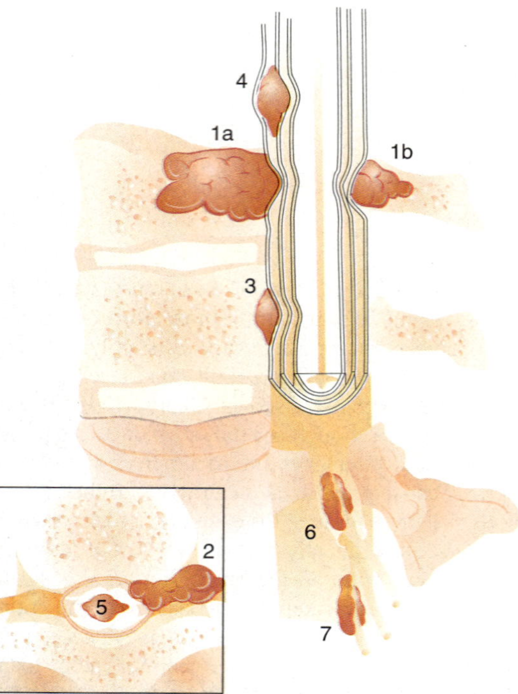

Figure 128-1 Neoplastic epidural spinal cord compression results from direct extension of a bony metastasis to the vertebral body (1a) or posterior elements (1b), by paraspinal neoplasm infiltrating through neural foramina (2), or a direct metastasis to the epidural space (3). Unusual causes of spinal metastases include subdural metastasis (4), intramedullary metastasis (5), and paraspinal metastasis to the radicular vessels (6) or root (7).

Pathophysiology of Spinal Cord Compression The mechanism(s) by which neurologic symptoms and signs are caused by SCC are not fully understood. The symptoms and signs depend on the level of compression (eg, cervical versus thoracic), but not on the site of compression in the transverse plane (eg, anterior, posterior or lateral).[1] In almost half of patients, epidural tumor is found both anterior and posterior to the spinal cord; in approximately one-fifth of patients, the tumor is circumferential.[22] Histologic studies show changes limited mainly to the lateral and posterior columns, while the central gray matter shows few abnormalities. The common abnormality is demyelination with infiltration by lipid-laden macrophages, interstitial edema, and focal axonal swelling, but infarction is rare, even in patients who develop the sudden onset of paraplegia. Traumatic injury causes a greater inflammatory response and more breakdown of the blood-CNS tissue barrier in spinal cord than in brain.[23] Compression of the epidural venous plexus (possibly contributing to spinal cord edema) occurs early in SCC, whereas obliteration of cord parenchymal vessels with decreased spinal cord blood flow takes place much later. These data suggest that cord ischemia is not a critical factor, at least in the early phases of SCC. Animal models of SCC demonstrate a disrupted blood–spinal cord barrier with vasogenic cord edema that decreases after corticosteroid administration. It is likely that mechanical pressure on the cord and its venous drainage in some manner produces a conduction block, with demyelination and spinal cord edema, resulting in symptomatic spinal cord dysfunction. Increasing evidence also suggests that release of potentially neurotoxic substances, including prostaglandins and serotonin, by compressed neural tissue may play a role in the development of neurologic disability.

Clinical Findings Back pain is the first symptom of SCC in virtually all patients (Table 128-4).[1] The pain may be local (at the involved area of the spine), radicular (radiating into arm, trunk, or leg), or both. The local pain is dull and aching; it is progressive and usually localizes within one or two segments of the involved area of the spine. Local pain caused by movement implies spinal instability. Radicular pain may be constant or brought on by movement. In the cervical and lumbosacral regions, radicular pain is often unilateral, but in the trunk, it is bilateral (band-like), a finding that is highly suggestive of epidural disease. Pain from SCC is typically worse when the patient is supine, so the patient may sleep sitting up. This feature may help to distinguish epidural tumor from a herniated disc where the pain improves when the patient is supine. The pain of SCC is exacerbated by coughing, straining, or flexion of the neck. During the examination, an attempt should be made to reproduce the patient's pain by spine percussion, gentle neck flexion, and straight leg raising. Pain may be absent in those patients whose SCC is identified incidentally on chest or abdominal computed tomography (CT) or magnetic resonance imaging (MRI) scans done to evaluate the patient's primary cancer.

Table 128-3 Primary Cancer Causing Symptomatic Spinal Cord Compression in 583 Patients at Memorial Sloan-Kettering Cancer Center (MSKCC)

Primary Tumor	Number of Patients
Breast	127
Lung	90
Prostate	58
Lymphoreticular	56
Sarcoma	52
Kidney	39
Gastrointestinal	29
Melanoma	23
Unknown primary	21
Head and neck	19
Miscellaneous	69
Total	583

Table 128-4 Symptoms and Signs of Spinal Cord Compression in 213 Patients at Memorial Sloan-Kettering Cancer Center (MSKCC)

	First Symptom		Present at Diagnosis	
	No.	%	No.	%
Pain	201	94	207	97
Weakness	7	3	157	74
Autonomic dysfunction	0	0	111	52
Sensory loss	1	0.5	112	53
Ataxia	2	0.9	8	4

Weakness is the second most common initial feature of epidural SCC; it usually follows the onset of pain by weeks to months. The weakness is most obvious in proximal muscles of the legs so that the patient may complain of difficulty when arising from a low chair or the toilet seat or when climbing stairs. By the time weakness occurs, tone in the lower extremities is usually increased, deep tendon reflexes are hyperactive, and the plantar responses are extensor. If the SCC occurs below the cord involving the cauda equina, hyporeflexia or areflexia is found. Proximal weakness might at first suggest a myopathy, but in that disorder, the proximal upper extremities are usually also weak, the tendon reflexes and muscle tone are normal, and sensory changes are absent. Strength in the legs can easily be tested by having the patients walk on their heels, walk on their toes, and do a deep knee bend. If all of these are performed easily, it is unlikely that the patient has significant weakness. If pain limits strength testing, analgesics should be administered to permit adequate evaluation.

Bowel and bladder dysfunction usually occur late in SCC. However, when the conus medullaris is the site of compression (vertebral lesions from T-10 to L-1), bladder dysfunction may be the first and only sign. Both the patient and the physician may fail to recognize that frequent small voidings may be a sign of urinary retention. The patient may be unaware of urinary retention because bladder sensation is lost. Palpation of the abdomen often reveals a distended bladder, and a post-void catheterization reveals urinary retention. The anal sphincter is usually flaccid, with loss of both voluntary and reflex constriction (anal wink).

Sensory symptoms include numbness and paresthesias that usually begin in the toes and spread proximally. Except in conus compression, the sacral segments may be spared, even when a sensory level to pinprick is found on the trunk. In a few patients, gait or truncal ataxia mimicking cerebellar disease may be the only neurologic finding although back pain usually precedes the ataxia. Varicella-zoster eruption may occur at the dermatomal level of epidural metastasis. If it precedes the diagnosis of the spinal metastasis, it can delay recognition of SCC.

None of the clinical signs or symptoms of epidural SCC are specific. Table 128-5 lists some of the disorders that can mimic SCC in patients with cancer. Some, such as lumbar strain, herniated disc, or spinal stenosis, are common in patients without cancer and may confuse the initial evaluation of an individual cancer patient. Others, such as epidural hematomas and abscesses, may be directly related to the cancer or its treatment. Metastases generally do not involve the intervertebral disc, and abnormalities at the disc space should raise the question of vertebral osteomyelitis or herniated disc. In most instances, evaluation with magnetic resonance imaging (MRI) is necessary and sufficient to establish the diagnosis.

Patients with cancer who develop back pain have SCC until proved otherwise (Figure 128-2). Evaluation should proceed urgently because patients with high-grade compression may develop abrupt compromise of the spinal cord and severe neurologic dysfunction. Risk factors for high-grade compression include (1) myelopathy on examination, (2) plain films revealing greater than 50% vertebral body collapse or pedicle erosion (three-fourths of patients with these radiographic findings have epidural disease), or (3) the presence of local and radicular pain (one-half of these patients have epidural disease).

The most sensitive and specific and usually the only necessary diagnostic test for spinal lesions caused by cancer is an MRI (Figure 128-3).[24–26] The entire spine should be imaged, but contrast is not necessary to detect spine metastasis or epidural tumor. However, contrast is essential to identify intramedullary spinal metastasis or leptomeningeal tumor. Those rare occasions when epidural mass lesions are missed by MRI appear to be a result of failure to examine the spine in its most lateral aspects and to obtain appropriate transverse, as well as sagittal, images. MR scans also distinguish malignant lesions from benign ones, such as disc herniation.

Table 128-5 Differential Diagnosis of Epidural Spinal Cord Compression

Diagnosis	Example(s)	Diagnostic Test
Intramedullary tumor	Glioma Metastasis	MRI with gadolinium
Extramedullary-intradural tumor	Meningioma Neurofibroma Drop metastasis from primary brain tumor Metastasis from systemic primary	MRI with gadolinium
Leptomeningeal tumor	Primary lymphoma Metastasis	MRI with gadolinium, CSF cytology
Radiation myelopathy	Previous RT to spine	MRI with gadolinium
Arteriovenous malformation		MRI with gadolinium, myelogram, arteriogram
Transverse myelopathy	Postinfectious myelopathy, multiple sclerosis	MRI with gadolinium
Epidural hematoma	Thrombocytopenia (history of lumbar puncture)	MRI or CT
Epidural abscess	Sepsis, epidural catheter (for pain control)	MRI with gadolinium/culture
Degenerative spinal disorder	Herniated disc, spinal stenosis	MRI
Osteoporosis	Vertebral collapse	MRI/biopsy

CSF = cerebrospinal fluid; CT = computed tomography; MRI = magnetic resonance imaging; RT = radiation therapy.
Adapted from Posner JB.[1]

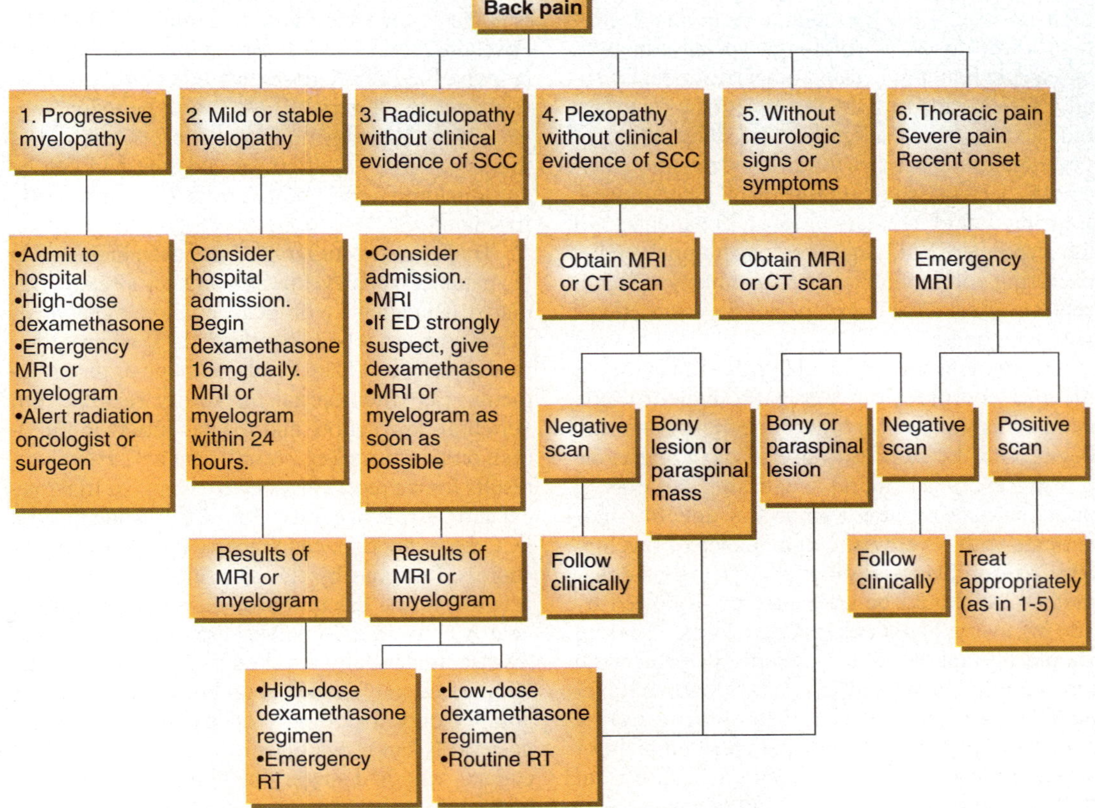

Figure 128-2 Algorithm for the management of back pain in cancer patients.

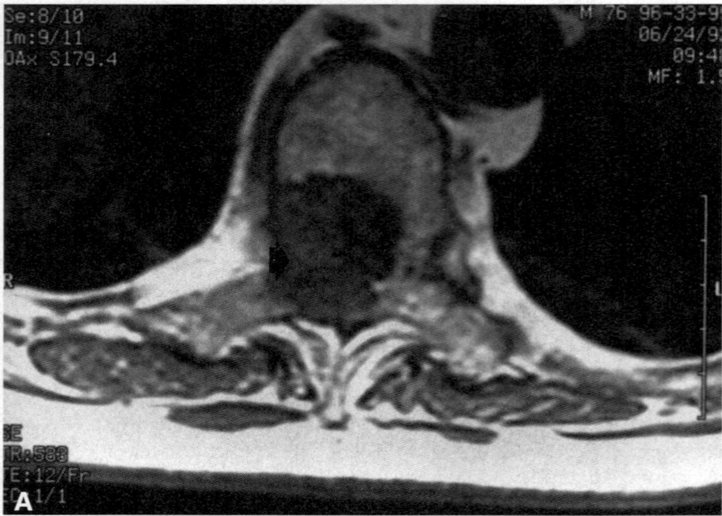
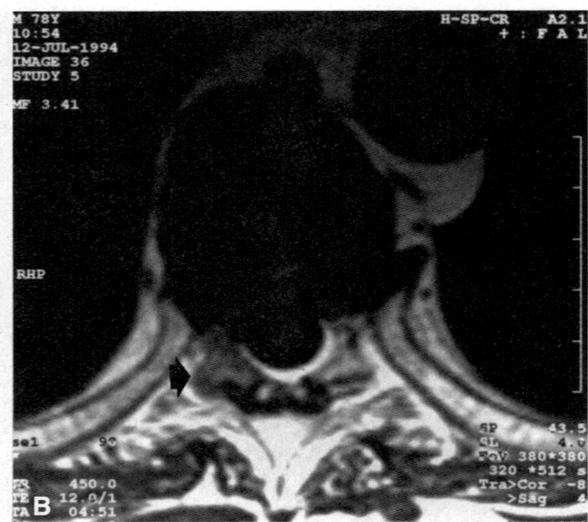

Figure 128-3 Magnetic resonance image demonstrating spinal cord compression from metastatic prostate cancer. **A,** Tumor *(arrowhead)* in the vertebral body and posterior elements compressing and distorting the spinal cord and pushing it to the left. **B,** Axial image at the same level after treatment with radiotherapy, demonstrating resolution of the cord compression and reduction of the tumor mass; residual tumor *(arrowhead).*

Treatment Spinal epidural disease requires urgent therapy directed at reduction of tumor mass and prevention of regrowth.[1,27] Radiation therapy is the primary treatment for most patients, but surgery and chemotherapy are important modalities in individual patients (see below). Re-evaluation during and following treatment is essential. Delay in diagnosis compromises therapy. Many patients present on Fridays suggesting that referral is often delayed.[28]

The initial treatment for all patients is corticosteroids. Corticosteroids have two effects: their oncolytic effect may relieve cord compression by shrinking tumors, especially lymphoma, but in most instances, their salutary effects probably result from their reduction of spinal cord edema. In experimental models, corticosteroids decreased cord edema and improved neurologic function, and higher doses have been found to be more effective than lower doses,[29,30] although not all clinicians agree.[31] In humans, because other treatment is usually started concurrently, the effect of corticosteroids is difficult to evaluate. In one study, 40 mg of dexamethasone per day, followed by radiation therapy (RT), resulted in "improvement" in neurologic function within 24 hours in 18 of 29 patients; 5 of the responders had lymphoma. Such improvement occurring within the first 24 h is unlikely to represent an effect of RT, except possibly in patients with lymphoma.

For patients with clinical or MR scan evidence of cord compression, but without neurologic symptoms except for moderate pain, one can begin with the standard dose of dexamethasone (16 mg every 24 hours), increasing the dose if pain persists or new symptoms develop. For patients with severe pain, or evidence of myelopathy, an intravenous bolus of 100 mg of dexamethasone should be administered, followed by 100 mg every 24 hours in divided doses. The drug should be tapered as the patient is treated with more definitive modalities (see below). Intravenous dexamethasone is infused slowly over a period of 5 to 10 min; some patients complain of severe genital burning as the drug is infused, but this lasts only a few minutes and is easily tolerated, particularly if the patient is forewarned.

Corticosteroids cause side effects, and some may be more prominent in patients with epidural SCC. Perforation of the gastrointestinal (GI) tract may occur in as many as 1% of patients; constipation, a frequent complication of SCC, appears to increase the risk of GI rupture. Postoperative infections may be more frequent in patients treated with corticosteroids.

Radiation therapy is the most common treatment for patients with SCC,[10] many of whom are poor surgical candidates because of advanced cancer or multiple vertebral body metastases. Radiotherapy is administered to a port that includes the site of compression and two vertebral bodies above and below that level. The width of the port depends on the amount of paraspinal disease. Variations in fractionation schedule do not influence outcome, and the standard schedule is 300 cGy for 10 fractions to a total of 3,000 cGy. A second course of RT for patients who initially respond but then relapse may be helpful and carries only modest risk.[32] Recent experience suggests that intensity-modulated stereotactic radiotherapy (IMRT) is effective and safe and can be administered with good results to a previously irradiated site.[33]

Traditionally, surgery[34,35] has been indicated in (1) patients who develop SCC at sites already irradiated, (2) patients with SCC in whom a diagnosis of cancer has not been established, (3) when epidural defects result from displaced bone or disc fragments, (4) when spinal instability results from vertebral destruction, and (5) patients with radioresistant tumors (eg, renal cancer). However, results from a recent prospective phase III trial may expand the role of surgery for SCC.[36] Patients with SCC were randomized to receive focal RT alone or surgery followed by RT. The surgical procedure was left to the discretion of the surgeon, but the goal was to do a complete resection of the local disease; this usually required an anterior approach with resection of the vertebral body in contrast to a laminectomy that simply opens the spinal canal posteriorly but rarely permits tumor removal. The patients who had surgery had a superior outcome with significantly better neurologic function for longer, including a greater proportion of patients who regained ambulation and continence. Length of survival was not significantly different between the two groups, but there was a trend towards longer survival with surgery (129 days vs 100 days, $p = .08$). These data suggest that surgery should be a consideration in all patients with SCC. However, the patients enrolled in the study were highly selected and it is not clear that the excellent outcome reported here can be expected for all patients with SCC.

The surgical approach depends in part on the location of the tumor, type of reconstruction necessary, and general condition of the patient.[35] Intraoperative radiation therapy has been reported to help control local recurrence,[37] but preoperative RT may lead to more surgical morbidity.[34] Vertebroplasty may be effective for treating pain, but is contraindicated in patients with SCC and can be complicated by extravasation of cement beyond the confines of the vertebra.[38]

Figure 128-2 illustrates our approach to the treatment of SCC. Regardless of treatment type, the majority of patients who are ambulatory at the beginning of therapy remain ambulatory. Some paraparetic patients will recover sufficient function to walk again, but only a few patients who are paraplegic recover useful function.

Chemotherapy, with or without radiation therapy, is useful in some patients with tumors that are sensitive, especially lymphoma and occasionally other solid tumors.[39–41] Excellent responses of SCC from chemosensitive tumors to appropriate chemotherapy are seen, but this approach is limited to those patients who have pain as the only symptom. If myelopathy is present, corticosteroids and RT or surgery must be the primary therapy.

Leptomeningeal Metastasis Leptomeningeal metastasis (LM), also called carcinomatous or neoplastic meningitis, is less frequent than brain metastasis or SCC, but it is becoming increasingly common, particularly in patients with small-cell lung, breast, and ovarian cancers.[42] Quality of life and duration of survival are both severely compromised by LM, and fewer than half of those treated by currently available therapy receive benefit.[43]

Table 128-6 Frequency of Leptomeningeal Metastases (LM) in Various Cancers

Cancer	Percent Developing LM	Features
Carcinoma		
Breast	5	Incidence may be increasing, more common with infiltrating lobular carcinoma
SCLC	9–25	Incidence is increasing, risk increases with duration of survival
NSCLC	?	Less common than breast, probably more common overall than SCLC LM
Melanoma	23	50% at autopsy
Leukemia		
AML	< 5	10% without prophylaxis, associated with high white blood count, elevated LDH, extramedullary disease at diagnosis, and with monocytic morphology
ALL	11	30% without prophylaxis, associated with T-cell phenotype, Burkitt's morphology and high white blood cell count at diagnosis
CLL	Rare	May occur during blast crisis
Lymphoma		
NHL	4–10	Associated with diffuse histiocytic and lymphocytic histology, bone marrow involvement
HD	Rare	
Overall	8.6	LM present at autopsy in 56 of 649 brains examined at Memorial Sloan-Kettering Cancer Center

Abbreviations: ALL = acute lymphocytic leukemia; AML = acute myelogenous leukemia; CLL = chronic lymphocytic leukemia; HD = Hodgkin's disease; LDH = lactic acid dehydrogenase; NHL = non-Hodgkin's lymphoma; NSCLC = non-small cell lung cancer; SCLC = small cell lung cancer.

Reliable estimates of the incidence of LM are difficult to obtain. Few studies of LM give incidence figures and the diagnosis is heavily dependent on the diligence with which it is pursued. Autopsies may double the number of clinically diagnosed cases of LM, but a routine autopsy may miss focal LM. Recognizing these limitations, Table 128-6 lists the reported frequency of LM in patients with various cancers. Overall, LM is probably found in approximately 5% of patients with metastatic cancer.

Pathophysiology Malignant cells may enter the subarachnoid space by several routes (Figure 128-4). Direct infiltration of the subarachnoid space from dural and bone-based lesions has been well documented. In an autopsy study of children with acute lymphocytic leukemia (ALL), early findings of subarachnoid invasion included infiltration of the wall of veins and of the marrow trabeculae[44]; infiltration via the bridging veins from the marrow of the skull also occurs. Studies with B16 melanoma clones that metastasize to the meninges of mice show that malignant cells attach to the walls of leptomeningeal capillaries and then move directly into the subarachnoid space.[45] Brain parenchymal lesions can erode into the ventricle or into the subarachnoid space or be spilled at surgery, causing LM.[46] LM develops in 40% of patients following resection of a cerebellar metastasis, but in only 2 to 3% of those who had resection of a supratentorial lesion presumably due to the large cerebrospinal fluid (CSF)-containing spaces in the posterior fossa. The choroid plexus is a route of entry in a few cases. Malignant cells may invade the subarachnoid space by direct infiltration along nerve roots, and possibly via epineural lymphatics.

Leptomeningeal metastasis is probably not a random metastatic event. Infiltrating lobular breast cancer often causes LM, whereas infiltrating ductal carcinoma metastasizes to the brain more commonly. Specific chromosomal abnormalities and eosinophilia in acute myelogenous leukemia (AML) appear to correlate with meningeal chloromas. Experimental B16 melanoma clones derived by serial re-inoculation of meningeal deposits eventually produce predominantly LM.[45]

At autopsy, the leptomeninges may be opacified by tumor, and the sulci may be obliterated. The inferior surface of the brain and the dorsal surface of the spinal cord and the cauda equina are commonly involved areas. Nodular deposits may be visible on nerve roots, especially in the cauda equina. Frequently, however, there is no grossly visible evidence of LM. Communicating hydrocephalus is present in some patients. Microscopically, tumor growth may be focal in any location of the subarachnoid space, or may infiltrate the leptomeninges diffusely. Blood vessels are often ensheathed by tumor, and superficial nodular deposits often form in the parenchyma of the brain and spinal cord via perivascular (Virchow–Robin) spaces. Ischemic changes may be seen superficially in the brain and cerebral infarction has been reported. Nerve roots may be either encased in tumor or directly infiltrated. Fibrosis of the arachnoid membranes is common. Inflammation may be florid but is often sparse or absent.

Leptomeningeal metastasis causes nervous system dysfunction by several mechanisms.[1,47,48] (1) There is often direct infiltration of malignant cells into the brain, spinal cord, or cranial nerves and spinal roots as they traverse the subarachnoid space. Such infiltration interferes with neural function. (2) Infiltration of the subarachnoid space by tumor interrupts CSF absorption and leads to hydrocephalus with its attendant symptoms of cognitive dysfunction, gait abnormalities, and incontinence. (3) Infiltration of tumor along the Virchow–Robin spaces may reduce blood supply to the brain, and cerebral infarction has been reported.[49] (4) By either infiltrating into neural parenchyma or lying on its surface, LM may interfere with neural metabolism. In an experimental model of LM, regional changes in cerebral glucose use have been identified.[50]

Symptoms and Signs Two clinical findings suggest LM. The first is synchronous symptoms or signs at multiple sites of the neuraxis.[1,42,51] This clinical pattern is a result of the multifocal or disseminated nature of the disease. The second is the presence of findings on neurologic examination without symptoms. An example is finding leg weakness or an absent ankle reflex in a patient complaining of diplopia or headache. Multifocal findings are not pathognomonic of LM, however, because multiple parenchymal metastases involving the central or peripheral nervous system can yield a similar clinical picture. Certain characteristic symptoms and signs should lead the physician to suspect LM. These include (1) headache, particularly early in the morning or posturally induced headache in the absence of CT or MRI evidence of cerebral metastases; (2) cranial nerve palsies, in particular, diplopia or facial weakness; (3) neck pain with or without nuchal rigidity in the absence of bony metastases of the cervical spine; (4) radicular pain in the upper or lower extremities, particularly when accompanied by weakness but not by local spine pain; (5) unexplained constipation, impotence, or urinary incontinence or retention (urinary retention is an early sign of LM); (6) asymmetric leg weakness and diminished reflexes in the absence of pain or sensory changes; and (7) confusion, memory loss, or other cognitive abnormalities.

Diagnosis The diagnosis of LM is usually established by the demonstration of malignant cells in the CSF. An MRI of the brain should be obtained prior to lumbar puncture. A cranial MRI suggests LM when either communicating hydrocephalus or meningeal enhancement is detected.[52] A gadolinium-enhanced spine MRI may demonstrate tumor nodules on spinal roots, particularly in the cauda equina, even when symptoms of nerve root dysfunction are absent (Figure 128-5). The whole neuraxis should be imaged to identify sites of bulky disease. When characteristic findings are identified, this may suffice to establish the diagnosis.[53–55] MRI is 76% sensitive and 77% specific.[52] When a lumbar puncture is performed, opening pressure measurement, cell count, protein, glucose, and bacterial and fungal studies should be obtained. The cytology specimen should contain at least 10 mL of CSF optimally, and should be processed quickly according to the laboratory's protocol.

Malignant cells are found in the initial CSF sample in 50 to 60% of patients with LM.[51] False-positives are rare, except in patients with lymphoma or leukemia, where the distinction between reactive and malignant cells may be difficult. Cytologic examination is 75% sensitive, but almost 100% specific.[52] In patients with subsequently documented LM and a negative first cytology, one or two additional samples increase the yield. In a few patients, cisternal CSF may be positive when lumbar CSF is negative. Likewise, cytology may be positive in ventricular fluid but negative in lum-

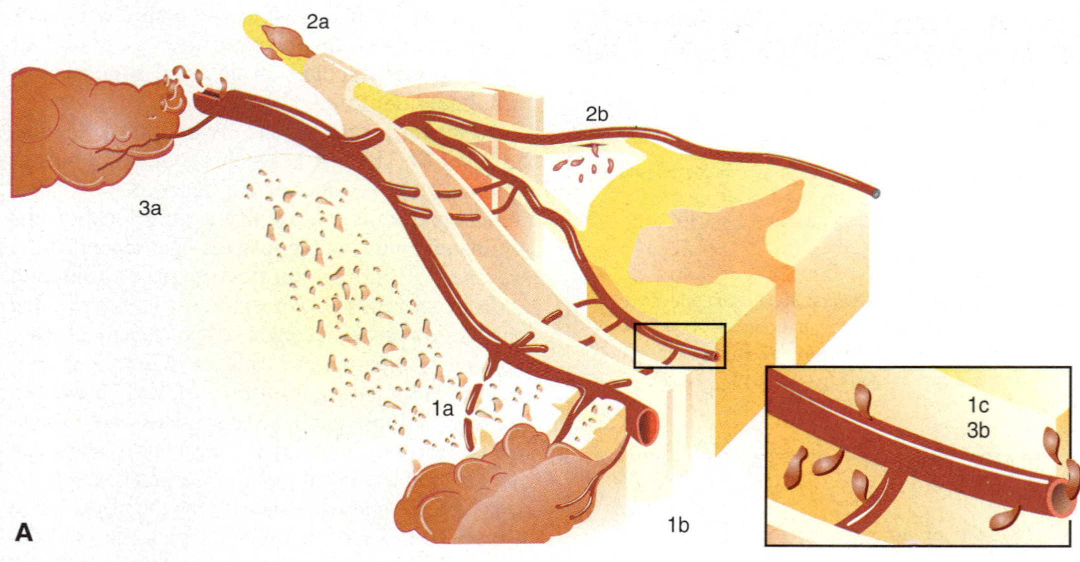

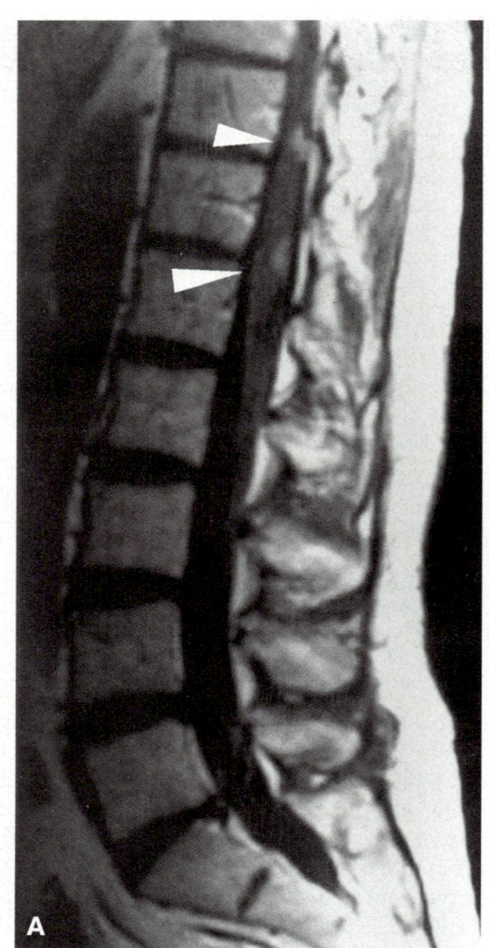

Figure 128-4 Pathophysiology of leptomeningeal metastases. **A,** Mechanisms of tumor cell entry into the spinal subarachnoid space. Tumor may invade the vertebral body (1a) and grow along vertebral veins (1b) into the subarachnoid space (1c). Tumor may invade peripheral nerves or nerve roots outside the vertebral canal (2a) and grow along the nerve sheath into the spinal canal to seed the leptomeninges (2b). The tumor can invade blood vessels outside the central nervous system (3a) and transverse subarachnoid veins into the subarachnoid space (3b). With permission from Posner JB.[1] **B,** Possible mechanisms of tumor entry into the cerebral subarachnoid space. Tumor may enter the cranial subarachnoid space via metastases either to the skull or brain, to the diploic veins of the skull, or directly from subarachnoid veins. The choroid plexus (not shown) is also an occasional site for the formation of leptomeningeal tumor.

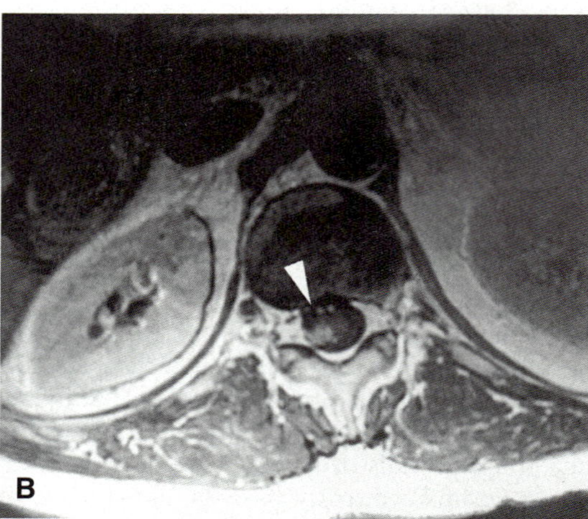

Figure 128-5 Gadolinium enhanced magnetic resonance imaging demonstrating leptomeningeal metastases from lung cancer. **A,** Sagittal and **B,** axial images demonstrating enhancing nodules within the thecal sac. This patient had a positive cerebrospinal fluid cytology for malignant cells.

bar fluid or vice versa.[56] In the remaining patients, the diagnosis must be supported by other tests. It is rare for a patient with LM to have an entirely normal initial lumbar puncture. Increased opening pressure, pleocytosis, increased CSF protein, and decreased CSF glucose are almost always present in some combination.[51]

Tumor markers,[42,43,57] deoxyribonucleic acid (DNA) studies, immunocytochemistry, and positron emission tomography (PET) scan[58] may help confirm LM when cytologic studies are negative. A tumor-associated antigen in the spinal fluid is virtually pathognomonic of LM. In the presence of a normal blood–brain barrier (suggested by a normal CSF protein concentration), the level of tumor antigens, such as carcinoembryonic antigen (CEA), beta human chorionic gonadotropin (βHCG), cancer antigen (CA) 125, breast cancer antigen, and prostate-specific antigen (PSA), should be no greater than 1% of the serum level. When that amount is exceeded, and particularly if the CSF level is higher than the serum level, the diagnosis is established, even in the absence of a positive cytology. Other markers, such as β-glucuronidase and β2-microglobulin, are less specific because inflammatory conditions frequently elevate these markers as well. If tumor markers are elevated in a patient with documented LM, they can also be used to follow disease status, provided the samples are always taken from the same site (ie, values from ventricular CSF cannot be compared with those from lumbar CSF). Table 128-7 lists tumor markers commonly employed in CSF studies.

An abnormal DNA content of cells in the CSF measured by flow cytometry or in situ hybridization[57] supports the diagnosis of LM. Fewer than 500 cells are necessary for analysis, so data can be obtained on almost all CSF samples (4 to 5 mL). When LM is suspected in patients with lymphoma or leukemia and the CSF contains cytologically nondiagnostic lymphocytes, immunohistochemistry, flow cytometry, or molecular markers[59] may demonstrate a clonal excess of cells similar to the phenotype of the systemic neoplasm, suggesting LM.

Treatment Untreated, LM usually causes relentless progression of neurologic dysfunction and death within weeks. Treatment is not very effective, and some believe that it does not reverse fixed neurologic deficits. Nevertheless, therapy alters the clinical course in about one-half of patients and often improves symptoms.[60] Occasionally, the course may be indolent especially in patients with LM from lymphoma or breast cancer.

Table 128-7 CSF Tumor Markers

CSF Tumor Marker	Comments
CEA	Above 1% of serum CEA[a] in colon and breast carcinoma
β-HCG	Choriocarcinoma, embryonal carcinoma, germ cell tumor
α-FP	Teratocarcinoma, yolk sac tumor, endodermal sinus tumor, embryonal carcinoma
CA 125	Ovarian carcinoma
CA 15-3	Breast cancer
β2-microglobulin	Above 2.0 mg/L.[a] Lymphoma (not specific), elevated by infection
β-glucuronidase	Above 80 mU/L[a] (not specific)
LDH	Isoenzyme 5 above 10% of total LDH[a] (not specific)
PSA	Prostate cancer

[a]Values suggestive of leptomeningeal metastasis.

Abbreviations: α-FP = α-fetoprotein; CEA = carcinoembryonic antigen; CSF = cerebrospinal fluid; HCG = human chorionic gonadotropin; LDH = lactic dehydrogenase; PSA = prostate specific antigen.

The type of primary cancer is the best predictor of response to treatment; the majority of lymphoma and breast cancer patients respond because these tumors are relatively sensitive to RT and the few chemotherapeutic agents that can be safely instilled into the CSF (see below). Patients with lung cancer or melanoma respond in about one-third and one-fifth of cases, respectively. Patients with severe neurologic disability from LM are less likely to derive benefit because neural damage is often irreversible. Correlations between CSF findings at diagnosis and subsequent response to therapy have been contradictory. Differences between chemotherapy administered intraventricularly and by lumbar puncture suggest that the intraventricular route is superior. Because LM disrupts the blood–brain barrier, systemic chemotherapy, particularly when administered in high doses, may also be effective.[61,62] If symptomatic hydrocephalus is present, a ventriculoperitoneal shunt should be considered.

Among patients receiving therapy for LM, survival is prolonged only in those whose disease responds to treatment.[60] Although this is not surprising, the inability to predict which patients will respond to treatment makes prognostication difficult. In addition to surviving longer (4 to 6 months median versus 1 to 2 months median in nonresponders), patients who respond to therapy are less likely to die as a result of their LM than are patients whose disease progresses despite therapy.

Radiation Therapy RT should be administered to symptomatic or radiologically involved areas of LM.[42] Symptomatic sites should be treated even if subarachnoid tumor is not evident radiographically at the symptomatic location. Entire neuraxis RT is rarely used because of its acute morbidity and myelosuppression that interferes with subsequent chemotherapy. Neuraxis RT is not used even when bulky LM is seen on MRI along the entire spinal axis; RT is still restricted to symptomatic areas. The brain is the most common site to which RT is administered, usually in a dose of 3,000 cGy, but the cauda equina is also a common location that produces symptoms requiring RT. Treatment ports should be generous, and for brain, RT should include the cribriform plate and the skull base. During cranial RT, patients often benefit symptomatically from dexamethasone, but corticosteroids do not relieve spinal symptoms. In a study of response of cranial nerve deficits from lymphoma and leukemia LM, early RT (3 days or less after onset of symptoms) resulted in more rapid improvement than treatment later in the course (more than 3 days), but the ultimate response rate was equal between the two treatment groups.[63]

Chemotherapy Intrathecal chemotherapy is used in conjunction with RT in the treatment of LM.[43,64] The most commonly used agent is methotrexate (MTX), which is active against breast cancer, lymphoma, and leukemia, but has poor activity against some of the other common cancers that cause LM, such as lung cancer.

The MTX is administered intrathecally to adults in doses of 12 to 15 mg, diluted in preservative-free saline. With this dose, MTX levels in the CSF exceed the therapeutic concentration of 10^{-6} M and remain above this level for about 36 to 48 hours.[65] Normal flow patterns of CSF may be altered by intradural deposits of tumor. Studies of CSF flow dynamics using indium[111]-DPTA (diethylenetriamine pentaacetic acid) cisternography have found some obstruction to CSF flow in a high percentage of patients with LM, raising the question of whether flow studies are required before starting treatment. Obstruction of CSF flow should be considered in patients with LM who develop focal leukoencephalopathy around the ventricular catheter track. Indium[111] studies do predict CSF MTX distribution and indicate that drug reaches all areas of the subarachnoid space unless a complete block is present.[43,66] Patients with impaired CSF flow have a worse prognosis, likely reflecting the extent of subarachnoid tumor, and increased incidence of leukoencephalopathy due to impaired egress of drug out of the ventricular system.

MTX appears in the serum for prolonged periods following intrathecal administration, and myelosuppression and stomatitis may result. Oral leucovorin can be administered to avert these complications starting 12 hours after MTX injection. Leucovorin does not appear in the CSF in appreciable amounts, but the active conversion product, 5-methyltetrahydrofolate (5-methylTHFA), does; however, the CSF levels of 5-methylTHFA are very low after oral leucovorin administration. High-dose intravenous MTX (eg, 3 to 8 g/m^2) may result in CSF MTX levels that exceed 10^{-6} M, and may represent an alternative to intrathecal delivery, particularly in patients with impaired CSF flow. Systemic drugs may also treat bulky LM, whereas intrathecal chemotherapy has insufficient penetration into tumor nodules. Other agents that can reach the CSF or have been reported effective for LM include high-dose cytarabine for hematologic malignancies and capecitabine for breast cancer.[67] Agents should be chosen on the basis of the likely sensitivity of the primary to a given drug.

Two studies have found that intrathecal MTX as a single agent is equal in efficacy to multi-agent intrathecal chemotherapy and has significantly less systemic toxicity. Patients treated with MTX plus RT respond more often than those treated with either alone. Cytarabine (cytosine arabinoside [ara-C]) and thiotepa and other agents may also be useful,[68] particularly in LM from lymphoma, leukemia, or breast cancer. Liposomal cytarabine has a long CSF half-life and can be given every 14 days; it has been reported effective against LM from solid tumors not usually considered sensitive to cytarabine.[69] Other agents have been used experimentally.[70–72]

Our approach is to irradiate symptomatic or radiologically involved areas, usually to 3,000 cGy over 2 weeks. An Ommaya reservoir is placed in the right lateral ventricle,[73] either before or after RT. After completion of RT, MTX (12 mg) is administered twice per week for six treatments, then once weekly for several weeks, depending on the clinical and CSF response. The treatments then are stretched out to once per month until relapse occurs or for a total treatment time of 6 months. At relapse, cytarabine (50 mg) or thiotepa (10 mg) can be considered for the appropriate primaries. There are few data to guide decisions regarding the duration of therapy in patients who are clinically stable and whose CSF remains free of malignant cells after 6 months of therapy. Neurotoxicity from intrathecal drug can occur and is discussed later in this chapter, (see "Nonmetastatic Complications of Cancer Therapy").

CRANIAL AND PERIPHERAL NERVE METASTASES

Incidence Lesions of cranial or peripheral nerves often cause severe pain and, depending on the nerve involved, substantial neurologic disability.[74] The frequency of metastatic disease causing cranial and peripheral nerve dysfunction is unknown because only a few studies address this issue in particular tumors. For example, facial nerve paralysis occurs in 5 to 25% of malignant parotid neoplasms, the lower figure associated with acinous cell carcinomas and the higher with undifferentiated neoplasms. Primary lung cancer arises in the superior sulcus in approximately 3%

of patients, the vast majority presenting with pain caused by infiltration of the brachial plexus (Pancoast syndrome). Abdominal and pelvic tumors may involve the lumbar or sacral plexus during the course of disease, but the precise incidence is not known. Individual nerves either alone or in combination (mononeuritis multiplex) may be compressed or invaded by tumor.

Pathogenesis Tumors affect cranial and peripheral nerves either by compression without directly breaching the epineurium or by invasion along perineurial and endoneurial planes. Pancoast tumors and breast carcinoma metastatic to supraclavicular lymph nodes compress the brachial plexus but usually do not invade it, whereas squamous cell carcinoma of the face, certain melanomas, and prostate cancer can be neurotropic, tracking microscopically along the course of a nerve,[74] often reaching the spinal canal or even the brainstem. The biologic factors that make these tumors neurotropic have not been established. A blood–nerve barrier similar to the blood–brain barrier may exclude water-soluble chemotherapeutic agents from nerve and provide a "sanctuary" for tumor cells.

Symptoms and Signs The specific symptoms and signs of cranial and peripheral nerve dysfunction depend on the nerves involved and the mechanism of involvement. With compressive lesions of nerves or plexuses, pain is usually the first symptom. The pain may be felt locally at the site of compression or more distantly in the sensory distribution of the nerve involved. Pain usually precedes other neurologic dysfunction by weeks to months. In invasive lesions of nerves, pain and neurologic dysfunction often occur simultaneously. In general, when mixed nerves are involved, motor function is affected out of proportion to sensory loss, no matter what the mechanism of nerve involvement. Examination of both motor and sensory functions will usually identify the nerves involved and pinpoint the location of the offending lesion. Compressive lesions of nerves can generally be identified by MR imaging studies directed at the area of dysfunction (Figure 128-6).[74–76] When the lesion is infiltrative instead of compressive, all imaging studies may be normal and the diagnosis must be established clinically or by biopsy. Occasionally infiltration of large nerves such as a plexus or root can be imaged by a coronal enhanced MRI.

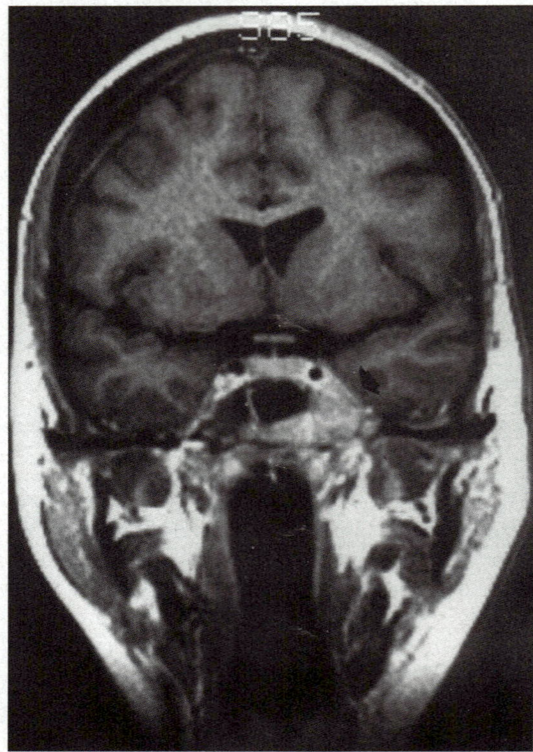

Figure 128-6 Coronal-enhanced magnetic resonance imaging demonstrating a metastasis to the left cavernous sinus *(arrowhead) from* breast carcinoma. Patient presented with retro-orbital pain and had evidence of a partial third, sixth, and V_1 palsy.

Cranial and peripheral neuropathies also occur as side effects of radiation or chemotherapy or as paraneoplastic syndromes (see section on nonmetastatic complications). It is frequently difficult to distinguish these nonmetastatic peripheral nerve lesions from those caused by metastases, but, in general, the latter tend to be painful whereas the former are usually painless. Furthermore, most paraneoplastic and drug-induced neuropathies are bilateral and symmetric, whereas metastatic neuropathies are unilateral or at least asymmetric. Recognizing that any nerve in the body can be affected by metastatic cancer, the following describes some of the more commonly encountered cranial and peripheral neuropathies associated with cancer, and the approach to diagnosis and treatment.

Cranial Neuropathies Cranial nerves may be affected by metastases at any point, from within the brainstem to their end organ (Table 128-8). Brainstem metastases occasionally cause isolated cranial nerve dysfunction, especially of the sixth cranial nerve, but usually other brainstem signs reveal the central location of the lesion. Leptomeningeal metastasis is a common cause of cranial neuropathies that are often multiple. Base of skull metastases often cause recognizable patterns of cranial nerve dysfunction that localize the lesion.[77] Finally, the cranial nerves may be damaged after exiting their foramina.

New-onset cranial neuropathy in a cancer patient should not be ascribed to toxic or idiopathic causes without thorough evaluation (Table 128-9). Evaluation should include an enhanced MRI to visualize the involved cranial nerve along its entire course.[78,79] Lumbar puncture should be performed in the evaluation of cranial neuropathies, and should be considered even when an appropriately placed skull metastasis is discovered, because LM may occur by local invasion from the skull metastasis or by extension along the nerve. If no diagnosis is apparent, empiric radiation therapy to the site of disease (eg, cavernous sinus syndrome) may be advisable in patients with rapidly advancing metastatic disease or with a primary that frequently metastasizes to bone or leptomeninges (eg, lymphoma, breast cancer).

Radiation therapy is usually employed for skull base and orbital metastases. Radiosurgery[80] or charged particle irradiation[81] is used in selected instances. Benefit can occasionally be obtained from surgical resection of a calvarial metastasis, but is almost never performed for a skull base metastasis. Chemotherapy can be used in appropriate circumstances.

Brachial Plexopathy Brachial plexopathy in cancer patients usually results from metastatic cancer in axillary or cervical lymph nodes or local bony structures (eg, clavicle), or from supe-

Table 128-8 Metastatic Lesions Causing Cranial Neuropathies

Lesion Site	Findings	Comments
Eye	Decreased visual acuity; retinal detachment	Choroidal lesions are more common than retinal; pain, proptosis and diplopia are rare; breast and lung cancer are common causes
Orbit	Pain, proptosis, diplopia; sensory loss V_1; decreased visual acuity in one-third of cases, usually late	Equally as common as choroidal metastases; breast and prostate cancer and lymphoma and neuroblastoma are common causes
Parasellar	Unilateral frontal headache, oculomotor palsies (III, IV, VI), sensory loss V_1	Vision rarely affected, no proptosis; lymphoma common
Sella	Diabetes insipidus	Anterior pituitary insufficiency and visual loss are rare; when present, they suggest a primary pituitary tumor. Breast common
Middle cranial fossa	Facial numbness ($V_{2,3}$), abducens palsy in some (VI)	Lightning-like facial pains (trigeminal neuralgia) rare in patients with neoplastic compression
Jugular foramen	Hoarseness, dysphagia, pain in pharynx (IX,X), sternocleidomastoid weakness (XI), occasionally tongue weakness (XII)	Papilledema may occur if a dominant jugular vein is compressed. Glossopharyngeal neuralgia is uncommon
Occipital condyle	Unilateral occipital pain and neck stiffness, unilateral tongue weakness (XII)	Pain may radiate to forehead
Mandible	Unilateral numb chin and gum ("mental neuropathy")	Also results from meningeal or skull base metastases; breast cancer and lymphoma are common causes
Carotid sinus or glossopharyngeal nerve	Syncope, pharynx or neck pain on swallowing	Cardioinhibitory, vasodepressor syncope, or both; head and neck cancer; indicates recurrent tumor; may be life-threatening

Table 128-9 Nonmetastatic Causes of Cranial Neuropathy in Cancer Patients

Cranial Nerve (Symptom)	Causes
II (unilateral vision loss)	Gallium, intra-arterial cisplatin, interferon alpha, RT, temporal arteritis, retinal diseases including hemorrhage
III (diplopia, ptosis)	Diabetes (usually spares pupil), aneurysm, increased intracranial pressure (uncal herniation); myasthenia gravis + Grave's disease[a]
IV (jaw pain; facial pain)	Vincristine, trigeminal neuralgia (sudden, lancinating pains without sensory loss)
VI (diplopia)	Vincristine, increased intracranial pressure, head trauma, diabetes, drug toxicity (eg, narcotics, anticonvulsants), strabismus
VII (facial weakness)	Bell's palsy (idiopathic), varicella-zoster infection (Ramsay Hunt syndrome), diabetes
VIII (hearing loss, dysequilibrium)	Cisplatin, aminoglycosides, degenerative disease, acoustic neuroma, RT-induced serous otitis
X (weak phonation, laryngeal paralysis)	Vincristine

RT = radiation therapy.
[a] = Common causes of diplopia, but are not cranial nerve diseases.

rior sulcus lung tumors.[76,82] Because most metastatic tumors compress the plexus from below, the initial symptom is usually pain in the posterior shoulder or pain radiating down the medial aspect of the arm, elbow, and forearm to the fourth and fifth fingers (C-8 or T-1 distribution). Weakness usually begins in the hand and sensory loss begins in the fourth and fifth fingers; both may progress to affect the entire arm. This initial presentation is helpful in distinguishing tumor from the more common cervical disc herniation where pain commonly affects the outer arm and dorsal surface of the forearm, with weakness in the triceps and wrist extensors (C-7 radiculopathy). Tumor masses are occasionally palpable in the axilla or supraclavicular area. When present, an ipsilateral Horner syndrome (ptosis, miosis, and anhydrosis) indicates the tumor has involved the stellate ganglion in the paraspinal region and, therefore, epidural extension must be sought on cervical MRI.

The differential diagnosis includes radiation-induced plexopathy,[83] trauma (eg, intraoperative positioning, or following central line placement), idiopathic plexopathy, and radiation-induced malignant peripheral nerve sheath tumor.[84] A common diagnostic dilemma is the differentiation of metastatic from radiation-induced plexopathy.[82] Clinical features that are helpful in distinguishing these two conditions include: (1) initial symptom of pain in metastatic plexopathy, and paresthesias in RT-induced plexopathy; the pain of metastatic disease may be accompanied by vasomotor and trophic changes in the arm[85]; (2) Horner syndrome, which is more consistent with metastatic plexopathy; (3) more rapid progression of symptoms and signs in metastatic plexopathy; (4) supraclavicular fullness in metastatic plexopathy; and (5) lymphedema, which suggests RT-induced plexopathy. Either CT or MRI may demonstrate a mass in the plexus (metastatic plexopathy) or loss of soft-tissue planes from fibrosis (RT-induced plexopathy). When findings are equivocal, a PET scan may help.[86]

Surgical exploration of the brachial plexus, once an important diagnostic procedure, is rarely necessary now that CT and MRI are available. Biopsy of the brachial plexus is still indicated when radiation-induced malignant peripheral nerve sheath tumors are suspected. Diagnostic imaging has also lessened the usefulness of electromyogram (EMG) studies, although the discovery of repetitive spontaneous motor unit discharges (myokymia) is pathognomonic of radiation-induced plexopathy and distinguishes it from metastatic plexopathy.[87] When metastases are paraspinal in location, epidural extension is common and should be excluded by MRI. The design of radiation treatment ports will also depend in part on this information.

Radiation therapy is the best available treatment for metastatic plexopathy; chemotherapy may be useful for some previously irradiated patients (eg, those with breast cancer or lymphoma). Some superior sulcus lung tumors that invade the brachial plexus can be resected with a combined thoracic and neurosurgical approach. There is no satisfactory treatment for radiation-induced plexopathy. Surgical lysis of fibrotic tissue surrounding the nerves has not been helpful, nor has systemic corticosteroid or local steroid injection. Treatments for pain include carbamazepine, opioids, gabapentin, and neurosurgical ablative procedures. Amputation of the limb does not relieve pain.

Lumbosacral Plexopathy The lumbosacral plexus is formed from spinal nerve roots L-2 to S-5. The upper lumbar portion (L-2 to L-4) exits the pelvis mainly as the obturator (adductor muscles) and femoral (quadriceps muscles) nerves, whereas the remainder of the leg is innervated by the sciatic nerve (L-5 to S-1). The bladder, rectum, and anus are innervated by roots S-3, S-4, and S-5. The lumbosacral plexus may be involved at any point along its course.[75] The femoral nerve may be compressed at the femoral canal by lymph node metastasis, the sciatic nerve may be affected by tumor extending from the pelvis into the sciatic notch, and the obturator nerve compressed in the pelvis or obturator foramen. The sacral plexus is often affected by a sacral bone metastasis or by a soft-tissue mass directly anterior to the sacrum. A difficult but critical problem with localization is differentiating between lesions of the lumbosacral plexus and the cauda equina resulting from epidural or meningeal metastases. Cauda equina involvement is more likely than plexopathy to cause bilateral symptoms and signs, although 25% of metastatic plexopathies were bilateral in one study.[88] Incontinence requires bilateral loss of innervation and, therefore, its presence suggests central (ie, cauda equina) or sacral involvement. Clear differentiation requires enhanced spinal MRI and CSF analysis.

Local extension of pelvic and abdominal tumors is the predominant cause of metastatic lumbosacral plexopathy. The differential includes herniated lumbar disc, epidural and meningeal metastases to the cauda equina, radiation-induced plexopathy (usually from brachytherapy for pelvic neoplasms), plexus injury from intra-arterial chemotherapy, intraoperative trauma, hematoma, abscess, and diabetic or idiopathic lumbosacral plexopathy.[89] The differential features of metastatic and radiation-induced plexopathy are similar to those for brachial plexopathy. CT or MRI often demonstrates a mass in the region of the lumbosacral plexus, and may also demonstrate hydronephrosis from ureteral obstruction. Biopsy is indicated if an abscess or a secondary tumor is suspected. Radiation therapy is the most commonly employed treatment for metastatic lumbosacral plexus. If metastatic disease approaches the spine, epidural disease may be present and should be included in the RT port.

Peripheral Neuropathy Single peripheral nerves are sometimes damaged by metastatic cancer, and more widespread invasion of peripheral nerves, causing either a mononeuritis multiplex or diffuse polyneuropathy, may complicate the course of leukemia or lymphoma. However, when polyneuropathy occurs in cancer patients, it usually results from toxin exposure or paraneoplastic disorders, both of which are discussed below.

NONMETASTATIC COMPLICATIONS OF CANCER THERAPY

Many cancer treatments are neurotoxic (Table 128-10). Some drugs (eg, vincristine) cause neurotoxicity even at low doses, whereas others (eg, cytarabine) cause neurotoxicity only during intensive therapy. Neurologic toxicity is a dose-limiting factor in several cancer treatments, such as RT, and patients may suffer more from these toxicities than from the cancer itself.[90–92] The more commonly encountered neurologic toxicities from cancer treatment are discussed below.

Chemotherapy **Vinca Alkaloids** Vinca alkaloids cause nerve damage by binding tubulin in peripheral nerves and disrupting the formation of microtubules that mediate fast axonal transport. Neurotoxicity is a dose-limiting side effect of all the vinca alkaloids, but especially of vincristine. Central neurotoxicity is rare because vincristine does not penetrate the normal blood–brain barrier[93]; however, accidental instillation directly into the CSF causes rapid axonal damage that is usually fatal.[94]

Vinca alkaloid neurotoxicity is age (more severe in adults) and dose dependent, and appears to be more prominent in patients with hepatic

Table 128-10 Neurotoxicity of Agents Commonly Used in Cancer Patients

Acute encephalopathy (delirium)	Headache without meningitis
Corticosteroids	Retinoic acid
Methotrexate (high-dose IV, IT)	Trimethoprim-sulfamethoxazole
Cisplatin	Cimetidine
Vincristine	Corticosteroids
Asparaginase	Tamoxifen
Procarbazine	Ondansetron
5-Fluorouracil (± levamisole)	Seizures
Cytarabine (high-dose IV, IT)	Methotrexate
Nitrosoureas (high-dose or arterial)	Etoposide (high-dose)
Ifosfamide/mesna	Cisplatin
Interferons	Vincristine
Chronic encephalopathy (dementia)	Asparaginase
Methotrexate	Nitrogen mustard
Carmustine	Carmustine
Cytarabine	Dacarbazine (intra-arterial or high-dose)
Fludarabine	Busulfan (high-dose)
Visual loss	Beta-lactam antibiotics
Tamoxifen	Iodinated contrast material (IV or IT)
Gallium nitrate	Myelopathy (intrathecal drugs)
Cisplatin	Methotrexate
Interferon alpha	Cytarabine
Cerebellar dysfunction/ataxia	Thiotepa
5-Fluorouracil (± levamisole)	Peripheral neuropathy
Cytarabine	Vinca alkaloids
Phenytoin	Cisplatin
Procarbazine	Etoposide
Aseptic meningitis	Teniposide
Trimethoprim-sulfamethoxazole (Cotrimoxazole)	Misonidazole
IVIg	Paclitaxel
NSAIDs	Suramin
Monoclonal antibodies	Docetaxel
Bortezomib	Bortezomib
Metrizamide	
Carbamazepine	
Cytarabine (IT)	
Methotrexate (IT)	
Corticosteroids (IT)	

IV = intravenous; IVIg = intravenous gammaglobulin; IT = intrathecal; NSAID = nonsteroidal anti-inflammatory drugs.
From Posner JB,[1] modified with permission.

dysfunction,[95] and in those who have received other potentially neurotoxic therapies.[96] Tingling paresthesias develop in the fingertips, and usually in the toes, of virtually all patients treated with vincristine, although clinically detectable sensory loss is often absent. Loss of ankle stretch reflexes is an early and almost universal sign, and with continued therapy, all reflexes may diminish or disappear. Weakness may occur as therapy continues. Weakness is of two types: (1) A generalized distal axonal neuropathy is the more common. When that weakness is mild, patients lose the ability to walk on their heels and lose strength in wrist extensors. More severely affected patients develop foot drop and slap their feet when they walk. Weakness can become severe enough to render the patient immobile or bedbound, but the drug should be discontinued prior to the development of such marked weakness. Pre-existing peripheral nerve diseases, especially Charcot–Marie–Tooth neuropathy[97] and probably other neuropathies (eg, diabetic polyneuropathy), increase the severity of vincristine neuropathy. (2) Some patients develop focal weakness, for example, unilateral foot drop or cranial nerve palsies, such as ptosis or extraocular muscle, facial, or laryngeal paralysis.[98] Although symptomatic toxicity is usually reversible after discontinuation of the drug, significant weakness may persist in severely affected patients. Autonomic dysfunction, particularly abdominal cramping and constipation, often occurs within hours to days of each dose. Adynamic ileus may result and can be life-threatening. A prophylactic bowel regimen or metoclopramide may reduce the severity of this complication. Impotence has been reported.

Less-common complications of vincristine administration include aching bone pain, sharp stabbing pain in the jaw or throat, or an increase in any pre-existing pain. These symptoms typically occur within hours of injection and subside over several days. The symptoms appear with the first or second dose, and rarely recur with subsequent doses. Hyponatremia from inappropriate secretion of antidiuretic hormone occurs within days of drug administration and may recur with subsequent doses.[96] Encephalopathy and seizures not related to hyponatremia have been reported to occur after vincristine administration, but are very rare. There is no effective treatment.

Methotrexate There are several clinically distinct forms of MTX toxicity.[90] An acute reaction with meningismus, confusion, fever, and CSF pleocytosis occurs 4 to 6 hours after intrathecal injection and resolves over several days. This syndrome is often confused with infectious meningitis, but the onset is too rapid after the injection for bacterial contamination; antibiotics are unnecessary unless Gram stain or cultures demonstrate organisms. Dexamethasone may relieve some of these symptoms. Mild acute toxicity occurs in as many as 10% of patients, but further doses of intrathecal MTX are usually uneventful. The cause of this syndrome is not known, although high CSF MTX levels may accompany the reaction.

An early delayed reaction follows high-dose intravenous infusion of MTX in about 4% of patients so treated.[99,100] The disorder usually occurs 7 to 10 days after the third or fourth treatment and is characterized by stupor or coma, often associated with lateralizing neurologic signs that change from hour to hour. Most patients recover completely and the disorder usually does not recur even if MTX is reinstituted. The pathogenesis of this syndrome is unknown.

Paraplegia may follow instillation of MTX or cytarabine by lumbar puncture.[101] The disorder is characterized by weakness and sensory loss in the legs, which evolves over several days to complete transverse myelopathy. Some patients recover, but most remain paraplegic. Extensive necrosis of the spinal cord is found at autopsy. The pathogenesis of the disorder is unknown, but it appears to be idiosyncratic rather than dose related.

MTX leukoencephalopathy occurs in patients who have received a high cumulative dose of intrathecal or systemic MTX[102] or MTX in combination with cranial RT.[42] Symptoms begin weeks or months after treatment and appear as focal neurologic deficits that sometimes progress to seizures, coma, and death. Such a severe outcome is uncommon and tends to occur in the pediatric population. More commonly in adults, progressive cognitive impairment in the absence of lateralizing signs may be seen in patients who survive > 6 months following treatment with systemic or intrathecal MTX ± RT. Leukoencephalopathy is always found on neuroimaging of these patients, but occasionally it may be found on MRI or at autopsy in asymptomatic patients. The neuropathologic findings consist of multifocal areas of coagulative necrosis in the white matter, often with extensive calcification. Unlike cerebral radionecrosis, fibrinoid necrosis of blood vessels is absent. The areas of necrosis may be randomly distributed in the white matter or be predominantly periventricular. The latter pattern may occur when MTX is injected into the ventricles of patients with abnormal outflow of ventricular CSF. Alternatively, focal leukoencephalopathy may develop around the catheter track.[103] When MTX is injected into ventricles with elevated pressure, the drug tracks along the catheter, producing focal leukoencephalopathy that mimics a mass lesion; MRI may show a hypointense enhancing mass (Figure 128-7). This may resolve on its own or require removal of the catheter.

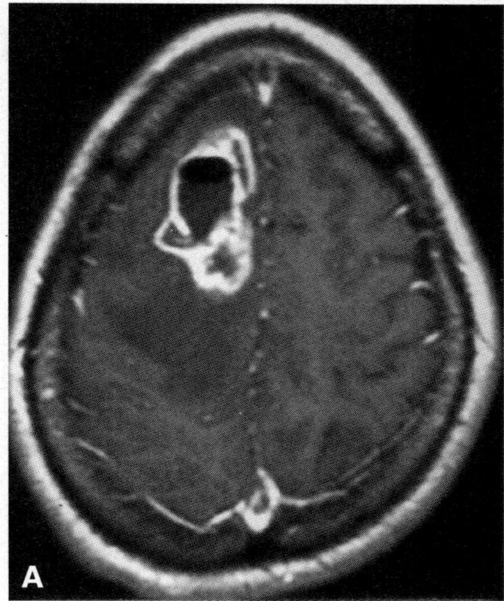
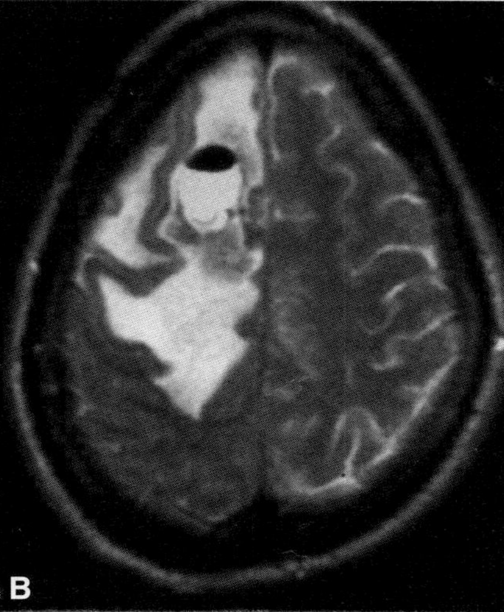

Figure 128-7 Gadolinium enhanced T_1-weighted **A,** and T_2-weighted **B,** magnetic resonance images of focal leukoencephalopathy in a patient with a malfunctioning Ommaya reservoir. This reservoir was obstructed but unrecognized. Multiple courses of methotrexate were instilled into the catheter. The drug dissected around the catheter and into the frontal lobe, causing a region of necrosis with prominent surrounding edema. Air can be seen in the central cavity of the lesion after a recent instillation. The patient presented with seizures and a left hemiparesis, both of which resolved with corticosteroids.

Platins Peripheral neuropathy is a dose-limiting toxicity of some platins, particularly cisplatin[90] and oxaliplatin.[104] Neuropathic symptoms begin as tingling paresthesias in the toes and fingers; loss of stretch reflexes and reduced vibratory and position sensation are found. Pain and temperature sensation and strength are unaffected. These findings and loss of sural (sensory) nerve conduction with preservation of motor nerve conduction indicate a large, myelinated sensory fiber neuropathy that impairs position sense and vibration. Severe, disabling sensory ataxia may result. Symptoms often begin after treatment has been completed, and can progress for months before stabilizing. Gradual resolution follows, although some patients are permanently disabled. Neurotrophic agents and amifostine[105] have both been reported to decrease cisplatin neurotoxicity, but the data are inconclusive.[106] Lhermitte sign, an electric sensation in the arms, back, or legs upon neck flexion, is an occasional manifestation of platin neurotoxicity.[104] Oxaliplatin may cause cold-induced paresthesias either during or shortly after an infusion.[107]

Ototoxicity caused by cisplatin is a result of damage to the organ of Corti. Toxicity severe enough to interfere with speech perception is uncommon, but hearing loss may or may not resolve. Cisplatin has been associated with optic neuropathy, especially after intracarotid infusion. Seizures and encephalopathy have been reported in patients receiving cisplatin. Cisplatin induces renal magnesium and calcium wasting, and although these disorders must be excluded when seizures or encephalopathy occur, they rarely contribute to platinum neurotoxicity.

Vascular disease producing neurologic symptoms has been reported as a late delayed effect of cisplatin-based chemotherapy. Many such patients develop Raynaud phenomenon, and a few have developed transient ischemic attacks or cerebral infarctions. Other platinum drugs are less neurotoxic.[108]

5-Fluorouracil Generalized encephalopathy has been seen in association with severe systemic toxicity during therapy, and may indicate an inherited deficiency of dihydropyrimidine dehydrogenase, the enzyme responsible for pyrimidine catabolism.[109]

Cytosine Arabinoside Intrathecal cytarabine can cause an acute chemical meningitis with confusion, fever and CSF pleocytosis. This occurs in almost all patients who receive the liposomal preparation (DepoCyte).[69] Dexamethasone should be administered for 2 days prior to and after every DepoCyte injection.

Intravenous high-dose cytarabine (eg, 3 g/m^2 every 12 hours for six doses) causes neurotoxicity in 10 to 25% of patients. The common form is pancerebellar dysfunction[110] starting several days after the initiation of therapy and worsening for several more days. Gradual recovery begins about 2 weeks after onset, but recovery may be incomplete in approximately 20% of patients, especially those in whom the neurologic disorder was severe. Pathologic changes include loss of cerebellar Purkinje cells and neurons in the deep cerebellar nuclei. Encephalopathy and seizures also occur, usually in the setting of cerebellar toxicity.[111] Neurotoxicity has been documented with minimum cumulative doses of 18 g/m^2, but higher doses (eg, 30 to 40 g/m^2) are associated with increasingly severe toxicity. Age older than 50 years and renal insufficiency predispose patients to more severe toxicity. A recrudescence of neurologic symptoms may occur with retreatment. Peripheral neuropathy is also a rare complication of high-dose cytarabine; in most patients, high-dose cytarabine was given with other potentially neurotoxic agents, such as fludarabine.[1]

Other Drugs Other commonly used drugs that cause neurotoxicity include the taxanes, bortezomib,[112] suramin, and procarbazine, all of which can cause peripheral neuropathy, although procarbazine does so rarely. High-dose busulfan therapy, used to prepare patients for bone marrow transplantation, can cause seizures. At standard doses the drug is not neurotoxic. Gemcitabine, in combination with abdominal radiation, has been reported to cause myositis with acute muscle pain and tenderness. It is responsive to steroids.[113] The drug has also been reported to cause a reversible posterior encephalopathy,[114] but this syndrome, characterized by headache, somnolence, seizures, and posterior hemisphere hyperintensities on MRI scans, is associated with a number of anticancer agents, including vincristine and cyclosporin. The clinical symptoms, which are usually reversible, are often associated with the development of severe hypertension that is likely critical to the pathophysiology of this disorder which is similar to hypertensive encephalopathy.

Corticosteroids Corticosteroids cause neurotoxicity in the form of myopathy[115] and alterations of mental status.[116] Myopathy affects most patients taking steroids for brain or spinal cord metastases. Patients develop symmetric, proximal weakness in their arms and legs within weeks after the institution of steroids. The weakness may progress, but very rarely renders the patient nonambulatory. Early symptoms include difficulty arising from chairs or toilet seats and climbing stairs. Muscle stretch reflexes are normal and sensation and bowel and bladder function are not affected. Respiratory function may be compromised,[115] resulting in exercise intolerance and dyspnea. The serum creatine phosphokinase (CPK) is not elevated. The differential diagnosis includes hypokalemia, thyroid dysfunction, polymyositis, Lambert–Eaton myasthenic syndrome (LEMS), and spinal cord compression. The only treatment is reduction or discontinuation of the steroids. Exercise and adequate protein intake may help.[117] Patients with hypoalbuminemia may be at higher risk for steroid myopathy.

Psychosis, delirium, euphoria, or dysphoria may complicate steroid therapy. Dose reduction or discontinuation is usually necessary, although neuroleptics or sedatives can be used in patients for whom continued therapy is critical.

Radiation Therapy Despite the fact that cells in the CNS turn over slowly or not at all, the brain, spinal cord, and, to a lesser degree, peripheral nerves are susceptible to damage by ionizing radiation that usually causes symptoms months or years after the radiation has been completed (Table 128-11).[90,118–120] With patients living longer after initial treatment, the problem of delayed radiation damage to the CNS is increasingly important.

Brain Toxicity Acute reactions, occurring within hours of a dose of RT, are rare with current fractionation schedules when patients are pretreated with dexamethasone.[1] Patients with large or multifocal tumors and cerebral edema, especially those with symptoms of increased intracranial pressure, are more likely to experience this side effect. Symptoms and signs of acute RT toxicity include worsening of existing deficits, headache, nausea and vomiting, lethargy, and somno-

Table 128-11 Neurological Complications of Central Nervous System Irradiation

Complication	Latency	Symptoms and Signs	Comments
Brain			
Acute	Hours	Increase in existing deficits, headache, nausea, vomiting, confusion, somnolence	Transient, corticosteroids help
Early delayed	Weeks to months	Malaise, increase in existing signs, increased seizures, somnolence	Resolves over days to weeks, steroids help
Delayed			
a. Radionecrosis	6 months to years	Focal mass lesion	Treatment includes steroids and surgery, tumor often coexists
b. Dementia	1 year	Loss of cognitive function	May be subtle
c. Endocrine	Years	Hypothyroidism, amenorrhea/galactorrhea, changes in libido, growth failure	Hypothalamic or pituitary in origin
d. Secondary tumors	10–40 years, earlier if radiated as a child	Symptoms of brain tumor	Meningioma, sarcoma, malignant glioma
e. Stroke	Years	Abrupt onset of neurologic dysfunction	Large or branch vessels
Spinal Cord			
Early	Weeks to months	Electric shocks with neck movement (Lhermitte's sign)	Usually transient
Delayed			
a. Myelopathy	Weeks to years	Progressive cord dysfunction, starts with sensory symptoms	Often fatal
b. Lower motor neuron syndrome	Months to years	Focal weakness and atrophy	May improve spontaneously

lence. These are usually transient and respond to increased doses of corticosteroids. The etiology has been ascribed to radiation-induced disruption of the blood–brain barrier with resulting cerebral edema. Occasionally, worsening perilesional edema may be seen on MRI scan.

Early delayed encephalopathy occurs a few weeks to a few months after RT. Patients may develop worsening of lateralizing signs or somnolence in the absence of focal deficits; the former predominates in adults treated for brain tumors and the latter in children treated prophylactically. Symptoms may persist for days to weeks, and are often relieved by corticosteroids; complete resolution is usual. Early delayed encephalopathy is often confused with progression of the primary brain tumor or metastasis being irradiated. An MRI scan reveals an enhancing lesion indistinguishable from progressive tumor. Clinical suspicion and resolution of symptoms over time may be the only real clue to the cause of the deterioration. The pathogenesis of early delayed encephalopathy is probably demyelination resulting from radiation injury to oligodendroglia.[121]

Delayed radiation toxicity is the most serious complication of brain RT,[122,123] and radionecrosis is its most common manifestation, arising months to years after treatment.[124] In one study, cerebral radionecrosis occurred in 6% of patients treated with 4,500 cGy or more.[125] The total dose is the most important factor in the development of cerebral radionecrosis; there is a threshold near 6,000 cGy above which radionecrosis becomes common. However, high daily fraction schedules also carry increased risk for radionecrosis. Headache, focal deficits, and seizures are the usual symptoms. CT/MRI reveals a contrast-enhancing lesion with surrounding edema producing mass effect; this radiographic appearance is indistinguishable from CNS tumor. PET or single-photon emission computed tomography (SPECT) scans may differentiate tumor that is hypermetabolic from necrosis that is hypometabolic. However, the differentiation between radionecrosis and tumor is often difficult, and biopsy may be required. Marked symptomatic improvement follows treatment with dexamethasone, and some patients remain well after steroids are discontinued. Surgical resection of the necrotic material is often necessary. Reports that anticoagulation[126] or hyperbaric oxygen[127] relieve symptoms require confirmation. Radiation may also cause dementia unassociated with evidence of necrosis.[128,129] The MRI may show only ventricular dilatation, sulcal atrophy, and white matter hyperintensity. Some of these patients respond to ventriculoperitoneal shunting[130] albeit incompletely and temporarily. This disorder is most common in patients who have received both RT and intensive systemic chemotherapy, and is likely a variant of delayed leukoencephalopathy.

Cerebral infarction may result from occlusion of cervical or intracranial arteries that have received large doses of RT.[131] Vascular malformations may appear and bleed many years after brain radiation therapy.[132] Complicated migraine-like episodes may occur in children after cranial irradiation.[133] Endocrinologic dysfunction may arise years after RT, resulting from either hypothalamic or pituitary failure.[134] Brain tumors may occur decades after cranial RT or radiosurgery[135] administered in adulthood, but latency is often much shorter (median 6 years) in those irradiated in childhood. Radiation-induced brain tumors include meningioma, sarcoma, and malignant glioma.[136,137]

Spinal Cord Toxicity Spinal cord damage caused by RT is uncommon. Transient, electric shock-like sensations following neck flexion (Lhermitte sign) may occur weeks to months after RT to the cervical cord,[138] including mantle RT for Hodgkin's disease. Spontaneous resolution is the rule. Progressive radiation myelopathy, on the other hand, is a devastating complication with onset months to years (median 20 months) following RT.[139] The incidence of radiation myelopathy is affected by the total RT dose and dose per fraction; an estimate of the ED5 (5% incidence of complication) is between 5,700 and 6,100 cGy for RT delivered in 200 cGy fractions. Symptoms of radiation myelopathy usually begin with sensory changes in the legs and gradually progress to sensory loss, weakness, and sphincter dysfunction. Pain may be present at the level of the cord damage. Dysesthetic pain below the level of cord injury may be prominent. Unlike epidural spinal cord compression, sensory and motor findings are often asymmetric at onset and a Brown–Sequard syndrome is often present. The MRI scan reveals either a normal, enlarged, or atrophic cord that may contrast-enhance, but extrinsic compression is absent (Figure 128-8). Steroids do not reverse the neurotoxic deficits. Anticoagulants and hyperbaric oxygen have been reported to be effective, but this has not been verified.[140,141] Spontaneous improvement sometimes occurs.[139] A lower motor neuron syndrome with weakness and muscle atrophy can occur after irradiation of the spinal cord. Although weakness is prominent, patients usually remain ambulatory; spontaneous improvement is occasionally seen.[142] Radiation-induced plexopathies were discussed in a previous section (see brachial plexopathy).

CEREBROVASCULAR COMPLICATIONS OF CANCER

Cerebrovascular lesions are the second most common neuropathologic finding, after metastases, in postmortem studies of cancer patients. Of 3,426 brains studied at autopsy, 15% contained vascular lesions.[143]

Cerebral hemorrhage can develop in any metastasis.[144] It is most commonly seen in lung cancer, but occurs proportionately more frequently in melanoma, thyroid, renal, and germ cell metastases. Intracerebral hemorrhages that are not associated with metastases are seen in patients with leukemia, thrombocytopenia, or coagulopathy. Intravascular leukostasis is not required for hemorrhage in leukemic patients.

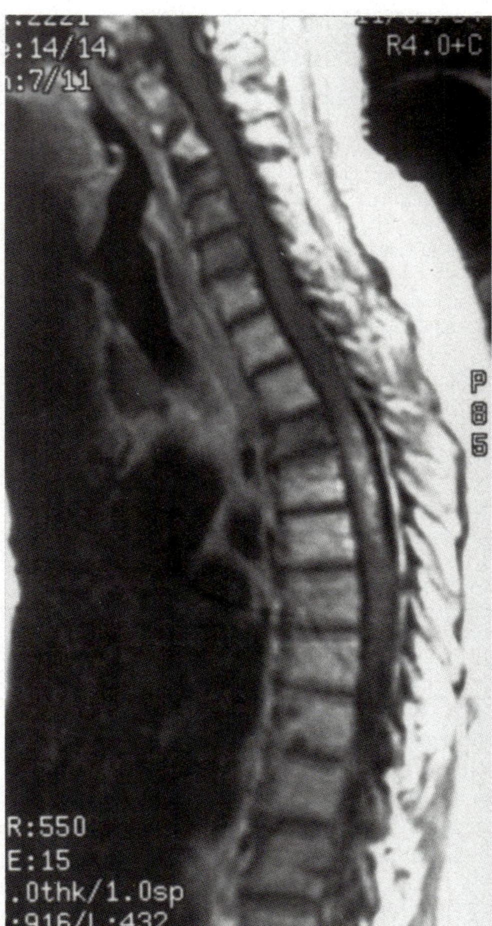

Figure 128-8 A magnetic resonance imaging scan demonstrating radiation myelopathy. The hypodense thoracic vertebral body is the site of a bone metastasis from breast cancer for which the patient was radiated. Some months later, the patient developed a myelopathy, and the contrast-enhancing lesion seen in the spinal cord represents radiation damage.

Subdural hemorrhage may occur in association with dural metastases or coagulopathy. A hemorrhage may cause abrupt neurologic deterioration or may be unsuspected prior to obtaining a brain scan. With large hemorrhages, patients experience an abrupt onset of headache, vomiting, lethargy, and focal deficits. For patients with intracerebral hemorrhage resulting from coagulopathy or thrombocytopenia, the underlying problem should be treated and the patient observed. Subdural hematomas and some hemorrhages into metastases may respond to surgical evacuation. Corticosteroids are useful in those patients who hemorrhage into an underlying brain metastasis but probably do not help hemorrhage into an otherwise normal brain.

Cerebral infarction is as common as hemorrhage.[143,145] Infarctions secondary to accelerated atherosclerosis take place decades following RT that has included cervical or cerebral vessels in the field.[146] Radiation therapy for head and neck cancer predisposes to carotid stenosis, and intracranial arterial stenosis with subsequent infarction may occur following cranial RT. Septic cerebral infarction is usually secondary to *Aspergillus, Candida,* or *Mucor.* These opportunistic organisms produce a vasculitis, and the infarctions are often multiple and hemorrhagic. *Aspergillus* is the most common causative agent and is always associated with pulmonary infection; discovery of the latter may be a clue to the correct diagnosis. Antifungal therapy is usually unsuccessful, and the outcome is often fatal.

Cerebral venous thrombosis (eg, superior sagittal sinus thrombosis) may result from compression or invasion of vascular structures by a metastasis, or from a coagulopathy.[147] Clinical features include worsening headache, focal deficits, and seizures. The diagnosis can be made by MRI combined with magnetic resonance venography. Lumbar puncture reveals an elevated opening pressure, and frequently red cells in the CSF. Spontaneous resolution usually occurs unless dural metastasis is the cause, in which case RT is required. Anticoagulation is safe and should be considered for progressive neurologic symptoms, even when due to hemorrhage from venous infarction; however, most patients recover fully without treatment.

Cerebral embolism accounts for more than half of strokes in patients with cancer.[145] It may be cardioembolic or result from nonbacterial thrombotic endocarditis (NBTE, marantic endocarditis).[148] Lung and GI carcinomas are the primary cancers most commonly associated with NBTE. Infarctions in patients with NBTE are often multiple and hemorrhagic. Diffuse encephalopathy and focal deficits usually coexist. Approximately one-third of patients with NBTE also have laboratory evidence of disseminated intravascular coagulation (DIC). Two-dimensional echocardiography is rarely helpful, but transesophageal echocardiography can demonstrate the valvular vegetations. Cerebral angiography demonstrates multiple arterial branch occlusions. Anticoagulation with heparin should be considered. Anecdotal evidence suggests that warfarin is not helpful. Tumor emboli[149] originate from pulmonary metastases in most circumstances. The patient develops a neurologic deficit, followed weeks to months later by progressive deficits referable to the same area of brain due to growth of the embolized tumor.

DIC may result in cerebrovascular thrombosis.[7] Neurologic symptoms, which usually begin abruptly with diffuse encephalopathy and fluctuating multifocal deficits, often precede laboratory evidence of DIC. Enhanced MRI is usually negative, although small foci of ischemia are occasionally seen and may be evident on diffusion-weighted sequences. Anticoagulation with heparin, but not warfarin, may prevent progressive neurologic dysfunction.[150]

METABOLIC ENCEPHALOPATHY

Diffuse encephalopathy with or without focal signs is a common and prominent sign of many of the neurologic complications of cancer,[151–153] including brain (usually multiple) or leptomeningeal metastases; neurotoxicity of many chemotherapeutic agents; vascular complications, particularly DIC; intracranial infections, and some paraneoplastic syndromes. However, most patients with encephalopathy do not suffer from one of these causes; instead, the disorder results from metabolic or nutritional abnormalities related to the underlying cancer or its treatment. Table 128-12 lists some of the causes of diffuse encephalopathy in cancer patients, but in most instances the disorder is either multifactorial or the underlying cause is never identified. Opioids or sedative drug overdose, hypoxia, or vital organ failure are the most frequently identified causes. In patients with multiple contributory causes, effective treatment of one factor may reverse the encephalopathy even though others cannot be treated. In patients in whom the cause is not identified, the symptoms often resolve spontaneously; however, the presence of delirium is associated with an overall poor prognosis.[154]

Table 128-12 Causes of Encephalopathy in Cancer Patients

Metabolic
Hypoxemia
Fever
Severe anemia
Uremia
Electrolyte imbalance—hypoglycemia
Metabolic acidosis
Hyperammonemia, hepatic failure
Hypercarbia (CO_2 narcosis)
Postanoxic encephalopathy
Thiamine deficiency (Wernicke's encephalopathy)
Thyroid disorders
Toxic
Sedative or opioid intoxication or withdrawal
Sepsis
Corticosteroids
Alcohol withdrawal
Anticholinergics
Chemotherapy agents (high-dose MTX, ifosfamide)
Anticonvulsants

Metabolic encephalopathy usually causes global impairment of attention, alertness, and cognition in the absence of lateralizing signs.[155,156] Focal neurologic findings may occur in metabolic encephalopathy, but their presence should prompt a search for structural lesions. The possibility of structural disease even in nonfocal, encephalopathic cancer patients should always be kept in mind; for example, multiple brain metastases may present only as a recent change in mental status. Nonconvulsive status epilepticus may cause encephalopathy without focal signs,[157] although careful observation will usually detect repetitive movements of eyes or extremities.

Investigation and treatment should proceed simultaneously. When the history does not immediately suggest the etiology (eg, opioid toxicity, sepsis), a stepwise investigation should be carried out to identify the cause. If the examination reveals focal neurologic findings, or if the patient is stuporous, an MRI with and without contrast should be obtained. Otherwise the scan may be deferred until the laboratory evaluation is available. The tests should cover each of the areas listed in Table 128-12. If no cause is apparent from these tests, a lumbar puncture should be considered.

Simultaneously with evaluation, treatment should be undertaken. General medical measures of

Table 128-13 Paraneoplastic Neurological Syndromes

Syndrome	Associated Cancer[a]	Clinical Features
Brain		
Limbic encephalopathy[b]	SCLC	Depression, memory loss, confusion, abnormal CSF
Brainstem encephalopathy[b]	SCLC	Ataxia, cranial nerve dysfunction, corticospinal dysfunction, abnormal CSF
Subacute cerebellar degeneration	Breast, ovary, SCLC, Hodgkin	Ataxia, dysarthria, nystagmus, normal CSF
Opsoclonus, myoclonus	Lung	Jerky, irregular movements of eyes and skeletal muscles
Optic neuritis, retinal degeneration	SCLC	Painless loss of vision, transient visual obscuration
Spinal cord		
Necrotizing myelopathy	SCLC, lymphoma, leukemia	Ascending myelopathy
Subacute motor neuronopathy	Hodgkin's and NHL	Patchy weakness, atrophy, and fasciculations
Dorsal root ganglia		
Subacute sensory neuronopathy[b]	SCLC	Dysesthesias, sensory ataxia, areflexia
Peripheral nerve		
Gammopathy associated neuropathy	Myeloma	Sensory loss, weakness, reflex loss
Acute polyradiculitis (Guillain-Barré)	Lymphoma	Cytochemical dissociation in CSF
Neuromuscular junction		
Eaton-Lambert myasthenic syndrome	SCLC	Proximal weakness, decreased reflexes, ocular muscles spared
Myasthenia gravis	Thymoma	Weakness, ocular muscles often involved
Muscle		
Dermatomyositis, polymyositis	Lung, breast, ovary, GI	Weakness, elevated CPK

CPK = creatine phosphokinase; CSF = cerebrospinal fluid; GI = gastrointestinal; NHL = non-Hodgkin's lymphoma; SCLC = small-cell-lung cancer.
[a] = The most commonly associated tumors are listed.
[b] = Often occur in association with each other.

oxygenation, blood pressure, temperature control, and hydration often improve mental function. In diabetic patients, dextrose should be administered while awaiting the results of laboratory tests. Medications that are not critical should be stopped. During the initial evaluation, symptomatic treatment with sedatives or neuroleptics should be avoided when possible, because these agents cloud the clinical picture and, therefore, may hamper diagnosis. Haloperidol or risperidone may help to control symptoms of agitation and hallucinations, if present, but should not be used in alcohol or sedative withdrawal (risk of seizures) or in anticholinergic intoxication. Benzodiazepines can be used in the former conditions and physostigmine in the latter. If opioid intoxication is suspected, and the patient's respiratory status is not compromised, it is best to let the intoxication resolve without specific treatment because naloxone administration may precipitate severe, abrupt withdrawal and its effect is short-lived. If naloxone is administered, the initial dose should be 0.2 mg (one-half vial) diluted in saline and administered slowly. Thiamine should be given intravenously to patients with severe malnutrition. Once identified, the underlying cause of the encephalopathy should be promptly treated. However, improvement of the encephalopathy may lag behind improvement in laboratory values, especially if the abnormality was gradual in development.

PARANEOPLASTIC NEUROLOGIC SYNDROMES

Paraneoplastic syndromes refer to disorders of unknown etiology that occur with increased frequency in patients with cancer.[1,8] Compared with known complications of cancer, paraneoplastic syndromes are rare, seen in less than 1% of patients with cancer. As paraneoplastic syndromes precede the diagnosis of cancer in about two-thirds of cases, prompt recognition may lead to early diagnosis and cure of the underlying neoplasm. These disorders often debilitate the patient to a greater degree than does the malignancy, but some of the syndromes are improved with successful treatment of the cancer. Table 128-13 lists some paraneoplastic syndromes. The primary cancers most commonly associated with each syndrome are also listed, but these associations are not absolute, because each syndrome has been observed with a variety of cancer types.

The etiologies of these syndromes are not well understood, but most are suspected to have an autoimmune basis. The strongest evidence for an autoimmune disorder is for the LEMs, in which autoantibodies inhibit the function of presynaptic calcium channels at the neuromuscular junction, resulting in weakness. Examination demonstrates an increase in muscle power after repetitive muscle contraction (the opposite of myasthenia gravis), and absent deep tendon reflexes. These findings, along with autonomic and sensory complaints of dry mouth, impotence, and thigh paresthesias, point to a nerve disorder. Electrodiagnostic tests of repetitive nerve stimulation reveal an increasing amplitude of the muscle action potential that is pathognomonic. Several other paraneoplastic syndromes are associated with the presence of specific antibodies, including subacute sensory neuronopathy, limbic encephalitis, subacute cerebellar degeneration, and gammopathy associated neuropathies. These specific antibodies serve as markers that not only identify the syndrome as paraneoplastic, but suggest the site of the underlying tumor.[8] The antibodies have not been proved to have an etiologic role in the pathogenesis of such syndromes.

A variety of therapies directed at immunomodulation, including plasmapheresis, corticosteroids and intravenous immunoglobin, have failed to reverse the neurologic impairment associated with paraneoplastic disorders. The exception is the LEMs, which responds well to immunosuppressive treatments. Some patients with paraneoplastic neurologic disorders have reversal or stabilization of their neurologic dysfunction when the underlying malignancy is effectively treated and this should be a therapeutic priority for all these patients.

REFERENCES

1. Posner JB. Neurologic complications of cancer. Philadelphia: F.A. Davis; 1995.
2. Boogerd W, Vos VW, Hart AAM, Baris G. Brain metastases in breast cancer; natural history, prognostic factors and outcome. J Neurooncol 1993;15:165–74.
3. Schiff D, Wen PY. Cancer Neurology in Clinical Practice. Totowa, New Jersey: Humana Press, 2003.
4. Delattre J-Y, Krol G, Thaler HT, Posner JB. Distribution of brain metastases. Arch Neurol 1988;45:741–4.
5. Osborn JL, Getzenberg RH, Trump DL. Spinal cord compression in prostate cancer. J Neurooncol 1995;23:135–47.
6. Hayashi T, Igarashi K, Tanizawa A, et al. Brain metastasis as a sole recurrence of prostate cancer after total prostatectomy. Urol Int 1998;60:121–3.
7. Levi M, ten Cate H. Review articles: disseminated intravascular coagulation. N Engl J Med 1999;341:586–92.
8. Dalmau J, Gultekin HS, Posner JB. Paraneoplastic neurologic syndromes: pathogenesis and physiopathology. Brain Pathol 1999;9:275–84.
9. Abrahm JL, ACP ASIM End Life Care Consensus Panel. Management of pain and spinal cord compression in patients with advanced cancer. Ann Intern Med 1999; 131:37–46.
10. Solberg A, Bremnes RM. Metastatic spinal cord compression: diagnostic delay, treatment, and outcome. Anti-cancer Res 1999;19:677–84.
11. Helweg-Larsen S, Sorensen PS, Kreiner S. Prognostic factors in metastatic spinal cord compression: a prospective study using multivariate analysis of variables influencing survival and gait function in 153 patients. Int J Radiat Oncol Biol Phys 2000;46:1163–9.
12. Kovner F, Spigel S, Rider I, et al. Radiation therapy of metastatic spinal cord compression—multidisciplinary team diagnosis and treatment. J Neurooncol 1999; 42:85–92.
13. Byrne TN. Spinal cord compression from epidural metastases. N Engl J Med 1992;327:614–9.
14. Walsh GL, Gokaslan ZL, McCutcheon IE, et al. Anterior approaches to the thoracic spine in patients with cancer: indications and results. Ann Thorac Surg 1997;64:1611–8.
15. Nishimura R, Nagao K, Miyayama H, et al. Diagnostic problems of evaluating vertebral metastasis from breast carcinoma with a higher degree of malignancy. Cancer 1999;85:1782–8.

16. Domchek SM, Younger J, Finkelstein DM, Seiden MV. Predictors of skeletal complications in patients with metastatic breast carcinoma. Cancer 2000;89:363–8.
17. Bubendorf L, Schopfer A, Wagner U, et al. Metastatic patterns of prostate cancer: an autopsy study of 1,589 patients. Hum Pathol 2000;31:578–83.
18. McDonald AC, Nicoll JAR, Rampling RP. Non-Hodgkin's lymphoma presenting with spinal cord compression; a clinicopathological review of 25 cases. Eur J Cancer 2000;36:207–13.
19. Oeppen RS, Tung K. Retrograde venous invasion causing vertebral metastases in renal cell carcinoma. Br J Radiol 2001;74:759–61.
20. Rades D, Bremer M, Goehde S, et al. Spondylodiscitis in patients with spinal cord compression: a possible pitfall in radiation oncology. Radiother Oncol 2001;59:307–9.
21. Schiff D, O'Neill BP, Wang CH, O'Fallon JR. Neuroimaging and treatment implications of patients with multiple epidural spinal metastases. Cancer 1998;83:1593–601.
22. Wang JC, Boland P, Mitra N, et al. Single-stage posterolateral transpedicular approach for resection of epidural metastatic spine tumors involving the vertebral body with circumferential reconstruction: results in 140 patients. Invited submission from the Joint Section Meeting on Disorders of the Spine and Peripheral Nerves, March 2004. J Neurosurg Spine 2004;1:287–98.
23. Schnell L, Fearn S, Klassen H, et al. Acute inflammatory responses to mechanical lesions in the CNS: differences between brain and spinal cord. Eur J Neurosci 1999;11:3648–58.
24. Traill ZC, Talbot D, Golding S, Gleeson FV. Magnetic resonance imaging versus radionuclide scintigraphy in screening for bone metastases. Clin Radiol 1999;54:448–51.
25. Khaw FM, Worthy SA, Gibson MJ, Gholkar A. The appearance on MRI of vertebrae in acute compression of the spinal cord due to metastases. J Bone Joint Surg Br 1999;81B:830–4.
26. Husband DJ, Grant KA, Romaniuk CS. MRI in the diagnosis and treatment of suspected malignant spinal cord compression. Br J Radiol 2001;74:15–23.
27. Loblaw DA, Laperriere NJ. Emergency treatment of malignant extradural spinal cord compression: an evidence-based guideline. J Clin Oncol 1998;16:1613–24.
28. Poortmans P, Vulto A, Raaijmakers E. Always on a Friday? Time pattern of referral for spinal cord compression. Acta Oncol 2001;40:88–91.
29. Delattre J-Y, Arbit E, Thaler HT, et al. A dose-response study of dexamethasone in a model of spinal cord compression caused by epidural tumor. J Neurosurg 1989;70:920–5.
30. Sorensen PS, Helweg-Larsen S, Mouridsen H, Hansen HH. Effect of high-dose dexamethasone in carcinomatous metastatic spinal cord compression treated with radiotherapy: a randomized trial. Eur J Cancer 1994;30A:22–7.
31. Vecht CJ, Haaxma-Reiche H, van Putten WLJ, et al. Initial bolus of conventional versus high-dose dexamethasone in metastatic spinal cord compression. Neurology 1989;39:1255–7.
32. Grosu AL, Andratschke N, Nieder C, Molls M. Retreatment of the spinal cord with palliative radiotherapy. Int J Radiat Oncol Biol Phys 2002;52:1288–92.
33. Bilsky MH, Yamada Y, Yenice KM, et al. Intensity-modulated stereotactic radiotherapy of paraspinal tumors: a preliminary report. Neurosurgery 2004;54:823–30.
34. Wise JJ, Fischgrund JS, Herkowitz HN, et al. Complication, survival rates, and risk factors of surgery for metastatic disease of the spine. Spine 1999;24:1943–51.
35. Bilsky MH, Boland P, Lis E, et al. Single-stage posterolateral transpedicle approach for spondylectomy, epidural decompression, and circumferential fusion of spinal metastases. Spine 2000;25:2240–9.
36. Patchell R, Tibbs PA, Regine WF, et al. A randomized trial of direct decompressive surgical resection in the treatment of spinal cord compression caused by metastasis. Proc ASCO 2003;22:1.
37. Seichi A, Kondoh T, Hozumi T, Karasawa K. Intraoperative radiation therapy for metastatic spinal tumors. Spine 1999;24:470–3.
38. Byrne TN. Metastatic epidural cord compression. Curr Neurol Neurosci Rep 2004;4:191–5.
39. Matsubara H, Watanabe K, Sakai H, et al. Rapid improvement of paraplegia caused by epidural involvements of Burkitt's lymphoma with chemotherapy. Spine 2004;29:4–6.
40. Katagiri H, Takahashi M, Inagaki J, et al. Clinical results of nonsurgical treatment for spinal metastases. Int J Radiat Oncol Biol Phys 1998;42:1127–32.
41. Wong ET, Portlock CS, O'Brien JP, DeAngelis LM. Chemosensitive epidural spinal cord disease in non-Hodgkin's lymphoma. Neurology 1996;46:1543–7.
42. Abrey LE, Chamberlain MC, Engelhard HH, editors. Leptomeningeal Metastases. Springer Science & Business Media, Norwell, Massachusetts, 2005.
43. DeAngelis LM. Current diagnosis and treatment of leptomeningeal metastasis. J Neurooncol 1998;38: 245–52.
44. Price RA, Johnson WW. The central nervous system in childhood leukemia. I. The arachnoid. Cancer 1973;31:520–33.
45. Nicolson GL, Kawaguchi T, Kawaguchi M, Van Pelt C. Brain surface invasion and metastasis of murine malignant melanoma variants. J Neurooncol 1987;4:209–18.
46. Van der Ree TC, Dippel DWJ, Avezaat CJJ, et al. Leptomeningeal metastasis after surgical resection of brain metastases. J Neurol Neurosurg Psychiatry 1999;66: 225–7.
47. Mareel M, Leroy A, Bracke M. Cellular and molecular mechanisms of metastasis as applied to carcinomatous meningitis. J Neurooncol 1998;38:97–102.
48. Kastenbauer S, Wiesmann M, Pfister HW. Cerebral vasculopathy and multiple infarctions in a woman with carcinomatous meningitis while on treatment with intrathecal methotrexate. J Neurooncol 2000;48:41–5.
49. Klein P, Haley EC, Wooten GF, VandenBerg SR. Focal cerebral infarctions associated with perivascular tumor infiltrates in carcinomatous leptomeningeal metastases. Arch Neurol 1989;46:1149–52.
50. Hiesiger EM, Picco-Del Bo A, Lipschutz LE, et al. Experimental meningeal carcinomatosis selectively depresses local cerebral glucose utilization in rat brain. Neurology 1989;39:90–5.
51. Van Oostenbrugge RJ, Twijnstra A. Presenting features and value of diagnostic procedures in leptomeningeal metastases. Neurology 1999;53:382–5.
52. Straathof CS, de Bruin HG, Dippel DW, Vecht CJ. The diagnostic accuracy of magnetic resonance imaging and cerebrospinal fluid cytology in leptomeningeal metastasis. J Neurol 1999;246:810–4.
53. Schumacher M, Orszagh M. Imaging techniques in neoplastic meningosis. J Neurooncol 1998;38:111–20.
54. Freilich RJ, Krol G, DeAngelis LM. Neuroimaging and cerebrospinal fluid cytology in the diagnosis of leptomeningeal metastasis. Ann Neurol 1995;38:51–7.
55. Collie DA, Brush JP, Lammie GA, et al. Imaging features of leptomeningeal metastases. Clin Radiol 1999;54: 765–71.
56. Chamberlain MC, Kormanik PA, Glantz MJ. A comparison between ventricular and lumbar cerebrospinal fluid cytology in adult patients with leptomeningeal metastases. J Neurooncol 2001;3:42–5.
57. Van Oostenbrugge RJ, Hopman AHN, Arends JW, et al. Treatment of leptomeningeal metastases evaluated by interphase cytogenetics. J Clin Oncol 2000;18:2053–8.
58. Padma MV, Jacobs M, Kraus G, et al. ^{11}C-methionine PET imaging of leptomeningeal metastases from primary breast cancer—a case report. J Neurooncol 2001; 55:39–44.
59. Gleissner B, Siehl J, Korfel A, et al. CSF evaluation in primary CNS lymphoma patients by PCR of the CDR III IgH genes. Neurology 2002;58:390–6.
60. Hildebrand J. Prophylaxis and treatment of leptomeningeal carcinomatosis in solid tumors of adulthood. J Neurooncol 1998;38:193–8.
61. Glantz MJ, Cole BF, Recht L, et al. High-dose intravenous methotrexate for patients with nonleukemic leptomeningeal cancer: is intrathecal chemotherapy necessary? J Clin Oncol 1998;16:1561–7.
62. Siegal T. Leptomeningeal metastases: rationale for systemic chemotherapy or what is the role of intra-CSF-chemotherapy? J Neurooncol 1998;38:151–7.
63. Gray JR, Wallner KE. Reversal of cranial nerve dysfunction with radiation therapy in adults with lymphoma and leukemia. Int J Radiat Oncol Biol Phys 1990;19:439–44.
64. Kerr JZ, Berg S, Blaney SM. Intrathecal chemotherapy. Crit Rev Oncol Hematol 2001;37:227–36.
65. Shapiro WR, Young DF, Mehta BM. Methotrexate: distribution in cerebrospinal fluid after intravenous, ventricular and lumbar injections. N Engl J Med 1975;293:161–6.
66. Mason WP, Yeh SD, DeAngelis LM: 111Indium-diethylenetriamine pentaacetic acid cerebrospinal fluid flow studies predict distribution of intrathecally administered chemotherapy and outcome in patients with leptomeningeal metastases. Neurology 1998;50:438–44.
67. Rogers LR, Remer Se, Tejwani S. Durable response of breast cancer leptomeningeal metastasis to capecitabine monotherapy. Neuro-oncol 2004;6:63–4.
68. Blaney SM, Poplack DG. New cytotoxic drugs for intrathecal administration. J Neurooncol 1998;38:219–23.
69. Glantz MJ, LaFollette S, Jaeckle KA, et al. Randomized trial of a slow-release versus a standard formulation of cytarabine for the intrathecal treatment of lymphomatous meningitis. J Clin Oncol 1999;17:3110–6.
70. Archer GE, Sampson JH, McLendon RE, et al. Intrathecal busulfan treatment of human neoplastic meningitis in athymic nude rats. J Neurooncol 1999;44:233–41.
71. Bergman I, Pohl CR, Venkataramanan R, et al. Intrathecal administration of an anti-ganglioside antibody results in specific accumulation within meningeal neoplastic xenografts in nude rats. J Immunother 1999;22:114–23.
72. Cokgor I, Akabani G, Friedman HS, et al. Long term response in a patient with neoplastic meningitis secondary to melanoma treated with ^{131}I-radiolabeled antichondroitin proteoglycan sulfate Mel-14 F(ab')2—a case study. Cancer 2001;91:1809–13.
73. Sandberg DI, Bilsky MH, Souweidane MM, et al. Ommaya reservoirs for the treatment of leptomeningeal metastases. Neurosurgery 2000;47:49–54.
74. Boerman RH, Maassen EM, Joosten J, et al. Trigeminal neuropathy secondary to perineural invasion of head and neck carcinomas. Neurology 1999;53:213–6.
75. Taylor BV, Kimmel DW, Krecke KN, Cascino TL. Magnetic resonance imaging in cancer-related lumbosacral plexopathy. Mayo Clin Proc 1997;72:823–9.
76. Kichari JR, Hussain SM, Den Hollander JC, Krestin GP. MR imaging of the brachial plexus: current imaging sequences, normal findings, and findings in a spectrum of focal lesions with MR-pathologic correlation. Curr Probl Diagn Radiol 2003;32:88–101.
77. Greenberg HS, Deck MD, Vikram B, et al. Metastasis to the base of the skull: clinical findings in 43 patients. Neurology 1981;31:530–7.
78. Jungehuelsing M, Sittel C, Fischbach R, et al. Limitations of magnetic resonance imaging in the evaluation of perineural tumor spread causing facial nerve paralysis. Arch Otolaryngol Head Neck Surg 2000;126:506–10.
79. Moore KR, Tsuruda JS, Dailey AT. The value of MR neurography for evaluating extraspinal neuropathic leg pain: a pictorial essay. AJNR Am J Neuroradiol 2001;22:786–94.
80. Cmelak AJ, Cox RS, Adler JR, et al. Radiosurgery for skull base malignancies and nasopharyngeal carcinoma. Int J Radiat Oncol Biol Phys 1997;37:997–1003.
81. Castro JR, Linstadt DE, Bahary J-P, et al. Experience in charged particle irradiation of tumors of the skull base: 1977–1992. Int J Radiat Oncol Biol Phys 1994;29:647–55.
82. Jaeckle KA. Neurological manifestations of neoplastic and radiation-induced plexopathies. Semin Neurol 2004;24:385–93.
83. Johansson S, Svensson H, Denekamp J. Dose response and latency for radiation-induced fibrosis, edema, and neuropathy in breast cancer patients. Int J Radiat Oncol Biol Phys 2002;52:1207–19.
84. Gorson KC, Musaphir S, Lathi ES, Wolfe G. Radiation-induced malignant fibrous histiocytoma of the brachial plexus. J Neurooncol 1995;26:73–7.
85. Ku A, Lachmann E, Tunkel R, Nagler W. Upper limb reflex sympathetic dystrophy associated with occult malignancy. Arch Phys Med Rehabil 1996;77:726–8.
86. Ahmad A, Barrington S, Maisey M, Rubens RD. Use of positron emission tomography in evaluation of brachial plexopathy in breast cancer patients. Br J Cancer 1999;79:478–82.
87. Boyaciyan A, Oge AE, Yazici J, Aslay I. Electrophysiological findings in patients who received radiation therapy over the brachial plexus: a magnetic stimulation study. Electroencephalogr Clin Neurophysiol 1996;101:483–90.
88. Jaeckle KA, Young DF, Foley KM. The natural history of lumbosacral plexopathy in cancer. Neurology 1985; 35:8–15.
89. Dyck PJ, Windebank AJ. Diabetic and nondiabetic lumbosacral radiculoplexus neuropathies: new insights into pathophysiology and treatment. Muscle Nerve 2002; 25:477–91.
90. Keime-Guibert F, Napolitano M, Delattre J-Y. Neurological complications of radiotherapy and chemotherapy. J Neurol 1998;245:695–708.
91. Lowenthal RM, Eaton K. Toxicity of chemotherapy. Hematol Oncol Clin North Am 1996;10:967–90.
92. Quasthoff S, Hartung HP. Chemotherapy-induced peripheral neuropathy. J Neurol 2002;249:9–17.
93. Kellie SJ, Barbaric D, Koopmans P, et al. Cerebrospinal fluid concentrations of vincristine after bolus intravenous dosing—a surrogate marker of brain penetration. Cancer 2002;94:1815–20.
94. Dettmeyer R, Driever F, Becker A, et al. Fatal myeloencephalopathy due to accidental intrathecal vincristine administration: a report of two cases. Forensic Sci Int 2001;122:60–4.

95. Donelli MG, Zucchetti M, Munzone E, et al. Pharmacokinetics of anticancer agents in patients with impaired liver function. Eur J Cancer 1998;34:33–46.
96. Gillies J, Hung KA, Fitzsimons E, Soutar R. Severe vincristine toxicity in combination with itraconazole. Clin Lab Haematol 1998;20:123–4.
97. Hildebrandt G, Holler E, Woenkhaus M, et al. Acute deterioration of Charcot–Marie–Tooth disease IA (CMT IA) following 2 mg of vincristine chemotherapy. Ann Oncol 2000;11:743–7.
98. Rezvani K, Bain BJ, Coulter CA. Loss of singing ability caused by vincristine. Clin Lab Haematol 1998;20: 47–8.
99. Mahoney DH Jr, Shuster JJ, Nitschke R, et al. Acute neurotoxicity in children with B-precursor acute lymphoid leukemia: an association with intermediate-dose intravenous methotrexate and intrathecal triple therapy—a Pediatric Oncology Group study. J Clin Oncol 1998;16:1712–22.
100. Genvresse I, Dietzmann A, Massenkeil G, et al. Subacute encephalopathy after combination chemotherapy including moderate-dose methotrexate in a patient with gastric cancer. Anticancer Drugs 1999;10:293–4.
101. Koh S, Nelson MD Jr, Kovanlikaya A, Chen LS. Anterior lumbosacral radiculopathy after intrathecal methotrexate treatment. Pediatr Neurol 1999;21:576–8.
102. Paakko E, Harila-Saari A, Vanionpaa L, et al. White matter changes on MRI during treatment in children with acute lymphoblastic leukemia: correlation with neuropsychological findings. Med Pediatr Oncol 2000;35:456–61.
103. Stone JA, Castillo M, Mukherji SK. Leukoencephalopathy complicating an Ommaya reservoir and chemotherapy. Neuroradiology 1999;41:134–6.
104. Taieb S, Trillet-Lenoir V, Rambaud L, et al. Lhermitte sign and urinary retention. Cancer 2002;94:2434–40.
105. DiPaola RS, Schuchter L. Neurologic protection by amifostine. Semin Oncol 1999;26(2 Suppl 7):82–8.
106. Hensley ML, Schuchter LM, Lindley C, et al. American Society of Clinical Oncology Clinical Practice Guidelines for the Use of Chemotherapy and Radiotherapy Protectants. J Clin Oncol 1999;17: 3333–55.
107. Wilson RH, Lehky T, Thomas RR, et al. Acute oxaliplatin-induced peripheral nerve hyperexcitability. J Clin Oncol 2002;20:1767–74.
108. McKeage MJ. Comparative adverse effect profiles of platinum drugs. Drug Saf 1995;13:228–44.
109. Johnson MR, Hageboutros A, Wang K, et al . Life-threatening toxicity in a dihydropyrimidine dehydrogenase-deficient patient after treatment with topical 5-fluorouracil. Clin Cancer Res 1999;5:2006–11.
110. Smith GA, Damon LE, Rugo HS, et al. High-dose cytarabine dose modification reduces the incidence of neurotoxicity in patients with renal insufficiency. J Clin Oncol 1997;15:833–9.
111. Courtney MJ, Coffey ET. The mechanism of ara-C–induced apoptosis of differentiating cerebellar granule neurons. Eur J Neurosci 1999;11:1073–84.
112. O'Connor OA, Wright J, Moskowitz C, et al. Phase II clinical experience with the novel proteasome inhibitor bortezomib in patients with indolent non-Hodgkin's lymphoma and mantle cell lymphoma. J Clin Oncol 2005;23:676–84.
113. Ganem G, Solal-Celigny P, Joffroy A, et al. Radiation myositis: the possible role of gemcitabine. Ann Oncol 2000;11:1615–6.
114. Russell MT, Nassif AS, Cacayorin ED, et al. Gemcitabine-associated posterior reversible encephalopathy syndrome: MR imaging and MR spectroscopy findings. Magn Reson Imaging 2001;19:129–32.
115. Zochodne D. Myopathies in the intensive care unit. Can J Neurol Sci 1998;25:S40–2.
116. De Kloet ER, Oitzl MS, Joels M. Stress and cognition: are corticosteroids good or bad guys? Trends Neurosci 1999;22:422–6.
117. LaPier TK. Glucocorticoid-induced muscle atrophy. The role of exercise in treatment and prevention. J Cardiopulm Rehabil 1997;17:76–84.
118. Belka C, Budach W, Kortmann R, Bamberg M. Radiation induced CNS toxicity—molecular and cellular mechanisms. Br J Cancer 2001;85(9):1233–9.
119. Cheng KM, Chan CM, Fu YT, et al. Acute hemorrhage in late radiation necrosis of the temporal lobe: report of five cases and review of the literature. J Neurooncol 2001;51:143–50.
120. Steen RG, Spence D, Wu SJ, Xiong XP, et al. Effect of therapeutic ionizing radiation on the human brain. Ann Neurol 2001;50:787–95.
121. Kleinschmidt-DeMasters BK. Necrotizing brainstem leukoencephalopathy six weeks following radiotherapy. Clin Neuropathol 1995;14:63–8.
122. Fonseca R, O'Neill BP, Foote RL, et al. Cerebral toxicity in patients treated for small cell carcinoma of the lung. Mayo Clin Proc 1999;74:461–5.
123. Regine WF, Scott C, Murray K, Curran W. Neurocognitive outcome in brain metastases patients treated with accelerated-fractionation vs accelerated-hyperfractionated radiotherapy: an analysis from Radiation Therapy Oncology Group study 91-04. Int J Radiat Oncol Biol Phys 2001;51:711–7.
124. Duffey P, Chari G, Cartlidge NEF, Shaw PJ. Progressive deterioration of intellect and motor function occurring several decades after cranial irradiation—a new facet in the clinical spectrum of radiation encephalopathy. Arch Neurol 1996;53:814–8.
125. Marks JE, Wong J. The risk of cerebral radionecrosis in relation to dose, time and fractionation: a follow-up study. Prog Exp Tumor Res 1985;29:210–8.
126. Glantz MJ, Burger PC, Friedman AH, et al. Treatment of radiation-induced nervous system injury with heparin and warfarin. Neurology 1994;44:2020–7.
127. Leber KA, Eder HG, Kovac H, et al. Treatment of cerebral radionecrosis by hyperbaric oxygen therapy. Stereotact Funct Neurosurg 1998;70 Suppl 1:229–36.
128. Meyers CA, Geara F, Wong PF, Morrison WH. Neurocognitive effects of therapeutic irradiation for base of skull tumors. Int J Radiat Oncol Biol Phys 2000;46:51–5.
129. Anderson VA, Godber T, Smibert E, et al. Cognitive and academic outcome following cranial irradiation and chemotherapy in children: a longitudinal study. Br J Cancer 2000;82:255–62.
130. Thiessen B, DeAngelis LM. Hydrocephalus in radiation leukoencephalopathy—results of ventriculoperitoneal shunting. Arch Neurol 1998;55:705–10.
131. O'Conner MM, Mayberg MR. Effects of radiation on cerebral vasculature. Neurosurgery 2000;46:138–51.
132. Larson JJ, Ball WS, Bove KE, et al. Formation of intracerebral cavernous malformations after radiation treatment for central nervous system neoplasia in children. J Neurosurg 1998;88:51–6.
133. Shuper A, Packer RJ, Vezina LG, et al. Complicated migraine-like episodes in children following cranial irradiation and chemotherapy. Neurology 1995;45:1837–40.
134. Brandes AA, Pasetto LM, Lumachi F, Monfardini S. Endocrine dysfunctions in patients treated for brain tumors: incidence and guidelines for management. J Neurooncol 2000;47:85–92.
135. Shamisa A, Bance M, Nag S, et al. Glioblastoma multiforme occurring in a patient treated with gamma knife surgery—case report and review of the literature. J Neurosurg 2001;94:816–21.
136. Nishio S, Morioka T, Inamura T, et al. Radiation-induced brain tumours: potential late complications of radiation therapy for brain tumours. Acta Neurochir (Wien) 1998;140:763–70.
137. Kubota M, Akiyama Y, Koishi S, et al. Second malignancy following treatment of acute lymphoblastic leukemia in children. Int J Hematol 1998;67:397–401.
138. Fein DA, Marcus RB Jr, Parsons JT, et al. Lhermitte's sign: incidence and treatment variables influencing risk after irradiation of the cervical spinal cord. Int J Radiat Oncol Biol Phys 1993;27:1029–33.
139. Esik O, Emri M, Csornai M, et al. Radiation myelopathy with partial functional recovery: PET evidence of long-term increased metabolic activity of the spinal cord. J Neurol Sci 1999;163:39–43.
140. Guy J, Schatz NJ. Hyperbaric oxygen in the treatment of radiation-induced optic neuropathy. Ophthalmology 1986;93:1083–8.
141. Liu CY, Yim BT, Wozniak AJ. Anticoagulation therapy for radiation-induced myelopathy. Ann Pharmacother 2001;35:188–91.
142. Tallaksen CME, Jetne V, Foss S. Postradiation lower motor neuron syndrome—a case report and brief literature review. Acta Oncol 1997;36:345–7.
143. Graus F, Rogers LR, Posner JB. Cerebrovascular complications in patients with cancer. Medicine 1985;64:16–35.
144. Lieu AS, Hwang SL, Howng SL, Chai CY. Brain tumors with hemorrhage. J Formos Med Assoc 1999;98:365–7.
145. Cestari DM, Weine Dm, Panageas KS, Segal AZ, DeAngelis LM. Stroke in patients with cancer. Incidence and etiology. Neurology 2004;62:2025–30.
146. Bowers DC, Mulne AF, Reisch JS, et al. Nonperioperative strokes in children with central nervous system tumors. Cancer 2002;94:1094–101.
147. Raizer JJ, DeAngelis LM: Cerebral sinus thrombosis in cancer patients. Neurology 2000;54:1222–6.
148. Vassallo R, Remstein ED, Parisi JE, et al. Multiple cerebral infarctions from nonbacterial thrombotic endocarditis mimicking cerebral vasculitis. Mayo Clin Proc 1999; 74:798–802.
149. O'Neill BP, DiNapoli RP, Okazaki H. Cerebral infarction as a result of tumor emboli. Cancer 1987;60:90–5.
150. Levi M, De Jonge E, van der Poll T, ten Cate H. Advances in the understanding of the pathogenetic pathways of disseminated intravascular coagulation result in more insight in the clinical picture and better management strategies. Semin Thromb Hemost 2001;27:569–75.
151. Tuma R, DeAngelis LM. Altered mental status in patients with cancer. Arch Neurol 2000;57:1727–31.
152. Amer PA. Practice guideline for the treatment of patients with delirium. Am J Psychiatry 1999;156:1–20.
153. Lawlor PG, Gagnon B, Mancini IL, et al. Occurrence, causes, and outcome of delirium in patients with advanced cancer—a prospective study. Arch Intern Med 2000;160:786–94.
154. Caraceni A, Nanni O, Maltoni M, et al. Impact of delirium on the short-term prognosis of advanced cancer patients. Cancer 2000;89:1145–9.
155. Ely EW, Margolin R, Francis J, et al. Evaluation of delirium in critically ill patients: validation of the confusion assessment method for the intensive care unit (CAM-ICU). Crit Care Med 2001;29:1370–9.
156. Inouye SK, Foreman MD, Mion LC, et al. Nurses' recognition of delirium and its symptoms—comparison of nurse and researcher ratings. Arch Intern Med 2001;161:2467–73.
157. Cocito L, Audenino D, Primavera A. Altered mental state and nonconvulsive status epilepticus in patients with cancer. Arch Neurol 2001;58:1310.

129

Dermatologic Complications of Cancer Chemotherapy

Joy H. Kunishige, MD
Narin Apisarnthanarax, MD
Madeleine M. Duvic, MD

Dermatologic complications of cancer chemotherapy have become increasingly significant, especially with the continued development of new antineoplastic agents. The frequency of mucocutaneous complications in cancer chemotherapy is a reflection of the increased proliferative nature of affected tissues, such as the mucous membranes, skin, hair, and nails, which renders them particularly susceptible to the actions of chemotherapeutic drugs. Diagnosis of cutaneous reactions in the cancer patient is complicated by the degree of their malignancy, concomitant diseases, polypharmacy, and immunosuppression. With the advances in bone marrow transplantation, graft-versus-host disease (GVHD) is also being seen more frequently and may mimic and complicate the diagnosis of chemotherapy-induced reactions. Thirteen major cutaneous reactions and a variety of miscellaneous reactions are discussed in this chapter and are listed in Table 129-1. As seen in Table 129-2, these reactions occur in varying degrees of frequency and severity among the classes of chemotherapeutic drugs. Although dermatologic complications are rarely fatal, it is important to recognize potential reactions as they may result in significant morbidity, cosmetic disfigurement, and psychological distress. Proper treatment of potentially dose-limiting cutaneous toxicity may also allow ideal durations of chemotherapy administration, and optimization of response.

ALOPECIA

Alopecia is the most common dermatologic complication associated with chemotherapy. Whereas most drug-induced alopecias involve a telogen effluvium pattern by inducing normal hairs into a premature resting phase, the anagen effluvium pattern of hair loss is the most common type of alopecia produced by chemotherapeutic agents, with the exception of interleukin-2 (IL-2) and interferon-α (IFN-α) therapy. In chemotherapy, anagen effluvium is caused by the abrupt cessation of the high mitotic activity of hair matrix cells in the anagen phase of hair follicles.[1] This type of alopecia can be seen to some degree in most antineoplastic therapies, depending on dosage and route of administration.[2,3] However, there are certain agents, such as doxorubicin, which induce alopecia more frequently and severely (Table 129-3).[2–6] These agents display a synergistic effect when used in combination and may cause severe and complete alopecia.[6] Anagen effluvium manifests within 1 to 2 weeks after the beginning of chemotherapy but is most noticeable 1 to 2 months later.[3] Initially, there may not be total hair loss, since approximately 10% of follicles will not be in anagen phase at the start of chemotherapy. However, total hair loss eventually occurs with prolonged therapy, which can also induce hair loss in other areas of the body. Hair regrowth can usually be expected 5 months after the end of chemotherapy, although hair color and texture may change.[7] Permanent alopecia has been reported with busulfan/cyclophosphamide therapy.[8]

Hair loss often has emotional impact on patients receiving chemotherapy. Unfortunately, there are currently no widely accepted methods of prevention and treatment for alopecia. To prevent alopecia, scalp hypothermia and tourniquets have been used with some demonstrated success. Drugs such as doxorubicin, vincristine, vinblastine, dactinomycin, and mechlorethamine, which have short administration periods and half-lives, are particularly well suited for scalp hypothermia.[2] Despite a reported 47% rate of success in preservation of hair, scalp cooling has been controversial. Widespread use of hypothermia has been limited by the possibility that the decreased scalp perfusion—and thereby decreased drug exposure—could increase the risk of scalp metastasis in certain patients with solid tumors.[7,9] However, confirmatory reports of this risk are lacking.[9] In patients with hematologic malignancies, scalp hypothermia is contraindicated. A small group of women with breast cancer applied topical 2% minoxidil and reported hastened regrowth (duration of alopecia decreased by an average of 50 days); unfortunately, the drug has no preventative effect.[10] Other therapies under investigation include cyclosporine A, FK506, 1,25-dihydroxyvitamin D_3, and parathyroid hormone antagonists.[11]

Table 129-1 Major Cutaneous Reactions Associated with Chemotherapy

1. Alopecia
2. Stomatitis
3. Nail reactions
4. Extravasation reactions
5. Hyperpigmentation
6. Radiation-associated reactions
7. Photosensitivity
8. Inflammation of keratoses
9. Hypersensitivity
10. Acral erythema
11. Neutrophilic eccrine hidradenitis
12. Eccrine squamous syringometaplasia
13. Cutaneous eruption of lymphocyte recovery
14. Miscellaneous reactions

Table 129-2 Most Common Mucocutaneous Reactions of the Major Classes of Chemotherapeutic Drugs

Alkylating Agents	Antibiotics
Hyperpigmentation Hypersensitivity	Alopecia Stomatitis Chemical cellulitis Hyperpigmentation Radiation-associated reactions
Vinca Alkaloids	**Antimetabolites**
Alopecia Chemical Cellulitis Inflammation of keratoses Neutrophilic eccrine hidradenitis	Acral erythema Alopecia Hyperpigmentation Radiation-associated reactions

Table 129-3 Chemotherapeutic Agents Associated with Alopecia

Most Common or Severe	Least Common or Severe
Bleomycin	Amsacrine
Cisplatin	Busulfan
Cyclophosphamide	Carboplatin
Cytarabine	Carmustine
Dacarbazine	Chlorambucil epirubicin
Dactinomycin	Gemcitabine
Daunorubicin	Hydroxyurea
Docetaxel	Melphalan
Doxorubicin	Mercaptopurine
Etoposide	Methotrexate
Fluorouracil	Mitomycin
Idarubicin	Procarbazine
Ifosfamide	Teniposide
Interferon-a	Vinorelbine
Irinotecan	
Mechlorethamine	
Nitrosoureas	
Paclitaxel	
Thiotepa	
Topotecan	
Vinblastine	
Vincristine	
Vindesine	

*Adapted from Susser WS et al.[5]

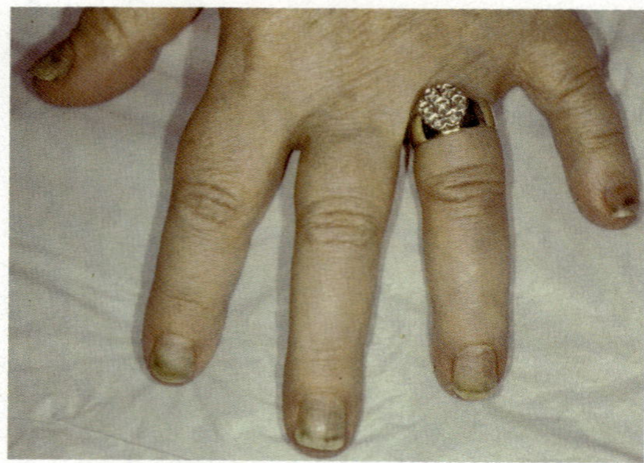

Figure 129-1 Docetaxel-induced nail hyperpigmentation and onychodystrophy.

STOMATITIS

Stomatitis and other oral complications of cancer chemotherapy are discussed in Chapters 136, "Gastrointestinal Complications," and 137, "Oral Complications."

NAIL REACTIONS

Hyperpigmentation is the most common nail abnormality encountered in patients receiving chemotherapy, particularly in dark-skinned patients.[2] Vertical bands, horizontal bands, or diffuse hyperpigmentation of nails has been associated with the following medications: bleomycin, cyclophosphamide, daunorubicin, doxorubicin, fluorouracil, hydroxyurea, aminoglutethimide, busulfan, cisplatin, dacarbazine, docetaxel, idarubicin, ifosfamide, melphalan, methotrexate, mitomycin, and mitoxantrone (Figure 129-1).[5] Hyperpigmentation due to chemotherapy-induced melanocyte stimulation should be distinguished from yellow nail syndrome (YNS). YNS nails have increased transverse curvature, absent lunulae, and no cuticle. Suggested etiologies include paraneoplastic process, AIDS-association, and drug-induction.[12]

Other common nail manifestations include horizontal depressions of the nail plate called *Beau's lines* (Figure 129-2), horizontal white discoloration of the entire width of the nail plate called *Mees lines*, horizontal white discoloration involving partial nail width called *leukonychia, onycholysis*, and *onychodystrophy*. Associations between bleomycin and nail loss; hydroxyurea and brittle nails; etoposide and nail bed pigmentation have also been reported in the literature.[2,5] Other onychopathies and their associated chemoagents are summarized in Table 129-4. Patients can be reassured that these nail changes are generally benign and resolve after discontinuation of the causative agent and the affected nails grow out. However, nails damaged by chemotherapy are more susceptible to infection by yeast, dermatophytes, and pseudomonas. Infections may cause lasting damage to the matrix that will not resolve.

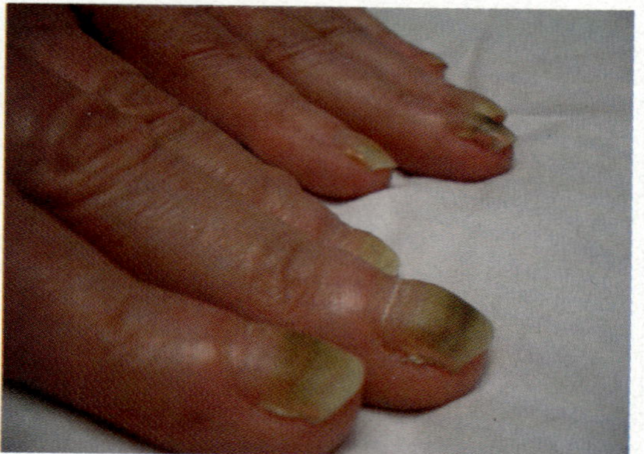

Figure 129-2 Hyperpigmentation and Beau's lines.

Table 129-4 Summary of Nail Abnormalities and Associated Chemoagents

Onychopathy	Associated Chemoagents
Beau's lines	Taxanes Bleomycin Cisplatin Doxorubicin Melphalan Vincristine
Transverse leukonychia	Adriamycin
Muehrcke's lines	Doxorubicin Cyclophosphamide Vincristine Leucovorin Levamisole Methotrexate
Onycholysis	Taxanes Doxorubicin Fluorouracil Mitoxantrone Bleomycin
Onychomadesis, defluvium unguium	Taxanes Bleomycin Fluorouracil Mercaptopurine Mitoxantrone
Ischemic changes	Bleomycin Taxanes
Melanonychia	Doxorubicin Methotrexate Nitrogen mustard Nitrosourea Etoposide Cyclophosphamide Busulfan Melphalan
Non-melanotic pigmentation	5-FU
Acute paronychia	Methotrexate Taxanes
Pyogenic granuloma	Cetuximab (C225) Gefitinib (Iressa)

EXTRAVASATION REACTIONS

Extravasation injury is a well-known adverse event that occurs when offending drugs escape from the veins or intravenous catheters into subcutaneous tissues. Accidental extravasation occurs in approximately 0.1 to 6% of patients receiving intravenous chemotherapy.[13] Cancer patients are inherently at high risk of extravasation for three reasons. First, these patients often require multiple venipuncture sites and have thin and fragile veins. Second, they may have concomitant peripheral vascular disease and be malnourished. Third, the number of optimal intravenous sites may be reduced due to previous chemotherapy, radiation therapy, surgery-related lymphedema.[2,14] The cutaneous manifestations of extravasation may range from discomfort and mild erythema to severely painful skin necrosis, ulcerations, and damage to deep tissue structures. Nerve and tendon damage leads to neurologic deficits, contractures, and joint stiffness. The extent of tissue damage in extravasation largely depends on the concentration, volume, and vesicant nature of the extravasated agent.[13,14]

Extravasated cytotoxic agents generally cause two types of local cutaneous reactions: irritant and vesicant reactions. Irritants cause a short-lived and self-limited phlebitis and tender, warm, erythematous reaction along the vein or at the site of intravenous administration. A variant of this local irritation is an erythematous and urticarial hypersensitivity flare reaction that has been associated with the anthracyclines. Vesicants initially cause a similar reaction; however the irritation may worsen, depending on the amount of drug that has extravasated.

Whereas small-volume extravasations cause limited erythema that resolves over a few weeks, large-volume extravasations may induce necrosis within a matter of days. Eschars are followed by painful ulcerations with red, raised edges. Antibiotics, such as doxorubicin, dactinomycin, daunorubicin, and mitomycin, are the most common, potent, and well-documented vesicants (Table 129-5). Though almost all vesicants cause some degree of irritation on a spectrum of injury, boplatin, cyclophosphamide, docetaxel, ifosfamide, menogaril, and thiotepa are known to produce irritation.[5] Paclitaxel can induce an extravasation recall reaction, in which extravasation of the agent at one site has induced a cutaneous reaction, ranging from erythema to ulcerations, at a previous extravasation site.[15] Drug administration through central venous catheters (CVCs) is less prone to extravasation; however central lines may dislodge, or venous vessels may be perforated with potentially disastrous consequences, including mediastinitis.[16] Thus, CVC extravasation should be considered in the setting of fever, severe pleuritic pain, upper extremity and neck swelling, and a widened mediastinum.

Table 129-5 Chemotherapeutic Agents Associated with Chemical Cellulitis

Most Common	Least Common	
Dactinomycin	Amsacrine	Melphalan
Daunorubicin	Bisantrene	Mechlor-ethamine
Doxorubicin	Bleomycin	Mitoxantrone
Mitomycin	Carmustine	Paclitaxel
	Chlorozotocin	Plicamycin
	Cisplatin	Pyrazofurin
	Dacarbazine	Streptozocin
	Epirubicin	Vinblastine
	Esorubicin	Vincristine
	Etoposide	Vindesine
	Fluorouracil	Vinorelbine
	Idarubicin	

Vesicant injury is sometimes referred to as chemical cellulitis. It displays poor healing and often continues to worsen, necessitating surgical intervention.[14] Vesicants delay fibroblastic wound contraction and have the ability to bind to DNA, possibly allowing them to be recycled and retained in the tissue to induce damage for a longer duration.[14] As it has been estimated that about one-third of all vesicant extravasations will develop into ulcerations, vigilant recognition and management of extravasation plays a major role in limiting tissue injury.[17] When extravasation is suspected, prompt discontinuation of the infusion is recommended, followed by aspiration of residual drug and removal of the catheter. Local cold application and elevation of the affected extremity are commonly used and helpful.[14] Intermittent local cooling alone has an 89.1% success rate in preventing ulceration.[18] For the vinca alkaloids, heat application is recommended instead, as cold application may actually induce ulceration.[17]

The use of antidotes is controversial, and some antidotes such as sodium bicarbonate may be harmful or ulcerative. Sodium thiosulfate and hyaluronidase have been recommended for mechlorethamine and vinca alkaloids, respectively. The success of locally injected corticosteroids has also been variable. As few inflammatory cells are involved in extravasation reactions, these reactions may not be inflammatory and would not, hypothetically, benefit from locally injected corticosteroids.[19] Locally injected granulocyte-macrophage colony stimulating factor, which has been used to promote healing of doxorubicin ulcerations, and pyridoxine, used to treat mitomycin extravasation, are both worthy of further study.[20,21] Whether a local antidote has a specific effect or acts as a diluent is hard to determine. Locally injected saline alone has proven successful in resolving extravasation reactions and preventing ulceration.[22] Although conservative treatment is preferable for most vesicant extravasations, early excision is sometimes favored, especially when the most potent vesicants are involved.[22,23] Surgical consultation for wide local excision and flap reconstruction is invariably necessary when ulcerations become evident, or if extravasation lesions prove unresponsive to therapy. For topical therapy, the free-radical scavenger dimethyl sulfoxide (DMSO) has shown consistent therapeutic success. In 1995, an analysis of 96 cumulative patients from multiple studies showed that DMSO protected 98.3% of extravasation cases from ulceration.[24]

HYPERPIGMENTATION

Hyperpigmentation is a common cutaneous manifestation that may be of cosmetic concern to patients. The skin, mucous membranes, hair, teeth, and nails may be affected, and the reaction may be diffuse or localized. Hyperpigmentation most commonly accompanies use of alkylating agents, antitumor antibiotics, and gemcitabine (Table 129-6).[5] Agents commonly associated with oral mucosal hyperpigmentation include busulfan, fluorouracil, tegafur, doxorubicin, hydroxyurea, cisplatin, and cyclophosphamide.[5] Among the antimetabolites, methotrexate may produce a characteristic hair "flag sign" with horizontal hyperpigmented bands alternating with normal hair color in light-haired individuals.[5] Tegafur can induce hyperpigmentation of the palms, soles, nails, and glans penis in a third of patients receiving the drug. A flagellate, band-like hyper-pigmentation in areas of trauma also occurs with high incidence in 8 to 20% of patients receiving bleomycin (Figure 129-3). Busulfan's hyperpigmentation can mimic Addison disease, with symptoms of weakness, weight loss, and diarrhea, but with normal melanocyte-stimulating hormone and adrenocorticotropic hormone serum levels.[7] Hyperpigmentation in areas of occlusion, such as cutaneous areas under electrocardiograph pads, tape, or dressings, with or without preceding erythema, has been reported with ifosfamide, topical carmustine, thiotepa, docetaxel, and combinations of etoposide and carboplatin with either cyclophosphamide or ifosfamide.[5] Finally, localized, serpentine, supravenous hyperpigmentation is often seen at the intravenous administration sites of fotemustine, fluorouracil, vinorelbine, and various combined chemotherapy regimens. The mechanism of chemotherapy-induced hyperpigmentation reactions is currently unknown but may involve direct toxicity, melanocyte stimulation, and post-inflammatory changes. Although these reactions may occasionally be permanent, in most cases, discoloration will gradually resolve after the discontinuation of the chemotherapy.

Table 129-6 Chemotherapeutic Agents Associated with Hyperpigmentation

Alkylating Agents	Antibiotics	Antimetabolites	Combined Regimens
Busulfan	Bleomycin	Fluorouracil	Bleomycin/doxorubicin/vincristine
Cisplatin	Dactinomycin	Methotrexate	Busulfan/cyclophosphamide
Cyclophosphamide	Daunorubicin	Tegafur	Cyclophosphamide/doxorubicin/vincristine/prednisone
Fotemustine	Doxorubicin	**Miscellaneous**	Cyclophosphamide/etoposide/carboplatin
Ifosfamide	Mitoxantrone	Brequinar sodium	Doxorubicin/bleomycin/vinblastine/dacarbazine
Thiotepa	Plicamycin	Docetaxel	Ifosfamide/carboplatin/etoposide
Topical carmustine	**Nucleoside Analogues**	Hydroxyurea	Methotrexate/cytarabine/L-asparaginase/daunorubicin/mercaptopurine/cyclophosphamide
Topical mechlorethamine	Gemcitabine	Procarbazine	
	Troxacitabine	Vinorelbine	

*Adapted from Susser WS et al.[5]

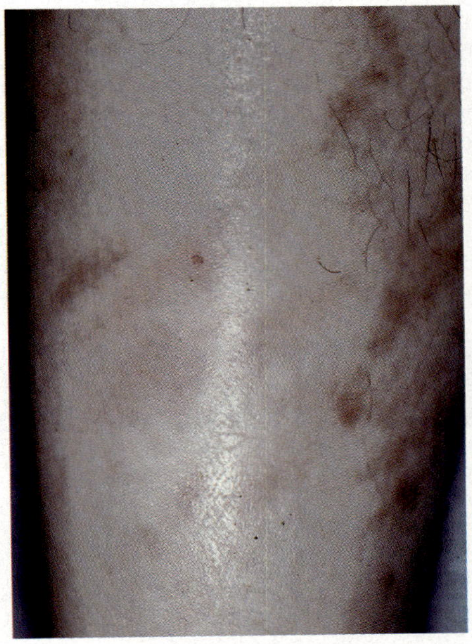

Figure 129-3 Cutaneous flagellate hyperpigmentation of bleomycin.

RADIATION-ASSOCIATION REACTIONS

With the widespread use of regimens combining chemotherapy and radiotherapy, two types of radiation-associated cutaneous reactions have been well described: radiation enhancement and radiation recall (Table 129-7). Radiation enhancement refers to the augmentation of radiation therapy effects, which may occur when both chemotherapy and radiation therapy are given within 1 week of each other. The agents most commonly

Table 129-7 Chemotherapeutic Agents Implicated in Radiation-Associated Reactions

Radiation Enhancement	Radiation Recall
Bleomycin	Bleomycin
Camptothecins	Cyclophosphamide
Chlorambucil	Cytarabine
Cisplatin*	Dactinomycin
Cyclophosphamide*	Daunorubicin
Dactinomycin	Doxorubicin
Doxorubicin	Docetaxel
Fluorouracil	Edatrexate
Hydroxyurea	Etoposide
Interferons	Fluorouracil
Mercaptopurine	Gemcitabine
Methotrexate	Hydroxyurea
Triazinate	Idarubicin
Vincristine*	Lomustine
	Melphalan
	Methotrexate
	Oxaliplatin
	Paclitaxel
	Tamoxifen
	Triazinate
	Trimetrexate
	Vinblastine

*Reported only in combination drug regimens.
Adapted from Susser WS et al.[5]

involved include bleomycin, dactinomycin, doxorubicin, fluorouracil, hydroxyurea, and methotrexate. Although other organs are also affected in this potentiation, the skin is the most common site of this toxicity. The reaction may appear as dry or moist desquamation, or as erythema and edema. When bullae, erosions, and ulcerations accompany erythema, Staphylococcus is usually the causative factor.[25] The degree of enhancement of radiation damage depends on, and is inversely related to, the time interval between administration of the drug and radiation. The less time there is between chemotherapy and irradiation, the greater the enhancement effect.[26] Enhancement is also dependent on drug dosage and the pharmacologic mechanism of the drug.[2]

Radiation recall is an erythematous inflammatory reaction in areas of previously irradiated skin. Severe radiation dermatitis can even spread to areas outside the portal as an id reaction. Radiation recall occurs from 8 days up to 15 years after radiation therapy and may also occur in other organs.[5] The most commonly associated agents are the antitumor antibiotics dactinomycin and doxorubicin.[27] Other agents are less frequently the culprit of radiation recall, including the new nucleoside analogue gemcitabine.[28,29] The radiation dosage and the time interval between radiation and chemotherapy determine the occurrence and severity of recall, respectively.[27] The mechanism of the recall reaction is currently unknown, although it has been theorized that impaired tissue repair may be a result of inadequate stem cell reserve or mutations in cells that survived radiation.[30] Generally, the treatment for radiation-associated reactions is symptomatic with an effort to avoid or treat secondary infections with appropriate antibiotics. Severe ulcerative and necrotic reactions may necessitate debridement. Topical mupirocin and systemic corticosteroids are mainstays in the treatment of radiation recall, and may even allow continuation of the offending drug without further recall effects.[30]

PHOTOSENSITIVITY REACTIONS

Cutaneous reactions related to chemotherapy and ultraviolet (UV) light exposure have been well documented, though they are relatively infrequent. Generally, most of these reactions involve exogenous phototoxicity with the agents acting as chromophores. Dacarbazine, fluorouracil, methotrexate, and vinblastine are the most common phototoxic antineoplastic agents (Table 129-8).[31] Both clinically and histologically, these phototoxic reactions appear as exaggerated sunburns.

Table 129-8 Chemotherapeutic Agents Associated with Phototoxicity

Brequinar sodium	Methotrexate
Dacarbazine	Mitomycin C
Dactinomycin	Porphyrins
Doxorubicin	Procarbazine
Fluorouracil	Tegafur
Flutamide	Thioguanine
Hydroxyurea	Vinblastine

Phototoxicity has also been reported to affect the nails in the form of mercaptopurine-induced photo-onycholysis, which is tender and usually involves the distal third of the nail. Hussain and colleagues reported onycholysis in five patients receiving paclitaxel that resolved when nails were shielded from the sun.[32]

Another form of photosensitivity is the photoallergy that has been described with flutamide and tegafur, in which the cutaneous reaction recurs with re-administration of the implicated agent.

A third type of photosensitivity, the UV recall reaction, is observed with suramin (35% incidence), methotrexate, and etoposide/cyclophosphamide therapy, which causes a sunburn reactivation if the drugs are administered within 1 week of obtaining a sunburn.[33] Photosensitivity is suspected when an eruption involves sun-exposed areas. Susceptibility to phototoxic reactions depends on both host and environmental factors and is hard to predict, with the exception of porphyrin drugs, such as hematoporphyrin derivative (74% incidence) and Photofrin polypophyrin (20–40% incidence).[31,34,35] Therapy for photosensitivity reactions is symptomatic with topical corticosteroids and antipruritics. Severe cases may require systemic steroids. Chloroquine and beta carotene have been used for prophylaxis but were not effective in controlled studies.[36] Furthermore, as the agent may remain in the patient's skin for several weeks, patients should be advised to take sun-avoidance measures.

INFLAMMATION OF KERATOSES

Several chemotherapeutic agents (Table 129-9) have been known to induce inflammation of preexisting skin disease. Inflammation of actinic keratoses (AKs) is known as an AK recall reaction and is common in elderly patients with fair complexion and history of sun damage. Suramin and cytarabine-induced inflammation of seborrheic keratosis and fludarabine-induced squamous cell carcinoma have also been reported. The association between systemic fluorouracil and the irritation of clinical and subclinical AKs is well known and resembles the effect produced by topical application of 5-fluorouracil (5-FU). AK recall reactions usually appear 1 week following the initiation of drug administration; reactions usually resolve 1 to 4 weeks following the end of therapy, although they may regress during therapy as well.[37] This recall reaction may be due to a process similar to radiation recall or increased DNA synthesis in AK lesions and consequently higher chemoagent uptake.[37,38] Although these lesions are self-limiting, superficial ulceration and staphylococcal colonization can occur and necessitate antibiotics or corticosteroids. The reaction may or may not recur with drug re-administration. Similar to the effect of topical 5-FU on AKs, systemic fluorouracil often clears the affected AKs after the inflammatory reaction resolves.[39]

Table 129-9 Chemotherapeutic Agents Associated with Inflammation of Actinic Keratoses

Dactinomycin/vincristine/dacarbazine
Docetaxel
Doxorubicin
Doxorubicin/cytarabine/thioguanine
Doxorubicin/vincristine
Fluorouracil
Fluorouracil/cisplatin
Pentostatin

Adapted from Susser WS et al.[5]

HYPERSENSITIVITY REACTIONS

Hypersensitivity reactions, mediated by types I, II, III, and IV immune-mediated allergy, can become dose limiting and are reported with most chemotherapeutic drugs. Although they are generally infrequent, these reactions occur more commonly with L-asparaginase, paclitaxel, docetaxel, teniposide, cisplatin (intravesical), procarbazine, and cytarabine.[40] The only cytotoxic drugs without reported hypersensitivity—when used as single agents—are the nitrosoureas, vinca alkaloids, altretamine, and dactinomycin.[40] Most reactions involve type I hypersensitivity with associated urticaria, angioedema, flushing, and pruritus. Severe anaphylactic reactions also occur, frequently causing shock, hypotension, and, occasionally, death.

L-asparaginase is most commonly associated with hypersensitivity, occurring in 10 to 25% of patients receiving the drug.[40] Hypersensitivity occurs less frequently when the drug is given in combination drug regimens, especially with vincristine and prednisone.[41] In up to 40% of patients, paclitaxel and docetaxel induce mild rashes and flushing, although premedication with antihistamines and corticosteroids reduces this frequency. Intravesically administered cisplatin in patients with bladder cancer seems to be more allergenic than when the drug is given intravenously and occurs with a 20% incidence.[42]

Maculopapular rashes are the most common manifestation of procarbazine hypersensitivity, although urticaria and angioedema, and type III hypersensitivity with immune complex deposition, manifesting as toxic epidermal necrolysis, may also occur. Maculopapular rash is also the most common manifestation of cytarabine type I hypersensitivity (5 to 30% incidence). The cytarabine syndrome presents with high fever, rigors, myalgia, arthralgias, and a diffuse erythematous maculopapular rash, and is postulated to be a type III hypersensitivity reaction.[43,44] Hypersensitivity reactions are generally responsive to corticosteroid therapy.

ACRAL ERYTHEMA

Acral erythema (AE) was first reported in association with chemotherapy by Zuehlke in 1974.[45] Other names include palmoplantar erythrodysesthesia, palmoplantar erythema, hand-foot syndrome, peculiar AE, and Burgdorf reaction. It commonly occurs with fluorouracil, capecitabine, cytarabine, clofarabine,[46] and doxorubicin (Table

Table 129-10 Chemotherapeutic Agents Associated with Inflammation of Acral Erythema

Most Common	Least Common	
Capecitabine	Cisplatin	Mercaptopurine
Cytarabine	Cyclophos-phamide	Methotrexate
Doxorubicin	Daunorubicin	Mitomycin
Fluorouracil	Docetaxel	Mitotane
	Doxifluridine	Paclitaxel
	Etoposide	Pegylated liposomal doxorubicin
	Floxuridine	Suramin
	Hydroxyurea	Troxacitabine
	Idarubicin	Tegafur
	Lomustine	Vincristine
	Melphalan	

Adapted from Susser WS et al.[5]

129-10). There is a prodrome of dysesthesia of the palms and soles, evolving into painful, tingling, symmetric, well-demarcated swelling and erythema (Figure 129-4), followed by a desquamative phase on resolution. Erythema and swelling usually appear on the thenar and hypothenar eminences, lateral aspect of the fingers, and the pads of the distal phalanges. The hands are more often affected than the feet. In its various manifestations, AE may appear as alternating bands of erythema and sparing and may also be accompanied by a mild erythema or a morbilliform eruption on the trunk, neck, chest, scalp, and extremities.[47] Methotrexate and cytarabine can reportedly induce a bullous variant of AE, which may progress to full-thickness epidermal necrosis before resolving.[48]

AE occurs with an incidence of 6 to 42% in different series, and occurs mostly in adults.[46] AE appears to be dose dependent on peak levels and total cumulative dose, as it occurs earlier and more severely after bolus infusions (24 hours to 3 weeks), as compared with continuous low-dose administration (2 to 10 months).[47,49] AE tends to persist and worsen with further continuation of chemotherapy and may be dose limiting, as the associated pain may progress to become physically and functionally limiting. Cyclosporine infusions have been shown to worsen the pain, possibly due to the therapy's high alcohol content.[50] With long-term chemotherapy, reversible palmoplantar kera-

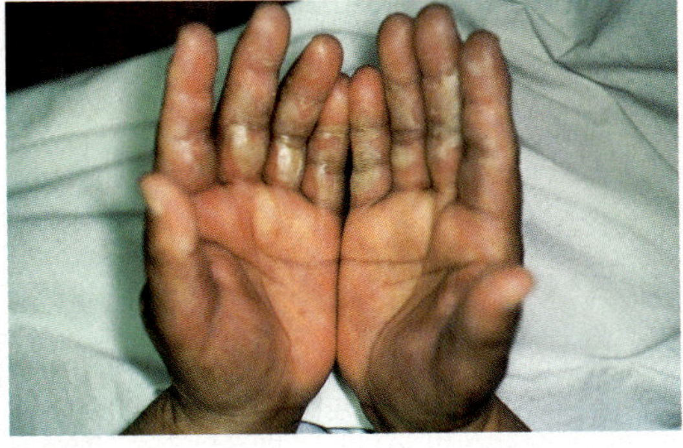

Figure 129-4 Chemo-induced acral erythema of the palms.

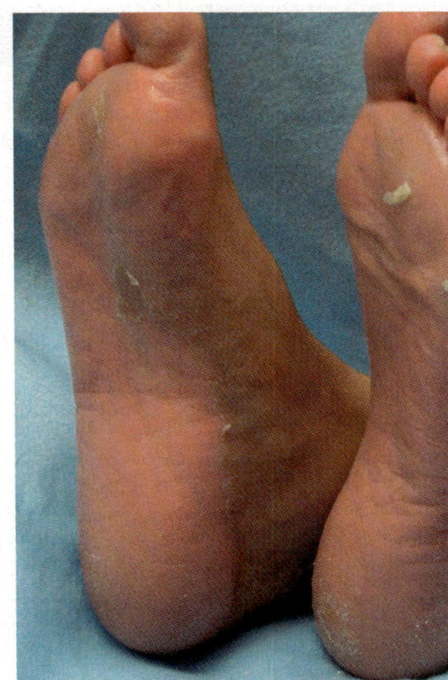

Figure 129-5 Desquamation phase of hand-and-foot syndrome, secondary to capecitabine.

toderma can also develop.[51] Cessation of the causative agent will allow resolution of AE in 1 to 2 weeks, with desquamation and re-epithelialization (Figure 129-5). AE may or may not recur with re-administration. The treatment of AE is symptomatic, aimed at increasing tolerability to allow continued chemotherapy. Corticosteroids have shown variable success. Supportive treatment includes topical wound care, elevation, and pain medication. Similar to the concept of scalp hypothermia for alopecia, the cooling of hands and feet may help prevent AE.[49,52] Pyridoxine may also reduce dysesthesia and pain to allow continuation of therapy.[53]

The pathogenesis of AE is currently unknown, but it is likely multifactorial. Theories are based on the fact that the reaction is usually limited to the palms and soles. Temperature gradients, vascular anatomy, the existence of rapidly dividing epidermal cells, and high concentration of eccrine glands are characteristics of these regions of the body and may play a role in pathogenesis. It is conceivable that AE may be related to a direct toxic effect. Biopsies of AE appear histologically nonspecific but are consistent with a toxic reaction.[49] In the setting of chemotherapy, diagnosis of AE is a relatively simple matter. However in bone marrow transplant (BMT) patients, it may be difficult to differentiate from acute graft-versus-host disease (GVHD). There is a 35% incidence of AE in BMT patients, which may be due to the use of higher doses of chemotherapy and total body irradiation.[54] There is a 10 to 80% incidence of acute GVHD in BMT patients, depending on degree of histoincompatibility between donor and recipient, the number of T-cells in the graft, the patient's age, and the GVHD prophylactic regimen.[55] Histologically and clinically, AE may resemble acute GVHD in the first 3 weeks: As in AE, the palms are commonly affected in acute GVHD although it usually progresses with involvement of other areas of the body. Since early biopsies of acute GVHD mimic AE, serial biopsies at 3- to 5-day intervals are helpful in establishing patterns of progression supportive of acute GVHD.[54] Distinguishing AE from acute GVHD is important because the latter requires greater intervention with further immunosuppression; without treatment it usually progresses and may be fatal.

NEUTROPHILIC ECCRINE HIDRADENITIS

Neutrophilic eccrine hidradenitis (NEH) has been associated with a variety of drugs and conditions including zidovudine, acetaminophen, granulocyte colony-stimulating factor, infections, and acute myelogenous leukemia.[5,56,57] NEH is most often observed with chemotherapy, and cytarabine is most frequently cited along with bleomycin, chlorambucil, cyclophosphamide, doxorubicin, lomustine, and mitoxantrone.[5] NEH manifests as erythematous to violaceous macules, papules, plaques, nodules, and pustules, which may be multiple or solitary, and painful or asymptomatic. Unusual presentations occur with involvement of the ears or periorbital inflammation.[57,58] NEH usually begins 2 days to 3 weeks following the initiation of chemotherapy, although it may occur as long as 2 years following therapy.[5] Fever may also accompany the reaction. Given the clinical variability of NEH, a skin biopsy is required for diagnosis. The histopathology shows necrosis of eccrine epithelial cells, and neutrophilic infiltrates centered on eccrine sweat glands and ducts, and possibly apocrine glands.[54] In neutropenic patients, these neutrophilic infiltrates may be sparse. Electron microscopic studies by Brehler and colleagues plus evidence of chemotherapeutic drug levels in sweat in a study by Madsen support the theory that chemotherapy-induced NEH is caused by direct toxicity of the sweat glands.[59,60] NEH is self-limited and resolves spontaneously without scarring within 1 to 4 weeks after the cessation of therapy. However, there is a 60% recurrence rate with the re-administration of the same drug or regimen.[5] Although therapy is rarely needed for NEH, treatment with ibuprofen and corticosteroids may alleviate the discomfort of fever and painful lesions. Dapsone, which has effects on neutrophil migration, has successfully prevented the recurrence of NEH in a case report.[58]

ECCRINE SQUAMOUS SYRINGOMETAPLASIA

Eccrine squamous syringometaplasia (ESS) is a relatively uncommon and benign cutaneous reaction, which is defined by pathognomonic noninflammatory metaplasia of the cuboidal epithelial cells of the eccrine sweat ducts. It differs from NEH by the absence of neutrophils on skin biopsy. Like NEH, the cutaneous manifestation of ESS is thought to result from a direct toxic effect. Clinically, ESS may give a presentation that is similar to NEH with erythematous macules, pap-

Table 129-11 Miscellaneous Reactions and Reactions Associated with Cytokine Therapy

- Flushing
  - L-Asparaginase
  - Bleomycin
  - Carboplatin
  - Carmustine (BCNU)
  - Cisplatin
  - Cyclophosphamide
  - Dacarbazine
  - Didemnin B
  - Diethylstilbestrol
  - Docetaxel
  - Doxorubicin
  - Etoposide
  - Fluorouracil
  - Flutamide
  - IL-2
  - Leuprolide
  - Lomustine
  - Paclitaxel
  - Plicamycin
  - Procarbazine
  - Suramin
  - Tamoxifen
  - Teniposide
  - Trimetrexate
- Folliculitis
  - Dactinomycin
  - Daunorubicin
  - Fluorouracil
  - Methotrexate
- Furunculosis
  - Fluoxymesterone
  - Methotrexate
- Acneiform eruptions
  - Dactinomycin
  - Fluoxymesterone
  - Medroxyprogesterone
  - Procarbazine
  - Vinblastine
  - C225 EGFR antibody[71]
  - OSI774 EGFR inhibitor[70]
- Dermatitis herpetiformis
  - Flare
  - Cyclophosphamide/doxorubicin/vincristine
- Raynaud phenomenon
  - Bleomycin
  - Cisplatin
  - Vincristine
- Drug-induced SLE
  - Aminoglutethimide
  - Diethylstilbestrol
  - Hydroxyurea
  - Leuprolide
  - Tegafur
  - IFN-α
- Dermatomyositis-like reaction
  - Hydroxyurea (long term)
  - Tamoxifen
  - Tegafur
- Sclerodermoid reaction
  - Bleomycin
  - Docetaxel
- Bullous pemphigoid
  - Dactinomycin/MTX
- Keratotic papules
  - Suramin
- Exfoliative dermatitis
  - Chlorambucil/busulfan
  - Cisplatin
  - Methotrexate
  - Mitomycin C (intravesical)
- Lichenoid eruptions
  - Hydroxyurea
  - Tegafur
- Capillaritis
  - Aminoglutethimide
- Telangiectasia
  - Carmustine (BCNU)
  - Fluorouracil (topical)
  - Hydroxyurea
  - IFN-α
- Erythema nodosum
  - Busulfan
  - Diethylstilbestrol
  - IL-2
- Exacerbation of seborrheic dermatitis
  - Fluorouracil
  - IL-2
  - INF-α
- Increased nonmelanoma skin cancer
  - Nitrogen mustard (topical)
- Acquired cutaneous adherence
  - Doxorubicin/ketoconazole
- Porphyria
  - Cisplatin
- Porphyria cutanea tarda
  - Busulfan
  - Cyclophosphamide
  - Diethylstilbestrol
  - Methotrexate
- Acute intermittent porphyria
  - Chlorambucil
  - Cyclophosphamide
- Other INF-α reactions
  - Eosinophilic fasciitis
  - Exacerbation of herpes labialis
  - Increased growth of eyelashes
  - Necrotizing vasculitis
  - Paraneoplastic pemphigus
  - Psoriasis exacerbation and de novo
  - Thyroiditis
- Other IL-2 reactions
  - Erosions in surgical scars
  - Hypersensitivity to iodine contrast dye
  - Linear IgA bullous dermatosis
  - Pemphigus vulgaris (de novo, recurrent)
  - Poly/Dermatomyositis exacerbation
  - Psoriasis exacerbation
  - Staphylococcal infections
  - TEN-like Bullous Desquamation
  - Vitiligo
- Fludarabine reactions
  - Paraneoplastic pemphigus[68]
  - Erythema multiforme[66]
  - Grover disease
- Pustular psoriasis
  - Aminoglutethimide
  - Pegylated liposomal doxorubicin[65]
- Cutaneous ulcers
  - Hydroxyurea
  - IFN-α, pegylated IFN-α
  - IL-2
  - Methotrexate
- Hirsutism
  - Diethylstilbestrol
  - Fluoxymesterone
  - Tamoxifen
- Hair color change
  - Bleomycin
  - Cisplatin
  - Cyclophosphamide
  - Methotrexate
  - Tamoxifen
- Fixed-drug eruption
  - Dacarbazine
  - Hydroxyurea
  - Paclitaxel (bullous)
  - Procarbazine

EGFR = epidermal growth factor receptor; IFN-α = interferon-α; IgA = immunoglobulin A; IL-2 = interleukin-2; MTX = methotrexate; SLE = systemic lupus erythematosus.

ules, plaques, or vesicles, which may be generalized or localized to the intertriginous areas or the palms and soles. Given these similarities to NEH, ESS is thought to represent the non-inflammatory end of the spectrum of chemotherapeutic eccrine gland reactions.[61] ESS reportedly appears 2 to 39 days after the initiation of chemotherapy and resolves spontaneously in 7 to 10 days.[62] It is not associated with any one particular cytotoxic agent. A histologic confirmation of ESS changes on biopsy can be a diagnostic aid in differentiating a chemotherapy-induced reaction from acute GVHD or other drug reactions. ESS deserves consideration in any erythematous eruption during chemotherapy.

CUTANEOUS ERUPTION OF LYMPHOCYTE RECOVERY

The cutaneous eruption of lymphocyte recovery (ELR) may be seen in patients receiving intensive marrow aplasia–inducing chemotherapy.[63] As with ESS, the ELR phenomenon has been observed with various cytotoxic agents but is not associated with a particular agent. Clinically, ELR has the appearance of variably distributed erythematous and pruritic macules, papules, and plaques, which may become confluent and erythrodermic, and is often associated with a couple days of fever. In the setting of chemotherapy, this reaction has been found to occur 6 to 21 days after the chemotherapy-induced nadir of the leukocyte count, which correlates with the time of the initial recovery of peripheral lymphocytes. ELR may reflect the return of highly alloreactive immunocompetent lymphocytes to the peripheral circulation and skin.[63] ELR is self-limited and resolves over several days with desquamation and mild residual hyperpigmentation. Given the nonspecific clinical manifestation of ELR, other causes of an erythematous exanthem must be considered in the differential diagnosis, particularly acute GVHD, sepsis, viral exanthem, leukemia or lymphoma cutis, ESS, and drug hypersensitivity. Of these types of eruptions, acute GVHD is similar in time of onset to ELR in the setting of bone marrow transplantation. The similarity with ELR is especially true in the case of autologous GVHD, as both involve a lymphocytic recovery in which histocompatibility is present. However, acute autologous GVHD cannot be reliably distinguished from ELR by skin biopsy.[64] As theorized by Horn, GVHD may represent a form of ELR.[65]

MISCELLANEOUS REACTIONS

A large number of miscellaneous cutaneous reactions have been reported in the literature as case reports. The reactions are uncommon or their incidence rates are mostly unknown. Table 129-11 lists and updates many of these reactions, including reactions to cytokines, novel pegylated and liposomal drugs, nucleoside analogues, and tyrosine kinase inhibitors.[5,66] This list continues to grow as new and investigational drugs continue to be developed.

CYTOKINES

With recent advances in biotechnology, there has been increased development of cytokines and immunotherapeutic agents, which target cancer at the cellular level. Roles have already been established for IL-2 as alternative treatment for

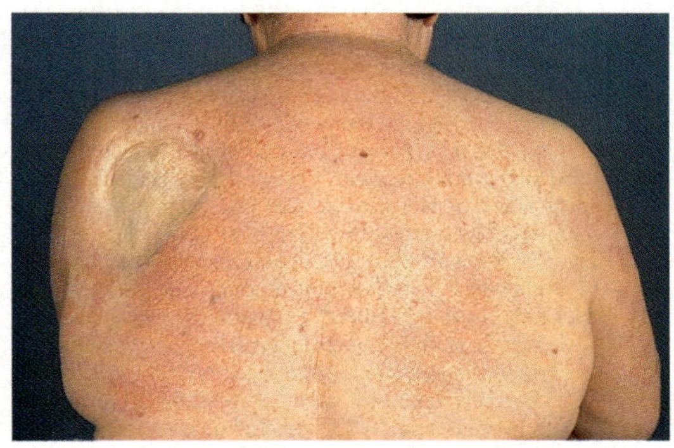

Figure 129-6 Erythematous rash associated with IL-2 therapy in a melanoma patient.

advanced metastatic melanoma and renal cell cancer and for IFN-α as standard treatment for chronic myelogenous leukemia, hairy-cell leukemia, cutaneous T-cell lymphoma, and Kaposi sarcoma. In addition to significant toxicities such as capillary leak syndrome, there is a 72% incidence of cutaneous reactions reported with IL-2.[67] Commonly, a pruritic diffuse erythroderma occurs 1 to 3 days after administration and resolves with desquamation 2 days after cessation of therapy (Figure 129-6).[67] This reaction is clinically similar to toxic shock syndrome and has been associated with staphylococcal sepsis in some patients. Intra-arterial IL-2 also causes hypersensitivity to iodine-containing contrast dyes in up to 30% of patients.[66] Of potential importance, one study of IL-2 for metastatic melanoma has reported a possible correlation between the development of vitiligo and good prognosis.[68] Although IFN-α is relatively less toxic than IL-2, several cutaneous reactions have been reported in the literature. Perhaps one-third of patients will develop a local injection-site reaction. In a study of 1,000 patients receiving IFN-α, alopecia and herpes labialis exacerbation were common with 10% and 5% incidence, respectively.[66,69] Both IFN-α and IL-2 also induce and/or exacerbate seborrheic dermatitis and psoriasis.[66]

PEGYLATED AND LIPOSOMAL MODIFIED DRUGS

Pegylation (polyethylene glycol) and liposomal modification of drugs are relatively recent innovations that are thought to increase the half-life of drugs and offer improved side-effect profiles. Pegylated IFN-α and pegylated liposomal doxorubicin are among the most well studied. Similar to non-modified recombinant IFN-α, pegylated IFN-α has been shown to cause local cutaneous ulcerations at sites of subcutaneous injection.[70] Cutaneous reactions have also been frequent with pegylated liposomal doxorubicin therapy, which has been shown to cause acral erythema in 40%, diffuse follicular rash in 10%, intertrigo-like eruption in 8%, and melanotic macule development in 5% of cases.[71] There has also been a report of the drug causing psoriasiform pustular eruptions.[72]

NUCLEOSIDE ANALOGUES

Some of the more recently developed nucleoside analogues have also been shown to produce reactions, particularly with 2-chlorodeoxyadenosine (2-CDA) or fludarabine, which may be associated with Grover's disease and severe adverse cutaneous reactions such as erythema multiforme, and paraneoplastic pemphigus.[73–75] In phase I trials, the new nucleoside analogue troxacitabine has been associated with drug eruptions, hyperpigmentation, and acral erythema.[76] At M. D. Anderson Cancer Center, there have been a number of cases of gemcitabine-induced hyperpigmentation, radiation recall, and cutaneous ulcerations in cutaneous T-cell lymphoma patients.[28,29]

TYROSINE KINASE INHIBITORS

Tyrosine kinase inhibitors include small molecules and targeted antibodies. Acne folliculitis is frequently observed during clinical trials of tarceva (OSI774), an epidermal growth factor receptor (EGFR) tyrosine kinase inhibitor, and cetuximab (C225), the monoclonal EGFR antibody. In phase I trials, OSI774 at the maximally tolerated dose induced a pustular acneiform eruption in 50% of cases during the second week of therapy.[77] Although the reaction usually resolves by the fourth week of therapy, the eruption is occasionally dose limiting. It may occur most severely in patients who have previously experienced cystic acne vulgaris. There is some suggestion that the acneiform eruption is associated with favorable clinical responses.

Likewise, C225 commonly produces an acneiform follicular eruption of the face, chest, and upper back, and is thought to be due to a direct follicular toxic effect (Figure 129-7).[78,79] Other C225 cutaneous reactions include paronychial inflammation of the toes and fingers and small oral aphthous ulcers.

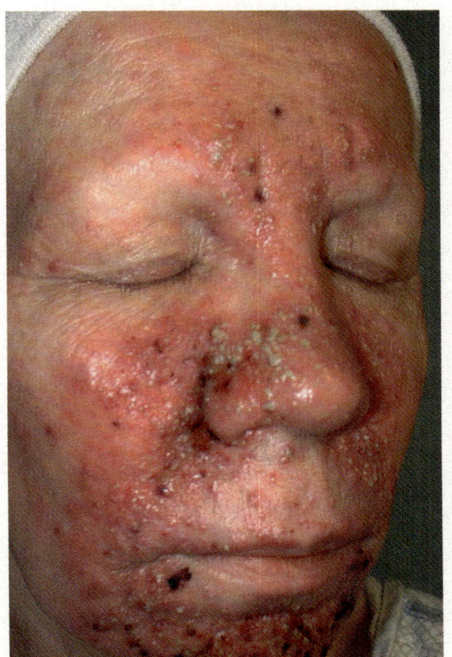

Figure 129-7 Acneiform eruption of the face associated with C225 therapy.

Another tyrosine kinase inhibitor, imatinib mesylate (STI571, Gleevec), targets the *BCR-ABL* gene and has been used in the treatment of chronic myeloid leukemia and acute lymphoblastic leukemia. Gleevec has been shown to frequently cause dose-dependent cutaneous reactions, including urticaria, dermatitis, and acute generalized exanthematous pustulosis (AGEP).[80,81] One patient developed an eczematous rash with histologic features of mycosis fungoides.[82]

Acute generalized exanthematous pustulosis (AGEP) is a cutaneous drug reaction characterized by acute development of dozens or hundreds of nonfollicular sterile pustules on an erythematous background. It usually begins on the face or intertriginous areas, perhaps with burning and itching. It can be accompanied by fever, neutrophilia, and eosinophilia.[83] Ninety percent of cases are drug induced, mostly with antibiotics such as betalactams, cephalosporins, fluconazole, nystatin, and terbinafine. Other reported triggers include imatinib, the histone deacetylase inhibitor bryostatin (personal observations by Duvic), mercury, thallium, iohexol, patch testing, pseudoephedrine, diltiazem, furosemide, and viral infections. Because of its severe appearance, it can be alarming. Confluence of pustules may mimic the positive Nikolsky's sign seen in toxic epidermal necrolysis (TEN). Rarely, AGEP can manifest as vesicles or targetoid lesions raising suspicion for Stevens-Johnson syndrome (SJS). However unlike SJS, AGEP affects the mucous membranes less often (only 20% of cases); involvement is usually mild and confined to the oral mucosa. Treatment of AGEP is to simply discontinue the offending agent and monitor for superinfection of the pustules. The macrophage migration inhibition factor (MIF) test, mast cell degranulation (MDC) test, and patch testing can help determine the causative agent. Lesions will spontaneously resolve in 4 to 14 days.[83]

REFERENCES

1. Crounse RG, Van Scott EJ. Changes in scalp hair roots as a measure of toxicity from cancer chemotherapeutic drugs. J Invest Dermatol 1960;35:83–90.
2. Fischer D, Knobf M, Durivage H. The cancer chemotherapy handbook. St. Louis: Mosby; 1997.
3. Hood AF. Dermatologic toxicity. In: Perry MC, editor. The chemotherapy source book. 2nd ed. Baltimore: Williams & Wilkins; 1996. p. 595–606.
4. Fitzpatrick JE, Yokel BE, Hood AF. Mucocutaneous complications of antineoplastic therapy. In: Freedberg IM, Eisen AZ, Wolff K, et al, editors. Fitzpatrick's dermatology in general medicine. 5th ed. New York: McGraw-Hill; 1999. p. 1642–53.
5. Susser WS, Whitaker-Worth DL, Grant-Kels JM. Mucocutaneous reactions to chemotherapy. J Am Acad Dermatol 1999;40:367–98.
6. Pillans P, Woods D. Drug-associated alopecia. Int J Dermatol 1995;34:149–58.
7. DeSpain JD. Dermatologic toxicity of chemotherapy. Semin Oncol 1992;19:501–7.
8. Baker B, Wilson C, Davis A, et al. Busulfan/cyclophosphamide conditioning for bone marrow transplantation may lead to failure of hair regrowth. Bone Marrow Transplant 1991;7:43–7.
9. Ron IG, Kalmus Y, Kalmus Z, et al. Scalp cooling in the prevention of alopecia in patients receiving depilating chemotherapy. Support Care Cancer 1997;5:136–8.

10. Duvic M, Lemak N, Valero V, et al. A randomized trial of minoxidil in chemotherapy-induced alopecia. J Am Acad Dermatol 1996;35:74–8.
11. Hesketh PJ, Batchelor D, Golant M, et al. Chemotherapy-induced alopecia: psychosocial impact and therapeutic approaches. Support Care Center 2004; 12:543–9.
12. Skarin A. Diagnosis in Oncology: Skin Lesions in Malignancy. J Clin Oncol 2001;19:2098–2102.
13. Clamon GH. Extravasation. In: Perry MC, editor. The chemotherapy source book. 2nd ed. Baltimore: Williams & Wilkins; 1996. p. 607–11.
14. Rudolph R, Larson DL. Etiology and treatment of chemotherapeutic agent extravasation injuries: a review. J Clin Oncol 1987;5:1116–26.
15. duBois A, Kommoss FG, Pfisterer J, et al. Paclitaxel-induced "recall" soft tissue ulcerations occurring at the site of previous subcutaneous administration of paclitaxel in low doses. Gynecol Oncol 1996;60:94–6.
16. Anderson CM, Walters RS, Hortobagyi GN. Mediastinitis related to probable central vinblastine extravasation in a woman undergoing adjuvant chemotherapy for early breast cancer. Am J Clin Oncol 1996;19:566–8.
17. Dorr RT. Antidotes to vesicant chemotherapy extravasations. Blood Rev 1990;4:41–60.
18. Larson DL. Treatment of tissue extravasation by antitumor agents. Cancer 1982;49:1796–9.
19. Luedke DW, Kennedy PS, Rietschel RL. Histopathogenesis of skin and subcutaneous injury induced by Adriamycin. Plast Reconstr Surg 1979;63:463–5.
20. Shamseddine AI, Khalil AM, Kibbi AG, et al. Granulocyte macrophage-colony stimulating factor for treatment of chemotherapy extravasation. Eur J Gynaecol Oncol 1998;19:479–81.
21. Rentschler R, Wilbur D. Pyridoxine: a potential local antidote for mitomycin-C extravasation. J Surg Oncol 1988; 37:269–71.
22. Scuderi N, Onesti MG. Antitumor agents: extravasation, management, and surgical treatment. Ann Plast Surg 1994;32:39–43.
23. Heitmann C, Durmus C, Ingianni G. Surgical management after doxorubicin and epirubicin extravasation. J Hand Surg [Am] 1998;23:666–8.
24. Bertelli G, Gozza A, Forno GB, et al. Topical dimethylsulfoxide for the prevention of soft tissue injury after extravasation of vesicant cytotoxic drugs: a prospective clinical study. J Clin Oncol 1995;13:2851–5.
25. Hill A, Hanson M, Bogle MA, Duvic M. Severe radiation dermatitis is related to Staphylococcus aureus. Am J Clin Oncol 2004;27:362–3.
26. Houtee PV, Danhier S, Mornex F. Toxicity of combined radiation and chemotherapy in non-small cell lung cancer. Lung Cancer 1994;10:S271–80.
27. Yeo W, Leung S, Johnson P. Radiation-recall dermatitis with docetaxel: establishment of a requisite radiation threshold. Eur J Cancer 1997;33:698–9.
28. Fogarty G, Ball D, Rischin D. Radiation recall reaction following gemcitabine. Lung Cancer 2001;33:299–302.
29. Talpur R, Apisarnthanarax N, Ward S, et al. Phase II evaluation of Gemcitabine as a single agent for cutaneous T-cell lymphoma. Poster presented to the American Society of Hematology, 2003.
30. Schweitzer VG, Juillard GJF, Bajada CL, Parker RG. Radiation recall dermatitis and pneumonitis in a patient treated with paclitaxel.
31. Gould JW, Mercurio MG, Elmets CA. Cutaneous photosensitivity diseases induced by exogenous agents. J Am Acad Dermatol 1995;33:551–73.
32. Hussain S, Anderson DN, et al. Onycholysis as a Complication of Systemic Chemotherapy: Report of Five Cases Associated with Prolonged Weekly Paclitaxel Therapy and Review of the Literature. Cancer 2000; 88:2367–71.
33. Lowitt M, Eisenberger M, Sina B, Kao G. Cutaneous eruptions from suramin: a clinical and histopathologic study of 60 patients. Arch Dermatol 1995;131:1128–53.
34. Wooten RS, Smith KC, Ahlquist DA, et al. Prospective study of cutaneous phototoxicity after systemic hematoporphyrin derivative. Lasers Surg Med 1988;8:294–300.
35. Dougherty TJ, Cooper MT, Mang TS. Cutaneous phototoxic occurrences in patients receiving Photofrin. Lasers Surg Med 1990;10:485–8.
36. Corbett MF, Hawk JLM, Herxheimer A, Magnus IA. Controlled therapeutic trials in polymorphic light eruption. Br J Dermatol 1982;107:571-81
37. Johnson T, Rapini R, Duvic M. Inflammation of actinic keratoses from systemic chemotherapy. J Am Acad Dermatol 1987;17:192–7.
38. Hardwick N, Murray A. Inflammation of actinic keratoses induced by cytotoxic drugs. Br J Dermatol 1986;114:639–40.
39. Bataille V, Cunningham D, Mansi J, Mortimer P. Inflammation of solar keratoses following systemic 5-fluorouracil. Br J Dermatol 1996;135:478–80.
40. Weiss RB. Hypersensitivity reactions. In: Perry MC, editor. The chemotherapy source book. 2nd ed. Baltimore: Williams & Wilkins; 1996. p. 595–606.
41. Harris RE, McCallister JA, Provisor DS, et al. Methotrexate/L-asparaginase combination chemotherapy for patients with acute leukemia in relapse: a study of 36 children. Cancer 1980;46:2004–8.
42. Blumenreich MS, Needles B, Yagoda A, et al. Intravesical cisplatin for superficial bladder tumors. Cancer 1982;50:863–5.
43. Castleberry RP, Crist WM, Holbrook T, et al. The cytosine arabinoside (Ara-C) syndrome. Med Pediatr Oncol 1989;9:257–64.
44. Williams SF, Larson RA. Hypersensitivity reaction to high-dose cytarabine. Br J Haematol 1989;73:274–5.
45. Zuehlke RL. Erythematous eruption of the palms and soles associated with mitotane therapy. Dermatologica 1974;148:90–2.
46. Chiao N, Bumgardner A, Duvic M. Clofarabine-induced acral erythema during the treatment of patients with myelodysplasia and acute leukemia: a report of two cases. Leuk Lymphoma 2003;44:1405–7.
47. Demircay Z, Gurbuz O, Alpdogan T, et al. Chemotherapy-induced acral erythema in leukemic patients: a report of 15 cases. Int J Dermatol 1997;36:593–8.
48. Hellier I, Bessis D, Sotto A, et al. High-dose methotrexate-induced bullous variant of acral erythema. Arch Dermatol 1996;132:590–1.
49. Baack BR, Burgdorf WHC. Chemotherapy-induced acral erythema. J Am Acad Dermatol 1991;24:457–61.
50. Kampmann KK, Graves T, Rogers SD. Acral erythema secondary to high-dose cytosine arabinoside with pain worsened by cyclosporin infusions. Cancer 1989;63:2482–5.
51. Jucgla A, Sais G, Navarro M, Peyri J. Palmoplantar keratoderma secondary to chronic acral erythema due to tegafur. Arch Dermatol 1995;131:364–5.
52. Zimmerman GC, Keeling JH, Burrris HA, et al. Acute cutaneous reactions to docetaxel: a new chemotherapeutic agent. Arch Dermatol 1995;131:202–6.
53. Vukelja SJ, Baker WJ, Burris HA III, et al. Pyridoxine therapy for palmar-plantar erythrodysesthesia associated with Taxotere. J Natl Cancer Inst 1993;85:1432.
54. Crider MK, Jansen J, Norins AL, McHale MS. Chemotherapy-induced acral erythema in patients receiving bone marrow transplantation. Arch Dermatol 1986;122:1023–7.
55. Deeg HJ, Cottler-Fox M. Clinical spectrum and pathophysiology of acute graft vs. host disease. In: Burakoff SJ, Deeg HJ, Ferrara J, Atkinson K editors. Graft vs. Host Disease: Immunology, Pathophysiology, and Treatment. New York: Marcel Dekker, Inc; 1990:539–55.
56. Harrist TJ, Fine JD, Berman RS, et al. Neutrophilic eccrine hidradenitis. Arch Dermatol 1982;118:263–6.
57. Ostlere LS, Wells J, Stevens HP, et al. Neutrophilic eccrine hidradenitis with an unusual presentation. Br J Dermatol 1993;128:696–8.
58. Shear NH, Knowles SR, Shapiro L, Poldre P. Dapsone in prevention of recurrent neutrophilic eccrine hidradenitis. J Am Acad Dermatol 1996;35:819–22.
59. Brehler R, Reimann S, Bonsmann G, Metze D. Neutrophilic hidradenitis induced by chemotherapy involves eccrine and apocrine glands. Am J Dermatopathol 1997;19:73–8.
60. Madsen ES, Larsen H. Excretion of mutagens in sweat from humans treated with anti-neoplastic drugs. Cancer Lett 1988;40:199–202.
61. Hurt MA, Halvorson RD, Petr FC Jr, et al. Eccrine squamous syringometaplasia: a cutaneous sweat gland reaction in the histologic spectrum of "chemotherapy-associated eccrine hidradenitis" and "neutrophilic eccrine hidradenitis." Arch Dermatol 1990;126:73–7.
62. Valks R, Fraga J, Porras-Luque J, et al. Chemotherapy-induced eccrine squamous syringometaplasia: a distinctive eruption in patients receiving hematopoietic progenitor cells. Arch Dermatol 1997;133:873–8.
63. Horn TD, Redd JV, Karp JE, et al. Cutaneous eruptions of lymphocyte recovery. Arch Dermatol 1989;215:1512–7.
64. Bauer DJ, Hood AF, Horn TD. Histologic comparison of autologous graft-vs-host reaction and cutaneous eruption of lymphocyte recovery. Arch Dermatol 1993;129:855–8.
65. Horn TD. Acute cutaneous eruptions after marrow ablation: roses by other names? J Cutan Pathol 1994;21:385–92.
66. Asnis LA, Gaspari AA. Cutaneous reactions to recombinant cytokine therapy. J Am Acad Dermatol 1995;33:393–410.
67. Wolkenstein P, Chosidow O, Wechsler J, et al. Cutaneous side effects associated with interleukin-2 administration for metastatic melanoma. J Am Acad Dermatol 1993;28:66–70.
68. Richards JM, Gilewksi TA, Ramming K, et al. Effective chemotherapy for melanoma after treatment with interleukin-2. Cancer 1992;69:427–9.
69. Jones GJ, Itri LM. Safety and tolerance of recombinant interferon a-2a (Roferon-A) in cancer patients. Cancer 1986;57:1709–15.
70. Heinzerling L, Dummer R, Wildberger H, Burg G. Cutaneous ulceration after injection of polyethylene-glycol-modified interferon alpha associated with visual disturbances in a melanoma patient. Dermatology 2000;201:154–7.
71. Lotem M, Hubert A, Lyass O, et al. Skin toxic effects of polyethylene glycol-coated liposomal doxorubicin. Arch Dermatol 2000;136:1285–80.
72. Kreuter A, Gambichler T, Schlottmann R, et al. Psoriasiform pustular eruptions from pegylated-liposomal doxorubicin in AIDS-related Kaposi's sarcoma. Acta Derm Venereol 2001;81:224.
73. Grey MR, Flanagan NG, Kelsey PR. Severe skin rash in two consecutive patients treated with 2-chlorodeoxyadenosine for hairy cell leukaemia at a single institution. Clin Lab Haematol 2000;22:111–3.
74. Cohen PR, Kurzrock R. Transient acantholytic dermatosis after treatment with 2-chlorodeoxyadenosine. Acta Derm Venereol 1977;77:412–3.
75. Gooptu C, Littlewood TJ, Frith P, et al. Paraneoplastic pemphigus: an association with fludarabine? Br J Dermatol 2001;144:1255–61.
76. DeBono JS, Stephenson J Jr, Baker SD, et al. Troxacitabine, an L-stereoisomeric nucleoside analog, on a five-times-daily schedule: a phase I and pharmacokinetic study in patients with advanced solid malignancies. J Clin Oncol 2002;20:96–109.
77. Hidalgo M, Siu LL, Nemunaitis J, et al. Phase I and pharmacologic study of OSI-774, an epidermal growth factor receptor tyrosine kinase inhibitor, in patients with advanced solid malignancies. J Clin Oncol 2001;19:3267–79.
78. Busam KJ, Capodieci P, Motzer P, et al. Cutaneous side-effects in cancer patients treated with the antiepidermal growth factor receptor antibody C225. Br J Dermatol 2001;144:1169–76.
79. Kimyai-Asadi AJ. Follicular toxic effects of chimeric anti-epidermal growth factor receptor antibody cetuximab used to treat human solid tumors. Arch Dermatol 2002;138:129–31.
80. Brouard M, Saurat JH. Cutaneous reactions to STI571 [letter]. N Engl J Med 2001;345:618–9.
81. Schwarz M, Kreuzer K, Baskaynak G, et al. Imatinib-induced acute generalized exanthematous pustulosis (AGEP) in two patients with chronic myeloid leukemia. Eur J Haematol 2002; 69:254–6.
82. Clark SH, Duvic M, Prieto V. Mycosis fungoides-like reaction in a patient treated with Gleevec. J Cutan Pathol 2003;30:279–81.
83. Sidoroff A, Halevy S, Bavinck JB, et al. Acute generalized exanthematous pustulosis (AGEP)—A clinical reaction pattern. J Cutan Pathol 2001; 28:113–9.

130

Skeletal Complications

Samuel Kenan, MD
Jeffrey I. Mechanick, MD

Cancer-associated morbidity remains a major public health problem. The development of bone metastases indicates that cure is unlikely, and management of symptoms becomes the focus of treatment. Following metastases to nodes, lung, and liver, the skeleton is the fourth most common site for metastases. A number of orthopedic complications may arise as a direct result of metastatic disease or as a result of the treatment itself, but skeletal metastases are by far the most common type of complication. Over the past several decades, an increase in the survival of patients with bone metastases has been achieved through earlier detection using improved diagnostic modalities and radiographic imaging techniques and through treatment advances in chemotherapy regimens and radiation therapy combined with better surgical approaches. In this chapter, the early and late skeletal complications of cancer are considered, as well as skeletal metastases and hypercalcemia of malignancy.

SKELETAL METASTASES

Skeletal metastases represent the major orthopedic complication of failed cancer treatment and are commonly associated with disabling pain and pathologic fracture. Treatment of all patients with metastatic disease involves a multidisciplinary team approach to include an oncologist, radiotherapist, and orthopedic surgeon. Advances in surgical techniques and internal fixation modalities have resulted in great improvement in pain control and management of patients with skeletal metastases. The main goals of treatment are to relieve pain, improve function, and return patients, as soon as possible, to their previous environment.

The vast majority of skeletal cancers are of metastatic origin rather than primary bone tumors. In the United States, it is estimated that there will be 1.4 million new cancer cases in 2006. It is estimated that one-third of these new cases eventually will develop metastatic bone disease. In contrast, there are only 5,000 primary soft tissue sarcomas and 2,000 cases of primary malignant bone tumors. In most cases, metastatic lesions are multifocal and show variable radiographic features, while primary bone tumors demonstrate a typical presentation by their anatomic site and radiographic features. The surgical approach for primary bone tumor is curative by wide surgical resection, while for metastatic disease, the surgical approach is palliative to restore function and relieve pain. In most instances of skeletal metastatic disease, the best treatment may not appreciably extend the life span of the patient.

Within the skeleton, the site of a metastatic lesion can be correlated with the activity of the bone marrow. The axial skeleton contains active hematopoietic (red) marrow, while the peripheral skeleton contains relatively avascular fatty (yellow) marrow.[1] The axial skeleton, especially the thoracolumbar spine, represents the most common site for metastases.[2] This is in part related to the paravertebral venous plexus system described by Batson.[3] Because of the relatively avascular marrow, metastases below the elbow and knee are relatively rare. At autopsy, 70% of patients who die of cancer have been shown to have skeletal metastases.[4] Many of these lesions are asymptomatic and are too small to be recognized radiographically. The proximal femur was found to be the site of metastatic lesions in 11% of all patients; however, when involved, they are often likely to fracture. Approximately 40% of all pathologic fractures occur in the proximal femur. The risk of pathologic fracture is correlated to the extent of the lesion, the type of destruction, and the anatomic location. Lesions in high-stress areas such as the lesser trochanter are very often associated with subsequent pathologic fracture. A high risk of fracture is particularly associated with highly anaplastic and rapidly growing vascular lesions, which are usually osteolytic.

Metastatic lesions that result in a net loss of bone are described as osteolytic, as can be seen in myeloma, metastatic renal cell carcinoma, and metastatic thyroid carcinoma (Figure 130-1). The mechanism of bone resorption is primarily osteoclast-mediated. Several known osteoclastic-stimulating factors associated with cancer play a significant role in the process of bone resorption.[6] Parathyroid hormone-related protein (PTHrP) is the most important molecule leading to bone resorption by transforming osteoblasts to osteoclasts. When the process involves bone formation as observed in metastatic prostate carcinoma, the net increase in bone results in blastic, sclerotic lesions (Figure 130-2). Transforming growth factor-β (TGF-β), expressed in abundant amount in prostate cancer cells has the ability to stimulate osteoblastic proliferation and increase bone formation. In cases in which there are lytic and blastic areas, as can be seen in some metastatic breast carcinomas, lesions are described radiographically as of mixed osteolytic osteoblastic type.

PATHOGENESIS OF METASTASES

Numerous pathologic events are required for a tumor cell to metastasize to bone and develop either osteolytic or osteoblastic lesions. The metastatic process depends on a successful interaction between tumor cells and bone marrow cells. Three events must occur to establish skeletal metastases:

1. A tumor cell must leave the primary site, travel to the skeleton, and occupy the osseous bone cavity.

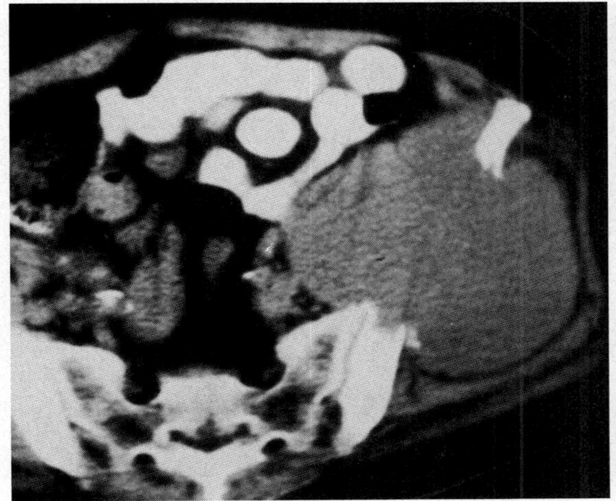

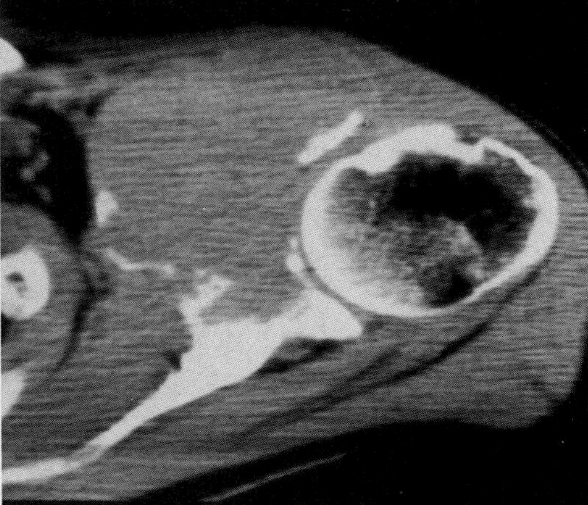

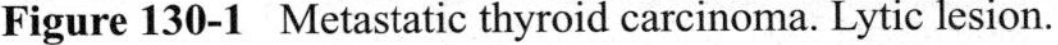

Figure 130-1 Metastatic thyroid carcinoma. Lytic lesion.

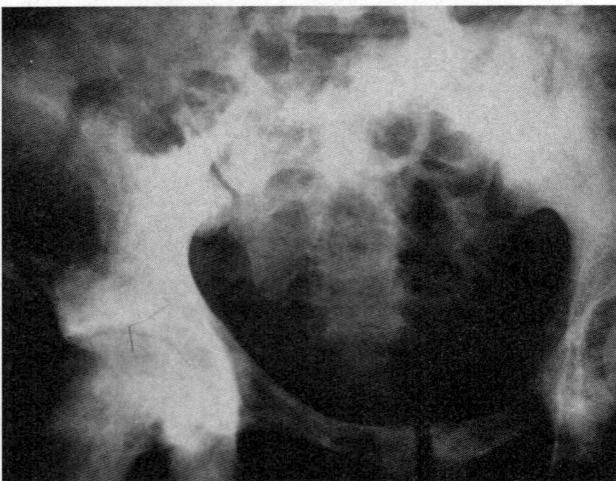
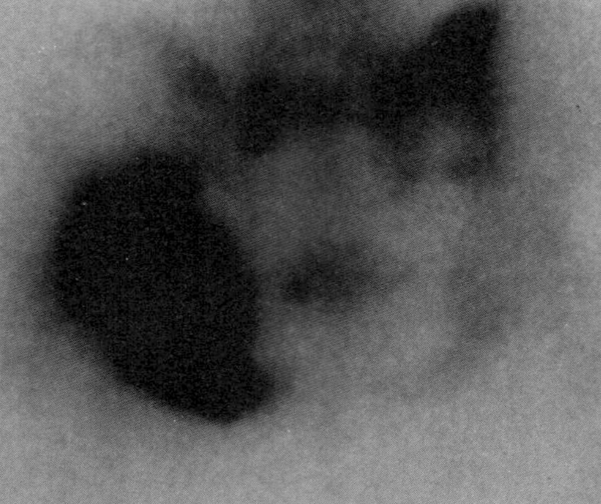

Figure 130-2 Metastatic prostate carcinoma. Sclerotic osteoblastic lesion of the acetabulum.

2. The tumor cell within the osseous cavity must adhere to extracellular matrix and cause bone destruction within the bone marrow compartment.
3. Tumor cells must interact with host cells to enhance tumor cell growth.

Several gene products have been identified in different tumors that have unique expression profiles that predict aggressiveness. Overexpression of gene products that facilitate cell cycling, angiogenesis, and invasion imply a more aggressive tumor. Bone marrow stromal cells and osteoblasts are important targets of tumor-derived factors. Osteoclasts are derived from hematopoietic monocytic macrophage precursors that are stimulated by macrophage colony-stimulating factors. Tumor cells interact with osteoblasts, which in turn stimulate osteoclasts to differentiate from hematopoietic precursors, resulting in increased osteoclastic bone resorption. Osteoclasts are the principal bone resorbing cell. Bone metastases involve a vicious cycle between tumor cells and bone. The main participants in this process are tumor cells, bone forming osteoblasts, bone destroying osteoclasts, and organic mineralized bone matrix.

Despite the fact that tumors originate from a single cell that lacks normal control mechanisms, tumors consist of vast numbers of cells that are not homogeneous. Only a limited number of cells may have the genetic potential to metastasize. Although numerous tumor cells gain access to the systemic circulation, only a small number of cells, probably less than 0.1%, survive the transport.[7] Although random sites of metastasis can occur, selectivity of the metastatic site depends on adhesion of molecules specific to the endothelium within the arterioles, capillaries, and postcapillary venules of particular organs.[8,9]

Complementary molecules characteristic of individual tumor types are permissive for attachment to the specific endothelium, initiating the metastatic cascade. Organ selectivity has been demonstrated in mice by the propensity of harvested metastatic tumor to return, after sequential transplantation, to the organ from which it had been harvested. The differential frequency with which human cancers metastasize to bone presumably represents the interaction between adhesion molecules on vascular endothelium of the skeleton and tumor cells of particular types.

SURGICAL MANAGEMENT

Treatment of patients with metastatic bone disease requires a multidisciplinary team approach, including the medical oncologist, radiation oncologist, and orthopedic oncologist. Patients should be analyzed based on the type of the tumor, anatomic location, and neurologic status. Surgical treatment should be individualized to each patient's medical circumstance and with consideration given to the anticipated impact on longevity. Good judgment and considerable experience are necessary in the selection of patients for surgery. The patient's general condition must allow the surgical procedure to be performed with reasonable expectation that the patient will survive long enough to benefit from the surgery. Patients should be informed and prepared prior to surgery concerning realistic expectations regarding relevant issues such as functional recovery, longevity, and cure. Preoperatively, patients should be evaluated and treated for dehydration, coagulopathies, anemia, and hypercalcemia of malignancy.

The primary goals of treatment of patients with painful skeletal metastatic lesions are to relieve pain, restore function, allow early mobilization, and ease nursing care. In general, before any surgical intervention, the underlying process must be confirmed as metastatic disease and not a primary malignant bone tumor. The diagnosis cannot be assumed and must be confirmed by biopsy before any irreversible procedure. The surgical modality should take into consideration the natural progress and biologic behavior of the underlying process. A reliable and reproducible fixation modality should be selected to allow immediate full weight bearing. It is prudent to intervene electively for impending fracture. Patients whose limbs were stabilized preventively had shorter hospitalizations and longer survival than patients with pathologic fractures. Pathologic fracture seems to be associated with an increased incidence of subsequent pulmonary metastases. Prophylactic fixation may reduce the incidence of lung metastases.[10]

Small lesions that do not present with an impending fracture, and which are radiosensitive, can be treated by radiotherapy alone to relieve pain[11] and to diminish progression of the radiated

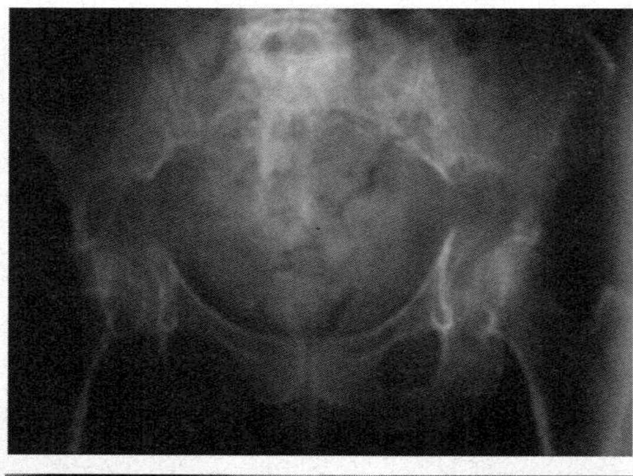
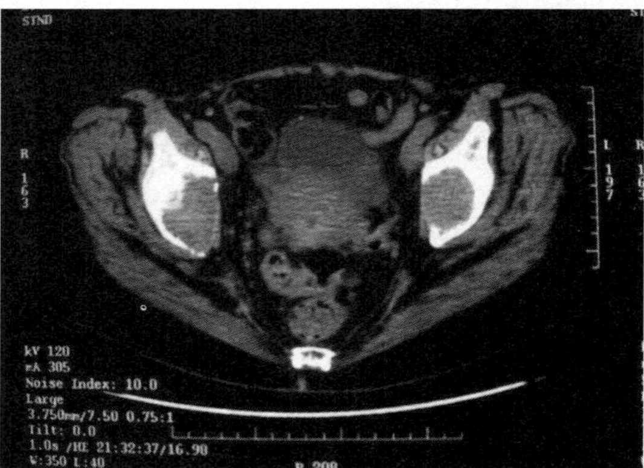

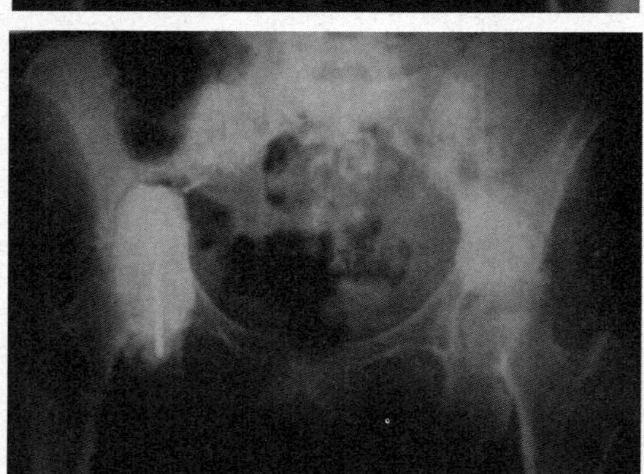
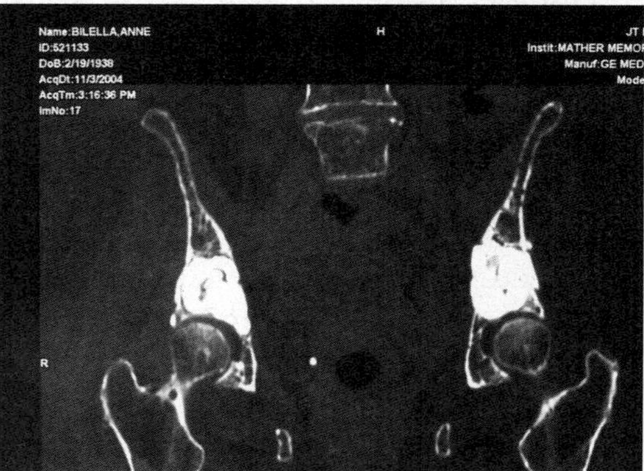

Figure 130-3 Sixty-five-year-old female with multiple myeloma involving both acetabuli. Treated by curettage and cement packing.

lesion. Radiation may cause hyperemia at the periphery of treated bone with short-lived softening, which may temporarily increase the risk of fracture. In lesions that may progress to impending fracture, blind intramedullary nailing with local irradiation may give good local control with pain relief. Irradiated pathologic fractures that lack rigid fixation show a higher rate of nonunion. In a larger osteolytic lesion, blind intramedullary nailing may not be sufficient because of mechanical failure and telescoping migration of the bone fragments.[12,13] In a significant number of patients with extensive destruction affecting the joint, particularly the hip or knee, segmental resection and prosthetic replacement may be indicated to allow immediate full weight bearing. The nature of metastatic cancer and the often relatively short survival generally make long-term durability of the prosthesis unimportant.

The most common metastatic tumors arise from carcinoma of the breast, a tumor that accounts for more than 50% of the cases requiring orthopedic intervention, followed by cancers of the lung, kidney, prostate, gastrointestinal tract, thyroid, and other miscellaneous sites. In patients who present with metastatic cancer of unknown primary site, the presence of bone metastases represents a sign of advanced disease with poor life expectancy.[14–16]

METASTATIC TUMORS TO THE ACETABULUM

The pelvis and acetabulum are common sites for skeletal metastasis. Periacetabular tumors may cause severe debilitating pain with hip dysfunction. Pathologic fractures often lead to protrusio acetabuli. Metastatic lesions to the acetabulum require a computed tomography (CT) scan for better evaluation of the extent of the lesion and to provide a guideline for the surgical approach. Highly vascular tumors such as renal cell carcinoma should be treated with preoperative arterial embolization to minimize intraoperative blood loss. Small metastatic lesions to the acetabulum may be managed by radiation alone. Larger lesions can be treated by intralesional curettage and cement packing (Figure 130-3). Joint instability with significant acetabular defect may require total hip replacement augmented by cement and screws fixation (Figure 130-4).

METASTATIC LESIONS TO THE FEMUR

The femur is a common place for metastatic lesions and pathologic fractures. The proximal femur is subjected to axial bending and shearing forces applied directly to any fixation device. Conventional fixation devices ultimately may fail. Surgical management should provide pain relief and immediate restoration of ambulation with unrestricted full weight bearing. A fracture is considered to be impending whenever there is a lesion greater than 50% of the bone diameter, or bigger than 2.5 cm, or whenever there is pathologic avulsion of the lesser trochanter or

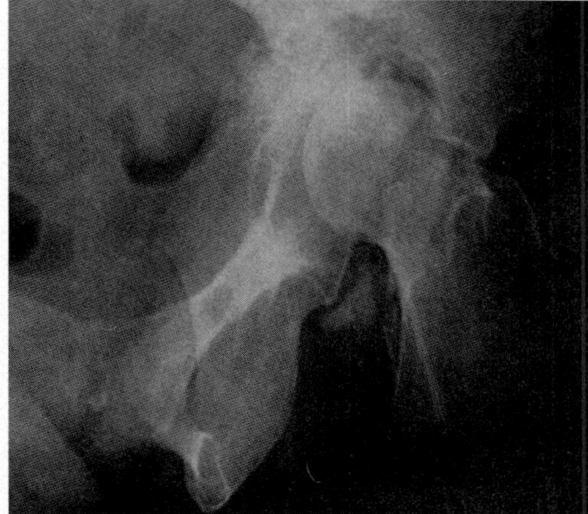
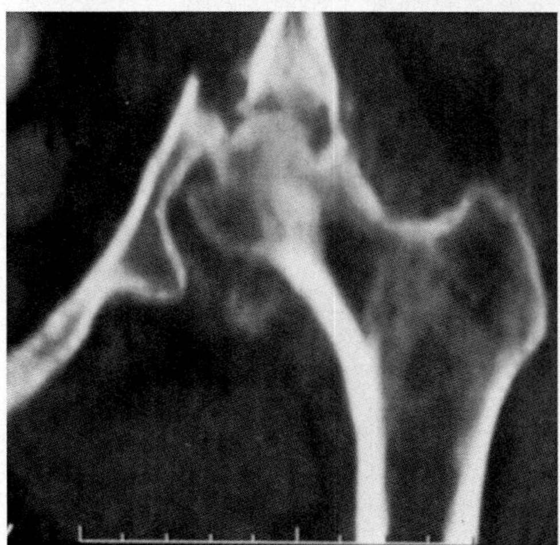
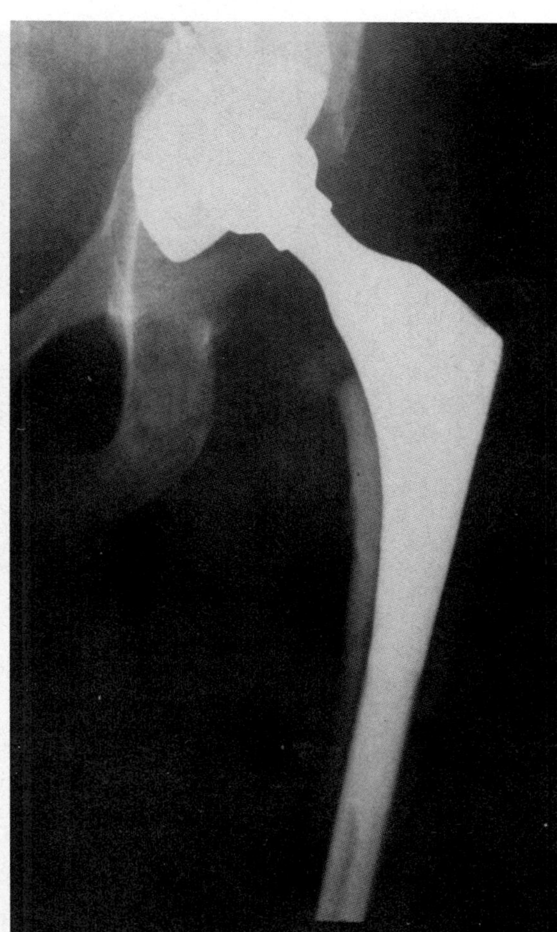

Figure 130-4 Fifty-eight-year-old female with a metastatic lesion to the left acetabulum. Treated by total hip replacement.

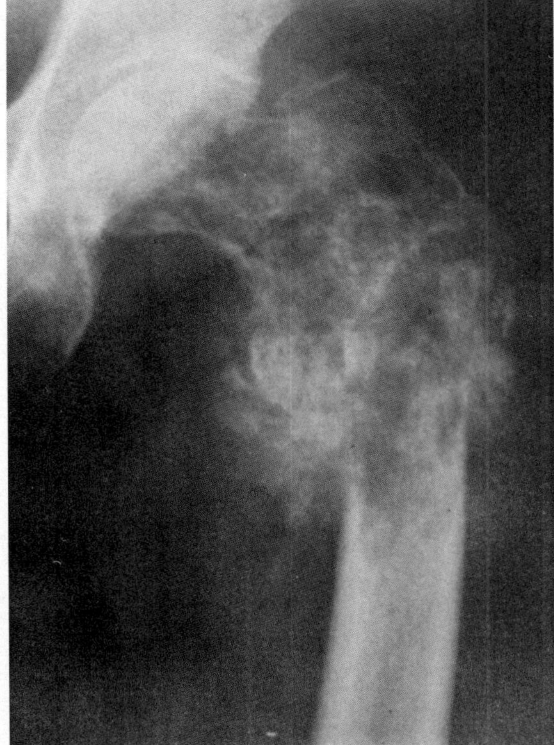
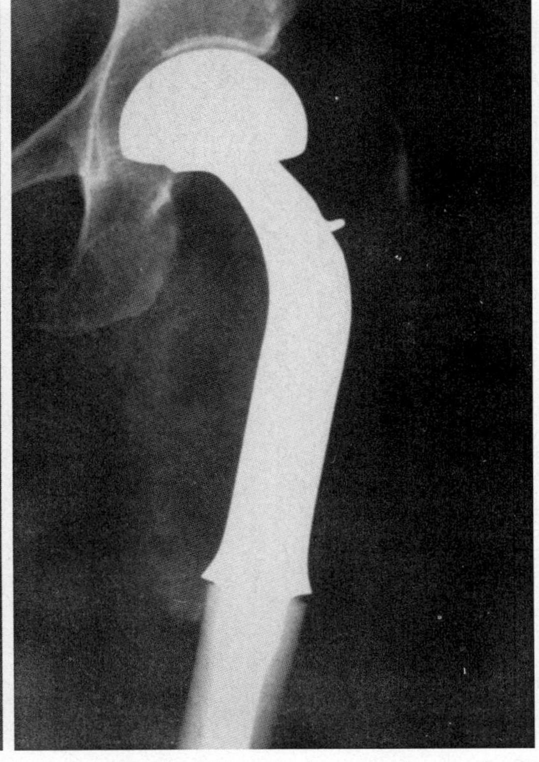

Figure 130-5 Fifty-five-year-old female with metastatic breast carcinoma of the left proximal femur with pathological fracture. Treated by wide proximal femur resection and replacement by custom prosthesis.

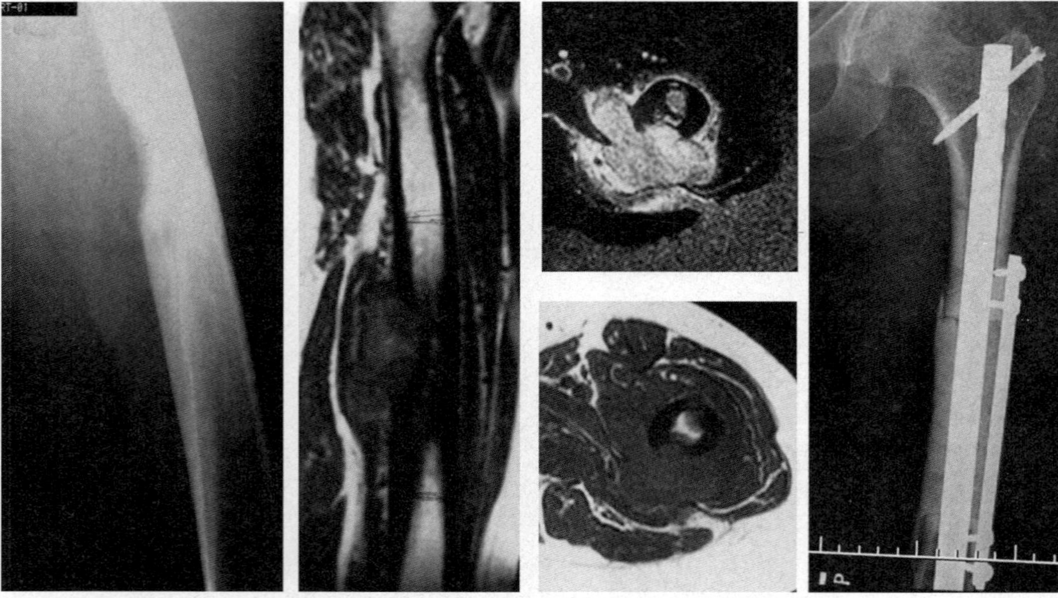

Figure 130-6 Sixty-year-old female with metastatic lung carcinoma to the midshaft of the femur with associated soft tissue mass. Treated by wide segmental resection and intramedullary rod augmented by cement spacer.

persistent pain. Methylmethacrylate is very resistant to compressive loading and provides an ideal substitute for deficient bone. Internal fixation of femoral neck fractures is often successful. Metastatic lesions to the femoral neck are best treated by resection and a bipolar prosthesis. Intralesional curettage and cement packing, supplemented by pin and plate fixation can treat metastatic disease to the trochanteric region. Larger lesions of the proximal femur with pathologic fracture are best treated by wide resection and proximal femur replacement (Figure 130-5).

Impending fractures of the femoral shaft are best treated by closed intramedullary locking nail, which provides rotational stability (Figure 130-6). Metastatic disease to the femoral condyle may be treated by intralesional curettage and cement packing (Figure 130-7). In those cases in which there is pathologic fracture, distal femur replacement may be indicated (Figure 130-8).[17]

The same could be applied to the tibia, where metastatic lesions could be treated by wide segmental resection, internal fixation, and cement spacer (Figure 130-9).

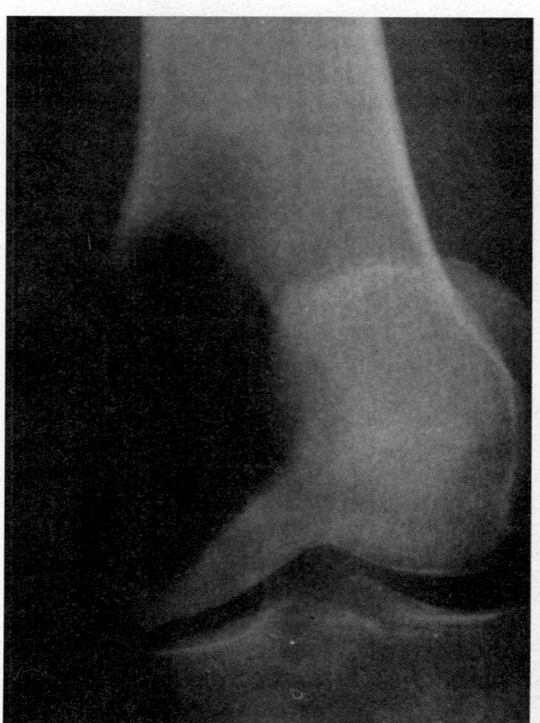

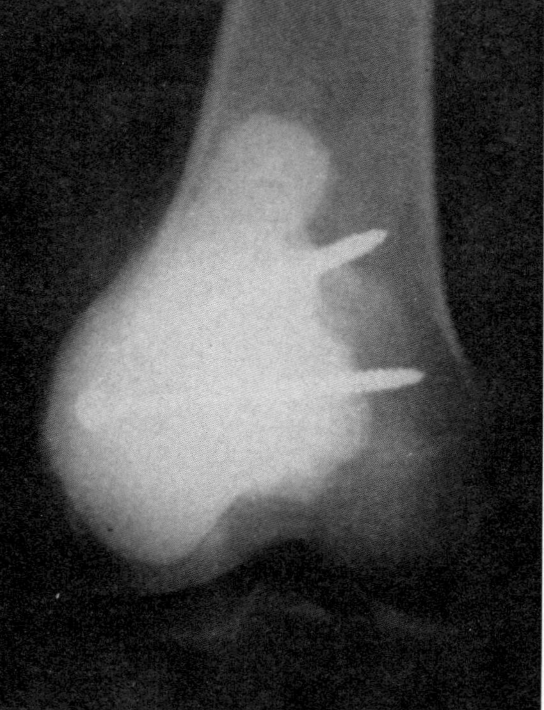

Figure 130-7 Sixty-seven-year-old female with metastatic renal cell carcinoma to the femoral condyle. Treated by intralesional curettage and cement augmentation.

METASTATIC LESIONS TO THE SCAPULA AND UPPER EXTREMITY

Conservative treatment of pathologic fracture of the humerus is often associated with persistent pain and shoulder stiffness. To provide immediate pain relief and restore shoulder mobility, internal fixation is recommended. Metastatic lesions to the scapula can be treated by partial or total scapulectomy (Figure 130-10). Pathologic fracture of the humeral head is best managed by endoprosthesis (Figure 130-11). Large lesions of the proximal humerus with or without pathological fracture are best treated by wide resection and replacement using a custom prosthesis (Figure 130-12). Cases with large segmental defects are best treated with wide resection and internal fixation using an intramedullary rod augmented by cement spacer (Figures 130-13 and 130-14). For better local control, radiation can be given 2 weeks postsurgery.[18] Metastatic tumors of the proximal ulna are best treated by wide segmental resection and internal fixation and cement augmentation (Figure130-15). For metastatic tumors of the radius or ulna shaft, an intramedullary rod is recommended (Figure 130-16).

METASTATIC LESIONS TO THE SPINE

The vertebral bodies are the most common site for metastatic lesions. Most vertebral metastases initially are occult and painless. The majority can be detected on routine bone scan. Metastatic lesions that do not compromise stability may remain asymptomatic. Pain typically occurs when a significant amount of bone destruction has occurred, leading to microfractures. Pathologic fractures of the vertebral bodies are of a compressive type and are usually stable. Patients with metastatic disease to the spine commonly develop back pain before any neurologic sequelae. MRI scan has replaced myelography as the method of choice to demonstrate local extension and extradural compression. In the absence of impingement on spinal cord or cauda equina, back pain may be alleviated by radiotherapy or by percutaneous vertebroplasty with polymethylmethacrylate. Spinal cord compression at the level of the cervical or thoracic spine can cause hyperreflexia and spasticity with complete paraplegia. Corticosteroids are indicated to reduce edema until emergency treatment is initiated for neurologic salvage. A radiosensitive metastatic condition, such as lymphoma, may be treated effectively by radiation therapy or chemotherapy. Surgical decompression may be indicated in those patients who do not respond to radiation therapy and who subsequently develop neurologic deterioration or where cord compression is already critical. Surgical treatment of metastatic conditions to the spine has improved significantly with the introduction of new surgical techniques and instrumentation. The result of anterior spinal decompression with vertebral body resection, replacement by a

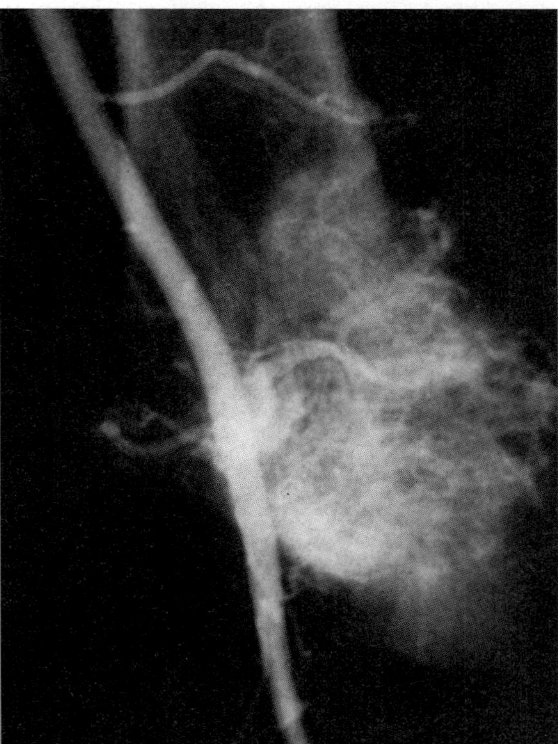
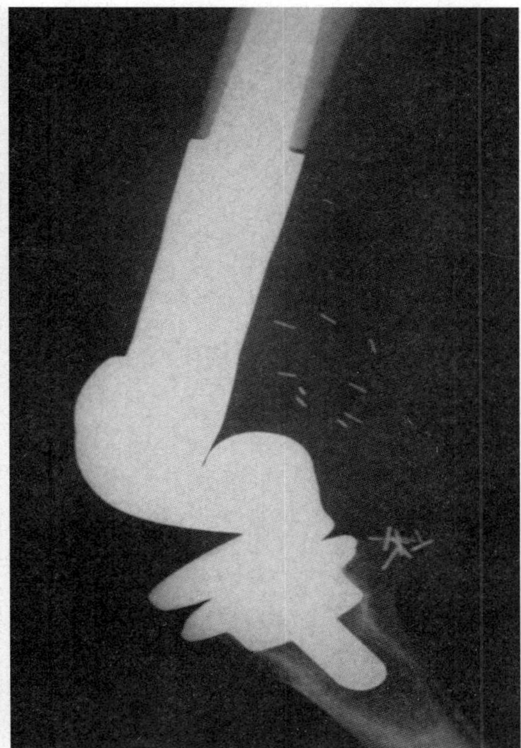

Figure 130-8 Seventy-year-old female with metastatic renal cell carcinoma of the distal femur. Treated by wide resection and prosthesis replacement.

cement spacer, and bracing has proved to be very effective in stabilizing the spine and preventing further neurologic deterioration[19,20] (Figure 130-17).

MEDICAL MANAGEMENT OF BONE METASTASES

The optimal management of bone metastases requires the coordinated efforts of various disciplines. In addition to systemic chemotherapy for bone metastases, endocrine interventions directed at bone metabolism have demonstrated effectiveness in controlling oncogenic bone pain, fracture risk, metastatic growth, and even in prolonging survival.

Bone metabolism is governed by a delicate, though highly regulated, balance between bone formation (by osteoblasts) and bone resorption (by osteoclasts). This results in an ongoing process of bone remodeling, which confers strength and decreased fracture risk. Bisphosphonates are the most efficacious antiresorptive agents available in the management of metabolic bone disease and bone metastases. These agents inhibit osteoclast function and interfere with recruitment and differentiation of osteoclast precursors. Bisphosphonates are pyrophosphate analogues with a high affinity for bone.[21] The non-nitrogen–containing bisphosphonates (etidronate and clodronate) are metabolized into cytotoxic analogues of ATP and are not considered to have antitumoral activity.[22] A growing body of experimental animal data demonstrates, however, antitumoral activity of the nitrogen-containing bisphosphonates (n-BP; pamidronate, ibandronate, zoledronate, risedronate, and alendronate). Their effect results in inhibition of tumor cell adhesion, inhibition of tumor cell invasion through the extracellular matrix, antiangiogenic effects (via vascular endothelial growth factor [VEGF]), and induction of tumor cell apoptosis.[23–25] n-BPs induce apoptosis of osteoclasts and antagonize osteoclastogenesis via (1) osteoblast secretion of an inhibitor of osteoclast recruitment; (2) altering osteoblast secretion of TGF-β, an osteoclast apoptosis signal; (3) inhibition of farnesyl diphosphate synthase, a key enzyme in the mevalonate pathway; (4) impaired prenylation (farnesylation) causing interference with small GTPases and intracellular signals such as Ras, Rho, and Rac (important for cancer cell migration and invasion); and (5) released mitochondrial cytochrome C and caspase activation.[26,27] Of interest, statins may potentiate n-BP inhibition of the mevalonate pathway.[28] n-BPs also affect expression of the antiapoptotic protein bcl-2, activate the p38 mitogen-activated protein kinase (MAPK) pathway, down-regulate integrins, and increase expression of osteoprotegerin.[23,29] Furthermore, n-BPs are broad-spectrum matrix metalloproteinase (MMP) inhibitors, which may prevent metastases into soft and hard tissue.[30]

In clinical studies, bisphosphonates are well tolerated with minimal acute side effects and only rare jaw necrosis, often after tooth extraction, as a putative chronic toxicity.[31] Patients may develop nausea, vomiting, and, with pamidronate, a posterior uveitis. Fever may occur after pamidronate owing to tumor necrosis factor (TNF)-α and IL-6 elaboration by γ/δ T cells, which may also be associated with antitumor activity.[32,33] Nephrotoxicity may be observed but is uncommon. Hypocalcemia and hypophosphatemia may also occur, particularly in patients with a vitamin D deficiency. The safety of long-term bisphosphonate administration (over 2 years) has been well documented.[21,34] The majority of an intravenously administered dose is deposited in the bone where it remains for extended periods of time. Oral absorption is only 1 to 3% of the administered dose. Bisphosphonates are not metabolized and are eliminated by renal excretion. In patients with renal failure, pamidronate may be dosed during, or within 24 hours before, hemodialysis. The antiresorptive response to bisphosphonates is best assessed with urine N-telopeptide (NTx) levels.[35] NTx is a bone-specific collagen breakdown that is also highly predictive of skeletal complications from metastatic bone disease, as well as of mortality.[36]

Figure 130-9 Fifty-year-old male with metastatic lung carcinoma of the midshaft tibia. Treated by wide segmental resection, internal fixation, and cement spacer augmentation.

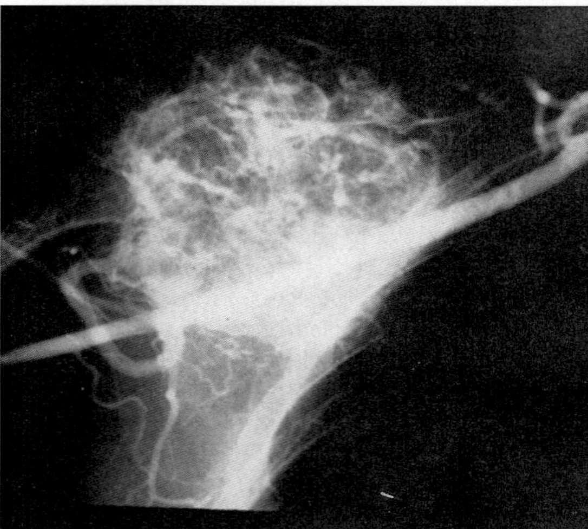
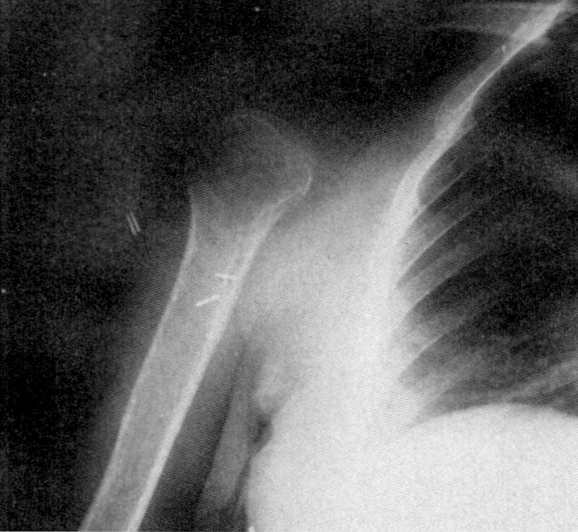

Figure 130-10 Sixty-two-year-old male with metastatic renal cell carcinoma of the scapula. Treated by total scapulectomy.

In malignant osteolytic bone disease, bisphosphonate administration has been associated with reduced skeletal-related events (SREs), including pain. Treatment protocols include (1) etidronate, 400 mg/day PO × 2 weeks; (2) alendronate, 70 mg PO weekly; (3) pamidronate 60 to 90 mg IV every 3 to 4 weeks; or (4) zoledronate, 4 mg IV every 3 to 4 weeks.[37–40] The shorter and more convenient infusion protocols, with comparable safety and potential advantages, favor zoledronate as the agent of choice. In a large metareview of 30 randomized, controlled trials involving 3,682 patients, bisphosphonate use was significantly more effective than placebo in providing pain relief from bone metastases.[41] Since pain relief might be delayed, bisphosphonate use should be combined with analgesics and/or radiotherapy when appropriate.[41] Moreover, various radiopharmaceuticals, such as rhenium-188, samarium-153, strontium-89, phosphorus-32, and tin-117m, show promise for palliation of bone pain from osseous metastases, albeit with varying levels of hematopoietic toxicity.[42]

The standard of care for the management of osteolytic lesions from breast cancer includes the use of intravenous pamidronate or zoledronate. Pamidronate, 45 mg IV every 3 weeks increased the median time to bone progression, improved pain control, reduced the need for radiotherapy, and increased the median time to radiotherapy with no serious adverse effects or worsening of chemotherapy-related toxicities.[43] These results were confirmed in a larger study of stage IV breast cancer patients with at least one lytic bone lesion given pamidronate, 90 mg IV over 2 hours every month for 12 cycles.[44] Furthermore, the effects of IV pamidronate in decreasing the risk of osteolytic bone lesion complications in women with breast cancer persists for at least 2 years.[45] On the other hand, in a study of 1,648 patients with either stage III multiple myeloma or advanced breast cancer, zoledronate, 4 mg IV over 15 minutes, was associated with more sustained beneficial effects on osteolytic bone lesions than 90 mg of IV pamidronate.[46] In a subsequent prospective randomized controlled study of 1,130 patients with breast cancer with at least one osteolytic lesion, 4 mg IV zoledronate was more effective than 90 mg IV pamidronate in reducing skeletal complications.[47] Overall, based on phase III studies involving over 3,000 patients with breast cancer, prostate cancer, lung cancer, multiple myeloma, and other cancers, 4 mg IV zoledronate dosing was safe and effective,[48] and in women with breast cancer, associated with increased health-related quality of life.[49]

Bisphosphonates are also used to manage cancer-treatment induced bone loss (CTIBL). This has particular application to patients undergoing hormonal therapies for breast and prostate cancers. Average rates of CTIBL owing to ovarian ablation are 1.4 to 5.9% (lumbar spine [LS]) and 0.34 to 2.7% (femoral neck [FN]); owing to LHRH agonist therapy, 5.3% (LS) and 3.2% (FN); owing to aromatase inhibitors, 2.6% (LS) and 1.7% (FN); and owing to androgen deprivation therapy for prostate cancer, 0.98 to 8% (LS) and 0.92 to 9.6% (FN).[50] In a study of women with breast cancer, oral risedronate, 30 mg/day × 2 weeks followed by 10 weeks of no drug, repeated for 8 12-week cycles, has been associated with prevention of trabecular and cortical bone loss.[51] Standard protocols for the use of bisphosphonates in the treatment of postmenopausal osteoporosis include alendronate, 70 mg/week PO or risedronate, 35 mg/week PO, with calcium, 1,200 to 1,500 mg/day and vitamin D, 600 to 800 units/day. Clinical trials have also demonstrated efficacy of pamidronate, 60 to 90 mg IV every 1 to 3 months[52,53] or zoledronate, 4 mg IV every 3 to 6 months[54–56] to manage CTIBL.

In prostate cancer, metabolic bone disease can result from direct effects of bone metastases, which have osteoblastic and osteoclastic components, or CTIBL. Fractures are an independent and adverse predictor of survival in prostate cancer patients.[53] Prostate cancer bone metastases produce MMPs, which promote osteolysis, and also the protein receptor activator of nuclear factor-κB ligand (RANKL), PTHrp, and interleukin (IL)-6, all of which induce osteoclastogenesis.[57] Of interest, osteoprotegerin is a soluble decoy receptor for RANKL that inhibits tumor-induced osteolysis.[57] The process of tumor-

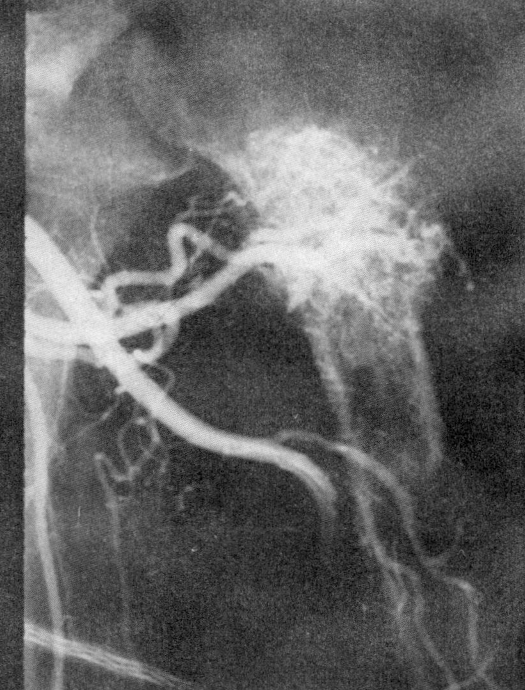

Figure 130-11 Metastatic renal cell carcinoma. Arteriogram demonstrates a highly vascular tumor, for which arterial embolization before surgery is recommended.

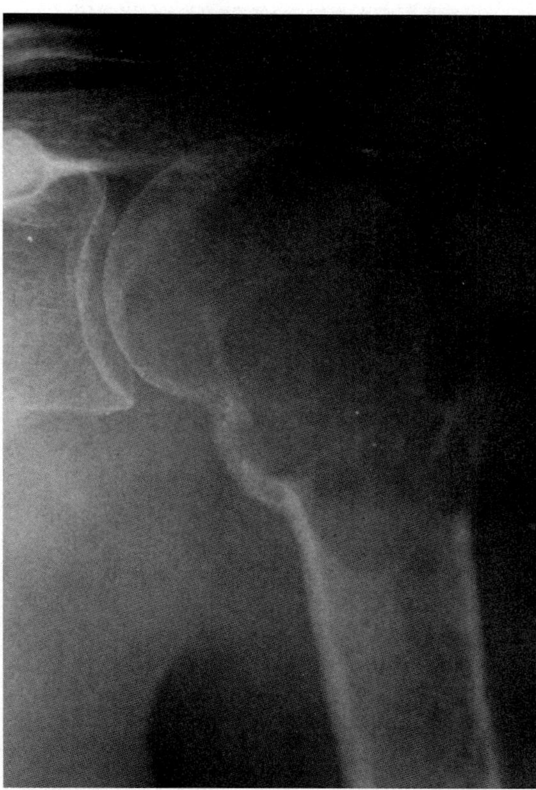
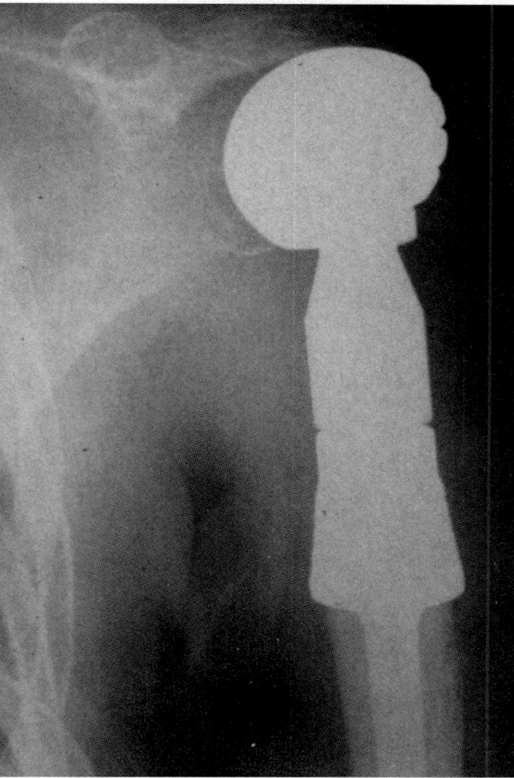

Figure 130-12 Metastatic breast carcinoma proximal humerus. Treated by wide resection and prosthesis replacement.

mediated local bone resorption can facilitate micrometastasis, tumor cell hiding, and eventual macrometastases.[58] Bisphosphonates can target this osteoclastic component of prostate cancer bone metastases as well as promote caspase-dependent apoptosis via G-protein geranylgeranylation.[59] However, pamidronate, 90 mg IV q 3 weeks × 27 weeks, was found to lack significant effects on skeletal-related events in men with metastatic prostate cancer.[60] On the other hand, zoledronate, 4 mg over 15 minutes every 3 weeks for 15 months was associated with decreased SREs in a prospective randomized controlled trial of 122 patients with metastatic hormone-refractory prostate cancer.[61] Nevertheless, in patients with progressive prostate cancer receiving zoledronate, 4 mg IV q month, the use of adjuvant calcitriol, with or without dexamethasone, was shown to have no antitumor effect.[62] Calcitriol has been shown to have differentiating and antiproliferating effects, as well as inducing apoptosis in experimental models of prostate cancer.[63,64] In small clinical trials, calcitriol slows the rate of prostatic-specific antigen rise.[65] This topic has led to an unresolved controversy: Is the antitumor effect of bisphosphonates mitigated by the antiresorptive (via RANKL stimulation) and tumor growth-promoting effects of calcitriol, or do bisphosphonates simply lack significant antitumor effects in prostate cancer?

Intravenous pamidronate or zoledronate has been used to reduce SREs in patients with multiple myeloma, as well as other malignancies.[66] Bisphosphonates may induce apoptosis in plasma cells; this antitumor effect is enhanced by dexamethasone and thalidomide,[67] but may diminish over time because of increased farnesyl pyrophosphate synthase activity.[68,69] Pamidronate, 90 mg over 4 hours IV every 4 weeks for 9 cycles, was associated with decreased bone pain without deterioration in performance status or quality of life in patients with multiple myeloma.[70] However, pamidronate therapy had no effect on progression-free survival in multiple myeloma.[71] Zoledronate, 2 to 4 mg over 5 minutes, demonstrated comparable efficacy in the management of multiple myeloma bone lesions.[72] Zoledronate has also been found to augment the antileukemic activity in vitro of several chemotherapeutic agents.[73]

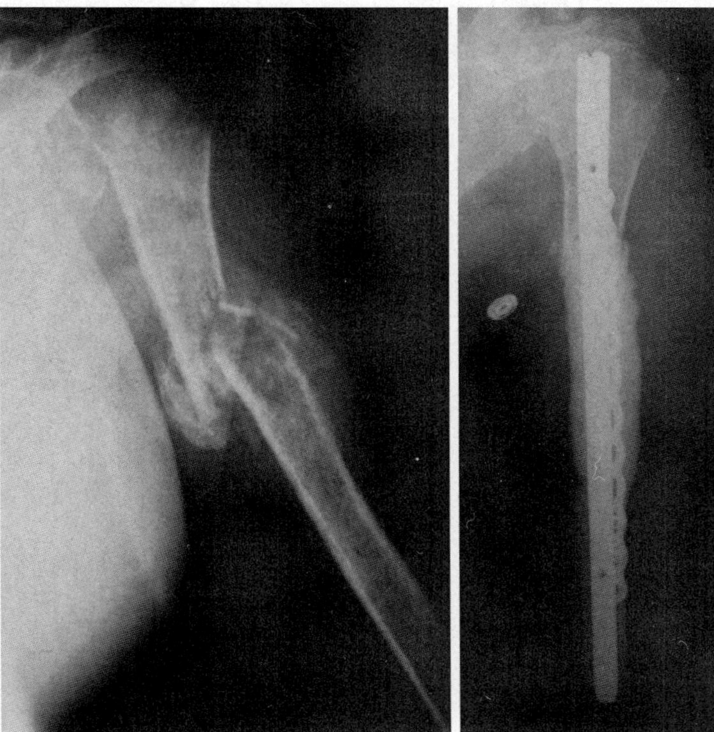

Figure 130-13 Seventy-year-old female with metastatic breast carcinoma midshaft humerus, associated with pathological fracture. Treated by wide segmental resection, intramedullary rod, and cement augmentation.

HYPERCALCEMIA OF MALIGNANCY

Hypercalcemia associated with skeletal metastases is a common metabolic complication and a life-threatening disorder. Symptoms include weakness, polyuria, nausea, vomiting, anorexia, dehydration, lethargy, confusion, stupor, and coma. Hypercalcemia of malignancy (HCM) is due to direct effects of local osteolytic factors derived from skeletal metastases (IL-1, TNF, TGF, and prostaglandins) or is due to production of systemic factors (PTHrp) secreted by the tumor that influence bone physiology. HCM is most common with multiple myeloma or breast cancer, but it can also occur with renal, ovarian, lung, and other cancers. The hypercalcemia associated with lymphomas is generally due to cytokines that stimulate osteoclastic bone resorption or is due to activation of ectopic 1α-hydroxylase activity, which converts 25-hydroxyvitamin D into the activated 1,25-dihydroxyvitamin D. The resultant hypervitaminosis D state causes increased gastrointestinal absorption of calcium. Medical management of HCM consists of the fol-

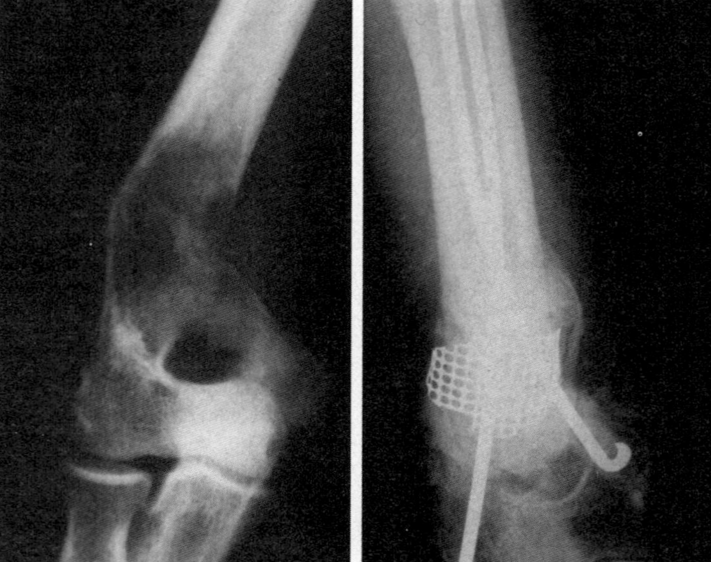

Figure 130-14 Seventy-year-old male with multiple myeloma. Pathological fracture of distal humerus. Treated by curettage, intramedullary rods, and cement augmentation.

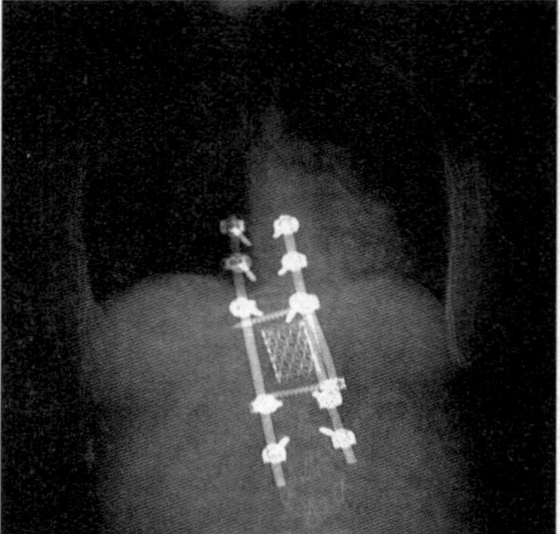

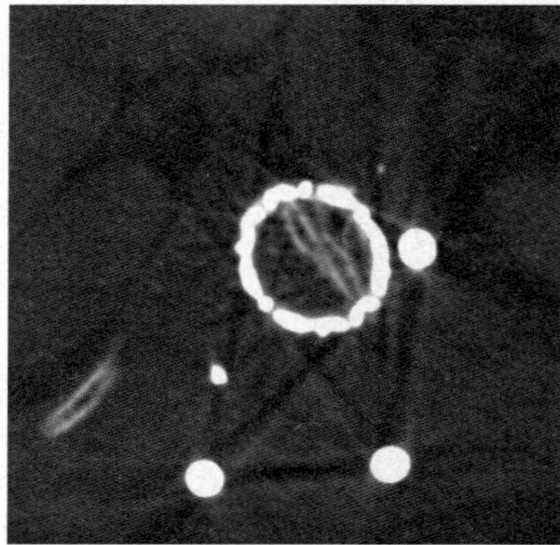

Figure 130-17 A patient with metastatic breast cancer and excruciating pain from vertebral collapse. Staged vertebral resection, posterior support first, with reconstruction of vertebral height with cage, cement, and external rods. The patient lived 4 more years.

lowing strategies: (1) promoting calciuresis with IV saline and using loop diuretics only if excessive fluid retention occurs; (2) using bisphosphonate (pamidronate, 90 mg over 4–24 hours IV) to inhibit bone resorption;[74] (3) discontinuing calcium and vitamin D supplementation (if any); and (4) consideration of glucocorticoids, which increase the effective circulatory volume, glomerular filtration rate, and calciuresis and suppress ectopic vitamin D activation. Calcitonin may also be used and can inhibit bone resorption to a lesser degree.

CORTICOSTEROID-INDUCED OSTEOPENIA

When glucocorticoids decrease the intestinal absorption of calcium, the 24-hour urinary calcium excretion rate will be low and calcium (1,200–1,500 mg/day) and vitamin D (600–1,000 units/day) may be provided orally. If glucocorticoids are increasing the urinary excretion of calcium, hydrochlorothiazide, 25 to 50 mg once or twice daily, may be used to reduce calciuresis. Negative calcium balance may be reflected by an

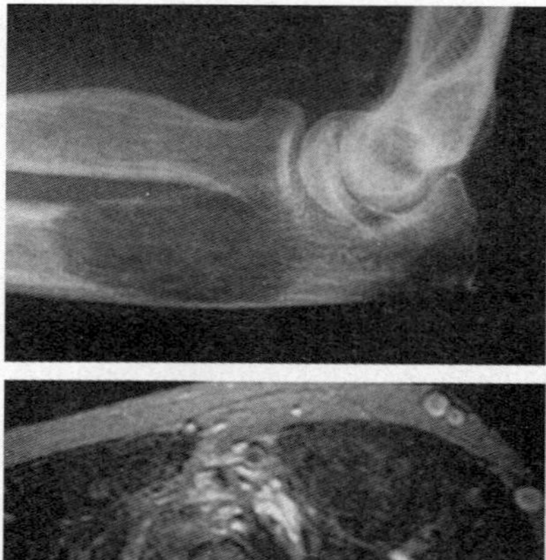

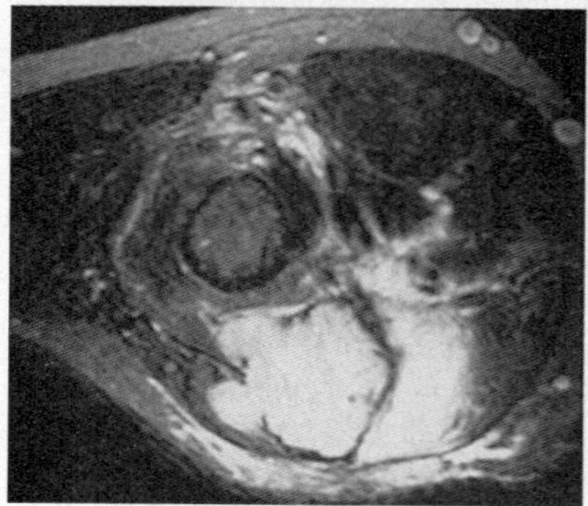

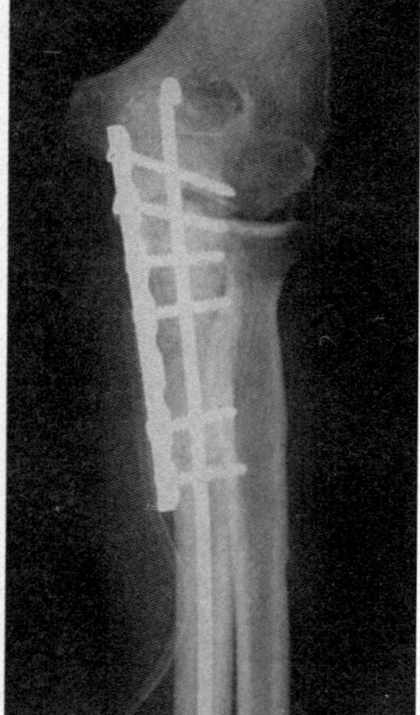

Figure 130-15 Fifty-five-year-old female with metastatic thyroid carcinoma of the proximal ulna with pathological fracture. Treated by wide resection, intramedullary nailing, and cement augmentation.

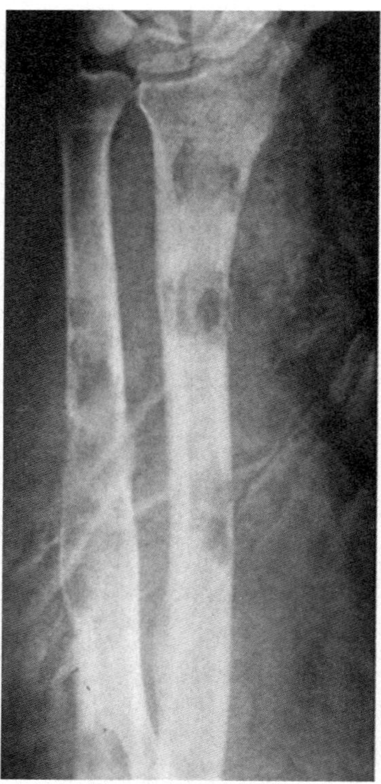

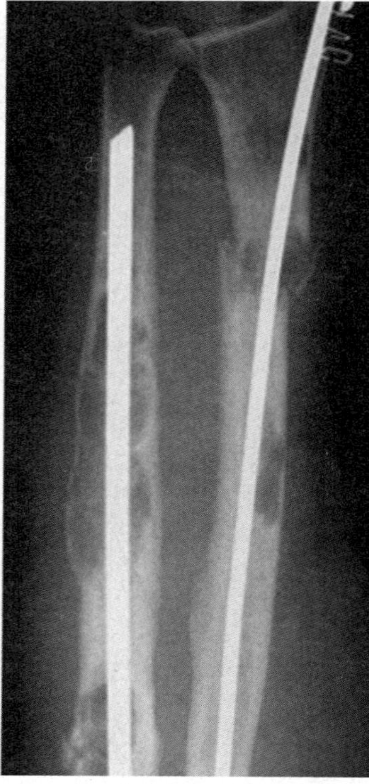

Figure 130-16 Multiple myeloma of radius and ulna with pathological fractures. Treated by intramedullary nailing.

elevated parathyroid hormone level (secondary hyperparathyroidism). The suppressive effect of glucocorticoids on osteoblastic bone formation may be reflected by low serum osteocalcin levels. Bisphosphonates can also prevent osteocyte and osteoblast apoptosis induced by glucocorticoids in experimental models.[75] Oral alendronate, 70 mg/week, or risedronate 35 mg/week, retards glucocorticoid-induced bone loss.[76,77]

REFERENCES

1. Boland PJ, Lane JM, Sundaresan N. Metastatic disease of the spine. Clin Orthop 1982;169:95–102.
2. Arguello F, Baggs RB, Duerst RE, et al. Pathogenesis of vertebral metastases and epidural spinal cord compression. Cancer 1990;65:98–106.
3. Batson OV. The role of the vertebral veins in metastatic processes. Ann Intern Med 1992;16:38–45.
4. Neff JR. Metastatic disease to bone. In: Lewis MM, editor. Musculoskeletal oncology: a multi-disciplinary approach. Philadelphia: Saunders; 1992. p. 377–99.
5. Galasko CSB. Mechanism of lytic and blastic metastatic disease of bone. Clin Orthop 1982;169:120–7.
6. Haberman ET, Lopez RA. Metastatic disease of bone and treatment of pathological fractures. Orthop Clin North Am 1989;20:469–86.
7. Folkman J. Tumor angiogenesis. Adv Cancer Res 1985;43:175–203.
8. Roos E, Dingemans KP. Mechanism of metastasis. Biochim Biophys Acta 1979;560:1335.
9. Springfield DS. Mechanisms of metastases. Clin Orthop 1982;169:15–9.
10. Bouma WH, Mulder JH, Hop WCJ. The influence of intramedullary nailing upon the development of metastases in the treatment of impending pathological fracture: an experimental study. Clin Exp Metastasis 1983;1:205–12.
11. Schocker JD, Brady LW. Radiation therapy for bone metastases. Clin Orthop 1982;169:38–43.
12. Fidler M. Prophylactic internal fixation of secondary neoplastic deposits in long bones. Br Med J 1973;1:341–3.
13. Ryan JR, Rowe DE, Salciccioli GG. Prophylactic internal fixation of the femur for neoplastic lesions. J Bone Joint Surg 1976;58A:1071.
14. Holmes FF, Fouts TL. Metastatic cancer of unknown primary site. Cancer 1970;26:816–20.
15. Moertel CG, Reitemeir RJ, Schutt AJ, Hahn RG. Treatment of patients with adenocarcinoma of unknown origin. Cancer 1972;30:1469–72.
16. Simon MD, Karluk BM. Skeletal metastases of unknown origin. Clin Orthop 1982;166:98–103.
17. Harrington KD, Sim FH, Ennis JE, et al. Methylmethacrylate as an adjunct in internal fixation of pathological fractures. J Bone Joint Surg 1976;58A:1047.
18. Sim FH, Pritchard DJ. Metastatic disease in the upper extremity. Clin Orthop 1982;169:83–94.
19. Siegal T, Siegal T. Current considerations in the management of neoplastic spinal cord compression. Spine 1989;14:223–8.
20. Sundaresan N, Sachdev VP, Holland JF, et al. Surgical treatment of metastatic spinal cord compression from epidural metastasis. J Clin Oncol 1995;139:2330–5.
21. Mundy GR, Martin TJ. The hypercalcemia of malignancy: pathogenesis and management. Metabolism 1982;31:1247–77.
22. Green JR. Antitumor effects of bisphosphonates. Cancer 2003;97(3 suppl):840–7.
23. Green JR. Clezardin P. Mechanisms of bisphosphonate effects on osteoclasts, tumor cell growth, and metastasis. Am J Clin Oncol 2002;25(6 suppl 1):S3–9.
24. Sebbah-Louriki M, Colombo BM, et al. A new phenylacetate-bisphosphonate inhibits breast cancer cell growth by proapoptotic and antiangiogenic effects. Anticancer Res 2002;22:3925–31.
25. Santini D, Vincenzi B, Avvisati G, et al. Pamidronate induces modifications of circulating angiogenetic factors in cancer patients. Clin Cancer Res 2002;8:1080–4.
26. Senaratne SG, Mansi JL, Colston KW. The bisphosphonate zoledronic acid impairs Ras membrane localization and induces cytochrome c release in breast cancer cells. Br J Cancer 2002;86:1479–86.
27. Smith MR. Antitumor activity of bisphosphonates. Clin Cancer Res 2003;9:5433–4.
28. Vincenzi B, Santini D, Avvisati G, et al. Statins may potentiate bisphosphonates anticancer properties: a new pharmacological approach? Med Hypoth 2003;61:98–101.
29. Merrell M, Suarez-Cuervo C, Harris KW, et al. Bisphosphonate induced growth inhibition of breast cancer cells augmented by p38 inhibition. Breast Cancer Res Treat 2003;81:231–41.
30. Heikkila P, Teronen O, Moilanen M, et al. Bisphosphonates inhibit stomelysin-1 (MMP-3), matrix metalloelastase (MMP-12), collagenase-3 (MMP-13), and enamelysin (MMP-20), but not urokinase-type plasminogen activator, and diminish invasion and migration of human malignant and endothelial cell lines. Anticancer Drugs 2002;13:245–54.
31. Ruggiero SL, Mehrota B, Rosenberg TJ, Engroff SL. Osteonecrosis of the jaws associated with the use of bisphosphomates: a review of 63 cases. J Oral Maxillofac Surg 2004;62:527–34.
32. DiCuonzo G, Vincenzi B, Santini D, et al. Fever after zoledronic acid administration is due to increase in TNF-α and IL-6. J Interferon Cytokine Res 2003;23:649–54.
33. Rischer M, Pscherer S, Duwe S, et al. Human γ/δ T cells as mediators of chimaeric-receptor redirected anti-tumour immunity. Br J Haematol 2004;126:583–92.
34. Ralston SH, Gallacher SJ, Patel U, et al. Cancer-associated hypercalcemia morbidity and mortality: clinical experience in 126 treated patients. Ann Intern Med 1990;112:499–504.
35. Vinholes JJ, Purohit OP, Abbey ME, et al. Relationship between biochemical and symptomatic response in a double-blind randomized trial of pamidronate for metastatic bone disease. Ann Oncol 1997;8:1243–50.
36. Brown JE, Thomson CS, Ellis SP, et al. Bone resorption predicts for skeletal complications in metastatic bone disease. Br J Cancer 2003;89:2031–7.
37. Rosen LS, Gordon D, Tchekmedyian NS, et al. Long-term efficacy and safety of zoledronic acid in the treatment of skeletal metastases in patients with nonsmall cell lung carcinoma and other solid tumors: a randomized, phase III, double-blind, placebo-controlled trial. Cancer 2004;100:2613–21.
38. Iwamoto J, Takedo T, Ichimura S. Treatment relief of metastatic cancer bone pain by oral administration of etidronate. J Bone Miner Metab 2002;20:228–34.
39. Koeberle D, Bacchus L, Thuerlimann B, et al. Pamidronate treatment in patients with malignant osteolytic bone disease and pain: a prospective randomized double-blind trial. Support Care Caner 1999;7:21–7.
40. Groff L, Zecca E, De Conno F, et al. The role of disodium pamidronate in the management of bone pain due to malignancy. Palliat Med 2001;15:297–307.
41. Wong R, Wiffen PJ. Bisphosphonates for the relief of pain secondary to bone metastases. Cochrane Database Syst Rev 2002;(2):CD002068.
42. Pandit-Taskar N, Batraki M, Divgi CR. Radiopharmaceutical therapy for palliation of bone pain from osseous metastases. J Nucl Med 2004;45:1358–65.
43. Conte PF, Giannessi PG, Latreille J, et al. Delayed progression of bone metastases with pamidronate therapy in breast cancer patients; a randomized, multicenter phase III trial. Ann Oncol 1994;5 suppl 7:S19–24.
44. Hortobagy GN, Theriault RL, Porter L, et al. Efficacy of pamidronate in reducing skeletal complications in patients with breast cancer and lytic bone metastases. Protocol 19 Aredia Breast Cancer Study Group. N Engl J Med 1996;335:1785–91.
45. Hortobagyi GN, Thieriault RL, Lipton A, et al. Long-term prevention of skeletal complications of metastatic breast cancer with pamidronate. Protocol 19 Aredia Breast Cancer Study Group. J Clin Oncol 1998;16:2038–44.
46. Rosen LS, Gordon D, Kaminski M, et al. Zoledronic acid versus pamidronate in the treatment of skeletal metastases in patients with breast cancer or osteolytic lesions of multiple myeloma: a phase III, double-blind, comparative trial. Cancer J 2001;7:377–87.
47. Rosen LS, Gordon DH, Dugan W, et al. Zoledronic acid is superior to pamidronate for the treatment of bone metastases in breast carcinoma patients with at least one osteolytic lesion. Cancer 2004;100:36–43.
48. Cameron D. Proven efficacy of zoledronic acid in the treatment of bone metastases in patients with breast cancer and other malignancies. Breast 2003;12 suppl 2:S22–9.
49. Weinfurt KP, Castel LD, Li Y, et al. Health-related quality of life among patients with breast cancer receiving zoledronic acid or pamidronate disodium for metastatic bone lesions. Med Care 2004;42:164–75.
50. Lipton A. Toward new horizons: the future of bisphosphonate therapy. Oncologist 2004;9 suppl 4:38–47.
51. Delmas PD, Balena R, Confravreux E, et al. Bisphosphonate risedronate prevents bone loss in women with artificial menopause due to chemotherapy of breast cancer: a double-blind, placebo-controlled study. J Clin Oncol 1997;15:955–62.
52. Smith MR, McGovern FJ, Zietman AL, et al. Pamidronate to prevent bone loss during androgen-deprivation therapy for prostate cancer. N Engl J Med 2001;345:948–55.
53. Diamond TH, Winters J, Smith A, et al. The antiosteoporotic efficacy of intravenous pamidronate in men with prostate carcinoma receiving combined androgen blockade: a double blind, randomized, placebo-controlled crossover study. Cancer 2001;92:1444–50.
54. Smith MR, Eastharn J, Gleason DM, et al. Randomized controlled trial of zoledronic acid to prevent bone loss in men receiving androgen deprivation therapy for nonmetastatic prostate cancer. J Urol 2003;169:2008–12.
55. Aapro MS. Long-term implications of bone loss in breast cancer. Breast 2004;13 suppl 1:S29–37.
56. Gnant M, Hausmaninger H, Samonigg H, et al. Changes in bone mineral density caused by anastrozole or tamoxifen in combination with goserelin (± zoledronate) as adjuvant treatment for hormone receptor-positive premenopausal breast cancer: results of a randomized multicenter trial. Presented at the 25th Annual San Antonio Breast Cancer Symposium, December 11–14, 2002, San Antonio, TX.
57. Keller ET. The role of osteoclastic activity in prostate cancer skeletal metastases. Drugs Today (Barc) 2002;38:91–102.
58. Karamanolakis D, Bogdanos J, Souria A, et al. Molecular evidence-based use of bone resorption-targeted therapy in prostate cancer patients at high risk for bone involvement. Mol Med 2002;8:667–75.
59. Coxon JP, Oades GM, Kirby RS, et al. Zoledronic acid induces apoptosis and inhibits adhesion to mineralized matrix in prostate cancer cells via inhibition of protein prenylation. Br J Urol 2004;94:164–70.
60. Small EJ, Smith MR, Seaman JJ, et al. Combined analysis of two multicenter, randomized, placebo-controlled studies of pamidronate disodium for the palliation of bone pain in men with metastatic prostate cancer. J Clin Oncol 2003;21:4277–84.
61. Saad F, Gleason DM, Murray R, et al. Long-term efficacy of zoledronic acid for the prevention of skeletal complications in patients with metastatic hormone-refractory prostate cancer. J Natl Cancer Inst 2004;96:879–82.
62. Morris MJ, Smaletz O, Solit D, et al. High-dose calcitriol, zoledronate, and dexamethasone for the treatment of progressive prostate carcinoma. Cancer 2004;100:1868–75.
63. Peehl DM, Skowronski RJ, Leung GK, et al. Antiproliferative effects of 1,25-vitamin D3 on primary cultures of human prostatic cells. Cancer Res 1994;54:805–10.
64. Guzey M, Kitada S, Reed JC. Apoptosis induction by 1-alpha, 25-dihydroxyvitamin D3 in prostate cancer. Mol Cancer Ther 2002;1:667–77.
65. Krishnan AV, Peehl DM, Feldman D. Inhibition of prostate cancer growth by vitamin D: regulation of target gene expression. J Cell Biochem 2003;88:363–71.
66. Rosen LS, Gordon D, Tchekmedyian S, et al. Zoledronic acid versus placebo in the treatment of skeletal metastases in patients with lung cancer and other solid tumors: phase III, double-blind, randomized trial—the Zoledronic Acid Lung Cancer and Other Solid Tumors Study Group. J Clin Oncol 2003;21:3150–7.
67. Ural AU, Yilmaz MI, Avcu F, et al. The bisphosphonate zoledronic acid induces cytotoxicity in human myeloma cell lines with enhancing effects of dexamethasone and thalidomide. Int J Hematol 2003;78:443–9.
68. Gordon S, Helfrich MH, Sati HI, et al. Pamidronate causes apoptosis of plasma cells in vivo in patients with multiple myeloma. Br J Haematol 2002;119:475–83.
69. Salomo M, Jurlander J, Nielsen LB, et al. How myeloma cells escape bisphosphonate-mediated killing: development of specific resistance with preserved sensitivity to conventional chemotherapeutics. Br J Haematol 2003;122:202–10.
70. Berenson JR, Lichtenstein A, Porter L, et al. Efficacy of pamidronate in reducing skeletal events in patients with advanced multiple myeloma. Myeloma Aredia Study Group. New Engl J Med 1996;334:488–93.
71. Musto P, Falcone A, Sampaolo G, et al. Pamidronate reduces skeletal events but does not improve progression-free survival in early-stage untreated myeloma: results of a randomized trial. Leuk Lymphoma 2003;44:1545–8.
72. Berenson JR, Rosen LS, Howell A, et al. Zoledronic acid reduces skeletal-related events in patients with osteolytic metastases. Cancer 2001;91:1191–200.
73. Kimura S, Kuroda J, Segawa H, et al. Antiproliferative effi-

cacy of the third-generation bisphosphonate zoledronic acid, combined with other anticancer drugs in leukemic cell lines. Int J Hematol 2004;79:37–43.
74. Saunders Y, Ross JR, Broadley KE, et al. Systemic review of bisphosphonates for hypercalcemia of malignancy. Palliat Med 2004;18:418–31.
75. Plorkin LI, Weinstein RS, Parfitt AM, et al. Prevention of osteocyte and osteoblast apoptosis by bisphosphonates and calcitonin. J Clin Invest 1999;104:1363–74.
76. Adachi JD, Saag KG, Delmas PD, et al. Two-year effects of alendronate on bone mineral density and vertebral fracture in patients receiving glucocorticoids: a randomized, double-blind, placebo-controlled extension trial. Arthritis Rheum 2001;44:202–11.
77. Wallach S, Cohen S, Reid DM, et al. Effects of risedronate treatment on bone density and vertebral fracture in patients on corticosteroid therapy. Calcif Tissue Int 2000;67:277–85.

131

Hematologic Complications and Blood Bank Support

Richard M. Kaufman, MD
Kenneth C. Anderson, MD

Hematologic complications occur commonly in patients with cancer, related either to the underlying disease or to its treatment.[1,2] Abnormalities in the red blood cell (RBC), leukocyte (WBC), and platelet number and function require transfusion medicine expertise for the provision of appropriate blood component support.[3,4] Indeed, the therapeutic advances made using high-dose combination chemotherapeutic approaches to date would not have been possible without the parallel development of technology to support patients through the hematologic complications of therapy. In addition, the blood component laboratory plays an increasingly central role in the cellular therapy of cancer, including the collection, processing, cryopreservation, infusion, and quality control of hematopoietic stem cells, donor lymphocytes, and dendritic cells for treatment protocols.[5]

NORMAL HEMATOPOIESIS

When considering the optimal strategy for supporting cellular blood component needs, a basic understanding of normal hematopoiesis, as well as the impact of cancer and its treatment on this process, is essential.[6] In human marrow, the most primitive clonogenic cell forms a colony of undifferentiated blasts in methylcellulose culture and is referred to as the "CFU-Blast," the majority of which are noncyclic under normal circumstances.[7] The individual cells of a blast cell colony can form a colony of granulocytes, erythroid cells, monocytes, and megakaryocytes (CFU-GEMM), which can give rise to secondary colonies of granulocytes and macrocytes (CFU-GM), erythroid cells arranged in clusters known as burst-forming units (BFU-E), megakaryocytes (CFU-Meg), eosinophils (CFU-Eo), or basophils (CFUBas) (Figure 131-1).

HEMATOPOIESIS

Although the CFU-GEMM is a cell that is multipotent by virtue of its ability to give rise to multiple cell lineages, it has very limited capacity for self-renewal and does not represent a true stem cell. This is further supported by the observation that CFU-GEMM may be almost eradicated from human bone marrow by in vitro purging with the active metabolite cyclophosphamide, 4-hydroperoxy-cyclophosphamide, yet the ability of that marrow to reconstitute a lethally irradiated recipient is unimpaired.[8] Colony-forming cells with a more restricted commitment status than the CFU-GEMM, such as the BFU-E or CFU-GM, lack self-renewal potential and are normally in an active cell cycle. On the basis of these observations, it has been proposed that normal hematopoiesis is characterized by the proliferation and commitment of small numbers of self-renewing, pluripotent, relatively quiescent progenitor cells that give rise to a succession of highly proliferative cells with more restrictive capacity for self-renewal (CFU-GEMM) and/or commitment (BFU-E, CFU-GM).

Hematopoietic progenitor cells proliferate and become committed to differentiate within a specialized environment that provides a supporting stroma on which the stem cells bind and receive regulatory signals required for stem cell growth. The viability and proliferation of bone marrow progenitor cells to form colonies of mature cells in semisolid medium requires the presence of one or more structurally heterogeneous glycoproteins termed "colony stimulatory factors" (CSFs). The cDNA for many of these factors have been cloned, their genes localized, and large amounts of purified factor have been produced through recombinant technology, thereby permitting delineation of their effects on marrow progenitor cells and their progeny, as well as their clinical utility.[6]

Of the many factors, those with clinical application affecting transfusion practice include erythropoietin (EPO), a glycoprotein produced in response to hypoxia in the kidney that induces red cell production by stimulating the mitotic activity of erythroid progenitor cells (BFU-E, CFU-Eo) and early erythroid progenitors in the bone marrow (see Figure 131-1).[9] Although granulocyte/macrophage (GM-CSF) was originally thought to stimulate the growth of relatively late myeloid progenitor cells such as CFU-GM and CFU-Eo, it may also support the growth of CFU-Blast, CFU-GEMM, BFU-E, and CFU-Meg, whereas granulocyte-CSF (G-CSF) has a more restricted action on myeloid lineage cells.[10] Although interleukin-11 (IL-11) and thrombopoietin both support megakaryocytopoiesis, only genetic elimination of the latter affects megakaryocyte and platelet production in vivo.[11–13] Normally, granulocytes, platelets, and red cells have half-lives of 4 to 10 hours, 4 to 5 days, and 50 to 65 days, respectively (Table 131-1).

CAUSES OF PANCYTOPENIA

Cancer and its treatment may alter normal hematopoiesis either by direct effects on hematopoietic stem cells or by inhibiting production of and responsiveness to hematopoietic growth factors (Table 131-2).

Disease Related Bone marrow hematopoietic cells can be replaced either by primary tumor in hematologic diseases, which are intrinsic to marrow, or by metastatic spread of tumor to the marrow from neoplasms of other organs. Hodgkin's, non-Hodgkin's lymphoma (NHL), malignant melanoma, neuroblastoma, as well as carcinoma of the breast, prostate, lung, adrenal, thyroid, and kidney commonly manifest marrow involvement. Although there may be associated symptomatology or radiographic abnormalities, these are commonly lacking. Leukoerythroblastic anemia, characterized by immature red cells and granulocytes in the peripheral blood, may be a signpost of tumor in the marrow.[14] Ultimately, diffuse involvement of marrow with tumor can lead to either marrow fibrosis or necrosis, which may be associated with splenomegaly, thrombocytopenia, and immature cells of all lineages in the peripheral blood.[15]

Chemotherapy Related The role of treatment in marrow injury and recovery varies both with the drugs employed and with the normal turnover rate of cells of different hematologic lineages. The bone marrow has a storage compartment that can supply mature cells to the peripheral blood for 8 to 10 days after the stem cell pool has ceased to function. Events in the peripheral blood are therefore a week behind the events in the bone marrow. In previously untreated patients, leukopenia and thrombocytopenia are described on days 9 or 10 after treatment, with the nadir of counts on days 14 to 18. Recovery of counts is evident by day 21 and complete by day 28. The cytotoxic dose-response effect is usually related to the nadir WBC and platelet count, not the duration of cytopenia. This is due to the resting state of the stem cells of normal bone marrow, which protects them from damage.

Route and schedule of drug administration, drug metabolism, and pattern of cell sensitivity may influence the pattern of marrow damage. Drugs act at specific points in the cell cycle and are classified on that basis; thus, hematopoietic stem cells may rebound after short-term exposure to a cell-cycle–specific agent, but prolonged administration results in permanent bone marrow suppression. For cell-cycle–specific agents, such as ara-C or methotrexate, recovery occurs rapidly

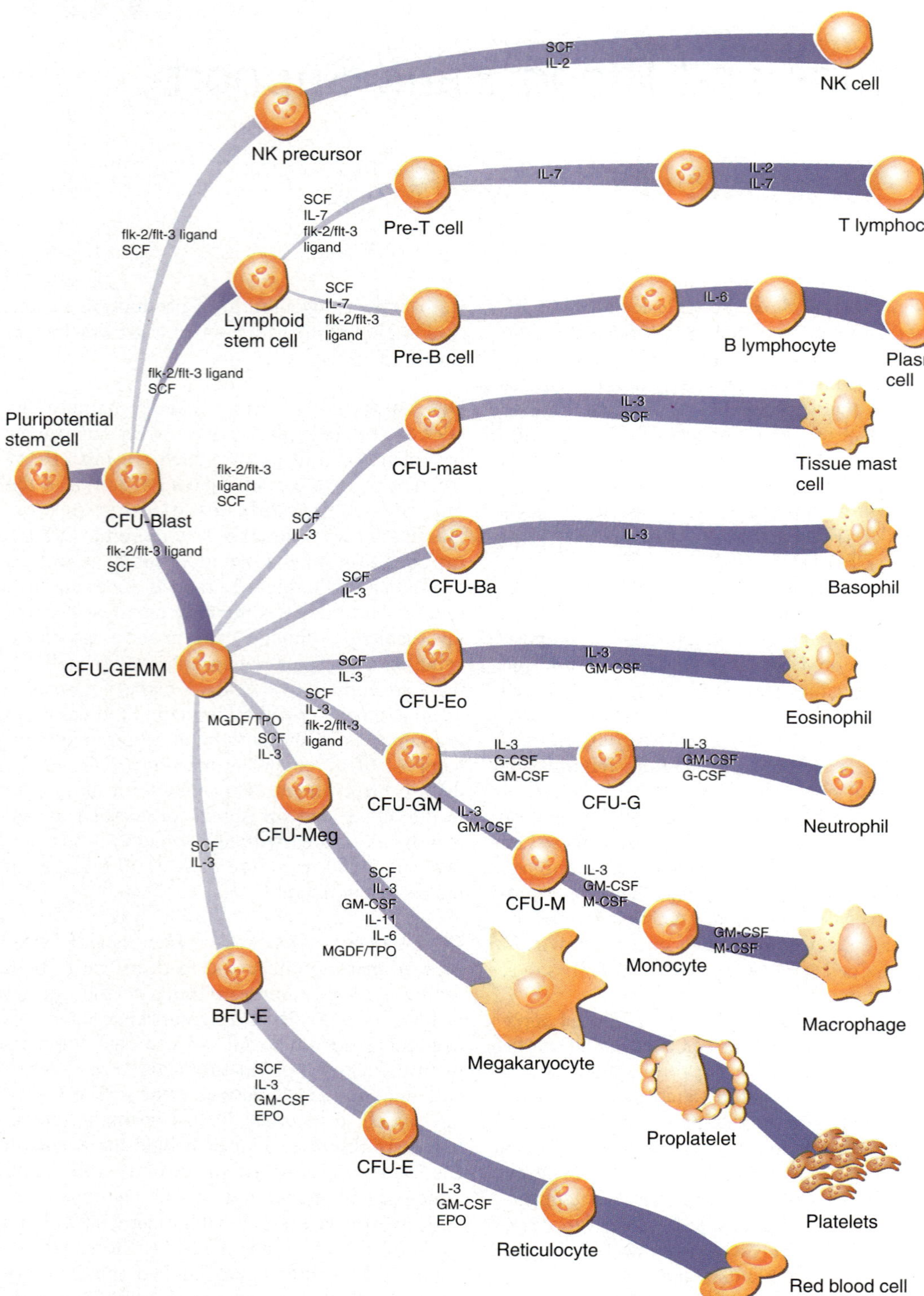

Figure 131-1 Hematopoiesis and its growth factors.

(7–14 days), whereas stem cell or G0-active agents, such as carmustine (BCNU) and busulfan, cause a much more delayed nadir (4–5 weeks) and recovery (6 weeks). Moreover, a chronic deficit in marrow reserve occurs fairly quickly with sequential BCNU therapy, but rarely, if ever, occurs after cell-cycle–specific agents such as ara-C. Bone marrow involvement with tumor may compromise bone marrow reserves, thereby shortening the time to leukopenia and thrombocytopenia and prolonging the recovery time. The characteristic effects of several drugs on marrow are shown in Table 131-3.

Gamma Radiation Related Cells damaged by irradiation may divide one time or more before all progeny are rendered reproductively sterile; thus, an irradiated cell will not appear damaged until it divides.[16] At the time of the first postirradiation subdivision, the cell may die, divide aberrantly and produce unusual forms, be unable to divide and remain physiologically functional, or give rise to one or more generation of progeny until cells become sterile. Since bone marrow stem cells have a very low capacity for repair of sublethal irradiation damage, multiple smaller radiation fractions may preserve other normal tissues (eg, lung, intestine), but will not spare bone marrow. During a course of fractionated irradiation, the ultimate effect on normal bone marrow will depend on whether there has been proliferation in the irradiated field between the fractions or migration of cells from unirradiated adjacent sites. Localized irradiation can cause a chronic lymphopenia (see Table 131-3). Finally, the effects of whole-body irradiation are qualitatively and quantitatively different from localized therapy. In particular, total-body irradiation causes profound suppression of humoral and cellular immune function.

Associated Processes It is essential to remain cognizant of derangements in normal physiology that may be occurring in the setting of cancer and/or treatment and that contribute to pancytopenia. These include nutritional factors, such as folate, iron, or vitamin deficiencies. There may be abnormal feedback loops in hematopoiesis, such as cell-mediated suppression of hematopoiesis in aplastic anemia or stimulation of thrombopoiesis in the set-

Table 131-2 Causes of Anemia, Thrombocytopenia, and Leukopenia in Cancer

- Bone marrow replacement by primary tumor (eg, leukemia)
- Bone marrow involvement by metastatic tumor (eg, breast, prostate)
- Derangement of normal physiology
  - Nutritional (eg, folate, iron, negative nitrogen balance)
  - Abnormal feedback (eg, stimulation/inhibition of hematopoiesis)
  - Bone marrow reaction (eg, fibrosis)
  - Peripheral destruction (eg, immune hemolysis, diffuse intravascular coagulation, splenomegaly)
  - Blood loss
- Myelosuppression by chemotherapy or radiotherapy

Table 131-1 Cellular Elements of Whole Blood

Total Blood	Total Body Pool	Circulating Pool	Half-Life in Circulation	Percentage of Volume Replaced Daily in Healthy Adults
Red blood cell ($\times 10^{10}$/kg)	33	33	50–65 days	0.8
Neutrophil ($\times 10^{7}$/kg)	70 (14–160)	31 (11–46)	6.7 (4–10 hours)	
Lymphocyte ($\times 10^{7}$/kg)	133–266	8–12	1 hour–1,500 days	230.0
Platelet ($\times 10^{10}$/kg)	2.8 (2.1–3.8)	2.1 (1.6–2.9)	4–5 days	10.0

Table 131-3 Characteristic Effects of Drugs and Treatments on Bone Marrow

Treatment	Hematologic Complication
Most chemotherapeutic agents	Leukopenia and thrombocytopenia at 9–10 days; nadir counts at 14–18 days; recovery of counts at 21–28 days
Nitrosourea	Myelosuppression at 4–6 weeks
Vincristine, L-asparaginase, bleomycin, methotrexate with leucovorin	No myelosuppression
Gamma irradiation	Chronic lymphopenia
Whole-body irradiation	Profound suppression of humoral and cellular immune response

ting of antibody-mediated platelet destruction.[17] Fibrosis can occur either as part of a disease process or as a reaction to therapy, thereby compromising bone marrow reserve. Immunologically mediated destruction of cells and other factors, such as splenomegaly, can result in cytopenias. Most important, occult bleeding must always be considered as a cause of persistent anemia and refractory thrombocytopenia. These clinical examples emphasize the importance of carefully assessing patients with cancer for treatable medical etiologies of their hematologic complications prior to attributing these effects to their underlying neoplasms.

ABNORMALITIES OF RED CELLS AND RED CELL SUPPORT

Anemia Anemia in patients with cancer can be mild to severe and may be attributable to many causes. Hematopoiesis in patients with early stages of cancer may be normal. On the other hand, replacement of marrow cells by tumor is not essential for the development of anemia, even in patients with metastatic cancer. Most commonly, the incidence and magnitude of anemia in patients with cancer increase as the disease progresses. This anemia is designated as anemia of chronic disease only if the cellular pattern in the marrow is nearly normal, the serum iron and iron-binding capacity are low, the iron content of the marrow is normal or increased, and the serum ferritin is elevated.[18] The coexistence of low plasma iron levels with adequate amounts of storage iron helps distinguish anemia of chronic disease from iron-deficiency anemia. Moreover, other causes of anemia, for example, overt hemolysis, bleeding, nutritional deficiency, or marrow replacement, must be ruled out. Finally, ^{51}chromium-labeled RBC studies suggest that RBC survival in patients with advanced cancer can be significantly shortened without classic clinical or laboratory evidence of hemolysis. In some patients, such as those with histiocytic medullary reticulosis or Hodgkin's disease (HD), erythrophagocytosis, or hypersplenism may account for this decrease in red cell survival, but in others its etiology is unclear.

Red Cell Growth Factors Serum erythropoietin (EPO) levels may be low for a given level of anemia in patients with cancer compared with a control population with anemias of other etiologies.[19] Moreover, increases in EPO serum levels expected for a given degree of anemia can be further blunted by chemotherapy regimens, with or without cisplatin. The inability to produce EPO in cancer patients is not absolute, however, since hypoxemia can restore EPO response. The exact nature of the EPO-producing cells in the kidney and liver is unclear, but it is possible that the EPO-producing cells are damaged by the chemotherapy and radiation therapy. This has been suggested as the etiology of the anemia associated with cisplatin chemotherapy, although direct erythroid marrow toxicity may play a role.[20] Since the endogenous EPO response is inappropriate in patients with cancer, treatment of the anemia of cancer with recombinant human (rH)EPO may be of value.[21,22] Randomized trials demonstrated that rHEPO corrected anemia and reduced homologous red cell transfusion requirements in patients receiving chemotherapy with and without cisplatin.[23–25] In addition to reducing transfusion requirements, a study of 2,370 outpatients with a variety of cancers who were also treated with rHEPO demonstrated a beneficial impact on patient-reported functional capacity and quality of life in patients who received chemotherapy independent of tumor response.[26] Endogenous EPO levels may also be low after autologous and allogeneic marrow transplantation and treatment with erythropoietin in this setting is also useful to accelerate erythropoiesis and reduce homologous red cell requirements.[27–30] One study suggests that patients with cancer who do not increase serum EPO levels to more than 100 mU/mL and hemoglobin (Hb) by at least 0.5 g/dL after 2 weeks of rHEPO therapy are likely unresponsive to treatment.[31]

Immune hemolytic anemias are associated with neoplasms of the lymphocytic and reticuloendothelial systems. Anemia is usually moderate to severe and is associated with jaundice, splenomegaly, and increased urine and fecal urobilinogen excretion. Red cell survival is decreased and the reticulocyte count increased unless erythropoiesis is profoundly impaired. Hemolytic anemia may be due to a warm-reacting immunoglobulin (IgG) with a positive direct antiglobulin (Coombs') test and positive reaction to antisera specific for IgG on the red cell. This occurs most commonly in chronic lymphocytic leukemia but has also been reported in patients with lymphomas, acute leukemias, myeloproliferative disorders, or carcinoma. Alternatively, IgM antibody can bind and cause agglutination in the cold. In either case, anemia occurs because of reticuloendothelial sequestration of red cells that are coated with antibody or complement components (extravascular hemolysis). Hemoglobinemia and hemoglobulinuria (intravascular hemolysis) occur very rarely and have been attributed to cold-reacting antibody. The production of inflammatory cytokines by phagocytes may mediate the symptomatology of IgG-mediated hemolytic transfusion reactions.[32]

Microangiopathic anemia, characterized by red cell distortion and fragmentation on smear (schistocytes) and intravascular hemolysis with associated thrombocytopenia, is uncommon, but when observed in oncology, it is usually evident in patients with metastatic adenocarcinomas of the stomach, breast, prostate, lung, pancreas, gallbladder, and colon, and in those with angiosarcomas.[33] Intravascular coagulation with low clotting factor levels, fibrinolysis, increased fibrin degradation products, and increased fibrin catabolism may be present. Red cell fragmentation may be due to deposition of fibrin within vessels, and/or intravascular coagulation may be initiated by the release of thromboplastins by the tumor cells. Finally, anemia may be related to pure red cell aplasia without associated leukocyte or platelet marrow abnormalities commonly associated with thymoma and rarely present in the setting of lymphoma or chronic lymphocytic leukemia.[34]

Red Cell Transfusion Red cell transfusions are indicated to increase oxygen carrying capacity in patients with anemia that is not adequately compensated by normal physiologic mechanisms. Sufficient oxygen-carrying capacity to maintain cardiopulmonary function can be met by a hemoglobin of 7 g/dL (a hematocrit of approximately 21%) when the intravascular volume is adequate for perfusion.[36] In a randomized multicenter study of critical care patients, a restrictive transfusion strategy (maintaining hemoglobin levels between 7 and 9 g/dL) was demonstrated to be at least as safe as a more liberal transfusion strategy, with the possible exception of patients with acute myocardial infarction or unstable angina.[37] However, there is no single hemoglobin level that can be universally applied as a "transfusion trigger." In deciding whether to transfuse a specific patient, the physician should consider the patient's age, degree of anemia, the intravascular volume, and the presence of coexisting cardiac, pulmonary, or vascular conditions.[38] To meet oxygen needs, some patients may require RBC transfusions at higher hemoglobin levels. In particular, hemoglobin levels are commonly maintained at levels of 8 g/dL in the setting of cancer and its therapy. Transfusing one unit of RBCs will usually increase the hemoglobin by 1 g/dL and the hematocrit by 2 to 3% in the average adult weighing 70 kg.

Red Cell Products In the United States, homologous red cell transfusion rates have fallen since 1986, with an associated increase in autologous blood usage.[39,40] However, autologous donations have not been universally accepted in patients with cancers and leukemias because of concern that there may be circulating tumor cells in peripheral blood. Packed red blood cells (PRBCs) are prepared from one unit of whole blood (WB) by the removal of plasma and are transfused for the maintenance of adequate oxygen-carrying capacity. Whole blood is rarely transfused, except to restore both volume and oxygen-carrying capacity in the setting of massive hemorrhage. Red cells can be depleted of leukocytes by filtration to produce leukoreduced red cells (LRBCs). Leukoreduction can prevent a significant percentage of febrile nonhemolytic transfusion reactions, alloimmunization, and cytomegalovirus infection in transfusion recipients.[41] Leukocyte reduction prior to storage can abrogate cytokine release and decrease transfusion reactions.[42] In the United States and around the world, there is a trend to universally transfuse leukoreduced cellular components to avoid the multiple adverse sequelae of leukocytes. Washed red blood cells (WRBCs) are prepared by further removal of plasma from PRBCs. These products are sometimes indicated to prevent allergic reactions to plasma proteins.[43] WRBCs may be useful in rare patients who are IgA deficient and have circulating anti-IgA antibodies, since these patients may have anaphylactic reactions if transfused with blood components containing IgA.

ABNORMALITIES OF WHITE CELLS AND WHITE CELL SUPPORT

Leukocytosis Peripheral blood leukocyte counts are usually normal in patients with cancer but may be slightly elevated in patients with lung cancer. Elevated circulating leukocyte counts > 50,000/mm^3 may occur in patients with cancer, are termed "leukemoid reactions," and can consist either of mature leukocytes or of early forms, such as myeloblasts and promyelocytes, in the peripheral blood.[44] Such reactions have been described most commonly in patients with metastatic tumors of the breast, lung, and stomach. They are distinguished from leukoerythroblastic reactions by the absence of nucleated red cells and the immature white cells. Lymphocytic leukemoid reactions occur most often in children and young adults with viral infections but rarely have been reported in association with cancer. Basophilia, frequently present in patients with myeloproliferative syndromes, is also uncommonly evident in patients with leukemoid reactions. Finally, eosinophilia has been reported in association with HD and mycosis fungoides, carcinomatosis, epithelial tumors, brain tumors, melanoma, lymphoma, acute lymphocytic leukemia, eosinophilic granuloma, and myeloproliferative disorders.

Leukopenia Leukopenia may occur related to cancer and its treatment. In 1965, Hersh and colleagues summarized the causes of death in patients with acute leukemia treated at the National Cancer Institute and noted a marked decline in fatal hemorrhage, due to the availability of platelet transfusions, with a concomitant increase in the occurrence of infection alone as a cause of death.[45]

A quantitative relationship between circulating leukocytes and infection was established in patients with leukemia; in particular, the probability of being infected is proportional to both the severity and duration of leukopenia.[46]

Associated Processes After profound marrow injury, monocytosis usually precedes neutrophilic recovery. Overshoot in the leukocyte count to 20,000/mm^3 to 30,000/mm^3 can occur before leveling out and return to normal leukocyte counts. The overshoot of leukocytes and platelets occurs much more frequently and is of greater magnitude in pediatric patients and young adults than in elderly patients, presumably reflecting marrow reserve capacity, differentiation rapidity, and hematopoietic homeostasis. Otherwise, elevated leukocyte counts in a cancer patient under observation should trigger an evaluation for an infectious cause. Defects in leukocyte function may be present with or without abnormalities in cell numbers. Patients with acute myelogenous leukemia, for example, have defects in phagocytosis or microbial killing that are not present in patients with acute lymphoblastic leukemia.[47]

Leukocyte Transfusion Therapeutic granulocytes were first utilized nearly 30 years ago in leukemic patients with leukopenia and serious infection. The earliest trials, which demonstrated the potential value of granulocyte transfusions, utilized granulocytes harvested from patients with chronic granulocytic leukemia and achieved cell dosages never approached when normal donors were utilized.[48] The importance of dose was defined: < 10^{10} granulocytes were ineffective, whereas > 10^{11} cells were effective. Indeed, in an afebrile, uninfected man, the half-life of granulocytes in the circulation is 6.7 (4–10) hours and the daily turnover rate is 230%; in the setting of fever and/or infection, this turnover rate can be severalfold higher.[49] Parallel work in canine models had also demonstrated that dogs deliberately made leukopenic by irradiation and given gram-negative bacteremia and pneumonia could be successfully treated with granulocyte transfusions.[50]

Clinical Studies The randomized prospective clinical trials of therapeutic leukocyte transfusions for leukopenic patients with established infections have been reviewed.[51] Early studies demonstrated benefit from leukocyte transfusions and defined several factors to be predictors of outcome: type of infecting organisms, the interval to bone marrow recovery, and the dose of granulocytes transfused. Granulocyte transfusion was not beneficial in the most controlled study, in which recipients were not tested for antileukocyte antibodies, lower numbers of leukocytes were transfused, and a much better survival was noted in the group treated with antibiotics alone.[52] Because of improved efficacy of antibiotics, therapeutic granulocytes are presently utilized only rarely, to treat refractory bacterial or fungal infection in a leukopenic patient who has reasonable expectation of marrow recovery. Five studies indicated a protective effect for leukocyte transfusions, although differences observed were significant in only two trials. Even this finite clinical need may be decreased with the use of recombinant growth factors, for example, GM-CSF or G-CSF, to stimulate normal myeloid recovery. Indeed, a recent retrospective analysis did not show a benefit for granulocyte transfusions for treatment of fungal infections in neutropenic patients following bone marrow transplantation.[53]

There have been six randomized prospective trials of prophylactic leukocyte transfusions given to prevent infections in leukopenic recipients.[49,51] However, none of the studies demonstrated improved survival because alloimmunization, transfusion reactions, cytomegalovirus infection, and pulmonary infiltrates occurred more frequently in the transfused group. These studies have been criticized methodologically because of inadequate donor-recipient matching and inadequate doses of granulocytes transfused; still, prophylactic granulocytes are not presently utilized in patients with cancer.

Leukocyte Collection and Administration Granulocytes are harvested in a leukopheresis procedure utilizing hydroxyethyl starch and sodium citrate, which usually takes 90 minutes to remove adequate granulocytes ($\geq 10^{10}$) while returning RBCs to the donor. The recent use of myeloid growth factors can facilitate the collection of large numbers of granulocytes from normal donors and warrant further study of the utility of granulocyte transfusions.[49,54–56] These leukocytes are obtained from ABO-compatible donors. A test for leukoagglutination using freshly obtained patient serum and donor white cells can be done prior to transfusion to assure compatibility and avoid leukoagglutinin-mediated pulmonary reactions in the recipient. Post-transfusion cytomegalovirus (CMV) interstitial pneumonitis is avoided through the use of only CMV-seronegative donors. Leukocytes are irradiated to prevent proliferation of T cells within the transfused product, which could potentially either engraft or induce graft-versus-host disease (GVHD) when transfused to an immunocompromised host.[57] It is important to note that despite earlier allegations, patients receiving amphotericin therapy are not at increased risk of transfusion-related pulmonary reactions.

Myeloid Growth Factors The development of recombinant myeloid growth factors, GM-CSF and G-CSF, has significantly shortened the period of leukopenia after high-dose therapies.[10] In particular, GM-CSF was first shown to accelerate myeloid recovery in patients with NHL, acute lymphoblastic leukemia, and HD undergoing autologous bone marrow transplantation (BMT).[58] G-CSF was shown to decrease the incidence of infection, as manifested by febrile neutropenia, in patients with nonmyeloid malignancies receiving myelosuppressive anticancer drugs associated with a significant incidence of severe neutropenia with fever.[59] Both have also been used, either alone or at the time of recovery from chemotherapy, to enhance collection of both autologous and allogeneic peripheral blood stem cells (PBSCs) for transplantation, and ongoing studies are evaluating their cost efficacy to enhance reconstitution post-transplantation.[10,60–64] As noted above, their availability has further decreased the need for therapeutic granulocyte transfusions, but they may facilitate collection of granulocytes from normal donors.[49,54,55] They should not be used in otherwise uncomplicated neutropenia and fever, but should be reserved for appropriate approved clinical settings.[62–65] Novel applications of these factors are emerging, that is, GM-CSF in vaccine and dendritic cell cancer therapies.[10]

ABNORMALITIES OF PLATELETS AND PLATELET SUPPORT

Thrombocytosis Primary thrombocytosis is noted not only in essential thrombocythemia, but also in polycythemia rubra vera, agnogenic myeloid metaplasia, and chronic myelogenous leukemia.[66] Related hemorrhage is usually from the skin or mucous membranes, and thrombosis involving the arterial and/or venous systems can also occur. Although an elevated whole-blood viscosity, intrinsic defects in platelets, and elevated platelet counts may all predispose to bleeding, it is difficult to assess risks in an asymptomatic patient. Therapy should be utilized for the symptomatic patient (eg, phlebotomy to correct polycythemia), which primarily consists of cytoreductive therapy of the underlying disorder.

Secondary or reactive thrombocytosis can also occur in other cancers, but is characterized by only mild elevations of platelet counts without associated changes in platelet morphology and function.[67] This can sometimes serve as a diagnostic clue and is not associated with Trousseau's syndrome of migratory thrombophlebitis. Indeed, persons with thrombocytosis over 400,000/mm^3 should be evaluated for chronic or acute inflammatory disorders, acute hemorrhage, anemia, iron deficiency, or neoplasm. After splenectomy, the platelet count rises in the first week to levels of 1×10^6/mm^3 or more, and then falls slowly to normal over 3 months.

Thrombocytopenia Thrombocytopenia in cancer patients is usually attributable to treatment with chemotherapy and radiotherapy. Impaired production of platelets owing to a decrease or absence of megakaryocytes is therefore the most common cause of thrombocytopenia in patients with cancer (Table 131-4). However, thrombocytopenia may also be due to splenic sequestration in patients who have splenomegaly as part of their primary neoplastic process. In this setting, increased numbers of megakaryocytes are evident unless extensive marrow infiltration is present. Immune-mediated thrombocytopenia may also occur related to antihuman leukocyte antigen (anti-HLA) or antiplatelet-specific alloantibodies. Interestingly, combination chemotherapy and pulsed high-dose dexamethasone therapy have been shown to be beneficial in some patients in whom immune thrombocytopenia is refractory to corticosteroids and splenectomy.[68,69] Finally, thrombocytopenia may be related to diffuse intravascular coagulation (DIC), especially in patients with acute myelocytic leukemias, lymphomas, and carcinoma of lung, breast, gastrointestinal, or urologic origin. DIC most commonly complicates acute promyelocytic leukemia because of the presence of both thromboplastic material and fibrinolytic proteases in the promyelocytic subcellular components.[70]

Table 131-4 Causes of Thrombocytopenia

Acute thrombocytopenia due to increased platelet depletion (utilization, sequestration, or destruction)
Massive blood replacement
Cardiac surgery
Splenomegaly
Immune destruction of platelets
Self-limited acute idiopathic thrombocytopenia purpura (ITP)
Post-transfusion purpura
Drug purpura
Chronic idiopathic thrombocytopenia purpura
Consumptive thrombocytopenia
Hereditary defects
Thrombocytopenia with decreased platelet production
Aplastic anemia
Acute leukemia
Idiopathic megakaryocytic aplasia
Marrow infiltration
Malignant
Nonmalignant—Gaucher disease, granulomatous diseases
Following radiation or myelosuppressive drugs
Drugs producing specific suppression of platelet production (eg, thiazides, ethanol, estrogens)
Nutritional deficiency—megaloblastic anemia, severe iron deficiency (rare)
Viral infections
Paroxysmal nocturnal hemoglobinuria

Abnormalities in Platelet Function Platelet function can be abnormal in several chronic myeloproliferative disorders. Although most bleeding in patients with acute myelogenous leukemia is related to thrombocytopenia, intrinsic abnormalities in platelet function have been described including decreased platelet procoagulant activity and decreased aggregation and serotonin release responses to ADP, epinephrine, or collagen.[71] These defects may reflect the fact that megakaryocytes have originated from a leukemic stem cell. Platelet transfusions, coupled with treatment of the underlying disease, remain the mainstay of therapy.

Platelet dysfunction is evident in a fraction of patients with IgA myeloma or Waldenström's macroglobulinemia, multiple myeloma, and monoclonal gammopathy of undetermined significance.[72] In addition to thrombocytopenia, the following factors may also predispose to bleeding: hyperviscosity, acquired factor X deficiency in the setting of amyloidosis, a circulating heparin-like anticoagulant, fibrinolysis, and interference by myeloma protein with fibrin polymerization and with the function of other coagulation proteins. Cytoreductive therapy is primary, with plasmapheresis reserved for acute bleeding.

Platelet Transfusion Support In 1910, fresh whole blood was first transfused to thrombocytopenic patients, resulting in a significant rise in the platelet count, hemostasis, and improvement of the bleeding time.[73] In the 1950s, platelets were first used for the treatment of thrombocytopenia related to combination chemotherapeutic treatments of leukemias.[74] Data from the National Cancer Institute in the early 1960s clearly demonstrated that leukemia patients died of hemorrhage during induction of remission with chemotherapy and established the quantitative relationship between platelet count and hemorrhage.[45,75] It was shown that platelet therapy could modify the course of hemorrhage in both pediatric and adult settings, the only difference being the doses required. In the 1970s, studies in children and adults confirmed the efficacy of platelet transfusion to prevent rather than control hemorrhage.[76,77]

Single- and Multiple-Donor Platelets One unit of platelet concentrate is obtained from one unit of whole blood by centrifugation and contains approximately 5.5×10^{10} platelets/unit. Concentrates from multiple (6–8) donors are pooled to produce a single component for transfusion. Currently, individual platelet concentrates can be stored for up to 5 days prior to pooling and transfusion. Apheresis technology has permitted harvesting the equivalent of several platelet concentrates from a single donor during a single donation.[78,79] A single-donor platelet unit typically contains at least 3×10^{11} platelets/unit. The major advantage of multiple-donor platelet concentrates is their availability, since they are derived from conventional whole blood donations. However, some studies suggest that alloimmunization can occur early in patients receiving multiple-donor platelets and that limiting the number of donors per transfusion may postpone the development of refractoriness to platelet transfusions in thrombocytopenic patients.[80,81] A second potential advantage of single-donor platelets stems from the decreased risk of infection when exposed to fewer donors. Indeed, the Retrovirus Epidemiology Donor Study demonstrated that the prevalence of any viral infection was 50% higher in whole blood donors as compared with apheresis donors.[82] The use of single-donor platelets is increasing; they are generally considered to be the platelet product of choice for patients being treated for malignancy.[40] Single-donor platelet collections are utilized to provide HLA-matched donors for alloimmunized recipients who have not responded to platelets from random donors.

Indications for Therapeutic and Prophylactic Platelet Transfusion A minority of patients with cancer require platelet transfusions; however, platelets are more commonly transfused to patients with cancer than to patients with any other category of disease. The majority of platelet transfusions are given prophylactically to prevent bleeding, as opposed to therapeutically, to treat active bleeding.[83] The appropriate indications for transfusion of platelets have been the subject of a National Institutes of Health Consensus Development Conference as well as a more recent American Society of Clinical Oncology clinical practice guideline.[84,85] At present, 6 to 8 units of random-donor platelet concentrates, or the equivalent platelet dose in the form of a single-donor apheresis platelet product, are often routinely transfused to cancer patients with platelet counts less than 10,000 to 20,000/mm^3 to prevent hemorrhage. Gmur and colleagues demonstrated that the threshold for prophylactic platelet transfusion can safely be set at 5×10^9/L in patients with acute leukemia without fever or bleeding manifestations and at 10×10^9/L in patients with such signs.[86] More recently, they have shown this policy to be safe in the outpatient management of patients with aplastic anemia. Prospective clinical trials have shown that the risk of major bleeding was similar whether 10×10^9/L or 20×10^9/L was used as the platelet-transfusion threshold in patients with acute leukemia, and that the lower threshold reduced platelet use.[87–89] The implications of thrombocytopenia as a risk factor for hemorrhage and therefore the timing and dose of prophylactic platelets may vary in different clinical settings. Moreover, the use of higher doses of platelets per transfusion may extend the interval until additional transfusions are needed.[90]

The risk of bleeding at a given platelet count may vary in distinct clinical settings. For example, patients with thrombocytopenia owing to acute myelocytic leukemia were reported to have increased bleeding at $<$ 10,000/mm^3 platelets, in contrast to patients with acute lymphoblastic leukemia, who had similar risk of hemorrhage at $<$ 20,000/mm^3 platelets.[91] Young platelets are more efficient at controlling hemorrhage, so the need for platelet transfusion will be greater if the count is falling after chemotherapy compared with a similar level during a rise from a nadir.[92] Patients with chronic thrombocytopenia owing to decreased platelet production (ie, myelodysplastic disorders) may require transfusions, in contrast to patients with accelerated destruction but active production of platelets (ie, idiopathic thrombocytopenic purpura), who may not require routine platelet transfusions. Moreover, patients with chronic thrombocytopenia may tolerate lower absolute platelet counts without transfusion. In patients with abnormalities of platelet function, it is not the absolute platelet count but rather the number of functional platelets that is important for the prevention of bleeding. Thus, it is difficult to define an absolute platelet threshold for transfusion for all patients, and both the timing and the dose of prophylactic platelet transfusion must therefore be determined on a clinical basis.[93–97]

Clinical and Laboratory Assessment of the Effectiveness of Platelet Transfusion The effectiveness of platelet transfusion can be assessed by laboratory parameters, the corrected increment (CCI) 10 minutes to 1 hour after transfusion and the bleeding time, as well as by the observed clinical outcome after transfusion.[98–101] The corrected platelet increment is defined as the increment in platelet counts from pre- to post-transfusion corrected for the number of units transfused and for the body surface area of the recipient. When low numbers of platelets are transfused, regression analysis of post-transfusion increments may provide a more accurate assessment than CCI.[102] Measurement of the bleeding time after transfusion serves as a measure of the number of functional platelets, particularly in patients known to have dysfunctional platelets. Techniques such as radio-labeling platelets can be utilized to diagnose and identify the site of accelerated platelet destruction, but the most important monitor of the effectiveness of platelet transfusion is critical clinical assessment for the presence and extent of hemorrhage.

Factors Adversely Affecting Platelet Recovery If an inappropriately low corrected platelet increment is noted at 1 hour after transfusion, the status of both the platelet product transfused and of the recipient must be examined for potential explanations. A corrected increment of 15,000/mm^3 to 20,000/mm^3 is usual at 18 to 24 hours, provided fresh, properly stored platelets have been transfused.[98] This translates into an absolute increment at 1 hour of approximately 7,000 to 11,000/mm^3 for each unit of platelet concentrate administered to an average-sized person with body surface area of 1.0 m^2.

Laboratory Factors Several factors involved in the harvesting and storage of platelets prior to transfusion might result in poor post-transfusion platelet survival: pH, number of contaminating leukocytes, concentration of platelets, plasma volume, temperature, time, and agitation during storage. With the quality control measures currently in practice in most blood banks, it is uncommon to identify a problem either in the harvesting or donation to account for a poor post-transfusion increment.

Clinical Factors If the survival of transfused platelets is compromised, several conditions in the transfusion recipients may be responsible.[103–107] First, patients with fevers and/or infections have increased consumption of platelets, even when there is no evidence of consumptive coagulopathy. Second, post-transfusion increments in platelet count may also be less than expected because of splenic sequestration, especially in the setting of splenomegaly.[108] Third, drug-induced platelet antibodies, which mediate immune destruction of platelets, have been demonstrated. Antibodies responsible for drug-induced thrombocytopenia may bind to platelets by their fragment-antigen binding (Fab) regions rather than by attaching nonspecifically as immune complexes.[109] Platelet membrane glycoproteins gpIb and gpIIb/IIIa appear to be the preferred targets, although gpV has also been implicated.[110–112] Drugs apparently bind to the platelet membrane, inducing a reversible structural change that provokes an antibody response. Drugs may also induce antibodies that mediate thrombocytopenia without direct drug-platelet interaction, for example, methyldopa.[113] Alternatively, drugs such as penicillin may bind covalently to the platelet membrane and induce hapten-dependent antibodies.[114] The survival of transfused platelets can be compromised if the recipient possesses antibodies against donor antigens (Ags) of HLA-A and HLA-B loci, the AB-H system, or platelet alloantigens. Response to platelet transfusion in recipients of hematopoietic stem cell transplantation has been specifically studied. One report identified high total bilirubin, total-body irradiation, and high serum cyclosporin A levels to be predictive of low CCI, whereas another found irradiation, post-transplant fever, and hepatic veno-occlusive disease to be associated with delayed platelet recovery.[105,106] A third study in patients who had undergone hematopoietic stem cell transplantation associated presence of lymphocytotoxic antibodies, male gender, large body surface area, concomitant red cell transfusion, concurrent steroids, major ABO incompatibility, and history of multiple recipient pregnancies with poor CCI postplatelet transfusion.[107]

Alloimmunization Platelets bear HLA-A and -B but lack HLA-C and -DR Ags, and there is a high correlation between the development of lymphocytotoxic anti-HLA antibodies in the recipient and refractoriness to random-donor platelets.[115] Anti-HLA antibodies are most easily detectable using the patient's serum and a panel of lymphocytes representing known HLA specificities. The incidence and the timing of production of anti-HLA antibodies after platelet transfusion remain controversial and may vary with the recipient population. Most studies document alloimmunization in 50 to 90% of multitransfused patients.[116] Some studies demonstrate that the rate of alloimmunization increases with the number of transfusions, whereas other reports find no relationship between the number of platelet transfusions given and the rate of alloimmunization.[117,118] Moreover, a fraction of patients with cancer never become sensitized.[119,120] Nonetheless, it is crucial to test for anti-HLA antibodies whenever recipients become refractory to random-donor platelet transfusion, since response to random-donor platelet transfusion is poor in the sensitized host, and HLA-matched or family-member platelets may be useful in this setting.[121–123] The panel reactive antibody (PRA) screen is usually performed in this context.

Yankee and colleagues[122] first demonstrated that platelets obtained from HLA-identical siblings or from unrelated donors matched at the HLA-A and -B loci (grade A or B matches) could result in satisfactory post-transfusion increments in alloimmunized recipients who were refractory to random-donor platelet transfusions.[122,123] Subsequently, Duquesnoy and colleagues found that donors whose HLA antigens were the same (B match) or cross-reactive with the patient's Ags (BX match) were equivalent.[124]

The evaluation of donors for the same or cross-reactive Ags became even more complex. For

Table 131-5 Trial to Reduce Alloimmunization to Platelets in Patients Undergoing Myeloablative Therapy for Myelocytic Leukemia

	Pooled Random Donor Concentrates %	Pooled Random Donor Concentrates Treated with UVB Irradiation %	Pooled Random Donor Platelets, White Cell Reduced by Filtration %	Single-Donor Platelets[a] %
Lymphocytotoxic antibodies and refractoriness to transfusion	13	5	3	4
Lymphocytotoxic antibodies only	45	21	18	17
Alloantibodies and refractoriness to transfusion	13	5	3	4
Alloantibodies only	11	7	6	7

[a]Prepared by apheresis in a white cell reduction protocol and further filtered to reduce contamination to the lowest possible amount.

example, platelets from donors lacking HLA-A2 who bear one of two (grade C match) or three of four (grade D match) Ags not present in the recipient may have favorable post-transfusion outcomes in alloimmunized recipients; in contrast, platelets from HLA-A2+ donors who were HLA-A and -B matches were unsuccessful.[124,125] Weak anti-HLA antibodies, which can cause platelet destruction in vivo, may not be detected by standard assays, and, alternatively, excellent platelet transfusion recoveries have been observed despite a positive lymphocytotoxicity crossmatch.[115,124] Additional crossmatching techniques may be required in those 20% of sensitized patients who remain refractory even to HLA-matched platelets.

The recognition of the refractoriness associated with the development of anti-HLA antibodies led to attempts to either avoid or delay alloimmunization by modifying the platelets to be transfused. Since HLA antigens are expressed on leukocytes, and platelets themselves are poor immunogens, investigators have attempted to (1) remove white blood cells from platelets or treat platelets with ultraviolet irradiation (UV) to abrogate the leukocyte antigen-presenting function, (2) use single rather than multiple donor platelets to minimize exposure to HLA, and (3) transfuse only HLA-matched or leukocyte-depleted HLA-matched platelets. Leukocyte-reduced platelets are prepared by filtration, which depletes white cells by 3 logs, with varying associated losses of platelets. Filtered platelets with no more than 10^6 contaminating leukocytes were found to reduce the likelihood of formation of anti-HLA antibodies; in contrast, transfusions of similar numbers of non-leukocyte–reduced platelets did sensitize recipients.[41,126] However, some reports suggest that neither bedside filtration nor UVB irradiation is effective in the prevention of alloimmunization to platelets.[127,128] In an animal model, prestorage, but not poststorage, leukodepletion did abrogate alloimmunization.[129]

Use of single-donor platelets or of ultraviolet irradiation of platelets has been evaluated in small studies to prevent the development of alloimmunization.[81,130] It is important to note that the Trial to Reduce Alloimmunization to Platelets (TRAP) showed that the incidence of anti-HLA and platelet-specific antibodies alone, as well as the incidence of antibodies associated with platelet refractoriness, were reduced in leukemic recipients who received either filtered or UV-treated pooled random-donor concentrates or filtered single-donor platelets compared with similar patients who received nonfiltered pooled random-donor concentrates (Table 131-5).[131] Only 13% of patients developed platelet refractoriness associated with lymphocytotoxic antibodies, suggesting that the majority of unresponsiveness to transfusion is related to other factors. A meta-analysis of seven randomized controlled trials published between 1983 and 1995 supports the TRAP findings and suggests that these findings can be extended to other than leukemic patients and applied to the prevention of platelet transfusion refractoriness.[126,132]

When sensitized recipients remain refractory to HLA-matched platelets, attempts have been made to carry out additional crossmatching to identify more compatible platelet donors.[112,133–135] These include leukoagglutination,[51] chromium-lysis, immunofluorescence, enzyme-linked immunosorbent assay (ELISA), assays of ^{131}iodine-labeled platelet-associated IgG, and platelet aggregometry. They have enjoyed variable success determining which platelets will be effective in refractory patients, and no one assay or combination of methods has been universally accepted to predict response to transfusion.

Potential mechanisms to explain unexpectedly suboptimal post-transfusion recoveries in patients receiving HLA-matched ABO-compatible platelet transfusions include unrecognized HLA specificities, circulating immune complexes, and antibodies to platelet-specific Ags. Plasma exchange or intravenous immunoglobulin therapy has been used prior to platelet transfusion in those patients who remain refractory to ABO-compatible HLA-matched platelets, with mixed benefit.[136,137]

The ABO blood group determinants, presumably absorbed from the plasma, are present on platelets with a structure similar to that on erythrocytes.[138] Major Ags of the Rh, Duffy, Kidd, Kell, and Lutheran systems, in contrast, are not expressed on the surface of human platelets.[139] Clinical studies have shown that platelet transfusions may induce the formation of isohemagglutinins because of a small number of contaminating erythrocytes, suggesting that ABO compatibility between donor and recipient is important.[140] However, in vitro studies have demonstrated that exposure of group A and AB platelets to the appropriate anti-A and anti-AB alloantibodies and complement does not cause ultrastructural damage to the platelets or induce platelet aggregation, suggesting that an ABO mismatch between donor and recipient is not an absolute contraindication to platelet transfusion.[141]

The need for ABO compatibility between platelet donor and recipient has been directly examined in several studies. A randomized trial of ABO-compatible versus ABO-incompatible platelets demonstrated that the corrected increments after the first transfusion were equivalent, but higher increments were noted after subsequent transfusion of ABO-compatible platelets in a subset of patients.[142] Rh-incompatible platelets may not be immunogenic in certain patients with cancer.[143] Therefore, ABO matching of donor and recipient is unimportant for the majority of platelet transfusions. The fact that transfusions that are not group specific are considered safe and clinically effective greatly expands the availability of platelets for transfusion. However, in specific clinical settings, donor and recipient ABO compatibility may be significant. For example, if HLA-matched but ABO-mismatched platelet transfusion does not result in a satisfactory increment after transfusion, HLA- and ABO-matched platelets may be of benefit.[144] Heal and colleagues have postulated that soluble plasma HLA-A and -B and ABO Ags contribute to the destruction of donor and sometimes recipient platelets by an immune complex or another "innocent bystander" mechanism.[145] Finally, hemolytic reactions caused by very high titers of isohemagglutinins present within the plasma in the transfused platelet concentrates, have very rarely been noted , but this is seldom a reason to provide only ABO-compatible platelets.[146]

Platelet Alloantigens There is now a variety of alloantigens implicated in alloimmune thrombocytopenia that have important biologic functions: platelet activation-dependent fibrinogen binding (gpIIb/IIIa complex), platelet/von Willebrand factor interactions (gpIb/IX complex), and platelet/collagen interactions (gpIa/IIa complex).[147,148] Antibodies directed at these Ags can cause immune-mediated destruction of platelets in the presence or absence of anti-HLA antibodies. Sensitization to these Ags is rarely the cause of refractory thrombocytopenia in patients with cancer.[112,131]

One clinical sequela of antibodies to platelet alloantigens is post-transfusion purpura, resulting from antibody directed at the PL^{A1} Ag. In post-transfusion purpura, profound thrombocytopenia develops approximately 1 week after transfusion, primarily in women who have been immunized either by earlier pregnancies or, less frequently, by a previous transfusion.[149,150] Almost all patients have been PL^{A1} negative with anti-PL^{A1} antibody in their plasma at the time of thrombocytopenia. Partial exchange transfusion, plasmapheresis, and high-dose IV immunoglobulin have all been used to accelerate recovery from posttransfusion purpura.[150] The abrupt onset of thrombocytopenia after transfusion can be related to passive alloimmune thrombocytopenia to HPA-1a and HPA-5b, and transplantation-associated alloimmune thrombocytopenia can result from residual host cells producing antibodies against donor platelet Ags (HPA-1).[148]

Alternatives to Platelet Transfusion

Studies to date have not shown reproducible effects of G-CSF or GM-CSF on recovery of platelets. However, numerous molecules have shown thrombopoietic effects in vitro and in vivo.[6,11,13] Examples of these include IL-1, IL-3, IL-6, IL-11, leukemia inhibitory factor (LIF), and c-Kit ligand (KL). Additionally, with the tools of recombinant DNA, there is the ability to "cut and splice" novel recombinant hybrid molecules that may possess thrombopoietic activity, such as the PIXY 321 molecule, which is a recombinant hybrid of the coding regions from the human *GM-CSF* and *IL3* genes. Although these growth factors do elevate platelet counts in patients, studies in humans to date suggest that fever and constitutional symptoms may be dose limiting for IL-1, IL-3, and IL-6. Interleukin-11 is now approved by the US Food and Drug Administration (FDA) as a platelet growth factor.[12] A most exciting development is the recent isolation of thrombopoietin, the c-Mpl ligand.[11,13] This promotes both megakaryocyte progenitor expansion and megakaryocyte differentiation, and its injection in nanogram quantities raises platelet levels of mice to three or four times the normal. Moreover, mice that are deficient in the c-Mpl receptor have few megakaryocytes and are profoundly thrombocytopenic but have normal numbers of other hematopoietic cell types.[151] Thrombopoietin may be useful to enhance collection of PBSCs and for ex vivo expansion of stem cells, but its future development to enhance platelet recovery is unclear, since its use in normal donors induced antibodies and related thrombocytopenia.

Attempts have also been made to develop alternatives to platelet transfusion.[152] Klein and colleagues have administered lyophilized whole platelets to treat thrombocytopenic bleeding in pediatric patients and observed clinical improvement in 50% of patients, suggesting that morphologic integrity of platelets might not be essential for their in vivo function.[153] Platelets preserved in gelatin also retain hemostatic efficacy.[154] New technologies for cryopreservation of platelets that achieve satisfactory platelet recovery after transfusion are being described.[155] Aldehyde-fixed, dried, and rehydrated platelets adhere to exposed subendothelium and may therefore remain hemostatically active.[156] By cross-linking argininenglycine-aspartic acid (RGD) tripeptides to erythrocytes, Coller and colleagues have produced "thromboerythrocytes" that interact with gpIIb/IIIa receptors on activated platelets.[157] Synthetic liposomes, composed of phospholipids and platelet glycoprotein complexes, can shorten prolonged bleeding times in thrombocytopenic animals.[158] Platelet membrane particles can normalize prolonged bleeding times in animal models and will soon undergo clinical testing.[159,160] Finally, synthetic phospholipids promote procoagulant activity on damaged vessels, suggesting their potential utility as platelet substitutes.[161,162] It is likely that cytokines and/or new products will be developed in the future to substitute for platelet transfusion therapy. The availability of new technology will then allow more effective strategies to both prevent thrombocytopenic hemorrhage and avoid the potential immunohematologic complications of platelet transfusion.

OTHER THERAPEUTIC MODALITIES

Transfusion of Fresh Frozen Plasma

Fresh frozen plasma is the fluid portion of 1 unit (450 mL) of whole blood that is centrifuged, separated, and frozen at –18°C or lower. It contains physiologic levels of coagulation factors. Fresh frozen plasma is utilized to correct coagulation factor deficiencies; to reverse warfarin effect; to correct coagulopathy of passive transfusion; for antithrombin III replacement; and to treat thrombotic thrombocytopenic purpura, disseminated intravascular coagulation, coagulopathy of liver disease, thrombolytic agent overdose, protein C or S deficiency, and hemolytic uremic syndrome.[163,164] In addition to the plasma obtained from donated whole blood, it can be collected using plasmapheresis procedures for the production of derivatives: coagulation factors (factors VIII and IX), immunoglobulin, and albumin preparations. Although solvent detergent-treated plasma is available, it is derived from pools of multiple donors and is active only against enveloped viruses and, therefore, of limited clinical utility.[165]

Therapeutic Pheresis Therapeutic cytapheresis is used in the setting of hyperleukocytic leukemias and lymphomas and in thrombocythemia to remove excess cells. In addition, therapeutic plasmapheresis or plasma exchange is useful in disorders associated with excess abnormal proteins in plasma. Therapeutic pheresis in a cancer patient does not alter the underlying condition; rather, it is utilized as an adjunct to conventional therapy.

Therapeutic leukopheresis can be done when hyperleukocytosis is present when first encountering a patient with leukemia who has clinical evidence of leukostasis or is threatened by a catastrophe from the hyperleukocytosis. Pulmonary sludging with related tachypnea and dyspnea, often with hypoxia and radiographic diffuse infiltration, is one indication. Torpor, headache, or confusion, suggesting the possibility of vascular invasion and related intracerebral hemorrhage, is another. Leukopheresis is also used to reduce tumor mass prior to chemotherapy and thereby to avoid treatment-related hyperuricemia and renal failure. It is indicated for patients with acute myelogenous leukemia (AML) or acute lymphoblastic leukemia (ALL) and white cell counts greater than 100 × 10^9/L and for patients with chronic myelogenous leukemia (CML) and counts greater than 300 × 10^9/L.[166] Leukopheresis has also been used to treat patients with chronic lymphocytic leukemia (CLL), hairy-cell leukemia, and Sézary syndrome.[167–169] However, leukopheresis remains expensive and time consuming and therefore is rarely utilized in place of cytotoxic therapy.

Plateletpheresis is commonly needed to provide single-donor platelets for patients undergoing therapy for leukemia or cancer. Plateletpheresis can also be utilized to reduce the elevated platelet counts present in the setting of thrombocythemia.[170] In these cases, there can be rapid relief of clinical sequelae, including cerebral and myocardial ischemia, gastrointestinal bleeding, and pulmonary embolism, before the effects of cytotoxic therapy become apparent.

Plasma exchange has been utilized in several oncologic settings. In patients receiving ABO-incompatible allogeneic marrow transplants, plasmapheresis has been utilized to remove high-titer isohemagglutinins.[171] Plasmapheresis has also been utilized to remove leukocyte antibodies from patients receiving granulocyte transfusions.[172] In patients refractory to platelet transfusion by virtue of sensitization to HLA, plasmapheresis has had variable success.[171] Finally, plasmapheresis has been used to deplete paraproteins and relieve hyperviscosity-related sludging and/or hemorrhage.[173] It is more commonly used to deplete IgM in Waldenström's macroglobulinemia than to remove paraprotein in myeloma, which is almost always non-IgM. Since the paraprotein reaccumulates, plasmapheresis is considered only an adjunct to cytotoxic therapy of the underlying disease.

EFFECTS OF TRANSFUSION ON THE IMMUNE SYSTEM

It is essential to emphasize that patients with cancer may be immunocompromised because of the neoplastic disease and/or its treatment. This may make any effects of transfusion on recipient immunity of particular importance in this patient population.

Alloimmunization The most firmly established effect of transfusion is the stimulation of antibodies in the recipient against Ags in the transfused products. Both cellular and plasma Ags in transfused blood expose the recipients to hundreds of known alloantigens.[174]

Over 400 RBC Ags have been identified, yet we routinely ensure compatibility for only three of them: A, B, and D. More than 100 HLA Ags, as well as granulocyte- and platelet-specific Ags, have also been identified. Genetic alleles can result in structural and therefore antigenic differences among all plasma proteins, leading to recipient alloantibodies to the donated immunoglobulins. Most alloantigens are ignored in transfusion therapy, since they are poor immunogens. However, studies clearly demonstrate that the development of recipient antibodies to Ags in transfused products relates not only to the number of transfusions but also to their timing. Specifically, individuals who receive equal numbers of transfusions are more likely to develop antibodies if the transfusions are given repeatedly over a long time period than if given within a shorter interval. Some cancer patients, by virtue of receiving repeated transfusions over a longer time period, may therefore be more likely to become alloimmunized. Alloantibodies to RBCs can lead to recipient morbidity and shortened RBC survival; antibodies to leukocytes are associated with febrile transfusion reactions and can impair effectiveness and survival of transfused granulocytes.[175] Anti-HLAA and -B antibodies as well as platelet-specific alloantibodies impair survival of transfused and autologous platelets.[126,132] Finally, anti-IgA sometimes causes anaphylactic reactions in IgA deficient recipients, but anti-IgG or -IgM or antilipoproteins are not clinically significant.[176]

Immunosuppression Transfusions may also have immunosuppressive effects on recipients. Animal models have demonstrated immune suppression and accelerated tumor growth in rats that received allogeneic transfusion.[177] In humans, patients who received multiple transfusions have decreased numbers of natural killer (NK) cells and increased circulating Ia+ T cells. T4:T8 ratios may also be decreased.[178,179] The decrease in NK cells is directly related to the number of RBC units received and is seen only in patients transfused within the past year. It has been reported that soluble HLA class I and II and well as Fas ligand accumulate in blood components, in relation to both the number of leukocytes and length of storage.[180] They may be immunoregulatory, evidenced by inhibition of in vitro allogeneic mixed lymphocyte responses and antigen-specific cytotoxic T-cell activity, as well as induction of apoptosis in Fas+ cells.

Research has demonstrated increased renal graft survival in patients who had been previously transfused with blood from donors who share at least one HLA-DR antigen.[181] More recently, both increased cancer recurrence rates and an increased incidence of postoperative infection have been noted following transfusion.[182] Specifically, nontransfused patients with a variety of stages and sites of large bowel cancer fared better in 11 of 14 retrospective studies; when multivariate analysis was done, transfusion was an independent unfavorable predictor of earlier recurrence or cancer-related deaths in 7 of 12 studies. Some studies suggest that recipients of homologous transfusions have higher recurrence rates than recipients of autologous transfusion.[183]

Transfused patients undergoing surgery for colorectal cancer have also been reported to have higher rates of postoperative infection than those who are not transfused, although this remains an area of investigation.[184,185] Overviews and meta-analyses confirm a lack of significant effect of perioperative transfusion on colorectal cancer recurrence or on postoperative septic complications.[186,187] However, given that patients are often immunosuppressed owing to their disease and/or its therapy, any immunosuppressive effect of transfusion further highlights the importance of justifying the medical and surgical indication for all transfusions.

Although the mechanisms of any transfusion-associated immunosuppressive effect in humans is unknown, cancer patients receiving only a small number of RBCs had fewer recurrences and improved survival compared with those receiving only whole blood or larger numbers of RBCs, suggesting that a factor present in whole blood, for example, plasma, is implicated.[182,188] However, in an animal model, transfused allogeneic lymphocytes appear to mediate an immunosuppressive effect, and prestorage, but not poststorage, leukodepletion abrogates this immunosuppressive effect, suggesting that a cytokine is the mediator of this effect.[189] Future studies are needed to define the precise relationship between transfusion, immunosuppression of the recipient, and cancer recurrence.

TRANSFUSION-ASSOCIATED GRAFT-VERSUS-HOST DISEASE

Historic Perspective Graft-versus-host disease is commonly observed after allogeneic BMT, but is rarely recognized after transfusion or transplantation of other organs. Transfusion-associated (TA)-GVHD usually occurs in the immunosuppressed recipient (eg, BMT recipients), but recent reports also involve more nearly immunocompetent recipients.[57,190] The clinical manifestations include fever and skin rash, anorexia, nausea, vomiting, and watery or bloody diarrhea with or without elevated liver enzymes and hyperbilirubinemia. Since there are no pathognomonic features of GVHD, this syndrome is sometimes difficult to distinguish from viral infections or drug eruptions. TA-GVHD is usually severe, and, unlike the situation after allogeneic BMT, it frequently results in pancytopenia secondary to marrow aplasia. The majority of reported cases of TA-GVHD have not responded to immunosuppressive therapies and have been fatal.

TA-GVHD has been reported after transfusion of unirradiated blood components to patients with severe combined immunodeficiency, thymic hypoplasia, and Wiskott-Aldrich syndrome; premature newborns and those with erythroblastosis fetalis; patients with hematologic neoplasms, including Hodgkin's and non-Hodgkin's lymphomas, acute myelocytic and lymphoblastic leukemias, chronic lymphocytic leukemia, and aplastic anemias; patients with carcinomas and sarcomas, including neuroblastomas, glioblastoma, rhabdomyosarcoma, cervical carcinoma, small-cell lung cancer, and germ cell tumor; patients after cardiac surgery and cholecystectomy; and pregnant women.[57,191] This syndrome has developed following exchange and intrauterine transfusions, and after transfusion of whole blood, plasma, red blood cells, and platelets. Leukocytes harvested from normal donors and from donors with chronic myelocytic leukemia have also been transfused to patients with hematologic neoplasms and been implicated in TA-GVHD.

Definition of Those at Risk In 1986, the National Institutes of Health Consensus Development Conference defined patients who have undergone BMT or those with other forms of immunodeficiency as candidates for irradiated platelet concentrates to avoid GVHD.[83] Patients with leukemias and other cancers who may be immunosuppressed secondary to chemotherapy and/or radiation therapy or because of intrinsic immune dysfunction (eg, HD), may be at risk of TA-GVHD.[192] Among patients with HD, it had previously been assumed that combined radiation and chemotherapy were necessary as predisposing factors for the development of TA-GVHD, but several cases of TA-GVHD have recently been documented in patients with HD who were treated with chemotherapy alone.[193] Patients receiving high-dose chemotherapy followed by autologous bone marrow support are also at risk of TA-GVHD.[194] Finally, immunocompetent patients who share an HLA haplotype with HLA-homozygous blood donors also appear to be at risk of TA-GVHD.[199,200] Homozygosity for HLA types is more likely to occur among first-degree family members (eg, parents, children, and siblings); it has, therefore, recently been recommended that cellular blood components from such donors be irradiated with at least 2,500 cGy prior to transfusion. Indeed, products from all family member-directed donors should be irradiated, given that TA-GVHD has now been reported after transfusion of blood from a second-degree relative.[196] Reports of TA-GVHD after transfusion of cellular blood components from homozygous blood donors to heterozygous non-blood relatives suggest that indications for gamma irradiation may need to be broadened.[195,200] The risk of transfusion of blood from HLA homozygous donors to unrelated HLA heterozygous patients is 1 in 874 in Japan and may be as high as 1 in 7,174 in the United States.[197] Finally, reports confirm that all HLA-matched cellular components should be irradiated.[57,198–200]

Strategies for Prevention The only currently effective method to prevent TA-GVHD is gamma irradiation of blood products prior to transfusion. Studies suggest that irradiation at 1,500 to 2,000 cGy can reduce mitogenresponsive lymphocytes by 5 to 6 logs compared with unirradiated controls.[201] However, the observation that a small percentage of lymphocytes survive irradiation at these doses, coupled with a single reported case of apparent TA-GVHD in a bone marrow transplant recipient who received only blood components irradiated at 2,000 cGy, suggest that existing blood product irradiation guidelines require reassessment.[202] Indeed, the standards of the American Association of Blood Banks (AABB), as well as those of the FDA, now require that blood and cellular components be irradiated with a midplane dose of a minimum of 2,500 cGy.[203] Studies to date suggest no adverse effects of irradiation on storage of platelets, but the clinical significance of potassium release on storage of irradiated red cells is not yet defined, and post-transfusion red cell recovery of irradiated units may be decreased.[204,205]

A potential alternative method to prevent TA-GVHD would be to deplete lymphocytes from blood products prior to transfusion; however, the number and precise T cells required to mediate TA-GVHD remain undefined, and it is unknown whether depletion of leukocytes using these currently available techniques would decrease the risk of TA-GVHD. Moreover, cases of TA-GVHD in recipients of filtered components have been reported.[206] Using a well-characterized parent to F1 hybrid murine transfusion model, it was shown that the depletion of recipient CD4+ cells increased the number of donor cells needed to induce GVHD, whereas depletion of recipient CD8+ cells decreased the number of donor cells needed to induce GVHD, suggesting the importance of CD8+ cells for their protective effect.[207] In this model, photochemical treatment with psoralen followed by long-wavelength UV treatment or cellular components before transfusion has been shown to prevent TA-GVHD, suggesting its potential clinical utility.[208]

Conclusions and Recommendations Patients who have congenital immunodeficiencies or those who undergo BMT should routinely receive only irradiated (2,500 cGy) blood components. Patients with cancer may be immunocompromised secondary to their underlying disease and/or chemoradiotherapy, but the frequency of occurrence and degree of immunosuppression predisposing to TA-GVHD in this population is not precisely defined. Within this group, however, patients receiving high-dose chemoradiotherapy (eg, in preparation for autologous BMT), those with HD, and patients receiving donations of cellular blood components from first-degree blood relatives should receive only irradiated blood components. Whole blood, packed red cells, granulocytes, platelets, and fresh plasma have all caused TA-GVHD, but fresh frozen plasma and frozen deglycerolized red cells have not yet been implicated. Platelets can be irradiated at the time of collection without adverse consequences, but the effects of irradiation and prolonged storage of red cells is not yet defined.

TRANSFUSION-RELATED INFECTIOUS DISEASES

Hepatitis B Although hepatitis B (HB) was formerly a common transfusion-related infection, the use of several generations of HB surface antigen assays to screen potential donors and the use of volunteer versus commercial donors has markedly reduced the incidence of HB transmitted by transfusion (Table 131-6).[209,210] It is of note that since the use of antibody to HB core (anti-HBc) as a surrogate test to screen potential donors for their ability to transmit non-A non-B hepatitis, the incidence of transfusion-related hepatitis B has fallen even further.[211,212] The current estimated per-unit risk of hepatitis B is approximately 1 in 200,000.[213]

Table 131-6 Risks of Transfusion

Complication	Frequency (Episode Unit)
Reactions	
Febrile nonhemolytic	1–4:100
Allergic	1–4:100
Transfusion-related acute lung injury	1:5,000
Acute hemolytic	1:250,000
Delayed hemolytic	1:1,000
Anaphylactic	1:150,000
Infections	
Hepatitis C	1:2,000,000
Hepatitis B	1:200,000
HIV-1	1:2,000,000
HIV-2	None reported
HTLV-I and II	1:250,000–1:2,000,000
Malaria	1:4,000,000
Bacteria red cells	1:500,000
Bacteria platelets	1:12,000
Other complications	
RBC allosensitization	1:100
HLA sensitization	1:10
Graft-versus-host disease	Rare

HIV = human immunodeficiency virus; HLA = human leukocyte antigen; HTLV = human T-cell leukemia/lymphoma virus; RBC = red blood cell.

Non-A Non-B Hepatitis Following the identification of hepatitis A virus and hepatitis B virus, it was quickly appreciated that neither agent was responsible for most cases of post-transfusion hepatitis. Thus, the term non-A non-B hepatitis (NANBH) was introduced. In the mid-1980s, donors were screened for alanine aminotransferase (ALT) as well as anti-HBc; these served as "surrogate" markers for individuals having a 20% chance of transmitting NANBH.[211,212] The advantage of surrogate marker testing was the potential reduction of transfusion-related NANBH cases by one-third; the disadvantage was that 70 to 80% donors with anti-HBc or elevated ALT do not transmit NANBH; moreover, 1 to 3% and 4 to 8% of donors are deferred because of elevated ALT and anti-HBc, respectively.[214]

The causative agent of NANBH was finally discovered by cloning a fragment of viral cDNA from a chimpanzee infected with NANBH.[215] Subsequently, the entire genome of what is now called hepatitis C virus (HCV) was cloned. A specific assay was developed for bloodborne NANBH, in which a recombinant HCV polypeptide is used to capture viral antibodies.[216] Subsequent testing using multiple-antigen HCV enzyme assays confirmed that nearly all cases of post-transfusion NANBH are caused by HCV. Uniform screening of blood donors for anti-HCV antibodies was implemented in 1990. Given that 90% of blood donors with anti-HCV have infective virus in their blood and that new generation assays for anti-HCV with enhanced sensitivity are available, lookback studies are currently under way to test patients who were transfused prior to the availability of current screening tests.[216–218] Nucleic acid amplification technology (NAT) is also being employed to enhance sensitivity in detecting infection.[219] Along with HIV (discussed below) all blood donations in the United States are now screened for HCV using NAT.[220] By narrowing the preseronconversion window period from about 75 days to less than 30, the use of NAT has reduced the per-unit risk of HCV to approximately 1 in 2,000,000.[213]

Hepatitis C can have important adverse sequelae in patients with cancer. Long-term leukemia survivors with chronic HCV infection may have more rapidly progressive liver disease.[221] As with blood transfusion, studies now document high rates of transmission of HCV from allogeneic marrow donors at the time of transplantation.[222] A retrospective review noted that patients with liver disease caused by HCV infection are at high risk of developing lethal veno-occlusive disease after bone marrow transplantation, demonstrating the importance of this pathogen in patients undergoing high-dose therapy.[223] Guidelines for the management of patient and donor in the setting of hepatitis infection have been reviewed.[224]

Hepatitis GB Virus Hepatitis GB virus (GBV) and GBV-C are ribonucleic acid (RNA) viruses of the Flaviviridae family, which are also transfusion transmitted.[225,226] However, studies suggest that this infection does not have significant clinical sequelae.[227]

Cytomegalovirus Cellular blood components transfused from cytomegalovirus (CMV)-seropositive donors to CMV-seronegative transplant recipients and neonates can cause CMV seroconversion and infection. In allogeneic BMT, transfusion with seronegative blood products (frozen deglycerolized RBCs and platelets drawn from CMV-seronegative donors) or treatment with immunoglobulin both appear to lessen CMV infection after allogeneic BMT when both donor and patient are seronegative but not when either is sero-

Table 131-7 Incidence and Actuarial Probability of CMV Infection and Disease by Study Arm

CMV Event	Seronegative Blood (n = 252)	Filtered Blood (n = 250)	p Value
Primary analysis (day 21–100)			
All CMV infections + disease	2 (1.3%)	3 (2.4%)	1.0
CMV disease only	0 (0%)	3 (1.2%)	.25
Secondary analysis (day 0–100)			
All CMV infections + disease	4 (1.4%)	6 (2.4%)	.5
CMV disease only	0 (0%)	6 (2.4%)	.03
Survival	79%	82%	.56

CMV = cytomegalovirus.

positive[228]; utilizing both immunoglobulin and CMV-seronegative blood products appears to confer no additional benefit. CMV infection is strongly associated with acute GVHD and may become less frequent because of the development of effective prophylaxis for GVHD.[229,230] In seropositive allogeneic BMT recipients, acyclovir therapy can lessen the incidence of CMV infection and related morbidity.[231] Although equivalent numbers of autologous and allogeneic BMT recipients either seroconvert to or excrete CMV, recipients of autologous BMT rarely develop clinical sequelae.[230]

Methods of CMV prophylaxis have therefore been reserved for allogeneic BMT when both donor and recipient are seronegative; they have not been used in autologous BMT. It should be noted, however, that CMV pneumonia developed in 11 of 159 autologous BMT recipients and was fatal in 9 cases, suggesting that these patients are also at risk of CMV visceral infection.[232]

The traditional CMV-seronegative blood products are red cells and platelets harvested from CMV-seronegative donors. Leukoreduced red cells and platelets have been shown to decrease transfusion-acquired CMV infection in infants, in patients undergoing treatment of acute leukemia, and in autologous and allogeneic BMT recipients.[228,233,234] The ability to utilize filtered blood products as if they were CMV seronegative would markedly expand the donor pool and thereby the supply of noninfectious components.[235] A multicenter randomized trial compared seronegative with filtered cellular blood components in CMV-seronegative patients undergoing autologous BMT and seronegative patients receiving allografts from CMV seronegative donors (Table 131-7).[228] Rates of CMV seroconversion and infection were equivalent in recipients of seronegative and filtered components, but significant clinical sequelae were noted only in those patients receiving filtered, unscreened components. These results suggest that filtering can markedly reduce CMV transmission, and filtered components are now considered "CMV safe"; however, it may be premature to conclude that filtered and seronegative components are equivalent. Transfer of CMV-specific clones of CD8+ T cells from the marrow donor has been shown to be a safe and effective way to reconstitute cellular immunity against CMV after allogeneic bone marrow transplantation.[236]

West Nile Virus West Nile virus (WNV) is a mosquitoborne flavivirus that can be transfusion-transmitted. The vast majority of WNV infections result from mosquito bites. About 80% of individuals infected with WNV are asymptomatic. Of the 20% who manifest symptoms, the vast majority will have a mild illness (West Nile virus fever). Less than 1% of infected individuals develop a severe meningo-encephalitis, with advanced age being the strongest risk factor.[237] WNV first appeared in the United States in 1999. In 2002, over 4,000 clinically significant cases of WNV were reported, including 23 cases determined to have been transfusion-associated. In 2003, nucleic acid testing of blood products was begun nationwide under an FDA investigational new drug (IND) protocol. This testing has eliminated most, although not all[238] of the risk of transfusion-transmitted WNV.

Bacterial Sepsis Bacteria very rarely survive in whole blood stored at 4°C. In contrast, platelets are stored at room temperature on an agitator and are a potential source of bacterial contamination, which can result in transfusion-related sepsis.[239] It is essential to systematically evaluate for transfusion-transmitted bacterial infections whenever a febrile transfusion reaction occurs. In vitro studies demonstrate that deliberate contamination of platelets with as few as 1/mL on day 0 (either gram-negative or -positive) can result in 10^8/mL or plateau phase growth after 48 to 72 hours' incubation. Storage of platelets for 5 days between harvest and transfusion is permitted; however, platelets should be utilized as soon after harvest as possible because of considerations related to in vitro function and recovery, as well as concern for bacterial contamination. Prestorage leukodepletion of platelet concentrates does not appear to increase the likelihood of transfusion-induced septicemia.[240] Screening platelets before transfusion using Gram staining has been shown to reduce transfusion-related infection in some, but not all, centers.[241,242] Blood collection facilities in the United States are now required by AABB to both detect and limit bacterial contamination of platelets.[203] A variety of techniques to address bacterial contamination within platelets, such as probes for bacterial ribosomal RNA, reagent strips for glucose and pH, and automated culture systems, are in use or are under development.[243–246]

Bacterial sepsis is a recognized but quite rare complication of red cell transfusion, owing to the fact that red cells, unlike platelets, are stored under refrigerated conditions. Pathogens such as *Yersinia enterocolitica* have been implicated in causing toxemia following transfusion of red cells.[247] Minimizing the storage time of red cells prior to transfusion or extending the screening process to exclude all potential donors with gastrointestinal symptoms or illness in the 4-week period before donation have been suggested as possible methods to minimize this problem, but it is felt to be a rare event.

Acquired Immunodeficiency Syndrome With the recognition in 1983 that acquired immunodeficiency syndrome (AIDS) may be transmitted via transfusion, several measures were implemented: (1) physicians were educated about the risk/benefits of transfusion, (2) autologous transfusion was recommended for elective surgery, and (3) questionnaires were used for anonymous self-deferral of high-risk donors. By mid-1983, pressures for "directed" donations from friends or family increased; however, directed donations are not safer than other donations. The use of autologous blood, especially in elective surgeries, is an effective way to avoid infections and other risks of transfusions; however, autologous blood in patients with cancer is not widely utilized because of fear of contaminating tumor cells.

Since 1985, all American blood donors have been screened for anti-HIV antibody using ELISA. Transfusion-transmitted HIV is now exceedingly rare; the few cases that do occur result almost exclusively from seronegative window period donations. Following the initial implementation of HIV antibody screening, improvements in the sensitivity of the HIV-1 and HIV-2 ELISAs limited the seronegative window period to approximately 22 days.[248]HIV p24 antigen screening was begun in 1996, shortening the window period to approximately 16 days.[248] The yield of HIV p24 antigen testing has been lower than predicted, perhaps because seroconverting donors may delay repeat donation because of symptoms of acute infection or concern over high-risk behavior.[249] All units donated in the United States are now tested by minipool nucleic acid testing (NAT). NAT testing is performed on pools of 16 to 24 samples; this technology shortens the window period to approximately 10 or 11 days from the time of exposure. In just over 1 year of testing, only 4 NAT-reactive, p24 antigen-negative/ELISA-negative units were identified out of 12.6 million donations screened (1/3,150,000).[219] It is estimated that the current residual per-unit risk of HIV transmission is less than 1 in 2,000,000.[220]

Human T-Cell Lymphotrophic Virus Type I Human T-cell lymphotrophic virus type 1 (HTLV-1) is associated with adult T-cell leukemia/lymphoma (ATL) and tropical spastic paresis (TSP)/HTLV-1–associated myelopathy (HAM), and clusters geographically in endemic areas such as parts of Japan and the Caribbean.[250, 251] In the United States, ATL incidence is similar to that in the Caribbean, since the cases in the United States are all among African Americans or in patients born outside the United States.[252,253] Most important, recent studies have found antibodies to HTLV-1 in intravenous drug users in New York and have shown that anti-HIV antibodies do not identify all individuals infected with HTLV-1.[254] Moreover, Minamoto and colleagues documented anti-HTLV-1 antibodies in 6 of 211 multitransfused patients with cancer: None of the HTLV-1–seropositive patients were HIV-1 seropositive; conversely, 18 patients were HIV-1 seropositive and HTLV-1 seronegative.[255]

In Japan, deferral of blood donors with antibodies to HTLV-1 has resulted in a lowering of the HTLV-1 seroconversion rate in transfusion recipients from 53.6 to 0.9%.[256] In the United States, screening of sera from 39,898 blood donors at eight blood centers in geographically distinct areas of the United States defined 10 donors (.025%) to have anti–HTLV-1 antibodies by ELISA, immunoblot, and radioimmunoprecipitation.[257] In accord with FDA guidelines, blood collection agencies, in November 1988, initiated testing of all blood donors for anti–HTLV-1 antibodies at the time of all donations, with permanent deferral of individuals with confirmed seropositivity. In addition, high-risk individuals who should not donate blood include patients with ATL or TSP, persons from HTLV-1–endemic areas, female sexual partners of infected men, IV drug abusers, recipients of seropositive cellular blood products, and homosexual men. Studies in the United States do, in fact, document that HTLV-1 has been transmitted via transfusion and demonstrate the efficacy of screening.[242,248,258] The risk per unit transfused is between 1 in 250,000 and 1 in 2,000,000.[259–261]

Other Viruses HTLV-2 is a retrovirus that was discovered in 1982 in a patient with hairy-cell leukemia of T cells.[252] No disease association (except for occasional cases of diverse malignant lymphoproliferative disease) or natural reservoir of infection (except drug abusers) has been found. Although there is serologic cross-reactivity between HTLV-1 and HTLV-2, type-specific identification of HTLVs can be achieved using the polymerase chain reaction.[262] HIV-2 screening of blood and plasma donated is routinely done in the United States, and no cases of transfusion-transmitted HIV-2 have occurred. It is now known that other herpesviruses, including human herpesviruses types 6, 7, and 8, are present in normal blood donors, and future studies will determine their pathogenic potential in immunocompromised recipients.[263]

Parasitic Diseases Since there is no practical laboratory screening test for malaria, exclusion of donors who have either traveled to or emigrated from endemic areas is the only effective measure to prevent transfusion-related infection. Other parasitic diseases, such as babesiosis or Lyme disease, can be transmitted by an asymptomatic donor who has been bitten by a tick and may be of particular importance in immunocompromised or asplenic patients. Although transmission of syphilis by transfusion is possible, it requires that blood be drawn during the rather short period of spirochetemia and that the organisms remain viable at the time of transfusion. Although performing a serologic test for syphilis does not prevent transmission of syphilis because this test does not become positive until well after the brief period of infectivity, US federal regulations do require its use as a screening test of potential donors.

Another recognized transfusion-related infection is Chagas' disease.[264] In Latin America, the risk of transmission is 13 to 23% for each unit of contaminated blood transfused, and most cases of illness associated with transfusion are mild. In the majority of cases, spontaneous resolution occurs, and patients enter the indeterminate phase with lifelong, low-grade parasitemia, antibodies to parasite antigens, and absence of symptoms. Between 10 and 30% of persons in the indeterminate phase eventually develop symptoms. However, in immunocompromised patients, this illness may take a more fulminant course. The diagnosis of acute infection is made by detection of parasites on blood smear and the diagnosis of chronic infection by the detection of serum antibodies. Neither test has the sensitivity or specificity necessary to be useful for screening blood donors at present. Potential blood donors immigrating from areas endemic for Chagas' disease are currently deferred.

Creutzfeldt–Jakob Disease Although there have been no cases of Creutzfeldt–Jakob disease (CJD) related to blood transfusion, prospective donors of blood products who have a familial history of dementia and have undergone corneal or brain surgery are deferred.[264–266] Because of the identification in 1996 of a variant CJD (vCJD), which may be associated with bovine spongiform encephalopathy (BSE), or "mad cow disease," potential donors who resided in the United Kingdom for 3 months from 1980 to 1996 are deferred from donating. Donors residing in Europe for 5 years cumulatively from 1980 onward are also deferred. These travel restrictions are expected to eliminate 90% of person-days of exposure to the causative agent of vCJD at a cost of eliminating 5% of US blood donors.[267] BSE has been transmitted from an infected sheep to a single other sheep by whole blood transfusion.[268] In the United Kingdom, a small number of human cases of transfusion-transmitted vCJD have been reported. Universal use of leukoreduced components for transfusion is being recommended in many countries, based on the fact that the vector for transmission of vCJD appears to be the B lymphocyte.

FUTURE DIRECTIONS IN BLOOD COMPONENT THERAPY

Increased Role in Primary Treatment of Cancer The blood component laboratory plays a role in the collection, cryopreservation, thawing, re-infusion, and quality control of PBSCs (Table 131-8).[5] A variety of strategies have been evaluated in the blood component laboratory evaluating the use of growth factors and standard versus large-volume apheresis to collect autologous and, more recently, allogeneic PBSCs.[6,61,269–271] Once collected, cryopreservation and thawing should be done so as to maintain both viability and sterility of PBSCs.[272–276] The blood component laboratory is also central to novel immune therapies based on adoptive immunotherapy and/or vaccines.[277–279] It is also the center for recruitment of donors for the National Marrow Donor Program to provide unrelated donor bone marrow and, more recently, PBSCs for transplantation. The blood component laboratory has also assumed an integral role in the management of programs for unrelated cord blood transplantation, which may permit partially matched unrelated donor transplantation, with less GVHD than has been noted after unrelated BMT.[279–283]

Table 131-8 The Role of the Blood Bank in Cellular Cancer Therapies

Allogeneic stem cell transplantation
HLA-matched sibling donors
Donor lymphocyte infusions
HLA-matched unrelated donors
Cord blood transplantation
Autologous stem cell transplantation
Optimal selection
Quality control
Positive selection
Negative selection
Post-transplantation immune therapies

HLA = human leukocyte antigen.

Hematopoietic Stem Cell Transplantation **Blood Component Support before Transplantation** Since many patients undergoing allogeneic BMT have received previous transfusions, sensitization to HLA may have occurred. The effect of HLA sensitization on marrow engraftment is most evident in the setting of aplastic anemia: Reported graft rejection rates range from 25 to 60% in multitransfused patients with aplastic anemia given HLA identical sibling marrow grafts.[284] The likelihood of sensitization to HLA after transfusion varies in different patient populations and, in some studies, appears to correlate with the number of donor exposures.[285] When HLA-matched allogeneic BMT is to be done, prior transfusions from family members and especially from the potential marrow donor should be avoided because of the risk of sensitization of the patient to both HLA and non-HLA antigens. Most studies also suggest that a patient's pretransplantation CMV status predicts for the likelihood of infection following transplantation, and efforts should be made not to infect the patient via transfusion, especially if both patient and donor are seronegative.

Blood Component Support Post-Transplantation After BMT, there is a period of pancytopenia when patients require multiple RBC and platelet transfusions. For example, patients with aplastic anemia undergoing allogeneic BMT received a median of 9 (1–82) and 44 (6–468) units of RBCs and platelets, respectively, primarily during the first 4 weeks after grafting.[286] Several donor and/or patient factors may influence hematologic engraftment and required blood product support after BMT.[5] In all recipients, engraftment may be compromised by disease- and/or treatment-related effects on the marrow microenvironment. Reconstitution after allogeneic BMT may be relatively enhanced since the donor marrow is healthy; however, the graft may be adversely affected by prophylaxis and treatment of GVHD. Moreover, in vitro T-cell depletion of donor marrow has in some patients resulted in failure to engraft and graft rejection. Autologous marrow may be intrinsically compromised by the patient's underlying disease and cytotoxic therapy received prior to marrow harvesting, in vitro techniques utilized for removal of tumor cells, or cryopreservation. In syngeneic BMT, donor marrow is histocompatible and healthy and is neither manipulated nor cryopreserved. However, the underlying disease and prior treatment of the recipient may, as is true in other types of BMT, compromise the marrow microenvironment and thereby adversely affect engraftment.

Testing for HLA compatibility between donor and recipient, combined with treatments to minimize and treat GVHD, has resulted in widespread utilization of allogeneic BMT. Although only 40% of patients have histocompatible related donors, the National Marrow Donor Program has recruited and collected unrelated histocompatible marrow for transplantation and shown very promising preliminary results.[287] Allogeneic PBSCs collected from normal donors are now in widespread use, suggesting an even more primary role of the blood bank in allograft stem cell transplantation.[61,271,288]

ABO incompatibility between marrow donor and recipient may be either major, with isohemagglutinin in the recipient directed against donor RBC antigens, or minor, with isohemagglutinin in the donor directed against recipient RBC antigens. Major ABO incompatibility has the potential risk of severe hemolytic reactions, graft rejection, or delayed engraftment.[289,290] Attempts to overcome major ABO incompatibility have included depletion of RBCs from the bone marrow graft prior to BMT and/or removal of isohemagglutinin from the recipient by large-volume plasma exchanges or immunoadsorption. In addition, some investigators have supplemented these techniques with pre-BMT transfusions of donor type blood or purified A or B substance to completely adsorb recipient isohemagglutinins. Although studies suggest that major ABO-incompatible HLA-matched transplants have resulted in no increase in patient mortality, incidence of rejection, delayed reconstitution, or GVHD compared with ABO-compatible controls, some reports suggest that RBC reconstitution can be delayed in this setting.[289,291–293] Red cell engraftment may be especially delayed in the setting of major ABO-incompatible nonmyeloablative stem cell transplantation, where host antidonor isohemagglutinin levels tend to decrease more slowly than in myeloablative BMT.[294] The current standard practice in major ABO-incompatible HLA-matched BMT is to deplete RBCs from marrow before BMT, to anticipate possible delayed erythropoiesis and hemolysis after BMT, and to utilize methods to deplete recipient isohemagglutinins when present in high (≥ 1:128) titer.

Potential adverse outcomes of minor ABO incompatibility between marrow donor and recipient include rapid immune hemolysis at the time of infusion of donor marrow resulting from passive transfer of isohemagglutinin in the marrow plasma, or delayed immune hemolysis caused by anti-RBC antibodies produced by donor lymphocytes.[5] There is no effect of minor ABO incompatibility on graft rejection, the incidence and severity of GVHD, or patient survival. Although exchange transfusion of the recipient before BMT using red cells of the donor's blood group has been utilized to prevent hemolysis caused by passive transfer of isohemagglutinin in the marrow product, this is rarely a clinically significant problem and can more easily be avoided by removing plasma from the marrow prior to infusion. Minor ABO incompatibility can result in adverse reactions owing to the production of anti-A and/or anti-B antibodies by donor marrow lymphocytes early (1–3 weeks) following transplantation, particularly in patients on cyclosporine therapy or those receiving T-cell–depleted allografts.[295,296] In this setting, transfusions of either group O or donor group RBCs are utilized to dilute the recipient red cells; in some cases, exchange transfusion has been required because of very rapid engraftment of donor lymphocytes and production of anti-RBC antibodies.

Peripheral Blood Stem Cell Autotransplantation The blood component laboratory plays a role in the collection, cryopreservation, thawing, re-infusion, and quality control of autologous hematopoietic stem cells for transplantation.[5] A variety of strategies have been analyzed in the blood component laboratory, evaluating the use of growth factors and standard versus large-volume apheresis to collect autologous PBSCs.[6,269,270] PBSCs must be collected, processed, cryopreserved, and thawed so as to maintain both their viability and their sterility.[272–276,297] Hematopoietic cell processing may consist of several steps: concentration and washing; sedimentation with hydroxyethyl starch, Ficoll-Hypaque, or Percoll; purging and washing; cryopreservation and storage; and thawing and reinfusion. The goal of hematopoietic cell processing is depletion of RBCs, plasma, and fat (from marrow), with minimal loss of progenitor cells. Although originally done manually by simple centrifugation, cell separators are now utilized for preferential concentration of progenitor cells with increased elimination of other hematopoietic cells. In addition, much work has been done to utilize large-volume leukapheresis and fewer procedures, or to compare various PBSC collection and processing technologies.[298–300] Processing may either purge tumor cells or enrich for normal hematopoietic progenitor cells (HPC) within autografts, or deplete T lymphocytes from allografts. Techniques have been developed to enrich and/or deplete cellular subsets via either positive or negative selection, increasing both the duration and complexity of the procedures performed in the cell processing laboratory, as well as the requirements for quality control. Moreover, specific cell populations are isolated for immune and gene-mediated therapies.[301]

Principles of current good manufacturing practice (cGMP) and total quality management (TQM) can be applied to HPC component processing. In 1991, the 14th edition of the American Association of Blood Banks (AABB) *Standards for Blood Banks and Transfusion Services* was extended to include hematopoietic stem cells. In 1996, the AABB published a separate *Standards for Hematopoietic Progenitor Cells* to expand and replace Section Q of the *Standards for Blood Banks and Transfusion Services*.[302] These standards include sections concerning donor selection, component collection, processing, testing, labeling, storage, transportation, issue, infusion, and record keeping for hematopoietic progenitor cells, including autologous as well as allogeneic bone marrow, peripheral blood progenitor cells, and cord blood. Furthermore, the Foundation for the Accreditation of Cellular Therapy (FACT), formed in 1993, has programs for inspection and accreditation of HPC collection and processing facilities as well as transplantation programs. The FACT Standards represent a consensus document of several organizations working together in the field of clinical conduct of hematopoietic progenitor cell transplantation, including the International Society for Hematotherapy and Graft Engineering (ISHAGE) and the American Society for Blood and Marrow Transplantation (ASBMT).[303] The FDA is currently reviewing the regulation of hematopoietic progenitor cell components and issued in February 1997 a comprehensive draft document concerning its approach to regulation.[304] The FDA has not yet finalized its approach to the regulation of this rapidly developing field but, as a first step, has proposed that all cell and tissue processing facilities register and report their activities.[305]

Leukopoor/Single-Donor Blood Components As noted above, potential adverse effects in recipients of transfused cellular blood components that have been attributed to WBCs include febrile nonhemolytic transfusion reactions (FNHTRs), alloimmunization, transmission of infectious diseases (eg, CMV), GVHD, transfusion-related acute lung injury, and immunomodulation.[40] Exclusive use of leukoreduced (leukopoor) components can decrease alloimmunization, CMV transmission, and FNHTRs.[126,234,306,307] Recent advances in filtration as well as apheresis techniques have allowed improvement in the extent of WBC reduction achievable in RBCs and platelets so that components with < 10^6 contaminating WBCs can be readily available. In addition, studies have examined the importance of the timing of WBC reduction. For example, in an animal model, prestorage WBC reduction of donor blood was associated with a significantly higher platelet survival and lower rate of refractoriness to allogeneic platelet transfusions than poststorage WBC reduction.[129] It has been reported that storage of platelet concentrates for 5 days results in highly increased levels of tumor necrosis factor-α (TFN-α) and IL-6, whereas prestorage WBC reduction by filtration, current apheresis technology, or buffy coat preparation of platelet concentrates resulted in leukoreduction and no increase in either TNF-α or IL-6.[308–313]Moreover, Stack and Snyder detected IL-8 in 59% of platelet concentrates sampled, at levels ranging from 30% of 2-day-old units to 83% of 5-day-old units.[314] Cytokines released from WBCs during component storage may, either directly or indirectly, mediate FNHTRs in transfusion recipients by acting on recipient cells and releasing pyrogens. Heddle and colleagues have shown first that IL-6 and IL-1B accumulate within the plasma of stored platelets, that FNHTRs are more common to plasma than to cellular fractions of stored products, and, more recently, that plasma depletion is more effective than poststorage leukoreduction in avoiding FNHTR, confirming the in vivo relevance of transfused cytokines in mediating adverse consequences in transfusion recipients.[307,315] Poststorage leukoreduction is not quality controlled and is ineffective, further supporting the use of prestorage leukodepleted components.[127] In addition, severe hypotension and respiratory distress have been observed after transfusion of components leukoreduced using negatively charged filters at the bedside (ie, poststorage), further limiting their utility. Interestingly, this reaction may be related to bradykinin release, which is of particular concern in patients on ACE inhibitors.[316,317] Another advantage of prestorage leukoreduction may be in the avoidance of transfusion-related infections. Since the concentration of bacteria in asymptomatic blood donors is thought to be very low, prestorage filtration of blood shortly after collection may represent a means by which the subsequent proliferation of organisms may be reduced or prevented.[318] Finally, B lymphocytes appear to be a vector of Creutzfeldt–Jakob disease infection in animal models, and therefore leukoreduction may decrease the risk of any theoretical transfusion-related infection.[259,265] On the basis of these multiple advantages, the United States and many countries around the world will likely utilize universally and exclusively prestorage leukoreduced components for transfusion.

CONCLUSION

The development and implementation of new and aggressive therapies for patients with cancer to date would not have been possible without parallel developments for the provision of blood component support. In the future, the blood component laboratory will provide specialized components, such as bone marrow and peripheral blood stem cells, to facilitate the use of new and promising transplantation and cellular therapies for patients with hitherto incurable diseases. Moreover, the advent of growth factor technology holds even greater potential for future treatment strategies, allowing more aggressive and specific therapies, while minimizing the need for homologous donor exposures.

REFERENCES

1. Anderson KC. Hematologic complications. In: Holland JF, Frei E III, Bast RC, et al, editors. Cancer medicine. 5th ed. Hamilton (ON): BC Decker; 1999.
2. Anderson KC, Ness PM. Scientific basis of transfusion medicine. Implications for clinical practice. 2nd ed. Philadelphia: WB Saunders; 1999.
3. Webb IJ, Anderson KC. Transfusion support in acute leukemias. Semin Oncol 1997;24:141–6.
4. Webb IJ, Anderson KC. Risks, costs, and alternatives to platelet transfusions. Leuk Lymphoma 1999;34:71–84.
5. Anderson KC. The role of the blood bank in hematopoietic stem cell transplantation. Transfusion 1992;32:272–85.
6. Ramsey G. Hematopoietic growth factors and transfusion medicine. Transfus Med Rev 1998;12:195–205.
7. Leary AG, Strauss LC, Civin CI, Ogawa M. Disparate differentiation in hematopoietic colonies derived from human paired progenitors. Blood 1985;66:327–32.
8. Rowley SD, Colvin OM, Stuart RK. Human multilineage progenitor cell sensitivity to 4-hydroxyperoxycyclophosphamide. Exp Hematol 1985;13:295–8.
9. Cazzola M, Mercuriali F, Brugnara C. Use of recombinant human erythropoietin outside the setting of uremia. Blood 1997;89:4248–67.
10. Armitage JO. Emerging applications of recombinant human granulocyte-macrophage colony-stimulating factor. Blood 1998;92:4491–508.
11. Kuter DJ, Cebon J, Harker LA, et al. Platelet growth factors. Potential impact on transfusion medicine. Transfusion 1999;39:321–32.
12. Du XX, Williams DA. Interleukin-11. A multifunctional growth factor derived from the hematopoietic microenvironment. Blood 1994;83:2023–30.
13. Kaushansky K. Thrombopoietin. N Engl J Med 1998;339:746–54.
14. Weick JK, Hagedorn AB, Linman JW. Leukoerythroblastosis. Diagnostic and prognostic significance. Mayo Clin Proc 1974;49:110–3.
15. Kiraly JF III, Wheby MS. Bone marrow necrosis. Am J Med 1976;60:361–8.
16. Mauch PM, Loeffler JS. Radiation oncology. Technology and biology. Philadelphia: WB Saunders; 1994. p. 594.
17. Zoumbos NC, Gascon P, Djeu JV, et al. Circulating activated suppressor T lymphocytes in aplastic anemia. N Engl J Med 1985;312:257–65.
18. Lee GR. The anemia of chronic disease. Semin Hematol 1983;20:61–80.
19. Miller CB, Jones RJ, Piantadosi S, et al. Decreased erythropoietin (EPO) response in patients with the anemia of cancer. N Engl J Med 1980;322:1689–92.
20. Rothmann SA, Paul P, Weick JK, et al. Effect of cisdiamin-odichloro-platinum on erythropoietin production and hematopoietic progenitor cells. Int J Cell Cloning 1985;3:415–23.
21. Spivak J. Recombinant human erythropoietin and the anemia of cancer. Blood 1994;84:997–1004.
22. Ludwig H, Fritz E, Kotzmann H, et al. Erythropoietin treatment of anemia associated with multiple myeloma. N Engl J Med 1990;322:1693–9.
23. Cascinu S, Fedeli A, Del Ferro E, et al. Recombinant human erythropoietin treatment in cisplatin-associated anemia. A randomized double-blind trial with placebo. J Clin Oncol 1994;12:1058–62.
24. Osterborg A, Boogaerts MA, Cimino R, et al. Recombinant human erythropoietin in transfusion-dependent anemic patients with multiple myeloma and non-Hodgkin's lymphoma—a randomized multicenter study. Blood 1996;87:2675–82.
25. Cazzola M, Messinger D, Battistel V, et al. Recombinant erythropoietin in the anemia associated with multiple myeloma or non-Hodgkin's lymphoma. Dose finding and identification of predictors of response. Blood 1995;86:4446–53.
26. Demetri G, Kris M, Wade J, et al. Quality of life benefit in chemotherapy patients treated with epoetin alpha is independent of disease response or tumor type. Results from a prospective community oncology study. J Clin Oncol 1998;16:3412–25.
27. Schapira L, Antin JH, Ransil BJ, et al. Serum erythropoietin levels in patients receiving intensive chemotherapy and radiotherapy. Blood 1990;76:2354–9.
28. Beguin Y, Clemons GK, Oris R, Fillet G. Circulating erythropoietin levels after bone marrow transplantation. Inappropriate response to anemia in allogeneic transplants. Blood 1991;77:868–73.
29. Ayash L, Elias A, Hunt M, et al. Recombinant human erythropoietin for the treatment of the anemia associated with autologous bone marrow transplantation. Br J Hematol 1994;87:153–61.
30. Link H, Boogaerts MA, Fauser AA, et al. A controlled trial of recombinant human erythropoietin after bone mar-row transplantation. Blood 1994;84:3327–35.
31. Ludwig H, Fritz E, Leitgeb C, et al. Prediction of response to erythropoietin treatment in chronic anemia of cancer. Blood 1994;84:1056–63.
32. Davenport RD, Burdick M, Moore SA, Kunkel SL. Cytokine production in IgG-mediated red cell incompatibility. Transfusion 1993;33:19–24.
33. Brain MC, Azzopardi JG, Baker LR, et al. Microangiopathic haemolytic anemia and mucin-forming adenocarcinoma. Br J Haematol 1970;18:183–93.
34. Hirst E, Robertson TI. The syndrome of thymoma and erythroblastopenic anemia. Medicine 1967;46:225–64.
35. Smith PJ, Edert H. Evidence of stem cell competition in children with malignant disease. A controlled study of hypertransfusion. Lancet 1976;1:776–9.
36. Audet AM, Goodnough LT. Practice strategies for elective red blood cell transfusion. Ann Intern Med 1992;116:403–6.
37. Hebert PC, Wells G, Blajchman MA, et al. A multicenter randomized, controlled clinical trial of transfusion requirements in critical care. Transfusion Requirements in Critical Care Investigators, Canadian Critical Care Trials Group. N Engl J Med 1999;340:409–17.
38. Stehling L, Luban NLC, Anderson KC. Guidelines for blood utilization review. Transfusion 1994;34:434–48.
39. Surgenor DM, Wallace EL, Hao SH, Chapman RH. Collection and transfusion of blood in the United States, 1982–1988. N Engl J Med 1990;322:1646–51.
40. Wallace EL, Surgenor DM, Hao HS, et al. Collection and transfusion of blood and blood components in the United States, 1989. Transfusion 1993;33:139–44.
41. Bordin JO, Heddle NM, Blajchman MA. Biologic effects of leukocytes present in transfused cellular blood products. Blood 1994;84:1703–21.
42. Dzieckowski JS, Barrett BB, Nester D, et al. Characterization of reactions after exclusive transfusion of white cell-reduced cellular blood components. Transfusion 1994;35:20–5.
43. Goldfinger D, Lowe C. Prevention of adverse reactions to blood transfusion by the administration of saline washed red cells. Transfusion 1981;21:277–80.
44. Hill JM, Duncan CN. Leukemoid reactions. Am J Med Sci 1941;201:847.
45. Hersh EM, Bodey GP, Nies BA, Freireich EJ. Causes of death in acute leukemia. A ten-year study of 414 patients from 1954–1963. JAMA 1965;193:105–9.
46. Bodey GP, Buckley M, Sathe YS, Freireich EJ. Quantitative relationships between circulating leukocytes and infection in patients with acute leukemia. Ann Intern Med 1966;64:328–40.
47. Solberg CO, Schreiner K, Hellum KB, Hamre E. Neutrophil granulocyte function in the early diagnosis of acute myelomonocyte and myeloblastic leukemia. Ann Intern Med 1975;64:328–40.
48. Freireich EJ, Leven RH, Whang J, et al. The function and fate of transfused leukocytes from donors with chronic myelocytic leukemia in leukopenic recipients. Ann N Y Acad Sci 1964;113:1081–9.
49. Strauss RG. Therapeutic granulocyte transfusions in 1993. Blood 1993;81:1675–8.
50. Applebaum FR, Bowles CA, Makuch RW, Deisseroth AB. Granulocyte transfusion therapy of experimental *Pseudomonas* septicemia. Study of cell dose and collection technique. Blood 1978;52:323–31.
51. Clift RA, Buckner CD. Granulocyte transfusions. Am J Med 1984;76:631–6.
52. Winston DJ, Ho WG, Gale RP. Therapeutic granulocyte transfusions for documented infections. A controlled trial in ninety-five infectious granulocytopenic episodes. Ann Intern Med 1982;97:509–15.
53. Bhatia S, McCullough J, Perry EH, et al. Granulocyte transfusions. Efficacy in treating fungal infections in neutropenic patients following bone marrow transplantation. Transfusion 1994;34:226–32.
54. Bensinger WI, Price TH, Dale DC, et al. The effects of daily recombinant human granulocyte colony-stimulating factor administration on normal granulocyte donors undergoing leukapheresis. Blood 1993;81:1883–8.

55. Adkins D, Ali S, Despotis G, et al. Granulocyte collection efficiency and yield are enhanced by the use of a higher inter-face offset during apheresis of donors given granulocyte colony–stimulating factor. Transfusion 1998;38:557–64.
56. Hubel K, Carter RA, Liles WC, et al. Granulocyte transfusion therapy for infections in candidates and recipients of HPC transplantation: a comparative analysis of feasibility and outcome for community donors versus related donors. Transfusion 2002;42:1393–5.
57. Anderson KC, Weinstein HC. Graft versus host disease after transfusion. N Engl J Med 1990;323:315–21.
58. Nemunaitis J, Rabinowe SN, Singer JW, et al. Recombinant granulocyte-macrophage colony–stimulating factor after autologous bone marrow transplantation for lymphoid cancer. N Engl J Med 1991;324:1773–6.
59. Crawford J, Ozer H, Stoller R, et al. Reduction by granulocyte colony-stimulating factor of fever and neutropenia induced by chemotherapy in patients with small cell lung cancer. N Engl J Med 1991;325:164–70.
60. Antman KS, Griffin JD, Elias A, et al. Effect of recombinant human granulocyte-macrophage colony-stimulating factor on chemotherapy-induced myelosuppression. N Engl J Med 1988;319:593–8.
61. Lane TA, Ho AD, Bashey A, et al. Mobilization of blood-derived stem and progenitor cells in normal subjects by granulocyte-macrophage- and granulocyte-colony-stimulating factors. Transfusion 1999;39:39–47.
62. Colby C, McAfee SL, Finkestein DM, Spitzer TR. Early vs delayed administration of G-CSF following autologous peripheral blood stem cell transplantation. Bone Marrow Transplant 1997;21:1005–10.
63. Hartmann LC, Tschetter LK, Habermann TM, et al. Granulocyte colony-stimulating factor in severe chemotherapy induced afebrile neutropenia. N Engl J Med 1997;336:1776–80.
64. Goodnough LT, Anderson KC, Kurtz S, et al. Instructions and guidelines for the use of hematopoietic growth factors. Transfusion 1993;33:944–59.
65. Bennett CL, Smith TJ, Weeks JC, et al. Use of hematopoietic colony-stimulating factors. The American Society of Clinical Oncology survey. J Clin Oncol 1996;14:2511–20.
66. Murphy S. Thrombocytosis and thrombocythaemia. Clin Haematol 1983;12:89–106.
67. Levin J, Conley CL. Thrombocytosis associated with malignant disease. Arch Intern Med 1964;114:497.
68. Figueroa M, Gehlsen J, Hammond D, et al. Combination chemotherapy in refractory immune thrombocytopenic purpura. N Engl J Med 1993;328:1226–9.
69. Andersen JC. Response of resistant idiopathic thrombocytopenic purpura to pulsed high-dose dexamethasone therapy. N Engl J Med 1994;330:1560–4.
70. Gralnick HR, Abrell E. Studies of the procoagulant and fibrinolytic activity of promyelocytes in acute promyelocytic leukemia. Br J Haematol 1973;24:89–99.
71. Cowan DH, Graham RC Jr, Baunach D. The platelet defect in leukemia. Platelet ultrastructure, adenine nucleotide metabolism, and the release reaction. J Clin Invest 1975;56:188–200.
72. Lackner H. Hemostatic abnormalities associated with dysproteinemias. Semin Hematol 1973;10:125–33.
73. Duke WW. The relation of blood platelets to hemorrhagic disease. Description of a method for determining the bleeding time and coagulation time and report of three cases of hemorrhagic disease relieved by transfusion. JAMA 1910;55:1185–92.
74. Farber S, Klein E. The nature and control of bleeding in acute leukemia and other thrombocytopenic states. A review of a 10-year program of research. Ann Paediatr Forum 1957;3:348.
75. Gaydos LA, Freireich EJ, Mantel N, et al. The quantitative relation between platelet count and hemorrhage in patients with acute leukemia. N Engl J Med 1962;266:905–9.
76. Murphy S, Litwin S, Herring LM, et al. Indications for platelet transfusion in children with acute leukemia. Am J Hematol 1982;12:347–56.
77. Higby DJ, Cohen E, Holland JF, et al. The prophylactic treatment of thrombocytopenic leukemic patients with platelets. A double blind study. Transfusion 1974;4:440–6.
78. Tullis JL, Eberle WG II, Baundanza P, Tinch R. Plateletpheresis. Description of a new technique. Transfusion 1968;8:154–64.
79. Kurtz SR, McMican A, Carciero R, et al. Plateletpheresis experience with the Haemonetics Blood Processor 30, the IBM Blood Processor 2997 and the Fenwal CS-3000 Blood Processor. Vox Sang 1981;41:212–8.
80. Sintnicolaas K, Vriesendorp HM, Sizoo W, Stenfert Kroese WF. Delayed alloimmunization by random single door platelet transfusions. A randomized study to compare single donor and multiple donor platelet transfusions in cancer patients with thrombocytopenia. Lancet 1981;1:750–4.
81. Gmur J, Von Felten A, Osterwalder B, et al. Delayed alloimmunization using random single donor platelet transfusions. A prospective study in thrombocytopenic patients with acute leukemia. Blood 1983;62:473–9.
82. Glynn SA, Schreiber GB, Busch MP, et al. Demographic characteristics, unreported risk behaviors, and prevalence and incidence of viral infections. A comparison of apheresis and whole-blood donors. Transfusion 1998;38:350–8.
83. Pisciotto PT, Benson K, Hume H, et al. Prophylactic versus therapeutic platelet transfusion practices in hematology/oncology patients. Transfusion 1995;35:498–502.
84. Consensus development conference on platelet transfusion therapy. JAMA 1987;258:1777–80.
85. Schiffer CA, Anderson KC, Bennett CL, et al. Platelet transfusion for patients with cancer: clinical practice guidelines of the American Society of Clinical Oncology. J Clin Oncol 2001;19:1519–38.
86. Gmur J, Burger J, Schanz U, et al. A safety of stringent prophylactic platelet transfusion policy for patients with acute leukemia. Lancet 1991;338:1223–6.
87. Rebulla P, Finazzi G, Marangoni F, et al. The threshold for prophylactic platelet transfusions in adults with acute myeloid leukemia. N Engl J Med 1997;337:1870–5.
88. Wandt H, Frank M, Ehninger G, et al. Safety and cost effectiveness of a 10×10^9/L trigger for prophylactic platelet transfusions compared with the traditional 20×10^9/L trigger. A prospective comparative trial in 105 patients with acute myeloid leukemia. Blood 1998;91:3601–6.
89. Heckman KD, Weiner GJ, Davis CS, et al. Randomized study of prophylactic platelet transfusion threshold during induction therapy for adult leukemia: 10,000/microL versus 20,000/microL. J Clin Oncol 1997;15:1143–9.
90. Norol F, Bierling P, Roudot Thoraval F, et al. Platelet transfusion. A dose-response study. Blood 1998;92:1448–52.
91. Aderka D, Praff G, Santo M, et al. Bleeding due to thrombocytopenia in acute leukemia and reevaluation of the prophylactic platelet transfusion policy. Am J Med Sci 1986;291:147–51.
92. Shulman NR, Watkins SP Jr, Itscoitz SB, Students AB. Evidence that the spleen retains the youngest and hemostatically most effective platelets. Trans Assoc Am Phys 1968;81:302–13.
93. Baer MR, Bloomfield CD. Controversies in transfusion medicine. Prophylactic platelet transfusion therapy: pro. Transfusion 1992;32:377–80.
94. Patten E. Controversies in transfusion medicine. Prophylactic platelet transfusion revisited after 25 years: con. Transfusion 1992;32:381–5.
95. Schiffer CA. Prophylactic platelet transfusion. Transfusion 1992;32:295–8.
96. Kretschmer V, Huss B, Dietrich G, et al. Determination of bleeding risk in thrombocytopenic patients receiving platelet substitution. Transfus Sci 1993;14:27–34.
97. Beutler E. Platelet transfusion. The 20,000/mL trigger. Blood 1993;81:1411–3.
98. Daly PA, Schiffer CA, Aisner J, Wiernik PH. Platelet transfusion therapy. One-hour post-transfusion increments are valuable in predicting the need for HLA-matched preparations. JAMA 1980;243:435–8.
99. Gorgone BC, Andersen JW, Anderson KC. Comparison of 15 min and 1H post-platelet counts in pediatric patients. Transfusion 1986;26:555.
100. O'Connell B, Lee EJ, Schiffer CA. The value of 10-minute posttransfusion platelet count. Transfusion 1988;28:66–7.
101. Harker LA, Slichter SJ. The bleeding time as a screening test for evaluation of platelet function. N Engl J Med 1972;287:155–9.
102. Davis KB, Slichter SJ, Corash L. Corrected count increment and percent platelet recovery as measures of post-transplantation platelet response. Problems and a solution. Transfusion 1999;39:586–92.
103. Bishop JF, McGrath K, Wolf MM, et al. Clinical factors influencing the efficacy of pooled platelet transfusions. Blood 1988;71:383–7.
104. Doughty HA, Murphy MF, Metcalfe P, et al. Relative importance of immune and non-immune causes of platelet refractoriness. Vox Sang 1994;66:200–5.
105. Ishida A, Handa M, Wakui M, et al. Clinical factors influencing posttransfusion platelet increment in patients undergoing hematopoietic cell transplantation—a prospective analysis. Transfusion 1998;38:839–47.
106. Bernstein SH, Nademanee AP, Vose JM, et al. A multicenter study of platelet recovery and utilization in patients after myeloablative therapy and hematopoietic stem cell transplantation. Blood 1998;91:3509–17.
107. Klumpp TR, Herman JH, Innis S, et al. Factors associated with response to platelet transfusion following hematopoietic stem cell transplantation. Bone Marrow Transplant 1996;17:1035–41.
108. Flatow FA, Freireich EJ. Effect of splenectomy on the response to platelet transfusion in three patients with aplastic anemia. N Engl J Med 1966;274:242–8.
109. Smith ME, Reid DM, Jones CE, et al. Binding of quinine- and quinidine-dependent drug antibodies to platelets is mediated by the Fab domain of the immunoglobulin G and is not Fc dependent. J Clin Invest 1987;79:912–7.
110. Stricker RB, Shuman MA. Quinidine purpura. Evidence that glycoprotein V is a target platelet antigen. Blood 1986;67:1377–81.
111. Fujisawa K, O'Toole TE, Tani P, et al. Autoantibodies to the presumptive cytoplasmic domain of platelet glycoprotein IIIa in patients with chronic immune thrombocytopenic purpura. Blood 1991;77:2207–13.
112. Kickler T, Kennedy SD, Braine HG. Alloimmunization to platelet specific antigens on glycoproteins IIb-IIIa and Ib/IX in multiply transfused thrombocytopenic patients. Transfusion 1990;30:622–5.
113. Shalev O, Brezis M. Methyldopa-induced thrombocytopenia in chronic lymphocytic leukemia. N Engl J Med 1977;297:1471.
114. Murphy MF, Riordan T, Minchinton RM. Demonstration of an immune-mediated mechanism of penicillin-induced neutropenia and thrombocytopenia. Br J Haematol 1983;1983:155–60.
115. Herzig RH, Terasaki PI, Trapani RJ, et al. The relationship between donor-recipient lymphocytotoxicity and the transfusion of response using HLA-matched platelet concentrates. Transfusion 1977;17:657–61.
116. Perkins HA. Immunologic effects of blood transfusion. In: Smith DM Jr, Silvergleid AJ, editors. Special considerations in transfusing the immunocompromised patient. Arlington (VA): American Association of Blood Banks; 1985. p. 1–10.
117. Van Eys J, Thomas D, Olivos B. Platelet use in pediatric oncology. A review of 393 transfusions. Transfusion 1978;18:169–73.
118. Dutcher JP, Schiffer CA, Aisner J, Wiernick PH. Alloimmunization following platelet transfusion. The absence of a dose–response relationship. Blood 1981;57:395–8.
119. Dutcher JP, Schiffer CA, Aisner J, Wiernick PH. Long-term follow-up of patients with leukemia receiving platelet transfusions. Identification of a large group of patients who do not become alloimmunized. Blood 1981;58:1007–11.
120. Holohan TV, Terasaki PI, Deisseroth AB. Suppression of transfusion-related alloimmunization in intensively treated cancer patients. Blood 1981;58:122–8.
121. Yankee RA, Grumet FC, Rogentine GN. Platelet transfusion therapy. The selection of compatible donors for refractory patients by lymphocyte HLA-typing. N Engl J Med 1969;281:1208–12.
122. Yankee RA, Graff KS, Dowling R, Henderson ES. Selection of unrelated compatible platelet donors by lymphocyte HLA matching. N Engl J Med 1973;288:760–4.
123. Lohrmann HP, Bull MI, Decter JA, et al. Platelet transfusions from HLA-compatible unrelated donors to alloimmunized patients. Ann Intern Med 1974;80:9–14.
124. Duquesnoy RJ, Filip DJ, Rodey GE, et al. Successful transfusion of platelets "mismatched" for HLA antigens to alloimmunized thrombocytopenic patients. Am J Hematol 1977;2:219–26.
125. Duquesnoy RJ, Filip DJ, Aster RH. Influence of HLA-A2 on the effectiveness of platelet transfusions in alloimmunized thrombocytopenic patients. Blood 1977;50:407–12.
126. Vamvakas EC. Meta-analysis of randomized controlled trials of the efficacy of white cell reduction in preventing HLA-alloimmunization and refractoriness to random-donor platelet transfusions. Transfus Med Rev 1998;12:258–70.
127. Williamson LM, Wimperis JZ, Williamson P, et al. Bedside filtration of blood products in the prevention of HLA alloimmunization—a prospective randomized study. Blood 1994;83:3028–35.
128. Grijzenhout MA, Aarts Riemens MI, de Gruijl FR, et al. UVB irradiation of human platelet concentrates does not prevent HLA alloimmunization in recipients. Blood 1994;84:3524–31.
129. Blajchman MA, Bardossy L, Carmen RA, et al. The effect of the time of leukodepletion. Blood 1992;79:1371–5.
130. Sherman L, Menitove J, Kagen LR. Ultraviolet-B irradiation of platelets. A preliminary trial of efficacy. Transfusion 1992;32:402–7.

131. Slichter SJ. Leukocyte reduction and ultraviolet B irradiation of platelets to prevent alloimmunization and refractoriness to platelet transfusions. N Engl J Med 1997;337:1861–9.
132. Novotny VMJ. Prevention and management of platelet transfusion refractoriness. Vox Sang 1996;76:1–13.
133. Moroff G, Garratty G, Heal JM, et al. Selection of platelets for refractory patients by HLA matching and prospective crossmatching. Transfusion 1992;32:633–40.
134. Friedberg RC, Donnelly SF, Boyd JC, et al. Clinical and blood bank factors in the management of platelet refractoriness and alloimmunization. Blood 1993;81:3428–34.
135. Friedberg RC, Donnelly SF, Mintz PD. Independent roles for platelet crossmatching and HLA in the selection of platelets for alloimmunized patients. Transfusion 1994;34:215–20.
136. Bensinger WI, Buckner CD, Clift RA, et al. Plasma exchange for platelet alloimmunization. Transplantation 1986;41:602–5.
137. Lee EJ, Norris D, Schiffer CA. Intravenous immune globulin for patients alloimmunized to random donor platelet transfusion. Transfusion 1987;27:245–7.
138. Murphy S. ABO blood groups and platelet transfusion. Transfusion 1988;28:401–2.
139. Dunstan RA, Simpson MB, Rosse WF. Erythrocyte antigens on human platelets. Absence of Rh, Duffy, Kell, Kidd and Lutheran antigens. Transfusion 1984;24:243–6.
140. McGinniss MH, Bronson WR, Freireich E, Kliman A. Formation of red cell antibodies in response to platelet transfusions. Transfusion 1963;3:426.
141. Skinnider LF, Taylor D. The in vitro effect of anti-A and anti-AB alloantibodies on group A and AB platelets. Transfusion 1981;21:706–8.
142. Lee EJ, Schiffer CA. ABO compatibility can influence the results of platelet transfusion: results of a randomized trial. Transfusion 1989;29:384–9.
143. Lichtiger B, Surgeon J, Rhorer S. Rh-incompatible platelet transfusion therapy in cancer patients: a study of 30 cases. Vox Sang 1983;43:139–43.
144. Brand A, Sintnicolaas K, Claas FH, Eernisse JG. ABH antibodies causing platelet transfusion refractoriness. Transfusion 1986;24:463–6.
145. Heal JM, Blumberg N, Masel D. An evaluation of crossmatching, HLA, and ABO matching for platelet transfusions to refractory patients. Blood 1987;70:23–30.
146. Pierce RN, Reich LM, Mayer K. Hemolysis following platelet transfusions from ABO-incompatible donors. Transfusion 1985;25:60–2.
147. Thompson CB, Jakubowski JA. The pathophysiology and clinical relevance of platelet heterogeneity. Blood 1988;72:1–8.
148. Warkentin TE, Smith JW. The alloimmune thrombocytopenic syndromes. Transfus Med Rev 1997;11:296–307.
149. Shulman NR, Aster RA, Leitner AL, Hiller MC. A new syndrome of post-transfusion purpura. J Clin Invest 1960;39:1028–9.
150. Cimo PL, Aster RH. Post-transfusion purpura. Successful treatment by exchange transfusion. N Engl J Med 1972;289:290–2.
151. Gurney AL, Carver-Moore K, de Sauvage FJ, Moore MW. Thrombocytopenia in c-mpl–deficient mice. Science 1994;255:1445–7.
152. Lee DH, Blajchman MA. Novel platelet products and substitutes. Transfus Med Rev 1998;12:175–87.
153. Klein E, Farber S, Djerassi I, et al. The preparation and clinical administration of lyophilized platelet material to children with acute leukemia and aplastic anemia. J Pediatr 1956;49:517.
154. Tullis JL, Surgenor DM, Baudanza P. Preserved platelets. Their preparation, storage and clinical use. Blood 1959;14:459.
155. Angelini A, Dragani A, Berardi A, et al. Evaluation of four different methods of platelet freezing. Vox Sang 1992;62:146–51.
156. Read MS, Bode AP, Reddick RL. Studies with dried and rehydrated platelets for transfusion products. FASEB J 1991;1:903a.
157. Coller BS, Springer KT, Beer JH, et al. In vitro studies of a potential autologous, semi-artificial alternative to platelet transfusions. J Clin Invest 1992;89:546–55.
158. Ryback ME, Renzulli L. A liposome based platelet substitute, the plateletsome, with hemostatic efficacy. Blood 1990;76:473a.
159. Chao FC, Kim BK, Houranieh AM, et al. Infusible platelet membrane microvesicles. A potential transfusion substitute for platelets. Transfusion 1996;36:536–42.
160. George JN, Thoi LL, McManus LM, Reimann TA. Isolation of human platelet membrane microparticles from plasma and serum. Blood 1982;60:834–40.
161. Galan AM, Hernandez MR, Bozzo J, et al. Preparations of synthetic phospholipids promote procoagulant activity on damaged vessels. Studies under flow conditions. Transfusion 1998;38:1004–10.
162. Alving B. Potential for synthetic phospholipids as partial platelet substitutes. Transfusion 1998;38:997–8.
163. Braunstein AH, Oberman HA. Transfusion of plasma components. Transfusion 1984;24:281–6.
164. Consensus Conference. Fresh frozen plasma. Indications and risks. JAMA 1985;253:551–3.
165. Horowitz B, Bonomo R, Prince AM. Solvent/detergent-treated plasma. A virus-inactivated substitute for fresh frozen plasma. Blood 1992;79:826–31.
166. Ventura GJ, Hester JP, Smith TL, Keating MJ. Acute myeloblastic leukemia with hyperleukocytosis. Risk factors for early mortality in induction. Am J Hematol 1988;27:34–7.
167. Curtis JE, Hersh EM, Freireich EJ. Leukapheresis therapy of chronic lymphocytic leukemia. Blood 1972;39:163–75.
168. Edelson R, Facktor M, Andrews A, et al. Successful management of the Sézary syndrome. Mobilization and removal of extravascular neoplastic T cells by leukapheresis. N Engl J Med 1974;291:293–4.
169. Fay JW, Moore JO, Logue GL, Huang AT. Leukapheresis therapy of leukemic reticuloendotheliosis (hairy cell leukemia). Blood 1979;54:747–9.
170. Taft EG, Babcock RB, Scharfman WB, Tartaglia AP. Plateletpheresis in the management of thrombocytosis. Blood 1979;50:927–33.
171. Bensinger WI, Baker DA, Buckner CD, et al. Immunoadsorption for removal of A and B blood group antibodies. N Engl J Med 1981;304:160–2.
172. Branda RF, Moldow CF, McCullough JJ, Jacob HS. Plasma exchange in the treatment of immune disease. Transfusion 1975;15:570–6.
173. Beck JR, Quinn BM, Meier FA, Rawnsley HM. Hyperviscosity syndrome in paraproteinemia managed by plasma exchange. Transfusion 1982;22:51–3.
174. Perkins HA, Payne R, Ferguson J, Wood M. Nonhemolytic febrile transfusion reactions. Quantitative effects of blood components with emphasis on isoantigenic incompatibility of leukocytes. Vox Sang 1966;11:578–600.
175. McCullough J, Weiblin BJ, Clay ME, Forstrom L. Effect of leukocyte antibodies on the fate in vivo of indium-111–labeled granulocytes. Blood 1981;58:164–70.
176. Vyas GN, Perkins HA, Fudenberg HH. Anaphylactoid transfusion reactions associated with anti-IgA. Lancet 1968;2:312–5.
177. Francis DM, Clunie GJ. Influence of the timing of blood transfusion on experimental tumor growth. J Surg Res 1993;54:237–41.
178. Gascon P, Zoumbos NC, Young NS. Immunologic abnormalities in patients receiving multiple blood transfusions. Ann Intern Med 1984;100:173–7.
179. Kaplan J, Sarnaik S, Gitlin J, Lusher J. Diminished helper/suppressor lymphocyte ratios and natural killer activity in recipients of repeated blood transfusions. Blood 1984;64:308–10.
180. Ghio M, Contini P, Mazzei C, et al. Soluble HLA Class I, HLA Class II, and fas ligand in blood components. A possible key to explain the immunomodulatory effects of allogeneic blood transfusions. Blood 1999;93:1770–7.
181. Lagaaij EL, Hennemann IP, Ruigrok M, et al. Effect of one HLA-DR antigen matched and completely HLA-DR-mismatched blood transfusions on survival of heart and kidney allografts. N Engl J Med 1989;321:701–5.
182. Blumberg N, Heal JM. Transfusion and host defenses against cancer recurrence and infection. Transfusion 1989;29:236–45.
183. Heiss MH, Mempel W, Delanoff C, et al. Blood transfusion-modulated tumor recurrence. First results of a randomized study of autologous versus allogeneic blood transfusion in colorectal cancer surgery. J Clin Oncol 1994;12:1859–67.
184. Tartter PI, Quintero S, Barron DM, et al. Perioperative blood transfusion associated with infectious complications after colorectal cancer operations. Am J Surg 1986;152:479–82.
185. Blajchman MA. Allogeneic blood transfusions, immunomodulation, and postoperative bacterial infection. Do we have the answers? Transfusion 1997;37:121–5.
186. Vamvakas EC, Moore SB. Perioperative blood transfusion and colorectal cancer recurrence. A qualitative statistical overview and meta-analysis. Transfusion 1993;33:754–65.
187. Vamvakas EC, Moore SB. Blood transfusion and postoperative septic complications. Transfusion 1994;34:714–27.
188. Blumberg N, Chuang-Stein C, Heal JM. The relationship of blood transfusion, tumor staging, and cancer recurrence. Transfusion 1990;30:291–4.
189. Bordin JO, Bardossy L, Blajchman MA. Growth enhancement of established tumors by allogeneic blood transfusion in experimental animals and its amelioration by leukodepletion. The importance of the timing of the leukodepletion. Blood 1994;84:344–8.
190. Shivdasani RA, Haluska FG, Dock NL, et al. Brief report. Graft-versus-host disease associated with transfusion of blood from unrelated HLA-homozygous donors. N Engl J Med 1993;328:766–70.
191. Anderson KC, Goodnough LT, Sayers M, et al. Variation in blood component irradiation practice: implications for prevention of transfusion associated graft versus host disease. Blood 1991;77:2096–102.
192. Twomey JJ, Rice L. Impact of Hodgkin's disease upon the immune system. Semin Oncol 1980;7:114–25.
193. Ekert H, Waters KD, Smith PJ, et al. Treatment with MOPP or ChIVPP chemotherapy only for all stages of childhood Hodgkin's disease. J Clin Oncol 1988;6:1845–50.
194. Postmus PE, Mulder NH, Elema JD. Graft versus host disease after transfusions of non-irradiated blood cells in patients having received autologous bone marrow. A report of 4 cases following ablative chemotherapy for solid tumors. Eur J Cancer Clin Oncol 1988;24:889–94.
195. Thaler M, Shamiss A, Orgad S, et al. The role of the blood from HLA-homozygous donors in fatal transfusion-associated graft-versus-host disease after open heart surgery. N Engl J Med 1989;321:25–8.
196. Petz LD, Calhoun L, Yam P, et al. Transfusion-associated graft-versus-host disease in immunocompetent patients. Report of a fatal case associated with transfusion of blood from a second-degree relative, and a survey of predisposing factors. Transfusion 1993;33:742–50.
197. Ohto H, Yasuda H, Noguchi M, Abe R. Risk of transfusion-associated graft-versus-host disease as a result of directed donations from relatives. Transfusion 1992;32:691–3.
198. Charpentier F, Bracq C, Bonin P, et al. HLA-matched blood products and post-transfusion graft-versus-host disease. Transfusion 1990;30:850.
199. Grishaber JE, Birney SM, Strauss RG. Potential for transfusion-associated graft-versus host disease due to apheresis platelets matched for HLA Class I antigens. Transfusion 1993;33:910–4.
200. Benson K, Marks AR, Marshall J, Goldstein JD. Fatal graft-versus-host disease associated with HLA-matched, HLA-homozygous platelet transfusions from unrelated donors. Transfusion 1994;34:432–7.
201. Pelszynski MM, Moroff G, Luban NLC, et al. Effect of y irradiation of red blood cell units on T-cell inactivation as assessed by limiting dilution analysis. Implications for preventing transfusion-associated graft-versus-host disease. Blood 1994;83:1683–8.
202. Drobyski W, Thibodeau S, Truitt RL, et al. Third party–mediated graft rejection and graft-versus-host disease after T cell depleted bone marrow transplantation, as demonstrated by hypervariable DNA probes and HLA-DR polymorphism. Blood 1989;74:2285–94.
203. Menitove J, editor. Standards for blood banks and transfusion services. 23rd ed. Bethesda (MD): American Associations of Blood Banks; 2005.
204. Read EJ, Kodis C, Carter CS, Leitman SF. Viability of platelets following storage in the irradiated state. A pair-controlled study. Transfusion 1988;28:446–50.
205. Davey RJ, McCoy NC, Yu M, et al. The effect of prestorage irradiation on posttransfusion red cell survival. Transfusion 1992;32:525–8.
206. Akahoshi M, Takanashi M, Masuda M, et al. A case of transfusion-associated graft-versus-host disease not prevented by white cell-reduction filters. Transfusion 1992;32:169–72.
207. Fast LD, Valeri CR, Crowley JP. Immune responses to major histocompatibility complex homozygous lymphoid cells in murine F1 hybrid recipients. Implications for transfusion-associated graft-versus-host disease. Blood 1995;86:3090–6.
208. Grass JA, Wafa T, Reames A, et al. Prevention of transfusion-associated graft-versus-host disease by photochemical treatment. Blood 1999;93:3140–7.
209. Hoofnagle J. Post-transfusion hepatitis B. Transfusion 1990;30:384–6.
210. Lee WM. Hepatitis B virus infection. N Engl J Med 1997;337:1733–45.
211. Koziol DE, Holland PV, Alling DW, et al. Antibody to hepatitis B core antigen as a paradoxical marker for non-A, non-B hepatitis agents in donated blood. Ann Intern Med 1986;104:488–95.
212. Stevens CE, Aach RD, Hollinger FB, et al. Hepatitis B virus antibody in blood donors and the occurrence of non-A, non-B hepatitis in transfusion recipients. An analysis of

the transfusion-transmitted viruses study. Ann Intern Med 1984;101:733–8.

213. Kline WE, Bowman RJ, McCurdy KK, et al. Hepatitis B core antibody (anti-BHc) in blood donors in the United States. Implications for surrogate testing programs. Transfusion 1987;27:99–102.
214. Choo QL, Kuo G, Weiner AJ, et al. Isolation of a cDNA clone derived from a blood borne non-A, non-B viral hepatitis genome. Science 1989;244:359–62.
215. Kuo G, Choo QL, Alter HJ, et al. An assay for circulating antibodies to a major etiologic virus of human non-A, non-B hepatitis. Science 1989;244:362–4.
216. Kleinman S, Alter H, Busch M, et al. Increased detection of hepatitis C virus (HCV)-infected blood donors by a multiple-antigen HCV enzyme immunoassay. Transfusion 1992;32:805–13.
217. Goldman M, Juodvalkis S, Gill P, Spurll G. Hepatitis C lookback. Transfus Med Rev 1998;12:84–93.
218. Flanagan P. Genomic screening of blood donations—the new dawn arrives. Vox Sang 1999;76:135–7.
219. Stramer SL, Caglioti S, Strong DM. NAT of the United States and Canadian blood supply. Transfusion 2000;40:1165–68.
220. Dodd RY, Notari EP, Stramer SL. Current prevalence and incidence of infectious disease markers and estimated window-period risk in the American Red Cross blood donor population. Transfusion 2000;42:975–9
221. Paul IM, Sanders J, Ruggiero F, et al. Chronic hepatitis C virus infections in leukemia survivors: prevalence, viral load, and severity of liver disease. Blood 1999;93:3672–7.
222. Shuhart MC, Myerson D, Childs BH, et al. Marrow transplantation from hepatitis C virus seropositive donors. Transmission rate and clinical course. Blood 1994;84:3229–35.
223. Frickhofen N, Wiesneth M, Jainta C, et al. Hepatitis C virus is a risk factor for liver failure from veno-occlusive disease after bone marrow transplantation. Blood 1994;83:1998–2004.
224. Strasser SI, McDonald GB. Hepatitis viruses and hematopoietic cell transplantation. A guide to patient and donor management. Blood 1999;93:1127–36.
225. Simons JN, Leary TP, Dawson GJ, et al. Isolation of novel virus-like sequences associated with human hepatitis. Nat Med 1995;1:564–9.
226. Linnen J, Wages JJ, Zhang-Keck Z-Y, et al. Molecular cloning and disease association of hepatitis G virus. A transfusion-transmissible agent. Science 1996;271:505–8.
227. Prati D, Zanella A, Bosoni P, et al. The incidence and natural course of transfusion-associated GB virus C/hepatitis G virus infection in a cohort of thalassemic patients. Blood 1998;91:774–7.
228. Bowden RA, Slichter SJ, Sayers M, et al. A comparison of filtered leukocyte-reduced and cytomegalovirus (CMV) seronegative blood products for the prevention of transfusion-associated CMV infection after marrow transplant. Blood 1995;86:3598–603.
229. Miller W, Flynn P, McCullough J, et al. Cytomegalovirus infection after bone marrow transplantation: association with acute graft-versus-host disease. Blood 1986;67:1162–7.
230. Wingard JR, Chen DV, Burns WH, et al. Cytomegalovirus infection after autologous bone marrow transplantation with comparison to infection after allogeneic bone marrow transplantation. Blood 1988;71:1432–7.
231. Prentice HG, Gluckman E, Powles CD, et al. Impact of long-term acyclovir on cytomegalovirus infection and survival after allogeneic bone marrow transplantation. Lancet 1994;343:749–53.
232. Reusser P, Fisher LD, Buckner CD, et al. Cytomegalovirus infection after autologous bone marrow transplantation. Occurrence of cytomegalovirus disease and effect on engraftment. Blood 1990;75:1888–94.
233. Gilbert GL, Hayes K, Hudson IL, James J. Prevention of transfusion-acquired cytomegalovirus infection in infants by blood filtration to remove leucocytes. Lancet 1989;1:1228–31.
234. DeGraan-Hentzen YC, Gratama JW, Mudde GC. Prevention of primary cytomegalovirus infection in patients with hematologic malignancies by intensive white cell depletion of blood products. Transfusion 1989;29:757–60.
235. Sayers MH, Anderson KC, Goodnough LT, et al. Reducing the risk for transfusion-transmitted cytomegalovirus infection. Ann Intern Med 1992;116:55–62.
236. Walter EA, Greenberg PD, Gilbert MJ, et al. Reconstruction of cellular immunity against cytomegalovirus in recipients of allogeneic bone marrow by transfer of T-cell clones from the donor. N Engl J Med 1995;333:1038–44.
237. Centers for Disease Control, Division of Vector-Borne Infectious Diseases. West Nile Virus 2005. Available at: http://www.cdc.gov/ncidod/dvbid/westnile/ (accessed July 20, 2005).
238. Macedo de Oliveira A, Beecham BD, Montgomery SP, et al. West Nile virus blood transfusion-related infection despite nucleic acid testing. Transfusion 2004;44:1695–9.
239. Klein HG, Dodd RY, Ness PM, et al. Current status of microbial contamination of blood components: summary of a conference. Transfusion 1997;37:95–101.
240. Heal JM, Cohen HJ. Do white cells in stored blood components reduce the likelihood of posttransfusion bacterial sepsis? Transfusion 1991;31:581–3.
241. Yomtovian R, Lazarus HM, Goodnough LT, et al. A prospective microbiologic surveillance program to detect and prevent the transfusion of bacterially contaminated platelets. Transfusion 1993;33:902–9.
242. Barrett BB, Andersen JW, Anderson KC. Strategies for the avoidance of bacterial contamination of blood components. Transfusion 1993;33:228–33.
243. Brecher ME, Hogan JJ, Boothe G, et al. Platelet bacterial contamination and the use of a chemiluminescence linked universal ribosomal RNA gene probe. Transfusion 1994;34:750–5.
244. Burstain JM, Brecher ME, Workman K, et al. Rapid identification of bacterially contaminated platelets using reagent strips: glucose and pH analysis as markers of bacterial metabolism. Transfusion 1997;37:255–8.
245. Wagner SJ, Robinette D. Evaluation of an automated microbiologic blood culture device for detection of bacteria in platelet components. Transfusion 1998;38:674–9.
246. Lin L, Londe H, Janda M, et al. Photochemical inactivation of pathogenic bacteria in human platelet concentrates. Blood 1994;83:2698–706.
247. Update. *Yersinia enterolitica* bacteremia and endotoxin shock associated with red blood cell transfusions—United States, 1991. MMWR Morb Mortal Wkly Rep 1991;40:176.
248. Busch MP, Alter HJ. Will human immunodeficiency virus p24 antigen screening increase the safety of the blood supply and, if so, at what cost? Transfusion 1995;35:536–9.
249. Schreiber GB, Glynn SA, Satten GA, et al. HIV seroconverting donors delay their return: screening test implications. Transfusion 2002;42:414–21.
250. Busch MP, Laycock M, Kleinman SH, et al. Accuracy of supplementary serologic testing for human T-lymphotropic virus types I and II in US blood donors. Blood 1994;83:1143–8.
251. Strong DM, Katz L. Blood-bank testing for infectious disease: how safe is blood transfusion? Trends Mol Med 2002;8:355–58.
252. Blattner WA. Human T-lymphotrophic viruses and diseases of long latency. Ann Intern Med 1989;111:4–6.
253. Blayney DW, Blattner WA, Robert-Guroff M, et al. The human T cell leukemia-lymphoma virus in the Southeastern United States. JAMA 1983;250:1048–52.
254. Robert-Guroff M, Weiss SH, Giron JA, et al. Prevalence of antibodies to HTLV-I, II, and III in intravenous drug abusers from AIDS endemic region. JAMA 1986;255:3133–7.
255. Minamoto GY, Gold JW, Scheinberg DA, et al. Infection with human T-cell leukemia virus type I in patients with leukemia. N Engl J Med 1988;318:219–22.
256. Kamihara S, Nakasima S, Oyakawa Y, et al. Transmission of human T-cell lymphotrophic virus type 1 by blood transfusion before and after mass screening of sera from seropositive donors. Vox Sang 1987;52:43–4.
257. Williams AE, Fang CT, Slamon DJ. Seroprevalence and epidemiological correlates of HTLV-I infection in US blood donors. Science 1988;240:643–6.
258. Donegan E, Lee H, Operskalski EA, et al. Transfusion transmission of retroviruses. Human T-lymphotropic virus types I and II compared with human immunodeficiency virus type I. Transfusion 1994;34:478–83.
259. Goodnough LT, Brecher ME, Kanter MH, Aubuchon JP. Blood transfusion. Part I. N Engl J Med 1999;340:438–47.
260. Goodnough LT, Brecher ME, Kanter MH, Aubuchon JP. Transfusion medicine (Part II). Blood conservation: preoperative autologous donation. N Engl J Med 1999;340:525–33.
261. Schreiber GB, Busch MP, Kleinman SH, Korelitz JJ. The risk of transfusion-transmitted viral infections. N Engl J Med 1996;334:1685–90.
262. Ehrlich GD, Glaser JB, LaVigne K, et al. Prevalence of human T-cell leukemia/lymphoma virus (HTLV) type II infection among high risk individuals. Type specific identification of HTLVs by polymerase chain reaction. Blood 1989;74:1658–64.
263. Krueger GR, Koch B, Leyssens N, et al. Comparison of seroprevalences of human herpesvirus-6 and -7 in healthy blood donors from nine countries. Vox Sang 1998;75:193–7.
264. Grant JH, Gold JW, Wittner M, et al. Transfusion-associated acute Chagas disease acquired in the United States. Ann Intern Med 1989;111:849–51.
265. Murphy MF. New variant Creutzfeldt–Jakob Disease (nvCJD). The risk of transmission by blood transfusion and the potential benefit of leukocyte-reduction of blood components. Transfus Med Rev 1999;13:75–83.
266. Johnson RT, Gibbs CJ. Creutzfeldt–Jakob disease and related transmissible spongiform encephalopathies. N Engl J Med 1998;339:1994–2004.
267. U.S. Dept. of Health and Human Services. Guidance for industry: revised preventative measures to reduce the possible risk of transmission of Creutzfeldt-Jakob disease (CJD) and variant Creutzfeldt-Jakob disease (vCJD) by blood and blood products.
268. Houston F, Foster JD, Chong A, et al. Transmission of BSE by blood transfusion in sheep. Lancet 2000;356:999–1000.
269. To LB, Haylock DN, Simmons PJ, Juttner CA. The biology and clinical uses of blood stem cells. Blood 1997;89:2233–58.
270. Gillespie TW, Hillyer CD. Peripheral blood progenitor cells for marrow reconstitution. Mobilization and collection strategies. Transfusion 1996;36:611–24.
271. Stroncek DF, Clay ME, Smith J, et al. Changes in blood counts after the administration of granulocyte colony-stimulating factor and the collection of peripheral blood stem cells from healthy donors. Transfusion 1996;36:596–600.
272. Prince HM, Page SR, Keating A, et al. Microbial contamination of harvested bone marrow and peripheral blood. Bone Marrow Transplant 1995;15:87–91.
273. Schwella N, Rick O, Heuft HG, et al. Bacterial contamination of autologous bone marrow. Re-infusion of culture-positive grafts does not result in clinical sequelae during the posttransplantation course. Vox Sang 1998;74:88–94.
274. Fountain D, Ralston M, Higgins N, et al. Liquid nitrogen freezers. A potential source of microbial contamination of hematopoietic stem cell components. Transfusion 1997;37:585–91.
275. Galmes A, Besalduch J, Bargay J, et al. Long-term storage at −80°C of hematopoietic progenitor cells with 5-percent dimethyl sulfoxide as the sole cryoprotectant. Transfusion 1999;39:70–3.
276. Webb IJ, Coral FS, Andersen JW, et al. Sources and sequelae of bacterial contamination of hematopoietic stem cell products. Implications for safety of hematotherapy and graft engineering. Transfusion 1996;36:782–8.
277. Hillyer CD, Klein HG. Immunotherapy and gene transfer in the treatment of the oncology patient. Role of transfusion medicine. Transfus Med Rev 1996;10:1–14.
278. Guillaume T, Rubinstein DB, Symann M. Immune reconstitution and immunotherapy after autologous hematopoietic stem cell transplantation. Blood 1998;92:1471–90.
279. Rubinstein P, Carrier C, Scaradavou A, et al. Outcomes among 562 recipients of placental-blood transplants from unrelated donors. N Engl J Med 1998;339:1565–77.
280. Gluckman E, Rocha V, Boyer-Chammard A, et al. Outcome of cord-blood transplantation from related and unrelated donors. N Engl J Med 1997;337:373–81.
281. Laporte J-P, Gorin N-C, Rubinstein P, et al. Cord-blood transplantation from an unrelated donor in an adult with chronic myelogenous leukemia. N Engl J Med 1996;335:167–70.
282. Kurtzberg J, Laughlin M, Graham ML, et al. Placental blood as a source of hematopoietic stem cells for transplantation into unrelated recipients. N Engl J Med 1996;335:157–66.
283. Cairo MS, Wagner JE. Placental and/or umbilical cord blood. An alternative source of hematopoietic stem cells for transplantation. Blood 1997;90:4665–78.
284. Storb R, Prentice RL, Thomas ED. Marrow transplantation for treatment of aplastic anemia. An analysis of factors associated with graft rejection. N Engl J Med 1977;296:61–6.
285. Klingemann HG, Self S, Banaji M, et al. Refractoriness to random donor platelet transfusions in patients with aplastic anemia. A multivariate analysis of data from 264 cases. Br J Haematol 1987;66:115–21.
286. Wulff JC, Santner TJ, Storb R, et al. Transfusion requirements after HLA identical marrow transplantation in 82 patients with aplastic anemia. Vox Sang 1983;44:366–74.
287. Kernan NA, Bartsch G, Ash RC, et al. Analysis of 462 transplantations from unrelated donors facilitated by the National Donor Program. N Engl J Med 1993;328:593–602.

288. Anderlini P, Donato M, Chan K-W, et al. Allogeneic blood progenitor cell collection in normal donors after mobilization with filgrastim. The M.D. Anderson Cancer Center experience. Transfusion 1999;39:555–60.
289. Benjamin RJ, Connors JM, McGurk S, et al. Prolonged erythroid aplasia after major ABO-mismatched trans-plantation for chronic myelogenous leukemia. Biol Blood Marrow Transplant 1998;4:151–6.
290. Lopez A, de la Rubia J, Arriaga F, et al. Severe hemolytic anemia due to multiple red cell alloantibodies after an ABO-incompatible allogeneic bone marrow transplant. Transfusion 1998;38:247–51.
291. Marmont AM, Damasio EE, Bacigalupo A, et al. A to O bone marrow transplantation in severe aplastic anemia. Dynamics of blood group conversion of early dyserythropoiesis in the engrafted marrow. Br J Haematol 1978;36:511–8.
292. Braine HG, Sensenbrenner LL, Wright SK, et al. Bone marrow transplantation with major ABO blood group incompatibility using erythrocyte depletion of marrow prior to infusion. Blood 1982;60:420–5.
293. Webb IJ, Soiffer RJ, Andersen JW, et al. In vivo adsorption of isohemagglutinins prior to major ABO incompatible bone marrow transplantation. Biol Blood Marrow Transplant 1997;3:267–72.
294. Bolan CD, Leitman SF, Griffith LM. Delayed donor red cell chimerism and pure red cell aplasia following major ABO-incompatible nonmyeloablative hematopoietic stem cell transplantation. Blood 2001;98:1687–94.
295. Hows J, Beddow K, Gordon-Smith E, et al. Donor-derived red blood cell antibodies and immune hemolysis after allogeneic bone marrow transplantation. Blood 1986;67:177–81.
296. Hazelhurst GR, Brenner MK, Wimperis JZ, et al. Hemolysis after T-cell depleted bone marrow transplantation. Scand J Haematol 1986;37:1–3.
297. Schwella N, Zimmerman R, Heuft HG, et al. Microbiologic contamination of peripheral blood stem cell autografts. Vox Sang 1994;67:32–5.
298. Pettengell R, Morgenstern GR, Woll PJ, et al. Peripheral blood progenitor cell transplantation in lymphoma and leukemia using a single apheresis. Blood 1993;82:3770–7.
299. Malachowski ME, Comenzo RL, Hillyer CD, et al. Large-volume leukapheresis for peripheral blood stem cell collection in patients with hematologic malignancies. Transfusion 1992;32:732–5.
300. Dzieczkowski JS, McGonigal M, Cook J, et al. A comparison of peripheral blood stem cell apheresis using the Fenwall CS3000 Plus and COBE Spectra. Transfus Sci 1995;16:71–7.
301. Klein HG. Cellular gene therapy. A credible odyssey. Transfusion 1997;37:675–7.
302. Menitove JE. Standards for hematopoietic progenitor cells. Bethesda (MD): American Association of Blood Banks; 1996.
303. Foundation for the Accreditation of Hematopoietic Cell Therapy. Standards for hematopoietic progenitor cell collection, processing, and transplantation. 1996.
304. Proposed approach to regulation of cellular and tissue-based products. Availability and public meeting. Fed Register 1997;62:9721–2.
305. Establishment registration and listing for manufacturers of human cellular and tissue-based products. Fed Register 1998;63:26744–55.
306. Slichter SJ. Leukocyte reduction and ultraviolet B irradiation of platelets to prevent alloimmunization and refractoriness to platelet transfusions. N Engl J Med 1997;337:1861–9.
307. Heddle NM, Klama L, Singer J, et al. The role of plasma supernatant from platelet concentrates in transfusion reactions. N Engl J Med 1994;331:625–8.
308. Muylle L, Peetermans ME. Effect of prestorage leukocyte removal on the cytokine levels in stored platelet concentrates. Vox Sang 1994;66:14–7.
309. Muylle L, Joos M, Wouters E, et al. Increased tumor necrosis factor α (TNFα), interleukin 1, and interleukin 6 (IL-6) levels in the plasma of stored platelet concentrates. Relationship between TNFα and IL-6 levels and febrile transfusion reactions. Transfusion 1993;33:195–9.
310. Zingsem J, Zimmermann R, Weisbach V, et al. Comparison of COBE white cell-reduction and standard plateletpheresis protocols in the same donors. Transfusion 1997;37:1045–9.
311. Moog R, Muller N. White cell reduction during plateletpheresis. A comparison of three blood cell separators. Transfusion 1999;39:572–7.
312. Palmer DS, Aye MT, Dumont L, et al. Prevention of cytokine accumulation in platelets obtained with the COBE Spectra apheresis system. Vox Sang 1998;75:115–23.
313. Chalandon Y, Mermillod B, Beris P, et al. Benefit of prestorage leukocyte depletion of single-donor platelet concentrates. Vox Sang 1999;76:27–37.
314. Stack G, Snyder EL. Cytokine generation in stored platelet concentrates. Transfusion 1994;34:20–5.
315. Heddle NM, Klama L, Meyer R, et al. A randomized controlled trial comparing plasma removal with white cell reduction to prevent reactions to platelets. Transfusion 1999;39:231–8.
316. Shiba M, Tadokoro K, Sawanobori M, et al. Activation of the contact system by filtration of platelet concentrates with a negatively charged white cell-removal filter and measurement of venous blood bradykinin level in patients who received filtered platelets. Transfusion 1997;37:457–62.
317. Hume H, Popovsky MA, Benson K, et al. Hypotensive reactions. A previously unrecognized complication of platelet transfusion. Transfusion 1996;36:904–9.
318. Wenz B, Ciavarella D, Freundlich L. Effect of prestorage white cell reduction on bacterial growth in platelet concentrates. Transfusion 1993;33:520–3.

Coagulopathic Complications of Cancer Patients

Maria T. DeSancho, MD
Jacob H. Rand, MD, FACP

Bleeding and thrombotic complications are important causes of morbidity and mortality in cancer patients. As a result of improvements in cancer treatment, the prevalence of these complications has been progressively increasing in recent years. Bleeding is common in patients with leukemias, particularly those with acute promyelocytic leukemia, where up to 90% of patients develop hemorrhage.[1] In general, bleeding complications occur relatively infrequently in patients with solid tumors, except those with melanoma, germ cell tumors, carcinoma of the cecum, and prostate cancer.[2] Thrombotic complications are common and may be a consequence of prothrombotic hemostatic changes that occur in more than 90% of cancer patients.[3] An indication of the frequency of thrombosis is the finding that venous thromboembolism is diagnosed postmortem in approximately 50% of cancer patients.[4,5]

This chapter reviews the physiology of normal hemostasis, and then discusses the relationship of the coagulation system and cancer, and the pathophysiology of bleeding and thrombosis in the cancer patient. Next, the diagnostic and treatment approaches to the disorders most frequently encountered in cancer patients are described. Finally, potential novel treatments such as recombinant factor VIIa concentrate; the synthetic pentasaccharide, fondaparinux; and the oral direct thrombin inhibitors are reviewed.

PHYSIOLOGY OF NORMAL HEMOSTASIS

Hemostasis is the physiologic mechanism that stems bleeding after injury to the vasculature. Normal hemostasis depends on both cellular components and soluble plasma proteins. Circulating platelets adhere and aggregate at sites of blood vessel injury. The adhesion is dependent on the presence of the von Willebrand's factor (vWF) and is followed by an aggregation response. Activation of platelets results in exposure of anionic phospholipids that serve as platforms for the assembly of blood coagulation enzyme complexes. The extrinsic pathway of blood coagulation is initiated when blood is exposed to tissue factor (TF), a transmembrane protein expressed in the deeper portions of the blood vessel wall that may also be present in stimulated endothelial cells. Thrombus propagation occurs via incorporation of active, blood-borne TF into the growing clot.[6] TF binds activated factor VII (factor VIIa) and the resulting complex activates factors X and IX. Activated factor IX (factor IXa) combines with factor VIIIa to provide

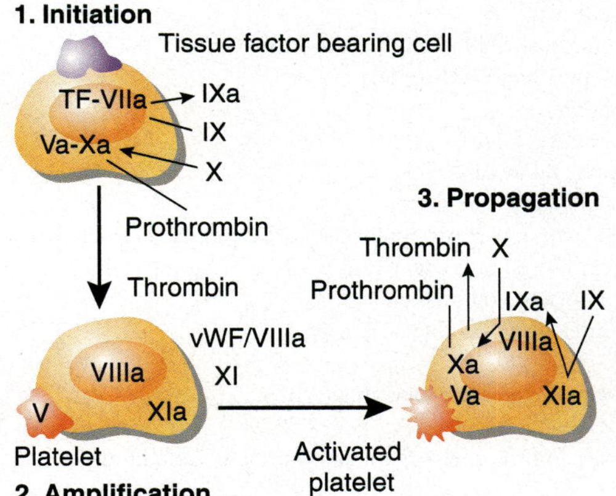

Figure 132-1 Tissue factor bearing membranes include stimulated monocytes, endothelial cells, circulating microparticles, vascular smooth muscle cells, brain cells, lung cells, placental mesenchymal cells and keratinocytes at the level of stratum granulosum.

a second pathway to activate factor X. Factor Xa complexes with factor Va and prothrombin to form prothrombinase, which cleaves prothrombin to generate thrombin, the key enzyme in hemostasis. In the final step of the coagulation cascade, thrombin cleaves fibrinogen to generate fibrin monomers, which then polymerize (Figure 132-1). This polymer is covalently cross-linked by factor XIIIa (itself generated from factor XIII by thrombin) to form a chemically stable clot. Thrombin also feeds back to activate cofactors V, VIII, and XI, further amplifying the coagulation system (Figure 132-2).

Fibrin deposition is limited by an endogenous anticoagulant system. Antithrombin (AT) is a plasma protein member of the serpin (serine protease inhibitor) family that inhibits the activities of all of the activated coagulation enzymes. Protein C is a vitamin K-dependent protein that proteolyses factor Va and factor VIIIa to inactive fragments. Protein C binds to an endothelial cell protein C receptor (EPCR) and is activated by thrombin bound to thrombomodulin, another endothelial cell membrane-based protein, in a reaction that is modulated by a cofactor, protein S. Tissue factor pathway inhibitor is a plasma protein that forms a quaternary complex with tissue factor, factor VIIa, and factor Xa, thereby inhibiting the extrinsic coagulation pathway.[5]

Finally, fibrin is digested by the fibrinolytic system, the major components of which are plasminogen and tissue-type plasminogen activator (tPA). Both of these proteins are incorporated into polymerizing fibrin, where they interact to generate plasmin, which, in turn, acts on fibrin to dissolve the preformed clot.[5,7] The fibrinolytic system is regulated by three serine proteinase inhibitors, namely, antiplasmin, plasminogen activator inhibitor-1 (PAI-1), and plasminogen activator inhibitor-2 (PAI-2).[7]

RELATIONSHIP OF COAGULATION SYSTEM AND CANCER

The earliest description of the relationship between blood coagulation and cancer in the medical literature dates back to the latter half of the nineteenth century when Trousseau reported the association of migratory thrombophlebitis and gastric carcinoma.[8] In 1878, Billroth demonstrated cancer cells within a thrombus and theorized that tumor cells were spread by thromboembolism.[9] The link between the coagulation system and cancer is supported by the demonstration of thromboplastic activity of circulating tumor cells, the discovery of a "cancer procoagulant factor," factor X activation and production of prothrombinase by tumor cells, and fibrin deposition in and around cancerous tissue.[10] These latter observations have prompted the investigational use of anticoagulants for the prevention and treatment of various cancers in animal models and in humans.[11] Platelets and fibrinogen have been shown to protect metastatic tumor cells from elimination by natural killer cells indicating a relevant mechanistic link between activation of the coagulation system and the spread of tumor metastases.[12]

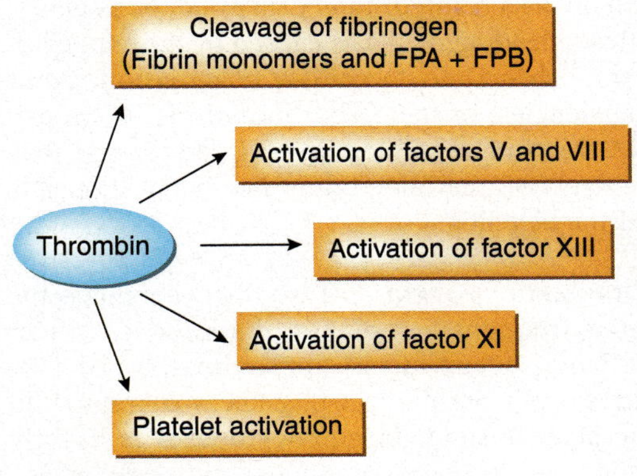

Figure 132-2

Table 132-1 Hemostatic Abnormalities in Cancer Patients

Abnormality	Mechanism
Platelets	
Thrombocytopenia	Marrow infiltration by tumor Chemotherapy effects Biological response modifiers Monoclonal antibodies and immunotoxins DIC Hypersplenism Immune mediated (autoimmune, alloimmune) Microangiopathic hemolytic anemia (TTP and HUS)
Thrombocytosis	Increased production: reactive, primary Myeloproliferative disorders
Platelet function abnormalities	Uremia Acquired von Willebrand's syndrome Myeloproliferative disorders
Abnormalities in coagulation factors and coagulation activation markers	
Hypofibrinogenemia	Asparaginase, DIC
Dysfibrinogenemia	Hepatocellular carcinoma
Factor X (decreased)	Amyloidosis
Decreased coagulation factors	Impairment in hepatic synthesis, DIC, vitamin K deficiency
Elevated prothrombin fragment 1+2	Disseminated malignancies
Elevated thrombin-antithrombin (TAT) complexes	Disseminated malignancies
Thrombus precursor protein (TpP)	Measures fibrin soluble polymers
Fibrinolysis	
Increased secretion of plasminogen activators	Acute promyelocytic leukemia (APL)
Overexpression of annexin II	APL
Decreased levels of plasminogen activator inhibitors	Increased fibrin(ogen) degradation products and D-dimer
Acquired thrombophilias	
Antithrombin deficiency	Impaired hepatic synthesis of anticoagulant proteins, DIC
Protein C deficiency	Impaired hepatic synthesis, DIC
Protein S deficiency	Impaired hepatic synthesis, DIC
Tissue factor pathway inhibitor deficiency (TFPI)	Impaired hepatic synthesis, DIC
Cytokines and hemostasis	
Proinflammatory cytokines (IL-1, IL-6, TNF)	Key role in tissue factor expression in monocytes and endothelial cells

DIC = disseminated intravascular coagulation; HUS = hemolytic uremic syndrome; IL = interleukin; TNF = tumor necrosis factor; TTP = thrombotic thrombocytopenic purpura.

Table 132-2 Differential Diagnosis of Thrombocytopenia in Cancer Patients

- Decreased platelet production
  - Metastases to bone marrow
  - Acute and chronic leukemias
  - Lymphomas
  - Plasma cell dyscrasias
  - Cytotoxic chemotherapy
  - Radiation therapy
- Platelet destruction
  - Medications
  - Immune mediated
  - Bacterial sepsis
  - Viral, fungal, and protozoal infections
  - DIC
  - TTP/HUS
- Splenic sequestration
  - Myeloproliferative disorders
  - Lymphomas
  - Chronic lymphocytic leukemias
- Combination of the above mechanisms

DIC = disseminated intravascular coagulation; HUS = hemolytic uremic syndrome; TTP = thrombotic thrombocytopenic purpura.

BLEEDING DISORDERS

Cancer can cause both quantitative and qualitative changes in platelets.[13] Reactive thrombocytosis occurs in approximately 60% of cancer patients, while thrombocytopenia occurs in up to 11% of patients with untreated malignancy (Table 132-1).

The major bleeding problems are commonly caused by tumor invasion of blood vessels and adjacent organs, complications of treatment, and vitamin K deficiency.[13] Bleeding in the cancer patient may present as either localized bleeding, usually as a result of tumor invasion, or as generalized bleeding diathesis caused by thrombocytopenia, thrombocytopathies, coagulation factor deficiencies, or increased fibrinolysis. Appropriate treatment of bleeding in cancer patients depends on the underlying disorder responsible for the bleeding.

Thrombocytopenia Thrombocytopenia is the most frequent hemostatic disorder in cancer patients, occurring in approximately 10% of cases, even prior to starting chemotherapy.[13] In the acute setting, thrombocytopenia is usually caused by decreased production either secondary to chemotherapy and/or radiation therapy, or bone marrow infiltration, platelet sequestration in the spleen, or increased peripheral[13] destruction, such as in sepsis, disseminated intravascular coagulation (DIC), and thrombotic thrombocytopenic purpura (TTP)/hemolytic uremic syndrome (HUS)[14] (Table 132-2). Thrombocytopenia has also been described with the use of cytokines such as interferon[15] and from treatment with certain monoclonal antibodies such as gemtuzumab ozogamicin (Mylotarg), a humanized monoclonal antibody that targets leukemia cells that express CD33.[16] Thrombocytopenia as a result of bone marrow infiltration commonly occurs in patients with small-cell lung cancer, breast cancer, and prostate cancer, as well as in patients with acute leukemia. On the other hand, thrombocytopenia secondary to splenic sequestration is usually observed with myeloproliferative disorders and less commonly with lymphomas and chronic lymphocytic leukemia (CLL). Clinically evident bleeding episodes are more likely to occur when thrombocytopenia is caused by diminished production of megakaryocytes rather than by immune system destruction.

The most common clinical manifestation of thrombocytopenia is mucocutaneous bleeding. This can occur in the form of petechiae, ecchymoses, epistaxis, oral, gastrointestinal, or genitourinary bleeding. Spontaneous bleeding usually does not occur unless the platelet count is less than 10,000/mm^3. However, in the presence of sepsis, uremia, trauma, or surgery, bleeding complications may occur with a higher platelet count.

The clinical history, physical examination, review of medications, and timing of prior chemotherapy or radiation therapy must be reviewed. In addition, examination of the peripheral blood smear is vital in the diagnostic work-up of thrombocytopenia in the cancer patient. The physician should exclude the possibility of spurious thrombocytopenia, which is manifested by platelet clumping on the peripheral smear or platelet satellitism (platelets surrounding the polymorphonuclear leukocytes).

The treatment of bleeding associated with thrombocytopenia in the cancer patient is often managed empirically even when a specifically defined cause cannot be identified. Table 132-3 lists the critical platelet counts in various situations and general guidelines for platelet transfusion.[17]

Table 132-3 Critical Platelet Counts and Recommendations for Transfusion in Cancer Patients[a]

Platelet Count Threshold	
Mucocutaneous or gastrointestinal bleeding	> 50,000
Leukemias	
Pre-induction chemotherapy	> 20,000
Acute promyelocytic leukemia	>5,000–10,000
Prophylaxis	
Asymptomatic	>5,000
Major surgery	>50,000
Invasive procedures	
Major	> 50,000
Minor	>20,000

[a]These are intended to serve as general guidelines. Actual treatment will vary depending on specific circumstances.

Prophylactic transfusion of platelets is not indicated in patients who are asymptomatic for bleeding unless the platelet count is below 5,000/mm^3.[18,19] However, in cancer patients undergoing chemotherapy and those with leukemia, prophylactic platelet transfusions are generally beneficial in decreasing the risk of bleeding when the platelet count is below 10,000/mm^3.[20,21] A few studies have supported the safety of a lower platelet transfusion threshold in the range of 5,000/mm^3 to 10,000/mm^3 in leukemic patients undergoing induction chemotherapy.[22] For cancer patients undergoing major surgery or invasive procedures such as central venous catheterization, bronchial or endoscopic biopsy, lumbar puncture, thoracentesis, thoracostomy tube placement, and abdominal paracentesis, it is generally recommended that platelet transfusions should be administered in thrombocytopenic patients to a target level of greater than 50,000/mm^3.[23] For minor invasive procedures, such as arterial puncture or cannulation, prophylactic transfusion is not necessary as long as the platelet count is at least 20,000/mm^3 and local pressure is applied at the puncture site until hemostasis is achieved. Platelet transfusions are usually indicated in thrombocytopenic patients to keep the platelet count above 50,000/mm^3 when evidence of microscopic or gross bleeding is detected, as manifested by either occult blood on stool guaiac tests and mucocutaneous bleeding. The risk of central nervous system (CNS) bleeding is generally low, and bleeding depends on several factors such as etiology of thrombocytopenia, coagulation abnormalities, impaired renal or hepatic function, severe sepsis, trauma, and the use of mechanical ventilation. Subdural hematomas occur in approximately 2.5 to 5%[24] of patients with leukemia following bone marrow transplantation (BMT), and intracerebral hematomas in 2%.[25,26] Comparative studies show that platelets derived from single or random donors produce similar post-transfusion increments, hemostatic benefits, and side effects. Single-donor platelets from selected donors are preferred when histocompatible platelet transfusions are needed.[27] Platelet transfusions should be individualized depending on the etiology of the thrombocytopenia and complicating factors, such as coagulation abnormalities, anticoagulant therapy, disruption of the vascular system, platelet dysfunction, and the anatomic location of tumors.[28]

Thrombocytopathies In addition to quantitative platelet changes, cancer can also cause qualitative platelet abnormalities. The main disorders are described below.

Acquired von Willebrand's Syndrome For a review, the reader is referred to an article by Federici and colleagues.[29] Several types of cancer have been reported in association with acquired von Willebrand's syndrome, including plasma cell dyscrasias, myeloproliferative disorders, leukemias, lymphomas, and solid tumors such as nephroblastoma, gastric carcinoma, and cancer of the adrenal gland.[30] The clinical manifestations of acquired von Willebrand's syndrome are similar to those seen in patients with the hereditary form of the disease, except for the notable absence of a family history or lifelong personal history for bleeding. Spontaneous mucocutaneous and gastrointestinal bleeding may be present. Postsurgical bleeding may also occur. Laboratory screening tests generally reveal a prolonged activated partial thromboplastin time (aPTT) and a normal or borderline prolonged bleeding time. Specific assays for plasma vWF antigen, vWF ristocetin cofactor activity, ristocetin-induced platelet aggregation, and vWF collagen-binding activity are generally decreased. Laboratory tests usually fail to demonstrate inhibitory activity against vWF or factor VIII. Treatment is directed to the underlying malignancy and supportive measures such as corticosteroids, deamino-8-D-arginine vasopressin (desmopressin acetate or DDAVP), factor VIII/vWF concentrate, and intravenous immunoglobulin.[31]

Acquired Hemophilia (Factor VIII Autoantibodies) Patients with solid tumors, plasma cell dyscrasias, and lymphoproliferative disorders may develop an acquired hemophilia as a consequence of inhibitors against factor VIII, also referred to as "spontaneous inhibitors," in contrast to the inhibitors that occur in patients with the hereditary form of hemophilia A. The inhibitors are autoantibodies and almost always immunoglobulin G (IgG) molecules. The most common presenting complaint is bleeding into the skin or muscles.[32] The hallmark of antibodies directed against factor VIII is a prolongation of the aPTT in the presence of a normal prothrombin time along with plasma mixing studies that demonstrate an aPTT that remains prolonged after incubation at 37°C for 1 to 2 hours. In contrast, in patients with coagulation factor deficiencies, plasma mixing studies normalize the aPTT. Contamination of the sample with heparin, which frequently is the inadvertent result of instillation for maintaining vascular access line patency, may artifactually prolong the aPTT and affect mixing tests. Heparin that has entered the sample may be removed with the enzyme reptilase or resin absorption, after which the plasma may be retested. A prolonged thrombin time in the presence of a normal reptilase time confirms the suspicion of heparin contamination. The objectives in the treatment of acquired factor VIII inhibitors in patients with cancer are twofold: (1) management of the acute bleeding and (2) elimination of the autoantibody against factor VIII. The acute bleeding can be managed with desmopressin acetate if there is a low inhibitor titer (< 5 Bethesda units [BU]) or with recombinant human factor VIII, porcine factor VIII, recombinant human factor VIIa, or activated prothrombin complex concentrate in case of moderate- to high-titer inhibitor (> 5 BU). Immunosuppressive therapy such as corticosteroids, cyclophosphamide, and intravenous immunoglobulin (IVIg) may be used in addition to the treatment of the underlying neoplasm.[33] Recently, the successful use of the anti-CD20 monoclonal antibody, rituximab in patients with acquired factor VIII inhibitors has been reported.[34]

Uremia Platelet dysfunction is common in cancer patients with chronic renal failure and causes significant bleeding. Treatment is recommended for patients with active bleeding or for those undergoing an invasive procedure, such as placement of a permanent intravenous catheter for hemodialysis. Patients usually respond to hemodialysis and administration of DDAVP. Occasionally, cryoprecipitate may be required. Recombinant erythropoietin has been shown to reduce and prevent bleeding in uremic patients and has a more sustained effect than either DDAVP or conjugated estrogens.[35,36] Darbepoetin alfa is an erythropoiesis-stimulating protein closely related to erythropoietin that has a threefold longer half-life than recombinant human erythropoietin (rHuEPO), allowing less-frequent dosing for treatment of anemia.[37,38]

Myeloproliferative Disorders Among the myeloproliferative conditions, polycythemia vera and essential thrombocythemia are the most likely to be associated with hemorrhagic and thrombotic complications. In a series of 74 young women with essential thrombocythemia, the incidence of hemorrhage was 26%. Most of these episodes were minor; however, major hemorrhagic events occurred in 4%.[39] The incidence of thrombosis was 18%, of which major episodes were found in 7% of the patients. Increasing age, a previous thrombotic event, and long duration of thrombocytosis were identified as major risk factors for thrombosis.[40] The template bleeding time is significantly prolonged in 7 to 19% of essential thrombocythemia patients; and several functional platelet abnormalities have been found in platelet structure, biochemistry, and survival. However, the attempt to relate these in vivo and in vitro abnormalities with diagnosis and clinical sequelae has been disappointing in most instances. Therefore, bleeding time and platelet function tests are not recommended in the initial evaluation or during follow-up of patients with essential thrombocythemia, unless in the setting of a clinical or biologic protocol.[41] An exception is represented by a subset of patients with a very high platelet count (> 1,500 × 10^9/L) and bleeding symptoms. These patients can have an acquired form of von Willebrand's disease. In these cases, prolonged bleeding time and abnormal multimeric pattern of vWF on electrophoresis are useful for diagnosing and monitoring this acquired hemorrhagic disease.[41]

Untreated patients with polycythemia vera do poorly, with the main cause of death being thrombosis. In a review of 253 patients with Budd-Chiari syndrome, polycythemia vera was found to be the etiology in approximately 10%.[42] Cytoreductive therapy with hydroxyurea and supplemental phlebotomy when required significantly diminish the risk of thrombosis when compared with a historical control group of patients treated with phlebotomy alone.[43] Aspirin is generally effective in relieving vasomotor and microvascular occlusive symptoms, but there is limited evidence that its use reduces large vessel thrombosis. Low-dose aspirin can also be used for low-risk patients such as patients younger than 60 years old with no previous history of thrombosis, no cardiovascular risk factors, and whose platelet counts are less than $1,500 \times 10^9$/L.[44]

COAGULATION FACTOR DEFICIENCIES

Cancer patients may develop various coagulation factor abnormalities resulting from vitamin K deficiency as a consequence of malnutrition, diarrhea, liver disease, biliary obstruction, use of oral anticoagulants, and antibiotic therapy. Patients with primary or metastatic hepatocellular carcinoma have deficiency of vitamin K–dependent factors (factors II, VII, IX, X, protein C, and S), similar to that seen with liver cirrhosis. These patients almost always have increased levels of fibrinogen, unlike patients with cirrhosis or acute liver failure who have decreased fibrinogen levels. Acquired inhibitors of coagulation factors are frequently seen in multiple myeloma and other dysproteinemias.

The treatment of cancer patients with coagulation factor deficiencies, aside from the treatment of the underlying neoplasm, is generally supportive and consists of vitamin K, fresh-frozen plasma, and cryoprecipitate. Oral vitamin K is the treatment of choice, and its administration is predictably effective and has the advantages of safety and convenience over parenteral routes.[45] However, vitamin K is usually administered via subcutaneous (SC) route. The response to subcutaneous vitamin K may be unpredictable and sometimes delayed.[46,47] Occasionally, an oncologist may want to achieve a rapid response by using IV vitamin K.[48] In that situation, it is generally advisable to give 1 to 2 mg of vitamin K by slow IV infusion (over at least 30 min) to minimize the risk of anaphylactic reactions and fatty emboli resulting from the lipid emulsion.[49] Fresh-frozen plasma should be transfused when immediate correction of coagulation factor deficiencies is required. The usual dose for fresh-frozen plasma is 10 to 15 mL/kg by IV infusion. Cryoprecipitate is the cold precipitable protein fraction derived from plasma, which is rich in vWF, fibrinogen, fibronectin, and factor XIII. It is indicated for hypofibrinogenemic states and also for some patients with renal failure. Cryoprecipitate is administered IV, generally at a dose of 1 unit of cryoprecipitate for every 5 kg of body weight.[50]

Amyloidosis Acquired factor X deficiency has been particularly described in patients with primary amyloidosis, although acquired deficiencies of factors II, V, IX, and X have all been reported.[51,52] It is believed to be caused by adsorption of factor X on amyloid fibrils in the liver and the spleen.[53] It is manifested as a serious bleeding disorder that is associated with a prolongation of the prothrombin time (PT) and the aPTT. Moreover, prolongations of the thrombin time (TT) and reptilase time (RT) have also been found; these are not dependent on the presence of heparin-like substances in the plasma or on fibrinogen levels.

DRUG EFFECTS (L-ASPARAGINASE)

L-Asparaginase is used in combination with other agents, for induction of remissions in acute lymphocytic leukemia. L-asparaginase can cause depletion of many of the coagulation factors with an associated risk of thrombosis and hemorrhage. Vitamin K–dependent proteins are significantly decreased during L-asparaginase therapy. The timing and severity of decrease vary among the proteins. The decrease in protein C and factors IX and X occur earlier than the decrease in protein S and factor II. This transient imbalance in the levels of plasma vitamin K–dependent proteins may contribute to the risk of thrombosis associated with L-asparaginase therapy.[54] Treatment with L-asparaginase also induces a marked decrease in fibrinogen and plasminogen levels.[55] In a study of 10 patients with acute lymphoblastic leukemia or lymphoma treated with L-asparaginase,[56] the following changes were observed: significant prolongation of the prothrombin time and activated partial thromboplastin time; markedly decreased fibrinogen level; and decreased antithrombin, protein C, protein S, plasminogen, and α-2-antiplasmin. Levels of tissue-type plasminogen activator and plasminogen activator inhibitor were increased during the treatment. Cross-linked fibrin degradation products remained within normal limits during treatment, excluding the presence of disseminated intravascular coagulation.

ACUTE PROMYELOCYTIC LEUKEMIA

Acute promyelocytic leukemia (APL)–associated hemostasis disorders result from at least two distinct mechanisms, the release of procoagulant activities and of plasminogen activators from the leukemic cells. It appears that plasmin-dependent primary fibrinogenolysis is the major etiologic factor for low fibrinogen levels in APL patients. In vivo differentiation therapy with all-*trans*-retinoic acid induces a rapid decrease in plasmin activation and a normalization of fibrinogen level, while DIC may persist in vivo for several weeks.[57] More recently, a receptor for fibrinolytic proteins, annexin A2 (previously known as annexin II), was described on cells from patients with APL and some other leukemias (Figure 132-3). Overexpression of annexin A2, with the resultant increased production of plasmin, appears to be a mechanism for excessive fibrin(ogen)olysis and the hemorrhagic complications in the 15;17 translocation subset of APL.[58]

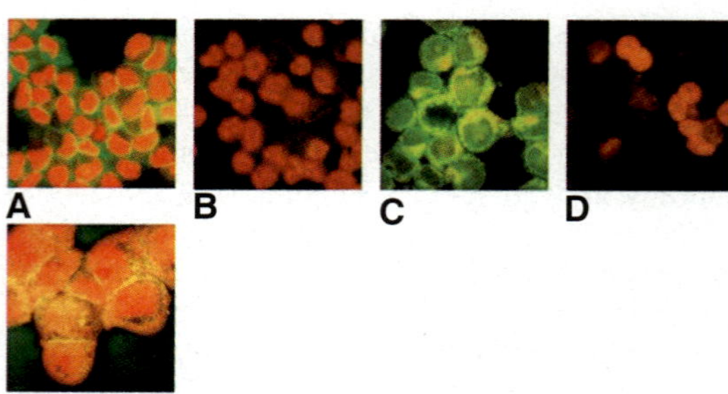

Figure 132-3 Immunofluorescence staining of APL cells with anti–annexin II antibodies. Cells from two patients with t (15;17)–positive APL (**A**, and **C**) and one patient with AML characterized by minimal myeloid differentiation (**D**) and cells from the t (15;17)–negative APL cell line (**E**) were stained with anti–annexin II (**A**, ×600; **C**, **D**, and **E**, ×1,000). The t (15;17)–positive APL cells shown in **A** were also stained with preimmune IgG (**B**, ×600). Cells were counterstained with propidium iodide (**A**, **B**, **D**, and **E**) or Evans blue (**C**).

THROMBOTIC COMPLICATIONS

Cancer patients frequently develop alterations in hemostasis, including platelet abnormalities, abnormal activation of the coagulation cascade, release of plasminogen activator, and decreased hepatic synthesis of anticoagulant and coagulant proteins (see Table 132-1).[59] Platelet aggregation and activation in cancer patients may be triggered by the shedding of membrane glycolipids into the host circulation by tumor cells.[60] Platelet activation by tumor cells also generates thrombin, which, in turn, stimulates platelets to supply factor V and the phospholipids necessary for the activation of factor X.[61]

Cancer causes an increase in coagulation factors V, VIII, IX, XI, and fibrinogen, and in fibrinogen degradation products.[62] The presence of increased levels of coagulation activation markers such as prothrombin fragment 1 + 2 (PF1 + 2), thrombin-antithrombin (TAT), fibrinogen/fibrin degradation products, and D-dimer in cancer patients that indicate a consumptive coagulation process is often seen in patients with malignancy.[63] These coagulation activation markers are increased in cancer patients with disseminated or extensive disease.[64] The thrombus precursor protein (TpP), which measures soluble fibrin polymers, is a sensitive marker of the prothrombotic process and may have the advantage of being more sensitive and specific than the D-dimer, TAT, and prothrombin fragment 1 + 2 to an active thrombotic event. An elevated TpP level may help to differentiate the hypercoagulable state of malignancy from that of actual fibrin formation and thrombosis.[65]

A variety of cancers may secrete plasminogen activators, which can increase the permeability of blood vessel walls and promote migration of tumor cells.[66] In addition, impaired fibrinolysis with increased levels of PAI-1 may be present in solid tumors.[67] Both plasminogen activators and their inhibitors are involved in the processes of tumor invasion, proliferation, and metastasis.[68]

Decreased hepatic synthesis of AT, protein C, and protein S have been demonstrated in cancer patients and correlate with serum albumin levels.[69] In addition, chemotherapy-induced reduction in these anticoagulant proteins is believed responsible for the thrombotic complications frequently observed in bone marrow transplant patients treated with high-dose regimens.[70] The decreased hepatic synthesis has been attributed to both hepatic metastases and the effect of cytokines involved in cancer cachexia, in particular, tumor necrosis factor (TNF).[13]

Table 132-4 Risk Factors for Bleeding and Thrombotic Complications in Cancer Patients

Use of indwelling catheters
Systemic inflammatory response syndrome (SIRS)
Sepsis
Prior chemotherapy and radiation treatment
Selective estrogen receptor modulators (SERMs): tamoxifen, raloxifene
Concomitant use of hormone replacement therapy or oral contraceptives
Metastatic disease to the liver and/or bone marrow
Vitamin K deficiency
Acute peptic ulcer
Slipped ligatures from recent surgery

Thrombotic complications in cancer patients have been attributed to multiple factors. These include increases in platelet aggregation and activation; tumor, chemotherapy, or hormonal adjuvant therapy-induced activation of the coagulation system; decreased hepatic synthesis or increased consumption of natural anticoagulant proteins; decreased hepatic clearance of activated coagulation factors; and autoimmune phenomena, such as the presence of antiphospholipid antibodies. Several factors contribute to the increased risk of bleeding and thrombotic complications in the cancer patient (Table 132-4).

Thrombotic manifestations in cancer patients may present as one of the following: migratory thrombophlebitis or Trousseau's syndrome, venous thromboembolism (VTE), thrombotic microangiopathy (TTP/HUS), arterial thrombosis, and DIC.

Migratory Thrombophlebitis (Trousseau's Syndrome) Trousseau's syndrome is a classically described variant form of venous thrombosis characterized by a recurrent and migratory pattern preferentially involving superficial veins of the arms and chest.[8] This syndrome should precipitate the search for an occult malignancy, especially in patients with recurrent and migratory venous thrombosis affecting unusual sites such as subclavian veins, or veins of upper extremities, axilla or neck.[71] Trousseau's syndrome is highly associated with adenocarcinomas and laboratory evidence of DIC. Migratory thrombophlebitis has also been associated with the use of somatostatin or octreotide therapy for malignant carcinoid syndrome.[72]

Venous Thromboembolism Venous thromboembolism (VTE), as manifested by deep venous thrombosis (DVT) and pulmonary embolism (PE), is diagnosed in up to 15% of cancer patients.[59] The overall incidence of cancer-related VTE in postmortem studies is much higher, however, ranging between 35 and 50%.[4] In patients presenting with de novo idiopathic VTE, there is a high risk of a concurrent cancer, especially within the first year after the diagnosis for the thromboembolism.[73] Cancer patients at greatest risk of VTE include those with mucin-secreting tumors (eg, pancreatic and gastrointestinal cancer), cancers of the lung, brain, prostate, breast, and ovary, and patients with acute promyelocytic leukemia and myeloproliferative disorders, specifically polycythemia vera and essential thrombocythemia.[74] VTE often complicates the care of cancer patients undergoing major surgery and of patients receiving chemotherapy and/or hormonal therapy.[75] The risk of developing thrombosis in cancer patients is influenced by the age and hormonal status of the patient. Postmenopausal women with advanced breast cancer receiving tamoxifen in addition to adjuvant chemotherapy have a higher risk of thrombotic events than do premenopausal women with breast cancer.[76] Thromboembolic events have been also reported with thalidomide therapy. During the first 18 months of US market availability, 27 spontaneous postmarketing reports of thromboembolic events were received for patients treated with thalidomide. Of these, 26 were received for patients being treated for cancer; 12 had multiple myeloma.[77] In one study, 100 patients with multiple myeloma were randomly assigned to receive thalidomide along with combination chemotherapy or chemotherapy alone. Fourteen of 50 patients receiving thalidomide developed DVT (28%), while DVT was diagnosed in only 2 of 50 patients who were not treated with that drug.[78] Further studies suggest that thalidomide may induce an acquired activated protein C resistance as a mechanism for thrombosis.[79] Bevacizumab, a monoclonal antibody to vascular endothelial growth factor has also been associated with an increased risk of thrombosis.[80]

In recent years, there have been major advances in the diagnosis of VTE. These include the development and validation of a standardized clinical model to determine the pretest probability of VTE, and the measurement of plasma D-dimer. The integration of these two advances has resulted in the formulation of safe, diagnostic algorithms that decrease the need for serial and/or invasive testing.[81] Of the various clinical models for DVT assessment, the model developed by Wells and colleagues has been validated for its reliability and accuracy.[82] In a clinical trial where this model was combined with compression ultrasonography, the need for venography and serial compression ultrasonography testing was decreased.[83] Laboratory testing for the measurement of D-dimer can be performed by enzyme-linked immunosorbent assay, latex agglutination assay, or by a rapid bedside whole-blood assay. Of the three assays, the whole-blood assay reportedly has the best predictive value with sensitivity rates in symptomatic general medical patients ranging from 85 to 95% and specificity rates of 65 to 68%.[84] However, a negative D-dimer in cancer patients does not reliably exclude VTE.[85] As with other patients, the majority of DVT in cancer patients originate in the ileofemoral venous system. Diagnostic imaging modalities for DVT include ascending contrast venography, compression ultrasonography, impedance plethysmography, and magnetic resonance venography. Ascending contrast venography remains the gold standard for diagnosing DVT, but this procedure is invasive and requires contrast material, which is frequently irritating and may result in complications. The finding of an intraluminal filling defect caused by thrombus surrounded by contrast is diagnostic for DVT. Noncompressibility of a proximal lower limb vein on compression ultrasonography has a diagnostic sensitivity rate of 97% and a specificity rate of 94%.[86] Although compression ultrasonography is highly sensitive for detecting proximal DVT, it is not as accurate for diagnosing isolated calf DVT. Magnetic resonance venography, a relatively new imaging modality that does not use contrast, has sensitivity and specificity rates > 95% for proximal DVT. It is potentially useful in diagnosing pelvic vein DVT, especially isolated iliac vein thrombosis, which is difficult to diagnose with compression ultrasonography.

Several studies conducted in patients with suspected DVT involving cancer have demonstrated that the combination of the following studies can reliably exclude DVT and decrease the need for invasive testing: a normal D-dimer level and a normal compression ultrasonogram,[87] a low pretest probability and normal compression ultrasonogram,[83] and a low pretest probability and a normal D-dimer level.

The standard treatment of VTE outside the setting of malignancy is to initiate anticoagulation with either intravenous or subcutaneous unfractionated heparin (UFH) or subcutaneous low-molecular-weight heparin (LMWH) at therapeutic doses followed by oral warfarin therapy for a minimum of 3 months to achieve an international normalized ratio (INR) between 2.0 and 3.0.[88] However, in patients with active cancer, the available evidence supports committing the patient to continued anticoagulation following the first episode of VTE.[89] Intravenous UFH is usually started with an initial bolus of 80 U/kg followed by a continuous IV infusion of 18 U/kg/h, adjusted to maintain the aPTT at 1.5 to 2.5 times the control value.[90] Alternatively, LMWH can be administered in weight-adjusted, once or twice daily subcutaneous doses without the need for laboratory monitoring. Warfarin therapy is commenced within 24 hours after heparin treatment is started.[91] Heparin therapy is continued for at least 5 days until the INR is within the therapeutic range for 2 consecutive days. However, in patients with large ileofemoral vein thrombosis or major pulmonary embolism, some investigators have recommended extending heparin treatment to 7 to 10 days.[92]

Studies conducted over the past decade show that LMWHs are as safe and effective as UFH in the initial treatment of VTE.[93] Preliminary evidence from meta-analyses of large randomized studies suggests that LMWHs may reduce mortality in cancer patients.[94] LMWHs have several advantages when compared with UFH: laboratory monitoring is not required, only subcutaneous injection is necessary, and there are lower incidences of bleeding, heparin-induced thrombocytopenia,[95] and osteoporosis.[96] Two recent clinical trials evaluated the use of long-term LMWH as an alternative to warfarin therapy in cancer patients with acute VTE. The CANTHANOX trial compared 3 months of warfarin versus enoxaparin anticoagulation in cancer patients with DVT and or PE. Although the risk of recurrent VTE was lower in the enoxaparin group, the difference was not statistically significant. Warfarin was associated with a high bleeding rate.[97] In the CLOT trial, the cumulative risk of recurrent VTE at 6 months was reduced from 17% in the oral anticoagulant group to 9% in the LMWH group, resulting in a statistically significant risk reduction for VTE.[98] Overall, there were no differences in bleeding between the groups. Therefore the current recommendation for treatment of VTE in cancer patients is LMWH for at least the first 3 to 6 months of long-term treatment.[99]

The use of IV thrombolytic agents such as streptokinase and tPA for VTE should be restricted to patients with massive ileofemoral DVT or massive pulmonary embolism and hemodynamic instability because of the significant risks of bleeding associated with thrombolysis.[99] Furthermore, studies have thus far not shown any survival benefit with thrombolytic agents despite their proven efficacy in achieving more rapid resolution of radiologic and hemodynamic abnormalities in patients with pulmonary embolism. Catheter-directed thrombolysis for initial treatment of VTE should be confined to selected patients requiring limb salvage. It is important to note that thrombolytic therapy is generally contraindicated in cancer patients with brain metastases who develop VTE because of their significant risk of intracranial bleeding.[100] Surgical thromboembolectomy is restricted to patients with massive pulmonary embolism who have contraindications to or who do not respond to thrombolysis, and to centers that have the available resources.[99] For cancer patients with VTE who have contraindications to anticoagulant therapy or those with recurrent VTE despite anticoagulation, placement of an inferior vena cava (IVC) filter is generally recommended. Although this may be necessary, because of the absence of other treatment options, it is important to note that recent data suggest that IVC filters do not have any survival benefit and are associated with undesirable side effects, such as debilitating leg symptoms caused by filter-related thrombosis.[101] Consequently, some investigators advocate against placement of IVC filters in cancer patients with metastatic disease and poor prognosis.[102]

The major concern about treatment of VTE in cancer patients is the higher risk of bleeding and VTE recurrence compared with noncancer patients.[103] A prospective cohort study demonstrated that the 12-month cumulative incidence of recurrent VTE in cancer patients was 20.7% versus 6.8% in patients without cancer, and the parallel estimate for major bleeding was 12.4% versus 4.9%, respectively.[104] Recurrence and bleeding were both related to cancer severity and occurred predominantly during the first month of anticoagulant therapy, but could not be explained by sub- or overanticoagulation. Based on current published data, the risk of recurrent VTE is two- to threefold higher and the risk of major bleeding is three- to sixfold higher in cancer patients than in patients without cancer.[105]

Previous studies demonstrated that for cancer patients with indwelling central venous catheters, routine prophylaxis with either low-dose warfarin (1 mg daily) or LMWH (dalteparin 2,500 anti-Xa U daily) was efficacious.[106,107] It appears that the incidence of catheter-related thrombosis (CRT) in cancer patients is much lower than previously reported.[108] Thus, routine prophylaxis with either warfarin 1 mg daily or LMWH (dalteparin 2,500 IU SC once a day) is not recommended.[109,110] Alteplase, a recombinant tPA, is effective in restoring flow to indwelling catheters occluded by thrombus; 1 to 2 mg per lumen of tPA is a suitable dose for catheter instillation.[111] Perioperative cancer patients, particularly those with breast cancer undergoing chemotherapy or on selective estrogen receptor modulators (SERMs) and patients with advanced cancers that are associated with high risk of VTE, such as brain tumors, and colorectal, pancreatic, lung, renal cell, and ovarian adenocarcinomas, should receive antithrombotic prophylaxis with intermittent pneumatic compression devices or compression elastic stockings and either subcutaneous UFH or LMWH.[112] The recommended doses are low-dose UFH 5,000 U SC every 8 hours or LMWH, either dalteparin 5,000 U SC daily, or enoxaparin 40 mg SC daily, starting 8 to 12 hours postoperatively.[109] Two recent trials in cancer patients undergoing surgery reported that continuation of LMWH prophylaxis for 3 weeks after hospital discharge reduced the risk of late venographic DVT by 60%.[113,114] Finally, cancer patients who are immobile or bedridden with an acute medical illness also should receive antithrombotic prophylaxis with low-dose UFH or LMWH. However, ambulatory cancer patients require no VTE prophylaxis.[109]

ANTICANCER EFFECTS OF ANTICOAGULATION TREATMENT

Experimental and indirect clinical evidence suggests that anticoagulants, particularly LMWH may have antineoplastic effects. It has been suggested that anticoagulants can interfere with tumor angiogenesis, proliferation potential of cancer cells and with the immune system by augmenting the antitumor activity of tumor necrosis factor and of interferon-mediated by natural killer cells.[115] Anticoagulants may also interfere with the various stages of the metastatic cascade. In recent clinical trials, the use of dalteparin was associated with a trend toward improved survival in cancer patients with early disease.[116,117] Additional studies are needed to confirm the antitumor effects of LMWH.

HEPARIN-INDUCED THROMBOCYTOPENIA

Approximately 1 to 5% of patients receiving heparin develop an immune-mediated thrombocytopenia.[118,119] The decrease in platelet count typically occurs after 5 to 10 days after starting heparin, but may develop within 24 hours if there has been exposure to heparin during the preceding 3 months. Sometimes, the platelet count begins to fall in heparin-induced thrombocytopenia (HIT) only after heparin has been stopped (delayed-onset HIT).[120] The frequency of HIT varies according to the type of heparin preparation (bovine UFH > porcine UFH > LMWH) and the exposed patient population (postoperative > medical > pregnancy).[121] HIT is caused by heparin-dependent, platelet-activating antibodies that recognize platelet factor 4 (PF4) bound to heparin.[120,122] The resulting platelet activation is associated with increased thrombin generation. The most common complications associated with HIT are DVT and PE. Additionally, arterial thrombosis and embolism with the "white clot syndrome," stroke, myocardial infarction, peripheral vascular gangrene, and limb loss can occur. HIT should be suspected and treatment rapidly instituted in a patient whose platelet count decreases by 30 to 50% from baseline during heparin therapy.[120] The gold standard test for laboratory diagnosis is the platelet serotonin release assay; however, this test is cumbersome and is performed only in a few specialized coagulation laboratories. Alternatively, assays for the presence of antibody to platelet factor 4 complexed to heparin may be used and allows results to be available more rapidly. Management consists of discontinuing all forms of heparin and using lepirudin or argatroban, both of which are direct thrombin inhibitors with no cross-reactivity to HIT antibodies. Lepirudin is excreted by the kidney, and thus should not be used in patients with renal failure, particularly if the creatinine clearance is < 20 mL/min. The approved dose is 0.4 mg/kg (IV bolus) followed by an initial infusion rate at 0.15 mg/kg/h targeting the aPTT to 1.5 to 2.5× baseline. Argatroban is safer to use in patients with renal failure but since it is metabolized by the liver, the dose should be reduced in patients with hepatic impairment. The usual dosage is 2 μg/kg per minute targeting the aPTT to 1.5 to 3× baseline. The starting dose should be reduced by 75% in a patient with significant liver dysfunction. In countries where danaparoid, a heparinoid, is available, this agent may also be used for the prevention and treatment of HIT complicated by thrombosis.[121] Warfarin should be avoided during the acute HIT episode because it decreases the level of protein C and predisposes to microvascular thrombosis, for example, warfarin-induced venous limb gangrene and skin necrosis syndromes.[120] For patients receiving warfarin at the time of diagnosis of HIT, reversal of warfarin anticoagulation with vitamin K is recommended.[121]

THROMBOTIC THROMBOCYTOPENIC PURPURA AND HEMOLYTIC UREMIC SYNDROME

TTP/HUS is characterized by a microangiopathic hemolytic anemia (Figure 132-4), thrombocytopenia, neurologic symptoms, renal dysfunction, and fever. The majority of TTP/HUS cases are

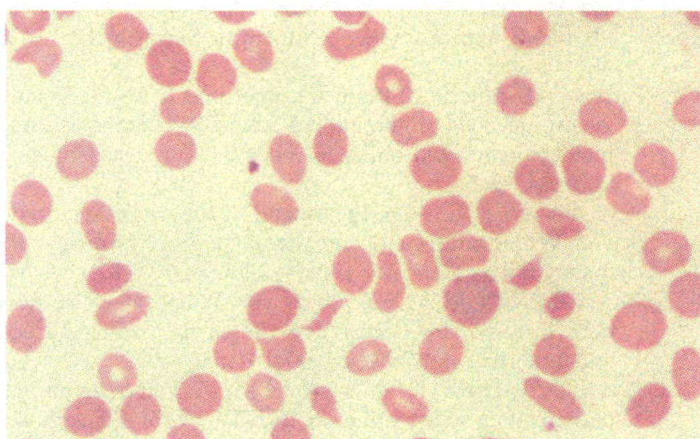

Figure 132-4

reported in patients with adenocarcinoma, particularly gastric cancer; however, TTP/HUS also occurs in patients with breast cancer and lung cancer, and in Hodgkin's and non-Hodgkin's lymphomas.[123] TTP/HUS also occurs in association with cancer chemotherapy, especially with mitomycin C, bleomycin, cisplatin, and tamoxifen,[124] use of cyclosporine,[125] and interferon,[126] as well as after bone marrow transplantation.[127]

The pathophysiology of cancer-associated TTP/HUS is postulated to be similar to that of usual primary TTP/HUS. It involves injury to vascular endothelium with release of ultralarge vWF multimers due to a deficiency of a vWF-cleaving protease (ADAMTS-13), causing platelet aggregation.[128,129]

The clinical manifestations of TTP/HUS in the cancer patient are often not readily obvious because they tend to occur in complicated patients often being treated with chemotherapy and/or radiation therapy with several comorbidities that may obscure the diagnosis. Typically, the microangiopathic hemolytic anemia and thrombocytopenia are severe and reticulocytosis is usually present, with increased levels of lactic acid dehydrogenase (LDH), reflecting intravascular hemolysis. The peripheral blood smear demonstrates numerous schistocytes. Renal failure and neurologic and pulmonary dysfunction are common. Neurologic signs and symptoms include headache, confusion, hemiplegia or hemiparesis, and coma. Rarely, severe acute respiratory distress syndrome may occur late in the disease process and is usually fatal.[130] Standard treatment of TTP is plasmapheresis. Other treatment modalities that may be used in refractory cases include vincristine, intravenous gamma globulin, rituximab, and splenectomy.[131,132] Platelet transfusions are contraindicated because infused platelets may amplify the extent and severity of the formation of microvascular thrombi.[133] Regardless of treatment, the prognosis of cancer patients with TTP/HUS is generally poor.

ARTERIAL THROMBOSIS AND NONBACTERIAL THROMBOTIC ENDOCARDITIS

Arterial thrombosis in cancer patients is much less frequent than venous thrombosis. It usually occurs as a complication of nonbacterial endocarditis and, rarely, in patients receiving chemotherapeutic agents such as cisplatin.[134] Episodes of arterial thromboses, including peripheral arterial thrombosis and cerebrovascular accidents, have been observed in breast cancer patients receiving adjuvant chemotherapy.[135] Nonbacterial thrombotic endocarditis (NBTE) represents a form of consumptive coagulopathy most commonly seen with adenocarcinomas of the lung and pancreas.[136] The diagnosis is made by echocardiography with the finding of sterile thrombotic vegetations on cardiac valves. In addition to vegetations, ventricular segmental wall motion abnormalities resulting from silent embolization to the coronary arteries has been reported in 18% of cancer patients with this diagnosis.[137] NBTE or "Libman-Sacks" endocarditis should be suspected in any cancer patient who presents with ischemic embolic events. Management is essentially supportive and similar to that of patients with chronic DIC or those with thromboembolic disease. Anticoagulant therapy may help some patients, and early diagnosis may prevent severe neurologic disability.[138]

DISSEMINATED INTRAVASCULAR COAGULATION

Patients with solid tumors (prostate, pancreas, lung, stomach, colon, and breast) and those with leukemia, especially APL, may be complicated by DIC that is manifested primarily by bleeding.[139] As previously described, one mechanism for the bleeding disorder in APL may be the abnormally high levels of expression of annexin A2 on APL cells, which leads to increased production of plasmin and ensuing bleeding from unopposed fibrinolysis.[140] Annexin A2 is a phospholipid-binding protein on the surface of endothelial cells that serves to bind plasminogen and its activator, tPA.[141]

The majority of cancer patients have an increased production of coagulation factors, however, which predisposes them to thrombotic complications. The thrombotic disorders associated with DIC include recurrent venous thrombosis, peripheral arterial thrombosis, cerebrovascular thrombosis, disseminated arterial disease with organ failure, peripheral limb ischemia, and gangrene.[75]

Chronic forms of DIC are characterized by less florid clinical findings and more subtle, but persistent, laboratory abnormalities. Metastatic cancer is a common cause of chronic DIC. Over time, approximately 25% of patients with metastatic cancer develop a thrombotic event.[142]

In cancer patients, the diagnosis of DIC is made clinically and corroborated by a constellation of laboratory abnormalities as shown in Table 132-5.[75] There is no unique laboratory test that can establish or exclude the diagnosis of DIC. In most cases, a combination of tests in a patient with a clinical condition that is associated with DIC can be used to diagnose the disorder with reasonable certainty. In the presence of an underlying disease associated with DIC, an initial platelet count of less than 100,000/mm^3 or a rapid decline in the platelet count, prolongation of the PT and aPTT, presence of fibrin(ogen) degradation products or D-dimers in plasma, and low plasma levels of coagulation inhibitors such as antithrombin are diagnostic of DIC. Fibrinogen levels may remain in the normal range in the face of its consumption because of increased synthesis of this acute-phase reactant. A finding of hypofibrinogenemia is only useful diagnostically in very severe cases of DIC. In patients with DIC, the peripheral blood smear may also demonstrate the presence of red cell fragmentation or schistocytes. More sophisticated laboratory tests useful in the diagnosis of DIC include the measurement of soluble fibrin and sensitive assays that can measure the generation of thrombin, such as prothrombin activation fragment F 1 + 2 and TAT complexes. The sensitivity and specificity of these assays for the diagnosis of DIC range from 80 to 90%; although helpful in complicated clinical situations, they are not essential in clinical practice.[143]

Table 132-5 Abnormalities in Cancer Patients with Disseminated Intravascular Coagulation

Thrombocytopenia
Prolongation of PT and aPTT
Hypofibrinogenemia
Decreased levels of factor V and factor VIII[a]
Presence of fibrin(ogen) degradation products and D-dimer[b]
Presence of schistocytes or fragmented red blood cells in the peripheral blood smear indicating microangiopathic hemolysis

[a]Factor VIII levels may be increased in some patients with early DIC because of thrombin activation of factor VIII.
[b]Plasma D-dimers are specific cross-linked fibrin derivative generated when the endogenous fibrinolytic system degrades fibrin.

In general, the treatment of DIC is directed against the underlying cancer and to either the bleeding or thrombotic manifestations that are clinically present.[144] Cancer patients with DIC who are bleeding should receive plasma and platelet transfusions to maintain the platelet count greater than 50,000/μL and fibrinogen level greater than 150 mg/dL, respectively. The administration of purified coagulation factor concentrates in DIC is not generally recommended because they may be contaminated with traces of activated coagulation factors, which could promote thrombosis.[144] The bleeding associated with DIC in APL often responds dramatically to treatment with all-*trans*-retinoic acid.[145]

Intravenous heparin may be tried in cancer patients with DIC-associated thrombosis for stabilization while the cancer is being treated unless moderate to severe thrombocytopenia is present. The recommended dosage of heparin is 15 U/kg/h (7.5 mg/kg/h for patients with APL by continuous IV infusion without a loading dose). In patients with DIC secondary to primary fibrinolysis (eg, prostate cancer), the fibrinolytic inhibitor, epsilon aminocaproic acid (Amicar), can be administered with an initial IV loading dosage of 4 to 6 g over 1 hour followed by an IV infusion of 1 g/h while monitoring the clinical response. The recommended oral dosage of aminocaproic acid is 50 to 60 mg/kg every 4 to 6 hours.[35] However, in those patients with a primary thrombotic presentation and secondary fibrinolysis, fibrinolytic inhibitors should be avoided until the thrombotic process is controlled.[75] Warfarin and/or antiplatelet drugs are generally ineffective for DIC states in cancer patients. LMWH, antithrombin, and protein C concentrates, hirudin, and plasmapheresis, all remain investigational and await prospective studies.

NOVEL DRUGS FOR TREATMENT OF BLEEDING AND THROMBOTIC DISORDERS

Recombinant Factor VIIa Recombinant factor VIIa (rFVIIa) is FDA approved for patients with bleeding secondary to hemophilia A or B who have inhibitors against factors VIII and IX.[146] It has also been shown to be effective in controlling bleeding due to thrombocytopenia, thrombocytopathies, acquired coagulation factor deficiencies, and in patients undergoing cancer surgery.[146] By enhancing thrombin generation on activated platelets, rFVIIa promotes the formation of a stable fibrin clot that is resistant to premature lysis. rFVIIa has a short half-life and is administered at doses of 90 to 120 mcg/kg every 2 hours and repeated as clinically warranted.[147] Caution should be undertaken in administering rFVIIa to patients with DIC, coronary artery disease, and severe sepsis because of their higher risk of thrombosis.

Factor Xa Inhibitors Fondaparinux, a synthetic pentasaccharide is an indirect factor Xa inhibitor that binds to antithrombin and has no activity against thrombin.[148] Fondaparinux is FDA approved for VTE prophylaxis in patients undergoing major knee and hip surgery at a dosage of 2.5 mg SC once daily.[149,150] Fondaparinux has also been recently approved for the treatment of VTE.[151] A potential limitation of fondaparinux is that it is not reversible with protamine sulfate, which may pose a problem in patients with life-threatening bleeding.

SUMMARY

Hemostatic alterations are common in cancer patients. Depending on the underlying disease and specific hemostatic abnormality, the cancer patient may develop bleeding, thrombosis, or both, such as in DIC. Bleeding complications usually result from abnormalities in platelets or deficiency of coagulation factors and require specific blood or coagulation factor replacement. Similarly, cancer patients are predisposed to VTE, including DVT, pulmonary embolism, and catheter-related thrombosis. Advances in diagnostic imaging and availability of newer and more potent anticoagulant agents have greatly facilitated the care of these patients. Ultimately, a thorough understanding of the various disturbances in hemostasis, innovative treatment approaches, and implementation of preventive strategies in cancer patients will lead to decreased morbidity and improvement in survival.

REFERENCES

1. Auger MJ, Mackie MJ. Haemostasis in malignant disease. J R Coll Physicians Lond 1988;22:74–9.
2. Goad KE, Gralnick HR. Coagulation disorders in cancer. Hematol Oncol Clin North Am 1996;10:457–84.
3. Rickles FR, Levine M, Edwards RL. Hemostatic alterations in cancer patients. Cancer Metastasis Rev 1992;11:237–48.
4. Francis JL, Biggerstaff J, Amirkhosravi A. Hemostasis and malignancy. Semin Thromb Hemost 1998;24:93–109.
5. Rosenberg RD, Aird WC. Vascular-bed-specific hemostasis and hypercoagulable states. N Engl J Med 1999;340:1555–64.
6. Giesen PL, Nemerson Y. Tissue factor on the loose. Semin Thromb Hemost 2000;26:379–84.
7. Wiman B. The fibrinolytic enzyme system. Basic principles and links to venous and arterial thrombosis. Hematol Oncol Clin North Am 2000;14:325–38, vii.
8. Trousseau A. Phlegmasia alba dolens. Lectures on clinical medicine, delivered at the Hotel-Dieu, Paris, New Sydenham Society 1877;281–95.
9. Billroth T. Lectures on surgical pathology and therapeutics: a handbook for students and practitioners. The New Sydemham Society 1877;1877–8.
10. Zacharski LR, Schned AR, Sorenson GD. Occurrence of fibrin and tissue factor antigen in human small cell carcinoma of the lung. Cancer Res 1983;43:3963–8.
11. Hejna M, Raderer M, Zielinski CC. Inhibition of metastases by anticoagulants. J Natl Cancer Inst 1999;91:22–36.
12. Palumbo JS, Talmage KE, Massari JV, et al. Platelets and fibrin(ogen) increase metastatic potential by impeding natural killer cell-mediated elimination of tumor cells. Blood 2005;105:178–85.
13. Johnson MJ. Bleeding, clotting and cancer. Clin Oncol (R Coll Radiol) 1997;9:294–301.
14. Schwartzberg LS, Holbert JM. Hemorrhagic and thrombotic abnormalities of cancer. Crit Care Clin 1988;4:107–28.
15. Dourakis SP, Deutsch M, Hadziyannis SJ. Immune thrombocytopenia and alpha-interferon therapy. J Hepatol 1996;25:972–5.
16. Leopold LH, Berger MS, Feingold J. Acute and long-term toxicities associated with gemtuzumab ozogamicin (Mylotarg[r]) therapy of acute myeloid leukemia. Clin Lymphoma 2002;2 Suppl 1:S29–34.
17. Benjamin RJ, Anderson KC. What is the proper threshold for platelet transfusion in patients with chemotherapy-induced thrombocytopenia? Crit Rev Oncol 2002;42:163–71.
18. Beutler E. Platelet transfusions: the 20,000/microL trigger. Blood 1993;81:1411–3.
19. Slichter SJ. Platelet transfusions a constantly evolving therapy. Thromb Haemost 1991;66:178–88.
20. Contreras M. Consensus conference on platelet transfusion. Final statement. Transfus Sci 1998;19:111–4.
21. Schiffer CA, Anderson KC, Bennett CL, et al. Platelet transfusion for patients with cancer: clinical practice guidelines of the American Society of Clinical Oncology. J Clin Oncol 2001;19:1519–38.
22. Gmur J, Burger J, Schanz U, et al. Safety of stringent prophylactic platelet transfusion policy for patients with acute leukaemia [comments]. Lancet 1991;338:1223–6.
23. Barrera R, Mina B, Huang Y, Groeger JS. Acute complications of central line placement in profoundly thrombocytopenic cancer patients. Cancer 1996;78:2025–30.
24. Colosimo M, McCarthy N, Jayasinghe R, et al. Diagnosis and management of subdural haematoma complicating bone marrow transplantation. Bone Marrow Transplant 2000;25:549–52.
25. Pomeranz S, Naparstek E, Ashkenazi E, et al. Intracranial haematomas following bone marrow transplantation. J Neurol 1994;241:252–6.
26. Graus F, Saiz A, Sierra J, et al. Neurologic complications of autologous and allogeneic bone marrow transplantation in patients with leukemia: a comparative study. Neurology 1996;46:1004–9.
27. Turner VS, Hawker RJ, Mitchell SG, Seymour MA. Paired in vivo and in vitro comparison of zpheresis and "recovered" platelet concentrates stored for 5 days. J Clin Apheresis 1994;9:189–94.
28. Wuest DL. Transfusion and stem cell support in cancer treatment. Hematol Oncol Clin North Am 1996;10:397–429.
29. Federici AB, Budde U, Rand JH. Acquired von Willebrand syndrome 2004: International Registry—diagnosis and management from online to bedside. Hamostaseologie 2004;24:50–5.
30. Veyradier A, Jenkins CS, Fressinaud E, Meyer D. Acquired von Willebrand syndrome: from pathophysiology to management. Thromb Haemost 2000;84:175–82.
31. Tefferi A, Nichols WL. Acquired von Willebrand disease: concise review of occurrence, diagnosis, pathogenesis, and treatment. Am J Med 1997;103:536–40.
32. Green D, Lechner K. A survey of 215 non-hemophilic patients with inhibitors to factor VIII. Thromb Haemost 1981;45:200–3.
33. Hauser I, Lechner K. Solid tumors and factor VIII antibodies [comments]. Thromb Haemost 1999;82:1005–7.
34. Stasi R, Brunetti M, Stipa E, Amadori S. Selective B-cell depletion with rituximab for the treatment of patients with acquired hemophilia. Blood 2004;103:4424–8.
35. Mannucci PM. Hemostatic drugs. N Engl J Med 1998;339:245–53.
36. el-Shahawy MA, Francis R, Akmal M, Massry SG. Recombinant human erythropoietin shortens the bleeding time and corrects the abnormal platelet aggregation in hemodialysis patients. Clin Nephrol 1994;41:308–13.
37. Nissenson AR. Novel erythropoiesis stimulating protein for managing the anemia of chronic kidney disease. Am J Kidney Dis 2001;38:1390–7.
38. Glaspy J. Introduction. Improving the standard of care in the management of cancer-related anaemia: focus on darbepoetin alfa, a novel erythropoiesis-stimulating protein. Br J Cancer 2001;84 Suppl 1:1–2.
39. Tefferi A, Solberg LA, Silverstein MN. A clinical update in polycythemia vera and essential thrombocythemia. Am J Med 2000;109:141–9.
40. Cortelazzo S, Viero P, Finazzi G, et al. Incidence and risk factors for thrombotic complications in a historical cohort of 100 patients with essential thrombocythemia. J Clin Oncol 1990;8:556–62.
41. Finazzi G, Budde U, Michiels JJ. Bleeding time and platelet function in essential thrombocythemia and other myeloproliferative syndromes. Leuk Lymphoma 1996;22 Suppl 1:71–8.
42. Mitchell MC, Boitnott JK, Kaufman S, et al. Budd-Chiari syndrome: etiology, diagnosis and management. Medicine (Baltimore) 1982;61:199–218.
43. Kaplan ME, Mack K, Goldberg JD, et al. Long-term management of polycythemia vera with hydroxyurea: a progress report. Semin Hematol 1986;23:167–71.
44. Solberg LA Jr. Therapeutic options for essential thrombocythemia and polycythemia vera. Semin Oncol 2002;29(3 Suppl 10):10–5.
45. Pengo V, Banzato A, Garelli E, et al. Reversal of excessive effect of regular anticoagulation: low oral dose of phytonadione (vitamin K1) compared with warfarin discontinuation. Blood Coagul Fibrinolysis 1993;4:739–41.
46. Raj G, Kumar R, McKinney WP. Time course of reversal of anticoagulant effect of warfarin by intravenous and subcutaneous phytonadione. Arch Intern Med 1999;159:2721–4.
47. Whitling AM, Bussey HI, Lyons RM. Comparing different routes and doses of phytonadione for reversing excessive anticoagulation. Arch Intern Med 1998;158:2136–40.
48. Hirsh J, Dalen J, Anderson DR, et al. Oral anticoagulants: mechanism of action, clinical effectiveness, and optimal therapeutic range. Chest 2001;119(1 Suppl):8S–21S.
49. Ansell J, Hirsh J, Dalen J, et al. Managing oral anticoagulant therapy. Chest 2001;119(1 Suppl):22S–38S.
50. Development Task Force of the College of American Pathologists. Practice parameter for the use of fresh-frozen plasma, cryoprecipitate, and platelets. Fresh-frozen plasma, cryoprecipitate, and platelets administration practice guidelines. JAMA 1994;271:777–81.
51. Greipp PR, Kyle RA, Bowie EJ. Factor-X deficiency in amyloidosis: a critical review. Am J Hematol 1981;11:443–50.
52. Gamba G, Montani N, Anesi E, et al. Clotting alterations in primary systemic amyloidosis. Haematologica 2000;85:289–92.
53. Furie B, Voo L, McAdam KP, Furie BC. Mechanism of factor X deficiency in systemic amyloidosis. N Engl J Med 1981;304:827–30.
54. Bezeaud A, Drouet L, Leverger G, et al. Effect of L-asparaginase therapy for acute lymphoblastic leukemia on plasma vitamin K-dependent coagulation factors and inhibitors. J Pediatr 1986;108(5 Pt 1):698–701.

55. Legnani C, Palareti G, Pession A, et al. Intravascular coagulation phenomena associated with prevalent fall in fibrinogen and plasminogen during L-asparaginase treatment in leukemic children. Haemostasis 1988;18:179–86.
56. Saito M, Asakura H, Jokaji H, et al. Changes in hemostatic and fibrinolytic proteins in patients receiving L-asparaginase therapy. Am J Hematol 1989;32:20–3.
57. Dombret H, Geiger S, Daniel MT, et al. Changes in microrheology of acute promyelocytic leukemia cells during all-trans retinoic acid (ATRA) differentiation therapy: a mechanism for ATRA-induced hyperleukocytosis? Leukemia 1995;9:1473–7.
58. Menell JS, Cesarman GM, Jacovina AT, et al. Annexin II and bleeding in acute promyelocytic leukemia. N Engl J Med 1999;340:994–1004.
59. Sun NC, McAfee WM, Hum GJ, Weiner JM. Hemostatic abnormalities in malignancy, a prospective study of one hundred eight patients. Part I. Coagulation studies. Am J Clin Pathol 1979;71:10–6.
60. Nand S, Messmore H. Hemostasis in malignancy [comments]. Am J Hematol 1990;35:45–55.
61. Johnson MJ. Bleeding, clotting and cancer. Clin Oncol (R Coll Radiol) 1997;9:294–301.
62. Miller SP, Sanchez-Avalos J, Stefanski T, Zuckerman L. Coagulation disorders in cancer. I. Clinical and laboratory studies. Cancer 1967;20:1452–65.
63. Rickles FR, Edwards RL, Barb C, Cronlund M. Abnormalities of blood coagulation in patients with cancer. Fibrinopeptide A generation and tumor growth. Cancer 1983;51:301–7.
64. Kakkar AK, DeRuvo N, Chinswangwatanakul V, et al. Extrinsic-pathway activation in cancer with high factor VIIa and tissue factor. Lancet 1995;346:1004–5.
65. LaCapra S, Arkel YS, Ku DH, et al. The use of thrombus precursor protein, D-dimer, prothrombin fragment 1.2, and thrombin antithrombin in the exclusion of proximal deep vein thrombosis and pulmonary embolism. Blood Coagul Fibrinolysis 2000;11:371–7.
66. Nand S, Fisher SG, Salgia R, Fisher RI. Hemostatic abnormalities in untreated cancer: incidence and correlation with thrombotic and hemorrhagic complications. J Clin Oncol 1987;5:1998–2003.
67. Rocha E, Paramo JA, Fernandez FJ, et al. Clotting activation and impairment of fibrinolysis in malignancy. Thromb Res 1989;54:699–707.
68. Falanga A. Mechanisms of hypercoagulation in malignancy and during chemotherapy. Haemostasis 1998;28 Suppl 3:50–60.
69. Honegger H, Anderson N, Hewitt LA, Tullis JL. Antithrombin III profiles in malignancy, relationship primary tumors and metastatic sites. Thromb Haemost 1981;46:500–3.
70. Harper PL, Jarvis J, Jennings I, et al. Changes in the natural anticoagulants following bone marrow transplantation. Bone Marrow Transplant 1990;5:39–42.
71. Rickles FR, Edwards RL. Activation of blood coagulation in cancer: Trousseau's syndrome revisited. Blood 1983;62:14–31.
72. Nathanson L, Sochet A, Williams ME. Migratory thrombophlebitis during sandostatin (SMS 201–995, Sandoz) therapy for malignant carcinoid syndrome. Invest New Drugs 1989;7:285–7.
73. Baron JA, Gridley G, Weiderpass E, et al. Venous thromboembolism and cancer [published erratum appears in Lancet 2000;355:758]. Lancet 1998;351:1077–80.
74. Bick RL. Coagulation abnormalities in malignancy: a review. Semin Thromb Hemost 1992;18:353–72.
75. Arkel YS. Thrombosis and cancer. Semin Oncol 2000;27:362–74.
76. Levine MN, Gent M, Hirsh J, et al. The thrombogenic effect of anticancer drug therapy in women with stage II breast cancer. N Engl J Med 1988;318:404–7.
77. Clark TE, Edom N, Larson J, Lindsey LJ. Thalomid (thalidomide) capsules: a review of the first 18 months of spontaneous postmarketing adverse event surveillance, including off-label prescribing. Drug Saf 1902;24:87–117.
78. Zangari M, Anaissie E, Barlogie B, et al. Increased risk of deep-vein thrombosis in patients with multiple myeloma receiving thalidomide and chemotherapy. Blood 2001;98:1614–5.
79. Zangari M, Saghafifar F, Anaissie E, et al. Activated protein C resistance in the absence of factor V Leiden mutation is a common finding in multiple myeloma and is associated with an increased risk of thrombotic complications. Blood Coagul Fibrinolysis 2002;13:187–92.
80. Kabbinavar F, Hurwitz HI, Fehrenbacher L, et al. Phase II, randomized trial comparing bevacizumab plus fluorouracil (FU)/leucovorin (LV) with FU/LV alone in patients with metastatic colorectal cancer. J Clin Oncol 2003;21:60–5.
81. Chunilal SD, Ginsberg JS. Strategies for the diagnosis of deep vein thrombosis and pulmonary embolism. Thromb Res 2000;97:V33–48.
82. Wells PS, Hirsh J, Anderson DR, et al. Accuracy of clinical assessment of deep-vein thrombosis [published erratum appears in Lancet 1995;346:516] [comments]. Lancet 1995;345:1326–30.
83. Wells PS, Anderson DR, Bormanis J, et al. Value of assessment of pretest probability of deep-vein thrombosis in clinical management [comments]. Lancet 1997;350:1795–8.
84. Ginsberg JS, Wells PS, Kearon C, et al. Sensitivity and specificity of a rapid whole-blood assay for D-dimer in the diagnosis of pulmonary embolism [comments]. Ann Intern Med 1998;129:1006–11.
85. Lee AY, Julian JA, Levine MN, et al. Clinical utility of a rapid whole-blood D-dimer assay in patients with cancer who present with suspected acute deep venous thrombosis. Ann Intern Med 1999;131:417–23.
86. Kearon C, Ginsberg JS, Hirsh J. The role of venous ultrasonography in the diagnosis of suspected deep venous thrombosis and pulmonary embolism. Ann Intern Med 1998;129:1044–9.
87. Ginsberg JS, Kearon C, Douketis J, et al. The use of D-dimer testing and impedance plethysmographic examination in patients with clinical indications of deep vein thrombosis [comments]. Arch Intern Med 1997;157:1077–81.
88. Ageno W. Treatment of venous thromboembolism. Thromb Res 2000;97:V63–72.
89. Anonymous.
90. Raschke RA, Reilly BM, Guidry JR, et al. The weight-based heparin dosing nomogram compared with a "standard care" nomogram. A randomized controlled trial [comments]. Ann Intern Med 1993;119:874–81.
91. Hull RD, Raskob GE, Rosenbloom D, et al. Heparin for 5 days as compared with 10 days in the initial treatment of proximal venous thrombosis [comments]. N Engl J Med 1990;322:1260–4.
92. Bates SM, Hirsh J. Treatment of venous thromboembolism. Thromb Haemost 1999;82:870–7.
93. Levine M, Gent M, Hirsh J, et al. A comparison of low-molecular-weight heparin administered primarily at home with unfractionated heparin administered in the hospital for proximal deep-vein thrombosis [comments]. N Engl J Med 1996;334:677–81.
94. Green D, Hull RD, Brant R, Pineo GF. Lower mortality in cancer patients treated with low-molecular-weight versus standard heparin [letter]. Lancet 1992;339:1476.
95. Warkentin TE, Levine MN, Hirsh J, et al. Heparin-induced thrombocytopenia in patients treated with low-molecular-weight heparin or unfractionated heparin [comments]. N Engl J Med 1995;332:1330–5.
96. Weitz JI. Low-molecular-weight heparins [published erratum appears in N Engl J Med 1997;337:1567] [comments]. N Engl J Med 1997;337:688–98.
97. Meyer G, Marjanovic Z, Valcke J, et al. Comparison of low-molecular-weight heparin and warfarin for the secondary prevention of venous thromboembolism in patients with cancer: a randomized controlled study. Arch Intern Med 2002;162:1729–35.
98. Lee AY, Levine MN, Baker RI, et al. Low-molecular-weight heparin versus a coumarin for the prevention of recurrent venous thromboembolism in patients with cancer. N Engl J Med 2003;349:146–53.
99. Buller HR, Agnelli G, Hull RD, et al. Antithrombotic therapy for venous thromboembolic disease: the Seventh ACCP Conference on Antithrombotic and Thrombolytic Therapy. Chest 2004;126(3 Suppl):401S–28S.
100. Goldhaber SZ. Thrombolytic therapy in venous thromboembolism. Clinical trials and current indications. Clin Chest Med 1995;16:307–20.
101. Decousus H, Leizorovicz A, Parent F, et al. A clinical trial of vena caval filters in the prevention of pulmonary embolism in patients with proximal deep-vein thrombosis. Prevention du Risque d'Embolie Pulmonaire par Interruption Cave Study Group [comments]. N Engl J Med 1998;338:409–15.
102. Walsh DB, Downing S, Nauta R, Gomes MN. Metastatic cancer. A relative contraindication to vena cava filter placement. Cancer 1987;59:161–3.
103. Prandoni P. Antithrombotic strategies in patients with cancer. Thromb Haemost 1997;78:141–4.
104. Prandoni P, Lensing AW, Piccioli A, et al. Recurrent venous thromboembolism and bleeding complications during anticoagulant treatment in patients with cancer and venous thrombosis. Blood 2002;100:3484–8.
105. Lee AY, Levine MN. Venous thromboembolism and cancer: risks and outcomes. Circulation 2003;107(23 Suppl 1):I17–21.
106. Bern MM, Lokich JJ, Wallach SR, et al. Very low doses of warfarin can prevent thrombosis in central venous catheters. A randomized prospective trial. Ann Intern Med 1990;112:423–8.
107. Monreal M, Alastrue A, Rull M, et al. Upper extremity deep venous thrombosis in cancer patients with venous access devices—prophylaxis with a low molecular weight heparin (Fragmin). Thromb Haemost 1996;75:251–3.
108. Walshe LJ, Malak SF, Eagan J, Sepkowitz KA. Complication rates among cancer patients with peripherally inserted central catheters. J Clin Oncol 2002;20:3276–81.
109. Geerts WH, Pineo GF, Heit JA, et al. Prevention of venous thromboembolism: the Seventh ACCP Conference on Antithrombotic and Thrombolytic Therapy. Chest 2004;126(3 Suppl):338S–400S.
110. Tesselaar ME, Ouwerkerk J, Nooy MA, et al. Risk factors for catheter-related thrombosis in cancer patients. Eur J Cancer 2004;40:2253–9.
111. Ponec D, Irwin D, Haire WD, et al. Recombinant tissue plasminogen activator (Alteplase) for restoration of flow in occluded central venous access devices: a double-blind placebo-controlled trial—the Cardiovascular Thrombolytic to Open Occluded Lines (COOL) efficacy trial. J Vasc Interv Radiol 2001;12:951–5.
112. Gallus AS. Prevention of post-operative deep leg vein thrombosis in patients with cancer. Thromb Haemost 1997;78:126–32.
113. Bergqvist D, Agnelli G, Cohen AT, et al. Duration of prophylaxis against venous thromboembolism with enoxaparin after surgery for cancer. N Engl J Med 2002;346:975–80.
114. Rasmussen MS. Preventing thromboembolic complications in cancer patients after surgery: a role for prolonged thromboprophylaxis. Cancer Treat Rev 2002;28:141–4.
115. Bobek V, Kovarik J. Antitumor and antimetastatic effect of warfarin and heparins. Biomed Pharmacother 2004;58:213–9.
116. Lee AY, Rickles FR, Julian JA, et al. Randomized comparison of low molecular weight heparin and coumarin derivatives on the survival of patients with cancer and venous thromboembolism. J Clin Oncol 2005;23:2123–9.
117. Kakkar AK, Levine MN, Kadziola Z, et al. Low molecular weight heparin, therapy with dalteparin, and survival in advanced cancer: the Fragmin Advanced Malignancy Outcome Study (FAMOUS). J Clin Oncol 2004;22:1944–8.
118. Warkentin TE. Heparin-induced thrombocytopenia. pathogenesis, frequency, avoidance and management. Drug Saf 1997;17:325–41.
119. Warkentin TE. Heparin-induced thrombocytopenia: a ten-year retrospective. Annu Rev Med 1999;50:129–47.
120. Warkentin TE. Heparin-induced thrombocytopenia: diagnosis and management. Circulation 2004;110:e454–8.
121. Warkentin TE, Greinacher A. Heparin-induced thrombocytopenia: recognition, treatment, and prevention: the Seventh ACCP Conference on Antithrombotic and Thrombolytic Therapy. Chest 2004;126(3 Suppl):311S–37S.
122. Amiral J, Bridey F, Dreyfus M, et al. Platelet factor 4 complexed to heparin is the target for antibodies generated in heparin-induced thrombocytopenia. Thromb Haemost 1992;68:95–6.
123. Kwaan HC, Gordon LI. Thrombotic microangiopathy in the cancer patient. Acta Haematol 2001;106:52–6.
124. Montes A, Powles TJ, O'Brien ME, et al. A toxic interaction between mitomycin C and tamoxifen causing the haemolytic uraemic syndrome. Eur J Cancer 1993;29A:1854–7.
125. Medina PJ, Sipols JM, George JN. Drug-associated thrombotic thrombocytopenic purpura-hemolytic uremic syndrome. Curr Opin Hematol 2001;8:286–93.
126. Lacotte L, Thierry A, Delwail V, et al. Thrombotic thrombocytopenic purpura during interferon alpha treatment for chronic myelogenous leukemia. Acta Haematol 2000;102:160–2.
127. Byrnes JJ, Hussein AM. Thrombotic microangiopathic syndromes after bone marrow transplantation [comments]. Cancer Invest 1996;14:151–7.
128. Tsai HM, Lian EC. Antibodies to von Willebrand factor-cleaving protease in acute thrombotic thrombocytopenic purpura [comments]. N Engl J Med 1998;339:1585–94.
129. Tripodi A, Chantarangkul V, Bohm M, et al. Measurement of von Willebrand factor cleaving protease (ADAMTS-13): results of an international collaborative study involving 11 methods testing the same set of coded plasmas. J Thromb Haemost 2004;2:1601–9.
130. Bone RC, Henry JE, Petterson J, Amare M. Respiratory dysfunction in thrombotic thrombocytopenic purpura. Am J Med 1978;65:262–70.

131. Veltman GA, Brand A, Leeksma OC, et al. The role of splenectomy in the treatment of relapsing thrombotic thrombocytopenic purpura. Ann Hematol 1995;70:231–6.
132. Reddy PS, Deauna-Limayo D, Cook JD, et al. Rituximab in the treatment of relapsed thrombotic thrombocytopenic purpura. Ann Hematol 2005;84:232–5.
133. Gordon LI, Kwaan HC. Cancer- and drug-associated thrombotic thrombocytopenic purpura and hemolytic uremic syndrome. Semin Hematol 1997;34:140–7.
134. Rohner RF, Prior JT, Sipple JH. Mucinous malignancies, venous thrombosis and terminal endocarditis with emboli. A syndrome. Cancer 1966;19:1805–12.
135. Wall JG, Weiss RB, Norton L, et al. Arterial thrombosis associated with adjuvant chemotherapy for breast carcinoma: a Cancer and Leukemia Group B Study. Am J Med 1989;87:501–4.
136. Kim HS, Suzuki M, Lie JT, Titus JL. Nonbacterial thrombotic endocarditis (NBTE) and disseminated intravascular coagulation (DIC): autopsy study of 36 patients. Arch Pathol Lab Med 1977;101:65–8.
137. Edoute Y, Haim N, Rinkevich D, et al. Cardiac valvular vegetations in cancer patients: a prospective echocardiographic study of 200 patients. Am J Med 1997;102:252–8.
138. Rogers LR, Cho ES, Kempin S, Posner JB. Cerebral infarction from non-bacterial thrombotic endocarditis. Clinical and pathological study including the effects of anticoagulation. Am J Med 1987;83:746–56.
139. Colman RW, Rubin RN. Disseminated intravascular coagulation due to malignancy. Semin Oncol 1990;17:172–86.
140. Menell JS, Cesarman GM, Jacovina AT, et al. Annexin II and bleeding in acute promyelocytic leukemia [comments]. N Engl J Med 1999;340:994–1004.
141. Hajjar KA, Menell JS. Annexin II: a novel mediator of cell surface plasmin generation. Ann N Y Acad Sci 1997;811:337–49.
142. Bick RL. Disseminated intravascular coagulation and related syndromes: a clinical review. Semin Thromb Hemost 1988;14:299–338.
143. Bauer KA, Rosenberg RD. The pathophysiology of the prethrombotic state in humans: insights fained from studies using markers of hemostatic system activation. Blood 1987;70:343–50.
144. Levi M, Ten Cate H. Disseminated intravascular coagulation [comments]. N Engl J Med 1999;341:586–92.
145. Dombret H, Scrobohaci ML, Daniel MT, et al. In vivo thrombin and plasmin activities in patients with acute promyelocytic leukemia (APL): effect of all-trans retinoic acid (ATRA) therapy. Leukemia 1995;9:19–24.
146. Hedner U. Recombinant factor VIIa (NovoSeven) as a hemostatic agent. Dis Mon 2003;49:39–48.
147. Hedner U. Dosing with recombinant factor VilIa based on current evidence. Semin Hematol 2004;41(1 Suppl 1):35–9.
148. Walenga JM, Jeske WP, Samama MM, et al. Fondaparinux: a synthetic heparin pentasaccharide as a new antithrombotic agent. Expert Opin Investig Drugs 2002;11:397–407.
149. Bauer KA, Eriksson BI, Lassen MR, Turpie AG. Fondaparinux compared with enoxaparin for the prevention of venous thromboembolism after elective major knee surgery. N Engl J Med 2001;345:1305–10.
150. Eriksson BI, Bauer KA, Lassen MR, Turpie AG. Fondaparinux compared with enoxaparin for the prevention of venous thromboembolism after hip-fracture surgery. N Engl J Med 2001;345:1298–304.
151. Buller HR, Davidson BL, Decousus H, et al. Subcutaneous fondaparinux versus intravenous unfractionated heparin in the initial treatment of pulmonary embolism. N Engl J Med 2003;349:1695–702.

Urologic Complications

Christopher J. Logothetis, MD
Diana M. Hey, PharmD

The appropriate anticipation and management of urologic complications of cancer and its therapy may significantly improve the opportunity for the treatment of patients with metastatic disease. The management of obstructive uropathy, the criteria for detection of drug-induced renal toxicity, and the management of such toxicity without excessive dose reduction are important ingredients that contribute to the successful treatment of cancer patients. Adjustment of the dose of different chemotherapeutic agents on the basis of renal function and interaction with other agents that may be delivered concomitantly is an essential component of oncologic practice. Furthermore, it is increasingly recognized that successful strategies require optimum control of the site of origin. Thus, for urologic malignancy, does not only control of the primary site not only reduce avoid local complication of cancer progression but may also be an essential component of a successful treatment strategy. This chapter reviews the most frequent urologic complications of cancers and therapy.

COMPLICATIONS RESULTING FROM PRIMARY CANCER PROGRESSION

Urinary Tract Obstruction Obstruction of the urinary tract may occur at multiple levels (ureter, bladder, and urethra). Large retroperitoneal tumors can produce ureteral obstruction, whereas urethral and outlet obstruction results from cancers involving the bladder, distal urethra, or prostate. Such involvement can be by direct extension, encasement, or invasion of these structures. Obstruction can also occur from metastatic deposits involving these same sites. The course and management of obstructive uropathy are determined by the primary tumor causing the obstruction. Factors that influence the treatment of obstructive uropathy include the anticipated benefit from therapy and the curability of the patient, sensitivity of the neoplasm to cytotoxic therapy, rapidity of response to therapy, and anatomic access to the obstruction. The development of newer imaging techniques and less invasive surgical approaches has increased the accuracy of our assessment and expanded the opportunities for intervention. These advances allow early discovery and intervention and have reduced the need for extensive surgery to palliate distal ureteral obstruction.

Ureteral Obstruction Ureteral obstruction most commonly occurs because of large periaortic nodal metastases in the retroperitoneal space adjacent to the ureters. Such obstructive uropathy is most frequently the result of either primary nodal diseases (lymphomas) or urologic neoplasms metastasizing to the periaortic nodes, particularly prostate cancer and germ cell tumors. Advanced retroperitoneal germ cell tumors and lymphomas are a unique subset of chemotherapy-sensitive tumors that frequently result in obstructive uropathy. These cancers best illustrate the different approaches that can be used to treat a particular urologic complication produced by different tumors. When the cancer has the typical pathologic and serologic markers of a seminoma, obstructive uropathy is frequently observed with regionally advanced disease, in the absence of distant metastases. Application of effective therapy targeting the cancer (radiation therapy or chemotherapy) can promptly relieve obstruction rapidly without requiring intervention to relieve obstruction. Another curable germ cell tumor, teratoma, is less likely to exhibit a rapid, gratifying reduction in size. Percutaneous nephrostomy is needed to ensure adequate renal function during cisplatin-based chemotherapy. Surgical resection of the teratoma can then follow. In both instances, high cure rates can be achieved.[1,2] The rapidity of the anticipated response and the degree of compromise in renal function often govern whether percutaneous nephrostomy is necessary or whether a reasonable expectation exists that relief of obstruction can be achieved with cytotoxic chemotherapy. Similar approaches can be used for the treatment of lymphomas in which one can anticipate a rapid response to therapy. For curable cancers that require therapies with essential components that are nephrotoxic: such as cisplatin, ifosfamide, and methotrexate (MTX). Attention to the prompt reversal of obstructive uropathy is important to permit renal excretion of the drug. Although a unilateral percutaneous nephrostomy may preserve adequate renal function, patients whose long-term disease-free survival is dependent on nephrotoxic therapy require maximal preservation of renal function. Bilateral percutaneous nephrostomy is often required in these settings. However, it should be recognized that percutaneous nephrostomies are a source of infection that may complicate, delay, and, ultimately, force modification of treatment plans. To avoid this undesired effect on therapy, attention to detail in the placement and care of nephrostomies is required. This includes the optimal placement of catheters to reduce pain, frequent changes of the catheter (approximately 3-month intervals), and care of the insertion site to reduce the impact on treatment.

In most patients with acute urinary tract obstruction treated with urinary diversion, retrograde stent placement is attempted initially. Large prostate or bladder tumors, multiple sites of ureteric obstruction, long occlusions, or a tortuous ureter may be indications to proceed directly with percutaneous nephrostomy.[3] During nephrostomy tube placement, the intrarenal collecting system must be properly imaged to select a site of renal entry. Unless the patient is azotemic or allergic to contrast material, the site of entry can be best determined fluoroscopically after intravenous urographic contrast. In experienced hands, an appropriate nephrostomy tract can be established in 98% of cases, with major complications occurring in approximately 4%.[4] Major complications include renal hemorrhage requiring transfusion (1–3%), vascular injury (0.5–1.0%), sepsis (1–2.5%), bowel injury (0.1%), lung injury (0.5–1.0%), and mortality (0.046–0.3%).[3] After the intrarenal collecting system and dilated ureter are allowed to decompress, an internal double-J stent is placed if cystoscopic management of the stent is anticipated. This is performed in an antegrade fashion using the nephrostomy. When cystoscopic management of the stent is inadequate or the stent fails rapidly after placement, permanent percutaneous nephrostomy with external drainage or an internal-external stent is preferred. Complications from such procedures may include infections, tube obstruction, and dislodgment.

Ureteral obstruction caused by retroperitoneal metastases from cervical or breast cancer or from retroperitoneal radiation fibrosis is often treated by stenting. The decision to stent the ureters is influenced by other considerations, including the potential response of the disease to available treatment and the presence of pain. The neoplasm causing the retroperitoneal ureteral obstruction often invades the lumbar or sacral nerve roots, leading to excruciating pain. The wisdom of substituting a prolonged painful death in a setting in which limited therapy options exist should be considered. It is clear that optimum use of this intervention will improve survival and avoid permanent renal compromise in patients with curative prospects. In settings in which limited therapy options exist, it is very clear that the optimum use of this intervention will improve survival and avoid permanent renal compromise in patients with curative prospects. Fortunately, with improved surgical technology, early detection of localized cancer this challenge is becoming less frequent.

Bladder Outlet Obstruction Bladder outlet obstruction as a result of a large prostate carcinoma can be rapidly palliated by hormonal therapy or radiation therapy. In a patient with prostate cancer who exhibits androgen-independent growth or progression after radiation therapy or in patients with primary urethral cancer, effective palliation is a much greater challenge. The symptoms resulting from small bladder capacity, bladder irritability, or outlet obstruction can substantially reduce the quality of life for such patients. If a decision has been made to attempt palliation with cytotoxic therapy, the judicious use of a percutaneous nephrostomy can be considered. If the cytotoxic agents used are not nephrotoxic or primarily dependent on renal metabolism for excretion, a unilateral nephrostomy is usually required to preserve sufficient renal function. If agents considered for use are either nephrotoxic or metabolized in the kidney, bilateral nephrostomy may be considered.

The decision to place percutaneous nephrostomies is simple for patients who have reversible and highly curable lesions obstructing the kidneys (lymphomas, seminomas, embryonal carcinomas, and other germ cell tumors). In addition, nephrostomies are a logical choice for patients in whom excellent and sustained palliation can be achieved (breast carcinoma and urothelial malignancies).[5] In patients with refractory tumors with limited therapeutic options, the implication of percutaneous nephrostomy placement without control of the primary tumor should be discussed before placement. Although obstructive uropathy can be relieved, control of symptoms related to the continued growth of the cancer within the pelvis is more challenging.

Pathologically, acute urinary tract obstruction results in increased central renal pressure and dilation of the ureter. This is reflected in the increased size and weight of the kidney. With persistent and progressive obstructive uropathy, irreversible injury finally manifests itself with renal cortical atrophy. The selection of a patient for percutaneous nephrostomy should be based, in part, on the cortical thickness. In the absence of significant atrophy, the obstructed kidney most likely will regain significant function, and percutaneous nephrostomy should be considered. Small atrophic kidneys caused by long-standing obstructive uropathy frequently do not benefit from percutaneous drainage. Placement of a percutaneous nephrostomy in a markedly atrophic kidney results in significant morbidity without benefit.

Following relief of obstructive uropathy, metabolic problems may occur. Difficulties in maximum concentration of urine and other tubular defects can result in a brisk postobstructive diuresis. This occurs most often after high-grade acute obstruction. Replacement of fluid and electrolytes is important until normal renal function returns.[6]

Lower Urinary Tract Obstruction Distal outlet obstructions by locally advancing tumors that invade the urethra or primary urethral, prostatic, or bladder tumors are frequently drained unsatisfactorily by placement of Foley catheters or suprapubic tubes. In general, a suprapubic tube is contraindicated in patients with urothelial malignancies, when there is curative intent, because it violates the normal anatomic barriers and increases the probability of regional spread of the disease. Urothelial malignancies that diffusely involve the bladder have a propensity to recur in surgical wounds. The inability to place a Foley catheter is sometimes a complication of primary urethral or prostatic tumors. In such instances, suprapubic catheter drainage can be used to relieve symptoms of acute obstruction. In patients with urinary frequency caused by bladder invasion or with bladder irritability as a consequence of treatment, Foley catheter placement to relieve symptoms can be attempted but has limited success.

Poorly controlled primary cancers of the bladder, prostate, or urethra frequently result in a debilitating dysuria, frequency, and nocturia that compromise the quality of life. The palliation of severe urinary tract symptoms infrequently requires permanent urinary diversion. Urethral and suprapubic catheters are sometimes associated with urethral discomfort, however. Under such circumstances, urinary diversion to reduce these symptoms is helpful. Because of the limited overall benefit patients can expect to achieve when they require diversion for advanced cancer, the method of diversion with the least morbidity is chosen. Thus, percutaneous nephrostomies are used more frequently than surgically constructed urinary diversion.

We attribute the apparent reduction in the frequency with which we encounter these events to earlier detection, improved anticipation of local progression, and more effective surgical techniques. The problem of locally advanced cancer limiting bladder outlet and results in symptoms has few effective palliative measures and is best avoided and justifies early intervention in properly selected patients. Locally advanced cancer is a major source of morbidity whose best solution is early effective intervention.

Diagnostic studies for the radiologic and urologic assessment of the lower urinary tract have changed little and provide detailed assessment of anatomic determinants of obstruction. The first indication of obstructive uropathy is frequently a rising serum creatinine level. Urinalysis may reveal isosthenuria, and the blood urea nitrogen (BUN) level may rise. Proteinuria is not uncommon in obstructive uropathy.[7] Difficulties sometimes exist in detecting small degrees of low-grade obstructive uropathy with equivocal radiographic abnormalities. In such rare circumstances, radionuclide scans with the use of diuretics may help distinguish between a vascular and an obstructive lesion. The mainstays for the study of obstructive uropathy are ultrasonography and computed tomography (CT). When ultrasonography cannot be effectively performed because of gaseous distention, CT scans can be helpful. The superiority of ultrasonography in such patients lies in its value for marking the area for percutaneous drainage of the kidney and in the absence of contrast material, which could be injurious to renal function. More recently, endoureteral ultrasonography has been used to define the anatomy of the obstruction.

Algorithm for the Management of Urinary Obstruction Pelvic tumors can produce urinary symptoms, obstruction, and renal failure. Urinary obstruction often requires palliation or urinary diversion before systemic therapy can be delivered. An algorithm for management of these complications based on factors such as sensitivity to chemotherapy and expected survival can be used to develop a reasoned approach to the management of pelvic disease. Before intervening in urinary obstruction, the first question that should always be asked is "To what end?" Relief of urinary obstruction does not relieve pelvic symptoms attributed to infiltration of tumor. Thus, the relief of urinary obstruction should principally be used in those subsets of patients in whom cancer control can be expected, or, at a minimum, the origin of the symptoms is judged to arise from the obstruction itself as opposed to pelvic or retroperitoneal infiltration of the cancer.

Methods for relief of urethral obstruction are principally retrograde or antegrade. Rarely, in the era of interventional radiology, is open surgical diversion considered a treatment option. Retrograde placement of urethral stints by cystoscopy is frequently used. The advantage of this approach is the avoidance of external catheters and urinary diversion. However, the success of such an approach frequently is difficult to assess. In some subsets of patients, ureteral stints cannot be placed because of acute angulation and lack of control of the primary tumor. The approach that is frequently used by many physicians is a percutaneous nephrostomy. Percutaneous nephrostomies are safe and reliable procedures when performed by experienced radiologists in properly selected patients. Bilateral percutaneous nephrostomies are best placed in renal failure when a delay in response to therapy is expected or nephrotoxic cytotoxic agents are used. Coagulopathy and patient preference are the two major contraindications to percutaneous nephrostomies. The risk of such procedures is exceedingly low, and complications as a consequence of malplacement occasionally occur, such as bleeding into the pelvocaliceal system, producing an obstructive uropathy. Both the percutaneous nephrostomy and retrograde ureteral stints often result in urinary tract infection.

On occasion, even with obstructive uropathy from urethral obstruction, expectant management could be considered, as in situations in which highly responsive tumors are expected to respond quickly and result in relief of urinary obstruction. Examples include lymphomas and germ cell tumors for which the placement of nephrostomy can be delayed in the hope of an excellent response resulting in response of the tumor. Tumors of an intermediate response rate that can produce obstructive uropathy and in which a nephrostomy is often considered are ovarian tumors, urothelial tumors, and, rarely, breast cancers. If bilateral obstructive uropathy is present, relief with percutaneous nephrostomy is generally recommended.

For patients with urethral obstruction, the symptoms are often more difficult to relieve. Although percutaneous nephrostomies can divert urinary drainage, they do not result in relief of the pelvic symptoms related to urgency, hematuria, dysuria, and frequency. In such instances, transurethral resection of the prostate can be considered, as can a simple placement of a percutaneous nephrostomy or suprapubic tube. Although relieving the urinary obstruction, such management often fails to relieve the severe pelvic symptoms related to progressive disease at this site. The management of these severe symptoms is a therapeutic challenge for clinicians.

Hemorrhagic Cystitis Hematuria is frequently a striking and frightening event in the course of cancer and its treatment. Hematuria can be a result of bleeding anywhere along the entire urinary tract. Gross hematuria frequently requires palliation. The characteristics of the hematuria often permit physicians to suspect the origin of the bleeding. Long, vermiform clots typically indicate upper tract bleeding and are a result of a ureteral cast (broader clots are occasionally difficult to evacuate and cause ureteral colic or are indicative of lower tract bleeding). Bright red blood without a clot that clears partially during urination usually indicates a lower tract bleed. Hemorrhage can be a result of drug- or radiation-induced effects or of progressive cancer.

Drug-Induced Hematuria Cyclophosphamide and ifosfamide are the most commonly used oxazaphosphorines. Both agents are metabolized to acrolein, the main urothelial toxic metabolite.[8,9] In addition to acrolein, thrombocytopenia tends to exacerbate the bleeding. Sterile hemorrhagic cystitis has been reported in up to 20% of patients receiving high doses of cyclophosphamide and in approximately 8% of patients receiving ifosfamide.[10] With conventional doses of cyclophosphamide, cystitis can be prevented by encouraging aggressive oral hydration at the time of chemotherapy. In the case of ifosfamide, this complication can be reduced with intravenous hyperhydration and the use of uroprotective mesna. Mesna is given as an intravenous bolus equal to 20% of the ifosfamide dose 15 minutes before ifosfamide administration, as well as 4 and 8 hours later (the total dose of mesna should be equivalent to 60% of the ifosfamide dose).[11] Mesna can also be given as a continuous infusion at a dose equal to the ifosfamide dose. Continuous infusion of mesna should be maintained for 4 to 8 hours after completion of the ifosfamide infusion. In the case of cyclophosphamide, mesna is given mainly with high-dose chemotherapy in bone marrow transplantation. The dose of mesna used is approximately 60 to 160% of the cyclophosphamide dose and is given intravenously in three to five divided doses or by continuous infusion.[10] Other agents that can produce gross hematuria include intravesical treatment with doxorubicin, mitomycin, and bacille Calmette-Guérin.[11]

With the use of high-dose chemotherapy, hemorrhagic cystitis occurs in approximately 2% of conditioning regimens without cyclophosphamide. This bleeding is most commonly associated with thrombocytopenia.[12] When cyclophosphamide is used, up to 20% of patients may develop macrohematuria.[13] Moreover, the use of busulfan in addition to cyclophosphamide in high-dose chemotherapy tends to increase the risk of bleeding.[14] Hemorrhagic cystitis in bone marrow transplantation can also be associated with infection from adenovirus[15] or BK human polyomavirus.[16]

Detailed care to ensure optimal delivery of the potentially offending agents must be taken to avoid these feared complications.

Radiation-Induced Hematuria From approximately 5.7 to 11.5% of patients treated with pelvic irradiation (median toxic dose of 80 Gy) can develop bladder complications.[17] Although less common, hemorrhagic cystitis can be seen in the treatment of pelvic neoplasms with both external beam radiation and brachytherapy. Up to 9% of these patients can develop hematuria,[18] and approximately 10% will have bleeding more than 6 months after treatment.[19] Total-body irradiation for bone marrow transplantation is associated with hemorrhagic cystitis in 10 to 17% of patients.[14,20] Symptoms include recurrent hemorrhage, urinary urgency, and pain. The patients at highest risk are those with previous operations and those receiving cyclophosphamide. It is important to note that approximately 85% of the patients who develop macrohematuria after radiation actually have a recurrence of their tumor.[19] The pathophysiology of radiation-induced cystitis involves damage to the vascular endothelium and endarteritis, causing progressive ischemia, inflammation, and fibrosis, with the end result being tissue necrosis. This is also complicated by infections that prevent proper healing.

Recurrence of Tumor Another important cause of gross hematuria is related to recurrence of bladder tumors or invasion by other pelvic neoplasms. Most of these patients have advanced disease. In many, the treatments are palliative and directed to the underlying malignancy and symptoms.

Treatment Clot retention is a painful complication of lower urinary tract bleeding. Intermittent bladder injections or constant two-channel bladder irrigation with antibiotic-containing saline or water usually can dissolve or dissociate clots. Cystoscopic evacuation of clots is sometimes required for palliation. In patients who have not been treated with radiation therapy for their bleeding tumors, radiation is a useful approach. Cyclophosphamide-, ifosfamide-, or radiation-induced cystitis and bleeding are far more challenging problems. Embolization of bladder vessels or instillation of steroids has occasionally palliated such patients, but treatment is frequently unsatisfactory. Diluted formaldehyde may denature and fix superficial tissue layers. Emergency cystectomy has been undertaken to avoid exsanguination. Other treatments include hyperhydration, bladder irrigation, intravesical alum,[20] and intravesical prostaglandins.[21] Experimental approaches include amifostine,[22] hyperbaric oxygenation,[23] conjugated estrogens,[24] and glucose-mannose binding plant lectins.[25]

Radiation Nephritis Radiation is frequently delivered to control nodal metastasis from radiation-sensitive tumors (eg, lymphomas and seminomas). The dose of radiation delivered to the kidneys can sometimes result in significant renal compromise from radiation-induced nephritis. The kidney is an important dose-limiting organ in radiation therapy. When both kidneys are radiated, the dose tolerance ($TD_{5/5}$) is 20 Gy in adults, and approximately 17% of patients will develop symptomatic renal disease. When only one kidney is irradiated, the tolerance increases. Glomerular function starts to decrease at 15 Gy, and function is completely lost at 25 to 30 Gy. Radiosensitizers such as cisplatin, carmustine (BCNU), and actinomycin D tend to lower normal tissue radiation tolerance. Symptoms are rarely seen acutely within 6 months of treatment. Subacute symptoms, such as anemia, hypertension, edema, albuminuria, active urinary sediment, and an increase in BUN and creatinine, are seen 6 to 12 months after radiation. In the chronic phase (> 12 months), benign or malignant hypertension is the most common finding. Eventually, the patient may develop hyperreninemic hypertension related to renal scarring, atrophy of cortical tubules, and glomerulosclerosis. Management involves decreasing the renal workload with salt and fluid restriction and a low-protein diet. Some patients may develop progressive deterioration of renal function requiring hemodialysis or renal transplantation.[26] Avoiding the debilitating complications of radiation injury to genitourinary tissue is an essential aspect to the good practice of oncology. Use of modern radiation techniques and an understanding of genitourinary tissue tolerance furnish the practicing physician with clear guidelines for the safe use of radiation therapy.

Long-term renal toxicity related to total-body irradiation in bone marrow transplantation is associated with hypertension, anemia, decreased glomerular filtration rate, hematuria, and proteinuria. These findings are caused by subendothelial widening of basement membrane, endothelial cell dropout, glomerular arteriolar intimal thickening, and tubular atrophy. These effects are dose dependent. In a review of bone marrow transplantation patients receiving total-body irradiation with 14 Gy, it was noted that the incidence of nephropathy decreased with increased shielding of the kidneys. Of the patients without shielding of the kidneys, 30% developed nephropathy. When the kidneys were partially shielded, reducing the dosage by 15%, the fraction of patients developing nephropathy decreased to 15%. When the shielding was increased and the dosage was reduced by 30%, none of the patients developed nephropathy.[27] These patients are more susceptible to radiation-induced renal injury secondary to the use of higher doses of chemotherapy, aminoglycosides, and antifungal medications, as well as infections and the development of graft-versus-host disease.

DIAGNOSIS, TREATMENT, AND PREVENTION OF NEPHROTOXICITY OF CANCER THERAPEUTIC AGENTS

With the advent of effective cytotoxic chemotherapy, attention has turned to the side effects of these widely used agents (Table 133-1). These side effects include tumor lysis syndrome, paraneoplastic glomerulonephritis, obstructive uropathy, and nephrotoxicity with renal failure and electrolyte disturbances. These are more common in the geriatric population secondary to polypharmacy or drug interactions and comorbid conditions. Also, nephrotoxicity with these agents is more common in bone marrow transplantation, secondary to high-dose chemotherapy, polypharmacy, and total-body irradiation. In the following sections, we describe commonly used agents that cause serious renal toxicity. Table 133-2 lists other agents that less commonly cause renal side effects. Table 133-3 lists the mechanism of renal injury for some of the drugs. Another important aspect related to prevention of nephrotoxicity involves the interaction among drugs. Drug interactions, by decreasing liver metabolism or renal clearance, can increase the serum concentration of antineoplastic agents. This increase can cause unexpected nephrotoxicity, even though the correct doses have been prescribed. A careful review of the patient's medications is essential in the prevention of renal toxicity. Table 133-4 describes some of these drug interactions. Also important is a baseline evaluation of the patient's renal function because several drugs may need a dose adjustment in the presence of renal insufficiency (Table 133-5).

Table 133-1 Therapy Agents Associated with Nephrotoxicity

Alkylating agents
AZQ (diaziquone)
Cisplatin
Cisplatin analogues
Oxaliplatin
Carboplatin
Ifosfamide
Nitrosoureas (streptozocin)
Antitumor antibiotics
Mitomycin C
Plicamycin
Antimetabolites
5-Azacytidine
High-dose methotrexate
Clofarabine
Folate antagonist
Pemetrexed
Monoclonal antibody
Bevacizumab
Cetuximab
Biologic agents
Interferon
Interleukin-2
Others
Gallium nitrate
Cyclosporine
Tacrolimus

Cisplatin The introduction of cisplatin to the clinic highlighted the hazards that follow failure to understand the renal complications of cytotoxic agents.[28] Effectively overcoming renal toxicity that is the principal toxicity of cisplatin has allowed significant benefit to patients with many types of cancer. Development of platinum analogues has, in part, been motivated by the renal toxicity associated with cisplatin. However, cisplatin continues to be widely used as a major cancer drug because of its differential antitumor activity when compared with the available analogues. The study of cisplatin, the modification of its delivery, and the anticipation of and screening for nephrotoxicity provide a paradigm for the study of nephrotoxic agents in general.

The principal excretion route of cisplatin is renal. However, only a small portion of the total cisplatin dose can be recovered in the urine in the first few days after therapy.[29] Much of the drug is irreversibly bound to protein, but active metabolites, the aquated diamino derivative, as well as the parent, dichlorodiammineplatinum, are found in the ultrafiltrable plasma fraction. This plasma clearance is triphasic, with nearly all of the drug gone in 4 hours, but it has a terminal half-life of over 24 hours. The primary lesion of cisplatin toxicity is necrosis of the proximal convoluted tubules. The severity of the nephrotoxicity can be modified by hydration. The strong emetic effects of cisplatin can, however, produce dehydration. These dual side effects—severe nausea and vomiting and primary nephrotoxicity exaggerated by dehydration—have been largely overcome with hydration schedules and the aggressive use of new antiemetics.[30,31]

A reduction in the glomerular filtration rate (GFR) is the primary cisplatin-induced injury that is measured clinically. Other complications include hypomagnesemia and modest amounts of proteinuria. The proteinuria associated with cisplatin nephrotoxicity is attributed to a tubular defect.[32] Hemolytic-uremic syndrome (HUS) has also been described, especially when cisplatin is combined with bleomycin.[33] Sequential measurement of the GFR is essential for monitoring of cisplatin toxicity. An accurate urine collection for inulin clearance is superior to 24-hour urine collection for creatinine clearance, but we have used the serum creatinine concentration and calculation of the creatinine clearance. Assay of electrolytes, including calcium, magnesium, and phosphorus, has also been routinely made. For patients treated at The University of Texas M. D. Anderson Cancer Center (UTMDACC) in the Department of Genitourinary Medical Oncology, electrolytes, BUN, and creatinine are monitored prior to each dose of therapy. There is a minimum interval of 7 days between cisplatin doses. This interval is important because maximal nephrotoxicity frequently does not manifest itself in less than 7 days. A significant decline in the creatinine clearance, as measured by the Cockroft formula, should result in a delay of therapy (Table 133-6).

Prevention of toxicity is important in patient care. Empiric observations, in both the laboratory and the clinic, demonstrate that hydration with the use of mannitol or hypertonic saline has significantly reduced the cisplatin-induced decline in renal function.[30,31] Although hypertonic saline is not commonly used, normal saline is important to provide abundant chloride ions. This diminishes the formation of the aquated species by mass action, thereby lessening the impact on renal function. Minimum urine flow should be sustained at 100 mL/h before cisplatin administration. Multiple clinical trials have demonstrated the effectiveness of using mannitol in different schedules. Conflicting reports exist regarding the use of furosemide (Lasix) and its ability to affect cisplatin's nephrotoxicity. Its use has generally been avoided at the UTMDACC.[34,35] More recently, amifostine (phosphorylated aminothiol prodrug) has been used in the prevention of nephrotoxicity by cisplatin. Amifostine is metabolized to WR-1065 and WR-33278, which reduce formation of deoxyribonucleic acid (DNA)–DNA crosslinks,[36] reverse platinum-DNA adducts,[37] and bind to oxygen free radicals. Several studies show that amifostine decreases the number of patients with a greater than 40% reduction in creatinine clearance or with a decrease in glomerular filtration secondary to cisplatin nephrotoxicity, from 30 to 40% to approximately 10%.[38–40] It has been noted that amifostine does not affect the response to chemotherapy. Certain chemotherapeutic agents and other nephrotoxic drugs can impact significantly on nephrotoxicity. Cisplatin is used frequently in combination with other agents, such as ifosfamide and MTX. The side effects seem to be greatly diminished by adequate hydration. Paclitaxel in combination with cisplatin has been associated with elevation of serum creatinine in the treatment of gynecologic cancers.[41] Concurrent aminoglycoside antibiotics have been reported to result in a significantly greater reduction in renal function.[42] Meticulous attention to detail, adequate hydration, and avoidance of these interactions are important.

Methotrexate MTX, an agent dependent on renal glomerular filtration as its principal excretory route, can also induce renal toxicity.[43,44] Renal toxicity can be particularly devastating because prolonged exposure to MTX at elevated levels substantially increases toxicity in the bone marrow and the oral cavity of the alimentary canal. The renal toxicity of MTX is a dose-dependent phenomenon. Renal failure has often been implicated in deaths associated with the use of this agent.

The nephrotoxicity of MTX is manifested primarily in the renal tubule, where extensive necrosis of the convoluted tubules occurs. The lesion has been termed crystalline hydronephrosis and

Table 133-2 Clinical and Pathologic Features of Chemotherapy-Associated Nephrotoxicity

Drug	Type of Injury	Clinical Features	Urine Analysis	Time of Toxicity	Treatment/Outcome	Prevention
5-Azacytidine	Acute tubular	Renal tubular acidosis	Bland, hypo-osmolar on therapy	Polyuria and rising creatinine 7–10 d post-dose	Replace HCO_3, PO_4, Mg; recovery is complete	Daily creatinine, BUN, and electrolytes
Bevacizumab	Glomerulopathy	Proteinuria	Proteinuria	Increasing with cumulative dose	Discontinue if nephrotic syndrome; hold therapy or urinary protein ≥ 2 gf in 24 h collection	Monitor regularly
Carboplatin	Tubular	Mg wasting	Bland	Rising creatinine 5–10 d after therapy	Cessation of drug; dialysis as necessary; recovery usually incomplete	Avoid other nephrotoxic drugs; Mg may increase in patients previously treated with cisplatin
Cisplatin	Acute tubular	Mg wasting	Bland	Rising creatinine with cumulative dose	Cessation of drug; dialysis as necessary; recovery usually incomplete	Vigorous hydration; Cl diuresis, mannitol diuresis, Na thiosulfate; avoid aminoglycosides
Cyclosporine	Tubular and afferent arteriole vasoconstriction	Increased K and decreased Mg; renal tubular acidosis; edema; hypertension	Proteinuria	Rising creatinine from days to months after initiation of therapy	Cessation of drug; dialysis as necessary; recovery usually complete	Periodic drug level; follow-up creatinine, BUN, and electrolytes
AZQ (diaziquone)	Tubular and glomerular	Anuria; proteinuria, and renal tubular acidosis	Proteinuria	Rising creatinine 5–10 d after therapy	Cessation of drug; dialysis as necessary; recovery usually complete	Avoid doses > 245 mg/m^2
Gallium nitrate	Glomerulopathy	Proteinuria and occasional azotemia	Proteinuria	Proteinuria followed by rising creatinine during and shortly after therapy days	Cessation of drug; recovery usually complete	Daily urine flow > 2 L; avoid doses > 300 mg/m^2/d for 7 consecutive d
Ifosfamide	Acute tubular	Oliguria	Bland	Rising creatinine within1–2 d after therapy	Supportive dialysis; recovery usually complete	Oliguria may be increased in patients with prior cisplatin therapy; mesna
Interleukin-2	Prerenal azotemia	Oliguria and hypotension	Proteinuria and hematuria	Rising creatinine during therapy	Stop drug when creatinine ≥ 4.5 mg/dL or > 4 mg/dL with acidosis, fluid overload or increased K; creatinine > 1.5 mg/dL with oliguria; recovery usually within 1–2 wk	Dopamine at renal doses and fluids
Methotrexate	Acute tubular	Oliguria	Bland	Rising creatinine within1–2 d of dose	High-dose leucovorin based on methotrexate level; high-volume urine output and alkalinization; recovery is complete	Vigorous hydration and urine alkalinization; dose reduction on renal dysfunction; avoid aminoglycosides and nonsteroidal anti-inflammatory; leucovorin
Plicamycin	Acute tubular	Abrupt renal failure	Mild proteinuria	Rising creatinine during dosing	Cessation of drug; re-treat, if recovery complete	Alternate-day dosing; check creatinine and BUN daily
Mitomycin C	Renal vascular lesions	Hypertension, anemia	Hematuria, proteinuria	Rising creatinine after 2 or more doses (12–40 wk from start)	Permanent cessation of drug; SPA immunoperfusion and dialysis; poor recovery	Stop drug at cumulative dose of 60 mg
Nitrosoureas	Interstitial fibrosis, glomerular sclerosis	Late complications	Bland	Rising creatinine months to years after therapy	Supportive dialysis; recovery is complete	Stop BCNU at cumulative dose of 1,200 mg/m^2
Streptozocin	Tubular	Proteinuria, occasionally severe	Proteinuria, aminoaciduria	Proteinuria followed by rising creatinine during dosing	Cessation of drug; recovery usually complete	Stop drug at first evidence of proteinuria; hydration will not prevent injury

BCNU = carmustine; BUN = blood urea nitrogen; SPA = staphylococcal protein A.

has been attributed to deposition of the agent. The precipitation of MTX and its less soluble principal metabolite, 7-hydroxy-MTX, in the renal tubule, results in changes in preglomerular vascular pressure and a direct decrease in glomerular filtration.

Avoidance of MTX nephrotoxicity can be accomplished by selecting patients with normal renal function, ensuring adequate hydration, and alkalinizing the urine to pH 7 or higher. Prior to administration of MTX at doses of 100 mg/m^2 or greater (and some doses are 100 to 200 times this amount), adequate renal function should be ensured by normal serum creatinine and minimum urinary flow of 100 mL/h. Urine should have a pH of 7 or higher, and leucovorin can be administered after MTX. MTX is highly protein bound and is not readily removed by dialysis.[33] Specific attention to interaction with other agents is important when administering MTX. Weak organic acids, such as salicylates or sulfisoxazole, increase MTX levels by displacing the drug from binding sites on plasma proteins. In addition, renal tubular transport is diminished by probenecid and salicylates. Specific avoidance of these agents reduces the risk of inducing nephrotoxicity or increasing other side effects.

Nitrosoureas Each of the nitrosoureas (lomustine [CCNU], methyl-CCNU, BCNU) was predicted to have significant nephrotoxicity.[45,46] Initial small phase I and II trials failed to reveal evidence of renal compromise, but with their use in large phase III trials, drug-induced nephrotoxicity was encountered.[47–49] Unlike the nephrotoxicity associated with MTX and cisplatin,

Table 133-3 Types of Renal Injury Caused by Cancer Chemotherapeutic Agents

Pathologic Finding	Causative Agent
Acute glomerulonephritis	None reported
Acute tubular necrosis	Plicamycin
	Cisplatin (?)
Interstitial nephritis	Nitrosoureas
Membranous glomerulonephritis (protein losing)	Gallium nitrate (?)
	AZQ (diaziquone)
	Bevacizumab
Obstructive uropathy	Methotrexate (?)
Renal tubular acidosis	5-Azacytidine
Renal vasculitis	Mitomycin C

nitrosoureas cause interstitial nephritis. The specific mechanism by which this occurs is unclear. At present, limiting the total cumulative dose of the agents is the only way of preventing this; hydration does not appear to alter it. Monitoring such patients with serial urinalysis and serum creatinine concentrations appears to be the most reliable way to screen for nephrotoxicity.

Mitomycin C Mitomycin C is an antibiotic isolated from *Streptomyces caespitosus.*

Although this agent has significant activity against a variety of tumors, it has received rather limited use because of prolonged thrombocytopenia and unpredictable side effects, which are dose limiting.

The unique clinical nephrotoxicity of mitomycin C is a striking HUS. This is sometimes manifested by early elevation of serum creatinine or anemia, with a rise in serum lactate acid dehydrogenase, indicating hemolysis. Patients receiving mitomycin C should be carefully monitored for HUS. Total cumulative doses of less than 30 mg/m^2 of body surface area are rarely, if ever, associated with HUS. The most difficult problem in managing the HUS of patients treated with mitomycin C is that it is sometimes difficult to anticipate because the onset can be delayed after the time of delivery of the agent.

Mitomycin C–induced nephrotoxicity can be prevented by limiting the cumulative dose to less than 30 mg/m^2 of body surface area. The use of steroids, which are believed to reduce the pulmonary toxicity of this agent, has not clearly demonstrated a role in reducing nephrotoxicity. Plasmapheresis appears to provide therapeutic benefit in selected patients, although only limited studies have been performed.[50,51] Small numbers of studies have been performed, but they seem to indicate that therapeutic benefit can be achieved in selected patients.

Immunologic Agents Interleukin-2 causes renal insufficiency by a direct toxic effect on the kidneys and by prerenal azotemia from capillary leak syndrome. This renal toxicity is commonly reversible after discontinuation of the drug, intravenous saline, albumin, pressors, and renal dose dopamine.[33]

Cyclosporine produces renal vasoconstriction primarily at the afferent arteriole, causing arterial

Table 133-4 Drug Interactions That Can Increase Serum Levels of Antineoplastic Agents or Add Renal Toxicity

Capecitabine	Leucovorin
Carboplatin	Cyclophosphamide, aminoglycosides, topotecan
Cisplatin	Any nephrotoxic agent,* melphalan, paclitaxel,† rituximab, topotecan†
Cladribine	Cyclophosphamide (high dose)
Cyclophosphamide	Allopurinol
Cyclosporine	Any nephrotoxic agent,* vancomycin, melphalan, cimetidine, potassium-sparing diuretics, naproxen, sulindac, diclofenac, allopurinol, cytochrome P-450 inhibitors,‡ methotrexate
Etoposide	Aprepitant, cyclosporine, valspodar
Gefitinib	Cytochrome P-450 3A4 inhibitors
Gemcitabine	5-Fluorouracil
Ifosfamide	Cytochrome P-450 inhibitors,‡ aprepitant
Interleukin-2	Any nephrotoxic agent*
Melphalan	Buthionine
Methotrexate	Organic acids, penicillins, cisplatin, NSAIDs, amiodarone, aspirin, ciprofloxacin, cotrimoxazole, cyclosporine, doxycycline, mercaptopurine, probenecid, procarbazine
Mercaptopurine	Allopurinol, methotrexate, TPMT inhibitors
Mitomycin	5-Fluorouracil–related hemolytic-uremic syndrome
Streptozocin	Any nephrotoxic agent*
Tacrolimus	Any nephrotoxic agent,* cyclosporine, cisplatin, drugs metabolized through cytochrome P-450 3A
Thioguanine	TPMT inhibitors
Topotecan	Cisplatin,† carboplatin†
Trimetrexate	Cimetidine, cytochrome P-450 inhibitors‡

NSAIDs = nonsteroidal anti-inflammatory drugs; TPMT = thiopurine methyltransferase.
*For example, aminoglycosides, amphotericin B, intravenous contrast, NSAIDs.
†Related to sequence of administration.
‡Azoles-antifungals, macrolides, calcium channel blockers, corticosteroids, grapefruit juice.

Table 133-5 Adjustment of Antineoplastic Agents Based on Renal Insufficiency

Azacytidine	Unexplained increases in creatinine or blood urea nitrogen; delay treatment until back to baseline, then reduce dose by 50%
Bleomycin	Creatinine clearance 10 to 50 mL/min: reduce dose by 25%
	Creatinine clearance < 10 mL/min: reduce dose by 50%
Capecitabine	Creatinine clearance 30–50 mL/min: reduce dose by 25%
	Creatinine clearance < 30 mL/min: not recommended
Carboplatin	Adjust according to Calvert formula
	Total dose (mg) = (target AUC) × (GFR + 25)
Cisplatin	Creatinine clearance 10–50 mL/min: decrease dose by 25%
	Creatinine clearance < 10 mL/min: decrease dose by 50%
	Some clinicians advocate no changes in dosing, independent of renal function
Clofarabine	Use with extreme caution
Cyclophosphamide	Creatinine clearance 10–50 mL/min: reduce dose by 25%
	Creatinine clearance < 10 mL/min: reduce dose by 50%
Cytarabine	Creatinine clearance < 60 mL/min; use caution: may decrease dose or change schedule
Daunorubicin	Creatinine > 3 mg/dL: decrease dose by 50%
Etoposide	Creatinine clearance 15–50 mL/min: decrease dose by 25%
	Creatinine clearance < 15 mL/min: consider 50% dose reduction
Fludarabine	Creatinine clearance 30–70 mL/min: decrease 20–50%
	Creatinine clearance < 30 mL/min: not recommended
Gefitinib	Use caution with severe renal impairment
Gemcitabine	Use caution with severe renal impairment
Ifosfamide	Use caution with renal impairment
Melphalan IV	BUN > 30 mg/dL or creatinine > 1.5 mg/dL: consider 50% dose reduction
Mercaptopurine	Consider decreasing dose when given with allopurinol (some clinicians recommend not giving these drugs together)
Methotrexate	Creatinine clearance 10–50 mL/min: reduce dose by 50%
	Creatinine clearance < 10 mL/min: avoid use
Nitrosoureas	Some clinicians recommend omitting doses when creatinine clearance < 60 mL/min
Oxaliplatin	Use with caution in mild to severe renal impairment
Pemetrexed	Hold therapy if creatinine clearance < 45 mL/min; patient with grade 3/4
	Nonhematologic toxicity should decrease dose by 25%
Plicamycin	Creatinine clearance 10–50 mL/min: reduce by 25%
	Creatinine clearance < 10 mL/min: reduce dose by 50–75%
Streptozocin	Use with caution
Topotecan	Creatinine clearance 20–39 mL/min: decrease dose to 0.75 mg/m^2
	Creatinine clearance < 20 mL/min: consider not to give dose
Thioguanine	Consider decreasing dose, no formal recommendation
Trimetrexate	Hold therapy if creatinine > 2.5 mg/dL; dose adjustment may be necessary in renal impairment

AUC = area under the curve; BUN = blood urea nitrogen; GFR = glomerular filtration rate; IV = intravenous.

hypertension, fluid retention, and, ultimately, renal dysfunction.[52] Acute nephrotoxicity is reversible with dose modification. In contrast, chronic administration may cause a slowly irreversible renal failure secondary to renal tubular fibrosis and afferent arteriopathy with proteinaceous material.[53]

Tacrolimus causes renal injury in a fashion similar to that of cyclosporine. In contrast to cyclosporine, however, it is less likely to cause arterial hypertension. Tacrolimus stimulates transforming growth factor α_1 expression and inhibits matrix protein degradation.[54]

Other Agents On the basis of preclinical studies, the anthracyclines daunorubicin and doxorubicin were predicted to cause renal toxicity.[55–57] Anthracycline-induced nephrotoxicity has not, however, been convincingly reported in clinical trials. Ifosfamide can cause proximal tubular dysfunction, distal renal tubular acidosis, nephrogenic diabetes insipidus, and the syndrome of inappropriate antidiuretic hormone release. Multiple new agents are associated with kidney toxicity, but data are limited. Fludarabine has been reported to cause urologic complications related to urinary tract infections in 12 to 22% of patients.[10,58,59] Abnormal renal function is observed in less than 5% of patients treated with fludarabine[10,59–61] and is related to tumor lysis syndrome. Paclitaxel has been associated with elevation of serum creatinine in about 18% of human immunodeficiency virus (HIV) patients treated for Kaposi's sarcoma.[10,62,63] Gemcitabine is linked to sporadic renal failure associated with thrombotic microangiopathy.[64] The increase in the number of new agents, including monoclonal antibodies, and small molecule inhibitors of tyrosine kinase inhibitors requires special considerations.

Several monoclonal antibodies have been approved for clinical trials. Bevacizumab is noteworthy for its nephrotoxic profile.

MONITORING FOR DRUG-INDUCED NEPHROTOXICITY

The principle that should guide clinicians in the use of potentially nephrotoxic agents in the treatment of cancer is close monitoring for the development of renal toxicity, its early detection, and its management. The wide range of renal insults induced by cytotoxic drugs complicates the selection of the appropriate study to monitor potential nephrotoxicity.[65] Clinicians apply similar screening studies to detect a wide range of renal insults from cytotoxic agents. The use of specific studies that focus on the nature of the cytotoxic injury induced by the specific agent is more likely to detect early injury. For example, tubular defects resulting from cisplatin nephrotoxicity are not directly correlated with reduction in the GFR, whereas hypermagnesiuria and hypomagnesemia are characteristic. Monitoring patients for nephrotoxicity for agents that can cause interstitial nephritis (nitrosoureas) or glomerular injury (mitomycin C) requires routine and frequent urinalyses. The appearance of microhematuria should lead physicians to further exclude drug-induced renal injury.

Table 133-6 Cockroft Formula

$$\frac{(140 - \text{age})\ \text{weight (kg)}}{72\ \times \text{serum creatinine}}$$

The most common renal functional abnormality as a result of cytotoxic therapy is a decline in GFR. The most frequently used measure of GFR is creatinine clearance. Creatinine clearance is less accurate than other measures of GFR but, for practical reasons, has been widely applied clinically.[66] A serial decline in creatinine clearance is a reliable index of worsening renal function. Significant limitations are encountered in estimating a creatinine clearance from serum creatinine alone, using predictive formulas (Cockroft; see Table 133-6). Use of such formulae has, however, been widely applied in clinical oncology, in view of the difficulties in collecting reliable 24-hour urine specimens. The 24-hour collection for creatinine clearance has been supplanted by the use of the Cockroft formula at UTMDACC in the Department of Genitourinary Medical Oncology. No increase in the frequency of renal compromise associated with cisplatin administration has been noted since this procedure was adopted. A practical approach has been to follow only the serum creatinine concentrations. In the absence of any change in the serum creatinine concentration or calculated clearance (Cockroft), no further study is required. In patients whose serum creatine concentration increases more than 0.4 mg/dL, further investigation of renal function is undertaken. An adjustment in dose or a change in therapy may then be ordered as required. Particular attention should be paid to the correct calculation of the renal function by adjusting for weight. The creatinine clearance calculated by the Cockroft formula is sufficient in patients of average body habitus but may result in erroneous predictions in patients who are emaciated or in those with a large muscle mass. The wide fluctuations in weight that occur in patients undergoing cancer therapy require that the patients be weighed before each dose of chemotherapy and that doses be adjusted for changes in weight.

REFERENCES

1. Logothetis CJ, Samuels ML, Ogden SL, et al. Cyclophosphamide and sequential cisplatin for advanced seminoma: long-term follow-up in 52 patients. J Urol 1987;138:789–94.
2. Logothetis CJ, Samuels ML, Selig DE, et al. Cyclic chemotherapy with cyclophosphamide, doxorubicin, and cisplatin plus vinblastine and bleomycin in advanced germinal tumors: results with 100 patients. Am J Med 1986;81:219–28.
3. Dyer RB, Assimos DG, Regan SD. Update on interventional uroradiology. Urol Clin North Am 1997;24:623–52.
4. Stables DP. Percutaneous nephrostomy: techniques, indications and results. Urol Clin North Am 1982;9:15–29.
5. Carrasco CH, Charnsangavej C, Richli WR, Wallace S. Percutaneous drainage. In: Hickey RC, editor. Current problems in cancer. Vol X, No 12. Chicago: Year Book; 1986. p. 599–600.
6. Gillenwater JY. The pathophysiology of urinary obstructions. In: Harrison JH, editor. Campbell's urology. 4th ed. Philadelphia: WB Saunders; 1979. p. 377.
7. Gutmann FD, Boxer RJ. Pathophysiology and management of urinary tract obstruction. In: Rieselbach RE, Garnick MB, editors. Cancer and the kidney. Philadelphia: Lea & Febiger; 1982. p. 594–624.
8. Cox PJ. Cyclophosphamide induced cystitis—identification of acrolein as the causative agent. Biochem Pharmacol 1979;28:2045–9.
9. Brade WP, Herdrich K, Varani, M. Ifosfamide—pharmacology, safety and therapeutic potential. Cancer Treat Rep 1985;12:1–47.
10. McEvoy GK. Drug information. Bethesda (MD): American Society of Health System Pharmacists; 1999.
11. Drake MJ, Nixon PM, Crew J. Drug-induced bladder and urinary disorders. Incidence, prevention and management. Drug Saf 1998;19:45–55.
12. Brugieres L, Hartmann O, Travagli JP, et al. Hemorrhagic cystitis following high-dose chemotherapy and bone marrow transplantation in children with malignancies: incidence, clinical course and outcome. J Clin Oncol 1989;7:194–9.
13. Klingemann JD, Sheperd DE, Reece MJ, et al. Regimen-related acute toxicities: pathophysiology, risk factors, clinical evaluation and preventive strategies. Bone Marrow Transplant 1994;14 Suppl 4:514–8.
14. Ringden Q, Remberger M, Ruutu T, et al. Increased risk of chronic graft-versus-host disease, obstructive bronchiolitis and alopecia with busulfan versus total-body irradiation. Blood 1999;93:2196–201.
15. Mufsen MA, Belshe RB. A review of adenoviruses in the etiology of acute hemorrhagic cystitis. J Urol 1976;115:191–4.
16. Bedi A, Miller, CB, Hanson, JL, et al. Association of BK virus with failure of prophylaxis against hemorrhagic cystitis following bone marrow transplantation. J Clin Oncol 1995;13:1103–9.
17. Burman C, Kutcher GJ, Goitein M. Fitting of normal tissue tolerance data to an analytic function. Int J Radiat Oncol Biol Phys 1991;21:123–35.
18. DeVries CR, Freiha, FS. Hemorrhagic cystitis: a review. J Urol 1990;143:1–9.
19. Dean RJ, Bernard L. Urologic complications of pelvic radiation. J Urol 1978;119:64–7.
20. Kohno A, Takeyama K, Narabajashi M, et al. Hemorrhagic cystitis associated with allogeneic and autologous bone marrow transplantation for malignant neoplasm in adults. Jpn J Clin Oncol 1993;23:46–52.
21. Miller LJ, Chandler SW, Ippolit CM. Treatment of cyclophosphamide-induced hemorrhagic cystitis with prostaglandins. Ann Pharmacother 1994;28:590–4.
22. Srivastava A, Nair SC, Srivastava VM, et al. Evaluation of uroprotective efficacy of amifostine against cyclophosphamide induced hemorrhagic cystitis. Bone Marrow Transplant 1999;23:463–7.
23. Yazawa H, Nakada T, Sasawaga I, et al. Hyperbaric oxygenation therapy for cyclophosphamide induced hemorrhagic cystitis. Int Urol Nephrol 1995;27:381–5.
24. Liu YK, Harty JI, Steinbok GS, et al. Treatment of radiation or cyclophosphamide induced cystitis using conjugated estrogens. J Urol 1990;144:41–3.
25. Assreuy AM, Martins GJ, Moreira ME. Prevention of cyclophosphamide-induced hemorrhagic cystitis by glucose-mannose binding plant lectins. J Urol 1999;161:1988–93.
26. Perez C, Brady L. Principles and practice of radiation oncology. 3rd ed. Philadelphia: Lippincott-Raven; 1998.
27. Lawton CA, Cohen EP, Murray KJ, et al. Long-term results of selective renal shielding in patients undergoing total-body irradiation in preparation for bone marrow transplantation. Bone Marrow Transplant 1997;20:1069–74.
28. Walker EM, Gale GR. Methods of reduction of cisplatin nephrotoxicity. Ann Clin Lab Sci 1981;11:397–410.
29. Speer RJ, Ridgway H, Hall LM. Coordination complexes of platinum as antitumor agents. Cancer Chemother Rep 1979;59:629–41.
30. Ozols RF, Cordon BJ, Jacobs J, et al. High-dose cisplatin in hypertonic saline. Ann Intern Med 1984;100:19–24.
31. Gonzales-Vitale JC, Hayes DM, Cvitkovic E, Sternberg SS. The renal pathology in clinical trial of cisplatinum (II) diamminodichloride. Cancer 1977;39:1362–71.
32. Buamah PK, Howell A, Whitby H, et al. Assessment of renal function during high-dose cisplatin therapy in patients with ovarian carcinoma. Cancer Chemother Pharmacol 1982;8:281–4.
33. Berns J, Ford P. Renal toxicities of antineoplastic drugs and bone marrow transplantation. Semin Nephrol 1997;17: 54–66.

34. Pera MF, Harder HC. Effects of furosemide- and mannitol-induced diuresis on the nephrotoxicity and physiologic disposition of cis-dichlorodiamminoplatinum in rats. Proc Am Assoc Cancer Res 1978;19:100.
35. Pera MF, Zook BC, Harder HC. Effects of mannitol or furosemide diuresis on the nephrotoxicity and physiological disposition of cisdiammineplatinum (II) in rats. Cancer Res 1979;29:1269–78.
36. De Neve WJ, Everett CK, Suminski JE, et al. Influence of WR-2721 on DNA's cross-linking by nitrogen mustard in normal mouse bone marrow and leukemia cells in vivo. Cancer Res 1988;48:6002–5.
37. Treskes M, Nijtmans LG, Fichtinger-Schepman AM, et al. Effects of the modulating agent WR 2721 and its main metabolites of the formation and stability of cisplatin DNA adducts in vitro in comparison to the effects of thiosulphate and diethylthiocarbamate. Biochem Pharmacol 1992;43:1013–9.
38. Kemp G, Rose P, Lurain J, et al. Amifostine pretreatment for protection against cyclophosphamide and cisplatin induced toxicities: results of a randomized control trial in patients with advanced ovarian cancer. J Clin Oncol 1996;14:2101–12.
39. Alberts DS, Green S, Hannigan EV, et al. Improved therapeutic index of carboplatin plus cyclophosphamide versus cisplatin plus cyclophosphamide: final report by the Southwest Oncology Group of a phase III randomized trial in stage IV ovarian cancer. J Clin Oncol 1992;10:706–17.
40. Schiller JH, Berry W, Storer B, et al. Phase II trial of amifostine, cisplatin and vinblastine for metastatic non-small cell lung cancer. Proc Am Soc Clin Oncol 1995;14:356.
41. Merouani A, Davidson SA, Schrier RW. Increased nephrotoxicity of combination Taxol and cisplatin chemotherapy in gynecologic cancers as compared to cisplatin alone. Am J Nephrol 1997;17:53–8.
42. Gonzales-Vitale JC, Hayes DM, Cvitkovic E, Sternberg SS. Acute renal failure after cis-dichlorodiammineplatinum (II) and gentamicin-cephalothin therapies. Cancer Treat Rep 1978;62:693–8.
43. Evans BD, Rajn KS, Calvert AH, et al. Phase II study of JM-8, a new platinum analog, in advanced ovarian carcinoma. Cancer Treat Rep 1983;67:997–1000.
44. Frei E. Methotrexate revisited. Med Pediatr Oncol 1976;2:227–41.
45. Denine EP, Harrison SD, Pechkam JC. Qualitative and quantitative toxicity of sublethal doses of methyl-CCNU in BDF1 mice. Cancer Treat Rep 1977;61:409–17.
46. Carter SK, Broder L, Friedman M. Streptozotocin and metastatic insulinoma. Ann Intern Med 1971;74:445–6.
47. Harmon WE, Cohen HJ, Schneeberger EE, Grupe WE. Chronic renal failure in children treated with methyl CCNU. N Engl J Med 1979;300:1200–3.
48. Berglund J. Progredierande njurinsufficiens efter CCNU-behandling. Lakartidningen 1980;77:1760.
49. Ellis ME, Weiss RB, Kuperminc M. Nephrotoxicity of lomustine. Cancer Chemother Pharmacol 1985;15:174–5.
50. Cantrell JE, Philips TM, Schein PS. Carcinoma-associated hemolytic-uremic syndrome: a complication of mitomycin C chemotherapy. J Clin Oncol 1985;3:723–34.
51. Lempert KD. Haemolysis and renal impairment syndrome in patients on 5-fluorouracil and mitomycin-C. Lancet 1980;ii:369–70.
52. Elzinga L, Kelley VE, Houghton DC, Bennett WM. Fish oil vehicle for cyclosporine lowers renal thromboxanes and reduces experimental nephrotoxicity. Transplant Proc 1987;19:1403–6.
53. Bennet WM, de Mattos A, Meyer MM, et al. Chronic cyclosporine nephropathy: the Achilles' heel of immunosuppressive therapy. Kidney Int 1996;50:1089–100.
54. Bennet WM. The nephrotoxicity of new and old immunosuppressive drugs. Ren Fail 1998;20:687–90.
55. Sternberg SS. Cross-striated fibrils and other ultra-structural alterations in glomeruli of rats with daunomycin nephrosis. Lab Invest 1970;23:39–51.
56. Buss H, Lamberts B. The kidney glomerulus of the rat during experimental daunomycin nephrosis. A comparative transmission-scanning electron microscopic study. Beitr Pathol 1973;148:360–87.
57. Serpick AA, Henderson ES. Observations on toxicity and clinical trials with daunomycin. Pathol Biol 1967;15:909–12.
58. Keating MJ, Kantarjian H, Talpaz M, et al. Fludarabine: a new agent with major activity against chronic lymphocytic leukemia. Blood 1989;74:19–25.
59. Puccio CA, Mittleman A, Lichtman SM, et al. A loading dose/continuous infusion schedule of fludarabine phosphate in chronic lymphocytic leukemia. J Clin Oncol 1991;9:1562–9.
60. Chun HG, Leylan-Jones B, Cheson BD. Fludarabine phosphate: a synthetic purine metabolite with significant activity against lymphoid malignancies. J Clin Oncol 1991;9:175–88.
61. List AF, Kummett TD, Adams JD, et al. Tumor lysis syndrome complicating chronic lymphocytic leukemia with fludarabine phosphate. Am J Med 1990;89:383–90.
62. Welles L, Saville MW, Lietzau J, et al. Phase II trial with dose titration of paclitaxel for the therapy of human immunodeficiency virus-associated Kaposi's sarcoma. J Clin Oncol 1998;16:1112–21.
63. Saville MW, Lietzau J, Pluda JM, et al. Treatment of HIV-associated Kaposi's sarcoma. Lancet 1995;346:26–8.
64. Flombaum CD, Mouradian JA, Casper ES, et al. Thrombotic microangiopathy as a complication of long-term therapy with gemcitabine. Am J Kidney Dis 1999;33:552–62.
65. Daugaard G, Abildgaard U. Evaluation of nephrotoxicity secondary to cytostatic agents. Clin Rev Oncol Hematol 1992;13:215–40.
66. Kassirer JP, Harrington JT. Laboratory evaluation of renal function. In: Schrier RW, Gottschalk CW, editors. Diseases of the kidney. Vol 1. Boston: Little, Brown; 1988. p. 393–441.

134

Cardiac Complications

Michael S. Ewer, MD, MPH, JD
Robert S. Benjamin, MD
Edward T.H. Yeh, MD

Patients with malignant neoplastic diseases often have cardiovascular disorders as well. These disorders may result from underlying conditions such as atherosclerosis, hypertension, or valvular abnormalities, or they may result directly from either the cancer or its treatment. Additionally, cardiovascular disorders that are unusual in patients not afflicted with cancer may be more common in cancer patients. At the same time, cardiovascular diseases common in the general population, such as atherosclerosis or hypertension, must not be overlooked in patients with cancer; the presentation of these entities may be altered, and thus the diagnosis more complex. Increased clinical scrutiny is therefore necessary in this population. Several clinical problems may also coexist and defy a simple explanation because of the complex interactions between the malignancy and the cardiovascular system; what affects the first often alters the second. This chapter will look at some of the more common cardiovascular complications and dilemmas found in cancer patients.

EVALUATION OF THE CARDIOVASCULAR SYSTEM IN THE CANCER PATIENT

Primary Medical Evaluation, Routine Laboratory Evaluation, Electrocardiogram, and Echocardiogram The evaluation of the cardiovascular system in patients with cancer begins with a detailed history and a complete physical examination of the cardiovascular structures.[1] Additionally, most patients require chest radiography and a standard 12-lead electrocardiogram. Echocardiography is the most widely used modality for diagnosing cardiomyopathy and assessing the integrity of cardiac structures.[2] A complete echocardiographic evaluation involves several complementary techniques, each providing information about a cardiac abnormality from a different vantage point. Transthoracic two-dimensional echocardiography is a totally safe and reproducible technique and is especially useful when serial studies are required. The two-dimensional echocardiogram provides information regarding a large region of the heart, and in some views, all four cardiac chambers can be seen and wall motion abnormalities reflecting global and regional dysfunction can be assessed. Asymmetric and localized or loculated pericardial effusions are also best evaluated with two-dimensional echocardiography. It is also the method of choice as a screening test for identifying and monitoring intracardiac masses; other imaging modalities, however, may be more useful in providing focused information regarding localization and structure.[3] In situations where ultrasound imaging is suboptimal, echo contrast agents may be employed to augment the echocardiographic interface. Such agents are increasingly being used and are generally regarded as safe.[4]

Spectral and color flow Doppler studies, which are usually performed as part of an echocardiographic evaluation, show the direction and velocity of blood flow in the cardiac chambers and across the valves. This information is graphically depicted and can be superimposed on the two-dimensional or M-mode echocardiogram. Valvular lesions, intracardiac shunts, turbulent blood movement, and abnormal direction of blood flow are best evaluated using the Doppler study. Doppler studies provide important information regarding diastolic cardiac function, an area of cardiac imaging that has become increasingly important; whereas two-dimensional echocardiography identifies anatomic relationships, the Doppler study provides vital supplemental information regarding blood flow and function.

Transesophageal echocardiography provides a more direct and focused view of cardiac structures than does the conventional transthoracic study. Although the technique is semi-invasive (the transducer has dimensions similar to those of a gastrointestinal endoscope and is passed into the midesophagus in a similar manner), the increased resolution of the transesophageal studies often offsets this disadvantage. Transesophageal studies are especially useful in identifying vegetations on cardiac valves, which may be extremely difficult to assess on transthoracic studies (Figure 134-1). They are also of great value in defining and moni-

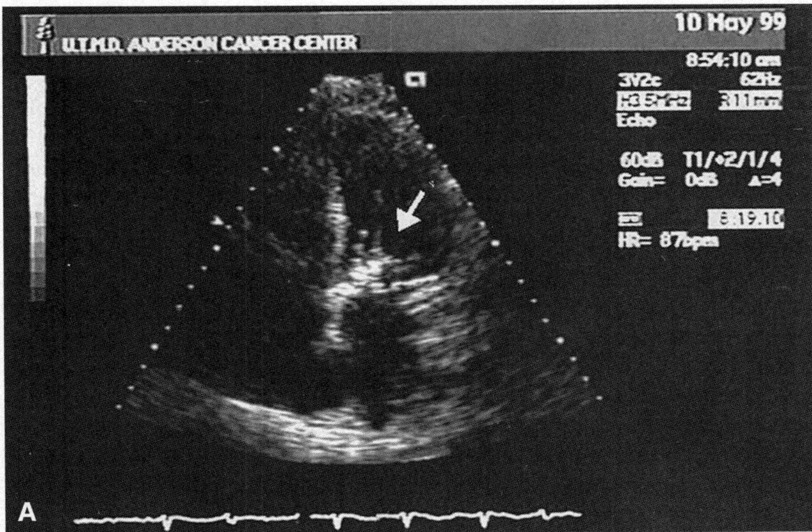

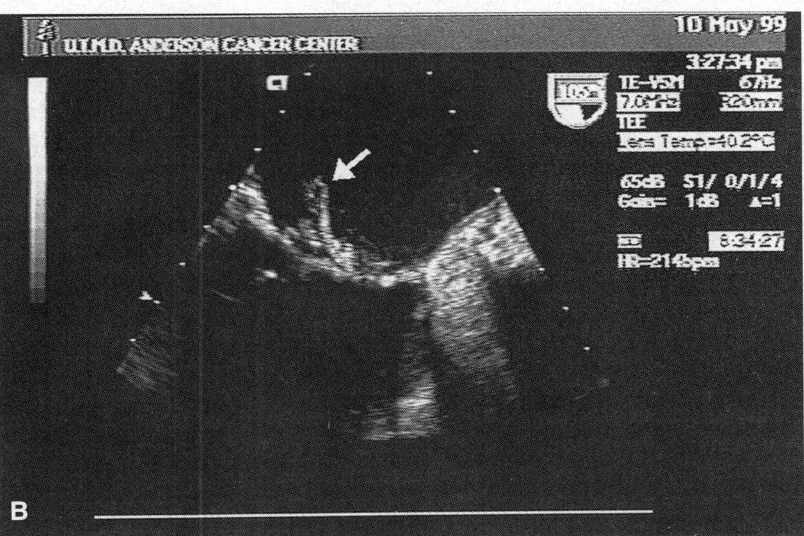

Figure 134-1 Echocardiogram frames of a patient with infective endocarditis involving the mitral valve. **A,** Nonspecific findings often seen on transthoracic studies, although suggestive of thickening of the leaflets, are not diagnostic for the valve infection, **B,** Transesophageal image from the same patient recorded the same day, clearly showing the infected mitral valve leaflet.

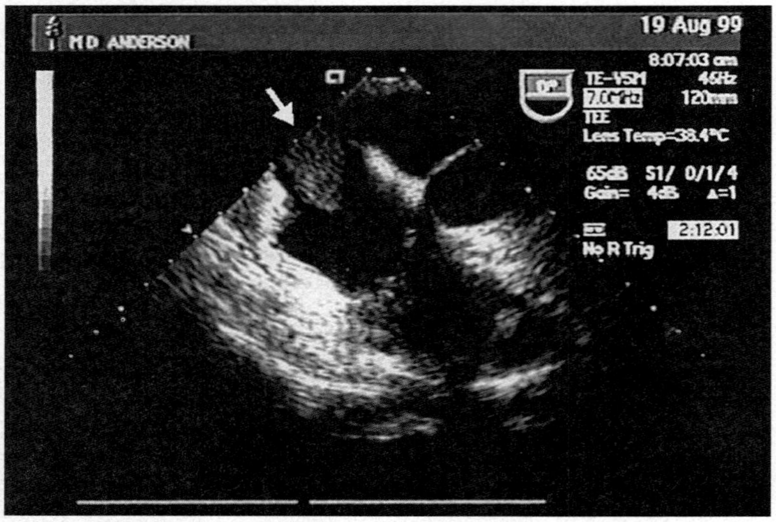

Figure 134-2 Frame from an intraoperative transesophageal echocardiogram showing spread of a renal cell carcinoma into the right atrium via the inferior vena cava.

toring intracardiac masses and thrombi. Intraoperative transesophageal echocardiography is helpful in documenting the extent of an inferior vena caval tumor as well as the result of resection of such tumors[5] (Figure 134-2). Three-dimensional echocardiography allows the two-dimensional image to be rotated around a selected axis. The technique provides images of excellent resolution and aids with spatial orientation of cardiac structures. It is anticipated that these techniques will enter into the mainstream of cardiac imaging in the near future.[6]

Nuclear Imaging Techniques Nuclear imaging techniques provide important information concerning both systolic and diastolic cardiac function. Nuclear studies are generally reproducible, are widely available, and remain a common assessment tool for following left ventricular ejection fraction in patients being treated with anthracyclines. Nuclear imaging derived ejection fractions may be estimated using any of a number of techniques. First-pass studies, in which a bolus of isotope is observed as it passes through the heart, identify changes in chamber dimensions during the cardiac cycle, and are used at some European centers; both left ventricular and right ventricular ejection fractions may be calculated accurately from these data.[7]

The most widely used nuclear technique for estimating cardiac function is the cardiac blood-pool scan, and it is used extensively in evaluating patients receiving anthracyclines. The technique requires electrocardiographic gating, and there is an acquisition time of several minutes during which data are accumulated in computer memory banks; these data can be then manipulated using one of several computer algorithms to provide an estimation of ejection fraction, information regarding wall-motion abnormalities, and parameters of cardiac relaxation (diastolic function). Because of the long acquisition time and the required gating, however, patients with cardiac rhythm disturbances and patients who cannot lie motionless often are better studied with real-time imaging techniques such as echocardiography. In interpreting the results of any estimation of cardiac function it must be emphasized that many noncardiac factors also affect cardiac function, and these studies must be interpreted with some caution.[8]

Other Imaging Techniques Magnetic resonance imaging (MRI) of the cardiovascular system can define pathologic lesions in and around the great vessels and can delineate intracardiac and pericardial masses. The technique is also useful in identifying constrictive pericarditis.[7,9] The cost of MRI is decreasing, but is still considerable; problems related to long imaging times are gradually being resolved.[10,11] Both rapid-acquisition MRI and cinenuclear angiography are making MRI techniques more suitable for routine use in cancer patients. Contrast-enhanced magnetic imaging of the heart is also expanding.[12] Such techniques as yet have not replaced echocardiography and radionuclide scanning techniques.[13] Nevertheless, magnetic resonance has become a much more readily available technique, and is now an established noninvasive imaging modality for the assessment of various cardiac disorders. To some extent it now can be considered the new gold standard for quantification of ventricular volumes, function and mass.[14–16] Positron emission tomography (PET) has theoretical advantages over more traditional imaging techniques and is gaining in acceptability and availability. It remains expensive and is not yet widely used to evaluate myocardial viability in the cancer patient.[17]

METASTATIC INVOLVEMENT OF CARDIAC STRUCTURES

Metastatic involvement of cardiac structures is common and is seen in approximately 8 to 10% of patients with cancer; there is a significant decrease in frequency in elderly patients.[18] Such involvement may constitute a subtle or incidental finding at autopsy or may be the initial catastrophic or life-threatening presentation of the cancer. There are wide variations among primary disease sites and tumor types.[19–22] Previously, it was unusual to diagnose cardiac involvement antemortem, except in cases of obvious pericardial tamponade. Newer imaging techniques have now made it possible to recognize cardiac involvement much earlier, often at a time when intervention can still be efficacious. Because of the high incidence of lung and breast cancers, these neoplasms are the most common source of metastatic lesions in cardiac structures. In one study, malignant melanoma, previously thought to be the tumor most likely to spread to cardiac structures,[23] was found in only 45% of cases at autopsy.[18] It should be kept in mind that the biologic behavior of some tumors is unpredictable and may lead to unusual metastatic sites; the heart should be included in routine examinations that seek metastatic involvement.[24] Hodgkin's and non-Hodgkin's lymphomas, leukemias, gastrointestinal or gynecologic cancers (especially ovarian), multiple myeloma, and sarcoma can also invade the pericardium.[25–27] In addition, renal cell cancer not infrequently spreads to the inferior vena cava and into the right atrium and right ventricle; these lesions often are amenable to surgical resection (see Figure 134-2).

Malignant Pericardial Effusion Malignant pericardial effusions demonstrate considerable variability with regard to both the quantity of fluid that accumulates as well as the pressure exerted on the pericardium and the cardiac chambers. The rate of accumulation and the distensibility of the pericardial sac determine the hemodynamic effect and the symptoms of these effusions.[28] For example, as little as 100 mL of fluid in the pericardial sac may cause symptoms in a patient with a scarred or infiltrated nondistensible parietal pericardium, whereas large effusions of as much as 1 L may remain relatively indolent when the pericardial sac is elastic and the effusion accumulates gradually.[29] Malignant pericardial effusion generally carries a poor prognosis.[30]

Normally, pericardial fluid is not static, but in equilibrium with other body fluids. Abnormal fluid build-up occurs when fluid enters the sac more rapidly than can be reabsorbed. This disequilibrium may occur when the efferent lymphatic vessels are obstructed, or when subcarinal lymph node metastases mechanically prevent effective drainage. Malignant effusions are usually serosanguinous or frankly bloody in content and often contain cytologically identifiable cancer cells. When chylous effusions are malignant, the most likely cause is lymphoma; chylous effusion have been reported as a complication of Behçet's disease and following radiation for gynecologic malignancy.[31–33]

The onset of symptoms in patients with pericardial effusion may be insidious. Indeed, many patients with large effusions are totally asymptomatic. Pericardial effusion may be suspected when the cardiac silhouette is enlarged on the chest radiograph. A decrease in the mean electrocardiographic QRS voltage also suggests a pericardial effusion, but other causes of decreased voltage are common in cancer patients, making such findings less useful. Pericardial effusions are often noted as incidental findings on radionuclide cardiac imaging studies, with the fluid appearing as a relatively inactive area separating the cardiac from the hepatic and pulmonary blood pools. Occasionally, a rocking motion of the heart suggesting hemodynamic compromise (cardiac tamponade) is noted on blood-pool scans. Computed tomographic (CT) images of the chest also may demonstrate pericardial effusions but are not especially helpful for estimating the volume. Because CT of the chest is frequently used to evaluate pulmonary or mediastinal tumor involvement, it may provide the first indication of an unsuspected pericardial effusion. Pericardioscopy has also been undertaken in the evaluation of patients with pericardial effusions.[34,35]

The diagnosis of pericardial effusion is usually confirmed by echocardiography.[2,36–38] Once an effusion has been diagnosed, its progression or resolution may be followed with serial echocardiograms.

Differential Diagnosis The etiology of a pericardial effusion in a cancer patient may not always be apparent,[39] It can result from various factors, and noninvasive evaluation may not be sufficient to establish the etiology. The patient's history is very helpful, and information regarding previous irradiation of the chest or previous nonspecific pericarditis with effusion is especially pertinent.[40] High fever, leukocytosis, and prostration suggest septic pericarditis, whereas recent myocardial infarction could suggest an association with the ischemic event. When the cause of a pericardial effusion remains unclear, diagnostic (cytologic, bacteriologic, chemical, and immunologic) analysis of a fluid specimen may be useful. In some instances, the etiology of pericardial effusion in a cancer patient remains elusive despite an aggressive attempt at evaluation; even pericardial biopsy does not always provide a definitive explanation. Interestingly, the serum cancer antigen 125 (CA 125) level may be elevated in patients with pericardial and pleural effusions, as well as in patients with heart failure, even in the absence of a gynecologic malignancy[41,42]; conditions that irritate or inflame serosal surfaces appear to induce apparently normal mesothelial cells to express this antigen.

Cardiac Tamponade The accumulation of pericardial fluid may increase intrapericardial pressure and compromise cardiac output, a condition known as cardiac tamponade.[43] Symptoms include dyspnea and exercise intolerance, and signs include tachycardia, neck-vein distention, and hepatomegaly.[44] Heart sounds are often, but not always, difficult to auscultate, and pericardial friction rubs may or may not be present.[45] Vague chest discomfort or fullness is frequently noted. Most patients with significantly increased intrapericardial pressure also demonstrate an exaggeration of the decrease in pulse pressure during inspiration (pulsus paradoxus). The Kussmaul sign (distention of the jugular veins on inspiration) is seen more commonly in the context of constrictive pericarditis or mediastinal tumors. A highly characteristic finding of cardiac tamponade is electrical alternans, in which the electrocardiographic QRS voltage becomes larger and smaller on alternate complexes.[46] This phenomenon is caused by physical movement of the heart toward and away from the electrode as the heart rocks back and forth within the fluid-containing pericardial sac. Cardiac tamponade can almost always be diagnosed on the basis of the physical findings and the findings from non-invasive studies. Echocardiography usually shows the effusion, which may vary considerably in size. Diastolic inward motion (collapse) of the right atrium is a sensitive but not specific finding; the finding is more specific when the collapse extends for more than one-third of the cardiac cycle. Diastolic collapse of the right ventricular wall becomes more pronounced as hemodynamic compromise progresses and is a much more specific finding. Doppler flow studies show exaggerated tricuspid and pulmonic flow velocities and reduced transmitral flow velocity with the onset of inspiration. Cardiac catheterization is usually not required to confirm the diagnosis, but may show a graphic representation of *pulsus paradoxus*, and there may be elevation and ultimate equalization of the diastolic pressures in the cardiac chambers as tamponade progresses. When frank tamponade ensues, the pulse becomes weak or totally absent during inspiration, and patients develop symptoms of low-output cardiogenic shock. Death, often preceded by profound bradycardia, ensues if the tamponade is not resolved promptly.

Management of Malignant Pericardial Effusion and Tamponade The management of malignant pericardial effusion depends on a number of factors, including the likelihood of the tumor responding to local (surgical, radiotherapeutic, or intracavitary) or systemic anticancer therapy; the extent of and the symptoms attributable to the effusion; and the overall anticipated survival of the patient.[47,48] Patients with tumors highly likely to respond to the systemic therapy may proceed with their treatment; sometimes the malignant effusion resolves in responses to the systemic anticancer therapy alone. Pericardial effusion in patients with tumors that are unlikely to respond to treatment, either because of the cell type or because the tumor has become refractory to chemotherapy, may require local intervention. In patients who have a more favorable oncologic prognosis and are sufficiently strong so as to undergo general anesthesia and surgery, creation of a pleuropericardial window is both effective and generally considered the procedure of choice. Although the transthoracic and the subxyphoid approaches are equally efficacious, in-hospital mortality was significantly greater for patients treated with the subxyphoid approach.[49,50] Using either approach, the communication formed usually remains patent, and the larger surface area available in the pleural space permits more effective resorption of the excess fluid. Pericardial needle drainage may be required prior to surgery as a stabilizing measure in patients who have very large effusions or pretamponade compromise of cardiac output. Symptoms often resolve dramatically after removal of the fluid, allowing patients to again engage in activities that had become impossible.

Needle drainage is now almost always undertaken with echocardiographic confirmation of the position of the draining catheter and is considered safe and effective.[51,52] Some patients experience transient left ventricular dysfunction after resolution of cardiac tamponade, and thus a period of careful monitoring is important.[53] The advantages of the pericardial window over percutaneous pericardiocentesis have not been fully evaluated, but some studies suggest little advantage to the more invasive pericardial window procedure. The advisability of routine drainage of large pericardial effusions in patients without tamponade has also been questioned; these authors point out the low diagnostic yield and the lack of therapeutic benefit.[54] The clinical management of such patients should be determined by their overall performance status, oncologic prognosis, and by the expertise at the treatment center.

Sclerosis may be considered following needle drainage. A number of sclerosing agents have been studied. These include hyperosmolar glucose, radioactive gold, bleomycin, sterile talc, doxycycline (Vibramycin), and triethylenethiophosphoramide (thio-TEPA).[55,56] Doxycycline, a semisynthetic tetracycline used at a dose of 250 to 500 mg, has received considerable attention as an effective sclerosing agent.[57] Sclerosis is carried out by instilling the sclerosing agent directly into the pericardial space; the procedure may be repeated every 24 to 48 hours until the pericardial fluid reaccumulation falls below 50 mL per day. For most patients, sclerosis of the pericardial sac will occur after three to five instillations. The likelihood of pericardial sclerosis succeeding in a specific patient is difficult to predict, but historically the procedure is helpful in more than half the patients.[58] It is clearly a useful adjunct because it may obviate the necessity for repeated pericardiocentesis and prevent recurrent cardiac tamponade. The procedure is usually well tolerated, although some patients experience considerable pain and discomfort that may require narcotic analgesia. In many instances daily draining the fluid until the residual effusion is less than 50 mL without instilling a sclerosing agent is also highly effective in preventing recurrent accumulations.[59]

Ziskind and colleagues have described using percutaneous pericardiotomy to relieve pericardial effusions.[60,61] In this technique, a balloon catheter is inserted so that the balloon crosses the pericardium. The balloon is then inflated, which tears the pericardium open, allowing the fluid to drain. The procedure may be quite painful, and patients require sedation and analgesia or anesthesia. Nonetheless, these authors reported success in 46 of 50 patients. Additional reports confirm that balloon intervention is a safe alternative to the creation of a pleuro-pericardial window.[61–63]

METASTATIC INVOLVEMENT OF THE MYOCARDIUM

The spread of malignant tumors to the myocardium is rarely recognized in vivo since most patients with myocardial metastases remain asymptomatic. It is not uncommon, however, to find significant and even extensive myocardial involvement at autopsy. Many patients in whom metastatic disease to the myocardium is sus-

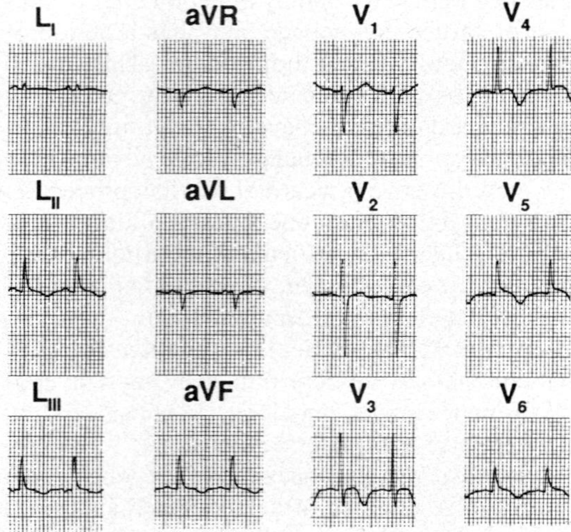

Figure 134-3 Electrocardiogram showing T-wave inversions suggesting ischemia or subendocardial infarction in a 26-year-old man with documented (by magnetic resonance imaging) myocardial metastatic disease and no history to suggest other causes of the electrocardiographic abnormality. Note T-wave inversions in the inferior leads (2, 3, and AVF) as well as in the precordial leads (V4–V6).

pected before death also have evidence of concomitant pericardial involvement.

The most dramatic manifestation of myocardial metastatic disease is a sudden abnormality of cardiac rhythm formation or conduction.[64] Sudden cardiac death can occur in this setting but is unusual. Cardiac perforation and erosion of the coronary vessels with hemorrhage or infarction may also occur but are exceedingly rare. More commonly, patients with myocardial involvement demonstrate signs of loss of functioning muscle mass and present with progressive shortness of breath and exercise intolerance; a decreased ejection fraction is seen on echocardiograms or nuclear imaging studies. It needs to be remembered, however, that the pattern of ischemia or infarction seen on a standard electrocardiogram in patients with large metastatic lesions may be indistinguishable from the electrocardiographic changes encountered with myocardial infarction due to coronary occlusion (Figure 134-3). ST segment elevations, T-wave inversions or Q waves may be seen in such cases, even when the coronary arteries are angiographically normal.[65,66]

The diagnosis of metastatic involvement of the myocardium is difficult to establish. A high degree of suspicion may prompt special imaging; MRI studies may be helpful in determining the presence and extent of metastatic myocardial disease. Although treatment of metastatic disease to the myocardium is usually supportive, large melanomas that had metastasized to the right ventricle have been successfully removed.[67,68]

CARDIAC EFFECTS OF MEDIATOR RELEASE FROM TUMORS

Metabolically active mediators are commonly associated with certain neoplastic diseases and frequently are the immediate cause of a patient's signs and symptoms.[69,70] Such mediator-associated diseases, or paraneoplastic syndromes, may have a direct or indirect effect on the cardiovascular system.

Carcinoid Heart Disease Carcinoid heart disease results from the long-term release of biologically active mediators that stimulate the formation of a distinctive fibromuscular plaque that destroys the integrity of the cardiac valves.[71–74] The carcinoid plaque is the characteristic lesion in carcinoid heart disease. Carcinoid heart disease is seen most commonly in patients who have ileocecal carcinoid tumors that have metastasized to the liver. Rarely, it occurs in patients with bronchial or ovarian carcinoid tumors, and in those instances carcinoid heart disease may develop in the absence of hepatic metastases. The exact mechanism of plaque formation and cardiac injury remains elusive, but a number of possible mediators, including the kinins, serotonin, 5-hydroxytryptophan, histamine, and prostaglandins, have been suggested; another as yet unidentified compound or combination of compounds may also be the cause.[75,76]

Mediator release into the hepatic vein from metastatic liver disease predisposes patients to right-sided cardiac lesions. The lesions generally appear along the intima of the great veins, the right atrium, and the coronary sinus. The margins and distal (ventricular or downstream) aspect of the tricuspid leaflets are often thickened, and the chordae tendineae may also be involved. The pulmonic valve is thickened and retracted. The damage appears to be aggravated by turbulent blood flow, which explains the characteristic location of the lesions. When the primary tumor or metastasis is in the lung, the mediators are released directly into the pulmonary venous bed and bypass the inactivating properties of lung tissue; left-sided valvular lesions are seen in such cases.[77] Left-sided lesions are less frequent than right-sided ones but are more likely to result in hemodynamic compromise. A review of surgically excised valves noted considerable variation in the histological appearance of the material; the excised valves predominantly (92%) came from the right side.[78]

The ultrastructure of the cardiac plaques has been studied extensively.[75] They are formed of smooth muscle cells embedded in a stroma of acid mucopolysaccharide and collagen and lack elastic fibers.[79] It has been postulated that the lesions, which resemble those seen after chronic endothelial irritation from long-term indwelling catheters, develop after repeated cycles of endothelial cell injury followed by healing.[80] Such lesions generally do not penetrate beyond the intima.

The most important consequence of carcinoid plaques is thickening and fibrosis of the valves with resultant distortion of the valvular apparatus and ring. Tricuspid regurgitation and pulmonic stenosis are typically seen, but in the case of progressive destruction, a rigid tricuspid valve with characteristic hemodynamic abnormalities reflecting both stenotic and regurgitant characteristics may be encountered. Significant pulmonic regurgitation is rare. Stiffening of the right atrium may be noted and contributes to the neck-vein distention commonly seen in patients with the carcinoid syndrome. Finally, a high-output state, probably due to mediator release, has also been described.[81,82]

The clinical manifestations of carcinoid heart disease vary considerably. Some patients are able to tolerate the hemodynamic consequences of their valvular lesions well, whereas symptoms develop early in others, especially the elderly or those with predisposing cardiac abnormalities.[83] Early symptoms include fatigue, dyspnea on exertion, and palpitations due to the high-output state, to dysrhythmias or to both. Later, symptoms of right-sided congestive heart failure, including edema, hepatomegaly, and sometimes ascites, predominate. Cardiac murmurs often predate symptoms, and the murmur of tricuspid regurgitation may be heard long before the hemodynamic effects become evident clinically. Most frequently, the murmur is appreciated as a loud, holosystolic, blowing sound heard along the left lower sternal border. The murmur may be augmented during inspiration. The murmur of pulmonic stenosis cannot always be distinguished from the often coexisting tricuspid regurgitation murmur; however the pulmonic mummer is usually harsher and is appreciated most prominently in the second left intercostal space.

The chest radiograph may reveal cardiomegaly with prominence of the right ventricle. Unlike congenital pulmonic stenosis, which often includes poststenotic dilatation of the pulmonary trunk, cardiomegaly is usually not seen in carcinoid heart disease. Electrocardiographic findings include changes of right ventricular volume or pressure overload with or without right atrial abnormalities, right ventricular hypertrophy, right bundle-branch block, and right axis deviation; low voltage in the standard (limb) leads may also be seen.

Echocardiography is the most useful noninvasive tool for diagnosing carcinoid heart disease (Figure 134-4). It not only identifies the valvular abnormality but, when coupled with Doppler ultrasonography studies, can also provide hemodynamic data for estimating the degree of valvular involvement.[84,85] Along with the thickening and loss of mobility of the tricuspid leaflets, increased flow velocity across the tricuspid valve during diastole is evident. A regurgitant jet can be seen in the right atrium during systole.[86,87] Furthermore, echocardiography can quantify the right atrial and right ventricular enlargement that are characteristic of this condition. Echocardiography has also been helpful in recognizing metastatic carcinoid tumors that involve the heart if those tumors are greater than 1 centimeter.[88]

The management of patients with carcinoid heart disease must be individualized and is often challenging. Although the carcinoid plaque is largely irreversible, controlling or eliminating the offending mediators can arrest its progression. In this respect, treatment of the primary tumor or metastatic disease is crucial. Once the diagnosis is established, carcinoid heart disease is initially

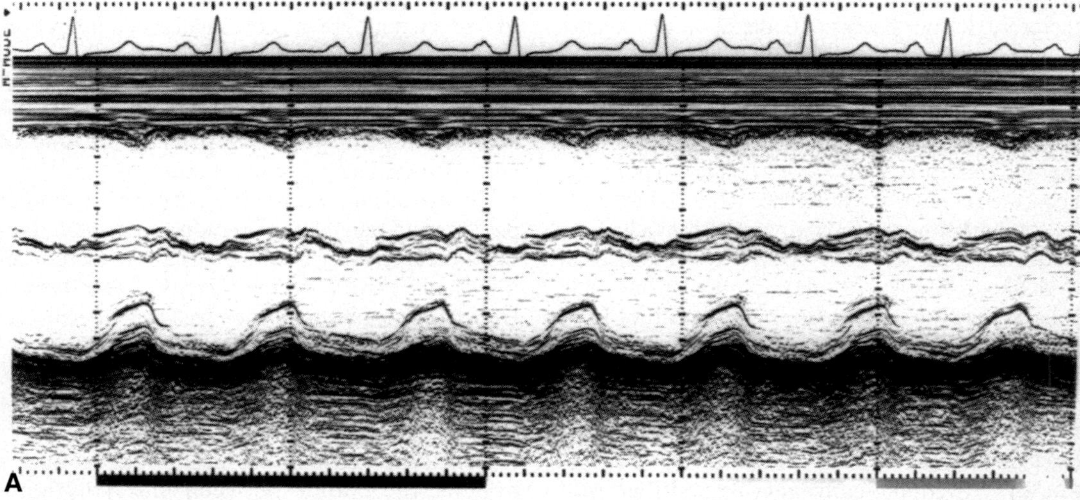

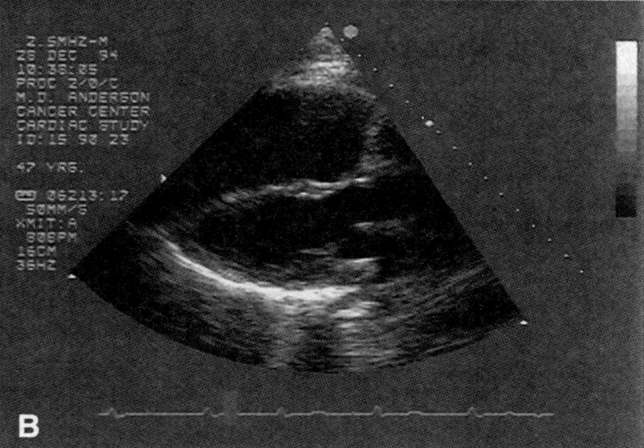

Figure 134-4 Echocardiogram of a 47-year-old woman with long-standing carcinoid heart disease. **A,** M-mode echocardiogram, showing right ventricle to be significantly enlarged and the septum showing paradoxical septal motion. These findings are characteristic of right ventricular volume and pressure overload. **B,** The long-axis projection of the two-dimensional study from the same patient.

managed pharmacologically with salt restriction, diuretics, and afterload reduction; the benefit of β-adrenergic blockade is unproven. Surgical intervention in the form of valvuloplasty or replacement becomes a consideration in patients with advanced disease and intractable heart failure; long-term survival has been achieved in carefully selected patients. Placement of a prosthetic tricuspid valve with either reconstruction or removal of the pulmonic valve has been successful.[89–91] These surgical procedures are often associated with significant morbidity and mortality.

High-Output States and High-Output Cardiac Failure Increased cardiac output occurs in many cancer patients and may be due to anemia, hyperthyroidism, primary or secondary aldosteronism, primary or secondary inappropriate antidiuretic hormone secretion, or the shunting of blood through tumors. High-output states are relatively common in patients with multiple myeloma.[92,93] Additionally, liver disease (nutritional cirrhosis or infectious hepatitis), fever, emotional excitement, and hypoxemia are also common causes of increased cardiac output and hyperdynamic states. High-output states are seen as well following treatment with a number of biologic response modifiers, including the interferons (possibly related to fever and the influenza-like reaction) and interleukins; the phenomenon is usually self-limited and of short duration.

High-output states are associated with a moderately increased heart rate (usually 85–110 beats per minute, but sometimes higher) and with increased stroke volume. Physical examination typically reveals neck veins of normal appearance, since the preload is usually not increased. Peripheral pulses, however, are often bounding and have a rapid upstroke and fall; systolic blood pressure is elevated, and diastolic blood pressure is reduced. Auscultation often reveals a systolic murmur and also may demonstrate a presystolic gallop. Pulmonary congestion is not uncommon in severe hyperdynamic states.

Echocardiography or radionuclide imaging is helpful in establishing the diagnosis. Two-dimensional studies show increased wall motion in the long-axis, short-axis, and four-chamber views. In extreme cases, the left ventricular cavity may appear almost to totally obliterate during systole; the ejection fraction is increased. Multi-gated cardiac blood-pool scans may also offer important data concerning the left ventricular ejection fraction and cardiac output. Right heart catheterization (most commonly undertaken with a flow-directed catheter) in conjunction with the measurement of cardiac output with thermodilution curves can confirm the diagnosis, but this procedure is rarely justified. It is important not to confuse this clinical picture with that of the more common low-output congestive heart failure, with which it shares a number of characteristics.

The treatment of high-output states should be directed toward the underlying cause, such as metastatic disease with or without shunting, hyperthyroidism, hypoxia, anemia, or infection. High-output states often respond to blood transfusion, diuretics, oxygen administration, or antipyretics. In selected cases, β-adrenergic blockers may be useful; digitalis preparations usually are not helpful, except as adjuncts in controlling the rate of ventricular response in patients with related or preexisting atrial fibrillation. Unless patients are symptomatic, the high-output state does not require specific therapy.

Cardiac Amyloidosis Amyloidosis is the deposition of amyloid, which may occur in a variety of organs. Amyloid deposits consist of twisted beta-pleated sheet fibrils formed from a variety of proteins.[94,95] Many organs, including the heart, may be involved, and a number of pathologic processes have been implicated.[95] Mild amyloid infiltration is often an incidental finding at autopsy. Clinically significant cancer-related amyloidosis is encountered in patients with multiple myeloma and, rarely, in patients with Hodgkin's disease; amyloidosis is also a nonspecific finding associated with chronic infection or inflammation.[96]

Clinically, patients with cardiac amyloidosis experience fatigue and show signs of decreased cardiac output. Conduction abnormalities are seen and may be symptomatic; stress-precipitated syncope may be a precursor of sudden cardiac death.[97,98] Both systolic and diastolic function may be impaired, the velocity of the ventricular contraction may be diminished, and diastolic relaxation may be incomplete. The pathophysiologic appearance is that of a restrictive cardiomyopathy, and the clinical picture may be indistinguishable from that of constrictive pericarditis. Even cardiac catheterization findings are not always conclusive in establishing the correct diagnosis. The chest radiograph shows a normal-sized or slightly enlarged heart shadow. When cardiac failure appears, pulmonary congestion or pleural effusion may be seen. The electrocardiogram characteristically shows decreased voltage, a pseudo-infarction pattern, and abnormalities of impulse formation or conduction. In one review, criteria for left-ventricular hypertrophy were observed in 16% of the cases.[99] The echocardiogram is often helpful in suggesting the diagnosis of amyloidosis: it shows a thickened septum and posterior wall with normal internal dimensions of the left ventricle; the diastolic relaxation is often impaired. In addition, a spotted or stippled appearance is often seen, and pericardial effusion is not uncommon (Figure 134-5). The paradox of a thickened and enlarged muscle mass with decreased electrocardiographic voltage should suggest cardiac amyloidosis.[100] Antimyosin scintigraphy, showing left ventricular thickening and diffuse myocardial antimyosin uptake, has been reported to be highly suggestive of amyloid heart disease.[101]

Cardiac catheterization demonstrates elevated intracardiac pressures in all chambers, with the minimum left ventricular pressure often increased to at least 10 mm Hg.[100] The "dip and plateau" pattern seen on intraventricular pressure tracings in patients with constrictive pericarditis may be

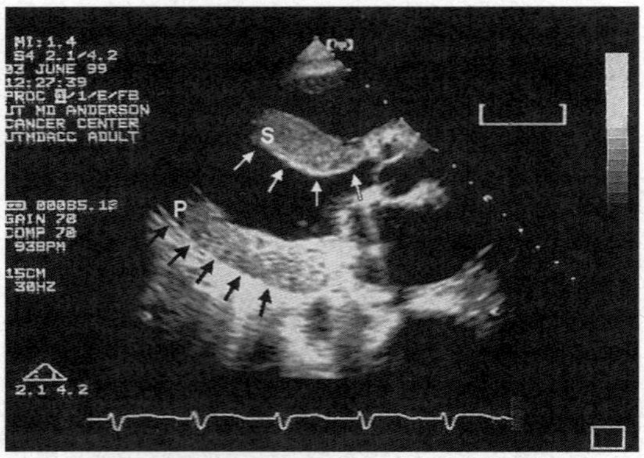

Figure 134-5 Long-axis view of a frame from the echocardiogram of a patient with cardiac amyloid infiltration. Note thickened septum (S) and posterior wall (P) with stippled appearance *(arrows)*.

absent. Prominent papillary muscles are demonstrated with angiography. Endomyocardial biopsy with Congo red staining may be helpful in establishing the diagnosis.[102]

The therapeutic interventions for cardiac amyloidosis are limited. Cardiac glycosides may reduce the symptoms of congestive failure, but dysrhythmia and sudden death have been reported following their use.[103,104] Preload and afterload reduction using diuretics alone or in combination with angiotensin-converting enzyme inhibitors, vasodilators, or long-acting nitroglycerin preparations also may be helpful. The use of β-adrenergic blockade has not been studied adequately. Clinical improvement may parallel control of the underlying process in patients with reactive forms of amyloidosis, and systemic treatment of the myeloma may delay or alleviate the symptoms of myeloma-related cardiac amyloidosis. Some authorities suggest anticoagulation in the presence of significant cardiac amyloidosis. Therapy with a number of antineoplastic agents, including melphalan, cyclophosphamide, carmustine, and vincristine, have been attempted, as has hematopoietic stem cell transplantation.[105] Restrictive cardiomyopathy due to light-chain deposition disease may be reversible.[106] Cardiac transplantation has been undertaken in a patient with senile systemic amyloidosis.[107]

CARDIAC DYSRHYTHMIA IN THE CANCER PATIENT

Cardiac rhythm disturbances are common in many patients with neoplastic diseases. These dysrhythmias may be caused by the tumor, by anticancer treatment, by metabolic abnormalities, or by underlying cardiac disease and are morphologically and functionally identical to the rhythm disturbances seen in non-cancer patients. In some settings, it is essential to suppress a cardiac dysrhythmia vigorously, whereas in others, rhythm disturbances may be a transient manifestation of a temporary disturbance in homeostasis requiring little or no intervention.[108,109]Many antineoplastic agents are associated with transient dysrhythmia, and because such rhythm disturbances are often asymptomatic the phenomenon is not fully appreciated. Most chemotherapy-related rhythm disturbances are of short duration and of little clinical importance; they, therefore, do not necessitate alteration of the chemotherapeutic regimen.

Clinical decisions regarding which patients to treat, at what point in their management to initiate therapy, how long to continue treatment, and what therapy (pharmacologic or electrical) to use have been the focus of considerable debate. The wide assortment of new antidysrhythmic drugs has not simplified these decisions. One useful approach is to distinguish dysrhythmias resulting from toxic substances or other metabolic abnormalities from those associated with primary or structural abnormalities of the heart itself.

Categories of Dysrhythmia: Primary (Structural) versus Secondary (Metabolic) Rhythm disturbances resulting from pathologic processes within the heart often behave as do dysrhythmias associated with the acute phase of myocardial infarction. The myocardium is unstable, and severe dysrhythmias, both supraventricular and ventricular, may appear with little warning and progress catastrophically to hemodynamic instability and sudden cardiac death. Such dysrhythmias may result from spread of the neoplastic process or from severe structural damage to the myocardium caused by the cancer treatment, such as may occur with established cardiomyopathy resulting from an anthracycline. Sudden arrhythmic death following cancer treatment is rare but has been reported following cardiotoxic chemotherapy and radiation injury. Sudden death is more common in the presence of infiltrative processes such as amyloidosis.

Dysrhythmias in cancer patients are often secondary to metabolic abnormalities or pharmacologic interventions and represent reactions of cardiac pacemaker tissue or of the conducting tracts to changes in the internal environment.[110,111] Electrolyte shifts are probably the most common cause, but the depletion or accumulation of physiologic products or metabolites is also associated with ectopy or conduction abnormalities. Metabolically active pathologic or pharmacologic substances may also cause dysrhythmia.

Treatment of Cardiac Rhythm Disturbances Rhythm disturbances that result from metabolic abnormalities and that are not life threatening may be managed conservatively; in such cases, careful observation during treatment of the underlying metabolic abnormality may suffice. Active intervention is required when the dysrhythmia results in significant hemodynamic embarrassment or when the rhythm disturbance becomes life threatening. As in acute myocardial infarction, control of a dysrhythmia in the structurally altered heart is often challenging. Hemodynamic instability, regardless of the underlying cause, constitutes a medical emergency requiring the use of advanced cardiac life-support protocols.[112,113]

Ventricular ectopy is common in cancer patients and ranges from benign accelerated idioventricular rhythm to malignant forms of ventricular tachycardia and ventricular fibrillation. Coexisting conditions, such as fever or debilitation, which may augment tissue hypoxia, especially in anemic patients, predispose patients to ventricular ectopy. Unexpected death in cancer patients is usually attributed to dysrhythmia.

Once the decision has been made to treat a patient, the choice between antiarrhythmic agent(s) or an implantable device generally follows the usual guidelines for these therapies. In difficult cases, electrophysiologic studies or pharmacologic threshold analysis may be useful. Implantable devices increasingly are being used in cancer patients, and malignant disease should not be considered a barrier to their use.

An ever-increasing number of drugs are being implicated in causing a well-recognized form of ventricular tachycardia known as torsades de pointes. This polymorphic ventricular tachycardia (Figure 134-6) is frequently accompanied by a prolonged QT interval. Antiarrhythmic drugs such as quinidine or procainamide hydrochloride characteristically produce prolonged QT intervals that may be associated with torsades as are some antibiotics (erythromycin, clarithromycin, and sulfamethoxazole-trimethoprim) and psychotropic drugs (haloperidol), high-dose chemotherapy, and bone marrow transplantation.[114–117] Arsenic trioxide, which is most commonly used in the treatment of acute promyelocytic leukemia, also prolongs the QT interval, and patients should be watched for this cardiac effect.[118,119] Prompt recognition of this potentially malignant dysrhythmia and withdrawal of the offending agent may be the most appropriate therapy. Anecdotally, torsade de pointes may be more likely in African-Americans; the QT prolongation has been reported to be more frequent in male patients and those with hypokalemia; serial monitoring of the QT interval is advised.[120]

Treatment of torsade de pointes with β blockers and phenytoin with phenobarbital, as well as maintenance of potassium and magnesium homeostasis may be helpful in preventing recurrences of the dysrhythmia; overdrive pacing, intravenous mag-

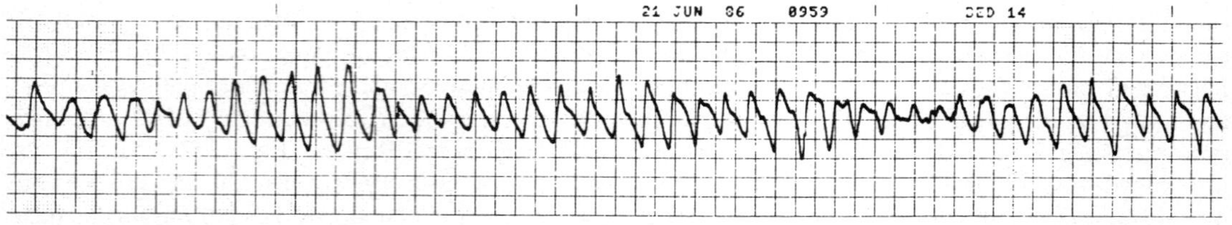

Figure 134-6 Rhythm strip of a patient with episodes of torsades de pointes, or polymorphic ventricular tachycardia. The previous rhythm strips showed prolongation of the QT interval.

nesium, or isoproterenol infusions may be used to convert the dysrhythmia back to a sinus .[121] Implantable defibrillators may be considered for patients in whom recurrent, hemodynamically significant tachydysrhythmias occur.[122]

CARDIAC COMPLICATIONS OF CANCER TREATMENT

Nonsurgical therapies used to treat patients with cancer can damage the heart in a variety of ways. These therapies consist of physical agents such as ionizing radiation and chemical agents (Table 134-1). Individual modalities and combinations may act independently or synergistically; for example, the combination of cardiac irradiation and anthracyclines produces additive or supra-additive toxicity. Damage resulting from cancer treatment may affect all cardiac structures: the pericardium, the myocardium, the vasculature, the conduction system, and the heart valves. Sometimes, the heart may incur subclinical damage, and a later insult or sequential stress may then trigger clinically relevant cardiac dysfunction.

Table 134-1 Anticancer Agents Associated with Cardiotoxicity

I. Drugs associated with type I myocardial depression
Anthracyclines
Doxorubicin (Adriamycin)
THP Adriamycin (Pirarubicin)
Idarubicin
Epirubicin (Ellence)
Daunorubicin
Other anthraquinones
Mitoxantrone
Potential toxicity intensifiers
Cyclophosphamide
Ifosfamide
Mitomycin c
Etoposide
Melphalan
Vincristine
Bleomycin
Paclitaxel
Toxicity inhibitors
Dexrazoxane (Zinocard, ICRF-187)
II. Other drugs associated with myocardial depression
Trastuzumab (Herceptin)
Other monoclonal antibodies
Cyclophosphamide (high dose)
α-Interferon
III. Antineoplastic agents associated with ischemia
5-Fluorouracil (5-FU)
Capecitabine
Vinblastine
Vincristine
Bleomycin
Cisplatin
Biological response modifiers
IV. Antineoplastic agents associated with hypotension
Interleukin-2
Homoharringtonine
V. Miscellaneous agents with known or suspected cardiac toxicity
Paclitaxel (associated with bradycardia)
Arsenic trioxide (associated with prolonged QT interval/torsades de pointes)
Bleomycin actinomycin D
Mitomycin C alkylating agents cyclophosphamide
Ifosfamide

CHEMOTHERAPEUTIC AGENTS **Agents with Myocardial Depressant Activity** Several antineoplastic agents have been implicated as etiologic factors that cause cardiomyopathies. The anthracyclines are the most common culprits, but other anthraquinones, and rarely other agents, have been implicated also. The effects of doxorubicin (Adriamycin) on the heart have been the most extensively studied and serve as a model for understanding anthracycline-associated and related cardiomyopathies.[123–165] Although the anthracyclines produce cardiac damage that is largely irreversible, other agents may demonstrate cardiotoxicity that is reversible. The mechanisms are different, and it has been proposed that the irreversible and reversible forms be recognized as type I and type II chemotherapy-related cardiac dysfunction.[166] The anthracyclines constitute type I dysfunction.

Doxorubicin Cardiotoxicity The cardiotoxicity caused by the anthracycline doxorubicin may occur early or late during a course of treatment, or it may appear months or even years after treatment has ended. Clinically relevant early toxicity is unusual, and when it occurs, it generally presents as a myopericarditis, which may progress to significant cardiac dysfunction within a few weeks of the first administration of the drug.[125] Early toxicity is more likely to occur in elderly patients or in patients who have received large single doses, and has been reported more commonly in patients treated with daunorubicin than with doxorubicin. Sudden death following doxorubicin administration also has been reported but is extremely rare. Both ventricular and supraventricular cardiac dysrhythmias are often seen during the administration of doxorubicin but are seldom life threatening. The mechanism of cardiac damage in patients with early toxicity is uncertain, and treatment is supportive. Of considerable interest however, is the finding that markers of acute cardiac damage such as troponin T are increased following exposure to doxorubicin. This suggests that early damage may be more important than had previously been appreciated, and marker release may be an indicator of the processes that give rise to the subsequent and more serious late cardiotoxicity.[167] Early elevations in troponin I has been shown to correlate with cardiac abnormalities observed later, and may allow the differentiation of patients who are at increased risk for subsequent cardiac dysfunction. Such a differentiation would allow for more careful monitoring of such patients, but perhaps more important, would provide the opportunity to alter potentially cardiotoxic therapy prior to the development of severe cardiac damage.[168] Although these strategies have great potential, they have not yet been incorporated into standard patient protocols.

Of greater clinical importance from the perspective of clinically relevant cardiac disease is chronic doxorubicin-associated cardiomyopathy, which once established reflects irreversible cell damage. Although the heart may adjust to the damage, and while patients may respond to appropriate medication, cardiac reserves remain diminished. Doxorubicin cardiotoxicity may lead to death from intractable congestive heart failure. The relationship to cumulative dose has been well established. Clinical manifestations of cardiomyopathy are unusual when the cumulative dose is below 400 mg/m^2, but the risk becomes greater as the cumulative dose exceeds 450 mg/m^2 administered by the usual rapid-infusion schedule.[123,124,128,169] Cardiomyopathy may occur at lower doses when other cardiotoxic drugs are administered concomitantly (see later discussion); there is considerable inter-patient variability.

The success of treatment of doxorubicin cardiotoxicity depends, in part, however, on the interval between the administration of the toxic drug and the appearance of cardiac dysfunction; if heart failure occurs less than 4 weeks from the last doxorubicin dose, it is much more likely to be fatal. Patients who experience this early form of toxicity probably have had more severe initial damage. Doxorubicin cardiomyopathy may become manifest months, and even years, after an uncomplicated course of chemotherapy at or near the usual maximum recommended dose. Such late cardiomyopathy may involve additional insults or stresses such as viral infections.[142] The sequential stress, whatever its nature, might not have been of importance were it not for the fact that there had been considerable preexisting heart disease and a lack of reserve to compensate for the additional injury. Cardiac biopsy findings are rarely helpful as the tissue specimens most frequently show nonspecific changes; the doxorubicin damage is no longer recognizable, and the sequential stress may not demonstrate structural changes. Sequential stress or injury may explain some of the cases heretofore thought of as "late" or "late-late" cardiotoxicity.[170]

As the anthracyclines have been in use for more than 30 years, some of the patients cured of leukemias, lymphomas, sarcomas, and breast cancer may harbor subclinical cardiac damage that now makes them particularly prone to symptomatic heart failure in the event of additional cardiac insult. The effect of doxorubicin exposure on the genesis of coronary artery disease, myocardial infarction, and other cardiac injuries that occur with aging is unknown. In one review, 12 of 43 patients with doxorubicin-induced cardiomyopathy died due to progressive cardiac dysfunction.[128] Our understanding of the facts that cardiac damage, albeit usually subclinical, probably takes place with the first exposure of an anthracycline, and the risk of subsequent or sequential stresses, makes the case for early and vigorous cardioprotection very compelling.[166]

Mechanism of Anthracycline-Associated Cardiotoxicity The mechanism of the cardiac damage caused by anthracycline exposure has not been fully elucidated, however free radical formation is believed to be an important factor. Free radicals can injure lipid structures in the myocardial cell, and the resultant peroxidation of these lipid structures impairs the function of the sarcoplasmic reticulum and mitochondria. Myocardial cells are more prone to these degenerative changes since they are less able to metabolize free radicals than are other cells. Cell necrosis is the end result of this damage. As noted above, following exposure to doxorubicin, cardiac troponin T-levels are elevated beyond the level expected from the malignancy itself.[133,167,171] The almost total absence of catalase and superoxide dismutase within cardiac muscle makes it very difficult for cardiac cells to counteract production of free-radicals through the normal scavenger mechanisms.[127] There is increasing evidence that the generation of the oxygen free radicals is mediated through an iron-doxorubicin complex.[137] Doxorubicinol, one of the principal metabolites of doxorubicin, has a greater effect on the calcium pump of the sarcoplasmic reticulum than does the parent doxorubicin, which suggests that the antitumor effect is distinct from the cardiotoxic effect.[135] It has been suggested that the level of atrial natriuretic peptide is increased in at least some patients with doxorubicin-associated cardiotoxicity, and this appears to correlate more with changes in diastolic than with changes in systolic function.[172]

Clinical Manifestations of Doxorubicin-Related Cardiomyopathy Doxorubicin produces a cardiomyopathy clinically indistinguishable from other forms of congestive heart failure. Patients may be asymptomatic in the early stages or may exhibit only minimal signs of cardiac dysfunction. In many patients, the first sign of a cardiac abnormality may be a failure to return to baseline cardiac rate in a timely manner following exertion; resting tachycardia in patients with a previously normal resting heart rate, and loss of respiratory variation in heart rate may also be seen. As cardiac damage progresses, patients experience increasing dyspnea, with dyspnea at rest a poor prognostic sign.

The cardiac examination of a patient with fully developed cardiomyopathy often reveals an S3 gallop, an enlarged area of cardiac dullness, an exaggerated increase in cardiac rate with minimal activity, and, when pulmonary congestion ensues, diffuse rales. The chest radiograph shows nonspecific findings of an increased cardiac silhouette and engorged vasculature. Various degrees of pleural effusion may be noted. The electrocardiogram shows nonspecific findings. Blood chemistry values are being increasingly explored as markers of cardiac damage. The plasma level of brain natriuretic peptide may also be a useful parameter of cardiac dysfunction.[173,174] Additionally, as noted above, serum levels of cardiac troponin T may detect cell damage at the time of injury.

The left ventricular ejection fraction remains the most frequently used noninvasive parameter with which to monitor the cardiac status in patients receiving doxorubicin or related agents. It is defined as the ratio of the quantity of blood in the left ventricle at the end of ventricular systole to the quantity of blood present at the end of diastole. The left ventricular ejection fraction is most commonly estimated from nuclear studies or echocardiography. Ultrasonography has the advantages of not using radiation and that data is accessed in real time, characteristics that are preferred by pediatricians. It is also less costly than the nuclear technique. On the other hand, because nuclear studies provide estimates derived from three-dimensional data, some consider such studies more accurate; nuclear studies are often preferred in clinical trials. The ultimate selection of one over the other of these techniques may well depend on the experience and resources available at any given center, and neither method is clearly recognized to be superior.

Estimates of left ventricular ejection fraction, however, are not infallible. The tests are associated with two factors that are problematic. First, they are influenced by many biologic variables in addition to the direct cardiac effects of the offending drugs. Second, the tests themselves are imperfect, and exhibit some degree of false-positive and false-negative results. Not infrequently, either biologic change or the study limitations may suggest a decrease in ejection fraction that is either real or artifactual, but that is unrelated to the drug under scrutiny. Serial and complementary determinations of ejection fraction are often useful. It must be pointed out, however, that ejection fraction measurements using various techniques are not interchangeable; wide variances in volumes and ejection fraction estimations between techniques have been noted. These differences are most marked in comparisons using cardiac ultrasound.[175]

Other measurements of cardiac function have also been used. Fractional shortening (derived from M-mode echocardiographic measurements) is often used in the pediatric population. Changes in diastolic function as an early sign of cardiotoxicity are also being used increasingly, and monitoring of these parameters following anthracycline therapy holds promise. None of these techniques, however, have yet been shown to have clear advantages over the commonly used ejection fractions.[176,177]

Roles of Cardiac Biopsy in Assessment of Cardiotoxicity The structural changes in myocardial tissue seen on examination of cardiac biopsy specimens can provide vital information concerning the toxicity of doxorubicin and related compounds.[126,178–190] Indeed, studying biopsy material is the best way to gauge cardiac damage at a time prior to the development of functional deterioration. Additionally, in highly selected patients, it provides the essential information needed to decide whether to continue or terminate chemotherapy that includes cardiotoxic drugs.

The procedure for obtaining myocardial tissue originated in Japan, where it was introduced in the early 1960s.[181] The technique was later modified by investigators at Stanford University, where the original work describing the structural changes in the heart associated with doxorubicin was undertaken.[182,183,191] Most laboratories in the United States obtain myocardial tissue from the right ventricle. The bioptome is inserted into the right internal jugular vein, and the biting jaw manipulated so that it passes through the right atrium and across the tricuspid valve to the apex of the right ventricle, from where specimens are taken. Some centers prefer to biopsy the left ventricle, in which case entry is by way of the femoral artery. The specimens, which are preserved in 5% buffered glutaraldehyde solution, are then prepared and examined under an electron microscope. Light microscopy is not useful. Patients report little or no sensation during tissue removal. Major complications are rare but include cardiac tamponade resulting from perforation of the free right ventricular wall or the coronary sinus. Pericarditis, dysrhythmia, vagal stimulation with associated hypotension and bradycardia, and local problems associated with the venous access site also occur. In one series of 1,350 procedures, however, cardiac perforation with tamponade occurred in less than 0.6% of the patients, minor problems were noted in 0.8% of the procedures, and there were no reported deaths.[184]

Cardiac biopsy specimens are graded according to ultrastructural changes seen by electron microscopy.[181,182,185,186] The original Billingham and colleagues grading system consisted of grade 0 (no evidence of anthracycline damage) to grade 3 (severe changes in most cells), with grade 1 and 2 constituting intermediate damage.[182] Later modifications to the scale by Billingham divided grade 2 into two subgroups, 2-A and 2-B.[187] The grading system was also modified by Mackay and colleagues, who added the intermediate grades of 0.5 and 1.5; grade 3 changes are rarely seen with careful dose limitation or continuous infusion schedules.[185] The Mackay grading system is semiquantitative, with both the degree and the extent of the abnormalities considered in determining the final grade; the grading scales are depicted in Table 134-2. A tissue grade of 0 is assigned to specimens with normal-appearing myocardial fibers, whereas higher grades indicate progressively increasing changes that include dilatation of the sarcoplasmic reticulum, myofibrillar dropout, and necrosis (Figure 134-7). However, because it is not unusual to find completely normal myocardial cells adjacent to markedly abnormal ones, adequate specimens and careful scrutiny of the material are essential to grade the tissue properly (see Table 134–2).

The biopsy grade does not take other causes of cardiac damage into account, therefore a combination of functional tests (ejection fraction) and morphologic studies (biopsy grade) is the most sensitive strategy for monitoring patients receiving unusually high cumulative doses of these drugs or with multifactorial myocardial dysfunction.[178–180] In larger studies, cardiac biopsy grades correlate well with cumulative doxorubicin dose. Among patients without histories of heart disease and no risk factors for toxicity, in those who received 200 to 400 mg/m^2 of doxorubicin by standard schedules the mean biopsy grade was 1. The mean biopsy grade was 1.5 in those who

Table 134-2 Morphologic Grading Systems for Anthracycline Cardiotoxicity*

	Billingham Scoring System		Mackay Scoring System†	
Grade	Morphologic Characteristics	Vacuoles[a]	Myofibrillar Dropout[a]	Necrosis[a]
0	Normal myocardial ultrastructural morphology			
0.5	Not completely normal but no evidence of anthracycline-specific damage	< 4	0	0
1.0	Isolated myocytes affected and/or early myofibrillar loss; damage to < 5% of all cells	4–10	< 3	0
1.5	Changes similar to grade 1 except damage involves 6–15% of all cells	> 10	3–5	< 2
2.0	Clusters of myocytes affected by myofibrillar loss and/or vacuolization, with damage to 16–25% of all cells	—[b]	6–8	2–5
2.5	Many myocytes (26–35% of all cells) affected by vacuolization and/or myofibrillar loss		—[c]	—[c]
3.0[d]	Severe, diffuse myocytes damage (> 35% of all cells)	—[b]	> 8	> 5

*Adapted from Mackay B et al,[185,186] Legha S et al,[190] and Billingham M.[191,281]
†Average number of abnormal muscle fibers per grid based on an examination of a minimum of six grids obtained from six blocks.
[a]The highest biopsy grade based on any one category is assigned. If two or more categories indicate the same grade, the grade is increased half a point.
[b]Any number of vacuoles.
[c]A grade of 2.5 is not included in the Mackay system.
[d]With present dosing and schedules, a biopsy grade of 3 is seldom achieved.

received 400 to 500 mg/m^2, and 2 in those who received more than 500 mg/m^2.[178] This dose/biopsy-grade relationship confirms the fact that morphologic changes in the myocardium are detectable at doses unlikely to be associated with clinically evident cardiac dysfunction. In addition, a high-grade cardiac biopsy grade (1.5 or higher) predicts a high risk of congestive heart failure developing with continued drug administration.[179] Thus, the biopsy grade not only measures the damage to the heart of an individual patient, it also serves as a damage scale against which the cardiotoxic effects of other anthracyclines or different dosage schedules can be measured and compared. For example, the cardiac damage scale has been used to compare extended-dose (continuous infusion) schedules with standard-infusion administration, as well as to compare other anthracyclines (epirubicin) or anthraquinones (mitoxantrone) with each other and with doxorubicin.[188–190] Such comparisons have contributed significantly to our understanding of the relative cardiotoxicities of different drugs and various administration schedules (Table 134-3). The need for cardiac biopsy in clinical settings has decreased significantly with the use of cardioprotective regimens, and even challenging patients can new be managed without biopsy; the procedure remains important for some research applications that seek to identify and quantify early cardiac damage.

Risk Factors for Anthracycline-Associated Cardiac Dysfunction Several groups of patients appear to be at greater risk of developing cardiac dysfunction at relatively low doses of anthracyclines. Extremes of age are an established risk factor for greater toxicity, and thus augmented surveillance and monitoring are essential in both the pediatric and geriatric populations.[124,126,192–195]

Some forms of underlying heart disease also predispose patients to increased damage, and there is evidence that the common denominator is increased left ventricular wall tension. Among frequently encountered entities that fall into this category are conditions involving gradients across the left ventricular outflow tract such as aortic stenosis, systemic hypertension, and cardiomyopathies of all types, including hypertrophic obstructive cardiomyopathy.[124] Ischemic heart disease may add some risk in that the increased metabolic needs produced by the chemotherapy may upset a precarious balance between oxygen supply and demand. Anecdotally, many patients with reduced baseline ejection fractions tolerate at least some doxorubicin, especially when used with adequate cardioprotection.[196] Despite some reports to the contrary, anthracyclines are generally not considered to be associated with coronary spasm or primary myocardial ischemia.[197]

Irradiation through portals that include the heart is a well-documented risk factor for cardiomyopathy developing at lower cumulative doses of doxorubicin than is usually seen, and patients who have undergone concomitant or sequential cardiac irradiation should be considered for cardioprotection or monitoring when high cumulative dosages are contemplated.[182,193]

A number of antineoplastic drugs have also been associated with increased anthracycline toxicity. Cyclophosphamide may augment the cardiotoxic effect of doxorubicin toxicity, a matter of particular clinical importance because the drugs are often used together. Although there is evidence both for and against the additive clinical cardiac toxicity of doxorubicin and cyclophosphamide in combination, cyclophosphamide at high doses is known to be independently cardiotoxic, and the combination is definitely more cardiotoxic in a monkey model.[124,198] Dactinomycin, plicamycin, dacarbazine, and mitomycin C, all reportedly augment doxorubicin toxicity, but the evidence for the first three

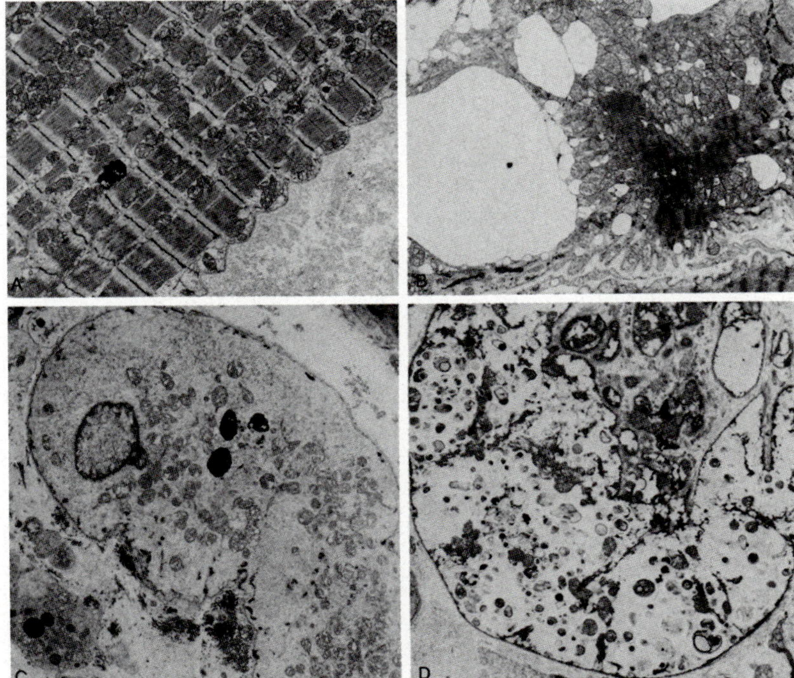

Figure 134-7 Electron micrographs of cardiac biopsy specimens. **A,** Normal heart. **B,** Vacuole formation. **C,** Myofibrillar dropout. **D,** Necrosis (×5,100 original magnification).

Table 134-3 Relative Toxicities of Anthracycline: A Comparison of Relative Toxicities of Different Cardiotoxic Drugs and Dosage Schedules

Drug	Schedule	Relative Myelosuppressive Potency of Single Dose Compared with Doxorubicin Administered by Standard Schedule	Approximate Relative Cardiotoxicity[a]	Cardiotoxicity Index Compared with Doxorubicin Administered by Standard Schedule[b]	Recommended Maximum Dose (mg/m^2)[c]
Doxorubicin	Rapid infusion (20 minutes)	1	1	1	400
Doxorubicin	Weekly	1	0.73	0.73	550
Doxorubicin	24-h infusion	1	0.73	0.73	550
Doxorubicin	48-h infusion	1	0.62	0.62	650[d]
Doxorubicin	96-h infusion	1	0.5	0.5	800–1,000[d]
Epirubicin	Rapid infusion	0.67	0.66	0.44	900
Mitoxantrone	Rapid infusion	5	0.5	2.5	160
Daunorubicin	Rapid infusion	0.67	0.75[e]	0.5[e]	800[e]
Idarubicin	Rapid infusion	5	0.53	2.67	150
Pirarubicin	Rapid infusion	1	0.62	0.62	650[e]
Doxorubicin + Dexrazoxane	Rapid infusion	1[e]	0.5	0.5[e]	800–1,000[e]
Doxorubicin, 300 mg/m^2 + dexrazoxane	Rapid infusion	1[e]	0.73[e]	0.73[e]	550[e]

[a]Factor by which the cardiotoxic effects of the cumulative dose of rapid infusion doxorubicin can be compared with the cumulative dose of the agent, combination and schedule listed, when given at an equivalent myelosuppressive dose.

[b]Derived by dividing 400 mg/m^2, the recommended maximum dose of rapid-infusion doxorubicin, by the recommended maximum dose for the agent in question. The cardiotoxicity index represents a factor by which to multiply the cumulative dose of a drug administered to obtain an approximation of toxicity that might be expected had the resultant amount of doxorubicin been given by rapid infusion. For example, if a cumulative dose of 120 mg/m^2 mitoxantrone had been administered, the patient would be expected to demonstrate cardiac damage approximately equal to 300 mg/m^2 of doxorubicin given by rapid infusion ($120 \times 2.5 = 300$). This value is useful when changing from one cardiotoxic regimen to another. When the sum of the products of the indexes and the cumulative doses administered exceeds 400, the risk of clinically significant cardiotoxicity exceeds 5%.

[c]Dose producing clinically significant congestive heart failure in 5% of patients.

[d]Less toxic by endomyocardial biopsy.

[e]Inadequate data.

has not been persuasive.[199,200] On the other hand, mitomycin C appears to add substantially to the toxicity of doxorubicin, even when given after the completion of doxorubicin therapy.[201] Paclitaxel has also been reported to increase the cardiotoxic effect of doxorubicin. In one study, however, patients receiving the combination at cumulative doses of doxorubicin of below 340 to 380 mg/m^2 did not appear to demonstrate the additive effect.[202] The higher incidence of cardiac toxicity observed when the two drugs are administered within a short time may be due to the fact that the paclitaxel interferes with the pharmacokinetics of doxorubicin, leading to higher systemic levels of both doxorubicin and doxorubicinol, a metabolic product.[203–205] Alternatively, the apparent increase in toxicity may simply be the result of increased surveillance using imperfect tests in patients undergoing frequent monitoring of cardiac function. Other anthracyclines and related agents, such as mitoxantrone (an anthraquinone), demonstrate intrinsic cardiac toxicity that is additive; as is noted below, changing from one anthracycline to another does not provide cardioprotection.[188,206]

Reducing the Cardiotoxic Effects of Doxorubicin A number of strategies can lower the extent of doxorubicin cardiotoxicity. Limiting the cumulative dose is a strategy that grew out of the observation that clinically apparent cardiotoxicity is unusual at cumulative doses of less than 300 mg/m^2 and that the incidence is about 5% at a cumulative dose of 400 mg/m^2. Limiting the cumulative doses to these levels in patients without risk factors will keep the cardiotoxicity within an acceptable range. Dose limitation also decreases the need for cardiac monitoring, as the likelihood of cardiotoxicity is quite low, and the risk of stopping effective therapy early because of false-positive testing results may exceed the benefits of such testing. Dose-limitation, however, does not take into consideration patients who are still responding after receiving the limiting dose. As noted above, most patients, even those with increased cardiac risk, usually tolerate 300 mg/m^2 of doxorubicin or the cardiotoxic equivalent of other anthracyclines.[207]

Encapsulating conventional anthracyclines in liposomes reduces the incidence and severity of cardiotoxicity.[208,209] Both pegylated and non-pegylated preparations have been studied, and the pegylated preparation is approved for the treatment of Kaposi's sarcoma and ovarian carcinoma in the United States under the trade name Doxil. Pegylated liposomal doxorubicin is also effective in the treatment of breast cancer; comparisons of liposome encapsulated and conventional doxorubicin in the treatment of that disease confirmed cardioprotection with comparable antitumor activity.[210–212] Pegylated liposomal doxorubicin appears to have a clinical spectrum similar to the parent compound in other diseases as well.[213] Both pegylated and non-pegylated liposomal doxorubicin are clearly cardioprotective. In the pegylated form, cardioprotection has been demonstrated both by cardiac biopsy as well as by non-invasive studies.[214,215] The degree of cardioprotection is difficult to quantify, but studies suggest that at least twice the number of cycles of pegylated liposomal doxorubicin can be given with the same degree of cardiotoxicity as is seen with the unprotected parent compound. The oncologic efficacy is not impaired, but the degree of stomatitis and hand-foot syndrome is reported to be higher.[216]

Modification of the dose schedule has been clearly shown to decrease anthracycline cardiotoxicity. Initially the effect was demonstrated for weekly administration; in comparison with the standard schedule (rapid-infusion, 21 to 28 day cycle), the weekly schedule allowed approximately 200 mg/m^2 more doxorubicin to be given than the usual amount tolerated. Subsequently, in two studies of 100 and 146 patients, highly significant decreases in cardiac toxicity were noted in cardiac biopsy specimens from patients treated with weekly doxorubicin schedules.[217,218] In one study, it was estimated that patients treated with the weekly doxorubicin schedule were able to receive an additional 168 mg/m^2.[217] The logical interpretation of the data was that doxorubicin cardiotoxicity is related to peak plasma levels. Since it was concluded that the best way to decrease peak levels was to prolong the infusion time, a series of trials of continuous-infusion doxorubicin were initiated using infusion times of 24 to 96 hours, gauging the cardiotoxicity on the basis of endomyocardial biopsy findings.[169,180,219,220] Patients treated with continuous infusions showed a significantly lower incidence of high-grade endomyocardial pathology in their biopsy specimens despite receiving a significantly higher cumulative dose. Further, the antitumor activity in patients with breast cancer or sarcoma was comparable to that seen in historic controls.[220–222] Randomized studies in patients with soft tissue sarcomas and sequential studies in patients with osteosarcoma confirmed the equivalent antitumor activity of continuous-infusion and bolus administration.[223,224] This has also been noted for lymphoma, myeloma, acute lymphocytic leukemia, and other cancers, but formal comparative trials in these patient populations have not been carried out.[132,138,139] In addition, the longer the infusion duration, the less the observed cardiac toxicity (see Table 134-3).[132,138,139,169,179] Infusions administered over 24 hours are similar to weekly administration and permit 150 to 200 mg/m^2 more doxorubicin to be administered with equivalent cardiotoxicity. Longer infusions allow still more doxorubicin to be administered before similar degrees of toxicity are evident. For example, 600 to 650 mg/m^2 can be given using 48-hour infusions and when 96-hour infusions are administered, 800 to 1,000 mg/m^2 of doxorubicin can be given; this is about twice the recommended maximal dose for bolus regimens (see Table 134-3).[179] The cardiotoxicity associated with prolonged (30 to 90 days) continuous infusions has not been well defined, but infusions of longer than 96 hours are limited by increasingly troublesome mucositis and hand-foot syndrome. Infusions shorter than 48 hours should be avoided unless mucositis necessitates this. The inconvenience of the portable infusion pumps and indwelling catheters that are required for continuous-infusion doxorubicin protocols has made many clinicians reluctant to use such schedules. Many oncologists continue to use conventional, less cumbersome schedules, less toxic alternatives or other strategies of cardioprotection.

The benefits of continuous-infusion schedules of doxorubicin in children were assessed in one prospective study of 121 pediatric patients with acute leukemia, that showed no difference in cardiotoxicity between the rapid-infusion and the 48-hour continuous-infusion subgroups on the basis of ultrasonography.[162] However, relatively low doses of doxorubicin were used in this study, and as a result relatively sparse episodes of true toxicity were to be expected. None of the patients experienced clinically evident cardiac disease after chemotherapy. In contrast, our experience in children indicated that continuous-infusion schedules of doxorubicin resulted in a lower incidence of cardiotoxicity.[157]

A number of compounds with possible cardioprotective properties have been investigated. Among them neither vitamin E (α-tocopherol) nor N-acetylcysteine has been found to confer clinically useful protection in human subjects.[134,136] The most useful cardiac protector to date is the iron chelator dexrazoxane (Zinocard, ICRF-187), which is a bisdiketopiperazine. In a study of 92 patients randomly assigned to receive a doxorubicin-containing regimen (50 mg/m^2 doxorubicin with 500 mg/m^2 cyclophosphamide and 500 mg/m^2 fluorouracil given every 21 days) or the same regimen together with dexrazoxane, the investigators found a significant decrease in cardiotoxic effects demonstrated by ejection fraction measurements, biopsy grades, and clinical signs or symptoms of cardiac dysfunction.[225,226] Other toxicities and antitumor effects were unaffected. However, at least one subsequent study, that confirmed the cardioprotective activity of dexrazoxane showed a possible decrease in antitumor effect as well.[143] There was no suggestion of diminished antineoplastic activity, however, in patients given dexrazoxane after they had received 300 mg/m^2 of doxorubicin.[144,145] Other studies have not found the efficacy of anthracyclines to be decreased by dexrazoxane. Clearly, additional studies are required before the relative risks and benefits of dexrazoxane can be placed in proper perspective. Although the data is not entirely firm, it is estimated that the degree of cardioprotection with dexrazoxane, were it to be given from the onset of therapy, is comparable with the protection provided by the 96-hour continuous-infusion doxorubicin schedule. Dexrazoxane has been approved in the United States for breast cancer patients who have previously received at least 300 mg/m^2 doxorubicin and who are to receive additional treatment with doxorubicin. The use of dexrazoxane in patients considered for re-treatment after initial primary or adjuvant treatment is under study. Additionally, dexrazoxane has been studied in conjunction with epirubicin and mitoxantrone.[147,227] These studies suggest that dexrazoxane also reduces the cardiotoxicity of agents other than doxorubicin.

Dexrazoxane is being increasingly used in children where there are special concerns regarding late toxicity.[149] The ultimate role of dexrazoxane in preventing doxorubicin cardiotoxicity has not been fully defined and requires further study. Recently, the cardioprotective ability of substances other than dexrazoxane has been studied in experimental animals.[150,151]

Cardiac Monitoring of Patients Receiving Doxorubicin As noted above, most patients undergoing treatment for cancer, even elderly patients and those with known cardiac disease, can tolerate at least some doxorubicin.[196] Patients with significant dilated cardiomyopathy and patients who have experienced cardiotoxicity from the prior use of an anthracycline or related drug are the major exceptions. Even patients with reduced ejection fractions as the result of prior myocardial infarctions seem to tolerate doxorubicin when it is given with some form of cardioprotection, and when the cumulative dose remains below 300 to 400 mg/m^2.

Patients being considered for doxorubicin therapy generally undergo a cardiac evaluation usually consisting of a complete medical history and physical examination, chest radiography, a determination of ejection fraction by using either a nuclear or ultrasonographic technique, and a standard electrocardiogram. The routine testing of ejection fraction, however, is being increasingly questioned, as basic studies and clinical assessment are usually sufficient in identifying patients at greatly increased risk.[152] Baseline measurements do provide useful data for later comparisons should they be needed. A recent analysis suggested that monitoring by nuclear scanning becomes cost-effective in patients older than 40 years of age scheduled to receive cumulative doses of greater than 350 mg/m^2.[161] When needed, echocardiographic studies are generally preferred in the pediatric population. Routine pretreatment evaluations in children without a history of cardiac abnormalities may not be necessary.[154]

Patients without risk factors need not be reassessed before receiving a cumulative dose of 300 to 350 mg/m^2 by standard infusion or its equivalent in a less cardiotoxic schedule (see Table 134-3). Thereafter, patients should be reassessed after each two additional cycles of treatment if doxorubicin treatment is continued beyond the doses recommended in Table 134-3. Patients with risk factors for early toxicity may be monitored more closely. The most important precaution, however, is keeping track of the cumulative dose, as, even within the dose range suggested in Table 134-3, the risk of heart failure approaches 5% in the absence of other cardiac risk factors when these cumulative dosages are exceeded.

Patients who continue to have an ejection fraction above the lower limit of normal for the laboratory conducting the study and who have not shown a decrease of more than 15% from the pretreatment value generally tolerate their next one or two cycles of doxorubicin well, up to a cumulative dosage of 400 mg/m^2. Patients whose ejection fractions fall below 45% are at considerably increased risk.[228] Patients with baseline ejection fractions between 45% and the lower limits of normal for the laboratory are considered at intermediate risk; in such patients, if the ejection fraction has not changed they may be treated up to 400 mg/m^2 with careful monitoring. For those whose ejection has either fallen by more than 15 percentage points or has fallen to a value below 45%, a strong consideration should be made to stop doxorubicin and substitute alternative therapy using noncardiotoxic agents. The rare patients requiring further cardiotoxic therapy should be considered for cardiac biopsy to evaluate structural changes. A biopsy grade of 1.5 or higher constitutes a contraindication to continued treatment with an anthracycline.[179]

Exercise test findings as a parameter of cardiac reserve in patients treated with anthracyclines were not found to correlate with cardiac biopsy results at our institution; however, other investigators consider exercise testing a useful modality. Although mean exercise ejection fractions do decrease with increasing cumulative dosages of anthracyclines, there is considerable overlap so as to preclude useful decision-making on the basis of these tests.[130,155,156,204,229] Some investigators have suggested that signal-averaged electrocardiography detect early cardiotoxicity damage in children.[158,160]

Other Anthracyclines and Related Agents Clinically, the cardiotoxic effects of daunorubicin, idarubicin, epirubicin, pirarubicin, and mitoxantrone are identical to those of doxorubicin. However, the cumulative dose that causes cardiotoxicity differs for each agent. The cardiotoxicity of these agents has not been studied as extensively as has that of doxorubicin. Nevertheless, on the basis of ejection fractions and findings from cardiac biopsy specimens, at equivalent oncologic doses, epirubicin is associated with a statistically significant decrease in the incidence of cardiac toxicity compared with that seen for doxorubicin given by rapid infusion (see Table 134-3).[131,230] The cardioprotection afforded by epirubicin, which is being used increasingly for the treatment of breast cancer, is at least equivalent to weekly doxorubicin, and may be more. Some investigations have suggested that the combination of paclitaxel and epirubicin causes less cardiotoxicity than the combination of doxorubicin and paclitaxel, and they attribute this to the fact the paclitaxel interferes less with the breakdown of epirubicin than with the parent compound.[148,164]

Mitoxantrone, an anthraquinone, has considerably less cardiotoxicity than does the parent compound.[129,188] Although idarubicin is the least studied commercially available anthracycline, available data suggest that 150 mg/m^2 is a safe cumulative dose for patients who have not yet been exposed to an anthracycline.[231] Preliminary data for pirarubicin (THP doxorubicin), a doxorubicin analogue used extensively in Japan and France, suggest that the agent is significantly less cardiotoxic than doxorubicin given by standard-infusion schedules.[140]

Switching from one agent to another does not offer protection, and considerable care must be exercised when considering a new cardiotoxic treatment in a patient who has previously been treated with other cardiotoxic agents. The best approach when prescribing cardiotoxic agents in sequence is to calculate the fraction of the recommended maximum cumulative dose of the agent that has already been administered and use that fraction to estimate the remaining dosage that can be safely administered. If the sum of the individual fractions remains below unity, the likelihood of cardiotoxicity will remain acceptable. Converting the various cardiotoxic drug doses to the corresponding doses of rapidly administered doxorubicin allows comparisons (see Table 134-3).

Other Drugs That Demonstrate a Decrease in Cardiac Function Significant decreases in myocardial function are occasionally noted for other agents. Alfa-interferon has been associated with a dramatic decrease in ejection fraction.[232] The mechanism is unknown; however, patients who survive the initial episode usually go on to recover cardiac function.[233] An unusual form of cardiac damage is associated with high-dose cyclophosphamide administration. When severe, the damage takes the form of a hemorrhagic myocarditis.[199,234,235] The process is often acute, is related to high individual doses (usually 4.5 g/m^2 or more) rather than to the cumulative dose, and is associated with decreased ejection fractions and mean QRS voltage. Although severe hemorrhagic myocarditis may be fatal, milder presentations may be asymptomatic and reversible.[235]

Trastuzumab (Herceptin), a humanized monoclonal antibody, is effective for the treatment of breast cancers that overexpress HER2, a characteristic present in about 25 to 30% of breast cancers. Cardiomyopathy with a clinical expression initially thought to be similar to that seen for the cardiomyopathy produced by anthracyclines, that is, a potentially progressive decrease in cardiac systolic function, was observed in early clinical studies with trastuzumab. In addition, cardiac dysfunction was noted in 28% of patients treated concomitantly with trastuzumab and doxorubicin, 19% of whom were deemed to have New York Heart Association class III or class IV dysfunction. Cardiac dysfunction was also noted in 11% of patients treated concurrently with trastuzumab and paclitaxel; 4% of patients in this group had New York Heart Association class III or IV dysfunction. The mechanism responsible for cardiac dysfunction and the clinical course of afflicted patients is now recognized to be sufficiently different from that associated with the anthracyclines that it should be considered a different entity, type II chemotherapy-related cardiac dysfunction.[166] The mechanism of trastuzumab-related cardiac dysfunction involves, at least in part, the Erb B-2 pathway. The agent binds to the extracellular domain of the HER2 protein and thus blocks Erb B-2 signaling required for the growth, repair and survival of cardiomyocytes, which help in maintaining cardiac contractility, function and structure.[236] HER2 activates transcription factors such as AP-1, which is involved in regulating cardiac hypertrophy, and nuclear factor-kappa B, which is involved in the cellular response to stress.[237] Erb B-2 signaling is highly complex, involving multiple ligand classes, cell systems, and pathway interactions. Erb B-2 signaling in cardiac muscle cells is essential for the prevention of dilated cardiomyopathy. Interestingly, on examination of cardiac biopsy material, no structural findings were evident. Additionally, it appears that many patients who experienced trastuzumab-related cardiac dysfunction and were rechallenged with the drug were able to tolerate the rechallenge without serious cardiac consequences. These observations add supporting evidence of the differences in clinical course and mechanism between trastuzumab cardiotoxicity and the toxicity related to anthracyclines.[238] It is apparent that Erb B-2 is essential for the preservation of cardiac muscle in vivo and that the temporary interruption of the Erb-B-2 signaling pathway by trastuzumab can cause myocytes to die and congestive heart failure to develop.[239]

The additive effects on cardiac function when trastuzumab is given to patients previously exposed to an anthracyclines is conjectured to constitute a sequential stress whereby the underlying damage, even in the absence of clear abnormalities in ejection fraction sets the stage for the subsequent cardiac insult. The component of cardiac dysfunction related to trastuzumab appears to be largely reversible.[240–242] Several multi-center trials are under way to define the extent and nature of trastuzumab-induced cardiotoxicity.

Management of Anticancer Treatment–Associated Cardiac Dysfunction The most important treatment consideration in patients who develop anthracycline-associated cardiac dysfunction is the avoidance of additional anthracyclines. Once established, anthracycline-associated cardiac dysfunction differs little from other forms of cardiomyopathy, and it is usually treated in a similar way. The American College of Cardiology and The American Heart Association have issued guidelines for the diagnosis and management of chronic heart failure in adults.[243] In terms of diagnosis, they recognize four stages of heart failure, A to D. A patient with stage A designation is at high risk for heart failure but has no structural disorder of the heart; stage B characterizes patients with a structural disorder of the heart but has never shown symptoms of heart failure. Asymptomatic patients who have received high cumulative doses of anthracyclines would fit into one of these two categories. Stage C denotes patients with past or current symptoms of an underlying structural heart disease, and stage D is applied to patients with end-stage disease who require specialized treatments such as mechanical devices, inotropic infusions, or transplantation. This staging of heart failure recognizes potential and actual cardiac changes earlier in the clinical course than does the New York Heart Association functional classes.

Patients who have been treated with anthracyclines but show no symptoms of cardiac dysfunction should have other conditions that exacerbate cardiac dysfunction aggressively treated. Hypertension should be controlled and lifestyle changes encouraged. Pharmacological intervention should also be considered for those who have ejection fractions below 40%. Angiotensin converting enzyme (ACE) inhibitors and β-adrenergic blockers may be appropriate for patients in stage A and stage B (Figure 134-8). For patients in stage C, salt restriction, and diuretics, may be added; Digitalis preparations may offer symptomatic relief, but probably do not prolong life. When the cardiac damage becomes moderate or severe, is associated with left ventricular dilatation, or causes persistent cardiac dysrhythmias, anticoagulation (warfarin sodium titrated to maintain the prothrombin time at least 1.5 times control) or anti-platelet therapy (enteric-coated aspirin, 81–324 mg) should be considered. There is no specific therapy for anthracycline-related cardiomyopathy. An underlying malignancy should not, however, be considered a contraindication to aggressive therapy, and, in selected patients, mechanical assist devices and continuous intravenous inotropic infusions may be helpful and should be employed; cardiac transplantation may be considered for those who have achieved oncologic stability or cure.[244]

As noted above, the cardiac failure associated with trastuzumab is different, in that there is evidence for recovery. Whether or not recovery is directly influenced by the specific therapy for

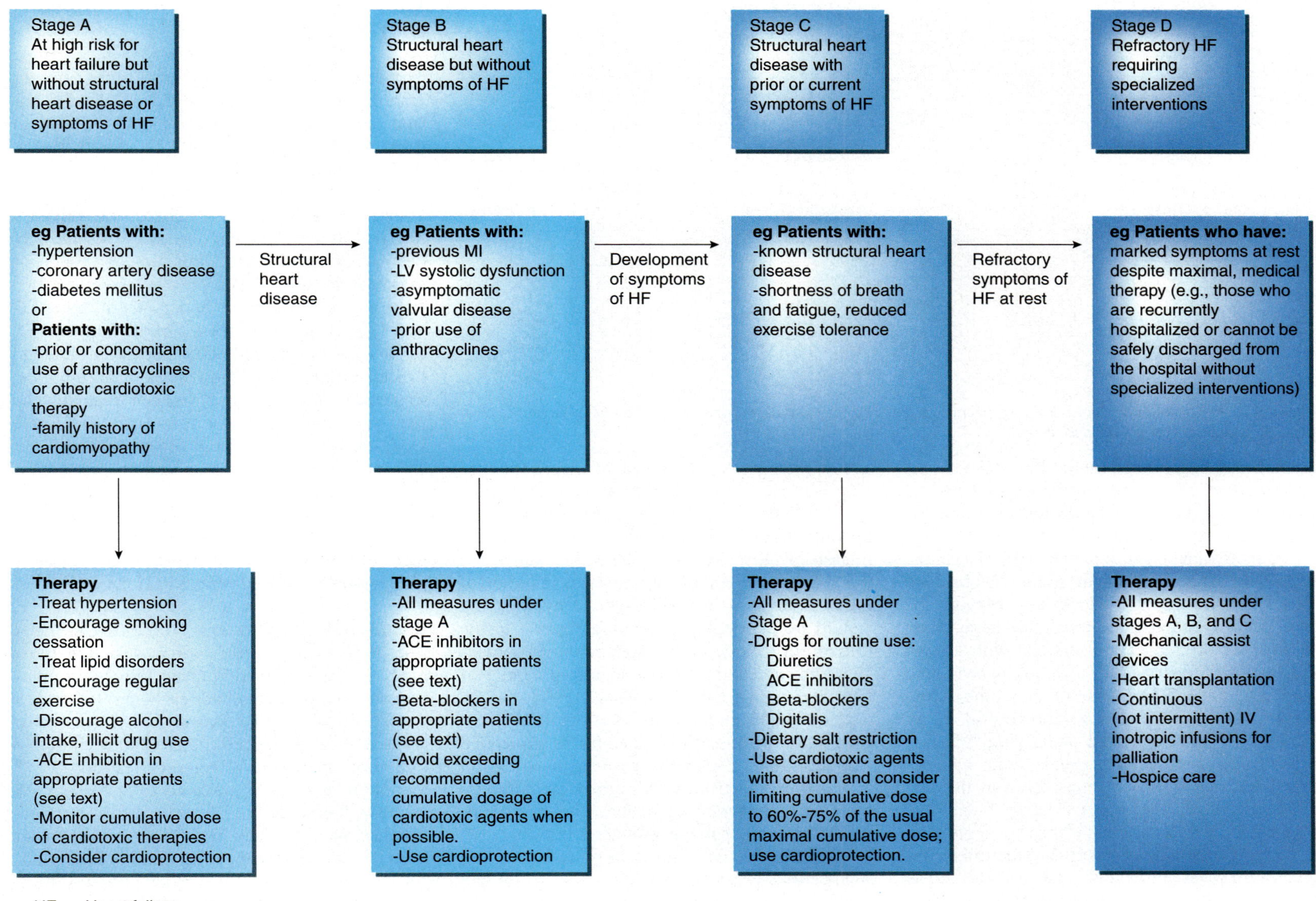

Figure 134-8 Stages and suggested management strategies for congestive heart failure. Adapted with permission from the American College of Cardiology/American Heart Association.[243]

congestive heart failure is uncertain; some patients have recovered without therapy. In any event, symptomatic patients should be treated aggressively.

Agents Associated with Myocardial Ischemia A number of agents have the potential to cause myocardial ischemia, with or without frank myocardial infarction. The most extensively studied agent that causes this is 5-fluorouracil, especially when the agent is administered in combination with cisplatin.[245,246] Isolated cases of myocardial ischemia have also occurred after the administration of vinblastine, vincristine, bleomycin, cisplatin, and biologic response modifiers. The wide spectrum of ischemic responses suggests that ischemia accompanying anti-cancer treatment is more common than is generally appreciated.

Nonspecific electrocardiographic changes may be seen in nearly half the patients treated with 5-fluorouracil, and as many as 16% show electrocardiographic evidence of ischemia including ST-segment depression or elevation and changes suggesting myocardial infarction (Figure 134-9).[246] Many of the affected patients have underlying coronary artery disease, which suggests that pre-existing coronary artery abnormalities augment the ischemic potential of 5-fluorouracil.

The mechanism of the ischemia is uncertain, but coronary artery vasoactivity or spasm probably plays a role; use of a calcium channel blocker has been reported to prevent the ischemia.[247] Selected patients may also be treated with intravenous nitroglycerin while receiving 5-fluorouracil to prevent myocardial ischemia or infarction.

Capecitabine, a fluoropyrimidine carbamate is currently used in the treatment of gastrointestinal and breast malignancy. It is an orally administered prodrug of 5-deoxy-5-fluorouridine (5DFUR) which is enzymatically converted to 5-FU. A number of reports of capecitabine causing angina as part of the acute coronary syndrome through a mechanism similar to that of 5-fluorouracil. Myocardial infarction has also been reported. Other adverse cardiac events associated with capecitabine include angina, myocardial infarction arrhythmias, ECG changes, and cardiomyopathy.[248,249]

High-output states may also result in myocardial ischemia in patients with fixed atherosclerotic lesions that preclude increasing the blood supply because the vessels cannot dilate. The interferons are especially likely to initiate ischemia in this manner. Ischemia may also result from fever, often produced by biologic agents, and from hyperthyroidism. Tumor necrosis factor has been associated with a hypercoagulable state, which suggests vascular occlusion as a possible alternative explanation for the ischemia that occurs in patients being treated with cytokines

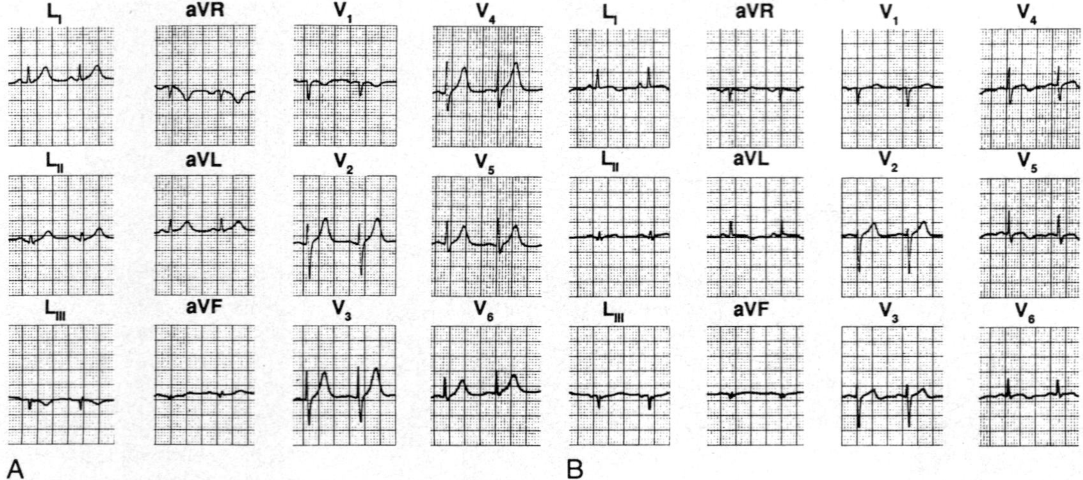

Figure 134-9 Electrocardiogram showing ischemic changes associated with 5-fluorouracil administration before treatment, **A**, and 2 days after treatment, **B**.

and other biologic response modifiers. Anemia is an important coexisting factor, as any cause of ischemia can be exacerbated by a diminished oxygen-carrying capacity.

Patients with evidence of myocardial ischemia, regardless of the mechanism, should be observed closely for rhythm abnormalities, although the level of observation and intervention depends on the overall prognosis. Individuals with known preexisting coronary artery disease can be treated with β-adrenergic blockers and/or a long-acting nitrate to help reduce the likelihood of an ischemic event. Controlled underlying ischemia or evidence of ischemia associated with a particular therapy should not be considered an absolute contraindication to further treatment with the implicated agent or agents. Cancer patients with underlying coronary artery disease are often candidates for revascularization, and stress testing as well as coronary angiography with appropriate interventions may significantly improve the patient's ability to tolerate therapy and to improve their overall quality of life.

Agents Associated with Hypotension and Vascular Toxicity Some degree of hypotension develops in many patients as a consequence of their chemotherapy. The most frequent cause is volume depletion, often as a result of nausea or vomiting. Other causes of hypotension related to chemotherapy are decreased cardiac output, loss of vascular tone, and increased permeability of the small vessels and capillaries (capillary leak). Most instances of hypotension in patients receiving chemotherapy are transient and can be managed with careful monitoring and the administration of fluids or vasopressor agents. Rare instances of profound hypotension, which may be life threatening, have been reported.

Interleukin-2 use is associated with significant, but usually transient, hypotension, frequently requiring pressor agents.[250,251] Capillary leak has been implicated. Interleukin-2–related myocardial ischemia, the exact mechanism of which has not yet been determined, is possibly related to the hypotension, although a direct toxic effect has not been excluded. Interleukin-2 is also associated with an increased incidence of supraventricular dysrhythmias and myocarditis.[251,252] The vasodilation that occurs in response to interleukin-2 appears to be mediated by the release of nitric oxide. Evidence has suggested that N^G-monomethyl-L-arginine, an inhibitor of nitric oxide synthase, reverses the hypotension caused by interleukin-2, lending support to the role of nitric oxide in the production of hypotension and indicating the therapeutic potential of N^G-monomethyl-L-arginine as well.[253]

Homoharringtonine, an investigational agent used in the treatment of leukemias, is associated with dose-related, sometimes severe, hypotension arising immediately after its intravenous administration.[254] Intravenous epinephrine has been helpful in stabilizing patients in this setting.

Considerable interest has surrounded the possible cardiac effects of paclitaxel (Taxol). In one study, asymptomatic bradycardia occurred in 29% of patients treated with maximally tolerated doses of paclitaxel. More severe rhythm abnormalities have also been reported, but they usually are seen in patients with underlying cardiac abnormalities or in the presence of electrolyte imbalance.[255] Serious cardiac problems are rare with paclitaxel, and most patients can be treated without special monitoring.[256,257] However, since patients with significant underlying cardiac disease have often been excluded from most paclitaxel trials, the safety of this drug in this population has yet to be fully defined. As described above, paclitaxel has also been reported to augment the cardiotoxic effects of doxorubicin when the two drugs are given together; at the same time, however, the efficacy of the combination is reportedly enhanced.[159,258] Hypersensitivity reactions are also known to occur.[259]

Cisplatin, an agent widely used to treat genitourinary malignancy, head and neck tumors, and non-small cell lung cancer is known to induce a toxic neuropathy. This phenomenon is also observed with thalidomide and Taxol. In the case of cisplatin, the toxic neuropathy associated with this agent is now believed to be caused by disruption of the nerve blood supply.[260]

EFFECTS OF IRRADIATION OF THE HEART

The heart, being composed of different tissues with different sensitivities to the effects of radiation, demonstrates a wide variety of clinical responses to radiation. The effects of radiation on the heart depend on many factors, including radiation energy, dose fraction, total dose, and the volume and structures included in the radiation portal Radiation effects on cardiac tissue may occur early, even before completion of a course of radiotherapy, or they can appear years later.[261,262]

Although radiation therapy to the chest is widely used to treat breast cancer, lung cancer, esophageal cancer, and other mediastinal tumors, the late effects of radiation on the heart are most frequent in patients who have been treated in the past with radiation for non-Hodgkin's and Hodgkin's lymphomas and breast cancer.[263,264] This is due to two factors: radiation portals that directed treatment through anterior/posterior fields that included heart, and the extended survival seen in large numbers of these patients.[264] Shielding as much of the heart as possible reduces the incidence of radiation-associated pericardial injury.[265–267]

Radiation Effects on the Pericardium

The pericardium is the cardiac structure most likely to show clinical damage following radiation and demonstrates both early and late radiation effects. The initial presentation of acute radiation-associated pericarditis is similar clinically to that of other types of acute pericarditis.[268,269] Symptoms may occur gradually or abruptly, with vague or focused, often dramatic diffuse substernal chest pain that may be difficult to distinguish from the pain of angina or myocardial infarction. As with myocardial infarction, patients often experience anxiety and fear of impending doom. Unlike myocardial ischemia, however, the discomfort of acute pericarditis is often increased with deep inspiration, movement, or recumbency.

Key to the diagnosis of radiation induced pericarditis is a review of the radiation portals to confirm inclusion of the heart in the radiation portal. If the heart is found to be included in the radiation field, radiation pericarditis should be considered in the differential diagnosis but only after myocardial infarction or other etiologies for the symptoms are excluded.

Damage is related to dose, volume and technique of radiation. Estimates of the relative risk for fatal cardiovascular events after mediastinal radiation for Hodgkin's disease ranged between 7.2 and 2.2, and 1.0 and 2.2 after radiation for left-sided breast cancer. Risk is life-long and absolute risk increases with time.[270] A clear association has been established between thoracic radiotherapy and ischemic heart disease among older clinical trials that involved radiotherapeutic techniques that are no longer standards of care. No increased risk of cardiac complications, however, has been seen with current radiotherapeutic approaches that carefully minimize cardiac dose and volume.[271] The severity of the fibrosis was correlated to radiation dose with moderate to severe changes noted after 30Gy.[272]

The physiological status of the heart, the patient, the size and weight of the organ, and the age of the patient will influence the radiosensitivity. Implicit among these factors is the percentage of the organ in the radiation field. Physiologic changes, including loss of oxygen diffusing capacity due to microvascular damage, affect tissue organization. The major contributing factor in the increase of organ weight is water content. The dissolved oxygen in cell water determines both the rate of metabolism and radiosensivity.[273] The TD_{50} evaluation with water content in 14 different human organs yielded a correlation coefficient of 0.60, which is consistent with values reported by others.

Pericardial friction rubs help to establish the diagnosis, but are not always present. Rubs are not a specific finding, however, as they may also be noted in patients following myocardial infarction. Ischemic infarction may also occur following radiation injury to the coronary vessels, a condition that adds to the dilemma of accurately differentiating infarction from pericarditis in the post-radiation period.

Cardiac symptoms induced by radiation should be a diagnosis of exclusion. Although radiation therapy is the most likely cause of constrictive pericarditis in cancer patients who have been radiated, the differential diagnosis also includes tuberculosis, chronic inflammation following infection of the pericardial sac, and the post-pericardiotomy syndrome. A clinically similar picture may also appear, without primary thickening of the pericardium itself, in patients with extensive tumor surrounding the heart.

Tolerance to radiation also depends on the type of tissue treated. There are two types of normal tissues. *Acute reacting tissues*, which are rapidly-proliferating tissues like mucosal surfaces, usually develop an inflammatory radiation reaction during the course of treatment. *Late reacting tissues*, which do not proliferate like brain, liver, and muscle [including the heart], generally do not develop a significant inflammatory reaction during the radiation course. Acute radiation reactions do not predict the extent of late radiation effects. Scar tissue is the most common form of late radiation effect. These effects are similar to those seen in wound healing.

Acute radiation-related pericarditis is usually treated with nonsteroidal anti-inflammatory drugs, such as ibuprofen, at a dosage of 400 mg three times a day. This usually results in prompt resolution of symptoms. In severe or refractory cases, corticosteroids are sometimes helpful, but, as in the case of other forms of pericarditis, it may be difficult to fully wean the patients from steroids. Once the inflammation is controlled, many patients can continue with their radiation therapy. Mild flare-ups of the inflammation with further radiation therapy can usually be prevented or treated with ibuprofen in the same dosage used to treat the initial episode.

A chronic effusive form of the disease, with intermittent acute exacerbations and spontaneous or pharmacologically induced remissions may develop over a period of months or years in some patients with radiation-associated pericarditis. Rarely, fibrous fusion of the parietal and visceral pericardia develops and can then evolve into the full clinical syndrome of constrictive pericarditis.

Hemodynamic alterations in patients with constrictive pericarditis result from the inability of blood to enter and thus be ejected from the heart. In some respects, the hemodynamic changes produced by cardiac tamponade and pericardial constriction are similar: both conditions demonstrate increased venous pressure and low cardiac output. Chest radiography or echocardiography may suggest pericardial calcification. Pericardial thickening and calcification may also be seen on CT studies. Classic cardiac enzymes levels are usually normal. CA-125 level may be elevated.[41]

The results of other diagnostic studies in patients with acute radiation-related pericarditis are usually nonspecific. The electrocardiogram often demonstrates elevations of the ST segments (classically, but not always in diffuse leads), so the initial impression based on the history of chest pain and the electrocardiogram may well be one of ischemic heart disease rather than of a complication of radiation. The echocardiogram may be completely normal or may demonstrate pericardial effusion; it may also show a thickened pericardium if the process has gone on for some time. The echocardiogram usually shows thickening of the pericardium and may show flattening of the posterior wall during diastole.

Cardiac catheterization may demonstrate the classic "square root" sign (dip and plateau), but differentiating constrictive pericarditis from infiltrative (restrictive) processes, such as amyloidosis, remains problematic.[45,274,275] Catheterization studies in patients with significant constriction usually show equalization and elevation of diastolic right and left ventricular pressures.

The treatment of radiation-associated constrictive pericarditis must be individualized, since surgery carries considerable risk and patients may have a life expectancy ranging from weeks to decades. When patients do not have extensive calcification, are not seriously debilitated, and do not have liver failure, surgery can usually be undertaken albeit with significant risk; even in skilled hands the mortality among some subgroups may be as high as 25%. Patients in whom symptomatic constriction develops following radiation present a major therapeutic dilemma. Removal of the pericardium for the management of established constrictive pericarditis is technically challenging and often requires cardiopulmonary bypass. To avoid this, many physicians prefer an aggressive approach earlier by removing a large portion of the pericardium before constriction develops.[276]

Radiation Effects on the Myocardium, Heart Valves, and Cardiac Vasculature

Radiation injuries to the myocardium, heart valves, and coronary vessels are seen occasionally. The symptoms may be confusing, and radiation injuries cannot be distinguished from other etiologies on purely clinical grounds. Radiation sensitivity can vary among patients, and radiation side effects are related to the total dose, what structures are included in the radiation field, and the age of the patient. The late effects of radiation to the heart require close followup among patients treated before 21 years of age.[270,272,277] Risk is life-long and absolute risk increases with time.[270] Abnormalities were identified in the EKG, chest radiograph, echocardiogram exercise stress test, or 24-hour Holter monitor among 49% of 41 patients who received chest radiation or chemotherapy (cyclophosphamide or Adriamycin) for childhood cancer.[278] Each additional year of follow-up was associated with a 1.3 times increase in risk for pathologic cardiac findings, and the risk for an abnormality on a diagnostic study was 12.8-fold higher for patients who had thoracic radiation.

Pancarditis with evidence of injury to virtually all cardiac tissue has also been reported.[279] Injury to the cardiac muscle is an infrequent clinical finding but has been noted in experimental animals.[280] Hyaline degeneration is the most characteristic feature. Although decreased ejection fractions have been noted following radiation in clinical studies, it is not altogether clear whether the decreased function is a result of muscle damage or is secondary to ischemia following injury to the small vessels.[281,282]

Radiation-associated vascular injury is a well-known phenomenon and has been noted in young persons with clinical or autopsy evidence of coronary occlusion, myocardial ischemia, or infarction.[262] At least two mechanisms appear to be involved in such injury. First, radiation induces thickening of the arterial wall secondary to intimal and adventitial proliferation; the luminal area is thereby reduced. Second, large doses of radiation greatly accelerate arteriosclerosis and act synergistically with that process to enhance cholesterol deposition and luminal ulceration.[283] Symptoms range from mild stable angina pectoris to extensive myocardial infarction causing sudden death.

The heart responds to radiation like a late-reacting tissue showing a chronic progressive decline with time and a direct correlation with radiation dose and fractionation. Animal models have demonstrated a radiation dose-dependent chronic congestive myocardial failure that follows radiation damage to the myocardial microvasculature and that indirectly damages the coronary macrovasulature when coupled with cholesterol feeding; histological examination shows a marked reduction in capillary density, myocardial degeneration and necrosis with interstitial fibrosis.[267,271] Cell kinetic studies show increased endothelial cell proliferation about 30 to 100 days postradiation. The morphologic changes in animal models parallel drops in cardiac output and left ventricular ejection fraction. The slightly reduced cardiac function is maintained for many weeks due to a compensatory up-regulation of cardiac beta-adrenergic receptors; in the denervated heart the stroke volume and cardiac contractility show rapid and steady deterioration.

Atrial natriuretic peptide (ANP) levels correlated with cardiac dysfunction in a study of 121 patients who had received cardiac radiation. The 73 Hodgkin's disease patients had 50–80% of the heart radiated, and the 48 breast cancers had 20–30% of the heart radiated. ANP levels were significantly elevated among the 121 patients when compared to age-matched controls. An age-related correlation was observed, for both Hodgkin's disease and breast cancer patients, with plasma ANP.[284] Patients with clinical symptoms of cardiovascular disease also had higher levels of ANP when compared to irradiated patients without symptoms. No correlation existed with ANP levels and time after treatment.

The treatment of radiation-associated vascular injury is similar to the conventional treatment of ischemic cardiac disease; nitrites, β-adrenergic blockers, platelet inhibitors, and calcium channel blockers are the mainstays of pharmacological therapy. Invasive approaches for the management of ischemic heart disease are also often helpful; balloon angioplasty, however, often requires inflation pressures that are higher than those ordinarily used, and longer periods of balloon inflation may be required. Bypass surgery may prove more difficult than usual from a technical standpoint because of the smaller vascular lumens and because the surgeon must work in a previously irradiated field. Nevertheless, bypass surgery remains an important option for these patients.

Radiation injury to the cardiac valves is occasionally noted at autopsy, but valvular problems resulting from radiation therapy usually are not clinically important. Histologically, the valves show endocardial thickening resembling fibroelastosis.[262]

Radiation injury to the cardiac conduction system has also been noted and is usually suggested by abnormalities on the electrocardiogram. Nonspecific changes involving the P wave are frequently seen but may be due, in part, to concomitant radiation injury of the lung. Prolongation of the PR interval is often seen, as are supranodal and infranodal atrioventricular blocks. Complete heart block is occasionally encountered, and pacemaker implantation may prove lifesaving for such patients.

Young patients who receive mediastinal radiation for lymphoma are at highest risk for cardiac complications because a significant volume of the heart is included in the radiation field and because lymphoma has high cure rates. About half of the patients, age 21–45 years, with followup ranging between 10 and 20 years after mantle radiotherapy alone for Hodgkin's disease had reduced systolic and diastolic function on myocardial scintigraphy. Valvular stenosis was not found but mild regurgitation of the aortic valve was present in 1/25, and 9/25 mitral valves, and 22/25 tricuspid valves based on the location of the radiation field.[285]

A wide variety of unsuspected, clinically significant cardiovascular abnormalities were identified in 48 long-term survivors of Hodgkin's disease treated with radiotherapy 14.3years (median; range 5.9 to 27.5 years) after diagnosis. All patients received mediastinal radiation (median 40 Gy; range 27 Gy to 51.7 Gy) at a median age of 16.5years (range 6.4 to 25 years), and four had received anthracycline chemotherapy. All patients were asymptomatic.[286] Restrictive cardiomyopathy was suggested by a reduced average left ventricular (LV) dimension and mass without increased LV thickness, 42% had significant valvular defects, and 75% had conduction defects. Autonomic dysfunction was evident by a monotonous heart rate in 57%, persistent tachycardia in 31% and blunted hemodynamic responses to exercise in 27%. Peak oxygen uptake during exercise was reduced in 30%, and it was associated with increased fatigue and dyspnea, and decreased physical function.

Cardiac dysfunction after breast cancer therapy is now rare because of modern radiation techniques that avoid treatment of the heart. The radiation fields used to treat lung cancer are now localized only to the primary tumor and the mediastinum is included only when there is primary disease extension. Also, the prognosis for lung cancer is poor and generally these patients do not survive long enough to develop long-term cardiac side effects from mediastinal radiation.

Cardiac complications now rarely occur after radiation for tumors located in the thorax because of modern radiation techniques. However, young lymphoma patients who require thoracic radiation are at highest risk for cardiac complications and require close follow-up especially when other cardiac risk factors, like a positive family history, are present.

REFERENCES

1. Braunwald E. Heart Disease: A Textbook of Cardiovascular Medicine. 6th ed. Philadelphia: WB Saunders; 2001.
2. Feigenbaum H. Echocardiography. 5th ed. Philadelphia: Lea & Febiger; 1995.
3. Errichetti A, Weyman A. Cardiac tumors and masses. In: Weyman, A. editor. Principles and Practice of Echocardiography, 2nd ed. Philadelphia: Williams and Wilkins; 1993. p. 11135–77.
4. Kirkpatrick J, Wong, T, Je B, et al. Differential diagnosis of cardiac masses using contrast echocardiographic perfusion imaging. J Am Coll Cardiol 2004;43:1412–9.
5. Huttemann E, Schelenz, C, Franke, U, et al. Transesophageal echocardiography and intraoperative management of patients with renal cell carcinoma and vena cava extension. Anaesthesist 2002;51:116–9.
6. Caiani EG, Corsi, C, Sugeng, L, et al. Improved quantification of left ventricular mass based on endo- and epicardial surface detection using real-time three-dimensional echocardiography. Heart 2005 (in press).
7. Dymond D, Elliot A, Stone D. Factors that affect the reproducibility of measurements of left ventricular function from first-pass radionuclide ventriculograms. Circulation 1982;65:311–22.
8. Ewer M, Benjamin R. Herceptin cardiotoxicity-inherent toxicity, sequential stress or artifact? Semin Oncol 1999;26(Suppl 26):96–101.
9. Francone M. Dymarkowski S, Kalantzi M, Bogaert J. Magnetic resonance imaging n the evaluation of the pericardium. A pictorial essay. Radiol Med 2005;109:64–74.
10. Higgins C, Holt W, Pflugfelde P, Sechtem U. Functional evaluation of the heart with magnetic resonance imaging. Magn Res Med 1988;6:121–39.
11. Jacobson H. Council of Scientific Affairs of the American Medical Association: Magnetic resonance of the cardiovascular system. JAMA 1988;259:253–9.
12. Edelman R. Contrast-enhanced MR imaging of the heart: overview of the literature. Radiology, 2004;232:653–68.
13. Lawson M, Blackwell G, Pohost G. Cardiovascular magnetic resonance imaging: A review of principles and utilities. Am Coll Cardial Curr J Rev1994;4:7.
14. Watzinger N, Maier R, Reiter U, et al. Clinical applications of cardiovascular magnetic resonance. Curr Pharm Des 2005;11:457–75.
15. Kramer C. Current and future applications of cardiovascular magnetic resonance imaging. Cardiol Rev 2000;8:216–22.
16. Lima J, Desai M. Cardiovascular magnetic resonance imaging: current and emerging applications. J Am Coll Cardiol 2004;44:1164–71.
17. Ritchie J, Bateman T, Bonow R. Guidelines for clinical use of cardiac radionuclide imaging. Report of the American College of Cardiology/American Heart Association Task Force on Assessment of Diagnostic and Therapeutic Cardiovascular Procedures (Committee on Radionuclide Imaging), developed in association with the American Society of Nuclear Cardiology. J Am Coll Cardiol 1995;25:521–47.
18. Silvestri F, Bussani R, Pavletic N, Mannone T. Metastases of the heart and pericardium. G Ital Cardiol 1997;27:1252–5.
19. Berge T, Sievers J. Myocardial metastases. A pathological and electrocardiographic study. Br Heart J 1968;30:383–90.
20. Hanfling S. Metastatic cancer to the heart: Review of the literature and report of 127 cases. Circulation 1960;22:474–83.
21. Spodick D. Neoplastic Pericardial Disease. In: Spodick D, editor. The Pericardium: A Comprehensive Textbook. New York: Dekkar; 1997. p. 301–13.
22. Sarjeant J, Butany J, Cusimano R. Cancer of the heart: epidemiology and management of primary tumors and metastases. Am J Cardiovasc Drugs 2003;6:407–21.
23. Glancy D, Roberts W. The heart in malignant melanoma: A study of 70 autopsy cases. Am J Cardiol 1968;21:555–71.
24. Savoia P, Fierro M, Zaccagna A, Bernengo M. Metastatic melanoma of the heart. J Surg Oncol 2000;75:203–7.
25. Kline I. Cardiac lymphatic involvement by metastatic tumor. Cancer 1972;29:799–808.
26. Onuigbo W. The spread of lung cancer to the heart, pericardium and great vessels. Jpn Heart J 1974;15:234–8.
27. Nour-Eddine M, Bensaid A, Tahiri A, Chraibi N. Malignant non-Hodgkin's lymphoma presenting with cardiac tamponade. Arch Mal Coeur Vaiss 2001;94:1112–6.
28. Kralstein J, Frishman W. Malignant pericardial diseases: diagnosis and treatment. Am Heart J 1987;113:785–90.
29. Shabetai R, Mangiardi L, Bhargava V. The pericardium and cardiac function. Prog Cardiovac Dis 1979;22:107–34.
30. Garcia-Riego A, Cuinas C, Vilanova J. Malignant pericardial effusion. Acta Cytol 2001;45:561–6.
31. Roberts W, Glancy D, DeVita V Jr. Heart in malignant lymphoma (Hodgkin's disease, lymphosarcoma, reticulum cell sarcoma and mycosis fungoides). A study of 196 autopsy cases. Am J Cardiol 1968;22:85–107.
32. Abadoglu O, Osma E, Ucan E, et al. Behçet's disease with pulmonary involvement, superior vena cava syndrome, chyloptysis and chylous ascites. Respir Med 1996;90:429–31.
33. Manolitsas T, Abdessalam S, Fowler J. Chylous ascites following treatment for gynecologic malignancies. Gynecol Oncol 2002;86:370–4.
34. Porte H, Janecki-Delebecq T, Finzi L, et al. Pericardioscopy for primary management of pericardial effusion in cancer patients. Eur J Cardiothorac Surg 1999;16:287–91.
35. Seferovic P, Ristic A, Maksimovic R, et al. Diagnostic value of pericardial biopsy: improvement with extensive sampling enabled by pericardioscopy. Circulation 2003;107:978–83.
36. Parameswaram R, Goldberg H. Echocardiographic quantitation of pericardial effusion. Chest 1983;83:767–70.
37. Come P, Riley M, Fortuin N. Echocardiographic mimicry of pericardial effusion. Am J Cardiol 1981;47:365–70.
38. Tominaga K, Shinkai T, Eguchi K, et al. The value of two-dimensional echocardiography in detecting malignant tumors of the heart. Cancer 1986;58:1641–7.
39. Nugue O, Millaire A. Neoplastic Versus Nonmalignant Pericardial Effusion in Patients with Malignancies: Etiology, Diagnostic Profile and Clinical Outcome. In: Seferociv D, Spodick D, Maisch B, editors. Pericardiology. Belgrade: Science Publishers; 2000. p. 339–44.
40. Posner M, Cohen G, Skarin A. Pericardial disease in patients with cancer: the differentiation of malignant from idiopathic and radiation-induced pericarditis. Am J Med 1981;71:407–13.
41. Eerdekens M, Nouwen E, Pollet D, et al. Placental alkaline phosphatase and cancer antigen-125 in sera of patients with benign and malignant diseases. Clin Chem 1985;31:687–90.
42. Nagele H, Bahlo M, Klapdor R, et al. CA 125 and its relation to cardiac function. Am Heart J 1999;137:1039–44.
43. Spodick D. Current concepts: acute cardiac tamponade. N Engl J Med 2003;349:684–90.
44. Reddy P, Curtiss E, O'Toole J, Shaver J. Cardiac tamponage: hemodynamic observations in man. Circulation 1978;58:265–72.
45. Tyberg T, Goodyer A, Langou R. Genesis of pericardial knock in constrictive pericarditis. Am J Cardiol 1980;46:570–5.
46. Spodick D. Truly total electric alternation of the heart. Clin Cardiol 1998;21:427–8.
47. Press O, Livingston R. Management of malignant pericardial effusion and tamponade. JAMA 1987;257:1088–92.

48. Vaitkus P, Herrmann H, LeWinter M. Treatment of malignant pericardial effusion. JAMA 1994;272:59–64.
49. Hill GI, Cohen B. Pleural pericardial window for the palliation of cardiac tamponade due to cancer. Cancer 1970;26:81–93.
50. Liberman M, Labos C, Sampalis J, et al. Ten-year surgical experience with nontraumatic pericardial effusions: a comparison between the subxyphoid and transthoracic approaches to pericardial window. Arch Surg 2005;140:191–5.
51. Tsang T, Seward J, Barnes M, et al. Outcomes of primary and secondary treatment of pericardial effusion in patients with malignancy. Mayo Clin Proc 2000;75:248–53.
52. Salem K, Mulji A, Loon E. Echocardiographically guided pericardiocentesis-the gold standard for the management of pericardial effusion and cardiac tamponade. Can J Cardiol 1999;15:1251–5.
53. Wolfe M, Edelman E. Transient systolic dysfunction after relief of cardiac tamponade. Ann Intern Med 1993;119:42–4.
54. Merce J, Sagrista-Sauleda J, Permanyer-Miralda G, Soler-Soler J. Should pericardial drainage be performed routinely in patients who have a large pericardial effusion without tamponade? Am J Med 1998;105:106–9.
55. Maher E, Shepherd F, Todd T. Pericardial sclerosis as the primary management of malignant pericardial effusion and cardiac tamponade. J Thorac Cardiovasc Surg 1996;112:637–43.
56. Martinoni A, Cipolla C, Carinale D, et al. Long-term results of intrapericardial chemotherapeutic treatment of malignant pericardial effusions with thiotepa. Chest 2004;126:1412–6.
57. Caliendo M, Lee D, Querioz R, Waldman D. Sclerotherapy with use of doxycycline after percutaneous drainage of postoperative lymphoceles. J Vasc Interv Radiol 2001;12:73–7.
58. Dollinger, M., Management of recurrent malignant effusions. CA Cancer J Clin 1972;22:138–47.
59. Marcy P, Bondiau P, Brunner P. Percutaneous treatment in patients presenting with malignant cardiac tamponade. Eur Radiol 2005;[Epub ahead of print].
60. Ziskind A, Pearc A, Lemmon C, et al. Percutaneous balloon pericardiotomy for the treatment of cardiac tamponade and large pericardial effusions: Descriptions of technique and report of the first 50 cases. J Am Coll Cardiol 1993;21:1–5.
61. Jalisi F, Morise A, Haque R, Jain A. Primary percutaneous balloon pericardiotomy. W V Med J 2004;100:102–5.
62. Galli M, Politi A, Pedretti F. Percutaneous balloon pericardiotomy for malignant pericardial tamponade. Chest 1995;108:1499–1501.
63. Ovune K, Aytemir K, Ozer N, et al. Percutaneous balloon pericardiotomy for patients with malignant pericardial effusion including three malignant pleural mesotheliomas. Angiology 2001;52:323–9.
64. Cates C, Virmani R, Vaughn W, Robertson R. Electrocardiographic markers of cardiac metastasis. Am Heart J 1986;112:1297–1303.
65. Vallot F, Berghmns T, Delhaye F, Dagnelie J, et al. Electrocardiographic manifestations of heart metastasis from a primary lung cancer. Support Care Cancer 2001;9:275–7.
66. Paliszewska L, Odyniec A. A case of metastasis of cancer of the kidney to the heart simulating myocardial infarction. Wiad Lek 1989;42:249–52.
67. Manner G, Harting M, Russo P, et al. Surgical management of metastatic melanoma to the ventricle. Tex Heart Inst J 2003;30:218–20.
68. Gibbs P, Cebon J, Calafiore P, Ropbinson W. Cardiac metastases from malignant melanoma. Cancer 1999;85:78–84.
69. Levin R, Meta S. A classification of ectopic hormone-producing tumors. Ann N Y Acad Sci 1974;230:533–46.
70. Dropcho E. Update on paraneoplastic syndromes. Curr Opin Neurol 2005;18:331–6.
71. Godwin J II. Carcinoid tumors: An analysis of 2,837 cases. Cancer 1975;36:560–9.
72. Ebagosti A, Favre R, Gueunoun M, Vitot P, et al. Carcinoid cardiopathy: value of ultrasonography and MRI. Apropos of a case related to bronchial tumor. A review of the literature. Ann Cardiol Angiol 1989;38:91–5.
73. Rajamannan N, Caplice N, Anthikad F, et al. Cell proliferation in carcinoid valve disease: a mechanism for serotonin effects. J Heart Valve Dis 2001;10:827–31.
74. Pearlman A. Carcinoid heart disease: echocardiographic recognition and differential diagnosis. Am Heart Hosp J 2005;3:132–5.
75. Ferrans V. The carcinoid endocardial plaque; an ultrastructural study. Hum Pathol 1976. 7:387–409.
76. Robiolio P, Rigolin V, Wilson J, et al. Carcinoid heart disease. Correlation of high serotonin levels with valvular abnormalities detected by cardiac catheterization and echocardiography. Circulation 1995;15:790–5.
77. Millward M, Blake M, Byrne M, et al. Left heart involvement with cardiac shunt complicating carcinoid heart disease. Aust N Z J Med 198919:716–7.
78. Simula D, Edwards W, Tazelaar H, et al. Surgical pathology of carcinoid heart disease: a study of 139 valves from 75 patients spanning 20 years. Mayo Clin Proc 2002;77:139–47.
79. Lundin L, Funa K, Hansson HE, et al. Histochemical and immunohistochemical morphology of carcinoid heart disease. Pathol Res Pract 1991;187:73–7.
80. Strickman NE, Rossi PA, Massumi A, Hall RJ. Carcinoid heart disease: a clinical, pathologic and therapeutic update. Curr Prob Cardiol 1982;6:1–41.
81. Rees L. The biosynthesis of hormones by non-endocrine tumours—A review. J Endocrinol 1975;67:143–75.
82. Yun D, Heywood JT. Metastatic carcinoid disease presenting solely as high-output heart failure. Ann Intern Med 1994;120:45–6.
83. Ewer M, Ali M, Balakrishnan P. Clinical recognition of carcinoid heart disease in the elderly. Geriatric Medicine Today 1985;4:23–30.
84. Tribouilly C, Slama M, Rey J, et al. Demonstration by Doppler echocardiography of multiple valvular involvement in carcinoid cardiopathy. Arch Mal Coeur Vaiss, 1989;82:109–14.
85. Pellikka PA, Tajik A, Khandheria B, et al. Carcinoid heart disease. Clinical and echocardiographic spectrum in 74 patients. Circulation 1993;87:1188–96.
86. Baker B, McNee V, Scovil J, et al. Tricuspid insufficiency in carcinoid heart disease: An echocardiographic description. Am Heart J 1981;101:107–8.
87. Callahan J, Wroblewski E, Reeder G, et al. Echocardiographic features of carcinoid heart disease. Am J Cardiol 1982;50:762–8.
88. Pandya UH, Pellikka P, Enriquez-Sarano M, et al. Metastatic carcinoid tumor to the heart: echocardiographic-pathologic study of 11 patients. J Am Coll Cardiol 2002;40:1328–32.
89. Hendel N, Leckie B, Richards J. Carcinoid heart disease. Eight-year survival following tricuspid valve replacement and pulmonary valvotomy. Ann Thorac Surg 1980;30:391–5.
90. Honey M, Paneth M. Carcinoid heart disease: Successful tricuspid valve replacement. Thorax 1975;30:464–9.
91. Connolly HM, Schaff H, Mullany C, et al. Carcinoid heart disease: impact of pulmonary valve replacement in right ventricular function and remodeling. Circulation 2002;106(12 Suppl 1):151–6.
92. McBride W, Jackman J, Gammon R, Willerson J. High-output cardiac failure in patients with multiple myeloma. N Engl J Med 1988;319:1651–3.
93. McBride W, Jackman JJ, Grayburn P. Prevalence and clinical characteristics of high cardiac output state in patients with multiple myeloma. Am J Med 1990;89:21–4.
94. Gertz M, Kyle R. Primary stemic amyloidosis-a diagnostic primer. Mayo Clin Proc 1989;64:1505–19.
95. Glenner G. Amyloid deposits and amyloidosis. [second of two parts]. N Engl J Med 1980;302:1333–43.
96. Stone M, Frenkel E. The clinical spectrum of light chain myeloma: A study of 35 patients with special reference to the occurrence of amyloidosis. Am J Med 1975;58:601–19.
97. Mathew V, Olson L, Gertz M, Hayes L. Symptomatic conduction systems disease in cardiac amyloidosis. Am J Cardiol 1997;49:9–13.
98. Chamarthi B, Dubrey S, Cha K, et al. Features and prognosis of exertional syncope in light-chain associated AL cardiac amyloidosis. Am J Cardiol 1997;80:963–5.
99. Murtagh B, Hammill S, Gertz M, et al. Electrocardiographic findings in primary systemic amyloidosis and biopsy-proven cardiac involvement. Am J Cardiol 2005;95:535–7.
100. Carroll J, Gaasch W, McAdam K. Amyloid cardiomyopathy: Characterization by a distinctive voltage/mass relation. Am J Cardiol 1982;49:9–13.
101. Lekakis J, Dimopolous M, Nanas J, et al. Antimyosin scintigraphy for detection of cardiac amyloidosis. Am J Cardiol 1997;80:963–5.
102. Tzankov A, Polzl G, Mairinger T. Congo red-positive cardiac kappa-AL amyloidosis in plasmacytoma–case report and review of the literature. Acta Med Austriaca 2003;30:29–32.
103. Chew C, Ziady G, Raphael M, Oakley C. The functional defect in amyloid heart disease. The "stiff heart" syndrome. Am J Cardiol 1975;36:438–44.
104. Rubinow A, Skinner M, Cohen AS. Digoxin sensitivity in amyloid cardiomyopathy. Circulation 1981;63:1285–8.
105. Gertz M, Lacy M, Dispenzieri A. Amyloidosis: recognition, confirmation, prognosis, and therapy. Mayo Clin Proc 1999;74:490–4.
106. Nakamura H, Hashimot T, Taguchi T, et al. Chemoembolization. Gan To Kagaku Ryoho 1987;14:1656–63.
107. Fuchs U, Zittermann A, Suhr O, et al. Heart transplantation in a 68-year-old patient with senile systemic amyloidosis. Am J Transplant 2005;5:1159–62.
108. Ali M, Ewer M. Cancer and the cardiopulmonary system. New York: Raven Press; 1984.
109. Ewer M, Ali M. Critical cardiologic considerations in the cancer patient. Crit Care Clin 1988;4:41–60.
110. Ewer M, Ali M, Mansour G, Balakrishnan P. Cardiac problems in ICU care of cancer patients. J Critical Illness 1989;4:37–44.
111. McLaughlin P, Salvador P, Banaillas F, Legha S. Ventricular fibrillation following AMSA. Uncomplicated retreatment following correction of hypokalemia. Cancer 1983;52:557–8.
112. Hazinski M, Cummins R, Field J, editors Handbook of emergency cardiovascular care for healthcare providers. Dallas: American Heart Association; 2000.
113. Kern K, Halperin J. New guidelines for cardiopulmonary resuscitation and emergency cardiac care: changes in the management of cardiac arrest. JAMA 2001;284:1267–9.
114. Tisdale J, Rasty S, Padhi I, et al. The effect of intravenous haloperidol on QT interval dispersion in critically ill patients: comparison with QT interval prolongation for assessment of risk of torsades de pointes. J Clin Pharmacol 2001;41:1310–8.
115. Guelon D, Bedock B, Chartier C, Haberer J. QT prolongation and recurrent "torsades de pointes" during erythromycin lactobionate infusion [letter]. Am J Cardiol 1986;58:666.
116. Lopez J, Harold J, Rosenthal M, et al. QT prolongation and torsades de pointes after administration of trimethoprim-sulfamethoxazole. Am J Cardiol 1987;59:376–7.
117. Frothingham R. Rates of torsades de pointes associated with ciprofloxacin, ofloxacin, levofloxacin, gatifloxacin, and moxifloxacin. Pharmacotherapy 2001;21:1468–72.
118. Kazunori O, Hitoshi Y, Kazuyuki S, et al. Prolongation of the QT interval and ventricular tachycardia in patients treated with arsenic trioxide for acute promyelocytic leukemia. Ann Intern Med 2001;133:881–5.
119. Unnikrishnan D, Dutcher J, Varshneya N, et al. Torsades de pointes in 3 patients with leukemia treated with arsenic trioxide. Blood 2001;97:1514–6.
120. Barbey JT, Pezzullo JC, Soignet SL. Effect of arsenic trioxide on QT interval in patients with advanced malignancies. J Clin Oncol 2003;21:3609–15.
121. Rinkenberger R, Naccarelli G. Evaluation and acute treatment of wide complex tachycardias. Crit Care Clin 1989;5:599–641.
122. Khan I. Long QT syndrome: diagnosis and management. Am Heart J 2002;143:7–14.
123. Gottlieb J, Lefrak E, O'Bryan R, Burgess M. Fatal Adriamycin cardiomyopathy (CMY): Prevention by dose limitation. Proc Am Assoc Cancer Res 1973;14:89.
124. Minow R, Benjamin R, Lee E, Gottlieb J. Adriamycin cardiomyopathy - risk factors. Cancer 1977;39:1397–1402.
125. Bristow M, Thompson P, Martin R, et al. Early anthracycline cardiotoxicity. Am J Med 1978;65:823–32.
126. Bristow M, Mason J, Billingham M, Daniels J. . Doxorubicin cardiomyopathy: evaluation by phonocardiography, endomyocardial biopsy, and cardiac catheterization. Ann Intern Med 1978;88:168–75.
127. Doroshow J, Locker G, Myers G. Enzymatic defenses of the mouse heart against reactive oxygen metabolites: Alterations produced by doxorubicin. J Clin Invest 1980;65:128-35.
128. Haq M, Legha S, Choksi J, et al. Doxorubicin-induced congestive heart failure in adults. Cancer 1985;56:1361–5.
129. Allegra J, Woodcock T, Woolf S, et al. A randomized trial comparing mitoxantrone with doxorubicin in patients with stage IV breast cancer. Invest New Drugs 1985;3:153–61.
130. Ewer M, Ali M, Chawla S, et al. A comparison of resting and exercise ejection fractions with cardiac biopsy grades in patients receiving Adriamycin. Proc Am Soc Clin Oncol 1985;4:27.
131. Jain K, Casper E, Geller N, et al. A prospective randomized comparison of epirubicin and doxorubicin in patients with advanced breast cancer. J Clin Oncol 1985;3:818–26.
132. Barlogie B, Alexanian R. Therapy of primary resistant and relapsed multiple myeloma. Onkologie 1986;9:210–4.
133. Herman E, Lipshultz S, Rifai N, et al. Use of cardiac troponin T levels as an indicator of doxorubicin-induced cardiotoxicity. Can Res 1998;38:195–7.
134. Myers C, Bonow R, Palmieri S, et al. A randomized controlled trial assessing the prevention of doxorubicin cardiomyopathy by *N*-acetylcysteine. Semin Oncol 1983;10:53–5.
135. Olson R, Mushlin P, Brenner D, et al. Doxorubicin cardiotoxicity may be caused by its metabolite, doxorubicinol. Proc Natl Acad Sci U S A 1988;85:3585–9.

136. Legha S, Wang Y, Mackay B, et al., Clinical and pharmacologic investigation of the effects of α-tocopherol on Adriamycin cardiotoxicity. Ann NY Acad Sci 1982;393:411-7.
137. Myers C. Role of iron in anthracycline action. In; Hacker M, Lazo J, Tritton T, editors. Organ Directed Toxicities of Anticancer Drugs Boston: Martinus Nijhoff; 1988. p. 17–30.
138. Cabanillas F, Rodriguez M, Swan FJ. Recent trends in the management of lymphomas at M.D. Anderson Cancer Center. Semin Oncol 1990;17:28–32.
139. Kantarjian H, Walters R, Keating M, et al. Results of the vincristine, doxorubicin, and dexamethasone regimen in adults with standard- and high-risk acute lymphocytic leukemia. J Clin Oncol 1990;8:994–1004.
140. Benjamin R, Fenogolio C, Hortobagyi G, et al. Cardiotoxicity of pirarubicin. Proc Am Assoc Cancer Res 1990;31:178.
141. Speyer J, Green M, Zeleniuch-Jacquotte A, et al. ICRF-187 permits longer treatment with doxorubicin in women with breast cancer. J Clin Oncol 1992;10:117–27.
142. Ali M, Ewer M, Gibbs H, et al. Late doxorubicin-associated cardiotoxicity in children: The possible role of intercurrent viral infection. Cancer 1994;74:182–8.
143. Swain S, Whaley F, Gerber M, et al. Cardioprotection with dexrazoxane for doxorubicin-containing chemotherapy in advanced breast cancer. J Clin Oncol 1997;15:1318–32.
144. Swain S, Whaley F, Gerber M, et al., Delayed administration of dexrazoxane provides cardioprotection for patients with advanced breast cancer treated with doxorubicin-containing chemotherapy. J Clin Oncol 1997;15:1333–40.
145. Speyer J, Wasserheit C. Strategies for reduction of anthracycline cardiac toxicity. Semin Oncol 1998;25:525–37.
146. Lopez M, Vici P. European trials with dexrazoxane in amelioration of doxorubicin and epirubicin-induced cardiotoxicity. Sem Oncol 1998;25:55–60.
147. Lemez P, Maresova J. Efficacy of dexrazoxane as cardioprotective agent in patients receiving mitoxantrone-and daunorubicin-based chemotherapy. Semin Oncol 1998;25(Suppl 10):61–5.
148. Gennari A, Salvadori B, Donati S, et al. Cardiotoxicity of epirubicin/paclitaxel-containing regimens: Role of cardiac risk factors. J Clin Oncol 1999;17:3596–602.
149. Iarussi D, Indolfi P, Casale F, et al. Recent advances in the prevention of anthracycline cardiotoxicity in childhood. Curr Med Chem 2001;8:1649–60.
150. Chakrabarti K, Hopewill J, Wilding D, Plowman P. Modification of doxorubicin-induced cardiotoxicity: Effect of essential fatty acids and ICRF-187 (dexrazoxane). Eur J Cancer 2001;37:1435–42.
151. van Acker F, Boven E, Kramer K, et al. Frederine, a new and promising protector against doxorubicin-induced cardiotoxicity. Clin Cancer Res 2001;7:1378–84.
152. Sabel M, Levine E, Hurd T, et al. Is MUGA scan necessary in patients with low-risk breast cancer before doxorubicin-based adjuvant therapy? Am J Clin Oncol 2001;4:425–8.
153. Meinardi M, van Veldhuisen D, Gietema J, et al. Prospective evaluation of early cardiac damage induced by epirubicin-containing adjuvant chemotherapy and locoregional radiotherapy in breast cancer patients. J Clin Oncol 2001;19:2746–53.
154. Porea T, Dreyer Z, Bricker J, Mahoney D. Evaluation of left ventricular function in asymptomatic children about to undergo anthracycline-based chemotherapy for acute leukemia: an outcome study. J Pediatr Hematol Oncol 2001;23:420–3.
155. Herth F, Schulz M, Manegold C, Becker H. Usefulness of stress echocardiography for early diagnosis of anthracycline-induced cardiomyopathy. Pneumologie 2001;55:385–9.
156. Hauser M, Gibson B, Wilson N. Diagnosis of anthracycline-induced late cardiomyopathy by exercise-spiroergometry and stress echocardiography. Eur J Pediatr 2001;160:601–10.
157. Berrak S, Ewer M, Jaffe N, et al. Doxorubicin cardiotoxicity in children: reduced incidence of cardiac dysfunction associated with continuous-infusion schedules. Oncol Rep 2001;8:611–4.
158. Vaksmann G, Gutierrez R, Duhamel A, et al. Signal averaged electrocardiography in children with anthracycline-induced cardiomyopathy. Pediatr Cardiol 2001;22:494–8.
159. Valero V, Perez E, Dieras V. Doxorubicin and taxane combination regimes for metastatic breast cancer: Focus on cardiac effects. Semin Oncol 2001;28(Suppl 12):15–23.
160. FukuMi D, Uchikoba Y, Maeda M, Ogawa S. Longitudinal evaluation of anthracycline cardiotoxicity by signal-averaged electrocardiography in children with cancer. Pediatr Int 2002;44:134–40.
161. Shureiqi I, Cantor S, Lippman S, et al. Clinical and economic impact of multiple gated acquisition scan monitoring during anthracycline therapy. Br J Cancer 2002;86:226–32.
162. Lipshultz S, Giantris A, Lipsitz S, et al. Doxorubicin administration by continuous infusion is not cardioprotective: the Dana-Farber 91-01 Acute Lymphoblastic protocol. J Clin Oncol 2002;20:1677–82.
163. Perez E, Russell C. Metastatic Breast Cancer. In: Jatoi I, editor. Manual of Breast Cancer. Philadelphia: Lippincott Williams & Wilkins, 2002. p. 365–87.
164. Danesi R, Fogli S, Gennari A. Pharmacokinetic-pharmacodynamic relationships of the anthracycline anticancer drugs. Clin Pharmacokinet 2002;41:431–44.
165. Swain S, Whaley F, Ewer M. Congestive heart failure in patients treated with doxorubicin: A retrospective analysis of three trials. Cancer 2003;97:2869–79.
166. Ewer M, Lippman S. Type II chemotherapy-related cardiac dysfunction: time to recognize a new entity. J Clin Oncol 2005;23[In press].
167. Ferretti G, Mandala M, Bria E, et al. Is cardiac troponin T serum level an accurate surrogate for acute doxorubicin-related myocardial injury? Ann Oncol 2005.
168. Cardinale D, Sandri M, Colombo A, et al. Prognostic value of troponin I in cardiac risk stratification of cancer patients undergoing high-dose chemotherapy. Circulation 2004;109:2749–54.
169. Benjamin R, Chawla S, Hortobagyi G, et al. Continuous-infusion Adriamycin. In: Rosenthal C, Rotman M, editors. Clinical Applications of Continuous Infusion Chemotherapy and Concomitant Radiation Therapy. New York: Plenum Press, 1986. p. 19–25.
170. Gottlieb SL, Edmiston WA Jr, Haywood LJ. Late, late doxorubicin cardiotoxicity. Chest 1980;78:880–2.
171. Herman E, Zhang J, Rifai N, et al. The use of serum levels of cardiac troponin T to compare the protective activity of dexrazoxane against doxorubicin- and mitoxantrone-induced cardiotoxicity. Cancer Chemother Pharmacol 2001;48:297–304.
172. Nousiainen T, Vanninen E, Jantunen E, et al. Natriuretic peptides during the development of doxorubicin-induced left ventricular diastolic dysfunction. J Intern Med 2002;251:228–34.
173. Okumura H, Iuchi K, Yoshida T, et al. Brain natriuretic peptide is a predictor of anthracycline-induced cardiotoxicity. Acta Haematol 2000;104:158–63.
174. Koh E, Nakamura T, Takahashi H. Troponin-T and brain natriuretic peptide as predictors for Adriamycin-induced cardiomyopathy in rats. Circ J 2004;68:163–7.
175. Bellenger N, Burgess M, Ray S, et al. Comparison of left ventricular ejection fraction and volumes in heart failure by echocardiography, radionuclide ventriculography and cardiovascular magnetic resonance; are they interchangeable? Eur Heart J 2000;16:1295–7.
176. Ewer M, Ali M, Gibbs H, et al. Cardiac diastolic function in pediatric patients receiving doxorubicin. Acta Oncol 1994;33:645–9.
177. Ocal B, Oguz D, Karademir S, et al. Myocardial performance index combining systolic and diastolic myocardial performance in doxorubicin-treated patients and its correlation to conventional echo/Doppler indices. Pediatr Cardiol 2002;23:522–7.
178. Ewer M, Ali M, Mackay B, et al. A comparison of cardiac biopsy grades and ejection fraction estimations in patients receiving Adriamycin. J Clin Oncol 1984;2:112–7.
179. Benjamin R, Chawla S, Ewer M. Adriamycin cardiac toxicity—an assessment of approaches to cardiac monitoring and cardioprotection. In: Hacker MP, Lazo JS, Tritton TR, editors. Organ Directed Toxicities of Anticancer Drugs. 1988, Boston: Martinus Nijhoff; 1988.p. 41–55.
180. Benjamin R, Ewer M, Mackay B, et al. An endomyocardial biopsy study of anthracycline-induced cardiomyopathy—detection, reversibility, and potential amelioration. Proc AACR/ASCO 1979;20:372.
181. Sakakibara S, Konno S. Endomyocardial biopsy. Japan Heart J 1962;3:537–43.
182. Billingham M, Bristow M, Glastein E, et al. Adriamycin cardiotoxicity: endomyocardial biopsy evidence of enhancement by irradiation. Am J Surg Pathol 1977;1:17–23.
183. Mason J. Techniques for right and left ventricular endomyocardial biopsy. Am J Cardiol 1978;41:887–92.
184. Ewer M, Carrasco C, Mackay B, et al., Cardiac biopsy procedures at a cancer center. Proc Am Soc Clin Oncol 1991;10:336.
185. Mackay B, Ewer M, Carasco C, Benjamin R. Assessment of anthracycline cardiomyopathy by endomyocardial biopsy. Ultrastructural Pathology 1994;18:203–11.
186. Mackay B, Keyes L, Benjamin R, et al. Cardiac biopsy. Texas Society for Electron Microscopy 1981;11:7–15.
187. Billingham M. Role of endomyocardial biopsy in diagnosis and treatment of heart disease. In: Silver M, editor. Cardiovascular Pathology. New York: Churchill Livingstone; 1991. p. 1465–8.
188. Benjamin R, Chawla S, Ewer M, et al. Evaluation of mitoxantrone cardiac toxicity by nuclear angiography and endomyocardial biopsy: an update. Invest New Drug 1985;3:117–21.
189. Chawla S, Benjamin R, Hortobagyi G, et al. Decreased cardiotoxicity of 96 hour continuous infusion Adriamycin compared with epirubicin. Proc Am Soc Clin Oncol 1986;5:44.
190. Legha S, Benjamin F, Mackay B, et al. Reduction of doxorubicin cardiotoxicity by prolonged continuous intravenous infusion. Ann Intern Med 1982;96:133–9.
191. Billingham M, Mason J, Bristow M, Daniels J. Anthracycline cardiomyopathy monitored by morphologic changes. Cancer Treat Rep 1978;62:865–72.
192. Ramos A, Meyer R, Korfhagen J, et al. Echocardiographic evaluation of Adriamycin cardiotoxicity in children. Cancer Treat Rep 1976;60:1281–4.
193. Von Hoff D, Layard M, Basa P, et al. Risk factors for doxorubicin-induced congestive heart failure. Ann Intern Med 1979;91:710–7.
194. Von Hoff D, Rozeneweig M, Layard M, et al. Daunomycin-induced cardiotoxicity in children and adults: A review of 110 cases. Am J Med 1977;62:200–8.
195. Pratt C, Ransom J, Evans W. Age-related Adriamycin cardiotoxicity in children. Cancer Treat Rep 1978;62:1381–5.
196. Ibrahim NK, Hortobagyi G, Ewer M, et al. Doxorubicin-induced congestive heart failure in elderly patients with metastatic breast cancer, with long-term follow-up: the M.D. Anderson experience. Cancer Chemother Pharmacol 1999;43:471–8.
197. Aydiner A, Bugra Z, Topuz E, Meric M. Acute myocardial infarction in man treated with epirubicin for non-Hodgkin lymphoma. Am J Clin Oncol 1995;18:444–8.
198. Appelbaum F, Strauchen J, Graw R Jr, et al. Acute lethal carditis caused by high-dose combination chemotherapy. A unique clinical and pathological entity. Lancet 1976;1:58–62.
199. Kushner J, Hansen V, Hammar S. Cardiomyopathy after widely separated courses of Adriamycin exacerbated by actinomycin-D and mithramycin. Cancer 1975;36:1577–84.
200. Beretta G, Villani F. Cardiomyopathy in adults after combination Adriamycin and DTIC. Cancer Treat Rep 1980;64:353.
201. Buzdar A, Legha S, Tashima C, et al. Adriamycin and mitomycin C: Possible synergistic cardiotoxicity. Cancer Treat Rep 1978;62:1005–8.
202. Gianni L, Dombernowsky P, Sledge G, et al. Cardiac function following combination therapy with paclitaxel and doxorubicin: an analysis of 657 women with advanced breast cancer. Ann Oncol 2001;12:1067–73.
203. Moreira A, Lobato R, Morais J, et al. Influence of the interval between the administration of doxorubicin and paclitaxel on the pharmacokinetics of these drugs in patients with locally advanced breast cancer. Cancer Chemother Pharmacol 2001;48:333–7.
204. Perez E. Doxorubicin and paclitaxel in the treatment of advanced breast cancer: efficacy and cardiac considerations. Cancer Invest 2001;19:155–64.
205. Minotti G, Ronchi R, Salvatorelli E, et al. Doxorubicin irreversibly inactivates iron regulatory proteins 1 and 2 in cardiomyocytes: evidence for distinct metabolic pathways and implications for iron-medicated cardiotoxicity of antitumor therapy. Cancer Res 2001;61:8422–8.
206. Schell F, Yap H. Potential cardiotoxicity with mitoxantrone. Cancer Treat Rep 1982;66:1641–3.
207. Ibrahim NK, Buzdar A, Asmar L, et al. Doxorubicin-based adjuvant chemotherapy in elderly breast cancer patients: the M.D. Anderson experience, with long-term follow-up. Ann Oncol 2000;11:1597–601.
208. Ewer M, Martin F, Henderson I, et al. Cardiac Safety of Liposomal Anthracyclines. Semin Oncol 2004;31(Suppl 13):161–81.
209. Theodoulou M, Hudis C. Cardiac profiles of liposomal anthracyclines: greater cardiac safety versus conventional doxorubicin? Cancer 2004;100:2052–63.
210. Harris L, Batist G, Belt R, et al. The TLC D-99 Study Group. Liposome-encapsulated doxorubicin compared with conventional doxorubicin in a randomized multicenter trial as first-line therapy of metastatic breast carcinoma. Cancer 2002;94:25–36.
211. Batist G, Ramakrishnan G, Rao C, et al. Reduced cardiotoxicity and preserved antitumor efficacy of liposome-encapsulated doxorubicin and cyclophosphamide in a randomized multicenter trial of metastatic breast cancer. J Clin Oncol 2001;19:1444–54.

212. Valero V, Buzdar A, Theriault R. Phase II trial of liposome-encapsulated doxorubicin, cyclophosphamide, and fluorouracil as first-line therapy in patients with metastatic breast cancer. J Clin Oncol 1999;17:1425–34.
213. Bafaloukos D, Papadimitriou C, Linardou H, et al. Combination of pegylated liposomal doxorubicin (PLD) and paclitaxel in patients with advanced soft tissue sarcoma: a phase II study of the Hellenic Cooperative Oncology Group. Br J Cancer 2004;91:1639–44.
214. Gabizon AA, Lyass O, Berry G, Wildgust M. Cardiac safety of pegylated liposomal doxorubicin (Doxil/Caelyx) demonstrated by endomyocardial biopsy in patients with advanced malignancies. Cancer Invest 2004;22:663–9.
215. Uyar D, Kulp B, Peterson G, et al. Cardiac safety profile of prolonged (> or = 6 cycles) pegylated liposomal doxorubicin administration in patients with gynecologic malignancies. Gynecol Oncol 2004;94:147–51.
216. O'Brian M, Wigler N, Inbar M, et al. Reduced cardiotoxicity and comparable efficacy in a phase III trial of pegylated liposomal doxorubicin HCL (CAELYX/Doxil) versus conventional doxorubicin for first-line treatment of metastatic breast cancer. Ann Oncol 2004;15:440–9.
217. Torti F, Bristow M, Howes A, et al., Reduced cardiotoxicity of doxorubicin delivered on a weekly schedule. Assessment by endomyocardial biopsy. Ann Intern Med 1983;99:745–9.
218. Valdivieso M, Burgess M, Ewer M, et al., Increased therapeutic index of weekly doxorubicin in the therapy of non-small cell lung cancer: a prospective randomized study. J Clin Oncol 1984;2:207–14.
219. Benjamin R, Legha S, Valdivieso M, et al. Reduction of Adriamycin cardiac toxicity by schedule manipulation, In: Muggia F, Young C, Carter S, editors. Anthracycline Antibiotics in Cancer Therapy. The Netherlands: Martinue Nijhoff; 1982. p. 352–7.
220. Hortobagyi G, Frye D, Buzdar A, et al. Decreased cardiac toxicity of doxorubicin administered by continuous intravenous infusion in combination chemotherapy for metastatic breast carcinoma. Cancer 1989;63:37–45.
221. Legha S, Benjamin R, Mackay B, et al. Adriamycin therapy by continuous intravenous infusion in patients with metastatic breast cancer. Cancer 1982;49:1762–6.
222. Benjamin R, Yap B. Infusion chemotherapy for soft tissue sarcomas. In: Baker L, editor. Soft Tissue Sarcoma. The Netherlands: Martinus Nijhoff; 1983. p. 109–15.
223. Zalupski, M, Metch B, Balcerzak S, et al. Phase III comparison of doxorubicin and dacarbazine given by bolus versus infusion in patients with soft-tissue sarcomas: a Southwest Oncology Group study. J Natl Cancer Inst 1991;83:926–32.
224. Bielack S, Bieling P, Fuchs N, et al. Can doxorubicin administration be altered from "bolus" to continuous infusion without compromising antineoplastic efficacy [abstract]. Proc 5th Intl Congress Anti-Cancer Chemotherapy 1995;5:167.
225. Speyer J, Green M, Kramer E, et al. Protective effect of the bispiperazinedione ICRF-187 against doxorubicin-induced cardiac toxicity in women with advanced breast cancer. N Engl J Med 1988;319:745–52.
226. Speyer J, Green M, Zeleniuch-Jacquotte A, et al. ICRF-187 permits longer treatment with doxorubicin in women with breast cancer. J Clin Oncol 1992;10:117–27.
227. Lopez M, Patrizia V. European trials with dexrazoxane in amelioration of doxorubicin and epirubicin-induced cardiotoxicity. Semin Oncol 1998;25(Suppl 10):55–60.
228. Alexander J, Dainiak N, Berger H, et al. Serial assessment of doxorubicin cardiotoxicity with quantitative radionuclide angiocardiography. N Engl J Med 1979;300:278–83.
229. Ewer M. Exercise echocardiography reflects cumulative anthracycline exposure during childhood [editorial]. Pediatric Blood & Cancer 2004;42:554–5.
230. Bonneterre J, Roche H, Kerbrat P, et al. Long-term cardiac follow-up in relapse-free patients after six courses of fluorouracil, epirubicin, and cyclophosphamide, with either 50 or 100 mg of epirubicin, as adjuvant therapy for node-positive breast cancer: French adjuvant study group. J Clin Oncol 2004;22:3070–9.
231. Anderlini P, Benjamin RS, Wong FC, et al. Idarubicin cardiotoxicity: a retrospective study in acute myeloid leukemia and myelodysplasia. J Clin Oncol 1995;13:2827–34.
232. Crum E. Biological-response modifier-induced emergencies. Semin Oncol 1989;16:579–87.
233. Angulo M, Navajas A, Galdeano J, et al. A reversible cardiomyopathy secondary to alpha-interferon in an infant. Pediatr Cardiol 1999;20:293–4.
234. Buja L, Ferrans V, Graw RJ. Cardiac pathologic findings in patients treated with bone marrow transplantation. Hum Pathol 1976;7:17–45.
235. Gottdiener J, et al. Cardiotoxicity associated with high dose cyclophosphamide therapy. Arch Intern Med 1981;141:758–63.
236. Negro A, Brar BK, Lee KF. Essential roles of Her2/erbB2 in cardiac development and function. Recent Prog Horm Res 2004;59:1–12.
237. Speyer J. Cardiac dysfunction in the trastuzumab clinical experience. J Clin Oncol 2002;20:1156–7.
238. Ewer M, Vooletich M, Durand J, et al. Reversibility of trastuzumab-related cardiotoxicity: new insights based on clinical course and response to medical treatment. J Clin Oncol 2005. [In Press].
239. Crone S, Zhao Y, Fan L, et al. ErbB2 is essential in the prevention of dilated cardiomyopathy. Nature Med 2002;8:459–65.
240. Ewer M, Gibbs H, Swafford J, Benjamin R. Cardiotoxicity in patients receiving trastuzumab (Herceptin): primary toxicity, synergistic or sequential stress, or surveillance artifact? Semin Oncol 1999;26(Suppl 12):96-101.
241. Seidman A, Hudis C, Pierri M, et al. Cardiac dysfunction in the trastuzumab clinical trials experience. J Clin Oncol 2002;20:1215–21.
242. Ewer M, Vooletich M, Valero V, et al. Trastuzumab (Herceptin) cardiotoxicity: clinical course and cardiac biopsy correlations. Proceedings ASCO 2002;21.
243. Hunt S, Baker D, Chin M, et al. ACC/AHA Guidelines for the evaluation and management of Chronic heart failure in the adult: executive summary: a report of the American College of Cardiology/American Heart Association Task Force on Practice Guidelines (Committee to Revise the 1995 Guidelines for the Evaluation and Management of Heart Failure). J Am Coll Cardiol 200138:2101–13.
244. Armitage JM, Kormor R, Griffith B, et al. Heart transplantation in patients with malignant disease. J Heart Transplant 1990;9:627–9.
245. Mancuso L, Bondi F, Marchi S, et al. Cardiac toxicity of 5-fluorouracil. Report of a case of spontaneous angina. Tumori 1986;72:121–4.
246. Ewer M, Benjamin R, Hong W, et al. Electrocardiographic changes in patients receiving chemotherapy with 5-fluorouracil and cisplatinum with and without diethyldithiocarbamate. Proc 15th Intl Cong Chemother 1987:203.
247. Oleksowicz L, Bruckner H. Prophylaxis of 5-fluorouracil induced coronary vasospasm with calcium channel blockers. Am J Med 1988;85:750–1.
248. Frickhofen N, et al. Capecitabine can induce acute coronary syndrome similar to 5-fluorouracil. Ann Oncol 2002;13:797–801.
249. Van Cutsem E, Hoff P, Blum J, et al. Incidence of cardiotoxicity with the oral fluoropyrimidine capecitabine is typical of that reported with 5-fluorouracil. Ann Oncol 2002;13:484–5.
250. Ognibene F, Rosenberg S, Lotze M, et al. Interleukin-2 administration causes reversible hemodynamic changes and left ventricular dysfunction similar to those seen in septic shock. Chest 1988;94:750–4.
251. Lee R, Lotze M, Skibber J, et al. Cardiorespiratory effects of immunotherapy with interleukin-2. J Clin Oncol 1989;7:7–20.
252. Margolin K, Rayner A, Hawkins M, et al. Interleukin-2 and lymphokine-activated killer cell therapy of solid tumors: Analysis of toxicity and management guidelines. J Clin Oncol 1989;7:486–98.
253. Kilbourn R, Fonesca GA, Griffith O, et al. N^G-monomethyl-L-arginine, an inhibitor of nitric oxide production, reversed interleukin-1-mediated hypotensions in humans. Crit Care Med 1995;23:1018–24.
254. Legha S, Keating M, Pickett S, et al. Phase I clinical investigation of homoharringtonine (NSC 141633). Cancer Treat Rep 1984;68:1085–91.
255. Rowinsky E, McGuire W, Guarnieri T, et al. Cardiac disturbances during the administration of Taxol. J Clin Oncol 1991;9:1704–12.
256. Rowinsky E, Eisenhauer E, Chaudhry V, et al. Clinical toxicities encountered with paclitaxel (TAXOL). Semin Oncol 1993;20:1–15.
257. Gibbs H, Ewer M, Holmes F, et al. Cardiac monitoring during administration of Taxol-doxorubicin chemotherapy in patients with metastatic breast cancer: A preliminary report. Proc Am Soc Clin Oncol 1992;11:87.
258. Gianni L, Munzone E, Capre G, et al. Paclitaxel by 3-hour infusion in combination with bolus doxorubicin in women with untreated metastatic breast cancer: High antitumor efficacy and cardiac effects in a dose-finding and sequence-finding study. J Clin Oncol 1995;13:2688–99.
259. Sendo T, Sakai N, Itoh Y, et al. Incidence and risk factors for paclitaxel hypersensitivity during ovarian cancer chemotherapy. Cancer Chemother Pharmacol 2005;56:91–6.
260. Kirchmair R, Walter D, Ii M, et al. Antiangiogenesis mediates cisplatin-induced peripheral neuropathy: attenuation or reversal by local vascular endothelial growth factor gene therapy without augmenting tumor growth. Circulation 2005;111:2662–70.
261. Stewart J, Fajardo L. Radiation-induced heart disease: Clinical and experimental aspects. Radiol Clin North Am 1971;9:511–31.
262. Brosius F III, Waller B, Roberts W. Radiation heart disease: Analysis of 16 young (aged 15-33 years) necropsy patients who received over 3,500 rads to the heart. Am J Med 1981;70:519–30.
263. Giraud P, Cosset JM. [Radiation toxicity to the heart: physiopathology and clinical data]. Bull Cancer 2004;91 Suppl 3:147–53.
264. Kaplan H. Radiotherapy, in Hodgkin's disease. H. Kaplan, Editor. 1972, Harvard Univ Press: Cambridge, MA.
265. Gagliardi G, Lax I, Rutqvist L. Partial irradiation of the heart. Semin Oncol 2001;11:224–33.
266. Ferri G, Dusi U. Radiazoni ionizzanti e cuore: Part I. Quad Radiol 1965;30:1007.
267. Schultz-Hector S. Radiation-induced heart disease: review of experimental data on dose response and pathogenesis. Int J Radiat Biol 199261:149–60.
268. Ali M, Ewer MS. Cardiovascular problems in the patient with cancer: effects of chemotherapy. Primary Care Cancer 1989;9:29–32.
269. Stewart J, Cohen K, Fajardo L, et al. Radiation-induced heart disease: a study of twenty-five patients. Radiology 1967;89:302–10.
270. Adams MJ, Hardenbergh PH, Constine LS, Lipshultz SE. Radiation-associated cardiovascular disease. Crit Rev Oncol Hematol 2003;45:55–75.
271. Corn BW, Trock BJ, Goodman RL. Irradiation-related ischemic heart disease. J Clin Oncol 1990;8:741–50.
272. Veinot JP, Edwards WD. Pathology of radiation-induced heart disease: a surgical and autopsy study of 27 cases. Hum Pathol 1996;27:766–73.
273. Akber SF. Correlation of radiation tolerance dose of normal human organs with organ weight, blood, and water content. Am J Clin Oncol 2000;23:345–48.
274. Meaney E, Shabetai R, Bhargava V, et al. Cardiac amyloidosis, constrictive pericarditis and restrictive cardiomyopathy. Am J Cardiol 1976;38:547–56.
275. Chambers C, Leaman D. Management of acute chest pain syndrome. Crit Care Clin 1989;5:415–34.
276. Miller J, Mansour K, Hatcher C. Pericardiectomy: current indications, concepts, and results in a university center. Ann Thorac Surg 1982;34:40–5.
277. Stewart JR, Fajardo LF, Gillette SM, Constine LS. Radiation injury to the heart. Int J Radiat Oncol Biol Phys 1995;31:1205–11.
278. Makinen L, Makipernaa A, Rautonen J, et al. Long-term cardiac sequelae after treatment of malignant tumors with radiotherapy or cytostatics in childhood. Cancer 1990;65:1913–17.
279. Cohn K, Stewart J, Fajardo L, Hancock E. Heart disease following radiation. Medicine 1967;46:281–98.
280. Moss AJ, Smith DW, Michaelson S, Schreiner BF Jr. Radiation technique for production of localized myocardial necrosis in the intact dog. Proc Soc Exp Biol Med 1963;112:903.
281. Botti RE, Driscol TE, Pearson OH, Smith JC. Radiation myocardial fibrosis simulating constrictive pericarditis. A review of the literature and a case report. Cancer 1968;22:1254–61.
282. Fajardo L, Stewart J. Pathogenesis of radiation-induced myocardial fibrosis. Lab Invest 1973;29:244–57.
283. Amromin G, Gildenhorn HL, Solomon RD, Nadkarni BB. The synergism of x-irradiation and cholesterol-fat feeding on the development of coronary artery lesions. J Atheroscler Res 1964;4:325–34.
284. Wondergem J, Strootman EG, Frolich M, et al. Circulating atrial natriuretic peptide plasma levels as a marker for cardiac damage after radiotherapy. Radiother Oncol 2001;58:295–301.
285. Gustavsson A, Eskilsson J, Landberg T, et al. Late cardiac effects after mantle radiotherapy in patients with Hodgkin's disease. Ann Oncol 1990;1:355–63.
286. Adams MJ, Lipsitz SR, Colan SD, et al. Cardiovascular status in long-term survivors of Hodgkin's disease treated with chest radiotherapy. J Clin Oncol 2004;22:3139–48.
287. Billingham M, Bristow M. Evaluation of anthracycline cardiotoxicity: predictive ability and functional correlation of endomyocardial biopsy. Cancer Treat Symp 1984;3:71–6.

Respiratory Complications

Vickie R. Shannon, MD
George A. Eapen, MD
Carlos A. Jimenez, MD
Rodolfo C. Morice, MD
Elizabeth L. Travis, PhD
Lara Bashoura, MD
Amar Safdar, MD, FACP
Roberto Adachi, MD
S. Egbert Pravinkumar, MD, FRCP
Burton F. Dickey, MD

INTRODUCTION

The respiratory system is particularly susceptible to complications of cancer and cancer therapy. This vulnerability arises from interactions among the stringent architectural requirements for gas exchange, the continuous exposure of the respiratory tract to the external environment, and the severe symptoms that accompany respiratory compromise. Effective gas exchange requires patent airways, a forceful respiratory pump composed of the musculoskeletal system of the chest and abdomen, a thin alveolocapillary membrane constituting a minimal barrier to efficient gas transfer, and adequate blood flow through the pulmonary circulation. In cancer patients, primary and metastatic tumors of the chest may compromise major airways, malignant pleural effusions may externally compress the lungs and impair diaphragmatic function, direct or lymphangitic spread of tumor to the lungs may replace functioning parenchyma, and radiation therapy or chemotherapy may diffusely injure the vulnerable alveolocapillary membrane. In addition, infection or the immune complications of stem cell transplantation may result in widespread lung injury, and tumors may directly or indirectly compromise function of the musculoskeletal pump. Finally, venous thromboembolism or pulmonary vasculopathy may result in obstruction of blood flow through the lungs.

The respiratory system in normal persons contains considerable physiologic reserve, such that surgical loss of one lung is generally well tolerated except with exertion. However, in cancer patients, insults to multiple components of the respiratory system often result in progressive loss of physiologic reserve and the development of increasing dyspnea. Dyspnea is a very distressing symptom that generally signals serious underlying pathophysiology. Treatment should be directed at the underlying pathophysiologic process whenever possible, but when reversal of the underlying processes is not possible, palliation of dyspnea is mandatory. In this chapter, we will discuss the pathophysiology, diagnosis, and management of the major respiratory complications of patients with cancer and patients who have undergone cancer therapy. We begin with the direct effects of cancer on the lungs (airspace compromise and malignant pleural effusion), then consider the effects of cancer therapy on the lungs (postoperative respiratory failure, chemotherapy- and radiation-induced lung injury, pneumonia, and the complications of stem cell transplantation), review major indirect effects of cancer on the lungs (thromboembolism and respiratory pump compromise), and end with the causes and treatment of respiratory failure in the cancer patient.

MALIGNANT AIRWAY OBSTRUCTION

Malignant airspace disease may be central or peripheral; focal or diffuse; endoluminal, extraluminal, or both. The dominant symptom complex associated with this process depends on the location and extent of disease, which also dictates therapy.

Common Cancer Types and Clinical Presentation The most common cause of malignant airway obstruction is direct extension from an adjacent tumor, particularly bronchogenic carcinoma. Esophageal and thyroid malignancies also frequently extend directly into the airways. Primary tumors of the major airways are relatively rare, with squamous cell carcinoma, adenoid cystic carcinoma, and carcinoid tumors most often implicated.[1] Airway obstruction can also occur secondary to metastatic malignancies from renal, breast, and thyroid sources. Lymphomatous involvement of the central airways and extrinsic compression by malignant lymphadenopathy causing obstruction has also been described. Both endoluminal disease and extrinsic compression by tumor may severely compromise airway luminal diameter. Reduction in airway caliber and architectural distortion synergistically impair airflow obstruction and mucus clearance, leading to increased work of breathing and dyspnea. Luminal narrowing of the trachea and mainstem bronchi in central airway obstruction leads to airflow limitation and an associated symptom complex that often includes dyspnea, cough, wheeze, stridor, and atelectasis. Airway obstruction beyond the mainstem bronchi usually results in atelectasis, post obstructive pneumonitis, cough, and dyspnea. Individual patient presentations range from asymptomatic discovery on staging work-up to frank respiratory failure due to critical airway obstruction.[2] Exertional dyspnea typically occurs when tracheal diameter is reduced below 8 mm. Further reductions in tracheal diameter to < 5 mm is usually associated with dyspnea at rest.[3] Chronic obstructive pulmonary disease (COPD) exacerbations or mucosal edema and increased secretions that accompany superimposed pneumonias may precipitate respiratory failure, even among patients with only moderate tumor-related airflow limitation. Symptoms may thus improve with measures directed at treating the infection or COPD exacerbation.

Differential Diagnosis Although critical airway obstruction is not usually a diagnostic challenge, the clinical presentation of subcritical obstruction can be. Stridor is usually pathognomonic of significant tracheal obstruction. Other findings, including dyspnea and wheezing, are prominent but nonspecific clinical symptoms that denote airflow limitation. Concurrent conditions, such as congestive heart failure, pleural effusions, and pulmonary emboli may produce similar symptoms, obscuring the diagnosis.

Diagnostic Evaluation The diagnostic work-up is aimed at establishing a definitive diagnosis, quantifying airflow limitation and delineating anatomic extent in an effort to optimize therapeutic strategies. The characteristic blunting noted in the flow volume loop upon pulmonary function testing often provides the earliest indication of tracheal obstruction. However, this is a relatively insensitive test, with positive findings noted only with tracheal diameters below 10 mm.[4] Spirometry may precipitate frank respiratory failure in patients with severe airway obstruction and, therefore, should also be used with caution in this subgroup of patients. Rarely, deviation or compression of the trachea may be seen on plain chest radiographs. Plain chest films are otherwise useless in defining the anatomic extent of tumor or therapeutic options. Standard chest computed tomography as well as the latest iterations of low-dose, multidetector scanners and advanced airway imaging techniques that allow multiplanar and three-dimensional reconstruction provide valuable additional information regarding the extent of the lesion and guidance in optimizing therapeutic strategies.[5] Bronchoscopy, either flexible or rigid, remains the gold standard in the work-up of airway obstruction. Histologic confirmation of malignancy can be obtained at the time of the examination. Furthermore, bronchoscopy offers direct visualization of the lesion, which permits precise characterization of tumor vascularity and the extent of obstruction, as well as the degree of obstruction attributable to endoluminal versus extraluminal disease. Recent reports have also supported the use of endobronchial ultrasonography as an adjunctive tool in treatment planning.[6]

Management of Malignant Airway Obstruction Tumor characteristics, including histologic type, stage and location, and patient attributes, such as urgency of presentation and performance status, dictate management. Therapeutic strategies vary based on the location and type of obstruction, as well as the local expertise and available institution-specific resources. Surgical resection provides the best prospect for long-term disease control and should be considered in all patients during the initial evaluation. Localized involvement of the small airways and lung parenchyma is best treated by surgical resection, if feasible. In many cases, however, external beam radiotherapy or systemic chemotherapy may be the only treatment options. Patients with central airway obstruction often present with either medically or surgically unresectable disease. Although a comprehensive review of the various modalities is beyond the scope of this chapter, some basic principles are outlined in Figure 135-1. In emergent cases, the barrel of the rigid bronchoscope may be used to mechanically core out the tumor and dilate the airways, providing palliation. Flexible bronchoscopy and balloon bronchoplasty may be used to dilate the airways in less urgent cases.[7] Electrocautery, argon plasma coagulation, laser therapy, cryotherapy, brachytherapy, and photodynamic therapy are reasonable approaches for predominantly endoluminal disease (Figure 135-2). Extraluminal-predominant disease may be best treated with external beam radiotherapy and endobronchial stent placement (Figure 135-3). Since most lesions are mixed with endo- and extraluminal components, multimodality therapy, using endobronchial laser therapy with mechanical debulking followed by stent placement and subsequent consolidation with external beam radiotherapy, for example, is quite common. Symptom palliation, resulting in reduction in levels of care, may be accomplished in most instances with the judicious application of endoscopic techniques. Patients should be carefully evaluated with an early referral to an experienced bronchoscopist who can match the various therapeutic modalities available to the individual patient.

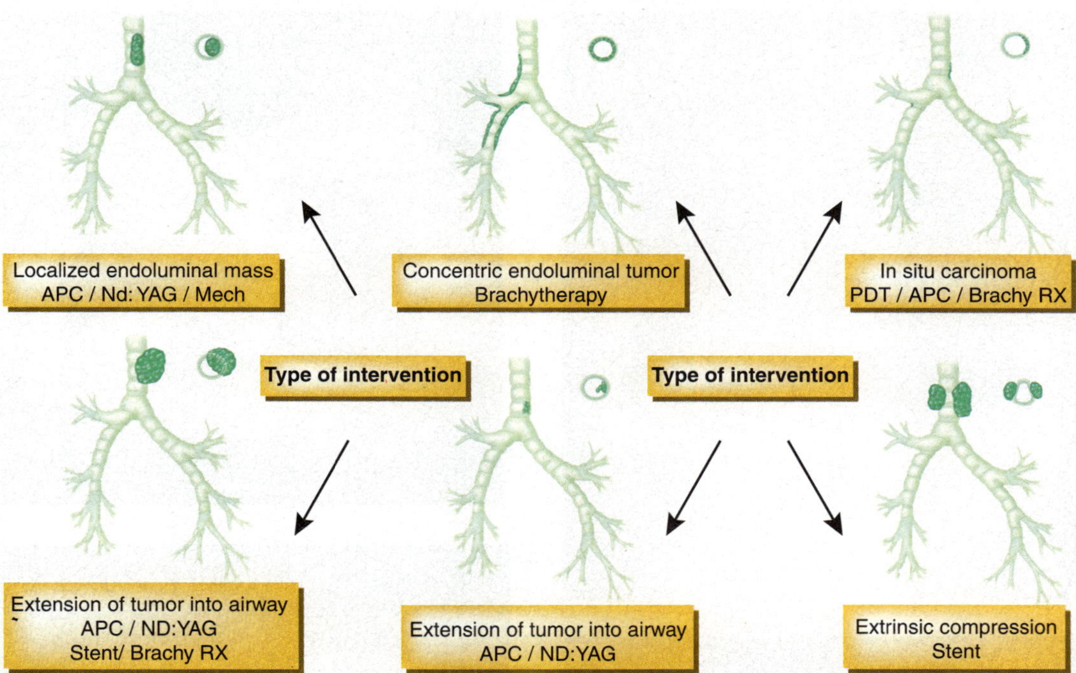

Figure 135-1 Approach to airway obstruction using interventional bronchoscopic therapy.

MALIGNANT PLEURAL EFFUSIONS

The presence of malignant cells in pleural fluid is a common clinical problem in the cancer setting that signifies distant spread of tumor and, hence, advanced disease. Malignant pleural effusions thus have significant therapeutic and prognostic implications. Estimates of the incidence of malignant pleural effusions in the United States approach 150,000 cases annually.[8] Malignant pleural involvement without effusion occurs in up to 45% of patients with metastatic disease to the pleura.[9] In primary pleural malignancies, such as malignant mesothelioma, pleural effusions may also be absent. Almost any type of neoplasm can affect the pleura. Lung cancer accounts for up to half of all malignant effusions, followed in frequency by breast carcinoma and lymphoma. In 5 to 10% of patients, a primary tumor cannot be identified.[10,11] The incidence of mesothelioma, the most common primary pleural malignancy in the United States, varies widely with geographic location. Most pleural malignancies arise from tumor emboli to the visceral pleura. The parietal pleura may be secondarily involved presumably by seeding from the visceral pleura. Direct extension of tumor from the lung, chest wall, mediastinal structures, or diaphragm, and hematogenous metastasis to the parietal pleura are other mechanisms that contribute to the genesis of malignant pleural fluid formation.[12] In addition to direct tumoral involvement of the pleura, malignant pleural effusions can result from lymphatic blockage anywhere between the parietal pleura and the mediastinal lymph nodes. Elevations in the local production of vascular endothelial growth factor (VGEF), a potent mediator of increased vascular permeability, also plays a significant role in the formation of malignant pleural effusions.[13,14]

Seventeen percent of all pleural effusions in patients with cancer are "paramalignant," a term used for effusions that occur in the setting of cancer that are not caused by direct malignant involvement of the pleural space.[12] These effusions develop as a result of local or systemic effects of the tumor, complications of cancer therapy, or concurrent nonmalignant disease.[15] Lymphatic obstruction is associated with both malignant and paramalignant effusions and is the most common cause of paramalignant effusions. Other common causes include bronchial obstruction, trapped lung, and pulmonary embolism.

Clinical Manifestations, Imaging Studies, and Diagnosis Patients most commonly present with symptoms of progressive exertional dyspnea. Cough may also be a troubling symptom with large effusions. Constitutional symptoms are common signals of advanced disease and thus malaise, weight loss, and poor appetite are recurrent complaints, which may become more frequent as the performance status worsens. Hemoptysis and chest wall pain are less common symptoms that indicate endobronchial malignant disease and tumoral invasion of the chest wall.

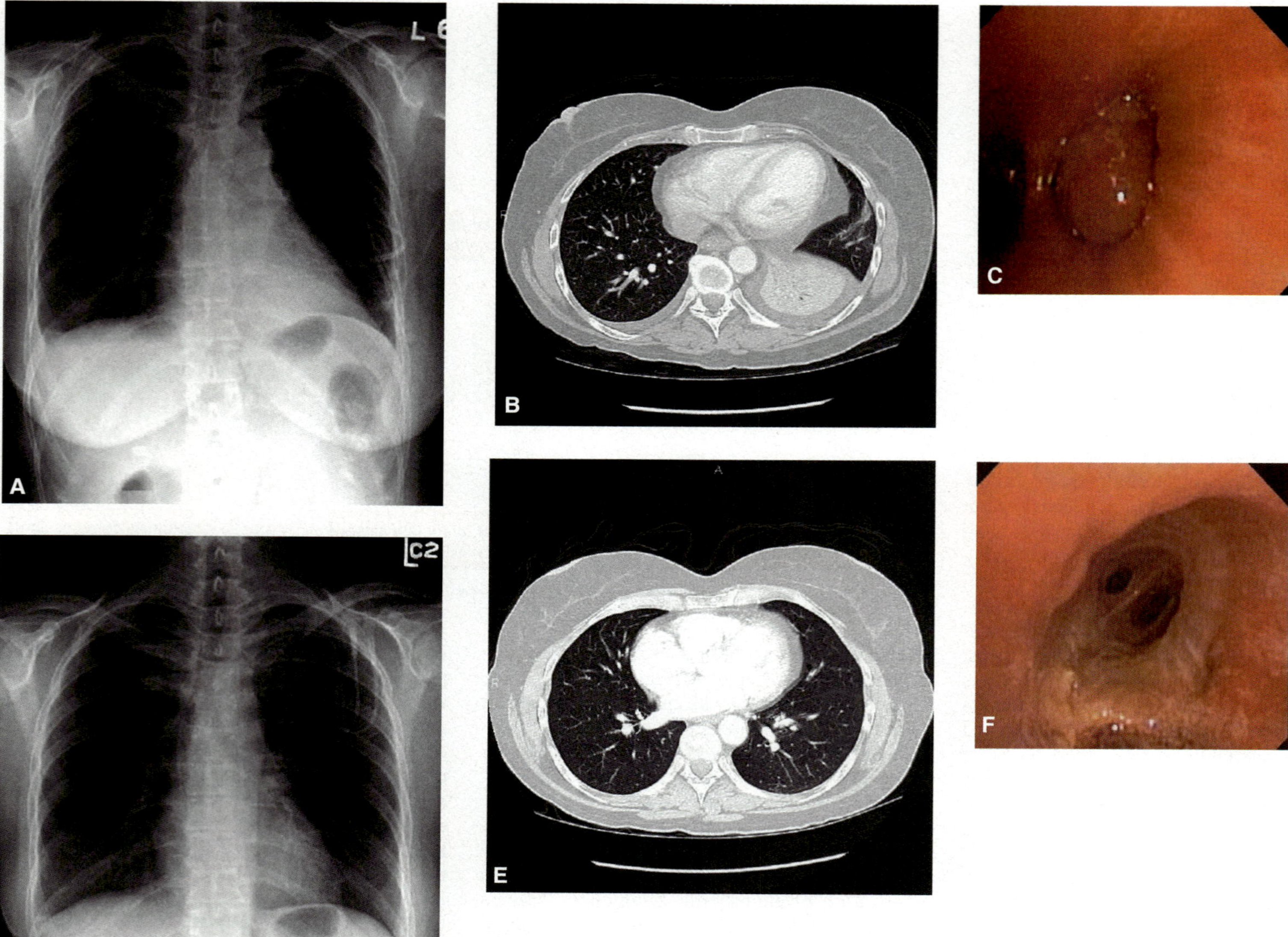

Figure 135-2 Left lower lobe (LLL) collapse secondary to metastatic sarcoma (**A** and **B**). Complete obstruction of the LLL basilar segments due to a large obstructing tumor was noted at bronchoscopy **(C)** which was removed using snare forceps and argon plasma coagulation, revealing reexpansion of the lung and a patent distal airway **(D–F)**.

Standard chest roentgenograms and bilateral decubitus films of the chest provide critical information in the initial evaluation of pleural effusions, including effusion size, position of the mediastinum and diaphragms, presence of loculations and air fluid levels within the pleural space, and characteristics of the underlying lung parenchyma. Lateral decubitus projections are useless in the evaluation of massive pleural effusions that obscure the entire hemithorax. Knowledge regarding the position of the mediastinum is imperative in therapeutic decision making. Large pleural effusions with contralateral mediastinal shift typically require prompt therapeutic thoracentesis, while those with a centered mediastinum or ipsilateral shift of the mediastinum should be approached cautiously (Figures 135-4 and 135-5). In addition to pleural effusions, other disease processes that may cause an ipsilateral shift of the mediastinum or a centered mediastinum with hemithorax opacification include a frozen mediastinum associated with malignant mesothelioma or lymphoma, atelectasis related to occlusion of the ipsilateral central airway, or extensive tumoral infiltration of the ipsilateral lung simulating a large effusion.[15] Computed tomography (CT) is especially valuable in delineating alternate diagnoses and in identifying loculated effusions. In addition, CT offers better anatomical information of the chest wall, parietal and visceral pleura, mediastinal structures, and lung parenchyma.[12] Ultrasonography is easy to learn and interpret and provides guidance in locating the optimal site for thoracentesis. This instrument is particularly helpful in the setting of loculated pleural effusions. Its utility in general practice, however, needs to be determined.[16] Positron emission tomography (PET) with 18-fluorodeoxyglucose is particularly helpful in highlighting extrapleural extension of disease associated with malignant mesothelioma. The utility of PET scanning in the evaluation of other malignant pleural diseases has not been established. Magnetic resonance imaging (MRI) also adds valuable information regarding extrapleural invasion of the chest wall, spine, nerves, or mediastinal vascular structures, which is particularly useful when planning complex surgical procedures.[17] Chemical analysis reveals an exudative effusion in most cases, with only 5% of malignant pleural effusions being transudates.[15] The diagnostic cornerstone of malignant pleural effusion is the cytologic demonstration of malignant cells in the pleural effusion. Positive pleural fluid cytology is noted in 62% of cases.[18] Tumor marker measurements using flow cytometry improve the diagnostic yield of cytologically negative effusions by 33% and are particularly valuable when lymphoma, leuke-

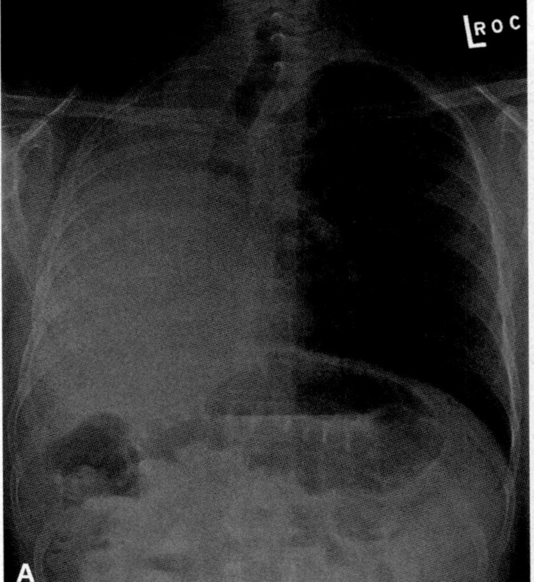

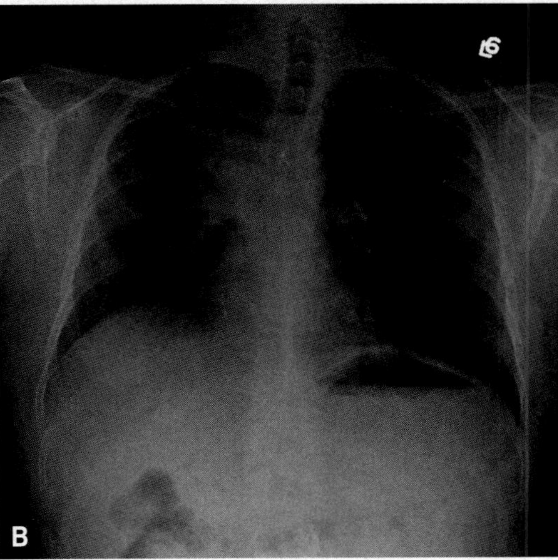

Figure 135-3 Complete opacification of the right thorax secondary to obstruction of the right mainstem bronchus by a large, predominantly extraluminal mass **(A)**. A wire stent was placed into the bronchus intermedius **(B)**, resulting in partial reexpansion of the right lung.

mia, or multiple myeloma are suspected.[19,20] Its role in the study of mesotheliomas remains controversial.[21] Pleural biopsies via pleuroscopy have a 95% sensitivity in the diagnosis of pleural malignancies. The diagnostic yield of pleuroscopy increases only incrementally (1%) when combined with pleural fluid cytology. By contrast, closed pleural biopsy has a diagnostic yield of only 44%, but improves to 77% when combined with an analysis of pleural fluid cytology.[22]

Management of Malignant Pleural Effusions Because malignant pleural effusions often signal advanced disease and incurability, treatment efforts are frequently directed toward palliation. Hence, awareness of available therapeutic options tailored to individual patient needs is important. The patient's performance status and information regarding prior thoracenteses, including the volume of fluid evacuated, whether lung reexpansion and symptom palliation were obtained, and the time interval between repeated taps, are important components of the evaluation that help to guide further therapy. Performance status is the best predictor of survival in patients with recurrent malignant pleural effusions.[23] The presence of local chest wall abnormalities, future cancer treatment plans, the patient's preferences, and the availability of family support also influence the approach to these patients.

Palliation with simple therapeutic thoracentesis represents a reasonable approach to patients with newly diagnosed chemo- or radiosensitive tumors, such as lymphoma, breast cancer, small-cell lung cancer, germ cell, ovarian, prostate, and thyroid neoplasms, while awaiting response to definitive therapy. After the initial clinical and roentgenographic evaluation, a symptom-limited therapeutic thoracentesis is recommended. A recent consensus statement by the American Thoracic Society and the European Respiratory Society recommends that not more than 1.0 to 1.5 liters of fluid be slowly evacuated from the pleural space in one sitting and that drainage should be discontinued if the patient develops symptoms of dyspnea, cough, or chest discomfort.[8] In our experience, patients with radiographic evidence of contralateral mediastinal shift from large pleural effusions may safely tolerate the removal of 2 to 2.5 liters of fluid in one sitting as long as there are no procedure-related symptoms of chest pain, cough, or dyspnea. However, large-volume pleural fluid drainage during a single procedure should be carried out cautiously, especially when radiological studies reveal a centered or ipsilaterally shifted mediastinum. Measurement of pleural pressures during the evacuation of large amounts of fluid may reduce procedure-related complications.[24] Lung reexpansion following thoracentesis may be assessed with posterior-anterior (PA) and lateral chest radiographs. Repeat thoracentesis spaced 1 to 2 days apart may be necessary to properly assess lung reexpansion associated with large effusions.[25] In 97% of patients, malignant pleural effusions will recur within 1 month, with most of these effusions reappearing within 1 to 3 days following fluid evacuation.[26] Patients with limited life expectancies (< 30 days), poor performance status, or those in which pleural fluid reaccumulation is slow are best treated with repeated therapeutic thoracentesis. Frequent thoracentesis may trigger the production of local cytokines and fibrin, resulting in pleural fluid loculation, which not only complicates further thoracenteses, but also obfuscates future modes of palliation.[27]

The use of indwelling pleural catheters has been increasingly accepted over the past few years as an alternative palliative option for patients with recurrent malignant effusions. Ideal candidates for this palliative modality include patients with a poor performance status, but with life expectancies in excess of 30 days, and in whom prior thoracenteses effected symptomatic relief. Considerations for pleural catheter implantation are valid in this group of patients regardless of lung reexpansion following thoracentesis. Indwelling pleural catheters may be placed in an outpatient setting. Following documentation of proper catheter position, the patient, trained family members, or caregivers may drain the fluid intermittently at home. Daily pleural fluid drainage is recommended initially. During each session, which typically lasts less than 15 minutes, drainage should be continued until the patient develops cough, chest discomfort, or fluid flow stops spontaneously, presumably because the

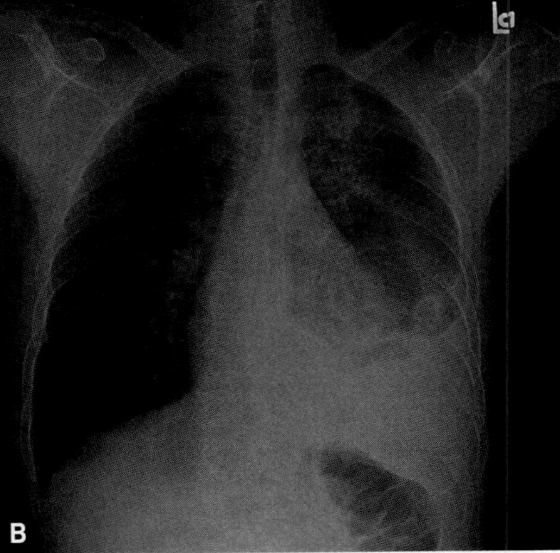

Figure 135-4 Large left sided pleural effusion causing opacification of the left hemithorax and contralateral shift of the mediastinum **(A)**. Following thoracentesis **(B)** the mediastinum shifted back to the midline.

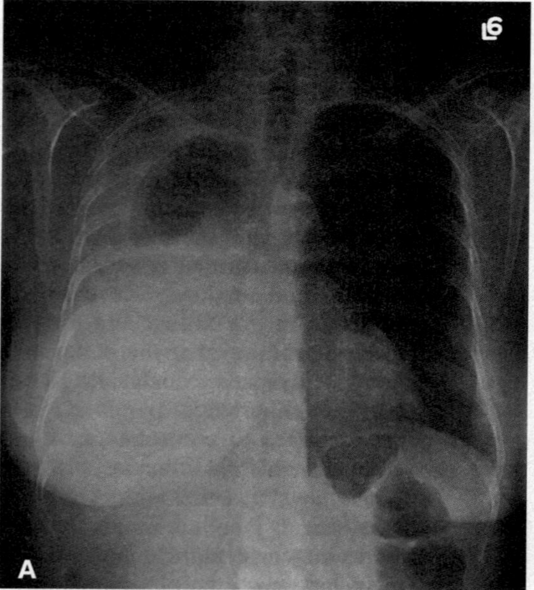

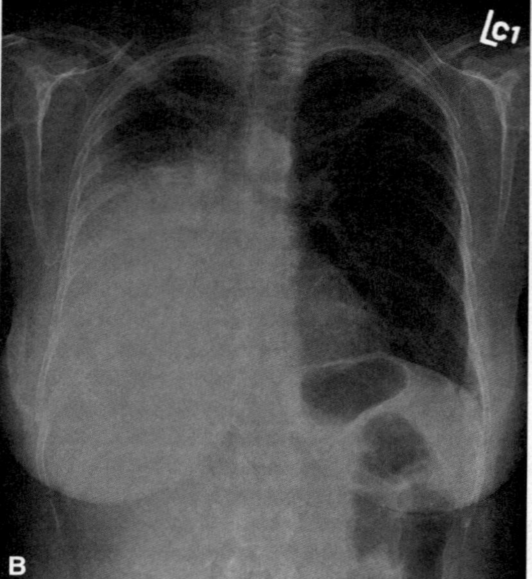

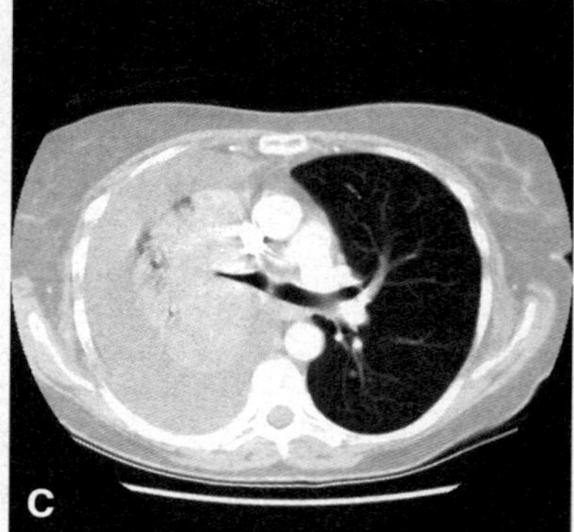

Figure 135-5 Large right sided pleural effusion **(A)** with ipsilateral shift of the mediastinum following thoracentesis **(B)**, indicating volume loss secondary to atelectasis or mass effect. A computed tomography scan of the chest **(C)** demonstrates a large mass compressing the right mainstem bronchus.

pleural space has been emptied. At our institution, 92% of patients treated with indwelling catheters reported significant relief of dyspnea, and 52% achieved effective pleurodesis. The mean time from catheter insertion to catheter removal was 32 days. Catheter-related complications were observed in only 4% of the patients, including one patient with empyema and two patients with persistent pain at the insertion site. Only 6% of patients required additional drainage of fluid following removal of the catheter.[28]

Chemical pleurodesis is the most widely used method to control recurrent malignant pleural effusions. Unfortunately, the lack of prospective studies precludes comparative analyses of efficacy, safety and cost of the existing chemical agents, and pleurodesis techniques. The results from available literature suggest that nonchemotherapeutic agents are more efficacious and the most cost-effective sclerosants.[8] Sterilized asbestos-free talc is the preferred pleurodesing agent. Complications vary with the dose, size, and surface characteristics of the talc particles. Administration of more than 5 g of talc during one session or simultaneous bilateral pleurodesis is not recommended. The use of talc particles that are less than 5 mm in size has been associated with pulmonary injury, including acute pneumonitis and respiratory failure associated with adult respiratory distress syndrome (ARDS), and should be avoided.[29] These safety concerns are being addressed in a European multicenter prospective trial, which is currently in process. The superiority of thoracoscopic talc insufflation over talc slurry as a method of administration of the sclerosant is a matter of debate. Success rates of > 90% have been reported for both techniques, without significant differences in the rate of overall complications or disease recurrence.[8] In a preliminary report of a prospective trial of 501 patients with a performance status of 1 or 2, limited data showed no difference in 30-day survival rates and pleurodesis success rates between chest tube talc slurry and thoracoscopic talc poudrage. Respiratory complications were greater with talc poudrage in this study, although symptoms of excess fatigue and pain were noted among recipients of talc slurry.[30] Based on the available information, our group considers all patients with a good performance status (ECOG 0, 1, or 2), and in whom symptomatic relief and lung reexpansion was achieved after initial drainage of the pleural fluid, for pleurodesis with pleuroscopic talc poudrage as the preferred modality of talc instillation.

Rarely, alternative modalities such as pleuroperitoneal shunts and parietal pleurectomy are used in the management of recurrent, symptomatic effusions following pleurodesis failures, or effusions associated with trapped lung.[31] Chylous effusions associated with malignancy may be palliated with pleuroperitoneal shunts. Prolonged loss of chyle, a protein-rich, fat-laden, and lymphocyte-predominant fluid, may result in lymphopenia, severe nutritional depletion, and water and electrolyte loss. Therefore, the preferred approach in the management of a chylous effusion is treatment of the underlying malignancy, followed by parenteral alimentation and talc pleurodesis for treatment failures.[32] In those cases where the effusion recurs after talc pleurodesis, pleuroperitoneal shunt placement is a reasonable therapeutic option. With pleuroperitoneal shunts, chyle is not lost but mobilized from the thorax to the peritoneum where it is reabsorbed, thus mitigating the risk of malnourishment and immune suppression. Unfortunately, the pleuroperitoneal shunt pump mechanism displaces only 1.5 to 2.5 mL at a time, making its use cumbersome. In addition, the incidence of obstruction of the pump is high. Peritoneal tumor seeding through the shunt is a theoretical concern, although this has not been clearly documented. Parietal pleurectomy, decortication, or pleuropneumonectomy are associated with high mortality rates and do not provide better symptom control than other palliative options.[8] The utilization of compounds to block vascular endothelial growth factor (VEGF) either alone or in combination with other palliative modalities is promising. Theoretically, decreasing the production of pleural fluid with VEGF blockade followed by drainage of the pleural effusion and instillation of a chemical agent to obtain pleural symphysis could accelerate pleurodesis and reduce hospital stay.[33]

In summary, in patients with limited life expectancies, modalities that offer the best chance for palliation of symptoms, the lowest procedure-related morbidity and mortality, and the shortest hospital stay represent a reasonable approach to the management of recurrent malignant effusions. A multidisciplinary approach (Figure 135-6), involving oncology, pulmonary medicine, interventional radiology, and thoracic surgery, offers the best opportunities to achieve these goals.

POSTSURGICAL RESPIRATORY INSUFFICIENCY

Acute Postoperative Respiratory Failure Cancer patients undergoing major abdominal or thoracic surgery, particularly those undergoing thoracotomy for lung or esophageal resection, are at greatest risk of postoperative acute respiratory failure (ARF). Diffuse pulmonary edema occurs in 5 to 10% of thoracotomy patients and may threaten the success of an otherwise uneventful surgery. Although pneumonia is frequently ascribed as the cause of respiratory failure in this setting, in many cases a microbial pathogen is never identified. Pulmo-

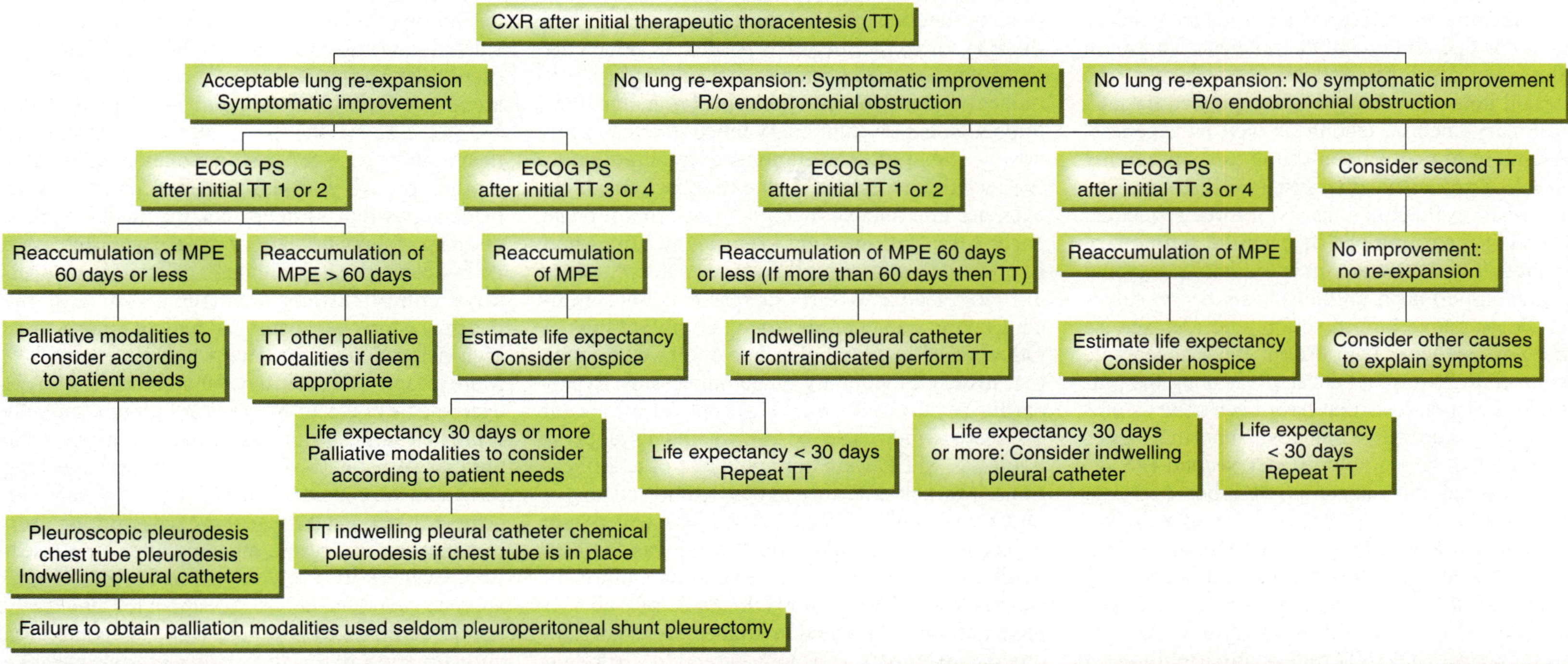

Figure 135-6 Management of malignant pleural effusions (MPE).

nary edema may be caused by a variety of factors that either increase capillary hydrostatic pressure or increase capillary permeability. Single lung ventilation and the associated high pulmonary pressures through the single ventilated lung during thoracic surgery is postulated to contribute to this disorder by increasing pulmonary capillary transmural pressures and damaging the pulmonary capillary endothelium, leading to edema formation. In addition, intraoperative ventilation with normal or near-normal tidal volumes, high inspired FIO_2 values to the single ventilated lung, microatelectasis, and lung ischemia-reperfusion injury caused by reduced blood flow to the collapsed lung may also contribute to postpneumonectomy pulmonary edema. Right-sided pneumonectomy confers a higher risk of postpneumonectomy pulmonary edema, presumably because of the increased risk of damage to the remaining (left) lung, which is smaller in volume. Patients typically present with severe dyspnea associated with pulmonary edema 48 to 72 hours after surgery, followed by respiratory failure (Figure 135-7). Despite aggressive supportive measures, mortality rates in excess of 50% have been reported.[34] Other etiologies of postoperative respiratory insufficiency include ventilatory failure, aspiration, airway obstruction, and pneumonia. Atelectasis and reduced functional residual capacity facilitate the development of pneumonia in up to 20% of patients following thoracic and upper abdominal cancer surgery, with an associated mortality rate of 50%.[35]

Chronic Postoperative Respiratory Failure In contrast to ARF following thoracic resection, which occurs sporadically, the development of chronic respiratory insufficiency tends to occur as a roughly predictable sequela of lung resection. Lung cancer is the leading cause of death from cancer in the United States and the world.[36] Surgical resection remains the treatment of choice for patients with resectable nonsmall-cell lung carcinoma and for selected cases of cancers metastatic to the lungs. Unfortunately, only 25% of patients with lung cancer have resectable disease at the time of diagnosis. Furthermore, most patients with lung cancer are smokers, and thus present with impaired pulmonary function associated with coexisting COPD, which augments perioperative risks and further reduces the proportion of patients who can be surgically treated. Thus, the selection of patients for resectional surgery requires careful evaluation of the preoperative surgical risk.

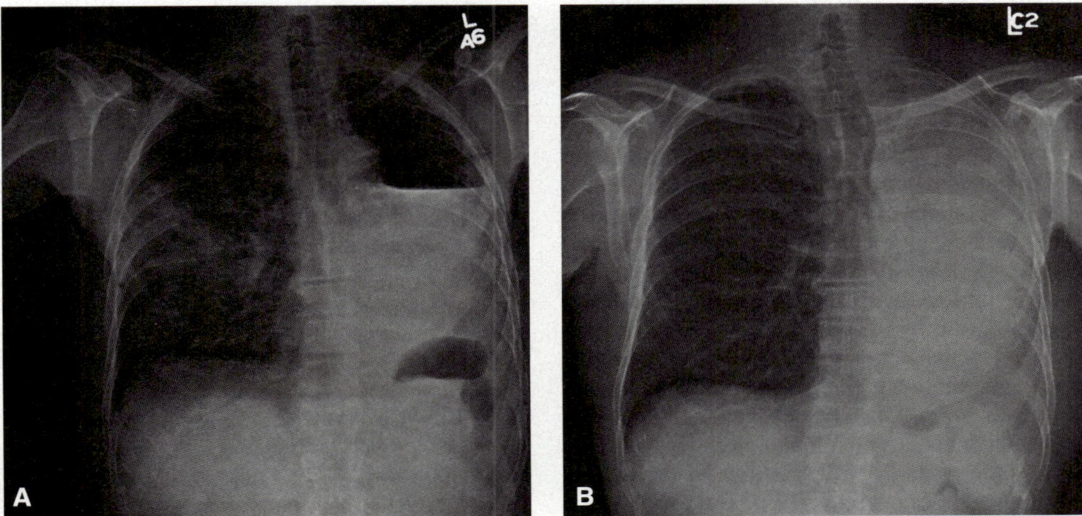

Figure 135-7 A 67-year-old man who underwent left pneumonectomy for treatment of nonsmall-cell carcinoma of the lung. Increased symptoms of cough and shortness of breath prompted a repeat chest radiograph 3 days later which showed consolidation throughout the right lung **(A)** in addition to an expected postpneumonectomy left-sided hydropneumothorax. The right-sided lung infiltrates resolved with aggressive diuresis **(B)**.

Diagnostic Evaluation The initial approach to the patient with an anatomically resectable tumor includes strategies to determine the patient's functional operability and the predicted long-term pulmonary disability following the loss of the resected lung. This may be accomplished through pulmonary-specific testing as well as a general assessment aimed at identifying and optimizing control of any coexisting systemic diseases. The pulmonary evaluation consists of three sequential steps: (1) measurement of baseline pulmonary function, (2) quantitative radionuclide regional ventilation-perfusion pulmonary studies to calculate postoperative lung function, and (3) exercise testing for patients who do not meet acceptable results on the two previous steps. Among the pulmonary function tests that have been used as predictors of postoperative outcome, abnormal values of forced expiratory volume in 1 second (FEV_1) and functional vital capacity (FVC) best correlate with severity of airway obstruction and/or reduction in lung volumes. The utility of maximal voluntary ventilation (MVV), an index of ventilatory muscle endurance, is limited by the patient's effort. Reduced values of the diffusing capacity for carbon monoxide (DLCO) reflect abnormalities in alveolar-capillary oxygen transfer. Hypercarbia ($pCO_2 > 45$ mm Hg) is a late manifestation of chronic ventilatory impairment. Thus, significant spirometric abnormalities precede the development of hypercarbia, which is rarely used as single criterion of inoperability. The following criteria have been reported as predictive of an acceptable risk of lung resection: FEV_1, > 60% of predicted; MVV, > 55% of predicted; DLCO, > 60% of predicted; and $pCO_2 < 45$ mm Hg.[37] Of these parameters, FEV_1 is the simplest, most reproducible, and most frequently used for predicting complications of lung resection. For decision making, values of FEV_1 reported as percent of predicted that take into account variations in patients' height, gender, and race are preferred over values reported in absolute units (L). In our laboratory, more than half of patients with an FEV_1 between 60% to 70% of predicted have an estimated postpneumonectomy FEV_1 by radionuclide studies that is below acceptable values for safe resection (< 40% of predicted). Therefore, we recommend that only those patients with baseline FEV_1 and DLCO ≥ 70% of predicted and no clinical evidence of contralateral pulmonary disease be considered for resection without further testing. All other patients should undergo a "split function" evaluation, which is a quantitative radionuclide assessment of regional lung ventilation and perfusion. In this study, the uptake of radioactive ions by various regions in each lung is measured by inhalation of ^{133}Xe and by intravenous administration of ^{133}Xe dissolved in saline or ^{99}Tc macroaggregates. The percentage of radioactivity contributed by each lung correlates with the contribution to the overall function by that lung. The predicted postoperative FEV_1 (FEV_1ppo) and predicted postoperative DLCO (DLCOppo) are calculated by subtracting the percent functional uptake of the region to be resected from the total uptake. Several investigators have documented the usefulness of split function studies for predicting both the risk of complications and the loss of pulmonary function after pulmonary resection.[38,39] In these studies, preoperative predicted values are closer to measured postoperative values for pneumonectomy and for resections involving more than three segments.[40] Pulmonary function remains relatively stable after pneumonectomy. Predictions for a smaller resection, such as a lobectomy, however, are less reliable owing to a disproportionate early loss, followed by significant functional improvement with time.[41] Kearney and colleagues also described a low FEV_1ppo as the only significant independent predictor of complications.[42] Other variables, including age ≥ 60 years, male sex, history of smoking, pneumonectomy, hypercarbia ($pCO_2 \geq 45$ mm Hg), desaturations on exercise oximetry ($SaO_2 \leq 90\%$), and a preoperative $FEV_1 \leq 1$ L were not predictive of complications. Markos and colleagues[43] reported that a DLCOppo < 40% of predicted was associated with higher morbidity and mortality and was the best predictor of postoperative respiratory failure. In summary, an FEV_1ppo and DLCOppo of ≥ 40% of predicted on split function studies represent safe preoperative criteria for lung resection, including pneumonectomy. Patients requiring lesser surgeries, such as a lobectomy, who do not meet these criteria, should undergo further evaluation with exercise testing before surgery can be undertaken.

The rationale for using exercise testing in these high-risk patients is based on two concepts: (1) lung function is not the only determinant of performance and (2) losses from lobectomies or lesser resections improve over time and tend to be overestimated by radiospirometric studies.[44] Exercise testing also offers the advantage of examining cardiopulmonary and musculoskeletal interactions during stress in a single study. The most validated form of exercise testing is cycle ergometry with incremental workloads to the symptom-limited maximum ($\dot{V}O_{2peak}$). Using this method, Smith and colleagues found that only 1 of 10 patients with a $\dot{V}O_{2peak} > 20$ mL/kg/min developed complications postoperatively, whereas all patients with a $\dot{V}O_{2peak} < 15$ mL/kg/min had complications.[45] We conducted two studies on patients who had been considered inoperable because of $FEV_1 \leq 40\%$ of predicted, FEV_1ppo ≤ 33 % of predicted, and/or arterial $PCO_2 \geq 45$ mm Hg. Patients who reached a $\dot{V}O_{2peak} \geq 15$ mL/kg/min underwent surgical treatment; others were referred to radiation and/or chemotherapy. All surgically treated patients were extubated within 24 hours, and the median time to discharge following surgery was 8 days. There were no in-hospital deaths, although reversible postoperative complications occurred in 40% of the patients. Moreover, a survival benefit among these high-risk patients treated surgically was noted.[46,47] More recently, we determined that values of $\dot{V}O_{2peak}$ expressed as percent of predicted more accurately estimated surgical risk and helped to maximize the number of patients who can safely undergo lung resection. We concluded that high-risk patients who achieve a $\dot{V}O_{2\,peak} \geq 60\%$ of predicted during exercise have an acceptable outcome after lung resection, even if $\dot{V}O_{2\,peak} < 15$ mL/kg/min.[48] Our approach to preoperative assessment for lung resection is summarized in Figure 135-8. In addition to an estimation of surgical risk and postoperative function, the goals of preoperative assessment include the development of strategies to reduce the risk and maximize the number of patients who can benefit from surgical therapy. Finally, one must keep in mind that there is no test that will predict all complications and that the patient and the surgeon should make the final decision regarding the risk-benefit of surgical treatment.

CHEMOTHERAPY-INDUCED LUNG INJURY

The lungs are frequent targets of chemotherapy-induced tissue injury. Because the response of the lungs to injury is limited, these agents give rise to a defined number of stereotyped lung injury patterns, including diffuse alveolar damage (DAD) with or without diffuse alveolar hemorrhage

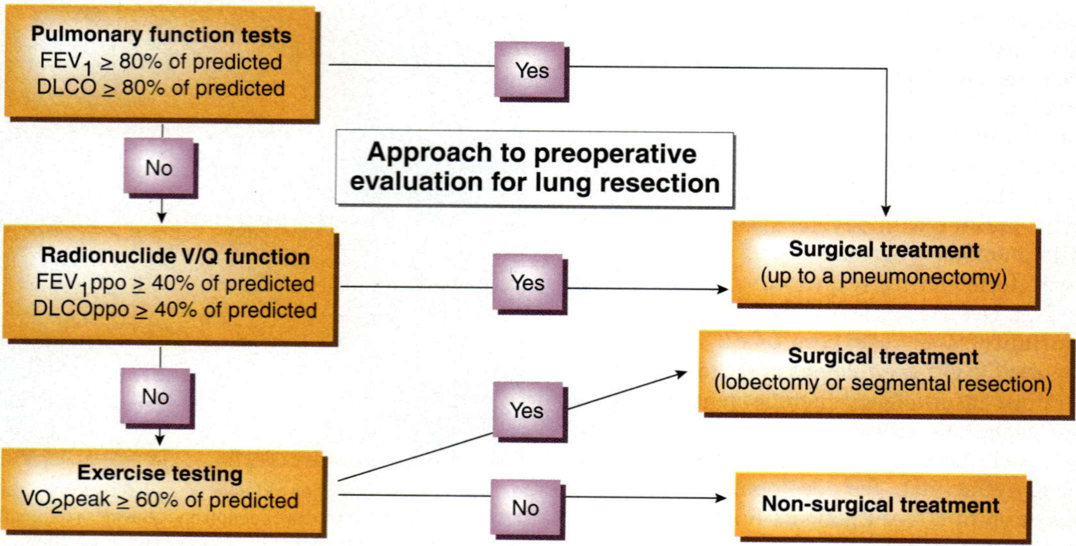

Figure 135-8 Approach to preoperative evaluation for lung resection.

Table 135-1 Major Clinical Syndromes and Histologic Patterns of Chemotherapy-Induced Lung Injury

Type of Lung Injury	Drug Class						
	Alkylating Agents	Antimetabolites/Purine Analogs	Cytotoxic Antibiotics	Nitrosoureas	Taxanes	Immunotoxins/BRMS	Other
ARDS	Busulfan, Cyclophosphamide	Methotrexate, Azathioprine, Ara-C, Fludarabine, Gemcitabine	Bleomycin Mitomycin C	BCNU, CCNU	Paclitaxel Docetaxel	Infliximab G-CSF, GM-CSF	ATRA
NCPE		Ara-C, Gemcitabine, Methotrexate, Pentostatin	Mitomycin C*		Paclitaxel, Docetaxel	IL-2, TNF, IFN-γ	
IP	Busulfan, Cyclophosphamide	Methotrexate, Azathioprine, Fludarabine, Gemcitabine	Bleomycin	BCNU, CCNU	Docetaxel, Paclitaxel	G-CSF, GM-CSF, IFN-γ, Gefitinib	Procarbazine, Irinotecan
HP	Cyclophosphamide	Methotrexate	Bleomycin	BCNU			Procarbazine
BOOP	Busulfan, Cyclophosphamide	Methotrexate	Bleomycin	BCNU, CCNU			IFN-γ
EP		Methotrexate, Fludarabine	Bleomycin			IL-2, Infliximab	
Pleural Disease	Cyclophosphamide	Methotrexate, Azathioprine, Gemcitabine	Bleomycin, Mitomycin C	BCNU	Docetaxel	IL-2, IFN-γ, G-CSF, GM-CSF	ATRA, Procarbazine
Airway Disease	Cyclophosphamide	Methotrexate, Gemcitabine	Bleomycin		Paclitaxel	Rituxan, IFN-αβ	Teniposide, Etoposide, Vinca alkaloids + mitomycin, L-Asparaginase
PVD		Zinostatin (PAH)	Bleomycin	BCNU (PVOD)		IL-2 (PAH), IFN-γ (PAH)	Tamoxifen (VTE), L-asparaginase (VTE), Thalidomide (VTE)

ARDS = acute respiratory distress syndrome; ATRA = all-trans-retinoic acid; BOOP = bronchiolitis obliterans with organizing pneumonia; BRMS = biologic response modifiers; EP = eosinophilic pneumonia; G-CSF = granulocyte-colony stimulating factor; GM-CSF = granulocyte macrophage colony stimulating factor; HP = hypersensitivity pneumonitis; IFN-γ = interferon-γ; IL-2 = interleukin-2; IP = interstitial pneumonitis; NCPE = noncardiogenic pulmonary edema; PAH = pulmonary arterial hypertension; PVD = pulmonary vascular disease; PVOD = pulmonary veno-occlusive disease; TNF = tumor necrosis factor.

(DAH), noncardiogenic pulmonary edema (NCPE), interstitial pneumonitis (IP), hypersensitivity pneumonitis (HP), and bronchiolitis obliterans with organizing pneumonia (BOOP). Diseases of the pleura and pulmonary vasculature may also emerge as sequelae of anticancer therapy. Finally, pneumonias are a well-known consequence of aggressive immunosuppressive therapy, and the specific immune defects induced by individual chemotherapeutic agents and the associated lung infections are discussed below in the section "Pulmonary Infections in HSCT Patients," as well as in Chapter 141, "Infections in Patients with Cancer." Precise estimates of the incidence of lung injury caused by individual chemotherapeutic agents are incomplete, owing in part to the frequent use of complex multidrug and multimodality regimens. In addition, overlapping clinical and radiographic manifestations of lung injury caused by drug toxicity, infection, and cancer relapse make clinical distinctions between these entities difficult. This section offers a brief overview of the clinically relevant pulmonary disease patterns induced by various chemotherapeutic agents (Table 135-1). Admittedly, the overview is neither comprehensive nor balanced and reflects our bias regarding certain chemotherapeutic agents and their propensity to cause lung injury.

Clinical Findings and Histopathologic Correlates **Diffuse Alveolar Damage (DAD)/ Adult Respiratory Distress Syndrome (ARDS) and Diffuse Alveolar Hemorrhage (DAH)** DAD, the histologic correlate of ARDS, frequently develops during severe lung injury. The most compelling causal associations of chemotherapy-induced DAD are with the alkylating agents (busulfan, cyclophosphamide), antibiotics (bleomycin, mitomycin C), antimetabolites (methotrexate, azathioprine, cytosine-arabinoside [Ara-C]), fludarabine, gemcitabine), and nitrosoureas (bischloroethyl nitrosourea [BCNU], chloroethylcyclohexyl nitrosourea [CCNU]). Bilateral heterogeneous ground-glass opacities are early radiographic findings of ARDS, which may progress to diffuse opacification with irreversible lung damage, marked by architectural distortion, fibrosis, and honeycomb lung. Multiagent protocols or the concurrent use of radiation or oxygen therapy potentiates both the risk and severity of lung injury, especially following therapy with bleomycin or busulfan.[49,50] Overall, the response to early drug withdrawal and initiation of corticosteroid therapy in the treatment of DAD has been variable. Progressive respiratory impairment, leading to respiratory failure and death, has been reported with some agents (busulfan, cyclophosphamide) despite drug withdrawal. Although drug-induced DAH may occur in association with capillaritis or as a consequence of bland alveolar hemorrhage without distortion of the lung architecture, most of the responsible cancer agents produce DAH as a result of toxicity to the alveolocapillary membrane. This type of injury produces the histologic lesion of DAD. Thus, many of the cytotoxic drugs that cause severe DAD may also trigger DAH. Bleeding commonly occurs during the early or exudative phase of DAD and originates from the alveolar capillaries. Despite massive bleeds, hemoptysis is seen only in approximately 25% of patients.[51,52] The diagnosis of DAH is made clinically by progressively more bloody aliquots of bronchoalveolar lavage (BAL) fluid and/or cytologic evidence of increased hemosiderin-laden macrophages in the setting of radiographic evidence of diffuse lung disease

Noncardiogenic Pulmonary Edema (NCPE) The antimetabolites (Ara-C, gemcitabine, methotrexate), all-*trans* retinoic acid (ATRA), and the biologic response modifiers (interleukin-2, tumor necrosis factor) are prominent causes of a bland pulmonary capillary leak syndrome. Drug-induced NCPE often occurs as an idiosyncratic reaction, unrelated to drug dosage or duration of therapy. Most reactions are mild and self-limited, although progression to ARDS with fatal outcomes occasionally occurs. The clinical and radiographic manifestations of NCPE are generally indistinguishable from other causes of pulmonary edema, although the presence of cardiomegaly, pulmonary vascular redistribution, and Kerley B lines on chest radiographs favor a cardiogenic etiology. Drug withdrawal, supplemental oxygen, and the judicious use of diuretics usually effect a rapid recovery. Rechallenge with the offending drug often results in recrudescence of symptoms.

Interstitial Pneumonitis (IP) An ever-enlarging list of chemotherapeutic agents has been associated with IP, of which bleomycin, busulfan, cyclophosphamide, carmustine, gemcitabine, methotrexate, and the tyrosine kinase inhibitor, gefitinib, have been most extensively studied.[53–56] Nonspecific interstitial pneumonia (NSIP) represents the most frequent morphologic pattern of drug-induced IP. In most patients, a nonproductive cough and dyspnea develop insidiously, usually within weeks to months following drug exposure. Radiographic changes typically lag behind clinical symptoms by days to weeks, but may occasionally occur as an early marker of lung injury. With the exception of methotrexate-associated hilar lymphadenopathy, the radiographic findings of IP are nonspecific for a particular chemotherapy agent.[50,57] Interstitial and mixed alveolar–interstitial abnormalities on chest imaging studies are the most frequent radiographic findings, which typically localize to the

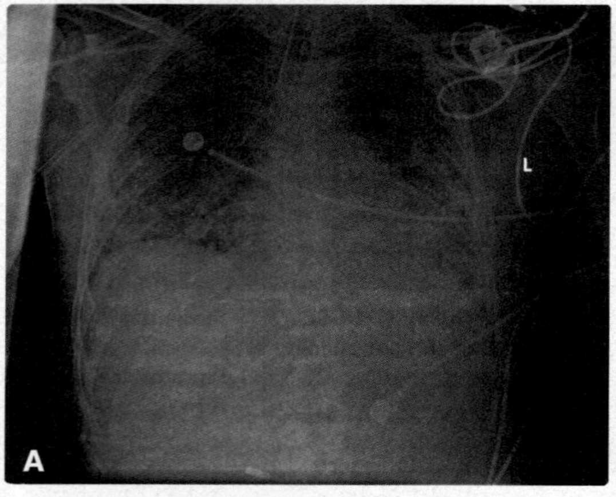

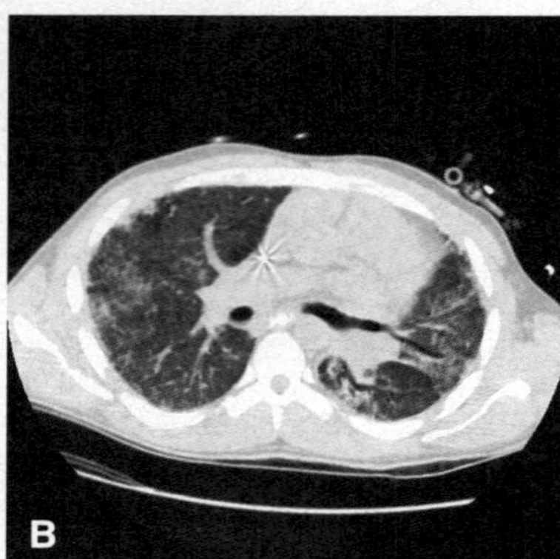

Figure 135-9 A 32-year-old man treated with bleomycin-based chemotherapy for germ cell tumor developed respiratory distress following surgical resection of retroperitoneal lymph nodes. CXR **(A)** and computed tomography scan of the chest **(B)** showed bilateral patchy reticulonodular and airspace disease. Work-up was consistent with adult respiratory distress syndrome associated with bleomycin toxicity, presumably triggered by hyperoxia during surgery.

peripheral and lower lung zones. Nodular lesions, reticular lines, septal thickening, mosaic patterns, and ground-glass attenuation are also observed (Figure 135-9). CT scan is far superior to plain films in identifying interstitial lung disease. Other supportive findings include a reduction in DLCO and a restrictive defect on pulmonary function testing. Risk factors for IP vary with individual agents, but, in general, include advanced age, concurrent radiation or multiagent therapy, and the need for high-inspired supplemental oxygen. This is particularly true following bleomycin or BCNU therapy, where the concomitant administration of high-inspired supplemental oxygen, other chemotherapeutic agents, or radiation significantly enhances the rate and severity of lung injury. Alveolar edema and DAD are usual features of advanced disease, which may progress to end-stage fibrotic lung despite corticosteroid therapy and drug withdrawal. IP associated with bleomycin and several other chemotherapeutic agents has been carefully scrutinized and deserves specific attention. Up to 20% of bleomycin-treated patients develop clinically significant lung disease. The incidence of bleomycin-induced lung injury appears to be dose related, with higher rates associated with total cumulative doses above 450 U. Mortality rates are low (1–3%) but increase to 10% among patients with cumulative doses above 550 U. BCNU also causes dose-dependent lung toxicity with rates as high as 50% among patients whose cumulative dose exceeds 1,500 mg/m^2.[58,59] The predilection for the middle and upper lobes distinguishes BCNU-induced IP. Intractable, upper-lobe predominant fibrosis and pneumothorax may occur years after completion of therapy.[60] Late onset pneumonitis following busulfan and cyclophosphamide administration has also been reported.

Hypersensitivity Pneumonitis (HP) HP has been most frequently described following treatment with methotrexate and bleomycin,[54,59,61–63] but also occurs with infliximab, fludarabine, and interleukin-2. Most patients present with fever, dyspnea, dry cough, and BAL lymphocytosis. Poorly formed noncaseating granulomas and mononuclear cell infiltration are typical histologic findings in subacute and chronic HP. Radiographic changes include homogeneous opacities with a predilection for the periphery and upper lobes, particularly in the chronic form of the disease. Histologic evidence of ill-defined granulomas, together with a skin rash and radiographic findings of hilar adenopathy or pleural effusions may help to distinguish methotrexate-induced lung injury from other types of drug-induced HP.

Bronchiolitis Obliterans with Organizing Pneumonia (BOOP) BOOP is suggested by radiographic evidence of patchy, widespread, migratory, pulmonary opacities, distributed predominantly in the lung periphery. Centrilobular nodules with linear opacities in a “tree-in-bud” pattern are also seen on CT.[64] Ascribing the appearance of BOOP to drug toxicity is often difficult, especially in the cancer setting where a variety of coexisting conditions, including background disease and graft-versus-host reactions may mimic the disease. Nevertheless, bleomycin, busulfan, BCNU, cyclophosphamide, methotrexate, and interferon-γ, are frequently cited as causative. Patients typically respond well to corticosteroid therapy and cessation of the offending agent.[65]

Eosinophilic Pneumonia Acute eosinophilic pneumonia is most frequently documented following therapy with fludarabine, interleukin-2, infliximab, methotrexate, and bleomycin. BAL or peripheral blood eosinophilia are prominent features, which may promptly resolve following corticosteroid therapy. Radiographic changes occur abruptly and include homogeneous opacities with a predilection for the periphery and upper lobes. The “reverse pulmonary edema pattern” is seen only in a minority of patients.[65] Drug withdrawal and initiation of high-dose steroids are typically associated with favorable outcomes, although occasionally rapid progression to respiratory failure may occur despite therapy.

Pleural Disease Drug-induced pleural disease is typically a component of a generalized pulmonary reaction that includes pulmonary infiltrates and effusions.[66] Pleuropulmonary reactions have been most frequently described following treatment with methotrexate, docetaxel, gemcitabine, azathioprine, mitomycin, interleukin-2, ATRA, and interferon-γ. Isolated pleural effusions are occasionally seen following methotrexate, docetaxel, and GCSF administration and may resolve with discontinuation of therapy.[67,68] Pleural thickening may accompany pulmonary fibrosis as a late manifestation of cyclophosphamide, BCNU, or bleomycin toxicity.

Pulmonary Vascular Disease (PVD) The adverse effects of chemotherapeutic agents on the pulmonary vasculature may result in thrombosis, pulmonary hypertension, or pulmonary veno-occlusive disease (PVOD). The diagnosis of PVD is suggested by an isolated reduction in DLCO or a DLCO that is disproportionately decreased relative to other lung function parameters on pulmonary function testing. The prothrombotic effects of tamoxifen appear to be related to drug-related decrements in protein C and antithrombin III levels.[69] Combined therapy with tamoxifen and other chemotherapeutic agents, such as cyclophosphamide, methotrexate and 5-flurouracil confers a 3-fold increased risk of thromboembolic phenomenon.[70,71] Thromboembolic events as high as 28 to 44% have been reported among recipients of thalidomide-based chemotherapy given in combination with doxorubicin or BCNU.[72,73] Zinostatin, a novel antitumor antibiotic, causes hypertrophy of the pulmonary vascular wall leading to pulmonary hypertension, possibly as a result of direct toxicity to the pulmonary endothelium.[65] More often, chemotherapy-related pulmonary hypertension emerges as a result of PVOD, a process characterized by fibrous obliteration of pulmonary venules and small pulmonary veins (see below). Although several drugs have been implicated in the development of PVOD, bleomycin and BCNU have been associated with the most incriminating data.[74,75]

Drug-Induced Airway Disease Alterations in airway function are typically a component of drug-induced parenchymal reactions, but occasionally may be seen as isolated airway disease. Direct degranulation of mast cells causes bronchospasm following paclitaxel administration; for many of the other agents, the mechanism underlying bronchospasm is unclear. Paclitaxel is formulated in a highly allergenic polyoxyethylated castor oil solvent (Cremophor EL), which may educe mast cell activation and histamine release, triggering type 1-hypersensitivity reactions. Standard prophylaxis with histamine receptor antagonists and steroids has reduced the incidence of paclitaxel-induced bronchospasm from 30 to 2%.[76] Teniposide, a podophyllotoxin formulated in Cremophor EL solvent, also causes prominent bronchospasm, presumably by the same mechanism.[77] Although the vinorelbine and other vinca alkaloids are rarely associated with lung toxicity, acute reactions characterized by cough, bronchospasm, flushing, dyspnea, abdominal pain, and hypotension have been described when these agents are given either concurrently or sequentially with mitomycin chemotherapy. Rituxan has been associated with symptoms of cough, rhinitis, bronchospasm, and dyspnea.[78,79] Drug withdrawal coupled with supplemental oxygen, antihistamines, steroids, and nebulized β-agonists generally result in favorable outcomes. Prophylaxis with steroids and antihistamines frequently permit successful rechallenge in selected cases.

PULMONARY COMPLICATIONS OF THORACIC RADIATION: RADIATION PNEUMONITIS AND FIBROSIS

Clinical Presentation A major dose-limiting organ to thoracic irradiation is the lung. Although the precise magnitude of lung injury attributable to radiation is unknown, clinically significant lung toxicity has been reported in 5 to 20% of patients following thoracic radiation. Recent reports suggest that the incidence may be marginally lower among patients treated with radiation for breast cancer, in part owing to the different radiation methods used.[80] Two clinically distinct clinical phases of radiation-induced lung damage are recognized: radiation pneumonitis and radiation fibrosis. Radiation pneumonitis most commonly occurs in its classic form, in which toxicity to the lung is confined to the irradiated field and lung damage occurs in a relatively predictable and dose-related manner. A less predictable or sporadic form of radiation pneumonitis has also been recognized.[81] The early phase of classic radiation pneumonitis is heralded by the development of fever, dyspnea, and nonproductive cough, which typically develop insidiously over the initial 1 to 3 months and peak at 3 to 4 months after radiotherapy. Measurable changes in pulmonary function tests, including a reduction in lung volumes and diffusing capacity may be seen as early as 2 to 3 months after irradiation. Pulmonary fibrosis appears as a late-phase sequela to chronic inflammation in these patients, usually at 6 months, and stabilizes over the ensuing year following thoracic irradiation. This phase of radiation lung injury is characterized histopathologically by collagen deposition in the alveolar walls, collapse of air spaces, and an attendant loss of lung volume. Radiographic and histologic evidence of fibrosis occurs following classical radiation pneumonitis regardless of prior clinical manifestations of pneumonitis. Sporadic pneumonitis occurs in a minority (5%) of patients and is thought to represent a type of hypersensitivity pneumonitis characterized by a bilateral CD_4+ T-lymphocytic alveolitis that diffusely involves both lung fields. Hence, radiation changes on imaging studies may extend well beyond the irradiated field. Patients present at 1 to 3 months following thoracic irradiation with symptoms of dyspnea and dry cough that are disproportionate to the volume of lung irradiated. This form of pneumonitis and its associated symptoms typically abate in 6 to 8 weeks without any long-term sequelae.[81–83]

Early changes on conventional chest radiographs that suggest classical radiation pneumonitis include diffuse haze and indistinct vascular margins within the irradiated field. Patchy areas of consolidation with or without air-bronchograms coalesce over time to conform to the treatment portals, defying anatomic boundaries. Later, radiation fibrosis is heralded by the appearance of a well-demarcated area of volume loss, linear densities, bronchiectasis, retraction of the lung parenchyma, tenting and elevation of the hemidiaphragm, and ipsilateral pleural thickening. Pneumothorax and occasionally small pleural effusions may occur on the irradiated side. Radiation-related pleural effusions typically develop within 6 months of completion of radiotherapy. This observation, coupled with the absence of malignant cells on pleural fluid cytology, and clinical and radiographic evidence of pneumonitis help to distinguish malignant from radiation-induced effusions. Pulmonary veno-occlusive disease has also been reported as a rare complication of radiation-induced lung toxicity. Recent reports of BOOP and eosinophilic pneumonia involving nonirradiated areas of the lung following breast radiation have also been documented.[84] Both entities may produce migratory pulmonary opacities on chest radiographs, which typically develop 1 to 3 months following radiotherapy. The presence of blood or tissue eosinophils, coupled with a prior history of asthma or atopy, favors the diagnosis of eosinophilic pneumonia.

Risk Factors Risk factors that influence the development of radiation injury to the lung include total dose, dose per fraction, irradiated lung volume, radiation portals and beam arrangements, as well as physical characteristics of the irradiation. Pulmonary damage is almost always radiographically apparent with total doses of radiation that exceed 4,000 cGy, whereas only subtle radiographic changes are seen at doses below 3,000 cGy.[80] Multimodality regimens that combine radiation with chemotherapeutic agents such as mitomycin, cyclophosphamide, vincristine, adriamycin, bleomycin, and actinomycin D not only potentiate an adverse radiation response in the lungs, but also shorten the latency period following radiation exposure.[85] Other factors affecting the development of lung injury and disease severity include preexisting lung disease, underlying pulmonary reserve, prior radiotherapy, and rapid steroid withdrawal.[86] Although data regarding optimal dose-fractionation and dose-volume relationships that mitigate lung injury are still evolving, it is generally agreed that a hyperfractionated course of radiation delivered to the smallest lung volume offers the lowest possibility of lung toxicity. Newer strategies, including conformal therapy and intensity-modulated radiation therapy (IMRT) have been developed to deliver adequate doses to the tumor while limiting exposure to normal lung. IMRT uses multiple radiation beams to generate dose distributions that tightly conform to irregularly shaped target volumes, ensuring that the entire tumor volume is adequately treated, while minimizing radiation to normal lung. Pneumonitis following IMRT does not appear as the traditional straight-edged infiltrate that is typically seen following conventional radiation and may, therefore, be more difficult to distinguish from competing disease entities such as infection or recurrence of the underlying malignancy.[87]

Pathophysiology The pathophysiology of radiation-induced changes in the lung is poorly understood because of the complexities of preexisting comorbidity, the use of multiple treatment modalities to achieve a high probability of cure, poor quantitation of the severity of the acute insult, and lack of knowledge of individual predisposing genetic factors. It is generally accepted that radiation-induced lung damage represents a continuum of changes initiated by an inflammatory pneumonitis, which progresses to fibrosis, although whether pneumonitis and fibrosis represent a continuum or separate entities has not been definitively resolved. Certain key regulatory genes and/or gene products, such as TGF-β, matrix metalloproteinases (MMPs), and TNF, are thought to be central in both pathological processes. TGF-β is a multifunctional cytokine regulator of cell growth and differentiation that stimulates the deposition of collagen and decreases its degradation, resulting in fibrosis. A clear relationship between plasma levels of TGF-β and radiation-induced pulmonary toxicity has been shown in preclinical and clinical studies.[88] In these studies, reductions in the expression of TGF-β_1 using various modifiers such as amifostine reduced the clinical and histologic manifestations of radiation pneumonitis and fibrosis.[89–91] More importantly, preselection of nonsmall-cell lung cancer patients for dose escalation using plasma TGF-β allowed identification of patients at low risk of complications to whom higher doses of radiation could be safely delivered.[88] One initiator of radiation lung damage that may be amenable to modulation is oxidative stress leading to the formation of reactive oxygen species.[90] Biological modifiers targeting oxidative damage, such as superoxide dismutase (SOD), a key enzyme in the defense against the superoxide radical, has been shown to protect the lung against radiation pneumonitis and fibrosis, most likely by removing free radicals. A postirradiation hypoxic environment in the lung may be permissive and mediate sustained expression of inflammatory and fibrogenic cytokines, accounting for the appearance of lung fibrosis months to years after irradiation.[92] A significant genetic component to radiation-induced lung damage has been demonstrated in mouse models and genetic loci associated with susceptibility to radiation-induced lung damage identified on specific chromosomes, although none of these "susceptibility" genes have yet been identified.[93,94] Currently, there are no effective strategies for predicting the response of individual patients to treatment. The identification of specific genes that confer an increased risk of radiation-induced lung damage in individual patients would allow stratification of patients by their risk of potential lung injury, permitting the use of more aggressive treatment protocols and higher tumor control in the less susceptible patients, while more susceptible patients could be treated with "targeted" therapies.

Management Fortunately, most cases of radiation pneumonitis are subclinical or mild and require only expectant management and occasional antipyretics, antitussives, and bronchodilators. Corticosteroids are indicated for moderate and severe cases and may result in dramatic improvements in symptoms. Although no large body of data detailing the efficacy of corticosteroids in the management of symptomatic radiation-induced lung disease is currently available, a long clinical history of successful steroid use in the treatment of this condition supports this practice. Guidelines for steroid administration in the treatment of radiation pneumonitis have not been firmly established, although a regimen of prednisone given at 0.5 to 1 mg/kg of body weight is generally accepted. Steroids should be initiated once the diagnosis is reasonably certain and tapered according to clinical response over the ensuing weeks. In light of reports suggesting that rapid steroid taper may unmask latent radiation injury to the lung, a slow steroid taper is recommended. The late phase of pneumonitis may be refractory to even high-dose steroids. No benefit of steroids in the treatment of fibrotic lung disease has been shown, and currently there are no effective strategies for intervening in this late sequela.

PULMONARY COMPLICATIONS OF HEMATOPOIETIC STEM CELL TRANSPLANTATION

Hematopoietic stem cell transplantation (HSCT) has become widely used in cancer therapy, and is the only curative option for many patients with relapsed and high-risk malignancies. Despite advances in treatment regimens and supportive care, pulmonary complications still occur in up to 60% of HSCT recipients, accounting for significant morbidity and mortality.[95,96] Like most aspects of transplantation care, pulmonary complications are conveniently divided into those that occur "early" (during the first 100 days after transplantation) and those that occur "late" (Table 135-2). These complications are mostly due to direct toxicities from conditioning regimens, delayed bone marrow recovery, prolonged immunosuppressive therapy, and graft-versus-host disease (GVHD). Infectious complications and constrictive bronchiolitis occur most commonly after allogeneic HSCT because of the high incidence of GVHD and prolonged use of immunosuppressive therapy, whereas noninfectious complications other than constrictive bronchiolitis occur with similar frequency after both allogeneic and autologous HSCT.

Table 135-2 Pulmonary Complications after Hematopoietic Stem Cell Transplantation

Early (< 100 Days)	Late (> 100 Days)
Infectious pneumonia	Infectious pneumonia
Pulmonary edema	Constrictive bronchiolitis
Engraftment syndrome	Cryptogenic organizing pneumonia
Idiopathic pneumonia syndrome/Diffuse alveolar hemorrhage	Delayed pulmonary toxicity syndrome
Pulmonary veno-occlusive disease	Post-transplant lymphoproliferative disorder
Pulmonary alveolar proteinosis	Lymphocytic interstitial pneumononitis

Pulmonary Infections in HSCT Patients Pneumonia is a major cause of morbidity and mortality in HSCT, occurring in a majority of patients.[97,98] Early after transplantation (within the first 100 days), host defense is compromised by neutropenia and the disruption of mucocutaneous barriers. Late after transplantation (> 100 days), host defense is compromised by the slow recovery of cellular immunity, hypogammaglobulinemia, and immunosuppressive treatment of GVHD.

Bacterial Pneumonias Bacterial pneumonias are most common during the neutropenic preengraftment period, though they can occur at any time after HSCT with an overall incidence of 15%. Gram-negative enteric organisms, such as *Pseudomonas aeruginosa*, *Klebsiella pneumoniae*, and *Enterobacter cloacae*, predominate during the first 100 days.[98] Gram-positive organisms, particularly *Staphylococcus aureus*, are also seen, but are usually associated with bacteremia from the universal use of central venous catheters. Encapsulated organisms such as *Streptococcus pneumoniae* and *Haemophilus influenzae* play a larger role in the postengraftment period owing to the prolonged impairment of humoral immunity. Hospital-acquired pneumonias are associated with higher mortality than community-acquired,[98] and *Legionella pneumophila* has been reported as a cause of severe nosocomial pneumonia by several transplant centers.[99,100] The diagnosis of bacterial pneumonia is often difficult because of the nonspecific clinical presentation and the long differential diagnosis in HSCT patients (see below). A chest radiograph is not a reliable method for primary detection of pneumonia because of its low sensitivity; a chest CT scan, in addition to being more sensitive for diagnosis, also helps direct the localization of invasive diagnostic procedures. Broad-spectrum antibiotics, including antipseudomonal coverage, should be initiated in all patients with suspected bacterial pneumonia, especially in the setting of neutropenia.

Viral Pneumonias Cytomegalovirus (CMV) pneumonia was a major infectious problem in the early days of HSCT. More recently, the incidence of CMV pneumonia early after transplantation has declined markedly because of effective prophylaxis and preemptive treatment;[101–103] however, it remains a problem during the late phase of HSCT, with a current incidence of 2% in both allogeneic and autologous transplants. CMV seropositive recipients are at highest risk, reflecting reactivation of latent virus.[103] Ganciclovir is currently the treatment of choice, and combination therapy with CMV immunoglobulin has improved survival in nonrandomized prospective studies.[104–106] Despite treatment, mortality rates remain high, especially in patients with associated respiratory failure. Community-acquired viral respiratory infections are also important in HSCT recipients, with respiratory syncytial virus (RSV) accounting for the majority.[107] Upper respiratory tract symptoms of fever, coryza, and cough may progress to pneumonia in half of HSCT patients, which usually occurs as an early complication following transplantation. Mortality rates among those with RSV pneumonia approaches 80%, and initiation of treatment with aerosolized ribavirin and intravenous immunoglobulin initiated at the stage of upper respiratory infection is recommended to avoid progression.[108] Less often, other viruses, such as parainfluenza, adenovirus, herpes simplex virus, and seasonal outbreaks of influenza virus, may affect the lungs. These can be diagnosed either by nasal washings or bronchoalveolar lavage.

Fungal Pneumonias Invasive aspergillosis remains an important problem among HSCT patients, with a rising incidence and high mortality. The major risk factors include allogeneic HSCT, immunosuppressive therapy, corticosteroid use, CMV disease, and GVHD.[109] The use of high-efficiency particulate air (HEPA) filters can decrease the risk of invasive aspergillosis.[110] A recent shift in the incidence of this disease from the pre- to the postengraftment period is attributed to the shorter duration of neutropenia and delayed onsets of GVHD and CMV infection.[109] Other fungal infections occur less commonly and are described below in the section "Indirect Effects of Cancer and Cancer Therapy on the Lungs."

Miscellaneous Lung Infections The widespread use of prophylactic trimethoprim-sulfamethoxazole during the early transplant period has resulted in a significant decline in the incidence of *Pneumocystis* pneumonia, which is now primarily seen among sulfa-allergic patients receiving less effective prophylaxis.[111] Indolent infections with nontuberculous mycobacteria are relatively common at some transplant centers.[112]

Early-Onset Noninfectious Complications of HSCT **Pulmonary Edema** Diffuse pulmonary edema is one of the most common early complications after transplantation. Etiologies include increased hydrostatic pressure associated with the administration of large volumes of fluid or chemoradiation-induced cardiac toxicity and increased pulmonary capillary permeability (ALI/ARDS) associated with fat embolism or DMSO administration during stem cell infusion, chemoradiation-induced lung toxicity, sepsis, stem cell engraftment, acute GVHD, or aspiration.[96] Hydrostatic and permeability etiologies are often simultaneously present. Pleural effusions may accompany pulmonary edema. Bilateral pleural effusions associated with weight gain may be approached conservatively without diagnostic thoracentesis.

Engraftment Syndrome This is characterized by fever, noncardiogenic pulmonary edema, erythematous skin rash, and hypoxemia, and occurs during the neutrophil recovery phase following HSCT. Hemorrhagic fluid may be recovered on bronchoalveolar lavage (see DAH, below). Although the pathophysiology is not precisely understood, it appears to involve the release of proinflammatory cytokines during engraftment. The reported incidence varies widely with disease definition and the population studied, but is generally around 10% when stringent diagnostic criteria are used. Rates of engraftment syndrome are similar among autologous and allogeneic transplant recipients.[113,114] Risk factors include the use of growth factors, number of infused mononuclear or CD34 positive cells, speed of neutrophil recovery, type of conditioning regimen, underlying disease, and peripheral blood as the source of stem cells. Some studies have shown improvement with corticosteroid therapy,[113] including a recent study in which corticosteroid prophylaxis decreased the risk of engraftment syndrome without increasing the risk of infection.[115] Whereas the NIH-sponsored Blood and Marrow Transplant Clinical Trials Network includes engraftment syndrome within the definition of idiopathic pneumonia syndrome (see below), there may be value to considering it separately because of its responsiveness to corticosteroid therapy.

Idiopathic Pneumonia Syndrome (IPS) In 1993, a panel convened by the NIH proposed a broad working definition of IPS reportedly as widespread nonlobar radiographic infiltrates in the absence of congestive heart failure or evidence of lower respiratory tract infection.[116] IPS occurs in 7 to 70% of HSCT recipients, usually 14 to 90 days following transplantation. Mortality rates range from 50 to 70%.[117,118] Risk factors include transplantation for malignancy other than leukemia, older age, total body irradiation, type of pretransplant chemotherapy, high-grade GVHD, CMV-seropositive donor, HLA disparity, and lower performance status.[118] The pathogenesis of IPS is thought to include direct toxic effects of the chemoradiation conditioning regimen, occult infection, and the release of inflammatory cytokines. The association of IPS with GVHD in several studies suggests the involvement of alloreactive T lymphocytes.[118] The clinical presentation is nonspecific, with symptoms of acute dyspnea, cough, and fever associated with diffuse infiltrates on chest radiograph. The diagnosis of IPS largely relies on the exclusion of infection on lower respiratory samples obtained from bronchoalveolar lavage. The nonspecific findings of diffuse alveolar damage and interstitial pneumonitis on histopathologic examination of tissue from lung biopsies are typically not helpful in directing therapy.[116,118] Although no randomized controlled trials of treatment of IPS are available, current standards include high-dose intravenous corticosteroids and supportive care, such as supplemental oxygen and broad-spectrum antibiotics. Recent preclinical and clinical data suggest a potential role for tumor necrosis factor-α (TNF-α) in the pathogenesis of IPS, and a randomized trial using etanercept, a TNF receptor fusion protein, is being conducted by the Blood and Marrow Transplant Clinical Trials Network.

Diffuse Alveolar Hemorrhage (DAH) Post-transplant DAH was initially defined in autologous HSCT recipients as widespread lung injury manifested as diffuse radiographic infiltrates that occurred in the absence of identifiable infection.[119] Bronchoscopic criteria included progressively bloodier returns on bronchoalveolar lavage taken from three or more subsegmental bronchi. DAH is now known to occur in both allogeneic and autologous transplant recipients with equal frequency,[120–123] and the bronchoscopic criteria have expanded to include cytologic evidence of > 20% hemosiderin-laden macrophages in the bronchoalveolar lavage fluid. These bronchoscopic criteria, however, may be seen in association with diffuse lung injury from a wide variety of causes in the post-transplant setting, and the diagnostic and therapeutic implications of DAH are unclear. In an autopsy study, bloody bronchoalveolar lavage fluid was neither sensitive nor specific for histologic evidence of DAH.[124] The severity of thrombocytopenia does not predict DAH, although most patients are thrombocytopenic at the time of study so the lack of correlation may be due to a threshold effect. The bronchoscopic findings of DAH may simply represent an index of severity of alveolar injury and concomitant hemostatic defects rather than a separate syndrome, with prognosis and therapy more importantly determined by the underlying pathophysiologic process (engraftment syndrome, idiopathic pneumonia syndrome, sepsis, etc). The Blood and Marrow Transplant Clinical Trials Network has adopted this view and includes DAH within the definition of idiopathic pneumonia syndrome.

Pulmonary Veno-Occlusive Disease (PVOD) PVOD is a rare complication of HSCT in which progressive occlusion of pulmonary veins and venules caused by intimal proliferation and fibrosis leads to pulmonary hypertension.[125] High-dose chemotherapy and infections are implicated as causes of PVOD. The onset is typically insidious, with progressive dyspnea and fatigue occurring 6 to 8 weeks after transplant.[75,126] The diagnosis and treatment of PVOD are further described below in the section "Pulmonary Hypertension in the Cancer Patient."

Pulmonary Alveolar Proteinosis (PAP) PAP is another rare complication that may occur within the first 3 months after HSCT.[127] Patients typically present with slowly progressive dyspnea and a nonproductive cough. Bilateral diffuse alveolar densities and diffuse ground-glass attenuation with superimposed interlobular septal thickening and intralobular lines suggesting a "crazy paving" pattern on chest CT are nonspecific, but supportive radiographic findings. Bronchoscopic examination demonstrates copious, milky BAL effluent, which on cytologic examination contains foamy macrophages engorged with periodic acid-Schiff positive intracellular inclusions and granular, acellular eosinophilic proteinaceous material. Concentrically laminated phospholipid lamellar bodies may be seen on electron microscopy, which is occasionally necessary to confirm the diagnosis. Spontaneous reversal of PAP in this population has been described after the resolution of neutropenia.

Late-Onset Noninfectious Complications of HSCT **Constrictive Bronchiolitis** Constrictive bronchiolitis (CB) is the most common noninfectious pulmonary complication among long-term survivors of HSCT. It is a late manifestation of GVHD that leads to progressive respiratory insufficiency, and sometimes causes death. CB almost never occurs in the absence of GVHD, and thus only affects patients undergoing allogeneic transplant.[95,128,129] Because of the lack of uniform diagnostic criteria, its reported incidence varies from 10 to 26%. CB affects small airways, causing chronic inflammation, epithelial mucous metaplasia, submucosal scarring, smooth muscle hypertrophy, and concentric bronchiolar fibrosis. The most commonly identified risk factors are chronic GVHD, older age, viral infections during the first 100 days after transplant, the presence of airflow limitation before transplant, low serum IgG, and the use of methotrexate or busulfan in the conditioning regimen. Allergic airway diseases (rhinosinusitis and asthma) have not previously been associated with CB in the literature, but we have observed a high rate of allergic symptoms, as well as laboratory findings consistent with allergy, such as elevated eosinophil and IgE levels. The pathophysiology is not completely understood, but owing to its strong association with GVHD, it is believed that the disorder occurs because of the recruitment of donor lymphocytes to the airways by viral infection or allergic inflammation, which then reacts against recipient alloantigens in host bronchiolar epithelial and mesenchymal cells. The onset of CB is typically insidious, affecting patients 3 to 12 months after HSCT. Up to 20% of patients can be asymptomatic, with the rest presenting with progressive dyspnea, cough, and wheezing. Chest radiographs are usually normal, but high-resolution CT scans may show evidence of air trapping, thickened or dilated small airways, and mosaic attenuation. Bronchoscopy with BAL and transbronchial lung biopsy is generally not helpful in establishing the diagnosis. Although nonhistopathological diagnostic criteria for CB have not been established, poorly reversible airflow obstruction in the appropriate clinical setting is the hallmark of the disorder and constitutes sufficient evidence to begin therapy. The clinical course and disease progression are variable, but persistent airflow obstruction is associated with a significantly increased risk of death.[128] No prospective clinical trial has addressed the management of CB. Augmentation of immunosuppressive therapy and systemic corticosteroids are widely used based on anecdotal experience. We have found inhaled steroids to be very helpful in dosages as high as 1 mg twice daily, with slow stepwise reductions when lung function and symptoms remain stable. If sputum is present, physical measures should be undertaken to clear it, such as the use of a flutter valve, nebulized saline solution, and a compressive vest as part of a pulmonary rehabilitation program. A recent observational study showed a beneficial effect of azithromycin, possibly because of its anti-inflammatory effects.[130] Lung transplantation is an option in selected patients.

Cryptogenic Organizing Pneumonitis (COP) Also known as idiopathic bronchiolitis obliterans with organizing pneumonia (BOOP), COP occurs mostly in allogeneic HSCT recipients with GVHD or following CMV pneumonitis.[129,131] It is less common than CB, with an incidence of 1 to 2% in long-term survivors. Dry cough and dyspnea accompanied by patchy infiltrates on chest radiograph and CT scan are the predominant presenting findings. The diagnosis is made with surgical lung biopsy. COP is usually responsive to corticosteroids. The prognosis is worse than COP unrelated to HSCT, with an overall case fatality of 20%.

Delayed Pulmonary Toxicity Syndrome This syndrome has been described in breast cancer patients undergoing autologous HSCT. It is characterized by interstitial pneumonitis and fibrosis, and is thought to be due to the toxic effects of high dose chemotherapy, including cyclophosphamide, cisplatin, and BCNU. Patients usually present around 10 to 14 weeks following transplantation with dry cough, dyspnea, and fever.[132] Pulmonary function testing reveals restrictive lung disease and a reduction in diffusing capacity. These patients respond favorably to steroid therapy, and the mortality rate is low.

Post-Transplant Lymphoproliferative Disorder (PTLD) PTLD is an uncontrolled expansion of donor-derived EBV-infected B lymphocytes that develops in response to inadequate cytotoxic T-cell function.[95,133] It occurs in approximately 1% of HSCT patients, usually within the first 4 to 12 months after transplant. The lung is involved only 20% of the time, most commonly with ill-defined nodular infiltrates. PTLD has been successfully treated with donor leukocytes.

Lymphocytic Interstitial Pneumonitis (LIP) LIP is a rare manifestation of GVHD of the lung that presents 1 year to several years after transplant.[131,134,135] The most prominent symptom is dyspnea, and radiographs show diffuse, predominantly basilar, reticular and reticulonodular infiltrates. Thoracoscopic or open biopsy is usually required to obtain sufficient tissue for confident diagnosis. Lymphocytic infiltration of airway walls may be present in addition to infiltration of the parenchymal interstitium. The response to treatment with steroids is usually poor. Additional immunosuppressive agents may be tried, although large therapeutic trials supporting the efficacy of this practice have not been done.

PNEUMONIA

Pulmonary infections frequently complicate cancer and its therapy.[136,137] Diminished host inflammatory responses and the emergence of multidrug-resistant (MDR) organisms associated with recurrent exposures to hospital environments may give rise to life-threatening infections and magnify the difficulty of diagnosing and treating pneumonia in the cancer setting. As a consequence of the blunted inflammatory response, the typical clinical observations of pneumonia, including purulent respiratory secretions and early radiographic findings may be conspicuously absent. Adding to this diagnostic challenge is the frequent colonization of the upper airway with nondisease-associated microorganisms, rendering the diagnosis of pneumonia by conventional culture techniques difficult. Conversely, sterile respiratory tract cultures do not exclude an infectious etiology, particularly in the setting of recent exposure to broad-spectrum antibiotics. Host susceptibility to infection is not only conditioned by the type and degree of immune suppression, but also by its duration. Multiple immune defects may coexist among patients with cancer, which adds to the conundrum and spectrum of opportunistic infections. Immune defects, including compromised acellular and cellular (alveolar macrophages, mast cells, neutrophils) innate immune responses, and altered adaptive immune function, leading to either inadequate immunoglobulin or defective T-cell mediated defenses may promote the development of specific types of pneumonia. In addition, treatment-induced disruption of the respiratory mucosa and ciliary dysfunction resulting in inadequate clearing and stagnation of bronchial secretions enhance the emergence of certain types of pneumonia. Hence, the predilection for pneumonia in the cancer setting is best understood by examining the effect of malignancy and its treatment on specific host immune defenses. Because the immune defect is often mixed, careful attention to clinical and radiographic features and recognition of community acquired versus nosocomial or health care-associated sources of the infection are critical additional pieces of information that may help in making the diagnosis and guiding empiric antimicrobial therapy.[138] Delays in appropriate antimicrobial therapy increase the risk of secondary complications and infection-associated deaths, especially in severely immunosuppressed individuals. Therefore, it is common practice to initiate empiric and/or preemptive antimicrobial therapy in patients in which the suspicion of infection is high. An approach to the diagnosis and treatment of cancer-related pneumonias based on the specific defects in the major arm(s) of host immunity and broad categories of infection source is emphasized in the early part of this section, followed by a more detailed discussion of selected pathogens that may cause fulminant infection in the cancer patient.

Specific Immune Defects Damage to local host airway defense mechanisms commonly follows cancer therapy and increases host vulnerability to infection. Breach of the respiratory mucosa and altered mucociliary function may occur as a direct result of cancer therapy. In addition, nasogastric and endotracheal tubes hinder coordinated glottic activities and mucociliary function and act as conduits for chronic colonization of pathogenic organisms.[139] Furthermore, impaired local innate airway defense mechanisms, including derangements in alveolar macrophage chemotaxis, phagocytosis, and killing, and compromised host defense caused by treatment-related alterations in mast cell, epithelial cell, and macrophage activities significantly heighten the risk of infection. Simultaneous alterations in systemic defense mechanisms, such as the innate immune system are common. Neutrophils are exquisitely sensitive to the cytotoxic effects of chemotherapy, which may induce an agranulocytosis by direct myelotoxicity, as well as functional neutropenia by interfering with the phagocytic and chemotactic activity of these cells.[140] In addition, neutrophil dysfunction as a corollary of radiation therapy, corticosteroid administration and common cancer-related disorders, such as hypovolemia, prolonged hypoxemia, acidosis, and poorly controlled hyperglycemia is a frequent problem. Severe neutropenia, defined as an absolute neutrophil count of ≤ 500/μL is associated with recalcitrant lung infections caused by bacterial and fungal organisms.[141] In addition, the rapidity of onset of neutropenia and delay in neutrophil recovery play a role in the infection severity. More than 10% of patients with febrile neutropenia present with pulmonary infiltrates, and infection remains the most frequent cause of radiographic abnormalities in these patients. The absence of pulmonary consolidations on chest radiographs does not exclude an evolving cryptic pneumonia, particularly in the setting of profound neutropenia (< 100 cells/μL). Severe pneumonias, including de novo infections and exacerbation of chronic lung infections may occur in the setting of neutropenia. Gram-negative bacilli, including Enterobacteriaceae (*Klebsiella*, *Escherichia coli*, *Enterobacter*, *Citrobacter*, *Serratia*), and *Proteus* species,[142] are the predominant source of pneumonias associated with neutropenic fever. MDR gram-positive bacteria such as methicillin-resistant *Staphylococcus aureus* (MRSA), and extended spectrum beta-lactamase producing Enterobacteriaceae are other bacterial pathogens in patients with pneumonias associated with febrile neutropenia. The incidence of pulmonary infections caused by gram-positive bacteria (*Staphylococcus aureus*, *Streptococcus* species, including *Streptococcus pneumoniae*) has decreased over the past 3 decades, while gram-negative pneumonias, particularly those caused by *Pseudomonas* species have become an increasing source of life-threatening infections.[143] Hematogenous dissemination represents another source of pneumonia, and bacteremia in febrile neutropenic patients may not present with an obvious primary site of origin. Initial antimicrobial therapy for febrile neutropenia in patients with pulmonary infiltrates should be broad in spectrum and provide antimicrobial activity against MDR strains of *S. aureus* and *Pseudomonas aeruginosa*. Early de-escalation therapy may be attempted in patients who have demonstrated prompt clinical response and in whom gran-

Table 135-3 Infections Causing Pneumonia in Cancer Patients Based on the Underlying Immune Defect

Immune Defect	Bacteria	Fungi	Parasites	Viruses
Granulocytopenia	*Staphylococcus aureus* *Streptococcus pneumoniae* *Streptococcus* spp *Pseudomonas aeruginosa* Enterobacteriaceae *Escherichia coli* *Klebsiella* spp *Stenotrophomonas maltophilia* *Acinetobacter species*	*Aspergillus fumigatus;* non-*fumigatus Aspergillus* Non-*Aspergillus* hyalohyphomycosis such as *Pseudallescheria boydii, Fusarium solani* *Mucorales* (zygomycoses) Dematiaceous (Black) fungi such as *Alternaria, Bipolaris, Curvularia, Scedosporium apiospermum* *Scedosporium prolificans*		Herpes simplex virus I & II Varicella-zoster virus
Cellular immune dysfunction	*Nocardia asteroids complex* *Salmonella typhimurium* *Salmonella enteritidis* *Rhodococcus equi* *Rhodococcus bronchialis* *Listeria monocytogenes* *Mycobacterium tuberculosis* Nontuberculous mycobacteria	*Aspergillus* and non-*Aspergillus* filamentous molds *Pneumocystis jiroveci (P. carinii)* *Cryptococcus neoformans* Endemic mycoses due to *Histoplasma capsulatum, Coccidioides immitis, Blastomyces dermatitidis*	*Toxoplasma gondii* *Microsporidium* spp *Leishmania donovani* *Leishmania infantum* *Strongyloides stercoralis*	Human cytomegalovirus Respiratory viruses Influenza A & Influenza B Parainfluenza type-3 Respiratory syncytial virus Adenovirus Varicella-zoster virus HHV-6 SARS-associated coronavirus? Paramyxovirus? Hantavirus?
Humoral immune dysfunction Splenectomy	*Streptococcus pneumoniae* *Haemophilus influenzae* *Neisseria meningitides* *Capnocytophaga canimorsus* *Campylobacter*	*Pneumocystis jiroveci (P. carinii)*?	*Giardia lamblia* *Babesia microti*	Varicella-zoster virus Echovirus Enterovirus
Mixed Defects	*Streptococcus pneumoniae* *Staphylococcus aureus* *Haemophilus influenzae* *Klebsiella pneumonia* *Pseudomonas aeruginosa* *Acinetobacter* spp *Enterobacter* spp *Stenotrophomonas maltophilia* *Nocardia* asteroids complex *Listeria monocytogenes* *Legionella* spp	*Pneumocystis jiroveci (P. carinii)* *Aspergillus* spp *Candida* spp *Cryptococcus neoformans* *Mucorales* (zygomycoses) Endemic mycoses (severe systemic dissemination)	*Toxoplasma gondii* *Strongyloides stercoralis*	Respiratory viruses Influenza Parainfluenza Respiratory syncytial virus Adenovirus Varicella-zoster virus

ulocyte recovery has occurred or is expected to occur in the near future. De-escalation should be undertaken with caution in high-risk patients with poor clinical response to antimicrobial therapy; persistent, severe, long-standing granulocytopenia; or patients on systemic immunosuppressive therapy.

In addition to neutropenia, cancer therapy and certain hematologic malignancies may cause severe depression of the humoral and cellular arms of adaptive immunity, resulting in inadequate immunoglobulin production and a variety of defective T- and B-cell–mediated defenses. For example, immunoglobulin dyscrasias associated with hypo-gammaglobulinemia and defects in opsonization owing to asplenism are frequent problems among patients with certain types of lymphoreticular malignancies, such as multiple myeloma, chronic lymphocytic leukemia, and Waldenström's macroglobulinemia. Hypocomplementemia associated with asplenism may lead to unchecked proliferation of encapsulated organisms that require opsonization with complement (C_3, C_5) for elimination. Furthermore, defects in antibody-dependent lymphocyte cytolytic activity may lead to fulminant parasitic infections. Altered T-cell numbers and activity is a frequent finding among patients with Hodgkin's disease, hairy-cell leukemia, adult T-cell leukemia, lymphocytic leukemia, and graft-versus-host disease (GVHD). In addition, viral illnesses, antineoplastic agents, and other immunosuppressive drugs (fludarabine, IL-2 inhibitors, antithymocyte globulins, calcineurin inhibitors, tacrolimus, glucocorticosteroids) that are commonly used in the armamentarium of cancer therapy may depress the cellular arm of the immune system by inducing profound lymphopenia and/or interrupting activated T-cell signal transduction pathways. Patients with cellular immune dysfunction are at increased risk of infection caused by intracellular organisms such as *Listeria monocytogenes*, *Salmonella*, *Legionella* spp, *Pneumocystis*, *Toxoplasma gondii*, invasive pulmonary mycoses, and opportunistic viruses due to human cytomegalovirus, human herpesvirus 6 (HHV-6) and varicella-zoster virus. Thus, all components of the host immune system may be assaulted by cancer and the simultaneous depression of more than one arm of host defense is common in this setting. The severe and oftentimes protracted immune suppression that follows encourages the development of unusual and intractable infections. Specific pathogens causing pneumonia that are commonly associated with depression of particular immune defects are listed in Table 135-3.

COMMUNITY-ACQUIRED PNEUMONIA Community acquired pneumonia (CAP), defined by the Infectious Disease Society of America (IDSA), refers to the radiographic and clinical appearance of pneumonia that develops among patients who have not been hospitalized or who have not resided in a nursing home for 14 or more days prior to the onset of symptoms.[138] The distinction of CAP from nosocomial or hospital-acquired pneumonia (HAP) is an important one that roughly permits prognostic estimations based on epidemiologic descriptions of the underlying cause and provides a framework for decisions regarding the diagnostic evaluation and empiric antimicrobial therapy.

The etiologic spectrum of bacterial pathogens causing CAP among those cancer patients with mild to moderate immunosuppression is similar to that of patients with no cancer history. However, a small microbial inoculum that typically would be of no clinical significance in the general population may cause severe infection among patients with underlying malignancy. *Streptococcus pneumoniae* remains the most commonly defined pathogen and the most frequent cause of lethal CAP.[138] Superinfection with multidrug-resistant organisms is an emerging problem and complicates the management of CAP. Other causative bacterial pathogens in CAP, including *Staphylococcus aureus*, nontypeable strains of *Haemophilus influenzae*, *Pseudomonas* pneumonia, and other gram-negative bacilli (GNB) may also cause life-threatening infections. Recently, other nonfermentative (NF)-GNB such as *Stenotrophomonas*, *Burkholderia*, *Chryseobacterium*, *Achromobacter*, and *Alcaligenes* species have been increasingly recognized as etiologic agents in both CAP and nosocomial infections.[144,145] Less frequently encountered are CAPs caused by *Streptococcus pyogenes*, *Neisseria meningitides*, and *Moraxella catarrhalis*. The frequency of CAP associated with the atypical agents, *Mycoplasma pneumoniae*, *Chlamydia pneumoniae*, and *Legionella* species varies widely with patient age and geographic location. Viral pneumonias, most commonly influenza, parainfluenza, and adenoviral infections are sources of CAP, which may cause severe pneumonias in the cancer setting.

Radiographic evidence of lobar consolidation is common in CAP. Diffuse, multicentric pulmonary disease may also be seen and, when present, heralds a poor outcome. The diagnosis of CAP is based on recovery of the likely agent from an uncontaminated specimen (blood, urine, pleural fluid), the isolation of an organism in respiratory secretions that does not normally colonize the respiratory tract, or positive results of selected serologic tests. Although the utility of Gram's staining and culture of expectorated sputum in the diagnosis of pneumonia has been debated for years, careful procurement of sputum specimens in which cytologic screening has confirmed the presence of lower-airway secretions appears to be diagnostically useful, particularly if obtained before the initiation of antimicrobial therapy. Early and accurate diagnoses are critical to a successful outcome, although treatment should not be withheld while diagnostic interventions are undertaken. Antimicrobial selections are based on knowledge of the infecting pathogen, if available, pneumonia severity, underlying immune status, and the presence of comorbid conditions.[146,147]

Hospital-Acquired Pneumonia Lung infections that occur more than 48 hours after hospital admission and in patients without antecedent clinical symptoms or radiographic findings suggestive of pneumonia are referred to as nosocomial pneumonia or HAP. HAP is a common complication in patients receiving therapy for cancer. Recently, the American Thoracic Society (ATS) and the IDSA recognized health care-associated pneumonia (HCAP) as a distinct entity within the spectrum of hospital-acquired pneumonia (HAP) and ventilator-associated pneumonia (VAP).[148] HCAP includes all patients hospitalized in an acute care hospital for 2 or more days within 90 days of the current infection; patients treated in a hospital or hemodialysis clinic within 30 days of the pneumonia diagnosis; residents of a nursing home or long-term care facility; and recipients of intravenous antibiotics, chemotherapy, or wound care within the past 30 days of the current infection. HAP, including HCAP and VAP, comprises the majority of pneumonias in the cancer setting. The spectrum of pathogens in HCAP more closely resembles late-onset HAP and VAP, particularly among elderly patients.[149] Thus, guidelines for the management of HCAP generally overlap with HAP and VAP. In the nonimmunosuppressed solid-organ cancer patient, HAP is most often seen in the intensive care units (ICUs). In fact, admission to the ICU increases the risk of pneumonia in these patients by nearly 20-fold. As many as 80% of ICU-related HAPs occur among patients receiving assisted ventilatory support, and the effect of ventilator-associated pneumonia (VAP) in increasing the length of ICU stay, days on the ventilator, and overall length of hospital admission and cost is well documented.[150] The etiologic spectrum of microbial pathogens causing HAP among low-risk solid-organ cancer patients with no recent antibiotic exposure is similar to that seen in the general population. *Haemophilus influenzae*, *Streptococcus pneumoniae*, *S. aureus*, and Enterobacteriaceae may be encountered. MRSA may cause recalcitrant HAP, especially among patients with prior community-acquired MRSA colonization antibiotic exposure, advanced age, and prolonged ventilatory support. Protracted mechanical ventilation and recent antibiotic administration are also associated with increased rates of HAP caused by *Pseudomonas aeruginosa*, *Acinetobacter baumannii* complex, *Enterobacter* spp, and emerging strains of MDR NF-GNB, such as *Stenotrophomonas maltophilia*, *Burkholderia cepacia* complex, and *Alcaligenes* (*Achromobacter*) species, which may be difficult to treat. Severe neutropenia remains an independent predictor of HAP and VAP due to NF-GNB. Mortality rates associated with nosocomial pneumonias due to MRSA or *Pseudomonas aeruginosa* are disproportionately higher than those caused by nosocomial lung infections due to other bacterial pathogens.[150] Polymicrobial isolates and MDR pathogens, including MRSA, are more common among patients with HAP, particularly when it occurs as a late complication during hospitalization. Recent evidence-based guidelines advocate the use of semiquantitative or quantitative lower respiratory tract cultures obtained either bronchoscopically or noninvasively as part of the initial evaluation of the patients with suspected HAP, VAP, or HCAP.[148]

Empiric antibiotic selections for HAP that develop within ≤ 7 days following hospitalization should target *H. influenzae*, *S. pneumoniae*, *S. aureus* (including MRSA), *Streptococcus* spp, and Enterobacteriaceae. Patients with late HAP (occurring > 1 week after hospitalization) should receive empiric antimicrobial therapy that includes coverage for MDR-GNB. The scope of alternative antimicrobial choices in patients with refractory or slow-to-respond HAP and/or VAP should be based on institution-dependent susceptibility profiles.

Pneumonias Caused by Aspiration and Bronchial Obstruction Aspiration of orointestinal contents and mechanical obstruction of the airways may create a favorable milieu for pneumonia caused by microaerophilic or anaerobic bacteria (*Peptostreptococcus* spp). A variety of factors, such as abnormal swallowing function, altered cough reflex, impaired respiratory mucociliary clearance, altered mental status, the frequent use of sedating medications, chemotherapy-induced mucositis, supine positioning, gastroparesis, the need for mechanical ventilation, and nasogastric tube feeding contribute to the increased predilection to aspirate in the cancer setting. Pneumonia associated with large-volume aspiration of gastric contents typically occurs as a late finding. The acidic gastric contents act as a poor medium for bacterial overgrowth. Thus, the earliest clinical response to gastric aspiration is due to the direct caustic effect of the acidic aspirate on the cells lining the alveolar-capillary interface. Pneumonia due to superimposed bacterial infection, if it occurs, presents as a late finding. ARDS, respiratory failure, and death may rapidly follow. Aspiration of oral contents, by contrast, results from inhalation of nonsterile oropharyngeal material. The clinical presentation is often insidious and the diagnosis is commonly inferred based on a compatible patient risk profile coupled with radiographic evidence of pneumonia. Chest radiographs may show areas of geographic abnormalities that correlate with the patient's position at the time of aspiration. For example, aspiration that occurs while the patient is in the upright position typically localizes to the basilar segments of the lower lobes, whereas the superior segments of the lower lobes and posterior segments of the upper lobes are more frequently affected following aspiration that occurs in the supine position. The major pathogens underlying nosocomial versus community-acquired aspiration pneumonias differ, and in a substantial portion of patients, a microbiologic diagnosis may not be established because of the limited yield of conventional anaerobic cultures. The management of patients with significant lung injury associated with the aspiration of gastric contents includes aggressive supportive care. Upper airway suctioning, pulmonary toileting, continuous positive airway pressure (CPAP), or mechanical ventilation with the application of positive end-expiratory pressure (PEEP) comprises the mainstay of therapy. Early and aggressive antimicrobial therapy is recommended for patients with pneumonia secondary to aspiration of oropharyngeal contents. Antimicrobial selections should be tailored according to the immune status of the patient and the setting in which the aspiration occurred (community versus nosocomial), but in general should be broad in spectrum and target gram-negative organisms with or without anaerobic coverage. Anaerobic coverage should be considered for patients with periodontal disease, putrid sputum, or evidence of necrotizing pneumonia.[151]

Carcinomas of the lung or metastatic lung lesions may cause partial obstruction of the airways and associated atelectasis and postobstructive pneumonia. Airway obstruction in this setting may be due to endobronchial tumor or a rapidly enlarging extraluminal mass. The associated pneumonias tend to be polymicrobial in etiology (gram-negative bacilli, staphylococci, anaerobes) and may require relief of the obstruction with chemoradiation therapy or invasive bronchoscopic measures (stent placement, tumor debulking, endobronchial brachytherapy) in addition to antimicrobial therapy to ensure adequate drainage and treatment of the affected lung.

Other Sources of Pneumonia The lungs may also become infected via septic emboli arising from suppurative endovascular bacterial and, rarely, fungal infections. Infected intravascular septic deep venous thrombi are increasingly recognized as a potential source of infection in patients with cancer. The radiographic pattern in these patients is distinctive and includes multicentric, pleomorphic lung nodules, with asymmetric, relatively small, thick-walled cavities.

SPECIFIC PATHOGENS

Nocardiosis *Nocardia asteroides* complex, including *Nocardia asteroides sensu stricto* and *Nocardia farcinica*, account for nearly 90% of *Nocardia* infections. Susceptibility profiles for *Nocardia* pneumonia include profound deficiency in cellular immunity, prolonged use of high-dose systemic corticosteroids, especially in the treatment of chronic lung diseases,[152] and the presence of GVHD. Infections are suppurative. Occasionally granulomatous reactions occur. Nodular pulmonary lesions are common, although reticulonodular or diffuse infiltrates are occasionally described. Solitary lung nodules associated with irregular, thick-walled cavities that mimic invasive pulmonary aspergillosis, necrotizing cancer, or chronic bacterial lung abscess have also been reported. Indolent *Nocardia* pneumonia is clinically indistinguishable from other actinomycetes infections and from pneumonias caused by pulmonary eumycetes infections. Severely immunosuppressed cancer patients with refractory leukemia or allogeneic HSCT may present with pulmonary nocardiosis, a rapidly progressive, often multicentric form of *Nocardia*. Concomitant brain involvement is common, and preemptive evaluation is recommended to diagnose asymptomatic brain abscesses. Trimethoprim-sulfamethoxazole (10–12 mg/kg daily) is effective against most *Nocardia* spp. Retrospective studies suggest improved outcome when the drug is given for an extended period of time (6–12 months).[153] Despite appropriate therapy, pulmonary nocardiosis carries a high mortality in high-risk cancer patients.[152]

Tuberculosis *Mycobacterium tuberculosis* is a rare cause of pulmonary infection in the developed world. It is occasionally found in severely immunosuppressed cancer patients and in foreign-born individuals receiving cancer care in nonendemic regions of the world. Patients with Hodgkin's disease and cancers of the head and neck, lung, and breast are considered at highest risk.[154] Most pulmonary tuberculous infections in oncology centers in the United States are caused by reactivation of a remotely acquired latent infection. Pulmonary tuberculosis may present as an insidious pneumonia that is difficult to distinguish from actinomycetes and eumycetes infection. Patients with impaired T-cell response may develop acute, rapidly progressive tuberculosis that may follow the course of a virulent bacterial infection. Systemic corticosteroid therapy is an independent predictor both of tuberculosis reactivation and of a suboptimal response to combination antimicrobial therapy. Hence, once the diagnosis of tuberculosis is established, every effort should be made to discontinue steroid therapy.[154]

Nontuberculous Mycobacteriosis Pulmonary nontuberculous mycobacteriosis (NTM) is classically caused by *Mycobacterium avium* intracellular complex and other slow-growing mycobacteria. These opportunistic pathogens can lead to chronic, indolent lung infections. In the United States, the rapidly growing mycobacteria, (particularly *Mycobacterium abscessus* and *Mycobacterium fortuitum*, *Mycobacterium smegmatis*, and *Mycobacterium gondii*) have emerged as less frequent causes of NTM infections. The diagnosis of pulmonary NTM remains a challenge, as identification of these mycobacteria in respiratory culture samples may result from colonization of the respiratory tract or environmental contamination. Causality is suggested by identification of NTM in sterile lower respiratory tract samples coupled with nonspecific clinical features, such as chronic nonproductive cough and exertional dyspnea. The cough may occasionally become productive, indicating underlying bronchiectasis. Fever, night sweats, weight loss, pleuritic chest pain, and pleural effusions are seldom seen. Radiographic features include nonspecific nodular lesions and small, thin-walled cavities. Chest CT findings, demonstrating the characteristic "tree-in-bud" appearance may also be seen in patients with chronic infection. Lady Windermere syndrome, characterized by relapsing or refractory pulmonary NTM due to slow-growing mycobacteria, may be seen in patients with defects in endogenous interferon-gamma activity.[155] NTM pulmonary infections are usually insidious, although rapidly progressive disease has been seen in patients with profound defects in helper T cells. Treatment should include at least two antimicrobial agents to which the mycobacterium is susceptible and should be given for 12 to 24 months. *Mycobacterium kansasii* is antigenically similar to *Mycobacterium tuberculosis* and causes lung disease that is clinically and radiographically indistinguishable from pulmonary tuberculosis. Endemic areas for *M. kansasii* infections in the United States include the urban southeast and midwestern states. Pneumoconiosis is a well-established predisposing condition. Upper lobe, thin-walled cavities are commonly present on chest radiographs. Prolonged therapy (12–18 months) with rifampin plus one or two other susceptible antimicrobials is recommended.

Pneumocystis Pneumonia (PCP) *Pneumocystis jiroveci* infections are primarily seen in patients with marked CD4 lymphocytopenia.[156] In most cancer patients, PCP presents as a slowly progressive infection accompanied by nonproductive cough, exertional dyspnea, and hypoxemia, although an acute form of PCP that rapidly progresses to respiratory failure and ARDS has been reported. CT evidence of perihilar infiltrates may be mistaken for pneumonitis caused by common community-acquired viral infections (RSV, influenza, parainfluenza type 3) or CMV during the early phase of the infection. Bronchoalveolar lavage has a high diagnostic yield. Lung biopsy is occasionally needed to establish the diagnosis in patients with chronic PCP, which is associated with a low fungal burden and false-negative BAL. High-dose trimethoprim-sulfamethoxazole given for 21 days is the treatment of choice. Adjuvant systemic corticosteroids should be administered to patients with severe hypoxemia ($PaO_2 < 70$, A-a gradient > 35). Oral atovaquone and parenteral pentamidine may be given to patients who are intolerant to sulfa-containing regimens.

Invasive Pulmonary Mycosis Invasive pulmonary aspergillosis is the most common fungal pneumonia in cancer patients. Susceptibility profiles for invasive pulmonary aspergillosis include patients with prolonged (> 1 week) and severe (< 100 cells/μL) neutropenia, refractory leukemia, allogeneic HSCT, GVHD immunosuppressive therapy, and those receiving high-dose systemic corticosteroids.[157,158] *Aspergillus fumigatus* is most prominent in this group. Amphotericin B-resistant *Aspergillus terreus* has recently emerged as the second most frequent *Aspergillus* spp in cancer patients.[159] The near-exponential rise in pulmonary invasive fungal infections due to non-*Aspergillus* molds such as *Fusarium*, *Pseudallescheria boydii*, *Scedosporium apiospermum*, *Scedosporium prolificans*, and the dematiaceous (black) molds that are often not susceptible to conventional antifungal agents pose a serious challenge in the selection of effective empiric and preemptive therapy. Fever, cough, and dyspnea, when present, suggest widespread lung infection. Hemoptysis may be a salient clinical feature. Chest imaging studies are frequently nonspecific, though CT scans may reveal a highly suggestive "halo sign" or "crescent sign." In most cases of pulmonary mycosis, the only radiographic findings at the time of presentation are peripheral, pleural-based lung nodules, with thick-walled regular or irregular cavities.[160] Diffuse alveolar hemorrhage may occasionally herald an underlying invasive pulmonary fungal infection.

A decline in the incidence of endemic mycoses, such as pulmonary histoplasmosis, blastomycosis, and coccidioidomycosis, as well as ubiquitous *Cryptococcus neoformans* infections, has been reported, which has largely been attributed to effective prophylaxis with fluconazole in immunosuppressed cancer patients. The incidence of zygomycosis, on the other hand, has increased at our institution. This rise in *Zygomycetes* infection rates is likely related to the increased utilization of the recently available antifungal agent, voriconazole, with a concomitant decline in the use of amphotericin B. *Zygomycetes* organisms typically show a high level of susceptibility to amphotericin B. With the decreased utilization of this agent, rates of fungal infections at our institution caused by zygomycosis, invasive aspergillosis, and Fusarium species during the years 2002 to 2004 were 0.095/1,000, 0.302/1,000, and 0.073/1,000 patient days, respectively.[161]

The diagnosis of pulmonary invasive fungal infection requires demonstration of fungal hyphae within the involved lung tissue and is often made by inference, as tissue biopsies are seldom available. It is important to note that the isolation of molds in patients from peripheral or central venous blood samples may not indicate disseminated mycosis, even in severely immunosuppressed allogeneic HSCT recipients.[162] Similarly, isolation of fungi in respiratory samples may misrepresent the etiology of underlying pulmonary infiltrates. Therefore, the current consensus for invasive fungal infections diagnosis includes: (1) evaluation of host's predisposing factors, such as prolonged granulocytopenia, high-risk HSCT, GVHD, and immunosuppressive therapy; (2) clinical features (less often seen in cancer and stem cell transplant recipients); (3) radiographic features (as mentioned earlier); and (4) isolation of pathogenic fungus from sterile respiratory sites. The measurement of fungal antigens such as serum galactomannan levels may be helpful in the detection of pulmonary mycosis. In a recent study of HSCT recipients, serum galactomannan levels were diagnostic in > 85% of patients. The diagnostic utility of this test, however, is markedly compromised in the setting of antifungal therapy.[163] Newer diagnostic tests, including mycotic DNA amplification in sterile samples are currently under investigation and need clinical validation before routine use is recommended.

The treatment of pulmonary mycosis has improved considerably in the past 5 years. In a recent study in which patients were randomized to receive voriconazole, a new broad-spectrum triazole agent or the "gold standard" amphotericin B as primary therapy for invasive pulmonary aspergillosis, voriconazole was shown to have superior efficacy and safety profiles.[164] In another study, salvage therapy with caspofungin, a new fungal cell-wall–lytic agent, in patients with refractory invasive aspergillosis or those intolerant to conventional antimicrobial therapy showed an encouraging 50% response rate.[165] Antifungal combinations may be prescribed for high-risk cancer patients and HSCT recipients with invasive mycosis. Because of the lack of prospective randomized trials, there is no consensus in recommending preferred antifungal combinations. A preliminary study using various antifungal combinations hinted modest superiority of caspofungin plus voriconazole in HSCT recipients with invasive fungal infections.[166] Restitution of the host's immune defects, including recovery of severe granulocytopenia remains the critical determinant in promoting resolution of invasive fungal infections and in the response to antifungal therapy. Donor granulocyte transfusions and adjuvant recombinant TH1 cytokines need prospective evaluation, albeit the results of preliminary observational studies among high-risk allogeneic HSCT recipients with disseminated mycosis appear promising.[167]

Viral Pneumonitis Human cytomegalovirus pneumonia is the most frequent cause of opportunistic viral complications in cancer patients with a defective cellular immune response. Pulmonary varicella-zoster virus (VZV) and human herpesvirus 6 (HHV-6) lung infections are difficult to distinguish from CMV pneumonitis. Seasonal respiratory viruses (RSV, influenza A and B, parainfluenza type 3, and adenovirus) may also lead to serious lower respiratory tract infections in immunosuppressed patients. Fever and nonproductive cough are prominent nonspecific features. In patients with extensive lung involvement, dyspnea may appear early in the course of infection. Viral antigen detection in nasal washes, tracheal aspirates, and bronchial specimens are most frequently used in determining active viral replication in the upper and lower respiratory tracts. Chest CT scans may show ground-glass infiltrates in the setting of a normal conventional chest radiograph. A normal chest CT scan in high-risk HSCT recipients with suspected viral pneumonitis excludes the possibility of infection in > 95% of cases. The presence of CMV viremia is another helpful indicator in determining the etiology of a pulmonary process. The isolation of CMV antigen from lower respiratory tract secretions may not necessarily indicate pulmonary infection, however, as patients with cellular immune defects may have intermittent low-level viral replication and shed virus without developing disease. Ganciclovir or foscarnet are commonly prescribed for systemic CMV and HHV-6 infections. Antiviral combinations with adjuvant immunoglobulin therapy is associated with variable results and presently not recommended for routine use.

Miscellaneous Pulmonary *Toxoplasma gondii* and *Listeria monocytogenes* infections can lead to serious, often life-threatening complications in patients with profound cellular immune dysfunction, and disease characteristics are described in detail elsewhere.[168]

VENOUS THROMBOEMBOLISM

Pulmonary embolism (PE) and deep venous thrombosis (DVT) are the two manifestations of venous thromboembolism (VTE), a common complication in cancer. Approximately 20% of VTE in the general population is associated with cancer, and cancer increases the risk of VTE about 5-fold. Therapy for cancer, including surgery, chemotherapy, hormonal therapy, growth factors, angiogenesis inhibitors, and central venous catheters (CVC), further heightens the risk of thrombosis.[169] For example, patients with cancer experience a 2- to 3-fold increase in the risk of VTE associated with any surgical procedure; the incidence of VTE in postmenopausal women receiving chemotherapy and tamoxifen for breast cancer is 10%, and in renal cancer patients receiving thalidomide-based chemotherapy regimens the incidence of VTE is more than 40%. Although fatality rates directly attributable to VTE among cancer patients have not been firmly established, prospective analyses have demonstrated a 4- to 8-fold increase in VTE-associated mortality over patients without cancer.[170]

VTE has many clinical presentations, most of which are not specific. Algorithms and "score" systems developed to assist in the estimation of a pretest probability of VTE in the general population are useless in the cancer population, in which the mere presence of malignancy entails such a

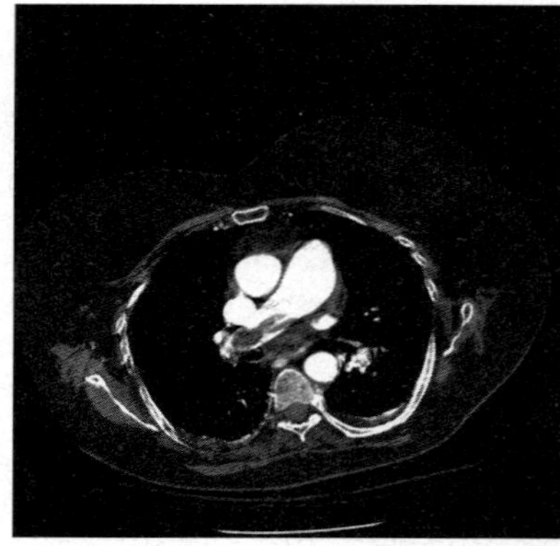

Figure 135-10 Computed tomography angiogram showing large central embolus in a patient treated with thalidomide for malignant melanoma.

high risk. D-dimer assays are helpful screening tests with an excellent negative predictive value in both the noncancer and cancer setting. The likelihood of finding a normal D-dimer level among cancer patients, however, is less than 30%, which significantly diminishes the utility of this examination in the cancer setting.[171] Venous ultrasound is the preferred method to diagnose DVT, although MRI and CT may be required in special circumstances, such as internal iliac vein or vena cava thrombosis. Perfusion/ventilation (V/Q) lung scans remain useful in the diagnosis of PE. The sensitivity and specificity of CT pulmonary angiography in the diagnosis of central thrombosis is equivalent if not superior to V/Q scans. Furthermore, CT angiography offers the advantage of providing additional information regarding competing thoracic pathology that may confound the diagnosis of PE (Figure 135-10).[172]

VTE prophylaxis is of proven efficacy among at-risk patients and should be considered in almost every patient with cancer.[173] Thromboprophylaxis among cancer patients should follow current recommendations for medical and surgical patients in the general population, although some cancer-specific recommendations do exist. Low molecular weight heparins (LMWH) are the most studied agents in this population, and their use is encouraged. Cancer patients undergoing abdominal or pelvic surgery should receive LMWH[174,175] prophylaxis for at least 4 weeks.[176] Results of studies evaluating prolonged prophylaxis after other surgical interventions are pending. In the past, fixed low-dose warfarin and LMWH were regularly used for the prevention of CVC thrombosis. This practice was based on the results of older, open-label investigations. More recent, larger, and better-controlled studies contradict these findings[177,178] and support the current opinion that no prophylaxis should be used for CVC thrombosis. Finally, the use of VTE prophylaxis during chemotherapy is currently being intensely evaluated with contradictory results.

Definitive therapy for established VTE follows general recommendations. Current recommendations include LMWH for most patients, UFH for patients with renal failure, thrombolysis in cases of massive PE, and IVC filters when there are clear contraindications for anticoagulation.[179] Based on recent evidence, the long-term treatment or secondary prophylaxis of VTE in cancer patients should include at least 6 months of LMWH instead of warfarin.[180] Whether there is any added benefit in extending therapy beyond 6 months is currently the subject of ongoing studies.

PULMONARY HYPERTENSION IN THE CANCER PATIENT

Pulmonary hypertension, defined as mean arterial pressures above 25 mm Hg at rest or 30 mm Hg during exercise, is a relatively common problem in the cancer setting. Echocardiographic evidence of an increased tricuspid regurgitant jet velocity, which reliably corresponds to elevated pulmonary artery pressures, is commonly used to diagnose pulmonary hypertension.[181] Cancer-related risk factors for pulmonary hypertension may be sorted according to those that predominantly affect the large pulmonary arteries (pulmonary embolic phenomenon), the pulmonary microcirculation (pulmonary arterial hypertension) and the pulmonary veins (pulmonary venous hypertension). Arterial thrombosis is a common and often life-threatening problem in the cancer setting and a frequent cause of pulmonary hypertension. Obstruction of the central pulmonary arteries is typically caused by clot, although tumor, air, and fat may also become trapped in the pulmonary circulation, with equally catastrophic consequences. Prolonged hypoxia, ARDS, sepsis, pneumonia, and treatment-related lung injury are prominent etiologies of pulmonary arterial hypertension (PAH) associated with microvascular arteriopathy. In addition, portal hypertension, and inflammatory or neoplastic processes that involve the pulmonary microcirculation, such as myeloproliferative disease and pulmonary hyperstasis with leukocytosis may also lead to PAH. Portal hypertension occurs in up to 17% of patients with certain types of myeloproliferative disorders, such as polycythemia vera, myelofibrosis with myeloid metaplasia, and essential thrombocythemia and its association with PH, are well described.[182] PAH associated with pulmonary leukocytosis typically occurs among leukemic patients with profound elevations in circulating myeloblasts or promyelocytes and is caused by sludging of white blood cells (WBCs) within the pulmonary microvasculature (the so-called "white clot" syndrome). The scourge of sepsis, arrhythmias, myocardial toxicity secondary to chemoradiation therapy, and the cancer itself, may instigate myocardial and/or valvular injury and associated pulmonary venous hypertension (PVH). In addition to primary cardiac disease, two other disorders, pulmonary veno-occlusive disease (PVOD) and PVH due to external compression and/or entrapment of large pulmonary veins by adenopathy, neoplasms, or mediastinal fibrosis are rare but life-threatening forms of PVH. These two disorders occur as a result of obstruction of the postcapillary pulmonary veins. Hodgkin's lymphoma and germ cell tumors underlie most causes of PVH due to mediastinal compression, although fibrosing mediastinitis related to infection and radiation has also been reported.[183–185] The distinction between PVOD and PAH is important, as pulmonary vasodilator therapy, which represents standard treatment of PAH may precipitate fulminant pulmonary edema in patients with PVOD. Most patients present with nonspecific complaints of exertional dyspnea and lethargy. As the disease progresses, cyanosis, chest pain, right upper quadrant pain associated with hepatic congestion, low-grade hemoptysis and exertional syncope may be noted. Diffuse alveolar hemorrhage and sudden death are more rare presentations that signal far advanced disease. Kerley B lines, septal thickening, and diffuse or mosaic ground-glass opacities are typical radiographic findings. Pleural effusion, an unusual feature of primary pulmonary hypertension, is seen in 50% of patients with PVOD, owing to postcapillary obstruction with associated elevations in pulmonary capillary and visceral pleural capillary hydrostatic pressures. The diagnosis of PVOD is suggested by the triad of severe pulmonary arterial hypertension, radiographic evidence of pulmonary edema, and a normal pulmonary artery occlusion pressure, though a substantial fraction of patients with PVOD do not have the full triad. A definitive diagnosis is rendered only by surgical lung biopsy. No randomized trials addressing treatment options for this rare condition are available. Immunosuppressive agents, including high-dose glucocorticoids and antimetabolites, and anticoagulant therapy have appeared to be effective in some cases. Arterial vasodilators should be used judiciously because of the association with massive pulmonary edema and death that has been reported.

VENTILATORY PUMP INSUFFICIENCY

In normal tidal breathing, approximately 5 liters of air are moved into and out of the chest each minute by the musculoskeletal ventilatory pump. Considerable ventilatory capacity can be lost before respiratory insufficiency begins to develop, but when vital capacity falls below 1 liter or maximal negative inspiratory pressure falls below 20 centimeters of water, frank ventilatory failure may be imminent. Changes in blood carbon dioxide level often do not occur until late in the course, and progressive respiratory insufficiency may be difficult to recognize until frank failure occurs, often in the setting of a second insult such as pneumonia. Thus, the early clinical signs of ventilatory insufficiency are often elusive and must be actively pursued. The major components of the ventilatory pump include the respiratory controllers of the drive to breathe located in the central nervous system (CNS), the chest wall (including the respiratory muscles), and the pathways that connect the central controllers with the respiratory muscles (spinal and peripheral nerves). Primary failure of alveolar ventilation, also referred to as type II respiratory failure or ventilatory pump insufficiency, occurs when there is sufficient compromise of any of the components of the ventilatory pump. In the cancer setting, multiple contributors to neural and musculoskeletal dysfunction underlie the frequent development of pump failure in this group of patients. Pulmonary rehabilitation has been increasingly used in the management of patients with chronic respiratory insufficiency associated with pump failure and will be discussed later in this section.

Causes of Pump Failure **Central Nervous System Disorders: Impaired Drive** Isolated central depression of ventilatory drive is a rare cause of pump failure that may result from insults to the central nervous system, such as medullary tumors or infarction, or sedating or narcotic medications. Acquired central hypoventilation may occur following neurosurgical procedures for brainstem tumors, particularly those that are close to the floor of the fourth ventricle. Radiation to the base of the skull may have similar adverse effects. Occult hypothyroidism may also contribute to central hypoventilation and ventilatory failure, particularly in elderly women and following treatment of head and neck carcinoma. More often, respiratory failure owing to depressed central drive occurs as an additional insult, superimposed on chronic respiratory insufficiency. In this setting, small doses of narcotic or sedating medications may have a profound effect on alveolar ventilation. Respiratory muscle fatigue may also contribute to central hypoventilation by sending inhibitory signals to the respiratory center in the CNS to reduce drive, thereby protecting the muscles from injury and mitigating further muscle fatigue.

Peripheral Nervous System Disorders: Inadequate Neuromuscular Competence Transmission of signals from the CNS to the respiratory muscles occurs via the spinal cord and peripheral nerves. Hence, conditions causing neuromuscular dysfunction, such as primary neurologic diseases, spinal cord lesions, neuromuscular blocking drugs, and muscle weakness may precipitate ventilatory failure. Systemic anesthetics cause potent neuromuscular blockade and ventilatory depression. Other agents, including sedatives, anxiolytics, hypnotics, and aminoglycosides typically produce severe respiratory depression only in the setting of preexisting neuromuscular diseases such as myasthenia gravis and myasthenic paraneoplastic syndrome or after massive overdose. One exception to this principle is methadone, which may cause ventilatory insufficiency with chronic administration. Muscular weakness and fatigue are prominent complaints that may emerge from diverse etiologies among patients with cancer. Malnutrition and cachexia are well-known complications of advanced cancer, affecting approximately 40 to 80% of this population and contributing to 22% of cancer-related deaths.[186,187] One of the most relevant manifestations of cancer cachexia is muscle wasting, which contributes to markedly depressed strength and endurance of the skeletal muscles, including the diaphragm.[188] Overinflation of the thorax and flattened diaphragms associated with COPD, a common comorbidity of lung cancer, further contributes to compromised respiratory muscle performance and ventilatory failure. Electrolyte disturbances such as hypophosphatemia, hypokalemia, and hypomagnesemia frequently complicate chemotherapy and may cause profound muscle weakness in the cancer patient. In addition, many of the drugs used in the treatment of ventilatory failure, including beta-agonists, diuretics, and corticosteroids may exacerbate hypophosphatemia and aggravate muscle weakness. The deleterious effects of chemotherapeutic agents and other drugs on the neuromuscular system are well described. Although corticosteroid-induced myopathy has been well described, the role of these drugs in potentiating respiratory muscle dysfunction has only recently been recognized.[189,190] Among the chemotherapeutic agents, vinca-alkyloids, cisplatin, and the taxanes are most frequently associated with peripheral neurotoxicity. The clinical manifestations of these drugs on lung function may be subtle in the absence of predisposing factors such as preexisting neuromuscular abnormalities. In addition to their CNS effects, the use of anesthetic agents, in particular halothane, propofol, and nitrous oxide may induce respiratory depression by decreasing diaphragmatic contractility.[191,192] Injury to the phrenic nerve following surgery for head and neck cancer, or surgery to the anterior mediastinum, esophagus, or lungs may cause persistent diaphragmatic dysfunction and ventilatory failure. Loss of diaphragmatic function from direct phrenic nerve invasion by tumor may also be seen, particularly among patients with lymphoma or cancers of the lung or head and neck. Diffuse neural dysfunction resulting from paraneoplastic syndromes is another cause of respiratory failure in the cancer setting. Lambert-Eaton myasthenic syndrome, which affects about 3% of patients with small-cell lung cancer; myasthenia gravis, which occurs in 10 to 15% of patients with thymoma; and demyelinating peripheral neuropathy, seen in 50% of patients with the osteosclerotic form of plasmacytoma are the most common types of paraneoplastic disorders of the peripheral nervous system. These disorders typically have a subacute and debilitating course that may lead to incipient ventilatory failure. Muscle fatigue, a pervasive problem in the cancer setting, is central to the development of respiratory failure. An extensive list of factors may potentiate cancer-related muscle fatigue and, thereby, respiratory failure, including hypoperfusion states (cardiogenic, septic or hemorrhagic shock), excess lactate or hydrogen ion production, and severe anemia.

Increased Work of Breathing: Increased Respiratory System Load and Chest Wall Abnormalities A variety of cancer-related factors may result in acute or chronic escalations in the respiratory system load. Elevation in resistive workload is a cardinal feature of COPD, airway inflammation, airway edema or physical obstruction by mucous, blood, or tumor. Upper airway obstruction caused by tracheal stenosis associated with prior intubation or radiation to the head and neck, and intubation with a small (< 7.5 mm internal diameter) endotracheal tube are significant sources of increased airflow resistance that may precipitate respiratory failure. Increased minute ventilation, owing to factors that contribute to excess carbon dioxide production (fever, respiratory distress, infection) or increased dead space ventilation (pulmonary embolism preexisting lung disease, hypovolemia, PEEP) are also implicated. Abnormalities involving the chest wall and thoracic spine caused by tumor, radiation, or surgery may cause increased chest wall elastic loads, increased work of breathing, and respiratory failure.

PULMONARY REHABILITATION

Dyspnea and fatigue are pervasive and frequently disabling symptoms that profoundly impact the quality of life of patients with cancer. Seventy percent of patients complain of fatigue during the course of cancer treatment, which may persist for years following the completion of therapy.[193,194] Rates of dyspnea approach 80% among patients with cancer and may be a marker of advanced disease.[195,196] The genesis of cancer-related dyspnea and fatigue emerges from overlapping and inherently multifactorial etiologies, including cancer and its therapy, hypoxia, anemia, inadequate nutrition, psychosocial factors, pain, altered energy and muscle metabolism, and the release of endogenous inflammatory cytokines. Optimal management thus requires a multifaceted approach. Pulmonary rehabilitation (PR) represents a multidisciplinary strategy that incorporates exercise training, patient and family education, psychosocial and behavioral interventions and outcome assessment in the management of patients with chronic dyspnea and fatigue. This approach has been consistently shown to improve dyspnea and fatigue among patients with chronic obstructive lung disease and in the lung transplant setting; however, the benefits of PR in the cancer setting is largely unstudied. Several small reports have suggested that PR may counter chemotherapy-related fatigue, ameliorate performance status, and reduce the length/frequency of hospitalizations among patients with cancer.[197–199] An increase in work rate and higher maximal oxygen consumption (VO_2max) claimed by recent studies have also been suggested.[200] These findings, although intriguing, have not been investigated in any large, controlled trials to determine their impact, if any, on improving surgical resectability or tolerance to aggressive chemoradiation therapy regimens. Such studies may expand the role of PR in the management of patients with cancer and endorse the benefits of such strategies in the cancer population.

RESPIRATORY FAILURE

The lung is frequently a target organ in life-threatening complications of cancer and its treatment, with acute respiratory failure (ARF) being the most common reason for ICU admission among adult patients with cancer. The mortality rate of critically ill cancer patients with respiratory failure is at least 3-fold higher than that of concurrently admitted cancer patients without respiratory failure.[201–203] Conditions common to the critically ill cancer patient, such as cardiovascular, renal or hepatic dysfunction, disseminated intravascular coagulation, hemodynamic instability, and the need for mechanical ventilation, are independent predictive variables that portend a poor outcome.[201,202,204] Mortality rates in excess of 90% have been reported among mechanically ventilated cancer patients with ARF in the past, especially those with hematologic malignancies and recipients of hematopoietic transplants.[205–208] More recent reports have offered a more favorable perspective, with mortality rates of 69 to 84%.[202,203,209] Survival gains may be attributable to better infection prophylaxis measures and improved transplantation techniques, standard use of preventive measures that mitigate aspiration, more aggressive use of hematopoietic growth factor support following transplantation, and trends toward the use of peripheral stem cells rather than bone marrow as a source of donor stem cells. In addition, the newer ventilation strategies, including noninvasive ventilation and lung protective ventilator strategies (eg, low tidal volumes with permissive hypercapnia), may play a role in improved survival.[203]

The predisposing conditions for both acute and chronic respiratory insufficiency can be divided into those that cause "lung" failure or "pump" failure. Lung failure is typically associated with ventilation/perfusion abnormalities, shunts, or alterations of alveolar-capillary diffusion and leads primarily to hypoxia, at least in its early stages. A classic example of lung failure is acute respiratory distress syndrome (ARDS). Many of the diverse causes of ARDS in cancer, including surgery, infection, chemotherapy, radiotherapy, and complications related to stem cell transplantation, have been discussed elsewhere in this chapter. Lung failure may also develop in the absence of ARDS as a consequence of ventilation/perfusion mismatch associated with pneumonia, atelectasis, or pulmonary embolism, or as a result of shunt associated with pulmonary edema. Other common causes of lung failure are listed in Table 135-4. Pump failure, by contrast, results from primary failure of alveolar ventilation and leads to severe hypercapnia and acidosis with only mild hypoxemia. Conditions that compromise specific components of the ventilatory pump, such as the peripheral nervous system (malnutrition, electrolyte disturbances, corticosteroids, chest wall disease, Eaton-Lambert syndrome), central nervous system (hypothyroidism, brain-stem lesions, sedating medications), and respiratory muscles (increased resistance loads due to COPD, asthma, obstructive sleep apnea, intrinsic/extrinsic obstruction of the large airways) are causes of pump failure, and have been discussed above. Multifactorial causes of ARF, such as severe COPD exacerbation with superimposed pneumonia may lead to both lung and pump failure. This mixed picture is a common source of respiratory failure in the cancer patient, which requires a systematic approach to each component of respiratory failure in an effort to logically devise treatment strategies. A discussion of "pump failure" is found above in the section "Ventilatory Pump Insufficiency." Major causes of lung failure are further discussed below.

PULMONARY EDEMA/ACUTE RESPIRATORY DISTRESS SYNDROME/ACUTE LUNG INJURY The predilection for pulmonary edema in the setting of cancer arises from a broad array of insults to the lungs that may be sorted according to the underlying permeability characteristics of the

Table 135-4 Lung versus Pump Failure in ARF: Characteristics and Underlying Causes

	Lung Failure	Ventilatory Failure
Characteristic feature(s)	Hypoxemia	Hypercapnia and acidosis Mild hypoxemia
Pathophysiology	Ventilation/perfusion mismatch Shunts Alterations in alveolar capillary membrane	Airflow obstruction Ventilatory pump dysfunction Extrapulmonary thoracic restriction
Underlying conditions	Acute lung injury/ARDS Pneumonia Atelectasis Pulmonary embolism/tumor emboli Lymphangitic spread of tumor Chemotherapy/radiation therapy Pulmonary leukostasis Transfusion-related lung injury Postoperative respiratory insufficiency	CNS depressant drugs CNS injury by cancer or cancer therapy Hypothyroidism Respiratory muscle fatigue Electrolyte disturbance Treatment related myopathy/neuropathy Diaphragmatic/phrenic nerve injury Paraneoplastic syndromes Bronchospasm Intrinsic or extrinsic airway compression Constrictive bronchiolitis Coexisting COPD/OSA Chest wall abnormalities

ARDS = adult respiratory distress syndrome; CNS = central nervous system; OSA = obstructive sleep apnea.

microcirculation and the presence or absence of diffuse alveolar damage histopathologically. In normal permeability pulmonary edema, increased hydrostatic pressure caused by an imbalance in Starling's forces leads to fluid filtration into the lungs. Pulmonary edema of cardiogenic and neurogenic etiologies, as well as lung edema caused by lung reexpansion, lymphatic obstruction, and relief of upper airway obstruction, are typically associated with normal microvascular permeability.

The histopathologic hallmark of increased microvascular permeability is the accumulation of proteinaceous fluid within the interstitium resulting from a breach in the integrity of the alveolar and microvascular surfaces. Increased permeability pulmonary edema occurring in the absence of diffuse alveolar damage is referred to as capillary leak syndrome. In the cancer setting this type of pulmonary edema may occur following the administration of cytokines such as interferon and IL-2, which disrupt capillary endothelial integrity. These drugs may also cause direct toxicity to the myocardium, resulting in mixed or overlap edema associated with normal and increased permeability etiologies. Neurogenic and reexpansion pulmonary edema represent two other causes of mixed edema, which are frequently observed in the cancer setting. The frequent need for transfused blood products in the cancer setting predisposes the cancer patient to the syndrome of transfusion-related lung injury (TRALI), another form of noncardiogenic pulmonary edema. TRALI is characterized by the development of fever, hypotension, severe hypoxemia, and bilateral lung infiltrates, which typically occur during or immediately following blood or blood product transfusion. Pulmonary hypertension with normal left ventricular end-diastolic pressures is also a cardinal feature of this syndrome. TRALI has been reported following transfusion of packed red blood cells, platelets, and granulocytes. The treatment is supportive. Resolution of clinical symptoms and radiographic changes typically occurs within 2 to 3 days of symptom onset without permanent pulmonary sequelae, although in 20% of patients symptoms and radiographic changes may persist for a week and be associated with lung injury (ALI/ARDS; see below).[210,211]

Acute lung injury (ALI) and ARDS are terms used for varying severity of pulmonary edema accompanying the histopathologic finding of diffuse alveolar damage. ARDS is reserved for severe lung injury in which bilateral pulmonary infiltrates and severe hypoxemia (as defined by a ratio of the partial pressure of arterial oxygen to the fraction of inspired oxygen [PaO_2/FiO_2] < 200) occur in the absence of clinical evidence of left atrial hypertension. ALI is reflective of a lesser injury, as indicated by a PaO_2/FiO_2 ratio between 200 to 300. The list of cancer-related precipitating conditions associated with ARDS is extensive. An etiological dichotomy that sorts the causes of ARDS into conditions that provoke direct lung injury (pneumonia, gastric aspiration) and those that are associated with systemic diseases that promote indirect lung injury (sepsis, transfusion-related lung injury) provides a simplistic approach to ARDS, but is confounded by the fact that the inciting events are often multifactorial or unknown. A complex interplay between humoral and cellular mediators and pro- and anti-inflammatory cytokines and chemokines has been implicated in the pathogenesis of ARDS. The proinflammatory cytokines tumor necrosis factor, interleukin- (IL) 1, 6, and 8 and the anti-inflammatory activities of tumor necrosis factor receptor (TNFr), interleukin-1 receptor antagonist, and interleukin-10 and 11 may modulate ARDS by either amplifying or dampening the inflammatory response.[212,213] In addition, variations in the levels of bioactive molecules such as activated protein C (APC) and high-mobility group B_1 protein ($HMGB_1$) may play a central role in the development of sepsis and sepsis-related ARDS.[214,215] Neutrophilic inflammation has been historically incriminated in the development of this disease; however, recent reports documenting ARDS in the setting of profound neutropenia[216,217] and the lack of evidence suggesting that the incidence or severity of lung injury is increased following neutrophil stimulation with granulocyte-colony stimulating factor[218] favors neutrophilic inflammation as the result rather than the cause of lung injury. Pathologically, ARDS is marked by three distinct stereotyped phases, regardless of the underlying cause—the acute or exudative phase (diffuse alveolar damage [DAD]), the fibroproliferative phase, and the recovery phase. Clinically, patients may present with acute respiratory failure and associated hypoxemia within 24 to 48 hours of the predisposing event. Fever and leukocytosis, owing to the inflammatory response associated with lung injury may be prominent findings, even in the absence of infection. Although the radiographic changes in ARDS are not distinctive, the CXR is nonetheless important in ruling out competing diagnoses such as pneumothorax, infections, and congestive heart failure. Patchy areas of lung involvement may be seen as ground-glass opacifications early on, which may progress to diffuse areas of consolidation. Radiographic findings suggestive of cardiogenic pulmonary edema such as Kerley B lines, cardiomegaly, and apical vascular redistribution are typically absent. Improvements in supportive care coupled with early identification and management of precipitating condition(s) and strategies that attenuate ventilator-associated lung injury have contributed to significant improvements in ARDS-related survival rates over the past decade.[219] The utility of anti-inflammatory agents, such as high-dose glucocorticoids, anti-TNF-α, and anti-interleukin-1 in attenuating lung injury has been investigated in small clinical trials and not found to be helpful, nor have other agents, including ketoconazole, prostaglandin E_1, prostacyclin, aerosolized surfactant, and inhaled nitric oxide. The effect of activated protein C administration in reducing sepsis-related ARDS mortality has been exciting,[220] though its use in thrombocytopenic cancer patients requires further study.

Progression to the fibroproliferative phase is common, resulting in persistent hypoxemia associated with poor lung compliance, increased dead space, ventilation-perfusion imbalance, and pulmonary hypertension. A salutary effect of high-dose glucocorticoids given during the fibroproliferative phase of ARDS was suggested in several small studies,[221,222] though not borne out in a multicenter NIH-sponsored trial (ARDS-Net).

Pulmonary Spread of Tumor: Lymphangitic Carcinomatosis and Pulmonary Leukostasis Tumoral involvement of the pulmonary vascular bed may present as macrovascular central tumor emboli or smaller tumor cell aggregates that occlude small vessels. The latter may occur with or

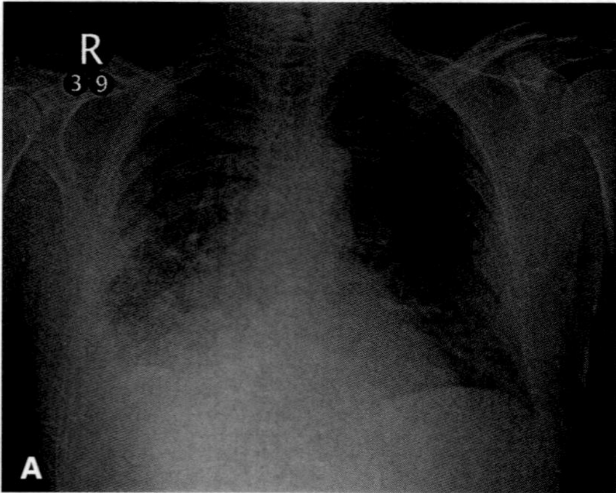

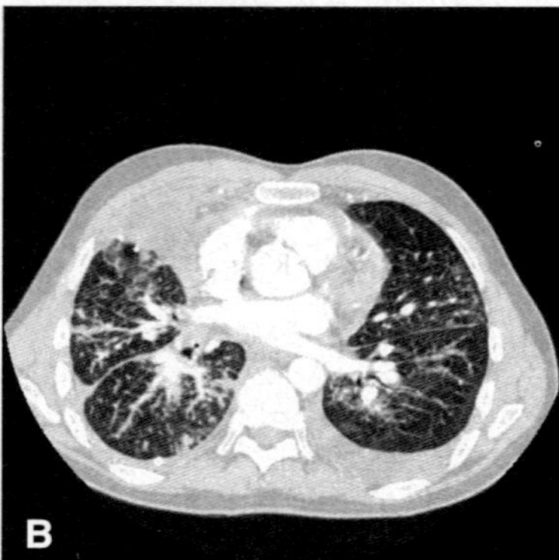

Figure 135-11 CXR **(A)** and chest computed tomography **(B)** of a patient with primary bronchogenic carcinoma. Nodular perivascular and septal thickening in the absence of architectural distortion of the lung parenchymal is typical of lymphangitic spread of tumor.

without lymphangitic spread of disease. Choriocarcinomas and mucinous tumors originating in the breast, lung, gastrointestinal tract, and kidneys are associated with the highest rates of tumor embolization. Leukemic sequestration and leukocyte thrombus formation within the pulmonary microvasculature are rare complications of hyperleukocytosis (WBC > 50,000/dL) and blast crisis associated with myeloid and lymphocytic leukemias. Patients typically present with dyspnea, nonproductive cough, and hypoxemia associated with interstitial infiltrates and signs of pulmonary hypertension and cor pulmonale. The clinical manifestations of macrovascular tumor emboli resemble acute pulmonary thromboembolic disease. Microvascular tumor embolization, however, typically presents with insidious symptoms of dyspnea, nonproductive cough, hypoxemia, and severe pulmonary artery pressure elevations. Cor pulmonale and diffuse interstitial infiltrates, suggestive of lymphangitic spread of disease, are common findings and heighten the already poor prognosis (Figure 135-11). Acute hypoxemic respiratory failure has also been reported following the initiation of chemotherapy for treatment of acute nonlymphocytic leukemia. This syndrome, known as leukemic cell lysis pneumopathy, typically occurs during the initial 48 hours of treatment and is thought to be caused by chemotherapy-induced pulmonary leukostasis and perivascular hemorrhage. Measured PaO_2 may be artificially low in patients with hyperleukocytic leukemias in the absence of lung involvement, owing to leukocyte metabolism of oxygen within the arterial blood gas syringe. In this setting oxygen saturations obtained by pulse oximetry are normal. Rapid analysis of the arterial blood gas specimen kept on ice or the addition of cyanide to the blood gas syringe eliminates this problem.

Management of Respiratory Failure The management of the critically ill cancer patient with respiratory failure involves aggressive supportive care as well as strategies that target the precipitating cause. Standard supportive measures include the provision of supplemental oxygen, inhaled bronchodilators, nutritional support, chest physiotherapy and pulmonary toilet, and the prudent use of diuretics, vasopressors, and antibiotics, where indicated. Although fluid loading augments oxygen consumption and tissue oxygen delivery, careful attention to fluid homeostasis is imperative because a persistent positive fluid balance has been associated with a poor outcome.[223,224] Assisted ventilation is often required to manage ARF that is nonresponsive to conservative medical therapy. Newer modes of mechanical ventilation as well as the use of noninvasive ventilation (NIV) have shown promising results and gained broad acceptance in the management of cancer patients with respiratory failure. The efficacy of NIV has been clearly demonstrated in several randomized, controlled studies in the management of pump failure[225,226] as well as selected cases of lung failure.[225] In a recent retrospective study of the outcome of cancer patients following ICU transfer for ARF, the use of NIV was associated with marked improvements in patient survival.[227] In addition, significant reductions in the need for conventional mechanical ventilation and declines in both ICU and post-ICU hospital mortality have been linked to the use of intermittent NIV during the early stages of hypoxemic ARF (PaO_2/FiO_2 ratio < 250).[228] Overdistension of the lungs at end inspiration and repetitive collapse of the lungs at end exhalation that occurs with conventional mechanical ventilation at high tidal volumes may trigger further lung injury. This observation prompted the development of lung-protective ventilator strategies that mitigate alveolar overdistension and enhance recruitment of atelectatic alveoli, thereby reducing the incidence of ventilator-induced lung injury. Convincing evidence favoring the use of protective ventilator strategies is derived from the National Institute of Heath ARDS Network trial where lower tidal volumes (6 mL/kg of predicted body weight) and limited static inspiratory pressures (< 30 cm H_2O) resulted in a 22% improved survival compared to patients mechanically ventilated using higher tidal volumes and inflation pressures.[229,230] Other adjuncts to ventilator management of patients with ARF, including airway pressure-release ventilation (APRV) jet and high-frequency oscillatory ventilation, extracorporeal membrane oxygenation (ECMO) and partial liquid ventilation (PLV), and prone positioning and surfactant instillation, have been proposed; however, the merits of these therapies over conventional treatment strategies have not been definitively proven.

REFERENCES

1. Wood KE. Major pulmonary embolism: review of a pathophysiologic approach to the golden hour of hemodynamically significant pulmonary embolism. Chest 2002;121:877–905.
2. Brichet A, Verkindre C, Dupont J, et al. Multidisciplinary approach to management of postintubation tracheal stenoses. Eur Respir J 1999;13:888–93.
3. Hollingsworth HM. Wheezing and stridor. Clin Chest Med 1987;8:231–40.
4. Miller RD, Hyatt RE. Evaluation of obstructing lesions of the trachea and larynx by flow-volume loops. Am Rev Respir Dis 1973;108:475–81.
5. LoCicero J 3rd, Costello P, Campos CT, et al. Spiral CT with multiplanar and three-dimensional reconstructions accurately predicts tracheobronchial pathology. Ann Thorac Surg 1996;62:818–22; discussion 822–3.
6. Kurimoto N, Hayashi K, Murayama M, Nishisaka T. Endobronchial ultrasonography for lung cancer. Nippon Geka Gakkai Zasshi 1999;100:724–8.
7. Hautmann H, Gamarra F, Pfeifer KJ, Huber RM. Fiberoptic bronchoscopic balloon dilatation in malignant tracheobronchial disease: indications and results. Chest 2001;120:43–9.
8. Antony VB, Loddenkemper R, Astoul P, et al. Management of malignant pleural effusions. Eur Respir J 2001;18:402–19.
9. Rodriguez-Panadero F, Lopez-Mejias J. Survival time of patients with pleural metastatic carcinoma predicted by glucose and pH studies. Chest 1989;95:320–4.
10. Johnston WW. The malignant pleural effusion. A review of cytopathologic diagnoses of 584 specimens from 472 consecutive patients. Cancer 1985;56:905–9.
11. Chernow B, Sahn S. Carcinomatous involvement of the pleura: an analysis of 96 patients. Am J Med 1977;63:695–702.
12. Rodriguez-Panadero F, Borderas Naranjo F. Benign pleural effusions in cancer patients. Frequency and etiopathogenic mechanism in a series of autopsy cases. Rev Clin Esp 1988;183:311–12.
13. Light RW, Hamm H. Malignant pleural effusion: would the real cause please stand up? Eur Respir J 1997;10:1907–13.
14. Zebrowski BK, Yano S, Liu W, et al. Vascular endothelial growth factor levels and induction of permeability in malignant pleural effusions. Clin Cancer Res 1999;5:3364–8.
15. Sahn S. Pleural diseases related to metastatic malignancies. Eur Respir J 1997;10:1907–13.
16. Doelken P, Strange C. Chest ultrasound for "Dummies." Chest 2003;123:332–3.
17. Evans AL, Gleeson FV. Radiology in pleural disease: state of the art. Respirology 2004;9:300–12.
18. Loddenkemper R. Thoracoscopy—state of the art. Eur Respir J 1998;11:213–21.
19. Porcel JM, Vives M, Esquerda A, et al. Use of a panel of tumor markers (carcinoembryonic antigen, cancer antigen 125, carbohydrate antigen 15-3, and cytokeratin 19 fragments) in pleural fluid for the differential diagnosis of benign and malignant effusions. Chest 2004;126:1757–63.
20. O'Hara MF, Cousar JB, Glick AD, Collins RD. Multiparameter approach to the diagnosis of hematopoietic-lymphoid neoplasms in body fluids. Diagn Cytopathol 1985;1:33–8.
21. Emri S, Akbulut H, Zorlu F, et al. Prognostic significance of flow cytometric DNA analysis in patients with malignant pleural mesothelioma. Lung Cancer 2001;33:109–14.
22. Loddenkemper R, Grosser H, Gabler A, et al. Prospective evaluation of biopsy methods in the diagnosis of malignant pleural effusions. Intrapatient comparison between pleural fluid cytology, blind needle biopsy and thoracoscopy. American Journal of Respiratory Diseases 1983;127(4 Suppl):114.
23. Burrows CM, Mathews WC, Colt HG. Predicting survival in patients with recurrent symptomatic malignant pleural effusions: an assessment of the prognostic values of

physiologic, morphologic, and quality of life measures of extent of disease. Chest 2000;117:73–8.
24. Villena V, Lopez-Encuentra A, Pozo F, et al. Measurement of pleural pressure during therapeutic thoracentesis. Am J Respir Crit Care Med 2000;162(4 Pt 1):1534–8.
25. De Campos J, Vargas F, DeCampos E, et al. Thoracoscopy talc poudrage: a 15-year experience. Chest 2001;119:801–6.
26. Anderson CB, Philpott GW, Ferguson TB. The treatment of malignant pleural effusions. Cancer 1974;33:916–22.
27. Chung CL, Chen YC, Chang SC. Effect of repeated thoracenteses on fluid characteristics, cytokines, and fibrinolytic activity in malignant pleural effusion. Chest 2003;123:1188–95.
28. Alinsonorin CY, Jimenez CA, Ersoy YM, et al. Indwelling pleural catheters for management of recurrent malignant pleural effusions. Am J Respir Crit Care Med 2003;167(7 Suppl):A901.
29. Ferrer J, Villarino MA, Tura JM, et al. Talc preparations used for pleurodesis vary markedly from one preparation to another. Chest 2001;119:1901–5.
30. Fleischman SB, Dresler C, Herndon JE, et al. Quality of life (QOL) advantage of sclerosis for malignant pleural effusion (MPE) via talc thoracoscopy over chest tube infusion of talc slurry: a Cancer and Leukemia Group B study [abstract]. Proc Am Soc Clin Oncol 2002;21:355a.
31. Schulze M, Boehle AS, Kurdow R, et al. Effective treatment of malignant pleural effusion by minimal invasive thoracic surgery: thoracoscopic talc pleurodesis and pleuroperitoneal shunts in 101 patients. Ann Thorac Surg 2001;71:1809–12.
32. Mares DC, Mathur PN. Medical thoracoscopic talc pleurodesis for chylothorax due to lymphoma: a case series. Chest 1998;114:731–5.
33. Verheul HM, Hoekman K, Jorna AS, et al. Targeting vascular endothelial growth factor blockade: ascites and pleural effusion formation. Oncologist 2000;5 Suppl 1:45–50.
34. Baudouin SV. Lung injury after thoracotomy. Br J Anaesth 2003;91:132–42.
35. Forshag MS, Cooper AD Jr. Postoperative care of the thoracotomy patient. Clin Chest Med 1992;13:33–45.
36. Landis SH, Murray T, Bolden S, Wingo PA. Cancer statistics, 1999. CA Cancer J Clin 1999;49:8–31
37. Datta D, Lahiri B. Preoperative evaluation of patients undergoing lung resection surgery. Chest 2003;123:2096–103.
38. Kristersson S, Lindell SE, Svanberg L. Prediction of pulmonary function loss due to pneumonectomy using 133 Xe-radiospirometry. Chest 1972;62:694–8.
39. Olsen GN, Block AJ, Tobias JA. Prediction of postpneumonectomy pulmonary function using quantitative macroaggregate lung scanning. Chest 1974;66:13–6.
40. Ali MK, Mountain CF, Ewer MS, et al. Predicting loss of pulmonary function after pulmonary resection for bronchogenic carcinoma. Chest 1980;77:337–42.
41. Ali MK, Ewer MS, Atallah MR, et al. Regional and overall pulmonary function changes in lung cancer. Correlations with tumor stage, extent of pulmonary resection, and patient survival. J Thorac Cardiovasc Surg 1983;86:1–8.
42. Kearney DJ, Lee TH, Reilly JJ, et al. Assessment of operative risk in patients undergoing lung resection. Importance of predicted pulmonary function. Chest 1994;105:753–9.
43. Markos J, Mullan BP, Hillman DR, et al. Preoperative assessment as a predictor of mortality and morbidity after lung resection. Am Rev Respir Dis 1989;139:902–10.
44. Bolliger CT, Wyser C, Roser H, et al. Lung scanning and exercise testing for the prediction of postoperative performance in lung resection candidates at increased risk for complications. Chest 1995;108:341–8.
45. Smith TP, Kinasewitz GT, Tucker WY, et al. Exercise capacity as a predictor of post-thoracotomy morbidity. Am Rev Respir Dis 1984;129:730–4.
46. Morice RC, Peters EJ, Ryan MB, et al. Exercise testing in the evaluation of patients at high risk for complications from lung resection. Chest 1992;101:356–61.
47. Walsh GL, Morice RC, Putnam JB Jr, et al. Resection of lung cancer is justified in high-risk patients selected by exercise oxygen consumption. Ann Thorac Surg 1994;58:704–10; discussion 711.
48. Ersoy Y, Alinsonrin C, Haque S, et al. A lower safe value of exercise oxygen consumption (VO2 peak) in patients at high-risk for lung resection. Am J Resp Crit Care 2003;1-351940:S167(7).
49. Shannon V, Price K. Pulmonary complications of cancer therapy. Anesthesiol Clin North Am 1998;16:563–85.
50. Cooper J. Drug-Induced Lung Disease. Adv Int Med 1997;42:231–268.
51. Hildebrand F, Rosenow EI, Haberman T. Pulmonary complications of leukemia. Chest 1998:1233–9.
52. Afessa B, Tefferi A, Litzow MR, et al. Diffuse alveolar hemorrhage in hematopoietic stem cell transplant recipients. Am J Respir Crit Care Med 2002;166:641–5.
53. Steijfer S. Bleomycin-induced pneumonitis. Chest 2001; 120:617–24.
54. Zisman DA, McCune WJ, Tino G, Lynch JP 3rd. Drug-induced pneumonitis: the role of methotrexate. Sarcoidosis Vasc Diffuse Lung Dis 2001;18:243–52.
55. Inoue A, Saijo Y, Maemondo M, et al. Severe acute interstitial pneumonia and gefitinib. Lancet 2003;361:137–9.
56. Kris MG, Natale RB, Herbst RS, et al. Efficacy of gefitinib, an inhibitor of the epidermal growth factor receptor tyrosine kinase, in symptomatic patients with non-small cell lung cancer: a randomized trial. JAMA 2003;290:2149–58.
57. Camus P, Bonniaud P, Fanton A, et al. Drug-induced and iatrogenic infiltrative lung disease. Clin Chest Med 2004;25:479–519.
58. Sleijfer S. Bleomycin-induced pneumonitis. Chest 2001; 120:617–24.
59. Parish JM, Muhm JR, Leslie KO. Upper lobe pulmonary fibrosis associated with high-dose chemotherapy containing BCNU for bone marrow transplantation. Mayo Clin Proc 2003;78:630–4.
60. O'Driscoll BR, Hasleton PS, Taylor PM, et al. Active lung fibrosis up to 17 years after chemotherapy with carmustine (BCNU) in childhood. N Engl J Med 1990;323:378–82.
61. Comis R. Bleomycin pulmonary toxicity: current status and future directions. Semin Oncol 1992;19(2 Suppl 5):64–70.
62. Willenbacher W, Mumm A, Bartsch HH. Late pulmonary toxicity of bleomycin. J Clin Oncol 1998;16:3205.
63. Rubio C, Hill M, O'Brien M, Cunningham D. Idiopathic pneumonia syndrome after high-dose chemotherapy for relapsed Hodgkin's disease. Br J Cancer 1997;75:1044–8.
64. Demedts M, Costabel U. ATS/ERS international multidisciplinary consensus classification of the idiopathic interstitial pneumonias. Eur Respir J 2002;19:794–6.
65. Rosenow E. Drug-induced pulmonary disease. Dis Mon 1994;40:253–310.
66. Huggins JT, Sahn SA. Drug-induced pleural disease. Clin Chest Med 2004;25:141–53.
67. Wohlrab J, Liu M, Anderson E, Kia Noury D. Docetaxel induced pleural effusions [abstract]. Chest 2002;122:94S–5S.
68. Busmanis IA, Beaty AE, Basser RL. Isolated pleural effusion with hematopoietic cells of mixed lineage in a patient receiving granulocyte-colony-stimulating factor after high-dose chemotherapy. Diagn Cytopathol 1998;18:204–7.
69. Rogers JI, Murgo A, Fontana J, Raich P. Chemotherapy for breast cancer decreased plasma protein C and protein S. J Clin Oncol 1988;6:276–81.
70. Pritchard KI, Paterson AH, Paul NA, et al. Increased thromboembolic complications with concurrent tamoxifen and chemotherapy in a randomized trial of adjuvant therapy for women with breast cancer. National Cancer Institute of Canada Clinical Trials Group Breast Cancer Site Group. J Clin Oncol 1996;14:2731–7.
71. Cuzick J, Forbes J, Edwards R, et al. First results from the International Breast Cancer Intervention Study (IBIS-I): a randomised prevention trial. Lancet 2002;360:817–24.
72. Fine HA, Wen PY, Maher EA, et al. Phase II trial of thalidomide and carmustine for patients with recurrent high-grade gliomas. J Clin Oncol 2003;21:2299–304.
73. Zangari M, Siegel E, Barlogie B, et al. Thrombogenic activity of doxorubicin in myeloma patients receiving thalidomide: implications for therapy. Blood 2002;100:1168–71.
74. Williams LM, Fussell S, Veith RW, et al. Pulmonary veno-occlusive disease in an adult following bone marrow transplantation. Case report and review of the literature. Chest 1996;109:1388–91.
75. Hackman R, Madtes D, Petersen F, Clark J. Pulmonary venoocclusive disease following bone marrow transplantation. Transplantation 1989;47:989–92.
76. Markman M. Management of toxicities associated with the administration of taxanes. Expert Opin Drug Saf 2003;2:141–6.
77. Szebeni J. Complement activation-related pseudoallergy caused by liposomes, micellar carriers of intravenous drugs, and radiocontrast agents. Crit Rev Ther Drug Carrier Syst 2001;18:567–606.
78. Piro LD, White CA, Grillo-Lopez AJ, et al. Extended Rituximab (anti-CD20 monoclonal antibody) therapy for relapsed or refractory low-grade or follicular non-Hodgkin's lymphoma. Ann Oncol 1999;10:655–61.
79. Davis TA, White CA, Grillo-Lopez AJ, et al. Single-agent monoclonal antibody efficacy in bulky non-Hodgkin's lymphoma: results of a phase II trial of rituximab. J Clin Oncol 1999;17:1851–7.
80. Marks LB, Yu X, Vujaskovic Z, et al. Radiation-induced lung injury. Semin Radiat Oncol 2003;13(3):333–45.
81. Abratt RP, Morgan GW. Lung toxicity following chest irradiation in patients with lung cancer. Lung Cancer 2002;35:103–9.
82. Smith JC. Radiation Pneumonitis. Case report of bilateral reaction after unilateral irradiation. Am Rev Respir Dis 1964;89:264–9.
83. Gibson PG, Bryant DH, Morgan GW, et al. Radiation-induced lung injury: a hypersensitivity pneumonitis? Ann Intern Med 1988;109:288–91.
84. Faller M, Quoix E, Popin E, et al. Migratory pulmonary infiltrates in a patient treated with sotalol. Eur Respir J 1997;10:2159–62.
85. Phillips TL. Effects of chemotherapy and irradiation on normal tissues. Front Radiat Ther Oncol 1992;26:45–54.
86. Movsas B, Raffin TA, Epstein AH, Link CJ Jr. Pulmonary radiation injury. Chest 1997;111:1061–76.
87. Liao ZX, Travis EL, Tucker SL. Damage and morbidity from pneumonitis after irradiation of partial volumes of mouse lung. Int J Radiat Oncol Biol Phys 1995;32:1359–70.
88. Anscher MS, Marks LB, Shafman TD, et al. Using plasma transforming growth factor beta-1 during radiotherapy to select patients for dose escalation. J Clin Oncol 2001;19:3758–65.
89. Vujaskovic Z, Feng QF, Rabbani ZN, et al. Assessment of the protective effect of amifostine on radiation-induced pulmonary toxicity. Exp Lung Res 2002;28:577–90.
90. Vujaskovic Z, Batinic-Haberle I, Rabbani ZN, et al. A small molecular weight catalytic metalloporphyrin antioxidant with superoxide dismutase (SOD) mimetic properties protects lungs from radiation-induced injury. Free Radic Biol Med 2002;33:857–63.
91. Vujaskovic Z, Feng QF, Rabbani ZN, et al. Radioprotection of lungs by amifostine is associated with reduction in profibrogenic cytokine activity. Radiat Res 2002;157:656–60.
92. Vujaskovic Z, Anscher MS, Feng QF, et al. Radiation-induced hypoxia may perpetuate late normal tissue injury. Int J Radiat Oncol Biol Phys 2001;50:851–5.
93. Haston CK, Travis EL. Murine susceptibility to radiation-induced pulmonary fibrosis is influenced by a genetic factor implicated in susceptibility to bleomycin-induced pulmonary fibrosis. Cancer Res 1997;57:5286–91.
94. Haston CK, Zhou X, Gumbiner-Russo L, et al. Universal and radiation-specific loci influence murine susceptibility to radiation-induced pulmonary fibrosis. Cancer Res 2002;62:3782–8.
95. Kotloff RM, Ahya VN, Crawford SW. Pulmonary complications of solid organ and hematopoietic stem cell transplantation. Am J Respir Crit Care Med 2004;170:22–48.
96. Soubani A, Miller K, Hassoun P. Pulmonary complications of bone marrow transplantation. Chest 1996;109:1066–77.
97. Roychowdhury M, Pambuccian SE, Aslan DL, et al. Pulmonary complications after bone marrow transplantation: an autopsy study from a large transplantation center. Arch Pathol Lab Med 2005;129:366–71.
98. Lossos IS, Breuer R, Or R, et al. Bacterial pneumonia in recipients of bone marrow transplantation. A five-year prospective study. Transplantation 1995;60:672–8.
99. Harrington RD, Woolfrey AE, Bowden R, et al. Legionellosis in a bone marrow transplant center. Bone Marrow Transplant 1996;18:361–8.
100. Kugler JW, Armitage JO, Helms CM, et al. Nosocomial legionnaires' disease. Occurrence in recipients of bone marrow transplants. Am J Med 1983;74:281–8.
101. Konoplev S, Champlin RE, Giralt S, et al. Cytomegalovirus pneumonia in adult autologous blood and marrow transplant recipients. Bone Marrow Transplant 2001;27:877–81.
102. Atkinson K, Nivison-Smith I, Dodds A, et al. A comparison of the pattern of interstitial pneumonitis following allogeneic bone marrow transplantation before and after the introduction of prophylactic ganciclovir therapy in 1989. Bone Marrow Transplant 1998;21:691–5.
103. Nguyen Q, Champlin R, Giralt S, et al. Late cytomegalovirus pneumonia in adult allogeneic blood and marrow transplant recipients. Clin Infect Dis 1999;28:618–23.
104. Reed E, Bowden R, Dandliker P, et al. Treatment of cytomegalovirus pneumonia with ganciclovir and intravenous

cytomegalovirus immunoglobulin in patients with bone marrow transplants. Ann Intern Med 1988;109:783–8.
105. Emanuel D, Cunningham I, Jules-Elysee K, et al. Cytomegalovirus pneumonia after bone marrow transplantation successfully treated with the combination of ganciclovir and high-dose intravenous immune globulin. Ann Intern Med 1988;109:777–82.
106. Ljungman P, Engelhard D, Link H, et al. Treatment of interstitial pneumonitis due to cytomegalovirus with ganciclovir and intravenous immune globulin: experience of European Bone Marrow Transplant Group. Clin Infect Dis 1992;14:831–5.
107. Bowden RA. Respiratory virus infections after marrow transplant: the Fred Hutchinson Cancer Research Center experience. Am J Med 1997;102:27–30; discussion 42–3.
108. Ghosh S, Champlin RE, Ueno NT, et al. Respiratory syncytial virus infections in autologous blood and marrow transplant recipients with breast cancer: combination therapy with aerosolized ribavirin and parenteral immunoglobulins. Bone Marrow Transplant 2001;28:271–5.
109. Fukuda T, Boeckh M, Carter RA, et al. Risks and outcomes of invasive fungal infections in recipients of allogeneic hematopoietic stem cell transplants after nonmyeloablative conditioning. Blood 2003;102:827–33.
110. Sherertz RJ, Belani A, Kramer BS, et al. Impact of air filtration on nosocomial Aspergillus infections. Unique risk of bone marrow transplant recipients. Am J Med 1987;83:709–18.
111. Souza JP, Boeckh M, Gooley TA, et al. High rates of *Pneumocystis carinii* pneumonia in allogeneic blood and marrow transplant recipients receiving dapsone prophylaxis. Clin Infect Dis 1999;29:1467–71.
112. Weinstock DM, Feinstein MB, Sepkowitz KA, Jakubowski A. High rates of infection and colonization by nontuberculous mycobacteria after allogeneic hematopoietic stem cell transplantation. Bone Marrow Transplant 2003;31:1015–21.
113. Spitzer TR. Engraftment syndrome following hematopoietic stem cell transplantation. Bone Marrow Transplant 2001;27:893–8.
114. Maiolino A, Biasoli I, Lima J, et al. Engraftment syndrome following autologous hematopoietic stem cell transplantation: definition of diagnostic criteria. Bone Marrow Transplant 2003;31:393–7.
115. Mossad S, Kalaycio M, Sobecks R, et al. Steroids prevent engraftment syndrome after autologous hematopoietic stem cell transplantation without increasing the risk of infection. Bone Marrow Transplant 2005;35:375–81.
116. Clark JG, Hansen JA, Hertz MI. Idiopathic pneumonia syndrome after bone marrow transplantation. Am Rev Respir Dis 1993;147:1601–6.
117. Kantrow SP, Hackman RC, Boeckh M, et al. Idiopathic pneumonia syndrome: changing spectrum of lung injury after marrow transplantation. Transplantation 1997;63:1079–86.
118. Yanik G, Hellerstedt B, Custer J, et al. Etanercept (Enbrel) administration for idiopathic pneumonia syndrome after allogeneic hematopoietic stem cell transplantation. Biol Blood Marrow Transplant 2002;8:395–400.
119. Robbins RA, Linder J, Stahl MG, et al. Diffuse alveolar hemorrhage in autologous bone marrow transplant recipients. Am J Med 1989;87:511–8.
120. Nevo S, Swan V, Enger C, et al. Acute bleeding after bone marrow transplantation (BMT)—incidence and effect on survival. A quantitative analysis in 1,402 patients. Blood 1998;91:1469–77.
121. Metcalf J, Rennard S, Reed E, et al. Corticosteroids as adjunctive therapy for diffuse alveolar hemorrhage associated with bone marrow transplantation. Am J Med 1994;94:327–34.
122. Jules-Elysee K, Stover D, Yahalom J, et al. Pulmonary complications in lymphoma patients treated with high-dose therapy and autologous bone marrow transplantation. Am Rev Respir Dis 1992;146:485.
123. Sisson J, Thompson A, Anderson J. Airway inflammation predicts diffuse alveolar hemorrhage during bone marrow transplantation in patients with Hodgkin disease. Am Rev Respir Dis 1992;146:439–43.
124. Agusti C, Ramirez J, Picado C, et al. Diffuse alveolar hemorrhage in allogeneic bone marrow transplantation. A postmortem study. Am J Respir Crit Care Med 1995;151:1006–10.
125. Salzman D, Adkins D, Freytes C, LeMaistre C. Malignancy-associated pulmonary veno-occlusive disease: report of a case following autologous bone marrow transplantation and review. Bone Marrow Transplant 1996;18:755–60.
126. Trobaugh-Lotrario AD, Greffe B, Deterding R, et al. Pulmonary veno-occlusive disease after autologous bone marrow transplant in a child with stage IV neuroblastoma: case report and literature review. J Pediatr Hematol Oncol 2003;25:405–9.
127. Krowka MJ, Rosenow EC, Hoagland HC. Pulmonary complications of bone marrow transplantation. Chest 1985;87:237–46.
128. Chien JW, Martin PJ, Gooley TA, et al. Airflow obstruction after myeloablative allogeneic hematopoietic stem cell transplantation. Am J Respir Crit Care Med 2003;168:208–14.
129. Afessa B, Litzow MR, Tefferi A. Bronchiolitis obliterans and other late onset non-infectious pulmonary complications in hematopoietic stem cell transplantation. Bone Marrow Transplant 2001;28:425–34.
130. Khalid M, Al Saghir A, Saleemi S, et al. Azithromycin in bronchiolitis obliterans complicating bone marrow transplantation: a preliminary study. Eur Respir J 2005;25:490–3.
131. Palmas A, Tefferi A, Myers JL, et al. Late-onset noninfectious pulmonary complications after allogeneic bone marrow transplantation. Br J Haematol 1998;100:680–7.
132. Wilczynski SW, Erasmus JJ, Petros WP. Delayed pulmonary toxicity syndrome following high-dose chemotherapy and bone marrow transplantation for breast cancer. Am J Respir Crit Care Med 1998;157:565–73.
133. Papadopoulos EB, Ladanyi M, Emanuel D, et al. Infusions of donor leukocytes to treat Epstein-Barr virus-associated lymphoproliferative disorders after allogeneic bone marrow transplantation. N Engl J Med 1994;330:1185–91.
134. Yousem SA. The histological spectrum of pulmonary graft-versus-host disease in bone marrow transplant recipients. Human Pathol 1995;26:668–75.
135. Perreault C, Cousineau S, D'Angelo G, et al. Lymphoid interstitial pneumonia after allogeneic bone marrow transplantation. A possible manifestation of chronic graft-versus-host disease. Cancer 1985;55:1–9.
136. Ahmed T, Ciavarella D, Feldman E. High-dose potentially myeloablative chemotherapy and autologous bone marrow transplantation for patients with advanced Hodgkin's disease. Leukemia 1989;3:223–9.
137. Safdar A, Armstrong D. Infectious morbidity in critically ill patients with cancer. Crit Care Clin 2001;17:531-70.
138. Bartlett JG. Community-acquired pneumonia. Int J Clin Pract Suppl 2000;115:18–22.
139. Ibrahim EH, Tracy L, Hill C, et al. The occurrence of ventilator-associated pneumonia in a community hospital: risk factors and clinical outcomes. Chest 2001;120:555–61.
140. Hubel K, Hegener K, Schnell R, et al. Suppressed neutrophil function as a risk factor for severe infection after cytotoxic chemotherapy in patients with acute nonlymphocytic leukemia. Ann Hematol 1999;78:73–7.
141. Bodey GP. Infectious complications of acute leukemia. Med Times 1966;94:1076–85.
142. Yadegarynia D, Tarrand J, Raad I, Rolston K. Current spectrum of bacterial infections in patients with cancer. Clin Infect Dis 2003;37:1144–5.
143. Chatzinikolaou I, Abi-Said D, Bodey GP, et al. Recent experience with Pseudomonas aeruginosa bacteremia in patients with cancer: retrospective analysis of 245 episodes. Arch Intern Med 2000;160:501–9.
144. Aisenberg G, Rolston KV, Safdar A. Bacteremia caused by Achromobacter and Alcaligenes species in 46 patients with cancer (1989–2003). Cancer 2004;101(9):2134–40.
145. Aisenberg G, Tarrand J, Rolston K, et al. Stenotrophomonas maltophilia: changing spectrum of bacterial pneumonia in cancer patients with low suspicion of S. maltophilia infection. 15th European Congress of Clinical Microbiology and Infectious Diseases (ECCMID) 2005, Copenhagen, Denmark.
146. Niederman MS, Mandell LA, Anzueto A, et al. Guidelines for the management of adults with community-acquired pneumonia. Diagnosis, assessment of severity, antimicrobial therapy, and prevention. Am J Respir Crit Care Med 2001;163:1730–54.
147. Mandell LA, Bartlett JG, Dowell SF, et al. Update of practice guidelines for the management of community-acquired pneumonia in immunocompetent adults. Clin Infect Dis 2003;37:1405–33.
148. American Thoracic Society, Infectious Diseases Society of America. Guidelines for the management of adults with hospital-acquired, ventilator-associated, and healthcare-associated pneumonia. Am J Respir Crit Care Med 2005;171:388–416.
149. El-Solh A, Aquilina A, Dhillon R, et al. Impact of invasive strategy on management of antimicrobial treatment failure in institutionalized older people with severe pneumonia. Am J Respir Crit Care Med 2002;166:1038–43.
150. Rello J, Ollendorf DA, Oster G, et al. Epidemiology and outcomes of ventilator-associated pneumonia in a large US database. Chest 2002;122:2115–21.
151. Marik PE. Aspiration pneumonitis and aspiration pneumonia. N Engl J Med 2001;344:665–71.
152. Torres HA, Reddy BT, Raad, II, et al. Nocardiosis in cancer patients. Medicine (Baltimore) 2002;81:388–97.
153. Uttamchandani RB, Daikos GL, Reyes RR, et al. Nocardiosis in 30 patients with advanced human immunodeficiency virus infection: clinical features and outcome. Clin Infect Dis 1994;18:348–53.
154. De La Rosa GR, Jacobson KL, Rolston KV, et al. Mycobacterium tuberculosis at a comprehensive cancer centre: active disease in patients with underlying malignancy during 1990–2000. Clin Microbiol Infect 2004;10:749–52.
155. Safdar A, White DA, Stover D, et al. Profound interferon gamma deficiency in patients with chronic pulmonary nontuberculous mycobacteriosis. Am J Med 2002;113:756–9.
156. Roblot F, Le Moal G, Godet C, et al. Pneumocystis carinii pneumonia in patients with hematologic malignancies: a descriptive study. J Infect 2003;47:19–27.
157. Marr KA, Carter RA, Crippa F, et al. Epidemiology and outcome of mould infections in hematopoietic stem cell transplant recipients. Clin Infect Dis 2002;34:909–17.
158. Marr KA, Patterson T, Denning D. Aspergillosis. Pathogenesis, clinical manifestations, and therapy. Infect Dis Clin North Am 2002;16:875–94.
159. Hachem RY, Kontoyiannis DP, Boktour MR, et al. Aspergillus terreus: an emerging amphotericin B-resistant opportunistic mold in patients with hematologic malignancies. Cancer 2004;101:1594–600.
160. Heussel CP, Kauczor HU, Heussel GE, et al. Pneumonia in febrile neutropenic patients and in bone marrow and blood stem-cell transplant recipients: use of high-resolution computed tomography. J Clin Oncol 1999;17:796–805.
161. Kontoyiannis DP, Lionakis MS, Lewis RE, et al. Zygomycosis in a tertiary-care cancer center in the era of Aspergillus-active antifungal therapy: a case-control observational study of 27 recent cases. J Infect Dis 2005;191:1350–60.
162. Safdar A, Singhal S, Mehta J. Clinical significance of non-Candida fungal blood isolation in patients undergoing high-risk allogeneic hematopoietic stem cell transplantation (1993–2001). Cancer 2004;100:2456–61.
163. Marr KA, Balajee SA, McLaughlin L, et al. Detection of galactomannan antigenemia by enzyme immunoassay for the diagnosis of invasive aspergillosis: variables that affect performance. J Infect Dis 2004;190:641–9.
164. Herbrecht R, Denning DW, Patterson TF, et al. Voriconazole versus amphotericin B for primary therapy of invasive aspergillosis. N Engl J Med 2002;347:408–15.
165. Maertens J, Raad I, Petrikkos G, et al. Efficacy and safety of caspofungin for treatment of invasive aspergillosis in patients refractory to or intolerant of conventional antifungal therapy. Clin Infect Dis 2004;39:1563–71.
166. Marr K. Combination antifungal therapy: where are we now, and where are we going? Oncology (Williston Park) 2004;18(13 Suppl 7):24–9.
167. Safdar A, Rodriguez G, Ohmagari N, et al. The safety of interferon-gamma-1b therapy for invasive fungal infections after hematopoietic stem cell transplantation. Cancer 2005;103:731–9.
168. Safdar A, Armstrong D. Listeriosis in patients at a comprehensive cancer center, 1955–1997. Clin Infect Dis 2003;37:359–64.
169. Bick RL. Cancer-associated thrombosis. N Engl J Med 2003;349:109–11.
170. Lee AY, Levine MN. Venous thromboembolism and cancer: risks and outcomes. Circulation 2003;107(23 Suppl 1):117–21.
171. ten Wolde M, Kraaijenhagen RA, Prins MH, Buller HR. The clinical usefulness of D-dimer testing in cancer patients with suspected deep venous thrombosis. Arch Intern Med 2002;162:1880–4.
172. Moores LK, Jackson WL Jr, Shorr AF, Jackson JL. Meta-analysis: outcomes in patients with suspected pulmonary embolism managed with computed tomographic pulmonary angiography. Ann Intern Med 2004;141:866–74.
173. Geerts WH, Pineo GF, Heit JA, et al. Prevention of venous thromboembolism: the Seventh ACCP Conference on Antithrombotic and Thrombolytic Therapy. Chest 2004;126(3 Suppl):338S–400S.
174. McLeod RS, Geerts WH, Sniderman KW, et al. Subcutaneous heparin versus low-molecular-weight heparin as thromboprophylaxis in patients undergoing colorectal surgery:

results of the Canadian colorectal DVT prophylaxis trial: a randomized, double-blind trial. Ann Surg 2001;233:438–44.
175. ENOXACAN Study Group. Efficacy and safety of enoxaparin versus unfractionated heparin for prevention of deep vein thrombosis in elective cancer surgery: a double-blind randomized multicentre trial with venographic assessment. Br J Surg 1997;84:1099–103.
176. Bergqvist D, Agnelli G, Cohen AT, et al. Duration of prophylaxis against venous thromboembolism with enoxaparin after surgery for cancer. N Engl J Med 2002;346:975–80.
177. Couban S, Goodyear M, Burnell M, et al. A randomized double-blind placebo controlled study of low dose warfarin for the prevention of symptomatic central venous catheter-associated thrombosis in patients with cancer [abstract]. Blood 2002;100:703A.
178. Agnelli G, Verso M, Gertoglio S, et al. A double-blind placebo-controlled randomized study on the efficacy and safety of enoxaparin for the prevention of upper limb deep vein thrombosis in cancer patients with central vein catheter [abstract]. Clin Oncol 2004;22:8021.
179. Buller HR, Agnelli G, Hull RD, et al. Antithrombotic therapy for venous thromboembolic disease: the Seventh ACCP Conference on Antithrombotic and Thrombolytic Therapy. Chest 2004;126(3 Suppl):401S–28S.
180. Lee AY, Levine MN, Baker RI, et al. Low-molecular-weight heparin versus a coumarin for the prevention of recurrent venous thromboembolism in patients with cancer. N Engl J Med 2003;349:146–53.
181. Rich S. Primary pulmonary hypertension: executive summary from the world symposium—primary pulmonary hypertension 1998. Evian France: World Health Organization; 1999.
182. Dingli D, Utz JP, Krowka MJ, et al. Unexplained pulmonary hypertension in chronic myeloproliferative disorders. Chest 2001;120:801–8.
183. Lee J, Kim Y, Lee K, Chung M. Tuberculous fibrosing mediastinitis: radiologic findings (letter). AJR Am J Roentgenol 1996;167:1598–99.
184. Lagerstrom C, Mitchell H, Graham B, Hammon JJ. Chronic fibrosing mediastinitis and superior vena caval obstruction from blastomycosis. Ann Thorac Surg 1992;54:764–65.
185. Mole T, Glover J, Sheppard M. Sclerosing mediastinitis: a report on 18 cases. Thorax 1995;50:280–3.
186. Ottery FD. Definition of standardized nutritional assessment and interventional pathways in oncology. Nutrition 1996;12(1 Suppl):S15–9.
187. Nitenberg G, Raynard B. Nutritional support of the cancer patient: issues and dilemmas. Crit Rev Oncol Hematol 2000;34:137–68.
188. Arora NS, Rochester DF. Effect of body weight and muscularity on human diaphragm muscle mass, thickness, and area. J Appl Physiol 1982;52:64–70.
189. Polla B, D'Antona G, Bottinelli R, Reggiani C. Respiratory muscle fibres: specialisation and plasticity. Thorax 2004;59:808–17.
190. van Balkom RH, van der Heijden HF, van Herwaarden CL, Dekhuijzen PN. Corticosteroid-induced myopathy of the respiratory muscles. Neth J Med 1994;45:114–22.
191. Fauroux B, Cordingley J, Hart N, et al. Depression of diaphragm contractility by nitrous oxide in humans [table of contents]. Anesth Analg 2002;94:340–5.
192. Shaw IC, Mills GH, Turnbull D. The effect of propofol on airway pressures generated by magnetic stimulation of the phrenic nerves. Intensive Care Med 2002;28:891–7.
193. Smets EM, Garssen B, Schuster-Uitterhoeve AL, de Haes JC. Fatigue in cancer patients. Br J Cancer 1993;68:220–4.
194. Andrykowski MA, Brady MJ, Greiner CB, et al. 'Returning to normal' following bone marrow transplantation: outcomes, expectations and informed consent. Bone Marrow Transplant 1995;15:573–81.
195. Edmonds P, Higginson I, Altmann D, et al. Is the presence of dyspnea a risk factor for morbidity in cancer patients? J Pain Symptom Manage 2000;19:15–22.
196. Dudgeon DJ, Lertzman M. Dyspnea in the advanced cancer patient. J Pain Symptom Manage 1998;16:212–9.
197. Winningham ML. Strategies for managing cancer-related fatigue syndrome: a rehabilitation approach. Cancer 2001;92(4 Suppl):988–97.
198. Dimeo F, Stieglitz RD, Novelli-Fischer U, et al. Correlation between physical performance and fatigue in cancer patients. Ann Oncol 1997;8:1251–5.
199. Dimeo FC. Effects of exercise on cancer-related fatigue. Cancer 2001;92(6 Suppl):1689–93.
200. Wijkstra PJ, van der Mark TW, Kraan J, et al. Long-term effects of home rehabilitation on physical performance in chronic obstructive pulmonary disease. Am J Respir Crit Care Med 1996;153(4 Pt 1):1234–41.
201. Groeger JS, Glassman J, Nierman DM, et al. Probability of mortality of critically ill cancer patients at 72 h of intensive care unit (ICU) management. Support Care Cancer 2003;11:686–95.
202. Groeger JS, White P Jr, Nierman DM, et al. Outcome for cancer patients requiring mechanical ventilation. J Clin Oncol 1999;17:991–7.
203. Azoulay E, Thiery G, Chevret S, et al. The prognosis of acute respiratory failure in critically ill cancer patients. Medicine (Baltimore) 2004;83:360–70.
204. Kress JP, Christenson J, Pohlman AS, et al. Outcomes of critically ill cancer patients in a university hospital setting. Am J Respir Crit Care Med 1999;160:1957–61.
205. Afessa B, Tefferi A, Hoagland HC, et al. Outcome of recipients of bone marrow transplants who require intensive-care unit support. Mayo Clin Proc 1992;67:117–22.
206. Price K, Thall P, Kish S, Shannon V. Prognostic indicators for blood and marrow transplant patients admitted to an intensive care unit. Am J Respir Crit Care Med 1998;158:876–84.
207. Tremblay LN, Hyland RH, Schouten BD, Hanly PJ. Survival of acute myelogenous leukemia patients requiring intubation/ventilatory support. Clin Invest Med 1995;18:19–24.
208. Crawford SW, Fisher L. Predictive value of pulmonary function tests before marrow transplantation. Chest 1992;101:1257–64.
209. Khassawneh BY, White P Jr, Anaissie EJ, et al. Outcome from mechanical ventilation after autologous peripheral blood stem cell transplantation. Chest 2002;121:185–8.
210. Goodnough LT, Brecher ME, Kanter MH, AuBuchon JP. Transfusion medicine. Second of two parts—blood conservation. N Engl J Med 1999;340:525–33.
211. Kopko PM, Marshall CS, MacKenzie MR, et al. Transfusion-related acute lung injury: report of a clinical look-back investigation. JAMA 2002;287:1968–71.
212. Hamacher J, Lucas R, Lijnen HR, et al. Tumor necrosis factor-alpha and angiostatin are mediators of endothelial cytotoxicity in bronchoalveolar lavages of patients with acute respiratory distress syndrome. Am J Respir Crit Care Med 2002;166:651–6.
213. Pittet JF, Mackersie RC, Martin TR, Matthay MA. Biological markers of acute lung injury: prognostic and pathogenetic significance. Am J Respir Crit Care Med 1997;155:1187–205.
214. Wang H, Yang H, Czura CJ, et al. HMGB1 as a late mediator of lethal systemic inflammation. Am J Respir Crit Care Med 2001;164(10 Pt 1):1768–73.
215. Abraham E, Arcaroli J, Carmody A, et al. HMG-1 as a mediator of acute lung inflammation. J Immunol 2000;165:2950–4.
216. Ware LB, Matthay MA. The acute respiratory distress syndrome. N Engl J Med 2000;342:1334–49.
217. Laufe MD, Simon RH, Flint A, Keller JB. Adult respiratory distress syndrome in neutropenic patients. Am J Med 1986;80:1022–6.
218. Nelson S. Novel nonantibiotic therapies for pneumonia: cytokines and host defense. Chest 2001;119:419S–25S.
219. Suchyta MR, Orme JF Jr, Morris AH. The changing face of organ failure in ARDS. Chest 2003;124:1871–9.
220. Bernard GR, Vincent JL, Laterre PF, et al. Efficacy and safety of recombinant human activated protein C for severe sepsis. N Engl J Med 2001;344:699–709.
221. Brun-Buisson C, Brochard L. Corticosteroid therapy in acute respiratory distress syndrome: better late than never? JAMA 1998;280:182–3.
222. Meduri GU, Headley AS, Golden E, et al. Effect of prolonged methylprednisolone therapy in unresolving acute respiratory distress syndrome: a randomized controlled trial. JAMA 1998;280:159–65.
223. Schuller D, Mitchell JP, Calandrino FS, Schuster DP. Fluid balance during pulmonary edema. Is fluid gain a marker or a cause of poor outcome? Chest 1991;100:1068–75.
224. Schuster DP. Fluid management in ARDS: "keep them dry" or does it matter? Intensive Care Med 1995;21:101–3.
225. Evans TW. International Consensus Conference in Intensive Care Medicine: noninvasive positive pressure ventilation in acute respiratory failure. Intensive Care Med 2001;27:166–78.
226. Kramer N, Meyer TJ, Meharg J, et al. Randomized, prospective trial of noninvasive positive pressure ventilation in acute respiratory failure. Am J Respir Crit Care Med 1995;151:1799–806.
227. Azoulay E, Alberti C, Bornstain C, et al. Improved survival in cancer patients requiring mechanical ventilatory support: impact of noninvasive mechanical ventilatory support. Crit Care Med 2001;29:519–25.
228. Hilbert G, Gruson D, Vargas F, et al. Noninvasive ventilation in immunosuppressed patients with pulmonary infiltrates, fever, and acute respiratory failure. N Engl J Med 2001;344:481–7.
229. ARDS Network. Ventilation with lower tidal volumes as compared with traditional tidal volumes for acute lung injury and the acute respiratory distress syndrome. N Engl J Med 2000;342:1301–8.
230. Brochard L, Roudot-Thoraval F, Roupie E, et al. Tidal volume reduction for prevention of ventilator-induced lung injury in acute respiratory distress syndrome. The Multicenter Trail Group on Tidal Volume reduction in ARDS. Am J Respir Crit Care Med 1998;158:1831–8.

136

Gastrointestinal and Hepatic Complications in Cancer Patients

Marta L. Davila, MD
Robert S. Bresalier, MD

Gastrointestinal complications are very common in patients undergoing cancer treatment. Some of these complications can be life threatening and require prompt and appropriate diagnosis and treatment. This chapter addresses important gastrointestinal issues for the patient with cancer, including those undergoing hematopoietic cell transplantation, and focuses on the evaluation and management of these problems.

MALIGNANT DYSPHAGIA

Patients with esophageal cancer will often present at an advanced, incurable stage. For those who are not candidates for surgical resection, palliation can be achieved by radiation with or without chemotherapy. Unfortunately, improvement of dysphagia by these methods may take several weeks during which patients may experience a decline in nutritional status and weight loss. For those who cannot tolerate chemoradiation or for those who develop recurrent dysphagia after treatment, a variety of endoscopic techniques have been developed to improve esophageal luminal patency (Table 136-1).

Esophageal Dilation Esophageal dilation with through-the-scope balloons, mercury-filled rubber bougies, or wire-guided bougies (Savary-Gilliard dilators) can provide safe, temporary relief of dysphagia until definitive treatment is initiated.[1–2] Dilation, to be successful, must be repeated every few weeks.[1–2] The procedure carries a small risk of perforation, particularly with blind passage of Maloney dilators or in patients receiving concurrent radiation therapy.[3]

Laser Therapy Laser energy produced by the neodymium:yttrium-aluminum-garnet crystal, or Nd:YAG has been extensively used for the palliation of esophageal cancer.[4–7] The technique involves administration of laser energy by way of a quartz fiber guided through the biopsy channel of an endoscope. The laser beam is directed at the tumor with the goal of vaporizing the tissue and restoring luminal patency.[4] Treatment is usually accomplished in a retrograde fashion so that the distal end of the tumor is treated first. This approach requires prior esophageal dilation to allow passage of the endoscope. Early experiences revealed that if the most proximal end of the tumor was treated first, acute tissue edema occurred leading to the inability to advance the endoscope distally and possible premature cessation of treatment. Treatments can be performed every 2 days and are usually completed in 3 to 4 sessions.[4] Luminal patency can be achieved in up to 97% of patients with functional success (or the ability to ingest all necessary calories) in 70%.[4,6] Major complications include esophageal perforation (in less than 5% of patients), development of tracheo-esophageal fistula, hemorrhage and bacteremia.[8] Disadvantages of Nd:YAG laser therapy include difficulties in treating long, tortuous lesions or lesions located in the proximal esophagus, number of treatment sessions required and high cost.[7]

Table 136-1 Endoscopic Options in the Treatment of Malignant Dysphagia
Esophageal dilation
Laser therapy with Nd:YAG
Photodynamic therapy
Self-expanding stents
Metal
Plastic

Photodynamic Therapy Photodynamic therapy (PDT) is another effective endoscopic technique used for palliation of esophageal cancer. PDT uses a photosensitizing agent and low power laser to achieve tumor necrosis and luminal patency. Porfimer sodium (Photofrin) is the only photosensitizer approved by the US Food and Drug Administration for the treatment of esophageal cancer. The usual Photofrin dose is 2 mg/kg of body weight given as an intravenous bolus over 3 to 5 minutes. After systemic injection, the photosensitizer is absorbed by most tissues, but for reasons not yet clearly understood, it is selectively retained at a higher concentration by neoplastic tissue. At approximately 48 hours after injection, the ratio of photosensitizer in neoplastic tissue compared to non-neoplastic tissue is approximately 2:1.[9] Some residual photosensitizer may remain in the skin for up to 45 days rendering the patient sensitive to ambient light and even strong indoor lighting. Thus, patients should be warned to avoid direct sunlight for up to 4 to 6 weeks after injection.

Approximately 48 hours after injection, patients are exposed to monochrome laser light at 630 nm via cylindrical diffuser attached to the tip of a quartz optical fiber placed through the accessory channel of an endoscope. The laser output is adjusted to deliver 300 J/cm of diffuser tip.[10] The tip of the diffusing fibers is provided in several lengths to better match the length of the lesion being treated.

Laser light will initiate a photochemical reaction in the tissue leading to the formation of oxygen radicals, ischemia and tumor necrosis.[11] In a study comparing PDT with Nd:YAG, PDT was found to be superior in treating circumferential lesions in the upper third of the esophagus. For tumors longer than 8 cm, PDT was twice as effective as Nd:YAG in eradicating tumor, and lumens remained patent for a longer period of time, especially in patients with esophageal adenocarcinoma.[11] In a prospective, randomized, multi-center study involving 218 patients, treatment with both PDT and Nd:YAG had similar improvement in dysphagia and equivalent objective tumor response at week 1. The objective tumor response was significantly higher in the PDT treated group (32%) at 1 month compared to the Nd:YAG-treated group (20%).[12] Trends for improved responses were seen with PDT for tumors located in the upper and lower third of the esophagus, in long tumors and in patients who had prior therapy. PDT was associated with significantly fewer perforations compared to Nd:YAG laser (1% vs 7%), although there were more minor complications in the PDT treated group, with complications related to photosensitivity in 19% of patients.[12]

Self-Expanding Stents Peroral insertion of a plastic or a stainless steel reinforced endoprostheses served as a useful option in patients in need of palliation of dysphagia for over two decades.[13] Esophageal dilation is required to properly prepare the esophageal lumen for prosthesis deployment. Unfortunately, insertion of this type of endoprostheses was associated with a high complication rate including obstruction (14.5%), migration (3%), and perforation (2%), with a procedure related mortality of approximately 7%.[13] Self-expanding metal stents (SEMS) were developed in the early 1990s in an attempt to decrease the complication rate and improve the ease of insertion.[14–16] In a study of 33 patients with inoperable esophageal cancer, all attempted insertions of expandable metal stents were successful, and the dysphagia scores were reduced from grades 3–4 to 0 or 1.[14] There were no perforations related to insertion, but dysphagia recurred in six patients (20%), due to stent migration, tumor overgrowth and food impaction. Similar results were seen in another study of 77 patients; with relief of dysphagia in over 90%, and a complication rate of 11%.[15] Advantages of SEMS include relative ease of insertion, larger stent diameters, and low risk of perforation with elimination of the need for excessive dilation. Disadvantages include high cost, tumor ingrowth and overgrowth, stent migration, maldeployment, inadequate expansion, airway obstruction and hemorrhage.[16] The rate of tumor ingrowth has now been reduced with the introduction of stents covered by a polyurethane coating.[17] Covered stents have now become the device of choice in the management of patients with tracheo-esophageal fistulas.[18] A recent additional option for palliation of esophageal cancer has resulted from the development of self-expanding plastic stents. These stents require fluoroscopic guidance for placement. The advantage for the operator is that these stents can be repositioned or removed if necessary. Self-expanding plastic stents have been reported to be as successful as metal stents in ease of deployment and palliation of dysphagia.[19] However, another study has reported a 25% deployment failure rate, and a 12.5% rate of early stent migration (within 72 hours).[20]

In summary, there are several endoscopic approaches to the palliation of malignant dysphagia. Covered stents are the therapy of choice in patients with tracheo-esophageal fistulas. In those without a fistula, endoscopic therapy should be individualized and based on location and features of the lesion, patient preference, and institutional expertise.

ESOPHAGITIS

Esophagitis can be caused by cytotoxic effects of chemotherapy, radiation, as well as by viral, fungal, and bacterial organisms. Other causes of esophagitis include acid reflux disease, pill-induced injury, and graft-versus-host disease (GVHD) in hematopoietic cell transplant recipients (Table 136-2). When esophagitis is suspected, particularly in an immuno-compromised patient, prompt evaluation with endoscopy with biopsies and/or brushings is indicated to allow for early diagnosis and therapy.[21]

Esophageal candidiasis is one of the most common infections in the immuno-compromised host. Patients usually complain of odynophagia (pain on swallowing) and/or dysphagia (difficulties swallowing). The absence of oral thrush does not preclude esophageal involvement. The diagnosis is usually made by endoscopic examination. On endoscopy, white plaque-like lesions with surrounding erythema can be seen covering the esophageal walls. Esophageal brushings confirm the presence of yeast or hyphal forms. The yeast may be seen invading mucosal cells on biopsy. Treatment requires systemic antifungal therapy. Fluconazole (100 to 200 mg daily for 14 to 21 days) is effective in eradicating the infection.[22] Itraconazole oral solution (200 mg daily) and voriconazole (200 mg twice daily) appear to be as effective as fluconazole in the treatment of esophageal candidiasis.[23,24] Furthermore, voriconazole may be used in the treatment of infections unresponsive or refractory to fluconazole therapy.[25] The new echinocandins (caspofungin, micafungin, and anidulafungin) are administered intravenously and are also effective for the treatment of *Candida* esophagitis.[26–28] Amphotericin B (0.3 to 0.7 mg/kg daily) has fallen out of favor because of its toxicity when compared to the other antifungal drugs.

Table 136-2 Causes of Esophagitis in the Cancer Patient

Acid related
Infection
Fungal—*Candida*
Viral—CMV, HSV, VZV
Bacterial—Polymicrobial from oral flora
Radiation
Pill-induced
Graft-versus-host disease

CMV = cytomegalovirus; HSV = herpes simplex virus; VZV = varicella-zoster virus.

Viral infections of the esophagus are caused by herpes simplex virus (HSV), cytomegalovirus (CMV) and, rarely, varicella-zoster virus (VZV).[21] Patients usually present with odynophagia and dysphagia. Less frequent symptoms include nausea, vomiting, heartburn, epigastric pain, and fever. In the case of HSV esophagitis, some patients may have coexistent herpes labialis or oropharyngeal ulcers.[29] Diagnosis is made by endoscopy and biopsy (Figure 136-1). HSV lesions in the early stage, may appear as small vesicles. The vesicles eventually coalesce to form large ulcers that are usually less than 2 cm in size. The ulcers are well circumscribed with normal appearing intervening mucosa.[30] CMV will cause ulcers which are linear or serpiginous and deeper than HSV-related ulcers. Exudates may also be present.[30] Biopsies taken from the edge of an HSV-related ulcer will show intranuclear inclusions and multinucleated giant cells. Inclusions can also be detected by immuno-histochemistry, using monoclonal antibodies to HSV.[30] Viral cultures are helpful in identifying resistant strains in patients who do not respond to acyclovir. VZV can produce esophagitis in adults with herpes zoster, usually in the setting of disseminated infection.[21] Endoscopically, VZV ulcers are similar to those seen with HSV. On biopsy specimens, distinction from HSV will require immuno-histochemistry or culture.

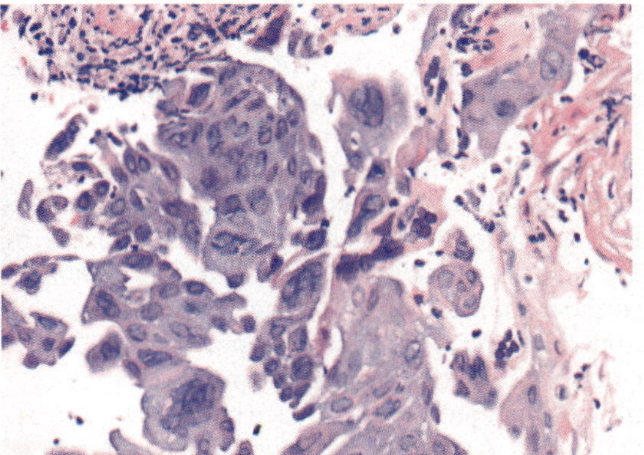

Figure 136-1 Herpes simplex virus (HSV) esophagitis. High power view of esophageal mucosa shows squamous cells with ground glass nuclear viral inclusions and multinucleated giant cells in a background of neutrophilic exudates. Courtesy of Dr. TT Wu, M.D. Anderson Cancer Center.

CMV infects endothelial cells and fibroblasts, but not epithelial cells as with HSV and VZV. Routine biopsies in a CMV-infected patient show intranuclear inclusions in fibroblasts and endothelial cells. Immuno-histochemistry with anti-CMV antibodies is also helpful for diagnosis.

For patients with HSV esophagitis, acyclovir (orally or intravenously) is the therapy of choice. Foscarnet is reserved for those patients who are known to be resistant or do not respond to acyclovir.[31] VZV esophagitis is treated with intravenous acyclovir because these patients usually will have disseminated infection. After initial clinical improvement, patients can be switched to an oral agent such as valacyclovir. There is limited clinical experience with either valacyclovir or famciclovir in the immuno-compromised host. However, there are data from immuno-competent adults that these drugs significantly accelerate the resolution of pain and reduce the duration of post-herpetic neuralgia when compared to acyclovir.[32,33] CMV esophagitis can be treated with intravenous ganciclovir (5 mg/kg bid) or foscarnet (90 mg/kg bid) for a total of 3 to 6 weeks.[34–36] There are anecdotal reports of oral valaciclovir being used effectively to treat CMV esophagitis once odynophagia has improved on IV ganciclovir and patients can tolerate oral medication. Additional studies are needed in this area to make specific recommendations.

Bacterial esophagitis can occur in the immuno-compromised patient and is usually polymicrobial, and derived from oral flora.[21] The diagnosis is made by endoscopic biopsies which demonstrate the presence of clusters of bacteria mixed with necrotic epithelial cells.[37] The treatment is broad-spectrum antibiotic therapy.

Radiation esophagitis usually occurs during treatment of lung and esophageal cancers. The severity of esophagitis increases with radiation dose and with the use of certain chemotherapeutic agents such as doxorubicin, bleomycin, cyclophosphamide, and cisplatin.[38,39] Patients may complain of odynophagia, dysphagia, and chest pain. Endoscopy may reveal erythema, edema and friability of the esophageal mucosa, as well as ulcerations with eventual stricture formation. Strictures can be managed with esophageal dilation. Medical therapy includes use of viscous lidocaine, H-2 blockers or proton pump inhibitors to prevent further acid-related injury.

Pill induced esophagitis can occur in patients taking medication at bedtime with insufficient liquid or in the recumbent position. The most common medications associated with this disorder include potassium chloride, tetracyclines, aspirin, nonsteroidal anti-inflammatory drugs,

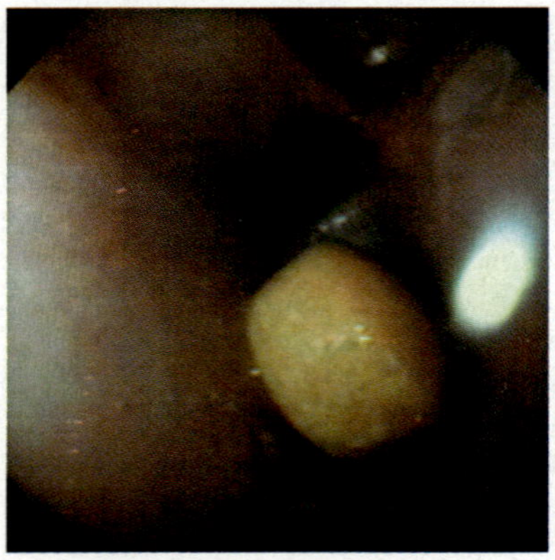

Figure 136-2 Pill-induced esophageal damage. A pill is seen at endoscopy lodged above an esophageal stricture.

quinidine, iron, and alendronate. Patients will often present with sudden onset of odynophagia that may be, severe enough to make even the swallowing of saliva difficult and painful. Endoscopy is helpful in making a diagnosis; but more important, it serves to rule out other diagnoses such as infectious esophagitis and malignancy. On endoscopy, there is usually a discrete, single ulcer located in the proximal esophagus.[40] On occasion, the injury appears as a nodular, polypoid lesion suggestive of a neoplasm, or as a stricture[41,42] (Figure 136-2). Esophageal biopsies are non-specific and may show acute inflammatory changes only. There is no specific therapy for this disorder, since pill-induced ulcerations can heal spontaneously within a few days without any intervention. Strictures will require endoscopic dilation. The only recommendation is to avoid the inciting agent, if possible. If a patient needs to continue on medication, he or she should be instructed on drinking plenty of liquids with the medicine and avoiding a recumbent position after ingestion.

TYPHLITIS

Typhlitis (from the Greek word *typhlon*) is a clinical syndrome in patients with neutropenia characterized by fever and right lower quadrant pain. This entity has received various names including necrotizing enterocolitis, neutropenic colitis, ileocecal syndrome, and cecitis.[43,44] Typhlitis was originally described in children following induction chemotherapy for acute leukemia.[45] It has subsequently been reported in adults with acute myeloid leukemia, acute lymphoblastic leukemia, multiple myeloma, aplastic anemia, myelodysplastic syndromes, granulocytopenias from other causes, acquired immuno-deficiency syndrome, and following immuno-suppressive therapy for solid malignancies and transplants.[46,47] The disease appears to be the result of a combination of factors including mucosal injury by cytotoxic drugs, neutropenia, and impaired host defense to intestinal organisms.[47] The cecum is almost always affected but the disease can often extend into the terminal ileum and right and left colon.[46] Pathology may reveal edema of the mucosa or entire intestinal wall, mucosal ulcerations, focal hemorrhage, and mucosal or transmural necrosis. Only rarely are leukemic or acute inflammatory infiltrates identified.[47] Various organisms alone, or in combination, have been identified in surgical specimens and peritoneal fluid, including gram-negative rods, gram-positive cocci, enterococci, *Clostridium septicum, Candida,* and CMV.[45,46] *Clostridium difficile* toxin is occasionally detected in the stools.[45] Bacteremia is frequently reported.[48]

Typhlitis should be suspected in any neutropenic patient presenting with fever and abdominal pain, particularly in the right lower quadrant, with or without rebound tenderness. Other presenting symptoms include abdominal distention, nausea, vomiting, and watery or bloody diarrhea. Peritoneal signs and shock can be present with bowel perforation. Symptoms often occur 10 to 14 days after initiation of cytotoxic chemotherapy.[49] Given that the clinical findings may be subtle and non-specific, one must consider other entities in the differential diagnosis, including pseudomembranous colitis, colonic pseudoobstruction, acute appendicitis, ischemic colitis, inflammatory bowel disease, and infectious colitis.

Imaging studies can be useful in supporting a diagnosis of typhlitis. CT is the preferred diagnostic modality over ultrasound and plain abdominal films.[45] Abnormal findings on CT imaging and ultrasonography include a fluid-filled, dilated cecum, a right lower quadrant inflammatory mass, and pericecal fluid or inflammatory changes in the pericecal soft tissues.[45] Plain films of the abdomen may be non-specific but, occasionally, a distended cecum with dilated adjacent small bowel loops, thumbprinting, or localized pneumatosis intestinalis is seen.[49] Barium enema or colonoscopy can be hazardous as they can precipitate perforation.

There have been no randomized trials on the treatment of typhlitis. Conservative management consists of bowel rest, nasogastric suction, intravenous fluids, and broad-spectrum antibiotic therapy.[45,50] Antibiotic coverage for *C. difficile* infection should be added if pseudomembranous colitis has not been excluded. Cytopenias and coagulopathy should be corrected. Recombinant granulocyte colony-stimulating factor (G-CSF) has been used to hasten recovery, since normalization of the leukocyte count may allow containment and healing of bowel lesions.[49,51] Surgery has been recommended for patients with gastrointestinal bleeding that persists despite correction of cytopenias and coagulopathy; for those with free intra-abdominal perforation or clinical deterioration during medical therapy, and to differentiate from other acute abdominal diseases for which surgery is indicated.[49,52] The standard surgical approach is a two-stage right hemicolectomy.[49] Some authors have reported significant complications when primary bowel anastomoses have been attempted in the face of ongoing leukopenia.[53,54] A surgeon must exert caution when dealing with edematous bowel without apparent gangrene, since mucosal necrosis may be present underneath very unimpressive serosal inflammation. Incomplete removal of all necrotic tissue may lead to death.[47]

Patients who develop typhlitis during chemotherapy are at risk for developing this complication during subsequent treatment. Patients should be allowed to heal completely and recover from typhlitis before chemotherapy is again administered.

DIARRHEA

Diarrhea is a common complication of cytotoxic therapy. It is most commonly described with fluoropyrimidines (particularly 5-fluorouracil [5-FU]), irinotecan, methotrexate and cisplatin. Chemotherapy-induced diarrhea can be debilitating and even life-threatening. It is the dose-limiting factor and the major toxicity of regimens containing a fluoropyrimidine and/or irinotecan. Severe diarrhea can lead to treatment delays, reduced quality of life, and diminished compliance with treatment regimens.

The incidence of diarrhea with 5-FU is increased by the addition of leucovorin. Diarrhea is worse when 5-FU is administered by bolus injection as opposed to protracted intravenous infusion.[55] The toxic effects of 5-FU also depend upon age and gender, being more common in women than men, and worse in women older than age 70 years.[56,57] Irinotecan can cause an early onset diarrhea accompanied by abdominal cramping, lacrimation, salivation, and other symptoms that appear cholinergic-mediated. These symptoms can be effectively treated with atropine as well as loperamide.[58] The late diarrhea associated with irinotecan is unpredictable and can occur at all dose levels, although it is severe at higher dose regimens. Significant diarrhea has been reported with a combination of irinotecan, 5-FU and leucovorin (IFL), compared to 5-FU and leucovorin alone.[59–62]

Radiation therapy can produce injury to the gastrointestinal mucosa that peaks 1 to 2 weeks after irradiation. Worsening diarrhea can be seen when radiation is given in combination with chemotherapy, such as 5-FU in the treatment of rectal cancer.[63]

The treatment of chemotherapy or radiation induced diarrhea involve aggressive fluid and electrolyte replacement and the use of pharmacologic agents to reduce fluid loss from the gut and decrease intestinal motility. Opioid agonists are the most commonly used agents in this setting. For mild to moderate diarrhea, loperamide (Imodium) 4 mg is given as the initial dose, followed by 2 mg every 4 hours or after every stool. A more aggressive regimen is often needed for patients with irinotecan-induced diarrhea with loperamide 4 mg initially followed by 2 mg every 2 hours or 4 mg every 4 hours until diarrhea-free for 12 hours.[64,65] Careful observation of patients receiving these drugs is warranted because of their impairment of intestinal motility. In patients with diarrhea refractory to opioid agonists, octreotide, a synthetic long-acting somatostatin analog, should be considered. Octreotide can reduce intestinal secretion, increase absorption of fluid and electrolytes and prolong intestinal transit time.[66] The recommended initial dose of octreotide is 100 to 150 μg subcutaneously or 25 to 50 µg over 1 hour IV, three times a day.[65,67] Higher doses (500 to 2,500 µg three times daily) may be effective in non-responders.[65,67–69] Other agents that have been used as adjunctive therapy in the treatment of mild to moderate chemotherapy induced diarrhea include absorbents such as kaolin and charcoal, deodorized tincture of opium (DTO), paregoric, and codeine. Guidelines from a consensus conference on the evaluation and management of patients with chemotherapy-induced diarrhea were published in 1998 and updated in 2004.[65] The guidelines emphasize assessment of symptoms including number of stools over baseline, stool composition, presence of nocturnal diarrhea, duration of symptoms, and the presence of added risk factors such as fever, abdominal pain and/or cramping, or neutropenia. Based on a detailed assessment, patients are classified as complicated or uncomplicated. Uncomplicated patients can be managed conservatively in the outpatient setting with oral rehydration and opioid agonists. Patients who have complications with severe diarrhea, nausea, vomiting, fever, or neutropenia, should be admitted to the hospital for a diagnostic work-up and treated aggressively with octreotide, intravenous fluids, and antibiotics.[65]

For patients undergoing hematopoietic stem cell transplantation, diarrhea may be due to the conditioning regimen, GVHD, or to an infection related to immuno-suppressive therapy (Table 136-3). Diarrhea in the immediate post-transplantation period is generally the result of injury to the intestinal mucosa caused by the conditioning regimen. This regimen includes total body irradiation and/or a combination of chemotherapy agents. Mucosal injury results in a secretory diarrhea that resolves with mucosal restitution, usually by the third week after treatment. After day 20, acute GVHD is the most common cause of diarrhea in this patients.[70] GVHD will be discussed separately in the next segment.

If diarrhea is not directly the result of chemotherapy or radiation and particularly if it occurs in a hospital setting, *C. difficile* infection should be considered since this is the most common cause of infectious diarrhea in hospitalized patients.[71] Although commonly associated with use of antibiotic therapy, risk factors for *C difficile* diarrhea or colitis also include bowel surgery, immunocompromised state and any process that suppresses the normal flora including anti-fungal and chemotherapeutic agents. Cancer patients receiving chemotherapy appear predisposed to *C. difficile*–induced diarrhea even in the absence of antibiotics.[72,73] In a study of such patients, methotrexate, doxorubicin, and cyclophosphamide were the drugs most frequently associated with *C. difficile* infection.[73] The diagnosis is established by detecting the presence of *C. difficile* toxin in stool or by identifying pseudomembranous colitis on endoscopic evaluation (Figure 136-3). The stool-cytotoxin test is a tissue culture assay based on the induction of cell rounding by *C. difficile* toxin in stool filtrate. This assay is the "gold standard" because of its high sensitivity (94–100%) and specificity (99%).[74,75] The disadvantages of this assay are its high cost and the time needed to complete the assay, typically two or three days. More rapid and inexpensive assays with similar sensitivity (70–90%) and specificity (99%) are provided by a number of enzyme linked immuno-sorbent assays (ELISAs).[76] A stool culture for *C. difficile* is a less efficient method of establishing a laboratory diagnosis, since some strains of *C. difficile* are non-toxicogenic. In pseudomembranous colitis caused by *C. difficile* infection, sigmoidoscopy or colonoscopy reveals characteristic adherent yellow plaques that vary in diameter from 2 to 10 mm. The intervening mucosa typically appears normal or only mildly erythematous.[71] The rectum and sigmoid colon are typically involved, but in approximately 10% of cases, colitis is confined to the more proximal colon and therefore may be missed during sigmoidoscopy.[77]

Table 136-3 Differential Diagnosis of Diarrhea in the Cancer and Hematopoietic Cell Transplant Patient
Chemotherapy-related (fluoropyrimidine, irinotecan, topotecan, methotrexate, cisplatin)
Radiation therapy
Conditioning regimen
Graft-versus-host disease
Infection
Bacterial (including *C. difficile*)
Viral (including CMV)
CMV = cytomegalovirus.

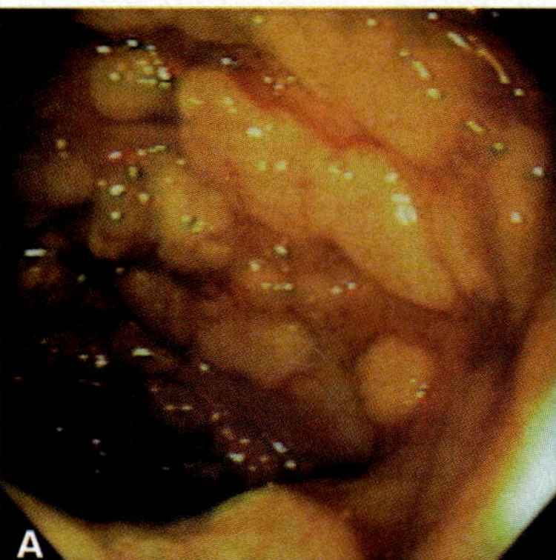

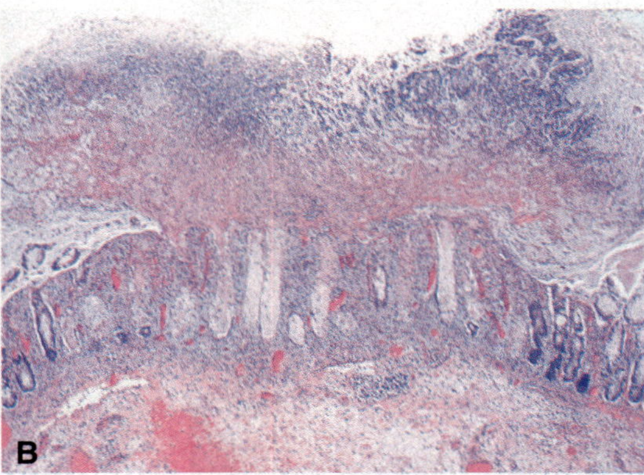

Figure 136-3 Pseudomembranous colitis. **A,** Pseudomembranes adherent to the colonic mucosa seen at colonoscopy. **B,** Low-power view of colonic mucosa shows a typical volcano (mushroom)-like appearance with luminal inflammatory exudates.

Oral metronidazole at a dose of 500 mg three times daily for 10 to 14 days given orally or intravenously appears to be as effective as vancomycin 125 mg given orally four times a day for 10 to 14 days for the treatment of *C. difficile*–associated diarrhea.[78,79] Symptomatic improvement can be expected within 72 hours, and diarrhea and colitis resolve completely in more than 95% of patients after 10 days of treatment. Metronidazole is considered by many the initial choice for treatment since it is much less expensive than vancomycin; and the use of vancomycin, even when administered orally, may lead to selection of vancomycin-resistant enterococci.

In patients with severe infection and signs of systemic toxicity, some experts recommend initial therapy with vancomycin 125 mg orally four times daily and escalating the dose at 48-hour intervals up to 500 mg four times daily if diarrhea, fever and leukocytosis fail to improve. When patients do not respond to oral vancomycin alone, they may benefit from the addition of intravenous metronidazole at a dose of 500 mg every 8 hours. Intravenous vancomycin has no role in the treatment of *C. difficile* colitis since it is not excreted into the colon. Successful treatment of severe cases has also been reported with the use of adjunctive intracolonic vancomycin therapy administered as retention enema (0.5–1 g of vancomycin dissolved in 1–2 L of normal saline every 4–12 hours).[80–82]

Relapse may occur in 10 to 25% of cases of diarrhea caused by *C. difficile*. Possible reasons for a relapse include a failure to eradicate the organism from the colon or reinfection from the environment.[71] Antibiotic resistance does not appear to be a factor in relapse.[83]

Relapses usually occur within 1 to 3 weeks after the termination of initial therapy, and further antibiotic therapy is not required to precipitate a relapse. The most reasonable regimen for a first relapse is to repeat a 10 to 14 day course of oral metronidazole or vancomycin.[71] If a patient relapses after a second course of metronidazole or vancomycin, various approaches have been suggested including tapering and pulsed antibiotic therapy,[84] the use of anion-binding resins (cholestyramine and cholestipol) alone[85] or in combination with vancomycin,[86] and treatment with the yeast *Saccharomyces boulardii*.[87] However, relapses from *C. difficile* infection have not been thoroughly studied in controlled trials, and the best therapeutic approach is not known.

In the post-hematopoietic cell transplant patient, infectious diarrhea is relatively uncommon. In a prospective study of 296 patients following bone marrow transplantation, 126 (43%) developed acute diarrhea. Intestinal infection was found in 13%, with viruses being the most common organisms found (astrovirus, adenovirus, CMV, and rotavirus), followed by nosocomially-acquired bacteria (*C. difficile* and *Aeromonas*).[88] CMV deserves a special mention since it can cause diarrhea and bleeding because of mucosal ulceration.[89] The diagnosis of CMV is made by endoscopic

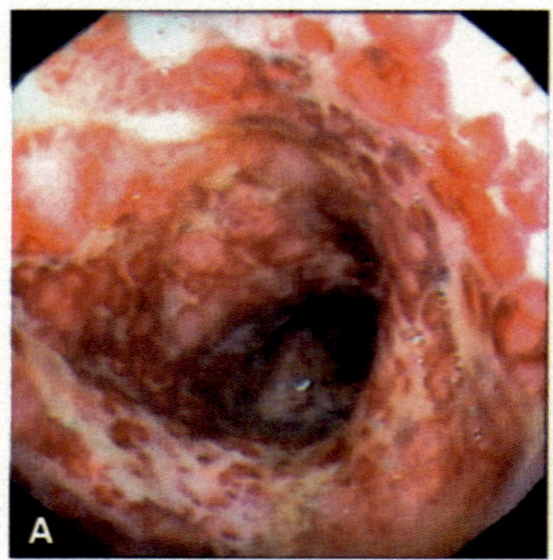

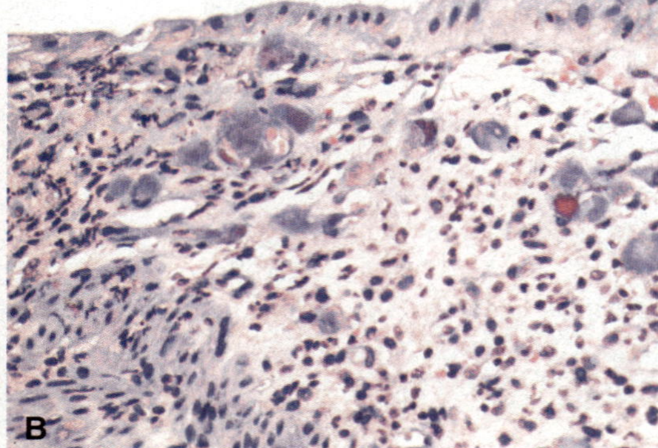

Figure 136-4 Cytomegalovirus (CMV) colitis. **A,** CMV colitis seen at endoscopy. **B,** High-power view of inflamed colonic mucosa demonstrates multiple viral inclusions in stroma cells.

biopsy (Figure 136-4), which should be sent for immuno-histochemistry and viral culture.[90] Infectious diarrhea related to *Salmonella*, *Shigella*, and *Campylobacter* species are very rare in hospitalized transplant patients. Parasites (*Cryptosporidium*, *Giardia lamblia*, *Entamoeba histolytica*) are also a rare cause of diarrhea, and most patients are infected pre-transplantation.[91–93]

GRAFT-VERSUS-HOST DISEASE

GVHD is divided into acute and chronic disease based upon the time of onset. Acute GVHD presents within the first 100 days of hematopoietic cell transplantation (HCT); whereas chronic GVHD is defined as the onset of disease after the first 100 days. The division at day 100 is artificial, and a continuum of clinical findings may be observed in patients with acute and chronic GVHD, as both commonly affect similar organs, principally the skin, liver, and gastrointestinal tract.

Acute Graft-Versus-Host Disease Clinically significant acute GVHD occurs in 20 to 50% of patients who receive an allogeneic hematopoietic cell transplant from a genotypically HLA-identical sibling.[94–96]

Risk factors for the development of acute GVHD include HLA mismatch, increasing dose of total body irradiation, increased donor or recipient age, female donor to male recipient, type and status of underlying disease, incomplete GVHD prophylaxis, and prior herpes infection in donor.[96–98] Involvement of the gastrointestinal tract is characterized by voluminous, watery diarrhea, and abdominal cramping. The diarrhea is secretory and occurs in the absence of oral intake, although such intake usually exacerbates the diarrhea. The diarrhea can frequently become bloody, resulting in significant transfusion requirements.[99] Patients can also present with upper gastrointestinal tract symptoms (such as dyspepsia, food intolerance, nausea, vomiting, and anorexia) in the absence of lower GI symptoms.[100] Apoptosis on a mucosal biopsy is required to make the diagnosis of gastrointestinal GVHD.[101] This finding, however, is not specific and can be seen in a variety of other conditions including CMV infection,[102] cryptosporidiosis,[103] inflammatory bowel disease,[104] and drug-induced colitis.[104–106] What area of the gastrointestinal tract to target for endoscopic biopsies continues to be a topic of debate. Some advocate directing the endoscopic evaluation based on the patient's gastrointestinal symptoms and the need to rule out infections and obstructing lesions.[107] Early literature relied on rectal biopsies for diagnosis (Figure 136-5),[108] and some centers continue to advocate this approach with a high diagnostic yield.[109] However, in another study involving 126 patients with diarrhea, gastric biopsies had the highest yield for the diagnosis of GVHD being positive in 22 of 26 patients, compared to 15 of 26 for duodenal and colonic biopsies.[88] Other studies have found that biopsies of the small bowel are the most sensitive tests in the diagnosis of GVHD regardless of whether the patient present with upper or lower GI symptoms.[110,111] The differences in results from these studies probably reflect a lack of a standardized approach to the diagnosis of gastrointestinal GVHD and the need for further studies. Until data from well-designed, prospective studies become available, it is best to routinely biopsy stomach, duodenum, and rectum when patients are referred for evaluation of potential acute GVHD.

In mild GVHD, the intestinal mucosa may appear grossly normal or have a mildly granular appearance.[112] Moderate to severe GVHD is associated with granular, erythematous, and edematous mucosa; and in severe cases, mucosal ulceration or large areas of mucosal sloughing may be present.[113,114] Still, endoscopic findings are usually reported as having no correlation with histologic or clinical grading of GVHD severity.[110,115]

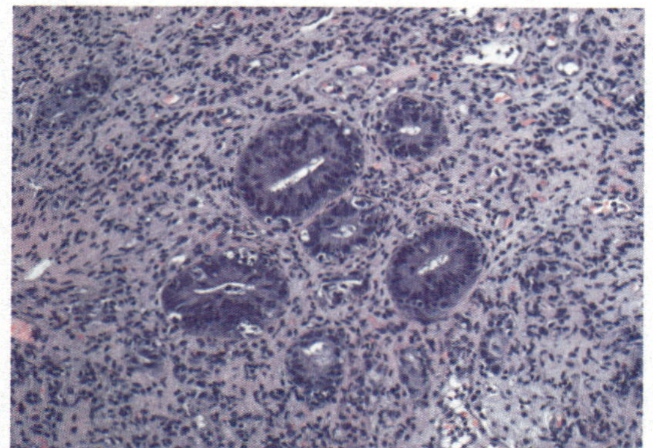

Figure 136-5 Graft-versus-host disease involving the colon. The colonic mucosa shows prominent crypt apoptosis and focal crypt dropouts in a background of granulation tissue. Courtesy of Dr. TT Wu, M.D. Anderson Cancer Center.

The liver is the second most commonly involved organ in acute GVHD. The earliest finding is commonly a rise in conjugated bilirubin and alkaline phosphatase. This reflects the underlying pathology in liver GVHD; that is, extensive bile duct damage with bile duct atypia and degeneration, epithelial cell dropout, and lymphocytic infiltration of small bile ducts leading to cholestasis.[116,117] Biopsy is the only method to diagnose GVHD of the liver, and to rule out other confounding diagnoses such veno-occlusive disease (VOD), infection, or drug toxicity. However, a liver biopsy may not be a feasible option because of the risk of bleeding due to thrombocytopenia soon after hematopoietic cell transplant. A transjugular liver biopsy might be the preferred option, if a liver biopsy is deemed necessary for diagnosis. But this is rarely the case, since biopsies from skin of gastrointestinal tract can be easily obtained, with less risk and a high diagnostic value.

For acute GVHD, the first and most effective treatment option is the use of corticosteroids.[107] Approximately 40% of patients will have a complete response.[118,119]

If high doses of steroids are not successful in controlling GVHD, second line treatments are less successful. These would include cyclosporine, tacrolimus, antithymocyte globulin, and mycophenolate mofetil.[120,121] In those with acute gastrointestinal GVHD, oral budesonide in addition to systemic steroids may confer some benefit, pushing complete response rated to 70% versus 40% with systemic steroids alone.[122,123] For symptoms relief, octreotide is reported to control diarrhea in some patients with GVHD.[124]

Chronic Graft-Versus-Host Disease The skin, liver, gastrointestinal tract, and lungs are the principal organs affected in patients with chronic GVHD. In this condition, liver histology will show lobular hepatitis, chronic hepatitis, and a reduction or absence of small bile ducts with cholestasis.[125] The liver function tests show elevations in bilirubin and alkaline phosphatase levels consistent with cholestasis. The oral mucosa is frequently involved and is commonly dry, resulting in ulceration and pain.[126] Involvement of the esophagus is the most common GI manifestation, with painful ulcerations, and formation of webs, rings, and strictures.[127,128] Involvement of small bowel and colon can occur, but it is significantly less frequent compared to the degree of involvement seen in acute GVHD. With intestinal involvement, patients can present with diarrhea, malabsorption, fibrosis of the submucosa, and sclerosis of the intestine.[128,129]

Treatment of chronic GVHD is beyond the scope of this review, but it should be mentioned that ursodeoxycholic acid (UDCA) has been used in the treatment of refractory chronic GVHD of the liver. The rationale for its use is that GVHD of the liver shares many characteristics of primary biliary cirrhosis, a disease known to respond to this therapy. In a study of 12 patients, treatment with UDCA resulted in a significant decrease in serum bilirubin, alkaline phosphatase and aspartate aminotransferase (AST) levels compared to baseline. Discontinuation of the drug resulted in prompt rise in the serum levels of all three markers.[130] The long-term efficacy of this treatment has not been studied.

RADIATION COLOPROCTITIS AND PROCTITIS

Patients receiving radiation therapy to the abdomen and pelvis for the treatment of gynecologic, genitourinary, gastrointestinal, and other malignancies are at risk for developing acute and chronic intestinal injury. Acute radiation injury usually occurs within six weeks of therapy. Patients will present with diarrhea, rectal urgency, tenesmus and less commonly rectal bleeding. These symptoms usually resolve without therapy within 6 months.[131] Chronic radiation proctitis or coloproctitis has a more delayed onset, occurring on average, a year or later after exposure. Chronic injury is due to epithelial atrophy and fibrosis associated with obliterative endarteritis and chronic mucosal ischemia.[131] The end result is an ischemic segment of bowel prone to stricture formation and bleeding. Patients may complain of diarrhea, difficulties with defecation, bleeding, tenesmus, rectal urgency, and, less commonly, fecal incontinence. The diagnosis is made by colonoscopy or sigmoidoscopy. Endoscopic findings include mucosal edema, erythema, friability and the presence of telangiectasias. Severe cases may show mucosal ulcerations with or without bleeding, and strictures.[131] There have been no large controlled trials in the treatment of radiation proctitis or coloproctitis. Information has been gathered mostly from case reports and small clinical trials. The use of aminosalicylate enemas has been disappointing.[132] Sucralfate, administered orally or topically, has been reported to improve symptoms, without causing significant adverse side effects,[133–135] but the data are limited and not definitive. Sucralfate enemas have been reported to be superior to a combination of oral sulfasalazine and prednisolone enemas for symptom control, but not in improving endoscopic appearance.[136] Other treatments that have shown some benefit in small clinical trials include the use of hyperbaric oxygen,[137] short-chain fatty acid enemas,[138] and rectal instillation of formaldehyde.[139–141] A number of endoscopic therapies have been used to treat bleeding in radiation proctitis or coloproctitis. Argon plasma coagulation (APC) is a modality that has gained wide acceptance in recent years in the treatment of bleeding telangiectasias of the gastrointestinal tract. APC uses energy transmitted to tissue by ionized gas. APC therapy can be administered with a probe inserted through an endoscope. The benefits of APC treatment in the setting of radiation proctitis have been shown in several case series.[142–145] APC treated patients will have improvement in bleeding and anemia after a median of 2.9 endoscopic sessions,[143] even when other treatment modalities have failed.[144,145] Lasers such as argon and Nd:YAG have also been used with good success to control bleeding.[146–148] Disadvantages of the lasers include lack of wide availability and high cost of equipment. Bipolar electrocoagulation (BiCAP) and heater probe are cautery devices that are inexpensive compared to lasers and have been extensively tested in other settings such as ulcer bleeding. They are effective in reducing bleeding and transfusion requirements in patients with radiation-induced damage to the bowel.[149] However, they may cause more tissue injury when compared to APC or lasers. Surgery should be reserved for patients with uncontrollable symptoms such as obstruction due to strictures, pain, or bleeding.

In summary, there are a number of medical, endoscopic, and surgical options for the treatment of radiation proctitis or coloproctitis, but definitive evidence of efficacy is limited. Selection of a treatment option should be based on type and severity of symptoms, and local expertise.

ACUTE PANCREATITIS

Acute pancreatitis in cancer and post hematopoietic cell transplant patients can be caused by conditions found in the general population such as gallstones or alcohol. However, when managing these patients, other etiologies should be taken into consideration including medications, chemotherapeutic agents, and infections. Drug-induced pancreatitis has no distinguishing clinical features. A careful drug history and the exclusion of other etiologies are essential to make a diagnosis. Some of the most common drugs involved include metronidazole, sulfonamides, tetracycline, furosemide, thiazides, estrogen, and tamoxifen.[150,151] The latter two may act via the induction of hypertriglyceridemia.[152,153] During the course of chemotherapy, pancreatitis has been reported with azathioprine,[154] ifosfamide,[155] prednisone,[156] cytosine arabinoside,[157] and various regimens of combination chemotherapy including vinca alkaloids, methotrexate, mitomycin C, 5-FU, cyclophosphamide, cisplatin, and bleomycin. Causes of pancreatitis in immuno-compromised patients include disseminated infections with CMV, VZV, adenovirus, and aspergillus.[158,159] Metastases to regional lymph nodes, producing ductal obstruction can cause pancreatitis, as can metastasis to the pancreas itself.[160,161]

In the evaluation of abdominal pain in patients with cancer, pancreatitis should be considered in the differential diagnosis. Evaluation should include a careful medication history, serum amylase and lipase levels, and imaging studies such as abdominal ultrasound to rule out gallstones or biliary obstruction, and CT scan to assess the severity of the inflammatory process and evaluate for associated complications.

VENO-OCCLUSIVE DISEASE

VOD is a clinical syndrome characterized by tender hepatomegaly, jaundice, and weight gain. It is more often seen in patients following hematopoietic cell transplantation, but it can also occur following use of chemotherapeutic agents in the non-transplant setting, ingestion of alkaloid toxins, and after high dose radiation therapy or liver transplantation.[162,163] In one report, the earliest signs of the disease were sudden weight gain and tender hepatomegaly occurring between days 3 and 6 following transplantation.[164] Peripheral edema and ascites were also present in a large proportion of patients. Liver function tests usually reveal an elevation in serum aminotransferases and conjugated bilirubin. In advanced cases, there will be deterioration of hepatic synthetic function. Hyperbilirubinemia tends to occur after the onset of weight gain and hepatomegaly. Patients with severe VOD had the greatest weight gain, developed hyperbilirubinemia early in their course, and were more likely to have edema and ascites. Severe VOD may be accompanied by renal insufficiency (similar to hepatorenal syndrome), confusion or disorientation, cardiac failure, and bleeding.[164]

The pathogenesis of VOD is not well understood but it is thought to begin with injury to the hepatic venous endothelium. Early changes include deposition of fibrinogen and factor VIII within the venular walls and liver sinusoids. Progressive venular occlusion occurs, leading to centrilobular hemorrhagic necrosis.[165–167] As disease progresses, pathology will reveal sclerosis of venular walls, fibrosis of venular lumens, and occlusion of terminal hepatic venules (Figure 136-6). The severity of clinical VOD appears to be proportional to the number and severity of histological changes noted and not due solely to occlusion of small hepatic venules.[167]

There are a number of risk factors associated with the development of VOD including: pre-existing liver disease, types of conditioning therapy prior to transplant, source of hematopoietic cells, degree of allogeneic match, female gender, use of certain antibiotics, and abnormal baseline lung diffusing capacity.[164,168–172]

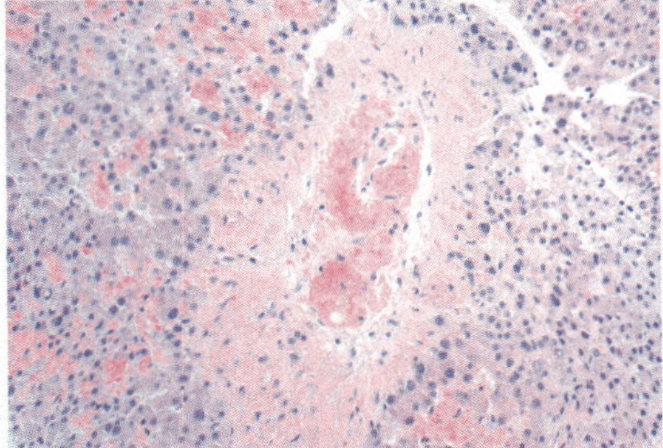

Figure 136-6 Veno-occlusive disease of the liver. The small hepatic vein demonstrates fibrous obliteration with fibrin deposits. The perivenular hepatocytes show prominent sinusoidal congestion. Courtesy of Dr. TT Wu, M. D. Anderson Cancer Center.

Most cases of VOD are diagnosed clinically. Two or more of the following (occurring within 20 days from transplant) have been proposed as clinical criteria for the diagnosis of VOD: (1) serum total bilirubin concentration greater than 2 mg/dL; (2) hepatomegaly or right upper quadrant pain; and (3) sudden weight gain due to fluid accumulation (greater than 5% of baseline).[165,173] However, the validity of this criteria has not been systematically tested.[173] There are a number of conditions that can mimic VOD including GVHD, hyperbilirubinemia associated with sepsis syndrome, passive congestion of the liver due to congestive heart failure, tumor infiltration of the liver, or a combination of these processes.[164] In patients for whom the diagnosis is in question, and GVHD or infection needs to be excluded, a liver biopsy may be necessary, but there is a high risk of bleeding in these patients given the concurrent thrombocytopenia and coagulopathy. A transjugular liver biopsy may be a safer approach, but in a study of 60 hematopoietic cell transplant patients who underwent transjugular liver biopsy, 11 patients (18%) had bleeding complications including three procedure-related deaths.[174] That same study reported on the utility of obtaining portal-hepatic venous pressure gradient for the diagnosis of VOD. A gradient >10 mm Hg correlated well with the histologic diagnosis of VOD, with a positive predictive value of 86% and a specificity of 91%.[174]

The clinical outcome of patients with VOD depends on the disease severity. Those with mild disease require no specific therapy despite evidence of liver biochemical abnormalities. Those with moderate disease will respond to sodium restriction, and diuretics. Severe VOD is associated with multi-organ failure and is usually fatal.[164] A number of treatment strategies have been used in severe VOD, including the use of alteplase (recombinant tissue-type plasminogen activator or tPA) in combination with heparin, and defibrotide. Treatment with alteplase and heparin have resulted in a response rate of approximately 30% but has been associated with a significant risk of life-threatening hemorrhage, particularly in patients with multi-organ failure.[175,176] Defibrotide is a polydeoxyribonucleotide that has been found to have anti-thrombotic, anti-ischemic and thrombolytic properties without causing significant anticoagulation. Defibrotide given intravenously in doses ranging from 5 to 60 mg/kg per day for a minimum of 14 days, results in a response in about 42 to 55% of patients, without any significant treatment-related toxicity.[177,178] Insertion of a transjugular intrahepatic portosystemic stent-shunt (TIPS) has been reported in small number of patients with severe VOD. TIPS was effective in improving portal pressure gradient; and in some patients, it was associated with clinical improvement of hepatic and renal symptoms. However, these effects may be transient and may not improve overall survival.[179–181]

In summary, there are limited options in the treatment of severe VOD, and further studies are needed to demonstrate the optimum treatment strategy.

DRUG HEPATOTOXICITY

Most hepatotoxic drug reactions are idiosyncratic, occurring because of either hypersensitivity mechanisms or host metabolic idiosyncrasy.[182] Chemotherapeutic agents may, however, possess predictable, dose-dependent, direct hepatotoxicity. Patients undergoing chemotherapy require careful assessment of liver function both prior to treatment and during therapy. If liver test findings are abnormal, the etiology must be defined promptly and as clearly as possible. In addition to drug reactions, there are multiple potential causes of abnormal liver test results in the population undergoing chemotherapy including tumor progression, infection, or the presence of coexisting hepatic disease (Table 136-4). Features suggestive of drug toxicity include the lack of abnormalities prior to the introduction of the drug, clinical illness, or biochemical abnormalities after drug administration, and resolution of those abnormalities after the drug is withdrawn.

Drug reactions can be classified as hepatocellular, cholestatic, or mixed, but these are generalizations that may not apply to all circumstances. Elevations of AST and ALT typically indicate hepatocellular injury, whereas increases in bilirubin and alkaline phosphatase suggest cholestasis. In addition to liver function tests, radiologic imaging such as abdominal ultrasound or computed tomography (CT) may be needed in the evaluation of these patients to rule out biliary, vascular, or tumor-related conditions.

Patients with pre-existing liver disease may be more susceptible to drug-induced hepatotoxicity. Chemotherapy (including the use of monoclonal antibodies) can lead to reactivation of hepatitis B.[183–185] Furthermore, the return of immune competence following chemotherapy may be associated with the development of clinical hepatitis and even liver failure.[186] Risk factors for reactivation include HepBsAg and HepBeAg seropositivity, detectable hepatitis B virus DNA prior to chemotherapy, male sex, diagnosis of lymphoma or breast cancer, and use of steroids.[183,187,188] Prophylactic treatment with lamivudine may be beneficial in preventing viral reactivation, or reducing its severity, in patients undergoing cytotoxic chemotherapy.[185,189] Hepatitis C infection also appears to have an impact in patients receiving chemotherapy, but the impact may be less than that seen in patients with hepatitis B virus.[190]

Table 136-4 Potential Causes of Hepatic Abnormalities in Cancer Patients

Direct effects of the tumor
Hepatic metastases
Portal vein thrombosis
Indirect effects of the tumor
Paraneoplastic syndromes
Preexisting liver disease
Coexisting medical conditions
Chemotherapeutic drugs
Graft-versus-host disease
Infection

Cytotoxic Drugs Very little is known regarding the hepatotoxic effects of most chemotherapeutic drugs, and mechanisms of injury are established for only a few agents. This section will discuss salient characteristics of hepatic injury by drug category.

Alkylating agents include a variety of drugs such cyclophosphamide, ifosfamide, melphalan, chlorambucil, busulfan, temozolomide, and the nitrosoureas. Although as a group, the mechanism of liver damage is unclear, depletion of glutathione, and oxidative injury have been implicated.[191] With the exception of cyclophosphamide and ifosfamide, patients receiving alkylating agents do not require a dose reduction. Cyclophosphamide at conventional dosage is uncommonly hepatotoxic and its effect is likely due to an idiosyncratic reaction. Diffuse hepatocellular destruction and massive hepatic necrosis have been described.[192]

The antimetabolites currently in clinical use include cytosine arabinoside (ara-C), 5-FU, 6-mercaptopurine (6-MP), azathioprine, 6-thioguanine and methotrexate. Hepatic metabolism plays an important role in the processing of these drugs, and dose reductions are usually necessary in patients with liver dysfunction. Ara-C, used in the treatment of acute myelogenous leukemia (AML), has been on rare occasions associated with cholestasis, which appears reversible.[193] Only rare reports of hepatotoxicity have been noted with intravenous 5-FU, but hepatotoxicity has been reported more commonly when 5-FU is administered in combination with levamisole.[194] Intra-arterial administration of the 5-FU metabolite floxuridine (fluorodeoxyuridine, FUdR) has been associated with two types of toxicity: one suggestive of hepatocellular injury, and the second one consistent with sclerosing cholangitis, with stricturing of the intra- and extra-hepatic bile ducts, and elevations of alkaline phosphatase and bilirubin.[195–197]

6-Mercaptopurine is often used for maintenance therapy in acute lymphoblastic leukemia (ALL). Two patterns of toxicity have been reported: hepatocellular injury and cholestasis.[198] Toxicity occurs more commonly when the daily dose of 2 mg/kg is exceeded. Azathioprine toxicity is less frequent and less dose-dependent compared with 6-mercaptopurine. Three different patterns of toxicity are described: a hypersensitivity reaction, an idiosyncratic cholestatic reaction, and endothelial cell injury with development of elevated portal pressures, VOD and peliosis hepatis.[199]

High-dose methotrexate (MTX) therapy has been associated with reversible elevations in aminotransferases,[200] and patients taking chronic low-dose methotrexate therapy for psoriasis or rheumatoid arthritis are at risk for developing hepatic fibrosis and cirrhosis. The risk is low in patients who receive less than 1.5 g of MTX as cumulative dose.[201]The antitumor antibiotics include doxorubicin and daunorubicin. Doxorubicin can cause hepatocellular injury and steatosis. Dose reduction has been recommended in patients with cholestasis to avoid greater toxicity.[202] Similar guidelines are followed for daunorubicin.

Table 136-5 Common Chemotherapeutic Agents That Produce Veno-Occlusive Disease
Dacarbazine
Azathioprine
6-Mercaptopurine
6-Thioguanine
Busulfan
Cyclophosphamide
ABVD (doxorubicin, bleomycin, vinblastine and dacarbazine)

VOD has been seen with dacarbazine,[203] 6-mercaptopurine,[204] azathioprine,[205,206] cyclophosphamide,[207] busulfan,[208] and following treatment with ABVD (doxorubicin, bleomycin, vinblastine, dacarbazine) for Hodgkin's disease (Table 136-5).[209]

In conclusion, chemotherapeutic agents alone or in combination with other drugs can cause a variety of toxic effects on the liver. Patients with underlying liver disease may be more susceptible to drug-induced hepatotoxicity. Careful monitoring of patients is critical in the prevention and treatment of hepatic complications of cancer chemotherapy.

REFERENCES

1. Heit HA, Johnson LF, Siegel SR, Boyce HW Jr. Palliative dilation for dysphagia in esophageal carcinoma. Ann Intern Med 1978;89:629–31.
2. Moses FM, Peura DA, Wong RK, Johnson LF. Palliative dilation of esophageal carcinoma. Gastrointest Endosc 1985;31:61–3.
3. Hernandez LV, Jacobson JW, Harris MS, Hernandez LJ. Comparison among the perforation rates of Maloney, balloon and Savary dilation of esophageal strictures. Gastrointest Endosc 2000;51:460–2.
4. Mellow MH, Pinkas H. Endoscopic laser therapy for malignancies affecting the esophagus and gastroesophageal junction. Arch Intern Med 1985;145:1443–46.
5. Murray FE, Bowers GJ, Birkett DH, Cave DR. Palliative laser therapy of advanced esophageal carcinoma: an alternative perspective. Am J Gastroenterol 1988;83:816–9.
6. Fleischer D, Kessler F. Endoscopic Nd:YAG laser therapy for carcinoma of the esophagus: a new form of palliative treatment. Gastroenterology 1983;85:600–6.
7. Fleischer D, Sivak MV Jr. Endoscopic Nd:YAG laser therapy as palliation for esophagogastric cancer. Parameters affecting initial outcome. Gastroenterology 1985;89:827–31.
8. Sander RR, Poesl H. Cancer of the oesophagus—palliation—laser treatment and combined procedures. Endoscopy 1993;25:679–82.
9. Nishioka, NS. Drug, light, and oxygen: a dynamic combination in the clinic. Gastroenterology 1998;114:604–6.
10. Haddad NG, Fleischer DE. Endoscopic laser therapy for esophageal cancer. Gastro Endo Clinics of North America 1994;4:863–74.
11. Marcon NE. Photodynamic therapy and cancer of the esophagus. Semin Oncol 1994;21:20–3.
12. Lightdale CJ, Heler SK, Marcon NE, et al. Photodynamic therapy with porfimer sodium versus thermal ablation therapy with Nd:YAG laser for palliation of esophageal cancer: a multicenter randomized trial. Gastrointest Endosc 1995;42:507–12.
13. Gasparri G, Casalegno PA, Camandona M, et al. Endoscopic insertion of 248 prostheses in inoperable carcinoma of the esophagus and cardia: short-term and long-term results. Gastrointest Endosc 1987;33:354–6.
14. Ellul JP, Watkinson A, Khan RJ, et al. Self-expanding metal stents for the palliation of dysphagia due to inoperable oesophageal carcinoma. Br J Surg 1995;82:1678–81.
15. Cowling MG, Hale H, Grundy A. Management of malignant oesophageal obstruction with self-expanding metallic stents. Br J Surg 1998;85:264–6.
16. Ell C, May A. Self-expanding metal stents for palliation of stenosing tumors of the esophagus and cardia: A critical review. Endoscopy 1997;29:392–8.
17. Morgan RA, Ellul JP, Denton ER et al. Malignant esophageal fistulas and perforations: Management with plastic covered metallic endoprostheses. Radiology 1997;204:527–32.
18. Raijman I, Siddique I, Ajani J, Lynch P. Palliation of malignant dysphagia and fistulae with coated expandable metal esophageal stents: experience with 101 patients. Gastrointest Endosc 1998;48:172–9.
19. Dormann AJ, Eisendrath P, Wigginghaus B, et al. Palliation of esophageal carcinoma with a new self-expanding plastic stent. Endoscopy 2003;35:207–11.
20. Costamagna G, Shah SK, Tringali A, et al. Prospective evaluation of a new self-expanding plastic stent for inoperable esophageal strictures. Surg Endosc 2003;17:891–5.
21. McDonald GB, Sharma P, Hackman RC, et al. Esophageal Infections in immunosuppressed patients after marrow transplantation. Gastroenterology 1985;88:1111–7.
22. Pappas PG, Rex JH, Sobel JD, et al. Guidelines for the treatment of candidiasis. Clin Infect Dis 2004;38:161–89.
23. Wilcox CM, Darouiche RO, Laine L, et al. A randomized, double-blind comparison of itraconazole oral solution and fluconazole tablets in the treatment of esophageal candidiasis. J Infect Dis 1997;176:227–32.
24. Ally R, Schurmann D, Kreisel W, et al. A randomized, double-blind, double-dummy, multicenter trial of voriconazole and fluconazole in the treatment of esophageal candidiasis in immunocompromised patients. Clin Infect Dis 2001;33:1447–54.
25. Perfect JR, Marr KA, Walsh TJ, et al. Voriconazole treatment for less-common, emerging, or refractory fungal infections. Clin Infect Dis 2003;36:1122–31.
26. Villanueva A, Gotuzzo E, Arathoon EG, et al. A randomized double-blind study of caspofungin versus fluconazole for the treatment of esophageal candidiasis. Am J Med 2002;113:294–9.
27. De Wet N, Llanos-Cuentas A, Suleiman J, et al. A randomized, double-blind, parallel-group, dose-response study of micafungin compared with fluconazole for the treatment of esophageal candidiasis in HIV-positive patients. Clin Infect Dis 2004;39:842–9.
28. Krause DS, Simjee AE, van Rensburg C, et al. A randomized, double-blind trial of anidulafungin versus fluconazole for the treatment of esophageal candidiasis. Clin Infect Dis 2004;39:770–5.
29. Baehr PH, McDonald GB. Esophageal infections: risk factors, presentation, diagnosis, and treatment. Gastroenterology 1994;106:509–32.
30. McBane RD, Gross JB Jr. Herpes esophagitis: Clinical syndrome, endoscopic appearance, and diagnosis in 23 patients. Gastrointest Endosc 1991;37:600–3
31. Erlich KS, Mills J, Chatis P, et al. Acyclovir-resistant herpes simplex virus infections in patients with the acquired immunodeficiency syndrome. N Engl J Med 1989;320:293–6.
32. Beutner KR, Friedman DJ, Forszpaniak C, et al. Valacyclovir compared with acyclovir for improved therapy for herpes zoster in immunocompetent adults. Antimicrob Agents Chemother 1995;39:1546–53.
33. Tyring S, Barbarash RA, Nahlik JE, et al. Famciclovir for the treatment of acute herpes zoster: effects on acute disease and postherpetic neuralgia. Ann Intern Med 1995;123:89–96.
34. Reed EC, Wolford JL, Kopecky KJ, et al. Ganciclovir for the treatment of cytomegalovirus gastroenteritis in bone marrow transplant patients. A randomized, placebo-controlled trial. Ann Intern Med 1990;112:505–10.
35. Blanshard C, Benhamou Y, Dohin E, et al. Treatment of AIDS-associated gastrointestinal cytomegalovirus infection with foscarnet and ganciclovir: A randomized comparison. J Infect Dis 1995;172:622–8.
36. Whitley RJ, Jacobson MA, Friedberg DN, et al. Guidelines for the treatment of cytomegalovirus diseases in patients with AIDS in the era of potent antiretroviral therapy: Recommendations of an international panel. Arch Intern Med 1998;158:957–69.
37. Walsh TJ, Belitsos NJ, Hamilton SR. Bacterial esophagitis in immunocompromised patients. Arch Intern Med 1986;146:1345–8.
38. Maguire PD, Sibley GS, Zhou SM, et al. Clinical and dosimetric predictors of radiation-induced esophageal toxicity. Int J Radiat Oncol Biol Phys 1999;45:97–103
39. Choy H, LaPorte K, Knill-Selby E, et al. Esophagitis in combined modality therapy for locally advanced non-small cell lung cancer. Semin Radiat Oncol 1999;9(2 Suppl 1):90–6.
40. Kikendall JW, Friedman AC, Oyewole MA, et al. Pill-induced esophageal injury: Case reports and review of the medical literature. Dig Dis Sci 1983;28:174–82.
41. Wong RK, Kikendall JW, Dachman AH. Quinaglute-induced esophagitis mimicking an esophageal mass. Ann Intern Med 1986;105:62–3.
42. Bonavina L, DeMeester TR, McChesney L, et al. Drug-induced esophageal strictures. Ann Surg 1987;206:173–83.
43. Alt B, Glass NR, Sollinger H. Neutropenic enterocolitis in adults. Review of the literature and assessment of surgical intervention. Am J Surg 1985;149:405–8.
44. Williams N, Scott AD. Neutropenic colitis: a continuing surgical challenge. Br J Surg 1997;84:1200–5.
45. Sloas MM, Flynn PM, Kaste SC, Patrick CC. Typhlitis in children with cancer: a 30-year experience. Clin Infect Dis 1993;17:484–90.
46. Katz JA, Wagner ML, Gresik MV, et al. Typhlitis. An 18-year experience and postmortem review. Cancer 1990;65:1041–7.
47. Urbach DR, Rotstein OD. Typhlitis. Can J Surg 1999;42:415–9.
48. Pokorney BH, Jones JM, Shaikh BS, Aber RC. Typhlitis: a treatable cause of recurrent septicemia. JAMA 1980;243:682–3.
49. Wade DS, Nava HR, Douglass HO. Neutropenic enterocolitis. Clinical diagnosis and treatment. Cancer 1992;69:17–23.
50. Kaste SC, Flynn PM, Furman WL. Acute lymphoblastic leukemia presenting with typhlitis. Med Pediatr Oncol 1997;28:209–12.
51. Kouroussis C, Samonis G, Androulakis N, et al. Successful conservative treatment of neutropenic enterocolitis complicating Taxane-based chemotherapy: a report of five cases. Am J Clin Oncol 2000;23:309–313.
52. Shamberger RC, Weinstein HJ, Delorey MJ, Levey RH. The medical and surgical management of typhlitis in children with acute nonlymphocytic (myelogenous) leukemia. Cancer 1986;57:603–9.
53. Villar HV, Warneke JA, Peck MD, et al. Role of surgical treatment in the management of complications of the gastrointestinal tract in patients with leukemia. Surg Gynecol Obstet 1987;165:217–22.
54. Glenn J, Funkhouser WK, Schneider PS. Acute illnesses necessitating urgent abdominal surgery in neutropenic cancer patients: Description o 14 cases and review of the literature. Surgery 1989;105:778–89.
55. Petrelli N, Douglass HO, Herrera L, et al. The modulation of fluorouracil with leucovorin in metastatic colorectal carcinoma: a prospective randomized phase III trial. Gastrointestinal Tumor Study Group. J Clin Oncol 1989;7:1419–26.
56. Stein BN, Petrelli NJ, Douglass HO, et al. Age and sex are independent predictors of 5-fluorouracil toxicity. Analysis of a large-scale phase III trial. Cancer 1995;75:11–7.
57. Sloan JA, Goldberg RM, Sargent DJ, et al. Women experience greater toxicity with fluorouracil-based chemotherapy for colorectal cancer. J Clin Oncol 2002;20:1491–8.
58. Abigerges D, Chabot GG, Armand JP, et al. Phase I and pharmacologic studies of the camptothecin analog irinotecan administered every 3 weeks in cancer patients. J Clin Oncol 1995;13:210–21.
59. Saltz LB, Cox JV, Blanke C, et al. Irinotecan plus fluorouracil and leucovorin for metastatic colorectal cancer. Irinotecan Study Group. N Engl J Med 2000;343:905–14.
60. Douillard JY, Cunningham D, Roth AD, et al. Irinotecan combined with fluorouracil compared with fluorouracil alone as first-line treatment for metastatic colorectal cancer: a multicenter randomized trial. Lancet 2000;355:1041–7.
61. Sargent DJ, Niedzwiecki D, O'Connell MJ, Schilsky RL. Recommendation for caution with irinotecan, fluorouracil and leucovorin for colorectal cancer. N Engl J Med 2001;345:144–5.
62. Rothenberg ML, Meropol NJ, Poplin EA, et al. Mortality associated with irinotecan plus bolus fluorouracil/leucovorin: summary findings of an independent panel. J Clin Oncol 2001;19:3801–7.
63. O'Connell MJ, Martenson JA, Wieand HS, et al. Improving adjuvant therapy for rectal cancer by combining protracted infusion fluorouracil with radiation therapy after curative surgery. N Engl J Med 1994;331:502–7.
64. Abigerges D, Armand JP, Chabot GG, et al. Irinotecan (CPT-11) high-dose escalation using intensive high-dose loperamide to control diarrhea. J Natl Cancer Inst 1994;86:446–9.
65. Benson AB, Ajani JA, Catalano RB, et al. Recommended guidelines for the treatment of cancer treatment-induced diarrhea. J Clin Oncol 2004;22:2918–26.
66. Lambert SW, van der Lely AJ, de Herder WW, et al. N Engl J Med 1996;334:246–54.
67. Harris AG, O'Dorisio TM, Woltering EA, et al. Consensus statement: octreotide dose titration in secretory diarrhea.

Diarrhea Management Consensus Development Panel. Dig Dis Sci 1995;40:1464–73.
68. Wadler S, Haynes H, Wiernik PH. Phase I trial of the somatostatin analog octreotide acetate in the treatment of fluoropyrimidine-induced diarrhea. J Clin Oncol 1995;13:222–6.
69. Barbounis V, Koumakis G, Vassilomanolakis M, et al. Control of irinotecan-induced diarrhea by octreotide after loperamide failure. Support Care Cancer 2001;9:258–60.
70. McDonald GB, Shulman HM, Sullivan KM, Spencer GD. Intestinal and hepatic complications of human bone marrow transplantation. Part I. Gastroenterology 1986;90:460–77.
71. Kelly CP, Pothoulakis C, LaMont JT. *Clostridium difficile* colitis. N Engl J Med 1994;330:257–62.
72. Cudmore MA, Silva J, Fekety R, et al. *Clostridium difficile* colitis associated with cancer chemotherapy. Arch Intern Med 1982;142:333–5.
73. Anand A, Glatt AE. *Clostridium difficile* infection associated with antineoplastic chemotherapy: a review. Clin Infect Dis 1993;17:109–13.
74. De Girolami PC, Hanff PA, Eichelberger K, et al. Multicenter evaluation of a new enzyme immunoassay for detection of *Clostridium difficile* enterotoxin A. J Clin Microbiol 1992;30:1085–1088.
75. Doern GV, Coughlin RT, Wu L. Laboratory diagnosis of *Clostridium difficile*–associated gastrointestinal disease: comparison of a monoclonal antibody enzyme immunoassay for toxins A and B with a monoclonal antibody enzyme immunoassay for toxin A only and two cytotoxicity assays. J Clin Microbiol 1992;30:2042–46.
76. Gerding DN, Johnson S, Peterson LR, et al. *Clostridium difficile*–associated diarrhea and colitis. Infect Control Hosp Epidemiol 1995;16:459–77.
77. Tedesco FJ, Corless JK, Brownstein RE. Rectal sparing in antibiotic-associated pseudomembranous colitis: a prospective study. Gastroenterology 1982;83:1259–60.
78. Teasley DG, Gerding DN, Olson MM, et al. Prospective randomized trial of metronidazole versus vancomycin for *Clostridium difficile*–associated diarrhoea and colitis. Lancet 1983;2:1043–46.
79. Bartlett JG. Antibiotic-associated diarrhea. N Engl J Med 2002;346:334–49.
80. Nathanson DR, Sheahan M, Chao L, Wallack MK. Intracolonic use of vancomycin for treatment of *Clostridium difficile* colitis in a patient with a diverted colon: report of a case. Dis Colon Rectum 2001;44:1871–2.
81. Shetler K, Nieuwenhuis R, Wren SM, Triadafilopoulos G. Decompressive colonoscopy with intracolonic vancomycin administration for the treatment of severe pseudomembranous colitis. Surg Endosc 2001;15:653–9.
82. Apisarnthanarak A, Razavi B, Mundy LM. Adjunctive intracolonic vancomycin for severe *Clostridium difficile* colitis: Case series and review of the literature. Clin Infect Dis 2002;35:690–6.
83. Bartlett JG, Tedesco FJ, Shull S, et al. Symptomatic relapse after oral vancomycin therapy of antibiotic-associated pseudomembranous colitis. Gastroenterology 1980;78:431–4.
84. Tedesco FJ, Gordon D, Fortson WC. Approach to patients with multiple relapses of antibiotic-associated pseudomembranous colitis. Am J Gastroenterol 1985;80:867–8.
85. Kreutzer EW, Milligan D. Treatment of antibiotic-associated pseudomembranous colitis with cholestyramine resin. Johns Hopkins Med J 1978;143:67–72.
86. Tedesco FJ. Treatment of recurrent antibiotic-associated pseudomembranous colitis. Am J Gastroenterol 1982;77:220–1.
87. McFarland LV, Surawicz CM, Greenberg RN, et al. A randomized placebo-controlled trial of *Saccharomyces boulardii* in combination with standard antibiotics or *Clostridium difficile* disease. JAMA 1994;271:1913–18.
88. Cox GJ, Matsui SM, Lo RS, et al. Etiology and outcome of diarrhea after marrow transplantation: a prospective study. Gastroenterology 1994;107:1398–407.
89. West JC, Armitage JO, Mitros FA, et al. Cytomegalovirus cecal erosion causing massive hemorrhage in a bone marrow transplant recipient. World J Surg 1982;6:251–5.
90. Hackman RC, Wolford JL, Leaves CA, et al. Recognition and rapid diagnosis of upper gastrointestinal cytomegalovirus infection in marrow transplant recipients. A comparison of seven virologic methods. Transplantation 1994;57:231–7.
91. Bromiker R, Korman SH, Or R, et al. Severe giardiasis in two patients undergoing bone marrow transplantation. Bone Marrow Transplant 1989;4:701–3.
92. Bavaro P, Di Girolamo G, Di Bartolomeo P, et al. Amebiasis after bone marrow transplantation. Bone Marrow Transplant 1994;13:213–4.
93. Collier AC, Miller RA, Meyers JD. Cryptosporidiosis after marrow transplantation: person-to-person transmission and treatment with spiramycin. Ann Intern Med 1984;101:205–6.
94. Gratwohl A, Hermans J, Apperley J, et al. Acute graft-versus-host disease: Grade and outcome in patients with chronic myelogenous leukemia. Blood 1995;86:813–8.
95. Champlin RE, Schmitz N, Horowitz MM, et al. Blood stem cells compared with bone marrow as a source of hematopoietic cells for allogeneic transplantation. Blood 2000;95:3702–9.
96. Remberger M, Persson U, Hauzenberger D, Ringden O. An association between human leukocyte antigen alleles and acute and chronic graft-versus-host disease after allogeneic haematopoietic stem cell transplantation. Br J Haematol 2002;119:751–9.
97. Tabbara IA, Zimmerman K, Morgan C, Nahleh Z. Allogeneic hematopoietic stem cell transplantation: complications and results. Arch Intern Med 2002;162:1558–66.
98. Nash RA, Pepe MS, Storb R, et al. Acute graft-versus-host disease: analysis of risk factors after allogeneic marrow transplantation and prophylaxis with cyclosporine and methotrexate. Blood 1992;80:1838–45.
99. Schwartz JM, Wolford JL, Thornquist MD, et al. Severe gastrointestinal bleeding after hematopoietic cell transplantation, 1987–1997: incidence, causes and outcome. Am J Gastroenterol 2001;96:385–93.
100. Weisdorf DJ, Snover DC, Haake R, et al. Acute upper gastrointestinal graft-versus-host disease: Clinical significance and response to immunosuppressive therapy. Blood 1990;76:624–9.
101. Snover DC, Weisdorf SA, Vercellotti GM, et al. A histopathologic study of gastric and small intestinal graft-versus-host disease following allogeneic bone marrow transplantation. Hum Pathol 1985;16:387–92.
102. Snover DC. Mucosal damage simulating graft-versus-host disease in cytomegalovirus colitis. Transplantation 1985;39:669–70.
103. Muller CI, Zeiser R, Grullich C, et al. Intestinal cryptosporidiosis mimicking acute graft-versus-host disease following matched unrelated hematopoietic stem cell transplantation. Transplantation 2004;77:1478–9.
104. Lee FD. Importance of apoptosis in the histopathology of drug related lesions in the large intestines. J Clin Pathol 1993;46:118–22.
105. Papadimitriou JC, Drachemberg LB, Beskow CO, et al. Graft-versus-host disease–like features in mycophenolate mofetil–related colitis. Transplant Proc 2001;33:2237–8.
106. Berrebi D, Sautet A, Flejou JF, et al. Ticlopidine induced colitis: a histopathological study including apoptosis. J Clin Pathol 1998;51:280–3.
107. Vogelsang GB, Lee L, Bensen-Kennedy DM. Pathogenesis and treatment of graft-versus-host disease after bone marrow transplant. Annu Rev Med 2003;54:29–52.
108. Sviland L, Pearson ADJ, Eastham EJ, et al. Histologic features of skin and rectal biopsy specimens after autologous and allogeneic bone marrow transplantation. J Clin Pathol 1988;41:148–54.
109. Schulenburg A, Turetschek K, Wrba F, et al. Early and late gastrointestinal complications after myeloablative and non-myeloablative allogeneic stem cell transplantation. Ann Hematol 2004;83:101–6.
110. Terdiman JP, Linker CA, Ries A, et al. The role of endoscopic evaluation in patients with suspected intestinal graft-versus-host disease after allogeneic bone-marrow transplantation. Endoscopy 1996;28:680–5.
111. Daneshpouy M, Socie G, Lemann M, et al. Activated eosinophils in upper gastrointestinal tract of patients with graft-versus-host disease. Blood 2002;99:3033–40.
112. Roy J, Snover D, Weisdorf S, et al. Simultaneous upper and lower endoscopic biopsy in the diagnosis of intestinal graft-versus-host disease. Transplantation 1991;51:642–6.
113. Spencer GD, Shulman HM, Myerson D, et al. Diffuse intestinal ulceration after marrow transplantation: a clinicopathologic study of 13 patients. Hum Pathol 1986;17:621–33.
114. Saito H, Oshimi K, Nagasako K, et al. Endoscopic appearance of the colon and small intestine of a patient with hemorrhagic enteric graft-vs.-host disease. Dis Colon Rectum 1990;33:695–7.
115. Ponec RJ, Hackman RC, McDonald GB. Endoscopic and histologic diagnosis of intestinal graft-versus-host disease after marrow transplantation. Gastrointest Endosc 1999;49:612–21.
116. Shulman HM, Sharma P, Amos D, et al. A coded histologic study of hepatic graft-versus-host disease after human bone marrow transplantation. Hepatology 1988;8:463–70.
117. Snover DC, Weisdorf SA, Ramsay NK, et al. Hepatic graft versus host disease: a study of the predictive value of liver biopsy in diagnosis. Hepatology 1984;4:123–30.
118. Hings IM, Severson R, Filipovich AH, et al. Treatment of moderate and severe acute GVHD after allogeneic bone marrow transplantation. Transplantation 1994;58:437–42.
119. Martin PJ, Schoch G, Fisher L, et al. A retrospective analysis of therapy for acute graft-versus-host disease: Secondary treatment. Blood 1991;77:1821–8.
120. Durrant S, Mollee P, Morton AJ, Irving I. Combination therapy with tacrolimus and antithymocyte globulin for the treatment of steroid-resistant acute graft-versus-host disease developing during cyclosporine prophylaxis. Br J Haematol 2001;113:217–23.
121. Couriel D, Caldera H, Champlin R, Komanduri K. Acute graft-versus-host disease: pathophysiology, clinical manifestations, and management. Cancer 2004;101:1936–46.
122. McDonald GB, Bouvier M, Hockenbery DM, et al. Oral beclomethasone dipropionate for treatment of intestinal graft-versus-host disease: a randomized, controlled trial. Gastroenterology 1998;115:28–35.
123. Bertz H, Afting M, Kreisel W, et al. Feasibility and response to budesonide as topical corticosteroids therapy for acute intestinal graft-versus-host disease. Bone Marrow Transplant 1999;24:1185–9.
124. Ippoliti C, Champlin R, Bugazia N, et al. Use of octreotide in the symptomatic management of diarrhea induced by graft-versus-host disease in patients with hematologic malignancies. J Clin Oncol 1997;15:3350–4.
125. Shulman HM, Sullivan KM, Weiden PL, et al. Chronic graft-versus-host syndrome in man. A long-term clinicopathologic study of 20 Seattle patients. Am J Med 1980;69:204–17.
126. Sullivan KM, Shulman HM, Storb R, et al. Chronic graft-versus-host disease in 52 patients: Adverse natural course and successful treatment with combination immunosuppression. Blood 1981;57:267–76.
127. McDonald GB, Sullivan KM, Plumley TF. Radiographic features of esophageal involvement in chronic graft-vs.-host disease. AJR Am J Roentgenol 1984;142:501–6.
128. Atkinson K. Chronic graft-versus-host disease. Bone Marrow Transplant 1990;5:69–82.
129. Akpek G, Chinratanalab W, Lee LA, et al. Gastrointestinal involvement in chronic graft-versus-host disease: a clinicopathologic study. Biol Blood Marrow Transplant 2003;9:46–51.
130. Fried RH, Murakami CS, Fisher LD, et al. Ursodeoxycholic acid treatment of refractory chronic graft-versus-host disease of the liver. Ann Intern Med 1992;116:624–9.
131. Babb RR. Radiation proctitis: A review. Am J Gastroenterol 1996;91:1309–11.
132. Baum CA, Biddle WL, Miner PB. Failure of 5-aminosalicylic acid enemas to improve chronic radiation proctitis. Dig Dis Sci 1989;34:758–60.
133. Kochhar R, Sriram PV, Sharma SC, et al. Natural history of late radiation proctosigmoiditis treated with topical sucralfate. Dig Dis Sci 1999;44:973–8.
134. Stockdale AD, Biswas A. Long-term control of radiation proctitis following treatment with sucralfate enemas. Br J Surg 1997;84:379.
135. Sasai T, Hiraishi H, Suzuki Y, et al. Treatment of chronic post-radiation proctitis with oral administration of sucralfate. Am J Gastroenterol 1998;93:1593–5.
136. Kochhar R, Patel F, Dhar A, et al. Radiation-induced proctosigmoiditis. Prospective, randomized, double-blind controlled trial of oral sulfasalazine plus rectal steroids versus rectal sucralfate. Dig Dis Sci 1991;36:103–7.
137. Mayer R, Klemen H, Quehenberger F, et al. Hyperbaric oxygen—an effective tool to treat radiation morbidity in prostate cancer. Radiother Oncol 2001;61:151–6.
138. al-Sabbagh R, Sinicrope FA, Sellin JH, et al. Evaluation of short-chain fatty acid enemas: treatment of radiation proctitis. Am J Gastroenterol 1996;91:1814–6.
139. Biswal BM, Lal P, Rath GK, Shukla NK, et al. Intrarectal formalin application, an effective treatment for grade III haemorrhagic radiation proctitis. Radiother Oncol 1995;35:212–5.
140. Counter SF, Froese DP, Hart MJ. Prospective evaluation of formalin therapy in radiation proctitis. Am J Surg 1999;177:396–8.
141. Parikh S, Hughes C, Salvati EP, et al. Treatment of hemorrhagic radiation proctitis with 4 percent formalin. Dis Colon Rectum 2003;46:596–600.
142. Fantin AC, Binek J, Suter WR, Meyenberger C. Argon beam coagulation or treatment of symptomatic radiation-induced proctitis. Gastrointest Endosc 1999;49:515–8.

143. Silva RA, Correia AJ, Dias LM, et al. Argon plasma coagulation therapy for hemorrhagic radiation proctosigmoiditis. Gastrointest Endosc 1999;50:221–4.
144. Tjandra JJ, Sengupta S. Argon plasma coagulation is an effective treatment for refractory hemorrhagic radiation proctitis. Dis Colon Rectum 2001;44:1759–65.
145. Taieb S, Rolachon A, Cenni JC, et al. Effective use of argon plasma coagulation in the treatment of severe radiation proctitis. Dis Colon Rectum 2001;44:1766–71.
146. Barbatzas C, Spencer GM, Thorpe SM, et al. Nd:YAG laser treatment or bleeding from radiation proctitis. Endoscopy 1996;28:497–500.
147. Viggiano TR, Zighelboim J, Ahlquist DA, et al. Endoscopic Nd:YAG laser coagulation of bleeding from radiation proctopathy. Gastrointest Endosc 199;39:513–7.
148. Taylor JG, DiSario JA, Buchi KN. Argon laser therapy for hemorrhagic radiation proctitis. Long-term results. Gastrointest Endosc 1993;39:641–5.
149. Jensen DM, Machicado GA, Cheng S, et al. A randomized prospective study of endoscopic bipolar electrocoagulation and heater probe treatment of chronic rectal bleeding from radiation telangiectasia. Gastrointest Endosc 1997;45:20–5.
150. Runzi M, Layer P. Drug-associated pancreatitis: facts and fiction. Pancreas 1996;13:100–9.
151. McArthur KE. Review article: drug-induced pancreatitis. Aliment Pharmacol Ther 1996;10:23–8.
152. Glueck CJ, Lang J, Hamer T, Tracy T. Severe hypertriglyceridemia and pancreatitis when estrogen replacement therapy is given to hypertriglyceridemia women. J Lab Clin Med 1994;123:59–64.
153. Hozumi Y, Kawano M, Saito T, Miyata M. Effect of tamoxifen on serum lipid metabolism. J Clin Endocrinol Metab 1998;83:1633–5.
154. Kawanishi H, Rudolph E, Bull FE. Azathioprine-induced acute pancreatitis. N Engl J Med 1973;289:357.
155. Izraeli S, Adamson PC. Blaney SM, Balis FM. Acute pancreatitis after ifosfamide therapy. Cancer 1994;74:1627–8.
156. Mallory A, Kern F. Drug-induced pancreatitis: a critical review. Gastroenterology 1980;78:813–20.
157. Siemers RF, Friedenberg WR, Norfleet RG. High-dose cytosine arabinoside-associated pancreatitis. Cancer 1985;56:1940–2.
158. Parenti DM, Steinberg W, Kang P. Infectious causes of acute pancreatitis. Pancreas 1996;13:356–71.
159. Wilcox CM, Forsmark CE, Grendell JH, et al. Cytomegalovirus-associated acute pancreatic disease in patients with acquired immunodeficiency syndrome. Report of two patients. Gastroenterology 1990;99:263–7.
160. Stewart KC, Dickout WJ, Urschel JD. Metastasis-induced acute pancreatitis as the initial manifestation of bronchogenic carcinoma. Chest 1993;104:98–100.
161. Gutman M, Inbar M, Klausner JM. Metastases-induced acute pancreatitis: a rare presentation of cancer. Eur J Surg Oncol 1993;19:302–4.
162. Kumar S, DeLeve LD, Kamath PS, Tefferi A. Hepatic veno-occlusive disease (sinusoidal obstruction syndrome) after hematopoietic stem cell transplantation. Mayo Clin Proc 2003;78:589–98.
163. Sebagh M, Debette M, Samuel D, et al. "Silent" presentation of veno-occlusive disease after liver transplantation as part of the process of cellular rejection with endothelial predilection. Hepatology 1999;30:1144–50.
164. McDonald GB, Hinds MS, Fisher LD, et al. Veno-occlusive disease of the liver and multiorgan failure after bone marrow transplantation: a cohort study of 355 patients. Ann Intern Med 1993;118:255–67.
165. McDonald GB, Sharma P, Mathews DE, et al. Veno-occlusive disease of the liver after bone marrow transplantation: Diagnosis, incidence and predisposing factors. Hepatology 1984;4:116–22.
166. Shulman HM, Gown AM, Nugent DJ. Hepatic veno-occlusive disease after bone marrow transplantation: Immunohistochemical identification o the material within occluded central venules. Am J Pathol 1987;127:549–58.
167. Shulman HM, Fisher LB, Schoch HG, et al. Venoocclusive disease of the liver after marrow transplantation: histological correlates of clinical signs and symptoms. Hepatology 1994;19:1171–80.
168. Dulley FL, Kanfer EJ, Appelbaum FR, et al. Venoocclusive disease of the liver after chemoradiotherapy and autologous bone marrow transplantation. Transplantation 1987;43:870–3.
169. Frickhofen N, Wiesneth M, Jainta C, et al. Hepatitis C virus infection is a risk factor for liver failure from veno-occlusive disease after bone marrow transplantation. Blood 1994;83:1998–2004
170. Girinsky T, Benhamou E, Bourhis JH, et al. Prospective randomized comparison of single-dose versus hyperfractionated total-body irradiation in patients with hematologic malignancies. J Clin Oncol 2000;18:981–6.
171. Shulman HM, Hinterberger W. Hepatic veno-occlusive disease liver toxicity syndrome after bone marrow transplantation. Bone Marrow Transplant 1992;10:197–214.
172. Matute-Bello G, McDonald GD, Hinds MS, et al. Association of pulmonary function testing abnormalities and severe veno-occlusive disease of the liver after marrow transplantation. Bone Marrow Transplant 1998;21:1125–30.
173. Carreras E, Grañena A, Navasa M, et al. On the reliability of clinical criteria for the diagnosis of hepatic veno-occlusive disease. Ann Hematol 1993;66:77–80.
174. Shulman HM, Gooley T, Dudley MD, et al. Utility of transvenous liver biopsies and wedged hepatic venous pressure measurements in sixty marrow transplant recipients. Transplantation 1995;59:1015–22.
175. Bearman SI, Shuhart MC, Hinds MS, McDonald GB. Recombinant human tissue plasminogen activator for the treatment of established severe venoocclusive disease of the liver after bone marrow transplantation. Blood 1992;80:2458–62.
176. Bearman SI, Lee JL, Baron AE, McDonald GB. Treatment of hepatic venoocclusive disease with recombinant human tissue plasminogen activator and heparin in 42 marrow transplant patients. Blood 1997;89:1501–6.
177. Richardson PG, Elias AD, Krishnan A, et al. Treatment of severe veno-occlusive disease with defibrotide: compassionate use results in response without significant toxicity in a high-risk population. Blood 1998;92:737–44.
178. Chopra R, Eaton JD, Grassi A, et al. Defibrotide for the treatment of hepatic veno-occlusive disease: results of the European compassionate-use study. Br J Haematol 2000;111:1122–9.
179. Lévy V, Azoulay D, Rio B, et al. Successful treatment of severe hepatic veno-occlusive disease after allogeneic bone marrow transplantation by transjugular intrahepatic portosystemic stent-shunt (TIPS). Bone Marrow Transplant 1996;18:443–5.
180. Fried MW, Connaghan DG, Sharma S, et al. Transjugular intrahepatic portosystemic shunt for the management of severe venoocclusive disease following bone marrow transplantation. Hepatology 1996;24:588–91.
181. Azoulay D, Castaing D, Lemoine A, et al. Transjugular intrahepatic portosystemic shunt (TIPS) for severe veno-occlusive disease of the liver following bone marrow transplantation. Bone Marrow Transplant 2000;25:987–92.
182. Lee WM. Drug-induced hepatotoxicity. N Engl J Med 1995;333:1118–27.
183. Lok AS, Liang RH, Chiu EK, et al. Reactivation of hepatitis B virus replication in patients receiving cytotoxic therapy. report of a prospective study. Gastroenterology 1991;100:182–8.
184. Liang R, Lau GK, Kwong YL. Chemotherapy and bone marrow transplantation for cancer patients who are also chronic hepatitis B carriers: a review of the problem. J Clin Oncol 1999;17:394–8.
185. Yeo W, Chan PK, Ho WM, et al. Lamivudine for the prevention of hepatitis B virus reactivation in hepatitis B s-Antigen seropositive cancer patients undergoing cytotoxic chemotherapy. J Clin Oncol 2004;22:927–34.
186. Nakamura Y, Motokura T, Fujita A, et al. Severe hepatitis related to chemotherapy in hepatitis B virus carriers with hematologic malignancies. Survey in Japan 1987–91. Cancer 1996;78:2210–5.
187. Yeo W, Chan PK, Zhong S, et al. Frequency of hepatitis B virus reactivation in cancer patients undergoing cytotoxic chemotherapy: A prospective study of 626 patients with identification of risk factors. J Med Virol 2000;62:299–307.
188. Yeo W, Zee B, Zhong S, et al. Comprehensive analysis of risk factors associating with Hepatitis B virus (HBV) reactivation in cancer patients undergoing cytotoxic chemotherapy. Br J Cancer 2004;90:1306–11.
189. Lau GK, Yiu HH, Fong DY, et al. Early is superior to deferred preemptive lamivudine therapy for hepatitis B patients undergoing chemotherapy. Gastroenterology 2003;125:1742–9.
190. Kawatani T, Suou T, Tajima F, et al. Incidence of hepatitis virus infection and severe liver dysfunction in patients receiving chemotherapy for hematologic malignancies. Eur J Haematol 2001;67:45–50.
191. Khan S, Ramwani JJ, O'Brien PJ. Hepatocyte toxicity of mechlorethamine and other alkylating anticancer drugs. Role of lipid peroxidation. Biochem Pharmacol 1992;43:1963–7.
192. Goldberg JW, Lidsky MD. Cyclophosphamide-associated hepatotoxicity. South Med J 1985;78:222–3.
193. George CB, Mansour RP, Redmond J, Gandara DR. Hepatic dysfunction and jaundice following high-dose cytosine arabinoside. Cancer 1984;54:2360–2.
194. Moertel CG, Fleming TR, MacDonald JS, et al. Hepatic toxicity associated with fluorouracil plus levamisole adjuvant therapy. J Clin Oncol 1993;11:2386–90.
195. Hohn D, Stagg RJ, Friedman MA, et al. A randomized trial of continuous intravenous versus hepatic intra-arterial floxuridine in patients with colorectal cancer metastatic to the liver: the Northern California Oncology Group trial. J Clin Oncol 1989;7:1646–54.
196. Kemeny N, Daly J, Reichman B, et al. Intrahepatic or systemic infusion of fluorodeoxyuridine in patients with liver metastases from colorectal carcinoma. Ann Intern Med 1987;107:459–65.
197. Chang AE, Schneider PD, Sugarbaker PH, et al. A prospective randomized trial of regional versus systemic continuous 5-fluorodeoxyuridine chemotherapy in the treatment of colorectal liver metastases. Ann Surg 1987;206:685–93.
198. Shorey J, Schenker S, Suki WN, Combes B. Hepatotoxicity of mercaptopurine. Arch Intern Med 1968;122:54–8.
199. Romagnuolo J, Sadowski DC, Lalor E, et al. Cholestatic hepatocellular injury with azathioprine: a case report and review of the mechanisms of hepatotoxicity. Can J Gastroenterol 1998;12:479–83.
200. Berkowitz RS, Goldstein DP, Bernstein MR. Ten year's experience with methotrexate and folinic acid as primary therapy for gestational trophoblastic disease. Gynecol Oncol 1986;23:111–8.
201. Roenigk HH, Auerback R, Maibach HI, Weinstein GD. Methotrexate guidelines: revised. J Am Acad Dermatol 1982;6:145–55.
202. Johnson PJ, Dobbs N, Kalayci C, et al. Clinical efficacy and toxicity of standard dose adriamycin in hyperbilirubinaemic patients with hepatocellular carcinoma: relation to liver tests and pharmacokinetic parameters. Br J Cancer 1992;65:751–5.
203. Erichsen C, Jonsson PE. Veno-occlusive liver disease after dacarbazine therapy (DTIC) for melanoma. J Surg Oncol 1984;27:268–70.
204. Stoneham S, Lennard L, Coen P, et al. Veno-occlusive disease in patients receiving thiopurines during maintenance therapy for childhood acute lymphoblastic leukaemia. Br J Haematol 2003;123:100–2.
205. Read AE, Wiesner RH, LaBrecque DR, et al. Hepatic veno-occlusive disease associated with renal transplantation and azathioprine therapy. Ann Intern Med 1986;104:651–5.
206. Sterneck M, Wiesner R, Ascher N, et al. Azathioprine hepatotoxicity after liver transplantation. Hepatology 1991;14:806–10.
207. Rollins BJ. Hepatic veno-occlusive disease. Am J Med 1986;81:297–306.
208. Vassal G, Hartmann O, Benhamou E. Busulfan and veno-occlusive disease of the liver. Ann Intern Med 1990;112:881.
209. Joensuu H, Soderstrom KO, Nikkanen V. Fatal necrosis of the liver during ABVD chemotherapy for Hodgkin's disease. A case report. Cancer 1986;58:1437–40.

Oral Complications of Cancer and Their Treatment

Stephen T. Sonis, DMD, DMSc

The oral cavity is a frequent site of undesirable side effects of cancer therapy that adversely affect patients' quality of life, ability to tolerate therapy, and overall cost of treatment. Stomatotoxicity, which leads to the disruption of the integrity of the oral mucosa, also results in the mouth serving as a source for systemic or distant infection. Unfortunately, oral complications of cancer therapy are common and their scope is increasing as innovative approaches to antineoplastic treatment evolve. In high-risk populations, such as patients receiving radiation therapy with or without concomitant chemotherapy for head and neck cancer or conditioning regimens for hematopoietic stem cell transplantation (HSCT) transplantation, almost all suffer some adverse oral event as a consequence of treatment.[1] Among patients receiving bisphosphonates as part of their treatment regimen, osteonecrosis of the jaw has become an increasing problem.[2]

Overall, about 40% of patients being treated for cancers not of the head and neck develop some form of mouth-related problem, which range from xerostomia to mucositis.[3] The symptomatic and functional consequences of oral complications associated with cancer treatment are associated with increased use of analgesics and antibiotics, increased length of hospital stays, hospitalization for pain and fluid management, more nursing resource use, and parenteral feeding. For example, an analysis of autologous bone marrow transplant recipients demonstrated that patients with mucositis had hospital stays that were 5 days longer than did patients without the condition.[4] In the past, oral complications were largely considered to inevitable, often they were not recognized early, and were treated retrospectively rather than in a prospective or preventive manner. Significant progress has been made in the past decade to better define the biology and epidemiology of oral complications of treatment. As a result, interventions that target mechanisms have evolved, as has a better understanding of at risk populations.

PRETREATMENT ASSESSMENT

There is no question that many of the side effects that impact the mouth can be prevented or minimized by the elimination of existing sites of dental disease before anticancer treated is initiated.[5–7] Thus, pretreatment oral assessment is strongly recommended. The primary objectives of such an evaluation are the identification and elimination of asymptomatic dental or periodontal infections, and sites of chronic irritation. For the patient about to undergo surgical intervention for tumors about the mouth, pretreatment evaluation is critical to optimize the fabrication of prostheses. The construction of protective appliances prior to the start of radiation therapy may reduce the impact of treatment on scatter-induced injury. Osteonecrosis of the jaws associated with bisphosphonate therapy seems to occur more often following dental surgical procedures or mucosal injury. Consequently, a thorough dental evaluation aimed at detecting subclinical dental disease is highly desirable since treatment can be completed before the start of cancer treatment.

In a study of the effectiveness of dental screening, Woods and Sonis found that 72% of patients screened prior to bone marrow transplantation demonstrated positive findings relative to latent dental infection, or mucosal irritation caused by faulty prostheses or dental restorations.[8] Results of another study in the same population suggested that one-third of the patients required oral care before transplantation.[9] Lockhart and Clark reported that 97% of patients about to undergo treatment for head and neck cancers required some dental care.[10] Epstein and Stevenson-Moore found that 68% of dentate patients screened prior to treatment for nasopharyngeal cancers required extractions, primarily because of periodontal disease. Surprisingly, these same investigators found that extractions were required in 28% of patients who reported regular dental care.[11] Studies by others further demonstrate that prechemotherapy intervention for abnormalities found on screening had a significant, favorable impact on morbidity relative to local infection and sepsis.[7] It has become increasingly clear that effective dental screening with appropriate treatment, prior to the onset of cancer therapy results in significant cost savings by reducing the incidence of infection during periods of granulocytopenia.[12]

Timing of Assessment and Dental Treatment If oral screening is performed so close to the initiation of cancer therapy as to preclude dental intervention, the value of the process is nullified. The ideal interval between the completion of dental treatment, particularly extraction, and the initiation of radiation therapy has been the subject of much debate.[13] Nonetheless, given the rate by which wounds of the mouth heal, particularly extraction sites, it appears that a minimum of 2 weeks is acceptable and 3 weeks desirable. For patients about to undergo chemotherapy, sufficient time between the completion of dental treatment and the patient's anticipated granulocyte nadir (< 500 cells/mL) is required. In general, non-emergent dental treatment should not be performed in a typical ambulatory setting if the patient is significantly thrombocytopenic (< 100,000 platelets/mL).

Because of the acute onset of some hematologic malignancies and the need for immediate chemotherapy, pre-treatment dental and oral screening in this high risk population may not be possible. In these cases, oral assessment should be performed as close to the initiation of therapy as possible for two reasons: first, such an examination provides an important baseline for oral health; and second, the finding and elimination of active oral infection in this markedly myeloablated group is often critical to their overall clinical course. Elimination of identified sources of ontogenic infection should not be delayed, as there is significant data to support the conclusion that dental extractions may be performed safely in this group if they are managed well, preferably in a hospital setting. The complication rate for extractions in patients with hematologic malignancies is reported to be 13%, with no effect on length of hospital stay or mortality. The most common complications include pain and bleeding. It is important to note that there is no evidence to suggest that an aggressive strategy of extraction of asymptomatic teeth has any benefit in the prevention of systemic infection.

Components of the pretreatment assessment include baseline data such as medical and dental histories; laboratory data—such as antibody status relative to herpes simplex type 1 virus—and a clinical assessment that should include an extraoral examination of the head and neck, intraoral soft tissue examination, periodontal disease screening, and dental evaluation.[14] Radiographic evaluation should include those films that are necessary to definitively diagnose periodontal disease and caries, periapical pathology and impacted teeth. It is also important to assess the patient's knowledge of, and motivation for dental maintenance. Teeth that demonstrate evidence of untreated periapical pathology, or advanced caries or periodontal disease should be eliminated.

Patients with removable prostheses should be encouraged to minimize their use or leave them out during their cancer therapy since even subtle mucosal trauma accelerates the risk and onset of mucositis. Similarly, the removal of orthodontic bands prior to the start of chemotherapy is an essential component to preventing trauma to atrophied mucosa.[15]

ORAL COMPLICATIONS OF RADIOTHERAPY

Oral complications of radiation therapy are primarily the result of acute and chronic local tissue injury. In addition, radiation-induced xerostomia may result in secondary effects on the teeth and periodontium. The dose rate, total dose of radiation, and the size and structures within the radiation field are the major determinants of oral toxicity. As a result, patients being treated for tumors of the mouth, oropharynx, tongue, nasopharynx, and salivary glands are at highest risk. Patients with hypopharyngeal or laryngeal tumors are also often affected, although at a slightly lower rate. Brachytherapy tends to be more stomatotoxic than external beam irradiation. Although intensity-modulated radiation therapy (IMRT) (Chapter 79, "Neoplasms of the Head and Neck") may spare some structures, its impact on oral mucosa is significant. Oral tissues that are directly affected by radiation include, mucosa (epithelium and tissues in the lamina propria), salivary glands, bone, and muscle. In children, radiation that includes the jaws negatively impacts on craniofacial and dental development.[16–18]

Mucositis Both radiation and chemotherapy can produce significant damage to the oral mucosa as a side effect of treatment. The term *mucositis* is preferred over *stomatitis* when describing mucosal injury caused by antineoplastic therapy as the latter is a generic term and can be associated with a range of infectious or traumatic etiologies unrelated to chemo- or radiotherapy. The severity and kinetics of radiation-induced oral mucositis are related to dose rate and total dose that target the oral mucosa. Local mucosal irritation, secondary infection, and xerostomia all are factors that amplify the damaging effects of radiation to the tissue.

Two themes have characterized thinking relative to mucositis in the past 5 years: first, the pathobiology has been more fully defined; and second, the commonality in mechanisms by which mucosal injury occurs has been applied to all parts of the alimentary canal.[19]

Historically, mucositis was viewed as the end result of direct radiation or chemotherapy mediated injury to stem cells in the basal layer of the oral mucosa. It was proposed that these rapidly dividing cells were indiscriminately damaged resulting in atrophy and subsequent ulceration. Simultaneously, connective tissue injury was thought to lead to an increase in vascular permeability and tissue edema.[20] However, studies defining the mechanisms by which mucositis occurs reveal a process that is biologically more complex. Although epithelial stem cells are the ultimate mediators of mucosal injury, it is now clear that their demise occurs by indirect, as well as direct, mechanisms.[21] In fact, direct clonogenic cell death of these cells is insufficient to produce the extent of clinical injury that is typically observed. Rather, a sequence of events[22] triggered by the generation of reactive species in cells of the lamina propria produce a cascade of events in the endothelium, connective tissue, extracellular matrix and the inflammatory infiltrate. This sequence begins almost immediately, following the initial exposure of the mucosa to radiation, and results in a range of molecular mediators and signals that permeate to the epithelium and cause injury, apoptosis, and necrosis.

Radiation-induced oral mucositis typically begins within the first two weeks of therapy, at cumulative doses of 10 to 20 Gy. Although clinical changes are observed at these doses, the cellular and tissue injury producing these changes begin almost immediately following initial dosing (see below). Mucosal erythema, mild epithelial sloughing, and the formation of islands of hyperkeratosis characterize early changes of mucositis. These changes are accompanied by relatively mild symptoms characterized by a painful burning sensation that is analogous to a food burn such as that caused by hot cheese. Patients often have difficulty tolerating spicy foods. With the exception of the dorsal surface of the tongue and the gingival, any mucosal surface of the mouth is susceptible. Most commonly affected areas are the buccal mucosa (cheeks), ventral and lateral surfaces of the tongue, and the floor of the mouth. The soft palate is also frequently involved. Consequently, patients may complain of a sore throat early in their treatment.

At cumulative doses of about 30 Gy, the integrity of the mucosa breaks down and ulceration occurs. Ulcers typically begin as isolated lesions, but then coalesce forming large, contiguous breaks in the mucosa, often covered by a collection of dead cells and bacteria in a pseudomembrane. In severe cases, the lesions may bleed. Ulcerative mucositis is extremely painful. Not only do ulcers cover large mucosal surface areas, but they are also deep. Patients who have undergone radiation therapy and have developed mucositis describe this complication as the most significant of their treatment.[23] In many cases, mucositis results in breaks in radiation treatment, hospitalization for fluid support or pain management, and the need for parenteral feeding.[24] It is important that patients about to begin treatment have some concept of the severity of mucosal injury that they are likely to develop. The typical pretreatment characterization of mucositis as "mouth sores" seems to trivialize their significance to patients. It seems likely that a more realistic description and management plan would be advantageous. In most patients, ulcerative mucositis is self-limiting and resolves spontaneously 2 to 3 weeks following the completion of radiation.

Evaluation of Mucositis Comparisons of the stomatotoxicity of treatment regimens and efficacy assessments of mucositis interventions have been hindered by the lack of a universally acceptable scoring system for the condition. A recent comprehensive review of mucositis by the Mucositis Study Section of the Multinational Association of Supportive Care in Cancer[19] lists 14 scales that are currently in use to grade mucositis. Measurement scales for mucositis fall into three major functional categories: those that are used to describe toxicity, those that are designed primarily for research, and those that are used as nursing management tools. Virtually all of the scales contain objective endpoints that focus on the extent of observed erythema and ulceration. Although some scales are limited to these objective findings, many add other elements that depend on symptomatic interpretation and patients' oral function, particularly associated with eating ability.

Currently, the grading systems most commonly used to describe oral mucosal toxicity are the World Health Organization (WHO) and National Cancer Institute's circulating tumor cell (NCI-CTC) scales. The WHO scale combines elements of objective findings of erythema and ulceration with the patients' ability to eat solids, liquids, or nothing by mouth. The complexity of mucositis assessment is reflected by the fact that the NCI CTC has multiple scales that separately grade objective and functional findings for different clinical situations (radiation, chemotherapy, and transplant). Establishment of a common, accepted scale is critical if there is to be uniformity in the assessment of the oral mucositis.

Prevention and Treatment There is currently no approved active preventive or treatment intervention for radiation-induced mucositis in the United States. There is general consensus that improved oral status may reduce the risk or severity of mucositis. Maintaining a high level of oral hygiene during treatment is thought to be beneficial.

Since mucosal injury is related to the extent of mucosa exposed to radiation, the use of midline radiation blocks[25] and three-dimensional radiation treatment[26] may reduce the extent of stomatotoxicity.

Benzydamine hydrochloride is a nonsteroidal rinse with anti-inflammatory, analgesic, and anesthetic properties that is approved for use in the prevention and treatment of radiation-induced mucositis in Canada, Australia and Europe. Results of a number of studies suggest its efficacy in this application.[27–31] The MASCC panel recommended the use of benzydamine among patients receiving moderate dose radiotherapy.[32]

A number of palliative barrier agents have been suggested to alleviate symptoms associated with oral mucositis. Gelclair, which has FDA approval as a device, purportedly forms a barrier on injured mucosa.[33] Sucralfate, an agent that has wide use in the treatment of gastric ulcers, forms a protein-drug complex on the site of ulcerated mucosa. Its use as a rinse in the treatment of mucositis has been reported in a number of studies, although its efficacy seems inconsistent.[34–37]

A variety of topical agents exist for pain management associated with mucositis. These include lidocaine viscous, benzocaine in Orabase, and suspensions of Benadryl in Kaopectate or milk of magnesia. In general, topical palliative rinses are only of value in mild forms of the condition. Systemic pain management, following the WHO pain ladder, is often necessary. Additionally, cold foods, such as ice cream or Popsicles, may be soothing. Patients should be instructed to remove dental prostheses.

The role of microbes on the severity and course of radiation-induced mucositis is unclear.[38] The strategy of mucosal decontamination as a mucositis intervention has produced conflicting results. Chlorhexidine gluconate rinses do not appear to have a role in mucositis prevention or treatment in radiation mucositis, although they may be used to help with oral hygiene.[32] Lozenges containing polymyxin E, tobramycin, and amphotericin have been studied and seem to of marginal value.[32]

The application of non-protein thiols as a mucositis intervention is currently under study.[39] Amifostine, which is approved as cytoprotective agent for xerostomia (see below), may be effective in modulating mucositis. N-acetyl cysteine, used as a topical rinse, is currently undergoing evaluation in the prevention and attenuation of radiation-induced oral mucositis. If these agents prove to be efficacious, it seems likely that their success is due to a combination of antioxidant and cytoprotective activities.

A wide range of agents is currently in different stages of development as possible interventions for radiation-induced mucositis. Among these are vitamin E, growth factors (GM-CSF and members of the FGF super family), anti-inflammatory drugs, prostaglandins and cyclo-oxygenase inhibitors.[40–43]

Xerostomia Xerostomia is one of the most consistent and bothersome side effects of radiation therapy in which the salivary glands are included in the field of treatment.[3,20] Concomitant chemotherapy may exacerbate the effect. The effects of radiation on salivary flow are variable and symptoms of dry mouth may not correspond to observed salivary flow. Xerostomia is caused by the effects of radiation on acinar cells, especially of the serous glands (parotid).[44] Consequently, inflammation, degeneration, and fibrosis of the glandular parenchyma occur. The extent, duration, and degree of recovery are functions of the dose rate, total dose, and radiation port. Onset of xerostomia may be noted as early as 1 week following the start of radiation (cumulative dose of 10 Gy).[45] The saliva turns thick and ropey as serous function is diminished, but mucous production remains. Patients whose radiation to the ear and neck in cumulative doses of 60 Gy more often develop irreversible xerostomia, with an 80% loss in salivary gland function.[46] Spontaneous recovery is unlikely for patients with xerostomia persisting for 12 months or longer.[47] With lesser doses of radiation, however, inflammation and edema of glandular tissue often spontaneously disappear within a year of the completion of treatment.[48]

In addition to functional changes caused by xerostomia, such as dysphasia and alteration in taste, loss of saliva is also associated with a reduction in oral clearance, diminished salivary immunoglobulin A (IgA) levels, and salivary antibacterial enzymes. Consequently, patients with xerostomia are susceptible to increases in local oral infections including caries, periodontal disease, and candidiasis.

Radiation-induced caries can be a common problem in patients with xerostomia.[49] Changes in salivary composition, decreases in buffering capacity, and loss of the cleansing action of saliva results in the accumulation of bacteria, increases in local cariogenic flora, and tooth decalcification with consequent caries development.[50–52] Typically, radiation caries presents with lesions at the cervical margins of teeth, which then rapidly progresses. Decalcification (white, chalky enamel) of the incisal edges of the teeth may also be noted. In addition to tooth loss, a major consequence of uncontrolled caries may be abscess formation in patients who are at risk for osteoradionecrosis.

Four goals should be considered for the prevention and treatment of xerostomia. Preservation of salivary function is critical. Whenever possible, tissue sparing techniques aimed at minimizing the amount of salivary tissues exposed to direct radiation should be used. Whereas bilateral field radiation may result in an 80% reduction of salivary flow, mantle irradiation typically causes only a 30 to 40% decrease. Parotid sparing using three-dimensional treatment or intensity-modulated radiotherapy techniques offers the greatest change of glandular repair.[26] Stimulation of salivary flow should start simultaneously with XRT, as should an anticaries regimen to protect the dentition. Replacement of reduced secretions may be introduced as soon as needed.

Stimulation of salivary flow may be accomplished through local or systemic means. Sucrose-free lemon drops or sugarless chewing gum may be used. Cinnamon- or mint-flavored mints or gum should be avoided as they may irritate the mucosa.

Drug therapy may also help to stimulate parotid flow.[54] Of the cholinergic agents, pilocarpine has been best studied and found to stimulate parotid function, but not submandibular or sublingual gland function in patients with Sjögren's syndrome and radiation-induced xerostomia.[55] Other agents such as bromhexine,[56] anetholtrithion,[57] bethanechol HCl, potassium iodide, neostigmine, and reserpine have been used for salivary stimulation,[54] but data substantiating their efficacy are scant. In contrast, substantial data exist to support the use of pilocarpine HCl tablets to stimulate salivary flow in patients with radiation-induced xerostomia.[58] In cases in which pilocarpine is used after patients have completed radiation treatment and are symptomatic, at least some residual salivary function must be present, and patients should be cautioned that clinically significant improvements in salivary flow may not be realized for up to 3 months following the initiation of treatment. Alternatively, pilocarpine may be prescribed to start simultaneous with radiation therapy. In either case, the typical dose of 5 mg given three times daily may be titrated depending on the patient's response and manifestation of side effects.

Amifostine, a non-protein, free-radical scavenger has been approved as a cytoprotective agent for salivary glands to prevent radiation-induced xerostomia.[59] The recommended dose for amifostine is 200 mg/m^2 administered once daily as a 3 minute infusion, starting 15 to 30 minutes prior to standard fraction radiation therapy.[60] The need for intravenous infusion, frequency of dosing, cost, and potential side effects have limited amifostine's adoption. A subcutaneous formulation is currently under study.[61]

Salivary replacement can be accomplished with the use of saliva substitutes or artificial saliva.[62] Most of these materials contain carboxymethylcellulose and may provide transient symptomatic relief of mucosal dryness. Saliva substitutes are available as over-the-counter rinses or sprays and are most effective if used before meals and at bedtime. A number of toothpastes and chewing gums have been developed specifically for use in patients with xerostomia.

Without question, the most effective protective agent for radiation-induced caries is the aggressive use of topical fluorides.[63] Topical fluoride supplements should be initiated at the start of radiation treatment. Continuation of fluoride following the completion of radiotherapy is critical, especially in patients who develop xerostomia. Fluorides for dental use come in three forms: rinses, gels applied by toothbrushing or in customized trays, and drops also used in trays that are molded to fit over patients' teeth. Patients in whom xerostomia is anticipated should have fluoride trays fabricated prior to the initiation of radiotherapy. Fluoride gel or drops are placed in the trays and applied by the patient each day. Use of tray-borne application can be supplemented with acidulated fluoride rinses; generally the use of rinses in the morning and trays before sleep is most effective and easiest for patients. Acidulated fluorides tend to work best, although neutral fluoride rinses are available for patients with mucositis in whom acidulated material might be irritating, or for patients with porcelain prostheses in whom pitting of the restorations might occur. Aggressive oral hygiene is to be encouraged, and patients should be seen by a dentist frequently. Regular dental visits are critical to insure early detection and intervention of caries and periodontal disease.

For patients who cannot tolerate trays because of gagging or mucositis, fluoride gels may be applied with a toothbrush, either as 1.1% sodium fluoride or 0.4% stannous fluoride. The latter appears to be more efficacious. Patients should be instructed to avoid sucrose.

Loss of taste is a transient, but bothersome sequelae of head and neck radiation. The severity of taste loss increases rapidly up to doses of 30 Gy, but then usually plateaus.[64] Patients who receive doses of 30 Gy or more may lose their ability to distinguish salt or sweet tastes. Fortunately, hypogeusia is typically transient and taste begins to return within 1 to 2 months after the completion of treatment. Total recovery may take up to a year. If there does not seem to be progression to improvement following radiotherapy, candidiasis should be ruled out.

Osteoradionecrosis Of all of the oral complications of head and neck radiation, perhaps the most significant is osteoradionecrosis (ORN).[65,66] First described in 1927, ORN results in the denudation of soft tissue and exposure and necrosis of bone.[67] Although not limited to the jaws, it frequently occurs at this site. ORN causes a painful, chronic, open, and foul-smelling wound that is typically of great distress to the patient. Most cases ultimately heal with conservative treatment, but the course is usually prolonged. Historically, ORN was attributed to a triad of trauma (often tooth extractions), radiation and infection.[68] Subsequent studies suggest, however, that ORN represents a defect in wound healing rather than a true osteomyelitis.[69] The etiology appears to relate to diminished vascularization as a consequence of XRT.[70] Histologic changes of thickened arterial and arteriolar walls substantiate this hypothesis,[71] and the lack of culturable pathogenic microorganisms from active ORN lesions suggest the noninfectious nature of the process.[72]

No consensus exists concerning the overall frequency of ORN. Although reported ranges vary between 4 and 44%, approximately 15% appears to be the preponderant experience.[65,66,71] The mandible is involved more often than the maxilla, which probably reflects the difference in blood supply and vascularity of the two bones. Time until onset of ORN following XRT is controversial. Some authors have described ORN as early as 2 weeks after XRT,[71] whereas others report it as a late condition.[72] Most cases occur within the first 3 years after XRT (74%). Equally controversial is the rate at which ORN risk diminishes with time after the completion of XRT, although it seems clear that the risk never reaches zero.[73]

A number of risk factors for ORN have been positively identified. Men have been reported to have a risk for ORN that is 3-fold higher than women.[65] Patients who are edentulous are twice as likely as patients with teeth to develop ORN.[74,75] Furthermore, the frequency of ORN increases dramatically in individuals with active dental disease (eg, periodontal disease, caries, periapical disease, poorly fitting prostheses).[74] Fifty percent of cases appear to be associated with tooth extraction following radiation. These findings strongly support pre-XRT dental evaluation and aggressive repair and removal of diseased teeth. The field size, dose rate, and total dose of XRT have a marked effect on the frequency of ORN. Patients who receive cumulative doses of 65 Gy or more to the mandible or maxilla are more likely to develop ORN than are patients receiving lesser doses.[66] For example, patients who receive 80 Gy or more are twice as likely to develop ORN compared to patients who are treated with 50 Gy to 60 Gy. Use of three-dimensional radiation techniques has resulted in a slight reduction in ORN risk.[76] Patients with tumors that are adjacent or contiguous with bone are also at higher ORN risk.[77] It is likely that this finding is due to the inclusion of bone in the radiated field since the volume of bone exposed to XRT has a direct impact on ORN risk. Poor nutrition and immune status also appear to predispose to the condition. Diagnosis of ORN is usually based on clinical findings. In cases in which the diagnosis is questionable, magnetic resonance imaging may be of value.[78] In contrast, although scintigraphy with 99m technetium Tc-HDP may demonstrate positive findings, the overall specificity of this technique for ORN (57%) makes it less desirable.[78]

Treatment of ORN is based on the severity and chronicity of the condition. Fortunately, most lesions (up to 60%) eventually heal in approximately 6 months with conservative therapy consisting of local debridement, saliva irrigation, and oral antibiotics.[79] Although potassium phenoxymethyl penicillin (500 mg every 6 hours) has demonstrated efficacy, the use of tetracycline (250 mg qid for 10 days followed by 250 mg bid for several months) has been suggested on the basis of tetracycline's predilection to be taken up by bone.[80]

Lesions that show no improvement or demonstrate progression require more aggressive therapy. For these cases, surgical debridement and hyperbaric oxygen (HBO) may be indicated.[81,82] In extensive cases, radical resection of involved bone with immediate microvascular reconstruction has been used successfully in patients who have failed more conservative treatment, including HBO.[83,84]

Because most cases of intraoral ORN are associated with dental disease and post-XRT extractions, eliminating potential sites of odontogenic pathology before the start of radiation is the basis for prevention. Teeth with periodontal disease, advanced caries with a risk of impingement on the dental pulp, fracture, or periapical disease should be removed before the initiation of XRT. Teeth adjacent to or involved in potential surgical sites (for tumor resection) also should be extracted. Because of the consequences of ORN, even suspiciously diseased teeth, especially in the XRT area, should be eliminated. The timing of dental extractions in patients being treated with XRT has been the subject of much analysis, discussion, and controversy; however, the consensus is that teeth should be extracted before XRT.[77] Ideally, a minimum 21-day healing period is desirable, although a shorter time may be dictated by circumstances. In either instance, extraction before XRT is much more desirable than extraction after the start of therapy, because a number of studies suggest that post-XRT extractions carry significant risk of ORN, no matter how long after XRT they are performed. In all cases, extraction should be performed as atraumatically as possible, with special care given to the soft tissue, primary closure if possible, and good local postoperative wound management. Perioperative use of antibiotics is also recommended.

Aggressive oral hygiene, use of fluorides, and dental care are important components in preventing the development of dental disease once XRT has started. If dental disease develops after XRT and a tooth is restorable, endodontic therapy is more desirable than extraction.[77] Inevitably, extractions are sometimes required of teeth in radiated fields. The risk of ORN in these cases has been reported to be reasonable (5.6%), even without the use of HBO. The efficacy of HBO in these cases is unresolved. One study found that, among patients having teeth removed within the first year following radiation, 98.5% of extraction sites treated pre- and post-operatively with HBO healed without complications. However, the efficacy of HBO reportedly decreased the farther out from radiation extractions were performed. On the other hand, a recent randomized, placebo-controlled, double-blind trial in which patients were treated pre- and postoperatively with HBO failed to demonstrate any benefit.[85] Thus, the use of HBO, with its incurred cost and multiple visits, warrants additional study.

ORAL COMPLICATIONS OF CHEMOTHERAPY

Oral complications of cancer chemotherapy result from the effects of the drug acting on the oral mucosa (direct or primary stomatotoxicity), the patients' inability to contain local, minor oral disease during myelosuppression (indirect or secondary stomatotoxicity), or some combination of the two.

Risk Factors Not all patients who undergo cancer chemotherapy are at equal risk to develop oral complications. A number of variables have been identified that bear on both the frequency and severity of oral problems associated with treatment. These can be divided into those that are associated with the patient and those that are related to the treatment regimen.[86]

Patient-related risk factors include tumor diagnosis, patient age, gender, body mass, genetics, the patient's oral condition before cancer therapy, the level of oral care during therapy, baseline xerostomia, and baseline neutrophil numbers. Patients with hematologic malignancies (ie, leukemia and lymphoma) are at greater risk of oral complications than are patients with non-head and neck solid tumors. For example, more than 66% of patients with leukemia and 33% of patients with non-Hodgkin lymphoma develop oral problems. It seems likely that tumor-related myelosuppression is at least partly the basis for this observation.[87] Almost all patients with tumors of the head and neck who receive local therapy develop problems after treatment.

The role of age as a risk factor for mucositis is unclear. There are few studies that compare the rate of mucositis among patients of varying ages with similar diagnoses. However, the rate of mucositis among children may be greater than among older patients being treated for the same diagnosis.[88] The observation that mitotic activity of oral mucosal cells in young patients is significantly greater than among older individuals may result in an increased stomatotoxic susceptibility of basal epithelium in younger patients.[89] Furthermore, quantification of epithelium-related growth factors has shown higher amounts in younger individuals,[90] which could, in part, be responsible for the rapidity with which these patients recover following ulcerative mucositis compared with older individuals. Among adult patients with solid tumors being treated with 5-fluorouracil (5-FU), mucositis appears to be more severe and persistent among older persons.

Gender may affect risk. There are reports to suggest that women are more likely to have toxicities associated with 5-FU than are men.[91] This observation has been limited and further studies are warranted to confirm this reported trend and, if correct, to determine its mechanism.

Genetics may affect risk of mucositis in two ways. Patients with genetic defects, which affect drug metabolism, are at increased risk for mucositis. For example, among a population of patients being treated with methotrexate for chronic myelogenous leukemia, increased toxicity (including mucositis) was observed in those individuals with lower methylenetetrahydrofolate reductase activity (TT genotype).[92] Similarly, deficiencies in dihydropyrimidine dehydrogenase (DPD) predisposes to toxicities mediated by 5-FU.[93] Alternatively, genetics may affect and regulate the mechanisms, which provide the biological basis for chemotherapy-induced mucosal injury. For example, pro-inflammatory cytokine production varies among the population and is genetically controlled. These cytokines play a role and track closely with non-hematologic toxicities. Consequently, patients who are predisposed to be high producers of these proteins may also be at increased risk for mucositis. Further study is needed to fully elucidate this hypothesis, but it promises to be important in determining both risk and predicting responsiveness to mechanism-based interventions.

It is generally agreed that patients whose pretreatment oral condition is poor are at greater risk for some, but not all, oral complications.[80,94] Chronic irritation for poorly fitting prostheses or faulty restorations predisposes patients to the development of ulcerative mucositis. Patients with advanced periodontal disease, pulpal disease, or low-grade soft-tissue infections such as those associated with partially erupted third molars (ie, wisdom teeth) are at increased risk for developing sepsis of oral origin once they become myelosuppressed. However, elevated risks of infection are not associated with asymptomatic radiographically demonstrable periapical lesions in endodontically treated teeth.[95]

The level of oral care during therapy has a marked influence on outcome relative to oral complications and infection.[96,97] The ability of the patient and his or her healthcare providers to reduce the load of oral bacterial flora favorably affects the risk of both local and systemic infection.[96] Aggressive techniques of oral hygiene, including mechanical debridement of the teeth and soft tissue, and antimicrobial rinses are effective.

Xerostomia prior to and during chemotherapy is associated with an increased risk of mucositis.[98] This observation may be the result of an alteration in the health of desiccated oral mucosa and an overall increase in the resident oral microflora, which is seen in patients without adequate salivary function. The value of salivary stimulation on the course of mucositis is unclear. The favorable effect of pilocarpine on chemotherapy-induced mucositis reported in one study was not replicated in a similar trial.[99] The extent of mucositis correlates negatively with neutropenia. Baseline neutrophil counts of < 4,000 are associated with higher rates of mucositis.[86] This finding may explain, in part, the observation of increased rates of mucositis among patients with hematologic malignancies.

Risk of complications also relates to the form, schedule, and dose of chemotherapy used.[19] Concomitant radiation, including TBI, also enhance the risk of oral problems. In general, the overall frequency of oral toxicities is under-reported.

Significant differences exist in the degree of stomatotoxicity of drugs used for chemotherapy.[19] Drugs or regimens containing anthracyclines, taxanes, platinum, and 5-FU are consistently stomatotoxic. Conditioning regimens in which TBI is used also cause mucositis at high rates. Among specific drugs or combinations in which oral mucositis rates (grade 3–4) affect a significant percentage of patients (> 25%) are[19]:

- Docetaxel/5-FU
- Docetaxel + XRT
- Paclitaxel + XRT
- Docetaxel + 5-FU
- Paclitaxel/5-FU + XRT
- Docetaxel/platinum + XRT
- Paclitaxel/platinum + XRT
- Docetaxel/platinum/5-FU
- Paclitaxel/platinum/5-FU
- Oxaliplatin + XRT
- Platinum/taxane + XRT
- Platinum/methotrexate/leucovorin
- 5-FU/platinum
- 5-FU/leucovorin/taxane
- Irinotecan/5-FU CI + XRT
- Ara-C/idarubicin/fludarabine
- Methotrexate
- Isofamide/etoposide
- Melphalan

In viewing the above list, it is important to remember that the incidence of oral complications, particularly mucositis, tends to be vastly under-reported both in terms of occurrence and severity. Virtually every chemotherapeutic agent in the current armamentarium has the potential to produce a stomatotoxic response in at least some portion of the treated population.

Repetitive, low-dose regimens tend to be less toxic than do bolus doses of the same agent. Toxicity that is secondary to radiation is dependent on cumulative dose; pulsed application of therapy does not significantly reduce stomatic changes.

Ulcerative mucositis usually occurs 5 to 8 days following the administration of chemotherapy and it lasts approximately 7 to 14 days. Lesions heal spontaneously and without scar formation. Chemotherapy-induced mucositis is confined to the movable oral mucosa: the mucosa of the cheeks, lateral and ventral tongue, inner aspects of the lips, floor of the mouth, and soft palate. Unlike radiation-induced mucositis, that produced by chemotherapy does not affect the hard palate or gingival. The dorsal surface of the tongue is not affected either. This observation is likely to be attributable to the differences in the character of the epithelium on each mucosal surface. Of the sites in the mouth, the buccal mucosa (cheeks), lateral and ventral surfaces of the tongue, and the floor of the mouth are the most commonly involved. In patients who receive multiple cycles of chemotherapy, lesions tend to reappear in the same sites. Numerous studies have confirmed that mucositis is not of infectious (particularly viral) origin. Although patients may also be at risk for herpes simplex infections, the lesions of viral stomatitis are quite distinct in appearance and behavior from those of mucositis.[100–102]

The biologic mechanisms, which underlie chemotherapy-induced mucositis, are currently the topic of intense investigation.[22] As noted above, mucositis was viewed as the result of non-specific toxicity of chemotherapy directed against the rapidly dividing cells of the oral basal epithelium. Although data exist to support the hypothesis, the observation that the course of mucositis could be altered by agents with little or no epithelial activity suggested a more broadly based pathogenesis. It appears that mucositis represents a clinical outcome due to a complex interaction of local tissue toxicity (endothelium, connective tissue, and epithelium), the level of myelosuppression and the local environment. Disruption of connective tissue and endothelial cells initiated by free radical formation likely leads to the activation of a range of transcription factors and increased expression of a number of genes that results in stimulation of pro-inflammatory cytokine production and tissue damage. Simultaneous activation of other signaling pathways and enzyme activation results in increases in ceramide, proteolytic enzymes, and other mediators of direct and indirect epithelial injury. Thus, in addition to clonogenic death of basal cells caused by direct DNA injury, secondary pathways produce a barrage of mechanisms that lead to apoptosis or necrosis. As a consequence, the epithelium first becomes atrophic, as its renewal ceases, and then eventually completely breaks down to form an ulcer. It is noteworthy that in some patients, the extent of cumulative injury to the basal epithelium does not reach the threshold needed for ulceration to occur. In these patients, the thinned mucosa is mildly to moderately symptomatic (grade 1 mucositis). In cases when ulceration does occur, secondary colonization by oral bacteria (both gram positives and gram negatives) occurs. Cell wall products from these bacteria make their way into the underlying connective tissue where they effectively stimulate additional proinflammatory cytokine production by infiltrating macrophages.

The better understanding of the pathobiology of mucositis has served as the basis for the development of interventions that are mechanistically based. The first of these agents to gain approval was palifermin (keratinocyte growth factor-1, Kepivance, Amgen) for the prevention and treatment of oral mucositis in patients receiving conditioning regimens in preparation for HSCT to treat hematologic malignancies. In a phase III trial in 212 HSCT recipients receiving a stomatotoxic conditioning regimen, palifermin, administered in multiple doses prior to and after transplantation was successful in significantly reducing the duration, incidence and severity of oral mucositis, favorably affecting patient-reported quality of life outcomes, and in reducing days of opioid use and fever.[103] It seems likely that palifermin's effect was the consequence, not only of its ability to stimulate epithelial proliferation, but also because of its cytoprotective activates mediated through increased expression of mediating transcription factors. FGF20, another growth factor in the same superclass, is currently in phase II trials.[104] Amifostine, a pleiotropic, free radical scavenger, has been reported to be efficacious in the HSCT population,[105] although other studies have not been positive. Of the 400,000 patients who develop mucositis each year in the United States, the HSCT population comprises only 5%. Consequently, extension of these, and other agents to other tumor populations is a major objective.

Low-level (helium-neon) laser ($\lambda = 632.8$ nm) therapy (LLLT) has demonstrated some efficacy in reducing the severity and symptoms associated with oral mucositis.[32] While additional studies are needed to confirm its value, the cost and logistics of LLLT may limit its overall utility.

A number of cytoprotective strategies and agents have been suggested as mucositis interventions. Oral cryotherapy is inexpensive and without risk, its use for 30 minutes starting 5 minutes before the infusion of bolus 5-FU or edatrexate may be helpful in reducing the severity of mucositis.[32] Allopurinol does not significantly reduce oral toxicity in patients being treated with 5-FU. Recently a new formulation of L-glutamine (Saforis) demonstrated modest, but significant, efficacy in a phase III trial in a population of patients being treated for breast cancer.[106] Pentoxifylline has been evaluated in a number of studies with mixed results. Similarly, antioxidant therapy with vitamin E and beta-carotene has produced inconsistent results. While anticholinergics, such as pilocarpine and Pro-Banthine, may be of benefit, it is likely that they function as salivary stimulants.

Because the presence of oral microorganisms is thought to adversely affect the course of mucositis, antimicrobial therapy has been studied extensively as an approach to intervention.[38] In general, the weight of data suggest that reduction of the oral bacterial load through medication does not bear significantly on the incidence or severity of mucositis. The use of topical antimicrobials such as chlorhexidine gluconate has consistently failed to improve the frequency or course of mucositis in randomized, blinded trials.[32,38]

Palliation has been the most widely used approach for the management of mucositis. Saline 0.9% has been used for years and is more effective than hydrogen peroxide, and at least as good as 'magic mouthwashes'.[107] Barrier type palliatives such as sucralfate suspension and Gelclair are available, although their benefit has not been convincingly shown. Topical lidocaine or Benadryl in Kaopectate or milk of magnesia may offer some topical relief, but often do not eliminate the need for parenteral analgesia.

OSTEONECROSIS

Bisphosphonate administration concomitant with chemotherapy has been introduced as a strategy to reduce metastases to bone. Among patients being treated in this way, osteonecrosis of the jaws, particularly of the maxilla has been reported with increasing frequency.[108] The presentation of osteonecrosis in this population varies in symptomatology. Although some patients experience pain, others do not. The majority of cases appear to be associated with dental manipulation, such as extraction, or soft tissue trauma. The mechanism underlying this pathology has yet to be defined, as is a full appreciation of the natural history of the condition. A variety of treatment approaches ranging from local debridement and antibiotic therapy to resection and HBO have been tried, but not in a disciplined way from which meaningful conclusions can made. Presently, the most judicious strategy is to assure aggressive dental screening and treatment prior to the initiation of treatment so that the possible need for dental intervention is minimized.

INFECTION

Simultaneous with the breakdown of the oral epithelium, the patients' ability to deal with the abundant oral microbial flora is compromised by their myelosuppression. Thus, the mouth becomes an important source of bacteremia and sepsis in the granulocytopenic cancer patient, as well as locoregional secondary infection.[109] These manifestations of indirect stomatotoxicity parallel the bone marrow status; hence, they are maximal at, or just proceeding the patient's granulocyte nadir. Systemic invasion of oral viridans streptococci are particularly common. Of these, *Streptococcus mitus* is associated with the most serious sequelae.

FUNGAL INFECTIONS Local oral infections in myelosuppressed patients are attributable to fungal, viral, and bacterial organisms, in order of descending frequency. Candidiasis is the most frequent oral infection and may appear in its characteristic white, curdy form or as erythematous, macular lesions.[110] It most frequently occurs on the palate, tongue, and corners of the mouth. Poorly controlled oral candidiasis increases the risk of aspiration and the development of candidal esophagitis or fungemia. In addition, aspergillosis and mucormycosis are not uncommon in myelosuppressed patients; these lesions can appear as invasive oral ulcerations that are painful and may involve bone.

Topical antifungal prophylaxis should be considered for all patients in whom granulocytopenia is anticipated. Although *Candida albicans* is a normal inhabitant of the oral flora in approximately 50% of the population, changes in salivary flow, granulocytopenia, and shifts in the oral bacterial flora predispose the patient with cancer to the development of clinical candidiasis.

The potential for regional or systemic spread of oropharyngeal candidal infection is significant. Systemic candidiasis is the cause of death in as many as one-third of immunocompromised patients.[111] Because of the morbidity and mortality that are associated with fungemia, candidal prophylaxis has been studied extensively but with unclear results. The polyene antifungal agents (eg, nystatin) are probably the most widely used form of topical therapy, although their efficacy in patients with marked neutropenia is not clear. Carpentieri and colleagues[112] reported a reduction in the clinical manifestations of candidal infection with nystatin, and Aviles[113] found a reduction in fatal candidiasis among individuals using topical nystatin. In contrast, other studies reported a 30% incidence of candidiasis in patients with leukemia despite nystatin use.

Of the imidazole agents, clotrimazole (Mycelex) is delivered as troches. Although it is doubtful that their efficacy is significantly better than that of nystatin,[114] patient compliance might be heightened, especially in patients with nausea. In addition, clotrimazole is significantly less expensive than nystatin.[115] Two other imidazoles also are available: ketoconazole (Nizoral) and fluconazole (Diflucan); both have demonstrated efficacy for the prophylaxis and treatment of existing disease.[116,117] The requirement of an acidic environment for ketoconazole, however, may limit its usefulness in patients who have difficulty eating. Azole resistance may be of relevance in the treatment of fungal infections. Some of the candida species such as *Candida glabriela an*d *Candida krusei* are inherently less sensitive to azole antifungal medications.[118]

The efficacy of chlorhexidine gluconate rinses as a topical antifungal agent is unclear.[116] Reports regarding its usefulness are inconsistent,[32] but in vivo data suggest that chlorhexidine reduces the activity of nystatin.[119,120] Hence, its simultaneous use with nystatin is not recommended.

Use of surveillance cultures for predicting the presence or course of fungal infection appears to have little value and generally is not recommended.[121]

VIRAL INFECTIONS Herpes simplex virus type 1 (HSV-1) is the most common oral viral infection in patients receiving chemotherapy or head and neck radiation. Oral infection by HSV-1 can result from a primary infection with the virus or the reactivation of latent virus in a previously exposed host. It is the latter which is most common in patients receiving cancer therapy. Individuals with prior HSV-1 exposure who are seropositive for the virus are at much greater risk than are patients who are negative.[122–124] The most common manifestation of infection with HSV-1 is oral ulceration, which clinically resembles other forms of mucositis. Additionally, extraoral or perioral vesiculation may occur. Determination of antibody status is therefore an important component of risk assessment for oral HSV-1 infection.

It appears that the timing of HSV-1 infection in patients receiving chemotherapy or bone marrow transplantation is quite consistent.[125] Lesions generally are seen approximately 18 days following the start of therapy. This temporal relationship is important in differentiating lesions that likely result from HSV-1 from those that result from direct stomatotoxicity, which are noted 5 to 7 days after the start of treatment, and from secondary surface infection (usually bacterial) that are seen at the patient's maximum myelosuppression (ie, granulocyte nadir), which occurs around 12 to 14 days. Viral culture is the most definitive way to diagnose HSV-1 infection, and aggressive culturing is recommended, especially in patients who are seropositive. Systemic acyclovir is the treatment of choice for prophylaxis and treatment of HSV infection.[122–124]

Herpes zoster also may present with oral lesions in patients who receive therapy for cancer. These lesions tend to be crop-like. Although they begin as vesicular lesions, they quickly rupture and form painful, small, ulcerative lesions. Unlike those from HSV-1, these lesions usually are unilateral and linear, often following one of the branches of the fifth cranial nerve.

Bacterial Infections The oral cavity may be a frequent source of local and systemic bacterial infection in the myelosuppressed patient with cancer, as evidenced by the increasing frequency of α-streptococcal infections among patients with granulocytopenic cancer.[126,127] Bacterial infections may be of soft tissue or gingival or odontogenic origin. Patients receiving cancer therapy often have increased numbers of oral organisms as a consequence of reduced hygiene and xerostomia. Additionally, the composition of the oral flora shifts from one in which gram-positive organisms predominate to one with an abundance of gram-negative pathogens.

Most often, odontogenic infections result from degeneration and infection of the dental pulp subsequent to bacterial invasion secondary to caries. Because of a patient's inability to mount an inflammatory response, conventional signs of dental infection (eg, abscess formation, swelling) are absent, and patients complain of localized tooth pain. Percussion or thermal sensitivity with clinical and/or radiographic evidence of caries progressing into the pulp is diagnostic. Neurotoxicity may cause dental pain that mimics odontogenic infection in patients receiving plant alkaloids. Odontogenic infections predominantly result from anaerobic species that are similar to those found in dental plaque. Treatment should consist of eliminating the source of infection, and in most cases, this involves tooth extraction. The safety of tooth extraction in the face of myelosuppression has been reported by a number of investigators.[128–130] These studies indicate that extraction may be performed with antibiotic coverage, platelet transfusion if needed, attention to tissue management, and good closure. Use of hemostatic agents such as Gelfoam in extraction sockets is discouraged, because they may act as foci of infection. Generally, platelet transfusion is not necessary for counts greater than 50,000 cells/mL. Systemic antibiotic coverage is indicated until the wound is epithelialized.

Gingival infections are relatively common in patients receiving myelosuppressive therapy. Some are localized, such as those that are associated with partially erupted third molars (ie, wisdom teeth), whereas others tend to be more diffuse. Acute gingival and periodontal infections are worse in patients with preexisting chronic gingival inflammation or periodontal disease. In addition, studies by Peterson[6] demonstrated that the periodontal health status of myelosuppressed patients influenced a shift from the normal oral flora to a composition rich in gram-negative bacteria.

The clinical appearance of acute gingival infections, which occur during periods of granulocytopenia, resembles that seen in acute necrotizing ulcerative gingivitis. Pain and loss of the gingival architecture, particularly necrosis of the interdental papillae, are characteristic. These lesions tend to be of a mixed bacterial nature, and they include a variety of pathogens, such as *Staphylococcus epidermidis, Pseudomonas aeruginosa,* and bacteria typically associated with periodontal disease such as *Bacteroides* and *Veillonella.*[6]

Treatment should include local debridement in addition to systemic antibiotics. Local culture of lesions may more useful than blood culture, because invasion of intact organisms may not occur. Empiric treatment is recommended regardless of culture results.

Mucosal infections in the myelosuppressed patient often are superimposed on ulcerated areas that have broken down as the result of direct stomatotoxicity. Ulcers may appear to be penetrating, with rounded borders and yellowish-white necrotic centers. Because of the lack of an inflammatory response, typical erythematous borders are usually absent. If the ulcerations are precipitated by trauma, secondary hematoma formation may occur in the patient with thrombocytopenia. Soft-tissue infections tend to be of gram-negative etiology, although HSV-1 must be ruled out. Treatment should include debridement, palliation, and antimicrobial therapy. Bacterial and viral cultures should be performed as well.

Preliminary data suggest that the mouth may seed indwelling lines with organisms, resulting in local-line infections and secondary sepsis. A correlation seems to exist between the presence of clinically significant mucositis α-hemolytic streptococcal positive blood cultures, and line infections and granulocytopenia.[131]

Strategies for the prevention of oral infection include eliminating sources of mucosal irritation and reducing the quantity of the local oral flora.[6] In addition, treatment of low-grade, asymptomatic infection before the start of therapy minimizes the risk of acute episodes once myelosuppression occurs.[132]

Reduction in the oral flora may be accomplished by mechanical and/or chemical means. Local debridement of the teeth can be accomplished with conventional toothbrushing; soft brushes should be used. Thrombocytopenia is not a contraindication to mechanical debridement if common sense is used. Brushing should be discontinued to the face of significant bleeding. Alternatively, cotton swabs or a towel-wrapped finger may be used to clean the teeth. Dental floss is an excellent adjuvant for cleaning but may be difficult for patients to use if they are unfamiliar with it. It also may be used until patients become profoundly thrombocytopenic. Essentially, anything that the patient or provider can use to physically wipe debris and microorganisms from the teeth will be beneficial. Cotton swabs, sponges, and rubber tips all may be of use.

Rinses are of varying degrees of help in maintaining oral hygiene. Any fluid that flushes the mouth, including water, will be of some help. Saline and diluted peroxide frequently are used. Generally, mouth rinses containing alcohol as their active agent cause burning of the atrophic mucosa and are not recommended. Mixed results have been reported with chlorhexidine gluconate rinses. No benefit of chlorhexidine over water was recently reported.[133] If chlorhexidine is used, its administration should be timed to avoid contact with nystatin, because the effects of the latter may be inactivated by chlorhexidine. Similarly, povidone-iodine rinses have demonstrated efficacy in reducing the resident oral flora. Other drugs have been tried as preventatives,[134] and fluoride rinses reduce the ability of oral bacteria to adhere to teeth. Consequently, they also may be helpful.

Patients with removable prostheses should be instructed to remove them during periods of myelosuppression. Oral bleeding during such periods most often is of gingival origin. Spontaneous gingival bleeding is a rare occurrence when platelet counts exceed 20,000 cells/mL. Slow oozing may be noted at lower platelet levels, especially in areas with pre-existing periodontal disease. Local treatment of gingival bleeding includes initial debridement, nondisturbance of formed clots, and topical application of thrombin under pressure. Gingival bleeding usually is interpreted as evidence that the platelet count is low enough to allow other, more threatening hemorrhage.

Hematoma formation often occurs in areas of trauma, especially the buccal mucosa, alveolar mucosa, or edentulous areas. Areas of submucosal hemorrhage form bluish, blister-like areas, which then form a yellowish-white, tumor-like mass of fibrin. Epithelialization occurs beneath the mass. If bleeding occurs before healing is complete, topical therapy may include thrombin, microfibrillar collagen, or other hemostatic gel. Before healing is complete, the clot may serve as a focus for microbial growth. It should be checked daily and removed as soon as epithelialization is complete. Unchecked sublingual bleeding may cause respiratory embarrassment by elevating the tongue.

ORAL COMPLICATIONS ASSOCIATED WITH HSCT

Mucositis Because of the intensity of HSCT conditioning regimens, mucositis is exceptionally frequent among this patient population. Although variation in the incidence of mucositis relates to the treatment protocol, at least three-quarters of patients in most cases can be expected to develop the condition. The inclusion of total-body irradiation does not seem to increase the risk of developing mucositis.[135] As with other forms of chemotherapy-induced mucositis, lesions are localized to the movable oral mucosa and are most frequent in the floor of the mouth, lingual frenum, and labial and buccal mucosae. There appears to be no significant difference in either the onset of mucositis following transplantation or the duration of mucositis among recipients of autologous or allogeneic HSCT. Woo and colleagues reported a mean time of mucositis onset as 5 days following HSCT for autologous recipients, as compared to 6 days for allogeneic recipients. The mean duration of mucositis for both groups was approximately 6 days, with resolution in 10 to 12 days. Importantly, no case of mucositis was noted in autologous recipients beyond day 22. There is a significant association between the absolute neutrophil count (ANC) and the presence of mucositis. Unless patients have extremely severe lesions or develop graft-versus-host disease (GVHD), mucositis resolves with ANC of greater than 500 cells/mL.

The mechanism of mucositis induction is discussed elsewhere in this chapter. It is important to note that the condition occurs independently of oral mucosal infections with either viral or fungal etiology. As noted above, palifermin has recently been approved for the prevention and treatment of oral mucositis in autologous HSCT recipients (see above).

Infection Oral infection is a major cause of morbidity among HSCT recipients. Of special importance in this patient population is the oral cavity as a source of systemic or distant infection. The incidence of streptococcal infections in HSCT recipients has increased dramatically. A recent study demonstrated that bacteria of the *Streptococcus viridans* group were frequent isolates from infections associated with indwelling lines.[131] Consequently, pretreatment screening to identify and eliminate asymptomatic, dormant, or potential sources of dental infection or irritation should be mandated for BMT recipients.

In addition to bacterial infections, HSCT recipients are at risk for oral viral and fungal infections during the period of their granulocytopenia. As with other myelosuppressed patients, the clinical presentation of these infections in the BMT population often varies from the classic descriptions typically associated with these lesions. Consequently, early and aggressive culturing is mandated. Members of the herpes group account for most viral infections; herpes simplex, varicella, and herpes zoster are associated with oral infections in HSCT patients. The routine practice of acyclovir prophylaxis, however, generally has been discontinued. In addition, acyclovir-resistant mucocutaneous herpes simplex infections have been reported in HSCT populations.[136] Candidiasis is the most common fungal infection, although both mucormycosis and aspergillosis have been reported. Lesions of the deep fungal infections generally present as nonhealing gingival ulcerations. Biopsy is the diagnostic method of choice.

Graft-Versus-Host Disease The mouth is a common site for manifestations of both acute and chronic GVHD.[137,138] Although there are relatively few reports on the oral manifestations of acute GVHD, three clinical patterns of oral lesions have been described by Barrett and Bilous[139] and are noted as early as 3 weeks following transplantation and almost 1 week after the onset of skin lesions. Initially, multiple, small, white, papillated lesions present on the movable mucosa. These progress to the development of keratotic, white, lacey lesions that clinically resemble lichen planus and, in fact, have been described as lichenoid in appearance. Desquamative lesions may then develop. These also are similar to the lesions of erosive or bullous lichen planus, and unlike the other two forms, these tend to be symptomatic and require intervention.

The oral lesions of chronic GVHD appear approximately 3 months or later following transplantation. Approximately 70% of patients with GVHD develop oral lesions, which most typically are lichenoid in appearance. Symptomatic lesions usually present as erosive, vesiculobullous lesions of the oral mucosa, with peripheral areas of keratotic striations. Additionally, xerostomia is a frequent finding among patients with chronic GVHD. Both mucosal and salivary gland changes result from lymphocytic infiltration; the resulting tissue changes are analogous to those seen in other autoimmune changes in the mouth.

Biopsy of the minor salivary glands of the lip appears to be an accurate and sensitive way to confirm the diagnosis of chronic GVHD, and it is more predictive than either biopsy of the buccal mucosa or the parotid gland.[140] Technically, minor salivary gland biopsy is easily performed in an office setting with local anesthesia and a minimum of tissue manipulation. Histologically, one notes acinar atrophy and/or destruction accompanied by a lymphocytic infiltrate that is rich in CD3+ T cells.

Lichenoid lesions generally respond to topical or systemic steroid therapy. Ultraviolet A light therapy reportedly has benefit in the treatment of severe, nonresponsive lesions.[141] Therapy for xerostomia was discussed earlier in this chapter. As with other patients having xerostomia, patients with GVHD are at increased risk for caries and should be managed accordingly.

Additional late effects of HSCT and GVHD also affect the mouth. Of sites for secondary malignancies in this population, the mouth is among the most common. Consequently, patients should receive routine and thorough oral examinations to screen for the development of squamous cell carcinoma. Pediatric HSCT has also been reported to be associated with significant long-term oral and craniofacial complications. Early referral and aggressive follow-up care by pediatric dental specialists is recommended.

REFERENCES

1. Sonis ST. Oral mucositis in cancer therapy. J Supportive Oncol 2004;2:3.
2. Lugassy G, Shaham R, Nemets A, et al. Severe osteomyelitis of the jaw in long-term survivors of multiple myeloma: a new clinical entity. Am J Med 2004;117:440.
3. Sonis ST, Sonis AL, Liberman A. Oral complications in patients receiving treatment for non-head and neck malignancies. J Am Dent Assoc 1978;97:468.
4. Avritscher EB, Cooksley CD, Elting LS. Scope and epidemiology of cancer therapy-induced oral and gastrointestinal mucositis. Semin Oncol Nurs 2004;20:3.
5. Friedman RB. Osteoradionecrosis: causes and prevention. Natl Cancer Inst Monogr 1990;9:45.
6. Peterson DE. Pretreatment strategies in infection prevention in chemotherapy patients. Natl Cancer Inst Monogr 1990:9:61.
7. Sonis ST, Kunz A. Impact of improved dental services on the frequency of oral complications of cancer therapy for patients with non-head and neck malignancies. Oral Surg Oral Med Oral Pathol 1988;65:19.
8. Woods P, Sonis ST. Dental problems among BMT recipients requiring pretreatment. J Dent Res 1989;68:253.
9. Heimdahl A, Matsson T, Dahilof G, et al. The oral cavity as a portal of entry for early infections in patients treated with bone marrow transplantation. Oral Surg Oral Med Oral Pathol 1989;68:711.
10. Lockhart PB, Clark J. Pretherapy dental status of patients with malignant conditions of the head and neck. Oral Surg Oral Med Oral Pathol 1994;77:236.
11. Epstein JB, Stevenson-Moore P. Periodontal disease and periodontal management in patients with cancer. Oral Oncol 2001;:613–9.
12. Sonis ST, Woods PD, White BA. Pretreatment oral assessment. Natl Cancer Inst Monogr 1990;9:29.
13. Stevenson-Moore P, Epstein JB. The management of teeth in irradiated sites. Oral Oncol 1993;29:338.
14. Stevenson-Moore P. Essential aspects of a pretreatment oral examination. Natl Cancer Inst Monogr 1990;9:33.
15. Sonis ST. Orthodontic management of selected medically compromised patients: cardiac disease, bleeding disorders, and asthma. Sem in Orthod 2004;10:277
16. Duggal MS, Curzon ME, Bailey CC, et al. Dental parameters in the long-term survivors of childhood cancers compared with siblings. Oral Oncol 1997;33:348.
17. Pajari U, Lanning M. Developmental defects of teeth in survivors of childhood ALL are related to the therapy and age at diagnosis. Med Pediatr Oncol 1995;24:30.
18. Sonis AL, Tarbell N, Valachovic RW, et al. Dentofacial development in long-term survivors of acute lymphoblastic leukemia. A comparison of two treatment modalities. Cancer 1990;66:2645.
19. Sonis ST, Elting LS, Keefe D, et al. Perspectives on cancer therapy-induced mucosal injury: pathogenesis, measurement, epidemiology and consequences for patients. Cancer 2004;100(9 Supp):1995.
20. Baker DG. The radiobiological basis for tissue reactions in the oral cavity following therapeutic x-irradiation. Arch Otolaryngol 1982;108:21.
21. Sonis ST. Mucositis as biological process: a new hypothesis for the development of chemotherapy-induced stomatotoxicity. Oral Oncol 1998;34:39.
22. Sonis ST. The pathobiology of mucositis. Nat Rev Cancer 2004;4:277.
23. Rose-Ped AM, Bellm LA, Epstein JB, et al. Complications of radiation therapy for head and neck cancers. The patient's perspective. Cancer Nurs 2002;25:461.
24. Trotti A, Bellm LA, Epstein JB, et al. Mucositis incidence, severity and associated outcomes in patients with head and neck cancer receiving radiotherapy with or without chemotherapy. Radiother Oncol 2003;66:253.
25. Perch SJ, Machtay M, Markiewicz DA, et al. Decreased acute toxicity by using midline mucosa-sparing blocks during radiation therapy for carcinoma of the oral cavity, oropharynx, and nasopharynx. Radiology 1995;197:863.
26. Malouf JG, Aragon C, Henson BS, et al. Influence of parotid-sparing radiotherapy on xerostomia in head and neck cancer patients. Cancer Detect and Prev 2003;27:305.
27. Epstein JB. Benzydamine HCl in prevention of oropharyngeal mucositis in radiation therapy: literature review and clinical study. Res Clin Forums 1988;10:91.
28. Kim JH, Chu FCH, Lakshimi V, Houde R. Benzydamine

HCl, a new agent for the treatment of radiation mucositis of the oropharynx. Am J Clin Oncol 1986;9:132.
29. Prada A, Chiesa F. Effects of benzydamine on the oral mucositis during antineoplastic radiotherapy and/or intra-arterial chemotherapy. Inst J Tissue React 1987;9:115.
30. Prada A, Lozza L, Moglila D, et al. Effects of benzydamine on radio-polychemotherapeutic mucositis of the oral cavity. Int J Tissue React 1985;7:237.
31. Epstein JB, Silverman S, Passiarino DA, et al. Benzydamine HCL for prophylaxis of radiation-induced oral mucositis: results from a multicenter, randomized, double-blind, placebo-controlled clinical trial. Cancer 2001;92;875–85.
32. Rubenstein EB, Peterson DE, Schubert M, et al. Clinical practice guidelines for the prevention and treatment of cancer therapy-induced oral and gastrointestinal mucositis. Cancer 2004;100 (9 Suppl):2026.
33. Smith T. Gelclair: managing the symptoms of oral mucositis. Hosp Med 2001;62:623–6.
34. Adams S, Toth B, Dudley BS. Evaluation of sucralfate as a compound oral suspension for the treatment of stomatitis. Clin Pharmacol Ther 1985;2:178.
35. Ferraro JM. Sucralfate suspension for mouth ulcers. Drug Intell Clin Pharmacol 1985;13:16–22.
36. Meredith R, Salter M, Kim R, et al. Sucralfate for radiation mucositis: results of a double-blind randomized trial. Int J Radiat Oncol Biol Phys 1997;37:275.
37. Dodd MJ, Miaskowski C, Greenspan D, et al. Radiation-induced mucositis: a randomized clinical trial of micronized sucralfate versus salt and soda mouthwashes. Cancer Invest 2003;21:21.
38. Donnelly JP, Bellm LA, Epstein JB, et al. Antimicrobial therapy to prevent or treat oral mucositis. Lancet Infect Dis 2003;3:405.
39. Hospers GA, Eisenhaurer EA, de Vries EG. The sulfhydryl containing compounds WR-2721 and glutathione as radio- and chemoprotective agents. A review, indications for use and prospects. Br J Cancer 1999;80:629.
40. Abdelaal AS, Barker DS, Ferguson MM. Treatment of irradiation-induced mucositis [letter]. Lancet 1989;1:97.
41. Pillsbury HC, Webster WP, Roseman JG. Prostaglandin inhibitor and radiotherapy in advanced head and neck cancers. Arch Otolaryngol Head Neck Surg 1986;112:552.
42. Morse S, Adamietz LA, Saran T, et al. Can prophylactic application of immunoglobulin decrease radiotherapy-induced oral mucositis? Am J Clin Oncol 1997;20:407.
43. Chi KH, Chen CCH, Chan WK, et al. Effect of granulocyte-macrophage colony-stimulating factor on oral mucositis in head and neck cancer patients after cisplatin, fluorouracil and leucovorin chemotherapy. J Clin Oncol 1995;13:2620.
44. Greenspan D. Management of salivary dysfunction. J Natl Cancer Inst 1990;9:159.
45. Dreizen S, Daly TE, Drane JB, Brown LR. Oral complications of cancer radiotherapy. Postgrad Med 1977;61:81.
46. Eneroth CM, Henrikson CO, Jakobsen PA. Effects of fractionated radiotherapy on salivary gland function. Cancer 1972;30:1147.
47. Kaplan P. Mantle irradiation of the major salivary glands. J Prosthet Dent 1985;54:681.
48. Schubert MM, Fzuitsu KT. Iatrogenic causes of salivary gland dysfunction. J Dent Res 1982;66:680.
49. Dreizen S, Brown LR, Daley TE, Drane JB. Prevention of xerostomia related dental caries in irradiated cancer patients. J Dent Res 1977;56:99.
50. Brown LR, Dreizen S, Handler S, Johnston DA. Effect of radiation-induced xerostomia on human oral microflora. J Dent Res 1975;24:740.
51. Brown LR, Dreizen S, Rider LJ, Johnston DA. The effect of radiation-induced xerostomia on saliva and serum lysozyme and immunoglobulin levels. Oral Surg Oral Med Oral Pathol 1976;41:83.
52. Edgar WM, Bowen DH, Cole MF. Development of rampant dental caries and composition of plaque fluid and saliva in irradiated primates. J Oral Pathol 1981;10:284.
53. Liu RP, Fleming TJ, Toth BB, Keene HJ. Salivary flow rates in patients with head and neck cancer 0.5 to 25 years after radiotherapy. Oral Surg Oral Med Oral Pathol 1990:70:724–9.
54. Vissink A, Burlage FR, Spijkervet FKL, et al. Prevention and treatment of the consequences of head and neck radiotherapy. Crit Rev Oral Biol Med 2003;14:213.
55. Taylor SE. Efficacy and economic evaluation of pilocarpine in treating radiation-induced xerostomia. Expert Opin Pharmacother 2003; 4:1489.
56. Manthorpe R, Frost-Larsen K, Isager H, Prause IU. Sjögren's syndrome treated with bromhexine: a reassessment. Br Med J 1980;281:1216.
57. Ukai Y, Taniguchi N, Takeshita K, et al. Chronic anethole trithione treatment enhances the salivary secretion and increases the muscarinic acetylcholine receptors in the rat submaxillary gland. Arch Int Pharmacodyn Ther 1984;271:206.
58. Johnson JT, Ferretti GA, Nethery WJ, et al. Oral pilocarpine for post-irradiation xerostomia in patients with head and neck cancer. N Engl J Med 1993;271:206.
59. Wasserman T. Radioprotective effects of amifostine. Semin Oncol 1999;26(2 Suppl 7):89.
60. Capizzi RL, Oster W. Chemoprotective and radioprotective effects of amifostine: an update of clinical trials. Int J Hematol 2000;72:425–35.
61. Thorstad WL, Chao KS, Haughey B. Toxicity and compliance of subcutaneous amifostine in patients undergoing postoperative intensity-modulated radiation therapy for head and neck cancer. Semin Oncol 2004;31:8.
62. Levine MJ, Aguirre A, Hatton MN, Tabak LA. Artificial salivas: present and future. J Dent Res 1987;66:693.
63. Lockhart PB. Oral complications of radiation therapy. In: Peterson D, Elias J, Sonis S, editors. Head and neck management of the cancer patient. Boston: Martinus Nijhoff; 1986. p. 444.
64. Conger AD. Loss and recovery of taste acuity in patients irradiated to the oral cavity. Radiat Res 1973;53:338.
65. Reuther T, Schuster T, Mende U, et al. Osteoradionecrosis of the jaws as a side effect of radiotherapy of head and neck tumour patients–a report of a thirty year retrospective review. Int J Oral Maxillofac Surg 2003;32:289.
66. Balogh JM, Sutherland SE. Osteoradionecrosis of the mandible: a review. J Otolaryngol 1989;18:245.
67. Regaud C. Sur la sensibili du tissu osseux normal visss-avis radiations X, et sur le mechanissme de Leosteoradionecrose. CR Soc Biol (Paris) 1922;87:629.
68. Meyer I. Osteoradionecrosis of the jaw. Pract Dent Monogr 1958;4:12.
69. Marx RE. Osteoradionecrosis: a new concept in its pathophysiology. J Oral Maxillofac Surg 1983;411:283.
70. Aitasolo K. Bone tissue response to irradiation and treatment model of mandibular irradiation injury. Acta Octolaryngol 1986;428 Suppl l.
71. Epstein JB, Wong FL, Stevenson-Moore P. Osteoradionecrosis: clinical experience and a proposal for classification. J Oral Maxillofac Surg 1987;45:104.
72. Zarem HA, Carr R. Salvage of the exposed irradiated mandible. Plast Reconstr Surg 1983;72:648.
73. Epstein J, van der Meij E, McKenzie W, et al. Postradiation osteonecrosis of the mandible: a long-term follow-up study. Oral Surg Oral Med Oral Pathol Oral Radiol Endod 1997;83:657.
74. Murray CG, Daly TE, Zimmerman SO. The relationship between dental disease and radiation necrosis of the mandible. Oral Surg Oral Med Oral Pathol 1980;49:99.
75. Murray CG, Herson J, Dally TE, Zimmerman S. Radiation necrosis of the mandible: a 10-year study. Part 1. Factors influencing the onset of necrosis. Int J Radiat Oncol Biol Phys 1980;6:543.
76. Studer G, et al. Osteoradionecrosis of the mandible in patients treated with different fractionations. Strahlenther Onkol 2004;180:233.
77. Beumer J III, Harrison R, Saunders B, Kurrasch M. Postradiation dental extractions: a review of the literature and a report of 72 episodes. Head Neck Surg 1983;6:581.
78. Bachman G, Rossler R, Klett R, et al. The role of magnetic resonance imaging and scintigraphy in the diagnosis of pathologic changes in the mandible after radiation therapy. Int J Oral Maxillofac Surg 1996;25:189.
79. Rothwell BR. Prevention and treatment of orofacial complications of radiotherapy. J Am Dent Assoc 1987;114:316.
80. Scully C, Epstein JB. Oral healthcare for the cancer patient. Oral Oncol 1996;25:189.
81. Cronje FJ. A review of the Marx protocols: prevention and management of osteoradionecrosis by combining surgery and hyperbaric oxygen therapy. South Afr Dent J 1998;53:469–71.
82. Mansfield MJ, Sanders DW, Heimback RD, Marx RE. Hyperbaric oxygen as an adjunct in the treatment of osteoradionecrosis of the mandible. J Oral Surg 1981;39:585.
83. Shaha AR, Cordiero PG, Hidalgo DA, et al. Resection and immediate microvascular reconstruction in the management of osteoradionecrosis of the mandible. Head Neck 1997;19:406.
84. Curi MM, Dib LL, Kowalski LP. Management of refractory osteoradionecrosis of the jaws with surgery and adjunctive hyperbaric oxygen therapy. Int J Oral Maxillofac Surg 2000;29:430–4.
85. Annane D, Depondt J, Anbert P, et al. Hyperbaric oxygen therapy for radionecrosis of the jaw: a randomized, placebo-controlled, double-blind trial from the ORN96 study group. J Clin Oncol 2004; 22:4893.
86. Barasch A, Peterson DE. Risk factors for ulcerative oral mucositis in cancer patients: unanswered questions. Oral Oncol 2003; 39:91.
87. Sonis ST, Koplovsky A, Mitus J, et al. Relationship of chemotherapy-induced mucositis and bone marrow cellularity in hamsters. Eur J Cancer Oral Oncol 1992;28B:43.
88. Sonis AL, Sonis ST. Oral complications of cancer therapy in pediatric patients. J Pedodontics 1979;3:122.
89. Guggenheimer J, Verbin RS, Appel BN, Schmutz J. Clinicopathologic effects of cancer chemotherapeutic agents in human buccal mucosa. Oral Surg Oral Med Oral Pathol 1977;44:58.
90. Waterfield MD. Epidermal growth factor and related molecules. Lancet 1989;i:1243.
91. Tsalic M, Bar-Sela G, Beny A, et al. Severe toxicity related to 5-fluorouracil/leucovorin combination (the Mayo Clinic regimen): a prospective study in colorectal cancer patients. Am J Clin Oncol 2003;26:103.
92. Ulrich CM, Yasui Y, Storb R, et al. Pharmacogenetics of methotrexate: toxicity among marrow transplantation patients varies with the methylenetetrahydrofolate reductase C677T polymorphism. Blood 2001;98:231.
93. Morrison GB, Bastian A, Dela Rosa T, et al. Dihydropyrimidine dehydrogenase deficiency: a pharmacogenetic defect causing severe adverse reactions to 5-fluorouracil-based chemotherapy. Oncol Nurs Forum 1997;24:83.
94. Bergman OJ. Oral infections and septicemia in immunocompromised patients with hematologic malignancies. J Clin Microbiol 1988;26:2105.
95. Peters E, Monopoli M, Woo SB, et al. Assessment of the need for treatment of postendodontic asymptomatic periapical radiolucencies in bone marrow transplant recipients. Oral Surg Oral Med Oral Pathol 1993;76:45.
96. Banier AR. Nursing management of acute oral complications in cancer. Natl Cancer Inst Monogr 1990;9:123.
97. Cho SY, Cheng AC, Cheng MCK. Oral care for children with leukemia. Hong Kong Med J 2000; 6:203–8.
98. McCarthy GM, Awde JD, Ghandi H, et al. Risk factors associated with mucositis in cancer patients receiving 5-fluorouracil. Oral Oncol 1998;34:484.
99. Awidi A, Homsi U, Kokail PI, et al. Double-blind, placebo-controlled cross-over study of oral pilocarpine for the prevention of chemotherapy-induced oral mucositis in adult patients with cancer. Eur J Cancer 2001;37:2010–4.
100. Montgomery MT, Redding SW, LeMaitre CF. The incidence of oral herpes simplex virus infection in patients undergoing cancer chemotherapy. Oral Surg Oral Med Oral Pathol 1986;61:238.
101. Seto BG, Kim M, Wolilnsky L, et al. Oral mucositis in patients undergoing bone marrow transplantation. Oral Surg Oral Med Oral Pathol 1985;60:493.
102. Woo SB, Sonis ST, Sonis AL. Oral herpes simplex virus infection in bone marrow transplant recipient. Cancer 1990;66:2375.
103. Spielberger R, Stiff P, Bensinger W, et al. Palifermin for oral mucositis after intensive therapy for hematologic cancers. N Engl J Med 2004; 16:2590.
104. Alvarez E, Fey EG, Valax P, et al. Preclinical characterization of CG 53135 (FGF-20) in radiation and concomitant chemotherapy/radiation-induced oral mucositis. Clin Cancer Res 2003;9:3454.
105. Spencer A, Horvath N, Gibson J, et al. Prospective randomized trial of amifostine cytoprotection in myeloma patients undergoing high-dose melphalan conditioned autologous stem cell transplantation. Bone Marrow Transplant 2005;35:971.
106. Peterson DE, Petit RG. Phase III study: AES-14 in patients at risk for mucositis secondary to anthracycline-based chemotherapy. J Clin Oncol 2004; 22 ASCO Annual Meeting Proc 8008.
107. Dodd MJ, Dibble SL, Miaskowski C, et al. Randomized clinical trial of the effectiveness of 3 commonly used mouthrinses to treat chemotherapy-induced mucositis. Oral Surg, Oral Med, Oral Pathol, Oral Radiol, Endo 2000; 90:39.
108. Ruggiero SL, Methrotra B, Rosenberg TJ, et al. Osteonecrosis of the jaws associated with the use of bisphosphonates: a review of 63 cases. J Oral Maxillofac Surg 2004; 62:527.
109. EORTC. International Antimicrobial Therapy Project Group. Three antibiotic regimens in the treatment of infection in febrile granulocytopenic patients with cancer. J Infect Dis 1978;137:14.
110. Dreizen S, Brown LR. Oral microbial changes and infections during cancer chemotherapy. In: Peterson DE,

Sonis ST, editors. Oral complications of cancer chemotherapy. New York: Martinus Nijhoff; 1983. p. 41.
111. Pizzo PA. Infectious complications in the child with cancer. J Pediatr 1981;98:513.
112. Carpentieri U, Haggard ME, Lockhart LH, et al. Clinical experience in prevention of candidiasis by nystatin in children with acute lymphocytic leukemia. J Pediatr 1975;92:593.
113. Aviles A. Clotrimazole treatment for prevention of oral candidiasis in patients with acute leukemia undergoing chemotherapy. Am J Med 1987;82:867.
114. Lawson RD, Bodey GP. Comparison of clotrimazole troche and nystatin vaginal tablet in the treatment of oropharyngeal candidiasis. Curr Ther Res 1980;27:774.
115. Gombert MG, duBouchet L, Aulianio TM, Butt KM. A comparative trial of clotrimazole troches and oral nystatin suspension in recipients of renal transplants. JAMA 1987;258:2553.
116. Dewit S, Weerts D, Gossens H, Cluneck N. Comparison of fluconazole and ketoconazole for oropharyngeal candidiasis in AIDS. Lancet 1989;8:746.
117. Munier F, Asan M, Gerard M. Therapy for oropharyngeal candidiasis in the immunocompromised host—a randomized double blind study of fluconazole and ketoconazole. Rev Infect Dis 1990;12 Suppl 35:364.
118. Ball K, Sweeney MP, Baxter WE, et al. Fluconazole sensitivities of *Candida* species isolated from the mouths of terminally ill cancer patients. Am J Hospice Palliat Care 1998;15:325–9.
119. Barkvoll P, Attramandal A. Effect of nystatin and chlorhexidine digluconate on *Candida albicans.* Oral Surg Oral Med Oral Pathol 1989;67:279.
120. Epstein JB, Hancock PJ, Nantel S. Oral candidiasis in hematopoietic cell transplantation patients: an outcome-based analysis. Oral Surg Oral Med Oral Pathol Oral Radiol Endo 2003;96:153.
121. Walsh TJ. Role of surveillance cultures in prevention and treatment of fungal infections. Natl Cancer Inst Monogr 1990;9:43.
122. Saral R, Burns WH, Prentice HG. Herpes virus infections. Clinical manifestations and therapeutic strategies in immunocompromised patients. Clin Haematol 1984; 13:645.
123. Wade JC, Day LM, Crowley JJ, Meyers JD. Recurrent infection with herpes simplex virus after marrow transplantation: role of specific immune response and acyclovir treatment. J Infect Dis 1984;149:750.
124. Wade JC, Newton B, McLaren C, et al. Intravenous acyclovir I to treat mucocutaneous herpes simplex virus infection after marrow transplantation: a double-blind trial. Ann Intern Med 1982;97:265.
125. Saral R, Burns WH, Laskin OL, et al. Acyclovir prophylaxis of herpes simplex virus infections. N Engl J Med 1981;305:63.
126. Beighton D, Carr AD, Oppenheim BA, et al. Identification of viridans streptococci associated with bacteraemia in neutropenic cancer patients. J Med Microbiol 1994;40:202.
127. Bochud PY, Eggiman P, Calandra T, et al. Bacteremia due to viridans streptococcus in neutropenic patients with cancer: clinical spectrum and risk factors. Clin Infect Dis 1994;18:25.
128. Overholser CD, Peterson DE, Bergman SA, Williams LT. Dental extractions in patients with acute nonlymphocytic leukemia. J Oral Maxillofac Surg 1982;40:296.
129. Williford SK, Salisbury PL, Peacock JE Jr, et al. The safety of dental extractions in patients with hematologic malignancies. J Clin Oncol 1989;7:798.
130. Raut A, Huryn JM, Hwang FR, et al. Sequelae and complications related to dental extractions in patients with hematologic malignancies and the impact on medical outcome. Oral Surg Oral Pathol Oral Med Oral Radiol Endo 2001;92:49.
131. Reuscher TJ, Sodufi A, Scrivani SJ, et al. The impact of mucositis on alpha-hemolytic streptococcal infection in patients undergoing autologous bone marrow transplantation for hematologic malignancies. Cancer 1998;82:2275.
132. Zerbe MB, Parkerson SG, Ortlieb ML, et al. Relationship between oral mucositis and treatment variables in bone marrow transplant patients. Cancer Nurs 1992;15:196.
133. Dodd MJ, Larson PJ, Dibble SL, et al. Randomized clinical trial of chlorhexidine versus placebo for prevention of oral mucositis in patients receiving chemotherapy. Oncol Nurs Forum 1996;23:921.
134. Ahmed T, Engelking C, Szalyga J, et al. Propantheline prevention of mucositis from etoposide. Bone Marrow Transplant 1993:12:131.
135. Woo SB, Sonis ST, Monopoli MM, et al. A longitudinal study of oral ulcerative mucositis in bone marrow transplant recipients. Cancer 1993;72:1612.
136. Darville JM, Lsy BE, Roome AP, Foot AB. Acyclovir-resistant herpes simplex virus infections in a bone marrow transplant population. Bone Marrow Transplant 1998;22:587.
137. Schubert M, Sullivan KM, Morton TM, et al. Oral manifestations and chronic graft-vs-host disease. Arch Intern Med 1984;144:1591.
138. Woo SB, Lee SJ, Schubert MM. Graft-vs-host disease. Crit Rev Oral Biol Med 1997;8:201.
139. Barrett AP, Bilous AM. Oral patterns of acute and chronic graft-vs-host disease. Arch Dermatol 1984;120:1461.
140. Hiroki A, Nakamura S. Shinohara M, et al. Significance of oral examination in chronic graft-versus-host disease. J Oral Pathol Med 1994;23:209.
141. Redding SW, Callander NS, Havernan CW, Lennard DL. Treatment of oral chronic graft-vs-host disease with PUVA therapy: case report and literature review. Oral Surg Oral Med Oral Pathol Oral Radiol Endodontol 1998;86:183.

138

Gonadal Complications

Catherine E. Klein, MD

The dramatic improvement in cancer therapy over the past 50 years is nowhere more evident than in the unprecedented survival now enjoyed by survivors of pediatric sarcomas and leukemias, and young adults with high-grade lymphomas, Hodgkin disease, and testicular tumors. Increasing, numbers of premenopausal women with breast cancer are undergoing adjuvant chemotherapy, extending their survival sufficiently to justify concerns about their long-term reproductive health. Many of the new therapies allowing large numbers of long-term survivors to reach adulthood, have been associated with both temporary and permanent alterations in gonadal function, now recognized as among the most frequent significant side effects of modern cancer therapy. Women surviving cancer face symptoms of premature gonadal failure, including menopause, sterility, and presumably accelerated osteoporosis and possible early heart disease. Men experience subnormal fertility with oligo-azoospermia and subclinical Leydig cell dysfunction which may correlate with the long-term effects of "andropause" including decreased bone density and lean muscle mass as well as decreased libido and increase in coronary heart disease risk. Recognition of these complications has resulted in better documentation of their frequency and severity, more effective patient counseling, and innovative approaches to attenuate or prevent the toxicity. Such interventions include hormonal manipulation, selection of alternative treatments, and pretreatment cryopreservation of germ cells, but they must be offered pre-therapy, and unfortunately many patients still report that they were uninformed of this potentially devastating outcome or of possible alternatives to the loss of fertility. As our cancer therapies continue to improve and the number of young cancer survivors increases, it will be vital for the practicing oncologist to address these issues in a timely and sensitive manner.

THE HYPOTHALAMIC-PITUITARY GONADAL AXIS

Regulation of the reproductive axis begins at the level of the hypothalamus, where neurosecretory cells synthesize and release gonadotropin-releasing hormone (GnRH) in pulsatile fashion into the hypothalamic-hypophysial-portal circulation. In response, gonadotropes in the anterior pituitary synthesize and release the gonadotropins follicle-stimulating hormone (FSH) and luteinizing hormone (LH), both of which ultimately control gonadal function. In women, ovarian follicles are stimulated by FSH to grow and mature; LH stimulates ovulation and corpus luteum formation. In men, FSH initiates, and in conjunction with high intratesticular testosterone, sustains spermatogenesis, whereas LH controls androgen synthesis by the testicular Leydig cells. In both men and women, gonadal failure results in increased LH, because of loss of the negative feedback of estrogen at the hypothalamus and pituitary in women and from decreases in both androgen and estrogen feedback in men. In response to decreased levels of sex steroids as well as the loss of inhibin, FSH levels are also elevated following gonadal damage. Serum gonadotropin and sex steroid values will differentiate between reproductive failure at the gonadal level or at the hypothalamic/pituitary level. Sex steroid levels will be low in both, but serum gonadotropin levels will be high in primary gonadal failure and low in those with hypothalamic or pituitary disease. Thus, the hallmark of primary gonadal failure from any cause is elevation of gonadotropin levels, and this is the usual state in postpubertal patients receiving substantial doses of antineoplastic agents. Cranial radiation, on the other hand, may result in significant hypothalamic-pituitary dysfunction and secondary gonadal failure with low serum levels of gonadotropins.

HISTORICAL BACKGROUND

The effects of radiation and chemotherapy on gonadal function were recognized a century ago. Radiation sensitivity of the testes was reported in 1903, and a large literature on the topic accumulated over the next 50 years. Atomic Energy Commission studies of normal men, completed in the 1960s, confirmed the extraordinary sensitivity of spermatogonia to as little as 10 cGy of irradiation, a dose one-third that required in mice to produce equivalent damage.[1] Oocytes were more resistant but nevertheless displayed a reproducible, dose-dependent radiation sensitivity, which resulted in sterility and premature menopause at a frequency that increased with age. Data reported in 1939 demonstrated that a dose of 500 cGy delivered to human ovaries was associated with predictable amenorrhea that persisted for up to 18 months. All women over the age of 40 became permanently infertile.[2]

Initial reports documenting the detrimental effects of chemotherapy on human reproductive function were confirmed by a pathologic study of the testes obtained from 30 men who received nitrogen mustard in the 1940s. Twenty-seven of these men had significant testicular atrophy and absent spermatogenesis.[3] The first convincing report of menstrual irregularities or amenorrhea in women in association with cancer therapy appeared in 1956.[4] Four young women treated with busulfan for chronic myelocytic leukemia developed menopausal symptoms within 3 months of starting therapy. Ovarian and endometrial histologic findings were consistent with primary ovarian failure. Soon after their introduction into medical use, nitrogen mustard, chlorambucil, and cyclophosphamide were recognized to do the same if administered in sufficient dose, and the list of chemotherapeutic agents with potential for testicular or ovarian toxicity continues to grow (Table 138-1).

PRECLINICAL STUDIES

Although the effects of chemotherapy and radiation therapy on gonadal function have been well documented in humans, a number of preclinical models have permitted more detailed investigations into the mechanism of germ cell damage and possible methods to prevent it. Alkylating agents have been extensively studied in male rodents where they produce marked inhibition of DNA synthesis in differentiating spermatogonia, but spare the slowly dividing stem spermatogonia.[5] Similar findings have been reported in dogs and monkeys. The post-stem spermatogonial population displays a distinct species-specific and drug-specific variation in drug susceptibility. Few animal studies evaluating ovarian function have been published, as there are no well-accepted, reliable animal models for drug-induced female infertility. In female rats, alkylating agents appear to selectively target the medium and large follicles. Once the animal has become hypogonadal, the compensatory pituitary increases in gonadotropins may recruit the relatively resistant small follicles into the more sensitive pool, and if alkylating agent administration continues, thereby aggravate the damage.

In most animal systems, male infertility is reversible. In contrast to other alkylators, however, long-term administration of procarbazine to male rats results in permanent sterility. Although all alkylating agents are toxic to human gonads, the very high frequency of long-term infertility seen in survivors of Hodgkin disease treated with the mechlorethamine, vincristine (Oncovin), procarbazine, prednisone (MOPP) regimen suggests that procarbazine may be particularly toxic in humans as well (Table 138-2). Less is known about other classes of drugs; most have not been well studied in animals. In a cross-sectional study on the effects of doxorubicin, cytosine arabinoside, bleomycin, cyclophosphamide, hydroxyurea, vinblastine, and vincristine given as single

Table 138-1 Probability of Decreased Gonadal Function Associated with Commonly Used Anti-Neoplastic Agents

Frequency	Men	Women
Common	Cyclophosphamide	Cyclophosphamide
	Nitrogen Mustard	Nitrogen Mustard
	Procarbazine	Procarbazine
	Nitrosoureas	Nitrosoureas
		Busulfan
		Melphalan
		Thalidomide
Possible	Vinblastine	Vinblastine
	Etoposide	Etoposide
	Cisplatin	Cisplatin
	Carboplatin	Carboplatin
	Corticosteroids	Chlorambucil
	Ifosfamide	Hydroxyurea
	Interferon	Actinomycin D
	Cytosine Arabinoside	Tamoxifen
	Thioguanine	Thioguanine
		Interferon
		Cytosine Arabinoside
Rare	Vincristine	Methotrexate
	Doxorubicin	Doxorubicin
	Bleomycin	Bleomycin
	Methotrexate	Vincristine
	5-Fluorouracil	5-Fluorouracil
	Azathioprine	Dacarbazine
Inadequate information	Navelbine	Navelbine
	Taxanes	Taxanes
	Gemcitabine	Gemcitabine
	Interleukin	Imatinib
	Gefitinib	Ifosfamide
	Alemtuzumab	Imatinib
		Gefitinib
		Alemtuzumab

injections to male mice, doxorubicin appeared to be the most toxic to stem cells. Presumably because of their relative specificity for the cell cycle S phase, antimetabolites have not been associated with long-term gonadal damage.

EFFECTS OF CHEMOTHERAPY ON GONADAL FUNCTION

Effects in Boys In contrast to the profound gonadal damage in adult men who receive nitrogen mustard therapy, early reports of therapy in prepubertal and pubertal boys suggested relative resistance of the less mature testicle to chemotherapy-induced effects. The reported frequency of significant testicular dysfunction, however, varies widely among studies. The vast majority of boys progress normally through puberty without the need for supplemental androgen.[6,7] Testicular volume may be reduced, however, and elevated LH levels attest to some degree of Leydig cell dysfunction.[8] The prevalence of normal adult sperm counts in these patients (treated with single-agent cyclophosphamide), even years after therapy, has been reported in small case series of heterogeneous patient populations to range between 0 and 100%.[9,10] A review of cyclophosphamide administered orally in cumulative doses of 0.7 to 52 g revealed gonadal damage in 10 (16%) of 63 pre-pubertal boys, whereas 10 (67%) of 15 pubertal boys had evidence of gonadal dysfunction.[11] Boys are not, however, immune to the damage. Chlorambucil given alone or in combination with prednisone and azathioprine for the treatment of renal disease in patients aged 6 to 15 years produced azoospermia in 17 of 21 patients for up to 11 years after cessation of treatment.[12] MOPP chemotherapy given to boys with Hodgkin disease produces significant impairment in spermatogenesis at the time of puberty, a defect reported to last for years.[7,13] In addition, although levels of LH, FSH, and serum testosterone following chemotherapy in prepubertal boys may be normal, testicular biopsies after combination chemotherapy for acute lymphoblastic leukemia or Hodgkin disease commonly show seminiferous tubular damage and interstitial fibrosis.[14]

Two major factors determine the degree of damage to testicular function among prepubertal boys receiving cytotoxic chemotherapy. The first is the cumulative dose of the drug administered, a relation especially clear for the alkylating agents. A meta-analysis was conducted of 30 studies comprising 456 patients who received cyclophosphamide alone or as part of combination chemotherapy for renal disease, Hodgkin disease, or leukemia, and who had no confounding exposure to either abdominal or gonadal irradiation. The analysis found that in addition to pubertal stage, the cumulative dose of cyclophosphamide profoundly affected the incidence of gonadal dysfunction assessed after reaching sexual maturity. Although fewer than 10% of prepubertal boys who received less than 400 mg/kg (total dose) of cyclophosphamide had gonadal dysfunction, the incidence rose to 30% in the group receiving 400 to 500 mg/kg and in the group receiving over 500 mg/kg.[15] The incidence of gonadal dysfunction ranged from 0 to 24% in prepubertal boys, but climbed to 68 to 95% in sexually mature men. Although a confounding effect of nutritional status may play some role, the critical factors in defining the extent of long-term damage to testicular spermatogenic epithelium in prepubertal boys undergoing chemotherapy with alkylating agents seems to be the drug dose and probably to a lesser extent the maturational stage of the testicle.

Unfortunately, there are many poorly understood exceptions to these general trends, and reliable predictions for any given patient are impossible. It cannot be assumed that even minimal doses of chemotherapy given to prepubertal children will not result in permanent sterility; the corollary is that infertility can not be assured either, and men wanting to avoid conception need to bear this in mind.

Whether the function of Leydig cells is affected by chemotherapy in pubertal males is less clear. Gynecomastia associated with elevated FSH and LH levels was reported in 9 of 13 pubertal boys who received MOPP treatment.[16] However, among four prepubertal boys similarly treated, all had normal basal and stimulated gonadotropin tests.[7] In addition, only two of 44 boys who recovered after therapy for acute lymphoblastic leukemia had abnormal testosterone responses to human chorionic gonadotropin (hCG) challenge, and gonadotropin secretion was normal in 29 of the 32 patients studied.[6] A more recent report on 40 men treated in childhood for Hodgkin disease found that 26 of 28 who received chemotherapy had elevated gonadotropin levels but normal serum testosterone levels and normal secondary sexual characteristics. Eleven of 13 tested were azoospermic. The study documented changes that persisted up to 17 years after therapy.[17] Follow-up of 17 adult survivors of childhood sarcoma documented azoospermia in 58%, oligospermia in another 30% and normal testosterone in 94%. LH was elevated, however in 40% of those with normal testosterone levels, and in 92% of their total cohort, suggesting some degree of Leydig cell insufficiency.[8] These data indicate that the seminiferous tubules are damaged by alkylating agents, generally in an age- and dose-dependent manner, and that Leydig cell function may be subclinically affected in a large portion of men who appear to have normal testosterone levels after chemotherapy for childhood cancer.

Effects in Men Administered as single agents, alkylating drugs produce permanent damage to the seminiferous epithelium. Cyclophosphamide administered in total doses of 9 g results in universal azoospermia. In total doses up to 18 g, the azoospermia is generally reversible.[18] As in animals, procarbazine appears to be the single most toxic chemotherapeutic agent to the adult male gonad. Although no studies of this drug as a single agent are available, inferences can be drawn from multiple studies in Hodgkin disease in which patients received combination chemother-

Table 138-2 Gonadal Effects of Combination Chemotherapy

Disease	Regimen	*n*	Azoospermia/ Amenorrhea (%)	Reference
Males				
Hodgkin disease	MOPP (adults)	150	73–95	15, 16, 20, 28
	(pubertal)	18	78	15
	(boys)	27	14–80	15, 138
	ABVD	13	0	15
	ChlVPP	13	87	17
	MVPP	210	84–100	22, 23, 26, 32
	PACEBOM	12	0	67
	NOVP	21	5	133
	Stanford V	79	< 85	29
Non-Hodgkin lymphoma	COPP	7	66–100	122
	VAPEC-B	14	14	30
	MACOP-B	15	0	67
Testis cancer	PVB	112	15–28	34, 139
	PVB+Dox	36	17–39	35, 36
	PEB	42	12	134
Acute leukemia	Standard dose	48	3–75	33
	High dose	104	14–32	33, 74
Sarcomas	Dox/MTX (rt)	222	6–90	41, 42, 140
Females				
Ovarian cancer	P+others	66	0–8	68, 70, 141
Breast cancer	L-pam +FU	98	21–72	52, 142
	CMF	549	54–96	135
	Mitomycin	15	26	50
Hodgkin disease	MOPP (adult)	95	55–71	135, 142
	(pubertal)	15	7	15
	MVPP	72	36	7
	ABVD	24	0	27
	PACE BOM	15	0	64
	Stanford V	63	<60	29
Acute leukemia	Various	47	15	142
Non-Hodgkin lymphoma	Various	36	44	142
	High-dose	Case reports of pregnancies		127, 136, 137, 142

ABVD = Adriamycin (doxorubicin), bleomycin, vinblastine, dacarbazine; ChlVPP = chlorambucil, vinblastine, prednisone, procarbazine; CMF = cyclophosphamide, methotrexate, 5-fluorouracil; COPP = cyclophosphamide, vincristine, prednisone, procarbazine; 5-FU = 5 fluorouracil; MACOP-B = methotrexate, doxorubicin (Adriamycin), cyclophosphamide, vincristine (Oncovin), prednisone, bleomycin; MOPP = mechlorethamine, Oncovin (vincristine), prednisone, procarbazine; MVPP = mechlorethamine, vinblastine, prednisone, procarbazine; NOVP = mitoxantrone, vinblastine, vincristine, prednisone; PACE BOM = doxorubicin, cyclophosphamide, etoposide, bleomycin, vincristine, methotrexate, prednisolone; PEB = cisplatin (Platinol), etoposide, bleomycin; L-PAM = L-phenylalanine mustard; PVB = Platinol (cisplatin), vinblastine, bleomycin; PVB + dox = cisplatin, vinblastine, bleomycin, doxorubicin; VAPEC-B = vincristine, doxorubicin, prednisone, etoposide, cyclophosphamide, bleomycin.

apy either with or without procarbazine. In one study all of 19 patients treated with the cyclophosphamide, vincristine (Oncovin), procarbazine, and prednisone (COPP) regimen remained oligospermic 11 years after therapy, whereas 7 of 10 treated with COPP minus the procarbazine had return of spermatogenesis within 3 years.[19,20]

Methotrexate causes minimal long-term reproductive toxicity. Little information is available with which to assess the potential harm from either vincristine or vinblastine, but that the former may be somewhat less toxic than the latter is inferred from the slightly lower incidence of infertility following MOPP therapy than that using mechlorethamine, vinblastine, procarbazine, and prednisone (MVPP). Although studies of single-agent daunorubicin are also not available, it appears to have minimal long-term effect when used in combination therapy not containing cyclophosphamide. When used with cyclophosphamide, however, daunorubicin appears to potentiate gonadal toxicity. Long-term administration of azathioprine to men with inflammatory bowel disease does not seem to affect semen quality. Hepatitis C patients treated long-term with interferon have been reported to have normal gonadal hormone levels.

With the advent of curative combination chemotherapy, multiple reports have appeared indicating permanent infertility among survivors particularly of Hodgkin disease and the nonseminomatous testicular cancers. Complicating the interpretation of published studies is observation that even prior to therapy as many as 30% of young men presenting with Hodgkin disease and 50% with germ cell tumors are oligospermic,[21] and disorders of sperm motility and morphology are even more common.[22,23] Multivariate analysis in one study from Germany has found that elevated erythrocyte sedimentation rate and advanced stage are the best predictors of pre-therapy infertility among Hodgkin disease patients.[24] Pretreatment FSH levels may provide a useful prognostic serum marker for subsequent spermatogenesis in young men with germ cell cancer.[25] MOPP or MOPP-like regimens to treat Hodgkin disease render all men infertile during therapy, and the recovery rate remains very poor (see Table 138-2). In a prospective study of 37 men receiving the MVPP combination, 12 had low sperm counts before beginning treatment, but all of 14 studied after two cycles were azoospermic. All of 27 remained azoospermic in the first 12 months after treatment.[26] Follow-up of men off therapy for more than 2 years finds only 5 to 15% ever regain spermatogenesis.[11] Studies comparing MOPP chemotherapy to that using doxorubicin (Adriamycin), bleomycin, vinblastine, and dacarbazine (ABVD) in the treatment of Hodgkin disease provide convincing evidence that the latter combination produces less gonadal toxicity.[27,28] Because it is equally effective in the induction of durable remissions, ABVD should be the treatment of choice for men who are concerned about preserving reproductive potential. Although there are many fewer data for treatment of non-Hodgkin lymphomas, there is some evidence that the cyclophosphamide, vinblastine, prednisone regimen may be less toxic than MOPP.[20] An update on the Stanford V regimen (vinblastine, doxorubicin, vincristine, bleomycin, mustard, etoposide and prednisone) recently reported 19 conceptions in 13 male survivors.[29] A recent analysis of 14 men treated with vincristine, doxorubicin, prednisone, etoposide, cyclophosphamide, and bleomycin suggests this may be an effective, relatively non-toxic regimen for non-Hodgkin lymphoma.[30]

Survivors of leukemia fare somewhat better, provided that abdominal or testicular irradiation is avoided.[31] Kreuser and colleagues found 100% recovery during the second year of maintenance therapy among 10 patients aged 14 to 38 years treated with combination chemotherapy for acute leukemia.[32] From limited data available, both allogeneic and autologous bone marrow transplantation for leukemia significantly increase the risk for long-term infertility.[33]

Among young men with testicular tumors, there is even greater evidence of spermatogenic dysfunction before therapy than there is among Hodgkin disease patients. In a series of 41 patients studied prospectively, Drasga and colleagues reported that 77% were oligoazoospermic and 17% were azoospermic, leaving only 6% with adequate sperm counts to consider cryopreservation.[34] Abnormalities of sperm motility are at least as prevalent. Pretreatment testicular histology demonstrates spermatogenic arrest, hyalinized tubules, or totally absent tubules with only Sertoli cells evident.

The etiology of this phenomenon is unknown, but a relation to elevated hCG levels with a subsequent increase in estrogen production or to the increased local heat from the tumor have been hypothesized. Sperm autoimmunity may also impair fertility in these men. It has been suggested that the altered blood-testis barrier associated with an invasive cancer may lead to circulating sperm antigen and antibody formation. In widespread cancer, generalized wasting may also contribute to impaired spermatogenesis. Nevertheless, recovery of spermatogenesis following chemotherapy for testis cancer is not uncommon. Following 2 months of therapy with cisplatin, vinblastine, and bleomycin, with or without doxorubicin, 94% of men in Drasga's study were azoospermic. However, in contrast to the MOPP-treated Hodgkin disease patients, most studies show a time-dependent recovery of spermatogenesis, with nearly 50% of patients recovering some sperm production after 2 years (see Table 138-2).[35,36] In a follow up survey of 59 patients treated with two cycles of cisplatin-based adjuvant chemotherapy for stage I nonseminomatous testis cancer, there appeared to be no adverse effects on fertility or sexual activity.[36] Recovery seems to be, at least in part, related to the cumulative dose of cisplatin. In men who receive more than 400 mg/m^2, permanent infertility should be anticipated. Limited data suggest that ifosfamide in this setting may cause less irreversible infertility than its similarity to cyclophosphamide might predict.[37,38] Japanese studies with high-dose chemotherapy including carboplatin, etoposide, and ifosfamide found recovery of spermatogenies in half of their small series of 27 patients and could find no association with the cumulative dose of drug administered.[39] Both abdominal radiation therapy and retroperitoneal lymph node dissection decrease further the likelihood of fertility in survivors of testicular tumors.

As in boys, Leydig cell function is more resistant and is usually well compensated; despite frequently elevated gonadotropin levels, few if any of these men require androgen replacement therapy.[13,20] Occasionally men with various forms of cancer develop gynecomastia as a result of cancer therapy, presumably from an imbalance of testosterone and estrogen production. Subclinical Leydig cell dysfunction may have poorly recognized sequelae, which are just now being considered. One Dutch center evaluated the cardiovascular morbidity in long-term survivors of metastatic testicular cancer and found an incidence of coronary heart disease seven times higher than expected, a high incidence of hypercholesterolemia and obesity, in conjunction with lower testosterone and elevated LH and FSH. They hypothesize a metabolic consequence of long-term gonadal toxicity from prior chemotherapy in this group of long-term survivors.[40]

Less well studied are the male survivors of other tumor types. Shamberger and colleagues reported that 3 of 5 patients who received adjuvant doxorubicin-based therapy for sarcoma recovered normal sperm counts, although concomitant irradiation of the abdomen and pelvis or thigh, or even more distant sites, reduced the recovery rate substantially in 20 other patients studied.[41] A similar study by Meistrich and colleagues estimated that 28% of men recovered adequate sperm counts after doxorubicin-based adjuvant treatment for osteosarcoma.[42]

Interferon-α therapy in men treated for hairy cell leukemia was associated with no change in serum gonadotropin levels or sexual function in 11 patients followed for a median of 10 months.[43] Interleukin-2 (IL-2) may suppress the hypothalamic-pituitary-gonadal axis.

In summary, most of the available data for adult male gonadal toxicity comes from studies of testicular cancer or lymphoma patients. A substantial portion of patients with Hodgkin disease or testicular tumors is sub-fertile before any therapy is given. The older MOPP-like regimens for Hodgkin disease uniformly produce azoospermia. Fewer than 15% regain adequate spermatogenesis. Fortunately, several newer regimens appear less toxic and equally therapeutic. Many patients treated for testicular cancer recover fertility within 1 to 2 years of completing chemotherapy, although the odds of full recovery decrease as the dose of cisplatin increases above 400 mg/m^2 and if surgery or radiation therapy is part of the treatment strategy.

Effect in Prepubertal Girls The ovarian effects of chemotherapy in prepubertal girls are variable and depend on the drug, dose, and duration of therapy. Unfortunately, much of the information comes from studies on survivors of childhood leukemias and brain tumors for which cranial radiation is part of the therapy, making hypothalamic disorders more difficult to exclude. Single-agent cyclophosphamide, used to treat non-malignant disorders, only rarely causes either a delay in puberty or permanent sterility.[44] Most girls treated with procarbazine and nitrosoureas for brain tumors show biochemical evidence of primary ovarian dysfunction, but essentially all enter and progress normally through puberty. Ovarian function appears to return to normal over a period of years, and elevated gonadotropin levels decrease to baseline in most women. Little is reported about the gonadal toxicity suffered by girls treated for lymphomas, but 80% of those surviving combination therapy for acute lymphoblastic leukemia also proceed normally through puberty. One study has suggested that despite evidence for primary gonadal damage, menarche may actually appear prematurely.[45]

Histologically, however, prepubertal ovaries are significantly damaged by cancer chemotherapy. Follicular maturation arrest, stromal fibrosis, and a partially depleted ova population have all been reported following single-agent cyclophosphamide as well as cytosine arabinoside (ara-C)-based antileukemic therapy.

Lasting effects on uterine function appear rare: successful pregnancy with no increased risk for miscarriage is the rule.

Effects in Women Because the human ovary is relatively inaccessible to biopsy, the effects of antineoplastic agents on the female gonad have been inferred from the incidence of amenorrhea, changes in gonadotropin levels, and long-term fertility rates and outcomes as measures of ovarian function. The few autopsy or biopsy series reported in women treated with cyclophosphamide for non-neoplastic diseases or with multiagent therapy for cancer consistently describe complete absence of ova and follicles, with tunica albuginea thickening and stromal hyalinization. One autopsy series of patients treated for acute leukemia showed no difference in the number of primary follicles, but secondary follicles were markedly depleted.[46] Clinically, women receiving these agents develop signs and symptoms of primary ovarian failure: vaginal dryness with dyspareunia, endometrial hypoplasia, decreased libido, hot flashes, oligomenorrhea evolving into amenorrhea, and low serum estrogen levels with compensatory elevations of serum FSH and LH levels.[47,48]

The precise frequency of permanent amenorrhea and infertility depends on the drug given and its total dose, concomitant radiation exposure, and the age of the patient at the time therapy is administered. Among the single agents studied, alkylating agents are the most consistently associated with premature ovarian failure, mutagenesis, and teratogenesis. Although mechlorethamine (nitrogen mustard) may be the most toxic, cyclophosphamide is the agent best studied in this regard. Most series report that 50 to 75% of women treated with cyclophosphamide develop amenorrhea within a month of starting therapy.[49] There is, however, a striking age-related susceptibility. In one study, the total dose of cyclophosphamide received before the onset of amenorrhea was 5.2 g for patients over 40 years of age, 9.3 g for patients aged 30 to 39, and 20.4 g for patients aged 20 to 29. Menses returned in 50% of those under 40 years of age.[50] For women under the age of 40, return of menstrual function seems closely correlated with the dose of cyclophosphamide administered after the cessation of menses. This same study has suggested a race-specific variation in sensitivity.

L-Phenylalanine mustard as adjuvant chemotherapy for women with premenopausal breast cancer causes significant, age-related loss of ovarian function. The National Surgical Adjuvant Breast and Bowel Project reported that 73% of the women between the ages of 40 and 49, but only 22% of the women under the age of 39, developed amenorrhea during therapy; elevated LH and FSH levels appeared only in the older age group.[51] Single-agent treatment with busulfan or chlorambucil is associated with well-documented ovarian toxicity that is also age and dose-related.[52,53] Amenorrhea among women undergoing adjuvant combination chemotherapy for breast cancer has been well described, but the absence of a uniform definition for menopause has complicated interpretation of these data. Bines and colleagues have reviewed the literature and found the average rate of amenorrhea among women treated with standard cyclophosphamide, methotrexate and fluorouracil (CMF) is about 68% but that the reported incidence ranges from 20 to 100%.[54] Most reports suggest that few women under the age of 30 treated with Adriamycin-containing regimens experience amenorrhea, but that about one-third of 30- to 40-year-old women and nearly all those over age 40 experience amenorrhea. Epirubicin-containing regimens are probably similar. One recent report of adjuvant Taxotere with Adriamycin and cyclophosphamide resulted in a 61% rate of amenorrhea.[55]

Small series of patients treated with high-dose methotrexate as adjuvant therapy for sarcomas report that associated amenorrhea even during therapy is uncommon and that serum gonadotropin levels remain normal during and after therapy.[41]

Given in low doses to women with gestational trophoblastic tumors, methotrexate appears to exert no significant toxicity. One large survey from the United Kingdom found that menopause occurred on average 3 years earlier in women who had received chemotherapy than in those who did not.[56] Fluorouracil, daunorubicin, and bleomycin as single agents are probably also well tolerated. Few data are available for etoposide, but some ovarian dysfunction has been reported among women receiving the drug for gestational tumors.[57] Vincristine and vinblastine likewise appear to be infrequent, reversible causes of amenorrhea. Reliable data on the taxanes are lacking.

The nonsteroidal antiestrogen tamoxifen, although not as well characterized, appears to exert a mild estrogenic effect associated with decreased gonadotropin levels in both premenopausal and postmenopausal women treated for breast cancer. Menstrual irregularities are common among the former, but the incidence of persistent amenorrhea is unclear. Data concerning the use of aromatase inhibitors in premenopausal cancer patients are scarce. Among children with precocious puberty, these drugs suppress estrogen levels in a safe and reversible manner, decreasing menses and bone maturation. Successful pregnancies are well documented following anastrazole treatment of endometriosis. Therapeutic doses of interferon-α are associated with attenuated menstrual cycling in monkeys, but there are little data available to assess its risk for humans. Successful pregnancies have been reported among women on chronic interferon therapy for a variety of malignant and nonmalignant diseases.[58] Anecdotal reports have been published of successful pregnancy in women previously treated with imatinib.[59] Reliable information about the ovarian effects of most small molecule, protein kinase inhibitors is unavailable. Similarly, there is no available information on the reproductive toxicity associated with angiogenesis inhibitors, farnesyl transferase inhibitors, or arsenic trioxide.

Most information concerning chemotherapeutic effects on gonadal function relates to combination chemotherapy. Best studied are women who have undergone chemotherapy for Hodgkin disease. The incidence of amenorrhea in women treated with MOPP, MVPP, or COPP ranges from 15 to 80%, with a median of 50% (see Table 138-2).[19,25,60–63] Two-thirds of those women develop amenorrhea during therapy, and in the rest, menses cease gradually over the next several years. A clear dose-response relationship remains to be fully established. In at least one study, there appeared to be no difference between women receiving three cycles of MOPP and those receiving six.[64] Age at the time of treatment, however, has been shown to be an important variable affecting the incidence and time of onset of permanent amenorrhea. In general, 60 to 100% of patients over the age of 25 develop permanent amenorrhea during therapy. Ovarian failure occurs with the initiation of therapy in 5 to 30% of women under the age of 25, and an additional percentage will cease menstruation over the next several months. Even younger women should anticipate a greater than 50% likelihood of premature menopause within 5 to 10 years of therapy.[65] Preliminary reports suggest that such alternative Hodgkin disease regimens as ABVD or doxorubicin, cyclophosphamide, etoposide, bleomycin, vincristine, methotrexate, and prednisolone may have lower rates of prolonged amenorrhea.[26,66] Horning and colleages have reported 24 conceptions among 19 women treated with the Stanford V regimen.[29] Women receiving methotrexate, doxorubicin cyclophosphamide, vincristine, prednisone, and bleomycin for aggressive lymphomas appear, in small series, to maintain fertility.[67]

Other forms of combination chemotherapy for ovarian germ cell tumors and some sarcomas have provided additional information on post-chemotherapy reproductive potential. Women receiving cisplatin-containing therapy for germ cell tumors typically become amenorrheic during treatment, but over 90% restart menstruation within a few months after completing treatment.[68–71] Among women with breast cancer, who may have age-related decreased reproductive potential to begin with, 80% receiving cyclophosphamide, methotrexate, and 5-fluorouracil (CMF) become menopausal within 10 months of beginning therapy[72,73] Those given doxorubicin and cyclophosphamide usually become anovulatory within 3 months, or sooner if they are perimenopausal.

FERTILITY FOLLOWING HIGH-DOSE CHEMOTHERAPY

As more young patients are undergoing high-dose, myeloablative chemotherapy, case reports and small series have documented the recovery of fertility in a few patients. Follow-up of 187 young women previously treated with bone marrow transplantation for either aplastic anemia or leukemia found the anticipated age-dependent effect of cyclophosphamide on ovarian function.[74] Patients with aplastic anemia overall retained fertility better than the leukemia patients, and those under 26 years of age had the best prognosis. One recent report evaluated 30 women who had survived at least 18 months following bone marrow transplantation for acute leukemia. Of the 10 who had received one transplant, 4 developed ovarian failure, 6 resumed spontaneous menstrual cycling, and 5 of those 6 became pregnant. Of the three pregnancies allowed to go to term, all resulted in a normal infant.[75] One small series has documented the recovery of spermatogenesis in 4 of 25 men aged 21 to 41 following allogeneic transplantation.[76]

Total-body irradiation in addition to chemotherapy is also a major risk factor for infertility.[74] Conditioning regimens without radiation should be considered when fertility is an issue and alternatives are available.

EFFECTS OF RADIATION THERAPY ON GONADAL FUNCTION

Effects in Men Information concerning the gonadal sequelae of therapeutic irradiation in boys comes from the population of long-term survivors of childhood leukemia, in whom the high incidence of testicular relapse once led to the common practice of gonadal irradiation. After it was demonstrated that doses below 1,200 cGy were insufficient to control disease, most protocols delivered 2,400 cGy to both testes. At these doses, permanent Leydig cell damage occurred, puberty was delayed, testosterone levels were frequently diminished, and gonadotropin levels were increased in most patients.[64,77] These data are in contrast to those showing effective control of testicular leukemia by high-dose methotrexate and normal progression through puberty, suggesting relatively normal Leydig cell function in boys receiving chemotherapy in childhood.[78]

In adults, single 400 to 600 cGy doses of testicular radiation may produce azoospermia 5 years or longer.[1] Scatter from fractionated radiation to the pelvis or lower extremities may result in substantial testicular doses as well. Berthelsen evaluated men undergoing prophylactic radiotherapy for seminoma and found that two-thirds became azoospermic from the scatter dose estimated to be between 20 and 130 cGy.[79] Shapiro and colleagues have documented oligospermia/azoospermia lasting up to 24 months after as little as 27 cGy.[80] Recovery occurs in the majority: series report 37 to 66% success rates in men wishing to conceive a pregnancy.[81] Adult Leydig cell dysfunction, with elevated LH values occurs at radiation doses greater than 2,000 to 3,000 cGy. Fractionated radiation appears to produce tubular damage similar to that seen with single doses. In adults, as in children, Leydig cell dysfunction after 2,400 to 3,000 cGy can be significant enough to require hormonal replacement. Total body irradiation for bone marrow transplantation conditioning is routinely associated with permanent azoospermia. Secondary infertility has been reported in association with radiation administered to the hypothalamus or pituitary in conjunction with chemotherapy for intracranial neoplasms.[82]

Whether there are permanent effects on the surviving germ cells of male patients receiving radiation therapy remains controversial. Animal models suggest an increased risk for common tumors following parental exposure to radiation and chemicals. Most studies have been unable to document equivalent findings in humans.[83]

Effects in Women The radiation sensitivity of the human ovary has not been defined as precisely as that of the male testis. Radiosensitivity is related to the oogonial developmental stage at the time of exposure. Small primordial oocytes are considerably more sensitive than large follicles. As in men, ovarian sensitivity to radiation is also dose-dependent and age-dependent. In children, the younger the age at exposure, the more primordial follicles present, and hence the longer time to loss of fertility. In adult women, single doses of 500 cGy produce menstrual irregularities in women of all ages. For women over the age of 40,600 cGy reliably induces menopause. Women aged 20 to 30 years can tolerate up to 3,000 cGy if the dose is fractionated over 6 weeks.[84]

Uterine radiation in childhood increases risk for nulliparity, spontaneous abortions, and intrauterine growth retardation, so fertility is not assured even if ovarian function is preserved.

PROTECTIVE MEASURES

Protection for Men Current information suggests that the toxic effects of chemotherapy are most pronounced for adult men, in whom spermatogenesis reflects a more brisk mitotic rate relative to the prepubertal testis or the adult female ovary, where the rate of germ cell mitosis is less. Such a differential susceptibility is consistent with the observation that the majority of chemotherapeutic agents affect the most rapidly dividing cells. This observation has led to speculation that halting spermatogenesis through hormonal manipulation might ameliorate testicular damage.

A number of animal studies have tested this hypothesis. Both GnRH analogues and sex steroids have been administered, and although the rate of spermatogenesis can be decreased, a protective effect has not been unequivocally documented. Although some degree of success has been reported in procarbazine rat, dog, and primate models, other studies have failed to demonstrate protection and have occasionally shown increased damage from such manipulation.[85–87] In clinical trials of men receiving chemotherapy for Hodgkin disease, two attempts using GnRH analogues have been unsuccessful.[88,89] Preserving fertility by hormonal manipulation has not been demonstrated. For men who desire fertility following combination chemotherapy for advanced Hodgkin disease, the ABVD regimen is clearly preferable to MOPP.[25]

For men anticipating cancer therapy, an alternative to in vivo protection is semen cryopreservation. Studies have shown that the process of sperm cryopreservation is no more detrimental to sperm quality in cancer patients that it is in noncancer controls.[90] In general, these men should bank semen every 3 days, or as often as possible, before anticancer therapy is initiated. Because of the high prevalence of abnormal pretherapy semen analyses, many patients have been considered inappropriate for this endeavor, but successful impregnation has been achieved following artificial insemination using semen with quite low sperm counts and poor sperm motility.[91] This requires careful, endocrinologically monitored timing with the woman's ovulation, and impeccable technique in freezing, storing, and thawing; if those conditions are met, fertilization may be effective in up to 45% of cases. Additionally, in vitro fertilization and subsequent implantation has been successful in cases of even lower sperm counts and motility.[92] With the advent of intracytoplasmic sperm injection the chance of conception can be greatly enhanced despite exceedingly low sperm counts. Most studies document a rate of azoospermia in cancer patients pretreatment on the order of 10%. Fertilization has been reported using spermatozoa retrieved by testicular biopsy and with sperm extracted from the vas deferens at the time of orchiectomy in several azoospermic testis cancer survivors.[93] Many centers nonetheless, report that the overall success rate among men who elect to preserve semen may be somewhat limited, and perhaps is influenced by factors other than semen quality. One series from Memorial Sloan-Kettering Cancer Center reported locating 48 of 69 men who had banked sperm, but at a median of 27 months post-treatment only 11 had attempted to use their sperm for artificial insemination. Of these, only three achieved successful pregnancies.[91,94] Other centers have documented even lower rates of cryopreserved sperm use.

Penile vibratory stimulation and electroejaculation may provide an option for pubertal boys.[95] Very preliminary studies of testicular circulatory isolation suggest that this mechanical procedure is protective in a rat model and might be feasible in human clinical trials .[96] None have been reported.

Testis sperm extraction is reported to recover spermatozoa in 55 to 85% of men with nonobstructive azoospermia of various etiologies. Damani and colleagues have reported a series of azoospermic men with a history of chemotherapy. Spermatozoa were found in 15 of 23 (65%). A total of 26 intracytoplasmic sperm injection cycles were performed in 12 couples. Fertilization rate was 65%. All babies born to date have had normal neonatal examinations.[97]

Testicular tissue biopsy and cryopreservation is experimental, as is isolation of germ cells from testicular tissue for storage.

Gonadal shielding remains the mainstay of protection from therapeutic radiation. No convincing studies to suggest benefit from scrotal cooling are currently available.

Table 138-3 Options for Preservation of Fertility in Patients with Cancer

	Males	Status	Females	Status
Children	Testicular tissue cryopreservation	Unproven	Ovarian tissue cryopreservation	Unproven
Adults	GnRH analogue	Unproven	GnRH analog suppression	?Effective
			OCP suppression	Unproven
	Sperm cryopreservation	Accepted	Oocyte cryopreservation	Experimental
	Testicular sperm extraction	Experimental	Ovarian tissue cryopreservation	Available
			Embryo cryopreservation	Available
			Ovarian tissue transposition	Experimental

GnRH analogue = gonadotropin-releasing hormone analogue; OCP = oral contraceptives.

Protection for Women Analogous to the hypothesis for men, it has also been proposed that suppression of ovarian function by oral contraceptives or GnRH analogue might offer gonadal protection to cycling women about to undergo potentially sterilizing radiation or chemotherapy. Some animal models have validated the hypothesis, both in protection from radiation and in chemotherapy-induced ovarian damage.[98] Results of such trials in humans have been conflicting, however, and the number of patients studied remains small. Most promising of these reports is that of Chapman and Sutcliffe, who administered oral contraceptives to women anticipating receiving MVPP therapy for Hodgkin disease. Five of 6 women had resumption of normal menses at a mean follow-up of 26 months.[99] One small study of patients with Hodgkin disease given the GnRH analogue buserelin for 1 week prior to initiation of MVPP failed to show any difference in amenorrhea or menopausal symptoms when compared to controls.[89] Pacheco and colleagues have administered leuprolide acetate to 12 patients aged 15 to 20 anticipating treatment for lymphoma.[100] Pretreatment suppression was instituted with both subcutaneous daily injections and the depot injection to overcome the delay in suppression of ovarian function. Suppression was continued monthly with depot administration until one month after cessation of chemotherapy. All twelve treated patients resumed normal menstrual cycling within 6 months, compared to none of the 4 women in this study who did not receive leuprolide suppression. Three pregnancies were reported. Although the short pretreatment interval may compromise the effect of ovarian suppression in some reported series, urgent cancer therapy often precludes a more lengthy delay. Protective benefit with administration of progesterone remains controversial.

The introduction of in vitro fertilization led to early optimism for the potential of ovarian tissue cryopreservation to preserve fertility, but oocyte cryopreservation has had very limited success and only an occasional successful pregnancy has been reported (Table 138-3). Although recent improvements in technology have increased oocyte survival rates and subsequent fertilization rates, at this time it is probably not a feasible option for women anticipating sterilizing therapy. Human ovarian cortical slices containing primordial ova have been obtained laparoscopically and cryopreserved successfully. Recent reports indicate that such tissue can be autografted subsequently and returned to patients, thus restoring fertility. Follicles can be retrieved from the orthotopic site.[101] No pregnancies in humans have been reported.

In women with stable relationships, embryo cryopreservation has been successful and has been offered to cancer patients. In general, superovulation is required before fertilization, and neither the time required nor the hormone manipulation necessary may be acceptable. In vitro fertilization without stimulation is a possible but less effective option. One case report of a woman with breast cancer who underwent successful in vitro fertilization and embryo cryopreservation after a natural cycle suggests that this might become a potential fertility-preserving tool. However, a number of ethical concerns remain to be addressed before this technique will gain widespread acceptance, including the appropriate disposal of unused "orphan" embryos, the potential for transmission of cancer, the use of donor sperm and various religious issues.[102] Oocyte donations have been used on occasion with subsequent in vitro fertilization and successful pregnancy. Sauer and colleagues have described a young woman, amenorrheic following therapy for Hodgkin disease, who was impregnated with a donor ovum recovered after insemination and uterine lavage.[103] Both oocyte and embryo cryopreservation require a significant delay in initiating cancer treatment while ovarian stimulation is undertaken, and in many situations this may be ethically unsound. Ovarian tissue preservation may prove an option that avoids this delay. Ovarian cortical tissue also has the advantage of containing large numbers of follicles and thereby increasing the potential for successful future pregnancies. The ovarian tissue can ultimately be transplanted back in to the patient thus restoring ongoing fertility. Transplanted tissue has been reported to restore normal menstrual cycling, but as of yet, no successful pregnancies have been reported.[104] This technique may ultimately offer an option for young girls as well as sexually mature young women. Risk of reseeding metastatic cancer needs to be defined carefully. Obviously, the ethical issues regarding the necessary clinical trials add further controversy to the technique.[105]

For patients undergoing pelvic radiation therapy, oophoropexy can be undertaken. Generally, this is done at the time of exploratory or staging laparotomy to move the ovaries either medially behind the uterine fundus or laterally out of the radiation port. Radiation exposure is decreased 90%, and hormonal function is preserved in 55 to 95% of patients; however, fertility is still compromised, possibly owing to the abnormal tuboovarian anatomy or radiation scatter. In a study of 22 patients with Hodgkin disease who had undergone oophoropexy, 1 of 2 receiving para-aortic and 1 of 12 receiving inverted-Y radiation therapy subsequently became pregnant.[106] In a study of 134 women who had undergone ovarian transposition, 126 of whom received radiation therapy, a total ovarian dose of 5 cGy was statistically associated with ovarian failure.[107] A small trial of laparoscopic propriosacral ovariopexy offers the possibility of a less invasive approach to fertility preservation.[108] Oktay and colleagues have recently reported the successful transplantation of ovarian tissue removed at the time of ovariectomy in a woman with cervical cancer. Frozen sections revealed no evident metastatic cancer, and fresh tissue was transplanted into her antecubital fossa before the initiation of her pelvic radiation. Follow-up determined that the tissue was cycling normally, oocytes were retrieved, but in vitro fertilization was not successful.[109] Specific ovarian shielding may be useful in some cases.

Protection for Children No proven methods for protection of future fertility in children are available at this time. Some centers offer ovarian tissue or testicular tissue cryopreservation as an experimental approach, but research in this area is fraught with ethical problems.

Many excellent reviews of the technical and ethical issues of fertility preservation are available.[105,110]

OUTCOMES OF PREGNANCY

Chemotherapy Case reports document successful conception and delivery of normal infants to patients who have received even the most aggressive of chemotherapy regimens; neither male nor female permanent infertility can be presumed following chemotherapy for cancer. This point must be reiterated in counseling both those patients who wish and those who do not wish to have children. For the latter, appropriate contraception should be encouraged. For those who do wish to have children, a common concern is for the potential adverse fetal outcomes. Several retrospective series have evaluated the outcome of pregnancy in women treated with chemotherapeutic agents as children or young adults who completed therapy and then became pregnant. Fewer data are available for women who conceived during active cancer treatment.

One large study evaluating offspring of children treated for a variety of cancers found that in a total of 286 subsequent pregnancies there was no increase in congenital anomalies, and chromosomal analysis was normal in 23 of 24 children tested.[111] Pregnancies in women previously treated for trophoblastic tumors also appear to have no associated increased risk of congenital anomalies, spontaneous abortions, or neonatal mortality.[112] Holmes and Holmes evaluated women treated for Hodgkin disease and compared the 93 pregnancies in their chemotherapy-treated patients to 288 sibling-control pregnancies. Overall there was no difference between the groups, although when the subgroup that received both radiation therapy and chemotherapy was analyzed separately, it appeared that combined treatment produced more spontaneous abortions in wives of male patients, and that female patients were slightly more likely to produce abnormal offspring than control women.[113] Offspring of fathers treated with prior chemotherapy likewise appear to be normal. When large series are combined, nearly 1,400 live-born children have been reported to have a congenital defect incidence of about 4%, not significantly different from the general population. Most of these anomalies represent common, nongenetic abnormalities.[114]

Further follow-up suggests that offspring growth, development, and school performance are probably normal. A National Cancer Institute study to address the question of cancer in offspring of treated patients found a slight and statistically insignificant excess of cancers in these children when compared to offspring of sibling-matched controls (0.3 vs 0.23%), numbers not different from those expected in the general population. When analyzed by age and sex, however, it appeared that there was an excess of cancers diagnosed in male offspring under age 5. Five cancers were detected in this group, compared to the 1.7 expected.[115] Some of these cancers may have represented familial clustering of known hereditary cancers, such as retinoblastoma or Wilms tumor.

Risk to the fetus exposed in utero to chemotherapy agents depends on gestational age and the drug and dose administered. Aminopterin, a known folate antagonist has been consistently associated with teratogenic effects, as would be predicted from the critical importance of folate in neurologic development. It may be concentrated in the amniotic fluid and is associated with up to a 100% incidence of fetal malformations, often in the central nervous system, when exposure occurs during the first trimester. Folate antagonists should not be administered during the first trimester. Other antimetabolites have rarely been associated with congenital abnormalities. First trimester exposure to 5-fluorouracil, cyclophosphamide, busulfan, and chlorambucil has been associated with low birth weight in infants and other abnormalities on rare occasion.[116] Fetal myocardial necrosis has been reported following maternal administration of anthracyclines.[117] Imatinib has demonstrated teratogenicity in animal models, but case reports have documented successful pregnancies in women who conceive during treatment.[118] Rituxan given unintentionally to a pregnant woman resulted in an uncomplicated pregnancy delivering an apparently healthy infant. Interferon-α has been given safely during pregnancy in a small number of women.[119]

Whether the risk to the fetus is further increased with drug combinations is uncertain. Case reports and small series indicate that exposure in the second and third trimesters is associated with minimal risk to the fetus and that long-term development of these offspring is normal.[120,121] One study of 16 children exposed to maternal antileukemic therapy could detect no difference in peripheral blood, bone marrow, cytogenetics, physical examination, neurologic assessment, school performance, or intelligence test results when compared to sibling controls.[122] Nonteratogenic effects including low birth weight, intrauterine growth retardation, and more subtle developmental abnormalities remain to be defined. In utero exposure to diethylstilbestrol has been linked to the development of genital clear cell carcinomas in the female offspring of these women, but other clear documentation of carcinogenesis from in utero exposure to chemotherapy is lacking. No information is available on the reproductive potential of these children.

Radiation Therapy Most of what is known about the genetic effects of radiation therapy is inferred from data on survivors of atomic bomb exposure. Although extensive data have been accumulated in their offspring, interpretation of the data is clouded by a variety of factors, particularly the calculation of the actual gonadal dose. Nevertheless, it is apparent that the increase in untoward pregnancy outcomes (major congenital defects, stillbirth, and death during the first week of life) is small, estimated at 0.00182/gonadal rem (roentgen-equivalent–man)—the quantity of any ionizing radiation equivalent to the biologic effect of 1 rad (cGy). Small head size has been reported in these offspring,[123] but has not been a consistent finding among offspring of women irradiated therapeutically during gestation.

Among women treated with radiation therapy below the diaphragm, preterm delivery in up to 20% of pregnancies and an excess of low-birth weight infants have been reported. That these adverse outcomes are often clustered in the first post-treatment year suggests they may result from local uterine or hormonal factors and may not be because of genetic defects.[123,124] One large study of Wilms tumor survivors found an increase in perinatal death and low-birth-weight infants, findings that contributed to an overall 30% adverse outcome in these patients. These abnormalities were limited to women who had received pelvic radiation therapy, and were not seen among those who had been treated with chemotherapy alone.

In utero exposure to irradiation produces the greatest risk of teratogenesis during the period of organogenesis from the second to the eighth week, with growth retardation, eye problems, and microcephaly appearing as the predominant abnormalities. A safe dose has not yet been defined, but generally, a therapeutic abortion is recommended for any uterine dose of 10 cGy during the first trimester. Supradiaphragmatic irradiation is associated with considerable scatter to the fetus, much of which can probably be prevented with abdominal shielding. Local irradiation of the neck and axilla may be safe during the first trimester.[116] Data on future fertility and the risks of malignancy in the offspring are unavailable.

PSYCHOSOCIAL ISSUES

The psychosocial issues of disfigurement, loss of fertility, anxiety about birth defects, sexual performance, and recurrence of tumor all have important impacts on the single patient facing dating and mate-selection issues, as well as on married patients in a stable relationship, for whom the separation rate may be four-fold of that of the general population.[125–127] Sildenafil for the treatment of erectile dysfunction appears to be useful for the treatment of men following radiation therapy for prostate cancer. Studies have shown that 70 to 80% of men treated with either external beam or brachytherapy respond favorably.[128,129] Loss of libido is particularly common in women; when associated with vaginal dryness and dyspareunia, vaginal lubricants, and estrogen creams may be helpful. Although many sexual side effects can be ameliorated (estrogen replacement, reconstructive surgery), many cannot be.[130,131] Effective counseling is critical in alleviating major morbidity in these patients and in allowing patients to feel open and hopeful regarding their problems. Early follow-up should include assessment of the hypothalamic-pituitary-gonadal axis (especially in total-body irradiated patients), thyroid function tests, and a check of serum gonadotropin levels to document spontaneous return of fertility. Excellent reviews are available for the interested reader seeking further information.[125,131,132]

For physician assessment of sexual functioning, Andersen[125] has proposed a model that helps the provider address many issues before they arise. It is only through specific inquiry and careful documentation of current and prior sexual functioning, including frequency of activity, libido, arousal, orgasm, and sensation of resolution, that the health professional can determine cancer therapy-related dysfunction. As in other areas of cancer medicine, such a role is highly demanding, but it often provides the patient much comfort and the caregiver great satisfaction, considering the challenges raised by the gonadal effects of cancer therapy.

REFERENCES

1. Clifton DK, Bremner WJ. The effect of testicular x-irradiation on spermatogenesis in man: a comparison with the mouse. J Androl 1983;4:387–92.
2. Jacox HW. Recovery following human ovum irradiation. Radiology 1939;32:538–45.
3. Gilman A. The initial clinical trial of nitrogen mustard. Am J Surg 1963;105:574.
4. Louis J, Limarzi LR, Best WR. Treatment of chronic granulocytic leukemia with myleran. Arch Intern Med 1956;97:299–307.
5. Gould SF, Powell D, Nett T, Glode LM. A rat model for chemotherapy-induced male infertility. Arch Androl 1983;11:141–50.
6. Shalet SM, Hann IM, Lendon M, et al. Testicular function after combination chemotherapy in childhood for acute lymphoblastic leukaemia. Arch Dis Child 1981;56:275–8.
7. Whitehead E, Shalet SM, Jones PH, et al. Gonadal function after combination chemotherapy for Hodgkin's disease in childhood. Arch Dis Child 1982;47:287–91.
8. Kenney LB, Laufer RR, Grant MR, Grier H, Diller L. High risk of infertility and long-term gonadal damage in males treated with high dose cyclophosphamide for sarcoma during childhood. Cancer 2001;91:613–21.
9. Watson AR, Rance CP, Bain J. Long-term effects of cyclophosphamide on testicular function. Br Med J 1985;291:1457–60.
10. Hsu AC, Folami AO, Bain J, Rance CP. Gonadal dysfunction in males treated with cyclophosphamide for nephrotic syndrome. Fertil Steril 1979;31:173–7.
11. Chapman RM. Gonadal injury resulting from chemotherapy. Am J Ind Med 1983;4:149–61.
12. Guesry P, Lenoir G, Broyer M. Gonadal effects of chlorambucil given to prepubertal and pubertal boys for nephrotic syndrome. J Pediatr 1978;92:299–303.
13. Aubier F, Flamant F, Caillaud JM, et al. Male gonadal function after chemotherapy for solid tumors in childhood. J Clin Oncol 1989;7:304–9.
14. Uderzo C, Locasciulli A, Mazorati R. Correlation of gonadal function with histology of testicular biopsies at treatment discontinuation in childhood acute leukemia. Med Pediatr Oncol 1984;12:97–100.
15. Rivkees SA, Crawford JD. The relationship of gonadal activity and chemotherapy-induced gonadal damage. JAMA 1988;259:2123–5.
16. Sherins RJ, Olweny CLM, Ziegler JL. Gynecomastia and gonadal dysfunction in adolescent boys treated with combination chemotherapy for Hodgkin's disease. N Engl J Med 1978;299:12–6.
17. Shafford EA, Kingston JE, Malpas JS, et al. Testicular function following the treatment of Hodgkin's disease in childhood. Br J Cancer 1993;68:1199–204.
18. Buchanan JD, Fairley KF, Barrie JU. Return of spermatogenesis after stopping cyclophosphamide therapy. Lancet 1975;2:156–7.
19. Kreuser ED, Ziros N, Hetzel WD, Heimple H. Reproductive and endocrine gonadal capacity in patients treated with COPP chemotherapy for Hodgkin's disease. J Cancer Res Clin Oncol 1987;113:260–6.
20. Roeser HP, Stocks AE, Smith AJ. Testicular damage due to cytotoxic drugs and recovery after cessation of therapy. Aust N Z J Med 1978;8:250–4.
21. Meirow D, Schenker JG. Cancer and male infertility. Hum Reprod 1995;10:2017–22.
22. Chapman RM, Sutcliffe SB, Malpas JS. Male gonadal dysfunction in Hodgkin's disease: a prospective study. JAMA 1981;245:1323–8.
23. Chapman RM, Sutcliffe SB, Reis LH, et al. Cyclical combination chemotherapy and gonadal function: retrospective study in males. Lancet 1979;1:285–9.
24. Rueffer U, Breuer K, Josting A, et al. Male gonadal dysfunction in patients with Hodgkin's disease prior to treatment. Ann Oncol 2001;12:1307–11.
25. Brennemann W, Stoffel-Wagner B, Wichers M, et al. Pretreatment follicle-stimulating hormone: a prognostic serum marker of spermatogenesis status in patients treated for germ cell cancer. J Urol 1998;159:1942–6.
26. Whitehead E, Shalet SM, Blackledge G, et al. The effects of Hodgkin's disease and combination chemotherapy on gonadal function in the adult male. Cancer 1982; 49:418–22.
27. Santoro A, Bonadonna G, Valagussa P, et al. Long-term results of combined chemotherapy-radiotherapy approach in Hodgkin's disease: superiority of ABVD plus radiotherapy versus MOPP plus radiotherapy. J Clin Oncol 1987;5:27–37.
28. Viviani S, Santoro A, Ragni G, et al. Gonadal toxicity after combination chemotherapy for Hodgkin's disease: comparative results of MOPP vs ABVD. Eur J Cancer Clin Oncol 1985;21:601–5.
29. Horning SJ, Hoppe RT, Breslin S, et al. Stanford V and radiotherapy for locally extensive and advanced Hodgkin's disease: mature results of a prospective clinical trial. J Clin Oncol 2002;20:630–7.
30. Radford JA, Clark S, Crowther D, Shalet SM. Male fertility after VAPEC-B chemotherapy for Hodgkin's disease and non-Hodgkin's lymphoma. Br J Cancer 1994;69:379–81.
31. Evenson DP, Arlin Z, Welt S. Male reproductive capacity may recover following drug treatment with the L-10 protocol for acute lymphocytic leukemia. Cancer 1984;53:30–6.
32. Kreuser ED, Hetzel WD, Wolfgang H, et al. Reproductive and endocrine gonadal functions in adults following multidrug chemotherapy for acute lymphoblastic or undifferentiated leukemia. J Clin Oncol 1988;6:588–95.
33. Zittoun R, Suciu S, Watson M, et al. Quality of life in patients with acute myelogenous leukemia in prolonged first complete remission after bone marrow transplantation (allogeneic or autologous) or chemotherapy: a cross sectional study of the EORTC-GIMEMA AML 8A trial. Bone Marrow Transplant 1997;20:307–15.
34. Drasga RE, Einhorn LH, Williams SD, et al. Fertility after chemotherapy for testicular cancer. J Clin Oncol 1983;1:179–83.
35. Kreuser ED, Harsch U, Hetzel WD, Schreml W. Chronic gonadal toxicity in patients with testicular cancer after chemotherapy. Eur J Cancer Clin Oncol 1986;22:289–94.
36. Hansen PV, Trykker H, Helkjaer PE, Andersen J. Testicular function in patients with testicular cancer treated with orchiectomy alone or orchiectomy plus cisplatin-based chemotherapy. J Natl Cancer Inst 1989;81:1246–50.
37. Dominik B, Burkhard FC, Mills R, et al. Fertility and sexual function following orchiectomy and 2 cycles of chemotherapy for stage I high risk nonseminomatous germ cell cancer. J Urol 2001;165:441–4.
38. Pont J, Albrecht W. Fertility after chemotherapy for testicular germ cell cancer. Fertil Steril 1997;68:1–5.
39. Ishikawa T, Kamidono S, Fujisawa M. Fertility after high-dose chemotherapy for testicular cancer. Urology 2004; 63:137–40.
40. Meinardi MT, Gietema JA, van der Graaf WTA, et al. Cardiovascular morbidity in long-term survivors of metastatic testicular cancer. J Clin Oncol 2000;18:1725–32.
41. Shamberger RC, Rosenberg SA, Siepp CA, Sherins RJ. Effects of high-dose methotrexate and vincristine on ovarian and testicular functions in patients undergoing post-operative adjuvant treatment of osteosarcoma. Cancer Treat Rep 1981;65:739–46.
42. Meistrich ML, Chawla SP, Cunha MF, et al. Recovery of sperm production after chemotherapy for osteosarcoma. Cancer 1989;63:2115–23.

43. Schilsky RL, Davidson HS, Magid D, et al. Gonadal and sexual function in male patients with hairy cell leukemia: lack of adverse effects of recombinant alpha 2-interferon treatment. Cancer Treat Rep 1987;71:179–81.
44. Pennisi TAJ, Grushkin CM, Lieberman E. Gonadal function in children with nephrosis treated with cyclophosphamide. Am J Dis Child 1975;129:315–8.
45. Quigley C, Cowell C, Jimenez M, et al. Normal or early development of puberty despite gonadal damage in children treated for acute lymphocytic leukemia. N Engl J Med 1989;321:143–51.
46. Himelstein-Braw R, Peters H, Faber M. Morphologic study of the ovaries of leukaemic children. Br J Cancer 1978;38:82–7.
47. Chapman RM, Rees LH, Sutcliffe SB, et al. Cyclical combination chemotherapy and gonadal function. Lancet 1979;1:285–9.
48. Chapman RM, Sutcliffe SB, Malpas JS. Cytotoxic-induced ovarian failure in women with Hodgkin's disease, I: hormone function. JAMA 1979;242:1877–81.
49. Schilsky RL, Lewis BJ, Sherins RJ. Gonadal dysfunction in patients receiving chemotherapy for cancer. Ann Intern Med 1980;93:109–14.
50. Koyama H, Wada T, Nishizawa Y, et al. Cyclophosphamide-induced ovarian failure and its therapeutic significance in patients with breast cancer. Cancer 1977;39:1403–9.
51. Fisher B, Sherman B, Rockette H. L-phenylalanine mustard in the management of premenopausal patients with primary breast cancer. Cancer 1979;44:847–57.
52. Belohorsky B, Sirack J, Sandor L, Klauber E. Comments on the development of amenorrhea caused by myleran in cases of chronic myelosis. Neoplasma 1960;7:397–403.
53. Freckman HA, Fry HL, Mendez ML, Maurer ER. Chlorambucil-prednisolone therapy for disseminated breast cancer. JAMA 1965;191:100–6.
54. Bines J, Oleske DM, Cobleigh MA. Ovarian function in premenopausal women treated with adjuvant chemotherapy for breast cancer. J Clin Oncol 1996;14:1718–29.
55. Martin M, Pienkowski T, Mackey J, et al. Adjuvant docetaxel for node-positive breast cancer. N Engl J Med 2005;352:2302–13.
56. Bower M, Rustin GJS, Newlands ES, et al. Chemotherapy for gestational trophoblastic tumours hastens menopause by 3 years. Eur J Cancer 1998;34:1204–7.
57. Choo YC, Chan SWY, Wong LC, Ma HK. Ovarian dysfunction in patients with gestational trophoblastic neoplasm treated with short intensive courses of etoposide. Cancer 1985;55:2348–52.
58. Lipton JH, Derzko CM, Curtis J. Alpha-interferon and pregnancy in a patient with CML. Hematol Oncol 1996;14:119–22.
59. Hensley ML, Ford JM. Imatinib treatment: specific issues related to safety, fertility, and pregnancy. Semin Hematol 2003;40(suppl 2):21–5.
60. King DJ, Ratcliffe MA, Dawson AA, et al. Fertility in young men and women after treatment for lymphoma: a population study. J Clin Pathol 1985;38:1247–51.
61. Lacher MJ, Toner K. Pregnancies and menstrual function before and after combined radiation and chemotherapy for Hodgkin's disease. Cancer Invest 1986;4:93–100.
62. Schilsky RL, Sherins RJ, Hubbard SM, et al. Long-term follow-up of ovarian function in women treated with MOPP chemotherapy for Hodgkin's disease. Am J Med 1981;71:552–6.
63. Horning SJ, Hoppe RT, Kaplan HS, Rosenberg SA. Female reproductive potential after treatment for Hodgkin's disease. N Engl J Med 1981;304:1377–82.
64. Sherins RJ, Winokur S, DeVita VT, Vaitukaitis J. Surprisingly high risk of functional castration in women receiving chemotherapy for lymphoma [abstract]. Clin Res 1975;23:343.
65. Waxman JHX, Terry YA, Wrigley PFM, et al. Gonadal function in Hodgkin's disease: long-term follow-up of chemotherapy. Br Med J 1982;285:1612–3.
66. Simmonds PD, Mead GM, Sweetenham JW, et al. PACE BOM chemotherapy: a 12-week regimen for advanced Hodgkin's disease. Ann Oncol 1997;8:259–66.
67. Muller U, Stahel RA. Gonadal function after MACOP-B or VACOP-B with or without dose intensification and ABMT in young patients with aggressive non-Hodgkin's lymphoma. Ann Oncol 1993;4:399–402.
68. Gershenson DM. Menstrual and reproductive function after treatment with combination chemotherapy for malignant ovarian germ cell tumors. J Clin Oncol 1988;6:270–5.
69. Marchetti M, Romagnolo C. Fertility after ovarian cancer treatment. Eur J Gynaecol Oncol 1992;13:498–501.
70. Pektasides D, Rustin GJS, Mewlands ES, et al. Fertility after chemotherapy for ovarian germ cell tumours. Br J Obstet Gynaecol 1987;94:477–9.
71. Pfleiderer A. Therapy of ovarian malignant germ cell tumors and granulosa tumors. Int J Gynecol Pathol 1993;12:162–5.
72. Dnistrian AM, Schwartz MK, Frecchia AA. Endocrine consequences of CMF adjuvant therapy in pre-menopausal and postmenopausal breast cancer patients. Cancer 1983:51:803–7.
73. Samaan NA, DeAsis DN, Bugdar AO. Pituitary-ovarian function in breast cancer patients on adjuvant chemoimmunotherapy. Cancer 1987;41:2082–7.
74. Sanders JE, Buckner CD, Amos D, et al. Ovarian function following marrow transplantation for aplastic anemia or leukemia. J Clin Oncol 1988;6:813–8.
75. Salooja N, Chatterjee R, McMillan AK, et al. Successful pregnancies in women following single autotransplantation for acute myeloid leukemia with a chemotherapy ablation protocol. Bone Marrow Transplant 1994;13:431–5.
76. Jacob A, Barker H, Goodman A, Holmes J. Recovery of spermatogenesis following bone marrow transplantation. Bone Marrow Transplant 1998;22:277–9.
77. Brauner R, Czernichow P, Cramer P. Leydig-cell function in children after direct testicular irradiation for acute lymphoblastic leukemia. N Engl J Med 1983;309:25–8.
78. Brecher ML, Weinberg V, Boyett JM. Intermediate dose methotrexate (IDM) in childhood acute lymphoblastic leukemia (ALL) resulting in decreased incidence of testicular relapse. Cancer 1986;58:1024–8.
79. Berthelsen JG. Sperm counts and serum follicle-stimulating hormone levels before and after radiotherapy and chemotherapy in men with testicular germ cell cancer. Fertil Steril 1984;41:281–6.
80. Shapiro E, Kinsella TJ, Makuch, RW, et al. Effects of fractionated irradiation on endocrine aspects of testicular function. J Clin Oncol 1985;3:1232–9.
81. Ohl DA, Sonksen J. What are the chances of fertility and should sperm be banked? Semin Urol Oncol 1996;14:36–44.
82. Rappaport R, Brauner R, Czernichow P. Effect of hypothalamic and pituitary irradiation on pubertal development in children with cranial tumours. J Clin Endocrinol Metab 1982;54:1164–8.
83. Hawkins MM. Is there evidence of a therapy-related increase in germ-cell mutation among childhood cancer survivors? J Natl Cancer Inst 1991;83:1643–50.
84. Lushbaugh C, Casarett GW. The effects of gonadal irradiation in clinical radiation therapy: a review. Cancer 1976;37:1111–20.
85. Glode LM, Shannon JM, Nett T. Protection of rat spermatogenic epithelium from damage induced by procarbazine chemotherapy. Br J Cancer 1990;62:61–4.
86. Lewis RW, Dowling KJ, Schally AV. D-tryptophan-6 analog of luteinizing hormone-releasing hormone as a protective agent against testicular damage caused by cyclophosphamide in baboons. Proc Natl Acad Sci U S A 1985;82:2977–9.
87. da Cunha MF, Meistrich ML, Nader S. Absence of testicular protection by a gonadotropin-releasing hormone analogue against cyclophosphamide-induced testicular cytotoxicity in the mouse. Cancer Res 1987;47:1093–7.
88. Johnson DH, Line R, Hainsworth JD, et al. Effects of luteinizing hormone releasing hormone agonist given during combination chemotherapy on post-therapy fertility in male patients with lymphoma: preliminary observations. Blood 1985;65:832–6.
89. Waxman JH, Ahmed R, Smith D, et al. Failure to preserve fertility in patients with Hodgkin's disease. Cancer Chemother Pharmacol 1987;19:159–62.
90. Hallak J, Kolettis PN, Sekhon VS. Thomas AJ, Agarwal A. Sperm cryopreservation in patients with testicular cancer. Urology 1999;54:894–9.
91. Redman JR, Bajorunas DR, Goldstein MC, et al. Semen cryopreservation and artificial insemination for Hodgkin's disease. J Clin Oncol 1987;5:233–8.
92. Davis OK, Graf MJ, Bedford JM. Pregnancy achieved through in vitro fertilization with cryopreserved semen from a man with Hodgkin's lymphoma. Fertil Steril 1990;53:377–8.
93. Naysmith TE, Blake DA, Harvey VH, Johnson NP. Do men undergoing sterilizing cancer treatments have a fertile future? Hum Reprod 1998;13:3250–5.
94. Reed E, Sanger WG, Armitage JO. Results of semen cryopreservation in young men with testicular carcinoma and lymphoma. J Clin Oncol 1986;4:537–9.
95. Schmiegelow ML, Sommer P, Carlson E, et al. Penile vibratory stimulation and electroejaculation before anti-cancer therapy in two pubertal boys. J Pediat Hematol Oncol 1998;20:429–30.
96. Gibbons JJ, Parra RO, Andriole GL, Johnson FE. Testicular circulatory isolation: a phase I study. Surg Oncol 1992;1:413–6.
97. Damani MN, Masters V, Meng MV, et al. Postchemotherapy ejaculatory azoospermia: fatherhood with sperm from testis tissue with intracytoplasmic sperm injection. J Clin Oncol 2002;20:930–6.
98. Jarrell J, YoungLai EV, McMahon A, et al. Effects of ionizing radiation and pretreatment with [D-Leu6, des-GlylO] luteinizing hormone-releasing hormone ethylamide on developing rat ovarian follicles. Cancer Res 1987; 47:5005–8.
99. Chapman R, Sutcliffe SB. Protection of ovarian function by oral contraceptives in women receiving chemotherapy for Hodgkin's disease. Blood 1981;58:849–51.
100. Pacheco BP, Ribas JMM, Milone G, et al. Use of GnRH analogs for functional protection of the ovary and preservation of fertility during cancer treatment in adolescents: a preliminary report. Gynecol Oncol 2001;81:391–7.
101. Oktay K, Karlikaya G. Ovarian function after transplantation of frozen, banked autologous ovarian tissue. N Engl J Med 2000;342:1919.
102. Abir R, Fisch B, Raz A, et al. Preservation of fertility in women undergoing chemotherapy: current approaches and future prospects. J Assist Reprod Genet 1998; 15:469–77.
103. Sauer MV, Guidice L, Macaso TM. Pregnancy following nonsurgical donor ovum transfer to a functionally agonadal woman. Fertil Steril 1987;48:324–5.
104. Tulandi T, Al-Shahrani AA. Laparoscopic fertility preservation. Obstet Gynecol Clin N Am 2004;31:611–8
105. Dudzinski JM. Ethical issues in fertility preservation for adolescent cancer survivors: oocyte and ovarian tissue cryopreservation. J Pediatr Adolesc Gynecol 2004;17:97–102
106. Gabriel D, Bernard S, Lambert J, Croom RD. Oophoropexy and the management of Hodgkin's disease. Arch Surg 1986;121:1083–5.
107. Haie-Meder C, Mlika-Cabanne N, Michel G, et al. Radiotherapy after ovarian transposition: ovarian function and fertility preservation. Int J Radiat Oncol Biol Phys 1993;25:419–24.
108. DeWilde RL, Hesseling M. No more radiogenic castration in women with Hodgkin's disease? Am J Obstet Gynecol 1995;173:1639.
109. Oktay K, Economos K, Kan M, et al. Endocrine function and oocyte retrieval after autologous transplantation of ovarian cortical strips to the forearm. JAMA 2001; 286:1490–3.
110. Pendse S, Ginsburg E, Singh AK. Strategies for preservation of ovarian and testicular function after immunosuppression. Am J Kidney Dis 2004;43:772–81.
111. Li FP, Fine W, Jaffe N. Offspring of patients treated for cancer in childhood. J Natl Cancer Inst 1979;62:1193–7.
112. Rustin GJS, Booth M, Dent J, et al. Pregnancy after cytotoxic chemotherapy for gestational trophoblastic tumours. Br Med J 1984;288:103–6.
113. Holmes GE, Holmes FF. Pregnancy outcome of patients treated for Hodgkin's disease. Cancer 1978;41: 1317–22.
114. Byrne J, Mulvihill JJ, Myers MH, et al. Effects of treatment on fertility in long-term survivors of childhood or adolescent cancer. N Engl J Med 1987;317:1315–21.
115. Mulvihill JJ, Connelly RR, Austin DF, et al. Cancer in offspring of long-term survivors of childhood and adolescent cancer. Lancet 1987;2:813–7.
116. Jacobs C, Donaldson SC, Rosenberg SA. Management of the pregnant patient with Hodgkin's disease. Ann Intern Med 1981;95:669–75.
117. Turchi JJ, Villasis C. Anthracyclines in the treatment of malignancy in pregnancy. Cancer 1988;61:435–40.
118. Heartin E, Walkinshaw S, Clark RE. Successful outcome of pregnancy in chronic myeloid leukaemia treated with imatinib. Leuk Lymph 2004;45;1307–8.
119. Hiratsuka M, Minakami H, Koshizuka S, Sato I. Administration of interferon-alpha during pregnancy: effects on the fetus. J Perinat Med 2000;28:372–6.
120. Blatt J, Mulvihill JJ, Ziegler JL, et al. Pregnancy outcome following cancer chemotherapy. Am J Med 1980; 69:828–32.
121. Doll DC, Ringenberg S, Yarbro JW. Management of cancer during pregnancy. Arch Intern Med 1988;148:2058–64.
122. Aviles A, Niz J. Long-term follow-up of children born to mothers with acute leukemia during pregnancy. Med Pediatr Oncol 1988;16:3–6.
123. Plummer G. Anomalies occurring in children exposed in utero to the atomic bomb at Hiroshima. Pediatrics 1952;10:687.

124. Mulvihill JJ, McKeen EA, Rosner F, Zarrabi MH. Pregnancy outcome in cancer patients. Cancer 1987;60:1143–50.
125. Andersen BL. How cancer affects sexual functioning. Oncology 1990;4:81–8.
126. Gritz ER, Wellisch DK, Wang H, et al. Long-term effects of testicular cancer on sexual functioning in married couples. Cancer 1989;64:1560–7.
127. Madorsky ML, Ashmalla MG, Schusler I. Post-prostatectomy impotence. J Urol 1976;115:401–3.
128. Zippe KS, Agarwal A, Nelson DR, Lakin MM. Treatment of erectile dysfunction with sildenafil citrate (Viagra) after radiation therapy for prostate cancer. Urology 1999;54:308–12.
129. Merrick GS, Butler WM, Lief JH, et al. Efficacy of sildenafil citrate in prostate brachytherapy patients with erectile dysfunction. Urology 1999;53:1112–6.
130. Andersen BL. Sexual functioning morbidity among cancer survivors. Cancer 1985;55:1835–42.
131. Maguire GP, Lee EG, Bevington DJ. Psychiatric problems in the first year after mastectomy. Br Med J 1978;1:963–5.
132. Morris T, Greer HS, White P. Psychological and social adjustment to mastectomy: a two-year follow-up study. Cancer 1977;40:2381–7.
133. Meistrich ML, Wilson G, Mathur K, et al. Rapid recovery of spermatogenesis after mitoxantrone, vincristine, vinblastine and prednisone chemotherapy for Hodgkin's disease. J Clin Oncol 1997;15;3488–95.
134. Pont J, Albrecht W, Postner G, et al. Adjuvant chemotherapy for high-risk clinical stage I nonseminomatous testicular germ cell cancer: long-term results of a prospective trial. J Clin Oncol 1996;14:441–8.
135. Bonnadonna G, Valagussa P. Adjuvant systemic therapy for resectable breast cancer. J. Clin Oncol 1985;3:259–75.
136. Meirow D. Ovarian injury and modern options to preserve fertility in female cancer patients treated with high-dose radio-chemotherapy for hemato-oncological neoplasms. Leuk Lymphoma 1999;33:65–76.
137. Jackson GH, Wood A, Taylor PRA, et al. Early high-dose chemotherapy intensification with autologous bone marrow transplantation in lymphoma associated with retention of fertility and normal pregnancies in females. Leuk Lymphoma 1997;28:127–32.
138. Ben Arush MW, Solt I, Lightman A, et al. Male gonadal function in survivors of childhood Hodgkin and non-Hodgkin lymphoma. Pediatr Hematol Oncol 2000; 17:239–45.
139. Bohlen D, Burkhard FC, Mills R, et al. Fertility and sexual function following orchiectomy and 2 cycles of chemotherapy for stage I high risk nonseminomatous germ cell cancer. J Urol 2001;165:441–4.
140. Bacci G, Ferrari S, Bertoni F, et al. Long-term outcome for patients with nonmetastatic osteosarcoma of the extremity treated at the Istituto Ortopedico Rizzoli according to the Instituto Ortopedico Rizzoli/Osteosarcoma-2 Protocol: an updated report. J Clin Oncol 2000;18:4016–27.
141. Yoshinaka A, Fukasawa I, Sakamoto T, et al. The fertility and pregnancy outcomes of the patients who underwent preservative operation followed by adjuvant chemotherapy for malignant ovarian tumors. Arch Gynecol Obstet 2000;264:124–7.
142. Meirow D. Reproduction post-chemotherapy in young cancer patients. Mol Cell Endocrinol 2000;169:123–31.

Endocrine Complications and Paraneoplastic Syndromes

Sai-Ching Jim Yeung, MD, PhD
Robert F. Gagel, MD

This chapter is divided in two major sections. The first focuses on endocrine complications in cancer patients; the second on paraneoplastic syndromes. Cancer and its treatment can lead to endocrine dysfunction or clinical and laboratory abnormalities that obscure or mimic endocrine diseases. Paraneoplastic syndromes are a group of diverse clinical syndromes seen in cancer patients caused by circulating biologic/humoral factors that include hormones, immunoglobulins, cytokines, and other agents.

ENDOCRINE COMPLICATIONS

Hypothalamic-Pituitary Dysfunction

Radiotherapy is a common cause of hypothalamic-pituitary dysfunction in cancer patients. There is no strong direct evidence to implicate chemotherapy as a cause of permanent dysfunction of the anterior pituitary. Metastasis to the hypothalamic region or the pituitary gland is uncommon,[1] and clinical manifestations of endocrine dysfunction because of metastatic disease in this region are rare. However, benign tumors such as pituitary tumors and craniopharyngiomas frequently affect this anatomic region and cause endocrine dysfunction.

Development of radiation-induced hypothalamic dysfunction is insidious; hormonal deficiency can manifest clinically years after radiation exposure. In general, the rapidity of onset and severity of dysfunction depend on the total dose of radiation and the rate of delivery. There is considerable variation in the sequence and frequency of hormonal dysfunction among the several axes of hypothalamic-pituitary functions. The somatotropic axis appears to be the most sensitive; the thyrotropic axis appears to be the least sensitive (Figure 139-1).[2–5] The diagnosis of hypothalamic-pituitary dysfunction requires vigilance of the physician because most of the presenting symptoms are nonspecific and can easily be attributed to other causes. For example, fatigue and weakness, symptoms of pituitary dysfunction, are common among cancer patients. A diagnostic screen for hypothalamic and pituitary dysfunction may include serum growth hormone (GH) and insulin-like growth factor-1 (IGF-1) measurement and evaluation for gonadal failure. Signs of overt hypopituitarism include hypoglycemia, hypotension, and hypothermia.

In children and teenagers, evaluation of sexual development is a useful diagnostic tool. The investigation should include staging of sexual development according to the Tanner staging criteria, examination of pubic and axillary hair, and review of menstrual history in girls and penile/testicular size in boys. In children who have had cranial irradiation, height and growth velocity should be measured at 6-month intervals. In children treated with spinal and craniospinal irradiation, local rather than general growth abnormalities may be present and, if so, require further specific evaluation. Foot size is a reliable indicator of growth that can be measured on a routine clinic visit.[6] A child whose growth rate is not within the limits of a normal growth curve should be evaluated for growth hormone deficiency, hypothyroidism, and adrenal insufficiency. If the initial evaluation of GH, IGF-1, thyrotropin (TSH) and free thyroxine (T_4) levels, and radiographic bone age reveal abnormality, then detailed dynamic testing to evaluate GH secretion (Table 139-1) and dynamic testing with corticotropin (ACTH), and gonadotropin-releasing hormone stimulation tests should be performed.

In adults who have received cranial or head and neck irradiation, detection of hypothalamic-pituitary abnormalities is more challenging. One strategy to detect hypothalamic-pituitary abnormalities in adults consists of routine screening for abnormal GH and IGF-1 levels and gonadal failure, the most sensitive indicators of radiation-induced hypothalamic-pituitary damage. It is recommended that measurements of IGF-1 and testosterone levels in males and documentation of menstrual history in females be obtained annually for 5 years, and then at 5-year intervals for another 10 years. Any abnormalities noted on the screening tests should be pursued with further dynamic testing to evaluate all the axes of hypothalamic-pituitary functions.

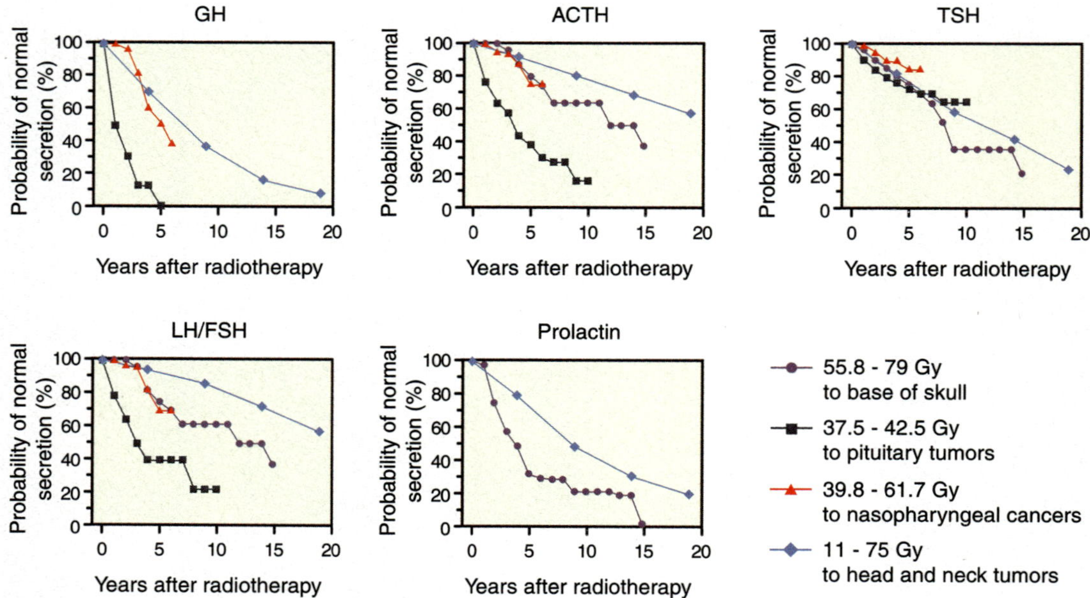

Figure 139-1 Probability of normal pituitary hormone secretion over time after radiation exposure to the hypothalamic–pituitary areas. Data from four studies were replotted on this single figure. The first set of values (*purple circle*) are from Pai HH et al,[3] where the patient received 55.8–79.0 Gy to the base of the skull. The second set of values (*gray square*) are from Shalet SM et al,[64] where patients with pituitary tumors were treated with 37.5–42.5 Gy. The third series (*red triangle*), from Lam KS et al,[2] shows the effect of radiation treatment of nasopharyngeal carcinoma with 39.8–61.7 Gy. The final series (*blue diamond*) represents data from Samaan NA et al,[4] in which 11.0–75.0 Gy was administered to treat of head and neck tumors.

Table 139-1 Dynamic Testing of the Growth Hormone Axis for the Diagnosis of Growth Hormone Deficiency

Test	Dose/Sampling	Contraindications
Insulin hypoglycemia	0.075–0.1 U regular insulin/kg IV to achieve glucose ≤ 40 mg/dL. Sample for glucose and GH at 0, 30, 45, 60, and 90 min	Coronary heart disease or seizures
Arginine	0.5 gm/kg (up to 30 gm) IV over 30 min. Sample for GH at 0, 30, 60, 90, and 120 min	Liver disease or renal disease
L-Dopa	500 mg by mouth. Sample for GH at 0, 30, 60, 90, and 120 min	Systolic blood pressure < 100 mm Hg or age > 60 years
Arginine and GHRH	Arginine dose as above. GHRH 1 μg/kg IV push. Sample for GH at 0, 30, 60, 90 and 120 min	Liver disease or renal disease

GH = growth hormone; GHRH = growth hormone-releasing hormone; IV = intravenous.

Thyroid Disorders Thyroid disorders and abnormalities in thyroid function are commonly associated with cancer and its therapy. These problems are discussed below.

Serum Thyroid Hormone-Binding Protein Abnormalities The levels of thyroid hormone-binding proteins (thyroxine-binding globulin [TBG], prealbumin, and albumin) can be modified by sex hormone levels and nutritional factors; abnormalities of both are encountered frequently in cancer patients. Several chemotherapy drugs affect thyroid function test results. L-Asparaginase appears to reversibly inhibit synthesis of albumin and TBG, resulting in low total thyroxine (T_4) but normal free T_4 levels.[7] The combination of podophyllin and alkylating agents has also been reported to decrease TBG.[8] Both 5-fluorouracil[9] and mitotane[10] increase the total T_4 and triiodothyronine (T_3) levels without suppressing TSH, suggesting that these drugs increase thyroid hormone binding capacity in the serum.

Euthyroid Sick Syndrome Alterations in thyroid hormone metabolism occur in patients with cancer and other serious systemic illnesses.[11] Low serum T_3 levels, which may be found in up to 70% of moderately to seriously ill cancer patients, are caused by a decrease in the extrathyroidal conversion of T_4 to T_3. Serum concentrations of free T_4 are usually normal or high, while concentrations of free T_3 are below normal or low. The patients are clinically euthyroid, and serum TSH level and TRH stimulation test results are normal.

In most patients with euthyroid sick syndrome, T_3, T_4, and TSH levels are normal. Clinical manifestations of hypothyroidism are usually absent, but assessment may be confounded by obtundation, edema, and hypothermia that may accompany severe illness. Low free T_4 levels in the context of euthyroid sick syndrome usually indicate a grave prognosis, with a mortality rate of more than 50%. Although it is generally accepted that thyroid hormone therapy has no benefit, in practice it is sometimes difficult to differentiate between the euthyroid sick syndrome and secondary hypothyroidism. Judicious replacement of thyroxine at physiologic levels in these uncommon patients may be appropriate if there are no contraindications (eg, coronary artery disease).

Hypothyroidism ***Thyroidectomy*** Thyroidectomy may be performed for a variety of oncologic reasons in the management of thyroid cancer, head and neck cancer, or thyroid metastasis. Thyroid replacement is needed in this group of patients. In thyroid cancer patients supraphysiologic doses of thyroid hormone are used routinely to maintain suppression of thyroid stimulating hormone (TSH). In others, replacement of thyroid hormone should be adjusted to maintain the serum TSH concentration in the normal range.

Radiation Irradiation is an important cause of hypothyroidism (primary, secondary, and tertiary). Radiation-induced primary hypothyroidism is caused by thyroid cell destruction, inhibition of cell division, vascular damage, and possibly an immune-mediated phenomenon. Factors that increase the risk of developing primary hypothyroidism include a high radiation dose to the vicinity of the thyroid gland, duration since therapy, lack of shielding of the thyroid during therapy, and combined irradiation and surgical treatments.[12]

The incidences of hypothyroidism after radiation therapy for various cancers and conditions are tabulated in Table 139-2.[4,12–22] A relationship between radiation dose and the prevalence of hypothyroidism is based on studies of patients with Hodgkin's disease.[15,18] Long-term follow-up of patients treated with low-dose radiotherapy suggests that the threshold for causing clinically evident hypothyroidism is approximately 10 Gy. For Hodgkin's disease patients who received > 30 Gy, the actuarial risk of hypothyroidism was up to 45% 20 years after irradiation.[15] Patients with frank or subclinical hypothyroidism should receive thyroid hormone replacement therapy.

Chemotherapy The diagnosis of hypothyroidism in 14% of bone marrow transplantation (BMT) patients who received chemotherapy but did not receive total-body irradiation[23] suggests a causal relation between hypothyroidism and high-dose combination cytotoxic chemotherapy. This notion is also supported by studies that showed an increased incidence of primary hypothyroidism in patients treated with multiple combination drug regimens[24,25] with or without radiation.[24] L-Asparaginase, in addition to inhibition of TBG synthesis discussed above, may also inhibit TSH synthesis reversibly and lead to temporary hypothyroidism with decreased free T_4 levels.[26]

Thyroid dysfunction is a recognized side effect of cytokine treatments. Treatment with interleukin-2 produces thyroid dysfunction in approximately 20 to 35% of patients.[27] These patients have hypothyroidism, hyperthyroidism, or hyperthyroidism followed by hypothyroidism.[28] Approximately 10% of interferon-treated patients develop primary hypothyroidism.[29] Patients with antithyroid antibodies before therapy are at higher risk of cytokine-induced thyroid dysfunction.

Retinoid X receptor (RXR) ligands may be used in the treatment of certain malignancies. Bexarotene (an RXR-selective ligand) caused secondary or pituitary hypothyroidism in patients treated for cutaneous T-cell lymphoma.[30] The effect is dose-related, and central hypothyroidism occurs less frequently with lower doses. In addition to suppressing transcription of TSH by an RXR-mediated thyroid hormone-independent mechanism, bexarotene also increases metabolic clearance of thyroid hormones.[30]

^{131}I-Containing Compounds The use of ^{131}I for treatment of thyroid cancer requires a high serum TSH level. High TSH level is achieved by either withholding thyroid hormone replacement or administration of recombinant human TSH. The use of ^{131}I-containing compounds in the treatment of other tumors may result in hypothyroidism. For instance, using high-dose (100–1,000 mCi) [^{131}I]-metaiodobenzylguanidine to treat unresectable pheochromocytoma may result in primary hypothyroidism.

Screening Children who have received either head-and-neck or cranial irradiation should have a free T_4 and a TSH measurement annually for 5 years and every 2 years thereafter. Early detection of abnormal T_4 and TSH levels will per-

Table 139-2 Incidence of Hypothyroidism (Including Compensated Hypothyroidism) after Radiotherapy[a]

Type of Malignancy or Conditions	Radiation Dose	% with Hypothyroidism
Hodgkin's disease	30–60 Gy	30–50
Head and neck cancer	40–72 Gy	25–50
Lymphoma	20–40 Gy (median 36 Gy)	30–42
Breast carcinoma	?	15–21
Total-body irradiation in BMT	13.75–15 Gy	15–43

BMT = bone marrow transplantation.
[a]Data based on refs. 4 and 12 to 22.

mit medical intervention before hypothyroidism adversely affects physical and intellectual development and growth. In adults, neck irradiation for treatment of lymphoma and various head and neck tumors is associated with a high incidence of primary hypothyroidism. Patients who have received irradiation should have free T_4 and TSH levels measured annually for 5 years, and then every other year for 10 years, and thereafter every 5 years for another 10 years. Once hypothyroidism is diagnosed, the patient should receive thyroid hormone replacement therapy.

Hyperthyroidism Radiation-induced painless thyroiditis with hyperthyroxinemia is an uncommon side effect of external beam radiotherapy to the head and neck area. Transient hyperthyroidism may occur as a result of inflammation and destruction of thyroid tissue with release of thyroglobulin (containing thyroxine or triiodothyronine) and is usually followed by hypothyroidism. Transient hyperthyroidism has been reported after mantle radiotherapy in Hodgkin's disease patients, and occurs usually within 18 months of treatment.[31] A low uptake of radioiodine in most of these cases suggests a diagnosis of silent thyroiditis, but some have Graves' disease. In one series of Hodgkin's disease patients treated with radiation, the risk of Graves' disease in these patients was estimated to be at least 7.2 times that in a healthy population.[15]

Ophthalmopathy similar to that in Graves' disease has been reported within 18 to 84 months of high-dose radiotherapy to the neck for lymphoma, breast cancer, and nasopharyngeal or laryngeal cancer. Ophthalmopathy may occur without hyperthyroidism and in the absence of the human leukocyte antigen-B8.[32] This suggests that radiation-induced thyroid injury may induce an autoimmune process that is similar to Graves' disease.

Thyroid Nodules It is well known that low-dose radiation increases the risk of thyroid nodules and cancer. High-dose radiation therapy is also associated with an increased prevalence of thyroid nodules.[33] In one study, 26 of 95 patients who had received high-dose radiotherapy for childhood malignancies had palpable thyroid nodules 5 to 34 years after therapy.[34] Radiation-induced thyroid nodules are common sequelae of head and neck cancer treatments and are also found in breast cancer patients whose radiation field included the lower neck. The frequency of palpable abnormalities increases with time after radiation, indicating a need for regular thyroid examination in such patients. Thyroid irregularities should be evaluated by ultrasonography and fine-needle aspiration biopsy. Figure 139-2 outlines the diagnostic approach to thyroid nodules in cancer patients.

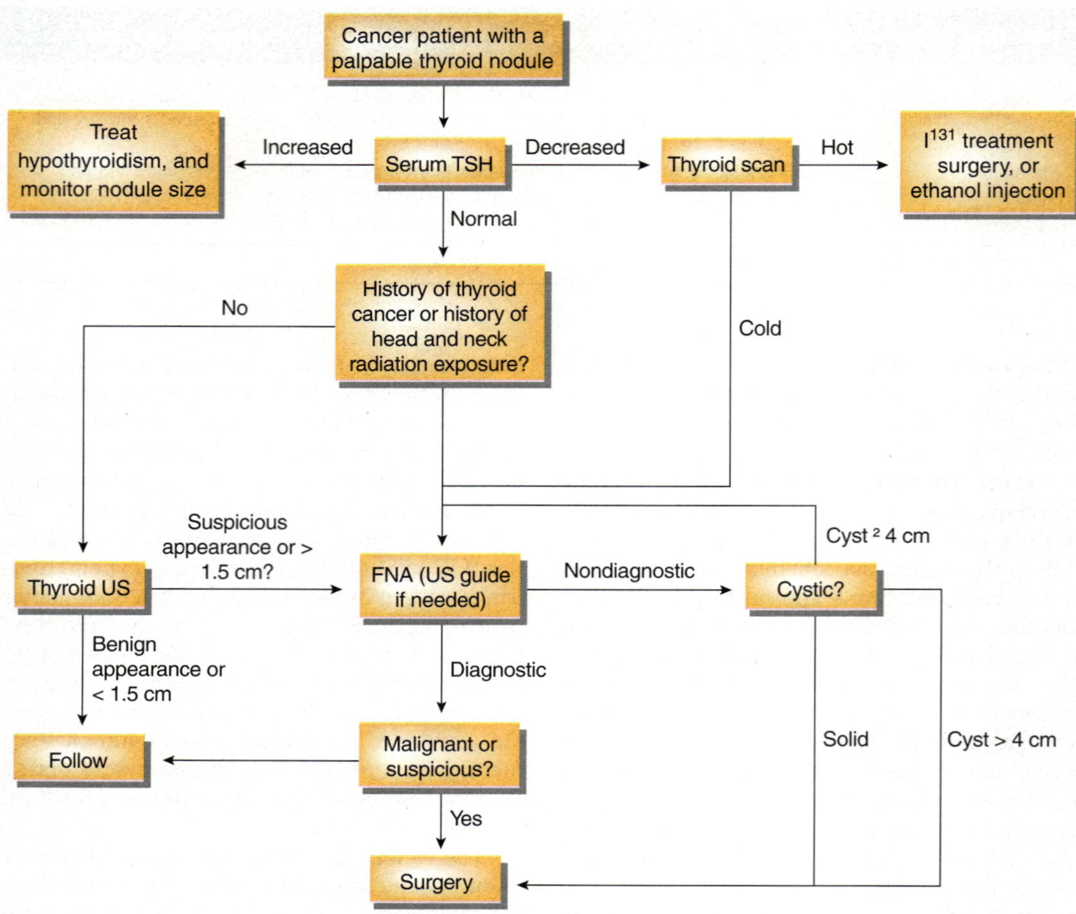

Figure 139-2 Approach to a cancer patient with a thyroid nodule.

The association between thyroid cancer and low-dose irradiation has been extensively examined[35] and is discussed in Chapter 76, "Neoplasm of the Thyroid." Thyroid cancer is increasingly recognized as a potential complication of high-dose radiation (> 40 Gy) exposure to the thyroid, which increases the risk of thyroid cancer by approximately 3-fold in adults,[36] and approximately 13-fold in children.[37] The latent period from radiotherapy to the diagnosis of thyroid cancer can be up to 30 years. Approximately 75 to 90% of radiation-induced thyroid cancers are papillary carcinomas.

Metastasis to the Thyroid In autopsy series, the incidence of metastasis to the thyroid gland varies from 1.25 to 24%. The primary tumor site includes the kidney (33%), lung (16%), breast (16%), esophagus (9%), and uterus (7%).[38] Hypothyroidism secondary to metastatic infiltration and replacement of the thyroid by cancer is extremely rare. Thyrotoxicosis has been reported in patients with thyroid metastasis from lymphoma and pancreatic cancer. In these cases, the etiology of thyrotoxicosis is probably follicular destruction resulting in unregulated release of thyroid hormone and thyroglobulin. Intrathyroidal metastasis is most commonly treated by surgical removal of the lobe containing the metastatic cancer.

Diabetes Mellitus The administration of glucocorticoids (eg, in combination therapy regimens, for edema of brain metastasis, for prevention of transplant rejection, for graft-versus-host disease in BMT, and for nausea/vomiting) is probably the most common cause of diabetes mellitus in cancer patients. Therefore, patients who receive glucocorticoids must be periodically screened for diabetes with evaluation of fasting glucose levels during therapy. Treatment with streptozotocin[39] or L-asparaginase[40] may result in insulin-deficient diabetes mellitus. Although there is no evidence of a delayed onset of diabetes mellitus following treatment with streptozotocin, follow-up has been limited and short-term. For long-term survivors treated with streptozotocin, periodic screening for delayed development of diabetes mellitus may be indicated. Diabetes mellitus may also develop as a consequence of serious pancreatitis secondary to treatment with L-asparaginase. Immunotherapy for cancer using cytokines such as interleukin-2 and interferons may cause toxicity to pancreatic β cells and lead to insulin-dependent diabetes.[41] Tacrolimus, an immunosuppressive agent used to prevent graft-versus-host disease in BMT, also increases the incidence of diabetes, perhaps by damaging pancreatic beta cells.[42] Patients who received allogenic BMT are likely to be receiving both glucocorticoids, cyclosporine A and tacrolimus, and are particularly at risk of developing diabetes mellitus.[43] Management of the blood glucose levels would depend on the severity of the blood glucose level abnormality and on the underlying pathophysiologic mechanism of the increase in blood sugar. In general, oral antidiabetic agents are unlikely to be effective in patients who are insulin-deficient.

There is recent evidence that outcomes in several malignancies (leukemia and colon cancer) is impacted negatively by the presence of hyperglycemia.[44] These findings suggest the possibility that hyperglycemia or hyperinsulinemia, often seen in insulin resistant patients (obesity or glucocorticoid therapy), may have an independent effect on neoplastic transformation. This may explain the higher than normal prevalence of cancer in obese and diabetic patients.[45] Prospective clinical trials are currently being performed to address the question of whether tight control of diabetes will improve clinical outcomes in patients with cancer.

Metabolic Bone Diseases **Osteoporosis** Normal bone remodeling involves a delicate balance between bone formation by osteoblasts and bone resorption by osteoclasts. Antineoplastic therapy is toxic to osteoblast function and decreases bone formation. Production by the tumor of hormonally active substances (eg, parathyroid hormone-related protein [PTHrP], lymphotoxin, interleukin-1, and interleukin-6) may contribute to the clinical picture of bone loss. In most cases, it is not clear whether bone loss is caused by antineoplastic therapy or by the underlying disease process and its effects (including cachexia, malnutrition, poor calcium and vitamin D intake, or a combination of these). In patients with breast or prostate cancer, sex steroid hormone deficiency is the most important cause of bone loss. Bone loss is prominent in patients with several disorders (myeloma, leukemia, lymphoma) disorders affecting hematopoietic cells, perhaps because of cytokine production and an intimate relationship of hematopoietic cells with bone-forming cells or the use of high-dose or prolonged therapy with glucocorticoids.

Nutritional deficiency and hypogonadism in teenagers and young adults result in lower bone mass. Attention to adequate calcium intake and vitamin D intake, prompt investigation of gonadal dysfunction in cancer survivors, and prompt replacement of gonadal steroids (in the absence of contraindications) in young hypogonadal men or women are recommended to decrease the risk of future bone fractures. The bone mass of long-term cancer survivors should be assessed when the patient is about 30 years old, the age at which most people have attained peak bone mass.[46] If bone mass is normal, no further evaluation is needed beyond the usual recommendations for prevention of osteoporosis. If it is abnormal (more than 2 standard deviations below normal), the patient should be referred for evaluation of the multiple reversible causes of osteoporosis.

Four groups of adult patients are at particular risk of osteoporosis. Women with breast cancer treated with cytotoxic chemotherapy frequently undergo an early menopause[47] and cannot receive estrogen-replacement therapy. Bone mass should be assessed (eg, by dual-energy x-ray absorptiometry), and alternative therapies such as bisphosphonates (alendronate or risedronate), calcitonin, or selective estrogen receptor modulators (SERMs) should be considered, in addition to a daily intake of 1,200 to 1,500 mg elemental calcium. Men with prostate cancer who are on antiandrogenic therapy and made hypogonadal are at equivalent risk of development of osteoporosis. Bisphosphonates are effective therapy for these patients. A third group at risk of bone loss are patients with lymphoma, myeloma, or leukemia. The common mechanisms shared by these entities include production of bone-resorbing cytokines secreted by the neoplastic cells and the use of high-dose glucocorticoids in treatment regimens. Osteoporosis in children with leukemia will frequently reverse because the children are in the formative years of bone development; in adults, more active measures such as bisphosphonate or teriparatide therapy may be indicated.

A number of drugs can induce osteoporosis.[48] In cancer patients, glucocorticoids, methotrexate and cytotoxic drugs that cause renal loss of calcium, magnesium, or phosphorus (eg, platinum compounds, cyclophosphamide, ifosfamide) have significant impact on bone density. Osteoporosis (generalized or localized) is observed in children receiving methotrexate therapy for acute lymphoblastic leukemia (ALL).[49] The osteoporosis improves significantly after cessation of methotrexate therapy. A longitudinal study of ALL patients showed that the leukemic process, high-dose glucocorticoids, and hypomagnesemia (due to renal wastage following cyclical glucocorticoid and nephrotoxic chemotherapy or anti-infective agents) contributed to the impairment of calcium and vitamin D metabolism and decrease in bone mass at different stages of the treatment process.[50] Adjuvant chemotherapy for breast cancer (usually involving 5-fluorouracil, cyclophosphamide, and doxorubicin or methotrexate) is associated with low bone mass in premenopausal patients.[51] Post-treatment hypogonadism appears to be a major factor in these adult patients with osteoporosis. BMT usually involves treatment with high-dose cytotoxic drug, glucocorticoids, and immunosuppressive agents. In 24 patients who underwent BMT with high-dose chemotherapy, profound effects on bone biomarkers were observed.[52]

A key point in the management of the osteoporosis syndrome in cancer patients is the use of bone mineral density measurement to assess fracture risk and to monitor the effects of therapy. This measurement should be performed early in the course of management of the malignancy so that appropriate preventive measures can be implemented. The oncologist who is prescribing medications that are likely to decrease bone mass should consider active use of antiresorptive therapy (estrogen, SERMs, or bisphosphonates) to prevent bone loss rather than waiting for the development of a fracture syndrome. Another key point is correction of abnormal mineral and vitamin D metabolism by dietary supplements. Treatment of hypocalcemia, hypomagnesemia, and vitamin D deficiency is integral to the successful therapy of osteoporosis in cancer patients. Recent studies document that clinically relevant vitamin D deficiency is present in 50% of the normal population; the percentage is almost certainly higher in patients undergoing cancer therapy.

Osteomalacia Osteomalacia, a condition characterized by unmineralized bone matrix, is a rare complication of chemotherapy, but should be considered in osteopenic patients and those with osteomalacic clinical syndrome (bone pain and proximal myopathy). The most common cause is a decrease in the serum calcium and/or phosphorus concentrations caused by nutritional deficiency and renal wasting of phosphorus and calcium. Patients who have received chemotherapeutic agents that cause hypophosphatemia, hypomagnesemia, or hypocalcemia are particularly at risk. Investigation of the levels of serum ionized calcium, phosphorus, magnesium, and vitamin D metabolites should be included in the initial evaluation. Appropriate replacement therapy of these vitamins and minerals should be instituted once deficiencies have been identified. Other contributing factors include systemic acidosis and drugs such as anticonvulsants and aluminum.[48] Tumor-induced osteomalacia will be addressed in the section that follows discussing paraneoplastic syndromes.

Ifosfamide causes tubular damage leading to renal phosphate wasting, hypophosphatemia, and rickets/osteomalacia.[53] The toxic effects of ifosfamide on renal tubular function include Fanconi syndrome in adults and children. Tubular damage is seen most commonly when ifosfamide is administered in doses of 50 g/m^2 or more, or when it is used in combination with cisplatin.[54] Rickets is reported most commonly in children. Estramustine, used in the treatment of prostate cancer, has been reported to increase bone resorption and at the same time cause hypocalcemia, hypophosphatemia, and secondary hyperparathyroidism.[55]

Adrenal Diseases **Adrenal Metastasis** Hematogenous metastasis to the adrenal glands is common, exceeded in frequency only by hematogenous metastasis to the lung, liver, and bone.[56] Autopsies have documented that 9 to 27% of patients who died from malignant illness had adrenal metastasis, with bilateral involvement in one-half to two-thirds of patients with adrenal metastasis.

The presence of adrenal metastasis may have important implications for diagnostic and therapeutic planning. When patients with cancer have an adrenal mass but no evidence of metastasis elsewhere, it is vital to determine whether this mass represents a metastatic deposit or a separate, unrelated adrenal lesion. Recent advances in imaging techniques have allowed the identification of adrenal lesions antemortem as part of the tumor-staging evaluation. The location of the adrenal glands in the perinephric fat allows the detection of almost all normal glands and contour-deforming masses as small as 5 to 10 mm. Computed tomography (CT) is a sensitive and specific method to detect adrenal masses. Characteristics on CT examination that suggest adrenal metastasis rather than primary adrenal disease include heterogeneity, contrast enhancement, bilaterality, and size greater than 3 cm.[57]

Without other evidence of metastatic disease, whether the adrenal mass is actually a metastatic tumor is critical information in determining the appropriate therapy for the cancer. Evaluation of a patient who has a malignant adrenal mass should include a history and physical examination to elicit evidence of adrenal insufficiency, Cushing's syndrome, mineralocorticoid excess, or pheochromocytoma. Biochemical assessment should include a short ACTH stimulation test to rule out adrenal sufficiency. A 24-hour urine collection should be obtained to measure urinary free cortisol, aldosterone, catecholamines, and metanephrines. Pheochromocytoma must be excluded, especially if there is hypertension or an operative procedure of any type is contemplated. It has been reported that one-half of the patients who had a clinically unsuspected pheochromocytoma had clinical deterioration or even death immediately following a nonadrenal-related surgical procedure.[58]

If the biochemical assessment for pheochromocytoma is negative, CT-guided fine-needle aspiration should be considered. This procedure has a sensitivity of 85% in detecting cancer.[59] Magnetic resonance imaging (MRI) may be helpful in the diagnosis of pheochromocytoma. Functional scintigraphy using ^{131}I-6-iodomethyl-19-*nor*-cholesterol (NP-59) may be used in conjunction with CT and MRI to aid in the diagnosis of a unilateral adrenal mass greater than 2 cm.[60]

Adrenal Insufficiency Despite the relatively high prevalence of adrenal infiltration by many common cancers, clinically evident adrenal hypofunction occurs infrequently, except when both adrenal glands are affected by metastatic disease.[61] It is estimated that more that 80% of adrenal tissue must be destroyed before corticosteroid production, under both basal and stress conditions, is impaired.[62] Because the clinical manifestations of adrenal insufficiency are nonspecific and overlap findings in cancer patients, a high index of suspicion is required to detect this treatable condition. The cachexia and weakness seen in patients with adrenal insufficiency can mimic the general wasting seen in patients with extensive metastatic disease. Electrolyte abnormalities can easily be explained by poor intake, malnutrition, side effects of chemotherapeutic agents, or paraneoplastic syndromes. Adrenal insufficiency may develop gradually and therefore be confused with cancer-associated cachexia.

Approximately 20 to 30% of the patients with bilateral adrenal metastasis will develop adrenal insufficiency.[61] These patients should all be evaluated by the ACTH stimulation test and should receive glucocorticoid and mineralocorticoid replacement therapy when adrenal insufficiency is suspected and until normal adrenal function is documented. Patients who are stable should receive 20 mg of hydrocortisone in the morning and 10 mg in the early afternoon. In the event of circulatory instability, sepsis, emergency surgery, or other major complications, stress dosages of parenteral glucocorticoid should be given (eg, hydrocortisone succinate 100 mg intravenously every 8 h).

Other causes of primary adrenal insufficiency in cancer patients include autoimmune adrenalitis, adrenal hemorrhage, and granulomatous diseases. Many cancer patients may be immunocompromised. For example, patients with leukemia or lymphoma or patients who have undergone BMT are immunocompromised. In these patients, infection of the adrenal glands by cytomegalovirus, mycobacteria, or fungi may lead to adrenal insufficiency.

Adrenal insufficiency may be drug-induced. Etomidate,[61] a common intravenous anesthetic, and ketoconazole, an antifungal drug, both inhibit the production of cytochrome P-450–dependent enzymes in the glucocorticoid synthetic pathway. Aminoglutethimide and metyrapone are drugs that inhibit enzymes in steroidogenesis, and may cause adrenal insufficiency when used in the treatment of prostate, breast, and adrenocortical cancers. Mitotane, structurally related to the insecticide dichlorodiphenyltrichloroethane (DDT), has selective toxicity for normal and neoplastic adrenocortical cells. Adrenal insufficiency is commonly observed when mitotane is administered in doses necessary to treat adrenocortical cancer; glucocorticoid replacement therapy is mandatory in such patients.[10] Increased protein binding may lead to an increased daily requirement of glucocorticoids during replacement therapy. Suramin, recently proposed as an anticancer agent based on its activity against the tumor growth factors, may also cause adrenal insufficiency.

Secondary adrenal insufficiency because of metastasis to the pituitary or hypothalamus may also occur. The most common cause of secondary adrenal hypofunction, however, is exogenous glucocorticoid therapy that suppresses the hypothalamic-pituitary adrenal axis. A prolonged course of therapy may lead to hypothalamic-pituitary suppression lasting for many months. Short periods of steroid therapy (ie, 1, 2, or 4 weeks) in patients with leukemia and lymphoma suppress adrenal function for 2 to 4 days in most patients, and for longer in some patients. In patients who have received glucocorticoids for more than 2 weeks, a tapering period of 10 to 14 days should be considered. This is especially true for chemotherapy regimens that included high-dose glucocorticoids, such as those used in the treatment of acute leukemia and lymphoma. In addition, patients who have been treated within the past year with prolonged glucocorticoid courses should receive stress dosages of glucocorticoid if acute medical or surgical complications occur (eg, neutropenic fever with hypotension, acute typhlitis). Irradiation of the hypothalamic-pituitary region causes ACTH deficiency and secondary adrenal insufficiency in 19 to 42% of treated patients (see Figure 139-1). Several diagnostic approaches have been used to evaluate secondary adrenal insufficiency, including basal 8 am serum cortisol measurements and dynamic tests with synthetic ACTH, insulin-induced hypoglycemia, or metyrapone.

Disorders of Growth Hormone Secretion and Growth Childhood cancer or its treatment commonly impairs growth. Medulloblastoma and ALL, common childhood malignancies, are frequently treated with cranial or craniospinal irradiation and/or chemotherapy. Close to 40% of adult survivors of childhood brain cancer are below the tenth population percentile for height, and the risk factors for short stature are young age at diagnosis and radiation treatment affecting the hypothalamic-pituitary axis.[63] GH-deficiency and damage to the osseous growth plates are two common mechanisms of growth retardation.

Cranial irradiation may cause hypothalamic or pituitary dysfunction. The hypothalamus appears to be more radiosensitive than does the pituitary gland and may be damaged by lower radiation doses (< 40 Gy). Higher doses (> 40 Gy) are likely to damage both hypothalamic and pituitary function. Deficiency of one or more pituitary hormones following irradiation of the hypothalamic/pituitary area occurs in almost 100% of patients 5 years after irradiation (see Figure 139-1).

GH deficiency is the most frequently noted deficiency and often the first deficiency to arise after cranial irradiation. Isolated GH deficiency following irradiation is common, and the effects are dose related. At lower doses (20–24 Gy), the only effect may be an altered GH secretory pattern and subnormal response to insulin-induced hypoglycemia. With intermediate and higher doses, the GH response to arginine is impaired, and the frequency and amplitude of pulsatile GH secretion is decreased.[5] At doses up to 30 Gy, abnormal GH secretion and growth retardation are observed in more than 35% of patients, necessitating GH treatment.[64]

In addition to growth retardation caused by GH deficiency, craniospinal or spinal irradiation for hematologic malignancy or central nervous system tumors and total-body irradiation prior to BMT may cause two other effects. First, irradiation affects the growth plates in vertebral bodies and in the pelvis and decreases vertebral growth. Second, irradiation causes resistance to GH or insulin-like growth factors.

Children treated with chemotherapy for malignancy frequently have a period of reduced growth velocity, followed by a "catch-up" growth phase. Systemic illness seems to be the most important component of growth retardation in these children, although chemotherapy may play a significant role. Both growth velocity and height are lower in children who are treated with higher doses of chemotherapy and for a longer duration with combination chemotherapy than in those who receive regular therapy or less-intensive chemotherapy. If there is no catch-up growth after 1.5 to 2 years, it is important to exclude GH deficiency.

In adults, GH deficiency is thought to cause decreased bone and muscle mass, lower exercise capacity, increased adipose tissue, fatigue, a poor sense of well-being, impaired myocardial function and increased cardiovascular risks. GH replacement may be indicated to improve the patients' quality of life and sense of well-being,[65] but the concern over IGF-1–induced reactivation of malignant disease should be factored into the decision.

Disorders of Electrolyte/Mineral Metabolism **Hyponatremia** In a prospective study of in-patient cancer patients, the incidence of hyponatraemia is 3.7% with sodium depletion and syndrome of inappropriate antidiuretic hormone (SIADH), each accounting for about one-third of all causes.[66] SIADH is characterized by low serum osmolality and inappropriately high urine osmolality in the absence of diuretics, heart failure, cirrhosis, adrenal insufficiency, and hypothyroidism. In cancer patients, SIADH may be caused by vasopressin secreted by tumors (eg, up to 15% of small-cell lung cancers), abnormal secretory stimuli (eg, intrathoracic infection, positive pressure ventilation), or cytotoxicity affecting paraventricular and supraoptic neurons. It is also possible that chemotherapy-induced lysis of vasopressin-containing cancer cells leads to or worsens SIADH. Drug-induced renal salt wasting or tumor-induced salt wasting (mediated by atrial natriuretic peptide)[67] can also cause hyponatremia, hypo-osmolality, elevated urinary sodium, and urinary osmolality. These SIADH-like syndromes are difficult to distinguish from SIADH when signs and symptoms of fluid volume depletion are subtle or absent. Nonetheless, there are convincing reports that provide evidence of chemotherapy-induced hypothalamic or pituitary damage in the context of SIADH. There are at least seven reports associating vincristine with SIADH, and some of these reports document inappropriately high serum levels of vasopressin.[68] Vinblastine has also been reported to cause severe hyponatremia and SIADH.[68] The presumed mechanism of vinca alkaloid-induced SIADH is paraventricular or supraoptic cell microtubular damage.

Cyclophosphamide therapy has been associated with hyponatremia and SIADH. Autopsy findings in a case of fatal hyponatremia induced by cyclophosphamide (1,800 mg/m^2) suggest that cyclophosphamide directly affects the hypothalamus.[69] Those findings included infundibular necrosis, decreased intraaxonal secretory granules, and depletion of posterior pituitary vasopressin. Patients treated with lower doses of cyclophosphamide also develop hyponatremia, hypotonicity, urinary hypertonicity, and increased plasma vasopressin levels. Damage to the renal tubules and resulting defects in salt and water transport may be the major cause of hyponatremia associated with low-dose cyclophosphamide therapy.[70]

There are many reports of cisplatin-induced hyponatremia caused by renal salt wasting.[71] Several reports claim that cisplatin induces SIADH. The mechanism of cisplatin-induced hyponatremia is unclear, but it has been suggested that renal toxic effects of cisplatin, that is, decreased papillary solute content, and maximal urinary osmolarity, are the major factors, rather than a direct effect of cisplatin on vasopressin secretion. In a majority of the patients who have elevated vasopressin levels, the vasopressin levels became suppressed after correction of hypovolemia.[71] Therefore, the stimulus for vasopressin release in these patients was probably hypovolemia caused by renal salt wasting. Figure 139-3 outlines the algorithm for evaluation and treatment of hyponatremia.

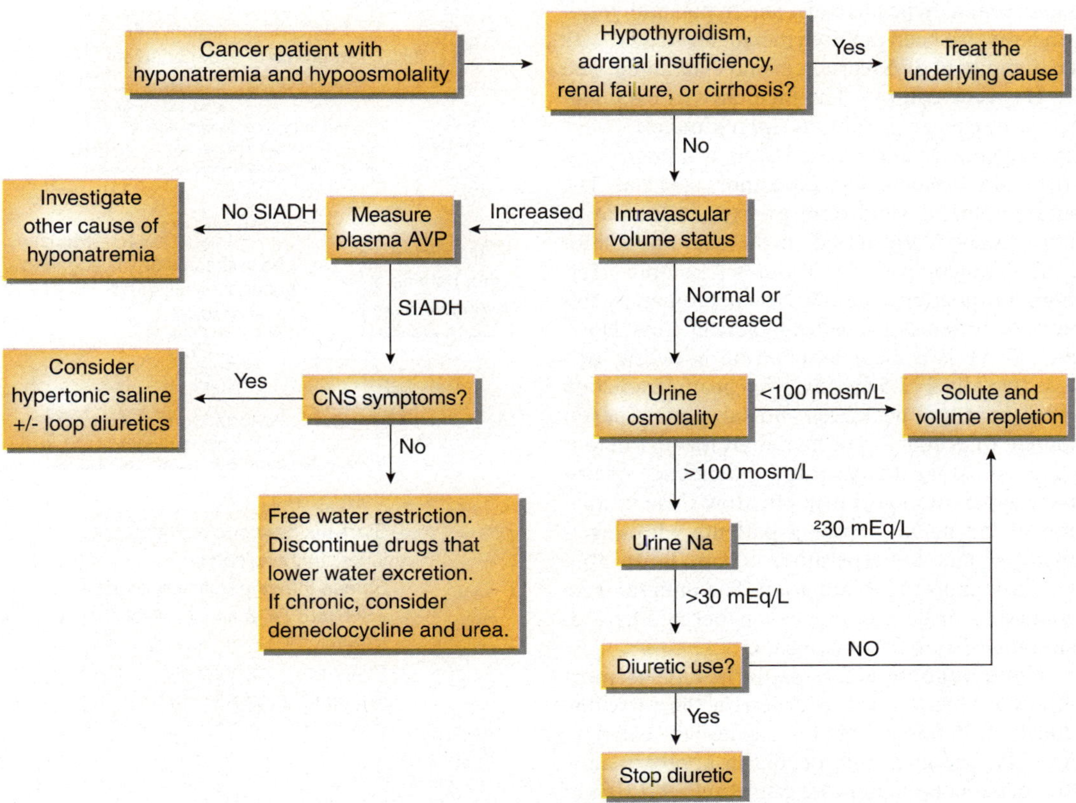

Figure 139-3 Approach to evaluation of hyponatremia in a cancer patient.

Hypernatremia Hypernatremia secondary to central diabetes insipidus occurs frequently as a complication of neurosurgery or destruction by the tumor of the anterior pituitary or the related hypothalamic nuclei. Nephrogenic diabetes insipidus can result from the effects of ifosfamide or streptozocin on tubular reabsorption of water. Ifosfamide has broad nephrotoxic effects, although tubular damage predominates. Distal tubular defects develop in about half of patients treated with ifosfamide. However, frank nephrogenic diabetes insipidus leading to hypernatremia is not common.[72] Streptozotocin is another nephrotoxic drug; in addition to causing glomerular defects (proteinuria) and tubular defects (Fanconi syndrome), streptozocin therapy has been reported to cause nephrogenic diabetes insipidus.[73]

Hypocalcemia Hypocalcemia may be one of the features of tumor lysis syndrome, which is discussed in Chapter 142, "Oncologic Emergencies." Hypocalcemia can also be caused by primary hypoparathyroidism after surgical procedures in the neck that sacrificed or damaged the parathyroid glands (eg, total laryngectomy, total thyroidectomy). Hypocalcemia is also a common complication of chemotherapy.[68] Hypocalcemia has been reported in 6 to 20% of cisplatin-treated patients. Effects of cisplatin on renal tubular function, magnesium metabolism, bone resorption, and vitamin D metabolism may explain the hypocalcemia. Hypomagnesemia may cause a decrease in the secretion of parathyroid hormone and a reduction in the calcium-mobilizing effects of parathyroid hormone. Hypomagnesemia also inhibits formation of 1,25-dihydroxy vitamin D_3 (1,25-dihydroxycholecalciferol). Cisplatin may inhibit the mitochondrial function in the kidneys and thereby inhibit conversion of 25-hydroxycholecalciferol to 1,25-dihydroxy cholecalciferol. In addition, cisplatin may have a direct inhibitory effect on bone resorption. Carboplatin therapy, similar to cisplatin therapy, is associated with a 16 to 31% incidence of hypocalcemia. Plicamycin (mithramycin) is an antitumor antibiotic that inhibits deoxyribonucleic acid (DNA)-dependent ribonucleic acid (RNA) polymerase. This drug has a major effect on calcium metabolism. At a dose of 25 mg/kg, which is below the dose needed for antineoplastic effects, it inhibits bone resorption and lowers serum calcium concentration within 24 to 48 hours. Plicamycin inhibits basal- and thyroid hormone-stimulated osteoclast function by a mechanism that is unclear. The effect of plicamycin on osteoclast function has made plicamycin useful for treating Paget's disease of the bone and osteoclast-mediated hypercalcemia associated with malignancy. The hypocalcemic effect of plicamycin, as well as its hepatic and renal toxicity, has limited usefulness as an anticancer agent. Dactinomycin is another antitumor antibiotic that blocks DNA-directed RNA synthesis, causing hypocalcemia in animals. Dactinomycin also abolishes the calcium-mobilizing effect of thyroid hormone, presumably by interfering with osteoclast-mediated bone resorption. Asymptomatic hypomagnesemia, hypocalcemia, and hypoparathyroidism have also been reported in patients treated with a combination of doxorubicin and cytarabine.

Hypercalcemia The incidence of hypercalcemia in cancer patients is approximately 1%.[74] Hypercalcemia in cancer patients is a poor prognostic sign associated with a short survival. The paraneoplastic syndrome of hypercalcemia of malignancy is discussed in the section "Endocrine Paraneoplastic Syndromes ('Ectopic' Hormone Production)" below. No chemotherapy has been identified as a cause of hypercalcemia. However, there is a clear association between low-dose (usually 2–7.5 Gy) external beam irradiation of the head and neck area and subsequent development of primary hyperparathyroidism. There is a 2.5- to 3-fold increase in the incidence of primary hyperparathyroidism after low-dose irradiation of the neck.[75] Among patients who developed primary hyperparathyroidism, 14 to 30% had prior exposure to radiation. The interval from irradiation to development of hyperparathyroidism ranges from 29 to 47 years.

Hypomagnesemia Cisplatin causes morphologic changes and necrosis in the proximal tubule, an important site of magnesium reabsorption. Hypomagnesemia occurs in approximately 90% of patients treated with cisplatin,[76] and 10% of the hypomagnesemic patients have symptoms of muscle weakness, tremors, and dizziness. Vigorous hydration and the use of osmotic diuretics such as mannitol may prevent renal failure, but has little effect on renal magnesium wasting. Hypomagnesemia may persist long after cessation of cisplatin therapy. There are no large series in the literature addressing the incidence of hypomagnesemia, but the information from the manufacturer indicates that 60% of those taking cisplatin may be affected. Hypomagnesemia also occurs in patients who receive cyclophosphamide and carboplatin.

Disorders of Lipid Metabolism Short-term lipid abnormalities caused by cancer therapy are generally of little clinical significance. However, major abnormalities can lead to acute complications. Interferons and vitamin A derivatives can cause significant increases in triglycerides that can lead to pancreatitis. Interferons cause hypertriglyceridemia by increasing hepatic and peripheral fatty acid production[77] and by suppressing hepatic triglyceride lipase.[78] Long-term treatment with interferon-α_2 causes hypertriglyceridemia in approximately one-third of patients, most of whom had previous serum lipid abnormalities. Serum triglyceride levels of more than 1,000 mg/dL are not unusual. In a case report, a therapeutic effect of diet and gemfibrozil was observed in the presence of continued interferon-α therapy.[79] All-*trans*-retinoic acid (tretinoin) and other derivatives, for example, 13-*cis*-retinoic acid (isotretinoin), have been used in the treatment of several malignancies, most notably head and neck cancers and acute promyelocytic leukemia. The effects on lipid metabolism are well characterized, although the mechanism of development of lipid abnormalities is less clear. These abnormalities include hypertriglyceridemia caused by elevated very-low-density lipoprotein levels, and hypercholesterolemia caused by increased low-density lipoprotein level. Retinoid-induced hypertriglyceridemia can cause stroke and pancreatitis. Hyperlipidemia associated with retinoid therapy has been treated with gemfibrozil or fish oil.

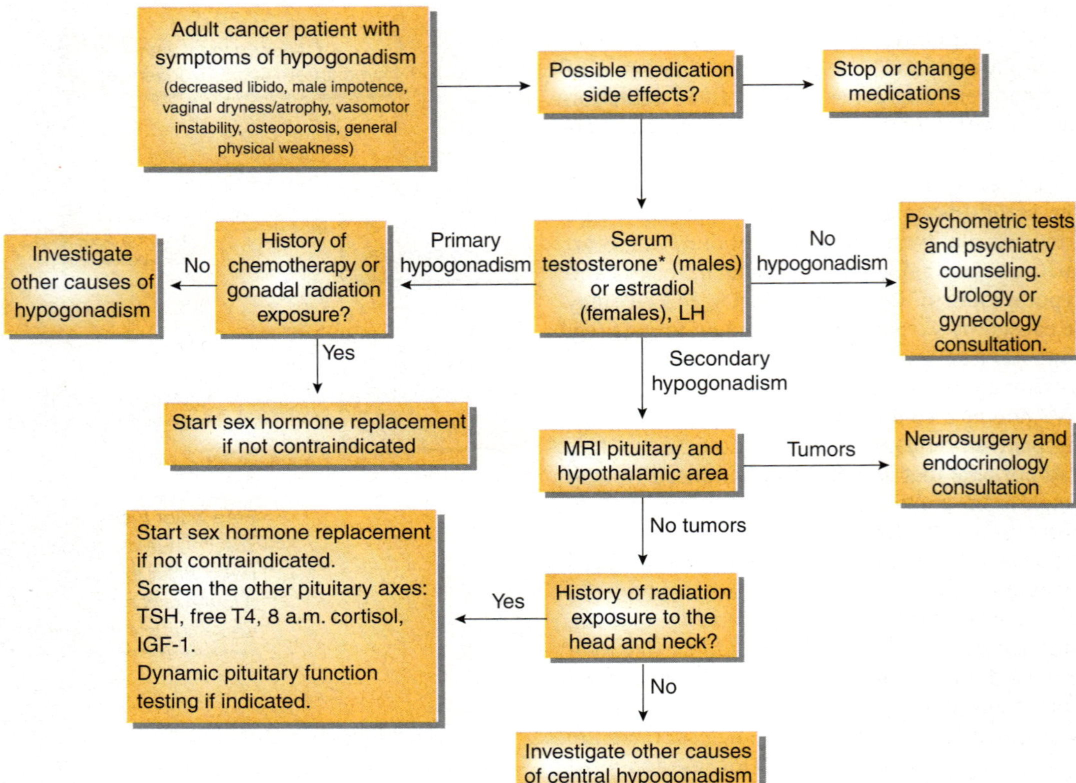

Figure 139-4 Approach to evaluation of hypogonadism in a cancer patient.

Sexual Dysfunction Radiation treatment to the head may cause a broad spectrum of hypothalamic-pituitary abnormalities (see Figure 139-1). The resultant thyroid, GH, or adrenal deficiency may indirectly affect reproductive function. Sexual function is directly affected by hyperprolactinemia or gonadotropin deficiency, commonly observed in patients treated with less than 40 Gy of cranial irradiation.

Hyperprolactinemia occurs commonly (up to 50% incidence within 2 years) following head and neck irradiation with a median hypothalamic-pituitary radiation exposure of 50 to 57 Gy.[4] Radiation damage to the hypothalamus leading to a loss of the normal inhibition of prolactin secretion is the proposed mechanism of hyperprolactinemia. Hyperprolactinemia inhibits the secretion of gonadotropin by the pituitary and decreases the responsiveness of the pituitary to gonadotropin-releasing hormone, thereby causing secondary hypogonadism. Dopaminergic therapy could reverse this process, and it may be reasonable to proceed with a therapeutic trial if other anterior pituitary functions are normal.

Gonadotropin deficiency occurs commonly (up to 61%) in patients treated with irradiation for brain tumors.[80] In children, delayed puberty, absent menarche, and inadequate sexual development are significant problems related to gonadotropin deficiency. Early or even precocious puberty has been reported in patients treated with combined chemotherapy and cranial irradiation for ALL[81] or cranial irradiation for brain tumor.[82] This phenomenon occurs more frequently in female patients. Concomitant GH deficiency is frequently noted, although its role in the development of precocious puberty is unclear.

In adults, gonadotropin deficiency may cause sex hormone deficiency and sexual dysfunction. Sex hormone deficiency may alter libido and adversely affect bone and lipid metabolism. Sexual dysfunction and impotence need to be evaluated and appropriately treated. Figure 139-4 outlines a diagnostic algorithm for the evaluation of hypogonadism.

Gonadal complications are discussed in Chapter 138, "Gonadal Complications," and gonadal dysfunction caused by anticancer therapy has been reviewed.[68]

ENDOCRINE PARANEOPLASTIC SYNDROMES ("ECTOPIC" HORMONE PRODUCTION)

Among the more interesting and protean manifestations of cancer is the production of hormonal substances that produce unique clinical syndromes. These syndromes can be classified broadly into several different types. The first is the production of a hormonal substance by a cell type that normally produces the hormone. Examples include parathyroid hormone production by a parathyroid cancer, production of calcitonin by medullary thyroid carcinoma, and serotonin by carcinoid tumors. In each of these examples a malignancy of a differentiated cell type continues to produce its normal product, but does so in a manner that is largely independent of the normal regulatory processes. These clinical syndromes are discussed in the relevant chapters in this text that discuss these malignancies. The second type, to be discussed in detail here, is the "ectopic" production of a hormone by a cell type that does not normally produce the hormonal substance or produces it normally at very low levels. In some examples, the cell may have produced the hormonal product at an earlier stage in its development. An example of this is PTHrP production by a squamous cell carcinoma. PTHrP is normally expressed in differentiating squamous cells, but is not expressed or is expressed at low levels in differentiated squamous epithelium.[83] A second type of ectopic hormone production occurs in a hormone-producing cell whose machinery has been co-opted to produce another hormone. An example of this is the production of ACTH by a wide spectrum of neuroendocrine tumor types including small-cell carcinoma of the lung.

Production of peptides by neuroendocrine tumors comprises the most common of the ectopic hormone syndromes. Neuroendocrine cells are dispersed throughout nearly all organs. Prominent are lung, gastrointestinal tract, pancreas, thyroid gland, adrenal medulla, breast, prostate, and skin. These cells are most commonly derived from neural crest and produce biogenic amines and polypeptide hormones. The list of hormones produced by tumors derived from members of this group of neuroendocrine cells includes ACTH, calcitonin, vasoactive intestinal peptide (VIP), bombesin, growth hormone-releasing hormone (GHRH), pancreatic polypeptide, corticotropin-releasing hormone (CRH), neurotensin, somatostatin (SRIH), and other small peptides.

Defined Clinical Syndromes There are clearly defined clinical ectopic hormone syndromes that occur with some frequency. It is important for the practicing oncologist to recognize these syndromes. Their recognition may help in the definition of the cancer type and lead to appropriate management approaches. In addition, these syndromes are a major cause of morbidity and mortality; treatment approaches are available for many of these syndromes.

Ectopic ACTH Production Inappropriate secretion of ACTH, although uncommon, is an important cause of morbidity and mortality in certain types of malignancies. There are at least two different mechanisms: ectopic ACTH production or ectopic production of CRH, the hypothalamic peptide that normally stimulates ACTH synthesis and release.

The most common cause of ectopic ACTH production is the expression of pro-opiomelanocortin (POMC) by a tumor. Post-translational processing of POMC normally proceeds down one of two mutually exclusive pathways.[84] The POMC precursor can be cleaved in two different ways to produce peptides with very different biologic activities. The pathway that leads to ACTH production and Cushing's syndrome is one in which POMC is cleaved to produce big melanocyte-stimulating hormone and ACTH. Fortunately for cancer patients, the enzymes that cleave POMC to produce ACTH are expressed uncommonly outside of the normal pituitary gland. As such, most malignant tumors expressing the *POMC* gene produce peptides that produce no identifiable clinical syndrome. The most common tumor associated with ACTH production is small-cell lung cancer (SCLC), although a broader spectrum of tumors including pulmonary carcinoid, medullary thyroid carcinoma, islet cell malignancy, pheochromocytoma, and occasional ganglioneuromas will produce this hormone. The clinical syndrome produced by "ectopic" production of ACTH is characterized by adrenal cortical hyperplasia and hypercortisolism.[85]

The second cause of excessive ACTH production is tumor production of corticotropin-releasing hormone.[86] Ectopic production of this peptide causes a clinical syndrome characterized by pituitary corticotrope hyperplasia leading to adrenal cortical hyperplasia and Cushing's syndrome. Identification of excessive CRH production requires that the clinician consider this possibility and measure CRH in blood. Neoplasms that can produce CRH include medullary thyroid carcinoma, paragangliomas, prostate cancer, and islet cell neoplasms. There are examples of cancers that produce both ACTH and CRH.

Patients with ectopic ACTH syndrome may present with clinical features of Cushing's syndrome—easy bruising, centripetal obesity, muscle wasting, hypertension, diabetes, and metabolic alkalosis predominate. Alternatively, patients with rapidly growing SCLC may present with a clinical syndrome characterized by wasting, muscle atrophy, profound hypokalemic metabolic alkalosis and hypertension without the other clinical findings of Cushing's syndrome.

The hallmark of ectopic ACTH syndrome is the finding of an elevated plasma ACTH concentration. However, in the differential diagnosis of hypercorticism with an elevated plasma ACTH concentration, the clinician should consider the possibility of an ACTH-producing pituitary tumor.[87] Differentiation between pituitary ACTH production and ectopic tumor production of ACTH or ectopic CRH production, mimicking a pituitary tumor, is among the most difficult diagnostic work-ups in the discipline of endocrinology. There are numerous examples where a patient with ectopic ACTH syndrome has been incorrectly labeled as pituitary Cushing's disease (ACTH production by a pituitary tumor).[88] In a similar manner, the oncologist confronted with a patient with a malignant neoplasm and clinical features of Cushing's syndrome should not assume a diagnosis of ectopic ACTH syndrome without considering other diagnostic possibilities that include primary adrenal corticosteroid production or a pituitary ACTH-producing tumor. In some cases, such as ectopic ACTH production by a SCLC, the clinical syndrome (hypokalemia, metabolic alkalosis, hypertension, exceedingly high plasma cortisol levels, and a rapidly growing tumor), the diagnosis will be straightforward.[89] In other cases, particularly those with tumors that have not been associated with frequent ectopic ACTH production, the diagnosis can be challenging and require the assistance of an endocrinologist experienced in this area and with full access to the full spectrum of interventional radiologic techniques used to differentiate pituitary from nonpituitary sources of ACTH.

The diagnostic evaluation is based on the measurement of plasma ACTH in a patient with hypercorticism (Figure 139-5). A plasma ACTH concentration greater than 100 pg/mL should prompt investigation for an ectopic source of ACTH.[90] In patients with an ACTH value below 10 pg/mL (collected under appropriate conditions to prevent degradation of ACTH), a primary adrenocortical process (adrenal adenoma or carcinoma) should be considered. The majority of patients will fall into the range of ACTH values between 10 and 100 pg/mL. The major differential diagnostic possibilities in these patients include a central (pituitary) or peripheral (ectopic) source of ACTH, with production of ectopic CRH by a tumor-producing central ACTH production a rare possibility. Differentiation between central and peripheral sources of ACTH is accomplished by several approaches. The identification of a pituitary tumor by MRI provides a presumptive diagnosis of a pituitary source, although pituitary tumors that are nonfunctional or produce another hormonal product occur with some frequency. For this reason petrosal venous sinus sampling is often employed.[91] The diagnosis of ectopic CRH production can only be made by suspecting this diagnosis and measuring the plasma concentration of this peptide. It is also possible to use other approaches to diagnose ectopic ACTH syndrome. ACTH production from a tumor is not generally suppressed by a high-dose of dexamethasone. In patients with an ACTH > 10 pg/mL, administration of a single 8 mg oral dose of dexamethasone at 11 pm followed with measurement of serum cortisol level at 8 am permits differentiation between central and peripheral sources.[85] In pituitary Cushing's syndrome, dexamethasone will generally suppress ACTH by 50%; this strategy will not generally suppress ACTH production by a tumor. False-positive or false-negative results occur with each of these testing procedures.

Surgical removal or treatment of the tumor with chemotherapeutic agents is the primary therapy for an ACTH- or CRH-producing tumor. Patients with these tumors should have electrolyte abnormalities, diabetes mellitus, and hypertension corrected prior to a planned surgical procedure. Patients with long-standing Cushing's syndrome and elevated plasma cortisol values have higher morbidity and mortality postoperatively. Preoperative treatment options include metyrapone (1–4 g/d orally), aminoglutethimide (250 mg orally four times per day with upward titration), or ketoconazole (200–400 mg twice a day orally).[92] Parenteral etomidate, used for sedation and induction of anesthesia, rapidly inhibits cortisol synthesis at sub-

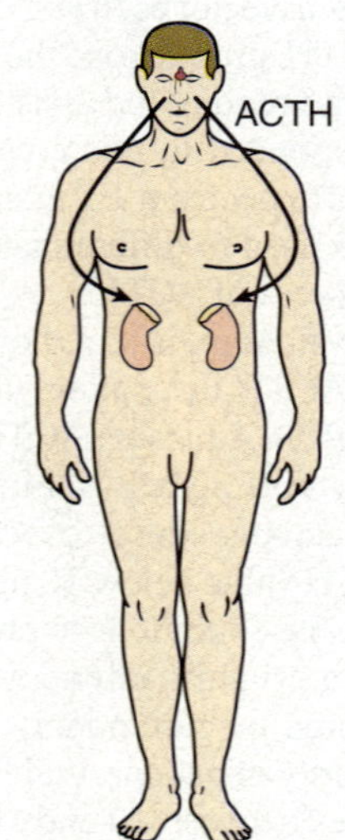

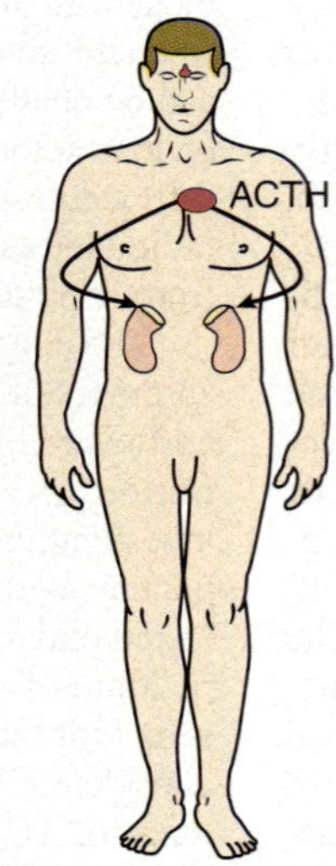

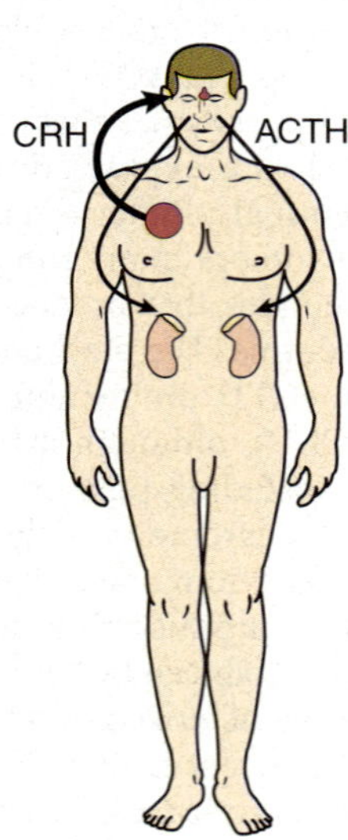

Figure 139-5 Differential diagnosis of adrenocorticotropin (ACTH)-dependent Cushing's syndrome. It is difficult to differentiate between a pituitary (left panel) and ectopic (midpanel) source of ACTH, the most common causes of ACTH-dependent Cushing's syndrome. To differentiate with certainty, placement of catheters in veins draining the pituitary gland (inferior petrosal sinuses) combined with stimulation by exogenous corticotropin-releasing hormone permits differentiation with certainty (discussed in text). Ectopic corticotropin-releasing hormone (CRH) production by a tumor results in increased ACTH production by the pituitary gland (right panel). It is difficult to differentiate between ectopic CRH production and pituitary-dependent Cushing's syndrome, necessitating the measurement of CRH in peripheral blood to make the diagnosis with certainty. Malignant tumors occasionally produce both CRH and ACTH, further complicating the diagnostic evaluation (not shown).

hypnotic concentrations.[93] It is titrated from 0.3 to 4 mg/kg/h to normalize serum cortisol measurements and has been used to rapidly reverse hypercorticism in a small number of patients. Replacement glucocorticoid therapy is needed when pharmacologic inhibitors of cortisol production are used to prevent adrenal insufficiency. If surgical removal of an ACTH- or CRH-producing tumor is not possible or inadvisable, chronic therapy with inhibitors of cortisol synthesis may be required. Alternatively, laparoscopic adrenalectomy with subsequent replacement of corticosteroids provides a rapid and generally safe approach to management of hypercorticism. This technique is probably underutilized as a therapeutic strategy for management of ectopic ACTH syndrome.

Patients with rapidly progressive SCLC and ectopic ACTH syndrome form a unique subset of patients because of the need to initiate chemotherapy on a timely basis. Unfortunately, these patients are also highly susceptible to opportunistic infections and initiation of therapy will often lead to death or serious morbidity related to infection.[94] The central dilemma in these patients is that a period of 1 to 2 weeks may be required for pharmacologic inhibitors of cortisol synthesis to normalize the serum cortisol (and a longer period may be required for normalization of immunity), a delay in the initiation of chemotherapy that is generally deemed unacceptable from an oncologic perspective. Laparoscopic adrenalectomy, a straightforward and well-tolerated technique following normalization of electrolyte abnormalities and hypertension, may provide a strategy for rapid normalization of excessive cortisol secretion. Prophylactic therapy for opportunistic infections caused by *Pneumocystis carinii* or fungi should be considered if chemotherapy is initiated shortly after normalization of the serum cortisol.

Hypercalcemia Caused by Malignancy Hypercalcemia is a common and serious cause of morbidity and mortality in cancer patients.

The most common causes of hypercalcemia in patients with cancer are parathyroid hormone-related protein (PTHrP)-mediated hypercalcemia; increased production of the active metabolite of vitamin D, calcitriol or 1,25 dihydroxy vitamin D3; and localized osteolytic hypercalcemia.[95,96] Ectopic production of PTH is a rare cause of cancer-associated hypercalcemia. Other causes of hypercalcemia, most notably primary hyperparathyroidism, should be considered in the cancer patient with hypercalcemia. Measurement of serum intact parathyroid hormone (iPTH) permits differentiation between hyperparathyroidism and a number of other causes of hypercalcemia. The combination of hypercalcemia and an elevated parathyroid hormone level combined with increased urinary calcium excretion provides reasonable evidence for primary hyperparathyroidism. Suppression of the iPTH below the normal range is found in PTHrP or calcitriol-mediated hypercalcemia. Other less common causes of hypercalcemia in cancer will be discussed below.

Parathyroid Hormone–Related Protein Parathyroid hormone-related protein (PTHrP) is a small peptide in which 8 of the first 16 amino acids are identical to PTH. This small peptide causes hypercalcemia by binding to the PTH receptor and activating the expression of an osteoblast-specific cell surface protein, RANK ligand (RANKL). Interaction between RANKL and the RANK receptor on the osteoclast precursor causes increased osteoclast differentiation, bone resorption, and hypercalcemia. Other PTH-like actions of PTHrp include hypophosphatemia and increased urinary calcium excretion. PTHrP-mediated hypercalcemia is characterized by a suppressed iPTH level and a low or normal calcitriol level. This contrasts with the finding of elevated iPTH and calcitriol levels in primary hyperparathyroidism. PTHrP production is found commonly in squamous cell carcinomas; other tumors that produce it include breast, neuroendocrine, renal, melanoma, and prostate tumors.

Calcitriol Production by Malignant Tumors Lymphoma commonly produces calcitriol, leading to increased gastrointestinal absorption of calcium. Lymphomatous tissue, like granulomatous tissue seen in sarcoid, berylliosis, tuberculosis, and fungal infection, expresses 1α-hydroxylase, the enzyme that converts 25 hydroxy vitamin D3 to calcitriol. Clinical studies show that a high percentage of lymphoma patients have hypercalciuria at the time of diagnosis; a smaller percentage have frank hypercalcemia.[97] The characteristic clinical features of hypercalcemia in the context of lymphoma include a suppressed serum iPTH, a normal or slightly increased phosphorus level (caused by the suppression of PTH), hypercalciuria, absence of bone metastasis, and an elevated serum calcitriol level in approximately one-half of hypercalcemic patients.[97]

Localized Osteolytic Bone Resorption Causing Hypercalcemia Certain malignancies metastasize to bone frequently and some cause hypercalcemia. Hypercalcemia associated with breast cancer and myeloma is common. In contrast, prostate cancer, despite its more frequent presence in bone, rarely produces hypercalcemia. Malignancies that cause hypercalcemia produce cytokines, PTHrP, or other factors that stimulate increased bone resorption.[95,96] Perhaps the best characterized is the production of PTHrP by breast carcinoma cells. There is compelling evidence in animal models that PTHrP production by breast cancer cells stimulates osteoclastic resorption and release of transforming growth factor (TGF)-β from normal bone. In this animal model TGF-β release from bone stimulates proliferation of breast carcinoma growth, setting up a loop in which PTHrP production not only stimulates increased osteoclastic resorption, but also accelerates growth of adjacent breast cancer.[98,99] Indeed, this thought process led to an examination of and subsequent approval of bisphosphonates, a class of drugs that inhibits osteoclast bone resorption, for prevention of breast cancer metastasis.[100]

In multiple myeloma, several factors contribute to localized osteolysis. Increased expression of RANKL, causing localized osteoclast proliferation, appears to be the most important cause. Other factors that may contribute to osteoclast proliferation in myeloma are interleukin-6 and macrophage inflammatory protein 1α, although they appear to be less important than RANKL.[96]

Impact of Malignancy-Related Hypercalcemia Severe hypercalcemia in the context of malignancy is associated with a shortened life span. The average survival for patients with severe and unresponsive hypercalcemia can be measured in weeks to months. The causes of death include complications of hypercalcemia (coma, renal failure) and progression of tumor. The development of hypercalcemia is often, although not always, an indicator of tumor progression in the face of adequate therapy. Since it is not always possible to predict which patients will respond to oncologic therapy, it is important to treat hypercalcemia in all newly diagnosed patients with cancer. Whether to continue to treat recurrent and/or refractory hypercalcemia is a decision that should be based on response of the causative tumor to oncologic therapy and the overall prognosis of the patient. Severe hypercalcemia frequently causes depression of cerebral function or coma, a clinical situation that may reduce suffering in a dying patient.

Therapy of Hypercalcemia Dehydration is a common finding in hypercalcemic patients. Increased urine excretion of calcium causes a concentrating defect leading to increased fluid loss. Initial management should focus on the reversal of dehydration by infusion of a solution of normal saline at rates between 100 and 300 mL/h. Hydration will commonly lower the serum calcium by 10 to 40% over a period of 6 to 12 hours. Patients with severe hypercalcemia, defined as a serum calcium concentration > 13 mg/dL (3.25 mmol/L), an alteration of mental status, or evidence of renal dysfunction attributable to hypercalcemia should be treated with either intravenous pamidronate (60–90 mg over 4 h) or zoledronate (4 mg over 30 min),[101] glucocorticoids (40–60 mg/d prednisone equivalent), or gallium nitrate (200 mg/m^2/d, infused daily for 7 days).[102,103] Salmon calcitonin may lower the serum calcium concentration by 1 to 2 mg/dL early in the treatment course, but is rarely effective long term. These drugs are sometimes used in combination or sequentially in a patient who is poorly responsive. Glucocorticoids, which inhibit calcium absorption, are most commonly used as primary therapy for lymphoma, whereas bisphosphonate therapy is more likely to be effective in hypercalcemia associated with solid tumors. Zoledronate is generally more effective than pamidronate because of its increased potency.[104]

There are several new therapies for treatment of hypercalcemia in early stages of development that show considerable promise. A monoclonal antibody directed against RANKL prevents its interaction with the RANK receptor on osteoclast precursors, thereby reducing osteoclast-mediated bone resorption.[105] Preliminary studies with this antibody (AMG 162) have shown it to be an effective inhibitor of bone resorption and clinical studies are currently underway to establish its efficacy in patients with hypercalcemia and bone metastasis. A second therapeutic approach undergoing clinical evaluation is the use of humanized PTHrP monoclonal antibodies.[106] Such an approach has potential not only to normalize PTHrP-mediated hypercalcemia, but also to prevent bone metastasis facilitated by PTHrP production by cancer cells.

Human Chorionic Gonadotropin Human chorionic gonadotropin (HCG) is formed from two different protein subunits encoded by separate genes. The first is the α subunit that is shared by all members of the pituitary class of glycoprotein hormones including HCG, luteinizing hormone (LH), follicle-stimulating hormone (FSH), and thyroid-stimulating hormone (TSH). The second, the β subunit, is unique for each of these hormones. Production of HCG is found in trophoblastic tumors (choriocarcinomas, testicular embryonal carcinomas, and seminomas) and, uncommonly, in tumors of the lung and pancreas. In younger children, precocious puberty, caused by HCG stimulation of ovarian function, is seen. In adult males, gynecomastia is a common occurrence. Hyperthyroidism may develop from an interaction of HCG with the thyroid-stimulating hormone receptor (TSHR) particularly when β-HCG is expressed at high levels.

Removal or effective therapy for the underlying tumor is the most effective therapy for clinical syndromes caused by excessive β-HCG production. Hyperthyroidism can be treated short term with thionamide therapy if there is belief that chemotherapy or other strategies to treat the underlying malignancy are likely to be effective. In patients with less responsive tumors, thyroidectomy or radioactive iodine may be required.

Hypoglycemia Tumor-induced hypoglycemia is an uncommon but challenging cause of morbidity for cancer patients. Three different clinical syndromes have been identified. First, insulin can be produced by islet cell malignancy. Islet cell tumors commonly produce low levels of insulin that are clinically insignificant until a large amount of tumor, most commonly in the form of hepatic metastasis, develops. A second cause is insufficient gluconeogenesis, seen in patients with near complete replacement of hepatic parenchyma by tumor, interfering with or eliminating enzymatic production of glucose. The third form is caused by increased concentrations of insulin-like growth factor II (IGF-II), a peptide that activates the insulin receptor. This syndrome is most commonly seen in patients with fibrosarcomas, hemangiopericytomas, or hepatomas. In these patients IGF-II levels are most commonly elevated, the result of a failure of IGF binding protein 3 (IGFBP3) and acid labile subunit to form a complex capable of binding IGF-II efficiently. The elevated circulating IGF-II activates the insulin receptor and causes hypoglycemia.[107–109]

The most common presentation for each of these clinical syndromes is fasting hypoglycemia, and patients are most likely to develop symptoms during normal periods of fasting, particularly during nocturnal hours. Measurement of a plasma insulin, proinsulin, and C-peptide during a period of hypoglycemia is the most important diagnostic tool for separating the first clinical type (insulin production) from the second (replacement of liver by tumor) and third (IGF-II) types. The finding of elevated insulin, proinsulin, and C-peptide in the face of hypoglycemia (and the absence of any drugs that might stimulate insulin release from normal pancreas) makes a compelling case for unregulated insulin production as a cause of the hypoglycemia. In contrast, insulin, proinsulin, and C-peptide levels will be low in tumor replacement of the liver or IGF-II–mediated hypoglycemia. Laboratory findings in IGF-II–mediated hypoglycemia include an elevated serum IGF-II; low or normal insulin, proinsulin, and C-peptide measurements; low IGF-I levels; and generally normal IGFBP3 or acid labile subunit measurements in the context of a large sarcoma or retroperitoneal tumor.

Surgical excision or antineoplastic therapy to reduce tumor mass is effective in insulin or IGF-II–mediated hypoglycemia; there is little effective therapy for hepatic replacement by tumor other than providing glucose. Hypoglycemia is treated with frequent meals. Patients may remain symptom-free by being awakened for caloric intake during nocturnal hours. A continuous infusion of 20% dextrose through a central venous line may be required to maintain normal blood glucose in patients, particularly those with hepatic replacement by tumors. Glucagon infusion (0.5–2 mg/h) to stimulate hepatic gluconeogenesis is also an effective therapy for patients with insulin-producing tumors or those with IGF-II–mediated hypoglycemia. It is important to document a response to glucagon (1 mg subcutaneously with measurement of plasma glucose at 30 and 60 min following injection) before trying this therapeutic approach. Glucagon can be administered in small volumes (1–5 mL over 24 h), making it possible to use small infusion pumps.[110] Patients treated with glucagon may develop the characteristic rash associated with glucagonoma, necessitating discontinuance of this treatment modality. Other therapies that have been applied with periodic success include recombinant growth hormone (3 to 6 μg/kg subcutaneously daily) or glucocorticoids (20–40 mg prednisone equivalents per day). Octreotide or lanreotide have been used in patients with insulin-producing islet cell tumors, generally without success. The lack of success may relate to the fact that somatostatin analogs currently available are more effective for inhibiting glucagon than insulin secretion. Diazoxide (3–8 mg/kg/d in 2–3 divided doses) has been used successfully to inhibit insulin secretion, but causes fluid retention, thereby limiting its usefulness at effective doses.

Hypoglycemia may also occur in patients with lactic acidosis in the context of end-stage leukemia or lymphoma. This clinical syndrome occurs in patients with end-stage or extensive disease and leukemic/lymphomatous involvement of the liver. It is hypothesized that lactic acid production by tumor cells exceeds the ability of the liver to clear it. The etiology of the hypoglycemia is unclear, but may result from impaired hepatic gluconeogenesis.[111]

Syndrome of Inappropriate Antidiuretic Hormone SIADH was discussed earlier (see "Disorders of Electrolyte/Mineral Metabolism: Hyponatremia") as a side effect of cancer therapy. In addition, approximately 15% of SCLC, 1% of other lung cancers, and 3% of squamous cell head and neck cancers produce vasopressin in an unregulated manner, leading to hyponatremia, hypo-osmolality, increased urine sodium excretion, and an inappropriately high urine osmolality relative to the plasma tonicity.[112] In addition, other benign or malignant neoplasms that include primary brain tumors, hematologic neoplasms, skin tumors, and gastrointestinal, gynecologic, breast, and prostate cancers, and sarcomas, can produce this clinical syndrome.

Most patients who develop this syndrome are asymptomatic. In cases where the serum sodium concentration falls below 120 mEq/L, altered mental status and seizures may develop. In particular, women of reproductive age who develop hyponatremia may develop profound cerebral degeneration. Fluid restriction can be used effectively for short-term management, but treatment with demeclocycline (150–300 mg/d), an agent that inhibits the effects of vasopressin on the kidney, is preferable for long-term treatment. Vasopressin receptor antagonists are in clinical trials but are not currently available.

OTHER ECTOPIC HORMONE SYNDROMES **Tumor-Induced Osteomalacia** Severe hypophosphatemia caused by renal phosphate wasting is the hallmark of tumor-induced osteomalacia. This clinical syndrome is characterized by osteomalacia, caused by inadequate mineralization of osteoid, and moderate to severe proximal myopathy.[113] Tumors that produce this clinical syndrome include mesenchymal tumors (osteoblastomas, giant cell osteosarcomas, hemangiopericytomas, hemangiomas, nonossifying fibromas)[114] and, rarely, malignant tumors such as prostate or lung cancer. There is evidence that fibroblast growth factor-23, a member of the fibroblast growth factor family that is mutated in autosomal dominant osteomalacia,[115] is overexpressed by some neoplasms causing tumor-induced osteomalacia.[116] Oral or intravenous supplementation of phosphate combined with vitamin D therapy is generally effective for eradicating or improving clinical symptoms. Complete surgical removal of the tumor is generally curative.

Erythropoietin, Thrombopoietin, Leukopoietin, or Colony-Stimulating Factor Production Polycythemia caused by ectopic erythropoietin production is a rare clinical syndrome. It is found in cerebellar hemangioblastoma, uterine fibroids, pheochromocytomas, and renal cell, ovarian and hepatic cancers.[117,118] Treatment can include surgical or chemotherapy reduction of tumor mass or phlebotomy. Other less well-defined syndromes include production of thrombopoietin, leukopoietin, or colony-stimulating factor by some tumors. These conditions are treated by appropriate chemotherapy to reduce its size or by surgical removal.

Renin Production Production of renin by renal (Wilms' tumor, renal cell carcinoma, or hemangiopericytoma), lung (SCLC, adenocarcinoma), hepatic, pancreatic, or ovarian carcinomas can produce a clinical syndrome characterized by hypertension, hypokalemia, and evidence of increased aldosterone production.[119] Therapy with spironolactone (Aldactone), angiotensin-converting enzyme, or angiotensin receptor antagonist inhibitors may lower the blood pressure and normalize electrolyte abnormalities in patients in whom the tumor cannot be resected.

Growth Hormone and Prolactin Acromegaly is a condition characterized by elevated growth hormone and IGF-1 values, most commonly caused by a pituitary tumor. There are uncommon examples of GH production by lung and gastric adenocarcinomas. Ectopic production of growth hormone releasing hormone, the hypothalamic peptide that normally regulates GH production by the pituitary,[120] has been demonstrated for islet cell tumors, bronchogenic carcinoids, and SCLC. Ectopic prolactin production is found rarely in gonadoblastoma,[121] lymphoma,[119] leukemia,[122] and colorectal cancer.[123] The clinical syndrome includes galactorrhea and amenorrhea in women and hypogonadism and gynecomastia in men. Dopamine agonists (bromocriptine, quinagolide, or cabergoline), effective for treatment of pituitary prolactinomas, are generally ineffective for treatment of ectopic prolactin production.

REFERENCES

1. Fassett DR, Couldwell WT. Metastases to the pituitary gland. Neurosurg Focus 2004;16:E8.
2. Lam KS, Tse VK, Wang C, et al. Effects of cranial irradiation on hypothalamic-pituitary function—a 5-year longitudinal study in patients with nasopharyngeal carcinoma. Q J Med 1991;78:165–76.
3. Pai HH, Thornton A, Katznelson L, et al. Hypothalamic/pituitary function following high-dose conformal radiotherapy to the base of skull: demonstration of a dose-effect relationship using dose-volume histogram analysis. Int J Radiat Oncol Biol Phys 2001;49:1079–92.
4. Samaan NA, Schultz PN, Yang KP, et al. Endocrine complications after radiotherapy for tumors of the head and neck. J Lab Clin Med 1987;109:364–72.
5. Shalet SM. Disorders of the endocrine system due to radiation and cytotoxic chemotherapy. Clin Endocrinol (Oxf) 1983;19:637–59.
6. Vassilopoulou-Sellin R, Klein MJ. Physical growth parameters in children treated for malignant diseases. Int J Hematol Oncol 1996;3:213–9.
7. Garnick MB, Larsen PR. Acute deficiency of thyroxine-binding globulin during L-asparaginase therapy. N Engl J Med 1979;301:252–3.
8. Djurica SN, Plecas V, Milojevic Z, et al. Direct effects of cytostatic therapy on the functional state of the thyroid gland and TBG in serum of patients. Exp Clin Endocrinol 1990;96:57–63.
9. Beex L, Ross A, Smals A, Kloppenborg P. 5-Fluorouracil-induced increase of total serum thyroxine and triiodothyronine. Cancer Treat Rep 1977;61:1291–5.
10. van Seters AP, Moolenaar AJ. Mitotane increases the blood levels of hormone-binding proteins. Acta Endocrinol (Copenh) 1991;124:526–33.
11. Chopra IJ. Clinical review 86: Euthyroid sick syndrome: is it a misnomer? J Clin Endocrinol Metab 1997;82:329–34.
12. Tami TA, Gomez P, Parker GS, et al. Thyroid dysfunction after radiation therapy in head and neck cancer patients. Am J Otolaryngol 1992;13:357–62.
13. Grande C. Hypothyroidism following radiotherapy for head and neck cancer: multivariate analysis of risk factors. Radiother Oncol 1992;25:31–6.
14. Tamura K, Shimaoka K, Friedman M. Thyroid abnormalities associated with treatment of malignant lymphoma. Cancer 1981;47:2704–11.
15. Hancock SL, Cox RS, McDougall IR. Thyroid diseases after treatment of Hodgkin's disease. N Engl J Med 1991;325:599–605.
16. Constine LS, Donaldson SS, McDougall IR, et al. Thyroid dysfunction after radiotherapy in children with Hodgkin's disease. Cancer 1984;53:878–83.
17. Devney RB, Sklar CA, Nesbit ME Jr, et al. Serial thyroid function measurements in children with Hodgkin disease. J Pediatr 1984;105:223–7.
18. Schimpff SC, Diggs CH, Wiswell JG, et al. Radiation-related thyroid dysfunction: implications for the treatment of Hodgkin's disease. Ann Int Med 1980;92:91–8.
19. Fuks Z, Glatstein E, Marsa GW, et al. Long-term effects on external radiation on the pituitary and thyroid glands. Cancer 1976;37:1152–61.
20. Joensuu H, Viikari J. Thyroid function after postoperative radiation therapy in patients with breast cancer. Acta Radiol Oncol 1986;25:167–70.
21. Sklar CA, Kim TH, Ramsay NK. Thyroid dysfunction among long-term survivors of bone marrow transplantation. Am J Med 1982;73:688–94.
22. Boulad F, Bromley M, Black P, et al. Thyroid dysfunction following bone marrow transplantation using hyperfractionated radiation. Bone Marrow Transplantation 1995;15:71–6.
23. Toubert ME, Socie G, Gluckman E, et al. Short- and long-term follow-up of thyroid dysfunction after allogeneic bone marrow transplantation without the use of preparative total body irradiation. Br J Haematol 1997;98:453–7.
24. Sutcliffe SB, Chapman R, Wrigley PF. Cyclical combination chemotherapy and thyroid function in patients with advanced Hodgkin's disease. Med Pediatr Oncol 1981;9:439–48.
25. Ogilvy-Stuart AL, Shalet SM, Gattamaneni HR. Thyroid function after treatment of brain tumors in children. J Pediatr 1991;119:733–7.
26. Heidemann PH, Stubbe P, Beck W. Transient secondary hypothyroidism and thyroxine binding globulin deficiency in leukemic children during polychemotherapy: an effect of L-asparaginase. Eur J Pediatr 1981;136:291–5.
27. Krouse RS, Royal RE, Heywood G, et al. Thyroid dysfunction in 281 patients with metastatic melanoma or renal carcinoma treated with interleukin-2 alone. J Immunother Emphasis Tumor Immunol 1995;18:272–8.
28. Vassilopoulou-Sellin R, Sella A, Dexeus FH, et al. Acute thyroid dysfunction (thyroiditis) after therapy with interleukin-2. Horm Metab Res 1992;24:434–8.
29. Baudin E, Marcellin P, Pouteau M, et al. Reversibility of thyroid dysfunction induced by recombinant alpha interferon in chronic hepatitis C. Clin Endocrinol (Oxf) 1993;39:657–61.
30. Sherman SI. Etiology, diagnosis, and treatment recommendations for central hypothyroidism associated with bexarotene therapy for cutaneous T-cell lymphoma. Clin Lymphoma 2003;3:249–52.
31. Petersen M, Keeling CA, McDougall IR. Hyperthyroidism with low radioiodine uptake after head and neck irradiation for Hodgkin's disease. J Nucl Med 1989;30:255–7.
32. Wasnich RD, Grumet FC, Payne RO, Kriss JP. Graves' ophthalmopathy following external neck irradiation for nonthyroidal neoplastic disease. J Clin Endocrinol Metab 1973;37:703–13.
33. Hancock SL, McDougall IR, Constine LS. Thyroid abnormalities after therapeutic external radiation. Int J Radiat Oncol Biol Phys 1995;31:1165–70.
34. Kaplan MM, Garnick MB, Gelber R, et al. Risk factors for thyroid abnormalities after neck irradiation for childhood cancer. Am J Med 1983;74:272–80.
35. Ron E, Lubin JH, Shore RE, et al. Thyroid cancer after exposure to external radiation: a pooled analysis of seven studies. Radiat Res 1995;141:259–77.
36. Hallquist A, Hardell L, Degerman A, et al. Medical diagnostic and therapeutic ionizing radiation and the risk for thyroid cancer: a case-control study. Eur J Cancer Prev 1994;3:259–67.
37. Tucker MA, Jones PH, Boice JD Jr, et al. Therapeutic radiation at a young age is linked to secondary thyroid cancer. The Late Effects Study Group. Cancer Res 1991;51:2885–8.
38. Nakhjavani MK, Gharib H, Goellner JR, van Heerden JA. Metastasis to the thyroid gland. A report of 43 cases. Cancer 1997;79:574–8.
39. Schein PS, O'Connell MJ, Blom J, et al. Clinical antitumor activity and toxicity of streptozotocin (NSC-85998). Cancer 1974;34:993–1000.
40. Gillette PC, Hill LL, Starling KA, Fernbach DJ. Transient diabetes mellitus secondary to L-asparaginase therapy in acute leukemia. J Pediatr 1972;81:109–11.
41. Almawi WY, Tamim H, Azar ST. Clinical review 103: T helper type 1 and 2 cytokines mediate the onset and progression of type I (insulin-dependent) diabetes. J Clin Endocrinol Metab 1999;84:1497–502.
42. Drachenberg CB, Klassen DK, Weir MR, et al. Islet cell damage associated with tacrolimus and cyclosporine: morphological features in pancreas allograft biopsies and clinical correlation. Transplantation 1999;68:396–402.
43. Jindal RM, Sidner RA, Milgrom ML. Post-transplant diabetes mellitus. The role of immunosuppression. Drug Saf 1997;16:242–57.
44. Weiser MA, Cabanillas ME, Konopleva M, et al. Relation between the duration of remission and hyperglycemia

during induction chemotherapy for acute lymphocytic leukemia with a hyperfractionated cyclophosphamide, vincristine, doxorubicin, and dexamethasone/methotrexate-cytarabine regimen. Cancer 2004;100:1179–85.

45. Calle EE, Rodriguez C, Walker-Thurmond K, Thun MJ. Overweight, obesity, and mortality from cancer in a prospectively studied cohort of U.S. adults. N Engl J Med 2003;348:1625–38.
46. Vassilopoulou-Sellin R, Brosnan P, Delpassand A, et al. Osteopenia in young adult survivors of childhood cancer. Med Pediatr Oncol 1999;32:272–8.
47. Headley JA, Theriault RL, LeBlanc AD, et al. Pilot study of bone mineral density in breast cancer patients treated with adjuvant chemotherapy. Cancer Invest 1998;16:6–11.
48. Jones G, Sambrook PN. Drug-induced disorders of bone metabolism. Incidence, management and avoidance. Drug Saf 1994;10:480–9.
49. Schwartz AM, Leonidas JC. Methotrexate osteopathy. Skeletal Radiol 1984;11:13–6.
50. Atkinson SA, Halton JM, Bradley C, et al. Bone and mineral abnormalities in childhood acute lymphoblastic leukemia: influence of disease, drugs and nutrition. Int J Cancer Suppl 1998;11:35–9.
51. Bruning PF, Pit MJ, de Jong-Bakker M, et al. Bone mineral density after adjuvant chemotherapy for premenopausal breast cancer. Br J Cancer 1990;61:308–10.
52. Carlson K, Simonsson B, Ljunghall S. Acute effects of high-dose chemotherapy followed by bone marrow transplantation on serum markers of bone metabolism. Calcif Tissue Int 1994;55:408–11.
53. Brade WP, Herdrich K, Kachel-Fischer U, Araujo CE. Dosing and side-effects of ifosfamide plus mesna. J Cancer Res Clin Oncol 1991;117 Suppl 4:S164–86.
54. Moncrieff M, Foot A. Fanconi syndrome after ifosfamide. Cancer Chemother Pharmacol 1989;23:121–2.
55. Citrin DL, Wallemark CB, Nadler R, et al. Estramustine affects bone mineral metabolism in metastatic prostate cancer. Cancer 1986;58:2208–13.
56. Abrams H, Spiro R, Goldstein N. Metastasis in carcinoma—one thousand autopsied cases. Cancer 1950;3:74
57. Hussain S, Belldegrun A, Seltzer SE, et al. CT diagnosis of adrenal abnormalities in patients with primary non-adrenal malignancies. Eur J Radiol 1986;6:127–31.
58. Platts JK, Drew PJ, Harvey JN. Death from phaeochromocytoma: lessons from a post-mortem survey. J R Coll Physicians Lond 1995;29:299–306.
59. Katz RL, Patel S, Mackay B, Zornoza J. Fine needle aspiration cytology of the adrenal gland. Acta Cytol 1984;28:269–82.
60. Francis IR, Smid A, Gross MD, et al. Adrenal masses in oncologic patients: functional and morphologic evaluation. Radiology 1988;166:353–6.
61. Redman BG, Pazdur R, Zingas AP, Loredo R. Prospective evaluation of adrenal insufficiency in patients with adrenal metastasis. Cancer 1987;60:103–7.
62. Cedermark BJ, Sjoberg HE. The clinical significance of metastases to the adrenal glands. Surg Gynecol Obstet 1981;152:607–10.
63. Gurney JG, Ness KK, Stovall M, et al. Final height and body mass index among adult survivors of childhood brain cancer: childhood cancer survivor study. J Clin Endocrinol Metab 2003;88:4731–9.
64. Shalet SM, Clayton PE, Price DA. Growth and pituitary function in children treated for brain tumours or acute lymphoblastic leukaemia. Horm Res 1988;30:53–61.
65. Burman P, Broman JE, Hetta J, et al. Quality of life in adults with growth hormone (GH) deficiency: response to treatment with recombinant human GH in a placebo-controlled 21-month trial. J Clin Endocrinol Metab 1995;80:3585–90.
66. Berghmans T, Paesmans M, Body JJ. A prospective study on hyponatraemia in medical cancer patients: epidemiology, aetiology and differential diagnosis. Support Care Cancer 2000;8:192–7.
67. Johnson BE, Damodaran A, Rushin J, et al. Ectopic production and processing of atrial natriuretic peptide in a small cell lung carcinoma cell line and tumor from a patient with hyponatremia. Cancer 1997;79:35–44.
68. Yeung SC, Chiu AC, Vassilopoulou-Sellin R, Gagel RF. The endocrine effects of nonhormonal antineoplastic therapy. Endocr Rev 1998;19:144–72.
69. Harlow PJ, DeClerck YA, Shore NA, et al. A fatal case of inappropriate ADH secretion induced by cyclophosphamide therapy. Cancer 1979;44:896–8.
70. Bode U, Seif SM, Levine AS. Studies on the antidiuretic effect of cyclophosphamide: vasopressin release and sodium excretion. Med Pediatr Oncol 1980;8:295–303.
71. Anand AJ, Bashey B. Newer insights into cisplatin nephrotoxicity. Ann Pharmacother 1993;27:1519–25.
72. Skinner R, Pearson AD, Price L, et al. Nephrotoxicity after ifosfamide. Arch Dis Child 1990;65:732–8.
73. Delaney V, de Pertuz Y, Nixon D, Bourke E. Indomethacin in streptozocin-induced nephrogenic diabetes insipidus. Am J Kidney Dis 1987;9:79–83.
74. Vassilopoulou-Sellin R, Newman BM, Taylor SH, Guinee VF. Incidence of hypercalcemia in patients with malignancy referred to a comprehensive cancer center. Cancer 1993;71:1309–12.
75. Cohen J, Gierlowski TC, Schneider AB. A prospective study of hyperparathyroidism in individuals exposed to radiation in childhood. JAMA 1990;264:581–4.
76. Stewart AF, Keating T, Schwartz PE. Magnesium homeostasis following chemotherapy with cisplatin: a prospective study. Am J Obstet Gynecol 1985;153:660–5.
77. Ehnholm C, Aho K, Huttunen JK, et al. Effect of interferon on plasma lipoproteins and on the activity of postheparin plasma lipases. Arteriosclerosis 1982;2:68–73.
78. Yamagishi S, Abe T, Sawada T. Human recombinant interferon alpha-2a (r IFN alpha-2a) therapy suppresses hepatic triglyceride lipase, leading to severe hypertriglyceridemia in a diabetic patient. Am J Gastroenterol 1994;89:2280.
79. Berruti A, Gorzegno G, Vitetta G, et al. Hypertriglyceridemia during long-term interferon-alpha therapy: efficacy of diet and gemfibrosil treatment. A case report. Tumori 1992;78:353–5.
80. Constine LS, Woolf PD, Cann D, et al. Hypothalamic-pituitary dysfunction after radiation for brain tumors. N Engl J Med 1993;328:87–94.
81. Quigley C, Cowell C, Jimenez M, et al. Normal or early development of puberty despite gonadal damage in children treated for acute lymphoblastic leukemia. N Engl J Med 1989;321:143–51.
82. Brauner R, Rappaport R. Precocious puberty secondary to cranial irradiation for tumors distant from the hypothalamo-pituitary area. Horm Res 1985;22:78–82.
83. Maioli E, Fortino V. The complexity of parathyroid hormone-related protein signalling. Cell Mol Life Sci 2004;61:257–62.
84. Eipper BA, Mains RE. Structure and biosynthesis of pro-adrenocorticotropin/endorphin and related peptides. Endocr Rev 1980;1:1–27.
85. Findling JW, Raff H. Diagnosis and differential diagnosis of Cushing's syndrome. Endocrinol Metab Clin North Am 2001;30:729–47.
86. O'Brien T, Young WF Jr, Davila DG, et al. Cushing's syndrome associated with ectopic production of corticotrophin-releasing hormone, corticotrophin and vasopressin by a phaeochromocytoma. Clin Endocrinol (Oxf) 1992;37:460–7.
87. Newell-Price J, Trainer P, Besser M, Grossman A. The diagnosis and differential diagnosis of Cushing's syndrome and pseudo-Cushing's states. Endocr Rev 1998;19:647–72.
88. Shrager JB, Wright CD, Wain JC, et al. Bronchopulmonary carcinoid tumors associated with Cushing's syndrome: a more aggressive variant of typical carcinoid. J Thorac Cardiovasc Surg 1997;114:367–75.
89. Islam M, Paul RV. Correction of metabolic alkalosis by potassium chloride in ectopic adrenocorticotropic hormone syndrome. Am J Kidney Dis 1996;28:610–3.
90. Cook DM, Loriaux DL. Cushing's: medical approach. Curr Ther Endocrinol Metab 1997;6:59–62.
91. Doppman JL, Oldfield EH, Nieman LK. Bilateral sampling of the internal jugular vein to distinguish between mechanisms of adrenocorticotropic hormone-dependent Cushing syndrome. Ann Intern Med 1998;128:33–6.
92. Winquist EW, Laskey J, Crump M, et al. Ketoconazole in the management of paraneoplastic Cushing's syndrome secondary to ectopic adrenocorticotropin production. J Clin Oncol 1995;13:157–64.
93. Schulte HM, Benker G, Reinwein D, et al. Infusion of low dose etomidate: correction of hypercortisolemia in patients with Cushing's syndrome and dose-response relationship in normal subjects. J Clin Endocrinol Metab 1990;70:1426–30.
94. Dimopoulos MA, Fernandez JF, Samaan NA, et al. Paraneoplastic Cushing's syndrome as an adverse prognostic factor in patients who die early with small cell lung cancer. Cancer 1992;69:66–71.
95. Stewart AF. Clinical practice. Hypercalcemia associated with cancer. N Engl J Med 2005;352:373–9.
96. Roodman GD. Mechanisms of bone metastasis. N Engl J Med 2004;350:1655–64.
97. Seymour JF, Gagel RF, Hagemeister FB, et al. Calcitriol production in hypercalcemic and normocalcemic patients with non-Hodgkin lymphoma. Ann Intern Med 1994;121:633–40.
98. Guise TA, Yin JJ, Thomas RJ, et al. Parathyroid hormone-related protein (PTHrP)-(1-139) isoform is efficiently secreted in vitro and enhances breast cancer metastasis to bone in vivo. Bone 2002;30:670–6.
99. Kakonen SM, Selander KS, Chirgwin JM, et al. Transforming growth factor-beta stimulates parathyroid hormone-related protein and osteolytic metastases via Smad and mitogen-activated protein kinase signaling pathways. J Biol Chem 2002;277:24571–8.
100. Hortobagyi GN, Theriault RL, Porter L, et al. Efficacy of pamidronate in reducing skeletal complications in patients with breast cancer and lytic bone metastases. Protocol 19 Aredia Breast Cancer Study Group. N Engl J Med 1996;335:1785–91.
101. Body JJ, Bartl R, Burckhardt P, et al. Current use of bisphosphonates in oncology. International Bone and Cancer Study Group. J Clin Oncol 1998;16:3890–9.
102. Chisholm MA, Mulloy AL, Taylor AT. Acute management of cancer-related hypercalcemia. Ann Pharmacother 1996;30:507–13.
103. Apseloff G. Therapeutic uses of gallium nitrate: past, present, and future. Am J Ther 1999;6:327–39.
104. Berenson JR, Rosen LS, Howell A, et al. Zoledronic acid reduces skeletal-related events in patients with osteolytic metastases. Cancer 2001;91:1191–200.
105. Bekker PJ, Holloway DL, Rasmussen AS, et al. A single-dose placebo-controlled study of AMG 162, a fully human monoclonal antibody to RANKL, in postmenopausal women. J Bone Miner Res 2004;19:1059–66.
106. Sato K, Yamakawa Y, Shizume K, et al. Passive immunization with anti-parathyroid hormone-related protein monoclonal antibody markedly prolongs survival time of hypercalcemic nude mice bearing transplanted human PTHrP-producing tumors. J Bone Miner Res 1993;8:849–60.
107. Baxter RC, Holman SR, Corbould A, et al. Regulation of the insulin-like growth factors and their binding proteins by glucocorticoid and growth hormone in nonislet cell tumor hypoglycemia. J Clin Endocrinol Metab 1995;80:2700–8.
108. Baxter RC. Insulin-like growth factor binding proteins as glucoregulators. Metabolism 1995;44:12–7.
109. Baxter RC. The role of insulin-like growth factors and their binding proteins in tumor hypoglycemia. Horm Res 1996;46:195–201.
110. Hoff AO, Vassilopoulou-Sellin R. The role of glucagon administration in the diagnosis and treatment of patients with tumor hypoglycemia. Cancer 1998;82:1585–92.
111. Sillos EM, Shenep JL, Burghen GA, et al. Lactic acidosis: a metabolic complication of hematologic malignancies: case report and review of the literature. Cancer 2001;92:2237–46.
112. Flombaum CD. Metabolic emergencies in the cancer patient. Semin Oncol 2000;27:322–34.
113. Kumar R. Tumor-induced osteomalacia and the regulation of phosphate homeostasis. Bone 2000;27:333–8.
114. Nuovo MA, Dorfman HD, Sun CC, Chalew SA. Tumor-induced osteomalacia and rickets. Am J Surg Pathol 1989;13:588–99.
115. Shimada T, Mizutani S, Muto T, et al. Cloning and characterization of FGF23 as a causative factor of tumor-induced osteomalacia. Proc Natl Acad Sci U S A 2001;98:6500–5.
116. Jonsson KB, Zahradnik R, Larsson T, et al. Fibroblast growth factor 23 in oncogenic osteomalacia and X-linked hypophosphatemia. N Engl J Med 2003;348:1656–63.
117. Suzuki M, Takamizawa S, Nomaguchi K, et al. Erythropoietin synthesis by tumour tissues in a patient with uterine myoma and erythrocytosis. Br J Haematol 2001;113:49–51.
118. Gold PJ, Fefer A, Thompson JA. Paraneoplastic manifestations of renal cell carcinoma. Semin Urol Oncol 1996;14:216–22.
119. Arbaiza D, Noriega K, Marcial J, et al. Ectopic production of prolactin in an infant with non-Hodgkin lymphoma. Med Pediatr Oncol 1999;32:311–2.
120. Doga M, Bonadonna S, Burattin A, Giustina A. Ectopic secretion of growth hormone-releasing hormone (GHRH) in neuroendocrine tumors: relevant clinical aspects. Ann Oncol 2001;12 Suppl 2:S89–94.
121. Hoffman WH, Gala RR, Kovacs K, Subramanian MG. Ectopic prolactin secretion from a gonadoblastoma. Cancer 1987;60:2690–5.
122. Hatfill SJ, Kirby R, Hanley M, et al. Hyperprolactinemia in acute myeloid leukemia and indication of ectopic expression of human prolactin in blast cells of a patient of subtype M4. Leuk Res 1990;14:57–62.
123. Bhatavdekar JM, Patel DD, Chikhlikar PR, et al. Ectopic production of prolactin by colorectal adenocarcinoma. Dis Colon Rectum 2001;44:119–27.

Treatment-Related Secondary Cancers

Susan R. Rheingold, MD
Alfred I. Neugut, MD, PhD
Anna T. Meadows, MD

Treatment-related secondary cancers have become an increasingly important concern in oncology during the last two decades.[1,2] This chapter discusses the prevalence and the etiologic factors responsible for treatment-related secondary malignant neoplasms (SMNs). Methods of long-term surveillance for individuals at high risk of developing SMN are also suggested.

What was formerly a problem primarily in pediatric cancer survivors and for the survivors of the more curable adult cancers has become a more universal problem in the present-day practice of oncology. Survivors of all cancers are living for longer periods, partly because of the more frequent use of effective therapy.[3] The formerly unacceptable toxicities of therapy are more readily controlled with better supportive care,[4] and more patients are receiving treatment and benefiting from it. When reviewing data on SMNs, consideration must be given to the definition. One can readily appreciate a "secondary cancer" as such when the secondary neoplasm differs histologically, or molecularly, from the primary neoplasm. Reports and analyses of data have emphasized the importance of ruling out metastatic disease when a new tumor arises, but, traditionally, many registries consider tumors of the same histologic type in the second of paired organs to be "secondary cancers." Reports of multiple primaries should clearly state whether secondary cancers include or exclude nonmetastatic neoplasms in paired organs.

The frequency of SMNs may be expressed as an actuarial risk within a given cohort, as a relative risk when compared with a standard population, or as an attributable risk, with the latter reflecting the additional cases associated with a specific exposure or other etiology. Each of these methods has inherent limitations when attempting to ascribe causation, especially when several factors are implicated.

SMNs are known to result from the radiation therapy and chemotherapy used to treat a primary cancer. Studies of pediatric cancer survivors have provided much information concerning the relationship of therapy to SMNs because of the young age at diagnosis and the high cure rates following successful therapy.[5,6] As therapy becomes more intensive for adults and children, and as cure rates increase, we may expect a resultant increase in toxicity, including SMN. Polymorphisms for metabolizing enzymes, such as those involved in detoxifying carcinogenic chemotherapeutic agents, are a critical category of etiologic factors that cannot yet be evaluated. For example, cytochrome P-450 and glutathione *S*-transferase variants may be important determinants of whether exposure to a specific agent or radiation is associated with an increased likelihood of developing SMN. These and other factors may play a role in determining therapy in the future.[7]

INCIDENCE OF SECONDARY CANCER

Overall, cancer is the second leading cause of death in the United States, exceeded only by heart disease.[8] It is estimated that within the next 10 to 15 years, cancer will overtake cardiovascular disease to become the most common cause of death in America.[9,10] Analyses from the US National Cancer Institute's Surveillance, Epidemiology, and End Results (SEER) Program in 1995 indicate that multiple primary neoplasms comprised 13.1% of cancers in men and 13.7% of cancers in women, a proportion that had doubled over the previous 20 years.[1,2] Not all of these additional neoplasms are treatment related, but it should be recognized that a cancer survivor has approximately twice the probability of developing a new primary cancer than a cancer-free individual of the same age and sex.[1,11]

A critical factor determining the increased risk of developing an SMN is the probability of surviving a first neoplasm and the age of the patient. The prevalence of SMNs in childhood cancer survivors, comprising more than 14,000 individuals diagnosed between 1970 and 1986 (the Childhood Cancer Survivor Study), was recently updated.[12,13] The cumulative incidence 20 years from diagnosis rose from 3.2 to 6.8% with longer follow-up.

CLINICAL CHARACTERISTICS

One question that often arises concerning SMNs is how do they differ clinically from their de novo counterparts. On the one hand, some SMNs are diagnosed earlier and thus have increased surveillance, better overall medical care, and a better outcome. Sadly, once cancer has been treated, some physicians focus on the primary neoplasm and neglect routine surveillance for secondary cancers.[14] Women who have survived cancer should at least have routine mammography screening, Papanicolaou (Pap) smears, and colorectal cancer screening, using the guidelines that would apply to any other woman in the general population. Men should undergo routine prostate and colorectal cancer screening. Counseling of survivors should include instructions for primary and secondary prevention of new malignancies and their risks.

Some SMNs appear to be less amenable to treatment than primary tumors of the same histologic type. The best example of this is therapy-related acute myelogenous leukemia (t-AML) for which the prognosis is worse than for de novo acute myelocytic leukemia.[15] However, a recent report suggests that if the treatment of secondary osteogenic sarcoma is no different from that of primary osteogenic sarcoma, the outcomes should also not differ.[16] Treatment for SMN must take into account the toxicity from the initial therapy. Robinson and colleagues explored the characteristics and stage distributions, as well as survival characteristics, of malignancies occurring as second primary tumors. For the most part, stage for stage, there do not appear to be major differences between SMNs and their de novo counterparts.[17–19]

IONIZING RADIATION

Radiation has long been associated with the development of primary cancers and, when used as treatment, imparts a risk of the development of a secondary cancer. Typically, secondary tumors occur within or at the margin of the radiated field. Bone and soft tissue sarcomas are the most frequent SMNs following radiation therapy, but skin, brain, thyroid, and breast cancers also can occur.[20] Radiation doses less than 30 Gy tend to be associated with skin, thyroid, and brain tumors, whereas doses greater than 30 Gy can evoke secondary sarcomas.[21,22] In the Late Effects Study Group, the median time to develop SMNs was 10 years following radiation, but some were seen as late as 34 years following exposure.[20] Similar results have been noted in major cohort studies by the United Kingdom's Childhood Cancer Research Group and a Nordic Cancer Registries review.[23–25] For many postradiation SMNs, the risk is higher if the radiation exposure occurs earlier in life or during periods of rapid growth of a tissue, such as bone sarcomas during adolescence. This is also seen with thyroid, breast, skin, brain, and stomach cancers.

Adolescent girls receiving mediastinal radiation therapy for Hodgkin's disease develop breast cancer more often than do their adult counterparts.[26,27] Cells that have matured and are no longer proliferating appear to be less susceptible to the effects of radiation, although lung cancer has been observed after chest irradiation[28,29] and bladder cancer after pelvic irradiation.[30,31] More recently, an association between radiation and gastrointestinal tract cancer has been observed.[32–34]

Dose-response relationships have been found between radiation dose and sarcomas. A 40-fold increase in the risk of bone sarcomas was observed following 60 Gy or more.[35] Tenfold increases in the risk of soft tissue sarcoma were seen in retinoblastoma (RB) patients receiving 60 Gy or more, but even 5 Gy increased the risk twofold for this genetically predisposed group.[36] High-dose radiation appears not to increase the risk of leukemia or thyroid cancer.[21] This may be a result of cell killing or inactivation, with cells losing their ability to proliferate and thus their ability to sustain a malignant transformation. As has been observed with other sources of radiation exposure, radiation therapy and cigarette smoking may act in a synergistic fashion.[37]

Dose-response relationships have also been noted in other radiation-induced secondary cancers. Young women with Hodgkin's disease who received doses as low as 4 Gy to the breast had a threefold increase in developing breast cancer. The risk increased to eightfold if doses of radiation were > 40 Gy.[26] Radiotherapy doses > 15 Gy increase the risk of developing a secondary melanoma versus no or low-dose radiation.[22] A dose response was also observed in the report by Guibout and colleagues in a small cohort of female childhood cancer survivors.[38] Breast cancer occurred following Hodgkin's disease after a mean dose of 11.84 Gy to the breast, with a higher risk when the dose was delivered in fewer than 20 fractions compared with 20 fractions or more. In that study, the report by Travis and colleagues, and a recent report from the Childhood Cancer Survivor Study, breast cancer risk was reduced following surgical castration or radiation to the pelvis.[26–29,39]

CHEMOTHERAPY

Leukemia is the most common secondary cancer following treatment with chemotherapy. Although acute myelogenous leukemia is the most common type of therapy-related leukemia, acute lymphocytic leukemia (ALL), chronic myelogenous leukemia, and myelodysplastic syndrome (MDS) have also been reported. Chemotherapy-induced myeloid leukemias are relatively resistant to subsequent therapy and have a cure rate of only 10 to 20%.[15]

Evidence is accumulating concerning the mechanisms of leukemogenesis by deoxyribonucleic acid (DNA) topoisomerase II inhibitors and alkylating agents.[40–42] Table 140-1 summarizes the features of these chemotherapy-related leukemias. Alkylating agents include cyclophosphamide, ifosfamide, cisplatin, carboplatin, chlorambucil, busulfan, melphalan, nitrogen mustard, and procarbazine. Alkylating agent–related t-AML is generally preceded by myelodysplasia and typically has a latency period of 3 to 7 years. Cytogenetic abnormalities demonstrate deletions on chromosome 5 or 7 and complex aberrant karyotypes. Topoisomerase inhibitors include the epipodophyllotoxins, etoposide, and teniposide, as well as the anthracycline doxorubicin and, presumptively, epirubicin. Leukemia following epipodophyllotoxin therapy has a shorter latency period (usually 1 to 3 years) and is primarily associated with translocation of the *MLL* gene at chromosome band 11q23. Chromosomal aberrations are usually balanced, and patients tend to have a more favorable response to treatment.[43]

Table 140-1 Secondary Acute Myelogenous Leukemia

	Alkylating Agent Related	Epipodophyllotoxin Related
Presentation	Myelodysplasia	M4/M5 AML, some M1, M2
Latency period	4–7 yr	1–3 yr
Cytogenetics	del (5q), del (7q), -5, -7	Translocations, usually involving 11q23
Frequency	1 to > 20%	2–12%
Outcome	Poor	Poor
Preleukemic phase	Common	Rare
Age	Typically older	Younger
Predisposition	Germline *TP53* and *NF1* mutations, *GSTT1* null genotype	Unknown

AML = acute myelogenous leukemia.

Treatment for solid tumors, such as Hodgkin's disease, Ewing's sarcoma, and rhabdomyosarcoma, is associated with a dose-response relationship for alkylators and the risk of leukemia. Alkylating agents increase the risk of leukemia almost 5-fold, but that risk increases to almost 24-fold in patients receiving the highest doses.[44,45] Doxorubicin, together with high-dose alkylating agents, increases that risk further. In one study of childhood solid tumor survivors, exposure to ≥ 170 mg/m^2 of anthracycline had a three-fold increase in the risk of developing secondary leukemia relative to those who received < 170 mg/m^2.[46]

A similar increase in risk of secondary leukemia has been reported with increasing doses of epipodophyllotoxins. t-AML is reported in fewer than 3% of germ cell tumor patients receiving doses of etoposide less than 2 g/m^2. This risk increased to more than 11% in patients receiving more than 2 g/m^2.[41] Compared with those who received no epipodophyllotoxins, children treated for a variety of malignancies had an increased risk of developing a secondary leukemia by a factor of 3.7, 5.7, and 93 for cumulative doses of 2 to 3, 3 to 6, and > 6 g/m^2, respectively.[46] The risk of secondary AML may also depend on the timing of epipodophyllotoxin administration. One study revealed an excess risk of leukemia in patients treated as children with weekly or twice-weekly epipodophyllotoxins compared with every other week, although more frequent dosing is associated with total higher dose.[47] Using data from the Cancer Therapy Evaluation Program, Smith and colleagues found neither a dose-response relationship for epipodophyllotoxin in solid tumors and secondary AML nor an increasing risk in patients who received up to 5 g/m^2 of etoposide.[42]

Two different studies have shown that alkylating agents may potentiate the risk of secondary bone cancers when used with radiation therapy.[25,35] The relative risk of secondary bone sarcomas following radiation therapy was 2.7, but when alkylating agents were used as well, the relative risk rose to 4.7.[35] Relling and colleagues found an increased risk of t-AML in children with ALL receiving granulocyte colony-stimulating factor while receiving St. Jude's Total-X ALL therapy with etoposide, doxorubicin, and cyclophosphamide.[48]

HIGH-DOSE THERAPY WITH RESCUE

In this section, high-dose therapy followed by stem cell rescue will be referred to as bone marrow transplantation (BMT). Although it is difficult to differentiate the role played by BMT compared with earlier therapy in the development of secondary cancers, several recent articles have attempted to shed light on the potentially important factors leading to cancer after autologous and allogenic BMT for both malignant and nonmalignant disease. Secondary solid tumors developed, on average, 4 to 6 years post-BMT (range 1–21 years) but were noted to occur as early as 1 year later.[49–51] Malignant tumors of the head; neck, skin, and gastrointestinal tract carcinomas; brain tumors; soft tissue and bone sarcomas; and breast, uterine, and liver tumors have been seen. The cumulative incidence rates of secondary solid tumors increase sharply with time; 10 years following BMT, the risk is 2 to 6%, and 15 years later, it increases to 7 to 15%.[49–51]

Risk factors for developing a secondary malignancy include age at the time of transplantation, development of graft-versus-host disease (GVHD), total-body irradiation, stem cell source, and type of primary cancer. Multiple studies have shown that children < 10 years of age with a variety of primary neoplasms have a 36 to 60 times higher risk of developing a secondary cancer when compared with older children undergoing BMT.[49,50,52] The risk of post-transplant malignancy in adults also appears to correlate inversely with age.[52] Some studies have shown a decreased risk of developing a secondary cancer in patients who develop moderate to severe chronic GVHD,[50] whereas others noted an increased risk of developing squamous cell carcinomas of the skin and buccal cavity.[49,51] It is hypothesized that the chronic inflammation associated with GVHD predisposes patients to secondary tumors. Several articles have noted an increased risk of developing a secondary neoplasm post-BMT when the primary diagnosis is acute or chronic leukemia.[51] Total-body irradiation at doses of 10 to 15 Gy is associated with head and neck carcinomas and skin cancers. The contribution of prior treatment, conditioning regimen, immunosuppression, and oncogenic viruses remains unclear.

Compared with allogenic BMT, autologous BMT (auto-BMT) is associated with an increased risk of therapy-related myelodysplastic syndrome (t-MDS)/AML.[52] Median time to developing t-MDS/AML was 2 years post-BMT (range 0.6–9 years).[52,53] Actuarial risk estimates of developing t-AML range from 3 to 20% in the first 5 years post-BMT for primary lymphomas and less for primary solid tumors. The use of autologous stimulated peripheral blood stem cells and pretransplantation use of high-risk alkylating agents have been found to be independent risk factors for the development of t-MDS/AML post–auto-BMT.

Post-transplant lymphoproliferative disease (PTLD) accounts for almost half of the secondary malignancies diagnosed post-BMT. The majority of cases occur within 6 to 12 months of transplantation, but latency periods have been reported as long as 5 years post-BMT.[50,52,54] Risk factors for PTLD include acute and chronic GVHD, unrelated or human leukocyte antigen–disparate related donor, primary diagnosis of an immune deficiency, T cell–depleted graft, and antithymocyte globulin therapy.

SECONDARY CANCERS RELATED TO PRIMARY NEOPLASMS

Hodgkin's Disease Patients with Hodgkin's disease treated with chemotherapy, radiation therapy, or a combination have an increased risk of developing SMNs.[55–59] Relative risks, based on comparison with cancer risk in age-matched individuals in the population, range from 2 to more than 50 and depend on the tissue of origin of the secondary cancer, as well as treatment.[29,55–58] The overall cumulative incidence of SMNs, the majority of which are solid neoplasms, after treatment for childhood Hodgkin's disease ranges between 2 and 27% by 30 years from diagnosis and depends primarily on the therapy received.

Thyroid cancer is the most common postradiation SMN in survivors of childhood and adolescent Hodgkin's disease.[12,13,21] As noted above, following radiation therapy, breast cancer is seen in females, with those over the age of 10 years being at greatest risk.[26,38,39,51,56–58] There is also an increased risk of skin cancer within the radiation field. Recently, many pediatric centers have altered their therapy of Hodgkin's disease to reflect differences in secondary cancer and gonadal toxicity in girls and boys, with girls receiving less chest irradiation and boys receiving less alkylating agent.[60]

Although radiation therapy for Hodgkin's disease is associated with secondary solid tumors, chemotherapy is associated with the development of secondary leukemia. As many as 25% of secondary malignancies following treatment for Hodgkin's disease are secondary leukemia or lymphoma.[29,57,58] Because MOPP (Mustargen [mechlorethamine], Oncovin [vincristine], procarbazine, and prednisone) regimens contain nitrogen mustard and procarbazine, they incur a greater risk of secondary leukemia than with either combination regimens containing cyclophosphamide or with ABVD (Adriamycin [doxorubicin], bleomycin, vinblastine, and dacarbazine).[60] Higher doses and multiple alkylating agents also increase that risk; hence, the incidence of secondary leukemia is higher in patients who suffer a recurrence of Hodgkin's disease and require retreatment. Radiation therapy alone does not appear to increase the secondary leukemia risk.

Retinoblastoma RB, although affecting only 1 in 20,000 children, is the prototype of heritable cancers. In 1986, the RB gene, *RB1*, on chromosome 13 became the first tumor suppressor gene to be cloned.[61] As Knudson had hypothesized in 1971, if both copies *of RB1* in a single retinoblast are lost or mutated, cancer develops.[62] In 40% of affected children, one copy of *RB1* is mutated prior to birth and is present in all cells of the body. This germline mutation results in RB in younger children (average age 10 months) and tends to be multifocal or bilateral.

Multiple tumors in both eyes and cancer in other organs, such as bone and soft tissue, have long been known in patients with the genetic form of this cancer. In an early study of RB survivors, Wong and colleagues reported 190 secondary cancers for a relative risk of 30 when compared with age-matched controls.[36] The cumulative incidence of secondary cancers for patients with hereditary RB was 51% at 50 years compared with 5% in 50 years for the nongenetic form of RB. Two-thirds of the secondary cancers were osteogenic or soft tissue sarcomas, and a radiation dose-response relationship was noted for all soft tissue sarcomas with as little as 5 Gy increasing the risk of secondary malignancy twofold. For those patients receiving over 60 Gy, there was a 10-fold increase in risk. A more recent report of this cohort with a longer follow-up also noted differences in the incidence of SMN at 50 years between RB survivors with the genetic form (36%) and those without evidence of the genetic form (6%).[63] When SMNs were analyzed for radiation, those who had received radiation therapy had a 40-year incidence of 30% compared with those who had not (9%). Patients with RB also appear to be at an increased risk of melanoma and brain tumors.[20,63] Another recent report of hereditary RB survivors who did not receive radiotherapy revealed an increased risk of secondary epithelial neoplasms, such as lung and bladder cancer, years after the initial diagnosis.[64] All children with bilateral disease and approximately 10 to 15% of those with unilateral tumor are gene carriers and should be monitored for life for the development of sarcomas, adult carcinomas, and other neoplasms. Mutation analysis is now possible to determine which children with a negative family history and unilateral tumor are genetically predisposed so that they may also be followed more closely.

Pediatric Sarcomas Recent studies show a consistent rate of secondary malignancies in patients treated with intensive chemotherapy for soft tissue and bone sarcomas. The cumulative risk of SMNs after therapy for Ewing's sarcoma ranged from 3% at 10 years to more than 20% at 20 years.[20,35,65,66] Patients developed AML, ALL, and MDS from 1 to 8 years after diagnosis. Secondary sarcomas, related to radiation therapy in a dose-dependent manner, were noted 7 to 11 years after diagnosis. Rhabdomyosarcoma survivors, similar to the Ewing's sarcoma cohorts, developed SMNs with an identical latency period and a similar cumulative risk.[67] The rates were highest for patients who received both alkylating agents and radiation therapy. Survivors of osteosarcoma who develop secondary cancers may be at increased risk of having germline *TP53* mutations, predisposing them to breast cancer and t-MDS/AML.[68]

Acute Lymphocytic Leukemia Several reports have been published analyzing the risk of secondary malignancies following therapy for childhood ALL.[47,69–73] Children treated on Children's Cancer Group (CCG) protocols, Berlin-Frankfurt-Munster (BFM) protocols, and Dana-Farber Cancer Institute protocols have an estimated cumulative risk of SMNs at 15 years to be 2.5 to 3.3%. In a review of seven large series of SMNs after ALL therapy, the most common SMNs were central nervous system (CNS) tumors (32%), t-MDS/AML (17%), thyroid cancer (10%), lymphoma (8%), and skin cancer (8%).[74] Patients who received craniospinal radiation were at increased risk of CNS tumors, skin cancer, and thyroid cancer.[6,70–72] Underlying genetic factors, such as *TP53* germline mutations, should be considered in children who develop SMNs following therapy for ALL.

Secondary brain tumors occurred after cranial radiation therapy for ALL in studies reported by the CCG and the St. Jude Children's Research Hospital.[69,72] In the latter report, the overall cumulative incidence was 1.4%. In multiple studies, a statistically significant increase in risk with increasing cranial radiation dose was noted.[6,72] Children treated on CCG protocols for ALL who received 18 Gy had a relative risk of developing a secondary brain tumor of 1.5, which increased to 3.9 in those who received 24 Gy.[6] Younger age increased the risk of secondary CNS tumors. Fortunately, in more recent pediatric ALL protocols, cranial radiation has been replaced by intensive intrathecal chemotherapy for children who have no evidence of CNS disease at diagnosis.[73]

The risk of t-MDS/AML in patients treated for ALL varies with the original protocol used and the dose and schedule of epipodophyllotoxins. Children receiving weekly or twice-weekly epipodophyllotoxins had a cumulative incidence of 12% of secondary AML.[47] In the BFM study, the development of t-AML was not associated with the use of any specific cytotoxic agent and 12 of 16 children with t-AML had not received epipodophyllotoxins.[71]

Wilms' Tumor The data from the National Wilms' Tumor Study Group found an eightfold increase in SMNs in children treated for Wilms' tumor between 1969 and 1991.[75] There was an excess of leukemia, as well as lymphomas and solid tumors. The secondary leukemias were primarily t-AML and were diagnosed 1 to 6 years after original therapy. Similar latency periods were seen for lymphomas. Secondary solid tumors following treatment for Wilms' tumor had a much longer latency period of 3 to 21 years. The solid tumors were primarily sarcomas and carcinomas (breast, thyroid, colon, hepatocellular, parotid), but there was also an increased incidence of brain tumors. Patients who had received abdominal radiation had twice the risk of secondary cancers compared with those who did not. The report also suggested that doxorubicin potentiates the radiation effect.

Neuroblastoma As survival improves in childhood high-risk neuroblastoma (NBL), more SMNs are being detected. The median time from NBL diagnosis to development of an SMN was almost 20 years, with a range of 7 to 38 years and a cumulative incidence of about 2.0% at 20 years.[13,76] SMNs include thyroid and breast carcinoma, sarcomas, and ALL and AML. In a multivariate analysis, treatment with radiation was associated with a relative risk of 4.3 of developing an SMN, but no increased risk was associated with the administration of chemotherapy.[76] An independent association between NBL and later development of thyroid carcinoma may exist because a fivefold excess of radiation-induced thyroid cancer is seen after therapy for NBL.[76,77] The role of autologous BMT and salvage metaiodobenzylguanidine 131 therapy in the development of SMNs is yet to be determined.

Brain and CNS Tumors Children and adolescents with primary brain tumors have a 15-year cumulative incidence of developing a secondary cancer of 5%.[78] Significantly elevated standardized incidence ratios (SIRs) have been noted for pathologically different brain tumors, t-MDS/AML, bone and soft tissue sarcomas, lymphomas, skin cancer, and salivary and thyroid gland carcinomas.[79] Development of secondary brain, bone, thyroid, and skin cancers is higher among patients whose up-front therapy included radiation.[79,80] Younger survivors of primary brain tumors are much more likely to develop secondary cancers than adults. One-third of children who developed secondary tumors had an underlying genetic predisposition, such as Li-Fraumeni syndrome (leukemia, sarcomas), neurofibromatosis (leukemia, brain tumors), Gorlin's syndrome (basal cell and brain tumors), and Gardner's syndrome (desmoid tumors).[78]

Breast Cancer Breast cancer is the most common malignancy diagnosed in women in the United States. Women with an initial breast cancer are at a significantly elevated risk of cancer in the contralateral breast. Antiestrogens can reduce the incidence of secondary malignancies and improve survival.[81,82] Disciplined systematic screening can identify a contralateral breast cancer at an early stage. New discoveries in breast cancer genetics also implicate mutations in *BRCA1* and *BRCA2* as risk factors for ovarian and breast cancer. Screening for ovarian and endometrial cancer, as well as colorectal cancer, should be done regularly in women with a history of breast cancer.[83–85]

The treatment used for breast cancer may have an impact on the subsequent risk of secondary malignancies. Studies show that postmastectomy radiation can elevate the subsequent risk of lung cancer, particularly in smokers.[37,86,87] In addition, similar increased risks have been observed for esophageal cancer following postmastectomy radiation.[88] If alkylating agents are used as adjuvant therapy, the risk of acute leukemia will also be increased, particularly if patients have also received postmastectomy radiation.[89] Postirradiation sarcomas may also occur in the treatment field, especially angiosarcomas.[90–92] Although tamoxifen acts as an antiestrogen with regard to breast cancer and significantly reduces the occurrence of contralateral breast cancer,[93] it acts as a weak estrogenic agent elsewhere, raising the risk of endometrial cancer.[81] Thus, patients who have received long-term adjuvant hormonal therapy should have regular endometrial screening by a gynecologist. Radiation therapy for an initial breast cancer does not appear to elevate the risk of contralateral breast cancer.[94]

Prostate Cancer Radiotherapy for prostate cancer slightly elevates the risk of bladder cancer after many years.[30] As described earlier, an association between prostate cancer and other malignancies has occasionally been found, for example, lung cancer or colorectal cancer, but these have usually been unidirectional and thus probably represent detection bias rather than some shared risk factor. One recent finding of interest was an increased risk of male breast cancer following prostate cancer[95]; whether this represents either a treatment-related, hormone-related, or shared risk factor, or detection bias, is unknown.

Testicular Cancer Testicular cancer is one of the most curable solid tumors, whether it occurs unilaterally or bilaterally.[96] Because etoposide is used as a major treatment modality in this disease and this chemotherapeutic agent is associated with acute leukemia, there may be some elevation in the risk of leukemia following successful therapy.[40,42,97] Furthermore, when radiation therapy is used in the primary management of testicular cancer, there may be elevated risks of other neoplasms in the pelvis.

Other Carcinomas The risk of esophageal cancer following lung cancer is increased by treatment of the initial lung cancer with radiation, strongly suggesting a carcinogenic effect of radiation in its etiology. Nonetheless, the risk of esophageal carcinoma is elevated following lung cancer even in the absence of radiation therapy.[98]

Because both pancreatic cancer and gastric cancer have a poor outlook, with few long-term survivors, it is difficult to know what secondary malignancies would be associated with these neoplasms. Both are associated with cigarette smoking, however; thus, one could speculate that when successful treatments are developed, other tobacco-related malignancies might be observed. Pancreatic cancer has occurred as a secondary malignancy in individuals with other smoking-related neoplasms.[99] No significant associations with gastric cancer were found in a recent report.[100]

Survivors of colorectal cancer are at elevated risk of secondary malignancies within the colon and rectum, as well as in the breast, uterus, and ovary.[84] In those patients with hereditary nonpolyposis colon cancer (HNPCC), there is an elevated risk of small bowel and endometrial cancers.

Survivors of endometrial cancer are at an elevated risk of ovarian and colorectal cancers, as well as breast cancer.[84,101] As a result, appropriate surveillance and screening should be performed in women with any of these neoplasms. If appropriate, bilateral oophorectomy should be considered at the time of hysterectomy to reduce the subsequent risk of ovarian cancer.

It has long been recognized that basal cell carcinomas and squamous cell carcinomas (nonmelanotic skin cancer) tend to occur in the same individuals.[102] This represents the impact of sun exposure, a shared risk factor. Thus, those who have nonmelanotic skin cancer should undergo regular surveillance for further skin malignancies and should avoid further sun exposure. Individuals with dysplastic nevi may develop multiple cutaneous melanomas and should undergo regular evaluations by experienced clinicians.[103] Certainly, those who survive an initial melanoma are also at an elevated risk (> 30-fold according to a recent report) for a secondary melanoma.[104]

CONCLUSION

Therapeutic options for secondary cancers are often compromised by the therapy for the first neoplasm, but early diagnosis can often lead to successful treatment of many secondary cancers. Identifying those who are at greater risk of multiple neoplasms can help health care providers institute more targeted monitoring for secondary neoplasms and counsel patients on the ways of reducing risks.

Many individuals at highest risk of therapy-related new cancers are already known, and several approaches to reducing their incidence are already under way. For instance, the knowledge that certain agents and regimens increase the risk of a secondary malignancy has prompted pediatric oncologists to modify therapy. Knowing that there are patients with genetic risk factors, such as those with the hereditary form of RB who are at high risk of developing sarcomas in the radiation field, has led to protocols using neoadjuvant chemotherapy and an emphasis on local treatment methods other than radiation therapy.[105]

For adult neoplasms, research that focuses on the avoidance of known environmental carcinogens offers the hope that some neoplasms in multiple sites can be prevented. In this regard, survivors of childhood cancer are an excellent population in which to study the effectiveness of educational intervention techniques. Finally, study of the genetic changes in cancer in families with many affected members and of individuals with more than one primary tumor can increase our knowledge of the nature of the changes leading to transformation of a normal cell to malignancy. This may lead to the identification of more susceptible individuals and to the development of appropriate methods of surveillance and counseling.

REFERENCES

1. Neugut AI, Meadows AT, Robinson E. Introduction. In: Neugut AI, Meadows AT, Robinson E, editors. Multiple primary cancers. Lippincott Williams & Wilkins, Philadelphia (PA):1999. p. 1–12.
2. Kosary CL, Ries LAG, Miller BA. SEER cancer statistics review 1973-1992: tables and graphs. Bethesda (MD): National Cancer Institute:1995.NIH Pub. No. 96-2789.
3. Hoel DG, Davis DL, Miller AB, et al. Trends in cancer mortality in 15 industrialized countries, 1969-1986. J Natl Cancer Inst 1992;84:313–20.
4. Schuchter LM, Hensley ML, Meropol NJ, Winer EP. 2002 update of recommendations for the use of chemotherapy and radiotherapy protectants: clinical practice guidelines of the American Society of Clinical Oncology. J Clin Oncol 2002;20:2895–903.
5. Meadows AT. Second tumours. Eur J Cancer 2001;37:2074–9; discussion 2079–81.
6. Bhatia S, Sklar C. Second cancers in survivors of childhood cancer. Nat Rev Cancer 2002;2:124–32.
7. Mertens AC, Mitby PA, Radloff G, et al. XRCC1 and glutathione-S-transferase gene polymorphisms and susceptibility to radiotherapy-related malignancies in survivors of Hodgkin disease. Cancer 2004;101:1463–72.
8. Jemal A, Murray T, Samuels A, et al. Cancer statistics, 2003. CA Cancer J Clin 2003;53:5–26.
9. Lopez AD. Competing causes of death. A review of recent trends in mortality in industrialized countries with special reference to cancer. Ann N Y Acad Sci 1990;609:58–74; discussion 74–56.
10. Bailar JC III, Gornik HL. Cancer undefeated. N Engl J Med 1997;336:1569–74.
11. Dong C, Hemminki K. Second primary neoplasms in 633,964 cancer patients in Sweden, 1958-1996. Int J Cancer 2001;93:155–61.
12. Friedman DL, Whitton J, Yasui Y, et al. Second malignant neoplasms in five-year survivors of childhood cancer: an update from the childhood cancer survivor study (CCSS). New Orleans (LA): American Society of Clinical Oncology; 2004.
13. Neglia JP, Friedman DL, Yasui Y, et al. Second malignant neoplasms in five-year survivors of childhood cancer: Childhood Cancer Survivor Study. J Natl Cancer Inst 2001;93:618–29.
14. Green RJ, Metlay JP, Propert K, et al. Surveillance for second primary colorectal cancer after adjuvant chemotherapy: an analysis of Intergroup 0089. Ann Intern Med 2002;136:261–9.
15. Josting A, Wiedenmann S, Franklin J, et al. Secondary myeloid leukemia and myelodysplastic syndromes in patients treated for Hodgkin's disease: a report from the German Hodgkin's Lymphoma Study Group. J Clin Oncol 2003;21:3440–6.
16. Bielack SS, Kempf-Bielack B, Delling G, et al. Prognostic factors in high-grade osteosarcoma of the extremities or trunk: an analysis of 1,702 patients treated on Neoadjuvant Cooperative Osteosarcoma Study Group protocols. J Clin Oncol 2002;20:776–90.
17. Robinson E, Neugut AI, Murray T, Rennert G. A comparison of the clinical characteristics of first and second primary head and neck cancers. A population-based study. Cancer 1991;68:189–92.
18. Robinson E, Rennert G, Rennert HS, Neugut AI. Survival of first and second primary breast cancer. Cancer 1993;71:172–6.
19. Robinson E, Neugut AI, Wylie P. Clinical aspects of postirradiation sarcomas. J Natl Cancer Inst 1988;80:233–40.
20. Meadows AT, Baum E, Fossati-Bellani F, et al. Second malignant neoplasms in children: an update from the Late Effects Study Group. J Clin Oncol 1985;3:532–8.
21. Sigurdson AJ, Ronckers CM, Mertens AC, et al. Primary thyroid cancer after a first tumour in childhood: (the Childhood Cancer Survivor Study). Lancet 2005;3651:2014–23.
22. Guerin S, Dupuy A, Anderson H, et al. Radiation dose as a risk factor for malignant melanoma following childhood cancer. Eur J Cancer 2003;39:2379–86.
23. Hawkins MM, Draper GJ, Kinstone JE. Incidence of second primary tumors among childhood cancer survivors. Br J Cancer 1987;56:339–47.
24. Olsen JH, Garwicz S, Hertz H, et al. Second malignant neoplasms after cancer in childhood or adolescence. Nordic Society of Paediatric Haematology and Oncology Association of the Nordic Cancer Registries. BMJ 1993;307:1030–6.
25. Menu-Branthomme A, Rubino C, Shamsaldin A, et al. Radiation dose, chemotherapy and risk of soft tissue sarcoma after solid tumours during childhood. Int J Cancer 2004;110:87–93.
26. Travis LB, Hill DA, Dores GM, et al. Breast cancer following radiotherapy and chemotherapy among young women with Hodgkin disease. JAMA 2003;290:465–75.
27. Bhatia S, Yasui Y, Robison LL, et al. High risk of subsequent neoplasms continues with extended follow-up of childhood Hodgkin's disease: report from the Late Effects Study Group. J Clin Oncol 2003;21:4386–94.
28. Travis LB, Gospodarowicz M, Curtis RE, et al. Lung cancer following chemotherapy and radiotherapy for Hodgkin's disease. J Natl Cancer Inst 2002;94:182–92.
29. Swerdlow AJ, Schoemaker MJ, Allerton R, et al. Lung cancer after Hodgkin's disease: a nested case-control study of the relation to treatment. J Clin Oncol 2001;19:1610–8.
30. Neugut AI, Ahsan H, Robinson E, Ennis RD. Bladder carcinoma and other second malignancies after radiotherapy for prostate carcinoma. Cancer 1997;79:1600–4.
31. Kleinerman RA, Boice JD Jr, Storm HH, et al. Second primary cancer after treatment for cervical cancer. An International Cancer Registries study. Cancer 1995;76:442–52.
32. Ahsan H, Neugut AI. Radiation therapy for breast cancer and increased risk for esophageal carcinoma. Ann Intern Med 1998;128:114–7.
33. Scholl B, Reis ED, Zouhair A, et al. Esophageal cancer as second primary tumor after breast cancer radiotherapy. Am J Surg 2001;182:476–80.
34. Palesty JA, Wang W, Javle MM, Yang GY. Side effects of therapy: case 3. Gastric cancer after radiotherapy of pediatric Hodgkin's disease. J Clin Oncol 2004;22:2507–9.
35. Tucker MA, D'Angio GJ, Boice JD, et al. Bone sarcomas linked to radiotherapy and chemotherapy in children. N Engl J Med 1987;317:588–93.
36. Wong FL, Boice JD Jr, Abramson DH, et al. Cancer incidence after retinoblastoma. Radiation dose and sarcoma risk. JAMA 1997;278:1262–7.
37. Neugut AI, Murray T, Santos J, et al. Increased risk of lung cancer after breast cancer radiation therapy in cigarette smokers. Cancer 1994;73:1615–20.
38. Guibout C, Adjadj E, Rubino C, et al. Malignant breast tumors after radiotherapy for a first cancer during childhood. J Clin Oncol 2005;23:197–204.
39. Kenney LB, Yasui Y, Inskip PD, et al. Breast cancer after childhood cancer: a report from the Childhood Cancer Survivor Study. Ann Intern Med 2004;141:590–7.
40. Felix CA. Chemotherapy-related second cancers. In: Neugut AL, Meadows AT, Robinson E, editors. Multiple primary cancers. Lippincott Williams & Wilkins, Philadelphia (PA): 1999. p. 137–64.
41. Hawkins MM, Wilson LM, Stovall MA, et al. Epipodophyllotoxins, alkylating agents, and radiation and risk of secondary leukaemia after childhood cancer. BMJ 1992;304:951–8.
42. Smith MA, Rubinstein L, Anderson JR, et al. Secondary leukemia or myelodysplastic syndrome after treatment with epipodophyllotoxins. J Clin Oncol 1999;17:569–77.
43. Schoch C, Kern W, Schnittger S, et al. Karyotype is an independent prognostic parameter in therapy-related acute myeloid leukemia (t-AML): an analysis of 93 patients with t-AML in comparison to 1091 patients with de novo AML. Leukemia 2004;18:120–5.
44. van Leeuwen FE, Chorus AM, van den Belt-Dusebout AW, et al. Leukemia risk following Hodgkin's disease: relation to cumulative dose of alkylating agents, treatment with teniposide combinations, number of episodes of chemotherapy, and bone marrow damage. J Clin Oncol 1994;12:1063–73.
45. Tucker MA, Meadows AT, Boice JD Jr, et al. Leukemia after therapy with alkylating agents for childhood cancer. J Natl Cancer Inst 1987;78:459–64.
46. Le Deley MC, Leblanc T, Shamsaldin A, et al. Risk of secondary leukemia after a solid tumor in childhood according to the dose of epipodophyllotoxins and anthracyclines: a case-control study by the Societe Francaise d'Oncologie Pediatrique. J Clin Oncol 2003;21:1074–81.
47. Pui CH, Ribeiro RC, Hancock ML, et al. Acute myeloid leukemia in children treated with epipodophyllotoxins for acute lymphoblastic leukemia. N Engl J Med 1991;325:1682–7.
48. Relling MV, Boyett JM, Blanco JG, et al. Granulocyte colony-stimulating factor and the risk of secondary myeloid malignancy after etoposide treatment. Blood 2003;101:3862–7.
49. Curtis RE, Rowlings PA, Deeg HJ, et al. Solid cancers after bone marrow transplantation. N Engl J Med 1997;336:897–904.
50. Socie G, Curtis RE, Deeg HJ, et al. New malignant diseases after allogeneic marrow transplantation for childhood acute leukemia. J Clin Oncol 2000;18:348–57.
51. Bhatia S, Louie AD, Bhatia R, et al. Solid cancers after bone marrow transplantation. J Clin Oncol 2001;19:464–71.
52. Baker KS, DeFor TE, Burns LJ, et al. New malignancies after blood or marrow stem-cell transplantation in children and adults: incidence and risk factors. J Clin Oncol 2003;21:1352–8.
53. Metayer C, Curtis RE, Vose J, et al. Myelodysplastic syndrome and acute myeloid leukemia after autotransplantation for lymphoma: a multicenter case-control study. Blood 2003;101:2015–23.
54. Curtis RE, Travis LB, Rowlings PA, et al. Risk of lymphoproliferative disorders after bone marrow transplantation: a multi-institutional study. Blood 1999;94:2208–16.
55. Green DM, Hyland A, Barcos MP, et al. Second malignant neoplasms after treatment for Hodgkin's disease in childhood or adolescence. J Clin Oncol 2000;18:1492–9.
56. Swerdlow AJ, Barber JA, Hudson GV, et al. Risk of second malignancy after Hodgkin's disease in a collaborative British cohort: the relation to age at treatment. J Clin Oncol 2000;18:498–509.
57. Metayer C, Lynch CF, Clarke EA, et al. Second cancers among long-term survivors of Hodgkin's disease diagnosed in childhood and adolescence. J Clin Oncol 2000;18:2435–43.
58. van Leeuwen FE, Klokman WJ, Veer MB, et al. Long-term risk of second malignancy in survivors of Hodgkin's disease treated during adolescence or young adulthood. J Clin Oncol 2000;18:487–97.
59. Chronowski GM, Wilder RB, Levy LB, et al. Second malignancies after chemotherapy and radiotherapy for Hodgkin disease. Am J Clin Oncol 2004;27:73–80.
60. Schellong G, Potter R, Bramswig J, et al. High cure rates and reduced long-term toxicity in pediatric Hodgkin's disease: the German-Austrian multicenter trial DAL-HD-90. German-Austrian Pediatric Hodgkin's Disease Study Group. J Clin Oncol 1999;17:3736–44.
61. Friend SH, Bernards R, Rogelj S, et al. A human DNA segment with properties of the gene that predisposes to retinoblastoma and osteosarcoma. Nature 1986;323:643–6.
62. Knudson AG Jr. Mutation and cancer: statistical study of retinoblastoma. Proc Natl Acad Sci U S A 1971;68:820–3.
63. Kleinerman RA, Tucker MA, Tarone RE, et al. Risk of new cancers after radiotherapy in long-term survivors of retinoblastoma: an extended follow-up. J Clin Oncol 2005;23:2272–9.
64. Fletcher O, Easton D, Anderson K, et al. Lifetime risks of common cancers among retinoblastoma survivors. J Natl Cancer Inst 2004;96:357–63.

65. Kuttesch JF Jr, Wexler LH, Marcus RB, et al. Second malignancies after Ewing's sarcoma: radiation dose-dependency of secondary sarcomas. J Clin Oncol 1996;14:2818–25.
66. Dunst J, Ahrens S, Paulussen M, et al. Second malignancies after treatment for Ewing's sarcoma: a report of the CESS-studies. Int J Radiat Oncol Biol Phys 1998;42:379–84.
67. Heyn R, Haeberlen V, Newton WA, et al. Second malignant neoplasms in children treated for rhabdomyosarcoma. Intergroup Rhabdomyosarcoma Study Committee. J Clin Oncol 1993;11:262–70.
68. Malkin D, Li FP, Strong LC, et al. Germ line p53 mutations in a familial syndrome of breast cancer, sarcomas, and other neoplasms. Science 1990;250:1233–8.
69. Neglia JP, Meadows AT, Robison LL, et al. Second neoplasms after acute lymphoblastic leukemia in childhood. N Engl J Med 1991;325:1330–6.
70. Kimball Dalton VM, Gelber RD, et al. Second malignancies in patients treated for childhood acute lymphoblastic leukemia. J Clin Oncol 1998;16:2848–53.
71. Loning L, Zimmermann M, Reiter A, et al. Secondary neoplasms subsequent to Berlin-Frankfurt-Munster therapy of acute lymphoblastic leukemia in childhood: significantly lower risk without cranial radiotherapy. Blood 2000;95:2770–5.
72. Walter AW, Hancock ML, Pui CH, et al. Secondary brain tumors in children treated for acute lymphoblastic leukemia at St Jude Children's Research Hospital. J Clin Oncol 1998;16:3761–7.
73. Bhatia S, Sather HN, Pabustan OB, et al. Low incidence of second neoplasms among children diagnosed with acute lymphoblastic leukemia after 1983. Blood 2002;99:4257–64.
74. Suarez CR, Bertolone SJ, Raj AB, Coventry S. Second malignant neoplasms in childhood acute lymphoblastic leukemia: primitive neuroectodermal tumor of the chest wall with germline p53 mutation as a second malignant neoplasm. Am J Hematol 2004;76:52–6.
75. Breslow NE, Takashima JR, Whitton JA, et al. Second malignant neoplasms following treatment for Wilms' tumor: a report from the National Wilms' Tumor Study Group. J Clin Oncol 1995;13:1851–9.
76. Rubino C, Adjadj E, Guerin S, et al. Long-term risk of second malignant neoplasms after neuroblastoma in childhood: role of treatment. Int J Cancer 2003;107:791–6.
77. de Vathaire F, Hardiman C, Shamsaldin A, et al. Thyroid carcinomas after irradiation for a first cancer during childhood. Arch Intern Med 1999;159:2713–9.
78. Broniscer A, Ke W, Fuller CE, et al. Second neoplasms in pediatric patients with primary central nervous system tumors: the St. Jude Children's Research Hospital experience. Cancer 2004;100:2246–52.
79. Inskip PD. Multiple primary tumors involving cancer of the brain and central nervous system as the first or subsequent cancer. Cancer 2003;98:562–70.
80. Devarahally SR, Severson RK, Chuba P, et al. Second malignant neoplasms after primary central nervous system malignancies of childhood and adolescence. Pediatr Hematol Oncol 2003;20:617–25.
81. Curtis RE, Boice JD Jr, Shriner DA, et al. Second cancers after adjuvant tamoxifen therapy for breast cancer. J Natl Cancer Inst 1996;88:832–4.
82. Li CI, Malone KE, Weiss NS, Daling JR. Tamoxifen therapy for primary breast cancer and risk of contralateral breast cancer. J Natl Cancer Inst 2001;93:1008–13.
83. Bond JH. Screening guidelines for colorectal cancer. Am J Med 1999;106:7S–10S.
84. Weinberg DS, Newschaffer CJ, Topham A. Risk for colorectal cancer after gynecologic cancer. Ann Intern Med 1999;131:189–93.
85. Metcalfe KA, Lynch HT, Ghadirian P, et al. The risk of ovarian cancer after breast cancer in BRCA1 and BRCA2 carriers. Gynecol Oncol 2005;96:222–6.
86. Inskip PD, Stovall M, Flannery JT. Lung cancer risk and radiation dose among women treated for breast cancer. J Natl Cancer Inst 1994;86:983–8.
87. Zablotska LB, Neugut AI. Lung cancer following breast cancer radiation therapy in women treated with lumpectomy or mastectomy. Cancer 2003;97:1404–11.
88. Zablotska LB, Chak A, Das A, Neugut AI. Increased risk of squamous cell esophageal cancer after adjuvant radiation therapy for primary breast cancer. Am J Epidemiol 2005;161:330–7.
89. Curtis RE, Boice JD Jr, Stovall M, et al. Risk of leukemia after chemotherapy and radiation treatment for breast cancer. N Engl J Med 1992;326:1745–51.
90. Yap J, Chuba PJ, Thomas R, et al. Sarcoma as a second malignancy after treatment for breast cancer. Int J Radiat Oncol Biol Phys 2002;52:1231–7.
91. Brady MS, Garfein CF, Petrek JA, Brennan MF. Post-treatment sarcoma in breast cancer patients. Ann Surg Oncol 1994;1:66–72.
92. Rubino C, Shamsaldin A, Le MG, et al. Radiation dose and risk of soft tissue and bone sarcoma after breast cancer treatment. Breast Cancer Res Treat 2005;89:277–88.
93. Early Breast Cancer Trialists' Collaborative Group. Effect of chemotherapy and hormonal therapy for early breast cancer on recurrence on 15-year survival: an overview of the randomised trials. Lancet 2005;365:1687–717.
94. Boice JD Jr, Harvey EB, Blettner M, et al. Cancer in the contralateral breast after radiotherapy for breast cancer. N Engl J Med 1992;326:781–5.
95. Thellenberg C, Malmer B, Tavelin B, Gronberg H. Second primary cancers in men with prostate cancer: an increased risk of male breast cancer. J Urol 2003;169:1345–8.
96. Travis LB, Curtis RE, Storm H, et al. Risk of second malignant neoplasms among long-term survivors of testicular cancer. J Natl Cancer Inst 1997;89:1429–39.
97. Chaudhary UB, Haldis JR. Long-term complications of chemotherapy for germ cell tumors. Drugs 2003;63:1565–77.
98. Ahsan H, Insel BJ, Neugut AI. Risk estimates for second primary cancers. In: Neugut AI, Meadows AT, Robinson E, editors. Multiple primary cancers. Lippincott Williams & Wilkins, Philadelphia (PA): 1999. p.27–53.
99. Neugut AI, Ahsan H, Robinson E. Pancreatic cancer as a second primary malignancy: a population based study. Cancer 1995;76:589–92.
100. Dinis-Ribeiro M, Lomba-Viana H, Silva R, et al. Associated primary tumors in patients with gastric cancer. J Clin Gastroenterol 2002;34:533–5.
101. Travis LB, Curtis RE, Boice JD Jr, et al. Second malignant neoplasms among long-term survivors of ovarian cancer. Cancer Res 1996;56:1564–70.
102. Berwick M. Skin cancers. In: Neugut AI, Meadows AT, Robinson E, editors. Multiple primary cancers. Lippincott Williams & Wilkins, Philadelphia (PA): 1999. p. 445–67.
103. Boland SL, Shaw HM, Milton GW. Multiple primary cancers in patients with malignant melanoma. Med J Aust 1976;1:517–9.
104. Schmid-Wendtner MH, Baumert J, Wendtner CM, et al. Risk of second primary malignancies in patients with cutaneous melanoma. Br J Dermatol 2001;145:981–5.
105. Friedman DL, Himelstein B, Shields CL, et al. Chemoreduction and local ophthalmic therapy for intraocular retinoblastoma. J Clin Oncol 2000;18:12–7.

INFECTION IN THE CANCER PATIENT

141

Infections in Patients with Cancer

Kenneth V.I. Rolston, MD, FACP
Gerald P. Bodey, MD

Infection continues to be a common problem in patients with cancer despite significant advances in supportive care.[1] The spectrum of infection continues to change, with newer opportunistic pathogens emerging.[2,3] Resistance among common bacterial and fungal pathogens is of concern, particularly because the pipeline for new drug development is relatively barren.[4] Fungal, viral, and some protozoal infections have increased in frequency, are often difficult to diagnose in a timely manner, are sometimes refractory to therapy, and are associated with substantial morbidity and mortality.[5,6] Consequently, infection prevention, and reversal of the immunologic deficit(s) leading to infection, are important aspects in the overall management of patients with cancer.

The frequency of infection is related to the type of underlying neoplastic disease. Approximately 80% of patients with acute leukemia, 75% of patients with lymphoma, and 50% of patients with multiple myeloma develop infection during the course of their disease.[7,8] Serious infections also occur in patients with solid tumors.[9] Multiple episodes of infection in the same patient are not uncommon. It is often not possible to make a specific diagnosis, and empiric therapy is generally administered in high-risk patients who are suspected of having an infection. A thorough knowledge of the factors that predispose these patients toward the development of infections is essential.

FACTORS RESPONSIBLE FOR INCREASED SUSCEPTIBILITY TO INFECTIONS

Many factors increase the susceptibility of patients with cancer to infection. Each is associated with a unique set of infections, although there is some overlap between predisposing factors and certain infections. Multiple predisposing factors might exist in the same patient, widening the spectrum. Table 141-1 lists the predominant defects in host defense mechanisms associated with various cancers and the infections associated with of those defects.

Neutropenia Neutropenia remains the most common predisposing factor. The relationship between neutropenia and infection has been studied most extensively in patients with acute leukemia.[10] Both the degree and the duration of neutropenia influence the development of infection. The currently accepted definition of neutropenia is an absolute neutrophil count of $\leq 500/mm^3$. Most serious infections, including bacteremias, develop during episodes of severe and prolonged neutropenia, (Figure 141-1). Patients with neutropenia often fail to develop the characteristic signs and symptoms of infection, because they are unable to mount an adequate inflammatory response.[11] Inflammatory exudates in patients with neutropenia may be devoid of neutrophils and may contain only a few lymphocytes and macrophages. Patients with neutropenia who develop pneumonia may not have pulmonary infiltrates on chest radiographs or may fail to demonstrate meningismus when they develop meningitis.

Common sites of infection in patients with neutropenia include the lung, oropharynx, blood, urinary tract, skin, and soft tissues, including the perirectal area. Infections are generally caused by organisms colonizing the patient, although some organisms are acquired after admission to the hospital. Hospital-acquired pathogens are more

Table 141-1 Defects in Host Defense Mechanisms and Common Infections Associated with Malignant Diseases

Disease	Prominent Defect	Predominant Infections
Acute leukemia, aplastic anemia	Neutropenia	Gram-positive cocci, gram-negative bacilli, *Candida, Aspergillus, Fusarium, Trichosporon*
Hairy cell leukemia	Neutropenia, impaired lymphocyte function	Gram-negative bacilli, gram-positive cocci, mycobacteria (including nontuberculous)
Chronic lymphatic leukemia, multiple myeloma	Hypogammaglobulinemia	Encapsulated organisms, *Streptococcus pneumoniae; Haemophilus influenzae; Neisseria meningitides*
Hodgkin disease	Impaired T-lymphocyte response	*Pneumocystis, Cryptococcus, mycobacteria, Toxoplasma, Listeria, Cryptosporidium, Candida*, cytomegalovirus
Bone marrow, transplant recipients	Neutropenia, impaired cellular and humoral immunity	Gram-positive cocci, gram-negative bacilli, cytomegalovirus, *Candida, Aspergillus*, herpes viruses
Breast cancer	Tissue necrosis	Gram-positive cocci, gram-negative bacilli, anaerobes
Lung cancer	Local obstruction, tissue necrosis	Gram-positive cocci, gram-negative bacilli, anaerobes
Gynecologic malignancy	Local obstruction, tissue necrosis	Mixed aerobic and anaerobic enteric flora

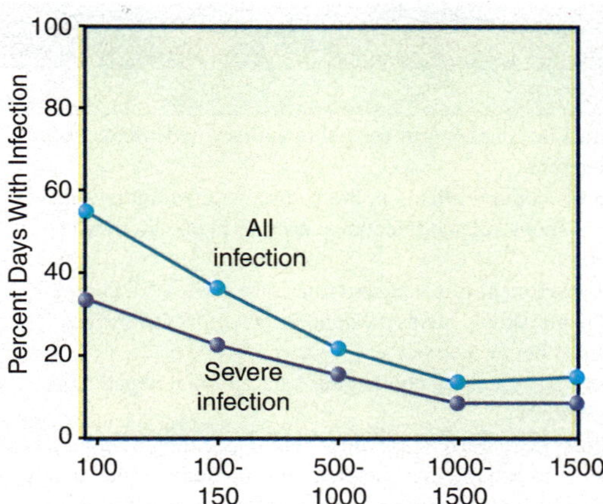

Figure 141-1 Relations between granulocyte count and infection in patients with acute leukemia. Percentage of days spent with infection is inversely related to the level of circulating granulocytes.

likely to be resistant to commonly used antimicrobial agents because of the pressure of heavy antibiotic usage.[12,13]

Patients with adequate levels of circulating neutrophils may be susceptible to infection because of impaired neutrophil function. Inadequate neutrophil function has been described in patients with acute and chronic leukemia and Hodgkin disease. Defects include the inability to migrate to sites of inflammation, impaired phagocytosis, and reduced killing of ingested bacteria.

Not all patients with neutropenia have the same risk for developing infection or serious complications when they become febrile. It is possible to recognize high-, moderate-, and low-risk patients with neutropenia by using clinical criteria and risk prediction rules during the initial phases of their febrile episode.[14,15] Many patients with solid tumors that are responding to antineoplastic therapy and in whom neutropenia is relatively short-lived (≤ 7 days) are considered low risk. These patients have a high response rate (> 95%) to antibacterial therapy and a low complication rate (< 2%). Strategies for their management, such as early discharge and outpatient antibiotic therapy, have been developed.[16–18] New strategies for predicting the degree and duration of neutropenia are being developed.[19] These will enhance our ability to differentiate high-risk from low-risk patients.

Cellular Immune Dysfunction Defects in the T lymphocyte and/or mononuclear phagocytic system result in an increased susceptibility to infection. Cell-mediated immunity plays a primary role in protecting against intracellular pathogens.[20] However, T4 lymphocytes have an impact on practically all aspects of immunity as a consequence of their ability to induce specific immune responses in other cells. Thus, the functions of B lymphocytes, which are primarily involved with maintaining humoral immunity, and granulocytes, which engulf and kill microorganisms, are regulated by T4 helper cells.

T-lymphocyte function is impaired in a variety of disorders. Patients with Hodgkin disease also have evidence of impaired cell-mediated immunity, and, to a lesser degree, so do patients with chronic and acute lymphocytic leukemia. Defects in the mononuclear phagocytic system have been described in patients with monocytic leukemia. Immunosuppressive therapy with agents such as cyclosporine, tacrolimus, azathioprine, corticosteroids, certain cytotoxic agents (fludarabine and other purine analogues), and irradiation produces dysfunction in cellular immunity. These patients are especially susceptible to infection with intracellular organisms such as those listed in Table 141-2.

Humoral Immune Dysfunction The immune response that is mediated by antibodies, which are immunoglobulins with a binding specificity for microbial antigens, is referred to as *humoral immunity.* B lymphocytes are responsible for anti-body production. In disorders such as multiple myeloma, Waldenstrom macroglobulinemia, and the various "heavy-chain diseases," overproduction of a specific subcomponent of an immunoglobulin occurs as a consequence of malignant proliferation of plasma cells or their precursors. As this pool of malignant plasma cells expands, it does so at the expense of normal cells, resulting in low levels of normal immunoglobulins. Hypogammaglobulinemia is also present in 30–40% of patients with chronic lymphocytic leukemia, and infection occurs in nearly 90% of these patients, as compared with only 15% in patients with normal gamma-globulin levels. Infection is the cause of death in approximately 60% of patients with multiple myeloma. Patients with multiple myeloma and chronic lymphocytic leukemia are especially susceptible to infections caused by encapsulated organisms such as *Streptococcus pneumoniae* and *Haemophilus influenzae* because specific opsonizing antibodies that play a major role in the defense against such pathogens are greatly reduced.

Marrow and Stem Cell Transplantation Infection is one of the major complications of bone marrow and/or hematopoietic stem cell transplantation. During the initial period of neutropenia, patients are at risk of developing bacterial infections. Fungal infections caused by *Candida* spp. and *Aspergillus* spp. also occur during this period. The risk of these infections decreases after recovery of the neutrophil count, but neutrophil and macrophage function remain abnormal. Patients undergoing allogeneic transplantation also have suppressed cell-mediated immunity. As a consequence, infections with herpes viruses, respiratory syncytial virus [RSV], and adenoviruses, protozoan organisms (such as *Pneumocystis carinii* and *Toxoplasma gondii),* bacteria (such as *Legionella* spp., and *S. pneumoniae)* and mould infections (aspergillosis) are common. These infections generally occur after the initial period of neutropenia has elapsed, and patients remain at risk until the regenerating immune system matures and restores normal immunity. This depends a great deal on whether or not graft-versus-host disease (GVHD) can be prevented or controlled. Multiple (polymicrobial) infections are not uncommon in this setting.

Table 141-2 Common Infectious Agents in Patients with Cancer

Neutropenia
Bacteria
Gram-positive organisms
Coagulase-negative staphylococci
Staphylococcus aureus (including MRSA)
Enterococcus species (including VRE)
Viridans group streptococci
β-Hemolytic streptococci
Corynebacterium jeikeium
Bacillus species
Stomatococcus mucilaginous
Micrococcus species
Gram-negative organisms
Escherichia coli
Klebsiella species
Pseudomonas aeruginosa
Enterobacter species
Citrobacter species
Serratia species
Pseudomonas (non-aeruginosa) species
Acinetobacter baumanni
Stenotrophomas maltophilia
Cellular Immune Dysfunction
Bacteria
Listeria monocytogenes
Rhodococcus equi
Salmonella spp.
Mycobacteria
Nocardia spp.
Legionella spp.
Fungi
Aspergillus spp.
Cryptococcus neoformans
Histoplasma capsulatum
Coccidioides immitis
Protozoa
Pneumocystis carinii (*P. jiroveci*)*
Toxoplasma gondii
Cryptosporidium spp.
Isospora belli
Viruses
Cytomegalovirus
Herpes simplex virus I and II
Varicella-zoster virus
Epstein-Barr virus
Human herpes virus-6
Community respiratory viruses
Helminth
Strongyloides stercoralis
Humoral immune dysfunction
Bacteria (encapsulated)
Streptococcus pneumoniae
Haemophilus influenzae

*Considered by some to be a fungus.

Local Factors Local factors, such as tumor metastases, that produce obstruction and operative procedures that result in disruption of normal anatomic barriers play an important role in infections occurring in patients with cancer. Pneumonia and pulmonary abscesses frequently develop distal to tumors, causing obstruction of major bronchi, and these infections respond poorly to antibiotic therapy, unless adequate drainage is established. Obstruction of the biliary tract secondary to cancer can result in ascending cholangitis.[21] Likewise, urinary tract infections are common in patients with tumors, such as bladder or prostatic carcinoma, that obstruct a ureter or the bladder neck causing retention of residual urine. Hydronephrosis, pyonephrosis, chronic pyelonephritis, and cystitis are not uncommon complications in patients with cancer of the genitourinary tract (Table 141-3). In these situations, the infection is generally caused by one or more of the microorganisms colonizing the site of obstruction.

Damage to mucosal surfaces (particularly the gastrointestinal mucosa) occurs frequently as a result of antineoplastic chemotherapy and provides a portal of entry for infecting organisms such as viridans group streptococci, VRE and *Candida* species. Radiation therapy results in depression of cell-mediated immunity, which can last for several months. Radiation also causes local tissue damage, which can predispose to secondary infection. Foreign bodies, such as urinary and venous catheters, also damage or circumvent normal anatomic barriers, thereby facilitating entry of microorganisms into tissues and the bloodstream.

Intravascular Devices Central venous catheters are used extensively in patients who require frequent vascular access. These catheters (Hickman, Broviac, and long lines) can have up to three lumens, greatly facilitate a variety of functions, including the drawing of blood, and may remain in the same location for prolonged periods, ranging from several weeks to months. Three separate types of device-related infection have been described: infection of the entry site, tunnel infection, and catheter-related bacteremia or fungemia.[22,23] Gram-positive organisms cause these infections most often, but gram-negative bacilli are not infrequent. Fungemia is most often caused by *Candida* spp. Localized *Aspergillus* infection has also been described. Infections of shunts, stents, and prosthetic devices are also common.

Splenectomy Patients who have undergone splenectomy are at risk of developing infections because the spleen performs several important host defense functions, including antibody production and the removal of poorly opsonized or unopsonized pathogens. The infections commonly seen in such patients are caused by *S. pneumoniae, H. influenzae, Neisseria meningitidis, Babesia* spp., and *Capnocytophaga* spp. These infections can be extremely severe. The syndrome of overwhelming pneumococcal sepsis, is much more common in splenectomized individuals and can be rapidly fatal. The emergence of penicillin-resistant pneumococci made this infection an even more serious problem. The newer fluoroquinolones might have a role instead of penicillin, for chemoprophylaxis. Patients should be given the pneumococcal polyvalent capsular polysaccharide vaccine prior to splenectomy and every 3 years thereafter. Vaccination with *H. influenzae* type B conjugated polysaccharide vaccine and yearly influenza vaccination are also recommended. Quadrivalent meningococcal vaccination should only be administered during an epidemic of meningococcal infection.

Table 141-3 Common Infections in Patients with Solid Tumors

Tumor Location	Infection Site or Type
Breast	Surgical wound infection; cellulitis or lymphangitis related to axillary node dissection; mastitis; breast abscess; bacteremia
Central nervous system (brain; meninges)	Surgical wound infection; epidural/subdural infection; brain abscess; meningitis/ventriculitis; proximal and distal end-shunt–related infections; aspiration pneumonia; urinary tract infection; bacteremia
Genitourinary and prostate	Cystitis; urethritis; acute/chronic pyelonephritis ± bacteremia; catheter-related complicated urinary tract infection (nephrostomy/stents); wound infection; acute/chronic prostatitis; epididymitis, orchitis; pelvic abscess
Hepatobiliary-pancreatic	Surgical wound infection; peritonitis; ascending cholangitis ± bacteremia; hepatic, pancreatic, or subdiaphragmatic abscess
Head and neck	Cellulitis; surgical wound infection; deep facial space infection; mastoiditis/osteomyelitis; sinusitis; aspiration/nosocomial pneumonia; bacteremia; suppurative intracranial phlebitis; meningitis; brain abscess; retropharyngeal and paravertebral abscesses
Musculoskeletal (muscles, bones, joints)	Surgical wound infections; skin and skin structure infection; pyomyositis; lymphangitis cartilage lymphadenitis; bursitis; synovitis; septic arthritis; osteomyelitis; wound infection; prosthesis related infections; bacteremia
Upper gastrointestinal	Esophagitis; tracheoesophageal fistula with pneumonitis/lung abscess; gastric perforation and abscess; feeding tube related infections; mediastinitis/osteomyelitis
Lower gastrointestinal	Surgical wound infection; intraabdominal or pelvic abscess; peritonitis (perforation); enterocolitis; urinary tract infection; perianal/perirectal infection; sacral/coccygeal osteomyelitis

Chemotherapeutic Agents Chemotherapeutic agents predispose to the development of infections in a variety of ways. Many agents produce mucositis, particularly of the gastrointestinal tract, facilitating entry of microorganisms into tissues and the bloodstream. Agents that are myelosuppressive produce neutropenia. Chemotherapeutic agents are also known to interfere with cell-mediated and humoral immunity even when administered in doses that do not generally produce significant myelosuppression. Some of the newer antitumor agents such as fludarabine and other purine analogues, and monoclonal antibodies such as rituximab and CAMPATH have profound effects on multiple components of host defenses.

BACTERIAL INFECTIONS

Current data from The University of Texas, M. D. Anderson Cancer Center indicate that gram-positive organisms cause approximately 50 to 55% of documented infections in patients who have neutropenia. (Table 141-4). Many other epidemiologic surveys focus only on bloodstream infections (EORTC, SCOPE).[3,24] These surveys give an incomplete and inaccurate picture of the overall spectrum because (1) bloodstream infections account for only 15 to 25% of infections (other common sites are the respiratory tract, the urinary tract, the gastrointestinal tract and skin/skin structure) (2) bloodstream infections are predominantly gram-positive (65–75%), whereas (3) infections at other sites are predominantly gram-negative or have mixed flora.

Additionally, 23% of bacterial infections in patients with hematologic malignancies, and 31% in patients with solid tumors are polymicrobial.[2] These infections including pneumonia, neutropenic enterocolitis, skin/skin structure infections (eg, perianal infections) are predominantly tissue based and are generally associated with greater morbidity and mortality than monomicrobial infections. When all sites (including monomicro-

Table 141-4 Distribution of Bacterial Infection in 5,445 Febrile Episodes in Patients with Cancer Who Are Neutropenic

	1975–1977		1986–1989		1994–1995		1999–2000		2002–2003	
Infection Type	No.	%	No.	%	No.	%	No.	%	No.	%
Microbiologically documented	318	31	344	27	189	28	207	30	262	26
Gram-positive	65	21	170	51	86	46	99	48	134	51
Gram-negative	201	63	110	33	54	28	51	25	51	20
Polymicrobial	42	13	54	16	49	26	51	25	71	27
Anaerobic	10	—	—	—	—	—	6	2	6	2
Clinically documented	227	22	248	20	107	16	93	13	210	21
Unexplained fever	481	47	644	53	373	56	390	57	521	53

bial and polymicrobial infections) are taken into account, a substantially different epidemiologic picture emerges, compared to that associated with bloodstream infections alone. The proportion of gram-positive infections decreases substantially (from 70 to 75% to 45 to 50%). This can influence the choice of agents used for prophylaxis and empiric therapy (eg. initial use of vancomycin, or monotherapy vs combination therapy). Consequently, clinicians should consider the entire spectrum of bacterial infections (not just bloodstream infections) when initiating empiric antibiotic therapy.[25]

SPECIFIC BACTERIAL PATHOGENS

***Staphylococcus* Species** Staphylococci are the most common organisms isolated from neutropenic and non-neutropenic cancer patients.[26,27] Coagulase-negative staphylococci (particularly *Staphylococcus epidermidis*) are isolated more often than *S. homins*, and *S. haemolyticus*. Increased use of medical devices and other conditions that usurp natural barriers to infection (surgery, trauma, radiation) are primarily responsible for increased recovery of these organisms. Antimicrobial prophylaxis with fluoroquinolones (to which these organisms are generally resistant) might also account for this increase. The gastrointestinal tract also serves as an important source for coagulase negative staphylococcus (CoNS) in febrile patients with neutropenia.

Staphylococcus aureus is the second most common gram-positive species isolated from patients with cancer. Of concern is the increasing rate of methicillin-resistance among *S. aureus* isolates which is now often > 50% at many cancer treatment centers. The countrywide increase in community acquired-methicillin-resistant *Staphylococcus aureus* (MRSA) (particularly organisms expressing the Panton Valentine Leucocydin gene) may require a change in guidelines and practice patterns for empiric therapy, and may result in an increased use of agents with activity against MRSA. Data from quantitative cultures indicate that the majority of infections caused by CoNS are low-grade (≤10 colony forming units/mL) and might be associated with lower morbidity and mortality than *S. aureus*, for which high-grade infections (≥ 500 CFU/mL) are far more common.[28] Bacteremia (including catheter-related infection) is the most common manifestation of staphylococcal infection. Skin and soft tissue infections, including surgical wound infections, are also relatively common. Serious complications including pneumonia, septic thrombophlebitis, endocarditis, lung and splenic abscesses, can occur, and occasionally can be fatal.

The treatment of staphylococcal infections should be guided by local susceptibility/resistance patterns. Most broad-spectrum agents used for empiric therapy in febrile patients with neutropenia are active against methicillin-susceptible isolates. Vancomycin remains the agent of choice for methicillin-resistant isolates although increasing numbers of vancomycin failures are being reported, even among vancomycin susceptible strains.[29] Older agents (tetracycline, clindamycin, rifampin, trimethoprim/sulfamethoxazole) and some newer agents (quinupristin/dalfopristin, linezolid, daptomycin, dalbavancin) are also useful for the treatment of staphylococcal infections, although many have not been evaluated in patients with neutropenia. Infected catheters should be removed, whenever feasible, although antibiotic therapy without catheter removal has also been shown to be successful. Recurrent infection will occur in 20 to 30% of patients in whom infected catheters are not removed.[30]

***Streptococcus* Species** Many streptococcal species are important pathogens in patients with cancer. *S. pneumoniae* causes infection primarily in patients who have undergone splenectomy, those with multiple myeloma, those with acute or chronic lymphocytic leukemia, and allogeneic bone marrow transplant (BMT) recipients.[31] The syndrome of overwhelming pneumococcal sepsis occurs in patients with splenectomy and often follows a fulminant course resulting in death. Disseminated intravascular coagulation may occur, and *S. pneumoniae* are often demonstrated in peripheral blood smears.[32] Defects in antibody formation and clearing of the organisms from the bloodstream are probably responsible for this clinical syndrome. Prompt and effective antimicrobial therapy is critical. Penicillin G remains the drug of choice for the treatment of pneumococcal infections caused by susceptible strains. However, penicillin-resistant pneumonococci are being reported with increasing frequency and need to be treated with alternative agents. Most penicillin-resistant strains are susceptible to the extended-spectrum cephalosporins (ceftriaxone, ceftazidime, cefepime). The carbapenems (imipenem, meropenem) have also been reported to be active against penicillin-resistant strains. These strains are uniformly susceptible to vancomycin, which is often included in empiric regimens until the results of susceptibility testing become available. Newer generation quinolones (gatifloxacin, moxifloxacin) have potent activity against penicillin-resistant pneumococci, and are being used with increasing frequency to treat these infections.[33,34]

Before the emergence of penicillin-resistance, high-risk patients were given a supply of antibiotics with antipneumococcal activity (eg, amoxicillin/clavulanic acid, Augmentin, which is also active against *H. influenzae)* so that they may initiate antibiotic therapy at the first sign of infection, prior to seeking medical attention. With current rates of penicillin-resistance running as high as 60%, the usefulness of this strategy has been severely limited. The newer generation quinolones have reliable activity against these organisms. Their use instead of amoxicillin/clavulanate might be prudent, but has not been fully evaluated.

Immunization with the polyvalent vaccine is recommended for high-risk individuals with a variety of chronic systemic illnesses and for persons 64 years or older. The highest levels of antibodies are developed by healthy young adults, and the existence of immunosuppressive disorders result in suboptimal antibody production. Vaccination should be given prior to splenectomy, if possible. Vaccination after splenectomy and in patients with continued immunosuppression results in low level antibody production but is still considered beneficial. The new conjugate pneumococcal vaccine is likely to be an improvement on the polyvalent vaccine.

α-Hemolytic (viridans) streptococci are important pathogens in patients with acute leukemia undergoing intensive chemotherapy and in allogeneic bone marrow transplant recipients.[35] α-Hemolytic streptococci colonize the oral cavity, and the most consistent predisposing factor for the development of infection appears to be high-dose chemotherapy with drugs, such as cytosine arabinoside, that induce severe mucosal damage, thereby facilitating entry of these organisms into the bloodstream. Other probable predisposing factors include antimicrobial prophylaxis, particularly with fluoroquinolones that might encourage the selection and overgrowth of these organisms, and the treatment of chemotherapy-induced gastritis with antacids or histamine type 2 (H2) antagonists.[36] *Streptococcus mitis, Streptococcus sanguis,* and *Streptococcus salivarius* are the predominant species. Bacteremia is the most common manifestation. In some patients, a rapidly progressive disseminated infection occurs involving the bloodstream, lungs, central nervous system, and skin (Figure 141-2). Septic shock is often present, and the clinical picture resembles that of staphylococcal "toxic shock syndrome." This syndrome (which is also caused by *Streptococcus pyogenes)* has been termed the "toxic-strep syndrome" or the streptococcal toxic shock syndrome. Overwhelming infection produces substantial morbidity, and mortality in the range of 25 to 35% occurs despite prompt and aggressive antibiotic therapy. The use of clindamycin that blocks toxin production is recommended.

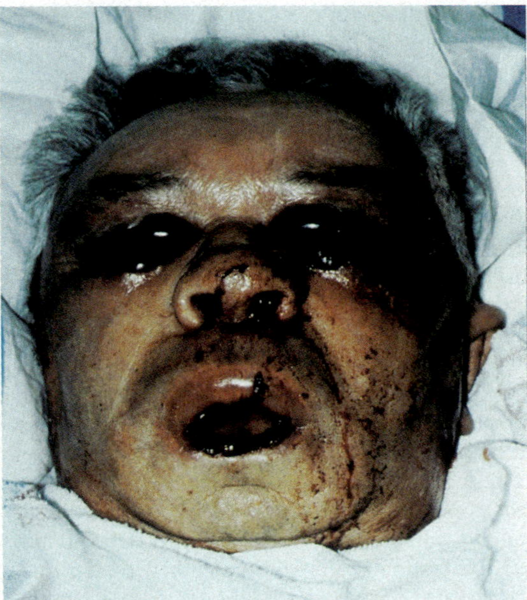

Figure 141-2 Invasive infection caused by α-hemolytic (viridans) streptococci. Note the hemorrhagic nature of the lesions in this patient with thrombocytopenia.

Of increasing concern are reports that 20 to 60% of α-hemolytic streptococci are now penicillin resistant at some institutions. This has limited the utility of penicillin G and other penicillins for the prevention and treatment of such infections. All isolates are currently susceptible to vancomycin, although tolerance has been described, and the use of antibiotic combinations (vancomycin + rifampin ± gentamicin) is sometimes necessary.[37] These organisms are also susceptible to the newer generation quinolones (gatifloxacin, moxifloxacin) daptomycin and linezolid, but clinical experience is limited.

β-Hemolytic streptococci belonging to Lancefield groups A, B, C, F, and G also cause infections in patients with cancer, but less often than *S. pneumoniae* and viridans streptococci. Like viridans streptococci, *S. pyogenes* has been associated with a rapidly progressive, toxic shock-like syndrome. The management of these infections is similar to that of other streptococcal infections. Penicillin G remains the drug of choice for susceptible isolates. Increasing resistance/tolerance to the penicillins is being described. Bactericidal combinations are recommended for the treatment of tolerant isolates.

***Enterococcus* Species** Enterococci are currently the third-most-common gram-positive organisms isolated from patients with neutropenia. This increased frequency is probably related to the increased use of extended-spectrum cephalosporins to which these organisms are intrinsically resistant.[38,39] The most common infections caused by enterococci are those of the bloodstream, urinary tract, wounds, and intra-abdominal infections, although occasionally endocarditis, meningitis, pneumonia, and other infections may be seen. *Enterococcus faecalis* is the predominant species accounting for 60 to 70% of clinical isolates. Most isolates of *E. faecalis* are susceptible to clinically achievable concentrations of penicillin, ampicillin, and vancomycin although these agents may lack bactericidal activity. Consequently, synergistic combinations of these agents with aminoglycosides, such as gentamicin, are recommended for serious enterococcal infections.

Infections caused by *Enterococcus faecium* are rising, particularly in patients who are neutropenic and other patients who are immunosuppressed.[39] These isolates often express high-level resistance to the aminoglycosides, thereby eliminating the synergistic interaction with the penicillins, high-level resistance to ampicillin, and (with increasing frequency) resistance to vancomycin. The most problematic infections occur when all these resistance patterns are seen within the same strains. Vancomycin resistance may now be seen in up to 35% of enterococcal isolates from high-risk populations. Risk factors for infection with vancomycin-resistant enterococci (VRE) include gastrointestinal colonization with these strains, and the use of antimicrobial agents with significant activity against anaerobes (metronidazole, clindamycin, imipenem). The administration of vancomycin (both oral and parenteral) is also a frequently cited risk factor for subsequent colonization with VRE.[40] Infections caused by VRE are much more common in patients with severe neutropenia (acute leukemia; bone marrow transplantation prior to engraftment) and are seldom seen in patients with solid tumors. VRE are associated more often with recurrent infections, higher rates of refractory infections, and serious morbidity and mortality.

There are two established therapeutic options: linezolid and quinupristin/dalfopristin (Synercid). Neither agent is bactericidal against VRE and response rates range from 55 to 65%, well below the 80 to 85% response rates seen with bactericidal combinations against susceptible enterococci.[41] Newer agents (daptomycin, dalbavancin) may have better bactericidal activity.

Attempts at eradicating gastrointestinal colonization with VRE have been singularly unsuccessful. Thus, infection control measures to reduce the transmission of VRE are of over-riding importance. These measures are more aggressive than standard infection control practices (Table 141-5) and strict compliance by hospital personnel is a prerequisite for their success.[42]

Table 141-5 Infection Control Measures Designed to Limit Nosocomial Spread of Vancomycin-Resistant Enterococci in High-Risk Areas (Oncology Units)

General measures
Development of a VRE explanatory brochure or video
Use of explanatory brochure/video for patient and staff orientation
Hand washing before and after patient contact
Development of hospital-wide policies for limiting the use of vancomycin
Substitution of metronidazole for oral vancomycin for the treatment of *Clostridium difficile* colitis
Infectious diseases consultation for appropriate antimicrobial management
Monitoring compliance of general and specific infection control measures
Keeping up the "background noise" with frequent educational activities
Specific measures
Environmental cultures from rooms housing patients who are VRE-positive, and room disinfection on patient discharge
Rectal swab cultures on admission and weekly
Separation of patients into three cohorts depending on VRE status: VRE-negative, VRE-positive, VRE-unknown
Use of gowns and gloves on entry into VRE-positive patient rooms and VRE- unknown patient rooms
Cohorting of staff for patients who are VRE-negative, VRE-positive, and VRE-unknown
Dedicated equipment (eg, stethoscopes) for VRE-positive rooms
Surveillance cultures of high-risk patients housed outside high-risk areas
Strict adherence to infection control measures

VRE = vancomycin-resistant enterococci.

Listeria Monocytogenes *Listeria monocytogenes* is a gram-positive bacillus that causes meningitis, encephalitis, septicemia, and endocarditis. Outbreaks have been reported following consumption of contaminated food products, such as milk, cheese, and coleslaw. The administration of fludarabine and prednisone is associated with an increased incidence of listeriosis in patients with chronic lymphocytic leukemia and may be the result of a depletion in CD4 cells.[43] Meningitis accounts for more than 60% of cases in patients with cancer, and septicemia without meningitis accounts for approximately 30%. Rarely, infections in other sites, such as pleural effusion or septic arthritis, are found. Meningismus is present in only one-half of the cancer patients with meningitis, and, occasionally, the cerebrospinal fluid is normal. When pleocytosis is present, either neutrophils or mononuclear cells predominate. The organisms may be initially difficult to culture from the cerebrospinal fluid and may be occasionally misidentified as either hemolytic streptococci or diphtheroids. Although these organisms are susceptible in vitro to various antibiotics, ampicillin or penicillin remains the drug of choice for therapy. These agents are frequently used in combination with an aminoglycoside, because experimental laboratory results have demonstrated synergism between penicillins and aminoglycosides against *L. monocytogenes.* If an aminoglycoside is administered for central nervous system infection, both systemic and intrathecal routes can be used. Although these organisms are susceptible, in vitro, to the extended-spectrum cephalosporins, these agents are not effective for the therapy of *L. monocytogenes* meningitis. Trimethoprim/sulfamethoxazole (TMP-SMX) is bactericidal against the majority of these isolates, and has been used successfully in patients with listeriosis who are allergic to penicillin, including those with *Listeria* meningitis. Several newer quinolones (gatifloxacin, moxifloxacin) are active against *L. monocytogenes,* but clinical experience with these agents is lacking.

Enterobacteriaceae The gastrointestinal tract serves as an important source of infection in patients who have neutropenia. Although the overall frequency of documented gram-negative infections has declined, the proportion of gram-negative infections caused by Enterobacteriaceae has remained remarkably constant.[44] Data from surveillance studies conducted at major cancer centers, both in the United States and Europe, indicate that Enterobacteriaceae cause approximately 65 to 80% of gram-negative infections in these patients, with *Escherichia coli and Klebsiella* spp. consistently being among the three most common species to be isolated. Thus, antimicrobial regimens used for prophylaxis and for empiric therapy in patients with neutropenia have stressed the need for potent activity against Enterobacteriaceae (and other gram-negative bacilli). The bloodstream is the most frequent site of infection, followed by the urinary tract and the lung. Central venous catheters and other vascular access devices can become secondarily seeded during episodes of bacteremia and can serve as a continuing source of infection. Fever is the only consistent manifestation of infection. Other manifestations depend on specific sites of infection (lung, urinary tract) and are often blunted in patients who are severely neutropenic and immunosuppressed. The majority of these infections respond to standard antimicrobial therapy. However, polymicrobial infections and infections that are complicated by deep tissue involvement (pneumonia, enterocolitis, perirectal infections), are associated with greater morbidity and mortality.[45,46] The emergence of resistance to β-lactam agents as a result of the production of type 1 and extended-spectrum β-lactamases is of great concern. The widespread use of fluoroquinolone prophylaxis has also resulted in the development of resistance among *E. coli* and other Enterobacteriaceae. Routine prophylaxis with the fluoroquinolones in patients with neutropenia is not recommended and should be considered only in patients whose risk of developing gram-negative infections is high.[47]

Pseudomonas Aeruginosa *Pseudomonas aeruginosa* has been a leading cause of infection in patients who have cancer with severe neutropenia. Pneumonia and bacteremia are the most common infections, but the urinary tract, skin and gastrointestinal tract are also sites of infection. It is also a cause of catheter-related infections. In recent years, there has been a decline in gram-negative bacteremias including *P. aeruginosa* among patients with neutropenia. However, the frequency of *P. aeruginosa* bacteremia among patients with acute leukemia has not changed.[48] This organism accounts for approximately 15 to 20% of gram-negative infections.[44]

Several reviews of *Pseudomonas* bacteremia in patients with cancer have been published.[48,49] The largest reviewed 410 episodes that occurred over a 10-year period. The overall rate of *Pseudomonas* bacteremia was 4.7 cases per 1,000 admissions. Neutropenia was the most important predisposing factor, with 69% having an initial neutrophil count of $< 1{,}000/mm^3$ and 40% being severely neutropenic with counts $< 100/mm^3$. Fever was present in approximately 95% of patients. A substantial number (33%) developed shock. Other sites of infection in patients with bacteremia included the respiratory and urinary tracts, the oropharynx, the skin, and soft-tissues, including the perianal region and catheter entry sites. A recent review from the same institution found a major increase in the frequency of community-acquired infections and a substantial decrease in complications such as disseminated intravascular coagulation and ecthyma gangrenosum.[48]

Skin lesions are present in approximately 20% of cases of bacteremia. Ecthyma gangrenosum, the characteristic skin lesion, may be located anywhere but is found most commonly in the axilla, groin, and perianal region. Single or multiple lesions at various stages might be present with extensive tissue damage (Figure 141-3). Ecthyma gangrenosum may occur in the absence of detectable bacteremia. *P. aeruginosa* can be cultured from these lesions, and histologically, the lesions represent a bacterial vasculitis without thrombosis, with dense bacillary infiltration of the media and adventitia of blood vessels.

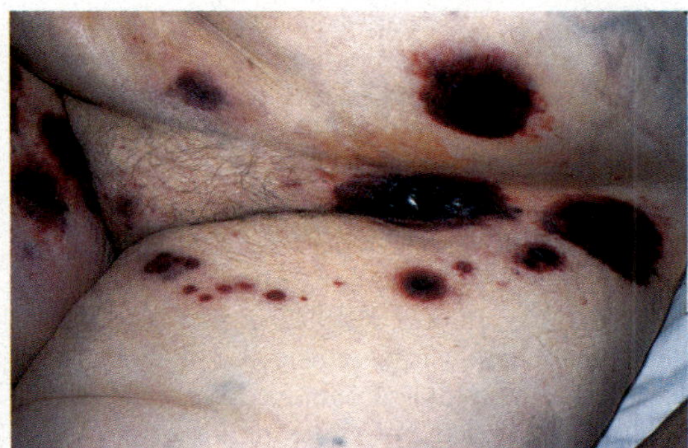

Figure 141-3 Multiple skin lesions (ecthyma gangrenosum) in a patient with *Pseudomonas aeruginosa* bacteremia.

P. aeruginosa is widespread in the hospital environment. It thrives in moist areas, such as faucets, sink drains, shower stalls, hydrotherapy tanks, and water pitchers, and in respiratory equipment, such as respirators and nebulizers. It can also persist in soaps, shampoos, germicidal solutions, and ophthalmic solutions. Epidemics of *P. aeruginosa* infection have been observed in patients with cancer. Approximately 25% of patients with acute leukemia are stool carriers of *P. aeruginosa*. The frequency of *Pseudomonas* infection is twice as high in carriers as in noncarriers. The greater the length of *Pseudomonas* carriage; the greater the chance is of acquiring infection. The widespread use of antimicrobial prophylaxis probably reduces *Pseudomonas* carriage substantially.

During the past 30 years, significant advances were made in the therapy of *P. aeruginosa* infections. Many potent anti-pseudomonal agents were developed including antipseudomonal penicillins (piperacillin ± tazobactam), extended spectrum cephalosporins (ceftazidime, cefepime), aminoglycosides (amikacin, tobramycin), monobactams (aztreonam), quinolones (ciprofloxacin), and carbapenems (imipenem, meropenem) The appropriate use of these agents resulted in response rates in the range of 80%.[48] Unfortunately, these advances are being eroded by the emergence of multidrug resistant *P. aeruginosa* isolates with unique mechanisms of resistance.[12,13] Some of these isolates are susceptible only to agents such as colistin and polymyxin B which are not particularly useful in patients with neutropenia.[25,50]

Stenotrophomonas *Stenotrophomonas maltophilia* are gram-negative bacilli that have emerged during the past decade as important nosocomial pathogens, particularly in patients with impaired host defense.[51] Moist hospital environments, such as sink drains and water faucets, are potential sources of infection. Broad-spectrum antimicrobial therapy and the presence of central venous catheters have been found to significantly increase the likelihood of infection. Patients previously colonized with *S. maltophilia* are at greater risk of developing infection than those not colonized.

Bacteremia (often related to central venous catheters) and pneumonia are the most common manifestations of infection. Urinary tract infection, skin and soft-tissue infection (including surgical wound infection), endocarditis, mastoiditis, and meningitis, have also been reported. Clinical manifestations of *S. maltophilia* infection are indistinguishable from those caused by other gram-negative rod infections. It is also often difficult to distinguish colonization from infection. Substantial mortality occurs in patients with neutropenia, especially if the infection goes unrecognized or a delay in appropriate antimicrobial therapy occurs. Monotherapy using broad-spectrum agents, such as the carbapenems (imipenem, meropenem), to which *S. maltophilia* isolates are generally resistant, is a common form of therapy in patients with neutropenia. Empiric coverage against *S. maltophilia* should be considered in patients who fail to respond to such regimens. Approximately 70% of strains are susceptible to TMP-SMX, although increasing resistance to this agent is being reported. Alternative agents include ticarcillin/clavulanate, minocycline, rifampin, the newer fluoroquinolones, and some extended-spectrum cephalosporins.[52] Most of these agents are less active than TMP-SMX, and susceptibility testing in each individual patient is recommended. Combination antibiotic therapy may be beneficial in patients from whom a relatively resistant strain has been isolated or who fail to respond to initial therapy with a single agent.[53] High-dose therapy with TMP/SMX as used for the treatment of *Pneumocystis carinii* pneumonia, might be beneficial in some patients.

***Acinetobacter* Species** *Acinetobacter* species are acknowledged opportunistic pathogens in patients who are debilitated, and in those with severe underlying conditions, including cancer. These organisms are widely distributed in nature and have the ability to colonize normal or devitalized tissue. They are often found in areas of moist skin, including the axilla, groin, and interdigital pockets. Although infections caused by *Acinetobacter* species are relatively infrequent (approximately 4% of all gram-negative infections in patients who have cancer), infections of nearly all body sites (lungs, meninges, skin, heart valves, biliary tract, urinary tract, bones and joints, peritoneum, skin and soft tissue, and blood) have been reported. It may be difficult to distinguish infection from colonization. In the past, the *anitratus* subspecies were reported to be more commonly associated with infection, whereas the *lwoffi* subspecies were reported more often from sites of colonization.[54] Recent data indicate that this trend has been maintained, and using current nomenclature, *A. baumannii* remain the predominant species isolated from clinical specimens.

Outbreaks of infection caused by *Acinetobacter* species have been traced to intravascular access devices, contaminated respiratory therapy equipment, and contaminated bedding materials. Transmission via the hands of hospital personnel has been documented. In patients with cancer, up to 80% of bacteremic infections caused by *Acinetobacter* species are related to indwelling central venous catheters. The most common clinical finding is the presence of fever. The clinical course may range from benign transient bacteremia to fulminant septic shock (< 5%), which is seen more often in patients with severe neutropenia. Polymicrobial infections from which *Acinetobacter* species are isolated appear to be increasing. Appropriate therapy includes the administration of antimicrobial agents to which the organisms are susceptible, and removal of the offending catheter in catheter-related infections. Multidrug resistance is common among these organisms and may complicate the treatment of serious infections.

***Salmonella* Species** There has been a substantial increase in the incidence of nontyphoidal *Salmonella* infections in the recent years. Fifteen to 25% of serious *Salmonella* infections occur in patients with cancer. Patients with lymphoma, leukemia, or carcinoma of the gastrointestinal and genitourinary tract are most susceptible. *Salmonella typhimurium and* *Salmonella enteritidis* are the most frequently isolated species. Although gastroenteritis, which is usually self-limited, does occur in patients with cancer, about one-half of the infections involve other organ systems. Pneumonia, urinary tract infection, peritonitis, osteomyelitis, meningitis, and wound infection have been observed. Bacteremia and disseminated infections occur more frequently in patients with cancer than other patients with salmonellosis. A small percentage of patients continue to harbor *Salmonella* in stools or urine for periods > 1 year following an acute infection, and are considered chronic carriers. Uncomplicated, nontyphoidal, *Salmonella* gastroenteritis generally requires no antibiotic therapy, but patients who are severely immunocompromised, who are at risk of developing bacteremia or disseminated infection might benefit from antibiotic therapy. The most reliable agents against *Salmonella* spp. are the fluoroquinolones, the extended-spectrum cephalosporins, and the carbapenems. Resistance to even these agents is being reported, and it may be prudent to administer more than one class of agent to seriously ill patients with salmonellosis until susceptibility determinations can be performed.

Mycobacterial Species Protection against mycobacterial infection is mediated by cellular immunity. Mycobacterial infections, therefore, occur more frequently in patients with impairment of the cellular component of the host defense mechanisms (ie, Hodgkin disease). The diagnosis of tuberculosis is often difficult to establish with certainty because the usual manifestations of fever, weight loss, pulmonary infiltrates, and hepatosplenomegaly may be a result of neoplastic disease. Furthermore, patients are often anergic to the tuberculin skin test. Tuberculosis is no more frequent in patients with leukemia than in the general population. However, when infection arises in these patients, it is likely to disseminate widely and rapidly. Substantial changes in the blood and bone marrow including lymphocytosis, monocytosis, eosinophilia, thrombocytopenia, and pancytopenia, may accompany tuberculous infection. In recent years, the spectrum of neoplastic diseases associated with tuberculosis has changed. Infection is frequent in patients with carcinoma of the head, neck, and lung and in patients with lymphoma.

Anergy frequently occurs in patients with cellular immune defects, and positive tuberculin skin tests may be seen in only 10 to 30% of patients. The acid-fast stain is the only widely available test for a rapid presumptive diagnosis of tuberculosis. Traditional culture techniques, followed by biochemical testing, take up to 4 to 8 weeks to identify *M. tuberculosis.* This process is shortened considerably (1 to 3 weeks) by the use of radiometric culture methods followed by a deoxyribonucleic acid (DNA) probe for an *M. tuberculosis*-specific ribosomal ribonucleic acid (RNA) sequence. The DNA probe can be used in mycobacterial cultures but is not sensitive enough to detect organisms in clinical samples. Newer methods based on polymerase chain reaction (PCR) offer great promise and have the potential of providing a specific diagnosis within 24 hours.

Standard therapy for drug-susceptible tuberculosis includes the administration of isoniazid, rifampin, and pyrazinamide daily for 2 months, followed by isoniazid and rifampin for 4 months, either daily or biweekly.[55] Cure rates of greater than 95% are achieved by this regimen. Treatment with isoniazid, rifampin, ethambutol, and pyrazinamide three times a week for a period of 6 months is also effective.[56] Because of the increasing frequency of drug resistance, the initial use of four-drug regimens is preferable until susceptibility determinations can be made. Cure rates of 90% can be achieved by using regimens containing isoniazid, rifampin, pyrazinamide, and ethambutol or streptomycin for 6 to 12 months in patients with an isoniazid-resistant isolate. Resistance to both isoniazid and rifampin markedly reduces the efficacy of therapeutic regimens, and failure rates of 40 to 70% have been reported. Quinolones, such as ofloxacin and ciprofloxacin, have been found to be useful in MDR tuberculosis. Individualized drug regimens, based on results of susceptibility testing, should be employed, generally using at least three drugs to which the isolate is susceptible.[55,57] Directly observed therapy is recommended for all drug-resistant tuberculosis and for patients who are known to be noncompliant or unreliable.

Some patients with cancer are prone to developing infection with mycobacteria other than *M. tuberculosis.* Patients with hairy cell leukemia are particularly prone to developing disseminated infection caused by *Mycobacterium avium intracellulare* complex (MAC).[58] Recent data indicate that MAC infections are not uncommon in patients with solid tumors as well.[59] Unlike MAC infection in patients with AIDS, patients with cancer predominantly present with pulmonary involvement. Bacteremia and disseminated disease are uncommon. In the past, disseminated MAC infections have been difficult to treat because the organisms are resistant to standard antitubercular agents. Commonly used agents include ethambutol, rifabutin, clarithromycin, azithromycin, and streptomycin.[60,61] Refractory cases may respond to therapy with interferon-γ (IFN-γ) in combination with drug therapy.[62]

Mycobacterium kansasii also causes infection both in patients with hematologic malignancies and in patients with solid tumors.[63] Most patients have pulmonary disease, which is indistinguishable from that caused by *M. tuberculosis.* The organisms are generally susceptible to standard antituberculous agents, and most patients respond to therapy.

The pathogenic, rapidly growing mycobacteria (*Mycobacterium chelonae abscessus, M. chelonae ssp. chelonae* and *Mycobacterium fortuitum*) are environmental organisms commonly found in water and soil. The two most common infections caused by these organisms in patients with cancer include catheter-related bacteremia and pulmonary infection.[64,65] In the former, antibiotic therapy in addition to catheter removal is generally effective. In pulmonary or disseminated infection, prolonged therapy with combination regimens is necessary.[66] The organisms have variable susceptibility to agents such as the quinolones, the tetracyclines, the macrolides, amikacin, cephalosporins, and TMP-SMX.

Disease caused by mycobacteria can mimic cancer or present a diagnostic problem in patients with cancer who have been effectively treated and subsequently present with a pulmonary lesion. The assumption that this lesion is a metastatic or recurrent neoplasm should not be made, and patients should be carefully evaluated for tuberculosis or fungal infection before cancer chemotherapy is instituted.

Legionella Pneumophila Since its initial description in 1976, *Legionella pneumophila* has been recognized as an important cause of community-acquired and nosocomial pneumonia in healthy and immunosuppressed persons, including bone marrow transplant recipients.[67] In addition, severe pneumonia, pleural effusion, empyema, and lung abscess formation, are recognized complications of *L. pneumophila* infection and occur more often in the immunosuppressed host.[68] Case fatality rates for treated legionnaires' disease depend on factors such as the immune status of the patient (higher case fatality in patients who are immunosuppressed), and whether the disease was acquired in the community, or in the hospital (nosocomial disease associated with greater fatality rates). Mortality rates as high as 80% have been documented in solid-organ transplant recipients and in others who are immunosuppressed.

A specific diagnosis *of L. pneumophila* infection might be difficult to establish. The organisms are fastidious and require selective culture media to promote growth (buffered charcoal yeast extract [BCYE] agar). Other diagnostic methods include serologic testing, direct fluorescent antibody staining, DNA probes, and the detection of urinary antigen.

Azithromycin is more active than erythromycin and clarithromycin, and should be used as a frontline agent for legionellosis.[69] The fluoroquinolones are also very active against *L. pneumophila* and are now the drugs of choice for the treatment of this infection.[69] Adding rifampin to azithromycin or a quinolone probably provides little further benefit. The quinolones are the agents of choice for the treatment of legionellosis in patients receiving immunosuppressive therapy with cyclosporin or tacrolimus, because they do not alter the metabolism of cyclosporin or tacrolimus.

FUNGAL INFECTIONS

Fungal infections began to emerge as a significant problem among patients with cancer once effective antibacterial agents became available. Initially, *Candida* spp. accounted for the vast majority of fungal infections, but in recent years, other organisms, especially *Aspergillus* spp., have been responsible for the continuing increased frequency. Most fungal infections occur in patients with hematologic neoplasms. Fungal infections occur in approximately 10% of patients with lymphoma but remain an infrequent complication in patients with metastatic carcinoma.

Fungemia is uncommon even in patients with disseminated infection. Most cases of fungemia are caused by *Candida* spp. In the past, the majority of infections were caused by *Candida albicans,* but in recent years *Candida tropicalis, Candida glabrata, Candida parapsilosis,* and other species have emerged as significant pathogens.[70] *Aspergillus* spp. and Mucorales are rarely cultured from the blood even in patients with widely disseminated infection. Fungi that are cultured from blood specimens of patients with disseminated infection include *Cryptococcus neoformans, H. capsulatum, Fusarium* spp., and *Trichosporon beigelii.* The extensive use of intravascular catheters has resulted in an increased frequency of fungemia, caused by *Candida* spp. Because 70 to 80% of these patients have evidence of deep-seated infection, all of these patients should be given antifungal therapy. The duration of fungemia during therapy is prolonged if intravascular catheters are not removed. If the infection is caused by *C. parapsilosis,* therapy is rarely effective without removal of the catheter.[71] Local infections caused by *Aspergillus* spp. and *Rhizopus* spp. may occur at catheter sites and progress to pulmonary or disseminated disease.

The setting in which fungal infection develops is complex, and multiple factors are responsible for the rapid increase in these infections. Frequently, this has been attributed to the widespread use of broad-spectrum antibiotics. Bacteria that inhibit the growth of *Candida* spp. are suppressed by antibiotic therapy permitting the overgrowth of *Candida* spp. Adrenal corticosteroids interfere with macrophage function, and the macrophage is one of the primary defenses against fungal invasion. Prolonged and severe neutropenia also predisposes to fungal infection. Neutrophils ingest and kill *Candida* spp. in vitro and serve as a major defense against systemic infection. The administration of adrenal corticosteroids interferes with macrophage function, allowing ingested spores to germinate. The administration of many cancer chemotherapeutic agents causes neutropenia, which facilitates establishment of infection by activated mycelia. The role of lymphocytes and lymphokines is complex and has not been fully elucidated.

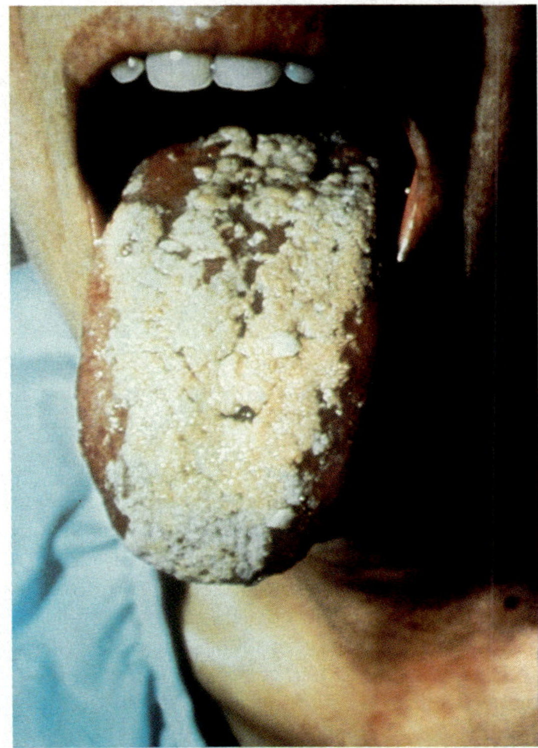

Figure 141-4 Severe oropharyngeal candidiasis in a patient with acquired immunodeficiency syndrome.

Fungal infections often become established at sites of previous infection or necrosis. For example, more than 70% of cases of pulmonary aspergillosis occur in association with a previous or concomitant bacterial pneumonia. *Candida* spp. often infect gastrointestinal ulcerations caused by antitumor agents, or herpes or bacterial infection. The availability of effective antitumor agents and supportive care measures has prolonged the survival of many patients with severely compromised host defense mechanisms, permitting the development of fungal infections in patients who previously would have died of bacterial infections.

***Candida* Species** Most superficial fungal infections of the oropharynx and gastrointestinal tract are caused by *C. albicans.* This infection is especially prevalent in patients receiving antitumor agents or radiotherapy that causes mucosal damage, patients receiving adrenal corticosteroids, and patients colonized with *Candida* spp. Patients with oropharyngeal candidiasis may have associated esophageal candidiasis that is asymptomatic.[72] The lesions appear as white or grayish white plaques surrounded by an erythematous halo (Figure 141-4). The plaques are friable with a freely bleeding base. These lesions may be difficult to differentiate from the necrotic mucosa caused by antitumor agents. Candida plaques may occur in association with herpes simplex infection. Topical agents, such as nystatin, are of minimum benefit. Fluconazole and itraconazole solution, are generally effective. Occasional patients may require a short course of parenteral amphotericin B (AMB), which produces dramatic improvement in most cases after the initial dose.

Candida esophagitis produces dysphagia, often accompanied by retrosternal pain, nausea, and vomiting, and occasionally, gastrointestinal bleeding. Rarely, this infection can lead to perforation. The pain during swallowing may become so severe that the patient is unable to eat. It may be present with or without oral candidiasis. A characteristic cobblestone or moth-eaten appearance of the esophageal mucosa is present on barium-contrast radiographic studies (Figure 141-5). However, these abnormalities may be caused by other organisms, such as herpes simplex and cytomegalovirus. Furthermore, in 25% of cases, the radiographic studies are negative. The diagnosis is established by esophagoscopy, which reveals characteristic ulcerations with pseudomembrane formation. Therapy consists of an orally absorbable antifungal agent, but some patients may have difficulty swallowing these medications. Parenteral amphotericin B is dramatically effective within 24 to 48 hours, and approximately 80% of patients respond after a 5-day course of therapy. Fluconazole is equally effective and less toxic. Because *Candida* spp. are the

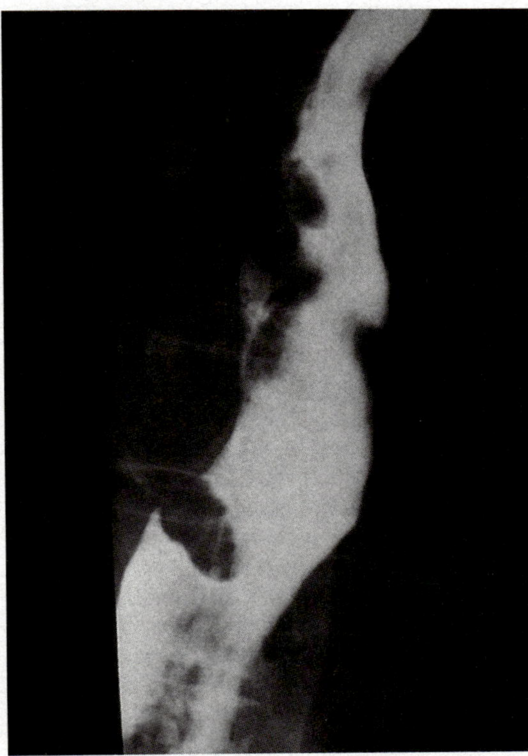

Figure 141-5 The characteristic "moth-eaten" appearance of the esophageal mucosa demonstrated on barium-swallow examination in a patient with esophageal candidiasis.

most common cause of infectious esophagitis, it is often appropriate to initiate antifungal therapy empirically and perform esophagoscopy if the patient fails to respond.

Systemic *Candida* infections may be localized to a single organ, but usually multiple organs are involved. Occasional cases of chronic laryngitis caused by *Candida* spp. have been recognized. Pulmonary infection is usually a manifestation of disseminated disease, but occasional primary infections of the lung occur because of aspiration of contaminated oropharyngeal secretions. It is difficult to establish the diagnosis of primary *Candida* pneumonia because there are no characteristic findings.[73] Isolation of *Candida* spp. from the sputum may represent contamination from the oropharynx. A substantial proportion of patients with urinary catheterization develop candiduria that often represents only colonization. Patients with surgery or abnormalities of the genitourinary tract, neutropenia or diabetes mellitus should always be treated with systemic therapy because they are at risk of serious *Candida* infection. *Candida* peritonitis may occur following intestinal perforation or in association with peritoneal catheters.

Disseminated candidiasis is found at autopsy examination in 20 to 30% of patients with acute leukemia, in 2% of patients with lymphoma, and in less than 1% of patients with metastatic cancer. Two patterns of organ involvement have been described. In one, occurring predominantly in patients with acute leukemia, the most frequent organs infected include the gastrointestinal tract, liver, spleen, and lungs. This pattern of involvement suggests the gastrointestinal tract as the primary site of origin. The second pattern of distribution predominantly involves the heart, kidneys, and lung, which is the pattern of distribution in animals following direct intravenous injection. There are no characteristic physical signs and symptoms of disseminated candidiasis. Some patients present with the acute onset of tachycardia, tachypnea, and hypotension. Often, the only indications of this infection are a gradual worsening of the patient's clinical condition, associated with fever which is unresponsive to antibiotic therapy. Some patients have ocular infection causing blurred vision, pain, scotomas, or loss of visual acuity. Ocular lesions include white fluffy retinal exudates with vitreous haze or hemorrhage, hypopyon, or iritis, but these lesions are rarely found in patients with neutropenia. Approximately 10% of patients, especially those with severe neutropenia, develop characteristic erythematous macronodular skin lesions. These lesions may be single or multiple, localized or diffuse, often resembling a drug rash. *Candida* organisms can be identified in the subcutaneous tissue of skin biopsies of these lesions and can be cultured from the tissue in 50% of cases. In occasional patients, these skin lesions are associated with a myositis in which the patient has exquisitely tender muscles.

A chronic form of *Candida* infection known as hepatosplenic candidiasis—or, more appropriately, chronic disseminated candidiasis—has been described.[74] This infection typically occurs in patients with acute leukemia undergoing chemotherapy while they are experiencing prolonged severe neutropenia. They develop fever that fails to respond to broad-spectrum antibiotics, as well as antifungal agents. After neutrophil recovery, they remain febrile and debilitated with substantial weight loss. Symptoms, including right upper quadrant or shoulder pain, may appear. Hepatosplenomegaly may be detected. Alkaline phosphatase concentration becomes highly elevated, and other liver function tests may also become abnormal. Ultrasonography, magnetic resonance imaging (MRI), or computed tomography (CT) of the liver and spleen reveals multiple lesions (Figure 141-6). Other organs may also be infected. Approximately 80% respond to fluconazole or lipid formulations of AMB.[75] Usually several weeks of therapy are required. This type of *Candida* infection has virtually disappeared from institutions where fluconazole is used prophylactically.

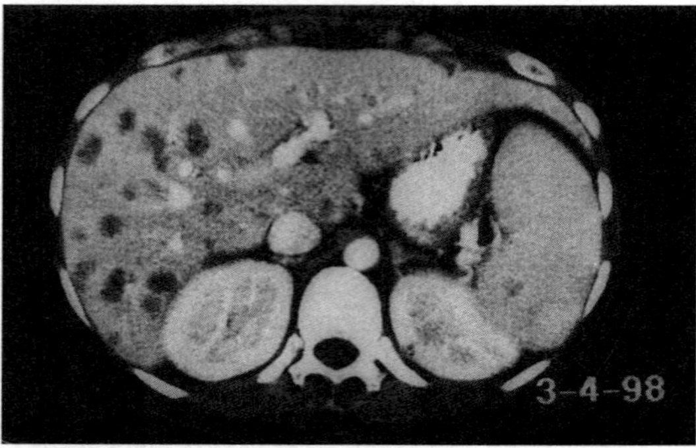

Figure 141-6 Multiple "punched-out" lesions in the liver, spleen, and kidneys in a patient with chronic disseminated candidiasis.

Because the frequency of infections caused by *Candida* spp. other than *C. albicans* has increased substantially in recent years, unique features of some of these infections have been recognized. At many institutions *C. tropicalis* has surpassed *C. albicans* as the most common cause of disseminated infection.[76] It appears to be more virulent because only 3 to 15% of neutropenic patients colonized by *C. albicans* subsequently develop disseminated infection, as compared to 40 to 80% of those colonized by *C. tropicalis.* Skin lesions and myositis are associated more often with *C. tropicalis* infection. *C. parapsilosis* is less virulent than *C. albicans,* and infection is nearly always associated with intravascular catheters and parenteral nutrition. Only 10% of patients with intravascular catheters who develop *C. parapsilosis* fungemia respond to antifungal therapy without removal of the catheter.[71]

Colonization and infection caused by *C. krusei* and *C. glabrata* are associated with the use of fluconazole prophylaxis.[77] Unlike other *Candida* spp., *C. krusei* has been isolated from many foods and beverages, but infrequently from healthy humans. It is resistant to fluconazole and variably susceptible to itraconazole. *C. glabrata* is a common contaminant of the skin and urine. It has variable susceptibility to fluconazole, and itraconazole, but many infections have been treated successfully with high doses of fluconazole. *C. glabrata* is often a cause of candidemia among patients already receiving fluconazole or AMB as therapy or prophylaxis.[78] Patients who are azole naïve may also develop infections caused by non-albicans candida species.[79]

The diagnosis of disseminated candidiasis is often not established before death. Only 50% of patients have abnormal chest radiographs at the onset of infection involving the lungs. *Candida* spp. are isolated from blood specimens of about 70% of patients with disseminated candidiasis using the most sensitive culture techniques such as lysis-centrifugation. A variety of nonculture methods, including monoclonal antibodies to detect mannoproteins, enzyme-linked immunosorbent assay (ELISA) techniques to detect enolase, and PCR analyses have been developed, but none are reliable.[80] The isolation of *C. albicans* from throat or urine specimens is of little diagnostic importance, whereas the isolation of *C. tropicalis* indicates the presence of infection in approximately 60% of patients with neutropenia.

AMB has been effective for the treatment of disseminated candidiasis in patients with adequate neutrophil counts, but it has undesirable acute toxicities including fever, chills, and headaches. Chronic administration often results in nephrotoxicity that is of concern in patients with cancer who often are receiving other nephrotoxic agents. The administration of AMB in lipid formulations reduces the frequency of nephrotoxicity and allows for the administration of much higher daily doses, but it is not clear that these higher doses result in enhanced efficacy. Combining AMB with 5-fluorocytosine may increase therapeutic efficacy, especially if the infection is caused by *C. tropicalis.* In vitro and animal studies indicate that these agents interact synergistically against *Candida* spp. The myelosuppressive toxicity of 5-fluorocytosine can be problematic in patients whose marrow function has been compromised already by chemotherapy. Fluconazole is as effective as AMB and is much less toxic.[81,82] *C. krusei* is inherently resistant to fluconazole and about 15% of isolates of *C. glabrata* are also resistant. Other agents available for therapy of *Candida* infections include itraconazole, voriconazole and caspofungin.[83] Newer agents such as micafungin, anidulafungin and posaconazole are in various stages of development.

The therapy of disseminated candidiasis in patients with neutropenia is often unsuccessful. The use of high-dose antifungal therapy (fluconazole, lipid preparations of amphotericin B) or combination therapy (eg, caspofungin and voriconazole) might offer some benefit in selected patients along with the use of hematopoietic growth factors (G-CSF, GM-CSF) and/or granulocyte transfusions.

***Aspergillus* Species** Aspergillosis is an increasing problem in patients with neutropenia and patients receiving chronic adrenal corticosteroid therapy. Recent studies report a frequency of 20 to 50% among patients with acute leukemia. This infection is also common in bone marrow transplant recipients during the posttransplant period when they are neutropenic and later if they develop graft-versus-host disease. The most common pathogen is *Aspergillus fumigatus*. Other human pathogens include *Aspergillus terreus, Aspergillus flavus, Aspergillus niger, Aspergillus glaucus,* and *Aspergillus nidulans*. Infection is usually acquired by inhalation of spores, which are deposited in the paranasal sinuses or lungs.[84] Outbreaks of aspergillosis have occurred on leukemic and bone marrow transplantation units, usually associated with construction within or adjacent to the hospital. Studies show that the concentration of *Aspergillus* spores is much higher at construction sites within the hospital than at other hospital sites. Disturbance of dust above false ceilings represents a significant risk to susceptible patients, and they should be protected from such exposure.

More than 70% of infections involve the lungs, and approximately 35% of patients with pulmonary aspergillosis have hematogenous dissemination to other organs. Pulmonary infection may be manifested as necrotizing bronchopneumonia, hemorrhagic pulmonary infarction, solitary or miliary lung abscesses, lobar pneumonia, or bronchitis. A few patients will develop exsanguinating pulmonary hemorrhage early in the course of their infection. The classic clinical presentation of pulmonary aspergillosis is the sudden onset of pleuritic chest pain with fever, hemoptysis, and a pleural friction rub suggestive of pulmonary embolus and infarction. Unfortunately, this classic syndrome occurs in less than 30% of patients. Often, the only evidence of infection is prolonged fever with pulmonary infiltrates that fail to respond to antibacterial therapy. The earliest abnormality on chest radiographic examination is the appearance of single or multiple rounded dense areas (Figure 141-7). Patients with symptoms of pulmonary infarction may develop typical wedge-shaped lesions. As the infection progresses, one of several patterns may emerge, including single or multiple abscesses with cavitation, lobar pneumonia, or patchy or diffuse pulmonary infiltrates located unilaterally or bilaterally. Patients whose infection is controlled often develop cavities with or without fungus balls. High-resolution CT scanning of the lung can be helpful in the early diagnosis of aspergillosis. Nodular lesions may be detected in the lungs of patients with normal chest radiographs. Characteristic findings in early stage disease are multiple nodules with a halo of surrounding ground-glass attenuation that represents hemorrhage surrounding a region of pulmonary infarction. As healing occurs, the infarcted tissue becomes necrotic and retracts from the viable tissue leaving an air crescent.[85]

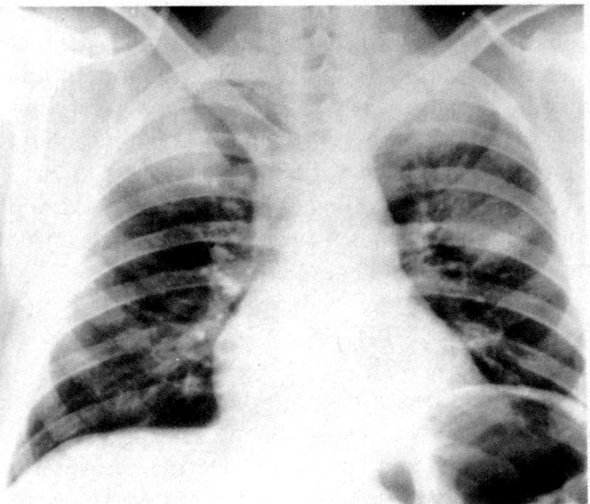

Figure 141-7 Multiple rounded pulmonary infiltrates compatible with invasive pulmonary aspergillosis.

Pathologically, pulmonary infection consists of nodular zones of consolidation surrounded by hemorrhage, abscess formation, or typical wedge-shaped infarcts. On microscopic examination, *Aspergillus* spp. appear as uniform septate hyphae, about 4 microns in diameter with dichotomous branching. These organisms have a propensity for invading blood vessels, causing thrombosis and infarction.

Aspergillus sino-orbital infection is being diagnosed with increasing frequency in patients with acute leukemia and in marrow transplant recipients, accounting for at least 15% of cases of aspergillosis (Figure 141-8). Signs and symptoms include fever, retro-orbital pain, headache, circumorbital erythema, nasal obstruction, and necrotic encrustation of the nasal septum, palate, or external nares. Infections may erode through the base of the skull and invade the brain or cause destruction of the paranasal and facial structures and the eye. About half the infections disseminate to other organs. The fungus can often be isolated from nasal cultures. It can be visualized histopathologically and often cultured from biopsy specimens.

Overall, approximately 35% of infections are widely disseminated. Organs involved include the lung, brain, gastrointestinal tract, liver, kidney, and thyroid. Aspergillus infection of the liver may cause multiple abscesses or vascular thrombosis and infarction, occasionally resulting in Budd–Chiari syndrome. The organism is seldom isolated from blood culture specimens of patients with disseminated disease.

Although central nervous system aspergillosis sometimes results from local extension of sinus infection, more often, it follows hematologic dissemination. Multiple lesions are usually present, with substantial vascular invasion leading to cerebral thrombosis, infarction, and abscess formation. These patients are lethargic and have focal neurologic signs indicative of the area of brain involvement. The cerebrospinal fluid is normal in most instances, although leukocytosis and increased protein concentrations may be found.

A localized form of aspergillosis has been described in association with intravascular catheters. *Aspergillus* spores may be deposited from the air at the time of insertion or may be impregnated in materials used for catheter dressings.[86] These infections are potentially serious because they can disseminate. Skin lesions, manifested as sharply defined black eschars, occur in about 5% of patients with disseminated infection. *Aspergillus stomatitis* occurs in patients with neutropenia.

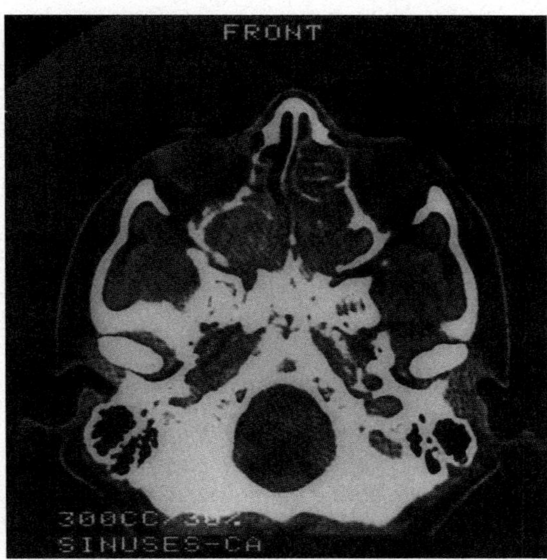

Figure 141-8 Pansinusitis caused by *Aspergillus* spp. in an allogeneic bone marrow transplant recipient with persistent fever.

Antemortem diagnosis of aspergillosis is difficult because the organism is cultured from clinical specimens of less than 30% of infected patients; hence, many infections are diagnosed only at autopsy examination. Although *Aspergillus* spp. can be cultured from normal, uninfected subjects and is a potential laboratory contaminant, if it is cultured from respiratory secretions of susceptible patients, there is a high probability of infection. Hyphal elements can be identified in infected sinus tissue biopsies, but the organism is cultured from only 75% of these cases. PCR and glucomannan detection by sandwich ELISA are promising noncultural methods for identifying infected patients.[87–89] Serial glucomannan assays may be useful for assessing response to therapy.

AMB is effective for the treatment of aspergillosis, provided the patient's underlying deficiency in host defense mechanisms has been corrected. Patients with persistent deficiencies in host defense mechanisms, especially neutropenia, seldom respond to therapy. Recovery often requires prolonged therapy with AMB, which usually causes dose-limiting nephrotoxicity, hence, a lipid formulation is preferable to AMB desoxycholate. Because substantially higher doses of AMB can be administered by the lipid formulations, they may be more effective, although the evidence is only suggestive.

Itraconazole is an azole compound that has activity against *Aspergillus* spp.[90] In the past, its use was limited because only an oral capsule was available and oral absorption was variable. Currently, an oral solution and an intravenous solution are available that provide more reliable serum concentrations. It appears to be as effective as AMB but no comparative trial has been conducted.

Two new agents are available for the treatment of aspergillosis.[91,92] Caspofungin has been demonstrated to be useful in the salvage treatment of invasive aspergillosis in patients refractory to or intolerant of conventional antifungal therapy.[90] Voriconazole therapy led to better responses, improved survival, and fewer side effects than AMB in patients with invasive aspergillosis.[92]

A major problem is the management of the patient who has recovered from pulmonary aspergillosis and who has a persistent cavity with or without a fungus ball. Acute pulmonary hemorrhage can occur, leading to death. Furthermore, the potential for reactivation of infection interferes with subsequent cancer chemotherapy. Surgical excision of the residual cavity should be given consideration, but that may not always be technically possible due to the presence of multiple cavities or the location of the lesion. Antifungal therapy should be administered during periods of neutropenia in patients with residual lesions to prevent reactivation. The appropriate duration of such therapy is unknown, but should be continued for a minimum of two courses.

***Cryptococcus* Species** Cryptococcosis is primarily a disease of patients with impaired cellular immunity; hence patients with lymphoma, Hodgkin disease, and other lymphatic malignancies are at risk from this infection. Occasionally, infection occurs in patients with solid tumors. The organism is ubiquitous in animals and soil specimens. Infection begins in the lungs, where in healthy humans, it may remain asymptomatic and resolve without therapy. Approximately 40% of infections in patients with cancer involve the lungs.[93] A variety of abnormalities may be found on chest radiographs, including miliary, nodular or cavitary lesions. On pathologic examination, the typical lesions have a gelatinous appearance. The lesions consist of aggregations of encapsulated budding yeast cells with minimal inflammatory response. Granulomas may be present in some cases. Primary cryptococcal pneumonia may follow a fulminant course, leading to the death of the patient within 1 to 2 weeks after onset of symptoms.

The most common form of cryptococcal infection is meningoencephalitis, accounting for approximately 50% of infections in patients with cancer.[93] It is a consequence of hematogenous dissemination from the lung where usually the infection is no longer apparent. Infection may be acute, subacute, or chronic, and may arise suddenly or insidiously. Symptoms of central nervous system infection include headache, vertigo, nausea, and vomiting; physical findings consist of fever, meningitis, stupor, signs of increased intracranial pressure, and focal neurologic defects. Leukocytosis (predominantly with lymphocytes), hypoglycorrhachia, and elevated protein concentrations are usually found in the cerebrospinal fluid. Yeast cells can be visualized in the cerebrospinal fluid of nearly 60% of patients. The organisms may be confused with mononuclear cells, but they can be differentiated by an India ink preparation that defines the capsule of the yeast cells. Although *Cryptococcus neoformans* usually is cultured easily from the cerebrospinal fluid of patients with meningitis, occasional patients with cancer have normal cerebrospinal fluid, and the organism cannot be isolated from repeated culture specimens. The serologic test for detection of cryptococcal antigen in cerebrospinal fluid and blood is useful for rapid diagnosis of this infection, especially in cases where the organism cannot be visualized.

Disseminated infection may involve multiple organs with the skin and bone being frequent sites. Skin lesions may be acneiform, nodular, pustular, plaque-like or ulcerated and are present in approximately 10% of patients with disseminated infection. Occasional patients develop a cryptococcal panniculitis. The yeast may be isolated from blood, urine, or sputum of patients with disseminated infection.

Initial therapy of meningitis should consist of AMB plus 5-fluorocytosine for about 2 weeks. Subsequently, therapy can be continued with fluconazole for at least 10 weeks. Fluconazole can also be used as primary therapy for subacute and chronic infections of other sites.

Other Opportunistic Fungi A variety of fungi of low pathogenicity have been recognized as cause of significant infection in patients with cancer. These organisms include *Trichosporon* spp., the Zygomycetes, *Blastoschizomyces capitatus, Fusarium* spp., *Scedosporium* spp., *Geotrichum candidum,* and *Malassezia furfur.* Most of these infections occur sporadically, although there have been clusters of *Fusarium* infections at some institutions. The majority of patients who are infected have hematologic neoplasms, especially acute leukemia.

Zygomycosis is a rare infection with the most common pathogens being Mucor, Rhizopus, Absidia, and Rhizomucor species.[94] Pneumonia is the most common form of infection in patients with cancer, and occurs primarily in patients with hematologic malignancies. Some patients develop sinopulmonary, rhinocerebral, gastrointestinal, cutaneous, or disseminated infection. The clinical presentation of zygomycosis is often indistinguishable from aspergillosis. Zygomycosis should be considered in patients who are immunosuppressed and who develop sinusitis or invasive fungal infection after prolonged exposure to voriconazole, which is not active against these organisms.[95]

Microscopically, these organisms appear as broad nonseptate branching hyphae. Like *Aspergillus* spp., Mucorales invade blood vessels, causing thrombosis and infarction. Most cases of mucormycosis in patients with cancer are diagnosed at autopsy; consequently, therapeutic measures have not been evaluated extensively. AMB is only marginally active against these fungi. Aggressive surgical debridement is an important component of the therapy of sino-orbital infection and should be considered in patients with residual lesions after pulmonary infection. Patients with neutropenia uniformly fail to respond to therapy unless neutrophil recovery occurs. Posaconazole is a new agent with promising activity against the Zygomycetes.

Trichosporon spp. cutaneum can cause disseminated infection, primarily in patients with hematologic neoplasms. The majority of patients have been severely neutropenic.[96] A few patients, especially those with adequate neutrophil counts, develop localized pneumonia without dissemination. There are no characteristic signs and symptoms suggestive of *Trichosporon* infection. A variety of skin lesions have been described, and skin lesions occur in approximately 30% of patients who are infected. Portals of entry include the gastrointestinal tract, respiratory tract, and intravenous catheter sites. *Trichosporon* infection is often associated with other concurrent opportunistic infections. Although these organisms may be susceptible to AMB, the azole compounds appear to be more effective therapeutic agents.

Fusarium spp. have emerged as significant pathogens in patients with neutropenia during the past decade.[97,98] These organisms produce a potent toxin that, when ingested, causes aplastic anemia. Localized infections of the lung, sinuses, and skin occur, but most patients have disseminated infection. Cutaneous and subcutaneous skin lesions are frequent in disseminated infection. Like *Aspergillus* spp., these organisms invade blood vessels, causing thrombosis and infarction. Usually *Fusarium* spp. can be isolated readily from blood culture or tissue specimens. It may be difficult to distinguish *Fusarium from* some other fungi on histopathologic examination. Recovery from this infection depends on resolution of neutropenia, and currently available antifungal agents are at best only marginally effective.

Empiric Therapy The high frequency of fungal infections in patients with neutropenia and the inadequacy of diagnostic procedures have led to empiric administration of antifungal agents in patients who are suspected of having these infections. Empiric therapy should be considered in patients with neutrophil counts of less than 100/mm^3 for greater than 1 week who develop fever that fails to respond to 4 to 7 days of broad-spectrum antibacterial therapy. Other supportive indications are indwelling catheters, chronic adrenal corticosteroid therapy, the presence of unexplained pulmonary infiltrates, and deteriorating renal or hepatic function. AMB has been used most often as empiric therapy, but other alternatives are effective, including lipid formulations of AMB, fluconazole, itraconazole, voriconazole and caspofungin. Fluconazole is less attractive than other agents for empiric therapy because it is not active against aspergillosis.[99,100] Patients who respond probably should remain on antifungal therapy for at least 1 or 2 weeks. Empiric antifungal therapy is not indicated for a majority of patients who have only transient or modest degrees of neutropenia.

VIRAL INFECTIONS

Viral infections are common following BMT/HSCT, and, to a lesser extent, among patients with leukemia and lymphoma. Herpes viruses are identified most frequently, especially herpes simplex virus (HSV), varicella zoster virus (VZV), and cytomegalovirus (CMV). Community respiratory viruses, including respiratory syncytial virus (RSV), influenza A and B, and parainfluenza viruses, are common among BMT recipients and patients with acute leukemia in whom upper respiratory tract infection can progress to pneumonitis, which is associated with a substantial mortality rate. Other viruses that can cause serious illness include Epstein-Barr virus (EBV), human herpes virus-6 (HHV-6), adenoviruses, hepatitis viruses, and polyoma viruses.[101–103]

HSV Infections caused by HSV are the most common viral infections in patients with lymphoma and acute leukemia. These infections occur predominantly in patients with preexistent antibodies to HSV, indicating that most represent reactivation of endogenous latent infection. More than 80% of bone marrow transplant recipients will have reactivation of latent HSV. Lesions caused by HSV are found most often on the lips and oral mucosa. In patients receiving antineoplastic chemotherapy, these lesions tend to become large and painful, and severe mucositis with extensive ulceration of the oral mucosa is not uncommon. Secondary infection with bacteria or fungi may occur. Localized bleeding may be a complication in patients with severe thrombocytopenia. Some patients develop chronic localized herpetic ulcers involving the nose, lips, or eyelids that begin as small papulovesicular lesions and gradually enlarge over several weeks. Herpetic lesions can extend from the oropharyngeal mucosa to involve the esophageal mucosa, producing symptoms that are indistinguishable from *Candida* esophagitis. Occasionally, esophagitis may occur without oropharyngeal lesions, and it may become necessary to perform invasive diagnostic procedures, such as endoscopy, and obtain a biopsy specimen in order to make an accurate diagnosis. Patients with herpetic esophagitis may also have lesions involving the larynx and trachea and occasionally may develop severe necrotizing tracheobronchitis. Localized HSV lesions may also be seen in other areas of the body, such as the genital and perianal areas, and may become quite destructive. Dissemination of HSV infection is uncommon and occurs most often in patients with Hodgkin disease. The liver, spleen, adrenal glands, kidneys, pancreas, lungs, brain, and gastrointestinal tract may be involved in disseminated infection. Acyclovir, famciclovir, and valacyclovir are effective for the treatment of these infections.[104–106] Because of the high frequency of mucocutaneous infections in acute leukemia patients undergoing induction chemotherapy and bone marrow transplant recipients who are seropositive, antiviral prophylaxis is indicated. Disseminated infection, encephalitis, and infection in immunocompromised patients generally require intravenous therapy with acyclovir (10 mg/kg q8h). Strains of HSV resistant to acyclovir may develop. In such cases, foscarnet is the treatment of choice. Cidofovir might also be useful in refractory infections.

VZV Primary infection with VZV causes approximately 4 million cases of chicken pox in the United States each year.[107] VZV remains latent in the sensory ganglia for the lifetime of the host, and reactivates in 15% of persons to cause herpes zoster.[108] Varicella has been recognized as a serious infection in children undergoing cancer chemotherapy. Because it is highly contagious, it is especially hazardous, and epidemics have occurred in pediatric cancer facilities. Serious complications arise in approximately 5% of otherwise healthy children who develop varicella, but the fatality rate is less than 0.5%. Approximately 30% of children receiving cancer chemotherapy develop serious complications during varicella infection, and the fatality rate is around 7%. Most serious complications and deaths occur in children with hematologic neoplasms. The severity of infection is related to the extent of the underlying cancer and to antitumor therapy.

Characteristic manifestations of varicella include a generalized vesicular rash and fever. Lesions appear initially on the face and scalp and subsequently spread to the trunk and extremities. New lesions continue to appear as older lesions crust. Infection may be unduly prolonged in patients with cancer. The vesicles become hemorrhagic and necrotic in patients with thrombocytopenia. Approximately 10% of children develop a bacterial superinfection. The disease is occasionally rapidly progressive, and in a few patients, can lead to circulatory collapse and death shortly after the appearance of the vesicles. Disseminated visceral infection may result in widespread pneumonia, and focal necrosis of the liver, pancreas, or adrenal glands. Fulminating encephalitis may develop. Dissemination generally develops within 1 week of the onset of skin lesions.

Herpes zoster occurs sporadically in the general adult population. Among patients with cancer, it occurs most often in those with lymphoproliferative disorders. The infection is characterized by a unilateral vesicular rash in the distribution of one or two adjacent sensory dermatomes (Figure 141-9). The thoracic, cervical, and lumbar dermatomes are most commonly involved. In approximately 20% of patients with cancer, herpes zoster lesions arise initially at sites where the tumor is in close proximity to a nerve trunk. In an additional 20% of the patients, eruption first appears at sites of recent radiation therapy. Initially, the lesions appear to be erythematous and maculopapular in nature but swiftly evolve into a vesicular rash. Vesicles may coalesce to form larger, bulbous lesions. Localized herpes zoster usually causes no unique problems in the cancer patient. Occasionally, the lesions heal slowly with necrosis and scarring. In others, lesion formation may continue for 10 to 15 days, and crusting or scabbing of lesions may not occur until approximately 3 to 4 weeks into the course of the disease. Occasionally, patients develop a generalized varicelliform eruption, without localization. The rash is accompanied by pain (zoster-associated pain) that often precedes the eruption by 2 to 3 days, and can last for several weeks or even months. Postherpetic neuralgia is zoster-associated pain that persists beyond 1 month.

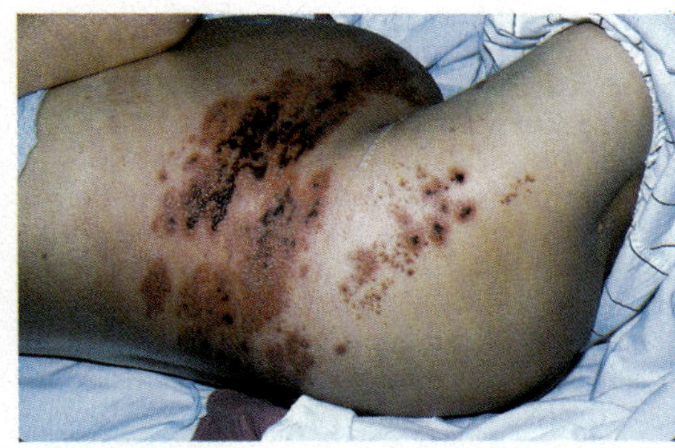

Figure 141-9 Typical vesicular rash caused by varicella-zoster virus. Note the dermatomal distribution, and the hemorrhagic nature of lesions in this patient with thrombocytopenia.

Cutaneous dissemination of herpes zoster occurs in approximately 35% of patients with cancer, as compared with only 4% of those without cancer. Therapy with adrenal corticosteroids, radiation, or antitumor agents facilitates dissemination. Localized skin lesions may precede cutaneous dissemination by 2 to 15 days. Lesions may appear in the mouth, pharynx, labia, or anus. Visceral dissemination occurs infrequently but then commonly involves the gastrointestinal tract, liver, adrenals, pancreas, lungs, and brain, resulting in hepatitis, pneumonitis, and meningoencephalitis. Muscular weakness, motor paralysis, and postherpetic neuralgia seem to be more common in patients with cancer. Multiple episodes of herpes zoster are much more common in immunosuppressed individuals than in persons who are immunocompetent.

Laboratory confirmation of the diagnosis is not required for most cases of varicella. VZV can be recovered from the vesicular fluid for a few days after the onset of the eruption but is recovered infrequently from other sites. Cultures are positive 30 to 60% of the time. Detection of VZV antigens in skin scrapings using fluorescence microscopy, and detection of VZV DNA, in the cerebrospinal fluid or other tissues, using PCR, are more rapid and sensitive diagnostic techniques.

Therapy of VZV infection shortens viral shedding, accelerates healing of lesions and reduces the frequency of visceral disease.[109,110] Oral famciclovir and valacyclovir are more effective than acyclovir. Severe infections such as meningoencephalitis and pneumonitis require intravenous acyclovir therapy along with skilled supportive therapy. Significant mortality may occur despite these measures. Therapy with foscarnet or combination therapy with foscarnet and acyclovir should be considered for patients who fail to respond to acyclovir alone.[111]

Zoster-associated pain represents a continuum that includes prodromal pain, acute phase pain, and chronic pain (commonly referred to as postherpetic neuralgia). All these appear to be more common in the elderly and in patients who are immunosuppressed. Although the role of adrenal corticosteroids to prevent this complication is controversial, one randomized study in patients older than age 50 years showed that acyclovir plus prednisone was more effective against zoster-associated pain than acyclovir alone.

The administration of varicella-zoster immune globulin is useful for postexposure prophylaxis in high-risk individuals and can also ameliorate established infection. Varicella-zoster immune globulin must be given within 96 hours of exposure to be effective. Varicella vaccine is available for universal immunization and postexposure prophylaxis. The vaccine is safe, immunogenic, and effective in leukemic children at risk for serious disease, if chemotherapy is interrupted for 1 week before and after administration. Approximately 50% developed a mild rash, of who 40% were treated with acyclovir.[112] A 1-week course of antiviral therapy following exposure may be useful for patients who are at risk.[113]

CMV Although CMV infections occur sporadically among patients with cancer, especially among those with hematologic malignancies, they are a significant complication among BMT recipients. Like other herpes viruses, CMV remains latent in tissues after recovery from initial infection. Up to 80% of patients who are seropositive and are undergoing BMT reactivate latent infection and approximately 30% of seronegative recipients with seropositive donors acquire infection. The most common forms of infection in patients with cancer are pneumonia and gastroenteritis, but other infections include esophagitis, myocarditis, hepatitis, encephalitis, and retinitis. Prior to the use of prophylaxis, most CMV infections occurred by day 60 after transplantation, but now it is diagnosed more often after day 100.

Early detection of CMV infection is critical to optimal management. The isolation of virus from body fluids or tissues indicates infection but not always symptomatic disease. The CMV pp65 antigenemia assay using infected white blood cells or serum is a reliable, rapid, and sensitive test that is cost-effective.[114] Real time PCR for detection of CMV DNA in blood is an alternative that is also rapid and sensitive and is useful for diagnosing active disease and monitoring response to therapy.[115]

The usual therapy for established CMV infection has been ganciclovir.[116] In combination with intravenous immunoglobulin, it has been shown to improve survival in transplant recipients with CMV pneumonia or gastroenteritis. The dose-limiting toxicity of ganciclovir is the development of neutropenia, which can increase the risk of bacterial and fungal superinfections. Resistance to ganciclovir may occur during therapy because of viral mutations. Foscarnet is an acceptable alternative that does not cause neutropenia but is associated with nephrotoxicity. It has also been used in combination with ganciclovir. Cidofovir can also be used for treatment, but like foscarnet, causes nephrotoxicity. Unfortunately, the treatment of established infections such as CMV pneumonitis is not very satisfactory. Among patients with leukemia, the mortality rate among treated patients was approximately 60%.[117]

Primary CMV infection can be prevented in CMV negative BMT recipients by using bone marrow and screened blood products from donors who are CMV negative. Because of the high risk of CMV infection in BMT recipients who are seropositive or whose donors are seropositive it is important to institute measures to prevent CMV disease. Two strategies are currently used to prevent CMV infection in patients who are seropositive and are at risk for reactivation. One is the prophylactic administration of ganciclovir. Although effective, prolonged ganciclovir administration often produces neutropenia. There is also evidence that prolonged ganciclovir prophylaxis inhibits the development of CMV-specific T-cell lymphocyte responses and promotes the occurrence of late CMV pneumonia.[118] The other approach involves preemptive therapy for subclinical CMV infection, on the basis of positive CMV antigenemia assays in blood or detection of CMV in bronchoalveolar lavage fluid.[119] This strategy has the advantage that it targets patients with subclinical CMV infection. However, a small percentage of patients may present with CMV pneumonia without prior detection of the virus. Foscarnet can be used as an alternative for prophylaxis. Valganciclovir is an oral prodrug of ganciclovir that may prove to be useful for prophylaxis in some high-risk patients.

HHV-6 HHV-6 is being recognized as an important pathogen in organ transplant (including bone marrow) recipients. Serologic reactivation accompanied by specific manifestations, including fever, rash, pneumonitis, hepatitis, myelosuppression, and neurologic dysfunction, have been described in recipients of bone marrow, kidney, and liver transplants. Ganciclovir and foscarnet inhibit viral replication, and therapy with these agents may be useful in patients with severe infections.[120]

EBV Reactivation of EBV may occur after HSCT or following chemotherapy with purine analogues such as fludarabine. EBV infection may be responsible for Richter transformation or development of Hodgkin disease in patients with chronic lymphocytic leukemia. In recipients of bone marrow or solid organ transplants, uncontrolled proliferation of EBV infected B cells may occur, producing post-transplant lymphoproliferative disorders. In younger patients, a mononucleosis-like syndrome is a common presentation. Fever, sore throat, and lymphadenopathy are typical findings. Dissemination can occur from localized nodular lesions, and can be fulminant and rapidly fatal.

Community Respiratory Viral Infections During the last decade, it became apparent that community respiratory viruses can cause significant infection in patients with leukemia who are receiving chemotherapy and in BMT recipients, accounting for approximately 30% of respiratory infections during the "flu" season. Although there are temporal and geographic variations, RSV accounts for approximately 35 to 50%, influenza 20 to 25%, and parainfluenza about 10 to 30% of infections. Rhinoviruses, picornaviruses, and adenoviruses have been detected less frequently. Strict infection control practices must be instituted to prevent the spread of these infections among patients, personnel, and visitors.

RSV Infection The presenting signs of RSV infection include fever, cough, rhinorrhea, and nasal congestion. Some patients demonstrate radiologic evidence of sinusitis. As many as 40 to 60% of hospitalized patients progress to pneumonitis, which is associated with a mortality rate of about 60%.[121] Early therapy should be instituted for RSV pneumonia with inhaled ribavirin and probably intravenous immunoglobulin. The role of palivizumab, a monoclonal antibody, for therapy in these patients is uncertain.

Influenza Most influenza infections are caused by influenza A. Approximately 60% of infections progress to pneumonia, and this is especially likely to occur among patients with severe lymphopenia.[122] A substantial proportion of these patients will have associated bacterial or fungal pneumonia. The mortality rate from influenza pneumonia is approximately 40% and is higher among elderly, patients with lymphopenia and those with concomitant infection. The impact of amantadine, rimantadine, oseltamivir and ribavirin therapy for influenza pneumonia in these patients is uncertain, but to be effective they must be administered early after onset. Annual immunization for patients, hospital staff and families is important. However, antibody response to vaccination in patients receiving chemotherapy is often suboptimal.

Parainfluenza Parainfluenza infections occur sporadically throughout the year. Infection progresses to pneumonia in 30 to 75% of patients who have leukemia and are and BMT recipients. As many as 30% of patients with pneumonia may not have upper respiratory symptoms. More than half of patients with pneumonia have concomitant pathogens. The mortality rate from pneumonia is 30 to 79%, and the efficacy of ribavirin is uncertain.

Hepatitis Viruses Hepatitis B virus (HBV) infection is the most common cause of acute liver disease worldwide, and more than 300 million people have chronic infection with HBV.[123] Chronic HBV infection leads to progressive liver disease, cirrhosis, and hepatocellular cancer. Hepatitis C virus (HCV) has been estimated to infect 100 million persons worldwide and 4 million in the United States.[124] Eventually 10 to 15% of these individuals will develop cirrhosis (chronic HCV infection is the leading indication for liver transplantation), and some will develop hepatocellular carcinoma.[125] Recently, an association with HCV and non-Hodgkin lymphoma has been established.[126] Many patients with cancer develop elevation of transaminase levels indicating the presence of hepatitis, but it is often difficult to determine whether the disease is viral or drug induced. Although the current risk of transmission of HBV and HCV infection by the transfusion of screened blood is negligible, patients with acute leukemia and others who receive multiple transfusions may be at greater risk. The greatest threat to the safety of the blood supply is seronegative donors who donate blood during the infectious window period when they are undergoing seroconversion.[127] However, the majority of HBV and HCV infections occur in individuals who use illegal drugs and/or engage in high-risk sexual behaviors.[127] Drug-induced hepatitis is exceedingly common and a large number of agents commonly used in medicine can inflict liver damage.

Hepatitis can be a serious problem in patients with cancer for various reasons. Patients with impaired host defense mechanisms are more likely to develop fulminant infections. The presence of hepatitis may result in substantial delays in the administration of antineoplastic therapy, and may further interfere with nutrition in a group of patients where nutritional status is already impaired. Several reports have focused on the phenomenon of reactivation of quiescent liver disease as a consequence of HBV following immunosuppressive or cytotoxic therapy.[128,129] The clinical picture is that of fulminant hepatic failure and some patients have required liver transplantation as a consequence. This syndrome has also been reported after withdrawal of low-dose methotrexate therapy, which has not been clearly established to be immunosuppressive.

Interferon-α (IFN-α) is currently the only approved treatment for HBV infection.[130] Recent evidence indicates that the oral nucleoside analogue lamivudine produces substantial histologic improvement in many patients with chronic hepatitis.[131] Long-term therapy with this drug may result in the emergence of resistant mutants. The combination of pegylated IFN-α plus ribavirin produces sustained virologic responses in hepatitis C; approximately 50% in genotype 1 infections and 80% in other genotype infections.[132] Pre-exposure vaccination of persons at risk using recombinant hepatitis B vaccines affords protection against hepatitis B infection. Postexposure prophylaxis includes the administration of hepatitis B vaccine and hepatitis B immunoglobulin. Measures for preventing hepatitis C need to be developed.

PROTOZOAL INFECTIONS

P. carinii and *T. gondii* are protozoal organisms (although *P. carinii* has been reclassified as a fungus) that are capable of causing serious infections in patients with cancer. Both organisms are ubiquitous and cause infection in a wide variety of animals. Antitumor agents and adrenal corticosteroids facilitate the establishment of these infections in experimental animals. In the past, the majority of patients with cancer who developed these protozoal infections had received antitumor agents and/or adrenal corticosteroids.

P. Carinii The first cases of *Pneumocystis carinii* pneumonia (PCP) were described in central Europe in the early 1950s and involved premature or debilitated infants. Prior to the acquired immunodeficiency syndrome (AIDS) epidemic, approximately 20% of *P. carinii* infections in the United States occurred in patients with leukemia, and 15% in patients with other cancers. Most patients who develop this infection have evidence of immunosuppression, including a substantial number of children with acute leukemia who were in remission. PCP most often represents reactivation of latent infection but occasionally represents newly acquired infection. An epidemic has been described among children with neoplastic diseases, and adults occupying the same hospital room have acquired the infection. There is also some evidence to indicate that the frequency of PCP in patients without AIDS increases during periods of normal contact (outpatient clinics, treatment rooms, hospital wards) with patients who have AIDS, suggesting person-to-person transfer of the organisms.[133] Recent reports indicate that cases of PCP in patients with solid tumors (breast cancer) who have not been treated with corticosteroids, appear to be increasing.[134,135]

PCP may be insidious in onset or may progress rapidly. The most frequent presenting symptoms are unexplained fever, a nonproductive cough, and shortness of breath. The shortness of breath may occur initially only with exertion, but as the infection progresses, it is also present at rest, and the patient characteristically develops tachypnea, cyanosis, and tachycardia.[136] Children may complain of anterior chest, substernal, or abdominal pain, associated with nausea or vomiting. Auscultatory findings are usually minimal. Bronchovesicular breathing is common. Dry rales may be heard, but findings indicative of consolidation are infrequent, except in advanced disease. The chest radiograph often reveals more extensive pulmonary involvement than is suggested by the clinical findings. The most common finding is that of a diffuse interstitial infiltration involving most portions of the lung relatively evenly, although asymmetry may occur. Pleural effusions are very uncommon and may indicate the presence of another disease process. In a small percentage of patients with proven PCP, the chest radiograph may be normal.

Abnormalities in lung function are common in patients with PCP. These include impairment in vital capacity and total lung diffusing capacity for carbon monoxide. Measurement of arterial blood gases is useful in determining the extent of pulmonary involvement. Hypoxemia is frequent, and an increased difference in the alveolar to arterial oxygen tension between rest and exercise measurements have also been described in patients with PCP.

In patients with normal chest radiographs and pulmonary function tests, whose symptoms are suggestive of PCP, gallium scanning has been found to be of use. There is generally diffuse uptake throughout the lung parenchyma, although focal uptake may also occur. These findings represent a fairly sensitive, but nonspecific test for the presence of PCP. Gallium scanning may also be helpful in determining relapse, when chest radiographic abnormalities cannot be determined to represent new or residual disease.

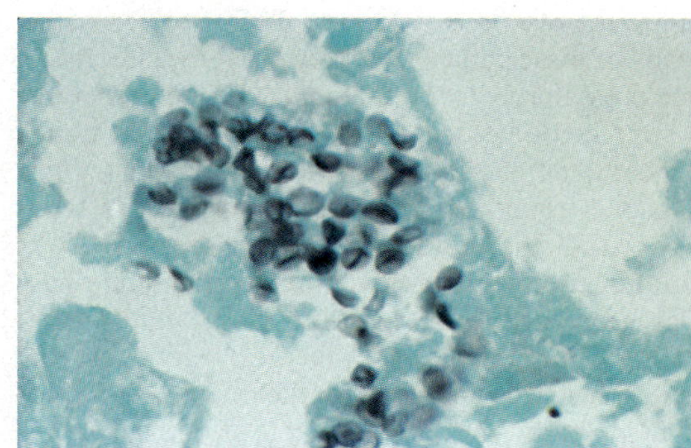

Figure 141-10 Gomori methenamine silver (GMS) stain from a bronchoalveolar lavage specimen demonstrating multiple organisms in an acquired immunodeficiency syndrome (AIDS) patient with *Pneumocystis carinii* pneumonia.

Several studies demonstrate that examination of sputum can provide a noninvasive and inexpensive means of diagnosing PCP, particularly in patients with AIDS. Most patients with PCP, however, have a dry cough and rarely produce sputum. Adequate amounts of sputum can be induced by having patients inhale a mist of hypertonic saline produced by an ultrasonic nebulizer for a period of 10 to 20 minutes. Staining of the sample can be done by a variety of stains that detect *P. carinii* (Gomori methenamine silver, toluidine blue O, Giemsa, polychrome methylene blue) (Figure 141-10). The sensitivity of this technique in a large number of AIDS patients is 79% with a negative predictive value of 61%. The use of a fluorescein-tagged monoclonal antibody increases the sensitivity of the procedure to around 92%.[137]

Various invasive techniques for establishing the diagnosis of PCP are available. These include fiberoptic bronchoscopy with bronchoalveolar lavage and/or transbronchial lung biopsy. Needle lung biopsy and open lung biopsy are rarely necessary. The sensitivity and specificity of these procedures are greater than noninvasive techniques, but they are associated with complications, such as bleeding and pneumothorax. Many patients with cancer who are suspected of having PCP are thrombocytopenic, and the hazards of performing invasive procedures in such patients are probably too great. Under these circumstances, a therapeutic trial may be indicated if the patient has the typical pulmonary infiltrates on the chest radiograph and has rapidly progressive dyspnea and hypoxemia.

TMP-SMX and pentamidine isethionate are effective for the treatment of PCP, both in patients with and without AIDS. In patients without AIDS, TMP-SMX represents the agent of choice because it is less toxic than pentamidine. The daily intravenous dosage of TMP-SMX recommended for the treatment of PCP is trimethoprim, 15 mg/kg, and sulfamethoxazole, 75 mg/kg. Pentamidine isethionate is administered by slow intravenous infusion at a dose of 4 mg/kg, as a single daily dose. Up to 50% of patients with AIDS experience untoward reactions related to TMP-SMX, and in many of these patients, therapy has to be discontinued prematurely.[138] For patients who are intolerant to, or who do not respond to, both TMP-SMX and pentamidine, the following alternatives exist. Oral dapsone-trimethoprim is useful in patients who have AIDS with mild to moderately severe PCP. A combination of clindamycin and primaquine has also been used to treat mild to moderately severe PCP in humans.[139] Another oral agent, atovaquone, has been approved for the treatment of mild to moderately severe PCP.[140] It is as efficacious as pentamidine and TMP-SMX in this setting and is less toxic.[141] The use of corticosteroids as adjunctive therapy for patients with moderate to severe PCP reduces the occurrence of respiratory failure and of mortality.[142] Prednisone is generally administered as follows: 40 mg PO, bid for 5 days followed by 40 mg PO daily for 5 days and then 20 mg PO daily until the end of treatment. TMP-SMX is highly successful in protecting children who are at high risk of acquiring PCP. It is also used frequently for this purpose in patients with AIDS. Aerosolized pentamidine has found widespread use for the prevention of PCP in patients with AIDS, particularly because it can be administered once a month. A small number of patients given aerosolized pentamidine will develop extrapulmonary (spleen, liver, bone marrow, eye) PCP. Other alternatives include intravenous pentamidine, dapsone, a combination of pyrimethamine and sulfadoxine (Fansidar), and atovaquone.

T. gondii *T. gondii,* an obligate intracellular protozoan parasite, is among the most prevalent causes of latent infection of the central nervous system. A variety of clinical syndromes have been described including asymptomatic infection, atypical pneumonia, chorioretinitis, congenital infection, encephalitis, and lymphadenitis. Lymphadenitis is common in systemic infection and frequently involves the cervical lymph nodes, although any lymph node group may be infected. Toxoplasmosis may first appear as myositis, myocarditis, hepatitis, pneumonitis, or encephalitis.

Cell-mediated immunity represents the primary arm of host defense against *T. gondii.* Serologic surveys in the United States indicate that up to 70% of healthy individuals have been infected with *T. gondii.* Patients with cancer, particularly those with defects in cell-mediated immunity, are at risk of reactivating latent infection or of developing newly acquired infection.[143] Infection can be acquired by the ingestion of improperly cooked meat products, including pork and lamb. Toxoplasmosis may also be transmitted by blood transfusion, including transfusion of whole blood, platelets, or white blood cells.

Toxoplasmosis is an infrequent infection even in patients who are immunosuppressed, except those with AIDS. Nearly half of the patients with cancer who develop toxoplasmosis have underlying Hodgkin disease. Sixty percent of patients with lymphoma who develop toxoplasmosis have central nervous system disease; although multiple other organs may be infected.[144] Central nervous system disease may present as a nonspecific encephalopathy, diffuse meningoencephalitis, or a syndrome compatible with multiple space-occupying lesions. The usual signs and symptoms include drowsiness, disorientation, headache, vomiting, seizures, visual disturbances, and paresis. Fever and nuchal rigidity are seen in less than 50% of patients. The cerebrospinal fluid may be completely normal, or may contain a few white blood cells (usually lymphocytes), and have normal or slightly elevated protein levels and slightly decreased glucose levels.[145]

In patients who present with symptoms of toxoplasmic encephalitis, the CT scan is usually abnormal. Typically, multiple intraparenchymal lesions involving cerebral hemispheres, thalamus, or cerebellum are seen. Contrast-enhancement may demonstrate a ring-like or nodular pattern.[146] Mild to moderate cerebral edema and a mass effect may be present. Occasionally solitary lesions may be present. Abnormalities demonstrated on the CT scan are not pathognomonic for toxoplasmosis, and similar lesions may be caused by other disease processes. MRI scanning appears to be more sensitive and may demonstrate the presence of lesions in patients with negative CT scans.

A specific diagnosis of toxoplasmosis is made by identification of the organisms in clinical specimens or by serologic methods. *T. gondii* have been identified microscopically in the blood, sputum, cerebrospinal fluid, and tissues of patients who are infected. Blood or body fluids may be inoculated into mice or tissue cultures and may demonstrate isolation of the organisms.[147] This may take up to 6 weeks and is rarely helpful in the initial management of the patient.

A large number of serologic tests for the detection of antibody to *T. gondii* are available. The most useful tests for the measurement of immunoglobulin (Ig)G antibody are the Sabin–Feldman dye test, the indirect fluorescent antibody (IFA) test, and the modified direct agglutination test. The methods available for detection of IgM antibodies include the IgM-IFA test and the double sandwich IgM-ELISA. IgG antibodies appear within 7 to 14 days of acquisition of infection, whereas IgM antibodies appear during the first week. IgG antibodies generally peak within 30 to 60 days and then begin to fall but persist for life. IgM antibodies rise rapidly, then fall to low levels, and disappear in a few months. Because the incidence of elevated antibody titers is high in the normal population, the diagnosis of toxoplasmosis can only be made if serial testing reveals increasing antibody titers. However, patients with cancer have had toxoplasmosis without producing increases in antibody titers. The diagnosis of toxoplasmosis can also be established by demonstrating trophozoites in tissues, such as brain biopsy or endomyocardial biopsy specimens.

Toxoplasmosis can be treated successfully with a combination of pyrimethamine and sulfadiazine (or trisulfapyrimidines). The initial loading dose of pyrimethamine is 100 to 200 mg. This is followed by 25 to 50 mg daily for a period of 4 to 6 weeks. Sulfadiazine or trisulfapyrimidines are given at a dose of 6 to 8 g/d in four divided doses for 4 to 6 weeks. Folinic acid, 5 mg every other day, is generally administered in an attempt to reduce the myelosuppression associated with this regimen. Clindamycin has shown promise as an alternative to sulfadiazine in patients with toxoplasmosis and sulfonamide intolerance.[148,149] It is well absorbed from the gut and has excellent tissue penetration, but achieves only erratic cerebrospinal fluid and brain concentrations. In combination with oral pyrimethamine, clindamycin seems comparable in efficacy to pyrimethamine and sulfadiazine. Atovaquone also appears promising for the treatment of cerebral toxoplasmosis, but relapse rates approach 50% when this agent is used alone. The new macrolides azithromycin, and clarithromycin have activity against *T. gondii,* but sufficient clinical data are lacking to recommend routine usage currently.

OTHER PARASITIC INFECTIONS

Opportunistic infections, including the syndrome of hyperinfection with the nematode *Strongyloides stercoralis,* occur most often in patients with T-lymphocyte impairment. Sporadic cases have been reported in patients with lymphoma and chronic lymphocytic leukemia. Infection with this parasite is common in the tropics, but it is worldwide in distribution. Usually, the parasite exists in the gut without causing severe disability. However, patients with impaired host defenses or those receiving antitumor and/or immunosuppressive agents may develop a serious infection. Large numbers of rhabditiform larvae may mature to filariform larvae and invade the gastrointestinal tract, causing ulceration. When hyperinfection occurs, pulmonary and gastrointestinal symptoms predominate.[150,151] Pulmonary manifestations include dyspnea, cough, hemoptysis, chest pain, and cyanosis. Migration of the larvae into the lungs produces a diffuse pulmonary infiltrate. Gastrointestinal manifestations include abdominal pain and/or distention, nausea, vomiting, diarrhea, hematochezia, and hematemesis. Fever, rash, headache, chills, and shock may also be present. Coexisting bacterial infections, which are generally caused by enteric gram-negative bacilli, are frequently present and may alert the astute clinician to the possibility of hyperinfection with *S. stercoralis.*

The crucial step in establishing the diagnosis of strongyloidiasis is the identification of larvae. They are usually demonstrated in stool samples and in pulmonary secretions. Duodenal aspiration might be necessary, if stool and pulmonary specimens fail to demonstrate larvae (Figure 141-11). Eosinophilia is present in up to 50% of patients. Various immunologic tests are available including complement fixation tests, precipitin tests, indirect fluorescent antibody techniques, and direct passive hemagglutination tests. These tests are generally sensitive and specific, but are limited by their lack of widespread availability. Thiabendazole (25 mg/kg twice daily for 2 days) is

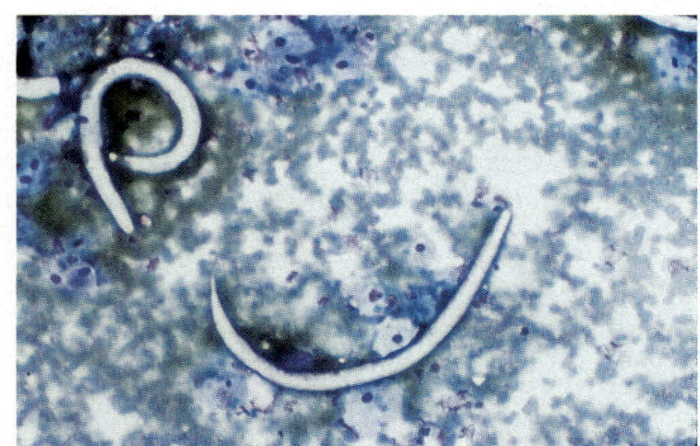

Figure 141-11 *Strongyloides stercoralis* larvae in a specimen obtained through duodenal aspiration. The patient had eosinophilia and chronic diarrhea.

the agent of choice for the treatment of strongyloidiasis.[152] A longer duration of therapy (5 to 14 days) may be necessary in seriously ill patients and those with hyperinfection. Ivermectin alone or in combination with thiabendazole may have a therapeutic role in refractory infections.[153]

PULMONARY INFECTIONS

The lung is a common site of infection in patients with cancer. The spectrum of pulmonary infection depends on the underlying immunologic deficit. In patients with neutropenia, bacterial infections predominate early. Most bacterial infections are mixed (polymicrobial) in nature with the following organisms being isolated frequently: *Staphylococcus aureus, Streptococcus pneumoniae*, the *Enterobacteriaceae, Pseudomonas aeruginosa*, and oral anaerobes. Secondary bacterial pathogens that emerge after prolonged antibacterial therapy include *Stenotrophomonas maltophilia, Acinetobacter* species, other non-fermentative gram-negative bacilli, and multidrug-resistant *Pseudomonas aeruginosa*. Fungal infections tend to occur more often in patients with persistent neutropenia and include molds such as *Aspergillus* species, *Fusarium* species, and the Zygomycetes.[154] Community respiratory viruses also cause infections in patients with neutropenia particularly in the preengraftment phase following HSCT.

The spectrum of pulmonary infection in patients with impaired cellular immunity is quite different. *Legionella* species are the most common bacterial pathogens although other bacteria including *Rhodococcus equi, Nocardia* species, and *Listeria monocytogenes* might occasionally be isolated. Mycobacterial infections (*M. tuberculosis* and nontuberculous mycobacteria) are also common particularly in patients with lymphoproliferative disorders, hairy cell leukemia, and those receiving cortisteroids or other immunosuppressive agents. *Aspergillus* species and the endemic fungi (*Cryptococcus neoformans, Histoplasma capsulatum, Coccoides imunitis*) cause most of the fungal infections in this setting. Viral infections are predominantly caused by the herpes group of viruses with CMV being the most frequent. The community respiratory viruses are now recognized as important causes of morbidity and mortality in high-risk subpopulations such as allogeneic HSCT recipients. Now regarded as fungi by some, *Pneumocystis jiroveci* also is a frequent cause of pneumonia in patients with impaired cellular immunity. Consequently, prophylaxis (usually with TMP-SMX) is recommended in patients at risk for this infection.

In patients with impaired humoral immunity, infections caused by encapsulated organisms such as *S. pneumoniae* and *H. influenzae* are common. Of concern is the increase in resistant pneumococcal isolates. Recent surveys at The University of Texas M. D. Anderson Cancer Center have indicated that 36 to 47% of *S. pneumoniae* are not susceptible to penicillin.[155,156]

Patients with carcinoma of the lung or metastatic lung disease often develop focal pulmonary infections. This is generally due to partial obstruction of the airways leading to atelectasis and post-obstructive pneumonia.[157] Occasionally, the infection may progress to empyema or lung abscess formation. These infections are predominantly polymicrobial (staphylococci, gram-negative bacilli, anaerobes) and are difficult to eradicate with antimicrobial therapy alone. Methods to overcome the obstruction (radiation, chemotherapy, stent placement, endobronchial brachytherapy) are usually necessary to ensure adequate drainage of the infected lung.

Patients with primary brain tumors or metastatic brain lesions often develop loss of the gag reflex that predisposes them to developing aspiration pneumonia. Damage to ciliary function, most often the result of radiation, also increases the likelihood of aspiration. These infections are also of mixed aerobic and anaerobic bacterial etiology and are caused by organisms colonizing the oropharynx and upper airways.[157]

Certain infections can produce clinical and radiographic findings that are indistinguishable from those associated with neoplasms. Fungal and mycobacterial pathogens head the list of such organisms. These may cause diagnostic challenges in two specific settings (1) patients with newly discovered pulmonary lesions in whom a neoplasm is suspected, and (2) patients with cancer who have received therapy, in whom a new pulmonary lesion (suspected to be metastatic) is seen.

For details of the various options and procedures commonly used to establish a diagnosis in patients with pulmonary infections, please refer to Chapter 135, "Respiratory Complications."

ABDOMINAL INFECTION

An acute abdomen is one of the most difficult problems for the physician caring for patients with cancer. Often, this occurs following the administration of chemotherapy when neutropenia and thrombocytopenia are complicating factors. Patients with neutropenia often cannot mount an adequate inflammatory response and, therefore, may have peritonitis without significant symptoms. Usually, they have abdominal pain, distention, and diminished to absent bowel sounds, but guarding and rebound may be absent. Adrenocorticosteroids can also mask the characteristic signs and symptoms of peritoneal inflammation. Some of the potential causes of acute abdomen in the immunocompromised host include appendicitis, cholecystitis, peritonitis, hepatic, splenic or ovarian abscesses, splenic infarcts, typhlitis, tumor lysis with perforation, and vinca alkaloid neuropathy.

Typhlitis or neutropenic enterocolitis is a disease that occurs in patients with neutropenia.[158] It was originally described in children with acute leukemia but now is recognized in adults with acute leukemia, and occasionally in patients undergoing intensive chemotherapy for metastatic carcinoma. The common presenting signs and symptoms include fever, abdominal pain, and diarrhea. More than 60% of patients have bloody diarrhea.[159] A substantial fraction of the patients have stomatitis, and 30% have vomiting. Physical examination reveals abdominal distention, tenderness often localized to the right lower quadrant, diminished to absent bowel sounds, and, infrequently, rebound tenderness. Septicemia is present in 70% of the patients, and the most common organisms are aerobic gram-negative bacteria. Some of the cases have been associated with infection caused by *Clostridium septicum*. Complications include perforation and peritonitis.

Pathologically, typhlitis is a patchy inflammation of the bowel wall with well-demarcated ulcers, hemorrhage, and masses of organisms with a paucity of inflammatory cells. Characteristically, the disease is limited to the cecum, but it can involve the entire lower gastrointestinal tract. The cause is unknown, but neutropenia is clearly a prerequisite. Chemotherapeutic agents may also play a role because they also cause mucosal ulceration.

Radiographic examination usually reveals evidence of a paralytic ileus with lack of bowel gas in the right lower quadrant, minimal distention of the terminal ileum, and thickening of the bowel wall. Ultrasonography or CT should be done to confirm the diagnosis and extent of disease. Initially, therapy should be supportive, consisting of nasogastric suction, intravenous fluids, and broad-spectrum antibiotics that include coverage for *P. aeruginosa* and anaerobes. Granulocyte transfusions can be an important component of the therapy, and because the infection may prove rapidly fatal, they may be administered simultaneously with antibiotics and not withheld until a response to antibiotic therapy alone is determined. Surgery is not indicated, unless it can be demonstrated that the process is localized and the patient is not responding to supportive therapy.[160] In a recent study, more than 70% of patients survived with medical therapy only.[159]

PERIANAL INFECTIONS

Perianal infections are estimated to occur in 6% of patients with hematologic neoplasms and in as many as 23% of patients with acute leukemia undergoing chemotherapy. They are especially common in patients with acute monocytic and acute myelomonocytic leukemia, suggesting that leukemic infiltration of the tissues may play a role. A common predisposing factor is neutropenia, which is found in more than 90% of these patients. The major presenting symptom is pain that is aggravated by defecation. Most patients are febrile. The lesion is erythematous, indurated, and ulcerated. Abscess formation occurs infrequently, but there may be extensive necrosis and sloughing extending into the rectum. Usually, the infection occurs at a site of a fissure or hemorrhoid, and, because of the absence of an inflammatory response, the extent of the infection may not be fully recognized.

The majority of these infections are caused by aerobic gram-negative bacilli, especially *P. aeruginosa* and *Escherichia coli. Pseudomonas* infection can be especially devastating because the organism invades blood vessel walls causing a vasculitis that can lead to tissue necrosis. Undoubtedly, anaerobic organisms play an important role in these infections, but are not often recognized because appropriate cultures have not been obtained. In most series, however, when septicemia occurs, anaerobes have only infrequently been cultured from the blood.

Initial therapy should be symptomatic, consisting of sitz baths or warm compresses, stool softeners, analgesics, and broad-spectrum antibiotics. Gut-sterilizing oral antibiotic regimens may be of some value in reducing contamination of ulcers by fecal flora. If an abscess is present, it should be incised and drained. Most physicians are reluctant to incise lesions without the presence of an abscess, but in one study, relief of symptoms and recovery were more likely to follow such an aggressive approach despite the absence of frank pus.[161] Even when only scant watery or serosanguineous fluid was drained, it resulted in resolution of fever and healing.

Mortality from these infections has varied from 10 to 35%, with most deaths being a result of septic shock. In the patient with neutropenia, resolution of infection often depends on recovery of the neutrophil count. Some patients may respond to initial antibiotic therapy, only to develop superinfection with a resistant organism. Patients with hematologic diseases who recover from perianal infections caused by hemorrhoids or anal fissures should undergo surgical correction when they achieve a remission of their underlying disease; otherwise, they may experience recurrent infections at a later date.[162]

SKIN INFECTIONS

Skin infections may occur secondary to necrotic tumor masses, postoperative wound infections, extravasation of vesicant drugs, infected intravascular catheters, folliculitis, infected decubitus ulcers, or as manifestations of systemic infection or embolic lesions secondary to endocarditis. Advanced squamous carcinomas of the skin, head and neck carcinomas, breast carcinomas, and sarcomas become necrotic and ulcerated and can serve as a focus of infection. Although initially these infections may be caused by gram-positive organisms, eventually superinfection with gram-negative bacilli occurs and is impossible to eradicate with antibiotic therapy alone. These infections can pose a serious threat to patients undergoing myelosuppressive chemotherapy because of the risk of septicemia when they become neutropenic.

Occasionally, patients develop gas-forming infections of large tumor masses, which may be caused by anaerobes, aerobic gram-negative bacilli, or mixed organisms.

Patients with neutropenia usually do not form abscesses at the site of skin infection but rather develop a spreading cellulitis, which often is associated with septicemia. A wide variety of aerobic gram-positive and gram-negative organisms can cause these infections, including skin contaminants such as *Bacillus* spp., *Corynebacterium jeikeium,* and *S. epidermidis.* Efforts should be made to aspirate material from these infected sites, although cultures are frequently negative.

Systemic infections in patients with cancer may be associated with skin lesions. An important skin lesion is ecthyma gangrenosum, which characteristically is found in the perianal area, groin, or axilla. Nearly always, it is caused by *P. aeruginosa,* but other gram-negative bacilli including *Aeromonas* and *Serratia,* fungi including *Aspergillus* or Mucorales, or *S. aureus* may be the cause.

Several fungi cause skin lesions as a manifestation of systemic infection. Approximately 10% of patients with disseminated candidiasis develop characteristic macronodular skin lesions (Figure 141-12). Disseminated aspergillosis and mucormycosis are infrequently associated with sharply demarcated lesions covered by a black eschar (Figure 141-13). Skin lesions occur in cryptococcosis and histoplasmosis but are not characteristic. *Fusarium* causes a fungal infection that is frequently associated with a variety of skin lesions.

CATHETER-RELATED INFECTIONS

Widespread use of intravascular catheters in patients with cancer has contributed to the changing spectrum of infection during the past decade. Whereas gram-positive infections accounted for less than 10% of cases of septicemia two decades ago, they now cause 60% of cases. *S. epidermidis* has emerged as an important pathogen, and the frequency of *S. aureus* infection has increased substantially. Some of these infections are caused by *Bacillus* spp., *Corynebacterium jeikeium, Enterococcus, Enterobacter* spp., *Acinetobacter,* and fungi. Despite the widespread use of catheters, the infection rate seldom exceeds 15%, even in patients with neutropenia.

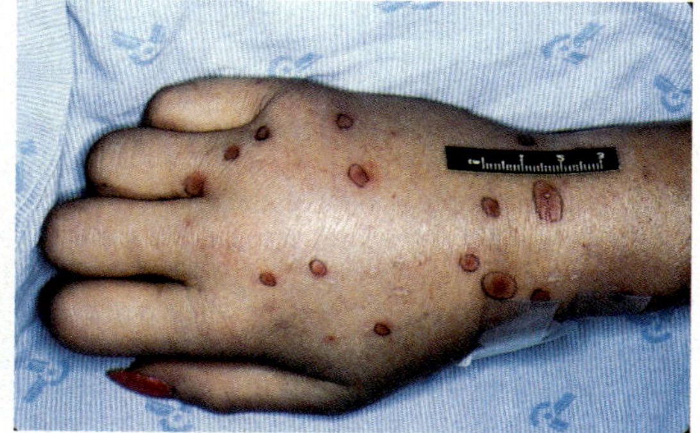

Figure 141-12 Characteristic macronodular cutaneous lesions in a patient with acute leukemia and disseminated *Candida krusei* infection.

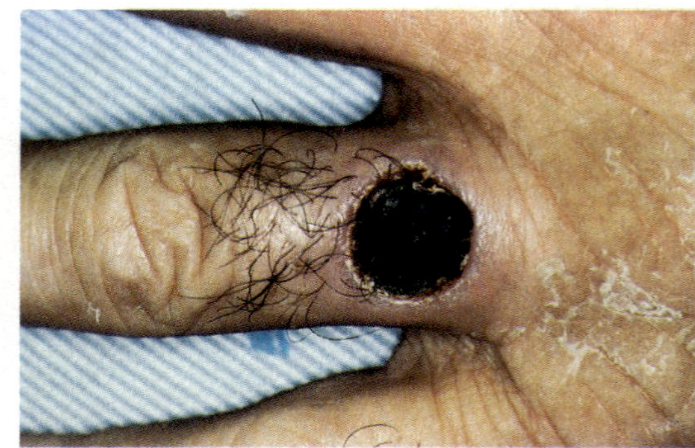

Figure 141-13 Disseminated aspergillosis and mucormycosis are infrequently associated with sharply demarcated lesions covered by a black eschar.

In the past, the recommended policy was to remove the catheter whenever a patient developed fever and especially when it was associated with septicemia. Recent experience indicates that many cases of septicemia can be successfully treated without the removal of the catheter. Exceptions include fungi, *S. aureus, Acinetobacter, Pseudomonas* spp. other than *P. aeruginosa,* the atypical mycobacteria, and whenever there is cellulitis at the catheter site. However, if fever or bacteremia persists despite antibiotic therapy, catheters must always be removed. Because many of the gram-positive organisms associated with catheter infections are resistant to methicillin, vancomycin has become an important component of antibiotic therapy.

The most serious catheter-related infections are septic thrombophlebitis and endocarditis. Septic thrombophlebitis is characterized by microabscess formation within a cannulated vein, which may be associated with repeated septic embolization. The majority of these infections are caused by *S. aureus, Streptococcus, Bacteroides* spp., and enteric gram-negative bacilli. As many as 70% of infections occur without local signs. Septic emboli occur in as many as 50% of the patients. This is a potentially life-threatening complication requiring prompt attention and should be suspected when a patient develops clinical evidence of sepsis with signs of local inflammation in the cannulated vein and positive blood cultures. The absence of pus within the vein does not preclude the diagnosis of septic phlebitis. Surgical exploration of the vein is necessary if the patient fails to respond to appropriate antibiotic therapy shortly after removal of the infected catheter. Endocarditis in the patient with cancer presents no unique manifestations. Because the risk of endocarditis is greater in patients with valvular heart disease, catheters should not be routinely used in these patients for the administration of chemotherapy. Recently, antimicrobial impregnated catheters have become available that reduce the frequency of catheter-associated infections during short-term use.

THERAPY OF INFECTIONS IN PATIENTS WITH NEUTROPENIA

General Principles The practice of initiating empiric broad-spectrum antimicrobial therapy when a neutropenic patient becomes febrile immediately after procuring all relevant cultures is now a well-accepted standard.[163–165] Antibiotic therapy should be administered promptly, via the intravenous route, and at maximal therapeutic doses in order to achieve maximal efficacy. A large number of antimicrobial agents are available that can be used effectively in empiric regimens, and no specific antibiotic or combination of antibiotics is considered optimal.[32,47] In general, an empiric regimen should provide a broad spectrum of activity against gram-negative organisms including *P. aeruginosa,* and gram-positive pathogens. This is usually achieved by administering antibiotic combinations (an aminoglycoside or quinolone plus an antipseudomonal β-lactam), or broad-spectrum drugs used as single agents (monotherapy). The recent increase in gram-positive infections has led to the inclusion of vancomycin in some empiric regimens.

A number of studies demonstrated that serum bactericidal activity is of great importance when treating infections in patients with neutropenia. In patients with neutropenia, a peak serum bactericidal titer of 1:16 or more was associated with a clinical success rate of 87%, whereas a peak serum bactericidal titer of 1:8 or less was associated with failure in 83% of bacteremias. The significant peak bactericidal titer for patients with adequate numbers of neutrophils was 1:8 with 98% success at or above this level and none below it.[166]

There is some evidence that antibiotic combinations that interact in a synergistic manner in vitro provide greater serum bactericidal activity and greater clinical efficacy than nonsynergistic combinations. Synergism may be of importance in patients with rapidly fatal underlying disease and severe and prolonged neutropenia who develop gram-negative septicemia. The enhanced activity of synergistic combinations is probably due to the lowering of the MIC of both drugs for the offending pathogen, thereby providing greater bactericidal activity in blood and tissues and, on occasion, rendering organisms that are resistant to the individual agents susceptible to the combination. Synergy occurs most often when an aminoglycoside is combined with an antipseudomonal penicillin and least often when two β-lactam antibiotics are used in combination.

The importance of synergy has been questioned by some investigators.[167] In many studies showing an advantage associated with synergistic combinations, often the nonsynergistic combination consisted of an aminoglycoside as the only agent to which the offending pathogen was susceptible. Several studies show that aminoglycosides are ineffective against gram-negative bacilli in patients with neutropenia, and should not be used alone. In patients who are severely neutropenic, better results may be obtained if the pathogen is susceptible to both agents of a combination rather than to only one, regardless of the presence or absence of synergy.

Antibiotic selection is also influenced by the potential toxicity associated with various agents. The aminoglycosides have long been associated with significant nephro- and ototoxicity and require frequent monitoring of renal function and serum levels, which can be expensive, time consuming, and uncomfortable to the patient. Elderly patients or those with preexisting renal insufficiency are at greater risk for developing aminoglycoside-associated toxicity. The toxicity of the aminoglycosides can also be potentiated by other agents frequently used in patients with cancer such as AMB, cisplatin, and cyclosporin. Although the β-lactam agents are associated with untoward reactions, such as hypersensitivity reactions and coagulation abnormalities, they are generally safer and better tolerated than aminoglycosides.

Local factors need to be considered when selecting antibiotics for initial empiric therapy. Certain pathogens may be endemic in a particular institution and must be included in the spectrum of the initial empiric regimen. Empiric therapy should include agents with antianaerobic activity in the case of intraabdominal and pelvic infections (Table141-6). In addition, the susceptibility of various organisms may differ from one institution to another, and local susceptibility/resistance patterns must be kept in mind when designing empiric regimens.

Patient Evaluation Antimicrobial therapy in febrile patients who are neutropenic needs to be administered promptly, and a delay of even a few hours can result in substantially increased mortality. Pretreatment evaluation of the patient should be performed as expeditiously as possible, yet it should be thorough. A careful interview for historic information and a physical examination must be performed. Particular attention should be paid to sites that are frequently infected, or serve as foci for the dissemination of infection. These include the oropharynx, lung, lower esophagus, perineum, paranasal sinuses, fingernails, and vascular catheter insertion sites. Prior to the initiation of empiric antibiotic therapy, at least two sets of blood cultures and cultures from other appropriate sites (ie, throat, urine, stool) should be obtained for bacterial and fungal pathogens. In patients with central venous catheters, cultures should be obtained from the catheters and from a peripheral site. Material exuding from infected catheter sites should also be sent for Gram staining and culture. All febrile neutropenic patients should undergo chest radiography to identify pulmonary lesions. In patients with neutropenia and pneumonia, radiographs may appear normal. However, CT scans of the chest or paranasal sinuses should be performed in patients in whom these sites are potential sources of infection. Other laboratory investigations include complete blood counts and determination of baseline values reflecting renal and hepatic function. These tests should be repeated at least twice a week while patients are receiving empiric antibiotic therapy. Imaging techniques, such as CT, MRI, ultrasonography, and radionuclide imaging, and invasive procedures, such as lung, liver, or skin biopsies, might be extremely useful at identifying sites of infection and isolating specific pathogens. The presence of thrombocytopenia often precludes the use of invasive diagnostic techniques. The absence of neutrophils precludes indium granulocyte localization studies. In this situation, gallium scanning may occasionally be helpful.

Table 141-6 Common Antibiotic Regimens in Patients with Neutropenia

Aminoglycoside-containing regimens
Aminoglycoside + antipseudomonal penicillin/β-lactamase inhibitors
Aminoglycoside + extended-spectrum cephalosporin
Aminoglycoside + carbapenem
Aminoglycoside + quinolone
Other regimens
Vancomycin + antipseudomonal penicillin/β-lactamase inhibitors
Vancomycin + extended-spectrum cephalosporin
Vancomycin + monobactam
Vancomycin + quinolone
Single-agent regimens (monotherapy)
Extended-spectrum cephalosporin
Carbapenems
Antipseudomonal penicillin/β-lactamase inhibitor

Initial Antibiotic Therapy Table 141-6 lists antibiotic regimens that are frequently deployed in febrile patients with neutropenia. These regimens provide broad-spectrum therapy and should be initiated promptly when patients with neutropenia develop an elevated temperature. No single regimen is optimal, and the various factors discussed above need to be carefully considered before making a specific choice. The initial regimen may also need to be altered during the course of the febrile episode, depending on the susceptibility of microorganisms isolated from clinical specimens, the development of bacterial, fungal, or viral superinfections, or lack of apparent efficacy after administration of the regimen for 3 days. Combinations of aminoglycosides and antipseudomonal penicillins have been extensively evaluated and are generally associated with overall response rates in the range of 65 to 85%. Amino-glycosides are often used in combination with extended-spectrum cephalosporins (ceftazidime, cefepime) and other β-lactam agents (aztreonam, ticarcillin + clavulanic acid, piperacillin + tazobactam).[47] The advantages of such combinations include the potential for synergy against gram-negative bacilli including *P. aeruginosa,* activity against many anaerobes, and minimal emergence of resistant organisms during therapy. Disadvantages of aminoglycoside–β-lactam combinations include the potential for oto- and nephrotoxicity (particularly with repeated use, in elderly patients or those with underlying renal insufficiency, and when other potentially nephrotoxic agents, such as AMB, are needed) and the lack of activity against many gram-positive organisms. Once-daily administration of aminoglycosides is associated with less toxicity than more frequent administration.[168] Care must be taken to ensure that the aminoglycoside is not the only active agent against any gram-negative bacilli that are isolated, because these agents are not effective by themselves in patients with neutropenia, even if the causative organisms are susceptible to them in vitro.

With the availability of broad-spectrum agents, such as carbapenems and extended-spectrum cephalosporins, it has become possible to initiate empiric therapy in febrile neutropenic patients using a single agent. Ceftazidime, imipenem/cilastatin, meropenem and piperacillin/tazobactam have been used alone as initial therapy and have produced response rates similar to those obtained with combination regimens (Table 141-7).[169–171] Patients on single-agent therapy need to be carefully monitored and antibiotic changes made if the clinical situation or microbiologic data indicate the need.

Table 141-7 Antimicrobial Agents Commonly Used in Patients with Neutropenia

Agent	Dose
Aminoglycosides	
Amikacin	5 mg/kg q8h or 15-20 g/kg/d (single dose)
Gentamicin	1.5 mg/kg q8h or 5 mg/kg/d (single dose)
Tobramycin	1.5 mg/kg q8h or 5 mg/kg/d (single dose)
Antipseudomonal penicillins + β-lactamase inhibitor	
Ticarcillin + clavulanate	3.1 g q4h, IV
Piperacillin + tazobactam	3.375 g q6h, IV
Extended-spectrum cephalosporins	
Cefepime	1–2 g q8h, IV
Carbapenem	
Imipenem/cilastatin	500 mg q6h, IV
Meropenem	1 g q8h, IV
Monobactam	
Aztreonam	1.5–2.0 g q6–8h, IV
Quinolones	
Ciprofloxacin	200–400 mg q8h, IV
Gatifloxacin	400 mg qd, IV
Moxifloxacin	400 mg qd, IV
Others	
Vancomycin	1 g q12h, IV
Clindamycin	900 mg q8h, IV
Nafcillin	2.0 g q4h, IV
Trimethoprim-sulfamethoxazole	2.0-20.0 mg/kg/d (trimethoprim) IV q6h
Metronidazole	500 mg IV q6-8h
Linezolid	600 mg IV q12h
Daptomycin	4-6 mg/kg/d IV
Quinupristin/dalfopristin	7.5 mg/kg q8h IV

IV = intravenously.

With the increased incidence of gram-positive infections, many of which are caused by multidrug-resistant organisms, the inclusion of vancomycin in the initial regimen might become necessary.[172,173] Most gram-positive infections are associated with low mortality, and several studies show that vancomycin can be safely added to the initial regimen if no response is obtained after 48 to 72 hours of therapy, or if a resistant organism is isolated, without adversely affecting the eventual outcome. This approach may reduce vancomycin-associated toxicity and costs and may decrease the potential for the emergence of vancomycin-resistant organisms. Fulminant gram-positive infections caused by α-hemolytic streptococci, *S. pyogenes,* or other gram-positive organisms have been described. It might be prudent to include vancomycin in the initial empiric regimen in institutions or specific patient populations (bone marrow transplant recipients) in whom these infections occur frequently.[173]

Recently, clinical vancomycin failures have been reported even in infections caused by organisms that are susceptible to it in vitro, presumably due to its diminishing bactericidal activity.[29,174] Newer agents with improved bactericidal activity (daptomycin, dalbavancin) are being developed, and need to be evaluated in patients who have cancer.

Low-Risk Patients Antibiotic therapy for febrile patients who are neutropenic has traditionally been administered in the hospital because of the risk of infection-related and other complications. Recently, simple clinical criteria and statistically derived risk prediction rules have made it possible to identify low-risk subsets among such patients at the onset of a febrile episode.[14,15] This has enabled clinicians to evaluate not only the nature of antibiotic therapy (eg, combinations vs monotherapy) but also the setting (hospital, clinic, office, home) in which it is delivered.[175] Several alternative treatment strategies in low-risk febrile patients with neutropenia have been evaluated including (1) hospital based oral antibiotic therapy[176,177] (2) initial hospitalization followed by early discharge on outpatient parenteral or oral antibiotics,[178] and (3) outpatient (parenteral or oral) antibiotic therapy for the entire febrile episode.[16,179,180]

This approach is associated with substantial cost saving, a lower incidence of nosocomial superinfections, and improved quality of life for patients and convenience for their families. Careful patient selection and daily follow-up are essential components of the success of this novel approach. The Infectious Diseases Society of America and the National Comprehensive Cancer Network recently published guidelines for the treatment of febrile patients with neutropenia, which include suggestions for the outpatient management of low-risk patients.[47,181]

DURATION OF THERAPY

Some authorities recommend continuation of antibiotic therapy in patients with documented infections until recovery of the neutrophil count. This approach is expensive, as it actually represents prophylaxis after resolution of infection and may result in an increased number of superinfections requiring numerous modifications of antibacterial therapy and/or the addition of antifungal therapy. Another approach is to continue antibiotics until all sites of infection have resolved, the causative pathogen, if isolated, has been eradicated, the patient has been treated for a minimum of 7 days and has remained free of significant symptoms or signs of infection for at least 4 days. Antibiotic therapy may be discontinued safely at this point despite the persistence of neutropenia. This approach may be associated with a low relapse rate and fewer superinfections.

Fever of Unexplained Origin The most perplexing group of patients are those with fever who display no clinical signs of infection and from whom no pathogen is isolated, that is, fever of unexplained origin. Many of these patients respond to the initial antibacterial regimens, suggesting that they do have bacterial infections. The widespread use of prophylactic antibiotics to an extent, may be responsible for the failure to isolate the offending pathogens in such patients. Patients who remain febrile despite antibacterial therapy pose a difficult diagnostic and therapeutic challenge. These patients may have bacterial infections that are resistant to therapy or infections by nonbacterial pathogens (fungi, viruses, parasites). Drug-related or tumor fever may also be present. Aggressive, often invasive, diagnostic maneuvers are sometimes necessary for the management of such patients. In patients unable to tolerate invasive diagnostic procedures, continuation of antibacterial therapy and the addition of empiric antifungal, antiviral, or antiparasitic therapy might be necessary.

Other Therapeutic Modalities Approximately 15 to 25% of infections occurring in patients with neutropenia fail to respond to appropriate antimicrobial therapy. In most cases, profound neutropenia persists, and patients remain febrile despite adjustments in antibacterial therapy and the addition of an antifungal agent. There was considerable interest in the use of white blood cell transfusions in the 1960s and 1970s. Early studies showed that optimum efficacy was achieved with the transfusion of 10^{11} neutrophils, an amount difficult to collect from normal donors. Dexamethasone was administered to donors to increase the number of neutrophils collected. Randomized trials in neutropenic patients with infections that failed to respond to appropriate therapy demonstrated that white blood cell transfusions increased the response rates. Interest in this therapeutic modality waned because of the difficulties in obtaining sufficient donors, alloimmunization of recipients when random donors were used, and the possibility of transmitting CMV infection from transfused cells. The availability of the hematopoietic growth factors has rekindled interest in this therapeutic modality because the administration of granulocyte colony-stimulating factor (G-CSF) to donors increases the number of neutrophils that can be collected. Preliminary clinical studies suggest that this approach to white blood cell collection has produced therapeutic benefit in about half the recipients.[182]

The administration of hematopoietic growth factors to patients receiving cancer chemotherapy reduces the severity and duration of neutropenia and, hence, the frequency of infectious complications. Guidelines for this use of these agents have been prepared by the American Society of Clinical Oncology.[183] The efficacy of these factors as adjuncts to antibiotic therapy for patients who are neutropenic after they have become infected has not been clearly established. It is reasonable to administer these agents to patients with neutrophil counts less than 500/mm^3 who develop pneumonia, septic shock, sepsis syndrome, or fungal infection, because these patients have a poor prognosis without recovery of their neutrophils. Also, these agents should be considered for patients with documented infections who are failing to respond to appropriate therapy after 24 to 48 hours. IFN-γ may be beneficial for therapy with nonviral infections that are not responding to appropriate therapy.[184,185]

INFECTION PREVENTION

The high frequency of infection in patients with cancer during periods of myelosuppression has led to the development of programs for the prevention of infection. The two main strategies that are used for infection prevention are directed toward suppressing the endogenous microflora and preventing the acquisition of new organisms from environmental sources. Suppression of the endogenous microflora is usually achieved by using prophylactic antibiotic regimens during periods of severe myelosuppression. In patients who are at risk for fungal, viral, or protozoal infections or in centers where such infections are relatively common, prophylactic regimens generally also include agents active against these groups of organisms. The prevention of acquisition of new organisms is accomplished by various techniques, including strict hand-washing precautions, use of well-cooked foods, which reduces contamination with gram-negative bacteria, and various isolation techniques or protected environments.[186]

Antimicrobial Prophylaxis Prophylactic antimicrobial regimens achieve a major reduction in the patients' microbial burden. TMP-SMX has been used in the past for this indication. Although most studies have shown a reduction in microbiologically documented infections and a reduction in the need for systemically administered antibiotics, the overall mortality has not been significantly altered. The use of TMP-SMX for prophylaxis has been associated with the emergence of resistant organisms, an increase in fungal colonization and infection, and prolongation of neutropenia.

The quinolones (ciprofloxacin, levofloxacin) are the most commonly used agents for antibacterial chemoprophylaxis. The use of these agents has been associated with significant reductions in the frequency of gram-negative infections, but they have had little impact on or, or may actually increase the frequency of gram-positive infections (eg, *Staphylococcus* spp., viridans group streptococci).[187–189] Newer quinolones (gatifloxacin, moxifloxacin) are more potent against most gram-positive organisms, and might be more suitable for prophylaxis than older agents.[190] Quinolone prophylaxis has also resulted in the emergence of quinolone resistance among enteric gram-negative bacilli including *E. coli.*[191] It is therefore not recommended for routine use in patients with neutropenia, but must be considered only in patients at high-risk for bacterial infection (ie, those with prolonged periods of neutropenia). TMP-SMX remains the agent of choice for PCP prophylaxis. Alternative (but less effective) agents include pentamidine, dapsone, and atovaquone.

ANTIFUNGAL AND ANTIVIRAL PROPHYLAXIS

Increasing frequency of invasive fungal infections in high-risk patients has led to the use of antifungal prophylaxis. Fluconazole (and itraconazole) prophylaxis has been shown to decrease both superficial colonization and systemic Candida infections.[192–195] The selection of resistant species (*C. krusei, C. glabratta*) is a potential problem, although these organisms are also seen in "azole naïve" patients.[196–198] As with antibacterial prophylaxis, the benefits of antifungal prophylaxis need to be weighed against the potential risks. Prophylaxis against molds including *Aspergillus* spp. is less successful although newer agents such as voriconazole and posaconazole, with more potent activity against most molds than older agents are being evaluated. Increased voriconazole administration has already been associated with the emergence of breakthrough zygomycotic infections, cautioning against the widespread adoption of this strategy.[95]

Prophylactic acyclovir has been shown to prevent reactivation of HSV infection in patients undergoing intensive chemotherapy (with or without radiation therapy) before HSCT or induction therapy for leukemia or lymphoma. Pre-emptive therapy (rather than prophylaxis) with ganciclovir or foscarnet is the current recommendation for high-risk patients with positive CMV antigenemia.[199]

Isolation Reduction of the acquisition of new organisms has been attempted by putting patients at risk into reverse isolation. Patients are also given well-cooked foods and are asked to avoid fresh fruits and vegetables (eg, tomatoes, salads) that are naturally contaminated with gram-negative bacilli such as *P. aeruginosa, Klebsiella pneumoniae,* and *E. coli.* More elaborate regimens are expensive and time consuming and have not been shown to be more effective than strict adherence to handwashing techniques.

Protected environments provide a combination of the two approaches, that is, the use of isolation units to protect the patient against nosocomial contamination plus antibiotic regimens to reduce the patient's endogenous flora. The protected environment generally consists of isolation units, which provide a barrier between the patient and the hospital environment, using aggressive decontamination techniques and filtered air. The most effective type of unit is the laminar airflow room, in which one wall or the ceiling comprises high efficiency air filters. Filtered air flows across the room with a laminar distribution, providing several hundred air exchanges per hour. All items used by the patient are sterilized before being placed in the unit, and various germicidal agents are used initially and during occupation of the units to maintain a sterile environment. The patient's food is specially prepared or sterilized to minimize contamination. Disinfection of the patient is achieved by using intensive regimens, which include oral nonabsorbable antibiotics. Patients bathe with germicidal soaps and apply topical antibiotic ointments or sprays to areas of heavy microbial contamination.

Because attempts at suppressing the endogenous microflora and those at preventing the acquisition of organisms have not been overwhelmingly successful, other means for infection prevention need to be developed. The hematopoietic growth factors (granulocyte-macrophage [GM]-CSF and G-CSF) have been demonstrated to shorten the duration of neutropenia and to reduce the number of febrile days and of documented infections in selected sub-populations of patients with neutropenia. Current guidelines suggest that the primary use of these agents is not indicated in patients who were previously untreated and receiving most chemotherapy regimens.[183] The secondary administration of growth factors can decrease the probability of febrile neutropenia after a documented occurrence in an earlier cycle. It can also reduce the period of neutropenia and the frequency of infectious complications in patients undergoing high-dose cytotoxic therapy with autologous marrow transplantation.

PERSPECTIVES

Despite substantial advances in supportive care, infection remains a serious complication for many patients with cancer. The spectrum of infection (bacterial, fungal, viral) continues to change, requiring continued vigilance, and new strategies for infection prevention and treatment. The emergence of multidrug resistant bacterial pathogens (eg, MRSA, VRE, *Pseudomonas aeruginosa, S. maltophilia*) has posed serious challenges, particularly in the area of new drug development as highlighted in the monograph published by the Infectious Diseases Society of America, entitled "Bad Bugs, No Drugs."[4] Disseminated fungal infections have become the leading cause of death in patients with hematologic malignancies, and in HSCT recipients. Although the armamentarium against fungi has expanded, resistant organisms (eg, *C. krusei, A. terreus*, Zygomycetes, *Scedosporium* spp., *Fusarium* spp.) have emerged. The early diagnosis and treatment of many invasive fungal infections, particularly in the setting of persistent neutropenia/immunosuppression remains unsatisfactory. Viral infections represent a growing threat particularly in patients with hematologic malignancies and HSCT recipients. Newly emerging global threats (such as SARS, avian influenza, West Nile virus, etc) can have a devastating impact on patients with cancer who are immunosuppressed. Reliable methods for the rapid diagnosis of these and other viral infections, and effective means for their prevention and treatment still need to be developed. Parasitic infections remain uncommon except in endemic areas. Although effective therapies are available, toxicity and the need for prolonged maintenance or suppressive therapy can be problematic.

The hematologic growth factors (G-CSF, GM-CSF) and other cytokines have had a significant impact in reducing the risk of infection in some patients with cancer. These agents may also be useful as therapeutic adjuncts in some infections that are refractory to antimicrobial therapy. Interest in granulocyte transfusions has been revived because it is now possible to transfer large numbers of granulocytes by stimulating their growth in normal donors using hematopoietic growth factors.

The development of risk assessment strategies has led to the recognition of a "low-risk" subset among patients with neutropenia. This has enabled clinicians to evaluate not only the nature of empiric therapy (eg. combination or monotherapy) but also the route of administration (IV or PO), and the setting in which such therapy is delivered (hospital, clinic, home). These strategies have resulted in substantial cost savings, reduction in healthcare associated (nosocomial) infections, and improved quality of life for patients and their families or caregivers. Protected environments, prophylactic programs, infection control strategies, and the CSFs have reduced the risk of infection in patients with cancer. The use of vaccines in high-risk patients affords protection against specific pathogens. Newer technologic advances should lead to further progress. However, the recognition, prevention, diagnosis, and treatment of infections in patients with cancer will continue to challenge us in the foreseeable future, as we work toward the larger goal of eliminating cancer.

REFERENCES

1. Bodey GP. Infections in cancer patients. A continuing association. Am J Med 1986;(81 Suppl 1A):11–26.
2 Yadegarynia D, Tarrand J, Raad I, Rolston K. Current spectrum of bacterial infections in cancer patients. Clin Infect Dis 2003;37:1144–5.
3. Wisplinghoff H, Seifert H, Wenzel RP, Edmond MB. Current trends in the epidemiology of nosocomial bloodstream infections in patients with hematological malignancies and solid neoplasms in hospitals in the United States. Clin Infect Dis 2003;36:1103–10.
4. Bad Bugs, No Drugs. Infectious Diseases Society of America, July 2004. Available at: http://www.idsociety.org/pa/IDSA_Paper4_final_web.pdf (accessed
5. Whimbey E, Englund JA, Couch RB. Community respiratory virus infections in immunocompromised patients with cancer. In: Whimbey E, Englund JA, Ljungman P, editors. Proceedings of a symposium. Am J Med 1997;102:10–8.
6. Kontoyiannis DP, Mantadakis E, Samonis G. Systemic mycoses in the immunocompromised host: an update in antifungal therapy. J Hosp Infect 2003:53:423–58.
7. Casazza AR, Duvall CP, Carbone PP. Infection in lymphoma—histology, treatment and duration in relation to incidence and survival. JAMA 1966;197:710–6.
8. Hersh EM, Bodey GP, Nies BA, Freireich EJ. Causes of death in acute leukemia. A ten-year study of 414 patients from 1954–1963. JAMA 1965;198:105–9.
9. Rolston KVI. Infections in patients with solid tumors. In: Glauser MP, Pizzo PA editors. Management of infections in immunocompromised patients. WB Saunders; London, 2000. pp. 117–40.
10. Bodey GP, Buckley M, Sathe YS, Freireich EJ. Quantitative relationships between circulating leukocytes and infection in patients with acute leukemia. Ann Intern Med 1966;64:328–40.
11. Sickles EA, Greene WH, Wiernik PH. Clinical presentation of infection in granulocytopenic patients. Arch Intern Med 1975;135:715–9.
12. Toleman MA, Rolston K, Jones RN, Walsh TR. Molecular and biochemical characterization of OXA-45, an extended-spectrum class 2d', β-lactamase in *Pseudomonas aeruginosa*. Antimicrob Agents Chemother 2003;47:2859–63.
13. Toleman MA, Rolston K, Jones RN, Walsh TR. *bla*$_{VIM-7}$, an evolutionarily distinct metallo-β-lactamase gene in a *Pseudomonas aeruginosa* isolate from the United States. Antimicrob Agents Chemother 2004;48:329–32.
14. Talcott JA, Siegel RD, Finberg R, Goldman L. Risk assessment in cancer patients with fever and neutropenia: a prospective, two center validation of a prediction rule. J Clin Oncol 1992;10:316–22.
15. Klastersky J, Paesmans M, Rubenstein E, et al. The MASCC Risk Index: A multinational scoring system to predict low-risk febrile neutropenic cancer patients. J Clin Oncol 2000;18:3038–51.
16. Rubenstein EB, Rolston K, Benjamin RS, et al. Outpatient treatment of febrile episodes in low-risk neutropenic patients with cancer. Cancer 1993;71:3640–6.
17. Rolston KVI, Rubenstein EB, Freifeld A. Early empiric antibiotic therapy for febrile neutropenia patients at "low-risk." In: Greene JN, Hiemenz JW, editors. Infectious disease clinics of North America. Philadelphia: WB Saunders; 1996. p. 223–37.
18. Rolston KVI. Expanding the options for risk-based therapy in febrile neutropenia. Diagn Microbiol Infect Dis 1998;31:411–6.
19. Rolston KVI. Prediction of neutropenia. International J Antimicrob Agents 2000;16:113–5.
20. Hahn H, Kaufmann SHE. The role of cell-mediated immunity in bacterial infections. Rev Infect Dis 1981;3:1221–50.
21. Rolston KVI, Dholakia N, Rodriguez S, Rubenstein EB. Nature and outcome of febrile episodes in patients with pancreatic and hepatobiliary cancer. Support Care Cancer 1995;3:414–7.
22. Raad II, Hanna HA. Intravascular catheter-related infections: new horizons and recent advances. Arch Intern Med 2002;162:871–8.
23. Maki DG. Infections associated with intravascular lines. In: Remington JS, Swartz MN, editors. Current clinical topics in infectious diseases, Vol. 3. New York: McGraw-Hill; 1980. p. 309–63.
24. Zinner SH. Changing epidemiology of infections in patients with neutropenia and cancer: emphasis on gram-positive and resistant bacteria. Clin Infect Dis 1999;29:490–4.
25. Rolston KVI. Challenges in the treatment of infections caused by gram-positive and gram-negative bacteria in patients with cancer and neutropenia. Clin Infect Dis 2005;40:S246–52.
26. Rolston KVI. Current spectrum of bacterial infection in patients with solid tumors [abstract] 7th International Symposium on Febrile Neutropenia. Seville, Spain, Jan 27–29, 2005.
27. Yadegarynia D, Rolston KV. Current spectrum of bacterial infections in patients with hematological malignancies [abstract]. 15th European Congress of Clinical Microbiology and Infectious Diseases; 2005 April 2–5; Copenhagen, Denmark.
28. Rolston KVI, Balakrishnan M, Elting LS, et al. Is quantitative variation in cancer patients with bacteremic infections linked to severity of infection [abstract]? 40th Interscience Conference on Antimicrobial Agents and Chemotherapy; 2000 Sept. 17–20; Toronto, Ontario, Canada.
29. Skaoulas G, Moise-Broder PA, Schentag J, et al. Relationship of MIC and bactericidal activity to efficacy of vancomycin for treatment of methicillin-resistant *Staphylococcus aureus* bacteremia. J Clin Microbiol 2004;42:2398–402.
30. Raad I, Davis S, Khan A, et al. Impact of central venous catheter removal on the recurrence of catheter-related coagulase-negative Staphylococci bacteremia. Infect Control Hosp Epidemiol 1992;13:215–21.
31. Tiera R, Tarrand J, Rolston K. Bacteremia due to penicillin susceptible (PSSP) and penicillin non-susceptible streptococcus pneumoniae (PNSP) in patients with cancer [abstract]. 4th International Symposium on Febrile Neutropenia; 1999 Dec 15–18; Brussels, Belgium.
32. Bisno AL, Freeman JC. The syndrome of asplenia, pneumococcal sepsis and disseminated intravascular coagulation. Ann Intern Med 1970;72:389–93.
33. Rolston KFI, Vaziri I, Frisbee-Hume S, et al. In vitro antimicrobial activity of gatifloxacin compared with other quinolones against clinical isolates from cancer patients. Chemotherapy 2004;50:214–20.
34. Rolston KVI, Frisbee-Hume S, LeBlanc B, et al. In vitro antimicrobial activity of moxifloxacin compared to other quinolones against recent clinical bacterial isolates from hospitalized and community-based cancer patients. Diagn Microbiol Infect Dis 2003;47:441–9.
35. Bochud P, Calandra T, Francoli P. Bacteremia due to viridans streptococci in neutropenic patients: a review. Am J Med 1994;97:256–64.
36. Elting LS, Bodey GP, Keefe BH. Septicemia and shock syndrome due to viridans streptococci: a case control study of predisposing factors. Clin Infect Dis 1992;14:1201–7.
37. Rolston KVI. The clinical significance of organisms tolerant to vancomycin [abstract]. 93rd Meeting of the American Society for Microbiology; 1993 May; Atlanta, GA.
38. Yu VL. Enterococcal superinfection and colonization after therapy with moxalactam, a new broad-spectrum antibiotic. Ann Intern Med 1981;94:784–5.
39. Edmond MB, Ober JF, Weinbaum DL, et al. Vancomycin resistant *Enterococcus faecium* bacteremia: risk factors for infection. Clin Infect Dis 1995;20:1126–33.
40. Murray BE. Vancomycin-resistant enterococci. Am J Med 1997;102:284–93.
41. Raad I, Hachem R, Hanna H, et al. Treatment of vancomycin-resistant enterococcal infections in the immunocompromised host: quinupristin-dalfopristin in combination with minocycline. Antimicrob Agents Chemother 2001;45:3202–4.
42. Montecalvo MA, Jarvis WR, Uman J, et al. Infection-control measures reduce transmission of vancomycin resistant enterococci in an endemic setting. Ann Intern Med 1999;131:269–72.
43. Anaissie E, Kontoyiannis DP, Kantarjian H, et al. Listeriosis in patients with chronic lymphocytic leukemia who were treated with fludarabine and prednisone. Ann Intern Med 1992;6:466–9.

44. Rolston KVI, Tarrand JJ. *Pseudomonas aeruginosa*—still *a* frequent pathogen in patients with cancer: 11-year experience at a comprehensive cancer center. Clin Infect Dis 1999;29:463–4.
45. Elting LS, Bodey GP, Fainstein V. Polymicrobial septicemia in the cancer patient. Medicine 1986;65:218–25.
46. Adachi JA, Yadegarynia D, Rolston K. Spectrum of polymicrobial bacterial infection in patients with cancer, 1975–2002 [abstract]. American Society for Microbiology. Polymicrobial Diseases; 2003 Oct. 19–23; Lake Tahoe, NV.
47. Hughes WT, Armstrong D, Bodey GP, et al.2002 Guidelines for the use of antimicrobial agents in neutropenic patients with cancer. Clin Infect Dis 2002;34:730–51.
48. Chatzinikolaou I, Abi-Said D, Bodey GP, et al. Recent experience in *Pseudomonas aeruginosa* bacteremia in cancer patients. Retrospective analysis of 245 episodes. Arch Intern Med 2000;160:501–9.
49. Bodey GP, Jadeja L, Elting L. *Pseudomonas* bacteremia: retrospective analysis of 410 episodes. Arch Intern Med 1985;145:1621–9.
50. Nguyen KA, Coyle EA, Tam VH, et al. Antibacterial activity of colistin (c) and Polymyxin B (PV) against multidrug-resistant (MDR) Pseudomonas aeruginosa (PSA), Alcalignes Xylosoxidans (AX), and Stenotrophomonas maltophilia (SM) at a cancer Center [abstract]. In: Program and abstracts for the 44th Interscience Conference on Antimicrobial Agents and Chemotherapy; 2004 Oct 30–Nov 4; Washington, D.C.
51. Rolston KVI. Stenotrophomonas maltophilia infection in cancer patients – frequency, spectrum of infections and antimicrobial susceptibility [abstract]. 13th European Congress of Clinical Microbiology and Infectious Diseases; 2003 May 10–13;Glasgow, UK.
52. Rolston KVI, Kontoyiannis DP, Yadegarynia D, Raad I. Nonfermentative gram-negative bacilli in cancer patients: increasing frequency of infection and antimicrobial susceptibility of clinical isolates to fluoroquinolones. Diag Microbiol Infect Dis 2005;51:215–8.
53. Vartivarian S, Anaissie E, Bodey GP, et al. A changing pattern of susceptibility of *Xanthomonas maltophilia* to antimicrobial agents: implications for therapy. Antimicrob Agents Chemother 1994;38:624–7.
54. Rolston KVI, Guan Z, Bodey GP, Elting L. *Acinetobacter calcoaceticus* septicemia in patients with cancer. South Med J 1985;78:647–51.
55. Barnes PF, Barrows SA. Tuberculosis in the 1990s. Ann Intern Med 1993;119:400–10.
56. Combs PL, O'Brien RJ, Geiter LJ. USPHS tuberculosis short course chemotherapy trial 21: effectiveness, toxicity, and acceptability. The report of final results. Ann Intern Med 1990;112:397–406.
57. Iseman MD. Treatment of multidrug-resistant tuberculosis. N Engl J Med 1993;329:784–91.
58. Husni R, Mouronte DA, Kantarjian H, Rolston K. Risk factors of infections in patients with hairy cell leukemia (HCL) [abstract]. 36th Annual Meeting of the Infectious Diseases Society of America; 1998 Nov 12–15; Denver, CO.
59. Infante R, Jacobson KL, Han HY. Mycobacterium intracellulare is a significant pathogen in cancer patients. [Abstract]. 40th Annual Meeting of the Infectious Diseases Society of America (IDSA). Chicago, IL, Sept. 27–30, 2002.
60. Griffith DE, Brown BA, Murphy DT, et al. Initial (6-month) results of three-times–weekly azithromycin in treatment regimens for *Mycobacterium avium complex* lung disease in human immunodeficiency virus-negative patients. J Infect Dis 1998;178:121–6.
61. Ward TT, Rimland D, Kauffman C. Randomized, open-label trial of azithromycin plus ethambutol vs clarithromycin plus ethambutol as therapy for *Mycobacterium avium* complex bacteremia in patients with human immunodeficiency virus infection. Clin Infect Dis 1998;27:1278–85.
62. Holland SM, Eisenstein EM, Kuhns DB, et al. Treatment of refractory disseminated nontuberculous mycobacterial infection with interferon gamma. N Engl J Med 1994;330:1348–55.
63. Jacobson K, Tiera R, Libshitz H, et al. *Mycobacterium kansasii* infections in patients with cancer. Clin Infect Dis 2000;30:965–9.
64. Hoy JF, Rolston KVI, Hopfer RL, Bodey GP. *Mycobacterium fortuitum* bacteremia in patients with cancer and long-term venous catheters. Am J Med 1987;83:213–7.
65. Rolston KVI, Jones PG, Fainstein V, Bodey GP. Pulmonary disease caused by rapidly growing mycobacteria in patients with cancer. Chest 1985;87:503–6.
66. Jongevos SF, Prens EP, Habets JMW. Successful triple-antibiotic therapy for cutaneous infection due to *Mycobacterium chelonae.* Clin Infect Dis 1999;28:145–6.
67. Tkatch LS, Kusni S, Irish WD, et al. Epidemiology of *Legionella pneumonia* and factors associated with *Legionella-related* mortality at a tertiary care center. Clin Infect Dis 1998;27:1479–86.
68. Benz-Lemoine E, Delwail V, Castel O, et al. Nosocomial Legionnaires' disease in a bone marrow transplant unit. Bone Marrow Transplant 1991;7:61–3.
69. Edelstein PH. Antimicrobial chemotherapy for Legionnaires disease: time for a change. Ann Intern Med 1998;129:328–30.
70. Pfaller MA, Jones RN, Doern GV, et al. Bloodstream infections due to *Candida* species: SENTRY antimicrobial surveillance program in North America and Latin America, 1997–1998. Antimicrob Agents Chemother 2000;44:747–51.
71. Giamaria C, Martino P, de Bernardis F, et al. Rising incidence of *Candida parapsilosis* fungemia in patients with hematologic malignancies: clinical aspects, predisposing factors, and differential pathogenicity of the causative strains. Clin Infect Dis 1996;23:506–14.
72. Samonis G, Skordilis P, Maraki S, et al. Oropharyngeal candidiasis as a marker for esophageal candidiasis in patients with cancer. Clin Infect Dis 1998;27:283–6.
73. Sobel J, Vazques J. Candidemia and systemic candidiasis. Semin Respir Infect 1990;5:123–37.
74. Haron E, Feld R, Tuffneff et al. Hepatic candidiasis: an increasing problem in immunocompromised hosts. Am J Med 1987;83:17–25.
75. Kauffman CA, Bradley SF, Ross SC, Weber DR. Hepatosplenic candidiasis: successful treatment with fluconazole. Am J Med 1991;91:137–41.
76. Winegard JR, Merz WG, Saral R. *Candida tropicalis*: a major pathogen in immunocompromised patients. Ann Intern Med 1979;91:539–43.
77. Wingard JR, Merz WG, Rinaldi MG, et al. Increase in *Candida krusei* infection among patients with bone marrow transplantation and neutropenia treated prophylactically with fluconazole. N Engl J Med 1991;325:1274–7.
78. Nguyen MH, Peacock JE Jr, Morris AJ, et al. The changing face of candidemia: emergence of *non-Candida albicans* species and antifungal resistance. Am J Med 1996;100:617–23.
79. Mullen CA, El-Baki H Abd., Samir H, Tarrand JJ, Rolston KV. Non-albicans *Candida* is the most common cause of candidemia in pediatric cancer patients. Support Care Cancer 2003;11:321–5.
80. Walsh TJ, Shanock SJ. Laboratory diagnosis of invasive candidiasis: a rationale for complementary use of culture- and nonculture-based detection system. Int J Infect Dis 1997;1:S11–9.
81. Rex JH, Bennet JE, Sugar AM, et al. A randomized trial comparing fluconazole with amphotericin B for the treatment of candidemia in patients without neutropenia. N Engl J Med 1994;331:1325–72.
82. Anaissie EJ, Darouiche RO, Abi-Said D, et al. Management of invasive candidal infections: results of a prospective, randomized, multicenter study of fluconazole versus amphotericin B and review of the literature. Clin Infect Dis 1996;23:964–72.
83. Mora-Durate J, Betts R, Rotstein C, et al. Comparison of caspofungin and amphotericin B for invasive candidiasis. N Engl J Med 2002;347:2020–9.
84. Bodey GP, Vartivarian S. Aspergillosis. Eur J Clin Microbiol Infect Dis 1989;8:413–37.
85. Caillot D, Couaillier JF, Bernard A, et al. Increasing volume and changing characteristics of invasive pulmonary aspergillosis on sequential thoracic computed tomography scans in patients with neutropenia. J Clin Oncol 2001;19:253–9.
86. Khardori N, Hayat S, Rolston K, Bodey GP: Cutaneous Rhizopus and Aspergillus infections in five cancer patients. Arch Derm 1989;125:952–6.
87. Kontoyiannis DP, Bodey GP. Invasive aspergillosis in 2002: an update. Eur J Clin Microbiol Infect Dis 2002;21:161–72.
88. Maertens J, Verhaegen J, Lagrou K, et al. Screening for circulating galactomannan as a noninvasive diagnostic tool for invasive aspergillosis in prolonged neutropenic patients and stem cell transplantation recipients: a prospective validation. Blood 2001;97:1604–10.
89. Herbrecht R, Letscher-Bru V, Oprea C, et al. Aspergillus galactomannan detection in the diagnosis of invasive aspergillosis in cancer patients. J Clin Oncol 2002;20:1898–1906.
90. Denning DW, Lee JY, Hostetler JS, et al. NIAID Mycoses Study Group multicenter trial of oral itraconazole therapy for invasive aspergillosis. Am J Med 1994;97:135–44.
91. Maertens J, Raad I, Petrikkos G, et al. Efficacy and safety of caspofungin for treatment of invasive aspergillosis in patients refractory to or intolerant of conventional antifungal therapy. Clin Infect Dis 2004;39:1563–71.
92. Herbrecht R, Denning DW, Patterson TF, et al. Voriconazole versus amphotericin B for primary therapy of invasive aspergillosis. N Engl J Med 2002;347:408–15.
93. Pappas PG, Perfect JR, Cloud GA, et al. Cryptococcosis in human immunodeficiency virus-negative patients in the era of effective azole therapy. Clin Infect Dis 2001;33:690–9.
94. Kontoyiannis DP, Wessel VC, Bodey GP, Rolston KVI. Zygomycosis in the 1990s in a tertiary-care center. Clin Infect Dis 2000;30:851–6.
95. Kontoyiannis DP, Lionakis MS, Lewis RE, et al. Zygomycosis in a tertiary-care cancer center in the era of Aspergillus-active antifungal therapy: A case-control observational study of 27 recent cases. J Infect Dis 2005;191:1350–60.
96. Hoy J, Hsu K, Rolston KVI, et al. *Trichosporon beigelii* infection: a review. Rev Infect Dis 1986;8:959–67.
97. Boutati EI, Anaissie EJ. Fusarium, a significant emerging pathogen in patients with hematologic malignancy: ten years' experience at a cancer center and implications for management. Blood 1997;90:999–1008.
98. Raad I, Tarrand J, Hanna H, et al. Epidemiology, molecular mycology, and environmental sources of Fusarium infection in patients with cancer. Infect Control Hosp Epidemiol 2002;23:532–7.
99. Walsh TJ, Teppler H, Donowitz GR, et al. Caspofungin versus liposomal amphotericin B for empirical antifungal therapy in patients with persistent fever and neutropenia. N Engl J Med 2004;351:1391–1402.
100. Walsh TJ, Pappas P, Winston DJ, et al. Voriconazole compared with liposomal amphotericin B for empirical antifungal therapy in patients with neutropenia and persistent fever. N Engl J Med 2002;346:225–34.
101. Whimbey E, Elting LS, Couch RB, et al. Influenza A virus infections among hospitalized adult bone marrow transplant recipients. Bone Marrow Transplant 1994;13:437–40.
102. Whimbey E, Vartivarian SE, Champlin RE, et al. Parainfluenzae virus infection in adult bone marrow transplant recipients. Eur J Clin Microbiol Infect Dis 1993;12:699–701.
103. Whimbey E, Bodey GP. Viral pneumonia in the immunocompromised adult with neoplastic disease; the role of community respiratory viruses. Semin Respir Infect 1992;7:122–33.
104. Gold D, Corey L. Acyclovir prophylaxis for herpes simplex virus infection. Antimicrob Agents Chemother 1987;31:361–7.
105. Perry CM, Faulds D. Valaciclovir. A review of its antiviral activity, pharmacokinetic properties and therapeutic efficacy in herpesvirus infection. Drugs 1996;52: 754–72.
106. Crumpacker C. The pharmacological profile of famciclovir. Semin Dermatol 1996;15(2 Suppl 1):14–26.
107. Straus SE, Ostrove JM, Inchauspe G, et al. NIH Conference. Varicella-zoster virus infections. Biology, natural history, treatment, and prevention. Ann Intern Med 1988;108:221–37.
108. Cohen JI, Brunell PA, Straus SE, Krause PR. NIH Conference. Recent advances in varicella-zoster virus infection. Ann Intern Med 1999;130:922–32.
109. Dunkle LM, Arvin AM, Whitley RJ, et al. A controlled trial of acyclovir for chickenpox in normal children. N Engl J Med 1991;325:1539–44.
110. Wood MJ, Johnson RW, McKendrick MW, et al. A randomized trial of acyclovir for 7 days or 21 days with and without prednisolone for treatment of acute herpes zoster. N Engl J Med 1994;330:896–900.
111. Wagstaff AJ, Bryson HM. Foscarnet. A reappraisal of its antiviral activity, pharmacokinetic properties and therapeutic use in immunocompromised patients with viral infections. Drugs 1994;48:199–226.
112. LaRussa P, Steinberg S, Gershon AA. Varicella vaccine for immunocompromised children: results of collaborative studies in the United States and Canada. J Infect Dis 1996;174 (Suppl 3):S320–3.
113. Asano Y, Yoshikawa T, Suga S, et al. Post exposure prophylaxis of varicella in family contact by oral acyclovir. Pediatrics 1993;92:219–22.
114. Erice A, Holm MA, Gill PC, et al. Cytomegalovirus (CMV) antigenemia assay is more sensitive than shell vial cultures for rapid detection of CMV in polymorphonuclear blood leukocytes. J Clin Microbiol 1992; 30:2822–5.
115. Prentice HG, Kho P. Clinical strategies for the management of cytomegalovirus infection and disease in allogeneic

bone marrow transplant. Bone Marrow Transplant 1997;19:135–42.

116. Vogel JU, Scholz M, Cinatl J Jr. Treatment of cytomegalovirus diseases. Intervirology 1997;40:357–67.

117. Nguyen Q, Estey E, Raad I, et al. Cytomegalovirus pneumonia in adults with leukemia: an emerging problem. Clin Infect Dis 2001;32:539–45.

118. Nguyen Q, Champlin R, Giralt S, et al. Late cytomegalovirus pneumonia in adult allogeneic blood and marrow transplant recipients. Clin Infect Dis 1999;28:618–23.

119. Zaia JA, Schmidt GM, Chao NJ, et al. Preemptive ganciclovir administration based solely on asymptomatic pulmonary cytomegalovirus infection in allogeneic bone marrow transplant recipients: long-term follow-up. Biol Blood Marrow Transplant 1995;1:188–93.

120. Cole PD, Stiles J, Boulad F, et al. Successful treatment of human herpes virus 6 encephalitis in a bone marrow transplant recipient. Clin Infect Dis 1998;27:653–4.

121. Whimbey E, Ghosh S. Respiratory syncytial virus infections in immunocompromised adults. In: Remington JS, Swartz MN, editors. Current clinical topics in infectious diseases. Boston: Blackwell Science; 2000. p. 232–55.

122. Yousuf H, Englund J, Couch R, et al. Influenza among hospitalized adults with leukemia. Clin Infect Dis 1997;24:1095–9.

123. Schreiber GB, Busch MP, Kleinman SH, Korelitz JJ. The risk of transfusion-transmitted viral infections. N Engl J Med 1996;334:1685–90.

124. Alter MJ, Kruszon-Moran D, Nainan OV, et al. The prevalence of hepatitis C virus infection in the United States, 1988 through 1994. N Engl J Med 1999;341:556–62.

125. Conry-Cantilena C, VanRaden M, Gibble J, et al. Routes of infection, viremia, and liver disease in blood donors found to have hepatitis C virus infection. N Engl J Med 1996;334:1691–6.

126. Vallisa D, Berte R, Rocca A, et al. Association between hepatitis C virus and non-Hodgkin's lymphoma, and effects of viral infection on histologic subtype and clinical course. Am J Med 1999;106:556–60.

127. Holland PV. Viral infections and the blood supply. N Engl J Med 1996;334:1734–5.

128. Galbraith RM, Eddleston AL, Williams R, Zuckerman AJ. Fulminant hepatic failure in leukemia and choriocarcinoma related to withdrawal of cytotoxic drug therapy. Lancet 1975;2:528–30.

129. Hanson CA, Sutherland DE, Snover DC. Fulminant hepatic failure in an HBsAg carrier renal transplant patient following cessation of immunosuppressive therapy. Transplantation 1985;39:311–2.

130. Omata M. Treatment of chronic hepatitis B infection. N Engl J Med 1998;339:114–5.

131. Lai CL, Chien RN, Leung NWY, et al. One year trial of lamivudine for chronic hepatitis B. N Engl J Med 1998;339:61–8.

132. Nguyen MH, Wright TL. Therapeutic advances in the management of hepatitis B and hepatitis C. Curr Opin Infect Dis 2001;14:593–601.

133. Haron E, Bodey GP, Luna MA, et al. Has the incidence of *Pneumocystis carinii* pneumonia in cancer patients increased with the AIDS epidemic? Lancet 1988;2:904–5.

134. Kulke MA, Vance EA. *Pneumocystis carinii* pneumonia in patients receiving chemotherapy for breast cancer. Clin Infect Dis 1997;25:215–8.

135. Walzer PD. Editorial response: *Pneumocystis carinii* pneumonia in patients without human immunodeficiency virus infection. Clin Infect Dis 1997;25:219–20.

136. Sepkowitz KA. *Pneumocystis carinii* pneumonia in patients without AIDS. Clin Infect Dis 1993;(17 Suppl 2):S416–22.

137. Kovacs JA, Ng VL, Masur H. Diagnosis of *Pneumocystis carinii* pneumonia. Improved detection in sputum with use of monoclonal antibodies. N Engl J Med 1988;318:589–93.

138. Moe AA, Hardy WD. *Pneumocystis carinii* infection in the HIV-seropositive patient. Infect Dis Clin North Am 1994;8:331–64.

139. Noskin GA, Murphy RL, Black JR, Phair JP. Salvage therapy with clindamycin/primaquine for *Pneumocystis carinii* pneumonia. Clin Infect Dis 1992;14:183–8.

140. Dohn MN, Weinberg WG, Torres RA, et al. Oral atovaquone compared with intravenous pentamidine for *Pneumocystis carinii* pneumonia in patients with AIDS. Ann Intern Med 1994;121:174–80.

141. Hughes W, Leoung G, Kramer F, et al. Comparison of atovaquone (S66C80) with trimethoprim-sulfamethoxazole to treat *Pneumocystis carinii* pneumonia in patients with AIDS. N Engl J Med 1993;328:1521–7.

142. Consensus statement on the use of corticosteroids as adjunctive therapy for *Pneumocystis pneumonia* in the acquired immunodeficiency syndrome. N Engl J Med 1990;323:1500–4.

143. Israelski DM, Remington JS. Toxoplasmosis in patients with cancer. Clin Infect Dis 1993;(17 Suppl 2):S424–35.

144. Vietzke WM, Gelderman AH, Grimley PM, Valsamis MD. Toxoplasmosis complicating malignancy: experience at the National Cancer Institute. Cancer 1968;21:816–27.

145. Luft BJ, Remington JS. Toxoplasmic encephalitis. J Infect Dis 1988;157:1–6.

146. Farkash AE, Maccabbee PJ, Sher JH. CNS toxoplasmosis in acquired immunodeficiency syndrome: a clinical pathological-radiological review of 12 cases. J Neurol Neurosurg Psychiatry 1986;49:744–8.

147. Hofflin JM, Remington JS. Tissue culture isolation of *Toxoplasma* from blood of a patient with AIDS. Arch Intern Med 1985;145:925–6.

148. Rolston KVI, Hoy JF. Role of clindamycin in the treatment of central nervous system toxoplasmosis. Am J Med 1987;83:551–4.

149. Rolston KVI. Treatment of acute toxoplasmosis with oral clindamycin. Eur J Clin Microbiol Infect Dis 1991;10:181–3.

150. Igra-Siegman Y, Kapila R, Sen P, et al. Syndrome of hyperinfection with *Strongyloides stercoralis.* Rev Infect Dis 1981;3:397–404.

151. Safdar A, Malathum K, Rodriguez SJ, et al. Strongyloidiasis in patients at a comprehensive cancer center in the United States. Cancer 2004;100:1531–6.

152. Drugs for parasitic infections. Med Lett Drugs Ther 1984;26:27–34.

153. Gann P, Neva F, Gamm A. A randomized trial of single- and two-dose ivermectin versus thiabendazole for treatment of strongyloidiasis. J Infect Dis 1994;169:1076–19.

154. Rolston KVI. The spectrum of pulmonary infections in cancer patients. Current Opinion in Oncology 2001;13:218–23.

155. Tierra, R Jacobson K, Tiera R, et al. *Mycobacterium kansasii* (MK) infections in cancer patients [abstract]. 35th Annual Meeting of the Infectious Diseases Society; 1997 Sept. 13–16; San Francisco, CA.

156. Kumashi P, Girgawy E, Tarrand JJ, et al. *Streptococcus pneumonia* bacteremia in patients with cancer: Disease characteristics and outcomes in the era of escalating drug resistance (1998–2002). Medicine. [In press]

157. Rolston KVI. Infections in patients with solid tumors. In: Rolston KVI, Rubenstein EB, editors. Textbook of febrile neutropenia. Martin Dunitz, London, U K, 2001, pp. 91–109.

158. Dosik GM, Luna M, Valdivieso M, et al. Necrotizing colitis in patients with cancer. Am J Med 1979;67:646–56.

159. Gomez L, Martin R, Rolston KV. Neutropenic enterocolitis: spectrum of the disease and comparison of definite and possible cases. Clin Infect Dis 1998;27:695–9.

160. Moir CR, Scudamore CH, Benny WB. Typhlitis: selective surgical management. Am J Surg 1986;151:563–6.

161. Barnes SG, Sattler FR, Ballard JO. Perirectal infections in acute leukemia. Improved survival after incision and debridement. Ann Intern Med 1984;100:515–8.

162. Rolston KVI, Bodey GP. Diagnosis and management of perianal and perirectal infection in the granulocytopenic patient. In: Remington J, Swartz MN, editors. Current clinical topics in infectious diseases. Boston: Blackwell Scientific; 1993. p. 164–71.

163. Bodey GP. Antibiotics in patients with neutropenia. Arch Intern Med 1984;144:1845–51.

164. Bodey GP. Empirical antibiotic therapy for fever in neutropenic patients. Clin Infect Dis 1993;17(Suppl 2): S378–84.

165. Pizzo PA. Empirical therapy and prevention of infection in the immunocompromised host. In: Mandell GL, Douglas RG Jr, Bennett JE, editors. Principles and practice of infectious diseases. 3rd ed. New York: Churchill Livingstone; 1990. p. 2303–12.

166. Sculier JP, Klastersky J. Significance of serum bactericidal activity in gram-negative bacillary bacteremia in patients with and without granulocytopenia. Am J Med 1984;76:429–35.

167. Bodey GP. Synergy. Should it determine antibiotic selection in neutropenic patients. Arch Intern Med 1985; 145:1964–6.

168. The International Antimicrobial Therapy Cooperative Group of the European Organization for Research and Treatment of Cancer. Efficacy and toxicity of single daily doses of amikacin and ceftriaxone versus multiple daily doses of amikacin and ceftazidime for infection in patients with cancer and granulocytopenia. Ann Intern Med 1993;119:584–93.

169. Rolston KVI, Berkey P, Bodey GP, et al. A comparison of imipenem to ceftazidime with or without amikacin as empiric therapy in febrile neutropenic patients. Arch Intern Med 1992;152:283–91.

170. Raad I, Escalante C, Hachem R, et al. Treatment of febrile neutropenic cancer patients requiring hospitalization: a prospective randomized study comparing imipenem and cefepime. Cancer 2003;98:1039–47.

171. Pizzo PA, Hathorn JW, Hiemenz J, et al. A randomized trial comparing ceftazidime alone with combination antibiotic therapy in cancer patients with fever and neutropenia. N Engl J Med 1986;315:552–8.

172. Karp JE, Dick JD, Angelopulos C, et al. Empiric use of vancomycin during prolonged treatment-induced granulocytopenia. Am J Med 1986;81:237–42.

173. Shenep J, Hughes WT, Roberson PK, et al. Vancomycin, ticarcillin and amikacin compared with ticarcillin clavulanate and amikacin in the empirical treatment of febrile, neutropenic children with cancer. N Engl J Med 1988;319:1053–8.

174. Safdar A, Rolston, KVI. Vancomycin-tolerant non-enterococcal gram-positive bacteremia- An emerging phenomenon in patients with cancer [abstract]. 13th International Symposium on Infections in the Immunocompromised Host; 2004 June 27–30; Granada, Spain.

175. Rolston K: New trends in patient management: Risk-based therapy for febrile patients with neutropenia. Clin Infect Dis 1999;29:515–21.

176. Freifeld A, Marchigiani D, Walsh T, et al. A double-blind comparison of empirical oral and intravenous antibiotic therapy for low-risk febrile patients with neutropenia during cancer chemotherapy. N Engl J Med 1999;341:305–11.

177. Kern WV, Cometta A, De Bock R, et al, for the International Antimicrobial Therapy Cooperative Group of the European Organization for Research and Treatment of Cancer. Oral versus intravenous empirical antimicrobial therapy for fever in patients with granulocytopenia who are receiving cancer chemotherapy. N Engl J Med 1999;341:312–8.

178. Rolston KVI. The Infectious Diseases Society of America 2002 Guidelines for the use of antimicrobial agents in patients with cancer and neutropenia: Salient features and comments. Clin Infect Dis 2004;39(Suppl 1):S44–8.

179. Rolston, Frisbee-Hume S, Manzullo E, Patel S, Benjamin R. Once daily, oral, outpatient, Quinolone monotherapy for low-risk, febrile neutropenic patients (FNP) [abstract]. 41st Annual Meeting of the Infectious Diseases Society of America; 2003 Oct. 9-12; San Diego, CA.

180. Malik IA, Wajahat A, Khan MD, et al. Feasibility of outpatient management of fever in cancer patients with low-risk neutropenia: results of a prospective randomized trial. Am J Med 1995;98:224–31.

181. NCCN practice guidelines for fever and neutropenia. Oncology 1999;13:197–257.

182. Dignani MC, Anaisise EJ, Hester JP, et al. Treatment of neutropenia-related fungal infections with granulocyte colony-stimulating factor-elicited white blood cell transfusions: a pilot study. Leukemia 1997;11:1621–30.

183. Update of recommendations for the use of hematopoietic colony-simulating factors: evidence-based clinical practice guidelines. J Clin Oncol 1996;14:1957–60.

184. Murray HW. Interferon-gamma and host antimicrobial defense: current and future clinical applications. Am J Med 1994;97:459–60.

185. Murray HW. Cytokines as antimicrobial therapy for the T-cell–deficient patient: prospects for treatment of nonviral opportunistic infections. Clin Infect Dis 1993;(17 Suppl 2):S407–13.

186. Verhoef J. Prevention of infections in the neutropenic patient. Clin Infect Dis 1993;(17 Suppl 2):S359–67.

187. Cruciani M, Rampazzo R, Malena M, et al. Prophylaxis with fluoroquinolones for bacterial infections in neutropenic patients. Clin Infect Dis 1996;23:795–805.

188. Tunkel AR, Sepkowitz KA. Infections caused by viridans streptococci in patients with neutropenia. Clin Infect Dis 2002;34:1524-9.

189. Razonable RR, Litzow MR, Khaliq Y, et al. Bacteremia due to viridans group streptococci with diminished susceptibility to levofloxacin among neutropenic patients receiving levofloxacin prophylaxis. Clin Infect Dis 2002;34:1469–74.

190. Rolston KVI, Yadegarynia D, Kontoyiannis DP, et al. The spectrum of gram-positive bloodstream infection in patients with hematologic malignancies, and the in-vitro activity of various quinolones against gram-positive bacteria isolated from cancer patients. Intern J Infect Dis (In Press)

191. Rolston KVI. Commentary: chemoprophylaxis and bacterial resistance in neutropenic patients. Infect Dis Clin Pract 1998;7:202–4.

192. Goodman JL, Winston DJ, Greenfield RA, , et al. A controlled trial of fluconazole to prevent fungal infections in patients undergoing bone marrow transplantation. New Engl L Med 1992;326:845–51.
193. Slavin MA, Osborne B, Adams R, et al. Efficacy and safety of fluconazole prophylaxis for fungal infections after marrow transplantation—a prospective, randomized, double-blind study. J Infect Dis 1995;171:1545-52.
194. Marr KA, Seidel K, Slavin MA, et al. Prolonged fluconazole prophylaxis is associated with persistent protection against candidiasis-related death in allogeneic marrow transplant recipients: long-term follow-up of a randomized, placebo-controlled trial. Blood 2000; 96:2055–61.
195. Winston DJ, Chandrasekar PH, Lazarus HM, , et al. Fluconazole prophylaxis of fungal infections in patients with acute leukemia. Annal Intern Med 1993;118:495–502.
196. Abi-Said D, Anaissie E, Uzun O, et al. The epidemiology of hematogenous candidiasis caused by different *Candida* species. Clin Infect Dis 1997;24:1122–8.
197. Wingard JR, Merz WG, Rinaldi MG, et al. Increase in *Candida krusei* infection among patients with bone marrow transplantation and neutropenia treated prophylactically with fluconazole. New Engl J Med 1991;325:1274–7.
198. Mullen CA, Abd El-Baki H, Samir H, et al. Non-albicans Candida is the most common cause of candidemia in pediatric cancer patients. Support Care Cancer 2003;11:321–5.
199. Goodrich JM, Mori M, Gleaves CA, et al. Early treatment with ganciclovir to prevent cytomegalovirus disease after allogeneic bone marrow transplantation. N Engl J Med 1991;325:1601–7.

Section 40

ONCOLOGIC EMERGENCIES

142

Oncologic Emergencies

Sai-Ching Jim Yeung, MD, PhD
Carmen P. Escalante, MD

Cancer patients are more likely than healthy individuals to require emergency health care. Accidents in everyday life (trauma, burn, electrocution, environmental stresses) can lead to emergencies in cancer patients. The debilitated physical status, altered hemostasis, and impaired immunity that can result from malignancy or treatment of malignancy make cancer patients more vulnerable to injuries than healthy people are. Moreover, cancer and its treatment can lead to emergency conditions. Because cancer patients have unique concerns different from those of the general population presenting to emergency care facilities, care providers need to adjust their routine practice patterns accordingly when caring for patients with cancer.

The care of cancer patients with emergency conditions is evolving into a hybrid discipline—a cross between oncology and emergency medicine. Cancer patients present to an emergency care facility for many types of problems, and an in-depth discussion fills a volume by itself.[1,2] Because of page constraints and the fact that some relevant topics are covered in other chapters of this book, this chapter can cover only a small number of selected topics. For some of the topics, the discussion is a condensed and updated version of the discussion in our book.[1]

An oncologic emergency may be defined as an acute condition that is caused by cancer or the treatment of cancer and that requires intervention as soon as possible to avoid mortality or severe permanent morbidity. During triage, serious emergencies in a cancer patient can be recognized by a brief assessment of vital signs and neurologic status. In the discussion that follows, we briefly review the general approach to acutely ill cancer patients, and we then review the causes, symptoms and signs, and treatment of selected oncologic emergencies.

APPROACH TO ACUTELY ILL CANCER PATIENTS

Cancer patients often have complex medical problems in addition to their cancer diagnosis—for example, coronary artery disease, diabetes mellitus, and chronic obstructive pulmonary disease. Some of these comorbid conditions may be attributable to the same risk factors that played a role in the development of cancer (ie, diet, cigarette smoking, or sedentary lifestyle). In addition, cancer patients are often older than the general population presenting to emergency care facilities, which can further increase the complexity of patient care.

Cancer patients presenting with acute emergencies should be approached in a manner similar to that used for patients without cancer. However, in addition to providing the usual emergency care, the care providers must rapidly assess the extent of the malignancy, the response of the malignancy to current treatment, the overall prognosis, and the patient's and family's wishes so that an appropriate treatment plan can be formulated and carried out (Figure 142-1).

First, the patient should be rapidly assessed. This assessment should include definition of the chief complaint, taking of a focused history, baseline assessment of vital signs, and quick overall physical assessment. If the patient is unable to relay the history, a family member or caregiver may be able to provide pertinent information. Unstable patients should be stabilized. In the case of cardiopulmonary arrest, appropriate guidelines should be followed (<http://www.acls.net>).[3] Patients with hypotension should be rapidly evaluated, and appropriate therapies should be instituted (ie, intravenous fluids, pericardial fluid drainage, vasopressors, etc). Once the patient is stabilized, a more thorough history and physical examination should be completed.

For most cancer patients with acute emergencies, a comprehensive evaluation is usually necessary. Depending on the clinical scenario, the acute event may be attributable to the malignancy itself, to treatment of the malignancy, or to a new or preexisting comorbid condition. These different possibilities should be considered when developing a differential diagnosis of the problem.

CIRCULATORY ONCOLOGIC EMERGENCIES

Sudden Cardiopulmonary Arrest Most deaths are preceded by cardiopulmonary arrest. Resuscitation is more likely to be successful when cardiopulmonary arrest results from an acute reversible insult (eg, pulmonary embolism, choking, aspiration, or cardiac arrhythmia) than when it results from a steady decline from an irreversible condition (eg, hypoxia because of diffuse infiltration of lungs by cancer). This is true in cancer patients as well as in patients with other diseases. The rate of success in resuscitating patients in cardiopulmonary arrest and the rate of resuscitated patients' being discharged from the hospital are similar for cancer patients and for noncancer patients.[4] A meta-analysis of inpatient resuscitation estimated that for patients overall, regardless of cancer status, the probability of surviving resuscitation is one in three, and the probability of being discharged alive is one in eight.[5] The mortality rate of cancer patients in the intensive care unit is about 50%, which is similar to the mortality rate of severely ill noncancer patients.[6]

If a cancer patient has a good performance status and is not expected to die soon, reluctance to resuscitate the patient or to admit the patient to an intensive care unit is unjustified. A non-end-stage cancer patient in cardiopulmonary arrest should be resuscitated with the same level of

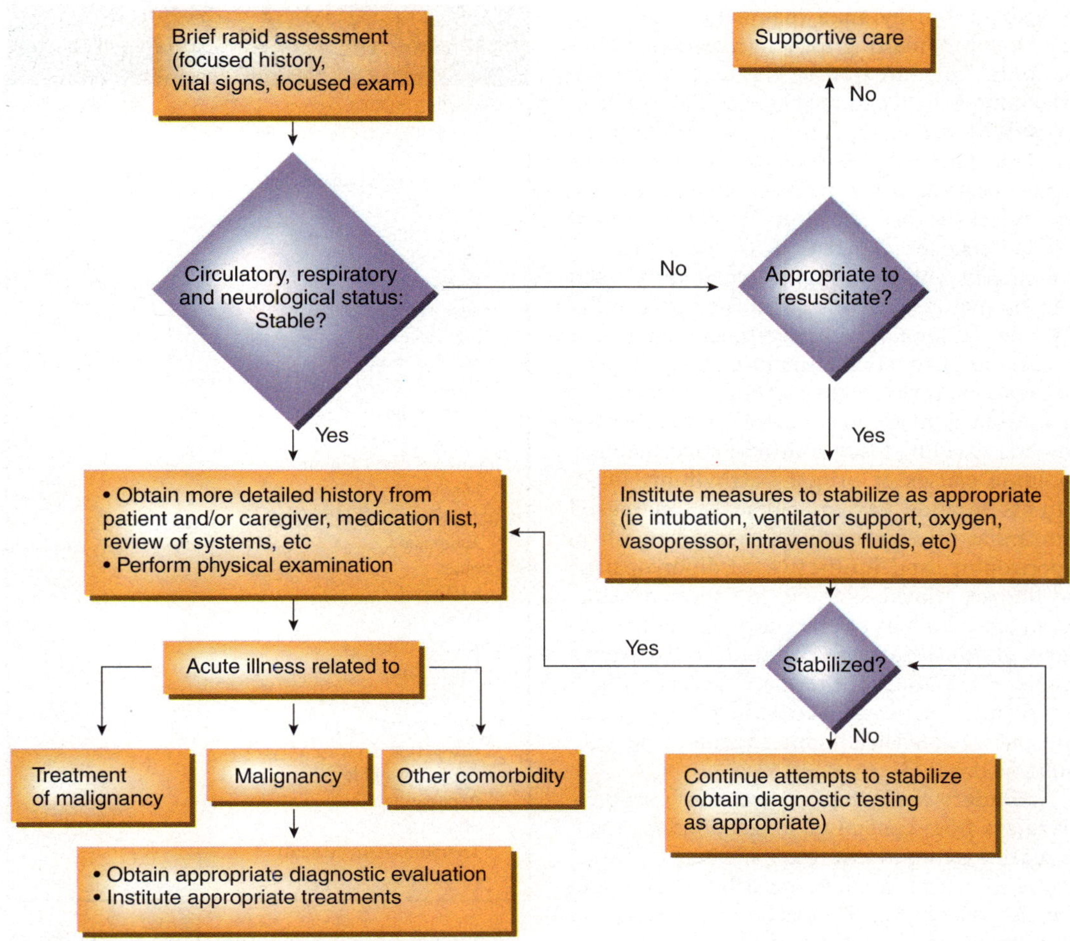

Figure 142-1 Approach to acutely ill cancer patients.

intense effort as any patient without cancer. However, when cardiopulmonary arrest occurs as the expected final episode of a gradual decline and disintegration of bodily functions caused by cancer, resuscitation generally will not succeed.

Oncologists should ensure that advance directives (medical power of attorney, living will, and out-of-hospital "do not resuscitate" [DNR] orders) are discussed with patients and their families. Oncologists should also ensure that such orders are provided as the patient and the family wish. DNR orders ensure that treatments will not be initiated if such efforts are fruitless and will only cause suffering. Many informed patients readily sign living wills or appoint health care proxies. Timely recommendation of DNR status may avoid unnecessary trauma to patients and anguish for family members. Timely recommendation of DNR status also provides time for open discussions to settle disagreements with patients or family.

When a cancer patient presents to a health care facility in cardiopulmonary arrest or impending arrest, the physician providing the emergency care may never have seen the patient before. In that situation, assessment of prognosis is difficult and quite often impossible. The decision to initiate or continue resuscitative efforts should be based on a rapid assessment of the patient's physical condition, a brief history of the events leading to or preceding the arrest, and any of the following factors that are known[7]: (1) duration of arrest; (2) initial cardiac rhythm; (3) rigor mortis or algor mortis; (4) type, stage, and prognosis of cancer; (5) history of cancer treatment and prospects for its success; (6) expressed directives of the patient or family; (7) comorbid conditions; (8) performance status and nutritional status; (9) potential quality of life if the patient survives; and (10) advanced age.

The fact that an emergency medical service has been summoned to transport the patient to an emergency care facility may indicate that death is unexpected, that the family has not yet accepted the patient's grave prognosis, or that the patient or family is seeking relief of symptoms or suffering at the last moments of life. Demands for resuscitation may be motivated by denial of the patient's terminal condition. In the absence of a clear advance directive from the patient, resuscitation may be needed to give the family "closure" by knowing that "everything possible was done." On the other hand, even in the absence of a clear advance directive, resuscitation of patients with advanced refractory malignancies may be inappropriate when intubation and resuscitation will only prolong pain and suffering and waste health care resources without affecting outcome.

Special Consideration in Resuscitation of Cancer Patients Most physicians and health care providers follow the resuscitation algorithms outlined in the advanced cardiac life-support protocols (<http://www.acls.net>).[3] However, identification of specific causes of cardiopulmonary arrest may enable physicians to tailor resuscitative efforts to reverse or control the specific causes of arrest.

Carcinoid crisis (also called "acute carcinoid syndrome") is a good example of an uncommon, but preventable and treatable cause of cardiopulmonary arrest in cancer patients. The crisis may be precipitated by anesthesia, biopsy, surgery, chemotherapy, or adrenergic drugs (eg, dopamine and epinephrine). Affected patients may develop refractory hypotension, arrhythmias, and bronchospasm attributable to massive release of serotonin and other vasoactive peptides from the tumor. Carcinoid crisis can be aborted or treated effectively with octreotide acetate (Sandostatin, Novartis Pharma, USA), a somatostatin analog, 150 to 500 μg intravenously.[8] Cardiac tamponade is another case in which knowledge of the precipitating cause would help the physician tailor the resuscitative effort to the patient's specific need. If a patient has pulseless electrical activity attributable to cardiac tamponade caused by malignant pericardial effusion, resuscitative efforts will not succeed until pericardiocentesis is performed to relieve the pressure on the cardiac chambers.

Causes of Cardiac Arrest in Cancer Patients Cardiopulmonary arrest in cancer patients may result from the neoplasm, from antineoplastic therapy, or from processes unrelated to cancer. In the general population, undiagnosed neoplasm is a rare cause of sudden death. In cancer patients, a review of causes of death found that 4% of patients died of cardiac problems and that 90% of those died from atherosclerosis-related ischemic heart disease.[9]

Tumor-Related Causes Tumor-related cardiac problems are usually the result of pericardial involvement. Neoplastic pericarditis and cardiac tamponade are good examples. Tumors can also induce arrhythmias because of the hormone mediators that they secrete (eg, catecholamines secreted by pheochromocytomas, and serotonin secreted by carcinoid tumors) or because of direct mechanical irritation of the heart or pericardium. Arrhythmias associated with myocardial tumors,[10] coronary obstruction by tumor,[11] and massive tumor embolization[12] have all been reported as causes of sudden cardiopulmonary arrest. Cardiac amyloidosis can also lead to intractable congestive heart failure, arrhythmias, conduction disturbances, and sudden death.[13] Other tumor-related causes of cardiopulmonary arrest include malignancy-induced hemorrhage and malignancy-induced loss of ventilatory function (lymphangitic spread of tumor, airway obstruction, and loss of brain stem function).

Chemotherapy-Related Causes Antineoplastic chemotherapeutic agents can cause complications leading to cardiopulmonary arrest. Angina, myocardial infarction, congestive heart failure, hypotension, arrhythmia, and sudden death have all been reported as complications of treatment with cytotoxic chemotherapy drugs.

Anthracyclines (doxorubicin, daunorubicin, idarubicin), mitoxantrone, and mitomycin are known to injure cardiomyocytes, leading to cardiomyopathy. The long-term cardiotoxicity of anthracyclines depends on the cumulative dose.[14] However, these drugs also cause acute side effects. Electrocardiographic and rhythm changes (mostly benign) have been noted in about 30% of patients treated with doxorubicin,[15] and sudden cardiopulmonary arrest has been reported in almost 1% of patients receiving doxorubicin.[16]

High-dose cyclophosphamide may cause acute problems of ventricular arrhythmia, cardiomyopathy, pericardial effusion, and cardiac arrest.[17] Fluorouracil has been associated with acute coronary vasospasm leading to angina and myocardial infarction.[18] Vasospasm or worsening angina in a patient receiving fluorouracil can be treated with calcium channel blockers. Hypotension, arrhythmia, and sudden death have also been reported with cytokines (interleukin-2 [IL-2], interferons [IFNs]) and monoclonal antibodies (discussed in the section "Systemic Reactions to Cytokines and Monoclonal Antibodies" later in this chapter).

Radiotherapy-Related Causes Radiotherapy to the chest has adverse effects on the pericardium and heart.[19] Pericarditis may occur shortly after exposure of the chest to radiation—or months or years afterward. Radiotherapy can lead to pericardial effusion, tamponade, or pericardial fibrosis. The direct toxic effect of radiation on the heart can lead to electrocardiographic changes, including T-wave abnormalities and atrial arrhythmias. Exposure of the heart to radiation is also associated with accelerated atherosclerosis, coronary artery endarteritis, medial fibrosis, intimal proliferation, myocardial infarction, and sudden death.[20] Restrictive cardiomyopathy, arrhythmia,[21] and valvular diseases[21] are also significant problems after irradiation of the chest.

Arrhythmia Arrhythmia is a common problem in cancer patients and often leads to emergent evaluation. As discussed earlier, arrhythmia can lead to cardiopulmonary arrest and death. Arrhythmia may be related to malignancy or treatment of the malignancy, or it may be the result of other unrelated medical problems.

Symptoms of arrhythmia can be subtle and intermittent. The symptoms are primarily attributable to the hemodynamic effects of the cardiac rhythm disturbance. Significant signs and symptoms include isolated or recurrent loss of consciousness (syncope), lightheadedness, dizziness, palpitation, chest pain, peripheral vascular embolization, dyspnea, and acute neurologic deficits (transient or persistent).

Sustained arrhythmia can be diagnosed electrographically with relative ease. However, arrhythmia is often transient, and transient or intermittent arrhythmia may present a diagnostic challenge. An electrocardiographic rhythm strip or a brief period of continuous monitoring does not exclude the possibility of a latent and potentially serious rhythm disturbance. When symptoms suggest arrhythmia (palpitation, syncope, etc), Holter monitoring for longer periods (24 to 48 hours) is indicated to try to capture the arrhythmic events and to diagnose the problem. Analysis of cardiac rhythm may be more complicated in cancer patients than in noncancer patients because cancer patients often have exaggerated respiratory variations of the electrical axis and changes in mean QRS voltage that can be confused with heart rhythm irregularity. Such changes may result from pleural or pericardial effusions, pulmonary surgery (pneumonectomy or lobectomy), or radiation-induced lung damage.

Primary Arrhythmia Primary arrhythmia arises from cardiac and pericardial structures and may be caused by focal or diffuse abnormalities. Common causes of primary arrhythmia in all patients include ischemic disease; increased intracardiac pressure and wall stress; congestive, hypertrophic, and infiltrative cardiomyopathy; and fibrosis related to aging. In cancer patients, the major causes of primary arrhythmia are primary or metastatic malignant intracardiac tumors,[22] amyloid infiltration,[23] myocarditis,[24] pericarditis,[25] pericardial constriction, and cardiomyopathy related to antitumor agents (especially anthracyclines).[15]

Secondary Arrhythmia Secondary arrhythmia arises from general toxic reactions to drugs; increased sympathetic states, such as those related to severe anxiety, hyperthyroidism, and mediator release (with pheochromocytomas and carcinoid tumors); derangements of electrolyte metabolism; and radiation-induced heart damage. Some cancer drugs are arrhythmogenic—examples include anthracyclines,[26] arsenic trioxide,[27] 5-fluorouracil,[28] irinotecan,[29] gemcitabine,[30] and interferon.[31] Table 142-1 shows a longer list of chemotherapeutic agents associated with arrhythmias. In addition to chemotherapeutic agents, antifungal agents,[32,33] antiprotozoals,[34] and antibiotics[35,36] have also been reported to be associated with rhythm disturbances.

Treatment of Arrhythmia Treatment of arrhythmia should be based on both urgency and cause. For hemodynamically stable arrhythmias that are secondary in origin, immediate treatment should aim to correct metabolic derangements (particularly to achieve homeostasis of potassium, calcium, and magnesium) and to discontinue culprit drugs or substances. Specific treatment aimed at reversing the causative factor should be administered. When treatment to control the cardiac rhythm is thought to be necessary, standard guidelines for management of arrhythmia may be followed.[3] Table 142-2 lists commonly used intravenous antiarrhythmic drugs and their dosages.

In a considerable proportion of cases, carotid sinus massage or other vagal maneuvers may convert paroxysmal supraventricular tachycardia back into sinus rhythm. Adenosine administered in one or two doses by rapid-infusion bolus under electrocardiographic monitoring is frequently effective in restoring normal heart rhythm. The drug is sometimes used to help determine the mechanism of the arrhythmia when the nature of the disturbance is unclear on electrocardiographic monitor strips. Careful analysis of standard electrocardiograms usually obviates the use of adenosine as a diagnostic tool.

Table 142-1 Chemotherapeutic Drugs Associated with Arrhythmias

- Alkylating Agents
  - Cisplatin
  - Ifosfamide
  - Cyclophosphamide
  - Busulfan
  - Carmustine
- Anthracyclines
  - Daunorubicin
  - Doxorubicin
  - Idarubicin
  - Mitoxantrone
- Anti-metabolites
  - 5-Fluorouracil
  - Gemcitabine
- Topoisomerase I Inhibitors
  - Irinotecan
- Topoisomerase II Inhibitors
  - Teniposide
- Taxanes
  - Paclitaxel
  - Docetaxel
- Vinca Alkaloids
  - Vincristine
  - Vinblastine
- Miscellaneous
  - Amsacrine
  - Arsenic trioxide
  - Asparaginase
  - Interferon
  - Tretinoin (retinoic acid)
  - Pentostatin

Stable secondary arrhythmia is unlikely to deteriorate into a life-threatening or catastrophic problem. Frequently, secondary arrhythmia presents as either ventricular ectopy, sometimes in bigeminy or trigeminy or other coupled patterns, or supraventricular ectopy, most often as intermittent or sustained supraventricular tachycardia.

Isolated premature ventricular complexes may not require treatment. More complex forms of ventricular ectopy are often controlled by beta-adrenergic blockers, which have no proarrhythmic properties. When control with a beta-blocker is not satisfactory and there are reasons to intervene, antiarrhythmic agents such as propafenone and acebutolol are preferred over amiodarone, which has an extremely long pharmacokinetic half-life. Nevertheless, amiodarone should be considered when short-acting agents have failed and in patients with a low left ventricular ejection fraction. Amiodarone should be used with caution in patients with hepatic insufficiency and patients with underlying thyroid disease. Rarely, amiodarone can cause hypotension, bradycardia, and QT prolongation that may precipitate episodes of torsades de pointes. Except for beta-adrenergic blockers, many antiarrhythmic drugs, especially those in types IA, IC, and III, are potentially proarrhythmic.[37] During initiation of antiarrhythmic therapy, cardiac monitoring should be con-

Table 142-2 Commonly Used Intravenous Antiarrhythmic Drugs

Name	Class	Dose[3]	Indication[3]
Adenosine	Nucleoside	6 mg IV over < 3 s, followed by NS 20 mL bolus; 2nd dose and 3rd dose of 12 mg, 2 min apart prn	Narrow complex PSVT; PSVT due to AV node or sinus node reentry
Amiodarone	Class III anti-arrhythmic	Cardiac arrest: 300 mg IVP; 150 mg IVP every 3–5 min up to 2.2 g/day	
		Stable wide complex tachycardia: 150 mg IV over 10 min; repeat every 10 min prn; maintenance infusion 0.5 mg/min; up to 2.2 g/day	Supraventricular or ventricular tachyarrhythmias; control of rapid atrial tachyarrhythmia in patients with low LVEF when digoxin is ineffective
Atropine	Anticholinergic	0.5–1 mg IVP every 3–5 min prn, up to 0.04 mg/kg	Symptomatic sinus bradycardia; Mobitz type I AV block; asystole
Digoxin	Digitalis glycoside	Loading dose: 10–15 μg/kg lean body weight in divided doses	To slow ventricular response in A. fib. or A. flutter; PSVT
Diltiazem	Calcium channel blocker	0.25 mg/kg IV over 2 min; 2nd dose 0.35 mg/kg IV over 2 min in 15 min prn; maintenance: 5–15 mg/h by titration	To slow ventricular response in A. fib. or A. flutter; PSVT; to terminate AV nodal reentrant tachycardia
Esmolol	Beta-blocker	0.5 mg/kg over 1 min; then infuse at 0.05 mg/kg/min; titrate up to maximum of 0.3 mg/kg/min	PSVT; A. fib. or A. flutter; reduce incidence of VF in MI or USA
Ibutilide	Class III anti-arrhythmic	1 mg IV over 10 min; repeat in 10 min prn	SVT including A. fib. or A. flutter; effective for conversion of A. fib. or flutter of relatively brief duration
Isoproterenol	Beta-agonist	Infuse 2–10 μg/min; titrate	Symptomatic bradycardia; torsades de pointes refractory to Mg; beta-blocker overdose
Lidocaine	Local anesthetic	1–1.5 mg/kg IVP; repeat 0.5–0.75 mg/kg IVP every 5–10 min up to total of 3 mg/kg prn; maintenance: 30–50 μg/kg/min IV	VT or VF; wide-complex tachycardia; significant ventricular ectopy; torsades de pointes
Metoprolol	Beta-blocker	5 mg slow IVP every 5 min up to a total dose of 15 mg	PSVT; A. fib. or flutter; reduce incidence of VF in MI or USA
Procainamide hydrochloride	Class IA anti-arrhythmic	20–50 mg/min up to a total dose of 17 mg/kg	Recurrent VF or VT
Propranolol	Beta-blocker	0.1 mg/kg slow IVP in 3 divided doses 2–3 min apart	PSVT; A. fib. or flutter; reduce incidence of VF in MI or USA
Quinidine gluconate	Class IA anti-arrhythmic	Intermittent bolus doses of 80 mg every 5–10 min or 10 mg/min intravenous infusion up to 400 mg	Supraventricular and ventricular arrhythmias
Verapamil	Calcium channel blocker	2.5–5 mg IV over 2 min; repeat every 15–30 min prn up to a total dose of 20 mg	PSVT; A. fib. or flutter

A. fib.= atrial fibrillation; A. flutter = atrial flutter; AV = atrioventricular; IV = intravenously; IVP = intravenous push; LVEF = left ventricular ejection fraction; MI = myocardial infarction; NS = normal saline; prn = as needed; PSVT = paroxysmal supraventricular tachycardia; SVT = supraventricular tachycardia; USA = unstable angina; VF = ventricular fibrillation; VT = ventricular tachycardia.

sidered, because metabolic derangements and the concomitant use of, or exposure to, other proarrhythmic agents confer increased susceptibility to proarrhythmic side effects in cancer patients.

Supraventricular tachycardia is the most common arrhythmia in cancer patients. In these patients, sustained supraventricular arrhythmia is often difficult to terminate with drug therapy. Pharmacologic agents are used to regulate or terminate the abnormal heart rhythm, but elective, synchronized cardioversion under conscious sedation should be considered early and planned appropriately. The initial energy level recommended by the American Heart Association for cardioversion is 100 joules, but that level may not be high enough to convert atrial fibrillation. Others have recommended an initial shock with an energy level of 200 joules for conversion of atrial fibrillation.[38] Higher energy levels are appropriate when cancer patients have concomitant effusions or are significantly overweight. Lower initial energy levels (ie, 50 to 100 joules) should be used to convert atrial flutter.

If sinus rhythm can be restored within 48 hours of the onset of supraventricular tachycardia, anticoagulation therapy may be avoided. However, the time of onset of the arrhythmia is not always clear, and the time of discovery of the arrhythmia cannot be presumed to be synchronous with the time of onset. In the absence of clear evidence as to the time of arrhythmia onset, anticoagulation therapy should be administered before cardioversion. Some authorities are using transesophageal echocardiography to exclude the presence of intracardiac thrombi before elective synchronized cardioversion.

Arrhythmias that originate from structural cardiac abnormalities are much more difficult to control than are arrhythmias arising from metabolic causes, and this situation is especially true in cancer patients. Arrhythmias related to structural abnormalities are likely to persist over long periods and to progress to higher-grade life-threatening arrhythmias. In the emergency setting, the therapeutic goals are stabilization of hemodynamic status and respiratory status, discovery of correctable pathologic conditions, and control of symptoms. Depending on the cause of the arrhythmia, emergent consultation with cardiologists and emergent diagnostic or interventional procedures may be required.

Patients with unstable arrhythmia should be treated with aggressive pharmacologic or electrical interventions that generally follow established algorithms or guidelines such as those recommended by the American Heart Association.[39] These interventions include administration of a vasopressor such as vasopressin or epinephrine to support blood pressure (if required); administration of antiarrhythmic drugs such as amiodarone, lidocaine, and procainamide; electrical cardioversion or defibrillation; airway management; ventilation with oxygen; administration of intravenous fluid; and chest compression (if required). Emergency treatment of torsades de pointes varies from the standard algorithms for other types of ventricular tachycardia: It entails expedient use of intravenous magnesium, electrical overdrive pacing or pharmacologic overdrive with isoproterenol, and administration of phenytoin or lidocaine.

Tumor Lysis Syndrome Tumor lysis syndrome (TLS) consists of severe hyperphosphatemia, hyperkalemia, hyperuricemia, azotemia, hypocalcemia, and metabolic acidosis (out of proportion to the degree of renal insufficiency) because of massive release of cell contents and degradation products of dead tumor cells into the bloodstream. Acute TLS is caused by the death of a large number of neoplastic cells.[40]

TLS usually occurs less than 72 hours after chemotherapy in patients with leukemia and lymphoma; however, new therapeutic regimens and methods may alter the time of onset of TLS. More effective new treatments have caused TLS in patients with chronic lymphocytic leukemia, which is an indolent and chronic disease.[41] TLS also has been reported in patients with nonhematologic malignancies, including small-cell carcinomas,[42] nonsmall-cell lung cancer,[43] breast cancer,[44] and ovarian cancer.[45]

The discussion of TLS immediately follows the discussion of arrhythmia because the main acute cause of death in patients with TLS is arrhythmia secondary to the severe electrolyte abnormalities (especially hyperkalemia) and renal failure associated with the syndrome. Early recognition of metabolic abnormalities and prompt treatment can avoid fatal outcomes.

The symptoms of TLS are nonspecific. Common symptoms include nausea, vomiting, cloudy urine, weakness, fatigue, and arthralgia. Other signs and symptoms related to metabolic and electrolyte abnormalities include neuromuscular irritability, seizures, muscle weakness, and arrhythmias. Arrhythmia may cause sudden death in patients with TLS.[46] Hyperuricemia, hyperkalemia, and hypocalcemia may lead to cardiac arrhythmia, tetany, and sudden death. Precipitation of uric acid or calcium phosphate in the renal tubules may lead to acute renal failure.

Factors associated with increased risk of TLS include the type of malignancy (eg, Burkitt's lymphoma), good responsiveness of the malignancy to therapy, rapid cell turnover, and large tumor burden. Other risk factors are pre-existing renal insufficiency, acute renal failure developing shortly after the initiation of treatment, and poor response to hydration. Pretreatment lactate dehydrogenase levels, which tend to correlate with tumor bulk in patients with stage C or D lymphoma, can predict the development of post-treatment azotemia, but pretreatment hyperuricemia is not predictive.

Diagnosis of TLS requires a high level of suspicion, because there are few or no signs or symptoms in the early stages. Routine uric acid and electrolyte screening (including measurement of calcium and phosphorus levels) is indicated in patients with high tumor bulk or hematologic malignancies. TLS can occur spontaneously, but it occurs most commonly after chemotherapy (including steroid use alone in some very sensitive lymphomas[47]), immunotherapy,[41] and radiotherapy.[48] Chemotherapy agents or regimens known to be involved are fludarabine, mitoxantrone, 6-mercaptopurine, methotrexate, chemotherapeutic conditioning or total-body irradiation for bone marrow transplantation, and various combination chemotherapy regimens.

Preventive measures should be started early in patients at risk for TLS. Aggressive hydration with crystalloid fluid or normal saline up to 3 L/m^2 daily may be required to maintain a urine output of at least 100 mL/h with or without the help of loop or osmotic diuretics. The xanthine oxidase inhibitor allopurinol (100 to 300 mg orally per day) may prevent severe hyperuricemia.

Patients with severe TLS should have their hemodynamic and electrocardiographic parameters continuously monitored in an intensive care unit. The allopurinol dose may be increased up to 900 mg daily. Increased intravenous fluid hydration may be coupled with promotion of diuresis by administration of loop diuretics (eg, 20 to 200 mg furosemide, intravenously [IV] every 4 to 6 hours) and acetazolamide (250 to 500 mg IV daily). If aciduria is present, sodium bicarbonate or acetate infusion may be used to maintain urine pH between 7.1 and 7.5. Recombinant urate oxidase (uricozyme or rasburicase, an enzyme that oxidizes uric acid to allantoin), 200 μg/kg IV over 30 minutes daily, may be used to prevent or treat urate nephropathy.[49] Frequent electrolyte measurements (every 4 to 6 hours) may be required. Hyperkalemia should be treated with insulin plus dextrose, calcium, and bicarbonate infusions, along with oral potassium ion-exchange resins (sodium polystyrene sulfonate—Kayexalate [Sanofi Winthrop, USA]). In hyperphosphatemic patients with hypocalcemia, the addition of an oral calcium-based compound—for example, calcium acetate (PhosLo) or calcium carbonate—will reduce phosphate absorption and enhance calcium absorption. Intravenous calcium infusion can potentially cause calcium phosphate precipitation in the presence of severe hyperphosphatemia and should therefore be used only with caution. Dialysis may be required for patients with symptomatic hypocalcemia and a serum phosphorus level greater than 3.3 mmol/L (>10.2 mg/dL). Other indications for dialysis include persistent azotemia; persistent hyperkalemia, hyperuricemia, oliguria, or anuria despite diuretic use; refractory acidemia; and volume overload. Dialysis should be instituted promptly, with continued careful monitoring until biochemical abnormalities resolve. Hemodialysis is the most common mode of dialysis; continuous arteriovenous hemodialysis with a high dialysate flow rate and continuous venovenous hemofiltration are also effective.

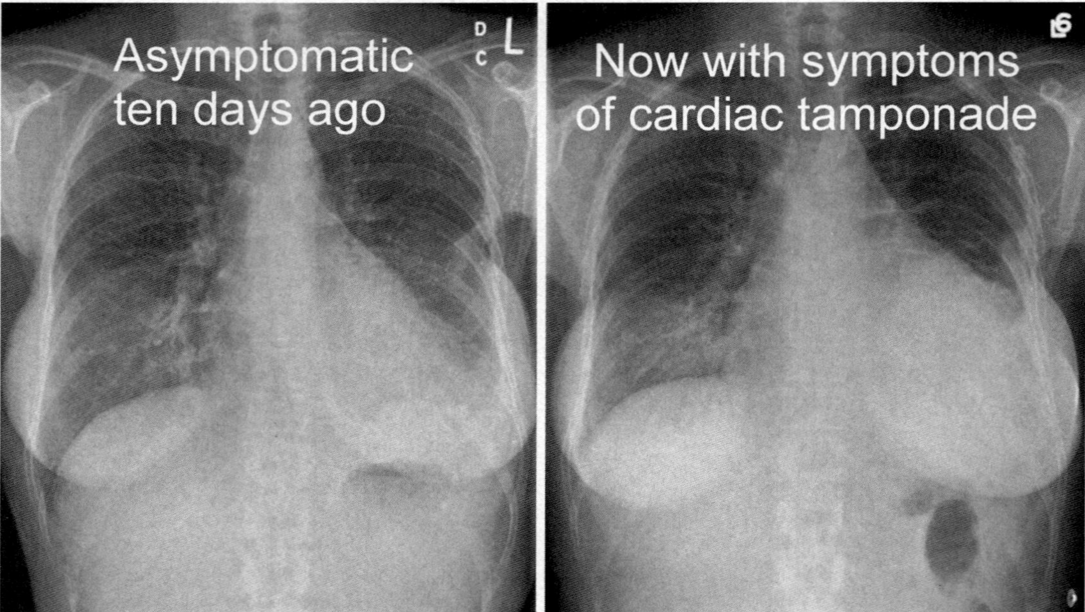

Figure 142-2 Chest radiographs of a breast cancer patient with pericardial tamponade. Widening of mediastinum and cardiac silhouette is evident when compared with an earlier chest radiograph.

Pericardial Tamponade Pericardial tamponade occurs when pericardial fluid accumulates to the point that hemodynamics are affected. Two mechanisms can lead to accumulation of excess fluid in the pericardial space in cancer patients: (1) obstruction of lymphatic drainage and (2) excess fluid secretion from tumor nodules on pericardial surfaces.

A number of tumors can lead to pericardial tamponade. Mesothelioma is the most common malignancy that arises from the pericardium. Carcinoma of the lung and malignant thymoma may involve the pericardium by direct extension. More frequently, malignancies arrive at the pericardium by retrograde lymphangitic spread or hematogenous dissemination (eg, carcinomas of the lung and breast). Malignant melanoma is the malignancy most likely to metastasize to the heart. Lymphomas (both Hodgkin's and non-Hodgkin's), leukemias, and gastrointestinal neoplasms may also cause pericardial effusions.[50]

Non-neoplastic causes of pericardial tamponade include pericardial abscess,[51] *Candida* pericarditis,[52] and complications of central venous catheterization.[53]

Although malignant pericardial effusion is occasionally the first clinical manifestation of malignancy, it is usually a late finding in patients with known metastatic disease. More than two-thirds of patients with malignant pericardial effusion are asymptomatic. In symptomatic patients, the most common complaints are shortness of breath, pleuritic chest pain, orthopnea, and general weakness. Findings on physical examination may vary from normal to hemodynamic collapse. Tachycardia, hypotension, jugular venous distention, organomegaly, and extremity edema may indicate compromised cardiac output. The classic findings of cardiac tamponade are determined by both the quantity of pericardial fluid and the rapidity of fluid accumulation. Pulsus paradoxus, an exaggeration of the usually normal decrease in systolic blood pressure with inspiration, is a classic but nonspecific finding of cardiac tamponade because it is seen also in patients with lung cancer, significant lung disease, or cor pulmonale.

Because the symptoms and physical findings associated with pericardial tamponade frequently are nonspecific, a definitive diagnosis usually requires additional testing. Electrical alternans in electrocardiographs, when present, is a very helpful finding. Plain chest radiographs may reveal widening of the mediastinum and cardiac silhouette (Figure 142-2). Computed tomography (CT) or magnetic resonance (MR) imaging studies frequently detect pericardial effusions as an incidental finding. Such studies provide information on the location (loculated or not) and size of pericar-

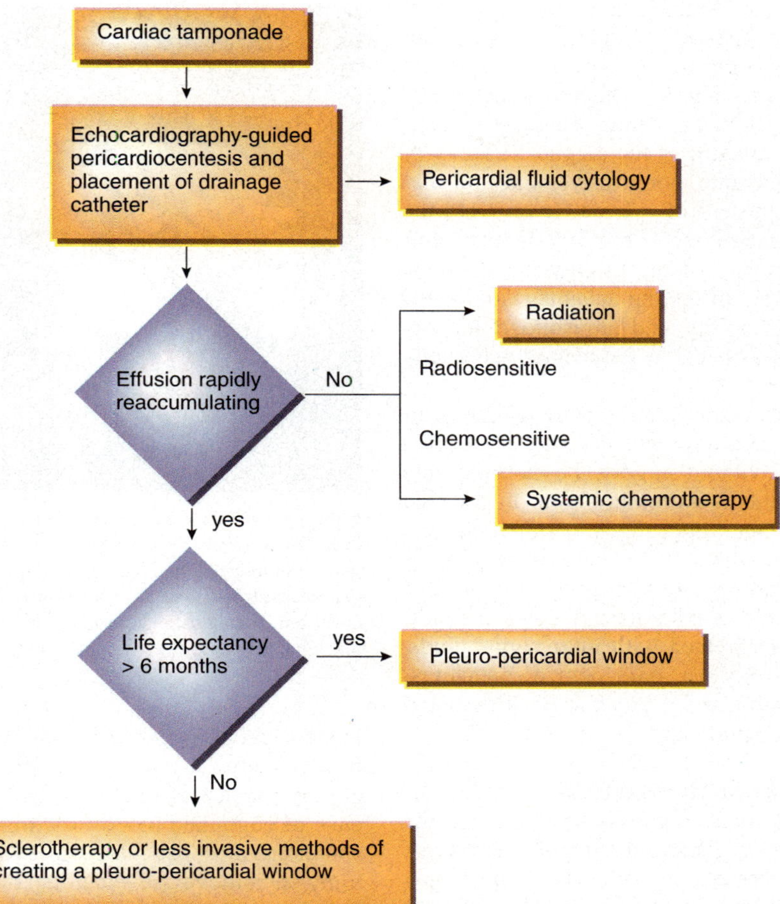

Figure 142-3 Algorithm for management of pericardial effusion.

dial effusions, but do not permit adequate assessment of their hemodynamic significance. Two-dimensional echocardiography is the most useful test for diagnosing and evaluating the hemodynamic significance of a pericardial effusion—that is, the presence or absence of cardiac tamponade. Collapse or compression of the right atrium, diastolic collapse of the right ventricle, and cardiac "rocking" (a side-to-side or front-to-back movement of the heart) are often observed in cardiac tamponade. Alterations in the respiratory variation of flow patterns across the mitral valve as measured by Doppler shift are helpful in evaluating the hemodynamic effects.

Initial management of a patient with malignant pericardial effusion depends on the patient's hemodynamic stability. Cytologic tests of pericardial fluid are positive for metastatic disease in 70% to 80% of patients with malignant pericardial effusion. In patients with hemodynamic compromise, echocardiography-guided pericardiocentesis, with placement of a drainage catheter into the pericardial space, may be performed emergently in the emergency center or intensive care unit (Figure 142-3). Complications are rare; they may include massive pericardial bleeding (when a coronary artery is damaged) and pneumothorax (especially in patients with emphysema). Pericardial fluid can be drained from the catheter, and the catheter can remain in place until less than 50 mL of fluid is drained over 24 hours. However, pericardial fluid frequently will reaccumulate after removal of the catheter.

Creation of a pleuropericardial window using one of a variety of approaches usually can avoid the need for repeated pericardiocentesis. The pleuropericardial window procedure is usually performed in an operating room, but can be performed in a hospital room or intensive care unit, using local anesthesia. A laparoscopic transdiaphragmatic approach to creating a pericardioperitoneal shunt has also been described.[54]

Long-term management of malignant pericardial effusion focuses on preventing the reaccumulation of fluid, which occurs in more than 50% of patients. Because, for most patients, long-term survival with malignant pericardial effusion is limited, an effective therapy that limits discomfort and that is not associated with excessive risk to the patient should be used. In patients with severe hemodynamic compromise and rapid fluid reaccumulation, the pleuropericardial window offers the most definitive therapy. In stable patients, systemic chemotherapy, pericardial radioactive colloid, or thoracic external-beam irradiation may be used for tumors that are still sensitive to these treatment modalities. Additional radiotherapy should be avoided in patients who have already had significant exposure of the heart to ionizing radiation. The use of local chemotherapeutic agents or agents given to sclerose the pericardium will prevent fluid reaccumulation in many patients.[55] Sclerotherapy can be very painful; adequate analgesia should be provided. The use of a percutaneous intrapericardial balloon catheter to create a pleuropericardial window has had some success,[56] but results from large series of patients treated with this modality are not yet available.

Acute Hemorrhage In cancer patients, acute hemorrhage may result from the underlying malignancy or the cancer treatment. Gastrointestinal bleeding and genitourinary bleeding are discussed in other chapters. Hemoptysis, which can rapidly compromise respiratory function, will be discussed later in the present chapter. This section covers some less-frequent serious bleeding events: carotid arterial rupture, splenic rupture, and retroperitoneal hemorrhage.

The manifestations of acute hemorrhage depend on the rate and the site of bleeding. In most cases, the site of bleeding is obvious, but sometimes bleeding can be occult. Some patients may have only nonspecific clinical manifestations related to the bleeding organ, and some patients with substantial blood loss may have only signs and symptoms of hypovolemia and hypoperfusion (eg, tachycardia, hypotension, oliguria, and depressed mental status). It may be difficult to diagnose internal bleeding. Very often, diagnostic imaging studies or procedures—for example, CT imaging, ultrasonography, arteriography, or endoscopy—are necessary to make the correct diagnosis.

The primary objectives of management of acute hemorrhage are to rapidly identify the bleeding source and to achieve hemostasis. In the acute setting, direct pressure to compress the bleeding vessel or site should be applied whenever feasible while the cardiopulmonary status is expeditiously assessed. Intravenous fluid resuscitation is vital in maintaining intravascular volume, cardiac output, and adequate vital organ perfusion. Isotonic crystalloid fluids (normal saline or lactated Ringer's solution, Plasmalyte [Baxter, USA], etc) should be used as first-line agents, because colloids (eg, hetastarch) have not been proven to improve mortality rates.[57] Coagulopathy or thrombocytopenia should be corrected immediately by transfusion of blood products. The decision to transfuse red blood cells depends on the hemodynamic stability of the patient, the persistence of hemorrhage, the estimated blood loss, and the presence of comorbid diseases (eg, coronary artery disease and cerebrovascular disease). Typed and cross-matched red blood cells are preferred, but noncross-matched type-specific blood or type O blood may have to be used in the case of massive, life-threatening hemorrhage. Specific therapeutic procedures to control bleeding, such as embolization, balloon tamponade, or surgery, should be performed in a timely manner.

Carotid Artery Rupture Most cases of carotid artery "blowout" or rupture occur in patients with head and neck cancers. Carotid artery rupture may be caused by direct tumor invasion or erosion into the carotid artery or by complications of cancer treatment—for example, post-surgical wound infection,[58] post-radiation necrosis,[59] or orocutaneous fistula.[60]

Carotid artery rupture usually occurs as a sudden and massive arterial spurting. Occasionally, ominous minor and transient bleeding episodes—so-called sentinel bleeds—herald the massive blowout. In some cases, bleeding through a fistula into the esophagus or trachea may manifest as massive hematemesis or hemoptysis. Without prompt management, the patient's condition will rapidly deteriorate to hypotension, hypovolemic shock, loss of consciousness, and death.

Hemostasis is of utmost importance. Because neck vessels are accessible to direct manual compression, continuous firm compression should be applied at the site of the carotid artery rupture until the patient arrives at the operating room for surgical treatment. Crystalloid intravenous fluid resuscitation, prompt transfusion of blood products, and administration of vasopressors should be performed to maintain perfusion of vital organs. Only very rarely does the bleeding stop spontaneously. Carotid artery rupture almost always requires surgical treatment. However, surgical ligation of the bleeding carotid artery is associated with high morbidity (25% of patients have neurologic sequelae) and high mortality (40%).[60] Intraluminal balloon occlusion with an intravascular catheter has been successful in controlling carotid bleeding in selected patients who are stable enough to undergo angiography.[61]

Splenic Rupture The spleen is a fragile intra-abdominal organ, vulnerable to rupture. In most cases, splenic rupture is the result of trauma. Spontaneous splenic rupture is often associated with development of splenomegaly secondary to malaria and infectious mononucleosis. Although the spleen is commonly involved in hematologic malignancies (leukemia and lymphoma), spontaneous splenic rupture is relatively rare in patients with those malignancies, and most cases have been reported in adults. Acute leukemia, non-Hodgkin's lymphoma, and chronic myelogenous leukemia are the most common malignancies associated with spontaneous splenic rupture. Other associated hematologic malignancies include hairy cell leukemia[62] and Hodgkin's lymphoma.[63] In patients with solid tumors such as gastric cancer,[64] prostate cancer,[65] and lung cancer,[66] metastases to the spleen can also cause rupture.

The mechanism of spontaneous splenic rupture is not clear. Minor trauma to the spleen may contribute in some cases. Other factors that may contribute include splenomegaly, infiltration of the splenic capsule by malignant cells, splenic infarction, thrombocytopenia, coagulopathy, anticoagulation therapy, and disseminated intravascular coagulation.

The typical clinical presentation of splenic rupture involves pain in the left shoulder or abdomen (left upper quadrant), tachycardia, and hypotension. The severity of the signs and symptoms may depend on the extent of bleeding. Definitive diagnosis of splenic rupture relies on imaging studies. Abdominal radiographs may reveal signs suggestive of splenic rupture, but these signs are neither sensitive nor specific enough to be very helpful. Diagnostic peritoneal lavage is rarely used in nontrauma cases. Contrast-enhanced CT imaging is the diagnostic study of choice. It is accurate, noninvasive, and informative about the extent of splenic rupture and the severity of intraperitoneal or retroperitoneal hemorrhage. Using ultrasonography to diagnose splenic rupture[67] offers the advantages of availability and portability, and ultrasonography can be performed at bedside for hemodynamically unstable patients.

For patients with splenic rupture and hematologic malignancies, prompt splenectomy is necessary, because, without surgery, the mortality rate for such patients is extremely high. In selected patients with contraindications to surgery, selective arterial embolization or external-beam irradiation of the rupture site may provide control of bleeding.[68] Patients who are not surgical candidates should be treated with intravenous fluids, supplemental oxygen, pain control measures, blood transfusion, and correction of thrombocytopenia and coagulopathy.

Retroperitoneal Hemorrhage Any damage to retroperitoneal organs or structures (ie, the kidneys, adrenal glands, duodenum, pancreas, major blood vessels, muscles, or bones) may cause retroperitoneal hemorrhage. Malignancies rarely cause spontaneous retroperitoneal hemorrhage. In the rare cases that are caused by malignancy, the culprit is usually renal-cell carcinoma (primary or metastatic)[69] or an adrenal-gland tumor.[70] Anticoagulation therapy, thrombocytopenia, and coagulopathy are predisposing factors for spontaneous retroperitoneal hemorrhage. Retroperitoneal or intraperitoneal invasive procedures and placement of a central venous catheter through a femoral vessel can also cause severe retroperitoneal hemorrhage.

Retroperitoneal hemorrhage causes nonspecific signs and symptoms that may vary according to the rate of bleeding and the underlying disease. Patients may present with abdominal pain, a tender mass in the flank, tachycardia, and hypotension. Some may have hematuria or hematochezia if the blood somehow finds its way into the ureter or gastrointestinal tract. It is difficult to establish a diagnosis of retroperitoneal hemorrhage on the basis of clinical findings. Maintaining a high level of clinical suspicion and performing early imaging studies are keys to the successful treatment of retroperitoneal hemorrhage. CT imaging of the abdomen and pelvis is the noninvasive study most commonly used to diagnose retroperitoneal bleeding (Figure 142-4). Ultrasonography performed at the bedside may be useful to rapidly diagnose retroperitoneal bleeding.

The management of retroperitoneal hemorrhage depends on the severity of bleeding and the underlying cause. Stabilizing treatments for acute hemorrhage—such as intravenous fluid resuscitation, blood transfusion, and correction of coagulopathy and thrombocytopenia—should be started immediately. The patient should be monitored closely for hemodynamic stability and the presence of continued blood loss. In life-threatening situations, most patients require emergent laparotomy to remove the bleeding tumor or organ. Renal-cell carcinomas are often hypervascular, and selective arterial embolization may control the bleeding of a renal lesion. External-beam radiation treatment of the bleeding tumor may be an option in hemodynamically stable patients with subacute bleeding and a relatively stable hematocrit.[71]

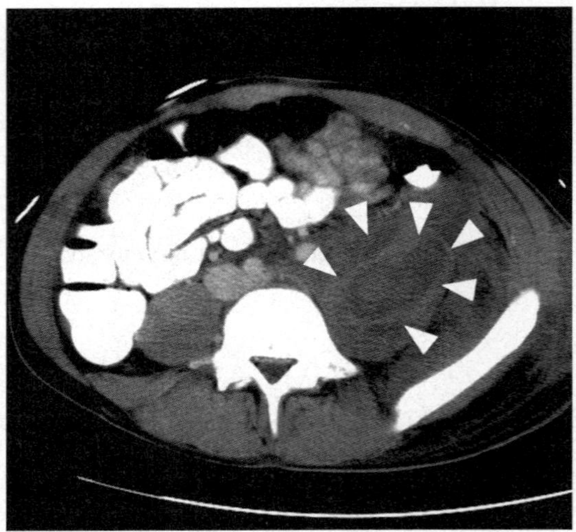

Figure 142-4 Retroperitoneal bleeding. This computed tomography scan of the abdomen and pelvis of a patient with thrombocytopenic leukemia showed a large inhomogeneous retroperitoneal collection (*white arrowheads*) consistent with a hematoma in the left psoas muscle displacing bowel loops to the right.

Superior Vena Cava Syndrome Superior vena cava (SVC) syndrome refers to a constellation of signs and symptoms resulting from partial or complete obstruction of blood flow through the SVC to the right atrium. The obstruction may be caused by compression, invasion, thrombosis, or fibrosis of the vessel. Although SVC syndrome is traditionally considered a medical emergency and continues to be discussed as such, it is also well recognized that SVC syndrome rarely causes immediate, life-threatening complications.

Lung cancer is the leading cause of SVC syndrome; non-Hodgkin's lymphoma is the second most common cause.[72] Although Hodgkin's lymphoma commonly involves the mediastinum, it rarely causes SVC syndrome. Primary mediastinal malignancies such as thymoma and germ-cell tumors account for fewer than 2% of cases of SVC syndrome. Breast cancer is the most common metastatic disease that causes SVC syndrome.[73] Other metastatic cancers that may cause SVC syndrome include gastrointestinal adenocarcinomas, prostate adenocarcinomas, sarcomas, and melanomas. Nonmalignant causes of SVC syndrome include retrosternal goiter, pyogenic infections, sarcoidosis, teratoma, pleural calcification, silicosis, post-radiation fibrosis, chemotherapy-induced fibrosis, constrictive pericarditis, and idiopathic mediastinal fibrosis.[72] An increasing cause of SVC syndrome in cancer patients is central venous catheter–induced thrombosis.

Obstruction of the SVC causes a rise in venous pressure in the SVC. Collateral venous circulation often flows through the azygos venous system. Obstruction below or at the entrance to the azygos veins forces blood to travel in the opposite direction down the azygos and chest wall veins to reach the inferior vena cava. Sudden obstruction of the SVC (which is rare) is a true emergency, because the rapid elevation of pressure in the SVC causes increased intracranial pressure, resulting in cerebral edema, intracranial thrombosis or bleeding, and death. However, SVC syndrome most often develops insidiously over a few weeks.

Common symptoms of SVC syndrome are a sensation of fullness and pressure in the head, cough, dyspnea, chest pain, and dysphagia. More significant symptoms include visual disturbances, hoarseness, stupor, seizure, and syncope. Typical signs include venous distention of the neck and chest wall, nonpitting edema of the neck, facial edema, facial plethora, tongue edema, proptosis, retinal vessel dilatation, stridor, and upper-extremity edema. The signs and symptoms are exacerbated by lowering the upper body relative to the heart (ie, bending forward, stooping, or lying down).

CT, especially contrast-enhanced spiral CT, is the most useful radiographic study for diagnosing SVC obstruction. CT imaging is able not only to reveal the site of obstruction and collateral flow, but also to differentiate extrinsic compression of SVC by tumor from intravascular thrombus formation. More importantly, CT imaging provides detailed information about the tumor mass and its relationship to mediastinal structures, helping to guide a fine-needle aspiration biopsy or other diagnostic procedure if a histologic diagnosis has not previously been established. Other critical structures, such as the bronchi and the spinal cord, are also visualized on a CT scan, and CT imaging can exclude other emergent complications—such as proximal airway obstruction and pericardial effusion—that frequently coexist with SVC obstruction. Radionuclide venograms are useful for identifying the site of obstruction and visualizing the collateral circulation. MR imaging may be used instead of CT imaging if intravenous iodine contrast is contraindicated. Three-dimensional contrast-enhanced MR venography may be superior to CT imaging, digital subtraction angiography, and Doppler ultrasonography in detecting and determining the extent of thrombo-occlusive disease in chest vessels.[74] Contrast angiography (with or without digital subtraction) for diagnosis of SVC syndrome is controversial and rarely indicated.

The method for establishing the histologic diagnosis of the malignancy may depend on the working diagnosis, location of the tumor, physical status of the patient, comorbid conditions, and available expertise of the health care facility. Percutaneous transthoracic biopsy with CT guidance is an effective and safe alternative to surgical biopsy by thoracotomy or mediastinoscopy. Percutaneous transthoracic biopsy provides a high diagnostic yield with low morbidity and mortality.[75] Bronchoscopy is another procedure commonly performed to diagnose the malignancy causing SVC syndrome. Bronchoscopy provides the diagnosis in up to 50% of patients with SVC syndrome and in most patients with SVC syndrome caused by small-cell lung cancer. If accessible lymph nodes are present, excisional lymph node biopsy can, in most cases, help to establish the diagnosis with minimal morbidity. Excisional biopsy is preferred over fine-needle aspiration if lymphoma is suspected, because the histologic classification of lymphoma is firmly based on lymph-node architecture. Needle aspiration can reveal only the cytologic features of the neoplastic cells.

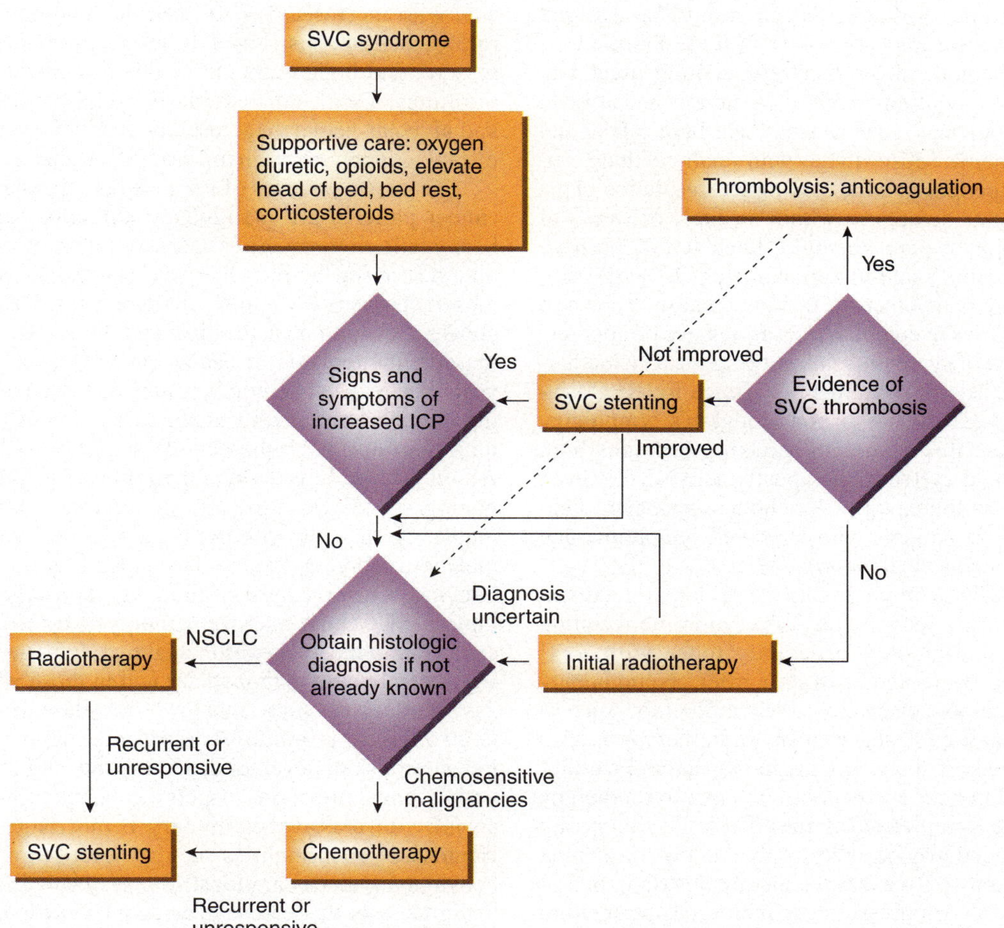

Figure 142-5 Algorithm for management of superior vena cava (SVC) syndrome. ICP = increased intracranial pressure; NSCLC = nonsmall-cell lung cancer.

More than 50% of patients with SVC syndrome become symptomatic before the primary diagnosis of malignancy is made. In management of SVC syndrome, the emphasis has shifted from empirical radiotherapy to methodical diagnostic evaluation, because emergent irradiation before biopsy may preclude proper interpretation of the biopsy specimen in 50% of cases (Figure 142-5).

The prognosis of patients with SVC syndrome primarily reflects the prognosis associated with the underlying disease. The common malignant causes of SVC syndrome, such as small-cell lung cancer and lymphoma, are chemosensitive and potentially curable even in the presence of SVC syndrome. The exception is that in rare emergent situations of impending airway obstruction or increased intracranial pressure, empiric radiotherapy or intravascular SVC stenting should be employed immediately. Supplemental oxygen, bed rest with upper body elevation, and sedation may help to lessen the symptoms by lowering venous pressure and cardiac output. The use of diuretics may transiently reduce edema, but the efficacy of diuretics has not been proven, and overdiuresis causes dehydration, which should be avoided to minimize the risk of thrombosis. Corticosteroids (eg, dexamethasone) may be useful in the presence of airway compromise or increased intracranial pressure.

Anticoagulation therapy in SVC syndrome is controversial despite the presence of superimposed thrombosis in up to 50% of patients. Anticoagulation and thrombolysis may be beneficial in certain situations, such as indwelling catheter–induced thrombosis or propagation of the thrombus into the brachiocephalic or subclavicular system. However, anticoagulation increases the risk of intracranial bleeding, especially when intracranial pressure is elevated, and anticoagulation may complicate or delay biopsy procedures for histologic diagnosis of the malignancy causing the syndrome. Anticoagulation should be avoided until a clear indication for its use is identified.

Chemotherapy is the preferred initial treatment of SVC syndrome caused by tumors sensitive to chemotherapy, such as small-cell lung cancer and lymphoma. Most patients with small-cell lung cancer experience partial or complete resolution of the signs and symptoms within a couple of weeks of initiation of chemotherapy. Although SVC obstruction occurs again in approximately 25% of cases, salvage chemotherapy or radiotherapy or the two modalities in combination can achieve prompt resolution of symptoms in most patients. Chemotherapy is also the treatment of choice for SVC syndrome secondary to non-Hodgkin's lymphoma, because this treatment modality provides both local and systemic therapeutic activity. However, local consolidation with radiotherapy may be beneficial in patients with large-cell lymphoma and large mediastinal masses.

Radiotherapy remains the principal treatment for many patients with SVC syndrome resulting from malignancy, especially those with SVC caused by recurrent disease after chemotherapy or by tumors insensitive to chemotherapy, such as nonsmall-cell lung cancer. Radiotherapy is also justified if a histologic diagnosis cannot be established in a timely manner. Emergent radiotherapy before completion of the histologic diagnostic evaluation may be indicated in rare, life-threatening situations—for example, airway obstruction, spinal cord compression, or increased intracranial pressure.[72] In general, external-beam radiotherapy for SVC syndrome is well tolerated, and most patients achieve relief of symptoms about 1 to 3 weeks after the beginning of radiotherapy.

SVC stenting provides rapid symptomatic relief within a couple of days in most patients; it also improves quality of life. In cancer patients with SVC syndrome, stents usually remain patent for the rest of the patient's life.[76] SVC stenting may provide relief of severe symptoms for patients while a histologic diagnosis of the malignancy causing the SVC obstruction is being actively pursued. Stenting may also be indicated in patients in whom radiation or chemotherapy has not yet taken effect or in whom those modalities have failed. Some authors recommend stenting as first-line treatment to be performed early in the treatment of SVC syndrome.[77]

RESPIRATORY ONCOLOGIC EMERGENCIES

MASSIVE HEMOPTYSIS Approximately 5% of hemoptysis episodes are considered massive. The definition of massive hemoptysis ranges from the expectoration of 100 mL of blood in a single episode to the expectoration of more than 600 mL of blood in 24 hours.[78,79] Airway bleeding leading to life-threatening airway obstruction, hypotension, aspiration, or anemia are also considered massive hemoptysis. Fatal hemorrhage occurs in about one-third of patients with massive hemoptysis.[80] The higher the amount of blood expectorated, the higher the risk of death.[80] Other factors associated with increased risk of death include higher rate of hemoptysis, lower baseline pulmonary reserve, and higher amount of blood retained in the lungs. Death attributable to endobronchial and alveolar hemorrhage usually occurs because of asphyxiation rather than exsanguination.

The primary causes of massive hemoptysis in cancer patients are malignancy, infection, and hemostatic abnormalities. Massive hemoptysis may be caused by bronchogenic carcinoma and lung metastases from other malignancies. Bronchogenic carcinoma is the most common cause of massive hemoptysis in cancer patients over 40 years of age. Fatal hemoptysis may be more common in necrotic squamous-cell carcinoma of the lung than in other subtypes of lung cancer.[80,81] About 3% of lung cancer patients have fatal hemoptysis.[81] Hemoptysis secondary to lung metastasis is most commonly associated with melanoma, breast, kidney, laryngeal, and colon cancers. Other tumors, such as esophageal tumors, may cause massive hemoptysis by direct extension to the tracheobronchial tree. In patients with hematologic malignancies and in those who have undergone bone-marrow transplantation, neutropenia or immunocompromise leads to increased risk of developing necrotizing, angioinvasive fungal infections (aspergillosis, mucormycosis) with massive pulmonary hemorrhage.[80] Hemostatic abnormalities such as severe thrombocytopenia and coagulopathy may result from malignancy or its treatments and contribute to the severity of pulmonary hemorrhage. Another factor that can contribute to massive pulmonary hemorrhage in cancer patients is lung injury from radiation or chemotherapeutic agents.

In addition to massive hemoptysis, the patient's symptoms may include hypotension, tachycardia, central cyanosis, clammy skin, dyspnea, or chest pain. The severity of the clinical presentation depends on several factors—namely, the rate and duration of the bleeding, the degree of airway obstruction and pulmonary involvement, the patient's underlying performance status, and the status of chronic comorbid conditions. The airway should be protected. Intubation is recommended in patients with rapid bleeding, hemodynamic instability, ventilatory impairment, severe dyspnea, or hypoxia.[78] Patients with hemodynamic instability may require volume resuscitation, administration of supplemental oxygen, correction of underlying coagulopathies, and cough suppressants. For patients bleeding from one lung, lateral decubitus positioning with the affected lung in the dependent position may help to minimize aspiration to the unaffected side.

In the management of massive hemoptysis, the site of bleeding must be first identified. For unstable patients, unilateral intubation via the bronchoscope is performed.[82] For massive right-sided pulmonary bleeding, the left mainstem bronchus is intubated over the bronchoscope.[83] Unilateral intubation of the right lung in patients with massive left-sided bleeding is not recommended because of the risk of right upper lobe occlusion. In this scenario, an alternative is to use a double-lumen endotracheal tube to isolate the unaffected lung.

Bronchoscopic treatments for massive hemoptysis include administration of topical agents (thrombin, fibrinogen–thrombin), iced saline lavage, endobronchial tamponade, laser photocoagulation, and electrocautery.[84–87] A balloon catheter may be used for endobronchial tamponade to alleviate bleeding. Rigid bronchoscopes offer both improved airway control and greater ability to suction; they are also more effective in removing large clots than are fiberoptic scopes. The advantage of fiberoptic scopes is improved access to, and visualization of, the distal airways. Laser photocoagulation and electrocautery have also been used to manage massive hemoptysis, with variable results. Neodymium-yttrium-garnet laser (Nd:YAG) phototherapy has been used for both palliative and curative treatment in patients with endobronchial tumors.[85,86] Argon plasma coagulation, a noncontact form of electrocoagulation, may be used for both palliative and curative treatment of hemoptysis secondary to proximal endobronchial lesions.

In the case of massive hemoptysis secondary to hemorrhage from the bronchial circulation, selective angiography is diagnostic in most patients. Embolization of the bleeding vessel may be performed with polyvinyl alcohol foam, Gianturco steel coils, isobutyl-2-cyanoacrylate, or absorbable gelatin pledgets.[88] Patients in whom embolization fails may benefit from radiotherapy.[89] Radiotherapy inhibits bleeding by causing vascular thrombosis and necrosis of contributing vessels. Surgical treatment is generally used in patients with refractory hemoptysis, in whom other treatment modalities have failed, and in patients with life-threatening cardiovascular compromise.[90]

MASSIVE PLEURAL EFFUSION Massive pleural effusions are described as those causing near-complete opacification of the hemithorax. Massive pleural effusions account for approximately 10% of effusions. About two-thirds of affected patients have underlying cancer.[91] Most patients with malignant pleural effusion have moderate- to large-volume effusions (500 to 2000 mL, Figure 142-6).

Most malignant pleural effusions (approximately 80% overall) are attributable to lung carcinoma (36%), breast carcinoma (25%), lymphoma (10%), and ovarian carcinoma (5%).[92] Adenocarcinoma accounts for 79% of cases of lung carcinoma that metastasize to the pleura.[93] In young adults, lymphoma is the most common cause of malignant pleural effusions.[93] After pneumonia, malignancy is the second leading cause of exudative pleural effusions, and malignancy is the cause of 8% to 20% of transudative pleural effusions.[94]

Conditions related to malignancy may also cause effusions; these conditions include local tumor effects (hilar and mediastinal lymphadenopathy causing impaired lymphatic drainage from the pleural space), systemic tumor effects, hypoalbuminemia, complications of cancer treatment (radiotherapy[95] and chemotherapy[96]—with,

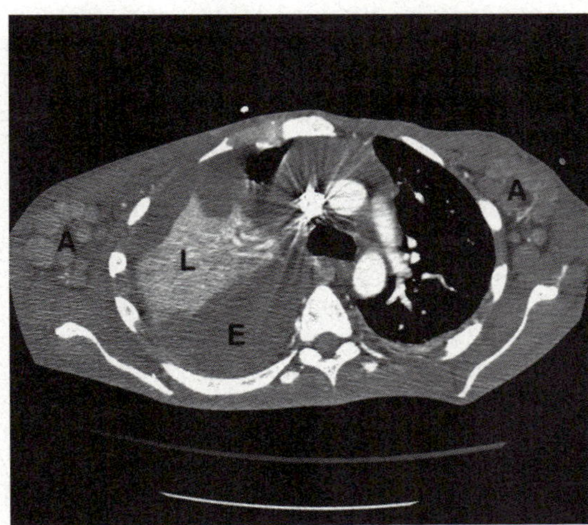

Figure 142-6 Massive pleural effusion. A computed tomography scan of the chest of a patient with a massive pleural effusion is shown. L = collapsed lung; E = pleural effusion; A = extensive axillary lymphadenopathy.

for example, methotrexate, procarbazine, cyclophosphamide, mitomycin, bleomycin, and interleukin-1), pneumonia (eg, postobstructive pneumonia), and congestive heart failure.

Malignant effusions may appear serous, serosanguinous, or bloody. In one-fourth of patients, the malignant pleural effusion causes no specific complaints or symptoms. However, these patients often have advanced cancer associated with substantial weight loss and debility. For some patients, pleural effusion may be the presenting sign of the malignancy. Common symptoms are cough, dyspnea, and orthopnea. The presence and severity of these symptoms depend on the volume and rapidity of the fluid accumulation. Fever is occasionally present and may result from atelectasis, infection, or pneumonia. Pleuritic chest pain and pleural friction rubs are not common; when present, they indicate extensive neoplastic involvement of the pleura, rib cage, and chest wall.

The presence of a pleural effusion is diagnosed by clinical examination and confirmed using radiography. On examination, patients with pleural effusion exhibit dullness to percussion, decreased breath sounds in the area of the effusion, and decreased diaphragmatic excursion and tactile and vocal fremitus on the affected side. Sometimes crackles may be auscultated immediately above the percussed dullness. Patients with large-volume effusions (>1500 mL) may have an inspiratory lag, contralateral tracheal deviation, and intercostal fullness. When the pleural effusion is caused by lung carcinoma, the effusion is generally on the same side as the primary lesion.[91]

The cause of a pleural effusion is generally diagnosed by thoracentesis.[97] Thoracentesis, generally a safe procedure, is easily performed. For symptomatic patients, partial removal of the effusion may alleviate symptoms. Fluid analysis discriminates between exudative and transudative effusions and may be helpful in identifying the cause of the effusion.[98] Cytology is more sensitive than percutaneous pleural biopsy.[93,99] If these two less-invasive procedures are nondiagnostic, other options for obtaining diagnostic material include bronchoscopy, pleuroscopy, video-assisted thoracoscopic surgery, and open pleural biopsy.

Treatment decisions are influenced by the severity of the symptoms, the rate of fluid accumulation, the overall prognosis, the patient's performance status, and the responsiveness of the malignancy to treatment. Patients with massive pleural effusion and hemodynamic instability, significant dyspnea, hypoxemia, or mediastinal shift should be treated emergently by thoracentesis. Thoracostomy may be indicated depending on the clinical and radiographic findings and the biochemical characteristics of the effusion.[100] Tube thoracostomy is recommended for patients with empyema or infected pleural fluid as confirmed by culture or microscopy (eg, Gram stain) and for patients with complicated parapneumonic effusions. Patients in whom thoracoscopic treatment fails and patients with chronic complicated parapneumonic effusions should be considered for open thoracotomy and decortication.

Pleurodesis may prevent effusions from recurring. In approximately 70% of patients with drainage of symptomatic malignant pleural effusion without pleurodesis, fluid reaccumulates within 30 days unless effective systemic chemotherapy is administered. Talc, tetracyclines, bleomycin, mechlorethamine (nitrogen mustard), minocycline, and 5-fluorouracil have all been used as sclerosing agents. Doxycycline, minocycline, bleomycin, and talc are the most effective agents, with success rates of 72% to 90%.[101,102] Pleurodesis should be considered in patients with symptomatic relief after thoracentesis. Life expectancy of more than several months should also be considered in deciding whether pleurodesis should be performed. Alternatives for patients with poor life expectancy may include repeated thoracentesis or placement of a chronic indwelling catheter (Denver catheter).[103]

Acute Airway Obstruction Acute airway obstruction usually involves the upper airway. Upper airway obstruction may result from malignant or nonmalignant causes. Tumors that can obstruct the upper airway by direct extension are primary tumors of the head and neck (base of tongue, larynx, hypopharynx, thyroid, or trachea) and lung. Tumors that can obstruct the upper airway by metastatic spread are tumors of the breast, esophagus, kidney, and colon; melanoma; sarcoma; and mediastinal lymphoma. Airway obstruction may also be caused by tumor encroachment and by tumor-associated airway edema or hemorrhage. Nonmalignant causes of airway obstruction in cancer patients include food or foreign body aspiration (Figure 142-7), airway edema, severe tracheomalacia, tracheal stenosis or stricture, and, rarely, infectious causes—fungal, viral, or bacterial. Severe acute upper airway obstruction can be caused by angioedema, an infrequent (affecting 2% to 3% of patients) side effect of paclitaxel administration.[104]

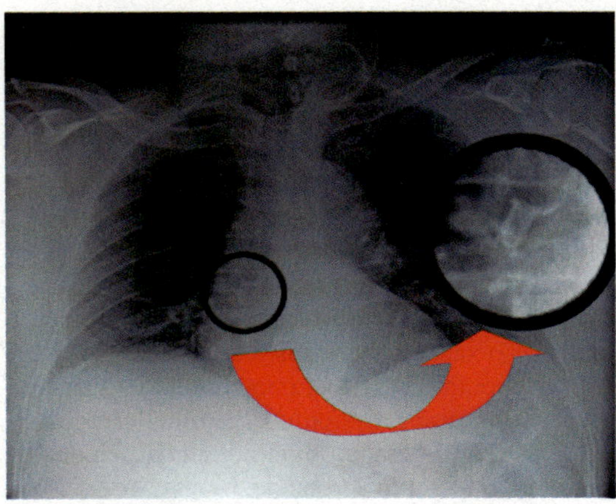

Figure 142-7 Foreign body in right mainstem bronchus. This patient underwent a laryngectomy for laryngeal cancer. He presented with a complaint of shortness of breath after his voice prosthesis fell inside his tracheal stoma. The prosthesis (*circled*) can be seen lodged in the right mainstem bronchus on this chest radiograph.

The most common cause of lower airway obstruction is primary bronchogenic carcinoma. Other, rare, causes of lower airway obstruction are metastases from cancers of the colon, breast, thyroid, and kidney; melanoma; lymphoma; and sarcoma. Patients with primary carcinoid tumors of the gastrointestinal tract may experience severe airway obstruction (bronchospasm) because of the release of hormone mediators.

Dyspnea may be the only early symptom of airway obstruction. When dyspnea occurs with exertion, the airway diameter is usually reduced to 8 mm; when dyspnea occurs while the patient is at rest, the airway diameter is usually reduced to 5 mm—a decrease that often coincides with the development of stridor. As upper airway obstruction progresses, wheezing, orthopnea, tachycardia, diaphoresis, stridor, and intracostal muscle retraction may be noted. Stridor is an ominous finding that may be rapidly followed by bradycardia, cyanosis, obtundation, and death.

For patients with upper airway obstruction, the clinical examination is often accompanied by direct visualization using either laryngoscopy or bronchoscopy depending on the location of the lesion. Biopsy may be required. For patients with lower airway obstruction, chest radiographs identify the obstruction in 75% of cases. Bronchoscopy or fine-needle aspiration may be considered.

The oral cavity should be quickly visualized to exclude foreign body aspiration. In most cases of upper airway obstruction, the clinical examination provides the diagnosis. Laryngoscopy or bronchoscopy may be necessary to guide the endotracheal tube. Patients with obstructions involving the upper third of the trachea may require a low tracheotomy. Other supportive therapies involve administration of corticosteroids, bronchodilators, and helium–oxygen mixtures. Other surgical interventions may be considered. They often depend on the extent of the disease, the responsiveness of the malignancy to treatment, the patient's performance status, and comorbid conditions. For central airway obstruction, interventional pulmonary treatments may use rigid or flexible bronchoscopes and may include balloon bronchoplasty,[105] placement of tracheobronchial stents,[87,106] laser bronchoscopy,[87] endobronchial argon plasma coagulation,[107] cryosurgery,[108] and brachytherapy.[109]

Pneumothorax Pneumothorax (air in the pleural space) occurs frequently in cancer patients. Most pneumothoraces in cancer patients are iatrogenic or occur spontaneously as a result of other medical conditions. Most pneumothoraces treated in hospitals are iatrogenic.[110] Procedures often associated with pneumothorax include percutaneous lung biopsy, transbronchial biopsy, insertion of central venous lines, and insertion of pulmonary artery catheters. Even nasogastric tube placement may occasionally cause pneumothorax. Secondary spontaneous pneumothorax is most commonly attributable to chronic obstructive pulmonary disease. Primary and metastatic pulmonary neoplasms may both result in pneumothorax. Chemotherapeutic agents associated with pneumothorax include bleomycin,[111] carmustine,[112] and lomustine. Infectious agents associated with pneumothorax include *Staphylococcus*, *Klebsiella*, and *Pseudomonas* species; *Pneumocystis carinii*; and *Mycobacterium* species. Rupture of mycetoma into the pleural space may result in pneumothorax and is associated with *Aspergillus fumigatus* infection, coccidioidomycosis, cryptococcosis, and mucormycosis.

The presence and severity of symptoms is related to the patient's underlying pulmonary status. Patients may present with respiratory distress, tachypnea, tachycardia, cyanosis, diaphoresis, and agitation. Patients with underlying lung disease are often unable to tolerate reductions in vital capacity or arterial PO_2 and are at higher risk for developing respiratory failure secondary to pneumothorax.

Dyspnea is often unrelated to the volume of the pneumothorax; however, dyspnea and chest pain are present in almost all patients with a significant pneumothorax. Chest pain is frequently acute in onset, pleuritic, and located on the affected side. Cough, hemoptysis, orthopnea, and Horner's syndrome are less frequent symptoms. Examination usually demonstrates tachycardia, absent tactile fremitus, hyperresonance, and absent or decreased breath sounds on auscultation of the affected side. Small pneumothoraces (< 20%) are usually undetectable on physical examination. Patients with large or tension pneumothoraces may have contralateral deviation of the trachea, asymmetrical hyperexpansion, and decreased movement of the affected hemithorax. Patients with a tension pneumothorax may have elevated central venous, pulmonary artery, and right atrial pressures. Hypotension, severe hypoxemia and respiratory acidosis occur when increased central venous and intrapleural pressures impede venous return.

The diagnosis of pneumothorax is confirmed when an upright chest radiograph reveals a visceral pleural line with absence of lung markings beyond the line. For patients with a small pneumothorax, the pleural line may be difficult to discern. A good-quality radiograph and a bright light for viewing are therefore needed to diagnose a small pneumothorax. Previous work has shown that one-third of pneumothoraces are undetected on semi-erect and supine films.[113] In some cases, expiratory films may be helpful.

Patients with small pneumothoraces and minor symptoms may require close observation and supplemental oxygen. Serial chest radiographs should be obtained 3 to 6 hours after the initial radiograph. If no expansion of the pneumothorax is seen, the patient may be discharged from observation with appropriate follow-up instructions, including scheduling for a repeat radiograph in 12 to 48 hours.[114]

For symptomatic pneumothoraces, rapidly expanding pneumothoraces, and pneumothoraces of more than 15% of the ipsilateral pleural space, catheter aspiration should be done. Patients with pneumothoraces that fail to re-expand or that recur following a successful catheter aspiration require chest tube thoracostomy. Heimlich valves are often used for that purpose. Tube thoracostomy is indicated from the start in patients with traumatic pneumothorax and hemothorax, patients with a pneumothorax occupying more than 15% of the ipsilateral pleural space with retained secretions, patients with lung infections on the affected side, and patients on mechanical ventilation. Patients with a persistent air leak because of a bronchopleural fistula and patients with only partial lung expansion 5 to 7 days after a tube thoracostomy should be considered for thoracotomy with surgical repair. Pleurodesis with talc or other drugs may be indicated to prevent recurrence.[115]

Pulmonary Embolism Pulmonary emboli can be difficult to diagnose in cancer patients because the signs and symptoms may be masked by the neoplastic process or by complications of cancer treatments. In the general population, patients at high risk for development of deep venous thrombosis are patients with major trauma, patients undergoing orthopedic surgery, and patients undergoing abdominal surgery. The risk of pulmonary embolism is increased in patients with advanced age, recent myocardial infarction, cerebral vascular accident, immobility, malignancy, obesity, or history of thrombosis.[116] Compared with patients without malignancies, patients with cancer have greater rates of initial thrombosis, thrombosis recurrence, and fatal pulmonary embolism.[117] Patients with malignancy and no other underlying comorbid condition have a 15% to 20% risk of developing thromboembolic disease. Compared with patients without cancer undergoing similar procedures, cancer patients undergoing surgical procedures have two to three times the risk of developing postoperative venous thrombosis.[118]

When massive pulmonary embolism occurs, increase in pulmonary vascular resistance and right ventricular afterload may occur. Increasing right ventricular afterload causes an increase in right ventricular wall tension and progressive dilation of the right ventricle, leading to right ventricular failure. Cardiovascular collapse may ultimately occur owing to development of ischemia, right ventricular dysfunction, tricuspid regurgitation, and forward flow failure. As cardiac output decreases, hypoperfusion, shock, and death may occur.

In most cases, symptoms of pulmonary embolism are vague. The most common presenting symptom is dyspnea. Dyspnea, pleuritic chest pain, and tachypnea were present in 97% of patients with pulmonary embolism documented by angiography in the Prospective Investigation of Pulmonary Embolism Diagnosis study.[119,120] Patients with massive pulmonary embolism may have syncope. Angina may occur secondary to right ventricular ischemia. Hemoptysis may occur on occasion and is associated with pulmonary infarction happening 12 to 36 hours after the thromboembolic event.

Most frequently, patients with pulmonary embolism have tachypnea and tachycardia. Sometimes, fever and a pleural rub may be detected. Deep venous thrombosis in the lower extremities occurs in fewer than half of all patients with pulmonary embolism.[121] However, clinical examination of the lower extremities for evidence of thrombosis should be performed. Patients with suspected pulmonary embolism should undergo an oxygen saturation measurement and may require measurement of arterial blood gases before supplemental oxygen is provided. A chest radiograph is most helpful in excluding other causes of pulmonary symptoms. An electrocardiogram commonly shows sinus tachycardia, inverted T waves, or nonspecific ST-T–wave abnormalities. Right-axis deviation, atrial arrhythmia, right bundle branch block, and P-pulmonale may occur, but the classical S_1-Q_3-T_3 pattern is unusual.

Radionuclide ventilation-perfusion (V/Q) imaging is usually the initial test for diagnosing pulmonary embolism. Pulmonary embolism is excluded when findings of a V/Q scan are normal.[122] Unfortunately, V/Q scans are often read as "intermediate probability," and this imprecision usually necessitates further diagnostic testing. Other tests that may be used for diagnosis are spiral CT imaging (Figure 142-8), MR imaging, and pulmonary angiography. Spiral CT and MR imaging are newer diagnostic modalities and have sensitivities and specificities of about 80% and 90% respectively.[123,124] The negative predictive value of spiral CT angiography for pulmonary embolism is 98%.[125] However, these modalities will not reliably detect thromboembolism in the distal pulmonary vasculature.[126] Patients in whom pulmonary embolism is strongly suspected and for whom findings on either spiral CT or MR imaging are negative should be considered for pulmonary angiography, the "gold standard" for diagnosis.

Hemodynamically unstable patients should be stabilized. Interventions for stabilization may include administration of fluids and inotropic

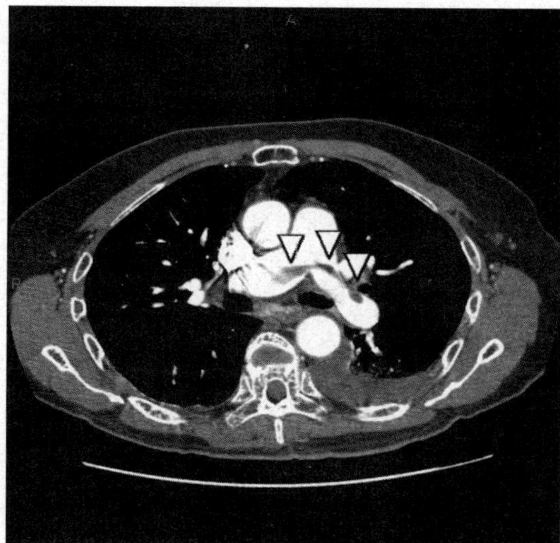

Figure 142-8 Saddle embolus. This computed tomography scan shows a saddle embolus (below the three arrowheads) at the bifurcation into the pulmonary arteries.

agents, usually guided by central venous monitoring in an intensive care setting. Oxygen administration by mask or endotracheal tube is necessary when massive pulmonary embolism occurs. In patients in whom pulmonary embolism is strongly suspected, heparin or low-molecular-weight heparin should be administered unless clinically contraindicated. When heparin is used, it is generally administered as a bolus injection of 5,000 to 10,000 U, followed by a continuous intravenous infusion of 1,000 to 1,500 U per hour with adjustments to maintain the activated partial thromboplastin time at 1.5 to 2.0 times the baseline control value.[127] Low-molecular-weight heparins may be used[128] and have the advantage of not requiring partial thromboplastin time monitoring and intravenous access. Moreover, the rate of bleeding complications with low-molecular-weight heparins is the same as or less than that seen with unfractionated heparin.[129] The goal of anticoagulation therapy is to prevent thromboembolic recurrence. For cancer patients, it is recommended that anticoagulation therapy be continued until the malignancy is no longer active,[130] and low-molecular-weight heparin may be superior to Coumadin in the prevention of recurrent venous thromboembolic events.[131]

Thrombolysis is generally considered in patients with massive pulmonary embolus and hemodynamic instability.[132] Indications for use of thrombolytics are occlusion of more than 40% of the pulmonary vasculature by the thrombus,[133] right ventricular dysfunction according to echocardiography, and severe hypoxemia.[134] Compared with heparin alone, thrombolytic agents are associated with twice the rate of major complications and intracranial hemorrhage.[135] Thrombolytic therapy has been shown to result in acceleration of fibrinolysis and clot dissolution and improvement in both early and late cardiopulmonary function; however, a definite beneficial effect on mortality has not yet been shown in large-scale studies.[136] Surgical and catheter embolectomy is reserved for patients in whom usual approaches of clot removal fail.

NEUROLOGIC ONCOLOGIC EMERGENCIES

Spinal Cord Compression Spinal cord compression occurs in 1% to 5% of cancer patients and should be considered an emergency.[137] Treatment delays may result in irreversible consequences, including paralysis. In 95% of cases, spinal cord compression is caused by extradural metastases from tumors involving the vertebral column. Of such cases, 70% involve the thoracic spine, 20% involve the lumbosacral spine, and 10% involve the cervical spine. Metastasis to the thoracic vertebrae often causes lesser symptoms than does metastasis to the lumbar or cervical vertebrae. However, thoracic spine metastasis is frequently more important because of the vulnerable blood supply in that region and the fact that the spinal canal is narrowest there. Spinal cord compression occurs more frequently in patients with lung, breast, unknown primary, prostate, and renal-cell cancer.

Back pain is the most common symptom in patients with spinal cord compression. Pain is often an early sign of spinal cord compression and may be present for months before the diagnosis. Patients may present with pain localized to the spine or radicular pain attributable to neural compression. The pain may worsen with movement, recumbency, coughing, sneezing, or straining. Pain that worsens with recumbency should increase the suspicion of epidural metastasis.

Muscle weakness follows pain and may be accompanied by sensory loss. Once symptoms of autonomic dysfunction, urinary retention, and constipation develop, spinal cord compression may result in rapid irreversible paralysis. Paralysis before treatment and urinary retention before treatment are the most significant factors associated with a poor outcome.

Tenderness and pain over the involved vertebral segments are elicited with palpation. Other clinical findings may include muscle weakness, abnormal muscle stretch reflexes and extensor plantar reflexes, and sensory loss in the distribution of the involved nerve roots. Leg ataxia may arise before muscle weakness and may occur without pain.[138] Sensory loss occurs below the involved segment. Patients with autonomic dysfunction may have a palpable bladder, an increased postvoid urinary volume, or decreased rectal tone.

An accurate history and physical examination are essential in diagnosing spinal cord compression. The neurologic examination often identifies the suspicious areas of the spine, allowing for focused imaging efforts. Patients with spinal cord compression often have abnormalities on plain radiographs of the spine. The abnormalities encountered may include bony erosion and pedicle loss, partial or complete vertebral collapse, and paraspinous soft-tissue masses. However, normal findings on spine films do not exclude epidural metastasis.

MR tomography of the spine is the best method for evaluating epidural spinal cord compression

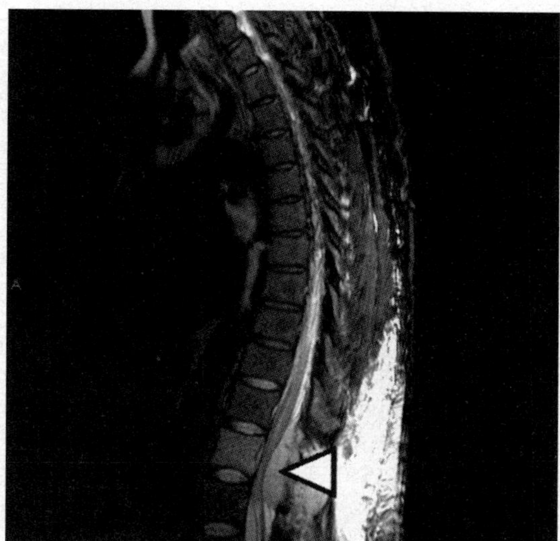

Figure 142-9 Spinal cord compression. Sagittal magnetic resonance imaging of the spine demonstrates compression of the lower portion of the spinal cord by tumor (*arrowhead*). Metastatic disease in the vertebral body is also seen.

(Figure 142-9). Gadolinium enhancement may be used when cord compression attributable to epidural abscess is suspected. Gadolinium enhances inflamed tissues and defines anatomic margins. Myelography requires an experienced physician. Myelography accompanied by CT imaging may be performed with minimum patient discomfort. However, when metastatic disease completely blocks the spinal cord, myelography does not allow definition of the upper margin of tumor involvement.

Treatment of spinal cord compression aims to maintain normal neurologic function (or, if symptoms are present, to improve neurologic function); to provide local tumor control; to stabilize the spine; and to provide appropriate pain control. Because bone is often affected and because bony metastases cause significant pain, analgesics, especially narcotics, should be administered promptly and judiciously. Appropriate physical examination and diagnostic imaging often are delayed if pain control is inadequate.

For patients with suspected spinal cord compression, corticosteroid therapy should be administered. Dexamethasone is often used because it has good gastrointestinal absorption and a 36-hour half-life. Controversy exists as to whether a high-dose (100 mg) intravenous bolus followed by maintenance doses (usually 16 mg every 6 hours) is necessary.[139] Other studies have suggested that lower doses are just as effective and cause fewer side effects.[140,141]

For most patients with spinal cord compression and a radiosensitive malignancy, radiotherapy alone is the standard initial treatment. The outcome of radiotherapy is directly related to the patient's neurologic status before treatment and the relative radiosensitivity of the malignancy.

Surgical decompression may also be an appropriate treatment option, especially in patients requiring spinal stability, in patients who have received radiotherapy in the area of the compression, when a tissue diagnosis is needed, and in patients with progression despite appropriate treatment with steroids and radiation. The status of the patient's malignancy should also be taken into account when decisions are made regarding the appropriateness of surgical decompression. Surgical decompression may not be appropriate for patients with advanced malignancy and a limited life expectancy. However, for some of those patients, surgical compression may afford an improved quality of life. Anterior vertebral body resection with stabilization may offer the best choice, but that procedure is a major surgery requiring a skilled neurosurgical team, uninvolved adjacent vertebral bodies for spinal canal stabilization, and a patient with a good performance status and acceptable operative risk.

Chemotherapy may be effective in patients with a chemosensitive malignancy. It may also be used in combination with other treatment modalities. Chemotherapy is sometimes used as a treatment alternative when other treatment choices are not appropriate. For example, chemotherapy may be administered when a patient has increased operative risk or when radiotherapy has previously been administered in the affected area.

Brain Herniation Patients with possible brain herniation should be rapidly assessed, and those with hemodynamic instability should be stabilized with appropriate therapies. Symptoms and physical findings suggestive of brain herniation include changes in the level of consciousness, papilledema, pupillary and eye movement irregularities, posturing, nausea, vomiting, and meningismus. Late clinical findings of brain herniation are hypertension, bradycardia, and the Cushing reflex. If findings are suggestive of herniation or increased intracranial pressure, imaging studies should be performed. The first study generally done is noncontrast CT imaging (to exclude hemorrhage). MR imaging is a better imaging technique when herniation is present, but if a patient is unstable, CT imaging may offer a safer venue until the patient is stabilized. In addition, CT imaging can be performed quickly.

If clinical findings suggest increased intracranial pressure and if the patient is unstable, treatment to reduce intracranial pressure should be instituted immediately, even before brain herniation is documented by imaging studies. Emergency treatments to ameliorate or prevent herniation are hyperventilation and administration of mannitol and steroids.

Hyperventilation lowers intracranial pressure the most rapidly. The patient must be sedated and intubated. Ventilation should achieve a PCO_2 of 25 to 30 mm Hg. This maneuver causes vasoconstriction, with decreased cerebral blood volume and, subsequently, decreased intracranial pressure. Decreased intracranial pressure secondary to hyperventilation is generally short-lived, and equilibration may occur within a few hours.

Mannitol, a hyperosmotic agent, becomes effective within minutes of administration and remains effective for several hours. Its usefulness may reflect formation of an osmotic gradient between blood and brain, driving water from the brain across the blood–brain barrier into the blood. This proposed mechanism is controversial. Solutions of 20% to 25% mannitol are administered IV at a rate of 0.5 to 2.0 g/kg over 20 to 30 minutes. Additional doses may be necessary if the patient's clinical condition continues to deteriorate. Mannitol may induce a rebound increase in intracranial pressure, and so it should be used cautiously.

Steroids should be administered and may be helpful especially when herniation is to the result of vasogenic edema. Dexamethasone is most commonly administered at an initial bolus dose of 40 to 100 mg IV, then 40 to 100 mg per day. Its onset of action occurs within hours, and its effect lasts several days. Dexamethasone may also be helpful in cancer patients when increased intracranial pressures are secondary to intracranial metastases or brain abscesses.[142] Neurosurgical intervention may be necessary if the patient has neurologic deterioration despite appropriate medical management. Treatment should be directed at the underlying cause once intracranial pressure is controlled.

Status Epilepticus Status epilepticus is defined as more than 30 minutes of continuous seizure activity or two or more sequential seizures without full recovery between seizures. It can lead to devastating neurologic and systemic consequences, such as neuronal injury and cell death, neurogenic pulmonary edema, and rhabdomyolysis with renal failure.

The cause of seizures in cancer patients may be structural, metabolic, infectious, or treatment-related. In a review of 50 cancer patients presenting to an emergency center with seizures, 16% had seizures because of a new structural lesion, and 52% had previously documented central nervous system lesions.[143] In patients with intracranial tumors, seizures commonly occur as a result of either metastatic disease or a primary brain tumor. The cancers that most commonly metastasize to the brain are lung cancer, breast cancer, melanoma, genitourinary malignancies, and gastrointestinal malignancies.

After a major seizure, neurologic function is suppressed, primarily owing to release of gamma-aminobutyric acid, an inhibitory endogenous neurotransmitter. Patients may be confused or unresponsive. They usually have a postictal phase that may last for 24 hours. Clinical findings after seizure activity may include bruising or tongue bites, signs of urinary or fecal incontinence, and increases in lactic acid and muscle enzyme levels. It is important to determine whether the patient has previously had seizures and, if so, the type of seizure and the medications used for control. The status, extent, and treatment of the malignancy should also be reviewed.

If the event precipitating seizure activity cannot easily be determined, a diagnostic workup should be initiated. Evaluation may include measurement of electrolytes, serum glucose, calcium, and magnesium, and testing of hepatic and renal function. A blood cell count, blood cultures, measurement of blood gases, electrocardiography, and drug screens may be appropriate. CT or MR imaging may be necessary. Lumbar puncture may also be indicated, depending on the suspected seizure precipitant, the patient's condition, and findings on imaging.[144]

Status epilepticus is a medical emergency. When patients present with status epilepticus, airway, breathing, and circulation should be assessed immediately (Figure 142-10). Anticonvulsant therapy with a short-acting intravenous benzodiazepine (lorazepam or diazepam) should then be administered to halt seizure activity. Generally, lorazepam is used because of its more rapid onset of action and longer period of efficacy. Patients with status epilepticus require other anticonvulsants, usually phenytoin. Fosphenytoin and phenobarbital are generally considered second-line and third-line agents, respectively. For patients with continuing seizure activity despite anticonvulsant treatment, combination anticonvulsant therapy with complete sedation is required. These patients will require intubation, monitoring (often in an intensive care setting), and electroencephalography.

Patients whose seizures are attributable to reversible medical causes should have the reversible cause corrected. These patients most likely will not require long-term anticonvulsant therapy. Patients whose status epilepticus is attributable to other causes will require prolonged treatment with an anticonvulsant. After a seizure, the unconscious patient should be placed in a side-lying position to help prevent aspiration and to improve oxygenation. Airway suctioning and supplemental oxygen may be required.

OTHER ONCOLOGIC EMERGENCIES

Perforated Bowel Perforation along the gastrointestinal tract is a serious emergency. In cancer patients, the most common causes of perforation are spontaneous perforation secondary to tumor (primary[145,146] or metastatic[147]) and iatrogenic perforation secondary to endoscopy or cancer treatment.[148,149] If the wall of the gastrointestinal tract is significantly infiltrated or replaced by tumor, tumor necrosis caused by radiotherapy or chemotherapy may lead to bowel perforation. Even when the wall of the gastrointestinal tract is not involved by tumor, severe gastroenteritis resulting from radiotherapy or chemotherapy may lead to severe bowel dilatation or distention and subsequent perforation. Bowel perforation can be caused by severe infections such as typhlitis and neutropenic enterocolitis.[150] Perforation can also be caused by disease processes unrelated to cancer. For example, appendicitis, diverticulitis, peptic ulcer disease, ischemic bowel disease, and inflammatory bowel disease can lead to bowel perforation in cancer patients as well as noncancer patients.

Typically, perforation of the gastrointestinal tract causes acute or sudden onset of pain that prompts emergent evaluation. In cases of cervical

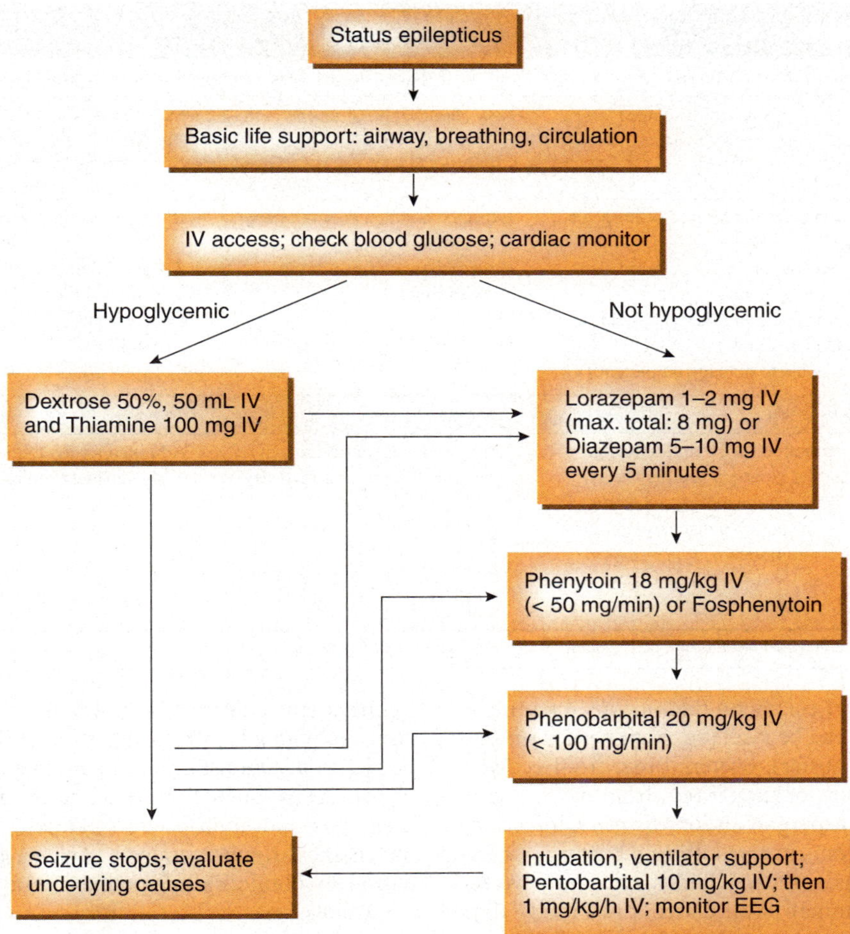

Figure 142-10 Algorithm for management of status epilepticus. IV = intravenous; EEG = electroencephalography.

esophageal perforation, symptoms at presentation may include neck pain, dysphagia, hoarseness, and subcutaneous emphysema. In thoracic esophageal perforation, upper abdominal rigidity, severe retrosternal chest pain, odynophagia, and hematemesis are common. In gastric perforation, acute onset of severe abdominal pain is usually the first symptom. The pain may be associated with nausea and vomiting. In about 15% of patients, significant bleeding is present. Radiation of abdominal pain to the shoulders may occur because of irritation of the diaphragm. In cases of free perforation into the peritoneal cavity, abdominal distension and signs of peritonitis (severe rebound abdominal tenderness, guarding, and absent bowel sounds) may be present. In peritonitis, abdominal rigidity and rebound tenderness are present. In diffuse peritonitis, auscultation of the abdomen may yield few or no bowel sounds.

Fever and leukocytosis with left shift may be present in patients with peritonitis, mediastinitis, or abscess. However, the white blood cell count should be interpreted in the context of recent cytotoxic chemotherapy or use of neutrophil-stimulating cytokines. Amylase levels may be high in intestinal, esophageal, and gastric perforation, and lipase levels may be high in gastric perforation.

In cervical perforation, a plain radiograph of the neck in the lateral view may show air in the deep cervical tissues. Plain radiographs of the chest are also valuable in esophageal perforation, because pneumomediastinum may be evident. Free air detected by plain radiographs (upright chest radiography or abdominal series with upright or decubitus views) can provide evidence of bowel perforation in the acute abdomen[151] (Figure 142-11). After a patient has been upright or in the left decubitus position for 10 minutes, a plain radiograph can detect as little as 1 to 2 mL of intraperitoneal free air.[152] With duodenal perforation, plain abdominal radiographs may show air in the retroperitoneal space or, if an oral contrast agent is used, retroperitoneal contrast collection. Other radiographic signs of perforation include outlining of both sides of the bowel wall by air and visualization of the hepatic ligament.

If bowel perforation is highly suspected clinically and if the initial studies do not show evidence of perforation, further study with oral contrast agents is indicated. A water-soluble contrast agent (eg, Gastrografin [Squibb Diagnostics, USA]) is used initially, because barium causes a severe inflammatory reaction when leaked into the peritoneal cavity. CT imaging is very accurate in diagnosing bowel perforation and can provide detailed information about the location of the perforation and the status of the surrounding structures.
Treatment of a perforated viscus can consist of expectant management, expectant management followed by surgery, or immediate surgery. The chosen course of action depends on the size and location of the perforating defect, the cause of the perforation, whether the perforation is free or contained, the clinical course (development of sepsis), the patient's performance status and quality of life before occurrence of the perforation, prognosis (based on the status of the malignant disease), and the presence of comorbid conditions that increase the risk of perioperative mortality. Nonsurgical treatment measures include nasogastric tube suction, administration of broad-spectrum intravenous antibiotics, intravenous hydration, parenteral nutrition, and close monitoring.[153] If the patient's condition deteriorates during expectant treatment, a decision to operate can be made. In general, perforations caused by peptic ulcer disease or by megacolon usually require emergent surgery. Factors associated with increased risk of perioperative mortality after peptic ulcer perforation include preoperative shock, long duration of perforation (> 24 hours), and major medical illness.[154]

Neutropenic Fever Neutropenic fever is a true medical emergency, and timely administration of antibiotics can potentially prevent development of sepsis syndrome and death. Neutro-

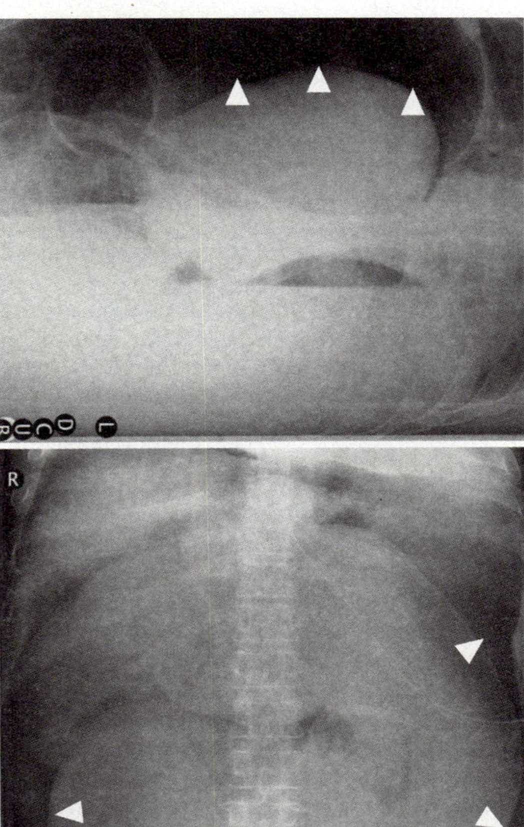

Figure 142-11 Pneumoperitoneum. A 53-year-old man with multiple myeloma and amyloidosis involving the gastrointestinal tract, undergoing treatment with thalidomide and dexamethasone, presented with acute abdominal pain and abdominal distention. Abdominal radiographs showed intraperitoneal free air (*white arrowheads*). Laparotomy revealed bowel perforation secondary to massive colonic distention.

Table 142-3 Five Risk-Based Pathways for the Care of Patients with Neutropenic Fever

Patients presenting in the emergency center with neutropenic fever are evaluated for placement on the neutropenic fever (NF) paths. There are five NF paths, and the patient eligibility criteria are as follows:

NF1 – Outpatient Oral Treatment (Solid Tumor)	NF2 – Outpatient IV Treatment (Solid Tumor)	NF3 – Inpatient IV Treatment (without Comorbidities)	NF4 – Inpatient IV Treatment (with Comorbidities)	NF5 – Inpatient IV Treatment (Hematology Patients)
Criteria	Criteria	Criteria	Criteria	Criteria
Expected duration of neutropenia < 1 week No concomitant comorbid conditions Normal liver and renal function Ability to take PO meds	Expected duration of neutropenia < 1 week No concomitant comorbid conditions Normal liver and renal function Unable to take PO meds Able to manage outpatient IVs	Expected duration of neutropenia < 1 week No concomitant comorbid conditions Normal liver and renal function Unable to take PO meds Unable to manage outpatient IVs	Expected duration of neutropenia > 1 week Concomitant comorbid conditions *Or* Failed outpatient treatment	BMT, leukemia, lymphoma Expected duration of neutropenia > 1 week Concomitant comorbid conditions
Treatment	Treatment	Treatment	Treatment	Treatment
PO antibiotics ×7 days Neutropenic fever workup on day 1 in the emergency center Clinic visits on days 2, 3, and 7 with CBC, Diff, Plt, Creat Telephone F/U on days 4, 5, and 6	IV antibiotics ×7 days in the home setting Clinic visits on days 2, 3, and 7 with CBC, Diff, Plt, Creat Telephone F/U on days 4, 5, and 6	Admitted for IV antibiotics in the inpatient setting Patient to be reassessed on day 4 for possible discharge on PO antibiotics	Admitted for IV antibiotics in the inpatient setting for 7 days	Admitted for IV antibiotics in the inpatient setting for 7 days

BMT = bone marrow transplant; CBC = complete blood count; Creat = creatinine; Diff = differential blood count; F/U = follow-up; IV = intravenous; Plt = platelet; PO = oral.

phils are phagocytic white blood cells that defend the human body against bacterial and fungal infections.[155] Neutropenia is defined as a neutrophil count of ≤1000 cells/μL, absolute neutropenia is defined as a neutrophil count of ≤500 cells/μL, and profound neutropenia is defined as a neutrophil count of ≤100 cells/μL.[155] Infection is the leading cause of morbidity and mortality in neutropenic patients. The risk of infection varies with the duration of neutropenia.[156]

The initial treatment of patients with a neutropenic febrile episode should be based on risk.[157,158] Table 142-3 shows an example of a risk stratification strategy. Subsequent treatment may be modified according to clinical response.[159]

The degree and duration of neutropenia are the most important risk factors for developing fever after chemotherapy. Before the mid-1980s, aerobic gram-negative bacteria were the most common pathogens in neutropenic patients, but now gram-positive cocci—especially *Staphylococcus aureus*, *Staphylococcus epidermidis*, and streptococcal species—have emerged as the most common pathogens in this population.

Factors that have contributed to the recent dominance of gram-positive bacterial infections are the increased use of chemotherapeutic agents that cause mucositis, increased use of central venous catheters, and the use prophylactic antibiotics against gram-negative bacteria. *Candida albicans* and non-*albicans* candidal species are important pathogens in patients with leukemia and in bone marrow transplant recipients. *Aspergillus* infection causes significant problems in patients with prolonged and profound neutropenia. Other fungi, such as *Fusarium* and *Trichosporon*, are emerging as important pathogens, perhaps owing to increased use of antifungal prophylaxis.

Neutropenic patients are immunocompromised and lack the ability to mount a full inflammatory response to infection. Any symptom or sign of infection in such patients should be investigated fully. Lesions on the mucous membranes and the skin can be viral (eg, from herpes simplex or varicella zoster), bacterial (eg, from ecthyma gangrenosum), or fungal (eg, from disseminated candidiasis, aspergillosis, or *Fusarium* infection). Sinus symptoms may result from bacterial or fungal infections, some of which may be invasive and fatal. Abdominal pain, distention, bloody diarrhea, nausea, and vomiting are typical findings in neutropenic enterocolitis.[150] Perianal symptoms may suggest the presence of a perianal abscess.

The spectrum of conditions that must be considered in the differential diagnosis of pulmonary disease in febrile neutropenic patients is broad: infection (viral, bacterial, fungal, and protozoan), radiation-induced pathologic conditions, chemotherapy-induced side effects, pulmonary hemorrhage, and pulmonary infarct. Physical findings in the chest are present in 30% of neutropenic patients with normal findings on chest radiography.[160] Correlation of pulmonary symptoms and findings on chest radiographs is a clinical challenge in neutropenic patients. In most cases, neutropenic fever occurs in the absence of any clinically evident source of infection. Bacteremia in these patients may have resulted from translocation of organisms from the gastrointestinal tracts. Thus, the organism cultured is usually the major organism that has colonized the gastrointestinal tract of the patient.

Blood cultures may be helpful in neutropenic patients. They may provide a definitive diagnosis of the organism causing the infection and information about the sensitivity of the pathogen to antimicrobial agents. However, in persistently febrile patients receiving broad-spectrum antimicrobial drugs, fewer than 1% of blood cultures yield organisms.[161] Sputum cultures should be obtained when a patient is expectorating. However, many neutropenic patients with documented pulmonary infection do not produce sputum. A positive sputum culture may provide a diagnosis of the agent causing the pulmonary infection. Any site with a localized sign of infection should be pursued with aspiration or biopsy for culture of pathogens. Such culture may lead to a definite diagnosis and appropriate treatment. However, coexisting thrombocytopenia can be a contraindication to obtaining specimens or biopsy from some sites.

Findings on chest radiography are abnormal in 17% to 25% of patients with neutropenic fever, despite the absence of pulmonary signs or symptoms.[160] Classic methods such as direct examination of stained specimens, culture, and testing of antibiotic sensitivities are now complemented by molecular methods (polymerase chain reaction, in particular) that detect microbial DNA and microbial antigens in body fluids or tissues. Polymerase chain reaction and antigen detection techniques for mycobacterial, *Aspergillus*, and some viral infections can help to diagnose a suspected infection early. These new detection methods offer rapid and sensitive diagnosis even after antimicrobial therapy has been started.[162] Serologic tests have also been helpful in identifying infections in neutropenic patients.

During the past few decades, the organisms predominantly isolated from neutropenic patients with fever have changed to gram-positive pathogens from gram-negative pathogens.[163] Because of the appearance of multi-drug–resistant organisms, antimicrobial therapy must be selected on the basis of the predominant pathogens and antimicrobial susceptibility patterns at each institution.[164]

Monotherapy with broad-spectrum beta-lactam antibiotics, including carbapenems or the fourth-generation cephalosporin cefepime, are established treatments. Empirical coverage for gram-negative bacilli is mandatory, because gram-negative sepsis is associated with high mortality. Double-agent therapy (aminoglycoside or fluoroquinolone plus beta-lactam) and monotherapy are both acceptable.[165] All of these regimens have an overall success rate of 60% to 80%. Empirical coverage for gram-positive organisms with vancomycin is acceptable if infection with a gram-positive organism (such as cellulitis or a central venous catheter–related infection), or severe mucositis is suspected or documented.

If a febrile neutropenic patient does not respond to the initial broad-spectrum antibiotic therapy, vancomycin can be added, because the presence of gram-positive bacterial infection is likely.[165] Teicoplanin and linezolid may be alternatives to vancomycin. If fever persists after 4 to 7 days of broad-spectrum antibiotics, antifungal therapy is recommended. Fluconazole may be used as initial empirical therapy in patients who have not received prior antifungal prophylaxis. Amphotericin B is beneficial to three groups of patients: patients with persistent fever during broad-spectrum antibiotic treatment who are not receiving antifungal prophylaxis, patients with persistent neutropenia for more than 15 days, and patients with a documented fungal infection. In some studies, hematopoietic growth factors shortened hospital stays and reduced the duration of neutropenia, but no reduction in the duration of fever or the rate of infection-related mortality was documented.[166,167]

Table 142-4 Recommendations for Acute Management of Anaphylaxis in Adults

1. Remove the antigen or delay absorption of the antigen.
2. Assess airway; intubate if there is evidence of laryngeal edema or impending severe airway obstruction.
3. Administer epinephrine.
   In case of a less severe episode:
   0.3 mg SQ, 1 mg/mL, repeated at 10- to 20-minute intervals.
   In case of a more severe episode:
   0.3 to 0.5 mg IM, 1 mg/mL, repeated at 5- to 10-minute intervals.
   In case of shock or airway obstruction:
   1 mg/100 mL IV, 0.01 to 0.02 mg/min, up to a total dose of 0.1 mg.
   In case of persistent shock:
   Repeat dose or start a drip. Add 1 mg to 500 mL normal saline and infuse at 2 to 10 μg/min.
   If patient is more than 50 years old or has a history of cardiac problems and if life-threatening symptoms exist:
   Test dose of 0.1 to 0.15 mg SQ or IM.
4. Administer IV crystalloid fluid (normal saline or lactated Ringer's solution).
   In case of hypotension, administer 1 L over 15 minutes, then reassess; repeat as needed up to 3 L.
5. Administer glucocorticoid:
   Methylprednisolone 125 mg IV push; may repeat every 4 hours if symptoms persist (alternative: hydrocortisone 500 mg, dexamethasone 20 mg, or other potent corticosteroids).
6. Administer antihistamine:
   Diphenhydramine 25 to 50 mg IV or IM; repeat every 2 to 4 hours as needed.
7. In case of resistant hypotension:
   Military antishock trousers and the Trendelenburg position may be helpful.
   Infuse dopamine 5 to 20 μg/kg/min IV by titration.
   Administer naloxone 0.4 to 2.0 mg IV every 2 minutes (maximum 10 mg).
   Administer cimetidine 300 mg IV or famotidine 20 mg IV.
8. In case of beta-blocker–accentuated epinephrine-resistant anaphylaxis:
   Administer glucagon 1 to 5 mg IV over 2 to 5 minutes.
   Administer terbutaline 0.25 mg SQ.
   Administer isoproterenol 2 to 10 μg/min IV by titration.

Adapted from Murrant T and Bihari D,[169] Gavalas M and colleagues,[170] and Brown AF.[171]
IM = intramuscularly; IV = intravenously; SQ = subcutaneously.

Anaphylactic Reactions to Chemotherapy Drugs Anaphylactic reactions to chemotherapy drugs are another important type of emergency in cancer patients. Urticaria and angioedema, the most common manifestations of anaphylaxis, occur in 90% of anaphylactic reactions. Other common manifestations are chest tightness, upper airway obstruction, abdominal pain, bronchospasm, and hypotension. Laryngeal edema causing upper airway obstruction is the most likely cause of death in anaphylaxis; hypotension is the second most likely cause.[168]

Routes of drug administration, in order of decreasing severity of associated reactions, are intravenous, intra-arterial, intramuscular, subcutaneous, intradermal, oral, vaginal, rectal, and dermal.[168] In addition to the route of administration, factors known to affect the incidence or severity of hypersensitivity reactions include the class of the offending agent, the dose, the rate of infusion, the interval between doses, the cumulative dose, the number of previous exposures to the drug, and administration of prophylactic agents (the dose and timing of administration of the prophylactic agents and the thoroughness of the prevention plan). The three important elements in the treatment of anaphylaxis are early recognition, airway maintenance, and hemodynamic support. Table 142-4 contains recommendations for treatment of anaphylaxis.[169–171]

L-Asparaginase L-Asparaginase is an enzyme of bacterial origin. Multiple antigenic sites on this bacterial protein stimulate production of immunoglobulins. The risk of hypersensitivity reactions increases by 5% to 8% with each subsequent exposure and reaches about 33% with the fourth dose.[172] Both the *Escherichia coli* and *Erwinia chrysanthemi* forms of L-asparaginase can cause anaphylactic reactions. Fortunately, anaphylaxis occurs in fewer than 10% of treated patients, and death occurs in fewer than 1% of treated patients.[173] Asparaginase covalently attached to polyethylene glycol (PEG-asparaginase) appears to decrease anaphylactic reactions.[174]

Risk factors for adverse reactions to L-asparaginase include high dosage (above 6,000 IU/m^2 daily),[175] previous exposure, intravenous administration,[176] a history of atopy or other drug allergy, and single-agent treatment with L-asparaginase.[177,178] Intradermal skin testing and test dosing are of no value in predicting adverse reactions to L-asparaginase.

Although reactions to L-asparaginase usually occur during the second week of treatment or later,[173] preparations for immediate treatment of hypersensitivity reactions must be in place before every dose, including the first. Intramuscular administration is recommended because, as compared with intravenous administration, that route is associated with a decreased incidence of anaphylactic reactions.[176] Reaction to one form of L-asparaginase should prompt a change to another, less immunogenic preparation.

Taxanes In early studies, the taxanes (paclitaxel and docetaxel) caused major hypersensitivity reactions in 10% to 30% of treated patients and minor reactions in approximately 40%.[179,180] The major hypersensitivity reactions are very similar to anaphylaxis (anaphylactoid reactions). Risk factors for hypersensitivity reactions with taxane infusion include short infusion schedule and fast infusion rate. Most major reactions occur within the first two doses. Reactions begin within 2 to 10 minutes of infusion and resolve within 15 minutes after the infusion is stopped. Manifestations of major hypersensitivity reactions are consistent with type I reactions and include urticaria, angioedema, dyspnea, bronchospasm, and hypotension.

Methods to prevent hypersensitivity reactions to taxanes include reducing the rate of infusion and administering prophylactic medications.[181] One study showed that infusion of paclitaxel over 96 hours without prophylactic premedication caused no major reactions.[182] With shorter infusion times of 24 hours, 3 hours, or 1 hour, prophylaxis with appropriate premedications (steroids and histamine type 1 and 2 receptor antagonists) reduced the incidence of major reactions to about 3%.[180,183]

Teniposide and Etoposide In adults, hypersensitivity reactions occur in about 7% of patients treated with teniposide[184] and about 3% of patients treated with etoposide.[185] Reactions to etoposide may occur more frequently in children than in adults.[186] Reactions can occur during the first exposure to these agents,[184] suggesting a nonimmunologic mechanism. On the other hand, the rate of reaction increases with increased cumulative doses,[187] suggesting development of an antibody-mediated reaction.[186] Reactions often occur during the first 10 minutes of infusion, sometimes after only a few milligrams have been infused, but they can also occur hours after administration. The hypersensitivity reactions seen are typical of a type I reaction, with angioedema, flushing, rashes, urticaria, bronchospasm, and hypotension. Teniposide can also cause a type II hemolytic reaction.[188] No hypersensitivity reactions have been reported with oral etoposide.[186]

Procarbazine Procarbazine causes type I hypersensitivity reactions in approximately 6% to 18% of treated patients,[189] and a case of type III reaction in the form of allergic alveolitis was reported.[190] Cutaneous manifestations are a maculopapular rash and urticaria typical of type I reactions. Patients who have a hypersensitivity reaction to procarbazine are unable to continue treatment because rechallenge causes[190] recurrence of symptoms.

Platinum Compounds Cisplatin produces type I and type II (hemolytic anemia) hypersensitivity reactions.[191] The incidence of hypersensitivity reactions appears to be between 1% and 20%[192] with intravenous administration and between 10% and 25% with intravesicular administration.[193] Carboplatin also produces type I hypersensitivity reactions.[194] The type I reactions of both cisplatin and carboplatin appear to be mediated by immunoglobulin E and may be caused by the platinum atom in those compounds.[195]

Cross-reactivity among platinum analogs is possible. One review has suggested that six or more doses may be necessary to produce a hypersensitivity reaction.[196] Manifestations of hypersensitivity reactions caused by cisplatin and its analogs include rashes, urticaria, bronchospasm, and hypotension. Anaphylaxis may occur in 5% of treated patients.

Cyclophosphamide and Ifosfamide Oral and intravenous cyclophosphamide and intravenous ifosfamide can produce type I reactions, which appear to be mediated by immunoglobulin E. Reactions to cyclophosphamide and ifosfamide may occur with the first or subsequent doses. Reported manifestations of cyclophosphamide- and ifosfamide-induced reactions include urticaria, rashes, angioedema, and anaphylaxis.[197–199]

Anthracyclines Reported manifestations of hypersensitivity reactions induced by anthracyclines include rash, pruritus, urticaria, hypotension, and anaphylaxis. Intravenous daunorubicin and doxorubicin can cause type I reactions,[200] and type I reactions have been reported with intravesicular doxorubicin.[201] Oral or intravenous idarubicin has not been reported to produce type I reactions. It appears that cross-reactivity between anthracyclines is uncommon.

Melphalan and Chlorambucil Reactions are uncommon when melphalan is given orally, but the incidence of type I hypersensitivity reactions when melphalan is given intravenously is approximately 2% to 4%.[202] Chlorambucil has also caused rare cases of type I hypersensitivity reactions.[203] Manifestations include urticaria and angioedema, but not hypotension or bronchospasm.[204] Toxic epidermal necrolysis,[205] hemolysis,[206] and pneumonitis[207] have been also reported with chlorambucil treatment.

Methotrexate Methotrexate can produce type I hypersensitivity reactions and possibly type III reactions in the form of acute pneumonitis or cutaneous vasculitis. Type I reactions manifest as generalized pruritus, rash, urticaria, angioedema, and hypotension. Type III reactions manifest as rash (vasculitic), lung eosinophilia, pleural effusion, and hilar lymphadenopathy.

Cytarabine Type I reactions to cytarabine are not common. There are no known risk factors for cytarabine-induced reactions. Manifestations of cytarabine-induced reactions that are mediated by immunoglobulin E include dyspnea, chest pain, fever, angioedema, urticaria, and hypotension.

Miscellaneous Antineoplastics Fluorouracil causes rare cases of angioedema and hypotension consistent with type I hypersensitivity reactions.[208] Diaziquone causes hypersensitivity reactions and anaphylaxis (urticaria, bronchospasm, and hypotension) in 1% to 2% of patients.[209] Bleomycin causes urticaria, periorbital edema, and bronchospasm.[210] In rare instances, hypersensitivity reactions to bleomycin have been fatal.[211]

Systemic Reactions to Cytokines and Monoclonal Antibodies Several cytokines (IFNs, interleukins) and monoclonal antibodies[212] have been approved for the treatment of specific malignancies. The toxic effects associated with cytokines may be serious. Monoclonal antibodies may induce massive release of cytokines, which may lead to fever, rigor, dyspnea, hypoxia, hypotension, or even death. Reactions to some of these biologic agents have recently been reviewed.[213]

Interferons IFNs are a family of proteins produced by cells in response to various stimuli. IFN-α is produced by macrophages and lymphocytes, IFN-β is produced by fibroblasts and epithelial cells, and IFN-γ is produced by natural killer cells, CD4- or CD8-positive lymphocytes, and lymphokine-activated killer cells. Recombinant forms of IFNs are used worldwide as therapy for viral infections, autoimmune diseases, and malignancies.

Acute adverse effects of IFN therapy occur during the first 2 to 8 hours after treatment, but these adverse effects rarely limit treatment. Flu-like symptoms,[214] hypotension or hypertension, tachycardia, nausea, and vomiting are common side effects. With chronic administration, fatigue and anorexia can become severe, and significant weight loss (>10% body weight) can occur.[215] Anxiety, agitation, seizures, and coma have been reported with high-dose schedules; all are reversible. These neurologic side effects and behavioral and cognitive changes may limit treatment. Mild granulocytopenia (about 50% reduction in cell counts) develops gradually after the first week of treatment and is rapidly reversible upon drug discontinuation. Autoimmune and immune hemolytic anemia, myelosuppression, and thrombocytopenia may be seen in rare instances. Flu-like side effects may be managed with acetaminophen or nonsteroidal anti-inflammatory drugs. Other supportive care measures may be provided depending on the symptoms. In most patients, symptoms lessen with subsequent doses of IFN.

Interleukin-2 IL-2 is approved for the treatment of patients with metastatic renal-cell carcinoma and melanoma. High-dose IL-2 therapy is associated with cardiovascular and hemodynamic adverse effects that resemble septic shock.[214] High-dose intravenous IL-2 therapy, which should be given in a hospital inpatient setting (sometimes with intensive care monitoring), can lead to hypotension, vascular leak syndrome, and respiratory insufficiency. Support of peripheral vascular resistance with vasopressors, endotracheal intubation, and fluid resuscitation may be necessary during therapy. Acute central nervous system side effects such as psychosis, disorientation, and behavioral changes may be seen with high-dose IL-2 therapy. Other neurologic side effects, such as seizures and coma, have been reported in patients with brain metastases. IL-2 treatment should be stopped as soon as neurologic side effects are observed. Guidelines for administration of high-dose IL-2 have been suggested.[216]

Lower-dose intravenous and subcutaneous IL-2 regimens can be administered in an ambulatory care setting with observation for several hours after administration. The severity of adverse effects of lower-dose therapy is dose dependent. Common symptoms include fever, chills, nausea, vomiting, anorexia, malaise, fatigue, myalgia, arthralgia, and pruritus. Prophylaxis includes acetaminophen 650 to 1,000 mg 1 hour before therapy and 4 and 8 hours later, and histamine type I and II receptor antagonists (eg, diphenhydramine 50 mg orally 1 hour before therapy and 25 mg 4, 8, and 12 hours later, plus cimetidine 800 mg orally before therapy). Meperidine (25 to 50 mg intravenously) may be given as needed for rigor and chills during therapy. Various antiemetics may be used as needed.

Monoclonal Antibodies Rituximab, a humanized monoclonal antibody directed against CD20, is used to treat B-cell lymphomas.[217] Transient nausea, headache, fever, chills, and fatigue are frequent complaints with the first dose. Other adverse effects, such as rash, pain at the tumor site, hypotension, arrhythmias, bronchospasm, and angioedema, may reflect immune responses to the murine immunoglobulin. Prophylactic treatment with acetaminophen and diphenhydramine may attenuate this antibody infusion syndrome. Reactions generally resolve with slowing or interruption of the infusion. The rituximab infusion may be interrupted and then restarted at 50% of the previous infusion rate when symptoms resolve.

Trastuzumab is a recombinant humanized monoclonal antibody against *HER2/neu* (c-*erb*-B2), a glycoprotein receptor with intrinsic tyrosine kinase activity and partial homology with the epidermal growth factor receptor.[218] Fever and chills during the first infusion are the most prominent symptoms. Other side effects are usually mild to moderate; they include nausea, vomiting, diarrhea, and pain at the tumor site.

Campath-1H is a humanized immunoglobulin G1 monoclonal antibody directed against CD52 antigen on the surface of malignant lymphocytes. The antibody binds to lymphomas and induces antibody-dependent lysis and cell killing. The first three or four infusions in each patient are associated with side effects such as nausea, vomiting, rigor, fever, facial flushing, hives, wheezing, diarrhea, and hypotension. However, these adverse effects become less severe or disappear with subsequent doses.

Gemtuzumab ozogamicin (Mylotarg [Wyeth-Ayerst, USA]) is a humanized anti-CD33 antibody conjugated with calicheamicin, which is an antineoplastic antibiotic 1,000 times more potent than doxorubicin.[219] Mylotarg is used in the treatment of selected patients with CD33-positive acute myeloid leukemia.[220] A post-infusion syndrome of fever and chills is commonly seen. Other adverse effects, often occurring within 4 hours of infusion, include nausea, vomiting, dyspnea, and hypotension. These reactions may be prevented or alleviated by prophylactic treatment with acetaminophen and diphenhydramine.[221]

Denileukin diftitox (Ontak [Ligand, USA]) is an IL-2–diphtheria toxin fusion protein. The IL-2 portion of the molecule targets lymphoma cells by binding to the IL-2 receptor on the plasma membrane. Upon endocytosis, the diphtheria toxin is delivered to the lymphoma cells. Common side effects are nausea and vomiting, fever, and flu-like symptoms. Other significant side effects include the cytokine release syndrome and vascular leak syndrome.[222] Acute complaints reported on the first day of treatment include back pain, shortness of breath, flushing, rash, chest pain, difficulty swallowing, dizziness, and fainting. Only 2% of patients experience severe reactions. Slowing or terminating the infusion and administering antihistamines, corticosteroids, and epinephrine can relieve these reactions. Prophylactic treatment with systemic corticosteroids is recommended.[223]

REFERENCES

1. Yeung SC, Escalante CP, editors. Oncologic emergencies. Hamilton, ON: BC Decker; 2002.
2. Johnston PG, Spence RAJ, editors. Oncologic emergencies. Oxford, UK: Oxford University Press; 2002.
3. ACLS provider manual. Dallas, TX: American Heart Association; 2001.
4. Hendrick JM, Pijls NH, van der Werf T, Crul JF Cardiopulmonary resuscitation on the general ward: no category of patients should be excluded in advance. Resuscitation 1990;20:163–171.
5. Ebell MH, Becker LA, Barry HC, Hagen M. Survival after in-hospital cardiopulmonary resuscitation. A meta-analysis. J Gen Intern Med 1998;13:805–16.
6. Staudinger T, Stoiser B, Mullner M, et al. Outcome and prognostic factors in critically ill cancer patients admitted to the intensive care unit. Crit Care Med 2000;28:1322–8.
7. Morris JC, Holland JF. Oncologic emergencies. In: Bast RC Jr, Kufe DW, Pollock RE, Weichselbaum R, Holland JF, Frei E III, editors. Cancer medicine. 5th ed. Hamilton, ON: BC Decker; 2000. p. 2433–53.
8. Kvols LK. Therapy of the malignant carcinoid syndrome. Endocrinol Metab Clin North Am 1989;18:557–68.
9. Inagaki J, Rodriguez V, Bodey GP. Proceedings: causes of death in cancer patients. Cancer, 1974;33:568–73.
10. Ottaviani G, Rossi L, Ramos SG, Matturri L. Pathology of the heart and conduction system in a case of sudden death due to a cardiac fibroma in a 6-month-old child. Cardiovasc Pathol 1999;8:109–12.
11. Bussani R, Silvestri F. Images in cardiovascular medicine. Sudden death in a woman with fibroelastoma of the aortic valve chronically occluding the right coronary ostium. Circulation 1999;100:2204.
12. Idir M, Oysel N, Guibaud JP, et al. Fragmentation of a right atrial myxoma presenting as a pulmonary embolism. J Am Soc Echocardiogr 2000;13:61–3.
13. King D, Sheard JD, Silas JH. Cardiac amyloidosis in the presence of Bence–Jones proteinuria and normal serum immunoglobulins. Br J Clin Pract 1993;47:336–7.
14. Steinherz L, Steinherz P. Delayed cardiac toxicity from anthracycline therapy. Pediatrician 1991;18:49–52.
15. Bristow MR, Billingham ME, Mason JW, Daniels JR. Clinical spectrum of anthracycline antibiotic cardiotoxicity. Cancer Treat Rep 1978;62:873–9.
16. Couch RD, Loh KK, Sugino J. Sudden cardiac death following Adriamycin therapy. Cancer 1981;48:38–9.
17. Mills BA, Roberts RW. Cyclophosphamide-induced cardiomyopathy: a report of two cases and review of the English literature. Cancer 1979;43:2223–6.
18. Gradishar W, Vokes E, Schilsky R, et al. Vascular events in patients receiving high-dose infusional 5-fluorouracil–based chemotherapy: the University of Chicago experience. Med Pediatr Oncol 1991;19:8–15.
19. Benoff LJ, Schweitzer P. Radiation therapy-induced cardiac injury. Am Heart J 1995;129:1193–6.
20. Gyenes G. Radiation-induced ischemic heart disease in breast cancer—a review. Acta Oncol 1998;37:241–6.
21. Knight CJ, Sutton GC. Complete heart block and severe tricuspid regurgitation after radiotherapy. Case report and review of the literature. Chest 1995;108:1748–51.
22. Lopez FF, Mangi A, Mylonakis E, et al. Atrial fibrillation and tumor emboli as manifestations of metastatic leiomyosarcoma to the heart and lung. Heart Lung 2000;29:47–9.
23. Mathew V, Olson LJ, Gertz MA, Hayes DL. Symptomatic conduction system disease in cardiac amyloidosis. Am J Cardiol 1997;80:1491–2.
24. Pentz WH. Advanced heart block as a manifestation of a paraneoplastic syndrome from malignant thymoma. Chest 1999;116:1135–6.
25. Donnelly MS, Weinberg DS, Skarin AT, Levine HD. Sick sinus syndrome with seroconstrictive pericarditis in malignant lymphoma involving the heart: a case report. Med Pediatr Oncol 1981:9:273–7.
26. Friess GG, Boyd JF, Geer MR, Garcia JC. Effects of first-dose doxorubicin on cardiac rhythm as evaluated by continuous 24-hour monitoring. Cancer 1985;56:2762–4.
27. Unnikrishnan D, Dutcher JP, Varshneya N, et al. Torsades de pointes in 3 patients with leukemia treated with arsenic trioxide. Blood 2001;97:1514–6.
28. Aziz SA, Tramboo NA, Mohi-ud-Din K, et al. Supraventricular arrhythmia: a complication of 5-fluorouracil therapy. Clin Oncol (R Coll Radiol) 1998;10:377–8.
29. Miya T, Fujikawa R, Fukushima J, et al. Bradycardia induced by irinotecan: a case report. Jpn J Clin Oncol 1998;28:709–11.
30. Santini D, Tonini G, Abbate A, et al. Gemcitabine-induced atrial fibrillation: a hitherto unreported manifestation of drug toxicity. Ann Oncol 2000;11:479–81.
31. Sonnenblick M, Rosin A. Cardiotoxicity of interferon. A review of 44 cases. Chest 1991;99:557–61.
32. Wassmann S, Nickenig G, Bohm M. Long QT syndrome and torsade de pointes in a patient receiving fluconazole. Ann Intern Med 1999;131:797.
33. Coley KC, Crain JL. Miconazole-induced fatal dysrhythmia. Pharmacotherapy 1997;17:379–82.
34. Otsuka M, Kanamori H, Sasaki S, et al. Torsades de pointes complicating pentamidine therapy of *Pneumocystis carinii* pneumonia in acute myelogenous leukemia. Intern Med 1997;36:705–8.
35. Anderson ME, Mazur A, Yang T, Roden DM. Potassium current antagonist properties and proarrhythmic consequences of quinolone antibiotics. J Pharmacol Exp Ther 2001;296:806–10.
36. Shaffer D, Singer S, Korvick J, Honig P. Concomitant risk factors in reports of torsades de pointes associated with macrolide use: review of the United States Food and Drug Administration Adverse Event Reporting System. Clin Infect Dis 2002;35:197–200.
37. Frumin H, Kerin NZ, Rubenfire M. Classification of antiarrhythmic drugs. J Clin Pharmacol 1989;29:387–94.
38. Gallagher MM, Guo XH, Poloniecki JD, et al. Initial energy setting, outcome and efficiency in direct current cardioversion of atrial fibrillation and flutter. J Am Coll Cardiol 2001;38:1498–504.
39. Kern KB, Halperin HR, Field J. New guidelines for cardiopulmonary resuscitation and emergency cardiac care: changes in the management of cardiac arrest. JAMA 2001;285:1267–9.
40. Flombaum CD. Metabolic emergencies in the cancer patient. Semin Oncol 2000;27:322–34.
41. Yang H, Rosove MH, Figlin RA. Tumor lysis syndrome occurring after the administration of rituximab in lymphoproliferative disorders: high-grade non-Hodgkin's lymphoma and chronic lymphocytic leukemia. Am J Hematol 1999;62:247–50.
42. Kalemkerian GP, Darwish B, Varterasian ML. Tumor lysis syndrome in small cell carcinoma and other solid tumors. Am J Med 1997;103:363–7.
43. Persons DA, Garst J, Vollmer R, Crawford J. Tumor lysis syndrome and acute renal failure after treatment of non-small-cell lung carcinoma with combination irinotecan and cisplatin. Am J Clin Oncol 1998;21:426–9.
44. Drakos P, Bar-Ziv J, Catane R. Tumor lysis syndrome in nonhematologic malignancies. Report of a case and review of the literature. Am J Clin Oncol 1994;17:502–5.
45. Bilgrami SF, Fallon BG. Tumor lysis syndrome after combination chemotherapy for ovarian cancer. Med Pediatr Oncol 1993;21:521–4.
46. Van Der Klooster JM, Van Der Wiel HE, Van Saase JL, Grootendorst AF. Asystole during combination chemotherapy for non-Hodgkin's lymphoma: the acute tumor lysis syndrome. Neth J Med 2000;56:147–52.
47. Loosveld OJ, Schouten HC, Gaillard CA, Blijham GH. Acute tumour lysis syndrome in a patient with acute lymphoblastic leukemia after a single dose of prednisone. Br J Haematol 1991;77:122–3.
48. Schifter T, Cohen A, Lewinski UH. Severe tumor lysis syndrome following splenic irradiation. Am J Hematol 1999;60:75–6.
49. Mahmoud HH, Leverger G, Patte C, et al. Advances in the management of malignancy-associated hyperuricaemia. Br J Cancer 1998;77:18–20.
50. McKenna RJ Jr, Ali MK, Ewer MS, Frazier OH. Pleural and pericardial effusions in cancer patients. Curr Probl Cancer 1985;9:1–44.
51. Muto M, Ohtsu A, Boku N, et al. *Streptococcus milleri* infection and pericardial abscess associated with esophageal carcinoma: report of two cases. Hepatogastroenterology 1999;46:1782–4.
52. Rabinovici R, Szewczyk D, Ovadia P, et al. *Candida* pericarditis: clinical profile and treatment. Ann Thorac Surg 1997;63:1200–4.
53. Murray BH, Cohle SD, Davison P. Pericardial tamponade and death from Hickman catheter perforation. Am Surg 1996;62:994–7.
54. Pataki N, Szelig L, Horvath OP, et al. Pericardial drainage using the transdiaphragmatic route: refinement of the laparoscopic technique. Surg Endosc 2002;16:1105.
55. Maher EA, Shepherd FA, Todd TJ. Pericardial sclerosis as the primary management of malignant pericardial effusion and cardiac tamponade. J Thorac Cardiovasc Surg 1996;112:637–43.
56. Galli M, Politi A, Pedretti F, et al. Percutaneous balloon pericardiotomy for malignant pericardial tamponade. Chest 1995;108:1499–501.
57. Bellomo R. Fluid resuscitation: colloids vs. crystalloids. Blood Purif 2002;20:239–42.
58. Friedman HD, Evangelisti PA, Emko P. Postoperative carotid artery rupture caused by *Actinomyces* infection. Otolaryngol Head Neck Surg 1996;114:145–7.
59. Okamura HO, Kamiyama R, Takiguchi Y, et al. Histopathological examination of ruptured carotid artery after irradiation. ORL J Otorhinolaryngol Relat Spec 2002;64:226–8.
60. Heller KS, Strong EW. Carotid arterial hemorrhage after radical head and neck surgery. Am J Surg 1979;138:607–10.
61. Morrissey DD, Andersen PE, Nesbit GM, et al. Endovascular management of hemorrhage in patients with head and neck cancer. Arch Otolaryngol Head Neck Surg 1997;123:15–9.
62. Von der Walde J, Mashiah A, Berrebi A. Spontaneous rupture of the spleen in hairy cell leukemia. Clin Oncol 1981;7:241–4.
63. Brissette M, Dhru RD. Hodgkin's disease presenting as spontaneous splenic rupture. Arch Pathol Lab Med 1992;116:1077–9.
64. Smart P, Cullinan M, Crosthwaite G. Spontaneous splenic rupture secondary to metastatic gastric carcinoma: case report and review. ANZ J Surg 2002;72:153–5.
65. Van Poppel H, Aswarie H, Vandenhove J, Baert L. Spontaneous rupture of splenomegaly due to disseminated bone metastases from prostatic carcinoma. Br J Urol 1991;67:653–4.
66. Massarweh S, Dhingra H. Unusual sites of malignancy: case 3. Solitary splenic metastasis in lung cancer with spontaneous rupture. J Clin Oncol 2001;19:1574–5.
67. Siniluoto TM, Paivansalo MJ, Lanning FP, et al. Ultrasonography in traumatic splenic rupture. Clin Radiol 1992;46:391–6.

68. Athale UH, Kaste SC, Bodner SM, Ribeiro RC. Splenic rupture in children with hematologic malignancies. Cancer 2000;88:480–90.
69. Heyman J, Leiter E. Spontaneous retroperitoneal hemorrhage: unusual presentation of renal cancer. Urology 1987;30:259–61.
70. Yamada AH, Sherrod AE, Boswell W, Skinner DG. Massive retroperitoneal hemorrhage from adrenal gland metastasis. Urology 1992;40:59–62.
71. Berney CR, Roth AD, Allal A, Rohner A. Spontaneous retroperitoneal hemorrhage due to adrenal metastasis for non-small cell lung cancer treated by radiation therapy. Acta Oncol 1997;36:91–3.
72. Yellin A, Rosen A, Reichert N, Lieberman Y. Superior vena cava syndrome. The myth–the facts. Am Rev Respir Dis 1990;141:1114–8.
73. Chen JC, Bongard F, Klein SR. A contemporary perspective on superior vena cava syndrome. Am J Surg 1990;160:207–11.
74. Kroencke TJ, Taupitz M, Arnold R, et al. Three-dimensional gadolinium-enhanced magnetic resonance venography in suspected thrombo-occlusive disease of the central chest veins. Chest 2001;120:1570–6.
75. Porte H, Metois D, Finzi L, et al. Superior vena cava syndrome of malignant origin. Which surgical procedure for which diagnosis? Eur J Cardiothorac Surg 2000;17:384–8.
76. Yim CD, Sane SS, Bjarnason H. Superior vena cava stenting. Radiol Clin North Am 2000;38:409–24.
77. Smayra T, Otal P, Chabbert V, et al. Long-term results of endovascular stent placement in the superior caval venous system. Cardiovasc Intervent Radiol 2001;24:388–94.
78. Cahill BC, Ingbar DH. Massive hemoptysis. Assessment and management. Clin Chest Med 1994;15:147–67.
79. Jean-Baptiste E. Clinical assessment and management of massive hemoptysis. Crit Care Med 2000;28:1642–7.
80. Panos RJ, Barr LF, Walsh TJ, Silverman HJ. Factors associated with fatal hemoptysis in cancer patients. Chest 1988;94:1008–13.
81. Miller RR, McGregor DH. Hemorrhage from carcinoma of the lung. Cancer 1980;46:200–5.
82. Karmy-Jones R, Cuschieri J, Vallieres E. Role of bronchoscopy in massive hemoptysis. Chest Surg Clin N Am 2001;11:873–906.
83. Ost D, Corbridge T. Independent lung ventilation. Clin Chest Med 1996;17:591–601.
84. Tsukamoto T, Sasaki H, Nakamura H. Treatment of hemoptysis patients by thrombin and fibrinogen–thrombin infusion therapy using a fiberoptic bronchoscope. Chest 1989;96:473–6.
85. Freitag L. Development of a new balloon catheter for management of hemoptysis with bronchofiberscopes. Chest 1993;103:593.
86. Colt HG. Laser bronchoscopy. Chest Surg Clin N Am 1996;6:277–91.
87. Lee P, Kupeli E, Mehta AC. Therapeutic bronchoscopy in lung cancer. Laser therapy, electrocautery, brachytherapy, stents, and photodynamic therapy. Clin Chest Med 2002;23:241–56.
88. Marshall TJ, Jackson JE. Vascular intervention in the thorax: bronchial artery embolization for haemoptysis. Eur Radiol 1997;7:1221–7.
89. Shneerson JM, Emerson PA, Phillips RH. Radiotherapy for massive haemoptysis from an aspergilloma. Thorax 1980;35:953–4.
90. Jougon J, Ballester M, Delcambre F, et al. Massive hemoptysis: what place for medical and surgical treatment. Eur J Cardiothorac Surg 2002;22:345.
91. Chernow B, Sahn SA. Carcinomatous involvement of the pleura: an analysis of 96 patients. Am J Med 1977;63:695–702.
92. Sahn S. Fishman's pulmonary diseases and disorders. 3rd ed. New York: McGraw–Hill; 1998. p. 1430.
93. Hsu C. Cytologic detection of malignancy in pleural effusion: a review of 5,255 samples from 3,811 patients. Diagn Cytopathol 1987;3:8–12.
94. Assi Z, Caruso JL, Herndon J, Patz EF Jr. Cytologically proved malignant pleural effusions: distribution of transudates and exudates. Chest 1998;113:1302–4.
95. Libshitz HI. Radiation changes in the lung. Semin Roentgenol 1993;28:303–32.
96. Morelock SY, Sahn SA. Drugs and the pleura. Chest 1999;116:212–21.
97. Light RW. Clinical practice. Pleural effusion. N Engl J Med 2002;346:1971–7.
98. Light RW, Erozan YS, Ball WC Jr. Cells in pleural fluid. Their value in differential diagnosis. Arch Intern Med 1973;132:854–60.
99. Prakash UB, Reiman HM. Comparison of needle biopsy with cytologic analysis for the evaluation of pleural effusion: analysis of 414 cases. Mayo Clin Proc 1985;60:158–64.
100. Heffner JE. Indications for draining a parapneumonic effusion: an evidence-based approach. Semin Respir Infect 1999;14:48–58.
101. Viallat JR, Rey F, Astoul P, Boutin C. Thoracoscopic talc poudrage pleurodesis for malignant effusions. A review of 360 cases. Chest 1996;110:1387–93.
102. de Campos JR, Vargas FS, de Campos Werebe E, et al. Thoracoscopy talc poudrage: a 15-year experience. Chest 2001;119:801–6.
103. Putnam JB Jr, Walsh GL, Swisher SG, et al. Outpatient management of malignant pleural effusion by a chronic indwelling pleural catheter. Ann Thorac Surg 2000;69:369–75.
104. Price KS, Castells MC. Taxol reactions. Allergy Asthma Proc 2002;23:205–8.
105. Sheski FD, Mathur PN. Long-term results of fiberoptic bronchoscopic balloon dilation in the management of benign tracheobronchial stenosis. Chest 1998;114:796–800.
106. Colt HG, Dumon JF. Airway stents. Present and future. Clin Chest Med 1995;16:465–78.
107. Morice RC, Ece T, Ece F, Keus L. Endobronchial argon plasma coagulation for treatment of hemoptysis and neoplastic airway obstruction. Chest 2001;119:781–7.
108. Walsh DA, Maiwand MO, Nath AR, et al. Bronchoscopic cryotherapy for advanced bronchial carcinoma. Thorax 1990;45:509–13.
109. Chella A, Ambrogi MC, Ribechini A, et al. Combined Nd-YAG laser/HDR brachytherapy versus Nd-YAG laser only in malignant central airway involvement: a prospective randomized study. Lung Cancer 2000;27:169–75.
110. Despars JA, Sassoon CS, Light RW. Significance of iatrogenic pneumothoraces. Chest 1994;105:1147–50.
111. Leeser JE, Carr D. Fatal pneumothorax following bleomycin and other cytotoxic drugs. Cancer Treat Rep 1985;69:344–5.
112. Wilson KS, Brigden ML, Alexander S, Worth A. Fatal pneumothorax in "BCNU lung." Med Pediatr Oncol 1982;10:195–9.
113. Tocino IM, Miller MH, Fairfax WR. Distribution of pneumothorax in the supine and semirecumbent critically ill adult. AJR Am J Roentgenol 1985;144:901–5.
114. Baumann MH, Strange C, Heffner JE, et al. Management of spontaneous pneumothorax: an American College of Chest Physicians Delphi consensus statement. Chest 2001;119:590–602.
115. Baumann MH. Treatment of spontaneous pneumothorax. Curr Opin Pulm Med 2000;6:275–80.
116. Bick RL, Haas SK. International consensus recommendations. Summary statement and additional suggested guidelines. European Consensus Conference November 1991. American College of Chest Physicians consensus statement of 1995. International Consensus Statement, 1997. Med Clin North Am 1998;82:613–33.
117. Levitan N, Dowlati A, Remick SC, et al. Rates of initial and recurrent thromboembolic disease among patients with malignancy versus those without malignancy. Risk analysis using Medicare claims data. Medicine (Baltimore) 1999;78:285–91.
118. Hirsh JD, Hull RD. Pathogenesis of venous thromboembolism and clinical risk factors. In: Venous thromboembolism: natural history, diagnosis and management. Boca Raton, FL: CRC Press; 1987. p. 5–16.
119. The PIOPED Investigators. Value of the ventilation/perfusion scan in acute pulmonary embolism. Results of the prospective investigation of pulmonary embolism diagnosis (PIOPED). JAMA 1990;263:2753–9.
120. Stein PD, Saltzman HA, Weg JG. Clinical characteristics of patients with acute pulmonary embolism. Am J Cardiol 1991;68:1723–4.
121. Davidson BL, Elliott CG, Lensing AW. Low accuracy of color Doppler ultrasound in the detection of proximal leg vein thrombosis in asymptomatic high-risk patients. The RD Heparin Arthroplasty Group. Ann Intern Med 1992;117:735–8.
122. Hull RD, Raskob GE, Coates G, Panju AA. Clinical validity of a normal perfusion lung scan in patients with suspected pulmonary embolism. Chest 1990;97:23–6.
123. Oudkerk M, van Beek EJ, Wielopolski P, et al. Comparison of contrast-enhanced magnetic resonance angiography and conventional pulmonary angiography for the diagnosis of pulmonary embolism: a prospective study. Lancet 2002;359:1643–7.
124. Herold CJ. Spiral computed tomography of pulmonary embolism. Eur Respir J Suppl 2002:35:13s–21s.
125. Tillie-Leblond I, Mastora I, Radenne F, et al. Risk of pulmonary embolism after a negative spiral CT angiogram in patients with pulmonary disease: 1-year clinical follow-up study. Radiology 2002;223:461–7.
126. Sostman HD, Layish DT, Tapson VF, et al. Prospective comparison of helical CT and MR imaging in clinically suspected acute pulmonary embolism. J Magn Reson Imaging 1996;6:275–81.
127. Hirsh J. Heparin. N Engl J Med 1991;324:1565–74.
128. The Columbus Investigators. Low-molecular-weight heparin in the treatment of patients with venous thromboembolism. N Engl J Med 1997;337:657–62.
129. Simonneau G, Sors H, Charbonnier B, et al. A comparison of low-molecular-weight heparin with unfractionated heparin for acute pulmonary embolism. The THESEE Study Group. Tinzaparine ou heparine standard: evaluations dans l'embolie pulmonaire. N Engl J Med 1997;337:663–9.
130. Schulman S, Granqvist S, Holmstrom M, et al. The duration of oral anticoagulant therapy after a second episode of venous thromboembolism. The Duration of Anticoagulation Trial Study Group. N Engl J Med 1997;336:393–8.
131. Lee AY, Levine MN, Baker RI, et al. Low-molecular-weight heparin versus a coumarin for the prevention of recurrent venous thromboembolism in patients with cancer. N Engl J Med 2003;349:146–53.
132. Dalen JE, Alpert JS, Hirsch J. Thrombolytic therapy for pulmonary embolism: is it effective? Is it safe? When is it indicated? Arch Intern Med 1997;157:2550–6.
133. Thrombolytic therapy in treatment: summary of an NIH consensus conference. Br Med J 1980;280:1585–7.
134. Goldhaber SZ, Haire WD, Feldstein ML, et al. Alteplase versus heparin in acute pulmonary embolism: randomised trial assessing right-ventricular function and pulmonary perfusion. Lancet 1993;341:507–11.
135. Marder VJ. Thrombolytic therapy: overview of results in major vascular occlusions. Thromb Haemost 1995;74:101–5.
136. Goldhaber SZ. Thrombolysis in pulmonary embolism: a debatable indication. Thromb Haemost 2001;86:444–51.
137. Byrne TN. Metastatic epidural cord compression. Curr Neurol Neurosci Rep, 2004;4:191–5.
138. Hainline B, Tuszynski MH, Posner JB. Ataxia in epidural spinal cord compression. Neurology 1992;42:2193–5.
139. Greenberg HS, Kim JH, Posner JB. Epidural spinal cord compression from metastatic tumor: results with a new treatment protocol. Ann Neurol 1980;8:361–6.
140. Vecht CJ, Haaxma-Reiche H, van Putten WL, et al. Initial bolus of conventional versus high-dose dexamethasone in metastatic spinal cord compression. Neurology 1989;39:1255–7.
141. Heimdal K, Hirschberg H, Slettebo H, et al. High incidence of serious side effects of high-dose dexamethasone treatment in patients with epidural spinal cord compression. J Neurooncol 1992;12:141–4.
142. Weissman DE. Glucocorticoid treatment for brain metastases and epidural spinal cord compression: a review. J Clin Oncol 1988;6:543–51.
143. Manzullo EF, Elting L, Forman A. Etiology and outcome of seizures in cancer patients. Proc Am Soc Clin Oncol 1994;13:466.
144. Roth HL, Drislane FW. Seizures. Neurol Clin 1998;16:257–84.
145. Kasakura Y, Ajani JA, Mochizuki F,. Outcomes after emergency surgery for gastric perforation or severe bleeding in patients with gastric cancer. J Surg Oncol 2002;80:181–5.
146. Yokota T, Yamada Y, Murakami Y, et al. Abdominal crisis caused by perforation of ileal lymphoma. Am J Emerg Med 2002;20:136–7.
147. Suzaki N, Hiraki A, Ueoka H, et al. Gastric perforation due to metastasis from adenocarcinoma of the lung. Anticancer Res 2002;22:1209–12.
148. Ramirez PT, Levenback C, Burke TW, et al. Sigmoid perforation following radiation therapy in patients with cervical cancer. Gynecol Oncol 2001;82:150–5.
149. Meloni MF, Goldberg SN, Moser V, et al. Colonic perforation and abscess following radiofrequency ablation treatment of hepatoma. Eur J Ultrasound 2002;15:73–6.
150. Bavaro MF. Neutropenic enterocolitis. Curr Gastroenterol Rep 2002;4:297–301.
151. Levine MS. Plain film diagnosis of the acute abdomen. Emerg Med Clin North Am 1985;3:541–62.
152. Miller RE, Nelson SW. The roentgenologic demonstration of tiny amounts of free intraperitoneal gas: experimental and clinical studies. Am J Roentgenol Radium Ther Nucl Med 1971;112:574–85.
153. Schlatter M, Snyder K, Freyer D. Successful nonoperative management of typhlitis in pediatric oncology patients. J Pediatr Surg 2002;37:1151–5.

154. Boey J, Choi SK, Poon A, Alagaratnam TT. Risk stratification in perforated duodenal ulcers. A prospective validation of predictive factors. Ann Surg 1987;205:22–6.
155. Bodey GP, Buckley M, Sathe YS, Freireich EJ. Quantitative relationships between circulating leukocytes and infection in patients with acute leukemia. Ann Intern Med 1966;64:328–40.
156. Rubin M, Hathorn JW, Pizzo PA. Controversies in the management of febrile neutropenic cancer patients. Cancer Invest 1988;6:167–84.
157. Kern WV. Risk assessment and risk-based therapeutic strategies in febrile neutropenia. Curr Opin Infect Dis 2001;14:415–22.
158. Paesmans M. Risk factors assessment in febrile neutropenia. Int J Antimicrob Agents 2000;16:107–11.
159. Kern WV. Modifications of therapy. Int J Antimicrob Agents 2000;16:139–41.
160. Donowitz GR, Harman C, Pope T, Stewart FM. The role of the chest roentgenogram in febrile neutropenic patients. Arch Intern Med 1991;151:701–4.
161. Donowitz GR. Fever in the compromised host. Infect Dis Clin North Am 1996;10:129–48.
162. Bille J. Laboratory diagnosis of infections in febrile neutropenic or immunocompromised patients. Int J Antimicrob Agents 2000;16:87–9.
163. Zinner SH. New pathogens in neutropenic patients with cancer: an update for the new millennium. Int J Antimicrob Agents 2000;16:97–101.
164. Bodey GP, Rolston KV. Management of fever in neutropenic patients. J Infect Chemother 2001;7:1–9.
165. Hughes WT, Armstrong D, Bodey GP, et al. 2002 guidelines for the use of antimicrobial agents in neutropenic patients with cancer. Clin Infect Dis 2002;34:730–51.
166. Papadimitris C, Dimopoulos MA, Kostis E, et al. Outpatient treatment of neutropenic fever with oral antibiotics and granulocyte colony-stimulating factor. Oncology 1999;57:127–30.
167. Nemunaitis J, Buckner CD, Dorsey KS, et al. Retrospective analysis of infectious disease in patients who received recombinant human granulocyte–macrophage colony-stimulating factor versus patients not receiving a cytokine who underwent autologous bone marrow transplantation for treatment of lymphoid cancer. Am J Clin Oncol 1998;21:341–6.
168. Smith PL, Kagey-Sobotka A, Bleecker ER, et al. Physiologic manifestations of human anaphylaxis. J Clin Invest 1980;66:1072–80.
169. Murrant T, Bihari D. Anaphylaxis and anaphylactoid reactions. Int J Clin Pract 2000;54:322–8.
170. Gavalas M, Sadana A, Metcalf S. Guidelines for the management of anaphylaxis in the emergency department. J Accid Emerg Med 1998;15:96–8.
171. Brown AF. Anaphylactic shock: mechanisms and treatment [see comments]. J Accid Emerg Med 1995;12:89–100.
172. Dellinger CT, Miale TD. Comparison of anaphylactic reactions to asparaginase derived from *Escherichia coli* and from *Erwinia* cultures. Cancer 1976;38:1843–6.
173. Jones B, Holland JF, Glidewell O, et al. Optimal use of L-asparaginase (NSC-109229) in acute lymphocytic leukemia. Med Pediatr Oncol 1977;3:387–400.
174. Holle LM. Pegaspargase: an alternative? Ann Pharmacother 1997;31:616–24.
175. Oettgen HF, Stephenson PA, Schwartz MK, et al. Toxicity of *E. coli* L-asparaginase in man. Cancer 1970;25:253–78.
176. Nesbit M, Chard R, Evans A, et al. Evaluation of intramuscular versus intravenous administration of L-asparaginase in childhood leukemia. Am J Pediatr Hematol Oncol 1979;1:9–13.
177. Peterson RG, Handschumacher RE, Mitchell MS. Immunological responses to L-asparaginase. J Clin Invest 1971;50:1080–90.
178. Capizzi RL, Bertino JR, Skeel RT, et al. L-Asparaginase: clinical, biochemical, pharmacological, and immunological studies. Ann Intern Med 1971;74:893–901.
179. Weiss RB, Donehower RC, Wiernik PH, et al. Hypersensitivity reactions from Taxol. J Clin Oncol 1990;8:1263–8.
180. Rowinsky EK, Eisenhauer EA, Chaudhry V, et al. Clinical toxicities encountered with paclitaxel (Taxol). Semin Oncol 1993;20:1–15.
181. Peereboom DM, Donehower RC, Eisenhauer EA, et al. Successful re-treatment with Taxol after major hypersensitivity reactions [see comments]. J Clin Oncol 1993;11:885–90.
182. Seidman AD, Hochhauser D, Gollub M, et al. Ninety-six-hour paclitaxel infusion after progression during short taxane exposure: a phase II pharmacokinetic and pharmacodynamic study in metastatic breast cancer. J Clin Oncol 1996;14:1877–84.
183. Greco FA, Thomas M, Hainsworth JD. One-hour paclitaxel infusions: review of safety and efficacy. Cancer J Sci Am 1999;5:179–91.
184. O'Dwyer PJ, King SA, Fortner CL, Leyland-Jones B. Hypersensitivity reactions to teniposide (VM-26): an analysis. J Clin Oncol 1986;4:1262–9.
185. de Souza P, Friedlander M, Wilde C, et al. Hypersensitivity reactions to etoposide. A report of three cases and review of the literature. Am J Clin Oncol 1994;17:387–9.
186. Kellie SJ, Crist WM, Pui CH, et al. Hypersensitivity reactions to epipodophyllotoxins in children with acute lymphoblastic leukemia. Cancer 1991;67:1070–5.
187. Cersosimo RJ, Calarese P, Karp DD. Acute hypotensive reaction to etoposide with successful rechallenge: case report and review of the literature. DICP 1989;23:876–7.
188. Habibi B, Lopez M, Serdaru M, et al. Immune hemolytic anemia and renal failure due to teniposide. N Engl J Med 1982;306:1091–3.
189. Glovsky MM, Braunwald J, Opelz G, Alenty A. Hypersensitivity to procarbazine associated with angioedema, urticaria, and low serum complement activity. J Allergy Clin Immunol 1976;57:134–140.
190. Brooks BJ Jr, Hendler NB, Alvarez S, et al. Delayed life-threatening pneumonitis secondary to procarbazine. Am J Clin Oncol 1990;13:244–6.
191. Getaz EP, Beckley S, Fitzpatrick J, Dozier A. Cisplatin-induced hemolysis. N Engl J Med 1980;302:334–5.
192. Cheng E, Cvitkovic E, Wittes RE, Golbey RB. Germ cell tumors (II): VAB II in metastatic testicular cancer. Cancer 1978;42:2162–8.
193. Blumenreich MS, Needles B, Yagoda A, et al. Intravesical cisplatin for superficial bladder tumors. Cancer 1982;50:863–5.
194. Markman M, Kennedy A, Webster K, et al. Clinical features of hypersensitivity reactions to carboplatin. J Clin Oncol 1999;17:1141.
195. Khan A, Hill JM, Grater W, et al. Atopic hypersensitivity to *cis*-dichlorodiammineplatinum(II) and other platinum complexes. Cancer Res 1975;35:2766–70.
196. Weiss RB. Hypersensitivity reactions. Semin Oncol 1992;19:458–77.
197. Jones JB, Purdy CY, Bailey RT. Cyclophosphamide anaphylaxis. DICP 1989;23:88–9.
198. Legha SS, Hall S. Acute cyclophosphamide hypersensitivity reaction: possible lack of cross-sensitivity to mechlorethamine and isophosphamide. Cancer Treat Rep 1978;62:180–1.
199. Lakin JD, Cahill RA. Generalized urticaria to cyclophosphamide: type I hypersensitivity to an immunosuppressive agent. J Allergy Clin Immunol 1976;58:160–71.
200. Solimando DA, Wilson JP. Doxorubicin-induced hypersensitivity reactions. Drug Intell Clin Pharm 1984;18:808–11.
201. Crawford ED, McKenzie D, Mansson W, et al. Adverse reactions to the intravesical administration of doxorubicin hydrochloride: report of 6 cases. J Urol 1986;136:668–9.
202. Cornwell GG, Pajak TF, McIntyre OR. Hypersensitivity reactions to IV melphalan during treatment of multiple myeloma: Cancer and Leukemia Group B experience. Cancer Treat Rep 1979;63:399–403.
203. Hitchins RN, Hocker GA, Thomson DB. Chlorambucil allergy—a series of three cases. Aust N Z J Med, 1987;17:600–2.
204. Peterman A, Braunstein B. Cutaneous reaction to chlorambucil therapy. Arch Dermatol 1986;122:1358–60.
205. Barone C, Cassano A, Astone A. Toxic epidermal necrolysis during chlorambucil therapy in chronic lymphocytic leukaemia. Eur J Cancer 1990;26:1262.
206. Thompson-Moya L, Martin T, Heuft HG, et al. Allergic reaction with immune hemolytic anemia resulting from chlorambucil. Am J Hematol 1989;32:230–1.
207. Crestani B, Jaccard A, Israel-Biet D, et al. Chlorambucil-associated pneumonitis. Chest 1994;105:634–6.
208. Sridhar KS. Allergic reaction to 5-fluorouracil infusion. Cancer 1986;58:862–4.
209. Posada JG, O'Dwyer PJ, Hoth DF. Anaphylactic reactions to diaziquone. Cancer Treat Rep 1984;68:1215–17.
210. Blum RH, Carter SK, Agre KA. Clinical review of bleomycin—a new antineoplastic agent. Cancer 1973;31:903–14.
211. Levy RL. Chiarillo S. Hyperpyrexia, allergic-type response and death occurring with low-dose bleomycin administration. Oncology 1980;37:316–7.
212. Levett M, Row M, Yeung SC. Miscellaneous oncologic emergencies. In: Yeung SC, Escalante CP, editors. Oncologic emergencies. Hamilton. ON: BC Decker; 2002. p. 441–55.
213. Albanell J, Baselga J. Systemic therapy emergencies. Semin Oncol 2000;27:347–61.
214. Vial T, Descotes J. Immune-mediated side-effects of cytokines in humans. Toxicology 1995;105:31–57.
215. Jones TH, Wadler S, Hupart KH. Endocrine-mediated mechanisms of fatigue during treatment with interferon-alpha. Semin Oncol 1998;25:54–63.
216. Schwartzentruber DJ. Guidelines for the safe administration of high-dose interleukin-2. J Immunother 2001;24:287–93.
217. Leget GA, Czuczman MS. Use of rituximab, the new FDA-approved antibody. Curr Opin Oncol 1998;10:548–51.
218. Stern DF. Tyrosine kinase signalling in breast cancer: ErbB family receptor tyrosine kinases. Breast Cancer Res 2000;2:176–83.
219. Bernstein ID. Monoclonal antibodies to the myeloid stem cells: therapeutic implications of CMA-676, a humanized anti-CD33 antibody calicheamicin conjugate. Leukemia 2000;14:474–5.
220. Gemtuzumab for relapsed acute myeloid leukemia. Med Lett Drugs Ther 2000;42:67–8.
221. Sievers EL, Appelbaum FR, Spielberger RT, et al. Selective ablation of acute myeloid leukemia using antibody-targeted chemotherapy: a phase I study of an anti-CD33 calicheamicin immunoconjugate. Blood 1999;93:3678–84.
222. Olsen E, Duvic M, Frankel A, et al. Pivotal phase III trial of two dose levels of denileukin diftitox for the treatment of cutaneous T-cell lymphoma. J Clin Oncol 2001;19:376–88.
223. Piascik P. FDA approves fusion protein for treatment of lymphoma. J Am Pharm Assoc (Wash) 1999;39:571–2.

Section 41
ONCOLOGY AND INFORMATICS

143

Oncology Informatics

Edward P. Ambinder, MD

HEALTH CARE POLICY AND INFORMATION TECHNOLOGY

As oncologists, we are experiencing unprecedented challenges to our research and therapeutic and practice management skills brought on by the necessity to manage the geometric increase in medical information and the striking changes in the clinical practice of oncology. The clinical oncologist must be a clinician, researcher, educator, businessperson, statistician, health care administrator, and informatician, who must interact with the whole patient, both as a specialist and as a primary-care physician. These skills must be assimilated into our daily clinical practice and research activities, while we continue to improve our quality for a much more sophisticated consumer and payer.

Information management has become the most frustrating aspect of our professional life. Cancer patients receive intricate multimodality therapies for their complex diseases, requiring greater access to, and tracking of, detailed medical data. Disease management clinical guidelines for cancer patients require micromanagement and economic awareness of patient care.[1] Clinical trials, which demand intense documentation, must not only show progression free and overall survival benefits, but now must also display cost effectiveness and patient satisfaction.[2,3]

The digitalization of information, the ability to network or connect computers, and the rapid electronic interchange of information on a worldwide basis are recognized as the hallmark of a new order in society (Figure 143-1). For oncologists to master these profound changes, it is necessary to embrace the medical tools of the Information Age. These tools include the computer, which acts as the information gateway and integrator, the Internet, which coordinates interactive information resources and personal communication, and the electronic medical record, which is the translator and repository of our clinical information gathering. Information technology and personal computers have transformed every other profession and are now revolutionizing medicine as well.

Our chaotic health care system continues to confound our nation with inadequate funding for clinical care, research, and teaching; continued dominance of managed care's flawed concepts; decreased reimbursements, especially for chemotherapy administration; a panoply of health care players with vested interests; and severe underuse of information technology. Despite all the money invested in research, little is used for the more prosaic technology needed for gathering, analyzing, and making use of the data collected. Oncologists remain uncomfortable with the nexus of technology and medicine. We are taught by observation and textbooks and by using our diagnostic skills with continued reliance on memory and experience.

Several recent influential groups, including the Institute of Medicine,[4–6] the President's Information Technology Advisory Committee,[7] and the President's Cancer Council,[8] have released assessments of our health care system that highlight its many inadequacies and the need to apply advances in information technology to improve administrative and clinical processes. The reports criticized the variation of cancer treatments by locale, the lack of using guidelines and care plans based on best available evidence, the absence of tools to measure and monitor quality of care using core sets of quality measures or an electronic medical record, and poor patient accrual to quality clinical trials. They also found major impediments for cancer patients to obtain compassionate psychosocial and palliative care. They stress the absence of any progress in restructuring health care to address both quality and cost concerns. Despite 10,000 clinical trials that are conducted annually that provide many medical advances, we do not efficiently translate this knowledge gained from research and development into routine clinical care, sometimes taking 15 to 20 years, and even then its adoption into routine clinical practice remains uneven. There is a convincing need for our health care system to methodically collect, analyze, and deliver medical evidence to physicians and patients.

Health care consumerism is an increasing fact of life that is fueled by the Internet and our economic prosperity. It is driven by individual autonomy; skepticism of the professional, governmental, managed care; and corporate dominance in health care, the women's health movement, complementary medicine, informed consent, increased malpractice litigation, Internet consumer information, consumer-directed drug advertisements, patient support groups, and patient-directed lab and procedure ordering. Consumers usually do not understand health care quality and true cost; however, and they cannot easily navigate the complex health care system. Consumers are always better served when they navigate the complex health care system with physician assistance.

The delivery of patient care in the United States is disjointed, especially when considering the mobile society, patients who change practitioners and health plans every 3 years on average, the absence of any coordination of the patient's longitudinal medical record, and the lip service given to screening and prevention of disease. Health care delivery automation, with the exceptions of practice management, results reporting and financial software, is shamelessly underused despite the nonmedical world's rapid acceptance of the tools of the Information Age. Similar changes will occur in health care delivery as computerization, electronic medical records, and the Internet permeate our profession. Although the delivery of oncology care is plodding along, there has been a spectacular increase in the knowledge base of oncology. Merging recent innovations in computerization and biomedical technologies,

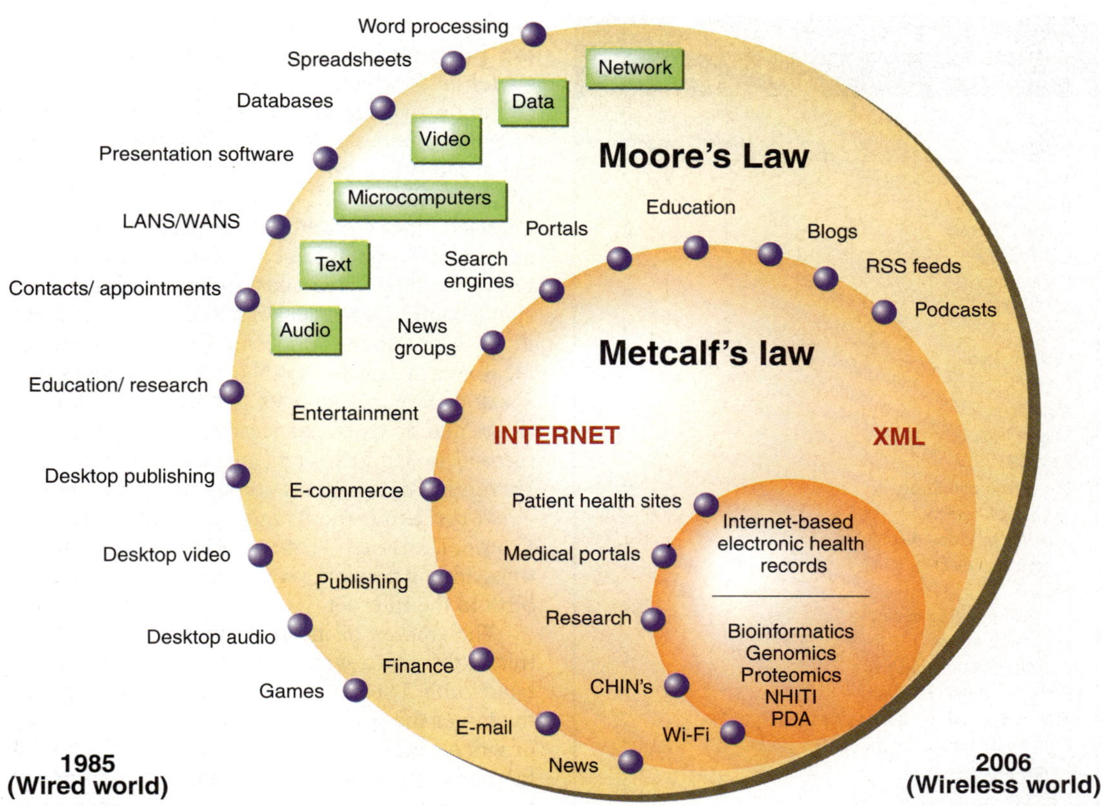

Figure 143-1 The digitalization of medicine 1985–2005. This figure depicts the swift chronologic evolution of the oncologist's personal, professional, and oncologic uses of information technology from 1985 through 2005 using the unprecedented improvements in computer hardware as predicted by Moore's law and the rapid increases in networking communication efficiency as predicted by Metcalf's law. CHIN = community health information networks; NANS = neighborhood area network system; NHITI = National Healthcare Information Technology Initiative; RSS = Really Simple Syndication; XML = Extensible Markup Language.

scientists have deciphered the human genome. Soon we may be able to inexpensively determine for each individual which of their 30,000 genes are missing, damaged, or overworking.[9] Medical illnesses and treatments will be discussed in relation to their genomic, genetic, proteomic, and polymorphism findings. Our medical system will be forced to put a greater emphasis on personal cancer prevention, health-risk appraisals, and predictive oncology based on a patient's genetic data. This may translate into lower health care costs through earlier detection of cancer.

If our health care system is to thrive in a rapidly changing medical universe, all the participants—providers, patients, administrators, researchers, educators, payers, industry, and the government—must understand the laws of the Information Age. By combining the huge cost-saving potential of computerization and Internet telecommunication, technology will provide a logical framework for health care.

With secured and confidential electronic medical records and the acceptance of community health information networks (CHINs) that electronically link, on a regional basis, all patients, practitioners, payers, hospitals, benefit managers, commercial laboratories, and drug stores, our health care system could become more cost-effective and efficient. Building on fundamental strengths and with a common spirit of compromise and sharing, we could look forward to a health care system that maintains its world leadership in the production of clinical and basic science oncologic research, and strives to achieve equivalent excellence in the delivery of oncologic health care and the oncologic education of health care providers and patients.

MEDICAL AND ONCOLOGIC INFORMATICS

Health care is an information-based science involving the gathering, synthesis, and implementation of information. Medical informatics is concerned with managing and using information in biomedicine and health care that is patient-specific (ie, electronic medical records [EMR]) and knowledge-based (ie, information retrieval and decision support tools). Medical informatics uses information science and its technologies to deal with the "cognitive, information processing and communication tasks of medical practice, education, and research."[10] Medical oncology, with its strong emphasis on data collection and analysis, is positioned at the forefront of clinical trials requiring quantitative methods to record clinical signs, symptoms, toxicity, and outcome. In its training programs, and carried over into clinical practice by its trainees, there is a heavy emphasis on research protocols requiring a time-oriented tabular flow sheet format that is ideal for computerization. Increasing documentation for cooperative groups, government bodies, insurance companies, pharmaceutical houses, and institutional review boards demands computerized records. Health care costs have escalated dramatically, particularly for cancer patients, who require complex diagnostic and therapeutic procedures, making them a prime target for cost-containment efforts by third-party payers and the federal government. Today, the computer is our most efficient tool for obtaining timely information. It has also become our most effective decision-making tool. The computer has become an integrated information device that has merged printers, scanners, facsimile machines (faxes), copiers, telephones, video and audio systems, and filing cabinets. Interested readers are referred to Shortliffe and Perreault for a comprehensive review of this field.[11]

As oncologists become more comfortable with computers and the electronic distribution of computer-based information, and as patients take more responsibility for their medical decisions, health care will use online computer-assisted communication among patients, medical databases, and physicians to replace a considerable part of the care now given in person.[12] Today's machines address the handling of data analysis by using intuitive interfaces. In the future, computers more nearly will simulate the "whole-person paradigm," whereby data can be input by voice, pointing, writing, or gestures, and different languages can be freely translated.

To understand how the decreasing cost and increasing efficiency of processing, storing, and transmitting information have changed more rapidly than any prior human endeavor, it is necessary to be familiar with the three basic laws that have governed the Information Age. Continuing unabated since 1950, Gordon Moore's law states that the performance of semiconductor technology, as exemplified by microprocessor chips where data are stored and manipulated, will double every 18 months while the cost of an equivalent computer will halve. As demonstrated by the Internet, Bob Metcalfe's law states that the power of a network rises by the square of the number of terminals attached to it. Finally, the law of the telecosm, as formulated by George Gilder, combines Metcalfe's law with Moore's law of the microcosm.[13] It ordains that the cost-effectiveness of computer terminals will rise by the square of the number of additional transistors integrated on a single chip. Amplified by the law of the microcosm, the law of the telecosm signifies a rise in the cost-effectiveness of a network in proportion to the resources deployed on it and the number of potential nodes and routers (connectors) available to it. In the 50 years since the development of ENIAC (Electronic Numerical Integrator and Computer), the first electronic computer, the efficiency of information technology has increased 100 octillion times.

OVERVIEW OF COMPUTERS

Computer Hardware and Software A computer receives information from the keyboard or mouse (input devices), stores it in its logic board (central processor) or hard disk (storage medium), manipulates the information in its logic board, and delivers it through its monitor (output device). The electronic currency of the computer is the electric signal, and it is based on binary mathematics: something is either positive or negative, 1 or 0, on or off, yes or no, black or white. In contrast, our numbering system relies on a base of 10 with 10 numbers (1 to 9 and 0) and is called the decimal system. Computers store information in "bits" (binary digits), which are defined as the smallest units of information. A bit can represent one of two states: 1 (on) or 0 (off). A bit can also represent a dot on a monitor screen (pixel), which is either turned on or turned off to represent black or white. Eight bits make a "byte" that can represent any of 256 values because its 8 bits can be on or off in 256 different combinations. Bytes can be used to represent a letter, number, symbol, or a horizontal row of eight pixels on a monitor as displayed in a paint or drawing program, or used as an aid for counting or summing. Finally, a byte can represent a code to tell the machine what to do, such as insert a carriage return or tab. A "word" is defined as a sequence of bits that can be assessed as a unit by the computer. Current computers can work with 4 bytes (32 bits) or 8 bytes (64 bits) of information at one time. The central processing unit (CPU) is the conductor of the computer that processes information. Its size determines the computer's speed and the amount of information that it can handle. Output devices deliver information to the user or to other computers and include the television screen or monitor, printer, modem (used to interface with the telephone or cable system), film processors, video recorders, or musical instruments. Storage devices, which include floppy disk drives, hard disk drives, tape drives, compact disk—read or write (CD), and digital video disk—read or write (DVD), keep programs and documents in permanent or transient memory. The user can enter data into the computer by writing, marking, typing, pointing, speaking, or using a direct link. Input devices, which accept information, can take audio, video, photographic, xerographic, radiographic, typographic, telephonic, or fax data and put the data in digital form for the computer's central processor to assimilate. Digital information is then transmitted to output devices that can display the information. Table 143-1 lists these devices. The computer itself, its electronic components, and the attached input/output and storage devices make up computer hardware. Software constitutes the instructions that tell the computer what to do. It is stored on disk media and read into random access memory (RAM) when needed for a particular application. Documents are words, numbers, or pictures created by the user. Table 143-2 summarizes the common types of software applications of interest to the oncologist.

Table 143-1 Input and Output Devices for the Computer

Device	Input Device	Output Device
35mm slides projector	*	*
Barcode reader	*	
Cellular Phone	*	*
CD-ROM	*	*
Digital Pen	*	
DVD-ROM	*	*
Fax	*	*
Graphic Pad	*	
Joystick	*	
Keyboard	*	
Microphone	*	
Keypad	*	
Music sound editing (MIDI, MP3)	*	*
Monitor or video display terminal (VDT)		*
Mouse	*	
Medical imaging devices	*	*
Other computers	*	*
Overhead projection pads		*
Personal video recorder	*	*
PDA (personal digital assistant)	*	*
Printer (laser, dot matrix, or ink-jet)		*
Plotters		*
Radio	*	*
Scanner	*	
Storage device (disk or tape)	*	*
Tape recorder	*	*
Telephone	*	*
Television	*	*
Touch screen	*	
Trackball (stationary mouse)	*	
Track pad (stationary mouse)	*	
Video, still camera	*	*
Video recorder	*	*

Personal Digital Assistants Personal digital assistants (PDAs) are hand-held devices that combine portability, computer processing power, pen-based interaction, and handwriting recognition. They also include personal organization programs, such as schedulers, calculators, reminder lists, address files, financial and travel tools, document and information retrieval capability, and wired and wireless communication by phone, modem, fax, or beeper. These devices can synchronize data with desktop computers and can use cellular modems for information updating and retrieval over the Internet to update all programs and databases. The oncologist uses these instruments to hold personal, financial, and patient medical data. Recently, all-in-one devices incorporating PDAs with cell phones, instant messaging, Web access, beepers, and digital and video cameras have become available, simplifying the oncologist's mobile communication needs. According to a recent American Society of Clinical Oncology survey, between 70 and 80% of members own and use PDAs.[14] An updated list of PDA programs generated from the survey is provided in Table 143-3.

Networks Networks allow one computer to talk to another computer, permitting electronic mail, exchanging files, sharing printers, telephony, videoconferencing, and accessing the Internet. For an orderly exchange of information to take place, office and home-based networks use the Ethernet protocol that combines "packet switching," which breaks data up into chunks containing an identifying address, and a single wire that broadcasts the same message to all computer addresses, but only the computer with the correct address will pick out the information intended for it. Currently, Ethernet communicates at up to 100 gigabits per second. As telephone-type wire supplanted coaxial cable and hub-and-spoke configurations proliferated, computer users in close proximity connected their computers to local area networks (LANs). For computers that speak different languages to communicate, even if situated at vast distances from one another, a method to send files and messages was needed. By routing data packets among different types of networks using the Transport Communication Protocol/Internet Protocol (TCP/IP), multiple links among networks were created, and this gave birth to the Internet.

The amount of information that can be transmitted through a wire is determined by the wire's bandwidth. The higher the number of messages or the larger the packet of information (ie, graphics or video), the slower is the network. Today, hospital networks that carry images of computed tomography (CT) scans, pathology pictures, or videoconferences, must have broader bandwidths that can carry data at a rate of 10 million bits per second with fast Ethernet. Packets can be any digital medium, such as voice, data, or video.

Because oncologists are always on the go, wireless communication and mobile PDAs have become indispensable tools. Desktop programs can now seamlessly link to the Internet and PDAs, providing selective information that is always available. As processing power and storage capabilities increase geometrically, any information available from computers or the Internet can be handled by these mobile devices. Recently, two inexpensive wireless protocols that facilitate wireless communications by defining protocols for security and authorization, and hardware and software designs, have become popular. The Bluetooth standard defines protocols for short-range communications between electronic devices; and the IEEE 802.11 or Wi-Fi (Wireless Fidelity) protocol defines a wireless local area network up to 1,500 feet per node, which permits access to the Internet at many public and corporate spaces at speeds up to 54 megabits per second in the 2.4 G Hz band. In the near future, a new technology named "Wimax" will become available, positioned as a wide-area version of Wi-Fi having a maximum range of 30 miles. Innovative individuals have been connecting 802.11 nodes building by building to create a free wireless network (NAN, neighborhood area network or nanny network) to the Internet for everyone.

INTERNET

World Wide Web No recent phenomenon has captured the world's and, in particular, the

Table 143-2 Medical Uses of the Computer

Medical uses of the computer	Examples	
Communications	Bulletin boards	Electronic mail
	Bibliographic databases	Electronic forums
	Voice mail	
Database management system		
Medical records	Admission/Discharges	Tumor registry
	Demographic information	Pain management tools
	Insurance eligibility	Protocol management
	Office records	Links to hospital databases
	Hospital records	Scheduling tests
	Bedside terminals	Cumulative drug dosing
	Patient monitoring	Orders
	Patient education/reminders	Blood products: history, matching, use
	Patient allergies	Flow sheets
	Body-surface-area calculation	Laboratory data
	Graphic data representation	Patient summaries
	Image analysis	Specialty encounters
	Integrated patient care plans	Malpractice documentation
	Clinical research protocols	Legal documentation
	Census reports	
Pharmacology Management	Drug–drug interactions	Drug monitoring
	Patient drug list	Antibiotic screening
	Drug ordering	
Clinical decision support	Artificial intelligence	Computer-aided treatment
	Natural language processing	Medical decision making
	Computer-aided diagnosis	Consultation
Laboratory monitoring	Control and data analysis	
	Physiologic monitoring	
Management systems	Practice management	Resource management
	Quality assurance	Usage review
Office Management	Electronic banking	Financial management
	Electronic billing	Inventory
	Accounts payable	Return visit reminders
	Accounts receivable	Patient schedules
	Financial analysis	Physician schedules
Graphics	Painting or bit-mapped	Drawing or vector-based or object-based
Image processing	Radiographic images	Pathologic images
	Radiation planning	
Presentation	Slides	Overhead projection pads
	Handouts	
	Television projection systems	
Scanning	Documents	Optical character recognition
	Graphics	
Statistics	Analysis of variance	Multivariate analysis
	Cluster analysis	Nonparametric tests
	Contingency tables	Path/latent variable analysis
	Correlation	
	Data handling	Regression
	Graphics	Reliability/test item analysis
	Linear programming	Survival analysis
Spreadsheets		
Word processing		
Publishing	Electronic textbooks	Electronic journals
Project Management		
Programming		
Grant proposals		
Handicapped patients	Input and output devices	
Music		
Organizational charts		
Text retrieval or search	Medical literature	Medical databases
	Medical textbooks	
Educational	Programmed instruction	Patient education
	Computer-aided instruction	Examinations
	Video simulation	Patient instructions
	Courseware	

medical establishment's attention more swiftly than the Internet. It is the "Information Superhighway," the World Wide Web (WWW), with its linked matrix of information resources and its ability to network different computer systems and networks, all using the same wired or wireless interconnection technologies. Wilkins and Hovhanesian describe attributes of the Internet that have produced a societal paradigm shift.[15] Its most basic attribute is the capability to publish information that was formerly paper-based. Making this information interactive allows obtaining information that is now current, easily accessible and at a single source. The information is stored in databases with self-servicing capabilities, whereby looking for information or filling out forms can take place without human assistance. Through two-way and real-time collaboration, the Internet becomes the virtual workplace where individual groups can share ideas synchronously in online meetings or asynchronously as in e-mail, bulletin boards, or news groups. With integration and knowledge management, information can finally be personalized, easily located, and encyclopedic. This permits the neophyte to have access to the same information available to the experts, thus forever changing the relationship between patient and physician. This will translate into a joint community relationship of patients and physicians who will share in the collection and storage of medical data, as well as prevention and screening reminders for disease, heralding the Internet-based electronic patient health care record. This vision can be facilitated by incentives such as reduced insurance premiums for patients who participate in screening programs and reduced malpractice premiums for physicians who use electronic records.

The Internet, with 813,000,000 users worldwide in December 2004,[16] and growing at a rate of 1% per month, is a global, independent, but cooperative network of government, university, research laboratory, corporate, and private computers communicating by e-mail, bulletin boards, and discussion groups. It has the capability of permitting searches of database files and of retrieving information and software programs. It is fast becoming a post office, telephone system, and research library for its users. The reader is referred to the articles "Computer Networks as a Medical Resource"[17] and "The Impact of the Internet on Cancer Outcomes"[18] and the editorial "The Next Transformation in the Delivery of Health Care"[12] for an excellent overview of the Internet's indispensability for oncologists and physicians.

For collaborative Internet efforts, Usenet acts as a bulletin-board system that groups together Internet messages that pertain to a given topic, making discussion groups, newsletters, focused scientific groups, and subscription lists a reality. The information can be threaded on a related topic, distributed automatically to specific groups, deleted selectively by the system administrator, and can have expiration dates attached.

The WWW uses a client-server networking scheme that allows remote requests for data from any client personal computer to the host computer, which treats the requesting computer as if it were on its own local network. The WWW displays its arrays of text, data, sounds, and video in an application called the browser. Microsoft's Explorer, the Mozilla Foundation's FireFox, Apple's Safari, and Netscape's Navigator are the

Table 143-3 PDA Applications of Interest to the Oncologist

Type	Application	Location for Obtaining	Comment	Cost
Drug Guides	Epocrates	http://www.epocrates.com	Combines drug information. Antibiotics, drug interactions, diagnostic information, clinical tables and clinical calculators	$
	Mobile PDR	http://www.pdr.net	Drug database & interactions	Free
	Mobile Micromedex	http://www.micromedex.com/mobilemicromedex	Drug database	$
	A to Z Drug facts	http://www.handheldmed.com (click on "products")	Drug database	$
	Lexi-Comp Onhand	http://www.store.lexi.com/lexistore	Drug database	$
	EDRUGSDATA HDB	http://www.pdacortex.com/eDrugsDataHDB_Pocket_PC_Download.htm	12,000 drugs. Requires HanDBase	$
Dosing, Protocols & Chemotherapy Regimens	OncoMD	http://www.medicine.jbpub.com/oncomed	Cancer chemotherapy	$
	ChemoRxPlus	http://www.chemorxplus.com	Dosing calculator and protocol guide	Free
	Guide to Cancer Chemotherapeutic Regimens	http://healthcareprofessionals.orthobiotech.com/services/download.jsp	Protocol guide by cancer type	Free
	CAChemoRx	http://www.skyscape.com/EStore/ProductDetail.aspx?ProductID=1009	From Handbook of Cancer Chemotherapy	$
Chemotherapy Regimens and Cancer Care	ChemoSrce	http://www.skyscape.com/EStore/ProductDetail.aspx?ProductID=1132&WT.mc_id=56789	Chemotherapy drugs, regimens and side effects	$
Clinical References	Journal Clinical Oncology	http://www.jco.org/misc/PDA.shtml	Tof C, Abstracts and Announcements	Subscription
	ASCO	http://www.asco.org/pda	PDA formatted site content	Members
	PIER PDA	http://www.acponline.org/pda/	The Physicians' Information and Education Resource from American College of Physicians. Has 355 diseases.	$
	JournaltoGo	http://www.journaltogo.com/	Find authoritative, evidence-based guidance to improve clinical care	Free
	5MCC/200	http://www.5mcc.com/handhelds.html or see Epocrates	Griffith's 5 Minute Clinical Consult 1000 medical conditions	$
	Washington Manual of Oncology	http://www.lww.com/pda		$
	NCI PDQ	http://www.cancer.gov	Download sections and place into PDA for a document reader (Silo at http://www.isilo.com)	Free
	Diagnosaurus	http://books.mcgraw-hill.com/medical/diagnosaurus/index.html	Differential diagnosis for medical and surgical conditions	Free
	Stedman's Medical Dictionary	http://www.Stedmans.com/product.cfm/320/210		$
	PocketMedicine	http://www.pocketmedicine.com	Clinical publications and treatment strategies	$
	Redi-reference Clinical Guidelines Handbook	http://www.redi-reference.com		$
	HaemOnc Rules	http://medeicine.com/my/palmsoft/	Collection of diagnostic and therapeutic algorithms and classifications	Free
	SurgOnco	http://www.pdamd.com/pdaorder/-/885030120699/item?oec-catalog-item-id=2492	MD Anderson Surgical Oncology Handbook	$
Staging	Cancer Staging and Treatment	http://www.palmgear.com search for "cancer staging"	Requires iSilo reader (http://www.isilo.com)	Free
	Cancer Staging Pocket Guide	http://healthcareprofessionals.orthobiotech.com/services/download.jsp		Free
	TNM Mobile Edition	http://www.wiley.com	Staging and staging Calculator	$
	AJCC TNM	http://www.skyscape.com	Staging (Springer-Verlag)	$
	EZTNM	http://www.skyscape.com	Staging Calculator (Springer-Verlag)	$
Prognosis & Risk Assessment	MSKCC: Prostate Cancer, RCC, Gastric Cancer & Sarcoma	http://www.mskcc.org/mskcc/html/5794.cfm	See also: http://www.nomograms.org	Free
	Cancer PRA	http://www.skyscape.com/EStore/ProductDetail.aspx?ProductID=1079	From The Handbook of Cancer Risk Assessment and Prevention	$
	MedRules	http://pbrain.hypermart.net/medrules.html		Free
	Adjuvant!	http://www.adjuvantonline.com	Breast and colon cancer	
	BreastCa	http://smi-web.stanford.edu/people/pcheng/breastca/index.html	Uses Gail and Claus models	Free
	BreastAssure	http://shop.store.yahoo.com/pilotgearsw/breastassure.html	Nottingham, Van Nuys Indices	$
	BRCA Guide	http://www.myriadtests.com/provider/brca.htm	Estimates probability of patient carrying BRCA1 or BRCA2 from Myriad genetic Laboratories	Free
	Lung Cancer Risk Assessment	http://www.mskcc.org/mskcc/html/12463.cfm	MSKCC	Free
	Partin Tables	http://urology.jhu.edu/Partin_tables	Prostate cancer	
Medical Calculators	MedMath	http://smi-web.stanford.edu/people/pcheng/medmath/index.html	Contains 30 formulas	Free
	MedCalc	http://www.med-ia.ch/medcalc/		Free
	ICU Math	http://www.freewarepalm.com/medical/icumath.shtml	50 calculators	Free

(Continued)

Table 143-3 PDA Applications of Interest to the Oncologist *(Continued)*

Type	Application	Location for Obtaining	Comment	Cost
	Ca-Tools	http://www.cancer.org/docroot/COM/content/div_TX/COM_5_1x_The_C-Tools_20.asp?SiteArea=	ACS & Texas Medical Assn Oncology items to prevent, diagnose and treat cancer	Free
	narcConvert	http://www.spazthecat.com	Converts one or more narcotics to equianalgesic doses of another drug	Free
Electronic Medical Records	Patientkeeper	http://www.patientkeeper.com		$
	ComChart	http://www.comchart.com		$
	ePatient	http://www.iatrosoft.com/		$
	eRecord System	http://www.erecordsystem.com/		$
Practice Management	STAT E&M Coder	http://pda.surfnet.nl/palm/preview/34396.html	Assists evaluation and management coding for Medicare	$
	Pocket Med	http://www.pocketmed.org/	Medical billing software	$
DataBase	HanDBase	http://www.ddhsoftware,com/handbase	Create templates for any purpose	$
Anatomy	Netter's Anatomy	http://www.medicalwizards.com/client/productdesc.aspx?productid=62	Flash cards anatomy images	$
Other Resources	pdaMD	http://www.pdamd.com		$
	AvantGo	http://avantgo.com		$
	Skyscape	http://www.skyscape.com		$
	Handheldmd.com	http://www.handheldmd.com		$
	Palmgear	http://www.palmgear.com		$
	Amazon	http://www.medicalamazon.com		$
	Collectivemed	http://www.collectivemed.com/pdasource.shtml		$
	Freewarepalm	http://www.freewarepalm.com		$
	MedicalPocketPC.com	http://www.medicalpocketpc.com		
	Health Palmpilot	http://www.healthypalmpilot.com		

most commonly used browsers. They use a graphical interface to search, retrieve, and display information from any Internet-linked source that is linked to the underlined words or images. They can also be used by anyone to publish information on the WWW. It has provided a unified interface to the diverse protocols, data formats, and information archives used on the Internet. It attaches the Internet address of the computer that stores the documents desired, the document's location on that computer, and the language that that computer understands to send the information back to the requester. Any information located anywhere in the world with an Internet connection can be interconnected, permitting users to travel through the information by clicking on the hyperlinked words. As of December 2004, the WWW had 46.5 million Web sites containing information and administrative content, with 77% of sites having commercial information, and 9% having scientific and educational content.[19]

The Internet has become the principal method for communicating between oncologists. Most cancer cooperative groups use it for communication among their investigators. Some oncologists send their patients' computerized medical records with all reports and actual imaging studies to other physicians and hospitals over the Internet. As the capability of sending 1 to 100 gigabytes per second of digital audio or video information on the Internet has become a reality, live transmission of scientific conferences on the Internet as virtual meetings with audio and video presentations and actual slides and posters are commonplace.

Electronic Publishing Electronic publishing over the WWW is now available; abstracts, selected articles, or entire journals are made available on the date of publication. Aside from archiving issues, some journals permit subscribers to do full text searches, set up personal archives for saving articles and search results, and download articles in a printed format identical to the typeset pages. PubMed (<http://www.ncbi.nlm.nih.gov/entrez/query.fcgi?CMD=Display&DB=pubmed>), a version of MEDLINE created by the National Library of Medicine, automatically links abstracts returned in searches with publishers' sites that provide full text versions of their journals. Varmus has summarized the potential advantages of electronic publishing: open access, rapid and wide dissemination, reduced costs, and flexible publication formats,[20] creating healthy debate among the medical establishment.[21] To expand access to research from the developing world, the Lancet has created an Electronic Research Archive and e-print server for international health articles that may be openly peer reviewed on the Internet by anyone prior to publication in the Lancet or just made available as a nonpeer-reviewed submission that can be updated at the discretion of the author.

Search Engines Internet portals are sites that consolidate, organize, and report data; assist with searching for data using search engines (Table 143-4); or assist with e-commerce and e-business, and they are fast achieving the status of an industrial utility. The most popular search engine is Google (<http://www.google.com>), which can search the Internet for text, images, newsgroup information, news, product information and pricing, catalogs, directories, and scholarly books. Text can include words or phrases segregated by languages, file formats, dates, occurrences, current news specificity, page-specificity, or topic specificity. Images can be searched for related words or phrases, image size, image file types, color, or domains. Already Google has branched beyond Web searching to assist users to find information in product databases, e-mail archives, their own hard drives, and the printed book. Future search engines will search instant messages, music, video, and even conversations using voice-over Internet protocol (VOIP). Other search sites are competing with Google to become more accurate in searching or more effective in presenting search results. Amazon's A9 search engine (<http://www.a9.com>) presents the user with multiple panes, each of which contains a different type of search on a term. For example, it will divide a search for a term into text, pictures, references in books, references in reference books, or database of movies. Past searches can be bookmarked for future reference. My Yahoo's Search (<http://mysearch.yahoo.com>) searches preselected highly relevant sites that can be customized by the user or chosen by Yahoo. Sites can be sorted by categories. Searches can also be saved and new searches can include saved searches. Clusty (<http://www.clusty.com>) groups searches into folders. Blinkx (<http://www.blinkx.com>) creates a toolbar on your desktop that automatically scans the WWW and places in its own window Web links to words you type into your word processor or e-mail program or that are on a Web page. Microsoft's search engine (<http://www.msn.com>) searches the Internet, news, encyclopedia, dictionary, stock quotes, movies, and shopping.

Health Care Portals Health care portals can be divided into three categories. First are the content-oriented sites, which divide nicely into four subgroups: patient-centric (<http://www.pwlc.org>), provider-centric (<http://www.asco.org>), hybrids such as WebMD (<http://www.webmd.com>), and companies that have a product to sell, such as A.D.A.

Table 143-4 Internet Portal Search Engines

Site	Description	URL
Alta-Vista	Fast free-text searching Divides search results by categories; can save searches for review and reexecute	http://www.altavista.com
Amazon's A9		http://www.a9.com
Anonymizer		http://anonymizer.com
Answers.com	Provides direct answers to search queries	http://www.answers.com
AOL	Searches websites, phone numbers, business information	http://search.aol.com
Ask	Ask Jeeves; can save searches for review and reexecute	http://www.ask.com
Blinkx	Automatically searches the internet for words you are typing or reading	http://www.blinkx.com
BrightPlanet	Finds databases that cannot be crawled or indexed by surface web search engines	http://completeplanet.com
Clusty	Divides search results into folders by categories and permits preview of pages	http://www.clusty.com
Dogpile	Searches multiple search engines	http://www.dogpile.com
Euroseek	European source	http://www.euroseek.com
Excite	Concept searching	http://www.excite.com
Google	Free-text, image searching; most popular site	http://www.google.com
Hotbot	Searches multiple search engines simultaneously	http://hotbot.lycos.com
Infoseek	Basic search engine	http://infoseek.go.com
Kartoo	Metasearch engine that searches other search sites and gives results in visual form	http://kartoo.com
Lycos		http://www.lycos.com
MelDex	Hum a tune, type in lyrics or play notes on virtual keyboard to find a song	http://www.sadl.uleth.ca/nz/cgibin/music/musiclibrary
Mooter	Categorizes search results in onscreen buttons and clusters	http://www.mooter.com
MSN	Searches internet, news, encyclopedia, dictionary, stock quotes, movies and shopping	http://www.msn.com
Northern Light	Free-text searches are categorized	http://www.northernlight.com
Profusion	Searches major search engines and filters the results	http://www.profusion.com
Rover	Provides customized information and maps based upon location of user	http://mindlab.umd.edu/research_rover.html
Shape	3D search engine that matches a drawn shape to images of similar forms	http://shape.cs.princeton.edu/search.html
Watson	Integrates search with user-interest profiles	http://www.openroad-tech.com
Webcrawler	Metasearch engine	http://www.webcrawler.com
Yahoo	Subject guide and free-text searching	http://mysearch.yahoo.com

M. Software's Interactive Anatomy 4 (<http://www.adam.com>). These companies are comparable to publishers and information media. Second are the commerce sites, including Internet drugstores and global health care marketplaces that offer medical products and services. These companies compare with stores. Third are the transaction-based companies such as WebMD that plan to reduce health care transaction costs by linking key health care constituencies, such as payers, providers, consumers, diagnostic agencies, and suppliers, providing patient enrollment, benefits administration, referral claims and tracking, third-party transactions, electronic prescriptions and reporting, and pharmacy benefit management.

Because the amount of information available on the Internet for oncologists and their patients is so vast and the quality of the material so varied, I have been working with ASCO to set up the ASCO Cancer Directories for ASCO members (<http://www.asco.org> click myASCO then Cancer Directories) listed by tumor type with filtered links to reliable cancer sources on the Internet that do not require payment for their use or a user name or password for access. It permits a one-click link to most of the useful Web-based cancer information resources. It will permit oncologists to seamlessly use this content in their electronic consultation notes and patient e-mails. Table 143-5 lists the topics available for each tumor type.

Because of the vastness, reliability, and ephemeral nature of Internet medical information, every oncologist needs to have an understanding of the basic issues related to information available on the Internet. It is important to know the expertise, conflicts of interests, and biases of the developers and sponsors of a site, as well as the site's purpose and intended audience. Is the original source of content identified, current, and valid? Is the user's confidentiality protected, and if not, who has access to information about the users?

PAGE DESCRIPTION LANGUAGES Page description languages define the appearance and user interface of the browser screen. They are derived

Table 143-5 Professional and Patient Cancer Information on the Internet

1. Overview for Professional and Patient Cancers by body location/system
   - Alphabetical list of cancers
2. Anatomy/Physiology
3. Genetics, genetic testing, and causes
4. Risk factors
5. Self-risk assessment
6. Detection/screening information
   - Specific tests
7. Prevention
8. Signs and symptoms
9. Diagnosis
   - Procedures
   - Imaging studies
   - Laboratory studies
10. Cell classification
11. Staging
12. Guidelines
13. Clinical trials
    - Open with eligibility and summary information
    - Closed with abstracts/full-text citations
    - Online access and data management
14. Types of therapy by stage/modality
15. Follow up
16. Statistics
    - Understanding
    - Data sources
    - By cancer type
17. Atlas incidence and mortality
18. Advocacy and support
19. Clinical research
20. Complementary and alternative medicine
21. Discussion groups
22. Disease classifications and coding
    - ICD-9
    - CPT
23. Educational programs/Meetings
24. Headline and archived news
25. Pharmaceutical information
26. Public policy
27. Practice management
28. Coping with cancer
    - Advanced directives
    - Supportive care and resources
    - Side effects of cancer
    - Complications caused by cancer
    - Sexuality
    - Survivorship
    - Caregiver
    - Financial
29. Toxicity criteria
30. Cancer literature
    - PubMed
    - Journal links
31. Research programs and funding
32. Patient tools
    - Questions for your oncologist
    - Medical record
    - Personal diary
    - Buddies
    - Calendar
    - Discussion groups
33. Resources
    - Cancer centers and hospitals
    - Foundations and Societies
    - Government Agencies
    - Medical dictionary
    - Physician and facility finder

from Standard Generalized Markup Language (SGML). This is a meta-language used by printers who originally scribbled notes on documents to instruct the typesetters and later codified these shortcuts for universal use. Hypertext Markup Language (HTML) was created as a computer-independent platform for the Internet, using tags to indicate the visual appearance and placement of text and pictures so all computer types see the same page. HTML uses angle-bracketed label tags that surround the text to which they apply and can be nested inside one another to multiple levels. For example, <BOLD>Name</BOLD> would produce **Name** on the screen. Although HTML is the most successful electronic publishing language to date, it can describe only the arrangement of text, images, and push buttons on a page. The deficiencies seen with HTML have all been rectified by the invention of Extensible Markup Language (XML), which combines more efficient processing and flexible linking.[22]

XML permits information to be self-describing, that is, what the information is, not just what it looks like. On the WWW, XML tags might tell the computer that a list of numbers represents the state of your bank account. Thus, the computer will know what the items are, how they are related, and how they should be dealt with. This opens up the possibility of facilitating the searching for and exchanging of scientific data, commercial products, and multilingual documents. It tells the computer how text, images, and video are placed on the screen, irrespective of whether the computer is a desktop PC or a PDA. Thus, the oncologist could pull up a list of medications that the patient is taking and e-mail the list to a colleague, who could then paste the list into his or her hospital's own database record for this patient.

Like HTML, XML uses tags, like parentheses, that must precede and follow the item described; and like quotation marks, tag pairs can be nested inside one another to multiple levels, like a tree structure used to designate hierarchical relationships. These tags are labels that point to a definition in a combined thesaurus and dictionary. To indicate that a patient has a drug allergy to a given drug, the following XML notation would be used: <patient> <name> xxx </name> <drug-allergy>xxx </drug-allergy> </patient>. XML will offer four benefits: (1) A better way to search: Today, a keyword search can return thousands of possibilities. XML tags will filter data and return only the results desired. (2) A better way to distribute and track information: Today, it is difficult to republish content across many sites, and more difficult to track who is reading it. XML will make both feasible. (3) A better way to do business: Today, one can browse through catalogs online. XML tags will allow data to be customized. (4) A better way to do business on the road: Today, WWW graphics bog down and slow Internet connections. With XML, your computer will download only material tagged as text. XML permits specialized markup languages, such as terms for medical record fields in a database or a chemical markup language that graphically renders a molecular structure when a markup term is used. It also allows a choice of multiple linked sites and automatic updating of all links to a given site when that site changes location. Thus, XML will permit a more powerful and useful WWW that will have great value in simplifying medical information management. Thus, computers filled with different kinds of information, run by different companies and connected to different Web sites could send messages behind the scenes to accomplish our tasks.

With XML as the alphabet and every item of information identified for its common meaning, every discipline, including medicine, will develop a specialized vocabulary for computers. By also having access to most of the information ever created, the Web will then become a semantic Web, as envisioned by its founder, Timothy Berners-Lee.[23] Thus the computer, already a master of mathematics, by using these Web agents, would understand not only the meaning of words and concepts, but also their logical relationships. This would also overcome our inability to easily translate jargon and significantly reduce foreign language barriers. As databases begin to use XML tags to give semantic meaning to their data fields, application programming interfaces (API) that are short hooks of computer code that allow smaller programs to communicate with larger software operating systems like Windows will permit programmers to allow the operating system to automatically interact with the database on the Web site. As large medical database repositories use this technology, innovative linking of their data to other databases like our desktop electronic medical records will occur and the Internet will not just be used for human users to call up preformatted documents, but computers will be able to share data with other computers.

Messaging Standards Messaging standards allow applications on the WWW to exchange information in a consistent and secure way. Computers have the capability to send the same information to individuals either in e-mail, fax, pager, or voice-mail format. E-mail can exchange letters and documents from within a word-processing application. Directory services allow a common point of information storage for access by groups of users. Authentication insures that all communications are kept secure and private by using encryption techniques. Digital signatures attach a reliable approval signature to documents. Thus, documents can be securely handled, reviewed, and approved among work groups, facilitating scientific collaboration.

Blogs Blogs—short for Web logs—and vlogs (video logs) are amateur Web sites that are easy to set up and are linkable to any other Web site. They provide information and opinion to audiences that are drawn by common interests. Blogs are rapidly becoming a genuine alternative to our mainstream information outlets. Suddenly everyone can become a publisher and a critic. Blogs have grown exponentially because of an innovation called the "permalink": a unique Web address for each posting, which remains accessible indefinitely, on every blog, not just the Web page, which can change frequently. Linking posts rapidly disseminates information, giving blogs almost a viral quality. With efficient blog search engines available, blogs have become a powerful "relationship generator" that can rapidly bring local, national, or worldwide attention to any subject. Blogs can host music, video, and photos. They are being used creatively as a substitute for e-mail, as project management software for collaborations in a company, as an up-to-date manual, and even by scientists as an experimental notebook since it is a written-down, date-stamped, and backed-up document. Blogs will rapidly become a major factor in medical communications. To locate blogs of interest, use <http://www.kinja.com>, <http://www.bloglines.com>, <http://www.feedster.com>, <http://www.technorati.com>, or <http://www.blogdex.net>. To create your own blog, go to Google's <http://www.blogger.com> or Microsoft's <http://www.Spaces.MSN.com> and create a free account. Name your blog, study the templates, and choose a template for your blog. Write something interesting and then register at <http://www.Feedburner.com> to find out if anyone's reading your blog and which posts are liked best.

Really Simple Syndication Using a software type known as RSS (Really Simple Syndication), custom-tailored bulletins that are continuously updated from thousands of sites can be linked to your blog or browser (Apple's *Safari*) without having to manually visit each site. By clicking on one of these headlines on your site that is linked to the parent site, one can get the full story. Thus the user, not the Web site, determines what information is seen and how often it is updated. RSS uses XML formats for the syndication of Web content that can be read by a newsreader that is either a standalone program or part of a browser. Newsreaders can bring together the latest postings from your favorite blogs in a single place. You can obtain RSS functionality by downloading a newsreader: (<http://www.feedDemon.com>, <http://www.newsGator.com>, <http://www.intraVnews.com>, Shrook 2 <http://www.fondantfancies.com>, NetNewsWire (<http://www.ranchero.com>), or use an online service such as myYahoo (<http://my.yahoo.com>) or Bloglines (<http://www.bloglines.com>). RSS technology could be used to send a physician medical alerts and reminders, and since RSS readers can be embedded into database applications, users can automate database searching that gives constantly updated reports.

Wiki A Wiki is a Web site on which anyone with appropriate authority can post material, do searches, and make changes fast, without using arcane commands, and with the ability to track changes and revisions. Volunteers have posted 500,000 articles in over 50 languages since 2001, creating the Wikipedia, the largest encyclopedia in the world. (<http://www.wikipedia.com>). This application can be used for creating textbooks, articles, manuals, catalogs, schedules, or structural database forms.

Health Care Applications Today, essential Internet health care applications include e-content with patients having almost equal access to medical information that professionals have; e-connectivity linking all health care participants for clinical objectives, such as diagnostic and laboratory test reporting, electronic medical records, prescriptions, e-mail, and administrative purposes with appointments, billing inquiries, claims processing, eligibility, and referral authorizations; e-commerce with purchasing of drugs and medical advice; and e-care management with disease management and home monitoring of patients. Sites such as RelayHealth (<http://www. relayhealth.com>) provide a secure and encrypted HIPAA-compliant site for e-mail with patients, e-prescriptions with drug–drug interactions, drug–disease interactions, and allergy checking, along with electronic billing for these services. In contrast to free-form messages, it can use customized clinically structured, branched questions that generate concise, structured messages. It includes the capability to collect fees from patients and reimbursements from payers. Messages can be triaged automatically. It should be noted that many national payers are beginning to permit e-mail interaction between patients and their physicians to be reimbursed based on a RelayHealth pilot.[24] Numerous academic health care networks have established Web sites that are providing Internet access for all transactions taking place between the patient, physician, hospital, clinic, commercial laboratory, imaging centers, and the payers, creating regional Community Health Information Networks. An example of such a site connecting patients and physicians that serves academic centers and hospitals is PatientSite (<http://patientsite.caregroup.org>). At the American Society of Clinical Oncology (ASCO), I have been working with the Information Technology Committee to enhance electronic communication between its members, our patients, and the public. By providing its members with a free customizable Web site for marketing and practice assistance and a unique customizable scrolling desktop screen consolidating oncologic, professional, and personal information portlets, e-mail, chat rooms, discussion forums, member finder, calendar, to-do lists, address books, mailing lists, bulletin boards, and user-defined links, the myASCO Web site could become a major Web oncology community resource for all oncologists.

Already, with the increasing consumerism of the Internet, personal electronic health records (PEHR) that are maintained by patients and electronic health records (EHR) that are maintained by physicians, cancer centers, and institutions have become available over the Internet to automatically synchronize updating and decision support reminders. This will permit the seamless electronic transfer of information from the patient to the physician for medical vetting and then on to all the other health care participants. Innovative desktop electronic records that permit easy customization for the physician's practice, Internet publishing, connectivity, and PDA synchronization are appearing. As nonemergency communication between physicians and patients becomes commonplace, it is imperative that oncologists understand their new security and documentation responsibilities. The American Medical Informatics Association has published guidelines for electronic communication with patients that summarize turnaround time, privacy issues, sensitivity of subject matter, identification, protocol, and behavior (<http://www.amia.org/pubs/fpubl.html>).[25] Although it is not a complete Web-based electronic medical record, the Society of Gynecologic Oncologists' database (<http://www.sgodb.com/>) is a basic tumor registry that allows oncologists to track patients in their office using an application service provider (ASP) that specializes in information technology management, software, and database development from a remote, secure server.

Oncologists are beginning to evaluate the use of the Internet by themselves and their patients. Pereira and colleagues explored the use of the Internet by breast cancer patients.[26] They found that of the 107 surveys returned, 74% came from patients and 26% from family members. The majority of Internet users desired more information on their cancer (91%), checked into information given to them by their provider (66%), researched other treatment options (63%), and obtained information on alternative therapies (61%). Most were satisfied with their Internet experience and spoke to their physician about their findings. Chen and Siu discussed the impact of the media and the Internet on information gathering by Canadian patients and oncologists.[27] They concluded that cancer patients in Canada commonly search for information on the Internet. It did not seem to affect the oncologist-patient relationship. Helft and colleagues surveyed ASCO members on their Internet use with patients.[28] Responding oncologists indicated that 30% of their patients used the Internet to gain cancer information, adding 10 minutes to the clinical encounter. Forty-four percent noted that they had difficulty discussing Internet information and 9% felt threatened.

Strategic assistance is needed to provide guidance for patients to better understand their cancer and interpret this information on the Internet more effectively. Bichakjian and colleagues warn patients that too many sites found through using search engines have sparse, and at times inaccurate, information about malignant melanoma.[29] They found that the majority of sites lacked complete basic melanoma information and 14% contained inaccuracies. It remains the duty of oncologists to be familiar with medical Internet sites and to educate their patients about linking to sites that have reputable information. A recent issue of the *British Medical Journal* is devoted to the theme of evaluating the quality of health information on the Internet.[30] Thus oncologists must be prepared to guide their patients on the Internet. The National Library of Medicine and the American College of Physicians, are using MedlinePlus (<http://www.medlineplus.gov>) as information, prepared therapy prescriptions to give patients appropriate Internet information for their medical conditions. People living with cancer (<http://www.plwc.org>), ASCO's site for cancer patients, is distributing cancer information prescription pads to oncologists to assist them with these endeavors.

Research Collaboration The Internet is acting as a potent catalyst for scientific advances by permitting new ties among researchers at any worldwide site. Marshall and Haley discuss their experience with this Internet technology for setting up a research collaboration with 15 laboratories and clinics, collecting and maintaining an Internet database that was more efficient and secure than through conventional methods of paper, filing cabinets, and locked doors.[31] Colleagues can, with permission, be linked directly or by e-mail or fax to any computer on the Internet. Mountains of data, large electronic meetings, bulletin boards where questions can be answered almost instantaneously, and electronic journal publications are commonplace.

File Sharing As online file sharing has evolved, new methods are emerging to make it readily possible to exchange material online without using a central file server. Currently, the Internet requires a host computer to deal with any request for information from all computers (client computers). In the near future, any computer will be able to talk directly to any other computer without a host computer connection. This peer-to-peer sharing of information is based on the Simple Object Access Protocol (SOAP), which enables the network to become the computer. An operating system spanning the Internet permits any computer connected to the Internet to connect directly to any other computer, eliminating the need for host computers and opening up the possibility of computers sharing their unused processing power with other Internet users.[32]

With appropriate adherence to HIPAA regulations, permission from the patient, the use of a controlled medical vocabulary like SNOMED, and universal identifiers for patients and physicians, it should be possible for a patient's latest medical data residing on multiple computers linked on the Internet to synchronize with a medical record in a given physician's office, giving the physician access to the latest patient medical data. Any doctor's office or hospital with a Web-connected computer will be able to share their stored records, via automated machine-to-machine processes, with any other doctor's office or hospital. An individual patient record would be maintained in a distributed fashion over the Internet, obtainable and aggregated into a complete whole automatically and immediately on demand by any authorized Web-connected computer at any time and from anywhere. The evolving electronic medical record will consist of many components linking patients, practices, clinics, imaging centers, hospitals, health plans, laboratories, and pharmacies over the Internet in a confidential, secure, and standardized format. We will use the Internet for practice management; scheduling, visits, procedures, and laboratory tests; documentation; referrals; prescriptions; patient eligibility; decision support; analyzing patterns of care; error checking; and e-mail communication.

INFORMATION MANAGEMENT

Medical Education Knowledge can be defined as the organization, analysis, and interpretation of data and observations that convey a higher degree of understanding. It is imperative that oncologists have direct access to knowledge for problem solving, and the ability to browse for curiosity's sake and to annotate and personalize knowledge. All major sources of oncologic information have become computerized. These include bibliographic information, such as CANCERLIT; factual information, such as Physician Data Query (PDQ); full text, such as this book; and knowledge bases, such as ONCOCIN.

Computerized Patient Records In 1989, in order to improve the usefulness of the medical record, the computer-based patient record (CPR) was coined and defined by a committee of the Institute of Medicine of the National Academy of Sciences. Clinical oncology, with its emphasis on clinical trials and longitudinal data for its patients, would seem to be a natural target for automated records. Today, however, most oncologists still do not use electronic medical records (EMR) because standards defining software tools, functions, or datasets are nonexistent; patient data remain insecure; physicians are expected to underwrite the costs of these technologies; software vendor viability is suspect; worries remain about how quickly programs can become obsolete; and one EMR program cannot easily exchange information with another.

Recently, government and other concerned private parties have finally begun addressing these problems. With the maturing of computer, communication and information technologies; acceptance by payers to reimburse for and the public to use electronic communication with their doctors; and the recognition of standards permitting cross-platform semantic understanding of data with information that is encrypted, secure, and authentic, oncologists must begin to participate in the defining of oncology tools, functions, and datasets as components of electronic medical records. Health care is being fundamentally changed by a coalition of forces, including employers reallocating benefit funding, health plan realignments, consumer action, and government mandates that will influence public policy to encourage the adoption of information and communication technologies. This will transform medicine by allowing gains in health care safety, efficiency, and cost savings.

Oncology practices have been hit hard by changes in Medicare and managed care. Oncologists are being forced to examine and control their costs, better track their inventories, and be more concerned with their billing and coding. They are also standardizing treatments, increasing documentation of the health care they provide, and measuring and collecting quality data for negotiations with payers—all processes requiring the right kind of computerized tools. As EMRs begin to address these requirements and seamlessly link with oncology-specific practice management software, all oncologists will have electronic medical records routinely deployed across all health care settings. The oncologist will be able to seamlessly create, maintain, edit, display, and manipulate all the data stored in the individual's record. Aggregates of data will be stored in a clinical data repository, which will serve as the storage facility database for CPRs, facilitating health research and clinical trials. Table 143-6 lists basic medical- and oncology-specific data elements for an electronic medical record.

The Institute of Medicine study listed 12 key attributes of the CPR that have become the gold standard by which all CPRs are judged. These are listed in Table 143-7. In addition to these 12 attributes, more recent underpinnings have been identified as enablers of a robust CPR. These include the need for a minimum standardized clinical data dictionary to define the data elements required in the CPR and the need to support a controlled vocabulary that defines precisely how a term is used so that there is a uniform understanding of its meaning in clinical medicine. Further provisions will require that ambulatory medical records be created in oncology offices and that they be integrated seamlessly with hospital information systems, such that there is a virtual longitudinal record. Most likely, the set of technologies that make up the Internet will be used to provide the foundation for creating the CPR that will be shared by the patient, provider, and payer, with appropriate encryption, security, confidentiality, and audit trails. Fortunately, clinical message sending is being standardized around the Health Level Seven (HL-7) version 3 standard and XML. HL-7 permits the transfer of information that is vendor-, application-, and foreign language-neutral.

As oncologists become more focused on cancer screening and prevention, and as data management of clinical trials becomes automated, disease management will become an accepted part of our practice management, and the CPR will become indispensable. We will see collaborative online efforts to develop clinical pathways (multidisciplinary plans of care that standardize patient treatment) and bring decision support to the oncologist at the point of care. This will assist us in practicing more evidence-based medicine (bringing current scientific knowledge to the oncologist for point-of-care decision making). To reduce errors and enforce documentation of chemotherapy administration, Prescher-Hughes describes the setting up of practice protocol guidelines for the oncologist's office that are stored on the computer.[33] Table 143-8 lists elements of this protocol list.

Recently, many Internet health care sites have put into place personal medical records that can be filled out and controlled by patients that are available to appropriate users given permission.[34] Thus, we are almost at a point where patients could self-manage their health information online by maintaining their record, choosing a physician, e-mailing their providers, making appointments online, refilling prescriptions, and receiving prevention and screening reminders. This portends a major power shift that will create new roles for providers and new responsibilities for patients. Masys has created a system called PCASSO, which gives patients completely secure access to their medical records via the Internet and has shown that patient access to their data did not cause undue alarm and that providers did not feel any reluctance to make detailed clinical notes.[35] In fact, as pointed out by Morrison, the physician of the future will have to play many new roles.[36]

Oncologists may be surprised that oncology and general medical practice have been criticized for not delivering state-of-the-art care. Specifically, these reports criticized the health care system for not using information technology effectively and not having a quality monitoring system capable of regular reporting on the quality of patient care. Government and payers, in their attempts to make health care more efficient, are also looking at patterns of health care treatment and how to define and measure quality health care. To answer our critics, ASCO's National Initiative on Cancer Care Quality (NICCQ) was set up to develop a prototype for a national system that could monitor the quality of cancer care.[37] As part of its mission, the NICCQ has been able to define a dataset (data dictionary) for common cancers that, along with other oncology datasets, could be used as an oncology component of an EMR. In addition, the program has created an innovative cancer medical record abstraction tool that could facilitate data collection in our offices.

To help oncologists begin to measure quality in their offices, ASCO set up the Quality Oncology Practice Initiative (QOPI) that included 15 practices and 376 physicians. The initiative assessed quality measures that included items derived from clinical guidelines, common sense items with high face validity and clinical relevance, and items related to physician-patient interactions. Its purpose was to become a tool for oncology offices to compare themselves with benchmarks reflecting quality cancer care and thereby become recognized by some type of certification. The presentation at ASCO's 2004 annual meeting used keypad technology to assess the interest of oncologists to measure quality care given in their offices by using computerized tools. Of the attendees, 50% already had a quality improvement effort, 13% used an EMR, 38% used some simple computer programs to gather patient data, 42% used 7 or more standing orders for administering chemotherapy with 56% using guidelines in their standing order, 76% would participate in future QOPI initiatives, 84% wanted help in collecting aggregate practice data and physician-specific data, and 88% had Internet access in their offices.

Although 80% of cancer care in the United States is provided in the community setting, very little of the data collected there is available. Thus

Table 143-6 Data Elements for Personal, Provider, and Oncology Medical Records

Common Data Elements	Personal Health Data Elements	Provider Data Elements	Oncology Data	Elements
Patient Identification elements	•	•	Historical	Surgery/Procedure
Emergency Contacts	•	•	Date diagnosis	Date
Lifetime health history	•	•	Cancer diagnosis	Procedure
Immunizations, allergies, family history,			Primary Site	Purpose
occupational history, environmental exposures,			Subsite	Hospital
social history, medical history, treatments,			Laterality	Sentinal nodes
procedures, medicines, outcomes			Prior Rx	Complications
Laboratory results	•	•	Staging primary disease	Operative findings
Emergency care information	•	•	Date staged	% Debulked
Provider identification and contact information	•	•	Geographic site	Surgeon
Treatment plans and instructions	•	•	Primary location size	Time Procedure
Health risk factor profile preventive services	•	•	Nodes	Estimated blood loss
and results			Metastatic sites	Transfusion
Health insurance coverage information	•	•	T | N | M	Radiation therapy
Correspondence	•	•	Stage	Purpose
Access and confidentiality information	•	•	Tumor status	Location
Audit log	•	•	Staging metastatic disease	Dose
Self-care trackers: nutrition, activity, medication	•	•	Date	Start/End date
Health care proxies, living wills, power of attorney	•	•	Site(s)	Response
Sociodemographic identifiers		•	Subsite	Progression date
gender, birthday, age, race/ethnicity, marital			Histology	Chemotherapy
status, living arrangement, educational level,			Same as primary	Protocol name
occupation			in situ	Group
Legal consents or permission		•	Residual	Protocol #
Referral information		•	Lesion size	Patient #
Reason for visit		•	Volume	Regimen (drugs)
External causes injury/illness		•	Status	Purpose
Symptoms		•	Link with Primary (?)	Start/End date
Physical exams		•	Pathology	Ht Wt BSA
Assessment of patient signs and symptoms		•	Date diagnosis	Response
Toxicity assessments		•	Site	Cycles #
Diagnoses		•	Gross	Cycle dates
Orders for lab, radiology and pharmacy		•	Morphology	Progression date
Laboratory results		•	Markers	Immunotherapy
Radiological images and interpretations		•	Histology	Protocol name
Records of alerts, warnings and reminders		•	Grade	Group
Operative reports		•	Maximum diameter	Protocol #
Vital signs		•	Volume	Patient #
Treatment plans and instructions		•	Vascular involvement	Regimen (drugs)
Progress notes		•	Lymph involvement	Purpose
Functional status		•	Margins	Start/End date
Discharge summaries		•	Character	Response
Outcome analyses		•	Size	# Cycles
Provider notes		•	Synchrony	Cycle length
Protocols		•	FISH	Progression date
Practice guidelines		•	DNA ploidy	Recurrence
Clinical decision-support programs		•	Receptors	rT | rN | rM
Referral history		•	Histochemistry	rStage
			Genetics	Date
			Currency	Site(s)
			Current Rx modalities	Subsite
			Status	Histology
			Response	Same as primary
			Rx intent	in situ
			Rx toleration	Residual
			Rx toxicity	Lesion size
			Performance status	Volume
			Pain level	Status
			Fatigue level	Link with Primary (?)
				Follow up
				Last date seen
				DNR
				Date of death
				Autopsy findings

there is a consensus among those of us in informatics and many governmental agencies (see below) that the time is right for the computer, communication, and information technologies available today to be harnessed, with appropriate financial incentives from the government and other payers, to provide a seamless, cost-effective approach to manage medical information that will benefit patients, providers, payers, government, and vendors.

In 2003, positive steps were first taken by the public and private sectors to assure the adoption

Table 143-7 Computer-Based Patient Record Attributes

1. Supports a problem list.
2. Has the ability to measure health status and functional levels.
3. Can document clinical reasoning and rationale.
4. Is a longitudinal computerized patient record (CPR) and has timely linkages with other patient records.
5. Guarantees confidentiality, privacy, and audit trails.
6. Offers continuous access for authorized users.
7. Supports simultaneously multiple user views into the CPR.
8. Supports timely access to local and remote information resources.
9. Facilitates clinical problem solving.
10. Supports direct data entry by physicians.
11. Supports practitioners in measuring costs and improving quality.
12. Has the flexibility to support existing or evolving needs of clinical specialties.

of EMRs into our offices within 5 to 8 years. Oncologists must begin to educate themselves about using this technology so they have a role in its dissemination. Initially, the DHHS agreed to adopt standards for transmitting electronic medical information. In its Consolidated Health Informatics (CHI) initiative, DHSS announced the five standards selected and mandated for sharing medical information among federal agencies: messaging standards from Health Level Seven Inc. (HL-7), retail pharmacy orders from the National Council for Prescription Drug Programs (NCDCP), the Institute of Electrical and Electronic Engineers (IEEE) 1073 series of standards for medical devices, Digital Imaging Communications in Medicine (DICOM) for images, and the Logical Observation Identifier Name codes (LOINC) for clinical laboratory results reporting. The National Library of Medicine (NLM) licensed SNOMED-CT (Systematized Nomenclature of Medicine-Clinical Terms), which is a machine-readable, clinically rich lexicon using a controlled clinical vocabulary dataset maintained by the College of American Pathologists to standardize clinical communication. The NLM and DHHS have made SNOMED-CT available free to all physicians. The idea is to use standardized terms in medical communication so that our computers and electronic files can talk to and understand each other. DHHS also announced that they will urge congress to use the government's fraud and abuse coffers to support a "mini Hill-Burton Foundation" for funding health care providers' information technology investments. The NCI's Cancer Trials Support Unit introduced its Online Regulatory Support System to be used by all cooperative groups and upcoming initiatives and to include online patient eligibility and data collection for clinical trials.

Table 143-8 Practice Protocol Items

Name of protocol
Diagnosis
Blood tests to be drawn and when
Source of drugs
Pre-treatment screen tests
Premedications
Chemotherapy drugs and formula for calculation
How to mix and dilute drugs, chose diluent, amount and IV fluid
Administration route, IV push or infusion and time infusion
Need for pump, special tubing and filter
Major side effects of drugs
Supportive drugs—post therapy
Number of office visits required to complete therapy
Time needed for each therapy
Prior authorization for drugs
Patient name, height, weight and M2
Central line placement (if needed)
Co-signatures for dose calculations
Physician signature

The NCI also updated terminology and the grading system for reporting adverse events covering medical, surgical, and radiation oncology events without regard to timing or cause of the event. This has become the standard dictionary for reporting adverse events and should become part of an oncology dataset for any oncologic EMR. In 2004, President Bush appointed Dr. David Brailer as National Coordinator for Health Information Technology to oversee health information technology initiatives by the federal government and the private sector and set a goal of having an electronic health care record in place for every American this decade. He released "The Decade of Health Information Technology: Delivering Consumer-centric and Information-rich Health Care" (<http://www.hhs.gov/onchit/framework>). Its key initiatives include working with the private sector for electronic health record product certification for minimal standards of functionality, security, and interoperability so physicians can make informed purchasing decisions; having CMS work on standards for electronic prescribing in Medicare for publication in 2005; and having Health Resources and Services Administration providing seed money for implementation of community-based health information exchanges. The National Health Care Information Technology Infrastructure is summarized by Yasnoff and colleagues.[38] This was followed immediately by CMS awarding a grant to the American Academy of Family Practitioners to create an open-source electronic medical record system to collect data on quality and performance, to deliver evidence-based guidelines and treatment information for selected diseases, and to ask the Veterans Administration to create a subset of their Vista Medical Record (Vista Office) to be made available free for the use of all physicians taking care of Medicare patients.

The ultimate goal of using these technologies is to have all of our medical information, practice management, and patient education needs in oncology accessible on our computer desktop; to reduce unnecessary paperwork; to be reimbursed fairly for our work; and to contribute to the development of an efficient health care system based on evidence-based data that is responsive to the needs of all health care constituents. We must be able to incorporate patient-specific decision support and physician reminders into our point-of-care patient activities. Electronic links across care settings will not only facilitate collaborative and coordinated approaches among care givers, but will also permit the real-time tracking and monitoring of the quality of our cancer care activities. The reader is referred to an excellent tutorial on the EMR at the American College of Physician's Website (<http://www.acponline.org/journals/news/apr04/emrs.htm#resources>), the *2004 Resource Guide* from Healthcare Informatics,[39] and the monthly newsletter *Medical Software Reviews*.[40]

Clinical Data Systems A clinical data system is a computer-based system that captures, stores, or communicates clinical data to enhance clinical decision making. Clinical information combines specific patient data (eg, history or laboratory data) and knowledge (facts about a cancer or how to interpret a laboratory result) that applies to many patients. Computers are essential for both types of data, with a computer-based patient record holding patient data and clinical databases and electronic medical textbooks containing clinical knowledge. Wyatt divides clinical data into five categories: identifiers (demographic data, identity numbers); patient findings (history and observations, including symptoms, clinical signs, and laboratory results); hypotheses (assessment and plan, such as diagnosis, stage, problem list, and possible tests or therapies); actions (therapy, referral, tests ordered, information given); and modifiers (who recorded data, when, certainty).[41] He identifies free text, diagrams, text, numerical reports, graphs, charts, photographs, and tracings as the different forms of clinical data that can be assimilated by the computer. The appearance of clinical data takes on added importance because of the ease of viewing and arranging data by the computer. Multiple small graphs printed on a laser printer can summarize a mass of clinical and laboratory data from a patient's clinical chart.[42] Numerical data can be plotted to reveal the course of an illness or the patient's response to treatment.

Hospital information systems can be divided into six levels of organization. Level 1 encompasses billing and accounting applications. Level 2 includes departmental applications such as laboratory, radiology, pharmacy, materials management, and order management. Level 3 covers clinical orders applications such as point-of-care charting, clinical process and provider profiling, and communication with ancillary services such as home care and practice management. Level 4 has enterprise clinical care charting that includes master patient index, data warehouses, electronic medical records, and ambulatory charting. Level 5 encompasses a repository of member financial, clinical, and demographic data in an electronic data repository. Finally, level 6 has applications for analyzing health care outcomes and disease management.

Wirtschafter and colleagues implemented a computerized consultant extender for a breast cancer clinical protocol that used algorithms to produce a 95% compliance rate among 75 local physicians who used the system, as compared with a 64% rate for cancer center physicians who did not use the automated system.[43] ONCOCIN is an expert system, in use at Stanford University, for assisting oncologists to manage patients on chemotherapy protocols.[44,45] It is both a medical record and an advice system that records the course of the patient on a protocol, and it can assume an active role in adapting the protocol to the individual patient. It can determine drug doses on the basis of time schedule, toxicity, and blood counts. When oncology patient care stipulated by the computer was compared with care given by oncology fellows, similar levels of competency were seen.

Numerous oncology medical records have been implemented at cancer centers to facilitate all aspects of patient care, to interact with hospital information systems and with data management offices, and to maintain patient and protocol charts. The CLIN system implemented at the Memorial Sloan-Kettering Cancer Center by Serber was one of the earliest systems that implemented an oncology protocol record with complete data management and statistical tools.[46] The OCIS (Oncology Clinical Information System) of the Johns Hopkins Hospital is a time-oriented tabular and graphic database with a meaningful grouping of related information that links patient data and procedural support.[47] It interconnects mainframe, minicomputers, and micro-computers effectively to automate all aspects of cancer patient management.

Clinical Trials To increase the number of patients accrued (now less than 3% of the national burden) and to simplify the data management requirements for cancer clinical trials, two recent innovations deserve comment. The National Cancer Institute's Cancer Informatics Infrastructure permits oncologists and their patients to use their computers over the Internet to identify appropriate cancer clinical trials for their specific cancer diagnosis and to facilitate patient registration (<http://cancertrials.nci.nih.gov>). Other useful sites include the American Cancer Society (<http://clinicaltrials.cancer.org>), and OncoLink (<http://cancer.med.upenn.edu:80>).

All phase I, II, and III cancer clinical trials approved by the NCI's Cancer Therapy Evaluation Program (CTEP) are now required to be reported to CTEP using the Clinical Data Update System (CDUS) that is based on coding standards approved by the International Conference on Harmonization Multidisciplinary Group 2 (<http://www.ich.org>). This group was established to recommend electronic standards for the transfer of regulatory information by evaluating and recommending open and nonproprietary standards that meet the requirements of regulatory authorities and pharmaceutical companies. The recommendations provide solutions for structured and personal messaging (free text), electronic data interchange, datasets, definitions that incorporate structured data formats, security to ensure confidentiality, data integrity, authentication, and nonrepudiation. The datasets include protocol administrative information, patient demographics, treatment information, toxicity information, and response information. Further information about CTEP is available at <http://ctep.info.nih.gov> and for CDUS at <http://ctep.cancer.gov/reporting/cdus.html>.

Clinical Practice Guidelines Clinical practice guidelines are systematically developed statements to assist the practitioner with clinical decisions about appropriate health care for specific clinical indications. With the upsurge in evidence-based medicine and systematic reviews, they have emerged as a health research tool to analyze and report patterns of care and clinical outcomes. In oncology, ASCO (<http://www.asco.org>) has developed clinical practice guidelines outlining appropriate methods of treatment and care that address specific clinical situations (disease-oriented) and the use of approved medical products, procedures, or tests (modality-oriented). In addition, ASCO has also published technology assessments that are used to determine if a procedure, device, or test is appropriate for broad-based conventional usage.

The National Comprehensive Cancer Network (NCCN) (<http://www.nccn.org>) has developed 90 specific guidelines for oncologic diseases, covering 93% of all tumor types and support modalities. The NCCN guidelines include screening, prevention, diagnosis, work-up, treatment, and follow-up components. The NCCN and the American Cancer Society have collaborated on patient education versions of the NCCN guidelines for the common cancer types (<http://www.nccn.org>).

The goal of these techniques is to provide a means to measure an improvement in clinical outcome, in terms of survival, quality of life, treatment toxicity, patient satisfaction, and cost-effectiveness. Clinical practice guidelines will be incorporated into point-of-care oncologic practice by integrating them into oncologic electronic patient records, permitting analysis of patterns of care. In addition, computers will give creators of guidelines instant feedback from users when guidelines are not followed so that guidelines can be constantly assessed. Another useful site that is acting as a clearinghouse for all guidelines is the National Guidelines Clearinghouse (<http://www.guidelines.gov>). Swanson and colleagues discuss using a practice-based computerized clinical information system to evaluate growth factor usage patterns and outcomes among oncologists in the community setting.[48] They found that ASCO's clinical guidelines were used mainly for reference purposes. They concluded that their system could accurately collect detailed information regarding practice patterns of oncologists and that ASCO's survey data significantly underreport the use of growth factors in the community and indicate that a substantial number of oncologists are not following these guidelines.

Information Refinement Computer technology today can increase accessibility to a collection of information. Tomorrow, it will make this information much more useful. Information refinement is an electronic, computer-based process that takes undifferentiated volumes of raw information and converts them into electronic form, extracts the content units, and recombines them into a new form that can be distributed in a variety of ways or recombined into new end products. Primitive refining today uses the literal terms of words, keywords, and synonym lists that rely on word indexes and the searching and indexing of keyword bases. It suffers from poor recall performance and poor precision. Future systems will be able to break all information into usable divisions, strip out the impurities, and turn the data into a basic form that can be reprocessed, refined, and transformed.

Unified Medical Language System Medical informatic standards will be required to simplify information management. The Unified Medical Language System (UMLS) project, undertaken by the National Library of Medicine, is designed to facilitate the retrieval and integration of information from many machine-readable information sources, including descriptions of the biomedical literature, clinical records, factual data banks, and medical knowledge bases. Further information is available at <http://umlsinfo.nlm.nih.gov>. Like MESH (Medical Subject Heading), which is a controlled vocabulary of 21,000 terms culled from the medical literature and arranged in a series of tree structures, the proposed UMLS is a highly structured language designed for a clinical database to define medical terminology more specifically. Thus, different software programs that describe signs and symptoms of a disease will use a common term and permit one program to communicate more easily with another. To the extent that an application conforms to the UMLS guidelines, it will be able to communicate with other UMLS systems.

Clinical Laboratory and Testing Standards A standard for exchange of laboratory data that will standardize the way all medical laboratories represent, store, and transmit data electronically has been defined by the American Society for Testing and Materials (ASTM).[49] Hospitals, the ASTM, and vendors have broadened these standards for similar handling of data for billing, admissions and discharges, orders, and laboratory reports in hospitals under the HL-7 guidelines. In addition, the American College of Radiology and the National Electronic Manufacturers Association have formalized the storing of digital radiographic images. This allows hospital, commercial, and physician office laboratories to communicate with each other and facilitate placing information on a patient's chart. Today, many innovative commercial laboratories and hospitals make laboratory and imaging results including actual x-ray and scanned images available in a secure manner over the Internet.

Text Retrieval Retrieval of information from computer databases uses either an exact match of

Table 143-9 Boolean Searching Examples

AND: Find all references to A AND B will bring all the records that contain A and that also contain B. Records containing only A or only B are excluded. It is used to limit a search (reduce the number of records found).

OR: Find all references to A OR B will bring all records that contain A, plus all the records that contain B, plus all the records that contain both A and B. It is used to expand a search (increase the number of records found).

AND NOT: Find all references to A AND NOT B will exclude topics that are not of interest. This means that all records that contain A but that do not contain B should be obtained.

WITHIN xx WORDS: (Proximity search) Find liver within three words of transplant will bring liver transplant, not transplant of the cornea or liver.

terms or phrases (keyword in context or "kwic") or a probabilistic scheme based on the appearance of terms or phrases.[50,51] Only exact matches are economically feasible with today's software. The combination of terms or phrases with the Boolean "AND," "OR," and "NOT" operations, together with adjacency or nearness of terms, serves as the basis for matching against a dictionary all the terms in the database, excluding certain STOP words, such as "the," "and," and "of" (Table 143-9). Keywords, such as MESH terms in MEDLARS, are assigned to citations by abstractors to help facilitate searching, since language is imprecise and exact terms may change with time. The oncologist will find invaluable a recent review by Lowe and Barnett on understanding and using the MESH vocabulary.[52] Full-text databases use proximity searching or the spatial relationships of words and phrases, along with synonyms to facilitate searching.

Initially, electronic databases used only Boolean algorithm searches. Although they reduce imprecision (the portion of retrieved items that are actually of interest) and increase recall (the portion of truly relevant items that are found), they require searching skills. Today databases are able to take a search query written in English, do a spelling check, remove words with low information content, extract root words from the words' different forms and create suffix variants, add synonyms from a thesaurus or MESH dictionary, deliver the articles in the order of importance, and reorder and redo the search when articles of low relevance are indicated by the searcher and the concept words are better defined. Finally, the articles may be presented in the decreasing order of the number of times the context words are repeated in the article.

MAJOR INTERNET RESOURCES OF INTEREST TO THE ONCOLOGIST

The reader is referred to DIRLINE (Directory of Information Resources Online), produced by the National Library of Medicine and available online at <http://www.nlm.nih.gov/pubs/factsheets/dirlinfs.html> for location and descriptive information about a wide variety of information resources, including organizations, research resources, projects, and databases concerned with health and biomedicine. More detailed summaries of the most popular medical and cancer-specific databases are given below.

Cancer Surveillance It is essential to be able to measure cancer-related risk factors, health behaviors, health services, clinical outcomes, and cost from cancer incidence, morbidity, mortality, and survival statistics. The information and computer technologies combining statistical methodologies and national databases evaluating these parameters are readily available for analysis and are available on the WWW.

SEER The NCI's Surveillance, Epidemiology, and End Results (SEER) tumor registry of cancer cases began in 1973 and collects cancer demographic information in the United States. The SEER program currently collects and publishes cancer incidence and survival data from 14 population-based cancer registries and 3 supplemental registries covering approximately 26% of the U.S. population. Information on more than 3 million in situ and invasive cancer cases is included in the SEER database, and approximately 170,000 new cases are added each year. The SEER registries routinely collect data on patient demographics, primary tumor site, morphology, stage at diagnosis, first course of treatment, and follow-up for vital status. The SEER program is the only comprehensive source of population-based information in the United States that includes stage of cancer at the time of diagnosis and survival rates within each stage. The mortality data reported by SEER are provided by the National Center for Health Statistics. It is located at <http://seer.cancer.gov>.

Medicare Claims Medical cost data can be obtained from the Center for Medicare and Medicaid Services database on medical care and Medicare claims (<http://www.cms.gov/>).

National Cancer Database The National Cancer Database collected by the American College of Surgeons Committee on Cancer and the American Cancer Society measures patterns of cancer care in the United States (<http://www.facs.org/dept/cancer/ncdb>).

Fraumeni and Rimer have inaugurated a series on the developing fields of cancer surveillance that uses these "geospatial databases," a term coined by them, to measure the progress of the National Cancer Program and to provide leads into the etiology and eventual control of cancer.[53] Researchers have combined the SEER database with the CMS Medicare claims files for the same patients.[54,55] This will help determine regional cancer treatment and staging procedure costs and the cost-effectiveness of screening and staging procedures, to compare hospital and outpatient costs of cancer care and to assist in outcome analyses and practice guidelines research.

Cancer.gov Cancer.gov (<http://www.cancer.gov/>) contains monthly updated information for professionals and patients on cancer, including PDQ, fact sheets, publications, and NCI news covering cancer treatment, detection, screening, prevention, rehabilitation, statistics, and quality-of-life issues, detailed information about ongoing clinical trials, selected information from the *Journal of the National Cancer Institute*, CANCERLIT topic searches, links to other NCI and government Web sites, and links to other organizations that provide cancer information and support services. In addition, summaries and fact sheets that have been added, changed, or deleted each month can be accessed for the oncologist's review.

CANCERLIT The CANCERLIT database (<http://www.cancer.gov/cancer_information/cancer_literature>), compiled since 1976, contains more than 1,800,000 citations from the world's cancer literature beginning from 1963, with more than 60% containing abstracts. Approximately 4,000 medical resources are currently indexed in CANCERLIT, including journals, meeting proceedings, symposia, books, doctoral theses, and research project summaries. Each year an additional 96,000 records are added. Each article is referenced with appropriate MESH terms. CANCERLIT can be searched for cancer literature, clinical trials, and genetic services (<http://www.cancer.gov/search/cancer_literature>) or by topics (<http://www.cancer.gov/search/cancer_literature/searchcancerlittopic.aspx>).

MEDLINE The MEDLINE database, compiled since 1966, contains more than 12,000,000 citations from the world's biomedical literature, with more than 60% containing abstracts since 1965 and 80% referring to English-language items. Approximately 4,500 of the world's 22,000 medical journals are currently indexed in MEDLINE. Each year 372,000 articles are added. Each article is referenced with carefully chosen key words and phrases from the National Library of Medicine's (NLM) MESH terms so that one can call up a list of relevant titles and then obtain the most appropriate abstracts. To assist with searching for evidence-based medicine, a search filter for "systematic reviews" was added in 2002. The most popular Internet location for MEDLINE is PubMed (<http://www.ncbi.nlm.nih.gov/entrez/query.fcgi>). The NLM links full text articles from about a quarter of the publishers represented on MEDLINE to PubMed. One of its most important features is the ability to search for "related articles" for more focused searching. The NLM Gateway site (<http://gateway.nlm.nih.gov/gw>) allows users to search multiple NLM databases simultaneously, including MEDLINE, PubMed, OLDMEDLINE, LOCATORplus, MEDLINEplus, DIRLINE, AIDS Meetings, and Health Services research meetings. A highly recommended tutorial for PubMed is located at <http://www.nlm.nih.gov/bsd/pubmed_tutorial/m1001.html>.

Cogent Medicine This is a site that merges MEDLINE with tools for searching and archiving citations to create an online, personalized reference system. One can create folders and subfolders for disease and other categories housing actual searches that can be reused, other search results found and expert commentary and citations covering these topics. Autoqueries can be set up to automatically generate periodic searching with notifications to the user by e-mail. It is free and located at <http://www.cogentmedicine.com>.

PubMed Central PubMed Central is a digital archive of full-text medical journals that agree to make their contents freely available. It also includes full-text from journals that are only published electronically (<http://www.pubmedcentral.nih.gov>).

Biosis Produced by Biosis.org, and available at <http://www.biosis.org>, this database contains 14.5 million citations from 1969 to the present, covering some 9,000 scientific journals and books, conferences, proceedings, and monographs.

Embase This is EXCERPTA MEDICA's online database produced by Embase.com, which screens 5,000 journals published since 1974, making available more than 13 million citations. It is located at <http://www.embase.com/>.

HealthSTAR This database includes patient outcomes and the effectiveness of procedures, programs, products, services, and processes, and nonclinical health care administration and planning aspects of health care delivery. It has 3.9 million records and adds 17,000 per month (<http://gateway.nlm.nih.gov/gw>).

National Cancer Database Produced by the Commission on Cancer of the American College of Surgeons and the American Cancer Society, this database collects cancer registry data from hospitals and helps oncologists compare trends in the treatment of cancer and its outcomes by individual hospital or by state, regional, or national patterns of care (<http://www.facs.org/dept/cancer/ncdb>).

ISI Journal Citation Reports The ISI journal citation reports (JCR) uses the Science Citation Index to determine the frequency of literature citations for a given article and permits the tracking of all articles that cite common references in order to trace common work. Journals indexed are selected on the basis of several criteria, including citation analysis, resulting in coverage of the most significant publications in the scientific, technical, and biomedical literature. In addition to the more conventional retrieval methods, the JCR offers citation indexing, which permits searching by cited references. It is available at <http://www.isinet.com/isi/products/citation/jcr/jcrweb/index.html>.

Physician Data Query Physician Data Query (PDQ) is the NCI's comprehensive database that contains information that has been evaluated by a panel of 70 experts and is updated on a quarterly basis. It contains the latest information about prognosis, staging, cellular classification, and state-of-the-art cancer treatments, clinical trials, screening, prevention, genetics, supportive care and complementary and alternative medicines. It gives detailed summaries for the physician or layperson of the 90 major tumor types. Tumors may be searched by body system/site or histologic tissue/type. It lists more than 2,000 currently active protocols that use mostly standardized formats and 13,000 closed-treatment protocols, with detailed information on the study objectives, patient entry criteria, treatment regimens, and demographic information for cooperative groups and physicians involved with the protocols. In addition, PDQ makes available demographic information for approximately 17,000 cancer specialists and more than 1,500 organizations affiliated with societies that are related to cancer. It is readily available to physicians and their patients through telecommunication facilities or telephone (1-800-4-CANCER). The reader is referred to two excellent reviews for further information.[56,57] Table 143-10 lists the major categories of PDQ. It is used primarily by oncologists to ensure that the most current treatment methods are used, to assist in making a clinical decision, and to find information about clinical trials. Less frequently, it is used to prepare for conferences or to confirm information from other sources. Other uses include referring a patient to an oncologic investigator in a specific location, finding an investigator who has access to a particular clinical trial, and seeking consultation from another physician (<http://cancer.gov/cancertopics/pdq>).

The Physicians' Information and Education Resource The Physicians' Information and Education Resource (PIER) is a practical, evidence-based medical knowledge and guidance resource for their members (<http://pier.acponline.org/index.html?hp>) It was developed by the American College of Physicians (ACP) as a member benefit with 130 modules, covering both common and uncommon diseases including modules dealing with prevention and screening, diagnosis, consultation for diagnosis, hospitalization, drug and nondrug therapies, patient education, consultation management, follow-up, case scenarios, clinical alerts, glossaries, and references, along with legal and ethical issues, complementary/alternative medicine procedures, and what's new for that disease. It is presented electronically in a unique layered and telegraphic format designed for rapid access to clinical information. PIER is linked to other resources at the ACP's Web site and to many other Internet resources. Its uniqueness relates to its intention to mirror the way a physician thinks through a problem. In the disease modules, for example, there is a logical flow of information from diagnosis through management. Its structure and format allows its content to be readily integrated into other applications such as electronic medical records.

Table 143-10 Physician Data Query (PDQ) Selections

Selections
1. Cancer Information
Treatment by body system/site
Treatment by histologic tissue type
Treatment of childhood cancer
Prognosis
Staging
Supportive care
Rare tumor
Design of clinical tools
Cancer screening/detection (testing)
Prevention
Genetics
Complementary and alternative medicine
2. Late-Breaking News in Oncology
3. Physicians
4. Organizations
5. Protocols
Open
Study objectives
Patient eligibility
Treatment regimens
Dose and schedule modifications
Names of principal investigators and institutions
Closed
Abstracts
6. Investigational Drug File
7. CANCERLIT searches

CCRIS The Chemical Carcinogenesis Research Information System (CCRIS) contains carcinogenicity, tumor promotion, tumor inhibition, and mutagenicity test results derived from the scanning of primary journals, current awareness tools, NCI technical reports, review articles, and International Agency for Research on Cancer monographs published since 1976. It is located at <http://toxnet.nlm.nih.gov/>.

CLINICAL AND RESEARCH AND OTHER USES OF COMPUTERS

Computer-Generated Media Computers integrate text, graphics, animation, audio, and video communication technologies into a potent method to deliver information. Oncologists now have a choice of media—print, slides, overhead, or live delivery from a computer screen. An idea can be drawn on paper and scanned into the computer, or drawn directly on the computer screen using up to 32 million colors, and even animated and given sound. Presentations using electronic links can have the input of many individuals and can be instantly altered for different audiences. Using a presentation program, like PowerPoint from Microsoft, for controlling external devices, such as a computer projector, one can integrate multimedia for live presentations.

Computers have replaced medical arts departments in medical schools. Oncologists can easily create graphics of their data and ideas and transmit them to an audio or video device. Changes can be reflected instantaneously. Laser printers can provide near–typeset-quality reproductions. Scanners replace paper images, such as photographs, illustrations, text, files, forms, and charts, with digitized images of the original, which, when converted into a computer document, can be customized for presentation. These images can be stored on magnetic media and transmitted over data communication networks. Thus, users can scan, store, retrieve, enhance, sort, and route these documents.

Document Imaging and Image Processing Because medical imaging plays such a major role in the oncologist's need to measure and define cancer, a method to acquire, display, analyze, store, and print digitized images becomes important. Radiographs, nuclear medicine scans, CT and magnetic resonance imaging (MRI) scans, and motion and still video films can all be viewed on the high resolution screens of personal computers so as to display images with the same clarity, resolution, and gray scale as the imaging systems' own consoles. Modern compression techniques can store up to 10,000 images on an optical disk for instantaneous retrieval for patient care, teaching, and documentation. Document imaging is the replacement of paper images and files with digitized images of the original, using a scanner. These images are stored on magnetic media and can be transmitted over data communication networks.

CT, MRI, ultrasonography, and PET scans remain the province of the radiologist. But now, from their desktop computers, oncologists are able to obtain these images; enhance, store, index, and transfer them to any computer worldwide; and manipulate them to make diagnosis and treatment planning easier. The computer is able to compare changes on different studies and give quantitative and qualitative information more accurately than can the human eye. Radiographs are now digitized for similar analyses.

Three-dimensional imaging has revolutionized radiation treatment planning. Two-dimensional digitized medical CT or MRI images can be combined with three-dimensional graphic programs to target tumor killing and minimize damage to normal tissue. By defining tumor location and anatomy, the computer can then design the proper radiation beam approaches and calculate the radiation dose distribution. Similar techniques will make surgical treatment more exacting. The iPod, which holds 60 gigabytes of data, is now being used to store medical images using OsiriX software to display and manipulate complex medical image data that is distributed free under Open Source licensing. Images can be seen on the iPod, a monitor, or TV screen in 2D, 3D, or 4D images. Large datasets can be transferred directly to the iPod through its firewire connection. OsiriX allows users to upload images to the Internet. It also supports iChat instant messaging, which is compatible with AOL instant messaging. This allows the user to take advantage of the video-conferencing capability. But instead of seeing the user's face on a Web cam, it is modified to show the user's screen at the other end of the conversation. The software can be downloaded at <http://www.homepage.mac.com/rossetantoine/osirix/>.

Presentation Devices Inexpensive projection pads permit projecting the computer image onto a screen, eliminating the need for slide film. Animated and audio presentations can be produced for educational and instructional purposes, and they can be transmitted to a television or video recorder. Cancer patients who have disabilities can use voice recognition software to control the computer. Textual material can be converted to speech by specialized software to assist the visually impaired.

Scanners Black-and-white or color scanners can convert photographs, line-art drawings, and gray-scale or halftone images into digital form for manipulation, visualization, and storage in the computer. These can then be used directly in a word-processing or page makeup program or placed in a presentation program for slides. Scanners can even take radiographic films and scan them into the computer.

Optical Character Recognition Optical character recognition (OCR) software can, with almost 100% accuracy, take typewritten or typeset text created with any font or font size, in any language; distinguish text from graphics and multiple columns of text in a table; and convert it into a digital form that can be manipulated by the computer. A scanner can easily put typewritten reports into an electronic medical record. A single typewritten page can be scanned in less than several seconds. Thus, large amounts of printed or faxed material can be easily and inexpensively stored, indexed, tracked, and made easily accessible.

Presentation Software Organization, outlining, graphic skills, and visual presentation are required to convey our thoughts to our colleagues. Presentation software such as PowerPoint from Microsoft or KeyNote from Apple can assist in creating, organizing, and producing presentations with the capability of easily making modifications for different audiences. Outliners can organize text into an outline form and transform it into bullet charts or organizational charts for onscreen or overhead slide presentations. Presentation programs control the font, size, style, and color of individual characters. One can scan into the computer diagrams, tables, graphs, or pictures; add text; modify the drawing; sort the slides; produce speaker notes; and then send the information to a desktop film recorder for slides, to a color ink-jet printer for handouts or overhead slides, or to service bureaus for professionally produced slides. One can even directly present what is seen on the computer monitor on a large screen, using a projection pad and an overhead projector.

Data Acquisition and Instrument Control Data acquisition requires taking measured experimental data in wavelengths or analog form and converting the data to digital form by an analog-to-digital converter. With specialized computer software, it is possible to have the computer read this information, display it, analyze it, and make appropriate decisions automatically. The computer, by transforming itself into a voltmeter, frequency counter, oscilloscope, spectrum analyzer, or x-y recorder, can record sound, heat, light, pressure, and electrical signals. The most popular instrument control program is Lab View (National Instruments Corp., Austin, TX).

Bioinformatics In the last few decades, advances in molecular biology and the equipment available for research in this field have allowed the increasingly rapid sequencing of complete genomes of several species, including man. Popular sequence databases, such as the National Center for Biotechnology Information's GenBank (<http://www.ncbi.nlm.nih.gov>) and the European Bioinformatics Institute's EMBL Nucleotide Sequence Database <http://www.embl.org/> have been growing at exponential rates. This deluge of information has necessitated the careful storage, organization, and indexing of sequence information, whereby information science has been applied to biology to produce the field called Bioinformatics.

The simplest tasks used in bioinformatics concern the creation and maintenance of databases of biologic information. Nucleic acid sequences (and the protein sequences derived from them) comprise the majority of such databases. Although the storage and organization of millions of nucleotides is far from trivial, designing a database and developing an interface whereby researchers can both access existing information and submit new entries is only the beginning. The most pressing tasks in bioinformatics involve the analysis of sequence information. Computational Biology is the name given to this process, and it involves finding the genes in the deoxyribonucleic acid (DNA) sequences of various organisms, developing methods to predict the structure and/or function of newly discovered proteins and structural ribonucleic acid (RNA) sequences, clustering protein sequences into families of related sequences and the development of protein models, and aligning similar proteins and generating phylogenetic trees to examine evolutionary relationships.

The process of evolution has produced DNA sequences that encode proteins with very specific functions. It is possible to predict the three-dimensional structure of a protein using algorithms that have been derived from our knowledge of physics, chemistry, and most importantly, from the analysis of other proteins with similar amino acid sequences. Using homology matrix analysis, the computer can compare sequences of numbers or letters. It, thus, can compare DNA sequences and perform DNA sequencing. Such an innovative program is Gene Construction Kit for Macintosh (Textco Biosoftware Inc., West Lebanon, NH). Users can represent DNA sequences graphically or as text. Recombinant DNA molecules can be constructed on the screen. The program has a database of restriction enzymes that can cut DNA at specific base pairs. Thus, one can cut and splice DNA sequences and then analyze the results in the model. It is a means to bring the world of desktop publishing into the molecular biologist's world. Another useful tool is Oncomine that was created by Dr. Arul Chinnaiyan and is a proprietary compilation of microarray datasets from over 100 cancer studies allowing researchers to analyze data from disparate sources by normalizing data and making qualitative comparisons across datasets (<http://www.oncomine.org>).[58]

GenMAPP (Gene MicroArray Pathway Profiler) is a free computer program available at

<http://www.genmapp.org> designed for viewing and analyzing gene expression data representing biological pathways and grouping of genes. It allows one to visualize gene expression data in a biological context with the graphical and more intuitive format of MAPPs that are computer generated files that graphically show the biological relationship between genes or gene products. MAPPs can be represented in GenMAPP as metabolic pathways, signal transduction cascades, subcellular locations, gene families, or lists of genes associated with Gene Ontology categories. Each MAPP contains gene objects, which represent biological genes or gene products such as receptors, membranes and ribosomes, and the relationships among the objects. Each gene object on a MAPP is identified by a gene identifier from one of the GenMAPP-accepted gene ID systems.

The reader is referred to an article by Buetow for a description of the NCI's Center for Bioinformatics program.[59] Information on the NCI's Cancer Biomedical Informatics Grid (CaBIG) can be found at <http://caBIG.nci.nih.gov>. For an excellent tutorial on how to use bioinformatics tools, the reader is referred to <http://www.ncbi.nlm.nih.gov/Coffeebreak>. For patients, an excellent resource that addresses the health implications of the Human Genome Project is the Genetics Home Reference (<http://ghr.nlm.nih.gov/ghr/page/Home>).[60]

STATISTICS There is a plethora of statistical programs that combine the major procedures used in most analyses with the ability to display results instantly as charts or plots. Most programs permit the data to be read in from other programs and to be stored in tables, rectangular files, or matrices. After analysis, the results can be exported to other programs. Data can be sorted, selected, and rotated on the basis of data values. Most programs include frequency distribution; data transformation; nonparametric statistics; cross-tabulation statistics; analysis of variance, correlation, and regression; and multivariate analysis.

All oncologists must become computer literate. A small investment in learning time and capital ($1,200 [US] to $3,000 [US]) will pay off handsomely. Oncologists will have easier access to patient data, less loss of records, greater medical knowledge, and more efficient updating of information. They would have immediate access to electronic textbooks and journals and easier communication from one's own office, using electronic mailboxes and modems, with other physicians' offices or the hospital. The computer has become the oncologist's "black bag."

REFERENCES

1. NCCN Guidelines. Cancer Control 2001;8(6 Suppl 2).
2. Gotay CC. Trial-related quality of life: using quality-of-life assessment to distinguish among cancer therapies. Monogr Natl Cancer Inst 1996;20:1–6.
3. Weeks J. Taking quality of life into account in health economic analyses. Monogr Natl Cancer Inst 1996;20:23–7.
4. Hewitt M, Simone J, editors. Ensuring quality cancer care. National Cancer Policy Board, Institute of Medicine and Commission on Life Sciences, National Research Council. Washington, DC: National Academy Press; 1999.
5. Kohn LT, Corrigan JM, Donaldson MS, editors. To err is human: building a safer health system. Committee on Quality of Health Care in America. Institute of Medicine. Washington, DC: National Academy Press; 1999.
6. Crossing the quality chasm: a new health system for the 21st century. Committee on Quality of Health Care in America. Institute of Medicine. Washington, DC: National Academy Press; 2001.
7. President's Information Technology Advisory Committee: Transforming health care through information technology. February 9, 2001. http://www.nitrd.gov/pubs/pitac/pitac-hc-9feb01.pdf (accessed June 23, 2005).
8. President's Cancer Panel: Voices of a broken system: real people, real problems. 2001. https://cissecure.nci.nih.gov/ncipubs/details.asp?pid=1060 (accessed June 23, 2005).
9. Stephenson J. Lab-on-a-chip shows promise in defining and diagnosing cancers. JAMA 1999;282:1801–2.
10. Greenes RA, Shortliffe EH. Medical informatics: an emerging academic discipline and institutional priority. JAMA 1990;263:1114–20.
11. Shortliffe EH, Perreault LE. Medical informatics: computer applications in health care and biomedicine (health care informatics). New York: Springer; 2000.
12. Kassirer JP. The next transformation in the delivery of health care [editorial]. N Engl J Med 1995;332:52–4.
13. Gilder G. The coming software shift. Forbes ASAP 1995;147–162.
14. Blumberg JW. PDA applications for physicians. ASCO Technology News January 2004; 4–6.
15. Wilkins A, Hovhanesian J. The virtual workplace. Healthcare Informatics November 1999;66–70.
16. Internet World Stats. Available at http://www.internetworldstats.com/stats.htm (accessed Dec 28, 2004)
17. Glowniak JV, Bushway MK. Computer networks as a medical resource. JAMA 1994;271:1934–9.
18. Eysenbach G. The impact of the Internet on cancer outcomes. CA Cancer J Clin 2003;53:356–71.
19. Whois Source. Available at http://www.whois.sc/internet-statistics/ (accessed Dec 28, 2004).
20. Varmus H. E-Biomed: a proposal for electronic publications in the biomedical sciences. http://www.nih.gov/about/director/ebiomed/ebi.htm (accessed June 23, 2005).
21. Relman AS. The NIH "E-BIOMED" proposal; a potential threat to the evaluation and orderly dissemination of new clinical studies. N Engl J Med 1999;340:1793–4.
22. Bosak J, Bray T. XML and the second-generation WEB. Sci Am 1999;269:89–93.
23. Berners-Lee T, Hendler J, Lassila O. The semantic Web. Sci Am 2001;284:35–43 and http://www.sciam.com/article.cfm?articleID=00048144-10D2-1C70-84A9809EC588EF21 (accessed June 23, 2005).
24. Carrns A. Employers urge doctors to make "visits" on line. Wall Street Journal 2001 March 21;Sect. B1.
25. Kane B, Sands DZ. Guidelines for the clinical use of electronic mail with patients. JAMIA 1998;5:104–11.
26. Pereira JL, Koski S, Hanson J, et al. Internet usage among women with breast cancer: an exploratory study. Clin Breast 2000;1:148–53.
27. Chen X, Siu LL. Impact of the media and the Internet on oncology: survey of cancer patients and oncologists in Canada. J Clin Oncol 2001;19:4291–7.
28. Helft PR, Hlubocky F, Daugherty CK. American oncologist's views of Internet use by cancer patients: a mail survey of American Society of Clinical Oncology members. J Clin Oncol 2003;21:942–7.
29. Bichakjian CK, Schwartz JL, Wang TS, et al. Melanoma information on the Internet: often incomplete—a public health opportunity? J Clin Oncol 2002;20:134–41.
30. Purcell GP, Wilson P. The quality of health information on the Internet. BMJ 2002;324:557–8.
31. Marshall WW, Haley RW. Use of a secure Internet Web site for collaborative medical research. JAMA 2000;284:1843–9.
32. Anderson DP, Kubiatowicz J. The worldwide computer. Sci Am 2002;286:40–42.
33. Prescher-Hughes DS. The nurse's forum: developing practice protocols. Oncologistics Fourth Quarter 2003, p. 11–3.
34. Kim MI, Johnson B. Personal health records: evaluation of functionality and utility. J Am Med Inform Assoc 2002;9:171–80.
35. Masys DR. Giving patients access to their medical records via the Internet: the PCASSO experience. CPRI-Mail 8:4 Dec 1999.
36. Morrison I. The future of physicians' time. Ann Intern Med 2000;132:80–4.
37. Schneider EC, Epstein AM, et al. Developing a system to assess the quality of cancer care: ASCO's National Initiative on Cancer Care Quality JCO 2004;22:2985–91.
38. Yasnoff WA, Humphreys BL, Overhage JM, et al. A consensus action agenda for achieving the national health information infrastructure. J Am Med Inform Assoc 2004;11:332–8.
39. 2004 Resource guide. Healthcare Inform Dec 2004;9–104.
40. Frisch S. Medical software reviews. Brooklyn (NY): Healthcare Computing Publications.
41. Wyatt JC. Clinical data system, part 1: data and medical records; part 2: components and techniques; part 3: development and evaluation. Lancet 1994;344:1543–7, 1609–14, 1682–8.
42. Powsner SM, Tufte ER. Graphical summary of patient status. Lancet 1994;344:386–9.
43. Wirtschafter DD, Gams R, Ferguson C, et al. Clinical protocol information system. In: O'Neill JT, editor. Proceedings, fourth annual symposium on computer applications in medical care. Washington, DC: IEEE Computer Society Press; 1980. p. 745.
44. Rennels GD, Shortliffe EH. Advanced computing for medicine. Sci Am 1987;257:154–61.
45. Shortliffe EH. Computer programs to support clinical decision making. JAMA 1987;258:61–6.
46. Serber MJ, Mackey R, Young CW. The Sloan-Kettering Information System for clinical oncology. In: O'Neill JT, editor. Proceedings, fourth annual symposium on computer applications in medical care. Washington, DC: IEEE Computer Society Press; 1980. p. 728.
47. Enterline JP, Lenhard RE Jr, Blum BI. A clinical information system for oncology. New York: Springer-Verlag; 1989.
48. Swanson G, Bergstrom K, Stump E, et al. Growth factor usage patterns and outcomes in the community setting: collection through a practice-based computerized clinical information system. J Clin Oncol 2000;18:1764–70.
49. McDonald CJ, Hammond WE. Standard formats for electronic transfer of clinical data. Ann Intern Med 1989;110:333–5.
50. Belkin NJ, Croft WB. Retrieval techniques. In: Williams ME, editor. Annual review of information science and technology. Amsterdam: Elsevier Science; 1987. p. 22.
51. Fenichel CH. The process of searching online bibliographic data bases: a review of research. Library Res 1980;2:107.
52. Lowe HJ, Barnett O. Understanding and using the medical subject headings (MESH) vocabulary to perform searches. JAMA 1994;272:1103–8.
53. Fraumeni JF, Rimer BK. Cancer surveillance series: inauguration. J Natl Cancer Inst 1999;91:1004.
54. Potosky AL, Riley GF, Lubitz JD, et al. Potential for cancer related health services research using a linked Medicare-tumor registry database. Med Care 1993;31:732–48.
55. Earle CC, Neuman PJ, Gelber RD, et al. Impact of referral patterns on the use of chemotherapy for lung cancer. J Clin Oncol 2002;20:1786–92.
56. Hubbard SM, Henney JE, DeVita VT Jr. A computer data base for information on cancer treatment. N Engl J Med 1987;316:315–8.
57. Hubbard SM. The physician data query (PDQ) cancer information system. Bull Cancer 1987;74:205:214.
58. Hampton T. Tool helps cancer scientists mine genes. JAMA. 2004;292:2073.
59. Buetow KH. The NCI Center for Bioinformatics (NCICB): Building a foundation for in silico biomedical research. Ca Inv 2004;22:117–22.
60. Mitchell JA, Fun J, McCray AT. Design of Genetics Home Reference: A new NLM consumer health resource. J Am Med Inform Assoc 2004;11:439–47.

Index

Note: Page numbers followed by *t* indicate tables; page numbers followed by *f* indicate figures.

A

AAV. *See* Adeno-associated virus (AAV)
ABC technique, 446
Abdomen
  biopsy, 496
  infection, 2239
Abelson-related gene, 729
Aberrant crypt focus, 1373–1374
ABL, 523–524
abl, 80, 82, 119
ABL tyrosine kinase
  CML, 723–724
Absolute risk, 348
Acetabulum
  metastatic tumor to, 2088
Acetyltransferase, 356
Acidification, 550
Acinetobacter, 2226–2227
Acinic cell carcinoma, 1155
Acoustic schwannoma
  magnetic resonance imaging, 461
Acquired immunodeficiency syndrome (AIDS)
  and cancer, 1887–1899a
    epidemiology, 1887–1888
  transfusion related, 2105
Acquired von Willebrand's syndrome, 2115
Acral erythema, 2080–2081, 2080t, 2081f
Acral-lentiginous melanoma, 1646
Acromegaly, 2215
  treatment, 1087f
ACTH. *See* Adrenocorticotropic hormone (ACTH)
Actinic keratoses, 1663–1664, 1664f
  inflammation, 2080, 2080t
Actinomycin D (Dactinomycin, Cosmegen), 693
  structure of, 693f
Active treatment
  adaptation to, 904
Activities of daily living (ADL), 922
Acupuncture
  education about, 963
  needles for, 961f
Acute emesis, 2055
Acute graft-vs-host disease (GVHD), 2178
Acute leukemia
  transcriptional repression and chromatin acetylation, 115
Acute lung injury, 2168–2170
Acutely ill, 2246, 2247f
Acute lymphoblastic leukemia. *See* Adult acute lymphoblastic leukemia (ALL)
Acute lymphocytic leukemia (ALL), 77
  chemotherapy, 578
  in children, 1934–1940
    bone marrow transplantation, 1938
    heterogeneity, 1934–1935
    induction, 1935
    minimal residual disease, 1936–1937
    ophthalmic neoplasms, 1078–1079
    outcome, 1935–1936
    parenteral methotrexate and rescue, 1937
    post induction intensification, 1937
    presymptomatic central nervous system therapy, 1937–1938
    relapse, 1938–1939
    treatment, 591t
  combination chemotherapy, 624–625
  corticosteroids for, 822
  transplantation for, 888
Acute lymphoid leukemia. *See* Acute lymphocytic leukemia (ALL)
Acute myelogenous leukemia. *See* Acute myeloid leukemia (AML)
Acute myeloid leukemia (AML), 1739–1755
  central nervous system, 1754
  chemotherapy, 578, 1748–1749
  in children, 1944–1948
    classification and diagnosis, 1945
    complications, 1947–1948
    cytogenic abnormalities, 1945t
    epidemiology, 1944
    etiology, 1944–1945
    presentation, 1945
    prognosis, 1947
    therapy, 1945–1947
  chromosomal abnormalities, 113–114
  classification, 1740–1745
  complications, 1753–1754
  corticosteroids for, 822
  drug resistance circumvention, 1752
  in elderly, 117
  etiology, 1739
  genetic basis, 230–231
  hematopoietic growth factor, 1751
  hyperleukocytosis, 1753–1754
  immune modulation, 1751–1752
  karyotype in, 109f
  metabolic abnormalities, 1755
  minimally differentiated, 1741–1742
  minimal residual disease, 1753
  ophthalmic complications, 1754
  peripheral blood, 1741
  point mutations and pathogenesis of, 116–117
  pregnancy, 1754–1755
  prognosis, 1753
  relapsed
    therapy, 1750–1751
  signs and symptoms, 1745–1746
  therapy, 1746–1751
  transplantation for, 887–888
Acute pancreatitis, 2179
Acute-phase protein response
  cachexia, 2044
Acute postoperative respiratory failure, 2154–2155
Acute progranulocytic leukemia (APL), 1752–1753
Acute promyelocytic leukemia, 2116
  immunofluorescence staining of, 2116f
  transcriptional regulation of, 114f
  translocations involving retinoic acid receptor alpha, 115
Acute respiratory distress syndrome, 2168–2170
Acute respiratory failure (ARF)
  lung *vs.* pump failure in, 2169t
Acyclovir, 669
Adamantinoma, 1685–1686, 1685f
Adaptation, 902–904
Adeno-associated virus (AAV)
  gene delivery, 862
Adenocarcinoma
  appendiceal, 1364
  of bladder, 1426
  of breast, 441f
  eervical, 265–266, 1500–1501
    risk factors, 1499
  clear cell
    vagina, 1494, 1495t
  colorectal, 1369–1372
    pathology, 1369
    staging, 1369
  endometrial, 1524
  endometrial papillary, 1524
  endometrioid, 1500
  of esophagus, 371
  of gallbladder, 1318
  of gastric cardia, 371
  of lung, 1185–1186
  mucinous
    cervix, 1500
  pancreatic, 1331f
    computed tomography, 474f
  papillary serous
    ovaries, 445f
  of prostate
    histology, 1435f, 1436f
  rectal
    therapy, 1382
  of small intestine, 1360–1361
    staging, 1361
  vaginal
    cause, 264
Adenocarcinomas
  bronchioalveolar, 1186
Adenoid cystic carcinoma, 1155
  of lacrimal gland, 1082f
Adenoma malignum
  of cervix, 1500–1501
Adenomas
  adrenal
    magnetic resonance imaging, 477f
  family history
    and colorectal cancer, 1377
  gonadotroph, 815

Adenomas—*continued*
hepatic
benign, 1300
pituitary. *See* Pituitary adenomas
prior history
and colorectal cancer, 1377
sebaceous, 1674
of small intestine, 1360
unknown primary site, 1906–1908
Adenomatous polyposis coli (APC), 92–94, 93–94, 94f, 218, 1372, 1694
gastric cancer, 1272
methylation, 355
Adenosquamous carcinoma
cervical, 1501
of endometrium, 1524
of lungs, 1186
Adenoviruses, 790
gene delivery, 861
oncolytic, 870–871
tumor-selective, 867–868
Adhesion, 149–150
Adhesion molecules
multiple myeloma, 1849–1850
Adhesion related kinase (Ark), 60
A-Difluoromethylornithine, 1504
Adjuvant chemotherapy, 565–566
randomized studies, 592
ADL, 922
Adolescents
Burkitt lymphoma in, 1966–1967, 1967f, 1967t
chemotherapy for, 2032
clinical trials for, 2033–2034, 2033f, 2034t
diagnosis in, 2030–2031, 2030f
etiology in, 2029–2030
incidence in, 2028–2029
psychosocial care, 2032–2033
radiation therapy, 2032
smoking cessation, 360
supportive care, 2032–2033
surgery, 2032
survival, 2034–2035, 2035t
treatment in, 2031–2033
Adoptive transfer, 791–792
Adrenal adenoma
magnetic resonance imaging, 477f
Adrenal androgen inhibitors, 858
Adrenal cortex
hormones, 817–826
steroid biosynthesis, 1104f
Adrenal cortex neoplasms, 1103–1108
aldosterone producing, 1104
benign *vs.* malignant, 1106f
diagnosis, 1103–1104
differential diagnosis, 1104
function inhibitors, 1107
imaging, 1104–1105
MacFarlane classification, 1105t
management, 1105–1107
algorithm, 1107f
metastasis site, 1106t
pathogenesis, 1103
pathologic diagnosis, 1105
staging, 1105
Adrenal diseases, 2207–2208
Adrenal insufficiency, 2208
Adrenal medullary implants, 994
Adrenocorticoids
biosynthesis, 818, 818f
Adrenocorticotropic hormone (ACTH), 817
ectopic syndrome, 2211–2212
secreting pituitary adenomas
ketoconazole, 1087–1088
for thymoma, 1241
Adriamycin
cardiotoxicity
childhood Hodgkin's disease, 1960
Hodgkin disease, 1863
Adult acute lymphoblastic leukemia (ALL), 1772–1781
with adult T-cell leukemia/lymphoma, 1772
adverse prognostic factors in, 1777t
allogeneic stem-cell transplantation, 1778
aneuploidy, 1775
autologous stem-cell transplantation, 1778–1779
chemotherapy of, 1777
chromosome 9p21 abnormalities, 1775
classification of, 1773–1776
clinical presentation of, 1772–1773
CNS prophylaxis, 1779
consolidation therapy of, 1777–1778
cytochemistry of, 1773
cytogenetic-molecular markers of, 1774–1775, 1774t
diagnosis of, 1773f
drug resistance, 1779
epidemiology of, 1772
epigenetic alterations in, 1776
etiology of, 1772
features of, 1773t
gene expression microarrays, 1776
immunophenotypic classification of, 1774t
immunophenotyping of, 1773–1774
laboratory abnormalities of, 1772–1773
maintenance therapy of, 1778
MLL rearrangements (11q23), 1775
morphology of, 1773
MRD in, 1779–1780
pH-positive, 1780
prognosis of, 1776
8q24 rearrangements, 1775
salvage therapy of, 1780–1781
stem-cell transplantation, 1778–1779
T-cell receptor gene rearrangements, 1775
transcription factor 3 gene rearrangements (19p13), 1775
translocation 5(12;21), 1775
translocation t(9;22), 1774–1775
treatment of, 1776–1780, 1781t
Adult respiratory distress syndrome (ARDS), 2157, 2158f
Adult T-cell leukemia/lymphoma (ATLL)
with adult acute lymphoblastic leukemia, 1772
Advance care documents, 1006–1007
Advanced practice
in oncology nursing, 919
Advocacy, 1020
Aflatoxins, 250
causing hepatocellular carcinoma, 324
in liver, 1293
Africa
bladder cancer in, 332
Age, 339–340
breast cancer, 260
colorectal cancer
incidence, 369f
incidence, 346f, 347f
invasive cancer, 344t
liver neoplasms, 1292
mortality, 344t, 345f
gastric cancer, 368f
mucositis, 2187
prostate neoplasms, 1431
schistosomiasis, 332
Agency for Health Care and Policy Research (AHCPR), 427a
clinical practice guidelines, 356
Agents
preparation for clinical trials, 608
Age of onset
skin cancer, 283
xeroderma pigmentosum, 284f
Aging, 949–954
biology, 949–950
impact on American population, 1031–1032
physiologic changes, 950
Agrin family, 60
AHCPR. *See* Agency for Health Care and Policy Research (AHCPR)
AHSCT. *See* Autologous hematopoietic stem cell transplantation (AHSCT)
AICAR, 638
AIDS. *See* Acquired immunodeficiency syndrome (AIDS)
Airway obstruction
acute, 2255, 2255f
bronchoscopic therapy for, 2151f
Akt, 48–49, 64
apoptosis substrates, 48f
ALCL. *See* Anaplastic large-cell lymphoma (ALCL)
Alcohol, 367
breast cancer, 369
colorectal cancer, 368, 1371
head and neck neoplasms, 1132
hepatitis B infection, 324
liver neoplasms, 1293
oral cancer, 368f
pancreatic neoplasms, 1332
Aldehyde dehydrogenase, 638
Aldosterone, 817
Alemtuzumab
for adult acute lymphoblastic leukemia, 1780
Alendronate, 2093
Alimentary tract
dysfunction
anorexia, 2039
ALK, 80
Alkylating agents, 638, 675–687
cellular resistance to, 678–679
chemistry, 675
clinical pharmacology, 680–681
cytotoxicity, 678
lung injury following, 1925
metabolism, 678
schedule effects, 593
toxicity, 681–684
toxicity of, 2180
in vivo resistance, 680

Alkyl sulfonates, 677
ALL. *See* Acute lymphocytic leukemia (ALL)
ALL1, 80
Allium vegetables, 374
Allogeneic hematopoietic transplantation, 880f
Allogeneic stem-cell transplantation
in adult acute lymphoblastic leukemia, 1778
multiple myeloma, 1860
Allogeneic transplantation, 880–881
donor selection, 881
engraftment of, 881–882
pretransplant therapy, 883–884
Allografting
multiple myeloma, 1863–1864
Alloimmunization, 2100–2101, 2101t
transfusion effect on, 2103
Allopurinol, 670, 2188
Alopecia, 2077
cause, 683
chemotherapeutic agents associated with, 2077, 2078t
Alpha-beta tubulin dimer, 699f
Alpha-fetoprotein
with testis cancer, 1472
Alpha-hemolytic streptococci, 2227–2228, 2228f
Alpha nu beta 3, 168
Alpha-particle radioimmunotherapy, 779
Alpha-reductase inhibitor, 854
Alprazolam
for nausea and vomiting, 2058
Alternative medicine, 960–961. *See also* Complementary/alternative medicine (CAM)
Alveolar soft part sarcoma
genomic alterations in, 127
Amenorrhea
in childhood cancer survivors, 1928
American Burkitt lymphoma, 337
American College of Physicians, 2274
EMR tutorial, 2277
American College of Radiology
breast imaging and reporting data system, 393t
American Joint Committee on Cancer (AJCC)
staging, 1473t
American Joint Committee on Cancer/Union Internationale Contre le Cancer, 1273, 1273t
American Medical Informatics Association (AMIA), 2274
American Society for Testing and Materials (ASTM), 2278
American Society of Anesthesiologists
physical stages classification, 510t, 511t
American Society of Clinical Oncology (ASCO)
Cancer Directories, 2272
website, 2274
Amifostine, 527, 2186
myelodysplastic syndrome, 1732
Aminoglutethimide, 819, 832, 854, 858
structure of, 833f
Aminoimadazole-4-carboxamide ribonucleoside (AICAR), 638
Aminopterin, 654–655
Amitriptyline, 987
AML. *See* Acute myeloid leukemia (AML)
Amphotericin B, 2232–2233, 2234
Amputation
radiotherapy, 1701–1704
soft-tissue sarcomas
extremities, 1700
Amyloidosis, 1866–1867, 2116
cardiac, 2135
Anabolic steroids
cachexia, 2046
Analgesics, 983t
Anal neoplasms, 1392–1398
anatomy, 1392
diagnosis, 1394
epidemiology, 1392
etiology, 1392–1393
external irradiation, 1396, 1396t
inguinal lymph node involvement, 1397
interstitial irradiation, 1396
metastatic disease, 1397
pathology, 1393–1394
radical surgery, 1396–1397
salvage treatment, 1397
staging, 1394
treatment, 1394–1395, 1395t
Anaphylaxis, 2261t
Anaplastic anemia (AA)
transplantation for, 891–892
Anaplastic astrocytoma, 1047–1052
Anaplastic large-cell lymphoma (ALCL)
in children, 1963, 1967–1969, 1968t, 1969f, 1970f
Anaplastic oligodendroglioma, 1052
Anaplastic thyroid carcinoma, 1100
Anastrozole, 834–835, 834t, 835–836
bone effects of, 837–838
for early disease, 836
effects on lipid, 838
tamoxifen, 837
Androgen receptor (AR) gene, 264
Androgens
deprivation strategies, 854–859
inhibitors, 858
lower circulating, 852–854
mechanism of action, 851–852
responsiveness, 850–851
synthesis-inhibiting agents, 854
systemic levels, 852
Anemia, 2097
anaplastic
transplantation for, 891–892
cachexia, 2044
causes, 2096t
Fanconi
genetic basis, 226
normochromic/normocytic, 2044
refractory, 112
sickle cell
transplantation for, 892
Anemia of chronic disease, 2044
Anesthesiologist, 937
Aneurysmal bone cysts, 1678–1679, 1678f, 1679f
Angiogenesis, 152, 157–180, 438–440
bone marrow, 178
childhood central nervous systems tumors, 1951–1952
circulating endothelial stem cells, 161–162
direct inhibitors, 165–166, 165t
gastric cancer, 1273
historic background, 157–158
indirect inhibitor, 164–165
indolent tumors, 178–179
in infants and children, 1952
inhibition
interferons, 737t
matrix protein, 175
metastasis, 160, 178
multiple myeloma, 1852–1853
nonendothelial host cells, 162
oncogenes, 165t
p53, 178
poorly vascularized, 179
promoters, 162, 163t
symptoms, 180
tumor growth, 157–160
Angiogenic switch, 161
Angiogenic therapy
microvessel density, 179
Angiomotin, 168
Angiopoietins, 63, 164
Angiosarcoma, 1246
cutaneous, 1673
head and neck, 1157
hepatic, 1300
peritoneum, 1365
Angiosarcomas
bone, 1688, 1688f
Angiostatin, 166–169
with endostatin, 172
formation, 167f
gene therapy, 168
pancreatic neoplasms, 1352–1353
protein therapy, 168–169
Animal pharmacology, 608
Animal toxicology studies, 609
Ann Arbor staging system
Hodgkin disease, 1862
Anoikis, 44
Anorexia, 2037–2049
vs. cachexia, 2038
etiology, 2037–2041
incidence, 2037
Anthracenediones, 692–693
Anthracyclines
activity of, 691–692
administration of, 691
for adult acute lymphoblastic leukemia, 1777
cardiac activity of, 692
cardiotoxicity, 2137–2139
causing anaphylaxis, 2261–2262
clinical pharmacology of, 691–692
coronary angiography, 1923–1924
dose of, 691
head and neck squamous cell carcinoma, 1163
historical development of, 690
mechanism of action, 690–691
mechanisms of resistance, 692
nephrotoxicity of, 2129
schedule effects, 593
structure of, 691f
targeting topoisomerases, 690–691
Antiadhesive agents, 153
invasion, 153

Antiandrogens, 853–854
prostate cancer, 857–858
Antiangiogenic therapy, 153–154, 177
invasion, 153–154
pancreatic neoplasms, 1352–1353
radiation therapy, 529–530
Anti-anxiety agents, 908t
Antiarrhythmic drugs, 2249t
Anticancer agents. *See* Chemotherapeutic agents
Anti-CD5, 771
Anti-CD10, 771
Anticipatory anxiety, 907
Anticipatory emesis, 2055
Anticipatory nausea and vomiting
treatment of, 2059
Anticoagulants
anticancer effects of, 2118
Anticonvulsants
for brain metastases, 1067
for cancer pain, 988
Anticorticosteroids, 825
Anticytokine antibodies
cachexia, 2047
Antidepressants, 909t, 987
for anxiety, 908
Antiemetics, 969t, 2055–2059
classes of, 2056–2057, 2058t
doses of, 2058t
Anti-endothelial antibodies, 773
Antiestrogens, 829–830
structure of, 830f
Antifolates
multitargeted, 735
Antifungal prophylaxis, 2243
Anti-ganglioside antibodies, 772–773
Antigens
broadly expressed, 195–196
detection, 447
human leukocyte, 319
prostate-specific, 5, 342
tumor. *See* Tumor antigens
tumor-associated, 786–787, 914
genes, 867
tumor-specific, 786
Antihistamines
for anxiety, 908
Anti-idiotypic antibodies, 770–771
Anti-invasion therapy, 154f
Antimetabolites, 638
toxicity of, 2180
Antimetastasis signal-transduction therapy, 154
Antimicrobial prophylaxis, 2243
Antineoplastic agents
adjustment for renal insufficiency, 2128t
drug interactions increasing levels of, 2128t
Antineoplastons, 961
Antisense, 865
Antisense oligonucleotides
non-Hodgkin's lymphoma, 1840
Anti-Tac(Fv)-PE-38, 781
Antitumor immunity defects, 209–211
Anti-vascular endothelial growth factor
antibodies, 773
Antiviral prophylaxis, 2243
Anxiety, 905, 907–908
anticipatory, 907
antidepressants for, 908
beta-blockers for, 908
buspirone for, 908
complementary and alternative medicine for, 958t
etiology of, 907t
treatment of, 908, 908t
APC. *See* Adenomatous polyposis coli (APC)
Aphasia, 927
Aphidicolin, 685
APL, 1752–1753
Apollon (Bruce), 46
Apoptosis, 41–49, 77, 145
caspases, 41–42
cell proliferation, 34
gene therapy, 864
glucocorticoid-induced, 826
pancreatic neoplasms, 1353
pathway, 44f
photosensitizers, 543
protein domains, 43–44
radiation, 270–271, 528
resistance to, 137–138
signal transduction, 48–49
therapeutic opportunities, 49
Apoptotic pathways
multidrug resistance, 635–636
Appendiceal neoplasms, 1363–1366
adenocarcinoma, 1364
carcinoids, 1363–1364
mucoceles, 1364
Application programming interfaces (API), 2273
Application service provider (ASP), 2274
Aprepitant
doses of, 2058t
for nausea and vomiting, 2058
Aprosodia, 927
APRT, 286
ARG (Abelson-related gene), 729
AR gene, 264
Argon plasma coagulation
for radiation coloproctitis, 2179
Arimidex
structure of, 833f
Ark, 60
Arm
magnetic resonance imaging, 481f
Aromatase
expression of, 828–829
Aromatase inhibitors, 832–838
adjuvant studies with, 836
bone effects of, 837–838
classification of, 833f
neoadjuvant studies with, 835–836
patient selection for, 838
postmenopausal women, 837t
structure of, 833f
tolerability of, 837–838
Aromatic amines, 249
Array comparative genomic hybridization (CGH), 110
Arresten, 175
Arrhenius relationship, 549–550
Arrhythmia, 2248–2249
chemotherapeutic drugs associated with, 2248t
Arsenic
adverse effects, 2136
liver neoplasms, 1294
Arsenical keratosis, 1664–1665, 1665f
Artemin (ART), 60
Arterial thrombosis, 2119
Artificial limbs, 933
Artificial sweeteners, 374
A rule, 286
Asbestos, 294
Ascites, 4
malignant
peritoneum, 1365–1366
ASCUS, 1502–1503
Asian herbal remedies, 962
Asparaginases. *See also* L-asparaginase (L-Asp)
Aspartame, 374
Aspergillosis
disseminated, 2240f
Aspergillus, 2233–2234
Aspergillus fumigatus fresenius, 176
Aspermia
after radiation therapy, 1483
Aspiration cytology, 445–446
Assisted suicide, 1008–1009
defined, 1008ft
Astrocytic tumors
in infants and children, 1952–1954
Astrocytoma, 462
anaplastic, 1047–1052
cerebellar
in children, 1952–1953
in children, 1952–1954
cerebellum, 1952–1953
spinal cord, 464
Astrocytomas
cerebellar
in infants and children, 1953
chiasmatic, 461
Ataxia-telangiectasia, 2220
genetic basis, 225
Atherosclerosis, 831
ATM, 31
ATP synthase, 168
Atrial myxoma, 1245
Attributable risk, 349
Atypical squamous cells of undetermined significance (ASCUS), 1502–1503
Atypical teratoid/rhabdoid tumor
in infants and children
imaging, 1955, 1955f
Autochthonous tumors
stroma generation, 439
Autocrine mode, 53
Autocrine stimulation, 71, 72f, 82f
Autografting
multiple myeloma, 1864–1865
Autologous stem cell transplantation
multiple myeloma, 1861
non-Hodgkin's lymphoma, 1839–1840
Autologous stem-cell transplantation
in adult acute lymphoblastic leukemia, 1778–1779
Autologous transplantation, 880
donor selection, 881
engraftment of, 881–882
pretransplant therapy, 883
tumor cell contamination and purging, 882

Autopsy pathologist
 role, 450
Avascular necrosis
 in childhood cancer survivors, 1929
Avidin-biotin complex (ABC) technique, 446
Avipox virus, 790
Axl, 60
Axl/Ufo family
 ligands, 59–60
Ayurveda, 960
Azacytidine, 38, 668
 adjustment for renal insufficiency, 2128t
 myelodysplastic syndrome, 1729
 nephrotoxicity of, 2127t
 structure, 668f
Azoospermia
 in childhood cancer survivors, 1927
AZQ (diaziquone)
 nephrotoxicity of, 2127t

B

Bacille Calmette-Guérin
 malignant melanoma, 1655–1656
Backache
 complementary and alternative medicine for, 958t
Back pain
 management, 2064f
Bacterial esophagitis, 2175
Bacterial infection, 2225–2230
 neutropenia, 2225t
Bacterial pneumonia
 with hematopoietic stem cell transplantation, 2160
Bacterial sepsis
 transfusion related, 2105
Baculovirus IAP repeat (BIR), 43
Bad news
 communicating, 967–968
Barium enema
 colon cancer, 398–399
Bartholin gland carcinoma, 1492
Basal cell carcinoma (BCC), 288–289, 1671f
 of eyelids, 1082–1083
 morphea-like, 1669
 pigmented, 1670f
 of skin, 1669–1670, 1669f
 of vulva, 1492
Basal cell nevus syndrome (BCN), 283, 1670–1671, 1671f, 1672f
Base excision repair, 251
Base pairing, 10, 11f
Basic fibroblast growth factor (bFGF), 35, 1273
 induced endothelial cell-cell adhesion loss prevention, 170
BCC. *See* Basal cell carcinoma (BCC)
B cells, 206–207
Bcl-2
 family protein, 47–48, 47f, 636
 homology, 43
 non-Hodgkin's lymphoma, 1840
BCN. *See* Basal cell nevus syndrome (BCN)
Bcr/abl, 80, 82
BCR-ABL tyrosine kinase
 CML, 723–724
BCRP, 631
Beckwith-Wiedemann syndrome, 325
Benign bone tumors, 1678–1685
Benign central nervous system tumors
 genomic alterations in, 122–123
Benign epithelial tumors
 genomic alterations in, 121–122
Benign mesenchymal tumors
 genomic alterations in, 122–123
Benign ovarian tumors
 genomic alterations in, 122
Benign prostate hyperplasia, 1431–1432
Benign solid tumors
 genomic alterations in, 120–121
Benign teratomas
 of mediastinum, 1249
Benzocaine
 mucositis, 2185
Benzydamine
 mucositis, 2185
Bereavement, 911–912
Berlin breakage syndrome
 genetic basis, 225
Best-interest standards, 1000
Beta-blockers
 for anxiety, 908
Beta carotene, 374
 head and neck neoplasms, 1133
Beta-cell lymphomas
 interferons, 738
Betacellulin, 57
Beta-hemolytic streptococci, 2228
Beta-large-cell lymphoma (B-LCL)
 in children, 1963, 1964–1965, 1966f
  cytogenetic features, 1965–1966
  outcome, 1965t
  pathology, 1965
  prognosis, 1965t
Betamethasone
 mucositis, 2185
Bevacizumab
 for lung cancer, 1213
 nephrotoxicity of, 2127t, 2129
Bexarotene (Targretin)
 mycosis fungoides/Sézary syndrome, 1842
Bexxar, 777
bFGF, 35, 170, 1273
Bicalutamide, 856
 prostate cancer, 1455
 withdrawal, 857
Bilateral modified radical mastectomy, 514f
Bilateral Wilms' tumor
 chemotherapy of, 1986
Bile duct cancer, 1322–1329
 chemotherapy, 1328
 clinical presentation, 1324
 diagnosis, 1324–1326
 etiology, 1323
 high-resolution helical computed tomography, 1324, 1325f
 magnetic resonance imaging, 1324
 palliation, 1328
 pathology, 1324
 radiotherapy, 1328–1329
 ultrasonography, 1324
Bilharzial bladder, 334f
 verrucous carcinoma, 333
Bilharziasis, 332
Biliary duct
 imaging, 476
 stents, 499
Billroth, Albert Theodore, 504
Billroth I gastroduodenostomy, 1279
Billroth II gastroduodenostomy, 1279
Bim, 48
Biochemistry, 135–145
Bioelectromagnetics, 960
Bioheat transfer, 556–557
Bioinformatics, 2281
Biomarkers, 199–202, 350
 application of, 199–200
 clinical trial validation of, 201–202
Biopsy, 507–508. *See also* Fine-needle aspiration (FNA)
 cardiac, 2138t
  cardiotoxicity, 2138
 cutting-core, 508
 excisional, 508
 incisional, 508
 incisions, 509f
 percutaneous, 496
 sentinel lymph node, 515
 sentinel node, 516f
 skeletal, 496
BIOSIS, 2280
BIR, 43
Bismuth-Corlette classification
 cholangiocarcinoma, 1328f
Bisphosphonates, 2093
 bone metastases, 2090–2091
 cancer pain, 988
 hypercalcemia, 1133
BL22, 781
Bladder cancer, 332–335, 1415–1426
 adenocarcinoma, 1426
 AJCC staging, 1418t
 biology, 1415–1416
 chemotherapy, 576
 diagnosis, 1416–1417
 epidemiology, 1415
 genomic alterations in, 123
 histologic distribution, 334t
 interventional radiology, 495
 metastatic
  chemotherapy, 1424–1426
 muscle-invasive, 1420–1424
 nutrition, 372
 pathology, 1416
 prevention, 384
 signs and symptoms, 1416
 squamous cell carcinoma, 1426
 superficial, 1417–1420
 TNM, 1417f
Bladder outlet obstruction, 2124
Bladder tumor
 recurrence of, 2125
B-LCL. *See* Beta-large-cell lymphoma (B-LCL)
Bleeding
 management, 1287–1288
Bleeding disorders, 2114–2116
 novel drug treatment, 2120
 risk factors for, 2117t
Bleomycin, 619
 adjustment for renal insufficiency, 2128t
 for disseminated germ cell tumors, 1478

Bleomycin—*continued*
head and neck squamous cell carcinoma, 1163
hyperpigmentation, 2079f
lung injury following, 1925
second malignancies after, 1482–1483
thyroid neoplasms, 1098
vascular toxicity of, 1482
Blogs, 2273
Blood
cellular elements, 2096t
Blood banks, 2106t
Blood component therapy
future directions, 2106–2107
Bloom syndrome, 2220
genetic basis, 225
Blue nevi, 1245
B-lymphoblastic lymphoma
precursor, 1829–1830
BNLI trial, 1813
Body cavity
cytology, 445
Bombesin
antagonists, 807–808
breast cancer, 811–812
structure, 807t
Bone
fibrous cortical defects, 1682
fibrous dysplasia, 1681, 1681f
osteofibroses dysplasia, 1685f
Bone cysts
aneurysmal, 1678–1679, 1678f, 1679f
Bone marrow
angiogenesis, 178
cytokinetics, 591
drug effects, 2097t
malignant cell elimination from, 774
myelodysplastic syndrome, 1724
Bone marrow transplantation, 879–892
childhood acute lymphoblastic leukemia, 1938
for chronic myeloid leukemia, 1765
dose effect, 592
graft-*versus*-host disease, 2190–2191
infection, 2224
non-Hodgkin's lymphoma, 1839
oral complications, 2190–2191
oral infection, 2190
Bone tumors, 1675–1692
angiosarcoma, 1688, 1688f
benign, 1678–1685
biopsy of, 1676
chemotherapy of, 1678
in childhood cancer survivors, 1922
in children, 2019–2402
epidemiology, 1918–1919
chondroblastoma, 1679, 1679f
chondromyxoid fibroma, 1679–1680
chondrosarcomas, 1686, 1686f
dedifferentiated chondrosarcomas, 1686–1687, 1687f
enchondroma, 1680, 1680f
eosinophilic granulomas, 1680–1681, 1681f
Ewing's sarcoma, 1687
giant cell tumor, 1681–1682, 1682f
hemangiopericytoma, 1687–1688
juxtacortical osteosarcoma, 1689–1690
limb salvage *vs.* amputation surgery, 1677–1678
lymphoma, 1688
malignant cartilage-producing, 1689f
malignant fibrous histiocytoma and fibrosarcoma, 1688–1689, 1689f
malignant hemangioendothelioma, 1688
malignant vascular tumors, 1687
mesenchymal chondrosarcomas, 1687, 1687f
metastatic
surgery of, 1678
multifocal sclerosing osteosarcomas, 1690–1691, 1690f
nonossifying fibroma, 1682
osteoblastoma, 1683–1684, 1683f, 1684f
osteochondromas, 1684, 1685f
osteoid osteoma, 1682–1683, 1683f
osteosarcomas, 1689–1690, 1690f, 1691f
peptide analogs, 814
postirradiation osteosarcomas, 1691–1692
radiation therapy of, 1678
reconstruction with, 1676–1677, 1677f
sarcomas
staging of, 1685t
staging of, 1675–1676, 1675t
surgery of, 1676
surgical sites, 1676t
WHO classification of, 1678t
Boolean searching examples, 2279, 2279t
Borrowed servant, 1018
Botanicals
interaction with cancer medications, 963t
Bourneville disease, 1041–1042
Bowen disease, 1667
Bowenoid papulosis, 1665
Boys
chemotherapy
gonadal complications, 2195–2196
Brachial plexopathy, 2068–2069
Brachytherapy, 519
cervical cancer, 1513
esophageal neoplasms, 1265
prostate cancer, 521f, 1445–1446, 1446f
retinoblastoma, 1075
Bradford-Hill criteria, 254
Bragg peak, 517
Brailer, David, 2277
Brain
herniation, 2258
neoplasm imaging, 460–464
radiation-induced injury, 2072–2073
Brain cancer
chemotherapy, 577
rehabilitation, 926–927
Brain metastases, 1065–1069
chemotherapy of, 1068–1069
magnetic resonance imaging, 1066–1067
prognosis of, 1069
radiation therapy of, 1067
radiosurgery of, 1067–1068
source of, 1065t
supportive care, 1067
surgery of, 1067
symptoms of, 1066, 1066t
treatment of, 1067–1069, 1067t
Brain metastasis
malignant melanoma, 1657
stereotactic radiosurgery, 521f
Brain stem gliomas (BSG)
in infants and children, 1954
Brain tumors
peptide analogs, 813–814
radioimmunotherapy, 778
Branched-chain amino acids
cachexia, 2047
BRCA1, 94–95, 217, 1544–1545, 2220
pancreatic neoplasms, 1331
BRCA2, 94–95, 217, 1544–1545, 2220
pancreatic neoplasms, 1331
Breakthrough nausea and vomiting
treatment of, 2059
Breast
adenocarcinoma, 441f
calcifications, 483–484
mammography, 485f, 486f
managing, 486f
terminology, 485f
ductal lavage, 514–515, 515f
imaging, 482–487
magnetic resonance imaging, 487
radionuclide imaging, 487
tissue composition, 483f
ultrasonography, 487f
Breast cancer
antiestrogens for
future of, 838–839
aromatase inhibitors for
future of, 838–839
chemoprevention
future of, 838–839
in childhood cancer survivors, 1921
genomic alterations in, 123–124
hormonal resistance, 839
Breast cancer resistance protein (BCRP), 631
Breast carcinoma
markers, 200–201
Breast International Group 1-98 (BIG 1-98), 836
Breast neoplasms, 392–396
advocacy, 1026–1027
age-adjusted mortality
nutrition, 371f
aspiration cytology, 445–446
chemotherapy, 574–576
combination therapy, 811
corticosteroids for, 823
estrogen receptor, 443–444
etiology, 259–261, 260t
familial, 2220
flow cytometry, 443
hepatic arterial infusion chemotherapy, 1308t
hyperthermia, 558–559
imaging-guided needle biopsy, 486–487
invasive
metastases prediction, 443–444
recurrence prediction, 443–444
metastatic, 2086f, 2088f, 2089f, 2091f, 2092f
methotrexate, 651
microvascular density, 444
nutrition, 368–369
occult, 457
peptide analogs, 811–812
during pregnancy, 942–943
prevention, 383–384
progesterone receptor, 443–444
progestin receptor, 846–847

radioimmunotherapy, 777
radiopaque, 483f
rehabilitation, 930–931
schistosomiasis, 335
screening, 392–396
evaluation, 394–395
physical examination, 395
randomized controlled trials, 394t
recommendations, 395–396
ultrasonography, 485–486
vaccine clinical trials, 792
Breast-ovarian cancer syndrome
genetic basis, 216–218
Breast self-examination (BSE), 392, 395
Breast tumors
estrogen synthesis in, 828
Broadly expressed antigens, 195–196
Bromocriptine
growth hormone secreting pituitary adenomas, 1087
Bromodeoxyuridine (BrdU), 213, 527
Bronchioalveolar adenocarcinomas, 1186
Bronchiolitis obliterans
in childhood cancer survivors, 1924
Bronchiolitis obliterans with organizing pneumonia (BOOP), 2158
Bronchogenic carcinoma, 2170f
Brown adipocytes, 2043
Bruce (apollon), 46
BSE, 392, 395, 1898
Buccal mucosa, 1141
Bupropion, 359
Burkitt's lymphoma, 336, 1830
with adult acute lymphoblastic leukemia, 1772
American, 337
in children and adolescents, 1966–1967, 1967f, 1967t
C-*myc* translocations, 77, 77f, 80, 80f
endemic, 336
Epstein-Barr virus, 312–313
genomic alterations in, 120
Burnout, 567–568
Buschke-Löwenstein tumor, 1462, 1463f, 1667
Buspirone
for anxiety, 908
Busulfan, 677
for chronic myeloid leukemia, 1764
clinical pharmacology, 681
lung injury following, 1925
neurotoxicity, 2071
structure, 678f

C

CA 19-9, 1375
CA 125, 408
Cabergoline
growth hormone secreting pituitary adenomas, 1087
c-Abl, 523–524
Cachexia, 2037–2049, 2042f
vs. anorexia, 2038
biochemical and metabolic derangement, 2039–2040
clinical manifestation, 2041–2042
enteral nutrition, 2048
etiology, 2037–2135
incidence, 2037
laboratory manifestations, 2042–2044
manifestations, 2041–2044
parenteral nutrition, 2048, 2048t
pharmacologic management, 2045–2048, 2045t
supportive care, 2044–2139
treatment, 2044–2139
Cadherins, 149–150
CAK, 29
Calcitonin
hypercalcemia, 1133
Calcitriol, 2213
Calcium, 373
colorectal cancer, 1371
CALGB trial, 1813
Calicheamicin, 775
CAM. *See* Complementary/alternative medicine (CAM)
Campath-1H, 771–772
systemic reaction to, 2262
Camptothecin, 694
pancreatic neoplasms, 1348
for small-cell lung cancer, 1217
structure of, 694f
Cancell, 961
Cancer
advocacy movement, 1026–1029
late effects in children and adolescents, 1921–1930
new cases, 343f
prevention, 254–256
temporal progression, 148f
Cancer and Leukemia Group B (CALGB) trial, 1813
Cancer care delivery
strategies for, 1334
Cancer cells
genetic alterations in, 140–141
phenotypic alterations, 136–137
Cancer cytogenetic aberrations, 106–107
Cancer Gene Census, 105
Cancer.gov, 2279
CANCERLIT, 2279
Cancer of unknown primary site (CUP)
adrenal metastasis, 458
bone metastasis, 458
imaging, 456–458
liver metastasis, 458
positron emission tomography, 457
skin metastases, 458
Cancer operations
types of, 511–512
Cancerophobia, 5
Cancer Outcomes Measurement Working Group (COMWG)
NCI, 426
Cancer Rehabilitation Evaluation System (CARES), 911
Cancer rehabilitation medicine, 922–935
Cancer Statistics Review, 340
Cancer surveillance
Internet, 2279–2280
Cancer therapy
cell differentiation, 38
Candida, 2231–2232
esophagitis, 2231
Candida albicans, 2189
Candidate genes
hormone-related cancer, 262t
Candidate tumor-suppressor genes, 98
Candidiasis
chronic disseminated, 2232, 2232f
disseminated, 2232
esophageal, 2231f
hepatosplenic, 2232
oropharyngeal, 2231f
Cannabinoids
cachexia, 2046
Canstatin, 175
Canvaxin vaccine
malignant melanoma, 1656
Capacitive coupling
deep heating, 555
Capacity, 998
Capecitabine, 666–667
adjustment for renal insufficiency, 2128t
colorectal cancer, 1390–1391, 1392
structure, 666f
Capillary hemangiomas
children, 1079
Captain-of-the-ship doctrine, 1018–1019
Carbamazepine
for brain metastases, 1067
cancer pain, 988
Carbohydrate metabolism
cachexia, 2043
Carboplatin, 686
adjustment for renal insufficiency, 2128t
colorectal metastases, 494
gastric cancer, 1285
nephrotoxicity of, 2127t
for nonsmall-cell lung cancer, 1210
pharmacodynamics, 624
Carboxyfluorescein succinimidyl ester (CFSE), 213
Carcinoembryonic antigens (CEA), 1374–1375
vaccine
colon cancer, 1389
Carcinogenesis
chemical, 246–256
examples, 246t
multistage chemical, 247f
radiation-induced
experimental, 275–276
genetic susceptibility, 276
human epidemiologic studies, 276–280
risk assessment, 279–280
Carcinogens, 294t
DNA dosimetry, 254
metabolism, 249–250
Carcinoid heart disease, 1115, 2133–2134
echocardiography, 2135f
Carcinoid syndrome, 1115
Carcinoid tumors, 1109, 1114–1115
age distribution of, 1114
appendiceal, 1363–1364
diagnosis of, 1115
of lungs, 1186
natural history, 1114
ovaries, 1567
prognosis of, 1115–1116
relative incidence of, 1113f
small intestine, 1361–1362

Carcinoma
in children, 1973–1974
Carcinoma ex pleomorphic adenoma, 1155
Carcinoma-in-situ, 3
penis, 1462
CARD, 42, 43
proteins, 45
Cardiac amyloidosis, 2135, 2135f
Cardiac arrest, 2247–2248
Cardiac biopsy, 2138t
cardiotoxicity, 2138
Cardiac blood-pool scan, 2131
Cardiac complications, 2131–2144
Cardiac conduction system injury
radiation-induced, 2144
Cardiac disease
childhood Hodgkin's disease, 1960
Cardiac dysrhythmia, 2135–2136
Cardiac tamponade, 2133
Cardiac tumors, 1245–1253
clinical features, 1245–1246
epidemiology, 1245
etiology, 1245
incidence, 1245
types, 1245t
Cardiac valvular injury
radiation-induced, 2144
Cardiotoxicity
cardiac biopsy, 2138
Cardiovascular system
corticosteroids, 821
evaluation, 2131
Caretaker genes, 248–249
Caries
radiation, 2186
Carmustine, 677
Carney complex, 1245
Carotenoids, 374
Carotid artery
rupture, 2251
Case control studies, 350–351, 391, 429
Caspase
activation pathways, 42–43, 42f
apoptosis, 41–42
suppression
IAP family protein, 46f
Caspase-8 antagonist, 49
Caspase recruitment domains (CARD), 42, 43
proteins, 45
Caspofungin, 2234
Castleman disease
multicentric
human herpesvirus 8, 314
Catalog of Chromosome Aberrations in Cancer, 120
Cataracts, 831–832
in childhood cancer survivors, 1929
Catenins, 1272
Catheters
causing infection, 2240
Causation, 1016
Cavernous sinus
metastases, 2068f
CBE, 392, 395
CBG, 819
CD5, 771
CD10, 771
CDC, 340
CDK, 29, 32–33
cDNA, 17–18
CEA. *See* Carcinoembryonic antigens (CEA)
Celecoxib, 171
Celiac axis block, 1287
Celiac sprue, 1361
Cell cycle
checkpoints, 33–34
control, 29–30
gene therapy, 864
cyclin-dependent kinase regulation, 29f
phases, 571–572
Cell death. *See also* Apoptosis
pathway, 44f
radiation, 270–271
Cell differentiation, 34–35, 142–143
cancer therapy, 38
cell proliferation, 34
extracellular factors controlling, 35–36
induction, 35t
Cell life
bcl-2, 73f
Cell membrane
changes, 138
Cell phones, 295
Cell proliferation, 27–38, 570–587
apoptosis, 34
cell differentiation, 34
tumor growth, 27–28
Cell survival
pathway, 44f
Cellular immune dysfunction, 2223–2224
Cellulitis
chemical, 2078
chemotherapeutic agents associated with, 2078, 2078t
Cementifying fibroma. *See* Cemento-ossifying fibroma
Centers for Disease Control and Prevention (CDC), 340
Central nervous system neoplasms, 1037–1064
in children, 1951–1956
biology, 1951–1952
epidemiology, 1917–1918
treatment, 1952
clinical presentation, 1044–1045
clinical trials, 1047
computed tomography, 1045
cortical mapping, 1047
corticosteroids, 821
corticosteroids for, 823–824
diagnostic neuroimaging, 1045–1046
epidemiology, 1037–1038
familial syndromes, 1041–1042, 1042t
gastrointestinal carcinoma, 463
in infants and children, 1951–1958
biology of, 1951–1952
epidemiology of, 1951
focal radiotherapy, 1952
invasion and metastasis, 1952
molecular genetic associations with, 1952f
treatment of, 1952
irradiation
neurologic complications, 2072–2073, 2072t
lymphoma, 463
with acquired immunodeficiency syndrome, 463
magnetic resonance imaging, 1045
melanoma, 463
metastasis to, 457–458
molecular genetics, 1039–1041
MRSI, 1046t
neuroepithelial
histopathology, 1042–1044
postoperative imaging, 1047
renal cell carcinoma, 463
risk factors, 1038–1039
surgical diagnosis and resection, 1046–1047
Central nervous system tumors
benign
genomic alterations in, 122–123
imaging, 460–464
in infants and children
novel treatment strategies of, 1953t
Central neurocytomas, 462
Centrosome, 699
Cereals, 366
Cerebellar astrocytomas
in infants and children, 1953
Cerebral embolism, 2073
Cerebral hemorrhage, 2073
Cerebral infarction, 2072–2073, 2073
Cerebral venous thrombosis, 2073
Cerebrospinal fluid
cytology, 445
tumor markers, 2067t
Cerebrovascular accidents
with cisplatin, 1482
Cerebrovascular complications, 2073
Cervical condyloma, 318f
Cervical conization, 1509
Cervical cytology
classification schemes, 407t
Cervical intraepithelial neoplasm
histopathology, 320f
Cervical neoplasms, 1497–1520
carcinoma in situ, 1514
cause, 265–266
chemotherapy, 576
epidemiology, 1497–1499
hyperthermia, 559–560
incidence, 341
invasive lesions, 1505–1510
diagnosis, 1506
evaluation and staging, 1506–1507, 1507t
patterns of spread, 1505
prognosis, 1507–1509
surgery, 1509–1510
symptoms, 1505–1506
magnetic resonance imaging, 477f
metastatic, 1517–1518
precancerous lesions, 1502–1505
during pregnancy, 943–944
radiation therapy, 1509–1514
outcomes, 1513–1514
recurrent, 1518–1519
relapse rates, 1506t
screening, 405–407
stage IA1, 1514
stage IA2, 1514
stage IB2, 1515–1517

stage IB1 and IIA, 1514–1515
stage IIB-IVA, 1517
Cervix
adenocarcinoma, 265–266
adenosquamous carcinoma, 1501
epithelial tumors
histologic classification, 1499–1501
lymphoepithelioma-like carcinoma, 1500
non-small-cell neuroendocrine carcinoma, 1501, 1502f
papillary squamous cell carcinoma, 1500
small-cell neuroendocrine carcinoma, 1501, 1502f
squamous cell carcinoma, 1499–1500, 1500f
verrucous carcinoma, 1500
Cetrorelix, 812
Cetuximab, 772
Chaplain, 924
Charcot-Marie-Tooth neuropathy, 2070
Checkpoints
cycle, 33–34
defects, 31–32
Checkup, 409–410
Chelators, 776
Chemical carcinogenesis, 246–256
examples, 246t
Chemical Carcinogenesis Research Information System (CCRIS), 2280
Chemical cellulitis, 2078
chemotherapeutic agents associated with, 2078, 2078t
Chemical hypophysectomy, 992
Chemical pleurodesis
for malignant pleural effusions, 2154
Chemoembolization, 492
complications, 493
Chemokines, 292f
Chemoprevention, 377–384
incidence, 384
trials, 379–384
Chemoradiotherapy
bleeding, 1287
Chemoreceptor trigger zone (CZT), 2055, 2056f
Chemotaxis, 55
Chemotherapeutic agents, 648–735. *See also* individual agents
activation, 618t
anaphylaxis, 2260–2261
cardiotoxicity, 2137t, 2139t
historical overview, 648
indications, 602t–607t
infection, 2225
mechanism of action, 648–649
neurotoxicity, 2070–2075, 2070t
potential of, 2057t
renal injury caused by, 2128t
stomatotoxicity, 2188t
Chemotherapy, 570–587
in adolescents, 2032
agents required for curve, 594t
with antiangiogenic therapy, 177
causing pancytopenia, 2096
chronic low-dose, 154
dermatologic complications, 2077–2083
differentiated thyroid carcinoma, 1098
hyperthermia, 553
mycosis fungoides/Sézary syndrome, 1843–1844
ophthalmic side effects, 1083, 1083f
oral complications, 2187–2190
pharmacodynamic modeling of, 624–625
pregnancy, 2199–2200
radiation therapy, 530t
secondary cancer, 2221–2222
trials, 565
Chemotherapy-induced lung injury, 2156–2159
syndromes of, 2157t
Chemotherapy-induced nausea and vomiting (CINV), 2055
pathophysiology of, 2055
prevention and treatment of, 2058–2059, 2058t
Chiasmatic astrocytomas, 461
Child development
parent's illness, 905t
Childhood cancer
auditory complications, 1929
cardiovascular function, 1923–1924
delivering survivorship care, 1929–1930
gastrointestinal function, 1925–1926
genitourinary abnormalities, 1926
gonadal function, 1927–1928
growth abnormalities, 1926–1927
musculoskeletal complications, 1929
neurocognitive sequelae of, 1923
ocular function, 1929
pregnancy outcome, 1928–1929
pulmonary function, 1924–1925
thyroid function, 1927
treatment of
late effects after, 1922t
Childhood cancer survivors, 1921t
amenorrhea in, 1928
azoospermia in, 1927
bone tumors, 1922
bronchiolitis obliterans in, 1924
cataracts, 1929
challenges, 1922t
future directions of, 1922t
future research opportunities for, 1930
late mortality among, 1921
second malignant neoplasms, 1921–1923
Childhood renal tumors, 1983–1987
chemotherapy of, 1985–1986
clinical presentation of, 1984
epidemiology of, 1983
genetics of, 1983–1984
long-term follow-up, 1987
molecular biology of, 1983–1984
pathology of, 1984
preoperative evaluation of, 1984–1985
prognosis of, 1987
radiation therapy of, 1985
recurrent disease
treatment of, 1987
staging of, 1985
surgery of, 1985
treatment, 1987f
treatment of, 1985–1987
Children. *See also* Adolescents; Pediatric oncology
anaplastic large-cell lymphoma, 1963, 1967
angiogenesis in, 1952
astrocytic tumors in, 1952–1954
astrocytoma
cerebellum, 1952–1953
atypical teratoid/rhabdoid tumor
imaging, 1955
beta-large-cell lymphoma, 1963
bone tumors, 2019–2402
capillary hemangiomas, 1079
carcinomas, 1973–1974
central nervous system neoplasms, 1951–1958
central nervous system tumors
novel treatment strategies of, 1953t
cerebellar astrocytomas, 1953
coping with parent's illness, 905t
dermoid cysts, 1079
epidemiology in, 1917–1919
Ewing sarcoma, 2024–2028, 2025f
exposed to cancer therapy in utero, 945
genetic testing, 1013
gonadal complications
protection from, 2199
Hodgkin disease, 1959–1960
incidence in, 1917–1919
liver tumors, 1972–1973
low-grade gliomas, 1055
lymphangioma, 1079
lymphoblastic lymphoma, 1969–1971
lymphocytic leukemia, 1934–1940
melanoma, 1973–1974
myeloid leukemia, 1944–1948
neuroblastoma, 1990–1999
non-Hodgkin lymphoma, 1962–1971
ophthalmic neoplasms, 1071–1079
origin in, 1917–1919
osteosarcomas, 2019–2024, 2021f
proptosis
causes, 1080t
retinoblastoma, 1968–1970
sarcomas, 1694
rhabdomyosarcoma, 1079–1080, 2007–2010
soft-tissue sarcomas, 2007–2381
tumors
chemotherapy, 577
Chimeric transcription factors, 78
Chiropractic education, 963
Chlamydia trachomatis, 1498
Chlorambucil, 676
causing anaphylaxis, 2262
chronic lymphocytic leukemia, 1794
clinical pharmacology, 681
metabolism, 678
Chlorhexidine, 2190
Cholangiocarcinoma, 1299, 1322–1323
Bismuth-Corlette classification, 1328f
computed tomography, 476f
distribution, 1323f
etiology, 1323
vs. hepatocellular carcinoma, 1323t
hilar, 1325–1328
intrahepatic
treatment, 1326
Cholangiography, 1325
Cholecystectomy, 1320–1322
Cholesterol, 374
Chondroblastomas
bone, 1679, 1679f

Chondroid tumors
genomic alterations in, 122
Chondromyxoid fibromas
bone, 1679–1680
Chondrosarcomas
bone, 1686, 1686f
genomic alterations in, 127
peptide analogs, 814
Choriocarcinomas, 461, 463, 1470–1471, 1470f
in children, 1971
methotrexate, 651
ovary, 1565
Choroidal melanoma, 1080–1081, 1081f
classification, 1082t
Choroidal nevi, 1080
Choroid plexus papillomas (CPP), 461
Chromatin, 10
Chromogranin A (CgA), 1110
Chromosomal aberrations, 104–130, 108f, 112
etiology of, 111–112
glossary, 104t
mechanisms of, 111–112
Chromosomal abnormalities
in acute myeloid leukemia, 113–114
radiation, 271–272
Chromosomal deletions, 1183
childhood neuroblastoma, 1992
Chromosomal rearrangements, 78
molecularly characterized, 76t, 79t
Chromosomal translocations, 81, 450t
Chromosome 11, 325
Chromosome 13, 87
Chromosome and genome analysis
newer method of, 107–111
Chromosome G banded karyotype
of metaphase chromosomes, 105f, 106f
Chromosome nomenclature, 106–107
Chromosome 9p21 abnormalities
in adult acute lymphoblastic leukemia, 1775
Chronic disseminated candidiasis, 2232, 2232f
Chronic graft-vs-host disease (GVHD), 2178–2179
Chronic inflammatory conditions, 293t
Chronic lymphocytic leukemia (CLL), 112, 1786–1797
anemia, 1796
chemoimmunotherapy, 1795
corticosteroids for, 822
cytogenetics, 1788
defective B- and T-cell functions, 1787–1788
differential diagnosis, 1789–1790
familial, 1786–1787
genetic basis, 231–232
historical perspective, 1786
infections in, 1796
lymphocytes, 1788–1789
minimal residual disease, 1795
in monozygotic twins, 1787
natural history, 1786
pathogenesis, 1786–1787
staging, 1791–1792
transplantation for, 889
treatment, 1792–1797
variants, 1796–1797
Chronic lymphoproliferative leukemia
genomic alterations in, 118
Chronic myeloid disorders
classification, 1874f
Chronic myeloid leukemia (CML), 82, 1761–1768, 1761f, 1762f
bone marrow transplantation for, 1765
BRC-ABL tyrosine kinase, 723–724
chemotherapy, 578
clinical characteristics of, 1761–1762
corticosteroids for, 822
cytogenetics of, 1762–1763
epidemiology of, 1761
etiology of, 1761
genomic alterations in, 117
Gleevec, 67
hematologic characteristics of, 1761–1762
incidence of, 1761
interferons, 737–738
long-term survival of, 1765f
molecular biology of, 1763–1764, 1763f
oncogenes, 80
pathophysiology of, 1762
prognosis of, 1762
transplantation for, 888–889
treatment of, 1764–1768
current recommendations, 1768
monitoring during, 1766–1767
recommendations for, 1768
Chronic myeloproliferative disorders
genomic alterations in, 117
Chronic pain
complementary and alternative medicine for, 958t
Chronic postoperative respiratory failure, 2155–2156
Chronomodulation
colorectal cancer, 1390
Cigarette smoke. *See* Tobacco smoke
Cigarette smoking, 341
pancreatic neoplasms, 1332
Cimetidine, 1406
Cingulotomy, 993
CIPER, 45
Circadian rhythm, 623
Circadian variations, 1390
Circulatory emergencies, 2246–2253
Cirrhosis
with hepatitis B infection, 324–325
liver neoplasms, 1293
Cisapride
cachexia, 2046
Cisplatin, 91, 527, 686, 1252
adjustment for renal insufficiency, 2128t
anal neoplasms, 1395
causing childhood renal damage, 1926
clinical trials, 684
colorectal metastases, 494
for disseminated germ cell tumors, 1478
emesis following, 2055
endocrine complications, 2210
esophageal neoplasms, 1266t
gastric cancer, 1284, 1286
head and neck squamous cell carcinoma, 1163, 1167–1168
hepatocellular carcinoma, 493
for nausea and vomiting, 2059
nephrotoxicity of, 2127t
nephrotoxicity with, 1482
neuroendocrine metastases, 495
neurotoxicity, 2071
neurotoxicity of, 1482
for nonsmall-cell lung cancer, 1210
with paclitaxel, 2126
pancreatic neoplasms, 1348, 1350
second malignancies after, 1482–1483
for small-cell lung cancer, 1217
toxicity, 638, 686–687
toxicity of, 2126
vascular toxicity of, 1482
Cisplatinum, 1153
c-Jun N-terminal kinase (JNK)/stress-activated protein kinase (SAPK), 65
Cladribine, 673
Clear cell carcinoma
endometrium, 1524
Clenbuterol
cachexia, 2048
Clinical breast examination (CBE), 392, 395
Clinical laboratory and testing standards, 2278
Clinical pathologist
role, 449
Clinical practice guidelines, 2278
Clinical protocol, 564t
Clinical research, 563–565, 1032, 1033–1034
Clinical syndrome, 1113f
Clinical trials, 411–425, 2278
adolescents, 2033–2034, 2033f, 2034t
categorical data, 419–420
characteristics, 413t
data collection, 415, 415t
data quality, 419
early, 609–613
early detection, 414
early stopping, 417–418
end points, 419
experimental design, 415–416, 416t
federal policies, 1029
incorrect conclusions, 414–415
older patient, 953
patient accounting, 419
phase I, 609–613
dose escalation, 610–612
patient selection, 612
schedule selection, 610
starting dose, 610
planning, 413–415
reporting, 418–421
statistical analysis, 419
statistical models, 421–422
survival data, 420–421
CLL. *See* Chronic lymphocytic leukemia (CLL)
Clodronate, 988
Clofarabine
adjustment for renal insufficiency, 2128t
for adult acute lymphoblastic leukemia, 1780
Clonal evolution, 252–253
Clonazepam
for anxiety, 908
Clonidine, 989
Clotrimazole, 2189
Cluster of differentiation 44, 1272–1273
Clusty, 2271
C-mer, 60
C-met, 59, 1273

CML. *See* Chronic myeloid leukemia (CML)
CMV. *See* Cytomegalovirus (CMV)
C-*myc* translocations
  Burkitt lymphoma, 77, 77f, 80, 80f
Coagulation factor deficiencies, 2116
Coagulation system
  relationship to cancer, 2113
Coagulopathic complications, 2113–2120
Cockayne syndrome, 283, 288
Cockroft formula, 2129, 2129t
Codeine, 983
Coding region, 9
Coffee
  pancreatic neoplasms, 1332
Cogent Medicine, 2279–2280
Cognition
  older patient, 951–952
Cognitive-behavioral therapy, 991
Cohort studies, 349–350
Colds
  complementary and alternative medicine for, 958t
Coley, William B., 505–506
Collaborative Ocular Melanoma Study, 1082t
Collagen XVIII, 175
Colon
  stents, 499
  surgical anatomy, 1378
Colon cancer. *See also* Colorectal neoplasms
  adjuvant treatment, 1387–1388
  BCG vaccination, 1388–1389
  immunotherapy, 1388–1389
  initiation, 82
  radiotherapy, 1386–1388
  somatic *APC* mutations, 93
  stage III, 1388t
Colonic adenomas
  genomic alterations in, 121–122
Colonic graft-vs-host disease (GVHD), 2178f
Colonoscopy
  colon cancer, 399
Colony stimulating factor (CSF), 2215
Colony stimulating factor 1 (CSF-1), 56
Colony-stimulating factor regimes, 764–765
Colorectal cancer
  development of, 81f
  genomic alterations in, 124
  oncogenes, 80–81
Colorectal carcinoma
  markers, 201
Colorectal neoplasms, 62
  age
    incidence, 369f
  chemoembolization, 1309
  chemotherapy, 576
  classification, 1370t
  combination chemotherapy, 1389t
  contiguous organ, 1380
  development, 82f
  epidemiology, 1369–1370
  family history of, 1377
  genetic basis, 218
  genetic pathways, 1373–1374
  hepatic resection, 1380–1381
  hormone replacement therapy, 1372
  imaging, 490
  incidence, 1370t
  laparoscopic colectomy, 1381
  location, 1370
  lymphadenectomy, 1379
  lymphatic mapping, 1379–1380
  management, 1378–1379
  metastatic
    treatment, 1305t
  molecular markers, 1375–1376
  mutator pathway, 1374
  nonsteroidal antiinflammatory drugs, 1373
  nutrition, 367–368
  obstruction, 1380
  occupational exposures, 1372–1373
  pathology, 1369t
  peptide analogs, 813
  perforation, 1380
  peritoneal disease, 1380
  preoperative workup, 1379
  prevention, 383, 396–400
  prognosis, 1375–1376
  radioimmunotherapy, 777
  resection margins, 1379
  risk, 370f
  risk factors, 1370–1371, 1377
  screening, 1376–1378
    guidelines, 400t
    recommendations, 399
  stage IV, 1389–1392
  surgery, 1379–1387
  tumor markers, 1374–1375
Color flow Doppler studies, 2131
Colostomy, 931
Colpostats, 1512f
Combination chemotherapy, 594–596
  cytokinetics, 594
  drug resistance, 594–595
  experimental models, 595–596
  vs. holotherapy, 595t
  modulation, 594
  synchronization, 594
Combined androgen blockade
  prostate cancer, 1454
Communication
  about bad news, 967–968
Community-acquired pneumonia (CAP), 2163–2164
Community-acquired respiratory viruses, 2236–2237
Comorbid medical conditions
  older patient, 951
Compact disk, 2268
Comparative genomic hybridization (CGH), 105, 109–110, 110f
  array, 110
Compensation
  for physicians, 1010–1011
    in managed care, 1020
Competitive aromatase inhibitors, 833
Complementary/alternative medicine (CAM), 958t
  for children, 959
  definitions of, 957
  evolution, 957
  health care system, 957
  mainstream disapproval, 959
  mainstream recognition, 959
  medical schools and centers, 959
  NIH, 959
  pharmacologic and biologic treatment, 961
  practitioners and practices, 963
  prevalence of, 957–958
  public access to information, 959
  research, 963
  terminology of, 957
  therapies and practitioners, 959–962
Complementary therapy, 957–963
Compliance, 416–417, 417t
Comprehensive geriatric model, 953f
Computed tomography (CT)-PET, 1032
Computer-generated media, 2280
Computerized patient records (CPR), 2275–2276
  attributes of, 2277t
  data elements for, 2276t
Computers, 2267–2268
  clinical and research use of, 2280–2281
  hardware, 2267–2268
  information refinement, 2278
  input and output devices for, 2268t
  medical uses of, 2269t
  software, 2267–2268
  statistics, 2282
Concomitant immunity, 166
Condyloma
  cervical, 318f
Confidentiality, 1011–1012
Conflicts of interest, 1010–1011
Confusion, 989
  management, 990t
Congenital metabolic disorders
  transplantation for, 892
Congenital nevi, 1645
Consent, 1018–1019
Consolidated Health Informatics (CHS), 2277
Constipation, 990
  complementary and alternative medicine for, 958t
Constitutive phosphorylation, 79
Constrictive bronchiolitis
  with hematopoietic stem cell transplantation, 2161–2162
Cooking methods
  carcinogens, 368
Coordination of care
  oncology nurse, 918
Coping, 902, 904t
Cordotomy, 993
Corticosteroid-binding globulin (CBG), 819
Corticosteroids, 817–826
  for adult acute lymphoblastic leukemia, 1777
  antiemetic action, 824
  antiinflammatory effects, 821
  for brain metastases, 1067
  cachexia, 2045–2046
  cancer pain, 988
  chronic lymphocytic leukemia, 1793
  for nausea and vomiting, 2058
  neoplasm treatment, 822–823
  neurotoxicity, 2072
  pharmaceutical derivatives, 819
  pharmacokinetics, 818–819
  pharmacology, 818–819
  physiologic and pharmacologic effects, 819–822
  potencies and equivalent doses, 820
  resistance, 825–826

Corticosteroids—*continued*
secretion, 817–818
spinal cord compression, 2063
symptomatic use of, 823–824
thymoma, 1241
Cortisol, 817
COSMIC (Catalogue of Somatic Mutations in Cancer), 105
Costimulatory genes, 866–867
Costimulatory molecule genes
direct injection of, 788
Costs, 431
Coumarin, 1406
Cowden disease, 1674
Cowden syndrome
genetic basis, 225
Cox survival models, 421–422
CPD, 284–285
Cranial nerve metastases, 2067–2068
Cranial neurectomy, 993
Cranial neuropathies, 2068, 2069t
CREB binding protein (CBP)
translocations involving transcriptional coactivators and chromatin modification, 116
Creutzfeldt-Jakob disease, 2106
Crises
normal responses to, 902
Crohn's disease, 1361, 1378
Cryotherapy
retinoblastoma, 1075
Cryptococcus, 2234
Cryptogenic organizing pneumonitis (COP)
with hematopoietic stem cell transplantation, 2162
Cryptorchidism
with testis cancer, 1468
Cryptorchid testes, 265
CSF-1. *See* Colony stimulating factor 1 (CSF-1)
CT antigens, 194–195
CTL, 41
CUP. *See* Cancer of unknown primary site (CUP)
Cushing syndrome, 1103, 2211, 2212f
Cutaneous angiosarcoma, 1673
Cutaneous eruption of lymphocyte recovery, 2081
Cutaneous lymphoscintigraphy
malignant melanoma, 1653
Cutaneous reactions, 2077–2083
causes, 2077t
radiation-associated, 2079–2080, 2079t
Cutting-core biopsy, 508
Cyclin D1
inhibition, 170
Cyclin-dependent kinase (CDK), 29
activation, 32–33
regulation, 29f
cell cycle, 29f
Cyclin-dependent kinase (CDK)-activating kinase (CAK), 29
Cyclobutane pyrimidine dimer (CPD), 284, 284f, 285f
Cyclooxygenase-2
colorectal cancer, 1392
Cyclopamine, 1670
Cyclophosphamide, 675–676
adjustment for renal insufficiency, 2128t
antidiuresis, 683
bladder toxicity, 495, 683
for Burkitt's acute lymphoblastic leukemia, 1780
cardiotoxicity, 683, 2141
causing anaphylaxis, 2261
causing childhood bladder damage, 1926
chronic lymphocytic leukemia, 1794
clinical pharmacology, 680–681
for drug-induced hematuria, 2125
endocrine complications, 2209
immunosuppression, 683–684
metabolism, 677f
for nausea and vomiting, 2059
for small-cell lung cancer, 1217
Cyclosporine
nephrotoxicity of, 2127t, 2128–2129
Cylindromas, 1155
CYP, 248–249, 255
CYP 1A1, 355–356
CYP 2B1, 864
CYP 2D6, 355
CYP 2E1, 356
Cyproheptadine
cachexia, 2046
Cyproterone acetate, 854
Cystadenocarcinoma
mucinous, 1548f
Cysticercus fasciolaris, 337
Cystitis
hemorrhagic
etiology, 683
Cysts
mammography, 484f
ultrasonography, 487f
Cytarabine
adjustment for renal insufficiency, 2128t
causing anaphylaxis, 2262
schedule effects, 592–593
Cytochrome P450 (CYP), 248–249, 255
Cytochrome P450 1A1 (CYP 1A1), 355–356
Cytochrome P450 2B1 (CYP 2B1), 864
Cytochrome P450 2D6 (CYP 2D6), 355
Cytochrome P450 2E1 (CYP 2E1), 356
Cytogenetic-molecular markers
of adult acute lymphoblastic leukemia, 1774–1775, 1774t
Cytogenetics
chronic lymphocytic leukemia, 1788
myelodysplastic syndrome, 1725–1726
Cytokine genes, 866
direct injection of, 788
Cytokine inhibitors
cachexia, 2047
Cytokines, 292f, 744–766
anorexia, 2038
cachexia, 2039, 2047
dermatologic complications, 2082
immunostimulants, 791
radiation, 527–528
receptor subunits shared among, 746t
stomatotoxicity, 2188
systemic reaction to, 2262
Cytokinetics
biologic diversity, 573–574
Cytologic specimens
microscopic interpretation, 444–445
preparation, 444
Cytolytic T cells (CTL), 41
Cytomegalovirus (CMV), 314, 2236
incidence, 2105t
transfusion related, 2104–2105
Cytomegalovirus (CMV) colitis, 2178f
Cytomegalovirus (CMV) esophagitis, 2175
Cytopathologist, 444
Cytosine arabinoside, 639, 667–668
metabolism, 639f
myelodysplastic syndrome, 1730
neurotoxicity, 2071
structure, 667f
Cytosine deaminase, 863–864
Cytotoxic drugs, 2180–2181
Cytotoxic therapy
reactions to, 2082t
Cytotoxic T lymphocytes, 205–206

D

Dacarbazine, 677
malignant melanoma, 1655
Dacryocystorhinostomy, 1153
Damages, 1016–1017
Damocles syndrome, 905
Danazol, 1731
DAP kinase, 44
Data
falsification, 424–425
Data acquisitions and instrument control, 2281
Daunomycin, 690–693
coronary angiography, 1923–1924
Daunorubicin (Cerubidine), 691
adjustment for renal insufficiency, 2128t
nephrotoxicity of, 2129
toxicity of, 2180
DCC
gastric cancer, 1272
DCIS, 392
DD, 43
proteins, 43–45
DDR, 63
DDTHF, 735
Death. *See also* End-of-life care
facing, 970
Death domains (DD), 43
proteins, 43–45
Death effector domains (DED), 42, 43, 45
Death-inducing signaling complex (DISC), 42
Decision, 1000
DED, 42, 43, 45
Dedifferentiated chondrosarcomas
bone, 1686–1687, 1687f
Deep heating, 555–556
Dehydroepiandrosterone sulfate, 1103
Delayed emesis, 2055
Delayed pulmonary toxicity syndrome
with hematopoietic stem cell transplantation, 2162
Delbruck-Luria model, 579
Deleted in colon cancer gene, 1374
Deletion, 18Q, 1376
Deletions, 107
Delirium, 910
behavioral symptoms of, 910t
etiology of, 910t
management, 990t
palliative care, 969
treatment of, 911t

Deltanoids, 379
Dendritic cells (DC), 207
Dendritic cell vaccines
  malignant melanoma, 1660
Denileukin diftitox, 781
  systemic reaction to, 2262
Deoxycoformycin, 671–672
Dephosphorylation, 144
Depression, 5, 902
  complementary and alternative medicine for, 958t
  predisposing factors for, 908t
  risk factors for, 909t
Dermatofibrosarcoma protuberans, 1667f, 1672–1673
  signal transduction inhibition, 1713–1714
Dermatologic complications, 2077–2083. *See also* Cutaneous reactions
  causes, 2077t
  radiation-associated, 2079–2080, 2079t
Dermoid cysts
  in children, 1079
Dermoids, 462
Dermoid tumors, 1249
Descriptive studies, 391
Desmoplastic infantile ganglioglioma (DIG), 462
Desmoplastic small round-cell tumors
  genomic alterations in, 129
Detectable preclinical phase, 389
Detection
  early. *See* Screening
Developmental stages, 903t
Dexamethasone
  bone toxicity following, 1929
  for Burkitt's acute lymphoblastic leukemia, 1780
  cancer pain, 988
  doses of, 2058t
  for nausea and vomiting, 2058, 2059
  spinal cord compression, 2063
Dexrazoxane, 2140
Dextromethorphan, 989
Diabetes mellitus, 2206
  pancreatic neoplasms, 1585
Diagnosis, 1033
  in adolescents, 2030–2031, 2030f
  reactions to, 902
Diagnostic mammography, 482
Diagnostic markers, 199
Dianhydrogalactitol, 676
Diarrhea, 2176–2178
  complementary and alternative medicine for, 958t
  differential diagnosis of, 2177t
Diaziquone, 676
Diazoxide
  for insulinoma, 1117
Dibromodulcitol, 676–677
Dideazatetrahydrofolate (DDTHF), 735
Diencephalic glioma
  in children, 1953
  in infants and children, 1953
Diencephalic syndrome
  cachexia, 2042
Diesel exhaust, 295
Diet, 363–365, 959–960
  assessment, 366t
  breast cancer, 260–261
  cervical cancer, 1499
  colorectal cancer, 1370
  head and neck neoplasms, 1133
  low-fat, 366
  prostate neoplasms, 1432
  secondary cancer, 2218
Dietary fat
  breast cancer, 261
  colorectal cancer, 1370
  pancreatic neoplasms, 1332
  prostate neoplasms, 1432
Dietary recalls, 365
Dietary supplements, 367
Diet histories, 365
Differentiated thyroid carcinoma, 1093–1098, 1093f, 1093t
  metastatic disease
    therapy, 1096–1098
  pathologic features, 1094, 1094f
  postoperative adjuvant therapy, 1095–1096
  in special populations, 1098
  surgery, 1094–1095
Differentiation antigens, 195
Diffuse alveolar damage (DAD), 2157
Diffuse alveolar hemorrhage (DAH), 2157
  with hematopoietic stem cell transplantation, 2161
Diffuse endocrine system (DES), 1109–1126
Diffuse large-B-cell lymphoma (DLBCL), 1828–1829, 1828f
  genomic alterations in, 120
Diffusion-weighted imaging (DWI), 461
Difluoromethylornithine, 379
DIG, 462
Digital clubbing
  with lung cancer, 1189
Digital rectal examination (DRE), 397, 402
Digital video disk (DVD), 2268
Dihydrofolate reductase, 648
Dihydropyrimidine dehydrogenase, 1376
Dimethyl-benzanthracene (DMBA), 81
Dimethylsulfoxide (DMSO), 2078
  myelodysplastic syndrome, 1729
Diphenhydramine, 2057
Directories
  American Society of Clinical Oncology, 2272
Direct patient care
  oncology nurse, 918
DIRLINE (Directory of Information Resources Online), 2279
DISC, 42
Disclosure, 998
Discodermolide, 714
  chemical structure, 713f
Discoidin domain receptors (DDR), 63
Discovery process
  clinical observation, 600
  evolution of, 600–603
  histocytotoxic effects, 600–603
Discrimination, 905
Disease occurrence, 339–340
Disseminated aspergillosis, 2240f
Disseminated candidiasis, 2232
Disseminated germ cell tumors
  bleomycin for, 1478
Disseminated intravascular coagulation, 2119–2120, 2119t
Distress
  anorexia, 2038
  factors contributing to, 970t
  screening for, 906
DLC, 48
DMBA, 81
DMSO, 2078
  myelodysplastic syndrome, 1729
DNA
  analysis, 13–14
  cell cycle phases, 571–572
  damage, 250–252
    radiation, 274
  damage-induced checkpoints, 31
  digestion, 12f
  flow cytometry, 572–573
  index
    childhood neuroblastoma, 1991
  ligases, 11
  methylation, 37–38, 141, 355
    genes silenced, 37t
  microarray analysis, 19, 19f
  mismatches, 252
  mismatch repair gene defects
    HNPCC, 97–98
  ploidy, 1375
  polymerase, 14f
    low-fidelity, 285–286
  polymorphisms, 14–16
  radiation-induced damage, 522
  recombinant, 10–11
  repair, 142
    genetic disorders, 287
    radiotherapy, 524–526
  repair genes, 97, 251t–252t
  repair pathways, 251
  sequencing, 15f
  sunlight-induced photoproducts, 283–284
DNA double-strand breaks, 690f
DNA microarray profiling, 202
DNA topoisomerases
  drugs targeting, 688–695
DNR, 567
Docetaxel, 706, 709
  administration, dose, schedule, 712–713
  causing nail hyperpigmentation, 2078f
  chemical structure, 706f
  gastric cancer, 1285, 1286
  head and neck squamous cell carcinoma, 1163
  for nonsmall-cell lung cancer, 1210
  ovarian cancer, 1555
  prostate cancer, 1457
  toxicity, 711–712
Doctor-patient relationship, 1017–1018
Document imaging, 2280–2281
Dolasetron
  doses of, 2058t
Do not resuscitate (DNR), 567
Dopamine, 362, 2055
Dopamine agonists
  pituitary adenomas, 1086
Dopamine receptor antagonists, 2057–2058
Dorsal column stimulation, 994
Dorsal rhizotomy, 993

Dorsal root entry zone lesion, 993
Dose, 590–592
Dose effect
  clinical trials, 591–592
  sensitive tumors, 592
Doxil, 1711
Doxorubicin, 527
  bile duct cancer, 1328
  cardiac monitoring, 2140
  cardiotoxicity, 2136–2141
  gastric cancer, 1284
  hepatocellular carcinoma, 493
  neuroendocrine metastases, 495
  pancreatic neoplasms, 1348
  soft-tissue sarcomas
    metastatic, 1711
  thyroid neoplasms, 1098
  uterine cervix carcinoma, 495
Doxorubicin (Adriamycin, Doxil, Rubex), 690–693
  for Burkitt's acute lymphoblastic leukemia, 1780
  congestive heart failure with, 692t
  coronary angiography, 1923–1924
  nephrotoxicity of, 2129
  for small-cell lung cancer, 1217
  toxicity of, 2180
DRE, 397, 402
Dronabinol, 968
  doses of, 2058t
Drug-conjugate export pumps
  multidrug resistance, 634–635
Drug discovery
  targeted, 607–608
Drug-drug interactions, 623
Drug effects, 2116
Drug hepatotoxicity, 2180–2181
Drug-induced airway disease, 2158–2159
Drug-induced hematuria, 2125
Drug-induced injury
  repair, 620
Drug-induced nephrotoxicity
  monitoring for, 2129
Drug-monoclonal antibody conjugates, 774–775
Drug resistance, 582–584, 591, 630–640
  overcoming, 636–637
  tumor cell heterogeneity, 594
Drugs
  action mechanisms, 617–620
  administration, 592–594
    continuous low-dose, 593–594
  decreased accumulation, 630–631
  intracellular activation, 618–619
  membrane transport, 617–618
  targets, 619–620
Ductal carcinoma in situ (DCIS), 392
Durable powers of attorney, 1006–1007
Dural tails, 460
Duty to warn, 1013
Dyclonine, 2188
  mucositis, 2185
Dying. *See also* End-of-life care
  facing, 970–973
Dynein light-chain (DLC), 48
Dysarthria, 927
Dysembryoplastic neuroepithelial tumors (DNET), 463
Dysgerminomas
  ovaries, 1560–1563
  pregnancy, 1563
Dysphagia, 927
  gastric cancer, 1288–1289
Dysplastic nevus syndrome, 1645
  with testis cancer, 1468
Dyspnea, 968
  causes, 969t
  lymphangitic carcinomatosis
    corticosteroids for, 824

E

Early aromatase inhibitors
  development of, 832
Early growth response (EGR-1) promoter, 868–869
Early response genes, 524
Early satiety, 2037–2041
East Asian distomiasis, 335–336
Eastern Cooperative Oncology Group (ECOG)
  performance scale, 510t
Eaton-Lambert syndrome, 1189
eBL, 336
EBRT. *See* External beam radiotherapy (EBRT)
EBV. *See* Epstein-Barr virus (EBV)
E-cadherin, 1272
Echocardiography, 2131
Ecteinascidin 743
  soft-tissue sarcomas
    metastatic, 1711
Ectopic ACTH syndrome, 2211–2212
Ectopic hormone production, 2210–2215
Edrecolomab, 772
E2F-1, 864
EGF, 56–57. *See* Epidermal growth factor (EGF)
  colorectal cancer, 1392
EGFR, 1273. *See* Epidermal growth factor receptor (EGFR)
  radiation, 527
EGFR tyrosine kinase
  inhibitors of, 1212–1213
EGFR tyrosine kinase response, 1213
EGR-1 promoter, 868–869
EIA protein
  adenoviral, 871
Eicosapentaenoic acid
  cachexia, 2047
Elderly. *See* Older patient
Electrolyte and water balance
  corticosteroids, 820
Electrolyte disorders, 2208–2209
Electrolytes
  cachexia, 2044
Electromagnetic fields (EMF), 295
Electromagnetic heating, 555–556
Electronic health records (EHR), 2274
Electronic medical records (EMR), 2267
Electronic publishing, 2271
Electron microscopist
  role, 448–449
Electrons, 517
Eleutherobin, 714
  chemical structure, 713f
ELISA, 22, 328
ELISPOT, 214
EMBASE, 2280
Embolism
  cerebral, 2073
Embolization, 492
  bleeding, 1287
Embolus, 2166f
Embryologic classification, 1111
Embryonal carcinoma, 1470, 1470f
  children, 1971
  ovaries, 1565
Embryonal tumors, 1951, 1954–1955
  in children, 1954–1956
Emergencies, 2246–2262
Emesis
  acute, 2055
  anticipatory, 2055
  types of, 2055
Emetic center, 2055
Emetogenic chemotherapy, 2055–2056
EMLA
  for cancer pain, 988
Emotional distress
  anorexia, 2038
Employee Retirement Income Security Act (ERISA), 1020
Encephalopathy
  cause, 2074t
  delayed, 2072
Enchondromas
  bone, 1680, 1680f
Endemic Burkitt lymphoma (eBL), 336
Endocarditis, 2240
Endocrine complications, 2204–2215
Endocrine glands, 1084–1089
  corticosteroids, 820–821
Endocrine paraneoplastic syndromes, 2210–2215
Endodermal sinus tumor
  children, 1971
Endodermal sinus tumors, 461
End-of-life care, 967t
  education and training for, 973
  guidelines in, 972–973
  physician competencies for, 973t
  practices, 1007
Endogenous retroviruses, 297, 306
Endometrial carcinoma
  with tamoxifen, 832
Endometrial hyperplasia, 1524
Endometrial neoplasms, 1522–1533
  clinical and molecular features, 1527t
  diagnosis, 1524–1525
  etiology, 262–263
  intensity modulated whole pelvic radiation therapy, 521f
  nutrition, 372
  oncogenes, 1527
  pathology, 1524–1525
  peptide analogs, 812
  prognosis, 1526–1527
  radiation therapy, 1528–1530
  risk factors, 1522–1524
  screening, 407–408
  staging, 1525–1526
  treatment, 1527–1533
    recurrent disease, 1530–1533
  tumor-suppressor, 1527

Endometrial papillary adenocarcinoma, 1524
Endometrioid adenocarcinoma
cervix, 1500
Endometrioid carcinoma, 1548f
Endometrium
adenocarcinoma, 1524
clear cell carcinoma, 1524
mitotic activity, 262
Endorectal coil magnetic resonance imaging
prostate, 1439
Endoscopic cytology, 445
Endoscopic retrograde cholangiopancreatogram (ERCP), 474, 1325, 1326f
Endoscopy
bleeding, 1287
Endostatin, 169–171
with angiostatin, 172
bolus *vs.* continuous administration, 172
with chemotherapy, radiotherapy, or immunotherapy, 172
clinical implications, 174–175
gene therapy, 171–172, 172–173
hypoxic down regulation, 171
integrin binding, 170
pancreatic neoplasms, 1352–1353
platelets, 171
production, 175
signaling network, 173–174
soluble recombinant, 172
thrombin, 171
vascular permeability, 171
Endothelial antibodies, 773
Endothelial cells
G1 arrest, 170
Endothelial nitric oxide
dephosphorylation, 170–171
Endpoints, 430
Energy
breast cancer, 368–369
colorectal cancer, 367
Energy expenditure
cachexia, 2042–2043
Engineered protein expression, 22
Engraftment syndrome
with hematopoietic stem cell transplantation, 2161
Enhancers, 9
ENIAC (Electronic Numerical Integrator and Computer), 2267
Eniluracil, 1391
Enneking system, 1675–1676, 1675t
Entelev, 961
Enteral nutrition
cachexia, 2048
Enterobacteriaceae, 2225–2226
Enterococcus, 2228–2229
Enucleation
retinoblastoma, 1075
Envelope, 299–300
Environmental factors
secondary cancer, 2218
Environmental tobacco smoke (ETS), 361–362, 1133
Enzyme
targets, 619
Enzyme-linked immunosorbent assay (ELISA), 22, 328
EOPPC
peritoneum, 1365
Eosinophilic granulomas
bone, 1680–1681, 1681f
Eosinophilic pneumonia, 2158
EPEC, 1007
Ependymal tumors
in infants and children
imaging, 1955–1956
Ependymomas, 461–462, 1055–1057
in children, 1956
in infants and children, 1951
Ephelides, 1245
Ephrin
signaling, 174
Ephrin family, 60
Epidemiology, 339–352
nutritional, 347
proof, 351–352
Epidermal growth factor (EGF), 53, 56–57
colorectal cancer, 1392
Epidermal growth factor receptor (EGFR), 53, 1273
lung cancer, 1182
radiation, 527
Epidermodysplasia verruciformis, 1665
Epinephrine
synthetic and metabolic pathways of, 1125f
Epipodophyllotoxins, 693–694
structure, 694f
Epiregulin, 57
Epirubicin (Ellence), 691–692
cardiotoxicity, 2140–2141, 2141
gastric cancer, 1284
Epithelial ovarian cancer, 1543–1560
etiology, 1543
genetic risk, 1543–1544
peptide analogs, 812
prevention, 1543
Epithelial tumors
benign
genomic alterations in, 121–122
Epithelioma cuniculatum, 1667
Epothilone, 714
chemical structure, 713f
Epoxide
structure, 678f
E-prescriptions, 2274
Epstein-Barr virus (EBV), 310–311, 1805f, 2236
with adult acute lymphoblastic leukemia, 1772
animal models, 312
Burkitt lymphoma, 312–313
cellular homologs, 311t
clinical aspects, 312
gene expression, 311–312
head and neck neoplasms, 1132
Hodgkin disease, 313, 1803
leiomyosarcoma, 313
lymphoproliferative disease, 312
nasopharyngeal carcinoma, 313
T-cell lymphoma, 313
Equipoise, 428
ERCC2, 355
ERCP, 474, 1325, 1326f
ERISA, 1020
ERK, 65
Erlotinib (Tarceva)
for lung adenocarcinoma, 105
for nonsmall-cell lung cancer, 1212–1213
Erythromelalgia, 1877f
Erythropoietin (EPO), 744–745, 746t, 765, 2215
myelodysplastic syndrome, 1732
Esophageal cancer
genomic alterations in, 124–125
Esophageal candidiasis, 2175
Esophageal dilation
for malignant dysphagia, 2174
Esophageal neoplasms, 1255–1268, 1256t
biologic staging, 1259
bone scintigraphy, 1259
bronchoscopy, 1258
cervical
surgery, 1263t
chemoradiotherapy, 1267
randomized trials, 1261t, 1262t
chemotherapy, 576–577, 1265–1267
computed tomography, 1258
contrast radiography, 1258
diagnosis, 1257
distribution, 1255f
endoscopy, 1258
epidemiology, 1256
etiology, 1256
hyperthermia, 559
imaging, 491
long-term outcome, 1260f
lymph node staging map, 1260f
magnetic resonance imaging, 1258
minimally invasive surgical staging, 1259
neck ultrasonography, 1259
neoadjuvant therapy, 1263
nutrition, 370–371
palliative therapy, 1267–1268
photodynamic therapy, 1267
positron emission tomography, 1258–1259
presentation, 1257
pretreatment assessment, 1257
prevention, 384
radiation therapy, 1264–1265, 1265t
brachytherapy, 1265
staging, 1257–1259
surgery, 1260–1263
therapy, 1260–1265
TNM staging, 1259, 1259t
treatment, 1257
algorithm, 1257f
Esophageal stents, 498–499
Esophagectomy, 1261t
lymphadenectomy, 1264f
reconstruction after, 1263–1264
resection, 1263f
results, 1263t
Esophagitis, 2175–2176
bacterial, 2175
Candida, 2231
etiology of, 2175t
Esophagus
adenocarcinoma, 371
anatomy and histology, 1255–1256
Essential thrombocythemia, 1875–1878, 1876f
pregnancy, 1878
Essiac, 961–962
Esterase D, 87

Esthesioneuroblastoma, 1154
Estradiol, 259f
Estramustine, 1457
Estrogen
 aromatase structure and regulation, 828
 biology of, 828–829
 biosynthesis of, 828
 role of, 828
Estrogen excess hypothesis, 265
Estrogen replacement therapy
 endometrial cancer, 262–263
Estrogens, 854
Ethernet protocol, 2268
Ethics, 998–1014
 genetics, 1012–1013
Ethmoid sinuses
 malignant primary tumors
  AJCC staging, 1152t
Ethnic groups, 343–345
 hepatitis C virus, 327
 incidence, 349t
 smoking cessation, 360
10-ethyl-10-deazaaminopterin, 655
Etidronate, 988, 2092
Etiology, 346
 in adolescents, 2029–2030
Etoposide, 693–694
 adjustment for renal insufficiency, 2128t
 causing anaphylaxis, 2261
 for disseminated germ cell tumors, 1478
 gastric cancer, 1286
 Hodgkin disease, 1863
 pharmacodynamics, 624
 schedule effects, 593
 second malignancies after, 1482–1483
 for small-cell lung cancer, 1217
Etoposide phosphate, 693–694
ETS, 361–362, 1133, 1386
European Organization for the Research and Treatment of Cancer H7F Trial, 1813
European Organization for the Research and Treatment of Cancer H9F Trial, 1814
Eutectic mixture of local anesthetic (EMLA)
 for cancer pain, 988
Euthanasia, 1008–1009, 1020
 defined, 1008t
Euthyroid sick syndrome, 2204
Ewing's sarcoma
 bone, 1687
 in children, 2024–2028, 2025f
  chemotherapy, 2025
  differential diagnosis, 2024
  epidemiology, 2024
  histologic findings, 2025
  localized disease, 2025–2026, 2026t
  metastatic disease, 2026, 2026t
  molecular diagnosis, 2025
  pathophysiology, 2024–2025
  presentation, 2024
  prognosis, 2027
  radiographic appearance, 2024
  second malignancy, 2027
  toxicity, 2026–2027
 genomic alterations in, 129
 transplantation for, 891
Excisional biopsy, 508
Excision margins, 442
Excision repair complementing group 2 (ERCC2), 355
Exemestane, 832–833, 834t, 836
 bone effects of, 837–838
Exenteration
 retinoblastoma, 1075
Exercise, 905
Exfoliative cytology, 445
Exons, 10
Experimentation
 strategy, 418
Expert witness, 1020
Exposure
 defined, 348
Expression cloning, 18
Extensible Markup Language (XML), 2273
External beam radiotherapy (EBRT), 518
 cervical cancer, 1511–1512
 differentiated thyroid carcinoma, 1096, 1098
 growth hormone secreting pituitary adenomas, 1087
 prostate cancer, 1445
 retinoblastoma, 1075
Extracellular matrix, 139–140
 cell invasion, 150f
Extracellular signal-regulated kinase (ERK), 65
Extracorporeal photopheresis
 mycosis fungoides/Sézary syndrome, 1844
Extrafascial hysterectomy, 1509
Extraglandular aromatase, 828
Extragonadal germ cell tumors, 1484–1485
Extramammary Paget disease, 1674
Extramucosal masses, 466–467
Extraovarian primary peritoneal carcinoma (EOPPC)
 peritoneum, 1365
Extrathymic tumors, 1239
Extravasation injury, 2078
Eyelid disease, 1082–1083

F

FAB M1, 1742
FAB M2, 1742, 1742f
FAB M4, 1743
FAB M5, 1743–1744
FAB M6, 1744
FAB M7, 1744–1745, 1745f
FAB M4EO, 1743
Face
 squamous cell carcinoma, 441f
Factor XA inhibitors, 2120
Fadrozole, 833–834
 structure of, 833f
Fallopian tube neoplasms, 1537–1540
 clinical presentation, 1537
 incidence and epidemiology, 1537
 patterns of spread, 1538
 preoperative diagnosis, 1537
 prognosis, 1538, 1540
 sarcoma, 1578–1579
 staging and classification, 1537–1538, 1538t
 treatment, 1538–1540, 1539f
Famciclovir, 327
Familial adenomatous polyposis (FAP), 92, 1271, 1377, 2220
 gastric cancer, 228
 genetic basis, 218
Familial atypical multiple-mole melanoma (FAMMM) syndrome, 1331
Familial chronic lymphocytic leukemia, 1786–1787
Familial gastric cancer, 227
Familial isolated pheochromocytoma, 1126
Familial juvenile polyposis coli
 genetic basis, 219
Familial medullary thyroid carcinoma (FMTC), 62, 1098–1099, 1123–1124, 1145–1148
Familial melanoma, 1645
Familial neuroblastoma
 genetic basis, 230
Familial pancreatic cancer
 genetic basis, 226–227
Familial prostate cancer, 228–230
Family
 distress
  factors contributing to, 971t
 genetic information, 1013
 grief, 912
 suffering, 970–971
Family history
 prostate neoplasms, 1431
Family issues, 911–912
FAMMM syndrome, 1331
Fanconi anemia
 genetic basis, 226
 transplantation for, 892
FAP. *See* Familial adenomatous polyposis (FAP)
Farnesyl transferase inhibitors
 pancreatic neoplasms, 1352
Fas, 43
Fasciola hepatica, 1323
Fat
 dietary. *See also* Dietary fat
 metabolism
  cachexia, 2043
Fatigue
 cachexia, 2042
Fatty acids, 374
FDG, 455, 474, 1439
Fecal occult blood testing (FOBT), 397
Federal policies
 research, 1029
Female reproductive tract
 imaging, 477
Femur
 magnetic resonance imaging, 479f
 metastatic tumor to, 2088
Fenretinide, 378, 1544
Fentanyl, 985
Fertility
 chemotherapy, 2198
 Hodgkin disease, 1863
  in children, 1960
 preservation, 2199t
Fetal liver kinase-2. *See* Flt3 ligand (Fms-like tyrosine kinase 3)
Fever
 cachexia, 2042

Fever of unexplained origin, 2242
Fever of unknown origin, 5
FGF, 35, 57–58, 162–163
FHIT, 82–83, 1272
Fiber
  colorectal cancer, 368, 1371
Fibroadenoma, 484f
Fibroblast growth factors (FGF), 35, 57–58, 162–163
Fibrosarcoma
  genomic alterations in, 127–128
FICTION, 108
Field cancer, 2218
Filgrastim, 1732
Financial incentives
  for physicians, 1010–1011
Finasteride, 379
Fine-needle aspiration (FNA), 508
Fish oil, 374
Flexible sigmoidoscopy
  colon cancer, 398
FLK-2 (Fetal liver kinase-2). *See* Flt3 ligand (Fms-like tyrosine kinase 3)
Flow cytometry-based assays, 213
Floxuridine (FUDR), 1405
  colorectal metastases, 494
  hepatic arterial infusion, 1306
FLT-3 ligand, 763–764, 764t
Flt3 receptor, 56
Flu
  complementary and alternative medicine for, 958t
Fluconazole, 2189
Fludara, 1794
Fludarabine, 672–673
  adjustment for renal insufficiency, 2128t
  nephrotoxicity of, 2129
Fluid attenuation inversion recovery (FLAIR), 461
Fluorescence in situ hybridization (FISH), 105
Fluorescence in situ hybridization (FISH)ISH, 107, 108, 108f, 199
Fluorescence spectroscopy, 1504
Fluorocytosine, 2234
Fluorodeoxy-D-glucose (FDG), 455, 474
  prostate, 1439
Fluoropyrimidines, 1389–1390
  colorectal cancer, 1390
  schedule effects, 593
5-fluorouracil, 661–665, 662f, 1153, 1347
  anabolism, 662–663
  anal neoplasms, 1395
  bile duct cancer, 1328
  cardiotoxicity, 2141
  catabolic reactions, 664
  cellular entry, 662
  colorectal cancer, 1388, 1391
  continuous infusion
    colorectal cancer, 1390
  gastric cancer, 1284, 1286
  head and neck squamous cell carcinoma, 1163
  mechanisms of action, 664–665
  metabolism, 639f
  neurotoxicity, 2071
  pancreatic neoplasms, 1348, 1349
  pharmacokinetics, 663–664
  renal carcinoma, 495
  resistance, 665
Flurbiprofen, 171
Flutamide, 856
  withdrawal, 857
FMTC, 62, 1098–1099, 1145–1148
FNA. *See* Fine-needle aspiration (FNA)
FNH, 1300
FOBT, 397
Focal nodular hyperplasia (FNH), 1300
Folate, 368, 373, 1371
Folic acid deficiency
  cachexia, 2042
Follicular cell tumorigenesis, 1094
Follicular large-cell lymphoma, 1838
Follicular lymphoma
  genomic alterations in, 120
Fondaparinux, 2120
Food
  additives, 374
  environmental contaminants, 374
  irradiation, 374
  natural, 374
  organic, 374
  preparation
    carcinogens, 368
  records, 365
Food-frequency questionnaires, 365
Food supplements
  regulation of, 962–963
  safety of, 962–963
Foot
  magnetic resonance imaging, 481f
Foregut carcinoid tumors, 1111
Foreign bodies, 292
Formestane, 832
Fractionation, 526
Frail older patient, 950
Free radical-mediated drug cytotoxicity, 637–638
Fresh frozen plasma
  transfusion, 2102
Fruit, 366
  breast cancer, 369
  colorectal cancer, 368
  head and neck neoplasms, 1133
FUDR, 1405. *See* Floxuridine (FUDR)
  colorectal metastases, 494
  hepatic arterial infusion, 1306
Fulvestrant (Faslodex), 831
Functional assessment, 924
Functional Assessment of Cancer Therapy (FACT), 911
Functional Living Index-Cancer (FLIC), 911
Fungal infections, 2189, 2230–2235
Fungal pneumonia
  with hematopoietic stem cell transplantation, 2160
Fusarium, 2235
Fusion genes, 78

G

Gabapentin, 988
Gag, 298–299
Gallbladder neoplasms, 1318–1322
  adenocarcinoma, 1318
  chemotherapy, 1322
  clinical presentation, 1319–1320
  diagnosis, 1320
  etiology, 1318
  high-resolution helical computed tomography, 1320f
  lymphatic drainage, 1319f
  palliation, 1322
  pathology, 1318–1319
  radiation therapy, 1322
  resection, 1320–1322
  staging, 1319t
  surgical decision making, 1321f
  treatment, 1320–1322
Gallium nitrate, 1133
  nephrotoxicity of, 2127t
Gallium scintigraphy, 489
Gallstones, 1318
Gamma radiation, 2096
Ganciclovir, 669
Ganglioside antibodies, 772–773
Gardner syndrome, 92, 1694
Garlic, 374
Gas chromatography/mass spectroscopy (GC/MS)
  tobacco smoke, 254–255
Gastrectomy, 1277–1278
Gastric carcinoids, 1115
Gastric cardia
  adenocarcinoma, 371
Gastric neoplasms, 1268–1289
  adjuvant therapy, 1280–1283, 1281t
  age-adjusted deaths, 368f
  cellular adhesion, 1272–1273
  chemoradiotherapy, 1280, 1282
    preoperative, 1283
  chemotherapy, 576–577, 1280–1282
    combination, 1285–1286
    preoperative, 1283
  clinical manifestations, 1270
  electron micrograph, 449f
  endoscopic mucosal resection, 1274
  epidemiology, 1268
  etiology, 1268–1269
  familial, 227
  familial adenomatous polyposis, 228
  genetic counseling, 228
  hereditary, 1270–1271
  histology, 1269–1270
  hypermethylation, 1271
  intraoperative radiotherapy, 1282–1283
  intraperitoneal therapy, 1282
  irradiation and supportive care, 1283
  localization, 1269t
  luminal resection, 1275
  microsatellites, 1271
  molecular biology, 1270–1273
  multivisceral resection, 1277
  node dissection, 1275–1277
  nutrition, 1289
  obstruction, 1288–1289
  palliative therapy, 1283–1284
  pathologic and clinical staging, 1273–1274
  peptide analogs, 813
  prevention, 384
  proximal, 1269
  reconstruction, 1279–1280
  SEER data, 1268f
  spread pattern, 1270

Gastric neoplasms—*continued*
surgical resection, 1274–1279
symptoms
management, 1286–1288
therapy, 1274–1275
tumor-suppressor genes, 1272
Gastric outlet obstruction
pancreatic neoplasms, 1345–1346
Gastrinoma, 1116–1117
tumor localization in, 1116t
vs. WDHHA syndrome, 1118
Gastrin-releasing peptide (GRP), 802, 807–808
structure, 807t
Gastroenteropancreatic (GEP) cells, 1109–1110
Gastroenteropancreatic neuroendocrine tumors (GEP-NET), 1109
adjuvant therapy for, 1121
biologic agents for, 1120
chemotherapy for, 1120–1121
classification of, 1111, 1111t
clinical features of, 1112–1114
computed tomography, 1113–1114
epidemiology of, 1113
external beam radiotherapy for, 1120
hepatic artery vaso-occlusive therapy for, 1119
hepatic resection for, 1119
hepatic transplantation for, 1119
high-dose somatostatin analogues for, 1120–1121
imaging of, 1113–1114
interferon for, 1120
magnetic resonance imaging, 1113–1114
MIBG, 1114
octreotide scanning, 1114, 1114f
peptide receptor radiotherapy for, 1120
somatostatin receptor scintigraphy, 1113–1114
treatment of, 1119–1120
Gastroenteropancreatic system
endocrine cells of, 1110t
Gastrohepatic ligament
incision, 1279f
Gastrointestinal complications, 2174–2181
Gastrointestinal neoplasms, 931–932
methotrexate, 651–652
vaccine clinical trials, 792
Gastrointestinal stromal tumors (GIST), 228, 1362–1363
imatinib, 727–728
KIT, 726–727
signal transduction inhibition, 1712–1714
Gastrointestinal tract
imaging, 475
Gatekeeper genes, 246, 248–249
Gatekeeper system, 1020
GBV
transfusion related, 2104
G0 checkpoint, 30–31
GC/MS
tobacco smoke, 254–255
GDNF, 60
Gefitinib (Iressa)
adjustment for renal insufficiency, 2128t
for lung adenocarcinoma, 105
for nonsmall-cell lung cancer, 1212–1213
Gelclair, 2188
Gel implants, 295
Gemcitabine, 619, 668–669
adjustment for renal insufficiency, 2128t
gallbladder cancer, 1322
nephrotoxicity of, 2129
neurotoxicity, 2071
for nonsmall-cell lung cancer, 1210
pancreatic neoplasms, 1343, 1347, 1349, 1353
schedule effects, 593
for testis cancer, 1481
Gemtuzumab ozogamycin, 775
acute myeloid leukemia, 1751
systemic reaction to, 2262
Gender
age
incidence, 347f
invasive cancer, 344t
liver neoplasms, 1292
malignant melanoma, 1647
mortality, 342t, 344t
schistosomiasis, 332
Gene(s)
activation, 78–79
amplification, 78
cloning, 11
delivery systems, 860–863
nonviral, 862–863
DNA methylation, 37t
expression, 9, 10f, 16–20, 20–21
fusion, 80–81, 80f
immunomodulatory, 866
probes, 12
radiation, 274, 276
structure, 9–10
Gene amplification, 81
Gene-environment interactions, 248, 255f
Gene expression microarrays
adult acute lymphoblastic leukemia, 1776
Gene expression profiling, 110–111
Gene fusion, 78f
Gene therapy, 860–873, 1052
angiostatin, 168
endostatin, 171–172, 172–173
hyperthermia, 553
intratumoral, 496
radiation therapy, 529
retroviral vectors, 306
Genetic counseling
algorithm, 234t
childhood retinoblastoma, 1968
gastric cancer, 228
Genetic ethics, 1012–1013
Genetic exceptionalism, 1012
Genetic information
family, 1013
Genetic medicolegal issues, 233–234
Genetic predisposition, 216–235, 347
breast cancer, 261–262
childhood neuroblastoma, 1990–1991
head and neck neoplasms, 1132
secondary cancer, 2218–2220
skin cancer, 284–287
tobacco addiction, 362
Genetic privacy
protection, 1013
Genetic risk
adaptation to, 906
Genetic screening, 1012–1013
Genetic testing
children, 1013
informed consent, 234t
research, 1013–1014
Gene transfer, 69
Genistein, 1432
Genital infections
defined, 318
Genital neoplasms, 932
Genitourinary neoplasms
methotrexate, 652
rehabilitation, 932
GenMAPP (Gene MicroArray Pathway Profiler), 2281–2282
Genomic alterations, 104–130, 112
in Burkitt's lymphoma, 120
glossary, 104t
Geographic variation, 347, 1431
Geriatric assessment, 950, 951–952
German Hodgkin's Study Group HD7 Trial, 1813–1814
German Hodgkin's Study Group HD10 Trial, 1814
Germ cell antigens, 194–195
Germ cell carcinoma
transplantation for, 891
Germ cell tumors, 461, 1240, 1469t
in children, 1956, 1971–1972
good-risk disseminated
treatment of, 1478
malignant, 1249–1253
markers, 200
mixed
ovaries, 1565
mixed malignant
in children, 1971
ovaries, 1560
poor-risk disseminated
treatment of, 1478–1479
primary, 1058–1059
Germ cell tumor syndrome, 1485
Germinomas, 461, 462
in children, 1971
Gestational trophoblastic disease, 1569–1574
classification, 1569–1570
diagnosis, 1571
epidemiology, 1569
historical perspective, 1569
markers, 200
molecular pathogenesis, 1570–1571
natural history, 1570–1571
subsequent pregnancies, 1574
therapy, 1571–1574
GGR, 285
Ghrelin, 809
GHRH. *See* Growth hormone-releasing hormone (GHRH)
Giant cell tumors
bone, 1681–1682, 1682f
Gingival infections, 2189
Gingival mucosa, 1141
Girdle pain
bilateral, 4
Girls
prepubertal
chemotherapy, 2197

GIST. *See* Gastrointestinal stromal tumors (GIST)
Glassy-cell carcinoma, 1502f
Gleevec, 67, 677
for cell-mediated lympholysis, 105
Glial cell line-derived neurotrophic factor (GDNF), 60
Glial tumors, 462
in infants and children, 1951–1952
Glioblastoma, 62
Glioblastoma multiforme, 1047–1052
hyperthermia, 559
Glioblastoma multiforme (GBM), 462
Glioma
brain stem
in children, 1954
diencephalic
in children, 1953
high-grade cortical
in children, 1954
low-grade, 1052–1055
in children, 1055
low-grade cortical
in children, 1953–1954
Gliomas
genomic alterations in, 128–129
Global genome repair (GGR), 285
Global tumor signature markers
validation of, 202
Glottic cancer, 1147–1149
Glucagonoma, 1118
Glucocorticoid-induced apoptosis, 826
Glucocorticoids, 858
mechanism of action, 824–825
myelodysplastic syndrome, 1730–1731
secretion, 817–818
for thymoma, 1241
Glucose
cachexia, 2039
Glutamine supplementation, 2188
Glutathione
alkylating agents, 679
Glutathione peroxidase (GSHPx), 637–638
Glutathione S-transferase (GST), 356
Glycolipids, 138
Glycoproteins, 138
Glycosyl transferase, 138–139
GM-CSF
in transplantation, 765
GNEF, 65
Goldie-Coldman model, 579–582
Gonadal complications, 2194–2200
protection from, 2198–2199
psychosocial issues, 2200
Gonadoblastomas
children, 1971
Gonadotroph adenomas, 815
Gonadotropin deficiency, 2210
Good death, 1008f
Google, 2271
Gordon Moore's law, 2267
Gorlin cyst. *See* Calcifying odontogenic cyst (COC)
Gorlin syndrome, 1670–1671
genetic basis, 224
Government, 1021–1030
Government funds
return on investment from, 1024–1025
Government policies
research, 1029
Government regulations, 1032
G1 phase checkpoint, 31f
Graft-vs-host disease (GVHD), 2178–2179
acute, 2178
bone marrow transplantation, 2190–2191
transfusion associated, 2103–2104
Grains, 366
Granisetron, 968
doses of, 2058t
Granulocyte colony-stimulating factor (G-CSF), 747, 747t
for adult acute lymphoblastic leukemia, 1777
in transplantation, 765
Granulocyte-macrophage colony-stimulating factor (GM-CSF), 745–747, 746t
biologic activities of, 745–746
clinical indications for, 746–747
in human disease, 746
Granulosa cell tumor, 1565f
Granulosa-stromal cell tumors, 1565–1566
Granzyme B, 42
Grb2, 63
Great vessels
tumors, 1246–1247
Greenfield filter, 496–497
Growth, 32t
biochemistry, 32
Growth curve analysis, 578–586
Growth factor(s)
abnormalities, 63–64
classification, 54–61
hepatitis B virus, 325
modes of action, 53f
multiple myeloma, 1850–1851
radiation, 527–528
Growth factor receptors, 71–72
aberrations, 62–63
tyrosine kinase, 54
Growth factors, 69–71
Growth fraction, 591
mass doubling time, 32t
Growth hormone, 2215
cachexia, 2048
deficiency, 2208, 2209t
secretion disorders, 2208
Growth hormone releasing factor (GRF), 1119
Growth hormone-releasing hormone (GHRH), 802
antagonists, 808–809, 808t
breast cancer, 811–812
cachexia, 2048
Growth stimulation plus two-step oncogenesis, 303f, 304–305
GRP, 802, 807–808
structure, 807t
GSHPx, 637–638
GST, 356
Guanine nucleotide exchange factor (GNEF), 65
Guidelines, 1034
Gut hormones
pancreatic neoplasms, 1351
GVHD. *See* Graft-*versus*-host disease (GVHD)
clinical staging of, 885t
Gynecologic oncologist, 939
Gynecologic sarcomas, 1576–1582
clinical profile, 1576–1577
nonuterine, 1578–1579
patterns of spread, 1577
prognosis, 1577–1578
sarcoma-like variants, 1577

H

Hairy cell leukemia
interferons, 737
Hallucinations, 989
Halo-orthosis, 928
Haloperidol, 968
for cancer pain, 988
for delirium, 910
doses of, 2058t
Halsted, William Stewart, 504
HAMA
mycosis fungoides/Sézary syndrome, 1844
Hamartomas, 1300
Hamartomatous polyposis syndrome, 1377
genetic basis, 220t
Haptophore, 779
HAT, 36
HAV, 329
HBIg, 326, 1294
HBsAG vaccines, 326
HBV. *See* Hepatitis B virus (HBV)
HBx protein, 325–326
HCC. *See* Hepatocellular carcinoma (HCC)
HCV. *See* Hepatitis C virus (HCV)
HDAC, 36
inhibitors, 37f, 49
HDV, 329
Head
lymph nodes, 1136f
Headache
complementary and alternative medicine for, 958t
Head and neck neoplasms, 1131–1169
accelerated and hyperfractionated radiotherapy, 1159–1161
anatomy, 1135–1136
carcinogenesis, 1133–1134
chemotherapy, 577, 1162
clinical tumor staging characteristics, 1138t
combined chemotherapy and radiotherapy, 1161
combined surgery and radiotherapy, 1161–1162
curative radiotherapy, 1158–1159
diagnosis and staging, 1137–1138
epidemiology, 1131–1135
genetic alterations, 1134
hyperthermia, 559
imaging, 464, 491
imaging of, 464–466
immunology, 1134–1135
incidence, 1131
intensity-modulated radiotherapy, 1158
methotrexate, 652
molecular biology, 1134
mortality, 1131
oral premalignancy, 379–381
pathologic assessment, 1136–1137
prevalence, 1131
prognosis, 1162
radiation therapy, 1157–1162

Head and neck neoplasms—*continued*
  rehabilitation, 929–930
  risk factors, 1131–1132
  sarcoma, 1156–1157
  treatment, 1138–1169
Head and neck squamous cell carcinoma (HNSCC), 1131–1169
  imaging, 464
  recurrent
    chemotherapy, 1162–1163
  survival, 1139t
Health care consumerism, 2266
Health care environment, 1031–1034
Health care portals, 2271–2272
Healthcare providers
  distress
    factors contributing to, 971t, 972t
Health care reform, 1031
  future directions in, 1034
Health Insurance Portability and Accountability Act (HIPPA), 1013, 1032
Health-related quality of life (HRQOL), 430
HealthSTAR, 2280
Hearing loss
  in childhood cancer survivors, 1929
Heart
  irradiation effects on, 2143–2144
  metastatic tumors to, 1246
Heartburn
  complementary and alternative medicine for, 958t
Heart disease
  carcinoid, 1115, 2133–2134
    echocardiography, 2135f
Heating
  step-down, 550
Heat shock proteins, 844
Heavy-chain diseases, 1866
Helicobacter pylori, 372, 1332
  head and neck neoplasms, 1132
Hemangioblastoma, 463
  spinal cord, 464
Hemangiocytomas, 462
Hemangiomas
  capillary
    children, 1079
  liver, 1300
  small intestine, 1360
Hemangiopericytoma, 1246
Hemangiopericytomas
  bone, 1687–1688
Hematologic complications, 2095–2108
  pharmacodynamic studies, 624t
Hematologic effects
  corticosteroids, 821
Hematologic malignancies, 1250–1251
  angiogenesis, 178
  genetic basis, 230
  radioimmunotherapy, 776
Hematoma, 2190
Hematopoiesis, 2095–2096
  growth factors, 744
Hematopoietic cancer, 112–117
  genomic alterations in, 117–120
Hematopoietic cell transplantation, 879–892, 879t
  autologous *vs.* allogeneic transplantation, 883
  donor selection, 881
  engraftment of, 881–887
  future directions of, 892
  indications for, 887–888
  late effects, 887
  methods of, 879–880
  pretransplant therapy, 883–884
Hematopoietic growth factor receptors, 745t
Hematopoietic growth factors, 744–766, 745f
  acute myeloid leukemia, 1751
  for adult acute lymphoblastic leukemia, 1777
  after chemotherapy, 764
  in aplastic anemia, 766
  in bone marrow failure states, 766
  in febrile and afebrile neutropenic patients, 764
  future of, 766
  and high-dose chemotherapy in solid tumors, 764
  in leukemic patients, 764
  in MDS, 766
  myelodysplastic syndrome, 1732
  in severe chronic neutropenia, 766
  in transplantation, 765
Hematopoietic stem cell transplantation
  autologous. *See* Autologous hematopoietic stem cell transplantation (AHSCT)
  future directions, 2106–2107
  pulmonary complications of, 2160–2166, 2160t
Hematopoietic transplantation
  allogeneic, 880f
  complications of, 884, 884t
  graft rejection and failure, 884–885
  graft-vs-host disease, 885–886
  hematologic complications, 886
  immunodeficiency and infections, 886–887
  regimen-related toxicity, 886
  treating malignancies, 880–881
Hemithorax, 2153f
Hemochromatosis
  liver neoplasms, 1293
Hemolytic streptococci, 2227–2228, 2228f
Hemolytic uremic syndrome, 2118–2119
Hemoptysis
  massive, 2253–2254
Hemorrhage
  acute, 2251
  cerebral, 2073
  management, 1287–1288
  retroperitoneal, 2252
Hemorrhagic cystitis, 2125
  etiology, 683
Hemostatic abnormalities, 2114t
Hemostasis
  physiology of, 2113
Heparin-induced thrombocytopenia, 2118
Hepatic adenomas
  benign, 1300
Hepatic angiosarcoma, 1300
Hepatic arterial infusion chemotherapy, 494, 1304–1306, 1305t, 1307t
  colorectal cancer, 1390
Hepatic arterial infusion floxuridine, 1306
Hepatic artery chemoembolization, 493
Hepatic catalase
  cachexia, 2044
Hepatic complications, 2174–2181
  etiology of, 2180t
Hepatic toxicity
  decrease, 1306–1307
Hepatitis A virus (HAV), 329
Hepatitis B immunoglobulin (HBIg), 326, 1294
Hepatitis B virus (HBV), 323–327, 2237
  DNA, 325
  hepatocellular carcinoma, 323–326
  hepatocytic hyperplasia, 326
  immunization, 1294
  liver neoplasms, 1292–1293
  treatment, 327
  vaccines, 326
Hepatitis C virus (HCV), 327–329
  hepatocellular carcinoma, 328
  liver neoplasms, 1293
  risk factors, 327–328
Hepatitis D virus (HDV), 329
Hepatitis E virus (HEV), 329
Hepatitis F virus (HFV), 329–330
Hepatitis G virus (HGV), 329–330
Hepatitis GV virus
  transfusion related, 2104
Hepatitis TT virus (HTTV), 329–330
Hepatitis viruses, 323–357, 324t
Hepatoblastoma
  in children, 1972
Hepatocellular carcinoma (HCC), 1295f
  chemoembolization, 493, 1310t
  chemotherapy, 1299f
  in children, 1972
  hepatitis B virus, 323–326
  interventional radiology, 493
  intraarterial chemotherapy, 1299t
  multifocal
    computed tomography, 475f
  peptide analogs, 814
  percutaneous ethanol injection, 493
  screening, 326–327
  serologic tests, 1295–1296
  staging, 1296t
  thermal ablation, 493
Hepatocyte growth factor (HGF), 59
Hepatoma
  chemotherapy, 576
Hepatopathy
  in childhood cancer survivors, 1925
Hepatosplenic candidiasis, 2232
Hepsulfam, 677
  structure, 678f
HER2 (ERBB2)
  lung cancer, 1182
Herbal remedies, 961–962
  Asian, 962
  regulation of, 962–963
  safety of, 962–963
Herbicides, 374
Herceptin
  cardiotoxicity, 2141
Herceptin, 67, 772
Hereditary cancer syndromes, 2219t
Hereditary diffuse gastric cancer, 227–228, 1270
Hereditary gastric carcinoma, 227
Hereditary nonpolyposis colorectal cancer (HNPCC), 2220
  definition, 221t

DNA mismatch repair gene defects, 97–98
genetic basis, 220–222
Hereditary nonpolyposis colorectal cancer syndrome, 1271, 1377
Hereditary papillary renal carcinoma (HPRC), 62
Her2/neu, 1273
pancreatic neoplasms, 1351
Herpes simplex viruses (HSV)
cervical cancer, 1498
gene delivery, 861–862
Herpes simplex viruses-1 (HSV-1), 2235
oral complications, 2189
Herpes Simplex virus (HSV) esophagitis, 2175f
Herpes simplex viruses -thymidine kinase (HSV-tk), 863
Herpesviruses, 310–314
oncogenic features, 310
properties, 310
Herpes zoster, 2235–2236
Heterocyclic amines, 250
HEV, 329
Hexamethylene bisacetamide (HMBA), 38
Hexamethylmelamine, 677–678
HFV, 329–330
HGF, 59
HGV, 329–330
High-dose chemotherapy
for disseminated germ cell tumors, 1479
High-dose therapy
stem cells, 592
High-fiber diet
breast cancer, 261
High-grade cortical glioma
in children, 1954
in infants and children, 1953–1954
Highly emetogenic chemotherapy, 2059
High-output states, 2134–2135
High-quality cancer care
barriers to achieving, 1032–1033
Hilar cholangiocarcinoma, 1325
liver transplantation, 1327–1328
prognosis, 1326–1327
resection, 1327
treatment, 1327–1328
HILP, 1707–1708
Hindgut carcinoid tumors, 1111
HIPAA, 2274
HIPPA, 1013
Hippocrates, 504
Histone acetyltransferases (HAT), 36
Histone deacetylase (HDAC), 36
inhibitors, 37f, 49
Histones
nucleosomes, 36f
HIV, 320
with adult acute lymphoblastic leukemia, 1772
cervical cancer, 1498
HLA, 319
HMBA, 38
HMO model, 1031, 1034
HN6600 (T-CRM107), 781
HNPCC. *See* Hereditary nonpolyposis colorectal cancer (HNPCC)
HNSCC. *See* Head and neck squamous cell carcinoma (HNSCC)
Hodgkin's disease
transplantation for, 890
Hodgkin's lymphoma, 1802–1822, 1862–1863
advanced
treatment, 1818–1822
AIDS, 1898–1899
chemotherapy, 577, 1814–1815, 1817–1818, 1819t, 1820t
combination, 1813–1814
in children, 1959–1960
biology, 1959
clinical presentation and staging, 1959
fertility, 1960
second malignant neoplasms, 1960
treatment, 1959–1960
computed tomography, 471f, 1810f
corticosteroids for, 822–823
CS I-11, 1813
prognosis, 1817–1818
epidemiology, 1803–1804
Epstein-Barr virus, 313
genetic basis, 232
history, 1802–1803
immunologic abnormalities, 1807
lymphocyte predominant, 1805f, 1807f
magnetic resonance imaging, 471f
mantle irradiation alone, 1815–1816
mortality, 1812t
nodular sclerosis, 1805f, 1806f
pathology, 1804–1809
during pregnancy, 944
radiation therapy alone, 1815
radiation therapy volume, 1818
randomized clinical trials, 1809–1818
Reed-Sternberg cells, 1804f, 1805
regional radiation alone, 1816
relapse patterns, 1808
stage I-II, 1809–1818
occult abdominal involvement, 1811
outcomes, 1811–1813
prognosis, 1810–1811, 1811t
stage III-IV
radiation therapy, 1820–1821
staging, 1807–1808, 1808–1809, 1808t
treatment
advanced, 1818–1822
stage I-II, 1809–1818
Holotherapy, 595–596
Homoharringtonine
cardiotoxicity, 2142
Homologous recombination, 274
Hormonal aberration
cachexia, 2041
Hormonal risk factors
candidate genes, 262t
endometrial cancer, 262t
ovarian cancer, 263t
Hormone(s)
myelodysplastic syndrome, 1730–1731
secondary cancer, 2218
Hormone replacement therapy (HRT)
breast cancer, 261, 261f
early *vs.* delayed
prostate cancer, 1454
malignant melanoma, 1661–1662
renal cell carcinoma, 1405
Hospital-acquired pneumonia (HAP), 2164
Hospital information systems, 2277
Host angiogenic response
genetically controlled, 178
Host defense, 2223t
Host immune response
effectors in, 205–207
Host-tumor drug interactions, 636
HPRC, 62
HPV. *See* Human papilloma virus (HPV)
H-RAS, 65
HRT. *See* Hormone replacement therapy (HRT)
HSV
cervical cancer, 1498
gene delivery, 861–862
HSV-1, 2235
oral complications, 2189
HSV esophagitis, 2175
HSV-tk, 863
HT3 antagonists, 2057
for nausea and vomiting, 2059
HTLV-2
transfusion related, 2105–2106
HTTV, 329–330
HuE10, 45
Human antimouse antibodies (HAMA)
mycosis fungoides/Sézary syndrome, 1844
Human chorionic gonadotrophin (hCG), 2214
Human Genome Project, 106
Human herpesvirus 8, 313
genes, 314t
Kaposi sarcoma, 314
multicentric Castleman disease, 314
primary effusion lymphoma, 314
Human immune virus (HIV), 320
cervical cancer, 1498
Human leukocyte antigen (HLA), 319
Human papilloma virus (HPV), 319–321, 319t, 320
anal neoplasms, 1392–1393
cervical cancer, 1497–1498
head and neck neoplasms, 1132
histopathology, 318f
penile, 320
premalignant papules, 1665
surrogate markers, 321
Human stem cell kinase-1. *See* Flt3 ligand (Fms-like tyrosine kinase 3)
Human subjects research, 1000–1001
Human T-cell lymphotrophic virus type I (HTLV-2)
transfusion related, 2105–2106
Human T-lymphotropic virus 1
with adult acute lymphoblastic leukemia, 1772
Humoral immune dysfunction, 2224
Hürthle cell neoplasms, 1094
Hybrid Capture II test, 321
Hybridization, 12
Hydration
palliative care, 969
Hydrazines, 677
Hydrazine sulfate
cachexia, 2046
Hydrocortisone replacement, 823
Hydromorphone, 984
Hydroxyurea, 527, 673–674, 677
for chronic myeloid leukemia, 1764

Hydroxyzine, 988
Hyperadrenalism, 5
Hyperbaric oxygen, 2187
Hypercalcemia, 823, 1131–1133, 2210, 2212–2213, 2213
Hypercalcemia of malignancy, 1189, 2093
Hypercortisolism, 1103
Hyperfractionation, 778
Hypernatremia, 2209
Hypernephroid tumors, 1401
Hypernephroma, 1401
Hyperparathyroidism, 5
Hyperpigmentation, 2079, 2079f, 2079t
Hyperplastic polyps, 228
Hyperprolactinemia, 2210
Hypersensitivity pneumonitis (HP), 2158
Hypersensitivity reactions, 2080
Hypertext Markup Language (HTML), 2273
Hyperthermia, 549–560
 biology, 549–550
 blood flow manipulation, 552
 chemotherapy, 553
 clinical, 557–560
 cytotoxicity, 550
 defined, 549
 gene therapy, 553
 metastases, 552
 normal tissue damage, 551
 physics, 553–557
 physiology, 550–551
 radiation, 552–553
 temperature measurement, 556–557
 tumor metabolism and oxygenation, 551
Hyperthermic isolated limb perfusion (HILP), 1707–1708
Hyperthyroidism, 2206
 in childhood cancer survivors, 1927
Hypertrophic pulmonary osteoarthropathy (HPO)
 with lung cancer, 1189
Hypoalbuminemia
 cachexia, 2044
Hypocalcemia, 2209–2210
Hypogammaglobulinemia, 1239
Hypogeusia, 2186
Hypoglycemia, 2043, 2214
Hypomagnesemia, 2210
Hyponatremia, 2044, 2208–2209, 2209f
Hypopharynx, 1143–1144
 primary tumor staging characteristics, 1143t
 squamous carcinoma
  survival, 1144t
Hypophysectomy
 chemical, 992
Hypothalamic astrocytomas, 461
Hypothalamic hormones, 802, 814–815
Hypothalamic-pituitary-gonadal axis, 2194
 dysfunction, 2204
Hypothalamic-pituitary-ovarian axis, 829f
Hypothalamo-hypophysial relationship, 802
Hypothyroidism, 2204–2206, 2205t
 in childhood cancer survivors, 1927
 in children and adolescents, 1960
Hysterectomy
 extrafascial, 1509
 radical, 1509

I

IAP, 34, 45–46
IARC, 340
 classification, 352
Ibuprofen
 cachexia, 2047
 pericarditis, 2144
Idarubicin
 cardiotoxicity, 2141
Idarubicin (Idamycin), 691–692
Ideal cancer biomarkers, 200
Idiopathic pneumonia syndrome
 with hematopoietic stem cell transplantation, 2161
Idiotype, 196
IFN. *See* Interferon (IFN)
Ifosfamide, 676
 adjustment for renal insufficiency, 2128t
 bladder toxicity, 683
 causing anaphylaxis, 2261
 causing childhood bladder damage, 1926
 causing childhood renal damage, 1926
 for disseminated germ cell tumors, 1479
 for drug-induced hematuria, 2125
 nephrotoxicity of, 2127t, 2129
IGF-1, 58
 prostate cancer, 350
IGFBP, 58
IGG-1, 764t
IgV gene mutation
 chronic lymphocytic leukemia, 1788
I1307K Ashkenazi mutation
 genetic basis, 219
IκB kinase (IKK), 64
IKK, 64
IL. *See* Interleukin (IL)
Ileostomy, 931–932
IL4(38-37)PE38KDEL, 781
Image processing, 2280–2281
Imaging, 455
Imatinib, 724–725, 725f
 for cell-mediated lympholysis, 105
 therapeutic trials, 728t
 toxicity, 729
Imatinib mesylate, 77
 for adult acute lymphoblastic leukemia, 1780
 adverse effects of, 1766, 1767t
 for chronic myeloid leukemia, 1766
 mode of action, 81f
 resistance to, 1767–1770
IMiD
 multiple myeloma, 1862
Immature teratomas
 children, 1971–1972
 ovaries, 1563–1564
Imminently dying
 sedation of, 994
Immune activation
 as danger to effector T cells, 210
Immune disorders
 transplantation for, 892
Immune effector cells, 205f, 736–737
Immune monitoring assays, 214f
Immune precipitation, 22
Immune response
 to cancer vaccines, 213–214
 cytokines, 207–208

Immune system
 corticosteroids, 821–822
Immunization
 strategies, 790–791
Immunoaugmentative therapy (IAT), 961
Immunobiology
 chronic lymphocytic leukemia, 1787
Immunoblotting, 20–22
Immunocytochemistry, 442
 limitations, 447–448
Immunocytoma, 1827
Immunoglobulin-M monoclonal gammopathy, 1865
Immunohistochemist
 role, 446
Immunohistochemistry
 common applications, 446t
Immunologic agents
 nephrotoxicity of, 2128–2129
Immunomodulatory analogs (IMiD)
 multiple myeloma, 1862
Immunomodulatory genes, 866
Immunoperoxidase staining
 unknown primary site, 1904–1906
Immunophenotype
 chronic lymphocytic leukemia, 1787
Immunophenotyping
 of adult acute lymphoblastic leukemia, 1773–1774
Immunostimulants, 791, 791t
Immunosuppression
 transfusion effect on, 2103
Immunotherapy
 chronic lymphocytic leukemia, 1795
 malignant melanoma, 1653–1654, 1655–1656, 1658
 problems, 787
Impotence
 in childhood cancer survivors, 1928
Improved aromatase inhibitors
 development of, 832
IMRT. *See* Intensity-modulated radiotherapy (IMRT)
Incapacity, 1000
Incidence
 in adolescents, 2028–2029
 age, 339f, 340–341, 341t, 346f, 347f, 2028t, 2031t
  colorectal cancer, 369f
 chemoprevention, 384
 ethnic groups, 349t
 race, 348f, 349t
Incisional biopsy, 508, 508f
Indium
 ^{131}I-tositumomab (Bexxar), 777
Indolent lymphoma
 non-Hodgkin's lymphoma, 1835–1836
Indomethacin
 cachexia, 2047
 mucositis, 2185
Inducible promoters, 868–869
Induction therapy
 acute myeloid leukemia, 1746–1747
Ineffective antigen-presenting cell function
 tumor-induced, 209–210
Infants
 angiogenesis in, 1952

astrocytic tumors in, 1952–1954
atypical teratoid/rhabdoid tumor imaging, 1955
brain stem gliomas in, 1954
central nervous system tumors
novel treatment strategies of, 1953t
cerebellar astrocytomas, 1953
Infants and children
central nervous system neoplasms, 1951–1958
Infection, 2222–2244
neutropenia, 2241–2243
prevention, 2243
susceptibility, 2222–2225
transfusion related, 2104–2108
Infectious agents, 292, 2224t
head and neck neoplasms, 1132
Infective endocarditis
echocardiography, 2132f
Inflammation, 292
Inflammatory conditions, 293t
Inflammatory myofibroblastic tumors
genomic alterations in, 123
Influenza, 2237
Informatics, 2266–2282
Information
communicating, 967–968
digitization of, 2266
Information management, 2275–2279
Information technology
and health care policy, 2266–2267
Informed consent, 998–999
genetic testing, 234t
legal cases, 999t
Infusion therapy, 492
Inhibitors-of-apoptosis (IAP), 34, 45–46
INK4A locus, 91–92
Inoperable Wilms' tumor
chemotherapy of, 1986
^{111}In-ProstaScint, 1439
Insertional activation, 303f, 304
Insertional mutagenesis, 71f
Institutional review board (IRB), 1001
Insulin, 58–59
anorexia, 2038
synthesis, 58
Insulin-growth factor-1 (IGF-1), 58
prostate cancer, 350
Insulin-like growth factor-binding proteins (IGFBP), 58
Insulinoma, 1117
Insulin receptor-related receptor (IRR), 59
Integrins, 150
Intensity-modulated radiotherapy (IMRT), 518–519, 520f, 1131–1169
childhood central nervous systems tumors, 1952
Interactive Anatomy 4, 2272
Intercalation, 619
Interferon (FN)
for chronic myeloid leukemia, 1764–1765
Interferon (IFN), 733–739
angiogenesis inhibition, 737t
antitumor action, 736–737
humans, 737–739
gene expression, 736t
induced genes, 734–736
induction, 733
pleiotropic biologic effects, 735t
receptors, 733–734
renal cell carcinoma, 1405–1406
research, 739t
side effects, 739, 739t
signal transduction, 734, 735f
systemic reaction to, 2262
Interferon alpha (IFN-alpha)
antiangiogenic activity, 180
cardiotoxicity, 2141
cutaneous reactions, 2082
hepatitis B virus, 327
hepatitis D virus, 329
mycosis fungoides/Sézary syndrome, 1844
renal carcinoma, 495
Interferon alpha2 (IFN-alpha2)
malignant melanoma, 1654–1655, 1658
Interferon alpha2a (IFN-alpha2a)
colorectal cancer, 1390
Interferon alpha2B (IFN-alpha2B)
multiple myeloma, 1859
Interferon gamma (IFN-gamma)
malignant melanoma, 1658–1659
Interleukin-1 (IL-1), 750–751, 750t
multiple myeloma, 1852
Interleukin-2 (IL-2), 751–752, 751t
cardiotoxicity, 2142
colon cancer, 1389
cutaneous reactions, 2082, 2083f
malignant melanoma, 1659–1660, 1660
nephrotoxicity of, 2127t, 2128
renal cell carcinoma, 1406
systemic reaction to, 2262
Interleukin-3 (IL-3), 752–753, 752t
myelodysplastic syndrome, 1732
Interleukin-4 (IL-4), 753, 753t
Interleukin-5 (IL-5), 753–754, 754t
Interleukin-6 (IL-6), 754–755, 754t
multiple myeloma, 1850–1851
Interleukin-7 (IL-7), 755, 755t
Interleukin-8 (IL-8), 755–756, 756t
Interleukin-9 (IL-9), 756, 756t
Interleukin-10 (IL-10), 756–757, 757t
Interleukin-11 (IL-11), 757–758, 757t, 765
Interleukin-12 (IL-12), 758–759, 758t
cachexia, 2047
Interleukin-13 (IL-13), 753, 753t
Interleukin-15 (IL-15), 759, 759t
cachexia, 2047
Interleukin-16 (IL-16), 759–760, 759t
Interleukin-17 (IL-17), 760, 760t
Interleukin-18 (IL-18), 760, 760t
Interleukin-19 (IL-19), 760, 761t
Interleukin-20 (IL-20), 760, 761t
Interleukin-21 (IL-21), 761, 761t
Interleukin-22 (IL-22), 761, 761t
Interleukin-24 (IL-24), 761–762
Interleukin-25 (IL-25), 762, 762t
Interleukin-26 (IL-26), 762, 762t
Interleukin-27 (IL-27), 762–763, 763t
Interleukin-28 (IL-28), 763, 763t
Interleukin-29 (IL-29), 763, 763t
Interleukin-31 (IL-31), 763, 763t
Intermittent dosing, 593
International Agency for Research on Cancer (IARC), 340
classification, 352
International Germ Cell Consensus Classification, 1478, 1478t
Internet, 2268–2275
file sharing, 2274–2275
health care applications, 2274
health information quality, 2274
for oncologists, 2279–2280
professional patient care information on, 2272t
research collaboration, 2274
Internet portal search engines, 2272t
Interstitial brachytherapy
cervical cancer, 1513
Interstitial pneumonitis (IP), 2157–2158
Interval failure rates
calculation, 422t
Interventional radiology, 492–500
Intraarterial therapy, 492–496
Intracavitary radiation therapy
cervical cancer, 1512–1513
Intracellular cytokine assays, 214
Intracellular regulators, 37
Intracellular signaling components
genetic alterations, 63t
Intracranial germ cell tumors (IGCT)
in infants and children
imaging, 1956
Intracranial metastases, 1065
Intracrine mode, 53
Intraepithelial neoplasia, 3
Intraoperative lymphatic mapping
malignant melanoma, 1653, 1653f
Intravascular devices
infection, 2224
Intravesical BCG
bladder cancer, 793
Introns, 10
Invasion, 148–154, 153–154
genetic regulation, 152
proteolysis, 150–151
Invasion-promoting genes, 152–153
Invasive ductal carcinoma
mammography, 484f
Invasive pulmonary mycosis, 2165–2166
Investigational New Drug application
preparation, 609, 609t
In vitro translation, 22
Iododeoxyuridine, 527
Ionizing radiation, 270–280
molecular events following, 521
secondary cancer, 2220–2221
IPod, 2281
I1317Q, 1372
IRB, 1001
Irinotecan, 620, 695
colorectal cancer, 1391, 1392
gastric cancer, 1286
Iris nevi, 1080
Iron
liver neoplasms, 1293
IRR, 59
IRS-1, 63
Iscador, 962
ISCN
abbreviated terms and symbols, 107f
ISI Journal Citation Reports, 2280
Islet-cell tumors. *See* Pancreatic neuroendocrine tumors (PNET)

Isochromosome 17, 82
Isolation, 2243
Isotretinoin, 1098
^{131}I-tositumomab, 777
Ivor Lewis procedure, 1275

J

Jaundice, 4
Jaw
  osteosarcoma of, 1692
Jejunal free flap, 514f
Jejunal interposition, 1279
JM-216, 686
JNK, 65
Jun N-terminal kinase (JNK)/stress-activated protein kinase (SAPK), 65
Juvenile pilocytic astrocytoma
  hematoxylin-eosin stained section of, 1953f
  magnetic resonance imaging, 1953f
Juvenile polyposis coli, 1377
  familial
    genetic basis, 219
Juxtacortical osteosarcomas
  bone, 1689–1690
Juxtamembrane sequence, 54

K

Kaposin, 313
Kaposi sarcoma, 1888–1893, 1890f
  human herpesvirus 8, 314
  interferons, 739
  treatment, 1891–1893
Kaposi sarcoma–associated herpes virus (KSHV), 1851
Karnofsky rating, 510t, 511t
Keratinizing and calcifying odontogenic cyst. *See* Calcifying odontogenic cyst (COC)
Keratoacanthoma, 1665–1666, 1666f
Ketamine, 992
Ketoconazole, 854, 2189
  ACTH secreting pituitary adenomas, 1087–1088
Kinases, 79
Ki-ras, 1375
KIT, 725–728
  GISTs, 726–727
  mutations, 727f
Kit ligand, 56
Klatskin tumors, 1299
KLG, 63
Klinefelter's syndrome
  with testis cancer, 1468
Klinefelter syndrome, 1250
K-*ras,* 83, 1374
  oncogene, 355
Krukenberg tumor
  ovaries, 1567
KSHV, 1851

L

Lacrimal gland
  adenoid cystic carcinoma, 1082f
  tumors, 1083–1082
Lactotrophs, 1086
LAMB (lentigines, atrial myxoma, mucocutaneous myxoma, blue nevi), 1245
Lambert-Eaton myasthenic syndrome (LEMS), 2072
Lamivudine
  hepatitis B virus, 327
Lanreotide
  for gastrinoma, 1117
Laparoscopic cholecystectomies, 1321
Large-cell carcinoma
  of lungs, 1186
Large-cell lymphoma (LCL)
  in children, 1963–1966
  follicular, 1838
Large-cell undifferentiated carcinoma
  of lung, 1186f
Large intestine cancer
  schistosomiasis, 335
Large-scale genomic analysis
  new markers from, 79
Laryngeal carcinoma
  imaging of, 466
Laryngopharyngeal reflux
  head and neck neoplasms, 1133
Larynx, 1144–1146
  advanced glottic lesions
    management algorithm, 1146f
  anatomy, 1135–1136
  early glottic lesions
    management algorithm, 1145f
  glottic
    survival, 1149f
  preservation
    randomized trials for, 1166
  primary tumor staging characteristics, 1144t
  supraglottic cancer
    management algorithm, 1148f
    squamous cell carcinoma survival, 1148f
Laser capture microdissection (LCM), 152–153
Laser therapy
  for malignant dysphagia, 2174
L-asparaginase, 2116
Lauren classification
  gastric cancer, 1269–1270
Law, 1015–1022
Law of therapeutics, 566–567
Law of the telecoms, 2267
LCL. *See* Large-cell lymphoma (LCL)
LCM, 152–153
Leader sequence, 298–299
Lead-time bias, 391
League table, 431
LEEP
  for HPV, 321
Legal complications
  preventing, 1017–1018
Legionella pneumophila, 2230
Leiomyoma
  small intestine, 1360
Leiomyosarcoma, 1246, 1697f
  Epstein-Barr virus, 313
  radiation therapy, 1580
LEMS, 2072
Length bias, 391
Lentigines, 1245
Lentigo maligna melanoma, 1646, 1647f
Leptin
  anorexia, 2038
Letrozole, 834t, 835, 836
  bone effects of, 837–838
  effects on lipid, 838
  post-tamoxifen treatment, 837
  structure of, 833f
Leucovorin, 666
  colorectal cancer, 1390
  gastric cancer, 1286
  pancreatic neoplasms, 1350
Leukapheresis therapy
  chronic lymphocytic leukemia, 1794
Leukemia
  acute
    methotrexate, 651
    transcriptional repression and chromatin acetylation, 115
  categorization, 447
  chemotherapy, 578
  children
    epidemiology, 1917
  hybrid, 1745
  monoclonal antibodies, 770–771
  ovaries, 1567
  during pregnancy, 944–945
  radiation-induced, 277
  targeted toxins, 781
Leukocytes
  collection and administration, 2098
  transfusion, 2098
Leukocyte tyrosine kinase (LTK), 63
Leukocytosis
  with chronic myeloid leukemia, 1761
Leukoencephalopathy, 2071
Leukopenia, 2098
  causes, 2096t
Leukoplakia, 1672, 1672f
Leukopoietin, 2215
Leukopoor/single-donor blood components, 2107–2108
Levamisole
  colon cancer, 1388, 1389
Lewis lung carcinoma, 439f
Leydig cell tumors, 1471
Lhermitte sign, 2071
LHRH. *See* Luteinizing hormone-releasing hormone (LHRH)
Liability, 1015–1016, 1018–1019
Lid disease, 1082–1083
Lidocaine, 2188
  for cancer pain, 988
  mucositis, 2185
LIF, 764t
Life expectancy, 949, 950t
Life support
  withdrawal of, 1020
Li-Fraumeni syndrome, 90–91, 1042, 1271, 1694, 2220
  genetic basis, 222
Limb amputation, 933
Limb cancer
  rehabilitation, 932
Limbs
  artificial, 933
Limb salvage *vs.* amputation surgery
  bone tumors, 1677–1678
Linear accelerator, 519f
Linoleic acid, 2043

Lipid
  anastrozole effects on, 838
  dietary
    colorectal cancer, 367
  metabolism
    cachexia, 2043
    disorders, 2210
Lipiodol, 492
  colorectal metastases, 494
Lipomas, 462
  genomic alterations in, 122
  small intestine, 1360
Liposarcoma
  CT, 507f
  genomic alterations in, 128
Liposomal modified
  dermatologic complications, 2082–2083
Liposome
  drug delivery, 551
Lips
  squamous cell carcinoma, 1139
Lisofylline
  cachexia, 2046–2047
Listeria monocytogenes, 2229
Listeria vectors, 790
Liver
  distomiasis, 335–336
  dysfunction score, 1298t
  hemangiomas, 1300
  radiofrequency ablation, 516f
Liver carcinogenesis
  with tamoxifen, 832
Liver cirrhosis
  in childhood cancer survivors, 1925
Liver fibrosis
  in childhood cancer survivors, 1925
Liver metastasis, 1555–1311
  adjuvant chemotherapy, 1304
  chemoembolization, 1309
  computed tomography, 1302f
  cryosurgery, 1307–1308
  embolization, 1308–1309
  imaging, 1555–1302
  magnetic resonance imaging, 1555
  neoadjuvant chemotherapy, 1304
  percutaneous ethanol injection, 1310
  positron emission tomography, 1555–1302
  primary site, 1555t
  radiation therapy, 1309–1310
  radiofrequency ablation, 1308
  resection, 1302–1304
  systemic chemotherapy, 1304–1305
  ultrasonography, 1555
Liver neoplasms, 1292–1300
  in children, 1972–1973
  clinical presentation, 1294
  epidemiology, 1292
  frequency, 1292t
  imaging, 475–476, 1296
  immunohistochemical staining, 1296t
  molecular pathogenesis, 1294
  nutrition, 372
  pathologic diagnosis, 1295
  prevention, 1294
  risk factors, 1292–1294
  schistosomiasis, 335
  staging and prognosis, 1295–1296, 1298t
  treatment, 1296–1299, 1297f
Liver transplantation
  hilar cholangiocarcinoma, 1327–1328
LMB-2 (anti-Tac(Fv)-PE-38), 781
Lobectomy
  for nonsmall-cell lung cancer, 1200–1201, 1201f
Loeb's rules of therapeutics, 566t
Logical Observation Identifier Name (LOINC), 2277
Logistic models, 421
Lomustine, 677
Long terminal repeat, 297–298
Loop electrical excision procedure (LEEP)
  for HPV, 321
Loop reconstruction, 1279
Lorazepam, 968
  for delirium, 910
  for nausea and vomiting, 2058
Loss of genomic imprinting, 141
Loss of heterozygosity, 141
Loss of heterozygosity (LOH), 105, 107
Lower urinary tract obstruction, 2124
Low-grade cortical glioma
  in children, 1953–1954
  in infants and children, 1953
Low-grade glioma
  children, 1055
Low-risk chemotherapy, 2059
LTK, 63
Lumbosacral plexopathy, 2069–2070
Lumpectomy
  for nonsmall-cell lung cancer, 1201
Lung
  adenocarcinoma of, 1185–1186
Lung cancer, 1179–1220
  angiogenesis inhibitors in, 1213–1214
  angiogenesis molecular markers, 1184
  autocrine-paracrine growth control, 1182
  bevacizumab for, 1213
  bronchoscopy, 1191
  cardiovascular manifestations, 1189–1190
  chest radiography, 1190
  in childhood cancer survivors, 1921–1922
  clinical manifestations of, 1188t
  computed tomography, 1190–1191
  cutaneous syndromes, 1189
  detection of, 1192–1193
  diagnosis of, 1190–1191
  distant metastases, 1188
  endocrine syndromes, 1188–1189
  environmental causes of, 1181
  epidemiology of, 1179
  etiology of, 1179
  familial predisposition to, 1180–1181
  fiberoptic bronchoscopy, 1191
  fine-needle aspiration biopsy, 1191
  gallium scintigraphy, 1191
  genomic alterations in, 125
  growth factors, 1182
  hematological manifestations, 1189–1190
  histopathogenesis of, 1185–1186
  imaging, 1190–1191
  integrated PET-CT, 1191
  invasive studies, 1191–1192
  magnetic resonance imaging, 1191
  mediastinoscopy, 1192
  molecular pathogenesis of, 1181–1182
  molecular premalignancy abnormalities, 1184
  molecular targeted therapy for, 1214t
  musculoskeletal syndromes, 1189
  neurologic syndromes, 1189
  noninvasive studies of, 1190–1191
  oncogenes, 80
  operative staging, 1192
  paraneoplastic manifestations of, 1189t
  paraneoplastic syndromes, 1188
  pathology of, 1184–1185
  positron emission tomography, 1191
  regional lymph nodes, 1193f
  scalene lymph node biopsy, 1192
  screening of, 1192–1193
  secondary primary cancers, 1184
  sequential pathogenic changes in, 1184f
  signs and symptoms of, 1188
  and smoking, 1179–1180
  sputum cytology, 1190
  staging of, 1190–1191
    guidelines for, 1196–1197
  staging systems, 1193–1197
  stem cell theory, 1185f
  subacute sensory neuropathy with, 1189
  thoracoscopy, 1192
  TNM subsets, 1194t
  transbronchial fine-needle aspiration biopsy, 1191–1192
  transthoracic percutaneous fine-needle aspiration biopsy, 1191
  tumor suppressor genes, 1182–1184
  WHO classification of, 1185t
  in women, 1180
Lung carcinoma
  markers, 201
Lung injury
  acute, 2168–2170
Lung metastases
  malignant melanoma, 1657
Lung neoplasms
  chemotherapy, 577
  chest film, 456f
  computed tomography, 401, 457f
  electron micrograph, 448f
  imaging, 468–470, 490
  incidence, 341
  initiation, 82
  metastatic, 2086f, 2090f
  methotrexate, 652
  nutrition, 370
  peptide analogs, 814
  polymerase chain reaction, 401
  prevention, 400–402
  primary
    prevention, 382
  rehabilitation, 930
  screening, 400–402
    recommendation, 402
  secondary
    prevention, 382–383
  undifferentiated, 441f
Lung premalignancy, 382
Lung resection, 2156
Lungs
  adenosquamous carcinoma of, 1186
  carcinoid tumors, 1186

Luteinizing hormone-releasing hormone (LHRH), 802
agonists, 802–803, 803t
breast cancer, 811–812
prostate cancer, 809–810
analogs
with cytotoxic radicals, 804
mode of action, 804–805
antagonists, 803–804, 803t
prostate cancer, 810
sustained-delivery systems, 802–803
Lvin (ML-IAP), 46
Lycopene, 374
prostate neoplasms, 1433
Lym-1, 777
Lymphadenectomy
malignant melanoma, 1652–1653
Lymphadenopathy, 466
Lymphangiography
hypothyroidism, 2205
Lymphangioma
children, 1079
small intestine, 1360
Lymphangitic carcinomatosis, 2169–2170
Lymph node map definitions, 1195t
Lymph nodes
axillary
metastasis, 1907
biopsy, 496
biopsy selection, 508
metastases
malignant melanoma, 1657
regional
clinical tumor staging characteristics, 1138t
Lymphoblastic leukemia. *See also* Adult acute lymphoblastic leukemia (ALL)
Lymphoblastic lymphoma, 1838
in children, 1963, 1969
advanced, 1969–1970
cytogenic features, 1971
pathology, 1970–1971
relapsed, 1970
Lymphocytic interstitial pneumonitis (LIP)
with hematopoietic stem cell transplantation, 2162
Lymphoepithelial thymoma, 1238f
Lymphoepithelioma-like carcinoma
cervix, 1500, 1501f
Lymphoid lineage malignancies
genomic alterations in, 117–120
Lymphokine-activated killer cells
malignant melanoma, 1659–1660
renal cell carcinoma, 1406
Lymphoma, 1240, 2087f
aggressive, 1836–1838
American Burkitt, 337
beta-cell
interferons, 738
biopsy, 496f
B-lymphoblastic
precursor, 1829–1830
bone, 1688
Burkitt. *See* Burkitt lymphoma
categorization, 447
causing ureteral obstruction, 2123
in children
anaplastic large-cell, 1967–1969
epidemiology, 1918
lymphoblastic, 1963
diffuse large B-cell, 1828–1829, 1828f
endemic Burkitt, 336
follicular
large-cell, 1838
Hodgkin
computed tomography, 471f
corticosteroids for, 822–823
magnetic resonance imaging, 471f
human herpesvirus 8, 314
imaging, 490–491
indolent
non-Hodgkin's lymphoma, 1835–1836
interferons, 738
lymphoblastic, 1838
lymphoplasmocytic, 1827
mantle cell, 1828
marginal zone, 1827–1828
methotrexate, 651
monoclonal antibodies, 770–771
non-Hodgkin. *See* Non-Hodgkin lymphoma
ovaries, 1567
peripheral T-cell, 1829
primary CNS, 1062
schistosomiasis, 335
small intestine, 1363
small lymphocytic, 1827, 1827f
targeted toxins, 781
T-cell
Epstein-Barr virus, 313
T-lymphoblastic, 1829f
precursor, 1829–1830
vaccines, 793
Lymphoplasmocytic lymphoma, 1827
Lymphoscintigraphy
cutaneous
malignant melanoma, 1653
Lyn, 523–524
Lynch syndrome
definition, 221t
genetic basis, 220–222
type II, 1544
Lytic enzymes, 140

M

MAC, 2230
Macroadenomas, 1085f
Macrobiotic diet, 960
Macrophage colony-stimulating factor (M-CSF), 747–748, 748t
in transplantation, 765
Macrophages, 206
Magnetic induction
deep heating, 555
Magnetic resonance imaging, 2131
endorectal coil
prostate, 1439
Major histocompatibility complex (MHC)
CTL, 193
Malaria, 336–337
Male breast cancer
aromatase inhibitors for, 838
Malignant airway obstruction, 2150–2151
diagnosis of, 2151
differential diagnosis of, 2150–2151
treatment of, 2151
Malignant bone tumors, 1685–1692
Malignant conversion, 247–248
Malignant dysphagia, 2174–2176
endoscopic options in, 2174t
Malignant effusion, 4
Malignant epithelial tumors
genomic alterations in, 123
Malignant fibrous histiocytoma, 1673
head and neck, 1157
Malignant fibrous histiocytoma and fibrosarcoma
bone, 1688–1689, 1689f
Malignant germ cell tumors, 1249–1253
clinical characteristics, 1250
epidemiology, 1249–1250
etiology, 1249
genomic alterations in, 128
Malignant hemangioendothelioma
bone, 1688
Malignant melanoma, 442f, 1644–1662, 1646f, 2131–2132
AJCC staging, 1648t
classification, 1646–1647
clinical characteristics, 1646–1647, 1646t
distant metastases
management, 1656–1662
prognosis, 1649
epidemiology and etiology, 1644–1645
genetic basis, 222
hyperthermia, 559
imaging, 490
invasion, 1647f
locally recurrent
management, 1655
management, 1649–1662, 1650f
precursor lesions, 1645–1646
prognosis, 1647–1648
recurrent, 1656f, 1657f
regional lymph node
management, 1652–1656
regional lymph node metastases
prognosis, 1648–1649, 1649t
Malignant mesenchymal tumors
genomic alterations in, 127
Malignant mesothelioma
vs. carcinomas, 447
Malignant neoplasms
pseudoencapsulation of, 511
second
following childhood Hodgkin's disease treatment, 1960
Malignant nervous system tumors
genomic alterations in, 128–129
Malignant pericardial effusion, 2132–2133
differential diagnosis, 2132
management, 2133
Malignant peripheral nerve sheath tumors (MPNST), 1694
Malignant pleural effusions, 2151–2154
chemical pleurodesis for, 2154
clinical manifestations of, 2151–2152
computed tomography of, 2152
diagnosis of, 2151–2152
imaging of, 2151–2152
magnetic resonance imaging of, 2152

PET of, 2152
studies of, 2151–2152
treatment of, 2153–2154, 2155f
tumor markers, 2152–2153
Malignant solid tumors
genomic alterations in, 123–130
recurrent chromosomal abnormalities in, 121t
Mammography, 392–394, 457
abnormal, 483–484
diagnostic, 482
normal, 483
postsurgical breast, 485
preoperative planning, 484–485
screening, 482
standardized reporting, 482–483
standard views, 482f
types, 482
Managed care, 1020
Manchester Pilot Study, 1813
Man-made mineral fibers (MMMF), 294
Mantle cell lymphoma, 1828
genomic alterations in, 119
Manual healing, 961
MAP, 699
MAPK
signaling, 523
MAP kinase kinase (MKK), 65
Marginal cost per year of life saved (MCYLS), 391
Marginal zone lymphoma, 1827–1828
Marijuana
head and neck neoplasms, 1133
Massage, 961
Mass doubling time
growth fraction, 32t
Mass spectrometry, 22, 23
Mast cell growth factor, 56
Mastectomy
bilateral modified radical, 514f
Matrix metalloproteinase inhibitors (MMPIs)
pancreatic neoplasms, 1352
Matrix metalloproteinases (MMP), 150–151
Matrix protein
angiogenesis inhibitors, 175
Mature B-cell lymphoma
genomic alterations in, 119, 119t
Mature cystic teratomas, 1249
Mature teratomas
children, 1971–1972
Maxillary sinuses
malignant primary tumors
AJCC staging, 1152t
Maxillectomy, 1153
McDowell, Ephraim, 504
MCYLS, 391
MDS. *See* Myelodysplastic syndromes (MDS)
Meat
colorectal cancer, 367–368, 1370
Mechanical bowel obstruction, 968
Mechanism-based aromatase inhibitors, 832–833
Mechlorethamine
for SCLC, 1217
Meclizine, 968
Mediastinal germ cell tumor
pretreatment evaluation and staging, 1251
Mediastinal masses
imaging, 470
Mediastinum
benign teratomas, 1249
poorly differentiated carcinoma, 1253
Mediators
cardiac effects of, 2133–2135
Medical art, 565
Medical decision making
for dying patient, 972
Medical education
information management, 2275
Medical informatics, 2267
Medical oncologist, 937–938
cancer prevention, 563
clinical responsibilities, 562–563
role, 562
Medical oncology, 562–569
Medicare claims
Internet, 2279
Medications. *See* Drugs
Medicine
digitization of, 2267f
MEDLARS, 2279
MEDLINE, 2279
MedlinePlus, 2274
Medroxyprogesterone, 844
cachexia, 2046
Medullary thyroid cancer (MTC), 1098–1100, 1099f, 1099t, 1133–1136, 1134f
adjuvant radiation therapy, 1099
algorithm, 1136f
calcitonin, 1100
familial, 1098–1099, 1145–1148
prophylactic surgery, 1100
Medullary thyroid carcinoma (MTC), 1109, 1123
histologic features of, 1124f
Medulloblastomas, 463
genomic alterations in, 129
in infants and children, 1951, 1954–1955, 1954f
magnetic resonance imaging, 1954f
Megace, 854
Megavitamins, 960
Megestrol, 834t, 854
Megestrol
cachexia, 2046
prostate cancer, 1455
MEK (mitogen/extracellular-signal-regulated kinase kinase), 65, 67
Melanocytes, 1645
Melanoma, 283, 463, 1397–1398
acral-lentiginous, 1646
chemotherapy, 577
children, 1973–1974
choroidal, 1080–1081, 1081f
classification, 1082t
familial, 1645
familial atypical multiple-mole, 1331
genomic alterations in, 130
lentigo maligna, 1646, 1647f
malignant. *See* Malignant melanoma
metastatic
interferons, 738
mucosal lentiginous, 1646–1647
nodular malignant, 1646, 1647f
oncogenes, 81
recurrent, 773f
screening, 409
superficial spreading, 1646
vaccine clinical trials, 792
vagina, 1494–1495
vulva, 1492–1493
Melatonin
cachexia, 2047–2048
Melphalan, 676
adjustment for renal insufficiency, 2128t
causing anaphylaxis, 2262
clinical pharmacology, 681
lung injury following, 1925
malignant melanoma, 1656
multiple myeloma, 1858
thyroid neoplasms, 1098
MEN. *See* Multiple endocrine neoplasia (MEN)
Men
gonadal complications
chemotherapy, 2196–2197
protection from, 2198–2199
gonadal function
radiation therapy, 2198
Menarche
breast cancer, 260
Meningioma, 1060–1061
magnetic resonance imaging, 460
spinal cord, 464
Meningiomas
genomic alterations in, 122–123
Meningitis, 1062–1064
methotrexate, 652
Meningoencephalitis, 2234
MEN-1 syndrome, 1122, 1122t
and gastrinoma, 1122–1123
and GEP-NET, 1122–1123
and parathyroid lesions, 1122
treatment of, 1123
MEN-2 syndrome, 1123
classification of, 1123t
Meperidine
for cancer pain, 985
Mercaptoethane sulfonate, 683
Mercaptopurine
adjustment for renal insufficiency, 2128t
toxicity of, 2180
6-Mercaptopurine (6-MP), 670
Merkel cell carcinoma, 1671–1672
Mesenchymal chondrosarcomas
bone, 1687, 1687f
Mesenchymal stem cells (MSC), 35
Mesenchymal tumors
benign
genomic alterations in, 122–123
MESH terms, 2279
Mesothelioma
computed tomography, 471f
malignant. *See* Malignant mesothelioma
peritoneum, 1365
Messaging standards, 2273
Met, 62
Meta-analysis, 422–424
Metabolic bone disease, 2206–2207
Metabolic derangement
cachexia, 2041
Metabolic detoxification, 960

Metabolic encephalopathy, 2073–2074
Metabolic therapy, 960
Metaiodobenzylguanidine, 489
Metallic stents, 497
Metalloproteinase
  inhibition, 170
Metallothionein, 685
Metastasis, 148–154
  adhesion, 149–150
  adrenal, 2207–2208
  angiogenesis, 160, 178
  axillary lymph node, 1907
  axillary lymph nodes, 1907
  axillary nodal, 457
  bone
    management, 2089–2093
  brain. *See* Brain metastasis
  breast neoplasms, 2086f, 2088f, 2089f, 2091f, 2092f
  colorectal, 494
  cranial nerve, 2067–2068
  gastrointestinal
    malignant melanoma, 1657–1658
  genetic regulation, 152
  hepatic, 494–495
  integrins, 150
  leptomeningeal, 2065–2067, 2067f
    chemotherapy, 2067
    diagnosis, 2066
    frequency, 2065t
    pathophysiology, 2065, 2066f
    radiation therapy, 2067
    signs and symptoms, 2065
    treatment, 2066–2067
  liver. *See* Liver metastasis
  lung
    malignant melanoma, 1657
  lymph node
    malignant melanoma, 1657
  melanoma
    interferons, 738
  microdissection, 152f
  neuroendocrine, 494–495
  novel technology, 152–153
  pathophysiology of, 1065–1066, 1066f
  patterns, 161t
  peripheral nerve, 2067–2068
  placental, 945t
  pulmonary. *See* Pulmonary metastasis
  site of origin, 446–447
  skeletal, 2085–2093
  spinal, 2061–2070
  therapeutic targets, 153t
  thyroid carcinoma, 2085f
  tumor-host interactions, 148–149, 149t
  tumor-stromal interactions, 148–149
Metastasis-suppressor genes, 152
Metastatic breast cancer
  potential sequential endocrine options for, 839f
Metastatic sarcoma, 2152f
Metcalfe's law, 2267
Methadone
  for cancer pain, 984
Methotrexate, 638
  adjustment for renal insufficiency, 2128t
  adverse effects, 652–653
  antifolate resistance, 653–735
  catabolism, 650f
  causing anaphylaxis, 2262
  childhood acute lymphoblastic leukemia, 1937
  clinical application, 650–653
  colorectal cancer, 1390
  combination chemotherapy with, 651t
  dosage scheduled, 651t
  drug interactions, 650
  head and neck squamous cell carcinoma, 1163
  inducing osteopathy, 2094
  leptomeningeal metastasis, 2067
  metabolism, 638f
  nephrotoxicity of, 2127t
  neurotoxicity, 2070–2071
  pharmacokinetics, 649–650
  schedule effects, 593
  sensitivity to, 654t
  sites of action, 649f
  supportive care, 652t
  toxicity of, 2126–2127, 2180
Methotrimeprazine
  for cancer pain, 988
Methoxyestradiol, 153
Metoclopramide, 968, 2057
  cachexia, 2046
  doses of, 2058t
  for nausea and vomiting, 2059
Metyrapone, 819
Mexiletine
  for cancer pain, 988
MGUS
  multiple myeloma, 1848
Microarray analysis
  DNA, 19
Microdissection
  invasion, 152f
Microsatellite instability, 1373, 1376
Microscopic sections
  preparation, 440
Microsoft's search engine, 2271
Microtubule-associated proteins (MAPs), 699
Microtubule-associated proteins kinase kinase (MKK), 65, 67
Microtubule organizing center (MTOC), 699
Microtubule-targeting natural products, 699–714
  novel compounds, 713–714
Midgut carcinoid tumors, 1111
Mifepristone, 825, 844
Migratory necrolytic erythema
  of glucagonoma syndrome, 1118f
Migratory thrombophlebitis (Trousseau's syndrome), 2117
Mind-body techniques, 960
Mineral metabolism disorders, 2208–2209
Mineralocorticoids, 818
  secretion, 818
Minerals, 373–374
Minimal deviation, 136
Minimally emetogenic chemotherapy, 2059
Mirtazapine
  for anxiety, 908
Mismatch DNA-repair genes, 248–249
Mismatch repair pathway, 98f
Mitelman Database of Chromosome Aberrations in Cancer, 105
Mithramycin
  hypercalcemia, 1133
Mitochondria
  apoptosis, 42
Mitogen activated protein kinase (MAPK) signaling, 523
Mitogen/extracellular-signal-regulated kinase kinase, 65, 67
Mitogenic signaling, 55
Mitomycin C, 527, 676
  bile duct cancer, 1328
  colorectal metastases, 494
  gastric cancer, 1284
  hepatocellular carcinoma, 493
  metabolism, 678
  nephrotoxicity of, 2127t, 2128
  pancreatic neoplasms, 1348
  renal carcinoma, 495
  structure, 677f
  uterine cervix carcinoma, 495
Mitosis, 573
Mitotane, 819
Mitotic cycle, 570–571, 571f
Mitotoxicity hypothesis, 586–587
Mitoxantrone, 692–693
  cardiotoxicity, 2141
  pancreatic neoplasms, 1350
  prostate cancer, 1457
  structure of, 692f
Mixed germ cell tumors
  ovaries, 1565
Mixed linkage leukemia (MLL)
  translocations involving chromatin remodeling proteins, 115–116
Mixed malignant germ cell tumors
  in children, 1971
MKK, 65, 67
ML-IAP, 46
M-mode echocardiography, 2131
MMP, 150–151
MMPIs
  pancreatic neoplasms, 1352
MMTV, 57–58
Modeling studies, 429–430
Moderately emetogenic chemotherapy, 2059
Modified radical mastectomy
  bilateral, 514f
Modified Stanford V, 1813
Modified vaccina Ankara (MVA), 790
Molecular pathologist
  role, 449–450
Molecular targets
  cancer treatment, 590t
Monoclonal antibodies, 770–773, 770t
  imaging, 489
  immunoperoxidase staining, 446f
  photoimmunotargeting, 548
  systemic reaction to, 2262
Monoclonal antibody 17-1A
  colon cancer, 1389
Monoclonal gammopathy of unclear significance (MGUS)
  multiple myeloma, 1848
Monoclonal serotherapy, 770–782
  barriers to, 773–774

Mood disorders, 908–909
Morphea-like basal cell carcinoma, 1669
Morphine
  for cancer pain, 984
Mortality, 341
  age, 339f, 340–341, 341t, 344t, 345f
    gastric cancer, 368f
  gender, 342t, 343f, 344t
  race, 348f, 350f
Morton, William T.G., 504
Mouse mammary tumor virus (MMTV), 57–58
Mouth
  floor, 1140–1141
    squamous cell carcinoma, 1141t
MPNST, 1694
MR angiography (MRA), 474
MRNA transcript analysis, 16–20
MRP, 631, 633
MR spectroscopy, 461
MSA, 58
MSC, 35
MSCT, 474
MTC. *See* Medullary thyroid cancer (MTC)
MTOC, 699
Mucinous adenocarcinoma
  cervix, 1500
Mucinous cystadenocarcinoma, 1548f
Mucins, 138, 139
Mucoceles
  appendiceal tumors, 1364
Mucocutaneous myxoma, 1245
Mucoepidermoid carcinoma, 1154–1155
Mucosa-associated lymphoid tissue lymphoma (MALT)
  genomic alterations in, 120
Mucosal infections
  myelosuppression, 2190
Mucosal lentiginous melanoma, 1646–1647
Mucositis, 2184–2185
  age, 2187
MUC1 tumor antigen
  tandem-repeat structure of, 196f
Muir-Torre syndrome, 1674
Multicentric Castleman disease
  human herpesvirus 8, 314
Multidisciplinary management, 935–945
Multidisciplinary planning, 1033
Multidisciplinary treatment, 1032
Multidrug resistance
  apoptotic pathways, 635–636
  drug-conjugate export pumps, 634–635
  refractory tumors, 635
  topoisomerase poisons, 633–634
Multidrug resistance protein (MRP), 631, 633
Multifocal myoclonus, 990
Multifocal sclerosing osteosarcomas
  bone, 1690–1691, 1690f
Multiple endocrine neoplasia (MEN), 62, 1143–1148, 1143t, 1144f, 2220
Multiple endocrine neoplasia (MEN) syndrome, 1109
Multiple endocrine neoplasia type 1 (MEN 1), 1143–1145
  genetic basis, 222–223
Multiple endocrine neoplasia type 2 (MEN 2)
  genetic basis, 223
Multiple endocrine neoplasia type 2a (MEN 2a), 78, 1145–1148
Multiple endocrine neoplasia type 2b (MEN 2b), 1145–1148, 1674
Multiple hamartoma syndrome
  genetic basis, 225–226
Multiple mucosal neuroma, 1674
Multiple myeloma, 1848–1867, 2092f
  apoptotic signaling, 1851f
  biology, 1849–1854
  chemotherapy, 577–578
  clinical features, 1848
  corticosteroids for, 823
  diagnosis, 1848
  epidemiology, 1848
  genetic basis, 232
  genomic alterations in, 120
  interferons, 738
  labeling index, 1855
  laboratory features, 1848–1849
  monoclonal gammopathy of unclear significance, 1848
  pedigree, 233f
  peripheral blood plasma cells, 1855
  prognosis, 1854–1857
  transplantation for, 890–891
  treatment, 1857–1865
Multiple recurrent germ cell cancer
  high-dose chemotherapy for, 1481
  salvage surgery for, 1481
  treatment of, 1481
Multiplex FISH (M-FISH), 107, 109–110, 109f
Multiplication stimulating activity (MSA), 58
Multislice computed tomography (MSCT), 474
Multistage chemical carcinogenesis, 247f
Multivitamins
  colorectal cancer, 1371
Musculoskeletal neoplasms
  corticosteroids, 821
  imaging, 479–481
Music therapy, 960
Mutagenesis
  radiation, 271
Mutated antigens, 196
Mutator phenotype, 251, 252
MVA, 790
Myasthenia gravis, 1239
Myc family, 1182
MYCN
  childhood neuroblastoma, 1991
Mycobacterial infection, 2229–2230
Mycobacterium avium-intracellulare complex (MAC), 2230
Mycobacterium kansasii, 2230
Mycosis fungoides, 1840f
Mycosis fungoides/Sézary syndrome, 1839–1844
  diagnosis, 1840–1841
  epidemiology, 1839
  natural history, 1840
  pathology, 1839–1840
  staging, 1841
  therapy, 1841–1844
Myelodysplastic syndrome
  azacytidine for, 1729
  transplantation for, 888
Myelodysplastic syndromes (MDS), 1721–1733
  bone marrow transplant, 1731–1732
  chemotherapy, 1731
  classification, 1721–1722
  clinical features, 1727–1728
  clonal origin, 1723
  etiology, 1722–1723
  history, 1721
  leukemia transformation, 1728–1729
  management, 1732–1733
  pathobiology, 1723–1731
  signal transduction, 1724–1725
Myelofibrosis
  with myeloid metaplasia, 1878–1881, 1879f, 1880f
Myeloid disorders
  recurrent chromosomal abnormalities in, 113t
Myeloid growth factors, 2098–2099
Myeloid lineage malignancies, 112–117
Myeloproliferative disorders, 2115–2116
Myelosuppression
  mucosal infections, 2190
Myocardial infarction
  with cisplatin, 1482
Myocardial ischemia
  with cisplatin, 1482
  drug-induced, 2141–2142
Myxoid liposarcoma, 81
Myxoid neurofibromata, 1245
Myxomas, 1245–1246
My Yahoo's Search, 2271

N

NAACCR, 340
N-acetylcysteine, 379
N-acetyltransferase-2 (NAT2), 356
Nails, 2077–2078
  hyperpigmentation, 2077, 2078f
NAME (nevi atrial myxoma, myxoid neurofibromata, ephelides), 1245
Nanoparticles, 295
Nasopharyngeal carcinoma
  Epstein-Barr virus, 313
Nasopharyngeal neoplasms
  imaging of, 465
Nasopharynx, 1149–1151
  imaging, 464
NAT2, 356
National Cancer Act, 1021, 1028–1029
National Cancer Advisory Board (NCAB), 1021
National Cancer Database, 2279, 2280
National Cancer Data Base (NCDB), 340
National Cancer Institute (NCI), 340
  Cancer Therapy Evaluation Program (CTEP), 2278
  funding, 1022–1024
  Gene Expression Data Portal, 110
National Cancer Institute Drug Discovery Program
  discovery process, 600
National Cancer Legislative Advisory Committee (NCLAC), 1028
National cancer program
  federal support for, 1022–1024
  legislative history of, 1021–1022, 1021t

National Comprehensive Cancer Network (NCCN), 2278
National Coordinator for Health Information Technology, 2277
National Dialogue on Cancer, 1027–1028
National Library of Medicine, 2274
National Library of Medicine Gene Expression Omnibus, 110
National Program of Cancer Registries (NPCR), 340
National Wilms Tumor Study
  treatment regimens used in, 1987f
Natural killer (NK) cells, 206
Natural killer (NK) cells, 41
Naturopathic education, 963
Nausea
  complementary and alternative medicine for, 958t
Nausea and vomiting, 968, 989–990. *See also* Chemotherapy-induced nausea and vomiting (CINV)
  alprazolam for, 2058
  anticipatory
    treatment of, 2059
  aprepitant for, 2058
  breakthrough
    treatment of, 2059
NB, 43
NCAB, 1021
NCDB, 340
NCI, 340
  funding, 1022–1024
NCI Cancer Genome Anatomy Project, 105
NCI/NIHGR Cancer Genome Project, 111
NCLAC, 1028
Neck. *See also* Head and neck
  anatomy, 1136
  lymph nodes, 1136f
Negligence, 1016
Neoadjuvant chemotherapy, 507f, 565–566
Neoplasms
  poorly differentiated, 1904–1906
Neoplastic cells
  evolution, 27f
Neoplastic meningitis, 1062–1064
  methotrexate, 652
Neoplastic spread patterns, 509t
Neoplastic transformation, 319
  in vitro, 272
Neovascularization, 152
Nephroblastoma, 1407
Nephrotoxicity
  diagnosis of, 2126–2129
  features of, 2127t
  prevention of, 2126–2129
  therapy agents associated with, 2126t
  treatment of, 2126–2129
NER, 285, 287
Nerve growth factor (NGF), 53
Netherlands
  euthanasia and assisted suicide, 1009
Networks, 2268
Neuroablation, 993
Neuroblastoma
  in children, 1990–1999
    chromosomal deletions, 1992
    classification, 1992t
    diagnosis and evaluation, 1993–1994
    diagnosis and staging, 1992–1993
    DNA index, 1991
    epidemiology, 1918, 1990
    genetics, 1990–1991
    molecular pathogenesis, 1990–1992
    MYCN, 1991
    neurotrophins, 1991
    paraneoplastic syndromes, 1993
    pathology, 1992
    prognosis, 1994–1995
    17Q unbalanced gain, 1991–1992
    screening, 1994
    staging, 1994, 1994t
    survival, 1990f
    therapy, 1995–1998
  familial
    genetic basis, 230
Neuroblastomas
  genomic alterations in, 129
  N-myc, 75t
  transplantation for, 891
Neuroendocrine çarcinoma, 1153–1154
Neuroendocrine carcinoma of unknown primary site, 1910–1912
Neuroendocrine cell, 1109
Neuroendocrine markers, 1109–1110
Neuroendocrine secretory protein-55 (NESP-55), 1110
Neuroendocrine system
  cachexia, 2044
Neuroendocrine tumor
  metastatic, 446f
Neuroepitheliomas
  genomic alterations in, 129
Neurofibromas
  genomic alterations in, 122–123
Neurofibromatosis, 96, 1041, 2219–2220
Neurofibromatosis type 1 (NF1), 1041
  genetic basis, 223
Neurofibromatosis type 2 (NF2), 96, 1041
  genetic basis, 223–224
Neuroleptics
  for anxiety, 908
Neurologic complications, 2061–2075, 2061t, 2062t
Neurologic emergencies, 2257–2258
Neuron-specific enolase (NSE), 1110
Neuropathic pain, 980
Neuropeptidergic circuit
  cachexia, 2041
Neuropeptidergic circuit dysregulation
  anorexia, 2038
Neurosurgeon, 939
Neurotrophin family, 59
Neurotrophins
  childhood neuroblastoma, 1991
Neurturin (NTN), 60
Neutrons, 517
Neutropenia, 2222–2223
  antibiotics, 2242t
  antimicrobial agents, 2241t
  bacterial infection, 2225t
  infection, 2241–2243
Neutropenic fever, 2259–2260, 2260t
Neutrophilic eccrine hidradenitis, 2081
Nevi
  congenital, 1645
Nevi atrial myxoma, 1245
Nevoid basal cell carcinoma
  genetic basis, 224
Nevus
  transformation to melanoma, 1081t
Nevus sebaceous, 1673–1674
New Affymetrix Gene Chip Human Mapping 100K Sets, 110
New anticancer agents, 600–613
New Drug application
  Investigational
    preparation, 609
News
  communicating, 967–968
Newsreader, 2273
New technology, 1032
NF1, 96, 1041
  genetic basis, 223
NF2, 96, 1041
  genetic basis, 223–224
NFKB, 48–49, 2188
  apoptosis-suppressing, 48f
NGF. *See* Nerve growth factor (NGF)
NHEJ, 274
Nicoderm, 358
Nicorette, 358
Nicotine, 354
Nicotine gum, 358
Nicotine nasal spray, 359
Nicotine replacement therapy (NRT), 358–359
Nicotine vapor inhaler, 359
Nicotrol, 358
Nicotrol NS, 359
Nijmegan breakage syndrome
  genetic basis, 225
Nilutamide
  prostate cancer, 1455
Nimustine, 677
Nitric oxide
  endothelial
    dephosphorylation, 170–171
Nitrogen mustard, 675–676
  alkylation mechanism, 676f
  mycosis fungoides/Sézary syndrome, 1841–1842
Nitrosoureas, 677
  adjustment for renal insufficiency, 2128t
  clinical pharmacology, 681
  nephrotoxicity of, 2127t
  renal toxicity, 683
  structure, 678f
  toxicity of, 2127–2128
Nitrous oxide, 992
NK. *See* Natural killer (NK) cells
NK-1 receptor antagonists
  for nausea and vomiting, 2058
NKT cells, 206
Nocardiosis, 2165
Nodular malignant melanoma, 1646, 1647f
Nomenclature, 568
Non-ablative allogeneic hematopoietic transplantation, 884f
Nonablative hematopoietic transplantation, 882–883
Non-A non-B hepatitis
  transfusion related, 2104

Nonbacterial thrombotic endocarditis (NBTE), 1189, 2119
Noncardiogenic pulmonary edema (NCPE), 2157
Nonepithelial ovarian cancer, 1560–1567
Nonfunctioning primitive neuroectodermal tumors (PNET), 1116
Nongerm cell cancers
  arising from germ cell tumors, 1471
Nonhematologic toxicity
  pharmacodynamic studies, 624t
Non-Hodgkin lymphoma
  chemotherapy, 577
  in children, 1962–1971, 1962t, 1963t
    classification, 1964t
    clinical presentation and staging, 1962–1963
    epidemiology, 1962
    pathology, 1962
    staging, 1964t
    treatment, 1964–1971
  corticosteroids for, 823
  genetic basis, 232
  during pregnancy, 944
  Rituxan, 771
Non-Hodgkin's lymphoma, 1825–1840
  AIDS, 1893–1898
    cytogenetics, 1830
    differential diagnosis, 1831–1832
    epidemiology, 1825–1826
    minimal residual disease, 1834–1835
    molecular basis, 1830–1831
    natural history, 1826–1830
    prognosis, 1833–1835
    recurrent
      treatment, 1838–1839
    serum markers, 1834
    staging, 1832–1833
    therapy, 1835–1840
  transplantation for, 889–890
Nonhomologous end-joining (NHEJ), 274
Nonintercalating topoisomerase-targeting drugs, 693–694
Nonmedical professionals, 940
Non-myeloid growth factors, 765
Nonopioid analgesics
  for cancer pain, 982, 983t
Nonossifying fibroma
  bone, 1682
Nonseminomatous germ cell tumor (NSGCT), 1469, 1470–1471
  Memorial Sloan-Kettering system for, 1473t
  treatment of, 1474f
Nonsmall-cell lung cancer (NSCLC)
  advanced
    chemotherapy, 1209–1210
    first-line therapy for, 1210
    second-line therapy for, 1210–1211
  anesthesia, 1199
  arterial blood gases, 1198
  brachytherapy, 1209
  cardiac function assessment, 1198
  chemotherapy of, 1209–1210
  chest exploration, 1200
  chest radiograph, 470f
  chromosomal deletions, 1183
  clinical target volume, 1203
  combination chemotherapy of, 1209–1210
  combination treatment of, 1214
  computed tomography, 468f, 469f
  diffusing capacity, 1199
  early-stage
    postoperative adjuvant chemotherapy of, 1212t
    stereotactic body radiation therapy for, 1205
  in elderly
    chemotherapy of, 1212
  extended surgical procedures, 1201–1202
  genetic aberrations in, 1181
  gross tumor volume, 1203
  high-risk surgery, 1203
  incisions, 1199–1200
  intensity modulated radiation therapy, 1204–1205
  internal target volume, 1204
  liver metastases, 469f
  malignant pleural effusions, 1203
  metastases
    surgery for, 1203
  molecular targeted therapy of, 1212–1213
  nodal metastases, 469f
  oxygen consumption study, 1198–1199
  planning target volume, 1203–1204
  positive margins, 1203
  preoperative and postoperative nodal irradiation, 1205–1206
  proton radiotherapy, 1204–1205
  pulmonary function assessment, 1198
  pulmonary hypertension, 1199
  pulmonary risk, 1199f
  radiotherapy, 1203
    techniques for, 1207
  satellite lesions, 1202
  stage I and II
    radiation therapy for, 1205
  stages IA and IB
    treatment of, 1197
  stages IIA and IIB
    treatment of, 1197
  stages IIIA
    treatment of, 1197
  stages IIIB
    treatment of, 1197
  stages IV
    treatment of, 1197
  staging of, 468–470, 1194
  standard surgical procedures, 1200–1201
  superior sulcus tumors, 1208–1209
  superior vena caval obstruction, 1207–1208
  surgery for N2 disease, 1202–1203
  surgical technique, 1199–1200
  surgical treatment of, 1198–1199
  synchronous and metachronous lung primaries, 1202
  treatment of, 1197–1214
  unresectable stage III
    radiation therapy for, 1206–1207
    treatment of, 1212
  xenon scanning, 1198
Non-small-cell neuroendocrine carcinoma
  cervix, 1501, 1502f
Nonsteroidal antiinflammatory drugs (NSAID), 379
  for cancer pain, 982–983
Nontuberculous mycobacteriosis, 2165
Norepinephrine
  synthetic and metabolic pathways of, 1125f
Normochromic/normocytic anemia, 2044
North American Association of Central Cancer Registries (NAACCR), 340
Northern blotting, 17
Norton-Simon model, 584–586
Nose, 1151–1154
  anatomy, 1136
  malignant tumor histology, 1153t
Novobiocin, 685
NPCR, 340
NPM, 80
NRT, 358–359
NSAID, 379
  for cancer pain, 982–983
NSCLC. *See* Nonsmall-cell lung cancer (NSCLC)
NTN, 60
Nuclear bodies (NB), 43
Nucleoside analogues
  cutaneous reactions, 2083, 2083f
Nucleosomes
  histones, 36f
Nucleotide excision repair, 251
Nucleotide excision repair (NER), 285, 287
Nucleotide sequences, 9, 13–14
Numorphan (oxymorphone)
  for cancer pain, 984
Nuremberg Code, 1000–1001
Nursing shortage, 919–920
Nutrition, 363–375, 959–960
  gastric cancer, 1289
  older patient, 951
  palliative care, 969
Nutritional deficiencies
  cachexia, 2042
Nutritionist, 923

O

Obesity
  breast cancer, 368–369
  pancreatic neoplasms, 1332
Observational studies, 428–429
Obsessive compulsive disorder (OCD), 907
Occupational exposure, 349–350
Occupational lung carcinogens, 1213
Occupational therapist, 923
Occupations
  head and neck neoplasms, 1133
Occurrence, 341
OCIS (Oncology Clinical Information System), 2278
Octreotide, 968
  for cancer pain, 989
  growth hormone secreting pituitary adenomas, 1087
  for insulinoma, 1117
Ocular diseases, 1080–1082
Ocular lymphoid tumors, 1082
Odds ratio, 348
OEPA (Oncovin, etoposide, prednisone, Adriamycin)
  Hodgkin disease, 1863
Olanzapine
  for anxiety, 908
  for delirium, 910

Older patient
acute myeloid leukemia in, 117
aggressive lymphoma
non-Hodgkin's lymphoma, 1838
assessment, 950, 951–952
chemotherapy, 954
clinical trials, 953
cognition, 951–952
comorbid medical conditions, 951
evaluation, 950
frail, 950
functional status, 950–951
nutrition, 951
polypharmacy, 952
psychological state and social support, 952
radiation therapy, 954
treatment tolerance, 953–954
Olfactory neuroblastoma, 1154
Oligodendroglioma
anaplastic, 1052
Oligodendrogliomas, 462
Oligosaccharide processing enzymes, 138–139
Olive oil, 374
Oltipraz, 379
Omega-3 fatty acids, 374
Omental bursectomy, 1277
Omeprazole
for gastrinoma, 1117
ONCOCIN, 2278
Oncogenes, 68–81, 70t, 75t, 253–254, 275, 1181–1182
activation of, 73–79, 74f
amplification, 78t
angiogenesis, 165t
capture, 302–304, 303f
chromosomal rearrangements, 75–76
discovery of, 68–69
endometrial cancer, 1527
function of, 69
gene activation, 77
gene amplification, 75, 75t
gene fusion, 77–78
hepatitis B virus, 325
identification of, 68–69
mutation, 77–78
myelodysplastic syndrome, 1726–1727
neoplasia, 79–81
Oncogenesis
mechanisms, 302–306
Oncologic informatics, 2267
Oncologist, 937–938
cancer prevention, 563
clinical responsibilities, 562–563
pain role, 966–967
role, 562
Oncology, 562–569
Oncology nurse, 915–921, 939
certification, 915–916
education, 916
health policy, 917
research, 916–917
role, 917–919
Oncology pharmacist, 939
Oncology staff
stress and burnout, 912
Oncolytic herpes simplex virus-1, 871–872
Oncolytic reovirus, 872
Oncovin
Hodgkin disease, 1863
Ondansetron, 968, 2057
doses of, 2058t
Oophorectomy, 1544
Operations
types of, 511–514
Ophthalmic neoplasms, 1071–1086, 1071t
children, 1071–1079
choroidal metastases, 1081–1082
metastatic disease, 1081–1082
Opioid analgesics
for cancer pain, 983–984, 984t
physical *vs.* psychological dependence, 990
side effects, 989–990
Opisthorchis sinensis, 1323
Opisthorchis viverrini, 335–336
Optical character recognition (OCR), 2281
Oral cancer
alcohol, 368f
nutrition, 370
screening, 409
smoking, 368f
Oral cavity
anatomy, 1135
Oral cavity carcinoma
primary tumor staging, 1140t
Oral cavity carcinoma (OCC)
imaging of, 465
Oral complications, 2184–2191
Oral contraceptives
breast cancer, 261
cervical cancer, 1499
colorectal cancer, 1372
endometrial cancer, 263, 1523
increasing risk of cervical neoplasia, 320
ovarian cancer, 264
Oral hygiene, 2186
Oral leukoplakia, 379
Oral mucosa
squamous cell carcinoma, 1667
Oral transmucosal fentanyl citrate (OTFC)
for cancer pain, 985, 985t
Orbital diseases, 1083–1082
Orbital tumors, 1083–1082, 1083t
diagnosis and treatment algorithm, 1082f
Oropharyngeal cancer
nutrition, 370
Oropharynx, 1141–1142
primary tumor staging, 1142t
Oropharynx carcinoma
imaging of, 465–466
Orphan receptors, 63
Orthomolecular therapy, 960
Orthotopic liver transplantation
cholangiocarcinoma, 1326
hepatitis B virus, 327
Ossifying fibroma. *See* Cemento-ossifying fibroma
Osteoblastoma
bone, 1683–1684, 1683f, 1684f
Osteochondromas, 1684, 1685f
Osteogenic sarcoma
head and neck, 1157
methotrexate, 652
peptide analogs, 814
Osteoid osteoma, 1682–1683, 1683f
Osteomalacia, 2207
tumor-induced, 2214–2215
Osteomyocutaneous composite tissue graft, 514f
Osteonecrosis, 2094
corticosteroid-induced, 2093–2094
Osteopenia
in childhood cancer survivors, 1929
corticosteroid-induced, 2093
Osteoporosis, 831, 2206–2207
Osteoprotegerin
hypercalcemia, 2213–2214
Osteoradionecrosis, 2186–2187
Osteosarcomas, 90–91, 1689–1690, 1690f, 1691f
cause, 266
in childhood cancer survivors, 1922
children, 2019–2024, 2021f
chemotherapy, 2021–2022
clinical trials, 2023t
epidemiology, 2019
histology, 2019–2020
pathogenesis, 2019
presentation, 2019–2020
prognosis, 2023
head and neck, 1157
magnetic resonance imaging, 480f
OTFC
for cancer pain, 985, 985t
Outcomes, 426–432, 426t, 1034
history of, 426–427
methods, 427–432
Ovarian cancer, 62, 1543–1567
adjuvant therapy, 1582
advanced
survival, 1559–1560
cause, 263–264
chemotherapy, 576, 1580–1581
classification, 1546–1547
clinical features, 1548
combination therapy, 1581–1582
complementary markers, 1549
diagnosis, 1548–1549
embryology, 1545
epithelial, 1543–1560
hormonal therapy, 1559
hormone therapy, 1580
immunotherapy, 1558–1559
malignant mixed müllerian tumors (MMT), 1580
nutrition, 372
palliative radiotherapy, 1559
patterns of spread, 1547–1548
postsurgical therapy, 1580
during pregnancy, 944
prognosis, 1545–1546
radioimmunotherapy, 777–778
risk, 1549–1550
screening, 408–409, 1549
staging, 1550–1551, 1550t
surgery, 1579
symptoms, 4
treatment, 1551–1556
Ovarian carcinoma
markers, 201
transplantation for, 891
Ovarian failure
in childhood cancer survivors, 1928

Ovarian tumors
  benign
    genomic alterations in, 122
Ovaries
  carcinoid, 1567
  choriocarcinoma, 1565
  dysgerminomas, 1560–1561, 1560–1563
  embryonal carcinoma, 1565
  estrogen biosynthesis, 828
  germ cell malignancies, 1560
  immature teratomas, 1563–1564
  Krukenberg tumor, 1567
  leukemia, 1567
  lymphoma, 1567
  mixed germ-cell tumors, 1565
  papillary carcinoma, 1548f
  papillary serous adenocarcinoma, 445f
  sarcomas, 1578–1579
  small cell carcinoma, 1566–1567
Ovary cancer
  progestin receptor, 847
Overdiagnosis, 391
Ovulation
  breast cancer, 260
Oxaliplatin, 686
  adjustment for renal insufficiency, 2128t
  colon cancer, 1388
  colorectal cancer, 1391–1392, 1392
  neurotoxicity, 2071
  for testis cancer, 1481
Oxidants, 292f
Oxycodone
  for cancer pain, 983–984
OxyContin
  for cancer pain, 984
Oxygen
  dosimetry, 546–547
Oxygen enhancement ration, 526
Oxymorphone (Numorphan)
  for cancer pain, 984

P

P21, 864
P53, 253–254, 254t, 864
  angiogenesis, 178
  gastric cancer, 1272
P53, 33, 90–91, 91f, 286
  chronic lymphocytic leukemia, 1788
P107, 90
P130, 90
Packet switching, 2268
Paclitaxel, 708
  administration, dose, schedule, 712
  anaplastic thyroid carcinoma, 1100
  cardiotoxicity, 2142–2143
  chemical structure, 706f
  gastric cancer, 1285, 1286
  head and neck squamous cell carcinoma, 1163
  nephrotoxicity of, 2129
  for nonsmall-cell lung cancer, 1210
  ovarian cancer, 1554–1555
  prostate cancer, 1457
  for SCLC, 1217
  toxicity, 710–711
Page description languages, 2272–2273
Paget's disease
  extramammary, 1674
    osteosarcoma arising in, 1692, 1692f
  vulva, 1489
Pain, 966–975
  behavioral approach, 991
  clinical assessment of, 981–982, 981t
  management, 979–994, 1287
    administration route, 986–987
    barriers to, 979, 979t
  mechanisms of, 979–980
  neurosurgical procedures for, 992–994, 992t
  psychological approach, 991
  research, 994
  types of, 980
Pain syndromes, 980, 981t
Palate
  soft, 1142–1143
Palliative care, 566
  adaptation to, 904
  corticosteroids for, 823
  legal mandate, 973
Palliative rehabilitation therapy, 923
Palmaz stent, 497
Palonosetron, 2056, 2057
  doses of, 2058t
Pamidronate, 2091
  for cancer pain, 988
  hypercalcemia, 2213
Pancarditis, 2144
Pancreas
  distomiasis, 335–336
Pancreatic cancer
  inflammation, 293f
Pancreatic neoplasms, 1585–1354
  adenocarcinoma, 1331f
    computed tomography, 474f
  adjuvant intraoperative radiation therapy, 1339–1340
  adjuvant therapy, 1341–1342
  biliary drainage, 1336
  chemoradiation therapy, 1342t
  chemotherapy, 576
  combination chemotherapy, 1348–1349
  diagnostic imaging, 1334–1336
  environmental factors, 1332
  epidemiology, 1585–1331
  exocrine
    peptide analogs, 812
  familial
    genetic basis, 226–227
  gastric outlet obstruction, 1345–1346
  hormonal therapy, 1350–1351
  imaging, 476
  immunotherapy, 1353
  interferons, 739
  localized potentially resectable disease
    treatment, 1336–1343
  locally advanced disease, 1345
    chemoradiation, 1343–1344
    down staging, 1344–1345
    intraoperative radiation therapy, 1345
  management algorithm, 1334f
  metastases, 1353–1354
    chemotherapy, 1347–1348
    treatment, 1346–1354
  neoadjuvant therapy, 1342–1343
  nutrition, 372
  pathology, 1332–1333
  prognosis, 1341
  pylorus preservation, 1339
  reconstruction, 1340
  regional chemotherapy, 1349–1350
  staging, 1340–1341, 1340t
  stents, 499f
  symptom patterns, 1333
  symptoms, 5
  treatment
    locally advanced disease, 1343–1346
  vascular resection, 1338–1339, 1339f
Pancreatic neuroendocrine tumors (PNET), 1109, 1116–1121
Pancreatic neuroprotective effects, 1116–1121
Pancreaticoduodenectomy, 1337–1338, 1338f
Pancreatitis
  acute, 2179
  pancreatic neoplasms, 1331
Pancytopenia
  causes, 2096–2097
PANOREX (edrecolomab), 772
Pansinusitis, 2233f
Papanicolaou smear, 321
Papillary carcinoma
  ovary, 1548f
Papillary fibroelastomas, 1246
Papillary serous adenocarcinoma
  ovaries, 445f
Papillary squamous cell carcinoma
  cervix, 1500, 1500f
Papillomaviruses, 318–321
PAR-4, 171
Paracrine stimulation, 72f, 82f
Parainfluenza, 2237
Paranasal sinuses, 1151–1154
  anatomy, 1136
  malignant tumor histology, 1153t
Paraneoplastic neurologic syndromes, 2074–2075, 2074t
Paraneoplastic syndromes, 5
Paraneoplastic visual loss, 1082
Paraplegia, 2070–2071
Parasites, 332–337
  animal cancer, 337
Parasitic disease
  transfusion related, 2106
Parasitism
  cachexia, 2041
Parathyroid carcinoma, 1121–1122
  biopsy of, 1121
  clinical features of, 1121
  epidemiology of, 1121
  etiology of, 1121
  imaging techniques of, 1121
  laboratory tests of, 1121
  nonfunctioning, 1131–1133
  noninvasive techniques of, 1121–1122
  treatment of, 1122
Parathyroid hormone-related protein (PTHrP), 2213, 2213f
Parathyroid tumors, 1109
Parenchyma, 437
Parenteral nutrition
  cachexia, 2048, 2048t
P19ARF, 91–92, 93f

Parity
 endometrial cancer, 263
 ovarian cancer, 263–264
Parotid glands, 1154
 carcinoma
  metastasis, 1156t
Paroxetine
 for cancer pain, 987
Paroxysmal supraventricular tachycardia, 2248
Particulate air pollution, 294
Passive smoking, 1180
Pathologist, 936–937
Pathology, 437–450
Pathways, 1034
Patient assessment
 oncology nurse, 917
Patient care
 oncology nurse, 918
Patient care delivery, 2266
Patient-controlled analgesia, 987
Patient education, 2278
 oncology nurse, 917–918
Patient Outcomes Research Teams (PORT), 427
Patient's Bill of Rights, 1020
Patient Self-Determination Act (PSDA), 972, 1007
PatientSite, 2274
Pau d'arco tea, 962
PCD, 41–49. *See also* Apoptosis
PCNSL, 1062
PCP, 1021
PC-SPES, 858
PDGF. *See* Platelet-derived growth factor family (PDGF)
Pediatric oncologist, 939
Pediatric oncology
 principles, 1914–1916
Pediatrics. *See* Children
Pediatric solid tumors
 transplantation for, 891
Pedigree analysis
 ovarian cancer, 1544
Pegylated drugs
 dermatologic complications, 2082
Pemetrexed
 adjustment for renal insufficiency, 2128t
 gastric cancer, 1284
Pemoline
 for cancer pain, 988
Penile cancer, 1462–1465
 histopathology, 1462
 prognosis, 1464–1465
 staging, 1463
 treatment, 1463–1464
Penile human papilloma virus (HPV), 320
Pentoxifylline
 cachexia, 2046
Peptide analogs, 809–814
 improvement, 811
Peptide hormones
 analogs, 802–804
Peptide-major histocompatibility complex (MHC), 213–214
Peptide receptor radiotherapy (PRRT), 1112
Percutaneous biopsy, 496
Perforated bowel, 2258–2259
Perianal infection, 2239–2240
Pericardial effusion
 malignant, 2132–2133
Pericardial tamponade, 2250–2251
Pericarditis
 radiation-induced, 2143–2144
Pericardium
 radiation effects on, 2143–2144
Peripheral blood stem cell
 autotransplantation, 2107
 dose effect, 592
Peripheral nerve blocks, 991
Peripheral nerve metastases, 2067–2068
Peripheral nerve sheath tumors (PNST)
 genomic alterations in, 129
Peripheral nerve stimulation, 993–994
Peripheral neurectomy, 993
Peripheral neuropathy, 2070
Peripheral T-cell lymphomas, 1829
Peritoneal carcinomatosis, 1906–1907
Peritoneum neoplasms, 1364–1366
Persephin (PSP), 60
Personal digital assistants (PDA), 2268
 applications of, 2270t–2271t
Personal electronic health records (PEHR), 2274
Pesticides, 374
PET, 1032. *See* Positron emission tomography (PET)
Peutz-Jeghers syndrome, 1331, 1361, 1377
 genetic basis, 219–220
PGK1, 286
P-glycoprotein-dependent multidrug resistance, 632–633, 633f, 636–637
Pharmacodynamic end points
 assays for, 608
Pharmacodynamics, 623–625
 defined, 623
Pharmacokinetics
 defined, 620–621
 interpatient variability, 622–623, 622t
 intrapatient variability, 623
 linear models, 621–622
 nonlinear models, 622
 principles, 620–623
Pharmacology, 617–625
Pharynx
 anatomy, 1135
 wall, 1142–1143
Phased array fields
 deep heating, 555
Phenobarbital
 for brain metastases, 1067
Phenylketonuria, 283
Phenytoin
 for brain metastases, 1067
Pheochromocytoma, 1109, 1124–1125, 1125f, 1136–1143, 1137f
 algorithm, 1141f
 biologic markers, 1138t
 diagnosis, 1139–1140
 epidemiology, 1137
 imaging of, 1126f
 MEN-2, 1126
 metastatic
  imaging, 1140f
 mutations in, 1126t
 natural history, 1137–1139
 survival, 1139f
 treatment, 1140–1143, 1143t
Pheresis
 therapeutic, 2102
Philadelphia chromosome, 77, 82
Philadelphia chromosome fragment, 105
Phosphorylation, 144
Photochemistry, 538–539
Photodynamic therapy (PDT), 537–550
 biologic mechanisms, 543–546
 delta-amino-levulinic acid, 541–542
 dosimetry, 546–547
 esophageal neoplasms, 1267
 history, 537
 indications, 539t
 for malignant dysphagia, 2174
 targeted molecular delivery systems, 547–549
Photoimmunotargeting, 547–548
Photons, 517
Photopheresis
 extracorporeal
  mycosis fungoides/Sézary syndrome, 1844
Photoproducts
 recognition, 287
Photosensitivity reactions, 2080, 2080t
Photosensitizers, 539–542
 anionic lipophilic, 539–540
 cationic, 540–541
 chemical structure, 538f
 dosimetry, 546
 transport, 542–543
Phototherapy
 mycosis fungoides/Sézary syndrome, 1842
Physiatrist, 923
Physical activity, 367
 colorectal cancer, 367, 1372
Physical carcinogens, 293
Physical therapist, 923
Physician-assisted suicide, 1020
Physician Data Query (PDQ), 2280, 2280t
Physicians
 challenges, 971–972
 compensation
  in managed care, 1020
 as expert witness, 1020
 features for dying patient care, 971–972
 financial incentives, 1010–1011
 suffering, 970–971
Physicians in End-of-Life Care, 1007
Physicians' Information and Education Resource (PIER), 2280
Phytochemicals, 374
PIGF. *See* Placenta-derived growth factor (PIGF)
PI-3-kinase
 signaling, 64
 survival signaling, 64
Pill induced esophagitis, 2175–2176, 2176f
Pilocarpine, 2186
Pilocytic astrocytoma, 462
Pindborg tumor. *See* Calcifying epithelial odontogenic tumor (CEOT)
Pineoblastomas, 461
P16INKA4, 91–92
Piritrexim, 655
Pituitary adenomas, 1084
 ACTH secreting, 1087–1088

gonadotropin secreting, 1088–1089
growth hormone secreting, 1086–1087
Hardy's classification, 1085f
prolactin-secreting, 1085–1086
TSH-secreting, 1089
PKC, 154
signaling, 523
P13K isoforms (P13K), 79
Placebo controls
ethics, 1003
Placenta-derived growth factor (PIGF), 56
Plasma
fresh frozen
transfusion, 2102
Plasma cell tumors, 1848–1867
Plasmacytoma, 1865
Plasmids, 11
Plasminogen activator family, 151
Plasmocytoma, 2088f
Platelet-derived growth factor (PDGF), 54–56, 69, 728, 1273
receptors, 728–729
Platelets
abnormalities, 2099
alloantigens, 2101–2102
endostatin, 171
transfusion, 2099
alternatives to, 2102
effectiveness, 2100
indications, 2100
Platins
neurotoxicity, 2071
Platinum
analogs, 686
Platinum antitumor agents, 684
cellular resistance to, 685–686
structure, 682f
Platinum compounds, 638
causing anaphylaxis, 2261
ovarian cancer, 1554
PLC-gamma, 63
Pleural disease, 2158
Pleural effusions, 2154f
massive, 2254–2255, 2254f
Pleural mesothelioma
malignant, 470–471
Pleurodesis, 2255
for malignant pleural effusions, 2154
Plicamycin
adjustment for renal insufficiency, 2128t
nephrotoxicity of, 2127t
P38 MAP kinase, 65
PML oncogenic domains (POD), 43
PML/RARA, 80
Pneumocystis carinii, 2237–2238, 2238f
Pneumocystis pneumonia (PCP), 2165
Pneumonia, 2162–2166
bacterial
with hematopoietic stem cell transplantation, 2160
caused by aspiration and bronchial obstruction, 2164–2165
Pneumonitis
in childhood cancer survivors, 1924
radiation
childhood Hodgkin's disease, 1960
Pneumothorax, 2255–2256
POD, 43
Podophyllotoxin
structure, 694f
Point mutations, 77f
proto-oncogenes, 73–75
Pol, 299
Pol H, 286
Polycyclic aromatic hydrocarbons, 354
Polycystic ovary syndrome, 1522
Polycythemia, 2215
Polycythemia vera, 1881–1884
Polymerase chain reaction, 14, 16f, 19–20
Polymorphisms
colorectal cancer, 1372
Polypharmacy
older patient, 952
Polyprenoic acid, 1294
Polyps, 396
Polysaccharide kureha (PSK), 962
POMC, 2211
Poorly differentiated carcinoma
of mediastinum, 1253
Poorly differentiated carcinoma of unknown primary site, 1909–1910
Porphyria, 283
Porphyrins
distribution, 543t
Portal vein embolization, 494
Positive predictive value
screening test, 390
Positive thinking, 902
Positron emission tomography (PET), 455, 489–490, 1325, 2131
prostate, 1439
Postchemotherapy surgery
for disseminated germ cell tumors, 1479–1480
Postirradiation osteosarcomas, 1691–1692
Postmenopausal women
aromatase inhibitors for, 838
with breast cancer, 834t
estrogen in, 829f
Postpneumonectomy hydropneumothorax, 2155f
Postsurgical respiratory insufficiency, 2154–2156
Post-tamoxifen treatment, 837
Posttranslational modifications, 20
Posttransplant lymphoproliferative disease (PTLD), 887
with hematopoietic stem cell transplantation, 2162
Pott, Percival, 504
Poxvirus, 790
Practice protocol items, 2277t
PRb protein, 89f
PRCA, 1239
Precisplatin
for disseminated testicular cancer, 1477
Precocious puberty, 2210
Prednisone, 858
for adult acute lymphoblastic leukemia, 1777
chronic lymphocytic leukemia, 1793
Hodgkin disease, 1863
hypercalcemia, 2213
multiple myeloma, 1858
Pregnancy, 941–945
cancer diagnosis and staging, 941
cancer treatment, 941–942
chemotherapy, 2199–2200
dysgerminomas, 1563
essential thrombocythemia, 1878
malignant melanoma, 1648
radiation therapy, 2200
smoking cessation, 360
tumor types, 942t
Premenopausal women
aromatase inhibitors for, 838
Preoperative planning
mammography, 484–485
Preoperative preparation, 510–511
Prepubertal girls
chemotherapy
gonadal complications, 2197
Presentation devices, 2281
Presentation software, 2281
President's Cancer Panel (PCP), 1021
Presymptomatic central nervous system therapy
childhood acute lymphoblastic leukemia, 1937–1938
Prevascular tumors
blood supply, 161
Prevention
public health guidelines, 364t, 365
Preventive rehabilitation therapy, 923
Primary CNS lymphoma (PCNSL), 1062
Primary germ cell tumors
of thorax, 1249–1253
Primary hyperparathyroidism
clinical features of, 1121t
Primary myelodysplastic syndrome (MDS), 112–113
Primary physician, 935–936
Primitive neuroectodermal tumor/medulloblastoma
in children, 1954–1955
Primitive neuroectodermal tumors (PNET), 461, 463
clinical presentation, 1116
diagnosis of, 1116
in infants and children, 1951, 1954–1955
surgery of, 1116
Privacy regulations
federal policies, 1029
Problem list, 907f
Procainamide
adverse effects, 2136
Procarbazine, 677
causing anaphylaxis, 2261
neurotoxicity, 2071
Prochlorperazine, 2057
doses of, 2058t
for nausea and vomiting, 2059
Progesterone
absorption, 843–844
PgR mutations, 845
target selection, 845
Progesterone receptors, 846
Progestin(s), 843–847
pharmacology, 843–846
physiology, 843
Progestin receptor, 846–847
Prognostic markers, 199

Programmed cell death (PCD), 41–49. *See also* Apoptosis
Programmed cell death regulation, 73
Progressive multifocal leukoencephalopathy, 2237
  cachexia, 2042
Prolactin, 2215
Proliferation assay, 213
Promoter region, 9
Promyelocytic leukemia. *See* Acute promyelocytic leukemia
Proopiomelanocortin (POMC), 2211
Proportional hazard models, 421–422
Proptosis, 1082
  causes
    children, 1080t
Prostaglandins
  cachexia, 2041
Prostate
  anatomy, 1434f
  cellular organization, 850
Prostate adenocarcinoma
  histology, 1435f, 1436f
Prostate cancer, 342, 1431–1459, 1451–1452
  adjuvant hormone therapy, 859
  androgen ablation timing, 858–859, 859t
  androgen deprivation, 854–856
  angiogenesis inhibitors, 1459
  antiandrogen withdrawal, 857
  apoptosis, 1458
  biology, 1433–1436
  bladder outlet obstruction from, 2124
  cause, 264
  chemoprevention, 1459
  chemotherapy, 576
  combined androgen blockade, 855–856
  diagnosis and staging, 1438–1439
  differentiation therapy, 1458
  disseminated
    treatment, 1453–1455
  epidemiology, 1431–1432
  estrogen, 856
  familial, 228–230
  genomic alterations in, 125–126
  hormonal agents, 853t
  hormonal therapy, 855f
  hormone-refractory, 1455–1458
  imaging, 477
  intermittent androgen suppression, 856
  interstitial brachytherapy, 521f
  latent, 1437
  LHRH agonists, 854–855
  localized
    management, 1440–1445
    prognosis, 1439–1440
  locally advanced
    treatment, 1452–1453
  metastatic, 2086f
  neoadjuvant hormone therapy, 859
  NSAID, 856
  nutrition, 369–370
  peptide analogs, 809–810
  prevention, 402–404
  radioimmunotherapy, 778
  schistosomiasis, 335
  screening, 402–404, 1436–1438
    recommendations, 404
  second-line hormone therapy, 857
  signal transduction inhibitors, 1458
  treatment, 1451–1458
  vaccine, 1458–1459
    clinical trials, 792–793
Prostate carcinoma
  markers, 201
Prostatectomy
  radical, 1442–1445
Prostate specific antigens (PSA), 5, 342, 402–404, 1436–1437
Prosthetist/orthotist, 923
PROSTVAC, 867
Protease inhibitors, 153
  invasion, 153
Protein
  analysis, 20–21
  identification and detection, 21f
  metabolism
    cachexia, 2043–2044
Proteinase-activated receptor-4 (PAR-4), 171
Protein kinase C (PKC), 154
  signaling, 523
Protein overexpression, 79
Protein phosphatase, 144–145
Protein therapy
  angiostatin, 168–169
Protein tyrosine phosphatases (PTP), 79
Proteoglycans, 138, 139
Proteolysis, 150–151
Proteolysis-mobilizing factor
  cachexia, 2041
Proteomic pattern profiling, 202
Protons, 517
Proto-oncogenes, 86
  function of, 69
  mutation, 73–75
Protozoal infection, 2237–2239
PS-341
  multiple myeloma, 1862
PSA. *See* Prostate specific antigens (PSA)
PSDA, 972, 1007
Pseudomembranous colitis, 2177f
Pseudomonas aeruginosa, 2226, 2226f
Pseudomyxoma peritonei
  peritoneum, 1365
PSP, 60
Psychiatric disorders, 906–910
Psychiatric interventions, 910–911
Psychological adjustment, 903t
Psychological responses, 902
Psychologist, 924
Psycho-oncologist, 939
Psycho-oncology, 901–912
  historical perspective of, 901–902, 901t
Psychosocial Adjustment to Illness Scale (PAIS), 911
Psychosocial care
  in adolescents, 2032–2033
Psychosocial interventions, 910–911
Psychosocial issues
  gonadal complications, 2200
Psychosocial sequelae
  in cancer survivors, 905t
Psychotherapy, 907–908
PTEN/MMAC tumor suppressor, 64
PTHrP, 2213, 2213f
PTSD, 903, 905, 907
Puberty
  precocious, 2210
Public attitudes, 1025–1026
PubMed Central, 2280
Pulmonary aspergillosis, 2233, 2233f
Pulmonary (tracheobronchial) carcinoids, 1115
Pulmonary chondroid hamartomas
  genomic alterations in, 122
Pulmonary edema, 2168–2170
  with hematopoietic stem cell transplantation, 2160–2161
Pulmonary embolism, 2256–2257, 2256f
Pulmonary fibrosis
  in childhood cancer survivors, 1924
Pulmonary hypertension, 2167
Pulmonary infection
  with hematopoietic stem cell transplantation, 2160
Pulmonary leukostasis, 2169–2170
Pulmonary neuroendocrine neoplasia
  of lungs, 1186
Pulmonary rehabilitation, 2168
Pulmonary toxicity
  childhood Hodgkin's disease, 1960
Pulmonary vascular disease (PVD), 2158
Pulmonary veno-occlusive disease
  with hematopoietic stem cell transplantation, 2161
Pure red cell aplasia (PRCA), 1239
Purine analogs, 669–674
  chronic lymphocytic leukemia, 1794
Purine antimetabolites, 669f
Purine nucleoside catabolism
  inhibitors, 671f
Purine synthesis
  inhibitors, 735
Pyrimidine, 287
Pyrimidine analogs, 661–669

Q

18Q deletion, 1376
Quality
  definition of, 1032–1033
  measures of, 431–432
Quality adjusted life years (QALYS), 429
Quality of care, 430
Quality of life, 430–431
Quality-of-life (QOL)
  assessment of, 911
  measurement, 911t
  research, 912f
Quality of Life Index (QL-index), 911
Quality Oncology Practice Initiative (QOPI), 2275
Questionnaires
  food-frequency, 365
Quetiapine
  for anxiety, 908
Quinidine
  adverse effects, 2136
17Q unbalanced gain
  childhood neuroblastoma, 1991–1992

R

Racial groups, 343–345, 351f
  incidence, 348f, 349t

mortality, 348f
prostate neoplasms, 1431
Radiation
absorbed dose, 518
bystander effects, 273–274, 274f
caries, 2186
cellular and tissue effects, 270–274
cellular response to, 520
dose response, 528–529
effects on heart, 2143–2144
growth, 522–523
head and neck neoplasms, 1133
hyperthermia, 552–553
induced carcinogenesis
experimental, 275–276
genetic susceptibility, 276
human epidemiologic studies, 276–280
risk assessment, 279–280
induced genomic instability, 272–273
injury, 270
leukemia, 277
low-dose exposures, 278–279
molecular mechanisms, 274–275
myelopathy
magnetic resonance imaging, 2073f
oncologist, 938–939
oncology, 517–531
clinical, 530
ophthalmic side effects, 1083, 1083f
pneumonitis
childhood Hodgkin's disease, 1960
during pregnancy, 942
response modifiers, 526–527
stress-signaling pathways, 522–523
survival analysis, 520–521
survival curve analysis, 521
types, 517–518
Radiation coloproctitis, 2179
argon plasma coagulation for, 2179
Radiation esophagitis, 2175
Radiation fibrosis, 2159–2160
Radiation-induced hematuria, 2125
Radiation-induced nausea and vomiting
treatment of, 2059
Radiation nephritis, 2125–2126
Radiation pneumonitis, 2159–2160
Radiation proctitis, 2179
Radiation therapy
adjuvant therapy, 530
in adolescents, 2032
antiangiogenic therapy, 529–530
biologic basis, 520–531
central nervous system
neurologic complications, 2072–2073, 2072t
chemotherapy, 530t
dermatologic complications, 2079–2080, 2079t
DNA repair, 524–526
dosing guidelines for, 1986–1987
gene therapy, 529
gonadal function, 2198
mycosis fungoides/Sézary syndrome, 1842–1843
oral complications, 2184–2185
palliative, 530
physical basis, 517–518
pregnancy, 2200
prophylactic, 530
prostate cancer, 1445–1451
complications, 1451
high-risk, 1448–1449
intermediate-risk, 1448
outcomes, 1446–1448
palliative, 1450–1451
post-prostatectomy, 1449–1450
sequelae, 530–531
skeletal complications of, 2094
Radical hysterectomy, 1509
Radical mastectomy
bilateral modified, 514f
Radiofrequency ablation, 515
liver, 516f
liver neoplasms, 1298
Radioimmunoguided surgery, 776
Radioimmunoscintigraphy, 776
Radioimmunotherapy, 775–780
alpha-particle, 779
improved, 778–779
pretargeting, 778–779
Radioiodine
differentiated thyroid carcinoma, 1095–1096, 1096–1097
Radioisotope
alpha emitters, 776
beta emitters, 775–776
selection, 775
Radiologist, 936
Radionuclide, 488–491
Raf, 65, 67
signaling, 523
Raloxifene (Evista), 379, 831
Raltitrexed
colorectal cancer, 1392
pancreatic neoplasms, 1348
Randomized clinical trials, 391–392
vs. nonrandomized, 411–413
Randomized controlled trials
ethics, 1002–1003
Randomized trials, 427–428
RAR, 36, 378
fusion proteins, 36f
RARA, 80
Ras, 64–65
MAP kinase cascade, 65–66
signaling, 523
signaling downstream, 65
Ras family, 1181–1182
Ras-raf-MAPK signaling pathway, 74, 74f
Rate difference, 348
Rate ratio, 348
Raynaud's phenomenon
with bleomycin, 1482
RB1, 87, 88f
cloning, 87–88
Rb growth control pathway
deregulation, 33f
Rb tumor-suppressor gene, 33
Really Simple Syndication (RSS), 2273
Recamier, Joseph, 504
Receptor tyrosine kinase (RTK), 54, 153
intracellular effects, 63f
invasion, 153
Recombinant DNA, 10–11
Recombinant factor VIIa (rFVIIa), 2120
Recombinant fused proteins
mycosis fungoides/Sézary syndrome, 1844
Recombinant HAV vaccine, 329
Recombinant immunoblot test (RIBA)
hepatitis C virus, 328
Recombinant proteins
large-scale production, 22–24
Recombinant vaccinia virus, 867
Reconstructive surgery, 512f, 514f
Recoverin, 1082
Recreational therapist, 924
Recruitment, 572
Rectal adenocarcinoma
therapy, 1382
Rectal neoplasms, 1381–1382
adjuvant chemotherapy, 1383, 1385–1386
adjuvant therapy
surgical prognosis, 1382
distal margin, 1381
extended lateral pelvic node dissection, 1382
intergroup postoperative trials, 1384
lymphovascular ligation, 1381
mesorectal excision, 1381–1382
metastases, 1386
NSABP postoperative trials, 1384
pelvic recurrence, 1382
postoperative chemoradiation, 1383–1384
preoperative chemoradiation, 1385
preoperative radiotherapy, 1385
preoperative *vs.* postoperative adjuvant chemoradiation, 1385
radiation therapy, 1383
radiotherapy, 1386
recurrence, 1383
recurrent, 1386
Rectum
surgical anatomy, 1378
Recurrence
prevention, 375
Recurrence and metastasis markers, 199–200
Red cell growth factors, 2097
Red cell hypoplasia, 1239
Red cells
abnormalities, 2097–2098
products, 2097–2098
transfusion, 2097
Red meat
colorectal cancer, 1370
Referrals
in managed care, 1020
Reflex sympathetic dystrophy, 927
Refractory anemia (RA), 112
Refractory sprue
cachexia, 2042
Refractory tumors
multidrug resistance, 635
Regulatory T cell-mediated suppression, 210
Regulatory T cells, 206
Rehabilitation oncology nurse, 923
Rehabilitation process, 924–926
Rehabilitation specialist, 939
Reimbursement, 1032
Relapse
childhood acute lymphoblastic leukemia, 1938–1939

Relative risk, 348
Relay-Health, 2274
Renal cell carcinoma, 463, 1401–1407
adjuvant therapy, 1404–1405
chemotherapy of, 1986–1987
clinical features, 1402
echocardiography, 2132f
embolization, 495
etiology, 1401
genetic basis, 230
genomic alterations in, 126
incidence, 1401
metastatic, 1405–1407, 2087f, 2090f, 2091f, 2092f
molecular biology, 1401–1402
pathogenesis, 1401
peptide analogs, 814
radiographic evaluation, 1402–1403
radioimmunotherapy, 778
staging and grading, 1403, 1403t, 1404t
surgery, 1403–1404
transplantation for, 891
Renal clear cell sarcoma
chemotherapy of, 1986
Renal insufficiency
antineoplastic agents with, 2128t
azacytidine, 2128t
bleomycin, 2128t
capecitabine, 2128t
carboplatin, 2128t
Renal oncocytoma, 1407
Renal pelvis/ureter neoplasms, 1410–1413
diagnosis, 1410–1411
etiology, 1410
histopathology, 1410
prognosis, 1412–1413
staging, 1411
treatment, 1411–1412
Renal rhabdoid tumor
chemotherapy of, 1986
Renal tumors. *See also* Childhood renal tumors
imaging, 476–477
Renin, 2215
Replication-competent viruses
combination chemotherapy/radiotherapy with, 873
therapeutic gene delivery with, 872–873
Reproductive factors
cervical cancer, 1498–1499
Reproductive tract
female
imaging, 477
Research
federal policies, 1029
funding, 1022
Research project grants
funding, 1023
Respiratory complications, 2150–2170
Respiratory depression, 989
Respiratory emergencies, 2253–2256
Respiratory failure, 2168–2170
acute postoperative, 2154–2155
treatment of, 2170
Restorative rehabilitation therapy, 923
Restriction endonucleases, 10–11
Restriction landmark genome scanning (RLGS), 107–108
Resuscitation, 567, 2247
Retina
vasculature development, 171
Retinoblastoma, 87–90, 1071–1078, 2219
central nervous system/distant metastases, 1076–1077
chemotherapy, 1077t
in children, 1968–1970
biology, 1968
clinical forms, 1968
clinical manifestations, 1969
epidemiology, 1918, 1968
evaluation, 1969
genetic counseling, 1968
pathology, 1968–1969
second malignant neoplasms, 1970–1971
staging, 1969–1970
treatment, 1970–1972
classification, 1074t
gene action, 1072f
genetic basis, 224
genetic counseling, 1072t
genomic alterations in, 129–130
lesions simulating, 1074–1075, 1075t
leukocoria, 1073f
molecular biology, 1072–1073
optic nerve/choroid invasion, 1076
second malignancies, 1077–1078
signs and symptoms, 1073–1074
staging, 1074
survivors, 1078t
systemic chemotherapy, 1075–1076
treatment, 1075–1078
algorithm, 1078f
Retinoblastoma protein, 88–90
Retinoic acid
myelodysplastic syndrome, 1730
Retinoic acid receptors (RAR), 36, 378
fusion proteins, 36f
Retinoids, 378, 1504
mycosis fungoides/Sézary syndrome, 1844
Retrograde ejaculation
in childhood cancer survivors, 1928
Retromolar trigone, 1141
Retroperitoneal germ cell tumors
causing ureteral obstruction, 2123
Retroperitoneal hemorrhage, 2252
Retroperitoneal metastases from cervical or breast cancer
causing ureteral obstruction, 2123
Retroviral oncogenes, 68
Retroviral transduction, 69f
Retroviral vectors, 306
Retroviruses
endogenous, 297, 306
gene delivery, 860–861
groups, 298t
life cycle, 300f
morphology, 298t
structure, 298f
Reverse transcriptase polymerase chain reaction (RT-PCR)
hepatitis C virus, 328
prostate, 1439
Reverse transcription, 301f
Reward deficiency syndrome, 362
Rhabdomyomas, 1246
Rhabdomyosarcoma, 1246
in children, 1079–1080, 2007–2010, 2008f, 2009t, 2010t
epidemiology, 1919
genomic alterations in, 128
head and neck, 1157
RIBA
hepatitis C virus, 328
Ribozymes, 20, 865–866
Right to refuse medical care, 1004
Rinses, 2190
Risedronate, 2093
Risk, 341
Risperidone
for anxiety, 908
Rituximab, 771
for adult acute lymphoblastic leukemia, 1780
systemic reaction to, 2262
RNA
5-fluorouracil, 664–665
RNA1, 866
RNA interference, 20
Robotic surgery, 515–516
Rogletimide
structure of, 833f
Ron/Stk, 59
Rous sarcoma virus (RSV), 2236–2237
oncogenic region, 85–86
Roux-en-Y reconstruction, 1279
RSV, 2236–2237
oncogenic region, 85–86
RTK. *See* Receptor tyrosine kinase (RTK)
RT-PCR
hepatitis C virus, 328
prostate, 1439
RU-486 (mifepristone), 844
RUNX3
gastric cancer, 1272
RYK, 63

S
S-1
colorectal cancer, 1392
Saccharin, 374
Sacrum
magnetic resonance imaging, 480f
SAGE, 18
Salivary gland adenomas
genomic alterations in, 122
Salivary glands, 1154–1155
anatomy, 1154
benign tumors, 1154t
chemotherapy, 1150t, 1156
histopathology, 1154–1155
malignant tumors, 1155t
neutron radiotherapy, 1156
primary tumors staging, 1155t
prognosis, 1155–1156
staging, 1155
Salivary substitute, 2186
Salmonella, 2227
vectors, 790
Salvage therapy
of adult acute lymphoblastic leukemia, 1780–1781

Hodgkin's disease, 1821–1822
non-Hodgkin's lymphoma, 1839
SAPK, 65
SARA, 825
Sarcoma, 81, 90–91, 1246
bone
staging of, 1685t
chemotherapy, 577
children
retinoblastoma, 1694
Ewing. *See* Ewing sarcoma
gynecologic. *See* Gynecologic sarcomas
head and neck, 1156–1157
of head and neck
imaging of, 467
Kaposi. *See* Kaposi sarcoma
osteogenic. *See* Osteogenic sarcoma
radiation associated, 1694
radiation-induced, 2094
of renal origin, 1407
retroperitoneal, 1714–1716
treatment
molecular, 1716–1717
outcome, 1716
vulva, 1493
Sarcotidicytin, 714
Scaffolding proteins, 63
Scanners, 2281
Scapula
metastatic tumor to, 2089
SCC. *See* Squamous cell carcinoma (SCC)
SCF. *See* Stem cell factor (SCF)
Schistosoma haematobium, 332, 1415
Schistosoma mansoni, 333
Schistosomiasis, 332–335
carcinogenicity, 335
metabolic observations, 334f
Schistosomiasis japonica, 1323
Schwannomas
cerebellar pontine angle, 461
genomic alterations in, 122–123
internal auditory canal, 461
SCLC. *See* Small-cell lung cancer (SCLC)
Sclerosing plasmocytoma, 2089f
Scoliosis
in childhood cancer survivors, 1929
Scopolamine, 968
Screening, 389–410
biases, 391–392
childhood neuroblastoma, 1994
cost effectiveness, 390–391
criteria, 389–391
hypothyroidism, 2205
recommendations, 396t
Screening mammography, 482
Screening test
effectiveness, 390
SCT. *See* Stem cell transplantation (SCT)
Search engines, 2271
Sebaceous gland adenoma, 1674
Sebaceous gland carcinoma, 1674
eyelids, 1082–1083
Secondary acute lymphocytic leukemia, 2221–2222
Secondary acute myelogenous leukemia, 2221t
and MDS, 117
Secondary breast cancer, 2222
Secondary cancer, 2216–2223
clinical characteristics, 2218
environmental factors, 2218
genetic factors, 2218–2220
incidence, 2216–2218
risk, 2217t
therapy related, 2220–2223
Secondary colorectal cancer, 2222
Secondary endometrial cancer, 2222
Secondary gastric cancer, 2222
Secondary Hodgkin's disease, 2221
Secondary ovarian cancer, 2222
Secondary pancreas cancer, 2222
Secondary pediatric sarcomas, 2222
Secondary prostate cancer, 2222
Secondary retinoblastoma, 2221
Secondary skin cancer, 2222–2223
Secondary structure, 17
Secondary testicular cancer, 2222
Secondary upper aerodigestive tract cancer, 2222
Secondary Wilms tumor, 2222
Second-generation nonsteroids, 833–834
Second-look operations, 513
Second malignancy
Ewing sarcoma
children, 2027
Sedation, 989
of imminently dying, 994
palliative care, 969–970
SEER, 340
SEER (Surveillance, Epidemiology, and End Results), 2279
Segmentectomy
for nonsmall-cell lung cancer, 1201
Seizures, 4
Selective aldosterone receptor antagonists (SARA), 825
Selective gene expression, 867–868
Selenium, 373
prostate cancer, 369
Self-expanding stents
for malignant dysphagia, 2174–2175
Seminoma, 1250
treatment, 1251–1252, 1251t
Seminomas, 1470, 1470f
chemotherapy of, 1480
salvage chemotherapy of, 1480
stage I
postorchiectomy chemotherapy of, 1476–1477
primary and adjuvant therapy, 1476
stage II
treatment of, 1477
standard salvage chemotherapy of, 1480–1481
Semliki forest virus, 790
Semustine, 677
Senile keratosis, 1663–1664
Sensitivity
screening test, 390
Sentinel lymphadenectomy
malignant melanoma, 1653
Sentinel lymph node biopsy, 515
Sentinel node biopsy, 516f
Sequencing, 22
Serial analysis of gene expression (SAGE), 18, 18f
Serotherapy
multiple myeloma, 1865
Serotonin, 362, 1109–1110, 2055
anorexia, 2037–2038
Serotonin reuptake inhibitors (SSRI)
for anxiety, 908
Sertoli cell tumors, 1471
Serum HCG
with testis cancer, 1472
Serum immunoassay markers, 200–201
Serum response element (SRE), 65
Serum response factor (SRF), 65
Serum thyroglobulin monitoring
differentiated thyroid carcinoma, 1096
Serum thyroid hormone-binding protein
abnormalities, 2204
Sex
mortality
age, 345f
Sex cord-stromal tumors, 1471, 1563t, 1565, 1565t
Sex hormones
pancreatic neoplasms, 1350–1351
Sexual behavior
cervical cancer, 1498
Sexual dysfunction, 2210, 2211f
Sexual maturation
in childhood cancer survivors, 1927
Sexual rehabilitation, 932
Sézary syndrome, 1840f. *See also* Mycosis fungoides/Sézary syndrome
SGA, 2041
Shark cartilage, 961
Sho-saiko-to, 962
SIADH, 2208–2209, 2214
Sickle cell anemia
transplantation for, 892
Sickness Impact Profile (SIP), 911
Sigmoidoscopy
flexible
colon cancer, 398
Signal transducers, 72
Signal transduction, 143–144
apoptosis, 48–49
cancer therapy, 65–66
Silica, 294
Simon Nitinol filter, 497
Simple Object Access Protocol (SOAP), 2274
Sindbis virus, 790
Single nucleotide polymorphism (SNP), 105, 110, 110f
Single nucleotide polymorphisms (SNPs), 16
Single-photon techniques, 488
Sinonasal cavity neoplasms
imaging of, 465
Sinus
malignant tumor distribution, 1152t
radiotherapy, 1153
SIR, 2217
SI units, 568, 568t
6-mercaptopurine (6-MP), 670
Sjögren syndrome, 2186
Skeletal complications, 2085–2094
of radiation therapy, 2094
steroid-induced, 2093–2094

Skeletal metastases, 2085–2093
pathogenesis, 2085–2086
patient evaluation, 2086–2087
surgery, 2087–2088
Skin complications. *See* Dermatologic complications
Skin infection, 2240
Skin neoplasms, 283–285, 1663t
age of onset, 283
basal cell carcinoma, 1669–1670, 1669f
genetic factors, 284–287
metastases to, 1674
prevention, 383
screening, 409
squamous cell carcinoma, 441f, 1667f
sunlight, 283–284
ultraviolet radiation genesis, 1663
verrucous carcinoma, 1667
Skin-related syndromes, 2220
Skipper-Schabel-Wilcox model, 578–579
Skull
osteosarcoma of, 1692
Sky, 60
Sleep problems
complementary and alternative medicine for, 958t
Sleeve pneumonectomy
for nonsmall-cell lung cancer, 1201f
SLF. *See* Steel factor (SLF)
Small bowel
stents, 499
Small bowel gastroenteropancreatic neuroendocrine tumors (GEP-NET), 1114–1115, 1115f
Small cell carcinoma
ovaries, 1566–1567
Small-cell lung cancer (SCLC), 1186–1187, 1187f
alternating chemotherapy and maintenance therapy, 1219
chemotherapy of, 1217–1218
in special clinical situations, 1219–1220
timing of, 1215–1216
chromosomal deletions, 1183
combination chemotherapy of, 1217–1218
dose intensity for, 1218–1219
genetic aberrations in, 1181
intrathoracic adenopathy, 470f
metastatic, 1068f
performance status, 1196
prognosis of, 1196
radiotherapy of, 1215
cranial, 1217
fractionation, 1216
timing of, 1215–1216
total tolerable of, 1216–1217
second-line therapy for, 1218
staging of, 1195–1196
surgery of, 1214–1215
transplantation for, 891
treatment of, 1214–1220, 1215f
future of, 1220
Small-cell neuroendocrine carcinoma
cervix, 1501, 1502f
Small intestine neoplasms, 1359–1363
clinical presentation, 1359
computed tomography, 1359–1360
diagnostic imaging, 1359–1360
endoscopic ultrasonography, 1359–1360
treatment, 1360–1361
Small lymphocytic lymphoma, 1827, 1827f
Smokeless tobacco
cessation, 361
Smoking, 354–363. *See also* Cigarette smoking
anal neoplasms, 1393
associated with HPV, 320
cervical cancer, 1499
liver neoplasms, 1293
oral cancer, 368f
in women, 1180
Smoking cessation, 356–361
clinics, 357
harm reduction, 359–360
pharmacological interventions, 358–359
physician-related interventions, 357–358, 358t
self-help methods, 356–357
special populations, 359–361
SNOMED, 2274
SNOMED-CT (Systematized Nomenclature of Medicine-Clinical Terms), 2277
SNPs, 16
Social worker, 924
Society, 903
Socioeconomic status, 343–345
Sodium dodecyl sulfate-polyacrylamide gel electrophoresis, 20
Soft-tissue sarcomas, 1694–1717
chemotherapy, 1704–1707
in children, 2007–2381, 2007f
classification, 1695–1697
etiology, 1694–1695
extremities
treatment, 1700–1707
imaging, 1697–1698
locally advanced disease
treatment, 1707–1708
metastatic
treatment, 1708–1712
screening, 1695
staging, 1698–1700
Sojourn time, 389
Solar keratosis, 1663–1664
Solid tumors
benign
genomic alterations in, 120–121
genomic alterations in, 120
infections, 2225t
radioimmunotherapy, 777
transplantation for, 891
Solitary pulmonary nodule (SPN), 1187–1190
clinical manifestations of, 1187–1190
clinical presentation of, 1187–1188
intrathoracic spread of, 1187–1188
Solitary thyroid nodule, 1093
diagnostic evaluation, 1093
differential diagnosis, 1093t
Somatic *APC* mutations
sporadic colon tumors, 93
Somatic cell genetic studies
tumorigenesis, 86–87
Somatic mutations, 85–86
Somatic pain, 980
Somatostatin (SST), 1112, 1112f
analogues of, 1119–1120
biology of, 1112
Somatostatin analogs, 805–807
breast cancer, 811–812
cytotoxic, 807
radiolabeled
local tumor therapy, 807
Somatostatin analogue binding affinities, 1112t
Somatostatinoma, 1118–1119
Somatostatin receptors (SSTR), 1112
biology of, 1112
Somatostatin receptor scintigraphy, 489
SOMI orthosis, 928
Southern blotting, 13, 13f
Southwest American Indians
gallbladder cancer, 1318
Southwest Oncology Cancer Group (SWOG) study, 1813
Soy, 373–374
prostate neoplasms, 1432
Specialized treatment, 1032
Specificity
screening test, 390
Specimens
handling, 440
obtaining, 440, 444
Spectral Doppler studies, 2131
Spectral karyotyping (SKY), 105, 109–110
Speech-language pathologist, 924
Speer-Retsky model, 584
Spermatocytic seminoma, 1469, 1471, 1471f
Spermatogenesis
in childhood cancer survivors, 1927
Spinal cord
imaging, 463–464
neoplasms
magnetic resonance imaging, 464
radiation-induced injury, 2073
Spinal cord compression, 2061–2065, 2062f, 2257–2258, 2257f
clinical findings, 2062–2063
differential diagnosis, 2063t
magnetic resonance imaging, 2064f
pathophysiology, 2062
radiation therapy, 2064
surgery, 2064
symptoms, 2063t
treatment, 2063
Spinal cord tumors, 1057–1058
Spindle-cell carcinoma
of lungs, 1186
Spindle-cell thymoma, 1237
Spine
metastatic tumor to, 2089
Spine cancer
rehabilitation, 927–929
Spirocerca lupi, 337
Spleen
rupture, 2251–2252
Splenectomy
chronic lymphocytic leukemia, 1794
infection, 2224–2225
Splicing, 16
Spreading pigmented actinic keratosis, 1664
Squamous cell carcinoma (SCC), 62, 288, 1185f
AIDS, 1899
anal
HPV DNA types, 1393t
bladder cancer, 1426

cervix, 1499–1500
computed tomography, 458f
eyelids, 1082–1083
head and neck
adjutant chemotherapy, 1168
combined chemoradiotherapy, 1167–1168
neoadjuvant chemotherapy, 1168
neoadjuvant therapy, 1165–1167, 1166t
primary chemotherapy, 1164–1165
randomized studies, 1164
recurrent
combined chemoradiotherapy, 1163–1164
of head and neck. *See* Head and neck squamous cell carcinoma (HNSCC)
imaging of, 464–465
inguinal lymph nodes, 1909
invasive, 1668f
of lung
histologic types of, 1185–1186
metastatic, 1909
oral mucosa, 1667
penis, 1462
PET, 457f
skin, 441f, 1666–1669, 1667f
surgery, 1153
of unknown primary site, 1908–1910
vagina
staging, 1494t
vulva, 1490
SRE, 65
SRF, 65
ST1571
action, 82f
Staging, 508–509, 509, 1033
American Joint Committee on Cancer, 1473t
Standard Generalized Markup Language (SGML), 2273
Standardized incidence ratio (SIR), 2217
Standardized information system, 1032
Standardized terminology, 2277.
Standard of care, 1015
Stanford Microarray Database, 110
Staphylococcus, 2228
Status epilepticus, 2258, 2259f
Steel factor (SLF), 56
Stem cell factor (SCF), 56, 748–749, 748t
Stem cells, 34–35
Stem cell transplantation (SCT)
acute myeloid leukemia, 1749–1750
for adult acute lymphoblastic leukemia, 1781
of adult acute lymphoblastic leukemia, 1778–1779
allogeneic
multiple myeloma, 1860
chronic lymphocytic leukemia, 1794–1795
multiple myeloma, 1860
Stenotrophomonas maltophilia, 2226
Stents
complications, 499
esophageal, 498–499
metallic, 497
for ureteral obstruction, 2123
Stereotactic radiosurgery, 519–520
Stereotactic radiotherapy, 519–520
Sterility
after radiation therapy, 1483
Sternal occipital mandibular immobilizer (SOMI orthosis), 928
Steroid(s)
inducing skeletal complications, 2093–2094
liver neoplasms, 1293
Steroid synthesis inhibitors, 819
STK-1 (human stem cell kinase-1). *See* Flt3 ligand (Fms-like tyrosine kinase 3)
Stomach
stents, 499
Stomach cancer
incidence, 341
nutrition, 371–372
Stomatitis, 2077, 2184–2185, 2185f
Stored tissue research
ethics, 1003
Streptococcus, 2227–2228
Streptozocin
adjustment for renal insufficiency, 2128t
nephrotoxicity of, 2127t
Streptozotocin
neuroendocrine metastases, 495
Stress, 818
causing cancer, 903
complementary and alternative medicine for, 958t
Stress-activated protein kinase (SAPK), 65, 523–524
Stroma, 437
generation, 438–439, 438f
Strongyloides stercoralis, 2239, 2239f
Study designs, 427–428
Study to Understand Prognoses and Preferences for Outcomes and Risks of Treatments (SUPPORT), 1007
Subependymal giant-cell astrocytoma (SEGA), 462
Subependymomas, 462
Subglottic cancer, 1147–1149
Subjective global assessment (SGA), 2041
Sublingual glands, 1154
Sublingual tablet, 359
Submandibular glands, 1154
Submaxillary glands, 1154
Substance P, 2055
Substituted judgment, 1000
Sucralfate, 2188
for radiation coloproctitis, 2179
Sudden cardiopulmonary arrest, 2246–2247
Suffering, 970–971
Sugar, 374
Suicide, 909–910, 910t
assisted, 1008–1009
defined, 1008ft
risk evaluation, 909t
risk factors for, 909t
Suicide genes, 864
Sunburn cell
apoptotic, 283
Sundowning, 910
Sunlight-induced photoproducts
DNA, 283–284
Sun Soup, 962
Superior sagittal sinus thrombosis, 2073
Superior sulcus tumors, 468f
Superior vena cava obstruction, 968
Superior vena cava syndrome, 498, 498f, 2252–2253
management, 2253f
SupF, 286
Supplements
dietary, 367
SUPPORT, 1007
Supportive care
in adolescents, 2032–2033
oncology nurse, 918–919
Supportive rehabilitation therapy, 923
Supraglottic cancer, 1146–1147
management algorithm, 1147f
Supratentorial primitive neuroectodermal tumor
in children, 1955–1956
Supratentorial primitive neuroectodermal tumors (PNET)
in infants and children
imaging, 1955
Supreme Court
euthanasia and assisted suicide, 1009
Suramin, 67
neurotoxicity, 2071
Surface-enhanced laser desorption ionization time of flight (SELDI-TOF), 202
Surgery
in adolescents, 2032
during pregnancy, 942
Surgical oncologist, 937
Surgical oncology, 501–506
biopsy, 507–508
contemporary role of, 505
future of, 514–515
historical development of, 501–503
landmark advances in, 504t
prevention, 507
Surgical pathologist
report, 444
role, 439–450
Surrogate consent, 1000
Surrogate end points, 566
Surveillance, 340–345
data validity, 341
Surveillance, Epidemiology, and End Results (SEER), 340
Survival, 345–346
adolescents, 2034–2035, 2035t
Survival models, 421–422
Survivor
adaptation to, 904–905
Survivorship, 919
diet, 374–375
Susceptibility
genetic variation, 355–356
SVC syndrome
with small-cell lung cancer, 1219–1220
Sweeteners
artificial, 374
SWOG study, 1813
Symptoms, 3–5
management, 968–969
oncology nurse, 918
Synatophysin, 1110
Syndrome of ectopic adrenocorticotropic hormone, 1188–1189

Syndrome of inappropriate secretion of antidiuretic hormone (SIADH), 1188
Synovial sarcoma
  genomic alterations in, 128
Synthetic angiogenesis inhibitors, 176
Systeme internationale (SI) units, 568, 568t
Systemic therapy
  during pregnancy, 942

T

T. gondii, 2238–2239
TAA, 786–787
  genes, 867
Taenia taeniaeformis, 337
Takeda neoplastic product-470 (TNP-470), 176
Tamoxifen, 49, 378, 829–830
  in adjuvant setting, 830
  in advanced breast cancer, 830
  anastrozole, 837
  clinical pharmacology of, 829–830
  endometrial cancer, 1523
  mode of action, 829
  ophthalmic effects of, 831–832
  plus chemotherapy, 830–831
  switching from, 837
  thromboembolic disorders with, 832
  uterine stimulation, 832
TAP1, 193
TAP2, 193
Targeted toxins, 779–782
  clinical trials, 780t
  ligands, 779t
  pharmacology, 782
Targretin (bexarotene)
  mycosis fungoides/Sézary syndrome, 1842
Taxanes, 706–713
  administration, dose, schedule, 712–713
  causing anaphylaxis, 2261
  clinical indications, 706
  clinical pharmacology, 708–709
  comparative pharmacokinetics, 708t
  drug interactions, 709–710
  mechanisms of action, 706–707
  mechanisms of resistance, 707–708
  neurotoxicity, 2071
  for small-cell lung cancer, 1217
  for testis cancer, 1481
  toxicity, 710–711
T-cell acute leukemia
  genomic alterations in, 118
T-cell acute lymphoblastic leukemia (T-ALL), 80
  c-myc, 77
T-cell costimulation, 791
T-cell lymphoma
  Epstein-Barr virus, 313
T-cell prolymphocytic leukemia (T-PLL)
  alemtuzumab, 771
T-cell receptor gene rearrangements
  in adult acute lymphoblastic leukemia, 1775
T-cell signaling defects, 210
Tcl-1, 80
TCR, 285
T-CRM107, 781
Tea, 374
Technetium-99m methoxyisobutyl isonitrile, 489
Teenagers. *See* Adolescents
Telesurgery, 515
Telomerase, 31, 141–142
Telomeres, 141–142
Temozolomide, 677
10-ethyl-10-deazaaminopterin, 655
Teniposide, 694
  causing anaphylaxis, 2261
TENS, 993
Teratoid/rhabdoid tumor
  atypical
    in infants and children, 1955, 1955f
Teratomas, 461, 1471, 1471f
  benign
    of mediastinum, 1249
  immature
    children, 1971–1972
    ovaries, 1563–1564
  mature
    children, 1971–1972
  mature cystic, 1249
Terminal illness, 1032
Terminating medical care, 1003–1004
  legal cases, 1005t–1006t
Testicular androgen suppression
  prostate cancer, 1453–1454
Testicular germ cell cancer
  markers, 200
Testicular germ cell tumors
  markers of, 1469t
Testicular neoplasms, 404–405
  cause, 264–265
  chemotherapy, 576
Testis cancer, 1468–1485
  alpha-fetoprotein with, 1472
  carcinoma in situ, 1473
  chemotherapy of
    fertility after, 1483
    long-term toxicity of, 1486–1487
    nephrotoxicity of, 1486
    neurotoxicity of, 1486
    second malignancies after, 1486–1487
    vascular toxicity of, 1486
  clinical presentation of, 1471–1473
  clinical stage I, 1475–1477
    treatment of, 1476
  CNS metastases, 1484
  diagnosis of, 1471–1472
  disseminated
    chemotherapy of, 1477–1478
    Indiana University Studies, 1477
    prognosis of, 1477–1478
    treatment of, 1477–1478
  early stage nonseminoma, 1473–1474
  epidemiology of, 1468–1469
  high-dose chemotherapy as initial salvage therapy, 1481
  incidence of, 1468–1469
  late relapse, 1481–1482
  molecular genetics, 1469–1471
  pathologic stage I
    treatment of, 1476
  pathology of, 1469–1471
  radiation therapy
    long-term toxicity of, 1483–1484
  radiotherapy of, 1475
  retroperitoneal lymph node dissection, 1474–1475
  risk factors of, 1468–1469
  sanctuary sites, 1484
  seminoma early stage
    treatment of, 1476
  staging of, 1473
  surveillance *vs.* RPLND, 1475–1477
  transplantation for, 891
  treatment of, 1473–1475
  tumor markers, 1472–1473
Tetracycline agents, 2187
Tetradecapeptide somatostatin, 805
Tetraphenylporphine axial disulfonate, 543
Tetraplatin, 686
Text retrieval, 2278–2279
TGF-alpha, 63
TGF-beta
  radiation, 527
Thalamic stimulation, 994
Thalassemia
  transplantation for, 892
Thalidomide, 177
  cachexia, 2047
Thallium-201, 489
T helper cells, 206
The March, 1027
Therapeutic genes, 863–864
Therapeutic touch, 961
Therapy selection and response markers, 199
Thermal cytotoxicity
  enhancing, 551–553
  modifiers, 550
Thermal isoeffect dose, 549–550
Thermometry
  noninvasive, 557
Thermotolerance, 550
Thioguanine, 670
  adjustment for renal insufficiency, 2128t
Thioinosine monophosphate (TIMP), 670
Thiopurines
  metabolic activation, 670f
Thiotepa, 676
  clinical pharmacology, 681
Thoracic radiation
  pulmonary complications of, 2159–2160
Thoracolumbar sacral orthosis (TLSO), 928–929
Thoracostomy, 2255
Thorax
  biopsy, 496
  imaging, 468–471
  primary germ cell tumors, 1249–1253
Thorotrast
  liver neoplasms, 1293
Thrombin
  central prothrombotic roles of, 2113f
  endostatin, 171
Thrombocythemia
  essential, 1875–1878, 1876f
    pregnancy, 1878
Thrombocytopathy, 2115
Thrombocytopenia, 2099, 2114–2115
  causes, 2096t, 2099t
  chronic lymphocytic leukemia, 1796
  differential diagnosis of, 2114t
Thrombocytosis, 2099
  interferons, 738
Thromboembolism
  occult malignancy, 458

Thrombopoietic agents
in the clinic, 765–766
Thrombopoietin, 749–750, 820t, 2215
Thrombospondin-1, 165
Thrombotic complications, 2116–2117
risk factors for, 2117t
Thrombotic disorders
novel drug treatment, 2120
Thrombotic thrombocytopenia purpura (TTP)
following transplantation, 886
Thrombotic thrombocytopenic purpura, 2118–2119
Thymic carcinoid tumors, 1240
chemotherapy, 1242
Thymic carcinoma, 1239–1240
Thymic tumors, 1237–1243, 1237t
Thymidine phosphorylase, 1376
Thymidylate synthase, 665, 1376
inhibition, 1347
colorectal cancer, 1392
inhibitors, 735
Thymomas, 1237–1243
anatomic pathogenesis, 1237–1238
associated paraneoplastic syndromes, 1239, 1239t
chemotherapy, 577
clinical features, 1238–1239
computed tomography, 471f
corticosteroids for, 823
diagnosis, 1239
differential diagnosis, 1239–1240
epidemiology and etiology, 1237
staging, 1240, 1240t
therapy, 1240–1242, 1241f
Thyroid
metastases to, 2206
Thyroid cancer
in childhood cancer survivors, 1922
genomic alterations in, 126
Thyroid carcinoma, 463
Thyroid disorders, 2204
Thyroid hormone
differentiated thyroid carcinoma, 1096
Thyroid neoplasms, 62, 1093–1100
anaplastic, 1100
biologic modifiers, 1097–1098
cause, 266
chemotherapy, 577, 1098
diagnostic imaging, 1096
differentiated. *See* Differentiated thyroid carcinoma
external beam radiotherapy, 1096, 1098
fine needle aspiration, 445
during pregnancy, 943
radiation-induced, 278
radioiodine, 1095–1096
radioiodine ^{131}I, 1096–1097, 1097f
serum thyroglobulin monitoring, 1096
staging, 1095t
thyroid hormone, 1096
TNM classification, 1095t
Thyroid nodules, 2206
Thyroid ophthalmopathy, 1083
Tibia
bone plates in, 1676f
bone tumors of, 1676f
TIE (tyrosine kinase with immunoglobulin and epidermal growth factor), 63
Time Without Symptoms and Toxicity (TWiST), 429–430
TIMP, 150–151, 670
Tingling paresthesia, 2070
Tissue-engineered vascularized osseus graft, 514f
Tissue factor bearing membranes, 2113f
Tissue inhibitor of metalloproteinase (TIMP), 150–151
Tissue sections
microscopic interpretation, 440–441
TLS, 1964
TLSO, 928–929
T-lymphoblastic lymphoma, 1829f
precursor, 1829–1830
TNF-alpha
cachexia, 2039–2040, 2047
TNF receptors, 42
TNM descriptors, 1194–1195, 1194t
TNP-470, 176
Tobacco, 1179–1180
carcinogenic effects, 354–355
colorectal cancer, 1371–1372
head and neck neoplasms, 1131–1132
secondary cancer, 2218
Tobacco addiction
genetics, 362
Tobacco-related cancer
prevention of, 354–363
Tobacco smoke, 90–91, 250
composition of, 1180
environmental, 361–362
head and neck neoplasms, 1133
gas chromatography/mass spectroscopy, 254–255
Tobacco-specific nitrosamines, 354
Tobacco use
prevention, 362–363
Tocopherols, 373
Tolerance, 990
Tongue
base, 1142
squamous cell carcinoma, 1139–1140
survival, 1140t
Tonsils, 1141–1142
squamous cell carcinoma
survival, 1142t
Tooth development
in childhood cancer survivors, 1929
Topoisomerase
biology of, 688
Topoisomerase II catalysis
model of, 689f
Topoisomerase II poisons, 637
Topoisomerase-mediated DNA damage
cellular response to, 689–690
Topoisomerase poisons
multidrug resistance, 633–634
Topoisomerases, 620
intercalating drugs targeting, 690–693
Topoisomerases I
DNA strand cleavage by, 688f
drugs poisoning, 688–689
Topoisomerase targeting
resistance to, 690
Topotecan, 620, 694–695
adjustment for renal insufficiency, 2128t
myelodysplastic syndrome, 1731
for small-cell lung cancer, 1217
Topotecan-DNA-topoisomerase I covalent complex, 689f
Toremifene (Fareston), 831
Torsades de pointes, 2136
Tositumomab (Bexxar), 777
Total gastrectomy, 1279–1280
TP53, 1375–1376
T-PLL
alemtuzumab, 771
Tracheal stomal recurrence
risk factors, 1146t
Traditional Chinese medicine, 960
TRAIL, 44
TRAIL receptors, 44f
Tramadol (Ultram)
for cancer pain, 983
Transactivation, 305–306
Transcriptionally targeted oncolytic viruses, 872
Transcription-coupled repair (TCR), 285
Transcription factor 3 gene rearrangements (19p13)
in adult acute lymphoblastic leukemia, 1775
Transcription factors, 72–73
Transcription therapy, 36
Transcriptome, 9
Transcutaneous electrical nerve stimulation (TENS), 993
Transdermal nicotine patch, 358–359
Transesophageal echocardiography, 2131
Transfection assay, 69, 71f
Transformation, 11
defined, 318
Transformed cells
immortality, 137
Transforming growth factor- alpha (TGF-alpha), 63
Transforming growth factor beta
multiple myeloma, 1851–1852
Transforming growth factor-beta, 35
Transforming growth factor-beta (TGF-beta)
radiation, 527
Transfusion
effect on immune system, 2102–2103
risks of, 2104t
Transfusions
recommendations for, 2114t
Transjugular intrahepatic portosystemic shunts, 499–500
Translocation 5(12;21)
in adult acute lymphoblastic leukemia, 1775
Translocations
involving core binding factors, 114–115
Translocation t(9;22)
in adult acute lymphoblastic leukemia, 1774–1775
Transmembrane domain, 54
Transplacental malignancy, 945, 945t
Transplantation. *See also* Bone marrow transplantation
for acute myeloid leukemia, 887–888
allogeneic, 880–881
donor selection, 881
engraftment of, 881–882
pretransplant therapy, 883–884

Transplantation—*continued*
allogeneic hematopoietic, 880f
for anaplastic anemia, 891–892
autologous, 880
donor selection, 881
engraftment of, 881–882
pretransplant therapy, 883
tumor cell contamination and purging, 882
for sickle cell anemia, 892
Transport Communication Protocol/Internet Protocol (TCP/IP), 2268
Transpupillary thermotherapy
retinoblastoma, 1075
Transrectal ultrasonography (TRUS)
prostate cancer, 402–404
Transsphenoidal surgery
growth hormone secreting pituitary adenomas, 1087
Transthoracic echocardiography, 2131
TrapEase, 497
Trastuzumab
systemic reaction to, 2262
Trastuzumab (Herceptin), 105
cardiotoxicity, 2141
Trauma, 292, 293
Trazodone
for anxiety, 908
Treatment
in adolescents, 2031–2033
Treatment guidelines, 906t
Tretinoin, 378
Triazenes, 677
Trichilemmoma, 1674
Trichosomoides crassi-cauda, 337
Trichosporon, 2234
Trichothiodystrophy (TTD), 283, 288
Trigger-point injection, 991
Trilostane (Modrenal), 831
Trimetrexate, 655
adjustment for renal insufficiency, 2128t
colorectal cancer, 1390
Triple-helix formation, 864–865
Trisomy 8, 82
Tropinin I, 176
TRUS, 477
prostate cancer, 402–404
Truth telling, 567
Tryptophan, 334
TTD, 283, 288
TT virus (TTV), 330
Tuberculosis, 2165
Tuberous sclerosis, 1041–1042
Tubulin binders
schedule effects, 593
Tubulin dimer, 699f
TUCAN, 45
Tumor(s)
grading, staging, prognosis, 442–443
structure, 437–438
Tumor antigens, 193–196
classification of, 194
Tumor-associated antigens (TAA), 786–787
in cancer vaccine clinical trials, 194t
genes, 867
Tumor blush, 460
Tumor burden, 590–591
Tumor cell migration, 151–152
Tumor cells
antibody-mediated killing, 207
cell-mediated killing, 207
checkpoint defects, 31–32
migration, 151–152
Tumor development
genetic basis, 85–86
Tumor expansion
prevascular phase, 160–161
Tumor growth
cell proliferation, 27–28
Tumor-host interactions, 148–149, 149t
Tumor hypoxia, 591
Tumorigenesis
somatic cell genetic studies, 86–87
Tumor-infiltrating lymphocytes
malignant melanoma, 1660
Tumor initiation, 246, 247
Tumor lysis syndrome, 1773, 2249–2250
Tumor lysis syndrome (TLS), 1964
Tumor markers
application of, 200t
cerebrospinal fluid, 2067t
colorectal cancer, 1374–1375
global profiling of, 202
Tumor necrosis factor
cardiotoxicity, 2142
Tumor necrosis factor alpha
multiple myeloma, 1851
Tumor necrosis factor-alpha (TNF-alpha), 764t
cachexia, 2039–2040, 2047
Tumor necrosis factor (TNF) receptors, 42
Tumor profiling
future of, 202
Tumor progression, 248, 253f
Tumor promotion, 247
Tumor registry, 2274
Tumors
unfavorable cytokine milieu, 209
withstanding immune-mediated destruction, 210
Tumor-selective adeno-associated viruses, 868
Tumor-selective promoters/enhancers, 868
Tumor-selective retroviruses, 867
Tumor-specific antigens, 786
Tumor spread
patterns, 509–510
Tumor spread patterns, 509–510
Tumor-stromal interactions, 148–149
Tumor suppressor
endometrial cancer, 1527
Tumor suppressor genes, 85–99, 253–254, 275
gastric cancer, 1272
hepatitis B virus, 325
protein function, 99t
Tumor viruses, 297–307
classification, 297
replication cycle, 300–302
structure, 297–300
Tumstatin, 175–176
Tuskegee Syphilis Study, 1001
TWIST (Time Without Symptoms or Toxicity), 911
Two-dimensional echocardiography, 2131
Typhlitis, 2176
Tyro3 (sky), 60
Tyrosine kinase inhibitors, 722–725, 723t
clinical trials, 729–730
cutaneous reactions, 2083
Tyrosine kinase receptor families, 72f
Tyrosine kinase receptors, 83f
signaling pathways, 63–66
Tyrosine kinases, 55f, 144, 1273
growth factor receptors, 54
Tyrosine kinase with immunoglobulin and epidermal growth factor, 63

U

Ufo, 60
Ulcerative colitis, 1361, 1378
Ulcerative mucositis, 2188
Ultram
for cancer pain, 983
Ultrasonography
breast, 487f
breast cancer, 485–486
cysts, 487f
Ultrasound heating, 556
Ultraviolet radiation (UVR)
carcinogenesis, 283–285
Ultraviolet recall reaction, 2080
Unbalanced gain
childhood neuroblastoma, 1991–1992
Understanding
legal requirement, 999–1000
Undifferentiated malignant tumors, 446
Unicameral bone cysts, 1684–1685
Unified Medical Language System (UMLS), 2278
Uniparental disomy (UPD), 110
Unique antigens, 196
United Nations Scientific Committee on the Effects of Atomic Radiation (UNSCEAR 2000), 276
Unknown primary site, 1904–1912
UNSCEAR 2000. *See* United Nations Scientific Committee on the Effects of Atomic Radiation (UNSCEAR 2000)
Upper extremities
metastatic tumor to, 2089
Uremia, 2115
Ureter
secondary tumors of, 1413
Ureteral obstruction, 2123–2124
Urethral carcinoma
female, 1465–1466
male, 1466
Urinary infection
schistosomiasis, 333
Urinary tract obstruction, 2123
treatment of, 2124–2125
Urologic complications, 2123–2129
from primary cancer progression, 2123–2124
Urothelium, 1410
Uterine cancer
genomic alterations in, 126–127
Uterine cervix
carcinoma
interventional radiology, 495–496
epithelial cancer
natural history, 1501–1502
Uterine leiomyomas
genomic alterations in, 122

Uterine myometrial tumors, 1577
Uterine neoplasms
chemotherapy, 576
incidence, 341
progestin receptor, 846
Uterine papillary serous carcinoma, 1524, 1524f
UV photoproducts
excision, 284–287
mutagenicity, 285–286
UVR
carcinogenesis, 283–285

V
Vaccines
agonist peptides, 789
allogeneic whole-tumor-cell, 788
antiidiotypes, 789
autologous whole-tumor-cell, 788
bacterial vectors, 790
CEA, 792
cervical neoplasia, 1504–1505
clinical trials, 792–793
combination therapy, 793
dendritic cell, 790
development, 787, 788t
DNA vectors, 790
fusion proteins, 790
immune response, 213–214
immunoglobulins, 790
malignant melanoma, 1653–1654
modalities, 789t
peptides, 788–789
proteins, 788
replication-competent vectors, 789–790
replication-defective, 790
RNA vectors, 790
targets, 786–793, 786t
vectors, 789–790
whole-tumor-cell, 788
Vaccinia virus, 790
recombinant, 867
Vagina
clear cell adenocarcinoma, 1494, 1495t
lymphatic drainage, 1494f
melanoma, 1494–1495
sarcoma, 1578
squamous cell carcinoma
staging, 1494t
Vaginal adenocarcinoma
cause, 264
Vaginal cancer, 1493–1495
treatment, 1494t
Vancomycin-resistant enterococci (VRE), 1374t, 2228
VAPEC-B chemotherapy, 1813
Varicella zoster virus (VZV), 2235–2236, 2235f
Vascular access, 514
Vascular endothelial growth factor (VEGF), 56, 1273
antibodies, 773
colorectal cancer, 1392
down regulation, 170
induced endothelial cell-cell adhesion loss prevention, 170
multiple myeloma, 1851
radiation therapy, 529–530
Vascular endothelial growth factor-A (VEGF-A), 438–440
Vascular endothelial growth factor (VEGF)-related factor (VRF), 56
Vascular injury
radiation-induced, 2144
Vascularized osseus graft, 515f
Vascular leak syndrome (VLS), 781–782
Vasogenic edema, 460
Vegetables, 366
breast cancer, 369
colorectal cancer, 368
head and neck neoplasms, 1133
pancreatic neoplasms, 1332
VEGF. *See* Vascular endothelial growth factor (VEGF)
Vena cava filters, 496–497
Venal caval syndrome, 498
Vena Tech filter, 497
Veno-occlusive disease (VOD), 2179–2180, 2179f
etiology of, 2181t
following transplantation, 886
Venous catheterization
complications, 514t
Venous stenosis, 498
Venous thromboembolism (VTE), 1189, 2117–2118, 2166–2167
Ventilatory pump insufficiency, 2167–2168
Verrucous carcinoma, 334f
bilharzial bladder, 333
cervix, 1500
penis, 1462, 1463f
skin, 1667
vulva, 1492
Vesical cancer
anatomic distribution, 333t
Vesicular monamine transporter protein, 1110
Vessel cooption, 162
Veterans Administration, 2277
VHL. *See* von Hippel-Lindau (VHL) syndrome
VHL, 96–97
Video logs, 2273
Vinblastine, 700, 703–704
neurotoxicity of, 1482
vascular toxicity of, 1482
Vinca alkaloids, 700–706
administration, dose and schedule, 705–706
chemical structure, 700f
clinical indications, 702–703
clinical pharmacology, 703–704
comparative pharmacokinetics, 703t
drug interactions, 704
mechanism of action, 700–701
mechanism of resistance, 701–702
toxicity, 704–705
Vincristine, 700, 703
for adult acute lymphoblastic leukemia, 1777
for Burkitt's acute lymphoblastic leukemia, 1780
neurotoxicity, 2070
for small-cell lung cancer, 1217
thyroid neoplasms, 1098
uterine cervix carcinoma, 495
Vindesine, 704
Vinorelbine, 700, 704
for nonsmall-cell lung cancer, 1210
Vinyl chloride
liver neoplasms, 1294
VIPoma (vasoactive intestinal polypeptide), 1117–1118
Viral hepatitis
in childhood cancer survivors, 1925
Viral infection, 2235–2237
oral complications, 2189
Viral-like particles (VLP), 321
electron micrography, 321f
Viral oncolysis, 869–873
Viral pneumonia
with hematopoietic stem cell transplantation, 2160
Viral pneumonitis, 2166
Viral proteins, 313–314
Virilization, 1103
Virus-directed enzyme/prodrug therapy, 863
Viscera
pain, 980
Vista Medical Record, 2277
Vitamin A, 373
head and neck neoplasms, 1133
Vitamin C, 373
Vitamin D, 379
colorectal cancer, 1371
prostate neoplasms, 1432
Vitamin E, 373
prostate cancer, 369
prostate neoplasms, 1432
Vitamin K deficiency
cachexia, 2042
VLP, 321
electron micrography, 321f
VLS, 781–782
Vocal cords
carcinoma in situ, 1149
Vocational counselor, 924
Voice-over Internet protocol (VOIP), 2271
Volume-outcome relationship, 1033
Voluntariness, 1000
Vomiting, 968, 989–990
Vomiting center, 2056f
von Hippel-Lindau (VHL) syndrome, 96–97, 1041
classification, 1043t
genetic basis, 224
Von Recklinghausen disease, 1041
Von Recklinghausen neurofibromatosis, 96
von Willebrand's syndrome
acquired, 2115
Voriconazole, 2234
Vorozole, 835
structure of, 833f
VP-16
for disseminated germ cell tumors, 1478
VRE, 1374t, 2228
VRF. *See* Vascular endothelial growth factor (VEGF)-related factor (VRF)
Vulva
basal cell carcinoma, 1492
melanoma, 1492–1493
Paget disease, 1489
sarcomas, 1493, 1578
squamous cell carcinoma, 1490
verrucous carcinoma, 1492
Vulva neoplasms, 1488–1493
invasive, 1489–1490

Vulvar atypias, 1488–1489, 1489t
VZV, 2235–2236, 2235f

W

Waldenstrom macroglobulinemia, 1865–1866
Wallstent, 497, 497f, 498
Warren, John Collins, 504
Water
  cachexia, 2044
Weber-Fergusson incision, 1152
Web logs, 2273
WebMD, 2271–2272
Wedge resection
  for nonsmall-cell lung cancer, 1201
Weight, 366–367
  breast cancer, 260, 368–369
  endometrial cancer, 263
Well-differentiated adenocarcinoma
  of lung, 1186f
Werner syndrome
  genetic basis, 226
White cells
  abnormalities, 2098
White clot syndrome, 2167
WHO. *See* World Health Organization (WHO)
Wi-Fi (Wireless Fidelity), 2268
Wiki, 2273
Wilms tumor, 95–96, 1407
  in children
    epidemiology, 1918
  genetic basis, 224–225
Wilms' tumor
  bilateral
    chemotherapy of, 1986
  chemotherapy of, 1986
Wilms' tumor (nephroblastoma)
  genomic alterations in, 130
Women
  chemotherapy
    gonadal complications, 2197–2198
  gonadal complications
    protection from, 2199
  with peritoneal carcinomatosis
    unknown primary site, 1906–1907
  radiation therapy
    gonadal function, 2198
  smoking cessation, 360
World Health Organization (WHO), 340
  classification, 1111
    bone tumors, 1678t
    central nervous system neoplasms
      neuroepithelial, 1043t
    gastric cancer, 1270
    germ cell tumors, 1060t
    low-grade gliomas, 1052t
  guidelines
    for cancer pain treatment, 982, 982f
  population nutrient goals, 365t
World Wide Web, 2268–2270
Wound healing
  vs. invasive tumor growth, 294f
  stroma generation, 439
WT1, 95–96

X

Xeroderma pigmentosum (XP), 283, 287–288, 287t
  age at onset, 284f
  DNA repair, 283
  genetic basis, 226
Xerostomia, 2185–2186
XIAP, 46
X-linked lymphoproliferative syndrome
  genetic basis, 232–233
XP. *See* Xeroderma pigmentosum (XP)
XPG protein, 287
X-ray cross-complementing group 1 (XRCC1), 355

Y

^{90}Y-iritumomab tiuxetan, 777
Yolk sac tumor
  in children, 1971
Yolk sac tumors, 1470, 1470f

Z

Zevalin (^{90}Y-iritumomab tiuxetan), 777
Zidovudine
  colorectal cancer, 1390
Zoledronate, 2091
  for cancer pain, 988
  hypercalcemia, 2213
Z stent, 497, 498

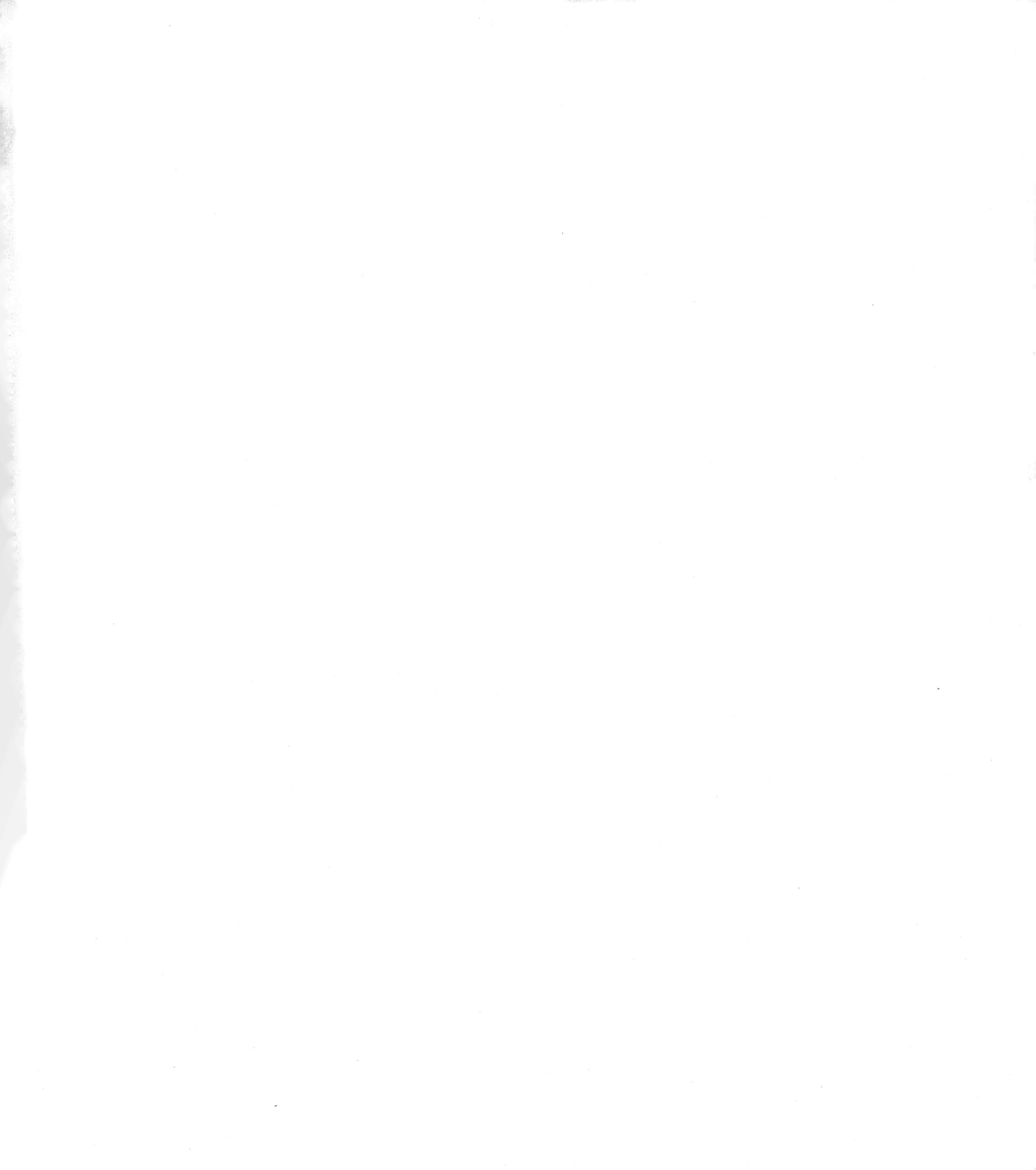